W I L L I A M S

HEMATOLOGY

S E V E N T H   E D I T I O N

NOTICE

WILLIAMS
HEMATOLOGY
SEVENTH EDITION

EDITORS

MARSHALL A. LICHTMAN, M.D.

Professor of Medicine and of Biochemistry and Biophysics
University of Rochester School of Medicine and Dentistry
Rochester, New York
Executive Vice President for Research and
Medical Programs
The Leukemia & Lymphoma Society
White Plains, New York

ERNEST BEUTLER, M.D.

Professor and Chairman
Department of Molecular and Experimental Medicine
The Scripps Research Institute
La Jolla, California
Senior Consultant
Division of Hematology Oncology
Scripps Clinic Medical Group, Inc.
Clinical Professor of Medicine
University of California, San Diego
La Jolla, California

THOMAS J. KIPPS, M.D., Ph.D.

Professor
Division of Hematology/Oncology
Deputy Director for Research Operations
Rebecca and John Moores UCSD Cancer Center
University of California, San Diego
La Jolla, California

URI SELIGSOHN, M.D.

Professor and Director
Amalia Biron Research Institute of
Thrombosis and Hemostasis
Department of Hematology
Chaim Sheba Medical Center
Tel-Hashomer and Sackler Faculty of Medicine
Tel Aviv University
Tel Aviv, Israel

KENNETH KAUSHANSKY, M.D.

Helen M. Ranney Professor and Chair
Department of Medicine
University of California, San Diego
San Diego, California

JOSEF T. PRCHAL, M.D.

Professor of Medicine and Pathology
Hematology Division
University of Utah
Salt Lake City, Utah
Department of Pathophysiology
First Faculty of Medicine
Charles University in Prague
Czech Republic

McGRAW-HILL
MEDICAL PUBLISHING DIVISION

New York / Chicago / San Francisco / Lisbon / London / Madrid / Mexico City
Milan / New Delhi / San Juan / Seoul / Singapore / Sydney / Toronto

Williams HEMATOLOGY, Seventh Edition

Copyright © 2006, by The McGraw-Hill Companies, Inc. All rights reserved. Printed in the United States of America. Except as permitted under the United States Copyright Act of 1976, no part of this publication may be reproduced or distributed in any form or by any means, or stored in a data base or retrieval system, without the prior written permission of the publisher.

2 3 4 5 6 7 8 9 0   DOW/DOW   0 9 8 7 6

ISBN: 0-07-143591-3

This book was set in Times Roman by Progressive.
The editors were Marc Strauss, Michelle Watt, Karen G. Edmonson, and Karen Davis.
The production supervisor was Sherri Souffrance.
The cover designer was Janice Bielawa.
The indexer was Kathleen Pitcoff.
RR Donnelley was printer and binder.

This book is printed on acid-free paper.

Library of Congress Cataloging-in-Publication Data

Williams hematology / edited by Marshall A. Lichtman ... [et al.].—7th ed.
    p. ; cm.
  Includes bibliographical references and index.
  ISBN 0-07-143591-3
    1. Blood—Diseases. 2. Hematology. I. Title: Hematology. II. Lichtman, Marshall
      A. III.
Williams, William J. (William Joseph), 1926–
  [DNLM: 1. Hematologic Diseases. WH 100 W721 2006]
RC633.H43 2006
616.1′5—dc22
                                                                              2004055200

C O N T E N T S

P A R T I

CLINICAL EVALUATION OF THE PATIENT

P A R T I I

GENERAL HEMATOLOGY

PART III

MOLECULAR AND CELLULAR HEMATOLOGY

P A R T V I

NEUTROPHILS, EOSINOPHILS, BASOPHILS, AND MAST CELLS

P A R T   V I I

MONOCYTES AND MACROPHAGES

PART VIII
LYMPHOCYTES AND PLASMA CELLS

PART IX
MALIGNANT DISEASES

PART X

HEMOSTASIS AND THROMBOSIS

P A R T   X I

TRANSFUSION MEDICINE

CONTRIBUTORS

CAMILLE N. ABBOUD, M.D. [4]
Professor of Medicine (Hematology-Oncology)
James P. Wilmot Cancer Center
University of Rochester Medical Center
Rochester, New York

CHARLES S. ABRAMS, M.D. [113]
Associate Professor of Medicine
Division of Hematology-Oncology
University of Pennsylvania School of Medicine
University of Pennsylvania Hospital
Philadelphia, Pennsylvania

ALICE ALEXANDER, PH.D. [103]
Research Service
Department of Medicine
New York Harbor Health Care Center
New York, New York

ELIAS ANAISSIE, M.D. [100]
Professor of Medicine
Director of Supportive Care
Myeloma Institute for Research and Therapy
University of Arkansas for Medical Sciences
    Medical Center
Little Rock, Arkansas

DANIEL A. ARBER, M.D. [63]
Director of Clinical Hematology
Clinical Laboratories
Stanford University Medical Center
Stanford, California

JOZEF ARNOUT, M.D. [119]
Associate Professor
Faculty of Medicine
Department of Molecular and Cardiovascular
    Research
University of Leuven, Belgium
Leuven, Belgium

BERNARD M. BABIOR, M.D., PH.D.* [39]
Professor and Head
Division of Biochemistry
Department of Molecular and Experimental
    Medicine
The Scripps Research Institute
La Jolla, California

DOROTHY F. BAINTON, M.D. [59]
Professor Emeritus
Department of Academic Affairs
University of California at San Francisco
    School of Medicine
San Francisco, California

STEPHEN M. BAIRD, M.D. [74, 98]
Professor of Clinical Pathology
University of California, San Diego Medical
    Center
Chief Pathology and Laboratory Medicine
VA Medical Center
San Diego, California

*Deceased.

KELTY R. BAKER, M.D. [49]
Assistant Professor of Medicine
Hematology/Oncology
Baylor College of Medicine
Houston, Texas

BART BARLOGIE, M.D., PH.D. [100]
Professor of Medicine and Pathology
Director, Myeloma Institute for Research &
    Therapy
University of Arkansas for Medical Sciences
Little Rock, Arkansas

JOEL S. BENNETT, M.D. [113]
Professor of Medicine and Pharmacology
Department of Medicine
University of Pennsylvania
Philadelphia, Pennsylvania

CAROLINA BERGER, M.D. [23]
Clinical Research/Immunology
Fred Hutchinson Cancer Research Center
Seattle, Washington

ROBERT F. BETTS, M.D. [84]
Professor of Medicine
Department of Medicine
Infectious Diseases Unit
University of Rochester School of Medicine
    and Dentistry
Rochester, New York

BRUCE BEUTLER, M.D. [17]
Professor
Department of Immunology
The Scripps Research Institute
La Jolla, California

ERNEST BEUTLER, M.D. [1, 9, 29, 31, 37, 38, 40,
    41, 45, 47, 48, 50, 51, 56, 58, 73, 131]
Professor and Chairman
Department of Molecular and Experimental
    Medicine
The Scripps Research Institute
La Jolla, California
Senior Consultant
Division of Hematology Oncology
Scripps Clinic Medical Group, Inc.
Clinical Professor of Medicine
University of California, San Diego
La Jolla, California

STEVEN M. BEUTLER, M.D. [20]
Assistant Clinical Professor of Medicine
University of California at Irvine
Irvine, California
Associate Director
Division of Infectious Diseases
Arrowhead Regional Medical Center
Colton, California

KARL G. BLUME, M.D. [22]
Professor of Medicine
Departments of Medicine and Bone Marrow
    Transplantation
Stanford University Medical Center
Stanford Hospitals and Clinics
Stanford, California

NIELS BORREGAARD, M.D. [66]
Professor of Hematology and Chief
Department of Hematology
University of Copenhagen
Copenhagen, Denmark

LAURENCE A. BOXER, M.D. [66]
Professor and Director of Pediatric
    Hematology/Oncology
University of Michigan Health System
Ann Arbor, Michigan

BRIAN S. BULL, M.D. [28]
Professor and Chair
Department of Pathology and Human Anatomy
Vice President and Dean
Loma Linda University
School of Medicine
Loma Linda, California

JOEL N. BUXBAUM, M.D. [101, 103]
Professor
Division of Rheumatology Research
Department of Molecular and Experimental
    Medicine
The Scripps Research Institute
La Jolla, California

LONI CALHOUN, M.D. [128]
Senior Technical Specialist
Department of Transfusion Medicine
University of California, Los Angeles Medical
    Center
Los Angeles, California

JAIME CARO, M.D. [35, 55]
Professor of Medicine
Jefferson Medical College of Thomas Jefferson
    University
Cardeza Foundation for Hematologic Research
Philadelphia, Pennsylvania

DENNIS A. CARSON, M.D. [12, 75]
Professor of Medicine
Department of Medicine
University of California, San Diego School of
    Medicine
Director of the Sam and Rose Stein Institute for
    Research on Aging
La Jolla, California

JANUARIO E. CASTRO, M.D. [26]
Assistant Clinical Professor
Division of Bone Marrow Transplantation
Rebecca and John Moores UCSD Cancer
    Center
University of California, San Diego
La Jolla, California

BRUCE A. CHABNER, M.D. [19]
Professor of Medicine
Harvard Medical School
Clinical Director
Massachusetts General Hospital Cancer Center
Chief, Division of Hematology and Oncology
Massachusetts General Hospital
Boston, Massachusetts

XIX

BARRY S. COLLER, M.D. [105, 112]
Professor
Laboratory of Blood and Vascular Medicine
Physician-in-Chief
Vice President for Medical Affairs
Hospital Medical Affairs
The Rockefeller University
New York, New York

MAX D. COOPER, M.D. [82]
Professor of Medicine
Howard Hughes Medical Institute
University of Alabama at Birmingham
Birmingham, Alabama

DAVID C. DALE, M.D. [65]
Professor of Medicine
Department of Medicine
University of Washington Medical Center
Seattle, Washington

PHILIP G. DE GROOT, PH.D. [120]
Professor, Department of Haematology
University Hospital of Utrecht
Utrecht, The Netherlands

MADHAV DHODAPKAR, M.D. [18]
Irene Diamond Associate Professor
Laboratory of Tumor Immunology &
    Immunotherapy
The Rockefeller University
New York, New York

JOEL E. DIMSDALE, M.D. [27]
Professor of Psychiatry
Department of Psychiatry
University of California, San Diego
La Jolla, California

REYHAN DIZ-KÜÇÜKKAYA, M.D. [110]
Associate Professor
Department of Internal Medicine
Division of Hematology
Ystanbul University
Ystanbul Faculty of Medicine
Ystanbul, Turkey

STEVEN D. DOUGLAS M.D. [67]
Professor of Pediatrics
Associate Chair, Academic Affairs
Chief, Section of Immunology
Director, Clinical Immunology Laboratories
The Children's Hospital of Philadelphia
Philadelphia, Pennsylvania

ANN M. DVORAK, M.D. [63]
Director, Electron Microscopy Unit
Senior Pathologist, Professor of Pathology
Department of Pathology
Beth Israel Deaconess Medical Center
Harvard Medical School
Boston, Massachusetts

JOSHUA EPSTEIN, DSc [100]
Research Professor
Myeloma Institute for Research and Therapy
University of Arkansas for Medical Sciences
    Medical Center
Little Rock, Arkansas

MIGUEL ESCOBAR, M.D. [115]
Clinical Instructor
Department of Medicine
University of North Carolina at Chapel Hill
University of North Carolina Hospitals
Chapel Hill, North Carolina

NAOMI L. ESMON, PH.D. [108]
OMRF Associate Professor
Department of Pathology
University of Oklahoma Health Sciences Center
Associate Member
Cardiovascular Biology Research Program
Oklahoma Medical Research Foundation
Oklahoma City, Oklahoma

RAYMOND E. FELGAR, M.D., PH.D. [3]
Associate Professor of Pathology and
    Laboratory Medicine
University of Rochester Medical Center
Rochester, New York

KENNETH A. FOON, M.D. [96]
Professor of Medicine
Department of Medicine
Division of Hematology/Oncology
Deputy Director for Clinical Investigations
Co-Director, Biological Therapeutics and
    Hematological Malignancy Programs
University of Pittsburgh Cancer Institute
Pittsburgh, Pennsylvania

CHARLES W. FRANCIS, M.D. [21, 127]
Professor of Medicine
Hematology/Oncology Unit
University of Rochester Medical Center
Rochester, New York

DEBORAH L. FRENCH, M.D. [112]
Assistant Professor
Department of Medicine
Mount Sinai School of Medicine
New York, New York

PATRICK G. GALLAGHER, M.D. [44]
Associate Professor
Department of Pediatrics
Yale University School of Medicine
Attending Physician
Department of Pediatrics
Yale-New Haven Hospital
New Haven, Connecticut

STEPHEN J. GALLI, M.D. [63]
Mary Hewitt Loveless, MD, Professor
Professor of Pathology and Microbiology and
    Immunology
Chair, Department of Pathology
Stanford University School of Medicine
Stanford University Medical Center
Stanford, California

RICHARD L. GALLO, M.D., PH.D. [114]
Associate Professor of Medicine and Pediatrics
University of California, San Diego
Section Chief, Division of Dermatology
VA San Diego Healthcare System
San Diego, California

TOMAS GANZ, PH.D., M.D. [43, 68, 69]
Professor of Medicine and Pathology
Department of Medicine
David Geffen School of Medicine at University
    of California, Los Angeles
Los Angeles, California

RANDY D. GASCOYNE, M.D., FRCPC [95]
Clinical Professor of Pathology
Department of Pathology
British Columbia Cancer Agency
University of British Columbia
Vancouver, British Columbia
Canada

LARISA J. GESKIN, M.D., FAAD [96]
Assistant Professor
Department of Dermatology
Director, Cutaneous Oncology Center and
    Photopheresis Unit
Pittsburgh, Pennsylvania

IRENE GHOBRIAL, M.D. [96]
Assistant Professor
Department of Medicine
University of Pittsburgh, School of Medicine
University of Pittsburgh Cancer Institute
Pittsburgh, Pennsylvania

DAVID GINSBURG, M.D. [118]
Professor, Department of Human Genetics
Professor, Internal Medicine; Molecular
    Medicine and Genetics
Research Professor, Life Sciences Institute
University of Michigan Medical School
Investigator
Howard Hughes Medical Institute
Ann Arbor, Michigan

LUCY A. GODLEY, M.D. [10]
Assistant Professor
Section of Hematology/Oncology
Department of Medicine
The University of Chicago Hospitals
Chicago, Illinois

ROBERTA A. GOTTLIEB, M.D. [11]
Associate Professor
Department of Molecular and Experimental
    Medicine
The Scripps Research Institute
La Jolla, California
Associate Professor (Adjunct)
Department of Medicine
University of California, San Diego
San Diego, California

XYLINA T. GREGG, M.D. [36]
Chief of Hematology/Oncology
Kelsey-Seybold Clinic and Assistant Professor
    of Medicine
Baylor College of Medicine
Houston, Texas

JOHN H. GRIFFIN, PH.D. [107, 122]
Professor
Department of Molecular and Experimental
    Medicine
The Scripps Research Institute
La Jolla, California

FRANCISCA C. GUSHIKEN, M.D. [110]
Assistant Professor
Department of Internal Medicine
Thrombosis Research Section
Baylor College of Medicine
Houston, Texas

KATHERINE A. HAJJAR, M.D. [108, 127]
Professor and Chairman
Department of Cell & Developmental Biology
Weill Medical College of Cornell University
Professor
Department of Pediatrics
New York-Presbyterian Hospital
New York, New York

ROBERT S. HILLMAN, M.D. [54]
Professor of Medicine
University of Vermont College of Medicine
Burlington, Vermont
Chairman Emeritus
Department of Medicine
Maine Medical Center
Portland, Maine

CHAIM HERSHKO, M.D. [54]
Professor of Medicine
Hebrew University Hadassah Medical School
    and Ben Gurion University School of
    Medicine
Shaare Zadek Medical Center
Jerusalem, Israel

WEN-ZHE HO, M.D. [67]
Associate Professor of Pediatrics
Division of Allergy & Immunology
The Children's Hospital of Philadelphia
Philadelphia, Pennsylvania

MAUREANE R. HOFFMAN, M.D. [106]
Associate Professor of Pathology
Assistant Professor of Immunology
Duke University
Director, Hematology and Blood Bank
Durham VA Medical Center
Durham, North Carolina

W. KEITH HOOTS, M.D. [121]
Professor
Gulf States Hemophilia and Thrombosis Center
University of Texas Health Science Center at
    Houston
Houston, Texas

SANDRA J. HORNING, M.D. [97]
Professor of Medicine
Oncology and Blood Marrow Transplantation
Stanford University Medical Center
Stanford Cancer Center
Stanford, California

RUSSELL D. HULL, M.D. [125]
Professor
Department of Medicine
University of Calgary
Active Staff
Department of General Internal Medicine
Foothills Hospital
Calgary, Alberta, Canada

AIDA INBAL, M.D. [116]
Acting Director
Institute of Thrombosis & Hemostasis
Sheba Medical Center
Tel Hashomer, Israel

SAMUEL A. JACOBS, M.D. [96]
Clinical Professor
Department of Medicine
University of Pittsburgh, School of Medicine
Associate Director for Clinical Investigations
University of Pittsburgh Cancer Institute
Pittsburgh, Pennsylvania

DANIEL R. JACOBSON, M.D. [101]
Chief of Oncology
VA Boston Healthcare System
Boston, Massachusetts

JILL JOHNSEN, M.D. [118]
Lecturer
Division of Hematology/Oncology
Department of Internal Medicine
University of Michigan Medical School
Ann Arbor, Michigan

MARSHALL E. KADIN, M.D. [94]
Professor of Pathology
Harvard Medical School
Director of Hematopathology
Beth Israel Deaconess Medical Center
Boston, Massachusetts

KAREN L. KAPLAN, M.D., PH.D. [21]
Professor of Medicine
Hematology/Oncology Unit
University of Rochester School of Medicine
    and Dentistry
Rochester, New York

KENNETH KAUSHANSKY, M.D. [13, 15, 104,
    109]
Helen M. Ranney Professor and Chair
Department of Medicine
University of California, San Diego
San Diego, California

THOMAS J. KIPPS, M.D., PH.D. [5, 14, 26, 75, 77,
    78, 80, 81, 90, 92, 102, 129]
Professor
Division of Hematology/Oncology
Deputy Director for Research Operations
Rebecca and John Moores UCSD Cancer
    Center
University of California, San Diego
La Jolla, California

LARRY W. KWAK, M.D., PH.D. [24]
Professor of Medicine
Chairman, Department of Lymphoma/Myeloma
Talpaz Chair in Immunology
Center for Cancer Immunology Research
University of Texas, M.D. Anderson Cancer
    Center
Houston, Texas

LEWIS L. LANIER, M.D. [79]
Professor and Vice-Chair
Department of Microbiology and Immunology
University of California, San Francisco
San Francisco, California

MICHELLE M. LE BEAU, PH.D. [10]
Professor of Medicine
Department of Medicine
Section of Hematology/Oncology
University of Chicago Hospitals
Chicago, Illinois

TUCKER W. LeBIEN, PH.D. [76]
Professor
Department of Laboratory Medicine/Pathology
University of Minnesota Medical School
Minneapolis, Minnesota

PHILLIP H. A. LEE, M.D. [114]
Post-Doctoral Fellow
Department of Medicine
Division of Dermatology
University of California, San Diego Medical
    Center
San Diego, California

ROBERT I. LEHRER, M.D. [68, 69]
Professor of Medicine
Department of Medicine
David Geffen School of Medicine at University
    of California, Los Angeles
Los Angeles, California

ALEXANDRA M. LEVINE, M.D. [83]
Distinguished Professor of Medicine
Chief, Division of Hematology
University of Southern California
Keck School of Medicine
Medical Director
USC/Norris Cancer Hospital
Los Angeles, California

MARSHALL A. LICHTMAN, M.D. [1, 4, 8, 33, 64,
    70, 71, 72, 85, 86, 87, 88, 89, 99]
Professor of Medicine and of Biochemistry and
    Biophysics
University of Rochester School of Medicine
    and Dentistry
Rochester, New York
Executive Vice President for Research and
    Medical Programs
The Leukemia & Lymphoma Society
White Plains, New York

JANE L. LIESVELD, M.D. [86, 87, 88]
Associate Professor of Medicine
University of Rochester Medical Center
Clinical Director, Leukemia/Blood and Marrow
    Transplantation Program
Department of Medicine/Hematology Oncology
Strong Memorial Hospital
J. P. Wilmot Cancer Center
Rochester, New York

SOON THYE LIM, M.D. [83]
Associate Consultant, Medical Oncology
National Cancer Centre
Singapore

WEONJEONG LIM, M.D. [27]
Research Scholar
Department of Psychiatry
University of California, San Diego
La Jolla, California
Assistant Professor
Department of Psychiatry
College of Medicine
Ewha Woman's University
Seoul, Republic of Korea

TON LISMAN, M.D. [120]
Thrombosis and Haemostasis Laboratory
Department of Haematology
University Hospital of Utrecht
Utrecht, The Netherlands

JOSÉ A. LÓPEZ, M.D. [110]
Professor of Medicine and Molecular and
    Human Genetics
Scientific Director, Thrombosis Research
    Section
Vice-Chairman of Medicine for Research
Baylor College of Medicine
Houston, Texas

THOMAS P. LOUGHRAN, M.D. [94]
Professor of Internal Medicine
University of South Florida School of Medicine
Program Leader, Hematologic Malignancies
H. Lee Moffitt Cancer Center & Research
    Institute
Tampa, Florida

NAOMI L.C. LUBAN, M.D. [53]
Professor, Pediatrics and Pathology
George Washington University School of
    Medicine
Chair, Laboratory Medicine & Pathology
Director, Transfusion Medicine / Donor Center
Children's National Medical Center
Washington, D.C.

AARON J. MARCUS, M.D. [108]
Professor of Medicine
Weill Medical College of Cornell University
Chief, Hematology-Oncology
New York DVA Medical Center
New York, New York

JEFFREY McCULLOUGH, M.D. [130]
Professor
Department of Laboratory Medicine and
    Pathology
Director, Division of Labaratory Medicine and
    Section of Transfusion Medicine
University of Minnesota Medical School
Minneapolis, Minnesota

BRUCE McLEOD, M.D. [25]
Professor of Medicine and Pathology
Rush Medical College
Director of Blood Center
Rush–Presbyterian–St. Luke's Medical Center
Chicago, Illinois

DEAN D. METCALFE, M.D. [63]
Chief, Laboratory of Allergic Diseases
NIAID/National Institute of Health
Bethesda, Maryland

MARTHA P. MIMS, M.D., PH.D. [7]
Assistant Professor
Department of Medicine, Hematology, and
    Oncology
Baylor College of Medicine
Houston, Texas

W. BEAU MITCHELL, M.D. [112]
Clinical Assistant
Department of Pediatrics
Mount Sinai Hospital
Instructor
Department of Pediatrics
Mount Sinai School of Medicine
New York, New York

JOEL MOAKE, M.D. [49]
Associate Director, Biomedical Engineering
    Laboratory
Rice University
Houston, Texas
Professor of Medicine
Department of Medicine, Hematology, and
    Oncology
Baylor College of Medicine
Houston, Texas

EMILE R. MOHLER III, M.D. [126]
Director, Vascular Medicine and Director,
    Vascular Diagnostic Center
Division of Cardiovascular Medicine
Department of Medicine
University of Pennsylvania School of Medicine
Director, Vascular Medicine Program
Presbyterian Medical Center
Philadelphia, Pennsylvania

DOUGALD M. MONROE III, PH.D. [106]
Associate Professor of Medicine
Division of Hematology-Oncology
University of North Carolina School of
    Medicine
Chapel Hill, North Carolina

MICHAEL W. MOSESSON, M.D. [117]
Professor
Department of Medicine
University of Wisconsin Medical School
Madison, Wisconsin
Senior Investigator
The Blood Research Institute
The Blood Center of Southeastern Wisconsin
Milwaukee, Wisconsin

WILLIAM MULLER, M.D., PH.D. [108]
Associate Professor
Department of Pathology
Weill Medical College of Cornell University
New York, New York

SCOTT MURPHY, M.D. [132]
Adjunct Professor of Medicine
Division of Hematology and Oncology
University of Pennsylvania School of Medicine
Chief Medical Officer
American Red Cross Services
Penn-Jersey Region
Philadelphia, Pennsylvania

ROBERT S. NEGRIN, M.D. [22]
Associate Professor of Medicine
Departments of Medicine and Bone Marrow
    Transplantation
Stanford University
Stanford Hospital and Clinics
Stanford, California

CHARLES H. PACKMAN, M.D. [52]
Clinical Professor of Medicine
University of North Carolina School of
    Medicine
Chapel Hill, North Carolina
Chief, Section of Hematology-Oncology
Department of Internal Medicine
Carolinas Medical Center
Charlotte, North Carolina

JAMES PALIS, M.D. [6]
Associate Professor of Pediatrics and Oncology
Biomedical Genetics, and Center for Human
    Genetics and Molecular Pediatric Disease
University of Rochester Medical Center
Rochester, New York

LESLIE V. PARISE, PH.D. [105]
Professor and Vice-Chair of Pharmacology
Department of Pharmacology
University of North Carolina at Chapel Hill
Chapel Hill, North Carolina

LAWRENCE D. PETZ, M.D. [128]
Medical Director, StemCyte, Inc.
Arcadia, California
Professor of Pathology and Laboratory
    Medicine
David Geffen School of Medicine at University
    of California, Los Angeles
Los Angeles, California

GRAHAM F. PINEO, M.D. [125]
Professor of Medicine
Department of Medicine and Oncology
University of Calgary
Department of Medicine
Foothills Hospital
Calgary, Alberta, Canada

MORTIMER PONCZ, M.D. [124]
Professor of Pediatrics
Department of Pediatics
University of Pennsylvania School of Medicine
The Children's Hospital of Philadelphia
Philadelphia, Pennsylvania

JOSEF T. PRCHAL, M.D. [7, 30, 32, 36, 42, 56]
Professor of Medicine and Pathology
Hematology Division
University of Utah
Salt Lake City, Utah
Department of Pathophysiology
First Faculty of Medicine
Charles University in Prague
Czech Republic

CHING-HON PUI, M.D. [91]
Professor of Pediatrics
University of Tennessee Health Sciences Center
Director, Leukemia/Lymphoma Division
St. Jude Children's Research Hospital
F.M. Kirby Clinical Research Professor
American Cancer Society
Memphis, Tennessee

JAYASHREE RAMASETHU, M.D. [53]
Assistant Professor of Pediatrics
Division of Neonatology
Department of Pediatrics
Georgetown University Hospital
Washington, D.C.

JACOB H. RAND, M.D. [123]
Professor of Pathology and Medicine
Director of Hematology Laboratory
Montefiore Medical Center
The University Hospital for the Albert Einstein
    College of Medicine
Bronx, New York

GARY E. RASKOB, PH.D. [125]
Dean, College of Public Health
Associate Vice President for Clinical Research
The University of Oklahoma Health Sciences
    Center
Oklahoma City, Oklahoma

MARION E. REID, PH.D. [128]
Immunology Laboratory
New York Blood Center
New York, New York

STANLEY RIDDELL, M.D. [23]
Immunology
Clinical Research Division
Fred Hutchinson Cancer Research Center
Seattle, Washington

HAROLD R. ROBERTS, M.D. [106, 115]
Sarah Graham Kenan Distinguished Professor
    of Medicine and Pathology
Division of Hematology
Department of Medicine
University of North Carolina at Chapel Hill
Attending Physician
Department of Medicine
University of North Carolina Hospitals
Chapel Hill, North Carolina

DANIEL H. RYAN, M.D. [2, 3]
Professor of Pathology and Laboratory
    Medicine
Director of Clinical Laboratories
University of Rochester Medical Center
Rochester, New York

J. EVAN SADLER, M.D., PH.D. [124]
Investigator
Howard Hughes Medical Institute
Professor
Division of Hematology
Department of Medicine
Washington University School of Medicine
St. Louis, Missouri

RALPH D. SANDERSON, PH.D. [100]
Professor of Pathology
Director of Research
Myeloma Institute for Research and Therapy
Arkansas Cancer Research Center
University of Arkansas for Medical Sciences
    Medical Center
Little Rock, Arkansas

SHIGERU SASSA, M.D., PH.D. [57]
Medical Director
Yamanouchi Pharmaceutical Co., Ltd.
Tokyo, Japan
Associate Professor and Physician
Emeritus and Head of Laboratory for
    Biochemical Hematology
The Rockefeller University
New York, New York

ALAN SAVEN, M.D. [93]
Adjunct Professor
Department of Molecular and Experimental
    Medicine
The Scripps Research Institute
Head, Division of Hematology/Oncology
Director, Ida M. and Cecil H. Green Cancer
    Center
La Jolla, California

ANDREW I. SCHAFER, M.D. [111, 126]
The Frank Wister Thomas Professor of
    Medicine
Chairman, Department of Medicine
University of Pennsylvania School of Medicine
Philadelphia, Pennsylvania

MATHIAS SCHMID, M.D. [12]
University of Ulm
Internal Medicine III
Hematology, Oncology, Rheumatology and
    Infectious Diseases
Ulm, Germany

HARRY W. SCHROEDER, JR. M.D., PH.D. [82]
Professor of Medicine
Division of Developmental and Clinical
    Immunology
Departments of Medicine, Microbiology, and
    Genetics
University of Alabama at Birmingham
Birmingham, Alabama

GEORGE B. SEGEL, M.D. [6, 33]
Professor of Pediatrics, Medicine, and
    Oncology
Vice-Chair, Department of Pediatrics
Chief, Pediatric Genetics
University of Rochester Medical Center
Rochester, New York

DAVID C. SELDIN, M.D., PH.D. [101]
Associate Professor of Medicine
Section of Hematology-Oncology
Boston University School of Medicine
Boston, Massachusetts

URI SELIGSOHN, M.D. [109, 116, 121, 122]
Professor and Director
Amalia Biron Research Institute of Thrombosis
    and Hemostasis
Department of Hematology
Chaim Sheba Medical Center
Tel-Hashomer and Sackler Faculty of Medicine
Tel Aviv University
Tel Aviv, Israel

LISA SENZEL, M.D., PH.D. [123]
Senior Resident
Department of Pathology
Montefiore Medical Center
Bronx, New York

SANFORD J. SHATTIL, M.D. [113]
Professor
Department of Vascular Biology
The Scripps Research Institute
La Jolla, California
Adjunct Professor of Medicine
University of California, San Diego
San Diego, California

JOHN SHAUGHNESSY, JR., PH.D. [100]
Associate Professor of Medicine
Director, Lambert Laboratory for Myeloma
    Genetics
Myeloma Institute for Research and Therapy
University of Arkansas for Medical Sciences
    Medical Center
Little Rock, Arkansas

MICHELLE SHAYNE, M.D. [8]
Senior Instructor in Medicine
James P. Wilmot Cancer Center
University of Rochester Medical Center
Rochester, New York

ARUN S. SHET, M.D. [105]
Research Associate/Clinical Scholar
Laboratory of Blood and Vascular Medicine
The Rockefeller University
New York, New York

BRIAN F. SKINNIDER, M.D. [95]
Clinical Assistant Professor
Department of Pathology and Laboratory
    Medicine
University of British Columbia
Pathologist
Department of Pathology
Vancouver Hospital and Health Sciences Center
    and British Columbia Cancer Agency
Vancouver, British Columbia
Canada

C. WAYNE SMITH, M.D. [60, 61]
Professor of Pediatrics–Leukocyte Biology
Departments of Pediatrics, Immunology, and
    Medicine
Baylor College of Medicine
Children's Nutrition Research Center
Houston, Texas

SUSAN S. SMYTH, M.D., PH.D. [105]
Research Assistant Professor of Medicine
Carolina Center for Cardiovascular Biology
Center for Thrombosis and Hemostasis
University of North Carolina School of
    Medicine
Chapel Hill, North Carolina

RALPH M. STEINMAN, M.D. [18]
Henry G. Kunkel Professor and Senior
    Physician
Laboratory of Cellular Physiology and
    Immunology
The Rockefeller University
New York, New York

KAREN A. SULLIVAN, PH.D. [129]
Research Professor of Medicine
Director, Histocompatibility and
    Immunogenetics Laboratory
Tulane University Health Sciences
    Center-School of Medicine
New Orleans, Louisiana

JEFFREY SUPKO, M.D. [19]
Assistant Professor of Medicine
Harvard Medical School
Director, Clinical Pharmacology Laboratory
Massachusetts General Hospital Cancer Center
Boston, Massachusetts

KaMaLa S. THOMAS, M.A. [27]
Doctoral Student, SDSU/UCSD Joint Doctoral
    Program in Clinical Psychology
University of California, San Diego
La Jolla, California

GUIDO TRICOT, M.D. [100]
Professor of Medicine and Pathology
University of Arkansas for Medical Sciences
Director of Clinical Research
Myeloma Institute for Research and Therapy
Little Rock, Arkansas

GIORGIO TRINCHIERI, M.D [79]
NIH Fogarty Scholar ORISE Senior Fellow
Laboratory of Parasitic Diseases
National Institute of Allergy and Infectious
    Diseases
Bethesda, Maryland

RALPH VASSALLO, JR., M.D. [132]
Medical Director
American Red Cross Services
Penn-Jersey Region
Philadelphia, Pennsylvania

JOZEF VERMYLEN, M.D. [119]
Professor of Medicine
University of Leuven, Belgium
Specialist in Internal Medicine
Head of the Division for Bleeding and Vascular
    Disorders
Center of Molecular & Vascular Research
University Hospital, Leuven
Leuven, Belgium

RONALD WALKER, M.D. [100]
Assistant Professor of Radiology
Co-Director, PET Facility and Research
University of Arkansas for Medical Sciences
    Medical Center
Myeloma Institute for Research and Therapy
Little Rock, Arkansas

PETER A. WARD, M.D. [16]
Godfrey D. Stobbe Professor of Pathology and
    Chairman
Department of Pathology
University of Michigan Medical School
Ann Arbor, Michigan

ANDREW WARDLAW, M.D., PH.D. [62]
Professor of Respiratory Medicine
Department of Infection, Immunity and
    Inflammation
Institute for Lung Health.
Leicester University Medical School
Glenfield Hospital
Leicester, United Kingdom

JEFFREY S. WARREN, M.D. [16]
Warthin-Weller Endowed Professor and
    Director
Division of Clinical Pathology
Department of Pathology
University of Michigan Medical Center
Ann Arbor, Michigan

SIR DAVID J. WEATHERALL, M.D. [46]
Regius Professor Emeritus of Medicine
University of Oxford
Emeritus Director of Weatherall Institute of
    Molecular Medicine
John Radcliffe Hospital
Headington, Oxford
United Kingdom

GILBERT C. WHITE II, M.D. [115]
John C. Parker Distinguished Professor of
    Medicine and Pharmacology
Division of Hematology-Oncology
Director, Center for Thrombosis and
    Hemostasis
University of North Carolina School of
    Medicine
Chapel Hill, North Carolina

WYNDHAM WILSON, M.D. [19]
Senior Investigator
Medical Branch
National Cancer Institute
National Institute of Health
Bethesda, Maryland

NEAL S. YOUNG, M.D. [34]
Chief, Hematology Branch
National Heart, Lung, and Blood Institute
National Institutes of Health
Bethesda, Maryland

ARIELLA ZIVELIN, M.D. [116]
Laboratory Manager
Institute of Thrombosis and Hemostasis
Sheba Medical Center
Tel Hashomer, Israel

The rate of growth in our understanding of diseases of blood cells and coagulation proteins provides a challenge for the editors of a comprehensive textbook of hematology. The completion of the genome project and the acquisition of knowledge in the fields of genomics and proteomics, as applied to hematologic disorders, have accelerated the understanding of the pathogenesis of the diseases of our interest. The rate at which basic knowledge in molecular and cell biology and molecular immunology has been translated into improved diagnostic and therapeutic methods is equally as impressive. The vision of specific molecular targets for therapy has become a reality for some diseases and more is sure to come.

In response to the increased number of facts amassed in hematology and the complexity of integrating these facts for the reader, the Editorial Board of Williams Hematology has added two new members, Josef T. Prchal and Kenneth Kaushansky. Drs. Prchal and Kaushansky bring special expertise in genetics, red cell and platelet disorders, hematopoiesis, and cell signaling, as well as a broad knowledge of clinical hematology, to our work. It is that combination of breadth and depth that permits them to have a significant impact on the quality of this textbook. In this transition, Barry Coller who participated in the 4th and 5th editions decided to retire from the Board as he took on new responsibilities at Rockefeller University.

Three past contributors died during the preparation of the book, Alan Erslev, Bernard Babior, and David Golde. Alan Erslev was a member of the editorial board for the first four editions of the book and continued as a contributor to the 5th and 6th editions. He was a person of intellect and integrity, which made his contributions especially meaningful. Each of these accomplished scholars was a friend, a colleague, and a valued participant. We share with their families and with their other friends and colleagues a deep sense of loss.

This edition of the book has undergone a significant reorganization. The section on Therapeutic Principles has been expanded to include new chapters: Principles of Antithrombotic Therapy, Immune Cell Therapy, and Vaccine Therapy, along with revised versions of Principles of Chemotherapy, Hematopoietic Stem Cell Transplantation, Hemapheresis, Gene Therapy, and Management of Infections in the Compromised Host. Other new chapters, "The Innate Immune System," "The Adaptive Immune System and Dendritic Cells," "Antibody-Mediated Coagulation Factor Deficiencies," "Antibody-Mediated Thrombotic Disorders," and "Hematologic Considerations in Pregnancy," have been added. Each chapter has been extensively revised or rewritten to provide the most current information available. Several areas in which there were separate chapters on basic science aspects of a topic and on relevant clinical disorders have been combined so that both basic and clinical material are found in one chapter. We believe that this organization makes it easier for readers to access the full range of information they may want, and it reduces duplication of text and references. These chapters include (a) the reorganization of material in separate chapters related to oral anticoagulant, heparin, and fibrinolytic therapy, and antiplatelet agents into a new chapter, "Principles of Antithrombotic Therapy," (b) the combination of the metabolism of folate and cobalamin and megaloblastic anemias into a single chapter, (c) the consolidation of iron metabolism, iron transport, iron deficiency, and iron storage diseases, (d) coupling energy metabolism of red cells with hemolytic anemia resulting from glucose-6-phosphate dehydrogenase and other enzyme deficiencies, (e) tying together the structure and biochemistry of the red cell membrane with hemolysis resulting from hereditary membrane disorders, (f) integrat-

ing hemoglobin structure and function with the inherited hemoglobin disorders, (g) combining traumatic, microangiopathic, march, and sports anemias into one unit, (h) condensing warm, cold, and drug-induced antibody-mediated hemolytic anemia into one chapter on immune hemolytic disorders, and (i) uniting the chapter on functions of neutrophils with qualitative abnormalities of the neutrophil.

Each chapter has a primary editor who interacts with the author and reviews the chapter, making suggestions ranging from grammar to organization to content. Thereafter, each of the other editors is sent the chapter and asked to comment. Suggestions are incorporated before the chapter is submitted to the publisher. This ensures that the author gets several reviews of the chapter, the assigned primary and secondary editor and any additional editors that may comment. The goal is to have each chapter (a) be informative in the fewest words possible, (b) avoid unnecessary duplication among chapters, (c) provide balance between basic science and clinical information, (d) contain cross-referencing to other relevant chapters, (e) include current and carefully selected references, (f) encourage the use of review articles among the references, and (g) display informative tables and figures. The production of this book required the timely cooperation of 150 contributors. We are grateful for their work in providing this comprehensive and up-to-date text. Despite the growth of both basic and clinical knowledge and the passion that each of our contributors brings to the topic of their chapter, we have been able to maintain the text in a single volume, through scrupulous attention to chapter length.

We also include twenty-five color plates that refer to blood, marrow, and lymph node pathology, cytogenetics, gene expression profiles, and patient clinical findings that are best illustrated in color. We thank Jean Shafer, B.S., M.A., of the University of Rochester Medical Center for providing the blood and marrow cell color images on Plates I through XXI-9; Bartel Barlogie and colleagues for providing the images of myeloma cells and gene expression profiles of normal plasma cells and myeloma cells for Plate XXI-10 through 13; Randy D. Gascogne, M.D., of the British Columbia Cancer Agency, for the images of lymph node pathology and gene expression profiling of lymphoma in Plate XXII-3 through 40; Michelle M. LeBeau, Ph.D., and Lucy A. Godley, M.D., Ph.D., of the University of Chicago Medical Center, for Plate XXIV on cytogenetics; Marissa Braff, M.D., Magdalene Dohil, M.D., Terrance O'Grady, M.D., Stephanie Sturgill, M.D., and William Sturgill, M.D., of the University of California, San Diego, for images on Plate XXV-6, 9, 13, 15, 25, 36, and 37, respectively; Virgil Fairbanks, M.D., of the Mayo Clinic, for image XXV-43; Karl Blume, M.D., of Stanford University for images on Plate XXV-44 and 45; Harold Roberts for image on Plate XXV-46; and Paul Schneiderman, M.D., Columbia University, for the other images of cutaneous abnormalities used in Plate XXV.

This edition represents the first that will be also available in electronic form on the McGraw-Hill Book Company website, AccessMedicine.com, which contains a variety of major textbooks and other sources. Periodic updates will enhance the timeliness of information available on this site. An extensive atlas of blood, marrow, lymph node, cytogenetic, and flow cytometric images relevant to hematologic diagnosis is planned for the site as well.

Each editor has had expert administrative assistance in the management of the manuscripts for which they were primarily responsible. We thank Mary Carpenter, Tracey Trettin, Jane Verenini, Catherine Worix, and Renee Johnson in La Jolla, and Orly Katz in Tel Aviv for their very helpful participation in the production of the book. Special thanks go to Susan Daley, in Rochester, who was responsible for coordinating the management of 132 chapters, including their figures and tables, and managing other administrative matters, a challenging task that Ms. Daley performed with skill and good humor. The Editors also acknowledge the interest and support of four staff in the Medical Division at McGraw-Hill: Marc Strauss, Editor-and-Chief; Michelle Watt, Developmental Editor; Karen Davis, Editorial Supervisor; and Karen Edmonson, Managing Editor.

Marshall A. Lichtman Uri Seligsohn
Ernest Beutler Kenneth Kaushansky
Thomas J. Kipps Josef T. Prchal

SI UNIT CONVERSION TABLE

CONSTITUENT[a]	TRADITIONAL UNITS	MULTIPLICATION FACTOR[b]	SI UNITS[c]
δ-Aminoleuvulinic acid (U)	mg per day	7.63	μmol per day
Bilirubin			
Direct (S)	mg per dl	17.1	μmol per liter
Total (S)	mg per dl	17.1	μmol per liter
Calcium (S)	mg per dl	0.25	mmol per liter
Coproporphyrin (U)	μg per dl	1.5	nmol per day
Erythrocyte count	number per μl	10^6	number per liter
Fibrinogen[d] (Factor I) (P)	mg per dl	0.01	g per liter
	mg per dl	0.029	μmol per liter
Folic acid (S)	ng per dl	1.0	μg per liter
	ng per dl	2.27	nmol per liter
Haptoglobin (S)	mg per dl	0.01	g per liter
Hematocrit (B)	%	0.01	ratio
Hemoglobin[e] (B)	g per dl	1.0	g per dl
Iron (S)	μg per dl	0.179	μmol per liter
Iron-binding capacity (S)	μg per dl	0.179	μmol per liter
Leukocyte count (B)	number per μl	10^6	number per liter
Mean corpuscular hemoglobin	pg	1.0	pg
Mean corpuscular hemoglobin concentration	%	1.0	g per dl
Mean corpuscular volume	μm^3	1.0	fl
Packed cell volume	%	0.01	ratio
Phosphorus (S)	mg per dl	0.323	mmol per liter
Platelet count (B)	number per μl	10^6	number per liter
Porphobilinogen (U)	mg per day	4.42	μmol per day
Protoporphyrin (erythrocyte)	μg per dl	0.018	μmol per liter
Reticulocyte count (B)	%	0.01	ratio
	number per μl	10^6	number per liter
Transferrin (S)	mg per dl	0.01	g per liter
Urea nitrogen (B)	mg per dl	0.36	mmol per liter
Uric acid	mg per dl	0.36	mmol per liter
Uroporphyrin (U)	μg per dl	1.2	nmol per day
Vitamin B_{12} (S)	pg per ml	1.0	ng per liter

[a] The following abbreviations are used: B = blood; S = serum; P = plasma; U = urine.

[b] Conventional units multiplied by this factor will yield SI units.

[c] The following units are used:

fl = femtoliter (10^{-15} liter)	fmol = femtomole	fg = femtogram
pl = picoliter (10^{-12} liter)	pmol = picomole	pg = picogram
nl = nanoliter (10^{-9} liter)	nmol = nanomole	ng = nanogram
μl = microliter (10^{-6} liter)	μmol = micromole	μg = microgram
ml = milliliter (10^{-3} liter)	mmol = millimole	mg = milligram
dl = deciliter (10^{-1} liter)		

[d] The molar concentration is calculated assuming a molecular weight of 340,000.

[e] Hemoglobin is not usually expressed in molar terms because of the uncertainty regarding the polymeric state of the molecule. If the unit molecular weight is assumed to be 16,000, the multiplication factor is 0.62 to convert g per dl to mmol per liter. If the molecular weight of 64,500 is assumed, the conversion factor is 0.1555.

SOURCES:

    Baron DN, Broughton PMG, Cohen M, Lansley TS, Lewis SM, Shinton NK: The use of SI units in reporting results obtained in hospital laboratories. *J Clin Pathol* 27:590, 1974.

    Young DS: "Normal laboratory values" (case records of the Massachusetts General Hospital) in SI units. *N Engl J Med* 292:795, 1975.

    Lehmann HP: Metrication of clinical laboratory data in SI units. *Am J Clin Pathol* 65:2, 1976.

CLINICAL EVALUATION OF THE PATIENT

INITIAL APPROACH TO THE PATIENT: HISTORY AND PHYSICAL EXAMINATION

MARSHALL A. LICHTMAN
ERNEST BEUTLER

The care of a patient with a suspected hematologic abnormality begins with a systematic attempt to determine the nature of the illness by eliciting an in-depth medical history and performing a physical examination. The physician should identify the patient's symptoms systematically and obtain as much relevant information as possible about the origin and evolution of the symptoms and about the general health of the patient by appropriate questions designed to explore the patient's recent and remote experience. Reviewing previous records may add important data for understanding the onset or progression of illness. Hereditary and environmental factors should be carefully sought and evaluated. The use of drugs and medications, nutritional patterns, and sexual behavior should be considered. The physician follows the medical history with a physical examination to obtain evidence for tissue and organ abnormalities that can be accessed through bedside observation to permit a careful search for signs of the illnesses suggested by the history. Skin changes and hepatic, splenic, or lymph nodal enlargement are a few findings that may be of considerable help in pointing toward a diagnosis. Additional history is obtained during the physical examination, as findings suggest an additional or alternative considerations. Thus, the history and physical examination should be considered as a unit, providing the basic information with which further diagnostic information is integrated: blood and marrow studies, imaging studies, and biopsies.

Primary hematologic diseases are common in the aggregate, but hematologic manifestations secondary to other diseases occur even more frequently. For example, the signs and symptoms of anemia and the presence of enlarged lymph nodes are common clinical findings that may be related to a hematologic disease but occur frequently as secondary manifestations of disorders not considered primarily hematologic. A wide variety of diseases may produce signs or symptoms of hematologic illness. Thus, in patients with a connective tissue disease, all the signs and symptoms of anemia may be elicited and lymphadenopathy may be notable, but additional findings are usually present that indicate primary involvement of some system besides the hematopoietic (marrow) or lymphopoietic (lymph nodes or other lymphatic sites). In this discussion, emphasis is placed on the clinical findings resulting from either primary hematologic disease or the complications of hematologic disorders in order to avoid presenting an extensive catalog of signs and symptoms encountered in general clinical medicine.

Acronyms and abbreviations that appear in this chapter include: Ig, immunoglobulin; PS, performance status.

In each discussion of specific diseases in subsequent chapters, the signs and symptoms that accompany the particular disorder are presented, and the clinical findings are covered in detail. In this chapter, a more general systematic approach is taken.

THE HEMATOLOGY CONSULTATION

Table 1-1 lists the major abnormalities that result in the evaluation of the patient by the hematologist. The signs indicated in Table 1-1 may reflect a primary or secondary hematologic problem. For example, immature granulocytes in the blood may be signs of myeloid diseases such as myelogenous leukemia or, depending on the frequency of these cells and the level of immaturity, the dislodgment of cells resulting from bone metastases of a carcinoma. Nucleated red cells in the blood may reflect the breakdown in the marrow–blood interface seen in idiopathic myelofibrosis or the hypoxia of congestive heart failure. Certain disorders have a propensity for secondary hematologic abnormalities; renal, liver, and connective tissue diseases are prominent among such abnormalities. Chronic alcoholism, nutritional fetishes, and use of certain medications can be causal factors in blood cell or coagulation protein disorders. Pregnancy and persons of older age are prone to certain hematologic disorders: anemia, thrombocytopenia, or disseminated coagulation in the former, and hematologic malignancies and pernicious anemia in the latter. The history and physical examination can provide vital clues to the possible diagnosis and also to the rational choice of laboratory tests.

HISTORY

In today's technology- and procedure-driven medical environment, the importance of carefully gathering information by patient inquiry and examination is at risk of losing its primacy. The history and physical examination remain the vital starting point for the evaluation of any clinical problem.[1, 3]

GENERAL SYMPTOMS

Performance status (PS) is a useful concept in establishing the seriousness of the patient's disability at the outset and in evaluating the effects of therapy.[4] Table 1-2 presents a well-founded set of criteria for evaluating PS.

Weight loss is a frequent accompaniment of many serious diseases, including primary hematologic entities, but it is not a prominent accompaniment of most hematologic disease. Many "wasting" diseases, such as disseminated carcinoma or tuberculosis, cause anemia, and pronounced emaciation should suggest one of these diseases rather than anemia as the primary disorder.

Fever is a common early manifestation of the aggressive lymphomas or acute leukemias as a result of the release of pyrogens as a reflection of the disease itself. After chemotherapy-induced cytopenias, or in the face of accompanying immunodeficiency, infection is usually the cause of fever. In patients with "fever of unknown origin," lymphoma, and particularly Hodgkin lymphoma, should be considered. Occasionally myelofibrosis and chronic lymphocytic leukemia may also cause fever. In rare patients with severe pernicious anemia or hemolytic anemia, fever may be present. *Chills* may accompany severe hemolytic processes and the bacteremia that may complicate the immunocompromised or neutropenic patient. *Night sweats* suggest the presence of low-grade fever and may occur in patients with lymphoma or leukemia.

Fatigue, malaise, and *lassitude* are such common accompaniments of both physical and emotional disorders that their evaluation is complex and often difficult. In patients with serious disease, these symp-

TABLE 1-1   FINDINGS THAT MAY LEAD TO A HEMATOLOGY CONSULTATION

Anemia
Polycythemia
Elevated serum ferritin level
Leukopenia or neutropenia
Immature granulocytes or nucleated red cells in the blood
Pancytopenia
Granulocytosis: neutrophilia, eosinophilia, basophilia, mastocytosis
Lymphocytosis
Lymphadenopathy
Splenomegaly
Hypergammaglobulinemia: monoclonal or polyclonal
Purpura
Thrombocytopenia
Thrombocythemia
Exaggerated bleeding: spontaneous or trauma-related
Prolonged partial thromboplastin or prothrombin time
Leg pain and deep venous thrombosis

toms may be readily explained by fever, muscle wasting, or other associated findings. Patients with anemia frequently complain of fatigue, malaise, or lassitude and these symptoms may accompany the hematologic malignancies. Fatigue or lassitude may occur also with iron deficiency even in the absence of sufficient anemia to account for the symptom. In slowly developing chronic anemias, the patient may not recognize, for example, reduced exercise tolerance, and the like, except in retrospect, after a remission has been induced by appropriate therapy. Anemia may be responsible for more symptoms than has been traditionally recognized, as suggested by the remarkable improvement in quality of life of most uremic patients treated with erythropoietin.

Weakness may accompany anemia or the wasting of malignant processes, in which cases it is manifest as a general loss of strength or reduced capacity for exercise. The weakness may be localized as a result of neurologic complications of hematologic disease. In pernicious anemia there may be weakness of the lower extremities, accompanied by numbness, tingling, and unsteadiness of gait. Peripheral neuropathy also occurs with dysproteinemias. Weakness of one or more extremities in patients with leukemia, myeloma, or lymphoma may

TABLE 1-2   CRITERIA OF PERFORMANCE STATUS

Able to carry on normal activity; no special care is needed

  100% Normal; no complaints, no evidence of disease
   90% Able to carry on normal activity; minor signs or symptoms of disease
   80% Normal activity with effort; some signs or symptoms of disease

Unable to work; able to live at home, care for most personal needs; a varying amount of assistance is needed

   70% Cares for self; unable to carry on normal activity or to do active work
   60% Requires occasional assistance but is able to care for most personal needs
   50% Requires considerable assistance and frequent medical care

Unable to care for self; requires equivalent of institutional or hospital care; disease may be progressing rapidly

   40% Disabled; requires special care and assistance
   30% Severely disabled; hospitalization is indicated although death not imminent
   20% Very sick; hospitalization necessary; active supportive treatment necessary
   10% Moribund; fatal processes progressing rapidly
    0% Dead

signify central or peripheral nervous system invasion or compression. Myopathy secondary to malignancy occurs with the hematologic malignancies and is usually manifest as weakness of proximal muscle groups. Foot drop or wrist drop may occur in lead poisoning, amyloidosis, systemic autoimmune diseases, or as a complication of vincristine therapy. Paralysis may occur in acute intermittent porphyria.

SPECIFIC SYMPTOMS

NERVOUS SYSTEM

Headache may be caused by a number of hematologic diseases. Anemia or polycythemia may cause mild to severe headache. Invasion or compression of the brain by leukemia or lymphoma, or opportunistic infection of the central nervous system by *Cryptococcus* or *Mycobacterium* species, may also cause headache in patients with hematologic malignancies. Hemorrhage into the brain or subarachnoid space in patients with thrombocytopenia or other bleeding disorders may cause sudden, severe headache.

Paresthesias may occur because of peripheral neuropathy in monclonal gammopathy, pernicious anemia, or secondary to hematologic malignancy or amyloidosis. They may also result from therapy with vincristine.

Confusion may accompany malignant or infectious processes involving the brain, sometimes as a result of the accompanying fever. Confusion may also occur with severe anemia, hypercalcemia (e.g., myeloma), or high-dose glucocorticoid therapy. Confusion or apparent senility may be a manifestation of pernicious anemia. Frank psychosis may develop in acute intermittent porphyria or with high-dose glucocorticoid therapy.

Impairment of consciousness may be caused by increased intracranial pressure secondary to hemorrhage or leukemia or lymphoma in the central nervous system. It may also accompany severe anemia, polycythemia, hyperviscosity secondary usually to an immunoglobulin (Ig) M paraprotein in the plasma, or a leukemic hyperleukocytosis syndrome, especially in chronic myelogenous leukemia.

EYES

Conjunctival plethora is a feature of polycythemia and pallor a result of anemia. Occasionally blindness may result from retinal hemorrhages secondary to severe anemia and thrombocytopenia or blurred vision resulting from severe hyperviscosity resulting from macroglobulinemia or extreme hyperleukocytosis of leukemia. Partial or complete visual loss can stem from retinal vein or artery thrombosis. Diplopia or disturbances of ocular movement may occur with orbital tumors or paralysis of the third, fourth, or sixth cranial nerves because of compression by tumor, especially extranodal lymphoma, extramedullary myeloma, or granulocytic sarcoma.

EARS

Vertigo, tinnitus, and "roaring" in the ears may occur with marked anemia, polycythemia, or macroglobulinemia-induced hyperviscosity.

NASOPHARYNX, OROPHARYNX, AND ORAL CAVITY

Epistaxis may occur in patients with thrombocytopenia, acquired or inherited platelet function disorders, and von Willebrand disease. *Anosmia* or *olfactory hallucinations* occur in pernicious anemia. The nasopharynx may be invaded by a granulocytic sarcoma or extranodal lymphoma; the symptoms are dependent on the structures invaded. The paranasal sinuses may be involved by opportunistic organisms, for example, fungal infection. *Sore tongue* occurs in pernicious anemia and may accompany severe iron deficiency or vitamin deficiencies. *Macroglossia* occurs in amyloidosis. *Bleeding gums* may occur with bleeding disorders. Infiltration of the gingiva with leukemic cells occurs notably in acute monocytic leukemia. *Ulceration* of the tongue or oral mucosa may be severe in the acute leukemias or in patients with severe neutropenia. *Dryness of the mouth* may be a result of hypercalcemia, secondary, for example, to myeloma. *Dysphagia* may be seen in patients with severe mucous membrane atrophy associated with chronic iron-deficiency anemia.

NECK

Painless swelling in the neck is characteristic of lymphoma but may be caused by a number of other diseases as well. Occasionally, the enlarged lymph nodes of lymphomas may be tender or painful because of secondary infection or rapid growth. Painful or tender lymphadenopathy is usually associated with inflammatory reactions such as infectious mononucleosis or suppurative adenitis. *Diffuse swelling* of the neck and face may occur with obstruction of the superior vena cava as a consequence of lymphoma.

CHEST AND HEART

Both *dyspnea* and *palpitations*, usually on effort but occasionally at rest, may occur because of anemia. *Congestive heart failure* may supervene, and *angina pectoris* may become manifest in anemic patients. The impact of anemia on the circulatory system depends in part on the rapidity with which it develops, and chronic anemia may become severe without producing major symptoms; with severe acute blood loss, the patient may develop shock with a nearly normal hemoglobin level, prior to compensatory hemodilution. *Cough* may result from enlarged mediastinal nodes. *Chest pain* may arise from involvement of the ribs or sternum with lymphoma or multiple myeloma, nerve-root invasion or compression, or herpes zoster; the pain of herpes zoster usually precedes the skin lesions by several days. *Tenderness of the sternum* may be quite pronounced in chronic myelogenous or acute leukemia, and occasionally in myelofibrosis, or if intramedullary lymphoma or myeloma proliferation is explosive.

GASTROINTESTINAL SYSTEM

Dysphagia was already mentioned earlier (see "Nasopharynx, Oropharynx, and Oral Cavity" above). *Anorexia* frequently occurs but usually has no specific diagnostic significance. Hypercalcemia and azotemia cause anorexia, nausea, and vomiting. A variety of ill-defined gastrointestinal complaints grouped under the heading "indigestion" may occur with hematologic diseases. *Abdominal fullness, premature satiety, belching,* or *discomfort* may occur because of a greatly enlarged spleen, but such splenomegaly may also be entirely asymptomatic. *Abdominal pain* may arise from intestinal obstruction by lymphoma, retroperitoneal bleeding, lead poisoning, ileus secondary to therapy with the *Vinca* alkaloids, acute hemolysis, allergic purpura, the abdominal crises of sickle cell disease, or acute intermittent porphyria. *Diarrhea* may occur in pernicious anemia. It also may be prominent in the various forms of intestinal malabsorption, although significant malabsorption may occur without diarrhea. In small-bowel malabsorption, steatorrhea may be a notable feature. Malabsorption may be a manifestation of small-bowel lymphoma. *Gastrointestinal bleeding* related to thrombocytopenia or other bleeding disorder may be entirely occult but often is manifest as *hematemesis* or *melena*. *Constipation* may occur in the patient with hypercalcemia or in one receiving treatment with the *Vinca* alkaloids.

GENITOURINARY AND REPRODUCTIVE SYSTEMS

Impotence or *bladder dysfunction* may occur with spinal cord or peripheral nerve damage as a result of one of the hematologic malignancies or with pernicious anemia. Priapism may occur in leukemia or sickle cell disease. *Hematuria* may be a manifestation of hemophilia A or B. *Red urine* may also occur with intravascular hemolysis (he-moglobinuria), myoglobinuria, or porphyrinuria. Injection of anthracycline drugs or ingestion of drugs such as phenazopyridine (Pyridium) regularly causes the urine to turn red. Beeturia also occurs as a benign genetic trait. Certain drugs, such as antimetabolites or alkylating agents, may also induce amenorrhea. *Menorrhagia* is a common cause of iron deficiency, and care must be taken to obtain an accurate history of the extent of menstrual blood loss. Semiquantification can be obtained from estimates of the number of days of heavy bleeding (usually 1 to 2), the number of days of any bleeding (usually 5 to 7), number of tampons or pads used (requirement for double pads suggests excessive bleeding), degree of blood soaking, and clots formed. Inquiries such as "Have you experienced a gush of blood when a tampon is removed?" are useful. Menorrhagia may occur in patients with bleeding disorders.

BACK AND EXTREMITIES

Back pain may accompany acute hemolytic reactions or be caused by involvement of bone or the nervous system in acute leukemia or aggressive lymphoma. It is one of the commonest manifestations of myeloma.

Arthritis or *arthralgia* may occur with gout secondary to increased uric acid production in patients with hematologic malignancies, myelofibrosis, myelodysplastic syndrome, or hemolytic anemia. They also occur in the plasma cell dyscrasias, acute leukemias, and sickle cell disease without evidence of gout, and in allergic purpura. Arthritis may accompany hemochromatosis. Hemarthroses in patients with severe bleeding disorders cause marked joint pain. Autoimmune diseases may present as anemia and/or thrombocytopenia, and arthritis appears as a later manifestation. *Shoulder pain* on the left may be a result of infarction of the spleen and on the right from gall bladder disease associated with chronic hemolytic anemia such as hereditary spherocytosis. *Bone pain* may occur with bone involvement by the hematologic malignancies; it is common in the congenital hemolytic anemias, such as sickle cell anemia, and may occur in myelofibrosis. In patients with Hodgkin lymphoma, ingestion of alcohol may induce pain at the site of any lesion, including those in bone. *Edema* of the lower extremities, sometimes unilateral, may occur because of obstruction to veins or lymphatics by enlarged lymph nodes. *Leg ulcers* are a common complaint in sickle cell anemia and occur rarely in other hereditary anemias.

SKIN

Skin manifestations of hematologic disease may be of great importance; they include changes in texture or color, itching, and the presence of specific or nonspecific lesions. The skin in iron-deficient patients may become dry, the hair dry and fine, and the nails brittle. In hypothyroidism, which may cause anemia, the skin is dry, coarse, and scaly. *Jaundice* may be apparent with pernicious anemia or congenital or acquired hemolytic anemia. The skin of patients with pernicious anemia is said to be "lemon yellow" because of the simultaneous appearance of jaundice and pallor. Jaundice may also occur in patients with hematologic malignancies as a result of liver involvement or biliary tract obstruction. *Pallor* is a common accompaniment of anemia, although some severely anemic patients may not appear pale. Erythromelalgia may be a troublesome complication of polycythemia vera. Widespread *erythroderma* occurs in cutaneous T cell cutaneous lymphoma (especially Sézary syndrome) and in some cases of chronic lymphocytic leukemia or lymphocytic lymphoma. The skin is often involved, sometimes severely, in graft-versus-host disease following marrow transplantation. Patients with hemochromatosis may have bronze or grayish pigmentation of the skin. *Cyanosis* occurs with methemoglobinemia, either hereditary or acquired, sulfhemoglobinemia, abnormal hemoglobins with low oxygen affinity, and primary and secondary polycythemia. Cyanosis of the ears or the fingertips may occur after exposure to cold in individuals with cryoglobulins or cold agglutinins.

Itching may occur in the absence of any visible skin lesions in Hodgkin lymphoma and may be extreme. Mycosis fungoides or other lymphomas with skin involvement may also present as itching. A significant number of patients with polycythemia vera will complain of itching after bathing.

Petechiae and *ecchymoses* are most often seen in the extremities in patients with thrombocytopenia, nonthrombocytopenic purpura, or acquired or inherited platelet function abnormalities and von Willebrand disease. These lesions usually are painless, although the lesions related to trauma, psychogenic purpura, or erythema nodosum are painful. *Easy bruising* is a common complaint, especially among women, and when no other hemorrhagic symptoms are present, usually no abnormalities are found after detailed study. This symptom may, however, indicate a mild hereditary bleeding disorder, such as von Willebrand disease or one of the platelet disorders.

Infiltrative lesions may occur in the leukemias (leukemia cutis) and lymphomas and are sometimes the presenting complaint. Monocytic leukemia has a higher frequency of skin infiltration than other forms of leukemia. *Necrotic lesions* may occur with intravascular coagulation, purpura fulminans, warfarin-induced skin necrosis, or rarely with exposure to cold in patients with circulating cryoproteins or cold agglutinins.

DRUGS AND CHEMICALS

DRUGS

Drug therapy, either self-prescribed or ordered by a physician, is extremely common in our society. Drugs often induce or aggravate hematologic disease, and it is therefore essential that a careful history of drug ingestion, including beneficial and adverse reactions, be obtained from all patients. Drugs taken regularly often become a part of the patient's way of life and are often forgotten or are not recognized as "drugs." Agents such as aspirin, laxatives, tranquilizers, medicinal iron, vitamins, other nutritional supplements, and sedatives belong to this category. Furthermore, drugs may be ingested in unrecognized form, such as antibiotics in food or quinine in tonic water. Specific, persistent questioning, often on several occasions, may be necessary before a complete history of drug use is obtained. It is very important to obtain detailed information on alcohol consumption from every patient. The four CAGE questions—about *c*utting down, being *a*nnoyed by criticism, having *g*uilt feelings, and needing an *e*yeopener—provide an effective approach to the history of alcohol use. Patients should also be asked about the use of recreational drugs. The use of "alternative medicines" and herbal medicines is common, and many patients will not consider these medications or may actively withhold information about their use. Nonjudgmental questioning may be successful in identifying agents in this category that the patient is taking. Some patients equate the term *drugs*, as opposed to *medicines*, with illicit drugs. Establishing that the examiner is interested in all forms of ingestants—prescribed drugs, self-remedies, alternative remedies, et cetera—is important to ensure that all the information required is obtained.

CHEMICALS

In addition to drugs, most people are exposed regularly to a variety of chemicals in the environment, some of which may be potentially harmful agents in hematologic disease. Similarly, occupational exposure to chemicals must be considered. When a toxin is suspected, the patient's daily activities and environment must be carefully reviewed, because significant exposure to toxic chemicals may occur incidentally.

VACCINATION

Vaccinations can exacerbate immune thrombocytopenia.

NUTRITION

Children who are breast-fed without iron supplementation may develop iron-deficiency anemia. Nutritional information can be useful in deducing the possible role of dietary deficiency in anemia. The avoidance of certain food groups, as might be the case with vegans, or the ingestion of uncooked fish can be clues to the pathogenesis of megaloblastic anemia.

FAMILY HISTORY

A carefully obtained family history may be of great importance in the study of patients with hematologic disease. In the case of hemolytic disorders, questions should be asked regarding jaundice, anemia, and gallstones in relatives. In patients with disorders of hemostasis or venous thrombosis, particular attention must be given to bleeding manifestations or venous thromboembolism in family members. In the case of autosomal recessive disorders such as pyruvate kinase deficiency the parents are usually not affected, but a similar clinical syndrome may have occurred in siblings. It is particularly important to inquire about siblings who may have died in infancy, because they may be forgotten, especially by older patients. When sex-linked inheritance is suspected, it is necessary to inquire about symptoms in the maternal grandfather, maternal uncles, male siblings, and nephews. In patients with disorders with dominant inheritance, such as hereditary spherocytosis, one may expect to find that one of the parents and possibly siblings and children of the patient have stigmata of the disease. Ethnic background may be important in the consideration of certain diseases such as thalassemia, sickle cell anemia, glucose-6-phosphate dehydrogenase deficiency, or other inherited disorders that are prevalent in geographic areas.

SEXUAL HISTORY

Because of the epidemic of infections with the human immunodeficiency viruses, it is important to ascertain the sexual behavior of the patient, especially risk factors for transmission of HIV.

PREVENTIVE HEMATOLOGY

Ideally, the physician's goal is to prevent illness, and opportunities exist for hematologists to prevent the development of hematologic disorders. These opportunities include identification of individual genetic risk factors and either avoidance of situations that may make a latent disorder manifest. Prophylactic therapy, as for example in avoiding venous stasis in patients heterozygous for protein C deficiency or administering prophylactic heparin at the time of major surgery, is a more immediate aspect of prevention because it depends on the physician's intervention. Hematologists may also prevent disease by reinforcing community medicine efforts. Examples include fostering the elimination of sources of environmental lead that may result in childhood anemia and fostering the careful regulation of environmental toxins, such as benzene, organochlorine and organophosphate pesticides, and phenoxyherbicides that increase the risk of lymphohematopoietic malignancies. Prenatal diagnosis of hematologic disorders can provide information to families as to whether a fetus is affected with a hematologic disorder.

PHYSICAL EXAMINATION

A detailed physical examination should be performed on every patient, with sufficient attention paid to all systems to obtain a full evaluation of the general health of the individual. Certain body areas are especially pertinent to hematologic disease and therefore deserve special attention. These are the skin, eyes, tongue, lymph nodes, skeleton, spleen and liver, and nervous system.

SKIN

PALLOR AND FLUSHING

The color of the skin is caused by the pigment contained therein and by the blood flowing through the skin capillaries. The component of skin color related to the blood may be a useful guide to anemia or polycythemia because pallor may result when the hemoglobin level is reduced and redness when the hemoglobin level is increased. The amount of pigment in the skin will modify skin color and may mislead the clinician, as in individuals with pallor as a result of decreased pigment, or make skin color useless as a guide because of the intense pigmentation present.

Alterations in blood flow and in hemoglobin content may change skin color; this, too, may mislead the clinician. Thus emotion may cause either pallor or blushing. Exposure of the skin to cold or heat may similarly cause pallor or blushing. Chronic exposure to wind or sun may lead to permanent redness of the skin, and chronic ingestion of alcohol to a flushed face. The degree of erythema of the skin can be evaluated by pressing the thumb firmly against the skin, for example, on the forehead, so that the capillaries are emptied, and comparing the color of the compressed spot with the surrounding skin immediately after the thumb is removed.

The mucous membranes and nail beds are usually more reliable guides to anemia or polycythemia than the skin. The conjunctivae and gums may be inflamed, however, and therefore not reflect the hemoglobin level, or the gums may appear pale because of pressure from the lips. The gums and the nail beds may also be pigmented and the capillaries correspondingly obscured. In some individuals, the color of the capillaries does not become fully visible through the nails unless pressure is applied to the fingertip, either laterally or on the end of the nail.

The palmar creases are useful guides to the hemoglobin level and appear pink in the fully opened hand unless the hemoglobin is 7 g/dl or less. Liver disease may induce flushing of the thenar and hypothenar eminences of the palm, even in patients with anemia.

CYANOSIS

The detection of cyanosis, like the detection of pallor, may be made difficult by skin pigmentation. Cyanosis is a function of the total amount of reduced hemoglobin, methemoglobin, or sulfhemoglobin present. The minimum amounts of these pigments that cause detectable cyanosis are about 5 g/dl blood of reduced hemoglobin, 1.5 to 2.0 g/dl of methemoglobin, and 0.5 g/dl of sulfhemoglobin.

JAUNDICE

Jaundice may be observed in the skin of individuals who are not otherwise deeply pigmented or in the sclerae or the mucous membranes. The patient should be examined in daylight rather than under incandescent or fluorescent light, because the yellow color of the latter masks the yellow color of the patient. Jaundice is caused by actual staining of the skin by bile pigment, and bilirubin glucuronide (direct-reacting or conjugated bilirubin) stains the skin more readily than the unconjugated form. Jaundice of the skin may not be visible if the bilirubin level is below 2 to 3 mg/dl. Yellow pigmentation of the skin may also occur with carotenemia, especially in young children.

PETECHIAE AND ECCHYMOSES

Petechiae are small (1 to 2 mm), round, red or brown lesions resulting from hemorrhage into the skin and are present primarily in areas with high venous pressure, such as the lower extremities. These lesions do not blanch on pressure, and this can be demonstrated most readily by compressing the skin with a glass microscope slide or magnifying lens. Petechiae may occasionally be elevated slightly, that is, palpable; this finding suggests vasculitis. Ecchymoses may be of various sizes and shapes and may be red, purple, blue, or yellowish green, depending on the intensity of the skin hemorrhage and its age. They may be flat or elevated; some are painful and tender. The lesions of hereditary hemorrhagic telangiectasia are small, flat, nonpulsatile, and violaceous. They blanch with pressure.

EXCORIATION

Itching may be intense in some hematologic disorders such as Hodgkin lymphoma, even in the absence of skin lesions. Excoriation of the skin from scratching is the only physical manifestation of this severe symptom.

LEG ULCERS

Open ulcers or scars from healed ulcers are often found in the region of the internal or external malleoli in patients with sickle cell anemia and, rarely, in other hereditary anemias.

NAILS

Detection of pallor or rubor by examining the nails was discussed earlier. The fingernails in chronic, severe iron-deficiency anemia may be ridged longitudinally and flattened or concave rather than convex. The latter change, concave-shaped nails, is referred to as *koilonychia* and is uncommon in present practice.

EYES

Jaundice, pallor, or *plethora* may be detected from examination of the eyes. Jaundice is usually more readily detected in the sclerae than in the skin. Ophthalmoscopic examination is also essential in patients with hematologic disease. *Retinal hemorrhages* and *exudates* occur in patients with severe anemia and thrombocytopenia. These hemorrhages are usually the typical "flame-shaped" hemorrhages, but they may be quite large and elevate the retina so that they may appear as a darkly colored tumor. Round hemorrhages with white centers are also often seen. *Dilatation of the veins* may be seen in polycythemia; in patients with macroglobulinemia, the veins are engorged and segmented, resembling link sausages.

MOUTH

Pallor of the mucosa has already been discussed. *Ulceration* of the oral mucosa occurs commonly in neutropenic patients. In leukemia there may also be infiltration of the gums with swelling, redness, and bleeding. *Bleeding* from the mucosa may occur with a hemorrhagic disease. A dark line of lead sulfide may be deposited in the gums at the base of the teeth in lead poisoning. The *tongue* may be completely smooth in pernicious anemia and iron-deficiency anemia. Patients with an upper dental prosthesis may also have papillary atrophy, presumably on a mechanical basis. The tongue may be smooth and red in patients with nutritional deficiencies. This may be accompanied by fissuring at the corners of the mouth, but fissuring may also be caused by ill-fitting dentures. An enlarged tongue, abnormally firm to palpation, may indicate the presence of primary amyloidosis.

LYMPH NODES

Lymph nodes are widely distributed in the body, and in disease any node or group of nodes may be involved. The major concern on physical examination is the detection of enlarged or tender nodes in the cervical, supraclavicular, axillary, epitrochlear, inguinal, or femoral regions. Under normal conditions in adults, the only readily palpable lymph nodes are in the inguinal region, where several firm nodes, 0.5 to 2.0 cm long, are normally attached to the dense fascia below the inguinal ligament and in the femoral triangle. In children, multiple small (0.5 to 1.0 cm) nodes may be palpated in the cervical region as well. Supraclavicular nodes may sometimes be palpable only when the patient performs the Valsalva maneuver.

Enlarged lymph nodes are ordinarily detected in the superficial areas by palpation, although they are sometimes large enough to be seen. Palpation should be gentle and is best performed with a circular motion of the fingertips, using slowly increasing pressure. Tender lymph nodes usually indicate an inflammatory etiology, although rapidly proliferative lymphoma may be tender to palpation.

Nodes too deep to palpate may be detected by specific imaging procedures, including computerized tomography, magnetic resonance imaging, ultrasonography studies, gallium scintography, and positron emission tomography.[5,6]

CHEST

Increased rib or sternal tenderness is an important physical sign that is often ignored. Increased bone pain may be generalized, as in leukemia, or spotty, as in plasma cell myeloma or in metastatic tumors. The superficial surfaces of all bones should be examined thoroughly by applying intermittent firm pressure with the fingertips to locate potential areas of disease.

SPLEEN

The normal adult spleen is usually not palpable on physical examination but occasionally the tip may be felt.[7] Palpability of the normal spleen may be related to body habitus, but there is disagreement on this point. Percussion, palpation, or a combination of these two methods may detect enlarged spleens.[8] Some enlarged spleens may be visible by protrusion of the abdominal wall.

The normal spleen weighs about 150 g and lies in the peritoneal cavity against the diaphragm and the posterolateral abdominal wall at the level of the lower three ribs. As it enlarges it remains close to the abdominal wall, while the lower pole moves downward, anteriorly, and to the right. Spleens enlarged only 40 percent above normal may be palpable, but significant splenic enlargement may occur and the organ still not be felt on physical examination. A good but imperfect correlation has been reported between spleen size estimated from radioisotope scanning or ultrasonography and spleen weight determined after splenectomy or at autopsy.[9] Although it is common to fail to palpate an enlarged spleen on physical examination, palpation of a normal-size spleen is unusual, and therefore a palpable spleen is usually a significant physical finding.

An enlarged spleen lies just beneath the abdominal wall and can be identified by its movement during respiration. The splenic notch may be evident if the organ is moderately enlarged. During the examination the patient lies in a relaxed, supine position. The examiner, standing on the patient's right, lightly palpates the left upper abdomen with the right hand while exerting pressure forward with the palm of the left hand placed over the lower ribs posterolaterally. This action permits the spleen to descend and be felt by the examiners fingers. If nothing is felt, the palpation should be performed repeatedly, moving the examining hand about 2 cm toward the inguinal ligament each time. It is often advantageous to carry out the examination initially with the patient lying on the right side with left knee flexed and to repeat it with the patient supine.

It is not always possible to be sure that a left upper quadrant mass is spleen; masses in the stomach, colon, kidney, or pancreas may mimic splenomegaly on physical examination. When there is uncertainty regarding the nature of a mass in the left upper quadrant, imaging procedures will usually permit accurate diagnosis.[9–11]

LIVER

Palpation of the edge of the liver in the right upper quadrant of the abdomen is commonly used to detect hepatic enlargement, even though the inaccuracies of this method have been demonstrated. To properly assess liver size, it is necessary to determine both the upper and lower borders of the liver by percussion.[12,13] The normal liver may be palpable as much as 4 to 5 cm below the right costal margin but is usually not palpable in the epigastrium. The height of liver dullness is best measured in a specific line 8, 10, or 12 cm to the right of the midline. Techniques should be standardized so that serial measurements can be made. The vertical span of the normal liver determined in this manner will range about 10 cm in an average-size man, and about 2 cm smaller in women. Because of variations introduced by technique, each physician should determine the normal area of liver dullness by his or her own procedure. Correlation of radioisotope imaging data with results from routine physical examinations indicates that often a normal-size liver is considered enlarged on physical examination and an enlarged liver is considered normal. Ultrasonography and computed tomography measurements are useful in determining size and demonstrating localized infiltrative lesions.[14–16]

NERVOUS SYSTEM

A thorough evaluation of neurologic function is necessary in many patients with hematologic disease. Vitamin B_{12} deficiency impairs cerebral, olfactory, spinal cord, and peripheral nerve function, and severe chronic deficiency may lead to irreversible neurologic degeneration. Leukemic meningitis is often manifested by headache, visual impairment, or cranial nerve dysfunction. Tumor growth in the brain or spinal cord compression may be caused by malignant lymphoma or plasma cell myeloma. A variety of neurologic abnormalities may develop in patients with leukemias, lymphomas, and myeloma as a consequence of tumor infiltration, bleeding, infection, or a paraneoplastic syndrome. Polyneuropathy is a feature of the POEMS (polyneuropathy, organomegaly, endocrinopathy, monoclonal gammopathy, and skin changes) syndrome.

JOINTS

Deformities of the knees, elbows, ankles, shoulders, wrists, or hips may be the result of repeated hemorrhage in patients with hemophilia A, hemophilia B, or severe factor VII deficiency. Often, a target joint is prominently affected.

REFERENCES

1. Bickley LS, Szilagyi PG: *Bates Guide to Physical Examination and History Taking*, 8th ed. Lippincott Williams & Wilkins, Philadelphia, 2002.
2. Sackett DL: A primer on the precision and accuracy of the clinical examination. *JAMA* 267:2638, 1992.
3. Enelow AJ, Forde DL, Brummel-Smith K: *Interviewing and Patient Care*, 4th ed. Oxford University Press, Oxford, 1996.
4. Mor V, Laliberte L, Morris JN, Wiemann M: The Karnovsky performance status scale: an examination of its reliability and validity in a research setting. *Cancer* 53:2002, 1984.
5. Grubnic S, Vinnicombe SJ, Norman AR, Husband JE: MR evaluation of normal retroperitoneal and pelvic lymph nodes. *Clin Radiol* 57:193, 2002.
6. Atula TS, Varpula MJ, Kurki TJI, et al: Assessment of cervical lymph node status in head and neck cancer patients: palpation, computed tomography and low-field magnetic resonance imaging compared with ultrasound-guided fine needle aspiration cytology. *Eur J Radiol* 25:152, 1997.
7. Arkles LB, Gill GD, Nolan MP: A palpable spleen is not necessarily enlarged or pathological. *Med J Aust* 145:15, 1986.

8. Barkun AN, Camus M, Green L, et al: The bedside assessment of splenic enlargement. *Am J Med* 91:512, 1991.

9. Downey MT: Estimation of splenic weight from ultrasonographic measurements. *Can Assn Radiol J* 43:273, 1992.

10. Lamb PM, Lund A, Kanagasbay RR, et al: Spleen size: how well do linear ultrasound measurements correlate with three-dimensional CT volume assessments? *Br J Radiol* 75:573, 2002.

11. Halpern S, Coel M, Ashburn W, et al: Correlation of liver and spleen size: determinations by nuclear medicine studies and physical examination. *Arch Intern Med* 134:123, 1974.

12. Castell DO, O'Brien KD, Muench H, Chalmers TC: Estimation of liver size by percussion in normal individuals. *Ann Intern Med* 70:1183, 1969.

13. Tucker WN, Saab S, Rickman LS, Mathews WC: The scratch test is unreliable for detecting the liver edge. *J Clin Gastroenterol* 25:410, 1997.

14. Bennett WF, Dova JG: Review of hepatic imaging and a problem-oriented approach to liver masses. *Hepatology* 12:761, 1990.

15. Barloon TJ, Brown BP, Abu-Yousef MM, et al: Teaching physical examination of the adult liver with the use of real-time sonography. *Acad Radiol* 5:101, 1998.

16. Elstein D, Hadas-Halpern I, Azuri Y, et al: Accuracy of ultrasonography in assessing spleen and liver size in patients with Gaucher disease: Comparison to computed tomographic measurements. *J Ultrasound Med* 16: 209, 1997.

EXAMINATION OF THE BLOOD

DANIEL H. RYAN

Examination of the blood is central to the diagnosis and management of hematologic diseases. In few other disciplines can the physician make a specific diagnosis and monitor therapy with easily accessible tissue samples and readily available methodologies, many of which can be performed in a physician's office. Assessment of the prevalence of red cells, of the several types of leukocytes, and of platelets, usually from automated particle counters, and examination of the blood film for qualitative changes in the appearance of red cells, leukocytes, and platelets, and the presence of marrow precursors, malignant cells, and intracellular parasites can be used to diagnose specific diseases, gain insight into pathophysiology, and measure the response to treatment.

The blood is examined in order to answer the questions: Is the marrow producing sufficient numbers of mature cells in the major hematopoietic lineages? and Is the development of each hematopoietic lineage qualitatively normal? Quantitative measures available from automated cell counters are generally reliable and provide a rapid and cost-effective way to screen for major disturbances of hematopoiesis. Morphologic observation of the blood film is essential to confirm certain quantitative results and to investigate qualitatively abnormal differentiation of the hematopoietic lineages. Based on examination of the blood, the physician is directed toward a more focused assessment of the marrow or to systemic disorders that secondarily involve the hematopoietic system. Table 2-1 lists blood cell values in a normal population.

The complete blood count is a necessary part of the diagnostic workup in a broad variety of clinical conditions. Similarly, the leukocyte differential count and examination of the blood film, in spite of limitations as a screening test for occult disease,[1] is important in initial consideration of the differential diagnosis in most ill patients. Quantitative and morphologic examination of the cells of the blood are considered separately in this chapter, but the distinction between these two is not absolute, and measures once considered "qualitative" can be quantified, as technology advances.

QUANTITATIVE MEASURES OF CELLS IN THE BLOOD

In a typical automated blood cell counter, the blood sample is aspirated and separated into two portions: one is lysed and diluted to permit measurement of hemoglobin concentration and leukocyte enumeration, and the other is diluted without lysis to enable counting and sizing of red cells and platelets.

Acronyms and abbreviations that appear in the chapter include: CHr, reticulocyte-specific hemoglobin content; EDTA, ethylenediaminetetraacetic acid; HCT, hematocrit; Ig, immunoglobulin; MCH, mean cell hemoglobin; MCHC, mean cell hemoglobin concentration; MCV, mean cell volume; MPV, mean platelet volume; NHANES, National Health and Nutrition Examination Survey; NK, natural killer; PDW, platelet volume distribution width; RBC, red blood cell; RDW, red cell distribution width.

RED CELLS

Most automated blood cell counters measure the number of red cells and the mean red cell volume (MCV) and hemoglobin concentration. The other red cell parameters, including the hematocrit, mean cell hemoglobin (MCH), and mean cell hemoglobin concentration (MCHC), are derived from these primary measurements. The classic method to count and determine the volume of a particle or a cell is electrical impedance in which a specific volume of an electrolyte solution containing a dilute suspension of blood cells is aspirated through a small orifice across which a current is flowing. The electrical impedance produced as a cell passes through the orifice is registered as a particle for counting purposes and the height of the pulse generated by the electrical impedance can be made proportional to the volume of the particle.[2] Automated hematology instruments today rely heavily on analysis of light scattered at different angles from an incident laser beam striking passing cells. Cell count, volume, and internal structure can be determined by multivariate analysis of these data.

MEASUREMENT OF THE RED CELL COUNT AND HEMATOCRIT

In electronic instruments, the hematocrit (HCT) (proportion of blood occupied by erythrocytes) is calculated from the product of direct measurements of the erythrocyte count and the MCV (HCT [μl/100 μl] = RBC [$\times$ 10^{-6}/μl] $\times$ MCV [fl]/10). Falsely elevated MCV and decreased red cell counts can be observed when red cell autoantibodies are present and retain binding capability at room temperature (cold agglutinins and some cases of autoimmune hemolytic anemia).[3] This causes red cells to clump and by affecting the accuracy of both red blood cell (RBC) count and MCV, also affects the resultant hematocrit.

The hematocrit may also be determined by subjecting the blood to sufficient centrifugal force to pack the cells while minimizing trapped extracellular fluid.[4] Before standardized methods for hemoglobin quantitation were available, the hematocrit was the best method of determining adequacy of red cell production. However, the "spun" hematocrit is a manual procedure not well adapted to routine processing in a high-volume clinical laboratory. The "spun" hematocrit includes plasma trapped between red cells in the packed cell volume,[5] typically about 2 to 3 percent of the packed volume.[6] Microhematocrits from polycythemic samples (HCT greater than 55) or blood containing abnormal erythrocytes (sickle cell anemia, thalassemia, iron deficiency, spherocytosis, macrocytosis) are increased because of enhanced plasma trapping that generally is caused by increased red cell rigidity.[6,7] Therefore, although automated hematocrit values are adjusted to be equivalent to spun hematocrit for normal samples, in abnormal samples, the spun hematocrit may be artifactually elevated (up to 6% in microcytosis[8]). In general, the automated hematocrit is more accurate and easier to obtain than the spun hematocrit, although the hemoglobin determination is preferred to either, because it is measured directly and is the best indicator of the oxygen-carrying capacity of the blood.

MEASUREMENT OF HEMOGLOBIN

Hemoglobin is intensely colored, and this property has been used in methods for estimating its concentration in blood. Erythrocytes contain a mixture of hemoglobin, oxyhemoglobin, carboxyhemoglobin, methemoglobin, and minor amounts of other forms of hemoglobin. To determine hemoglobin concentration in the blood, red cells are lysed and hemoglobin variants are converted to the stable compound cyanmethemoglobin for quantitation by absorption at 540 nm.[9] All forms of hemoglobin are readily converted to cyanmethemoglobin except sulfhemoglobin, which is rarely present in significant amounts. In automated blood cell counters, hemoglobin is measured accurately;

age, when the polymorphonuclear leukocyte again becomes the predominant cell and remains so throughout the rest of childhood and adult life. The leukocyte count in the older persons is discussed in Chap. 8. The leukocyte count may decrease slightly in older subjects because of a fall in the lymphocyte count. The reference range for neutrophil counts is lower in African American, African, Afro-Caribbean, and some Middle Eastern populations than in persons of European descent.[53–56]

PLATELETS

PLATELET COUNT

Platelets are usually counted electronically by enumerating particles in the unlysed sample within a specified volume window (e.g., 2–20 fl), where volume may be measured by electrical impedance or light scatter. The platelet count was more difficult to automate than the red cell count because of the small size, tendency to aggregate, and potential overlap of platelets with more numerous smaller red cells. Current instruments typically construct a platelet volume histogram based on measured platelet size within the platelet volume window and mathematically extrapolate this histogram to account for platelets whose size overlaps with debris or small red cells. Some analyzers compare platelet counts determined by both impedance and light scatter measurements to improve accuracy, especially in patients with thrombocytopenia. The normal platelet count is lower in individuals of African ethnic origin[56] (Table 2-3).

Because platelet volumes in health or disease follow a log-normal distribution,[57] volume histograms inconsistent with such a distribution are flagged for manual review. Automated platelet counting by current instrumentation is accurate and reliable, even in the thrombocytopenic range,[58] and far more precise than manual methods.[58] Platelet counts by either manual or automated methods may be falsely decreased if the sample is incompletely anticoagulated (often indicated by small clots in the specimen or fibrin strands on the stained film). Infrequently, it may be necessary to confirm automated results by a manual (phase contrast) platelet count or platelet estimate from the blood film when potential interferences are present. These include severe microcytosis and leukocyte fragmentation (falsely elevated count) or platelet clumping or "satellitism" (falsely decreased count). Automated analyzers use a variety of proprietary techniques, including comparison of optical and electrical impedance measurements, to identify and flag such samples for manual review.[10] Platelet clumping, or platelet "satellitism" (adherence of platelets to neutrophils), may occur as a result of platelet-reactive antibodies,[59] which typically cause no clinical symptoms. These antibodies recognize epitopes on adhesion molecules which are exposed in the absence of divalent cations, and so become activated in EDTA- or citrate-anticoagulated blood specimens.[59] This condition occurs in approximately 0.1 percent of hospitalized patients

and the origin of the thrombocytopenia in such cases can be suspected by the appearance of small particles (representing the platelet clumps) on the leukocyte volume histogram.[60] Platelet counting under these conditions is difficult, but can be minimized by collecting blood in citrate[60] or estimating platelet count from a freshly prepared fingerstick blood smear.

The mean platelet volume (MPV) has been proposed as a useful clinical tool in the differential diagnosis of thrombocytopenias.[61] Increased MPV may be related in a complex way to thrombopoietic stimulus,[62] and not platelet age per se.[63] However, in spite of the known association of increased platelet size on blood films with consumptive thrombocytopenias, platelet size is a difficult parameter to accurately quantitate and use diagnostically because of a wide physiologic variation of the MPV in normal subjects (i.e., Mediterranean macrothrombocytopenia[64,65]) and susceptibility of anticoagulated platelets to time-dependent swelling in vitro.[66] Mediterranean macrothrombocytopenia is prevalent in Greeks and Italians and is distinguished by larger-than-normal platelet volume, lower-than-normal platelet counts, normal platelet biomass concentration, and normal hemostasis.[64,65] A platelet volume distribution width (PDW) can be calculated just as the RDW, and is correlated with platelet count and MPV.[67] This measurement has yet to find a clinical use.

The number of platelets with high RNA content ("reticulated platelets"), measured using RNA-binding fluorescent dyes such as thiazole orange, is a marker of marrow megakaryopoiesis and has been proposed as a way of differentiating hypoproductive from destructive causes of thrombocytopenia, in an analogous fashion to the reticulocyte count. The percentage, but not the absolute number, of reticulated platelets is increased in destructive thrombocytopenias, whereas the absolute number, but not percentage, is decreased in hypoproductive states.[68] Reticulated platelet number or RNA correlates with imminent platelet recovery after chemotherapy.[69]

REFERENCE RANGES

The use of reference ranges for quantitative hematology measurements deserves some additional comment. The physiologic variation of certain blood cell counts is notably higher than usually found in blood chemistry analytes. This is presumably a reflection of the adaptive responsiveness of the marrow and other tissues to cytokine and hormonal signaling. For instance, the leukocyte and differential counts are affected by stress, diurnal variation, smoking history, and ethnic origin. Platelet count and MPV are typically inversely related in normal individuals, and also show substantial ethnic variation.[70] In contrast, the MCV is rather stable within an individual; in fact, most variables show more stability within an individual than between individuals,[71] illustrating one reason for the lack of sensitivity and specificity of any test "cutoff" that is designed for a population rather

TABLE 2-3 ETHNIC DIFFERENCES IN NORMAL BLOOD CELL VALUES

	MEN			WOMEN		
	EUROPEAN DESCENT N = 100	AFRO-CARRIBEAN N = 51	AFRICAN N = 65	EUROPEAN DESCENT N = 100	AFRO-CARRIBEAN N = 51	AFRICAN N = 50
White cell count*	5.7 (3.6–9.2)	5.2 (2.8–9.5)	4.5 (2.8–7.2)	6.2 (3.5–10.8)	5.7 (3.3–9.9)	5.0 (3.2–7.8)
Neutrophil count	3.2 (1.7–6.1)	2.5 (1.0–5.8)	2.0 (0.9–4.2)	3.6 (1.7–7.5)	3.0 (1.4–6.5)	2.4 (1.3–4.2)
Lymphocyte count	1.7 (1.0–2.9)	1.9 (1.0–3.6)	1.8 (1.0–3.2)	1.8 (1.0–3.5)	2.0 (1.2–3.4)	2.0 (1.1–3.6)
Monocyte count	0.34 (0.18–0.62)	0.33 (0.18–0.52)	0.29 (0.15–0.58)	0.30 (0.14–0.61)	0.31 (0.16–0.59)	0.28 (0.15–0.39)
Eosinophil count	0.12 (0.03–0.48)	0.13 (0.03–0.58)	0.12 (0.02–0.79)	0.13 (0.04–0.44)	0.10 (0.03–0.33)	0.10 (0.02–0.41)
Platelet count	218 (143–332)	196 (122–313)	183 (115–290)	246 (169–358)	236 (149–374)	207 (125–342)

* All counts expressed in thousands per μl; geometric mean and 95 percent reference range, with studies performed on the Bayer-Technicon H.2 counter. This table is provided as a guide. Normal ranges should be validated by the clinical laboratory for the specific methods in use. See reference 56.

than for an individual person. Normal ranges for hematocrit and hemoglobin can be problematic if individuals with occult iron deficiency are not excluded, and this is difficult to do in a large study, particularly considering the frequency of mild iron deficiency in a supposedly "normal" population of women. For instance, in defining the upper range of hematocrit and hemoglobin in relation to a possible diagnosis of polycythemia, one has to carefully weigh the likelihood that a "normal-range" study has adequately excluded iron-deficient subjects.[72,73] With the newer parameters, such as the reticulocyte indices, lack of methodological standardization is a big issue. Finally, when one observes significant changes in reference ranges based on age, there is the question of whether this is physiologic or a result of undiagnosed occult disease. The results of the National Health and Nutrition Examination Survey (NHANES) III, which excludes a number of clinically evident disorders, but not iron deficiency, have been published and compared with published normal ranges.[76]

MORPHOLOGIC EXAMINATION OF THE BLOOD

Microscopic examination of the blood spread on a glass slide or coverslip yields useful information regarding all the formed elements of the blood. The process of preparing a thin blood film causes mechanical trauma to the cells. Also, the cells flatten on the glass during drying, and the fixation and staining involve exposure to methanol and water. Some artifacts are inevitably introduced, but these can be minimized by good technique. The optimal part of the stained blood film to use for morphologic examination of the blood cells should be sufficiently thin that only a few erythrocytes in a ×100 field touch each other, but not so thin that no red cells are touching. Selection of a portion of the blood film for analysis that is too thick or too thin for proper morphologic evaluation is by far the most common error in blood film interpretation. For example, leukemic blasts may appear dense and rounded and lose their characteristic features when viewed in the thick part of the film. For specific purposes, the thick portion or side and "feathered" edges of the film are of interest (for instance, to detect microfilariae and malarial parasites or to search for large abnormal cells and platelet clumps).

The blood film is first scanned at low magnification (×200) to confirm reasonably even distribution of leukocytes, and check for abnormally large or immature cells in the side and feathered edges of the film. The feathered edge is examined for platelet clumps. Abnormal cells, red cell aggregation or rouleaux, background bluish staining consistent with paraproteinemia, and parasites are all findings that can be suggested by medium magnification examination (×400). The optimal portion of the film is then examined at high magnification (×1000, oil immersion) to systematically assess the size, shape, and morphology of the major cell lineages.

RED CELL MORPHOLOGY

Normal erythrocytes on dried films are nearly uniform in size, with a normal distribution of about a mean diameter of 7.2 to 7.9 μm. The normal-sized erythrocyte is about the diameter of the nucleus of a small lymphocyte. The MCV is a more sensitive measure of red cell volume than the red cell diameter. However, an experienced observer should be able to recognize abnormalities in average red cell size when the MCV is significantly elevated or decreased. *Anisocytosis* is the term that describes variation in erythrocyte size, and is the morphologic correlate of the RDW. The *macrocyte*, a red cell larger than normal, may be seen in a number of disease states, for example, folic acid or vitamin B_{12} deficiency. Cells are considered to be macrocytes if they are well hemoglobinized and their diameters exceed 9 μm. Early ("shift" or "stress") *reticulocytes* (i.e., those with the most re-

sidual RNA) appear in stained films as large, bluish cells, referred to as *polychromatophilic* cells. These cells roughly correspond to those quantitated by automated analyzers as the immature reticulocyte fraction. *Microcyte*, a red cell smaller than normal, is the term used to describe a cell less than 6 μm in diameter.

The normal erythrocyte on a blood film is round with central pallor. *Poikilocytosis* is a term used to describe variations in the shape of erythrocytes. The predominant appearance of a specific abnormality in red cell shape can be an important diagnostic clue in patients with anemia. These are described in detail in Chap. 28. Erythrocytes with evenly spaced spikes (crenated cells) can be an artifact caused by prolonged storage, or may reflect metabolic erythrocyte abnormalities.

The normal erythrocyte appears as a disc with a rim of hemoglobin and a clear central area. The central pallor normally occupies less than one-half the diameter of the cells. Increased central pallor (*hypochromia*) is associated with disorders characterized by diminished hemoglobin synthesis. Evaluation of red cell hemoglobinization, as well as red cell size, is dependent on examining the proper part of the blood film. Cells at the far "feathered edge" will always be large and lack central pallor, whereas cells in the thick part of the film will look small and rounded and will also lack central pallor. A sharp refractile border demarcating the central area of pallor is an artifact secondary to inadequate drying of the film before staining (because of high humidity; more common in anemic samples). *Spherocytes* are more densely stained and appear smaller because of their rounded shape; they show decreased or absent central pallor. The hemoglobin may appear to be abnormally distributed in erythrocytes, particularly in a form of cell in which there is a spot or disc of hemoglobin in the center surrounded by a clear area which is, in turn, surrounded by a rim of hemoglobin at the outer edge of the cell, giving the appearance of a target—a *target cell*. This is in reality a cup-shaped cell that is distorted as it is flattened on the glass slide. These cells are typically found in disorders of hemoglobin synthesis (e.g., thalassemia, iron deficiency), where the cell-surface-to-cell-volume ratio is high. Some common red cell morphologic abnormalities and associated diseases are diagrammatically illustrated in Fig. 2-1.

Erythrocytes are usually distributed evenly throughout the blood film. In some cases the cells become aligned in overlapping stacks,

	Name	Characteristic	Also seen in
	Spherocyte	Hereditary spherocytosis, immune hemolytic anemia	Clostridial sepsis, hemolytic anemia of Wilson disease, hemoglobin CC disease
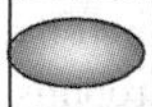	Elliptocyte	Hereditary elliptocytosis (HE)	Iron deficiency, MDS, megaloblastic anemia, thalassemias,
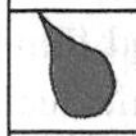	Dacrocyte	Hemolytic hereditary elliptocytosis, hereditary pyropoikilocytosis	Severe iron deficiency, megaloblastic anemia, thalassemias, myelofibrosis, MDS
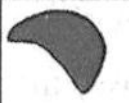	Schistocyte	Microangiopathic and fragmentation hemolytic anemias	
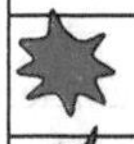	Echinocyte	Renal failure, malnutrition	Common in vitro artifact after blood storage
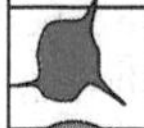	Acanthocyte	Spur cell anemia, abetalipoproteinemia	Splenectomy
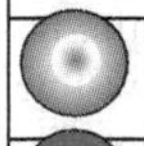	Target cell	Cholestasis, hemoglobin C trait and CC disease	Iron deficiency, thalassemias
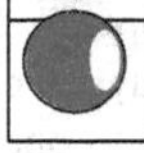	Stomatocyte	Hereditary stomatocytosis	Alcoholism

FIGURE 2-1 Disorders associated with common red cell morphologic changes.

referred to as rouleaux, resembling overlapping rows of coins. Such rouleaux formation is normal in the thicker part of the film; when found in the optimal viewing portion of the film, it may be a result of the presence of an increase in immunoglobulin (Ig), especially IgM, and suggests the diagnosis of macroglobulinemia. Occasionally, very high concentrations of IgA or IgG may produce noticeable pathologic rouleaux, as a manifestation of myeloma.

Inclusions that may be observed in erythrocytes on films stained with Wright stain are described in Chap. 28. Nucleated red cells are not normally observed in blood films but may be found in newborns, particularly if physiologically stressed, and in a variety of disorders, including severe hemolytic anemia, myeloproliferative disorders, and infiltrative disease of the marrow.

PLATELET MORPHOLOGY

Platelets appear in normal stained blood film as small blue or colorless bodies with red or purple granules. Normal platelets average about 1 to 2 μm in diameter but show wide variation in shape, from round to elongated, cigar-shaped forms. A rough estimate of the platelet count can be made by observation of the stained blood film. If the platelet count is normal, approximately 8 to 15 platelets (individually or in small clumps) should be visible in each oil-immersion ($\times$1000) field. There should be 1 platelet present for about every 20 erythrocytes. This is a valuable check when the automated platelet count is in question or an unexpected result is obtained.

In improperly prepared films, platelets may form large aggregates in some areas and appear to be diminished or absent in others. The occurrence of giant platelets or platelet masses may indicate a myeloproliferative disorder or improper collection of the blood specimen. The latter circumstance can occur when venipuncture technique is faulty and platelets become activated before the blood sample is thoroughly mixed with anticoagulant. These platelet masses are apparent typically in the thin "feathered edge" of the film. This maldistribution may create a mistaken impression of thrombocytopenia if the aggregates are not detected. Platelet clumping throughout the blood film, or platelet "satellitism" (adherence of platelets to neutrophils), may be due to platelet agglutinins as previously discussed.

A platelet will occasionally overlie an erythrocyte, where it may be mistaken for an inclusion body or a parasite. The differentiation depends on the observation of a halo around the platelet, determination that it lies above the plane of the erythrocyte, and observation of the characteristics of a normal platelet in the "inclusion."

LEUKOCYTE MORPHOLOGY

The distribution of leukocytes on glass slides is not uniform, and the larger cells, such as monocytes and polymorphonuclear neutrophils, tend to be concentrated on the edges and thin end of the blood film. The cells that are normally found in blood are polymorphonuclear leukocytes of the neutrophilic, eosinophilic, and basophilic types; lymphocytes; and monocytes. These cell types are described below, and Table 2-2 presents normal values for the differential count.

Neutrophils are round cells ranging from 10 to 14 μm in diameter (see Color Plate VII). The nucleus is lobulated, with two to five lobes connected by a thin chromatin thread. The defining feature of the segmented neutrophil is the round lobes with condensed chromatin, because the chromatin thread may overlie the nucleus and not be visible. The chromatin stains purple and is coarse and arranged in clumps. The nucleus of 1 to 16 percent of the neutrophils from females may have an appendage that is shaped like a drumstick and is attached to one lobe by a strand of chromatin. The cytoplasm is clear and contains many small, tan to pink granules distributed evenly throughout the cell, although they may not be apparent when they lie over the nucleus.

Bands are identical to mature polymorphonuclear leukocytes except that the nucleus is U-shaped or has rudimentary lobes connected by a band containing chromatin rather than by a thin thread (see Color Plate X-6). The nuclear chromatin is slightly less condensed than the mature neutrophil.

Eosinophils are on the average slightly larger than neutrophils. The nucleus usually has only two lobes. The chromatin pattern is the same as that in the neutrophil, but the nucleus tends to be more lightly stained. The differentiating characteristic of these cells is the presence of many refractile, orange-red granules that are distributed evenly throughout the cell and may be visible overlying the nucleus (see Color Plate VII-3). These granules are larger than those in the neutrophil and are more uniform in size. Occasionally, some of the granules in eosinophils stain light blue rather than orange-red.

Basophils are similar to the other polymorphonuclear cells and are slightly smaller than neutrophils. The nucleus may stain more faintly and usually is less segmented and has less distinct chromatin condensation than is the case in neutrophils. The large deeply basophilic granules are fewer in number and less regular in size and shape than in the eosinophil. The granules are visible overlying the nucleus and, in some cells, almost completely obscure the lightly stained nuclear chromatin. Because the granular constituents are water soluble, some granules may stain only faintly or not at all (see Color Plate VII-4).

Lymphocytes on blood films are usually small, about 10 μm in diameter, but larger forms up to 20 μm in diameter are seen. The small lymphocyte, the predominant type in normal blood, is round and contains a relatively large, round, densely stained nucleus (see Color Plates VII 1–4). The cytoplasm is scanty and stains pale to dark blue. In the large lymphocytes, the nuclear:cytoplasmic ratio is lower and the chromatin is less condensed than in the small lymphocytes. The nucleus is usually round but may be oval or indented. The cytoplasm is abundant and may contain a few azurophilic granules. Large lymphocytes containing azurophilic granules and relatively abundant cytoplasm are designated *large granular lymphocytes*, and generally represent cytotoxic T cells or natural killer (NK) cells. *Reactive lymphocytes*, as seen in viral infections caused by Epstein-Barr virus, cytomegalovirus, adenovirus, or other organisms, are large with indented nuclei and abundant blue cytoplasm. Nuclear chromatin condensation is variable, and nucleoli may be evident. A low nuclear:cytoplasmic ratio distinguishes these reactive T lymphocytes from neoplastic cells.

Monocytes are the largest normal cells in the blood, usually measuring from 15 to 22 μm in diameter. The nucleus is of various shapes—round, kidney-shaped, oval, or lobulated—and frequently appears to be folded (see Color Plates VII-1,2). The chromatin is arranged in fine strands with sharply defined margins. The cytoplasm is light blue or gray, contains variable numbers of fine lilac or purple granules, and is frequently vacuolated, especially in films made from blood anticoagulated with EDTA. The gray (as opposed to blue) color of monocyte cytoplasm is a result of fine granules (staining pink) seen on the background of RNA-containing cytoplasm (staining blue), and helps to distinguish between monocytes and reactive lymphocytes. The monocyte nuclear chromatin contains a fine, string-like structure as opposed to the smudgy-appearing clumps of the lymphoid chromatin. Nuclear shape and cytoplasmic vacuolation are less reliable distinguishing features between monocytic and lymphoid cells.

LEUKOCYTE INCLUSIONS

Leukocytes may contain abnormal inclusions as a result of genetic or acquired disorders.

ABNORMAL GRANULES

In patients with conditions associated with a systemic inflammatory reaction, neutrophil granules may appear larger than normal and stain more darkly, often assuming a dark blue-black color. This has been called *toxic granulation*. These granules can be confused with the larger granules of basophils. In *mucopolysaccharidoses*, coarse, dark granules may be found in the neutrophils (the Alder-Reilly anomaly) and large azurophilic granules are often found in some lymphocytes (Gasser cells) and monocytes. Huge misshapen granules are found in the polymorphonuclear leukocytes, and giant azurophilic granules are present in the lymphocytes of patients exhibiting the *Chédiak-Higashi* anomaly (see Chaps. 59 and 66).[74] *Auer rods* are sharply outlined, red-staining rods found in the cytoplasm in blast cells, and occasionally in more mature leukemic cells, in the blood of some patients with acute myelogenous leukemia (see Color Plates XVI-2 and 3).

ABNORMAL RNA AGGREGATIONS
Light blue round or oval *Döhle bodies*, about 1 to 2 μm in diameter, may be seen in the cytoplasm of neutrophils of patients with infections, burns, and other inflammatory states. The blue staining is caused by RNA of the rough-surfaced endoplasmic reticulum contained in Döhle bodies. Similar blue inclusions are seen in patients with the *May-Hegglin* anomaly. The staining of May-Hegglin inclusions is also attributable to RNA, but ultrastructurally they differ from Döhle bodies, suggesting alterations in the RNA.[75]

LEUKOCYTE ARTIFACTS

CRUSHED ("SMUDGE," "BASKET") CELLS
During the process of preparing the film, leukocytes may be damaged, with consequent alteration in their appearance and staining. In some damaged leukocytes the nucleus appears enlarged, with alteration of the chromatin so that the strands appear more homogeneous, stain with a distinct reddish hue, and are more widely separated; the cytoplasm may or may not appear intact. Such cells may appear to have a large blue nucleolus. There is no specific association with disease other than chronic lymphocytic leukemia, where the neoplastic lymphocytes are fragile and "smudge" cells are frequent.

RADIAL NUCLEAR SEGMENTATION
This refers to abnormal segmentation of the nuclei of leukocytes on the blood film, in which the lobes appear to radiate from a single point, giving a cloverleaf or cartwheel picture. This change is common in cytocentrifuged preparations (i.e., from a body fluid), EDTA anticoagulated blood after excessive storage, or samples collected in oxalate.

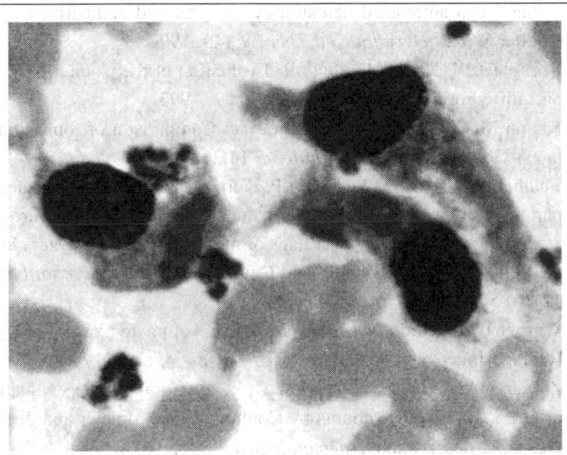

FIGURE 2-2 Endothelial cells in blood film. (Courtesy of Dr. H.A. Wurzel.)

TABLE 2-4 CONDITIONS IN WHICH THE BLOOD COUNT MAY BE RELATIVELY UNREMARKABLE BUT EXAMINATION OF THE BLOOD FILM WILL SUGGEST OR CONFIRM THE DISORDER

DISEASE	FINDINGS ON BLOOD FILM
Compensated immune hemolytic anemia	Spherocytosis, polychromatophilia; erythrocyte agglutination if immune mediated
Hereditary spherocytosis	Spherocytosis, polychromatophilia
Hemoglobin C disease	Target cells
Elliptocytosis	Elliptocytes
Lead poisoning	Basophilic stippling (not a sensitive indicator)
Macroglobulinemia, myeloma	Rouleaux formation
Malaria, babesiosis	Parasites in the erythrocytes
Disseminated intravascular coagulation	Schizocytes (not a sensitive indicator)
Hemolysis related to physical injury to red cells	Schizocytes
Severe bacterial infection	Neutrophilia with band neutrophils; Döhle bodies, neutrophil vacuoles
Infectious mononucleosis	Reactive lymphocytes

VACUOLATION
Vacuoles may develop in the nucleus and cytoplasm of leukocytes, especially monocytes and neutrophils, with prolonged storage in EDTA anticoagulated blood. Vacuoles may be associated with swelling of the nuclei and loss of granules from the cytoplasm. In blood films prepared without anticoagulation, vacuoles in neutrophils suggest sepsis.

ENDOTHELIAL CELLS
If the blood film is prepared from the first drop of blood issuing from the microsampling wound, endothelial cells may be present singly or in clumps. Figure 2-2 illustrates such cells. These cells appear quite immature and may be misinterpreted as blasts or metastatic tumor cells.

THE NEED FOR EXAMINATION OF THE BLOOD FILM
The quantitative determinations discussed earlier in this chapter describe the blood in sufficient detail that the physician will often recognize the need for further laboratory and clinical workup. Quantitative analysis of the blood may suggest certain diseases involving erythrocytes, leukocytes, and/or platelets that should be confirmed by examination of a stained blood film. Table 2-4 lists a number of diseases in which the blood counts may be relatively unremarkable but in which examination of the blood film will suggest the disorder. Based on the quantitative and morphologic examination of the blood, the physician can assess the need for direct examination of the marrow, as described in Chap. 3.

REFERENCES
1. Shapiro MF, Hatch RL, Greenfield S: Cost containment and labor-intensive tests. The case of the leukocyte differential count. *JAMA* 252:231, 1984.
2. Coulter WH: High speed automatic blood cell counter and cell size analyzer. *Proc Natl Elect Conf* 12:1034, 1956.
3. Bessman JD, Banks D: Spurious macrocytosis, a common clue to erythrocyte cold agglutinins. *Am J Clin Pathol* 74:797, 1980.
4. Wintrobe MM: Macroscopic examination of the blood. *Am J Med Sci* 185:58, 1933.

5.   England JM, Walford DM, Waters DA: Re-assessment of the reliability of the haematocrit. *Br J Haematol* 23:247, 1972.

6.   Fairbanks VF: Nonequivalence of automated and manual hematocrit and erythrocyte indices. *Am J Clin Pathol* 73:55, 1980.

7.   Pearson TC, Guthrie DL: Trapped plasma in the microhematocrit. *Am J Clin Pathol* 78:770, 1982.

8.   England JM: *Blood Cell Sizing.* Churchill Livingstone, New York, 1991.

9.   Recommendations for reference method for haemoglobinometry in human blood (ICSH standard 1986) and specifications for international haemiglobincyanide reference preparation (3rd edition). International Committee for Standardization in Haematology; Expert Panel on Haemoglobinometry. *Clin Lab Haematol* 9:73, 1987.

10. Kickler TS: Clinical analyzers. Advances in automated cell counting. *Anal Chem* 71:363R, 1999.

11. Dallman PR, Bart GD, Allen CM, et al: Hemoglobin concentration in white, black and Oriental children: is there a need for separate criteria in screening for anemia? *Am J Clin Nutr* 31:377, 1978.

12. Dallman PR, Siimes MA: Percentile curves for hemoglobin and red cell volume in infancy and childhood. *J Pediatr* 94:26, 1979.

13. Wintrobe MM: Anemia: classification and treatment on the basis of differences in the average volume and hemoglobin content of the red corpuscles. *Arch Intern Med* 54:256, 1934.

14. Hillman RS: After sixty years: the MCV is still alive and well. *J Gen Intern Med* 5:264, 1990.

15. Rund D, Filon D, Strauss N, et al: Mean corpuscular volume of heterozygotes for beta-thalassemia correlates with the severity of mutations. *Blood* 79:238, 1992.

16. Mach-Pascual S, Darbellay R, Pilotto PA, et al: Investigation of microcytosis: a comprehensive approach. *Eur J Haematol* 57:54, 1996.

17. Griner PF, Oranburg PR: Predictive values of erythrocyte indices for tests of iron, folic acid, and vitamin B_{12} deficiency. *Am J Clin Pathol* 70:748, 1978.

18. Seward SJ, Safran C, Marton KI, et al: Does the mean corpuscular volume help physicians evaluate hospitalized patients with anemia? *J Gen Intern Med* 5:187, 1990.

19. Carmel R: Pernicious anemia. The expected findings of very low serum cobalamin levels, anemia, and macrocytosis are often lacking. *Arch Intern Med* 148:1712, 1988.

20. Mahmoud MY, Lugon M, Anderson CC: Unexplained macrocytosis in elderly patients. *Age Ageing* 25:310, 1996.

21. Eldibany MM, Totonchi KF, Joseph NJ, et al: Usefulness of certain red blood cell indices in diagnosing and differentiating thalassemia trait from iron-deficiency anemia. *Am J Clin Pathol* 111:676, 1999.

22. Lafferty JD, Crowther MA, Ali MA, et al: The evaluation of various mathematical RBC indices and their efficacy in discriminating between thalassemic and non-thalassemic microcytosis. *Am J Clin Pathol* 106: 201, 1996.

23. Michaels LA, Cohen AR, Zhao H, et al: Screening for hereditary spherocytosis by use of automated erythrocyte indexes. *J Pediatr* 130:957, 1997.

24. Bentley SA, Ayscue LH, Watson JM, et al: The clinical utility of discriminant functions for the differential diagnosis of microcytic anemias. *Blood Cells* 15:575; discussion 583, 1989.

25. Mahu JL, Leclercq C, Suquet JP: Usefulness of red cell distribution width in association with biological parameters in an epidemiological survey of iron deficiency in children. *Int J Epidemiol* 19:646, 1990.

26. Rose MS: Epitaph for the M.C.H.C. *Br Med J* 4:169, 1971.

27. McClure S, Custer E, Bessman JD: Improved detection of early iron deficiency in nonanemic subjects. *JAMA* 253:1021, 1985.

28. Patton WN, Cave RJ, Harris RI: A study of changes in red cell volume and haemoglobin concentration during phlebotomy induced iron deficiency and iron repletion using the Technicon H1. *Clin Lab Haematol* 13:153, 1991.

29. Bessman JD, Gilmer PR Jr, Gardner FH: Improved classification of anemias by MCV and RDW. *Am J Clin Pathol* 80:322, 1983.

30. Flynn MM, Reppun TS, Bhagavan NV: Limitations of red blood cell distribution width (RDW) in evaluation of microcytosis. *Am J Clin Pathol* 85:445, 1986.

31. Riley RS, Ben-Ezra JM, Tidwell A, et al: Reticulocyte analysis by flow cytometry and other techniques. *Hematol Oncol Clin North Am* 16:373, 2002.

32. Buttarello M, Bulian P, Farina G, et al: Flow cytometric reticulocyte counting. Parallel evaluation of five fully automated analyzers: an NCCLS-ICSH approach. *Am J Clin Pathol* 115:100, 2001.

33. Buttarello M, Temporin V, Ceravolo R, et al: The new reticulocyte parameter (RET-Y) of the Sysmex XE 2100: its use in the diagnosis and monitoring of posttreatment sideropenic anemia. *Am J Clin Pathol* 121: 489, 2004.

34. Chuang CL, Liu RS, Wei YH, et al: Early prediction of response to intravenous iron supplementation by reticulocyte haemoglobin content and high-fluorescence reticulocyte count in haemodialysis patients. *Nephrol Dial Transplant* 18:370, 2003.

35. Fishbane S, Shapiro W, Dutka P, et al: A randomized trial of iron deficiency testing strategies in hemodialysis patients. *Kidney Int* 60:2406, 2001.

36. Kaneko Y, Miyazaki S, Hirasawa Y, et al: Transferrin saturation versus reticulocyte hemoglobin content for iron deficiency in Japanese hemodialysis patients. *Kidney Int* 63:1086, 2003.

37. Mast AE, Blinder MA, Lu Q, et al: Clinical utility of the reticulocyte hemoglobin content in the diagnosis of iron deficiency. *Blood* 99:1489, 2002.

38. Noronha JF, De Souza CA, Vigorito AC, et al: Immature reticulocytes as an early predictor of engraftment in autologous and allogeneic bone marrow transplantation. *Clin Lab Haematol* 25:47, 2003.

39. Torres Gomez A, Casano J, Sanchez J, et al: Utility of reticulocyte maturation parameters in the differential diagnosis of macrocytic anemias. *Clin Lab Haematol* 25:283, 2003.

40. Buttarello M, Bulian P, Farina G, et al: Five fully automated methods for performing immature reticulocyte fraction: comparison in diagnosis of bone marrow aplasia. *Am J Clin Pathol* 117:871, 2002.

41. Gulati GL, Hyun BH, Gagaldon H: Falsely elevated automated leukocyte count on cryoglobulinemic and/or cryofibrinogenic blood samples. *Lab Med* 8:14, 1977.

42. Williams LJ: Cell histograms: New trends in data interpretation and classification. *J Med Technol* 1:189, 1984.

43. Lombarts AJ, deKieviet W: Recognition and prevention of pseudothrombocytopenia and consomitant pseudoleukocytosis. *Am J Clin Pathol* 89:534, 1988.

44. Ferrero-Vacher C, Sudaka I, Jambou D, et al: Evaluation of the ABX Cobas Vega automated hematology analyzer and comparison with the Coulter STKS. *Hematol Cell Ther* 39:149, 1997.

45. Cornbleet PJ, Myrick D, Levy R: Evaluation of the Coulter STKS five-part differential. *Am J Clin Pathol* 99:72, 1993.

46. Koenn ME, Kirby BA, Cook LL, et al: Comparison of four automated hematology analyzers. *Clin Lab Sci* 14:238, 2001.

47. Thalhammer-Scherrer R, Knobl P, Korninger L, et al: Automated five-part white blood cell differential counts. Efficiency of software-generated white blood cell suspect flags of the hematology analyzers Sysmex SE-9000, Sysmex NE-8000, and Coulter STKS. *Arch Pathol Lab Med* 121(6):573, 1997.

48. Warner BA, Reardon DM, Marshall DP: Automated haematology analysers: a four-way comparison. *Med Lab Sci* 47:285, 1990.

49. Zaccaria A, Celso B, Raspadori D, et al: Comparative evaluation of differential leukocyte counts by Coulter VCS cytometer and direct microscopic observation. *Haematologica* 75:412, 1990.

50. Ruzicka K, Veitl M, Thalhammer-Scherrer R, et al: The new hematology analyzer Sysmex XE-2100: performance evaluation of a novel white

blood cell differential technology. *Arch Pathol Lab Med* 125:391-396, 2001.

51. Aulesa C, Pastor I, Naranjo D, et al: Application of receiver operating characteristics curve (ROC) analysis when definitive and suspect morphologic flags appear in the new Coulter LH 750 analyzer. *Lab Hematol* 10:14, 2004.

52. Atwater S, Corash L: Advances in leukocyte differential and peripheral blood stem cell enumeration. *Curr Opin Hematol* 3:71, 1996.

53. Reed WW: Leukopenia, neutropenia, and reduced hemoglobin levels in healthy American blacks. *Arch Intern Med* 151:501, 1991.

54. Haddy TB, Rana SR, Castro O: Benign ethnic neutropenia: what is a normal absolute neutrophil count? *J Lab Clin Med* 133:15, 1999.

55. Caramihai E, Karayalcin G, Aballi AJ, et al: Leukocyte count differences in healthy white and black children 1 to 5 years of age. *J Pediatr* 86:252, 1975.

56. Bain BJ: Ethnic and sex differences in the total and differential white cell count and platelet count. *J Clin Pathol* 49:664, 1996.

57. Paulus JM: Platelet size in man. *Blood* 46:321, 1975.

58. Lawrence JB, Yomtovian RA, Dillman C, et al: Reliability of automated platelet counts: comparison with manual method and utility for prediction of clinical bleeding. *Am J Hematol* 48:244, 1995.

59. Fiorin F, Steffan A, Pradella P, et al: IgG platelet antibodies in EDTA-dependent pseudothrombocytopenia bind to platelet membrane glycoprotein IIb. *Am J Clin Pathol* 110(2):178, 1998.

60. Bartels PC, Schoorl M, Lombarts AJ: Screening for EDTA-dependent deviations in platelet counts and abnormalities in platelet distribution histograms in pseudothrombocytopenia. *Scand J Clin Lab Invest* 57:629, 1997.

61. Levin J, Bessman JD: The inverse relation between platelet volume and platelet number. Abnormalities in hematologic disease and evidence that platelet size does not correlate with platelet age. *J Lab Clin Med* 101:295, 1983.

62. Bessman JD: The relation of megakaryocyte ploidy to platelet volume. *Am J Hematol* 16:161, 1984.

63. Thompson CB, Love DG, Quinn PG, et al: Platelet size does not correlate with platelet age. *Blood* 62:487, 1983.

64. Behrens WE: Mediterranean macrothrombocytopenia. *Blood* 46:199, 1975.

65. Altes A, Pujol-Moix N, Muniz-Diaz E, et al: Hereditary macrothrombocytopenia and pregnancy. *Thromb Haemost* 76:29, 1996.

66. O'Malley T, Ludlam CA, Fox KA, et al: Measurement of platelet volume using a variety of different anticoagulant and antiplatelet mixtures. *Blood Coagul Fibrinolysis* 7:431, 1996.

67. Osselaer JC, Jamart J, Scheiff JM: Platelet distribution width for differential diagnosis of thrombocytosis. *Clin Chem* 43(6 Pt 1):1072, 1997.

68. Kurata Y, Hayashi S, Kiyoi T, et al: Diagnostic value of tests for reticulated platelets, plasma glycocalicin, and thrombopoietin levels for discriminating between hyperdestructive and hypoplastic thrombocytopenia. *Am J Clin Pathol* 115:656, 2001.

69. Wang C, Smith BR, Ault KA, et al: Reticulated platelets predict platelet count recovery following chemotherapy. *Transfusion* 42:368, 2002.

70. Peng L, Yang J, Lu X, et al: Effects of biological variations on platelet count in healthy subjects in China. *Thromb Haemost* 91:367, 2004.

71. Fraser CG, Wilkinson SP, Neville RG, et al: Biologic variation of common hematologic laboratory quantities in the elderly. *Am J Clin Pathol* 92:465, 1989.

72. Fairbanks VF, Tefferi A: Normal ranges for packed cell volume and hemoglobin concentration in adults: relevance to "apparent polycythemia." *Eur J Haematol* 65:285, 2000.

73. Pearson TC: Normal ranges for packed cell volume and hemoglobin concentration in adults: relevance to "apparent polycythemia." *Eur J Haematol* 67:56, 2001.

74. Brunning RD: Morphologic alterations in nucleated blood and marrow cells in genetic disorders. *Hum Pathol* 1:99, 1970.

75. Jenis EH, Takeuchi A, Dillon DE, et al: The May-Hegglin anomaly: Ultrastructure of the granulocytic inclusion. *Am J Clin Pathol* 55:187, 1971.

76. Cheng CK, Chan J, Cembrowski GS, et al: Complete blood count reference interval diagrams derived from NHANES III: Stratification by age, sex, and race. *Lab Hematol* 10:42, 2004.

EXAMINATION OF THE MARROW

DANIEL H. RYAN

RAYMOND E. FELGAR

Microscopic examination of the marrow is a mainstay of hematologic diagnosis. Even with the advent of specialized biochemical and molecular assays that capitalize on advances in our understanding of the cell biology of hematopoiesis, the primary diagnosis of hematologic malignancies and many non-neoplastic hematologic disorders relies upon examination of the cells in the marrow. Aspirate and biopsy of marrow can be obtained with minimal risk and only minor discomfort and are quickly and easily processed for examination. The marrow should be examined when the clinical history, blood cell counts, blood film, or laboratory test results suggest the possibility of a primary or secondary hematologic disorder for which morphologic analysis or special studies of the marrow would aid in the diagnosis. Leukopenia, thrombocytopenia, bicytopenia, or tricytopenia nearly always require a marrow examination for diagnosis. Nonhemolytic anemia that is not readily diagnosed as iron deficiency, thalassemia, vitamin B_{12} deficiency, folate deficiency, or another type of anemia defined by blood cell examination and supporting laboratory tests often requires a marrow examination. Abnormal cells in the blood, such as blast cells, may require a marrow examination. In addition to determining the cellularity and morphology of precursor cells or the presence of nonhematopoietic cells, the study provides marrow cells for immunophenotyping by cell flow analysis, for cytogenetic studies, and in special cases for marrow cell culture. Granulomatous and storage diseases may be found in the marrow, and the marrow can be used to culture fastidious organisms such as fungi and mycobacteria.

HISTORY OF THE MARROW EXAMINATION

The first recorded examinations of marrow in living patients occurred in the first decade of the 10th century. The sample was obtained from the tibial tubercle. Biopsy of the tibia using drill-like devices was reported in the next decade. Open biopsy also was proposed. Neither technique led to routine examination of the marrow because in the former case the tibia usually was hypocellular in adults and in the latter case because of the invasiveness of an open procedure and the discomfort and risk of infection and bleeding.[1] In 1923, Arinkin,[2] who was working in Leningrad, devised the marrow aspiration technique, which was the prototype for our current aspiration procedure. Thirty gyears passed before the suggestion that the pelvis might be preferable to the sternum gained hold, and another 10 years passed before a practical marrow biopsy instrument was put to use.[1] Regular use of the posterior iliac crest for aspiration and biopsy and regular use of biopsy to complement aspiration did not occur until the 1970s, when staging

of lymphoma made biopsy a frequent procedure and new simpler biopsy instruments became readily available.

INDICATIONS FOR MARROW ASPIRATE OR BIOPSY

Although marrow aspiration and biopsy techniques are safe, they should be performed with a clear idea as to how the results will help distinguish the differential diagnoses under consideration or provide follow-up of treatment.[3–5] In most hematologic disorders, such as most cases of iron deficiency anemia, thalassemia, and acquired and inherited hemolytic anemia, examination of the blood and specialized laboratory tests may suffice to make the diagnosis without the need for a marrow examination.

When examination of the marrow is indicated, the decision as to whether an aspirate only or an aspirate plus biopsy is desired must be made. Aspiration is always performed because of the superior morphology offered by examination of the aspirate smear. However, a marrow biopsy is superior to the aspirate in quantitating marrow cellularity and diagnosing infiltrative diseases of the marrow and should be performed when these conditions are part of the differential diagnosis.[6–10] In low-grade lymphoma, the marrow frequently is involved at the time of diagnosis, and this involvement is most sensitively detected by marrow biopsy.[11] Marrow biopsy is useful for diagnosing and following the course of disorders that are commonly associated with reticulin fibrosis, such as megakaryoblastic leukemia, hairy cell leukemia, and the chronic myeloproliferative disorders.[12,13] In myelodysplastic syndromes, marrow biopsy is useful for evaluating abnormal localization of immature precursor cells and abnormal megakaryocytes.[12] Marrow necrosis and gelatinous transformation are more readily detected in marrow sections than in aspirate films. Marrow aspirate alone may be appropriate in some clinical settings where the diagnostic question is very targeted, such as diagnosis of childhood immune thrombocytopenia purpura or routine surveillance follow-up of leukemia patients.

Depending on the diagnostic question, availability of material, and expected frequency of the abnormal cells, an appropriate selection of specialized diagnostic methods may be needed to support the clinical diagnosis. Morphology is still the gold standard for diagnosis of malignancy and allows construction of a good differential diagnosis for nonmalignant disorders. Immunocytochemistry provides excellent phenotype–morphology correlation on an individual cell basis but is limited to epitopes that resist fixation and/or drying. Flow cytometry allows study of almost any surface or intracellular protein, with the added ability to detect important quantitative changes in cellular proteins and simultaneous determination of multiple proteins within the same cell. However, flow cytometry requires that cells be viable and dissociated from tissue. Gene expression arrays allow analysis of complex patterns of RNA expression by sophisticated mathematical algorithms to detect diagnostic patterns based on the broadest range of cellular gene products, but with relatively less ability to study small subpopulations. Attempts at clinical validation of gene expression data are significant and ongoing. Classic metaphase cytogenetics, fluorescence *in situ* hybridization (FISH), and reverse transcriptase polymerase chain reaction (PCR) each assesses the underlying oncogenetic mechanisms involved in hematopoietic malignancies. In the order given, these techniques are characterized by increasing ability to detect rare malignant cells but increasingly limited sequences of DNA queried.

MARROW ASPIRATION TECHNIQUE

At birth, all bones contain hematopoietic marrow. Fat cells begin to replace hemopoietic marrow in the extremities in the fifth to seventh year. By adulthood, the hemopoietic marrow is limited to the axial skeleton and the proximal portions of the extremities (see Chaps. 4 and 8). Chapter 4 discusses the structure and function of the marrow

Acronyms and abbreviations that appear in this chapter include: CD, cluster of differentiation; EDTA, ethylenediaminetetraacetic acid; FISH, fluorescence *in situ* hybridization; HLA, human leukocyte antigen; PCR, polymerase chain reaction; PNH, paroxysmal nocturnal hemoglobinuria.

and the distribution of marrow in the skeleton. Fatty marrow appears yellow, whereas hematopoietic marrow is red. Red marrow contains fat, however, and fat droplets are visible grossly in aspirated marrow specimens. Histologically, yellow marrow consists almost entirely of fat cells and supporting connective tissue. Red marrow contains an abundance of hemopoietic cells, fat cells, and connective tissue. The marrow fills the spaces between the trabeculae of bone in the marrow cavity. Marrow is soft and friable and can be readily aspirated or biopsied with a needle.

The posterior iliac crest (Fig. 3-1) is the preferred site for marrow aspiration and biopsy. In adults, the sternum and the anterior iliac crest also can be utilized (Fig. 3-2). The sternum should be used for aspiration only. The anterior iliac crest is less preferred than the posterior crest in adults because of the crest's thick cortical bone. The anteromedial surface of the tibia is an option for infants younger than 1 year old (particularly newborns), but the posterior iliac crest is still the preferred site. The spinous processes of the vertebrae, the ribs, or other marrow-containing bones are rarely used. Serious adverse outcomes after marrow aspiration or biopsy are rare, probably less than 0.05 percent, and most frequently involve hemorrhage, which is associated more with platelet function impairment than thrombocytopenia or coagulation factor defect.[14] Infection and reactions to anesthetic agents

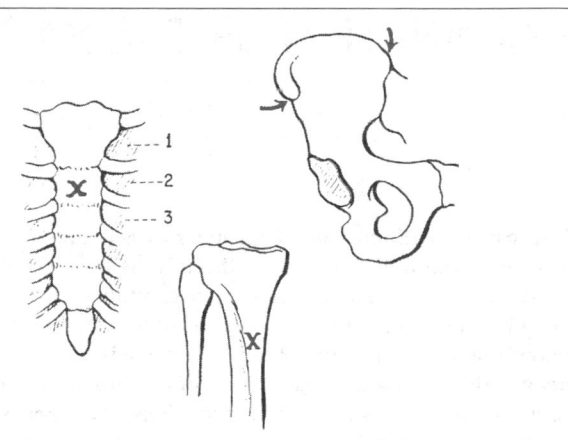

FIGURE 3-2   Sites used for marrow aspiration. (Modified from SO Schwartz, WH Hartz Jr, and JH Robbins, *Hematology in Practice*, part 1, p 36. McGraw-Hill, New York, 1961.)

may occur. Penetration of the bone with damage to the underlying structures is possible with all marrow aspirations, but the hazard is greatest in sternal aspirations because the sternum at the second interspace is only approximately 1 cm thick in adults.

For either a marrow biopsy or aspiration, sedation minimizes anxiety and pain,[15] particularly in children.[16,17] However, the sedation must be performed with proper monitoring to minimize risk.[18] Marrow biopsies and aspirations for staging purposes often can be performed while the patient is under anesthesia for other procedures. Several different types of needles, most of which are satisfactory, are available for marrow aspiration.[5] For adults, an 18-gauge needle is sufficiently large to permit aspiration of adequate specimens; larger needles are unnecessary. The patient is prone or in the left or right lateral decubitus position. Sterile precautions must be observed. The skin over the puncture site is shaved if necessary and cleansed with a disinfectant solution. The skin, subcutaneous tissues, and periosteum are infiltrated with a local anesthetic solution, such as 1 percent lidocaine. Adequate infiltration of the anesthetic at the periosteal surface is important, but no more than 20 ml of 1 percent lidocaine should be used in an adult.[19] An air gun can be used to anesthetize the skin surface prior to application of anesthetic to the periosteal surface by injection. After the anesthesia has taken effect, the marrow needle is inserted through the skin, subcutaneous tissue, and cortex of the bone using a slight twisting motion. In obese patients, the length of the needle must be sufficient to reach the iliac crest. The stylet should be locked into place on the hub of the needle to prevent plugging of the needle with tissue prior to needle entry into the marrow cavity. Penetration of the cortex can be sensed by a slight, rapid forward movement accompanied by a sudden increase in the ease of advancing the needle. The stylet of the needle is removed promptly, the hub is attached to a 10- or 20-ml syringe, and approximately 0.2 to 0.5 ml of fluid is aspirated. The actual aspiration of the marrow causes a transient painful sensation for most patients. If additional specimen volume is required, another syringe is fitted on the marrow needle, and marrow is aspirated. The stylet may be reinserted and the marrow needle slightly repositioned between aspirations. When aspiration is complete, the stylet is reinserted and the needle immediately removed from the bone. Pressure is applied to the skin over the aspiration site for at least 5 minutes to minimize bruising at the site. In a thrombocytopenic patient, firm pressure should be applied for at least 10 to 15 minutes. The bloody fluid that is aspirated contains light-colored particles of marrow approximately 0.5 to 1 mm in diameter. They often are readily visible in the syringe but may not be detected until the syringe contents are discharged on glass slides for film preparation.

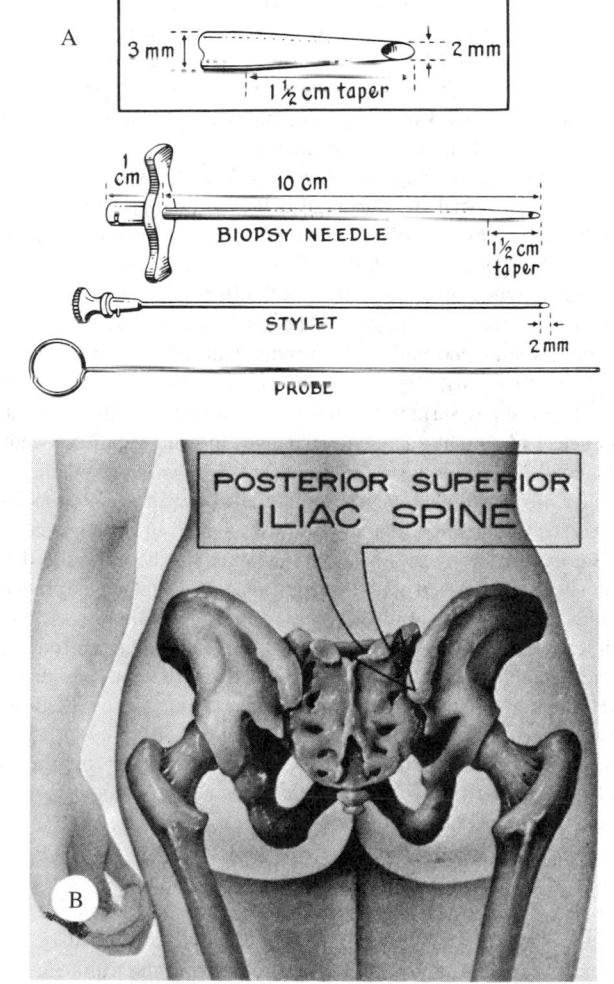

FIGURE 3-1   *(A)* Jamshidi biopsy instrument. (From K Jamshidi and WR Swaim,[20] with permission.) *(B)* Site of marrow biopsy. (From Ellis et al,[6] with permission.)

If nothing enters the syringe when aspiration is performed, the needle was not properly placed in the marrow cavity. The needle can be cautiously advanced 1 to 2 mm after reinsertion of the stylet and aspiration attempted again. Perhaps as a more desired alternative, the needle can be removed from the bone and reinserted in a nearby site in the anesthetized area. The thickness of the bone must be considered when the needle is being adjusted in the bone. Occasionally the needle must be rotated on its longitudinal axis, or in a larger orbit, in order to loosen the marrow mechanically before the marrow can be aspirated. If a small amount of blood has been aspirated, a new needle should be used because of the probability of clotting of the aspirate when it finally is obtained. Aspiration with a 50-ml syringe may succeed if use of a smaller syringe failed. Leukemic marrow may be so densely packed in the bone as to resist all attempts at aspiration, in which case biopsy is necessary. Fibrotic marrow may be impossible to aspirate. The most common cause of failure to obtain marrow is faulty positioning of the needle, and a second attempt at aspiration usually succeeds.

NEEDLE BIOPSY TECHNIQUE

Needle biopsy usually is performed with the Jamshidi needle,[20] using the same preparation as described above in "Marrow Aspiration Technique." The Jamshidi instrument (see Fig. 3-1) consists of a cylindrical needle with constant bore, except for a concentrically tapered distal portion ending in a sharp, beveled cutting tip. The stylet fits precisely inside the opening at the tapered tip, interlocks at the hub of the needle, and extends 1 to 2 mm beyond the end of the needle. An 11-gauge needle is most commonly used in the United States. After the skin and the periosteum of the biopsy site are anesthetized, a 3-mm incision is made in the skin. The needle, with obturator in place, is inserted into the skin incision and through the subcutaneous tissue to the cortex of the bone. The needle is directed toward the posterior iliac spine and advanced with a twisting motion. Penetration of the cortex is sensed by a decreased resistance to forward movement of the needle. The obturator is removed, and the needle is slowly advanced with reciprocal clockwise–counterclockwise twisting motions around the long axis. After sufficient penetration of the bone (up to approximately 3 cm), the needle is rotated several times on its axis and withdrawn approximately 2 to 3 mm. The needle is reinserted to the original depth at a slightly different angle, taking care not to bend the needle, and rotated several times to free the specimen from attachments in the marrow cavity. The needle is slowly withdrawn, with the same twisting motion used during insertion. The core of marrow inside the needle is removed by inserting the probe through the cutting tip and extruding the specimen through the hub of the needle. The smaller size of the cutting aperture relative to the bore of the shaft of the Jamshidi instrument yields a specimen that fits loosely inside the needle and therefore is less subject to compression, distortion, or fragmentation. The technique reliably produces good-quality biopsy specimens. Marrow biopsy should be performed before marrow aspiration is attempted (or in a slightly different site on the iliac crest) to avoid hemorrhage and distorted marrow architecture in the biopsy core. With the availability of the biopsy needles described in this section, open (surgical) biopsies rarely are necessary but may be performed, for example, for diagnosis of deeply situated bone lesions or at the time of a surgical procedure performed for related indications (e.g., staging).

PREPARATION OF MARROW SPECIMENS FOR STUDY

Several types of preparations can be made from the marrow aspirate to maximize use of the diagnostic material. Most important is the *direct film*, which is made immediately from the unmanipulated aspirate.

This preparation is the best for evaluating cellular morphology and differential counts of the marrow. The *particle film* is best for estimating marrow cellularity and megakaryocyte abundance, but morphology is obscured in the thicker parts of the film. A *concentrate film*, which is prepared from a buffy coat of the marrow, is useful for detecting low-abundance cells, such as megakaryocytes and metastatic tumor, or when the marrow is hypocellular. However, the relative proportions of cell lineages are not reliably maintained in the concentrate film preparation (often erythroid precursors are relatively enriched). In addition, this preparation is subject to anticoagulant-induced changes in nuclear morphology or cytoplasmic vacuolation. The *touch imprint* from the biopsy is essential for evaluating cellular morphology in case of a "dry tap"[21] and provides cytologic detail of cells that may not appear in the aspirate specimen.[22]

MARROW FILMS

After aspiration, approximately 0.5 ml of marrow is placed on a glass slide, the rest is mixed into a tube containing ethylenediaminetetraacetic acid (EDTA) solution. The marrow specimen is examined to ensure the presence of "spicules" or particles of marrow containing bony or fatty pieces, indicating successful aspiration of the marrow cavity. Direct marrow films are immediately prepared by transferring drops of the unanticoagulated marrow pool to fresh slides and making push films with coverslips. Sufficient films should be made for special stains. Heparinization of the aspirate is not necessary if the operator works rapidly and should be avoided because heparinization may introduce artifacts.

A useful technique is preparing a thick film of marrow by discharging a drop or two of the aspirate on a slide, covering the aspirate with a second slide, gently pressing the slides together to express most of the blood into a gauze sponge, and then pulling the slides apart longitudinally. Such preparations may contain an increased number of broken cells if too much pressure is applied, but they provide a large number of particles from which marrow cellularity can be estimated and which are useful for estimating the amount of hemosiderin present.

The EDTA-anticoagulated sample is centrifuged (1500g for 10 minutes) in a Wintrobe tube to concentrate the cellular elements of the marrow. After centrifugation, the fatty layer and plasma are removed, and the "buffy coat" is mixed with an equal amount of plasma. Multiple films of this preparation are made. These films should be air dried, labeled, and retained as unstained preparations in case special stains are required.

TOUCH PREPARATIONS

After a biopsy specimen is obtained using the Jamshidi needle, the specimen should be extruded through the hub of the needle and then gently rolled across a glass slide (using an applicator stick to move the specimen) before it is placed in fixative, taking care to avoid crushing. The touch preparations are allowed to dry and are stained in the same manner as films.

SPECIAL STUDIES

It is essential to formulate the diagnostic question before performing a marrow aspiration to ensure an adequate sample is obtained for all the special studies that may be needed to make the correct diagnosis. A sterile anticoagulated sample containing viable unfixed cells in single-cell suspension is the best substrate for nearly all special studies of a marrow sample that likely will be required. Specifically, flow cytometry is best performed on an EDTA- or heparin-anticoagulated aspirate specimen, which is stable for at least 24 hours at room temperature. For cytogenetic or cell culture analysis, anticoagulated marrow should be added to tissue culture medium and analyzed as soon as possible to maintain optimal cell viability. Cytogenetic samples are generally not adversely affected by overnight incubation.[23]

For molecular analysis of genomic DNA in fresh specimens, sample preparation and storage as described for cell marker studies are adequate because DNA is relatively stable. EDTA is the preferred anticoagulant because heparin can interfere with some molecular assays. Messenger RNA (mRNA) has a variable half-life in an intact cell and is degraded rapidly (on the order of seconds to minutes) in a cell lysate by ubiquitous RNAses. Sample storage prior to RNA isolation should be minimized.[24] For maximal mRNA recovery, cell suspensions (typically buffy coat or mononuclear cell preparations) should be lysed in an appropriate RNAse inhibitor containing buffer as soon as possible after sampling. DNA and mRNA can be extracted and analyzed from paraffin-embedded tissue sections[25,26] and dried stained films,[27] but degradation is significant, and its impact is proportional to the length of sequence required.

Archival storage of marrow specimens is important in light of advances in molecular diagnosis that may necessitate validation studies using samples of known origin or testing of diagnostic material from a patient now in remission. Isolated DNA or RNA can be stored for long periods at −70°C, whereas viable, intact cells can be reliably preserved only by controlled rate freezing in dimethylsulfoxide (DMSO) and storage in liquid nitrogen.

HISTOLOGIC SECTIONS

A variety of techniques for preparing aspirated material for histologic study have been advocated. All of the techniques are designed to collect a sufficient number of marrow particles in a small volume so that adequate sections can be prepared. This goal can be accomplished by discharging the marrow aspirate onto a glass slide, allowing the particles to settle for a few seconds, and then gently tilting the slide so that the excess blood runs off. The particles then are pushed together with an applicator stick, and the remaining blood is allowed to clot. The clot is promptly fixed in Zenker solution, B5, or buffered formalin[28] for tissue processing and sectioning. An alternative method using filtration of the anticoagulated aspirate specimen has been described.[29]

The core marrow biopsy specimen is processed for histologic examination by fixation in Zenker solution, B5 fixative, or neutral buffered formalin, followed by decalcification and embedding in paraffin. Sections of high quality cut at 4 μm and stained with hematoxylin and eosin or with Giemsa are eminently satisfactory for routine work. Refinements in fixation and embedding techniques have enabled use of most immunologic markers in decalcified paraffin-embedded marrow biopsy specimens.[29] Fixation in neutral buffered formalin and embedding in plastic have the advantage of superior morphology[30] and suitability for most immunochemical procedures,[31] but the method is technically more demanding and expensive.[32]

MORPHOLOGIC INTERPRETATION OF MARROW PREPARATIONS

OVERVIEW

The Wright-Giemsa–stained direct marrow aspirate film should be examined as quickly as possible to provide a preliminary assessment of the marrow morphology and allow setup of specialized testing based on this preliminary evaluation while the sample is fresh. Final interpretation of the marrow biopsy and aspirate should be integrated with results from the clinical history, blood film, cell counts, laboratory data, cell marker studies, and molecular or cytogenetic data. No other histologic specimen exists in which a state-of-the-art interpretation is

dependent on such an array of supportive data. This results from the wealth of basic biologic information gained from *in vitro* studies of blood cells, which has been translated into useful diagnostic tests. The challenge for the hematopathologist and hematologist is to understand the advantages and limitations of each diagnostic approach so that apparently conflicting results can be reconciled and placed into perspective.

ADEQUACY OF THE MARROW SAMPLE

The first question in interpreting the marrow is whether the sample is adequate for diagnosis. At the time of the procedure, the presence of marrow particles in the aspirate is the best indicator that the needle entered the medullary cavity and marrow was successfully withdrawn. Marrow particles are bony with a glistening appearance caused by fat in the particles. Specimens containing cortical bone, muscle, or other tissue with little or no medullary bone are inadequate for marrow interpretation but may provide other information. Samples with extensive crush artifact or hemorrhage also are inadequate, underscoring the importance of proper technique in obtaining a useful sample. An unspoken assumption is that the piece of marrow provided for diagnostic evaluation is representative of the marrow as a whole. Based on reproducibility of bilateral biopsies, this more likely is true in leukemia and myeloma than in lymphoma and metastatic tumor.[33] A biopsy specimen should contain at least a 0.5-cm length of marrow cavity. However, for detection of lymphoma or metastatic tumor, current recommendations suggest a biopsy length of 1.6 to 2.0 cm,[34] with examination of two to four deeper sections to maximize sensitivity.[35]

The marrow cavity was entered if the aspirate contains marrow particles or hematopoietic precursors (e.g., megakaryocytes, nucleated red cells) not found in the blood film. However, this finding does not ensure the specimen is adequate for diagnosis, because the amount of marrow actually aspirated can vary significantly in disease states.[36] Also, some cell types, notably fibroblasts and metastatic tumor cells, are not as readily removed from the marrow space by aspiration as are normal precursors. Lack of particles or precursor cells does not prove the marrow cavity was not entered, because marrow packed with leukemic cells or infiltrated with fibroblasts may yield a "dry tap."[21] Marrow aspirations resulting in a "dry tap" usually are a consequence of significant pathology (only 7 percent show normal histology on biopsy)[21] and indicate the need to examine a biopsy specimen.

MARROW CELLULARITY

The "gold standard" for overall marrow cellularity is examination of an adequate marrow biopsy specimen.[37,38] The normal cellularity (percentage of nonbony marrow space occupied by hematopoietic cells as opposed to fatty and nonhematopoietic tissue) of iliac crest marrow decreases from a mean of 80 percent in early childhood to 50 percent by age 30 years, with further decreases after age 70 years.[39] Therefore, marrow cellularity should be evaluated with reference to normal individuals of the same age as the patient.[40] The normal range of iliac crest marrow cellularity is broader than expected.[39] When evaluating cellularity, remember that marrow spaces directly adjacent to cortical bone frequently are fatty in the elderly and are not representative of the cellularity of the deeper marrow spaces.[41]

Cellularity assessment by examination of the direct marrow aspirate film is more difficult because of loss of histologic structure and mixture with peripheral blood. The aspirate may suggest the marrow is more hypocellular than indicated by the biopsy.[38] Marrow particles (seen in the direct film or a particle preparation) are the best indicators of cellularity. These particles are like "mini-biopsies" and contain sufficient hematopoietic and fatty elements to give some idea of marrow cellularity. Cellularity estimates based on careful examination of par-

TABLE 3-1 NORMAL VALUES FOR MARROW DIFFERENTIAL CELL COUNT AT DIFFERENT AGES (PERCENT OF CELLS)

	ROSSE ET AL[65] INFANTS TIBIAL MARROW			GLASER ET AL[76] SUBJECTS AGED 1–20 YEARS STERNAL MARROW, 1 ML ASPIRATED	BAIN[45] SUBJECTS AGED 21–56 YEARS ILIAC MARROW, 0.1–0.2 ML ASPIRATED	
TYPE OF CELL	<1 MONTH (n = 57)	1 MONTH (n = 7)	18 MONTHS (n = 19)		Men (n = 30)	Women (n = 20)
Myeloblast	—	—	—	1.2 (0–3)	1.4 (0–3.0)	
Promyelocyte	0.79 ± 0.91	0.76 ± 0.65	0.64 ± 0.59	1.8 (0–4)	7.8 (3.2–12.4)	
Myelocyte	3.95 ± 2.93	2.50 ± 1.48	2.49 ± 1.39	16.5 (8–25)		
Neutrophilic					7.6 (3.7–10.0)	
Eosinophilic					1.3 (0–2.8)	
Basophilic						
Metamyelocyte	19.37 ± 4.84	11.34 ± 3.59	12.42 ± 4.15	23 (14–34)	4.1 (2.3–5.9)	
Band form	28.89 ± 7.56	14.10 ± 4.63	14.20 ± 5.63	—	**	
Segmented						
Neutrophil	7.37 ± 4.64	3.64 ± 2.97	6.31 ± 3.91	12.9 (4.5–29)	32.1 (21.9–42.3)	37.4 (28.8–45.9)
Eosinophil	2.70 ± 1.27	2.61 ± 1.40	2.70 ± 2.16	—	2.2 (0.3–4.2)	
Basophil	0.12 ± 0.20	0.07 ± 0.16	0.10 ± 0.12	—	0.1 (0–0.4)	
Lymphocyte	14.42 ± 5.54	47.05 ± 9.24	43.55 ± 8.56	16 (5–36)	13.1 (6.0–20.0)	
Monocyte	0.88 ± 0.85	1.01 ± 0.89	2.12 ± 1.59	—	1.3 (0–2.6)	
Plasma cell	0.00 ± 0.02	0.02 ± 0.06	0.06 ± 0.08	—	0.6 (0–1.2)	
Proerythroblast	0.02 ± 0.06	0.10 ± 0.14	0.08 ± 0.13	0.5 (0–1.5)		
Erythroblast					28.1 (16.2–40.1)[§]	22.5 (13.0–32.0)[§]
Basophilic	0.24 ± 0.25	0.34 ± 0.33	0.50 ± 0.34	1.7 (0–5)		
Polychromatophilic	13.06 ± 6.78	6.90 ± 4.45	6.97 ± 3.56	18 (5–34)		
Orthochromatic	0.09 ± 0.73	0.54 ± 1.88	0.44 + 0.49	2.7 (0–8)		
Megakaryocyte	0.06 ± 0.15	0.05 ± 0.09	0.07 ± 0.12	—	31 (6–77)[‡]	
Macrophage					0.4 (0–1.3)	
Others					[¶]	
Transitional cells*	1.18 ± 1.13	1.95 ± 0.94	1.99 ± 1.00	—		
Broken cell	5.79 ± 2.78	5.50 ± 2.46	5.05 ± 2.15	—		
M/E ratio	4.4:1	4.4:1	4.8:1	2.9:1 (1:1–5:1)	2.1 (1.1–4.1)	2.8 (1.6–5.2)

* Immature lymphoid cells.
** Bands included in segmented neutrophil count.
§ All erythroblast forms (basophilic, polychromatophilic, orthochromatic) grouped together.
‡ Number of megakaryocytes near the advancing edge of the film (mean, range).
¶ Osteoclasts noted in 8/50 subjects, osteoblasts in 5/50, no mast cells observed.

ticles in the aspirate preparation agree well with cellularity estimated from the marrow biopsy.[40]

The degree of dilution of marrow aspirate specimens with blood during the aspiration is variable and may affect interpretation of marrow cellularity. Adult marrows with greater than 30 percent lymphocytes plus monocytes likely are substantially admixed with peripheral blood, as shown by cytokinetic studies of paired marrow aspirate and biopsy preparations.[42] Radiolabeled erythrocytes and serum albumin have been used to estimate the admixture of nucleated cells from blood with those from marrow in sternal marrow aspirates.[36] In patients with hematologic disease, from 6 to 93 percent of the nucleated cells were derived from the blood.[36] The greatest admixture was observed in patients with leukemia. Substantial dilution with blood may occur in aspirates that were difficult to obtain or when multiple draws were taken from the same puncture site. Based on cell markers and progenitor assays, the first 1.0 ml of marrow aspirated from healthy donors was only 8 percent contaminated with peripheral blood nucleated cells. In contrast, subsequent aspirates obtained for marrow harvesting were 20 percent contaminated with nucleated peripheral cells.[43] Interestingly, the bulk volume of the "marrow" aspirate (i.e., plasma, red cells) is almost completely derived from blood, even if the nucleated cells are mostly marrow derived.[43] Assessment of marrow cellularity by measuring the "buffy coat" observed after centrifugation of the aspirate specimen is unreliable.[38]

Cellularity of individual lineages is best assessed by examination of the biopsy specimen. Erythroid cells typically are arranged in clusters, whereas megakaryocytes are scattered throughout the biopsy. Erythroid and megakaryocytic cellularity is best appreciated at low power. In the aspirate, a myeloid to erythroid (M/E) ratio frequently is calculated to give some impression of the relative cellularity of these two major lineages. As a rule of thumb, the M/E ratio normally should be between 2:1 and 4:1 (Table 3-1 lists the normal ranges in men and women). The relative proportions of cell types should be assessed only on the direct marrow film or particle preparation, not a "concentrate" film, which has been manipulated by centrifugation. A decreased M/E ratio can be interpreted as either myeloid hypocellularity or erythroid hyperplasia, depending on the overall marrow cellularity. Advances in automated hematology instruments offer the possibility of performing automated marrow erythroid and myeloid cell counts.[44] Megakaryocyte numbers can be assessed from the direct marrow aspirate film, where at least five megakaryocytes should be present in the optimal portion of the film. In the particle preparation, most large particles should contain one or more megakaryocytes. Megakaryocyte number varies markedly in direct marrow aspirate films of normal subjects[45]

(Table 3-1) and depends on the degree of admixture of the specimen with peripheral blood. Megakaryocytes are variably enriched in the feathered edge of concentrate films.

INFILTRATIVE DISEASES OF THE MARROW

MALIGNANT NEOPLASMS

Metastatic nonhematopoietic tumor in the marrow biopsy is characterized by disruption of the marrow architecture with groups of cytologically abnormal cells. Assessment of the tissue of origin is primarily based on morphology, clinical history, and immunocytochemical staining. The tendency of carcinoma cells to form tightly adherent clusters frequently is helpful in recognizing these neoplasms (see Color Plate XV). The clumps can appear on the marrow aspirate, but the aspirate is less sensitive than the biopsy for detecting metastatic tumor. Tumor clumps may occur infrequently in the aspirate, often appearing only on side or feathered edges of the film or only in the concentrate preparation. These tumor clumps must be distinguished from clumps of damaged hematopoietic cells, which commonly appear in aspirate preparations, especially the concentrate. The distinction is best accomplished by examining cells at the periphery of the clumps to determine if the cells show the morphology of hematopoietic precursors or cytologically atypical cells. Isolated nonhematopoietic tumor cells are seen infrequently in aspirate preparations, even when tumor is obvious in the biopsy, because of the adherent nature of most nonhematopoietic tumors. Examination of multiple films may be necessary to find isolated tumor cell clumps.[46] Rare metastatic carcinoma cells can be identified by immunocytochemical staining for epithelial markers, such as cytokeratins, not found on normal hematopoietic cells. The presence of such cells in node-negative breast cancer conveys a negative prognostic risk,[47] although full-blown metastatic disease does not always occur. Molecular evidence suggests that tumor cells in breast cancer may disseminate in a far less progressed genomic state than previously thought, and that the tumor cells acquire genomic aberrations typical of metastatic cells thereafter.[48] This finding may explain the variable clinical outcome of micrometastatic disease.

Myeloma[49] and lymphomas[11] are more reliably detected on the biopsy preparation, where the typical aggregation pattern of abnormal lymphoid cells can be appreciated (see Color Plates XIV-5 and 6 and XXI-10). Abnormal lymphoid aggregates must be distinguished from lymphoid aggregates found in reactive conditions or in older patients.[50] Neoplastic aggregates more likely show cytologic atypia and monomorphous cellular population, and they often are adjacent to bony trabeculae, but the distinction can be difficult in some cases. The cellular morphology often can be better appreciated on the marrow aspirate, but the key histologic features are lost. Lymphoma cells do not form the tight clusters seen in nonhematopoietic tumors on the marrow aspirate film. In hairy cell leukemia, however, the hematopoietic cells are sufficiently adherent to each other and the marrow matrix that the aspirate specimen is often markedly hypocellular, which is refered to as a "dry tap," whereas biopsy specimens show extensive infiltration with tumor. Special studies, such as *in situ* hybridization for κ versus λ light-chain mRNA[51] or immunohistochemistry/flow cytometry to determine cell lineage and demonstrate surface light-chain restriction, may be necessary to distinguish a reactive process from malignant lymphoma. Detection of clonal immunoglobulin H rearrangements by PCR amplification of mRNA transcripts may be used for this purpose, but clinical interpretation of the results can be problematic, and morphology remains the gold standard in evaluating marrow involvement by lymphoma.[52]

FIBROSIS

Marrow fibrosis typically is recognizable only on a marrow biopsy specimen; the aspirate merely shows reduced or absent recovery of hematopoietic cells. Early stages of fibrosis are characterized by increased stainable marrow reticulin fibers (see Color Plate XIV-12). Fibrosis may accompany either primary hematopoietic disorders (e.g., myelofibrosis) or infiltrative diseases such as metastatic tumor.

STORAGE DISEASES

Storage disorders, such as Gaucher and Niemann-Pick diseases (see Chap. 73), are characterized by abnormal macrophages containing stored material in various forms.[53] These cells can be appreciated on both the biopsy and aspirate specimens (see Color Plates IX-4 and 5). In the latter preparation, they typically are more common in the feathered edge of the films. Reactive cells, such as the histiocytes with "sea-blue" inclusion granules or pseudo-Gaucher cells associated with chronic myelogenous leukemia,[54] can resemble the cells seen in storage disorders (see Color Plates IX-6 and 9).

INFECTIONS

Infectious organisms with an intracellular location, such as *Leishmania*,[55] *Histoplasma*, and *Toxoplasma*[56] can be visualized in monocytic cells by morphologic examination of the marrow (see Plates IX-8 and XXIII-5). Identification of mycobacterial organisms in the marrow by acid-fast staining lacks sensitivity but allows early diagnosis in one third of cases with HIV-related mycobacterium avium complex infection.[57] Morphologic examination and culture of the marrow is the most sensitive diagnostic test for disseminated leishmaniasis, a troublesome problem in HIV-infected patients exposed to this organism.[58] Marrow morphology also is a sensitive diagnostic tool for detecting disseminated histoplasmosis in patients with AIDS.[59] However, marrow culture has a low diagnostic yield in the workup of fever of unknown origin in nonimmunosuppressed patients.[60] The presence of marrow granulomas, recognizable only on biopsy specimens, necessitates examination by special stains for fungal and mycobacterial organisms, but the differential diagnosis is extensive.[53,61]

NECROSIS AND GELATINOUS TRANSFORMATION

Marrow necrosis may occur in a variety of disorders, particularly sickle cell disease and neoplastic processes involving the marrow.[62] Aspirates of necrotic marrow stained with polychrome stains contain cells with indistinct margins and smudged basophilic nuclei surrounded by acidophilic material. Sections of marrow stained with hematoxylin and eosin or with polychrome stains show loss of normal marrow architecture, indistinct cellular margins, and a background of amorphous eosinophilic material. Patients with severe weight loss may develop *gelatinous transformation* of the marrow, characterized by amorphous extracellular material (proteoglycans), fat atrophy, and marrow hypoplasia.[63] The findings of gelatinous transformation are reversible.[64]

MORPHOLOGIC DIFFERENTIATION OF HEMATOPOIETIC LINEAGES

OVERVIEW

Marrow aspirate films should be examined under low-power magnification to assess the relative amounts of fat and hemopoietic cells in particles and the number of megakaryocytes, plasma cells, and mast cells present. Low-power examination also permits detection of osteoclasts or osteoblasts (see Color Plates XV-1, 2, and 3), groups of malignant cells (see Color Plates XV-4, 5, 6, and 7), Gaucher cells (see Color Plate IX-5), lymphoid follicles (see Color Plate XIV-5), and granulomas. The entire film should be examined, including the particles, and higher magnification should be used to study any abnormalities discovered. Similarly, biopsy sections are examined at low power to assess adequacy, overall cellularity, presence of infiltrative disease, and cellularity of the major hematopoietic lineages.

After the low-power survey, the films should be examined at higher power and under oil-immersion magnification to determine the various hemopoietic cell types present and assess adequacy of differentiation in each hematopoietic lineage. For most diagnostic questions, careful and systematic visual examination of the marrow is sufficient to assess differentiation, but a marrow differential count can be performed to quantify the status of hematopoietic differentiation, particularly in the granulocytic lineages. Because a large variety of cell types normally are present in the marrow and their distribution is irregular, accurate marrow differential count requires examination of 300 to 500 nucleated cells. Table 3-1 lists the normal values for these determinations, including data for infants from birth to age 18 months.[65] Between birth and age 1 month, lymphocytes increase and erythroid and granulocytic precursors decrease. After 1 month, the marrow differential count varies little to age 18 months, the duration of the study.[65] The proportion of segmented neutrophils increases with large volumes of aspirate, probably because of dilution of marrow cells by mature granulocytes in the blood.[66] The range of normal for all cell types is broad, and differential counts and M/E ratios should be considered rough guides to the character of the marrow as a whole.

Morphologically recognizable cells in the normal marrow include mature granulocytes and their precursors, erythroid precursors, lymphocytes in varying stages of development, plasma cells, monocytes, macrophages (histiocytes), stromal cells, megakaryocytes, and mast cells. Typically only the later stages of differentiation, in which progenitors become fully committed to a given lineage, are morphologically recognizable. Progenitors of all lineages typically are unremarkable cells without distinctive morphologic attributes. The next stage of maturation precursor cells take on identifiable morphologic features, can be identified in marrow samples, and provide essential evidence for diagnosis of many hematologic diseases.

The characteristics of each cell type are briefly described, and the nomenclature is discussed. Further details of the morphology of these cells are discussed in other chapters of this book (see Chap. 28 for discussion of erythrocyte precursors; Chap. 59 for granulocyte series; Chap. 67 for monocyte series; and Chap. 74 for lymphocytes and plasma cells).

GRANULOCYTES

The term *granulocytes* refers to the precursors and mature forms of leukocytes characterized by neutrophilic, eosinophilic, or basophilic granules in their cytoplasm in the more mature stages of development. This series sometimes is referred to as the *myeloid series*. The overall trend is a gradual decrease in nuclear size and enhanced clumping of nuclear chromatin as cells lose proliferative capacity, while granules of varying types progressively appear in the cytoplasm.

The *myeloblast* (see Color Plate X-1) is round and large, approximately 14 to 18 μm in diameter on a dried film. The nucleus occupies most of the cell. The nuclear chromatin is very fine, and two to five nucleoli are present. The cytoplasm is basophilic but less so than the cytoplasm of the erythroid series. No granules are present.

The *promyelocyte* (progranulocyte) (see Color Plate X-2) is larger than the myeloblast. The chromatin pattern is coarser than that of the myeloblast, but nucleoli usually are present. The cytoplasm is basophilic with a clear Golgi area and is characterized by a small number of prominent, large red granules—the primary, nonspecific, or azurophilic granules. In the marrow, the granules usually mark the cell as a granulocyte precursor, although similar-appearing granules (with different enzymatic composition) may occur in large lymphocytes.

The *myelocyte* (see Color Plates X-3, 4, and 7) is slightly smaller than the promyelocyte. The myelocyte is the most mature mitotic cell

in the myeloid lineage. Its nucleus is round or oval and often eccentrically located. The chromatin pattern is coarser than that of the promyelocyte, and nucleoli usually are not visible. The defining feature is the presence of specific granules in the cytoplasm, which identify the cell lineage. The granules may be neutrophilic (fine, variable size, lilac color), eosinophilic (larger, round, orange–red), or basophilic (larger still, irregular in size, deep blue). The granules first appear in the perinuclear area. The cytoplasm is only slightly basophilic.

The *metamyelocyte* (see Color Plates X-5 and 8) is about the same size as the myelocyte and resembles it closely, except that the nucleus is indented, the chromatin is more coarse, and the cytoplasm is less basophilic.

The *band cell* (see Color Plates X-6, 7, and 8) is characterized by a nucleus that is horseshoe shaped or lobulated but is not segmented in that the rudimentary lobes are connected by a thick band of chromatin rather than the thin thread or filament characterizing the mature polymorphonuclear leukocyte. The cytoplasm is yellowish–pink or nearly colorless. Lineage specific granules are abundant in the cytoplasm. Nuclear chromatin is dense but less so than in the segmented granulocyte.

Segmented (polymorphonuclear) granulocytes (see Color Plates X-6, 7, and 8) differ from band cells by the multilobed character of the nucleus. At least two separate lobes are defined by a complete rounded shape, whether or not the thin filament joining them is seen. Nuclear chromatin is very dense. The mature eosinophil typically has only two lobes, whereas the nuclei of most neutrophils have two to four lobes. Basophil nuclei often are obscured by the abundant basophilic granules.

MONOCYTES

Monocytes in normal marrow are identical morphologically to those in the blood (see Color Plates VII-1 and 2) (see Chap. 67). Promonocytes have more delicate chromatin, visible nucleoli, often a few fine granules, and somewhat more basophilic cytoplasm.

MACROPHAGES (HISTIOCYTES)

These cells are derived from monocytes but are larger, reaching 20 to 30 μm in the longest dimension (see Color Plate IX). The nucleus is oval with delicate reticular chromatin and one or two small nucleoli. The cytoplasm ranges from blue–gray to pale and colorless and often contains phagocytosed cells, degenerating cell debris, and vacuoles. Normally, intact red cells are rarely visible inside marrow histiocytes. However, uncontrolled activation of histiocytic cells leads to a "hemophagocytic syndrome," which is associated with a variety of neoplastic, viral, and reactive conditions[67] (see Chap. 72).

ERYTHROID CELLS

During erythroid differentiation, the nucleus progressively becomes smaller and nuclear chromatin more condensed, as the cell's proliferative capacity decreases. The cytoplasm gradually loses the bluish color imparted by RNA, which is replaced by the pink-staining hemoglobin. Cells in the erythroid series are termed "erythroblasts" or "normoblasts." The latter term was used to distinguish the normal sequence from the sequence observed in megaloblastic anemia, in which the erythroid precursors are called "megaloblasts" because of their large size (see Color Plate VI). The term "normoblast" is obsolete. These stages are arbitrary divisions within a continuum of differentiation. Chapter 28 provides more detailed descriptions of normal red cell precursors.

The *proerythroblast* (see Color Plate V-1) is a large round cell measuring from 15 to 20 μm in diameter. The nucleus occupies most of the cell. The chromatin is present in a fine reticular or stippled pattern but is more densely stained than the chromatin of the myeloblast. Nucleoli are present and often are bluish. The cytoplasm typically is more basophilic than the myeloblast.

The *basophilic erythroblast* (see Color Plate V-2) is smaller than the proerythroblast, and the nucleus occupies less of the cell. The chromatin pattern is stippled, and the small, condensed masses of chromatin are sharply defined and separated by pale parachromatin. The cytoplasm is deeply basophilic.

The *polychromatophilic erythroblast* (see Color Plate V-3) is smaller than the basophilic erythroblast. The nucleus occupies even less of the cell, and the chromatin pattern is more condensed, with larger masses of chromatin sharply defined by pale parachromatin. The cytoplasm is gray or grayish–pink because of the increasing amounts of hemoglobin.

The *orthochromatic erythroblast* (see Color Plate V-4) is only slightly larger than the mature erythrocyte. The nucleus is small and pyknotic. The cytoplasm is red, like that of the mature erythrocyte.

The *erythrocyte* (see Color Plate I-1) is the mature anucleate red cell. *Polychromatophilic erythrocytes* are mature anucleate red cells that are just released from the marrow and still have sufficient residual RNA to impart a slight grayish tinge to the cytoplasm (see Color Plate I-4). The gray color of the cytoplasm results from a combination of cytoplasmic RNA and hemoglobin.

EVALUATION OF IRON STORES

Marrow examination should include evaluation of the iron stores, especially if the patient is anemic. The examination is accomplished by staining a marrow film or section by the Prussian blue technique. Because decalcification of marrow biopsy specimens results in decreased recovery of stainable iron,[68] a nondecalcified specimen should be stained when evaluating iron stores in the differential diagnosis of anemia. Marrow macrophages (seen best in the aspirate particle preparation) are evaluated for storage iron, and erythroblasts (best evaluated in the direct film or concentrate) are examined for the presence of iron granules in the cytoplasm (sideroblasts). Late erythroblasts are readily identified by their small size and the size, shape, and chromatin pattern of the nucleus. The proportion of late erythroblasts that contain one or more Prussian blue granules is extremely variable (3–69%) in normal subjects.[45] Abnormal sideroblasts are characterized by increased number (>5) or size of iron granules, particularly if the sideroblasts are arranged in a ring around the nucleus, reflecting accumulation of iron in mitochondria.

MEGAKARYOCYTES

Chapter 104 discusses in detail the megakaryocyte (see Color Plate XII). Megakaryocytes are large cells (30–150 μm) with darkly stained, irregularly lobed nuclei. The cytoplasm is blue "cotton candy" textured, and the more mature cells contain many red granules. About half the megakaryocytes should have platelets adjacent to their periphery.

LYMPHOCYTES

In normal marrow, lymphocytes similar to those found in the blood occur in variable numbers, depending on the degree of blood contamination of the marrow. Immature lymphoid cells with a very high nuclear to cytoplasmic ratio and moderately dense but finely distributed chromatin often are seen in marrow aspirates of children. The immature lymphoid cells may cause diagnostic difficulty in some clinical settings, such as the "rebound" lymphocytosis that occurs after cessation of maintenance chemotherapy for acute lymphoblastic leukemia.[69] These lymphocytes mostly represent varying stages of B cell precursor development.[70] Mature lymphocytes and smaller numbers of immature lymphoid forms are prominent in infant marrows but diminish in number with age.

PLASMA CELLS

Normal plasma cells vary in size but usually are 12 to 16 μm in diameter when spread on a slide (see Chap. 74). They are round or oval. The nucleus is small, round, eccentrically placed, and stained densely purple. The chromatin is coarse and clumped. Nucleoli are not visible. The cytoplasm is deep blue, often with a paranuclear clear zone (see Color Plate XXI). Binuclate forms may be found in normal marrow.

OTHER CELL TYPES

Mast cells are readily recognized by their content of dark-blue granules, which usually completely fill the cytoplasm and may obscure the nucleus (see Color Plate VII-5). The cells are round or spindle shaped and often are located deep in the particles, frequently lying along blood vessels. The nucleus often is not visible but when seen is round or oval with a vesicular chromatin pattern.

Osteoclasts and *osteoblasts* are uncommon. They are seen more frequently in marrow obtained from children and from adults with hyperparathyroidism or osteoblastic reactions to tumors. Osteoclasts are large cells and may be larger than 100 μm in diameter (see Color Plates XV-1 and 2). They superficially resemble megakaryocytes but contain multiple separated nuclei that have a moderately fine chromatin pattern with nucleoli. The cytoplasm varies from slightly basophilic to intensely acidophilic because of the content of acidophilic granules. Osteoclasts may contain coarse basophilic debris.

Osteoblasts usually are oval cells up to 30 μm in the longest diameter (see Color Plate XV-3). They often occur in groups. The nucleus usually is quite eccentric and may seem to be spilling out of the cell. The chromatin pattern is uniform, and one to three nucleoli are present. The cytoplasm is light blue and may contain a few red granules. Osteoblasts may be mistaken for plasma cells. In osteoblasts, the pale centrosomal region of the cytoplasm is separated from the nucleus, in contrast to that of the plasma cell, in which the centrosomal region directly abuts the nucleus.

PRINCIPLES OF FLOW CYTOMETRY INTERPRETATION

With implementation of the World Health Organization Classification of Hematologic Malignancies,[71] immunophenotypic data have become an integral part of the diagnosis and classification of many marrow-based malignancies. As a consequence, phenotypic assessment of marrow cells by flow cytometry provides information that is complementary to morphologic evaluation and other special studies. Typically, the diagnostic question relates to the differentiation stage and lineage assignment of leukemias or lymphomas. Flow cytometry is increasingly used in the assessment and diagnosis of myelodysplastic and myeloproliferative disorders, but this diagnostic application is controversial. Only the basic principles of marrow analysis are described in this chapter. The specific morphologic and cell marker phenotypes seen in hematopoietic disorders are described in greater detail in other chapters of this book.

METHODOLOGY

The specific details of flow cytometry instrumentation and staining methods are beyond the scope of this chapter. However, in brief, a single-cell suspension is aspirated into a laminar flow of isotonic diluent that passes in front of one or more laser beams. Light scatter and fluorescence data are collected using specific photomultiplier tubes and dichroic filters that eliminate extraneous wavelengths. In most instruments used for clinical immunophenotypic analysis, light scatter information is collected at two angles: (1) forward-angle light scatter, which correlates with cell surface area and hence indirectly with cell size, and (2) 90-degree light scatter (orthogonal or side scatter), which correlates with cellular complexity. For practical purposes in evaluating hematologic samples such as marrow, orthogonal light scatter indicates cellular granularity, with neutrophils and myeloid progenitors having greater side scatter than lymphocytes or monocytes.

Immunophenotyping can be achieved by using monoclonal antibodies specific to certain cell surface proteins, most of which have cluster of differentiation (CD) designations, which are periodically updated by international workshops (see Chap. 14).[72] The monoclonal antibodies used can be directly tagged with fluorochrome molecules that emit light at specific wavelengths, thereby allowing correlation of the signal emitted with expression of the corresponding cell protein. By using fluorochromes that are excited at similar wavelengths (allowing use of one or two lasers) but emit light at relatively nonoverlapping wavelengths, multiple markers in a single stained sample can be assessed and information gained about the marker profile of a specific neoplasm or cell type.

A primary requirement for flow cytometry analysis is that cells must be viable and in single-cell suspension prior to staining.[73] This requirement makes flow cytometry especially useful for evaluating blood and marrow samples. In a well-equipped and appropriately staffed clinical laboratory, preliminary information often can be provided within 3 to 4 hours after the initial sample collection, thereby facilitating institution of appropriate therapy (e.g., in the case of newly diagnosed acute leukemias).

Four-color marker analysis has become the norm for most routine clinical laboratories, and five- or six-color analysis likely will be widely used in the next few years. For research purposes, simultaneous analysis of up to 14 or more markers is possible. Most markers are analyzed as cell surface proteins by directly adding conjugated antibodies to cell suspension, followed by washing and lysis of red cells.[73] However, assessment of intracytoplasmic and nuclear-associated proteins is fairly easy by first fixing cells in suspension and adding the relevant antibodies in conjunction with a membrane permeabilizing agent (usually a weak detergent added at low concentration). Commercial kits for cytoplasmic staining are readily available from a number of vendors. Fluorescence and light scatter data are stored electronically as list mode data files that can be archived on compact disk or digital video disk and later reanalyzed using appropriate software.

GATING STRATEGIES

In heterogeneous specimens such as marrow, in which the relevant clinical population (such as blasts) may be a minor population overall, a strategy for specifically identifying the population(s) of interest is necessary. So-called "cluster analysis," which involves examination of all data points using multicolor displays, or analysis that selects for specific populations based on light scatter features and/or expression of specific surface markers (a concept known as gating) can be used.[74] For samples with low cell viability, gating strategies based on light scatter and/or vital exclusion dyes such as 7-α-actinomycin-D to limit analysis to the viable cell population only may be used.[73]

Although light scatter alone may be sufficient for selecting the relevant cell population for analysis in homogeneous populations such as cell lines, tissue suspensions, and blood, a more powerful gating method for marrows involves CD45 (leukocyte common antigen) in conjunction with 90-degree (orthogonal) light scatter (see Color Plate VII-6). This strategy permits identification of blast and other populations that compose as little as 1 percent of all cell events analyzed. In most samples, lymphocytes, monocytes, myeloid progenitors, and blasts are easily separated by this method. However,

the major disadvantage is that one of the available fluorochrome channels is needed for the specific marker used in gating (usually CD45), thereby effectively limiting four-color methods to three-color evaluation.

Another advantage to CD45-based gating is the easier exclusion of populations such as monocytes that express high-affinity surface Fc receptors, which nonspecifically bind antibodies and may cause falsely-positive fluorescence signals. CD45-negative populations may indicate the presence of poorly differentiated metastatic tumors of nonhematopoietic origin. Nonhematopoietic or metastatic tumor cells in marrow samples may occasionally be more specifically characterized with epithelial-associated, fluorochrome-labeled antibodies such as anticytokeratin antibodies.

DETERMINING THE IMMUNOPHENOTYPE OF AN ABNORMAL POPULATION

Once an abnormal population is identified for analysis, its phenotypic profile can be characterized by simultaneous analysis of various cell surface markers, to determine cell lineage (lymphoid, B cell, T cell, myeloid, monocytic) and stage of differentiation. The determination can be achieved by examining lineage-specific markers or markers expressed only at specific stages of cell maturation. For instance, in marrow, immature cell populations can be identified by expression of antigens such as CD34 (an early progenitor marker) and terminal deoxynucleotidyl transferase. In some instances, the stage of differentiation can be determined using combinations of markers that are expressed only during certain phases of differentiation (e.g., dual expression of CD4 and CD8 in an immature T precursor population). This method also may allow identification of abnormal phenotypes not seen in normal samples, thereby providing indirect evidence of malignancy. For example, expression of the immature T cell marker CD1a in an otherwise mature T cell population or expression of human leukocyte antigen (HLA)-DR on myeloid cells that express later-appearing myeloid markers may be seen. HLA-DR is a class II major histocompatibility protein that is expressed in early myeloid progenitors but is lost by the promyelocyte stage of differentiation in normal samples.

In some samples, loss of expected light scatter features may provide clues to diagnosis. Loss of 90-degree light scatter in myeloid populations often correlates with the hypogranularity that can be seen in myelodysplasia. Increased forward-angle light scatter (an indicator of cell size) may be seen in some blast populations, large cell lymphomas, and metastatic tumors of nonhematopoietic origin.

OTHER COMMON FLOW CYTOMETRY APPLICATIONS

Clonality of immunoglobulin-expressing B cell malignancies involving marrow (e.g., chronic lymphocytic leukemia and lymphoplasmacytic lymphoma) can be assessed by simultaneous assessment of surface κ and λ immunoglobulin light-chain expression.[75] Cytoplasmic κ and λ assessment can be useful in establishing the clonality of plasma cell dyscrasias in marrow.

Flow cytometry is used to enumerate CD34+ progenitors when evaluating the adequacy of blood stem cell collections (see Chap. 25). Lymphocyte subset quantitation is diagnostically important in acquired and congenital immunodeficiency states. Diagnosis of paroxysmal nocturnal hemoglobinuria (PNH) by flow cytometry is accomplished by measuring expression of multiple glycophosphatidylinositol-linked proteins in different cell lineages, providing a more sensitive detection method than traditional *in vitro* assays. Most flow cytometry–based PNH assays are performed on blood and not marrow because of the requirement for concomitant comparison to a normal control sample.

REFERENCES

1. Arinkin M: Die intravital Untersuchungsmethodik des Knockenmarks. *Folia Haematol (Frankf)* 38:233, 1929, reproduced in Lichtman MA, Spivak JL, Boxer LA, et al: *Hematology: Landmark papers of the Twentieth Century.* English translation p 824. Academic Press, New York, 2000.
2. Custer RP, Ahlfeldt FE: Studies on the structure and function of bone marrow: II. Variations in cellularity in various bones with advancing years of life and their relative response to stimuli. *J Lab Clin Med* 17:960, 1932.
3. Bain BJ: Bone marrow trephine biopsy. *J Clin Pathol* 54:737, 2001.
4. Bain BJ: Bone marrow aspiration. *J Clin Pathol* 54:657, 2001.
5. Riley RS, Hogan TF, Pavot DR, et al: A pathologist's perspective on bone marrow aspiration and biopsy: I. Performing a bone marrow examination. *J Clin Lab Anal* 18:70, 2004.
6. Ellis LD, Jensen WN, Westerman MP: Needle biopsy of bone marrow: An experience with 1,445 biopsies. *Arch Intern Med* 114:213, 1964.
7. Sabharwal BD, Malhotra V, Aruna S, et al: Comparative evaluation of bone marrow aspirate particle smears, imprints, and biopsy sections. *J Postgrad Med* 36:194, 1990.
8. Bearden JD, Ratkin GA, Coltman CA: Comparison of the diagnostic value of bone marrow biopsy and bone marrow aspiration in neoplastic disease. *J Clin Pathol* 27:738, 1974.
9. Pasquale D, Chikkappa G: Comparative evaluation of bone marrow aspirate particle smears, biopsy imprints, and biopsy sections. *Am J Hematol* 22:381, 1986.
10. Kidd PG, Saminathan T, Drachtman RA, et al: Comparison of the cellularity and presence of residual leukemia in bone marrow aspirate and biopsy specimens in pediatric patients with acute lymphoblastic leukemia (ALL) at day 7-14 of chemotherapy. *Med Pediatr Oncol* 29:541, 1997.
11. Montserrat E, Villamor N, Reverter JC, et al: Bone marrow assessment in B-cell chronic lymphocytic leukaemia: Aspirate or biopsy? A comparative study in 258 patients. *Br J Haematol* 93:111, 1996.
12. Winfield DA, Polacarz SU: Bone marrow histology 3: Value of bone marrow core biopsies in acute leukemia, myelodysplastic syndromes, and chronic myeloid leukemia. *J Clin Pathol* 45:855, 1992.
13. Bartl R, Frisch B, Wilmanns W: Potential of bone marrow biopsy in chronic myeloproliferative disorders (MPD). *Eur J Haematol* 50:41, 1993.
14. Bain BJ: Bone marrow biopsy morbidity and mortality. *Br J Haematol* 121:949, 2003.
15. Dunlop TJ, Deen C, Lind S, et al: Use of combined oral narcotic and benzodiazepine for control of pain associated with bone marrow examination. *South Med J* 92:477, 1999.
16. Hertzog JH, Dalton HJ, Anderson BD, et al: Prospective evaluation of propofol anesthesia in the pediatric intensive care unit for elective oncology procedures in ambulatory and hospitalized children. *Pediatrics* 106:742, 2000.
17. Holdsworth MT, Raisch DW, Winter SS, et al: Pain and distress from bone marrow aspirations and lumbar punctures. *Ann Pharmacother* 37:17, 2003.
18. Reeves ST, Havidich JE, Tobin DP: Conscious sedation of children with propofol is anything but conscious. *Pediatrics* 114:E74, 2004.
19. Cannell H: Evidence for safety margins of lignocaine local anaesthetics for peri-oral use [review]. *Br Dent J* 181:243, 1996.
20. Jamshidi K, Swaim WR: Bone marrow biopsy with unaltered architecture: A new biopsy device. *J Lab Clin Med* 77:335, 1971.
21. Humphries J: Dry tap bone marrow aspiration: Clinical significance. *Am J Hematol* 247, 1990.
22. James L, Stass S, Schumacher H: Value of imprint preparation of bone marrow biopsies in hematologic diagnosis. *Cancer* 46:173, 1980.
23. Dewald G, Allen JE, Strutzenberg DK: A cytogenetic method for mailed in bone marrow specimens for the study of hematologic disorders. *Lab Med* 13:225, 1982.
24. Breit S, Nees M, Schaefer U, et al: Impact of pre-analytical handling on bone marrow mRNA gene expression. *Br J Haematol* 126:231, 2004.
25. Wickham CL, Boyce M, Joyner MV, et al: Amplification of PCR products in excess of 600 base pairs using DNA extracted from decalcified, paraffin wax embedded bone marrow trephine biopsies. *Mol Pathol* 53:19, 2000.
26. Bock O, Lehmann U, Kreipe H: Quantitative intra-individual monitoring of BCR-ABL transcript levels in archival bone marrow trephines of patients with chronic myeloid leukemia. *J Mol Diagn* 5:54, 2003.
27. Akoury DA, Seo JJ, James CD, et al: RT-PCR detection of mRNA recovered from archival glass slide smears. *Mod Pathol* 6:195, 1993.
28. Lillie RD, Fullmer HM: *Histopathologic Technic and Practical Histochemistry.* McGraw-Hill, New York, 1976.
29. Hyun BH, Stevenson AJ, Hanau CA: Fundamentals of bone marrow examination. *Hematol Oncol Clin North Am* 8:651, 1994.
30. Moosavi H, Lichtman MA, Donnelly JA, et al: Plastic-embedded human marrow biopsy specimens: Improved histochemical methods. *Arch Pathol Lab Med* 105:269, 1981.
31. Blythe D, Hand NM, Jackson P, et al: Use of methyl methacrylate resin for embedding bone marrow trephine biopsy specimens. *J Clin Pathol* 50:45, 1997.
32. Brown DC, Gatter KC: The bone marrow trephine biopsy. A review of normal histology. *Histopathology* 22:411, 1992.
33. Wang J, Weiss LM, Chang KL, et al: Diagnostic utility of bilateral bone marrow examination: Significance of morphologic and ancillary technique study in malignant. *Cancer* 94:1522, 2002.
34. Cheson BD, Horning SJ, Coiffier B, et al: Report of an international workshop to standardize response criteria for non-Hodgkin's lymphomas. NCI Sponsored International Working Group. *J Clin Oncol* 17:1244, 1999.
35. Campbell JK, Matthews JP, Seymour JF, et al: Optimum trephine length in the assessment of bone marrow involvement in patients with diffuse large cell lymphoma. *Ann Oncol* 14:273, 2003.
36. Holdrinet RSG, Egmond J, Wessels JMC, et al: A method for quantification of peripheral blood admixture in bone marrow aspirates. *Exp Hematol* 8:103, 1980.
37. Ozkaynak MF, Scribano P, Gomperts E, et al: Comparative evaluation of the bone marrow by the volumetric method, particle smears, and biopsies in pediatric disorders. *Am J Hematol* 29:144, 1988.
38. Gruppo RA, Lampkin BC, Granger S: Bone marrow cellularity determination: Comparison of the biopsy, aspirate, and buffy coat. *Blood* 49:29, 1977.
39. Hartsock RJ, Smith EB, Petty CS: Normal variations with aging of the amount of hemopoietic tissue in bone marrow from the anterior iliac crest. *Am J Clin Pathol* 43:326, 1965.
40. Tuzuner N, Cox C, Rowe JM, et al: Bone marrow cellularity in myeloid stem cell disorders: Impact of age correction. *Leuk Res* 18:559, 1994.
41. Wilkins BS: Histology of normal haemopoiesis: Bone marrow histology I. *J Clin Pathol* 45:645, 1992.
42. Abrahamsen JF, Lund-Johansen F, Laerum OD, et al: Flow cytometric assessment of peripheral blood contamination and proliferative activity of human bone marrow cell populations. *Cytometry* 19:77, 1995.
43. Batinic D, Marusic M, Pavletic Z, et al: Relationship between differing volumes of bone marrow aspirates and their cellular composition. *Bone Marrow Transplant* 6:103, 1990.
44. Mori Y, Mizukami T, Hamaguchi Y, et al: Automation of bone marrow aspirate examination using the XE-2100 automated hematology analyzer. *Cytometry* 58B:25, 2004.
45. Bain BJ: The bone marrow aspirate of healthy subjects. *Br J Haematol* 94:206, 1996.

46. Atac B, Lawrence C, Goldberg S: Metastatic tumor: The complementary role of the marrow aspirate and biopsy. *Am J Med Sci* 302:211, 1991.

47. Braun S, Pantel K, Muller P, et al: Cytokeratin-positive cells in the bone marrow and survival of patients with stage I, II, or III breast cancer. *N Engl J Med* 342:525, 2000.

48. Schmidt-Kittler O, Ragg T, Daskalakis A, et al: From latent disseminated cells to overt metastasis: Genetic analysis of systemic breast cancer progression. *Proc Natl Acad Sci U S A* 100:7737, 2003.

49. Terpstra W, Lokhorst H, Blomjous F: Comparison of plasma cell infiltration in bone marrow biopsies and aspirates in patients with multiple myeloma. *Br J Haematol* 82:46, 1992.

50. Navone R, Valpreda M, Pich A: Lymphoid nodules and nodular lymphoid hyperplasia in bone marrow biopsies. *Acta Haematol* 74:19, 1985.

51. Erber WN, Asbahr HD, Phelps PN: In situ hybridization of immunoglobulin light chain mRNA on bone marrow trephines using biotinylated probes and the APAAP method. *Pathology* 25:63, 1993.

52. Kang YH, Park CJ, Seo EJ, et al: Polymerase chain reaction-based diagnosis of bone marrow involvement in 170 cases of non-Hodgkin lymphoma. *Cancer* 94:3073, 2002.

53. Chang KL, Gaal KK, Huang Q, et al: Histiocytic lesions involving the bone marrow. *Semin Diagn Pathol* 20:226, 2003.

54. Anastasi J, Musvee T, Roulston D, et al: Pseudo-Gaucher histiocytes identified up to 1 year after transplantation for CML are BCR/ABL-positive. *Leukemia* 12:233, 1998.

55. Magill AJ, Grogl M, Gasser RA Jr, et al: Visceral infection caused by Leishmania tropica in veterans of Operation Desert Storm. *N Engl J Med* 328:1383, 1993.

56. Brouland JP, Audouin J, Hofman P, et al: Bone marrow involvement by disseminated toxoplasmosis in acquired immunodeficiency syndrome: The value of bone marrow trephine biopsy and immunohistochemistry for the diagnosis. *Hum Pathol* 27:302, 1996.

57. Hussong J, Peterson LR, Warren JR, et al: Detecting disseminated Mycobacterium avium complex infections in HIV-positive patients. The usefulness of bone marrow trephine biopsy specimens, aspirate cultures, and blood cultures. *Am J Clin Pathol* 110:806, 1998.

58. Agostoni C, Dorigoni N, Malfitano A, et al: Mediterranean leishmaniasis in HIV-infected patients: Epidemiological, clinical, and diagnostic features of 22 cases. *Infection* 26:93, 1998.

59. Neubauer MA, Bodensteiner DC: Disseminated histoplasmosis in patients with AIDS. *South Med J* 85:1166, 1992.

60. Mourad O, Palda V, Detsky AS: A comprehensive evidence-based approach to fever of unknown origin. *Arch Intern Med* 163:545, 2003.

61. Eid A, Carion W, Nystrom JS: Differential diagnoses of bone marrow granuloma. *West J Med* 164:510, 1996.

62. Norgard MJ, Carpenter JTJ, Conrad ME. Bone marrow necrosis and degeneration. *Arch Intern Med* 139:905, 1979.

63. Seaman JP, Kjeldsberg CR, Linker A: Gelatinous transformation of the bone marrow. *Hum Pathol* 9:685, 1978.

64. Tavassoli M, Eastlund DT, Yam LT, et al: Gelatinous transformation of bone marrow in prolonged self-induced starvation. *Scand J Haematol* 16:311, 1976.

65. Rosse C, Krauner MJ, Dillon TL, et al: Bone marrow cell populations of normal infants: The predominance of lymphocytes. *J Lab Clin Med* 89:1225, 1977.

66. Dresch C, Faille A, Poirier O, et al: The cellular composition of the granulocyte series in the normal human bone marrow according to the volume of the sample. *J Clin Pathol* 27:106, 1974.

67. Janka G, Imashuku S, Elinder G, et al: Infection- and malignancy-associated hemophagocytic syndromes. Secondary hemophagocytic lymphohistiocytosis. *Hematol Oncol Clin North Am* 12:435, 1998.

68. DePalma L: The effect of decalcification and choice of fixative on histiocytic iron in bone marrow core biopsies. *Biotech Histochem* 71:57, 1996.

69. Pritchard-Jones K, Toogood IR, Rice MS: The significance of an M2 bone marrow at cessation of chemotherapy in childhood acute lymphoblastic leukemia. *Am J Pediatr Hematol Oncol* 10:292, 1988.

70. Longacre TA, Foucar K, Crago S, et al: Hematogones: A multiparameter analysis of bone marrow precursor cells. *Blood* 73:543, 1989.

71. Jaffe ES, Harris NL, Stein H, et al: *World Health Organization Classification of Tumours: Pathology and Genetics: Tumours of Haematopoietic and Lymphoid Tissues.* IARC Press, Lyon, 2001.

72. Zola H, Swart B, Boumsell L, et al: Human leucocyte differentiation antigen nomenclature: Update on CD nomenclature. Report of IUIS/WHO Subcommittee. *J Immunol Methods* 275:1, 2003.

73. Stelzer GT, Marti G, Hurley A, et al: U.S.-Canadian Consensus recommendations on the immunophenotypic analysis of hematologic neoplasia by flow cytometry: Standardization and validation of laboratory procedures. *Cytometry* 30:214, 1997.

74. Kerin DF, McCoy JP Jr, Carey JL: *Flow Cytometry in Clinical Diagnosis.* ASCP Press, Chicago, 2001.

75. Kawano-Yamamoto C, Muroi K, Izumi T, et al: Two-color flow cytometry with a CD19 gate for the evaluation of bone marrow involvement of B-cell lymphoma. *Leuk Lymphoma* 43:2133, 2002.

76. Glaser K, Limarzi LR, Poncher G: Cellular composition of the bone marrow in normal infants and children. *Pediatrics* 6:789, 1950.

PART II

GENERAL HEMATOLOGY

STRUCTURE OF THE MARROW AND THE HEMATOPOIETIC MICROENVIRONMENT

CAMILLE N. ABBOUD

MARSHALL A. LICHTMAN

The marrow, located in the medullary cavity of bone, is the sole site of effective hematopoiesis in humans. The marrow produces approximately six billion cells per kilogram of body weight per day. Hematopoietically active (red) marrow regresses after birth until late adolescence, after which it is focused in the lower skull, vertebrae, shoulder and pelvic girdles, ribs, and sternum. Fat cells replace hematopoietic cells in the bones of the hands, feet, legs, and arms (yellow marrow). Fat occupies approximately 50 percent of the space of red marrow in the adult. Further fatty metamorphosis continues slowly with aging. In very old individuals, a gelatinous transformation of fat to a mucoid material may occur (white marrow). Yellow marrow can revert to hematopoietically active marrow if prolonged demand is present, as in chronic hemolytic anemia. Thus, hematopoiesis can be expanded by increasing the volume of red marrow and decreasing the development (transit) time from progenitor to mature cell.

The marrow stroma consists principally of a network of sinuses that originate at the endosteum from cortical capillaries and terminate in collecting vessels that enter the systemic venous circulation. The trilaminar sinus wall is composed of endothelial cells; an underdeveloped, thin basement membrane; and adventitial reticular cells that are fibroblasts capable of transforming into adipocytes. The endothelium and reticular cells are sources of hematopoietic cytokines. Hematopoiesis occurs in the intersinus spaces and is controlled by a complex array of stimulatory and inhibitory cytokines, cell–cell contacts, and the effects of extracellular matrix components on proximate cells. In this unique environment, lymphohematopoietic stem cells differentiate into all the blood cell lineages. Mature cells are produced and released to maintain steady-state blood cell levels. The system also can respond to meet increased demands for additional cells as a result of blood loss, hemolysis, inflammation, immune cytopenias, and other causes. Stem cells can leave and reenter marrow as part of their normal circulation. Their extramedullary circulation can be increased by exogenous cytokines and chemokines.

The evolutionary factors that led to confinement of hematopoiesis to the medullary cavity of bone are not fully understood. Two relationships that may underlie this requirement for proximity are the biochemical and receptor contributions of osteoblasts to hematopoiesis and the homing of hematopoietic stem cells to endosteum.

HISTORY AND GENERAL CONSIDERATIONS

The marrow, one of the largest organs in the human body, is the principal site for blood cell formation. In the normal adult, daily marrow production amounts to approximately 2.5 billion red cells, 2.5 billion platelets, and 1.0 billion granulocytes per kilogram of body weight. The rate of production adjusts to actual needs and can vary from nearly zero to many times normal.[1] Until the late 19th century, blood cell formation was thought to be the prerogative of the lymph nodes or the liver and spleen. In 1868, Neuman[2] and Bizzozero[3] independently observed nucleated blood cells in material squeezed from the ribs of human cadavers and proposed that the marrow is the major source of blood cells.[4] The first in vivo marrow biopsy probably was done in 1876 by Mosler,[5] who used a regular wood drill to obtain marrow particles from a patient with leukemia. Fifty years later, studies by Arinkin[6] in 1929 established marrow aspiration as a safe, easy, and useful technique.

Kinetic studies of marrow cells, using radioisotopes and in vitro cultures, have shown that cell lines consist of mature end cells with a finite functional life span. The cells are capable of limited proliferation before they reach full maturation but do not have the capacity for self-renewal. On the other hand, sustained cellular production depends on the presence of pools of primordial cells capable of both differentiation and self-replication.[7] The most primitive pool consists of pluripotential stem cells with the capacity for continuous self-renewal. The more mature pools consist of differentiated unipotential progenitor cells, with their maturation restricted to single cell lines and no capacity for self-renewal. The proliferative activity of these pools involves humoral feedback from peripheral target tissues[8] and cell–cell and cell–matrix interactions within the microenvironment of the marrow.[9] The marrow stroma has evolved to provide a unique structural and chemical environment (niches) to support the survival, differentiation, and proliferation of pluripotential lymphohematopoietic stem cells. Primitive hematopoietic stem cell interactive niches[10] have been identified at the structural and molecular[11] levels and are dynamically controlled by bone morphogenetic protein[12] and factors regulating intramedullary osteoblastic cells.[13] Early stem cells can be identified and isolated using a unique array of surface antigen-receptor expressions (CD34+/−, Thy-1lo, c-kit+, CD38−, CD33−, vascular endothelial [VE]-cadherin+, KDR/FLK1+, FLK2−/FLT3−, CD133+/−)[14–19] and have a unique molecular signature.[20,21] Isolated cell populations enriched in stem cells can be quantified using in vitro long-term progenitor assays[22–25] and surrogate in vivo repopulating assays in severely immunodeficient mice and xenogeneic animal models[26–28] (see Chap. 15).

Acronyms and abbreviations that appear in this chapter include: AGM, aorta-gonad-mesonephros; bFGF, basic fibroblast growth factor; BMP, bone morphogenetic protein; CFU-E, colony forming unit–erythroid; CFU-S, colony forming unit-spleen; ECM, extracellular matrix protein; ELAM, endothelial leukocyte adhesion molecule; GAG, glycosaminoglycan; G-CSF, granulocyte colony stimulating factor; G-CSF-R, granulocyte colony stimulating factor receptor; GM-CSF, granulocyte-macrophage colony stimulating factor; HCA, hematopoietic cell antigen; HCAM, homing cell adhesion molecule; HGF, hepatocyte growth factor; HLA, human leukocyte antigen; HPP-CFC, high proliferative potential–colony forming cell; IAP, integrin-associated protein; ICAM, intercellular adhesion molecule; IIICS, type III connecting segment; IL, interleukin; LIF, leukemia inhibitory factor; M-CSF, macrophage colony stimulating factor; MIP, macrophage inflammatory protein; MMP, matrix metalloproteinase; NF-κB, nuclear factor κB; NFAT, nuclear factor of activated T cells; NK, natural killer; ODF, osteoclast differentiation and activation factor; OPG, osteoprotegrin; PCLP, podocalyxin; PDGF, platelet-derived growth factor; PRR2, poliovirus receptor-related–2 protein; PSGL, P-selectin glycoprotein ligand; RANTES, regulated on activation, normal T cell expressed, presumed secreted; SDF, stromal cell-derived factor; SHP-1, Src homology 2 domain-bearing protein tyrosine phosphatase-1; SP, side population; TGF-β, transforming growth factor beta; TPO, thrombopoietin; TSP, thrombospondin; VAP, vascular adhesion protein; VCAM, vascular cell adhesion molecule; VEGF, vascular endothelial growth factor; VLA, very late antigen.

SITES OF HEMATOPOIESIS

EMBRYOGENESIS AND EARLY STEM CELL DEVELOPMENT

Dominant anatomical sites of hematopoiesis change during ontogeny. The yolk sac and later the fetal liver are sites of early erythropoiesis and contain cells with multilineage differentiation capabilities beginning at day 8 of gestation (yolk sac)[29] (Fig. 4-1). Non–yolk sac regions such as the paraaortic splanchnopleura give rise to B cell progenitors when transplanted into mice with severe combined immunodeficiency.[30] Pluripotential hematopoietic stem cells are generated in the intrabody portion of the mouse embryo, the aorta-gonad-mesonephros (AGM) region, and sublocalize to the dorsal aorta.[31,32] Stem cells in the AGM region appear before the fetal liver, indicating the importance of this mesodermal region of the embryo in stem cell migration.[33] Early lymphoid precursors have been identified in the day 8 yolk sac[34] and the body of embryos beginning at the 10- to 12-somite stage.[35] The earliest repopulating lymphohematopoietic stem cells in the day 9 yolk sac have been detected *in vivo* using primary conditioned newborn mice[36] and *in vitro* using high proliferative potential–colony forming cell (HPP-CFC) assays[37] (see Chap. 6).

The early inductive microenvironment for pluripotential stem cells elaborates kit ligand, encoded by the Sl locus. A later transition from early independent to the late kit ligand-dependent fetal hematopoiesis in the embryo occurs.[38] Similarly, kit-negative stem cells give rise to kit-positive cells with pluripotential stem cell activity.[39] Murine embryonic stem cells require multiple growth factors such as leukemia inhibitory factor (LIF), kit ligand, and basic fibroblast growth factor (bFGF) acting in concert.[40,41] Direct interactions and soluble growth factors from AGM and urogenital ridge stromal[42] or endothelial cells[43] and marrow-derived stromal cells improve the survival of primitive hematopoiesis.[44] This action is exerted via intimate cell–cell interactions of CD34-positive stem cells, which are human leukocyte antigen (HLA)-DR negative and uncommitted, with adventitial reticular cells.[44] Transcription factor (Runx1, TEL/ETV6) expression governs hematopoietic stem cell, endothelial cell, and mesenchymal cell development in the embryo, yolk sac, and marrow.[45–49] Uniquely expressed surface receptors Delta-like (DLK) preadipocyte factor-1,[50–52] Notch ligands (Delta-1, Jagged-1),[53] signaling molecules WNT,[54] Hedgehog,[31,55] stromal-derived growth factors (BMPs, granulocyte colony stimulating factor [G-CSF], LIF, stem cell factor, thrombopoietin [TPO]),[56] and chemokines such as stromal cell-derived factor (SDF)-1[57] explain differences in stem cell supportive functions of these stromal/endothelial cells[58] of early blood islands and those of marrow or spleen.[59]

Morphologic studies of marrow recovering from aplasia show that early hematopoiesis is localized to the endosteum and vascular endothelium.[60] The intimate relationship of angiogenesis and early hematopoiesis is validated by the demonstration that AGM-derived single cells at day 10.5 post coitum express the receptor tyrosine kinase TEK and give rise to hematopoietic cells in the presence of interleukin (IL)-3 and endothelial cells when exposed to angiopoietin-1, defining them as hemangioblasts.[61] Podocalyxin-1 (PCLP1), a highly glycosylated protein with similarity to CD34, a high-endothelial venule ligand for L-selectin, has been found on AGM-derived hemangioblasts.[62] These PCLP1-positive, CD45-negative cells give rise to hematopoietic cells and endothelial cells when cultured over stromal cells.[62] Expression of α_4-integrin in CD45-negative VE-cadherin–positive or VE-cadherin–negative cells defines the earliest precursor of hematopoietic cell lineage diverged from endothelial cells.[63,64]

STEM CELL AND MESENCHYMAL CELL PLASTICITY

Primitive stem cells obtained from human fetal liver or marrow reconstitute all lymphohematopoietic-derived cells and part of the stromal microenvironment in *in vivo* repopulation assays.[65] These observations are consistent with the early derivation of hematopoietic, vascular, and stromal cells from a CD34-negative, vascular endothelial cell growth factor-2 receptor (known as *KDR*)-positive, multipotential mesenchymal stem cell.[15–17,28] Identification of AC133-positive, CD34-negative, CD7-negative hematopoietic stem cells[66] and demonstration of endothelial precursors in AC133-positive progenitor cells[67] underscore the crosstalk between hematopoiesis and angiogenesis signaling pathways and establish the functional role of hemangioblasts in ontogeny.[68–71] As early fetal hematopoiesis is established, the yolk sac vascular networks remain active sites of progenitor production and hematopoiesis.[72] Long-term reconstituting hematopoietic stem cells express two members of the ATP-binding cassette genes (ABCG-2 and P-glycoprotein), allowing the efflux of mitochondrial vital dyes such as Hoescht 33342 and rhodamine 123 and their isolation by multiparameter flow cytometry based on their low side scatter (side population [SP] cells).[73–76]

Early hematopoietic stem cells have been found in skeletal tissue[77] and in brain-derived neural cells,[78] indicating the widespread tissue distribution of these totipotential cells. Heterogeneity in SP and non-SP marrow-derived progenitor cells within muscle shows SP cells are incorporated into endothelial structure during vasculogenesis whereas non-SP cells differentiate into smooth muscle.[79] These findings confirm the intimate overlap of hematopoietic stem cells and hemangioblast activity[70] while showing that resident marrow-derived stem mesenchymal cell progenitors can differentiate into nonhematopoietic tissue cell types.[79] The plasticity of mesenchymal cells is accepted and is evident in several tissues (bone, muscle, brain, cardiac, hepatic, smooth muscle) when repair homeostatic mechanisms are triggered following acute injury.[80–86] Derivation of hematopoietic cells from adult tissue (muscle, liver) has been attributed to resident marrow-derived stem cells in these tissues.[87,88] Tissue (muscle, neural, hepatic) committed stem cells have been detected in CD34+, AC133+, CXCR4-positive marrow cell populations, providing an explanation for the cells' ability to be mobilized after growth factor administration and to participate in distal organ regeneration.[89] The exact contribution of marrow-derived stem cells to this process is debatable in some cases showing localized cell–cell fusion versus true stem cell transdifferentiation (open chromatin hypothesis)[90–96] (see Chap. 15).

HISTOGENESIS

Cavities within bone occur in the human being at about the fifth fetal month and soon become the exclusive site for granulocytic and megakaryocytic proliferation. Erythropoietic activity at the time is

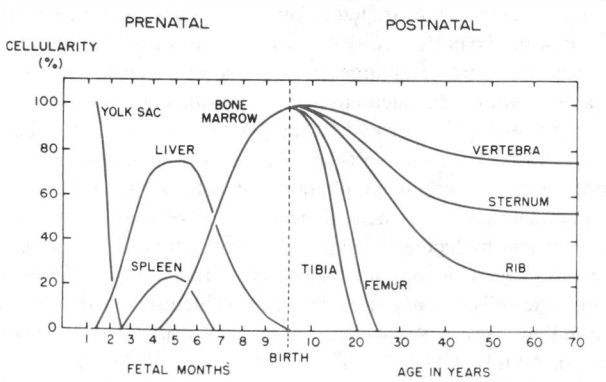

FIGURE 4-1   Expansion and recession of hematopoietic activity in extramedullary and medullary sites. For details regarding the nature of yolk sac and hepatic hematopoiesis, see "Sites of Hematopoiesis: Embryogenesis and Early Stem Cell Development." Chapter 6 provides a more comprehensive treatment of this topic (see Fig. 6-1).

confined to the liver. The microenvironment in the marrow becomes supportive of erythroblasts only toward the end of the last trimester (see Fig. 4-1). At birth, the bone cavities are the only sites of significant hematopoietic activity and are completely engorged with hematopoietic cells.[97] The sequential appearance and disappearance of hematopoietic activity is governed by signaling via chemokine receptors (CXCR4) for SDF-1[98,99] and cellular adhesion molecule–ligand pair interactions, such as α_4-integrin with vascular cell adhesion molecule-1 (VCAM-1) or α_4-integrin with fibronectin.[100,101]

By the fourth year of life, a significant number of fat cells have appeared in the diaphysis of the human long bones.[102] These cells slowly replace hematopoietic elements and expand centripetally until, at approximately age 18 years, hematopoietic marrow is found only in the vertebrae, ribs, skull, pelvis, and proximal epiphyses of the femora and humeri. Direct measurements of the volume of bone cavities reveal bone cavity volume increases from 1.4 percent of body weight at birth to 4.8 percent in the adult,[102] whereas blood volume decreases from 8 percent of body weight in the newborn to approximately 7 percent in the adult.[103] Expansion of marrow space continues throughout life, resulting in a further gradual increase in the amount of fatty tissue in all bone cavities, especially in the long bones.[104,105] The preference of hematopoietic tissue for centrally located bones has been ascribed to higher central tissue temperature with greater vascularity.[106] However, because complete reactivation of fatty marrow can occur in experimental animals in which hematopoietic expansion is induced, other factors (cytokines, hormonal signals) must be involved.[107–110]

MARROW STRUCTURE

VASCULATURE

The blood supply to the marrow comes from two major sources. The nutrient artery, the principal source, penetrates the cortex through the nutrient canal. In the marrow cavity, the nutrient artery bifurcates into ascending and descending medullary arteries from which radial branches travel to the inner face of the cortex. After repenetrating the endosteum, the radial vessels diminish in caliber to structures of capillary size that course within the canalicular system of the cortex. Here arterial blood from the nutrient artery mixes with blood that enters the cortical capillary system from the periosteal capillaries derived from muscular arteries.[111] After reentering the marrow cavity, the cortical capillaries form a sinusoidal network (Fig. 4-2). Hematopoietic cells are located in the intersinusoidal tissue spaces. Some arteries have specialized, thin-walled segments that arise abruptly as continuations of arteries with walls of normal thickness.[112] These vessels give off nearly perpendicular branches analogous to the arterial branching observed in the spleen and kidney, permitting volume compensation for changes in intramedullary pressure. In the marrow cavity, blood flows through a highly branching network of medullary sinuses. These sinuses collect into a large central sinus from which the blood enters the systemic venous circulation through emissary veins.

Vascular networks consisting of cells expressing CD31, CD34, and CD105 (endoglin) but lacking intercellular adhesion molecule (ICAM)-1, ICAM-2, ICAM-3, or endothelial leukocyte adhesion molecule (ELAM)-1 (E-selectin) can form within the stroma of long-term marrow cultures. These findings underscore the intimate relationship of blood vessels to hematopoietic activity.[113] A study of early hematopoiesis of human marrow from long bones (ages 6–28 weeks) has shown an absence of CD34-positive hematopoietic progenitors before onset of hematopoiesis, a predominance of CD68-positive cells mediating chondrolysis, and CD34-positive endothelial cells developing into specific vascular structures organized by endothelial cells and myoid cells.[114] Vascular endothelial growth factor (VEGF) receptors

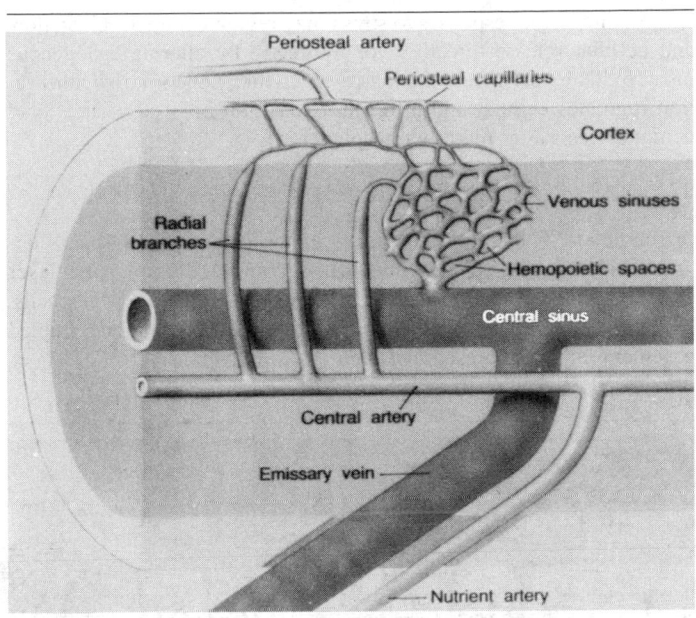

FIGURE 4-2   Schematic diagram of the marrow circulation (see "Marrow Structure" for further explanation).

found on CD34-positive cells[17] and AGM primitive stem cells underscore the common ontogeny.[115,116] Subsets of CD34-positive cells expressing the AC133 antigen and the human VEGF receptor-2 define the functional endothelial precursor phenotype.[117] Endothelial progenitors residing in the CD34+, CD11b+ subsets are capable of producing and binding angiopoietins,[118] and fibronectin enhances VEGF-induced CD34 cell differentiation into endothelial cells.[119]

INNERVATION

Myelinated and nonmyelinated nerve fibers are present in periarterial sheaths in marrow,[120] where they are believed to regulate arterial vessel tone. Nerve terminals are distributed between layers of periarterial adventitial cells or localize next to arterial smooth muscle cells.[121] Nonmyelinated fibers terminate in the hematopoietic spaces, implying that neurohumors elaborated from free-nerve terminals affect hematopoiesis. Intimate cell–cell communication between sympathetic nerve cells and structural elements within the marrow sinuses occurs at less than 5 percent of nerve terminals that terminate within the hematopoietic parenchyma or on sinus walls. This anatomical unit, termed a *neuroreticular complex*, consists of efferent (autonomic) nerves and marrow stromal cells connected by gap junctions.[121] The marrow is supplied by sensory and autonomic innovation seen by glyoxylic acid-induced fluorescence histochemistry of catecholaminergic nerve fibers and nerve fibers exhibiting cholinacetyltransferase immunoreactivity.[122] Bone also is highly innervated, as shown by the localization of substance P and neurokinin-1 receptors.[123] Osteoblasts and osteoclasts express glutamate receptors and transporters, as underscored by the bone loss induced by sciatic neurectomy resulting in decreased glutaminergic innervation.[124]

Nerve growth factor receptor antibody reacts with adventitial reticular cells.[125] Tachykinins have demonstrated stimulatory and inhibitory hematopoietic activities within the marrow microenvironment.[126] Substance P stimulates primitive hematopoietic progenitors[127] and CD34-positive cell proliferation by modulating stromal cell release of stem cell factor and cytokines such as IL-1,[126] IL-3, IL-6, G-CSF, granulocyte-macrophage colony stimulating factor (GM-CSF), and kit ligand.[128] Neurokinin-1 receptors for substance P are present on marrow vascular endothelium[129] and regulate blood flow and angiogenesis.[130] Adrenergic responses to stress may regulate marrow blood flow and cellular release directly[131] or indirectly by altering endogenous nitric oxide levels within the marrow.[132] Thus, bone marrow innervation regulates cellular and progenitor retention in steady state[133] and hematopoiesis after marrow transplantation.[134]

SINUS ARCHITECTURE AND CELLULAR ORGANIZATION

In mammals, hematopoiesis occurs in the extravascular spaces between marrow sinuses. The sinus wall is composed of a luminal layer of endothelial cells and an abluminal coat of adventitial reticular cells, which forms an incomplete outer lining (Fig. 4-3). A thin, interrupted basement lamina is present between the cell layers.

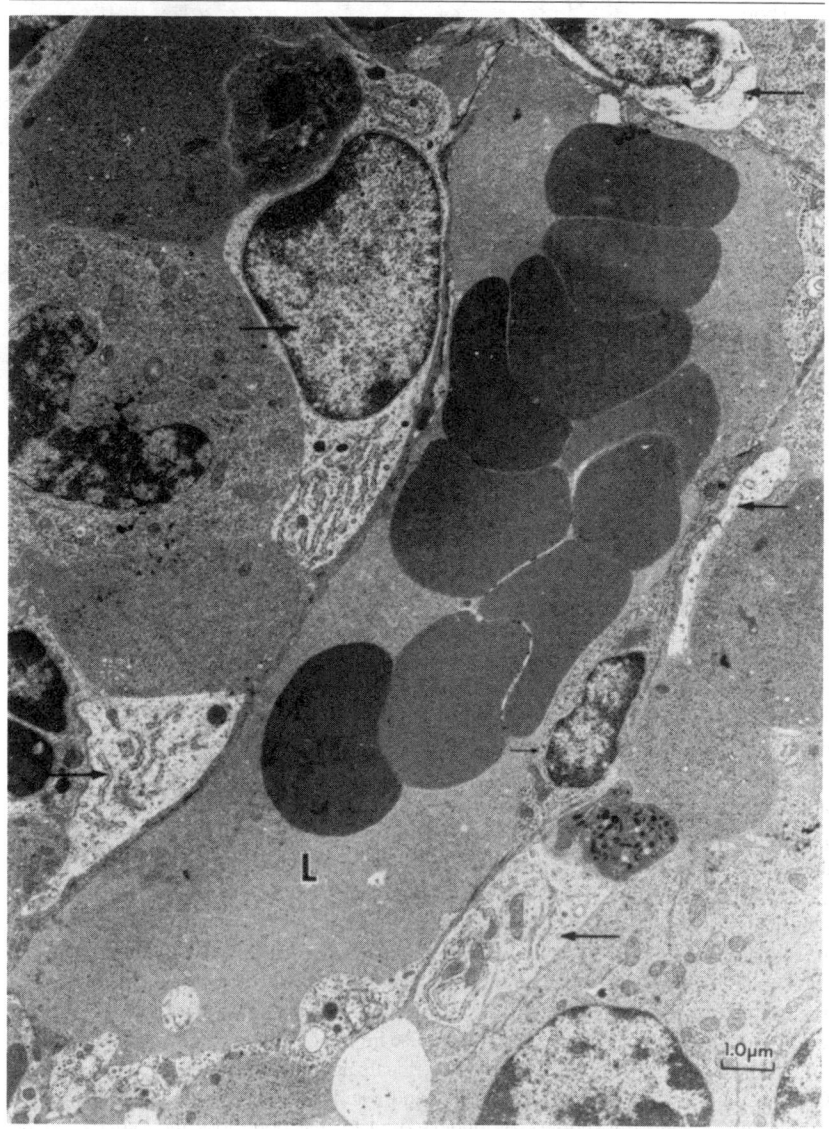

FIGURE 4-3   Transmission electron micrograph of a mouse marrow sinus. The *small arrow* in the sinus lumen (L) indicates the perikaryon of an endothelial cell. Several endothelial cell junctions are present along the circumference of the sinus endothelial wall. Thus, the wall is composed of the cytoplasm of endothelial cells that overlap or interdigitate. Two adventitial reticular cells are identified by *arrows* at the top and upper left of the sinus. The cytoplasm of the adventitial reticular cells is discontinuous as it is followed around the sinus. Four cytoplasmic processes of adventitial reticular cells are indicated by *arrows*. Other, smaller processes of reticular cell cytoplasm are found upon close inspection of the sinus periphery and the hematopoietic spaces. The scattered rough endoplasmic reticulum and dense bodies are characteristic of the reticular cell cytoplasm. (From Lichtman,[120] with permission.)

ENDOTHELIAL CELLS

Endothelial cells are broad flat cells that completely cover the inner surface of the sinus.[135] They form the major barrier and control the system for chemicals and particles entering and leaving the hematopoietic spaces, with overlapping or interdigitating unions permitting volume expansion.[136] The endothelium of marrow sinusoids is actively endocytic and contains clathrin-coated pits, clathrin-coated vesicles, lysosomes, phagosomes, transfer tubules, and diaphragmed fenestrae.[137,138] Particles are endocytosed by endothelial cells primarily through clathrin-coated pits.[139] Such endocytic features are in accordance with studies demonstrating colony stimulating factor receptors on endothelial cells[140] and their shared antigenic determinants with macrophages.[141,142] Marrow endothelial cells express von Willebrand factor antigen,[143] type IV collagen, and laminin.[144] They also constitutively express adhesion molecules: ICAM3,[145] VCAM-1, and E-selectin.[146] The distribution of sialic acid and other carbohydrates on the luminal surface of marrow sinus endothelium is discontinued at diaphragmed fenestrae and coated pits, suggesting such sugars play a role in endothelial membrane function and cellular interactions.[139] Marrow microvascular endothelium can be isolated using *Ulex europaeus* lectin[147] and CD34 monoclonal antibodies.[148]

Marrow endothelial cells via direct cell–cell contacts and secreted peptides uniquely influence osteoprogenitor cell differentiation[149,150] and regulate hematopoiesis by elaborating cytokines such as IL-5,[151] negative regulators thymosin β4, AsSDKP,[152] and transforming growth factor beta (TGF-β) antagonists such as B-type natriuretic peptide.[153] Reciprocal regulation of CD34 expression and adhesion molecules by vascular endothelial cells exposed to inflammatory stimuli such as IL-1, interferon-γ, and tumor necrosis factor alpha (TNF-α) is observed.[154] Receptors for the complement component C1q are up-regulated on marrow microvascular endothelium by inflammatory cytokines.[155] Endothelial cells regulate cellular trafficking into and out of the marrow sinusoidal spaces by altering their permeability and reorganizing their cytoskeleton by ICAM-3, by VE-cadherin mediated cell–cell contacts,[145,156] and via specialized heparin sulfate proteoglycans,[157] SDF-1 bound to surface proteoglycans,[158] and chemokines/chemokine receptors[159,160] such as fractalkine, a membrane-bound chemokine with a mucin stalk expressed in activated vascular beds.[161] Marrow sinusoidal endothelium specifically expresses sialylated CD22 ligands, which are homing receptors for recirculating B lymphocytes.[162]

ADVENTITIAL RETICULAR CELLS

The abluminal or adventitial surface of the vascular sinus is composed of reticular cells.[135,163,164] The reticular cell bodies are contiguous with the sinus, forming part of its adventitial coat (see Fig. 4-3). Their extensive branching cytoplasmic processes envelop the outer wall of the sinus to form an adventitial sheath. The sheath is interrupted and is estimated to cover approximately two thirds of the abluminal surface area of sinuses. The reticular cells synthesize reticular (argentophilic) fibers that, with their cytoplasmic processes, extend into the hematopoietic compartments and form a meshwork on which hematopoietic cells rest (Figs. 4-4 and 4-5). The cell bodies, their broad processes, and their fibers constitute the reticulum of the marrow.

Adventitial reticular cells have a high concentration of alkaline phosphatase in their membranes, express CD10, CD13, and class I HLA antigens,[135] react with the 6/19 and STRO-1 monoclonal antibodies,[165,166] and express all neurotrophin receptors including the low-affinity nerve growth factor receptor (p75LNGFR) and the Trk receptors (TrkA, TrkB, and TrkC),[167] even though nerve growth factor is not a growth factor for STRO-1–derived stromal cells.[168] These adventitial reticular cells can differentiate along the smooth muscle pathway and contain α smooth muscle actin, vimentin, laminin, fibronectin, and collagens I, III, and IV.[169,170] Unlike embryonic fibroblasts,[171] adventitial reticular cells usually are CD34-negative.[136,169,172] Stromal cells display cell–cell contacts via connexin-43 gap junctions, which are critical for normal hematopoiesis.[173,174] These gap junctions are localized to areas of adherence of stromal cells and hematopoietic cells in marrow recovering from cytotoxic injury.[175] The importance of direct cell–cell communication between progenitors and stromal cells remains unclear, because the hematopoietic capacity of connexin-43 wild-type and knockout fetal liver cells does not differ on wild-type stroma.[176] Marrow-derived stromal cell lines display heterogeneity at the molecular level (expression of cytokines such as kit ligand, TPO, and flt3 or differentiation regulatory genes such as human Jagged-1) and at the functional level (cobblestone formation, CD34+ cell proliferation), with variable expression of ICAM-1, VCAM-1, and collagens I, III, and IV.[177]

More specialized contractile reticular "barrier cells" have been described in mouse spleen and marrow after hematopoietic stress, such as malarial infection or administration of IL-1.[178] Barrier cells increase in number and seem to enclose developing hematopoietic progenitors in these animals. The cells may regulate the release of precursors into the circulation.[178] Human counterparts of barrier cells are α smooth muscle-positive cells that appear in culture after 2 weeks and are represented by myoid cells lining sinuses at the abluminal side of endothelial cells in marrow biopsies.[169] These cells also have been described in fetal marrow and are increased in areas of active marrow proliferation after inflammation.[178]

Mesenchymal cell stem cell plasticity (fibroblast, adipocyte,[179] endothelial, muscle, neural cell, osteoblasts, chondrocytes) has been extensively demonstrated *in vitro*[180,181] and by single-cell microarray gene analysis.[182] The process is regulated by the dynamic interplay of various cell–cell interactions, growth factors, and chemical mediators and leads to formation of specialized microenvironmental niches that support spatial expansion of hematopoietic cells.[183]

ADIPOCYTES

Adipocytes in marrow develop by lipogenesis in fibroblast-like cells, most likely the adventitial reticular cells (Fig. 4-6). Reticular cells in mouse and human marrow can undergo transformation to fat cells *in vitro* and can revert into fibroblasts in culture by lipolysis.[135,179] Marrow fat cells are relatively resistant to lipolysis during starvation. Their proportion of saturated fatty acids is lower than in other fat deposits, but their composition depends on whether they are located in red, hematopoietically active, or yellow, hematopoietically inactive, marrow.[179] Adipocytes express leptin, osteocalcin, and increased prolactin receptors during differentiation, thereby promoting hematopoiesis and influencing osteogenesis.[184–186] Adipocyte maturation *in vitro* is inhib

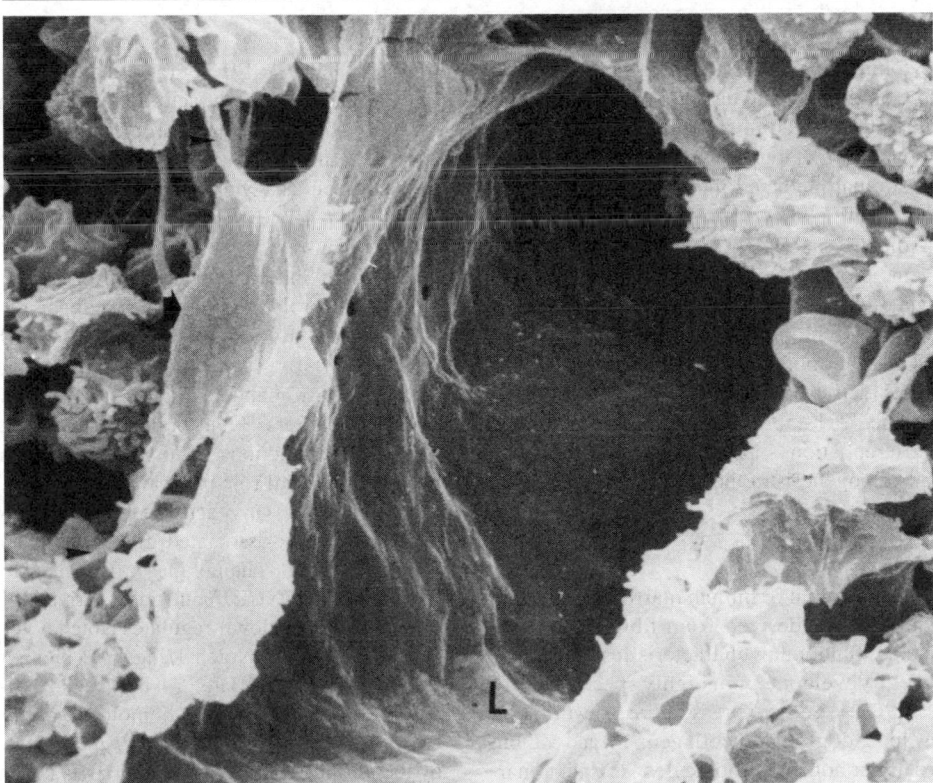

FIGURE 4-4   Scanning electron micrograph of rat marrow sinus. The floor of the lumen (L) is indicated. The *arrow on the left* indicates the cell body of an adventitial reticular cell, which is just beneath the endothelial cell layer. Reticular cell processes can be seen coursing between the sinus wall and the hematopoietic compartment (*small arrows*). (From Lichtman,[120] with permission.)

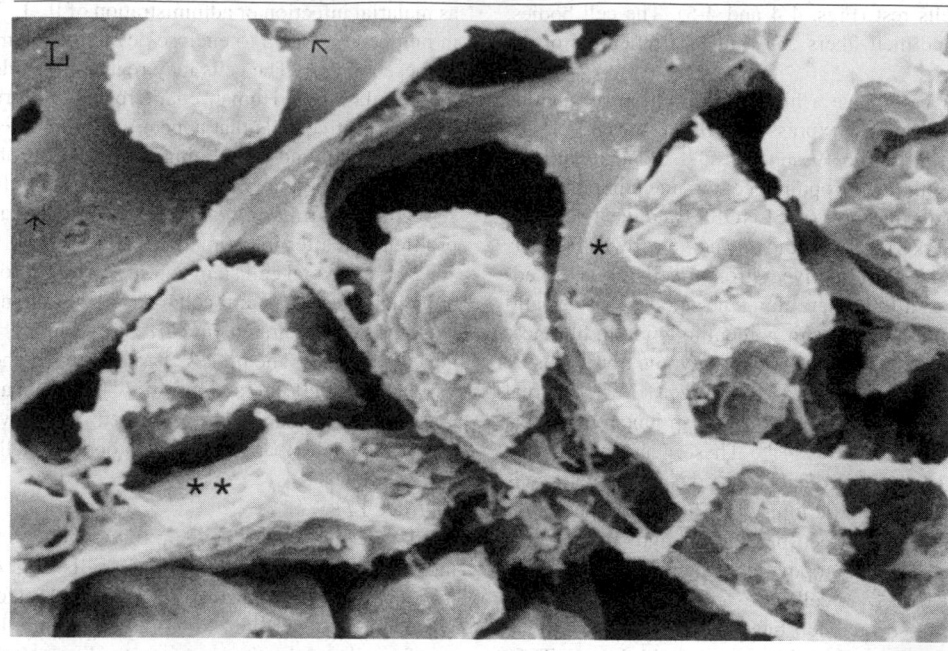

FIGURE 4-5   Scanning electron micrograph of rat femoral marrow sinus. The lumen (L) of an exposed sinus that has been cut open is indicated. The *single asterisk* indicates the process of an adventitial reticular cell and the intimate contact it makes with a hematopoietic cell. To the left of this process are adventitial reticular cell fibers, which form a scaffold for hematopoietic cells. The *double asterisk* identifies a portion of a reticular cell. The hole in the sinus floor is an artifact of preparation or a migration channel bereft of the emigrating cell. Empty spaces between cells and fibers are artifacts of preparation. The *arrow to the left* points to thin-walled fenestrae in the endothelial cytoplasm. The *arrow to the right* identifies the portion of a reticulocyte that may be penetrating the sinus wall, early in egress (see Fig. 4-7A).

ited by stromal-derived cytokines such as IL-1 and IL-11.[187,188] Marrow brown fat[179] is a source of leptin[189] and an adipocyte-derived hormone adiponectin,[190] which inhibit preadipocyte differentiation and B lymphopoiesis while supporting myeloid hematopoietic progenitor growth *in vitro*.[191,192] This stromal-mediated inhibition of B cell lymphopoiesis is mediated by activation of cyclooxygenase pathways and prostaglandin release.[193] Adiponectin, which is present at a low level in obesity, has antiangiogenic properties and induces apoptosis of endothelial cells.[194] Adipocyte differentiation by marrow stromal cells is modulated in a dose-dependent fashion by TGF-β[195] and bone morphogenetic proteins.[196,197] Other hormonal signaling pathways, such as the peroxisome proliferators activated receptor gamma 2 (PPAR-gamma2),[198] growth hormone,[199] 1,25(OH)$_2$D$_3$,[200] and estrogens,[201] also influence adipocyte differentiation, supporting the reciprocal regulation of osteogenesis and adipogenesis in the marrow microenvironment.[202]

STROMAL CELLS

Stromal cells are obtained from animal or human marrow and studied in cultures.[203] They presumably are derived from fibroblasts. They have unique phenotypic and functional characteristics that allow them to nurture hematopoietic development in highly specialized microenvironmental niches.[204] These cells express nerve growth factor receptor, VCAM-1, tenascin, endoglin, and collagens IV and VI, but they do not express intercellular adhesion molecules.[205] Unlike marrow fibroblasts, marrow stromal cells fail to up-regulate collagenase when exposed to IL-1.[206] Stromal cells and cell lines differ in their capacities to support the growth of myeloid,[207,208] pro-B,[209,210] and T cell precursors.[211] This hematopoietic nurturing function of stromal cells parallels growth factor expression such as flt3 ligand,[212] kit

ligand,[213] TPO,[214] LIF,[215] IL-6 and soluble IL-6 receptor,[216,217] IL-7,[218] insulinlike growth factor I,[219] early-acting growth arrest-specific gene-6 (a ligand for the Axl, Sky, and Mer families of tyrosine kinases),[220] and chemokines.[221] Other interactions that regulate hematopoietic cell survival and differentiation are mediated by cell–cell contact via negative regulators of hematopoiesis such as TGF-β, which down-regulates c-*kit* expression[222]; the Notch/Jagged pathway, which inhibits myeloid differentiation[223]; specific receptors (e.g., WNT protein family[224] or angiogenins such as neuropilin-1[225]) and adhesion molecules (MUC18, CD164, hematopoietic cell antigen [HCA]) on stromal cells and hematopoietic CD34-positive cells.[226–228] Stromal cells produce nerve growth factor[229] and express neuronal markers[230] and brain natriuretic peptide, a potent vasodilator. These functions underscore their versatile differentiative capacity and crucial role in repair mechanisms.[231] Human stromal cells and cell lines *in vitro* activate CD14+ monocytes to secrete osteopontin (a matrix-associated glycoprotein important for T cell activation)[232] and chemokines (CXCL1/growth-related oncogene [GROα], and CXCL7/neutrophil-activating protein NAP-2).[233] Osteopontin in turn down-regulates Notch-1 gene expression in CD34+ cells[233] modifying Notch-1/Jagged-1 signaling and their capacity to expand and differentiate.[234] The stromal cell-derived membrane protein mKirre (a mammalian homologue of the genkirre of *Drosophila melanogaster*) encodes a type Ia membrane protein that is cleaved by metalloproteinases and supports via its extracellular domain hematopoietic stem cells in a murine stromal cell line (OP9).[235] Another example of cellular interactions between adipocytes and stromal cells involves a transmembrane protein with epidermal growth factor-like repeat motifs dlk (delta-like),[50] which inhibits stromal cell adipogenesis and promotes cobblestone area colony formation, bypassing the IL-7 requirement for B lymphopoiesis. This function underscores the complexity and redundancy of microenvironmental signals regulating hematopoiesis.[236,237]

BONE CELLS

Osteoblasts, osteoclasts, and elongated flat cells with a spindle-shaped nucleus form the marrow endosteal lining.[238] Resting endosteal cells express vimentin, tenascin, α smooth muscle actin, osteocalcin, CD51, and CD56. They do not react with CD3, CD15, CD20, CD34, CD45, CD68, or CD117.[239] Enriched CD56-positive, CD45-negative, CD34-negative endosteal cells grown in the presence of cytokines (insulin growth factor I, bFGF, kit ligand, IL-3, GM-CSF) do not give rise to hematopoietic cells, which suggests they are not totipotent mesenchymal stem cells in these culture conditions.[239] Cultured human bone cells have high levels of the integrins $\alpha_1\beta_1$, $\alpha_3\beta_1$, $\alpha_5\beta_1$, and $\alpha_v\beta_5$.[240] Endosteal cells are a rich source of stem cells (using the *in vivo* colony-forming unit-spleen (CFU-S) assay; see Chap. 15)[241] and provide a homing niche for newly transplanted early hematopoietic stem cells expressing hyaluronic acid.[242] Mesenchymal stem cells positive for the STRO-1 antibody can differentiate into adipocyte, chondrocytic, and osteogenic cells.[243–245] Similar osteogenic potential is found in STRO-1–positive vascular pericytes.[246] Mesenchymal stem cell to osteogenic differentiation is associated with loss of the activated leukocyte adhesion molecule (CD166).[247]

OSTEOBLASTS

Hematopoietic cells and osteoblasts are derived from a common marrow progenitor after bone marrow transplantation.[248] Bone-forming osteoblast progenitor cells, like stromal precursors, reside in the CD34-negative, STRO-1–positive nonadherent marrow cell population.[249,250] Bone morphogenic protein 2,[251] bFGF,[252] hepatocyte growth factor (HGF),[253] and endothelin-1[254] promote osteoblast growth, whereas TGF-β[255] affects their differentiation.[249,255] Osteoblasts expand early hematopoietic progenitor survival in long-term cultures and secrete hematopoietic growth factors such as macrophage colony stimulating factor (M-CSF), G-CSF, GM-CSF, IL-1, and IL-6.[256,257] Osteoblasts also produce hematopoietic cell cycle inhibitory factors such as TGF-β, which may contribute to their intimate role in stem cell regulation within the marrow microenvironment.[258] These cells can be transplanted in nonablated mouse[259] and facilitate engraftment of purified allogeneic hematopoietic stem cells, which is in keeping with their ability to support hematopoiesis.[260] Subcapsular renal explants of bone can form a suitable hematopoietic microenvironment for early stem cells, underscoring the potential for osteoblasts to nurture hematopoiesis.[261] Direct cell–cell communication has been shown in marrow and in osteoblastic cell networks,[262] indicating a potential regulatory role for these anatomical gap junctions in hematopoiesis.[173,174] *In vivo*, the size of stem cell niches increases after osteoblastic expansion and Notch activation in transgenic models.[12,13] However, in another model, intramedullary hematopoiesis and stem cell numbers are severely diminished following *in vivo* ablation of osteoblasts,[263] underscoring the importance of this cell type to the marrow hematopoietic inductive microenvironment.[264]

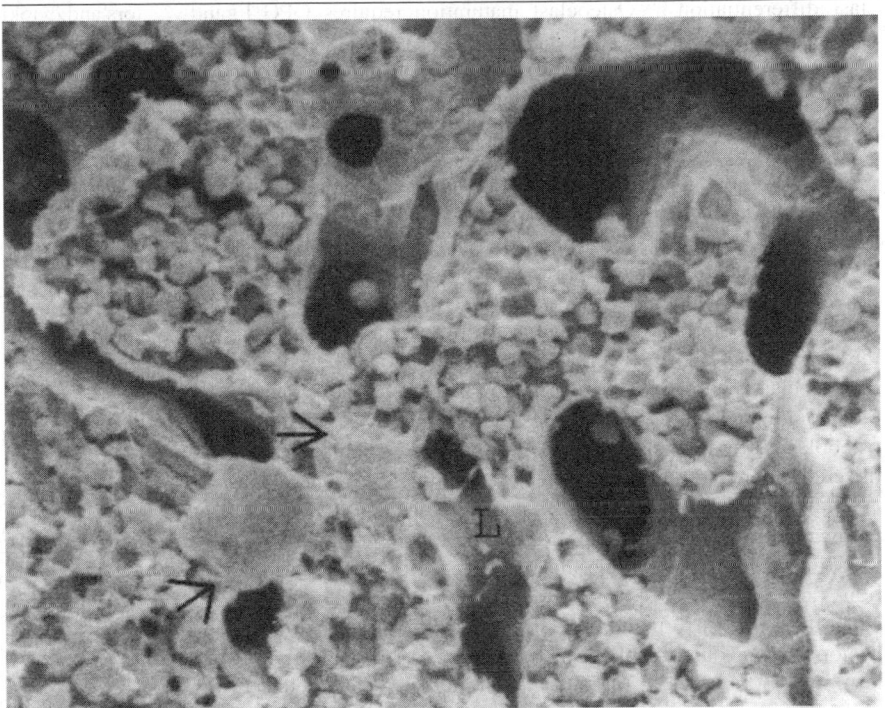

FIGURE 4-6 Scanning electron micrograph of rat femoral marrow. Several sinuses and the intervening hematopoietic cords are evident. The exposed lumen (L) of one branching sinus is indicated. The sinus, just above the L, contains a bean-shaped proplatelet with an attenuated strand connected to a separating smaller proplatelet fragment. Smaller proplatelet fragments are below the L. The *short horizontal arrow* points to the cytoplasm of a transected megakaryocyte. The *lower arrow* points to a fat cell. The rat femoral marrow contains a modest number of fat cells. Spaces in the hematopoietic cords are artifacts of transecting the femur. (From Lichtman,[120] with permission.)

OSTEOCLASTS

Mature osteoclasts are multinucleated giant cells derived from hematopoietic progenitors (CD34-positive, STRO-1–negative) branching from the monocyte-macrophage lineage early during differentiation.[265,266] The flt3-expanded macrophage precursors can differentiate sequentially into osteoclasts, dendritic cells, and microglia.[267] Osteoclasts are highly motile cells involved in bone resorption and remodeling. They require the Wiskott-Aldrich syndrome protein during clustering and fusion of actin-based adhesion structures named *podosomes*.[268] Osteoclasts also can be derived from pro-B cells, as shown by Pax-5 knockout mice, which have increased osteoclasts and severe osteopenia.[269] Secreted M-CSF (CSF-1) is essential for osteoclastogenesis, as demonstrated by the op/op mouse, which has osteopetrosis and congenital deficiency of M-CSF that improves after M-CSF treatment.[270] Cell surface expression of CSF-1 in transgenic *Csf1op/Csf1op* mice leads to incomplete restoration of osteopetrosis and hematologic abmormalities.[271] The KIT ligand and M-CSF act synergistically on osteoclast maturation.[272] M-CSF is essential for proliferation and maturation of osteoclast progenitors.[273] Membrane-bound M-CSF and soluble M-CSF are synergistic in stimulating osteoclast formation.[274] The major form of secreted M-CSF is a proteoglycan that binds to bone-derived collagens and can be extracted from the bone matrix, indicating a local role for this factor in bone development and remodeling.[275] The anti-inflammatory cytokine IL-4 abrogates osteoclast differentiation by STAT6-dependent inhibition of nuclear factor-κB (NF-κB).[276] Targeted disruption of oncogenes such as c-*fos*[277] and pp60 c-*src*[278] prevents osteoclast differentiation leading to osteopetrosis. Osteoprotegrin (OPG), or osteoclastogenesis inhibitory factor, is a cytokine of the TNF receptor superfamily that inhibits osteoclast differentiation.[279] Osteoclast maturation requires OPG ligand (TRANCE/RANKL), an osteoclast differentiation and activation factor (ODF) elaborated by stromal cells and osteoblasts.[280] RANKL (ODF)-regulated osteoclast differentiation requires c-Jun signaling in cooperation with nuclear factor of activated T cells (NFAT).[281] ODF with M-CSF induces osteoclast formation without requiring stromal cells.[282] Proinflammatory cytokine IL-1–induced osteoclastogenesis requires RANKL and is amplified by M-CSF but does not depend on TNF-α.[283] Cross-linking antibodies to the adhesion receptor CD44 inhibit osteoclast formation in primary marrow cultures treated with $1\alpha,25$-dihydroxyvitamin D_3.[284]

Osteoblast/stromal cells regulate differentiation of osteoclasts through intimate cell–cell contacts. They are found in direct apposition to osteoclasts with coated pit formation, suggesting accumulation of receptor–ligand complexes in endocytic vesicles.[285] OPG produced by osteoblasts/stromal cells[286] and megakaryocytes[287] inhibits osteoclast differentiation and function. Osteoclasts produce HGF and express c-Met, the HGF receptor, implying a paracrine and autocrine regulatory pathway between them and adjoining osteoblasts.[253,288] Similarly, blocking expression of cadherin-6 interferes with heterotypic interactions between osteoclasts and stromal cells, impairing their ability to support osteoclast formation.[289] CD9, a tetraspan transmembrane adhesion protein on stromal cells,[290] influences myelopoiesis in long-term marrow cultures.[291] Inhibition of stromal cell CD9-mediated signaling by a blocking antibody reduces ODF transcription, leading to reduced osteoclastogenesis.[292] Macrophage-stimulating protein, a hepatocyte growth factor-like protein, signals through the stem cell-derived tyrosine kinase (STK), a member of the HGF receptor family. It also stimulates osteoclast bone-resorbing activity by enhanced cytoskeletal reorganization without affecting proliferation of osteoclast precursors.[293,294] Osteoclast differentiation is influenced by monocytes expressing ADAM-8 (CD156), a protein of the disintegrin and metalloproteinase family,[295] and eosinophil chemotactic factor-L (ECF-L),[296] characterizing complex cell–cell, cell adhesion protein, stromal cell cytokine, and chemokine signals within the marrow microenvironment.

MACROPHAGES AND LYMPHOCYTES

Macrophages and lymphocytes form part of the marrow microenvironment through growth factor production (IL-3, macrophage inflammatory protein [MIP]-1α) and cell–cell interactions with developing progenitors.[120,135,297–300] Macrophages[301] and lymphocytes[302] are an integral part of the adherent monolayer found in long-term lymphohematopoietic cultures. Mature T and B lymphocytes and plasma cells are found near foci of granulopoiesis in the adherent layers of long-term cultures in humans.[303] Marrow stroma can support thymocyte differentiation,[304] and an early T cell progenitor maturation pathway occurs in the marrow.[305] Marrow stroma regulates B lymphopoiesis by different stromal cell niches and homing receptors (VCAM-1) and by production of cytokines such as flt3 ligand, kit ligand, IL-7, and TGF-β.[306–308] Stromal cells facilitate the maturation of natural killer (NK) cells,[309] an effect likely mediated by stromal-derived flt3 ligand and IL-15.[310]

Stromal cells elaborate and respond to protein growth factors, such as platelet-derived growth factor (PDGF).[311] PDGF up-regulates M-CSF secretion by stromal cells, establishing a paracrine stimulatory loop between the two cell types.[312] Addition of PDGF to macrophages expressing PDGF receptors up-regulates IL-1 secretion and thereby activates primitive hematopoietic cells.[313] Macrophages also modulate the structure and composition of the extracellular matrix and its fibronectin content.[314] Marrow macrophage phenotype[315] is regulated by adjoining stromal cell–accessory cell–derived colony-stimulating factors and cytokines,[316] such as M-CSF up-regulation of $\alpha_4\beta_1$- and $\alpha_5\beta_1$-integrin expression[317] and flt3 ligand-promoting macrophage outgrowth with B cell-associated antigens.[318] Macrophages express sialic acid-binding receptors[319] and play an integral role in erythropoiesis.[320]

EXTRACELLULAR MATRIX

Mesenchymal cells forming the cellular stroma in marrow are active in laying down a rich carpet of extracellular matrix proteins (ECMs),[321] such as proteoglycans or glycosaminoglycans (GAGs),[321,322] fibronectin,[321,323] tenascin,[321,324] collagen,[321,324] laminin,[324] hemonectin,[325] and thrombospondin (TSP).[321,326] Localizing signals are provided by stromal–ECM hematopoietic cell adhesive interactions,[327,328] in concert with chemokines[329] and cytokines, bound to heparin-like structures in the GAGs.[330] These interactions form specialized niches that may facilitate lymphocytic (B and T) or lineage-specific development along the erythroid, myeloid, or megakaryocytic pathways.[331,332] Other functions of these niches include stem cell survival[333] and quiescence.[331,334] Table 4-1 lists the cytokines that are presented on the surface of stromal cells and matrix-binding chemokines and cytokines.[330,335–347] Sl/Sl^d mice that have a deficient hematopoietic microenvironment as a result of a deficiency in kit ligand[348] processing or membrane presentation are anemic and have altered extracellular matrix composition.[349] Addition of hemonectin improves stem cell adhesion to a stromal line derived from Sl/Sl^d mice.[350]

In long-term marrow cultures, collagen, fibronectin, and laminin are secreted early, and extracellular deposition of these proteins coincides with active hematopoiesis.[349] Antibodies to GM-CSF stain adipocyte membranes.[351] Cultures actively generating granulocyte-macrophage precursors produce M-CSF, GM-CSF, and, to a lesser extent, kit ligand and G-CSF within the adherent layer.[352] GM-CSF, G-CSF, and bFGF are detected on the surface of endothelial cells and fibroblasts. GM-CSF localizes to the extracellular matrix, as shown by double labeling of heparan sulfate proteoglycans and GM-CSF.[353] Negative regulators such as TGF-β exert their effects early on long-term

TABLE 4-1 CELL MEMBRANE PRESENTATION AND MATRIX ASSOCIATION OF CYTOKINES AND CHEMOKINES

CELL MEMBRANE	MATRIX ASSOCIATION
Chemokine	*Chemokine*
Fractalkine	RANTES, PF-4, IP-10, IL-8
	Macrophage inflammatory proteins (MIP-1α, MIP-1β)
	Stromal cell-derived growth factor-1 (SDF-1α, SDF-1β)
	Monocyte chemoattractant protein-1 (MCP-1)
Cytokine	*Cytokine*
c-KIT ligand	Granulocyte-macrophage colony-stimulating factor
Tumor necrosis factor alpha (TNF-α)	Interferon gamma (IFN-γ)
Interleukin-1 (IL-1)	Leukemia inhibitory factor (LIF)
Macrophage colony stimulating factor (M-CSF)	Interleukins (IL-1α, IL-1β, IL-2, IL-3, IL-4, IL-5, IL-6, IL-7, IL-12)
	Basic fibroblast growth factor (bFGF)
Transforming growth factor alpha (TGF-α)	Hepatocyte growth factor (HGF)
	Transforming growth factor beta (TGF-β) (binding to endoglin and heparan sulfate)

IP-10, interferon inducible protein 10; PF-4, platelet factor 4; RANTES, *r*egulated upon *a*ctivation *n*ormal *T* cell *e*xpressed, presumed *s*ecreted.

marrow cultures by limiting megakaryocyte progenitor and stem cell expansion.[354]

PROTEOGLYCANS

Proteoglycans are polyanionic macromolecules (heparan sulfate, dermatan, chondroitin sulfate, hyaluronic acid) that are distributed on the surface of adventitial reticular cells and within the extracellular matrix.[321,355] Heparan sulfate is the main cell-surface GAG in long-term marrow cultures, and chondroitin sulfate is the major secreted species.[349,356] D-xylosides, which stimulate artificial sulfated GAG synthesis, increase chondroitin sulfate synthesis and hematopoietic cell production.[356] Hyaluronic acid and chondroitin sulfate-containing proteoglycans are prominent in the adherent and nonadherent compartments of long-term marrow cultures.[355] Heparin-containing and heparan sulfate-containing proteoglycans interact with laminin and type IV collagen[357] and may play a role in cell–cell interactions, cytokine presentation, and cell differentiation.[358–361] They also mediate progenitor cell binding to stroma and other extracellular matrix molecules such as fibronectin.[362–366]

Another important lymphocyte–progenitor cell–associated proteoglycan, CD44, uses hyaluronate as a ligand and promotes stromal adhesive interactions.[302,367] A binding site for lymphocyte CD44 on the carboxy-terminal heparin-binding domain of fibronectin is present,[368] and neutralizing antibodies to CD44 inhibit hematopoiesis in long-term marrow cultures.[369] Cytokines (GM-CSF, IL-3, KIT ligand) rapidly induce CD44 expression and increase CD44-mediated adhesion of CD34-positive hematopoietic progenitors to hyaluronan.[370] Chondroitin sulfates A and B mediate monocyte and B cell activation via a CD44-dependent pathway.[371] Hyaluronate, the CD44 ligand, enhances hematopoiesis by releasing IL-1 (CD44-dependent) and IL-6 (CD44-independent pathway), supporting the important role of this proteoglycan receptor in hematopoiesis.[372]

Heparan sulfate mediates IL-7–dependent lymphopoiesis[344] and modulates hematopoiesis and stromal cell–matrix remodeling[373] by anchoring HGF[345,374] and bFGF.[373,375,376] Marrow stromal cell surface heparan sulfate-containing proteoglycans consist mainly of syndecan-3, syndecan-4, and glypican-1. The major extracellular matrix-associated form is perlecan.[377] Syndecan-3 is expressed in marrow stromal cells as a variant form with a core protein of 50 to 55 kDa, suggesting syndecan-3 plays a role in hematopoiesis.[377] Perlecan promotes bFGF receptor binding and mitogenesis and can bind GM-CSF.[371,378] Heparan sulfate expression is induced on the cell surface in early erythroid differentiation of multipotential hematopoietic stem cells.[379] Glypican-4, another member of this family, is found on marrow stromal cells and progenitor cells.[380] Syndecan-1 expression in B lymphoid cells is reduced by IL-6, which implies similar regulatory pathways in other cell types.[381] Biglycan, a matrix glycoprotein *sc1*, with homology to osteonectin, and the molecule SIM selectively increase IL-7–dependent proliferation of B cells.[382] Interactions of B cells with other components of the immune system are mediated by syndecan-4, which facilitates the formation of dendritic processes[383] and regulates focal adhesion, stress fiber formation, and cell migration.[384] Taken together, these observations underscore the major contribution of proteoglycans in the formation of specialized microenvironmental niches to promote lineage-specific hematopoiesis.

FIBRONECTIN

Fibronectin localizes at sites of attachment of hematopoietic cells and marrow stromal cells *in vitro*,[323,385] at sites of interaction between these cells and developing granulocytes or monocytes.[386] Early erythroid progenitors attach to the cell-binding domain of fibronectin.[387,388] This association can be inhibited by blocking antibodies to the fibronectin integrin receptors $\alpha_5\beta_1$ and $\alpha_4\beta_1$.[389] Adhesion of hematopoietic progenitor cells to stroma is partly mediated by fibronectin.[362,390] This binding can be enhanced by protein kinase C activators such as phorbol esters, suggesting the involvement of integrin receptors in the process.[391–393] The alternatively spliced form of fibronectin (type III connecting segment [IIICS]) is expressed uniquely within the marrow microenvironment[393] and associates with the $\alpha_4\beta_1$-integrin receptor on hematopoietic stem cells.[394] Additional IIICS fibronectin variants have been detected in marrow stroma, providing for a fine control using mRNA splicing of progenitor–stem cell interactions.[395] Fibronectin adhesion to peptide domains, such as the CS1 domain (which activates α_4-integrins) or stromal cells, has dual effects of stimulation and inhibition of hematopoietic progenitor growth.[396–399]

The integrins very late antigen (VLA)-4 and VLA-5, and CD44, cooperate to promote fibronectin adhesive interactions.[396,400–402] Cytokines such as IL-3, KIT ligand, and TPO augment the magnitude of fibronectin mediated hematopoietic progenitor cell adhesion and migration.[403–406] Fibronectin facilitates maturation of CD34-positive progenitor-derived dendritic cells[407] and is involved in adhesion of mature cells, including megakaryocytes,[408,409] mast cells,[410] chemokine-activated T lymphocytes,[411] eosinophils,[412] and neutrophils.[413] Fibronectin is required for expression of gelatinase in macrophages[414] and regulates cytokine release by M-CSF–activated macrophages[415] and chondrocytes.[416] These interactions of fibronectin and its integrin counter-receptors on hematopoietic cells are associated with activation of the sodium–hydrogen exchanger and result in improved cell survival or stimulation.[417]

TENASCIN

Tenascin is an extracellular matrix glycoprotein family consisting of three members: tenascin-C, tenascin-R (restrictin), and tenascin-X.[324,418] Tenascin-C is expressed on the surface of stromal cells in the marrow. Like fibronectin and collagen III, tenascin-C is found in the microenvironment surrounding maturing hematopoietic cells.[321,419] In a long-term marrow culture system (Whitlock-Witte), thiol 2-mercaptoethanol induced expression of tenascin-C and improved lymphoid-lineage differentiation.[420] Glucocorticoids, on the other hand, promote myeloid differentiation in long-term marrow cultures and down-regulate tenascin expression.[421] Tenascin-C has distinct functional domains that promote hematopoietic cell adhesion to stroma or extracellular matrix proteins or mediate a strong mitogenic signal to marrow mononuclear cells.[422] In tenascin-C–deficient mutant mice, the colony-forming capacity of marrow is markedly decreased.[423] Long-term marrow cultures from these tenascin-deficient animals result in decreased progenitor cell output.[423] Addition of tenascin-C to these cultures restores hematopoietic cell production.[423] Mutant tenascin-C–deficient animals also display decreased fibronectin in their marrow, suggesting a possible mechanistic interaction between tenascin-C and fibronectin in the marrow microenvironment.[424] These studies underscore the important role of extracellular matrix proteins such as fibronectin and tenascin-C in hematopoiesis.

COLLAGEN

Collagen types I and III are associated with microvascular walls, whereas collagen type IV is confined to basal lamina beneath endothelial cells.[142,349,425] Marrow-derived capillary networks grow in collagen gel cultures,[426] and inhibition of collagen synthesis reduces hematopoiesis *in vitro*,[427] underscoring the importance of the underlying matrix in reconstituting an intact hematopoietic microenvironment.[428] Erythroid and granulocytic progenitors adhere to collagen type I *in vitro*,[429] and a low molecular weight collagen has been described in lithium-stimulated marrow cultures,[430] emphasizing the effects of induction on matrix composition and stromal support of hematopoiesis.[431] Marrow-derived fibroblasts and stromal cells synthesize collagens I, III, IV, V, and VI.[432] Collagen VI is a strong cytoadhesive component of the marrow microenvironment. Collagen VI binds von Willebrand factor.[433] Collagen type XIV, another fibril-associated collagen, promotes hematopoietic cell adhesion of myeloid and lymphoid cell lines.[434] Collagen-induced, intracellular calcium-mediated signaling events occur in megakaryocytes.[435] *In situ* immunolocalization of ECMs in murine marrow showed that collagen types I and IV and fibronectin localize to the endosteum.[436] The distinct spatial distribution of these matrix proteins underscores their role in the preferential homing of engrafted hematopoietic stem cells to marrow.[242]

LAMININ

Laminin is a multidomain glycoprotein with mitogenic and adhesive sites. It is a major component of the extracellular matrix and basement membranes.[349,437] Laminin interacts with collagen type IV and basement membrane components such as proteoglycans and entactin[438] and thus can regulate leukocyte chemotaxis.[439,440] Similarly, CD34-positive granulocytic progenitors,[441] mature monocytes,[442] and neutrophils[443] adhere to laminin. Its role within the cytomatrix may be to strengthen adhesive interactions with the integrin receptors $\alpha_5\beta_1$ (VLA-5) and $\alpha_6\beta_1$ (VLA-6) on hematopoietic cells.[444] Integrins $\alpha_6\beta_1$ and $\alpha_6\beta_4$ are receptors for laminin-10/11 and laminin-8.[445] Laminin-10/11 ($\alpha_5\beta_1\gamma_1/\gamma_5\beta_2\gamma_1$) and fibronectin bind CD34-positive and CD34-positive CD38-negative progenitors, whereas laminin-8 ($\alpha_4\beta_1\gamma_1$) and laminin 10/11 facilitate SDF-1-α–stimulated transmigration of CD34-positive cells.[445] VLA-6 mediates mast cell adhesion to laminin,[446] whereas the Lutheran blood group glycoproteins serve as laminin receptors on erythroid cells.[447] A 67-kDa laminin receptor has been identified on acute myeloid leukemia cells displaying monocytic differentiation. Laminins are heterodimers composed of α, β, and γ polypeptides. Laminin-1 ($\alpha_1\beta_1\gamma_1$) is not expressed in marrow, which expresses laminin-2 ($\alpha_2\beta_1\gamma_1$), laminin-8 ($\alpha_4\beta_1\gamma_1$), and laminin-10 ($\alpha_5\beta_1\gamma_1$).[448] Laminins containing the α_5-chain bind to multipotential hematopoietic cells (FDCP-mix cells), in contrast to laminin-1 heterodimers.[449] Stromal cells in cultures and cytokine-expanded CD34-positive cells also express laminin β_2, which is found in the pericellular space in marrow and intracellularly in megakaryocytes.[448,450] Laminin promotes the M-CSF–dependent proliferation of marrow-derived macrophages and macrophage cell lines. This effect is partially mediated via an α_6-integrin subunit.[451] Laminin γ_2-chain expression is unique to bone marrow-derived stromal cells. It colocalizes with α smooth muscle actin in marrow and is not expressed in endothelial cells or megakaryocytes.[452]

HEMONECTIN

Hemonectin, a 60-kDa glycoprotein, mediates the attachment of granulocytes to marrow.[325] This protein is expressed in hematopoietic tissues as they develop in murine embryos.[453] Hemonectin is related to the plasma glycoprotein fetuin.[454] Granulocytic adhesion to marrow-derived hemonectin is mediated by galactose and mannose.[455] The exact nature of this molecule and its receptor has not been identified; therefore, the role of hemonectin in the marrow hematopoietic microenvironment remains unclear.

THROMBOSPONDIN

The TSPs are a small family of secreted matricellular glycoproteins that modulate cell function by altering cell–matrix interactions.[456] Thrombospondin-1 (TSP1) is a 450-kDa multifunctional extracellular matrix protein, initially identified in platelet α-granules. TSP1 has domains that interact with collagen and fibronectin and may participate in stem cell lodgement.[457] Receptors on hematopoietic and nonhematopoietic cells can interact with TSP, including CD36[458] and the CLA-1 protein of the CD36/LIMP II gene family.[459] Perlecan mediates the binding of TSP to endothelial cells.[460] The TSP receptor CD36 is expressed during erythroid (CFU-E stage) and megakaryocytic maturation.[461] TSP binds to matrix heparan sulfates[271] and inhibits *in vitro* megakaryopoiesis via CD36.[462] Mature megakaryocytes require thrombospondin-2 (TSP2) for normal hemostasis, as shown in mice lacking TSP2.[463] TSP2 is a matrix-associated protein necessary for the release of functionally competent platelets by megakaryocytes. TSP2 is taken up in an integrin-dependent manner from the marrow milieu, illustrating another important function of this matricellular protein.[463] TSP has a stimulatory effect on NK cells by activating latent TGF-β.[464,465] All-*trans*-retinoic acid–induced granulocytic differentiation of HL-60 cells is associated with increased TSP secretion. The process is delayed by a blocking anti-TSP antibody.[466] TSP decreases the proliferation and promotes the differentiation of HL-60 cells; these effects are not mediated by latent TGF-β activation.[466] A 140-kDa fragment of TSP1 binds bFGF, and TSP1 acts as a scavenger for matrix-associated angiogenic factors (FGF2, VEGF, HGF), underscoring its antiangiogenic properties.[467,468] Endothelial cell TSP expression is inhibited by proangiogenic inflammatory cytokines such as IL-1 and TNF-α.[469] TSP stimulates matrix metalloproteinase-9 activity in endothelial cells[470] and is chemotactic to monocytes[471] and neutrophil-like HL-60 cells.[472]

VITRONECTIN

Vitronectin, also known as *serum spreading factor*, is a 75-kDa protein present in plasma, platelets, and connective tissue.[324] Vitronectin, a major cytoadhesive glycoprotein, binds to the specific integrin $\alpha_v\beta_3$ receptor (CD51) on fibroblasts, endothelial cells, mature hematopoietic cells,[473] including platelets and megakaryocytes,[474] mast cells,[475] and bone cells[476] such as osteoblasts and osteoclasts.[477,478] The vitronectin receptor CD51 cooperates with c-Fms in osteoclast differentiation[479] and contributes to cell fusion and bone resorption in osteoclasts stimulated by TGF-β.[480] CD51 ($\alpha_v\beta_3$) is expressed on monocyte-macrophages and neutrophils and mediates their transendothelial migration.[481,482] Metargidin (ADAM-15) is a type I transmembrane glycoprotein (ADAM, a disintegrin and metalloprotease domain) that binds the $\alpha_v\beta_3$ receptor on a monocytic cell line.[483] It uses a different integrin receptor ($\alpha_5\beta_1$) to mediate adhesion of a lymphoid cell line, underscoring the complexity of cell adhesive interactions in different hematopoietic cells. The vitronectin receptor cooperates with TSP and CD36 in the recognition and phagocytosis of apoptotic cells by neutrophils, macrophages, and dendritic cells.[484–486] Vitronectin and the platelet-derived GAG serglycin augment megakaryocyte proplatelet formation.[487,488] Soluble vitronectin inhibits bFGF-mediated endothelial cell adhesion by interfering with its interaction with the $\alpha_v\beta_3$ receptor.[489] Cytotoxic T lymphocytes,[490] γ/δ-lymphocytes,[491] and NK cells[492] utilize the $\alpha_v\beta_3$ vitronectin receptor as a costimulatory molecule mediating activation signals and cell proliferation. The TSP receptor integrin-associated protein CD47 and the $\alpha_v\beta_3$ vitronectin receptor mediate monocyte activation and cytokine release after interacting with soluble CD23.[493] Hence, vitronectin appears to contribute mainly to terminal megakaryocyte maturation and platelet formation, while exerting a major role in apoptotic cell clearance, cellular activation, and trafficking to areas of inflammation, bone remodeling, and angiogenesis.

HEMATOPOIETIC CELL ORGANIZATION

The hematopoietic cells lie in cords or wedges between the vascular sinuses.

ERYTHROBLASTS

Erythroblasts are arranged against the outside surface of the vascular sinuses in distinctive clusters, called *erythroblastic islands*,[494] which consist of one or more concentric circles of erythroblasts closely surrounding a macrophage. The inner erythroblastic cells are less mature than the peripheral cells. The central macrophage sends out extensive slender membranous processes that envelop each erythroblast and may phagocytize defective erythroblasts and extruded nuclei.[495] Macrophage-stimulating protein boosts the effect of erythropoietin on erythroid progenitor cells *in vitro*.[496] The optimal microenvironmental niche for the terminal erythroid maturation into erythroblasts and erythrocytes consists of closely associated fibroblasts, macrophages, and endothelial cells.[497] Erythropoiesis is stimulated by stromal cell-derived stem cell factor[498] and activin A,[499] a member of the TGF-β family, whereas mesodermal erythroid islands are induced by stromal cell-derived growth factors acting in concert, BMP-4 plus activin A or bFGF.[500] The complex regulation of red blood cell formation also is demonstrated by the enhanced actions of bFGF and HGF on erythropoiesis (see Chap. 30).[501,502]

MEGAKARYOCYTES AND GRANULOCYTES

Megakaryocytes lie directly outside the vascular wall[503] in normal and myeloproliferative diseases,[504] whereas granulocytes mature deeper in the hematopoietic cords, away from the vascular sinuses. Such discrete spatial structural distribution may be determined by specific adhesive interactions and the provision of specific growth factors for a given cell lineage.[505–507] The intimate relation of megakaryocyte to sinus endothelium is explained by their expression of CXCR4, the receptor for the marrow endothelial cell-derived chemokine SDF-1.[508] SDF-1 increases transendothelial migration of megakaryocytes and, unlike TPO, enhances platelet formation.[509,510] Thrombopoiesis also is regulated by locally produced synergistic cytokines such as IL-11,[511] kit ligand,[512] IL-6,[513] and LIF.[514] These factors either increase the expression of TPO[511,513,515] or potentiate its activity.[512,514] TPO increases stem cell number (see Chap. 15), and antibodies to TPO cause neutropenia and thrombocytopenia or frank aplastic anemia in human subjects.[809,810] Stem cells and granulocytic progenitor cells are concentrated in the subcortical regions of the hematopoietic cords.[516]

LYMPHOCYTES AND MACROPHAGES

Lymphocytes and macrophages concentrate around arterial vessels, near the center of the hematopoietic cords.

Macrophages are an integral component of the local microenvironment and regulate hematopoiesis via a complex array of dually acting stem cell stimulatory and inhibitory factors, such as IL-1, MIP-1α, TNF-α, and TGF-β.[517–523] Stromal cells and accessory cells are needed for optimum hematopoietic cell development.[524] Signals regulating the pluripotential hematopoietic stem cells are not entirely defined but require intimate cell–cell contact for signaling through cytokine–chemokine receptors, integrin receptors, alone or together with heparan sulfate or chondroitin sulfate-containing glycoproteins.

This regulatory paradigm is underscored by several studies. (1) A neutralizing antibody to KIT, although able to abrogate myelopoiesis in stromal–stem cell cocultures, did not affect stem cell survival.[525] (2) Stromal-cell-derived BMPs (BMP-2, BMP-4, BMP-7) regulate the proliferation and differentiation of CD34-positive, CD38-negative, lineage-negative cells, with high amounts of BMP-2 and BMP-7 inhibiting proliferation and maintaining repopulating capacity, whereas BMP-4 at higher concentrations extends the survival of these repopulating cells *ex vivo*.[526] (3) Several adhesion receptors of the sialomucin family mediate inhibitory signals to limit stem cell expansion or differentiation.[527] (4) Direct contact of enriched CD34-positive, lineage-negative cells and stroma induces a soluble factor that increases primitive hematopoietic cell production.[528]

THREE-DIMENSIONAL ORGANIZATION

Computer-assisted three-dimensional reconstruction analysis of human marrow confirms the megakaryocyte apposition against the sinus wall and the position of granulocytic cells along the wall of the central arteriole.[529] Erythropoietic cells located mainly around the sinus wall form a continuous network or cord instead of separate "islands." On this basis, the unitary structure of marrow has been defined as a hematopoietic cord with a central arteriole and surrounded by sinuses.[529] A similar structure termed a *hematon* serves as a multicellular functional unit of marrow and contains adipocytes, stromal elements, macrophages, and hematopoietic stem cells in a compact spheroid.[530]

CELL ADHESION AND HOMING

Hematopoietic stem progenitor cells (mostly expressing the CD34 antigen[14]) have multiple adhesion and cytokine receptors. The receptors allow the cells to attach to cellular and matrix components within the marrow sinusoidal spaces.[389–394] Such attachment facilitates their homing and lodgment in the marrow and provide the close cell–cell contacts required for cell survival and regulated steady-state proliferation,[529] as shown by the membrane-bound KIT ligand in regulating the lodgment of stem cells within the endosteal marrow region.[531] Table 4-2 lists the adhesive receptors and their ligands, present on hematopoietic stem progenitor cells, and components of the hematopoietic microenvironment. Six subgroups of receptors, the integrins,[193,532] immunoglobulins,[529,533] lectins (selectins),[534,535] sialomucins,[536–538] hyaladherin (CD44, H-CAM),[539,540] and other receptors such as CD38 (ADP-ribosyl cyclase),[541] CD144 (cadherin),[542] and CD157 (BST-1),[543] are shown, listing mostly interactions involving CD34-positive cells and progenitors.[531,544] Thus, receptor–ligand interactions that regulate the trafficking of mature leukocytes are not included exhaustively.[545,546]

INTEGRINS

Members of the integrin family are divalent cation-requiring heterodimeric proteins (17 α-subunits and eight β-subunits). Integrins mediate important cellular functions, which include embryonic development, cell differentiation, and adhesive interactions between hematopoietic cells and inflammatory cells and surrounding vascular and stromal microenvironment.[393,547] They are subdivided based on the β-chain composition. Table 4-2 indicates that α-chains can associate with more than one β-chain subunit. The principal integrin receptors of the β_1 subgroup involved in hematopoietic stem cells' endothelial and stromal interactions are $\alpha_4\beta_1$ (VLA-4), $\alpha_5\beta_1$ (VLA-5), and $\alpha_L\beta_2$ (LFA-1) of the β_2 subgroup. $\alpha_4\beta_1$-based stromal adhesion events *in vitro*[548] or *in vivo*,[549] alone or in conjunction with the integrin-associated protein ([IAP] CD47),[550] regulate erythropoiesis. This receptor also stimulates granulopoiesis over established marrow stromal cells in cooperation with PECAM-1 (CD31), an immunoglobulin superfamily member,[551] and is essential for pre-B cell growth and differentiation over stromal cells expressing IL-7, kit ligand, and flt3 ligand.[552–555] An acquired defect in stromal function, characterized by a deficiency in VCAM-1 and IL-7 expression,[556–558] accounts for the delayed B lymphoid reconstitution seen after marrow transplantation. Integrin $\alpha_4\beta_7$ and its counterreceptor MAdCAM-1, like the integrin $\alpha_4\beta_1$/VCAM-1 receptor, contribute equally to the homing of hematopoietic progenitors to the marrow.[559]

TABLE 4-2   HEMATOPOIETIC AND MICROENVIRONMENT ADHESION RECEPTORS AND THEIR LIGANDS

RECEPTOR SUBGROUPS	RECEPTOR	CELLULAR DISTRIBUTION	LIGAND
Integrins			
β_1 subgroup (CD29)	CD49d, $\alpha_4\beta_1$ (VLA-4)	CD34+ cells, (erythroid, and lymphomyeloid progenitors)	VCAM-1 (CD106), FN, TSP
	CD49e, $\alpha_5\beta_1$ (VLA-5)	CD34+ cells, bone cells	FN, laminin
	CD49f, $\alpha_6\beta_1$ (VLA-6)	Rare CD34+ cells, monocytes	Collagen, laminin
β_2 subgroup (CD18)	CD11a/CD18, $\alpha_L\beta_2$ (LFA-1)	CD34+ cell subsets, not on repopulating stem cells	ICAM-1, ICAM-2, ICAM-3, DYNAM-1
	CD11b/CD18, $M\beta_2$ (Mac-1)	CD34+ subsets, monocytes	ICAM-1, ICAM-2, iC3b, fibrinogen
β_3 subgroup	$V\beta_3$ (VNR)	Megakaryocytes, osteoclast	FN, TSP, CD31
β_7 subgroup	$\alpha_4\beta_7$ (LPAM-1)	Lymphoid and myeloid progenitor cells, mature myeloid cells	MAdCAM-1, VCAM-1, FN
Immunoglobulins			
	CD31 (PECAM-1)	ECs, CD34+ cells, monocytes	CD31 homophilic adhesion, $\alpha V\beta_3$ (VNR), CD38
	CD50 (ICAM-3, ICAM-R)	CD34+ cells, monocytes	$\alpha L\beta_2$ (LFA-1), CD11d/CD18 ($\alpha D\beta_2$)
	CD54 (ICAM-1)	CD34+ cells, stroma, activated ECs	$\alpha L\beta_2$ (LFA-1), $\alpha M\beta_2$ (Mac-1)
	CD58 (LFA-3)	CD34+ progenitors, stroma, ECs	CD2
	CD102 (ICAM-2)	ECs, monocytes	$\alpha L\beta_2$ (LFA-1)
	CD106 (VCAM-1)	Stroma, activated ECs	$\alpha_4\beta_1$ (VLA-4), $\alpha_4\beta_7$ (LPAM-1)
	CD117 (*c-kit*)	CD34+ progenitors	Membrane kit ligand
	PRR2 (related to CD155, the poliovirus receptor)	CD34+, CD33+, CD41+, myelomonocytic cells, megakaryocytic cells, ECs	PRR2 homophilic adhesion
Lectins			
	CD62L (L-selectin)	Stroma, CD34+ cells	GlyCAM-1, MAdCAM-1, CD162, CD34, s-Lex, PCLP1
	CD62E (E-selectin)	Activated ECs, (marrow ECs express CD62E constitutively)	CD15, s-Lea, CD162, CLA, s-Lex
	CD62P (P-selectin)	Activated ECs	CD162, s-Lex, CD24 (HSA)
Sialomucins			
	CD34	CD34+ cells, endothelial cells	Selectins, other ligands?
	CD43	CD34+, monocytes, NK cells	CD54 (ICAM-1)
	CD162 (PSGL-1)	CD34+ cells, endothelial cells	CD62L, CD62E, CD62P
	CD164 (MGC-24v)	CD34+ cells, stroma, monocytes	Unknown
	CD166 (HCA, ALCAM)	CD34+ cells, stromal cells, ECs	CD6, CD166
Hyaladherin			
	CD44	CD34+ cells, broad distribution	Hyaluronan, bFGF, HGF
Other			
	CD38	CD34+ subsets, early T and B cells, plasma cells, thymocytes	CD31, hyaluronan
	CD144 (VE-cadherin)	CFU-E, stromal cells, ECs	E-cadherin
	CD157 (BST-1)	Stroma, T and B cells, myeloid cells	Unknown

ALCAM, activated leukocyte adhesion molecule; bFGF, basic fibroblast growth factor; CD, cluster designation; CFU-E, colony forming unit–erythroid; CLA, cutaneous lymphocyte antigen; EC, endothelial cell; FN, fibronectin; GlyCAM, glycosylation-dependent cell adhesion molecule; HCA, hematopoietic cell antigen; HGF, hepatocyte growth factor; HSA, heat-stable antigen; ICAM, intercellular adhesion molecule; iC3b, inactive complement 3b complex; LFA, lymphocyte function antigen; LPAM, lymphocyte Peyer patch specific adhesion molecule; MAdCAM, mucosal addressin cell adhesion molecule; MGC-24, multiglycosylated core of 24 kDa; PCLP, podocalyxin-like protein; PECAM, platelet/endothelial cell adhesion molecule; PRR2, poliovirus receptor-related protein2; PSGL-P, selectin glycoprotein ligand; s-Le, sialyl Lewis; TSP, thrombospondin; VLA, very late antigen; VCAM, vascular cell adhesion molecule; VNR, vitronectin receptor.

Integrins are signaling molecules.[560,561] After engaging their ligands, or subsequent to activation by monoclonal antibodies, multiple events (tyrosine phosphorylation of focal adhesion kinase, paxillin, and ERK-2) are triggered (inside–out signaling), culminating with Ras activation.[562–566] Integrin receptor cross-talk[567] with other adhesive receptor members, such as the immunoglobulin superfamily [NK cell–T cell ($\alpha_L\beta_2$/DYNAM-1), CD34-positive–endothelial cell PECAM-1,[568–571] or selectins[572]], also results from outside–in signaling events that regulate receptor-binding affinity[554,573] and mediates inhibitory signals for erythroid, myeloid, and lymphoid progenitor growth.[574–578] Integrin binding to their counterreceptors, such as $\alpha_4\beta_1$/VCAM-1[579] or $\alpha_4\beta_1$/FN,[395] in early CD34-positive progenitors is associated with a decreased rate of apoptosis. Unchecked tyrosine kinase activation, as in chronic myeloid leukemia cells,[580] alters integrin affinity and allows the cells to egress from the marrow.[581] Inhibition of *Abl* kinase activity directly,[582] or indirectly, using α-interferon,[583] restores the adhesive properties of these progenitors.

IMMUNOGLOBULIN SUPERFAMILY

The immunoglobulin superfamily[327] designates a group of molecules containing one or more amino acid repeats also found in immunoglobulins and consists of PECAM-1 (CD31), ICAM-3/R (CD50) and ICAM-1 (CD54), LFA-3 (CD58), ICAM-2 (CD102), VCAM-1 (CD106), KIT (CD117),[584–604] and poliovirus receptor-related–2 protein (PRR2), a molecule related to CD155, which serves as a poliovirus receptor[605] (see Table 4-2). VCAM-1 is up-regulated by inflammatory cytokines (IL-4, IL-13).[602,603] Immunoglobulin-like adhesion molecules also include NCAM, a neural adhesion molecule that binds lymphocytes but not hematopoietic progenitors; Thy-1, a stem cell antigen MHC classes I and II; and CD2, CD4, and CD8[327] (see Table 4-2).

LECTINS (SELECTINS)

Homing of stem cells requires lectin receptors with galactosyl and mannosyl specificities.[606,607] The selectins are a family of adhesion molecules, each containing type C lectin structures. The leukocyte selectin (L-selectin, CD62L) is expressed on hematopoietic stem-progenitors[608] and mediates adhesive interactions with other receptors (addressins), such as the CD34 sialomucin present on specialized endothelium, using sialylated fucosyl-glucoconjugates (see Table 4-2). The CD34 receptor on stem cells, however, does not bind L-selectin,[608] as a putative L-selectin ligand yet to be defined exists on these cells. The selectin family also contains CD62E, an E-selectin constitutively expressed on marrow sinusoidal endothelium that regulates transmigration of leukocytes and CD34-positive stem cell homing. The third member of this family is P-selectin, which is found on platelets. P-selectin can bind hematopoietic stem cells using a mucin receptor, the P-selectin glycoprotein ligand (PSGL)-1, which binds to all three selectins (see Table 4-2). These proteins are responsible for leukocyte rolling over endothelial surfaces and tethering, thereby allowing integrin-mediated firm adhesion to the endothelium and mediating cellular homing events using specialized high endothelial venule lymphocyte homing sites.[609–617] E-selectin– and P-selectin–mediated growth inhibition and apoptosis of hematopoietic progenitors is another important negative regulatory pathway for intramedullary hematopoiesis.[614,618]

SIALOMUCINS

The mucin family includes the CD34 stem cell antigen,[619,620] not an L-selectin ligand on these cells,[621] and CD43, an antiadhesion large glycoprotein (leukosialin)[622] able to regulate hematopoietic progenitor survival.[623] CD34 and CD43 signal via tyrosine kinases when capping their surface receptors[619,624,625] and, in the case of CD43, clustering of cytoskeleton with CD44 and ICAM-2.[674] CD162 (PSGL-1) is important in cell trafficking and stem cell homing.[626–632] CD164 (MGC-24v), another sialomucin receptor,[633] transmits inhibitory signals to stem progenitor cells such as CD162 and CD34.[327] CD166 (HCA, ALCAM) forms homodimers (CD166) and heterodimers with CD6.[634,635]

HYALADHERIN

The fifth subgroup listed in Table 4-2 is the cartilage-related proteoglycan, CD44, also known as the *lymphocyte homing cell adhesion molecule* (HCAM). This adhesion receptor is expressed on hematopoietic stem progenitor cells and facilitates their homing and adhesion to marrow in concert with VLA-4, ICAM-1, and ICAM-3. Several isoforms of CD44 are expressed in normal and tumor tissues. The CD44 variant v10 regulates hematopoietic progenitor mobilization, underscoring its importance in mediating cellular matrix-stromal cell adhesion.[636–639]

OTHER ADHESION MOLECULES

CD38 is a newly recognized adhesion receptor that binds the CD31 receptor and matrix hyaluronan. It is expressed on early T and B cells and subsets of CD34-positive hematopoietic progenitors.[640,641] Cadherins are large molecules involved in cell–cell junctions and vascular integrity. CD144 (E-cadherin) is expressed on CD34-positive progenitors, marrow stroma, and endothelial cells, thereby providing another

pathway for stem cell lodgement.[642] Down-regulation of VE-cadherin is associated with cross-linking of VCAM-1, resulting in enhanced transendothelial migration of CD34-positive cells in response to SDF-1.[156] The stromal adhesion receptor BST-1 (CD157) is an ADP-ribosyl cyclase with similarity to CD38. CD157 is expressed on marrow stroma, T and B cells, and myeloid cells. It promotes pre-B cell adhesion and growth.[643–646]

CELLULAR HOMING

Control of lymphocyte and leukocyte cellular trafficking[647,648] is a multistep process that involves (1) selectin-mediated tethering and rolling over vascular endothelial cells expressing in a tissue-specific distribution selectin-binding sialomucins such as GlyCAM-1 on lymphatic tissue high endothelial venules,[649] MAdCAM-1 on Peyer patch endothelium,[650] peripheral lymph node addressin PNAd,[651] and vascular adhesion protein (VAP)-1[652] molecule (both mediating CD8 T lymphocyte migration)[653]; (2) a triggering step, at sites of inflammation, by short-acting signals such as platelet-activating factor,[654] cytokine,[655,656] or chemokine-activating[657,658] integrins; (3) tight adhesion and spreading of cells over endothelial surfaces mediated by the immunoglobulin receptors (ICAM-1, ICAM-2, VCAM-1)[658–660]; and (4) CD31-mediated diapedesis,[661] in concert with selectin-mediated tethering at vascular endothelial cell junctions.[662] Other molecules can promote rolling of cells, such as tenascin.[663] Cooperation between different adhesion receptors is frequently seen during the transmigration process.[664]

Chemokines bind heparan sulfate proteoglycans and thereby play a central role in directing cellular trafficking at sites of inflammation.[335–340,665] In the case of SDF-1,[341] chemokines regulate cellular trafficking under steady-state conditions. Fractalkine, an endothelial transmembrane mucin–chemokine hybrid molecule, is strategically placed on the surface of activated endothelium and mediates the rapid capture, firm adhesion, and activation under physiologic flow of circulating monocytes, resting or IL-2–activated CD8 lymphocytes, and NK cells.[666] The cytokines TNF-α and IL-1 up-regulate fractalkine, in keeping with the need to recruit effector cells rapidly at sites of inflammation.[667] Tissue-restricted chemokines modulate hematopoietic cell adhesive interactions by providing local activation signals, thereby enhancing the specificity of cellular trafficking.[329]

Unlike lymph nodes, no specific marrow sinusoidal addressins have been defined. A study comparing the adhesive capacity of human marrow or umbilical cord-derived endothelial cell lines[668] did not show any major differences in CD34-positive progenitor adhesion. This interaction is blocked to varying degrees by combinations of monoclonal antibodies against $\alpha_4\beta_1$, CD18, and/or E-selectin.[668] These findings support the concept of a complex stem cell homing and lodgment process that relies on several short-range signals, that is, adhesive interactions between homing CD34-positive cells and marrow sinusoidal endothelial cells.[669,670]

Thus, stem cell homing and lodgment appear to rely on the distinct characteristics of marrow endothelium and stroma and intrinsic properties of hematopoietic stem and progenitor cells. Marrow sinusoidal endothelial cells constitutively express E-selectin. Upon activation, both E-selectin and P-selectin are up-regulated.[671] They also express VCAM-1.[672] The homing CD34-positive progenitors express PSGL-1 (CD162), a highly glycosylated sialomucin that binds all selectins,[626] and the integrin receptor $\alpha_4\beta_1$, which engages VCAM-1.[554] PSGL-1 is expressed in a nonfunctional form in early CD34-positive CD38-low/negative cells displaying reduced rolling on bone marrow endothelium.[627] L-selectin on CD34-positive progenitors[673] may influence the engraftment process by providing a carbohydrate interaction with sinus cavity E-selectin[612] and with underlying stroma. L-selectin may improve progenitor survival as shown by its ability to improve the clonogenic potential of CD34-positive cells.[674,675] Although the sinusoidal endothelial cells rarely express PSGL-1 (CD162), they display other L-selectin ligands such as chondroitin sulfate[676] and heparan sulfate proteoglycans,[677] and VEGF-driven E-selectin.[678] Stromal cells and bone marrow endothelial cells constitutively express CXCL12 (SDF-1), a potent chemokine that enhances integrin activation,[678] and mediate endothelial CD34-positive cell arrest under flow,[679] thereby enhancing CD34-positive cell transmigration.[672,678] The final element in this complex homing process is based upon the constitutive stromal cell expression of VCAM-1,[675] leading to $\alpha_4\beta_1$-integrin–mediated firm adhesion to marrow stroma,[675] of $\alpha_4\beta_1$-positive early reconstituting hematopoietic stem cells,[63] and of CD34-positive progenitor cells.[100,101] G-CSF increases stromal VCAM-1 expression by activating p38 mitogen-activated kinase, thereby promoting adhesion of CD34-positive cells under flow conditions and enhancing the homing of stem cells.[680]

Additional homing signals result from $\alpha_5\beta_1$-integrin binding to fibronectin[391,405]; CD44 and hyaluronic acid on sinusoidal endothelium and endosteum colocalizing with SDF-1 and enhancing intramedullary transmigration[370,681,682]; ubiquitin binding sites on stroma cells interacting with progenitors[683]; and L-selectin interacting with PCLP1.[62,617] This heterotypic adhesion occurs because CD34-positive stem cells and endothelial cells express this receptor/ligand pair. Other immunoglobulin superfamily receptors—PECAM-1 (CD31), ICAM-1, ICAM-2 (CD54, CD102), and CD117—also participate in the stem cell lodgment process.[529] CD117 (KIT) can interact with membrane-bound kit ligand to promote adhesion and cross-activate other integrin receptors.[529]

Another homotypic adhesion receptor in this family is human PRR2, which is expressed on endothelial cells at the intercellular junctions, on the majority of CD34-positive cells, and on hematopoietic precursors differentiating along the myelomonocytic and megakaryocytic lineages (CD33-positive and CD41-positive).[605] PRR2 isoforms can homodimerize or heterodimerize, on the cell surface of endothelial cells, in a fashion similar to PECAM-1 (CD31)–mediated aggregation. The latter PECAM-1 signaling events involve phosphorylation of tyrosine on the receptor's intracytoplasmic tail and recruitment and activation of Src homology 2 domain-bearing protein tyrosine phosphatase-1 (SHP-1) and SHP-2.[684]

This cellular trafficking model is supported by experiments in mutant mice deficient in E-selectin and P-selectin[675] showing decreased marrow progenitor homing *in vivo*. Similar results are obtained after administration of blocking antibodies to VLA-4/VCAM-1 or SDF-1/CXCR4[685] or in genetic studies of α_4-null mice.[669] These events result in decreased stromal–stem cell adhesion[554] and diminished CD34-positive cell–endothelial cell transmigration,[99,686] leading to impaired homing of transplanted stem cells.[685]

CELL PROLIFERATION AND MATURATION

The earliest stem cells are pluripotential and capable of differentiating to either lymphopoietic or hematopoietic multipotential stem cells (see Chap. 15). The pluripotential stem cells and progenitor cells are in a dormant state[14,20] and can withstand the normal hypoxic milieu within the marrow sinusoidal spaces.[687] Hematopoietic stem progenitor cells are prevented from unchecked proliferation by matrix-associated negative regulators such as BMPs[528] and TGF-β,[688–690] alone or in combination with locally induced inhibitory chemokines such as MIP-1α and MCP-1.[691–693] Direct inhibitory signals also are triggered by stromal–hematopoietic progenitor binding using sialomucins such as CD34,[529] CD162,[618] and CD164.[227,613]

Later unipotential progenitor cells respond to lineage-specific cytokines and mature into precursor cells that may undergo four or five cell divisions before terminating in functional blood cells (see Chap. 15). Hematopoietic growth factors and cytokines are produced locally by stromal cells and other cellular elements of marrow. Factors such as kit ligand are expressed in a membrane-bound form,[213] bind to proteoglycans and heparan sulfate moieties within the cytomatrix, and mediate hematopoietic cell attachment, where they are presented in an active form to receptor-bearing hematopoietic progenitors[694] (see "Extracellular Matrix" above and Table 4-1). Cellular attachment to the marrow cytomatrix is an active process leading to signaling and activation of focal adhesion kinases within regions of integrin receptor clustering.[695] These properties explain the ability of stromal cells to promote the self-renewal of stem cells[696] and inhibit apoptosis of hematopoietic cells.[697,698]

After committed progenitor cells mature, the erythroid and granulocytic blast cells undergo four to five mitotic divisions, whereas megakaryocytic blast cells divide perhaps once and then undergo five or six endomitotic divisions (see Chap. 104). The number of precursor cells in the marrow of humans has been calculated primarily through the study of marrow films and sections relating differential counts of marrow samples to their content of injected radioactive iron. A number of assumptions and approximations are made,[699] but the summary data (Table 4-3) agree well with many other observations on the cellular content and kinetics of normal marrows.

CELLULAR RELEASE

Cell migration occurs between adventitial cells but through endothelial cell channels that develop at the time of cell transit. Migrating cells make the hole that develops in the endothelial cell cytoplasm. A number of releasing factors have been implicated in the initiation of marrow egress. The best characterized releasing factors are those for granulocytes, which include G-CSF,[700,701] GM-CSF,[702] the C3$_e$ component of complement,[703] zymosan-activated plasma-containing complement fragments,[704] glucocorticoid hormones,[705] androgenic steroids,[706] and endotoxin.[707] Cellular migration is under the complex control of a family of small cytokines termed *chemokines* with overlapping tissue and target cell specificity, allowing them to regulate effector cell trafficking throughout the body. The chemokine superfamily has several branches based on the cysteine motifs: the "C-X-C" family (platelet factor 4, IL-8, melanocyte growth-stimulating activity/GROα, neutrophil activating protein-2, granulocyte chemotactic protein-2), which all mediate neutrophil migration and activation; and the "C-C" family (MIP-1α, MIP-1β, RANTES [regulated on activation, normal T cell expressed, presumed secreted], MCP-1 through MCP-5), which mediate mostly monocyte and in some cases lymphocyte chemotaxis.[329,667] Neutrophils residing in the marrow venous sinusoids are

TABLE 4-3   NORMAL PRECURSOR CELL KINETICS

CELL TYPE	MARROW		
	NUMBER (CELLS/KG)	TRANSIT TIME (DAYS)	PRODUCTION RATE (CELLS/KG/DAY)
I. Red cells			
Erythroblasts	5.3×10^9	~5.0	3.0×10^9
Reticulocytes	8.2×10^9	2.8	3.0×10^9
II. Megakaryocytes	15.0×10^6	~7.0	2.0×10^6
III. Granulocytes			
Proliferation pool	2.1×10^9	~5.0	0.85×10^9
Postmitotic pool	5.6×10^9	6.6	0.85×10^9

SOURCE: Finch, Harker, and Cook,[699] with permission.

rapidly released into the circulation by IL-8.[708] Eosinophil and eosinophil progenitors are recruited from marrow selectively in allergic states, after exposure to IL-5,[709] by the chemokines eotaxin[710] or RANTES.[711] In the two systems, migration is inhibited by blocking the β_2-integrin CD18, underscoring the importance of integrin activation and surface proteolytic activation in mediating transendothelial migration.[711,712] The CXCR4/CXCL12 (SDF-1) chemokine axis regulates neutrophil homeostasis as the marrow sequesters 60 percent of postmitotic pool resting neutrophils expressing CXCR4, as demonstrated by antibody blockade.[713] Similarly, SDF-1 and kit ligand cooperate to enhance hematopoietic progenitor chemotaxis.[714] Table 4-4 gives a detailed listing of chemokine receptors and the cellular targets and ligands interacting with each receptor subgroup.[715–718] Chemokines capable of enhancing transendothelial migration of human CD34-positive cells include the CC, CXC, and CX3C classes (Table 4-4).[719]

Releasing factors for reticulocytes and platelets have been more difficult to identify. They may be of less biologic significance because early release of these cells has little impact on the large pool of circulating cells. Erythropoietin therapy in uremic patients accelerates the egress of reticulocytes.[720] Adventitial reticular cell cytoplasm is a barrier to the reticulocytes on the abluminal surface of the endothelium.[721] Phlebotomy, phenylhydrazine induced hemolytic anemia, and erythropoietin result in marked reduction of the adventitial cell cover of the sinus, a process that is thought to facilitate cell egress through the endothelium.[722] To leave the marrow, the reticulocyte depends on a pressure gradient across the membrane to drive it through the pore[721,722] (Fig. 4-7). The pressures within the marrow sinuses are pulsatile, and pressures sufficient to cause egress may be transient.[723] Anemia and erythropoietin administration markedly increase blood flow to marrow and bone,[724] whereas G-CSF increases blood flow to marrow only.[725] This effect is not blocked by denervation[726] and may explain the egress of cells after G-CSF administration.[725]

Electron micrographs of leukocytes partially translocated across endothelium indicate that marked deformation of these cells occurs as they penetrate the cytoplasm of the endothelial cell and enter the sinus lumen (Fig. 4-8).[727] As with reticulocytes, egress occurs adjacent to junctions of endothelial cells.[495] The nucleus of the granulocyte, usually segmented, does not require as marked a deformation to traverse

TABLE 4-4   CHEMOKINE RECEPTORS, INTERACTING CHEMOKINE LIGANDS, AND CELLULAR SPECIFICITY

RECEPTORS	RECEPTOR EXPRESSION	CHEMOKINE LIGANDS
CXCR1	Neutrophils (Neu)	CXCL8 (IL-8), CXCL6 (GCP-2)
CXCR2	Neutrophils, IL-5–primed Eos	CXCL8, CXCL1,2,3 (GROα/β/γ), CXCL5 (ENA78), CXCL6,CXCL7 (NAP-2)
CXCR3	Activated memory and naive T cells, NK cells; T (preferentially Th1) cells	CXCL9 (MIG), CXCL10 (IP-10), CXCL11 (I-TAC)
CXCR4	Neutrophils, monocytes, megakaryocytes, CD34+ and pre-B cell precursors, resting and activated T cells	CXCL12 (SDF-1α, SDF-1β, stromal cell derived factor)
CXCR5	B lymphocytes	CXCL13 (BCA-1/BLC)
CX3CR1	Monocytes, DCs, CD34+ cells, NK cells; in nodal tissues activated T helper lymphocytes, activated B cells, and follicular DCs	CXCL1 (fractalkine/neurotactin)
XCR1	Resting T cells, NK cells	XCL1 (lymphotactin/SCM-1α/ATAC) XCL2 (SCM-1β)
CCR1	Monocytes, Eos, basophils, activated Neu and T cells, CD34+ cells, immature DCs	CCL5 (RANTES), CCL3 (MIP-1α), MIP-5, CCL7 (MCP-3), CCL8 (MCP-2), CCL14 (MCP-4), CCL23 (CK-β8/CK-β8-1/MPIF-1)
	Monocytes, T cells (not Neu, Eos, or B cells)	CKCCL14 (HCC-1), CCL16 (HCC-4/LEC), CCL15 (HCC-2/MIP-1δ)
CCR2	Monocytes, basophils, DCs, T cells, activated memory CD4 T cells, NK cells	CCL2(MCP-1), CCL7 (MCP-3), CCL8 (MCP-2), CCL13 (MCP-4), CCL12 (MCP-5), CCL5 (RANTES), CCL11 (Eotaxin-1), CCL24 (Eotaxin-2/MPIF-2)
CCR3	Eos, thymocytes, basophils, DCs, activated memory CD4 T cells	CCL11, CCL24, CCL26 (Eotaxin-3), CCL5, MCP-2, MCP-3, MCP-4, MIP-5, vMIP-II
CCR4	Activated T cells, immature DCs	CCL17 (TARC)
	Monocyte-derived DCs, activated NK cells	CCL22 (MDC)
	Thymocytes (CD3+, CD4+, CD8^{low})	CCL22 (MDC)
CCR5	Monocytes, activated memory CD4 T cells	CCL5 (RANTES), MCP-2, MCP-3, MCP-4
	Immature DCs, CD34+ cells, NK cells	CCL3 (MIP-1α), CCL4 (MIP-1β)
	Human thymocytes	CCL4 (MIP-1β)
CCR6	T cells, CD34+–derived dendritic cells	CCL20 (MIP-3α/LARC/exodus-1)
CCR7	Activated T (naive and memory T cells) > B lymphocytes, NK cells subsets, CD34+ macrophage progenitors, mature DCs	CCL19 (MIP-3β/ELC/CK-β11/exodus-3), CL21 (SLC/exodus-2/TCA4/6Ckine) (6Ckine inactive on B cells)
CCR8	Monocytes, T (Th2) cells	CCL1 (I309), CCL17 (TARC), vMIP-1, vMIP-II
CCR9	Thymocytes (CD4+/CD8+, CD4+/CD8−), activated macrophages	CCL25 (TECK)
CCR10	Skin-homing memory T cells, CD4/CD8 cells	CCL27 (CTACK/ILC/ESkine)
CCR1 and CCR3	Neutrophils, monocytes, lymphocytes	CCL15 (Leutactin-1/HCC-2/MIP1δ)
Not known	Resting T cells	CCL18 (DC-CK1/PARC)
CCR3/CCR10	Memory lymphocytes, Eos, IgA plasmablasts	CCL28 (MEC)

BLC, B cell homing chemokine that activates Burkitt lymphoma receptor 1 (BLR1); CTACK, cutaneous T cell-attracting chemokine; DC, dendritic cell; DC-CK-1, dendritic cell chemokine-1; ELC, EBI1-ligand chemokine; EOS, eosinophil; HCC, human, hemofiltrate C-C-chemokine; IL-8 is also chemotactic for a specific subset of (CD3+, CD8+, CD56+, CD26-) T cells; I-TAC, interferon inducible T cell alpha chemoattractant; LARC, liver and activation-regulated chemokine; Lkn-1 (leukotactin-1), beta chemokine, identical to CK-β8, CK-β8-1 is alternatively spliced, Ck-β8 is 17 amino acids shorter; MCP-3 binding does not transduce a signal and is a natural antagonist of the CCR5 receptor; MDC, macrophage-derived chemokine, MDC is chemotactic to eosinophils, in a CCR3- and CCR4-independent manner; MEC-mucosae-associated epithelial chemokine; MPIF-1, -2, myeloid progenitor inhibitory factor 1, 2 (MPIF-1 is identical to CKβ-8 and MIP-3, MPIF-2 is also known as CKβ-6 or eotaxin-2); NK, natural killer; PARC, pulmonary and activation-regulated chemokine; SLC, secondary lymphoid-tissue chemokine, also known as exodus-2 and 6Ckine; TARC, thymus and activation-regulated chemokine; TECK, thymus-expressed chemokine; vMIP-II is a human herpes virus-8–encoded chemokine antagonist of CC, CXC, and CXCR1 receptors.

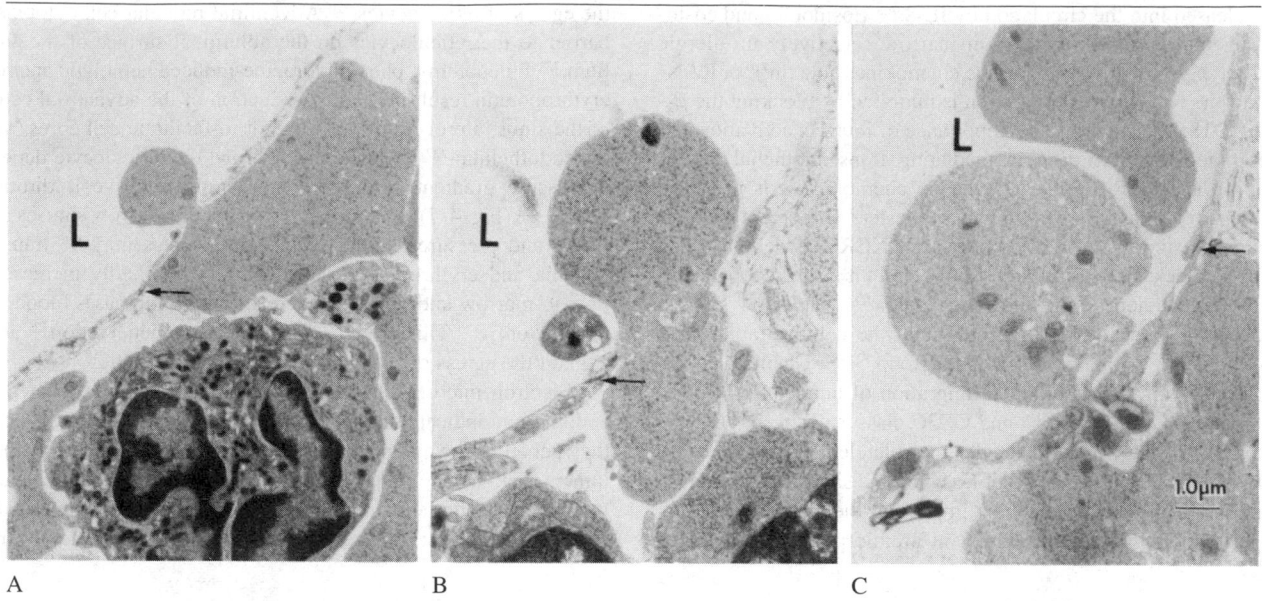

FIGURE 4-7   Transmission electron micrograph of mouse femoral marrow. Composite of reticulocytes in egress. *(A)* Small protrusion of marrow reticulocyte into sinus lumen (L). *(B)* Reticulocyte in egress, with approximately half the cell in the sinus lumen. *(C)* Reticulocyte virtually in the sinus. Egress occurs through a migration pore that is parajunctional in position (*arrows* point to endothelial cell junctions). (From Lichtman and Waugh,[495] with permission.)

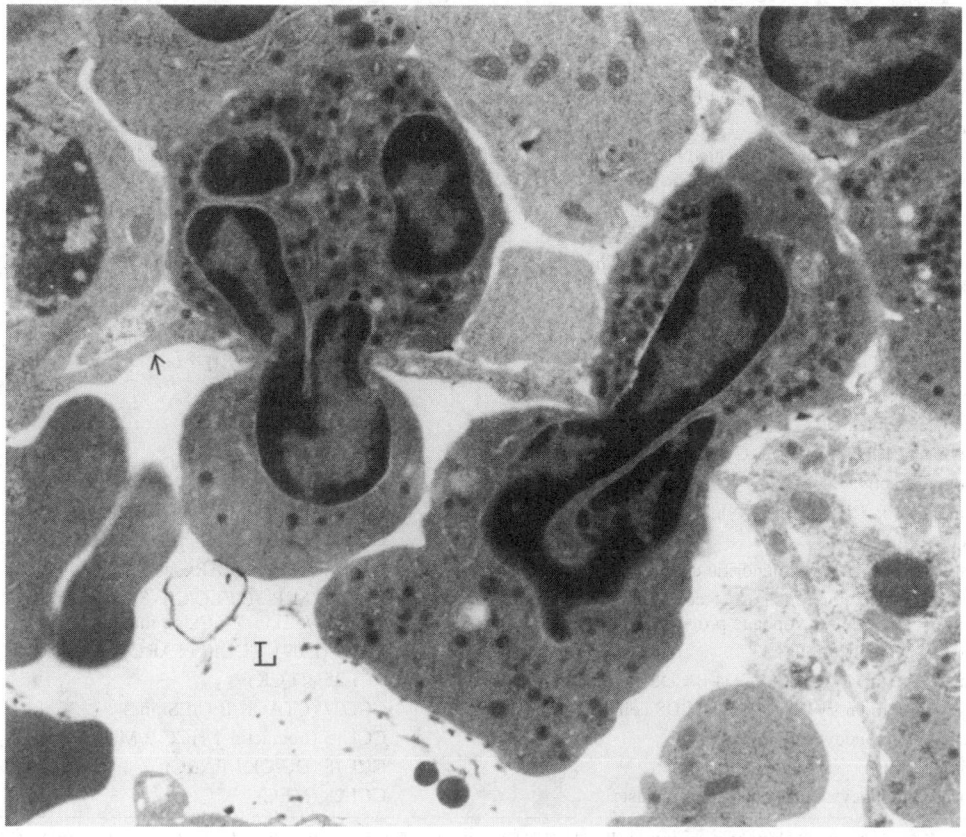

FIGURE 4-8   Transmission electron micrograph of mouse femoral marrow. The lumen (L) of a sinus is indicated. Endothelial cell cytoplasm separates the sinus lumen from the hematopoietic spaces *(arrow)*. Two neutrophils are evident traversing the sinus wall. Note deformation of the cell producing a narrow waist where the cell passes through endothelium. The luminal portion of the migrating cells is granule-poor. The remainder of the cytoplasm is granule-rich, possibly reflecting gel-sol transformation during pseudopod formation.

the migration pore as do the nuclei of monocytes and lymphocytes.[727] The immature granulocytes in marrow are anchored to adventitial reticular cells through lectin-like adhesion molecules. Gradual loss of these molecules (e.g., shedding of L-selectin) during maturation or after activation could permit movement toward the sinus wall.[728] Transient changes in surface glycoproteins (up-regulation of α-2,6 sialylation of CD11b and CD18) of maturing marrow myeloid cells lead to decreased stromal and fibronectin adhesion and may favor contact with endothelium and cell egress.[729] Activated neutrophils can adhere under flow using the VLA-4 integrin pathway.[730] Neutrophil egress occurs mostly at the endothelial cell borders and is entirely P-selectin mediated.[731] C5a and G-CSF administration recruit neutrophils by altering integrins (low CD11a with G-CSF) and decreased L-selectin expression (with both agents).[732,733] Similar findings obtained in mice lacking two or all three selectins underscore the essential role of selectins in neutrophil recruitment.[734]

Platelet release is initiated by megakaryocyte cytoplasm invaginating the abluminal surface of the marrow sinus endothelial cell until a pore is made (Fig. 4-9). Cytoplasm flows through this pore into the marrow sinus and eventually is separated from the body of the megakaryocyte, resulting in a multiplatelet fragment or proplatelet (Fig. 4-10).[503,735] The proplatelets often are stringbean-shaped structures and are found in the marrow sinus lumen. Eventually they fragment into single platelets.[487,488] Megakaryocyte nuclei are left in marrow after platelet release and are degraded and phagocytized there.[736] The entry of either nuclear remnants or entire megakaryocytes with residual cytoplasm has been observed in both normal individuals[737] and in patients with marrow disorders.[738] Megakaryocyte transendothelial migration and proplatelet formation are enhanced by CXCL12 (SDF-1).[509]

Occasional immature granulocytes and megakaryocyte nuclei or whole megakaryocytes are present in cell concentrates of normal blood.[737] Nucleated red cells rarely escape from the marrow under normal conditions. The absence of circulating erythroblasts may relate to the spleen's capacity to sequester and enucleate circulating erythroblasts. The late myelocytes and metamyelocytes have the capacity to move, respond to chemoattractants, and deform, albeit less well than the mature neutrophils, and thus occasionally exit marrow by normal mechanisms. Invasion of marrow by neoplastic cells or replacement of marrow by fibrous tissue is associated with an increased prevalence of immature cells in the circulation. Damage to the architecture of marrow with a breakdown of the integrity of sinus walls may allow cells to enter the circulation less discriminately. Tumor cells elaborate chemoattractive cytokines (chemokines), thus explaining their ability to facilitate cell egress from marrow.[739]

Intramedullary expression of CXCL12 (SDF-1) and kit ligand may allow stem cells to localize to that space.[531,740] The kit ligand up-regulates CXCR4 (CXCL12/SDF-1 receptor) expression on CD34-positive cells, enhancing their chemotactic response.[741] Similarly, mobilized blood CD34-positive progenitors exposed to complement activation

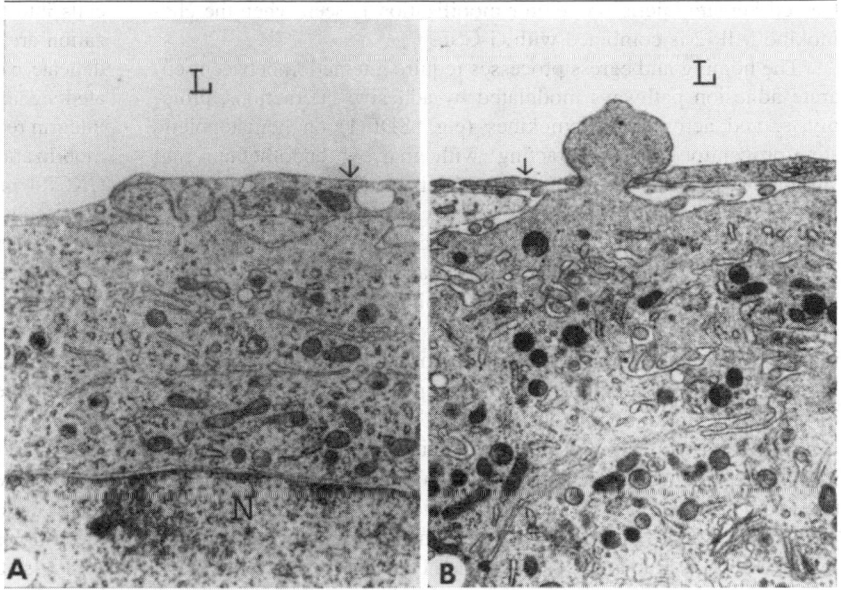

FIGURE 4-9   Transmission electron micrograph of mouse femoral marrow. *(A)* The lumen (L) of a marrow sinus is indicated. The *arrow* points to the thin endothelial cytoplasmic lining of the sinus. The nucleus of a megakaryocyte (N) is indicated, with the cytoplasm of the megakaryocyte invaginating the endothelial cell cytoplasm in three places below the lumen. *(B)* The arrow indicates the thin endothelial cell cytoplasmic lining of the sinus. The endothelium is attenuated to a double membrane in two places. A small process of megakaryocyte cytoplasm has formed a pore in the endothelial cell and has entered the sinus lumen (L). Cytoplasm flows through such pores and delivers proplatelets to the sinus lumen.

display functional receptors for C3a anaphylatoxin,[742] which enhances their homing responses to intramedullary SDF-1–mediated signals.[742] CXCR4 is expressed on early lymphohematopoietic progenitors,[743] providing a model in which mobilized CD34-positive cells have altered an adhesion repertoire and chemotactic capacities, allowing them to leave their sinusoidal niches to the peripheral circulation.[744] En-

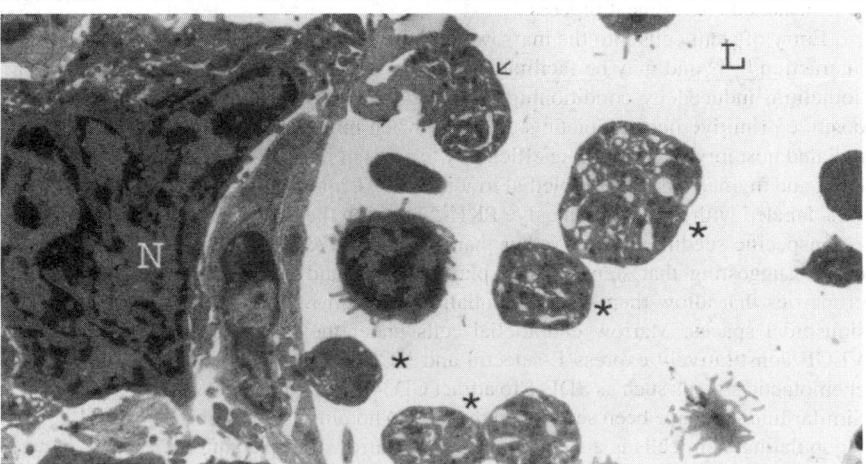

FIGURE 4-10   Transmission electron micrograph of mouse femoral marrow. The marrow sinus lumen (L) and a megakaryocyte nucleus (N) virtually denuded of cytoplasm are indicated. The megakaryocyte nucleus abuts the nucleus of an adventitial reticular cell; the latter is separated from the lumen by the very thin endothelial cell cytoplasm. A portion of residual megakaryocyte cytoplasm (proplatelet) can be seen streaming into the lumen *(arrow)*. The lumen contains several proplatelets *(asterisks)*. Compare the size of the proplatelets to that of lymphocyte in the sinus. The bean-shaped, three-dimensional appearance of the proplatelets can be seen in the scanning micrograph shown in Fig. 4-6.

hanced hematopoietic progenitor mobilization is seen when the chemokine MIP-2 is combined with G-CSF.[745]

The homing and egress processes require interaction between separate adhesion pathways modulated by adhesive interactions, proteolysis, and activating chemokines (e.g., SDF-1) on hematopoietic stem/progenitor cells interacting with marrow endothelium and stroma, as shown in several *in vivo* models using chemokines, monoclonal antibodies and integrin, G-CSF receptor (G-CSF-R), and elastase knockout mice.[746–748] Marrow stem cell homing depends on the $\alpha_4\beta_1$/VCAM-1 adhesion pathway, whereas CD44/hyaluronan affects homing to marrow[242] and spleen.[242,749] Inhibition of CD44 and/or $\alpha_4\beta_1$ adhesion rapidly mobilizes stem cells.[749] The CS1 domain FN fragment did not mobilize progenitors, and antibody to $\alpha_5\beta_1$ did not alter homing.[750] G-CSF augments the mobilizing action of $\alpha_4\beta_1$/VCAM-1 integrin-blocking antibodies in primates,[751] and kit signaling cooperates with this integrin-based mobilization process.[752] Chemokine signals that regulate adhesion, migration *in vivo* and in a spheroid three-dimensional model, and mobilization of hematopoietic stem/progenitor cells are mediated by G-protein–coupled receptors and are regulated by the Rac and Cdc42 small GTPases.[753–755]

STEM CELL CIRCULATION

Fetal and mature hematopoietic stem cells circulate in the blood throughout ontogeny, responding to kit ligand that acts synergistically with SDF-1 to promote stem cell seeding of the spleen and marrow as suitable niches are formed in the sinusoidal cords.[756,757] Whole-body irradiation of an animal with shielding of a single bone results in repopulation of the irradiated marrow, strongly implying transfer of stem cells from shielded marrow into irradiated marrow.[758] Marrow or blood cells from a syngeneic or histocompatible allogeneic donor can reenter marrow and reconstitute hematopoiesis of an animal or human recipient.[748] Expression of L-selectin and CD44 in blood CD34-positive progenitors seems to correlate with faster engraftment and platelet recovery.[759,760] High proliferative potential colony forming cells in the CD34-positive, CD38-negative subgroup are detectable in the circulation, very early after allogeneic transplantation. This finding coincides with rapid recovery of blood counts and implies a role for *in vivo* stem cell recirculation leading to a sustained engraftment process.[761]

Entry of stem cells into the marrow is mediated by a lectin–sugar interaction[762,763] and may be facilitated by alterations in the sinus endothelium induced by conditioning therapy.[764,765] However, c-*KIT*-positive primitive hematopoietic stem cells, when infused in a nonirradiated host model, home more efficiently to areas of marrow, spleen, lung, and thymus than after sublethal irradiation.[766] Unpurified marrow cells labeled with the membrane dye PKH-2 appear to be governed by a nonspecific seeding process rather than by a selective homing signal,[767] suggesting that stem cells display adhesive and chemotactic properties that allow them to preferentially seek marrow endothelial sinusoidal spaces. Marrow endothelial cells under the influence of VEGF constitutively express E-selectin and VCAM-1 and elaborate chemotactic signals such as SDF-1 to attract CD34-positive cells.[768,769] Similar findings have been seen when the *in vivo* homing of long-term repopulating stem cells is analyzed in a serial marrow transplantation model.[770] CD8-positive but not CD4-positive T cells facilitate the engraftment process by heterologous cell–cell cooperation resulting in enhanced motility and transendothelial migration of CD34-positive stem cells.[771]

Blood stem cell mobilization for marrow transplantation has been facilitated by improvements in CD34 cell collection and processing and the demonstrated ability of recombinant cytokines such as the early-acting flt3 ligand, KIT ligand, IL-3, IL-7, and TPO, and the late-acting GM-CSF and G-CSF, all of which enhance the release of stem cells into the circulation.[772–779] The mechanisms of stem cell mobilization are complex and vary with each modality utilized, keeping a delicate balance between adhesive interactions and chemokine-mediated signals affecting CXCR4/SDF-1 levels and the activated state of integrin receptors on the cell surface.[748,780,781] G-CSF induces stem cell mobilization by down-regulating CXCL12 (SDF-1) and up-regulating CXCR4 on CD34-positive cells, thereby reducing the adhesion of these cells to membrane- and cytomatrix-associated KIT ligand.[782] This process explains the propensity of KIT ligand to mobilize stem cells, since it can alter receptor affinity and/or density and thus decrease the anchorage of stem cells to the membrane-bound KIT ligand on marrow stromal cells.[744,781,782]

CD44-mediated adhesion and $\alpha_4\beta_1$/VCAM-1 interactions affect hematopoietic stem cell egress and homing.[539,639] CD44v7 isoforms expressed on stromal cells support progenitor homing and marrow repopulation.[783] Antibodies directed to the CD44v10 isoform release hematopoietic progenitors into the circulation.[639] Moreover, intracellular pools of hyaluronate receptor (RHAMM) and CD44 have been identified in early stem cells (CD34-positive, CD45-low/medium). Steady-state marrow CD34-positive progenitors have larger intracellular CD44 and intracellular RHAMM pools than do cells obtained from G-CSF–mobilized blood collections, which show a depleted intracellular RHAMM compartment.[784] Progenitor adhesion is blocked by anti-CD44 and anti-β_1-integrin antibodies, whereas motility is inhibited by antibodies to β_1-integrin and RHAMM, suggesting a reciprocal role between these two molecules during stem cell trafficking.

Table 4-5 details a working model of stem cell egress.[748] This complex process does not rely on any one feature of stem cells and the marrow microenvironment. Rather, the process assumes a continuous series of interactions involving blood flow[725]; adventitial reticular cell–microvascular endothelial cell contraction[785]; altered integrin, se-

TABLE 4-5   FACTORS REGULATING MARROW STEM CELL EGRESS

A.   Increased marrow blood flow[725]

B.   Adventitial reticular cell/microvascular endothelial cell contraction[785]

C.   Altered adhesive interactions of CD34 cells and underlying cytomatrix

   1. Integrin receptor ($\alpha_4\beta_1$) affinity[655,656] and expression ($\alpha4$ null mice[669] or blocking antibody)[748,751,752]

   2. Decreased L-selectin affinity and expression[673]

   3. c-*KIT*–KIT ligand interactions[531,744,748,751]

   4. β_1-mediated integrin–cytoskeletal interactions[656,746,748]

   5. Alteration in intracellular hyaluronan receptor (RHAMM) and CD44 pools[784]

   6. CD44v10 blocking antibody, progenitor egress with CD44v10 receptor globulin[639,749]

D. Increased enzyme production by

   1. CD34 cells (gelatinase A [MMP-2] and gelatinase B [MMP-9])[748,801,802]

   2. Neutrophils activated by cytomatrix adherence, CXCL8 (IL-8), and/or G-CSF (elastase and gelatinase B)[800,802]

E.   Chemokine gradient(s) across sinusoidal barrier

   1. Heparan sulfate containing matrix proteins binding to chemokines[335–343,681]

   2. Decreased CXCR4 receptor expression and CXCL12 (SDF-1) expression by stromal cell or microvascular endothelial cell[748,780–782]

   3. Proteolytic degradation of CXCL12 and VCAM-1 anchoring molecules[748,781,782]

F.   Stem cell motility

   1. Differential expression of proteins regulating motility in primitive stem cells[807]

   2. Stem and progenitor trafficking to areas of injury[807] regulated by hypoxic gradients and expression of hypoxia-inducible factor-1 (HIF-1), which induces SDF-1 expression in ischemic tissue[808]

lectin, cytokine, and cytoskeletal receptor expression[784]; or functional activation.[748,781] Chemokines such as CXCL8 (IL-8) can efficiently mobilize hematopoietic stem cells *in vivo*, a process that requires the presence of neutrophils.[786,787] IL-8, a potent activator of neutrophil integrin function, causes shedding of L-selectin and degranulation, exposing nearby matrix components to proteolytic enzymes such as elastase and gelatinase B, also known as *matrix metalloproteinase-9* (MMP-9).[535,788] Antibodies against gelatinase B inhibit stem cell mobilization in this model.[789] G-CSF administration *in vivo* is accompanied by a surge in IL-8 that may potentiate stem cell release.[790] This action is indirect, as long-term repopulating stem cells mobilized by IL-8 do not express $\alpha_L\beta_1$,[791] whereas administration of anti-$\alpha_L\beta_1$ antibody blocks IL-8–induced stem cell egress.[792]

Another example of cooperation between cytokines and chemoattractants is provided by the study of G-CSF-R–deficient neutrophils, showing that a functional G-CSF-R is needed for β-integrin activation.[793] In that G-CSF-R knockout model, flt3 ligand mobilizes progenitors, whereas IL-8 fails to do so.[794] Indeed, a functional G-CSF-R is needed to activate β_2-integrins and mediate the CXCL8 (IL-8) activation process, with subsequent gelatinase B release.[795] The inhibitory effects of anti-$\alpha_L\beta_1$ antibodies and the requirement for a functional G-CSF-R imply this mobilization process involves intramedullary activation of neutrophils, leading to enhanced stem cell egress.[792] This localized proteolysis (elastase, gelatinase B) is necessary for active cell migration[796] and is enhanced by cooperating signals from CXCL8-, G-CSF–activated neutrophils adhering to matrix heparan sulfates.[797–800] CD34-positive progenitor cells elaborate gelatinase A and B, a process also augmented by cytokines.[801] Studies in protease-deficient mice reveal both protease-dependent and protease-independent pathways for G-CSF hematopoietic progenitor mobilization.[802]

Stem cell egress is affected by gelatinase expression coupled with altered integrin-, hyaluronan-based anchorage-migration ($\alpha_4\beta_1$/VCAM-1, CD44), by cytokine enhanced blood flow, by $\alpha_M\beta_2$ anchoring,[803] and by E-selectin/chemokine–driven transendothelial migration.[804] This model (see Table 4-5)[804] also takes into account the ability of antibody to gelatinase B and β_2-integrin to block the CXCL8 (IL-8) mobilization cascade. Integrin signaling and cross-talk with CD44 and the localized production of cytokines (such as KIT ligand, flt3 ligand, G-CSF, TPO) create a complex matrix of interactions resulting in up-modulation (or down-regulation) of CD34 active chemokine–chemokine receptors (CXCL12/CXCR4, CXCL8/CXCR2, CCL5/CCR1, CCL3/CCR1, CCL21/CCR7), thereby setting the stage for multiple stem cell mobilization strategies.[748,804] The central role of CXCL12/CXCR4 in anchoring stem cells is underscored by the rapid mobilization of CD34-positive cells following administration of the CXCR4 antagonist AMD3100 to normal subjects and to patients undergoing peripheral blood autologous stem cell transplantation.[804–806] In preclinical models, G-CSF administration combined with chemokine agonists such as AMD3100 augments the peripheral blood progenitor mobilization process.[804] Clinical trials currently underway are testing this hypothesis in normal donors and in patients undergoing autologous or allogeneic peripheral stem cell transplantation. Table 4-5 lists the expression of motility genes, which is characteristic of early stem cells,[807] in keeping with their migration out of the marrow to areas of ischemic injury to mediate localized tissue repair. The process is highly regulated, requiring hypoxia-inducible factor-1 induction of CXCL12 (SDF-1).[808]

REFERENCES

1. Testa NG, Molineux G: *Haemopoiesis: A Practical Approach*. IRL Press at Oxford University Press, New York, 1993.
2. Neuman E: Ueber die Bedeutung des Knochenmarks für die Blutbildung. *Cbl Med Wiss* 6:689, 1868.
3. Bizzozero G: Sulla fungione ematopoietica del midollo delle ossa. *Gazz Med Ital-Lomb*, 46, 1868.
4. Neuman E: Du Role de la möelle des os dans la formation du sang. *C R Acad Sci (Paris)* 68:1112, 1869.
5. Mosler F: Klinische Symptome und Therapie der medullalären Leukemi. *Berl Klin Wochenschr* 13:233, 1876.
6. Arinkin MJ: Die intravitale Untersuchungsmetodik des Knochenmarks. *Folia Haematol Int Mag Klin Morphol Blutforsch (Leipzig)* 38:233, 1929.
7. Lajtha LG: The common ancestral cell, in *Blood Pure and Eloquent*, edited by MM Wintrobe, p 81. McGraw-Hill, New York, 1980.
8. Erslev AJ: Feedback circuits in the control of stem cell differentiation. *Am J Pathol* 65:629, 1971.
9. Trentin JJ: Determination of bone marrow stem cell differentiation by stroma hemopoietic inductive microenvironment (HIM). *Am J Pathol* 65:621, 1971.
10. Lemischka IR, Moore KA: Stem cells: Interactive niches. *Nature* 425:778, 2003.
11. Hackney JA, Charbord P, Brunk BP, et al: A molecular profile of a hematopoietic stem cell niche. *Proc Natl Acad Sci U S A* 99:13061, 2002.
12. Zhang J, Niu C, Ye L, et al: Identification of the haematopoietic stem cell niche and control of the niche size. *Nature* 425:836, 2003.
13. Calvi LM, Adams GB, Weibrecht KW, et al: Osteoblastic cells regulate the haematopoietic stem cell niche. *Nature* 425:841, 2003.
14. Weissman IL, Anderson DJ, Gage F: Stem and progenitor cells: Origins, phenotypes, lineage commitments, and transdifferentiations. *Annu Rev Cell Dev Biol* 17:387, 2001.
15. Dao MA, Arevalo J, Nolta JA: Reversibility of CD34 expression on human hematopoietic stem cells that retain the capacity for secondary reconstitution. *Blood* 112, 2003.
16. Kuci S, Wessels JT, Buhring HJ, et al: Identification of a novel class of human adherent CD34-stem cells that give rise to SCID-repopulating cells. *Blood* 101:869, 2003.
17. Ziegler BL, Valtieri M, Almeida-Porada G, et al: KDR receptor: A key marker defining hematopoietic stem cells. *Science* 285:1553, 1999.
18. Christensen JL, Weissman IL: Flk-2 is a marker in hematopoietic stem cell differentiation: A simple method to isolate long-term stem cells. *Proc Natl Acad Sci U S A* 98:14541, 2001.
19. Bhatia M: AC133 expression in human stem cells. *Leukemia* 15:1686, 2001.
20. Steidl U, Krovenwett R, Rohr UP, et al: Gene expression profiling identifies significant differences between the molecular phenotypes of bone marrow-derived and circulating human CD34+ hematopoietic stem cells. *Blood* 99:2037, 2002.
21. Ivanova NB, Dimos JT, Schaniel C, et al: A stem cell molecular signature. *Science* 298:601, 2002.
22. Bertoncello I, Bradford GB: Surrogate assays for hematopoietic stem cell activity, in *Colony-Stimulating Factors: Molecular and Cellular Biology*, edited by JM Garland, PJ Quesenberry, DJ Hilton, p 35. Marcel Dekker, New York, 1997.
23. Fujisaki T, Berger MG, Rose-John S, Eaves CJ: Rapid differentiation of a rare subset of adult human Lin- CD34- CD38- cells stimulated by multiple growth factors *in vitro*. *Blood* 94:1926, 1999.
24. Punzel M, Wissink SD, Miller JS, et al: The myeloid-lymphoid initiating cell (ML-IC) assay assesses the fate of multipotent human progenitors *in vitro*. *Blood* 93:3750, 1999.
25. Forraz N, Pettengell R, McGuckin CP: Characterization of a lineage-negative stem-progenitor cell population optimized for ex vivo expansion and enriched for LTC-IC. *Stem Cells* 22:100, 2004.
26. Bahtia M, Bonnet D, Murdoch B, et al: A newly discovered class of human hematopoietic cells with SCID-repopulating activity. *Nat Med* 4:1038, 1998.

27. Mazurier F, Doedens M, Gan OI, et al: Rapid myeloerythroid repopulation after intrafemoral transplantation of NOD-SCID mice reveals a new class of human stem cells. *Nat Med* 9:959, 2003.

28. Zanjani ED, Almeida-Porada G, Livingston AG, et al: Reversible expression of CD34 by adult human bone marrow long-term engrafting hematopoietic stem cells. *Exp Hematol* 31:406, 2003.

29. Palis J, Yoder MC: Yolk-sac hematopoiesis: The first blood cells of mouse and man. *Exp Hematol* 29:927, 2001.

30. Godin IE, Garcia-Porrero JA, Coutinho A, et al: Para-aortic splanchnopleura from early mouse embryos contains B1a cell progenitors. *Nature* 364:67, 1993.

31. Baron MH: Embryonic origins of mammalian hematopoiesis. *Exp Hematol* 31:1160, 2003.

32. Galloway JL, Zon LI: Ontogeny of hematopoiesis: Examining the emergence of hematopoietic cells in the vertebrate embryo. *Curr Top Dev Bio* 53:139, 2003.

33. Medvinski A, Dzierzak EA: Definitive hematopoiesis is autonomously initiated by the AGM region. *Cell* 86:897, 1996.

34. Yoder MC, Hiatt K, Dutt P, et al: Characterization of definitive lymphohematopoietic stem cells in the day 9 murine yolk sac. *Immunity* 7:335, 1997.

35. Cumano A, Furlonger C, Paige CG: Differentiation and characterization of B-cell precursors detected in the yolk sac and embryo body of embryos beginning at the 10- to 12-somite stage. *Proc Natl Acad Sci U S A* 90:6429, 1993.

36. Yoder MC, Hiatt K, Mukherjee P: In vivo repopulating hematopoietic stem cells are present in the murine yolk sac at day 9.0 postcoitus. *Proc Natl Acad Sci U S A* 94:6776, 1997.

37. Palis J, Chan RJ, Koniski A, et al: Spatial and temporal emergence of high proliferative potential hematopoietic precursors during murine embryogenesis. *Proc Natl Acad Sci U S A* 98:4528, 2001.

38. Ogawa M, Nishikawa S, Yoshinaga K, et al: Expression and function of c-Kit in fetal hemopoietic progenitor cells: Transition from the early c-Kit-independent to the late c-Kit-dependent wave of hematopoiesis in the murine embryo. *Development* 117:1089, 1993.

39. Ortiz M, Wine JW, Lohrey N, et al: Functional characterization of a novel hematopoietic stem cell and its place in the c-Kit maturation pathway in bone marrow cell development. *Immunity* 10:173, 1999.

40. Matsui Y, Zsebo K, Hogan BL: Derivation of pluripotential embryonic stem cells from murine primordial germ cells in culture. *Cell* 70:841, 1992.

41. Conquet F, Brulet P: Developmental expression of myeloid leukemia inhibitory factor gene in preimplantation blastocysts and in extraembryonic tissue of mouse embryos. *Mol Cell Biol* 10:3801, 1990.

42. Xu MJ, Tsuji K, Ueda T, et al: Stimulation of mouse and human primitive hematopoiesis by murine embryonic aorta-gonad-mesonephros-derived stromal cell lines. *Blood* 92:2032, 1998.

43. Ohneda O, Fennie C, Zheng Z, et al: Hematopoietic stem cell maintenance and differentiation are supported by embryonic aorta-gonad-mesonephros region-derived endothelium. *Blood* 92:908, 1998.

44. Verfaille CM: Soluble factor(s) produced by human bone marrow stroma increase cytokine-induced proliferation and maturation of primitive hematopoietic progenitors while preventing their terminal differentiation. *Blood* 82:2045, 1993.

45. Lacaud G, Kouskoff V, Trumble A, et al: Haploinsufficiency of Runx1 results in the acceleration of mesodermal development and hemangioblast specification upon in vitro differentiation of ES cells. *Blood* 103:886, 2004.

46. Lorsbach RB, Moore J, Ang SO, et al: Role of RUNX1 in adult hematopoiesis: Analysis of RUNX1-IRES-GFP knock-in mice reveals differential lineage expression. *Blood* 103:2522, 2004.

47. North TE, Stacy T, Matheny CJ, et al: Runx1 is expressed in adult mouse hematopoietic stem cells and differentiating myeloid and lymphoid cells, but not in maturing erythroid cells. *Stem Cells* 22:158, 2004.

48. Lacaud G, Robertson S, Palis J, et al: Regulation of hemangioblast development. *Ann N Y Acad Sci* 938:96, 2001.

49. Wang LC, Swat W, Fujiwara Y, et al: The TEL/ETV6 gene is required specifically for hematopoiesis in the bone marrow. *Genes Dev* 12:2392, 1998.

50. Moore KA, Pytowski B, Witte L, et al: Hematopoietic activity of a stromal cell transmembrane protein containing epidermal growth factor-like repeat motifs. *Proc Natl Acad Sci U S A* 94:4011, 1997.

51. Laborda J: The role of the epidermal growth factor-like protein dlk in cell differentiation. *Histol Histopathol* 15:119, 2000.

52. Moore KA, Lin L: Comparative expression analyses of hematopoietic stem cell supporting stromal cell lines. *Blood* 102(part 1):361a, 1312, 2003.

53. Ohishi K, Katayama N, Shiku H, et al: Notch signaling in hematopoiesis. *Semin Cell Dev Biol* 14:143, 2003.

54. Murdoch B, Chadwick K, Martin M, et al: Wnt-5A augments repopulating capacity and primitive hematopoietic development of human blood stem cells in vivo. *Proc Natl Acad Sci U S A* 100:3422, 2003.

55. Bhardwaj G, Murdoch B, Wu D, et al: Sonic hedgehog induces the proliferation of primitive human hematopoietic cells via BMP regulation. *Nat Immunol* 2:172, 2001.

56. Ara T, Tokoyada K, Sugiyama T, et al: Long-term hematopoietic stem cells require stromal cell-derived factor-1 for colonizing bone marrow during ontogeny. *Immunity* 19:257, 2003.

57. Dormandy SP, Bashayan O, Dougherty R, et al: Immortalized multipotential mesenchymal cells and the hematopoietic microenvironment. *J Hematother Stem Cell Res* 10:125, 2001.

58. Charbord P, Oostendorp R, Pang W, et al: Comparative study of stromal cell lines derived from embryonic, fetal, and postnatal mouse blood-forming tissues. *Exp Hematol* 30:1202, 2002.

59. Fukushima N, Nishina H, Koishihara Y, Ohkawa H: Enhanced hematopoiesis in vivo and in vitro by splenic stromal cells derived from the mouse with recombinant granulocyte colony-stimulating factor. *Blood* 80:1914, 1992.

60. Islam A, Glomski C, Henderson ES: Endothelial cells and hematopoiesis: A light microscopic study of fetal, normal, and pathologic human bone marrow in plastic-embedded sections. *Anat Rec* 233:440, 1992.

61. Hamaguchi I, Huang X-L, Takakura N, et al: In vitro hematopoietic and endothelial cell development from cells expressing TEK receptor in murine aorta-gonad-mesonephros region. *Blood* 93:1549, 1999.

62. Hara T, Nakano Y-K, Tanaka M, et al: Identification of podocalyxin-like protein 1 as a novel cell surface marker for hemangioblasts in the murine aorta-gonad-mesonephros region. *Immunity* 11:567, 1999.

63. Ogawa M, Kizumoto M, Nishikawa S, et al: Expression of α4-integrin defines the earliest precursor of hematopoietic cell lineage diverged from endothelial cells. *Blood* 93:1168, 1999.

64. Kuci S, Wessels JT, Buhring HJ, et al: Identification of a novel class of human adherent CD34- stem cells that give rise to SCID-repopulating cells. *Blood* 101:869, 2003.

65. Almeida-Porada GD, Hoffman R, Manalo P, et al: Detection of human cells in human/sheep chimeric lambs with in vitro human stroma-forming potential. *Exp Hematol* 24:482, 1996.

66. Gallacher L, Murdoch B, Wu DM, et al: Isolation and characterization of human CD34(-)Lin(-) and CD34(+)Lin(-) hematopoietic stem cells using cell surface markers AC133 and CD7. *Blood* 95:2813, 2000.

67. Gehling UM, Ergun S, Schumacher U, et al: In vitro differentiation of endothelial cells from AC133-positive progenitor cells. *Blood* 95:3106, 2000.

68. Takakura N, Watanabe T, Suenobu S, et al: A role for hematopoietic stem cells in promoting angiogenesis. *Cell* 102:199, 2000.

69. Wang L, Li L, Shojaei F, et al: Endothelial and hematopoietic cell fate of human embryonic stem cells originates from primitive endothelium with hemangioblastic properties. *Immunity* 21:31, 2004.

70. Cogle CR, Wainman DA, Jorgensen ML, et al: Adult human hematopoietic cells provide functional hemangioblast activity. *Blood* 103:133, 2004.

71. Bailey AS, Jiang S, Afentoulis M, et al: Transplanted adult hematopoietic stems cells differentiate into functional endothelial cells. *Blood* 103:13, 2004.

72. McGrath KE, Koniski AD, Malik J, Palis J: Circulation is established in a stepwise pattern in the mammalian embryo. *Blood* 101:1669, 2003.

73. Nadin BM, Goodell MA, Hirschi KK: Phenotype and hematopoietic potential of side population cells throughout embryonic development. *Blood* 102:2436, 2003.

74. Scharenberg CW, Harkey MA, Tork-Storb B: The ABCG2 transporter is an efficient Hoechst 33342 efflux pump and is preferentially expressed by immature human progenitors. *Blood* 99:507, 2002.

75. Pearce DJ, Ridler CM, Simpson C, Bonnet D: Multiparameter analysis of murine bone marrow side population cells. *Blood* 103:2541, 2004.

76. Eaker SS, Hawley TS, Ramezani A, Hawley RG: Detection and enrichment of hematopoietic stem cells by side population phenotype. *Methods Mol Biol* 263:161, 2004.

77. Jackson KA, Mi T, Goodell MA: Hematopoietic potential of stem cells isolated from murine skeletal muscle. *Proc Natl Acad Sci U S A* 96:14482, 1999.

78. Bjornson CR, Rietze RL, Reynolds BA, et al: Turning brain into blood: A hematopoietic fate adopted by adult neural stem cells in vivo. *Science* 283:534, 1999.

79. Majka SM, Jackson KA, Kienstra KA, et al: Distinct progenitor populations in skeletal muscle are bone marrow derived and exhibit different cell fates during vascular regeneration. *J Clin Invest* 111:71, 2003.

80. Ahdjoudj S, Fromigue O, Marie PJ: Plasticity and regulation of human bone marrow stromal osteoprogenitor cells: Potential implication in the treatment of age-related bone loss. *Histol Histopathol* 19:151, 2004.

81. Chapel A, Bertho JM, Bensidhoum M, et al: Mesenchymal stem cells home to injured tissues when co-infused with hematopoietic cells to treat a radiation-induced multi-organ failure syndrome. *J Gene Med* 5:1028, 2003.

82. Orlic D: Adult bone marrow stem cells regenerate myocardium in ischemic heart disease. *Ann N Y Acad Sci* 996:152, 2003.

83. Jiang Y, Vaessen B, Lenvik T, et al: Multipotent progenitor cells can be isolated from postnatal murine bone marrow, muscle, and brain. *Exp Hematol* 30:896, 2002.

84. Zhao LR, Duan WM, Reyes M, et al: Human bone marrow stem cells exhibit neural phenotypes and ameliorate neurological deficits after grafting into the ischemic brain of rats. *Exp Neurol* 174:11, 2002.

85. Yamamoto N, Terai S, Ohata S, et al: A subpopulation of bone marrow cells depleted by a novel antibody, anti-Liv8, is useful for cell therapy to repair damaged liver. *Biochem Biophys Res Commun* 313:1110, 2004.

86. Kashiwakura Y, Katoh Y, Tamayose K, et al: Isolation of bone marrow stromal cell-derived smooth muscle cells by a human SM22alpha promoter: In vitro differentiation of putative smooth muscle progenitor cells of bone marrow. *Circulation* 107:2078, 2003.

87. Geiger H, True JM, Grimes B, et al: Analysis of the hematopoietic potential of muscle-derived cells in mice. *Blood* 100:721, 2002.

88. Issarachai S, Priestley GV, Nakamoto B, Papayannopoulou T: Cells with hemopoietic potential residing in muscle are itinerant bone marrow-derived cells. *Exp Hematol* 30:366, 2002.

89. Ratajczak MZ, Kucia M, Reca R, et al: Stem cell plasticity revisited: CXCR4-positive cells expressing mRNA for early muscle, liver and neural cells "hide out" in the bone marrow. *Leukemia* 18:29, 2004.

90. Wagers AJ, Sherwood RI, Christensen JL, Weissman IL: Little evidence for developmental plasticity of adult hematopoietic stem cells. *Science* 297:2256, 2002.

91. Wang X, Willenbring H, Akkari Y, et al: Cell fusion is the principal source of bone-marrow-derived hepatocytes. *Nature* 422:897, 2003.

92. Alvarez-Dolado M, Pardal R, Garcia-Verdugo JM, et al: Fusion of bone-marrow-derived cells with Purkinje neurons, cardiomyocytes and hepatocytes. *Nature* 425:968, 2003.

93. Camargo FD, Chambers SM, Goodell MA: Stem cell plasticity: From transdifferentiation to macrophage fusion. *Cell Prolif* 37:55, 2004.

94. Abedi M, Greer DA, Colvin GA, et al: Tissue injury in marrow transdifferentiation. *Blood Cells Mol Dis* 32:42, 2004.

95. Quesenberry PJ, Abedi M, Aliotta J, et al: Stem cell plasticity: An overview. *Blood Cells Mol Dis* 32:1, 2004.

96. Heike T, Nakahata T: Stem cell plasticity in the hematopoietic system. *Int J Hematol* 79:7, 2004.

97. Hudson G: Bone marrow volume in the human fetus and newborn. *Br J Haematol* 11:446, 1965.

98. Nagasawa T, Hirota S, Tachibana K, et al: Defects of B-cell lymphopoiesis and bone marrow myelopoiesis in mice lacking the CXC chemokine PBSF/SDF-1. *Nature* 382:635, 1996.

99. Imai K, Kobayashi M, Wang J, et al: Selective transendothelial migration of hematopoietic progenitor cells: A role in homing of progenitor cells. *Blood* 93:149, 1999.

100. Arroyo AG, Yang JT, Rayburn H, et al: α4 integrins regulate the proliferation/differentiation balance of multilineage hematopoietic progenitors in vivo. *Immunity* 11:555, 1999.

101. Roy V, Verfaille CM: Expression and function of cell adhesion molecules on fetal liver, cord blood and bone marrow hematopoietic progenitors: Implications for anatomical localization and developmental stage specific regulation of hematopoiesis. *Exp Hematol* 27:302, 1999.

102. Custer RP, Ahlfeldt FE: Studies on the structure and function of the bone marrow. *J Lab Clin Med* 17:960, 1932.

103. Gregersen MI, Rawson RA: Blood volume. *Physiol Rev* 39:307, 1969.

104. Christy M: Active marrow distribution as a function of age in humans. *Phys Med Biol* 26:389, 1981.

105. Babyn PS, Ranson M, McCarvelle ME: Normal bone marrow signal characteristics and fatty conversion. *Med Clin North Am* 6:473, 1998.

106. Huggins C, Blocksom BH Jr: Changes in outlying bone marrow accompanying a local increase in temperature within physiologic limits. *J Exp Med* 64:253, 1936.

107. Maniatis A, Tavassoli M, Crosby WH: Factors affecting the conversion of yellow to red marrow. *Blood* 37:581, 1971.

108. Crosby WH: Experience with injured and implanted bone marrow: Relation of function to structure, in *Hemopoietic Cellular Proliferation*, edited by F Stohlman Jr, p 87. Grune & Stratton, New York, 1970.

109. Ji X, Chen D, Xu C, et al: Patterns of gene expression associated with BMP-2-induced osteoblast and adipocyte differentiation of mesenchymal progenitor cell 3T3-F442A. *J Bone Miner Metab* 18:132, 2000.

110. Martin RB, Chow BD, Lucas PA: Bone marrow fat content in relation to bone remodeling and serum chemistry in intact and ovariectomized dogs. *Calcif Tissue Int* 46:189, 1990.

111. Brookes M: *The Blood Supply of Bone*. Butterworth, London, 1971.

112. Tavassoli M: Arterial structure of the bone marrow in rabbits with special reference to thin walled arteries. *Acta Anat (Basel)* 90:608, 1974.

113. Wilkins BS, Jones DB: Vascular networks within the stroma of human long-term bone marrow cultures. *J Pathol* 177:295, 1995.

114. Charbord P, Tavian M, Humeau L, Peault B: Early ontogeny of the human marrow from long bones: An immunohistochemical study of hematopoiesis and its microenvironment. *Blood* 87:4109, 1996.

115. Eichman A, Corbel C, Nataf V, et al: Ligand-dependent development of the endothelial and hematopoietic lineages from embryonic mesodermal cells expressing vascular endothelial growth factor receptor 2. *Proc Natl Acad Sci U S A* 94:141, 1997.

116. Marshall CJ, Moore RL, Thorogood P, et al: Detailed characterization of the human aorta-gonad-mesonephros region reveals morphological polarity resembling a hematopoietic stromal layer. *Dev Dyn* 215:139, 1999.

117. Peichev M, Naiyer AJ, Pereira D, et al: Expression of VEGFR-2 and AC133 by circulating human CD34(+) cells identifies a population of functional endothelial precursors. *Blood* 95:952, 2000.

118. Hildebrand P, Cirulli V, Prinsen RC, et al: The role of angiopoietins in the development of endothelial cells from cord blood CD34+ progenitors. *Blood* 104:2010, 2004.

119. Wijelath ES, Rahman S, Murray J, et al: Fibronectin promotes VEGF-induced CD34 cell differentiation into endothelial cells. *J Vasc Surg* 39: 655, 2004.

120. Lichtman MA: The ultrastructure of the hemopoietic environment of the marrow: A review. *Exp Hematol* 9:391, 1981.

121. Yamazaki K, Allen TD: Ultrastructural morphometric study of efferent nerve terminals on murine bone marrow stromal cells, and the recognition of a novel anatomical unit: The "neuro-reticular complex." *Am J Anat* 187:261, 1990.

122. Artico M, Bosco S, Cavallotti C, et al: Noradrenergic and cholinergic innervation of the bone marrow. *Int J Mol Med* 10:77, 2002.

123. Goto T, Yamaza T, Kido MA, et al: Light- and electron microscopy study of the distribution of axon containing substance-P and the localization of neurokinin-1 receptor in bone. *Cell Tissue Res* 293:87, 1998.

124. Chenu C: Glutaminergic innervation in bone. *Microsc Res Tech* 58:70, 2002.

125. Cattoretti G, Schiro R, Orazi A, et al: Bone marrow stroma in humans: Anti-nerve growth factor receptor antibodies selectively stain reticular cells *in vivo* and *in vitro*. *Blood* 81:1726, 1993.

126. Rameshwar P, Gascon P: Substance P (SP) mediates production of stem cell factor and interleukin-1 in bone marrow stroma: Potential autoregulatory role for these cytokines in SP receptor expression and induction. *Blood* 86:482, 1995.

127. Rameshwar P, Zhu G, Donelly RJ, et al: The dynamics of bone marrow stromal cells in the proliferation of multipotent hematopoietic progenitors by substance P: An understanding of the effects of a neurotransmitter on the differentiating hematopoietic stem cell. *J Neuroimmunol* 121:22, 2001.

128. Hiramoto M, Aizawa S, Iwase O, et al: Stimulatory effects of substance P on CD34 positive cell proliferation and differentiation in vitro are mediated by the modulation of stromal cell function. *Int J Mol Med* 1: 347, 1998.

129. Greeno EW, Mantyh P, Vercellotti GM, Moldow CF: Functional neurokin 1 receptors for substance P are expressed by human vascular endothelium. *J Exp Med* 177:1269, 1993.

130. Pelletier L, Angonin R, Regnard J, et al: Human bone marrow angiogenesis: In vitro modulation by substance P and neurokinin A. *Br J Haematol* 119:1083, 2002.

131. Tang Y, Shankar R, Gamelli R, Jones S: Dynamic norepinephrine alterations in bone marrow: Evidence of functional innervation. *J Neuroimmunol* 96:182, 1999.

132. Iversen PO, Nicolaysen G, Benestad HB: Endogenous nitric oxide causes vasodilatation in rat bone marrow, bone, and spleen during accelerated hematopoiesis. *Exp Hematol* 22:1297, 1994.

133. Afran AM, Broome CS, Nicholls SE, et al: Bone marrow innervation regulates cellular retention in the murine haematopoietic system. *Br J Haematol* 98:569, 1997.

134. Maestroni GJM, Conti A, Pedrinis E: Effect of adrenergic agents on hematopoiesis after syngeneic bone marrow transplantation in mice. *Blood* 80:1178, 1992.

135. Abboud CN, Liesveld JL, Lichtman MA: The architecture of marrow and its role in hematopoietic cell lodgement, in *The Hematopoietic Microenvironment*, edited by MW Long, MS Wicha, p 2. Johns Hopkins University Press, Baltimore and London, 1993.

136. Tavassoli M, Shaklai M: Absence of tight junctions in endothelium of marrow sinuses: Possible significance for marrow cell egress. *Br J Haematol* 41:303, 1979.

137. Bankston PW, DeBruyn PPH: The permeability to carbon of the sinusoidal lining cells of the embryonic rat liver and rat bone marrow. *Am J Anat* 141:281, 1974.

138. Lichtman MA, Packman CH, Constine LS: Molecular and cellular traffic across the marrow sinus wall, in *Blood Cell Formation: The Role of Hemopoietic Microenvironment*, edited by M. Tavassoli, p 87. Humana Press, Clifton, NJ, 1989.

139. Kataoka M, Tavassoli M: Identification of lectin-like substances recognizing galactosyl residues of glycoconjugates on the plasma membrane of marrow sinus endothelium. *Blood* 65:1163, 1985.

140. Bussolino F, Colotta F, Bocchietto E, et al: Recent developments in the cell biology of granulocyte-macrophage colony-stimulating factor and granulocyte colony-stimulating factor: Activities on endothelial cells. *Int J Clin Lab Res* 23:8, 1993.

141. Koch AE, Burrows JC, Domer PH, et al: Monoclonal antibodies defining shared human macrophage-endothelial antigens. *Pathobiology* 60:59, 1992.

142. Penn PE, Jiang D-Z, Fei R-G, et al: Dissecting the hematopoietic microenvironment: IX. Further characterization of murine bone marrow stromal cells. *Blood* 81:1205, 1993.

143. Hasthorpe S, Bogdanovski M, Rogerson J, Radley JM: Characterization of endothelial cells in murine long-term marrow culture: Implication for hemopoietic regulation. *Exp Hematol* 20:386, 1992.

144. Perkins S, Fleischman RA: Stromal cell progeny of murine bone marrow fibroblast colony-forming units are clonal endothelial-like cells that express collagen IV and laminin. *Blood* 75:620, 1990.

145. van Buul JD, Mul FP, Van der Schoot CE, Hordijk PL: ICAM-3 activation modulates cell-cell contacts of human bone marrow endothelial cells. *J Vasc Res* 41:28, 2004.

146. Schweitzer KM, Drager AM, Van der Valk P, et al: Constitutive expression of E-selectin and vascular cell adhesion molecule-1 on endothelial cells of hematopoietic tissues. *Am J Pathol* 148:165, 1996.

147. Masek LC, Sweetenham JW, Whitehouse JMA, Schumacher U: Immuno-, lectin-, and enzyme-histochemical characterization of human bone marrow endothelium. *Exp Hematol* 22:1203, 1994.

148. Rafii S, Shapiro F, Rimarachin J, et al: Isolation and characterization of human bone marrow microvascular endothelial cells: Hematopoietic progenitor adhesion. *Blood* 84:10, 1994.

149. Villars F, Guillotin B, Amedee T, et al: Effect of HUVEC on human osteoprogenitor cell differentiation needs heterotypic gap junction communication. *Am J Physiol Cell Physiol* 282:C775, 2002.

150. Guillotin B, Bourget C, Remy-Zolgadri M, et al: Human primary endothelial cells stimulate human osteoprogenitor cell differentiation. *Cell Physiol Biochem* 14:325, 2004.

151. Mohle R, Salemi P, Moore MA, Rafii S: Expression of interleukin-5 by human bone marrow microvascular endothelail cells: Implications for the regulation of eosinophilopoiesis in vivo. *Br J Haematol* 99:732, 1997.

152. Huang WQ, Wang QR: Bone marrow endothelial cells secrete thymosin beta4 and AcSDKP. *Exp Hematol* 29:12, 2001.

153. Bordenave L, Georges A, Bareille R, et al: Human bone marrow endothelial cells: A new identified source of B-type natriuretic peptide. *Peptides* 23:935, 2002.

154. Delia D, Lampugnani MG, Resnati M, et al: CD34 expression is regulated reciprocally with adhesion molecules in vascular cells in vitro. *Blood* 81:1001, 1993.

155. Guo WX, Ghebrehiwet B, Weksler B, et al: Up-regulation of endothelial cell binding proteins/receptors for complement component C1q by inflammatory cytokines. *J Lab Clin Med* 133:541, 1999.

156. van Buul JD, Voermans C, Van den Berg V, et al: Migration of human hematopoietic progenitor cells across bone marrow endothelium is regulated by vascular endothelial cadherin. *J Immunol* 168:588, 2002.

157. Netelenbos T, Van den Born J, Kessler FL, et al: In vitro model for hematopoietic progenitor cell homing reveals endothelial heparan sulfate proteoglycans as direct adhesive ligands. *J Leukoc Biol* 74:1035, 2003.

158. Netelenbos T, Van den Born J, Kessler FL, et al: Proteoglycans on bone marrow endothelial cells bind and present SDF-1 towards hematopoietic progenitor cells. *Leukemia* 17:175, 2003.

159. Hillyer P, Mordelet E, Flynn G, Male D: Chemokines, chemokine receptors and adhesion molecules on different human endothelia: Discriminating the tissue-specific functions that affect leucocyte migration. *Clin Exp Immunol* 134:431, 2003.

160. Yun HJ, Jo DY: Production of stromal cell-derived factor-1 (SDF-1) and expression of CXCR4 in human bone marrow endothelial cells. *J Korean Med Sci* 18:679, 2003.

161. Imai T, Hieshima K, Haskell C, et al: Identification and molecular characterization of fractalkine receptor CX3CR1, which mediates both leukocyte migration and adhesion. *Cell* 91:521, 1997.

162. Nitschke L, Floyd H, Ferguson DJ, Crocker PR: Identification of CD22 ligands on bone marrow sinusoidal endothelium implicated in CD22-dependent homing of recirculating B cells *J Exp Med* 189:1513, 1999.

163. Weiss L, Chen L-T: The organization of hemopoietic cords and vascular sinuses in bone marrow. *Blood Cells* 1:617, 1975.

164. Leblond PF, Chamberlain JK, Weed RI: Scanning electron microscopy of erythropoietin-stimulated bone marrow. *Blood Cells* 1:639, 1975.

165. Abboud CN, Duerst RE, Frantz CN, et al: Lysis of human fibroblast colony-forming cells and endothelial cells by monoclonal antibody (6-19) and complement. *Blood* 68:1196, 1986.

166. Simmons PJ, Torok-Storb B: Identification of stromal cell precursors in human bone marrow by a novel monoclonal antibody, STRO-1. *Blood* 78:55, 1991.

167. Labouyrie E, Dubus P, Groppi A, et al: Expression of neurotrophins and their receptors in human bone marrow. *Am J Pathol* 154:405, 1999.

168. Gronthos S, Simmons PJ: The growth factor requirements of STRO-1-positive human bone marrow stromal precursors under serum-deprived conditions in vitro. *Blood* 85:929, 1995.

169. Galmiche MC, Koteliansky VE, Briere J, et al: Stromal cells from human long-term marrow cultures are mesenchymal cells that differentiate following a vascular smooth muscle differentiation pathway. *Blood* 82:66, 1993.

170. Dennis JE, Charbord P: Origin and differentiation of human and murine stroma. *Stem Cells* 20:205, 2002.

171. Brown J, Greaves MF, Molgaard HV: The gene encoding the stem cell antigen, CD34, is conserved in mouse and expressed in haemopoietic progenitor cell lines, brain, and embryonic fibroblasts. *Int Immunol* 3:175, 1991.

172. Simmons PJ, Torok-Storb B: CD34 expression by stromal precursors in normal adult bone marrow. *Blood* 78:2848, 1991.

173. Dorshkind K, Green L, Godwin A, Fletcher WH: Connexin-43-type gap junctions mediate communication between bone marrow stromal cells. *Blood* 82:38, 1993.

174. Montecino RE, Leathers H, Dorshkind K: Expression of connexin 43 (Gx43) is critical for normal hematopoiesis. *Blood* 96:917, 2000.

175. Durig J, Rosenthal C, Halfmeyer K, et al: Intercellular communication between bone marrow stromal cell and CD34+ haematopoietic progenitor cells is mediated by connexin 43-type gap junctions. *Br J Haematol* 111:416, 2000.

176. Rosendaal M, Jopling C: Hematopoietic capacity of connexin43 wild-type and knock-out fetal liver cells not different on wild-type stroma. *Blood* 101:2996, 2003.

177. Torok-Storb B, Iwata M, Graf L, et al: Dissecting the marrow microenvironment. *Ann N Y Acad Sci* 872:164, 1999.

178. Weiss L, Geduldig U: Barrier cells: Stromal regulation of hematopoiesis and blood cell release in normal and stressed murine bone marrow. *Blood* 78:975, 1991.

179. Tavassoli M: Fatty evolution of marrow and the role of adipose tissue in hematopoiesis, in *Handbook of the Hemopoietic Microenvironment*, edited by M Tavassoli, p 157. Humana Press, Clifton, NJ, 1989.

180. Dominici M, Hofmann TJ, Horwitz EM: Bone marrow mesenchymal cells: Biological properties and clinical applications. *J Biol Regul Homeost Agents* 15:28, 2001.

181. D'Ippolito G, Diabira S, Howard GA, et al: Marrow-isolated adult multilineage inducible (MIAMI) cells, a unique population of postnatal young and old human cells with extensive expansion and differentiation potential. *J Cell Sci* 117:2971, 2004.

182. Seshi B, Kumar S, King D: Multilineage gene expression in human bone marrow stromal cells as evidenced by single-cell microarray analysis. *Blood Cells Mol Dis* 31:268, 2003.

183. Moore KA: Recent advances in defining the hematopoietic stem cell niche. *Curr Opin Hematol* 11:107, 2004.

184. Laharrague P, Larrouy D, Fontanilles AM, et al: High expression of leptin by human bone marrow adipocytes in primary cultures. *FASEB J* 12:747, 1998.

185. Benayahu D, Shamay A, Wientroub S: Osteocalcin (BGP), gene expression, and protein production by marrow stromal adipocytes. *Biochem Biophys Res Commun* 13:442, 1997.

186. McAveny KM, Gimble JM, Yu-Lee L: Prolactin receptor expression during adipocyte differentiation of bone marrow stroma. *Endocrinology* 137:5723, 1996.

187. Delikat S, Harris RJ, Galvani DW: Il.-1 beta inhibits adipocyte formation in human long-term bone marrow culture. *Exp Hematol* 21:31, 1993.

188. Keller DC, Du XX, Srour EF, et al: Interleukin-11 inhibits adipogenesis and stimulates myelopoiesis in human long-term marrow cultures. *Blood* 82:1428, 1993.

189. Fantuzzi G, Faggioni R: Leptin in the regulation of immunity, inflammation, and hematopoiesis. *J Leukoc Biol* 68:437, 2000.

190. Yokota T, Meka CS, Kouro T, et al: Adiponectin, a fat cell product, influences the earliest lymphocyte precursors in bone marrow cultures by activation of the cyclooxygenase-prostaglandin pathway in stromal cells. *J Immunol* 171:5091, 2003.

191. Thomas T, Gori F, Khosla S, et al: Leptin acts on human marrow stromal cells to enhance differentiation to osteoblasts and to inhibit differentiation to adipocytes. *Endocrinology* 140:1630, 1999.

192. Yokota T, Meka CS, Medina KL, et al: Paracrine regulation of fat cell formation in bone marrow cultures via adiponectin and prostaglandins. *J Clin Invest* 109:1303, 2002.

193. Yokota T, Meka CS, Kouro T, et al: Adiponectin, a fat cell product, influences the earliest lymphocyte precursors in bone marrow cultures by activation of the cyclooxygenase-protaglandin pathway in stromal cells. *J Immunol* 171:5091, 2003.

194. Brakenhielm E, Veitonmaki N, Cao R, et al: Adiponectin-induced antiangiogenesis and antitumor activity involve caspase-mediated endothelial cell apoptosis. *Proc Natl Acad Sci U S A* 101:2476, 2004.

195. Zhou S, Eid K, Glowacki J: Cooperation between TGF-beta and Wnt pathways during chondrocyte and adipocyte differentiation of human marrow stromal cells. *J Bone Miner Res* 19:463, 2004.

196. Gimble JM, Morgan C, Kelly K, et al: Bone morphogenetic proteins inhibit adipocyte differentiation by bone marrow stromal cells. *J Cell Biochem* 58:393, 1995.

197. Chen TL, Shen WJ, Kraemer FB: Human BMP-7/OP-1 induces the growth and differentiation of adipocytes and osteoblasts in bone marrow stromal cell cultures. *J Cell Biochem* 82:187, 2001.

198. Li X, Cui Q, Kao C, et al: Lovastatin inhibits adipogenic and stimulates osteogenic differentiation by suppressing PPARgamma2 and increasing Cbfa1/Runx2 expression in bone marrow mesenchymal cell cultures. *Bone* 33:652, 2003.

199. Gevers EF, Loveridge N, Robinson IC: Bone marrow adipocytes: A ne-glected target tissue for growth hormone. *Endocrinology* 143:4065, 2002.

200. Duque G, Macoritto M, Kremer R: 1,25(OH)2D3 inhibits bone marrow adipogenesis in senescence accelerated mice (SAM-P/6) by decreasing the expression of peroxisome proliferators-activated receptor gamma 2 (PPARgamma2). *Exp Gerontol* 39:333, 2004.

201. Okazaki R, Inoue D, Shibata M, et al: Estrogen promotes early osteo-blast differentiation and inhibits adipocyte differentiation in mouse bone marrow stromal cell lines that express estrogen receptor (ER) alpha or beta. *Endocrinology* 143:2349, 2002.

202. Nuttal ME, Gimble JM: Controlling the balance between osteoblasto-genesis and adipogenesis and the consequent therapeutic implications. *Curr Opin Pharmacol* 4:290, 2004.

203. Lichtman MA: The relationship of stromal cells to hemopoietic cells in marrow, in *Long-Term Bone Marrow Culture*, edited by DG Wright, JS Greenberger, p 3. Liss, New York, 1984.

204. Seshi B, Kumar S, Sellers D: Human bone marrow stromal cell: Coex-pression of markers specific for multiple mesenchymal cell lineages. *Blood Cells Mol Dis* 26:234, 2000.

205. Wilkins BS, Jones DB: Immunophenotypic characterization of stromal cells in aspirated human bone marrow samples. *Exp Hematol* 26:1061, 1998.

206. Takahashi GW, Moran D, Andrews DF III, Singer JW: Differential ex-pression of collagenase by human fibroblasts and bone marrow stromal cells. *Leukemia* 8:305, 1994.

207. Liesveld JL, Abboud CN, Duerst RE, et al: Characterization of human marrow stromal cells: Role in progenitor cell binding and granulo-poiesis. *Blood* 73:1794, 1989.

208. Li J, Sensebe L, Herve P, Charbord P: Nontransformed colony-derived stromal cell lines from normal human marrows: III. The maintenance of hematopoiesis from CD34+ cell populations. *Exp Hematol* 25:582, 1997.

209. Osmond DG, Kim N, Manoukina R, et al: Dynamics and localization of early B-lymphocyte precursor cells (pro-B cells) in the bone marrow of scid mice. *Blood* 79:1695, 1992.

210. Moreau I, Duvert V, Caux C, et al: Myofibroblastic stromal cells isolated from human bone marrow induce the proliferation of both early myeloid and B lymphoid cells. *Blood* 82:2396, 1993.

211. Tamir M, Eren R, Globerson A, et al: Selective accumulation of lym-phocyte precursor cells mediated by stromal cells of hemopoietic origin. *Exp Hematol* 18:332, 1990.

212. Lisovsky M, Braun SE, Ge Y, et al: Flt3-ligand production by human bone marrow stromal cells. *Leukemia* 10:1012, 1996.

213. Besmer P: Kit-ligand-stem cell factor, in *Colony-Stimulating Factors: Molecular and Cellular Biology*, edited by JM Garland, PJ Quesenberry, DJ Hilton, p 369. Marcel Dekker, New York, 1997.

214. Guerriero A, Worford L, Holland HK, et al: Thrombopoietin is synthe-sized by bone marrow stromal cells. *Blood* 90:3444, 1997.

215. Waring PM: Leukemia inhibitory factor, in *Colony-Stimulating Factors: Molecular and Cellular Biology*, edited by JM Garland, PJ Quesenberry, DJ Hilton, p 467. Marcel Dekker, New York, 1997.

216. Rodriguez Mdel C, Bernad A, Aracil M: Interleukin-6 deficiency affects bone marrow stromal precursors, resulting in defective hematopoietic support. *Blood* 103:3349, 2004.

217. Ueda T, Tsuji K, Yoshino H, et al: Expansion of human NOD/SCID-repopulating cells by stem cell factor, Flk2/Flt3 ligand, thrombopoietin, Il-6, and soluble Il-6 receptor. *J Clin Invest* 105:1013, 2000.

218. Iwata M, Graf L, Awaya N, Torok-Storb B: Functional interleukin-7 receptors (IL-7Rs) are expressed by marrow stromal cells: Binding of IL-7 increases levels of IL-6 mRNA and secreted protein. *Blood* 100:1318, 2002.

219. Abboud SL, Bethel CR, Aron DC: Secretion of insulinlike growth factor I and insulinlike growth factor-binding proteins by murine bone marrow stromal cells. *J Clin Invest* 88:470, 1991.

220. Dormady SP, Zhang X-M, Basch RS: Hematopoietic progenitor cells grow on 3T3 fibroblast monolayers that overexpress growth arrest-spe-cific gene-6 (GAS6). *Proc Natl Acad Sci U S A* 97:12260, 2000.

221. Hidalgo A, Sanz-Rodriguez F, Rodriguez-Fernandez JL, et al: Chemo-kine stromal cell-derived factor-1alpha modulates VLA-4 integrin-de-pendent adhesion to fibronectin and VCAM-1 on bone marrow hema-topoietic progenitor cells. *Exp Hematol* 29:345, 2001.

222. Heberlein C, Friel J, Laker C, et al: Downregulation of c-kit (stem cell factor receptor) in transformed hematopoietic precursor cells by stroma cells. *Blood* 93:554, 1999.

223. Walker L, Lynch M, Silverman S, et al: The Notch/Jagged pathway inhibits proliferation of human hematopoietic progenitors in vitro. *Stem Cells* 17:162, 1999.

224. Van Den Berg DJ, Sharma AK, Bruno E, Hoffman R: Role of members of the Wnt gene family in human hematopoiesis. *Blood* 92:89, 1998.

225. Tordjman R, Ortega N, Coulombel L, et al: Neuropilin-1 is expressed on bone marrow stromal cells: A novel interaction with hematopoietic cells? *Blood* 94:2301, 1999.

226. Filshie RJ, Zannettino AC, Makrynikola V, et al: MUC18, a member of the immunoglobulin superfamily, is expressed on bone marrow fibro-blasts and a subset of hematological malignancies. *Leukemia* 12:414, 1998.

227. Zannettino ACW, Buhring H-J, Niutta S, et al: The sialomucin CD164 (MCG-24v) is an adhesive glycoprotein expressed by human hemato-poietic progenitors and bone marrow stromal cells that serves as a potent negative regulator of hematopoiesis. *Blood* 92:2613, 1998.

228. Cortes F, Deschaseaux F, Uchida N, et al: HCA, an immunoglobulin-like adhesion molecule present on the earliest human hematopoietic pre-cursor cells, is also expressed by stromal cells in blood-forming tissues. *Blood* 93:826, 1999.

229. Garcia R, Agular J, Alberti E, et al: Bone marrow stromal cells produce nerve growth factor and glial cell line–derived neurotrophic factors. *Biochem Biophys Res Commun* 316:753, 2004.

230. Padovan CS, Jahn K, Birnbaum T, et al: Expression of neuronal markers in differentiated marrow stromal cells and CD133+ stem-like cells. *Cell Transplant* 12:839, 2003.

231. Song S, Kamath S, Mosquera D, et al: Expression of brain natriuretic peptide by human bone marrow stromal cells. *Exp Neurol* 185:191, 2004.

232. Denhardt DT, Noda M, O'Regan AW, et al: Osteopontin as a means to cope with environmental insults: Regulation of inflammation, tissue re-modeling, and cell survival. *J Clin Invest* 107:1055, 2001.

233. Iwata M, Awaya N, Graf L, et al: Human marrow stromal cells activate monocytes to secrete osteopontin, which down-regulates Notch 1 gene expression in CD34+ cells. *Blood* 103:4496, 2004.

234. Kumano K, Chiba S, Kunisato A, et al: Notch1 but not Notch2 is es-sential for generating hematopoietic stem cells from endothelial cells. *Immunity* 18:699, 2003.

235. Ueno H, Sakita-Ishikawa M, Morikawa Y, et al: A stromal cell-derived membrane protein that supports hematopoietic stem cells. *Nat Immunol* 4:457, 2003.

236. Bauer SR, Ruiz-Hidalgo MJ, Rudikoff EK, et al: Modulated expression of the epidermal growth factor-like homeotic protein dlk influences stromal-cell-pre-B-cell interactions, stromal cell adipogenesis, and pre-B-cell interleukin-7 requirements. *Mol Cell Biol* 18:5247, 1998.

237. Ohno N, Izawaa A, Hattori M, et al: Dlk inhibits stem cell factor-induced colony formation of murine hematopoietic progenitors. Hes-1 indepen-dent effects. *Stem Cells* 19:7109, 2001.

238. Miller SC, De Saint-Georges L, Bowman BM, Jee WS: Bone lining cells: Structure and function. *Scanning Microsc* 3:953, 1989.

239. Sillaber C, Walchshofer S, Mosberger I, et al: Immunophenotypic char-acterization of human bone marrow endosteal cells. *Tissue Antigens* 53:559, 1999.

240. Saito T, Albelda SM, Brighton CT: Identification of integrin receptors on cultured human bone cells. *J Orthop Res* 12:384, 1994.

241. Gong J: Endosteal marrow: A rich source of hematopoietic stem cells. *Science* 199:1443, 1978.

242. Nilsson SK, Haylock DN, Johnston HM, et al: Hyaluronan is synthesized by primitive hemopoietic cells, participates in their lodgement at the endosteum following transplantation, and is involved in the regulation of their proliferation and differentiation in vitro. *Blood* 101:856, 2003.

243. Park SR, Oreffo RO, Triffitt JT: Interconversion potential of cloned human marrow adipocytes in vitro. *Bone* 24:549, 1999.

244. Pittenger MF, Mackay AM, Beck SC, et al: Multilineage potential of adult human mesenchymal stem cells. *Science* 284:143, 1999.

245. Oyajobi BO, Lomri A, Hott M, Marie PJ: Isolation and characterization of human clonogenic osteoblast progenitors immunoselected from fetal bone marrow stroma using STRO-1 monoclonal antibody. *J Bone Miner Res* 14:351, 1999.

246. Doherty MJ, Ashton BA, Walsh S, et al: Vascular pericytes express osteogenic potential in vitro and in vivo. *J Bone Miner Res* 13:828, 1999.

247. Bruder SP, Ricalton NS, Boynton RE, et al: Mesenchymal stem cell surface antigen SB-10 corresponds to activated leukocyte cell adhesion molecule and is involved in osteogenic differentiation. *J Bone Miner Res* 13:655, 1998.

248. Dominici M, Pritchard C, Garlits JE, et al: Hematopoietic cells and osteoblasts are derived from a common marrow progenitor after bone marrow transplantation. *Proc Natl Acad Sci U S A* 101:11761, 2004.

249. Long MW, Robinson JA, Ashcraft EA, Mann KG: Regulation of human bone marrow-derived osteoprogenitor cells by osteogenic growth factors. *J Clin Invest* 95:881, 1995.

250. Gronthos S, Zannettino AC, Graves SE, et al: Differential cell surface expression of the STRO-1 and alkaline phosphatase antigens on discrete developmental stages in primary cultures of human bone cells. *J Bone Miner Res* 14:47, 1999.

251. Hanada K, Dennis JE, Caplan AI: Stimulatory effects of basic fibroblast growth factor and bone morphogenetic protein-2 on osteogenic differentiation of rat bone marrow-derived mesenchymal stem cells. *J Bone Miner Res* 12:1606, 1997.

252. Blanquaert F, Delany AM, Canalis E: Fibroblast growth factor-2 induces hepatocyte growth factor/scatter factor expression in osteoblasts. *Endocrinology* 140:1069, 1999.

253. Grano M, Galimi F, Zambonin G, et al: Hepatocyte growth factor is a coupling factor for osteoclasts and osteoblasts in vitro. *Proc Natl Acad Sci U S A* 93:7644, 1996.

254. Yin JJ, Mohammad KS, Kakonen SM, et al: A causal role for endothelin-1 in the pathogenesis of osteoblastic bone metastases. *Proc Natl Acad Sci U S A* 100:10954, 2003.

255. Erlebacher A, Filvaroff EH, Ye J-Q, Derynck R: Osteoblastic responses to TGF-β during bone remodeling. *Mol Biol Cell* 9:1903, 1998.

256. Taichman RS, Emerson SG: The role of osteoblasts in the hematopoietic microenvironment. *Stem Cells* 16:7, 1998.

257. Ahmed N, Khokher MA, Hassan HT: Cytokine-induced expansion of human CD34+ stem/progenitor and CD34+CD41+ early megakaryocytic marrow cells cultured on normal osteoblasts. *Stem Cells* 17:92, 1999.

258. Gehron Robey P, Young MF, Flanders KC, et al: Osteoblasts synthesize and respond to transforming growth factor-type β (TGF-beta) in vitro. *J Cell Biol* 105:457, 1987.

259. Nilsson SK, Dooner MS, Weier HU, et al: Cells capable of bone production engraft from whole bone marrow transplants in nonablated mice. *J Exp Med* 189:729, 1999.

260. El-Badri NS, Wang B-Y, Cherry, Good RA: Osteoblasts promote engraftment of allogeneic hematopoietic stem cells. *Exp Hematol* 26:110, 1998.

261. Gurevitch O, Fabian I: Ability of the hemopoietic microenvironment in the induced bone to maintain the proliferative potential of early hemopoietic precursors. *Stem Cells* 11:56, 1993.

262. Civitelli R, Beyer EC, Warlow PM, et al: Connexin43 mediates direct intercellular communication in human osteoblastic cell networks. *J Clin Invest* 91:1888, 1993.

263. Visnjic D, Kalajzic Z, Rowe DW, et al: Hematopoiesis is severely altered in mice with an induced osteoblast deficiency. *Blood* 103, 3258, 2004.

264. Zhu J, Emerson SG: A new bone to pick: Osteoblasts and the haematopoietic stem-cell niche. *Bioessays* 26:595, 2004.

265. Matayoshi A, Brown C, DiPersio JF, et al: Human blood-mobilized hematopoietic precursors differentiate into osteoclasts in the absence of stromal cells. *Proc Natl Acad Sci U S A* 93:10785, 1996.

266. Roodman GD: Cell biology of the osteoclast. *Exp Hematol* 27:1229, 1999.

267. Servet-Delprat C, Arnaud S, Jurdic P, et al: Flt3+ macrophage precursors commit sequentially to osteoclasts, dendritic cells and microglia. *BMC Immunol* 3:15, 2002.

268. Calle Y, Jones GE, Jagger C, et al: WASp deficiency in mice results in failure to form osteoclast sealing zones and defects in bone resorption. *Blood* 103:3552, 2004.

269. Horowitz MC, Lorenzo JA: The origins of osteoclasts. *Curr Opin Rheumatol* 16:464, 2004.

270. Wiktor-Jedrzejczak W, Urbanowska E, Aukerman SL, et al: Correction by CSF-1 of defects in the osteopetrotic op/op mouse suggests local, developmental, and humoral requirements for this growth factor. *Exp Hematol* 19:1049, 1991.

271. Dai X-M, Zong X-H, Sylvestre V, Stanley R: Incomplete restoration of colony-stimulating factor 1 (CSF-1) function in CSF-1-deficient Csf1op/Csf1op mice by transgenic expression of cell surface CSF-1. *Blood* 103:1114, 2004.

272. Demulder A, Suggs SV, Zsebo KM, et al: Effects of stem cell factor on osteoclast-like cell formation in long-term human marrow cultures. *J Bone Miner Res* 7:1337, 1992.

273. Tanaka S, Takahashi N, Udagawa N, et al: Macrophage colony-stimulating factor is indispensable for both proliferation and differentiation of osteoclast progenitors. *J Clin Invest* 91:257, 1993.

274. Yao GQ, Sun BH, Weir EC, Insogna KL: A role for cell-surface CSF-1 in osteoclast-mediated osteoclastogenesis. *Calcif Tissue Int* 70:339, 2002.

275. Ohtsuki T, Suzu S, Hatake K, et al: A proteoglycan form of macrophage colony-stimulating factor that binds to bone-derived collagens and can be extracted from bone matrix. *Biochem Biophys Res Commun* 190:215, 1993.

276. Abu-Amer Y: IL-4 abrogates osteoclastogenesis through STAT6-dependent inhibition of NF-κB. *J Clin Invest* 107:1375, 2001.

277. Grigoriadis AE, Wang ZQ, Ceccini MG, et al: C-Fos a key regulator of osteoclast-macrophage lineage determination and bone remodeling. *Science* 266:443, 1994.

278. Soriano P, Montgomery C, Geske R, Bradley A: Targeted disruption of the c-src proto-oncogene leads to osteopetrosis in mice. *Cell* 64:693, 1991.

279. Shalhoub V, Faust J, Boyle WJ, et al: Osteoprotegrin and osteoprotegrin ligand effects on osteoclast formation from human peripheral blood mononuclear cell precursors. *J Cell Biochem* 72:251, 1999.

280. Takahashi N, Udagawa N, Suda T: A new member of tumor necrosis factor ligand family, ODF/OPGL/TRANCE/RANKL, regulates osteoclast differentiation and function. *Biochem Biophys Res Commun* 256:449, 1999.

281. Ikeda F, Nishimura R, Matsubara T, et al: Critical roles of c-Jun signaling in regulation of NFAT family and RANKL-regulated osteoclast differentiation. *J Clin Invest* 114:475, 2004.

282. Hsu H, Lacey DL, Dunstan CR, et al: Tumor necrosis factor receptor family member RANK mediates osteoclast differentiation and activation induced by osteoprotegrin ligand. *Proc Natl Acad Sci U S A* 96:3540, 1999.

283. Ma T, Miyanishi K, Suen A, et al: Human interleukin-1-induced murine osteoclatogenesis is dependent on RANKL, but independent of TNF-alpha. *Cytokine* 26:138, 2004.

284. Kania JR, Kehat-Stadler T, Kupfer SR: CD44 antibodies inhibit osteoclast formation. *J Bone Miner Res* 12:1155, 1997.

285. Udagawa N, Takahashi N, Yasuda H, et al: Osteoprotegrin produced by osteoblasts is an important regulator of osteoclast development and function. *Endocrinology* 141:3478, 2000.

286. Domon T, Yamazaki Y, Fukui A, et al: Ultrastructural study of cell-cell interaction between osteoclasts osteoblasts/stroma cells in vitro. *Ann Anat* 184:221, 2002.

287. Bord S, Frith E, Ireland DC, et al: Synthesis of osteoprotegerin and RANKL by megakaryocytes is modulated by oestrogen. *Br J Haematol* 126:244, 2004.

288. Jimi E, Nakamura I, Amano H, et al; Osteoblast function is activated by osteoblastic cells through a mechanism involving cell-to-cell contact. *Endocrinology* 137:2187, 1996.

289. Mbalaviele G, Nishimura R, Myoi A, et al: Cadherin-6 mediates the heterotypic interactions between the hemopoietic osteoclast cell lineage and stromal cells in a murine model of osteoclast differentiation. *J Cell Biol* 141:1467, 1998.

290. Hayashi S, Miyake K, Kincade PW: The CD9 molecule on stromal cells. *Leuk Lymphoma* 38:265, 2000.

291. Oritani K, Wu X, Medina K, et al: Antibody ligation of CD9 modifies production of myeloid cells in long-term cultures. *Blood* 87:2252, 1996.

292. Tanio Y, Yamazaki H, Kunisada T, et al: CD9 molecule expressed on stromal cells is involved in osteoclastogenesis. *Exp Hematol* 27:853, 1999.

293. Iwama A, Yamaguchi N, Suda T: STK/RON receptor tyrosine kinase mediates both apoptotic and growth signals via the multifunctional docking site conserved in the HGF receptor family. *EMBO J* 15:5866, 1996.

294. Kurihara N, Tatsumi J, Arai F, et al: Macrophage-stimulating protein (MSP) and its receptor, RON, stimulate human osteoclast activity but not proliferation: Effect of MSP distinct from that of hepatocyte growth factor. *Exp Hematol* 26:1080, 1998.

295. Choi SJ, Han JH, Roodman GD: ADAM8: A novel osteoclast stimulating factor. *J Bone Miner Res* 16:814, 2001.

296. Oba Y, Chung HY, Choi SJ, Roodman GD: Eosinophil chemotactic factor-L (ECF-L): A novel osteoclast stimulating factor. *J Bone Miner Res* 18:1332, 2003.

297. Quesenberry PJ, Crittenden RB, Lowry P, et al: In vitro and in vivo studies of stromal niches. *Blood Cells* 20:97, 1994.

298. Gibson FM, Scopes J, Daly S, et al: IL-3 is produced by normal stroma in long-term bone marrow cultures. *Br J Haematol* 90:518, 1995.

299. Verfaillie CM, Catanzarro PM, Li WN: Macrophage inflammatory protein 1 alpha, interleukin-3 and diffusible marrow stromal factors maintain human hematopoietic stem cells for at least eight weeks in vitro. *J Exp Med* 179:643, 1994.

300. Crocker PR, Morris L, Gordon S: Novel cell surface adhesion receptors involved in interactions between stromal macrophages and haematopoietic cells. *J Cell Sci* 9(suppl):185, 1988.

301. Wang QR, Wolf NS: Dissecting the hematopoietic microenvironment: VIII. Clonal isolation and identification of cell types in murine CFU-F colonies by limiting dilution. *Exp Hematol* 18:355, 1990.

302. Kincade PW: Cell interaction molecules and cytokines which participate in B lymphopoiesis. *Baillieres Clin Haematol* 5:575, 1992.

303. Berneman ZN, Chen ZZ, Van Bockstaele D, et al: The nature of the adherent hemopoietic cells in human long-term bone marrow cultures (HLTBMCs): Presence of lymphocytes and plasma cells next to the myelomonocytic population. *Leukemia* 9:648, 1989.

304. Tong J, Kishi H, Matsuda T, Muraguchi A: A bone marrow-derived stroma line, ST2, can support the differentiation of fetal thymocytes from CD4+ CD8+ double negative to the CD4+ CD8+ double positive differentiation stage in vitro. *Immunology* 97:672, 1999.

305. Dejbakhsh-Jones S, Strober S: Identification of an early T cell progenitor for a pathway of T cell maturation in the bone marrow. *Proc Natl Acad Sci U S A* 96:14493, 1999.

306. Kurosaka D, LeBien TW, Priby JAR: Comparative studies of different stromal cell microenvironments in support of human B-cell development. *Exp Hematol* 27:1271, 1999.

307. Funk PE, Stephan RP, Witte PL: Vascular adhesion molecule-1-positive reticular cells express interleukin-7 and stem cell factor in the bone marrow. *Blood* 86:2661, 1995.

308. Tang J, Nuccie BL, Ritterman I, et al: TGF-beta down-regulates stromal IL-7 secretion and inhibits proliferation of human B cell precursors. *J Immunol* 159:117, 1997.

309. Tsuji JM, Pollack SB: Maturation of murine natural killer precursor cells in the absence of exogenous cytokines requires contact with bone marrow stroma. *Nat Immunol* 14:44, 1995.

310. Yu H, Fehniger TA, Fuschsuber P, et al: Flt3 ligand promotes the generation of a distinct CD34(+) human natural killer cell progenitor that responds to interleukin-15. *Blood* 92:3647, 1998.

311. Abboud SL: A bone marrow stromal cell line is a source and target for platelet-derived growth factor. *Blood* 81:2547, 1993.

312. Abboud SL, Pinzani M: Peptide growth factors stimulate macrophage colony-stimulating factor in murine stromal cells. *Blood* 78:103, 1991.

313. Yan XQ, Brady G, Iscove NN: Platelet-derived growth factor (PDGF) activates primitive hematopoietic precursors (pre-CFCmulti) by upregulating IL-1 in PDGF receptor-expressing macrophages. *J Immunol* 150:2440, 1993.

314. Lerat H, Lissitzky JC, Singer JW, et al: Role of stromal cells and macrophages in fibronectin biosynthesis and matrix assembly in human long-term marrow cultures. *Blood* 82:1480, 1993.

315. Baldus SE, Wickenhauser C, Stefanovic A, et al: Enrichment of human bone marrow mononuclear phagocytes and characterization of macrophage subpopulations by immunoenzymatic double staining. *Histochem J* 30:285, 1998.

316. Wijffels JF, De Rover Z, Kraal G, Beelen RH: Macrophage phenotype regulation by colony-stimulating factors at bone marrow level. *J Leukoc Biol* 53:249, 1993.

317. Shima M, Teitelbaum SL, Holers VM, et al: Macrophage-colony-stimulating factor regulates expression of the integrins alpha 4 beta 1 and alpha 5 beta 1 by murine marrow macrophages. *Proc Natl Acad Sci U S A* 92:5179, 1995.

318. Dannaeus K, Johannisson A, Nilsson K, Jonsson JI: Flt3 ligand induces the outgrowth of Mac-1+ B22+ mouse bone marrow progenitor cells restricted to macrophage differentiation that coexpress early B cell-associated genes. *Exp Hematol* 27:1646, 1999.

319. Munday J, Floyd H, Criker PR: Sialic acid binding receptors (siglecs) expressed by macrophages. *J Leukoc Biol* 66:705, 1999.

320. Sadahira Y, Mori M: Role of the macrophage in erythropoiesis. *Pathol Int* 49:841, 1999.

321. Klein G: The extracellular matrix of the hematopoietic microenvironment. *Experimentia* 51:914, 1995.

322. Singer JW, Keating A, Wright TN: The human haemopoietic microenvironment, in *Recent Advances in Haematology*, edited by AV Hoffbrand, p 1. Churchill Livingstone, London, 1985.

323. Bentley SA, Tralka TS: Fibronectin-mediated attachment of hematopoietic cells to stromal elements in continuous bone marrow culture. *Exp Hematol* 11:129, 1983.

324. Postlethwaite A, Kang AH: Fibroblasts and matrix proteins, in *Inflammation Basic Principles and Clinical Correlates*, 3rd ed, edited by JI Gallin, R Snyderman, p 227. Lippincott Williams & Wilkins, Philadelphia, 1999.

325. Campbell AD, Long MW, Wicha MS: Haemonectin: A bone marrow adhesion protein specific for cells of granulocytic lineage. *Nature* 329: 445, 1987.

326. Lawler J: The structural and functional properties of thrombospondin. *Blood* 67:1197, 1986.

327. Simmons PJ, Levesque JP, Zannettino AC: Adhesion molecules in haemopoiesis. *Baillieres Clin Haematol* 10:485, 1997.

328. Verfaille CM: Adhesion receptors as regulators of the hematopoietic process. *Blood* 92:2609, 1998.

329. Broxmeyer HE, Kim CH: Regulation of hematopoiesis in a sea of chemokine family members with a plethora of redundant activities. *Exp Hematol* 27:1113, 1999.

330. Gordon MY: Extracellular matrix- and membrane-bound cytokines, in *Colony-Stimulating Factors: Molecular and Cellular Biology*, edited by JM Garland, PJ Quesenberry, DJ Hilton, p 133, Marcel Dekker, New York, 1997.

331. Long MW: Hematopoietic microenvironments, in *Colony-Stimulating Factors: Molecular and Cellular Biology*, edited by JM Garland, PJ Quesenberry, DJ Hilton, p 117. Marcel Dekker, New York, 1997.

332. Oritani K, Kanakura Y, Aoyama K, et al: Matrix glycoprotein SC1/ECM2 augments B lymphopoiesis. *Blood* 90:3404, 1997.

333. Koller MR, Oxender M, Jensen TC, et al: Direct contact between CD34+ lin- cells and stroma induces a soluble activity that specifically increases primitive hematopoietic cell production. *Exp Hematol* 27:734, 1999.

334. Varnum-Finney B, Purton LE, Yu M, et al: The Notch ligand, Jagged-1, influences the development of primitive hematopoietic precursor cells. *Blood* 91:4084, 1998.

335. Hoogewerf AJ, Kuschert GS, Proudfoot AE, et al: Glycosaminoglycans mediate cell surface oligomerization of chemokines. *Biochemistry* 36: 13570, 1997.

336. Luster AD, Greenberg SM, Leder P: The IP-10 chemokine binds to a specific cell surface heparan sulfate site shared with platelet factor 4 and inhibits endothelial cell proliferation. *J Exp Med* 182:219, 1995.

337. Tanaka T, Adams DH, Hubscher S, et al: T-cell adhesion induced by proteoglycan immobilized cytokine MIP-1β. *Nature* 361:78, 1993.

338. Chakravarty L, Rogers L, Quach T, et al: Lysine 58 and histidine 66 at the C terminal alpha-helix of monocyte chemoattractant protein-1 are essential for glycosaminoglycan binding. *J Biol Chem* 273:29641, 1998.

339. Spillman D, Witt D, Lindahl U: Defining the interleukin-8-binding domain of heparan sulfate. *J Biol Chem* 273:15487, 1998.

340. Koopman W, Ediriwickrema C, Krangel MS: Structure and function of the glycosaminoglycan binding site of chemokine macrophage-inflammatory protein-1 beta. *J Immunol* 163:2120, 1999.

341. Amara A, Lorthioir O, Valenzuela A, et al: Stromal cell derived factor-1 alpha associates with heparan sulfates through the first beta-strand of the chemokine. *J Cell Biol Chem* 274:23916, 1999.

342. Wolff EA, Greenfield B, Taub DD, et al: Generation of artificial proteoglycans containing glycosaminoglycan-modified CD44. Demonstration of the interaction between rantes and chondroitin sulfate. *J Biol Chem* 274:2518, 1999.

343. Lipscombe RJ, Nakhoul AM, Sanderson CJ, Coombe DR: Interleukin-5 binds to heparin/heparan sulfate. A model for an interaction with extracellular matrix. *J Leukoc Biol* 63:342, 1998.

344. Borghesi LA, Yamashita Y, Kincade PW: Heparan sulfate proteoglycans mediate interleukin-7-dependent B lymphopoiesis. *Blood* 93:140, 1999.

345. Lyon M, Deakin JA, Nakamura T, Gallagher JT: Interaction of hepatocyte growth factor with heparan sulfate. Elucidation of major heparan sulfate structural determinants. *J Biol Chem* 269:11216, 1994.

346. Kiefer MC, Stephans JC, Crawford K, et al: Ligand-affinity cloning and structure of a cell surface heparan sulfate proteoglycan that binds basic fibroblast growth factor. *Proc Natl Acad Sci U S A* 87:6985, 1990.

347. Robledo MM, Ursa MA, Sanchez-Madrid F, Teixido J: Associations between TGF-beta1 receptors in human bone marrow stromal cells. *Br J Haematol* 102:804, 1998.

348. Kapur R, Cooper R, Xiao X, et al: The presence of novel amino acids in the cytoplasmic domain of stem cell factor results in hematopoietic defects in the *Steel^{17H}* mice. *Blood* 94:1915, 1999.

349. Gay RE, Prince CW, Zuckerman KS, Gay S: The collagenous hemopoietic microenvironment, in *Handbook of the Hemopoietic Microenvironment*, edited by M Tavassoli, p 369. Humana Press, Clifton, NJ, 1989.

350. Anklesaria P, Greenberger JS, Fitzgerald TJ, et al: Hemonectin mediates adhesion of engrafted murine progenitors to a clonal bone marrow stromal cell line from *Sl/Sl^d* mice. *Blood* 77:1691, 1991.

351. De Wynter E, Allen T, Coutinho L, et al: Localization of granulocytic macrophage colony-stimulating factor in human long-term bone marrow cultures. Biological and immunocytochemical characterization. *J Cell Sci* 106:761, 1993.

352. Deschaseaux ML, Herve P, Charbord P: The detection of colony-stimulating factors and steel factor in adherent layers of human long-term marrow cultures using reverse-transcriptase polymerase chain reaction. *Leukemia* 8:513, 1994.

353. Liu J, De Wynter E, Testa NG, et al: Immunoelectron microscopic localization of growth factors and other markers of human long-term bone marrow cultures. *Chin Med Sci J* 11:129, 1996.

354. Waegell WO, Higley HR, Kincade PW, Dasch JR: Growth acceleration and stem cell expansion in Dexter-type cultures by neutralization of TGF-beta. *Exp Hematol* 22:1051, 1994.

355. Wight TN, Kinsella MG, Keating A, Singer JW: Proteoglycans in human long-term bone marrow cultures: Biochemical and ultrastructural analyses. *Blood* 67:1333, 1986.

356. Allen TD, Dexter TM, Simmons PJ: Marrow biology and stem cells, in *Colony Stimulating Factors, Molecular and Cellular Biology, Immunology Series*, vol 49, edited by TM Dexter, JM Garland, NG Testa, p 1. Marcel Dekker, New York, 1990.

357. Yurchenco PD, Schittny JC: Molecular architecture of basement membranes. *FASEB J* 4:1577, 1990.

358. Keating A, Gordon MY: Hierarchical organization of hematopoietic microenvironments: Role of proteoglycans. *Leukemia* 2:766, 1988.

359. Gordon MY, Riley GP, Clarke D: Heparan sulfate is necessary for adhesive interactions between human early hemopoietic progenitor cells and the extracellular matrix of the marrow microenvironment. *Leukemia* 2:804, 1988.

360. Uhlman DL, Luikart SD: The role of proteoglycans in the adhesion and differentiation of hematopoietic cells, in *The Hematopoietic Microenvironment*, edited by MW Long, MS Wicha, p 232. Johns Hopkins University Press, Baltimore and London, 1993.

361. Bruno E, Luikart SD, Long MW, Hoffman R: Marrow-derived heparan sulfate proteoglycan mediates the adhesion of hematopoietic progenitor cells to cytokines. *Exp Hematol* 23:1212, 1995.

362. Minguell JJ, Hardy C, Tavassoli M: Membrane-associated chondroitin sulfate proteoglycan and fibronectin mediate the binding of hemopoietic progenitor cells to stromal cells. *Exp Cell Res* 201:200, 1992.

363. Han ZC, Bellucci S, Shen ZX, et al: Glycosaminoglycans enhance megakaryopoiesis by modifying the activities of hematopoietic growth regulators. *J Cell Physiol* 168:97, 1996.

364. Gordon MY, Lewis JL, Marley SB, et al: Stromal cells negatively regulate primitive haematopoietic progenitor cell activation via a phosphatidylinositol-anchored cell adhesion/signaling mechanism. *Br J Haematol* 96:647, 1997.

365. Gupta P, Oegema TR Jr, Brazil JJ, et al: Structurally specific heparan sulfates support primitive human hematopoiesis by formation of a multimolecular stem cell niche. *Blood* 92:4641,1998.

366. Da Prato I, Valentini P, Testi R, et al: Differential activity of glycosaminoglycans on colony-forming cells from cord blood. Preliminary results. *Leuk Res* 23:1015, 1999.

367. Lewinsohn DM, Nagler A, Ginzton N, et al: Hematopoietic progenitor cell expression of the H-CAM (CD44) homing-associated adhesion molecule. *Blood* 75:589, 1990.

368. Jalkanen S, Jalkanen M: Lymphocyte CD44 binds the COOH-terminal heparin-binding domain of fibronectin. *J Cell Biol* 116:817, 1992.

369. Miyake K, Medina KL, Mayashi S-I, et al: Monoclonal antibodies to Pgp-1/CD44 block lympho-hemopoiesis in long-term bone marrow cultures. *J Exp Med* 171:477, 1990.

370. Legras S, Levesque JP, Charrad R, et al: CD44-mediated adhesiveness of human hematopoietic progenitors to hyaluronan is modulated by cytokines. *Blood* 89:1905, 1997.

371. Rachmilewitz J, Tykocinski ML: Differential effects of chondroitin sulfates A and B on monocyte and B cell activation: Evidence for B-cell activation via a CD44-dependent pathway. *Blood* 92:223, 1998.

372. Khaldoyanidi S, Moll J, Karakhanova S, et al: Hyaluronate-enhanced hematopoiesis: Two different receptors trigger the release of interleukin-1β and interleukin-6 from bone marrow macrophages. *Blood* 94:940, 1999.

373. Sternberg D, Peled A, Shezen E, et al: Control of stroma-dependent hematopoiesis by basic fibroblast growth factor: Stromal phenotypic plasticity and modified myelopoietic functions. *Cytokines Mol Ther* 2:29, 1996.

374. Weimar IS, Miranda N, Muller EJ, et al: Hepatocyte growth factor/scatter factor (HGF/SF) is produced by bone marrow stromal cells and promotes proliferation, adhesion and survival of human hematopoietic progenitor cells (CD34+). *Exp Hematol* 26:885, 1998.

375. Pivak-Kroizman T, Lemmon MA, Dikic I, et al: Heparin-induced oligomerization of FGF molecules is responsible for FGF receptor dimerization, activation, and cell proliferation. *Cell* 79:1015, 1994.

376. Ratajczak MZ, Ratajczak J, Slorska M, et al: Effect of basic (FGF-2) and acidic (FGF-1) fibroblast growth factors on early haematopoietic cell development. *Br J Haematol* 93:772, 1996.

377. Schofield KP, Gallagher JT, David G: Expression of proteoglycan core proteins in human bone marrow stroma. *Biochem J* 343:663, 1999.

378. Klein G, Conzelmann S, Beck S, et al: Perlecan in human bone marrow: A growth-factor-presenting, but anti-adhesive, extracellular matrix component for hematopoietic cells. *Matrix Biol* 14:457, 1995.

379. Drzeniek Z, Stoocker G, Siebertz B, et al: Heparan sulfate proteoglycan expression is induced during early erythroid differentiation of multipotential hematopoietic stem cells. *Blood* 93:2884, 1999.

380. Siebertz B, Stocker G, Drzeniek Z, et al: Expression of glypican-4 in haematopoietic-progenitor and bone-marrow-stromal cells. *Biochem J* 344:937, 1999.

381. Sneed TB, Stanley DJ, Young LA, Sanderson RD: Interleukin-6 regulates expression of the syndecan-1 proteoglycan on B lymphoid cells. *Cell Immunol* 153:456, 1994.

382. Oritani K, Kincade PW: Identification of stromal cell products that interact with pre-B cells. *J Cell Biol* 134:771, 1996.

383. Yamashita Y, Oritani K, Miyoshi EK, et al: Syndecan-4 is expressed by B lineage lymphocytes and can transmit a signal for formation of dendritic processes. *J Immunol* 162:5940, 1999.

384. Longley RL, Woods A, Fleetwood A, et al: Control of morphology, cytoskeleton and migration by syndecan-4. *J Cell Sci* 112:3421, 1999.

385. Zukerman KS, Wicha MS: Extracellular matrix production by the adherent cells of long-term murine bone marrow cultures. *Blood* 61:540, 1983.

386. Sorrel JM: Ultrastructural localization of fibronectin in bone marrow of the embryonic chick and its relationship to granulopoiesis. *Cell Tissue Res* 252:565, 1988.

387. Tsai S, Patel V, Beaumont E, et al: Differential binding of erythroid and myeloid progenitors to fibroblasts and fibronectin. *Blood* 69:1587, 1987.

388. Vuillet-Gaugler MH, Breton-Gorius J, Vainchenker W, et al: Loss of attachment to fibronectin with terminal human erythroid differentiation. *Blood* 75:865, 1990.

389. Rosemblatt M, Vuillet-Gaugler MH, Leroy C, Coulombel L: Coexpression of two fibronectin receptors, VLA-4 and VLA-5, by immature human erythroblastic precursor cells. *J Clin Invest* 87:6, 1991.

390. Liesveld JL, Winslow J, Kempski MC, et al: Adhesive interactions of normal and leukemic human CD34+ myeloid progenitors: Role of marrow stroma, fibroblasts and cytomatrix components. *Exp Hematol* 19:63, 1991.

391. Kerst JM, Sanders JB, Slaper Cortenbach IC, et al: Alpha 4 beta 1 and alpha 5 beta 1 are differentially expressed during myelopoiesis and mediate the adherence of human CD34+ cells to fibronectin in an activation-dependent way. *Blood* 81:344, 1993.

392. Ryan DH, Nuccie BL, Abboud CN, Winslow JM: Vascular cell adhesion molecule-1 and the integrin VLA-4 mediate adhesion of human B cell precursors to cultured bone marrow adherent cells. *J Clin Invest* 88:995, 1991.

393. Hynes RO: Integrins: Versatility, modulation, and signaling in cell adhesion. *Cell* 69:11, 1992.

394. Williams DA, Rios M, Stephens C, Patel VP: Fibronectin and VLA-4 in haematopoietic stem cell-microenvironment interactions. *Nature* 352:438, 1991.

395. Schofield KP, Humphries MJ: Identification of fibronectin IIICS variants in human bone marrow stroma. *Blood* 93:410, 1999.

396. Verfaillie CM, Benis A, Iida J, et al: Adhesion of committed human hematopoietic progenitors to synthetic peptides from the C-terminal heparin-binding domain of fibronectin: Cooperation between the integrin alpha 4 beta 1 and the CD44 adhesion receptor. *Blood* 84:1802, 1994.

397. Hassan HT, Sadovinkova EY, Drize NJ, et al: Fibronectin increases both non-adherent cells and CFU-GM while collagen increases adherent cells in human normal long-term bone marrow cultures. *Haematologica (Budap)* 28:77, 1997.

398. Yokota T, Oritani K, Mitsui H, et al: Growth-supporting activities of fibronectin on hematopoietic stem/progenitor cells in vitro and in vivo: Structural requirements for fibronectin activities of CS1 and cell-binding domains. *Blood* 91:3263, 1998.

399. Hurley RW, McCarthy JB, Verfaillie CM: Direct adhesion to bone marrow stroma via fibronectin receptors inhibits hematopoietic progenitor proliferation. *J Clin Invest* 96:511, 1995.

400. Goltry KL, Patel VP: Specific domains of fibronectin mediate adhesion and migration of early murine erythroid progenitors. *Blood* 90:138, 1997.

401. Van der Loo JC, Xiao X, McMillin D, et al: VLA-5 is expressed by mouse and human long-term repopulating hematopoietic cells and mediates adhesion to extracellular matrix protein fibronectin. *J Clin Invest* 102:1051, 1998.

402. Robledo MM, Sanz-Rodrigues F, Hidalgo A, Teixido J: Differential use of very late antigen-4 and -5 integrins by hematopoietic precursors and myeloma cells to adhere to transforming growth factor-beta-1-treated bone marrow stroma. *J Biol Chem* 273:12056, 1998.

403. Schofield KP, Rushton G, Humphries MJ, et al: Influence of interleukin-3 and other growth factors on alpha$_4$beta$_1$ integrin-mediated adhesion and migration of human hematopoietic progenitor cells. *Blood* 90:1858, 1997.

404. Levesque JP, Haylock DN, Simmons PJ: Cytokine regulation of proliferation and cell adhesion are correlated events in human CD34+ hemopoietic progenitors. *Blood* 88:1168, 1996.

405. Cui L, Ramsfjell V, Borge OJ, et al: Thrombopoietin promotes adhesion of primitive human hemopoietic cells to fibronectin and vascular cell adhesion molecule-1: Role of activation of very late antigen (VLA)-4 and VLA-5. *J Immunol* 159:1961, 1997.

406. Schofield KP, Humphries MJ, De Wynter E, et al: The effect of α4β1-integrin binding sequences of fibronectin on growth of cells from human hematopoietic progenitors. *Blood* 91:3230, 1998.

407. Staquet MJ, Jacquet C, Dezutter-Dambuyant C, Schmitt D: Fibronectin upregulates in vitro generation of dendritic Langerhans cells from human cord blood CD34+ progenitors. *J Invest Dermatol* 109:738, 1997.

408. Berthier R, Jacquier-Sarlin M, Schweitzer A, et al: Adhesion of mature polypoid megakaryocytes to fibronectin is mediated by beta 1 integrins and leads to cell damage. *Exp Cell Res* 242:315, 1998.

409. Schick PK, Wojenski CM, He X, et al: Integrins involved in the adhesion of megakaryocytes to fibronectin and fibrinogen. *Blood* 92:2650, 1998.

410. Krugger-Krasagakes S, Grutzkau A, Krasagakis K, et al: Adhesion of human mast cells to extracellular matrix provides a co-stimulatory signal for cytokine production. *Immunology* 98:253, 1999.

411. Lloyd AR, Oppenheim JJ, Kelvin DJ, Taub DD: Chemokines regulate T cell adherence to recombinant adhesion molecules and extracellular matrix proteins. *J Immunol* 156:932, 1996.

412. Higashimoto I, Chihara J, Kawabata M, et al: Adhesion to fibronectin regulates expression of intercellular adhesion molecule-1 on eosinophilic cells. *Int Arch Allergy Immunol* 120 (suppl 1):34, 1999.

413. Xu X, Hakansson L: Simultaneous analysis of eosinophil and neutrophil adhesion to plasma and tissue fibronectin, fibrinogen, and albumin. *J Immunol Methods* 226:93, 1999.

414. Xie B, Laouar A, Huberman E: Fibronectin-mediated cell adhesion is required for induction of 92-kDa type IV collagenase/gelatinase (MMP-9) gene expression during macrophage differentiation. The signaling role of protein kinase C-beta. *J Biol Chem* 273:11576, 1998.

415. Kremlev SG, Chapoval AI, Evans R: Cytokine release by macrophages after interacting with CSF-1 and extracellular matrix proteins: Characteristics of a mouse model of inflammatory responses in vitro. *Cell Immunol* 185:59, 1998.

416. Yonezawa I, Kato K, Yagita H, et al: VLA-5-mediated interactions with fibronectin induces cytokine production by human chondrocytes. *Biochem Biophys Res Commun* 219:261, 1996.

417. Rich IN, Brackmann I, Worthington-White D, Dewey MJ: Activation of sodium/hydrogen exchanger via the fibronectin-integrin pathway results in hematopoietic stimulation. *J Cell Physiol* 177:109, 1998.

418. Klein G, Beck S, Muller CA: Tenascin is a cytoadhesive extracellular matrix component of the human hematopoietic microenvironment. *J Cell Biol* 123:1027, 1993.

419. Chiquet-Ehrismann R, Matsuoka Y, Hofer U, et al: Tenascin variants: Differential binding to fibronectin and distinct distribution in cell cultures and tissues. *Cell Regul* 2:927, 1991.

420. Sakai T, Ohta M, Kawakatsu H, et al: Tenascin-C induction in Whitlock-Witte culture: A relevant role of the thiol moiety in lymphoid-lineage differentiation. *Exp Cell Res* 217:395, 1995.

421. Ekblom M, Fassler R, Tomasini-Johansson B, et al: Downregulation of tenascin expression by glucocorticoids in bone marrow stromal cells and in fibroblasts. *J Cell Biol* 123:1037, 1993.

422. Seiffert M, Beck SC, Schermutzki F, et al: Mitogenic and adhesive effects of tenascin-C on human hematopoietic cells are mediated by various functional domains. *Matrix Biol* 17:47, 1998.

423. Ohta M, Sakai T, Saga Y, et al: Suppression of hematopoietic activity in tenascin-C-deficient mice. *Blood* 91:4074, 1998.

424. Mackie EJ, Tucker RP: The tenascin-C knockout revisited. *J Cell Sci* 112:3847, 1999.

425. Bentley SA: Collagen synthesis by bone marrow stromal cells: A quantitative study. *Br J Haematol* 50:491, 1982.

426. Mori M, Sadahira Y, Kawasaki S, et al: Formation of capillary networks from bone marrow cultured in collagen gel. *Cell Struct Funct* 14:393, 1989.

427. Zukerman KS, Rhodes RK, Goodrum DD, et al: Inhibition of collagen deposition in the extracellular matrix prevents the establishment of a stroma supportive of hematopoiesis in long-term murine bone marrow cultures. *J Clin Invest* 75:970, 1985.

428. Zukerman KS, Prince CW, Gay S: The hemopoietic extracellular matrix, in *Handbook of the Hemopoietic Microenvironment*, edited by M Tavassoli, p 399. Humana Press, Clifton, NJ, 1989.

429. Koenigsmann M, Griffin JD, DiCarlo J, Cannistra SA: Myeloid and erythroid progenitor cells from normal bone marrow adhere to collagen type I. *Blood* 79:657, 1992.

430. Waterhouse EJ, Quesenberry PJ, Balian G: Collagen synthesis by murine bone marrow cell culture. *J Cell Physiol* 127:397, 1987.

431. Charbord P, Tamayo E, Saeland S, et al: Granulocyte-macrophage colony-stimulating factor (GM-CSF) in human long-term bone marrow cultures: Endogenous production in the adherent layer and effect on exogenous GM-CSF on granulomonopoiesis. *Blood* 78:1230, 1991.

432. Chichester CO, Fernández M, Minguel JJ: Extracellular matrix gene expression by human bone marrow stroma and by marrow fibroblasts. *Cell Adhes Commun* 1:93, 1993.

433. Klein G, Muller CA, Tillet E, et al: Collagen type VI in the human bone marrow microenvironment: A strong cytoadhesive component. *Blood* 86:1740, 1995.

434. Klein G, Kibler C, Schermutzki F, et al: Cell binding properties of collagen type XIV for human hematopoietic cells. *Matrix Biol* 16:307, 1998.

435. Briddon SJ, Melford SK, Turner M, et al: Collagen mediates changes in intracellular calcium in primary mouse megakaryocytes through syk-dependent and -independent pathways. *Blood* 93:3847, 1999.

436. Nilsson SK, Debatis ME, Dooner MS, et al: Imunofluorescence characterization of key extracellular matrix proteins in murine bone marrow in situ. *J Histochem Cytochem* 46:371, 1998.

437. Kleinman HK, Weeks BS: Laminin: Structure, function and receptors. *Curr Opin Cell Biol* 1:964, 1989.

438. Senior RM, Gresham HD, Griffin GL, et al: Entactin stimulates neutrophil adhesion and chemotaxis through interactions between its Arg-Gly-Asp (RGD) domain and the leukocyte response integrin. *J Clin Invest* 90:2251, 1992.

439. Bryant G, Rao CN, Brentani M, et al: A role for the laminin receptor in leukocyte chemotaxis. *J Leukoc Biol* 41:220, 1987.

440. Lundgren-Akerlund E, Olofsson AM, Berger E, Arfors KE: CD11b/CD18-dependent polymorphonuclear leucocyte interaction with matrix proteins in adhesion and migration. *Scand J Immunol* 37:569, 1993.

441. Liesveld JL, Ryan DH, Kempski MC, et al: Quantitation of the binding of human CD34 positive myeloid progenitors to marrow stroma fibroblasts, and components of the extracellular matrix, in *Hematopoiesis, UCLA Symposia on Molecular and Cellular Biology New Series*, edited by SC Clark, DW Golde, p 157. Wiley-Liss, New York, 1990.

442. Tobias JW, Bern MM, Netland PA, Zetter BR: Monocyte adhesion to subendothelial components. *Blood* 69:1265, 1987.

443. Bohnsack JF, Akiyama SK, Damsky CH, et al: Human neutrophil adherence to laminin in vitro: Evidence for a distinct neutrophil integrin receptor for laminin. *J Exp Med* 171:1221, 1990.

444. Bohnsack JF: CD11/CD18-independent neutrophil adherence to laminin is mediated by the integrin VLA-6. *Blood* 79:1545, 1992.

445. Gu Y-C, Kortesmaa J, Tryggvason K, et al: Laminin isoform-specific promotion of adhesion and migration of human bone marrow progenitor cells. *Blood* 101:877, 2003.

446. Fehlner-Gardiner C, Uniyal S, Von Ballestrem C, et al: Integrin VLA-6 (alpha 6 beta 1) mediates adhesion of mouse bone marrow-derived mast cells to laminin. *Allergy* 51:650, 1996.

447. El-Nemer W, Gane P, Colin Y, et al: The Lutheran blood group glycoproteins, the erythroid receptors for laminin, are adhesion molecules. *J Biol Chem* 273:16686, 1998.

448. Monturi N, Selleri C, Risitano AM, et al: Expression of the 67-kDa laminin receptor in acute myeloid leukemia cells mediates adhesion to laminin and is frequently associated with monocytic differentiation. *Clin Cancer Res* 5:1465, 1999.

449. Gu Y, Sorokin L, Durbeej M, et al: Characterization of bone marrow laminins and identification of α5-containing laminins as adhesive proteins for multipotent hematopoietic FDCP-mix cells. *Blood* 93:2533, 1999.

450. Vogel W, Kanz L, Brugger W, et al: Expression of laminin β2 chain in normal human bone marrow. *Blood* 94:1143, 1999.

451. Ohki K, Kohashi O: Laminin promotes proliferation of bone marrow-derived macrophages and macrophage cell lines. *Cell Struct Funct* 19:63, 1994.

452. Siler U, Roussell P, Muller CA, Klein G: Laminin gamma2 chain is a stromal cell marker of the human bone marrow microenvironment. *Br J Haematol* 119:212, 2002.

453. Peters C, O'Shea KS, Campbell AD, et al: Fetal expression of hemonectin: An extracellular matrix hematopoietic cytoadhesion molecule. *Blood* 75:357, 1990.

454. White H, Totty N, Panayotou G: Haemonectin, a granulocyte-cell-binding protein, is related to the plasma glycoprotein fetuin. *Eur J Biochem* 213:523, 1993.

455. Sullenbarger BA, Petitt MS, Chong P, et al: Murine granulocytic cell adhesion to bone marrow hemonectin is mediated by mannose and galactose. *Blood* 86:135, 1995.

456. Bornstein P: Thrombospondins as matricellular modulators of cell function. *J Clin Invest* 107:929, 2001.

457. Long MW, Dixit VM: Thrombospondin functions as a cytoadhesion molecule for human hematopoietic progenitor cells. *Blood* 75:2311, 1990.

458. Li WX, Howard RJ, Leung LL: Identification of SVTCG in thrombospondin as the conformation-dependent, high affinity binding site for its receptor, CD36. *J Biol Chem* 268:16179, 1993.

459. Calvo D, Vega MA: Identification, primary structure, and distribution of CLA-1, a novel member of the CD36/LIMPII gene family. *J Biol Chem* 268:18929, 1993.

460. Vischer P, Feitsma K, Schon P, Volker W: Perlecan is responsible for thrombospondin 1 binding on the surface of cultured porcine endothelial cells. *Eur J Cell Biol* 73:332, 1997.

461. Nakahata T, Okumura N: Cell surface antigen expression in human erythroid progenitors: Erythroid and megakaryocytic markers. *Leuk Lymphoma* 13:401, 1994.

462. Yang M, Li K, Ng MH, et al: Thrombospondin-1 inhibits in vitro megakaryocytopoiesis via CD36. *Thromb Res* 109:47, 2003.

463. Kyriakides TR, Rojnuckarin P, Reidy MA, et al: Megakaryocytes require thrombospondin-2 for normal platelet formation and function. *Blood* 101:3915, 2003.

464. Pierson BA, Gupta K, Hu WS, Miller JS: Human natural killer cell expansion is regulated by thrombospondin-mediated activation of transforming growth factor-beta 1 and independent accessory cell-derived contact and soluble factors. *Blood* 87:180, 1996.

465. Crawford SE, Stellmach V, Murphy-Ullrich JE, et al: Thrombospondin-1 is a major activator of TGF-beta 1 in vivo. *Cell* 93:1159, 1998.

466. Touhami M, Fauvel-Lafeve F, Da Silva N, et al: Induction of thrombospondin-1 by all-*trans* retinoic acid modulates growth and differentiation of HL-60 myeloid leukemia cells. *Leukemia* 11:2137, 1997.

467. Taraboletti G, Belotti D, Borsotti P, et al: The 140-kilodalton antiangiogenic fragment of thrombospondin-1 binds to basic fibroblast growth factor. *Cell Growth Differ* 8:471, 1997.

468. Margosio B, Marchetti D, Vergani V, et al: Thrombospondin 1 as a scavenger for matrix-associated fibroblast growth factor 2. *Blood* 102:4399, 2003.

469. Loganadane LD, Berge N, Legrand C, Fauvel-Lafeve F: Endothelial cell proliferation regulated by cytokines modulates thrombospondin-1 secretion into the subendothelium. *Cytokine* 9:740, 1997.

470. Qian X, Wang TN, Rothman VL, et al: Thrombospondin-1 modulates angiogenesis in vitro by up-regulation of matrix metalloproteinase-9 in endothelial cells. *Exp Cell Res* 235:403, 1997.

471. Mansfield PJ, Suchard SJ: Thrombospondin promotes both chemotaxis and haptotaxis of human peripheral blood monocytes. *J Immunol* 153:4219, 1994.

472. Mansfield PJ, Suchard SJ: Thrombospondin promotes both chemotaxis and haptotaxis in neutrophil-like HL-60 cells. *J Immunol* 150:1959, 1993.

473. Horton MA: The alpha$_v$beta$_3$ integrin "vitronectin receptor." *Int J Biochem Cell Biol* 29:721, 1997.

474. Poujol C, Nurden AT, Nurden P: Ultrastructural analysis of the distribution of vitronectin receptor (alpha v beta 3) in human platelets and megakaryocytes reveals an intracellular pool and labeling of the alpha-granule membrane. *Br J Haematol* 96:823, 1997.

475. Shimizu Y, Irani AM, Brown EJ, et al: Human mast cells derived from fetal liver cells cultured with stem cell factor express a functional CD51/CD61 (alpha$_v$beta$_3$) integrin. *Blood* 86:930, 1995.

476. Hughes DE, Salter DM, Dedhar S, Simpson R: Integrin expression in human bone. *J Bone Miner Res* 8:527, 1993.

477. Mbalaviele G, Jaiswal N, Meng A, et al: Human mesenchymal stem cells promote human osteoclast differentiation from CD34+ bone marrow hematopoietic progenitors. *Endocrinology* 140:3736, 1999.

478. Boissy P, Machuca I, Pfaff M, et al: Aggregation of mononucleated precursors triggers cell surface expression of alpha$_v$beta$_3$ integrin, essential to formation of osteoclast-like multinucleated cells. *J Cell Sci* 111:2563, 1998.

479. Faccio R, Takeshita S, Zallone A, et al: C-Fms and the $\alpha_v\beta_3$ integrin collaborate during osteoclast differentiation. *J Clin Invest* 111:749, 2003.

480. Chin SL, Johnson SA, Quinn J, et al: A role for alpha V integrin subunit in TGF-beta-stimulated osteoclastogenesis. *Biochem Biophys Res Commun* 307:1051, 2003.

481. Weerasinghe D, McHugh KP, Ross FP, et al: A role for the alpha$_v$beta$_3$ integrin in the transmigration of monocytes. *J Cell Biol* 142:595, 1998.

482. Rainger GE, Buckley CD, Simmons DL, Nash GB: Neutrophils sense flow-generated stress and direct their migration through alpha$_v$beta$_3$-integrin. *Am J Physiol* 276:H858, 1999.

483. Nath D, Slocombe PM, Stephens PE, et al: Interactions of metargidin (ADAM-15) with alpha$_v$beta$_3$ and alpha$_5$beta$_1$ integrins on different haemopoietic cells. *J Cell Sci* 112:579, 1999.

484. Savill J, Hogg N, Ren Y, Haslett C: Thrombospondin cooperates with CD36 and the vitronectin receptor in macrophage recognition of neutrophils undergoing apoptosis. *J Clin Invest* 90:1513, 1992.

485. Fadok VA, Warner ML, Bratton DL, Henson PM: CD36 is required for phagocytosis of apoptotic cells by human macrophages that use either a phosphatidylserine receptor or the vitronectin receptor (alpha$_v$beta$_3$). *J Immunol* 161:6250, 1998.

486. Rubartelli A, Poggi A, Zocchi MR: The selective engulfment of apoptotic bodies by dendritic cells is mediated by the alpha$_{(v)}$beta$_3$ integrin and requires intracellular calcium and extracellular calcium. *Eur J Immunol* 27:1893, 1997.

487. Hunt P, Hokom MM, Hornkohl A, et al: The effect of platelet-derived glycosaminoglycan serglycin on in vitro proplatelet-like process formation. *Exp Hematol* 21:1295, 1993.

488. Leven RM: Differential regulation of integrin-mediated proplatelet formation and megakaryocyte spreading. *J Cell Physiol* 163:597, 1995.

489. Rusnati M, Tanghetti E, Dell'Era P, et al: Alpha,beta$_3$ integrin mediates the cell-adhesive capacity and biological activity of basic fibroblast growth factor (FGF-2) in cultured endothelial cells. *Mol Cell Biol* 8: 2449, 1997.

490. Ybarrondo B, O'Rourke AM, McCarthy JB, Mescher MF: Cytotoxic T-lymphocyte interaction with fibronectin and vitronectin: Activated adhesion and cosignalling. *Immunology* 91:186, 1997.

491. Roberts K, Yokoyama WM, Kehn PJ, Shevach EM: The vitronectin receptor serves as an accessory molecule for the activation of a subset of gamma/delta T cells. *J Exp Med* 173:231, 1991.

492. Rabinowich H, Lin WC, Amoscato A, et al: Expression of vitronectin receptor on human NK cells and its role in protein phosphorylation, cytokine production, and cell proliferation. *J Immunol* 154:1124, 1995.

493. Hermann P, Armant M, Brown E, et al: The vitronectin receptor and its associated CD47 molecule mediates proinflammatory cytokine synthesis in human monocytes by interactions with soluble CD23. *J Cell Biol* 144: 767, 1999.

494. Bessis M: L'ilot èrythroblastique, unitè fonctionelle de le moelle os seuse. *Rev Hematol* 13:8, 1958.

495. Lichtman MA, Waugh RE: Red cell egress from the marrow: Ultrastructural and biophysical aspects, in *Regulation of Erythropoiesis*, edited by ED Zanjani, M Tavassoli, J Ascencao, p 15. PMA Literary & Film Management, Great Neck, NY, 1989.

496. Teal HE, Craici A, Paulson RF, Corell PH: Macrophage-stimulating protein cooperates with erythropoietin to induce colony formation and MAP kinase activation in primary erythroid progenitor cells. *J Hematother Stem Cell Res* 12:165, 2003.

497. Zuhrie SR, Wickramasinghe SN: Stromal cell-dependent terminal maturation of K562 erythroleukemia cells. *Leuk Res* 15.975, 1991.

498. Kapur R, Zhang L: A novel mechanism of cooperation between c-Kit and erythropoietin receptor. Stem cell factor induces the expression of Stat5 and erythropoietin receptor, resulting in efficient proliferation and survival by erythropoietin. *J Biol Chem* 276:1099, 2001.

499. Yu AW, Shao LE, Frigon NL Jr, Yu J: Detection of functional and dimeric activin A in human marrow microenvironment. Implications for the modulation of erythropoiesis. *Ann N Y Acad Sci* 718:285, 1994.

500. Huber TL, Zhou Y, Mead PE, Zon LI: Cooperative effects of growth factors involved in the induction of hematopoietic mesoderm. *Blood* 92: 4128, 1998.

501. Koristschoner NP, Bartunek P, Knespel S, et al: The fibroblast growth factor receptor FGFR-4 acts as a ligand dependent modulator of erythroid cell proliferation. *Oncogene* 18:5904,1999.

502. Iguchi T, Sogo S, Hisha H, et al: HGF activates signal transduction from EPO receptor on human cord blood CD34+/CD45+ cells. *Stem Cells* 17:82, 1999.

503. Lichtman MA, Chamberlain JK, Simon W, et al: Parasinusoidal location of megakaryocytes in marrow: A determinant of platelet release. *Am J Hematol* 4:303, 1978.

504. Thiele J, Galle R, Sander C, Fischer R: Interactions between megakaryocytes and sinus wall: An ultrastructural study of bone marrow tissue in primary (essential) thrombocythemia. *J Submicrosc Cytol Pathol* 23: 595, 1991.

505. Avraham H, Cowley S, Chi SY, et al: Characterization of adhesive interactions between human endothelial cells and megakaryocytes. *J Clin Invest* 91:2378, 1993.

506. Zweegman S, Veenhof MA, Huijgens PC, et al: Regulation of megakaryopoiesis in an in vitro stroma model: Preferential adhesion of megakaryocytic progenitors and subsequent inhibition of maturation. *Exp Hematol* 28:401, 2000.

507. Yang M, Li K, Lam AC, et al: Platelet-derived growth factor enhances granulopoiesis via bone marrow stromal cells. *Int J Hematol* 73:327, 2001.

508. Riviere C, Subra F, Cohen-Solal K, et al: Phenotypic and functional evidence for the expression of CXCR4 receptor during megakaryopoiesis. *Blood* 93:1511, 1999.

509. Hamada T, Mohle R, Hesselgesser J, et al: Transendothelial migration of megakaryocytes in response to stromal cell-derived factor 1 (SDF-1) enhances platelet formation. *J Exp Med* 188:539, 1998.

510. Ito T, Ishida Y, Kashiwagi R, Kuriya S: Recombinant human c-Mpl ligand is not a direct stimulator of proplatelet formation in mature human megakaryocytes. *Br J Haematol* 94:387, 1996.

511. Bruno E, Briddell RA, Cooper RJ, Hoffman R: Effects of recombinant interleukin 11 on human megakaryocyte progenitor cells. *Exp Hematol* 19:378, 1991.

512. Gordon MS, Hoffman R: Growth factors affecting human thrombopoiesis: Potential agents for the treatment of thrombocythemia. *Blood* 80:302, 1992.

513. Ishibashi T, Kimura H, Shikama Y, et al: Interleukin-6 is a potent thrombopoietic factor in vivo in mice. *Blood* 74:1241, 1989.

514. Metcalf D, Hilton D, Nicola NA: Leukemia inhibitory factor can potentiate murine megakaryocyte production in vitro. *Blood* 77:2150, 1991.

515. Kaushansky K: Thrombopoietin. *N Engl J Med* 339:746, 1998.

516. Lambertsen RH, Weiss L: A model of intramedullary hemopoietic microenvironments based on stereologic study of the distribution of endoclonal colonies. *Blood* 63:287, 1984.

517. Wright EC, Pragnell IB: Stem cell proliferation inhibitors. *Baillieres Clin Haematol* 5:723, 1992.

518. Su S, Mukaida N, Wang J, et al: Inhibition of immature progenitor cell proliferation by 1macrophage inflammatory protein-1 alpha by interacting mainly with a C-C chemokine receptor, CCR1. *Blood* 90:605, 1997.

519. Jacobsen SEW, Ruscetti FW, Dubois CM, Keller JR: Tumor necrosis factor α directly and indirectly regulates hematopoietic progenitor cell proliferation: Role of colony-stimulating factor receptor modulation. *J Exp Med* 175:1759, 1992.

520. Dufour C, Corcione A, Svahn J, et al: TNF-alpha and IFN-gamma are overexpressed in the bone marrow of Fanconi anemia patients and TNF-alpha suppresses erythropoiesis in vitro. *Blood* 102:2053, 2003.

521. Rogers JA, Berman JW: A tumor necrosis factor-responsive long-term-culture-initiating cell is associated with the stromal layer of mouse long-term bone marrow cultures. *Proc Natl Acad Sci U S A* 90:5777, 1993.

522. Akel S, Petrow-Sadowski C, Laughlin MJ, Ruscetti FW: Neutralizing of autocrine transforming growth factor-beta in human cord blood CD34(+)CD38(-)Lin(-) cells promotes stem cell factor-mediated erythropoietin-independent early erythroid progenitor development and reduces terminal differentiation. *Stem Cells* 21:557, 2003.

523. Bohmer RM: IL-3-dependent early erythropoiesis is stimulated by autocrine transforming growth factor beta. *Stem Cells* 22:216, 2004.

524. Knospe WH, Husseini SG, Zipori D, Fried W: Hematopoiesis on cellulose ester membranes: XIII. A combination of cloned stromal cells is needed to establish a hematopoietic microenvironment supportive of trilineal hematopoiesis. *Exp Hematol* 21:257, 1993.

525. Winerman JP, Nishikawa S, Muller-Sieburg CE: Maintenance of high levels of pluripotent hematopoietic stem cells in vitro: Effect of stromal cells and c-kit. *Blood* 81:365, 1993.

526. Bhatia M, Bonnet D, Wu D, et al: Bone morphogenetic proteins regulate the developmental program of human hematopoietic stem cells. *J Exp Med* 189:1139, 1999.

527. Simmons PJ, Zannettino A, Gronthos S, Leavesley D: Potential adhesion mechanisms for localization of haemopoietic progenitors to bone marrow stroma. *Leuk Lymphoma* 12:353, 1994.

528. Koller MR, Oxender M, Jensen TC, et al: Direct contact between CD34+ lin- cells and stroma induces a soluble activity that specifically increases primitive hematopoietic cell production. *Exp Hematol* 27:734, 1999.

529. Naito K, Tamahashi N, Chiba T, et al: The microvasculature of the human bone marrow correlated with the distribution of hematopoietic cells: A computer-assisted three-dimensional reconstruction study. *Tohoku J Exp Med* 166:439, 1992.

530. Blazsek I, Misset JL, Benavides M, et al: Hematon, a multicellular functional unit in normal human bone marrow: Structural organization, hemopoietic activity, and its relationship to myelodysplasia and myeloid leukemias. *Exp Hematol* 18:259, 1990.

531. Driessen RL, Johnston HM, Nilsson SK: Membrane bound stem cell factor is a key regulator in the initial lodgement of stem cells within the endosteal marrow region. *Exp Hematol* 31:1284, 2003.

532. Coulombel L, Auffray I, Gaugler MH, Rosemblatt M: Expression and function of integrins on hematopoietic progenitor cells. *Acta Haematol* 97:13, 1997.

533. Wang J, Springer TA: Structural specializations of immunoglobulin superfamily members for adhesion to integrins and viruses. *Immunol Rev* 163:197, 1998.

534. Kansas GS: Selectins and their ligands: Current concepts and controversies. *Blood* 88:3259, 1996.

535. Robinson LA, Steeber DA, Tedder TA: The selectins in inflammation, in *Inflammation Basic Principles and Clinical Correlates*, 3rd ed, edited by JI Gallin, R Snyderman, p 571. Lippincott Williams & Wilkins, Philadelphia, 1999.

536. Lasky LA: Sialomucin ligands for selectins: A new family of cell adhesion molecules. *Princess Takamatsu Symp* 24:81, 1994.

537. Butcher EC, Picker LJ: Lymphocyte homing and homeostasis. *Science* 272:60, 1996.

538. Watt SM, Buhring HJ, Rappold I, et al: CD164, a novel sialomucin on CD34(+) and erythroid subsets, is located on human chromosome 6q21. *Blood* 92:849, 1998.

539. Lesley J, Hyman R, Kincade PW: CD44 and its interaction with extracellular matrix. *Adv Immunol* 54:271, 1993.

540. Borland G, Ross JA, Guy K: Forms and functions of CD44. *Immunology* 93:139, 1998.

541. Deaglio S, Morra M, Mallone R, et al: Human CD38 (ADP-ribosyl cyclase) is a counter-receptor of CD31, an Ig superfamily member. *J Immunol* 160:395, 1998.

542. Hynes RO: Specificity of cell adhesion in development: The cadherin superfamily. *Curr Opin Genet Dev* 2:621, 1992.

543. Okuyama Y, Ishihara K, Kimura N, et al: Human BST-1 expressed on myeloid cells functions as a receptor molecule. *Biochem Biophys Res Commun* 228:838, 1996.

544. Liesveld JL, DiPersio JF, Abboud CN: Integrins and adhesive receptors in normal and leukemic CD34+ progenitor cells: Potential regulatory checkpoints for cellular traffic. *Leuk Lymphoma* 14:19, 1994.

545. Kishimoto TK, Baldwin ET, Anderson DC: The role of β_2 integrins in inflammation, in *Inflammation Basic Principles and Clinical Correlates*, 3rd ed, edited by JI Gallin, R Snyderman, p 537. Lippincott Williams & Wilkins, Philadelphia, 1999.

546. Lasky LA: Selectin-carbohydrate interactions and the initiation of the inflammatory response. *Annu Rev Biochem* 64:113, 1995.

547. Ruoslahti E: Integrins. *J Clin Invest* 87:1, 1991.

548. Yanai N, Sekine C, Yagita H, Obinata M: Roles for integrin very late activation antigen-4 in stroma-dependent erythropoiesis. *Blood* 83:2844, 1994.

549. Hamamura K, Matsuda H, Takeuchi Y, et al: A critical role of VLA-4 in erythropoiesis in vivo. *Blood* 87:2513, 1996.

550. Furasawa T, Yanai N, Hara T, et al: Integrin-associated protein (IAP, also termed CD47) is involved in stroma-supported erythropoiesis. *J Biochem (Tokyo)* 123:101, 1998.

551. Iguchi A, Okuyama R, Koguma M, et al: Selective stimulation of granulopoiesis in vitro by established bone marrow stromal cells. *Cell Struct Funct* 22:357, 1997.

552. Dittel BN, McCarthy JB, Wayner EA, LeBien TW: Regulation of human B-cell precursor adhesion to bone marrow stromal cells by cytokines that exert opposing effects on the expression of vascular cell adhesion molecule-1 (VCAM-1). *Blood* 81:2272, 1993.

553. Ryan DH, Nuccie BL, Ritterman I, et al: Cytokine regulation of early human lymphopoiesis. *J Immunol* 152:5250, 1994.

554. Oostendorp RA, Dormer P: VLA-4-mediated interactions between normal human hematopoietic progenitors and stromal cells. *Leuk Lymphoma* 24:423, 1997.

555. Ryan DH, Nuccie BL, Ritterman I, et al: Expression of interleukin-7 receptor by lineage-negative human bone marrow progenitors with enhanced lymphoid proliferative potential and B-lineage differentiation capacity. *Blood* 89:929, 1997.

556. Dittel BN, LeBien TW: Reduced expression of vascular cell adhesion molecule-1 on bone marrow stromal cells isolated from marrow transplant recipients correlates with a reduced capacity to support human B lymphopoiesis in vitro. *Blood* 86:2833, 1995.

557. Funk PE, Stephan RP, Witte PL: Vascular cell adhesion molecule 1-positive reticular cells express interleukin-7 and stem cell factor in the bone marrow. *Blood* 86:2661, 1995.

558. Galotto M, Berisso G, Delfino L, et al: Stromal damage as a consequence of high-dose chemo/radiotherapy in bone marrow transplant recipients. *Exp Hematol* 27:1460, 1999.

559. Katayama Y, Hildalgo A, Peired A, Frenette PS: $\alpha 4\beta 7$ and its counter-receptor MAdCAM-1 contribute to hematopoietic progenitor recruitment into bone marrow following transplantation. *Blood* 104:2020, 2004.

560. Dedhar S: Integrins and signal transduction. *Curr Opin Hematol* 6:37, 1999.

561. Lowell CA, Berton G: Integrin signal transduction in myeloid leukocytes. *J Leukoc Biol* 65:313, 1999.

562. Aplin AE, Howe A, Alahari SK, Juliano RL: Signal transduction and signal modulation by cell adhesion receptors: The role of integrins, cadherins, immunoglobulin-cell adhesion molecules and selectins. *Pharmacol Rev* 50:197, 1998.

563. Jarvis LJ, Maguire JE, LeBien TW: Contact between human bone marrow stromal cells and B lymphocytes enhances very late antigen-4/vascular cell adhesion molecule-1-independent tyrosine phosphorylation of focal adhesion kinase, paxillin, and ERK-2 in stromal cells. *Blood* 90:1626, 1997.

564. Shibayama H, Anzai N, Braun SE, et al: H-Ras is involved in the inside-out signaling pathway of interleukin-3-induced integrin activation. *Blood* 93:1540, 1999.

565. Levesque JP, Simmons PJ: Cytoskeleton and integrin-mediated adhesion signaling in human CD34+ hemopoietic progenitor cells. *Exp Hematol* 27:579, 1999.

566. Arai A, Nosaka Y, Kohsaka H, et al: CrkL activates integrin-mediated hematopoietic cell adhesion through the guanine nucleotide exchange factor C3G. *Blood* 93:3713, 1999.

567. Porter JC, Hogg N: Integrin cross talk: Activation of lymphocyte function-associated antigen-1 on human T cells alters alpha$_4$beta$_1$- and alpha$_5$beta$_1$-mediated function. *J Cell Biol* 138:1437, 1997.

568. Shibuya A, Campbell D, Hannum C, et al: DYNAM-1, a novel adhesion molecule involved in the cytolytic function of T lymphocytes. *Immunity* 4:573, 1996.

569. Shibuya K, Lanier LL, Phillips JH, et al: Physical and functional association of LFA-1 with DYNAM-1 adhesion molecule. *Immunity* 11:615, 1999.

570. Rodriguez-Fernandez JL, Gomez M, Luque A, et al: The interaction of activated integrin lymphocyte function-associated antigen 1 with ligand intercellular adhesion molecule 1 induces activation and redistribution of focal adhesion kinase and proline-rich tyrosine kinase 2 in T lymphocytes. *Mol Biol Cell* 10:1891, 1999.

571. Leavesley DI, Oliver JM, Swart BW, et al: Signals from platelet/endothelial cell adhesion molecule enhance the adhesive activity of the very late antigen-4 integrin of human CD34+ hematopoietic progenitor cells. *J Immunol* 153:4673, 1994.

572. Vestweber D, Blanks JE: Mechanisms that regulate the function of the selectins and their ligands. *Physiol Rev* 79:181, 1999.

573. Gotoh A, Ritchie A, Takahira H, Broxmeyer HE: Thrombopoietin and erythropoietin activate inside-out signaling of integrin and enhance adhesion to immobilized fibronectin in human growth-factor-dependent hematopoietic cells. *Ann Hematol* 75:207, 1997.

574. Liesveld JL, Winslow JM, Frediani KE, et al: Expression of integrins and examination of their adhesive function in normal and leukemic hematopoietic cells. *Blood* 81:112, 1993.

575. Ryan DH, Nuccie BL, Abboud CN: Inhibition of human bone marrow lymphoid progenitor colonies by antibodies to VLA integrins. *J Immunol* 149:3759, 1992.

576. Sugahara H, Kanakura Y, Furitsu T, et al: Induction of programmed cell death in human hematopoietic cell lines by fibronectin via its interaction with very late antigen 5. *J Exp Med* 179:1757, 1994.

577. Hurley RW, McCarthy JB, Wayner EA, Verfaillie CM: Monoclonal antibody crosslinking of the alpha 4 beta 1 integrin inhibits committed clonogenic hematopoietic progenitor proliferation. *Exp Hematol* 25:321, 1997.

578. Oostendorp RA, Spitzer E, Reisbach G, Dormer P: Antibodies to the beta 1-integrin chain, CD44, or ICAM-3 stimulate adhesion of blast colony-forming cells and may inhibit their growth. *Exp Hematol* 25:345, 1997.

579. Wang MW, Consoli U, Lane CM, et al: Rescue from apoptosis in early (CD34-selected) versus late (non-CD34-selected) human hematopoietic cells by very late antigen 4- and vascular cell adhesion molecule (VCAM) 1-dependent adhesion to bone marrow stromal cells. *Cell Growth Differ* 9:105, 1998.

580. Bhatia R, Munthe HA, Verfaillie CM: Role of abnormal integrin-cytoskeletal interactions in impaired $\beta1$ integrin function in chronic myelogenous leukemia hematopoietic progenitors. *Exp Hematol* 27:1384, 1999.

581. Verfaillie CM, Hurley R, Zhao RC, et al: Pathophysiology of CML: Do defects in integrin function contribute to the premature circulation and massive expansion of the BCR/ABL positive clone? *J Lab Clin Med* 129:584, 1997.

582. Bahtia R, Munthe HA, Verfaillie CM: Tyrphostin AG957, a tyrosine kinase inhibitor with anti-BCR/ABL tyrosine kinase activity restores beta$_1$ integrin-mediated adhesion and inhibitory signaling in chronic myelogenous leukemia hematopoietic progenitors. *Leukemia* 12:1708, 1998.

583. Bahtia R, Verfaillie CM: The effect of interferon-alpha on beta-1 integrin mediated adhesion and growth regulation in chronic myelogenous leukemia. *Leuk Lymphoma* 28:241, 1998.

584. Sun QH, Paddock C, Visentin GP, et al: Cell surface glycosaminoglycans do not serve as ligands for PECAM-1. PECAM-1 is not a heparin-binding protein. *J Biol Chem* 273:11483, 1998.

585. Muller WA, Randolph GJ: Migration of leukocytes across endothelium and beyond: Molecules involved in the transmigration and fate of monocytes. *J Leukoc Biol* 66:698, 1999.

586. Chiba R, Nakagawa N, Kurasawa K, et al: Ligation of CD31 (PECAM-1) on endothelial cells increases adhesive function of $\alpha_v\beta_3$ integrin and enhances β_1 integrin-mediated adhesion of eosinophils to endothelial cells. *Blood* 94:1319, 1999.

587. Duncan GS, Andrew DP, Takimoto H, et al: Genetic evidence for functional redundancy of platelet/endothelial cell adhesion molecule-1 (PECAM-1): CD31-deficient mice reveal PECAM-1-dependent and PECAM-1-independent functions. *J Immunol* 162:3022, 1999.

588. Nakada MT, Amin K, Christofidou-Solomidou M, et al: Antibodies against the first Ig-like domain of human platelet endothelial cell adhesion molecule-1 (PECAM-1) that inhibit PECAM-1-dependent homophilic adhesion block in vivo neutrophil recruitment. *J Immunol* 164:452, 2000.

589. Arkin S, Naprstek B, Guarini L, et al: Expression of intercellular adhesion molecule-1 (CD54) on hematopoietic progenitors. *Blood* 77:948, 1991.

590. Gunji Y, Nakamura M, Hagiwara T, et al: Expression and function of adhesion molecules on human hematopoietic stem cells: CD34+ LFA-1(neg) cells are more primitive than CD34+ LFA-1+ cells. *Blood* 80:429, 1992.

591. Makgoba MW, Sanders ME, Ginther Luce GE, et al: ICAM-1, a ligand for LFA-1-dependent adhesion of B T and myeloid cells. *Nature* 331:86, 1988.

592. Rao SG, Chitnis VS, Deora A, et al: An ICAM-1-like cell adhesion molecule is responsible for CD34-positive haemopoietic stem cells adhesion to bone-marrow stroma. *Cell Biol Int* 20:255, 1996.

593. Staunton DE, Dustin ML, Springer TA: Functional cloning of ICAM-2, a cell adhesion ligand for LFA-1 homologous to ICAM-1. *Nature* 339:61, 1989.

594. Fawcett J, Holness CLL, Needham LA, et al: Molecular cloning of ICAM-3, a third ligand for LFA-1, constitutively expressed on resting leukocytes. *Nature* 360:481, 1992.

595. Campanero MR, Sanchez-Mateos P, del Pozo MA, Sanchez-Madrid F: ICAM-3 regulates lymphocyte morphology and integrin-mediated T cell interactions with endothelial cell and extracellular matrix ligands. *J Cell Biol* 127:867, 1994.

596. Wang JH, Smolyar A, Tan K, et al: Structure of a heterophilic adhesion complex between the human CD2 and CD58 (LFA-3) counterreceptors. *Cell* 97:791, 1999.

597. Nielsen M, Gerwien J, Geisler C, et al: MHC class II ligation induces CD58 (LFA-3)-mediated adhesion in human T cells. *Exp Clin Immunogenet* 15:61, 1998.

598. LeGuiner S, Le Drean E, Labarriere N, et al: LFA-3 co-stimulates cytokine secretion by cytotoxic T lymphocytes by providing a TCR-independent activation signal. *Eur J Immunol* 28:1322, 1998.

599. Itzhaky D, Raz N, Hollander N: The glycosylphosphatidylinositol-anchored form and the transmembrane form of CD58 associate with protein kinases. *J Immunol* 60:4361,1998.

600. Kirby AC, Cahen P, Porter SR, Olsen I: LFA-3 (CD58) mediates T-lymphocyte adhesion in chronic inflammatory infiltrates. *Scand J Immunol* 50:469, 1999.

601. De Waele M, Renmans W, Jochmans K, et al: Different expression of adhesion molecules on CD34+ cells in AML and B lineage ALL and their normal bone marrow counterparts. *Eur J Haematol* 63:192, 1999.

602. McCarty JM, Yee EK, Deisher TA, et al: Interleukin-4 induces endothelial vascular cell adhesion molecule-1 (VCAM-1) by an NF-kappa b-independent mechanism. *FEBS Lett* 372:194, 1995.

603. Bochner BS, Klunk DA, Sterbinsky SA, et al: IL-13 selectively induces vascular cell adhesion molecule-1 expression in human endothelial cells. *J Immunol* 154:799, 1995.

604. Kinashi T, Springer TA: Regulation of cell-matrix adhesion by receptor tyrosine kinases. *Leuk Lymphoma* 18:203, 1995.

605. Lopez M, Aoubala M, Jordier F, et al: The human poliovirus receptor related 2 protein is a new hematopoietic/endothelial homophilic adhesion molecule. *Blood* 92:4602, 1998.

606. Aizawa S, Tavassoli M: In vitro homing of hemopoietic stem cells mediated by a recognition system with galactosyl and mannosyl specificities. *Proc Natl Acad Sci U S A* 84:4485, 1987.

607. Tavassoli M, Hardy CL: Molecular basis of homing of intravenously transplanted stem cells. *Blood* 76:1059, 1990.

608. Sackstein R: Expression of an L-selectin ligand on hematopoietic progenitor cells. *Acta Haematol* 97:22, 1997.

609. Tu L, Murphy PG, Li X, Tedder TF: L-selectin ligands expressed by human leukocytes are HECA-452 antibody-defined carbohydrate epi-

topes preferentially displayed by P-selectin glycoprotein ligand-1. *J Immunol* 161:1140, 1998.

610. Mazo IB, Gutierrez-Ramos JC, Frenette PS, et al: Hematopoietic progenitor cell rolling in bone marrow microvessels: Parallel contributions by endothelial selectins and vascular cell adhesion molecule 1. *J Exp Med* 188:465, 1998.

611. Zollner O, Lenter MC, Blanks JE, et al: L-selectin from human, but not mouse, neutrophils binds directly to E-selectin. *J Cell Biol* 136:707, 1997.

612. Von Andrian UH, M-Rini C: In situ analysis of lymphocyte migration to lymph nodes. *Cell Adhes Commun* 6:85, 1998.

613. Levesque J-P, Zannettino ACW, Pudney M, et al: PSGL-1-mediated adhesion of human hematopoietic progenitors to P-selectin results in suppression of hematopoiesis. *Immunity* 11:369, 1999.

614. Van der Merwe PA: Leukocyte adhesion: High-speed cells with ABS. *Curr Biol* 9:R419, 1999.

615. Vestweber D, Blanks JE: Mechanisms that regulate the function of the selectins and their ligands. *Physiol Rev* 79:181, 1999.

616. Puri KD, Finger EB, Gaudernack G, Springer TA: Sialomucin CD34 is the major L-selectin ligand in human tonsil high endothelial venules. *J Cell Biol* 131:261, 1995.

617. Sassetti C, Tangemann K, Singer MS, et al: Identification of podocalyxin-like protein as a high endothelial venule ligand for L-selectin: Parallels to CD34. *J Exp Med* 187:1965, 1998.

618. Winkler IG, Snapp KR, Simmons PJ, Levesque JP: Adhesion to E-selectin promotes growth inhibition and apoptosis of human and murine hematopoietic progenitor cells independent of PSGL-1. *Blood* 103:1685, 2004.

619. Tada J, Omine M, Suda T, Yamaguchi N: A common signaling pathway via *Syk* and *Lyn* tyrosine kinases generated from capping of the sialomucins CD34 and CD43 in immature hematopoietic cells. *Blood* 93:3723, 1999.

620. Young PE, Baumhueter S, Lasky LA: The sialomucin CD34 is expressed on hematopoietic cells and blood vessels during murine development. *Blood* 85:96, 1995.

621. Oxley SM, Sackstein R: Detection of an L-selectin ligand on a hematopoietic progenitor cell line. *Blood* 84:3299, 1994.

622. Stockton BM, Cheng G, Manjunath N, et al: Negative regulation of T cell homing by CD43. *Immunity* 8:373, 1998.

623. Bazil V, Brandt J, Chen S, et al: A monoclonal antibody recognizing CD43 (leukosialin) initiates apoptosis of human hematopoietic progenitor cells but not stem cells. *Blood* 87:1272, 1996.

624. Yonemura S, Hirao M, Doi Y, et al: Ezrin/radixin/moesin (ERM) proteins bind to a positively charged amino acid cluster in the juxta-membrane cytoplasmic domain of CD44, CD43, and ICAM-2. *J Cell Biol* 140:885, 1998.

625. Anzai N, Gotoh A, Shibayama H, Broxmeyer HE: Modulation of integrin function in hematopoietic progenitor cells by CD43 engagement: Possible involvement of protein tyrosine kinase and phospholipase C-γ. *Blood* 93:3317, 1999.

626. Spertini O, Cordey AS, Monai N, et al: P-selectin glycoprotein ligand 1 is a ligand for L-selectin on neutrophils, monocytes, and CD34+ hematopoietic progenitor cells. *J Cell Biol* 135:523, 1996.

627. Hidalgo A, Weiss LA, Frenette PS: Functional selectin ligands mediating human CD34+ cell interactions with bone marrow endothelium are enhamced postnatally. *J Clin Invest* 110:559, 2002.

628. Zannettino AC, Berndt MC, Butcher C, et al: Primitive human hematopoietic progenitors adhere to P-selectin (CD62P). *Blood* 85:3466, 1995.

629. Blanks JE, Moll T, Eytner R, Vestweber D: Stimulation of P-selectin glycoprotein ligand-1 on mouse neutrophils activates beta 2-integrin mediated cell attachment to ICAM-1. *Eur J Immunol* 28:433, 1998.

630. Yang J, Hirata T, Croce K, et al: Targeted gene disruption demonstrates that P-selectin glycoprotein ligand 1 (PSGL-1) is required for P-selectin-mediated but not E-selectin-mediated neutrophil rolling and migration. *J Exp Med* 190:1769, 1999.

631. Fuhbridge RC, Kieffer JD, Armerding D, Kupper TS: Cutaneous lymphocyte antigen is a specialized form of PSGL-1 expressed on skin-homing T cells. *Nature* 389:978, 1997.

632. Aigner S, Sthoeger ZM, Fogel M, et al: CD24, a mucin-type glycoprotein, is a ligand for P-selectin on human tumor cells. *Blood* 89:3385, 1997.

633. Watt SM, Butler LH, Tavian M, et al: Functionally defined CD164 epitopes are expressed on CD34(+) cells throughout ontogeny but display distinct distribution patterns in adult hematopoietic and nonhematopoietic tissues. *Blood* 95:3113, 2000.

634. Bowen MA, Aruffo A: Adhesion molecules, their receptors, and their regulation: Analysis of CD6-activated leukocyte cell-adhesion molecule (ALCAM/CD166) interactions. *Transplant Proc* 31:795, 1999.

635. Ohneda O, Ohneda K, Arai F, et al: ALCAM (CD166): Its role in hematopoietic and endothelial development. *Blood* 98:2134, 2001.

636. Stamenkovin I, Aruffo A, Amiot M, Seed B: The hematopoietic and epithelial forms of CD44 are distinct polypeptides with different adhesion potentials for hyaluronate-bearing cells. *EMBO J* 10:343, 1991.

637. Dougherty GJ, Lansdorp PM, Cooper DL, Humphries RK: Molecular cloning of CD44R1 and CD44R2, two novel isoforms of the human CD44 lymphocyte "homing" receptor expressed by hemopoietic cells. *J Exp Med* 174:1, 1991.

638. Herrlich P, Zöller M, Pals ST, Ponta H: CD44 splice variants: Metastases meet lymphocytes. *Immunol Today* 14:395, 1993.

639. Rosel M, Khaldoyanidi S, Zawadski V, Zoller M: Involvement of CD44 variant isoform v10 in progenitor cell adhesion and maturation. *Exp Hematol* 27:698, 1999.

640. Funaro A, Malavasi F: Human CD38, a surface receptor, an enzyme, an adhesion molecule and not a simple marker. *J Biol Regul Homeost Agents* 13:54, 1999.

641. Hoenstein AL, Stokinger H, Imhof BA, Malavasi F: CD38 binding to human myeloid cells is mediated by mouse and human CD31. *Biochem J* 330:1129, 1998.

642. Turel KR, Rao SG: Expression of the cell adhesion molecule E-cadherin by the human bone marrow stromal cells and its probable role in CD34(+) stem cell adhesion. *Cell Biol Int* 22:641, 1998.

643. Hirata Y, Kimura N, Sato K, et al: ADP ribosyl cyclase activity of a novel bone marrow stromal cell surface molecule, BST-1. *FEBS Lett* 356:244, 1994.

644. Kaisho T, Ishikawa J, Oritani K, et al: BST-1, a surface molecule of bone marrow stromal cell lines that facilitates pre-B-cell growth. *Proc Natl Acad Sci U S A* 91:5325, 1994.

645. Vicari AP, Bean AG, Zlotnik A: A role for BP-3/BST-1 antigen in early T cell development. *Int Immunol* 8:183, 1996.

646. Okuyama Y, Ishihara K, Kimura N, et al: Human BST-1 expressed on myeloid cells functions as a receptor molecule. *Biochem Biophys Res Commun* 228:838, 1996.

647. Springer TA: Traffic signals for lymphocyte recirculation and leukocyte emigration: The multistep paradigm. *Cell* 76:301, 1994.

648. Steeber DA, Tedder TF: Molecular basis of lymphocyte migration, in *Inflammation Basic Principles and Clinical Correlates*, 3rd ed, edited by JI Gallin, R Snyderman, p 593. Lippincott Williams & Wilkins, Philadelphia, 1999.

649. Imai Y, Lasky LA, Rosen SD: Sulphation requirement for GlyCAM-1, an endothelial ligand for L-selectin. *Nature* 361:555, 1993.

650. Berg EL, McEvoy LM, Berlin C, et al: L-selectin-mediated lymphocyte rolling on MAdCAM-1. *Nature* 366:695, 1993.

651. Lawrence MB, Berg EL, Butcher EC, Springer TA: Rolling of lymphocytes and neutrophils on peripheral node addressin and subsequent arrest on ICAM-1 in shear flow. *Eur J Immunol* 25:1025, 1995.

652. Salmi M, Hellman J, Jalkanen S: The role of two distinct endothelial molecules, vascular adhesion protein-1 and peripheral lymph node addressin, in the binding of lymphocyte subsets to human lymph nodes. *J Immunol* 160:5629, 1998.

653. Weber C, Springer TA. Neutrophil accumulation on activated, surface-adherent platelets in flow is mediated by interaction of Mac-1 with fibrinogen bound to alphaIIbbeta3 and stimulated by platelet-activating factor. *J Clin Invest* 100:2085, 1997.

654. Kovach NL, Lin N, Yednock T, et al: Stem cell factor modulates avidity of alpha 4 beta 1 and alpha 5 beta 1 integrins expressed on hematopoietic cell lines. *Blood* 85:159, 1995.

655. Levesque JP, Leavesley DI, Niutta S, et al: Cytokines increase human hemopoietic cell adhesiveness by activation of very late antigen (VLA)-4 and VLA-5 integrins. *J Exp Med* 181:1805, 1995.

656. Weber C, Alon R, Moser B, Springer TA: Sequential regulation of alpha 4 beta 1 and alpha 5 beta 1 integrin avidity by CC chemokines in monocytes: Implications for transendothelial chemotaxis. *J Cell Biol* 134:1063, 1996.

657. Suehiro Y, Muta K, Umemura T, et al: Macrophage inflammatory protein 1alpha enhances in a different manner adhesion of hematopoietic progenitor cells from bone marrow, cord blood, and mobilized peripheral blood. *Exp Hematol* 27:1637,1999.

658. Issekutz AC, Rowter D, Springer TA: Role of ICAM-1 and ICAM-2 and alternate CD11/CD18 ligands in neutrophil transendothelial migration. *J Leukoc Biol* 65:117, 1999.

659. Meerschaert J, Furie MB: The adhesion molecules used by monocytes for migration across endothelium include CD11a/CD18, CD11b/CD18, and VLA-4 on monocytes and ICAM-1, VCAM-1, and other ligands on endothelium. *J Immunol* 154:4099, 1995.

660. Weber C, Springer TA: Interaction of very late antigen-4 with VCAM-1 supports transendothelial chemotaxis of monocytes by facilitating lateral migration. *J Immunol* 161:6825, 1998.

661. Yong KL, Watts M, Shaun TN, et al: Transmigration of CD34+ cells across specialized and non-specialized endothelium requires prior activation by growth factors and is mediated by PECAM-1 (CD31). *Blood* 91:1196, 1998.

662. Muller WA: The role of PECAM-1 (CD31) in leukocyte emigration: Studies in vitro and in vivo. *J Leukoc Biol* 57:523, 1995.

663. Clark RA, Erickson HP, Springer TA: Tenascin supports lymphocyte rolling. *J Cell Biol* 137:755, 1997.

664. Imhof BA, Weerasinghe D, Brown EJ, et al: Cross talk between alpha(v)beta3 and alpha4beta1 integrins regulates lymphocyte migration on vascular cell adhesion molecule 1. *Eur J Immunol* 27:3242, 1997.

665. Muller WA: Leukocyte-endothelial cell adhesion molecules in transendothelial migration, in *Inflammation Basic Principles and Clinical Correlates*, 3rd ed, edited by JI Gallin, R Snyderman, p 585. Lippincott Williams & Wilkins, Philadelphia, 1999.

666. Fong AM, Robinson LA, Steeber DA, et al: Fractalkine and CX3CR1 mediate a novel mechanism of leukocyte capture, firm adhesion, and activation under physiologic flow. *J Exp Med* 188:1413, 1998.

667. Bacon KB, Greaves DR, Dairaghi DJ, Schall TJ: The expanding universe of C, CX3C and CC chemokines, in *The Cytokine Handbook*, 3rd ed, edited by AW Thompson, p 753. Academic Press, San Diego, 1998.

668. Rood PML, Gerristen WR, Kramer D, et al: Adhesion of hematopoietic progenitor cell to human bone marrow or umbilical vein derived endothelial cell lines: A comparison. *Exp Hematol* 27:1306, 1999.

669. Scott LM, Priestley GV, Papayannopoulou T: Deletion of alpha4 integrin from adult hematopoietic cells reveals roles in homeostasis, regeneration, and homing. *Mol Cell Biol* 23:9349, 2003.

670. Voermans C, van Hennik PB, van der Schoot CE: Homing of human hematopoietic stem and progenitor cells: New insights, new challenges? *J Hematother Stem Cell Res* 10:725, 2001.

671. Mazo IB, von Andrian UH: Adhesion and homing of blood-borne cells in bone marrow microvessels. *J Leukoc Biol* 66:25, 1999.

672. Schweitzer KM, Vicart P, Delouis C, et al: Characterization of a newly established human bone marrow endothelial cell line: Distinct adhesive properties for hematopoietic progenitors compared with human umbilical vein endothelial cells. *Lab Invest* 76:25, 1997.

673. Mohle R, Murea S, Kirsch M, Haas R: Differential expression of L-selectin, VLA-4, from LFA-1 on CD34+ progenitor cells from bone marrow and peripheral blood during G-CSF-enhanced recovery. *Exp Hematol* 23:1535, 1995.

674. Koenig JM, Baron S, Luo D, et al: L-selectin expression enhances clonogenesis of CD34+ cord blood progenitors. *Pediatr Res* 45:867, 1999.

675. Frenette PS, Subbarao S, Mazo IB, et al: Endothelial selectins and vascular cell adhesion molecule-1 promote hematopoietic progenitor homing to bone marrow. *Proc Natl Acad Sci U S A* 95:14423, 1998.

676. Derry CJ, Faveeuw C, Mordsley KR, Ager A: Novel chondroitin sulfate-modified ligands for L-selectin on lymph node high endothelial venules. *Eur J Immunol* 29:419, 1999.

677. Norgard-Sumnicht K, Varki A: Endothelial heparan sulfate proteoglycans that bind to L-selectin have glucosamine residues with unsubstituted amino groups. *J Biol Chem* 270:12012, 1995.

678. Naiyer AJ, Jo DY, Ahn J, et al: Stromal derived factor-1-induced chemokinesis of cord blood CD34(+) cells (long-term culture-initiating cells) through endothelial cells is mediated by E-selectin. *Blood* 94:4011, 1999.

679. Peled A, Grabovsky V, Habler L, et al: The chemokine SDF-1 stimulates integrin-mediated arrest of CD34(+) cells on vascular endothelium under shear flow. *J Clin Invest* 104:1199, 1999.

680. Fuste B, Escolar G, Marin P, et al: G-CSF increases the expression of VCAM-1 on stromal cells promoting the adhesion of CD34+ hematopoietic cells: Studies under flow conditions. *Exp Hematol* 32:765, 2004.

681. Avigdor A, Goichberg P, Shivtiel S, et al: CD44 and hyaluronic acid cooperate with SDF-1 in the trafficking of human CD34+ stem/progenitor cells to the bone marrow. *Blood* 103.2981, 2004.

682. Sbaa-Ketata E, Courel MN, Delpech B, Vannier JP: Hyaluronan-derived oligosaccharides enhance SDF-1 dependent chemotactic effect on peripheral blood hematopoietic CD34+ cells. *Stem Cells* 20:585, 2002.

683. Parakh KA, Kannan K: Demonstration of a ubiquitin binding site on murine haemopoietic progenitor cells: Implications of ubiquitin in homing and adhesion. *Br J Haematol* 84:212, 1993.

684. Hua CT, Gamble JR, Vadas MA, Jackson DE: Recruitment and activation of SHP-1 protein-tyrosine kinase phosphatase by human platelet endothelial cell adhesion molecule-1 (PECAM-1). Identification of immunoreceptor tyrosine-based inhibitory motif-like binding motifs and substrates. *J Biol Chem* 273:28332, 1998.

685. Peled A, Petit I, Kollet O, et al: Dependence of human stem cell engraftment and repopulation of NOD/SCID mice on CXCR4. *Science* 283:845, 1999.

686. Mohle R, Bautz F, Rafii S, et al: The chemokine receptor CXCR-4 is expressed on CD34+ hematopoietic progenitors and leukemic cells and mediates transendothelial migration induced by stromal cell-derived factor-1. *Blood* 91:4523, 1998.

687. Cipolleschi MG, Dello Sbarba P, Olivotto M: The role of hypoxia in the maintenance of hematopoietic stem cells. *Blood* 82:2031, 1993.

688. Jacobsen SE, Ruscetti FW, Ortiz M, et al: The growth response of Lin-Thy1+ hematopoietic progenitors to cytokines is determined by the balance between synergy of multiple stimulators and negative cooperation of multiple inhibitors. *Exp Hematol* 22:985, 1994.

689. Tang J, Nuccie BL, Ritterman I, et al: TGF-beta down-regulates stromal IL-7 secretion and inhibits proliferation of human B cell precursors. *J Immunol* 159:117, 1997.

690. Sakamaki S, Hirayama Y, Matsunaga T, et al: Transforming growth factor-β1 (TGF-β1) induces thrombopoietin from bone marrow stromal

cells which stimulates the expression of TGF-β receptor on megakaryocytes and, in turn, renders them susceptible to suppression by TGF-β itself with high specificity. *Blood* 94:1961, 1999.

691. Cashman JD, Clark-Lewis I, Eaves AC, Eaves CJ: Differentiation stage-specific regulation of primitive human hematopoietic progenitor cycling by exogenous and endogenous inhibitors in an in vivo model. *Blood* 94:3722, 1999.

692. Cashman JD, Eaves CJ, Sarris AH, Eaves AC: MCP-1, not MIP-1alpha, is the endogenous chemokine that cooperates with TGF-beta to inhibit the cycling of primitive normal but not leukemic (CML) progenitors in long-term human marrow cultures. *Blood* 92:2338, 1998.

693. Liesveld JL, Harbol AW, Belanger T, et al: MIP-1alpha and TGF-beta production in CD34+ progenitor-stroma cell coculture systems: Effects of progenitor isolation method and cell contact. *Blood Cells Mol Dis* 26:261, 2000.

694. Kinashi T, Springer TA: Steel factor and c-kit regulate cell matrix adhesion. *Blood* 83:1033, 1994.

695. Juliano RL, Haskill S: Signal transduction from the extracellular matrix. *J Cell Biol* 120:577, 1993.

696. Issaad C, Croisille L, Katz A, et al: A murine stromal cell line allows the proliferation of very primitive human CD34++/CD38- progenitor cells in long-term cultures and semisolid assays. *Blood* 81:2916, 1993.

697. Liesveld JL, Harbol AW, Abboud CN: Stem cell factor and stromal cell co-culture prevent apoptosis in a subculture of the megakaryoblastic cell line, UT-7. *Leuk Res* 20:591, 1996.

698. Borge OJ, Ramsfjell V, Cui L, Jacobsen SE: Ability of early acting cytokines to directly promote survival and suppress apoptosis of human primitive CD34+CD38- bone marrow cells with multilineage potential at the single-cell level: Key role of thrombopoietin. *Blood* 90:2282, 1997.

699. Finch CA, Harker LA, Cook JD: Kinetics of the formed elements of human blood. *Blood* 50:699, 1977.

700. Yong KL: Granulocyte colony-stimulating factor (G-CSF) increases neutrophil migration across vascular endothelium independent of an effect on adhesion: Comparison with granulocyte-macrophage colony-stimulating factor (GM-CSF). *Br J Haematol* 94:40, 1996.

701. Ulich TR, Del Castillo J, Souza L: Kinetics and mechanisms of recombinant human granulocyte-colony stimulating factor-induced neutrophilia. *Am J Pathol* 133:630, 1988.

702. DiPersio JF, Abboud CN: Activation of neutrophils by granulocyte-macrophage colony-stimulating factor, in *Granulocyte Responses to Cytokines: Basic and Clinical Research, Immunology Series*, vol 57, edited by RG Coffey, p 457. Marcel Dekker, New York, 1992.

703. Ghebrehiwet B, Muller-Eberhard HJ: C3e: An acidic fragment of human C3 with leukocytosis-inducing activity. *J Immunol* 123:616, 1979.

704. Kubo H, Graham L, Doyle NA, et al: Complement fragment-induced release of neutrophils from bone marrow and sequestration within pulmonary capillaries in rabbits. *Blood* 92:283, 1998.

705. Deinard AS, Page AR: A study of steroid-induced granulocytosis. *Br J Haematol* 28:333, 1974.

706. Vogel MJ, Yankee RA, Kimball HR, et al: The effect of etiocholanolone on granulocyte kinetics. *Blood* 30:474, 1967.

707. Cybulsky MI, McComb DJ, Movat HZ: Neutrophil leukocyte emigration induced by endotoxin: Mediator roles of interleukin-1 and tumor necrosis factor alpha. *J Immunol* 140:3144, 1988.

708. Terashima T, English D, Hogg JC, Van Eeden SF: Release of polymorphonuclear leukocytes from the bone marrow by interleukin-8. *Blood* 92:1062, 1998.

709. Wang JM, Rambaldi A, Biondi A, et al: Recombinant human interleukin 5 is a selective eosinophil chemoattractant. *Eur J Immunol* 19:701, 1989.

710. Palframan RT, Collins PD, Williams TJ, Rankin SM: Eotaxin induces a rapid release of eosinophils and their progenitors from the bone marrow. *Blood* 91:2240, 1998.

711. Ebisawa M, Yamada T, Bickel C, et al: Eosinophil transendothelial migration induced by cytokines: III. Effect of the chemokine RANTES. *J Immunol* 153:2153, 1994.

712. Lundahl J, Moshfegh A, Gronneberg R, Hallden G: Eotaxin increases the expression of CD11b/CD18 and adhesion properties in IL-5, but not fMLP-prestimulated human peripheral blood eosinophils. *Inflammation* 22:123, 1998.

713. Suratt BT, Petty JM, Young SK, et al: Role of the CXCR4/SDF-1 chemokine axis in circulating neutrophil homeostasis. *Blood* 104:565, 2004.

714. Dutt P, Wang JF, Groopman JE: Stromal cell-derived factor-1 alpha and stem cell factor/kit ligand share signaling pathways in hemopoietic progenitors: A potential mechanism for cooperative induction of chemotaxis. *J Immunol* 161:3652, 1998.

715. Zlotnik A, Yoshie O: Chemokines: A new classification system and their role in immunity. *Immunity* 12:121, 2000.

716. Gerard C, Rollins BJ: Chemokines and disease. *Nat Immunol* 2:108, 2001.

717. Moser B, Wolf M, Walz A, Loetscher P: Chemokines: Multiple levels of leukocyte migration control. *Trends Immunol* 25:75, 2004.

718. Hieshima K, Kawasaki Y, Hanamoto H, et al: CC chemokine ligands 25 and 28 play essential roles in intestinal extravation of IgA antibody-secreting cells. *J Immunol* 173:3668, 2004.

719. Liesveld JL, Rosell K, Panoskaltsis N, et al: Response of human CD34+ cells to CXC, CC, and CX3C chemokines: Implications for cell migration and activation. *J Hematother Stem Cell Res* 10:643, 2001.

720. Tanaka H, Tatsumi N, Kan E, et al: EPO test in hemodialysis patients. *Biomater Artif Cells Immobil Biotechnol* 21:221, 1993.

721. Chamberlain JK, Weiss L, Weed RI: Bone marrow sinus cell packing: A determinant of cell release. *Blood* 46:91, 1975.

722. Waugh RE, Sassi M: An in vitro model of erythroid egress in bone marrow. *Blood* 68:250, 1986.

723. Dabrowski A, Szygula Z, Miszta H: Do changes in bone marrow pressure contribute to the egress of cells from the bone marrow? *Acta Physiol Pol* 32:729, 1981.

724. Iversen PO, Nicolaysen G, Benestad HB: Blood flow to bone marrow during development of anemia or polycythemia in the rat. *Blood* 79:594, 1992.

725. Iversen PO, Nicolaysen G, Benestad HB: The leukopoietic cytokine granulocyte colony-stimulating factor increases blood flow to rat bone marrow. *Exp Hematol* 21:231, 1993.

726. Iversen PO: Blood flow to the haemopoietic bone marrow. *Acta Physiol Scand* 159:269, 1997.

727. Lichtman MA, Chamberlain JK, Santillo PA: Factors thought to contribute to the regulation of egress of cells from marrow, in *The Year in Hematology 1978*, edited by R Silber, J LoBue, A Gordon, p 243. Plenum Press, New York, 1978.

728. Van Eeden SF, Miyagashima R, Haley L, Hogg JC: A possible role for L-selectin in the release of polymorphonuclear leukocytes from bone marrow. *Am J Physiol* 272:H1717, 1997.

729. LeMarer N, Skacel PO: Up-regulation of alpha2,6 sialylation during myeloid maturation: A potential role in myeloid cell release from the bone marrow. *J Cell Physiol* 179:315, 1999.

730. Reinhardt PH, Elliott JF, Kubes P: Neutrophils can adhere via alpha$_2$-beta$_1$-integrin under flow conditions. *Blood* 89:3837, 1997.

731. Burns AR, Bowden RA, Abe Y, et al: P-selectin mediates neutrophil adhesion to endothelial cell borders. *J Leukoc Biol* 65:299, 1999

732. Jagels MA, Chambers JD, Arfors KE, Hugli TE: C5a- and tumor necrosis factor-alpha-induced leukocytosis occurs independently of beta 2 integrins and L-selectin: Differential effects on neutrophil adhesion molecule expression in vivo. *Blood* 85:2900, 1995.

733. Stroncek DF, Kaszcz W, Herr GP, et al: Expression of neutrophil antigens after 10 days of granulocyte-colony-stimulating factor. *Transfusion* 38:663, 1998.

734. Jung U, Ley K: Mice lacking two or all three selectins demonstrate overlapping and distinct functions for each selectin. *J Immunol* 162: 6755, 1999.

735. Scurfield G, Radley JM: Aspects of platelet formation and release. *Am J Hematol* 10:285, 1981.

736. Radley JM, Haller CJ: Fate of senescent megakaryocytes in bone marrow. *Br J Haematol* 53:277, 1983.

737. Efrati P, Rozenszajn L: The morphology of buffy coats in normal human adults. *Blood* 16:1012, 1960.

738. Tinggaard-Pedersen N, Laursen B: Megakaryocytes in cubital venous blood in patients with chronic myeloproliferative diseases. *Scand J Haematol* 30:50, 1983.

739. Mantovani A, Vecchi A, Sozzani S, et al: Tumors as a paradigm for the in vivo role of chemokines in leukocyte recruitment, in *Chemokines and Cancer, Contemporary Cancer Research*, edited by BJ Rollins, p 35. Humana Press, Totowa, NJ, 1999.

740. Kim CH, Broxmeyer HE: In vitro behavior of hematopoietic progenitor cells under the influence of chemoattractants: Stromal cell-derived factor-1, steel factor, and the bone marrow environment. *Blood* 91:100, 1998.

741. Aiuti A, Webb IJ, Bleul C, et al: The chemokine SDF-1 is a chemoattractant for human hematopoietic progenitor cells and provides a new mechanism to explain the mobilization of CD34+ progenitors to peripheral blood. *J Exp Med* 185:111, 1997.

742. Reca R, Mastellos D, Majka M, et al: Functional receptor for C3a anaphylatoxin is expressed by normal hematopoietic stem/progenitor cells, and C3a enhances their homing-related responses to SDF-1. *Blood* 101: 3784, 2003.

743. Aiuti A, Tavian M, Cipponi A, et al: Expression of CXCR4, the receptor for stromal cell-derived factor-1 on fetal and adult human lympho-hematopoietic progenitors. *Eur J Immunol* 29:1823, 1999.

744. Roberts MM, Swart BW, Simmons PJ, et al: Prolonged release and c kit expression of haemopoietic precursor cells mobilized by stem cell factor and granulocyte colony stimulating factor. *Br J Haematol* 104: 778, 1999.

745. Wang JB, Mukaida N, Zhang Y, et al: Enhanced mobilization of hematopoietic progenitor cells by mouse MIP-2 and granulocyte colony-stimulating factor. *J Leukoc Biol* 62:503, 1997.

746. Papayannopoulou T, Priestley GV, Nakamoto B, et al: Synergistic mobilization of hemopoietic progenitor cells using concurrent beta1 and beta2 integrin blockade or beta2-deficient mice. *Blood* 97:1282, 2001.

747. Sweeney EA, Papayannopoulou T: Increase in circulating SDF-1 after treatment with sulfated glycans. The role of SDF-1 in mobilization. *Ann N Y Acad Sci* 938:48, 2001.

748. Papayannopoulou T: Current mechanistic scenarios in hematopoietic stem/progenitor cell mobilization. *Blood* 103:1580, 2004.

749. Vermeulen M, Le Pesteur F, Gagnerault MC, et al: Role of adhesion molecules in the homing and mobilization of murine hematopoietic stem and progenitor cells. *Blood* 92:894, 1998.

750. Craddock CF, Nakamoto B, Elices M, Papayannopoulou TH: The role of CS1 moiety of fibronectin in VLA mediated haemopoietic progenitor trafficking. *Br J Haematol* 98:828, 1997.

751. Craddock CF, Nakamoto B, Andrews RG, et al: Antibodies to VLA4 integrin mobilize long-term repopulating cells and augment cytokine-induced mobilization in primates and mice. *Blood* 90:4779, 1997.

752. Papayannopoulou T, Priestley GV, Nakamoto B: Anti-VLA4/VCAM-1-induced mobilization requires cooperative signaling through the kit/mkit ligand pathway. *Blood* 91:2231, 1998.

753. Yang F-C, Atkinson SJ, Gu Y, et al: Rac and Cdc42 GTPases control hematopoietic stem cell shape, adhesion, migration and mobilization. *Proc Natl Acad Sci U S A* 98:5614, 2001.

754. Bug G, Rossmanith T, Henschler R, et al: Rho family small GTPases control migration of hematopoietic progenitor cells into multicellular spheroids of bone marrow stroma. *J Leukoc Biol* 72:837, 2002.

755. Papayannopoulou T, Priestley GV, Bonig H, Nakamoto B: The role of G-protein signaling in hematopoietic stem/progenitor cell mobilization. *Blood* 101:4739, 2003.

756. Christensen JL, Wright DE, Wagers AJ, Weismann IL: Circulation and chemotaxis of fetal hematopoietic stem cells. *PLoS Biology* 2:368, 2004.

757. Preffer FI, Dombkowski D, Sykes M, et al: Lineage-negative side-population (SP) cells with restricted hematopoietic capacity circulate in normal human adult blood: Immunophenotypic and functional characterization. *Stem Cells* 20:417, 2002.

758. Maloney MA, Patt HM: Migration of cells from shielded to irradiated marrow. *Blood* 39:804, 1972.

759. Dercksen MW, Gerristen WR, Rodenhuis S, et al: Expression of adhesion molecules on CD34+ cells: CD34+ L-selectin+ cells predict a rapid platelet recovery after blood stem cell transplantation. *Blood* 85: 3313, 1995.

760. Watanabe T, Dave B, Heiman DG, et al: Cell adhesion molecule expression on CD34+ cells in grafts and time to myeloid and platelet recovery after autologous stem cell transplantation. *Exp Hematol* 26:10, 1998.

761. Katayama Y, Mahmut N, Takimoto H, et al: Hematopoietic progenitor cells from allogeneic bone marrow transplant donors circulate in the very early post-transplant period. *Bone Marrow Transplant* 23:659, 1999.

762. Hardy CL: The homing of hematopoietic stem cells to the bone marrow. *Am J Med Sci* 309:260, 1995.

763. Pipia GG, Long MW: Human hematopoietic progenitor cell isolation based on galactose-specific cell surface binding. *Nat Biotechnol* 15: 1007, 1997.

764. Shirota T, Tavassoli M: Alterations of bone marrow sinus endothelium induced by ionizing irradiation: Implications in homing of intravenously transplanted marrow cells. *Blood Cells* 18:197, 1992.

765. Yamazaki K, Allen TD: The structure and function of the blood-marrow barrier: Early ultrastructural changes in irradiated bone marrow sinus endothelial cells detected by vascular perfusion fixation [comment]. *Blood Cells* 18:215, 1992.

766. Bolante-Cervantes R, Li S, Sahota A, et al: Pattern of localization of primitive hematopoietic cells in vivo using a novel mouse model. *Exp Hematol* 27:1346, 1999.

767. Cui J, Wahl RL, Shen T, et al: Bone marrow cell trafficking following intravenous administration. *Br J Haematol* 107:895, 1999.

768. Imai K, Kobayashi M, Wang J, et al: Selective secretion of chemoattractants for haemopoietic progenitor cells by bone marrow endothelial cells: A possible role in homing of haemopoietic progenitor cells to bone marrow. *Br J Haematol* 106:905, 1999.

769. Jo DY, Rafii S, Hamada T, Moore MA: Chemotaxis of primitive hematopoietic cells is in response to stromal cell-derived factor-1. *J Clin Invest* 105:101, 2000.

770. Lanzkron SM, Collector MI, Sharkis SJ: Hematopoietic stem cell trafficking in vivo: A comparison of short-term and long-term repopulating cells. *Blood* 93:1916, 1999.

771. Adams GB, Chabner KT, Foxall RB, et al: Heterologous cells cooperate to augment stem cell migration, homing and engraftment. *Blood* 101: 45, 2003.

772. Olavarria E, Kanfer EJ: Selection and use of chemotherapy with hematopoietic growth factors for mobilization of peripheral blood progenitor cells. *Curr Opin Hematol* 7:191, 2000.

773. Korbling M: Collection of allogeneic peripheral blood stem cells. *Baillieres Best Pract Res Clin Haematol* 12:41, 1999.

774. Facon T, Harousseau JL, Maloisel F, et al: Stem cell factor in combination with filgastrim after chemotherapy improves peripheral blood progenitor cell yield and reduces apheresis requirements in multiple myeloma patients: A randomized, controlled trial. *Blood* 94:1218, 1999.

775. MacVittie TJ, Farese AM, Davis TA, et al: Myelopoietin, a chimeric agonist of human interleukin 3 and granulocyte colony-stimulating factor receptors, mobilizes CD34+ cells that rapidly engraft lethally x-irradiated nonhuman primates. *Exp Hematol* 27:1557, 1999.

776. Grzegorwski KJ, Komschlies Kl, Franco JL, et al: Quantitative and cell-cycle differences in progenitor cells mobilized by recombinant human interleukin-7 and recombinant human granulocyte colony-stimulating factor. *Blood* 88:4139, 1996.

777. Somlo G, Sniecinski I, Ter Veer A, et al: Recombinant human thrombopoietin in combination with granulocyte colony-stimulating factor enhances mobilization of peripheral blood progenitor cells, increases peripheral blood platelet concentration, and accelerates hematopoietic recovery following high-dose chemotherapy. *Blood* 93:2798, 1999.

778. Siena S, Bregni M, Gianni AM: Mobilization of peripheral blood progenitor cells for autografting: Chemotherapy and G-CSF or GM-CSF. *Baillieres Best Pract Res Clin Haematol* 12:27, 1999.

779. Gazitt Y: Comparison between granulocyte colony-stimulating factor and granulocyte-macrophage colony-stimulating factor in the mobilization of peripheral blood stem cells. *Curr Opin Hematol* 9:190, 2002.

780. Lapidot T, Petit I: Current understanding of stem cell mobilization: The roles of chemokines, proteolytic enzymes, adhesion molecules, cytokines, and stromal cells. *Exp Hematol* 30:973, 2002.

781. Cottler-Fox MH, Lapidot T, Petit I, et al: Stem cell mobilization. *Hematology (Am Soc Hematol Educ Program)* 419, 2003.

782. Petit I, Szyper-Kravitz M, Nagler A, et al: G-CSF induces stem cell mobilization by decreasing bone marrow SDF-1 and up-regulating CXCR4. *Nat Immunol* 3:687, 2002.

783. Christ O, Gunthert U, Haas R, Zoller M: Importance of CD44v7 isoforms for homing and seeding of hematopoietic progenitor cells. *J Leukoc Biol* 69:343, 2001.

784. Pilarski LM, Pruski E, Wizniak J, et al: Potential role for hyaluronan and the hyaluronan receptor RHAMM in mobilization and trafficking of hematopoietic progenitor cells. *Blood* 93:2918, 1999.

785. Chamberlain JK, Leblond PF, Weed RI: Reduction of adventitial cell cover: An early direct effect of erythropoietin on bone marrow ultrastructure. *Blood Cells* 1:655, 1975.

786. Pruijt JFM, Williamze R, Fibbe WE: Mechanisms underlying hematopoietic stem cell mobilization induced by the CXC chemokine interleukin-8. *Curr Opin Hematol* 6:152, 1999.

787. Pruijt JFM, Verzaal P, Van Ros R, et al: Neutrophils are indispensable for hematopoietic stem cell mobilization by interleukin-8 in mice. *Proc Natl Acad Sci U S A* 99:6228, 2002.

788. Starckx S, Van den Steen PE, Wuyts A, et al: Neutrophil gelatinase B and chemokines in leukocytosis and stem cell mobilization. *Leuk Lymphoma* 43:233, 2002.

789. Pruijt JFM, Fibbe WE, Laterveer L, et al: Prevention of interleukin-8-induced mobilization of hematopoietic progenitor cells in rhesus monkeys by inhibitory antibodies against the metalloproteinase gelatinase B (MMP-9). *Proc Natl Acad Sci U S A* 96:10863, 1999.

790. Watanabe T, Kawano Y, Kanamaru S, et al: Endogenous interleukin-8 (IL-8) surge in granulocyte colony-stimulating factor-induced peripheral blood stem cell mobilization. *Blood* 93:1157, 1999.

791. Pruijt JFM, Van Kooyk Y, Figdor CG, et al: Murine hematopoietic progenitor cells with colony-forming or radioprotective capacity lack expression of the beta 2-integrin LFA-1. *Blood* 93:107, 1999.

792. Pruijt JFM, Van Kooyk Y, Figdor CG, et al: Anti-LFA-1 blocking antibodies prevent mobilization of hematopoietic progenitor cells induced by interleukin-8. *Blood* 91:4099, 1998.

793. Semerad, CL, Poursine-Laurent J, Liu F, et al: A role for G-CSF receptor signaling in the regulation of hematopoietic cell function but not lineage commitment or differentiation. *Immunity* 11:153, 1999.

794. Liu F, Poursine-Laurent J, Link D: The granulocyte colony-stimulating factor receptor is required for the mobilization of murine hematopoietic progenitors into peripheral blood by cyclophosphamide or interleukin-8 but not Flt-3 ligand. *Blood* 90:2522, 1997.

795. Betsuyaku T, Liu F, Senior RM, et al: A functional granulocyte-macrophage colony-stimulating factor receptor is required for normal chemoattractant-induced neutrophil activation. *J Clin Invest* 103:825, 1999.

796. Murphy G, Gavrilovic J: Proteolysis and cell migration: Creating a path? *Curr Opin Cell Biol* 11:614, 1999.

797. Webb LM, Ehrengruber MU, Clark-Lewis I, et al: Binding of heparan sulfate or heparin enhances neutrophil responses to interleukin-8. *Proc Natl Acad Sci U S A* 90:7158, 1993.

798. Dias Baruffi M, Pereira-da-Silva G, Jamur MC, Roque-Barreira MC: Heparin potentiates in vivo neutrophil migration induced by IL-8. *Glyconj J* 15:523, 1998.

799. Rainger GE, Rowley AF, Nash GB: Adhesion-dependent release of elastase from human neutrophils in a novel, flow-based model: Specificity of different chemotactic agents. *Blood* 92:4819, 1998.

800. Wize J, Sopata I, Smerdel A, Maslinski S: Ligation of selectin L and integrin CD11b/CD18 (Mac-1) induces release of gelatinase B (MMP-9) from human neutrophils. *Inflamm Res* 47:325, 1998.

801. Janowska-Wieczorek A, Marquez LA, Nabholtz J-M, et al: Growth factors and cytokines upregulate gelatinase expression in bone marrow CD34+ cells and their transmigration through reconstituted basement membrane. *Blood* 93:3379, 1999.

802. Levesque J-P, Liu F, Simmons PJ, et al: Characterization of hematopoietic progenitor mobilization in protease-deficient mice. *Blood* 104: 65, 2004.

803. Hidalgo A, Peired AJ, Weiss LA, et al: The integrin aMb2 anchors hematopoietic progenitors in the bone marrow during enforced mobilization. *Blood* 104:993, 2004.

804. Fruehauf S, Seggewiss R: Its moving day: Factors affecting peripheral blood stem cell mobilization and strategies for improvement. *Br J Haematol* 122:360, 2003.

805. Liles WC, Broxmeyer HE, Rodger E, et al: Mobilization of hematopoietic progenitor cells in healthy volunterrs by AMD3100, a CXCR4 antagonist. *Blood* 102:2728, 2003.

806. Devine SM, Flomenberg N, Vesole DH, et al: Rapid mobilization of CD34+ cells following administration of the CXCR4 antagonist AMD3100 to patients with multiple myeloma and non-Hodgkins lymphoma. *J Clin Oncol* 22:1095, 2004.

807. Evans CA, Tonge R, Blinco D, et al: Comparative proteomics of primitive hematopoietic cell populations reveal differences in expression of proteins regulating motility. *Blood* 103:3751, 2004.

808. Ceradini DJ, Kulkarni AR, Callaghan MJ, et al: Progenitor cell trafficking is regulated by hypoxic gradients through HIF-1 induction of SDF-1. *Nat Med* 10:858, 2004.

809. Basser RL, O'Flaherty E, Green M, et al: Development of pancytopenia with neutralizing antibodies to thrombopoietin after multicycle chemotherapy supported by megakaryocyte growth and development factor. *Blood* 99:2599, 2002.

810. Kuter DJ, Begley G: Recombinant human thrombopoietin: Basic biology and evaluation of clinical studies. *Blood* 100:3457, 2002.

THE LYMPHOID TISSUES

THOMAS J. KIPPS

The lymphoid tissues can be divided into primary and second- ary lymphoid organs. Primary lymphoid tissues are sites where lymphocytes develop from progenitor cells into functional and mature lymphocytes. The major primary lymphoid tissue is the marrow, the site where all lymphocyte progenitor cells reside and initially differentiate. This organ is discussed in Chap. 4. The other primary lymphoid tissue is the thymus, the site where progenitor cells from the marrow differentiate into mature thymus-derived (T) cells. Secondary lymphoid tissues are sites where lymphocytes interact with each other and nonlymphoid cells to generate immune responses to antigens. These include the spleen, lymph nodes, and mucosa-associated lymphoid tis- sues (MALT). The structure of these tissues provides insight into how the immune system discriminates between self anti- gens and foreign antigens and develops the capacity to orches- trate a variety of specific and nonspecific defenses against in- vading pathogens.

THE THYMUS

The thymus is the site for development of thymic-dependent lympho- cytes (T cells). It is a primary lymphoid organ in that it is a major site of lymphopoiesis (lymphocyte development). In this organ, develop- ing T cells, called *thymocytes*, differentiate from lymphoid stem cells derived from the marrow into functional, mature T cells.[1] It is here that T cells acquire their repertoire of specific antigen receptors to cope with the antigenic challenges received throughout one's life span. Once they have completed their maturation, the T cells leave the thymus and circulate in the blood and through secondary lymphoid tissues.

THYMIC ANATOMY

The thymus is located in the superior mediastinum, overlying, in order, the left brachiocephalic (or innominate) vein, the innominate artery, the left common carotid artery, and the trachea. It overlaps the upper limit of the pericardial sac below and extends into the neck beneath the upper anterior ribs. It receives its blood supply from the internal thoracic arteries. Venous blood from the thymus drains into the bra- chiocephalic and internal thoracic veins, which communicate above with the inferior thyroid veins.

Arising from the third and fourth brachial pouches as an epithelial organ populated by lymphoid cells and endoderm-derived thymic ep- ithelial cells, the thymus develops at about the eighth week of gesta- tion.[2] The thymus increases in size through fetal and postnatal life and remains ample into puberty,[3] when it weighs about 40 g. Thereafter, the size progressively decreases with aging as a consequence of thymic involution.[4–6]

Acronyms and abbreviations that appear in this chapter include: CT, computed tomography; GALT, gut-associated lymphoid tissue; Ig, immunoglobulin; MALT, mucosa-associated lymphoid tissues; MHC, major histocompatibility complex; PALS, periarteriolar lymphoid sheath; T, thymus-derived; TCR, T cell receptor.

The volume of the thymus can be estimated by sonography. In one study of 149 healthy term infants within 1 week of birth, there was a significant correlation between the estimated thymic volume and the weight of the infant.[7] However, no correlation was apparent between the estimated thymic volume and the infant's sex, length, or gestational age. Also, there was no apparent correlation between estimated volume and the proportions of CD4+ T cells or CD8+ T cells found in the blood. The estimated thymic volume of healthy infants increases from birth to between 4 and 8 months of age and then decreases.[3] Most of the individual variation at 4 and 10 months of age appears to correlate with breast-feeding status, body size, and, to a lesser extent, illness. Breast-fed infants at 4 months of age have significantly larger esti- mated thymic volumes than do age-matched formula-fed infants with similar thymic volumes at birth.[8]

THYMIC STRUCTURE

A longitudinal fissure divides the thymus into two asymmetric lobes— a larger right and a smaller left—that are derived from the right and left brachial pouches, respectively. These two developmentally sepa- rate parts of the thymus are easily separated from each other by blunt dissection.

Each lobe of the thymus is divided into multiple lobules by fibrous septa. Each lobule consists of an outer cortex and an inner medulla. The cortex contains dense collections of thymocytes that appear as lymphocytes of slightly variable size with scattered, rare mitoses. The lighter-staining medulla is more sparsely populated with cells. It con- tains loosely arranged mature thymocytes and characteristic tightly packed whorls of squamous-appearing epithelial cells, called Hassall concentric corpuscles. These appear to be remnants of degenerating cells and are rich in high molecular weight cytokeratins.

The thymus contains several other important cell types in addition to thymocytes. There are three types of specialized epithelial cells within the thymus: the medullary epithelial cells, which are organized into clusters; the cortical epithelial cells, which form an epithelial net- work; and the epithelial cells of the outer cortex.[9] The epithelial cells in the cortex and medulla often have a stellate shape, display desmo- somal connections to one another, and may function as nurse cells to developing thymocytes. In addition, the thymus contains marrow-de- rived antigen-presenting cells, primarily interdigitating dendritic cells and macrophages, particularly at the corticomedullary junction.

After puberty, thymic involution begins within the cortex. This region may disappear completely with aging, whereas medullary rem- nants persist throughout life. Glucocorticoids also may induce atrophy of the cortex secondary to glucocorticoid-induced apoptosis of cortical thymocytes.[10] This also may be seen in conditions that are associated with increases in circulating steroids, for example, pregnancy or stress.[11,12]

THYMIC IMMUNE FUNCTION

Prothymocytes originate in the marrow and migrate to the thymus, where they mature into T cells (see Chaps. 76 and 78). Maturation of T cells is accompanied by the sequential acquisition by thymocytes of the various T-cell markers (Fig. 5-1).[13] Terminal deoxynucleotidyl transferase is found in prothymocytes and immature thymocytes but is absent in mature T cells.

Pre-T cells enter the cortex via small blood vessels and are double negative for CD4 and CD8 antigens.[1] One of the earliest identifiable T-cell membrane antigens is CD2. As the thymocytes proliferate and differentiate in the cortex, they acquire CD4 and CD8 antigens. They subsequently acquire the CD3 antigen and the T-cell receptor for an- tigen as they migrate toward the medulla.

Positive and negative selection of maturing T cells takes place in the thymus.[14] "Double-positive" (CD4+ and CD8+) thymocytes un- dergo an initial positive selection step that is mediated exclusively by

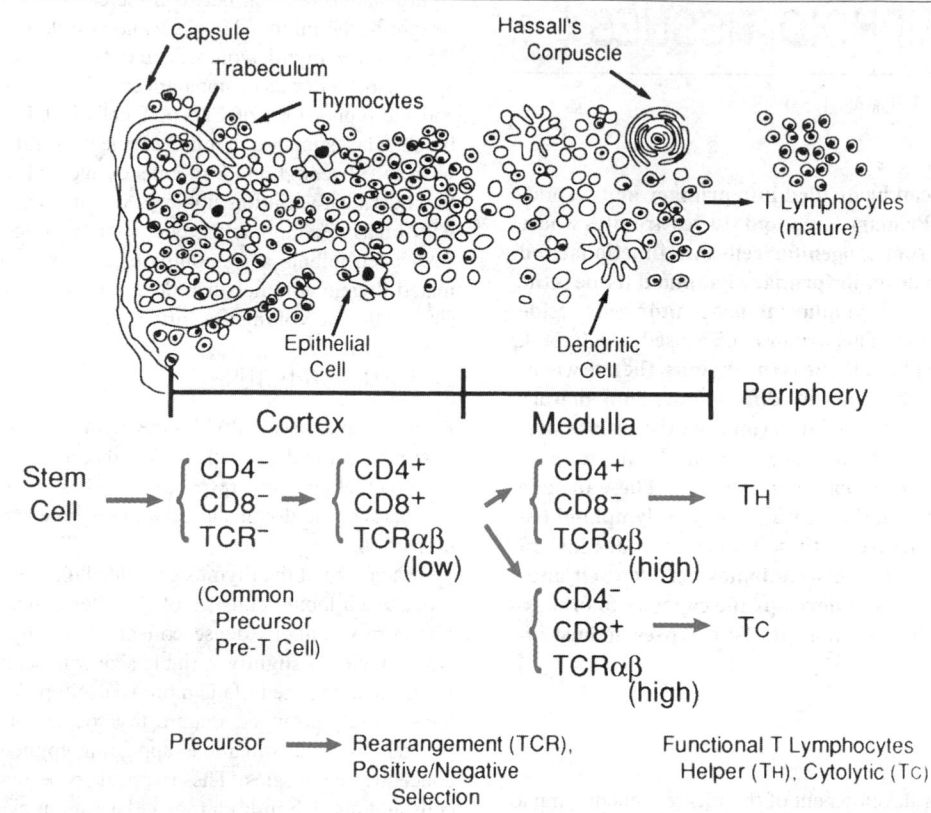

FIGURE 5-1 Structure of the thymus. The top half of the figure provides a cross section of a thymic lobule, indicating the outer cortex (*left*), inner medulla (*center*), and periphery (*far right*). The marked arrows indicate various structures and cell types. As thymocytes mature, they migrate from the cortex toward the medullary region and acquire phenotypic features that are outlined at the bottom of the figure, as described in the text (see Chap. 76).

thymic cortical epithelium.[15] Thymocytes that have T cell receptors (TCRs) capable of interacting with the major histocompatibility complex (MHC) molecules expressed by thymic cortical epithelial cells will undergo expansion, whereas thymocytes with defective TCRs will undergo apoptosis.[16–18] As these positively selected cells migrate toward the medulla, they experience negative selection. Those thymocytes that have TCRs that react too vigorously with the MHC molecules of the medullary epithelium and marrow-derived cells will undergo apoptosis.[17,19,20] Most of the developing thymocytes are destroyed. In this way, only those T cells that have the appropriate level of low affinity for self-MHC molecules will reach the final maturation stages and be allowed to exit the thymus.

The selected thymocytes enter the thymic medulla, where they further mature and differentiate to become "single positive" for either CD4 or CD8 and acquire the capacity for future helper and cytolytic functions, respectively[1] (see Chaps. 76 and 78). Here they also may interact with scattered B cells during their final stages of thymic education. A small percentage of the lymphocytes produced in the thymus finally exit the medulla via efferent lymphatics as mature, naive T cells.

THE SPLEEN

The spleen is a secondary lymphoid organ. Secondary lymphoid tissues provide an environment in which the cells of the immune system can interact with antigen and with one another to develop an immune response to antigen. The spleen is a major site of immune response to blood-borne antigens. In addition, the splenic red pulp contains macrophages that are responsible for clearing the blood of unwanted for-

eign substances and senescent erythrocytes, even in the absence of specific immunity. Thus, it acts as a filter for the blood.

SPLENIC ANATOMY

The spleen is located within the peritoneum in the left upper quadrant of the abdomen between the fundus of the stomach and the diaphragm. It receives its blood supply from the systemic circulation via the splenic artery, which branches off the celiac trunk, and the left gastroepiploic artery.[21] The blood returning from the spleen drains into the portal circulation via the splenic vein. Consequently, the spleen can become congested with blood and increase in size when there is portal hypertension (see Chap. 55).

Approximately 10 percent of individuals have one or more accessory spleens. Accessory spleens are usually 1 cm in diameter and resemble lymph nodes. However, they usually are covered with peritoneum, as is the spleen itself. Accessory spleens typically lie along the course of the splenic artery or its gastroepiploic branch, but they may be elsewhere.[22] The commonest location is near the hilus of the spleen, but approximately one in six accessory spleens can be found embedded in the tail of the pancreas, where they may be occasionally mistaken for a pancreatic mass lesion.[23–27]

The average weight of the spleen in the adult human is 135 g, ranging from 100 to 250 g. However, when emptied of blood it weighs only about 80 g. On autopsy of 539 subjects with normal spleens, there was a positive correlation between the spleen weight and both the degree of acute splenic congestion and the subject's height and weight, but not with the subject's sex or age.[28]

The splenic volume can be estimated by computed tomography (CT) of the abdomen. In one study,[29,30] the splenic volume was calculated from the linear and the maximal cross-sectional area measurements of the spleen, using the following formula: splenic volume = 30 cm³ + 0.58 × the product of the width, length, and thickness of the spleen measured in centimeters.[29] Using this formula, the mean value of the calculated splenic volume for 47 normal subjects was 214.6 cm³, with a range from 107.2 to 314.5 cm³. The calculated splenic volume did not appear to vary significantly with the subject's age, gender, height, weight, body mass index, or the diameter of the first lumbar vertebra, the latter being considered representative of body habitus on CT.

The splenic volume also can be estimated by sonography. In one study of 32 normal spleens from adult corpses, the ultrasound measurements of maximal height, width, and thickness of the spleen were compared with the actual volume displaced by the excised organ.[31] The mean actual splenic volume was approximately 148 cm³ (± 81 cm³ SD), whereas mean splenic volume estimated from ultrasonography was 284 cm³ (± 168 cm³ SD). Despite the differences between the actual and estimated volumes, these investigators did find a roughly linear correlation between actual splenic volume and the estimated splenic volume measured by ultrasonography. However, there may be operator-to-operator variation in measurement of the estimated splenic volume, making the use of sonography in longitudinal studies technically demanding.

SPLENIC STRUCTURE

The spleen has an "open" circulation that lacks endothelial continuity from artery to vein.[32] When isolated spleens are perfused in washout studies, erythrocytes that appear in the splenic vein appear to be flushed out from three compartments. The red cells that are flushed out first come from a compartment that presumably is formed by the splenic vessels. The erythrocytes that are flushed out next come from a second compartment, where they presumably are loosely held within the filtration beds. The erythrocytes that are flushed out last presumably were adherent to cells of the filtration beds. Although 90 percent of the blood flow passes through the splenic vessels, only approximately 10 percent of the total splenic red cells are found within this first compartment. The second compartment is perfused by 9 percent of the total inflow yet contains 70 percent of the splenic red cells. The last compartment is perfused by only 1 percent of the inflow but contains 20 percent of the splenic red cells.

These compartments reflect the anatomy of the spleen and its stroma. The stroma is composed of branched, fibroblast-like cells called reticular cells. These cells produce slender collagen fibers, the reticular fibers, which are rich in type IV collagen. The reticular cells and fibers form a meshwork, or reticulum, which filters the blood. Three major types of filtration beds can be distinguished by their structure and content: the white pulp, the marginal zone, and the red pulp.

WHITE PULP

The white pulp contains the lymphocytes and other mononuclear cells that surround the arterioles branching off the splenic artery. After the splenic artery pierces the splenic capsule at the hilum, it divides into progressively smaller branches. Each branch is called a central artery because it runs through the central longitudinal axis of a distinctive filtration bed that surrounds each central artery (Fig. 5-2). This is com-

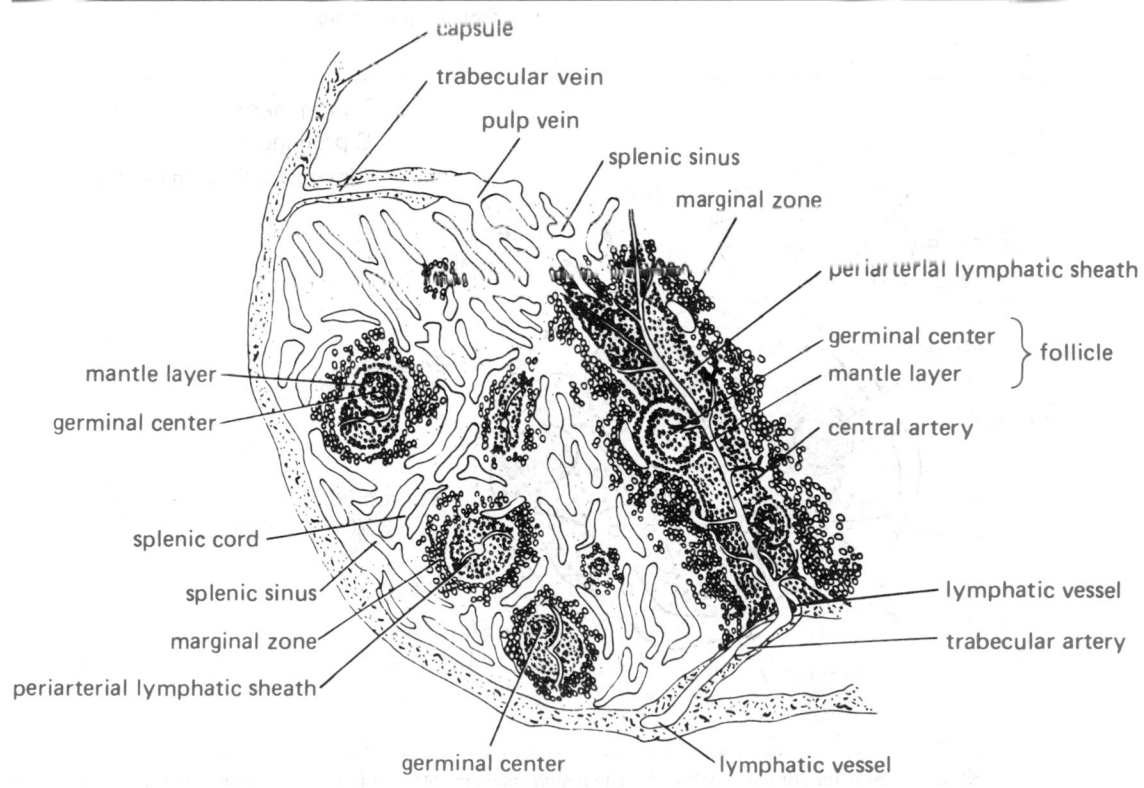

FIGURE 5-2   Structure of the spleen. A branch of the splenic artery enters the pulp and becomes a central artery. Surrounding the central artery is a periarteriolar lymphoid sheath (PALS). At the circumference of the PALS is the marginal zone, which generally separates the white pulp of the PALS from the red pulp. Follicles of B cells with occasional germinal centers (Malpighian corpuscles) are located at the outer margins of the PALS for the depicted central artery and the PALS of central arteries that are in a different plane from that of the figure.

posed of a cuff of lymphocytes called the *periarteriolar lymphoid sheath* (PALS). The PALS is composed mostly of T lymphocytes, about two-thirds of which are CD4+ T cells. The PALS around white pulp arterioles of the human spleen is not continuous.[33] Indeed, segments of the central arterioles might not be surrounded by T cells in areas where they run through lymphoid follicles containing pale kernels of activated B lymphocytes interspersed with large, pale macrophages and dendritic cells.[1] On gross inspection of the surface of a freshly cut spleen, these follicles appear as white dots referred to as *Malpighian corpuscles*. These corpuscles predominantly contain a germinal center and have the same anatomic features and functions as secondary follicles in the lymph node (Fig. 5-3).

Branches coming off the central artery deliver disproportionate amounts of plasma and lymphocytes to the rims of the PALS. These branches tend to run at acute angles, leading to a selective loss of plasma from the blood, a phenomenon referred to as skimming. After becoming relatively depleted of plasma, the arterioles then carry high-hematocrit blood into the filtration beds of the red pulp and marginal zone. As a result, the red pulp and marginal zone beds contain relatively high concentrations of red cells.

THE MARGINAL ZONE

The marginal zone surrounds the PALS and follicles. It is composed of reticulum, which forms a finely meshed filtration bed, serving as a vestibule for much of the blood that flows through the spleen. The marginal zone surrounds the white pulp and merges imperceptibly into the red pulp. It contains more lymphocytes than the red pulp. These are primarily memory B cells and CD4+ T cells that appear especially well equipped for rapid antibody immune responses to blood-borne antigens.[34–39] However, like the red pulp, the marginal zone may become congested and clear imperfect and senescent red cells and parasites.

THE RED PULP

The red pulp of the spleen is composed of a reticular meshwork, called the *splenic cords of Billroth*, and splenic sinuses.[40] This region predominantly contains erythrocytes but has large numbers of macrophages and dendritic cells. There are relatively few lymphocytes and plasma cells in this area.

As the central arteries branch and decrease in size, the PALS also branches and decreases in diameter to but a few cells surrounding the arteriole. The small arteriole finally emerges from its sheath and then terminates in either the marginal zone or the red pulp. Here these vessels are suspended and anchored by adventitial reticular cells in the periarterial beds. They often terminate abruptly as arteriolar capillaries or as vessels with a trumpet-like flare with widened slits called *interendothelial slits*. The blood flows through these slits into filtration beds composed of large-meshed loculi that open to one another.

The blood in the red pulp and marginal zone drains into venous sinuses that form anastomosing, blind-ending vessels. These venous sinuses actually are specialized postcapillary venules. The endothelial cells are shaped as tapered rods that are stiffened by basal, longitudinal, intermediate cytoskeletal filaments and by contractile filaments of actin and myosin. These intracellular contractile filaments can shorten the vein, causing the endothelium to buckle and form interendothelial gaps, favoring transmural passage.

The endothelial cells are attached to a basement membrane. While this appears to be fashioned of fibers, the basement membrane actually is an extracellular membranous wall with large, regular defects that expose considerable basal endothelial surface. This includes the interendothelial slits, through which blood may flow from the filtration bed and into the vein. Ordinarily the interendothelial slits are narrow, or even closed, unless forced apart by cells in transmural transit or by endothelial contraction.

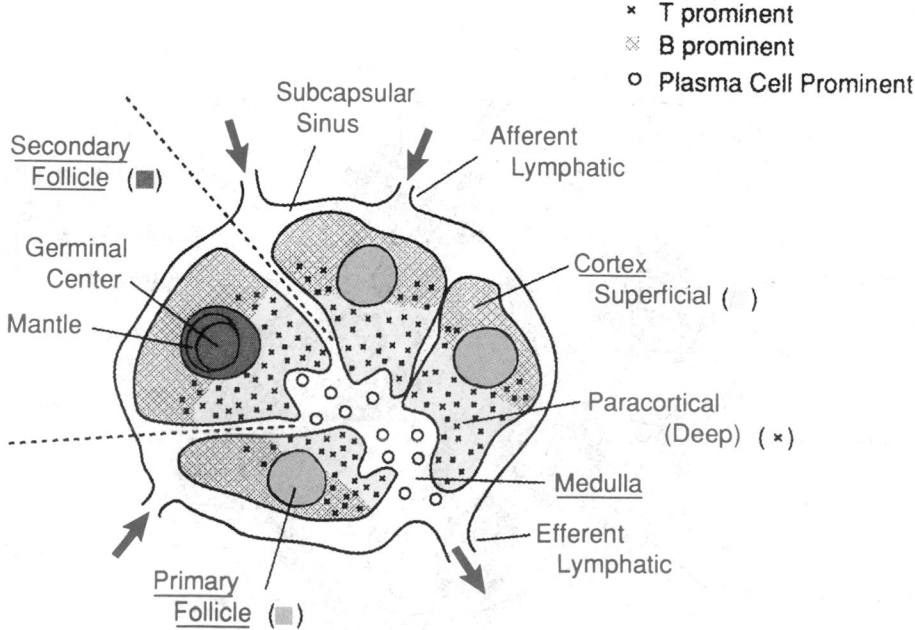

FIGURE 5-3　Structure of the lymph node. The lymph enters via afferent lymphatic channels and exits via the efferent lymphatic channel. The *large arrows* indicate the direction of the lymphatic flow into and out of the lymph node. The legend shows the symbols used for the T cell zone (**x**) and the B cell zone (*shaded*) of each follicle. The follicle in the lower left part of the node contains a primary follicle lacking a germinal center. The follicle immediately above this follicle contains a germinal center. Thus, the entire follicle delineated by the *dashed lines* is a secondary follicle. The cortex, paracortical area, and medulla are also shown.

Splenic arterioles terminate at varied distances from the walls of venous vessels. Blood flowing from arterioles that terminate at the venous vessel wall may flow directly into the splenic vein. However, blood flowing from arterioles that terminate at a distance from a vein must traffic through the spleen. In so doing, the blood either may pass quickly through a nonsinusal venous aperture or slowly through sinusal interendothelial slits and the fibroblast stroma.

The fibroblast stroma contains reticular cells and myofibroblast cells, also called *barrier cells*.[41] The latter may fuse with each other to form a syncytial membrane that connects the arterial terminals with venous interendothelial slits or apertures. Like other myofibroblasts, these cells contain actin and myosin and may contract, thereby approximating splenic arterial and venous vessels with one another. Thus, the fibroblast stroma may affect the relative proportion of blood that flows through the stroma or the sinusal interendothelial slits. Such redistribution might occur during periods of acute physiologic stress, allow for increased expulsion of red cells from the spleen, and account for some of the slight increase in hematocrit observed during strenuous exercise.[42]

SPLENIC FUNCTION

RED CELL CLEARANCE

Mixed within the stroma of the red pulp and marginal zone are monocytes and macrophages. As the blood passes through the stroma, monocytes may be held on the stroma, where the microenvironment is conducive to their maturation into macrophages and large, dendritic, lysosome-rich phagocytes. These cells may assist the reticular cells in mechanical filtration. More important, these cells have phagocytic activity that allows them to ingest imperfect erythrocytes, store platelets, and remove infectious agents, such as *Plasmodium*, from the circulation.[43] In addition, these cells have nonphagocytic functions, such as the presentation of antigens to T cells or the elaboration of certain cytokines.

Collectively, the anatomy of the spleen allows the marginal zone and red pulp to cull defective erythrocytes. As the blood passes slowly through the sinusal interendothelial slits and the fibroblast stroma, the erythrocytes must undergo alterations in shape to squeeze through the mechanical barrier generated by this filtration compartment. Normal red cells that are supple can pass through readily because the interendothelial slits can open to about 0.5 μm. However, blood cells containing large, rigid inclusions, such as *Plasmodium*-containing erythrocytes, are delayed or sequestered.[44]

Splenic macrophages residing within these filtration beds also can sequester erythrocytes that are coated with antibody. Polymorphisms of Fcα-RII (CD32) or Fcα-RIII (CD16) that affect immunoglobulin (Ig) G binding in vitro can alter the efficiency of clearance of antibody-coated red cells in vivo.[45]

When these filtration beds sequester imperfect red cells, the blood pools inside the spleen, causing stasis and congestion. This stimulates sphincter-like contraction of the distal vein, resulting in proximal plasma transudation that produces a viscous luminal mass of high-hematocrit blood. During episodes of enhanced red cell sequestration, as occur during malarial crises or hemolytic episodes in sickle cell disease, the splenic volume and weight may increase ten- to twenty-fold.[46,47] Although the white pulp may enlarge, particularly in germinal centers, the marginal zones and red pulp become greatly widened with pooled erythrocytes and macrophages in this setting.

SPLENIC IMMUNE FUNCTION

The spleen and its responses to antigens are similar to those of lymph nodes, the major difference being that the spleen is the major site of immune responses to blood-borne antigens, while lymph nodes are involved in responses to antigens in the lymph.[40] Antigens and lymphocytes enter the spleen through the vascular sinusoids because the spleen lacks high endothelial venules. Upon entry, the lymphocytes home to the white pulp. T cells migrate to the PALS and B cells to the lymphoid nodules. T cells and B cells migrate within these compartments for about 5 and 7 h, respectively. In the absence of an immune response, these cells migrate through a reticulum arranged around the circumference of the central artery.

Upon immune activation in response to antigen, the lymphocytes may remain in the spleen to sustain a primary or secondary immune response. Activation of B cells is initiated in the marginal zones that are adjacent to CD4+ T cells in the PALS. Activated B cells then migrate into germinal centers or into the red pulp.[48] Lymphoid nodules appear and expand by recruiting lymphocytes from the blood and the peripheral zone of the follicles, termed the *mantle zone*. These cells then proliferate and differentiate in the center of a lymphoid nodule, forming a germinal center.[49] In their path from the marginal zone to the follicles, B cells pass the PALS, where they remain in contact with T lymphocytes for a few hours, allowing ample time for T-B cell interaction in response to antigens. If they are not recruited in an immune response to antigen, both T and B lymphocytes exit the spleen via deep efferent lymphatics, not the splenic veins.

These efferent lymphatics are not distinguished as separate structures within the PALS, being quite thin-walled and often packed with efferent lymphocytes. However, they are important in moving nonreactive lymphocytes out of the spleen and in producing high-hematocrit pulp blood. After leaving the spleen, the efferent lymphocytes become the afferent lymphatics of the perisplenic mesenteric lymph nodes or empty into the thoracic duct. This duct empties into the left subclavian vein, thus returning the lymphocytes to the venous circulation.

LYMPH NODES

The lymphoid nodes are secondary lymphoid tissues. They form part of a network that filters antigens from the interstitial tissue fluid and lymph during its passage from the periphery to the thoracic duct. Thus, the lymph nodes are the primary sites of immune response to tissue antigens.

LYMPH NODE ANATOMY

The lymph nodes are round or kidney-shaped clusters of mononuclear cells that normally are less than 1 cm in diameter. A collagenous capsule surrounds a typical lymph node and has an indentation called the *hilus* where blood vessels enter and leave.

Lymph nodes typically are present at the branches of the lymphatic vessels and form part of the extensive network of lymphatic channels that extends throughout the body. Several afferent lymphatic channels that drain lymph from regional tissues into the lymph node perforate the capsule of each lymph node. The lymph draining from the node leaves through one efferent lymphatic vessel at the hilus. The lymph from the node, in turn, empties into efferent lymphatic vessels that eventually drain into larger lymphatic channels leading eventually to the thoracic duct. The thoracic duct, in turn, drains into the left subclavian vein, thus returning lymph into the systemic circulation.

Clusters of lymph nodes are placed strategically in areas that drain various superficial and deep regions of the body, such as the neck, axillae, groin, mediastinum, and abdominal cavity. The lymph nodes that receive lymph that drains from the skin, termed *somatic nodes*, are superficial. The lymph nodes that receive their lymph from the mucosal surface of the respiratory, digestive, or genitourinary tract, termed *visceral nodes*, are usually deep within body cavities.

LYMPH NODE STRUCTURE

Beneath the collagenous capsule is the subcapsular sinus, into which the afferent lymphatic channels drain (see Fig. 5-3). This sinus is lined with phagocytic cells. Fibrous trabeculae radiate from the medulla adjacent to the hilus of the node to the subcapsular sinus, thus breaking the node into several follicles, called cortical follicles. These trabeculae, together with the capsule and a network of reticulin fibers, support the various cellular components of the node and serve as the scaffolding for lymphatic spaces, namely, the subcapsular and cortical sinuses. These lymphatic spaces are continuous with medullary sinuses and the solitary efferent lymphatic channel exiting the hilus.

Each cortical follicle contains dense collections of small, mature, recirculating lymphocytes. These consist of a B cell area (cortex), a T cell area (paracortex), and a central medulla with cellular cords that contain T cells, B cells, plasma cells, and macrophages.[1] Some follicles contain lightly staining areas of 1 to 2 mm in diameter, called *germinal centers*. Germinal centers are the specialized sites for the generation of memory B cells and antibody affinity maturation via the process of immunoglobulin variable-region somatic hypermutation.[50,51] Follicles without germinal centers are called *primary follicles*, and those with germinal centers are called *secondary follicles*. Primary lymphoid follicles contain nodules that consist predominantly of small, mature, recirculating B lymphocytes.

Within 1 week after antigenic stimulation, secondary follicles develop a germinal center, which contains proliferating B cells and macrophages.[52,53] The small, nonreactive B cells are apparently forced to the periphery of the follicle, where they form a dense follicular mantle. Conversely, the B cells within the germinal center are highly activated, typically forming lymphoblasts that have abundant cytoplasm and round, cleaved, or convoluted shapes. Follicular dendritic cells also are found within the germinal centers. These cells can trap and retain antigens for months, possibly in the form of immune complexes.[54] The germinal centers of the secondary follicle may gradually regress after the antigenic stimulus is eliminated.

Surrounding the lymphoid follicles of the superficial cortex are sheets of lymphocytes that extend to the deep cortex, the so-called paracortex, that blend into medullary cords of cells. The paracortical zones are formed mostly of T cells. The ratio of T cells to B cells in these zones is about 3:1. The medulla, however, contains scattered B cells, dendritic cells, macrophages, and, during an immune response, plasma cells. The superficial cortex and medulla of the lymph nodes are the thymic-independent areas, whereas the deep cortex is particularly enriched with T cells, forming an area that sometimes is referred to as the thymic-dependent area. The major T cell population found within the lymph node consists of CD4+ T cells. The scattering of CD4+ T cells in the follicles, and in more prominent numbers in the interfollicular zones, reveals the proximity of CD4+ T and B cells important for T-B cooperation during proliferation and maturation of antigen-stimulated B cells.[55]

Lymphocytes primarily enter lymphatic tissues from the blood by migrating across the tall, active endothelium of specialized postcapillary venules called *high endothelial venules*.[56] Cellular adhesion molecules and various chemokines are responsible for the pattern of lymphocyte trafficking and determine the microanatomy of the lymphoid tissues.[57]

LYMPH NODE FUNCTION

The lymph node is the site where different types of lymphocytes, macrophages, and dendritic cells can interact with one another to generate an immune response to antigens carried within the lymph. As the lymph passes across the nodes from afferent to efferent lymphatic vessels, particulate antigens are removed by the phagocytic cells and transported into the lymphoid tissue of the lymph node.[1] Abnormal cells within the lymph, such as neoplastic cells, also can be trapped within the lymph node.

Within the lymph node, antigen is presented to T cells as processed peptides by major histocompatibility complex (MHC) molecules of antigen-presenting cells (see Chap. 78). T cell recognition is mediated by the TCR for antigen. Which T cells are activated is determined by the specificity of the TCRs, the structure of MHC molecules, and the nature of antigen-presenting cells, including the dendritic reticular cells, macrophages, and B cells.

However, along with TCR recognition of processed antigen presented in the MHC of the antigen-presenting cell, adequate T cell activation requires second signals, or costimulation, delivered through accessory molecules, such as CD28 on T cells (see Chap. 78).[58] Without these second signals, the T cells may become anergic, or specifically nonresponsive to antigen stimulation.[59] This specific suppression is thought to play an important regulatory role in the maintenance of self-tolerance.[60,61]

T cell recognition of specific antigen may induce release of soluble factors, such as the interleukins, that can activate T cells, B cells, and/or monocytes.[62–65] Also, the activated T cells express surface molecules, such as CD40 ligand, that also can activate B cells, dendritic cells, or macrophages.[66,67]

The T-dependent immune response includes the formation of early germinal centers within days after antigen exposure. There is a mixture of B cells and activated CD4+ T cells in the lymphoid follicles. T-B cooperation involves the accessory B cell antigen CD40 and the CD40 ligand expressed on activated T cells. Activated B cells become blasts and comprise the largest numbers of cells in the early germinal center.[52] Subsequently, B cell lymphoblasts give rise to smaller B cells, the *centrocytes*. B cells undergo affinity maturation within the germinal center. During this process, the genes encoding the surface immunoglobulin of B cells undergo high rates of mutation, called *somatic hypermutation*.[49,67] B cells, including the centrocytes, that express immunoglobulin with little or no affinity for antigen undergo apoptosis.[68] The resulting cellular debris is *tingible*, or capable of being stained, and is found prominently within macrophages specifically designated tingible body macrophages. Conversely, B cells expressing surface immunoglobulin with a high affinity for antigen are selected to proliferate and differentiate to memory B cells or plasma cells.[69] As well as promoting activation of B cells, CD4+ T cells, and CD8+ T cells, the T cell limb of the primary immune response may generate circulating CD4+ and CD8+ memory T cells[70,71] (see Chap. 78).

Following release of specific antibody, antigen–antibody complexes may form and become sequestered on the surface of follicular dendritic cells within the germinal centers. These antigen–antibody complexes produce a coating of small, bead-like, immune complex-coated bodies called *iccosomes*. Iccosomes can be presented to CD4+ T cells by B cells and dendritic cells. Iccosomes also appear to assist in anamnestic recall of high levels of antibody following reentry of antigen in the host.[72] T cell and B cell memory functions and self-tolerance depend on persistence of antigen.[70,73–75]

PERIPHERAL LYMPHOID TISSUES

MUCOSA-ASSOCIATED LYMPHOID TISSUES

MALT are diffusely organized aggregates of lymphocytes that protect the respiratory and gastrointestinal epithelium.[76] The lymphoid aggregates associated with the respiratory epithelium are sometimes referred to as the bronchial-associated lymphoid tissue. The lymphoid aggregates associated with the intestinal epithelium are sometimes referred to as the gut-associated lymphoid tissue (GALT). These tissues include the tonsils, adenoids, appendix, and specialized structures called Peyer patches found in the ileum, and they collect antigen from the epithelial surfaces of the gastrointestinal tract.

Solitary lymph nodules with follicular and germinal center structures occur in the mucosa and submucosa of the respiratory tract, the gastrointestinal tract (particularly within the ileum), the urinary tract, and the vagina. During states of chronic inflammation, lymphoid nodules may form as a localized center of lymphocytes with marked follicular activity. The Waldeyer ring of pharyngeal lymphoid tissues and Peyer patches in the ileum contain prominent aggregated nodular lymphoid tissue. No capsule or efferent or afferent lymphatic vessels are present in these accessory lymphoid tissues.

These MALT are rich in plasma cells and eosinophils. The plasma cells are a source of secretory immunoglobulin that is transferred into the lumina of the bronchi and gastrointestinal tract. The majority of plasma cells in the mucosa of the bronchi and gut contain IgA. IgA is released from the plasma cell and then combines with a secretory piece synthesized within the mucosal epithelium to become secretory IgA (see Chap. 77). Secretory IgA then is secreted across the microvilli of mucosal epithelium into the lumen, where it may prevent colonization of mucosal membranes by pathogens. Lymphoid nodules along mucosa-lined tracts serve as precursors of IgA-producing cells. These nodules form a barrier against many microorganisms and antigens. Microfolds overlying specialized epithelial cells in the gut transport antigenic material by pinocytosis, with subsequent immunization and IgA secretion.

PEYER PATCHES

Peyer patches are the most important and highly organized of the GALT.[76] They are found in the lamina propria of the small intestine (beneath the mucosa near the ileocolonic junction) and consist of up to 50 or more lymphoid nodules covered by a single layer of columnar epithelium. They are well developed in youth and regress with age. Antigens from the intestinal epithelium are collected by specialized epithelial cells called M cells, allowing for generation of specific immune responses against intestinal pathogens.[77] Peyer patches are the sites at which B cells differentiate, in response to these antigens, into the plasma cells found within the intestine.[78]

TONSILS

The tonsils are the major component of the Waldeyer ring of pharyngeal lymphoid tissues. They are covered by variable epithelial surfaces that have deep, branching depressions called crypts. Fused lymphatic nodules lie adjacent to the crypts, and germinal centers are prominent. A pseudocapsule of condensed connective tissue surrounds the tonsils, and septae within the structures form lobulations. Together with the other lymphoid tissues of the Waldeyer ring, the tonsils provide the initial barrier to pathogens entering the oral pharynx.

REFERENCES

1. Crivellato E, Vacca A, Ribatti D: Setting the stage: An anatomist's view of the immune system. *Trends Immunol* 25:210, 2004.

2. Blackburn CC, Manley NR: Developing a new paradigm for thymus organogenesis. *Nat Rev Immunol* 4:278, 2004.

3. Hasselbalch H, Jeppesen DL, Ersbøll AK, et al: Thymus size evaluated by sonography. A longitudinal study on infants during the first year of life. *Acta Radiol* 38:222, 1997.

4. Pawelec G, Adibzadeh M, Solana R, Beckman I: The T cell in the ageing individual. *Mech Ageing Dev* 93:35, 1997.

5. Haynes BF, Hale LP: The human thymus. A chimeric organ comprised of central and peripheral lymphoid components [corrected and repub-

lished article originally printed in *Immunol Res* 18(2):61, 1998]. *Immunol Res* 18:175, 1998.

6. Linton PJ, Dorshkind K: Age-related changes in lymphocyte development and function. *Nat Immunol* 5:133, 2004.

7. Hasselbalch H, Jeppesen DL, Ersbøll AK, et al: Sonographic measurement of thymic size in healthy neonates. Relation to clinical variables. *Acta Radiol* 38:95, 1997.

8. Hasselbalch H, Jeppesen DL, Engelmann MD, et al: Decreased thymus size in formula-fed infants compared with breastfed infants. *Acta Paediatr* 85:1029, 1996.

9. Röpke C: Thymic epithelial cell culture. *Microsc Res Tech* 38:276, 1997.

10. Cifone MG, Migliorati G, Parroni R, et al: Dexamethasone-induced thymocyte apoptosis: apoptotic signal involves the sequential activation of phosphoinositide-specific phospholipase C, acidic sphingomyelinase, and caspases. *Blood* 93:2282, 1999.

11. Rijhsinghani AG, Thompson K, Bhatia SK, Waldschmidt TJ: Estrogen blocks early T cell development in the thymus. *Am J Reprod Immunol* 36:269, 1996.

12. Ayala A, Herdon CD, Lehman DL, et al: Differential induction of apoptosis in lymphoid tissues during sepsis: Variation in onset, frequency, and the nature of the mediators. *Blood* 87:4261, 1996.

13. Hale LP: Histologic and molecular assessment of human thymus. *Ann Diagn Pathol* 8:50, 2004.

14. Starr TK, Jameson SC, Hogquist KA: Positive and negative selection of T cells. *Annu Rev Immunol* 21:139, 2003.

15. Laufer TM, Glimcher LH, Lo D: Using thymus anatomy to dissect T cell repertoire selection. *Semin Immunol* 11:65, 1999.

16. Blackman M, Kappler J, Marrack P: The role of the T cell receptor in positive and negative selection of developing T cells. *Science* 248.1335, 1990.

17. Müller-Hermelink HK, Wilisch A, Schultz A, Marx A: Characterization of the human thymic microenvironment: lymphoepithelial interaction in normal thymus and thymoma. *Arch Histol Cytol* 60:9, 1997.

18. Nikolich-Žugich J, Slifka MK, Messaoudi I: The many important facets of T-cell repertoire diversity. *Nat Rev Immunol* 4:123, 2004.

19. Takahama Y, Shores EW, Singer A: Negative selection of precursor thymocytes before their differentiation into CD4+CD8+ cells. *Science* 258:653, 1992.

20. Oukka M, Colucci-Guyon E, Tran PL, et al: CD4 T cell tolerance to nuclear proteins induced by medullary thymic epithelium. *Immunity* 4: 545, 1996.

21. Romero-Torres R: The true splenic blood supply and its surgical applications. *Hepatogastroenterology* 45:885, 1998.

22. Paul R, Bielmeier J, Breul J, et al: Accessory spleen of the spermatic cord. *Urologe A* 36:262, 1997.

23. Takayama T, Shimada K, Inoue K, et al: Intrapancreatic Accessory Spleen. *Lancet* 344:957, 1994.

24. Harris GN, Kase DJ, Bradnock H, McKinley MJ: Accessory spleen causing a mass in the tail of the pancreas—MR imaging findings. *AJR Am J Roentgenol* 163:1120, 1994.

25. Ota T, Tei M, Yoshioka A, et al: Intrapancreatic accessory spleen diagnosed by technetium-99m heat-damaged red blood cell SPECT. *J Nucl Med* 38:494, 1997.

26. Churei H, Inoue H, Nakajo M: Intrapancreatic accessory spleen: Case report. *Abdom Imaging* 23:191, 1998.

27. Lauffer JM, Baer HU, Maurer CA, et al: Intrapancreatic accessory spleen—A rare cause of a pancreatic mass. *Int J Pancreatol* 25:65, 1999.

28. Sprogøe-Jakobsen S, Sprogøe-Jakobsen U: The weight of the normal spleen. *Forensic Sci Int* 88:215, 1997.

29. Prassopoulos P, Daskalogiannaki M, Raissaki M, et al: Determination of normal splenic volume on computed tomography in relation to age, gender and body habitus. *Eur Radiol* 7:246, 1997.

30. Watanabe Y, Todani T, Noda T, Yamamoto S: Standard splenic volume in children and young adults measured from CT images. *Surg Today* 27: 726, 1997.

31. Rodrigues Júnior AJ, Rodrigues CJ, Germano MA, et al: Sonographic assessment of normal spleen volume. *Clin Anat* 8:252, 1995.

32. Skandalakis PN, Colborn GL, Skandalakis LJ, et al. The surgical anatomy of the spleen. *Surg Clin North Am* 73:747, 1993.

33. Steiniger B, Ruttinger L, Barth PJ: The three-dimensional structure of human splenic white pulp compartments. *J Histochem Cytochem* 51: 655, 2003.

34. Spencer J, Perry ME, Dunn-Walters DK: Human marginal-zone B cells. *Immunol Today* 19:421, 1998.

35. Tierens A, Delabie J, Michiels L, et al.: Marginal-zone B cells in the human lymph node and spleen show somatic hypermutations and display clonal expansion. *Blood* 93:226, 1999.

36. Kurtin PJ: Marginal zone B cells, monocytoid B cells, and the follicular microenvironment. Determinants of morphologic features in a subset of low-grade B-cell lymphomas. *Am J Clin Pathol* 114:505, 2000.

37. Martin F, Kearney JF: Marginal-zone B cells. *Nat Rev Immunol* 2:323, 2002.

38. Zandvoort A, Timens W: The dual function of the splenic marginal zone: Essential for initiation of anti-TI-2 responses but also vital in the general first-line defense against blood-borne antigens. *Clin Exp Immunol* 130: 4, 2002.

39. Weller S, Faili A, Aoufouchi S, et al: Hypermutation in human B cells in vivo and in vitro. *Ann N Y Acad Sci* 987:158, 2003.

40. Kraus MD: Splenic histology and histopathology: An update. *Semin Diagn Pathol* 20:84, 2003.

41. Weiss L: Barrier cells in the spleen. *Immunol Today* 12:24, 1991.

42. Stewart IB, McKenzie DC: The human spleen during physiological stress. *Sports Med* 32:361, 2002.

43. Chotivanich K, Udomsangpetch R, McGready R, et al: Central role of the spleen in malaria parasite clearance. *J Infect Dis* 185:1538, 2002.

44. Suwanarusk R, Cooke BM, Dondorp AM, et al: The deformability of red blood cells parasitized by *Plasmodium falciparum* and *P. vivax*. *J Infect Dis* 189:190, 2004.

45. Kumpel BM, De Haas M, Koene HR, et al: Clearance of red cells by monoclonal IgG3 anti-D in vivo is affected by the VF polymorphism of Fcgamma RIIIa (CD16). *Clin Exp Immunol* 132:81, 2003.

46. Weiss L, Geduldig U, Weidanz W: Mechanisms of splenic control of murine malaria: reticular cell activation and the development of a blood-spleen barrier. *Am J Anat* 176:251, 1986.

47. Smith NC, Fell A, Good MF: The immune response to asexual blood stages of malaria parasites. *Chem Immunol* 70:144, 1998.

48. Rizzo LV, Secord EA, Tsiagbe VK, et al: Components essential for the generation of germinal centers. *Dev Immunol* 6:325, 1998.

49. Hollowood K, Goodlad JR: Germinal centre cell kinetics. *J Pathol* 185: 229, 1998.

50. Varade WS, Insel RA: Isolation of germinal center-like events from human spleen RNA—somatic hypermutation of a clonally related VH6DJH rearrangement expressed with IgM, IgG, and IgA. *J Clin Invest* 91:1838, 1993.

51. Han S, Zheng B, Takahashi Y, Kelsoe G: Distinctive characteristics of germinal center B cells. *Semin Immunol* 9:255, 1997.

52. Tarlinton D: Germinal centers: Form and function. *Curr Opin Immunol* 10:245, 1998.

53. Dunn-Walters DK, Isaacson PG, Spencer J: Analysis of mutations in immunoglobulin heavy chain variable region genes of microdissected marginal zone (MGZ) B cells suggests that the MGZ of human spleen is a reservoir of memory B cells. *J Exp Med* 182:559, 1995.

54. Burton GF, Masuda A, Heath SL, et al: Follicular dendritic cells (FDC) in retroviral infection: Host/pathogen perspectives. *Immunol Rev* 156: 185, 1997.

55. Gulbranson-Judge A, Casamayor-Palleja M, MacLennan IC: Mutually dependent T and B cell responses in germinal centers. *Ann N Y Acad Sci* 815:199, 1997.

56. Butcher EC, Williams M, Youngman K, et al: Lymphocyte trafficking and regional immunity. *Adv Immunol* 72:209, 1999.

57. Warnock RA, Askari S, Butcher EC, Von Andrian UH: Molecular mechanisms of lymphocyte homing to peripheral lymph nodes. *J Exp Med* 187:205, 1998.

58. Greenfield EA, Nguyen KA, Kuchroo VK: CD28/B7 costimulation: A review. *Crit Rev Immunol* 18:389, 1998.

59. Schwartz RH: T cell anergy. *Annu Rev Immunol* 21:305, 2003.

60. Van Parijs L, Abbas AK: Homeostasis and self-tolerance in the immune system: Turning lymphocytes off. *Science* 280:243, 1998.

61. Malvey EN, Telander DG, Vanasek TL, Mueller DL: The role of clonal anergy in the avoidance of autoimmunity: Inactivation of autocrine growth without loss of effector function. *Immunol Rev* 165:301, 1998.

62. Mosmann TR, Li L, Hengartner H, et al: Differentiation and functions of T cell subsets. *Ciba Found Symp* 204:148, 1997.

63. Mosmann TR, Li L, Sad S: Functions of CD8 T-cell subsets secreting different cytokine patterns. *Semin Immunol* 9:87, 1997.

64. Takatsu K: Cytokines involved in B-cell differentiation and their sites of action. *Proc Soc Exp Biol Med* 215:121, 1997.

65. Seder RA, Gazzinelli RT: Cytokines are critical in linking the innate and adaptive immune responses to bacterial, fungal, and parasitic infection. *Adv Intern Med* 44:353, 1999.

66. Grewal IS, Flavell RA: CD40 and CD154 in cell-mediated immunity. *Annu Rev Immunol* 16:111, 1998.

67. Vora KA, Ravetch JV, Manser T: Insights into the mechanisms of antibody-affinity maturation and the generation of the memory B-cell compartment using genetically altered mice. *Dev Immunol* 6:305, 1998.

68. Liu YJ, De Bouteiller O, Fugier-Vivier I: Mechanisms of selection and differentiation in germinal centers. *Curr Opin Immunol* 9:256, 1997.

69. Przylepa J, Himes C, Kelsoe G: Lymphocyte development and selection in germinal centers. *Curr Top Microbiol Immunol* 229:85, 1998.

70. Doherty PC, Topham DJ, Tripp RA: Establishment and persistence of virus-specific CD4+ and CD8+ T cell memory. *Immunol Rev* 150:23, 1996.

71. Callan MF, Annels N, Steven N, et al: T cell selection during the evolution of CD8+ T cell memory in vivo. *Eur J Immunol* 28:4382, 1998.

72. Liu YJ, Grouard G, De Bouteiller O, Bancherau J: Follicular dendritic cells and germinal centers. *Int Rev Cytol* 166:139, 1996.

73. Choe J, Kim HS, Armitage RJ, Choi YS: The functional role of B cell antigen receptor stimulation and IL-4 in the generation of human memory B cells from germinal center B cells. *J Immunol* 159:3757, 1997.

74. Freitas AA, Rocha B: Peripheral T cell survival. *Curr Opin Immunol* 11:152, 1999.

75. Slifka MK, Ahmed R: Long-lived plasma cells: A mechanism for maintaining persistent antibody production. *Curr Opin Immunol* 10:252, 1998.

76. MacDonald TT: The mucosal immune system. *Parasite Immunol* 25: 235, 2003.

77. Clark MA, Jepson MA: Intestinal M cells and their role in bacterial infection. *Int J Med Microbiol* 293:17, 2003.

78. Dunn-Walters DK, Isaacson PG, Spencer J: Sequence analysis of human IgV_H genes indicates that ileal lamina propria plasma cells are derived from Peyer's patches. *Eur J Immunol* 27:463, 1997.

C H A P T E R   6

HEMATOLOGY OF THE
NEWBORN

GEORGE B. SEGEL
JAMES PALIS

During embryogenesis, hematopoiesis occurs in spatially and temporally distinct sites, including the extraembryonic yolk sac, the fetal liver, and the preterm bone marrow. The development of primitive erythroblasts in the yolk sac is critical for embryonic survival. Primitive erythroblasts differentiate within the vascular network rather than in the extravascular space and circulate as nucleated cells. While it is widely assumed that primitive red cells remain nucleated throughout their life span, it is likely that many ultimately enucleate upon terminal differentiation. After 7 weeks' gestation, hematopoietic progenitors are no longer detected in the yolk sac. The liver serves as the primary source of red cells from the 9th to the 24th week of gestation. Like primitive erythropoiesis in the yolk sac, definitive erythropoiesis in the fetal liver is necessary for continued survival of the embryo. In contrast to the yolk sac, where hematopoiesis is restricted to maturing primitive erythroid, macrophage, and megakaryocytic cells, hematopoiesis in the fetal liver consists of definitive erythroid, megakaryocyte, and multiple myeloid, as well as lymphoid, lineages. Hematopoietic cells are first seen in the marrow of the 10- to 11-week embryo, and they remain confined to the diaphyseal regions of long bones until 15 weeks' gestation. Lymphopoiesis is present in the lymph plexuses and the thymus beginning at 9 weeks' gestation. Yolk sac stem cells were first thought to seed the liver and eventually the bone marrow. However, later experiments in avian and amphibian embryos indicate that the hematopoietic stem cells that seed the marrow arise within the body of the embryo proper rather than from the yolk sac. Prior to the fetal liver, the aorta-gonad-mesonephros (AGM) region of the embryo proper contains stem cells capable of engrafting myeloablated adult recipients. Studies suggest that the AGM-region-derived stem cells seed the liver and the marrow to provide lifelong hematopoiesis. Hb Gower-1 ($\zeta_2\varepsilon_2$) is the major hemoglobin in embryos younger than 5 weeks. Hb F ($\alpha_2\gamma_2$) is the major hemoglobin of fetal life. The fetal hemoglobin concentration in blood decreases after birth by approximately 3 percent per week and is generally less than 2 to 3 percent of

the total hemoglobin by 6 months of age. The mean hemoglobin level in cord blood at term is 16.8 g/dl, with 95 percent of the values falling between 13.7 and 20.1 g/dl. The red cells of the newborn are macrocytic, with a mean cell volume (MCV) in excess of 110 fl/cell. The red cell, hemoglobin, and hematocrit values decrease only slightly during the first week, but decline more rapidly in the following 5 to 8 weeks, producing the physiologic anemia of the newborn. The absolute number of neutrophils in the blood of term and premature infants is usually greater than that found in older children. Segmented neutrophils are the predominant leukocytes in the first few days after birth. As their number decreases, the lymphocyte becomes the most numerous cell and remains so during the first postnatal 4 years. Phagocytosis of bacteria and latex granules by neutrophils from premature and term infants is normal. Bactericidal activity varies according to the conditions of testing and the clinical status of the neonates. The platelet counts in term and preterm infants are between 150 and 400 × 10⁹/liter (150,000 to 400,000/µl), comparable to adult values. The absolute number of lymphocytes in the newborn is equivalent to that in older children, with lower values in premature infants at birth. The absolute number of CD3+ and CD4+ (helper/inducer phenotype) T cell subsets in blood of newborns is significantly higher than in adults. Humoral (B cell) immunity also develops early in gestation, but it is not fully active until after birth. In the newborn, approximately 15 percent of lymphocytes have immunoglobulin on their surface, with all immunoglobulin (Ig) isotypes represented. The term newborn has reduced mean plasma levels (<60% of adult levels) of factors II, IX, X, XI, and XII, prekallikrein, and high molecular weight kininogen. In contrast, the plasma concentration of factor VIII is similar and von Willebrand factor is increased compared to older children and adults.

FETAL HEMATOLYMPHOPOIESIS

PRODUCTION OF EMBRYONIC AND FETAL HEMATOPOIETIC CELLS

During embryogenesis, hematopoiesis occurs in spatially and temporally distinct sites, including the extraembryonic yolk sac, the fetal liver, and the preterm bone marrow. Erythropoiesis is established soon after implantation of the blastocyst, with primitive erythroid cells appearing in yolk sac blood islands by day 18 of gestation.[1] The initial origin of hematopoietic cells in mammals is tied closely to gastrulation and the formation of mesoderm. Yolk sac erythroblasts arise in close association with the first embryonic blood vessels, suggesting that endothelial cells and blood cells arise from a common hemangioblast precursor.[2] "Primitive" red cells derived from the yolk sac constitute a distinct transient erythroid lineage that differs from "definitive" red cells that subsequently mature in the fetal liver and bone marrow (Fig. 6-1).[3]

YOLK SAC HEMATOPOIESIS
The development of primitive erythroblasts in the yolk sac is critical for embryonic survival. In the mouse, targeted disruption of the transcription factors SCL (TAL1), LM02 (RBTN2), and GATA-1 each abrogates primitive erythropoiesis in the yolk sac and leads to early embryonic death.[4–6] Primitive erythroblasts begin to enter the embryo proper at days 21 to 22 of gestation with the onset of cardiac contractions[7,8] and circulate until approximately 12 weeks of gestation. Yolk sac erythroblasts have several characteristics distinguishing them from their later definitive counterparts. Primitive erythroblasts circulate as nucleated cells, accumulating embryonic hemoglobins and completing

Acronyms and abbreviations that appear in this chapter include: ADP, adenosine diphosphate; AGM, aorta-gonad-mesonephros; ATP, adenosine triphosphate; ATPase, adenosine triphosphatase; BFU-E, burst forming unit–erythroid; BPG, bisphosphoglycerate; cAMP, cyclic adenosine monophosphate; CFU-E, colony forming unit–erythroid; CFU-GEMM, colony forming unit–granulocyte-erythroid-monocyte-macrophage; CFU-GM, colony forming unit–granulocyte-monocyte; CFU-Meg, colony forming unit–megakaryocyte; G-CSF, granulocyte colony stimulating factor; GM-CSF, granulocyte-monocyte colony stimulating factor; IL, interleukin; MCV, mean cell volume; NADPH, nicotinamide adenine dinucleotide phosphate; NBT, nitroblue tetrazolium; NK, natural killer; RDW, red cell distribution width; SIDS, sudden infant death syndrome; TNF, tumor necrosis factor; TPO, thrombopoietin.

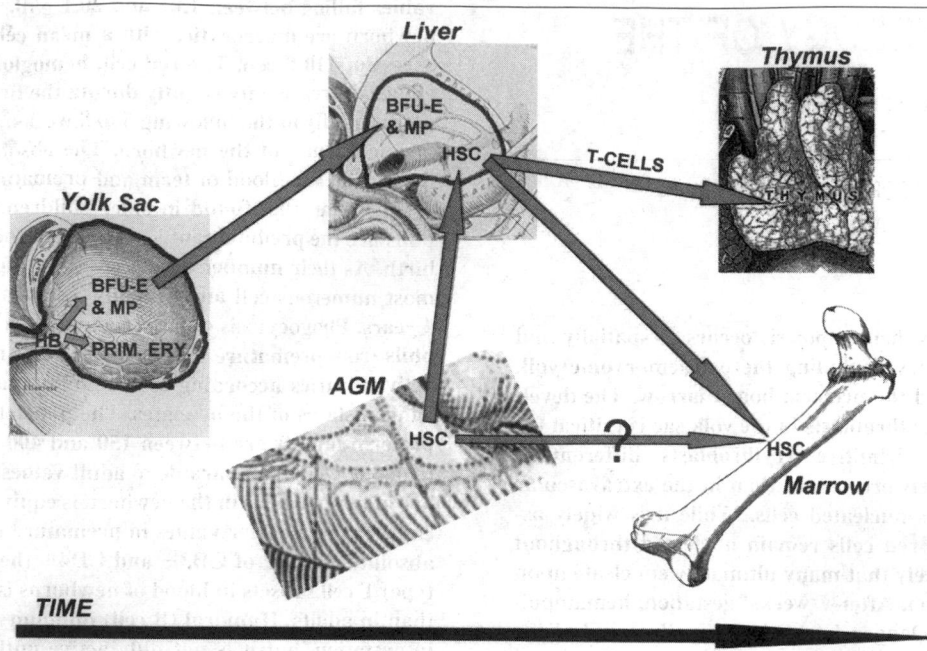

FIGURE 6-1   Hypothetical model of human hematopoietic ontogeny based on amphibian, avian, murine and human developmental data. The yolk sac provides two transient populations of committed progenitors that are thought to arise from a mesoderm derived hemangioblast (HB) precursor. The first wave of proliferation produces primitive erythroblasts (PRIM. ERY.) (see text). The second wave produces BFU-E and several myeloid precursors (MP) that are thought to seed the liver. A long term hematopoietic stem cell (HSC) arises later in the aorta-gonad-mesonephros region (AGM) that subsequently populates the liver and ultimately the marrow to generate the full panoply of definitive hematopoiesis. The HSC from liver also provide naïve lymphoid cells to the thymus, and T-lineage maturation occurs there. [The figure is constructed from illustrations obtained from the World Wide Web and are modified from those by M. Drodel in *Cullen's Embryology, Anatomy and Diseases of the Umbilicus* (www.netembryo.org) and those appearing in *Gray's Anatomy* (http://education.yahoo.com/reference/gray/).

terminal differentiation within the vascular network.[9] Yolk sac erythroblasts are extremely large red cells (megaloblasts) with an estimated MCV of >400 fl/cell. Although it is widely assumed that primitive red cells remain nucleated throughout their life span, it is likely that many ultimately enucleate upon terminal differentiation.[3,10,11]

In the mouse, primitive red cells are derived from a transient population of primitive erythroid progenitors that is confined to the yolk sac.[12] Ultrastructural examination of the human yolk sac reveals the presence, not only of primitive erythroblasts, but also of macrophage cells and megakaryocytes.[11] These findings are consistent with hematopoietic progenitor studies in the mouse embryo suggesting that primitive hematopoiesis in the yolk sac includes the primitive erythroid, macrophage and megakaryocyte lineages.[12,13]

The initial wave of primitive erythroid progenitors is followed by a second wave of yolk sac-derived definitive erythroid progenitors, termed burst forming units–erythroid (BFU-E). BFU-E are present in the human yolk sac as early as 4 weeks' gestation and are found in the fetal liver by 5 weeks' gestation.[14] These findings suggest that the fetal liver is initially seeded by hematopoietic progenitors derived from the yolk sac. Erythroid and nonerythroid progenitors are evident also in the nonliver regions of the embryo proper.[15] After 7 weeks' gestation, hematopoietic progenitors are no longer detected in the yolk sac.[16]

HEPATIC HEMATOPOIESIS

The liver serves as the primary source of red cells from the 9th to the 24th weeks of gestation. Between 7 and 15 weeks' gestation, 60 percent of the liver cells are hematopoietic.[17] Erythroid cells differentiate in close association with macrophages and extrude their nuclei prior to entering the bloodstream. These fetal liver-derived definitive "macrocytes" are smaller than yolk sac-derived primitive megaloblasts and contain one-third the amount of hemoglobin. Differentiation of erythroid cells in the fetal liver is dependent on erythropoietin signaling through its receptor and the Janus kinase 2 (JAK2).[18,19] Fetal liver-derived erythroid progenitors will differentiate in vitro with erythropoietin alone, in contrast to adult bone marrow-derived BFU-E which require erythropoietin plus interleukin (IL)-3.[20,21] Erythropoietin transcripts are present during the first trimester in the liver.[14] The liver remains the primary site of erythropoietin transcription throughout fetal life.[22] Erythropoietin transcripts also are present in the developing human kidney as early as 17 weeks' gestation and increase after 30 weeks.[22] Like primitive erythropoiesis in the yolk sac, definitive erythropoiesis in the fetal liver is necessary for continued survival of the embryo. Targeted disruption of the c-myb and EKLF transcription factors in the mouse each blocks fetal liver erythropoiesis and leads to fetal death.[23,24] These mutations do not effect yolk sac erythropoiesis, indicating fundamental differences in the transcriptional regulation of these distinct forms of erythropoiesis.

In contrast to the yolk sac, where hematopoiesis is restricted to maturing primitive erythroid, macrophage, and megakaryocytic cells, hematopoiesis in the fetal liver consists of definitive erythroid, megakaryocyte, and multiple myeloid, as well as lymphoid, lineages. Megakaryocytes are present in the liver by 6 weeks' gestation. Platelets are first evident in the circulation at 8 to 9 weeks' gestation.[17] Small numbers of circulating leukocytes are present at the 11th week of gestation.[2] Granulopoiesis is present in the liver parenchyma and in some areas of connective tissue as early as 7 weeks' gestation. Despite the low number and immature appearance of hepatic neutrophils, the fetal liver contains abundant hematopoietic progenitor cells, including the multipotential colony forming unit–granulocyte-erythroid-monocyte-macrophage (CFU-GEMM) and colony forming unit–granulocyte-monocyte (CFU-GM).[25,26] CFU-GM growth depends upon several cytokines, including granulocyte colony stimulating factor (G-CSF), granulocyte-monocyte colony stimulating factor (GM-CSF), and interleukins.[27] When compared to adult bone marrow-derived myeloid progenitors, these fetal-liver-derived myeloid progenitors have a similar dose response in vitro to G-CSF.[28] G-CSF is expressed by hepatocytes at 14 weeks' gestation.[29]

MARROW HEMATOPOIESIS

Hematopoietic cells are first seen in the marrow of the 10- to 11-week embryo,[1,2] and they remain confined to the diaphyseal regions of long bones until 15 weeks' gestation.[30] Initially there are approximately equal numbers of myeloid and erythroid cells in the fetal marrow. However, myeloid cells predominate by 12 weeks' gestation, and the myeloid-to-erythroid ratio approaches the adult level of 3:1 by 21 weeks' gestation.[17] Macrophage cells in the fetal marrow, but not in the fetal liver, express the lipopolysaccharide receptor CD14.[29] The marrow becomes the major site of hematopoiesis after the 24th week of gestation.

LYMPHOPOIESIS

Lymphopoiesis is present in the lymph plexuses and the thymus beginning at 9 weeks' gestation.[17] B cells with surface IgM are present in the liver, and circulating lymphocytes also are seen at 9 weeks' gestation.[2] T lymphocytes are found only rarely before 12 weeks' gestation.[31] Lymphocyte subpopulations are detected by 13 weeks' gestation in fetal liver.[32] Absolute numbers of major lymphoid subsets in 20- to 26-week-old fetuses, as defined by the antigens CD2, CD3, CD4, CD8, CD16, CD19, and CD20 (see Chap. 14 for functional significance of these phenotypes), are similar to those in newborns (see "Neonatal Lymphopoiesis" below).[33,34]

ONTOGENY OF HEMATOPOIETIC STEM CELLS

The reconstitution of hematopoiesis by transplantation with cord blood indicates that hematopoietic stem cells are present at birth.[35] However, the developmental origin of hematopoietic stem cells has not yet been defined. It was first postulated that hematopoietic stem cells originate independently in each hematopoietic site (yolk sac, liver, and marrow) of the embryo.[36] However, experiments in the mammalian embryo indicate that the liver rudiment is seeded by exogenous hematopoietic cells.[37,38] The marrow also is seeded by exogenously derived blood cells. Fetal liver provides a source of stem cells for myeloid and lymphoid reconstitution of fetal sheep and monkey transplant recipients.[39] The immunologic reconstitution of an immunodeficient human fetus with fetal liver-derived cells also indicates that hematopoietic stem cells exist in the fetal liver.[40]

Yolk sac stem cells were first thought to seed the liver and eventually the bone marrow.[41] However, later experiments in avian and amphibian embryos indicated that the hematopoietic stem cells that seed the marrow arise within the body of the embryo proper rather than from the yolk sac.[42,43] Investigations in the mouse embryo also suggest that prior to the fetal liver, the AGM region of the embryo proper contains stem cells capable of engrafting myeloablated adult recipients.[44] This correlates anatomically with the transient appearance of CD34+ blood cells closely associated with the ventral wall of the aorta in several mammalian species, including the 5 weeks' gestation human embryo.[45,46] These studies suggest that the AGM-region-derived stem cells seed the liver and the marrow to provide lifelong hematopoiesis. The underlying relationship of primitive hematopoiesis in the yolk sac to definitive hematopoiesis in the fetal liver and the marrow remains unclear.

SYNTHESIS OF FETAL HEMOGLOBINS

Human hemoglobin (Hb) is a tetramer composed of two α-type and two β-type globin chains (Table 6-1). The α-globin gene cluster is located on chromosome 16 and contains the ζ gene 5' to the pair of α-globin genes. The β-globin gene cluster is located on chromosome 11 and contains five globin genes oriented 5' to 3' as ε-γ^A-γ^G-δ-β.[47] During embryogenesis the genes on both chromosomes are activated sequentially from the 5' to the 3' end. This globin "switching" is related not only to the relative positions of the globin genes within their respective chromosomal clusters, but also to interacting upstream "locus control regions."[48]

Hb Gower-1 ($\zeta_2\varepsilon_2$) is the major hemoglobin in embryos younger than 5 weeks' gestation (see Table 6-1).[49] Hb Gower-2 ($\alpha_2\varepsilon_2$) has been found in embryos with a gestational age as young as 4 weeks and is absent in embryos older than 13 weeks.[50] Hb Portland ($\zeta_2\gamma_2$) is found in young embryos but persists in infants with homozygous α-thalassemia. Synthesis of the ζ and ε chains decreases as that of α and γ chains increases (Fig. 6-2). The ζ-to-α-globin switch precedes the ε-to-γ-globin switch as the liver replaces the yolk sac as the main site of erythropoiesis.[51,52]

Hb F ($\alpha_2\gamma_2$) is the major hemoglobin of fetal life[53] (see Fig. 6-2). Synthesis of Hb A can be demonstrated in fetuses as young as 9 weeks' gestation.[54,55] In fetuses of 9 to 21 weeks' gestation, the amount of Hb A ($\alpha_2\beta_2$) rises from 4 to 13 percent of the total hemoglobin.[55] These levels of Hb A have enabled the antenatal diagnosis of β-thalassemia using globin chain synthesis. After 34 to 36 weeks' gestation the percentage of Hb A rises, whereas that of Hb F decreases (see Fig. 6-2). The mean synthesis of Hb F in term infants was 59.0 ± 10 percent (1 SD) of total hemoglobin synthesis as assessed by ^{14}C-leucine uptake.[56] The amount of Hb F in blood varies in term infants from 53 to 95 percent of total hemoglobin.[57,58]

The fetal hemoglobin concentration in blood decreases after birth by approximately 3 percent per week and is generally less than 2 to 3 percent of the total hemoglobin by 6 months of age. This rate of decrease in Hb F production is closely related to the gestational age of the infant and is not affected by the changes in environment and oxygen tension that occur at the time of birth.[59] Hb A_2 ($\alpha_2\delta_2$) has not been detected in fetuses. Normal adult levels of Hb A_2 are achieved by 4 months of age.[60] Increased proportions of Hb F at birth have been reported in infants who are small for gestational age, who have experienced chronic intrauterine hypoxia, who have trisomy 13, or who have died from the sudden infant death syndrome (SIDS).[61–65] Decreased levels of Hb F at birth are found in trisomy 21.[66]

TABLE 6-1 EMBRYONIC HEMOGLOBINS

HEMOGLOBIN	CHAIN COMPOSITION	PRIMARY SITE	APPEARANCE
Gower-1	$\zeta_2\varepsilon_2$	Yolk sac	<5–6 weeks
Gower-2	$\alpha_2\varepsilon_2$	Yolk sac	4–13 weeks
Portland	$\zeta_2\gamma_2$	Yolk sac	4–13 weeks
Fetal (F)	$\alpha_2\gamma_2$	Liver	Early, 53–95% at term
Adult (A)	$\alpha_2\beta_2$	Marrow	9 weeks, 5–45% at term

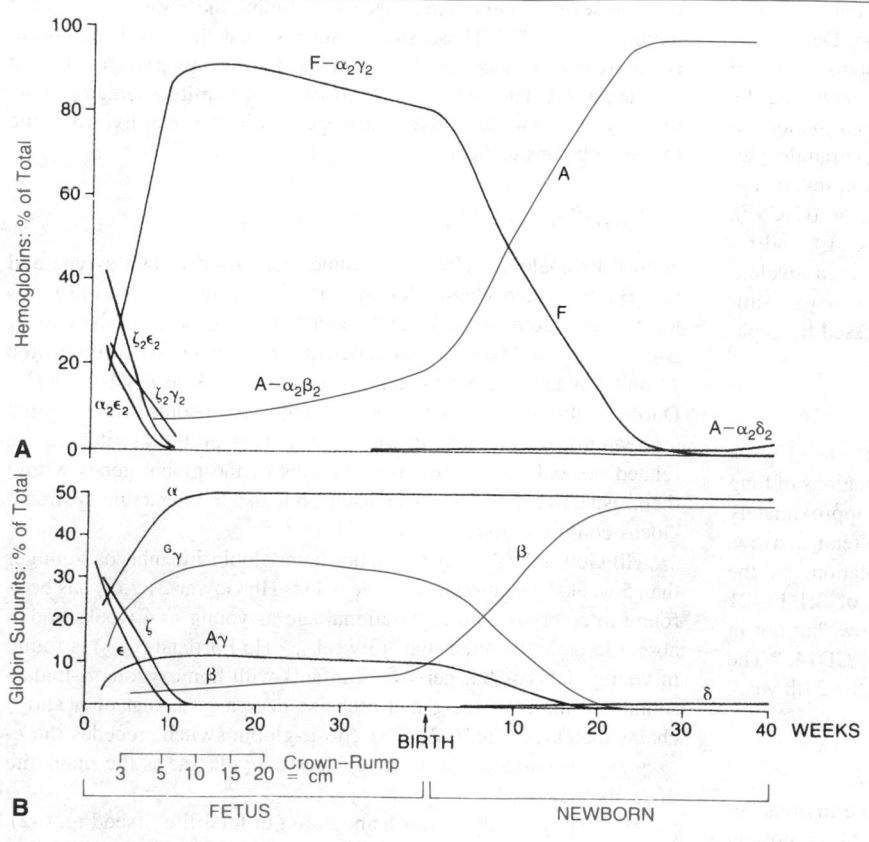

FIGURE 6-2 Changes in hemoglobin tetramers (A) and in globin subunits (B) during human development from embryo to early infancy. (Reproduced from Bunn HF, Forget BG: *Hemoglobin: Molecular, Genetic and Clinical Aspects.* WB Saunders, Philadelphia, 1986, p 68, with permission.)

FETAL BLOOD

The fetal blood composition changes markedly during the second and third trimesters. The mean hemoglobin in fetuses progressively increases from 9.0 ± 2.8 g/dl at age 10 weeks to 16.5 ± 4.0 g/dl at 39 weeks.[67] There is a concomitant decrease in the MCV of fetal red cells from a mean of 134 fl/cell at 18 weeks to 118 fl/cell at 30 weeks' gestation.[68] The total white blood cell count averages 2×10^9/liter between 10 and 17 weeks of gestation[31] and increases during the middle trimester to between 4 and 4.5×10^9/liter, with an 80 to 85 percent preponderance of lymphocytes and 5 to 10 percent neutrophils.[68] The percentage of circulating nucleated red cells decreases from a mean of 12 percent at 18 weeks to 4 percent at 30 weeks.[68] The platelet count remains greater than 150,000/μl from 15 weeks' gestation to term.[68,69]

Large numbers of committed hematopoietic progenitors circulate in the fetal blood. Blood samples obtained by fetoscopy at 12 to 19 weeks of gestation reveal a mean of 20,450 BFU-E/ml and 12,490 CFU-GM/ml.[70] This is in striking contrast to adult blood, which contains many fewer erythroid progenitors and 30 to 250 CFU-GM/ml.[71] The cycling rate of 26 to 28 weeks' gestation fetal hematopoietic progenitors is nearly maximal (70–80%) compared to the relative quiescence (0–5%) of adult marrow-derived progenitors.[71]

NEONATAL HEMATOPOIESIS

NEONATAL ERYTHROPOIESIS AND RED CELLS

HEMOGLOBIN, HEMATOCRIT, AND INDICES
The mean hemoglobin level in cord blood at term is 16.8 g/dl, with 95 percent of the values falling between 13.7 and 20.1 g/dl.[72] This

variation reflects perinatal events, particularly asphyxia,[73] and also the amount of blood transferred from the placenta to the infant after delivery. Early cord clamping appears to heighten the occurrence of anemia at 2 months and to impair cardiopulmonary adaptation.[74,75] Delay of cord clamping may increase the blood volume and red cell mass of the infant by as much as 55 percent.[76,77] This results in fewer transfusions and fewer days requiring oxygen and ventilation in preterm infants.[74,75] The mean total blood volume after birth is 86.3 ml/kg for the term infant and 89.4 ml/kg for the premature infant.[78] The blood volume per kilogram decreases over the ensuing weeks, reaching a mean value of about 65 ml/kg by 3 to 4 months of age.

Normally the hemoglobin and hematocrit values rise in the first several hours after birth because of the movement of plasma from the intravascular to the extravascular space.[79] A venous hemoglobin concentration of less than 14 g/dl in a term infant and/or a fall in hemoglobin or hematocrit level in the first postnatal day are abnormal. Table 6-2 shows the normal red cell values from capillary blood samples for term infants in the first 12 weeks after birth.[80] Capillary hematocrit values in newborns are higher than those in simultaneous venous samples, particularly during the first postnatal days, and the capillary-to-venous ratio is approximately 1.1:1.[81] This difference reflects circulatory factors and is greater in preterm and sick infants.

The red cells of the newborn are macrocytic, with an MCV in excess of 110 fl/cell. The MCV begins to fall after the first week, reaching adult values by the ninth week (see Table 6-2).[80,82] The blood film from a newborn infant shows macrocytic normochromic cells, polychromasia, and a few nucleated red blood cells. Even in healthy infants there may be mild anisocytosis and poikilocytosis.[83] Three to 5 percent of the red cells may be fragments, target cells, or distorted. By 3 to 5 days after birth, nucleated red blood cells are not found normally in the blood of term or premature infants, but they may be present in markedly elevated numbers in the presence of hemolysis or hypoxic stress. As expected from these findings, the red cell distribution width (RDW) is markedly elevated in the newborn period.[84]

There are significant numbers of circulating progenitor cells in cord blood.[85–88] Cord blood BFU-E and CFU-E differentiate more rapidly than their adult counterparts.[89] Furthermore, the proportion of cord blood hematopoietic progenitors in the mitotic cycle is approximately 50 percent, intermediate between the proportions found in fetal and adult progenitor cells.[87]

In several,[90,91] but not all, studies[92] premature infants at birth had lower hemoglobin levels, higher reticulocyte counts, and higher nucleated red cell counts than did the term infants. The reticulocyte counts of premature infants are inversely proportional to their gestational age, with a mean of 8 percent reticulocytes evident at 32 weeks' gestation and 4 to 5 percent at term.[93] Infants who are small for their gestational ages have higher red cell counts, hematocrit levels, and hemoglobin concentrations as compared with infants whose size is appropriate for their gestational age.[91,94]

Erythropoietin and Physiologic Anemia of the Newborn Erythropoietin is the primary regulator of erythropoiesis. Although erythropoietin is present in cord blood, it falls to undetectable levels after birth in healthy infants.[95] Subsequently, the reticulocyte count falls to less than 1 percent by the sixth day after birth.[96] Erythropoietin with-

TABLE 6-2   RED CELL VALUES FOR TERM INFANTS DURING THE FIRST 12 WEEKS AFTER BIRTH*

AGE	HB, G/DL ± SD	RBC × 10¹²/LITER ± SD	HEMATOCRIT, % ± SD	MCV, FL ± SD	MCHC, G/DL ± SD	RETICULOCYTES, % ± SD
Days						
1	19.3 ± 2.2	5.14 ± 0.7	61 ± 7.4	119 ± 9.4	31.6 ± 1.9	3.2 ± 1.4
2	19.0 ± 1.9	5.15 ± 0.8	60 ± 6.4	115 ± 7.0	31.6 ± 1.4	3.2 ± 1.3
3	18.8 ± 2.0	5.11 ± 0.7	62 ± 9.3	116 ± 5.3	31.1 ± 2.8	2.8 ± 1.7
4	18.6 ± 2.1	5.00 ± 0.6	57 ± 8.1	114 ± 7.5	32.6 ± 1.5	1.8 ± 1.1
5	17.6 ± 1.1	4.97 ± 0.4	57 ± 7.3	114 ± 8.9	30.9 ± 2.2	1.2 ± 0.2
6	17.4 ± 2.2	5.00 ± 0.7	54 ± 7.2	113 ± 10.0	32.2 ± 1.6	0.6 ± 0.2
7	17.9 ± 2.5	4.86 ± 0.6	56 ± 9.4	118 ± 11.2	32.0 ± 1.6	0.5 ± 0.4
Weeks						
1–2	17.3 ± 2.3	4.80 ± 0.8	54 ± 8.3	112 ± 19.0	32.1 ± 2.9	0.5 ± 0.3
2–3	15.6 ± 2.6	4.20 ± 0.6	46 ± 7.3	111 ± 8.2	33.9 ± 1.9	0.8 ± 0.6
3–4	14.2 ± 2.1	4.00 ± 0.6	43 ± 5.7	105 ± 7.5	33.5 ± 1.6	0.6 ± 0.3
4–5	12.7 ± 1.6	3.60 ± 0.4	36 ± 4.8	101 ± 8.1	34.9 ± 1.6	0.9 ± 0.8
5–6	11.9 ± 1.5	3.55 ± 0.2	36 ± 6.2	102 ± 10.2	34.1 ± 2.9	1.0 ± 0.7
6–7	12.0 ± 1.5	3.40 ± 0.4	36 ± 4.8	105 ± 12.0	33.8 ± 2.3	1.2 ± 0.7
7–8	11.1 ± 1.1	3.40 ± 0.4	33 ± 3.7	100 ± 13.0	33.7 ± 2.6	1.5 ± 0.7
8–9	10.7 ± 0.9	3.40 ± 0.5	31 ± 2.5	93 ± 12.0	34.1 ± 2.2	1.8 ± 1.0
9–10	11.2 ± 0.9	3.60 ± 0.3	32 ± 2.7	91 ± 9.3	34.3 ± 2.9	1.2 ± 0.6
10–11	11.4 ± 0.9	3.70 ± 0.4	34 ± 2.1	91 ± 7.7	33.2 ± 2.4	1.2 ± 0.7
11–12	11.3 ± 0.9	3.70 ± 0.3	33 ± 3.3	88 ± 7.9	34.8 ± 2.2	0.7 ± 0.3

* Capillary blood samples. The RBC count and MCV measurements were made on an electronic counter.
MCHC = mean corpuscular hemoglobin concentration; MCV = mean cell volume; RBC = red blood cell.
SOURCE: Adapted from Matoth et al.[80]

drawal also may increase the destruction of red cells at the endothelial–macrophage interface. This process is called *neocytolysis* and results from heightened macrophage phagocytosis of the youngest circulating red cells.[97] The red cell, hemoglobin, and hematocrit values decrease only slightly during the first week, but decline more rapidly in the following 5 to 8 weeks (see Table 6-2),[80] producing the physiologic anemia of the newborn. The lowest hemoglobin values in the term infant occur at about 2 months of age.[82] When the hemoglobin concentration falls below 11 g/dl, erythropoietic activity begins to increase. Erythropoietin can be measured after the 60th postnatal day,[98] corresponding to the recovery from physiologic anemia. If there is sufficient stimulus, such as hemolytic anemia or cyanotic heart disease, the newborn infant is able to produce erythropoietin during the first several months after birth.[95]

The fall in hemoglobin level is more pronounced in the premature infant. In one study of premature infants the mean hemoglobin level at 2 months was 9.4 g/dl, with a 95 percent range of 7.2 to 11.7 g/dl.[99] In healthy premature infants erythropoietin becomes detectable when the hemoglobin level falls to about 12 g/dl. In infants with a lower percentage of Hb F (as from transfusion) and consequently better oxygen delivery, erythropoietin does not rise until the hemoglobin falls to about 9.5 g/dl.[100] The mean values for iron-sufficient premature infants reached those of term infants by 4 months for red cell count, 5 months for hemoglobin level, and 6 months for mean corpuscular volume and mean corpuscular hemoglobin.[99]

Blood Viscosity   The viscosity of blood increases logarithmically in relation to the hematocrit.[101,102] Hyperviscosity was found in 5 percent of infants in one series[103] and in 18 percent of infants who were small for gestational age in another.[104] Newborn infants with hematocrit values of greater than 65 to 70 percent may become symptomatic because of increased viscosity.[105] Of 45 infants with documented hyperviscosity and a mean hematocrit greater than 65 percent, 17 (38%) had symptoms of irritability, hypotonia, tremors, or poor suck reflex.[106] Partial plasma exchange transfusion reduced blood viscosity, improved cerebral blood flow, and relieved the symptoms. However, cerebral blood flow was normal in the asymptomatic infants with hyperviscosity, and there consequently was no benefit from exchange transfusion.[106]

Red Cell Antigens   The blood group antigens on neonatal red cells differ from those of the older child and adult. The i antigen is expressed strongly while the I antigen and the A and B antigens are expressed only weakly on neonatal red cells. The i antigen is a straight-chain carbohydrate that is replaced by the branched-chain derivative, I antigen, as a result of the developmental acquisition of a glycosyltransferase.[107] By 1 year of age the i antigen is undetectable, and the ABH antigens increase to adult levels by age 3 years. The ABH, Kell, Duffy, and Vel antigens can be detected on the cells of the fetus in the first trimester and are present at birth.[108] The Lua and Lub antigens also are detectable on fetal red cells and are more weakly expressed at birth, increasing to adult levels by age 15 years.[108] The Xg antigen is variably expressed in the fetus and is weaker on newborn than on adult red cells. Moreover, particularly poor expression of Xg has been noted in newborns with trisomy 13, 18, and 21.[108] The Lewis group (Lea/Leb) antigens are adsorbed on the red cell membrane and become detectable within 1 to 2 weeks after birth as the receptor sites develop. Anti-A and anti-B as isohemagglutinins develop during the first 6 postnatal months, reaching adult levels by 2 years of age.

Red Cell Life Span   The life span of the red cells in the newborn infant is shorter than that of red cells in the adult. The average of several studies of mean half-life of newborn red cells labeled with chromium was 23.3 days in term infants and 16.6 days in premature infants. When corrected for the elution rate of chromium from newborn cells, the estimate of mean red cell survival in the newborn is 60 to 80 days.[109] The reasons for this shortened survival are unclear, but the known susceptibility to oxidant injury of newborn red cells may be a contributing factor.

Iron and Transferrin   The serum iron level in cord blood of the normal infant is elevated compared to maternal levels. The mean value is about 150 ± 40 μg/dl (1 SD).[110] Infants on an iron-supplemented diet have a median serum iron level of 125 μg/dl at 1 month of age and of about 75 μg/dl at 6 months of age. The total iron-binding capacity rises throughout the first year. The median transferrin saturation falls from almost 65 percent at 2 weeks to 25 percent at 1 year, and saturations as low as 10 percent may be observed in the absence of iron deficiency.[111] The mean serum ferritin levels in iron-sufficient infants are high at birth, 160 μg/l, rise further during the first month, and then fall to a mean of 30 μg/l by 1 year of age.[112] The amount of stainable iron in the marrow at birth is small but increases in both term and premature infants during the first weeks after birth. Stainable marrow iron begins to decrease after 2 months and is gone by 4 to 6 months in term infants and earlier in premature infants.[113] Iron is preferentially allocated to erythropoiesis if the availability of iron is limited.[114] This makes the availability of adequate iron particularly important to avoid iron lack in the brain, heart, and skeletal muscle.

RED CELL FUNCTIONS

Oxygen Delivery The oxygen affinity of cord blood is greater than that of maternal blood, because the affinity of Hb F for 2,3-bisphosphoglycerate (2,3-BPG) is less than that of Hb A.[115] Levels of 2,3-BPG are lower in newborn red cells than in adult cells and even more decreased in the red cells of premature infants,[116] and this low 2,3-BPG level further heightens the oxygen affinity of newborn red cells. Consequently, the red cell oxygen equilibrium curve of the newborn is shifted to the left of that of the adult (Fig. 6-3). The mean partial pressure of oxygen at which hemoglobin is 50 percent saturated with oxygen at 1 day of age in term infants is 19.4 ± 1.8 torr, as compared with the normal adult value of 27.0 ± 1.1 torr.[117] This results in a decrease in the oxygen released at the tissue level, as shown in Figure 6-3. As the PO_2 falls from 90 torr in arterial to 40 torr in the venous blood, 3.0 ml/dl of oxygen are released from newborn blood, whereas 4.5 ml/dl are released from adult Hb A-containing blood. The shift to the left of the oxygen equilibrium curve is even more pronounced in the premature infant, requiring a larger fall in PO_2 to release an equivalent amount of oxygen. After birth the oxygen equilibrium curve shifts gradually to the right, reaching the position of the adult curve by 6 months of age. The position of the curve in the premature

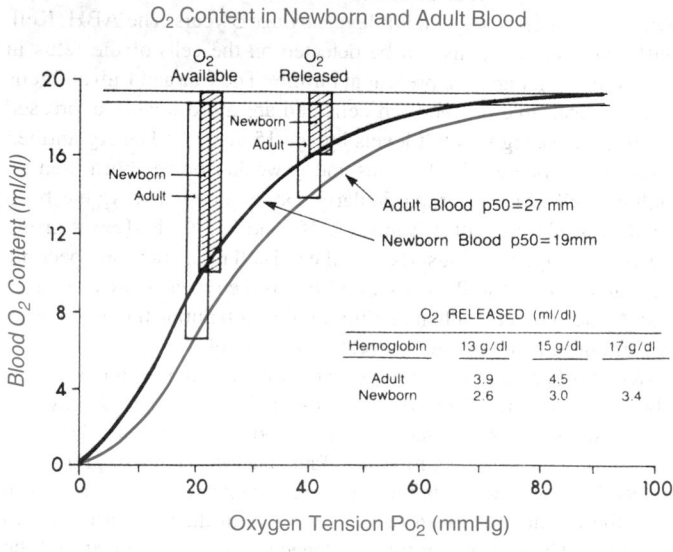

FIGURE 6-3 The oxygen equilibrium curves are based on the assumption that the Hb concentration is 15 g/dl and that there is full O_2 saturation of Hb at a PaO_2 of 100 torr. The O_2 released is the difference in O_2 content between a PaO_2 of 90 torr and the mixed venous PaO_2 of 40 torr. The O_2 available is the difference in O_2 content between a PaO_2 of 90 torr and a mixed venous PaO_2 of 20 torr. This is the maximum O_2 available without evoking compensatory mechanisms such as increased cardiac output.

infant correlates with gestational age rather than with postnatal age,[117] and its shift to the adult position is more gradual.

Metabolism Many differences have been found between the metabolism of the red cells of newborn infants and that of adults.[118,119] Some of the differences may be explained by the younger mean cell age in the newborn, but others seem to be properties of the fetal cell. The glucose consumption in newborn cells is lower than that in adult cells.[120] Elevated levels of glucose phosphate isomerase, glyceraldehyde-3-phosphate dehydrogenase, phosphoglycerate kinase, and enolase beyond those explainable by the young cell age have been found in neonatal cells.[116,121] The level of phosphofructokinase is low in red cells of term and premature infants.[116,121,122] The pentose phosphate shunt is active in red cells of term and premature infants,[123] but there is glutathione instability and a heightened susceptibility to oxidant injury. The result of oxidant stress is depletion of adenosine triphosphate (ATP) and adenine nucleotides leading to iron release, denaturing of membrane proteins, and hemoglobin and membrane peroxidation.[124] Furthermore, there is relative instability of the 2,3-BPG concentration. Lower-than-adult activities have been found for several other red cell enzymes, including nicotinamide adenine dinucleotide (NADH)-dependent methemoglobin reductase[125] and glutathione peroxidase.[126] The levels of ATP and adenosine diphosphate (ADP) are higher in the red cells of term and preterm infants[122] but may merely reflect the younger age of the erythrocyte population.[127]

Membrane The membrane of the newborn red cell also is different from that of the adult red cell. Ouabain-sensitive adenosine triphosphatase (ATPase) is decreased,[128] and active potassium influx is significantly less in neonatal red cells.[129] Newborn cells are more sensitive to osmotic hemolysis and to oxidant injury than are adult cells. Newborn red cell membranes have higher total lipid, phospholipid, and cholesterol per cell than adult red cells.[130,131] The patterns of phospholipid and phospholipid fatty acid composition also differ from those in adult red cells. Red cells of newborns have the same pattern of membrane proteins on polyacrylamide gel electrophoresis[132] and the same rate of mobility in an electric field[133] as do red cells from adults. After trypsin treatment of newborn and adult cells, however, there is a difference in electrophoretic mobility, indicating that the surface trypsin-resistant proteins are different.[133] The relationship of the metabolic and membrane alterations in neonatal red cells to their shorter life span is not clear.

WHITE CELLS

GRANULOCYTOPOIESIS AND MONOCYTOPOIESIS

Colony-Stimulating Factors and Granulomonopoiesis The absolute number of neutrophils in the blood of term and premature infants is usually greater than that found in older children (Table 6-3).[134] The neutrophil count tends to be lower in the premature than in the term infant, and the proportion of myelocytes and band neutrophils is higher.[135] Serum and urinary colony-stimulating activity are elevated during the period of neutrophilia.[136,137] When granulopoiesis was studied in cord blood, blood, and marrow of infants, the macrophage colony forming unit was predominant despite the clinical neutrophilia, and this pattern was not altered by different sources of colony-stimulating factors.[138,139] The endogenous cytokines produced by mononuclear cells from cord or systemic venous blood support the growth of neutrophil colonies in assays using marrow from adults.[138] However, there is diminished GM-CSF, G-CSF, and IL-3 production and diminished messenger RNA (mRNA) expression in stimulated newborn compared to adult mononuclear cells,[140–142] which may limit the response to bacterial infection in the newborn. Furthermore, preterm infants have a reduced neutrophil storage pool and a restricted capacity to increase their progenitor proliferation, and their neutrophil count

TABLE 6-3   THE WHITE CELL COUNT AND THE DIFFERENTIAL COUNT DURING THE FIRST 2 WEEKS AFTER BIRTH*

| AGE | LEUKOCYTES | NEUTROPHILS | | | EOSINOPHILS | BASOPHILS | LYMPHOCYTES | MONOCYTES |
		TOTAL	SEGMENTED	BAND				
Birth								
Mean	18.0	11.0	9.4	1.6	0.40	0.10	0.5	1.05
Range	9.0–30.0	6.0–26.0	—	—	0.02–0.85	0–0.64	2.0–11.0	0.4–3.1
Mean %	—	61	52	9	2.2	0.6	31	5.8
7 days								
Mean	12.2	5.5	4.7	0.83	0.50	0.05	5.0	1.1
Range	5.0–21.0	1.5–10.0	—	—	0.07–1.1	0–0.25	2.0–17.0	0.3–2.7
Mean %	—	45	39	6	4.1	0.4	41	9.1
14 days								
Mean	11.4	4.5	3.9	0.63	0.35	0.05	5.5	1.0
Range	5.0–20.0	1.0–9.5	—	—	0.07–1.0	0–0.23	2.0–17.0	0.2–2.4
Mean %	—	40	34	5.5	3.1	0.4	48	8.8

* All white cell counts are expressed as cells $\times 10^9$/liter.
SOURCE: From Altman and Dittmer,[134] with permission.

may fall precipitously with neonatal bacterial infection.[143] Dysregulation as well as diminished capacity of neonatal granulopoiesis may impair the neonatal response to infection.[144] Smaller numbers of CFU-GM colonies were observed in the blood of sick infants, who also have diminished endogenous production of colony-stimulating factors in culture.[139] The administration of stem cell factor with G-CSF to newborn rats reduces the mortality of experimental group B streptococcal infection; this approach may be useful in human disease.[145] The clinical use of cytokines to treat neonatal sepsis remains controversial,[146] but circulating neutrophils are increased in preterm infants treated with recombinant G-CSF, and their length of stay in the neonatal intensive care unit is shortened.[147]

White Cell and Differential Counts   Table 6-3 gives the values for the white cell and differential counts during the first 2 weeks after birth. The absolute number of segmented neutrophils rises in both term and premature infants in the first 24 h.[148] In term infants, the mean value increases from 8×10^9/liter (8000/μl) to a peak of 13×10^9/liter (13,000/μl) and then falls to 4×10^9/liter (4000/μl) by 72 h of age, remaining at this level through the following 7 days. In the premature infant, the mean values for neutrophils are 5×10^9/liter (5000/μl) at birth, 8×10^9/liter (8000/μl) at 12 h, and 4×10^9/liter (4000/μl) at 72 h. The mean count then falls gradually to 2.5×10^9/liter (2500/μl) by the 28th postnatal day. The level after the first 72 h is very stable for an individual infant, whether term or premature. Immature forms, including an occasional promyelocyte and blast cell, may be seen in the blood of healthy infants in the first few days of life and are more frequent in premature infants than in term infants.[148] Segmented granulocytes are the predominant cells in the first few days after birth. As their number decreases, the lymphocyte becomes the most numerous cell and remains so during the first 4 years of life. An absolute eosinophil count of greater than 0.7×10^9/liter (700/μl) was found in 76 percent of premature infants at 2 to 3 weeks of age. The onset of the eosinophilia coincided with the establishment of steady weight gain in the infants.[149] It is increased by the use of total parenteral nutrition, endotracheal intubation, and blood transfusions.

PHAGOCYTE FUNCTIONS

Bacterial infections are a major cause of morbidity and mortality in the newborn period.[150] The infections are frequently caused by organisms of low virulence in normal children and adults, including *Staphylococcus*, Lancefield group B β-hemolytic streptococci, *Pseudomonas*, and other gram-negative bacilli. Cellular defense mechanisms

and humoral immunity of the newborn differ from those found later in life, and these undoubtedly contribute to the unusual susceptibility to infection noted in the neonatal period.[150]

Opsonins and Complement   Engulfment and destruction of bacteria by neutrophils depend on opsonic activity of the plasma and on chemotaxis, phagocytosis, and the bacteriocidal capacity of the leukocyte. The serum factors necessary for optimal phagocytosis (opsonins) include the immunoglobulins and complement components. In term infants, opsonic activity is normal for *Staphylococcus aureus*,[151,152] but it is low for yeast[153] and *Escherichia coli*.[152] Diminished opsonic antibody is associated with group B streptococcal infection and represents one risk factor for neonatal infection.[154]

In premature infants, opsonic activity is low for *S. aureus* and *Serratia marcescens*,[151] but is normal for *Pseudomonas aeruginosa*.[155] When serum concentrations of fibronectin and IgG subclasses C3 and C4 were measured at birth, 1 month, 3 months, and 6 months, early gestational age was correlated with lower initial levels.[156] The decreased opsonic activity for some organisms in premature infants has been attributed to diminished IgG levels, because additional IgG will correct the opsonic defect both in vivo and in vitro.[151] The added IgG improves bacterial opsonization by serum of premature infants in part because complement consumption and deposition of C3 on the bacterial surface are augmented.[157,158]

Complement components appear in fetal blood before 20 weeks' gestation and increase markedly during the third trimester. However, in many newborns both the classical and alternative complement pathways are decreased in activity and in levels of individual components.[159] The mean level of C3, the first common component of the two pathways of complement activation, is approximately 65 percent of that in normal adults.[160–162] There is no transplacental transfer of this protein, and levels in infants are lower than those in their mothers.[160] Total serum hemolytic complement (CH_{50}) and alternative pathway activity (PH_{50}) in newborns are lower than in adults, as are mean levels of C1q, C2–C9, properdin, and factors B, I, and H.[161–163] In general, the mean levels in full-term infants are greater than 50 percent of those in normal adult controls and may be somewhat less in premature infants. There is considerable overlap, however, between levels in infants and in controls. A functional deficiency in the alternative pathway has been detected in infants.[164]

Fibronectin mediates more efficient interactions between phagocytes and infectious agents. Fibronectin, a 450-kDa glycoprotein found in plasma and in the intercellular matrix, promotes the attachment of staphylococci to neutrophils[165] and enhances opsonic activity of antibodies against group B streptococci.[166] Because both these bacteria are common pathogens for neonates, the deficiency in fibronectin observed in neonates[167] may further compromise opsonic capacity and hence bactericidal activity in the neonate.

The administration of intravenous IgG may be useful in the treatment or prophylaxis of infection in preterm infants based on the reduced placental transfer of maternal antibody and the restricted endogenous synthesis of IgG.[168] IgG administered to septic neonates appears to enhance serum opsonic capacity as well as to increase the quantity of circulating neutrophils.[169] Added IgG heightens phagocytosis of granulocytes from premature neonates,[170] and intravenous IgG has been reported to effectively treat infected premature neonates, but these reports involved small numbers of subjects.[171,172] The clinical efficacy of IgG prophylaxis against neonatal pathogens is not firmly established.[173–175] New IgG preparations with consistent, adequate levels of antibodies directed against neonatal pathogens can be achieved by selection of sera with high levels of functional antibodies,[176] or potentially by the addition of monoclonal antibodies, and these may prove more effective.

Chemotaxis Chemotactic function of leukocytes is low in neonates, whereas random motility is normal.[177–179] Neonatal serum does not generate as much chemotactic factor as does adult serum, even after the addition of purified C3. The defect in chemotaxis may be related to decreased granulocyte deformability and impaired capping of cell surface receptors.[180] The role of observed cyclic adenosine monophosphate (cAMP) and membrane potential alterations in the defective chemotaxis is not clear.[180] The ability of neutrophils to roll along the blood vessel endothelium also is impaired in neonates. Diminished up-regulation and surface migration of β_2-integrins and fewer L-selectin receptors reduce the ability of neonatal neutrophils to interact with adhesion molecules on the endothelium.[143]

The densities of the C3bi receptor (CD11b/CD18) and of the low-affinity receptor for immunoglobulin, FcRIII (CD16), are decreased on neutrophils of premature infants, whereas term infants' cells show a lesser impairment.[181–184] The deficient up-regulation of C3bi correlates with decreased adherence and chemotaxis by neonatal neutrophils.[185] Low FcRIII is associated with impaired chemotaxis of neonatal neutrophils,[186] although decreased FcRIII might also be responsible for subtle defects in adherence and subsequent phagocytosis of opsonized[176] and unopsonized[187] organisms by neutrophils.

Phagocytic and Bactericidal Activity Phagocytosis of bacteria and latex granules by neutrophils from premature and term infants is normal.[151,155,188,189] Bactericidal activity varies according to the conditions of testing and the clinical status of the neonates. The intracellular killing of *S. aureus* and *S. marcescens* in cells from most term and low-birth-weight infants is normal,[151,190] as is that of *E. coli* in term infants.[152] Similar studies have shown defective bactericidal activity against *S. aureus* in some infants in the first 12 h of life,[188] *P. aeruginosa* in cells from premature infants,[155] and *Candida albicans* in granulocytes from term and premature infants.[191] With bacteria-to-neutrophil ratios of 1:1, newborn cells kill *S. aureus* and *E. coli* as effectively as controls; however, at the higher ratio of 100:1, killing and oxidative response as measured by chemiluminescence are markedly depressed, although phagocytosis is normal.[189] Depressed activity also has been found in cells from newborns who have had clinical stress, either from infection or other disorders, shown both as decreased chemiluminescence and impaired bactericidal activity against *S. aureus*, *E. coli*, and group B streptococci.[192–194] The decreased granulocyte function shown in these studies also is found in liquid culture, where neutrophils from newborns do not survive as long as those from adults, perhaps because of decreased resistance to autoxidation.[195] Although superoxide dismutase levels are normal and superoxide pro-

duction is normal or increased in neutrophils from newborns, glutathione peroxidase and catalase levels are decreased.[196,197] The relationship of these in vitro cellular defects to bacterial infections in the newborn is still not clear.

Monocytes from newborn infants have normal nitroblue tetrazolium (NBT) reduction,[198] normal antibody-dependent cellular cytotoxicity,[199] and normal in vitro killing of *S. aureus* and *E. coli*.[200] However, they are slower than monocytes from adults in phagocytosis of polystyrene spheres,[201] and they have reduced ATP production.[202] Furthermore, chemotaxis to serum-derived factors is decreased, as is monocyte appearance in skin windows.[203] These functional aspects may contribute to the observed susceptibility of newborns to a variety of infectious agents.

Cytokine Effects on Neonatal Phagocytic Function There is a complex interaction between cytokines produced by lymphocytes and macrophages, and the activation status of neutrophils during infection. There is decreased production of γ-interferon by neonatal leukocytes.[204–206] γ-Interferon causes the up-regulation of the C3bi receptor and induces the surface expression of the high-affinity immunoglobulin receptor FcRI (CD64)[207] on neutrophils. C3bi is required for adherence and efficient chemotaxis by neutrophils. Low levels of this receptor also impair complement-mediated phagocytosis and oxidative metabolism. FcRI mediates oxidative responses as well, and appears on neutrophils of adults during infection. The diminished production of G-CSF and GM-CSF by neonatal mononuclear cells[140–142] may not only limit progenitor colony growth, but may also impair neonatal neutrophil functions, including chemotaxis, superoxide production, and C3bi expression, which are enhanced by these factors.[208,209] Tumor necrosis factor alpha (TNF-α) and IL-4, cytokines that modulate neutrophil functions, also may be produced at lower levels in neonates.[210] IL-8, a cytokine that enhances neutrophil functions, has not been adequately studied in neonates.

THROMBOPOIESIS AND PLATELETS

The platelet counts in term and preterm infants are between 150 and 400×10^9/liter (150,000 to 400,000/μl), comparable to adult values.[211,212] Thrombocytopenia of less than 100×10^9/liter (100,000/μl) may occur in high-risk infants with respiratory distress or sepsis,[213] small-for-date infants,[214] and newborns with trisomy syndromes.[215] Even normal newborns are unable to regulate thrombopoiesis and myelopoiesis in a wholly effective manner.[216] Although committed megakaryocyte progenitors (colony forming unit–megakaryocyte [CFU-Meg]) are increased in the marrow and cord blood of newborns, they are less able to produce adequate numbers of platelets when severely stressed. Reduced levels of G-CSF, GM-CSF, and IL-3 may play a role in the impaired response.[217] Thrombopoietin (TPO) is a major regulator of platelet production in adults. TPO transcripts have been detected as early as 6 weeks postconception and the primary source of TPO in the fetus and neonate is thought to be the liver.[218] Serum TPO levels are higher in preterm and term neonates compared to adults. However, thrombocytopenic newborns do not increase serum TPO levels as robustly as thrombocytopenic adults, which may contribute to the high incidence of thrombocytopenia seen in sick infants.[218]

PLATELET FUNCTIONS

Bleeding Time and Closure Time The expected inverse relationship between the platelet count and bleeding time has been described in term and preterm newborns.[219] However, the bleeding time often is longer than would be predicted by the platelet count because of sepsis or respiratory distress resulting in impaired platelet function, aggravating the effects of thrombocytopenia.

The bleeding time reflects platelet function and capillary integrity, as well as the platelet count, and traditionally has been used to assess these parameters. However, there are technical difficulties in applying a technique for measuring bleeding time to neonates or preterm infants because of the need for venous occlusion of the forearm, where the test normally is performed, and for a minimal incision to avoid scarring of the skin. Bleeding times were measured using an automatic device to minimize trauma in normal neonates, with venous occlusion of 20 torr for infants who weigh less than 1000 g, 25 torr for those who weigh 1000 to 2000 g, and 30 torr for those who weigh more than 2000 g. In 82 observations, 97 percent of the measurements were below 3.5 min, which was suggested as the upper limit for normal in these infants.[220] A similar upper limit (200 s) for the bleeding time of normal infants has been obtained using an automated device and vertical incisions.[221] Generally, newborn infants have shorter bleeding times than do children and adults, which may reflect their higher hematocrit, increased concentration of von Willebrand factor, and higher proportion of high molecular weight multimers of von Willebrand factor.[222] Children have longer bleeding times than either adults or newborns,[223] and the upper limit measured with an automated pediatric device may be as high as 13 min before age 10 years, compared to an upper limit of 7 min in adults measured with the same device.[223]

The bleeding times in newborns may be prolonged for a variety of reasons, including neonatal infection and respiratory distress syndrome, which do not necessarily result in thrombocytopenia.[224] The use of indomethacin for treatment of patent ductus arteriosus in preterm infants has been questioned because this agent interferes with prostaglandin metabolism and the production of thromboxane A_2, an important initiator of platelet aggregation. Although bleeding times are prolonged from a normal 3.5 min to approximately 9 min in indomethacin-treated patients,[225] indomethacin did not result in an increase in periventricular or intraventricular hemorrhage in preterm infants treated for patent ductus arteriosus.

A new technique to assess platelet function, the *closure time*, may replace the bleeding time, particularly for neonates and young children in whom bleeding times are difficult to perform and interpret. The closure time is measured using the PFA-100 system (Dade-Behring Inc., Deerfield, IL) and employs a fine capillary attached to membranes containing collagen-epinephrine and collagen-ADP, combinations of agents that activate platelets. An anticoagulated (3.2% sodium citrate) blood sample is passed through the capillary, and the time to occlusion of the membrane with each agent is measured as the closure time. Newborn infants have closure times that are shorter than those of adults, likely related to their higher hematocrits, increased ristocetin cofactor, and higher leukocyte counts.[226–228] The normal adult value for collagen-epinephrine closure time is less than 164 s, and for collagen-ADP closure time is less than 116 s. However, each laboratory must determine its own normal range for these tests.

Platelet Aggregation and Metabolism A variety of differences have been described in the platelet function of neonates. These include decreased ADP release, platelet factor 3 activity, platelet adhesiveness, and platelet aggregation in response to ADP, epinephrine, collagen, or thrombin.[229,230] These defects result from intrinsic differences in neonatal compared to adult platelets.[231] Paradoxically, these insufficiencies have little effect on the bleeding time of neonates. The in vitro findings do not appear related to a significant defect in prostaglandin synthesis or to storage pool deficiency of adenine nucleotides.[229] Furthermore, electron micrographs of neonatal platelets do not differ from those of platelets from normal adults.[232] This leaves unexplained the in vitro observations in neonatal platelets, which may be related to platelet membrane immaturity. These in vitro abnormalities may aggravate the impairment in platelet function and the predisposition to

bleeding that results from neonatal diseases, particularly respiratory distress syndrome and sepsis.

Maternal aspirin ingestion also results in abnormalities in platelet aggregation in the newborn in response to collagen.[233,234] However, aspirin has been studied extensively in patients with preeclampsia, and there is no significant bleeding in the fetus or newborn.[235,236]

Newborn infants commonly have petechiae, particularly on the head, neck, and shoulders, after vertex deliveries. They are presumably caused by trauma associated with passage through the birth canal and disappear within a few days. Petechiae usually are not present in infants delivered by cesarean section.

Platelet Antigens and Glycoproteins The glycoprotein complex GPIIb/IIIa represents approximately 15 percent of platelet surface protein and exhibits two allelic forms, Pl^{A1} and Pl^{A2}.[237] The Pl^{A1} antigen can be identified on fetal platelets by 16 weeks' gestation.[229] Pl^{A1} antigen is observed in a higher percentage of fetuses between 18 and 26 weeks' gestation than in adults. Approximately 2 percent of the population in the United States of European descent is homozygous for Pl^{A2} and hence are Pl^{A1}-negative. The complete expression of the Pl^{A1} antigen during early gestation likely permits sensitization in women who are Pl^{A1}-negative even during their first pregnancy.[238] The membrane glycoprotein GPIb, as well as the GPIIb/IIIa complex, is expressed by 18 weeks of gestation.[238] The gene for GPIIb/IIIa has been cloned, and the difference between Pl^{A1} and Pl^{A2} is a leucine 33–proline 33 amino acid polymorphism in glycoprotein IIIA.[237] Prenatal diagnosis of the glycoprotein genotype using DNA from amniocytes and the polymerase chain reaction can establish the potential for neonatal alloimmune thrombocytopenia[239] as well as the diagnosis of Glanzmann thrombasthenia. Rarely, other fetal platelet antigens such as Pl^{E2}, DUZO^a, Ko^u, and Bak^a have caused maternal sensitization and neonatal alloimmune thrombocytopenia.[240] The gestational ages for expression of these antigens have not been defined but are sufficiently early to permit sensitization.

NEONATAL LYMPHOPOIESIS

T-LYMPHOCYTE FUNCTIONS—CELLULAR IMMUNITY

The absolute number of lymphocytes in the newborn is equivalent to that in older children (Table 6-4), with lower values in premature infants at birth. Thymus-derived cells (T cells) develop early in gestation.[241] Table 6-4 shows the various lymphocyte subsets in infants.[242] The absolute number of CD3+ and CD4+ (helper/inducer phenotype) T-cell subsets in blood of newborns is significantly higher than in adults.[243] This is a result of an increased total lymphocyte count in neonates (and older children) as compared with adults.[244] The percentages of major lymphoid subsets (CD2, CD3, CD4, CD8, CD19) are not markedly different in neonates, children, and adults when measured by flow cytometry methods.[245] While the numbers of T and B lymphocytes are sustained or increased during the first 2 postnatal months, there is a marked decrease in the natural killer (NK) cell population.[246] There is a trend toward increased CD4 and decreased CD8 lymphocytes in newborns and children, resulting in an increased CD4/CD8 ratio.[247,248] In spite of this, T-cell suppressor activity may be increased in newborns.[249] Most responses of the cellular immunity system, such as antigen recognition and binding, antibody-dependent cytotoxicity, and graft-versus-host reactivity are present in the newborn,[249] although some are decreased in comparison with adults.[250] The in vitro response to phytohemagglutinin of cord blood lymphocytes is increased,[251,252] but the response of the newborn to 2,4-dinitrofluorobenzene, a potent inducer of delayed hypersensitivity, is not as consistent as that seen in older children.[253] Impaired T-cell production of γ-interferon and other lymphokines may be related to immature macrophage rather than to T-lymphocyte function, because intercellular

TABLE 6-4 LYMPHOCYTE SUBSETS

LYMPHOCYTE SUBSET	MEAN (25–75 PERCENTILE RANGE)		
	INFANTS (2 DAYS–11 MONTHS)	CHILDREN* (1–6 YEARS)	ADULTS (18–70 YEARS)
Lymphocytes, total	47% (39–59)	46 (38–53)	32 (28–39)
	4.1×10^9/liter (2.7–5.4)	3.6 (2.9–5.1)	2.1 (1.6–2.4)
CD3	64% (58–67)	64 (62–69)	72 (67–76)
	2.5×10^9/liter (1.7–3.6)	2.5 (1.8–3.0)	1.4 (1.1–1.7)
CD4	41% (38–50)	37 (30–40)	42 (38–46)
	2.2×10^9/liter (1.7–2.8)	1.6 (1.0–1.8)	0.8 (0.7–1.1)
CD8	21% (18–25)	29 (25–32)	35 (31–40)
	0.9×10^9/liter (0.8–1.2)	0.9 (0.8–1.5)	0.7 (0.5–0.9)
CD4/CD8 ratio	1.9 (1.5–2.9)	1.3 (1.0–1.6)	1.2 (1.0–1.5)
NK (CD3−/CD16+ or CD56+)	11% (8.0–17)	11 (8.0–15)	14 (10–19)
	0.5×10^9/liter (0.3–0.7)	0.4 (0.2–0.6)	0.3 (0.2–0.4)
CD20	23% (19–31)	16 (12–22)	13 (11–16)
	0.9×10^9/liter (0.5–1.5)	0.4 (0.3–0.5)	0.3 (0.2–0.4)

* Age 7–17 years, similar to adults.
SOURCE: Based on Erkeller-Yuksel et al.[242]

cooperation is a requisite for these processes.[254] Furthermore, cord blood T lymphocytes form a functional IL-2 receptor complex and have normal IL-2 receptors, but they do not up-regulate γ-interferon in response to IL-2.[255]

B-LYMPHOCYTE FUNCTIONS–HUMORAL IMMUNITY

Humoral (B-cell) immunity also develops early in gestation,[241] but it is not fully active until after birth. In the newborn, approximately 15 percent of lymphocytes have immunoglobulin on their surface, with all Ig isotypes represented.[256] A percentage of these cells are CD5+ B cells (B-1 cells), which produce polyreactive autoantibodies whose function is yet unclear.[257] The proportion of CD5+ B cells is markedly higher in the fetus compared to adults. The percentages of B cells expressing specific immunoglobulin isotypes are not related to the plasma levels of those isotypes. Variation in antibody response to specific antigens relates to the interaction of macrophages, T cells, and B cells; B lymphocytes are well represented in newborns.[258]

Fetal lymphocytes synthesize little immunoglobulin, presumably because of the sheltered environment in utero. Animals kept germ-free after birth have few plasma cells and markedly decreased production of immunoglobulins.[259] IgG levels of term infants are similar to maternal levels because of transplacental transfer.[260] IgM, IgD, and IgE do not cross the placenta,[260,261] and the levels of these immunoglobulins and of IgA are low or not detectable at birth. Breast feeding provides some transfer of antibodies, particularly secretory IgA, lysozyme, and lactoferrin. Large numbers of lymphocytes and monocytes (106 cells/ml) are found in colostrum and milk during the first 2 months postpartum.[262] These may provide local gastrointestinal protection against infection,[263] and there is some evidence for absorption of immunoglobulin and transfer of tuberculin sensitivity to the infant.

Although the newborn infant can produce specific IgG antibody,[264] only small amounts of IgG are usually produced by the fetus. IgG levels in premature infants are reduced in relation to gestational age because of the low placental transport early in pregnancy.[265–267] The ability of the fetus to produce IgM and IgA with appropriate stimuli is indicated by the presence of these antibodies in many newborn infants who have had prenatal infections[268] and by the presence of IgM isohemagglutinins in more than half of term newborn infants.[269] In human newborns and in fetal animals, the IgM response is predominant, and the appearance of IgG after exposure to specific antigens is delayed. These differences from the adult may relate to functional

immaturity of B and T lymphocytes,[270–272] to increased activity of suppressor T cells,[259,270] and perhaps to altered macrophage function.[273]

Newborns also may have relative splenic hypofunction, suggested by the large number of "pocked" red cells seen in the blood films of neonates, particularly premature infants. These "pocks" represent residual intraerythrocyte inclusions, which remain because of monocyte and macrophage hypofunction.[274,275]

COAGULATION IN THE NEONATE

PLASMA COAGULATION FACTORS

When the term newborn is compared to older children and adults, several differences in the coagulation and fibrinolytic systems have been described.[276–281] A comprehensive evaluation of the developmental changes in the levels of clotting factors and coagulation tests in preterm and term infants has been published.[282,283] The term newborn has reduced mean plasma levels (<60% of adult levels) of factors II, IX, X, XI, XII, prekallikrein, and high molecular weight kininogen (Table 6-5). This is not a result of impaired mRNA expression, at least in the case of factors II and X.[284] In contrast, the plasma concentration of factor VIII is similar and von Willebrand factor is increased compared to that of older children and adults. In spite of the lower levels of factors, the functional tests (prothrombin and partial thromboplastin times) are only slightly prolonged compared to adult normal values (see Table 6-5). Although different coagulation factors show different postnatal patterns of maturation, near-adult values are achieved for most components by 6 months of life.[279]

Factors II (prothrombin), VII, IX, and X require vitamin K for the final gamma glutamyl carboxylation step in their synthesis.[285] These factors decrease during the first 3 to 4 days after birth. This fall may be lessened by administration of vitamin K,[286] effectively preventing classic, early occurring (first few days after birth) hemorrhagic disease of the newborn. Inactive prothrombin molecules have been found in the plasma of some newborns, but they disappear after administration of vitamin K.[287] Early occurring hemorrhagic disease is most often associated with maternal administration of medications such as phenytoin (Dilantin)[288] and warfarin,[289] which reduce the vitamin K-dependent factors. In rare cases, no contributing factor is found.

A hemorrhagic diathesis also may occur later, 2 to 12 weeks after birth, as a result of lack of vitamin K, and is called *late hemorrhagic disease of the newborn* or *acquired prothrombin complex deficiency*.[290,291] The etiology of the vitamin K lack is unclear but may result from poor dietary intake, particularly related to breast feeding, alterations in liver function with cholestasis and decreased vitamin K absorption, or a toxic or infectious impairment of hepatic utilization.[290] Unfortunately, intracranial hemorrhage frequently is the presenting event in this condition. This problem can be prevented by parenteral or oral vitamin K, but the preferred route of administration remains controversial.[292] The parenteral route may result rarely in neuromuscular complications,[293] and an association of intramuscular vitamin K prophylaxis and cancer in infancy was suggested but not substantiated. Oral administration, however, appears less reliable and may require repeated doses.[290] The current recommendation of the American Academy of Pediatrics suggests that vitamin K_1, 0.5 to 1 mg, be administered intramuscularly at birth.[294] A new mixed micellar vitamin K_1 preparation is particularly well absorbed and may permit prophylaxis with a single oral dose,[295] but the efficacy and safety of oral prophylaxis require further study.[294]

TABLE 6-5 REFERENCE VALUES FOR COAGULATION TESTS IN PRETERM AND FULL-TERM INFANTS*

Coagulation Test	Preterm 28–31-Week Infants Day 1	Preterm 30–36-Week Infants			Full-Term Infants			Adults
		Day 1	Day 30	Day 180	Day 1	Day 30	Day 180	
PT (s)	15.4 (14.6–16.9)	13.0 (10.6–16.2)	11.8 (10.0–13.6)	12.5 (10.0–15.0)	13.0 (10.1–15.9)	11.8 (10.0–14.3)	12.3 (10.7–13.9)	12.4 (10.8–13.9)
INR	1.0 (0.61–1.70)	1.00 (0.53–1.62)	0.79 (0.53–1.11)	0.91 (0.53–1.48)	1.00 (0.53–1.26)	0.79 (0.53–1.26)	0.88 (0.61–1.17)	0.89 (0.64–1.17)
APTT (s)	108 (80.0–168)	53.6 (27.5–79.4)	44.7 (26.9–62.5)	37.5 (27.2–53.5)	42.9 (31.3–54.5)	40.4 (32.0–55.2)	35.5 (28.1–42.9)	33.5 (26.6–40.3)
TCT (s)	24.8 (19.2–30.4)	24.8 (19.2–30.4)	24.4 (18.8–29.9)	25.2 (18.9–31.5)	23.5 (19.0–28.3)	24.3 (19.4–29.2)	25.5 (19.8–31.2)	25.0 (19.7–30.3)
Fibrinogen (g/liter)	2.56 (1.60–5.50)	2.43 (1.50–3.73)	2.54 (1.50–4.14)	2.28 (1.50–3.60)	2.83 (1.67–3.99)	2.70 (1.62–3.78)	2.51 (1.50–3.87)	2.78 (1.56–4.00)
II (U/ml)	0.31 (0.19–0.54)	0.45 (0.20–0.77)	0.57 (0.36–0.95)	0.87 (0.51–1.23)	0.48 (0.26–0.70)	0.68 (0.34–1.02)	0.88 (0.60–1.16)	1.08 (0.70–1.46)
V (U/ml)	0.65 (0.43–0.80)	0.88 (0.41–1.44)	1.02 (0.48–1.56)	1.02 (0.58–1.46)	0.72 (0.34–1.08)	0.98 (0.62–1.34)	0.91 (0.55–1.27)	1.06 (0.62–1.50)
VII (U/ml)	0.37 (0.24–0.76)	0.67 (0.21–1.13)	0.83 (0.21–1.45)	0.99 (0.47–1.51)	0.66 (0.28–1.04)	0.90 (0.42–1.38)	0.87 (0.47–1.27)	1.05 (0.67–1.43)
VIII (U/ml)	0.79 (0.37–1.26)	1.11 (0.50–2.13)	1.11 (0.50–1.99)	0.99 (0.50–1.87)	1.00 (0.50–1.78)	0.91 (0.50–1.57)	0.73 (0.50–1.09)	0.99 (0.50–1.49)
vWF (U/ml)	1.41 (0.83–2.23)	1.36 (0.78–2.10)	1.36 (0.66–2.16)	0.98 (0.54–1.58)	1.53 (0.50–2.87)	1.28 (0.50–2.46)	1.07 (0.50–1.97)	0.92 (0.50–1.58)
IX (U/ml)	0.18 (0.17–0.20)	0.35 (0.19–0.65)	0.44 (0.13–0.80)	0.81 (0.50–1.20)	0.53 (0.15–0.91)	0.51 (0.21–0.81)	0.86 (0.36–1.36)	1.09 (0.55–1.63)
X (U/ml)	0.36 (0.25–0.64)	0.41 (0.11–0.71)	0.56 (0.20–0.92)	0.77 (0.35–1.19)	0.40 (0.12–0.68)	0.59 (0.31–0.87)	0.78 (0.38–1.18)	1.06 (0.70–1.52)
XI (U/ml)	0.23 (0.11–0.33)	0.30 (0.08–0.52)	0.43 (0.15–0.71)	0.78 (0.46–1.10)	0.38 (0.10–0.66)	0.53 (0.27–0.79)	0.86 (0.49–1.34)	0.97 (0.67–1.27)
XII (U/ml)	0.25 (0.05–0.35)	0.38 (0.10–0.66)	0.43 (0.11–0.75)	0.82 (0.22–1.42)	0.53 (0.13–0.93)	0.49 (0.17–0.81)	0.77 (0.39–1.15)	1.08 (0.52–1.64)
PK (U/ml)	0.26 (0.15–0.32)	0.33 (0.09–0.57)	0.59 (0.31–0.87)	0.78 (0.40–1.16)	0.37 (0.18–0.69)	0.57 (0.23–0.91)	0.86 (0.56–1.16)	1.12 (0.62–1.62)
HK (U/ml)	0.32 (0.19–0.52)	0.49 (0.09–0.89)	0.64 (0.16–1.12)	0.83 (0.41–1.25)	0.54 (0.06–1.02)	0.77 (0.33–1.21)	0.82 (0.36–1.28)	0.92 (0.50–1.36)
XIIIa (U/ml)		0.70 (0.32–1.08)	0.99 (0.51–1.47)	1.13 (0.65–1.61)	0.79 (0.27–1.31)	0.93 (0.39–1.47)	1.04 (0.46–1.62)	1.05 (0.55–1.55)
XIIIb (U/ml)		0.81 (0.35–1.27)	1.07 (0.57–1.57)	1.15 (0.67–1.63)	0.76 (0.30–1.22)	1.11 (0.39–1.73)	1.10 (0.50–1.70)	0.97 (0.57–1.37)

* All factors except fibrinogen are expressed as units per milliliter (U/ml), where pooled plasma contains 1.0 U/ml. All values are expressed as the mean of 40 to 77 samples for each population. The range of values encompassing 95% of the population is shown in parentheses.

ABBREVIATIONS: APTT, activated partial thromboplastin time; HK, high molecular weight kininogen; INR, international normalized ratio; PK, prekallikrein; PT, prothrombin time; TCT, thrombin clotting time; vWF, von Willebrand factor.

SOURCE: Modified from Andrew et al[279,282] with permission.

TABLE 6-6 REFERENCE VALUES FOR INHIBITORS OF COAGULATION IN PRETERM AND FULL-TERM INFANTS*

INHIBITOR LEVELS	PRETERM 30–36-WEEK INFANTS			FULL-TERM INFANTS			
	DAY 1	DAY 30	DAY 180	DAY 1	DAY 30	DAY 180	ADULTS
AT (U/ml)	0.38 (0.14–0.62)	0.59 (0.37–0.81)	0.90 (0.52–1.28)	0.63 (0.39–0.87)	0.78 (0.48–1.08)	1.04 (0.84–1.24)	1.05 (0.79–1.31)
α_2M (U/ml)	1.10 (0.56–1.82)	1.38 (0.72–2.04)	2.09 (1.10–3.21)	1.39 (0.95–1.83)	1.50 (1.06–1.94)	1.91 (1.49–2.33)	0.86 (0.52–1.20)
C_1E-INH (U/ml)	0.65 (0.31–0.99)	0.74 (0.40–1.24)	1.40 (0.96–2.04)	0.72 (0.36–1.08)	0.89 (0.47–1.31)	1.41 (0.89–1.93)	1.01 (0.71–1.31)
α_1AT (U/ml)	0.90 (0.36–1.44)	0.76 (0.38–1.12)	0.82 (0.48–1.16)	0.93 (0.49–1.37)	0.62 (0.36–0.88)	0.77 (0.47–1.07)	0.93 (0.55–1.31)
HCll (U/ml)	0.32 (0.10–0.60)	0.43 (0.15–0.71)	0.89 (0.45–1.40)	0.43 (0.10–0.93)	0.47 (0.10–0.87)	1.20 (0.50–1.90)	0.96 (0.66–1.26)
Protein C (U/ml)	0.28 (0.12–0.44)	0.37 (0.15–0.59)	0.57 (0.31–0.83)	0.35 (0.17–0.53)	0.43 (0.21–0.65)	0.59 (0.37–0.81)	0.96 (0.64–1.28)
Protein S (U/ml)	0.26 (0.14–0.38)	0.56 (0.22–0.90)	0.82 (0.44–1.20)	0.36 (0.12–0.60)	0.63 (0.33–0.93)	0.87 (0.55–1.19)	0.92 (0.60–1.24)

* All values are expressed in units per milliliter (U/ml) where pooled plasma contains 1.0 U/ml. All values are expressed as the mean of 40 to 75 samples for each population. The range of values encompassing 95% of the population is shown in parentheses.
ABBREVIATIONS: α_1AT, α_1-antitrypsin; AT, antithrombin; α_2M, α_2-macroglobulin; C_1E-INH, C_1 esterase inhibitor; HCll, heparin cofactor II.
SOURCE: Modified from Andrew et al[279,282] with permission.

Table 6-5 shows the values for coagulation factors in healthy 30- to 36-week-gestation premature infants. More prominent decreases in factors IX, XI, and XII are noted, which tend to prolong the partial thromboplastin time. Table 6-5 also shows the values for coagulation factors in 28- to 31-week-gestation infants. All of the coagulation factors are lower at earlier gestational ages.

There are no significant differences in mean prothrombin time determinations between 30- to 36-week premature and full-term infants who have not received vitamin K.[296] Premature infants given vitamin K have a longer mean prothrombin time than do term infants similarly treated. In some small infants there is no improvement in prothrombin time or levels of prothrombin, and factors VII and X after the intramuscular administration of vitamin K.[286,297] These results suggest a greater degree of "immaturity" of the liver in the small infants.

BLEEDING AND THROMBOSIS

Significant bleeding occurs more often in low-birth-weight infants than in term newborn infants. Increased capillary fragility is frequently found in premature infants in the first 2 days after birth and is not associated with thrombocytopenia.[286] Bleeding under the scalp or in other superficial areas may be caused by trauma coupled with increased capillary fragility. The more serious disorders of periventricular–intraventricular hemorrhage and pulmonary hemorrhage probably are not primarily caused by coagulation disorders, although such disorders may increase the bleeding.[298] Hypoxia seems to affect the clotting status of low-birth-weight infants.[299] Many infants with markedly abnormal prothrombin times have had hypoxia during delivery or shortly thereafter.[296] Cardiovascular collapse seen with episodes of cardiac arrest or with profound shock may cause disseminated intravascular coagulation and generalized bleeding. In many sick premature infants, a combination of shock, sepsis, liver immaturity, hypoxia, and other factors may contribute to the pathogenesis of coagulation abnormalities.

Arterial and venous thromboses are relatively frequent in newborns as compared to other age groups, but greater than 90 percent of arterial and greater than 80 percent of venous clots are related to catheters. Spontaneous thromboses are much less common, and most involve the renal veins or, rarely, the pulmonary vasculature.[300] Relative hypercoagulability in the newborn could result from a difference in the vascular endothelium, activation of the coagulation cascade, diminished coagulation inhibitor activity, or a defect in fibrinolysis. Inhibitors of coagulation include antithrombin, heparin cofactor II, protein C, and protein S.[283,301] The levels of proteins C and S, which are vitamin K-dependent, as well as antithrombin and heparin cofactor II, are low in the newborn; they are in a range associated with thrombotic episodes in adults with inherited deficiencies.[301] In addition, the presence of factor V Leiden may occur in as many as 6 percent of newborns.[302] This produces resistance to the action of protein C and may heighten the susceptibility to thrombosis. Hyperprothrombinemia caused by the 20210A allele prothrombin gene may affect 1 percent of the population,[303] but the elevated prothrombin level predisposing to thrombosis occurs in older patients.[304] The combined deficiency of these anticoagulant proteins may further intensify the thrombotic risk. However, the precise role of these inhibitors of coagulation in newborn hypercoagulability is uncertain because a proportionate decrease in vitamin K-dependent procoagulant factors (II, VII, IX, X) also is present, and an additional inhibitor, α_2-macroglobulin, is increased. Table 6-6 shows the values for plasma inhibitors of coagulation in premature and term infants.

HEMATOLOGIC EFFECTS OF MATERNAL DRUGS ON THE FETUS AND NEWBORN

HEMOSTATIC EFFECTS

A number of maternally administered pharmacologic agents have been implicated in hematologic abnormalities of the fetus or newborn (Table 6-7). Maternal aspirin ingestion results in impaired platelet aggregation but does not foster neonatal bleeding. Other agents taken by the mother, including diazoxide and thiazides, may be associated with neonatal thrombocytopenia.[305–307]

The newborn's plasma coagulation factors may be depressed by maternal warfarin ingestion.[289] This drug is best avoided during pregnancy because it is teratogenic (first trimester) and may cause growth retardation of the fetus as well as bleeding.[289] In contrast, heparin does not cross the placenta, and maternal treatment with heparin appears to be safe for the fetus.[308]

Phenytoin (Dilantin) and/or phenobarbital also may reduce the newborn's vitamin K-dependent factors, possibly by microsomal enzyme induction, which enhances their degradation.[288] Furthermore, phenytoin may depress the platelet count as a result of prenatal exposure[309] and cause teratogenic effects, for example, the fetal hydantoin syndrome.[310] The decision to use this agent during pregnancy should reflect an assessment of the need for this specific drug, and also the risk of maternal seizures to the fetus and mother versus the potential side effects of treatment. Newborns of mothers taking rifampin and isoniazid also may have depressed vitamin K-dependent factors.[311]

BILIRUBIN/KERNICTERUS

Nitrofurantoin and nalidixic acid may cause oxidant injury to the red cell membrane and hemoglobin.[312,313] If there is glucose-6-phosphate dehydrogenase deficiency, or if reduced glutathione is diminished, as in newborn red cells, these drugs have the potential to induce hemol-

TABLE 6-7 HEMATOLOGIC EFFECTS OF MATERNAL DRUGS ON THE FETUS AND NEWBORN

DRUG	EFFECT	CERTAINTY*	MECHANISM	REFERENCE
Aspirin	Bleeding	Known	Interference with platelet function	229, 233, 124
	Kernicterus	Potential	Displacement of bilirubin from albumin	315
Warfarin (Coumadin)	Bleeding	Known	Known depletion of vitamin K-dependent coagulation factors by blocking carboxylation	288, 289
Diazoxide	Bleeding	Questionable	Thrombocytopenia	305
Phenytoin (Dilantin)/ phenobarbitol	Bleeding	Suspected	Depletion of vitamin K-dependent coagulation factors by hepatic enzyme induction and factor degradation	288
		Questionable	Thrombocytopenia	309
Nalidixic acid	Hyperbilirubinemia	Potential	Oxidant damage to hemoglobin	313
Nitrofurantoin	Hyperbilirubinemia	Potential	Oxidant damage to hemoglobin	312, 314
Rifampin/isoniazid	Bleeding	Suspected	Depletion of vitamin K-dependent coagulation factors	311
Sulfonamides	Kernicterus	Known	Displacement of bilirubin from albumin	315
Thiazides	Bleeding	Suspected	Thrombocytopenia	306, 307

* Certainty reflects the level of confidence in the data, assigned in increasing order from potential through questionable, suspected, and known.
SOURCE: Based on Miller et al.**305**

ysis and heighten neonatal hyperbilirubinemia. Although this problem has not been documented by transplacental transfer of nitrofurantoin or nalidixic acid, hemolysis has occurred in glucose-6-phosphate dehydrogenase-deficient infants who acquired the drugs from breast milk.[313,314] Alternatively, sulfonamides may cause displacement of bilirubin bound to albumin and heighten the risk of kernicterus.[315] Salicylates, phenylbutazone, and naproxen may have a similar effect at very high plasma concentrations.[315]

Ideally, all these medications should be avoided during pregnancy unless their indication outweighs the potential risk to the fetus and newborn.

REFERENCES

1. Bloom W, Bartelmez GW: Hematopoiesis in young human embryos. *Am J Anat* 67:21, 1940.
2. Huber TL, Kouskoff V, Fehling HJ, et al: Haemangioblast commitment is initiated in the primitive streak of the mouse embryo. *Nature* 432: 625, 2004.
3. Kingsley PD, Malik J, Fantauzzo KA, Palis J: Yolk sac derived primitive erythroblasts enucleate during mammalian embryogenesis. *Blood* 104: 19, 2004.
4. Shivdasani RA, Mayer EL, Orkin SH: Absence of blood formation in mice lacking T-cell leukemia oncoprotein tal-1/SCL. *Nature* 373:432, 1995.
5. Warren AJ, Colledge WH, Carlton MBL, et al: The oncogenic cysteine-rich LIM domain protein is essential for erythroid development. *Cell* 78:45, 1994.
6. Fujiwara Y, Browne CP, Cuniff K, Goff SC, Orkin SH: Arrested development of embryonic red cell precursors in mouse embryos lacking transcription factor GATA-1. *Proc Natl Acad Sci U S A* 93:12355, 1996.
7. de Vries PA, Saunders JB: Development of the ventricles and spiral outflow tract in the human heart. *Carnegie Inst Wash Publ 621, Contrib Embryol* 37:87, 1962.
8. Tavian M, Hallais M-F, Peault B: Emergence of intraembryonic hematopoietic precursors in the pre-liver human embryo. *Development* 126: 793, 1999.
9. Peschle C, Mavilio F, Care A, et al: Haemoglobin switching in human embryos: Asynchrony of zeta > alpha and epsilon > gamma-globin switches in primitive and definite erythropoietic lineage. *Nature* 313: 235, 1985.
10. Knoll W: Blut und blutbildende organe menschlicher embryonen. *Denkschriften der Schweizerischen Naturforschenden Gesellschaft* 64:1, 1927.

11. Fukuda T: Fetal hemopoiesis. I. Electron microscopic studies on human yolk sac hemopoiesis. *Virchows Archiv B Cell Pathol* 14:197, 1973.
12. Palis J, Robertson S, Kennedy M, Wall C, Keller G: Development of erythroid and myeloid progenitors in the yolk sac and embryo proper of the mouse. *Development* 126:5073, 1999.
13. Xu M-J, Matsuoka S, Yang F-C, et al: Evidence for the presence of megakaryocytopoiesis in the early yolk sac. *Blood* 97:2016, 2001.
14. Migliaccio G, Migliaccio AR, Petti S, et al: Human embryonic hemopoiesis. Kinetics of progenitors and precursors underlying the yolk sac—liver transition. *J Clin Invest* 78:51, 1986.
15. Huyhn A, Dommergues M, Izac B, et al: Characterization of hematopoietic progenitors from human yolk sacs and embryos. *Blood* 86:4474, 1995.
16. Dommergues M, Aubeny E, Dumez Y, et al: Hematopoiesis in the human yolk sac: Quantitation of erythroid and granulopoietic progenitors between 3.5 and 8 weeks of development. *Bone Marrow Transplant* 9: 23, 1992.
17. Keleman E, Calvo W, Fliedner TM: *Atlas of Human Hemopoietic Development*. Springer-Verlag, Berlin, 1979.
18. Lin C-S, Lim S-K, D'Agati V, Constantini F: Differential effects of an erythropoietin receptor gene disruption on primitive and definitive erythropoiesis. *Genes Dev* 10:154, 1996.
19. Neubauer H, Cumano A, Muller M, et al: Jak2 deficiency defines an essential developmental checkpoint in definitive hematopoiesis. *Cell* 93: 397, 1998.
20. Valtieri M, Gabbianelli M, Pelosi E, et al: Erythropoietin alone induces erythroid burst formation by human embryonic but not adult BFU-E in unicellular serum-free culture. *Blood* 74:460, 1989.
21. Emerson SG, Shanti T, Ferrara JL, Greenstein JL: Developmental regulation of erythropoiesis by hematopoietic growth factors: analysis on populations of BFU-E from bone marrow, peripheral blood, and fetal liver. *Blood* 74:49, 1989.
22. Dame C, Fahnenstich H, Feitag P, et al: Erythropoietin mRNA expression in human fetal and neonatal tissue. *Blood* 92:3218, 1998.
23. Mucenski ML, McLain K, Kier AB, et al: A functional c-myb gene is required for normal murine fetal hepatic hematopoiesis. *Cell* 65:677, 1991.
24. Nuez B, Michalovich D, Bygrave A, et al: Defective haematopoiesis in fetal liver resulting from inactivation of the EKLF gene. *Nature* 375: 316, 1995.
25. Hann IM, Bodger MP, Hoffbrand AV: Development of pluripotent hematopoietic progenitor cells in the human fetus. *Blood* 62:118, 1983.
26. Porcellini A, Manna A, Manna M, et al: Ontogeny of granulocyte macrophage progenitor cells in the human fetus. *Int J Cell Cloning* 1:92, 1983.

27. Nicola NA, Metcalf D: Specificity of action of colony-stimulating factors in the differentiation of granulocytes and macrophages. *CIBA Found Symp* 118:7, 1986.

28. Ohls RK, Li Y, Abdel-Mageed A, et al: Neutrophil pool sizes and granulocyte colony-stimulating factor production in human mid-trimester fetuses. *Pediatr Res* 37:806, 1995.

29. Slayton WB, Juul SE, Calhoun DA, et al: Hematopoiesis in the liver and marrow of human fetuses at 5 to 16 weeks postconception: quantitative assessment of macrophage and neutrophil populations. *Pediatr Res* 43: 774, 1998.

30. Charbord P, Tavian M, Humeau L, Peault B: Early ontogeny of the human marrow from long bones: An immunohistochemical study of hematopoiesis and its microenvironment. *Blood* 87:4109, 1996.

31. Pahal GS, Jauniaux E, Kinnon C, et al: Normal development of human hematopoiesis between eight and seventeen weeks' gestation. *Am J Obstet Gynecol* 183:1029, 2000.

32. Gupta S, Pahwa R, O'Reilly R, et al: Ontogeny of lymphocyte subpopulation in human fetal liver. *Proc Natl Acad Sci U S A* 73:919, 1976.

33. Rainaut M, Pagniez M, Hercend T, et al: Characterization of mononuclear cell subpopulations in normal fetal peripheral blood. *Hum Immunol* 18:331, 1987.

34. Hann IM, Gibson BES, Letsky EA: *Fetal and Neonatal Haematology.* Baillaire Tindale, Philadelphia, 1991.

35. Cairo MS, Wagner JE: Placental and/or umbilical cord blood: an alternative source of hematopoietic stem cells for transplantation. *J Am Soc Hematol* 90:4665, 1997.

36. Maximow AA: Relation of blood cells to connective tissues and endothelium. *Physiol Rev* IV(4):532, 1924.

37. Houssaint E: Differentiation of the mouse hepatic primordium. II. Extrinsic origin of the haemopoietic cell line. *Cell Differ* 10:243, 1981.

38. Cudennec CA, Thiery J-P, Le Douarin N-M: In vitro induction of adult erythropoiesis in early mouse yolk sac. *Proc Natl Acad Sci U S A* 78: 2412, 1981.

39. Zanjani ED, Ascensao JL, Flake AW, et al: The fetus as an optimal donor and recipient of hemopoietic stem cells. *Bone Marrow Transplant* 10:107(suppl 1), 1992.

40. Touraine JL, Raudrant D, Laplace S: Transplantation of hemopoietic cells from the fetal liver to treat patients with congenital diseases postnatally or prenatally. *Transplant Proc* 29:712, 1997.

41. Moore MAS, Owen JJT: Stem-cell migration in developing myeloid and lymphoid systems. *Lancet* i:658, 1967.

42. Dieterlen-Lievre F: On the origin of hematopoietic stem cells in the avian embryo: An experimental approach. *J Embryol Exp Morphol* 33: 607, 1975.

43. Carpenter KL, Turpen JB: Experimental studies on hemopoiesis in the pronephros of *Rana pipiens. Differentiation* 14:167, 1979.

44. Muller AM, Medvinsky A, Strouboulis J, et al: Development of hematopoietic stem cell activity in the mouse embryo. *Immunity* 1:291, 1994.

45. Smith RA, Glomski CA: "Hemogenic endothelium" of the embryonic aorta: Does it exist? *Dev Comp Immunol* 6:359, 1982.

46. Tavian M, Coulombel L, Luton D, et al: Aorta-associated CD-34+ hematopoietic cells in the early human embryo. *Blood* 87:67, 1996.

47. Proudfoot NJ, Shander MH, Manley JL, et al: Structure and in vitro transcription of human globin genes. *Science* 209:1329, 1980.

48. Grosveld F, Van Assendelft GB, Greaves DR, Kolias B: Position independent, high-level expression of the human β globin gene in transgenic mice. *Cell* 51:975, 1987.

49. Hecht F, Motulsky AG, Lemire RJ, et al: Predominance of hemoglobin Gower 1 in early human embryonic development. *Science* 152:91, 1966.

50. Huehns ER, Dance N, Beaven GH, et al: Human embryonic hemoglobins. *Cold Spring Harbor Symp Quant Biol* 29:327, 1964.

51. Gale RE, Clegg JB, Huehns ER: Human embryonic haemoglobins Gower 1 and Gower 2. *Nature* 280:162, 1979.

52. Peschle C, Mavilio F, Care A, et al: Haemoglobin switching in human embryos: asynchrony of the ζ to α and ε to γ globin switches in primitive and definitive erythropoietic lineage. *Nature* 313:235, 1985.

53. Pataryas HA, Stomatoyannopoulos G: Hemoglobins in human fetuses: Evidence of adult hemoglobin production after the 11th gestational week. *Blood* 39:688, 1972.

54. Thomas ED, Lochte HL Jr, Greenough WB III, et al: In vitro synthesis of foetal and adult haemoglobin by foetal haematopoietic tissues. *Nature* 185:396, 1960.

55. Kazazian HH, Woodhead AP: Hemoglobin A synthesis in the developing fetus. *N Engl J Med* 289:58, 1973.

56. Bard H: The effect of placental insufficiency on fetal and adult hemoglobin synthesis. *Am J Obstet Gynecol* 120:67, 1974.

57. Kirschbaum T: Fetal hemoglobin content of cord blood determined by column chromatography. *Am J Obstet Gynecol* 84:1375, 1962.

58. Armstrong D, Schroeder WA, Fenninger W: A comparison of the percentage of fetal hemoglobin in human umbilical cord blood as determined by chromatography and by alkali denaturation. *Blood* 22:554, 1963.

59. Bard H: Postnatal fetal and adult hemoglobin synthesis in early preterm newborn infants. *J Clin Invest* 60:1789, 1973.

60. Metaxotou-Mavromati AD, Antonopoulou HK, Laskari SA, et al: Developmental changes in hemoglobin F levels during the first two years of life in normal and heterozygous β-thalassemia infants. *Pediatrics* 69: 734, 1982.

61. Bard H, Makowski EL, Meschia G, et al: The relative rates of synthesis of hemoglobins A and F in red cells of newborn infants. *Pediatrics* 45: 766, 1970.

62. Bromberg YN, Abrahamov A, Salzberger M: The effect of maternal anoxemia on the foetal haemoglobin of the newborn. *J Obstet Gynaecol Br Commonw* 63:875, 1956.

63. Huehns ER, Hecht F, Keil JV, et al: Developmental hemoglobin anomalies in a chromosomal triplication. *Proc Natl Acad Sci U S A* 51:89, 1964.

64. Lee CSN, Boyer SH, Bowen P, et al: The D1 trisomy syndrome: three subjects with unequally advancing development. *Johns Hopkins Med J* 118:374, 1966.

65. Giulian GG, Gilbert EF, Moss RL: Elevated fetal hemoglobin levels in sudden infant death syndrome. *N Engl J Med* 316:1122, 1987.

66. Wilson MG, Schroeder WA, Graves DA: Postnatal change of hemoglobins F and A2 in infants with Down's syndrome (G trisomy). *Pediatrics* 42:349, 1968.

67. Brown MS: Fetal and neonatal erythropoieses, in *Developmental and Neonatal Hematology,* edited by JA Stockman, III, C Pochedly, p 39. Raven Press, New York, 1988.

68. Forestier F, Daffos F, Galacteros F, et al: Haematological values of 163 normal fetuses between 18 and 30 weeks of gestation. *Pediatr Res* 20: 342, 1986.

69. Millar DS, Davis LR, Rodich CH, et al: Normal blood cell values in the early midtrimester fetus. *Prenat Diagn* 5:367, 1985.

70. Linch DC, Knott LJ, Rodech CH, et al: Studies of circulating hemopoietic progenitor cells in human fetal blood. *Blood* 59:976, 1982.

71. Christensen RD: Hematopoiesis in the fetus and neonate. *Pediatr Res* 26:531, 1989.

72. Marks J, Gairdner D, Roscoe JD: Blood formation in infancy. III. Cord blood. *Arch Dis Child* 30:117, 1955.

73. Linderkamp O, Versmold HT, Messow-Zahn K, et al: The effect of intrapartum and intra-uterine asphyxia on placental transfusion in premature and full-term infants. *Eur J Pediatr* 127:91, 1978.

74. Mercer JS: Current best evidence: A review of the literature on umbilical cord clamping. *J Midwifery Women's Health* 46:402, 2001.

75. Mercer JS, Skovgaard RL: Neonatal transitional physiology: A new paradigm. *J Perinat Neonatal Nurs* 15:56, 2002.

76. Yao AC, Hirvensalo M, Lind J: Placental transfusion rate and uterine contraction. *Lancet* 1:380, 1968.

77. Usher R, Shepard M, Lind J, et al: The blood volume of the newborn and placental transfusion. *Acta Paediatr* 52:497, 1963.

78. Bratteby LE: Studies on erythro-kinetics in infancy. XI. The change in circulating red cell volume during the first five months of life. *Acta Paediatr Scand* 57:215, 1968.

79. McCue CM, Garner FB, Hurt WG, et al: Placental transfusion. *J Pediatr* 72:15, 1968.

80. Matoth Y, Zaizor R, Varsano I: Postnatal changes in some red cell parameters. *Acta Paediatr Scand* 60:317, 1971.

81. Linderkamp O, Versmold HT, Strohhacker I, et al: Capillary-venous hematocrit differences in newborn infants. *Eur J Pediatr* 127:9, 1977.

82. Saarinen UM, Simmes MA: Developmental changes in red blood cell counts and indices of infants after exclusion of iron deficiency by laboratory criteria and continuous iron supplementation. *J Pediatr* 92:412, 1978.

83. Zipursky A, Brown E, Palko J, et al: The erythrocyte differential count in newborn infants. *Am J Pediatr Hematol Oncol* 5:45, 1983.

84. Alter BP, Goldberg JD, Berkowitz RL: Red cell size heterogeneity during ontogeny. *Am J Pediatr Hematol Oncol* 10:279, 1988.

85. Shannon KM, Naylor GS, Torkildson JC, et al: Circulating erythroid progenitors in the anemia of prematurity. *N Engl J Med* 317:728, 1987.

86. Linch DC, Knott LJ, Rodeck CH, Huehns ER: Studies of circulating hemopoietic progenitor cells in human fetal blood. *Blood* 59:976, 1983.

87. Christensen RD: Circulating pluripotent hematopoietic progenitor cells in neonates. *J Pediatr* 11:622, 1987.

88. Clapp DW, Baley JE, Gerson SL: Gestational age dependent changes in circulating hematopoietic stem cells in newborn infants. *J Lab Clin Med* 113:422, 1989.

89. Holbrook SR, Christensen RD, Rothstein G: Erythroid colonies derived from fetal blood display different growth patterns from those derived from adult marrow. *Pediatr Res* 24:605, 1988.

90. Burman D, Morris AF: Cord hemoglobin in low birth weight infants. *Arch Dis Child* 49:382, 1974.

91. Meberg A: Haemoglobin concentrations and erythropoietin levels in appropriate and small for gestational age infants. *Scand J Haematol* 24:162, 1980.

92. Zaizov R, Matoth Y: Red cell values on the first postnatal day during the last 16 weeks of gestation. *Am J Hematol* 1:275, 1976.

93. Lockridge S, Pass R, Cassidy G: Reticulocyte counts in intrauterine growth retardation. *Pediatrics* 47:919, 1971.

94. Humbert JR, Abelson H, Hathaway WE, et al: Polycythemia in small for gestational age infants. *J Pediatr* 75:1812, 1969.

95. Halvorsen S, Finne PH: Erythropoietin production in the human fetus and newborn. *Ann N Y Acad Sci* 149:576, 1968.

96. Seip M: The reticulocyte level and the erythrocyte production judged from reticulocyte studies in newborn infants during the first week of life. *Acta Paediatr Scand* 44:355, 1955.

97. Trial J, Rice L: Erythropoietin withdrawal leads to the destruction of young red cells at the endothelial-macrophage interface. *Curr Pharm Des* 10:183, 2004.

98. Mann DL, Sites ML, Donati RM, et al: Erythropoietic stimulating activity during the first ninety days of life. *Proc Soc Exp Biol Med* 118:212, 1965.

99. Lundstrom U, Simmes MA: Red blood cell values in low-birth-weight infants: Ages at which values become equivalent to those of term infants. *J Pediatr* 96:1040, 1980.

100. Stockman JA III, Garcia JF, Oski FA: The anemia of prematurity: factors governing the erythropoietin response. *N Engl J Med* 296:647, 1977.

101. MackIntosh TF, Walker CHM: Blood viscosity in the newborn. *Arch Dis Child* 48:547, 1973.

102. Bergqvist G: Viscosity of the blood in the newborn infant. *Acta Paediatr Scand* 63:858, 1974.

103. Wirth FH, Goldberg WR, Lubchenco L: Neonatal hyperviscosity. I. Incidence. *Pediatrics* 63:833, 1979.

104. Hakanson DO, Oh W: Hyperviscosity in the small-for-gestational age infant. *Biol Neonate* 37:190, 1980.

105. Ramamurthy RS, Berlanga M: Postnatal alteration in hematocrit and viscosity in normal and polycythemic infants. *J Pediatr* 110:929, 1987.

106. Bada HS, Korones SB, Pourcyrous M, et al: Asymptomatic syndrome of polycythemic hyperviscosity: Effect of partial plasma exchange transfusion. *J Pediatr* 120:579, 1992.

107. Bierhuizen MF, Mattei MG, Fukuda M: Expression of the developmental I antigen by a cloned human cDNA encoding a member of a beta-1,6-N-acetylglucosaminyltransferase gene family. *Gene Dev* 7:468, 1993.

108. Race RR, Sanger R: *Blood Groups in Man*, 6th ed. Blackwell Scientific Publications, London, 1975.

109. Pearson HA: Life-span of the fetal red blood cell. *J Pediatr* 70:166, 1967.

110. Weipple G, Pantlitschko M, Bauer P, et al: Normal values and distribution of serum iron in cord blood. *Clin Chim Acta* 44:147, 1973.

111. Saarinen UM, Siimes MA: Developmental changes in serum iron, total iron-binding capacity, and transferrin saturation in infancy. *J Pediatr* 91:875, 1977.

112. Saarinen UM, Siimes MA: Serum ferritin in assessment of iron nutrition in healthy infants. *Acta Paediatr Scand* 67:745, 1978.

113. Seip M, Halvorsen S: Erythrocyte production and iron stores in premature infants during the first months of life. The anemia of prematurity—etiology, pathogenesis, iron requirement. *Acta Paediatr Scand* 45:600, 1956.

114. Rao R, Georgieff MK: Perinatal aspects of iron metabolism. *Acta Paediatr Suppl* 91:124, 2002.

115. Bauer C, Ludwig I, Ludwig M: Different effects of 2,3-diphosphoglycerate and adenosine triphosphate on oxygen affinity of adult and fetal hemoglobin. *Life Sci* 7:1339, 1968.

116. Oski FA: Red cell metabolism in the newborn infant. V. Glycolytic intermediates and glycolytic enzymes. *Pediatrics* 44:84, 1969.

117. Oski FA, Delivoria-Papadopoulos M: The red cell, 2, 3-diphosphoglycerate, and tissue oxygen release. *J Pediatr* 77:941, 1970.

118. Zipursky A: The erythrocytes of the newborn infant. *Semin Hematol* 2:167, 1965.

119. Oski FA, Komazawa M: Metabolism of the erythrocytes of the newborn infant. *Semin Hematol* 12:209, 1975.

120. Oski FA, Smith CA: Red cell metabolism in the premature infant. III. Apparent inappropriate glucose consumption for cell age. *Pediatrics* 41:473, 1968.

121. Konrad PN, Valentine WN, Paglia DE: Enzymatic activities and glutathione content of erythrocytes in the newborn: comparison with red cells of older normal subjects and those with comparable reticulocytosis. *Acta Haematol* 48:193, 1972.

122. Gross RT, Schroeder EAR, Brounstein SA: Energy metabolism in the erythrocytes of premature infants compared to full term newborn infants and adults. *Blood* 21:755, 1963.

123. Oski FA: Red cell metabolism in the premature infant. II. The pentose phosphate pathway. *Pediatrics* 39:689, 1967.

124. Bracci R, Perrone S, Buonocore G: Oxidant injury in neonatal erythrocytes during the neonatal period. *Acta Paediatr Suppl* 91:130, 2002.

125. Ross JD: Deficient activity of DPNH-dependent methemoglobin diaphorase in cord blood erythrocytes. *Blood* 21:51, 1963.

126. Gross RT, Bracci R, Rudolph N, et al: Hydrogen peroxide toxicity and detoxification in erythrocytes of newborn infants. *Blood* 29:481, 1967.

127. Travis SF, Kumar SP, Delivoria-Papadopoulos M: Red cell metabolic alterations in postnatal life in term infants: glycolytic intermediates and adenosine triphosphate. *Pediatr Res* 15:34, 1981.

128. Whaun JM, Oski FA: Red cell stromal adenosine triphosphatase (ATP-ase) of newborn infants. *Pediatr Res* 3:105, 1969.

129. Blum SF, Oski FA: Red cell metabolism in the newborn infant. IV. Transmembrane potassium flux. *Pediatrics* 43:396, 1969.

130. Crowley J, Ways P, Jones JW: Human fetal erythrocyte and plasma lipids. *J Clin Invest* 44:989, 1965.

131. Neerhout RC: Erythrocyte lipids in the neonate. *Pediatr Res* 2:172, 1968.

132. Shapiro DL, Pasqualini P: Erythrocyte membrane proteins of premature and full-term infants. *Pediatr Res* 12:176, 1978.

133. Kosztolanyi G, Jobst K: Electrokinetic analysis of the fetal erythrocyte membrane after trypsin digestion. *Pediatr Res* 14:138, 1980.

134. Altman PL, Dittmer, DS: *Blood and Other Body Fluids*. Federation of American Societies for Experimental Biology, Washington, DC, 1961.

135. Coulombel L, Dehan M, Tchernia G, et al: The number of polymorpho-nuclear leukocytes in relation to gestational age in the newborn. *Acta Paediatr Scand* 68:709, 1979.

136. Barak Y, Blachar Y, Levin S: Neonatal neutrophilia: Possible role of a humoral granulopoietic factor. *Pediatr Res* 14:1026, 1980.

137. Laver J, Duncan E, Abboud M, et al: High levels of granulocyte and granulocyte-macrophage colony-stimulating factors in cord blood of normal full-term neonates. *J Pediatr* 116:627, 1990.

138. Ijima H, Suda T, Miura Y: Predominance of macrophage-colony for-mation in human cord blood. *Exp Hematol* 10:234, 1982.

139. Prindull G, Ben-Ishay Z, Gabriel M, et al: A comparison of spontaneous and CSF added CFU-MG colony formation in healthy, sick and hypo-trophic pre-term infants. *Blut* 45:167, 1982.

140. Cairo MS, Suen Y, Knoppel E, et al: Decreased stimulated GM-CSF production and GM-CSF gene expression but normal numbers of GM-CSF receptors in human term newborns compared with adults. *Pediatr Res* 30:362, 1991.

141. English BK, Hammond WP, Lewis DB, et al: Decreased granulocyte-macrophage colony-stimulating factor production by human neonatal blood mononuclear cells and T cells. *Pediatr Res* 31:211, 1992.

142. Cairo MS, Suen Y, Knoppel E, et al: Decreased G-CSF and IL-3 pro-duction and gene expression from mononuclear cells of newborn infants. *Pediatr Res* 31:574, 1992.

143. Carr R: Neutrophil production and function in newborn infants. *Br J Haematol* 110:18, 2000.

144. Rosenthal J, Cairo MS: The role of cytokines in modulating neonatal myelopoiesis and host defense. *Cytokines Mol Ther* 1:165, 1995.

145. Cairo MS, Plunkett JM, Nguyen A, Van De Ven C: Effect of stem cell factor with and without granulocyte colony-stimulating factor on neo-natal hematopoiesis: In vivo induction of newborn myelopoiesis and reduction of mortality during experimental group B streptococcal sepsis. *Blood* 80:96, 1992.

146. Banerjea MC, Speer CP: The current role of colony-stimulating factors in prevention and treatment of neonatal sepsis. *Semin Neonatol* 7:335, 2002.

147. Kucukoduk S, Sezer T, Yildiran A, et al: Randomized, double-blinded, placebo-controlled trial of early administration of recombinant human granulocyte colony-stimulating factor to non-neutropenic preterm new-borns between 33 and 36 weeks with presumed sepsis. *Scand J Infec Dis* 34:893, 2002.

148. Xanthou M: Leucocyte blood picture in healthy full-term and premature babies during neonatal period. *Arch Dis Child* 45:242, 1970.

149. Gibson EL, Vaucher Y, Corrigan JJ Jr: Eosinophilia in premature in-fants. Relationship to weight gain. *J Pediatr* 95:99, 1979.

150. Siegel JD, McCracken GH Jr: Sepsis neonatorum. *N Engl J Med* 304:642, 1981.

151. Forman ML, Stiehm ER: Impaired opsonic activity but normal phago-cytosis in low-birth-weight infants. *N Engl J Med* 281:926, 1969.

152. Dossett JH, Williams RC Jr, Quie PG: Studies on interaction of bacteria, serum factors and polymorphonuclear leukocytes in mothers and new-borns. *Pediatrics* 44:49, 1969.

153. Miller ME: Phagocytosis in the newborn infant: Humoral and cellular factors. *J Pediatr* 74:255, 1969.

154. Hill HR, Shigeoka AO, Pincus S, Christensen RD: Intravenous IgG in combination with other modalities in the treatment of neonatal infection. *Pediatr Infect Dis* 5:180, 1986.

155. Cocchi P, Marianelli L: Phagocytosis and intracellular killing of *Pseu-domonas aeruginosa* in premature infants. *Helv Paediatr Acta* 22:110, 1967.

156. Drossou V, Kanakoudi F, Diamanti E, et al: Concentrations of main serum opsonins in early infancy. *Arch Dis Child* 72:F172, 1995.

157. Yang KD, Bathras JM, Shigeoka AO, et al: Mechanisms of bacterial opsonization by immune globulin intravenous correlation of comple-ment consumption with opsonic activity and protective efficacy. *J Infect Dis* 159:701, 1989.

158. Shaio MF, Yang KD, Bohnsack JF, Hill HR: Effect of immune globulin intravenous on opsonization of bacteria by classic and alternative com-plement pathways in premature serum. *Pediatr Res* 25:634, 1989.

159. Hill H: Host defenses in the neonate: prospects for enhancement. *Semin Perinatol* 9:2, 1985.

160. Propp RP, Alper CA: C3 synthesis in the human fetus and lack of trans-placental passage. *Science* 162:672, 1968.

161. Johnston RB Jr, Altenburger KM, Atkinson AW Jr, et al: Complement in the newborn infant. *Pediatrics* 64:781, 1979.

162. Strunk RC, Fenton LJ, Gaines JA: Alternative pathway of complement activation in full term and premature infants. *Pediatr Res* 13:641, 1979.

163. Davis CA, Vallota EH, Forristal J: Serum complement levels in infancy: Age related changes. *Pediatr Res* 13:1043, 1979.

164. Mills EL, Bjorksten B, Quie PG: Deficient alternative complement path-way activity in newborn sera. *Pediatr Res* 13:1341, 1979.

165. Proctor RA, Prendergast E, Mosher DF: Fibronectin mediates attach-ment of *Staphylococcus aureus* to human neutrophils. *Blood* 59:681, 1982.

166. Hill HR, Shigeoka AO, Augustine NH, et al: Fibronectin enhances the opsonic and protective activity of monoclonal and polyclonal antibody against group B streptococci. *J Exp Med* 159:1618, 1984.

167. Harris MC, Levitt J, Douglas SD, et al: Effect of fibronectin on adher-ence of neutrophils from newborn infants. *J Clin Microbiol* 21:243, 1985.

168. Hill HR, Shigeoka AO, Gonzales LA, Christensen RD: Intravenous im-mune globulin use in newborns. *J Allergy Clin Immunol* 84:617, 1989.

169. Christensen RD, Brown MS, Hall DC, et al: Effect on neutrophil kinetics and serum opsonic capacity of intravenous administration of immune globulin to neonates with clinical signs of early-onset sepsis. *J Pediatr* 118:606, 1991.

170. Fujiwara T, Taniuchi S, Hattori K, et al: Effect of immunoglobulin ther-apy on phagocytosis by polymorphonuclear leukocytes in whole blood of neonates. *Clin Exp Immunol* 107:435, 1997.

171. Weisman LE, Stoll BJ, Kueser TJ, et al: Intravenous immune globulin therapy for early-onset sepsis in premature neonates. *J Pediatr* 121:434, 1992.

172. Schreiber JR, Berger M: Intravenous immune globulin therapy for sepsis in premature neonates. *J Pediatr* 121:401, 1992.

173. Baker CJ, Melish ME, Hall RT, et al: Intravenous immune globulin for the prevention of nosocomial infection in low-birth-weight infants. *N Engl J Med* 327:213, 1992.

174. Fanaroff A, Wright E, Korones S, Wright L: A controlled trial of pro-phylactic intravenous immunoglobulin to reduce nosocomial infections in VLBW infants. *Pediatr Res* 31:202A, 1992.

175. Suri M, Harrison L, Van de Ven C, et al: Immunotherapy in the pro-phylaxis of neonatal sepsis. *Curr Opin Pediatr* 15:155, 2003.

176. Fischer GW, Weisman LE, Hemming VG: Directed immune globulin for the prevention or treatment of neonatal group B streptococcal infections: A review. *Clin Immunol Immunopathol* 62:S92, 1992.

177. Miller ME: Chemotactic function in the neonate. Humoral and cellular aspects. *Pediatr Res* 5:487, 1971.

178. Klei RB, Fischer TJ, Gard SE, et al: Decreased mononuclear and polymorphonuclear chemotaxis in human newborns, infants, and young children. *Pediatrics* 60:467, 1977.

179. Tono-oka T, Nakayama M, Uehara H, et al: Characteristics of impaired chemotactic function in cord blood leukocytes. *Pediatr Res* 13:148, 1979.

180. Hill HR, Augustine NH, Newton JA, et al: Correction of a developmental defect in neutrophil activation and movement. *Am J Pathol* 128:307, 1987.

181. Bruce MC, Baley JE, Medvik KA, et al: Impaired surface membrane expression of C3bi but not C3b receptors on neonatal neutrophils. *Pediatr Res* 21:306, 1987.

182. Anderson DC, Freeman KLB, Heerdt B, et al: Abnormal stimulated adherence of neonatal granulocytes: impaired induction of surface MAC-1 by chemotactic factors or secretagogues. *Blood* 70:740, 1987.

183. Smith JB, Campbell DE, Ludomirsky A, et al: Expression of the complement receptors CR1 and CR3 and the type III Pc-gamma receptor on neutrophils from newborn infants and from fetuses with Rh disease. *Pediatr Res* 28:120, 1990.

184. Carr R, Davies JM: Abnormal PcRIII expression by neutrophils from very preterm neonates. *Blood* 76:607, 1990.

185. Anderson DC, Rothlein R, Marlin SD, et al: Impaired transendothelial migration by neonatal neutrophils: Abnormalities of Mac-1(CD11b/CD18)-dependent adherence reactions. *Blood* 76:2613, 1990.

186. Masuda K, Kinoshita Y, Kobayashi Y: Heterogeneity of Fc expression in chemotaxis and adherence of neonatal neutrophils. *Pediatr Res* 25:6, 1989.

187. Tosi MF, Berger M: Functional differences between the 40 kDa and 50 kDa IgG Fc receptors on human neutrophils revealed by elastase treatment and antireceptor antibodies. *J Immunol* 141:2097, 1988.

188. Coen R, Grush O, Kander E: Studies of bactericidal activity and metabolism of the leukocyte in full-term neonates. *J Pediatr* 78:400, 1969.

189. Mills EL, Thompson T, Bjorksten B, et al: The chemiluminescence response and bactericidal activity of polymorphonuclear neutrophils from newborns and their mothers. *Pediatrics* 63:429, 1979.

190. Park BH, Holmes B, Good RA: Metabolic activities in leukocytes of newborn infants. *J Pediatr* 76:237, 1970.

191. Xanthou M, Valassi-Adam E, Kintronidou E, et al: Phagocytosis and killing ability of *Candida albicans* by blood leucocytes of healthy term and preterm babies. *Arch Dis Child* 50:72, 1975.

192. Wright WC Jr, Ank BJ, Herbert J, et al: Decreased bactericidal activity of leukocytes of stressed newborn infants. *Pediatrics* 56:569, 1975.

193. Shigeoka AO, Santos JI, Hill HR: Functional analysis of neutrophil granulocytes from healthy, infected, and stressed neonates. *J Pediatr* 95:454, 1979.

194. Shigeoka AO, Charette RP, Wyman ML, et al: Defective oxidative metabolic responses of neutrophils from stressed neonates. *J Pediatr* 98:392, 1981.

195. Strauss RG, Snyder EL: Neutrophils from human infants exhibit decreased viability. *Pediatr Res* 15:794, 1981.

196. Strauss RG, Snyder EL, Wallace PO, et al: Oxygen-detoxifying enzymes in neutrophils of infants and their mothers. *J Lab Clin Med* 95:897, 1980.

197. Yamazaki M, Matsuoka T, Yasui K, et al: Increased production of superoxide anion by neonatal polymorphonuclear leukocytes stimulated with a chemotactic peptide. *Am J Hematol* 27:169, 1988.

198. Kretschmer RR, Papierniak CK, Stewardson-Krieger P, et al: Quantitative nitroblue tetrazolium reduction by normal newborn monocytes. *J Pediatr* 91:306, 1977.

199. Milgrom H, Shore SL: Assessment of monocyte function in the normal newborn infant by antibody-dependent cellular cytotoxicity. *J Pediatr* 91:612, 1977.

200. Orlowski JP, Sieger L, Anthony BF: Bactericidal capacity of monocytes of newborn infants. *J Pediatr* 89:797, 1976.

201. Schuit KE, Powell DA: Phagocytic dysfunction in monocytes of normal newborn infants. *Pediatrics* 65:501, 1980.

202. Das M, Henderson T, Feig SA: Neonatal mononuclear cell metabolism: Further evidence for diminished monocyte function in the neonate. *Pediatr Res* 13:632, 1979.

203. Mills EL: Mononuclear phagocytes in the newborn: Their relation to the state of relative immunodeficiency. *Am J Pediatr Hematol* 5:189, 1983.

204. Bryson YJ, Winter HS, Gard SE, et al: Deficiency of immune interferon production by leukocytes of normal newborns. *Cell Immunol* 55:191, 1987.

205. Frenkel L, Bryson YJ: Ontogeny of phytohemagglutinin-induced gamma interferon by leukocytes of healthy infants and children: Evidence for decreased production in infants younger than 2 months of age. *J Pediatr* 111:97, 1987.

206. Wilson CB, Westall J, Johnston L, et al: Decreased production of interferon-gamma by human neonatal cells. *J Clin Invest* 77:860, 1986.

207. Perussia B, Dayton ET, Lazarus R, et al: Immune interferon induces the receptor for monomeric IgG on human monocytic and myeloid cells. *J Exp Med* 158:1092, 1983.

208. Cairo MS: Review of G-CSF and GM-CSF effects on neonatal neutrophil kinetics. *Am J Pediatr Hematol Oncol* 11:238, 1989.

209. Cairo MS, VandeVen C, Toy C, et al: GM-CSF primes and modulates neonatal PMN motility: Up-regulation of C3bi (Mol) expression with alteration in PMN adherence and aggregation. *Am J Pediatr Hematol Oncol* 13:249, 1991.

210. Sautois B, Fillet G, Beguin Y: Comparative cytokine production by in vitro stimulated mononucleated cells from cord blood and adult blood. *Exp Hematol* 25:103, 1997.

211. Fogel BJ, Arais D, Kung F: Platelet counts in healthy premature infants. *J Pediatr* 73:108, 1968.

212. Sell EJ, Corrigan JJ: Platelet counts, fibrinogen concentrations and factor V and factor VIII levels in healthy infants according to gestational age. *J Pediatr* 82:1028, 1973.

213. Mehta P, Vasa R, Neumann L, Karpatkin M: Thrombocytopenia in the high-risk infant. *J Pediatr* 97:791, 1980.

214. Meberg A, Halvorsen S, Orstavik I: Transitory thrombocytopenia in small-for-dates infants, possibly related to maternal smoking. *Lancet* 2:303, 1977.

215. Thuring W, Tonz O: Neonatale Thrombozytenwerbe: Kindern mit Down-Syndrom und anderen autosomalen Trisomien. *Helv Paediatr Acta* 34:545, 1979.

216. Cairo, MS: The regulation of hematopoietic growth factor production from cord mononuclear cells and its effect on newborn rat hematopoiesis. *J Hematother* 2:217, 1993.

217. Suen Y, Chang M, Lee SM, et al: Regulation of interleukin-11 protein and mRNA expression in neonatal and adult fibroblasts and endothelial cells. *Blood* 84:4125, 1994.

218. Murray NA, Watts TL, Roberts IAG: Thrombopoietin in the fetus and neonate. *Early Hum Dev* 59:1, 2000.

219. Feusner JH: Normal and abnormal bleeding times in neonates and young children utilizing a fully standardized template technic. *Am Soc Clin Pathol* 74:73, 1980.

220. Rennie JM, Gibson T, Cooke RWI: Micromethod for bleeding time in the newborn. *Arch Dis Child* 60:51, 1985.

221. Andrew M, Paes B, Bowker J, Vegh P: Evaluation of an automated bleeding time device in the newborn. *Am J Hematol* 35:275, 1990.

222. Weinstein MJ, Blanchard R, Moake JL, et al: Fetal and neonatal von Willebrand factor (vWF) is unusually large and similar to the vWF in

patients with thrombotic thrombocytopenic purpura. *Br J Haematol* 72: 68, 1989.

223. Andrew M, Vegh P, Johnston M, et al: Maturation of the hemostatic system during childhood. *Blood* 80:1998, 1992.

224. Andrew M, Castle V, Saigal S, et al: Clinical impact of neonatal thrombocytopenia. *J Pediatr* 110:457, 1987.

225. Corazza MS, Davis RF, Merritt TA, et al: Prolonged bleeding time in preterm infants receiving indomethacin for patent ductus arteriosus. *J Pediatr* 105:292, 1984.

226. Israels SJ, Cheang T, McMillan-Ward EM, et al: Evaluation of primary hemostasis in neonates with a new in vitro platelet function analyzer. *J Pediatr* 138:116, 2001.

227. Knofler R, Weissbach G, Kuhlisch E: Platelet function tests in childhood. Measuring aggregation and release reaction in whole blood. *Semin Thromb Hemost* 24:513, 1998.

228. Carcao MD, Blanchette VS, Dean JA, et al: The platelet function analyzer (PFA-100): A novel in-vitro system for evaluation of primary hemostasis in children. *Br J Haematol* 101:70, 1998.

229. Stuart MJ: Platelet function in the neonate. *Am J Pediatr Hematol Oncol* 1:227, 1979.

230. Israels SJ, Daniels M, McMillan EM: Deficient collagen-induced activation in the newborn platelet. *Pediatr Res* 27:337, 1990.

231. Rajasekhar D, Kestin AS, Bednarek FJ, et al: Neonatal platelets are less reactive than adult platelets to physiological agonists in whole blood. *Thromb Haemost* 72:957, 1994.

232. Ts'ao C, Green D, Schultz K: Function and ultrastructure of platelets of neonates; enhanced ristocetin aggregation of neonatal platelets. *Br J Haematol* 32:225, 1976.

233. Blieyer WA, Breckenridge RT: Studies on the detection of adverse drug reactions in the newborn. II. The effects of prenatal aspirin on newborn hemostasis. *JAMA* 213:2049, 1970.

234. Corby DG, Schulman I: The effects of antenatal drug administration on aggregation of platelets of newborn infants. *J Pediatr* 79:307, 1971.

235. Hauth JC, Goldenberg RL, Parker CR Jr, et al: Low-dose aspirin: Lack of association with an increase in abruptio placentae or perinatal mortality. *Obstet Gynecol* 85:1055, 1995.

236. Sibai BM, Caritis SN, Thom E, et al: Low-dose aspirin in nulliparous women: Safety of continuous epidural block and correlation between bleeding time and maternal-neonatal bleeding complications. National Institute of Child Health and Human Developmental Maternal–Fetal Medicine Network. *Am J Obstet Gynecol* 172:1553, 1995.

237. Newman PJ, Derbes RS, Aster RH: The human platelet alloantigens, PLA1 and PLA2, are associated with a leucine 33/proline 33 amino acid polymorphism in membrane glycoprotein IIIa, and are distinguishable by DNA typing. *J Clin Invest* 83:1778, 1989.

238. Gruel Y, Boizard B, Daffos F, et al: Determination of platelet antigens and glycoproteins in the human fetus. *Blood* 68:488, 1986.

239. McFarland JG, Aster RH, Bussel JB, et al: Prenatal diagnosis of neonatal alloimmune thrombocytopenia using allele-specific oligonucleotide probes. *Blood* 78:2276, 1991.

240. Shulman NR, Jordan JV Jr: Platelet immunology, in *Hemostasis and Thrombosis: Basic Principles and Clinical Practice*, 2nd ed, edited by RW Colman, J Hirsh, VJ Marder, EW Salzman, pp 476–483. JB Lippincott, Philadelphia, 1987.

241. Pabst HF: Ontogeny of the immune response as a basis of childhood diseases. *J Pediatr* 97:519, 1980.

242. Erkeller-Yuksel FM, Deneys V, Yuksel B, et al: Age related changes in human blood lymphocyte subpopulations. *J Pediatr* 120:216, 1992.

243. De Waele M, Foulon W, Renmans W, et al: Hematologic values and lymphocyte subsets in fetal blood. *Am J Clin Pathol* 89:742, 1988.

244. Hicks MJ, Jones JF, Minnich LL, et al: Age-related changes in T- and B-lymphocyte subpopulations in the peripheral blood. *Arch Pathol Lab Med* 107:518, 1983.

245. Kotylo PA, Baenzinger JC, Yoder MC, et al: Rapid analysis of lymphocyte subsets in cord blood. *Am J Clin Pathol* 93:263, 1990.

246. Comans-Bitter WM, de Groot R, van den Beemd R, et al: Immunophenotyping of blood lymphocytes in childhood. Reference values for lymphocyte subpopulations. *J Pediatr* 130:388, 1997.

247. Slukvin II, Chernishov VP: Two-color flow cytometric analysis of natural killer and cytotoxic T-lymphocyte subsets in peripheral blood of normal human neonates. *Biol Neonate* 61:156, 1992.

248. Neubert R, Delgado I, Abraham K, et al: Evaluation of the age-dependent development of lymphocyte surface receptors in children. *Life Sci* 62:1099, 1998.

249. Miller ME: Immune-inflammatory response in the human neonate. *Am J Pediatr Hematol* 3:199, 1981.

250. Stiehm ER, Winter HS, Bryson YF: Cellular (T cell) immunity in the human newborn. *Pediatrics* 64:814, 1979.

251. Carr MC, Stites DP, Fudenberg HH: Cellular immune aspects of the human fetal-maternal relationship. I. In vitro response of cord blood lymphocytes to phytohemagglutinin. *Cell Immunol* 5:21, 1972.

252. Papiernick M: Comparison of human foetal with child blood lymphocytic kinetics. *Biol Neonate* 19:163, 1971.

253. Uhr JW, Dancis J, Newmann CG: Delayed-type hypersensitivity in premature neonatal humans. *Nature* 187:1130, 1960.

254. Blaese RM, Poplack DG, Muchmore AV: The mononuclear phagocyte system: Role in expression of immunocompetence in neonatal and adult life. *Pediatrics* 64(suppl):829, 1979.

255. Von Freeden U, Zessack N, Van Valen F, Burdach S: Defective interferon gamma production in neonatal T cells is independent of interleukin-2 receptor binding. *Pediatr Res* 30:270, 1991.

256. Sterm CMM: Changes in lymphocytes subpopulations in the blood of healthy and sick newborn infants. *Pediatr Res* 13:792, 1979.

257. Raveche ES: Possible immunoregulatory role for CD5+ B cells. *Clin Immunol Immunopathol* 56:135, 1990.

258. Lawton AR, Cooper MD: B cell ontogeny: immunoglobulin genes and their expression. *Pediatrics* 64:750, 1979.

259. Gustafsson BE, Laurell CB: Gamma globulin production in germ free rats after bacterial contamination. *J Exp Med* 110:675, 1959.

260. Gitlin D: The differentiation and maturation of specific immune mechanisms. *Acta Pediatr Scand* 172(suppl):60, 1967.

261. Stiehm ER: Fetal defense mechanisms. *Am J Dis Child* 129:438, 1975.

262. Goldman AS, Garza C, Nichols BL, Goldblum RM: Immunological factors in human milk during the first year of lactation. *J Pediatr* 100:563, 1982.

263. Goldman AS, Ham Pong AJ, Goldblum RM: Host defenses: Development and maternal contributions. *Adv Pediatr* 32:71, 1985.

264. Rothberg RM: Immunoglobulin and specific antibody synthesis during the first weeks of life of premature infants. *J Pediatr* 75:391, 1969.

265. Harworth JC, Norris M, Dilling L: A study of the immunoglobulins in premature infants. *Arch Dis Child* 40:243, 1965.

266. Thom H, McKay E, Gray DWG: Protein concentrations in the umbilical cord plasma of premature and mature infants. *Clin Sci* 33:433, 1967.

267. Yeung CY, Hoffs JR: Serum gamma-G-globulin levels in normal, premature, postmature, and "small-for-dates" newborn babies. *Lancet* 1: 1167, 1968.

268. Sever JH: Immunological responses to perinatal responses to perinatal infections. *J Pediatr* 75:1111, 1969.

269. Thomaidis T, Agathopoulos A, Matsaniotis N: Natural isohemagglutinin production by the fetus. *J Pediatr* 74:39, 1969.

270. Morito T, Bankhurst AD, Williams RC Jr: Studies of human cord blood and adult lymphocyte interactions with in vitro immunoglobulin production. *J Clin Invest* 64:990, 1979.

271. Miyagawa Y, Sugita K, Komiyama A, et al: Delayed in vitro immunoglobulin production by cord lymphocytes. *Pediatrics* 65:497, 1980.

272. Ferguson AC, Cheung SC: Modulation of immunoglobulin M and G synthesis by monocytes and T lymphocytes in the newborn infant. *J Pediatr* 98:385, 1981.

273. Blaese RM, Poplack DG, Muchmore AV: The mononuclear phagocyte system: role in expression of immunocompetence in neonatal and adult life. *Pediatrics* 64:829, 1977.

274. Holroyde CP, Oski FA, Gardner FH: The "pocked" erythrocyte. *N Engl J Med* 281:516, 1969.

275. Freedman RM, Johnston D, Mahoney MJ, et al: Development of splenic reticuloendothelial function in neonates. *J Pediatr* 96:466, 1980.

276. Gross SJ, Stuart MJ: Hemostasis in the premature infant. *Clin Perinatol* 4:259, 1977.

277. Barnard DR, Hathaway WE: Neonatal thrombosis. *Am J Pediatr Hematol Oncol* 1:235, 1979.

278. Bleyer WA, Hakami N, Shepard TH: The development of hemostasis in the human fetus and newborn infant. *J Pediatr* 79:838, 1971.

279. Andrew M, Paes B, Milner B, et al: Development of the human coagulation system in the full-term infant. *Blood* 70:165, 1987.

280. Andrew M, Paes B, Milner R, et al: Development of the human coagulation system in the healthy premature infant. *Blood* 72:1651, 1988.

281. Corrigan JJ Jr: Neonatal thrombosis and the thrombolytic system: Pathophysiology and therapy. *Am J Pediatr Hematol Oncol* 10:83, 1988.

282. Andrew M, Paes B, Johnston M: Development of the hemostatic system in the neonate and young infant. *Am J Pediatr Hematol Oncol* 12:95, 1990.

283. Andrew M: The relevance of developmental hemostasis to hemorrhagic disorders of newborns. *Semin Perinatol* 21:70, 1997.

284. Karpatkin M, Lee M, Cohen L, et al: Synthesis of coagulation proteins in the fetus and neonate. *J Pediatr Hematol Oncol* 22:276, 2000.

285. Furie B, Furie BC: Molecular basis of gamma-carboxylation. Role of the propeptide in the vitamin K-dependent proteins. *Ann N Y Acad Sci* 614:1, 1991.

286. Aballi AJ, deLamerens S: Coagulation changes in the neonatal period and in early infancy. *Pediatr Clin North Am* 9:785, 1962.

287. Muntean W, Petek W, Rosanelli K, et al: Immunologic studies of prothrombin in newborns. *Pediatr Res* 13:1262, 1979.

288. Lane PA, Hathaway WE: Vitamin K in infancy. *J Pediatr* 106:351, 1985.

289. Stevenson RE, Burton OM, Ferlauto GJ, et al: Hazards of oral anticoagulants during pregnancy. *JAMA* 243:1549, 1980.

290. Shearer MJ: Annotation: Vitamin K and vitamin K-dependent proteins. *Br J Haematol* 75:156, 1990.

291. von Kries R, Hanawa Y: Neonatal vitamin K prophylaxis. Report of Scientific and Standardization Subcommittee on Perinatal Haemostasis. *Thromb Haemost* 69:293, 1993.

292. Sutor AH, Gobel U, Kries RV, et al: Vitamin K prophylaxis in the newborn. *Blut* 60:275, 1990.

293. Hathaway WE, Isarangkura PB, Mahasandana C, et al: Comparison of oral and parenteral vitamin K prophylaxis for prevention of late hemorrhagic disease of the newborn. *J Pediatr* 119:461, 1991.

294. Blackmon L, Batton DG, Bell EF, et al: Controversies concerning vitamin K and the newborn. American Academy of Pediatrics Policy Statement. *Pediatrics* 112:191, 2003.

295. Amadee-Manesme O, Labert WE, Alagille D, De Leenheer AP: Pharmacokinetics and safety of a new solution of vitamin K₁ (20) in children with cholestasis. *J Pediatr Gastroenterol Nutr* 14:160, 1996.

296. Aballi AJ: The action of vitamin K in the neonatal period. *South Med J* 58:48, 1965.

297. Gray OP, Ackerman A, Fraser AJ: Intracranial haemorrhage and clotting in low birth weight infants. *Lancet* 1:543, 1968.

298. Volpe JJ: Neonatal intraventricular hemorrhage. *N Engl J Med* 304:886, 1981.

299. Appleyard WJ, Cottom DG: Effect of asphyxia on Thrombotest values in low birthweight infants. *Arch Dis Child* 45:705, 1970.

300. Schmidt B, Zipursky A: Thrombotic disease in newborn infants. *Clin Perinatol* 2:461, 1984.

301. Rodgers GM, Shuman MA: Congenital thrombotic disorders. *Am J Hematol* 21:419, 1986.

302. Sifontes MT, Nuss R, Hunger SP, et al: Correlation between the functional assay for activated protein C resistance and factor V Leiden in the neonate. *Pediatr Res* 42:776, 1997.

303. Leroyer C, Mercier B, Oger E, et al: Prevalence of 20210 A allele of the prothrombin gene in venous thromboembolism patients. *Thromb Haemost* 80:49, 1998.

304. Poort SR, Rosendaal FR, Reitsma PH, Bertina RM: A common genetic variation in the 3'-untranslated region of the prothrombin gene is associated with elevated plasma prothrombin levels and an increase in venous thrombosis. *Blood* 88:3698, 1996.

305. Miller RK, Kellogg CR, Saltzman RA: Reproductive and perinatal toxicology, in *Handbook of Toxicology*, edited by TJ Haley, WO Berndt, pp 195–309. Hemisphere Publishing, Washington, DC, 1987.

306. Gray MJ: Use and abuse of thiazides in pregnancy. *Clin Obstet Gynecol* 11:568, 1968.

307. Leikin SL: Thiazide and neonatal thrombocytopenia. *N Engl J Med* 271:161, 1964.

308. Ginsberg JS, Kowalchuk G, Hirsh J, Brill-Edwards P, Burrows R: Heparin therapy during pregnancy. *Arch Intern Med* 149:2233, 1989.

309. Page TE, Hoyme HE, Markarian M, et al: Neonatal hemorrhage secondary to thrombocytopenia: an occasional effect of prenatal hydantoin exposure. *Birth Defects* 18:47, 1982.

310. Hanson JW, Buehler BA: Fetal hydantoin syndrome: current status. *J Pediatr* 101:816, 1982.

311. Eggermont E, Logghe N, van de Casseye W, et al: Haemorrhagic disease of the newborn in the offspring of rifampin and isoniazid treated mothers. *Acta Pediatr Belg* 29:87, 1976.

312. Powell RD, DeGowin RL, Alving AS, et al: Nitrofurantoin-induced hemolysis. *J Lab Clin Med* 62:1002, 1963.

313. Belton EM, Jones RV: Haemolytic anaemia due to nalidixic acid. *Lancet* 2:691, 1965.

314. Varsano I, Fischl J, Tikvah P, et al: The excretion of orally ingested nitrofurantoin in human milk. *J Pediatr* 82:886, 1973.

315. Brodersen R: Prevention of kernicterus, based on recent progress in bilirubin chemistry. *Acta Paediatr* 66:625, 1977.

HEMATOLOGY DURING PREGNANCY

MARTHA P. MIMS

JOSEF T. PRCHAL

Normal pregnancy involves many changes in maternal physiology including alterations in hematologic parameters. These changes include expansion in maternal blood and plasma volume and a decrease in hematocrit, as well as an increase in the levels of some plasma proteins that alters the balance of coagulation and fibrinolysis. Worldwide, the predominant cause of anemia in pregnancy is iron deficiency. Fetal requirements for iron are met despite maternal deficiency, but maternal iron deficiency has a number of adverse consequences, including preterm delivery and low-birth-weight infants. Bleeding disorders in pregnancy are a common reason for hematologic consultation and evoke concern for both the mother and child. Life-threatening bleeding as a consequence of disseminated intravascular coagulation is seen with some complications unique to pregnancy, including placental abruption, retained dead fetus, and amniotic fluid embolism. Von Willebrand disease is the commonest inherited bleeding disorder, but because of increases in factor VIIIc and von Willebrand factor (vWF) during pregnancy, excessive bleeding at delivery is rarely a problem. Factor levels fall rapidly postpartum and serious hemorrhage can occur during this period. Carriers of hemophilia A and B should be monitored during pregnancy to determine if factor levels will be adequate for delivery at term. Caution should be exercised at delivery and during the first few days of life with offspring of hemophilia carriers until hemophilia testing is completed and the infant's status is known. Acquired hemophilia caused by factor VIII autoantibodies is rare, but can occur during pregnancy or the puerperium. Thrombocytopenia is not uncommon in pregnancy and its causes include several conditions that are unique to pregnancy. Idiopathic thrombocytopenic purpura (ITP) is common and is managed conservatively if possible; close follow-up of newborns of mothers with ITP is essential. Hemolysis, elevated liver enzymes, and low platelets (HELLP) syndrome and thrombotic thrombocytopenic purpura and hemolytic uremic syndrome (TTP-HUS) are also seen in pregnancy and the puerperium. HELLP syndrome is managed with delivery if possible, whereas TTP requires plasma exchange. Inherited and acquired prothrombotic conditions can be exacerbated by pregnancy and can result in adverse reproductive outcomes as well as venous thromboembolism. Although the strongest evidence for an association between a thrombophilia and recurrent fetal loss exists for antiphospholipid antibody syndrome, evidence is mounting for a connection between inherited thrombophilias and the severity of some complications of pregnancy. Inherited thrombophilias increase the risk of venous thromboembolism in pregnancy. Treatment of hematologic malignancies in pregnancy can present a difficult dilemma, both in terms of staging studies and management. In many cases of Hodgkin lymphoma, treatment can be delayed safely until after delivery. In aggressive lymphomas and acute leukemias, however, rapid initiation of chemotherapy is often necessary to save the life of the mother. In general, the teratogenic effects of chemotherapy are greatest in the first trimester; however, care must be taken in later trimesters to avoid cytopenias at delivery. Hemorrhagic and thrombotic complications associated with pregnancy in females with essential thrombocythemia and polycythemia vera present a unique challenge because of the lack of controlled trials in these situations.

HEMATOLOGIC ADAPTATIONS TO PREGNANCY

BLOOD VOLUME, CELL COUNTS, AND ERYTHROPOIETIN LEVEL

Maternal blood volume increases by an average of 40 to 50 percent above the nonpregnant level.[1] Plasma volume begins to rise early in pregnancy with most of the escalation taking place in the second trimester and prior to week 32 of gestation.[2] Red cell mass increases significantly beginning in the second trimester and continues to expand throughout pregnancy, but to a lesser extent than plasma volume.[2] Erythropoietin levels increase throughout pregnancy, reaching approximately 150 percent of their prepregnancy levels at term.[3,4] The overall effect of these changes in most women is a slight drop in hematocrit which is most pronounced in the second trimester and slowly improves approaching term. The effect of pregnancy on maternal platelet count is somewhat more controversial; some studies demonstrate a mild decline in platelet count over the course of gestation,[5] whereas others do not.[6] In general, white cell counts rise during pregnancy with the occasional appearance of myelocytes or metamyelocytes in the blood.[7] During labor and the early puerperium, there is a rise in the leukocyte count. Leukocytosis appears to be linearly related to the duration of labor.[8]

PLASMA PROTEINS

Levels of some plasma proteins also increase during pregnancy. In particular, C-reactive protein concentration is higher in pregnant women and rises even further during labor.[9] Erythrocyte sedimentation rates (ESRs) rise during pregnancy, and are affected by both hemoglobin concentration and gestational age.[10] The rise in ESR during pregnancy, in large part a result of an increase in levels of plasma globulins and fibrinogen, makes its use as a marker of inflammation difficult. As discussed in more detail below, the levels of many of the procoagulant factors increase during pregnancy whereas activity of the fibrinolytic system diminishes in preparation for the hemostatic challenge of delivery. Plasma levels of vWF, fibrinogen, and factors VII, VIII, IX, and X all increase markedly while factors II, V, and XII are essentially unchanged and factors XI and XIII decline.[11] Levels of protein C and antithrombin remain stable throughout pregnancy whereas total and free protein S fall with increasing gestation.[12] Fibrinolysis is also impaired by increases in plasminogen activator inhibitors I and II, the latter a product of the placenta.[13]

ANEMIA IN PREGNANCY

IRON DEFICIENCY

Worldwide the contribution of anemia to maternal and fetal morbidity and mortality is well recognized; in some parts of Africa, more than 75 percent of pregnant women are anemic and there is a significant correlation between maternal mortality and anemia.[14] In pregnant women, anemia is defined as a hemoglobin concentration of less than 11g/dl in the first and third trimesters, and less than 10.5 g/dl in the second trimester.[15] In both the industrialized and the developing world, iron-deficiency anemia (see Chap. 40) is the commonest cause of anemia.[16] On average approximately 1 g of iron is required during a normal pregnancy; 300 mg of iron are required by the fetus and the placenta, whereas expansion of the maternal red blood cell (RBC) mass requires 500 mg, and 200 mg are lost via excretion.[17] These requirements exceed the iron storage (~300 mg) of most young women, and in general cannot be met by the diet. Even in cases of maternal iron deficiency, the fetal requirements for iron are always met, thus there is no correlation between the hematocrit of the fetus and that of the mother.[18]

Iron-deficiency anemia during the first two trimesters of pregnancy is associated with a twofold increased risk for preterm delivery and a threefold increased risk for delivery of a low-birth-weight infant.[19] However, a large randomized trial comparing routine iron prophylaxis in pregnancy versus iron supplementation given only as needed demonstrated no significant differences in adverse maternal or fetal outcomes.[20] As in nonpregnant individuals, iron-deficiency anemia can generally be diagnosed using laboratory values such as serum ferritin, and transferrin levels (see Chap. 40). *Pica*, the ingestion of nonnutritive substances, is said to be more common among iron-deficient pregnant women than among other populations with iron deficiency. Ice, clay or dirt, and starch are the most frequent substances ingested (see Chap. 40); to some extent, however, the choice appears to be cultural and much more widespread than most practitioners realize.[21]

FOLATE AND VITAMIN B$_{12}$ DEFICIENCY

Apart from iron deficiency, folate deficiency is the next most frequent nutritional deficiency leading to anemia in pregnant women. In the United States, where foodstuffs are supplemented with folate and the level of awareness of the association between folate deficiency and neural tube defects is high, folate deficiency is relatively unusual. Folate requirements in pregnancy are roughly twice those in the nonpregnant state (800 μg/day vs. 400 μg/day), and if diet is insufficient may exceed the body's stores of folate (5–10 mg) in short order.[22] Anemia related to folate deficiency most often presents in the third trimester and responds to folate supplementation with reticulocytosis within 24 to 72 hours.[16] Reports of severe pancytopenia and even states resembling the HELLP syndrome as a result of folate deficiency in pregnancy have appeared in the literature.[23,24] Despite these case reports, a review of 21 trials measuring the effect of folate supplementation on biochemical and hematologic parameters and pregnancy outcome (excluding neural tube defects) revealed improvement in low hemoglobin level in late pregnancy, but had no measurable effect on any substantive measures of pregnancy outcome (see Chap. 39).[25]

Vitamin B$_{12}$ deficiency during pregnancy is rare, in part because deficiency of this vitamin leads to infertility. Serum cobalamin levels are known to fall during pregnancy.[26] A shift from the serum to tissue stores is proposed to account for the drop in serum B$_{12}$ levels. However, values less than 180 pmol/liter are not observed in healthy women, and these low normal levels are not accompanied by increased levels of methylmalonic acid (see Chap. 39).[27]

RED CELL APLASIA

A rarer, but well-recognized cause of anemia in pregnancy is pure red cell aplasia (see Chap. 34). In pure red cell aplasia, anemia tends to occur early in pregnancy and often resolves within weeks of delivery. The anemia does not appear to be transferred to the fetus, but does tend to recur in subsequent pregnancies.[28,29] Conservative treatment, if feasible, is probably best until delivery; successful prenatal treatments with steroids and with intravenous immunoglobulin have been reported.[30,31]

BLEEDING DISORDERS AND CAUSES OF THROMBOCYTOPENIA

Bleeding disorders in pregnancy require consideration of maternal bleeding and hemorrhagic complications in the newborn. Data on the fetus is often lacking and the practitioner must base decisions on past experience and the mother's previous reproductive history.

DISSEMINATED INTRAVASCULAR COAGULATION

Life-threatening bleeding is seen with some pregnancy-unique complications resulting in disseminated intravascular coagulation (DIC) stemming from placental abruption, a retained dead fetus, and amniotic fluid embolism (see Chap. 121). Although amniotic fluid embolism is a significant cause of maternal death in developed countries, in recent years, the mortality decreased from 86 percent in 1979 to less than 30 percent in 1994 and 1995.[32] Amniotic fluid embolism is heralded by maternal vascular collapse with dyspnea, hypotension, and cardiac arrhythmias followed by DIC that is manifested by oozing from intravenous lines, hematuria, hemoptysis, and excessive uterine bleeding. Cryptic cases have also been reported in which there is rapid deterioration of an intrauterine fetus followed by maternal deterioration postpartum with development of DIC.[33]

DIC is thought to arise from the procoagulant properties of amniotic fluid containing vernix, caseosa, and fetal squamous epithelial cells in the pulmonary circulation followed by a secondary fibrinolytic response.[34] Treatment from the point of view of the hematologist is not significantly different than in other cases of DIC with bleeding (see Chap. 121); however, there are some reports of successful management with uterine artery embolization.[35] Placental abruption has also led to development of DIC and the spectrum of hemostatic failure is broad and appears to be related to the degree of placental separation.[36] Volume resuscitation, delivery of the fetus, and infusion of blood products to correct the maternal coagulation defect are indicated. Regional anesthesia is contraindicated because of the risk of bleeding in the epidural space and of the pooling of blood in the lower limb vascular bed, which could worsen hypovolemia.[36] Finally, intrauterine fetal death can also lead to DIC. Thromboplastic substances released from dead fetal tissues into the maternal circulation are thought to trigger DIC; however, this is not usually detectable by laboratory tests until 3 or 4 weeks after fetal demise. Overt DIC is present in approximately 50 percent of women who retain a dead fetus for 5 weeks or longer.[37]

VON WILLEBRAND DISEASE

Although von Willebrand disease (vWD) is transmitted in an autosomal dominant fashion, women appear to be disproportionately affected with bleeding symptoms; primarily menorrhagia and postpartum hemorrhage (see Chap. 118). In normal women and in types 1 and 2 (but not type 3) vWD patients, levels of factor VIIIc and vWF rise during pregnancy, with the most pronounced increase in the third trimester.[38] As a result, prophylactic administration of vWF-containing factor concentrates at delivery is often unnecessary in type 1 and type 2 vWD patients; however, the risk of postpartum hemorrhage is significant (13–29 percent) as levels fall rapidly after birth.[39] Thus in type 1 patients, factor VIIIc levels should be tested not only late in the third trimester, but also for 1 to 2 weeks postpartum. These patients should be monitored for increases in menstrual blood flow for at least 1 month. Risk of bleeding appears to be minimal when factor VIIIc levels are greater than 40 U/dl. The literature contains several reports of severe thrombocytopenia developing late in pregnancy in patients with type 2B vWD[40,41] and at least one of these patients developed a pulmonary embolus while receiving cryoprecipitate for postpartum hemorrhage. Despite the possible risk of thrombus, these patients may require treatment with plasma-derived vWF-containing concentrates at delivery or postpartum if there is abnormal bleeding, and with platelets if thrombocytopenic bleeding is not controlled with infusion of vWF concentrate. Type 3 vWD patients require infusion of a plasma-derived vWF-containing concentrate at delivery, typically 40 to 80 IU/kg, followed by doses of 20 to 40 IU/kg daily for a week then tapered over the next few weeks.[42] Use of desmopressin acetate (DDAVP) antepartum is controversial because of the theoretical risk of vasoconstriction and placental insufficiency and the risk of maternal hyponatremia; however, a systematic review of its use to treat diabetes insipidus during pregnancy revealed no evidence of adverse outcome for either mother or child.[43]

COAGULATION FACTOR DEFICIENCIES (SEE CHAP. 116)

Carriers of hemophilia A generally have levels of factor VIII that are 50 percent or less of normal, whereas the range is somewhat broader in factor IX carriers. Ideally, carriers are identified before pregnancy when prenatal counseling can be offered. Baseline factor levels should be tested at the first visit during pregnancy and again in the third trimester, but it should be noted that factor IX levels generally do not rise during the course of the pregnancy.[44] At a minimum, the sex of the fetus should be determined to guide the obstetrician at delivery. In general, cesarean section is not indicated if there are no complications, and a factor VIII or IX level of 40 IU/dl is generally safe for a normal vaginal delivery.[45] To protect a potentially affected or known hemophiliac fetus, vacuum extraction should be avoided at delivery and forceps should be used only with caution. All intramuscular injections should be withheld from the newborn until hemophilia testing is completed. Testing should be done on cord blood to avoid potential bleeding or bruising after a blood draw.[46] The mother's factor level should be followed for a few days after delivery and menstrual bleeding should be monitored to ensure adequate hemostasis. There is also an association between pregnancy and acquired hemophilia caused by factor VIII autoantibodies. This condition usually appears 1 to 4 months postpartum, but emerges during pregnancy in up to 14 percent of patients.[47] In general, the Bethesda titer of the inhibitor is low and in most cases the inhibitor disappears spontaneously. Inhibitors can recur in subsequent pregnancies.[48]

Rarely, obstetric patients with factor deficiencies other than factor VIII and factor IX may be identified. The most important of these to recognize is deficiency of factor XIII, which is associated with habitual hemorrhagic abortions and postpartum hemorrhage. In rare pregnancies reaching term, bleeding complications, including intracranial hemorrhage in the infant, have been observed.[49,50] Treatment of this deficiency with fresh-frozen plasma, cryoprecipitate, or plasma-derived factor XIII concentrates is thought to prevent abortion in women, although there are no controlled studies to confirm this impression.[51] Most authorities recommend more frequent prophylactic therapy during pregnancy (every 3 weeks vs. every 5–6 weeks) with booster doses during labor or before cesarean section to ensure a level of 5 percent or greater.[52]

THROMBOCYTOPENIA

Thrombocytopenia in pregnancy is relatively common with up to 5 percent of all pregnant women exhibiting asymptomatic thrombocytopenia.[53] Many of the causes of thrombocytopenia in pregnancy are identical to those seen in the nonpregnant state, with some predisposing to bleeding whereas others predispose to clotting. However, there are several conditions leading to thrombocytopenia that are unique to pregnancy, including gestational thrombocytopenia, preeclampsia/HELLP syndrome/eclampsia, and acute fatty liver of pregnancy.

GESTATIONAL AND IMMUNE THROMBOCYTOPENIA

Gestational thrombocytopenia and idiopathic thrombocytopenic purpura (ITP) are best discussed together as they can be difficult to differentiate and may in fact be two extremes of a spectrum of disease. In general, gestational thrombocytopenia is asymptomatic and is said to occur later in pregnancy and be less severe than ITP. Most sources suggest that gestational thrombocytopenia occurs in the second and third trimesters, with platelet counts rarely falling below 70,000/μl.[54] Gestational thrombocytopenia can sometimes be diagnosed with certainty only after delivery; usually there is no past history of low platelets, except perhaps with previous pregnancies, the platelet count returns to normal after delivery, and there is no association with fetal thrombocytopenia. Gestational thrombocytopenia is benign and does not require intervention (see Chap. 52).

In contrast to gestational thrombocytopenia, ITP can occur at any point in pregnancy and the fall in platelet count can be severe. Diagnosis is essentially the same as it would be in any patient in that alternative causes of thrombocytopenia must be ruled out. As in other cases, treatment of ITP in pregnancy must take into account the severity of the thrombocytopenia and the presence or absence of symptoms. In general, platelet counts less than 10,000/μl require treatment regardless of the trimester; platelet counts of 30,000 to 50,000/μl without bleeding require no treatment, and platelet counts of 10,000 to 30,000/μl in later trimesters or in the presence of bleeding require treatment. Although glucocorticoid and intravenous immunoglobulin (IVIg) are safe in pregnancy, it should be recognized that they may have no effect on fetal counts and should only be used to treat the mother.[55] Splenectomy for ITP in pregnancy is best done in the second trimester if platelet counts are extremely low and unresponsive to treatment.[54] Maternal platelet counts of greater than 50,000/μl are safe for both vaginal and cesarean delivery. In terms of predicting fetal platelet count, it should be noted that less than 5 percent of babies born to mothers with ITP have platelet counts less than 20,000/μl, although there does seem to be some correlation between very severely depressed maternal platelet count and thrombocytopenia in the newborn.[56] No clear recommendations can be given for measuring fetal platelet count prior to or at delivery as measurements are fraught with error; however, if the fetal platelet count is known to be less than 20,000/μl, cesarean section is probably reasonable. Newborns of mothers with ITP should be monitored for 5 to 7 days after delivery to ensure that the platelet count does not drop (see Chap. 52).

ECLAMPSIA AND HELLP SYNDROME

The spectrum of hypertensive disorders of pregnancy ranging from preeclampsia to severe preeclampsia and HELLP syndrome to eclampsia may also result in thrombocytopenia, although clotting is more of an issue than is bleeding. There is some debate in the literature as to whether thrombocytopenia can be diagnosed in preeclampsia without HELLP syndrome; however, data from one large study[53] demonstrate that approximately 15 percent of cases of preeclampsia are complicated by thrombocytopenia. In general the symptoms of preeclampsia, including hematologic manifestations, resolve with delivery; however, in a small proportion of cases they persist, worsen, or even develop immediately postpartum. When symptoms persist postpartum, the differentiation from TTP-HUS becomes more difficult. Some data suggests that maternal recovery from the HELLP syndrome is accelerated by administration of intravenous dexamethasone[57]; however, a recent meta-analysis demonstrated no clear advantage to the use of glucocorticoids in terms of maternal or perinatal morbidity or mortality.[58] Observation or treatment of HELLP with steroids alone postpartum should probably not persist beyond the third postpartum day. If the patient is not clearly improving, plasma exchange should be initiated as one would do for TTP.[59,60] Although not associated with hypertension, acute fatty liver of pregnancy is another rare disorder that can present in the third trimester with severe liver dysfunction, but thrombocytopenia, if present, is generally mild and does not require treatment (see Chap. 49).

THROMBOPHILIA

FETAL LOSS AND COMPLICATIONS

Pregnancy is a prothrombotic state. Inherited prothrombotic conditions contribute to 50 percent of the cases of venous thromboembolism and pulmonary embolism, as well as to stroke in pregnancy and the puerperium. Evidence is mounting that congenital thrombophilias (see Chap. 122) may also predispose to fetal loss through placental vascular disorders. The best evidence for an association between a thrombophilia, albeit acquired, and recurrent fetal loss exists for antiphospholipid antibody syndrome in which the association between the antibodies and pregnancy loss has been recognized for more than 20 years.[61] As many as 20 percent of women with recurrent fetal loss have antiphospholipid antibodies[62] and studies show that without treatment, up to 90 percent will experience fetal loss.[63] In a randomized controlled trial including 90 women with a history of recurrent miscarriage associated with phospholipid antibodies (or antiphospholipid antibodies), lupus anticoagulant, and cardiolipin antibodies (or anticardiolipin antibodies), the rate of live births with low-dose aspirin (75 mg/day) and unfractionated heparin (5000 U subcutaneously twice per day) was 71 percent (32/45 pregnancies) and 42 percent (19/45 pregnancies) with low-dose aspirin alone (odds ratio, 3.37 [95 percent confidence interval 1.40 to 8.10]).[64] Although an association between inherited thrombophilias and pregnancy loss has been elusive and there are inconsistencies between studies, there does appear to be an association between factor V Leiden and recurrent fetal loss.[65,66] Less convincing data exist for prothrombin 20210A, but there is no clear association with methionine tetrahydrofolate reductase C677T polymorphism (hyperhomocysteinemia).[67] No controlled studies have examined the benefit of aspirin or heparin in patients with inherited thrombophilias to prevent recurrent pregnancy loss. Studies evaluating a role for inherited thrombophilias in preeclampsia and intrauterine growth retardation indicate that these factors may not be causative, but may contribute to disease severity.[68,69]

THROMBOEMBOLIC EVENTS

Risk Factors Estimates place the risk of venous thromboembolism (VTE) in pregnant women (see Chaps. 122 and 125) at two to six times that of nonpregnant women.[70,71] Factors specific to pregnancy that increase the risk of VTE include obstruction of venous return by the gravid uterus, acquired prothrombotic changes in hemostatic proteins, and venous atonia caused by hormonal factors.[72] Additional risk factors include cesarean section (especially emergency), obesity, and increasing age. Approximately 80 percent of deep vein thromboses (DVTs) in pregnancy occur in the iliofemoral veins on the left, probably as a consequence of compression of the left iliac vein by the right

iliac and ovarian arteries.[73,74] Rates of VTE immediately postpartum are difficult to assess as many occur after the patient is discharged; however, some studies suggest that postpartum rates may be even higher than antepartum rates.[75,76] Inherited thrombophilia plays a role in VTE in pregnancy. The highest rates occur with inherited antithrombin deficiency where it has been estimated that in the absence of anticoagulation, 32 to 44 percent of patients will experience thromboembolism.[75] In a large retrospective study of more than 70,000 pregnancies,[77] the risk of VTE in pregnancy was estimated at about 1 in 437 for carriers of factor V Leiden, 1 in 113 for protein C deficiency, and 1 in 2.8 for type I antithrombin deficiency. Based on results from other studies, the risk for carriers of protein S deficiency appears to be similar to that for protein C deficiency, and risk for carriers of the prothrombin 20210A gene mutation is similar to or lower than that of factor V Leiden carriers.[78–80]

Diagnostic Methods Diagnosis of VTE in pregnancy is complicated both because the presenting complaints—leg edema, back pain, and chest pain—are common in pregnancy, and because radiologic studies used to make the diagnosis in nonpregnant individuals are relatively contraindicated in pregnant women. Compression ultrasonography is the initial test of choice in pregnant women. If this test is nondiagnostic, several other tests may be considered. If pulmonary embolus is suspected, lung ventilation perfusion scanning, which gives relatively low-dose radiation, may be used. Magnetic resonance imaging or magnetic resonance venography are also informative if available. Measurement of D-dimers is a useful adjunct in nonpregnant patients to rule out VTE (D-dimers are sensitive, but not specific, for VTE). However, D-dimer levels rise over the course of normal pregnancy[81,82] and with several complications of pregnancy, including preterm labor, hypertension, and placental abruption,[83] and thus may not be useful in excluding VTE.

Prophylaxis Prophylaxis for VTE is a controversial issue as only a few prospective studies have been done to assess the risk of use.[84,85] There is general agreement, however, that because of its teratogenic potential, warfarin should not be used during pregnancy and that low molecular weight heparins are the anticoagulant of choice because they do not cross the placenta and have a lower risk of osteoporosis and heparin-induced thrombocytopenia.[86] Most experts agree that women with low risk, including those with no prior history of VTE and a confirmed hypercoagulable state or with a single prior VTE associated with a transient risk factor, can be managed with careful surveillance during pregnancy (except for patients with antithrombin deficiency and antiphospholipid syndrome who should receive prophylactic doses of low molecular weight heparin or unfractionated heparin during pregnancy). Postpartum risk increases somewhat, and anticoagulation should be continued for 6 to 8 weeks. Some experts recommend initiating anticoagulation for patients with protein C or S deficiency during this period. Treatment of patients with a single previous thromboembolism and a hypercoagulable state not on warfarin at conception is more controversial. Some recommend careful clinical surveillance, whereas others counsel use of prophylactic low molecular weight heparins antepartum; postpartum most experts recommend 6 to 8 weeks of prophylaxis for all patients in this category. Patients with two or more episodes of VTE should be treated throughout pregnancy and the puerperium.[87–91] Treatment of VTE in pregnancy should be with full-dose low molecular weight heparin. Ideally, women on treatment doses of heparin have elective induction of labor. Heparin is usually discontinued 24 h prior to induction; however, women deemed to be at very high risk of recurrent VTE can then receive IV heparin up to 4 to 6 hours prior to delivery.[87,90] Great care should be taken with epidural anesthesia and it should be avoided if there is any question of a significant anticoagulant effect. Heparins and warfarin are safe postpartum, even when breast-feeding.[92]

TREATMENT OF HEMATOLOGIC MALIGNANCIES IN PREGNANCY

Although not common, leukemias and lymphomas do occur in pregnancy and present problems with proper diagnosis, staging, and treatment (see Chaps. 87, 88, 96, and 97). The literature suggests that the incidence of Hodgkin lymphoma is 1:1000 to 1:6000 pregnancies, whereas the incidence of non-Hodgkin lymphoma is many-fold lower.[93] Leukemia in pregnancy is uncommon.

HODGKIN LYMPHOMA

A review of the literature suggests that neither the histology nor the outcome of patients who present during pregnancy is worse than that of other patients.[94] Diagnosis, usually by biopsy of a lymph node, is usually not problematic, but staging can be difficult. Posterior–anterior chest films with abdominal shielding and marrow biopsy should be done and present little risk to the fetus. Laboratory studies, including blood counts, liver functions tests, and ESR, should be done, but care should be taken in interpreting the alkaline phosphatase and ESR measurements, which both rise during the course of a normal pregnancy. Evaluation for the presence of abdominopelvic disease is difficult because computed tomography imaging is contraindicated in pregnant women. Abdominal ultrasonograms are safe, but provide limited information. If necessary, magnetic resonance imaging scans can probably be done safely in pregnancy; however, this is rarely necessary. The toxicities of treatment and the risks of delaying treatment until later in pregnancy or postpartum need to be considered carefully in each case. Fetal risks of chemotherapy are greatest in the first trimester during the period of organogenesis, with folate antagonists and antimetabolites carrying the largest risk.[95] Despite the changes in physiology that occur during pregnancy, there is no evidence that dosing should be changed. If chemotherapy is indicated, it should be delayed until the second trimester; however, single-agent vinblastine has been given in the first trimester with a low incidence of fetal abnormalities.[96] Treatment should be timed so that there is the maximum amount of time possible between the last dose of chemotherapy and delivery to avoid cytopenias in either the mother or the fetus. In some cases, radiotherapy may be a feasible alternative in the second and third trimesters of pregnancy. Of 16 patients who received radiotherapy for supradiaphragmatic Hodgkin disease (clinical stages IA and IIA) during pregnancy, 11 received full mantle irradiation, and all patients had lead shielding of the uterus.[97] All 16 pregnancies were carried to completion with full-term deliveries of normal infants. However, a review of the records of 382 women treated with radiotherapy for Hodgkin lymphoma suggests that the risk of breast cancer after radiation therapy is nearly sevenfold greater with irradiation around the time of pregnancy.[98] Additional studies are needed to confirm these findings, but this potential risk should be borne in mind by the clinician when making therapeutic decisions. Relapse of Hodgkin lymphoma usually occurs within the first 2 years following treatment, and patients are counseled to avoid pregnancy during this period. Vigilance for second cancers in these patients is also advised as is monitoring for hypothyroidism in those who receive radiation therapy, especially during subsequent pregnancies when hypothyroidism could have profound maternal and fetal effects.

NON-HODGKIN LYMPHOMA

As compared with Hodgkin lymphoma, other lymphomas are less frequent in pregnancy, tend to present with a higher stage disease, and have a poorer prognosis.[99] Burkitt or Burkitt-like lymphoma can involve the breasts of young pregnant or lactating women and typically behaves aggressively.[100,101] In patients with high-grade lymphomas, chemotherapy often cannot be delayed and difficult decisions must be made. However, in one report of 16 pregnant patients who received aggressive chemotherapy for non-Hodgkin lymphoma during their pregnancies, all survived to delivery.[102] Half of the 16 patients received chemotherapy in their first trimester and all 16 delivered healthy infants despite episodes of myelosuppression during the pregnancies. In a subsequent report, the health of 84 children born to mothers who received chemotherapy for hematologic malignancies during pregnancy revealed no abnormalities in physical or cognitive development and no increase in cancers at a median followup of 18.7 years.[103] Rituximab in pregnancy both as a single agent and in combination with chemotherapy has not been associated with abnormalities of the newborn when given in the first, second, or third trimester.[104,105]

ACUTE LEUKEMIA

Leukemia is distinctly uncommon in pregnancy; estimates derived from studies beginning in the 1950s place the incidence at about 1:75,000 pregnancies.[106,107] Acute leukemias make up nearly 90 percent of the total, followed by chronic myeloid leukemia, which comprises an additional 10 percent; chronic lymphocytic leukemia is extremely rare.[108] The acute leukemias require urgent treatment, and while pregnancy itself does not alter the course of the leukemia, the outcome is much worse if treatment is delayed.[109] A summary of data on 96 pregnant women reported in the literature from 1983 to 1995 who were treated with cytotoxic chemotherapy for leukemias (most of which were acute) revealed that most patients received regimens that included multiple drugs and were not different from those given to nonpregnant patients.[110] Nearly one-third of patients were treated in the first trimester of pregnancy. Among the 96 pregnancies, there were 2 maternal deaths, 2 children were stillborn, 2 therapeutic abortions were performed, 1 child had chromosomal abnormalities, and 8 had congenital defects. Seven of the eight children born with congenital defects were born to mothers who had been treated in the first trimester. It was not possible to identify a drug (or drugs) that was most likely responsible for adverse outcomes. Treatment in the first trimester carries a high risk of fetal anomaly or miscarriage. Case reports of treatment of acute promyelocytic leukemia in pregnancy with all-*trans*-retinoic acid[111–113] suggest that it may be safe after the first trimester. For patients who require chemotherapy postpartum, breast-feeding is not recommended, so as to avoid exposure of the newborn to cytotoxic drugs in the breast milk.[114] Patients with chronic myeloid leukemia have been successfully treated in pregnancy with interferon alpha, hydroxyurea, leukapheresis, and even busulfan.[115–117] However, imatinib should be avoided as a dose of >100 mg/kg/day in rats, which is equivalent to 800 mg/day in humans, uniformly causes birth defects.[118]

ESSENTIAL THROMBOCYTHEMIA AND POLYCYTHEMIA VERA

ESSENTIAL THROMBOCYTHEMIA

The management of pregnant patients with essential thrombocythemia (ET) is a challenge because thrombosis is the main complication of ET (see Chap. 111) and is accentuated by the prothrombotic state of pregnancy. In addition, of all the myeloproliferative disorders, ET has the highest proportion of affected females of child-bearing age. One study reviewed 155 pregnancies in 86 women with ET, and only 59 percent of these pregnancies resulted in a live neonate.[119] First-trimester abortion was seen in 31 percent of pregnancies, the main cause being placental infarction. Maternal thrombotic or hemorrhagic complications were infrequent, but were more common than in normal pregnancy. Pregnancy did not appear to adversely affect the course and prognosis of ET.

A meta-analysis claimed to reveal a benefit for aspirin treatment, while the benefit of heparin prophylaxis has not been established, but may have a role in selected cases.[122] If cytoreductive therapy becomes necessary, interferon alpha is the drug of choice. A similar incidence of ET pregnancy complications was reported in a series from the Mayo clinic.[120] Another large single institution study of 68 young ET patients demonstrated that for both polycythemia vera (PV) and ET, most thromboses in young patients occurred at the time of diagnosis and also suggested, but did not prove, the benefit of aspirin.[121] The most detailed analysis was published by the Italian Society of Hematology in its guidelines.[122] The Society's report analyzed pooled outcome data from 461 pregnancies in women with ET. The mean age of the pregnant patients was 29 years, and the mean platelet count at the beginning of pregnancy was 1000×10^9/liter, which declined to 400×10^9/liter in the second trimester. This decrease in the platelet count during pregnancy documented for the first time the anecdotal observation that some women with ET spontaneously normalize their platelet count during their pregnancy (the authors of this chapter have rarely observed this phenomenon; however, in one of their ET patients a spontaneous, but transient, ET remission occurred in the first pregnancy, but not in the following pregnancy). The Italian study found that 44 percent of pregnancies were unsuccessful in women with ET, a figure that is threefold higher than in the general population. Among the 461 pregnancies there were 13 pre- or postpartum bleeding events. The median duration of gestation was 38 weeks because of abortions and preterm deliveries. Cesarean section was necessary in 15 percent of the patients. The platelet count at the beginning of pregnancy did not predict pregnancy outcome. Placental infarctions were reported in 18 pregnancies and these were associated with intrauterine fetal growth retardation (11 pregnancies). Placental abruption was reported in 3.6 percent of ET pregnancies compared to 1 percent in the non-ET population. Preeclampsia was seen at a rate equal to that seen in non-ET pregnancies. Postpartum thrombotic episodes were reported in 5.2 percent of the pregnancies and included venous thrombosis, pulmonary embolism, sagittal sinus thrombosis, transient ischemic attacks, and Budd-Chiari syndrome (rates for all problems were significantly higher than in non-ET pregnancies). The impact of therapy was difficult to evaluate because management of ET pregnancies was heterogeneous; no specific therapy for ET was given in 48 percent of the pregnancies. Aspirin therapy at doses ranging from 75 mg to 500 mg per day was used in 106 pregnancies, low molecular weight heparin (pre-/postpartum) was used in 26, interferon alpha was used in 19 pregnancies, and a handful of patients had various chemotherapies and radioactive phosphorus. When the outcome of the ET pregnancies was reviewed, 74 percent of patients treated with aspirin during pregnancy had successful pregnancies, whereas 55 percent of the patients not receiving aspirin had successful pregnancies. Based on the detailed analyses of all variables, this panel of experts felt that there was no direct evidence of the efficacy of aspirin in pregnant ET women, but that "it seems possible that aspirin increases the rate of successful pregnancies." The panel also recommended that ET patients with a thrombotic episode (peripheral or placental) during pregnancy should receive low molecular weight heparin at therapeutic doses and oral anticoagulant therapy (prothrombin time international normalized ratio [INR] 2–3) for at least 6 weeks postpartum. Longer periods of anticoagulation were recommended for patients with familial thrombophilia. Pregnant women deemed candidates for platelet-lowering therapy (a history of major thrombosis, or of major bleeding, platelet count greater than 1000×10^9/liter, familial thrombophilia or cardiovascular risk factors) should receive interferon. The Italian panel also recommended avoidance of anagrelide in pregnancy because of uncertainty about its teratogenic potential; however, several normal infants have been born to women who inadvertently took this drug during pregnancy (FDA documents submitted by the manufacturer). Although the risk of congenital anomalies among infants of women treated with hydroxyurea during pregnancy was thought to be substantial, of 15 infants born to women treated with hydroxyurea at conception and/or during pregnancy, no malformations were observed, and only one stillbirth was reported in a woman who also had eclampsia.

POLYCYTHEMIA VERA

There is significant overlap in the clinical features of PV and ET; however, there are some noteworthy differences (see Chap. 56). In PV, the number of reported pregnancies is low because most PV patients are past child-bearing age, and comorbid conditions are more frequent. One authoritative review suggests maintaining the hematocrit below 45 percent[123] in pregnancy and another recommends using interferon alpha when myelosuppression is indicated.[124] Another noted authority in PV recommends that the hematocrit be kept lower than 35 percent in pregnancy.[125] However, because of a dearth of data and controlled studies, optimal management of PV pregnancies is poorly defined and agreed upon protocols are not available. Thus, none of the available information allows definite therapeutic recommendations.[126]

HEMOGLOBINOPATHIES

SICKLE SYNDROMES

Although pregnancy in patients with sickle cell trait is typically uneventful, these patients probably have an increased risk for urinary tract infection.[127] Earlier studies suggested an increased risk for preeclampsia in patients with sickle cell trait, but a recent large study demonstrated that sickle cell trait is not an independent risk factor for preeclampsia (see Chap. 47).[128]

Sickle cell patients should receive at least 1 mg of folate per day; however, they should not receive iron supplementation until a ferritin level is checked and iron deficiency is documented.[129] Because of the risk of fetal malformation, hydroxyurea should be discontinued at least 3 months before pregnancy. However, successful outcomes have been reported in sickle cell disease patients who were exposed to the drug while pregnant.[130] Women with sickle cell anemia and their fetuses have an increased risk of complications during pregnancy. In a retrospective review of 127 deliveries of women with sickle cell disease,[131] nearly 50 percent of women with SS disease experienced pain crises during pregnancy. As compared with deliveries among women with hemoglobin AA, deliveries among women with sickle cell disease were at increased risk for intrauterine growth restriction, low birth weight, prematurity, and preterm labor. In general, these risks were lower for patients with SC disease than with SS disease. More than half of the patients with SS disease in this study had received a blood transfusion during pregnancy. The issue of prophylactic versus need-based transfusion in sickle cell patients is controversial. The single randomized study to address this issue demonstrated no difference in perinatal outcome between the offspring of mothers with sickle cell disease who were assigned to treatment with prophylactic transfusions and those who were not.[132]

Although the incidence of cesarean section in sickle cell patients is reported to be as high as 36 percent,[133] delivery can generally be accomplished vaginally. Most experts recommend avoiding induction of labor as this can lead to sickle crisis.[134] Epidural anesthesia is reported to be safe and to decrease the risk of peripartum painful crises.[135]

THALASSEMIA SYNDROMES

β-THALASSEMIA SYNDROMES

Preconception evaluation of patients with β-thalassemia syndromes is recommended and should include assessment of transfusion needs, chelation therapy, body iron status and organ function, and the presence of antibodies to red cell antigens.[136] Patients with β-thalassemia minor generally tolerate pregnancy well; however, doses of at least 4 mg of folate per day are recommended in the preconception period and the first trimester as there is some data to suggest an increased risk of neural tube defects in their offspring.[137] Transfusion and iron chelation therapy has improved both life expectancy and fertility in patients with β-thalassemia intermedia and major, and successful pregnancies have been reported in both disorders.[138] During pregnancy, regular transfusions are recommended to keep the hemoglobin level at 10 mg/dl.[139] Iron-chelation therapy with deferoxamine in pregnancy is controversial and most authorities recommend a hiatus during pregnancy; however, no fetal abnormalities have been reported in pregnancies in which it was continued.[140]

α-THALASSEMIA SYNDROMES

Patients with the silent carrier state or α-thalassemia trait have no increase in pregnancy complications; however, identification of patients with heterozygous α-thalassemia trait is important in assessing the risk of having a fetus that has hemoglobin H or hemoglobin Bart's. Although women with hemoglobin H are generally able to have successful pregnancies, the chronic anemia often worsens, requiring blood transfusion. Patients with hemoglobin H are sensitive to oxidizing compounds and medications, which should be borne in mind, particularly during pregnancy (see Chap. 46).

REFERENCES

1. Pritchard JA: Changes in blood volume during pregnancy and delivery. *Anesthesiology* 26:393, 1965.
2. Scott D: Anemia in pregnancy: *Obstet Gynecol Ann* 1:219, 1972.
3. Harstad TW, Mason RA, Cox SM: Serum erythropoietin quantitation in pregnancy using an enzyme linked immunoassay. *Am J Perinatol* 9:233, 1992.
4. McMullin MF, White R, Lappin T, et al: Haemoglobin during pregnancy: Relationship to erythropoietin and haematinic status. *Eur J Haematol* 71:44, 2003.
5. Pitkin RM, Witte DL: Platelet and leukocyte counts in pregnancy. *JAMA* 242:2696, 1979.
6. van Buul EJA, Steeggers EAP, Jongsma HW, et al: Haematological and biochemical profile of uncomplicated pregnancy in nulliparous women: A longitudinal study. *Neth J Med* 46:73, 1995.
7. England JM, Bain BJ: Total and differential leucocyte count. *Br J Haematol* 33:1, 1976.
8. Acker DB, Johnson MP, Sachs BP, Friedman EA: The leukocyte count in labor. *Am J Obstet Gynecol* 153:737, 1985.
9. Watts, DH, Krohn MA, Wener MH, Eschenbach DA: C-reactive protein in normal pregnancy. *Obstet Gynecol* 77:176, 1991.
10. van den Broe NR, Letsky EA: Pregnancy and the erythrocyte sedimentation rate. *Br J Obstet Gynaecol* 108:1164, 2001.
11. Greer IA: Thrombosis in pregnancy: Maternal and fetal issues. *Lancet* 353:1258, 1999.
12. Clark P, Brennand J, Conkie JA, et al: Activated protein C sensitivity, protein C, protein S and coagulation in normal pregnancy. *Thromb Haemost* 79:1166, 1998.
13. Halligan A, Bonnar J, Sheppard B, et al: Haemostatic, fibrinolytic and endothelial variables in normal pregnancies and pre-eclampsia. *Br J Obstet Gynaecol* 101:488, 1992.
14. Brabin BJ, Hakimi M, Pelletier D: An analysis of anemia and pregnancy-related maternal mortality. *J Nutr* 131:604S, 2001.
15. Centers for Disease Control and Prevention: CDC criteria for anemia in children and childbearing-aged women. *MMWR Morb Mortal Wkly Rep* 38:400, 1989.
16. Sifakis S, Pharmakides G: Anemia in pregnancy. *Ann N Y Acad Sci* 900: 125, 2000.
17. FAO/WHO: *Joint Expert Consultation Report; Requirements of Vitamin A, Iron, Folate, and Vitamin B$_{12}$. FAO Food and Nutrition Series 23.* Rome: FAO, 1988.
18. Harthoorn-Lasthuizen EJ, Lindemans J, Langenhuijsen MM: Does iron-deficient erythropoiesis in pregnancy influence fetal iron supply? *Acta Obstet Gynecol Scand* 80:392, 2001.
19. Scholl TO, Hediger ML, Fischer RL, Shearer JW: Anemia vs iron deficiency: Increased risk of preterm delivery in a prospective study. *Am J Clin Nutr* 55:985, 1992.
20. Hemminki E, Rimpela U: A randomized comparison of routine versus selective iron supplementation during pregnancy. *J Am Coll Nutr* 10:3, 1991.
21. Horner RD, Lackey CJ, Kolasa K, Warren K: Pica practices of pregnant women. *J Am Diet Assoc* 91:34, 1991.
22. Shojania AM: Folic acid and vitamin B$_{12}$ deficiency in pregnancy and in the neonatal period. *Clin Perinatol* 11:433, 1984.
23. Walker SP, Wein P, Ihle BU: Severe folate deficiency masquerading as the syndrome of hemolysis, elevated liver enzymes and low platelets. *Obstet Gynecol* 90:655, 1997.
24. Van de Velde A, Van Droogenbroeck J, Tjalma W, et al: Folate and vitamin B$_{12}$ deficiency presenting as pancytopenia in pregnancy: A case report and review of the literature. *Eur J Obstet Gynecol Reprod Biol* 100:251, 2002.
25. Mahomed K: Folate supplementation in pregnancy. *Cochrane Database Syst Rev* 2:CD000183, 2000.
26. Bruinse HW, van den Berg H: Changes of some vitamin levels during and after normal pregnancy. *Eur J Obstet Gynecol Reprod Biol* 61:31, 1995.
27. Frenkel EP, Yardley DA: Clinical and laboratory features and sequelae of deficiency of folic acid (folate) and vitamin B$_{12}$ (cobalamin) in pregnancy and gynecology. *Hematol Oncol Clin North Am* 14:1079, 2000.
28. Baker RI, Manoharan A, de Luca E, Begley CG: Pure red cell aplasia of pregnancy: A distinct clinical entity. *Br J Haematol* 85:619, 1993.
29. Aggio MC, Zunini C: Reversible pure red-cell aplasia in pregnancy. *N Engl J Med* 297:221, 1977.
30. Makino Y, Nagano M, Tamura K, Kawarabayashi T: Pregnancy complicated with pure red cell aplasia: A case report. *J Perinat Med* 31:530, 2003.
31. Mant MJ: Chronic idiopathic pure red cell aplasia: Successful treatment during pregnancy and durable response to intravenous immunoglobulin. *J Intern Med* 23:593, 1994.
32. Tuffnell DJ: Amniotic fluid embolism. *Curr Opin Obstet Gynecol* 15: 119, 2003.
33. Awad IT, Shorten GD: Amniotic fluid embolism and isolated coagulopathy: Atypical presentation of amniotic fluid embolism. *Eur J Anaesthesiol* 18:410, 2001.
34. Bick RL: Syndromes of disseminated intravascular coagulation in obstetrics, pregnancy, and gynecology. Objective criteria for diagnosis and management. *Hematol Oncol Clin North Am* 14:999, 2000.
35. Goldszmidt E, Davies S: Two cases of hemorrhage secondary to amniotic fluid embolus managed with uterine artery embolization. *Can J Anaesth* 50:917, 2003.
36. Letsky EA: Disseminated intravascular coagulation. *Best Pract Res Clin Obstet Gynaecol* 15:623, 2001.
37. Romero R, Copel JA, Hobbins JC: Intrauterine fetal demise and hemostatic failure: The fetal death syndrome. *Clin Obstet Gynecol* 28:24, 1985.
38. Conti M, Mari D, Conti E, et al: Pregnancy in women with different types of von Willebrand disease. *Obstet Gynecol* 68:282, 1986.
39. Batlle J, Noya MS, Giangrande P, Lopez-Fernandez MF: Advances in the therapy of von Willebrand disease. *Haemophilia* 8:301, 2002.

40. Mathew P, Greist A, Maahs JA, et al: Type 2B vWD: The varied clinical manifestations in two kindreds. *Haemophilia* 9:137, 2003.

41. Rick ME, Williams SB, Sacher RA, McKeown LP: Thrombocytopenia associated with pregnancy in a patient with type IIB von Willebrand's disease. *Blood* 69:786, 1987.

42. Foster PA: On behalf of the subcommittee on von Willebrand factor of the Scientific and Standardization Committee of the ISTH. The reproductive health of women with von Willebrand disease unresponsive to DDAVP: Results of an international survey. *Thromb Haemost* 74:784, 1995.

43. Ray JG: DDAVP use during pregnancy: An analysis of its safety for mother and child. *Obstet Gynecol Surv* 53:450, 1998.

44. Briet E, Reisner HM, Blatt PM: Factor IX levels during pregnancy in a woman with hemophilia B. *Haemostasis* 11:87, 1982.

45. Ljung R, Lindgren A-C, Petrini P, Tengborn L: Normal vaginal delivery is to be recommended for haemophilia carrier gravidae. *Acta Paediatr* 83:609, 1994.

46. Giangrande PLF: Management of pregnancy in carriers of haemophilia. *Haemophilia* 4:779, 1998.

47. Michiels JJ, Hamulyak K, Nieuwenhuis, HK, et al: Acquired haemophilia A in women postpartum: Management of bleeding episodes and natural history of the factor VIII inhibitor. *Eur J Haematol* 59:105, 1997.

48. Solymuss S: Postpartum acquired factor VIII inhibitors: Results of a survey. *Am J Hematol* 59:1, 1998.

49. Kobayashi T, Terao T, Kojima T, et al: Congenital factor XIII deficiency with treatment of factor XIII concentrate and normal vaginal delivery. *Gynecol Obstet Invest* 29:235, 1990.

50. Rodeghiero F, Castaman GC, Di Bona E, et al: Successful pregnancy in a woman with congenital factor XIII deficiency treated with substitutive therapy. *Blut* 55:45, 1987.

51. Burrows RF, Ray JG, Burrows EA: Bleeding risk and reproductive capacity among patients with factor XIII deficiency: A case presentation and review of the literature. *Obstet Gynecol Surv* 55:103, 2000.

52. Anwar R, Miloszewski KJA: Factor XIII deficiency. *Br J Haematol* 107:468, 1999.

53. Burrows RF, Kelton JG: Fetal thrombocytopenia and its relation to maternal thrombocytopenia. *N Engl J Med* 329:1463, 1993.

54. George JN, Woolf SH, Raskob GE, et al: Idiopathic thrombocytopenic purpura: A practice guideline developed by explicit methods for the American Society of Hematology. *Blood* 88:3, 1996.

55. Kaplan C, Daffos F, Forestier F, et al: Fetal platelet counts in thrombocytopenic pregnancy. *Lancet* 336:979, 1990.

56. Valat AS, Caulier MT, Devos P, et al: Relationships between severe neonatal thrombocytopenia and maternal characteristics in pregnancies associated with autoimmune thrombocytopenia. *Br J Haematol* 103:397, 1998.

57. Martin JN Jr, Perry KG Jr, Blake PG, et al: Better maternal outcomes are achieved with dexamethasone therapy for postpartum HELLP (hemolysis, elevated liver enzymes, and thrombocytopenia) syndrome. *Am J Obstet Gynecol* 177:1011, 1997.

58. Matchaba P, Moodley J: Corticosteroids for HELLP syndrome in pregnancy. *Cochrane Database Syst Rev* CD002076, 2004.

59. Martin JN Jr, Blake PG, Perry KG Jr, et al: The natural history of HELLP syndrome: Patterns of disease progression and regression. *Am J Obstet Gynecol* 164:1500, 1991.

60. Martin JN Jr, Files JC, Blake PG, et al: Postpartum plasma exchange for atypical preeclampsia-eclampsia as HELLP (hemolysis, elevated liver enzymes, and low platelets) syndrome. *Am J Obstet Gynecol* 172:1107, 1995.

61. Rouget JP, Goudemand J, Ducloux G, et al: [Circulating anticoagulant, recurrent abortions and venous thrombosis: A new entity or a pre-lupus syndrome? 2 cases.] *Ann Med Interne (Paris)* 134:111, 1983.

62. Kutteh WH: Antiphospholipid antibodies and reproduction. *J Reprod Immunol* 35:151, 1997.

63. Rai RS, Clifford K, Cohen H, Regan L: High prospective fetal loss rate in untreated pregnancies of women with recurrent miscarriage and antiphospholipid antibodies. *Hum Reprod* 10:3301, 1995.

64. Rai R, Cohen H, Dave M, Regan L: Randomised controlled trial of aspirin and aspirin plus heparin in pregnant women with recurrent miscarriage associated with phospholipid antibodies (or antiphospholipid antibodies). *BMJ* 314:253, 1997.

65. Martinelli I, Taioli E, Cetin I, et al: Mutations in coagulation factors in women with unexplained late fetal loss. *N Engl J Med* 343:1015, 2000.

66. Ridker PM, Miletich JP, Buring JE, et al: Factor V Leiden mutation as a risk factor for recurrent pregnancy loss. *Ann Intern Med* 128:1000, 1998.

67. Rey E, Kahn SR, David M, Shrier I: Thrombophilic disorders and fetal loss: A meta-analysis. *Lancet* 361:901, 2003.

68. Morrison ER, Miedzybrodzka ZH, Campbell DM, et al: Prothrombotic genotypes are not associated with pre-eclampsia and gestational hypertension: Results from a large population-based study and systematic review. *Thromb Haemost* 87:779, 2002.

69. Greer IA: Thrombophilia: Implications for pregnancy outcome. *Thromb Res* 109:73, 2003.

70. Greer IA: Thrombosis in pregnancy: Maternal and fetal issues. *Lancet* 353:1258, 1999.

71. Gerhardt A, Scharf RE, Beckmann MW, et al: Prothrombin and factor V mutations in women with a history of thrombosis during pregnancy and the puerperium. *N Engl J Med* 342:374, 2000.

72. Macklon NS, Greer IA, Bowman AW: An ultrasound study of gestational and postural changes in the deep venous system of the leg in pregnancy. *Br J Obstet Gynaecol* 104:191, 1997.

73. Cockett FB, Thomas ML: The iliac compression syndrome. *Br J Surg* 52:816, 1965.

74. Ginsberg JS, Brill-Edwards P, Burrows RF: DVT during pregnancy: Leg and trimester of presentation. *Thromb Haemost* 67:519, 1992.

75. Conard J, Horellou MH, van Dreden P, et al: Thrombosis in pregnancy and congenital deficiencies in AT III, protein C or protein S: Study of 78 women. *Thromb Haemost* 63:319, 1990.

76. Paninger I and the Study Group on Natural Inhibitors: Thrombotic risk in hereditary anti-thrombin III, protein C or protein S deficiency. *Arterioscler Thromb Vasc Biol* 16:742, 1996.

77. McColl MD, Ramsay JE, Tait RC, et al: Risk factors for pregnancy associated venous thromboembolism. *Thromb Haemost* 78:1183, 1997.

78. DeStefano V, Leone G, Masterangela S, et al: Thrombosis during pregnancy and surgery in patients with congenital deficiency of antithrombin III, protein C-protein S. *Thromb Haemost* 71:799, 1994.

79. Grandone E, Margaglione M, Colaizzo D, et al: Genetic susceptibility to pregnancy-related venous thromboembolism: Roles of factor V Leiden, prothrombin G20210A, and methylenetetrahydrofolate reductase C677T mutations. *Am J Obstet Gynecol* 179:1324, 1998.

80. Martinelli I, DeStefano V, Taioli E, et al: Inherited thrombophilias and first venous thromboembolism during pregnancy and puerperium. *Thromb Haemost* 87:791, 2002.

81. Paniccia R, Prisco D, Bandinelli B, et al: Plasma and serum levels of D-dimer and their correlations with other hemostatic parameters in pregnancy. *Thromb Res* 105:257, 2002.

82. Chabloz P, Reber G, Boehlen F, et al: TAFI antigen and D-dimer levels during normal pregnancy and at delivery. *Br J Haematol* 115:150, 2001.

83. Kobayashi T, Tokunaga N, Sugimura M, et al: Coagulation/fibrinolysis disorder in patients with severe preeclampsia. *Semin Thromb Hemost* 25:451, 1999.

84. Brill-Edwards P, Ginsberg JS, Gent M, et al., for the Recurrence of Clot In This Pregnancy (ROCIT) Study Group: Safety of withholding antepartum heparin in women with a previous episode of venous thromboembolism. *N Engl J Med* 343:1439, 2000.

85. Pabinger I, Grafenhofer H, Kyrle PA, et al: Temporary increase in the risk for recurrence during pregnancy in women with a history of venous thromboembolism. *Blood* 100:1060, 2002.

86. Ageno W, Crotti S, Turpie AG: The safety of antithrombotic therapy during pregnancy. *Expert Opin Drug Saf* 3:113, 2004.

87. Ginsberg JS, Bates SM: Management of venous thromboembolism during pregnancy. *J Thromb Haemost* 1:1435, 2003.

88. Bauer KA: Management of thrombophilia. *J Thromb Haemost* 1:1429, 2003.

89. Bowles L, Cohen H: Inherited thrombophilias and anticoagulation in pregnancy. *Best Pract Res Clin Obstet Gynaecol* 17:471, 2003.

90. Kearon C, Crowther M, Hirsh J: Management of patients with hereditary hypercoagulable disorders. *Annu Rev Med* 51:169, 2000.

91. Schafer AI, Levine MN, Konkle BA, Kearon C: Thrombotic disorders: Diagnosis and treatment. *Hematology (Am Soc Hematol Educ Program)* 520, 2003.

92. Clark SL, Porter TF, West FG: Coumarin derivatives and breast-feeding. *Obstet Gynecol* 95:938, 2000.

93. Ward FT, Weiss RB: Lymphoma and pregnancy. *Semin Oncol* 16:397, 1989.

94. Lishner M, Zemlickis D, Sutcliffe SB, Koren G: Non-Hodgkin's lymphoma and pregnancy. *Leuk Lymphoma* 14:411, 1994.

95. Doll DC, Ringenberg QS, Yarbro JW: Antineoplastic agents and pregnancy. *Semin Oncol* 16:337, 1989.

96. Nisce LZ, Tome MA, He S, et al: Management of coexisting Hodgkin's disease and pregnancy. *Am J Clin Oncol* 9:146, 1986.

97. Woo SY, Fuller LM, Cundiff JH, et al: Radiotherapy during pregnancy for clinical stages IA-IIA Hodgkin's disease. *Int J Radiation Biol Phys* 23:407, 1992.

98. Chen J, Lee RJ, Tsodikov A, et al: Does radiotherapy around the time of pregnancy for Hodgkin's disease modify the risk of breast cancer? *Int J Radiation Biol Phys* 58:1474, 2004.

99. Gelb AB, van de Rijn M, Warnke RA, Kamel OW: Pregnancy-associated lymphomas. A clinicopathologic study. *Cancer* 78:304, 1996.

100. Brogi E, Harris NL: Lymphomas of the breast: Pathology and clinical behavior. *Semin Oncol* 26:357, 1999.

101. Bobrow LG, Richards MA, Happerfield LC, et al: Breast lymphomas: A clinicopathologic review. *Hum Pathol* 24:274, 1993.

102. Aviles A, Diaz-Maqueo JC, Talavera A, et al: Growth and development of children of mothers treated with chemotherapy during pregnancy: Current status of 43 children. *Am J Hematol* 36:243, 1991.

103. Aviles A, Neri N: Hematological malignancies and pregnancy: A final report of 84 children who received chemotherapy in utero. *Clin Lymphoma* 2:173, 2001.

104. Kimby E, Sverrisdottir A, Elinder G: Safety of rituximab therapy during the first trimester of pregnancy: A case history. *Eur J Haematol* 72:292, 2004.

105. Herold M, Schnohr S, Bittrich H: Efficacy and safety of a combined rituximab chemotherapy during pregnancy. *J Clin Oncol* 19:3438, 2001.

106. Yahia C, Hyman GA, Phillips LL: Acute Leukemia and pregnancy. *Obstet Gynecol Surv* 13:1, 1958.

107. Catanzarite VA, Ferguson JE 2nd: Acute leukemia and pregnancy: A review of management and outcome, 1972–1982. *Obstet Gynecol Surv* 39:663, 1984.

108. Pavlidis NA: Coexistence of pregnancy and malignancy. *Oncologist* 7: 279, 2002.

109. Kawamura S, Yoshiike M, Shimoyama T, et al: Management of acute leukemia during pregnancy: From the results of a nationwide questionnaire survey and literature survey. *Tohoku J Exp Med* 174:167, 1994.

110. Ebert U, Loffler H, Kirch W: Cytotoxic therapy and pregnancy. *Pharmacol Ther* 74:207, 1997.

111. Giagounidis AA, Beckmann MW, Giagounidis AS, et al: Acute promyelocytic leukemia and pregnancy. *Eur J Haemotol* 64:267, 2000.

112. Delgado-Lamas JL, Garces-Ruiz OM: Malignancy: Case report: Acute promyelocytic leukemia in late pregnancy. Successful treatment with all-*trans*-retinoic acid (ATRA) and chemotherapy. *Hematology* 4:415, 2000.

113. Lipovsky MM, Biesma DH, Christiaens GC, Petersen EJ: Successful treatment of acute promyelocytic leukaemia with all-*trans*-retinoic-acid during late pregnancy. *Br J Haematol* 94:699, 1996.

114. Pejovic T, Schwartz PE: Leukemias. *Clin Obstet Gynecol* 45:866, 2002.

115. Baer MR, Ozer H, Foon KA: Interferon-alpha therapy during pregnancy in chronic myelogenous leukaemia and hairy cell leukaemia. *Br J Haematol* 81:167, 1992.

116. Bazarbashi MS, Smith MR, Karanes C, et al: Successful management of Ph chromosome chronic myelogenous leukemia with leukapheresis during pregnancy. *Am J Hematol* 38:235, 1991.

117. Delmer A, Rio B, Bauduer F, et al: Pregnancy during myelosuppressive treatment for chronic myelogenous leukemia. *Br J Haematol* 82:783, 1992.

118. Gleevec package insert, Novartis Pharmaceuticals, East Hanover, NJ, 2001.

119. Griesshammer M, Grunewald M, Michiels JJ: Acquired thrombophilia in pregnancy: Essential thrombocythemia. *Semin Thromb Hemost* 2:205, 2003.

120. Elliott MA, Tefferi A: Thrombocythaemia and pregnancy. *Best Pract Res Clin Haematol* 2:227, 2003.

121. Randi ML, Rossi C, Fabris F, Girolami A: Essential thrombocythemia in young adults: Major thrombotic complications and complications during pregnancy—a follow-up study in 68 patients. *Clin Appl Thromb Hemost* 6:31, 2000.

122. Barbui T, Barosi G, Grossi A, et al: Practice guidelines for the therapy of essential thrombocythemia. A consensus statement from the Italian Society of Hematology, the Italian Society of Experimental Hematology and the Italian Group for Bone Marrow Transplantation. *Haematologica* 89:215, 2004.

123. Griesshammer M, Bergmann L, Pearson T: Fertility, pregnancy and the management of myeloproliferative disorders. *Baillieres Clin Haematol* 11:859, 1998.

124. Silver RT: Interferon alfa: Effects of long-term treatment for polycythemia vera. *Semin Hematol* 34:40, 1997.

125. Spivak JL: Polycythemia vera: Myths, mechanisms, and management. *Blood* 100:4272, 2002.

126. Elliott MA, Tefferi A: Interferon-alpha therapy in polycythemia vera and essential thrombocythemia. *Semin Thromb Hemost* 23:463, 1997.

127. Pastore LM, Savitz DA, Thorp JM Jr: Predictors of urinary tract infection at first prenatal visit. *Epidemiology* 10:282, 1999.

128. Stamilio DM, Sehdev HM, Macones GA: Pregnant women with the sickle cell trait are not at increased risk for developing preeclampsia. *Am J Perinatol* 20:41, 2003.

129. Thinkhamrop J, Apiwantanakul S, Lumbiganon P, et al: Iron status in anemic pregnant women. *J Obstet Gynaecol* 29:160, 2003.

130. Diav-Citrin O, Hunnisett L, Sher GD, Kore G: Hydroxyurea use during pregnancy: A case report in sickle cell disease and review of the literature. *Am J Hematol* 60:148, 1999.

131. Sun PM, Wilburn W, Raynor BD, Jamieson D: Sickle cell disease in pregnancy: Twenty years of experience at Grady Memorial Hospital, Atlanta, Georgia. *Am J Obstet Gynecol* 184:1127, 2001.

132. Koshy M, Burd L, Wallace D, et al: Prophylactic red-cell transfusions in pregnant patients with sickle cell disease. A randomized cooperative study. *N Engl J Med* 319:1447, 1988.

133. Koshy M, Burd L: Management of pregnancy in sickle cell syndromes. *Hematol Oncol Clin North Am* 5:484, 1991.

134. Rappaport VJ, Velazquez M, Williams K: Hemoglobinopathies in pregnancy. *Obstet Gynecol Clin North Am* 31:287, 2004.

135. Finer P, Blair J, Rowe P: Epidural analgesia in the management of labor pain and sickle cell crisis. *Anesthesiology* 68:799, 1988.

136. Aessopos A, Karabatsos F, Farmakis D, et al: Pregnancy in patients with well-treated β thalassemia: Outcome for mothers and newborn infants. *Am J Obstet Gynecol* 180:360, 1999.

137. Ibba RM, Zoppi MA, Floris M, et al: Neural tube effects in the offspring of thalassemia carriers. *Fetal Diagn Ther* 18:5, 2003.

138. Tamakoudis P, Tsatalas C, Mamopoulos M, et al: Transfusion-dependent homozygous beta-thalassemia major: Successful pregnancy in five cases. *Eur J Obstet Gynecol Reprod Biol* 74:127, 1997.

139. Kumar RM, Rizk DE, Khuranna A: Beta-thalassemia major and successful pregnancy. *J Reprod Med* 42:294, 1997.

140. Singer ST, Vichinsky EP: Deferoxamine treatment during pregnancy: Is it harmful? *Am J Hematol* 60:24, 1999.

HEMATOLOGY IN OLDER PERSONS

MICHELLE SHAYNE
MARSHALL A. LICHTMAN

The hematopoietic system is modestly affected by aging, but these effects become particularly notable after age 65 years. There is a continuous decrease in the volume of the hematopoietic marrow with age, which does not cause significant alterations in either granulocyte, monocyte, or platelet counts, although a slight (≤ 1.0 g/dl) decrease in population mean hemoglobin concentration in men occurs. While the population mean vitamin B_{12} and folate levels decrease with age, these changes do not result in decreased hematopoiesis as judged by blood counts, except in individuals with significant deficiencies of these vitamins. Anemia in older individuals should be evaluated in the same manner as anemia in younger individuals. Increased platelet aggregation in vitro is a feature of the blood in older individuals. In addition, certain plasma coagulation proteins increase significantly with age (e.g., factors VII and VIIIC, von Willebrand factor, and fibrinogen). Activated peptides of prothrombin, factor VII, factor IX, and factor X, are also increased in the plasma. Changes occurring in the fibrinolytic system with aging are ambiguous. Higher D-dimer and plasmin–antiplasmin complexes reflect enhanced fibrinolysis while increased levels of tissue-plasminogen activator inhibitor and thrombin-activatable fibrinolysis inhibitor are compatible with reduced fibrinolytic activity. Decreased immune cell function is the most consistent change in older persons, and perhaps the most important functionally. Although there is a tendency toward decreased lymphocyte counts in the blood, the major effects are mediated by dysregulation of T lymphocyte function, perhaps as a result of the prolonged period since thymic atrophy in older subjects. This change in the adaptive immune system affects both cellular and antibody responses to antigens because of the T helper cell function required for the latter responses. Abnormalities in neutrophils are also responsible for a compromise of the innate immune system of older individuals. Neutrophil count, adhesion, and degranulation are preserved in older individuals, whereas rates of phagocytosis and superoxide generation are decreased. An age-related effect on neutrophil chemotaxis is controversial.

Acronyms and abbreviations that appear in this chapter include: ATP, adenosine triphosphate; BPG, bisphosphoglycerate; CD, cluster of differentiation; CFU-E, colony forming unit–erythroid; fMLP, N-formyl-methionyl-leucyl-phenylalanine; G-CSF, granulocyte colony stimulating factor; GM-CSF, granulocyte-monocyte colony stimulating factor; Ig, immunoglobulin; IL, interleukin; LDL, low-density lipoprotein; MCHC, mean corpuscular hemoglobin concentration; MCV, mean corpuscular volume; MIP, macrophage inflammatory protein; mRNA, messenger RNA; mt, mitochondrial; NK, natural killer; NO, nitric oxide; RANTES, regulated on activation, normal T cell expressed and secreted; rRNA, recombinant RNA; SEER, National Cancer Institute Surveillance Epidemiology End Results; TAFI, thrombin-activatable lysis inhibitor; TNF, tumor necrosis factor; t-PA, tissue-plasminogen activator; tRNA, transfer RNA.

In 2000, there were 39.3 million individuals 65 years of age or older in the United States, representing 12.6 percent of the population; this group is expected to grow to 23 percent of the population by the year 2040. Currently, there are 4 million people in the United States who are age 85 years old or older.[1] Mean life expectancy at age 65 years is 14 years for males and 18 years for females in most developed countries.[2] As a result, physicians increasingly are caring for older patients and are being called upon to interpret hematologic data in the context of the age of the patient. Age-related effects on DNA result in a dramatic increase in the incidence of clonal hematopoietic diseases, especially leukemia, lymphoma, myeloma, and closely related diseases in the decades after age 50 years. In addition, the decrease in immune function has an impact on vaccine use and resistance to infection in older individuals.

AGING AND HEMATOPOIESIS

Throughout embryogenesis and early infancy nearly all cells of the body have mitotic capacity. Subsequently, certain cells of the body lose their ability to divide (e.g., nervous tissue, muscles).[3] Others continue to divide until full growth has been achieved. Thereafter, cells usually do not divide at a significant rate except under conditions of stress, when they become capable of rapid cell division. These cells are said to be "potentially mitotic" or "discontinuous replicators," as exemplified by hepatic cells and renal tubular cells.[3] Cells of organs that require continuous self-renewal, such as the marrow, the scalp hair follicles, and the gastrointestinal mucosa, are continuously mitotic throughout life.[3]

Studies of diploid human cells maintained in continuous culture have led to the assertion that there is a limit to the number of divisions a cell may undergo,[4–6] a state of replication senescence, which may be related in part to telomere shortening.[7] Additional mechanisms contributing to cellular senescence include extended exposure to reactive oxygen species[8] and the accumulation of numbers of mutations in genomic and mitochondrial DNA.[9,10] The proliferative capacity of marrow cells from older animals and humans has been studied by a variety of techniques, both in vivo and in vitro. Most studies indicate that marrow can sustain normal blood cell counts in older animals,[11–17] but the reserve capacity may be limited during periods of exaggerated demand.[13,18–21] The hematopoietic limitations observed in older animals could be intrinsic to marrow stem cells or to cells of the hematopoietic stroma and/or their cytokine production.[12,15,16,22] The short-term hematopoietic responses to the growth factors granulocyte-monocyte colony stimulating factor (GM-CSF), interleukin-3 (IL-3), and erythropoietin are well maintained in older subjects[23,24]; however, the response of multipotential (CD34+) cells to granulocyte colony stimulating factor (G-CSF) in culture in older patients is decreased, and the mobilization of neutrophils by G-CSF in vivo is diminished.[24,25]

Although a positive association exists in healthy subjects between age and dyshematopoiesis,[26] there is no evidence that the effects of aging on marrow proliferative capacity, or, ultimately on steady-state blood cell levels, are clinically significant within existing life spans.[27–30]

Although the evidence strongly argues against an exhaustion of human pluripotential stem cells during the human life span, even in the face of intensive chemotherapy in older individuals, there is an apparent alteration in stem cell behavior with aging that has clinical relevance.[31] In older women, studies show a dramatic increase in extreme skewing of X chromosome inactivation patterns.[31,32] Clonal myeloid diseases occur in older subjects with a high frequency and, in some cases, determination of clonality may be required for the diagnosis. Thus, the extreme skewing of X chromosome inactivation patterns (greater than 90%) in as many as 30 percent of healthy older women makes interpretation difficult. This late-in-life extreme skewing occurs in myeloid cells but not in T lymphocytes. This has been interpreted as reflecting the marked reduction in T lymphocyte production in older persons (see "Immunosenescence" below), resulting in a pattern that could be misinterpreted as reflecting a clonal myeloid disease. Older women with extreme skewing have neither cytopenias, other evidence of disease, nor mutations in the *RAS* gene, the latter making clinically inapparent (embryonal) myelodysplasia very unlikely. The latter disease has an expected frequency of RAS mutations of about 25 percent. A change in stem cell usage with aging, leading to preferential loss of cells with the active X chromosome derived from one parent, and expressing its allele, could explain the phenomenon.[31] This would require stem cells to be capable of both asymmetric and symmetric division. In the latter case, there would be no heir to that pattern of X chromosome activation because both daughter cells would differentiate. If a sufficient proportion of such events involving stem cells with the same active X chromosome occurred, skewing of the X chromosome inactivation pattern in hematopoietic stem cells could be acquired with age.

MARROW CELLULARITY

The cellularity of the marrow decreases with aging, as estimated from studies of histologic sections.[33–35] Studies of marrow from the anterior iliac crest demonstrate a progressive decrease in cellularity from approximately 90 percent to approximately 50 percent over the first 30 years of life. Cellularity of approximately 40 percent has been found in sternal marrow from normal adults.[36] In iliac crest marrow there is a plateau of approximately 50 percent cellularity to age 65 years, after which a decrease in cellularity to approximately 30 percent occurs over the succeeding decade.[34] Magnetic resonance imaging confirms an age-related reduction in marrow cellularity.[37] The apparent decline in cellularity, evident both with aging and osteoporosis, is accompanied by an age-related increase in marrow adipose tissue volume fraction and a concomitant decrease in trabecular bone volume fraction. Osteoblasts and adipocytes share a common mesenchymal stem cell origin in marrow stroma and effects of aging may favor adipogenesis over osteogenesis.[38] These changes may account for the more pronounced marrow hypocellularity in the subcortical zone.

GENETIC ALTERATIONS

Four principal genetic changes in hematopoietic cells have been identified in relationship to human aging: loss of nuclear chromosomes, increased micronucleus formation, mitochondrial (mt) DNA mutations, and telomere shortening.

CHROMOSOME LOSS

There is an exponential increase during aging in the proportion of adult women whose phytohemagglutinin-stimulated blood lymphocytes display X chromosome aneuploidy as a result of X chromosome loss. Thus, the proportion of women with X chromosome aneuploidy increases from approximately 1 percent of women younger than age 25 years to approximately 15 percent of women older than 45 years of age.[39,40] This alteration is not evident, however, in marrow erythroid or granulocytic cells. Loss of the Y chromosome also increases with age and is a feature of marrow hematopoietic cells. Y chromosome loss is very unusual in persons younger than age 50 years, but occurs in approximately 10 percent of men older than age 50 years, with a continuously increasing frequency each decade between 50 and 90 years of age.[41] Loss of the Y chromosome as the sole cytogenetic abnormality in 81 percent of metaphase cells from unstimulated cultures, in one study, yielded a combined sensitivity and specificity of 28 percent and 100 percent, respectively, for predicting a hematologic disease. A loss of the Y chromosome from at least 75 percent of cells provided the best estimate of hematologic disease risk.[42] Autosome

loss also increases in frequency with age. Autosomes contain genes necessary for cell survival. Hence, although loss of autosomes may occur at the same frequency as that of sex chromosomes, autosome loss can trigger cell death.[43] Smaller chromosomes are lost more frequently than larger chromosomes.[40] An increase in stable aberrations of chromosomes, including insertions, translocations, and dicentric and acentric chromosome fragments, is evident with aging.[44,45] An increase in somatic mutations occurs with age when studied in blood lymphocytes, but this may reflect an accumulation with time rather than an age-dependent increase in mutation rate.[46]

MICRONUCLEI FORMATION

Micronuclei are cytoplasmic inclusions formed when chromosome fragments without spindle attachments are excluded from the nucleus of daughter cells during mitosis. An increase in micronuclei is evident in the blood lymphocytes of older as compared with younger individuals.[45] The frequency of X and Y aneuploidy, which increases with age in women and men, respectively, correlates with an increase in micronuclei frequency in both sexes.[47,48]

MUTATIONS IN MITOCHONDRIAL DNA

Stochastic somatic mutations of mitochondrial DNA (mtDNA) are associated with aging in humans.[49] mtDNA is particularly susceptible to mutations. DNA repair mechanisms are less efficient in mitochondria than in nuclei. Mitochondria also lack the protection conferred by histones, beaded proteins around which DNA is tightly coiled in chromatin nucleosomes. Frequent mutations arise from damage incurred with exposure to reactive oxygen species, free radical byproducts of the neighboring mitochondrial respiratory chain.[50] The mitochondrial genome is a 16.6-kb molecule that codes for 2 recombinant RNAs (rRNAs), 22 transfer RNAs (tRNAs), and 13 proteins. These proteins comprise the subunits of the respiratory chain. Mutations in a structural mtDNA gene can compromise an enzyme complex, whereas mutations in a tRNA gene can impair translation of all 13 mitochondrial proteins because all 22 tRNAs are essential.[49] Clonal expansion of a single mutated mtDNA molecule may then occur via random drift.[51] The resultant impaired mitochondrial adenosine triphosphate (ATP) generation can undermine genomic stability. Thus, mtDNA mutations may contribute to malignant transformation.[52] Up to 40 percent of patients with both acute and chronic leukemias have leukemic cells containing somatic mutations in mtDNA.[53] Accumulation of certain mtDNA mutations is also believed to contribute to normal cell aging. A deletion of 4977 base pairs in length known as the *common deletion* is present with increased frequency in the blood and marrow cells of hematologically normal older individuals, but the deletion is not detected in patients with myelodysplastic syndromes, acute myelogenous leukemia, or chronic myelogenous leukemia.[54]

TELOMERE SHORTENING

The termini of chromosomes contain telomeres consisting of unique proteins and tandem-repeat sequences of DNA, specifically, TTAGGG, that prevent degradation or fusion of chromosomes. Telomerase is a ribonucleoprotein that functions as a reverse transcriptase, synthesizing DNA from an RNA template. It adds telomere repeat sequences to the 3' end of DNA strands. This permits DNA polymerase to complete the synthesis of the incomplete ends of the opposing strand. Telomeres shorten during mitosis of cells in culture and in the cells of humans (and other species) as they age.[55] When telomere length is decreased to a critical point, cell division ceases. Aging of hematopoietic tissues is complex because of the potential lengthy dormancy and the self-renewal capability of stem cells, whereas their derivative cells die and are replaced in relatively short periods of time. Telomerase activity is not present in neutrophils[56] and is barely detectable in unstimulated B or T lymphocytes.[57] However, lymphocytes stimulated with mitogens or antigens have a marked increase in telomerase activity.[57] Human neutrophil telomeres shorten at the rate of about 35 base pairs per year, a reflection of the shortening in the hematopoietic stem (CD34+,CD38−) cell.[58–60] Neutrophil telomere length of the subject under study at any age is about 750 base pairs less than that in CD34+ cells, reflecting the approximately 15 to 20 mitotic events prior to the formation of a neutrophil. Neutrophils and naive T cells have a biphasic decline in telomere length over 90 years of the human life span. Loss of telomere length is rapid in the first few years of life and continues to decline at a much slower rate over eight decades.[61,62] This pattern indicates a marked reduction in hematopoietic stem cell turnover after infancy. The rate of telomere shortening in human lymphocytes over eight decades of life is different among CD4+ and CD8+ T lymphocytes and B lymphocytes.[61] The rate of telomere shortening is most rapid in CD4+ T cells and least rapid in B cells. CD8+ lymphocytes have an intermediate rate of shortening over the eight decades of age of study subjects, presumably reflecting differences in their biologic functions and mitotic events.

Telomere length is genetically determined[63,64] and varies widely among individuals of the same age.[65] For example, the range in a sample of blood cells in 80-year-old individuals is from 4 to 10 kilobases. Telomere length in blood cells is inversely correlated with age in both sexes, but at a given age blood cell telomeres are longer in women than in men.[66] Telomere length in humans is a predictor of vascular disease and longevity.[65–67] Persons with longer blood cell telomeres have longer life spans and have fewer indicators of deleterious cardiovascular alterations.

ERYTHROCYTES

HEMOGLOBIN LEVEL

Conflicting results have been reported regarding the relationship between age and hemoglobin level. Most studies show that the mean hemoglobin level or hematocrit[68–72] for a population of men falls slightly after middle age. Although statistically significant in some cases, mean hemoglobin levels decrease by less than 1.0 g/dl in the sixth through eighth decades.[68–74] In a group of men age 96 to 106 years the mean hemoglobin level was 12.4 g/dl,[75] but a later report of centenarians did not find a decrease in mean hemoglobin as compared with other men.[76] In a group of men age 84 to 98 years the mean hemoglobin level was 14.8 g/dl, only 0.8 g/dl less than that of a younger comparison group.[70] The lowest levels, however, were found in the oldest patients.[71,72,77] The hemoglobin levels in women may increase slightly with age[68,73,78] or remain unchanged.[79] In contrast, studies with smaller numbers of subjects demonstrated small mean decreases in hemoglobin levels in older women.[69,71,72,74,75] In studies that identified a decrease in hemoglobin level of both men and women, the decrease was less in women than in men. The narrowing of the difference in hemoglobin level between older men and older women may be the result of decreased androgen levels in older men and decreased estrogen levels in older women. Several mechanisms may account for anemia attributable solely to advancing age in otherwise healthy individuals. These include a reduction in hematopoietic progenitor cells and a diminished response to stimulatory cytokines. In addition, dysregulation of proinflammatory cytokines such as IL-1, IL-6, and tumor necrosis factor alpha (TNF-α) may play a role. These cytokines are thought to act both at the molecular and cellular levels via inhibition of erythropoietin gene expression and messenger RNA (mRNA), and by interfering with colony forming unit–erythroid (CFU-E) maturation and iron metabolism, respectively.[80] IL-6 exerts these effects via hepcidin, an iron-regulating protein (see Chap. 43).

Iron deficiency and the anemia of chronic disease have usually been responsible for low hemoglobin levels in the majority of asymptomatic older people.[69,77,81–83] Iron absorption is not impaired in the elderly, but use of orally administered iron for hemoglobin production is reduced.[84] Because hemoglobin concentration does not decrease significantly with age, elderly patients with anemia should be evaluated for a cause (e.g., iron, folate, or vitamin B_{12} deficiency or underlying malignancy or renal disease) before ascribing it to age.[85–87]

Unexplained anemia is also frequently observed in studies of older people.[61,69,74] One set of studies found that the red cells of older individuals separated in vitro had a greater proportion of dense cells in each density fraction, a greater proportion of reticulocytes, and an increase in autologous immunoglobulin (Ig) G antibodies per cell. In vitro erythrophagocytosis by macrophages was increased when red cells from older individuals were the target particles.[88,89] The inference drawn was that shortened red cell survival may play a role in the unexplained mild decrease in hemoglobin concentration in some older individuals.

2,3-BISPHOSPHOGLYCERATE CONCENTRATION

The erythrocyte 2,3-bisphosphoglycerate (2,3-BPG) level has been reported to fall with age from a mean value of 14.9 μmol/g hemoglobin at ages 18 to 24 years to 13.9 μmol/g hemoglobin at ages 75 to 84 years.[90,91] This decrease is statistically significant and accounts for a slight increase in oxygen affinity of hemoglobin, but is of doubtful physiologic significance.

OSMOTIC FRAGILITY

Erythrocyte osmotic fragility is increased in older individuals in comparison with younger subjects.[92,93] This phenomenon is associated with an increased mean corpuscular volume (MCV) and decreased mean corpuscular hemoglobin concentration (MCHC) of the red cells of older people.[93]

SERUM IRON, IRON-BINDING CAPACITY, AND FERRITIN LEVELS

In individuals of both sexes with normal hemoglobin levels, and presumably with normal iron stores, the serum iron level falls after the ages of 20 to 30 years.[78,94] In one study the values fell from a mean of about 130 μg/dl (28 μmol/liter) in men and 116 μg/dl (21 μmol/liter) in women to a mean at age 71 to 80 years of about 75 μg/dl (13 μmol/liter) in men and 66 μg/dl (12 μmol/liter) in women.[94] Levels of 50 μg/dl (9 μmol/liter) or less were found in 40 percent of men and women older than the age of 50 years.[95] The iron-binding capacity also falls in the elderly.[78,96,97]

Serum ferritin levels rise from a median of 25 μg/liter to 94 μg/liter in men in the third decade and then to a median of 124 μg/liter after age 45 years.[98] Ferritin levels in women remain low until middle age and then increase from a median of 25 μg/liter to 89 μg/liter in women after menopause.[99] In a study of centiles for the distribution of transferrin saturation and ferritin values for healthy men and women of European descent age 25 years and older, the most prominent age-related trend occurs with women whose serum ferritin increases strikingly as they progress through menopause, whereas percent saturation of transferrin did not change over the age range studied, implying that serum iron rose proportionately to iron-binding capacity.[237] Serum ferritin levels continue to reflect iron stores in older persons.[81,99] Because iron deficiency and concomitant inflammatory disease states may be more prevalent in older persons, some investigators suggest adding an assay for plasma transferrin receptors to aid in differentiating between the two.[100,101] Alternatively, a ferritin level of less than 45 μg/liter has been proposed as optimal for maximizing the detection of iron deficiency in older persons with possible coexisting inflammatory states.[102] Chapter 40, "Disorders of Iron Metabolism," discusses these approaches and the serum transferrin receptor:serum ferritin ratio[103] and red cell ferritin in considering the effects of inflammation on the diagnosis of iron deficiency.[103]

SERUM ERYTHROPOIETIN CONCENTRATION

Serum erythropoietin levels in nonanemic elderly individuals appear to be the same as those found in younger people,[104–107] although elevated levels were found in one study[94] and lower levels in another.[108] Serum erythropoietin levels are generally inversely related to hemoglobin levels,[104–106] suggesting that the erythropoietin response in older persons is the same as that in younger individuals. The peak and trough of the diurnal variation in erythropoietin levels is the same in younger and older individuals.[99,103]

SERUM VITAMIN B$_{12}$ AND FOLATE LEVELS

Low serum vitamin B$_{12}$ levels are found in a significant number of older individuals who do not have clinical findings of vitamin B$_{12}$ deficiency (i.e., anemia or a neurologic disorder).[109–115] They are very nonspecific screening measurements. The absorption of pure vitamin B$_{12}$ (Schilling test) is normal in older individuals,[97] but absorption of protein-bound vitamin B$_{12}$ may be reduced[116] in apparently healthy adults older than 55 years of age.[117] Reexamination, however, showed normal absorption of free and protein-bound cobalamin in older subjects.[118] Conversely, untreated patients with pernicious anemia may have only a moderate reduction in the serum vitamin B$_{12}$ level and not have anemia or macrocytosis.[119] These data require that reductions in the serum vitamin B$_{12}$ level in older subjects be evaluated carefully.[119–121] Some individuals with low serum vitamin B$_{12}$ levels have been followed for a 4-year period without developing anemia or other signs of vitamin B$_{12}$ deficiency.[122] Serum and urine methylmalonic acid and serum homocysteine assays are helpful in assessing such patients. Patients with metabolically significant decreases in plasma vitamin B$_{12}$ concentration will usually have elevated levels of methylmalonic acid and homocysteine, and their levels decrease to normal after vitamin B$_{12}$ replacement (see Chap. 39).

Both serum[74,114,120] and red cell[74] folate levels are below the usual lower limit of normal (3 μg/liter) in a small proportion (3–7%) of both males and females older than age 65 years. Low values of serum folate were found in individuals in the eighth decade compared to younger subjects.[121–124] However, low levels of serum folate can be found in healthy younger persons on a normal diet.[123,125] None of the subjects with low serum folate were anemic, highlighting the importance of the red cell folate as a measure of tissue folate content.

The MCV increases slightly but significantly with age.[70,78–81,126–128] Cigarette smoking may also cause an increase in the MCV,[127,128] and it has been reported that older persons who smoke may have an MCV of 100 fl or more in the absence of any demonstrable cause of macrocytosis.[128]

LEUKOCYTES

There is no consistent, significant variation in the total leukocyte count in older subjects. Normal leukocyte and neutrophil counts are present in nonagenarian[75] and centenarian populations.[76] Some investigators have found that after age 65 years the total leukocyte count tends to be lower in both sexes,[77] primarily as a result of a decrease in the lymphocyte count.[129–134] Others report a decrease in the leukocyte count as a result of a fall in the lymphocyte and the neutrophil counts

in women, but not in men, after age 50 years.[135,136] The absolute lymphocyte count has also been reported to be unchanged in older persons.[137–139]

IMMUNOSENESCENCE

Infectious diseases cause significant morbidity and mortality in older persons. Influenza and other pneumonias were the fifth most common cause of death in older persons in the United States in 2001, resulting in 55,518 deaths. Septicemia claimed another 25,418 lives that year.[140] The increased susceptibility of older persons to infection is ascribed to an imbalance in the interdependent adaptive and innate components of the immune system. Table 8-1 summarizes observations of what occurs in the immune system with aging.

ADAPTIVE IMMUNE SYSTEM

The adaptive immune system (see Chap. 18) is primarily mediated by T lymphocytes and their reduced competency with aging accounts for increased susceptibility to viral infections as well as a dampened protective antibody response to vaccination.[141,142] Total thymic atrophy occurs by late middle age. Thymic-mediated T lymphocyte development disappears, and at this age, and thereafter, individuals depend on their existing T lymphocyte pool to mediate T cell-dependent immune responses.[137–139,143,144]

T cells in older patients have impaired responsiveness to mitogens and antigens,[145,146] in part because of a decrease in expression of CD28 costimulator on the cell surface.[146] The age-associated decrease in CD28 expression is further correlated with increased T cell apoptosis.[147] T cell activation is also impaired in the elderly as evidenced by reduced surface expression of the activation marker CD69 in CD4+ cells, altered expression of the inflammatory cytokine interferon gamma (INF-γ), and subsequent diminished proliferation of both T cell subsets.[148] The clonal expansion of T cells in culture is decreased, reflecting a diminished response to antigen stimulation. T cell clones do not reach full development as a result of fewer doublings when T cells are obtained from older individuals.[149,150] In the absence of thymic function, the number of naive T cells decreases in older individuals; memory T cells predominate.[151] Spontaneous T cell clonal expansion is a feature of older individuals and may occur among CD4+[152,153] and CD8+ cell subsets.[153] Although likened to benign monoclonal gammopathy, the T cell clones may be stable and less prone to malignant progression.[153]

B lymphocyte function is dependent on T cell accessory roles, and the decreased ability to generate antibody responses, especially to primary antigens,[139,154,155] may be the result of T cell inadequacies rather than an intrinsic fault of B lymphocytes. The response to T cell-dependent antigens is characterized by the formation of low-affinity antibodies and antiidiotypic autoantibodies.[155] In addition, the age-associated decline in B cell antibody repertoire diversity may be the result of B cell clonal expansions.[156] Although variable from study to study, total B lymphocyte,[76,157] as well as T lymphocyte[76,157] and T lymphocyte subset,[76,158,159] concentrations in the blood are decreased in older individuals. Serum IgM and IgG concentrations either do not change significantly[160] or are reduced in older subjects,[161] whereas serum IgA levels increase with age.[161,162] An increased prevalence of autoantibodies (e.g., anti-IgG rheumatoid factor) occurs in older persons.[131,154,162] An increased frequency of somatic mutations in the IgV$_H$ gene of blood B cells of older individuals may decrease IgG antibody affinity.[163] Monoclonal plasma immunoglobulins (essential monoclonal gammopathy) are found with increasing frequency with age, reaching 3 percent in people older than age 70 years and nearly 6 percent in those between the ages of 80 and 89 years[164,165] (see Chap. 99). Not

TABLE 8-1   THE IMMUNE SYSTEM IN OLDER PERSONS

OBSERVATION	REFERENCE
ADAPTIVE IMMUNE SYSTEM	
T Lymphocytes	
Impaired response to mitogens or antigens	145, 146
Thymic atrophy results in decrease in naïve T cell numbers with predominance of memory T cells	151
Increased CD28-mediated T cell apoptosis	147
Diminished response to mitogenic stimulation	148
Diminished response to antigen stimulation	149, 150
B Lymphocytes	
Decreased ability to generate an antibody response	139, 154, 155
Increased generation of low-affinity antibodies and antiidiotype autoantibodies	155
Decrease in antibody repertoire diversity	156
INNATE IMMUNE SYSTEM	
Neutrophils	
Normal chemotaxis	173, 174
Impaired chemotaxis	171, 176
Normal endothelial cell adhesion	173
Normal granule content and degranulation	173
Decreased phagocytosis	175, 176
Bacteria-induced superoxide generation is normal with particulate stimulants and reduced with soluble stimulants	174, 177, 236
Reduced capacity to inhibit Fas-mediated apoptosis in the presence of proinflammatory inhibitors*	180, 181
Increased ADP-ribosylated proteins involved in signal transduction	230
Monocytes	
Decrease in number of plasmacytoid dendritic cells with resultant reduction in interferon-α	231
Dendritic cell function is preserved	232
Chronically activated (associated with inflammatory states)	233
Dysregulated cytokine production (increased IL-1β, IL-1 receptor antagonist, IL-6)	233
Increased MCP-1 (involved in monocyte recruitment); functions, in part, in an autocrine fashion, however, it is also produced by other cell types	234
Decreased inducibility of heat shock protein 70 with resultant decrease in cell's ability to withstand adverse conditions*	235
Natural Killer Cells	
Compromised function	76, 157, 182, 183, 236
Decreased NK cell production of MIP-1α, RANTES, and IL-8 causing impaired cytolytic activity of infected cells	184

* Also in lymphocytes. ADP, adenosine diphosphate; IL, interleukin; MCP-1, monocyte chemoattractant protein; NK, natural killer; MIP, macrophage inflammatory protein; RANTES, regulated on activation normal T cell expressed and secreted.

unexpectedly, delayed hypersensitivity reactions are also reduced in the elderly.[166-169] These immunologic deficits are correlated with overall mortality in individuals older than age 60 years.[170]

INNATE IMMUNE SYSTEM

Neutrophils play a key role in the innate immune system (see Chap. 17) as the primary defense against bacteria and fungi. Neutrophil numbers are maintained in older individuals.[171,172] An age-related effect on chemotaxis is controversial because studies demonstrate both a normal response[173,174] and a reduced response.[175,176] There is no age-related

change in neutrophil endothelial adhesion.[173] In keeping with this, adhesion molecule CD15 and CD11b expression are slightly increased in older subjects.[174] Granule content and degranulation do not change with increasing age,[173] whereas Fc-mediated phagocytosis decreases.[175,176] The bactericidal function of superoxide generation as a function of aging is complex because the release of reactive oxygen species from neutrophils of elderly subjects varies, depending on the stimulant.[174,177] Particulate stimulants such as *Candida albicans* produced no significant difference in neutrophil release of reactive oxygen species of older subjects compared to young controls, whereas subjecting neutrophils of older subjects to soluble stimulants such as N-formyl-methionyl-leucyl-phenylalanine (fMLP) results in a significant reduction in oxidative burst compared with young controls.[177] Neither spontaneous nor AP01/Fas (CD95)-linked apoptosis contributes significantly to compromised neutrophil function.[178,179] Neutrophils from older subjects do, however, demonstrate a reduced capacity to inhibit Fas-mediated apoptosis in the presence of proinflammatory mediators such as GM-CSF and bacterial lipopolysaccharide.[180,181] Ordinarily, this means of temporarily interfering with apoptosis facilitates extension of functional viability under special conditions such as bacterial infection, effectively conferring a host advantage. Neutrophils of older patients, lacking such an advantage, may render older patients more susceptible to life-threatening infections. Natural killer cells, large granular lymphocytes expressing CD16 and CD56, but not CD3, are increased in number, but their function is disturbed.[75,157,182,183] For example, cytolytic activity per cell was decreased in older as compared to younger individuals. The decreased production of the chemokines (1) macrophage inflammatory protein (MIP)-1α, (2) regulated on activation, normal T cell expressed and secreted (RANTES), and (3) IL-8 from natural killer (NK) cells in nonagenarians, as compared to younger individuals, may result in impaired cytolytic activity of infected cells.[184]

PLATELETS

The platelet count does not change with age.[76,77] Increased plasma levels of two platelet α-granule constituents—β-thromboglobulin and platelet factor 4—have been found in individuals older than 65 years of age in comparison with younger individuals.[185,186] Enhanced in vitro reactivity to platelet-aggregating agents has been observed.[187-192] Decreased platelet membrane protein kinase C activity and translocation to the cytosol after platelet activation was noted in platelets from older subjects.[193] The enhanced platelet sensitivity seen in older subjects may be the result of diminished antioxidant protective mechanisms. These include decreased scavenger nitric oxide (NO) bioavailability mediated by oxidative low-density lipoprotein (LDL)[194] and/or increased sensitivity to serotonin.[195] Platelet levels of sialic acid are lower in older individuals as compared with younger individuals. This result of oxidative stress, which is abrogated by exposure to the antioxidant 2-mercatoethanol, could, in turn, modulate platelet aggregation.[196] Higher intraplatelet calcium levels and more pronounced platelet membrane rigidity may also contribute to the increased platelet aggregation seen in older individuals.[197] (See Chap. 105 for further discussion of platelet biochemistry.)

PLASMA COAGULATION FACTORS

Several studies have emphasized the changes with human aging in the level of proteins involved in the formation or dissolution of fibrin.[198-200] Plasma concentrations of factor VII coagulant activity and antigen,[198-202] and factor VIIIC,[198,199,203] as well as von Willebrand factor,[198,203] fibrinogen,[198,199,201,204] fibrinopeptide A,[198,199,205] and tissue plasminogen activator antigen[198,206-208] increase with age. Fibrinogen level is a risk factor for thrombotic vascular disease.[204] In healthy centenarians, levels of activated factor VII, activation peptides of pro-thrombin, factors IX and X, and thrombin–antithrombin complex concentration were increased, which are signs of higher-than-expected coagulation enzyme activity.[199] Age-associated increases in levels of protein C occur in both sexes. Aging is also associated with increasing levels of free protein S.[200] In contrast, antithrombin III tends to decrease with age in males and increases with age in females following menopause.[209] Higher D-dimer and plasmin–antiplasmin complexes indicate an accompanying increase in fibrinolytic activity.[199,210] In contrast, plasma tissue-plasminogen activator (t-PA) inhibitor levels increase with increasing age, as do levels of thrombin-activatable fibrinolysis inhibitor (TAFI) in women[211] and its proenzyme form, procarboxypeptidase U in both sexes.[212] These latter findings are suggestive of a possible age-dependent compromise in fibrinolytic activity.[213] Thus, procoagulant and, in some studies, fibrinolytic activities appear to be increased in older subjects by both in vitro[199,214–217] and in vivo studies.[205,218] Older patients may show an exaggerated anticoagulant response to warfarin.[219] (See Chap. 106 for discussion of coagulation factor biochemistry and Chap. 127 for discussion of fibrinolysis.)

ERYTHROCYTE SEDIMENTATION RATE AND C-REACTIVE PROTEIN

The erythrocyte sedimentation rate increases significantly with age.[70,220–223] Hypercholesterolemia further enhances the erythrocyte

sedimentation rate in older individuals.[224] Mean values of 14 mm/h (Westergren) and individual values as high as 69 mm/h were found in healthy women age 70 to 89 years who were followed for 3 to 11 years.[223–225] The erythrocyte sedimentation rate is of limited value in detecting disease in elderly patients. Estimation of levels of acute-phase proteins appears to offer no advantage over the erythrocyte sedimentation rate.[226,227] The C-reactive protein content of serum also is mildly elevated in older individuals without an apparent inflammatory process.[228,229]

THE INCIDENCE OF CLONAL HEMOPATHIES

Several hematologic diseases (e.g., pernicious anemia) increase in frequency with age. The notable increase in clonal (neoplastic) diseases of hematopoiesis is shown in Fig. 8-1, which depicts the rate of occurrence of the leukemias (the aggregate of the four major types), lymphoma, and myeloma at 5-year intervals. The inclusion of acute lymphocytic leukemia, which has a mode at about 3.5 years, decreases, and then increases in frequency again after middle age, does not dampen the dramatic age-dependent incidence rate. Age-dependent increases in other neoplastic diseases such as polycythemia, idiopathic myelofibrosis, and clonal cytopenias (myelodysplastic syndromes) are striking as well. The curves do not provide insight into the cause of the relationship, which could reflect the accumulated injury resulting from external factors, the accumulated effects of spontaneous somatic mutations, or some combination of these events.

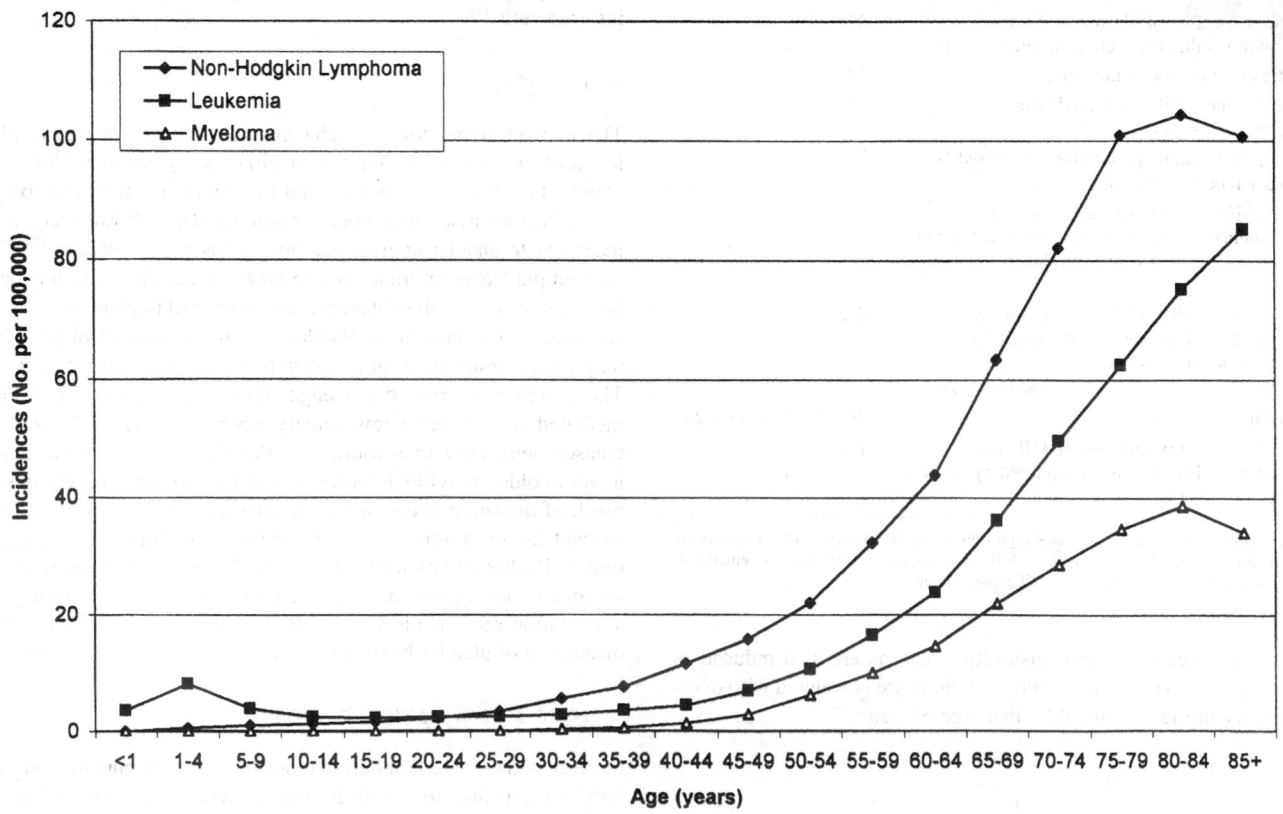

FIGURE 8-1 Age-specific incidence rates, 1997–2001. The abscissa depicts age in intervals of 5 years. The ordinate represents the incidence per 100,000 Americans of myeloma, lymphoma, and leukemia. The rates for each of the four major leukemias and the various subtypes of lymphoma are aggregated. The increment at 1 to 4 years among the leukemias reflects a mode in acute lymphocytic leukemia at that age. These data were obtained from the National Cancer Institute Surveillance Epidemiology End Results (SEER) Program.

REFERENCES

1. www.census.gov/population/estimates/nation/intfile2-1.txt

2. Kinsella KG: Changes in life expectancy 1900–1990. *Am J Clin Nutr* 55:1196S, 1992.

3. Lansdorp PM: Self-renewal of stem cells. *Biol Blood Marrow Transplant* 3:171, 1997.

4. Hayflick L: Mortality and immortality at the cellular level. A review. *Biochemistry* 62:1180, 1997.

5. Perillo NL, Walford RL, Newman MA, Effros RB: Human T lymphocytes possess a limited in vitro life span. *Exp Gerontol* 24:177, 1989.

6. Kirkland JL: The biochemistry of mammalian senescence. *Clin Biochem* 25:61, 1992.

7. Rubin H: Cell aging in vivo and vitro. *Mech Ageing Dev* 100:209, 1998.

8. Hyland P, Barnett C, Pawelec G, Barnett Y: Age-related accumulation of oxidative DNA damage and alterations in levels of $p16^{ink4a/CDKN2a}$, $p21^{WAF1/CIPA/SDI1}$ and $p27^{KIP1}$ in human CD4+ T cell clones in vitro. *Mech Ageing Dev* 122:1151, 2001.

9. Geiger H, Van Zant G: The aging of lympho-hematopoietic stem cells. *Nat Immunol* 3:329, 2002.

10. Barnett YA, Barnett CR: DNA damage and mutation: contributors to the age-related alterations in T cell-mediated immune responses? *Mech Ageing Dev* 102:165, 1998.

11. Schofield R, Dexter TM, Lord BI, Tasta NG: Comparison of haemopoiesis in young and old mice. *Mech Ageing Dev* 34:1, 1986.

12. Boggs D, Patrene K, Steinberg H: Aging and hematopoiesis. VI. Neutrophilia and other leukocyte changes in aged mice. *Exp Hematol* 14:372, 1986.

13. Williams LH, Udupa KB, Lipschitz DA: Evaluation of the effect of age on hematopoiesis in the C57BL/6 mouse. *Exp Hematol* 14:827, 1986.

14. Maggio-Price L, Wolf NS, Priestley GV, et al: Evaluation of stem cell reserve using serial bone marrow transplantation and competitive repopulation in a murine model of chronic hemolytic anemia. *Exp Hematol* 16:653, 1988.

15. Harrison DE, Astle CM, Stone M: Numbers and functions of transplantable primitive immunohematopoietic stem cells: effects of age. *J Immunol* 142:3833, 1989.

16. Sharp A, Zipori D, Toledo J, et al: Age related changes in hemopoietic capacity of bone marrow cells. *Mech Ageing Dev* 48:91, 1989.

17. Egusa Y, Fujiwara Y, Syahrrudin E, et al: Effect of age on human peripheral blood stem cells. *Oncol Rep* 5:398, 1998.

18. Udupa KB, Lipschitz DA: Erythropoiesis in the aged mouse. II. Response to stimulation in vitro. *J Lab Clin Med* 103:581, 1984.

19. Boggs DR, Patrene KD: Hematopoiesis and aging. III. Anemia and a blunted erythropoietic response to hemorrhage in aged mice. *Am J Hematol* 19:327, 1985.

20. Kamminga LM, van Os R, Ausema A, et al: Impaired hematopoietic stem cell functioning after serial transplantation and during normal aging. *Stem Cells* 23:82, 2005.

21. Globerson A: Hematopoietic stem cells and aging. *Exp Gerontol* 34:137, 1999.

22. Lee MA, Segal GM, Bagby GC: The hematopoietic microenvironment in the elderly: defects in IL-1-induced CSF expression in vitro. *Exp Hematol* 17:952, 1989.

23. Shank WA Jr, Balducci L: Recombinant hemopoietic growth factors: comparative hemopoietic response in younger and older subjects. *J Am Geriatr Soc* 40:151, 1992.

24. Chatta GS, Andrews RG, Rodger E, et al: Hematopoietic progenitors and aging: alterations in granulocyte precursors and responsiveness to recombinant human G-CSF, GM-CSF, and IL-3. *J Gerontol* 48:M207, 1993.

25. Chatta GS, Price TH, Dale DC, et al: The effects of in vivo rhG-CSF on the neutrophil response in healthy young and elderly volunteers. *Blood* 84:2923, 1994.

26. Fernandez-Ferrer S, Ramos F: Dyshaemopoietic bone marrow features in healthy subjects are related to age. *Leuk Res* 25:187, 2001.

27. Lajtha LB, Schofield R: Regulation of stem cell renewal and differentiation of possible significance in aging. *Adv Gerontol Res* 3:131, 1971.

28. Harrison DE: Normal production of erythrocytes by mouse marrow continuous for 73 months. *Proc Natl Acad Sci U S A* 70:3184, 1973.

29. Relucke U, Burlington H, Cronkite EP, Laissue J: Hayflick's hypothesis: An approach to in vivo testing. *Fed Proc* 34:71, 1975.

30. Harrison DE: Normal function of transplanted marrow cell lines from aged mice. *J Gerontol* 30:279, 1975.

31. Gale RE, Fielding AK, Harrison CN, Linch DC: Acquired skewing of X-chromosome inactivation patterns in myeloid cells of the elderly suggests stochastic clonal loss with age. *Br J Haematol* 98:512, 1997.

32. El-Kassar N, Hetet G, Briere J, Grandchamp B: X-chromosome inactivation in healthy females: Incidence of excessive lyonization with age and comparison of assays involving DNA methylation and transcript polymorphisms. *Clin Chem* 44:61, 1998.

33. Custer RP, Ahlfeldt FE: Studies on the structure and function of the bone marrow. *J Lab Clin Med* 17:960, 1932.

34. Hartsock RJ, Smith EB, Petty CS: Normal variations with aging on the amount of hematopoietic tissue in bone marrow from the anterior iliac crest. *Am J Clin Pathol* 43:326, 1965.

35. Kricun ME: Red-yellow marrow conversion: Its effect on location of some solitary bone lesions. *Skeletal Radiol* 14:10, 1985.

36. Beutler E, Drennan W, Block M: The bone marrow and liver in iron-deficiency anemia: A histopathologic study of sections with special reference to the stainable iron content. *J Lab Clin Med* 43:427, 1954.

37. Ricci C, Cova M, Kang YS, et al: Normal age-related patterns of cellular and fatty bone marrow distribution in the axial skeleton: MR imaging study. *Radiology* 177:83, 1990.

38. Justesen J, Stenderup K, Ebbesen EN, et al: Adipocyte tissue volume in bone marrow is increased with aging and in patients with osteoporosis. *Biogerontology* 2:165, 2001.

39. Nowinski GP, Van Dyke DL, Tilley BC, et al: The frequency of aneuploidy in cultured lymphocytes is correlated with age and gender but not with reproductive history. *Am J Hum Genet* 46:1101, 1990.

40. Stone JF, Sandberg AA: Sex chromosome aneuploidy and aging. *Mutat Res* 338:107, 1995.

41. United Kingdom Cancer Cytogenetics Group: Loss of Y chromosome from normal and neoplastic bone marrow. *Genes Chromosomes Cancer* 5:83, 1992.

42. Wiktor A, Rybicki BA, Piao ZS, et al: Clinical significance of Y chromosome loss in hematologic disease. *Genes Chromosomes Cancer* 27:11, 2000.

43. Hando JC, Nath J, Tucker JD: Sex chromosomes, micronuclei and aging in women. *Chromosoma* 103:186, 1994.

44. Ramsey MJ, Moore DH II, Briner JF, et al: The effects of age and lifestyle factors on the accumulation of cytogenetic damage as measured by chromosome painting. *Mutat Res* 338:95, 1995.

45. Bolognesi C, Abbondandolo A, Barale R, et al: Age-related increase of baseline frequencies of sister chromatid exchanges, chromosome aberrations, and micronuclei in human lymphocytes. *Cancer Epidemiol Biomarkers Prev* 6:249, 1997.

46. Grist SA, Mccarron M, Kutlaca A, et al: In vivo human somatic mutation: Frequency and spectrum with age. *Mutat Res* 266:189, 1992.

47. Bukvic N, Gentile M, Susca F, et al: Sex chromosome loss, micronuclei, sister chromatid exchange and aging: a study including 16 centenarians. *Mutat Res* 498:159, 2001.

48. Catalan J, Autio K, Wessman M, et al: Age-associated micronuclei containing centromeres and the X chromosome in lymphocytes of women. *Cytogenet Cell Genet* 68:11, 1995.

49. Kadenbach B, Munscher C, Frank V, et al: Human aging is associated with stochastic somatic mutations of mitochondrial DNA. *Mutat Res* 338:161, 1995.

50. Yakes FM, van Houten B: Mitochondria DNA damage is more extensive and persists longer than nuclear DNA damage in human cells following oxidative stress. *Proc Natl Acad Sci U S A* 94:514, 1997.

51. Chinnery PF, Samuels DC, Elson J, Turnbull DM: Accumulation of mitochondrial DNA mutations in ageing, cancer, and mitochondrial disease: Is there a common mechanism? *Lancet* 360:1323, 2002.

52. Gattermann N: Mitochondrial DNA mutations in the hematopoietic system. *Leukemia* 18:18, 2004.

53. He L, Luo L, Proctor SJ, et al: Somatic mitochondrial DNA mutations in adult-onset leukaemia. *Leukemia* 17:2487, 2003.

54. Gattermann N, Berneburg M, Heinisch J, et al: Detection of the ageing-associated 5-Kb common deletion of mitochondrial DNA in blood and bone marrow of hematologically normal adults. Absence of the deletion in clonal bone marrow disorders. *Leukemia* 9:1704, 1995.

55. Greider CW: Telomeres and senescence. *Curr Biol* 8:R178, 1998.

56. Robertson JD, Gale RE, Wynn RF, et al: Dynamics of telomere shortening in neutrophils and T lymphocytes during ageing and the relationship to skewed X chromosome inactivation patterns. *Br J Haematol* 109:272, 2000.

57. Son NH, Murray S, Yanovisky J, et al: Lineage-specific telomere shortening and unaltered capacity for telomerase expression in human T and B lymphocytes. *J Immunol* 165:1191, 2000.

58. Engelhardt M, Kumar R, Albanell J, et al: Telomerase regulation, cell cycle, and telomere stability in primitive hematopoietic cells. *Blood* 90:182, 1997.

59. Vaziri H, Dragowski W, Allsopp RC, et al: Evidence for a mitotic clock in hematopoietic stem cells. *Proc Natl Acad Sci U S A* 91:9857, 1994.

60. Notario R, Cimmino A, Tabarini D, et al. In vivo telomere dynamics of human hematopoietic stem cells. *Proc Natl Acad Sci U S A* 94:13782, 1997.

61. Rufer N, Brummendorf TH, Kolvraa S, et al: Telomerase fluorescence measurements in granulocytes and T lymphocyte subsets point to a high turnover of hematopoietic stem cells and memory T cells in early childhood. *J Exp Med* 190:157, 1999.

62. Frenck RW Jr, Blackburn EH, Shannon KM: The rate of telomere sequence loss in human leukocyte varies with age. *Proc Natl Acad Sci U S A* 95:5607, 1998.

63. Jeanclos E, Schork NJ, Kyvik KO, et al: Telomere length inversely correlates with pulse pressure and is highly familial. *Hypertension* 36:195, 2000.

64. Slagboom PE, Droog S, Boomsma DI: Genetic determination of telomere size in humans: twin studies of three age groups. *Am J Hum Genet* 55:876, 1994.

65. Cawthon RM, Smith KR, O'Brien E, et al: Association between telomere length in blood and mortality in people aged 60 years and older. *Lancet* 361:393, 2003.

66. Benetos A, Okuda K, Lajemi M, et al: Telomere length as an indicator of biological aging: the gender effect and relation with pulse pressure and pulse wave velocity. *Hypertension* 37:381, 2001.

67. Samani NJ, Boultby R, Butler R, et al: Telomere shortening in atherosclerosis. *Lancet* 358:472, 2001.

68. McDonough JR, Hames CG, Garrison GE, et al: The relationship of hematocrit to cardiovascular states of health in the negro and white population of Evans County, Georgia. *J Chronic Dis* 18:243, 1965.

69. McLennan WJ, Andrews GR, Macleod C, Caird FI: Anaemia in the elderly. *Q J Med* 42:1, 1973.

70. Zauber NP, Zauber AG: Hematologic data of healthy very old people. *JAMA* 257:2181, 1987.

71. Nilsson-Ehle H, Jagenburg R, Landahl S, et al: Decline of blood haemoglobin in the aged: a longitudinal study of an urban Swedish population from age 70 to 81. *Br J Haematol* 71:437, 1989.

72. Salive ME, Cornoni-Huntley J, Guralnik JM, et al: Anemia and hemoglobin level in older persons: Relationship with age, gender, and health status. *J Am Geriatr Soc* 40:489, 1992.

73. Cruickshank JM: Some variations in the normal haemoglobin concentration. *Br J Haematol* 18:523, 1970.

74. Elwood PC, Shinton NK, Wilson CD, et al: Haemoglobin, vitamin B$_{12}$ and folate levels in the elderly. *Br J Haematol* 21:557, 1971.

75. Zaino EC: Blood counts in the nonagenarian. *N Y State J Med* 81:1199, 1981.

76. Sansoni P, Cossarizza A, Brianti V, et al: Lymphocyte subsets and natural killer cell activity in healthy old people and centenarians. *Blood* 82:2767, 1993.

77. Nilsson-Ehle H, Jagenburg R, Landahl S, et al: Haematological abnormalities and reference intervals in the elderly: A cross-sectional comparative study of three Swedish population samples aged 70, 78 and 81 years. *Acta Med Scand* 224:595, 1988.

78. Yip R, Johnson C, Dallman PR: Age-related changes in laboratory values used in the diagnosis of anemia and iron deficiency. *Am J Clin Nutr* 39:427, 1984.

79. Jernigan JA, Gudat JC, Blake JL, et al: Reference values for blood findings in relatively fit elderly persons. *J Am Geriatr Soc* 28:308, 1980.

80. Ershler WB: Biological interactions of aging and anemia: A focus on cytokines. *J Am Geriatr Soc* 51(suppl):518, 2003.

81. Kelly A, Munan L: Haematologic profile of natural populations: Red cell parameters. *Br J Haematol* 35:153, 1977.

82. Htoo MSH, Kofkoff RL, Freedman ML: Erythrocyte parameters in the elderly: An argument against new geriatric normal values. *J Am Geriatr Soc* 27:547, 1979.

83. Lipschitz DA, Mitchell CO, Thompson C: The anemia of senescence. *Am J Hematol* 11:47, 1981.

84. Marx JJM: Normal iron absorption and decreased red cell iron uptake in the aged. *Blood* 53:204, 1979.

85. Garry PJ, Goodwin JS, Hunt WC: Iron status and anemia in the elderly: New findings and a review of previous studies. *J Am Geriatr Soc* 31:389, 1983.

86. Timiras ML, Brownstein H: Prevalence of anemia and correlation of hemoglobin with age in a geriatric screening clinic population. *J Am Geriatr Soc* 35:639, 1987.

87. Baldwin JG: Hematopoietic function in the elderly. *Arch Intern Med* 148:2544, 1988.

88. Glass GA, Gershon D, Gershon H: Some characteristics of the human erythrocyte as a function of donor and cell age. *Exp Hematol* 13:1122, 1978.

89. Sheibon E, Gershon H: Recognition and sequestration of young and old erythrocytes from young and elderly human donors: In vitro studies. *J Lab Clin Med* 121:493, 1993.

90. Purcell Y, Brozovic B: Red cell 2,3-diphosphoglycerate concentration in man decreases with age. *Nature* 241:511, 1974.

91. Kalofoutis A, Paterakis S, Koutselenis A, Spanos V: Relationship between erythrocyte 2,3-diphosphoglycerate and age in a normal population. *Clin Chem* 22:1918, 1976.

92. Detraglia M, Cook FB, Stasiw DM, Cerny LC: Erythrocyte fragility in aging. *Biochim Biophys Acta* 345:213, 1974.

93. Araki K, Rifkind JM: Age dependent changes in osmotic hemolysis of human erythrocyte. *J Gerontol* 35:499, 1980.

94. Pirrie R: The influence of age upon serum iron in normal subjects. *J Clin Pathol* 5:10, 1952.

95. Powell DEB, Thomas JH, Mills P: Serum iron in elderly hospital patients. *Gerontol Clin (Basel)* 10:21, 1968.

96. Rechenberger J: über die Eisenbildungskapazität des Blutserums in den verscheidenen Lebensaltern. *Z Alternsforsch* 9:98, 1955.

97. Powell DEB, Thomas JH: The iron-binding capacity of serum in elderly hospital patients. *Gerontol Clin (Basel)* 11:36, 1969.

98. Cook JD, Finch CA, Smith NJ: Evaluation of the iron status of a population. *Blood* 48:449, 1976.

99. Guyatt GH, Patterson C, Ali M, et al: Diagnosis of iron deficiency anemia in the elderly. *Am J Med* 88:205, 1990.

100. Lammi-Keefe CL, Lickteig ES, Ghluwalia N, Haley NR: Day-to-day variation in iron status indexes is similar for most measures in elderly women with and without rheumatoid arthritis. *J Am Diet Assoc* 96:247, 1996.

101. Kohgo Y, Nitsu Y, Kondo H, et al: Serum transferrin receptor as a new index of erythropoiesis. *Blood* 70:1955, 1987.

102. Guyatt GH, Patterson C, Ali M, et al: Diagnosis of iron-deficiency anemia in the elderly. *Am J Med* 88:205, 1990.

103. Pasqualetti P, Casale R: No influence of aging on the circadian rhythm of erythropoietin in healthy subjects. *Gerontology* 43:206, 1997.

104. Mori M, Murai Y, Hirai M, et al: Serum erythropoietin titers in the aged. *Mech Ageing Dev* 46:105, 1988.

105. Powers JS, Lichtenstein MJ, Collins JC, et al: Serum erythropoietin in healthy older persons. *J Am Geriatr Soc* 37:388, 1989.

106. Powers JS, Krantz SB, Collins JC, et al: Erythropoietin response to anemia as a function of age. *J Am Geriatr Soc* 39:30, 1991.

107. Kario K, Matsuo T, Nakao K: Serum erythropoietin levels in the elderly. *Gerontology* 37:345, 1991.

108. Pasqualetti P, Casale R: No influence of aging on the circadian rhythm of erythropoietin in healthy subjects. *Gerontology* 43:206, 1997.

109. Henderson JG, Strachen RW, Swanson Beck J, et al: The antigastrin-antibody test as a screening procedure for vitamin B_{12} deficiency in psychiatric practice. *Lancet* 2:809, 1966.

110. Schilling RF, Fairbanks VF, Miller R, et al: "Improved" vitamin B_{12} assays: A report on two commercial kits. *Clin Chem* 29:582, 1983

111. Cooper BA, Fehedy V, Blanshay P: Recognition of deficiency of vitamin B_{12} using measurement of serum concentration. *J Lab Clin Med* 107: 447, 1986.

112. Thompson WG, Babitz L, Cassino C, et al: Evaluation of current criteria used to measure vitamin B_{12} levels. *Am J Med* 82:291, 1987.

113. Nilsson-Ehle H, Landahl S, Lindstedt G, et al: Low serum cobalamin levels in a population study of 70- and 75-year-old subjects: gastrointestinal causes and hematologic effects. *Dig Dis Sci* 34:716, 1989.

114. Lindenbaum J, Rosenberg IH, Wilson PWF, et al: Prevalence of cobalamin deficiency in the Framingham elderly population. *Am J Clin Nutr* 60:2, 1994.

115. Carmel R: Cobalamin, the stomach and aging. *Am J Clin Nutr* 66:750, 1997.

116. Carmel R, Sinow RM, Siegel ME, Samloff IM: Food cobalamin malabsorption occurs frequently in patients with unexplained low serum cobalamin levels. *Arch Intern Med* 148:1715, 1988.

117. Scarlett JD, Read H, O'Dea K: Protein-bound cobalamin absorption declines in the elderly. *Am J Hematol* 39:79, 1992.

118. van Asselt DZ, van den Broek MJ, Lamers CB, et al: Free and protein-bound cobalamin absorption in healthy middle-aged and older subjects. *J Am Geriatr Soc* 44:949, 1996.

119. Carmel R: Pernicious anemia. The expected findings of very low serum cobalamin levels, anemia, and macrocytosis are often lacking. *Arch Intern Med* 148:1712, 1988.

120. Herbert V: Don't ignore low serum cobalamin (vitamin B_{12}) levels. *Arch Intern Med* 148:1705, 1988.

121. Carmel R, Sinow RM, Karnaze DS: Atypical cobalamin deficiency: Subtle biochemical evidence of deficiency is commonly demonstrable in patients with megaloblastic anemia and is often associated with protein-bound cobalamin malabsorption. *J Lab Clin Med* 109:454, 1987.

122. Pathy MS, Newcombe RG: Temporal variation of serum levels of vitamin B_{12}, folate, iron, and total iron-binding capacity. *Gerontology* 26: 34, 1980.

123. Girdwood RH, Thompson AD, Williamson J: Folate status in the elderly. *Br Med J* 2:670, 1967.

124. Osterlind PO, Alafuzoff I, Lofgren A-C, et al: Blood components in an elderly population. *Gerontology* 30:247, 1984.

125. Hall CA, Bardwell SA, Allen ES, Rappazzo ME: Variation in plasma folate levels among groups of healthy persons. *Am J Clin Nutr* 28:854, 1975.

126. Okuno T: Red cell size as measured by the Coulter model S. *J Clin Pathol* 25:599, 1972.

127. Okuno T: Smoking and blood changes. *JAMA* 225:1387, 1973.

128. Helman N, Rubenstein LS: The effects of age, sex, and smoking on erythrocytes and leukocytes. *Am J Clin Pathol* 63:35, 1975.

129. Caird FI, Andrews GR, Gallie TB: The leukocyte count in old age. *Age Ageing* 1:239, 1972.

130. Conrad RA, Demoise CF, Scott WA, Makar M: Immunohematological studies of Marshall Islanders sixteen years after fallout radiation exposure. *J Gerontol* 26:28, 1971.

131. Diaz-Jouanen E, Strickland RG, Williams RC Jr: Studies of human lymphocytes in the newborn and the aged. *Am J Med* 58:620, 1975.

132. MacKinney AA Jr: Effect of aging on the peripheral blood lymphocyte count. *J Gerontol* 33:213, 1978.

133. Jamil NAK, Millard RE: Studies of T, B, and "null" blood lymphocytes in normal persons of different age groups. *Gerontology* 27:79, 1981.

134. Polednak AP: Age changes in differential leukocyte count among female adults. *Hum Biol* 50:30, 1978.

135. Allan RN, Alexander MK: A sex difference in the leukocyte count. *J Clin Pathol* 21:691, 1968.

136. Cruickshank JM, Alexander MK: The effect of age, sex, parity, haemoglobin level, and oral contraceptive preparations on the normal leukocyte count. *Br J Haematol* 18:541, 1970.

137. Globerson A: T lymphocytes and aging. *Int Arch Allergy Immunol* 107: 491, 1995.

138. Miller RA: The aging immune system. *Science* 273:70, 1996.

139. Wick G, Grubeck-Loebenstein B: The aging immune system: primary and secondary alterations of immune reactivity in elderly. *Exp Gerontol* 32:401,1997.

140. www.cdc.gov/nchs/data/hus/tables/2003/03hus032.pdf.

141. Arreaza EE, Gibbons JJ, Siskind GW, Weksler ME: Lower antibody response to tetanus toxoid associated with higher auto-anti-idiotypic antibody in old compared with young humans. *Clin Exp Immunol* 92:169, 1993.

142. Powers DC: Influenza: a virus specific cytotoxic T lymphocyte activity declines with advancing age. *J Am Geriatr Soc* 41:887, 1993.

143. Grubeck-Loebenstein B: Changes in the aging immune system. *Biologicals* 25:205, 1997.

144. Yoshikawa TT: Perspective: Aging and infectious diseases: past, present and future. *J Infect Dis* 176:1053, 1997.

145. Song L, Kim YH, Chopra RK, et al: Age-related effects in T cell activation and proliferation. *Exp Gerontol* 28:313, 1993.

146. Effros RB, Boucher N, Porter V, et al: Decline in CD2 T cells in centenarians and in long-term T cell cultures: A possible cause for both in vivo and in vitro immunosenescence. *Exp Gerontol* 29:60, 1994.

147. Dennett NS, Barcia RN, McLeod JD: Age associated decline in CD25 and CD28 expression correlate with an increased susceptibility to CD95 mediated apoptosis in T cells. *Exp Gerontol* 37:271, 2002.

148. Schindowski K, Frohlich L, Maurer K, et al: Age-related impairment of human T lymphocytes' activation: Specific differences between CD14+ and CD8+ subsets. *Mech Ageing Dev* 123:375, 2002.

149. Grubeck-Loebenstein B, Lechner H, Trieb K: Long-term in vitro growth of human T cell clones: Can postmitotic senescent cell population be defined? *Int Arch Allergy Immunol* 110:238, 1996.

150. Lechner H, Amort M, Steger MM, et al: Regulation of CD95 (APO-1) expression and the induction of apoptosis in human T cells: Changes in old age. *Int Arch Allergy Immunol* 110:238, 1996.

151. Cossarizza A, Ortolani C, Paganelli R, et al: CD4 isoform expression on CD4+ and CD8+ T cells throughout life, from newborn to centenarians. Implication for T cell memory. *Mech Aging Dev* 86:173, 1996.

152. Posnett DN, Sinka R, Kabak S, Russo C: Clonal populations of T cells in normal elderly humans: The T cell equivalent to "benign monoclonal gammopathy." *J Exp Med* 179:609, 1994.

153. Schwab R, Szabo P, Manavalan JS, et al: Expanded CD4+ and CD8+ T cell clones in elderly humans. *J Immunol* 158:4493, 1997.

154. Schulze DH, Goidl EA: Age-associated changes in antibody-forming cells (B cells). *Proc Soc Exp Biol Med* 196:253, 1991.

155. Powers DC: Immunological principles and emerging strategies of vaccination for the elderly. *J Am Geriatr Soc* 40:81, 1992.

156. Ghia P, Prato G, Scieizo C, et al: Monoclonal CD5+ and CD5− B-lymphocyte expansions are frequent in the peripheral blood of the elderly. *Blood* 103:2337, 2004.

157. McArthur WP, Bloom K, Taylor M, et al: Peripheral blood leukocyte populations in the elderly with and without periodontal disease. *J Clin Periodontol* 23:846, 1996.

158. Miyaji C, Watanabe H, Minagawa M, et al: Numerical and functional characteristics of lymphocyte subsets in centenarians. *J Clin Immunol* 17:420, 1997.

159. Ruiz M, Esparza B, Perez C, et al: CD8+ T cell subsets in aging. *Immunol Invest* 24:891, 1995.

160. Ritchie RF, Palomaki GE, Neveux LM, et al: Reference distributions for immunoglobulins A, G, and M: a practical, simple, and clinically relevant approach in a large cohort. *J Clin Lab Anal* 12:363, 1998.

161. Lock RJ, Unsworth DJ: Immunoglobulins and immunoglobulin subclasses in the elderly. *Ann Clin Biochem* 40:143, 2003.

162. Lichtman MA, Vaughn JH, Hames CG: The distribution of serum immunoglobulins, anti-gamma G globulins ("rheumatoid factors"), and antinuclear antibodies in Evans County, Georgia. *Arthritis Rheum* 10:204, 1967.

163. Chong A, Ikematsu H, Yamaji K, et al: Age-related accumulation of Ig V_H gene somatic mutations in peripheral B cells from aged humans. *Clin Exp Immunol* 133:59, 2003.

164. Axelsson U, Bachmann R, Hällén J: Frequency of pathological proteins (M-components) in 6995 sera from an adult population. *Acta Med Scand* 179:235, 1966.

165. Hällén J: Frequency of "abnormal" serum globulins (M-components) in the aged. *Acta Med Scand* 173:737, 1963.

166. Moesgaard F, Nielsen ML, Larsen N, et al: Cell-mediated immunity assessed by skin testing (Multitest). I. Normal values in healthy Danish adults. *Allergy* 42:591, 1987.

167. Stead WW, To T: Significance of the tuberculin skin test in elderly patients. *Ann Intern Med* 107:837, 1987.

168. Marrie TJ, Johnson S, Durant H: Cell-mediated immunity of healthy adult Nova Scotians in various age groups compared with nursing home and hospitalized senior citizens. *J Allergy Clin Immunol* 81:836, 1988.

169. Castle SC, Norman DC, Perls TT, et al: Analysis of cutaneous delayed-type hypersensitivity reaction and T cell proliferative response in elderly nursing home patients: An approach to identifying immunodeficient patients. *Gerontology* 36:217, 1990.

170. Wayne SJ, Rhyne RL, Garry PJ, Goodwin JS: Cell-mediated immunity as a predictor of morbidity and mortality in subjects over 60. *J Gerontol* 45:M45, 1990.

171. Chatta GS, Andrews RG, Rodger E, et al: Hematopoietic progenitors and aging: alterations in granulycytic precursors and responsiveness to recombinant human G-CSF, GM-CSF, and IL-3. *J Gerontol* 48:M207, 1993.

172. Angelis P, Scharf S, and Christophidis N: Effects of age on neutrophil function and its relevance to bacterial infections in the elderly. *J Clin Lab Immunol* 49:33, 1997.

173. MacGregor RR, Shalit M: Neutrophil function in healthy elderly subjects. *J Gerontol* 45:M55, 1990.

174. Esparza B, Sanchez H, Ruiz M, et al: Neutrophil function in elderly person assessed by flow cytometry. *Immunol Invest* 25:185, 1996.

175. Wenish C, Patruta S, Daxbock F, et al: Effect of age on human neutrophil function. *J Leuk Biol* 67:40, 2000.

176. Butcher SK, Chahal H, Nayak L, et al: Senescence in innate immune responses: reduced neutrophil phagocytic capacity and CD16 expression in elderly humans. *J Leuk Biol* 70:881, 2001.

177. Braga PC, Sala MT, Dal Sasso M, et al: Age-associated differences in neutrophil oxidative burst (chemiluminescence). *Exp Gerontol* 33:477, 1998.

178. Tortorella C, Piazzolla G, Napoli N, Antonaci S: Neutrophil apoptotic cell death: does it contributed to the increased infectious risk in aging? *Microbios* 106:129, 2001.

179. Di Lorenzo G, Balistreri CR, Candore G, et al: Granulocyte and natural killer activity in the elderly. *Mech Ageing Dev* 108:25, 1999.

180. Tortorella C, Piazzola G, Spaccavento F, et al: Spontaneous and Fas-induced apoptotic cell death in aged neutrophils. *J Clin Immunol* 18:321, 1998.

181. Fülöp T, Fouquet C, Allaire P, et al: Changes in apoptosis of human polymorphonuclear granulocytes with aging. *Mech Ageing Dev* 96:15, 1997.

182. McNerlan SE, Rea IM, Alexander HD, Morris TCM: Changes in natural killer cells, the CD57CD8 subset, and related cytokines in healthy aging. *J Clin Immunol* 18:31, 1998.

183. Solana R, Alonso MC, Pena J: Natural killer cells in healthy aging. *Exp Gerontol* 34:435, 1999.

184. Mariani E, Meneghetti A, Neri S, et al: Chemokine production by natural killer cells from nonagenarians. *Eur J Immunol* 32:1524, 2002.

185. Van Rensburg EJ, Heyns A du P: The effect of age, arteriosclerosis and hypercholesterolemia on platelet function tests, in *Thrombotic and Haemorrhagic Disorders,* Springer-Verlag, New York, 1990.

186. Zahavi J, Jones NRG, Leyton J, et al: Enhanced in vivo platelet "release reaction" in old healthy individuals. *Thromb Res* 17:329, 1980.

187. Fetkovska N, Amstein R, Ferraein F, et al: 5HT-kinetics and sensitivity of human blood platelets: Variations with age, gender and platelet number. *Thromb Haemost* 60:486, 1988.

188. Kasjanovova D, Balaz V: Age-related changes in human platelet function in vitro. *Mech Ageing Dev* 37:175, 1986.

189. Winther K, Naesh O: Aging and platelet β-adrenoceptor function. *Eur J Pharmacol* 136:219, 1987.

190. Vericel E, Croset M, Sedivy P, et al: Platelets and aging. I. Aggregation, arachidonate metabolism and antioxidant status. *Thromb Res* 49:331, 1988.

191. Winther K, Naesh O: Platelet alpha-adrenoreceptor function and aging. *Thromb Res* 46:677, 1987.

192. Bastyr EJ, Kadrofske MM, Vinik AI: Platelet activity and phosphoinositide turnover increase with advancing age. *Am J Med* 88:601, 1990.

193. Wang H-Y, Bashore TR, Friedman E: Exercise reduces age-dependent decrease in platelet protein kinase C activity and translocation. *J Gerontol* 50A:M12, 1995.

194. Di Massimo C, Penco M, Serri F, Tozzi-Ciancarelli MG: Possible involvement of increased susceptibility of LDL to oxidation in age-related platelet activation. *Clin Hemorheol Microcirc* 25:13, 2001.

195. Fornitz GG: Platelet function and fibrinolytic activity in borderline and mild hypertension. *Dan Med Bull* 49:210, 2002.

196. Goswami K, Koner BC: Level of sialic acid residues in platelet proteins in diabetes, aging, and Hodgkin's lymphoma: A potential role of free radicals in desialyation. *Biochem Biophys Res Com* 297:502, 2002.

197. Massimo CD, Taglieri G, Penco M, Tozzi-Ciancarelli MG: Influence of aging and exercise-induced stress on human platelet function. *Clin Hemorheol Microcirc* 20:105, 1999.

198. Kario K, Matsuo T, Kobayashi H, et al: Close relationship between hemostatic factors and acute-phase reaction as normal aging process. *J Am Geriatr Soc* 44:614, 1996.

199. Mari D, Mannucci PM, Coppola R, et al: Hypercoagulability in centenarians: The paradox of successful aging. *Blood* 85:3144, 1995.

200. Haverkate F, Thompson SG, Duckert F: Haemostasis factors in angina pectoris: relation to gender, age and acute phase reaction: results from the ECAT Angina Pectoris Study Group. *Thromb Haemost* 73:561, 1995.

201. Balleisen L, Bailey J, Epping P-H, et al: Epidemiological study on factor VII, factor VIII and fibrinogen in an industrial population. I. Baseline data on the relation to age, gender, body weight, smoking, alcohol, pill-using, and menopause. *Thromb Haemost* 54:475, 1985.

202. Scarabin PY, Van Dreden P, Bonithon-Kop C, et al: Age-related changes in factor VII activation in healthy women. *Clin Sci* 75:341, 1988.

203. Conlan MG, Folsom AR, Finch A, et al: Associations of Factor VIII and von Willebrand factor with age, race, sex, and risk factors for atherosclerosis. *Thromb Haemost* 70:380, 1993.

204. Ernst E, Rosch KL: Fibrinogen as a cardiovascular risk factor: A meta-analysis and review of the literature. *Ann Intern Med* 118:956, 1993.

205. Bauer KA, Weiss LM, Sparrow D, et al: Aging associated changes in indices of thrombin generation and protein C activation in humans: Normative aging study. *J Clin Invest* 80:1527, 1987.

206. Sundell B, Nilsson TK, Rainby M, et al: Fibrinolytic variables are related to age, sex, blood pressure, and body build measurements: A cross-sectional study in Norsjo, Sweden. *J Clin Epidemiol* 42:719, 1989.

207. Gudnason T, Hrafnkelsdottir T, Wall U, et al: Fibrinolytic capacity increases with age in healthy humans, while endothelium-dependent vasodilation is unaffected. *Thromb Haemost* 89:374, 2003.

208. Cadroy Y, Daviaud P, Saivin S, et al: Distribution of 16 hemostatic laboratory variables assayed in 100 blood donors. *Nouv Rev Fr Hematol* 32:259, 1990.

209. Dolan G, Neal K, Cooper P, et al: Protein C, antithrombin III and plasminogen: Effect of age, sex and blood group. *Brit J Haematol* 86:798, 1994.

210. Pieper CF, Murali K, Rao K, et al: Age, functional status and racial differences in plasma D-dimer levels in community-dwelling elderly persons. *J Gerontol A Biol Sci Med Sci* 55A:M649, 2000.

211. Juhan-Vague I, Renucci JF, Grimaus M, et al: Thrombin-activated fibrinolysis inhibitor antigen levels and cardiovascular risk factors. *Arterioscler Thromb Vasc Biol* 20:2156, 2000.

212. Schatteman KA, Goossens FJ, Scharpé SS, et al: Assay of procarboxypeptidase U, a novel determinant of the fibrinolytic cascade, in human plasma. *Clin Chem* 45:807, 1999.

213. Mehta J, Mehta P, Lawson D, Saldeen T: Plasma tissue plasminogen activator inhibitor levels in coronary artery disease: correlation with age and serum triglyceride concentrations. *J Am Coll Cardiol* 9:263, 1987.

214. Eliasson M, Evrin PE, Lundblad D, et al: Influence of gender, age, sampling time on fibrinolytic variables and fibrinogen. A population study. *Fibrinolysis* 7:316, 1993.

215. Siegert G, Bergmann S, Jaross W: Influence of age, gender and lipoprotein metabolism parameters on the activity of plasminogen activator inhibitor and the fibrinogen concentration. *Fibrinolysis* 6(suppl 3):47, 1992.

216. Cawkwell RC: Patient's age and the activated partial thromboplastin time test. *Thromb Haemost* 39:780, 1978.

217. Ibbotson SH, Tate GM, Davies JA: Thrombin activity by intrinsic activation of plasma in vitro accelerates with increasing age of the donor. *Thromb Haemost* 67:377, 1992.

218. Kario K, Matsuo T, Kobayashi H: Which factors affect high D-dimer levels in the elderly? *Thromb Res* 62:501, 1991.

219. Gurwitz JH, Avorn J, Ross-Oegnan D, et al: Aging and the anticoagulant response to warfarin therapy. *Ann Intern Med* 116:901, 1992.

220. Boyd RV, Hoffbrand BI: Erythrocyte sedimentation rate in elderly hospital in-patients. *Br Med J* 1:901, 1966.

221. Böttiger LE, Svedberg CA: Normal erythrocyte sedimentation rate and age. *Br Med J* 2:85, 1967.

222. Sharland DE: Erythrocyte sedimentation rate: The normal range in the elderly. *J Am Geriatr Soc* 28:346, 1980.

223. Sparrow D, Rowe JW, Silbert JE: Cross-sectional and longitudinal changes in the erythrocyte sedimentation rate in man. *J Gerontol* 36:180, 1981.

224. Choi JW, Pai SH: Influences of hypercholesterolemia on red cell indices and erythrocyte sedimentation rate in elderly persons. *Clin Chim Acta* 341:117, 2004.

225. Shearn MA, Kang IY: Effect of age and sex on the erythrocyte sedimentation rate. *J Rheumatol* 13:297, 1986.

226. Katz PR, Gutman SJ, Richman, et al: Erythrocyte sedimentation rate and C-reactive protein compared in the elderly. *Clin Chem* 35:466, 1989.

227. Katz PR, Karuza J, Gutman SI, et al: A comparison between erythrocyte sedimentation rate (ESR) and selected acute-phase proteins in the elderly. *Am J Clin Pathol* 94:637, 1990.

228. Ballou SP, Lozanski GP, Hadder S, et al: Quantitative and qualitative alterations of acute phase proteins in healthy elderly persons. *Age Ageing* 25:224, 1996.

229. Caswell M, Pike LA, Bull BS: Effect of patients' age on tests of the acute-phase response. *Arch Pathol Lab Med* 117:906, 1993.

230. Fulop T, Barabas G, Zsuzsa V, et al: Age-dependent changes in transmembrane signaling: Identification of g proteins in human lymphocytes and polymorphonuclear leukocytes. *Cell Signal* 5:593, 1993.

231. Shodell M, Siegal FP: Circulating, interferon-producing plasmacytoid dendritic cells decline during human ageing. *Scand J Immunol* 56:518, 2002.

232. Lung TL, Saurwein-Teissl M, Parson W, et al: Unimpaired dendritic cells can be derived from monocytes in old age and can mobilize residual function in senescent T cells. *Vaccine* 18:1606, 2000.

233. Sadeghi HM, Schnelle JF, Thomas JK, et al: Phenotypic and functional characteristics of circulating monocytes of elderly persons. *Exp Gerontol* 34:959, 1999.

234. Inadera H, Egashira K, Takemoto M, et al: Increase in circulating levels of monocyte chemoattractant protien-1 with aging. *J Interferon Cytokine Res* 19:1179, 1999.

235. Njemini R, Abeele MV, Demanet C, et al: Age-related decrease in the inducibility of heat-shock protein 70 in human peripheral blood mononuclear cells. *J Clin Immunol* 22:195, 2002.

236. Pawelec G, Solana R, Remarque E, Mariani E: Impact of aging on innate immunity. *J Leuk Biol* 64:703, 1998.

237. Koziol JA, Ho NJ, Felitti VJ, Beutler E: Reference centiles for serum ferritin and percent of transferrin saturation, with application to mutations of the *HFE* gene. *Clin Chem* 47:1804, 2001.

MOLECULAR
AND
CELLULAR
HEMATOLOGY

C H A P T E R 9

GENETIC PRINCIPLES AND MOLECULAR BIOLOGY

ERNEST BEUTLER

The understanding of hematology is more than ever dependent upon an appreciation of genetic principles and the tools that can be used to study genetic variation. All of the genetic information that makes up an organism is encoded in the DNA. This information is *transcribed* into RNA and then the triplet code of the RNA is *translated* into protein. Changes that affect the DNA or RNA sequence, either in the germ line or acquired after birth, can cause many hematologic disorders. These may be mutations that change the DNA sequence, including single base changes, deletions, insertions, or duplications, or they may be epigenetic changes that affect gene expression without any change in the DNA sequence.

The detection of defined mutations that cause a variety of diseases is now possible and has become a routine method for the diagnosis of some disorders, particularly prenatally. The development of methods to disrupt or to prevent expression of specific genes has made it possible to produce mouse models of human hematologic diseases, and such models have the potential to serve as means to better understand pathophysiology and to study treatment strategies.

Inheritance patterns depend upon the biologic effect and chromosomal location of the mutation. Common autosomal recessive hematologic diseases include sickle cell disease, the thalassemias, and Gaucher disease. Hereditary spherocytosis, thrombophilia caused by factor V Leiden, most forms of von Willebrand disease, and acute intermittent porphyria are characterized by autosomal dominant inheritance. Mutations that cause glucose-6-phosphate dehydrogenase deficiency, hemophilia A and B, and the most common form of chronic granulomatous disease are all carried on the X chromosome and therefore manifest X-linked inheritance, with transmission of the disease state from a heterozygous mother to her son. Understanding of the genetics of a disorder is necessary for accurate genetic counseling.

Many of the hematologic diseases described in this text have a genetic basis. Often the disease is caused by a mutation in a single gene. Some of these disorders, such as sickle cell disease (Chap. 47), thalassemia (Chap. 46), glucose-6-phosphate dehydrogenase deficiency (Chap. 45), and factor V Leiden (Chap. 116), are extremely common. Others such as congenital dyserythropoietic anemia type I (Chap. 37), chronic granulomatous disease (Chap. 66), and afibrinogenemia (Chap. 117) are rare, but all are caused by mutations in a gene that result in the formation of a defective protein or an insufficient amount of a normal protein. The principal focus of this chapter is such genetic disorders. However, a number of acquired hematologic diseases, including lymphomas, leukemias, and paroxysmal nocturnal hemoglobinuria, are the consequence of acquired damage to the genetic apparatus. Understanding these diseases requires an appreciation of how the genetic apparatus functions.

All of the information required for the development of a complete adult organism is encoded in the DNA of a single cell, the zygote. This information, designated the *genome*, includes the data needed for the synthesis of all enzymes; all the plasma proteins, including the clotting factors, complement components, and the transport proteins; all the membrane proteins, including receptors; and all of the cytoskeletal proteins. The units of information into which the genome is organized are the *genes*. Genetic diseases are the result of changes, or *mutations*, in these genes.

THE PATTERN OF INHERITANCE

The inheritance of each genetic disease follows a distinctive pattern. The concept of dominant and recessive inheritance is one of the most deeply ingrained in our genetic thinking. It has long played a primary role in the introduction of every high school student of biology to genetics and is used extensively in the classification of genetic disease. A dominant disease is one that is expressed when the patient has only a single copy of the mutant gene, that is, in the heterozygous state. A recessive disease, on the other hand, is expressed only when both copies of the gene are abnormal. If the mutations on both alleles are the same, the patient is said to be *homozygous*. If two different abnormal alleles have been inherited, then the patient is designated as being a *compound heterozygote*. It is often implied that genes are dominant or recessive. This is incorrect. It is disease states or phenotypes that are dominant or recessive. The gene for sickle cell hemoglobin is expressed in the heterozygous state, so that the carrier of this gene has sickle cell trait. Sickle cell trait is therefore dominant, but sickle cell disease, which occurs in the homozygote, is recessive. By definition, the phenotype of an individual heterozygous for a mutation causing recessive disease does not differ from the phenotype of an individual homozygous for the normal gene.

The principles of dominant and recessive disease can be readily applied to mutations occurring on the *autosomes* (chromosomes other than the X chromosome), but the situation is somewhat different when dealing with genes on the X chromosome. Although the X chromosome is involved in the sex determination process, most of the genes on the X chromosome have nothing whatsoever to do with sex determination. Some of the hematologically more important of these "X-linked" genes include those which code for glucose-6-phosphate dehydrogenase (G-6-PD), phosphoglycerate kinase, factor VIII, factor IX, Bruton-type agammaglobulinemia, one form of chronic granulomatous disease, and one of the enzymes required for the synthesis of the phosphatidylinositol anchor that is involved in the etiology of paroxysmal nocturnal hemoglobinemia (PNH).

THE FAMILY HISTORY

A carefully taken family history can give a physician considerable insight into the nature of a hematologic disorder. One should ascertain whether another member of the family has had a similar disease. In the case of patients with anemia, this is often difficult, because so many women have a history of anemia, usually as a result of iron deficiency. To estimate the severity of anemia, it is particularly germane to inquire whether transfusion was required. A history of gallstones, particularly at an early age, may indicate that a hemolytic disorder was present. Similarly, episodes of jaundice in family members may be the only clue to the existence of familial hemolytic anemia.

Presence of the disease in one of the parents strongly suggests a dominant mode of transmission. If neither parent is affected, but one or more siblings have the disease, an autosomal recessive transmission is more likely. Consanguinity of the patient's parents makes it highly probable that a disease is an autosomal recessive disorder. Occurrence primarily in male siblings and maternal uncles, with mild or absent manifestations of the disease in the mother, suggests a X-linked mode of inheritance. Father-to-son transmission rules out X linkage.

Lack of any family history does not rule out the genetic basis of a disease. In some instances, the disease may be so mild in other family members that it is not recognized. Whenever possible, the family members should be examined, rather than relying solely on history. In some instances, of course, the gene mutation causing the disorder may have arisen in the generation in which the disease presents.

Once the mode of genetic transmission is clear, the diagnostic alternatives are narrowed considerably. For example, methemoglobinemia transmitted as an autosomal dominant disorder is caused by hemoglobin M, whereas methemoglobinemia transmitted as an autosomal recessive disorder is caused by NADH diaphorase (cytochrome b5 reductase) deficiency. Hemolytic anemia with autosomal dominant transmission is likely to be caused by hereditary spherocytosis, but sex-linked transmission of the hemolytic state suggests a deficiency of G-6-PD or, more rarely, phosphoglycerate kinase. A bleeding disorder that is transmitted in a sex-linked fashion may be caused by a deficiency of factor VIII or factor IX, but autosomal recessive inheritance should suggest to the physician a deficiency of other clotting factors, such as V, X, or XI. Careful analysis of the family history not only will make possible more appropriate genetic counseling to the patient and family, but also will shorten the road to a correct diagnosis.

LINKAGE

In human somatic cells chromosomes are present in pairs—1 pair of sex chromosomes (two X chromosomes in females and an X and Y in males) and 22 pairs of autosomes. One chromosome of each pair is distributed into the gametes, so that eggs and sperm of humans each contain 23 chromosomes.

If two genes are located on different chromosomes or are far apart on the same chromosome, they are said to be unlinked. This means the chance of inheriting each of the genes is independent of the other. For example, if a parent is a carrier of pyruvate kinase deficiency and sickle cell trait, which are caused by genes on different autosomes, the chance of an offspring inheriting pyruvate kinase deficiency is 1 in 2 and the chance of an offspring inheriting sickle cell trait is 1 in 2. Therefore one-fourth of the offspring will inherit both pyruvate kinase deficiency and sickle cell trait, one-fourth the offspring will inherit neither, one-fourth will inherit only sickle cell trait, and one-fourth will inherit only pyruvate kinase deficiency.

If the two genes in question are close together on the same chromosome, however, the situation may be quite different. For example, the genes encoding glucocerebrosidase (Gaucher disease) and pyruvate kinase are both on the long arm of chromosome 1. If a mother carries mutations in both these genes on the same chromosome, the proba-

bility of her child's inheriting either both of the abnormal genes or neither of the abnormal genes is much greater than the probability of the child's inheriting one or the other. Yet the inheritance of only one of these two genes is not an impossibility because of the phenomenon of crossing-over during meiosis. In the course of the formation of germ cells, homologous pairs of chromosomes come into side-by-side apposition and regularly exchange chromosomal material. Thus two genes that were originally on the same chromosome may find themselves on separate chromosomes after germ cell formation (Fig. 9-1). The probability of their being separated during meiosis is a function of their distance from one another on the chromosome, and this distance is expressed in terms of map units or Morgans. One-hundredth of a Morgan, a centimorgan (cM), represents the genetic distance that gives a 1 percent probability per generation of a crossover between the two genes. A rule of thumb is that this corresponds to a physical distance of 1 megabase (1,000,000 base pairs), but the actual physical distance represented by a centimorgan varies a great deal from one location in the genome to another. In fact, the correlation between physical distance and recombination distance varies a great deal even at the same location between the sexes.

It is not unusual for genes on the same chromosome to be so far apart that the probability of their finding themselves in separate germ cells is just as great as though they had been on separate chromosomes. The genes encoding red cell pyruvate kinase and glucocerebrosidase are very tightly linked[1] and, not surprisingly, the physical distance between their 5′ ends is only 71,000 base pairs.[2]

X LINKAGE AND X INACTIVATION

The chromosomal complement of males differs from that of females in that males have one X chromosome and one Y chromosome, whereas females have two X chromosomes. However, early in embryonic development, one of the two X chromosomes of somatic cells of female mammals becomes transcriptionally inactive. In some cells, the paternally derived chromosome is inactivated; in others, the maternally derived chromosome is inactivated.[3,4] Inactivation remains fixed, so that all the progeny of the cell in which the maternally derived X chromosome is inactive show only the gene products from the paternal X. Female heterozygotes for X-linked genes such as G-6-PD deficiency, phosphoglycerate kinase deficiency, factor VIII, or factor IX deficiency are therefore a mosaic of cells, some of which manifest the full-blown deficiency, as it is found in affected males, and some of which are normal. Inactivation is a process controlled by the XIST gene[5]; the final proportion of cells with one or the other X chromosome active depends upon random factors, and on selection between cell populations which may occur following the inactivation process.[6,7] The process of X inactivation is not only useful in understanding the ex-

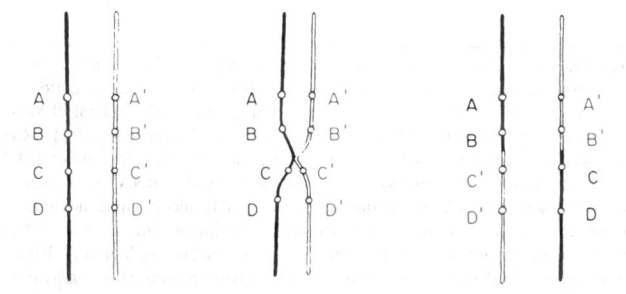

FIGURE 9-1   Representation of equal crossing-over during meiosis. There has been an exchange of chromosomal material between the maternally derived and paternally derived chromosome, but all genes are represented on the products of the crossover.

pression of X-linked diseases in women, but is valuable in studying the possible clonal origin of a variety of disorders. As shown in Fig. 9-2, the progeny of a single cell of a female heterozygous for an X-linked gene will manifest only the phenotype of the original cell. Examination of electrophoretically distinguishable variants of G-6-PD has made it possible to demonstrate that the red cells are a clone in chronic myelogenous leukemia,[8] in paroxysmal nocturnal hemoglobinuria, [9] and probably in acute myelogenous leukemia.[10,11] This implies that each of these disorders arises through transformation of a single cell and that, in the case of the leukemias, erythroid cells as well as leukocytes are part of the malignant clone.

The development of DNA-based technology has made it possible to use X-linked genes as a clonal marker even when there is not a different protein product from the two alleles. A different pattern of methylation of cytidines distinguishes the active from the inactive X chromosome.[12] This fact, together with the existence of restriction endonucleases that distinguish methylated from unmethylated cytidine, has made it possible to use restriction fragment length polymorphisms to determine the clonal origin of neoplasms,[13,14] even when no polymorphism involving an X-linked enzyme is available. The existence of polymorphisms involving the coding region of genes also makes possible the detection of clones by reverse transcription and amplification of messenger RNA (mRNA).[15,16]

The pattern of genetic transmission of X-linked genes is characteristic: a father cannot transmit an X-linked gene to his son; the offspring is a boy by virtue of the fact that he inherited the father's Y chromosome, not his X chromosome. Conversely, it is a truism that males always inherit X-linked genes from their mother and that the mother must therefore be either heterozygous or homozygous for the gene. Because X inactivation is random, however, the degree of expression of mutant alleles of X-linked genes in females is highly variable. This is why, even with the most sophisticated phenotypic assessment, it is not always possible to detect the heterozygous state in the mother of an affected individual. It also explains why even twin carriers of diseases such as factor VIII deficiency can have very different levels of the clotting factor.

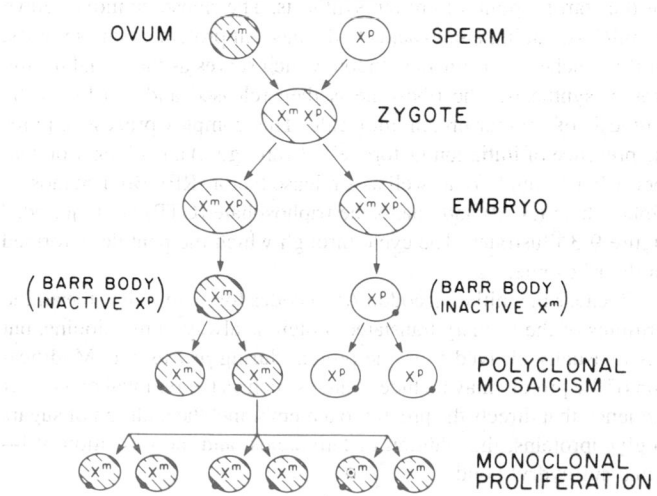

FIGURE 9-2   At fertilization, the female zygote inherits one maternal chromosome (X^m) and one paternal X chromosome (X^p). At some time early in embryogenesis, one X in each cell is inactivated at random and condenses to form the Barr body. The active X remains active not only for the lifetime of that cell but for the lifetime of all of its progeny. A tumor with a clonal origin will consist entirely of cells in all of which either X^m or X^p is active. A tumor with a multicentric origin may contain both X^m and X^p cells.

MITOCHONDRIAL INHERITANCE

The vast majority of the genetic material in cells is encoded in the chromosomal nuclear DNA. However, mitochondria have their own replicating DNA. Apparently having arisen from symbiotic bacteria over a billion years ago, the DNA of mitochondrial DNA (mtDNA) exists as a closed circular molecule of 16,569 nucleotides. This DNA encodes 13 polypeptides, all of which are subunits of the mitochondrial energy-producing pathway, a small and a large ribosomal RNA, and 22 transfer RNAs.[17] Some proteins found in mitochondria are, however, encoded in nuclear DNA. Mitochondria are transmitted through the egg; thus inheritance is entirely maternal.[18,19] Cells contain several hundred mitochondria, each with several copies of mtDNA. To become clinically significant, mitochondrial mutations must confer some selective advantage upon the mitochondrion with the mutation; mutations that affect only a few of the hundreds of mitochondria in each cell are unlikely to produce a phenotype. Mitochondrial mutations, often consisting of deletions, are responsible for a number of neurologic diseases.[18] Some of the childhood myelodysplastic syndromes,[20,21] particularly Pearson marrow-pancreas syndrome,[22] are hematologic manifestations of mitochondrial mutations.

EPIGENETICS

Even genetically identical individuals may differ in their phenotype. For example, genetically identical mice homozygous for the agouti gene may differ markedly in their coat color, and this has been attributed to random inactivation of an upstream retrotransposon.[23] The inactivation of the X-chromosome by *XIST*[5] is another example. Relatively little is understood of the factors that produce epigenetic changes, but most attention has been paid to methylation of CpG dinucleotides and the acetylation of histones.[24]

DNA AND THE GENETIC CODE

Understanding how the massive amount of information required to allow a complex organism to grow and survive is coded is one of the major advances of modern biology. The information is all contained in the polynucleotide, DNA. DNA contains only four different bases—adenine (A), guanine (G), thymine (T), and cytosine (C). DNA exists as a double helix in which A is always paired with T, and G is always paired with C.

The two ends of a strand of DNA are not the same. The nucleosides that make up each strand are linked to each other through a molecule of phosphoric acid, attached to the 3' carbon of the deoxyribose of one nucleoside and to the 5' carbon of the next one. A linear strand of DNA thus has one end in which the hydroxyl group attached to the 5' carbon is free; at the other end the hydroxyl group attached to the 3' carbon is not involved in a link. These ends are designated the 5' and 3' ends, respectively, and, by convention, the 5' end is drawn at the left and is called the "upstream" end. The 3' end is designated as "downstream." In the pairing of two complementary strands of DNA, the polarity of the two strands is opposite (antiparallel); that is, the 5' end of each strand is paired with the 3' end of the other. By convention, the strand shown at the top is the coding, or "sense" strand, but the strand at the bottom is the one that actually serves as a template for RNA synthesis. Thus the sequence of the mRNA corresponds to that of the top strand, and the triplet code may be read from this strand.

It is the faithful pairing of A with T and C with G in double-stranded DNA that makes possible the accurate replication of the genetic code. When cells divide, the two DNA strands separate. As this occurs, the bases of the separate strands pair with the complementary purine or pyrimidine nucleotide which become linked to each other, forming a complementary strand of nucleotides. In this way, the cell forms two double strands that are identical with the original double strand.

The sequence of base pairs in the DNA strand specifies the sequence of amino acids in proteins. Each base cannot represent a single amino acid, because only four bases are found in DNA and there are 20 commonly occurring amino acids in proteins. Similarly, pairs of bases are not sufficient; they could code for only 16 amino acids. A triplet code is therefore the minimum number of bases that is required to code for 20 amino acids. The genetic code has been found, in fact, to consist of triplets: each amino acid is specified by one or more sequences of three bases. Long stretches of the triplet code are colinear with the amino acid sequence of the protein whose synthesis the gene specifies, but these stretches are separated by intervening sequences or introns that do not encode the amino acid sequence of the protein. Moreover, DNA does not directly assemble amino acids into protein. This is achieved through a mechanism that involves another polynucleotide, RNA. There are two differences between DNA and RNA. First, the nucleotide units contain ribose instead of deoxyribose. Second, in RNA uridine (U) is used instead of the thymidine (T) component of DNA. mRNA is synthesized with a base sequence determined by the DNA, which serves as a template in a copying process that is designated as *transcription*. The mRNA is then *translated* into protein.

TRANSCRIPTION

The transcription of DNA into mRNA is the first step in gene expression. For a gene to be transcribed, a promoter must be located "upstream" (i.e., in the 5′ direction) from the coding region. Typical promoters have certain sequences in common. These include a "CAT box," the cytosine- and guanine-rich CCAAT sequence, and a TAATA box, an adenine- and thymine-rich sequence. Mutations in these regions impair transcription of a gene; such lesions have been identified as causes of the thalassemias, and are discussed in greater detail in Chap. 46. The effectiveness of a promoter may be increased by more distant DNA sequences, known as *enhancers*, which may be either upstream or downstream of the gene. The identification of sequences that enhance expression of the globin genes has been of particular importance in designing vectors for gene transfer to remedy the hemoglobinopathies (see Chap. 26).[25,26]

RNA PROCESSING

The mRNA that is formed on the DNA template by RNA polymerase is not ready to be translated to a polypeptide. First it must be processed, adding a cap to the 3′ end and a poly-A tail to the 5′ end and by removing introns. Capping consists of formation of an atypical 5′ to 5′ triphosphate bond between the 5′ terminus of the mRNA and a molecule of 7-methylguanosine. The addition of a poly-A tail serves to stabilize the mRNA. Recognition of a sequence (AAUAAA) serves as a signal that a poly-A tail should be added at a point that is approximately 15 bases downstream from the signal when another consensus sequence, YGTGTTYY (where Y stands for a pyrimidine, i.e., thymine or cytidine), is present further downstream. Sometimes more than one adenylation signal is present, and then additional species of mRNA with 3′ portions differing in length are formed.

Excision of introns is particularly important, because they interrupt the coding sequence. The first (5′) bases of the intron are always GpU and the last (3′) bases are always ApG (the p represents the phosphate bond between the nucleosides). But there are many such couplets in the RNA and additional information is required for an actual splice site to exist. The nature of this information has not been clearly defined, but a "consensus" sequence that most splice sites resemble closely has been defined. Removal of the intron is a complex enzymatic process.[27] Splicing of a given normal mRNA does not always occur in the same manner. Sometimes "alternative splicing" occurs, so that after processing, some of the mRNA molecules contain an exon that is missing from other messenger molecules. This is a powerful mechanism that allows a single gene to direct the synthesis of more than one polypeptide. Potentially the type of polypeptide made can be modulated according to need, and different tissues and different developmental stages may utilize different splice sites to make tissue-specific polypeptides. Alternative splicing has been important, for example, in producing different forms of erythrocyte membrane band 4.1[28] and different forms of pyruvate kinase for the liver and for the erythrocyte.[29] It is a powerful mechanisms that allows that body to produce more than 100,000 proteins from some 30,000 genes. On the other hand, mutations may cause missplicing. Usually this results in decreased protein production, as in hemoglobin E disease, no protein production, as in some Gaucher disease mutations and thalassemia (see Chap. 46), and, in rare cases, increased protein production, as in dominant thrombocythemia.[30]

TRANSLATION

Processed mRNA contains the code for the synthesis of proteins, and an elaborate mechanism has evolved for the *translation* of the triplet code in the mRNA into protein. A ribosomal complex, consisting of ribosomal RNA (rRNA) subunits and protein components, attaches to the 5′ end of the mRNA. The transport of the needed amino acids to the ribosomal complex is achieved by clover-shaped RNA molecules designated transfer RNA (tRNA). tRNA molecules contain a recognition site that binds to a triplet on mRNA and a site that carries the amino acid appropriate for that triplet to the mRNA, where the ribosomal complex creates the peptide bond between it and the amino acid that is immediately 5′ to it. The initiation of protein synthesis is almost always at an AUG codon,[31] usually one quite near the 5′ end of the messenger RNA. A consensus sequence around this codon marks it for the starting point of protein synthesis. The ribosome moves down the mRNA, adding amino acids to the nascent protein chain as it goes, until it reaches a termination codon, which serves as the signal to stop protein synthesis. The ribosome is then released and can begin the synthesis of another protein molecule. This complex process requires the presence of initiation factors (eIF-1 through 6) and elongation factors (EF-1 through 3), as well as a release factor (RF). Both adenosine triphosphate (ATP) and guanosine triphosphate (GTP) are required.[32] Figure 9-3 illustrates. The cycle through which the peptide is formed on the ribosome.

Because the initiation codon AUG codes for methionine, the amino terminus of the primary translated protein is always a methionine, but this is usually cleaved from the protein during *processing*. Modification of the protein may include changes such as the removal of a leader sequence that directs the protein to a membrane, the addition of sugars to glycoproteins, the addition of fatty acids, and the formation of internal sulfhydryl bonds.

REGULATION

Many genes are highly specialized in their function. Hemoglobin is made only by erythrocyte precursors, crystallin only by the lens, and immunoglobulins only by lymphoid cells. Such genes must be silenced in other types of cells. On the other hand, so-called *housekeeping genes* produce their products in all cells. The latter include the enzymes of

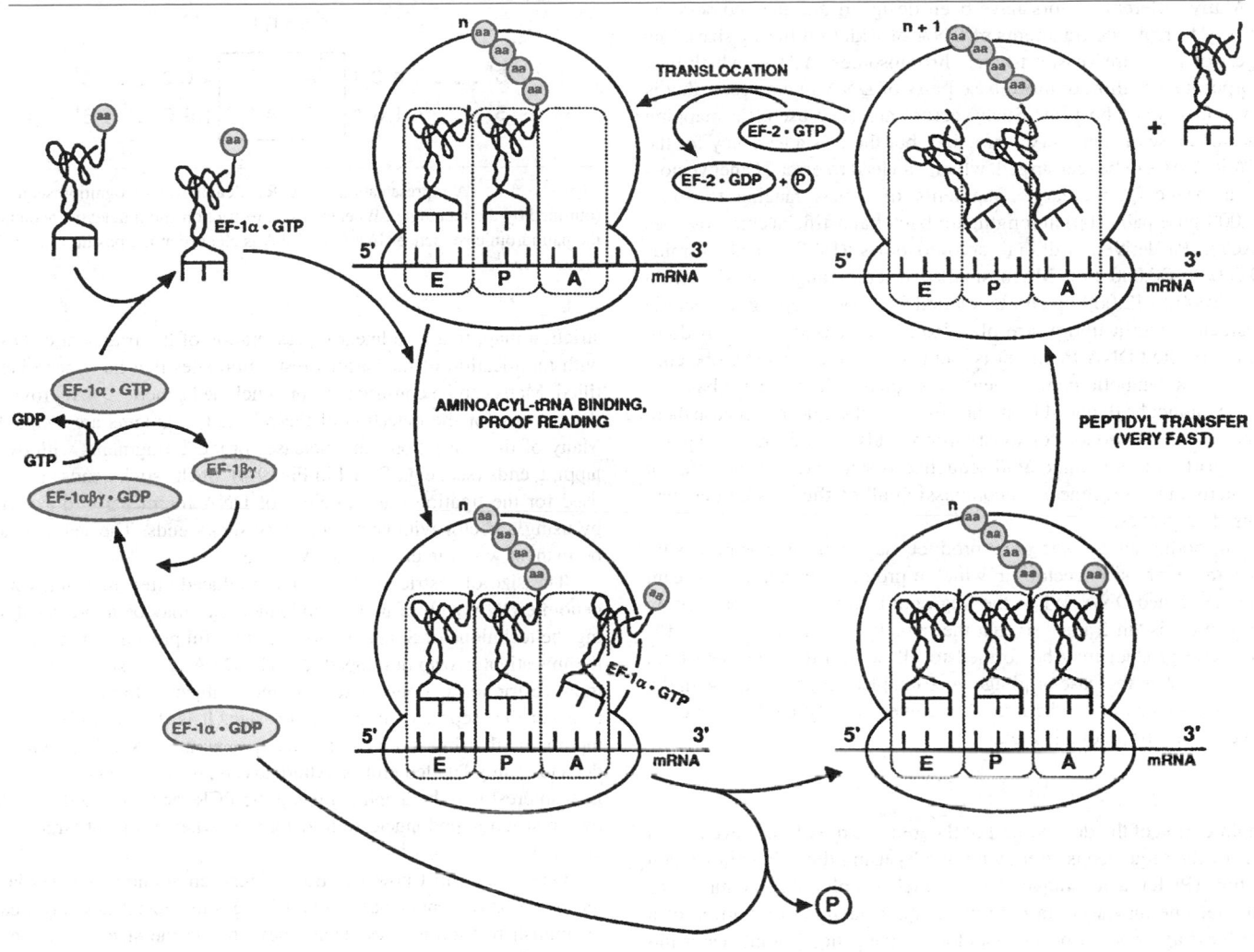

FIGURE 9-3 The elongation of a polypeptide as the ribosome moves down the mRNA. Each amino acid (*aa*) is added to the preceding one by the coordinated activity of elongation factors (*EF*). From Merrick[32] with permission.

the basic metabolic processes that provide energy to all cells, such as hexokinase, phosphoglycerate kinase, and G-6-PD, or genes that encode basic structural proteins.

Clearly, an elaborate system for the regulation of protein production exists in all organisms, and this system is only beginning to be understood. Regulation of transcription determines to a large extent whether a protein will be synthesized.[33] Promoters and enhancers are activated by transcription factors that are produced by the cell. Such factors, in turn, may be activated or inactivated by phosphorylation and by other processes. How enhancers act at a distance to increase the activity of promoters is not well understood, and the locus control region of the globin genes is serving as a paradigm in gaining understanding of possible interactions between transcription factors, enhancers, and promoters. Regulation also occurs at the translational level. The mRNA of ferritin contains an iron-responsive element that binds to an 87-kDa regulatory protein in the absence of iron, effectively shutting off translation.[34] The same type of binding site in the 3' untranslated region of the transferrin receptor mRNA serves to stabilize the message by allowing the protein to bind in the absence of iron.[35] Similarly, a UA-rich portion in the 3' untranslated portion of the tumor necrosis factor gene serves to inhibit translation of that mRNA.[36] It is also likely that the stability of the mRNA itself is regulated by nucleases.[37,38]

THE METHODS OF MOLECULAR BIOLOGY

CLONING DNA

The sequencing of DNA and the preparation of probes require that a fragment of DNA is amplified manyfold to provide a relatively pure sample for study. The classic method by which this is achieved, cloning, is one of the central techniques of molecular biology. It is generally accomplished by inserting the DNA into a vector, a bacteriophage or plasmid, that normally replicates within a bacterial cell. When such a phage or plasmid contains a foreign DNA fragment, the fragment also undergoes replication and can then be purified in greatly amplified form.

If the DNA is not available in pure form to begin with, it must be purified from a collection of DNA fragments that is designated a *library*. An adequate genomic library consists of millions of fragments of the genetic material of a cell that have been ligated into a suitable vector. Another valuable type of library is made by transcribing mRNA from a tissue into complementary DNA (cDNA) using the enzyme reverse transcriptase. Such a cDNA library is particularly useful for the isolation of genes because in it are represented only the intron-free portions of genes that are being actively transcribed in a tissue. In contrast, a genomic library represents all of the genetic material, coded and noncoded, transcribed and nontranscribed.

Many different vectors have been designed and they possess the capacity to replicate fragments of DNA of widely differing sizes. The largest of these are yeast artificial chromosomes (YACs), which may incorporate a million or more base pairs of DNA into a vector that is grown in a yeast host.[39,40] Such vectors are very useful in mapping genes because of their very large size, but there is a tendency for the DNA in YACs to be rearranged, which can lead to errors. Other vectors that also incorporate large fragments of DNA, ranging to about 100,000 base pairs (bp) in length, are bacterial artificial chromosomes (BACs), P1-derived artificial chromosomes (PACs), and cosmids (20,000 to 30,000 bp). Much smaller inserts, ranging in size from about 3000 to 12,000 bp can be cloned into bacteriophages. Bacteria transfected with a library are plated on a semisolid culture medium and the desired DNA fragment is identified with a labeled probe consisting of a synthetic complementary sequence. The precise base sequence cannot be deduced from the amino acid sequence because there is more than one codon for most amino acids. However, if an appropriate portion of an amino acid sequence is selected, several different complementary sequences, encompassing all of the possibilities may be used as probes.

Antibodies against the gene product may also serve as probes by using an "expression vector" in which a promoter is present upstream from the cloned DNA. When the fragment is in the correct orientation and when it is "in frame" so that the triplets are read correctly, sufficient gene product may be formed to allow immunologic detection. Colonies (or, in the case of phage vectors, plaques) that react with the probe are picked and subcultured at lower density until a single reactive colony or plaque is isolated.

THE POLYMERASE CHAIN REACTION

Amplification of the desired part of the genome may be achieved when some of the sequence is already known by using the polymerase chain reaction (PCR), a technique that is much simpler than cloning. For example, one may wish to determine the sequence of a portion of a gene for diagnostic purposes, but cloning the gene(s) of interest is too time-consuming and labor intensive to be practical. Two primers, matching opposite strands of DNA on either side of the region of interest, are used to amplify the intervening segment of DNA by more than a million fold. Successive cycles of DNA synthesis from the primers and chain separation by heating between the cycles are the basis of this powerful technique.[41,42] The polymerase chain reaction is so sensitive that under optimal conditions the DNA from a single cell may be amplified. Moreover, the stability of DNA is such that very old preserved material may be used. Thus, it is possible to amplify the DNA from blood smears,[43] mummies, and even from insects preserved in amber for more than 25,000,000 years.[44] Amplifying by PCR cDNA produced by reverse-transcribing mRNA in tissue extracts (reverse transcriptase polymerase chain reaction [RT-PCR]) provides a very sensitive means for measuring the expression of genes in tissues.

CUTTING DNA WITH RESTRICTION ENDONUCLEASES

The discovery that many bacteria elaborate enzymes that cleave double-stranded DNA at the sites of very specific sequences greatly facilitated the study of DNA. Such enzymes generally recognize palindromes, that is, DNA sequences that read the same in one direction on the upper strand and in the opposite direction in the lower strand. Figure 9-4 illustrates how one such palindrome is cleaved by the commonly used restriction endonuclease, EcoRI. Several hundred restriction endonucleases are now commercially available.

Restriction endonucleases are useful both for cloning DNA and for analyzing its structure. By digesting DNA with various endonucleases and combinations of endonucleases one may construct a re-

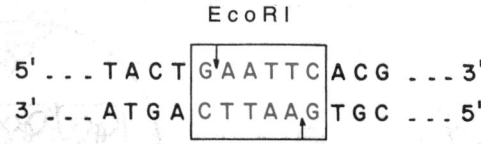

FIGURE 9-4 A representation of EcoR1 cleaving its recognition sequence (outlined by the rectangle). Whenever this restriction endonuclease encounters the palindromic sequence GAATTC, DNA is cleaved at the position shown by the *arrows.*

striction map, that is, a linear representation of the fragment of DNA with the location of the various restriction sites that have been identified. Maps can be constructed from uncloned genetic DNA, provided that probes for the detection of the relevant fragments are available. Many of the restriction endonucleases produce fragments with overlapping ends (see, e.g., EcoRI in Fig. 9-4). Such "sticky ends" may be used for the ligation (i.e., splicing) of DNA fragments into a vector by using a vector with complementary sticky ends. The seal is made permanent with the enzyme DNA ligase.

The size of restriction fragments produced after digesting whole genomic DNA with restriction endonucleases may be appreciated using the technique of Southern blotting, a useful procedure named after the investigator who developed it.[45] The DNA is digested with one or more restriction endonucleases and then subjected to electrophoresis in a gel that separates fragments by size. It is then transferred to a membrane that binds DNA, and the appropriate DNA fragments are detected using labeled probes. Alternatively, the segment of DNA that is of interest may be amplified using the PCR technique and digested by a restriction endonuclease to determine whether or not target sites are present.

One of the most powerful uses of restriction endonucleases is in the detection of genetic variability. Changes in nucleotides may create or abolish restriction sites. Thus, they change the size of fragments that are formed when the DNA is digested. Such areas of variability represent restriction fragment length polymorphisms (RFLPs). In some cases, the changes in nucleotide sequence may be the ones that cause the disease itself. For example, the sickle cell mutation causes disappearance of a restriction site recognized by the enzyme *Mst* II[46] and the G-6-PD A mutation causes the formation of a restriction site recognized by *Nla* III; such changes are valuable in diagnosis (see Chaps. 45 and 47).

Deletions of chromosomal material, as occur in α-thalassemia, also produce changes in fragment sizes. Larger fragments may appear if the deleted fragment contains a restriction site or smaller fragments if it does not. If the area covered by the probe is deleted in its entirety, as occurs in hydrops fetalis, no band will be seen at all. Even when the lesion that causes the disease does not directly affect a restriction site, RLFPs may be valuable in disease detection by virtue of close linkage to a disease-causing gene. Multiple restriction sites near the gene of interest produce haplotypes that may unequivocally identify a chromosome. Such haplotypes are particularly useful in the prenatal diagnosis of the thalassemias (see Chap. 46).

SEQUENCING

The chain termination technique[47] is commonly used to determine the sequence of DNA. It depends on synthesizing a labeled strand of DNA, with the DNA to be sequenced serving as the template. The mixture of nucleotides used contains, in addition to the native deoxynucleotides, a nucleotide analogue that results in chain termination when incorporated. The normal nucleotides are present in excess, and therefore chain termination occurs only sporadically, but always when the analogue is incorporated. Four different incubation mixtures are used, each with an analogue of one of the four nucleotides. Gel electrophoresis of the labeled products produces "ladders" of polynucleotides. The size of each fragment depends on the point at which there exists a nucleotide corresponding to the chain terminating analogue in the mixture. Sequencing can now be carried out rapidly and accurately by automated methods in which the elongation of the strand is terminated by a fluorescent nucleotide.[48]

Although DNA sequencing formerly required cloning of the fragment to be studied, amplification by PCR serves as a simpler alternative when the surrounding sequences are known.

DETECTING MUTATIONS IN INDIVIDUAL PATIENTS

The cloning and sequencing of DNA is too time-consuming to permit application for diagnostic purposes for individual patients. Fortunately, there are shortcuts that can be used when the nature of the lesion is known and a yes-or-no answer is sought with regard to the existence of a certain substitution. The value of restriction sites was discussed above (see "Cutting DNA with Restriction Endonucleases"), but because many substitutions neither abolish nor create restriction sites, the use of restriction endonucleases is not feasible in every case. However, a mismatch in one of the primers used in amplifying DNA by PCR, selected so as to create a restriction site where none existed before, is a technique that has been used successfully to detect mutations.[49] Using amplifying primers that fit one genotype but not the other has been used in "color PCR"[50] and in the "amplification refractory mutation system (ARMS)."[51] The failure of fragments of DNA to ligate when aligned on a template in which there is a misfit of the terminal nucleotide also has been used to detect mutations.[52] The hybridization of labeled oligonucleotide probes with a defined sequence to an amplified DNA target, a method designated allele-specific oligonucleotide hybridization (ASOH), is also very useful.[53] Probes containing approximately 17 nucleotides fitting either the normal or the mutant sequence are hybridized to PCR-amplified DNA. A single mismatch in an oligonucleotide of this size produces a sufficient change in melting temperature (i.e., the temperature at which the strands of DNA separate) that the two sequences can be distinguished from one another.

When the mutation is not known, other techniques may prove useful. Single-stranded conformation polymorphism (SSCP) analysis takes advantage of the fact that a single base substitution will usually change the conformation of single-stranded DNA and change its migration in a gel when subjected to electrophoresis. Denaturing high-pressure liquid chromatography is a more recent embodiment of this technique that appears to be highly efficient in detecting mutations.[54]

EXPERIMENTAL INTERFERENCE WITH GENE EXPRESSION

It is possible to interdict the expression of a gene at several different levels. Genes can be interrupted in murine embryonic stem cells by the process of *targeted disruption*, destroying their function.[55,56] Such knockout mice (a subset of *transgenic* mice, see below) can provide valuable insights into the function of genes and serve as animal models of human disease.

The translation of mRNA can be inhibited and the RNA degraded by placing *antisense* RNA or DNA into cells; these molecules have a sequence complementary to the mRNA that is to be inactivated. When such oligonucleotides are present, they inhibit gene expression through a variety of mechanisms. For example, they form a double strand with the RNA, just as two complementary strands of DNA will hybridize to form the normal double-stranded form of DNA. Because the double-stranded form cannot be translated and is probably degraded rapidly,

the production of its protein product is inhibited specifically. Because antisense RNA can be produced in vivo by transcribing the complementary strand of a gene, it may represent a natural regulatory mechanism.[57-59] In experimental systems, antisense DNA or stable DNA analogues such as the methylphosphonates[60] can be transfected directly into cells, or the RNA can be made by a plasmid with the appropriate DNA template and a promoter. Some of the uses of this approach include the suppression of lymphoma growth with DNA oligonucleotides antisense to introns of the oncogene c-myc,[61] the suppression of the growth of marrow cells from patients with chronic myelogenous leukemia by antisense DNA directed at the BCR-ABL junction,[62] the down-regulation of growth of BCL-2-positive lymphoma cells in culture by BCL-2 antisense,[63] and the inhibition of Friend murine erythroleukemia cell growth by transfection with a plasmid that produced antisense to c-jun.[64] Small interfering RNAs (siRNAs) and the closely related microRNAs (miRNAs) represent a more recently discovered mechanism for silencing of genes.[65,66] Double-stranded RNA is cleaved by an enzyme designated "dicer" into approximately 22-base pair segments that trigger the destruction of the homologous mRNA[67] in the case of siRNA, or interfere with translation in the case of miRNA.[65] Because siRNA molecules can act as primers to make additional double-stranded RNA, again converted to siRNA by dicer, the suppression of mRNA can be very long-lasting. This mechanism seems to be widely used as a gene regulatory and antiviral measure. Evidence has been presented that suggests that miRNA may play an important role in hematopoietic differentiation.[68] Moreover, the use of siRNA has become very useful to molecular biologists as an alternative method for the down-regulation of genes in experimental systems.

The discovery of the enzymatic activity of certain forms of RNA represents a major advance in our understanding of how life may have originated on earth. Cleaving RNA at defined sequences, much as restriction endonucleases cleave DNA, is one of the known enzymatic functions of RNA, and this function provides a means by which the expression of a gene can be interdicted in experimental systems. This *ribozyme* approach has been used, for example, in preventing replication of the HIV-1 virus[69,70] and by cleaving BCR-ABL with a view to developing a treatment for chronic myelogenous leukemia.[71]

The mechanical insertion of DNA fragments into the nucleus of a fertilized ovum provides a means for altering the genetic constitution of animals. Animals engineered in this manner are referred to as *transgenic*. The use of promoters that are inducible or tissue specific permits studies of the effect of a gene product that might be lethal if expressed in all tissues or at all times during embryogenesis. Transgenic mice that carry the human sickle β-globin gene have been produced,[72,73] and when superimposed on a murine thalassemic genotype, produce high enough levels of human hemoglobin S to have some potential as an animal model of sickle disease.

Another valuable technique for the study of gene function is targeted disruption ("knocking out") of genes. In this technique, a DNA construct that contains regions homologous to the gene being targeted and selectable markers is transfected into an embryonic mouse stem cell. Once a cell in which recombination has occurred within a gene is found, it can be implanted into a blastocyst, with the hope that some of the progeny of the implanted cell will become germ cells. If this does occur, the knockout can be propagated and homozygous animals bred. The value of the technique is often limited by the fact that the knockout may be lethal (e.g., G6PD[74] deficiency and Gaucher disease[75]) or may not have any abnormal phenotype. But in some diseases, such as hemochromatosis,[76,77] the knockout model is a valuable resource for study of the disease. In situations in which a knockout proves to be lethal, or where it would be useful to limit the deficiency to a single organ system, the Cre/LoxP site-specific recombination system is very useful.[78] The LoxP sequence, a 13-base pair inverted repeat, is inserted so that it flanks the gene that is to be removed. Site-specific recombination is catalyzed by the P-1 bacteriophage Cre-recombinase, excising the intervening DNA targeted by the LoxP sequence and ligating the remaining 5′ and 3′ DNA. Tissue-specific excision can be achieved by inserting the Cre-recombinase downstream from a tissue-specific promoter.

MUTATIONS

TYPES OF MUTATIONS

Mutations can occur in structural genes (the part of the DNA that specifies the amino acid sequence of protein), in the poorly understood regulatory apparatus that determines whether or not a gene will be available for transcription, in introns, or in portions of the DNA between genes that have no known function. As Table 9-1 shows, hematologic diseases provide examples of every known mechanism for causing mutations.

A change of one nucleotide to another without a change in the number of nucleotides in the sequence is called a *point mutation* or a *single nucleotide polymorphism* (SNP). Other types of mutations are deletions, and insertions (e.g., duplication of stretches of DNA in a gene). Mutations do not occur at random. Changes in the dinucleotide CpG to TpG are particularly common because invertebrate DNA cytidines followed by guanine are often methylated and the methylcytosine formed is susceptible to oxidation to thymine. Thus an unusually high proportion of point mutations are found in CpG dinucleotides in both hemophilia A[79] and G-6-PD deficiency.[80] Deletions or dupli-

cations of portions of genes tend to occur in areas in which the same sequence is repeated more than once. Thus, there are "hot spots" in the genome in which, for one reason or another, mutations are particularly likely to occur.

Another mechanism by which mutation appears to occur is that of *gene conversion*. This poorly understood phenomenon results in the sequence of one gene being transferred *en bloc* to another. This phenomenon is thought to account for the maintenance of identical sequence between duplicated genes.[81]

Many mutations affect the amount of processed mRNA that is formed. For example, mutations that cause abnormal splicing may produce a messenger that cannot be translated. Regulatory mutations that impair the rate at which a gene is transcribed into mRNA can be the consequence of mutations in promoter or enhancer elements, with mutations that cause thalassemia by impairing transcription of the hemoglobin-β locus being the best characterized (Chap. 46). However, most mutations causing hematologic disease seem to be structural mutations, those in which the sequence of the coding region of the gene is altered.

Errors in the coding sequence of a gene may result in failure to form any of the protein, in the formation of a very unstable protein that may never appear in the fully assembled form, or in the formation of an abnormal protein. The latter circumstance appears to be the most common. The abnormal protein may maintain all, some, or none of the functional properties of the normal protein. Even when it has lost the functional properties of the original protein, it may retain its antigenic properties, and it is then designated *cross-reacting material* (CRM). Mutations that result in the formation of stable proteins with normal functional properties are not clinically significant, but they may be very valuable from the point of view of population and family studies, or as genetic markers for various types of biologic investigations. Some "deficiencies" of enzymes are also clinically harmless. For example, genetic absence of the glycosyl transferases that convert the H antigen to the A or B antigen (see Chap. 128) results in the appearance of blood group O, surely a clinical state that cannot be considered a disease. Genetic variants that reach a frequency of more than 1 percent in a population are known as *polymorphisms*. Sometimes genetic variants such as the sickle cell gene or the G-6-PD deficiency gene reach polymorphic levels because the deleterious effects that they may have are counterbalanced by beneficial effects on survival, such as increased resistance to malaria. They are known as *balanced polymorphisms*.

All cells receive the same complement of genes. Nonetheless some proteins are tissue specific. Several circumstances can account for this. Some enzymes that appear to perform the same function are encoded by different genes in different tissues. For example, the pyruvate kinase of leukocytes and that of erythrocytes are under separate genetic control (see Chap. 45). In other cases, alternative splicing of the primary mRNA can produce different polypeptides.[82,83] Differences in posttranslational processing, including proteolysis and glycosylation of the same polypeptide by different enzymes in different tissues, can lead to different final products. However, in most instances a mutation that affects an enzyme in one type of blood cell will also affect the same enzyme in other blood cells, in liver, in brain, and in other tissues.

The types of enzyme deficiencies encountered clinically are limited by the ability of the affected individual to survive. Thus complete absence of a key glycolytic enzyme from all tissues is incompatible with the basic process of energy metabolism and would almost surely be lethal long before birth. In contrast, the inheritance of enzyme deficiencies that are manifested only in erythrocytes are apparently quite compatible with survival and thus, many of the enzyme defects that are observed in humans are ones that only affect the red blood cell.

TABLE 9-1   EXAMPLES OF GENETIC MECHANISMS IN HEMATOLOGIC DISEASE

MECHANISM		WHERE DISCUSSED
Diseases caused by inherited mitochondrial mutations		
Myelodysplastic syndromes	del	Chap. 86
Diseases caused by inherited X-linked mutations mutations		
Glucose-6-phosphate dehydrogenase deficiency	del, spl, pm	Chap. 45
Chronic granulomatous disease	pm, del, spl, ins	Chap. 66
Bruton agammaglobulinemia	pm, del, spl, ins	Chap. 82
Hemophilia	pm, del, spl, ins, tr	Chap. 115
Inherited autosomal dominant diseases		
Hereditary spherocytosis	pm, del, spl, ins	Chap. 44
Unstable hemoglobinopathies	pm, del	Chap. 47
Acute intermittent porphyria	pm, del, spl, ins	Chap. 57
von Willebrand disease	pm, del, ins	Chap. 118
Factor V Leiden	pm	Chap. 122
Inherited autosomal recessive diseases		
Pyruvate kinase deficiency	pm, del, spl, ins	Chap. 45
Thalassemia major	pm, del, spl, ins	Chap. 46
Sickle cell disease	pm	Chap. 47
Gaucher disease	pm, del, spl, ins, tr	Chap. 73
Diseases caused by acquired X-linked mutations		
Paroxysmal nocturnal hemoglobinuria	pm, del, spl, ins	Chap. 38
Diseases caused by acquired autosomal dominant mutations		
Chronic granulocytic leukemia	tr	Chap. 88

del = deletion; ins = insertion; pm = point mutation; spl = splicing mutation; tr = translocation.

MUTATION NOMENCLATURE

Historically, mutations were first detected by sequencing the protein, usually hemoglobin. Indeed, the mutation in sickle cell disease was described before the genetic code had been deciphered. Thus, mutations were designated by indicating the amino acid change. Amino acid-based nomenclature does not unambiguously define the mutation, because the same amino acid substitution can be caused by different nucleotide substitutions. Further ambiguity is introduced by the fact that three different starting points for the numbering of amino acids in protein are commonly employed: (1) the methionine start codon; (2) the amino acid after the methionine start codon; and (3) the amino-terminal amino acid of the processed protein. Finally, there are many mutations, such as those that change splice sites or promoters that cannot be designated by an amino acid substitution. Nonetheless, amino acid-based mutations have been so widely used that they serve as useful "nicknames" for mutations; the nucleotide-based designation would simply not be recognized by workers in the field. Moreover, knowing the amino acid change sometimes provides valuable information regarding the effect of the mutation at the protein level. Therefore, while the more robust nucleotide-based notation is preferred in this text, the amino acid-based notation is used when it is the one that is generally recognized. Standards have been established for the different notations that are in use.[84–87]

GENE DUPLICATION

Crossing-over during meiosis usually occurs with great precision. Homologous genes pair with each other, and although genes which were together on the chromosome before meiosis may now be on opposite chromosomes of the pair, each chromosome still contains a complete set of genes (see Fig. 9-1). Occasionally, however, an error occurs and pairing during meiosis is imperfect. Under these circumstances—unequal crossing over (see Fig. 46-6)—one of the daughter chromosomes contains a duplicated gene, while the other one exists with a gene deleted.

Once a duplication has occurred, further duplications occur more readily, because pairing of the first of the duplicate genes on one chromosome with the second gene of the duplicate on the other produces one chromosome with a triplicate gene and one with a single gene. Duplication has probably played a very important role in the course of evolution,[88] because the presence of two genes with the same function allows experiments of nature: mutations can accumulate on one of the genes while the original function is still provided by the duplicate. Examples of the results of gene duplication abound in hematology, particularly with respect to the hemoglobin loci. The α-chain loci are duplicated, and there are also two nearly identical copies of the γ-chain locus (see Chap. 46). Furthermore, the close similarity of their amino acid sequence and the fact that they are tightly linked indicate that the β, γ, and δ loci represent the result of duplication of a single ancestral gene. The process of unequal crossing-over takes place not only between genes, but also within genes. When this occurs, one would anticipate that a portion of the amino acid sequence of a protein is represented twice on one chromosome and is missing on the other. The Lepore hemoglobins, leading to a thalassemic clinical state, are an example of this type of unequal crossing-over (see Fig. 46-6). These abnormal hemoglobins have the amino acid sequence of the δ-chain at the amino end, and the sequence of the β-chain at the carboxyl end. The complement to this kind of abnormality, the "anti-Lepore" hemoglobin, also has been found (see Chap. 46). Similarly, a mutation of the glucocerebrosidase gene that causes Gaucher disease was found to be the result of a crossover between the active gene and the pseudogene.[89] The two types of haptoglobin represent an ancestral gene and one in which a major part of that gene has been duplicated.[90]

PSEUDOGENES

Pseudogenes are DNA sequences that resemble the corresponding functional genes, but do not form a gene product. Pseudogenes exist, for example, for the β-globin chain, von Willebrand factor, ferritin, and glucocerebrosidase. These pseudogenes apparently arose by gene duplication and simulate the true gene, even in having introns. They apparently have lost their ability to function, either through mutations in the coding region or in their promoters. Some pseudogenes are devoid of introns. They may well have arisen in evolution as a result of the reverse transcription of a processed mRNA by retroviral reverse transcriptase. Unlike genes that arose by tandem duplication as a result of unequal crossover, such pseudogenes can be found anywhere in the genome. For example, a functional glutathione-S-transferase gene is on chromosome 11 and a pseudogene is located on chromosome 12.[91]

GENOTYPE—PHENOTYPE CORRELATIONS

Even before it was feasible to detect mutations at the DNA level, clinicians could deduce that the same genotype did not always produce the same clinical disease picture (phenotype). Sibs inheriting autosomal recessive disorders from their parents often are observed to have discordant clinical presentations—one severely affected, one mildly so—even though the same pair of disease-producing genes were inherited. With the development of the ability to define genotypes directly, the great degree of genotype–phenotype dissociation is even more evident. Thus, persons inheriting the same sickle, G-6-PD, factor VIII, or glucocerebrosidase mutations may have mild or severe sickle disease, hemolytic anemia, hemophilia A, or Gaucher disease, respectively. The factors that modify disease expression are usually not understood.[92] In the case of G-6-PD deficiency, a second mutation, one in the uridine diphosphate (UDP) glucuronyltransferase-1 gene, has been shown to determine whether severe jaundice will be present.[93,94] Thrombophilia is much more likely to occur in patients with factor V Leiden if a second mutation of a gene encoding another coagulation factor such as protein C is co-inherited.[95,96] Environmental factors may play a role; clinically significant hemochromatosis is probably more common in alcoholics. Epigenetic factors are important in the case of imprinted genes, such as the KCNQ1OT1 gene of Beckwith-Wiedemann syndrome.[97]

GENOMICS AND PROTEOMICS

Genomics and proteomics are catch-phrases used to describe the large-scale analysis of gene sequence and protein production, respectively. Much, but contrary to common belief, far from all of the human genome sequence is known. There are many areas with extensive duplications in which the sequence is incorrect and there are large gaps. Nonetheless, much of the sequence is accurate and it is now possible to use powerful computer programs to search for new members of gene families that are important, or DNA or amino acid sequence motifs that are known or believed to serve specific functions. Another application of genomics is the hybridization of the mRNA from a tissue with microarrays of fragments of thousands of DNA sequences. This technology, known as *expression profiling*, is used to characterize gene expression in tissues or cells under different conditions. These data may sometimes be useful in understanding a disease state, and this approach has been used, for example, in an attempt to provide predictive data about lymphomas.[98]

Gene sequences only predict the unprocessed sequence of a protein and give only indirect information about the important posttranslational changes that create the final functional protein. Proteomics provides techniques for the separation of proteins and for their rapid identification by means such as the characterization of tryptic fragments by mass spectrometry and their comparison with a large computerized library of data.[94]

REFERENCES

1. Glenn D, Gelbart T, Beutler E: Tight linkage of pyruvate kinase (*PKLR*) and glucocerebrosidase (*GBA*) genes. *Hum Genet* 93:635, 1994.
2. Demina A, Boas E, Beutler E: Structure and linkage relationships of the region containing the human L-type pyruvate kinase (*PKLR*) and glucocerebrosidase (*GBA*) genes. *Hematopathol Mol Hematol* 11:63, 1998.
3. Beutler E, Yeh M, Fairbanks VF: The normal human female as a mosaic of X-chromosome activity: Studies using the gene for G-6-PD deficiency as a marker. *Proc Natl Acad Sci U S A* 48:9, 1962.
4. Lyon MF: Sex chromatin and gene action in the mammalian X-chromosome. *Am J Hum Genet* 14:135, 1962.
5. Hall LL, Byron M, Sakai K, et al: An ectopic human XIST gene can induce chromosome inactivation in postdifferentiation human HT-1080 cells. *Proc Natl Acad Sci U S A* 99:8677, 2002.
6. Gartler SM, Linder D: Developmental and evolutionary implications of the mosaic nature of the G-6-PD system. *Cold Spring Harb Symp Quant Biol* 29:253, 1964.
7. Beutler E: The distribution of gene products among populations of cells in heterozygous humans. *Cold Spring Harb Symp Quant Biol* 29:261, 1964.
8. Fialkow PJ, Gartler SM, Yoshida A: Clonal origin of chronic myelocytic leukemia in man. *Proc Natl Acad Sci U S A* 58:1468, 1967.
9. Oni SB, Osunkoya BO, Luzzatto L: Paroxysmal nocturnal hemoglobinuria: Evidence for monoclonal origin of abnormal red cells. *Blood* 36:145, 1970.
10. Beutler E, West C, Johnson C: Involvement of the erythroid series in acute myeloid leukemia. *Blood* 53:1203, 1979.
11. Fialkow PJ, Singer JW, Raskind WH, et al: Clonal development, stem-cell differentiation, and clinical remissions in acute nonlymphocytic leukemia. *N Engl J Med* 317:468, 1987.
12. Lindsay S, Monk M, Holliday R, et al: Differences in methylation on the active and inactive human X chromosomes. *Ann Hum Genet* 49:115, 1985.
13. Gilliland DG, Blanchard KL, Bunn HF: Clonality in acquired hematologic disorders. *Annu Rev Med* 42:491, 1991.
14. Gilliland DG, Blanchard KL, Levy J, et al: Clonality in myeloproliferative disorders: analysis by means of the polymerase chain reaction. *Proc Natl Acad Sci U S A* 88:6848, 1991.
15. Curnutte JT, Hopkins PJ, Kuhl W, Beutler E: Studying X-inactivation. *Lancet* 339:749, 1992.
16. Prchal JT, Guan YL, Prchal JF, Barany F: Transcriptional analysis of the active X-chromosome in normal and clonal hematopoiesis. *Blood* 81:269, 1993.
17. Wallace DC: Mitochondrial DNA sequence variation in human evolution and disease. *Proc Natl Acad Sci U S A* 91:8739, 1994.
18. Marsh WL, Nelson DP, Koenig HM: Free erythrocyte protoporphyrin (FEP) I. Normal values for adults and evaluation of the hematofluorometer. *Am J Clin Pathol* 79:655, 1983.
19. Mager J, Glaser G, Razin A, et al: Metabolic effects of pyrimidines derived from fava bean glycosides on human erythrocytes deficient in glucose-6-phosphate dehydrogenase. *Biochem Biophys Res Commun* 20:235, 1965.
20. Bader-Meunier B, Rotig A, Mielot F, et al: Refractory anaemia and mitochondrial cytopathy in childhood. *Br J Haematol* 87:381, 1994.
21. Superti-Furga A, Schoenle E, Tuchschmid P, et al: Pearson bone marrow-pancreas syndrome with insulin-dependent diabetes, progressive renal tubulopathy, organic aciduria and elevated fetal haemoglobin caused by deletion and duplication of mitochondrial DNA. *Eur J Pediatr* 152:44, 1993.
22. Cormier V, Rötig A, Quartino AR, et al: Widespread multi-tissue deletions of the mitochondrial genome in the Pearson marrow-pancreas syndrome. *J Pediatr* 117:599, 1990.
23. Whitelaw E, Martin DI: Retrotransposons as epigenetic mediators of phenotypic variation in mammals. *Nat Genet* 27:361, 2001.
24. Ordway JM, Curran T: Methylation matters: modeling a manageable genome. *Cell Growth Differ* 13:149, 2002.
25. Jarman AP, Wood WG, Sharpe JA, et al: Characterization of the major regulatory element upstream of the human alpha-globin gene cluster. *Mol Cell Biol* 11:4679, 1991.
26. Orkin SH: Globin gene regulation and switching: circa 1990. *Cell* 63:665, 1990.
27. Faustino NA, Cooper TA: Pre-mRNA splicing and human disease. *Genes Dev* 17:419, 2003.
28. Conboy JG, Chan J, Mohandas N, Kan YW: Multiple protein 4.1 isoforms produced by alternative splicing in human erythroid cells. *Proc Natl Acad Sci U S A* 85:9062, 1988.
29. Noguchi T, Yamada K, Inoue H, et al: The L- and R-type isozymes of rat pyruvate kinase are produced from a single gene by use of different promoters. *J Biol Chem* 262:14366, 1987.
30. Wiestner A, Schlemper RJ, van der Maas AP, Skoda RC: An activating splice donor mutation in the thrombopoietin gene causes hereditary thrombocythaemia. *Nat Genet* 18:49, 1998.
31. Kozak M: Compilation and analysis of sequences upstream from the translational start site in eukaryotic mRNAs. *Nucleic Acids Res* 12:857, 1984.
32. Merrick WC: Mechanism and regulation of eukaryotic protein synthesis. *Microbiol Rev* 56:291, 1992.
33. Maniatis T, Goodbourn S, Fischer JA: Regulation of inducible and tissue-specific gene expression. *Science* 236:1237, 1987.
34. Cazzola M, Skoda RC: Translational pathophysiology: A novel molecular mechanism of human disease. *Blood* 95:3280, 2000.
35. Rouault T, Klausner R: Regulation of iron metabolism in eukaryotes. *Curr Top Cell Regul* 35:1, 1997.
36. Han J, Brown T, Beutler B: Endotoxin-responsive sequences control cachectin/tumor necrosis factor biosynthesis at the translational level. *J Exp Med* 171:465, 1990.
37. Han J, Beutler B, Huez G: Complex regulation of tumor necrosis factor mRNA turnover in lipopolysaccharide-activated macrophages. *Biochim Biophys Acta* 1090:22, 1991.
38. Liebhaber SA: mRNA stability and the control of gene expression. *Nucleic Acids Symp Ser* 36:29, 1997.
39. Burt MJ, Smit DJ, Pyper WR, et al: A 4.5-megabase YAC contig and physical map over the hemochromatosis gene region. *Genomics* 33:153, 1996.
40. Schuler GD, Boguski MS, Stewart EA, et al: A gene map of the human genome. *Science* 274:540, 1996.
41. Amplification of nucleic acid sequences: The choices multiply. *J NIH Res* 3:81, 1991.
42. Innis MA, Gelfand DH, Sninsky JJ, White TJ: *PCR Protocols: A Guide to Methods and Applications.* Academic Press, San Diego, 1990.
43. De Melo MB, Sales TSI, Lorand-Metze I, Costa FF: Rapid method for isolation of DNA from glass slide smears for PCR. *Acta Haematol (Basel)* 87:214, 1992.

44. DeSalle R, Gatesy J, Wheeler W, Grimaldi D: DNA sequences from a fossil termite in Oligo-Miocene amber and their phylogenetic implications. *Science* 257:1933, 1992.

45. Southern E: Gel electrophoresis of restriction fragments. *Methods Enzymol* 68:152, 1979.

46. Chang JC, Kan YW: Antenatal diagnosis of sickle cell anaemia by direct analysis of the sickle mutation. *Lancet* 2:1127, 1981.

47. Sanger F, Nicklen S, Coulson AR: DNA sequencing with chain-terminating inhibitors. *Proc Natl Acad Sci U S A* 74:5463, 1977.

48. Sterky F, Lundeberg J: Sequence analysis of genes and genomes. *J Biotechnol* 76:1, 2000.

49. Kumar R, Dunn LL: Designed diagnostic restriction fragment length polymorphisms for the detection of point mutations in ras oncogenes. *Oncogene Res* 4:235, 1989.

50. Chehab FF, Kan YW: Detection of specific DNA sequences by fluorescence amplification: A color complementation assay. *Proc Natl Acad Sci U S A* 86:9178, 1989.

51. Mistry PK, Smith SJ, Ali M, et al: Genetic diagnosis of Gaucher's disease. *Lancet* 339:889, 1992.

52. Kalin I, Shephard S, Candrian U: Evaluation of the ligase chain reaction (LCR) for the detection of point mutations. *Mutat Res* 283:119, 1992.

53. Beutler E, Gelbart T: Large-scale screening for HFE mutations: Methodology and cost. *Genet Test* 4:131, 2000.

54. Fruchon S, Bensaid M, Borot N, et al: Use of denaturing HPLC and a heteroduplex generator to detect the HFE C282Y mutation associated with genetic hemochromatosis. *Clin Chem* 49:822, 2003.

55. Gridley T: Insertional versus targeted mutagenesis in mice. *New Biol* 3:1025, 1991.

56. Waldman AS: Targeted homologous recombination in mammalian cells. *Crit Rev Oncol Hematol* 12:49, 1992.

57. Weintraub HM: Antisense RNA and DNA. *Sci Am* 262:40, 1990.

58. Simons RW: Naturally occurring antisense RNA control—a brief review. *Gene* 72:35, 1988.

59. Weintraub LR, Goral A, Grasso J, et al: Pathogenesis of hepatic fibrosis in experimental iron overload. *Br J Haematol* 59:321, 1985.

60. Smith CC, Aurelian L, Reddy MP, et al: Antiviral effect of an oligo(nucleoside methylphosphonate) complementary to the splice junction of herpes simplex virus type 1 immediate early pre-mRNAs 4 and 5. *Proc Natl Acad Sci U S A* 83:2787, 1986.

61. McManaway ME, Neckers LM, Loke SL, et al: Tumour-specific inhibition of lymphoma growth by an antisense oligodeoxynucleotide. *Lancet* 335:808, 1990.

62. Szczylik C, Skorski T, Nicolaides NC, et al: Selective inhibition of leukemia cell proliferation by BCR-ABL antisense oligodeoxynucleotides. *Science* 253:562, 1991.

63. Cotter FE, Johnson P, Hall P, et al: Antisense oligonucleotides suppress B-cell lymphoma growth in a SCID-hu mouse model. *Oncogene* 9:3049, 1994.

64. Smith MJ, Prochownik EV: Inhibition of c-jun causes reversible proliferative arrest and withdrawal from the cell cycle. *Blood* 79:2107, 1992.

65. Khvorova A, Reynolds A, Jayasena SD: Functional siRNAs and miRNAs exhibit strand bias. *Cell* 115:209, 2003.

66. Couzin J: Breakthrough of the year. Small RNAs make big splash. *Science* 298:2296, 2002.

67. Scherr M, Morgan MA, Eder M: Gene silencing mediated by small interfering RNAs in mammalian cells. *Curr Med Chem* 10:245, 2003.

68. Chen CZ, Li L, Lodish HF, Bartel DP: MicroRNAs modulate hematopoietic lineage differentiation. *Science* 303:83, 2004.

69. Chen CJ, Banerjea AC, Harmison GG, et al: Multitarget-ribozyme directed to cleave at up to nine highly conserved HIV-1 env RNA regions inhibits HIV-1 replication—potential effectiveness against

70. Heidenreich O, Eckstein F: Hammerhead ribozyme-mediated cleavage of the long terminal repeat RNA of human immunodeficiency virus type 1. *J Biol Chem* 267:1904, 1992.

71. Kuwabara T, Warashina M, Tanabe T, et al: Comparison of the specificities and catalytic activities of hammerhead ribozymes and DNA enzymes with respect to the cleavage of BCR-ABL chimeric L6 (b2a2) mRNA. *Nucleic Acids Res* 25:3074, 1997.

72. Pawliuk R, Westerman KA, Fabry ME, et al: Correction of sickle cell disease in transgenic mouse models by gene therapy. *Science* 294:2368, 2001.

73. Belcher JD, Bryant CJ, Nguyen J, et al: Transgenic sickle mice have vascular inflammation. *Blood* 101:3953, 2003.

74. Longo L, Vanegas OC, Patel M, et al: Maternally transmitted severe glucose 6-phosphate dehydrogenase deficiency is an embryonic lethal. *EMBO J* 21:4229, 2002.

75. Tybulewicz VLJ, Tremblay ML, LaMarca ME, et al: Animal model of Gaucher's disease from targeted disruption of the mouse glucocerebrosidase gene. *Nature* 357:407, 1992.

76. Zhou XY, Tomatsu S, Fleming RE, et al: HFE gene knockout produces mouse model of hereditary hemochromatosis. *Proc Natl Acad Sci U S A* 95:2492, 1998.

77. Nicolas G, Bennoun M, Devaux I, et al: Lack of hepcidin gene expression and severe tissue iron overload in upstream stimulatory factor 2 (USF2) knockout mice. *Proc Natl Acad Sci U S A* 98:8780, 2001.

78. Yu Y, Bradley A: Engineering chromosomal rearrangements in mice. *Nat Rev Genet* 2:780, 2001.

79. Youssoufian H, Kazazian HHJr, Phillips DG, et al: Recurrent mutations in haemophilia A give evidence for CpG mutation hotspots. *Nature* 324:380, 1986.

80. Vulliamy TJ, D'Urso M, Battistuzzi G, et al: Diverse point mutations in the human glucose 6-phosphate dehydrogenase gene cause enzyme deficiency and mild or severe hemolytic anemia. *Proc Natl Acad Sci U S A* 85:5171, 1988.

81. Hess JF, Schmid CW, Shen CK: A gradient of sequence divergence in the human adult alpha-globin duplication units. *Science* 226:67, 1984.

82. Amara SG, Jonas V, Rosenfeld MG, et al: Alternative RNA processing in calcitonin gene expression generates mRNAs encoding different polypeptide products. *Nature* 298:240, 1982.

83. Pihlajaniemi T, Myllyla R, Seyer J, et al: Partial characterization of a low molecular weight human collagen that undergoes alternative splicing. *Proc Natl Acad Sci U S A* 84:940, 1987.

84. Ad Hoc Committee on Mutation Nomenclature: Update on nomenclature for human gene mutations. *Hum Mutat* 8:197, 1996.

85. Antonarakis SE: Recommendations for a nomenclature system for human gene mutations. Nomenclature Working Group. *Hum Mutat* 11:1, 1998.

86. den Dunnen JT, Antonarakis SE: Mutation nomenclature extensions and suggestions to describe complex mutations: a discussion. *Hum Mutat* 15:7, 2000.

87. Beutler E, McKusick VA, Motulsky AG, et al: Mutation nomenclature: Nicknames, systematic names, and unique identifiers. *Hum Mutat* 8:203, 1996.

88. Ohno S: *Evolution by Gene Duplication.* Springer Verlag, Berlin, 1970.

89. Zimran A, Sorge J, Gross E, et al: A glucocerebrosidase fusion gene in Gaucher disease. Implications for the molecular anatomy, pathogenesis and diagnosis of this disorder. *J Clin Invest* 85:219, 1990.

90. Manoharan A: Congenital haptoglobin deficiency. *Blood* 90:1709, 1997.

91. Board PG, Coggan M, Woodcock DM: The human Pi class glutathione transferase sequence at 12q13-q14 is a reverse-transcribed pseudogene. *Genomics* 14:470, 1992.

92. Beutler E: Discrepancies between genotype and phenotype in hematology: an important frontier. *Blood* 98:2597, 2001.

93. Kaplan M, Renbaum P, Levy-Lahad E, et al: Gilbert syndrome and glucose-6-phosphate dehydrogenase deficiency: A dose-dependent genetic interaction crucial to neonatal hyperbilirubinemia. *Proc Natl Acad Sci U S A* 94:12128, 1997.

94. Sampietro M, Lupica L, Perrero L, et al: The expression of uridine diphosphate glucuronosyltransferase gene is a major determinant of bil-irubin level in heterozygous beta-thalassaemia and in glucose-6-phosphate dehydrogenase deficiency. *Br J Haematol* 99:437, 1997.

95. Lane DA, Grant PJ: Role of hemostatic gene polymorphisms in venous and arterial thrombotic disease. *Blood* 95:1517, 2000.

96. Rosendaal FR: Venous thrombosis: A multicausal disease. *Lancet* 353: 1167, 1999.

97. Weksberg R, Shuman C, Caluseriu O, et al: Discordant KCNQ1OT1 imprinting in sets of monozygotic twins discordant for Beckwith-Wiedemann syndrome. *Hum Mol Genet* 11:1317, 2002.

98. Lossos IS, Levy R: Diffuse large B-cell lymphoma: insights gained from gene expression profiling. *Int J Hematol* 77:321, 2003.

CYTOGENETICS AND GENE REARRANGEMENT

LUCY A. GODLEY

MICHELLE M. LE BEAU

Cytogenetic analysis provides pathologists and clinicians with a powerful tool for the diagnosis and classification of hematologic malignant diseases. The detection of an acquired, clonal, somatic mutation establishes the diagnosis of a neoplastic disorder and rules out hyperplasia, dysplasia, metaplasia, and aplasia, morphologic changes that may be a result of toxic injury, inflammation, degeneration, or vitamin deficiency. A number of specific cytogenetic abnormalities have been identified that are very closely, and sometimes uniquely, associated with morphologically and clinically distinct subsets of leukemia or lymphoma, enabling clinicians to predict their clinical course and likelihood of responding to particular treatments. The detection of one of these recurring abnormalities is helpful in establishing the diagnosis and adds information of prognostic importance. In many cases, the prognostic information derived from cytogenetic analysis is independent of that provided by other clinical features. Patients with favorable prognostic features benefit from standard therapies with well-known spectra of toxicities, whereas those with less favorable clinical and cytogenetic characteristics may be better treated with more intensive or investigational therapies. Pretreatment cytogenetic analysis also can be useful in choosing between postremission therapies that differ widely in cost, acute and chronic morbidity, and effectiveness. The appearance of new abnormalities in the karyotype of a patient under observation often signals clonal evolution and more aggressive behavior. The disappearance of a chromosomal abnormality present at diagnosis is an important indicator of complete remission following treatment, and its reappearance invariably heralds relapse of the disease.

GENETIC CONSEQUENCES OF GENOMIC REARRANGEMENTS

Over the past decade, the genes that are located at the breakpoints of a number of the recurring chromosomal translocations have been identified.[1-5] Alterations in the expression of the genes or in the properties of the encoded proteins resulting from the rearrangement play an integral role in the process of malignant transformation.[2,6] The altered genes fall into several functional classes, including tyrosine or serine protein kinases, cell surface receptors, and growth factors. However, the largest class are transcriptional regulating factors. These proteins are involved in the induction or repression of gene transcription, often functioning in a tissue-specific fashion to regulate growth and differentiation.

There are two general mechanisms by which chromosomal translocations result in altered gene function. The first is deregulation of gene expression. This mechanism is characteristic of the translocations in lymphoid neoplasms that involve the immunoglobulin genes in B lineage tumors and the T cell receptor genes in T lineage tumors. These rearrangements result in the inappropriate or constitutive expression of an oncogene. The second mechanism is the expression of a novel fusion protein, resulting from the juxtaposition of coding sequences from two genes that are normally located on different chromosomes. Such chimeric proteins are "tumor-specific" in that the fusion gene typically does not exist in nonmalignant cells. Thus, the detection of such a fusion gene and fusion protein can be important in diagnosis and in the detection of residual disease or early relapse. Moreover, it may also be an appropriate target for tumor specific therapies. An example is the chimeric BCR-ABL protein resulting from the t(9;22) in chronic myeloid leukemia (see "Methods of Cell Preparation" below). All of the translocations cloned to date in the myeloid leukemias result in a fusion protein.

Chromosomal translocations result in the activation of genes in a dominant fashion. A number of human tumors are believed to result from homozygous, recessive mutations. These mutations lead to the *absence* of a functional protein product, suggesting that these genes function as "suppressor" genes whose normal role is to limit cellular proliferation. The hallmark of tumor suppressor genes is the loss of genetic material in malignant cells, resulting from chromosomal loss or deletion, as well as by other genetic mechanisms.[1]

Extensive experimental evidence indicates that more than one mutation is required for the pathogenesis of hematologic malignancies; that is, expression of translocation-specific fusion genes or deregulated expression of oncogenes is required, but is insufficient by itself to induce leukemia. Thus, an important aspect of leukemia biology is the elucidation of the spectrum of chromosomal abnormalities and molecular mutations that cooperate in the pathways leading to leukemogenesis. Where known, we have described the cooperating mutations associated with specific cytogenetic subsets of leukemia or lymphoma.

METHODS OF CELL PREPARATION

Cytogenetic analysis of malignant diseases must be based on the study of the tumor cells themselves. In leukemia, the specimen is usually obtained by marrow aspiration and is either processed immediately (direct preparation) or cultured for 24 to 72 hours. When a marrow aspirate cannot be obtained, a marrow biopsy (bone core specimen) or a blood sample from patients who have circulating immature myeloid or lymphoid cells can often be processed successfully. An involved lymph node or tumor mass specimen may be processed similarly for the analysis of lymphomas.

Acronyms and abbreviations that appear in this chapter include: AIDS, acquired immunodeficiency syndrome; ALCL, anaplastic large-cell lymphoma; ALL, acute lymphoblastic leukemia; AML, acute myelogenous leukemia; AML-M2, acute myelogenous leukemia with maturation; AMMoL-M4Eo, acute myelomonocytic leukemia with abnormal eosinophils; APL, acute promyelocytic leukemia; BL, Burkitt lymphoma; CALLA, common acute lymphoblastic leukemia antigen; CD30, cluster of differentiation; CLL, chronic lymphocytic leukemia; CML, chronic myelogenous leukemia; CMMoL, chronic myelomonocytic leukemia; CNS, central nervous system; CTCL, cutaneous T cell lymphoma; DLBCL, diffuse large B cell lymphoma; EBV, Epstein-Barr virus; EFS, event-free survival; FAB, French-American-British; FISH, fluorescence *in situ* hybridization; FITC, fluorescein isothiocyanate; HDAC, histone deacetylase; IgH, immunoglobulin heavy-chain; IgHv, immunoglobulin heavy-chain variable region; ITD, internal tandem duplication; LPL, lymphoplasmacytoid lymphoma; MALT, mucosa-associated lymphoid tumor; MCL, mantle cell lymphoma; MDS, myelodysplastic syndrome; MGUS, monoclonal gammopathy of undetermined significance; MPD, myeloproliferative disease; mRNA, messenger RNA; NHL, non-Hodgkin lymphoma; PML, promyelocytic leukemia; PML-RARA, promyelocytic leukemia-retinoic acid receptor-alpha protein; Q-PCR, quantitative polymerase chain reaction; RA, refractory anemia; RAEB, refractory anemia with excess blasts; RAEB-T, refractory anemia with excess blasts in transformation; RARS, refractory anemia with ringed sideroblasts; RT-PCR, reverse transcriptase polymerase chain reaction; SIg, surface immunoglobulin; SLL, small lymphocytic lymphoma; t-AML, therapy-related acute myelogenous leukemia; t-MDS, therapy-related myelodysplastic syndrome; WBC, white blood cell.

For specimen collection, 1 to 5 ml of marrow is aspirated asepticelly into a syringe coated with preservative-free sodium heparin (preservatives in heparin suppress cell growth) and transferred to a sterile 15 ml centrifuge tube containing 5 ml of culture medium (Roswell Park Memorial Institute [RPMI] 1640, 100 U sodium heparin). If a marrow aspirate cannot be obtained, a marrow biopsy may be taken and placed into the collection tube. For blood specimens, 10 ml are drawn aseptically by venipuncture into a syringe coated with preservative-free heparin (the use of Vacutainer tubes should be avoided because the heparin contains preservatives). To avoid loss of cell viability, it is critical that the specimen be transported at room temperature to the cytogenetics laboratory without delay. Overnight shipment of specimens frequently results in loss of cell viability, and most laboratories experience a high proportion (25–50%) of inadequate analyses using such specimens. For optimally handled specimens, approximately 95 percent of all cases should be adequate for cytogenetic analysis. Inadequate cases generally represent samples from patients with hypocellular marrows. Overall, approximately 75 percent of marrow biopsies will yield adequate numbers of metaphase cells for complete analysis.

FLUORESCENCE *IN SITU* HYBRIDIZATION AND POLYMERASE CHAIN REACTION

Cytogenetic analysis of human tumors is often technically difficult because of the presence of multiple abnormalities and requires highly skilled personnel. These factors have led investigators to seek alternative methods for identifying chromosomal abnormalities, such as fluorescence *in situ* hybridization (FISH).[7] The FISH technique is based on the same principle as Southern blot analysis, namely, the ability of single-stranded DNA to anneal to complementary DNA.[7] In the case of FISH, the target DNA is the nuclear DNA of interphase cells, or the DNA of metaphase chromosomes that are affixed to a glass microscope slide (FISH can also be accomplished with marrow or blood smears, or fixed and sectioned tissue). The test probe is labeled with biotin- or digoxigenin-labeled nucleotides, and detected with fluorescein isothiocyanate (FITC)- or CY3-conjugated avidin, or rhodamine-labeled antidigoxigenin antibodies. Commercially available probes are often directly labeled with fluorochrome, which simplifies the technique by eliminating the detection by probe steps. With the development of dual- and triple-pass filters, most laboratories now have the capacity to hybridize and detect two to three probes simultaneously. Table 10-1 lists FISH probes used to detect recurring chromosomal abnormalities.

Several types of probes can be used to detect chromosomal abnormalities by FISH. Table 10-1 summarizes the commercially available probes. FISH techniques have a number of applications (Table 10-2). In some cases, FISH analysis provides more sensitivity in that cytogenetic abnormalities have been identified by FISH in samples that appeared to be normal by morphologic and conventional cytogenetic analyses. FISH is most powerful when the analysis is targeted toward those abnormalities that are known to be associated with a particular tumor or disease. The following is an example of how FISH could be used in a clinical setting. Cytogenetic analysis could be performed at the time of diagnosis to identify the chromosomal abnormalities in an individual patient's malignant cells. Thereafter, FISH with the appropriate probes could be used to detect residual disease or early relapse, and to assess the efficacy of therapeutic regimens. For example, the use of FISH to detect the t(9;22) in chronic myelogenous leukemia (CML) patients following transplantation or imatinib therapy, or sex chromosome determination after a sex-mismatched transplant, is widespread. Hybridization of centromere-specific probes has been used to detect monosomy, trisomy, and other aneuploidies in both

leukemias and solid tumors, as well as the sex chromosome complement in the transplant setting (Color Plate XXIII). Chromosome-specific libraries, which paint the chromosomes, are particularly useful in identifying marker chromosomes (rearranged chromosomes of unidentified origin), or structural rearrangements, such as translocations. Translocations and deletions can also be identified in interphase or metaphase cells by using genomic probes that are derived from the breakpoints of recurring translocations or within the deleted segment (Color Plate XXIV). The innovation in FISH technology is spectral karyotyping, also known as multiplex FISH.[8] Using this approach, 24 differentially labeled painting probes representing each chromosome are cohybridized. Fourier spectroscopy is used to distinguish each spectrally overlapping probe, and imaging software assigns a unique color to each chromosome (Color Plate XXIV). Often referred to as "color karyotyping," this method is applicable to the identification of numerical abnormalities, as well as many structural abnormalities. Table 10-3 summarizes the applications and limitations of spectral karyotyping.

QUANTITATIVE POLYMERASE CHAIN REACTION AND GENE EXPRESSION PROFILES

The detection of chromosomal abnormalities in hematopoietic malignancies is relatively straightforward, because large numbers of malignant cells can be isolated from marrow or blood. The malignant cells can be analyzed by Southern blot analysis of DNA, reverse transcription polymerase chain reaction (RT-PCR) analysis of RNA, FISH, or standard cytogenetic methods. Material from patients newly presenting are often analyzed most efficiently by conventional cytogenetic analysis, possibly combined with RT-PCR analysis if a specific chromosome rearrangement is suspected, for example, a *BCR-ABL* fusion. Emerging technologies that are likely to play a major role in the future diagnosis and management of hematologic disorders include RT-PCR and quantitative RT-PCR (Q-PCR), microarray-based gene expression profiling, and proteomic analysis.[9] Q-PCR is being studied extensively as a means of measuring minimal residual disease, although it remains a research-based technique. Virtually all of the hematopoietic malignancies have been studied by microarray technology, revealing complex, but unique, expression profiles for each disease subtype, suggesting that future diagnostic tests and management decisions will be based on the initial gene expression profiling of individual patients. The fingerprint of proteins expressed within malignant cells can be revealed by proteomic patterns in a manner similar to the way gene expression levels can be measured by microarray analysis. To date, all such studies have been research-based, and no microarray or proteomic technologies are available for routine patient evaluation.

CHROMOSOME NOMENCLATURE

Chromosomal abnormalities are described according to the International System for Human Cytogenetic Nomenclature (Table 10-4).[10] To describe the chromosomal complement, the total chromosome number is listed first, followed by the sex chromosomes, and numerical and structural abnormalities in ascending order. The observation of at least two cells with the same structural rearrangement (for example, translocations, deletions or inversions, gain of the same chromosome, or three cells each showing loss of the same chromosome) is considered evidence for the presence of an abnormal clone. However, one cell with a normal karyotype is considered evidence for the presence of a normal cell line. Patients whose cells show no alteration or nonclonal (single cell) abnormalities are considered to be normal. An exception to this is a single cell characterized by a recurring structural abnormality. In such instances, it is likely that this represents the karyotype of the malignant cells in that particular patient.

TABLE 10-1 FISH PROBES TO DETECT RECURRING CHROMOSOMAL ABNORMALITIES

DISEASE	ABNORMALITY	PROBE	FORMAT*	VENDOR†
AML-M2	t(8;21)	RUNX1/ETO	Two-color dual fusion	Vysis
AML-M4Eo	inv(16)/t(16;16)	CBFB	Two-color break-apart	Vysis, Ventana
AML-M3	t(15;17)	PML/RARA	Two-color single fusion	Vysis, Ventana
AML	t(11q23)	MLL	Two-color break-apart Single color	Vysis, Ventana
AML/MDS	−5/del(5q)	EGR1/5p	Two-color deletion	Vysis
		CSF1R/5p	Two-color deletion	Vysis
	−7/del(7q)	D7S522/CEP7	Two-color deletion	Vysis
		D7S486/CEP7	Two-color deletion	Vysis
	del(20q)	D20S108	Single color	Vysis
	+8	CEP8	Single color	Vysis, Cytocell
CML	t(9;22)	BCR/ABL	Two-color single fusion	Vysis
		BCR/ABL ES	Two-color extra signal	Vysis
		BCR/ABL	Two color dual fusion	Vysis
		MBCR/ABL	Two-color single fusion	Ventana
		BCR/ABL	Two-color dual fusion	Ventana
	+8	CEP8	Single color	Vysis, Cytocell
	i(17q)	HER2/CEP17	Two-color (17q/centromere)	Vysis, Ventana
ALL	t(12;21)	TEL/AML1	Two-color extra signal	Vysis
	t(11q23)	MLL	Two-color break-apart	Vysis
	t(8;14)	IGH/MYC/CEP8	Tri-color dual fusion	Vysis
	t(9;22)	BCR/ABL ES	Two-color extra signal	Vysis
		BCR/ABL	Two-color single fusion	Vysis
		BCR/ABL	Two-color dual fusion	Vysis
		MBCR/ABL	Two-color single fusion	Ventana
		mBCR/ABL	Two-color single fusion	Ventana
	del(9p)/t(9p)	CDKN2A(p16)/CEP9	Dual color	Vysis
CLL, Myeloma	+12	CEP12	Single color	Vysis
	del(13q)	D13S319/13q34	Two color	Vysis
		RB1/13q34	Two color	Vysis
	del(11q)	ATM	Single color	Vysis
	−17/del(17p)	TP53	Single color	Vysis
	t(14q32)	IGH	Two-color break-apart	Vysis
Myeloma	t(4;14)	IGH/FGFR3	Two-color dual fusion	Vysis
NHL	t(11;18)	BIRC3/MALT1	Two-color dual fusion	Vysis
	t(14;18)	IGH/BCL2	Two-color dual fusion	Vysis
	t(8;14)	IGH/MYC	Two-color dual fusion	Vysis
		MYC	Two-color break-apart	Vysis
	t(14q32)	IGH	Two-color break-apart	Vysis
ALCL	t(2;5)	ALK	Two-color break-apart	Vysis
MCL, Myeloma	t(11;14)	CCND1/IGH	Two-color dual fusion	Vysis
Miscellaneous				
Bone marrow transplants		CEPX/CEPY	Single color or two color	Vysis
Subtelomeric—each chromosomal arm			Single color	Vysis
			Two color	Cytocell

ALCL, anaplastic large-cell lymphoma; ALL, acute lymphoblastic leukemia; AML, acute myelogenous leukemia; CLL, chronic lymphocytic leukemia; CML, chronic myelogenous leukemia; MCL, mantle cell lymphoma; MDS, myelodysplastic syndrome; MM, multiple myeloma; NHL, non-Hodgkin lymphoma.
* In two-color break-apart probes, DNA sequences from the 5' and 3' regions of a single gene are labeled and detected with red and green fluorochromes. In the germ line configuration, a yellow fusion signal is observed, whereas individual red and green signals are observed when the sequences are separated as a result of a translocation. With two-color fusion probes, DNA sequences flanking the breakpoints of the involved genes are brought together to form either one (single-fusion probes) or two (dual-fusion probes) yellow fusion signal(s). With the two-color extra-signal probes, DNA sequences flanking the breakpoint on the partner chromosomes are brought together to form a fusion yellow signal; however, part of the DNA sequences recognized by one of the probes may remain at the original site, giving rise to an extra signal in a single color.
† Vysis, Downers Grove, IL (www.vysis.com); Ventana Medical Systems, Tucson, AZ, (www.ventanamed.com); Cytocell, Banbury, England (www.cytocell.co.uk).

SPECIFIC CLONAL DISORDERS

CHRONIC MYELOGENOUS LEUKEMIA

The first consistent chromosome abnormality in any malignant disease was identified in chronic myelogenous leukemia (CML). The Philadelphia (Ph) chromosome results from a translocation involving chromosomes 9 and 22 [t(9;22)(q34;q11.2)] (Fig. 10-1A), and arises in a pluripotential stem cell that gives rise to both lymphoid and myeloid lineage cells (see Chap. 88). The standard t(9;22) is identified in approximately 92 percent of CML patients, whereas 6 percent have variant translocations that involve a third chromosome in addition to chromosomes 9 and 22. The genetic consequence of the t(9;22) or the complex translocations is to move the Abelson (ABL) oncogene on chromosome 9 next to the BCR gene on 22. Analyses of leukemia cells

TABLE 10-2   APPLICATIONS AND ADVANTAGES OF FISH

Applications

Detection of numerical and structural chromosomal abnormalities

Identification of marker chromosomes (rearranged chromosomes of uncertain origin)

Monitoring the effects of therapy and detection of minimal residual disease or early relapse

Identification of the origin of marrow cells following marrow transplantation

Identification of the lineage of neoplastic cells

Examination of the karyotypic pattern of nondividing or interphase cells

Detection of gene amplification

Advantages

Rapid technique; large numbers of cells can be analyzed in a short time

The efficiency of hybridization and detection is high

The sensitivity and specificity are very high

Cytogenetic data can be obtained from nondividing or terminally differentiated cells, from tumors with a low mitotic index (e.g., chronic lymphocytic leukemia), or from posttreatment samples that contain too few cells for routine cytogenetic studies

Permits the direct correlation of cytogenetic and cytologic/morphologic features, which enables pathologists to differentiate malignant from benign conditions in equivocal cases

Automated systems for analysis of hybridized slides are available

from rare patients with typical CML who lack the t(9;22) reveal a rearrangement involving *ABL* and *BCR* that is detectable only at the molecular level (1–2% of cases).[11,12]

The t(9;22) and resultant *BCR-ABL* fusion is the genetic *sine qua non* of CML.[12] The BCR-ABL fusion protein is located on the cytoplasmic surface of the cell membrane and acquires a novel function in transmitting growth-regulatory signals to the nucleus via the RAS/MAPK, PI3K/AKT, and JAK/STAT signal transduction pathways. The tyrosine kinase activity of the BCR-ABL fusion protein can be specifically inhibited by imatinib mesylate.[13] Imatinib has shown remarkable activity in all phases of CML and is the preferred therapy for most patients with newly diagnosed CML.[14,15] The *BCR-ABL* fusion gene can be detected by Southern blot analysis of DNA or by RT-PCR analysis of messenger RNA (mRNA) for diagnosis and detection of residual disease. Studies of patients treated with imatinib show a strong correlation between *BCR-ABL* levels as measured in the blood by Q-PCR and the percentage of Ph+ cells in the marrow.[16,17] Examination of patients by Q-PCR remains a research endeavor, and most CML patients are followed by marrow cytogenetic analysis or by FISH analysis of blood or marrow.

Several types of genetic changes are associated with imatinib resistance, including point mutations leading to amino acid substitutions in the BCR-ABL kinase domain that interfere with imatinib binding, as well as the acquisition of additional copies of the Ph chromosome or *BCR-ABL* gene amplification, both of which can be detected by FISH.[18] Patients on imatinib may acquire chromosomal abnormalities in Ph– cells that herald disease progression or that may be of unclear clinical significance. In a recent series, 15 percent of patients who had achieved a complete cytogenetic response on imatinib showed clonal karyotypic abnormalities, most commonly +8, –7, or del(20q), and some of them had clinical features of a myelodysplastic syndrome.[19] The significance of these early findings will be elucidated by the analysis of a large number of patients who have had complete cytogenetic responses to imatinib and are being followed prospectively.

As they enter the more aggressive stages of accelerated and blast phase disease, most CML patients (80%) show karyotypic evolution with the appearance of new chromosomal abnormalities in very distinct patterns in addition to the Ph chromosome.[11] A change in the karyotype is considered to be a grave prognostic sign.[11] With the exception of an isochromosome of the long arm of chromosome 17 [i(17)(q10)], which is usually associated with myeloid blast transformation, there is no association of a particular karyotype with lymphoid or myeloid blast transformation. The most common changes, a gain of chromosomes 8 or 19, or a second Ph (by gain of the first), or an i(17q), frequently occur in combination to produce modal chromosome numbers of 47 to 50. Other genetic changes identified in CML in blast crisis include mutations in the *TP53, RB1, MYC, CDKN2A(p16), KRAS1/NRAS,* or *RUNX1/AML1* genes.

Rarely, marrow biopsies from patients will appear similar to those patients with CML, but will lack a Ph chromosome or the *BCR-ABL* fusion. Most often these patients have a clonal myeloid disorder, most commonly chronic myelomonocytic leukemia, refractory anemia with excess blasts, or the poorly understood disorder of "atypical CML." Cytogenetic analysis of marrow biopsies from these patients commonly have a normal karyotype, +8, +13, del(20q), or i(17q). These patients have a substantially shorter survival than do those patients whose cells have the t(9;22). Because imatinib inhibits the tyrosine kinase activity of several proteins in addition to BCR-ABL, imatinib has proved effective in other disorders, including chronic clonal myeloid diseases with platelet-derived growth factor receptor β rearrangements,[20] a subset of hypereosinophilic syndrome that expresses the FIP1L1-PDGFRα fusion protein,[21,22] and in patients with mast cell malignancies that demonstrate *KIT* activation but who lack *KIT* mutations that inhibit imatinib binding.[23]

OTHER CHRONIC CLONAL MYELOID DISORDERS

A cytogenetically abnormal clone is present in 15 percent of untreated polycythemia vera patients compared with 40 percent of treated patients.[24] When the disease transforms to acute myeloid leukemia (AML), virtually all patients have an abnormal clone. The presence of

TABLE 10-3   APPLICATIONS AND LIMITATIONS OF SPECTRAL KARYOTYPING

Cancer diagnostics

Detection of numerical and structural chromosomal abnormalities

Identification of marker chromosomes (rearranged chromosomes of uncertain origin)

Identification of some cryptic rearrangements

Identification of the chromosomal origin of amplified sequences

Research applications

Molecular analysis of chromosomal abnormalities in human tumors

Characterization of somatic cell hybrids

Phylogenetic studies to determine the location and extent of synteny between species

Detection of amplified genes

Examination of the organization of chromosomal domains or multigene families in interphase nuclei as a function of tissue type, developmental status, cell cycle stage, or disease state (three-dimensional reconstruction)

Analysis of chromosome aberrations in genetic toxicology studies

Limitations

Costly procedure (reagent costs are ~$165 per slide)

Requires dedicated spectral karyotype imaging system ($80,000)

Labor intensive (analysis of >10 cells per case is prohibitive)

Does not detect some structural rearrangements, e.g., small cryptic translocations, paracentric inversions, small deletions, and small duplications

Does not provide information on breakpoints or involved chromosomal segment

TABLE 10-4 GLOSSARY OF CYTOGENETIC TERMINOLOGY

Aneuploidy An abnormal chromosome number caused by either gain or loss of chromosomes.

Banded chromosomes Chromosomes with alternating dark and light segments as a result of special stains or pretreatment of metaphase cells with enzymes before staining. Each chromosome pair has a unique pattern of bands.

Breakpoint A specific site on a chromosome containing a DNA break that is involved in a structural rearrangement, such as a translocation or deletion.

Centromere The constriction along the length of the chromosome that is the site of the spindle fiber attachment. The position of the centromere determines whether chromosomes are *metacentric* (X-shaped, e.g., chromosomes 1–3, 6–12, X, 16, 19, 20) or *acrocentric* (inverted V-shaped, e.g., chromosomes 13–15, 21, 22, Y). During mitosis, the two exact copies of the DNA in each chromosome are separated by shortening of the spindle fibers attached to opposite sides of the dividing cell.

Clone In the cytogenetic sense, this is defined as two cells with the same additional or structurally rearranged chromosome or three cells with loss of the same chromosome.

Deletion A segment of a chromosome is missing as the result of two breaks and loss of the intervening piece (interstitial deletion). Molecular studies of many recurring chromosomal deletions have shown that, in each case, the deletions were interstitial, rather than terminal (single break with loss of the terminal segment).

Diploid Normal chromosome number and composition of chromosomes.

Haploid Only one-half the normal complement, that is, 23 chromosomes.

Hyperdiploid Additional chromosomes; therefore, the modal number is 47 or greater.

Hypodiploid Loss of chromosomes with a modal number of 45 or less.

Inversion Two breaks occur in the same chromosome with rotation of the intervening segment. If both breaks occur on the same side of the centromere, it is called a *paracentric inversion*. If they occur on opposite sides, it is called a *pericentric inversion*.

Isochromosome A chromosome that consists of identical copies of one chromosome arm with loss of the other arm. Thus, an isochromosome for the long arm of chromosome 17 [i(17)(q10)] contains two copies of the long arm (separated by the centromere) with loss of the short arm of the chromosome.

Karyotype Arrangement of chromosomes from a particular cell according to a internationally established system such that the largest chromosomes are first and the smallest ones are last. A normal female karyotype is described as 46,XX and a normal male karyotype is 46,XY. An *idiogram* is an idealized representation (diagram) of the chromosomes.

Pseudodiploid A diploid number of chromosomes accompanied by structural chromosomal abnormalities.

Recurring abnormality A numerical or structural abnormality noted in multiple patients who have a similar neoplasm. Such abnormalities are characteristic or diagnostic of distinct subtypes of leukemia and lymphoma that have unique morphologic and/or immunophenotypic features. Recurring abnormalities represent genetic mutations that are involved in the pathogenesis of the corresponding diseases; many recurring abnormalities have prognostic significance.

Translocation A break in at least two chromosomes with exchange of material. In a reciprocal translocation, there is no obvious loss of chromosomal material. Translocations are indicated by t; the chromosomes involved are noted in the first set of parentheses and the breakpoints in the second set of parentheses. For example, the Ph translocation is t(9;22)(q34;q11.2).

Nomenclature symbols:

p Short arm

q Long arm

+ If before the chromosome, indicates a gain of a whole chromosome (e.g., +8).

− If before the chromosome, indicates a loss of a whole chromosome (e.g., −7); if after the chromosome, indicates loss of part of the chromosome (e.g., 5q−, loss of part of the long arm of chromosome 5)

? Indicates uncertainty about the identity of the chromosome or band listed just after the ?.

t Translocation

del Deletion

inv Inversion

i Isochromosome

mar Marker chromosome

r Ring chromosome

SOURCE: Modified from Rowley JD: Chromosome abnormalities in human cancer, in *Practice and Principles of Oncology*, 3rd ed, edited by VT De Vita, S Hellman, S Rosenberg. JP Lippincott, Philadelphia, 1991.

a chromosome abnormality at diagnosis does not necessarily predict a short survival or the development of leukemia. However, a change in the karyotype may be an ominous sign. Marrow cells frequently contain additional chromosomes (+8 or +9). Trisomy 8 and 9 may occur together, which is otherwise rare.[24] Structural rearrangements most often involve a del(13q) or del(20q), which is noted in 30 percent of patients. Loss of chromosome 7 (20%) and del(5q) (40%) is often observed in the leukemic phase, and may be related to the prior treatment received by these patients.

Cytogenetic analysis of cells from patients with idiopathic myelofibrosis (see Chap. 89) has revealed clonal abnormalities in 60 percent of patients.[24] These abnormalities are similar to those noted in other myeloid disorders. The most common anomalies are +8, −7, or a del(7q), del(11q), del(13q), and del(20q).[24] A change in the karyotype may signal evolution to AML. Fewer than 10 percent of patients with essential thrombocythemia have an abnormal clone. Recurring abnormalities include +8 and del(13q). Although del(5q) and inv(3)/t(3;3) are associated with thrombocytosis, they are characteristic of myelodysplastic syndrome (MDS) or AML, rather than essential thrombocythemia.

CLONAL CYTOPENIAS AND OLIGOBLASTIC MYELOGENOUS LEUKEMIA (MYELODYSPLASTIC DISORDERS)

The MDSs are a heterogeneous group of clonal myeloid diseases that span the spectrum from clonal cytopenias to oligoblastic myelogenous leukemia and are discussed in Chap. 86. They include refractory anemia (RA), refractory anemia with ringed sideroblasts (RARS), refractory cytopenias with multilineage dysplasia (RCMD), RCMD with ringed sideroblasts (RCMD-RS), refractory anemia with excess blasts (RAEB), unclassified MDS, and MDS with isolated del(5q). Clonal chromosome abnormalities can be detected in marrow cells of 40 to

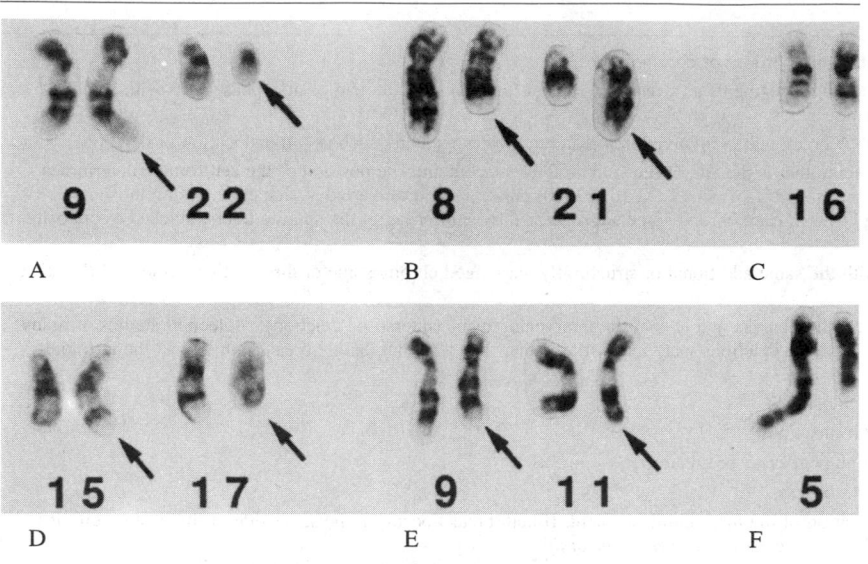

FIGURE 10-1   Partial karyotypes from trypsin-Giemsa-banded metaphase cells depicting recurring chromosomal rearrangements observed in myeloid leukemias. (A) t(9;22)(q34;q11.2), CML. (B) t(8;21)(q22;q22), AML-M2. (C) inv(16)(p13.1;q22), AMMoL-M4Eo. (D) t(15;17)(q22;q11.2-12), APL. (E) t(9;11)(p22;q23), AMoL-M5. (F) del(5)(q13q33), t-AML. The rearranged chromosomes are identified with *arrows*.

100 percent of patients with primary MDS at diagnosis (RA, 25%; RARS, 10%; RCMD, 50%; RAEB, 50–70%; MDS with isolated del(5q), 100%).[25,26] The proportion varies with the risk that a subtype will transform to AML, which is highest for RCMD and RAEB. The common chromosome changes, +8, −5/del(5q), −7/del(7q), and del(20q), are similar to those seen in AML *de novo*. The recurring translocations that are closely associated with the distinct morphologic subsets of AML *de novo* are almost never seen in MDS. With the exception of MDS with isolated del(5q), the chromosome changes show no close association with the specific subtypes of MDS. MDS with isolated del(5q) occurs in a subset of older patients with RA, frequently women, generally low blast counts, and normal or elevated platelet counts.[27] These patients have an interstitial deletion of 5q, typically as the sole abnormality. The deletions vary in size, but are similar to those noted in AML. These patients can have a relatively benign course that extends over several years (see Chap. 86).

Cytogenetic abnormalities in MDS are predictive of survival and progression to AML.[26] Patients with a "good outcome" have normal karyotypes, −Y alone, del(5q) alone, or del(20q) alone; those with an "intermediate outcome" have other abnormalities; and those with a "poor outcome" have complex karyotypes (more than three abnormalities, typically with abnormalities of chromosome 5 and/or 7) or chromosome 7 abnormalities.[26]

ACUTE MYELOGENOUS LEUKEMIA *DE NOVO*

Clonal chromosomal abnormalities are detected in 80 to 90 percent of patients with AML. The most frequent abnormalities are +8 and −7, which are seen in most subtypes of AML.[1,3] Specific rearrangements are closely associated with particular phenotypic (morphologic) subtypes of AML as defined by the French-American-British (FAB) classification (Table 10-5).[1,28] A new scoring system established by the World Health Organization (WHO) uses cytogenetic abnormalities as a criterion for AML classification.[29]

The 8;21 translocation [t(8;21)(q22;q22)], described in 1973, was the first translocation identified in AML (see Fig. 10-1B). The t(8;21) is common and is observed in 5 to 10 percent of all AML cases with

an abnormal karyotype and in 10 percent of M2 patients.[30] This translocation is the most frequent abnormality in children with AML and occurs in 15 to 20 percent of karyotypically abnormal cases. Loss of a sex chromosome (−Y in males, −X in females) accompanies the t(8;21) in 75 percent of cases. The presence of the t(8;21) identifies a morphologically and clinically distinct subset of AML, and most cases with the t(8;21) are classified as AML with maturation (M2). AML with the t(8;21) has a favorable prognosis in adults (overall 5-year survival of 70%), but the outcome in children is poor.[28] At the molecular level, the t(8;21) involves the *RUNX1/AML1* gene, which encodes a transcription factor, also known as core-binding factor, that is essential for hematopoiesis.[30] The *RUNX1* gene on chromosome 21 is fused to the *ETO* gene on chromosome 8 and results in an AML1-ETO chimeric protein.[30] Transformation by AML1-ETO likely results from transcriptional repression of normal AML1 target genes via aberrant recruitment of nuclear transcriptional corepressor complexes.

Another clinical–cytogenetic association involves acute myelomonocytic (M4) leukemia with abnormal eosinophils, including large and irregular basophilic granules, and positive reactions with periodic-acid Schiff and chloroacetate esterase (AMMoL-M4Eo). Most patients have an inversion of chromosome 16, inv(16)(p13.1q22) (see Fig. 10-1C), but some have a t(16;16)(p13.1;q22). These aberrations are relatively common, occurring in 5 percent of AML and 25 percent of AMMoL patients.[1,28] These patients have a good response to intensive chemotherapy with a complete remission rate of approximately 90 percent and an overall 5-year survival of 60 percent.[28] The breakpoint at 16q22 occurs within the *CBFB* gene, which encodes one subunit of the RUNX1/CBFB transcription factor. Thus, like the t(8;21), the inv(16) disrupts the RUNX1/AML1 pathway regulating hematopoiesis.[30] Secondary cooperating mutations of *KRAS1* or *NRAS* are common in core-binding factor-associated leukemias.

The t(15;17)(q22;q11.2-12) (see Fig. 10-1D) is highly specific for acute promyelocytic leukemia (APL) and has not been found in any other disease.[31] Although the t(15;17) was believed to be present in all cases of APL initially, it is now recognized that there are rare variant translocations that occur in less than 2 percent of cases. These include the t(11;17)(q23;q11.2-12) and t(5;17)(q34;q11.2-12), which result in the PLZF-RARA and NPM-RARA fusion proteins, respectively. Establishing the diagnosis of APL with the typical t(15;17) is important, because this disease is sensitive to therapy with all-*trans* retinoic acid, whereas other cases of AML and some of the APL-like disorders associated with the variant translocations do not respond to this treatment. The t(15;17) results in a fusion promyelocytic leukemia-retinoic acid receptor-alpha protein (PML-RARA). The oncogenic potential of the APL fusion proteins appears to result from the aberrant repression of retinoic acid receptor-mediated gene transcription through histone deacetylase (HDAC)-dependent chromatin remodeling. Genetic mutations that cooperate with PML-RARA in mediating leukemogenesis include *FLT3* internal tandem duplications, which are observed in 35 percent of patients.

Recurring translocations involving 11q23 are seen in approximately 35 percent of M5 patients and are of importance in acute leukemia for at least three reasons.[1,32,33] First, there are at least 47 different recurring rearrangements that involve 11q23 and, thus, along with 14q32, 11q23 is one of the bands most frequently involved in rearrangements in human tumor cells.[1,33] The breakpoints in the translo-

TABLE 10-5 RECURRING CHROMOSOME ABNORMALITIES IN MALIGNANT MYELOID DISEASES

DISEASE	CHROMOSOME ABNORMALITY	FREQUENCY*	INVOLVED GENES†		CONSEQUENCE
CML	t(9;22)(q34;q11.2)	98% (100%)‡	ABL	BCR	Fusion protein—altered cytokine signaling pathways
CML blast phase	t(9;22) with +8, +Ph, +19, or i(17q)	~70%			
AML-M2	t(8;21)(q22;q22)	18% (30%)	ETO	RUNX1/AML1	Fusion protein—altered transcriptional regulation
AML-M3, M3V	t(15;17)(q22;q11.2−12)	14% (98%)	PML	RARA	Fusion protein—altered transcriptional regulation
AMMoL-M4Eo	inv(16)(p13.1;q22) or t(16;16)(p13.1;q22)	8% (~100%)	MYH11	CBFB	Fusion protein—altered transcriptional regulation
AMMoL- M4, AMoL- M5	t(9;11)(p22;q23)	11% (30%) for all t(11q23)	AF9	MLL	MLL fusion proteins—altered transcriptional regulation
	t(10;11)(p11-p15;q23)		AF10	MLL	
	t(11;17)(q23;q25)		MLL	AF17	
	t(11;19)(q23;p13.3)		MLL	ENL	
	t(11;19)(q23;p13.1)		MLL	ELL	
	t(6;11)(q27;q23)		AF6	MLL	
	Other t(11q23)		MLL		
	del(11)(q23)				
AML	+8	10%			
	+11	1–2%	MLL		Internal tandem duplication
	−7 or del(7q)	10%			
	−5 or del (5q)	10%			
	t(6;9)(p23;q34)	1%	DEK	NUP214	
	inv(3)(q21q26.2) or t(3;3)	2%	EVI1		
	del(20q)	5%			
	t(12p) or del(12p)	2%			
Therapy-related AML	−7 or del(7q) and/or −5 or del(5q)	75%			
	der(1;7)(q10;p10)	2%			
	t(9;11)(p22;q23)/t(11q23)	3%	MLL		MLL fusion protein—altered transcriptional regulation
	t(21q22)	2%	RUNX1/AML1		Fusion protein—altered transcriptional regulation
CMMoL	t(5;12)(q33;p12)	2–5%	PDGFRB	ETV6/TEL	Fusion protein—altered signaling pathways

AML-M2, acute myeloblastic leukemia with maturation; AMMoL, acute myelomonocytic leukemia; AMMoL-M4Eo, acute myelomonocytic leukemia with abnormal eosinophils; AMoL, acute monoblastic leukemia; AML, acute myeloid leukemia; APL-M3, M3V, hypergranular (M3) and microgranular (M3V) acute promyelocytic leukemia; CML, chronic myelogenous leukemia; CMMoL, chronic myelomonocytic leukemia.

* The percentage refer to the frequency within the disease overall. The numbers in the parentheses refer to the frequency within the morphologic or immunologic subtype of the disease.
† Genes are listed in order of citation in the karyotype; e.g., for CML, ABL is at 9q34 and BCR at 22q11.2.
‡ Some patients with CML have an insertion of ABL adjacent to BCR in a normal-appearing chromosome 22.

cation partners include 1p32, 4q21, and 19p13.3 in acute lymphoblastic leukemia (ALL), and 1q21, 2q21, 6q27, 9p22, 10p11, 17q25, 19p13.3, and 19p13.1 in AML. Second, these translocations occur in both lymphoid and myeloid leukemias. One common translocation in infants, t(4;11)(q21;q23), has a lymphoblastic phenotype, whereas other translocations, such as the t(9;11)(p22;q23) (see Fig. 10-1E) and t(11;19)(q23;p13.1), are common in monoblastic leukemias. Translocations involving 11q23 have a very unusual age distribution, comprising approximately 75 percent of the chromosome abnormalities in leukemia cells of children younger than 1 year of age.[33] With the exception of the t(9;11), which may have an intermediate outcome, translocations of 11q23 are associated with a poor outcome.[28] Translocations of 11q23 involve MLL, a very large gene (>100 kb) with multiple transcripts of 12 to 15 kb.[32] The MLL protein is a histone methyltransferase that assembles in protein complexes that regulate gene transcription via chromatin remodeling. All of the MLL translocations identified to date result in fusion proteins.

Trisomy 11 is a rare abnormality, noted as a sole aberration in 1 to 2 percent of MDS or AML, and confers an unfavorable outcome.[34] It is notable that duplications of the MLL gene are detected in 90 percent of AMLs with +11 as the sole abnormality, and in 10 percent of AML cases with an apparently normal karyotype. The rearrangement is the result of a partial tandem duplication of MLL exons 2 to

6 or 2 to 8 mediated by recombination between Alu repetitive elements, which may produce a partially duplicated protein.

Each of the other recurring rearrangements in AML occur in fewer than 3 percent of patients. A unique feature of abnormalities involving the long arm of chromosome 3 [inv(3)(q21q26.2) or t(3;3)(q21;q26.2)] is the presence of platelet counts above 1000×10^9/liter and an increase in marrow megakaryocytes, especially micromegakaryocytes.[1] Most of the recurring translocations described above occur in younger patients with a median age in the thirties, whereas other abnormalities, such as −5/del(5q) or −7/del(7q), occur in patients with a median age greater than 50 years. Moreover, many of the latter patients have occupational exposure to mutagenic agents such as solvents, petroleum, and pesticides.

Some of the most common genetic changes involved in the pathogenesis of AML are mutations of individual genes. Mutations of the FMS-like tyrosine kinase 3 (FLT3) gene, including both point mutations within the kinase domain and internal tandem duplications (ITDs), are among the most common genetic changes seen in AML, occurring in 15 to 35 percent of cases.[35] FLT3-ITD mutations are associated with a poor prognosis, particularly in those cases with loss of the remaining wild-type FLT3 allele.[35] Activation of KIT occurs in 5 percent of AML cases through similar mechanisms, as well as through in-frame insertion and deletion mutations.[36] Point mutations of a number of the genes that encode transcription factors important for hematopoiesis, for example, *RUNX1/AML1*, *GATA1*, *PU.1*, and *C/EBPA*, have been identified in AML.[6] Some of these are associated with particular forms of AML. For example, *GATA1* mutations have been found to date only in Down syndrome-associated megakaryoblastic leukemia or transient MPD,[37] and *C/EBPA* mutations seem to be particularly common in AML cases with a normal karyotype, where they confer a favorable prognosis.[38] Figure 10-2 shows the relative frequency of recurring cytogenetic abnormalities in AML.

ACUTE MYELOGENOUS LEUKEMIA AND MYELODYSPLASTIC SYNDROMES ASSOCIATED WITH PRIOR CYTOTOXIC TREATMENT

Therapy-related myelodysplastic syndrome (t-MDS) and therapy-related acute myelogenous leukemia (t-AML) are recognized as late complications of cytotoxic therapy used in the treatment of both malignant and nonmalignant diseases.[39] In patients who received alkylating agents, the characteristic recurring chromosome abnormalities observed are loss of part or all of chromosomes 5 and/or 7 [−5/del(5q) or −7/del(7q)] (see Fig. 10-1F). In our experience, 92 percent of t-MDS/t-AML patients had an abnormal karyotype and 70 percent had an abnormality of either chromosome 5 or 7 or both[40]; other series have confirmed these observations.[41] In contrast, only approximately 16 percent of patients with AML *de novo* have a similar abnormality of chromosome 5 or 7 or both.[1]

By cytogenetic analysis of 177 patients with malignant myeloid diseases and a del(5q), we identified a small segment of 5q, consisting of band 5q31, that was deleted in each patient.[42] This segment has been termed the commonly deleted segment. By molecular analyses, we have narrowed the commonly deleted segment to a region of 1.5 Mb that contains 21 genes.[42] Parallel studies have revealed a 2.5-Mb commonly deleted segment within 7q22 that contains 16 genes. We have not detected any mutations of the genes within these regions, which suggests that novel tumor suppressor genes are located in 5q31 or 7q22, or that a novel mechanism is involved in the pathogenesis of t-AML, for example, promoter hypermethylation or haploinsufficiency (gene dosage effect resulting from loss of one allele).

A second subtype of t-AML has been identified that is distinctly different from the more common leukemia that follows alkylating agents or irradiation. This type of t-AML is seen in patients receiving drugs known to inhibit topoisomerase II such as etoposide, teniposide, and doxorubicin.[39] Clinically, these patients have a shorter latency period (1–2 years), present with overt leukemia, often with monocytic features, without a preceding myelodysplastic phase, and have a more favorable response to intensive induction therapy. Balanced translocations involving the *MLL* gene at 11q23 or the *RUNX1/AML1* gene at 21q22 are common in this subgroup.[39] Figure 10-2 shows the relative frequency of recurring cytogenetic abnormalities in AML.

ACUTE LYMPHOBLASTIC LEUKEMIA

ALL is the most frequent leukemia in children (see Chap. 91). The most useful prognostic indicators are karyotype (including ploidy), age, white blood cell count, sex, and response to initial therapy.[1,4,43] Children who are between the ages of 2 and 10 years old, who have a white blood cell count of less than 10×10^9/liter, and whose leukemia cells express the common acute lymphoblastic leukemia antigen (CALLA, CD10) have the best prognosis. In both childhood and adult ALL, the identification of prognostic subgroups based on recurring cytogenetic abnormalities (Table 10-6) and molecular markers has resulted in the application of risk-adapted therapies.[2,4]

The incidence of the t(9;22) in ALL is 30 percent in adults (the incidence may approach 50 percent in adults older than 60 years of age) and 5 percent in children. Thus, the Ph chromosome is the most frequent rearrangement in adult ALL. Approximately 70 percent of the patients show additional abnormalities, a frequency that is substantially higher than that observed in CML with +der(22)t(9;22),+21, abnormalities of 9p, +8, −7, and +X (noted in descending frequency). Monosomy 7 is associated with a poorer outcome.[44] A chromosomally normal cell line is frequently noted in the marrow of Ph+ ALL patients (70%), but is rare in untreated CML. Most cases have an early pre-B phenotype. However, some cases have had both B cell and myeloid markers. The disease in both adults and children is characterized by high white blood cell counts, a high percentage

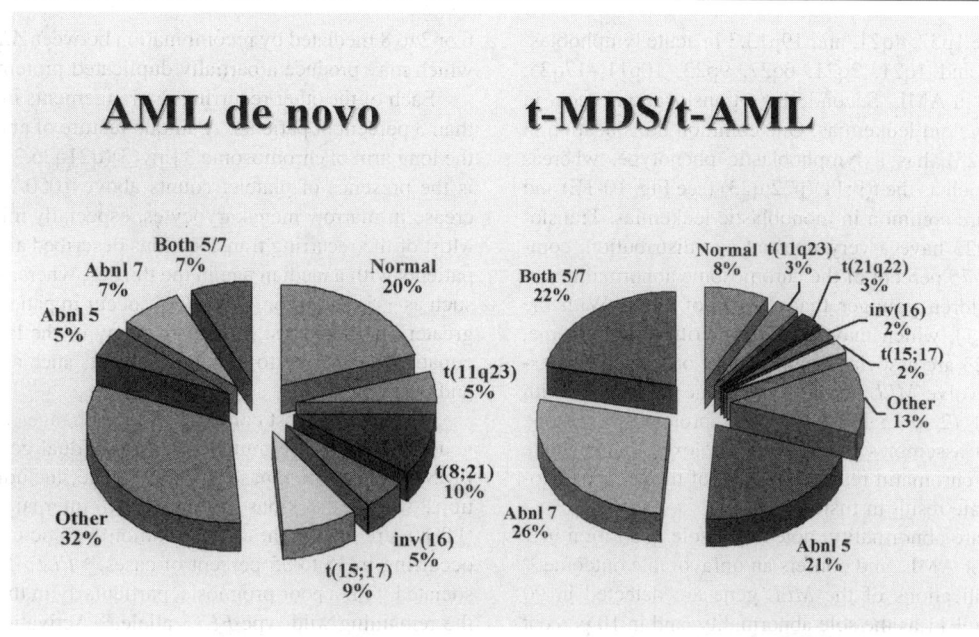

FIGURE 10-2   Frequency of recurring cytogenetic abnormalities in clonal myeloid diseases. Abnl, abnormal.

TABLE 10-6 CYTOGENETIC–IMUNOPHENOTYPIC CORRELATIONS IN MALIGNANT LYMPHOID DISEASES

DISEASE	CHROMOSOME ABNORMALITY	FREQUENCY*	INVOLVED GENES†		CONSEQUENCE‡
Acute lymphoblastic leukemia					
Precursor B	t(12;21)(p12;q22)	25%	ETV6/TEL	RUNX1/AML1	Fusion protein—TF
	t(9;22)(q34;q11.2)	10%‡	ABL	BCR	Fusion protein—altered cytokine signaling pathways
	t(4;11)(q21;q23)	5%	AF4	MLL	Fusion protein—TF
	t(17;19)(q21−22;p13.3)	1%	HLF	TCF3 (E2A)	Fusion protein—TF
	t(11;19)(q23;p13.3)	1%	MLL	ENL	Fusion protein—TF
Pre-B	t(1;19)(q23;p13.3)	6% (30%)	PBX1	TCF3 (E2A)	Fusion protein—TF
B(SIg+)	t(8;14)(q24.1;q32)	5% (95%)	MYC	IGH	Deregulated expression—TF
	t(2;8)(p12;q24.1)	<1% (1%)	IGK	MYC	Deregulated expression—TF
	t(8;22)(q24.1;q11.2)	<1% (4%)	MYC	IGL	Deregulated expression—TF
Other	Hyperdiploidy (50–60)	10%			
	del(12p),t(12p)	10%			
T	t(11;14)(p15;q11.2)	1%	RBTN1	TCRA	Deregulated expression—TF
	t(11;14)(p13;q11.2)	3%	RBTN2	TCRA	Deregulated expression—TF
	t(8;14)(q24.1;q11.2)	<1%	MYC	TCRA	Deregulated expression—TF
	inv(14)(q11.2;q32)	<1%	TCRA	TCL1	Deregulated expression—TF
	t(10;14)(q24;q11.2)	3%	HOX11	TCRA	Deregulated expression—TF
	t(1;14)(p32;q11.2)	1%	TALI	TCRD	Deregulated expression—TF
	t(7;9)(q34;q32)		TCRB	TAN1	Deregulated expression—TF
	t(7;9)(q34;q34)	2%	TCRB	NOTCH1	Deregulated expression—TF
	t(7;19)(q34;p13.3)	<1%			
	del(9p),t(9p)	<1% (10%)	CDKN2A,B		Tumor-suppressor gene—cell cycle regulation
Non-Hodgkin lymphoma					
B cell NHL					
Burkitt	t(8;14)(q24.1;q32)	95%	MYC	IGH	Deregulated expression—TF
	t(2;8)(p12;q24.1)	1%	IGK	MYC	Deregulated expression—TF
	t(8;22)(q24.1;q11.2)	4%	MYC	IGL	Deregulated expression—TF
Follicular SNCL	t(14;18)(q32;q21.3)	80%	IGH	BCL2	Deregulated expression—antiapoptosis protein
DLBCL	t(14;18)(q32;q21)	20%			
DLBCL	t(3;22)(q27;q11.2)	45% for both	BCL6	IGL	Deregulated expression—TF
	t(3;14)(q27;q32)		BCL6	IGH	Deregulated expression—TF
MCL	t(11;14)(q13;q32)	~100%	CCND1	IGH	Deregulated expression—TF
LPL	t(9;14)(p13;q32)		PAX5	IGH	Deregulated expression—TF
SLL	t(14;19)(q32;q13.3)		IGH	BCL3	Deregulated expression—TF
MALT	t(11;18)(q21;q21)	40-50%	BIRC3/API2	MALT1	Fusion protein—increased NFκB activation
	t(1;14)(p22;q32)	10%	BCL10	IGH	Deregulated expression—increased NFκB activation
T cell NHL					
(Ki-1+) ALCL	t(2;5)(p23;q35)	75%	ALK	NPM	Deregulated expression—tyrosine kinase
Chronic lymphocytic leukemia					
B	t(11;14)(q13;q32)	10%	CCND1	IGH	Deregulated expression—cell cycle regulation
	t(14;19)(q32;q13.2)	10%	IGH	BCL3	Deregulated expression—increased NFκB activation
	t(2;14)(p13;q32)	5%		IGH	
	t(14q32)	20%			
	del(13q)	30%			
	+12	30%			
T	t(8;14)(q24.1;q11.2)	5%	MYC	TCRA	Deregulated expression—TF
	inv(14)(q11.2q32)	5%	TCRA/D	IGH	Deregulated expression
	inv(14)(q11.2q32)	5%	TCRA/D	TCL1	Deregulated expression—TF
Myeloma					
B	−13/del(13q)	40%			
	t(4;14)(p16;q32)	15%	FGFR3	IGH	Deregulated expression—growth factor receptor
	t(14;16)(q32;q23)	5%	IGH	MAF	Deregulated expression—TF
	t(6;14)(p21;q32)	4%	CCND3	IGH	Deregulated expression—cell cycle regulation
	t(11;14)(q13;q32)	15%	CCND1	IGH	Deregulated expression—cell cycle regulation
	t(14q32)	50%	IGH		
	Hyperdiploidy, +3,+7	20%			
Adult T-cell leukemia/lymphoma					
	t(14;14)(q11.2;q32)		TCRA	IGH	Deregulated expression
	inv(14)(q11.2q32)		TCRA/D	IGH	Deregulated expression
	+3				

ALCL, anaplastic large-cell lymphoma; CTCL, cutaneous T cell lymphoma; DLBCL, diffuse large B cell lymphoma; Ki-1, anti-CD30 antibody; LPL, lymphoplasmacytoid lymphoma; MALT, mucosa-associated lymphoid tumor; MCL, mantle cell lymphoma; SIg, surface immunoglobulin; SLL, small-cell lymphocytic lymphoma.

* The percentage refers to the frequency within the disease overall. The number in the parentheses refers to the frequency within the morphologic or immunologic subtype of the disease.
† Genes are listed in order of citation in karyotype; for example, for precursor B ALL, ETV6/TEL is at 12p12 and RUNX1/AML1 is at 21q22.
‡ By cytogenetic analysis, the frequency in children is approximately 5 percent, and in adults it is approximately 25 percent; using molecular probes, this frequency is 30 percent in adults overall, and 50 percent in adults older than 60 years of age.

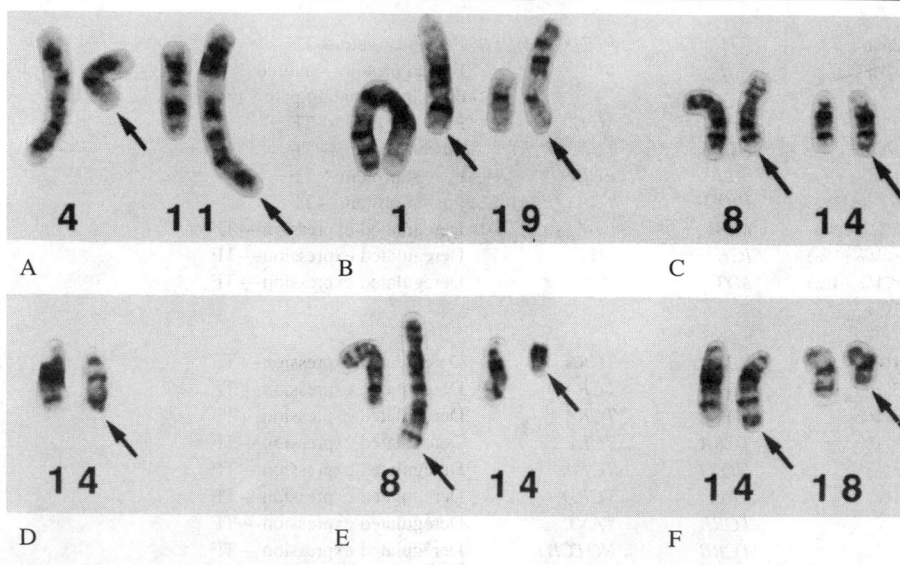

FIGURE 10-3 Partial karyotypes of trypsin-Giemsa-banded metaphase cells depicting recurring chromosomal rearrangements observed in lymphoid malignant diseases. (A) t(4;11)(q21;q23) in ALL. (B) t(1;19)(q21;p13.3) in pre-B cell ALL. (C) t(8;14)(q24.1;q32) in B cell ALL and Burkitt lymphoma. (D) inv(14)(q11.2q32) in T cell leukemia/lymphoma. (E) t(8;14)(q24.1;q11.2) in T cell leukemia/lymphoma. (F) t(14;18)(q32;q21.3) in B cell non-Hodgkin lymphoma. The rearranged chromosomes are identified with *arrows*.

of circulating blasts, and a poor prognosis. As in CML, the t(9;22) in ALL results in a *BCR-ABL*^{p210} fusion gene. However, in more than half of patients the break in *BCR* is more proximal, resulting in a smaller fusion protein with even greater tyrosine kinase activity (BCR-ABL^{p190}).

Translocations involving the *MLL* gene at 11q23 are observed in 5 percent of ALL patients.[1,45] Of these, the most common is the t(4;11)(q21;q23) (Fig. 10-3A). The t(11;19)(q23;p13.3) is second in frequency. However, this rearrangement is not limited to ALL in that approximately 50 percent of these cases have AML, usually monoblastic. Of note is the high frequency of translocations involving 11q23 in infant ALL (60–80%). Patients with the t(4;11) have a pro-B phenotype (CD10−, CD19+), with coexpression of monocytic (CD15+) or, less commonly, T cell markers. Clinically, they have aggressive features with hyperleukocytosis, extramedullary disease, and a poor response to conventional chemotherapy. Adults with the t(4;11) have a remission rate of 75 percent, but a median event-free survival (EFS) of only 7 months.[4] Children with the t(4;11) have a similarly poor outcome.[45] Rearrangements affecting *MLL* represent a major class of mutations in acute leukemia and identify patients with a poor outcome.

The t(12;21)(p12;q22) has been identified in a high proportion (~25%) of childhood precursor B leukemia.[46] The translocation is not easily detected by cytogenetic analysis because of the similarity in size and banding pattern of 12p and 21q. However, the rearrangement can be detected reliably using RT-PCR or FISH analysis. The t(12;21) defines a distinct subgroup of patients characterized by an age between 1 and 10 years, B lineage immunophenotype (CD10+, CD19+, HLA-DR+), and a favorable outcome. It is not seen in T cell ALL and is uncommon in adults (~4% of ALL cases). In a recent series, patients with the t(12;21) had a 5-year EFS of 91 percent as compared with 65 percent for patients without this rearrangement. However, the t(12;21) may be associated with late disease recurrences. The t(12;21) results in a fusion protein containing the *N*-terminus of ETV6/TEL, a transcriptional repressor of the ETS family, and most of the RUNX1/AML1 transcription factor.

The leukemia cells of some patients with ALL are characterized by a gain of many chromosomes. Two distinct subgroups are recognized: a group with 1 to 4 extra chromosomes (47 to 50), and the more common group with more than 50 chromosomes. Chromosome numbers usually range from 51 to 60, and a few patients may have up to 65 chromosomes. Hyperdiploidy (>50 chromosomes) is common in children (~30%), but is rarely observed in adults (<5%). Certain additional chromosomes are common (X chromosome, and chromosomes 4, 6, 10, 14, 17, 18, and 21). Chromosome 21 is gained most frequently (100% of cases). Patients who have hyperdiploidy with more than 50 chromosomes have all of the previously recognized clinical factors that indicate a good prognosis, including age between 1 and 9 years, low white blood cell count (median 6,700/μl), and favorable immunophenotype (early pre-B or pre-B).[47] The favorable prognosis associated with high hyperdiploidy is associated with gains of chromosomes 4, 10, 6, and 17, whereas a gain of chromosome 5 and i(17q) are associated with a poor outcome.[47]

The t(1;19)(q23;p13.3) has been identified in approximately 25 percent of patients with a pre-B phenotype. The leukemia cells have cytoplasmic immunoglobulin and are CD10+, CD34−, and CD20− (see Fig. 10-3B). A reciprocal translocation involving the long arms of chromosomes 8 and 14 [t(8;14)(q24;q32)] is observed in mature B cell ALL (see Fig. 10-3C).[4,43] These patients have a high incidence of central nervous system involvement and/or abdominal nodal involvement at diagnosis. The use of high-intensity chemotherapy has markedly improved the previously poor outcome for both children and adults with a t(8;14), especially in children (EFS of 80% in children).[43]

T CELL ACUTE LYMPHOBLASTIC LEUKEMIA

Precursor T cell neoplasms have a distinct pattern of recurring karyotypic abnormalities.[1] Rearrangements involving 14q11.2 (see Fig. 10-3D) and two regions of chromosome 7 (7q34 and 7p14) are particularly frequent in T-cell malignancies (see Table 10-6). The most common are the t(11;14)(p13;q11.2) (~3%, *RBTN2* gene), t(10;11)(q24;q11.2) (~3%, *HOX11* gene), and t(7;9)(q34;q34) (~2%, *NOTCH1* gene). Patients with T cell ALL are most often young males and often have a mediastinal tumor mass, high white blood cell count, and leukemia cells in the cerebrospinal fluid. These same clinical characteristics are associated with lymphoblastic lymphoma, another T cell malignancy.

CHRONIC LYMPHOCYTIC LEUKEMIA

The chromosomal abnormalities associated with CLL have been delineated through the use of FISH.[48] When conventional cytogenetic techniques are used, only 50 percent of CLL patients have detectable chromosomal abnormalities (see Chap. 92). The most common abnormality is trisomy 12, followed by structural abnormalities of 13q and 14q.[49] However, when FISH analysis is used to study specific abnormalities, chromosomal abnormalities can be detected in greater than 80 percent of patients.[49] The most frequent chromosomal changes seen by FISH are deletion of 13q (55%); deletion of 11q, the location of the *ATM* gene (18%); trisomy of 12q (16%); deletion of 17p, the location of the *TP53* gene (7%); and deletion of 6q (6%).[49] Patient survival correlates with cytogenetic subtype, with a shorter median survival observed in patients with 17p (32 months) or 11q (79 months) deletions, than in those with no detectable abnormality (111 months), trisomy of 12q (114 months), or −13/del(13q) (133 months).[49] FISH probes capable of detecting the deletions of 11q, 13q, and 17p, trisomy 12, and *IGH* translocations are now commercially available and may facilitate the application of risk-adapted treatment strategies.

The prognosis of patients with CLL is also determined by two other molecular abnormalities: the status of the immunoglobulin heavy-chain variable region (*IgHv*) and the expression level of CD38. Patients whose CLL cells express *IgHv* genes containing somatic mutations have a 24-year median survival compared to only 6 to 8 years in those patients who do not have somatic *IGHV* gene mutations.[50,51] This simple grouping of patients based on the mutation status of the *IGHV* gene may reflect the fact that CLL cells that have few or no *IgHv* mutations also often contain chromosomal aberrations that confer a poor prognosis, for example, deletions of 11q or 17p, whereas CLL cells with *IgHv* mutations often contain deletions of 13q, which confer a more favorable clinical course. Unfortunately, testing for somatic mutations in the *IgH* gene is not currently commercially available. ZAP-70, an enzyme normally expressed in T lymphocytes and critical for T cell activation, is up-regulated in CLL cells that contain unmutated *IgHv* genes, conferring a poor prognosis.[52] CD38, a membrane protein with signaling activity, is often expressed in CLL cells that contain *IgHv* mutations; consequently, the presence of CD38 staining on CLL cells confers a favorable prognosis.[50]

T cell CLL and large granular lymphocytic leukemia are uncommon disorders in which the malignant lymphocytes have a T cell immunophenotype. Rearrangements involving band 14q11.2 with or without an accompanying break in 14q32 have been reported in T cell CLL as well as in T cell lymphomas (see Table 10-6).[1] The most common is inv(14)(q11.2q32).

NON-HODGKIN LYMPHOMA

Cytogenetic analyses of non-Hodgkin lymphoma (NHL) have been reported in a number of large series (see Chaps. 95 and 96).[53] These investigations demonstrate that greater than 90 percent of cases are characterized by clonal chromosomal abnormalities and, more importantly, many of the recurring abnormalities correlate with histology and immunophenotype (see Table 10-6). For example, the t(14;18) is observed in a high proportion of follicular small cleaved cell lymphomas (70–90%); most patients with a t(3;22)(q27;q11.2) or t(3;14)(q27; q32) have diffuse large B cell lymphomas (DLBCLs), and patients with a t(8;14)(q24.1;q32) have either small noncleaved cell lymphomas or DLBCLs. Band 14q32, the location of *IGH*, is frequently involved in translocations in B cell neoplasms (~70%). In contrast, a large proportion of T cell neoplasms are characterized by rearrangements that involve 14q11.2, 7q34, or 7p14, the locations of the T cell receptor genes.

The t(8;14) is characteristic of both endemic and nonendemic Burkitt tumors, as well as Epstein-Barr virus (EBV)-negative and EBV-positive tumors (see Fig. 10-3E). Moreover, the t(8;14) has also been observed in other lymphomas, particularly small noncleaved cell (non-Burkitt) and large cell immunoblastic lymphomas, AIDS-associated Burkitt lymphoma (BL) (100%) and AIDS-related DLBCL (30%).[53,54] Two other variant translocations also occur in BL: t(2; 8)(p12;q24.1) and t(8;22)(q24.1;q11.2). All three translocations involve chromosome band 8q24. As discussed in "Acute Lymphoblastic Leukemia," these same translocations have been seen in some patients with B cell ALL. The t(8;14) involves a break within the *IGH* locus on chromosome 14 and a break either 5′ or within *MYC* on chromosome 8, and relocates the *MYC* coding exons to chromosome 14. MYC

is a transcription factor that plays a role in a number of cellular processes including proliferation and apoptosis, and its oncogenic properties are due to its constitutive expression.

Between 80 and 90 percent of follicular lymphomas and 20 percent of DLBCLs have the t(14;18) (see Fig. 10-3F), in which the *BCL2* gene at 18q21.3 is juxtaposed to the *IgH* J segment, leading to the deregulated expression of *BCL2*.[53–55] Common secondary abnormalities include −7, +18, and del(6q). Other malignancies that overexpress *BCL2* but do not harbor the t(14;18), include hairy cell leukemia and CLL. The *BCL2* gene encodes a 26 kDa membrane protein that functions to increase cell survival (antiapoptosis). Thus, this class of oncogene contributes to the development of a neoplastic state by preventing programmed cell death, rather than promoting proliferation.

The t(11;14)(q13;q32) is observed in virtually all cases of mantle cell lymphoma.[56] Besides mantle cell lymphomas, the t(11;14) has also been reported in 3 percent of multiple myeloma, and up to 20 percent of prolymphocytic leukemias.[57] Many cases also have deletions or point mutations of the *ATM* gene (11q22). Mantle cell lymphomas are currently regarded as a poor prognostic group with a median survival from diagnosis of 3 years. This translocation results in the activation of the cyclin D1 (*CCND1*) gene by the *IgH* gene (J region).[56] Interestingly, the *CCND1* gene is located 100 to 130 kb away from the breakpoint on 11q13. The D-type cyclins act as growth factor sensors, causing cells to go through the restriction start point of the cell cycle at G_1 and committing them to divide via phosphorylation and inactivation of RB1.

The *BCL6* gene was cloned from the recurring breakpoint at 3q27 in cells characterized by a t(3;22)(q27;q11.2), t(3;14)(q27;q32), or, rarely, t(2;3)(p12;q27).[53] *BCL6* rearrangements occur in 40 percent of DLBCLs and, in some series, up to 10 percent of follicular lymphomas. The translocations lead to the truncation of the *BCL6* gene within the first exon or the first intron, substitution of its promoter sequences with an *IG* promoter, and deregulated expression. The *BCL6* gene product is a 96-kDa POZ/Zn finger, nuclear protein that acts as a potent transcriptional repressor. It is predominantly expressed in the B cell lineage, particularly in mature B cells, and may suppress genes involved in lymphocyte activation, differentiation, cell cycle arrest, and apoptosis. Somatic mutations have been identified in the 5′ regulatory regions of *BCL6* in approximately 20 percent of DLBCLs without translocations leading to deregulation of *BCL6*, suggesting that overexpression of *BCL6* is more broadly involved than initially recognized.[58]

Extranodal marginal zone B cell lymphomas of mucosa-associated lymphoid tissue (MALT) are comprised of several genetic subgroups, one characterized by trisomy 3 plus other abnormalities (60%) and another by the t(11;18)(q21;q21)(25–50%).[59] Of note is that the t(11; 18) is not observed in primary large B cell gastric lymphoma. The t(11;18) results in the fusion of the apoptosis-inhibitor gene *BIRC3* (*API2*) to a novel gene at 18q21, *MALT1*.

A number of recurring chromosomal abnormalities have been recognized in T cell leukemias and lymphomas (see Table 10-6). Similar to B cell neoplasms, in which rearrangements frequently involve the chromosomal bands containing the immunoglobulin gene loci, T cell neoplasms often have rearrangements involving band 14q11.2, the site of the T cell receptor α-chain (*TCRA*) and δ-chain (*TCRD*) genes, or, less often, one of two regions of chromosome 7 (7q34 and 7p14) to which the T cell receptor β-chain (*TCRB*) and γ-chain (*TCRG*) genes have been localized, respectively.[53] These translocations result from aberrant V-D-J recombination events (see Chap. 18). With few exceptions, the involved gene on the partner chromosome encodes a transcription factor, whose expression is deregulated or activated as a result of the rearrangement (see Table 10-6). A chromosomal re-

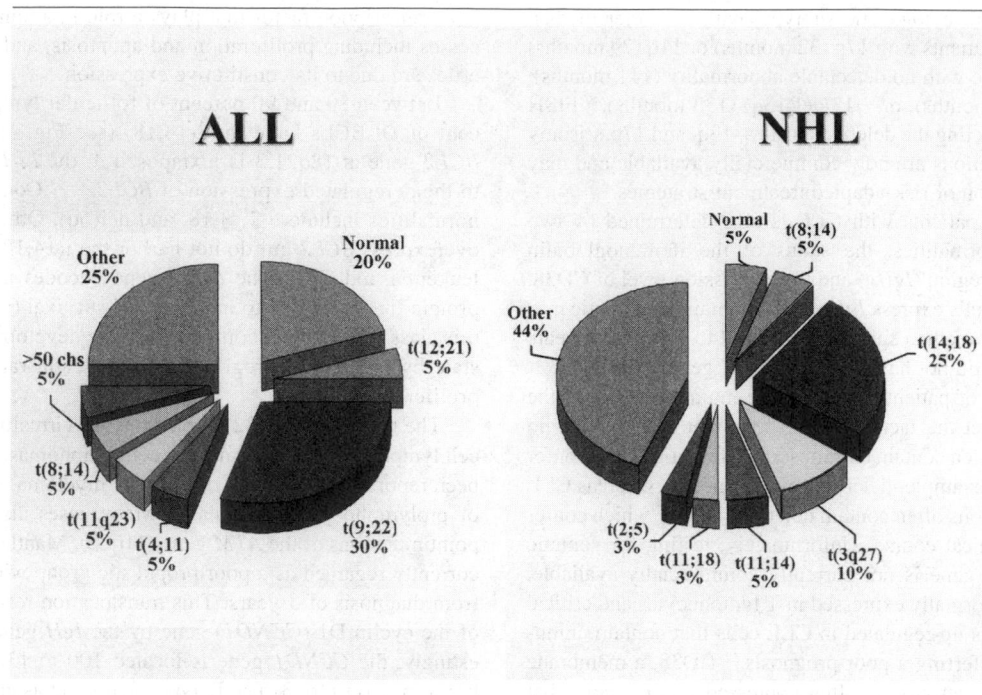

FIGURE 10-4 Frequency of recurring cytogenetic abnormalities in clonal lymphoid diseases. (>50 chs refers to 5% of patients with greater than 50 chromosomes.)

arrangement that brings an oncogene under the controlling influence of promoters or enhancers that are active for immunoglobulin synthesis in B cells or T cell receptor synthesis in T cells may, as a consequence, impart a proliferative advantage to that cell and result in malignant clonal expansion.

A distinctive subtype of NHL, namely, anaplastic large-cell lymphoma (ALCL), is characterized by a young age at presentation and skin and/or lymph node infiltration by large, often bizarre lymphoma cells, which preferentially involve the paracortical areas and lymph node sinuses. The majority of such tumors express one or more T cell antigens, a minority express B cell antigens, and some express both T and B cell antigens (the null phenotype). A reciprocal translocation, t(2;5)(p23;q35), or variant rearrangement involving the *ALK* tyrosine kinase gene at 2p23 appears to be restricted to ALCL of either T cell or null phenotype, and is present in a high percentage of these cases.[53] The tumor cells are positive for CD30 on the cell membrane and in the Golgi region, and ALK expression is detectable in 60 to 85 percent of cases, where it confers a more favorable outcome (5-year survival, 80% in ALK+ vs. 40% in ALK− tumors). The t(2;5) has also been found in CD30+ primary cutaneous lymphomas. Figure 10-4 shows the relative frequency of recurring cytogenetic abnormalities in clonal lymphoid diseases.

MYELOMA

As in CLL, the application of molecular cytogenetic tools, such as FISH, has led to the discovery of numerous chromosomal abnormalities in myeloma (see Chap. 100), its precursor, essential monoclonal gammopathy (see Chap. 99), and plasma cell leukemia.[57,60] Essential monoclonal gammopathy is characterized by chromosomal aneuploidy, *IGH* translocations (45% of patients), and deletions of 13q (15–50%). Myeloma is a malignancy of postfollicular B cells and is characterized by the acquisition of complex chromosomal rearrangements. As in monoclonal gammopathy, the earliest changes involve deletions of 13q14 and translocations of the *IGH* gene, which deregulate the

expression of oncogenes located near the translocation breakpoints. Loss of chromosome 13 or a del(13q) is the most frequently observed chromosomal losses in myeloma and confers a poor prognosis.[60] With the use of FISH, deletions of 13q are detected in 40 to 50 percent of patients with myeloma and may be associated with specific 14q translocations.

Among the most frequent chromosomal rearrangements noted in plasma cell malignancies are translocations involving the *IgH* locus on 14q32. *IgH* translocations are detectable by interphase FISH analysis in approximately 50 percent of patients with essential monoclonal gammopathy, in 60 to 75 percent of patients with myeloma, and in more than 80 percent of patients with plasma cell leukemia.[60] The t(11;14)(q13;q32) is found in 15 percent of cases and results in cyclin D1 overexpression; it also may deregulate expression of *MYEOV* (*myeloma overexpressed gene*). The t(4;14)(p16;q32) is noted in approximately 15 percent of patients and deregulates the expression of the fibroblast growth factor receptor 3 gene *(FGFR3)* on the der(14)/chromosome and the *MMSET* domain on the der(4) chromosome. The t(14;16)(q32;q23), noted in 5 percent of cases, results in the overexpression of the *MAF* transcription factor gene. Cyclin D3 overexpression occurs in the context of the t(6;14)(p21;q32), observed in 4 percent of patients. The translocation partners for the remaining 40 percent of myeloma cases are currently unknown. The t(4;14) and t(14;16) are both associated with a poor clinical outcome, whereas the t(11;14) confers a favorable prognosis. Translocations involving unknown partners confer an intermediate prognosis.

Additional events occur with disease progression, including mutations of *NRAS* and *KRAS1*, *MYC* deregulation, and epigenetic alterations. *NRAS* codon 61 mutations were identified in a subpopulation of plasma cells in all patients examined at diagnosis.[61] In another study, *NRAS* and/or *KRAS1* mutations were found in 55 percent of patients at diagnosis and in more than 80 percent of patients who relapsed.[62] Several genes are silenced through aberrant promoter hypermethylation in both MGUS and myeloma, including *DAPK* (67%), *SOCS1, p15 (CDKN2B)*, and *p16 (CDKN2A)*.[60]

REFERENCES

1. Bain BJ: Overview. Cytogenetic analysis in haematology. *Best Pract Res Clin Haematol* 14.463, 2001.

2. Gilliland DG: Molecular genetics of human leukemias: New insights into therapy. *Semin Hematol* 39:6, 2002.

3. Kebriaei P, Anastasi J, Larson RA: Acute lymphoblastic leukaemia: Diagnosis and classification. *Best Pract Res Clin Haematol* 15:597, 2002.

4. Falini B, Mason DY: Proteins encoded by genes involved in chromosomal alterations in lymphoma and leukemia: Clinical value of their detection by immunocytochemistry. *Blood* 99:409, 2002.

5. Tenen DG: Disruption of differentiation in human cancer: AML shows the way. *Nat Rev Cancer* 3:89, 2003.

6. Le Beau MM, Larson RA: Cytogenetics and neoplasia, in *Hematology: Basic Principles and Practices*, 3rd ed, edited by R Hoffman, EJ Benz, SJ Shattil, B Furie, HJ Cohen, LE Silberstein, P McGlave, p 848. Churchill-Livingstone, New York, 2000.

7. Gozzetti A, Le Beau MM: Fluorescence *in situ* hybridization: Uses and limitations. *Semin Hematol* 37:320, 2000.

8. Schrock E, Padilla-Nash H: Spectral karyotyping and multicolor fluorescence *in situ* hybridization reveal new tumor-specific chromosomal aberrations. *Semin Hematol* 37:334, 2000.

9. Braziel RM, Shipp MA, Feldman AL, et al: Molecular diagnostics. *Hematology (Am Soc Hematol Educ Program)* p 279, 2003.

10. Mitelman F: *An International System for Human Cytogenetic Nomenclature.* Karger, Basel, 1995.

11. Barnes DJ, Melo JV: Cytogenetic and molecular genetic aspects of chronic myeloid leukaemia. *Acta Haematol* 108:180, 2002.

12. Goldman JM, Melo JV: Chronic myeloid leukemia—Advances in biology and new approaches to treatment. *N Engl J Med* 349:1451, 2003.

13. Mauro MJ, O'Dwyer M, Heinrich MC, Druker BJ: STI571: A paradigm of new agents for cancer therapeutics. *J Clin Oncol* 20:325, 2002.

14. O'Brien SG, Guilhot F, Larson RA, et al: Imatinib compared with interferon and low-dose cytarabine for newly diagnosed chronic-phase chronic myeloid leukemia. *N Engl J Med* 348:994, 2003.

15. Druker BJ, Sawyers CL, Kantarjian H, et al: Activity of a specific inhibitor of the BCR-ABL tyrosine kinase in the blast crisis of chronic myeloid leukemia and acute lymphoblastic leukemia with the Philadelphia chromosome. *N Engl J Med* 344:1038, 2001.

16. Merx K, Muller MC, Kreil S, et al: Early reduction of BCR-ABL mRNA transcript levels predicts cytogenetic response in chronic phase CML patients treated with imatinib after failure of interferon alpha. *Leukemia* 16:1579, 2002.

17. Wang L, Pearson K, Pillitteri L, et al: Serial monitoring of BCR-ABL by peripheral blood real-time polymerase chain reaction predicts the marrow cytogenetic response to imatinib mesylate in chronic myeloid leukaemia. *Br J Haematol* 118:771, 2002.

18. Nardi V, Azam M, Daley GQ: Mechanisms and implications of imatinib resistance mutations in BCR-ABL. *Curr Opin Hematol* 11:35, 2004.

19. Bumm T, Muller C, Al-Ali HK, et al: Emergence of clonal cytogenetic abnormalities in Ph− cells in some CML patients in cytogenetic remission to imatinib but restoration of polyclonal hematopoiesis in the majority. *Blood* 101:1941, 2003.

20. Apperley JF, Gardembas M, Melo JV, et al: Response to imatinib mesylate in patients with chronic myeloproliferative diseases with rearrangements of the platelet-derived growth factor receptor beta. *N Engl J Med* 347:481, 2002.

21. Cools J, DeAngelo DJ, Gotlib J, et al: A tyrosine kinase created by fusion of the PDGFRA and FIP1L1 genes as a therapeutic target of imatinib in idiopathic hypereosinophilic syndrome. *N Engl J Med* 348:1201, 2003.

22. Klion AD, Robyn J, Akin C, et al: Molecular remission and reversal of myelofibrosis in response to imatinib mesylate treatment in patients with the myeloproliferative variant of hypereosinophilic syndrome. *Blood* 103:473, 2004.

23. Tefferi A: Treatment of systemic mast cell disease: beyond interferon. *Leuk Res* 28:223, 2004.

24. Adeyinka A, Dewald GW: Cytogenetics of chronic myeloproliferative disorders and related myelodysplastic syndromes. *Hematol Oncol Clin North Am* 17:1129, 2003.

25. Olney HJ, Le Beau MM: The cytogenetics of myelodysplastic syndromes. *Best Pract Res Clin Haematol* 14:479, 2001.

26. Greenberg P, Cox C, LeBeau MM, et al: International scoring system for evaluating prognosis in myelodysplastic syndromes. *Blood* 89:2079, 1997.

27. Boultwood J, Lewis S, Wainscoat JS: The 5q-syndrome. *Blood* 84:3253, 1994.

28. Mrozek K, Heinonen K, Bloomfield CD: Clinical importance of cytogenetics in acute myeloid leukaemia. *Best Pract Res Clin Haematol* 14:19, 2001.

29. Vardiman JW, Harris NL, Brunning RD: The World Health Organization (WHO) classification of the myeloid neoplasms. *Blood* 100:2292, 2002.

30. Speck NA, Gilliland DG: Core-binding factors in haematopoiesis and leukaemia. *Nat Rev Cancer* 2:502, 2002.

31. Mistry AR, Pedersen EW, Solomon E, Grimwade D: The molecular pathogenesis of acute promyelocytic leukaemia: Implications for the clinical management of the disease. *Blood Rev* 17:71, 2003.

32. Ernst P, Wang J, Korsmeyer SJ: The role of MLL in hematopoiesis and leukemia. *Curr Opin Hematol* 9:282, 2002.

33. Olney HJ, Mitelman F, Johansson B, et al: Unique balanced chromosome abnormalities in treatment-related myelodysplastic syndromes and acute myeloid leukemia: Report from an international workshop. *Genes Chromosomes Cancer* 33:413, 2002.

34. Farag SS, Archer KJ, Mrozek K, et al: Isolated trisomy of chromosomes 8, 11, 13 and 21 is an adverse prognostic factor in adults with de novo acute myeloid leukemia: Results from Cancer and Leukemia Group B 8461. *Int J Oncol* 21:1041, 2002.

35. Stirewalt DL, Radich JP: The role of FLT3 in haematopoietic malignancies. *Nat Rev Cancer* 3:650, 2003.

36. Longley BJ, Reguera MJ, Ma Y: Classes of c-KIT activating mutations: Proposed mechanisms of action and implications for disease classification and therapy. *Leuk Res* 25:571, 2001.

37. Gurbuxani S, Vyas P, Crispino JD: Recent insights into the mechanisms of myeloid leukemogenesis in Down syndrome. *Blood* 103:399, 2004.

38. Frohling S, Schlenk RF, Stolze I, et al: CEBPA mutations in younger adults with acute myeloid leukemia and normal cytogenetics: prognostic relevance and analysis of cooperating mutations. *J Clin Oncol* 22:624, 2004.

39. Godley LA, Larson RA: The syndrome of therapy-related myelodysplasia and myeloid leukemia, in *The Myelodysplastic Syndromes: Pathobiology and Clinical Management*, edited by JM Bennett, p 139. Marcel Dekker, New York, 2002.

40. Smith SM, Le Beau MM, Huo D, et al: Clinical-cytogenetic associations in 306 patients with therapy-related myelodysplasia and myeloid leukemia: The University of Chicago series. *Blood* 102:43, 2003.

41. Pedersen-Bjergaard J, Andersen MK, Christiansen DH: Therapy-related acute myeloid leukemia and myelodysplasia after high-dose chemotherapy and autologous stem cell transplantation. *Blood* 95:3273, 2000.

42. Lai F, Godley LA, Joslin J, et al: Transcript map and comparative analysis of the 1.5-Mb commonly deleted segment of human 5q31 in malignant myeloid diseases with a del(5q). *Genomics* 71:235, 2001.

43. Faderl S, Jeha S, Kantarjian HM: The biology and therapy of adult acute lymphoblastic leukemia. *Cancer* 98:1337, 2003.

44. Wetzler M, Dodge RK, Mrozek K, et al: Additional cytogenetic abnormalities in adults with Philadelphia chromosome-positive acute lymphoblastic leukemia: A study of the Cancer and Leukaemia Group B. *Br J Haematol* 124:275, 2004.

45. Pui CH, Chessells JM, Camitta B, et al: Clinical heterogeneity in childhood acute lymphoblastic leukemia with 11q23 rearrangements. *Leukemia* 17:700, 2003.

46. Rubnitz JE, Downing JR, Pui CH, et al: TEL gene rearrangement in acute lymphoblastic leukemia: A new genetic marker with prognostic significance. *J Clin Oncol* 15:1150, 1997.

47. Heerema NA, Sather HN, Sensel MG, et al: Prognostic impact of trisomies of chromosomes 10, 17, and 5 among children with acute lymphoblastic leukemia and high hyperdiploidy (>50 chromosomes). *J Clin Oncol* 18:1876, 2000.

48. Shanafelt TD, Geyer SM, Kay NE: Prognosis at diagnosis: integrating molecular biologic insights into clinical practice for patients with CLL. *Blood* 103:1202, 2004.

49. Dohner H, Stilgenbauer S, Benner A, et al: Genomic aberrations and survival in chronic lymphocytic leukemia. *N Engl J Med* 343:1910, 2000.

50. Damle RN, Wasil T, Fais F, et al: Ig V gene mutation status and CD38 expression as novel prognostic indicators in chronic lymphocytic leukemia. *Blood* 94:1840, 1999.

51. Hamblin TJ, Davis Z, Gardiner A, et al: Unmutated Ig V(H) genes are associated with a more aggressive form of chronic lymphocytic leukemia. *Blood* 94:1848, 1999.

52. Crespo M, Bosch F, Villamor N, et al: ZAP-70 expression as a surrogate for immunoglobulin-variable-region mutations in chronic lymphocytic leukemia. *N Engl J Med* 348:1764, 2003.

53. Ong ST, Le Beau MM: Chromosomal abnormalities and molecular genetics of non-Hodgkin's lymphoma. *Semin Oncol* 25:447, 1998.

54. Offit K, Wong G, Filippa DA, et al: Cytogenetic analysis of 434 consecutively ascertained specimens of non-Hodgkin's lymphoma: clinical correlations. *Blood* 77:1508, 1991.

55. Viardot A, Barth TF, Moller P, et al: Cytogenetic evolution of follicular lymphoma. *Semin Cancer Biol* 13:183, 2003.

56. Bertoni F, Zucca E, Cotter FE: Molecular basis of mantle cell lymphoma. *Br J Haematol* 124:130, 2004.

57. Kuehl WM, Bergsagel PL: Multiple myeloma: Evolving genetic events and host interactions. *Nat Rev Cancer* 2:177, 2002.

58. Pasqualucci L, Migliazza A, Basso K, et al: Mutations of the BCL6 proto-oncogene disrupt its negative autoregulation in diffuse large B-cell lymphoma. *Blood* 101:2914, 2003.

59. Starostik P, Patzner J, Greiner A, et al: Gastric marginal zone B-cell lymphomas of MALT type develop along 2 distinct pathogenetic pathways. *Blood* 99:3, 2002.

60. Seidl S, Kaufmann H, Drach J: New insights into the pathophysiology of multiple myeloma. *Lancet Oncol* 4:557, 2003.

61. Kalakonda N, Rothwell DG, Scarffe JH, Norton JD: Detection of N-Ras codon 61 mutations in subpopulations of tumor cells in multiple myeloma at presentation. *Blood* 98:1555, 2001.

62. Bezieau S, Devilder MC, Avet-Loiseau H, et al: High incidence of N and K-Ras activating mutations in multiple myeloma and primary plasma cell leukemia at diagnosis. *Hum Mutat* 18:212, 2001.

APOPTOSIS

ROBERTA A. GOTTLIEB

> **Apoptosis is a physiologic form of cell death that has evolved in multicellular organisms as a mechanism of eliminating unwanted cells. Apoptosis is a cell-autonomous process that may be triggered through a receptor or through the detection of cellular damage. It involves a coordinated series of enzymatic steps orchestrated by activation of a special class of proteases (caspases) and is controlled by inhibitors at each step, conferring tight control over this lethal process. The cell destruction process is accompanied by alterations in most organelles, particularly mitochondria, as well as changes to the cytoskeleton, plasma membrane, and ion transport systems, and culminates in the degradation of nuclear DNA through the action of endonucleases.**

Apoptosis is a term originally coined by Wyllie, Kerr, and Currie[1] to describe a form of cell death characterized by cell shrinkage and nuclear condensation, and is derived from the Greek term for the shedding of leaves or petals. This physiologic, tightly regulated process is initiated by eukaryotic cells in response to internal or external cues. Apoptosis occurs in all multicellular organisms as the means to balance cell proliferation in continuously renewing tissues in order to maintain a constant organ size.

In the hematopoietic system, cell production is delicately balanced against cell death and removal through the monocyte–macrophage system.

A panoply of cytokines and growth factors regulate cell survival, proliferation, and apoptosis.[2] Stem cell factor, Flt ligand, thrombopoietin, and interleukin (IL)-3 suppress apoptosis, whereas IL-6 and IL-11 stimulate proliferation of early progenitors. Granulocyte-macrophage colony stimulating factor (GM-CSF) can both suppress apoptosis and trigger proliferation. Tumor necrosis factor alpha (TNF-α), Fas ligand, TNF-related apoptosis-inducing ligand (TRAIL), and interferon gamma promote apoptosis of cells expressing the appropriate receptors.

Apoptosis occurs at defined times and locations during development, thus earning it the name *programmed cell death*. It is a critical process during embryogenesis, where remodeling requires highly regulated cell death. Programmed cell death takes place during the elimination of interdigital webs in mammalian development, and in the regression of the tadpole's tail as it develops into a frog. Our understanding of apoptosis has been greatly advanced by detailed studies in the nematode *Caenorhabditis elegans*. Three of the most important genes that control apoptosis have been identified through studies of development in *C. elegans*. Two of them, designated *ced-3* and *ced-4* (*C. elegans* death gene), are essential for programmed cell death to occur, and one gene, *ced-9*, is essential for opposing cell death.[3,4] These genes are conserved throughout evolution and are represented by large families of mammalian homologues. Ced-3 is a cysteine protease with the unusual characteristic of cleaving peptides after aspartic acid residues. The first mammalian homologue of Ced-3 to be identified was interleukin-1β–converting enzyme (ICE). Subsequently, a family of more than 10 related cysteine proteases ("death proteases") was identified; they are designated caspases, for cysteine aspartases.[5] The nematode death gene, *ced-4*, encodes a protein that controls the activation of the caspase, Ced-3. Ced-4 is, in turn, regulated through interaction with Ced-9.[6] Apaf-1 is the mammalian homologue of Ced-4. Bcl-2 is the mammalian homologue of the antiapoptosis gene, *ced-9*, and was first identified as an oncogene created by a chromosomal 8;14 translocation in B-cell lymphoma.[7] Studies of the mammalian homologues of the *C. elegans* death genes have led to an understanding of the critical elements of the "death machinery" of apoptosis.

FEATURES OF PROGRAMMED CELL DEATH

Mitochondrial alterations, caspase activation, and chromatin fragmentation are among the key events that characterize apoptosis and are discussed in greater detail below. Upon initiation of the death program, cells undergo dramatic volume loss, membrane blebbing, cytoplasmic acidification, rearrangement of the cytoskeleton, and loss of contact with adjacent cells and extracellular matrix. Cells exhibit disordered ion homeostasis characterized by diminished proton elimination (and/or increased proton production), and volume loss accomplished largely through potassium and chloride efflux, which is accompanied by water loss. Calcium homeostasis is also disturbed, because mitochondrial sequestration of calcium is impaired. Membrane blebbing and phosphatidylserine externalization are attributed to proteolytic cleavage of the membrane cytoskeletal protein fodrin (a spectrin homologue) and to activation of the phospholipid scramblase, which is activated by low pH and elevated calcium levels. Cytoskeletal alterations are partly caused by proteolytic cleavage of actin, as well as to changes in the activity of kinases and G proteins that regulate the state of assembly of cytoskeletal components. A variety of signaling pathways that participate in survival signaling are proteolytically inactivated.[8]

The cell is marked for ingestion by neighboring cells or professional phagocytes through the up-regulation of certain adhesion markers and through the externalization of phosphatidylserine. In the intact organism, apoptotic cells are removed before membrane integrity is lost, thereby preventing spillage of cellular contents. The magnitude of this clearance process is demonstrated by the clearance of inflammatory cells during the resolution of pneumonia.[9]

MITOCHONDRIAL ALTERATIONS

The mitochondria are complex organelles consisting of an outer membrane, an inner membrane, an intermembrane space, and the matrix, which is enclosed by the inner membrane. The outer membrane is permeable to small molecules, while the inner membrane is highly impermeable and able to maintain a proton gradient equivalent to 1 pH unit. The electron transport system is embedded in the inner membrane and oxidizes substrates in order to move protons across the inner membrane. This proton gradient is the driving force for ATP synthesis.

Acronyms and abbreviations that appear in this chapter include: ADP, adenosine diphosphate; AIF, apoptosis-inducing factor; AML, acute myelogenous leukemia; ANCA, antineutrophil cytoplasmic autoantibody; ATP, adenosine triphosphate; ATPase, adenosine triphosphatase; BAFF, B cell activation factor; B-CLL, B cell chronic lymphocytic leukemia; CAD, caspase-activated DNase; CARD, caspase activation and recruitment domain; CML, chronic myelogenous leukemia; dATP, deoxyadenosine triphosphate; DFF, DNA fragmentation factor; dUTP, deoxyuridine triphosphate; FADD, Fas-associated death domain; GM-CSF, granulocyte-macrophage colony stimulating factor; IAP, inhibitor of apoptosis protein; ICAD, caspase-activated DNase inhibitor; ICE, interleukin-1β–converting enzyme; IL, interleukin; MDS, myelodysplastic syndrome; MTP, mitochondrial permeability transition pore (MPTP); Smac/DIABLO, second mitochondrial activator of caspases/direct IAP binding protein with low pI; TNF-α, tumor necrosis factor alpha; TRADD, TNF receptor associated death domain; TRAIL, TNF-related apoptosis-inducing ligand; TUNEL, terminal transferase dUTP nick end labeling.

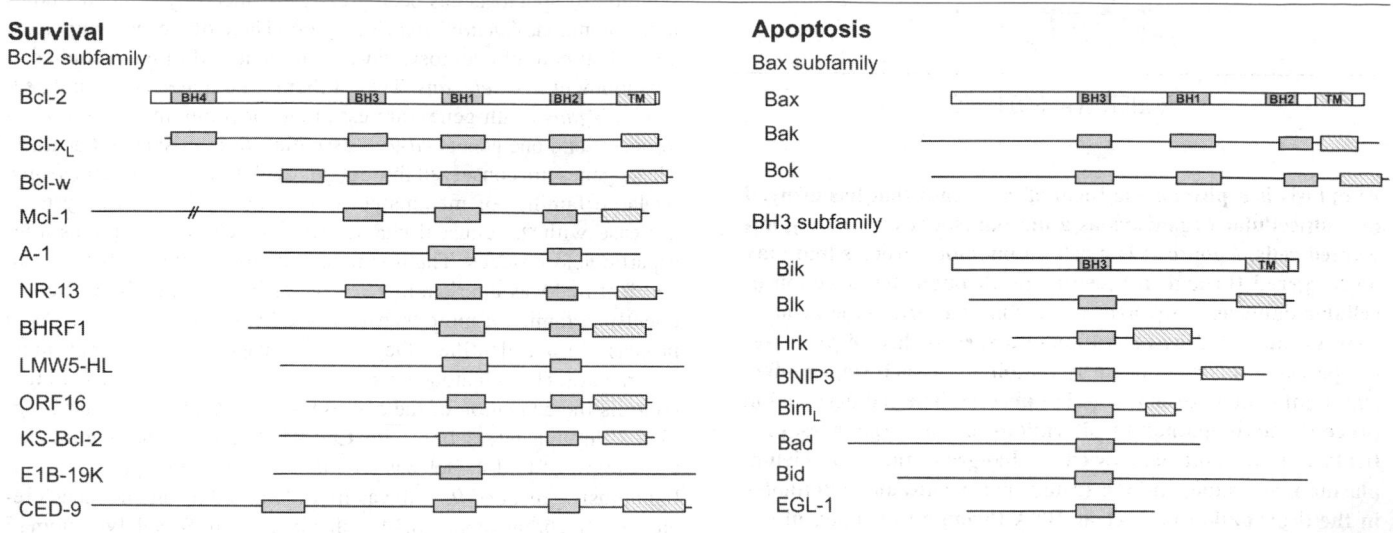

FIGURE 11-1   Bcl-2 family members and their role in apoptosis regulation. Bcl-2 homology (BH) domains represent conserved sequences among family members. TM designates the transmembrane domain. The Bcl-2 subfamily promotes cell survival. Proapoptotic members are grouped into the Bax subfamily and the BH3 subfamily, which has high sequence divergence outside the BH3 domain. (Adapted from JM Adams and S Cory,[44] with permission.)

The inner membrane, which has extensive infoldings (cristae) to increase the available sites for ATP synthesis on the matrix face of the inner membrane, has a much greater surface area than does the outer membrane. Cytochrome c, which serves as an electron carrier, is located in the intermembrane space and is electrostatically associated with the inner membrane.

In addition to their role in ATP production, the mitochondria play a key role in the regulation of apoptosis. Sequestered in the space between the inner and outer mitochondrial membranes are cytochrome c, which is a cofactor for caspase activation; Smac/DIABLO (second mitochondrial activator of caspases/direct inhibitor of apoptosis protein binding protein with a low isoelectric point [pI]), a factor that relieves the inhibition of caspases by inhibitor of apoptosis protein (IAP); Omi/HtrA2, a serine protease that may also interact with IAPs; and apoptosis-inducing factor (AIF) and endonuclease G, both of which promote DNA fragmentation and chromatin condensation.[10]

Two major mitochondrial alterations occur in apoptosis: loss of cytochrome c and depolarization of the inner membrane. The earliest event is the dissociation of cytochrome c from the electron transport chain, followed somewhat later by its release from the mitochondria to the cytosol, where it may participate in caspase activation. Loss of cytochrome c from its normal association with the electron transport chain prevents delivery of electrons to complex IV and thence to oxygen. However, it may be possible for electrons to "bleed off" at the upstream site of ubiquinone, leading to superoxide production. This may explain the production of free radicals frequently observed in apoptosis. Effective mitochondrial respiration is shut down, and dissipation of the proton gradient may result in loss of membrane potential across the inner membrane. In some cases, the F0F1 ATPase may run in reverse, hydrolyzing any available ATP so as to maintain mitochondrial inner membrane potential through proton pumping. The mitochondria also become engaged in futile calcium cycling (uptake and release); the combination of the two processes may lead to a crisis state for the mitochondria, at which point the inner mitochondrial membrane becomes freely permeable to solutes, resulting in loss of mitochondrial membrane potential. This is often referred to as opening of the mitochondrial permeability transition pore (MPTP), although the event may be less specific than the term *pore* implies. Loss of ion

homeostasis across the inner mitochondrial membrane may lead to swelling of the mitochondrial matrix compartment and eventual rupture of the outer mitochondrial membrane, leading to release of cytochrome c, Smac/DIABLO, and AIF.

The participation of the mitochondria in these apoptotic events is regulated by members of the Bcl-2 family, some of which oppose apoptosis while others promote apoptosis. Bcl-2, some of which opposes apoptosis, is able to prevent the release of cytochrome c from mitochondria, while the proapoptotic Bax promotes cytochrome c release.[11,12] Proteolytic processing of Bid, or dephosphorylation of Bad, results in their translocation to the mitochondria, where they cause cytochrome c release. Bax also translocates from cytosol to mitochondria during apoptosis. Because these molecules bear structural similarity to the pore-forming colicins, much attention has been directed toward their potential role as pore formers in the outer mitochondrial membrane. They may interact with the voltage-dependent anion channel, a large-conductance porin in the outer mitochondrial membrane, as well as with the adenine nucleotide transporter, an inner-membrane protein believed to be a component of the MPT pore in addition to its primary role in ATP–ADP exchange.[13] Bcl-2 family members are extremely important in the regulation of cell death. Bcl-2 family members and their function (pro- or antiapoptotic) are shown in Fig. 11-1 and reviewed in ref. 14.

CASPASE ACTIVATION

The caspases can now be grouped into three functional categories. The first group includes ICE (also designated caspase-1) and two related caspases: caspase-4 and caspase-5. Although ICE primarily participates in cytokine processing, the function of the other members of this group is not clear. The second group consists of the effector caspases, such as caspase-3, which possess a short prodomain (<3 kDa). The effector caspases are responsible for cleaving many of the important intracellular protein substrates that are degraded during apoptosis.[15] The third, and perhaps most interesting, group includes the signaling caspases, which possess a large prodomain. Most cells express multiple caspases, probably related to the observed redundancy in pathways that initiate cell death; it also appears that the caspases may work in a cascade fashion, perhaps anal-

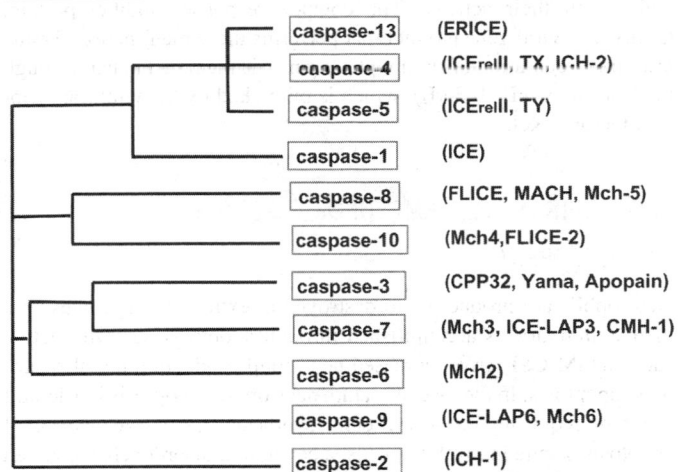

FIGURE 11-2   Phylogenetic tree for the caspase family. Caspase designations and their aliases are shown. (Adapted from Wang and Gu,[45] with permission.)

ogous to the amplification seen in the clotting system. The caspase family is diagrammed in Fig. 11-2.

Caspases are synthesized as proenzymes with an amino-terminal prodomain that is removed by proteolytic processing. The enzyme is further processed into large ($\approx$20 kDa) and small ($\approx$10 kDa) fragments that form a heterodimer. Two heterodimers assemble to form the active tetrameric protease (Fig. 11-3). Caspases are capable of autoprocessing under certain circumstances. While effector caspases are dependent on proteolytic activation, the signaling caspases depend

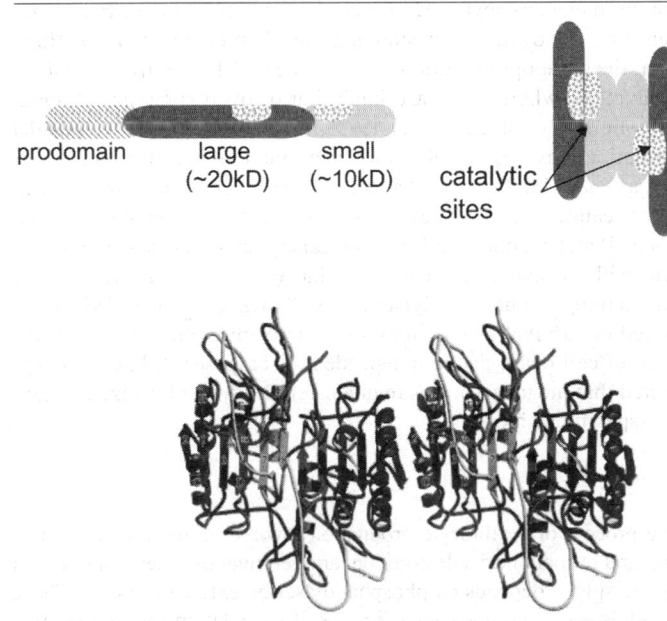

FIGURE 11-3   Diagram of caspase processing and assembly. Members of the cysteine aspartate protease (caspase) family are characterized by an amino-terminal prodomain (*hatched area*) and a catalytic domain (*dotted area*), which is processed by cleavage after Asp residues to release large ($\approx$20 kDa) and small ($\approx$10 kDa) subunits. The two fragments assemble into a heterodimer. Two heterodimers form a tetramer in the active form of the caspase. A stereo pair image of the crystal structure of a typical caspase is shown.[46]

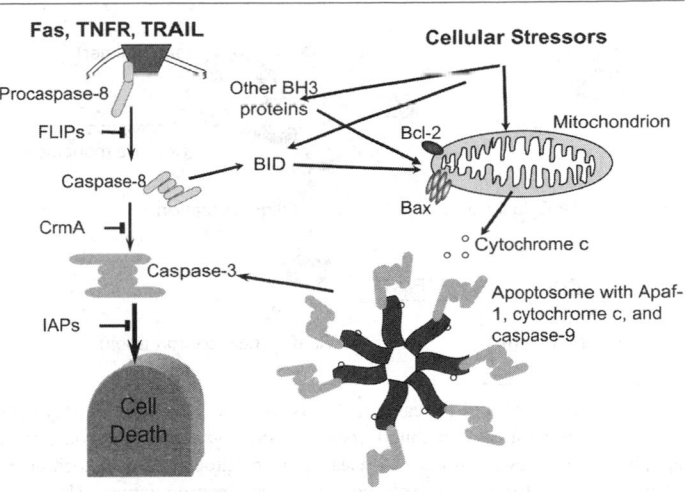

FIGURE 11-4   Two main signaling cascades lead to caspase activation. Extracellular signaling from the death receptors tumor necrosis factor receptor (TNFR), Fas, and TRAIL lead to activation of caspase-8 and/or caspase-10, which leads to activation of caspase-3 and other end effectors of apoptosis. Caspase-8 and caspase-10 are inhibited by CrmA. Cell stressors and related signals lead to mitochondrial alterations resulting in caspase-3 activation through the interaction of Apaf-1, cytochrome c, and caspase-9. Bcl-2 opposes the pathway that involves mitochondria.

on interaction with a cofactor, as exemplified by the interaction of caspase-9 with Apaf-1.[16,17]

Activation of caspases may be accomplished through multiple pathways, two of which have been worked out in detail (Fig. 11-4). The receptor-mediated pathway involves a cell surface receptor, such as Fas or the receptor for TNF-α. Occupancy of the receptor with its ligand causes recruitment of a cytosolic adapter molecule containing a protein-protein interaction region termed the death domain. The adapter molecule (e.g., Fas-associated death domain [FADD] or TNFR-associated death domain [TRADD]) then recruits a signaling procaspase such as caspase-8 or caspase-10 that docks with the adapter molecule and undergoes proximity-induced processing. Caspase-8 or caspase-10 may directly activate caspase-3 and related effector caspases.[18]

An alternative pathway exists involving activation of caspase-9 through interaction of Apaf-1, which must bind cytochrome c and deoxyadenosine triphosphate (dATP) or ATP (Fig. 11-5).[19] Apaf-1, which has homology to Ced-4, is present in the cytosol and inactive until cytochrome c is available for interaction. It possesses a caspase activation and recruitment domain (CARD) that is essential for its function. Additional Apaf-1-like molecules are now being identified that presumably will be activated through different pathways.

Cytotoxic T lymphocytes inject granzyme B into cells to trigger apoptosis. Granzyme B is a serine protease that cleaves caspases after Asp residues to generate active caspases. The introduction of granzyme B into the cytosol of target cells results in the rapid activation of caspase-3 and subsequent cell death. Granzyme B also cleaves Bid to an active fragment, thereby triggering the mitochondrial pathway. Cytotoxic T lymphocytes are protected from their own granzyme B by expression of a serpin (serine protease inhibitor protein), and adenovirus type 5 also encodes an inhibitor of granzyme B, thereby allowing escape from this mechanism of immune surveillance.

It is generally believed that activation of proteases constitutes an irreversible event and that the caspases are the ultimate effectors of apoptotic cell destruction. There are, however, exceptions. For example, caspase-3 is activated in a subset of T cells and participates in

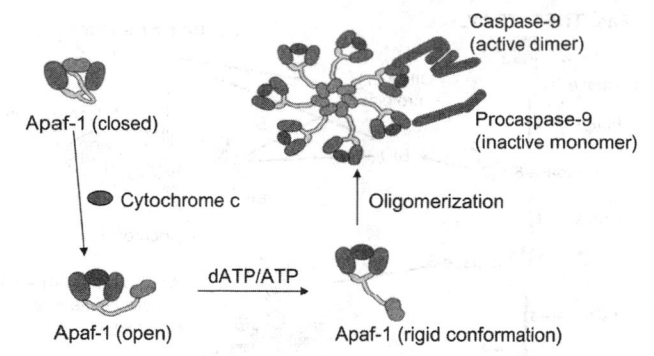

FIGURE 11-5   Model for caspase-9 activation by Apaf-1. In healthy cells, Apaf-1 exists in an autoinhibited conformation (*top left*). In response to an apoptotic signal, cytochrome c is released from mitochondria. Cytochrome c converts Apaf-1 from a "closed" monomer to an open conformer. The subsequent binding of dATP/ATP results in oligomerization to a heptamer that recruits procaspase-9. An inactive procaspase-9 monomer on one spoke of the apoptosome is presumed to recruit another monomer to create the asymmetric dimer having a single active site. (Adapted from Acehan et al.,[47] and Adams and Cory,[48] with permission.)

processing of IL-16 without leading to apoptosis. Conversely, inhibition of caspases may not always prevent cell death. Because multiple enzymatic pathways are activated in apoptosis, it is reasonable to think that completion of any subset of processes will result in the death of the cell or, at the very least, in loss of its ability to divide.

NUCLEAR ALTERATIONS

The classic histologic manifestations of apoptosis are the condensation of nuclear chromatin and fragmentation of the nucleus. DNA condensation and classic apoptotic body formation depend on proteolysis of lamin by one or more caspases.[20] DNA digestion is accomplished by several distinct endonucleases, eventually resulting in fragments representing multiples of the approximately 200-bp nucleosome (the so-called nucleosomal ladder). The search for the responsible endonucleases has yielded several candidates, including DNase I and DNase II. DNA fragmentation factor (DFF) consists of a 40-kDa caspase-activated DNase (CAD) bound to its 45-kDa inhibitor (ICAD). Cleavage of CAD releases it from ICAD, thereby enabling it to function as an endonuclease.[21] AIF and endonuclease G can also mediate DNA fragmentation. Although DNA fragmentation is commonly observed in apoptosis, it is not an essential feature.

In addition to the characteristic morphologic changes in the nucleus, it is possible to detect DNA fragmentation using a histologic method known as terminal deoxynucleotidyl transferase deoxyuridine triphosphate (dUTP) nick end labeling (TUNEL), in which labeled deoxynucleotides are incorporated into nuclear DNA at sites of nicking. The incorporated nucleotides are then detected using conventional histochemical staining or fluorescence detection. This method is widely used to detect DNA fragmentation in tissue sections and in cell suspensions evaluated by flow cytometry. DNA fragmentation is also reflected by a subdiploid DNA content.

ENDOGENOUS PREVENTION OF APOPTOSIS

Cells have evolved a variety of safeguards to prevent inappropriate apoptosis. Viruses have also exploited these safeguards to prevent the cell from undergoing apoptosis in response to the presence of the virus. Bcl-2, which opposes apoptosis, has corresponding viral homologues, including E1B-19K. The cell also has IAPs, which bind to caspases

and inhibit their activity. The cowpox response modifier protein, CrmA, is a viral gene product that performs the same function. Transcriptional regulation of antiapoptotic genes is mediated in part through nuclear factor-κB (NF-κB), which is mimicked by the viral transcription factor v-Rel.

APOPTOSIS IN THE HEMATOPOIETIC SYSTEM

NEUTROPHILS

Neutrophils are produced and destroyed at extremely high rates, and their elimination is accomplished through apoptosis. Growth factors such as GM-CSF drive increased neutrophil production but also suppress apoptosis. In the case of mature neutrophils, apoptosis is a default program requiring no new protein synthesis. Excessive neutrophil apoptosis occurs in myelokathexis, a congenital disorder characterized by severe chronic leukopenia and neutropenia. Defective expression of Bcl-x_L has been implicated in this disorder.[22] Excessive apoptosis of myeloid progenitor cells has been described in cyclic neutropenia and severe congenital neutropenia (Kostmann syndrome), as well as in myelokathexis.

Delayed neutrophil apoptosis is observed in chronic neutrophilic leukemia and chronic myelogenous leukemia. Inefficient clearance of apoptotic neutrophils contributes to inflammation in rheumatoid arthritis and systemic lupus erythematosus, and may predispose to formation of autoantibodies against neutrophil granule proteins (antineutrophil cytoplasmic autoantibodies [ANCAs]). Defective clearance of neutrophils from airways may exacerbate inflammation in cystic fibrosis and bronchiectasis and may permit survival of ingested pathogens.

PLATELETS

Maximal platelet production coincides with the onset of apoptosis in mature megakaryocytes. However, detailed studies have been hampered by the difficulty of studying megakaryocytes in vitro. However, the proapoptotic stimuli nitric oxide and TNF-α trigger platelet production, whereas caspase inhibition or overexpression of antiapoptotic Bcl-x_L block proplatelet formation. The process of platelet formation may require additional coordination, because staurosporine, a kinase inhibitor that triggers apoptosis in a wide range of cell types, causes megakaryocyte apoptosis without proplatelet formation.[23] Platelets, once shed from megakaryocytes, possess mitochondria with normal membrane potential, exhibit normal transbilayer orientation of phosphatidylserine, and lack caspase-9. When deprived of survival factors in plasma, these enucleate cells undergo a form of cell death that is independent of caspases. It has been suggested that megakaryocytes regulate cell death in a localized, organelle-specific fashion.[24]

ERYTHROCYTES

The process of erythrocyte production involves chromatin condensation and mitochondrial destruction, and removal of senescent red cells by the spleen depends on phosphatidylserine externalization.[25] These parallels with apoptosis have prompted speculation that erythrocyte maturation and senescence represent "apoptosis in slow motion." In support of that notion, it has been shown that Raf-1 suppresses caspase activation in erythroid progenitors, and that Raf-1 down-regulation and caspase activation are required for red cell production.[26] Erythropoietin, which stimulates erythropoiesis, also prolongs red cell survival by inhibiting a volume-sensitive cation channel that activates phosphatidylserine externalization.

APOPTOSIS IN HUMAN DISEASE

The occurrence of apoptosis in pathophysiologic settings, or its absence in physiologic settings, results in human disease. More simply, diseases can be grouped according to whether there is too much apoptosis or too little.

INSUFFICIENT APOPTOSIS

Because apoptosis must occur at defined times during development, a failure of apoptosis to occur in the appropriate settings would be expected to give rise to developmental defects. However, genetically defined abnormalities in known elements of the process of apoptosis have not been identified in human developmental disorders. Some insights have been derived from gene knockout studies in mice. Deletion of the gene encoding caspase-3, arguably the most important death protease, results in mice that die in utero or soon after birth with an excess of brain tissue, owing to a failure of normal programmed cell death during neural development.

In the immune system, deletion of self-reactive T cells is essential to prevent autoimmune disorders.[27] Signaling for lymphocyte deletion is accomplished through engagement of one or more cell surface receptors, including a molecule known as Fas/APO-1/CD95. Engagement of Fas by its ligand results in aggregation of proteins (FADD and caspase-8) through self-association regions known as death domains, culminating in caspase activation and death of the cell. Fas expression on lymphocytes provides a means by which unwanted T cells can be eliminated. Mutation of Fas or its ligand in mice results in a disease that strongly resembles systemic lupus erythematosus. In humans, mutations of Fas occur in the heritable autoimmune lymphoproliferative syndrome, in which CD3+CD4−CD8− T cells fail to undergo apoptosis and contribute to autoimmune disease.[28] Interestingly, many of the cellular proteins that are autoantigens are selectively cleaved by granzyme B to generate unique fragments.[29] However, it is not yet clear whether cleavage by granzyme B contributes to their autoantigenic properties.

In areas of immune sanctuary, such as the testis, Sertoli cells express high levels of Fas ligand to prevent invading T cells from surviving long enough to mount an immune response against sperm cells (which the body recognizes as foreign). A similar mechanism of protection is involved in limiting inflammatory responses in viral infections in sensitive organs such as the eye. Immune-mediated rejection of transplanted organs rests in part on the induction of apoptosis in the foreign cells. This mechanism has been exploited by genetic manipulation to express Fas ligand on pancreatic islet cells to prevent induction of apoptosis in the transplanted cells, with resulting prolonged survival of the allograft.

A number of viral proteins block apoptosis signaling or effector pathways. Baculovirus p35 and cowpox viral protein CrmA directly inhibit caspases; adenovirus E1B inhibits caspase-3 activation, and herpesvirus-poxvirus caspase-8 inhibitor proteins block downstream death domain signaling. The function of these proteins may be critical to viral virulence by blocking host defense against viral replication; infected cells engage the apoptotic machinery and mark themselves for phagocytic ingestion, thus limiting the extent of viral infection. Numerous Bcl-2 homologues have been identified in γ-herpesviruses, thus explaining their persistence and propensity for malignant transformation.[30]

Polycythemia vera is characterized by an abnormal clone of erythroid progenitors capable of proliferating independently of erythropoietin. These clonal cells overexpress Bcl-x$_L$, which prevents apoptosis and may contribute to the survival of erythroid progenitors in the absence of erythropoietin.[31]

Tumor growth rate is determined by the imbalance between apoptosis and mitosis. For example, the function of the Bcl-2 gene product was discovered because its overexpression prevents the normal death of B cells, leading to a lymphoma associated with a normal rate of proliferation but reduced apoptosis.[32] Epstein-Barr virus encodes at least two Bcl-2 homologues and is associated with Burkitt lymphoma, Hodgkin disease, AIDS-related lymphoma, and nasopharyngeal carcinoma. Human herpesvirus 8 expresses a Bcl-2 homologue and is associated with AIDS-related Kaposi sarcoma. A malignant cell may arise when a cell fails to undergo apoptosis when it should have. Loss of a necessary growth factor or removal from the normal extracellular matrix should trigger a cell to commit suicide. If, however, the cell fails to die, it may survive and proliferate sufficiently for its progeny to acquire other mutations, including loss of p53 and activation of other oncogenes. Thus, the first step in oncogenesis may be a failure of apoptosis. The tumor suppressor p53 gene product is a transcription factor activated by DNA damage to induce a family of p53-dependent genes that regulate the cell cycle and induce apoptosis.[33] While mutations of p53 have been found in many malignant tumors and in some families with hereditary cancer syndromes, it is mutated in <20% of hematologic malignancies, most commonly in acute myelogenous leukemia (AML), myelodysplastic syndrome (MDS), and chronic myelogenous leukemia (CML) in blast crisis.[34] This suggests that p53 is a relatively weak apoptosis regulator in myeloid cells, or that hematopoietic cells can override p53-mediated death signals.

In B cell chronic lymphocytic leukemia (B-CLL), small mature B cells accumulate as a result of diminished apoptosis. In part this is mediated through an autocrine loop involving survival factors of the tumor necrosis factor family, such as B cell activation factor (BAFF). These autocrine factors are secreted by B-CLL cells and bind to their receptors to suppress apoptosis, drive proliferation, and increase resistance to chemotherapeutic drugs.[35] Disruption of this autocrine loop may represent an effective therapeutic approach in B-CLL.

Modulation of apoptosis is widely considered a key target for cancer therapy.[36] In CML the activity of the BCR-ABL oncogene prevents apoptosis. Imatinib mesylate, a potent and selective inhibitor of the BCR-ABL tyrosine kinase, shows promise in the treatment of CML.[37] Although malignant cells are generally considered more resistant to the induction of apoptosis, they still possess the necessary cellular machinery and, when exposed to appropriate chemotherapeutic agents (or radiation), usually die by apoptosis, not necrosis.[38] Efforts to decrease their resistance to apoptosis are directed at targets such as Bcl-2 or disruption of autonomous survival pathways.[39] Evaluation of apoptosis in response to chemotherapeutic agents may correlate with prognosis and might eventually direct the selection of agents on an individualized basis.

One hypothesis about mechanisms of aging is that too little apoptosis occurs, permitting the survival of cells that have sustained DNA damage. Such damaged cells would function inefficiently at best, owing to the accumulation of mutations in essential genes, and could undergo malignant transformation. Eventually, such marginally functioning and precancerous cells would predominate, with more generalized cellular dysfunction as time went on.

EXCESSIVE APOPTOSIS

Excessive cell death is of particular concern in organs that are populated by terminally differentiated, nondividing cells. Any cells lost, whether by apoptosis or necrosis, are irreplaceable. In settings where cell death is inevitable, inhibiting the enzymatic processes of apoptosis may not salvage the cell but may merely convert its demise to a necrotic form. However, if a cell is damaged beyond repair, a tidy, non-inflammatory apoptotic death may still be preferable, avoiding collateral damage from inflammation.

Excessive apoptosis is now being recognized in a variety of hematopoietic disorders. Megaloblastic anemia as a result of deficiency of folate or vitamin B_{12} is characterized by ineffective erythropoiesis with increased early erythrocyte progenitors and failure to mature into reticulocytes. Animal studies reveal that folate deficiency results in insufficient purines for DNA synthesis. Erythroblasts fail to progress through S phase and instead undergo apoptosis, which can be rescued by providing thymidine.[40,41]

In some cases, excessive apoptosis may be a result of unavailability of a necessary growth factor, an inability to respond to the growth factor, or alterations in the balance of proapoptotic and antiapoptotic Bcl-2 family members. The myelodysplastic syndrome, which is characterized by peripheral cytopenias and (at least in the early stages) marrow hyperplasia, is associated with defects in DNA repair or cell cycle regulation. It is also associated with excessive apoptosis throughout myeloid differentiation, resulting in ineffective myelopoiesis.[42] Stromal cells also show increased apoptosis. Therapy aimed at increasing cell survival or blocking apoptosis improves the hematologic picture. However, in the natural course of the disease, apoptosis-resistant clones eventually emerge, with concomitant progression to acute myelogenous leukemia. Fanconi's anemia is accompanied by increased susceptibility to apoptosis mediated by Fas and TNF-α. It seems likely that additional myeloid disorders will be recognized to possess abnormalities in apoptosis.[43]

REFERENCES

1. Wyllie AH, Kerr JFR, Currie AR: Cell death: the significance of apoptosis. *Int Rev Cytol* 68:251, 1980.
2. Wickremasinghe RG, Hoffbrand AV: Biochemical and genetic control of apoptosis: Relevance to normal hematopoiesis and hematological malignancies. *Blood* 93:3587, 1999.
3. Ellis HM, Horvitz HR: Genetic control of programmed cell death in the nematode *C. elegans*. *Cell* 44:817, 1986.
4. Metzstein MM, Stanfield GM, Horvitz HR: Genetics of programmed cell death in *C. elegans*: Past, present and future. *Trends Genet* 14:410, 1998.
5. Alnemri ES, Livingston DJ, Nicholson DW, et al: Human ICE/CED-3 protease nomenclature [letter]. *Cell* 87:171, 1996.
6. Putcha GV, Johnson EM: "Men are but worms": Neuronal cell death in *C. elegans* and vertebrates. *Cell Death Differ* 11:38, 2004.
7. Korsmeyer SJ: Chromosomal translocations in lymphoid malignancies reveal novel proto-oncogenes. *Annu Rev Immunol* 10:785, 1992.
8. Wolf BB, Green DR: Suicidal tendencies: Apoptotic cell death by caspase family proteinases. *J Biol Chem* 274:20049, 1999.
9. Savill J, Haslett C: Granulocyte clearance by apoptosis in the resolution of inflammation. *Semin Cell Biol* 6:385, 1995.
10. Festjens N, van Gurp M, van Loo G, et al: Bcl-2 family members as sentinels of cellular integrity and role of mitochondrial intermembrane space proteins in apoptotic cell death. *Acta Haematol* 111:7-27, 2004.
11. Kluck RM, Bossy-Wetzel E, Green DR, Newmeyer DD: The release of cytochrome c from mitochondria: a primary site for Bcl-2 regulation of apoptosis. *Science* 275:1132, 1997.
12. Yang J, Liu X, Bhalla K, et al: Prevention of apoptosis by Bcl-2: Release of cytochrome c from mitochondria blocked. *Science* 275:1129, 1997.
13. Tsujimoto Y: Role of Bcl-2 family proteins in apoptosis: Apoptosomes or mitochondria? *Genes Cells* 3:697, 1998.
14. Cory S, Huang DC, Adams JM: The Bcl-2 family: Roles in cell survival and oncogenesis. *Oncogene* 22:8590, 2003.
15. Tewari M, Quan LT, O'Rourke K, et al: Yama/CPP32, a mammalian homolog of CED-3, is a Crm-A-inhibitable protease that cleaves the death substrate poly(ADP-ribose) polymerase. *Cell* 81:801, 1995.
16. Creagh EM, Martin SJ: Caspases: cellular demolition experts. *Biochem Soc Trans* 29:696, 2001.
17. Boatright KM, Salvesen GS: Mechanisms of caspase activation. *Curr Opin Cell Biol* 15:725, 2003.
18. Ashkenazi A, Dixit VM: Death receptors: signaling and modulation. *Science* 281:1305, 1998.
19. Li P, Nijhawan D, Budihardjo I, et al: Cytochrome c and dATP-dependent formation of Apaf-1/caspase-9 complex initiates an apoptotic protease cascade. *Cell* 91:479, 1997.
20. Lazebnik YA, Takahashi A, Moir RD, et al: Studies of the lamin proteinase reveal multiple parallel biochemical pathways during apoptotic execution. *Proc Natl Acad Sci U S A* 92:9042, 1995.
21. Sakahira H, Enari M, Nagata S: Cleavage of CAD inhibitor in CAD activation and DNA degradation during apoptosis. *Nature* 391:96, 1998.
22. Aprikyan AA, Liles WD, Park JR, et al: Myelokathexis, a congenital disorder of severe neutropenia characterized by accelerated apoptosis and defective expression of bcl-x in neutrophil precursors. *Blood* 95:320, 2000.
23. De Botton S, Sabri S, Daugas E, et al: Platelet formation is the consequence of caspase activation within megakaryocytes. *Blood* 100:1310, 2002.
24. Kaluzhny Y, Ravid K: Role of apoptotic processes in platelet biogenesis. *Acta Haematol* 111:67, 2004.
25. Boas FE, Forman L, Beutler E: Phosphatidylserine exposure and red cell viability in red cell aging and in hemolytic anemia. *Proc Natl Acad Sci U S A* 95:3077, 1998.
26. Kolbus A, Pilat S, Husak Z, et al: Raf-1 antagonizes erythroid differentiation by restraining caspase activation. *J Exp Med* 196:1347, 2002.
27. Los M, Wesselborg S, Schulze-Osthoff K: The role of caspases in development, immunity, and apoptotic signal transduction: lessons from knockout mice. *Immunity* 10:629, 1999.
28. Straus SE, Sneller M, Lenardo MJ, et al: An inherited disorder of lymphocyte apoptosis: the autoimmune lymphoproliferative syndrome. *Ann Intern Med* 130:591, 1999.
29. Andrade F, Cascioloa-Rosen LA, Rosen A: Granzyme B-induced apoptosis. *Acta Haematol* 111:28, 2004.
30. Ivanovska I, Galonek HL, Hildeman DA, Hardwick JM: Regulation of cell death in the lymphoid system by Bcl-2 family proteins. *Acta Haematol* 111:42, 2004.
31. Fernandez-Luna JL: Apoptosis and polycythemia vera. *Curr Opin Hematol* 6:94, 1999.
32. Hockenbery DM, Nunez G, Milliman C, et al: Bcl-2 is an inner mitochondrial membrane protein that blocks programmed cell death. *Nature* 348:334, 1990.
33. el-Deiry WS: Regulation of p53 downstream genes. *Semin Cancer Biol* 8:345, 1998.
34. Boyapati A, Kanbe E, Zhang D-E: p53 alterations in myeloid leukemia. *Acta Haematol* 111:100, 2004.
35. Kern C, Cornuel J-F, Billard C, et al: Involvement of BAFF and APRIL in the resistance to apoptosis of B-CLL through an autocrine pathway. *Blood* 103:679, 2004.
36. Hannun YA: Apoptosis and the dilemma of cancer chemotherapy. *Blood* 89:1845, 1997.
37. O'Brien SG, Guilhot F, Larson RA, et al: Imatinib compared with interferon and low-dose cytarabine for newly diagnosed chronic-phase chronic myeloid leukemia. *N Engl J Med* 348:994, 2003.
38. Brown JM, Wouters BG: Apoptosis, p53, and tumor cell sensitivity to anticancer agents. *Cancer Res* 59:1391, 1999.
39. Adachi S, Leoni LM, Carson DA, Nakahata T: Apoptosis induced by

molecular targeting therapy in hematological malignancies. *Acta Haematol* 111:107, 2004.

40. Koury MJ, Price JO, Hicks GG: Apoptosis in megaloblastic anemia occurs during DNA synthesis by a p53-independent, nucleoside-reversible mechanism. *Blood* 96:3249, 2000.

41. Koury MJ, Horne DW: Apoptosis mediates and thymidine prevents erythroblast destruction in folate deficiency anemia. *Proc Natl Acad Sci U S A* 91:4067, 1994.

42. Parker JE, Mufti GJ: The myelodysplastic syndromes: A matter of life or death. *Acta Haematol* 111:78, 2004.

43. Haurie C, Dale DC, Mackey MC: Cyclical neutropenia and other periodic hematological disorders: A review of mechanisms and mathematical models. *Blood* 92:2629, 1998.

44. Adams JM, Cory S: The Bcl-2 protein family: Arbiters of cell survival. *Science* 281:1322, 1998.

45. Wang Y, Gu X: Functional divergence in the caspase gene family and altered functional constraints: Statistical analysis and prediction. *Genetics* 158:1311, 2001.

46. Riedl SJ, Fuentes-Prior P, Renatus M, et al: Structural basis for the activation of human procaspase-7. *Proc Natl Acad Sci U S A* 98:14790, 2001.

47. Acehan D, Jiang X, Morgan DG, et al: Three-dimensional structure of the apoptosome: Implications for assembly, procaspase-9 binding, and activation. *Mol Cell* 9:423, 2002.

48. Adams JM, Cory S: Apoptosomes: Engines for caspase activation. *Curr Opin Cell Biol* 14:715, 2002.

CELL CYCLE REGULATION AND HEMATOLOGIC DISORDERS

MATHIAS SCHMID
DENNIS A. CARSON

Complex feedback pathways regulate the passage of cells through the G_1, S, G_2, and M phases of the growth cycle. Two key checkpoints control the commitment of cells to replicate DNA synthesis and to mitosis. Many oncogenes and tumor-suppressor genes promote malignant change by stimulating cell cycle entry, or disrupting the checkpoint response to DNA damage. Advances in the understanding of epigenetic gene expression regulation provide the basis for novel therapeutic approaches. This chapter presents the pathways as well as the genetic and epigenetic alterations that regulate cell replication and tabulates the various oncogenes and tumor-suppressor genes that are involved in hematologic malignancies.

INTRODUCTION

Cell mitosis is the final step of a defined program—the cell cycle—which can be separated into four phases: the G_1, S, G_2, and M phases (Fig. 12-1). A number of surveillance systems (checkpoints) control the cell cycle and interrupt its progression when DNA damage occurs or when the cells have failed to complete a necessary event.[1] These checkpoints have been given an empirical definition: When the occurrence of an event B is dependent on the completion of prior event A, the dependence is a result of a checkpoint if a loss-of-function mutation can be found that relieves the dependence.[1] Three major cell cycle checkpoints have been discovered: the DNA damage checkpoint, the spindle checkpoint, and the spindle pole body duplication checkpoint.[2–4]

The functional consequence of cell cycle checkpoint failure is usually death by apoptosis. However, small numbers of genetically altered cells may survive. Cells with defective checkpoints have an advantage when selection favors multiple genetic changes. Cancer cells are often missing one or more checkpoints, which facilitates a greater rate of genomic evolution.[5]

Most of the basic principles of cell cycle regulation were worked out in yeast, but the underlying principles are equally applicable to the mammalian cell cycle. A disturbance of cell cycle regulation is an important pathway in the development of many hematologic malignancies as a result of mutations in tumor-suppressor genes or oncogenes. Until the end of the 20th century, it was believed that the only mechanism by which the "gatekeepers" of the cell cycle could be inactivated was deletion or mutation (gain-of-function or loss-of-function mutations). Progress in the understanding of the regulation of gene expression put emphasis on another mechanism of gene inactivation, called *epigenetic regulation*. This term summarizes several molecular modifications including histone deacetylation, CpG-island hypermethylation, ubiquitination, and phosphorylation.

CYCLINS AND CYCLIN-DEPENDENT KINASES (TABLE 12-1)

Early experiments on the control of mitosis in human cells provided evidence for the existence of factors called *M-phase* and *S-phase promoting factors* (MPF, SPF).[10] The key element of SPF was thought to be cdc2. Experiments performed in *Xenopus* eggs showed that cdc2 is an M-phase-specific histone H1 kinase,[11] but is just one subunit of a regulatory complex. A second component is cyclin B, which is synthesized in interphase and degraded in mitosis. At least eight members of the mammalian cyclin family have been cloned (cyclins A to H). Each of these cyclins interacts with a group of cdc2-related kinases called *cyclin-dependent kinases* (cdks).[12,13] The cyclin/cdk complex is the mammalian counterpart of the cdc2/cdc13 complex in yeast. Phosphorylation of tyrosine 15 is the key event in regulating human cdc2 activity. Threonine 14 also is phosphorylated in G_2 phase. Both phosphorylation sites are required for mitotic initiation. Cdc2 interacts with cyclin B in mitosis, whereas the cdc2/cyclin A complex is formed before mitosis and probably is required for progression through late G_2 phase.[14] Thus, cyclins A and B are also called the *mitotic* cyclins, because they are up-regulated in late G_2 or G_2/M phase and undergo proteolysis in M phase.

The exit from mitosis is characterized by the abrupt ubiquitination and subsequent degradation of cyclin B. Cells with a defective cyclin B degradation mechanism or without mitotic cyclin B easily become aneuploid. The exact role of the other mitotic cyclin, cyclin A, is still unclear. There is evidence that it both acts at the G_2/M transition and binds cdk2 in S phase. Overexpression of cyclin A in G_1 phase leads to an accelerated entry into S phase.[15] Because cdc2 is able to interact with mitotic and G_1 cyclins, it is likely that one protein kinase potentially can fulfill several different functions in the cell cycle at various checkpoints. The redundancy of cyclin functions makes it difficult to ascertain the exact function of each protein in all cell types.

There are several cdc2-related protein kinases in humans that interact with the corresponding cyclins. Originally, three cdc2-related proteins were isolated, which were able to replace deficient cdc28 function in budding yeast: cdk1, cdk2, and cdk3.[16–18] Another group of cdks that bind to cyclin D (a G_1 cyclin) are named cdk4,[19] cdk5,[20] and cdk6.[21] Cdk4 has been in the focus of tumor-suppressor gene research for the past several years, because it complexes with cyclin D1. This complex is an important element in the $p16^{INK4A}$-retinoblastoma (RB) gene pathway, which is commonly disrupted in cancer (see below). Three other cyclin-dependent kinases have been partially characterized: cdk7 ($p40^{MO15}$) interacts with cyclin H and is responsible for phosphorylating pcdc2 on threonine 161.[22,23] Cdk8 interacts with cyclin C and is associated with RNA polymerase II.[24,25] Cdk9 binds cyclin T1 and displays a tissue-specific expression pattern.[26,27] That cdk9/cyclin T1 specifically interacts with the tat element of the human immunodeficiency virus 1 (HIV-1) links this cyclin-dependent kinase directly to the replication pathway of HIV, and circumstantially to HIV-1-related malignancies (e.g., Kaposi sarcoma).[28,29]

Acronyms and abbreviations that appear in this chapter include: AML, acute myelogenous leukemia; APL, acute promyelocytic leukemia; ATRA, all-*trans*-retinoic acid; CDI, cyclin-dependent kinase inhibitor; CDK, cyclin-dependent kinase; CML, chronic myelogenous leukemia; HAT, histone acetylases; HDAC, histone deacetylase; HDACi, histone deacetylase inhibitor; HIV, human immunodeficiency virus 1; INK4, inhibitor of kinase 4; MPF, M-phase promoting factor; MTAP, methylthioadenosine phosphorylase; PLZF, promyelocytic leukemia Kruppel-like zinc finger; P-TEFb positive transcription elongation factor b; RA, retinoic acid; RARA, retinoic acid receptor-alpha; rPTK, receptor protein-tyrosine kinase; SCID, severe combined immune deficiency; SPF, S-phase promoting factor; T-ALL, T cell acute lymphoblastic leukemia; TAR, transactivation response element; TGF-β, transforming growth factor β; TNF-α, tumor necrosis factor alpha; TRAF2, tumor receptor-associated factor 2; vAPL, variant form of acute promyelocytic leukemia.

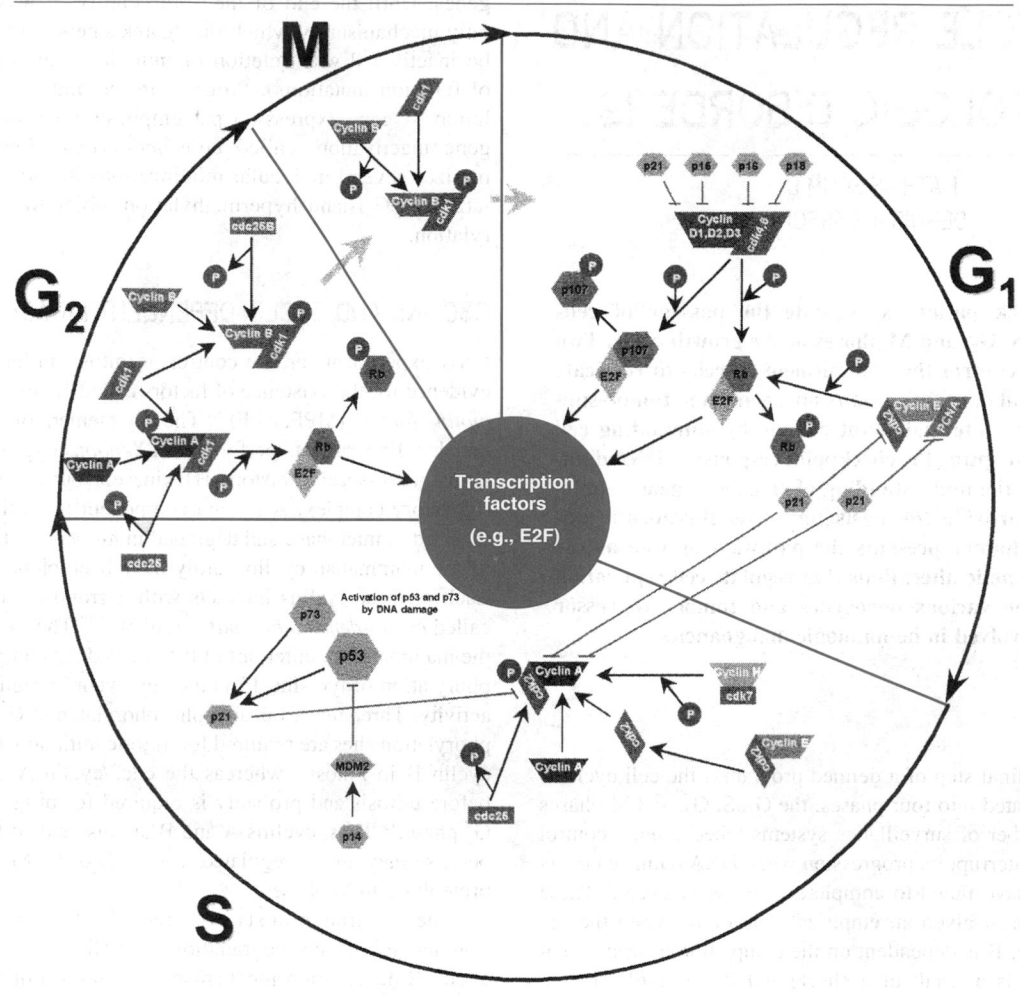

FIGURE 12-1 Cell cycle regulation in mammalian cells.

Cdk10[6,7] and cdk11[8,9] define a novel class of cyclin-dependent kinases, because no corresponding cyclin has been yet identified. Both cdks interact with apoptosis-related factors[8,9] or transcription factors such as ets.[7]

All cyclins share an approximately 150-amino-acid region, called the *cyclin box*, which interacts with the cdks.[30] The G_1 cyclins (C, D, and E) and the mitotic cyclins (A and B)[31] form distinct categories, although cyclin H and the type T cyclins (T_1, T_2a, and T_2b) fall outside these two major groups.

Cyclin A binds and activates cdk2 mainly in S phase. However, microinjection of anticyclin A antibodies into cells causes cell cycle arrest just before S phase.[14] The integration of the hepatitis B virus into the cellular genome is accompanied by the formation of a chimeric cyclin A, lacking the cyclin destruction box, and with a prolonged half-life.[32] This observation, together with the finding that overexpression of cyclin A leads to accelerated S-phase entry, suggests that cyclin A is involved in transformation.[15] Cyclin E, the other cyclin that interacts with cdk2, may control the progression from G_1 to S phase, but the exact time point when cdk2 "switches" from cyclin E to cyclin A binding is unknown. Cdk2/cyclin E activity peaks during late G_1 phase, and declines in early S phase.[33] Cells overexpressing cyclin E progress much faster through G_1 into S phase, but the time required for DNA synthesis remains normal.[34] Cyclin E levels also are regulated by environmental factors, including transforming growth factor β (TGF-β) and irradiation. These effects are, in part, mediated by small proteins, the cyclin-dependent kinase inhibitors (CDIs). In addition to its role at the G_1/S boundary, cyclin A acts in late G_2 phase, where it complexes with cdk1. It has been suggested that this interaction might be necessary for the reorganization of the cytoskeleton prior to mitosis.[35]

TABLE 12-1 CDKs, ASSOCIATED CYCLINS, AND THE STAGE OF THE CELL CYCLE WHERE THEY ACT

CDK	ASSOCIATED CYCLIN	CELL CYCLE STAGE
CdK1	Cyclin A, B	G_2/M
Cdk2	Cyclin A, D, E; cyclin H?	G_1/S; S; G_2/M?
Cdk3	Ik3-1, Ik3-2	G_1
Cdk4	Cyclin D	G_1/S; S
Cdk5	Cyclin D	G_1/S
Cdk6	Cyclin D	G_1/S; S
Cdk7	Cyclin H	G_1/S; transcriptional regulation
Cdk8	Cyclin C	G_1/S; G_2/M, transcriptional regulation
Cdk9	Cyclin T1, T2	Acts on differentiation, interaction with tat, the transcriptional regulator of the HIV virus
Cdk10	Interacts with ets-2[6]	G_2/M[7]
Cdk11	RanBPM, RNPS1[8] casein kinase[9], cyclin L	Promotes apoptosis

The B-type cyclins associate with cdk1 and cdk2 to form the classical mitotic cyclin/cdk complexes.[36] Cyclin B is synthesized in S phase and accumulates together with cdk2, is ubiquitinated, which is followed by degradation, allowing the cell to exit from mitosis. The cyclin B/cdk2 checkpoint is very often defective in malignant cells, leading to uncontrolled M-phase entry and aneuploidy. The cellular localization of the cdk1-cyclin B complexes also is strictly cell-cycle−dependent. Although the complexes accumulate in the cytoplasm during G_2 and S phase, they move to the nucleus in mitosis and bind to the mitotic spindle.[37,38]

The three cyclin D molecules—D_1, D_2, and D_3—function mainly in late G_1 phase, where they bind cdk4 and cdk6. These complexes phosphorylate RB, restraining its inhibitory effects on E2F and related transcription factors. Cyclin D_1 is the major D cyclin in most cell types. All three cyclin D molecules act in late G phase, just before entry into S phase. Forced overexpression of cyclin D_1 shortens the G_1 phase. Many tumors have high cyclin D_1 levels without amplification or mutation of the cyclin D_1 structural gene. Instead, cyclin D levels may be regulated by a feedback loop dependent on RB. Alterations of the RB gene in cancer may secondarily cause up-regulation of cyclin D transcription.

Another member of the cdk family, cdk9, partners with cyclin T, an 87-kDa cyclin C-type protein with three subunits.[26] Cdk9 and its binding partner cyclin T1 comprise the positive transcription elongation factor b (P-TEFb).[39] P-TEFb can hyperphosphorylate the C-terminal domain of RNA polymerase II, similar to the cyclin H/cdk7/MAT1 complex.[28] In addition, P-TEFβ forms a complex with the HIV tat protein that binds the transactivation response element (TAR). The modification of RNA polymerase II by cdk9/cyclin T facilitates the efficient multiplication of the viral genome.[40,41] The fact that the cyclin T1/cdk9 complex is up-regulated during T cell activation enables the HIV to use this complex for replication.[42] Other binding partners of cdk9 include tumor necrosis factor signal transducer molecule and tumor receptor-associated factor 2,[43] as well as MAQ1 and 7SK RNA.[44] It has been shown that cdk9 is expressed throughout the cell cycle[45]; other postulated mechanisms are reviewed in reference 46.

The cdk10 gene encodes two different CDK-like putative kinases; it is postulated that they exert their function at the G_2/M transition.[6] These two isoforms predominate in human tissues, except in brain and muscle, and the relative isoform levels do not vary during the cell cycle.[6] Cdk10 interacts with the N-terminus of the Ets2 transcription factor, which contains the highly conserved pointed transactivation domain. The pointed domain is implicated in protein−protein interactions and Ets2 requires an intact pointed domain to bind Cdk10, which inhibits Ets2 transactivation in mammalian cells.[7] This could be an important factor for the development of follicular lymphoma, because it could be shown that cdk10 is overexpressed in this entity.[47]

Cdk11 is associated with cyclin L.[9] It is part of the large family of p34(cdc2)-related kinases whose functions appear to be linked with cell cycle progression, tumorigenesis, and apoptotic signaling. Cdk11 interacts with the p47 subunit of eukaryotic initiation factor 3 during apoptosis and is therefore directly involved in cell death mechanisms.[48] Casein kinase 2 phosphorylates the cdk11 amino-terminal domain, suggesting that cdk11 participates in signaling pathways that include casein kinase 2 and that its function may help to coordinate the regulation of RNA transcription and processing events.[9] So far two isoforms of cdk11 have been identified, a larger p110 and a smaller p46 isoform. During Fas- or tumor necrosis factor alpha (TNF-α)-induced apoptosis, the caspase-processed p46 isoform is generated from the larger p110 isoform and it promotes apoptosis when it is ectopically expressed in human cells.

SUBSTRATES AND INHIBITORS OF CYCLIN-DEPENDENT KINASES

Many cyclin-cdk substrates have been identified by immunoprecipitation or two-hybrid assays, but only a few of them are thought to exert a direct function in cell cycle control. The regulation of the cell cycle has been studied extensively during the last decade and a consensus paradigm of cell cycle regulation has been suggested.[49,50] According to this consensus paradigm, the important switch of the cell cycle is the RB family of proteins (Fig. 12-2). In its hypophosphorylated state, RB binds to and inhibits a class of transcription factors, of which the best characterized is the E2F transcription factor. Hyperphosphorylation causes RB to detach from its binding site, permitting transcriptional activation of genes necessary for DNA synthesis and cell division. This phosphorylation of RB is regulated in a cell-cycle−dependent manner.[51,52] Interference with RB function impairs G_1 checkpoint regulation, fosters unrestrained cell growth, and is a nearly universal characteristic of malignancy. Causes of reduced RB activity include changes in the structural gene, the sequestration and inactivation of the protein by viral oncogene products, and hyperphosphorylation of RB as a result of increased cdk4 and cyclin D activity or deletion of the gene for the $p16^{INK4A}$ inhibitor of cdk4. Deletions, mutations, and translocations of RB are common in various malignancies, while homozygous deletions of the $p16^{INK4A}$ gene are even more frequent. Many different transforming viruses, such as papilloma virus and simian virus 40, produce proteins that interact with RB. Both cyclin D_1/cdk4 and cyclin D_1(D_2, D_3)/cdk6 complexes are able to phosphorylate the RB.[53,54] The time point of RB phosphorylation correlates strongly with the appearance of the cyclin D_1/cdk4 complex. The link between RB and cyclin D is supported by the observation that loss of RB function leads to a decrease in the cellular cyclin D level.[55,56] However, cyclin D may not be the only cyclin that is involved in the RB regulatory pathway.[57,58] Ectopic expression of both cyclin A and cyclin E restores RB hyperphosphorylation and causes cell cycle arrest in cancer cell lines. Perhaps the cdk2-cyclin A complex contributes to additional phosphorylation of RB, whereas cdk2/cyclin E prolongs the phosphorylation time.[57] The key regulatory element for the G_1 to S transition is the RB:E2F complex. After RB is phosphorylated by cdk4 and/or cdk6 complexes (e.g., cyclin D1/cdk4) during G_1 phase and cdk2 at G_1/S interphase, E2F proteins are released and then promote the transcription of genes essential for the transition to S phase.[59,60] As mentioned above the $p16^{INK4A}$/cyclin D_1/cdk4/RB/E2F cascade is probably one of the most important cascades in cell cycle control, and is therefore also frequently affected in human cancer. We could show that this pathway is defective in nearly 100 percent of acute myelogenous leukemia (AML) cell lines and most of the primary AML samples, although the exact mechanism of inactivation is not always clear. Two RB-related proteins, p107 and p130, form complexes with the transcription factor E2F,[56,61] bind to the region of the adenovirus E1A protein required for transformation, and are able to induce G_1 arrest when they are overexpressed in human malignant cell lines.[62,63] Unlike the RB, the p107 and p130 proteins contain a so-called spacer region that interacts with cdk2/cyclin A and cdk2/cyclin E,[64,65] although it seems to be unlikely that these two complexes regulate the activity of p107 and p130.[57] Instead, p107 may bind and inactivate the cyclin A and cyclin E complexes. Thus, p107 may regulate the cell cycle by several different mechanisms. Because both p107 and p130 are regulated through phosphorylation, efficient cell cycle entry is accompanied by phosphorylation of all the RB-related proteins.

RB has not only cell cycle regulatory properties but it also influences hematopoietic differentiation. RB interacts with the transcription factor PU.1, which blocks erythroid differentiation in the proerythro-

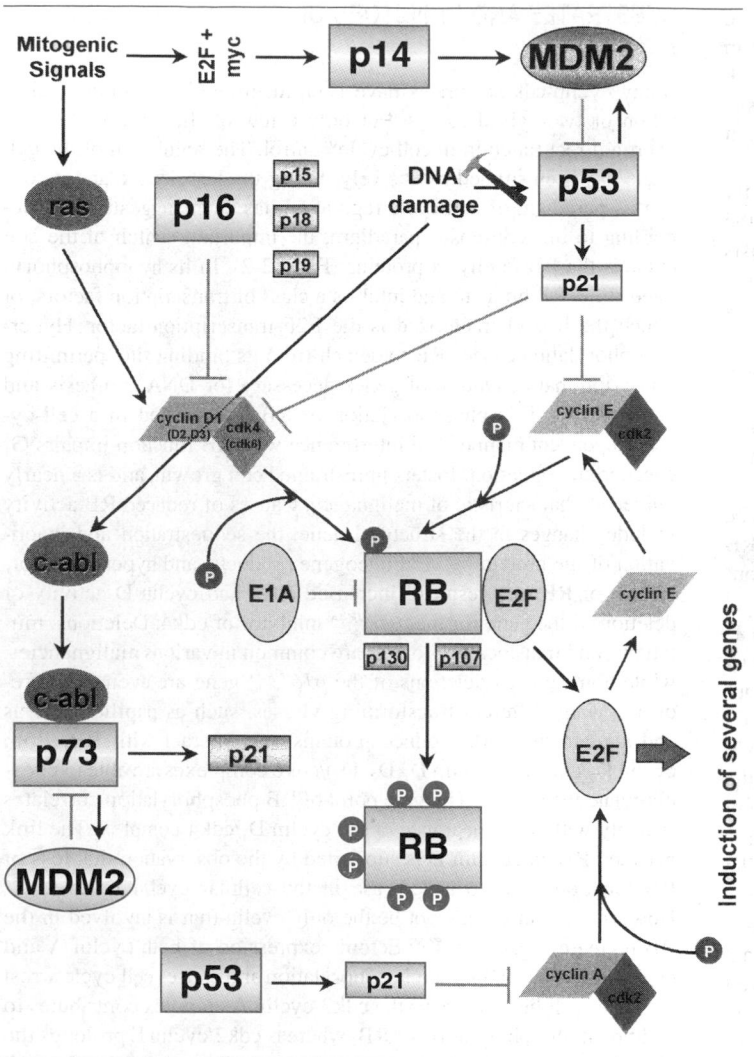

FIGURE 12-2   Interactions between cyclin-dependent kinase inhibitors (p16, p14, p21), p53, and the retinoblastoma protein (RB).

blast stage when ectopically overexpressed in bone marrow cells,[66,67] and represses GATA-1 activity.[68] In addition, hypophosphorylated RB promotes monocytic differentiation in favor of neutrophilic differentiation, but this completely switches toward neutrophilic differentiation if RB expression is inhibited. This clearly demonstrates that RB acts also independent of cell cycle control.[69]

The cyclin-dependent kinases themselves are also controlled by several different mechanisms. Besides their regulation by phosphorylation, specific protein inhibitors of enzyme activity have been identified.[70,71] The cyclin-dependent kinase inhibitors cause cells to arrest in G_1 phase, followed by differentiation and/or senescence. The first cyclin-dependent kinase inhibitor identified was p21cip1.[72] It binds to several cyclin/cdk complexes, including cyclin A/cdk2, cyclin D/cdk4, and cyclin E/cdk2 (see Fig. 12-2).[51,73–75] Several different cell cycle regulatory pathways involve p21cip1. This molecule has a p53 binding site in its promoter, and an increase in p53 levels results in transcriptional activation of p21cip1, slowing down cell cycle progression. The p21cip1 cyclin-dependent kinase inhibitor also plays a role in cellular differentiation in myoblasts.[76] Several binding partners of p21cip1, for example, pim-1, have been identified. Pim-1 associates with and phosphorylates p21cip1 in vivo, which influences the subcellular localization of p21cip1.[77] The p21cip1 is also regulated by several different mechanisms, including mutation and histone deacetylation (see "The Role

of Histone Deacetylases in Cell Cycle Regulation"). Other members of the p21cip1 family of cyclin-dependent kinase inhibitors include p27kip1 and p57kip1.[53,54] High-level expression of p27kip1 leads to a cell cycle block in G_1 phase after treatment of cells with TGF-β. One major difference between p21cip1 and p27kip1 is that the former binds predominantly to cdk2 whereas the latter binds cdk4. Cyclin concentrations are regulated by ubiquitination and subsequent proteolysis. The formation of ubiquitin/protein complexes requires a ubiquitin-activating enzyme, a ubiquitin-conjugating enzyme, and a so-called specificity factor, which permits substrate recognition. Polyubiquitinated proteins are degraded by the 26S proteasome complex. There are two major ubiquitination systems in the cell, designated *SCF* and *APC*.[62–64] SCF is named for three of its core components, Skp1, Cdc53, and an F-box-containing protein. Important examples of SCF substrates are Cln1, Sic1, Wee1 Cdc6/Cdc18, E2F, cyclin D_1, cyclin E, p21cip1, p27kip1, and p57kip2.[65]

The second group of cyclin-dependent kinase inhibitors belong to the inhibitor of the kinase 4 (INK4) family and include *p15INK4B*, *p16INK4A*, p18INK4C, and p19INK4D.[55,57,58,61,78] They all bind and inhibit the cyclin D_1/cdk4 and/or cyclin D_1/cdk6 complex, which regulates cell cycle progression via the RB.[55,58,78] TGF-β also is a potent inducer of *p15INK4B*.[55] *p16INK4A* is probably the most important cyclin-dependent kinase inhibitor, because the *p16INK4A* gene is inactivated by several mechanisms (deletion, mutation, hypermethylation) in many different human cancers. Surprisingly, *p16INK4A* and *p14ARF* are overexpressed in some cases of human hematologic malignancies.[79] This overexpression is probably a result of defects downstream of *p16INK4A*, particularly caused by mutations in the RB gene. The alterations of the INK4-locus genes are excellently reviewed in reference 80. In hematologic malignancies, the highest frequencies of *p14ARF*, *p15INK4B*, or *p16INK4A* are found in T cell acute lymphoblastic leukemia (T-ALL), secondary high-grade lymphomas, and mantle cell lymphomas.[81,82] The potency of *p14ARF* and *p16INK4A* in terms of tumorigenicity becomes obvious by the fact that the reexpression of both genes by either retroviral transfection or demethylation of the promoter regions result in a complete conversion of the malignant phenotype.[83–86]

ONCOGENES (TABLE 12-2)

The complicated cell cycle network has its parallel in the several different oncogenes and tumor suppressor genes that influence carcinogenesis and tumor progression. The products of oncogenes, the oncoproteins, lead to or facilitate the transformation of a normal into a malignant cell. Oncogenes can be carried into the cell by viruses or they can arise from mutations in normal cellular genes. In addition, they can also arise from leukemia- or lymphoma-associated translocations where two usually separated genes are fused together and form a novel fusion protein. The familiar concept of this kind of protooncogene activation can be blurred by the fusion proteins because they possess unique capabilities not shared by either of the individual fusion partners. Oncoproteins can interact directly with cell cycle regulatory proteins or control their activity by phosphorylation and dephosphorylation. Not all mutations in oncogenes lead to an altered function of the resulting product. The nomenclature in the oncogene tumor suppressor gene field is not always clear. As a general guideline, if a mutation causes a functional loss of the gene product (loss of function), and the recessive loss of function leads directly to uncontrolled cell division, the underlying gene can be named a *tumor suppressor gene*. On the other hand, if the mutation leads to an altered gene product (gain of function) that interacts abnormally with other proteins to in-

TABLE 12-2 ONCOGENES INVOLVED IN HUMAN HEMATOLOGIC MALIGNANCIES AND THEIR CHROMOSOMAL LOCALIZATION

Oncogene	Description	Locus	Function	Associated Malignancies
ab11; ab12	Abelson murine leukemia virus	9q34.1; 1q24-q25	tyr protein kinase	Lymphoid and myeloid neoplasms
akt1; akt2	Murine thymoma virus	14q32.3; 19q13.1	ser/thr kinase	Breast cancer, thymoma
am11	AML-associated protein	21q22.3	Transcription factor	Acute myeloid leukemia
bc12, bc13	B cell leukemia-associated oncogenes	18q21; 19q13.1-q13.2	Apoptosis regulation	B cell leukemias, lymphomas
EGFR	Epidermal growth factor receptor	7p12	Growth factor receptor	Several human neoplasms
erb	Avian erythroblastic leukemia viral oncogene	17q21.1	EGF receptor	Brain tumors, breast cancer, several others
erg	v-ets avian erythroblastosis virus	21q22.3	Transcription factor	Acute myeloid leukemia
eto	Involved in the t(8;21) in acute myeloid leukemia	8q22	Transcription factor?	Acute myeloid leukemia
fgr	Gardner-Rasheed feline sarcoma virus	1p36.2-p36.1	tyr kinase	Myeloid leukemias
fos	Murine osteosarcoma virus	14q24.3	Transcription factor	Several human neoplasms
fyn	Oncogene related to src, fgr yes	6q21	tyr kinase	Several human neoplasms
jun	Avian sarcoma virus 17	1p32-p31	Transcription factor	Ovarian, breast, colon, lung, leukemia, several others
kit	Hardy-Zuckerman 4 feline sarcoma virus	4p11-p12	Receptor tyr kinase	Acute myeloid leukemia
lyn	Yamaguchi sarcoma virus related	8q13	tyr kinase	Lymphoid and myeloid neoplasms
myb	Avian myeloblastosis virus	6q22-q23	Transcription factor	Hematologic disorders, several human neoplasms
myc	MC29 myelocytoma virus	8q24.12-q24.13	Transcription factor	Myeloid, lymphatic neoplasms, renal cancer
npm1	Nucleophosmin (nuclear phosphoprotein)	5q35	tyr kinase	Childhood acute myeloid leukemia
pim1	Murine leukemia virus	6p21.2	ser/thr kinase	T cell lymphoma
pml	Involved in t(15;17) in promyelocytic leukemia	15q22	Transcription factor	Promyelocytic leukemia
raf	Murine leukemia virus	3p25	ser/thr kinase	Several human neoplasms
rar	Retinoic acid receptor	17q12	Transcription factor	(Pro-)myelocytic leukemia
ras	Harvey sarcoma viral oncogene	Several	G-protein	Myeloid neoplasms, several human neoplasms
spi	Spleen focus forming virus	11p12-p11.22	Transcription factor	Myeloid leukemias, lymphomas?
src	Rous sarcoma virus	20q11.2-q12	tyr kinase	Lymphomas
tax1	Human T cell leukemia virus-binding protein	7q13	Binding protein	Acute T cell leukemia
tel	t(5;12) involved oncogene	12p13	Transcription factor	Myeloid leukemia
tm11	TCL1/ MTCP1-like protein	14q32.1	?	T cell leukemia, lymphoma

fluence the cell cycle, this gene is an *oncogene*, acting in a dominant fashion. Mutations are found in both oncogenes and tumor suppressor genes. Translocations are typical of oncogenes, whereas homozygous deletions and hypermethylation of CpG-nucleotide repeats are characteristic features of tumor suppressor genes.

Probably more than 100 oncogenes and oncogene candidates have been described in the literature, most of them are involved in the pathogenesis and development of all kinds of tumors, especially the hematologic malignancies. Among the chromosomal translocations, the most well-studied are found in AML. They include t(8;21)(q22;q22), t(15;17)(q22;12), inv16(p13;q22), t(9;11)(p22;q23), t(9;22)(q34;q11), t(3;3)(q21;q26), t(8;16)(p11;p13), t(6;9)(p23;q34), t(7;11)(p15;p15), t(6;11)(q27;q23), t(11;19)(q23;p13.1), t(11;19)(q23;p13.3), t(16;16)(p13;q22), t(16;21)(p11;q22), and t(1;22)(p13;q13).[87] In contrast, in secondary myeloid leukemias recurrent numerical and unbalanced cytogenetic abnormalities predominate such as del(5q), del(7q), −7, or del(20q) and are often associated with a bad prognosis.[88] Table 12-2 lists some of the fusion partners. Next to the chromosomal translocations in AML as described above, there also aberrant fusion proteins in acute lymphoblastic leukemia (ALL) such as t(9;21), which is also found in chronic myelogenous leukemia (CML), and t(4;11). Some lymphomas are characterized by t(8;14), t(11;14), or t(14;18) (for a review see reference 89).

The exact mechanism by which the fusion proteins lead to tumorigenesis is not well understood for most of the above described translocations. Nevertheless, it could be shown in AML that AML1 is able to promote cell cycle progression by shortening G_1-phase and it also represses p21[cip1] promoter activity. In contrast, the fusion product AML1/ETO, derived from the t(8;21), slows down cell cycle progression, suggesting that one gene in different "fusion situations" can cause different effects on the cell cycle.[90] Activation of the AML1-repression domain or fusing AML1 to ETO results in down-regulation of cdk4 and myc, directly linking this fusion protein to cell cycle checkpoints.[90] Another interesting fusion product with relation to cell cycle control is found in acute promyelocytic leukemia (APL) or its variant form (vAPL). The promyelocytic leukemia-retinoic acid receptor-alpha, PML-RARA, which results from t(15;17)(q22;12), up-regulates cyclin A1 expression, whereas PML itself seems to be a negative regulator of cell growth because PML overexpression leads to growth suppression and G_1 arrest in a variety of different cell types.[91,92] PML is crucial for the growth-inhibiting activity of retinoic acid (RA) and its absence abrogates the retinoic acid-dependent transactivation of p21[WAF/cip1].[93] Consequently, PML by itself is a tumor suppressor gene that positively regulates cell cycle progression. Further evidence for a tumor suppressor gene function of PML comes from transgenic mice models where PML[−/−] mouse embryonic fibroblasts are enriched in S phase and the G_0/G_1 phase is minimized.[91] In APL, this regulatory role is disrupted by the fusion to RARA. One mechanism by which this fusion protein (and also the [PLZF]-RARA fusion derived from the rare t(11;17)) affects cell cycle control is its strong interaction with SMRT or N-CoR, two corepressor elements that are important for the recruitment of histone deacetylases as described in "The Role of Histone Deacetylases in Cell Cycle Regulation" below.[92]

In accordance with this is the finding that retrovirally transduced PML-RARA induces a maturation stop in the corresponding cells, implying that these cells are unable to express certain transcription factors as a consequence of the conformational changes caused by the recruitment of the histone deacetylases (HDACs).[90] A variant of this chromosomal translocation results in a fusion protein between RARA and the promyelocytic leukemia Kruppel-like zinc finger (PLZF) protein, which is observed in a subset of patients with APL.[94]

The translocation t(9:22), which fuses the *BCR* gene to the c-*ABL* gene, is a characteristic feature of CML (see Chap. 88). It is also found in some cases of ALL and in occasional cases of AML.[95,96] *BCR-ABL* not only regulates cell proliferation, apoptosis, differentiation, and adhesion, but also induces resistance to cytostatic drugs by modulation of DNA repair mechanisms, cell cycle checkpoints, and Bcl-2 protein family members. Upon DNA damage bcr/abl enhances repair of DNA lesions and prolongs activation of cell cycle checkpoints (e.g., G_2/M), providing more time for repair of otherwise lethal lesions, so that these cells have a significant survival advantage.[96] The BCR-ABL fusion product is so far the only oncogenic product that is sufficient to induce malignant growth *in vivo* without the presence of other abnormal molecular changes. Several reports have shown that bcr/abl-positive cells display pronounced G_2/M delay in response to various chemotherapeutics and in some cases also to irradiation. The exact mechanism of G_2/M delay in bcr/abl-positive cells has not been characterized in detail but it seems that the cdc2-cyclin B1 regulation is affected. In addition, there is no direct evidence that the abnormal bcr/abl product affects the M checkpoint itself, but some data suggest that bcr/abl-positive CML cells contain elevated MAD2 and BUB1-levels. Both genes inhibit the anaphase-promoting complex and therefore cause mitotic spindle arrest.[96] Amplification of the fusion sequence is frequently used to detect minimal residual disease in patients under therapy with interferon alpha, the tyrosine kinase inhibitor STI571,[97] and after marrow or stem cell transplantation.[98] Other oncogenes that belong to this family are Ret (mutations in Ret cause multiple endocrine neoplasia types 2A and 2B),[99] and c-Cbl, the homolog of the *Caenorhabditis elegans* gene *Sli1*.[100]

Mutant-activated receptor protein-tyrosine kinases (rPTK) comprise a family of very-well-characterized oncogenes. The constitutive activation of rPTK usually is achieved by mutations that lead to the dimerization and activation of their cytoplasmic catalytic domains.[101] Prominent examples include Neu/ERbB and CSF-1 oncogenes. NeuERbB2 is frequently mutated in breast cancer as well as in brain tumors.[102,103] Another possible cause of rPTK dimerization is chromosomal translocations that create chimeric proteins. In the t(2;5) translocation, found in several anaplastic large-cell lymphomas, N-terminal nucleophosmin sequences on the long arm of chromosome 5 are fused to the cytoplasmic domain of the Alk protein on chromosome 2.[104,105] The characteristic translocation of chronic myelomonocytic leukemia (CMMoL), t(5;12), fuses sequences from the transcription factor Tel to the cytoplasmic domain of the platelet-derived growth factor β receptor (*TEL-PDGFβR*), resulting in the formation of a TEL-PDGFβR fusion protein and the constitutive activation of the PTK.[106] The chromosomal area surrounding the *TEL* gene is a fragile site, because the Tel gene is involved in several other translocations in human acute leukemias [e.g., t(12;9)]. For several years, oncogene research focused on growth factor receptors because of the possibilities for therapeutic intervention. For example, the murine myeloproliferative leukemia virus protein (v-Mpl) is actually a mutant form of the human thrombopoietin receptor (c-Mpl). v-Mpl has part of the viral Env protein fused to the C-terminal end of c-Mpl and is activated through dimerization. This blocks normal differentiation and leads to uncontrolled cell growth. One of the TGF-β receptors also is involved in oncogenesis, because mutations are frequently found in colon cancer. TGF-β receptor signaling acts through the Smad family of transcription factors.

Two important oncogene families encode the Ras and Rho family

proteins. Ras itself is a G-protein, and activating mutations in H-Ras, K-Ras, and N-Ras have been found in nearly all kinds of human cancers. Several different ras mutations are able to transform normal cells in tissue culture.[107–109] Mutations in many different Ras family members have been identified in cancer (e.g., Raf1, p110 PI3 kinase, Rin1, Mekk1), but the exact downstream signaling effects of each mutation are still unclear. The Ras and the Rho families of oncoproteins are linked by a small G-protein called *Rac*, which is required for transformation by Ras.[110,111] The Rho family of small G-proteins also regulates actin stress fiber formation.[112] The regular formation of actin filaments is required for G_1/S-phase entry. Thus, alterations in the Rho pathway may lead to premature entry into S phase by interference with cytoskeletal organization. The NF2 tumor suppressor gene also encodes a cytoskeletal protein.[113]

The Ras/Raf/Mek/Erk cascade couples signals from the surface to the intracellular space and therefore triggers cell proliferation signals that influence the cell cycle. Abnormal activation of this cascade occurs in several leukemias because of activating mutations in the ras protooncogene.[114] Ectopic overexpression of Raf proteins is associated with cell proliferation whereas overexpression of activated Raf is associated with cell cycle arrest in G_1 phase.[115] Different raf genes have different functions in the cells. A-Raf is able to upregulate the expression of cyclin D_1, cdk2, cyclin e, and cdk4, whereas B-Raf and Raf-1 induce p21^{cip1}, leading to a G_1 arrest.[114] The mode of action of these raf-molecules is not fully understood but one explanation why they act differently may be because they activate different downstream pathways, namely the mitogen-activated protein (MAP) kinases (MEK [MAP/ERK kinase]). The three different MAP kinase cascades are the ERK-, JNK/SAPK-, and the p38 pathways. The MAP kinase pathways consist of three types of kinases in a series, MAPK, MAPKK, and MAPKKK. The MAP kinase cascades all transmit responses from several different surface receptors to the nucleus.[116] The next downstream kinase below MEK is ERK, which by itself activates c-myc via phosphorylation on serine 62.[117,118] Repression of c-MYC is required for terminal differentiation of many cell types, including hematopoietic cells. Deregulated expression of c-Myc in both M1 myeloid leukemic cells and normal myeloid cells derived from murine bone marrow, blocks terminal differentiation and its associated growth arrest, and also induces apoptosis, which is dependent on the Fas/CD95 pathway. Several different transcription factors have been implicated in the down-regulation of c-myc expression during differentiation, including C/EBPalpha, CTCF, BLIMP-1, and RFX1. Alterations in the expression and/or function of these transcription factors, or of the c-Myc and Max interacting proteins, such as MM-1 and Mxi1, can influence the neoplastic process.[118]

Experiments on oncoproteins have focused on apoptosis, the lethal response of a cell to either DNA damage or to signaling through cell surface "death" receptors. Key regulators of apoptosis induced by DNA damage are the multiple members of the bcl family of proteins, which include bcl, bcl-X_L, bax, and bad. Bcl-2 is involved in the t(14;18) chromosomal translocation, which is found in many leukemias and lymphomas of B cell origin.[119,120] The disruption of these loci increases expression of bcl, and results in the uncontrolled accumulation of malignant B cells, because of an impaired balance between growth and apoptosis.[121,122] Apoptosis also is controlled by certain tumor suppressor genes, such as p53, that influence the cellular response to DNA damage. The nuclear histone deacetylase complex, which regulates the structural conformation of DNA and therefore the activation of several genes, is targeted by ETO, the fusion partner of the acute myelogenous leukemia AML1 gene. The t(8;21) translocation that occurs in acute myelogenous leukemia allows the formation of a stable complex between the histone deacetylase complex and ETO, with resultant leukemogenesis.[123–125] PLZF, PLZF-

RARA, and BCL-6 are other oncogenes that target the histone deacetylase complex.[126,127]

TUMOR SUPPRESSOR GENES (TABLE 12-3)

Almost every cancer harbors one or more abnormalities of tumor suppressor genes. These include mutations, translocations, or deletions. In addition, at least two epigenetic mechanisms—the hypermethylation of CpG islands in the promoter and the aberrant acetylation of histones (especially histone H4)—can silence tumor suppressor genes in a variety of human cancer cell lines and primary tumors.

The products of the three most important tumor suppressor genes (RB, P53, and p16[INK4A]) are interconnected biochemically. The RB gene maps to chromosome 13q14 and has several downstream effectors, among which the transcription factor E2F is the best characterized.[128] The RB gene family consists of three closely related proteins, RB, p107, and p130. All three proteins are able to interact with several E2F family members.

Transcriptional activation and repression are mediated via complexes consisting of RB family members, E2F family members, and so-called DP proteins.[129] Besides its role in cell cycle control, RB can modulate RNA polymerase activity, thus linking cell cycle progression to transcriptional regulation. More than 30 separate cellular proteins have been identified that bind to RB. These proteins can be divided into different groups, including transcription factors, growth factors, protein kinases, protein phosphatases, and nuclear matrix proteins. Mutations of RB are frequent in leukemias; soft-tissue sarcomas; and breast, esophagus, prostate, and renal carcinomas.[130] Several viral or oncoproteins can bind to and inactivate RB.[131,132]

The p53 gene has been called a "guardian" of the genome because it transmits signals arising from various forms of DNA damage, leading to cell cycle arrest or apoptosis. The major regulator of p53 expression is MDM2. The MDM2 protein inhibits p53 transcription and stimulates p53 degradation.[133,134] The MDM2 binding region includes several phosphorylation sites, although the exact mechanism by which MDM2 regulates p53 degradation is still not clear.[133–135] The recently discovered p14[ARF] tumor suppressor gene, which is encoded within the p16[INK4A] locus by alternate splicing, controls MDM2 activity.[136] The p14[ARF] gene shares exons 2 and 3 with p16[INK4A] but has a distinct exon 1. The discovery that two important tumor suppressor genes are encoded by the same chromosomal locus and share several exons was unexpected and is unique in human biology. The p16[INK4A] gene function depends on p53, because overexpression of p16[INK4A] causes cell cycle arrest in p53 wild-type cells but not in p53-dependent cells.[137] The transcription of p16[INK4A] is regulated by E2F, which is under the control of RB.[138] This indicates the existence of yet another feedback loop, which links the RB pathway to p53.[139] The Ras protein is another recently identified p16[INK4A] factor involved in MDM2-p53-p21-RB regulation.[140,141]

Abnormalities of p53 are found in slightly more than 50 percent of all human tumors and, surprisingly, even in some normal cells. It is unclear if these "normal" cells represent a pool of premalignant cells in an otherwise healthy body or if p53 changes are just one step in multistage tumorigenesis. A human p53 homologue, p73, has been described, which has DNA binding, transactivation, and oligomerization domains similar to p53. The p73 gene has been localized to chromosome 1p36, a common region of cytogenetic changes in cancer. If p73 is overexpressed, the pzl cyclin-dependent kinase inhibitor, a downstream element in the p53 pathway, is also up-regulated.[142] The p73 protein also can bind p53, inhibiting its transcriptional regulatory activity.[143] Although p53 mutations are found in many cancers, p73 mutations apparently are much more rare. However, the p73 gene is inactivated by hypermethylation of CpG islands in its promoter region

TABLE 12-3   CHARACTERIZATION OF HUMAN TUMOR SUPPRESSOR GENES

TUMOR SUPPRESSOR GENE	CHROMOSOME LOCUS	DISEASES	MAJOR MECHANISM(S) OF INACTIVATION
Cadherin 1 (E cadherin)	16q22.1	Malignomas of the gastrointestinal tract	Hypermethylation of CpG islands, mutation
CDKN1A (p21, Cip1)	6p21.2	Several human malignant and nonmalignant diseases	Homozygous deletion?
CDKN1C (p57, Kip2)	11p15.5	Breast cancer?, Wilms tumor	Hypermethylation of CpG islands, mutations?
CDKN2A (p16)	9p21	Several human cancers	Homozygous deletion, hypermethylation of CpG islands, mutations
CDKN2B (p15)	9p21	Several human cancers	Homozygous deletion, hypermethylation of CpG islands
p14[ARF]	9p21	Several human cancers	Homozygous deletion, hypermethylation of CpG islands, mutations
p53	17p13.1	Several human cancers	Mutations
WT1	11p13	Wilms tumor, nephroblastoma	Homozygous deletion, mutation
DMBT1	10q25.3-26.1	Malignant brain tumors	Homozygous deletion
PTEN	10q23	Glioblastoma, breast cancer	Mutation
p73	1p36	Leukemia, lymphoma	Hypermethylation of CpG islands, mutation?
VHL	3p	von Hippel-Lindau disease	Hypermethylation of CpG islands
H19	11p15.5	Hepatoblastoma, Wilms tumor	Hypermethylation of CpG islands
HIC1	17p13	AML, HCC, breast cancer	Hypermethylation of CpG islands
Rb	13q14.2	Several human cancers	Mutation
nm23	17q21.3-22	Neuroblastoma, breast, prostate cancer, melanoma	Mutation, hypermethylation of CpG islands?
H-cadherin	16q24	Lung cancer	Hypermethylation of CpG islands
N33	8p22	Glioblastoma multiforme	Hypermethylation of CpG-islands, mutation
S100A2	1q21	Breast cancer	Hypermethylation of CpG-islands, mutation
APC	5q21-q22	Adenomatosis polyposis coli	Homozygous deletion, mutation hypermethylation of CpG islands,
NF-1, NF-2	17q11.2, 22q12.2	Neurofibromatosis, bilateral acoustic neuroma	Mutation

in both leukemias and lymphomas.[144] This finding supports the hypothesis that p73 is a tumor suppressor gene on chromosome 1p36.

Homozygous deletions of the *p16^INK4A*/*p14^ARF* gene locus on human chromosome 9p21 have been detected in gliomas,[61,145,146] primary cancers of the lung,[61,147] bladder,[148,149] and head and neck,[150,151] as well as in acute T cell leukemias[152–154] and mesotheliomas.[155] Because inherited mutations of *p16^INK4A* exon 2 may interfere with its expression and/or function, without causing an amino acid change in *p14^ARF*, it is clear that *p16^INK4A* inactivation alone is an important step in the evolution of malignant disease. However, in established tumor cell lines, nearly all chromosome 9p21 deletions disable the entire *p16^INK4A*/*p14^IARF* locus. Both proteins act as suppressors of the G$_1$-S transition, even though they function in two different pathways where *p16^INK4A* acts as an inhibitor of cyclin D$_1$/cdk4(6) complexes while *p14^ARF* stabilizes p53 by inhibition of MDM2.[132] Several models provide insight into the different modes of action of *p16^INK4A* and *p14^ARF* on cell cycle regulation. Interestingly, if the entire p19^ARF/p16^INK4A locus is disrupted in mice (the mouse homologue of p14^ARF is p19^ARF), the mice develop lymphomas, lymphoid leukemias, and sarcomas, suggesting that these tumor suppressor genes do not act in a lineage-specific manner on cell cycle regulation but in a more general one. Retroviral expression of p16^INK4A restores the normal phenotype in some cell types underlining the strong tumorigenic potency of p16^INK4A. The *p15^INK4B* gene, also located on chromosome 9p21, about 20 kDa centromeric of *p16^INK4A*, is deleted somewhat less frequently. Analyses of primary tumors, however, show that not all 9p21 deletions encompass these three tumor suppressor genes. One mechanism for disruption of the *p15^INK4B*/*p14^ARF*/*p16^INKA* region in T cell leukemias may be the action of an illegitimate V(D)J recombinase.[156]

The p15^INK4B/p16^INK4A/p14^ARF locus on chromosome 9p21 is a real hotspot in the development of human cancer and approximately 50 percent of all human malignancies show abnormalities in at least one of these tumor suppressor genes. Another gene lies about 100 kb telomeric of p16^INK4A, and this gene, methylthioadenosine phosphorylase (MTAP), encodes an important enzyme in the purine metabolism. Some early gliomas show MTAP deletions without deletions of other genes on 9p21, suggesting that MTAP by itself has tumor suppressor properties. The re-expression of MTAP in breast cancer cells severely inhibits their ability to form colonies in soft agar or collagen, supporting this hypothesis.[157] In addition, MTAP-expressing cells are suppressed for tumor formation when implanted into severe combined immune deficiency (SCID) mice. The molecular basis for this tumor suppressor gene mechanism is barely understood, but recent findings that the enzyme ornithine decarboxylase is overexpressed in MTAP-deleted tumors provide evidence for a new pathway in tumorigenesis. Overexpression of ornithine decarboxylase has been observed in many tumors and is linked to the ras pathway.[158] Re-expression of MTAP in ornithine decarboxylase overexpressing cells decreases ornithine decarboxylase levels and inhibits tumor cell growth.[159] These findings emphasize the importance of this locus on the chromosomal band 9p21 in carcinogenesis.

The mechanisms by which the above-mentioned genes are inactivated are rather different. Especially in permanent cell lines, *p15^INK4B*/*p14^ARF*/*p16^INKA* and MTAP are homozygously deleted. We could show that MTAP is also heterozygously deleted in AML lines but not in primary AML samples. Mutations in *p15^INK4B*/*p14^ARF*/*p16^INKA* genes are rare, and if present, occur in exon 2. Hypermethylation of CpG islands in the promoter areas of both *p15^INK4B*/*p14^ARF*/*p16^INKA* are frequently found in hematological malignancies.[80,160–163] The availability of demethylating agents such as 5-aza-2′-deoxycytidine (decitabine) makes this phenomenon an interesting target for chemotherapy.[83,164] Decitabine has been used to treat patients suffering from different hematologic malignancies and was reported to

have activity in advanced myelodysplastic syndrome, accompanied by demethylation of the *p16^INK4A* promoter.[165–167] Transcriptional regulation by methylation is mediated by a multiprotein complex consisting of a MeCP2, a methylcytosine-binding protein with a transcriptional repressor domain that binds the corepressor mSin3A, which is itself one element of a multiprotein complex that includes HDAC1 and HDAC2.[168,169] Therefore, re-expression of silenced genes can be achieved by demethylating DNA or by destabilizing HDACs, and it could be demonstrated that both mechanisms are tightly linked. Histone deacetylase inhibitors and demethylating agents act synergistically to induce genes silenced in cancer by hypermethylation.[84]

THE ROLE OF HISTONE DEACETYLASES IN CELL CYCLE REGULATION

HDACs catalyze the deacetylation of lysine residues in the histone N-terminal tails and are found in large multiprotein complexes with transcriptional corepressors. Human HDACs are grouped into three classes based on their similarity to known yeast factors: class I HDACs are similar to the yeast transcriptional repressor yRPD3; class II HDACs are similar to the yeast transcriptional repressor yHDA1; and class III HDACs are similar to the yeast transcriptional repressor ySIR2 (Table 12-4, Fig. 12-3).[170–172]

Eleven different HDACs have been identified so far. The physiologic counterparts of the HDACs are histone acetylases (HATs). In the nucleosome, positively charged hypoacetylated histones bind tightly to the phosphate backbone of the DNA and maintain the chromatin in an inactive, silent state. Both HAT and HDAC activities are recruited to target genes in complexes with sequence-specific transcription factors and their cofactors. Examples of these cofactors include NCoR or SMRT (see Fig. 12-4). Several different transcription factors are assembled with these complexes, including bcl-6, Mad-1, PML, or ETO.[170] Gene silencing by HDAC complexes is an important mechanism in the development of acute myelogenous leukemia, most no-

TABLE 12-4 DIFFERENT TYPES AND CLASSES OF HISTONE DEACETYLASES

ENZYME	MECHANISM OF DEACETYLASE ACTIVITY	TISSUE EXPRESSION	INTERACTING PROTEIN
Class I			
HDAC1	Zn^{2+} dependent	Ubiquitous	RB, p53, MYOD, NF-κB, DNMT1, DNMT3A, MBD2, SP1, BRCA1, MeCP2, ATM
HDAC2	Zn^{2+} dependent	Ubiquitous	RB, NF-κB, BRCA1, DNMT1
HDAC3	Zn^{2+} dependent	Ubiquitous	RB, NF-κB
HDAC8	Zn^{2+} dependent	Ubiquitous	?
HDAC11	Zn^{2+} dependent?	Tissue specific	?
Class II			
HDAC4	Zn^{2+} dependent	Tissue specific	MEF2
HDAC5	Zn^{2+} dependent	Tissue specific	MEF2
HDAC6	Zn^{2+} dependent	Tissue specific	?
HDAC7	Zn^{2+} dependent	Tissue specific	MEF2
HDAC9	Zn^{2+} dependent?	Tissue specific	MEF2
HDAC10	Zn^{2+} dependent?	Ubiquitous	RB
Class III			
Sirt1-7	NAD$^+$ dependent	?	p53

HDAC, histone deacetylase; NF-κB, nuclear factor kappa B; NAD, nicotinamide adenine dinucleotide; RB, retinoblastoma.

tably acute promyelocytic leukemia. The PML–RARA fusion protein is an oncoprotein which represses retinoic acid-dependent transcription by recruitment of HDAC to RAR-regulated genes (Fig. 12-4B), causing a maturation stop because of cell cycle arrest in these myeloid cells. In the PML–RARA fusion protein, the RARA is not responsive to physiologic concentrations of retinoic acid and supraphysiologic doses of all-*trans*-retinoic acid are necessary to overcome the tight HDAC-recruitment and the consequent cell cycle block.[170] The rare translocation t(11;17) fuses the RARA gene to the PLZF gene, which directly interacts with the NCoR-mSin3a-HDAC complex to suppress gene transcription. This block can only be overcome by the addition of a histone deacetylase inhibitor (HDACi). Another well-known example of transcriptional silencing by the recruitment of an HDAC repressor is the AML1-ETO fusion protein which results from the t(8;21) translocation. As already described, the addition of an HDACi can relieve ETO-mediated transcriptional repression.[173] Although 11 HDACs have been described so far, only limited information is available about their redundant biologic and physiologic functions. As shown in Fig. 12-4B, inhibitors of HDAC activity lead to the re-expression of silenced genes and to the induction of differentiation. Most of these inhibitors do not exhibit isoenzyme selectivity and are therefore of limited therapeutic value. However, HDACi valproic acid is the first drug within this group that selectively inhibits one HDAC, namely HDAC2.[174] Valproic acid induces proteasomal degradation of HDAC2. Basal and valproic acid-induced HDAC2 turnover strongly depend on the E2 ubiquitin conjugase Ubc8 and the E3 ubiquitin ligase RLIM. Thus, polyubiquitination and proteasomal degradation provide an isoenzyme-selective mechanism for down-regulation of HDAC2.[174] This also underlines the importance of another cell cycle element and leads to the last part of this chapter, to the proteasome.

THE PROTEASOME: THE RECYCLING MACHINERY

The proteasome is a large, multicentric protease complex with an important role in cellular protein regulation. Its structure consists of a cylindrical core, the so-called 20S particle, composed of four stacked rings with a total of seven proteins in each ring. The second part of the proteasome, two copies of the so-called 19S particle are bound to the 20S core. Only proteins that have been ubiquitinated can be degraded in the proteasome. The ubiquitin-proteasome pathway plays a critical role in the degradation of intracellular proteins involved in cell cycle control, transcription factor activation, apoptosis, and tumor growth through an adenosine triphosphate (ATP)-dependent mechanism (the proteasome-ubiquitin pathway).[175] Proteins such as HDAC2 are tagged with several ubiquitin molecules and then degraded in the machinery.[174] Several tumors depend on rapid cell cycling, which requires expression and degradation of numerous regulatory proteins. Some of the proteins that undergo degradation include the cyclins and cdk inhibitors. The rapid turnover of these genes triggers the fast growth rate of certain human malignomas, thus the proteasome is an excellent new target for the development of new drugs, such as the proteasome inhibitors. These

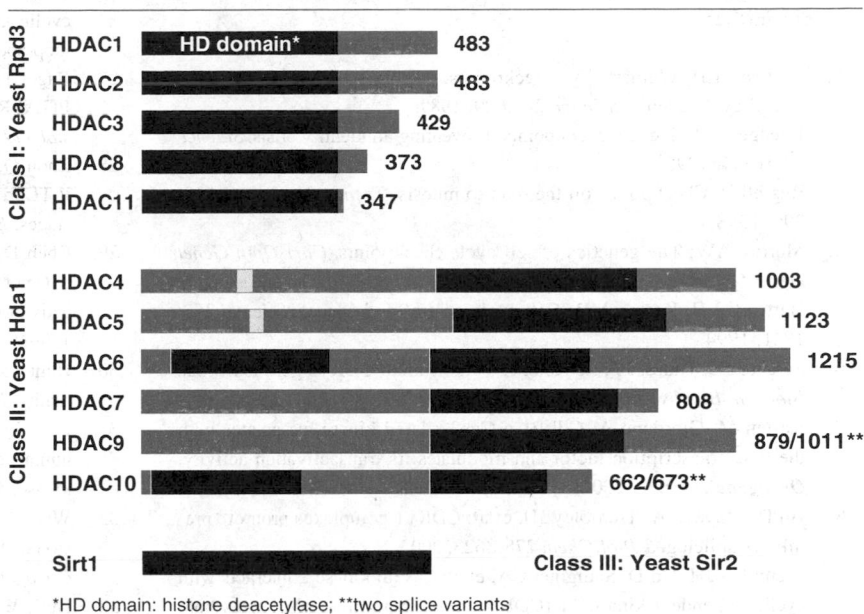

Class I: Yeast Rpd3	HDAC1	HD domain*	483
	HDAC2		483
	HDAC3		429
	HDAC8		373
	HDAC11		347
Class II: Yeast Hda1	HDAC4		1003
	HDAC5		1123
	HDAC6		1215
	HDAC7		808
	HDAC9		879/1011**
	HDAC10		662/673**
	Sirt1		Class III: Yeast Sir2

*HD domain: histone deacetylase; **two splice variants

FIGURE 12-3   Classes of human histone deacetylases.

substances inhibit or at least slow down the proteolytic activity of the proteasome and the cells accumulate in the G_2-M phase of the cell cycle with a decrease of cells in G_1.[176,177]

The proteasome is also required for activation of the nuclear transcription factor nuclear factor-κB, which plays a role in maintaining cell viability through the transcription of inhibitors of apoptosis in response to environmental stress or cytotoxic agents. Based on these observations, targeting the proteasome has become a novel new approach to cancer therapy and with a better understanding of the human cell cycle machinery it will be possible in the future to identify new targets for antineoplastic therapies.

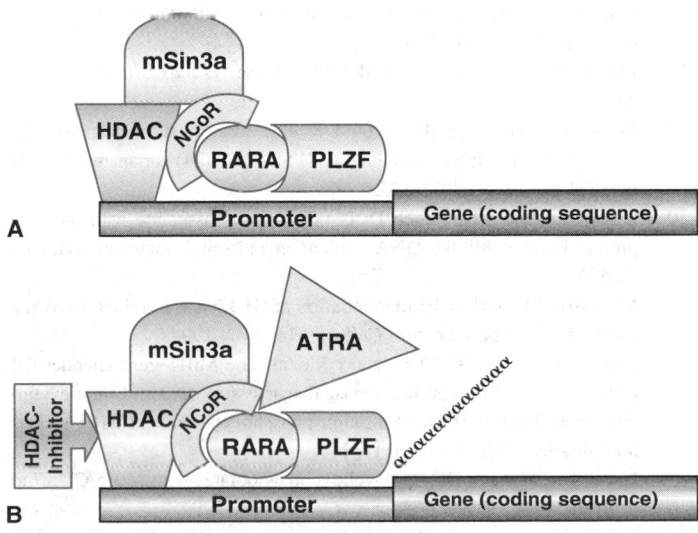

FIGURE 12-4   (A) Transcriptional silencing by the recruitment of histone deacetylases in AML with t(11;17). See text for further description. (B) Transcriptional reactivation and induction of differentiation by histone deacetylase inhibitors and all-*trans*-retinoic acid in AML with t(11;17). See text for further description.

REFERENCES

1. Hartwell LH, Weinert TA: Checkpoints: Controls that ensure the order of cell cycle events. *Science* 246:629, 1989.

2. Elledge SJ: Cell cycle checkpoints: Preventing an identity crisis. *Science* 274:1664, 1996.

3. Russell P: Checkpoints on the road to mitosis. *Trends Biochem Sci* 23: 399, 1998.

4. Murray AW: The genetics of cell cycle checkpoints. *Curr Opin Genet Dev* 5:5, 1995.

5. Hartwell LH, Kastan MB: Cell cycle control and cancer. *Science* 266: 1821, 1994.

6. Sergere JC, Thuret JY, Le Roux G, et al: Human CDK10 gene isoforms. *Biochem Biophys Res Commun* 276:271, 2000.

7. Kasten M, Giordano A: Cdk10, a Cdc2-related kinase, associates with the Ets2 transcription factor and modulates its transactivation activity. *Oncogene* 20:1832, 2001.

8. Hu D, Mayeda A, Trembley JH, et al: CDK11 complexes promote pre-mRNA splicing. *J Biol Chem* 278:8623, 2003.

9. Trembley JH, Hu D, Slaughter CA, et al: Casein kinase 2 interacts with cyclin-dependent kinase 11 (CDK11) *in vivo* and phosphorylates both the RNA polymerase II carboxyl-terminal domain and CDK11 *in vitro*. *J Biol Chem* 278:2265, 2003.

10. Rao PN, Johnson RT: Mammalian cell fusion: Studies on the regulation of DNA synthesis and mitosis. *Nature* 225:159, 1970.

11. Lohka MJ, Hayes MK, Maller JL: Purification of maturation-promoting factor, an intracellular regulator of early mitotic events. *Proc Natl Acad Sci U S A* 85:3009, 1988.

12. Sherr CJ: Mammalian G1 cyclins. *Cell* 73:1059, 1993.

13. Pines J: Cyclins and cyclin-dependent kinases: Take your partners. *Trends Biochem Sci* 18:195, 1993.

14. Pagano M, Pepperkok R, Verde F, et al: Cyclin A is required at two points in the human cell cycle. *EMBO J* 11:961, 1992.

15. Resnitzky D, Hengst L, Reed SI: Cyclin A-associated kinase activity is rate limiting for entrance into S phase and is negatively regulated in G1 by p27Kip1. *Mol Cell Biol* 15:4347, 1995.

16. Meyerson M, Enders GH, Wu CL, et al: A family of human cdc2-related protein kinases. *EMBO J* 11:2909, 1992.

17. Solomon MJ: Activation of the various cyclin/cdc2 protein kinases. *Curr Opin Cell Biol* 5:180, 1993.

18. Lew J, Wang JH: Neuronal cdc2-like kinase. *Trends Biochem Sci* 20: 33, 1995.

19. Matsushime H, Ewen ME, Strom DK, et al: Identification and properties of an atypical catalytic subunit (p34PSK- J3/cdk4) for mammalian D type G1 cyclins. *Cell* 71:323, 1992.

20. Xiong Y, Zhang H, Beach D: D type cyclins associate with multiple protein kinases and the DNA replication and repair factor PCNA. *Cell* 71:505, 1992.

21. Meyerson M, Harlow E: Identification of G1 kinase activity for cdk6, a novel cyclin D partner. *Mol Cell Biol* 14:2077, 1994.

22. Fesquet D, Labbe JC, Derancourt J, et al: The M015 gene encodes the catalytic subunit of a protein kinase that activates cdc2 and other cyclin-dependent kinases (CDKs) through phosphorylation of Thr161 and its homologues. *EMBO J* 12:3111, 1993.

23. Fisher RP, Morgan DO. A novel cyclin associates with M015/CDK7 to form the CDK-activating kinase. *Cell* 78:713, 1994.

24. Tassan JP, Jaquenoud M, Leopold P, et al: Identification of human cyclin-dependent kinase 8, a putative protein kinase partner for cyclin C. *Proc Natl Acad Sci U S A* 92:8871, 1995.

25. Rickert P, Seghezzi W, Shanahan F, et al: Cyclin C/CDK8 is a novel CTD kinase associated with RNA polymerase II. *Oncogene* 12:2631, 1996.

26. Wei P, Garber ME, Fang SM, et al: A novel CDK9-associated C-type cyclin interacts directly with HIV-1 Tat and mediates its high-affinity, loop-specific binding to TAR RNA. *Cell* 92:451, 1998.

27. Bagella L, MacLachlan TK, Buono RJ, et al: Cloning of murine CDK9/ PITALRE and its tissue-specific expression in development. *J Cell Physiol* 177:206, 1998.

28. Zhou Q, Chen D, Pierstorff E, Luo K: Transcription elongation factor P-TEFb mediates Tat activation of HIV-1 transcription at multiple stages. *EMBO J* 17:3681, 1998.

29. Chen D, Fong Y, Zhou Q: Specific interaction of Tat with the human but not rodent P-TEFb complex mediates the species-specific Tat activation of HIV-1 transcription. *Proc Natl Acad Sci U S A* 96:2728, 1999.

30. Hunt T: Cyclins and their partners: From a simple idea to complicated reality. *Semin Cell Biol* 2:213, 1991.

31. Lees EM, Harlow E: Sequences within the conserved cyclin box of human cyclin A are sufficient for binding to and activation of cdc2 kinase. *Mol Cell Biol* 13:1194, 1993.

32. Wang J, Zindy F, Chenivesse X, et al: Modification of cyclin A expression by hepatitis B virus DNA integration in a hepatocellular carcinoma. *Oncogene* 7:1653, 1992.

33. Dulic V, Lees E, Reed SI: Association of human cyclin E with a periodic G1-S phase protein kinase. *Science* 257:1958, 1992.

34. Ohtsubo M, Roberts JM: Cyclin-dependent regulation of G1 in mammalian fibroblasts. *Science* 259:1908, 1993.

35. Verde F, Dogterom M, Stelzer E, et al: Control of microtubule dynamics and length by cyclin A- and cyclin B-dependent kinases in Xenopus egg extracts. *J Cell Biol* 118:1097, 1992.

36. McGowan CH, Russell P, Reed SI: Periodic biosynthesis of the human M-phase promoting factor catalytic subunit p34 during the cell cycle. *Mol Cell Biol* 10:3847, 1990.

37. Buendia B, Draetta G, Karsenti E: Regulation of the microtubule nucleating activity of centrosomes in Xenopus egg extracts: Role of cyclin A-associated protein kinase. *J Cell Biol* 116:1431, 1992.

38. Gallant P, Nigg EA: Cyclin B2 undergoes cell cycle-dependent nuclear translocation and, when expressed as a non-destructible mutant, causes mitotic arrest in HeLa cells. *J Cell Biol* 117:213, 1992.

39. Peng J, Zhu Y, Milton JT, Price DH: Identification of multiple cyclin subunits of human P-TEFb. *Genes Dev* 12:755, 1998.

40. Fujinaga K, Cujec TP, Peng J, et al: The ability of positive transcription elongation factor B to transactivate human immunodeficiency virus transcription depends on a functional kinase domain, cyclin T1, and Tat. *J Virol* 72:7154, 1998.

41. Isel C, Karn J: Direct evidence that HIV-1 Tat stimulates RNA polymerase II carboxyl-terminal domain hyperphosphorylation during transcriptional elongation. *J Mol Biol* 290:929, 1999.

42. Garriga J, Peng J, Parreno M, et al:. Upregulation of cyclin T1/CDK9 complexes during T cell activation. *Oncogene* 17:3093, 1998.

43. MacLachlan TK, Sang N, De Luca A, et al: Binding of CDK9 to TRAF2. *J Cell Biochem* 71:467, 1998.

44. Michels AA, Nguyen VT, Fraldi A, et al: MAQ1 and 7SK RNA interact with CDK9/cyclin T complexes in a transcription-dependent manner. *Mol Cell Biol* 23:4859, 2003.

45. Garriga J, Bhattacharya S, Calbo J, et al: CDK9 is constitutively expressed throughout the cell cycle, and its steady-state expression is independent of SKP2. *Mol Cell Biol* 23:5165, 2003.

46. De Falco G, Giordano A: CDK9: From basal transcription to cancer and AIDS. *Cancer Biol Ther* 1:342, 2002.

47. Husson H, Carideo EG, Neuberg D, et al: Gene expression profiling of follicular lymphoma and normal germinal center B cells using cDNA arrays. *Blood* 99:282, 2002.

48. Shi J, Feng Y, Goulet AC, et al: The p34cdc2-related cyclin-dependent kinase 11 interacts with the p47 subunit of eukaryotic initiation factor 3 during apoptosis. *J Biol Chem* 278:5062, 2003.

49. Pines J: The cell cycle kinases. *Semin Cancer Biol* 5:305, 1994.
50. Sherr CJ: Cancer cell cycles. *Science* 274:1672, 1996.
51. Gu Y, Turck CW, Morgan DO: Inhibition of CDK2 activity *in vivo* by an associated 20K regulatory subunit. *Nature* 366:707, 1993.
52. Harper JW, Adami GR, Wei N, et al: The p21 Cdk-interacting protein Cip1 is a potent inhibitor of G1 cyclin-dependent kinases. *Cell* 75:805, 1993.
53. Nourse J, Firpo E, Flanagan WM, et al: Interleukin-2-mediated elimination of the p27Kip1 cyclin-dependent kinase inhibitor prevented by rapamycin. *Nature* 372:570, 1994.
54. Kato JY, Matsuoka M, Polyak K, et al: Cyclic AMP-induced G1 phase arrest mediated by an inhibitor (p27Kip1) of cyclin-dependent kinase 4 activation. *Cell* 79:487, 1994.
55. Serrano M, Hannon GJ, Beach D: A new regulatory motif in cell-cycle control causing specific inhibition of cyclin D/CDK4 [see comments]. *Nature* 366:704, 1993.
56. Guan KL, Jenkins CW, Li Y, Nichols MA, et al: Growth suppression by p18, a p16INK4/MTS1 and p14INK4B/MTS2-related CDK6 inhibitor, correlates with wild-type pRb function. *Genes Dev* 8:2939, 1994.
57. Chan FK, Zhang J, Cheng L, et al: Identification of human and mouse p19, a novel CDK4 and CDK6 inhibitor with homology to p16ink4. *Mol Cell Biol* 15:2682, 1995.
58. Hirai H, Roussel MF, Kato JY, et al: Novel INK4 proteins, p19 and p18, are specific inhibitors of the cyclin D-dependent kinases CDK4 and CDK6. *Mol Cell Biol* 15:2672, 1995.
59. DeGregori J, Leone G, Ohtani K, et al: E2F-1 accumulation bypasses a G1 arrest resulting from the inhibition of G1 cyclin-dependent kinase activity. *Genes Dev* 9:2873, 1995.
60. Lees JA, Saito M, Vidal M, et al: The retinoblastoma protein binds to a family of E2F transcription factors. *Mol Cell Biol* 13:7813, 1993.
61. Nobori T, Miura K, Wu DJ, et al: Deletions of the cyclin-dependent kinase-4 inhibitor gene in multiple human cancers. *Nature* 368:753, 1994.
62. Bai C, Sen P, Hofmann K, et al: SKP1 connects cell cycle regulators to the ubiquitin proteolysis machinery through a novel motif, the F-box. *Cell* 86:263, 1996.
63. Feldman RM, Correll CC, Kaplan KB, Deshaies RJ: A complex of Cdc4p, Skp1p, and Cdc53p/cullin catalyzes ubiquitination of the phosphorylated CDK inhibitor Sic1p [see comments]. *Cell* 91:221, 1997.
64. Skowyra D, Koepp DM, Kamura T, et al: Reconstitution of G1 cyclin ubiquitination with complexes containing SCFGrr1 and Rbx1 [see comments]. *Science* 284:662, 1999.
65. Koepp DM, Harper JW, Elledge SJ: How the cyclin became a cyclin: Regulated proteolysis in the cell cycle. *Cell* 97:431, 1999.
66. Hagemeier C, Bannister AJ, Cook A, Kouzarides T: The activation domain of transcription factor PU.1 binds the retinoblastoma (RB) protein and the transcription factor TFIID *in vitro*: RB shows sequence similarity to TFIID and TFIIB. *Proc Natl Acad Sci U S A* 90:1580, 1993.
67. Schuetze S, Stenberg PE, Kabat D: The Ets-related transcription factor PU.1 immortalizes erythroblasts. *Mol Cell Biol* 13:5670, 1993.
68. Zhang P, Zhang X, Iwama A, et al: PU.1 inhibits GATA-1 function and erythroid differentiation by blocking GATA-1 DNA binding. *Blood* 96:2641, 2000.
69. Bergh G, Ehinger M, Olsson I, et al: Involvement of the retinoblastoma protein in monocytic and neutrophilic lineage commitment of human bone marrow progenitor cells. *Blood* 94:1971, 1999.
70. Hunter T, Pines J: Cyclins and cancer. II: Cyclin D and CDK inhibitors come of age [see comments]. *Cell* 79:573, 1994.
71. Sherr CJ, Roberts JM: Inhibitors of mammalian G1 cyclin-dependent kinases. *Genes Dev* 9:1149, 1995.
72. Zhang H, Xiong Y, Beach D: Proliferating cell nuclear antigen and p21 are components of multiple cell cycle kinase complexes. *Mol Biol Cell* 4:897, 1993.
73. Xiong Y, Hannon GJ, Zhang H, et al: p21 is a universal inhibitor of cyclin kinases [see comments]. *Nature* 366:701, 1993.
74. El-Deiry WS, Harper JW, PM OC, et al: WAF1/CIP1 is induced in p53-mediated G1 arrest and apoptosis. *Cancer Res* 54:1169, 1994.
75. Li Y, Jenkins CW, Nichols MA, Xiong Y: Cell cycle expression and p53 regulation of the cyclin-dependent kinase inhibitor p21. *Oncogene* 9:2261, 1994.
76. Deng C, Zhang P, Harper JW, et al: Mice lacking p21CIP1/WAF1 undergo normal development, but are defective in G1 checkpoint control. *Cell* 82:675, 1995.
77. Wang Z, Bhattacharya N, Mixter PF, et al: Phosphorylation of the cell cycle inhibitor p21Cip1/WAF1 by Pim-1 kinase. *Biochim Biophys Acta* 1593:45, 2002.
78. Hannon GJ, Beach D: p15ink4b is a potential effector of Tgf-beta-induced cell cycle arrest [see comments]. *Nature* 371:257, 1994.
79. Lee YK, Park JY, Kang HJ, Cho HC: Overexpression of p16INK4A and p14ARF in haematological malignancies. *Clin Lab Haematol* 25:233, 2003.
80. Drexler HG: Review of alterations of the cyclin-dependent kinase inhibitor INK4 family genes p15, p16, p18 and p19 in human leukemia-lymphoma cells. *Leukemia* 12:845, 1998.
81. Dreyling MH, Roulston D, Bohlander SK, et al: Codeletion of CDKN2 and MTAP genes in a subset of non-Hodgkin's lymphoma may be associated with histologic transformation from low- grade to diffuse large-cell lymphoma. *Genes Chromosomes Cancer* 22:72, 1998.
82. Diccianni MB, Batova A, Yu J, et al: Shortened survival after relapse in T-cell acute lymphoblastic leukemia patients with p16/p15 deletions. *Leuk Res* 21:549, 1997.
83. Bender CM, Pao MM, Jones PA: Inhibition of DNA methylation by 5-aza-2'-deoxycytidine suppresses the growth of human tumor cell lines. *Cancer Res* 58:95, 1998.
84. Cameron EE, Bachman KE, Myohanen S, et al: Synergy of demethylation and histone deacetylase inhibition in the re-expression of genes silenced in cancer. *Nat Genet* 21:103, 1999.
85. Chin L, Pomerantz J, DePinho RA: The INK4a/ARF tumor suppressor: One gene—two products—two pathways. *Trends Biochem Sci* 23:291, 1998.
86. Grim J, A DA, Frizelle S, et al: Adenovirus-mediated delivery of p16 to p16-deficient human bladder cancer cells confers chemoresistance to cisplatin and paclitaxel. *Clin Cancer Res* 3:2415, 1997.
87. Mrozek K, Heinonen K, Bloomfield CD: Clinical importance of cytogenetics in acute myeloid leukaemia. *Best Pract Res Clin Haematol* 14:19, 2001.
88. Dann EJ, Rowe JM. Biology and therapy of secondary leukaemias. *Baillieres Best Pract Res Clin Haematol* 14:119, 2001.
89. Vega F, Medeiros LJ: Chromosomal translocations involved in non-Hodgkin lymphomas. *Arch Pathol Lab Med* 127:1148, 2003.
90. Scandura JM, Boccuni P, Cammenga J, Nimer SD: Transcription factor fusions in acute leukemia: Variations on a theme. *Oncogene* 21:3422, 2002.
91. Salomoni P, Pandolfi PP: The role of PML in tumor suppression. *Cell* 108:165, 2002.
92. Lin RJ, Sternsdorf T, Tini M, Evans RM: Transcriptional regulation in acute promyelocytic leukemia. *Oncogene* 20:7204, 2001.
93. Le XF, Vallian S, Mu ZM, et al: Recombinant PML adenovirus suppresses growth and tumorigenicity of human breast cancer cells by inducing G1 cell cycle arrest and apoptosis. *Oncogene* 16:1839, 1998.
94. Chen Z, Brand NJ, Chen A, et al: Fusion between a novel Kruppel-like zinc finger gene and the retinoic acid receptor-alpha locus due to a variant t(11;17) translocation associated with acute promyelocytic leukaemia. *EMBO J* 12:1161, 1993.
95. Gleissner B, Thiel E: Molecular genetic events in adult acute lymphoblastic leukemia. *Expert Rev Mol Diagn* 3:339, 2003.

96. Skorski T: BCR/ABL regulates response to DNA damage: The role in resistance to genotoxic treatment and in genomic instability. *Oncogene* 21:8591, 2002.

97. Fabbro D, Ruetz S, Buchdunger E, et al: Protein kinases as targets for anticancer agents: From inhibitors to useful drugs. *Pharmacol Ther* 93:79, 2002.

98. Mitterbauer G, Nemeth P, Wacha S, et al: Quantification of minimal residual disease in patients with BCR-ABL-positive acute lymphoblastic leukaemia using quantitative competitive polymerase chain reaction. *Br J Haematol* 106:634, 1999.

99. Hoppener JW, Lips CJ: RET receptor tyrosine kinase gene mutations: Molecular biological, physiological and clinical aspects. *Eur J Clin Invest* 26:613, 1996.

100. Galisteo ML, Dikic I, Batzer AG, et al: Tyrosine phosphorylation of the c-cbl proto-oncogene protein product and association with epidermal growth factor (EGF) receptor upon EGF stimulation. *J Biol Chem* 270:20242, 1995.

101. Rodrigues GA, Park M: Dimerization mediated through a leucine zipper activates the oncogenic potential of the met receptor tyrosine kinase. *Mol Cell Biol* 13:6711, 1993.

102. Mezzelani A, Alasio L, Bartoli C, et al: c-erbB2/neu gene and chromosome 17 analysis in breast cancer by Fish on archival cytological fine-needle aspirates. *Br J Cancer* 80:519, 1999.

103. Haapasalo H, Hyytinen E, Sallinen P, et al: c-erbB-2 in astrocytomas: Infrequent overexpression by immunohistochemistry and absence of gene amplification by fluorescence in situ hybridization. *Br J Cancer* 73:620, 1996.

104. Morris SW, Kirstein MN, Valentine MB, et al: Fusion of a kinase gene, ALK, to a nucleolar protein gene, NPM, in non-Hodgkin's lymphoma [published erratum appears in *Science* 267:316, 1995;]. *Science* 263:1281, 1994.

105. Fujimoto J, Shiota M, Iwahara T, et al: Characterization of the transforming activity of p80, a hyperphosphorylated protein in a Ki-1 lymphoma cell line with chromosomal translocation t(2;5). *Proc Natl Acad Sci U S A* 93:4181, 1996.

106. Golub TR, Barker GF, Lovett M, Gilliland DG: Fusion of PDGF receptor beta to a novel ets-like gene, tel, in chronic myelomonocytic leukemia with t(5;12) chromosomal translocation. *Cell* 77:307, 1994.

107. Graham SM, Cox AD, Drivas G, et al: Aberrant function of the Ras-related protein TC21/R-Ras2 triggers malignant transformation. *Mol Cell Biol* 14:4108, 1994.

108. Graham SM, Oldham SM, Martin CB, et al: TC21 and Ras share indistinguishable transforming and differentiating activities. *Oncogene* 18:2107, 1999.

109. Saez R, Chan AM, Miki T, Aaronson SA: Oncogenic activation of human R-ras by point mutations analogous to those of prototype H-ras oncogenes. *Oncogene* 9:2977, 1994.

110. Khosravi-Far R, Solski PA, Clark GJ, et al: Activation of Rac1, RhoA, and mitogen-activated protein kinases is required for Ras transformation. *Mol Cell Biol* 15:6443, 1995.

111. Qiu RG, Chen J, McCormick F, Symons M: A role for Rho in Ras transformation. *Proc Natl Acad Sci U S A* 92:11781, 1995.

112. Nobes CD, Hall A: Rho, rac, and cdc42 GTPases regulate the assembly of multimolecular focal complexes associated with actin stress fibers, lamellipodia, and filopodia. *Cell* 81:53, 1995.

113. Belliveau MJ, Lutchman M, Claudio JO, et al: Schwannomin: New insights into this member of the band 4.1 superfamily. *Biochem Cell Biol* 73:733, 1995.

114. Chang F, Steelman LS, Lee JT, et al: Signal transduction mediated by the Ras/Raf/MEK/ERK pathway from cytokine receptors to TF: Potential targeting for therapeutic intervention. *Leukemia* 17:1263, 2003.

115. Crump M: Inhibition of raf kinase in the treatment of myeloid leukemia. *Curr Pharm Des* 8:2243, 2002.

116. Johnson NL, Gardner AM, Diener KM, et al: Signal transduction pathways regulated by mitogen-activated/extracellular response kinase kinase induce cell death. *J Biol Chem* 271:3229, 1996.

117. Seth A, Gonzalez FA, Gupta S, et al: Signal transduction within the nucleus by mitogen-activated protein kinase. *J Biol Chem* 267:24796, 1992.

118. Hoffman B, Amanullah A, Shafarenko M, Liebermann DA. The proto-oncogene c-myc in hematopoietic development and leukemogenesis. *Oncogene* 21:3414, 2002.

119. Monni O, Franssila K, Joensuu H, Knuutila S: BCL2 overexpression in diffuse large B-cell lymphoma. *Leuk Lymphoma* 34:45, 1999.

120. Kramer MH, Hermans J, Wijburg E, et al: Clinical relevance of BCL2, BCL6, and MYC rearrangements in diffuse large B-cell lymphoma. *Blood* 92:3152, 1998.

121. Bonnotte B, Favre N, Moutet M, et al: Bcl-2-mediated inhibition of apoptosis prevents immunogenicity and restores tumorigenicity of spontaneously regressive tumors. *J Immunol* 161:1433, 1998.

122. Yin DX, Schimke RT: Inhibition of apoptosis by overexpressing Bcl-2 enhances gene amplification by a mechanism independent of aphidicolin pretreatment. *Proc Natl Acad Sci U S A* 93:3394, 1996.

123. Gelmetti V, Zhang J, Fanelli M, et al: Aberrant recruitment of the nuclear receptor corepressor-histone deacetylase complex by the acute myeloid leukemia fusion partner ETO. *Mol Cell Biol* 18:7185, 1998.

124. Lutterbach B, Westendorf JJ, Linggi B, et al: ETO, a target of t(8;21) in acute leukemia, interacts with the N-CoR and mSin3 corepressors. *Mol Cell Biol* 18:7176, 1998.

125. Wang J, Hoshino T, Redner RL, et al: ETO, fusion partner in t(8;21) acute myeloid leukemia, represses transcription by interaction with the human N-CoR/mSin3/HDAC1 complex. *Proc Natl Acad Sci U S A* 95:10860, 1998.

126. Wong CW, Privalsky ML: Components of the SMRT corepressor complex exhibit distinctive interactions with the POZ domain oncoproteins PLZF, PLZF-RARalpha, and BCL-6. *J Biol Chem* 273:27695, 1998.

127. David G, Alland L, Hong SH, et al: Histone deacetylase associated with mSin3A mediates repression by the acute promyelocytic leukemia-associated PLZF protein. *Oncogene* 16:2549, 1998.

128. Yunis JJ, Ramsay N: Retinoblastoma and subband deletion of chr 13. *Am J Dis Child* 132:161, 1978.

129. Grana X, Garriga J, Mayol X: Role of the retinoblastoma protein family, pRB, p107 and p130 in the negative control of cell growth. *Oncogene* 17:3365, 1998.

130. Bookstein R, Lee WH: Molecular genetics of the retinoblastoma suppressor gene. *Crit Rev Oncog* 2:211, 1991.

131. Chellappan S, Kraus VB, Kroger B, et al: Adenovirus E1A, simian virus 40 tumor antigen, and human papillomavirus E7 protein share the capacity to disrupt the interaction between transcription factor E2F and the retinoblastoma gene product. *Proc Natl Acad Sci U S A* 89:4549, 1992.

132. Krug U, Ganser A, Koeffler HP: Tumor suppressor genes in normal and malignant hematopoiesis. *Oncogene* 21:3475, 2002.

133. Haupt Y, Maya R, Kazaz A, Oren M: Mdm2 promotes the rapid degradation of p53. *Nature* 387:296, 1997.

134. Kubbutat MH, Jones SN, Vousden KH: Regulation of p53 stability by Mdm2. *Nature* 387:299, 1997.

135. Roth J, Dobbelstein M, Freedman DA, et al: Nucleo-cytoplasmic shuttling of the hdm2 oncoprotein regulates the levels of the p53 protein via a pathway used by the HI virus rev protein. *EMBO J* 17:554, 1998.

136. Quelle DE, Zindy F, Ashmun RA, Sherr CJ: Alternative reading frames of the INK4a tumor suppressor gene encode two unrelated proteins capable of inducing cell cycle arrest. *Cell* 83:993, 1995.

137. Kamijo T, Zindy F, Roussel MF, et al: Tumor suppression at the mouse INK4a locus mediated by the alternative reading frame product p19ARF. *Cell* 91:649, 1997.

138. Bates S, Phillips AC, Clark PA, et al: p14arf links the tumour suppressors Rb and p53 [letter]. *Nature* 395:124, 1998.

139. Palmero I, Pantoja C, Serrano M: p19arf links the tumour suppressor p53 to Ras [letter]. *Nature* 395:125, 1998.

140. Prives C: Signaling to p53: Breaking the MDM2-p53 circuit. *Cell* 95:5, 1998.

141. Sherr CJ: Tumor surveillance via the ARF-p53 pathway. *Genes Dev* 12:2984, 1998.

142. Jost CA, Marin MC, Kaelin WGJr: p73 is a simian [correction of human] p53-related protein that can induce apoptosis [see comments] [published erratum appears in *Nature* 399:817, 1999]. *Nature* 389:191, 1997.

143. Di Como CJ, Gaiddon C, Prives C: p73 function is inhibited by tumor-derived p53 mutants in mammalian cells. *Mol Cell Biol* 19:1438, 1999.

144. Kawano S, Miller CW, Gombart AF, et al: Loss of p73 gene expression in leukemias/lymphomas due to hypermethylation. *Blood* 94:1113, 1999.

145. Nishikawa R, Furnari FB, Lin H, et al: Loss of P16INK4 expression is frequent in high grade gliomas. *Cancer Res* 55:1941, 1995.

146. Olopade OI, Jenkins RB, Ransom DT, et al: Molecular analysis of deletions of the short arm of chromosome 9 in human gliomas. *Cancer Res* 52:2523, 1992.

147. Schmid M, Malicki D, Nobori T, et al: Homozygous deletions of methylthioadenosine phosphorylase (MTAP) are more frequent than p16INK4A (CDKN2) homozygous deletions in primary non-small cell lung cancers (NSCLC). *Oncogene* 17:2669, 1998.

148. Stadler WM, Olopade OI: The 9p21 region in bladder cancer cell lines: Large homozygous deletions inactivate the CDKN2, CDKN2B and MTAP genes. *Urol Res* 24:239, 1996.

149. Orlow I, Lacombe L, Hannon GJ, et al: Deletion of the p16 and p15 genes in human bladder tumors [see comments]. *J Natl Cancer Inst* 87:1524, 1995.

150. Gonzalez MV, Pello MF, Lopez-Larrea C, et al: Deletion and methylation of the tumour suppressor gene p16/CDKN2 in primary head and neck squamous cell carcinoma. *J Clin Pathol* 50:509, 1997.

151. Matsuura K, Shiga K, Yokoyama J, et al: Loss of heterozygosity of chromosome 9p21 and 7q31 is correlated with high incidence of recurrent tumor in head and neck squamous cell carcinoma. *Anticancer Res* 18:453, 1998.

152. Yamada Y, Hatta Y, Murata K, et al: Deletions of p15 and/or p16 genes as a poor-prognosis factor in adult T-cell leukemia. *J Clin Oncol* 15:1778, 1997.

153. Hatta Y, Hirama T, Miller CW, et al: Homozygous deletions of the p15 (MTS2) and p16 (CDKN2/MTS1) genes in adult T-cell leukemia. *Blood* 85:2699, 1995.

154. Hori Y, Hori H, Yamada Y, et al: The methylthioadenosine phosphorylase gene is frequently co-deleted with the p16INK4a gene in acute type adult T-cell leukemia. *Int J Cancer* 75:51, 1998.

155. Kratzke RA, Otterson GA, Lincoln CE, et al:. Immunohistochemical analysis of the p16INK4 cyclin-dependent kinase inhibitor in malignant mesothelioma. *J Natl Cancer Inst* 87:1870, 1995.

156. Cayuela JM, Gardie B, Sigaux F: Disruption of the multiple tumor suppressor gene MTS1/p16(INK4a)/CDKN2 by illegitimate V(D)J recombinase activity in T-cell acute lymphoblastic leukemias. *Blood* 90:3720, 1997.

157. Christopher SA, Diegelman P, Porter CW, Kruger WD: Methylthioadenosine phosphorylase, a gene frequently codeleted with p16(cdkN2a/ARF), acts as a tumor suppressor in a breast cancer cell line. *Cancer Res* 62:6639, 2002.

158. Lan L, Trempus C, Gilmour SK: Inhibition of ornithine decarboxylase (ODC) decreases tumor vascularization and reverses spontaneous tumors in ODC/Ras transgenic mice. *Cancer Res* 60:5696, 2000.

159. Subhi AL, Diegelman P, Porter CW, et al: Methylthioadenosine phosphorylase regulates ornithine decarboxylase by production of downstream metabolites. *J Biol Chem* 2323, 2003.

160. Jaffrain-Rea ML, Ferretti E, Toniato E, et al: p16 (Ink4a, Mts-1) gene polymorphism and methylation status in human pituitary tumours. *Clin Endocrinol (Oxf)* 51:317, 1999.

161. Melki JR, Vincent PC, Clark SJ: Concurrent DNA hypermethylation of multiple genes in acute myeloid leukemia. *Cancer Res* 59:3730, 1999.

162. Nakamura M, Sugita K, Inukai T, et al: p16/Mts1/Ink4a gene is frequently inactivated by hypermethylation in childhood acute lymphoblastic leukemia with 11q23 translocation. *Leukemia* 13:884, 1999.

163. Baylin SB, Herman JG, Graff JR, et al: Alterations in DNA methylation: A fundamental aspect of neoplasia. *Adv Cancer Res* 72:141, 1998.

164. Timmermann S, Hinds PW, Munger K: Re-expression of endogenous p16ink4a in oral squamous cell carcinoma lines by 5-aza-2'-deoxycytidine treatment induces a senescence-like state. *Oncogene* 17:3445, 1998.

165. Kantarjian HM, Keating M, Beran M, et al: Results of decitabine therapy in the accelerated and blastic phases of chronic myelogenous leukemia. *Leukemia* 11:1617, 1997.

166. Petti MC, Mandelli F, Zagonel V, et al: Pilot study of 5-aza-2'-deoxycytidine (Decitabine) in the treatment of poor prognosis acute myelogenous leukemia patients: Preliminary results. *Leukemia* 7 (Suppl 1):36, 1993.

167. Quesnel B, Guillerm G, Vereecque R, et al: Methylation of the p15(INK4b) gene in myelodysplastic syndromes is frequent and acquired during disease progression. *Blood* 91:2985, 1998.

168. Razin A: CpG methylation, chromatin structure and gene silencing—a three-way connection. *EMBO J* 17:4905, 1998.

169. Jones PL, Veenstra GJ, Wade PA, et al: Methylated DNA and MeCP2 recruit histone deacetylase to repress transcription. *Nat Genet* 19:187, 1998.

170. Vigushin DM, Coombes RC: Histone deacetylase inhibitors in cancer treatment. *Anticancer Drugs* 13:1, 2002.

171. Verdin E, Dequiedt F, Kasler HG: Class II histone deacetylases: Versatile regulators. *Trends Genet* 19:286, 2003.

172. Thiagalingam S, Cheng KH, Lee HJ, et al: Histone deacetylases: Unique players in shaping the epigenetic histone code. *Ann N Y Acad Sci* 983:84, 2003.

173. Wang J, Saunthararajah Y, Redner RL, Liu JM: Inhibitors of histone deacetylase relieve ETO-mediated repression and induce differentiation of AML1-ETO leukemia cells. *Cancer Res* 59:2766, 1999.

174. Kramer OH, Zhu P, Ostendorff HP, et al: The histone deacetylase inhibitor valproic acid selectively induces proteasomal degradation of HDAC2. *EMBO J* 22:3411, 2003.

175. McBride WH, Iwamoto KS, Syljuasen R, et al: The role of the ubiquitin/proteasome system in cellular responses to radiation. *Oncogene* 22:5755, 2003.

176. Elliott PJ, Ross JS: The proteasome: A new target for novel drug therapies. *Am J Clin Pathol* 116:637, 2001.

177. Adams J, Palombella VJ, Elliott PJ: Proteasome inhibition: A new strategy in cancer treatment. *Invest New Drugs* 18:109, 2000.

SIGNAL TRANSDUCTION PATHWAYS

KENNETH KAUSHANSKY

Essentially all external influences on cells of any organ are mediated by biochemical and molecular mechanisms that are triggered by interactions with membrane, cytoplasmic, or nuclear receptors. Recently, our understanding of the receptors and the intermediate molecules that couple them with cellular pathways that influence the proliferation, activation, differentiation, or survival of hematopoietic cells has expanded significantly. This chapter discusses the receptors that influence blood cell production and function, the secondary mediators and the biochemical modifications they undergo to alert the cell to an external influence, the molecular mechanisms that allow for the coordination of multiple signals impacting a cell simultaneously, and the processes that they impact.

AN OVERVIEW OF CELL SIGNALING

Blood cells and their marrow-based progenitors are exquisitely responsive to their environment. A wide variety of cues are detected by mature blood cells that impact significantly on their function. For example, leukocytes respond to noxious stimuli by chemokine-induced migration toward inflammatory stimuli, cross endothelial cell barriers and the extracellular matrix by engaging integrins, and then engulf microorganisms on encountering bacterial products. Likewise, platelets adhere to reactive endothelial surfaces or denuded subendothelial cell matrix by engagement of extracellular adhesive proteins. Bound platelets can also recruit additional platelets and aggregate with them through interactions with platelet integrins, and then contract to strengthen the platelet plug by engagement of numerous granule substances. Even the anucleate erythrocyte responds to mechanical deformation and hypoxemia with adenosine triphosphate (ATP) release. Adrenergic receptors also play important roles in the normal erythro-

Acronyms and abbreviations that appear in this chapter include: ATP, adenosine triphosphate; BCR, B cell receptor; BMP, bone morphogenic protein; CNTF, ciliary neurotrophic factor; CT-1, cardiotrophin-1; DD, death domain; DR, death receptor; Epo, erythropoietin; EpoR, erythropoietin receptor; ERK, extracellular response kinase; FADD, Fas-associated death domain; FAK, focal adhesion kinase; Gab, Grb-associated binding; G-CSF, granulocyte colony stimulating factor; GH, growth hormone; GPCR, G-protein coupled receptor; HCR, hematopoietic cytokine receptor; IKK, IκB kinase; IL, interleukin; IRS, Insulin receptor substrate; ITAM, immunoreceptor tyrosine-based activation motif; ITIM, immunoreceptor tyrosine-based inhibitory motif; JAK, Janus family kinase; JNK, c-Jun N-terminal kinase; LIF, leukemia inhibitory factor; MAPK, mitogen activated protein kinase; M-CSF, macrophage colony stimulating factor; NR, nuclear receptor; OSM, oncostatin M; PIAS, protein inhibitor of activated STATs; PIP, phosphoinositol phosphate; PI3K, phosphoinositol 3 kinase; PKC, protein kinase C; PTP, protein tyrosine phosphatase; RACK, receptor for activated C kinase; RTK, receptor tyrosine kinase; SCID, severe combined immunodeficiency; SH2, Src homology 2; SOCS, suppressors of cytokine signaling; STATs, signal transducers and activators of transcription; SUMO, small ubiquitin-like modifier; TGF, transforming growth factor; TM, transmembrane; TNF, tumor necrosis factor; TPO, thrombopoietin; TRADD, tumor necrosis factor receptor death domain; TRAF, tumor necrosis factor receptor associated factor.

cyte response to parasitic infection or in the pathologic red cell (e.g., patients with hemoglobinopathies) interactions with endothelial cell surfaces. Each of these events induces an intracellular signal that leads to further cellular reactivity toward the initiating stimulus, or that prepares the cell for subsequent functional events. Like the functional activation of mature blood cells, the generation of blood cells is under tight regulation, mediated by both soluble growth factors and components of the marrow microenvironment. Here again, the response to anemia is sensed by hematopoietic progenitor cell surface receptors; their coordinated response involves a myriad of signals that impact on the survival, growth, and differentiation of both undifferentiated and lineage-committed cells. Although anemia induces red cell production and inflammation leads to the production and functional activation of leukocytes, many of the intracellular signals that mediate these two responses overlap substantially. This chapter illustrates a number of principles that mediate each of the growth and functional responses of blood cells and their progenitors in health and disease. A better understanding of how blood cells respond to their environment can lead to improved strategies to intervene in pathologic processes in which too many or too few blood cells are produced, or in which the functional activation of blood cells is insufficient or overly exuberant and leads to disease. Moreover, a thorough knowledge of how the signaling pathways that mediate growth and cell survival are disrupted in the hematologic malignancies has begun to allow the rational intervention in such diseases.

TYPES OF RECEPTORS AND THEIR MECHANISMS OF ACTIVATION

THE TYPE I HEMATOPOIETIC CYTOKINE RECEPTORS

The erythropoietin receptor (EpoR) was cloned in 1989,[1] settling several controversies and setting many important paradigms in receptor biology. Like other hematopoietic cytokines of this class (granulocyte colony stimulating factor [G-CSF], thrombopoietin [TPO], and growth hormone [GH]), erythropoietin (Epo) binds to a homodimeric receptor[2,3] with picomolar affinity.[4] Numerous studies in these and multiple other cell-signaling systems demonstrate the importance of phosphorylation of vital cytoplasmic mediators in signal transduction,[5-7] yet one initial conundrum was that the cloned EpoR bears no kinase domain.[1] Rather, subsequent studies revealed that the EpoR employs a cytoplasmic kinase of the Janus family (JAK) to initiate signaling.[8] Although cytokine binding to the receptor was initially thought to recruit JAKs to the cytoplasmic domain motifs termed *Box1* and *Box2* domains, it is almost certain that inactive kinase molecules are tethered to the receptor prior to ligand engagement. This information, along with the availability of the tertiary structure of EpoR and of Epo bound to EpoR,[9,10] has provided a key insight into the initiation of signal transduction. EpoR exists as a preformed cell surface dimer (see Fig. 13-1), in a conformation that separates the two cytoplasmic domains of the subunits (and hence the two tethered JAK molecules) by 78 Å. Epo binds sequentially to the two subunits of the preformed EpoR dimer at two distinct faces of the molecule, first to one subunit with the high-affinity face of the ligand (also termed *site I*), and then to the second subunit of EpoR with a lower-affinity face (termed *site II*), but an interaction that reduces the off-rate of the ligand. Upon engagement of the two EpoR subunits, a stunning conformational change ensues, shifting the distance between the two cytoplasmic domains of the receptor subunits from 78 Å to 39 Å, a shift that brings the two inactive JAK molecules into sufficiently close juxtaposition to allow cross-phosphorylation and kinase activation. Once the two tethered JAK molecules are active, multiple additional tyrosine residues become phosphorylated, residues of the receptor itself and those on a number of tethered signaling molecules, events that trigger the totality of cel-

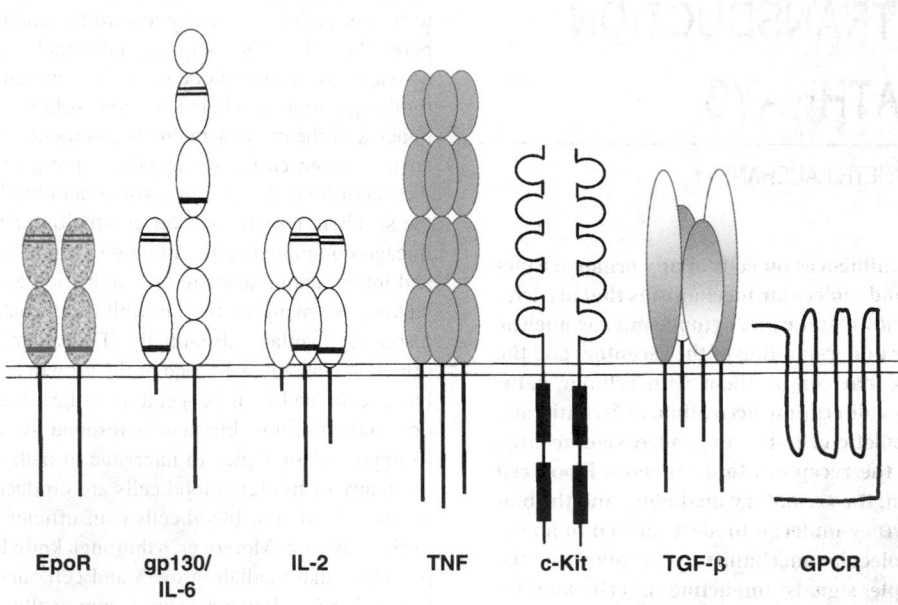

FIGURE 13-1   An illustration of cell surface receptors. Each member of the cell surface receptors is depicted as an extracellular region of one or multiple domains, with conserved disulfide bonds indicated by *thin cross lines*, and the conserved WS box indicated by a *thick cross line*. The founding member of each receptor class is indicated. EpoR, erythropoietin receptor; GPCR, G-protein couple receptor; gp130, glycoprotein 130; IL, interleukin; TGF, transforming growth factor; TNF, tumor necrosis factor.

lular Epo responses. Although direct proof for this model of signal initiation is not available for other cytokines of this class, it is widely assumed that a variety of growth factors, interleukins, and hormones activate cellular events in the same manner.

The understanding that a single molecule of Epo can bind simultaneously to two EpoR molecules has allowed for therapeutic engineering of cytokines into antagonists. Following Epo binding to a first molecule of EpoR through site I, the receptor conformational change becomes dependent on binding of Epo site II to a second EpoR subunit. By altering the residues at site II, it is possible to block this engagement, and if site I is altered to increase its affinity for binding to a first receptor subunit so that the affinity of the mutant protein rivals that of the intact molecule, a potent rationally designed antagonist is generated. This strategy has been successfully employed to create pegvisomant, a GH antagonist useful for the treatment of acromegaly, and a forerunner of the interleukin (IL)-5 antagonists for eosinophil-mediated disorders currently under development.

The engagement of two receptor subunits by cognate ligand is one mechanism of inducing the receptor conformational change necessary for JAK activation, but several other mechanisms exist that have been exploited by man and nature. Small molecules and dimeric antibodies can induce signaling through the EpoR and at least for the former, can serve as Epo mimetics for therapeutic use.[11] Moreover, the 55-kDa glycoprotein (gp55) of the Friend erythroleukemia virus hijacks the EpoR for virus-induced proliferation[12] by directly binding to EpoR and (presumably) by inducing the same receptor conformational changes as induced by the authentic hormone. Thus, there are many ways to activate EpoR, and many subtleties dependent on the actual tertiary structural changes induced.[13]

The IL-6 family of cytokine receptors displays several properties distinct from those of EpoR and its related receptors.[14,15] Unlike the receptors discussed thus far, the IL-6R is composed of a heterodimer. One subunit is termed IL-6Rα, which binds IL-6 with modest affinity,

but despite a short cytoplasmic domain IL-6Rα plays no role in signaling. Instead, the second receptor subunit, termed gp130 based on its apparent molecular weight (M_r), a molecule that alone has no affinity for IL-6 but together with IL-6Rα enhances the binding affinity of the heterodimeric receptor, is responsible for initiating signal transduction in the presence of ligand. In addition, soluble forms of the IL-6R, if loaded with IL-6, can bind to cells bearing only gp130 and activate the latter.[16] Like EpoR and other members of that subfamily, gp130 engages JAKs to initiate signal transduction.[17] Moreover, it is almost certain that the mature IL-6R complex is composed of at least two molecules of IL-6R and two of gp130,[18] the latter required to bring the requisite two JAK molecules to the signaling complex. An additional feature of the IL-6 family is that gp130 serves as the signaling receptor subunit for several cytokines, including IL-11, oncostatin M (OSM), leukemia inhibitory factor (LIF), ciliary neurotrophic factor (CNTF), and cardiotrophin-1 (CT-1). Similar to its role in the IL-6R, gp130 binds to each of these ligands only in the additional presence of a cytokine-specific receptor subunit (e.g., IL-11R, LIF-R) to form the holoreceptor. As a consequence of this shared coreceptor physiology, when two or more of the cytokine-specific receptors are present on a cell, the two corresponding ligands can compete for a limiting amount of gp130, and hence for cytokine-specific signaling. Moreover, the physiology allows therapeutically engineered cytokine-receptor complexes to stimulate signaling in all cells that express gp130.[19] Furthermore, the same principles that allow the rationale design of an Epo or GH antagonist can be used to engineer IL-6 antagonists for treatment of pathologic states dependent on interactions with receptors that require gp130 for receptor signaling.[20,21]

The IL-2 family of receptors is also quite complex, in most cases sharing one and even two subunits with receptors for other cytokines of the same class (see Fig. 13-1). IL-2Rβ is shared with the IL-15R, and IL-2Rγ (also termed $γ_C$ [for common]) is shared with the IL-4, IL-7, IL-9, IL-15, and IL-21 receptors.[22] Another feature of the IL-2R not yet discussed for the EpoR or IL-6R families is that of a devoted JAK. While JAK2 is employed by all the EpoR subfamily members along with some of the IL-6R subfamily members, and JAK1 and TYK2 are also shared amongst these latter receptors, the fourth and final JAK family member, JAK3, is engaged only by γ_C. In addition to providing a more fundamental understanding of the principles of signal transduction, careful investigation of the IL-2 family of receptors also has afforded detailed insights into a number of clinically important immunodeficiency states.[23] The complexity of this family of receptors was illustrated by the progressive investigation into the origins of severe combined immunodeficiency (SCID).[24] As is discussed in Chapter 82, SCID is a severe loss of natural killer (NK) and T lymphocytes and has been traced to deficiencies of either γ_C or JAK3, a phenotype recapitulated quite well (but not perfectly) by genetic elimination of the same molecules in mice. However, genetic elimination of IL-2 leads to a phenotype quite different than the disease in humans or engineered mice. Instead, of the multiple cytokines for which γ_C and JAK3 support signaling, only elimination of IL-7 or the IL-7R recapitulates the phenotype,[25,26] a finding now consistent with the finding that IL-7 affects common lymphoid progenitors, while other cytokines in the family affect more differentiated lymphoid cells.

THE TUMOR NECROSIS FACTOR RECEPTOR SUPERFAMILY

At present the tumor necrosis factor (TNF) superfamily of receptors and ligands comprises 29 receptors and 19 ligands,[27,28] and illustrates several novel points in signal transduction pathways: trimeric binding (see Fig. 13-1), receptor promiscuity, and decoy receptors. Although many TNF ligand family members (TNF-α, TNF-β, CD40L [CD154], receptor activator of nuclear factor κB ligand [RANKL; osteoprotegerin ligand (OPGL)], OX40L, etc.) can bind to several receptors, the ligands are, for the most part, subfamily specific. For example, TNF-α only binds to the six TNF-α receptors and tumor necrosis factor-related apoptosis-inducing ligand (TRAIL) binds to the five TRAIL receptors,[29] although it can also bind to the receptor termed *osteoprotegerin* (OPG).[30] Ligands in this family bind as trimers to homotrimeric receptors, leading to recruitment of secondary signaling molecules to the cytoplasmic domain of the receptors. In general, there are two classes of cytoplasmic domains in these receptors, based on whether they contain the death domain (DD), a region capable of binding signaling mediators that initiate apoptosis (see Chap. 11). As such, receptors that do not contain a DD or other signaling domain can function as "decoy receptors," diverting ligand from initiating programmed cell death in the target cell. For example, among the TNF-α receptors, TNFRI (DR2) contains a DD, and among the five TRAIL receptors, DR4 and DR5 contain DDs, whereas TNFR2 and DcR1, DcR2 and OPG act as decoy receptors for TNF and TRAIL, respectively. The biologic consequences of ligand binding to individual TNFR family members depend on the relative affinity of their cytoplasmic domains for multiple adaptor proteins; TRADD (tumor necrosis factor receptor death domain) and FADD (Fas-associated death domain) engagement trigger apoptosis pathways, whereas recruitment of one of the six TRAF (TNF receptor associated factor) family members leads to activation of transcription factors such as nuclear factor-κB (NF κB) and kinases such as JNK (c-Jun N-terminal kinase) that lead to cell survival, proliferation, and activation of inflammation.

THE RECEPTOR TYROSINE KINASES

The receptor tyrosine kinases (RTKs) comprise another class of receptors that contains members vital for hematopoiesis and mature blood cell function (see Fig. 13-1). The first isolated hematopoietic member of this family was the eukaryotic version of the *v-fms* oncogene, designated *c-fms*. Further study revealed that the protooncogene is the sole receptor for macrophage colony stimulating factor (M-CSF),[31] and although somewhat distinct in possessing a split kinase domain, was immediately grouped with other RTKs, such as the receptors for insulin, vascular endothelial cell growth factor and epidermal growth factor, among several others. More recently, two additional hematopoietic receptor family members have been identified, namely c-Kit and Flt-3. These receptors were each cloned based on their homology to the viral oncogene *v-kit* or *c-fms*, respectively.[32,33] Like all other members of the family, upon engagement of their cognate ligand the kinase domains of homodimeric RTKs become activated, leading to the phosphorylation of receptor cytoplasmic domain tyrosine residues and other tethered substrates. In an apparent example of convergent evolution, like members of the hematopoietic cytokine receptor (HCR) family, RTKs were also found to employ JAKs in their signaling pathways[34]; as a result many of the same secondary signaling pathways are activated by both classes of receptors. But perhaps serving as an even more striking example of convergent evolution, the tertiary structure of the index ligand for a hematopoietic RTK, M-CSF, bears substantial homology to essentially all the ligands of the hematopoietic cytokine receptor family, such as GM-CSF.[35]

TRANSFORMING GROWTH FACTOR β RECEPTORS

The TGF receptor family consists of seven type I and five type II receptors that heterodimerize to form receptors for multiple TGF-β family members, including the TGF-β/activin/nodal and bone morphogenic protein (BMP) subfamilies. The precise stoichiometry of binding involves a ligand dimer, stabilized by disulfide and/or hydrophobic bonds, and two type I and two type II subunits (see Fig. 13-1); the tertiary structure of the complex has been carefully investigated.[36] Both type I and type II receptors contain an N-terminal ligand binding, transmembrane, and cytoplasmic ser/thr kinase domains, and the type I receptors additionally contain a Gly/Ser (GS)-rich domain.[36] For TGF-β subfamily members, the type II subunit bears a high-affinity ligand binding site, which on TGF-β or activin engagement recruits type I receptors, bringing the two cytoplasmic domains into close juxtaposition, enabling the type II kinase to phosphorylate Ser residues on the type I receptor GS domain, and thereby activating the type I kinase. Cell surface bound coreceptors also exist and aid in generating the signaling complex for TGF-β, but not activin or BMP ligands. For BMP family members, the type I receptor bears the high-affinity ligand binding site, such that BMP initially binds to type I receptor, with the type II subunit subsequently recruited to form the signaling complex. Once the two receptor kinases are activated, they recruit and phosphorylate the SMAD adaptor proteins, allowing their nuclear translocation and transcriptional activation. However, SMAD-independent TGF-β signaling pathways also exist.[37]

G-PROTEIN COUPLED RECEPTORS

Several molecules that play essential roles in blood cell development or function signal by engaging G-protein coupled receptors (GPCRs), clearly the largest family of cell surface receptors in organisms as diverse as yeast and humans, estimated to comprise approximately 1000 distinct gene products, or approximately 3 percent of the human genome. Also termed *serpentine* or *heptahelical receptors* (for their seven transmembrane domains that form four extracellular and three intracellular loops; see Fig. 13-1), GPCRs are so named because of their use of three small "G" proteins (G_α, G_β, and G_γ) for signal transduction. In the unstimulated state, all three G proteins bind to the intracellular loops of the receptor. Individual ligands engage GPCR in one of many different ways. For example, small lipophilic molecules (e.g. epinephrine) bind to transmembrane (TM) domains of the receptor, disrupting the interactions between TM3 and TM6, leading to conformational changes that alter G protein binding.[38] Other GPCRs use additional extracellular domains (e.g., the "Venus flytrap" domain)[39] to bind and dimerize receptors. Still others, which are engaged by proteases, are activated by protease cleavage of the receptor amino terminus, leading to the "unmasking" of a hexapeptide at the new amino terminus, which then interacts with one of the receptor extracellular or transmembrane domains.[40] By each of these and other mechanisms a conformational change occurs in the GPCR, allowing monomeric G_α and dimeric $G_{\beta\gamma}$ to dissociate from the intracellular loops and each to engage secondary signaling pathways.[41] Examples of critical molecules that that employ GPCRs and display hematologic activity are thrombin, adrenergic hormones, and chemokines. The outcomes of such engagement include cellular growth and survival, functional activation, and migration.

INTEGRINS AND OTHER ADHESION MOLECULES

Although adhesion molecules play a vital structural role in tissue cohesion, physically bridging cells in the marrow with each other and with extracellular matrix macromolecules, and at sites at which mature blood cells interact with the endothelium, engagement of blood and progenitor cell integrins and other adhesion molecules also generates vital signals within the cell that affect its survival, proliferation, and functional activation.[42–44] In fibroblasts, cell adhesion is most clearly manifest at contact sites termed focal adhesions, and the signaling complexes that form on cytoplasmic domains of the integrins that support them are termed focal adhesion complexes.[45] Within such complexes are components of the actin cytoskeleton, kinases both specific for focal adhesions and several others found in other cytoplasmic sites,[46–48] and a number of scaffolding molecules upon which adhesion strengthening and signaling take place. Thus, adhesion molecules must also be considered as signaling receptors.

NUCLEAR RECEPTORS

Nuclear receptors (NRs) are nascent transcription factors that play a wide variety of roles in cellular physiology by binding small lipophilic hormones. Some NRs, such as steroid hormone receptors, remain sequestered in the cytoplasm in the absence of their cognate ligand, and upon ligand engagement translocate to the nucleus and bind and activate palindromic, direct repeat, or inverted palindromic sequences that comprise nucleotide hormone response elements.[49] Other NRs, such as receptors for vitamin A metabolites (retinoids), remain bound to nuclear DNA and repress transcription, until engaged by ligand upon which nuclear coactivators are recruited leading to enhancement of gene transcription.[50–52] Although sex steroids and thyroid hormones may play subtle roles in blood cell biology, retinoid receptors, which most commonly bind as heterodimers with the RXR receptor to retinoid response elements of the form PuGTTCA(N)2,5PuGTTCA, play vital developmental roles in a myriad of cell systems, and play similar roles in hematopoiesis. Amongst the hematopoietic targets of retinoid receptors are c-myc, C/EBPε, and p21.[53] However, because this class of receptors represents a nearly direct pathway from stimulus to response, without intervening signaling, they are not discussed further in this chapter.

THE DIVERSITY OF DOWNSTREAM SIGNALS

PROTEIN PHOSPHORYLATION

Protein phosphorylation is the critical first and vital response to engagement of signaling molecules of nearly all classes of cell surface receptors, including those that affect blood cell production and function. Numerous studies reveal that protein tyrosine phosphorylation is

detectible within a minute of the addition of a wide variety of hematopoietic cytokines to blood cells and their progenitors. Evidence from nearly all studies employing chemical inhibitors of kinase function or various knock-out and knock-in strategies shows that JAK activation is critical for hematopoietic cell survival, growth, and differentiation, and mature cell response to a wide range of stimuli (Fig. 13-2).[54] Among the phosphorylation targets of JAKs and other immediately responsive kinases are the signaling receptor itself, perhaps the rate-limiting step in signaling,[55] adaptor molecules (Shc, Grb2, IRS, Gab) that once modified recruit additional signaling substrates, regulatory subunits of secondary kinases (p85 phosphoinositol 3 kinase [PI3K]), latent transcription factors (signal transducers and activators of transcription [STATs]), and several phosphatases (SHP2, SHIP). By phosphorylating Tyr residues present in certain receptor motifs, the modified protein acquires the capacity to bind Src homology (SH)-2 domain-containing proteins. Several similar substrates exist for receptor tyrosine kinases, including JAKs and STAT proteins, and several distinct targets for Ser/Thr phosphorylation exist for activated TGF-β receptors.

MEMBRANE LIPID MODIFICATION

Upon recruitment to a doubly phosphorylated receptor cytoplasmic domain or adapter protein the regulatory subunit of PI3K undergoes conformational changes enabling the binding of its 110-kDa kinase subunit, resulting in activation of the kinase (see Fig. 13-2).[56] The major target of PI3K is membrane inositols, perhaps most importantly $PI_{4,5}$ phosphate (PIP2), converting the latter into $PI_{3,4,5}P$ (PIP3). Once present in adequate amounts, PIP3 recruits proteins with pleckstrin homology domains to the inner cytoplasmic membrane, which become phosphorylated by their juxtaposition to another PH domain containing kinase, PDK.[57] Among the best known of the recruited proteins are protein kinase B (also termed Akt), a kinase that phosphorylates a broad range of substrates in a wide variety of cells, all with the ultimate effect of enhancing cell survival and/or cell cycling.[58] For example, Akt phosphorylates Bad, a proapoptotic protein that once so modified is targeted for degradation.[59] Akt indirectly activates NF-κB,[59] a transcription factor that influences several cell cycle and survival proteins,[60] including the antiapoptotic Bcl and IAP (inhibitors of apoptosis) proteins and the cell cycle activators c-Myc and cyclin D. In addition, forkhead family members, which when present enhance transcription of cell cycle inhibitors such as p27 and the proapoptotic protein Fas ligand, are phosphorylated and inactivated by Akt.[61] Of interest, Akt is activated by the bcr-abl oncogene in blood cells of patients with chronic myelogenous leukemia (CML), and blockade of PI3K reduces their proliferation substantially.[62]

NUCLEAR TRANSLOCATION

In addition to the posttranslational modification of signaling molecules illustrated in the preceding examples, relocalization of signaling molecules is also a vital process that conveys information within the cell. This cellular strategy is well illustrated by the activation of NF-κB,[60] a family of transcription factors that affect genes vital for cell survival and growth. In the unstimulated cell, NF-κB subunits reside in the cytoplasm, sequestered from their nuclear targets by virtue of its binding to I-κB. Upon cellular activation of Akt, I-κB kinase is activated by phosphorylation, which then phosphorylates I-κB, thereby releasing NF-κB and targeting I-κB for proteosomal destruction, allowing NK-κB to translocate to the nucleus and bind and activate target genes. A second example of cytoplasmic sequestration blocking nuclear function involves the SMAD proteins that mediate TGF-β receptor signaling.[36] Once recruited to the phosphorylated type I TGF-β receptor, SMAD2 is phosphorylated, reducing its affinity for SARA, a molecule that helps tether SMAD2 to the receptor. Once free of SARA, a SMAD2/SMAD4 complex forms, which is competent to translocate to the nucleus, either by the generation of a nuclear localization signal or because of the elimination of the SARA blockade of the SMAD2 nuclear pore complex interaction site. In addition to ingress, the formation of a SMAD2/SMAD4 complex also blocks a nuclear export signal present on the latter.[63]

ENGAGEMENT OF ADAPTOR PROTEINS

Another general theme to emerge from numerous studies on signal transduction is that multimolecular complexes of signaling intermediaries often assemble on scaffolding or adaptor proteins, which develop the capacity to assemble signaling complexes upon phosphorylation.[64] Insulin receptor substrates (IRSs) were the first such adaptors identified, and are phosphorylated by the activated insulin receptor.[65] More recently, IRS proteins were found to be modified by several other receptor-activated kinases, including JAKs.[54] Grb-binding (Gab) proteins are a family of at least three adapters, so named because of their ability to bind to the adaptor Grb2, a signaling intermediate necessary for Ras activation.[66] Both IRS and Gab proteins present

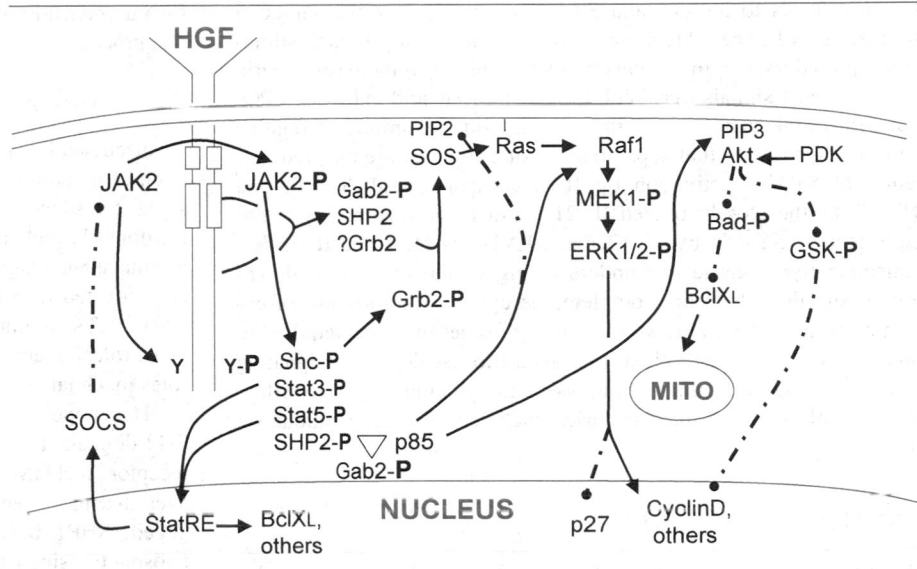

FIGURE 13-2   An illustration of signal transduction pathways. Signal transduction ensues when a hematopoietic growth factor (HGF) binds to its cognate receptor, resulting in a change in receptor conformation bringing two tethered JAK molecules into close proximity (attachment site to receptor is indicated by two *blue boxes*, representing the box1 and box2 motifs). Molecules that become phosphorylated upon activation are indicated by **P**. A multiprotein complex that forms on a scaffolding molecule, such as Gab2, is indicated by the *triangle*. Stimulatory pathways (vis-à-vis cell proliferation) are indicated by *solid lines with arrow heads*. Inhibitory pathways are indicated by *broken lines with ball heads*. The nucleus and the mitochondria (MITO) are indicated.

multiple sites for phosphorylation, and once so modified present numerous SH2-binding and other protein–protein interacting motifs (see Fig. 13-2), which allow assembly of signaling complexes. Additional molecules serve this function in other signaling receptors, such as paxillin binding on the cytoplasmic tails of α-integrin.[48] Paxillin presents four different types of protein–protein interaction domains (SH3, SH2, LD [Leu-Asp], and LIM [lin-11/Isl-1/Mec-3]) enabling it to bind downstream kinases (focal adhesion kinase [FAK], the related Pyk2 kinase, Src kinase, and paxillin-associated kinase [PAK]), other adaptor molecules (Crk, PIX, PKL), and phosphatases (PTP PEST). As many cellular kinases can phosphorylate adaptor proteins (e.g., in addition to integrin engagement, GH binding leads to paxillin phosphorylation), such complexes can function as a nexus to coordinate multiple cellular stimuli into a concerted response.

Another example of the capacity of adaptor proteins to translate extracellular signals into intracellular physiologic change is found in the response to TNF ligands. The capacity of receptors that bear DDs to induce apoptosis is dependent on the binding of the adaptor protein FADD to the cytoplasmic domain of TNFR, which then recruits and activates the initiating caspases 8 and 10, leading to activation of the executioner caspases 3, 6, and 7 (see Chap. 11).[28,29,67] This extracellular signal-mediated apoptotic pathway stands in contrast to a second, cell-intrinsic apoptosis pathway, in which DNA damage, cell cycle checkpoint defects, or loss of survival factors leads to enhanced expression of proapoptotic bcl family members (bax, bad, bclXs, bid). Once proapoptotic proteins overcome the level of antiapoptotic family members (bc12, BclXL), mitochondrial transmembrane potential declines, leading to leakage of cytochrome c and SMAC, the former engaging the apoptotic protease-activating factor (APAF) adaptor, thereby activating caspase 9 and, subsequently, the executioner family of caspases, the latter inhibiting members of the IAP family that otherwise attenuate caspase action. It should also be noted that although these two apoptosis pathways can be discussed as distinct entities, merging at the level of caspase 3, they interact. For example, activation

of caspase 8 by TNF family members can also cleave Bid to cause mitochondrial leakage of cytochrome c, thereby engaging the cell intrinsic pathway, serving to amplify the extracellular signal pathway to programmed cell death.

Binding of TNF family members to their receptors does not always result in apoptosis. Although there are likely many mechanisms for this finding, one is mediated by the binding of adaptors. Different TNF family receptors employ one of six TRAFs to engage and activate I-κB kinase (IKK), which leads to the release of NF-κB, a transcription factor that induces expression of several prosurvival and proliferation-associated genes.[60]

SIGNALING SPECIFICITY WITHIN EACH RECEPTOR FAMILY

Once a large number of receptor/cytokine systems were identified and tools to study their downstream signaling events developed, it became clear that most cytokine receptors stimulate a very similar cadre of signaling events as other members of the same family. For example, Epo, TPO, GH, GM-CSF, IL-6, and leptin all stimulate the phosphorylation of JAK2, yet lead to quite different cellular effects. One theory of hematopoiesis posits that growth factors merely serve to prevent apoptosis; the stochastic induction of one or another set of transcription factors is responsible for the distinct lineage differentiation events of hematopoiesis.[68] If this is true, then overlapping signaling events supported by a diverse range of cytokines might not be surprising as they would subserve the same end point, inhibition of programmed cell death. However, it is also clear that some cytokines and extracellular stimuli induce changes in critical transcription factors, and that the fate of multipotent progenitor cells can be influenced by the cytokines to which they are exposed; if so, each cytokine would need to induce distinct signals. Careful studies of signaling events have supported this hypothesis. For example, JAK3 is engaged only by cytokine receptors that use γ_C,[69] and although Epo activates the same JAK as TPO (JAK2), the former leads to activation of STAT5,[70] whereas the latter leads to STAT5 and STAT3 activation,[71] which targets a different set of genes. Moreover, engagement of integrin $\alpha_5\beta_1$ stimulates Epo-induced erythroid development, while stimulation of integrin $\alpha_4\beta_1$ mediates signals that inhibit erythropoiesis and enhances TPO-induced megakaryocyte growth.[72,73] Additional examples of relative signaling specificity that separates sets of cytokines are the predominance of STAT5 activation by IL-2, compared with STAT1 and STAT3 by the closely related IL-21,[74] and the almost exclusive engagement of STAT4 by IL-12 and STAT6 by IL-4 and IL-13.[75,76] Consequently, because our understanding of the entirety of downstream signals is far from complete, the cytoplasmic domains of cytokine receptors bear almost no homology other than that required to engage JAKs, and there already exists a modest degree of signaling specificity, it is likely that although several cytokines engage overlapping sets of signaling intermediaries, each will result in a unique set of signaling events.

SIGNALING INSULATION

Many of the kinases and other intermediaries that play important roles in signal transduction are not absolutely substrate specific; nevertheless, they do participate in specific pathways free from interference from other pathways. Perhaps the best example of this is found in the mitogen-activated protein kinase (MAPK) pathway.[77] At least three major MAPK pathways operate in most cells, the p42/p44 ERK (extracellular response kinase), p38, and JNK, each of which is triggered by distinct stimuli (mitogens such as cytokines for ERK, inflammatory mediators and hypoxia for p38, and stress and noxious stimuli for JNK), but all of which eventuate in the activation of a cascade of kinases, a MAPK kinase kinase (also termed MEKK), which phosphorylates and activates a MAPK kinase (also termed a MEK), and finally the MAPK. The MAPKKK for ERK1/2 is Raf-1 and the MAPKK for ERK1/2 is MEK1, the MAPKKK for p38 is MEKK1 and the MAPKK is MKK3, and for JNK they are MEKK1 and MKK4 or MKK7, respectively. Because each of these kinases display only limited substrate specificity *in vitro*, it would be difficult to explain how MEKK1 activation does not lead to ERK activation without some mechanism to insulate the signals. Recently, several scaffolding proteins have been identified that assemble specific MAPKKK, MAPKK, and MAPKs.[78] By forming complexes of the cascade on pathway-specific scaffolding molecules, signaling integrity is preserved. Moreover, once the MAPK is activated, additional scaffolding molecules can link the specific MAPK to its target transcription factors.[79] Additional examples of "insulating" signaling scaffolds include those for NF-κB and the TNF receptor,[80] the B cell antigen receptor (termed BLNK),[81] and protein kinase C and integrins (termed RACKs).[82]

EXTINGUISHING SIGNALS

In addition to initiating signaling by extracellular ligands, the cell must also be able to extinguish the stimulus to prepare for additional events and to guard against continuous cell growth. Several mechanisms have been identified that extinguish the signals initiated by extracellular stimuli.

RECEPTOR DOWN-MODULATION

Shortly after binding to ligand, hematopoietic cytokine receptors and receptor tyrosine kinases are rapidly internalized,[83] serving to down-modulate further signaling.[84] Receptor internalization is dependent on membrane clathrin,[84] which represents a major mechanism of endocytosis of cell surface proteins, and on at least one element of ligand-induced signaling.[85] The sites on hematopoietic receptors responsible for internalization are mapped,[86] potentially allowing intervention in this process.

PHOSPHATASES

As discussed in "The Diversity of Downstream Signals," phosphorylation of numerous proteins and membrane lipids plays a vital role in signal transduction within the cell. Thus, elimination of these modifications through the action of phosphatases would be expected to terminate such signals. Moreover, because some of the same signals are activated in malignant transformation, protein tyrosine phosphatases (PTPs) might also be expected to play an important antioncogenic role. Several cellular phosphatases have been identified that play roles in signal termination and as tumor suppressors.

Hematopoietic cell phosphatase (also termed SHP1) bears two SH2 domains that interact with cytokine and inhibitory immune coreceptors at ITIM (immunoreceptor tyrosine-based inhibitory motif) sites that have been modified by Tyr phosphorylation. Once so engaged, SHP1 becomes activated and dephosphorylates associated phosphotyrosine activation sites on receptors, adaptor molecules, and their associated kinases.[87] One of the earliest clues that SHP1 plays an important role in hematopoietic signaling came from the discovery that the moth-eaten mouse phenotype is a result of a genetic loss of function of SHP1.[88] These mice demonstrate a massive expansion and tissue accumulation of monocytes and myeloid cells, resulting in chronic inflammation, massive immune defects and premature death. Careful analysis of the mice revealed they manifest defective controls over the cellular activation and proliferation response to exogenous stimuli, such as that induced by engagement of the B cell antigen receptor (BCR) complex. At steady state SHP1 is thought to engage the BCR (through presently unclear mechanisms) and maintains the antigen binding subunits (Igα and Igβ) in a dephosphorylated, quiescent state. The phosphatase is displaced from the complex upon antigen engagement, but is later re-recruited to the complex once ITIM containing inhibitory coreceptors such as CD22, PIR-B, CD72, and FcγRIIb are phosphorylated and recruited to the activated complex.[89] Once recruited to the BCR complex, SHP1 removes the activating Tyr phosphate sites on the ITAM (immunoreceptor tyrosine-based activation motif) sites of Igα/β, the coreceptor CD19, the adaptor BLNK and Lyn kinase, and the BCR returns to its quiescent state. Similar roles for SHP1 have been identified in T cells,[90] NK cells,[91] monocytes and macrophages,[92] and erythroid cells.[93] The latter is of particular interest, as mutation of the site on EpoR to which SHP1 binds causes familial erythrocytosis, due to reduction of Epo signaling. Of interest, this mutation was identified in a family containing a two-time Olympic gold medalist.[94]

SOCS PROTEINS

Another mechanism of growth factor signal termination is mediated by the suppressors of cytokine signaling (SOCS) proteins. The cloning of a STAT-inducible gene, CIS,[95] and several additional genes that bear substantial sequence homology,[96,97] has yielded a family of proteins that can directly suppress growth factor receptor-induced signals. The engagement of either hematopoietic cytokine receptors or receptor tyrosine kinases leads to STAT activation, as in "The Diversity of Downsteam Signals." One of the transcriptional targets of STATs are the SOCS and PIAS (protein inhibitor of activated STATs) genes (see Fig. 13-2), which upon transcription and translation bind to phosphotyrosine residues and inhibit either JAK kinases, STATs, or the phosphorylated receptors themselves, blocking recruitment of signaling adaptor molecules.[98] More recently, ubiquitin and SUMO (small ubiquitin-like modifier) also have been shown to play a vital role in SOCS- and PIAS-mediated repression of cytokine signaling.[98,99]

INHIBITORY SIGNALS

Finally, some signals impact adversely on signals derived from alternate receptors. One example is the interaction of growth factors and TGF-β-derived signals. One of the major hematopoietic effects of TGF-β on hematopoietic stem cells is to reduce cell cycling. In contrast, many growth factors, such as SCF, Flt3 ligand, and TPO enhance stem cell cycling and induce their proliferation. As TGF-β is constitutively expressed in the marrow stroma, one mechanism by which growth factors can overcome cell cycle suppression is mediated by growth factor-induced ERK1/2 activation. The cell cycling effects of TGF-β are mediated by nuclear SMAD2–SMAD4, and nuclear localization of the complex is determined, at least in part, by the blockade of a nuclear export signal on the complex. As growth factor-induced MAPK leads to the phosphorylation of several sites on the linker region of SMAD2, the balance of nuclear and cytoplasmic SMAD is tipped toward the latter, leading to reduced suppressive effects of TGF-β on the cell cycle.[100] Another form of this type of cross-talk between cytokines is illustrated by TPO and interferon alpha (IFN-α), the latter suppressing megakaryopoiesis driven by the former. By induction of SOCS-1, not usually induced by TPO, IFN-α inhibits TPO mediated signaling.[101]

SIGNAL COORDINATION AND CROSS-TALK

In the foregoing discussion several examples of the convergence of signaling pathways and receptor cross-talk were summarized. Over the past decade, two types of cell membrane-based supramolecular organizations have been identified, lipid rafts and tetraspanin webs. In their seminal fluid–mosaic model of the cell membrane, Singer and Nicolson posited that integral membrane proteins float in a random array of membrane lipids.[102] This model was modified to account for local heterogeneity of the lipid bilayer. Lipid rafts, local concentrations of specific membrane lipids and proteins, are defined by the methods to isolate them—the insoluble components of a cold detergent extraction in which raft components "float" to the top of a density gradient.[103] Upon discovery that many of the proteins present in such rafts were involved in signal transduction, it became apparent that these membrane subdomains could represent a structural basis for communication between seemingly disparate components of the signal transduction apparatus. This hypothesis was best validated in hematopoietic cells.[37,104,105]

A second level of membrane-based structural organization of signaling molecules has been elucidated—the tetraspanin-enriched microdomain or "web." The tetraspanin family of membrane proteins is characterized by four transmembrane domains punctuating two extracellular regions, a CCG motif, and several other conserved cysteine residues in the extracellular domain. The tetraspanins now include more than 30 members,[106] most or all of which interact with other cell surface molecules, and have been functionally linked to cell adhesion, migration, differentiation, and signal transduction. Members of this family are thought to act as molecular facilitators of protein–protein interaction by associating with "partners," the bimolecular complexes then interact with others in a slightly less avid manner, and the complexes loosely associate in microdomains. CD9, CD63, and CD81 are the tetraspanins most closely linked to hematopoietic cell function, are usually found in association with β_1 and β_3 integrins,[107] affect many hematopoietic cell types,[108–110] and act in concert with multiple signaling receptors, kinases, and phosphatases.[111,112]

REFERENCES

1. D'Andrea AD, Lodish HF, Wong GG: Expression cloning of the murine erythropoietin receptor. *Cell* 57:277, 1989.

2. Watowich SS, Hilton DJ, Lodish HF: Activation and inhibition of erythropoietin receptor function: Role of receptor dimerization. *Mol Cell Biol* 14:3535, 1994.

3. Livnah O, Stura EA, Middleton SA, et al: Crystallographic evidence for preformed dimers of erythropoietin receptor before ligand activation. *Science* 283:987, 1999.

4. Broudy VC, Lin N, Egrie J, et al: Identification of the receptor for erythropoietin on human and murine erythroleukemia cells and modulation by phorbol ester and dimethyl sulfoxide. *Proc Natl Acad Sci U S A* 85:6513, 1988.

5. Kanakura Y, Druker B, Cannistra SA, et al: Signal transduction of the human granulocyte-macrophage colony-stimulating factor and interleukin-3 receptors involves tyrosine phosphorylation of a common set of cytoplasmic proteins. *Blood* 76:706, 1990.

6. Spivak JL, Fisher J, Isaacs MA, et al: Protein kinases and phosphatases are involved in erythropoietin-mediated signal transduction. *Exp Hematol* 20:500, 1992.

7. Otani H, Erdos M, Leonard WJ: Tyrosine kinase(s) regulate apoptosis and bcl-2 expression in a growth factor-dependent cell line. *J Biol Chem* 268:22733, 1993.

8. Witthuhn BA, Quelle FW, Silvennoinen O, et al: JAK2 associates with the erythropoietin receptor and is tyrosine phosphorylated and activated following stimulation with erythropoietin. *Cell* 74:227, 1993.

9. Syed RS, Reid SW, Li C, et al: Efficiency of signalling through cytokine receptors depends critically on receptor orientation. *Nature* 395:511, 1998.

10. Cheetham JC, Smith DM, Aoki KH, et al: NMR structure of human erythropoietin and a comparison with its receptor bound conformation. *Nat Struct Biol* 5:861, 1998.

11. Wrighton NC, Farrell FX, Chang R, et al: Small peptides as potent mimetics of the protein hormone erythropoietin. *Science* 273:458, 1996.

12. Li JP, D'Andrea AD, Lodish HF, et al: Activation of cell growth by binding of Friend spleen focus-forming virus gp55 glycoprotein to the erythropoietin receptor. *Nature* 343:762, 1990.

13. Livnah O, Johnson DL, Stura EA, et al: An antagonist peptide-EPO receptor complex suggests that receptor dimerization is not sufficient for activation. *Nat Struct Biol* 5:993, 1998.

14. Taga T, Kishimoto T: Gp130 and the interleukin-6 family of cytokines. *Annu Rev Immunol* 15:797, 1997.

15. Hirano T: Interleukin 6 and its receptor: Ten years later. *Int Rev Immunol* 16:249, 1998.

16. Jones SA, Rose-John S: The role of soluble receptors in cytokine biology: The agonistic properties of the sIL-6R/IL-6 complex. *Biochim Biophys Acta* 1592:251, 2002.

17. Stahl N, Boulton TG, Farruggella T, et al: Association and activation of Jak-Tyk kinases by CNTF-LIF-OSM-IL-6 beta receptor components. *Science* 263:92, 1994.

18. Pflanz S, Kurth I, Grotzinger J, et al: Two different epitopes of the signal transducer gp130 sequentially cooperate on IL-6-induced receptor activation. *J Immunol* 165:7042, 2000.

19. Baiocchi M, Marcucci I, Rose-John S, et al: An IL-6/IL-6 soluble receptor (IL-6R) hybrid protein (H-IL-6) induces EPO-independent erythroid differentiation in human CD34(+) cells. *Cytokine* 12:1395, 2000.

20. Savino R, Ciapponi L, Lahm A, et al: Rational design of a receptor super-antagonist of human interleukin-6. *EMBO J* 13:5863, 1994.

21. Tassone P, Galea E, Forciniti S, et al: The IL-6 receptor super-antagonist Sant7 enhances antiproliferative and apoptotic effects induced by dexamethasone and zoledronic acid on multiple myeloma cells. *Int J Oncol* 21:867, 2002.

22. Waldmann TA: T-cell receptors for cytokines: Targets for immunotherapy of leukemia/lymphoma. *Ann Oncol* 11(Suppl 1):101, 2000.

23. Leonard WJ: The molecular basis of X-linked severe combined immunodeficiency: Defective cytokine receptor signaling. *Annu Rev Med* 47:229, 1996.

24. Uribe L, Weinberg KI: X-linked SCID and other defects of cytokine pathways. *Semin Hematol* 35:299, 1998.

25. von Freeden-Jeffry U, Vieira P, Lucian LA, et al: Lymphopenia in interleukin (IL)-7 gene-deleted mice identifies IL-7 as a nonredundant cytokine. *J Exp Med* 181:1519, 1995.

26. Appasamy PM: Biological and clinical implications of interleukin-7 and lymphopoiesis. *Cytokines Cell Mol Ther* 5:25, 1999.

27. Ashkenazi A: Targeting death and decoy receptors of the tumour-necrosis factor superfamily. *Nat Rev Cancer* 2:420, 2002.

28. Aggarwal BB: Signalling pathways of the TNF superfamily: A double-edged sword. *Nat Rev Immunol* 3:745, 2003.

29. Wang S, El-Deiry WS: TRAIL and apoptosis induction by TNF-family death receptors. *Oncogene* 22:8628, 2003.

30. Emery JG, McDonnell P, Burke MB, et al: Osteoprotegerin is a receptor for the cytotoxic ligand TRAIL. *J Biol Chem* 273:14363, 1998.

31. Sherr CJ: The role of the CSF-1 receptor gene (C-fms) in cell transformation. *Leukemia* 2:132S, 1988.

32. Lyman SD, Jacobsen SE: c-Kit ligand and Flt3 ligand: Stem/progenitor cell factors with overlapping yet distinct activities. *Blood* 91:1101, 1998.

33. Broudy VC: Stem cell factor and hematopoiesis. *Blood* 90:1345, 1997.

34. Linnekin D: Early signaling pathways activated by c-Kit in hematopoietic cells. *Int J Biochem Cell Biol* 31:1053, 1999.

35. Pandit J, Bohm A, Jancarik J, et al: Three-dimensional structure of dimeric human recombinant macrophage colony-stimulating factor. *Science* 258:1358, 1992.

36. Shi Y, Massague J: Mechanisms of TGF-beta signaling from cell membrane to the nucleus. *Cell* 113:685, 2003.

37. Derynck R, Zhang YE: Smad-dependent and Smad-independent pathways in TGF-beta family signalling. *Nature* 425:577, 2003.

38. Chen S, Lin F, Xu M, et al: Phe(303) in TMVI of the alpha(1B)-adrenergic receptor is a key residue coupling TM helical movements to G-protein activation. *Biochemistry* 41:588, 2002.

39. Bessis AS, Rondard P, Gaven F, et al: Closure of the Venus flytrap module of mGlu8 receptor and the activation process: Insights from mutations converting antagonists into agonists. *Proc Natl Acad Sci U S A* 99:11097, 2002.

40. Coughlin SR: Thrombin signalling and protease-activated receptors. *Nature* 407:258, 2000.

41. Slupsky JR, Quitterer U, Weber CK, et al: Binding of Gbetagamma subunits to cRaf1 downregulates G-protein-coupled receptor signalling. *Curr Biol* 9:971, 1999.

42. Levesque JP, Simmons PJ: Cytoskeleton and integrin-mediated adhesion signaling in human CD34+ hemopoietic progenitor cells. *Exp Hematol* 27:579, 1999.

43. Martin KH, Slack JK, Boerner SA, et al: Integrin connections map: To infinity and beyond. *Science* 296:1652, 2002.

44. Rose DM, Han J, Ginsberg MH: Alpha4 integrins and the immune response. *Immunol Rev* 186:118, 2002.

45. Parsons JT, Martin KH, Slack JK, et al: Focal adhesion kinase: A regulator of focal adhesion dynamics and cell movement. *Oncogene* 19:5606, 2000.

46. Sastry SK, Burridge K: Focal adhesions: A nexus for intracellular signaling and cytoskeletal dynamics. *Exp Cell Res* 261:25, 2000.

47. Schwartz MA, Ginsberg MH: Networks and crosstalk: Integrin signalling spreads. *Nat Cell Biol* 4:E65, 2002.

48. Schaller MD: Paxillin: A focal adhesion-associated adaptor protein. *Oncogene* 20:6459, 2001.

49. Aranda A, Pascual A: Nuclear hormone receptors and gene expression. *Physiol Rev* 81:1269, 2001.

50. Mehta K: Retinoids as regulators of gene transcription. *J Biol Regul Homeost Agents* 17:1, 2003.

51. Ahuja HS, Szanto A, Nagy L, et al: The retinoid X receptor and its ligands: Versatile regulators of metabolic function, cell differentiation and cell death. *J Biol Regul Homeost Agents* 17:29, 2003.

52. Carlberg C: Current understanding of the function of the nuclear vitamin D receptor in response to its natural and synthetic ligands. *Recent Results Cancer Res* 164:29, 2003.

53. Collins SJ: The role of retinoids and retinoic acid receptors in normal hematopoiesis. *Leukemia* 16:1896, 2002.

54. Ihle JN, Kerr IM: Jaks and Stats in signaling by the cytokine receptor superfamily. *Trends Genet* 11:69, 1995.

55. Rane SG, Reddy EP: Janus kinases: Components of multiple signaling pathways. *Oncogene* 19:5662, 2000.

56. Rameh LE, Cantley LC: The role of phosphoinositide 3-kinase lipid products in cell function. *J Biol Chem* 274:8347, 1999.

57. Vanhaesebroeck B, Alessi DR: The PI3K-PDK1 connection: More than just a road to PKB. *Biochem J* 346 Pt 3:561, 2000.

58. Chang F, Lee JT, Navolanic PM, et al: Involvement of PI3K/Akt pathway in cell cycle progression, apoptosis, and neoplastic transformation: A target for cancer chemotherapy. *Leukemia* 17:590, 2003.

59. Datta SR, Brunet A, Greenberg ME: Cellular survival: A play in three Akts. *Genes Dev* 13:2905, 1999.

60. Karin M, Lin A: NF-kappaB at the crossroads of life and death. *Nat Immunol* 3:221, 2002.

61. Birkenkamp KU, Coffer PJ: FOXO transcription factors as regulators of immune homeostasis: Molecules to die for? *J Immunol* 171:1623, 2003.

62. Kawauchi K, Ogasawara T, Yasuyama M, et al: Involvement of Akt kinase in the action of STI571 on chronic myelogenous leukemia cells. *Blood Cells Mol Dis* 31:11, 2003.

63. Inman GJ, Nicolas FJ, Hill CS: Nucleocytoplasmic shuttling of Smads 2, 3, and 4 permits sensing of TGF-beta receptor activity. *Mol Cell* 10:283, 2002.

64. Pawson T, Scott JD: Signaling through scaffold, anchoring, and adaptor proteins. *Science* 278:2075, 1997.

65. White MF: The IRS-1 signaling system. *Curr Opin Genet Dev* 4:47, 1994.

66. Gu H, Neel BG: The "Gab" in signal transduction. *Trends Cell Biol* 13:122, 2003.

67. Micheau O, Tschopp J: Induction of TNF receptor I-mediated apoptosis via two sequential signaling complexes. *Cell* 114:181, 2003.

68. Cantor AB, Orkin SH: Hematopoietic development: A balancing act. *Curr Opin Genet Dev* 11:513, 2001.

69. Liu KD, Gaffen SL, Goldsmith MA, et al: Janus kinases in interleukin-2-mediated signaling: JAK1 and JAK3 are differentially regulated by tyrosine phosphorylation. *Curr Biol* 7:817, 1997.

70. Wakao H, Harada N, Kitamura T, et al: Interleukin 2 and erythropoietin activate STAT5/MGF via distinct pathways. *EMBO J* 14:2527, 1995.

71. Drachman JG, Sabath DF, Fox NE, et al: Thrombopoietin signal transduction in purified murine megakaryocytes. *Blood* 89:483, 1997.

72. Kapur R, Cooper R, Zhang L, et al: Cross-talk between alpha(4)beta(1)/alpha(5)beta(1) and c-Kit results in opposing effect on growth and survival of hematopoietic cells via the activation of focal adhesion kinase, mitogen-activated protein kinase, and Akt signaling pathways. *Blood* 97:1975, 2001.

73. Fox N, Kaushansky K: Engagement of integrin alpha 4 beta 1 but not alpha 5 beta 1 enhances thrombopoietin (TPO)-induced megakaryocyte (MK) growth. *Blood* 98:292a, 2001.

74. Habib T, Nelson A, Kaushansky K: IL-21: A novel IL-2-family lymphokine that modulates B, T, and natural killer cell responses. *J Allergy Clin Immunol* 112:1033, 2003.

75. Bacon CM, Petricoin EF 3rd, Ortaldo JR, et al: Interleukin 12 induces tyrosine phosphorylation and activation of STAT4 in human lymphocytes. *Proc Natl Acad Sci U S A* 92:7307, 1995.

76. Quelle FW, Shimoda K, Thierfelder W, et al: Cloning of murine Stat6 and human Stat6, Stat proteins that are tyrosine phosphorylated in responses to IL-4 and IL-3 but are not required for mitogenesis. *Mol Cell Biol* 15:3336, 1995.

77. Cobb MH, Goldsmith EJ: How MAP kinases are regulated. *J Biol Chem* 270:14843, 1995.

78. Whitmarsh AJ, Davis RJ: Structural organization of MAP-kinase signaling modules by scaffold proteins in yeast and mammals. *Trends Biochem Sci* 23:481, 1998.

79. Lee CM, Onesime D, Reddy CD, et al: JLP: A scaffolding protein that tethers JNK/p38MAPK signaling modules and transcription factors. *Proc Natl Acad Sci U S A* 99:14189, 2002.

80. Soond SM, Terry JL, Colbert JD, et al: TRUSS, a novel tumor necrosis factor receptor 1 scaffolding protein that mediates activation of the transcription factor NF-kappaB. *Mol Cell Biol* 23:8334, 2003.

81. Chiu CW, Dalton M, Ishiai M, et al: BLNK: Molecular scaffolding through "cis"-mediated organization of signaling proteins. *EMBO J* 21:6461, 2002.

82. Besson A, Wilson TL, Yong VW: The anchoring protein RACK1 links protein kinase Cepsilon to integrin beta chains. Requirements for adhesion and motility. *J Biol Chem* 277:22073, 2002.

83. Yee NS, Langen H, Besmer P: Mechanism of kit ligand, phorbol ester, and calcium-induced down-regulation of c-kit receptors in mast cells. *J Biol Chem* 268:14189, 1993.

84. Vieira AV, Lamaze C, Schmid SL: Control of EGF receptor signaling by clathrin-mediated endocytosis. *Science* 274:2086, 1996.

85. Broudy VC, Lin NL, Liles WC, et al: Signaling via Src family kinases is required for normal internalization of the receptor c-Kit. *Blood* 94:1979, 1999.

86. Dahlen DD, Broudy VC, Drachman JG: Internalization of the thrombopoietin receptor is regulated by 2 cytoplasmic motifs. *Blood* 102:102, 2003.

87. Zhang J, Somani AK, Siminovitch KA: Roles of the SHP-1 tyrosine phosphatase in the negative regulation of cell signalling. *Semin Immunol* 12:361, 2000.

88. Tsui HW, Siminovitch KA, De Souza L, et al: Motheaten and viable motheaten mice have mutations in the haematopoietic cell phosphatase gene. *Nat Genet* 4:124, 1993.

89. Otipoby KL, Draves KE, Clark EA: CD22 regulates B cell receptor-mediated signals via two domains that independently recruit Grb2 and SHP-1. *J Biol Chem* 276:44315, 2001.

90. Pani G, Fischer KD, Mlinaric-Rascan I, et al: Signaling capacity of the T cell antigen receptor is negatively regulated by the PTP1C tyrosine phosphatase. *J Exp Med* 184:839, 1996.

91. Binstadt BA, Brumbaugh KM, Dick CJ, et al: Sequential involvement of Lck and SHP-1 with MHC-recognizing receptors on NK cells inhibits FcR-initiated tyrosine kinase activation. *Immunity* 5:629, 1996.

92. Kim CH, Qu CK, Hangoc G, et al: Abnormal chemokine-induced responses of immature and mature hematopoietic cells from motheaten mice implicate the protein tyrosine phosphatase SHP-1 in chemokine responses. *J Exp Med* 190:681, 1999.

93. Sharlow ER, Pacifici R, Crouse J, et al: Hematopoietic cell phosphatase negatively regulates erythropoietin-induced hemoglobinization in erythroleukemic SKT6 cells. *Blood* 90:2175, 1997.

94. Longmore GD: Erythropoietin receptor mutations and Olympic glory. *Nat Genet* 4:108, 1993.

95. Yoshimura A, Ohkubo T, Kiguchi T, et al: A novel cytokine-inducible gene CIS encodes an SH2-containing protein that binds to tyrosine-phosphorylated interleukin 3 and erythropoietin receptors. *EMBO* 14:2816, 1995.

96. Naka T, Narazaki M, Hirata M, et al: Structure and function of a new STAT-induced STAT inhibitor. *Nature* 387:924, 1997.

97. Starr R, Willson TA, Viney EM, et al: A family of cytokine-inducible inhibitors of signalling. *Nature* 387:917, 1997.

98. Wormald S, Hilton DJ: Inhibitors of cytokine signal transduction. *J Biol Chem* 279:821, 2004.

99. Schmidt D, Muller S: PIAS/SUMO: New partners in transcriptional regulation. *Cell Mol Life Sci* 60:2561, 2003.

100. Grimm OH, Gurdon JB: Nuclear exclusion of Smad2 is a mechanism leading to loss of competence. *Nat Cell Biol* 4:519, 2002.

101. Wang Q, Miyakawa Y, Fox N, et al: Interferon-alpha directly represses megakaryopoiesis by inhibiting thrombopoietin-induced signaling through induction of SOCS-1. *Blood* 96:2093, 2000.

102. Singer SJ, Nicolson GL: The fluid mosaic model of the structure of cell membranes. *Science* 175:720, 1972.

103. Brown DA, Rose JK: Sorting of GPI-anchored proteins to glycolipid-enriched membrane subdomains during transport to the apical cell surface. *Cell* 68:533, 1992.

104. Viola A, Schroeder S, Sakakibara Y, et al: T lymphocyte costimulation mediated by reorganization of membrane microdomains. *Science* 283:680, 1999.

105. Bodin S, Viala C, Ragab A, et al: A critical role of lipid rafts in the organization of a key FcgammaRIIa-mediated signaling pathway in human platelets. *Thromb Haemost* 89:318, 2003.

106. Hemler ME: Tetraspanin proteins mediate cellular penetration, invasion, and fusion events and define a novel type of membrane microdomain. *Annu Rev Cell Dev Biol* 19:397, 2003.

107. Cook GA, Longhurst CM, Grgurevich S, et al: Identification of CD9 extracellular domains important in regulation of CHO cell adhesion to fibronectin and fibronectin pericellular matrix assembly. *Blood* 100:4502, 2002.

108. Miyazaki T, Muller U, Campbell KS: Normal development but differentially altered proliferative responses of lymphocytes in mice lacking CD81. *EMBO J* 16:4217, 1997.

109. Clay D, Rubinstein E, Mishal Z, et al: CD9 and megakaryocyte differentiation. *Blood* 97:1982, 2001.

110. Anzai N, Lee Y, Youn BS, et al: C-kit associated with the transmembrane 4 superfamily proteins constitutes a functionally distinct subunit in human hematopoietic progenitors. *Blood* 99:4413, 2002.

111. Skubitz KM, Campbell KD, Iida J, et al: CD63 associates with tyrosine kinase activity and CD11/CD18, and transmits an activation signal in neutrophils. *J Immunol* 157:3617, 1996.

112. Kurita-Taniguchi M, Hazeki K, Murabayashi N, et al: Molecular assembly of CD46 with CD9, alpha3-beta1 integrin and protein tyrosine phosphatase SHP-1 in human macrophages through differentiation by GM-CSF. *Mol Immunol* 38:689, 2002.

CHAPTER 14

THE CLUSTER OF DIFFERENTIATION (CD) ANTIGENS

THOMAS J. KIPPS

The cluster of differentiation (CD) antigens are cellular molecules that are each recognized by monoclonal antibodies (MAbs) that allow for the identification each molecule's biochemical properties and cellular distribution. The CD number for each molecule is defined at international workshops that exchange such Mabs and compare their ability to react with human cells and/or human cell molecules. This chapter provides an overview of the nearly 250 CD antigens defined as of the seventh international workshop, listing the other names for these CD antigens along with their biochemistry, membrane-orientation, genetics, and cellular distribution on hematopoietic cells.

Acronyms and abbreviations that appear in this chapter include: act., activated; ADAM, a disintegrin and metalloprotease; Ag, antigen; ALK, anaplastic lymphoma kinase; ALL, acute lymphocytic leukemia; APC, antigen-presenting cell; APO-1, apoptosis antigen ligand 1; CA, carcinoma; CALLA, common acute leukemia antigen; CEA, carcinoembryonic antigen; CD, cluster of differentiation; CTLA-4, cytotoxic T lymphocyte-associated protein-4; DAF, decay accelerating factor; DC, dendritic cells; DNAM, DNAX accessory molecule; ELAM, endothelial leukocyte adhesion molecule; eos, eosinophils; EBV, Epstein-Barr virus; FDC, follicular dendritic cells; G-CSF, granulocyte colony stimulating factor; GM-CSF, granulocyte-macrophage colony stimulating factor; GP, glycoprotein; GPI, glycosylphosphatidylinositol; HA, hyaluronan; HCL, hairy cell leukemia; HEV, high endothelial venules; HIV, human immunodeficiency virus; HLA, human leukocyte antigen; HML, human mucosal lymphocyte; IAP, integrin associated protein; ICAM, intercellular adhesion molecule; IFN, interferon; IGF, insulin-like growth factor; IgSF, immunoglobulin super family; IL, interleukin; ITAM, immune tyrosine-based activating motifs; ITGAE, integrin alpha E; ITIM, immune tyrosine-based inhibitory motifs; KIR, killer cell inhibitory receptor; LAMP, lysosomal membrane-associated glycoprotein; LECAM, leukocyte endothelial cell adhesion molecule; LFA, leukocyte function antigen; LGL, large granular lymphocyte; LPS, lipopolysaccharide; MAb, monoclonal antibody; MCP, monocyte chemoattractant protein; MDR, multidrug resistance; MHC, major histocompatibility complex; MIP-1, macrophage inflammatory protein; MMP, matrix metalloproteinase; MRP, mobility-related protein; MUC-1, mucin-1; MØ, macrophages; NCAM, neural cell adhesion molecule; NK, natural killer; O, orientation/anchorage of the antigen in the plasma membrane; PDGF, platelet-derived growth factor; PECAM, platelet endothelial cell adhesion molecule; PHN, paroxysmal nocturnal hemoglobinuria; PI-PLC, phosphatidylinositol phospholipase C; plts, platelets; PMN, polymorphonuclear leukocytes; RANTES, regulated on activation normal T expressed and secreted protein; RBC, red blood cells; Rc, receptor; RGD, amino acid sequence, arginine-glycine-aspartic acid; SCR, steel factor receptor; Sema, semaphorin; sIg, surface immunoglobulin; Siglec, sialic acid-binding immunoglobulin-like lectin; SLC, secondary lymphoid tissue chemokine; TACTILE, T cell activation increased late expression; TALLA-1, T cell–acute lymphoblastic leukemia antigen-1; TAPA, target of antiproliferative antibody; Tet, tetraspan; TGF, transforming growth factor; TLX, trophoblast leukocyte-common antigen; TNF, tumor necrosis factor; TNFR, tumor necrosis factor receptor; uPA, urokinase plasminogen activator; VCAM, vascular cell adhesion molecule; VLA, very late antigen; vWF, von Willebrand factor; WBC, white blood cells.

DEFINITION AND HISTORY

The advent of monoclonal antibody (MAb) technology revolutionized the classification of cell surface antigens. The availability of virtually unlimited quantities of monospecific typing reagents permitted the identification and study of previously unrecognized lymphoid and myeloid-specific surface proteins. However, as the number of MAbs detecting cell surface differentiation antigens grew, the need for an international standardization became apparent.

Accordingly, seven international workshops have been held to exchange MAbs to compare their ability to react with human cells and/or human cell proteins.[1-3] MAbs having similar patterns of reactivity with various tissues or cell types are assigned to a cluster group. An antigen that is recognized by a cluster of antibodies can be assigned a "cluster of differentiation" (CD) number. If only one MAb defines a cluster or if all MAbs defining a cluster originate from the same laboratory, a suffix "w" is added to the CD designation. The last conference, held in Harrogate, United Kingdom, in June 2000, compiled the data obtained from testing hundreds of different MAbs.[3] The conference culminated in the classification of scores of new CD antigens.

Table 14-1 presents all CD antigens defined at this and previous workshops and any common names used before a CD number was assigned (column marked "Other Names"). Table 14-1 summarizes what is known about each CD antigen's molecular size(s) ("Size"), orientation or attachment to the plasma membrane ("O"), tissue distribution ("Distribution"), and known or suspected physiology ("Physiology"). Table 14-1 also indicates the chromosomal location of the gene(s) encoding each CD antigen and the GenBank accession number of the reference cDNA encoding the antigen ("Genetics"). "Selected References" cites a few key papers and review articles for each CD antigen.

Additional information regarding the CD antigens can be found on the Internet. The accession numbers provided in the "Genetics" column can be used to obtain the primary nucleic acid and protein sequences of each CD antigen using the GenBank web site on the Internet (available at *http://www.ncbi.nlm.nih.gov*) or by e-mail at *retrieve@ncbi.nlm.nih.gov*. Other useful web sites for analyzing protein or genomic structure are SWISSPROT protein structure database (available at *http://us.expasy.org*), or the central repository for genomic mapping data from the Human Genome Initiative (available at *http://gdbwww.gdb.org/*). A complete listing of the MAbs used to define the CD antigens is available at *http://www.mh-hannover.de/aktuelles/projekete/hlda7/hldabase/cdindex.htm*. A comprehensive list of other useful servers provided by SWISSPROT is available at *http://us.expasy.org/links.html*.

GENERAL STRUCTURE OF MEMBRANE ANTIGENS

Membrane antigens are classified into different groups, depending on how they orient or anchor themselves to the plasma membrane (Fig. 14-1).[4]

TYPE I TRANSMEMBRANE PROTEINS (I)

Type I transmembrane molecules have their COOH-termini in the cytoplasm and their NH$_2$-termini outside the cell. Each of these molecules generally has a signal sequence at the NH$_2$-terminus that is cleaved off after the molecule passes into the endoplasmic reticulum. Afterward, it may be glycosylated in the Golgi apparatus (if it contains glycosylation sites) and then expressed on the cell surface. These proteins commonly serve as cell surface receptors and/or ligands. Many belong to the immunoglobulin superfamily (see Chaps. 77 and 78).

Each type I protein generally has a transmembrane domain of approximately 25 hydrophobic amino acid residues followed by a cluster of basic amino acids that bind the protein to phospholipid head groups

TABLE 14-1 CLUSTER OF DIFFERENTIATION ANTIGENS DEFINED AS OF THE SEVENTH INTERNATIONAL WORKSHOP ON LEUKOCYTE TYPING

ANTIGEN	OTHER NAMES	SIZE	O	GENETICS	DISTRIBUTION	PHYSIOLOGY	SELECTED REFERENCES
CD1a–e	T6	43–49	I	1q22-23 X04450 . . . 1a M28826 . . . 1b M28827 . . . 1c J04142 . . . 1d X14975 . . . 1e	Cortical thymocytes, DC, Langerhans cells (CD1a), brain astrocytes, dermal cells, some B cells (CD1c, d)	Six different isoforms exist, with functional domains of each encoded by separate exons. Each is involved in presentation of "nonclassic"antigens, including lipids and glycolipids.	Curr Opin Immunol 11:100, 1999 Curr Opin Microbiol 2:89, 1999 Immunol Today 19:362, 1998 J Clin Invest 113:701, 2004
CD2	Sheep red blood cell Rc, leukocyte function antigen-2 (LFA-2), Leu-5, T11, Tp50	45–58	I	1p13 M16445	Thymocytes, T cells, NK cells	Serves as a ligand for CD48 and CD58 (LFA-3), which enhances adhesion between T cells and antigen-presenting cells (APC) and plays a role in signal transduction.	Immunol Rev 163:217, 1998 J Biol Chem 278:22396, 2003 Blood 102:1745, 2003
CD3	CD3γ	25–28	I	11q23 X04145	Pan T cell	Defines a family of proteins that, together with CD247, forms the signal transduction complex for T cell Rc for antigen (see Chap. 78).	Adv Immunol 72:103, 1999 Semin Hematol 35:310, 1998 Scand J Immunol 56:436, 2002 N Engl J Med 349:1821, 2003
	CD3δ	20	I	11q23 X03934			
	CD3ε	20	I	11q23 X03884			
CD4	T4, Leu-3, L3T4	55	I	12pter-p12 M12807	Thymocytes, helper/inducer T cells, monocytes, MØ, DC	Serves as a Rc for class II MHC, which facilitates recognition of peptide antigens. It also is a co-Rc for HIV gp120.	Transplant Proc 31:820, 1999 Int J Biochem Cell Bio 29:871, 1997 Curr Top Microbiol Immunol 205, 1996
CD5	Tp67, Leu-1, T1	67	I	11q13 M15177	T cells and some B cells	Scaveger Rc previously thought to serve as ligand for CD72, which modulates signals transduced by the Rc for antigen.	Cur Opin Hematol 6:30, 1999 Immunol Today 19:106, 1998 Science 269:535, 1995
CD6	T12, Tp120	105, 130	I	11q13 U66142	T cells, some B cells, medullary thymocytes, some cortical thymocytes, brain	Scavenger Rc that serves as ligand for CD166, which plays role in T cell development.	Transplant Proc 31:795, 1999 J Exp Med 181:2213, 1995 Immunol Today 18:498, 1997
CD7	gp40, Tp41	40	I	17q25.2-q25.3 X06180	Some hemopoietic stem cells (denotes commitment to B or NK cells), some T cells, monocytes, NK cells	Associates with PI3 kinase via YXXM motif upon cross-linking, implying that it may be involved in cell activation and serves as a cognate Rc of K12 protein.	J Biol Chem 275:3431, 2000 Blood 101:576, 2003 Eur J Immunol 33:46, 2003 Immunol Res 24:46, 2001
CD8α	T8, Leu-2 α-chain	68 (32–34)	I	2p12 M27161	Cytotoxic/suppressor T cells, some NK cells, most thymocytes	Forms a heterodimer with CD8β to form Rc for class I MHC to facilitate recognition of peptide antigens presented in the context of MHC class I antigens.	Sem Immunol 9:87, 1997 J Immunol 157:4287, 1996
CD8β	β-chain of CD8 heterodimer	68 (32–34)	I	2p12 X13444	Same as CD8α	Forms a heterodimer with CD8α to act as Rc for class I MHC (see above).	Immnol Res 19:201, 1999
CD9	p24, DRAP-27, MRP-1	24	III Tet	12p13 M38690	Plts, pre-B, act. T cells, eos, basophils, endothelial and epithelial cells, brain	Plays role in signal transduction leading to cell activation, adhesion, and/or aggregation. Associates with other tetraspan proteins (CD63, CD81, CD82).	Leuk Lymphoma 38:147, 2000 Mol Biol Cell 7:193, 1996 Semin Thromb Hemast 21:10, 1995
CD10	CALLA, neutral endopeptidase, enkephalinase, metalloendopeptidase	95–100	II	3q21-27 Y00811	Pre-B and pre-T cells, germinal center B cells, some PMN, epithelial cells	Zinc-binding metalloprotease that cleaves peptides on the amino side of hydrophobic amino acids, thereby reducing the local concentration of peptide hormones.	J Exp Med 181:2271, 1995 Blood 82:1052, 1993 Allergy 53:1023, 1998
CD11a	αL-chain of β2-integrins, leukocyte function antigen-1 (LFA-1)	180	I	16p13.1-11 Y00796	Lymphocytes, PMN, monocytes, MØ	Associates with CD18 to form Rc for CD50, CD54, or CD102, thereby facilitating homotypic or heterotypic adhesion and cell activation.	Curr Opin Cell Biol 9:643, 1997 Immunol Rev 146:82, 1995 Eur J Biochem 270:1710, 2003
CD11b	Complement Rc 3 (CR3), C3biR, Mac-1, Mo-1, αM-chain of β2-integrins	165–170	I	16p13.1-11 J03925	Monocytes, MØ, PMN, DC, some B and T cells, NK cells	Assembles with CD18 to form a Rc for C3bi, clotting factor X, fibrinogen, CD54, or CD102, thereby facilitating homotypic or heterotypic adhesion, cell activation, phagocytosis, and/or chemotaxis.	Structure 3:1333, 1995 Cell 80:631, 1995 Immunol Today 14:145, 1996 J Immunol 171:2003
CD11c	gp150/95, αX-chain of β2-integrins, Leu M5, CR4, Axb2	145–150	I	16p13.1-11 M81695	Monocytes, MØ, PMN, NK cells, some B and T cells	Assembles with CD18 to form an adhesion Rc for fibrinogen and Rc for C3bi. Binding of ligand to heterodimer induces cellular activation and helps trigger neutrophil respiratory burst.	Immunol Today 17:209, 1996 Immunity 5:653, 1996 J Immunol 156:3780, 1996
CD11d	Integrin αD-subunit	150	I	16p13.1-11 U37028	Red pulp MØ (strong), blood WBC (moderate)	Forms a heterodimer with CD18 to make a Rc that binds CD50 (ICAM-3), but not CD54 or CD106.	Immunity 3:683, 1995 J Immunol 173:297, 2004
CDw12		150–160 (120)			Monocytes, PMN, NK cells (weak)	Phosphoprotein of unknown function.	Leucocyte Typing VI, Garland Scientific Publishing, NY, p 961, 1998
CD13	Aminopeptidase N (EC 3.4.11.2), gp150	150–170	II	15q25-26 X13276	Myeloid cells, enthothelial and epithelial cells, osteoclasts, marrow stroma	A zinc-binding metalloprotease that catalyses removal of NH2-terminal amino acids from peptides, thereby reducing local concentration of peptide hormones.	J Exp Med 184:183, 1996 J Exp Med 194:1183, 1996 Adv Exp Med Biol 477:25, 2000
CD14	gp55, GPI-liked glycoprotein, LPS Rc	53–55	V GPI	5q31 X06882	Monocytes, DC Nurse-like cells	Rc for lipopolysaccharide (LPS) that can transduce signal(s), leading to oxidative burst and/or synthesis of tumor necrosis factor alpha.	Infect Dis Clin North Am 13:341, 1999 Curr Opin Immunol 11:19, 1999 Biochem Soc Trans 26:644, 1998 Blood 99:1030, 2002

TABLE 14-1   CLUSTER OF DIFFERENTIATION ANTIGENS DEFINED AS OF THE SEVENTH INTERNATIONAL WORKSHOP ON LEUKOCYTE TYPING (*CONTINUED*)

ANTIGEN	OTHER NAMES	SIZE	O	GENETICS	DISTRIBUTION	PHYSIOLOGY	SELECTED REFERENCES
CD15	Lewis x (LeX), 3-fucosyl-N-acetyl-lactosamine (3-FAL)	185–260			PMN, eos, monocytes	Carbohydrate determinant found on several glycoproteins (e.g. CD11/CD18, CD66) and is dependent on the activity of alpha (1,3)-fucosyltransferase (FucT-IV).	Histo Histopathol 11:1007, 1996 J Biol Chem 274.24838, 1999 Leucocyte Typing VII, Oxford University Press, Oxford, p 178, 2002
CD15s	sialyl Lewis x (sLeX)	185–260			PMN, basophils, monocytes, myeloid cells, some T cells (weak), myelomonocytic leukemias, some adenoCA	Sialyated form of CD15 is a ligand for CD62E (ELAM-1) and is dependent upon fucosyl transferase VII (FucT-VII).	Am J Pathol 143:1220, 1993 J Leukoc Biol 53:541, 1993 Leucocyte Typing VII, Oxford University Press, Oxford, p 178, 2002
CD15su	6-Sulfo-sialyl Lewis x	185–260			Similar to CD15s	Structurally the same as CD15 except that it possesses a sulfate group on GlcNAc.	Leucocyte Typing VII, Oxford University Press, Oxford, p 178, 2002
CD15u	3′-Sulfo Lewis x	185–260			Similar to CD15s	Structurally the same as CD15 except that it possesses a sulfate group on the terminal galactose.	Leucocyte Typing VII, Oxford University Press, Oxford, p 178, 2002
CD16a	Transmembrane form of FcγRIIIA (low-affinity FcRc)	50–65	I	1q23 X52645	NK cells, MØ, mast cells	Low-affinity Rc for aggregated IgG that also may be involved in lysis of cells independent of IgG. CD16 (A) associates with the FcϵRIγ, CD3ζ, or FcϵRI β-chain (mast cells) for signal transduction.	J Immunol 162:735, 1999 Proc Natl Acad Sci U S A 96:5640, 1999 J Clin Invest 100:1059, 1997
CD16b	GPI anchored form of FcγRIII (low-affinity FcRc), FcγRIIIB	48–60	V GPI	1q23 X16863	PMN	GPI isoform of CD16 that is deficient in patients with PNH. Cross-linking CD16B may transduce a different signal than that of CD16A.	J Leukoc Biol 65:875, 1999 Transfusion 39:593, 1999 J Biol Chem 271:3659, 1996
CDw17	Lactosylceramide (LacCer)	150–160 (120)			PMN, basophils, plts, monocytes, some B cells	Glycosphingolipid that may play role in granule content packaging, exocytosis, and signaling. Binds some bacteria and may function in phagocytosis.	J Biol Chem 273:34349, 1998 Circ Res 82:540, 1998
CD18	Beta-chain of the β_2 integrins	90–95	I	21q22.3 M15395	Same as CD11a–d combined	Assembles into a heterodimer with one of several α-chains (CD11a–d) and appears responsible for signal transduction via the heterodimer.	Int J Biochem Cell Biol 30:179, 1998 Curr Opin Cell Biol 9:643, 1997 Eur J Biochem 245:215, 1997
CD19	B4	120 (95)	I	16p11.2 M28170	All B cells and B cell precursors, some FDC	Forms a noncovalent complex with CD21, CD81, Leu 13, which modulates signal transduction by the B cell receptor for antigen.	Curr Opin Immunol 8:378, 1996 Sem Immunol 10:267, 1998 Curr Opin Immunol 9:324, 1997
CD20	B1, Bp35	33, 35, 37	III Tet.	11q13 X12530	B cells but not plasma cells	May act as a Ca^{2+} channel involved in regulating cell cycle progression, which can be targeted by MAb for therapy of B cell lymphomas.	Biochem Soc Trans 25:705, 1997 Curr Opin Hematol 5:237, 1998
CD21	CR2, EBV-Rc, C3d-Rc	145	I	1q32 M26004	B cells, FDC, pharyngeal and cervical epithelial cells, some T cells, astrocytes	Rc for C3d and Epstein-Barr virus. Binding of C3d to CD21 enhances B cell antigen receptor signal transduction. In concert with CD23, it may regulate production of IgE.	Adv Exp Med Biol 452:181, 1998 Semin Immunol 10:279, 1998 Immunol Lett 54:201, 1996 Immunol Today 14:56, 1993
CD22	Bgp135, B lymphocyte cell adhesion molecule (BL-CAM), Leu-14, Lyb-8	110–130	I	19p13.1 X52785-a X59350-b	Mature B cells but not plasma cells	Binds sialoglycoconjugates (NeuAcα2->6Galβ1->4GlcNAc) on some CD45 isoforms and glycoproteins to modulate B cell signal transduction. Two isoforms (α/β) are formed by alternative splicing.	Adv Exp Med Biol 452:181, 1998 Curr Opin Immunol 8:378, 1996 Annu Rev Immunol 15:481, 1997 Immunity 6:509, 1997
CD23	FcϵRII, BLAST-2, (alternatively spliced forms are called FcϵRIIa and FcϵRIIb), Leu 20, B6	45–50	II	19p13.3 M15059	sIgM$^+$/sIgD$^+$ B cells, monocytes, some T cells, FDC, eos, NK cells, plts	Ca^{2+}-dependent (C-type) lectin with low affinity for IgE, CD21, CD11a, and CD11b, which plays a role in regulation of IgE synthesis and in cell–cell adhesion. Secreted form of CD23 may act as growth factor.	Int Rev Immunol 16:113, 1997 Biochem Soc Trans 25:393, 1997 Curr Opin Immunol 7:355, 1995 Immunol Today 19:313, 1998
CD24	Heat-stable antigen (HSA), BA-1	35–45	V GPI	6q21 M58664 L33930	B cells, pre-B cells, PMN, epithelium, ≤2% of thymocytes	May play a role in regulation of B cell proliferation and/or differentiation and serve as a ligand for CD62P.	Blood 89:3385, 1997 J Immunol 170:252, 2003
CD25	IL-2 Rc, TAC-antigen, α-chain of IL-2 Rc	55	I	10p14-15 X01057	Act. T and act. B cells, some thymocytes, early myeloid cells	Low-affinity Rc for IL-2 that can associate with CD122 and CD132 to form a heterotrimeric Rc with high affinity for IL-2.	Adv Immunol 59:225, 1995 Cell 75:5, 1995 J Biol Chem 278:10239, 2003
CD26	Dipeptylpeptidase IV (EC 3.4.14.5), adenosine deaminase-binding protein	110, 120	II	2q24.3 X60708	Intestinal epithelial cells, renal proximal tubule, bile duct, prostate, memory or act. T cells, medullary thymocytes, some B cells, NK cells	Serine-type exopeptidase that cleaves dipeptides from the amino-termini of proteins with a penultimate proline residue. With an intracellular domain that associates with adenosine deaminase, it also can function as a T cell costimulatory molecule.	Immunol Rev 161:43, 1998 Curr Med Chem 6:311, 1999 Int J Oncol 22:481, 2003 Blood 103:1002, 2004
CD27	S152, T14	110 (55)	I	12p13 M63928	Some T cells, memory-type B cells, NK cells, medullary thymocytes	Ligand for CD70 and member of the nerve growth factor receptor superfamily, plays a role in generation of memory T and B cells.	Semin Immunol 10:491, 1998 Immunol Lett 89:251, 2003 Nat Immunol 1:433, 2000

(Continued)

TABLE 14-1　CLUSTER OF DIFFERENTIATION ANTIGENS DEFINED AS OF THE SEVENTH INTERNATIONAL WORKSHOP ON LEUKOCYTE TYPING (*Continued*)

Antigen	Other Names	Size	O	Genetics	Distribution	Physiology	Selected References
CD28	Tp44 antigen	90 (44)	I	2q33 *J02988*	95% of CD4 T cells, 50% of CD8 T cells, most plasma cells	Interacts with CD80 and CD86. Cross-linking CD28 serves as costimulatory signal and enhances transcription and stability of IL-2 mRNA.	*Immunol Rev 165:287, 1998* *Crit Rev Immunol 18:389, 1998* *Adv Immunol 62:131, 1996*
CD29	VLA β-chain, platelet GPIIa, integrin β_1-subunit	110–130	I	10p11.2 *X07979*	Plts and all leukocytes with higher levels on memory T cells	Assembles into a heterodimer with one of several α-chains (CD49a->f or $\alpha1$->$\alpha6$) to form Rc involved in cell–cell or cell–matrix adhesion. Highly conserved cytoplasmic domain can interact with cytoskeleton.	*Int J Biochem Cell Biol 30:179, 1998* *Artifi Organs 20:828, 1996* *Annu Rev Cell Dev Biol 11:549, 1995* *J Cell Biol 132:211, 1996*
CD30	Ki-1 antigen, Ber-H2	120 (105)	I	1p36 *M83554*	Act. T, B, and NK cells, monocytes, Reed-Sternberg cells, embryonal CA	Member of the nerve growth factor receptor superfamily that may play a role in cell activation and/or differentiation.	*Sem Immunol 10:457, 1998* *APMIS 106:169, 1998*
CD31	Platelet endothelial cell adhesion molecule-1 (PECAM-1), endocam	130–140	I	17q23-ter *M28526* *M37780*	Monocytes, myeloid cells, plts, cell–cell junctions of endothelium, some T cells	Interacts with itself and with integrin $\alpha V/\beta3$ and glycosaminoglycans. Ligation of CD31 activates leukocyte integrins and may play a role in diapedesis.	*J Clin Invest 99:3, 1997* *N Engl J Med 334:286, 1996* *J Exp Med 184:229, 1996*
CD32	FcγRII, gp40, isoforms (A, B1->3, and C) arise through alternative splicing.	40	I	1 q23 *M31932 . . . A* *M31935 . . . B1* *M31934 . . . B2* *M31933 . . . B3* *X17652 . . . C*	Monocytes, MØ, plts; B cells express only the B isoforms, whereas PMN express isoforms A and C.	Rc for aggregated IgG that can trigger IgG-mediated phagocytosis and oxidative burst. Transduces an inhibitory signal on B cells and its expression on placental epithelia suggests a role in transport of IgG.	*Biomembranes 3:269, 1996* *Adv Immunol 57:1, 1994* *J Immunol 171:3296, 2003*
CD33	gp67	150 (67)	I	19q13.3 *M23197*	Cells of myelomonocytic lineage but not stem cells	Binds to sialoglycoconjugates NeuAc$\alpha2$->3Gal$\beta1$->3(4)GlcNAc and NeuAc$\alpha2$->3Gal$\beta1$->3GalNAc and may mediate cell–cell adhesion.	*Blood 85:2005, 1995* *Biochem Soc Trans 24:150, 1996*
CD34	My10, Spg90	105–120	I	1q32 *M81104*	1–4% of marrow cells including hematopoietic stem cell, endothelium	May play a role in signal transduction or leukocyte-endothelial interactions through its ability to interact with CD62L, CD62P, and CD62E.	*Blood 87:3550, 1996* *Blood 87:479, 1996* *Acta Haematol 97:22, 1997*
CD35	CR1, C3b/C4b Rc	160–285	I	1q32 *Y00816* *X05309*	Monocytes, PMN, DC, RBC, B cells, some T cells, some astrocytes, glomerular podocytes	Facilitates phagocytosis and/or binding to immune complexes or cells coated with C3b or C4b. CD35 is one of the few CD antigens with allotypic polymorphism resulting in varied molecular sizes.	*J Immunol 157:1242, 1996* *J Hematother 4:357, 1995* *Proc Natl Acad Sci U S A 93:3357, 1996*
CD36	Platelet GPIV, GPIIIb, OKM5, PASIV	78–90	I	7q11.2 *M24795*	Plts, monocytes, MØ, adipocytes, some epithelial, endothelial cells, some DC	Signal-transducing scavenger Rc for thrombospondin, collagen, oxidized low-density lipoprotein, fatty acids, anionic phospholipids, *Plasmodium falciparum* infected RBC.	*J Biol Chem 7635271:22315, 1996* *Platelets 7:117, 1996* *J Biol chem 278:2003*
CD37	gp52-40	40–52	III Tet.	19p13-q13.4 *X14046*	Mature B cells, some T cells/ monocytes (weak)	Associates with MHC class II, CD19, CD21, CD53, CD81, and CD82 in B cell membrane and may play a regulatory role in T cell proliferation.	*J Immunol 172:2953, 2003* *Mol Immunol 33:867, 1996*
CD38	T10, ADP-ribosyl cyclase	39–45	II	4p15 *M34461*	Plasma cells, early or act. B and T cells, thymocytes, monocytes, NK cells, brain, myeloid progenitors	Can synthesize cyclic ADP-ribose (ADPR) from nicotinamide adenine dinucleotide and hydrolyze cADPR to ADP-ribose. May play a role in cell activation, proliferation, or survival.	*Immunol Today 16:469, 1995* *FASEB J 10:1408, 1996* *J Immunol 15:741, 1997*
CD39	Vascular ATP diphospho-hydrolase, ATPDase apyrase	78		10q24 *S73813*	Endothelial cells, MØ, DC, act. cells of the NK, B, or T cell lineage (not on resting cells or germinal center B cells)	Ecto-apyrase that may inhibit platelet adhesion and aggregation by digesting ADP and protect activated cells through hydrolysis of extracellular ATP.	*Platelet 14:47, 2003* *Mol Med 6:591, 2000* *Biochem Biophys Res Commun 218: 916, 1996*
CD40	Bp50	85 (48)	I	20q12-13.2 *X60592*	Mature B cells, monocytes, MØ, DC, some epithelial cells, CD34 stem cells, nurse-like cells	Member of the nerve growth factor receptor superfamily that induces cell activation and/or differentiation upon binding its ligand, CD154.	*Adv Immunol 61:1, 1996* *Int J Mol Med 3:343, 1999* *Immunol Today 19:502, 1998* *Blood 99:1030, 2002*
CD41	GPIIb of the GPIIb/ GPIIIa complex, αIIβ integrin	135 (120, 23)	I	17q21.32 *J02764*	Plts and megakaryocytes	Associates with CD61 to form Rc for fibrinogen, fibronectin, vitronectin, vWF, and thrombospondin to facilitate platelet adhesion and aggregation.	*N Engl J Med 332:1553, 1995* *J Biol Chem 271:6017, 1996* *J Biol Chem 271:18610, 1996*
CD42a	GPIX	17–22	I	17pter-p12 *X52997*	Plts and megakaryocytes	GPIbα, GPIbβ, GPIX, and GPV form a complex with 2:2:2:1 stoichiometry, making the GP1b complex that binds to subendothelial vWF, allowing for platelet adhesion to damaged blood vessels.	*Blood 87:1377, 1996* *J Biol Chem 277:47080, 2002* *J Biol Chem 278:21744, 2003*
CD42b	CD42bα, GPIbα, glycocalicin	160 (145)	I	17pter-p12 *J02940*	Plts and megakaryocytes	Mucin that serves as binding site of the GP1b complex for vWF by forming disulfide-linked heterodimer with CD42c, which noncovalently associates with CD42a and CD42d.	*J Biol Chem 269:23716, 1996* *J Biol Chem 278:45375, 2003* *Science 301:222, 2003* *Science 301:218, 2003*

TABLE 14-1 CLUSTER OF DIFFERENTIATION ANTIGENS DEFINED AS OF THE SEVENTH INTERNATIONAL WORKSHOP ON LEUKOCYTE TYPING (*Continued*)

Antigen	Other Names	Size	O	Genetics	Distribution	Physiology	Selected References
CD42c	CD42bβ, GPIbβ, GPIBB	160 (24)	I	17pter-p12 JO3259	Plts and megakaryocytes	Forms disulfide-linked heterodimer with CD42b that associates with CD42a and CD42d to form a Rc for vWF.	*Blood 89:2404, 1997* *Thromb Haemost 88:1026, 2002*
CD42d	Glycoprotein V (GPV)	82	I	3q29 Z23091	Plts and megakaryocytes	Associates with CD42a, CD42b, and CD42c to form Rc for vWF and thrombin.	*Biochemistry 35:906, 1996* *Thromb Haemost 86:1065, 2001*
CD43	Leukosialin, sialophorin, leukocyte sialoglycoprotein	95–135	I	16p11.2 J04168	Thymocytes, T cells, PMN, MØ, monocytes, NK cells, plts, brain, act. B cells (weak), plasma cells, hemopoietic stem cells	Sialoglycoprotein that may interact with CD54 or albumin and function as an antiadhesion molecule, inhibiting T cell interactions, including T cell killing. May play a costimulatory role on T cells. Soluble form is present in human serum.	*Immunol Today 19:546, 1998* *Tumour Biol 23:193, 2002* *J Immunol 171:1901, 2003* *Oncogene 23:2523, 2004*
CD44	Phagocytic glycoprotein-1 (Pgp-1), Hermes antigen, extracellular matrix Rc type III (ECMRIII), Hutch-1	85	I	11pter-p13 M59040	Most cell types except plts, hepatocytes, cardiac muscle, renal tubular epithelium, testis	Rc for hyaluronate that facilitates lymphocyte binding to high endothelial venules (HEV). Variants of CD44 have attached chrondroitin sulfate and are able to bind fibronectin, laminin, and collagen. Rc for chemotactic cytokine osteopontin.	*Exp Hematol 27:978, 1999* *Immuology 93:139, 1998* *Int J Biochem Cell Biol 30:299, 1998* *Mol Pathol 51:191, 1998* *Science 271:509, 1996*
CD44R	CD44R1, restricted (exon 9 of CD44), CD44v	85–200	I	11pter-p13 X56794	Epithelial cells, RBC, monocytes, act. leukocytes	Serves as the protein backbone of RBC Lutheran antigen and, like CD44, may be involved in leukocyte attachment and rolling on endothelium for homing to lymphoid tissue and sites of inflammation.	*Blood 103:2981, 2004* *J Cell Biol 279:25745, 2004* *J Immunol 156:1557, 1996*
CD45	T200, leukocyte common antigen (LCA)	180–240	I	1q31-32 Y00638	All hematopoietic cells except RBC	Tyrosine phosphatase that modulates signal transduction by surface antigen Rc. Changes in the extracellular domain do not affect the intracellular phosphatase activity of the cytoplasmic domain.	*Immunol Res 16:101, 1997* *Adv Immunol 66:1, 1997* *Immunol Cell Biol 75:430, 1997*
CD45RA	B220	220	I	1q31-32 Y00638	B cells, subset of naive CD4 T cells, monocytes	Formed by joining the 8 amino acid NH2-terminal sequence to that encoded by exons A, B, and C. This is the largest of the CD45 isoforms.	*Immunology 2:246, 1999* *Eur J Immunol 29:2098, 1999* *Int Immunol 10:1837, 1998*
CD45RB	T200	205, 220	I	1q31-32 Y00638	Memory T cell subset, monocytes, PMN (weak)	Formed by joining the 8 amino acid NH2-terminal sequence to that encoded by exon B and C.	*Eur J Immunol 28:3435, 1998* *Cell Immunol 167:56, 1996* *Annu Rev Immunol 21:107, 2003*
CD45RC		190, 205, 220	I	1q31-32 Y00638	Some T cells	Formed by joining the 8 amino acid NH2-terminal sequence to that encoded by exon C.	*Immunol Rev 146:82, 1995*
CD45RO	Restricted T200	180	I	1q31-32 Y00638	Thymocytes act., some memory T-cells	Formed by joining the 8 amino acid NH2-terminal sequence to the CD45 backbone without A, B, or C. Is the smallest of the CD45 isoforms.	*Leuk Lymphoma 28:583, 1998* *Eur J Immunol 29:2098, 1999* *Annu Rev Immunol 21:107, 2003*
CD46	Membrane cofactor protein (MCP), HuLy-m5, trophoblast leukocyte-common antigen (TLX)	46–63 (51 68)	I	1q32 M58050	Endothelial cells, epithelial cells, fibroblasts, placenta, sperm, all blood cells except RBC	Acts as a cofactor that binds to CD3b or CD4b, thereby permitting factor I, a serine protease, to convert them into inactive complement fragments. CD46 may be the Rc used by measles virus.	*Int J Mol Med 1:809, 1998* *Virus Res 48:1, 1997* *Int J Hematol 64:101, 1996*
CD47	Integrin-associated protein (IAP), ovarian CA antigen (OA3), Rh-associated antigen	47–55 (≈50)	III Tet.	3q13.1-2 Z25521	All hematopoietic cells	Associates with CD61 integrins to form Rc for thrombospondin, suggesting a role in chemotaxis and cell-cell adhesion. Forms part of the Rh complex on RBC and is not expressed on Rh_null RBC.	*Blood 103:1131, 2004* *J Biol Chem 279:17301, 2004* *J Biol Chem 279:14542, 2004*
CD48	HuLy-m3, Blast-1, BCM1, MEM-102, OX-45	45	V GPI	1q21-23 M37766	All hematopoietic cells except PMN, plts, or RBC	Low-affinity ligand for CD2 that may play role in signal transduction and intercellular adhesion. On T cells, the cytoplasmic domain associates with the lck and fyn tyrosine kinases.	*Immunol Today 17:177, 1996* *Immunogenetics 42:59, 1995* *J Immunol 170:294, 2003*
CD49a	Very late antigen (VLA)-1 α-subunit, integrin α1-subunit	200 (210)	I	5q11.2 X68742	Monocytes, endothelium, smooth muscle, act. T and B cells	Assembles into a heterodimer with CD29 to form a Rc for collagen and laminin.	*J Mol Biol 327:1031, 2003* *J Biol Chem 276:48206, 2001*
CD49b	Very late antigen (VLA)-2 α-subunit, integrin α2-subunit; Ia subunit of platelet glycoprotein Ia–IIa, ECMRI, collagen Rc	160	I	5q23-q31 X17033	Monocytes, plts, T, B, and NK cells, thymocytes, fibroblasts, endothelium, osteoclasts, epithelium	Assembles with CD29 to form a Rc for laminin and collagen types I, II, III and IV that is responsible for Mg^{2+}-dependent adhesion of platelets to collagen.	*J Biol Chem 279:11632, 2004* *J Biol Chem 279:8056, 2004* *Blood 103:1333, 2004* *J Biol Chem 278:48633, 2003*
CD49c	Very late antigen (VLA)-3 α-subunit, integrin α3-subunit	150 (25/130)	I	17q21.33 M59911	Monocytes, T and B cells, kidney glomerulus, thyroid, some basement membranes	Assembles with CD29 to form an Rc for laminin-5 and epilgrin (kalinin) that also binds weakly to collagen and fibronectin, suggesting a role in cell–cell adhesion.	*J Cell Biol 163:1167, 2003* *J Biol Chem 179:5184, 2004* *Mol Biol Cell 7:194, 1996*

(Continued)

TABLE 14-1 CLUSTER OF DIFFERENTIATION ANTIGENS DEFINED AS OF THE SEVENTH INTERNATIONAL WORKSHOP ON LEUKOCYTE TYPING (*CONTINUED*)

ANTIGEN	OTHER NAMES	SIZE	O	GENETICS	DISTRIBUTION	PHYSIOLOGY	SELECTED REFERENCES
CD49d	Very late antigen (VLA)-4α subunit, integrin α_4 subunit	180 (150)	I	2q31-32 X16983	T, B, and NK cells, eos, monocytes, erythroblasts, thymocytes, mast cells, DC, basophils, myeloblasts	Assembles with CD29 or β7 integrin to form VLA-4 or α4β7, respectively. These integrins bind VCAM-1 (CD106) and some forms of fibronectin. α4β7 also binds mucosal addressin MAdCAM-1. These integrins help mediate cell arrest and adhesion to endothelium.	Circ Res 94:462, 2004 J Biol Chem 278:38174, 2003 J Biol Chem 278:34845, 2003 J Immunol 170:5912, 2003
CD49e	Very late antigen (VLA)-5 α-subunit, Integrin α_5-subunit, Ic subunit of GPIc-IIa	155 (135/25)	I	12q11-q13 X06256	Thymocytes, T cells, monocytes, plts, act. or very early B cells	Assembles with CD29 to form an Rc for fibronectin and invasin via binding to RGD. Upon binding, it activates the Na^+/H^+ antiporter and may act as accessory molecule for T cell activation.	Biochemistry 42:12950, 2003 EMBO J 22:4607, 2003 J Biol Chem 279:4862, 2004
CD49f	Very late antigen (VLA)-6 α-subunit, Integrin α_6-subunit, subunit of laminin Rc, platelet GPIc	140 (120/30)	I	2p31.1 X53586	Plts, MØ, monocytes, thymocytes, T cells, adherent epithelia	Assembles with CD29 or the β4 integrin chain (CD104) to form a Rc for laminin on basement membranes of vessels and thrombospondin-1 and -2.	J Biol Chem 162:1189, 2003 J Biol Chem 278:40679, 2003 Dev Cell 5:695, 2003
CD50	Intercellular adhesion molecule-3 (ICAM-3)	120–160	I	19p13.3-2 X69711	Thymocytes, T and B cells, monocytes, PMN, endothelial cells, Langerhans cells	CD50 is a ligand for activated LFA-1 (CD11a/CD18) and that, when engaged, can provide a costimulatory signal for cell activation and/or HIV replication	Biochem Soc Trans 26:644, 1998 J Virol 78:6692, 2004 J Vasc Res 41:28, 2004
CD51	Vitronectin Rc α-chain, αv subunit of αVβ3 integrin (CD51/CD61)	150 (125/24)	I	2q31-32 M14648	Endothelial cells, monocytes, MØ, plts (weak), some B cells (weak)	Assembles with CD61(β3) to form an Rc for vitronectin, vWF, thrombospondin, fibrinogen, and collagen. These Rc facilitate plt aggregation and/or endothelial cell adhesion and may play a role in monocyte migration through subendothelium. CD51 also can associate with the β5 integrin to form an alternate vitronectin Rc.	Exp Cell Res 295:48, 2004 J Biol Chem 279:23996, 2004 J Biol Chem 279:17731, 2004 FEBS Lett 557:159, 2004
CD52	CAMPATH-1	21–28	V GPI	1p36 X62466	Lymphocytes, monocytes, PMN (weak), eos (strong), seminal vesicles, epididymis, spermatozoa	Some anti-CD52 mAbs are strongly mitogenic, suggesting CD52 plays a role in signal transduction.	Biochim Biophys Acta 1446:334, 1999 Eur J Immunol 21:1677, 1991 Transplantation 54:97, 1992
CD53	OX-44	35–42	III Tet.	1p12-13.3 M37033	Leukocytes	Can transduce signals in B cells, monocytes, and PMN, leading to cell activation and/or survival.	J Cell Sci 114:4143, 2001 Oncogene 22:1219, 2003
CD54	Intercellular adhesion molecule-1 (ICAM-1)	90	I	19p13.3-2 X06990	Leukocytes, endothelial and epithelial cells, expression increased with activation	Functions as a ligand for LFA-1 (CD11a/CD18), Mac-1 (CD11b/CD18), and CD11c/CD18 (p150,95). CD54 also is Rc for rhinovirus, can bind CD43, and can bind to *Plasmodium falciparum*-infected RBC.	J Exp Med 182:1231, 1995 J Immunol 171:6135, 2003 Lancet 362:1723, 2003
CD55	Decay accelerating factor (DAF)	55–70	V GPI	1q32 M35156	All cells in contact with serum, CNS, epithelial cells	Neutralizes complement activation on autologous tissue by preventing assembly of C3 convertase or accelerating disassembly of pre-formed convertase.	Pharmacol Rev 50:59, 1998 Adv Immunol 61:201, 1996
CD56	Neural cell adhesion molecule-1 (NCAM), Leu 19, NKH1	175–220	I or V GPI	11q23.1 X16841	NK cells, embryonic cells, muscle, neural cells, epithelium, some act. T cells	Facilitates homotypic adhesion and may play a role in contact-dependent growth inhibition and NK cell cytotoxicity.	Ann Hematol 74:51, 1997 Proc Natl Acad Sci U S A 93:6421, 1996 Neuron 17:413, 1996
CD57	Human natural killer-1 (HNK-1), Leu 7	110			NK cells, some T, few B, some Schwann cells	A carbohydrate antigen that may be a marker of senescence when expressed by CD8 T cells.	Blood 101:2711, 2003 J Biol Chem 279:22693, 2004
CD58	Leukocyte function associated-3 (LFA-3)	45–70	I or V GPI	1p13.1 Y00636	Most hemopoietic cells, fibroblasts; endothelial and epithelial cells.	Binds CD2 and enhances T cell Ag recognition. The CD58 homologue on sheep RBC allows these cells to form rosettes with human T cells.	Cell 97:791, 1999 Proc Natl Acad Sci U S A 96:4289, 1999
CD59	Complement protectin, MIRL, H19, MACIF, HRF20, P-18, IF-5Ag	19	V GPI	11p13 X16447	Leukocytes, RBC, endothelial and epithelial cells, placenta, spermatozoa, body fluids	Inhibits complement membrane attack by binding to activated C8 and C9. It also is a minor ligand for CD2 and may be involved in T cell signal transduction.	Int J Oncol 13:305, 1998 Adv Immunol 61:201, 1996
CD60a	GD3	—	—	—	Neuroectodermal cells, thymocytes, melanocytes, weak on some B cells, plts	Oligosaccharide sequence of the ganglioside GD3: NeuAcα2-NeuAcα2-3Galβ1-4Glcβ1-Cer.	Science 277:1652, 1997 Med Oncol 15:191, 1998
CD60b	9-O-acetyl GD3	—	—	—	Some T cells, act. B cells, neuroectodermal cells	Epitope formed by 9-O-acetylated disialosyl groups linked to lactosylceramide or its analogues.	Cell Immunol 187:117, 1998 Cell Biol 110:217, 1998
CD60c	7-O-acetyl GD3	—	—	—	T cells	Epitope formed by 7-O-acetylated disialosyl groups linked either to lactosylceramide or its analogues.	Blood 82:1776, 1993
CD61	GPIIIa, β_3 integrin, vitronectin Rc β chain, 9-O-acetyl-GD3	90 (110)	I	17q21.3 J02703	Plts, megakaryocytes, monocytes, MØ, endothelial cells, some B cells	Associates with CD41 to form the GPIIb-IIIa heterodimer that facilitates plt aggregation, or with CD51 to form a Rc for vitronectin.	Blood 88:1666, 1996 Curr Pharm Des 10:1567, 2004
CD62E	E-Selectin, endothelial leukocyte adhesion molecule-1 (ELAM-1), LECAM-2	115 (97)	I	1q23-25 M30640	Endothelium	Facilitates adhesion of PMN, monocytes, and some T cells to vascular endothelium by binding sialyl Lewis X, sialyl Lewis A and related fucosylated N-acetyl-lactosamines of leukocyte glycolipids and glycoproteins.	Cell 84:563, 1996 Proc Natl Acad Sci U S A 101:8005, 2004 Blood 103:1685, 2004

TABLE 14-1   CLUSTER OF DIFFERENTIATION ANTIGENS DEFINED AS OF THE SEVENTH INTERNATIONAL WORKSHOP ON LEUKOCYTE TYPING (*CONTINUED*)

ANTIGEN	OTHER NAMES	SIZE	O	GENETICS	DISTRIBUTION	PHYSIOLOGY	SELECTED REFERENCES
CD62L	L-Selectin, TQ1, gp90[MEL-14], leukocyte adhesion molecule-1 (LAM-1), LECAM-1, Leu-8	65 (74–95)	I	1q23-25 M25280	B cells, T cells, PMN, thymocytes monocytes, eos, basophils, erythroid and myeloid progenitor cells, NK cells.	Functions as a peripheral lymph node homing Rc. Facilitates binding to endothelium at inflammatory sites or at high endothelial venules (HEV) of peripheral lymph nodes by binding to endothelial heparin-like chains and the vascular sialomucin, CD34. Involved in leukocyte rolling in mesenteric venules.	*Cell Immunol 215:219, 2002* *J Immunol 169:4542, 2002* *J Immunol 170:28, 2003* *Science 299:405, 2003* *Blood 101:4245, 2003*
CD62P	P-Selectin, GMP-140, LECAM-3, PADGEM, CD62	130–150	I	1q21-24 M25322	Plts, endothelial cells, megakaryocytes	Facilitates adhesion of monocytes and neutrophils to activated platelets and endothelial cells by binding sialylated, fucosylated lactosaminoglycans, including sialyl Lewis X, on neutrophils.	*Curr Biol 6:261, 1996* *Science 273:252, 1996* *Blood 103:3789, 2004* *J Biol Chem 279:21984, 2004*
CD63	Lysosomal membrane-associated glycoprotein 3 (LAMP 3), LIMP, granulophysin	40–60	III Tet.	12q12-13 X07982	Act. plts, monocytes, MØ, secretory granules of vascular endothelial cells, platelet dense granules	Lysosomal protein that translocates to the cell surface upon cellular activation and may facilitate adhesion to activated endothelium.	*Biochem Biophys Res Commun 246: 841, 1998* *Immunol Today 15:588, 1994* *J Immunol 157:2039, 1996*
CD64	FcγRI, FcRI	72	I	1q21.1 X14356 . . . A M91615 . . . B M91647 . . . C	Monocytes (B and C forms), MØ, act. PMN	At least three isoforms (A, B, C) exist, each acting as a high-affinity Rc for IgG and mediating release of cytokines, including IL-1, IL-6, and TNF-α.	*Mol Immunol 35:989, 1998* *J Immunol 157:541, 1996* *Immunol Today 14:215, 1994*
CD65	Ceramide-dodecasaccharide 4c, VIM-2	—	—	—	Myeloid cells, some monocytic cells	CD65 is a carbohydrate determinant with a minimal epitope consisting of NeuAcα2->3Galβ1->4GlcNAcβ1->3Galβ1->4GlcNAc(Fucα1->3)β1->3Galβ. Associated glycoprotein is involved in signal transduction leading to formation of the respiratory burst.	*J Biochem 119:456, 1996* *J Biol Chem 263:10186, 1988*
CD66a	Phosphorylated glycoprotein, biliary glycoprotein-1 (BGP-1), nonspecific cross-reacting antigen-160 (NCA-160)	140–180 (113, 96, 74)	I	19q13.1-2 X16354	PMN, histiocytes, some myeloid progenitor cells, brush border of colonic epithelial cells	Biliary glycoprotein member of the carcinoembryonic antigen family of adhesion molecules that facilitates Ca²⁺-independent homotypic and heterotypic adhesion and neutrophil activation. CD66 possesses Lewis X and sialyl Lewis X determinants.	*Eur J Immunol 28:3664, 1998* *Am J Pathol 152:1401, 1998* *J Histochem Cytochem 45:957, 1997* *J Histochem Cytochem 44:35, 1996*
CD66b	Formerly CD67, CGM6, p100, nonspecific cross-reacting antigen-95 (NCA-95)	95–100	GPI	19q13.1-2 X52378	Granulocytes	CD66b is one GPI isoform of CD66. Cross-linking of CD66b induces aggregation and activation, possibly via binding to CD62E.	*Blood 91:663, 1998* *J Leukoc Biol 60:106, 1996*
CD66c	Nonspecific cross-reacting antigen-90 (NCA-90)	90	GPI	19q13.1-2 M29541	Myeloid and epithelial cells	CD66c is another GPI isoform of CD66. Cross-linking of CD66c induces aggregation and activation possibly via binding to CD62E.	*Leukemia 13:779, 1999* *Tissue Antigens 52:1, 1998*
CD66d	CGM1	35	I	19q13.1-2 L00692	Granulocytes	Member of carcinoembryonic antigen family of adhesion molecules that facilitates homotypic adhesion and neutrophil activation.	*J Leukoc Biol 60:106, 1996*
CD66e	Carcinoembryonic antigen (CEA)	180–200	GPI	19q13.1-2 M17303	Tissues derived from all three germ layers during embryogenesis; adult colon epithelial cells (very weak)	May facilitate Ca²⁺-independent homotypic and heterotypic adhesion during embryogenesis. CD66e binds weakly to other nonspecific cross-reacting antigens CD66a–c.	*Semin Cancer Biol 9:67, 1999* *Cancer Res 55:3873, 1995* *Cancer Res 56:4805, 1996*
CD66f	PSG (pregnancy-specific glycoprotein), SP-1	54–72	GPI	19q13.1-2 U18469	Tissues derived from all three germ layers during embryogenesis; adult colon epithelial cells (very weak)	Function unknown but appears necessary for successful pregnancy and may be involved in protection of fetus from maternal immune recognition.	*Semin Cancer Biol 9:67, 1999* *Cancer Res 55:3873, 1995* *Cancer Res 56:4805, 1996*
CD68	gp110, macrosialin (mouse)	110	I	17p13 S57235	Monocytes/MØ, DC, granulocytes, osteoclasts, mast cells, act. lymphocytes, myeloid progenitor cells, nurse-like cells	Sialomucin belonging to a family of highly glycosylated, acidic lysosomal glycoproteins (LGPs) that include LAMP-1 (CD107a), and LAMP-2 (CD107b). May protect lysosomal membranes from attack by hydrolases.	*Proc Natl Acad Sci U S A 93: 14833, 1996* *Genomics 54:165, 1998* *Proc Natl Acad Sci U S A 92:9580, 1995* *Am J Clin Pathol 103:425, 1995* *Blood 99:1030, 2002*
CD69	Activation inducer molecule (AIM), early activation antigen (EA 1), MLR-3, gp34/28, Leu-23	60 (28/33)	II	12p12.3-13.2 L07555	Plts, act. lymphocytes, act. granulocytes, CD4⁺ or CD8⁺ thymocytes,	Member of the Ca²⁺-dependent (C-type) lectin superfamily of type II transmembrane proteins. Forms a homodimer that may function as signal transducer enhancing cell activation and/or platelet aggregation.	*J Immunol 162:3978, 1999* *Clin Exp Immunol 114:66, 1998* *Scand J Immunol 48:196, 1998*
CD70	Ki-24 antigen, CD27-ligand	29	II	19p13.3 L08096	Act. B cells, some act. T cells	Member of TNF family that binds CD27 and may provide costimulatory signal for T cell activation.	*Semin Immunol 10:491, 1998*
CD71	Transferrin Rc, T9	190 (95)	II	3q26.2-qter X01060	Act. or proliferating cells, reticulocytes, brain capillary endothelium	Binds serum iron transport protein ferrotransferrin at neutral pH and iron-free apotransferrin at acidic intracellular pH to facilitate cellular iron uptake.	*Proc Natl Acad Sci U S A 93:8175, 1996* *Crit Rev Oncog 4:241, 1993*
CD72	Lyb-2, Ly-32.2	86 (39/43)	II	9p13.2 M54992	All B cells (except plasma cells), MØ (weak)	May be involved in B cell activation. Binding of CD72 by CD5 remains controversial.	*Eur J Immunol 28:3003, 1998* *J Immunol 160:4662, 1998*

TABLE 14-1   CLUSTER OF DIFFERENTIATION ANTIGENS DEFINED AS OF THE SEVENTH INTERNATIONAL WORKSHOP ON LEUKOCYTE TYPING (*Continued*)

Antigen	Other Names	Size	O	Genetics	Distribution	Physiology	Selected References
CD73	Ecto-5′-nucleotidase	69–72	GPI	6q14-21 X55740	Some B cells, some T cells, thymocytes (weak), some epithelial and endothelial cells, FDC	Catalyzes 5′-dephosphorylation of pyrimidine and purine ribo- and deoxyribonucleoside monophosphates to nucleosides.	*Immunol Rev 161:95, 1998* *Blood 82:1052, 1993* *Mol Cell Biochem 232:113, 2002*
CD74	Class II-specific chaperone, invariant chain, Ii	33–35 (41)	II	5q32 X03339 X03340	B cells, monocytes (weak), DC, act. T cells	Associates with the α- and β-chains of MHC class II proteins in endoplasmic reticulum to prevent binding of endogenous peptides. Released from MHC protein in the acidic lysosomal compartment	*Hum Immunol 54:159, 1997* *J Exp Med 197:1467, 2003*
CD75 (CD75s)	NeuAc α-2,6 Galβ 1,4 GlcNAc core epitope	53, 87	II	3q27-28 (SiaT-1) X54363	Few T cells, RBC, most mature B cells but not plasma cells	Ligand for CD22 that requires β-galactoside α2,6-sialyltransferase (SiaT-1) activity in the Golgi to produce the α-2,6-sialylated form of CD75, which is designated CD75s.	*Biochem Biophys Res Commun 309: 32, 2003* *Glycobiology 14:39, 2004* *Glycobiology 9:907, 1999*
CDw76		85/67			Mature B cells (strong, particularly on mantle zone B cells), some T cells (weak), melanocytes, endothelial cells, hepatocytes, kidney tubules	Neuraminidase-sensitive carbohydrate determinant (NeuAcα2-6Galβ1-4GlcNAcβ1-3Galβ1-4Glc-β1-1′Cer) found on glycosphingolipids and glycoproteins that is dependent on β-galactoside α2,6-sialyltransferase activity in the Golgi.	*Blood 87:5113, 1996* *Eur J Immunol 22:2777, 1992*
CD77	Globotriaocylceramide (Gβ3), Pᵏ blood group, Burkitt lymphoma associated antigen (BLA), ceramide trihexoside			22q13.2 AB041418	Germinal center B cells, FDC, endothelium, some epithelial cells	Formed by action of a-1,4-galactosyltransferase, which transfers a galactose to the a-1,4 postion of lactosylceramide to form globotriaosylceramide of CD77. May serve as Rc for vero toxin of *E. coli* and the Shiga toxin of *Shigella dysenteriae*. Ligation may induce apoptosis.	*J Biol Chem 278:44429, 2003* *J Biol Chem 275:15152, 2000* *J Biol Chem 275:16723, 2000*
CDw78	Epitope of HLA class II molecules				B cells (increased after activation), tissue MØ	Provisional designation dropped since MAbs assigned to this specificity were found to recognize epitopes on HLA class II molecules.	*Leucocyte Typing VII, Oxford University Press, Oxford, p. 82, 2002*
CD79a	MB-1, Igα	82–95 (32–33)	I	19q13.2 L32754	B cells	Accessory molecule that mediates sIg expression and B cell Rc signal transduction (see Chap. 77).	*Curr Opin Cell Biol 7:163, 1995*
CD79b	B29, Igβ	82–95 (37–39)	I	17q23 L27587	B cells	An accessory molecule that mediates sIg expression and B cell Rc signal transduction (see Chap. 77)	*Immunity 4:145, 1996*
CD80	B7, B7-1, BB1	60	I	3q21 M27533	Act. B cells, monocytes, FDC	Interacts with CD28 or CD152 (CTLA-4) for costimulation or inhibition of T cells, respectively.	*Annu Rev Immunol 14:233, 1996* *Curr Opin Immunol 9:858, 1997*
CD81	Target of anti-proliferative antibody-1 (TAPA-1)	22	III Tet.	11p15.5 M33680	Many cell types including lymphocytes	Member of the CD19/CD21/Leu-13 signal transduction complex that is involved in B cell signaling. Can serve as the Rc for hepatitis C virus.	*Annu Rev Immunol 16:89, 1998* *Science 282:938, 1998*
CD82	R2, IA4, 4F9, KAI1	50–53	III Tet.	11p11.2 X53795	Epithelia, endothelium, monocytes, PMN, plt, act. lymphocytes	Member of tetraspanin family that plays a role in signal transduction.	*Immunol Today 15:588, 1994* *Biochem Biophys Acta 1287:67, 1996* *J Cell Sci 116:4557, 2003*
CD83	HB15	43	I	6p23-21.3 Z11697	DC (not FDC), Langerhans cells, B cells (weak), interdigitating reticular cells	May play a role in antigen presentation or cellular interactions that follow lymphocyte activation. Currently one of the best markers for mature DC.	*J Immunol 154:3821, 1995* *J Immunol 156:541, 1996*
CD84	SLAM family, member 5 (SLAMF5)	68–80 (72–86)	I	1q24 U82988	Monocytes, MØ, germinal center B cells (strong), mantle zone B cells (weak), plts	Member of IgSF that may be involved in signal transduction. Soluble form may inhibit T cell activation.	*J Immunol 171:2485, 2003* *Leuk Res 28:237, 2004* *Blood 103:4207, 2004*
CD85 (CD85j)	ILT2, LIR1, MIR7, now designated CD85j	110 (83)	I	19q13.4	NK cells, plasma cells (strong), B cells, monocytes, HCL	IgSF member that belongs to a family of related molecules with immune tyrosine-based inhibitory motifs (ITIMs) and serves as inhibitory Rc for HLA class I molecules, including HLA-A, -B, G1, -E.	*Leucocyte Typing VII, Oxford University Press, Oxford, p 295, 2002* *Immunogenetics 53:270, 2001* *Immunobiology 202:34, 2000*
CD85a	ILT5, LIR3, HL9	110	I	19q13.4	Monocytes, MØ, DC, PMN, and some T cells	Highly polymorphic inhibitory Rc for HLA class I molecules.	*Leucocyte Typing VII, Oxford University Press, Oxford, p 289, 2002*
CD85d	ILT4, LIR2, MIR10	110	I	19q13.4	Myeloid cells, PMN (weak)	Inhibitory Rc for HLA class I molecules, including HLA-A, -B, G1, and –E. Also binds UL18, a class-I-like molecule of cytomegalovirus.	*Leucocyte Typing VII, Oxford University Press, Oxford, p 296, 2002*
CD85k	ILT3, LIR5, HM18	60	I	19q13.4	Myeloid cells, DC, MØ	Inhibitory Rc with cytoplasmic ITIM.	*Leucocyte Typing VII, Oxford University Press, Oxford, p 296, 2002*
CD86	B7-2, B70	80	I	3q13-23 U404343	Monocytes, act. B and T cells, DC	Interacts with CD28 to provide a costimulatory signal or with CD152 (CTLA-4) to provide an inhibitory signal for T cell activation.	*Annu Rev Immunol 14:233, 1996* *J Biol Chem 271:26762, 1996*

TABLE 14-1 CLUSTER OF DIFFERENTIATION ANTIGENS DEFINED AS OF THE SEVENTH INTERNATIONAL WORKSHOP ON LEUKOCYTE TYPING (*Continued*)

Antigen	Other Names	Size	O	Genetics	Distribution	Physiology	Selected References
CD87	Urokinase plasminogen activator Rc (uPAR), Mo3	50–65	GPI	19q13 M83246	Monocytes, PMN, act. NK and LGL cells	Rc for uPA, which can retain and concentrate uPA at the plasma membrane, allowing for local conversion of plasminogen to plasmin.	J Immunol 156:297, 1996 J Immunol 152:505, 1994 J Biol Chem 279:1400, 2004
CD88	Rc for C5a (C5aR)	40	III	19q13.3-13.4 X57250	PMN, MØ, eos, mast cells, hepatocytes, smooth muscle, endothelium	G protein-coupled Rc that triggers chemotaxis, activation, respiratory burst, and degranulation, upon binding to C5a.	Nature 383:86, 1996 J Immunol 162:6510, 1999 J Immunol 170:6115, 2003
CD89	FcRc for IgA, FcαR,	55–75	I	19q13.4 X54150	PMN, monocytes, MØ, mucosa, some T and B cells	Binds Fc of IgA1 or IgA2 with high affinity to trigger granulocyte respiratory burst. As such, it amplifies the protective effects of IgA.	Scand J Immunol 57:506, 2003 J Biol Chem 278:27966, 2003 Nature 423:614, 2003 J Mol Biol 327:645, 2003
CD90	Thy-1, theta	18	V GPI	11q23.3 M11749	Prothymocytes, brain, other nonlymphoid tissues	May contribute to formation of neuron memory and to growth regulation of hematopoietic stem cells.	Nature 379:826, 1996 Science 216:696, 1982
CD91	Rc for α₂-macroglobulin, low-density lipoprotein (LDL) Rc-associated protein	600 (515/85)	I	12q13.1-13.3 X13916	Monocytic and macrophage phagocytes, astrocytes, fibroblasts, epithelial cells	Member of the low-density lipoprotein Rc family that binds to α₂ macroglobulin, is involved in lipoprotein metabolism, and interacts with the human frizzled-1 to down-regulate canonical Wnt signaling pathway.	J Biol Chem 279:22595, 2004 J Biol Chem 279:17535, 2004 J Biol Chem 279:10005, 2004 J Biol Chem 279:4260, 2004 Nat Med 9:1313, 2003
CDw92	Choline transporter-like protein 1 (CTL1)	70	III	9q31.2 AJ245620	Monocytes, blood-derived DC, lymphocytes (weak), PMN, endothelium (weak)	Member of choline transporter-like protein family that may help regulate leukocyte function.	J Immunol 167:5795, 2001 Proc Natl Acad Sci U S A 97:1835, 2000 Nat Genet 36:40, 2004
CDw93		110–120			PMN, monocytes, endothelial cells	O-sialoglycoprotein of unknown function.	Leucocyte Typing VI, Garland Scientific Publishing, NY, p 1032, 1998
CD94	Kp43	70 (30,43)	II	12p12.3-13.1 U30610	NK (increased upon activation), few T cells	Plays role in NK recognition of MHC class I molecules. Ligation on NK cells can inhibit target cell killing.	Immunity 5:163, 1996 J Immunol 157:4741, 1996
CD95	Apo-1, FAS, TNFRSF6, APT1	42	I	10q 24.1 M67454	Act. lymphocytes, fibroblasts, monocytes, PMN, liver	Cross linking CD95 can induce apoptosis.	Curr Opin Immunol 8:355, 1996 Cell 85:781, 1996
CD96	T cell activation increased late expression (TACTILE)	240/180/160 (160)	I	M88282	T and NK cells (increased upon activation)	Expressed primarily upon activation, suggesting it may have binding activity for some unknown ligand. CD96 may promote NK cell–target adhesion by interacting with CD155.	J Immunol 148:2600, 1992 J Immunol 172:3994, 2004
CD97		74,80,89	III	19p13.12-2 X94630	PMN, monocytes, DC, most T cells, few act. B cells, thyroid and colon CA	G protein-coupled Rc with 7 potential membrane spanning domains and 5 extracellular EGF domains with 1 RGD sequence.	J Exp Med 184:1185, 1996 Tissue Antigens 57:325, 2001 Am J Pathol 161:1657, 2002
CD98	4F2, FRP-1, RL-388	125 (45/80)	II	11q13 AB018010	Strong on monocytes, myocardial, act. T cells, but weak on T, B, and NK cells	Potential amino acid transporter that may be involved in the regulation of cellular activation. Together with CD54 may regulate the amino acids transporter (LAT-2) activity.	Blood 87:3676, 1996 J Biol Chem 278:23672, 2003 Mol Biol Cell 13:2841, 2002
CD99	MIC2, E2, 12E7, HuLym6, FMC29, CD99R	32	I	Xp22.32 and Yp11.3 X16006	All WBC, especially thymocytes, CD99 is found on surface of Xg(a+) RBC and in cytoplasm of Xg(a-) RBC.	Involved in rosette formation with sheep RBC. The gene encoding CD99 is pseudoautosomal. MIC2Y or MIC2X is expressed by males or females, respectively. MIC2X does not undergo X inactivation. CD99 signaling may enhance apoptosis.	Immunol Invest 24:173, 1995 FEBS Lett 554:478, 2003 FEBS Lett 546:379, 2003
CD100	Semaphorin 4D, SEMA4D, collapsin 4, Coll4	300 (150)	I	9q22-q31 U60800	B, T, and NK cells, most myeloid cells, expression increases upon activation	Semaphorin (Sema) Rc for plexin B1 that plays a role in lymphocyte activation by modifying the signaling of other Rc, such as CD40 or CD45, and down-regulates B cell expression of CD23.	Proc Natl Acad Sci U S A 93:11780, 1996 Blood 101:1962, 2002 J Immunol 172:1246, 2004 Nat Med 9:191, 2003
CD101	IGSF2, V7, p126	200 (126)	I	1p13 Z33642	PMN, monocytes, some mucosal T cells, act. T	May play costimulatory role in T cell activation.	J Immunol 157:3366, 1996
CD102	ICAM-2 (intercellular adhesion molecule-2)	54–68	I	17q23-25 X15606	Endothelial cells (strong), plts (strong), subset of lymphocytes, monocytes, DC, splenic sinusoids	Acts as a ligand for LFA-1 (CD11a/CD18) but, unlike CD54, does not bind to Mac-1 (CD11b/CD18) or undergo up-regulation upon cellular activation. May facilitate re-circulation of memory T cells.	Immunol Res 17:313, 1998 Proc Natl Acad Sci U S A 96:3017, 1999 J Biol Chem 279:19122, 2004
CD103	ITGAE, human mucosal lymphocyte-1 integrin (HML-1), integrin αE-chain	175 (150,25)	I	17p13 L25851	Intraepithelial, 1–2% of blood lymphocytes, testis, prostate ovary, pancreas	Associates with β₇ integrin to form an Rc that binds E-cadherin to facilitate adhesion to epithelia.	J Cell Sci 115:4505, 2002 J Biol Chem 269:6016, 1994 Semin Immunol 7:335, 1995
CD104	Integrin β4-subunit of laminin Rc, TSP-1180	210 (220)	I	17q11-qter X51841	Epithelia, thymocytes, few neuronal cells, basement membranes, Schwann cells	Associates with α6 (CD49f) to form an Rc for laminin (and possibly epiligrin), facilitating adhesion of cells to the extracellular matrix.	J Cell Biol 162:1189, 2003 J Biol Chem 278:49406, 2003
CD105	Endoglin, Rc for transforming growth factor-beta (TGF-β) types I and III	170 (95)	II	9q34.1 X72012	Endothelium, act. monocytes, MØ, proerythroblasts, FDC, tumor-associated angiogenic blood vessels	Has binding activity for TGF-β1 and TGF-β3 in association with TGF-β Rc I and Rc II and is involved in regulation of cell differentiation and migration.	Nat Genet 8:345, 1994 J Cell Biol 133:1109, 1996 Oncogene 22:6557, 2003

(Continued)

TABLE 14-1 CLUSTER OF DIFFERENTIATION ANTIGENS DEFINED AS OF THE SEVENTH INTERNATIONAL WORKSHOP ON LEUKOCYTE TYPING (*CONTINUED*)

ANTIGEN	OTHER NAMES	SIZE	O	GENETICS	DISTRIBUTION	PHYSIOLOGY	SELECTED REFERENCES
CD106	Vascular cell adhesion molecule-1 (VCAM-1), INCAM-110	100–110	I	1p31-32 M73255	Act. endothelial cells, MØ, FDC, marrow stroma, myoblasts, some MØ, myotubes	Serves as a ligand for VLA-4 ($\alpha_4\beta_1$ integrin or CD49d/CD29) and, to a lesser degree, $\alpha_4\beta_2$ integrin. CD106 facilitates recruitment of leukocytes to sites of inflammation and is involved in lymphocyte–dendritic cell interactions and in myogenesis.	*Nature 373:539, 1995* *J Immunol 156:2851, 1996* *Blood 84:2068, 1994*
CD107a	Lysosome-associated membrane protein-1 (LAMP-1)	120	I	13q34 J04182	Act. plts, PMN, T cells, MØ, DC, endothelial cells, tonsillar epithelium	Serves as ligand for galaptin, an S-type lectin (galectin) in the extracellular matrix. Contains sialylated Lewis X (sLe X) structures that can bind CD62E.	*J Biol Chem 266:21327, 1991* *J Biol Regul Homeost Agents 16: 147, 2002*
CD107b	Lysosome-associated membrane protein-2 (LAMP-2)	120	I	Xq24 J04183	Act. plts, PMN, act. endothelial cells, tonsillar epithelium, melanoma	Same as CD107a.	*J Biol Chem 266:21327, 1991* *J Biol Regul Homeost Agents 16: 147, 2002*
CD108	SEMA7A, John-Milton-Hagen rbc blood group antigen	75 (80)	V GPI	15q22.3-q23 NM003612	Some act. lymphocytes, RBC, myeloid, stromal cells	Membrane-bound semaphorin that plays a role in cellular activation.	*J Immunol 162:4094, 1999* *Scand J Immunol 56:270, 2002*
CD109	Gov$^{a/b}$ alloantigen, 8A3, E123, 7D1	175	V GPI	6q14.1 AF410459	Endothelium, plts, act.T cell, hematopoietic and mesenchymal stem cells	Member of the α2-macroglobulin/C3, C4, C5 family of thioester-containing proteins.	*Gene 327:171, 2004* *Ann N Y Acad Sci 996:227, 2003* *Blood 99:1683, 2002*
CD110	Thrombopoietin Rc, c-MPL, TPO-R	85–92	I	1p34 U68159	Hematopoietic stem cells, megakaryocytes, plts	Rc for thrombopoietin that signals for megakaryocyte proliferation and differentiation or stem cell survival.	*Blood 86:419, 1995* *Curr Opin Hematol 7:183, 2000* *Semin Hematol 37:41, 2000*
CD111	PRR1, Nectin-1, HevC, HIgR	75	I	11q23-q24 AF110314	Myelomonocytic cells, megakaryocytes, plts, epithelial and neuronal cells	Adhesion molecule of the "nectin" family that also serves as one of several Rc for herpes simplex virus 1 and 2.	*J Virol 74:3909, 2000* *Science 280:1618, 1998* *J Cell Biol 150:1161, 2000*
CD112	PRR2, Nectin-2, HVEB	72, 64	I	19q13.2-q13.4 AF044962	Hematopoietic, endothelial, epithelial, and neuronal cells	"Nectin" family adhesion ligand for CD226 that also can serve as Rc for some herpes simplex viruses.	*Blood 92:4602, 2000* *Int Immunol 16:533, 2004* *J Exp Med 198:557, 2003*
CD113	Reserved						
CD114	Granulocyte colony stimulating factor Rc	150	I	1p35-34.3 X55721	Monocytes, MØ, PMN and their precursors	Class I cytokine receptor for G-CSF that plays a role in the regulation of myeloid proliferation and differentiation.	*Blood 101:4615, 2003* *Biochemistry 43:2458, 2004*
CD115	Colony stimulating factor (CSF)-1 Rc, c-*fms* proto-oncogene	150	I	5q33.2-33.3 X03663	Placenta, MØ, monocytes and their precursors	Class III cytokine Rc for macrophage-CSF. M-CSF induces tyrosine phosphorylation of CD115, leading to proliferation and differentiation of monocytes and their progenitors.	*Leukemia 17:98, 2003* *EMBO J 22: 2798, 2003* *J Cell Biochem 85:10, 2002* *Genes Chromosome Cancer 22:251, 1998*
CD116	Rc for granulocyte-macrophage colony stimulating factor (GM-CSFR), CSF-1 R, HGM-CSFR	70–85	I	Xp22.32; Yp11.3; pseudo-autosomal X17648	Monocytes, PMN, endothelial cells, DC, fibroblasts	CD116 is the Rc for GM-CSF. The low affinity of the α-subunit for GM-CSF is increased when it forms a heterodimer with a 120–140 kDa β-subunit common to IL3-Rc (CD123) and IL5-Rc (CD125). Binding of CD116 to GM-CSF induces NF-κB and stimulates cell proliferation and differentiation.	*Blood 103:507, 2004* *Blood 102:192, 2003* *Blood 101:1308, 2003* *J Biol Chem 269:10905, 1994*
CD117	Rc for stem cell factor (SCFR), c-*kit*, steel factor Rc (SCR)	145	I	4q11-q12 X06182	Hematopoietic progenitors, mast cells, melanocytes, spermatogonia, oocytes, some NK cells	Class III cytokine Rc for "steel factor" that induces its tyrosine kinase activity, leading to cellular proliferation and/or differentiation. CD117 is commonly altered in various neoplasms.	*Oncogene 23:588, 2004* *Biochim Biophys Acta 1688:250, 2004* *Am J Pathol 164:305, 2004*
CDw119	Rc for interferon (IFN)-γ (IFNγ-R)	90–100	I	6q23-q24 J03143	MØ, monocytes, T, B, and NK cells, PMN, epithelial cells, endothelium, fibroblasts	Class II cytokine Rc for IFN-γ that is responsible for binding IFN-γ, but cannot transduce a signal in transfected cell lines without IFN-γ accessory factor-1 (AF-1).	*Annu Rev Immunol 11:571, 1993* *Cell 76:793, 1994* *Am J Hum Genet 72:448, 2003*
CD120a	55-kDa Rc for tumor necrosis factor alpha (TNF-α), TNFRI	55	I	12p13.2 M33294	Many cell types; highest levels on epithelial cells, germinal center dendritic reticulum cells	Functions as high-affinity Rc for TNF-α and TNF-β.	*Cell 114:181, 2003* *Cell 114:148, 2003* *Arthritis Rheum 50:413, 2004*
CD120b	75-kDa Rc for TNF-α, TNFRII	75	I	1p36.3-p36.2 M35857	Many cell types; highest levels on epithelial cells, germinal center dendritic reticulum cells	Functions as high-affinity Rc for TNF-α and TNF-β or lymphotoxin alpha.	*J Biol Chem 278:51613, 2003* *J Leukoc Biol 74:572, 2003*
CDw121a	Rc for IL-1 (type I), IL-1R	80	I	2q12 M27492	T cells, thymocytes, chondrocytes, synovial cells, endothelial cells, fibroblasts, keratinocytes, hepatocytes	Rc for interleukin-1 alpha (IL-1α) and interleukin-1 beta (IL-1β) that induces cellular proliferation and/ or activation upon binding IL-1.	*Arch Biochem Biophys 413:229, 2003* *J Rheumatol 29:1404, 2002* *J Immunol 169:393, 2002*
CDw121b	Rc for IL-1 (type II), IL-1R	68	I	2q12 M59770	B cells, monocytes, PMN, MØ	Nonsignal transducing Rc for IL-1α and IL-1β that may inhibit IL-1 effects by competing with CD120a for IL-1 binding. Soluble form acts as an antagonist.	*J Immunol 170:5999, 2003* *Immunity 18:87, 2003* *J Leukoc Biol 72:643, 2002*
CD122	β-Chain of the IL-2 Rc, p75, IL-2R-β	75	I	22q11.2-q13 M26062	Act. T cells, B cells, monocytes, NK cells	Associates with CD25 and CD132 to form a heterotrimeric Rc with high affinity for IL-2.	*J Biol Chem 278:22868, 2003* *Cytokine Growth Factor Rev 13:27, 2002*
CD123	IL-3 Rc α-chain	70	I	Xp22.3, Yp13.3 M74782	Pluripotent stem cells, committed hemopoietic progenitor cells	Low-affinity Rc for IL-3 that associates with CDw131 to form a high-affinity Rc for IL-3 that, upon binding to IL-3, stimulates proliferation and/or differentiation.	*Leukemia 18:219, 2004* *J Biol Chem 270:22422, 1995*

TABLE 14-1 CLUSTER OF DIFFERENTIATION ANTIGENS DEFINED AS OF THE SEVENTH INTERNATIONAL WORKSHOP ON LEUKOCYTE TYPING (*CONTINUED*)

ANTIGEN	OTHER NAMES	SIZE	O	GENETICS	DISTRIBUTION	PHYSIOLOGY	SELECTED REFERENCES
CD124	HIL-4R, IL-4 Rc α-chain	140	I	16p11.2-p12.1 X52425	Mature B cells, T cells, epithelium, endothelium, hematopoietic precursors, fibroblasts	Rc for IL-4 that forms a heterodimer with CD132 to induce cellular differentiation and/or activation upon binding IL-4.	*Hum Genet 114:391, 2004* *J Biol Chem 278:3903, 2003*
CDw125	IL-5 Rc α-chain	55–60	I	3p26 X61176-8 X62156	Eos, basophils, act. B cells	Associates with CDw131 to form the IL-5 Rc that stimulates proliferation and/or differentiation upon binding IL-5.	*EMBO J 14:3395, 1995* *Immunity 4:483, 1996*
CD126	IL-6 Rc α-chain	80	I	1q21 X12830	Plasma cells (high), act. B (high), WBC (weak), epithelial cells, fibroblasts, neural cells, hepatocytes	Associates with CD130 to form IL-6 Rc that stimulates cell growth and/or differentiation upon binding IL-6. Soluble CD126 can be generated by selected matrix metalloproteinases.	*Annu Rev Immunol 15:797, 1997* *J Biol Chem 278:179, 2003* *Clin Exp Med 3:27, 2003* *FEBS Lett 538:113, 2003*
CD127	HIL-7R, IL-7 Rc α-chain, p90 IL-7R	75	I	5p13 M29696	B cell precursors, thymocytes, mature T cells, monocytes	Specific Rc for IL-7. Forms functional high-affinity complex in association with γc-chain (CD132). Critical role for IL-7/IL-7R system in lymphoid development.	*Leucocyte Typing VII, Oxford University Press, Oxford, p 866, 2002* *Histol Histopathol 18:911, 2003* *Proc Natl Acad Sci U S A 99: 13759, 2002*
CDw128a	IL-8 Rc A, CXCR1, IL-8 Rc A (IL-8RA)	58–67	III	2q35 L19592	PMN, basophils, monocytes, keratinocytes, some T cells	G protein-coupled CXC Rc for IL-8 that induces chemotaxis and/or cell activation upon binding IL-8.	*Leucocyte Typing VII, Oxford University Press, Oxford, p 866, 2002* *Semin Immunol 11:95, 1999* *Crit Rev Immunol 19:1, 1999*
CDw128b	IL-8 Rc B (IL-8RB), CXCR2	58–67	III	2q35	PMN, basophils, monocytes, keratinocytes, some T cells	G protein-coupled CXC Rc for IL-8 that induces chemotaxis and/or cell activation upon binding IL-8.	*Leucocyte Typing VII, Oxford University Press, Oxford, p 867, 2002* *Semin Immunol 11:95, 1999* *Crit Rev Immunol 19:1, 1999*
CD129	IL-9 Rc	64	I	Xq28, Yq12 M84747	Act. T cells, B cells, myeloid and erythroid precursors, mast cells	Associates with CD132 to form an Rc for IL-9 that stimulates cell growth and/or differentiation.	*J Biol Chem 273:9255, 1998* *Adv Immunol 54:79, 1993*
CD130	gp130, subunit of Rc for IL-6, oncostatin-M, leukemia inhibitory factor, IL-11, ciliary neurotrophic factor	130–140	I	5q11 M57230	Most WBC, epithelial cells, fibroblasts, hepatocytes, neural cells	Low-affinity Rc for oncostatin-M. Together with each respective specific α-chain, forms high-affinity Rc for IL-6, oncostatin-M, leukemia inhibitory factor, IL-11, ciliary neurotrophic factor, or cardiotrophin I.	*Annu Rev Immunol 15:797, 1997* *Science 300:2101, 2003* *Cancer Res 63:2948, 2003*
CDw131	IL-3 Rc common β-chain	140	I	22q12.2-13.1 M59941	Myeloid, blood, and progenitor cells, neutrophils, some B cells	Common β-subunit of IL-3, IL-5, GM-CSF Rc.	*J Leukoc Biol 72:1246, 2002* *Blood 101:1308, 2003* *Blood 100:3164, 2002*
CD132	IL-2 Rc common γ-chain	64	I	Xq13 D11086	Thymocytes, most WBC, increased with activation	Common γ-subunit for IL-2, IL-4, IL-7, IL-9, IL-15 Rc.	*Immunol Today 20:71, 1999* *Crit Rev Immunol 18:503, 1998*
CD133	AC133, PROML1, hematopoietic stem cell antigen, prominin-like I	120	III	4p16.2-p12 AF027208	Hematopoietic tissues especially stem cells, epithelial cells,	Pentaspan membrane protein that can be used for positive selection of hematopoietic stem cells.	*J Biol Regul Homeost Agents 15: 101, 2001* *Leukemia 15:1685, 2001*
CD134	MRC OX40, Rc for OX40-ligand	50	I	1p36 X7562	Medullary thymocytes, act. CD4 T cells	Member of TNF-Rc family that is the Rc for OX40-ligand. Costimulatory molecule for B cell activation.	*J Immunol 163:3007, 1999* *J Exp Med 183:979, 1996* *Adv Immunol 61:1, 1996*
CD135	STK-1, FLT3, flk-2	130 (160)	I	13q12 U02687	Hematopoietic stem cell	Type III Rc tyrosine kinase that is the Rc for FLT3-ligand. Mutations in CD135 are associated with acquired drug resistance in acute leukemia.	*Blood 103:3544, 2004* *Blood 103:2266, 2004* *Leukemia 17:2492, 2003*
CDw136	Récepteur d'Origine Nantaise (RON)	180 (150/40)	I	3p21.3 X70040	Monocytes, epithelial cells	Heterodimeric Rc tyrosine kinase that provides signal transduction, leading to cell growth and differentiation.	*J Biol Chem 279:3726, 2004* *Dev Cell 5:257, 2003* *Oncogene 22:186, 2003*
CDw137	4-1BB, ILA (induced by lymphocyte act.)	85 (39)	I	1p36 U03397	Act. T cells, thymocytes, some non-lymphoid cells	Member of TNF-Rc family that is the Rc for 4-1BBL that serves as costimulatory signal for T cell growth.	*Eur J Immunol 33:446, 2003* *Eur J Immunol 32:3617, 2003* *Blood 100:3253, 2002*
CD138	Syndecan-1, heparan sulfate proteoglycan	80–250	I	2p23 J05392	Pre-B, immature B, plasma cells, epithelial, mesenchymal cells	Extracellular matrix Rc that can serve as co-Rc for fibroblast growth factor-2, fibronectin, collagen, thrombospondin, and antithrombin III, which facilitates cell spreading.	*J Cell Biochem 61:578, 1996* *J Biol Chem 278:46607, 2003* *J Biol Chem 278:44168, 2003* *Exp Cell Res 286:219, 2003*
CD139		209 (228)			B cells, monocytes, FDC, PMN, endothelial cells	Unknown.	*Leucocyte Typing VII, Oxford University Press, Oxford, p 875, 2002*
CD140a	α-chain of Rc for platelet-derived growth factor (PDGF)	160, 175	I	4q11-12 Y10208	Mesenchymal cells, plts, various cancers	Split-tyrosine kinase that serves as Rc for PDGF, which is involved in signal transduction induced by binding PDGF.	*Arterioscler Thromb Vasc Biol 19: 900, 1999* *Proc Natl Acad Sci U S A 93:2884, 1996* *FASEB J 18:341, 2003*
CD140b	β-chain of Rc for platelet-derived growth factor	160, 180	I	5q23-31	Mesenchymal cells, monocytes, PMN, various cancers	Same as CD140a.	*Biochim Biophys Acta 1305:63, 1996* *J Biol Chem 279:19732, 2004*
CD141	Thrombomodulin, fetomodulin	75 (105)	I	20p12-cen AF495471	Endothelial cells, PMN, keratinocytes, smooth muscle, megakaryocytes, monocytes, synovial lining	C-type lectin critical for activation of protein C and may play a role in cell adhesion.	*Hematol Rev 9:251, 1996* *J Biol Chem 278:46750, 2003* *Blood 89:652, 1997*

(Continued)

TABLE 14-1   CLUSTER OF DIFFERENTIATION ANTIGENS DEFINED AS OF THE SEVENTH INTERNATIONAL WORKSHOP ON LEUKOCYTE TYPING (*Continued*)

ANTIGEN	OTHER NAMES	SIZE	O	GENETICS	DISTRIBUTION	PHYSIOLOGY	SELECTED REFERENCES
CD142	Tissue factor, thromboplastin, coagulation factor III, F3	45–47	I	1p22-p21 AF540377	Keratinocyte, epithelia, adventitia, stromal cells, act. monocytes and endothelial cells, some PMN	Serine protease cofactor that acts as major initiator of clotting in normal hemostasis and thrombotic diseases.	FASEB J 9:883, 1995 J Thromb Haemost 1:1920, 2003 Blood 102:3998, 2003
CD143	Peptidyl dipeptidase A, ACE (angiotensin-converting enzyme), kininase II	170	I	17q23 P12821	Endothelial cells, proximal renal tubules, neuronal cells, mesenchymal tissues, some T cells	Acts as a peptidyl dipeptide hydrolase to metabolize angiotensin II, bradykinin, substance P, LH-RH, other dipeptides	J Hypertens 13:S3, 1995 J Biol Chem 269:26806, 1994
CD144	VE-cadherin, cadherin-5	135	I	16q22.1 AB035304	Endothelium	Involved in homotypic binding and maintenance of endothelial barrier function.	J Biol Chem 278:19199, 2003 Am J Physiol Lung Cell Mol Physiol 285:L434, 2003
CDw145		110, 90, 25			Endothelium, stromal cells	Unknown.	Leucocyte Typing VI, Garland Scientific Publishing, NY, p 754, 1998
CD146	Melanoma cell adhesion molecule (MCAM), Muc 18, S-ENDO, Mel-CAM, A32	118 (130)	I	11q23.3 BC056418	Endothelium, sm. muscle, subset act. T cells, FDC	Potential adhesion molecule, esp. of neural crest cells during development.	Curr Topics Micobiol Immunol 213: 95, 1996 Thromb Haemost 90:915, 2003 Cytogenet Cell Genet 87:258, 1999
CD147	M6, EMMPRIN (extracellular matrix metaloproteinase inducer)	54 (65)	I	19p13.3 X64364	Act. lymphocytes, monocytes, resting WBC (weak)	Binds unknown ligand on fibroblasts to induce production of collagenase and extracellular MMP.	Cancer Res 55:434, 1995 Biochem Biophys Res Commun 224: 33, 1996
CD148	HTPT-η, DEP-1 (high cell density-enhanced phosphotyrosine phosphatase-1), p260	220–250	I	11p11.2 D37781	PMN, monocytes, plts, fibroblasts, DC, nerve cells	Phosphotyrosine phosphatase that increases on contact between cells and may be involved in contact inhibition, lymphocyte signal transduction, and T cell activation.	J Immunol 161:3249, 1998 Blood 91:2800, 1998 Cancer Res 56:4236, 1996
CDw149	MEM-133			see CD47	Blood lymphocytes, weakly on plt, PMN, monocytes	MAbs that defined this specificity actually recognize CD47 with low affinity (see CD47).	Leucocyte Typing VII, Oxford University Press, Oxford, p 462, 2002
CD150	SLAM, IPO-3	70	I	Unknown U33017	Thymocytes, some memory T, some B, act. lymphocytes	IgSF that associates with protein kinases and CD45, which may function as costimulatory molecule that also modulates sensitivity to apoptosis.	J Immunol 162:5719, 1999 Nature 376:260, 1995 Immunol Today 17:177, 1996
CD151	PETA-3, SFA-1	32	III Tet.	Unknown U14650	Plt, megakaryocytes, monocytes, epithelial and endothelial cells	May play role in platelet activation, integrin Rc signaling, tumor cell migration, and metastasis.	Cancer Res 59:3812, 1999 J Cell Biol 146:477, 1999 Blood 86:1348, 1995 J Histochem Cytochem 45:515, 1997
CD152	CTLA-4	50 (33)	I	2q33 M74363	Act. T cells	Ligand for CD80 and CD86 that negatively regulates T cell activation.	Science 271:1734, 1996 J Exp Med 185:393, 1997
CD153	CD30-ligand	40	II	9q33 L09753	Act. T cells, act. MØ, neutrophils, B cells	TNF family member that serves as ligand for CD30.	Blood 85:3378, 1995
CD154	CD40-ligand, gp39	39	II	Xq26.3-27.1 Z15017	Act. CD4+ T cells, few act. CD8+ T cells	Ligand for CD40 that induces activation, proliferation and/or differentiation of CD40-expressing cells.	Adv Immunol 61:1, 1996 Annu Rev Immunol 14:591, 1996
CD155	Poliovirus Rc	80–90	I	19q13 P15151	Monocytes	Can serve as Rc for poliovirus, possibly in association with CD44, and ligand for CD226.	Virology 195:798, 1993
CD156a	ADAM 8	69	I	10q26.3 P78325	Monocytes, PMN	A disintegrin and metalloprotease (ADAM) possibly involved in leukocyte extravasation.	Leucocyte Typing VI, Garland Scientific Publishing, NY, p 1083, 1998
CD156b	ADAM 8, MS2, TACE	69	I	10q26.3 P78325	Monocytes, PMN	A disintegrin and metalloprotease (ADAM) that can cleave membrane-bound TNF into a soluble cytokine.	Leucocyte Typing VI, Garland Scientific Publishing, NY, p 1083, 1998
CD157	Mo5, BST-1, BP-3	42–45	V GPI	4p15 Q10588	Monocytes, PMN, marrow stroma, FDC, synovial cells, endothelial cells	ADP-ribosyl cyclase and cADP-ribose hydrolase.	Int Immunol 8:1395, 1996 Int Immunol 8:183, 1996
CD158a	Killer cell inhibitory receptor (KIR)-cl.42, NKAT1, p58.1, EB6-reactive	58/50	I	19q13.4 L41267	Subset of NK cells, some T cells	Ligand for HLA-Cw2, 3, 4, 5, and 6 that regulates NK-mediated cytotoxicity (p58 is inhibitory and p50 is activating.	Annu Rev Immunol 14:619, 1996 Annu Rev Immunol 16:359, 1998 Science 268:405, 1995
CD158b	Killer cell inhibitory receptor (KIR)-cl.6, NKAT2, p58.2, p50.2, GL183-reactive	58/50	I	19q13.4 L41268	Subset of NK cells, some T cells	Ligand for HLA-Cw1, 3, 7, and 8 that regulates NK-mediated cytotoxicity (p58 is inhibitory and p50 is activating).	Annu Rev Immunol 14:619, 1996 Immunological Reviews, Vol. 155, 1997
CD158d	KIRDL1, p70	70	I	19q13.4 P43629	Subset of NK cells, some T cells	Ligand for HLA-B molecules of the Bw4 serologic group that inhibits NK-mediated cytotoxicity.	Annu Rev Immunol 14:619, 1996 Immunol Rev 155:5, 1997 Annu Rev Immunol 16:359, 1998
CD158h	KIRDS4, PAX, p50.3	50	I	19q13.4 P43632	Subset of NK cells, some T cells	Probable ligand for some HLA-C molecules that activates NK cell function.	Annu Rev Immunol 14:619, 1996 Immunol Rev 155:5, 1997 Annu Rev Immunol 16:359, 1998
CD158j	KIRDL2, p140	140	I	19q13.4 P43630	Subset of NK cells, some T cells	Probable ligand for some HLA molecules that may inhibit NK-mediated cytotoxicity.	Annu Rev Immunol 14:619, 1996 Immunol Rev 155:5, 1997 Annu Rev Immunol 16:359, 1998
CD160	BY55, NK1, NK28	27	V GPI	1q42.3 AF060981	Subset of NK cells and CD8 T cells with cytolytic activity, intestinal intraepithelial lymphocytes	Ligand for classic and nonclassic HLA class I molecules that serves as costimulatory molecules for cytotoxic effector cells.	J Immunol 162:1223, 1999 J Immunol 161:2780, 1998
CD161	NKR-P1A	80–85 (40–44)	II	12p12.3-p13.1 U11276	NK cells, weakly on some T cells, monocytes	Group V C-type lectin that may function as a specific Rc for certain NK cell targets.	Annu Rev Immunol 11:613, 1993

TABLE 14-1   CLUSTER OF DIFFERENTIATION ANTIGENS DEFINED AS OF THE SEVENTH INTERNATIONAL WORKSHOP ON LEUKOCYTE TYPING (*Continued*)

ANTIGEN	OTHER NAMES	SIZE	O	GENETICS	DISTRIBUTION	PHYSIOLOGY	SELECTED REFERENCES
CD162	P-selectin glycoprotein ligand-1	220 (120)	I	12q24 U02297	PMN, monocytes, most lymphocytes	Binds to CD62P, CD62E, and CD62L, helps mediate cell migration.	*J Biol Chem* 271:6342, 1996 *Curr Biol* 6:261, 1996
CD163	M130 antigen, GHI/61, Ber-Mac3, Ki-M8, SM4	110 (130)	I	Unknown Z22971	Monocytes, MØ	Scavenger Rc group B family member that may play a role in regulation of immune response in inflammatory processes.	*Biochem Biophys Res Commun* 260: 466, 1999 *J Immunol* 161:1883, 1998 *Eur J Immunol* 23:2320, 1993
CD164	MUC-24, multiglycosylated core protein 24 (MGC-24)	160 (80)	I	6q21 Q04900	Epithelial cells, monocytes, marrow stroma	Mucin-like molecule that may mediate adhesion between marrow stroma and hemopoietic progenitors and may be involved in negatively regulating CD34$^+$ hematopoietic progenitor cell growth.	*Blood* 92:849, 1998 *Blood*, 92:2613, 1998 *J Biochem Tokyo* 112:609, 1992
CD165	AD2, gp37	37 (42)			Plts, thymocytes, T, B, and NK cells, few monocytes,	May play a role in intercellular adhesion between thymocytes and thymic epithelial cells.	*J Immunol* 154:2012, 1995
CD166	ALCAM, CD6L, BEN, SC-1, DM-GRASP, neurolin, Kg-CAM	105	I	3q13.1-2 L38608	Thymic epithelial cells, act. T cells, CD34$^+$ marrow cells, endothelial cells	May interact with CD6 and play a role in T cell development.	*Blood* 93:826, 1999 *J Exp Med* 181:2213 1995
CD167a	DDR1, tyrosine kinase Rc E (trkE), cell adhesion kinase (cak)	54 (α), 67 (β)	I	6p21.3 U48705	Mammary glands, kidney, lung, colon, thyroid, brain, islets of Langerhans	*P53*-regulated tyrosine kinase that binds various types of collagens, possibly acting to regulate synthesis of collagens and their degrading enzymes.	*FASEB J* 13:S77, 1999 *FASEB J* 14:973, 2000 *Oncogene* 10:609, 1995
CD168	RHAMM, IHABP, HMMR	88, 84		5q33.2 U29343	Subset of thymocytes, act. T and B cells, monocytes, G-CSF mobilized blood cells	Hyaluronan (HA)-binding Rc involved in HA-dependent cell motility.	*Dev Immunol* 7:209, 2000 *J Cell Biochem* 61:569, 1996 *Blood* 87:1891, 1999
CD169	Sialoadhesin, Siglec-1	180–200	I	20p13 AF230073	Stromal MØ, particularly those in spleen, lymph nodes, and marrow	Sialoadhesin that binds sialylated ligands (e.g., MUC-1), especially sialic acid in the α2,3-glycosidic linkage on N- and O-glycans, thereby enhancing cell–cell adhesion.	*Biochem Soc Trans* 24:150, 1996 *Glycoconj J* 14:601, 1997 *J Biol Chem* 275:8633, 2000
CD170	OB binding protein-2, CD33L2, Siglec-5	140 (70)	I	19q13.3 U71383	Monocytes, PMN	Cell adhesion molecule highly related to CD33 that is involved in signal transduction and cell–cell adhesions.	*J Biol Chem* 274:22729, 1999 *Exp Hematol* 31:382, 2003 *Blood* 92:2123, 1998
CD171	L1 cell adhesion molecule, L1CAM	190–220	I	Xq28 NM000425	Neurons, CD4 T cells, some B cells, monocytes, DC	Cell adhesion molecule that facilitates cell–cell interactions and may function as a T cell costimulatory molecule.	*Dev Dyn* 218:260, 2000 *Neuron* 17:587, 1996 *Mol Cell Neurosci* 15:1, 2000
CD172	Signal regulatory protein alpha (SIRP-α), brain Ig-like molecule with tyrosine-based activation motifs	90	I	20p13 AB023430	Myelomonocytic cells, hematopoietic stem/ progenitor cells, brain neurons	Member of the signal regulatory protein family and IgSF involved in negative regulation of receptor tyrosine kinase-coupled signaling processes.	*Cancer Res* 64:117, 2004 *J Neurochem* 72:1402, 1999 *Blood* 94:3633, 1999 *J Biol Chem* 273:22719, 1998
CD173	Blood group H type 2				Carcinomas, endothelial cells, RBC	Carbohydrate specificity regulated in its expression by the fucosyltransferase FUT-1.	*Leucocyte Typing VII, Oxford University Press, Oxford, p 162, 2002*
CD174	Lewis y (Le^y)				Epithelial cells and hematopoietic stem cells	Difucosylated tetrasaccharide found on type 2 blood group oligosaccharides on glycolipids/ proteins formed by α1,2 and α1,3 fucosyltransferases.	*Leucocyte Typing VII, Oxford University Press, Oxford, p 199, 2002*
CD175	Tn				Hematopoietic cells, leukemia cell lines, adenoCA	Carbohydrate specificity consisting of a monosaccharde attached in an O-linked fashion.	*Leucocyte Typing VII, Oxford University Press, Oxford, p 201, 2002*
CD175s	Sialyl-Tn				Hematopoietic cells especially in CFU-E to erythroblasts	Carbohydrate specificity dependent upon sialyltransferase ST6GalNAcI.	*Leucocyte Typing VII, Oxford University Press, Oxford, p 162, 2002* *Blood* 83:84, 1994
CD176	Thomsen-Friedenreich (TF) Ag, pan-CA Ag				Epithelium, hematopoietic cells, various adenoCA, leukemia cell lines	Disaccharide, Galβ1-3GalNAcα1-, attached to various protein carriers via O-glycosyl linkage that binds to asialoglycoprotein Rc on hepatocytes.	*Leucocyte Typing VII, Oxford University Press, Oxford, p 202, 2002* *J Mol Med* 75:594, 1997 *Cancer* 76:1700, 1995
CD177	NB1	56–64	V GPI	19q13.2 AJ290452	PMN and some neutrophil precursors	Member of leukocyte Ag (Ly-6) superfamily involved in neutrophil proliferation and polycythemia vera.	*Br J Haematol* 126:252, 2004 *J Transl Med* 2:8, 2004 *Eur J Immunol* 31:1301, 2001
CD178	Fas ligand, APO-1, TNFSF6	70 (40–42)	II	1q23 NM000639	Act. T cells, NK, neutrophils, eye parenchyma, astrocytes, placenta	Member of TNF superfamily that induces ligation of CD95 (Fas).	*Immunol Today* 9:121, 1998 *Annu Rev Genet* 33:29, 1999 *Immunol Today* 20:46, 1999
CD179a	Vpre-B	16–18		22q11.22 S74019	Pro-B and pre-B cells	Associates noncovalently with CD179b to form an Ig light chain-like structure on developing pro-B and pre-B cell that plays a critical role in early B cell differentiation.	*Adv Immunol* 63:1, 1996 *Proc Natl Acad Sci U S A* 96:2571, 1999
CD179b	Lambda5	22		22q11.23 M27749	Pro-B and early pre-B cells	Associates noncovalently with CD179a to form an Ig light chain-like structure on developing pro-B and pre-B cell that plays a critical role in early B cell differentiation.	*Adv Immunol* 63:1, 1996 *Proc Natl Acad Sci U S A* 96:2571, 1999
CD180	RP105, LY64, Bgp95	95–105	I	5q12 NM005582	Mantle zone and marginal zone B cells, monocytes, DC	Toll-like Rc that, upon ligation, induces activation leading to up-regulation of CD80 and CD86 and increase in cell size.	*J Exp Med* 188:93, 1998 *J Exp Med* 187:663, 1998 *Blood* 92:2815, 1998

(Continued)

TABLE 14-1   CLUSTER OF DIFFERENTIATION ANTIGENS DEFINED AS OF THE SEVENTH INTERNATIONAL WORKSHOP ON LEUKOCYTE TYPING (*Continued*)

ANTIGEN	OTHER NAMES	SIZE	O	GENETICS	DISTRIBUTION	PHYSIOLOGY	SELECTED REFERENCES
CD183	CXCR3, GPR9, CXC-L2, IP10-R, Mig-R	41	III	Xq13 X95876	Act. T cells, some B and NK cells, plasmacytoid DC, eos	G protein-coupled Rc for CXC chemokines IP10 (INF-γ inducible 10-kDa protein), Mig (monokine induced by IFN-γ), and I-TAC (IFN-inducible T cell α-chemoattractant).	*Adv Immunol 74:127, 2000* *Pharmacol Rev 52:145, 2000* *Crit Rev Immunol 19:1, 1999*
CD184	CXCR4, Fusin, LESTR, NPY3R, HM89, FB22, LCR1, HUMSTR	40	III	2q21 AF005058	B and T cells, monocytes, MØ, DC, PMN, endothelial and epitheial cells, astrocytes	G protein-coupled Rc for CXC chemokine CXCL12, also known as stromal derived factor 1-alpha (SDF-1α).	*Ann Rev Immunol 17:657, 1999* *Adv Immunol 74:127, 2000* *Pharmacol Rev 52:145, 2000*
CD195	C-C motif chemokine Rc 5 (CCR5)	37	III	3q21 NM000579	T cells, MØ, monocytes, endothelial/epithelial cells, some neurons, astrocytes	G protein-coupled Rc for C-C type chemokines (e.g., MCP-2, MIP-1α, MIP-1β, RANTES) that also may play a role in cell proliferation/differentiation.	*Biochemisry 35:3362, 1996* *Proc Natl Acad Sci U S A 96:7922, 1999* *Eur J Biochem 263:746, 1999*
CDw197	C-C motif chemokine Rc 7 (CCR7), BLR2, EBI1	40	III	17q12-q21.2 NM001838	Lymphocytes, thymus, blood-derived DC, MØ, monocytes	G protein-coupled Rc for C-C type chemokines (e.g., CCL19/ECL or MIP-3β, SLC) that is up-regulated by infection with Epstein-Barr virus.	*J Biol Chem 272:13803, 1997* *J Immunol 161:2580, 1998* *Immunity 12:121, 2000*
CD200	OX2	40–50	I		Thymocytes, B cells, act. T cells, FDC, neurons, endothelium, kidney glomeruli, smooth muscle	Member of IgSF that serves as ligand for OX2 Rc found on MØ, PMN, monocytes, DC, and microglia involved in intercellular signaling.	*EMBO J 4:113, 1985* *Leucocyte Typing VII, Oxford University Press, Oxford, p 471, 2002*
CD201	Endothelial protein C Rc (EPCR)	30–40	I	20q11,2 BC014451	Endothelium of large vessels	Binds to activated protein C to augment its activation by the thrombin–thrombomodulin complex. A soluble form in plasma can inhibit anticoagulant activity of protein C.	*J Thromb Haemost 1:495, 2003* *Biochem J 373:65, 2003* *Blood 101:4797, 2003*
CD202b	Tyrosine kinase with Ig and EGF homology domains (Tie2), tunica interna endothelial cell kinase (tek)	140	I	9p21	Endothelial cells, angioblasts	Rc for angiopoietin-1, -2, and -4, which are involved in vascular development.	*Mol Cell Biol 12:1698, 1992* *Proc Natl Acad Sci U S A 96:1904, 1999* *Hum Pathol 35:176, 2004* *Arthritis Rheum 48:2461, 2003*
CD203c	E-NPP3 (nucleotide pyrophosphatase 3), B10, Gp130RB13-6	270 (130, 150)	II	6q22 AF005632	Basophils, mast cells, uterus, pancreas, intestine, liver, immature glial cells	Ectoenzyme that catalyzes hydrolysis of extracellular nucleotides (e.g., nucleoside phosphates, NAD, and oligonucleotides).	*J Leukoc Biol 67:285, 2000* *Immunol Rev 161:11, 1998* *Immunol Rev 161:5, 1998*
CD204	Class A MØ scavenger Rc	220	I	8q22 D13263	Tissue MØ	Rc for low-density lipoproteins that also functions in recognition of pathogenic microorganisms.	*J Biol Chem 278:34219, 2003* *J Biol Chem 268:2120, 1993*
CD205	DEC205, gp200-MR6, LY75	200	I	2q24 AF011333	Tingible body MØ, interdigitating and blood-derived DC, criptic epithelia	Involved in Ag uptake and Ag processing.	*Immunogenetics 47:442, 1998* *J Biol Chem 278:34035, 2003*
CD206	MMR (macrophage mannose Rc), mannose Rc, C-type lectin, MRC1	162–175	I	10p13 J05550	Subset of mononuclear phagocytes, endothelial cells, some DC, retinal epithelium	Rc for glycans and sulfated sugars involved in phagocytosis and endocytosis.	*Adv Exp Med Biol 479:1, 2000* *Curr Opin Immunol 10:50, 1998* *Immunol Rev 163:19, 1998*
CD207	Langerin	40–45	II	2p13 AJ242859	Langerhans DC	C-type lectin with mannose-binding activity that may facilitate internalization of Ag into Birbeck granules for nonclassical antigen presentation.	*Immunity 12:71, 2000* *Eur J Immunol 29:2695, 1999* *J Clin Invest 113:701, 2004*
CD208	DC lysosomal-associated protein (DC-LAMP)	50	I	3q26.3-q27 AJ005766	DC and CD40-activated B cells	Lysosomal associated protein that may facilitate Ag processing.	*Immunity 9:325, 1998* *Cancer Res 58:3499, 1998*
CD209	DC-SIGN (DC-specific ICAM-3 grabbing nonintegrin)	45	II	19p13 AF290886	DC and small subset of blood CD14+ mononuclear cells	Rc for ICAM-3 (CD50), ICAM-2 (CD102), HIV-1 gp120.	*Cell 100:575, 2000* *Cell 100:587, 2000* *Am J Pathol 164:1587, 2004*
CDw210	IL-10 Rc, IL10R1	70–75	I	11q23 U00672	Hematopoietic cells, lymphocytes, monocytes, MØ	Rc for IL-10 that can trigger tyrosine phosphrylation of JAK1 and TYK2 kinases.	*Proc Natl Acad Sci U S A 99:9409, 2002* *J Immunol 170:5578, 2003*
CD212	IL-12 Rc β-component	85	I	19p13.1 U03187	Act. T cells, NK cells, and some monocytes	Binds IL-12 with low affinity and serves as part of the high-affinity Rc for IL-12.	*Ann N Y Acad Sci 31:36, 1996* *Hum Genet 112:237, 2003*
CD213a1	IL-13 Rc α 1	65	I	Xq24 Y10659	Some lymphocytes, immature DC, heart, liver, ovary	α-Subunit of Rc for IL-13 that may mediate signaling via JAK1, STAT3, and STAT6.	*Imunogenetics 51:1499, 2000* *FEBS Lett 550:139, 2003*
CD213a2	IL-13 Rc α 2	50	I	Xq13.1-q28 Y08768	Some lymphocytes, immature DC	β-Subunit of Rc for IL-13 that lacks a cytoplasmic domain, but with CD213a plays a role in binding and internalization of IL-13.	*J Biol Chem 276:25114, 2001* *Genomics 42:141, 1997* *Immunol Rev 202:191, 2004*
CDw217	IL-17 Rc	120	I	22q11.1 BC011624	Thymocytes, leukocytes, fibroblast-like synoviocytes	Low affinity Rc for IL-17.	*Clin Exp Immunol 127:539, 2002* *Nature 402:489, 2000*
CD220	Insulin Rc	84, 70	I	19p13.3-p13.2 M10051	Widely expressed on many tissues	High-affinity Rc for insulin with low affinity for insulin-like growth factors that stimulates glucose uptake.	*J Biol Chem 277:39684, 2002* *J Biol Chem 277:47380, 2002*
CD221	Type I insulin-like growth factor Rc (IGF1 Rc)	80, 71	I	15q26.3 X04434	Widely expressed on many tissues and overexpressed in many cancers	High-affinity Rc for insulin-like growth factors with low affinity for insulin that stimulates glucose uptake.	*Proc Natl Acad Sci U S A 101: 2076, 2004* *Am J Physiol Endocrinol Metab 286:E896, 2004*
CD222	Man-6p Rc, Insulin-like growth factor type-2 Rc (IGFII-R)	230, 250, 280, 300	I	6q26-q27 J03528	Ubiquitous	Rc for insulin-like growth factor type 2 that internalizes or sorts lysosomal enzymes and other M6P-containing proteins (e.g., latent transforming growth factor-β).	*Biochem Soc Trans 24:136, 1996* *FASEB J 11:60, 1997* *Annu Rev Biochem 61:307, 1992*

TABLE 14-1   CLUSTER OF DIFFERENTIATION ANTIGENS DEFINED AS OF THE SEVENTH INTERNATIONAL WORKSHOP ON LEUKOCYTE TYPING (*Continued*)

ANTIGEN	OTHER NAMES	SIZE	O	GENETICS	DISTRIBUTION	PHYSIOLOGY	SELECTED REFERENCES
CD223	Lymphocyte-activation protein (LAG-3)	70	I	12p13.32 X51985	NK, some T cells	Rc for MHC class II that is stucturally related to CD4 and may serve as costimulatory/ adhesion molecule in Ag presentation.	*Trends Immunol 24:619, 2003* *DNA Seq 14:79, 2003* *Blood 102:2130, 2003*
CD224	Gamma-glutamyltransferase 1 (GGT), EC2.3.2.2	62–68, 22	II	22q11.23 X60069	Some B and T cells, hematopoietic precursors	Ectoenzyme involved in degradation and neosynthesis of glutathione.	*Mol Cell Biochem 232:160, 2002* *Biochem J 297:503, 1994*
CD225	Leu13, interferon-induced transmembrane protein	16–18	I	11p15.5 J04164	B and T cells, NK, vascular endothelial cells	Noncovalently associates with CD81 to form a signaling complex that triggers diverse biologic responses.	*J Biol Chem 270:23860, 1995* *Radiat Res 160:302, 2003*
CD226	DNAM-1, platelet and T cell activation antigen 1 (PTA1), TLisA1	≈65	I	18q22.3 U56102	Act. T cells, NK cells, plts, monocytes, and some B cells and thymocytes	IgSF member that associates with CD11a/CD18, serves as adhesion Rc for CD155 and CD112, and facilitates NK or T cell mediated cytotoxicity or plt adhesion.	*J Biol Chem 272:21735, 1997* *Immunity 11:615, 1999* *J Exp Med 199:1331, 2004*
CD227	MUC1, episialin, DF3, H23	220–700	I	1q21 M61170	Apical surface of all glandular epithelial cells, act. T cells, monocytes, some B cells, FDC, some hematopoietic cells	Transmembrane epithelial mucin that can bind various other proteins (e.g., CD54, selectins, CD169, Grb2, β-catenin, GSK-3β) involved in multiple signal transduction pathways.	*Immunol Rev 145:61, 1995* *Annu Rev Physiol 57:607, 1995* *Glycobiology 10:439, 2000*
CD228	Melanotransferrin	97	V GPI	3q28-q29 AH002920	Melanomas, myoepithelial cells, liver parachyma, brain capillary endothelium	Structurally related to transferrin, may help sequester iron at the cell surface membrane.	*Blood 102:1723, 2002* *Eur J Biochem 269:4435, 2002*
CD229	Ly9	120	I	1q21.2-q22 AF244129	Mature T and B cells	Cytoplasmic tail contains 2 tyrosine-based motifs, inferring that CD229 plays a role in cell signaling.	*Immunogenetics 43:13, 1996* *Leucocyte Typing VII, Oxford University Press, Oxford, p 505, 2002*
CD230	Prion protein	33–37	V GPI	20pter-p12 M13899	Widely expressed on most cell types, expecially on neurons	Sialoglycoprotein that can assume a conformational change to aggregate into protease resistant prions-proteinacous particles seen in prion diseases.	*Leucocyte Typing VII, Oxford University Press, Oxford, p 507, 2002* *J Biol Chem 279:18008, 2004* *J Biol Chem 278:50175, 2003*
CD231	TALLA-1, SN1, SN1a	150 (28–45)	III Tet.	Xq11 NM004615	T cell ALL, neurons, neuroblastoma	Tetraspan protein identified as marker for T cell ALL.	*J Immunol 229:35, 1999* *Tissue Antigens 48:460, 1996*
CD232	Virus-encoded semaphorin protein Rc (VESP Rc), plexin C1	300 (150)	I	12q23.3 AF030339	Lymphocytes (weak), monocytes, PMN, some DC	Rc that binds a semaphorin derived from a virus and may play a role in immune modulation.	*Cell 99:71, 1999* *Immunity 8:473, 1998*
CD233	Band 3, SLC4A1, anion exchange protein (AE1), Diego blood group, EPB3	95–110	III	17q21-q22 S68680	RBC; a truncated form is expressed in the renal distal tubules	Functions as a bicarbonate transporter/anion exchanger and as attachment site for RBC cytoskeleton. Mutations in CD233 can result in hereditary spherocytosis, renal tubular acidosis, or novel RBC antigens (e.g., Diego blood group).	*Mol Membr Biol 14:155, 1997* *Blood 96:2925, 2000* *Biochemistry 43:1633, 2004*
CD234	Fu-glycoprotein, Duffy Ag	35–43	III	1q21-q22 BC017817	RBC, postcapillary venules, high-endothelial venules, endothelium of spleen and marrow, Purkinje cells, renal collecting ducts, lung alveoli	Rc for CC chemokines (RANTES, MCP-1) and CXC (IL-8, MSGA) that also bind *Plasmodium vivax*.	*J Immunol 170:5244, 2003* *Am J Hum Genet 70:369, 2002* *Proc Natl Acad Sci U S A 90: 10793, 1993*
CD235a	Glycophorin A, GYPA		I	4q28.2-q31.1 L31860	RBC	Major sialoglycoprotein that bears the antigenic determinants of the MN and Ss blood groups and binds some strains of *Plasmodium falciparum*.	*J Biol Chem 278:3254, 2003* *Mol Biol Evol 19.223, 2002* *Transfus Clin Biol 4:357, 1997*
CD235b	Glycophorin B		I	4q28.2-q31 J02982	RBC	Major sialoglycoprotein that bears the antigenic determinants of the MN and Ss blood groups.	*Transfus Clin Biol 4:357, 1997* *J Biol Chem 269:10804, 1994*
CD236	Glycophorin C	40	I	2q14-q21 X12496	RBC	Glycoprotein that bears the antigenic determinants of the Berbich blood groups system, can serve as Rc for *Plasmodium falciparum*.	*Blood 101:4628, 2003* *Nat Med 9:87, 2002*
CD236c/d	Glycophorin C/D, glycophorin D	30	I	2q14-q21 X12496	RBC	Truncated form of CD236 because of mutation, resulting in loss of the first 21 N-terminal amino acids, forming the Webb and Duch antigens.	*Blood 82:3198, 1993* *Transfus Clin Biol 9:121, 2002*
CD238	Kell	93	II	7q33 M64934	RBC, testis, weak on various other tissues (e.g., brain, heart, skeletal muscle)	Member of the neprilysin family of zinc metalloproteases that acts on big endothelin-3, a potent vasoconstrictor.	*Blood 102:3028, 2003* *Blood 85:912, 1995*
CD239	B cell adhesion molecule (B-CAM), Lutheran blood group	85, 78	I	19q13.2 BC050450	RBC, basal epithelium, endothelium, weak on many other cell types	Member of IgSF that may play a role in terminal RBC differentiation.	*Blood 89:19, 1997* *Am J Hematol 75:63, 2004*
CD240CE	Rh30CE, RHCE	30	III	1p36.11 AB030388	RBC	Forms part of Rh complex on RBC membrane composed of two CD240 chains and CD241, CD47, CD235B, and CD242 that may play a role in ammonium transport	*Transfusion 44:407, 2004* *Proc Natl Acad Sci U S A 100: 8793, 2003* *J Biol Chem 277:12499, 2002* *Br J Haematol 122:333, 2003*
CD240D	Rh30D, RHD	32	III	1p36.11 AB018969	RBC	Loss of CD240D results in Rh-negative RBC phenotype.	*Blood 100:1038, 2002* *Transfusion 42:627, 2002*

(Continued)

TABLE 14-1   CLUSTER OF DIFFERENTIATION ANTIGENS DEFINED AS OF THE SEVENTH INTERNATIONAL WORKSHOP ON LEUKOCYTE TYPING (*CONTINUED*)

ANTIGEN	OTHER NAMES	SIZE	O	GENETICS	DISTRIBUTION	PHYSIOLOGY	SELECTED REFERENCES
CD241	RhAg, Rh50	32 (45–100)	III	6p11-p21.1 X64594	RBC, express the glycosylated antigen of 45–100 μDa	Forms part of Rh complex on RBC membrane; also is composed of two CD240 chains, CD47, CD235B, and CD242 and may play a role in ammonium transport.	Br J Haematol 122:333, 2003 Blood 100:1038, 2002 J Biol Chem 277:12499, 2002
CD242	ICAM-4, Landsteiner-Wiener blood group	37–43	I	19p13.2-cen X93093	RBC	Member of intercellular adhesion molecule (ICAM) family that forms part of Rh complex on RBC membrane and may be involved in integrin adhesion.	Blood 103:1503, 2004 Eur J Biochem 270:1710, 2003
CD243	Multidrug resistance-1 (MDR-1)	170	III	7q21.1 M14758	Widely expressed on epithelia and endothelia	Member of ATP-binding cassette (ABC) transporters involved in transport of various molecules across membranes and multidrug resistance.	Gut 52:759, 2003 Cancer Sci 94;9, 2003
CD244	NK cell Rc 2B4, NK activation-inducing ligand (NAIL), p38	38	I	1q23.1 AF11711	NK cell, γδ T cells, some CD8 thymocytes and subsets of CD8 cytotoxic T cells	Rc of IgSF that carries tyrosine-based signaling motifs that can enhance NK cell activation, cytotoxicity, and function.	Mol Cell Biol 24:5144, 2004 J Exp Med 197:77, 2003 J Immunol 167:6210, 2001
CD245	P220/240	220–240			Mononuclear leukocytes, PMN (weak), plt (weak)	May be involved in signal transduction and co-stimulation of T and NK cells.	Leucocyte Typing VII, Oxford University Press, Oxford, p 691, 2002
CD246	Anaplastic lymphoma kinase (ALK), Ki-1	200	I	2p23 U66559	Scattered cells in the adult brain; otherwise absent from normal adult tissues	Single-chain Rc tyrosine kinase that serves as an Rc for growth factor pleiotrophin and can form oncogenic fusion proteins resulting from translocations.	Am J Pathol 156:1711, 2000 J Biol Chem 276:16772, 2001 Blood 94:3265, 1999
CD247	Zeta chain, CD3ζ	16	I	1q22-q23 J04132	T cells	Zeta chain of the CD3 T cell receptor complex (see Chap. 78)	Biochemistry 43:2049, 2004 J Biol Chem 279:7760, 2004

The CD designation is listed in the far left column labeled "Antigen." Common names of an antigen before it was given CD status are listed in the column labeled "Other Names." The molecular size(s) of the nonreduced CD antigen is listed in the column labeled "Size." If the molecular size(s) of the reduced CD antigen is different, then the size is provided in parentheses. The orientation or anchorage to the plasma membrane of each protein is listed in the column labeled "O." The chromosomal location of the gene(s) encoding a surface antigen and the GenBank Accession number of the cDNA encoding the molecule are listed in the column labeled "Genetics." Tissue and cell types that are known to express a particular CD are listed in the column marked "Distribution." The proposed or known physiology of a CD antigen is listed in the column labeled "Physiology." A few key references and/or reviews concerning each CD antigen are listed in the column labeled "Selected References."

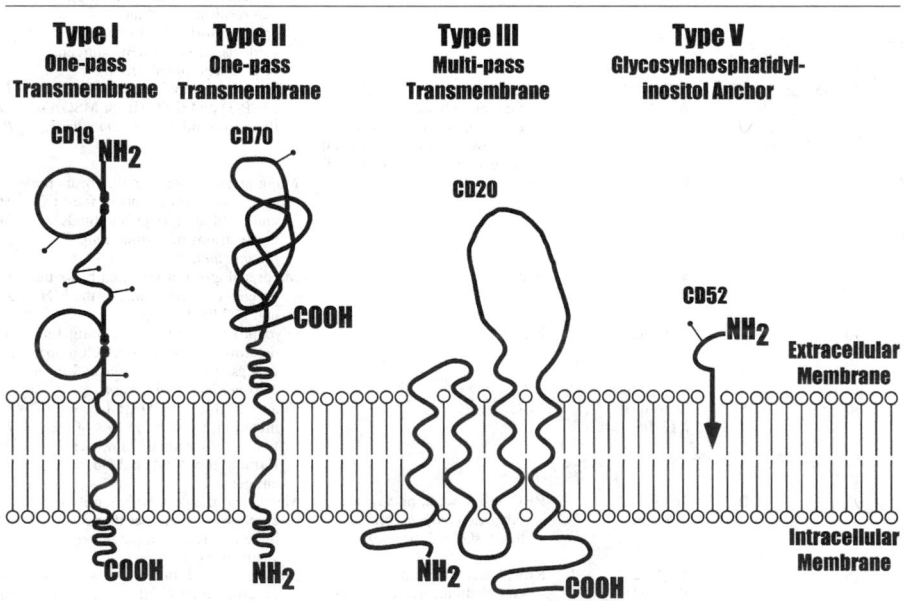

FIGURE 14-1   Major different types of surface proteins with respect to how they integrate into the membrane bilayer. The types of membrane protein are indicated at the *top*. The *straight lines* attached to the *open circles* represent the lipid bilayer. The *colored lines* represent the polypeptide backbones. The *thin pegs* extending from the polypeptide backbone represent carbohydrates. CD19 (*far left*) is a type I transmembrane protein that passes through the membrane once. It has its C-terminus (COOH) in the cytoplasm and N-terminus (NH₂) outside the cell. CD70 (*second from left*) is a type II single-pass transmembrane protein with the N-terminus inside the cell. CD20 (*second from right*) is a type III multispan protein that also is a tetraspan molecule in that it traverses the lipid bilayer four times. The tetraspan proteins have both the N-terminus and C-terminus in the cytoplasm. CD52 (*far right*) is a glycosylphosphatidyl-inositol (GPI) anchored protein. *Labels at the far right* indicate the extracellular and intracellular membranes.

inside the surface membrane bilayer. The transmembrane domain does not contain any charged amino acid residues, such as Arg, Asn, Asp, Glu, Gln, His, or Lys, except when it associates with the transmembrane domain of another cell surface protein(s) to form a multimeric complex. An example of this formation is the multimeric complex formed by the CD3 proteins, CD247, and the two chains of the T cell receptor for antigen (see Chap. 78).

TYPE II TRANSMEMBRANE PROTEINS (II)

Type II transmembrane proteins have an orientation opposite to that of type I transmembrane proteins. The NH_2-terminus is located inside the cell and the COOH-terminus is located extracellularly. These proteins often have uncleaved signal sequences for transmembrane domains, allowing for their cleavage and release from the cell surface. As such, these proteins may double as cell surface antigens and plasma proteins, each often having a physiologic effect(s) on cells bearing the respective ligand(s).

TYPE III TRANSMEMBRANE PROTEINS (III)

Type III transmembrane proteins cross the plasma membrane more than once. Some pass through the bilayer as many as 12 times, such as the multidrug resistance transporter protein MDR-1, now designated as CD243. Because these proteins cross the membrane multiple times, the molecules can form channels that often are used to transport ions or small molecules through the lipid bilayer. An important subgroup of type III transmembrane proteins that commonly are found on leukocytes is the tetraspan family. These proteins each pass through the surface bilayer four times and have both COOH-termini and NH_2-termini inside the cell. Many of the type III transmembrane proteins listed in Table 14-1 belong to this family. An example is CD20, a molecule postulated to form a calcium channel for B lymphocytes that is required for B cell activation.

TYPE IV TRANSMEMBRANE PROTEINS (IV)

Type IV proteins can be distinguished from type III proteins by the presence of a water-filled transmembrane channel. None of the current CD antigens have such a membrane organization.

TYPE V GLYCOSYL-PHOSPHATIDYLINOSITOL ANCHORED PROTEINS

Type V proteins use lipid to attach themselves to the plasma membrane. The most common attachment for extracellular proteins in this category is the glycosyl-phosphatidylinositol (GPI) anchor. The GPI anchor can be cleaved by the bacterial enzyme phosphatidylinositol phospholipase C (PI-PLC). Release of an antigen from the cell surface by treatment with PI-PLC often is used to verify that the surface protein has a GPI anchor. However, this criterion is not absolute, as some GPI-anchored proteins are resistant to PI-PLC.

Newly synthesized proteins destined to receive a GPI anchor each contains a secretion signal sequence at the NH_2-terminus and another signal sequence at the COOH-terminus. The latter directs cleavage and subsequent appendage of a GPI anchor soon after the molecule's biosynthesis and extrusion into the endoplasmic reticulum. This biosynthetic pathway is defective in paroxysmal nocturnal hemoglobinuria (PNH) (see Chap. 38).

The site of attachment for GPI generally precedes a hydrophobic domain of seven to 20 amino acids that sometimes doubles as an actual transmembrane domain. In this case, the molecule may exist as either of two isoforms, one attached to the membrane via a GPI anchor and another as a type I transmembrane protein. Because GPI-anchored proteins associate specifically with sphingomyelin lipids, follow a different path of transport to the cell surface than type I transmembrane proteins, are excluded from coated pits, and are not able to associate directly with intracellular proteins, a GPI isoform of a given surface protein usually has a physiology that is distinct from that of its respective type I transmembrane isoform.

TISSUE DISTRIBUTION OF MEMBRANE ANTIGENS

The tissue distributions for each CD antigen listed in Table 14-1 summarize the work of many laboratories. However, comprehensive analysis of the full gamut of different tissues has not been performed for most CD antigens. Therefore, failure to list in Table 14-1 a cell type for a particular CD antigen does not necessarily mean that cell type does not express that antigen. A complete review of the tissue distributions of the CD antigens is given in the summary books published after each workshop.[1-3] References to these books are implied, but not necessarily cited, for each CD antigen listed.

Some surface antigens are useful for delineating the cell lineage of leukocytes. Unique assignment of a surface antigen to a particular lineage is best when the antigen is related to a unique functional property of a given cell type. The CD3 surface antigens form part of the T cell receptor complex for antigen (see Chap. 78). As such, CD3 is expressed exclusively by mature lymphocytes of the T cell lineage. In a similar vein, surface immunoglobulin (sIg) is a B cell lineage specific marker. The presence of sIg on a given cell may be misleading, however, because of expression on diffuse cell types of Fc receptors for soluble and/or aggregated Ig. Instead, expression of CD79α and CD79β, two chains that associate with sIg to form part of the B cell surface antigen receptor, may be more precise in defining B lineage cells (see Chap. 77). In addition, CD20 is another antigen found exclusively on lymphocytes of the B cell lineage.

Many CD antigens are expressed at varying levels by many different cell types. Rather than the exclusive expression of a single CD antigen with a particular cell type, the peculiar constellation of surface antigens expressed by a given cell helps assign the cell to a particular lineage or sublineage of cells. Increasingly, the resolution of many important cell subpopulations requires two or more color multiparameter flow cytometric analyses.

REFERENCES

1. Schlossman SF, Boumsell L, Gilks W, et al: *Leucocyte Typing V, White Cell Differentiation Antigens.* Oxford University Press, Oxford, 1995.
2. Kishimoto T, Kikutani H, von dem Borne AE, et al: *Leucocyte Typing VI, White Cell Differentiation Antigens.* Garland Science Publishing, New York, 1998.
3. Mason D, André P, Bensussan A, et al: *Leucocyte Typing VII, White Cell Differentiation Antigens.* Oxford University Press, Oxford, 2002.
4. Barclay AN, Brown MH, McKnight AJ, et al: *The Leucocyte Antigen Facts Book,* 2nd ed. Academic Press, San Diego, 1997.

HEMATOPOIETIC STEM CELLS, PROGENITORS, AND CYTOKINES

KENNETH KAUSHANSKY

Blood cell production is an enormously complex process in which a small number of hematopoietic stem cells (HSCs) expand and differentiate into an excess of 10^{11} cells each day. Based on a number of strategies available to the experimental hematologist a hierarchy of hematopoietic stem, progenitor, and mature blood cells is emerging in which each successive developmental stage loses the potential to differentiate into a specific type or class of cells. The characteristics of the stem and progenitor cells that give rise to the formed elements of the blood are the subject of this chapter, including the roles played by transcription factors and external signals in lineage fate determination, the cytokines and cell adhesion molecules that support cell survival, self-renewal, expansion and differentiation, and the cell surface properties that allow for their purification, and biochemical and genetic characterization. A thorough understanding of hematopoietic stem and progenitor cells and their supportive microenvironment can provide critical insights into developmental biology of multiple cell systems, favorably impact blood cell development for therapeutic benefit, impact genetic therapy for a number of blood and other disorders of man, and potentially even provide the tools necessary to allow the regeneration of multiple organs.

AN OVERVIEW OF HEMATOPOIESIS

Blood cell production is an enormous and complex process. Based on the adult blood volume (5 liters), the number of each of the blood cell types per microliter of blood, and their circulatory half-life, it can be calculated that each day an adult human produces 2×10^{11} erythrocytes, 1×10^{11} leukocytes, and 1×10^{11} platelets. Over the past 4 decades experimental hematologists have developed a model of blood cell production in which a hierarchical developmental progression of primitive, multipotential HSCs gradually lose one or more developmental potentials and ultimately become committed to a single cell lineage, which matures into the corresponding blood cell type.[1] Perhaps one of the most compelling arguments supporting this model of hematopoiesis is derived from extensive purification schemes using cell surface markers that yield cells at each predicted developmental stage[2] (Fig. 15-1). Although hematopoietic development is considered by most investigators as an irreversible stepwise and progressive loss of developmental potentials, studies now suggest that cells undergoing apparent differentiation steps might oscillate between different stages depending on their position in the cell cycle.[3] But regardless of the precise relationships between different stages of hematopoietic development, the availability of this model and the data leading to its construction have provided important insights into the biology and clinical uses of hematopoietic stem and progenitor cells. This chapter focuses on our understanding of the molecular basis for blood cell development, beginning with the HSC and its offspring, the lineage-committed progenitor cells.

DEVELOPMENTAL BIOLOGY OF HEMATOPOIESIS

Blood cell production begins in the yolk sac,[4] where extraembryonic mesoderm develops into angioblasts and primitive erythroid precursors at day 7 postcoitum of the mouse; cells of the outer layer of the undifferentiated mesoderm at this time flatten and become endothelial cells, and the inner cells round up to become clusters of erythroid precursors,[5] termed *blood islands*. Like in the embryo proper, there is much evidence to suggest that these two cells are derived from a common precursor (the hemangioblast).[6] Once adjacent blood islands begin to coalesce on day 8, the endothelial cells form vascular channels, which by day 8.5 connect with the embryonic vasculature, allowing yolk sac blood cells to exit the blood islands, complete their maturation, and enucleate in the embryonic bloodstream.[7] In both mouse and man there is a stage of embryonic development where both primitive erythrocytes (as characterized by ζ globin phenotype) and definitive red cells are produced in the yolk sac, although the former appear only very transiently. Although not as well characterized, yolk sac myelopoiesis and thrombopoiesis also occur, perhaps as part of the development of multipotent progenitors that appear by day 8.5 postcoitum. Cells capable of differentiating into multiple cell lineages become recognizable early during yolk sac hematopoiesis.[8] However, such cells reproducibly engraft only in the marrow of myeloablated embryonic animals and not in adults,[9] making it unlikely that such cells are true HSCs, although this topic remains controversial. By day 11 postcoitum repopulating HSCs are clearly present in the yolk sac, but the relationship of these cells and the HSCs that are clearly demonstrable a day earlier in the aorta-gonad-mesonephros (AGM) region (see below) is uncertain. By day 12.5 postcoitum hematopoiesis in the murine yolk sac is eliminated.

Although it was long believed that the developmental origin of the adult mammalian hematopoietic system was the yolk sac, subsequent research has shown that the first adult-type HSCs are derived from mesodermal cells within the AGM region of the embryonic paraaortic splanchnopleure, particularly from the ventral wall of the dorsal aorta.[10-12] The AGM remains a source of hematopoiesis between days 9.5 to 11.5 postcoitum in the mouse and days 30 to 37 in the human.[13,14] Of interest, the development of hematopoietic cells in this region (as well as in the yolk sac) occurs in a "reverse" direction, that is, single lineage-committed progenitors appear prior to multilineage progenitors, which appear prior to stem cells. In this region there are also cells that express a number of molecules in common with endothelial cells, including CD34, the transcription factors SCL and GATA-2, and the receptors c-kit and FLK-1.[15] Moreover, cell culture experiments have established that such cells display combined endothelial and hematopoietic potential, establishing them as "hemangiob-

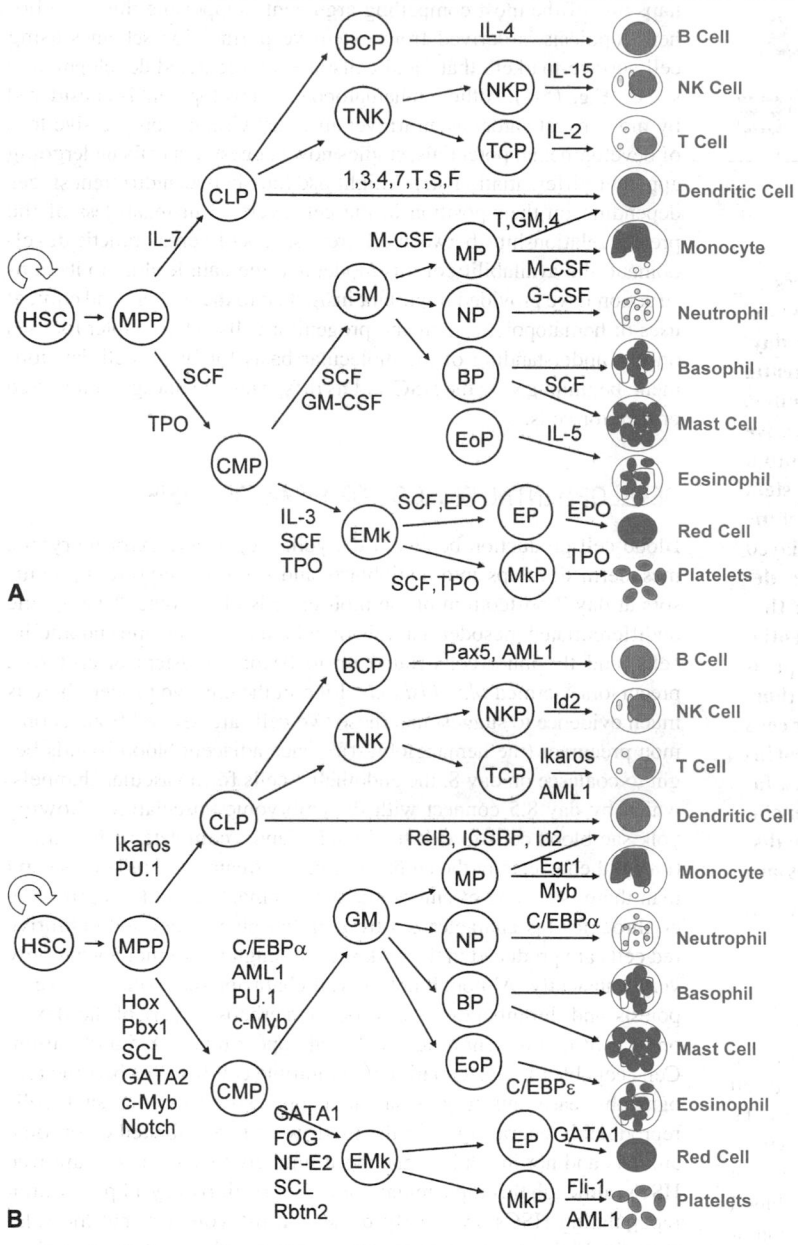

FIGURE 15-1 The figure displays the hematopoietic progenitors that have been defined by *in vitro* assays or by more complex tissue-based assays. In (*A*) the growth factors responsible for cell survival and proliferation at each corresponding stage of hematopoietic development are shown, and in (*B*) the corresponding transcription factors are illustrated. See text for definitions, except that T,GM,4 represents tumor necrosis factor alpha (TNF-α), GM-CSF, and IL-4, and 1,3,4,7,T,S,F represents IL-1, IL-3, IL-4, IL-7, TNF-α, SCF, and Flt3 ligand. Although a single type of macrophage is illustrated, the blood monocyte can differentiate into a plethora of tissue specific macrophage types, including the hepatic Kupffer cell, the brain microglia, and the bone osteoclast (see Chaps. 67 and 69 for details). Similarly, a single dendritic cell is shown, but of two distinct origins, lymphoid or myeloid (see Chap. 18).

lasts," the postulated combined endothelial cell/hematopoietic precursors.[16]

Approximately 2 days following the appearance of HSCs in the AGM region, hematopoiesis begins in the fetal liver. Careful dissection experiments of the 1970s indicate that fetal liver hematopoiesis is dependent on an exogenous source of hematopoietic cells,[17] which populate the fetal liver in two waves, consisting of erythroid and multilineage progenitors around day 9 of murine gestation and committed

progenitors and true HSCs at day 11.[18] Although there is no direct proof, the temporal appearance of these cell types in the AGM approximately 1 to 2 days prior to their appearance in the fetal liver strongly suggests that the former is the source for populating the latter. In humans the fetal liver becomes the major source of blood cells around 5 weeks' gestation, and the marrow begins to populate with hematopoietic cells at 8 weeks' gestation. Unlike the random pattern of cells see in the yolk sac, hematopoiesis in the fetal liver is well organized; erythroid cells are usually found in clusters surrounding a central macrophage and CD15+ myelopoietic cells localize mainly around portal triad vessels, although lymphoid precursors fail to demonstrate a specific localization pattern and are randomly found amongst hepatocytes.[19] Up to 50 percent of the fetal liver is composed of hematopoietic cells at days 12 to 14 of murine embryonic life, a proportion that begins to decrease as hepatocytes replace hematopoietic cells and the latter shift to the marrow, prior to birth.

The final shift in the site of hematopoiesis occurs before birth; although the marrow begins to populate with liver-derived hematopoietic cells at day 16 in the mouse and at 8 weeks' gestation in the human, it is mostly myeloid in nature and contributes little to the circulating blood until just before birth.[20] Hematopoietic stem and progenitor cells circulate in large numbers during fetal life, as clinically witnessed by the use of umbilical cord blood as a rich source of HSCs for transplantation. However, shortly after birth neonatal blood has very few primitive hematopoietic cells, as they begin to home to and lodge in the marrow. Genetic studies have revealed that marrow localization of HSCs is dependent on stromal cell-derived factor (SDF)-1[21] as elimination of the chemokine or its receptor (CXCR4) leads to marrow hypoplasia.[22] The shifts in localization of hematopoiesis during mammalian development are likely the result of changes both in the cell surface adhesion molecules on hematopoietic stem and progenitors that occur during ontogeny, and in the characteristics of stromal cells of the yolk sac, AGM, fetal liver, and adult marrow that provide the microenvironmental support of HSC survival, homing and lodgment, self-renewal, proliferative expansion, and differentiation.

THE HEMATOPOIETIC STEM CELL

FUNCTIONAL DEFINITION

Although the concept of a common "mother cell" of all blood elements in the adult dates to Maximov in 1909, and its potential for participation in disease as proposed by Danchakoff in 1916,[23] the basic concepts of a hierarchical organization of stem and progenitor cells leading to mature blood cell production were experimentally verified by Till and McCulloch using a spleen colony forming assay.[24] The capacity to transplant marrow cells and reconstitute all aspects of hematopoiesis in myeloablated recipients provided an *in vivo* assay for the HSC, but it was not until the development of clonal *in vitro* assays of lineage-committed progenitors that a coherent model of blood cell production emerged. The pioneering work of Pluznik and Sachs[25] and of Bradley and Metcalf[26] provided methods to enumerate and characterize marrow cells committed to the hematopoietic lineage. These investigators independently developed culture conditions that allowed colonies of leukocytes to develop from single progenitors. However, as a result of the more fastidious conditions required for erythropoiesis and megakaryopoiesis *in vitro*, the description of methods to culture these progenitors did not occur for another decade or more.[27-31] Recent work using density fractionation, cell sorting, and fluorescent dye exclusion methods have yielded purified populations of stem cells,[32-35] common myeloid[36] and lymphoid[37] progenitors, and lineage-restricted hematopoietic progenitors,[38,39] methods that have greatly advanced our understanding of the cell and molecular biology of blood cell development. Figure 15-1 depicts a working model of this process.

STEM CELL KINETICS

Based on transplantation data indicating that there are a remarkably similar total body number of HSCs in mice and cats, it has been estimated that all mammals, including humans, possess 2×10^4 stem cells,[40] and because only a small fraction of these are cycling (and therefore contributing to blood cell production) at any given time, it is also clear that daily blood cell development from the few cycling stem cells to produce the approximately 4×10^{11} mature blood cells represents a massive amplification process.

Another measure of stem cell kinetics is the time it takes for transplanted marrow cells to repopulate a lethally irradiated animal. Studies using retroviral markers suggest that HSCs can be divided into short-term and long-term repopulating cells, based on the timing of their appearance in the blood following intravenous transplantation (fewer than or more than 3 months following transplantation in mice).[41] This conclusion was verified using a lentiviral marking system,[42] an advantageous experimental strategy because of less cell manipulation. However, a rapidly repopulating stem cell has been identified using a direct marrow injection strategy, a cell capable of generating large numbers of erythroid and myeloid cells within 2 weeks of injection.[43] Moreover, by transplanting luciferase-labeled single stem cells, a strategy that allows the serial tracking of the cells during life, initially detected foci were found to expand locally, seed other sites in the marrow or spleen, and then recede with different kinetics.[44] From these experimental approaches it is clear that hematopoietic stem cells are heterogeneous.

STEM CELL ASSAYS

TRANSPLANTATION ASSAYS

Assays of Murine Stem Cells Experimental transplantation in animals affords the clearest estimation of HSC properties as the capacity to durably regenerate all of hematopoiesis in an otherwise lethally irradiated animal remains the gold standard for the field; moreover, the technique can be made quantitative. Typically, either 1×10^5 genetically marked, whole murine marrow cells or reduced numbers of variably purified cells are infused intravenously into recipient animals who had previously received 90 to 110 cGy of whole-body irradiation. Blood cells and marrow are monitored for hematopoietic recovery in the following weeks and months, and the success of the transplant is measured by survival and long-range contribution to hematopoiesis in the recipient. The contribution of donor cells to recovery is established by analysis of the posttransplant blood or marrow cells; the most common method of distinguishing donor from residual recipient blood and marrow cells is the use of flow cytometry against isoforms of the cell membrane-bound phosphatase CD45, present on virtually all hematopoietic cells. In a more quantitative embodiment of the strategy, limiting numbers of the genetically distinct cells (e.g., CD45.1$^+$) are mixed with a "just adequate" (for full recovery) number of alternately marked cells (e.g., CD45.2$^+$) and the proportion of CD45.1 to total CD45.1$^+$ plus CD45.2$^+$ cells is assessed following

transplantation, yielding a calculation of the number of stem cells in the initial inoculum, an approach termed *competitive repopulation*.[45] Because there exist both "short-term" and "long-term" repopulating cells, the degree of donor cell chimerism is tested 3 or more months following transplantation, to be certain that only the latter are evaluated. This approach allows an assessment of the numbers or "quality" of HSCs in the test population (i.e., some genetically altered stem cell populations repopulate less robustly than wild-type cells as a consequence of defects in cytokine receptors or other genes that affect the self-renewal, survival, or proliferation of stem cells). Based on the use of these experimental tools, we know most about murine stem cells. Obviously, this approach is not available to assess human HSCs. Instead, a number of alternate experimental approaches have been developed.

Assays of Human HSCs Severely immunocompromised mice can be engrafted by human HSCs, provided their survival can be supported in a strictly controlled animal care environment and that the experiments take place prior to the development of other untoward effects in such animals (e.g., tumor formation). The first assay employing this strategy relies on the combined immunodeficiency created by the severe combined immunodeficiency (SCID) and nonobese diabetic (NOD) genetic mutations.[46] More recently, these mice were found to bear some ability to reject or alter the developmental characteristics of human cell repopulation, leading other investigators to add genetic defects to the NOD-SCID background that improve the engraftment of normal and pathologic human marrow cells, such as β_2-microglobulin nu11,[47] γC nu11,[48] or crossing with mice that also express human hematopoietic cytokines.[49,50] Such animal models have allowed (a) the assessment of stem cell numbers in human CD34$^+$ cells from mobilized peripheral blood or umbilical cord blood,[51] (b) assessment of the effects of gene therapy vectors,[52,53] cell cycle inhibitors,[54] or cytokine cocktails designed to expand stem cell numbers[51,55-57] on the retention of repopulating capacity, or (c) the study of fundamental biological properties of human HSCs *in vivo*, such as the cell cycle restriction of repopulating cells.[58]

IN VITRO COLONY ASSAYS

Although *in vivo* assays remain the gold standard, NOD-SCID and more severely immunocompromised mice are difficult to maintain and remain expensive and quite cumbersome methods to assess human HSC quality and quantity. As a result, a number of culture-based methods have been developed to more quickly and quantitatively evaluate human HSC function. Generally, each relies on long-term cell growth in culture and other special features to establish its validity as a model of the human HSC.

The ability to grow marrow cells in culture for extended periods of time provided an important tool to explore HSC biology.[59] In long-term cultures human or murine marrow is incubated in serum-containing medium under defined conditions, and after several weeks the stromal layer that has developed is recharged with fresh marrow cells, which then produce mature blood cells and their progenitors for many months. Cell fractionation studies show that the HSC resides adherent to the stromal cell layer in such cultures,[60] and that enzymatic disruption of the stromal layer will allow one to reseed a secondary stromal cell layer with the capacity to produce hematopoietic cells for a period of weeks to months, thereby defining an *in vitro* assayable cell termed the *long-term culture-initiating cell* (LTC-IC).[61] A second assay that has been developed based on similar principles is the cobblestone area forming cell (CAFC), which, when evaluated by phase-contrast microscopy, gives rise to complex colonies of multiple hematopoietic cell types under the stromal cell layer of long-term cultures.[62] Unfortunately, when careful comparisons are made between these assays and transplantation studies, the true HSCs comprise only a fraction of the repopulating cells found in marrow. Thus, conclusions about stem cell behavior from such *in vitro* assays cannot be considered rigorous.

CELL SURFACE PHENOTYPE

Numerous investigators have used monoclonal antibodies to an increasing number of hematopoietic cell surface proteins to negatively and/or positively enrich for stem and primitive hematopoietic progenitor cells. Although the function of only a few of these stem cell markers is known, it has not impeded their use for research and/or therapeutic benefit. Others have taken advantage of the capacity of primitive hematopoietic cells to extrude fluorescent organic chemicals or on their buoyant density to obtain purified populations of these scarce marrow cells (see below); most successful stem cell purification strategies employ several such techniques.

The antigenic proteins and glycoproteins exclusively or predominantly present on HSCs include (a) CD34, a 90- to 110-kDa type I glycoprotein that is postulated to mediate cell adhesion and/or cell cycle arrest[63-65]; (b) Thy1 (CD90),[66] a heavily glycosylated glycophosphoinositol-linked protein that participates in T cell adhesion to stromal cells[67]; (c) the c-Kit receptor (CD117),[68] which supports primitive hematopoietic cell survival and proliferation[69,70]; (d) AA4,[34] a murine molecule homologous to the human phagocyte C1q complement receptor[71]; (e) Sca1,[72] a murine surface molecule shown by knockout studies to be necessary for normal stem cell development[73]; (f) CD133,[74] a 115-kDa pentaspan cell surface glycoprotein expressed on the apical surface of neuroepithelial and HSCs that has been proposed to function in establishing or maintaining plasma membrane protrusions[75]; (g) CD164,[76] a cell surface sialomucin that is present in several alternately spliced isoforms and that enhances blood cell homing and inhibits CD34$^+$/CD38$^-$ cell proliferation[77]; and (h) the thrombopoietin (TPO) receptor c-Mpl (CD110)[78] shown to be present on virtually all repopulating HSCs,[79] and established to be vital for human HSC physiology as genetic elimination of the receptor leads to congenital amegakaryocytic thrombocytopenia at birth and aplastic anemia shortly thereafter.[80]

Many or most of the surface membrane proteins found on HSCs are also present on cells that have begun to differentiate toward specific lineages, precluding the exclusive use of positive selection alone for stem cell purification. Thus, a number of stem cell purification strategies include negative selection, based on cell surface markers absent on HSCs but present on mature blood cells and their corresponding unilineage-committed progenitors. Typically, cocktails of negatively selecting antibodies include CD38, HLA-DR, CD3, CD4, CD5 or CD8 for T lymphocytes; CD11b, CD14 or Gr-1 to exclude macrophages and granulocytes; CD10, CD19, CD20 or B220 to eliminate B lymphocytes; and glycophorin A or Ter119 to remove erythroid cells. The products that result from the use of such combinations of negative-selecting antibodies are termed Lin$^-$ cells.

A particularly difficult problem is presented by separating true HSCs from their progeny committed to the lymphoid or myeloid lineage, but not differentiated beyond that stage. Recent studies clarify the cell surface profile of the common lymphoid progenitor (CLP) as Lin$^-$/interlekin (IL)-7R(receptor)α^+/Thy1$^-$/Sca-110^w/ c-kit^{low37} and the common myeloid progenitor (CMP) as Lin$^-$/IL-7Rα^-/c-Kit$^+$/Sca-1$^-$.[36] The cell surface phenotype of human HSCs includes CD34$^+$/CD38$^-$/KDR(VEGFR2)$^+$/Thy1$^+$/CD133$^+$/Lin^{-2}, although most of these markers require careful clinical assessment before their widespread use in patients can be considered.

STEM CELL INTEGRINS

Integrins are a family of heterodimeric single pass transmembrane proteins (18 α and 8 β subunits form more than 20 different cell surface adhesion receptors in humans) characterized by multiple immunoglobin (Ig)-like extracellular domains that allow two-way communication between a cell and its environment.[81] A large number of cell types require contact for survival; *in vitro*, this is usually manifest as integrin-dependent cell adhesion, either to extracellular matrix protein(s) or to other cells. In such cultures, disruption of adherence causes programmed cell death; for example, endothelial cells undergo apoptosis upon forced detachment *in vitro*, as a result of disruption of multiple integrins.[82] Integrins also influence the proliferation of cells by affecting the G$_1$ to S phase transition of the cell cycle.[83] These effects also operate *in vivo*; α_1 integrin (a component of the $\alpha_1\beta_1$ collagen receptor) null mice have a hypoplastic dermis, and the growth of α_1 $-/-$ fibroblasts on collagen is substantially reduced.[84]

Hematopoietic stem and progenitor cells express multiple integrins, including $\alpha_4\beta_1$ (also termed very late antigen [VLA] 4), which binds to either vascular cell adhesion molecule (VCAM) 1 or fibronectin, and $\alpha_5\beta_1$ (VLA5), which binds to a region of fibronectin distinct from the $\beta_1\beta_1$ binding domain. Moreover, primitive hematopoietic cells are thought to express integrin αIIbβ_3, the platelet fibrinogen receptor, based on the death of multiple hematopoietic lineages in mice expressing a suicide transgene under control of the integrin αIIb promoter.[85] However, the physiologic significance of this finding is uncertain at present.

The avidity of progenitor cell-integrin interactions can be altered by external effectors; numerous cytokines and chemokines, including cytokines critical for stem cell function (stem cell factor [SCF], TPO and SDF-1), enhance integrin-mediated binding.[86-88] Counterreceptors for both integrins, such as VCAM1 and fibronectin (FN), are highly expressed in the marrow matrix and on marrow stromal cells (see below). Integrin-based interactions with the stroma are responsible for homing and retention of stem and primitive progenitor cells in the marrow, as antibodies that interfere with the interaction can mobilize stem and progenitor cells into the peripheral blood.[89] However, it is uncertain whether integrins can influence the survival or growth of HSCs, or affect their ultimate developmental fate.

METABOLISM-BASED CHARACTERISTICS

One of the hallmarks of HSCs is their resistance to chemotherapy-induced cytotoxicity. A primary reason for this property is high-level expression of drug efflux pumps of the multidrug resistance class of proteins.[90,91] The presence of these verapamil-sensitive efflux pumps has enabled the separation of HSCs based on their low-level retention of various fluorescent markers such as rhodamine 123 and Hoechst 33342, the "Rh^{lo}/Ho^{lo}" population of murine cells,[92] and the side population (SP) of cells in human marrow.[93] However, before such maneuvers can be used for clinical stem cell enrichment procedures, the lack of toxicity of the fluorescent dyes must be confirmed. Nevertheless, such experimental strategies continue to shed important insights into HSC biology.

CELL CYCLE CHARACTERISTICS

Adult hematopoietic cells display altered engraftment capacity dependent on their phase in the cell cycle. Using primitive hematopoietic cell populations, several investigators have demonstrated that only quiescent G$_0$/G$_1$ phase cells engraft into lethally irradiated recipient animals; that cells in the S and early G$_2$ phase display minimal engraftment capacity,[94,95] a situation that can be experimentally manipulated;

and that elimination of p21, a key cell cycle progression gene, enhances stem cell expansion.[96] These findings correlate well with findings that the profile of expressed genes in a highly selected population of primitive hematopoietic cells shifts when they are induced from $G_{0/1}$ phase into the cell cycle.[97] However, although this cell cycle dependence of engraftment of stem cells is true for adult cells, the corresponding cell populations derived from umbilical cord blood or fetal liver is not cell-cycle–dependent.[98] A better understanding of these findings is very likely to shed important new insights into the genes that regulate engraftment.

GENE EXPRESSION PROFILE

It can be argued that the most critical feature of the HSC is its ability to quantitatively balance its three fates, apoptosis, self-renewal, and differentiation into the mature elements of the blood. Moreover, the undifferentiated cell must express (at the least) the initiating genes responsible for all possible developmental lineages. A useful conceptual framework for this process can be constructed by considering the gene expression profiles of stem and committed hematopoietic progenitors that develop into the multiple hematopoietic differentiation pathways. At each developmental step genes associated with the adopted pathway should remain expressed or be up-regulated, while the genes that specify the alternate lineage(s) are likely silenced. A thorough understanding of these gene expression profiles should help to explain the circuitry of specific aspects of hematopoiesis, and of developmental biology in general.

Initial studies using immortalized multipotent hematopoietic cell lines reinforced this conceptual framework; pluripotency is characterized by the expression of multiple genes associated with multiple cell fates.[99] Studies of purified HSCs and lineage-committed progenitors have also strengthened this hypothesis, revealing coexpression of several different lineage-affiliated gene sets in single primitive hematopoietic cells.[100] In contrast, the downstream progenitors of HSCs were found to express only lineage-appropriate transcripts, such as for the granulocyte colony stimulating factor receptor (G-CSF-R) in committed granulocyte-macrophage (GM) progenitors, or β-globin and the erythropoietin receptor (EpoR) in committed erythroid progenitors.[36] Similar findings were reported for lymphoid committed cells, although some promiscuity was detected in B cell progenitors.[101]

With these principles established, more ambitious efforts to catalogue all the genes expressed by each stage of hematopoietic development have been made possible by advances in microarray approaches to gene expression.[102] On an even broader scale, and as might be expected, comparisons of different types of stem cells reveals an overlap in the expressed genes, supporting the hypothesis that the mechanisms responsible for critical stem cell properties, such as self-renewal, are shared among the cells derived from multiple organs.[103] This observation also provides a powerful tool to identify such proteins. Such studies have also begun to identify novel genes expressed in HSCs, potentially allowing our better understanding of their role in hematopoiesis.

TRANSCRIPTION FACTOR PROFILE

An important goal of modern cell biology is to provide a molecular explanation for the gene or sets of genes required to orchestrate specific developmental events. Fundamental to this process is an understanding of the proteins present in cells that regulate gene transcription in a lineage-, ontogenic stage-, and developmental level-specific manner. Several transcription factors have been identified in stem cell populations or have been shown to affect stem cell differentiation into the lymphoid and myeloid lineages.

HSC SELF-RENEWAL AND EXPANSION

Members of the Hox family of transcription factors likely serve as master regulators of hematopoietic cell fate decisions, at least at the level of self-renewal/expansion, based on (a) a similar role in multiple organ systems[104]; (b) their lineage- and differentiation-stage-specific expression pattern in hematopoietic cells[105]; (c) disruption of their usual level or pattern of expression leads to hematologic expansion or malignancies[106,107]; and (d) their elimination,[108] or elimination of the gene(s) that regulate them,[109] leads to significant defects in hematopoiesis. In addition, members of the extradenticle family of homeodomain-containing proteins serve as cofactors for Hox proteins, altering their cellular localization, DNA binding affinities, and specificities. Like Hox genes, genetic elimination of some of these cofactor proteins can lead to hematopoietic stem cell defects. For example, Pbx1 null mice display greatly reduced numbers of CMPs,[110] and overexpression or altered expression of MEIS1 is associated with hematologic malignancy.[111]

HSC TO COMMON LYMPHOID PROGENITOR COMMITMENT

The *Ikaros* gene encodes a family of lymphoid-restricted zinc-finger transcription factors related to the *Drosophila hunchback* gene.[112] All isoforms of Ikaros contain a highly conserved C-terminal activation domain and two zinc-finger domains that mediate their dimerization. However, only isoforms 1 to 3 of the six known alternately spliced forms contain more than 3 of the four N-terminal zinc fingers required for DNA binding to the consensus DNA core motif GGGA.[113] The PU.1 gene is 1 of approximately 30 members of the Ets family of transcription factors that bind to the purine-rich sequence 5'-GGAA-3'.[112] Genetic elimination of the *Ikaros* and *PU.1* genes have established their critical role in commitment of HSCs to the lymphoid lineage; fetal stem cells in *Ikaros* −/− mice fail to generate any definitive T or B lymphocyte precursors,[114] and although thymocyte precursors can be identified postnatally, they undergo aberrant differentiation or fail to develop into the CD4, dendritic and some $\gamma\delta$T cell subsets in adult mice. Thus, *Ikaros* is essential to all of lymphopoiesis early during ontogeny, and for several subsets of lymphocytes later in life. In a similar fashion, *PU.1*-deficient mice also lack any definitive T and B cell precursors in their lymphoid organs at birth,[115] and if knockout mice are maintained on antibiotics and survive the first 48 hours of life, they begin to develop normal-appearing T cells 3 to 5 days later. In contrast, mature B cells and macrophages remain undetectable in the older mice, indicating absolute tissue dependence for this lineage.

HSC TO COMMON MYELOID PROGENITOR COMMITMENT

The *SCL* gene encodes one of the transcription factors responsible for the initial stages of myeloid development, a gene first identified at the site of chromosomal rearrangement in a patient with stem cell leukemia.[116] SCL belongs to the helix-loop-helix family of transcription factors, which form dimers and bind DNA at consensus E-box motifs (CANNTG).[117] Although initially identified as a gene rearranged in T cell acute lymphocytic leukemia, an essential role for SCL in hematopoietic development was established by gene ablation studies, which revealed a complete absence of primitive blood cells and lethality in *scl* −/− embryos at day 9.5 postcoitum.[118] Consistent with this panhematopoietic phenotype, previous studies showed that SCL is down-regulated in differentiating granulocytic and monocytic progenitor cells and that forced expression of the gene in hematopoietic cell lines inhibits cytokine-induced granulocytic and monocytic differentiation.[119,120] Consistent with their respective roles in promoting stem cell and mature cell survival and proliferation, SCF sustains *SCL* expression in primary CD34$^+$ cells, maintaining them in an undifferentiated state, whereas granulocyte-monocyte colony stimulating factor (GM-CSF) down-regulates SCL levels and favors granulocyte and monocyte differentiation.[107,121] Together, these results suggest that *SCL* expression is required for HSC and CMP maintenance, and that down-modulation of the transcription factor is essential for myeloid differentiation.

The GATA transcription factor family contains six members possessing a highly related DNA-binding domain composed of two conserved zinc-finger motifs.[122] GATA1 and GATA2 are present in hematopoietic cells, GATA2 is found in the same cells as SCL, with GATA1 expression restricted to latter stages of erythroid/megakaryocytic (EMK) differentiation. Because genetic elimination of GATA2 is lethal as a result of numerous nonhematopoietic defects, and because lineage-specific knockouts have not yet been engineered, the role of GATA2 in early hematopoiesis is uncertain. However, like SCL, elimination of GATA2 expression is required for hematopoietic cell maturation.[123]

As noted above numerous lines of evidence indicate that hematopoietic stem cells express the TPO receptor, c-Mpl, as best exemplified by its expression on all AA4+/Sca+ cells that are capable of long-term hematopoietic repopulation.[79] Several investigators have shown that the 5′ flanking region of the *c-mpl* gene contains a functionally important GATA site and that GATA1 *trans*-activates the gene in hematopoietic cell lines.[124,125] Because GATA1 does not appear in hematopoietic cells until they have lost their repopulating capacity, it is possible that GATA2 fulfills this role in HSCs, although there is no evidence yet available establishing that this protein can *trans*-activate the *c-mpl* GATA site.[126]

THE HEMATOPOIETIC MICROENVIRONMENT

It has been estimated that the concentration of cells within the marrow is 10^9/ml; as a result, multiple cell–cell and cell–matrix interactions occur.[127] A major advance in experimental hematology has been the capacity to grow hematopoietic cells in long-term culture.[128] When high concentrations of marrow cells are placed in serum-containing cultures, a stromal cell layer and extracellular proteinaceous matrix form, and when subsequently recharged with fresh marrow cells, these long-term cultures (LTCs) are capable of supporting hematopoiesis for months with simple demi-depletion and replacement of culture medium. It is assumed that the cell–cell and cell–matrix interactions that develop in such cultures more closely resemble those found *in vivo*, helping to explain the longevity of such cultures and their capacity to maintain hematopoietic stem and primitive progenitor cells far longer *ex vivo* than do nonstromal cell-containing cultures. The molecular basis for the improved hematopoietic environment of LTCs is thought to rely on stromal cell surface molecules that promote cell–cell contact, prevent programmed cell death, and regulate growth.

The microenvironmental effects on stem cells have far reaching clinical implications as well; our ability to mobilize marrow stem cells for transplantation has greatly changed the way we treat hematologic and other malignancies, and ultimate success in the efforts of experimental hematologists to expand HSCs *ex vivo* with cocktails of cytokines and stromal cells for applications in gene therapy and regenerative medicine will undoubtedly derive only from a thorough understanding of the molecular bases for the interaction of HSCs with their microenvironment.

Marrow stromal cells influence hematopoiesis in a number of ways, by producing several cytokines that positively or negatively affect hematopoietic cell growth,[129–132] including some, like SCF, that are expressed on their cell surfaces, resulting in enhanced biologic activity.[133] Stromal cells are the origin of a number of extracellular matrix proteins that either directly affect hematopoietic cells, or do so indirectly by binding growth factors and presenting them in a functional context.[134] They also bear the Jagged/Delta family ligands that

stimulate Notch proteins to undergo cleavage and translocation into the nucleus, events that are critical mediators of cell fate decision making,[135,136] including for hematopoietic cells.[137] Cell–cell interactions mediated by integrins present on hematopoietic cells and counterreceptors on stromal cells are also very important for hematopoiesis[65]; in addition to bringing hematopoietic cells into close proximity to cells producing soluble or cell-bound cytokines, and hence raising the local concentration of these growth promoting proteins, integrin engagement leads to intracellular signaling, usually promoting entry into the cell cycle and preventing programmed cell death.[138] Reflecting the vital and sometimes lineage-specific roles of the hematopoietic microenvironment, the extracellular matrix and stromal cells reside in a highly organized structure.

ANATOMY

Hematopoiesis is highly compartmentalized within areas of red marrow, with erythropoiesis occurring in clusters surrounding a central macrophage,[139] granulocyte development being associated with stromal cells,[140] and megakaryopoiesis occurring adjacent to the endothelial sinusoidal cells (Chap. 4).[141] In the adult marrow, the specialized niche in which HSCs develop into differentiated progeny has been termed the hematon by Peault, a structure that includes Str01+ mesenchymal cells, desmin-positive perivascular lipocytes, Flk1+ endothelial cells, macrophages, and hematopoietic progenitors.[142] From these structures can be derived all lineages of committed colony-forming cells (e.g., colony forming unit–granulocyte-macrophage [CFU-GM] and burst forming unit–erythroid [BFU-E]) and primitive cells that score positive in CAFC assays, LTC-IC, and high proliferative potential colony-forming cell assays (see Chap. 4).

STROMAL CELLS

Fibroblasts are perhaps the best-studied of the marrow stromal cells, and can bind to primitive hematopoietic cells[143] by engaging cell surface integrins.[144] Marrow endothelial cells also support primitive hematopoietic cells, including LTC-IC.[145] Moreover, osteoblasts, which line trabecular bone and reside adjacent to primitive hematopoietic cells,[146] have been identified as contributing to the HSC supportive niche.[147–149] Each of these cells is known to produce a number of cytokines critical for primitive and mature hematopoietic cell development. For example, although a number of organs produce TPO constitutively,[148] marrow stromal cells are induced to produce the hormone in states of thrombocytopenia.[149,150] Stromal cells produce SCF constitutively in both soluble and membrane-bound forms,[69] and flt3 ligand (FL) is produced both constitutively and can be induced to high levels in the presence of pancytopenia by stromal cells and lymphocytes.[151]

Besides growth factor production, stromal cells are also known to display counterreceptors for the integrins present on hematopoietic cells, including VCAM1,[152] interactions which promote cell survival and proliferation in several ways.[153] Stromal cells also elaborate extracellular matrix components including collagen, laminin, fibronectin, heparins, hyaluronan, and tenascins. These substances, in turn, also engage a number of HSC integrins and other cell surface molecules, and form a solid matrix on which hematopoietic cells firmly attach. Of considerable clinical interest, it appears that interference with cell–matrix interactions,[154] or digestion of the extracellular matrix itself,[155,156] is involved in mobilizing HSCs by some agents such as granulocyte colony stimulating factor (G-CSF) and IL-8.

CYTOKINES

The regulation of stem cell survival, proliferation, and differentiation has been difficult to address due to the rarity of stem cells and the requirement that they be assessed using cumbersome transplantation assays. Several cytokines are able to exert effects on HSCs. The pursuit of the cytokines that affect HSCs is of more than pure physiologic interest, as the availability of the right combination of such proteins could allow expansion of the cells for therapeutic use without sacrificing their pluripotent and self-renewal capacities. Three proteins, SCF, FL, and TPO, and their corresponding receptors (c-Kit, Flt3, and c-Mpl, respectively) exert important effects on the number and/or growth of HSCs both *in vitro* and *in vivo* (Table 15-1).

Stem Cell Factor The molecule termed SCF, steel factor, mast cell growth factor, or c-Kit ligand, was cloned by several groups based on its binding to a cell surface receptor encoded by the protooncogene *c-Kit*,[69] previously identified as responsible for the severe defects in hematopoiesis, pigmentation, and gametogenesis in *W* mice. As the phenotype of mice bearing alleles of *W* was quite similar to those of *steel* (*Sl*), but in transplantation studies one strain displayed a stem cell autonomous defect (*W*) while the other did not (*Sl*), it had been hypothesized that the two genes represented the receptor for a growth factor and the cytokine itself, respectively,[157] a tenet proven true with the cloning of SCF.

SCF is synthesized by marrow fibroblasts and other cell types. Soluble SCF is a highly glycosylated 36-kDa protein released from its initial site on the cell membrane by proteolytic processing. An alternatively spliced form of SCF messenger RNA (mRNA), that does not encode the cleavage site, remains on the cell membrane, and is a more potent stimulus of c-Kit-receptor-bearing cells.[130] The ratio of soluble to membrane encoding SCF mRNA varies widely in different tissues, ranging from 10:1 in the brain, to 4:1 in the bone marrow, to 0.4:1 in the testis.[130,158]

TABLE 15-1 CYTOKINES AND HORMONES ACTIVE ON STEM CELLS AND PROGENITORS

CYTOKINE	PRINCIPAL ACTIVITIES
IL-1	Induces production of other cytokines from many cells, works in synergy with other cytokines on primitive hematopoietic cells
IL-2	T cell growth factor
IL-3	Stimulates the growth of multiple myeloid cell types, involved in delayed type hypersensitivity
IL-4	Stimulates B cell growth and modulates the immune response by affecting immunoglobulin class switching
IL-5*	Eosinophil growth factor and affects mature cell function
IL-6	Stimulates B lymphocyte growth, works in synergy with other cytokines on megakaryocytic progenitors
IL-7*	Principal regulator of early lymphocyte growth
IL-9	Produced by Th2 lymphocytes, costimulates the growth of multiple myeloid cell types
IL-11	Shares activities with IL-6, also affects the gut mucosa
IL-15*	Modulates T lymphocyte activity and stimulates NK cell proliferation
IL-21	Affects growth and maturation of B, T, and NK cells
SCF*	Affects primitive hematopoietic cells of all lineages and the growth of basophils and mast cells
Epo*	Stimulates the proliferation of erythroid progenitors
M-CSF*	Promotes the proliferation of monocytic progenitors
G-CSF*	Stimulates growth of neutrophilic progenitors, acts in synergy with IL-3 on primitive myeloid cells, and activates mature neutrophils
GM-CSF	Affects granulocyte and macrophage progenitors and activates macrophages
TPO*	Affects hematopoietic stem cells and megakaryocytic progenitors

* Primary regulator of the corresponding cell lineage

The importance of SCF to hematopoiesis is easily demonstrated; although nullizygous mice (*Sl/Sl*) are embryonic lethal because of a number of developmental defects, the presence of a partially functional allele (*Sl^d*) allows compound heterozygotes (*Sl/Sl^d*) to survive into adulthood, albeit with severe anemia[157] because of diminished numbers/quality of HSCs.[159] In addition to its critical role in the development of embryonic and fetal hematopoiesis, treatment of adult mice with an antibody that neutralizes the SCF receptor, c-Kit, also results in severe pancytopenia,[160] indicating an important hematopoietic role for the receptor/ligand pair throughout life.

When present in culture SCF alone can maintain the long-term repopulating ability of murine Sca-1+/Rh^lo/Lin− hematopoietic cells, suggesting that the cytokine can promote the survival of hematopoietic stem cells *in vitro*.[161] However, alone, SCF is only a weak stimulator of cell proliferation, primarily inducing the development of mast cells both *in vitro* and *in vivo*. Nevertheless, in the additional presence of IL-3, IL-6, IL-11, G-CSF, or TPO, SCF exerts profound effects on the generation of hematopoietic progenitor cells of all lineages,[162–164] pointing to primitive hematopoietic cells as critical targets. The molecular mechanisms of such synergy are beginning to emerge. A physical association of c-Kit and EpoR has been detected following SCF stimulation of cells bearing both receptors, an event that is essential for their functional synergy.[165]

Flt3 Ligand FL was cloned as the binding partner for a then newly identified novel orphan receptor,[166] a protein most closely related to the receptors for macrophage colony stimulating factor (M-CSF) (hence the term flt = *fms like tyrosine kinase*), and c-Kit. FL is expressed by T lymphocytes and marrow stromal cells.[151,166] The Flt3 receptor is a 160-kDa cell surface molecule expressed primarily on primitive hematopoietic cells.[167] Of considerable clinical interest, from 11 percent to 25 percent of the abnormal cells from patients with myelodysplastic syndromes or acute myelogenous leukemia express an aberrant form of Flt3 receptor which bears an internal tandem duplication,[168–170] resulting in the constitutive activation of the receptor and a reduced likelihood of patient survival. This observation has led to an attempt to control the growth of such mutant receptor bearing cells with a specific Flt3 kinase inhibitor.[171]

FL was initially cloned utilizing a soluble form of the receptor to identify ligand bearing cells.[172] As their receptors bear a number of common structural features, it was not surprising to find that FL shares significant structural homology, as well as biologic properties, with both M-CSF and SCF. Like the other two cytokines, FL displays a four α-helix bundle tertiary structure and exists in both membrane-bound and soluble states, the result of alternate splicing of the primary transcript that does or does not include a cleavage site for its release from the cell membrane.[173]

Unlike SCF levels, which remain relatively static regardless of peripheral blood cell counts,[69] blood concentrations of FL can rise more than 25-fold in response to pancytopenia.[174] Interestingly, only pancytopenia, and not individual lineage deficiencies, causes an increase in blood FL concentrations, suggesting that the cytokine is a bone fide regulator of stem or primitive hematopoietic cells. Consistent with this conclusion, transplantation data indicate that HSCs from Flt3-deficient mice do not effectively reconstitute the hematopoietic system,[175] being three- to eightfold less efficient in repopulation as wild-type cells, a conclusion reinforced by its genetic combination with c-Kit mutant mice.[175]

Like SCF, FL appears to act on HSCs only in synergy with other hematopoietic cytokines,[176,177] a finding particularly true for its combination with TPO.[178,179] In addition, FL is a potent stimulus of B lymphopoiesis and granulocyte-macrophage proliferation and development, particularly of the latter toward the dendritic cell lineage.[180,181]

Thrombopoietin Thrombopoietin is a 45- to 70-kDa hormone, which was first cloned by both traditional biochemical purification and expression cloning strategies based on the use of a then orphan class I cytokine receptor, first identified as the cellular homologue of the murine-transforming oncogene *v-mp1*.[182] Thrombopoietin bears extensive sequence homology to Epo, sharing 20 percent identity and an additional 25 percent similarity. The hormone is produced in several organs, including the liver, kidney, skeletal muscle, and the marrow stroma. Based on murine liver transplantation studies about half of steady-state TPO production occurs in that organ,[183] but in states of thrombocytopenia the marrow stroma increases production impressively.[149,150] The hormone acts on megakaryocyte (Meg) progenitors to enhance their survival and proliferation and on immature megakaryocytes to promote their differentiation, but surprisingly not on mature cells during platelet formation.[184] Multiple lines of evidence also indicate that TPO can exert profound effects on the HSC. The hormone has been shown to support the survival of candidate HSC populations, and acts in synergy with IL-3 and SCF to induce these cells into the cell cycle and increase their output of both primitive and committed hematopoietic progenitor cells of all lineages.[185,186] These properties are also seen *in vivo*. For example, administration of the hormone to myelosuppressed animals leads to more rapid recovery of all hematopoietic lineages, including primitive cells,[187–190] and genetic elimination of *TPO* or its receptor severely reduces the number of marrow stem and progenitor cells of all lineages to 15 to 25 percent of normal values.[79,191,192] In addition, as noted above, TPO acts in synergy with FL to expand primitive hematopoietic cells in suspension culture, and when used to supplement LTC the hormone was found to maintain HSC numbers for up to 2 months,[192] compared to standard LTCs in which repopulating HSCs are no longer detectable at this time.

The mechanisms by which these cytokines exert their effects on HSCs are only now beginning to be understood at the molecular level, but it is already clear that effects on the transcription factors that govern HSC survival, self-renewal, and expansion likely play critical roles. At least three such mechanisms have now been identified.

As discussed above in "HSC to Common Myeloid Progenitor Commitment," SCL is a helix-loop-helix transcription factor critical for hematopoiesis. SCF enhances the survival of primitive hematopoietic cells in culture by maintaining their expression of SCL,[121] which enhances expression of the SCF receptor c-Kit.[193] Two additional transcription factors that play vital roles in HSC expansion, HOXB4 and HOXA9, are both affected by cytokines. Exogenous expression of HOXB4 to levels only twice normal is associated with a marked and rapid expansion of transduced HSCs on their transplantation into lethally irradiated recipients.[106] In both model cell lines and primitive hematopoietic cells TPO doubles the expression of HOXB4, in a p38 mitogen-activated protein kinase (MAPK) fashion.[194] Of probably greater significance is the effect of TPO on HOXA9, a gene that also induces rapid expansion of HSCs on its introduction into these cells, and whose genetic elimination leads to a profound deficit in numbers of HSC *in vivo*.[108] Although the hormone fails to affect total cellular levels of HOXA9 in either model cells or primary primitive murine HSC populations, TPO greatly enhances HOXA9 nuclear translocation by inducing expression of its translocation partner, MEIS1, and leading to ERK1/2 MAPK-induced MEIS1 phosphorylation.[195]

MATRIX PROTEINS

FIBRONECTIN

Fibronectin is a 450-kDa fibril-forming glycoprotein composed of two subunits that is a major component of the hematopoietic microenvironment. Fibronectin is produced by both marrow stromal (endothelial cells and fibroblasts) and blood cells,[196] and is implicated in marrow homing of hematopoietic cells.[197] Distinct domains of fibronectin have been identified that interact with different integrins, for example, those for integrin $\alpha_4\beta_1$ and for integrin $\alpha_5\beta_1$.[138] HSCs display multiple integrins and their engagement contributes to cell survival and/or expansion. For example, *ex vivo* culture of human CD34+ cells on fibronectin maintains the repopulating capacity of HSCs, whereas growing the cells in suspension obliterates their ability to repopulate hematopoiesis.[198] Fibronectin binding to $\beta_1\beta_1$ binding also enhances the generation of large numbers of committed hematopoietic progenitors[199] and LTC-IC[200] from primitive precursors. Multiple molecular mechanisms for the effects of fibronectin on integrin bearing cells have been identified, and serve as a paradigm for the supportive effects of this entire class of microenvironmental signals.

Integrin engagement by fibronectin triggers a number of intracellular signaling events that affect the cellular cytoskeleton and transcriptional events. Complexes composed of kinases, adaptors, and cytoskeletal components are recruited to sites of integrin engagement, initiated by interactions with integrin cytoplasmic domains.[81] A critical molecule for integrin-based signaling is paxillin, a 68-kDa protein that contains a number of protein–protein binding domains, and which binds to the cytoplasmic domain of the integrin.[201] Additional binding partners also help trigger intracellular signaling, including focal adhesion kinase (FAK) and the closely related Pyk2 kinase. Upon recruitment, FAK and Pyk2 are activated and initiate Tyr phosphorylation of paxillin and other associated molecules, creating additional protein binding sites and activating tethered secondary messenger molecules. One vital signaling pathway downstream of FAK and Pyk2 is PI3K, which is mediated by the association of its regulatory p85 subunit with the adhesion kinases[202] (see Chap. 13). FAK also directly activates a pathway that results in up-regulation of the cyclin D promoter,[203] affecting cell proliferation. Integrin engagement also leads to Src activation, engagement of Grb2, and activation of Ras,[204] pathways also activated by SCF and TPO, and potentially provides a mechanism by which diverse extrinsic stimuli of HSCs may converge.

HYALURONAN

Another stromal cell matrix glycoprotein is hyaluronan, which binds to two hematopoietic cell surface receptors, RHAMM and CD44. Although most CD34+ marrow cells express CD44, only a fraction of them adhere to hyaluronan,[205] a process that can be mediated by cytokines, due either to increased surface expression of CD44 or an alteration in its conformation. Consistent with the latter notion, certain epitopes on CD44 have been shown to be inducible,[206] and antibodies to CD44 can alter the adherence of CD34+ cells to bone marrow stroma.[207] Nevertheless, other data suggests that RHAMM is the primary receptor for hyaluronan.[208] It is also of considerable interest that primitive hematopoietic cells also express hyaluronan, and that it plays an important role in their lodgment in the marrow and subsequent proliferation.[209]

HEPARAN SULFATE

Long-term cultures that support hematopoiesis develop a heparan sulfate proteoglycan layer. Immunochemical analysis has shown that marrow stromal cell lines synthesize and secrete numerous members of the syndecan family of heparan sulfate, including glypican, betaglycan, and perlecan.[18] Evidence is accumulating that heparan sulfate-containing proteoglycans may be vital components of the stem cell niche. For example, the structure of the heparan sulfate secreted from stromal cell lines that support long-term hematopoiesis is significantly larger and more highly sulfated than heparan sulfate from nonsupportive stromal cell lines, and when used alone in long-term cultures, the former can support LTC-IC whereas desulfated heparan sulfate cannot.[210]

TENASCIN

Tenascins are large, extracellular matrix (ECM) glycoproteins found in several tissues, synthesis of which is up-regulated in response to tissue regeneration. Tenascins are multimeric proteins composed of numerous modules. For example, tenascin-C is composed of six subunits linked like spokes in a wheel by their C-terminal fibrinogen-like domains, each subunit being composed of multiple endothelial growth factor (EGF)-like and fibronectin type III modules. Two forms of tenascin of M_r 280 and 220 kDa are also expressed at high levels by marrow stromal cells.[211] Bone marrow cells can adhere to tenascin-C within the fibrinogen-like domains and to two sets of the fibronectin type III-like repeats, and when so engaged, they undergo a proliferative response.[212] Genetic elimination of tenascin leads to modest deficiencies in marrow hematopoietic progenitor cells,[213] although as the levels of fibronectin in such mice are also reduced, it is unclear if direct tenascin engagement of hematopoietic cells is responsible, or the defect is a result of the secondary reduction of fibronectin engagement of $\beta_1\beta_1$ or $\alpha_5\beta_1$ integrins.

LAMININS

Laminins are heterotrimeric ($\alpha\beta\gamma$) extracellular proteins that regulate cellular function by adhesion to integrin and nonintegrin receptors. At present, 5 α chains, 3 β chains, and 2 γ chains have been characterized, which combine to form at least 12 distinct laminin isoforms.[214] Laminins containing γ_2 and either β_1 and α_5 chains are expressed in bone marrow, but only the latter (laminin-10/11) binds to $\alpha_6\beta_1$ integrin on primitive hematopoietic cell lines[215] and to primary human CD34$^+$/ CD38$^-$ stem and progenitor cells.[216] A second, nonintegrin laminin receptor (LR) also binds laminins, as well as other components of the extracellular matrix such as fibronectin, collagen, and elastin, and is composed of an acylated dimer of 32-kDa subunits.[217] Although not an integrin, the LR associates with integrins (e.g., integrin $\alpha_6\beta_4$) to modulate laminin binding.[218] Functionally, laminin-10/11 facilitates SDF-1α-stimulated transmigration of CD34$^+$ cells,[219] and displays mitogenic activity toward human hematopoietic progenitor cells.[214] The nonintegrin LR associates with the GM-CSF-R to modulate its signaling properties, down-modulating receptor signaling in the absence of laminin, and releasing the inhibition when bound by its ligand.[220] This arrangement could provide a novel molecular explanation for how laminins affect cell proliferation; whether this physiology extends to other cytokines that affect HSCs is under investigation.

COLLAGEN TYPES I, III, V, AND VI

Collagen types I, III, IV, and VI have been identified in LTC or in situ from marrow sections by a number of methods.[35,221] Most of the marrow-derived collagen types are assembled into long fibrils, which form the fine, background reticulin staining seen on marrow biopsies, although type IV collagen is assembled into a meshwork seen most commonly as part of basement membranes. Collagens also interact with laminins in the marrow. Collagen types I and VI are strong adhesive substrates for various hematopoietic cell lines and marrow mononuclear cells, including committed myeloid and erythroid progenitors.[221,222] Classic collagen receptors on blood cells are of two types, the β_1 integrins $\alpha_1\beta_1$ and $\alpha_2\beta_1$, and the nonintegrin glycoprotein VI, present predominantly on platelets.

CONTROVERSIES IN HEMATOPOIESIS

LINEAGE FATE DETERMINATION

One of the most contentious issues in hematopoiesis is the origin of stem cell commitment to specific blood cell lineages. Two schools of thought exist: extrinsic and intrinsic control. The former, championed by Metcalf and others,[223] argues that cytokines, extracellular matrix, or other stimuli instruct the hematopoietic stem or progenitor cell to differentiate into specific cell types. In contrast, Dexter and others[224] argue that a hierarchy of transcription factors direct a cell toward a specific lineage, mechanistically explained by a stochastic rise in one or more of a mutually antagonistic set of transcription factors that drive developmental pathways by enhancing expression of the genes that characterize that pathway, and by interfering with the levels or function of the transcription factors that drive the alternate lineage fate choice.

THE CASE FOR TRANSCRIPTION FACTORS

A strong case has been made for intrinsic control of stem cell lineage determination.[224] As Enver and colleagues state: "Simply put, the question is this: is unilineage commitment the result of a cell-autonomous, internally driven program, or rather is it the consequence of a cell responding to an external, environmentally imposed agenda?" These and several other investigators argue that the stochastic rise in one or another lineage determining transcription factor in the multilineage progenitor leads to its ultimate lineage commitment.

It is abundantly clear that transcription factors can direct lineage commitment in hematopoietic cells. A partial list of transcription factors restricted to specific hematopoietic lineages includes Pax5 (B cells),[225] Ikaros (B/T cells),[226] PU.1 and C/EBPα (myeloid and B cells),[227,228] GATA1 (erythrocytes and megakaryocytes),[122,229] Fli1 (megakaryocytes),[230] and C/EBPε (granulocytes).[231] A number of loss-of-function studies have revealed the nonredundant role of these proteins in development of the corresponding cell lineage. For example, genetic elimination of Pax5 eliminates B cells[232,233]; elimination of Ikaros leave a mouse devoid of fetal T cells, fetal and adult B cells, and their progenitors[114]; and loss of C/EBPα leads to absolute neutropenia.[234] Moreover, the exogenous expression of several transcription factors in lineage-committed progenitor cells can redirect cell fate. For example, C/EBPα is expressed in myeloid progenitor cells, and introduction of a regulatable C/EBPα gene into purified erythroid progenitors caused their switch to the myeloid lineage.[235] In further support of this hypothesis, several lines of evidence have been gathered, including the finding that forced expression of the antiapoptotic gene bcl2 in a growth factor-dependent multipotential hematopoietic cell line resulted in growth factor independence and spontaneous differentiation into all of the possible cell lineages that develop when the corresponding growth factor(s) are added to the wild-type cells.[236]

In addition to providing these and other arguments in favor of a transcription factor-based intrinsic regulatory mechanism of stem cell fate, proponents of the intrinsic hypothesis point to feed-forward switch-like molecular mechanisms in which a stochastic increase in one of a binary set of such transcription factors reduces the level or activity of those transcription factors responsible for alternate cell fates. An example of this physiology is illustrated by the mutually antagonistic effects of the erythroid transcription factor GATA1 and the myeloid transcription factor PU.1; GATA1 acts to inhibit the myeloid activation potential of PU.1,[237] and PU.1 blocks the binding of GATA1 to its genetic target sites.[238] For example, should the level of GATA1 stochastically rise above that of PU.1 in a CMP, the GM potential would be extinguished and the EMK potential of the cell would march forward, unfettered.

THE CASE FOR HUMORAL MEDIATORS

Although much evidence has been garnered in favor of an intrinsic mechanism of stem and progenitor cell fate determination, proponents of an extrinsic instructive hypothesis have also generated a large amount of compelling evidence in favor of the importance of extrinsic signals. One illustrative example of the capacity of certain extrinsic signals to impact specific patterns of differentiation is that the exogenous expression of an IL-2Rβ transgene in CLPs induces their differentiation into myeloid cells.[239] Subsequent studies revealed that the presence of the exogenous receptor leads to up-regulation of the GM-CSF-R in the CLP, and that exogenous expression of GM-CSF-R could also lead a CLP toward monocyte/macrophage development.[2] In separate studies, other cytokines were shown to direct myeloid lineage fate determination; compared to the differentiation profile seen when marrow cells were cultured with SCF alone, an antiapoptotic stimulus, the addition of IL-5 greatly enhanced the number of marrow progenitor cells that gave rise to eosinophilic colonies, whereas the addition of TPO induced a predominance of megakaryocytic colonies, without significant changes in the number of apoptotic cells in any of the three culture conditions. These results were interpreted to indicate that while the SCF could keep nearly all progenitor cells alive under the cell culture conditions employed, the second cytokine directed the multilineage progenitors into specific cell fates.[240]

More recently a number of external signaling events have been found to directly impact the transcriptional apparatus of the cell. For example, as previously noted, two transcription factors that lead to the self-renewal and expansion of HSCs, HOXB4 and HOXA9, are induced to higher levels of expression or to translocate into the nucleus of stem cells in response to TPO.[194,195] Moreover, SCL, a transcription factor that when expressed in maturing hematopoietic cells inhibits cytokine-induced granulocytic and monocytic differentiation, maintaining them in an undifferentiated state, is enhanced by SCF and down-modulated by GM-CSF.[121] Thus, strong evidence supporting both extrinsic and intrinsic control of lineage determination has been presented, and like the case for most conflicts in biology, it is most likely that elements of both mechanisms operate in hematopoiesis.

STEM CELL EXPANSION, SELF-RENEWAL, OR DIFFERENTIATION

The ability to divide symmetrically to generate identical daughters is a feature of most cells, including HSCs. However, the multipotent stem cell possesses an added ability to undergo asymmetric cell divisions, yielding one committed progenitor daughter and one stem cell daughter, or two differentiating progeny; regulating the balance between symmetric and asymmetric stem cell divisions becomes critical in maintaining proper HSC numbers and in meeting the demand for differentiated cells. A question related to the previous discussion of whether intrinsic or extrinsic factors determine HSC lineage fate is whether intrinsic or extrinsic factors determine the possible outcomes for a dividing HSC (two HSC progeny [stem cell expansion], one HSC and one differentiating cell [a self-renewal division], or two differentiating progeny). It is clear that feedback mechanisms exist that govern the size of the stem cell pool, as following myeloablation and transplantation of a limited number of HSCs the pool expands toward that seen in a normal individual but not beyond, even when subjected to forced overexpression of genes that enhance HSC expansion.[241] HSCs do not appear to have a limit on their capacity for expansion; experiments utilizing serial transplantation of marrow cells revealed that even after four such maneuvers the transplantation of a limiting number of HSCs was associated with a tenfold expansion in the recipient,[242] a level of expansion remarkably consistent from one serial transplant to the next. Thus, there does not appear to be an intrinsic limit on HSC expansion that sets the size of the stem cell pool. Rather, evidence from quantitative transplants suggests that there exist both intrinsic and extrinsic controls on the size of the stem cell pool.

Using a competitive repopulation strategy Pawliuk and colleagues have shown that following transplantation the degree to which a limiting number of transplanted HSCs expand depends on the source of the cells, fetal liver cells expand to a far greater degree than a similar

number of adult marrow-derived HSCs,[243] suggesting to these investigators that an intrinsic mechanism governs stem cell expansion divisions. However, evidence for an extrinsic mechanism that regulates stem cell expansion also exists, as the transplantation of a smaller number of either fetal liver or adult marrow HSCs resulted in slower marrow recovery but ultimately greater levels of HSC expansion than did infusion of larger numbers of cells. These results were interpreted to suggest that the more rapid recovery of marrow function associated with the administration of a larger marrow inoculum, with its increased numbers of stem cells, prematurely shut down HSC expansion, calling attention to an extrinsic regulatory mechanism. Moreover, the differences in expansion capacity among fetal and adult stem cells might also reflect the influence of extrinsic factors. It was recently shown that when adult human marrow cells are transplanted, they retain their stem cell capacity only if quiescent at the time of transfer.[244] In contrast, fetal liver and cord blood stem cells contribute to long-term hematopoiesis regardless of the phase of the cell cycle in which they reside at the time of harvest.[245] It is postulated that this latter property of fetal stem cells depends on the fetal hematopoietic microenvironment, making it likely that extrinsic factors play the key role in the decision to self-renew or differentiate.

Clues from the developmental biology of lower organisms may shed important insights into the mechanisms that regulate the decision between stem cell expansion, self-renewal, and differentiation.[246] Within the niche of developing *Drosophila* gonadal tissue exist hierarchies of cells. When female gonadal stem cells divide, the cell directly contacting the niche supportive cells remains a stem cell, the daughter that loses contact differentiates and initiates oogenesis. A similar niche architecture also sets the stage for gonadal stem cell retention in the fly testis and in many tissues of many organisms. The developing principle is that a stem cell in contact with the stem cell determining niche stromal cell, or residing in a region of the niche possessing the highest concentration of a stem cell determining soluble factor, will remain a stem cell, and those removed from contact or soluble factor will differentiate. In such a niche, the axis of stem cell division then determines cell fate; if the axis of cell division is parallel to the front of stem cell determining contact or soluble mediator gradient, the proximal cell will remain a stem cell while the distal cell differentiates; if the axis of cell division is perpendicular, both cells will remain under the influence of the "stemness" factor(s), and remain stem cells. Consequently, spindle-polarizing signals could be responsible for the fate of the daughters of stem cell division, a focus of much research, but at present, few established mechanisms.

STEM CELL PLASTICITY

A remarkable observation has been repeatedly made in patients who had undergone sex-mismatched (male into female) bone marrow transplantation, subsequent organ damage, and careful study at the time of their eventual death. In such settings, Y chromosome-bearing cells were identified at the site of repair of previous myocardial infarctions, strokes, and other organ damage. These observations suggest that hematopoietic cells can contribute to the replacement of damaged cells of multiple organs. More direct experimentation has lent additional support to this idea; several investigators have found that marrow cells are capable of giving rise to cells of multiple organs, including nerve,[247,248] liver,[249,250] skeletal muscle,[251] and cardiac muscle,[252] in a process termed *transdifferentiation*. However, direct evidence establishing this conclusion is lacking, as most such studies have assayed only partially purified cell populations that might also contain alternate types of stem cells,[253] and almost none have been performed using single cells, a requirement for robust proof of their multipotency. An alternate explanation for the presence of marked hematopoietic cells at nonhematopoietic sites of organ damage has been termed *cell fusion*. It has long been appreciated that marrow cells (especially macrophages) can fuse with other cells, and spontaneous *in vitro* fusion of embryonic stem cells with marrow-derived cells yields hybrids that display stem cell function[254,255]; further experimentation is required to prove or disprove the concept of HSC plasticity,[256] a proof that will have far-reaching implications for regenerative medicine.

HEMATOPOIETIC PROGENITORS

The loss of one or more developmental potentials of the HSC results in a progenitor committed to any number of specific hematopoietic cell lineages. Besides the loss of pluripotency, committed hematopoietic progenitors display a number of characteristics that differ from their parents, including the lack of capacity for self-renewal, a higher fraction of cells traversing the cell cycle, reduced ability to efflux foreign substances, and a change in their surface protein profile. On the genetic level, the transition of HSCs to committed progenitors is marked by the down-regulation of a large number of HSC-associated genes and progressive up-regulation of a limited number of lineage-specific genes. This section highlights some of the features of specific lineage-committed progenitors that allow for their purification, characterization, and, potentially, their manipulation for therapeutic benefit. Details of the morphologic, biochemical, and genetic aspects of the differentiation of each of these progenitors are found in the chapters corresponding to their mature blood cell types.

PROGENITOR CELL ASSAYS

Assays for most hematopoietic progenitor cells consist of marrow or (occasionally) peripheral blood cells, either unfractionated or purified to varying degrees, a semisolid support (either methylcellulose or agar, which prevents cellular migration), and a source of hematopoietic growth factors. The cultures are incubated in a humidified environment at 37°C (98.6°F) for 2 to 7 days for murine cells, or 5 to 14 days for human cells, during which time the vast majority of the cells that began culture as mature blood cells die, allowing the few hematopoietic progenitors present to proliferate and differentiate into mature blood cells. As the cells in such culture systems are immobilized by the semisolid supporting matrix, all of the progeny in the resultant colonies are derived from a single progenitor, allowing one to retrospectively determine the developmental capacity of that cell, termed a colony-forming cell (CFC) or unit (CFU). The requirement for a source of hematopoietic growth factors was initially fulfilled by using cellular underlayers containing fibroblasts, lymphocytes, or monocytes, or tissue culture medium conditioned by a variety of normal and neoplastic cellular sources, but more recently essentially all the requisite growth factors are available in purified recombinant form. Despite substantial progress in our understanding of the developmental requirements of committed hematopoietic progenitors, we still do not have an adequate *in vitro* colony-forming assay for some well-characterized hematopoietic progenitor cells (e.g., those committed to the T lymphocytic or NK cell lineages) that still require more complex assays (e.g., fetal thymus explant assay).

CHARACTERISTICS OF SPECIFIC PROGENITOR CELL TYPES

LYMPHOID PROGENITORS

Common Lymphoid Progenitors The existence of a population of cells committed to all lymphoid lineages but devoid of myeloid capacity was theorized to exist based on a number of analyses. For example, patients with adenosine deaminase deficiency, or mice with genetic elimination of the γ_C receptor, the signaling kinase JAK3, or the transcription factor Ikaros lack T and B lymphocytes and have few,

if any, myeloid defects, arguing that the defects in these disorders might affect a CLP; however, this does not prove the existence of a cell common for all. Work using cell sorting for CD10+/CD34+/Thy-/c-Kit-/Lin- human marrow cells revealed the capacity to develop into T, B, NK, and lymphoid dendritic cell progenitors,[256] but the report did not demonstrate a common progenitor capable of giving rise to each lineage on a clonal level.

More recent work, based upon the importance of IL-7 for all single-lineage lymphoid progenitor cells, and on the severe lymphopenia seen when the gene was eliminated in mice,[257] has indicated that the IL-7R marks a CLP that can be used in flow cytometry to isolate a population of IL7R+/Lin-/Thy-/Sca^lo/Kit^lo cells that engraft all of lymphopoiesis but no myelopoiesis in congenic mice.[37] For example, the injection of 2000 such CD45.1+ cells plus 1×10^5 whole-marrow CD45.2+ cells into lethally irradiated CD45.2 recipients lead to 3 to 20 percent CD45.1+ B and T lymphocytes, which disappear after about 6 months. In contrast, this strategy never results in the appearance of CD45.1+ myeloid cells. When limiting dilution studies were performed, about 1 in 20 such cells could give rise to short-term B-lymphopoiesis when injected intravenously, and an equal number could give rise to T-lymphopoiesis when injected into the thymus. In colony-forming assays using IL-7, SCF, and FL, approximately 20 percent of such cells gave rise to pre-B and pro-B cell colonies *in vitro*. Thus, given the low likelihood of proper homing when injected into mice, it is almost certain that the CLP exists and is IL7R+/Lin-/Thy-/Sca^lo/Kit^lo. When a genetic expression analysis was performed comparing HSC to CLP, the latter demonstrated a down-modulation of many molecules associated with HSCs, such as the cell surface receptors c-Mpl, β_1 integrin, and Tie2 and the transcription factors HOXA9 and EGR1, and up-regulation of the IL-7R and the recombination activating protein RAG2.[258]

T Lymphocyte/NK Cell, T Lymphocyte, and NK Cell Progenitors Simple colony-forming assays for mixed T/NK cell progenitors have not been developed, but the existence of the bipotent progenitor can be inferred from studies in which CD44+/CD25-/FcγRII/III- fetal thymic cells are cultured with genetically marked, deoxyguanosine-treated fetal thymic lobes under 70 percent oxygen at 37°C (98.6°F). Without cytokine supplementation, such cultures yield primarily CD3+/Thy1+ T cells, but if IL-2 plus IL-15 are added, the NK cell potential (CD3-/NK1.1+) of these cells is realized, and if IL-7 is also added, the number of single cells that yield cells of both lineages increases significantly.[259] As this type of readout is possible from single day 12 fetal thymus cells, such studies establish that bipotent T/NK cell progenitors exist.

E-box binding proteins consisting of HEB, E2-2, and the E2A gene products E12 and E47 form a distinct subgroup within the large family of basic helix-loop-helix transcription factors.[260] Heterodimers or homodimers form between family members through their HLH region, and through their basic regions bind to canonical E-box DNA sequences and thereby affect gene expression, including T cell targets such as CD4[261] and the pre-Tα,[262] and assist in recombination of the γδ T cell receptors.[263] It is now clear that E2A is required for the transition from the bipotent T/NK progenitor to committed T cell progenitors as its genetic elimination leads to preservation of the former but elimination of the latter.[259]

Another important subgroup of HLH proteins is the Id family, which contain an HLH region but lack a DNA binding domain, thereby acting as a sink for functional HLH proteins and thus negatively regulating the function of E proteins.[264] Id proteins appear to be essential for NK cell development, as genetic elimination of Id2 leads to a profound loss of NK cell progenitors[265] and forced overexpression of Id3 leads to a shift of T/NK cells preferentially into the NK cell lineage.[266]

It is also clear that Notch activation plays a vital role in T cell lineage commitment from the CLP. Overexpression of active Notch1 directs marrow stem cells into immature CD4+/CD8+ T cells and inhibits B lymphocyte development.[267] Overexpression of Notch1 in RAG-deficient precursors also results in differentiation to the T cell lineage, although only to the immature CD4−/CD8− stage, indicating that Notch cannot substitute for pre-T cell receptor signaling.[268]

B Lymphocyte Progenitors B cell progenitors include the pro-B cell, the earliest cell irreversibly committed to the lineage, which is CD34+/CD10+/CD38+/CD1910/CD2010, the pre-B cell, which displays the initial stages of Ig rearrangement, expresses immunoglobulin heavy chains in the cytoplasm and is CD34−/CD1010/CD19+/CD2010/CD38−, and immature B cells, which begins immunoglobulin light chain production, express cell surface IgM, and is CD10+/CD19+/CD20+. Pro-B cells can be detected in a simple colony-forming assay.[269] Normally, B cell precursor development occurs in contact with the hematopoietic microenvironment, mediated by precursor cell integrin $\beta_1\beta_1$ and stromal cell VCAM or matrix fibronectin. A number of cytokines affect B cell progenitor proliferation,[270] including IL-7,[271] insulin-like growth factor (IGF)-1,[272] SDF1,[273] and SCF,[274] although based on genetic knockout studies, B cells are absolutely dependent only on IL-7[257] and SDF1.[22]

A number of cytokines also inhibit B precursor cell development, including interferon alpha/beta (IFN-α/β),[275] IFN-γ,[276] IL-4,[277] and transforming growth factor (TGF)-β.[278] The role of these and other inhibitory cytokines in B lymphopoiesis is complex, as in some situations a cytokine can inhibit one stage and stimulate another stage of development, and some might act indirectly.

A number of transcription factors are required for mature B cell function, including PU.1, NF-κB, early B cell factor (EBF), interferon regulatory factor 4 (IRF4), and Oct2, many of which bind to the promoters and enhancers involved in immunoglobulin gene expression. In contrast to these relatively later stage effects, E2A is required for commitment to the lineage.[279] The marrow of E2A-deficient mice is devoid of CD19 B cells, as well as most B lineage-specific genes, including *Rag1/2, Pax5, EBF,* and *VpreB*. Moreover, no immunoglobulin rearrangement is detectable, and there are no IL-7-responsive cells. Reintroduction of E2A into the marrow cells of null mice reconstitutes pre-B cell development.[280] E2A sits upon a hierarchy of B cell lineage-specific genes and transcription factors[281]; E2A directly regulates the expression of Rag1, λ5, D-J$_H$, V-Jκ, and the transcription factor EBF, the latter in turn regulating VpreB, mb-1, D-J$_H$, V-Jκ, and the transcription factor Pax5, which, in turn, regulates CD19 and LEF1 and shuts down genes associated with alternate lineages, such as M-CSF-R (monocytic), myeloperoxidase (neutrophilic), GATA1 (EMeg), and pTα (T lymphocytic). As noted earlier in "T Lymphocyte/NK Cell, T Lymphocyte, and NK Cell Progenitors," a critical condition for B cell commitment is the absence of Notch signaling.

MYELOID PROGENITORS

Common Myeloid Progenitors Flow cytometry has also been extensively used to purify myeloid progenitors; an IL-7Rα−/Lin−/c-Kit+/Sca-1− population of murine marrow cells, which by virtue of being Sca1− exclude HSCs, develop into all myeloid lineages.[36] Based on expression of CD34 and the FcγRII/III, three distinct subpopulations can be identified by further flow cytometry, IL-7Rα−/Lin−/c-Kit+/Sca-1−/CD34+/FcRγlo, IL-7Rα−/Lin−/c-Kit+/Sca-1−/CD34−/FcRγlo, and IL-7Rα−/Lin−/c-Kit+/Sca-1−/CD34+/FcRγhi. When tested in colony-forming assays in the presence of SCF, FL, IL-11, IL-3, GM-CSF, Epo, and TPO, each cell population yielded distinct mature cell types.[36] IL-7Rα−/Lin−/c-Kit+/Sca-1−/CD34+/FcRγlo cells give rise to all myeloid colony types, including CFU-Mix, BFU-E, CFU–megakaryocyte (CFU-Meg), CFU–erythroid/megakaryocyte

(CFU-EMK), CFU–granulocyte/macrophage (CFU-GM), CFU–granulocyte (CFU-G), and CFU–macrophage (CFU-M), consistent with that expected for the CMP. In contrast, IL-7Rα−/Lin−/c-Kit+/Sca-1−/CD34+/FcRγhi cells form only CFU-M-, CFU-G-, and CFU-GM-derived colonies in response to any of the growth factors, alone or in combination, and thus represent granulocyte/macrophage lineage-restricted progenitors (GMP). Finally, IL-7Rα−/Lin−/c-Kit+/Sca-1−/CD34−/FcRγlo cells form only BFU-E-, CFU-Meg-, and CFU-EMK-derived colonies, leading to their designation as erythroid/megakaryocytic lineage-restricted progenitors (EMP, also termed EMK). To demonstrate their capacity to differentiate *in vivo*, limiting numbers of each cell population were transplanted into congenic mice; in such studies, cell fate outcomes correspond strictly with those of the *in vitro* colony assays. For example, 6 days after injection of 5000 CMPs, both donor-derived Gr-1+/Mac-1+ myelomonocytic cells and TER119+ erythroid cells were detectable in recipients. In contrast, when 5000 GMPs were transplanted, only Gr-1+/Mac-1+ cells were recovered, and only for a transient period of time. Likewise, EMPs reconstituted only TER119+ cells in similar experiments, and the genetically marked progeny from each of these progenitor populations disappear within four weeks of transplantation, indicating their limited self-renewal capacity.

Erythroid/Megakaryopoietic, Erythroid, and Megakaryopoietic Progenitors Culture conditions necessary for *in vitro* erythropoiesis have been known for 30 years,[282,283] with colony morphologies ranging from small compact clusters of 20 to 50 erythrocytes developing with 2 to 5 days in murine and human marrow plasma clot cultures (CFU-E) to large highly complex colonies containing up to thousands of cells taking from 7 to 14 days to develop in methylcellulose or agar (BFU-E). The cytokine requirement for the former is simple—Epo, whereas a cytokine that stimulates earlier cells, such as IL-3 or SCF, is required for the latter progenitor cell type.

Culture conditions that support the proliferation of Meg progenitors have been established for both mouse and man.[29,31] Using either methylcellulose, agar, or a plasma clot, two colony morphologies that contain exclusively megakaryocytes have been described. The CFU-Meg is a cell that develops into a simple colony containing from 3 to 50 mature Megs, larger, more complex colonies that include satellite collections of Megs and contain up to several hundred cells are derived from the burst forming unit–megakaryocyte (BFU-Meg). Because of the difference in their proliferative potential and by analogy to erythroid progenitors, BFU-Meg and CFU-Meg are thought to represent primitive and mature progenitors restricted to the Meg lineage. And like their erythroid counterparts, the cytokine requirements for CFU-Meg are simple: TPO stimulates the growth of 75 percent of all CFU-Meg, with IL-3 being required along with TPO for the remainder,[70] whereas IL-3 or SCF is required alone with TPO for more complex, larger Meg colony formation from their more primitive progenitors.

Progenitors for erythrocytes and Megs display many common features: they share a number of transcription factors (SCL, GATA1, GATA2, NF-E2), cell surface molecules (TER119), and cytokine receptors (for IL-3, SCF, Epo, and TPO), and most erythroid and Meg leukemia cell lines display or can be induced to display features of the alternate lineage.[284] Moreover, the cytokines most responsible for development of these two lineages—Epo and TPO—are the two most closely related proteins in the hematopoietic cytokine family[148] and display synergy in stimulating the growth of progenitors of both lineages.[70] For these and other reasons it has been postulated that erythropoiesis and megakaryopoiesis share a common progenitor cell,[285] a hypothesis now established[36] with the identification of IL-7Rα−/Lin−/c-Kit+/Sca-1−/CD34−/FcRγlo cells.

Like other primitive hematopoietic cells, bipotent EMK progenitors resemble small lymphocytes but can be distinguished by a specific pattern of cell surface protein display. As noted above, EMKs are IL-7Rα^-/Lin$^-$/c-Kit$^+$/Sca-1$^-$/CD34$^-$/FcRγ^{lo}. Cells committed to the Meg lineage then begin to express CD41 and CD61 (integrin αIIbβ_3), CD42 (glycoprotein Ib), and glycoprotein V. Those that are committed to the erythroid lineage begin to express CD41 and the transferrin receptor (CD71), and as they mature lose CD41 expression but express the thrombospondin receptor (CD36), glycophorin, and, ultimately, globin.[286] These and other cell surface markers provide experimental hematologists several strategies to purify committed Meg[39,287] and erythroid[288] progenitors. Another useful method to identify megakaryoblasts is histochemical staining for von Willebrand factor, and in rodents, acetylcholinesterase.[289]

The transcription factors expressed by erythroid and Meg progenitors that allow for their commitment to the lineage are becoming increasingly well understood. GATA1 is an X-linked gene encoding a 50-kDa polypeptide that contains two zinc fingers required for DNA binding.[229] Genetic elimination of the transcription factor established the critical role of this transcription factor in hematopoiesis; GATA1 $-/-$ mice are embryonic lethal as a consequence of failure of erythropoiesis,[290] and Meg-specific elimination of GATA1 leads to severe thrombocytopenia as a consequence of dysmegakaryopoiesis.[291] GATA1 acts in concert with another protein that affects transcription without binding to DNA, Friend of GATA (FOG).[292] The importance of this interaction to megakaryopoiesis is clear: several different mutations of the site on GATA1 responsible for FOG binding lead to congenital thrombocytopenia.[293]

The ets family of transcription factors includes about 30 members that bind to a purine box sequence, proteins that interact in both positive and antagonistic ways. For example, PU.1, initially termed Spi-1 based on its association with spleen focus-forming virus-induced erythroleukemias, blocks erythroid differentiation, although it appears important for megakaryocyte development.[294] Moreover, the ets factor Fli-1 is essential for megakaryopoiesis[295] and mutations in the transcription factor are also associated with congenital thrombocytopenia in man.[230]

Granulocyte/Monocytic, Granulocyte, and Monocytic Progenitors As noted above, GMPs (CFU-GM) are IL-7Rα^-/Lin$^-$/c-Kit$^+$/Sca-1$^-$/CD34$^+$/FcRγ^{hi}, reflecting their beginning differentiation toward phagocytic cells (i.e., FcRγ positive). In the human, GMPs are CD34$^+$/CD33$^+$/CD13$^+$ markers, which are of clinical significance. For example, CD33 is also termed Siglec-2, a member of a family of sialic-acid-binding surface membrane proteins of the immunoglobulin superfamily that are involved in cell–cell interactions and signaling. Although the role of CD33 is not yet known with certainty, it has become a therapeutic target because of its high-level expression on the blasts of several forms of acute myelogenous leukemia[296]; the use of gemtuzumab ozogamicin, in which a humanized anti-CD33 monoclonal antibody has been fused to *N*-acetyl-gamma calicheamicin 1,2-dimethyl hydrazine dichloride, a potent antitumor antibiotic, has resulted in a complete remission rate of 15 to 20 percent as a single agent in patients with relapsed disease. These initial successes have prompted its testing in earlier stage disease along with other active agents. When marrow grafts are purged of CD33-bearing cells, durable engraftment occurs but is often quite delayed, indicating that CD33 is not present on the HSC but that the presence of GMPs in a transplantation product is vital for rapid engraftment.

CD13 is also termed aminopeptidase N, an ectopeptidase present in many organs other than the marrow and a member of a family of proteases that play an important role in cell growth by virtue of their cleavage of biologically important peptides, in some cases inactivating, and in some cases activating them, and by serving a cell adhesive function as well. CD13 is present on early hematopoietic cells, including myeloid and lymphoid lineage progenitors, but disappears

from the latter class of cells and its expression rises as monocytes mature. Although it functions to scavenge peptides in the intestinal brush border and degrade endorphins and enkephalins in the synaptic cleft, its role in hematopoiesis is less clear, although IL-8 is a substrate of its proteolytic activity.

Once bipotent GMPs differentiate, they further restrict their developmental potential. Monocytic progenitors are characterized by a predominance of PU.1, whereas granulocytic cells by members of the C/EBP family—C/EBPα and C/EBPϵ—are vital for the expression of neutrophil and eosinophil granule proteins.[297,231] A recent study suggests that the developmental decision of a bipotent GMP into each of the two lineages might be mediated by alterations in the relative levels of PU.1 and C/EBP expression;[298] haploinsufficiency of PU.1 (*PU.1$^{+/-}$*) results in a reduction in CFU-M frequency in the marrow and an increase in CFU-G levels, even ameliorating the neutropenia seen in *G-CSF* null mice. Moreover, by increasing expression of C/EBPα, a transcription factor that drives granulocytic differentiation, G-CSF further influences the choice between the granulocytic and monocytic lineages. However, it is also clear that PU.1 plays an important role in both lineages, and it is likely that additional investigation will yield new insights into the molecular mechanisms that establish the ordered process we term myelopoiesis.

REFERENCES

1. Ogawa M: Differentiation and proliferation of hematopoietic stem cells. *Blood* 81:2844, 1993.
2. Kondo M, Wagers AJ, Manz MG, et al: Biology of hematopoietic stem cells and progenitors: Implications for clinical application. *Annu Rev Immunol* 21:759, 2003.
3. Colvin GA, Lambert JF, Moore BE, et al: Intrinsic hematopoietic stem cell/progenitor plasticity: Inversions. *J Cell Physiol* 199:20, 2004.
4. Moore MA, Metcalf D: Ontogeny of the haemopoietic system: Yolk sac origin of *in vivo* and *in vitro* colony forming cells in the developing mouse embryo. *Br J Haematol* 18:279, 1970.
5. Flamme I, Frolich T, Risau W: Molecular mechanisms of vasculogenesis and embryonic angiogenesis. *J Cell Physiol* 173:206, 1997.
6. Jaffredo T, Gautier R, Eichmann A, et al: Intraaortic hemopoietic cells are derived from endothelial cells during ontogeny. *Development* 125:4575, 1998.
7. Palis J, Yoder MC: Yolk-sac hematopoiesis: The first blood cells of mouse and man. *Exp Hematol* 29:927, 2001.
8. Huang H, Zettergren LD, Auerbach R: *In vitro* differentiation of B cells and myeloid cells from the early mouse embryo and its extraembryonic yolk sac. *Exp Hematol* 22:19, 1994.
9. Cumano A, Dieterlen-Lievre F, Godin I: Lymphoid potential, probed before circulation in mouse, is restricted to caudal intraembryonic splanchnopleura. *Cell* 86:907, 1996.
10. Peault B, Oberlin E, Tavian M: Emergence of hematopoietic stem cells in the human embryo. *C R Biol* 325:1021, 2002.
11. Robin C, Ottersbach K, de Bruijn M, et al: Developmental origins of hematopoietic stem cells. *Oncol Res* 13:315, 2003.
12. Galloway JL, Zon LI: Ontogeny of hematopoiesis: Examining the emergence of hematopoietic cells in the vertebrate embryo. *Curr Top Dev Biol* 53:139, 2003.
13. Wood HB, May G, Healy L, et al: CD34 expression patterns during early mouse development are related to modes of blood vessel formation and reveal additional sites of hematopoiesis. *Blood* 90:2300, 1997.
14. Tavian M, Coulombel L, Luton D, et al: Aorta-associated CD34+ hematopoietic cells in the early human embryo. *Blood* 87:67, 1996.
15. Marshall CJ, Moore RL, Thorogood P, et al: Detailed characterization of the human aorta-gonad-mesonephros region reveals morphological

polarity resembling a hematopoietic stromal layer. *Dev Dyn* 215:139, 1999.

16. Marshall CJ, Kinnon C, Thrasher AJ: Polarized expression of bone morphogenetic protein-4 in the human aorta-gonad-mesonephros region. *Blood* 96:1591, 2000.

17. Johnson GR, Moore MA: Role of stem cell migration in initiation of mouse foetal liver haemopoiesis. *Nature* 258:726, 1975.

18. Dzierzak E, Medvinsky A: Mouse embryonic hematopoiesis. *Trends Genet* 11(9):359, 1995.

19. Timens W, Kamps WA: Hemopoiesis in human fetal and embryonic liver. *Microsc Res Tech* 39:387, 1997.

20. Clapp DW, Freie B, Lee WH, et al: Molecular evidence that in situ-transduced fetal liver hematopoietic stem/progenitor cells give rise to medullary hematopoiesis in adult rats. *Blood* 86:2113, 1995.

21. Ara T, Tokoyoda K, Sugiyama T, et al: Long-term hematopoietic stem cells require stromal cell-derived factor-1 for colonizing bone marrow during ontogeny. *Immunity* 19:257, 2003.

22. Nagasawa T, Hirota S, Tachibana K, et al: Defects of B-cell lymphopoiesis and bone-marrow myelopoiesis in mice lacking the CXC chemokine PBSF/SDF-1. *Nature* 382:635, 1996.

23. Danchakoff V: Origin of the blood cells. Development of the haematopoietic organs and regeneration of the blood cells from the standpoint of the monophyletic school. *Anat Rec* 10:397, 1916.

24. Till JE, McCulloch CE: A direct measurement of the radiation sensitivity of normal mouse bone marrow cells. *Radiat Res* 14:213, 1961.

25. Pluznik DH, Sachs L: The cloning of normal "mast" cells in tissue culture. *J Cell Physiol* 66:319, 1965.

26. Bradley TR, Metcalf D: The growth of mouse bone marrow cells *in vitro*. *Aust J Exp Biol Med Sci* 44:287, 1966.

27. Silver RK, Erslev AJ: The action of erythropoietin on erythroid cells *in vitro*. *Scand J Haematol* 13:338, 1974.

28. Hara H, Ogawa M: Erthropoietic precursors in mice with phenylhydrazine-induced anemia. *Am J Hematol* 1:453, 1976.

29. Metcalf D, MacDonald HR, Odartchenko N, et al: Growth of mouse megakaryocyte colonies *in vitro*. *Proc Natl Acad Sci U S A* 72:1744, 1975.

30. McLeod DL, Shreve MM, Axelrad AA. Induction of megakaryocyte colonies with platelet formation *in vitro*. *Nature* 261:492, 1976.

31. Vainchenker W, Bouguet J, Guichard J, et al: Megakaryocyte colony formation from human bone marrow precursors. *Blood* 54:940, 1979.

32. Spangrude GJ, Heimfeld S, Weissman IL. Purification and characterization of mouse hematopoietic stem cells. *Science* 241:58, 1988.

33. Civin CI, Strauss LC, Fackler MJ, et al: Positive stem cell selection—Basic science. *Prog Clin Biol Res* 333:387; discussion 402, 1990.

34. Matthews W, Jordan CT, Wiegand GW, et al: A receptor tyrosine kinase specific to hematopoietic stem and progenitor cell-enriched populations. *Cell* 65:1143, 1991.

35. Penn PE, Jiang DZ, Fei RG, et al: Dissecting the hematopoietic microenvironment. IX. Further characterization of murine bone marrow stromal cells. *Blood* 81:1205, 1993.

36. Akashi K, Traver D, Miyamoto T, et al: A clonogenic common myeloid progenitor that gives rise to all myeloid lineages. *Nature* 404:193, 2000.

37. Kondo M, Weissman IL, Akashi K: Identification of clonogenic common lymphoid progenitors in mouse bone marrow. *Cell* 91:661, 1997.

38. Muta K, Krantz SB, Bondurant MC, et al: Distinct roles of erythropoietin, insulin-like growth factor I, and stem cell factor in the development of erythroid progenitor cells. *J Clin Invest* 94:34, 1994.

39. Nakorn TN, Miyamoto T, Weissman IL: Characterization of mouse clonogenic megakaryocyte progenitors. *Proc Natl Acad Sci U S A* 100:205, 2003.

40. Abkowitz JL, Catlin SN, McCallie MT, et al: Evidence that the number of hematopoietic stem cells per animal is conserved in mammals. *Blood* 100:2665, 2002.

41. Guenechea G, Gan OI, Dorrell C, et al: Distinct classes of human stem cells that differ in proliferative and self-renewal potential. *Nat Immunol* 2:75, 2001.

42. Mazurier F, Gan OI, McKenzie JL, et al: Lentivector-mediated clonal tracking reveals intrinsic heterogeneity in the human hematopoietic stem cell compartment and culture-induced stem cell impairment. *Blood* 103:545, 2004.

43. Mazurier F, Doedens M, Gan OI, et al: Rapid myeloerythroid repopulation after intrafemoral transplantation of NOD-SCID mice reveals a new class of human stem cells. *Nat Med* 9:959, 2003.

44. Cao YA, Wagers AJ, Beilhack A, et al: Shifting foci of hematopoiesis during reconstitution from single stem cells. *Proc Natl Acad Sci U S A* 101:221, 2004.

45. Harrison DE: Competitive repopulation: A new assay for long-term stem cell functional capacity. *Blood* 55:77, 1980.

46. Larochelle A, Vormoor J, Hanenberg H, et al: Identification of primitive human hematopoietic cells capable of repopulating NOD/SCID mouse bone marrow: Implications for gene therapy. *Nat Med* 2:1329, 1996.

47. Thanopoulou E, Cashman J, Kakagianne T, et al: Engraftment of NOD/SCID–β_2 microglobulin null mice with multi-lineage neoplastic cells from patients with myelodysplastic syndrome. *Blood* 103:4285, 2004.

48. Ito M, Hiramatsu H, Kobayashi K, et al: NOD/SCID/gamma(c)(null) mouse: An excellent recipient mouse model for engraftment of human cells. *Blood* 100:3175, 2002.

49. Feuring-Buske M, Gerhard B, Cashman J, et al: Improved engraftment of human acute myeloid leukemia progenitor cells in beta 2-microglobulin-deficient NOD/SCID mice and in NOD/SCID mice transgenic for human growth factors. *Leukemia* 17:760, 2003.

50. Punzon I, Criado LM, Serrano A, et al: Highly efficient lentiviral-mediated human cytokine transgenesis on the NOD/scid background. *Blood* 103:580, 2004.

51. Tanavde VM, Malehorn MT, Lumkul R, et al: Human stem-progenitor cells from neonatal cord blood have greater hematopoietic expansion capacity than those from mobilized adult blood. *Exp Hematol* 30:816, 2002.

52. Miyoshi H, Smith KA, Mosier DE, et al: Transduction of human CD34+ cells that mediate long-term engraftment of NOD/SCID mice by HIV vectors. *Science* 283:682, 1999.

53. Scherr M, Battmer K, Blomer U, et al: Lentiviral gene transfer into peripheral blood-derived CD34+ NOD/SCID-repopulating cells. *Blood* 99:709, 2002.

54. Cashman J, Dykstra B, Clark-Lewis I, et al: Changes in the proliferative activity of human hematopoietic stem cells in NOD/SCID mice and enhancement of their transplantability after *in vivo* treatment with cell cycle inhibitors. *J Exp Med* 196:1141, 2002.

55. Guenechea G, Segovia JC, Albella B, et al: Delayed engraftment of nonobese diabetic/severe combined immunodeficient mice transplanted with *ex vivo*-expanded human CD34(+) cord blood cells. *Blood* 93:1097, 1999.

56. Ueda T, Tsuji K, Yoshino H, et al: Expansion of human NOD/SCID-repopulating cells by stem cell factor, Flk2/Flt3 ligand, thrombopoietin, IL-6, and soluble IL-6 receptor. *J Clin Invest* 105:1013, 2000.

57. Zielske SP, Gerson SL: Cytokines, including stem cell factor alone, enhance lentiviral transduction in nondividing human LTCIC and NOD/SCID repopulating cells. *Mol Ther* 7:325, 2003.

58. Glimm H, Oh IH, Eaves CJ: Human hematopoietic stem cells stimulated to proliferate *in vitro* lose engraftment potential during their S/G(2)/M transit and do not reenter G(0). *Blood* 96:4185, 2000.

59. Dexter TM, Allen TD, Lajtha LG: Conditions controlling the proliferation of haemopoietic stem cells *in vitro*. *J Cell Physiol* 91:335, 1977.

60. Coulombel L, Eaves AC, Eaves CJ. Enzymatic treatment of long-term human marrow cultures reveals the preferential location of primitive hemopoietic progenitors in the adherent layer. *Blood* 62:291, 1983.

61. Sutherland HJ, Lansdorp PM, Henkelman DH, et al: Functional characterization of individual human hematopoietic stem cells cultured at limiting dilution on supportive marrow stromal layers. *Proc Natl Acad Sci U S A* 87:3584, 1990.

62. Ploemacher RE, Van der Sluijs JP, Voerman JS, et al: An *in vitro* limiting-dilution assay of long-term repopulating hematopoietic stem cells in the mouse. *Blood* 74:2755, 1989.

63. Fackler MJ, Krause DS, Smith OM, et al: Full-length but not truncated CD34 inhibits hematopoietic cell differentiation of M1 cells. *Blood* 85: 3040, 1995.

64. Krause DS, Fackler MJ, Civin CI, et al: CD34: Structure, biology, and clinical utility. *Blood* 87:1, 1996.

65. Verfaillie CM: Adhesion receptors as regulators of the hematopoietic process. *Blood* 92:2609, 1998.

66. Baum CM, Weissman IL, Tsukamoto AS, et al: Isolation of a candidate human hematopoietic stem-cell population. *Proc Natl Acad Sci U S A* 89:2804, 1992.

67. Barda-Saad M, Rozenszajn LA, Ashush H, et al: Adhesion molecules involved in the interactions between early T cells and mesenchymal bone marrow stromal cells. *Exp Hematol* 27:834, 1999.

68. Sanchez MJ, Holmes A, Miles C, et al: Characterization of the first definitive hematopoietic stem cells in the AGM and liver of the mouse embryo. *Immunity* 5:513, 1996.

69. Broudy VC: Stem cell factor and hematopoiesis. *Blood* 90:1345, 1997.

70. Broudy VC, Lin NL, Kaushansky K: Thrombopoietin (c-mpl ligand) acts synergistically with erythropoietin, stem cell factor, and interleukin-11 to enhance murine megakaryocyte colony growth and increases megakaryocyte ploidy *in vitro*. *Blood* 85:1719, 1995.

71. Dean YD, McGreal EP, Akatsu H, et al: Molecular and cellular properties of the rat AA4 antigen, a C-type lectin-like receptor with structural homology to thrombomodulin. *J Biol Chem* 275:34382, 2000.

72. Uchida N, Weissman IL: Searching for hematopoietic stem cells: Evidence that Thy-1.1lo Lin− Sca-1+ cells are the only stem cells in C57BL/Ka-Thy-1.1 bone marrow. *J Exp Med* 175:175, 1992.

73. Ito CY, Li CY, Bernstein A, et al: Hematopoietic stem cell and progenitor defects in Sca-1/Ly-6A-null mice. *Blood* 101:517, 2003.

74. Miraglia S, Godfrey W, Yin AH, et al: A novel five-transmembrane hematopoietic stem cell antigen: Isolation, characterization, and molecular cloning. *Blood* 90:5013, 1997.

75. Fargeas CA, Florek M, Huttner WB, et al: Characterization of prominin-2, a new member of the prominin family of pentaspan membrane glycoproteins. *J Biol Chem* 278:8586, 2003.

76. Watt SM, Buhring HJ, Rappold I, et al: CD164, a novel sialomucin on CD34(+) and erythroid subsets, is located on human chromosome 6q21. *Blood* 92:849, 1998.

77. Zannettino AC, Buhring HJ, Niutta S, et al: The sialomucin CD164 (MGC-24v) is an adhesive glycoprotein expressed by human hematopoietic progenitors and bone marrow stromal cells that serves as a potent negative regulator of hematopoiesis. *Blood* 92:2613, 1998.

78. Zeigler FC, de Sauvage F, Widmer HR, et al: *In vitro* megakaryocytopoietic and thrombopoietic activity of c-mpl ligand (TPO) on purified murine hematopoietic stem cells. *Blood* 84:4045, 1994.

79. Solar GP, Kerr WG, Zeigler FC, et al: Role of c-mpl in early hematopoiesis. *Blood* 92:4, 1998.

80. Ballmaier M, Germeshausen M, Schulze H, et al: C-mpl mutations are the cause of congenital amegakaryocytic thrombocytopenia. *Blood* 97: 139, 2001.

81. Hynes RO: Integrins: Versatility, modulation, and signaling in cell adhesion. *Cell* 69:11, 1992.

82. Fukai F, Mashimo M, Akiyama K, et al: Modulation of apoptotic cell death by extracellular matrix proteins and a fibronectin-derived antiadhesive peptide. *Exp Cell Res* 242:92, 1998.

83. Fang F, Orend G, Watanabe N, et al: Dependence of cyclin E-CDK2 kinase activity on cell anchorage. *Science* 271:499, 1996.

84. Pozzi A, Wary KK, Giancotti FG, et al: Integrin alpha1beta1 mediates a unique collagen-dependent proliferation pathway *in vivo*. *J Cell Biol* 142:587, 1998.

85. Tropel P, Roullot V, Vernet M, et al: A 2.7-kb portion of the 5′ flanking region of the murine glycoprotein alphaIIb gene is transcriptionally active in primitive hematopoietic progenitor cells. *Blood* 90:2995, 1997.

86. Kovach NL, Lin N, Yednock T, et al: Stem cell factor modulates avidity of alpha 4 beta 1 and alpha 5 beta 1 integrins expressed on hematopoietic cell lines. *Blood* 85:159, 1995.

87. Zauli G, Bassini A, Vitale M, et al: Thrombopoietin enhances the alpha IIb beta 3-dependent adhesion of megakaryocytic cells to fibrinogen or fibronectin through PI 3 kinase. *Blood* 89:883, 1997.

88. Peled A, Kollet O, Ponomaryov T, et al: The chemokine SDF-1 activates the integrins LFA-1, VLA-4, and VLA-5 on immature human CD34(+) cells: Role in transendothelial/stromal migration and engraftment of NOD/SCID mice. *Blood* 95:3289, 2000.

89. Papayannopoulou T: Mechanisms of stem-/progenitor-cell mobilization: The anti-VLA-4 paradigm. *Semin Hematol* 37:11, 2000.

90. Chaudhary PM, Roninson IB: Expression and activity of P-glycoprotein, a multidrug efflux pump, in human hematopoietic stem cells. *Cell* 66: 85, 1991.

91. Scharenberg CW, Harkey MA, Torok Storb B: The ABCG2 transporter is an efficient Hoechst 33342 efflux pump and is preferentially expressed by immature human hematopoietic progenitors. *Blood* 99:507, 2002.

92. Wolf NS, Kone A, Priestley GV, et al: *In vivo* and *in vitro* characterization of long-term repopulating primitive hematopoietic cells isolated by sequential Hoechst 33342-rhodamine 123 FACS selection. *Exp Hematol* 21:614, 1993.

93. Uchida N, Fujisaki T, Eaves AC, et al: Transplantable hematopoietic stem cells in human fetal liver have a CD34(+) side population (SP) phenotype. *J Clin Invest* 108:1071, 2001.

94. Habibian HK, Peters SO, Hsieh CC, et al: The fluctuating phenotype of the lymphohematopoietic stem cell with cell cycle transit. *J Exp Med* 188:393, 1998.

95. Orschell-Traycoff CM, Hiatt K, Dagher RN, et al: Homing and engraftment potential of Sca-1(+)lin(−) cells fractionated on the basis of adhesion molecule expression and position in cell cycle. *Blood* 96:1380, 2000.

96. Stier S, Cheng T, Forkert R, et al: *Ex vivo* targeting of p21Cip1/Waf1 permits relative expansion of human hematopoietic stem cells. *Blood* 102:1260, 2003.

97. Lambert JF, Liu M, Colvin GA, et al: Marrow stem cells shift gene expression and engraftment phenotype with cell cycle transit. *J Exp Med* 197:1563, 2003.

98. Wilpshaar J, Falkenburg JH, Tong X, et al: Similar repopulating capacity of mitotically active and resting umbilical cord blood CD34(+) cells in NOD/SCID mice. *Blood* 96:2100, 2000.

99. Hu M, Krause D, Greaves M, et al: Multilineage gene expression precedes commitment in the hemopoietic system. *Genes Dev* 11:774, 1997.

100. Miyamoto T, Iwasaki H, Reizis B, et al: Myeloid or lymphoid promiscuity as a critical step in hematopoietic lineage commitment. *Dev Cell* 3:137, 2002.

101. Nutt SL, Heavey B, Rolink AG, et al: Commitment to the B-lymphoid lineage depends on the transcription factor Pax5. *Nature* 401:556, 1999.

102. Phillips RL, Ernst RE, Brunk B, et al: The genetic program of hematopoietic stem cells. *Science* 288:1635, 2000.

103. Terskikh AV, Easterday MC, Li L, et al: From hematopoiesis to neuropoiesis: Evidence of overlapping genetic programs. *Proc Natl Acad Sci U S A* 98:7934, 2001.

104. Cillo C, Cantile M, Faiella A, et al: Homeobox genes in normal and malignant cells. *J Cell Physiol* 188:161, 2001.

105. Magli MC, Largman C, Lawrence HJ: Effects of HOX homeobox genes in blood cell differentiation. *J Cell Physiol* 173:168, 1997.

106. Sauvageau G, Thorsteinsdottir U, Eaves CJ, et al: Overexpression of HOXB4 in hematopoietic cells causes the selective expansion of more primitive populations *in vitro* and *in vivo*. *Genes Dev* 9:1753, 1995.

107. Buske C, Humphries RK: Homeobox genes in leukemogenesis. *Int J Hematol* 71:301, 2000.

108. Lawrence HJ, Helgason CD, Sauvageau G, et al: Mice bearing a targeted interruption of the homeobox gene HOXA9 have defects in myeloid, erythroid, and lymphoid hematopoiesis. *Blood* 89:1922, 1997.

109. Yagi H, Deguchi K, Aono A, et al: Growth disturbance in fetal liver hematopoiesis of Mll-mutant mice. *Blood* 92:108, 1998.

110. DiMartino JF, Selleri L, Traver D, et al: The Hox cofactor and proto-oncogene Pbx1 is required for maintenance of definitive hematopoiesis in the fetal liver. *Blood* 98:618, 2001.

111. Calvo KR, Knoepfler PS, Sykes DB, et al: Meis1a suppresses differentiation by G-CSF and promotes proliferation by SCF: Potential mechanisms of cooperativity with Hoxa9 in myeloid leukemia. *Proc Natl Acad Sci U S A* 98:13120, 2001.

112. Georgopoulos K: Transcription factors required for lymphoid lineage commitment. *Curr Opin Immunol* 9:222, 1997.

113. Molnar A, Georgopoulos K: The Ikaros gene encodes a family of functionally diverse zinc finger DNA-binding proteins. *Mol Cell Biol* 14:8292, 1994.

114. Wang JH, Nichogiannopoulou A, Wu L, et al: Selective defects in the development of the fetal and adult lymphoid system in mice with an Ikaros null mutation. *Immunity* 5:537, 1996.

115. McKercher SR, Torbett BE, Anderson KL, et al: Targeted disruption of the PU.1 gene results in multiple hematopoietic abnormalities. *EMBO J* 15:5647, 1996.

116. Begley CG, Aplan PD, Denning SM, et al: The gene SCL is expressed during early hematopoiesis and encodes a differentiation-related DNA-binding motif. *Proc Natl Acad Sci U S A* 86:10128, 1989.

117. Lecuyer E, Hoang T: SCL: From the origin of hematopoiesis to stem cells and leukemia. *Exp Hematol* 32:11, 2004.

118. Shivdasani RA, Mayer EL, Orkin SH: Absence of blood formation in mice lacking the T-cell leukaemia oncoprotein tal-1/SCL. *Nature* 373:432, 1995.

119. Brady G, Billia F, Knox J, et al: Analysis of gene expression in a complex differentiation hierarchy by global amplification of cDNA from single cells. *Curr Biol* 5:909, 1995.

120. Hoang T, Paradis E, Brady G, et al: Opposing effects of the basic helix-loop-helix transcription factor SCL on erythroid and monocytic differentiation. *Blood* 87:102, 1996.

121. Caceres-Cortes JR, Krosl G, Tessier N, et al: Steel factor sustains SCL expression and the survival of purified CD34+ bone marrow cells in the absence of detectable cell differentiation. *Stem Cells* 19:59, 2001.

122. Martin DI, Tsai SF, Orkin SH: Increased gamma-globin expression in a nondeletion HPFH mediated by an erythroid-specific DNA-binding factor. *Nature* 338:435, 1989.

123. Persons DA, Allay JA, Allay ER, et al: Enforced expression of the GATA-2 transcription factor blocks normal hematopoiesis. *Blood* 93:488, 1999.

124. Deveaux S, Filipe A, Lemarchandel V, et al: Analysis of the thrombopoietin receptor (MPL) promoter implicates GATA and Ets proteins in the coregulation of megakaryocyte-specific genes. *Blood* 87:4678, 1996.

125. Yamaguchi Y, Zon LI, Ackerman SJ, et al: Forced GATA-1 expression in the murine myeloid cell line M1: Induction of c-Mpl expression and megakaryocytic/erythroid differentiation. *Blood* 91:450, 1998.

126. Yamaguchi Y, Ackerman SJ, Minegishi N, et al: Mechanisms of transcription in eosinophils: GATA-1, but not GATA-2, transactivates the promoter of the eosinophil granule major basic protein gene. *Blood* 91:3447, 1998.

127. Long MW: Blood cell cytoadhesion molecules. *Exp Hematol* 20:288, 1992.

128. Dexter TM: Haemopoiesis in long-term bone marrow cultures. A review. *Acta Haematol* 62:299, 1979.

129. Kaushansky K, Lin N, Adamson JW: Interleukin 1 stimulates fibroblasts to synthesize granulocyte-macrophage and granulocyte colony-stimulating factors. Mechanism for the hematopoietic response to inflammation. *J Clin Invest* 81:92, 1988.

130. Toksoz D, Zsebo KM, Smith KA, et al: Support of human hematopoiesis in long-term bone marrow cultures by murine stromal cells selectively expressing the membrane-bound and secreted forms of the human homolog of the steel gene product, stem cell factor. *Proc Natl Acad Sci U S A* 89:7350, 1992.

131. Selleri C, Maciejewski JP, Sato T, et al: Interferon-gamma constitutively expressed in the stromal microenvironment of human marrow cultures mediates potent hematopoietic inhibition. *Blood* 87:4149, 1996.

132. Guerriero A, Worford L, Holland HK, et al: Thrombopoietin is synthesized by bone marrow stromal cells. *Blood* 90:3444, 1997.

133. Miyazawa K, Williams DA, Gotoh A, et al: Membrane-bound Steel factor induces more persistent tyrosine kinase activation and longer life span of c-kit gene-encoded protein than its soluble form. *Blood* 85:641, 1995.

134. Gordon MY, Riley GP, Watt SM, et al: Compartmentalization of a haematopoietic growth factor (GM-CSF) by glycosaminoglycans in the bone marrow microenvironment. *Nature* 326:403, 1987.

135. Artavanis-Tsakonas S, Matsuno K, Fortini ME: Notch signaling. *Science* 268:225, 1995.

136. Nye JS, Kopan R: Developmental signaling. Vertebrate ligands for Notch. *Curr Biol* 5:966, 1995.

137. Karanu FN, Murdoch B, Miyabayashi T, et al: Human homologues of Delta-1 and Delta-4 function as mitogenic regulators of primitive human hematopoietic cells. *Blood* 97:1960, 2001.

138. Kapur R, Cooper R, Zhang L, et al: Cross-talk between alpha(4)beta(1)/alpha(5)beta(1) and c-Kit results in opposing effect on growth and survival of hematopoietic cells via the activation of focal adhesion kinase, mitogen-activated protein kinase, and Akt signaling pathways. *Blood* 97:1975, 2001.

139. Shaklai M, Tavassoli M: Cellular relationship in the rat bone marrow studied by freeze fracture and lanthanum impregnation thin-sectioning electron microscopy. *J Ultrastruct Res* 69:343, 1979.

140. Westen H, Bainton DF: Association of alkaline-phosphatase-positive reticulum cells in bone marrow with granulocytic precursors. *J Exp Med* 150:919, 1979.

141. Tavassoli M, Aoki M: Localization of megakaryocytes in the bone marrow. *Blood Cells* 15:3, 1989.

142. Blazsek I, Chagraoui J, Peault B: Ontogenic emergence of the hematon, a morphogenetic stromal unit that supports multipotential hematopoietic progenitors in mouse bone marrow. *Blood* 96:3763, 2000.

143. Verfaillie C, Blakolmer K, McGlave P: Purified primitive human hematopoietic progenitor cells with long-term *in vitro* repopulating capacity adhere selectively to irradiated bone marrow stroma. *J Exp Med* 172:509, 1990.

144. Simmons PJ, Masinovsky B, Longenecker BM, et al: Vascular cell adhesion molecule-1 expressed by bone marrow stromal cells mediates the binding of hematopoietic progenitor cells. *Blood* 80:388, 1992.

145. Rafii S, Shapiro F, Pettengell R, et al: Human bone marrow microvascular endothelial cells support long-term proliferation and differentiation of myeloid and megakaryocytic progenitors. *Blood* 86:3353, 1995.

146. Islam A, Glomski C, Henderson ES: Bone lining (endosteal) cells and hematopoiesis: A light microscopic study of normal and pathologic human bone marrow in plastic-embedded sections. *Anat Rec* 227:300, 1990.

147. Calvi LM, Adams GB, Weibrecht KW, et al: Osteoblastic cells regulate the haematopoietic stem cell niche. *Nature* 425:841, 2003.

148. Lok S, Kaushansky K, Holly RD, et al: Cloning and expression of murine thrombopoietin cDNA and stimulation of platelet production *in vivo*. *Nature* 369:565, 1994.

149. McCarty JM, Sprugel KH, Fox NE, et al: Murine thrombopoietin mRNA levels are modulated by platelet count. *Blood* 86:3668, 1995.

150. Sungaran R, Markovic B, Chong BH: Localization and regulation of thrombopoietin mRNa expression in human kidney, liver, bone marrow, and spleen using in situ hybridization. *Blood* 89:101, 1997.

151. Solanilla A, Dechanet J, El Andaloussi A, et al: CD40-ligand stimulates myelopoiesis by regulating flt3-ligand and thrombopoietin production in bone marrow stromal cells. *Blood* 95:3758, 2000.

152. Quirici N, Soligo D, Caneva L, et al: Differentiation and expansion of endothelial cells from human bone marrow CD133(+) cells. *Br J Haematol* 115:186, 2001.

153. Yanai N, Sekine C, Yagita H, et al: Roles for integrin very late activation antigen-4 in stroma-dependent erythropoiesis. *Blood* 83:2844, 1994.

154. Scott LM, Priestley GV, Papayannopoulou T: Deletion of alpha 4 integrins from adult hematopoietic cells reveals roles in homeostasis, regeneration and homing. *Mol Cell Biol* 23:9349, 2003.

155. Carstanjen D, Ulbricht N, Iacone A, et al: Matrix metalloproteinase-9 (gelatinase B) is elevated during mobilization of peripheral blood progenitor cells by G-CSF. *Transfusion* 42:588, 2002.

156. Fibbe WE, Pruijt JF, van Kooyk Y, et al: The role of metalloproteinases and adhesion molecules in interleukin-8-induced stem-cell mobilization. *Semin Hematol* 37:19, 2000.

157. Russell ES: Hereditary anemias of the mouse: A review for geneticists. *Adv Genet* 20:357, 1979.

158. Huang EJ, Nocka KH, Buck J, et al: Differential expression and processing of two cell associated forms of the kit-ligand: KL-1 and KL-2. *Mol Biol Cell* 3:349, 1992.

159. Miller CL, Rebel VI, Helgason CD, et al: Impaired steel factor responsiveness differentially affects the detection and long-term maintenance of fetal liver hematopoietic stem cells *in vivo*. *Blood* 89:1214, 1997.

160. Ogawa M, Matsuzaki Y, Nishikawa S, et al: Expression and function of c-kit in hemopoietic progenitor cells. *J Exp Med* 174:63, 1991.

161. Li CL, Johnson GR: Stem cell factor enhances the survival but not the self-renewal of murine hematopoietic long-term repopulating cells. *Blood* 84:408, 1994.

162. Bernstein ID, Andrews RG, Zsebo KM: Recombinant human stem-cell factor enhances the formation of colonies by CD34+ and CD34+Lin− cells, and the generation of colony-forming cell progeny from CD34+Lin− cells cultured with interleukin-3, granulocyte colony-stimulating factor, or granulocyte-macrophage colony-stimulating factor. *Blood* 77:2316, 1991.

163. Brandt J, Briddell RA, Srour EF, et al: Role of c-Kit ligand in the expansion of human hematopoietic progenitor cells. *Blood* 79:634, 1992.

164. Ariyama Y, Misawa S, Sonoda Y: Synergistic effects of stem-cell factor and interleukin-6 or interleukin-11 on the expansion of murine hematopoietic progenitors in liquid suspension-culture. *Stem Cells* 13:404, 1995.

165. Wu H, Klingmuller U, Acurio A, et al: Functional interaction of erythropoietin and stem cell factor receptors is essential for erythroid colony formation. *Proc Natl Acad Sci U S A* 94:1806, 1997.

166. Lyman SD, James L, Johnson L, et al: Cloning of the human homolog of the murine Flt3 ligand—A growth-factor for early hematopoietic progenitor cells. *Blood* 83:2795, 1994.

167. Rosnet O, Schiff C, Pebusque MJ, et al: Human Flt3/Flk2 gene—CDNA cloning and expression in hematopoietic cells. *Blood* 82:1110, 1993.

168. Yokota S, Kiyoi H, Nakao M, et al: Internal tandem duplication of the FLT3 gene is preferentially seen in acute myeloid leukemia and myelodysplastic syndrome among various hematological malignancies. A

study on a large series of patients and cell lines. *Leukemia* 11:1605, 1997.

169. Thiede C, Steudel C, Mohr B, et al: Analysis of FLT3-activating mutations in 979 patients with acute myelogenous leukemia: Association with FAB subtypes and identification of subgroups with poor prognosis. *Blood* 99:4326, 2002.

170. Zwaan CM, Meshinchi S, Radich JP, et al: FLT3 internal tandem duplication in 234 children with acute myeloid leukemia: Prognostic significance and relation to cellular drug resistance. *Blood* 102:2387, 2003.

171. O'Farrell AM, Foran JM, Fiedler W, et al: An innovative phase I clinical study demonstrates inhibition of FLT3 phosphorylation by SU11248 in acute myeloid leukemia patients. *Clin Cancer Res* 9:5465, 2003.

172. Lyman SD, James L, Vanden Bos T, et al: Molecular cloning of a ligand for the flt3/flk-2 tyrosine kinase receptor: A proliferative factor for primitive hematopoietic cells. *Cell* 75:1157, 1993.

173. Lyman SD, James L, Escobar S, et al: Identification of soluble and membrane-bound isoforms of the murine flt3 ligand generated by alternative splicing of mRNAs. *Oncogene* 10:149, 1995.

174. Lyman SD, Seaberg M, Hanna R, et al: Plasma/serum levels of flt3 ligand are low in normal individuals and highly elevated in patients with Fanconi anemia and acquired aplastic anemia. *Blood* 86:4091, 1995.

175. Mackarehtschian K, Hardin JD, Moore KA, et al: Targeted disruption of the flk2/flt3 gene leads to deficiencies in primitive hematopoietic progenitors. *Immunity* 3:147, 1995.

176. Rasko JE, Metcalf D, Rossner MT, et al: The flt3/flk-2 ligand: Receptor distribution and action on murine haemopoietic cell survival and proliferation. *Leukemia* 9:2058, 1995.

177. Robinson S, Mosley RL, Parajuli P, et al: Comparison of the hematopoietic activity of flt-3 ligand and granulocyte-macrophage colony-stimulating factor acting alone or in combination. *J Hematother Stem Cell Res* 9:711, 2000.

178. Kobayashi M, Laver JH, Kato T, et al: Thrombopoietin supports proliferation of human primitive hematopoietic cells in synergy with steel factor and/or interleukin-3. *Blood* 88:429, 1996.

179. Piacibello W, Sanavio F, Garetto L, et al: Extensive amplification and self-renewal of human primitive hematopoietic stem cells from cord blood. *Blood* 89:2644, 1997.

180. Namikawa R, Muench MO, De Vries JE, et al: The FLK2/FLT3 ligand synergizes with interleukin-7 in promoting stromal-cell-independent expansion and differentiation of human fetal pro-B cells *in vitro*. *Blood* 87:1881, 1996.

181. Strobl H, Bello-Fernandez C, Riedl E, et al: Flt3 ligand in cooperation with transforming growth factor-beta1 potentiates *in vitro* development of Langerhans-type dendritic cells and allows single-cell dendritic cell cluster formation under serum-free conditions. *Blood* 90:1425, 1997.

182. Kaushansky K: Thrombopoietin: The primary regulator of platelet production. *Blood* 86:419, 1995.

183. Qian S, Fu F, Li W, et al: Primary role of the liver in thrombopoietin production shown by tissue-specific knockout. *Blood* 92:2189, 1998.

184. Kaushansky K: Thrombopoietin. *N Engl J Med* 339:746, 1998.

185. Sitnicka E, Lin N, Priestley GV, et al: The effect of thrombopoietin on the proliferation and differentiation of murine hematopoietic stem cells. *Blood* 87:4998, 1996.

186. Kobayashi M, Laver JH, Kato T, et al: Recombinant human thrombopoietin (Mpl ligand) enhances proliferation of erythroid progenitors. *Blood* 86:2494, 1995.

187. Kaushansky K, Broudy VC, Grossmann A, et al: Thrombopoietin expands erythroid progenitors, increases red cell production, and enhances erythroid recovery after myelosuppressive therapy. *J Clin Invest* 96: 1683, 1995.

188. Akahori H, Shibuya K, Obuchi M, et al: Effect of recombinant human thrombopoietin in nonhuman primates with chemotherapy-induced thrombocytopenia. *Br J Haematol* 94:722, 1996.

189. Neelis KJ, Hartong SC, Egeland T, et al: The efficacy of single-dose administration of thrombopoietin with coadministration of either granulocyte/macrophage or granulocyte colony-stimulating factor in myelosuppressed rhesus monkeys. *Blood* 90:2565, 1997.

190. Farese AM, Hunt P, Grab LB, et al: Combined administration of recombinant human megakaryocyte growth and development factor and granulocyte colony-stimulating factor enhances multilineage hematopoietic reconstitution in nonhuman primates after radiation-induced marrow aplasia. *J Clin Invest* 97:2145, 1996.

191. Alexander WS, Roberts AW, Nicola NA, et al: Deficiencies in progenitor cells of multiple hematopoietic lineages and defective megakaryocytopoiesis in mice lacking the thrombopoietic receptor c-Mpl. *Blood* 87:2162, 1996.

192. Yagi M, Ritchie KA, Sitnicka E, et al: Sustained *ex vivo* expansion of hematopoietic stem cells mediated by thrombopoietin. *Proc Natl Acad Sci U S A* 96:8126, 1999.

193. Krosl G, He G, Lefrancois M, et al: Transcription factor SCL is required for c-kit expression and c-Kit function in hemopoietic cells. *J Exp Med* 188:439, 1998.

194. Kirito K, Fox N, Kaushansky K: Thrombopoietin stimulates Hoxb4 expression: An explanation for the favorable effects of TPO on hematopoietic stem cells. *Blood* 102:3172, 2003.

195. Kirito K, Kaushansky K: *Thrombopoietin (TPO) Favorably Affects Hematopoietic Stem Cell (HSC) Expansion by Inducing the Nuclear Translocation of HoxA9, and Its Interaction with Pbx and Meis1.* American Society of Hematology, San Diego, CA, 2003.

196. Schick PK, Wojenski CM, Bennett VD, et al: The synthesis and localization of alternatively spliced fibronectin EIIIB in resting and thrombin-treated megakaryocytes. *Blood* 87:1817, 1996.

197. Prosper F, Stroncek D, McCarthy JB, et al: Mobilization and homing of peripheral blood progenitors is related to reversible downregulation of alpha4 beta1 integrin expression and function. *J Clin Invest* 101:2456, 1998.

198. Dao MA, Hashino K, Kato I, et al: Adhesion to fibronectin maintains regenerative capacity during *ex vivo* culture and transduction of human hematopoietic stem and progenitor cells. *Blood* 92:4612, 1998.

199. Yokota T, Oritani K, Mitsui H, et al: Growth-supporting activities of fibronectin on hematopoietic stem/progenitor cells *in vitro* and *in vivo*: Structural requirement for fibronectin activities of CS1 and cell-binding domains. *Blood* 91:3263, 1998.

200. Bhatia R, Williams AD, Munthe HA: Contact with fibronectin enhances preservation of normal but not chronic myelogenous leukemia primitive hematopoietic progenitors. *Exp Hematol* 30:324, 2002.

201. Liu S, Kiosses WB, Rose DM, et al: A fragment of paxillin binds the alpha 4 integrin cytoplasmic domain (tail) and selectively inhibits alpha 4-mediated cell migration. *J Biol Chem* 277:20887, 2002.

202. Sarkar S, Svoboda M, de Beaumont R, et al: The role of Aktand RAFTK in beta1 integrin mediated survival of precursor B-acute lymphoblastic leukemia cells. *Leuk Lymphoma* 43:1663, 2002.

203. Zhao J, Bian ZC, Yee K, et al: Identification of transcription factor KLF8 as a downstream target of focal adhesion kinase in its regulation of cyclin D1 and cell cycle progression. *Mol Cell* 11:1503, 2003.

204. Schlaepfer DD, Hunter T: Focal adhesion kinase overexpression enhances ras-dependent integrin signaling to ERK2/mitogen-activated protein kinase through interactions with and activation of c-Src. *J Biol Chem* 272:13189, 1997.

205. Legras S, Levesque JP, Charrad R, et al: CD44-mediated adhesiveness of human hematopoietic progenitors to hyaluronan is modulated by cytokines. *Blood* 89:1905, 1997.

206. Bendall LJ, James A, Zannettino A, et al: A novel CD44 antibody identifies an epitope that is aberrantly expressed on acute lymphoblastic leukaemia cells. *Immunol Cell Biol* 81:311, 2003.

207. Bendall LJ, Kirkness J, Hutchinson A, et al: Antibodies to CD44 enhance adhesion of normal CD34+ cells and acute myeloblastic but not lymphoblastic leukaemia cells to bone marrow stroma. *Br J Haematol* 98:828, 1997.

208. Pilarski LM, Pruski E, Wizniak J, et al: Potential role for hyaluronan and the hyaluronan receptor RHAMM in mobilization and trafficking of hematopoietic progenitor cells. *Blood* 93:2918, 1999.

209. Nilsson SK, Haylock DN, Johnston HM, et al: Hyaluronan is synthesized by primitive hemopoietic cells, participates in their lodgment at the endosteum following transplantation, and is involved in the regulation of their proliferation and differentiation *in vitro*. *Blood* 101:856, 2003.

210. Gupta P, Oegema TR Jr, Brazil JJ, et al: Structurally specific heparan sulfates support primitive human hematopoiesis by formation of a multimolecular stem cell niche. *Blood* 92:4641, 1998.

211. Klein G, Beck S, Muller CA: Tenascin is a cytoadhesive extracellular matrix component of the human hematopoietic microenvironment. *J Cell Biol* 123:1027, 1993.

212. Seiffert M, Beck SC, Schermutzki F, et al: Mitogenic and adhesive effects of tenascin-C on human hematopoietic cells are mediated by various functional domains. *Matrix Biol* 17:47, 1998.

213. Ohta M, Sakai T, Saga Y, et al: Suppression of hematopoietic activity in tenascin-C-deficient mice. *Blood* 91:4074, 1998.

214. Siler U, Seiffert M, Puch S, et al: Characterization and functional analysis of laminin isoforms in human bone marrow. *Blood* 96:4194, 2000.

215. Gu Y, Sorokin L, Durbeej M, et al: Characterization of bone marrow laminins and identification of alpha5-containing laminins as adhesive proteins for multipotent hematopoietic FDCP-Mix cells. *Blood* 93:2533, 1999.

216. Siler U, Rousselle P, Muller CA, et al: Laminin gamma2 chain as a stromal cell marker of the human bone marrow microenvironment. *Br J Haematol* 119:212, 2002.

217. Landowski TH, Dratz EA, Starkey JR: Studies of the structure of the metastasis-associated 67 kDa laminin binding protein: Fatty acid acylation and evidence supporting dimerization of the 32 kDa gene product to form the mature protein. *Biochemistry* 34:11276, 1995.

218. Ardini E, Tagliabue E, Magnifico A, et al: Co-regulation and physical association of the 67-kDa monomeric laminin receptor and the alpha6beta4 integrin. *J Biol Chem* 272:2342, 1997.

219. Gu YC, Kortesmaa J, Tryggvason K, et al: Laminin isoform-specific promotion of adhesion and migration of human bone marrow progenitor cells. *Blood* 101:877, 2003.

220. Chen J, Carcamo JM, Borquez-Ojeda O, et al: The laminin receptor modulates granulocyte-macrophage colony-stimulating factor receptor complex formation and modulates its signaling. *Proc Natl Acad Sci U S A* 100:14000, 2003.

221. Klein G, Muller CA, Tillet E, et al: Collagen type VI in the human bone marrow microenvironment: A strong cytoadhesive component. *Blood* 86:1740, 1995.

222. Koenigsmann M, Griffin JD, DiCarlo J, et al: Myeloid and erythroid progenitor cells from normal bone marrow adhere to collagen type I. *Blood* 79:657, 1992.

223. Metcalf D: Lineage commitment and maturation in hematopoietic cells: The case for extrinsic regulation. *Blood* 92:345; discussion 352, 1998.

224. Enver T, Heyworth CM, Dexter TM: Do stem cells play dice? *Blood* 92:348; discussion 352, 1998.

225. Souabni A, Cobaleda C, Schebesta M, et al: Pax5 promotes B lymphopoiesis and blocks T cell development by repressing Notch1. *Immunity* 17:781, 2002.

226. Georgopoulos K, Moore DD, Derfler B: Ikaros, an early lymphoid-specific transcription factor and a putative mediator for T cell commitment. *Science* 258:808, 1992.

227. Hromas R, Orazi A, Neiman RS, et al: Hematopoietic lineage- and stage-restricted expression of the ETS oncogene family member PU.1. *Blood* 82:2998, 1993.

228. Hohaus S, Petrovick MS, Voso MT, et al: PU.1 (Spi-1) and C/EBP alpha regulate expression of the granulocyte-macrophage colony-stimulating factor receptor alpha gene. *Mol Cell Biol* 15:5830, 1995.

229. Martin DI, Zon LI, Mutter G, et al: Expression of an erythroid transcription factor in megakaryocytic and mast cell lineages. *Nature* 344:444, 1990.

230. Hart A, Melet F, Grossfeld P, et al: Fli-1 is required for murine vascular and megakaryocytic development and is hemizygously deleted in patients with thrombocytopenia. *Immunity* 13:167, 2000.

231. Gombart AF, Kwok SH, Anderson KL, et al: Regulation of neutrophil and eosinophil secondary granule gene expression by transcription factors C/EBP epsilon and PU.1. *Blood* 101:3265, 2003.

232. Thevenin C, Nutt SL, Busslinger M: Early function of Pax5 (BSAP) before the pre-B cell receptor stage of B lymphopoiesis. *J Exp Med* 188:735, 1998.

233. Enver T: B-cell commitment: Pax5 is the deciding factor. *Curr Biol* 9:R933, 1999.

234. Zhang DE, Zhang P, Wang ND, et al: Absence of granulocyte colony-stimulating factor signaling and neutrophil development in CCAAT enhancer binding protein alpha-deficient mice. *Proc Natl Acad Sci U S A* 94:569, 1997.

235. Cammenga J, Mulloy JC, Berguido FJ, et al: Induction of C/EBPalpha activity alters gene expression and differentiation of human CD34+ cells. *Blood* 101:2206, 2003.

236. Fairbairn LJ, Cowling GJ, Reipert BM, et al: Suppression of apoptosis allows differentiation and development of a multipotent hemopoietic cell line in the absence of added growth factors. *Cell* 74:823, 1993.

237. Nerlov C, Querfurth E, Kulessa H, et al: GATA-1 interacts with the myeloid PU.1 transcription factor and represses PU.1-dependent transcription. *Blood* 95:2543, 2000.

238. Zhang P, Zhang X, Iwama A, et al: PU.1 inhibits GATA-1 function and erythroid differentiation by blocking GATA-1 DNA binding. *Blood* 96:2641, 2000.

239. Kondo M, Scherer DC, Miyamoto T, et al: Cell-fate conversion of lymphoid-committed progenitors by instructive actions of cytokines. *Nature* 407:383, 2000.

240. Metcalf D: Lineage commitment in the progeny of murine hematopoietic preprogenitor cells: Influence of thrombopoietin and interleukin 5. *Proc Natl Acad Sci U S A* 95:6408, 1998.

241. Thorsteinsdottir U, Sauvageau G, Humphries RK: Enhanced *in vivo* regenerative potential of HOXB4-transduced hematopoietic stem cells with regulation of their pool size. *Blood* 94:2605, 1999.

242. Iscove NN, Nawa K. Hematopoietic stem cells expand during serial transplantation *in vivo* without apparent exhaustion. *Curr Biol* 7:805, 1997.

243. Pawliuk R, Eaves C, Humphries RK: Evidence of both ontogeny and transplant dose-regulated expansion of hematopoietic stem cells *in vivo*. *Blood* 88:2852, 1996.

244. Gothot A, van der Loo JC, Clapp DW, et al: Cell cycle-related changes in repopulating capacity of human mobilized peripheral blood CD34(+) cells in non-obese diabetic/severe combined immune-deficient mice. *Blood* 92:2641, 1998.

245. Wilpshaar J, Bhatia M, Kanhai HH, et al: Engraftment potential of human fetal hematopoietic cells in NOD/SCID mice is not restricted to mitotically quiescent cells. *Blood* 100:120, 2002.

246. Fuchs E, Tumbar T, Guasch G: Socializing with the neighbors: Stem cells and their niche. *Cell* 116:769, 2004.

247. Mezey E, Chandross KJ, Harta G, et al: Turning blood into brain: Cells bearing neuronal antigens generated *in vivo* from bone marrow. *Science* 290:1779, 2000.

248. Brazelton TR, Rossi FM, Keshet GI, et al: From marrow to brain: Expression of neuronal phenotypes in adult mice. *Science* 290:1775, a 2000.

249. Lagasse E, Connors H, Al-Dhalimy M, et al: Purified hematopoietic stem cells can differentiate into hepatocytes *in vivo*. *Nat Med* 6:1229, 2000.

250. Alison MR, Poulsom R, Jeffery R, et al: Hepatocytes from non-hepatic adult stem cells. *Nature* 406:257, 2000.

251. Ferrari G, Cusella-De Angelis G, Coletta M, et al: Muscle regeneration by bone marrow-derived myogenic progenitors. *Science* 279:1528, 1998.

252. Orlic D, Kajstura J, Chimenti S, et al: Bone marrow cells regenerate infarcted myocardium. *Nature* 410:701, 2001.

253. Jiang Y, Jahagirdar BN, Reinhardt RL, et al: Pluripotency of mesenchymal stem cells derived from adult marrow. *Nature* 418:41, 2002.

254. Ying QL, Nichols J, Evans EP, et al: Changing potency by spontaneous fusion. *Nature* 416:545, 2002.

255. Terada N, Hamazaki T, Oka M, et al: Bone marrow cells adopt the phenotype of other cells by spontaneous cell fusion. *Nature* 416:542, 2002.

256. Galy A, Travis M, Cen D, et al: Human T, B, natural killer, and dendritic cells arise from a common bone marrow progenitor cell subset. *Immunity* 3:459, 1995.

257. von Freeden-Jeffry U, Vieira P, Lucian LA, et al: Lymphopenia in interleukin (IL)-7 gene-deleted mice identifies IL-7 as a nonredundant cytokine. *J Exp Med* 181:1519, 1995.

258. Terskikh AV, Miyamoto T, Chang C, et al: Gene expression analysis of purified hematopoietic stem cells and committed progenitors. *Blood* 102:94, 2003.

259. Ikawa T, Kawamoto H, Fujimoto S, et al: Commitment of common T/Natural killer (NK) progenitors to unipotent T and NK progenitors in the murine fetal thymus revealed by a single progenitor assay. *J Exp Med* 190:1617, 1999.

260. Massari ME, Murre C: Helix-loop-helix proteins: Regulators of transcription in eucaryotic organisms. *Mol Cell Biol* 20:429, 2000.

261. Sawada S, Littman DR: A heterodimer of HEB and an E12-related protein interacts with the CD4 enhancer and regulates its activity in T-cell lines. *Mol Cell Biol* 13:5620, 1993.

262. Takeuchi A, Yamasaki S, Takase K, et al: E2A and HEB activate the pre-TCR alpha promoter during immature T cell development. *J Immunol* 167:2157, 2001.

263. Bain G, Romanow WJ, Albers K, et al: Positive and negative regulation of V(D)J recombination by the E2A proteins. *J Exp Med* 189:289, 1999.

264. Norton JD: ID helix-loop-helix proteins in cell growth, differentiation and tumorigenesis. *J Cell Sci* 113 Pt 22:3897, 2000.

265. Yokota Y, Mansouri A, Mori S, et al: Development of peripheral lymphoid organs and natural killer cells depends on the helix-loop-helix inhibitor Id2. *Nature* 397:702, 1999.

266. Heemskerk MH, Blom B, Nolan G, et al: Inhibition of T cell and promotion of natural killer cell development by the dominant negative helix loop helix factor Id3. *J Exp Med* 186:1597, 1997.

267. Pui JC, Allman D, Xu L, et al: Notch1 expression in early lymphopoiesis influences B versus T lineage determination. *Immunity* 11:299, 1999.

268. Allman D, Karnell FG, Punt JA, et al: Separation of Notch1 promoted lineage commitment and expansion/transformation in developing T cells. *J Exp Med* 194:99, 2001.

269. Denis KA, Witte ON: *In vitro* development of B lymphocytes from long-term cultured precursor cells. *Proc Natl Acad Sci U S A* 83:441, 1986.

270. Takatsu K: Cytokines involved in B-cell differentiation and their sites of action. *Proc Soc Exp Biol Med* 215:121, 1997.

271. Namen AE, Lupton S, Hjerrild K, et al: Stimulation of B-cell progenitors by cloned murine interleukin-7. *Nature* 333:571, 1988.

272. Gibson LF, Piktel D, Landreth KS: Insulin-like growth factor-1 potentiates expansion of interleukin-7-dependent pro-B cells. *Blood* 82:3005, 1993.

273. Nagasawa T, Kikutani H, Kishimoto T: Molecular cloning and structure of a pre-B-cell growth-stimulating factor. *Proc Natl Acad Sci U S A* 91: 2305, 1994.

274. McNiece IK, Langley KE, Zsebo KM: The role of recombinant stem cell factor in early B cell development. Synergistic interaction with IL-7. *J Immunol* 146:3785, 1991.

275. Gongora R, Stephan RP, Zhang Z, et al: An essential role for Daxx in the inhibition of B lymphopoiesis by type I interferons. *Immunity* 14: 727, 2001.

276. Yoshikawa H, Nakajima Y, Tasaka K: IFN-gamma induces the apoptosis of WEHI 279 and normal pre-B cell lines by expressing direct inhibitor of apoptosis protein binding protein with low pI. *J Immunol* 167:2487, 2001.

277. Mitchell PL, Clutterbuck RD, Powles RL, et al: Interleukin-4 enhances the survival of severe combined immunodeficient mice engrafted with human B-cell precursor leukemia. *Blood* 87:4797, 1996.

278. Lee G, Namen AE, Gillis S, et al: Normal B cell precursors responsive to recombinant murine IL-7 and inhibition of IL-7 activity by transforming growth factor-beta. *J Immunol* 142:3875, 1989.

279. Bain G, Maandag EC, Izon DJ, et al: E2A proteins are required for proper B cell development and initiation of immunoglobulin gene rearrangements. *Cell* 79:885, 1994.

280. Bain G, Robanus Maandag EC, te Riele HP, et al: Both E12 and E47 allow commitment to the B cell lineage. *Immunity* 6:145, 1997.

281. Kee BL, Quong MW, Murre C: E2A proteins: Essential regulators at multiple stages of B-cell development. *Immunol Rev* 175:138, 2000.

282. Iscove NN, Sieber F: Erythroid progenitors in mouse bone marrow detected by macroscopic colony formation in culture. *Exp Hematol* 3:32, 1975.

283. Clarke BJ, Housman D: Characterization of an erythroid precursor cell of high proliferative capacity in normal human peripheral blood. *Proc Natl Acad Sci U S A* 74:1105, 1977.

284. Long MW, Heffner CH, Williams JL, et al: Regulation of megakaryocyte phenotype in human erythroleukemia cells. *J Clin Invest* 85:1072, 1990.

285. McDonald TP, Sullivan PS: Megakaryocytic and erythrocytic cell lines share a common precursor cell. *Exp Hematol* 21:1316, 1993.

286. Nakahata T, Okumura N: Cell surface antigen expression in human erythroid progenitors: Erythroid and megakaryocytic markers. *Leuk Lymphoma* 13:401, 1994.

287. Hodohara K, Fujii N, Yamamoto N, et al: Stromal cell-derived factor-1 (SDF-1) acts together with thrombopoietin to enhance the development of megakaryocytic progenitor cells (CFU-MK). *Blood* 95:769, 2000.

288. Sawada K, Krantz SB, Dai CH, et al: Purification of human blood burst-forming units-erythroid and demonstration of the evolution of erythropoietin receptors. *J Cell Physiol* 142:219, 1990.

289. Sporn LA, Chavin SI, Marder VJ, et al: Biosynthesis of von Willebrand protein by human megakaryocytes. *J Clin Invest* 76:1102, 1985.

290. Pevny L, Simon MC, Robertson E, et al: Erythroid differentiation in chimaeric mice blocked by a targeted mutation in the gene for transcription factor GATA-1. *Nature* 349:257, 1991.

291. Shivdasani RA, Fujiwara Y, McDevitt MA, et al: A lineage-selective knockout establishes the critical role of transcription factor GATA-1 in megakaryocyte growth and platelet development. *EMBO J* 16:3965, 1997.

292. Tsang AP, Visvader JE, Turner CA, et al: FOG, a multitype zinc finger protein, acts as a cofactor for transcription factor GATA-1 in erythroid and megakaryocytic differentiation. *Cell* 90:109, 1997.

293. Nichols KE, Crispino JD, Poncz M, et al: Familial dyserythropoietic anaemia and thrombocytopenia due to an inherited mutation in GATA1. *Nat Genet* 24:266, 2000.

294. Doubeikovski A, Uzan G, Doubeikovski Z, et al: Thrombopoietin-induced expression of the glycoprotein IIb gene involves the transcription factor PU.1/Spi-1 in UT7-Mpl cells. *J Biol Chem* 272:24300, 1997.

295. Athanasiou M, Clausen PA, Mavrothalassitis GJ, et al: Increased expression of the ETS-related transcription factor FLI-1/ERGB correlates with and can induce the megakaryocytic phenotype. *Cell Growth Differ* 7:1525, 1996.

296. Giles F, Estey E, O'Brien S: Gemtuzumab ozogamicin in the treatment of acute myeloid leukemia. *Cancer* 98:2095, 2003.

297. Khanna-Gupta A, Zibello T, Sun H, et al: C/EBP epsilon mediates myeloid differentiation and is regulated by the CCAAT displacement protein (CDP/cut). *Proc Natl Acad Sci U S A* 98:8000, 2001.

298. Dahl R, Walsh JC, Lancki D, et al: Regulation of macrophage and neutrophil cell fates by the PU.1:C/EBPalpha ratio and granulocyte colony-stimulating factor. *Nat Immunol* 4:1029, 2003.

THE INFLAMMATORY RESPONSE

JEFFREY S. WARREN

PETER A. WARD

The inflammatory response is characterized by a rapid but relatively short-lived increase in local blood flow, an increase in microvascular permeability, and the sequential recruitment of different types of leukocytes. Superimposed is a series of reparative processes (e.g., parenchymal regeneration, angiogenesis, production of extracellular matrix, and scar formation). The early hemodynamic changes at a site of inflammation establish conditions that enable marginated leukocytes to engage in low-affinity selectin-mediated rolling interactions with endothelial cells. In response to locally produced soluble and cell surface mediators, endothelial cells and rolling leukocytes become activated and sequentially express sets of complementary adhesion molecules that include β_2 integrins, selectins, and members of the immunoglobulin superfamily. Leukocyte and endothelial cell adhesion molecules mediate the high-affinity adhesive interactions necessary for leukocyte emigration from the vascular space and along chemotactic gradients. Analogous, temporally regulated, soluble mediators and cellular adhesion molecules also orchestrate succeeding monocyte- and lymphocyte-rich chronic inflammatory responses. This basic paradigm is modulated by a large number of surface-active and soluble inflammatory mediators. Both recruited leukocytes and cells indigenous to the anatomic site of inflammation play critical roles in host defense and tissue repair.

HISTORY

The sentinel clinical features of acute inflammation, rubor, calor, tumor, and dolor, have been recognized for 5000 years. Dr. John Hunter, the renowned late 18th century Scottish surgeon, observed that the inflammatory response is not a disease per se but rather a nonspecific and salutary response to a variety of insults. Through his microscopic examinations of transparent vital membrane preparations, Julius Cohnheim concluded that the inflammatory response is fundamentally a vascular phenomenon. Phagocytosis was discovered late in the 19th century by Eli Metchnikoff and his colleagues. Morphologic studies, using both live animals and fixed histologic preparations, transformed our understanding of inflammation and led to the currently held concepts of inflammation-associated hemodynamic alterations, "acute" inflammation, and "chronic" inflammation.[1] It has been during the past 50 years that the modern techniques of biochemistry, tissue culture, monoclonal antibody production, recombinant DNA technology, and the genetic manipulation of isolated cells and whole animals, have enabled a more detailed understanding of the cellular and molecular mechanisms which characterize the inflammatory response. These studies, in concert with "experiments of nature" such as chronic granulomatous disease (see Chap. 66) and the leukocyte adhesion deficiency disorders (see Chap. 66), have provided for the formulation of complex, yet elegant, models of acute and chronic inflammation and led to the promise of incisive therapeutic approaches. A vast array of human diseases is marked by either defects in the development of the inflammatory response or the deleterious effects of the inflammatory response itself.

GENERAL CHARACTERISTICS OF INFLAMMATION

While necessarily contrived, it is useful to consider inflammation as an acute or chronic process. "Acute" inflammation lasts from minutes to a few days and is characterized by local hemodynamic and microvascular changes and leukocyte accumulation.[2] The acute inflammatory response is consistently marked by microvascular leakage and the accumulation of neutrophils. The four cardinal signs of inflammation, alluded to above, can be accounted for within the physiologic terms of acute inflammation.

In contrast, the chronic inflammatory response, which lasts much longer and is more varied in its effects, is also marked by the proliferation of resident fibroblasts and the growth of new capillaries.[2] Cellular infiltrates include primarily lymphocytes and monocytes but there are many variations in the cellular composition, anatomic distribution, and tempo of development of chronic inflammatory lesions. Chronic inflammatory processes are classified according to these variations. For example, granulomatous inflammation is a chronic process marked by nodular aggregates of mononuclear phagocytes that have become "transformed" into so-called epithelioid histiocytes because of their similar appearance to epithelial cells. Granulomas may be distributed along blood vessels (e.g., angiocentric), along airways (e.g., bronchocentric), or randomly throughout the interstitium or parenchyma of an organ. Other chronic inflammatory processes are marked by a preponderance of plasma cells or eosinophils. In contrast to the more stereotyped appearance of an acute inflammatory lesion, the particular appearance of a chronic inflammatory lesion can sometimes provide insight into its cause (e.g., caseating granulomas in tuberculosis, eosinophil-rich infiltrates in a parasitic infection, and plasma-cell-rich infiltrates in viral hepatitis).

Superimposed upon the acute and chronic inflammatory response is repair.[2] Repair may entail the regeneration of parenchymal cells damaged as the direct result of an insult per se or as "bystanders" to the inflammatory response. Repair is characterized by the growth of new capillaries (angiogenesis) and the activation of fibroblasts which produce extracellular matrix molecules (e.g., scar tissue). In some circumstances an acute inflammatory response is self-limited (e.g., sunburn), whereas in other situations the response becomes chronic and can persist for years (e.g., tuberculous granulomas).

This chapter first addresses acute inflammation, which encompasses localized changes in blood flow, alterations in microvascular permeability, and neutrophil exudation. There has been great progress in understanding of the processes of endothelial cell activation, leukocyte–endothelial cell rolling, and so-called stationary adhesive interactions, leukocyte emigration, leukocyte activation, and the subsequent dampening of an inflammatory response. The second section of this chapter introduces the vast array of soluble and surface-active mediators that orchestrate both acute and chronic inflammatory responses. These mediators include substances that range from short-lived reactive oxygen and nitrogen intermediates to entire regulatory

Acronyms and abbreviations that appear in this chapter include: BPI, bactericidal/permeability increasing protein; CAP37, cationic antimicrobial protein; CD, cluster of differentiation; eNOS, endothelial nitric oxide synthase; HPETE, hydroperoxyeicosatetraenoic acid; ICAM, intercellular adhesion molecule; Ig, immunoglobulin; IL, interleukin; iNOS, inducible nitric oxide synthase; LT, leukotriene; LTB$_4$ / C$_4$ / D$_4$ / E$_4$, leukotriene B4 / C4 / D4 / E4; MASP, mannan-binding lectin-associated serine protease; MBL, mannan-binding lectin; NADPH, reduced nicotinamide adenine dinucleotide phospate; nNOS, neuronal nitric oxide synthase; NO, nitric oxide; NOS, nitric oxide synthase; PAF, platelet-activating factor; PSGL-1, P-selectin glycoprotein ligand-1; RGD, arginine-glycine-aspartic acid peptide sequence; TNF, tumor necrosis factor; VCAM, vascular cell adhesion molecule; VLA, very late antigen.

systems (e.g., complement system and coagulation cascade). Finally, a brief overview of chronic inflammation and tissue repair is provided. This chapter provides a framework for understanding the basic processes of inflammation while promoting an appreciation for the highly complex and integrated nature of the regulated inflammatory response.

ACUTE INFLAMMATION

HEMODYNAMIC CHANGES

The hemodynamic changes that occur early in the acute phase of inflammation include arteriolar vasodilatation and a localized increase in microvascular permeability (Fig. 16-1). In many circumstances, arteriolar vasodilatation follows a rapid and transient period of vasoconstriction.[3] Arteriolar vasodilatation results in increased blood flow, thus explaining the familiar redness and warmth which characterize a site of acute inflammation. The increase in blood flow, coupled with

increases in microvascular permeability, results in hemoconcentration and a localized increase in blood viscosity. These localized hemodynamic changes are critical to subsequent leukocyte emigration because selectin-mediated, low-affinity, rolling leukocyte–endothelial adhesive interactions can efficiently occur only under conditions of reduced shear force. Experimental studies using in vitro flow chambers and live animals indicate that selectin-mediated leukocyte–endothelial rolling adhesive interactions cannot occur in the face of the shear forces exerted by normal blood flow. Increased microvascular permeability leads to protein-rich plasma exudation, which is characteristic of acute inflammation. Microvascular leakage occurs through a variety of mechanisms, including venular endothelial cell contraction, which is accompanied by widening of intercellular junctions; so-called endothelial cell retraction, which is not well understood but involves cytoskeletal changes; leukocyte-mediated endothelial cell injury; direct endothelial injury; and leakage via new capillaries that do not yet possess fully "closed" intercellular junctions.[3] An increase in the rate of transcytosis in which plasma constituents cross endothelial cells in vesicles or vacuoles has a role in neoplastic blood vessels and may play a role in inflammation.[4] Alterations in local blood flow occur at the level of arterioles, which are regulated largely by the autonomic nervous system, vasoactive peptides, and eicosanoids. A variety of soluble mediators can induce increases in microvascular permeability through several of the above-mentioned mechanisms.

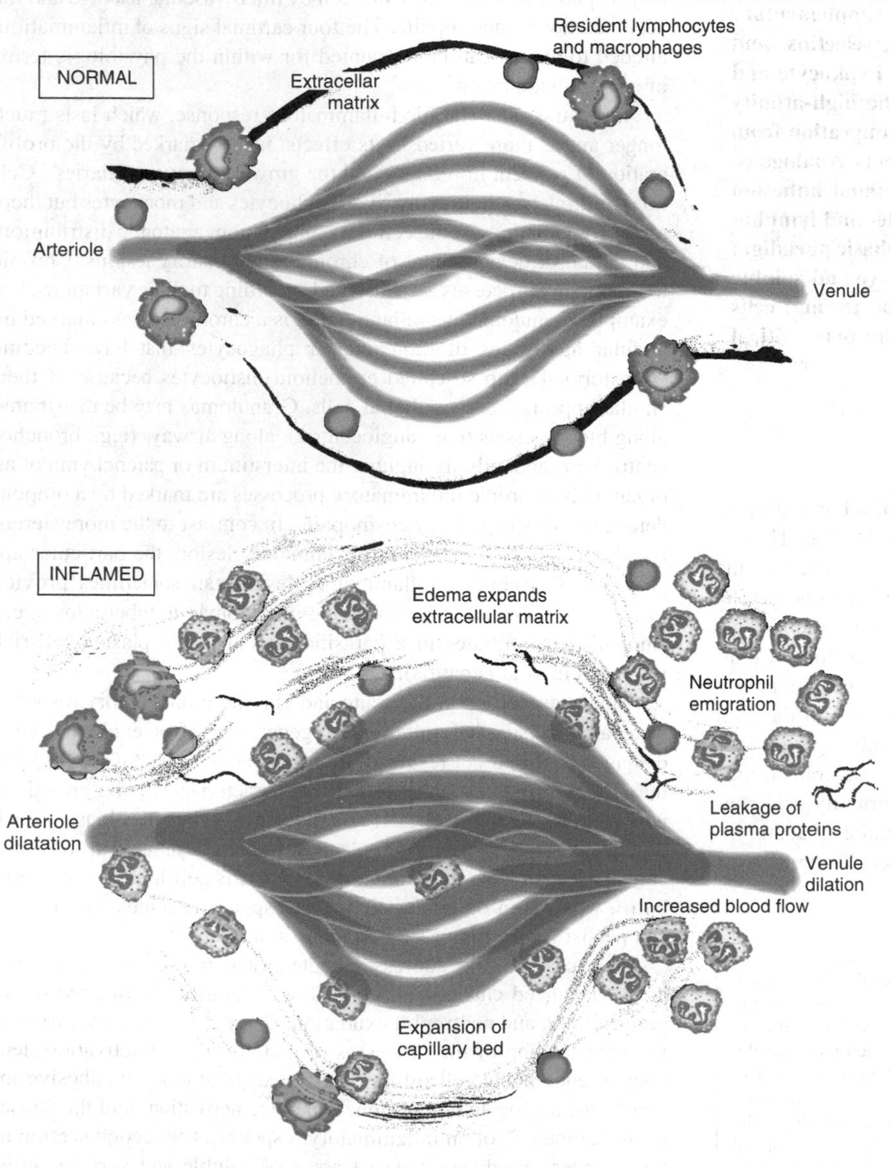

LEUKOCYTE RECRUITMENT

The orchestrated recruitment of leukocytes into a site of inflammation is a fundamental characteristic of the inflammatory response.[5] The importance of white blood cells in host defense is highlighted in patients with genetic defects in white cell function. Leukocytes are critical because of their central role in the phagocytosis and containment or killing of microbes and in the digestion of necrotic tissue debris. Leukocyte-derived products such as proteolytic enzymes and reactive oxygen intermediates contribute to tissue injury.

LEUKOCYTE ADHESION AND TRANSMIGRATION

When vascular stasis occurs as the result of the hemodynamic changes of early acute inflammation, leukocytes are displaced from the central axial column of blood cells to a position along the endothelial surface. This process is enhanced under conditions of slowed blood flow.[2] Individual leukocytes adhere transiently and weakly to the endothelial surface. Studies using vital membrane preparations and flow chamber studies using endothelial cell monolayers and suspensions of purified leukocytes reveal that cells roll along the endothelial surface.[6] Rolling neutrophil–endothelial adhesive interactions occur within minutes of the initiation of an acute inflammatory response and can, depending on the time within the evolution of an inflammatory response, involve neutrophils, lymphocytes, monocytes, basophils, or eosinophils. The leu-

FIGURE 16-1   Early hemodynamic events in acute inflammation. Vascular dilatation, increased microvascular permeability, fluid transudation, and leukocyte recruitment and emigration occur after a transient period of arteriolar vasoconstriction. (Modified and redrawn with permission from *Robbins Pathologic Basis of Disease*, 6th ed. WB Saunders, Philadelphia, 1999.)

TABLE 16-1   ADHESION MOLECULES IN INFLAMMATION

FAMILY	STRUCTURE	MEMBERS	TISSUE DISTRIBUTION	COUNTERRECEPTOR
Selectin	N-terminal lectin domain, epidermal growth factor domain, multiple complement regulatory repeats, transmembrane, and short cytoplasmic tail	P-selectin E-selectin L-selectin	Endothelium, platelets Endothelium Leukocytes	PSGL-1, Sle^X glycoprotein PSGL-1, SLe^X glycoprotein PSGL-1
Immunoglobulin superfamily	Multiple immunoglobulin domains, transmembrane region and cytoplasmic tail	ICAM-1 ICAM-2 ICAM-3 VCAM-1	Endothelium Endothelium	CD11a/CD18 CD11b/CD18 VLA-4
Integrin (β_2; leukocyte)	Heterodimers: distinct α subunits with common β subunits	CD11a/CD18 (LFA-1) CD11b/CD18 (Mac-1) VLA-4	Neutrophils, monocytes, macrophages, and lymphocytes Neutrophils, monocytes, and macrophages Monocytes and lymphocytes	ICAM-1 ICAM-2 ICAM-3 ICAM-1, iC3b, LPS, and fibronectin VCAM-1 and fibronectin

CD, cluster of differentiation; ICAM, intercellular adhesion molecule; LPS, lipopolysaccharide; PSGL-1, P-selectin glycoprotein ligand-1; VCAM, vascular cell adhesion molecule; VLA, very late antigen.

kocyte–endothelial cell rolling adhesive interaction is a specific and necessary step that precedes high-affinity, or so-called stationary, adhesion and emigration.[6,7] Early rolling adhesive interactions are mediated largely by selectins and their counterreceptors.[6] In turn, the cell surface expression of selectins (and other intercellular adhesion molecules, see below) is regulated by a number of locally produced proinflammatory mediators.[6,7]

Selectins contain an extracellular N-terminal carbohydrate-binding region that is homologous to mammalian lectins, an epidermal growth factor-like domain, a series of complement regulatory domains, and a lipophilic transmembrane domain (Table 16-1).[8,9] P-selectin is expressed by endothelial cells and platelets, E-selectin by endothelial cells, and L-selectin by most white blood cells. P-selectin is stored in endothelial intracytoplasmic granules called Weibel-Palade bodies. [9–11] When endothelial cells are exposed to histamine, thrombin, or platelet-activating factor (PAF), P-selectin is rapidly (within minutes) translocated to the endothelial surface where it engages marginated leukocytes via carbohydrate moieties that contain sialic acid residues (e.g., P-selectin glycoprotein ligand-1 [PSGL-1]).[8–11] This transient, low-affinity, binding interaction, which can withstand only the low-flow shear force conditions found in stasis, accounts in part for the early rolling interactions (Fig. 16-2). The development of single knockout mice (i.e., lack individual selectins [P−/−; E−/−; L−/−]), double knockout mice (e.g., E/P−/−), and even triple knockout mice, has confirmed that rolling can be almost completely accounted for by selectins.[46,47] Exposure of endothelial cells to tumor necrosis factor alpha (TNF-α) or interleukin (IL)-β results in protein synthesis-dependent expression of E-selectin, a response that occurs within 1 to 2 hours and peaks at 4 to 6 hours.[6,12] As in the case of P-selectin–mediated leukocyte adhesion, E-selectin–mediated adhesion occurs via a series of sialylated and fucosylated carbohydrate moieties related to the sialyl Lewis^X and sialyl Lewis^A blood group antigens on leukocytes (Table 16-1).[13,14] L-selectin is constitutively expressed by leukocytes, participates in white blood cell–endothelial cell and leukocyte–leukocyte adhesive interactions via mucin-like glycoproteins (e.g., PSGL-1 and other

SLe^X-bearing molecules), and is shed when the leukocyte is activated (Table 16-1).[9,10,14] L-selectin shedding facilitates leukocyte emigration by allowing the white blood cell to detach from the endothelium. Low-affinity rolling adhesive interactions set the stage for β-integrin and immunoglobulin superfamily mediated, high-affinity adhesive interactions and leukocyte transmigration.[6,8,9]

Relatively weak selectin-mediated and high-affinity stationary adhesive interactions are not temporally or mechanistically discrete. For example, TNF-α and IL-β induce both E-selectin, which is not expressed by quiescent cells, and increases in endothelial expression of intercellular adhesion molecule (ICAM)-1 and vascular cell adhesion molecule (VCAM)-1, which are constitutively expressed in low concentrations and, in the case of ICAM-1, are involved in the recruitment of all types of leukocytes, and in the case of VCAM-1, are involved in the recruitment of all types of chronic inflammatory leukocytes (lymphocytes, monocytes, eosinophils, and basophils).[5] ICAM-1 binds to β_2 (leukocyte) integrins, which are heterodimeric structures that contain varied alpha chains (CD11a, CD11b, CD11c, CD11d) and a common beta chain (CD18).[15,16] VCAM-1 binds to β_1 integrins (e.g., VLA-4/$\alpha_4\beta_1$) (see Table 16-1).[5,7] Activated endothelial cells secrete

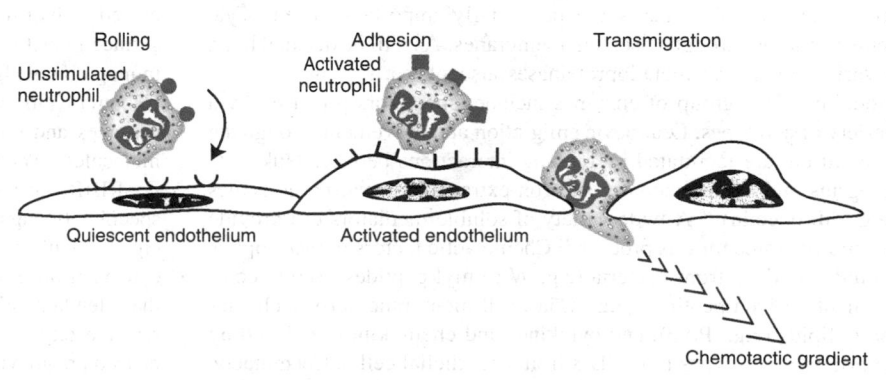

FIGURE 16-2   Leukocyte–endothelial adhesive interactions. Early in the acute inflammatory response, marginated leukocytes engage in transient, low-affinity, selectin-mediated adhesive interactions with endothelial cells. As the response evolves, activated leukocytes and endothelial cells engage in high-affinity β_2-integrin and immunoglobulin superfamily-mediated adhesive interactions. A variety of chemotactic factors can provide the motive force for leukocyte emigration. (Modified and redrawn from multiple references.)

platelet-activating factor and IL-8, which activate overlying leukocytes.[15] Leukocyte CD11b/CD18 (Mac-1) is up-regulated in terms of number and undergoes a transient conformational change that increases its binding affinity for endothelial ICAM-1. CD11a/CD18 also exhibits an increase in binding avidity, but there is no increase in number of surface molecules. CD11c/CD18 binds to iC3b (see below) and initiates phagocytosis, but plays a lesser role in neutrophils than do CD11a/CD18 and CD11b/CD18. Intercellular adhesion molecules are found on a variety of cell types aside from endothelial cells.[7] CD11a/CD18 interacts with both ICAM-1 and ICAM-2, whereas CD11b/CD18 binds to ICAM-1 and the complement activation product, iC3b (see below). The roles of CD11c/CD18, CD11d/CD18, and ICAM-3 in leukocyte–endothelial adhesion are less well established. β_1 Integrins, notably very late antigen (VLA)-4, are found on chronic inflammatory leukocytes (e.g., lymphocytes, monocytes, basophils, and eosinophils) and mediate leukocyte binding via VCAM-1.[17] β_1-integrin–mediated adhesive interactions occur via arginine-glycine-aspartic acid peptide sequences (RGDs) within VCAM-1 as well as matrix molecules (e.g., fibronectin). β_2-Integrin-ICAM– and β_1-VCAM-1–mediated adhesive interactions occur later (hours to days) in the inflammatory response than do selectin-mediated interactions. Additional adhesive interactions are also involved in leukocyte transmigration.[5] The functional importance of the various complementary leukocyte–endothelial adhesive interactions has been clarified by *in vitro* leukocyte–endothelial binding studies and *in vivo* studies that employed neutralizing antibodies directed against adhesion molecules, pharmacologic antagonists of adhesion molecules, and knockout mice.[18–20] The functional importance of leukocyte integrins (CD11a/CD18, CD11b/CD18, CD11c/CD18) has also been highlighted by clinical and experimental observations in patients with leukocyte adhesion deficiencies (see Chap. 66). The life span of neutrophils, normally 4 to 10 hours, can be greatly extended (up to 48 hours) following emigration into an inflammatory site. Various soluble cytokines (see "Leukocyte Chemotaxis and Activation," below) can alter the basal rate of neutrophil apoptosis, thus providing a means for localized increases or decreases in duration of survival.

LEUKOCYTE CHEMOTAXIS AND ACTIVATION

Leukocytes that are tightly bound to endothelium emigrate from the vascular space into the interstitium by extending pseudopods between intercellular junctions (see Fig. 16-2). Secreted neutral proteases, such as elastase, cathepsin G, and proteinase 3, play a role in the passage or "invasion" of leukocytes through subendothelial extracellular matrix material. Collagenases are particularly important in leukocyte transmigration through basement membranes. As will be detailed later, a variety of matrix metalloproteinases also play a role in tissue remodeling. This group of enzymes includes mediators produced by a variety of cell types. Leukocyte emigration and movement through the interstitium are facilitated by binding interactions between leukocyte integrins and complementary sites on extracellular matrix molecules (e.g., fibronectin).[21] A wide variety of soluble mediators can provide the motive force for this process.[21] Chemotactic factors for neutrophils include peptides from bacteria (e.g., N-formyl peptides), serum complement-derived peptides (e.g., C5a), cell membrane-derived chemotactic lipids (e.g., PAF), and cytokines and chemokines produced by a variety of cell types (e.g., IL-8 from endothelial cells). Chemotactic factors vary with respect to their specificity for different types of leukocytes. For example, C5a and N-formyl peptides both induce neutrophil and monocyte chemotaxis, IL-8 induces neutrophil chemotaxis, and monocyte chemoattractant protein-1 induces chemotactic responses in monocytes and a specific subset of memory T lymphocytes. Each of these chemotactic factors activates "target" cells by engaging specific cell surface receptors, which, in turn, are linked to the con-

tractile cell motility apparatus.[21] In addition to chemotaxis, soluble and cell surface mediators induce leukocyte activation, which is manifested by a wide array of changes in cellular function (e.g., adhesion molecule up-regulation and increased adhesion molecule binding avidity [e.g., CD11a/CD18], selectin shedding [e.g., L-selectin], lysosome degranulation, and initiation of the respiratory burst). Great advances in understanding of the biochemical pathways involved in chemotaxis, cell activation, and degranulation have occurred. Although there are many nuances in the signal transduction pathways involved in these processes, several themes have emerged. Cell surface receptors are activated by specific ligands (e.g., C5a, leukotriene B4 [LTB$_4$], IL-8) and receptor activation is transduced via specific G proteins and membrane-associated phospholipases, which lead to mobilization of intracellular calcium, influx of extracellular calcium, and protein phosphorylation. Genetic defects in the regulation of many of these processes are detailed elsewhere throughout this text.

The principal result of neutrophil and monocyte recruitment is to provide: (1) high concentrations of activated leukocytes that can release lytic substances and reactive oxygen and nitrogen intermediates needed to destroy foreign invaders, and (2) a vehicle to contain foreign particulates through phagocytosis. The products and functions of activated inflammatory cells are at once salutary because they contain and destroy invaders and deleterious because they cause tissue damage.

Leukocyte activation, especially that of neutrophils and mononuclear phagocytes, results in the secretion of many microbicidal peptides (e.g., defensins, serprocidins, bactericidal/permeability-increasing protein [BPI], cationic antimicrobial protein [CAP37]) and lytic enzymes (e.g., myeloperoxidase, elastase, cathepsin G).[22] The release of such granular constituents is accompanied by the generation of reactive oxygen and nitrogen intermediates (e.g., O_2^-, H_2O_2, NO), the generation of arachidonate metabolites (e.g., leukotrienes and prostaglandins), and the production of other mediators (see below).[22,23] In some circumstances these materials are released into phagolysosomes, where they contribute to the destruction of engulfed microbes, while in other circumstances they are secreted into the extracellular milieu, where they amplify the inflammatory response and cause tissue damage. The different types of neutrophil granules (primary azurophilic, secondary specific, tertiary gelatinase-containing, and secretory vesicles) are released in a coordinated differential fashion.[22]

Phagocytosis involves three distinct steps: recognition and attachment, engulfment, and degradation (killing) of the ingested material.[24] Phagocytosis is enhanced greatly when particles (e.g., bacteria) are coated with opsonins, which, in turn, function as ligands for leukocyte surface receptors. The major opsonins include the Fc domain of immunoglobulin (Ig) G and IgM and the complement-derived fragments C3b and iC3b, which are generated via activation of the complement cascades and covalently bond to the surfaces of particles and large molecules. There are a variety of Fc receptors (FcγRI, FcγRII, FcγRIIIB, etc.) and complement receptors (e.g., CR1, CR3, CR4) that specifically engage their respective opsonins when the latter coat foreign particulates.[25] In addition to facilitating receptor-mediated phagocytosis of opsonized particles, Fc receptors trigger cell activation with the attendant release of granular constituents and the generation of reactive oxygen intermediates.[25] As noted in Table 16-1, some enhanced phagocytic reactions occur independently of opsonins. The engulfment, degranulation, and oxidative burst triggered as the result of engagement of FcR is enhanced by the concurrent engagement of complement receptors. In some circumstances, engulfment is enhanced by the simultaneous binding of the leukocyte to specific extracellular matrix molecules (e.g., fibronectin) or soluble cytokines. Engulfment results in the formation of phagosomes, which fuse with lysosomes to form phagolysosomes in which the foreign particle is oxidized and

TABLE 16-2 KILLING AND DEGRADATION OF MICROORGANISMS IN PHAGOCYTES

Oxygen-Dependent		Oxygen-Independent
Superoxide anion	(O_2)	Arachidonate metabolites (prostaglandins, leukotrienes)
Hydrogen peroxide	(H_2O_2)	Platelet-activating factor
Hydroxyl radical	$(HO\cdot)$	Lysosomal proteases
Singlet oxygen	$(^1O_2)$	Lactoferrin
N-chloramines	$(R\text{-}NHC1, R\text{-}NCl_2)$	Lysozyme
Hypohalous acids	$(HO\text{-}X)$	Cationic proteins (e.g., major basic protein, defensins)
Nitric oxide	(NO)	
Peroxynitrite	$(ONOO^-)$	

degraded. Numerous mechanisms for killing and/or degradation of microbes have been elucidated (Table 16-2). Although these mechanisms are classified as either oxygen-dependent or oxygen-independent, both types of processes may be involved in the destruction of a given microorganism, and a given microorganism may vary greatly in its susceptibility to various mechanisms of destruction.[22-25]

REGULATION OF THE INFLAMMATORY RESPONSE

The foregoing sections provide a conceptual framework for the inflammatory response, specifically, the hemodynamic alterations, mechanisms of specific leukocyte–endothelial adhesive interactions, chemotaxis, and leukocyte activation and phagocytosis. The many steps that constitute this paradigm are regulated by a variety of soluble mediators that are produced by endothelial cells and leukocytes at a site of inflammation, by other resident cells (e.g., tissue macrophages, fibroblasts, mast cells), and as by-products of blood-borne proteins (e.g., complement system, coagulation cascade) (Table 16-3).

REACTIVE OXYGEN INTERMEDIATES

Since the early 1970s it has been recognized that activated phagocytes exhibit a transient but marked increase in oxygen consumption and in the generation of reduced oxygen metabolites.[23] Although small quan-

tities of reactive oxygen intermediates are produced as by-products of a variety of biochemical pathways, the chief source is the leukocyte membrane-associated reduced nicotinamide adenine dinucleotide phospate (NADPH) oxidase, an enzyme complex that is defective in patients with chronic granulomatous disease (see Chap. 66). Reactive oxygen intermediates include superoxide anion (O_2^-), hydrogen peroxide (H_2O_2), hydroxyl radical (HO·), and singlet oxygen ($^1O_2$). These reduced oxygen products play a major role in intraphagolysosomal killing of microorganisms and when released extracellularly are directly or indirectly responsible for a variety of inflammatory processes, including endothelial cell lysis, extracellular matrix degradation, activation of latent proteolytic enzymes (collagenase, gelatinase), inactivation of antiproteases, interaction with toxic metabolites of L-arginine, and generation of chemotactic factors from arachidonic acid and the complement component C5.[23] In addition to their role in endothelial cytotoxicity, reactive oxygen intermediates are cytotoxic for fibroblasts, erythrocytes, tumor cells, and various parenchymal cells.[23] The biochemical mechanisms implicated include lipid peroxidation, formation of carbonyl moieties and nitrosylation products, intracellular enzyme inactivation, protein oxidation, and oxidant-mediated DNA damage. Reactive oxygen intermediates (e.g., O_2^-) can also undergo reactions with reactive nitrogen intermediates (e.g., nitric oxide [NO]; see "Reactive Nitrogen Intermediates," below) to generate toxic NO derivatives.

REACTIVE NITROGEN INTERMEDIATES

Described in 1980 as endothelium-derived relaxing factor, NO is the soluble, short-acting biosynthetic product of L-arginine, O_2, NADPH, and nitric oxide synthase (NOS).[26,27] As suggested by its original name, NO mediates vascular smooth muscle relaxation. NO binds to the heme moiety of guanylyl cyclase to trigger the generation of intracytoplasmic cGMP and, through the activation of a series of kinases, induces smooth-muscle relaxation and vasodilatation.[26,27] Three different forms of NOS have been characterized[27]: endothelial (eNOS), neuronal (nNOS), and inducible (iNOS). Nitric oxide can be produced either constitutively (cNOS, nNOS) or induced (iNOS) in a wide variety of cell types (e.g., endothelial cells, neurons, macrophages, respectively). Nitric oxide produced by eNOS plays a particularly important role in the localized regulation of vascular tone, whereas NO

TABLE 16-3 INFLAMMATORY MEDIATOR SYSTEMS

Mediator System	Source	Major Actions
Reactive oxygen intermediates (O_2^-, H_2O_2, HOX, HO)	Leukocytes, endothelial cells	Tissue damage through cytolysis, matrix degradation, activation of complement, and generation of chemotactic lipids
Reactive nitrogen intermediates (NO, $ONOO^-$, NO_2^-, NO_3^-)	Monocytes, macrophages, lymphocytes, endothelial cells	Cytostasis of cells, inhibition of DNA synthesis, inhibition of mitochondrial respiration, and formation of OH
Lysosomal granule constituents (proteases, lysozyme, lactoferrin, cationic proteins)	Neutrophils, monocytes	Tissue damage through proteolysis, matrix degradation, and catalysis of oxidant-generating reactions
Cytokines and chemokines (TNF, IL-1, IL-8, MCP-1, etc.)	Monocytes, macrophages, and endothelial cells	Cell activation, induction of adhesion, chemotaxis, fever, and acute-phase response
Platelet-activating factor	Leukocytes, endothelial cells	Vascular permeability and cell activation
Arachidonic acid metabolites (prostaglandins, 5-HPETE, leukotrienes)	Cell membranes (endothelial cells, platelets, leukocytes)	Coagulation, vasodilatation, vascular permeability, cell activation, and chemotaxis
Kinins (bradykinin, kallikrein)	Plasma	Pain, vascular permeability, and vasodilatation
Vasoactive amines (serotonin, histamine)	Platelets, mast cells, and basophils	Vascular permeability, induction of adhesion
Complement	Plasma, macrophages	Chemotaxis, vascular permeability, and cell activation
Coagulation	Plasma	Chemotaxis, vascular permeability, and complement activation

5-HPETE, 5 hydroperoxyeicosatetraenoic acid; MCP-1, monocyte chemoattractant protein-1.

derived from nNOS is important in neuronal signal transduction.[2,27] NO also plays important roles in the inhibition of smooth-muscle proliferation and in inflammation. The roles of NO in inflammation include inhibition of most cell-mediated inflammation, reduction in platelet aggregation and adhesion, and as a regulator of leukocyte recruitment.[2] Specifically, NO produced by cytokine-iNOS reduces leukocyte recruitment into sites of inflammation.[2,27] NO can react with reactive oxygen intermediates to form both reactive oxygen and nitrogen species (e.g., $NO + O_2^- \rightarrow NO_2^- + HO\cdot$), it can inhibit DNA synthesis, it can directly kill microbes and tumor cells, and it can inactivate cytosolic glutathione and a number of sulfhydryl enzymes. *In vivo* studies confirm that inhibition of NO synthesis with antagonistic L-arginine analogues can reduce tissue injury in models of inflammation.[28,29]

LYSOSOMAL GRANULE CONSTITUENTS

The activation of neutrophils, monocytes, and macrophages results in the release, either through exocytosis or as the result of cell death, of a wide variety of proinflammatory mediators that have important roles in the inflammatory response. Neutrophils contain three major types of granules and also secretory vesicles (see Chaps. 59 and 60).[22] Large, primary (azurophilic) granules contain myeloperoxidase, lysozyme, a variety of cationic proteins, defensins, phospholipase, acid hydrolases, and neutral proteases (e.g., proteinase 3, collagenases, elastase). Smaller, secondary (specific) granules contain lactoferrin, lysozyme, type IV collagenase, subunits of NADPH oxidase, and the β_2-integrin CD11b/CD18. Tertiary granules contain gelatinase, subunits of NADPH oxidase, and CD11b/CD18. Acid proteases function most efficiently within phagolysosomes where the pH is low, whereas neutral proteases can function efficiently within extracellular inflammatory exudates. Lysosomal granule constituents contribute to the inflammatory response and tissue injury through a wide array of mechanisms (e.g., degradation of extracellular matrix, proteolytic generation of chemotactic peptide, and catalysis of reactive oxygen and nitrogen metabolite generation).

CYTOKINES AND CHEMOKINES

Cytokines are relatively small (5–20-kDa) proteins that are produced by many cell types and modulate the function of other cell types. Individual cells may produce many different cytokines, and an individual cytokine may exert a wide variety of effects; they are pleiotropic. A large number of cytokines and chemokines have been identified and characterized.[30] In addition to their important roles in regulating various aspects of the immune response (e.g., lymphocyte activation and differentiation), many cytokines participate in natural immunity (e.g., TNF-α, IL-1α, type I interferons), activate inflammatory cells (e.g., γ-interferon), and participate in hematopoiesis (e.g., IL-3, granulocyte-monocyte colony stimulating factor, granulocyte colony stimulating factor, macrophage colony stimulating factor).[30] Among the most thoroughly characterized cytokines are IL-1 and TNF-α. IL-1 and TNF-α are structurally dissimilar but share many biologic activities and can function as autocrine, paracrine, and endocrine mediators (Table 16-4). IL-1 and TNF-α are produced by various cell types and are pleiotropic. Their most important functions in inflammation include endothelial, leukocyte, and fibroblast activation.

IL-1 and TNF-α are key proximal mediators of the "acute-phase response." Stimuli such as bacterial endotoxin (lipopolysaccharide), toxins, immune complexes, and physical factors (e.g., heat or trauma) can induce macrophages (and other cell types) to secrete IL-1 and TNF-α. In turn, IL-1 and TNF-α mediate fever, somnolence, increased production of proteins such as α_1-antiprotease and α_2-macroglobulin, and decreased production of proteins such as albumin and transferrin. The acute phase response is a stereotyped host metabolic response to

TABLE 16-4 INTERLEUKIN-1 AND TUMOR NECROSIS FACTOR IN INFLAMMATION

Acute-phase response
Fever
Shock
Neutrophilia
Somnolence
Anorexia
Acute-phase proteins
Endothelial activation
Induction of IL-1, IL-6, IL-8
Procoagulant phenotype
Leukocyte adherence
Fibroblast activation
Proliferation
Collagen synthesis
Collagenase and protease induction

a wide variety of insults. In clinical medicine, the above changes in specific protein synthesis yield a characteristic set of changes visible by serum protein electrophoresis. In addition to the systemic acute-phase response, IL-1 and TNF-α induce endothelial activation marked by increases in leukocyte adherence and a procoagulant state, leukocyte activation marked by cytokine secretion, and fibroblast activation marked by proliferation, collagen synthesis, and collagenase production. These actions are critical components of inflammation and wound healing, and they exemplify the linkage between the inflammatory response and the coagulation system.

IL-1, which exhibits a wide variety of biologic activities, was initially termed *endogenous pyrogen* because of its ability to induce temperature elevation and the acute-phase response.[30] IL-1 is now known to be relevant to acute inflammation because of its ability to induce cytokine production in monocytes, macrophages, fibroblasts, and endothelial cells (TNF-α, IL-1, and IL-6). IL-1 can also induce NOS. As noted previously, IL-1 can activate endothelial cells, resulting in the expression of adhesion molecules and a procoagulant phenotype.

TNF-α, originally identified as *cachectin*, can induce cytokine production in a variety of cells. TNF-α can induce neutrophil activation and the expression of adhesion molecules on endothelial cells.[31] In contrast to IL-1, TNF-α also possesses potent cytotoxic activities for certain types of cells. Both IL-1 and TNF-α are produced in response to endotoxemia and both can mediate a systemic shock-like response.

Chemokines, or *intercrines*, are small proteins, which, in addition to the more general properties of cytokines, exhibit prominent chemotactic activities.[32] They were recently grouped into four classes based on the arrangements of conserved cysteine (C) residues in mature peptides.[2] The two most studied subfamilies include the alpha, or -C-X-C- chemokines, and the beta, or C-C chemokines. "C-X-C" chemokines are so designated because the first two N-terminal cystine residues are separated by a single amino acid. Alpha chemokines, of which IL-8 is the prototype, consistently exhibit neutrophil chemotactic activity, whereas the beta, or -C-C chemokines, of which monocyte chemoattractant protein-1 (MCP-1) is the prototype, exhibit monocyte chemotactic activity (Table 16-5). Both *in vitro* and *in vivo* studies have provided insight into the roles of chemokines in inflammation. For example, MCP-1 knockout mice (MCP-1 −/−) exhibit reductions in monocyte influx into sites of experimentally induced peritonitis and delayed-type hypersensitivity.[48] Complementary studies using knockout mice devoid of the MCP-1 receptor CCR2 (C-C chemokine receptor 2), do not form typical granulomas.[49] These types of studies, as well as many studies that have employed specific chemokine-neutral-

TABLE 16-5   CHEMOKINES

FAMILY	MEMBERS	ABBREVIATIONS	PRIMARY TARGET CELLS
α-Chemokines (C-X-C)	Interleukin-8	IL-8	Neutrophils
	Platelet factor 4	PF4	Neutrophils
	Melanocyte growth-stimulatory activity	MGSA or GROα	Neutrophils
	Neutrophil-activating peptide-2	NAP-2	Neutrophils
	γ-Interferon-inducible protein	γ-IP-10	Neutrophils
β-Chemokines (C-C)	Monocyte chemoattractant protein-1	MCP-1/MCAF or JE	Monocytes, basophils
	Regulated on activation, normal T cell expressed and presumably secreted	RANTES	Monocytes, eosinophils, basophils
	Macrophage inflammatory protein-1α	MIP-1α	Monocytes, eosinophils
	Macrophage inflammatory protein-1β	MIP-1β	Monocytes

izing antibodies or soluble chemokine receptor antagonists, have provided valuable insight into the pathophysiology of inflammation. Seemingly contradictory experimental results suggest that leukocyte recruitment mechanisms are multiple, overlapping, or redundant, and certainly not completely understood. For instance, a recent knockout mouse study of wound healing revealed no difference in macrophage numbers between MCP-1 (−/−) mice and their MCP-1 (+/+) controls.[50] Chemokines activate leukocytes through a family of membrane receptors (serpentines) that contain seven transmembrane domains and are linked to heterotrimeric G proteins.[32-34,48-50]

INFLAMMATORY LIPIDS
Arachidonic acid, a 20-carbon polyunsaturated fatty acid (5,8,11,14-eicosatetraenoic acid) derived either from dietary sources or by conversion from linoleic acid, is maintained in cell membranes as an esterified phospholipid.[35] The two families of inflammatory mediators derived from arachidonic acid are generated via the cyclooxygenase and lipoxygenase pathways (resulting in the appearance of prostaglandins and leukotrienes, respectively).[35] Cell activation or mechanical stress can result in the release of arachidonic acid. Activation of the cyclooxygenase family of phospholipases results in prostaglandin synthesis. Members of this group of mediators exhibit several proinflammatory activities, including vasodilatation, vasoconstriction, increases in permeability, and platelet activation (aggregation). Activation of the lipoxygenase pathway results in the synthesis of 5-hydroperoxyeicosatetraenoic acid (5-HPETE), which is a potent chemoattractant of neutrophils and can be modified to yield a series of other leukotrienes. LTB$_4$ induces neutrophil chemotaxis, aggregation, degranulation, and adherence, while LTC$_4$, LTD$_4$, and LTE$_4$ trigger smooth-muscle constriction and increases in vascular permeability. Members of both of these families of lipid-derived mediators have been detected in inflammatory exudates. The effectiveness of nonsteroidal antiinflammatory agents and aspirin, which inhibit cyclooxygenase, highlight the importance of these mediators in the development of an acute inflammatory response.

PAF is a potent proinflammatory lipid produced by a variety of cell types, including neutrophils, monocytes, endothelial cells, and IgE-sensitized basophils.[36] Derived from the cell membrane constituent choline phosphoglyceride, PAF is an acetyl glycerol ether phosphocholine that is synthesized following the activation of phospholipase A$_2$. PAF triggers platelet aggregation and degranulation, increases vascular permeability, and promotes leukocyte accumulation and activation. In vivo studies using specific PAF antagonists have suggested a role for PAF in a variety of acute inflammatory lesions.[36]

KININS
The kinin system is activated by contact activation of clotting factor XII (Hageman factor) (see Chaps. 106 and 107).[37] Activation of the kinin system results in the generation of bradykinin, the nine-amino-acid vasoactive peptide. Bradykinin possesses several activities, including the capacity to increase vascular permeability, to induce smooth-muscle contraction, to trigger vasodilation, and to cause pain.[37] Activated Hageman factor (factor XIIa), also known as the prekallikrein activator, converts plasma prekallikrein to kallikrein. Kallikrein cleaves high molecular weight kininogen to produce bradykinin. Models of septic shock reveal decreases in plasma kininogen that parallel decreases in peripheral arterial resistance.[37]

VASOACTIVE AMINES
Histamine and serotonin (5-hydroxytryptamine) are low molecular weight vasoactive amines. Histamine is contained in mast cell and basophil granules, whereas platelets are the chief source of serotonin.[38] Localized release of histamine results in wheal formation as a consequence of increases in vascular permeability. Histamine induces the formation of reversible openings in endothelial tight junctions, triggers the formation of prostacyclin by endothelial cells, and induces NO release from the endothelium. In addition, histamine, like thrombin, can induce the rapid up-regulation of endothelial P-selectin.[38] Serotonin, which acts through receptors on vascular smooth-muscle cells, is responsible for vasoconstriction, whereas interaction with endothelial receptors results in vasodilation (via release of NO) and increased permeability. Release of histamine and serotonin from mast cells and platelets can be triggered by IgE-mediated type I hypersensitivity reactions, directly by C3a or C5a, and directly by neutrophil granule-derived cationic proteins.

COMPLEMENT
The complement system, including its soluble and cell membrane-associated regulators, consists of nearly two dozen plasma proteins that give rise to mediators of chemotaxis, increased vascular permeability, opsonic activity, phagocytic activation, and cytolysis.[39,40] In a manner analogous to coagulation, the complement system is activated through a cascade of proteolytic cleavage reactions. There are three convergent pathways (Fig. 16-3). The first of these, the classical pathway, is initiated primarily by complement-fixing immune complexes (IgG and IgM), whereas the second, the alternative pathway, is triggered by a variety of substances that include IgA aggregates, endotoxin, cobra venom factor, and the polysaccharide components of some bacterial and fungal cell walls. The third pathway, the mannan-binding lectin (MBL) pathway, is activated when MBL binds to a carbohydrate-coated microorganism. Upon binding, mannan-binding lectin activates MBL-associated serine proteases (e.g., MASP-1, MASP-2), which function in a manner analogous to C1r and C1s of the classical pathway. Mannan-binding lectin recognizes carbohydrate moieties infrequently present in mammalian hosts, thus constituting a system for recognizing foreign particulates. The classical pathway is initiated by

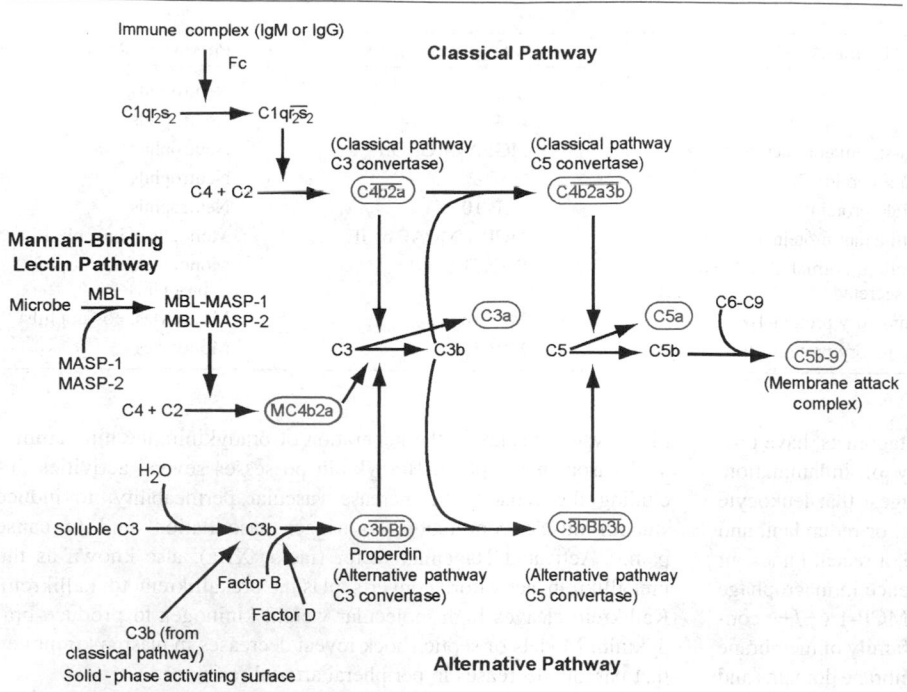

FIGURE 16-3 The complement system. The complement system consists of a series of soluble and surface-associated mediators that are functionally organized into the classical, alternative, and mannan-binding lectin (MBL) pathways. The three pathways of complement converge and lead to the production of the pore-forming membrane attack complex. The classical pathway is most often activated by IgG- and IgM-containing immune complexes, the alternative pathway can be activated by a variety of particulates, and the MBL pathway by various carbohydrate surfaces. In all three cases, complex multicomponent enzyme complexes, called C3 and C5 convertases, are formed. A variety of proinflammatory peptide fragments (e.g., C3a, C5a) are generated as a result of complement activation.

the fixation of C1 (C1qr$_2$s$_2$) by the Fc portion of surface-bound IgG or IgM immunoglobulins. Activated C1 (C1qr$_2$s$_2$) cleaves C2 and C4, which leads to the formation of the "classical pathway" C3 convertase C4b2a. Activation of the alternative pathway results in the formation of an "alternative pathway" C3 convertase following direct cleavage of C3 and subsequent interactions of C3b with factors B and D in the presence of Mg^{2+}. The resulting complex, C3bBb, is stabilized by properdin, leading to the stable C3 convertase C3bBbP. C3 convertases generated via each of the three pathways can cleave C3 to form C3a and C3b. C3b can bind to either the classical or alternative pathway C3 convertase to form a C5 convertase, which cleaves C5 into C5a and C5b. C5a is released into the fluid phase, like C3a, whereas C5b combines first with C6 and then C7 to form C5b-7, which, in turn, binds with C8 and multiple C9 molecules to form C5b-9, the membrane attack complex. In addition to the cell-activating and cytolytic activities of C5b-9, individual complement cleavage products and complexes perform a variety of specific and potent proinflammatory activities.[39,40] These various functions, combined with the rapid amplification in numbers of complement-derived mediators, emphasize the vital role of complement in acute inflammation. The most important activation products of complement appear to be C5a, the major chemotactic factor, and the anaphylatoxins (C3a, C4a, C5a), of which C3a is the most abundant. C5b-9 appears to be a major cytotoxic product, provided that this complex is assembled on the surface of a susceptible cell (e.g., bacterium). A series of soluble and cell membrane-associated complement proteins play important roles in the regulation of the complement cascade.[39,40]

COAGULATION SYSTEM

The coagulation system is reviewed in detail in Chaps. 106, 107, and 127. The interrelationships among the coagulation system and inflammatory mediator systems are important in the context of host defense and the pathophysiology of septic shock. Activation of the clotting cascade results in the generation of fibrinopeptides which increase vascular permeability and are chemotactic for leukocytes. Thrombin induces endothelial expression of P-selectin, resulting in increased neutrophil adhesion.[41] In addition, plasmin is responsible for the activation of Hageman factor, which then can activate the kinin system, and can cleave C3 into its active components. It can also generate fibrin-split products. The induction of procoagulant activity in endothelial cells exposed to TNF-α and IL-1 further links the coagulation system to the inflammatory response.[42]

CHRONIC INFLAMMATION AND REPAIR

The chronic inflammatory response and repair processes are, like the acute inflammatory response, highly regulated. By definition, *chronic* inflammation connotes a process that lasts for weeks to months, and sometimes for years.[2] Chronic inflammation is characterized by the recruitment of mononuclear cells including lymphocytes, monocytes, and plasma cells as well as by the proliferation of new capillaries (angiogenesis) and increases in the deposition of extracellular matrix molecules.[2] Replacement of damaged tissue by new small blood vessels and extracellular matrix constitutes a fundamental aspect of chronic inflammation and, simultaneously, is an integral part of wound healing and repair. The recruitment of this wide variety of cell types is achieved by a complex interaction among cytokines, chemokines, and indigenous cells. Great advances in understanding of angiogenesis and extracellular matrix molecule metabolism have been made in recent years.

Chronic inflammation can be caused by persistent infections with a wide variety of microorganisms (e.g., *Treponema pallidum, Mycobacterium tuberculosis*). In contrast to highly virulent organisms that trigger acute pyogenic infections (e.g., *Streptococcus pneumoniae, Haemophilus influenzae*), organisms that induce chronic inflammation typically exhibit relatively low intrinsic toxicity, are poorly cleared, and provoke a delayed-type hypersensitivity reaction. Chronic inflammation is also triggered by long-term exposure to insoluble exogenous particles (e.g., carbon dust, silica).[2] The initiation of other chronic inflammatory processes such as atherosclerosis and autoimmune diseases (e.g., rheumatoid arthritis, systemic lupus erythematosus) is less well understood, but it is clear that a variety of environmental factors (e.g., diet in atherosclerosis) and genetic factors (e.g., HLA-linked susceptibility is rheumatoid arthritis) are important. The characteristics of individual chronic inflammatory responses are dependent on the location of the injury and the type of injurious agent. As noted throughout this chapter, the recruitment of mononuclear cells into an inflammatory lesion is governed by the same types of mechanisms that orchestrate the recruitment of neutrophils into sites of acute inflammation. Unlike most acute conditions, chronic inflammatory processes are often marked by a relatively specific morphology (e.g., granuloma formation in tuberculosis, eosinophil infiltration in parasitic infections) and by the coexistence of tissue repair (i.e., angiogenesis and extracellular matrix production). A key cell type in chronic inflammatory processes is the macrophage.[43] Tissue macrophages are derived from circulating blood monocytes and can adopt relatively specific functions based on their differentiation in selected body sites (e.g., hepatic Kupffer cells, alveolar macrophages, central nervous system microglia). In the setting of chronic inflammation, tissue macrophages can be activated by immunologic means (γ-interferon secreted by antigen-activated T lymphocytes) and by nonimmunologic means (microbial endotoxin, extracellular matrix proteins, and foreign particulates). In turn, activated macrophages enlarge, become more metabolically active, exhibit enhanced phagocytosis, and secrete a large array of mediators.[43] Mediators secreted by activated macrophages include proteases, reactive oxygen and nitrogen intermediates, coagulation factors, arachidonic acid-derived lipids, and cytokines. These mediators, as detailed in preceding sections, participate in inflammation. Activated macrophages also secrete collagenases that participate in tissue remodeling, angiogenic factors (e.g., fibroblast growth factor), and profibrogenic growth factors (fibroblast growth factor, transforming growth factor-β, platelet-derived growth factor).[43] Consequently, activated tissue macrophages participate in inflammation per se, tissue remodeling, angiogenesis, and fibrosis.

While macrophages play a central role in all facets of chronic inflammation, other cell types are also important. Lymphocytes, both B and T cells, are recruited into chronic inflammatory lesions via leukocyte–endothelial adhesive interactions and via chemotactic mechanisms analogous to those involved in neutrophil recruitment. Antigen-activated T lymphocytes produce γ-interferon, which, as discussed above, is an important soluble activator of tissue macrophages. Activated lymphocytes produce a variety of proinflammatory mediators that are involved in lymphocyte proliferation (e.g., IL-2) and in immune regulation (e.g., IL-5 in IgE production).

Eosinophils and mast cells also play important roles in some types of chronic inflammation. Mast cells, which tend to be distributed along small blood vessels, possess high-affinity FcεRI receptors for IgE.[44,45] Engagement of mast cell-bound IgE triggers degranulation that leads to histamine and arachidonic acid-derived lipid release. Eosinophils are characteristically formed in IgE-mediated allergic reactions and in parasitic infections. Eotaxin, a C-C chemokine, binds to and activates eosinophils via CCR3.[44,45] Recruited eosinophils secrete various granule proteins that help kill parasites, but which can also cause tissue damage. As inferred above, the histopathologic appearance of many chronic inflammatory lesions can provide insight into their pathogenesis and cause. A variety of poorly degraded, intrinsically low toxicity agents can induce granulomatous inflammation (e.g., *Mycobacterium tuberculosis*). Many parasites induce an eosinophilic response (e.g., *Toxocara canis*). Finally, the induction of tissue remodeling, angiogenesis, and fibrosis can contribute to both tissue damage and repair, and can also suggest underlying etiology (e.g., lung fibrosis associated with asbestos.) The tremendous advances in understanding of the inflammatory response hold great promise for the future of both diagnostics and therapeutics.

REFERENCES

1. Weissman G: Inflammation: Historical perspectives, in *Inflammation: Basic Principles and Clinical Correlates*, 2d ed, edited by JJ Gallin, IM Goldstein, R Snyderman, p 5. Raven Press, New York, 1992.

2. Acute and chronic inflammation, in *Robbins and Cotran Pathologic Basis of Disease*, 7th ed, edited by V Kumar, AK Abbas, N Fausto, p 50. Saunders Elsevier, Philadelphia, 2005.

3. Majno G: The capillary then and now: An overview of capillary pathology. *Mod Pathol* 5:9, 1992.

4. Lampugnani MG, Dejana E: Interendothelial junctions: Structure, signaling and functional roles. *Curr Opin Cell Biol* 9:674, 1997.

5. Cotran RS, Mayadas TN: Endothelial adhesion molecules in health and disease. *Pathol Biol* 46:164, 1998.

6. Chen S, Springer TA: Selectin receptor-ligand bonds: Formation limited by shear rate and dissociation governed by the Bell model. *Proc Natl Acad Sci U S A* 98:950, 2001.

7. Dustin ML, Springer TA: Intercellular adhesion molecules (ICAMs), in *Guidebook to the Extracellular Matrix and Adhesion Proteins*, edited by T Kreis, R Vale, page 46. Sambrook and Tooze, New York, 1999.

8. McEver RP: Perspectives series: Cell adhesion in vascular biology: Role in PSGL-1 binding to selectins in leukocyte recruitment. *J Clin Invest* 100:485, 1997.

9. Bevilacqua MP, Nelson RM: Selectins. *J Clin Invest* 91:379, 1993.

10. Ley K, Gaehtgens P, Fennie C, et al: Lectin-like cell adhesion molecule 1 mediates leukocyte rolling in mesenteric venules in vivo. *Blood* 77:2553, 1991.

11. Lorant DE, Topham MK, Whatley RE, et al: Inflammatory roles of P-selectin. *J Clin Invest* 92:559, 1993.

12. Bevilacqua MP, Stengelin S, Gimbrone MAJ, Seed B: Endothelial leukocyte adhesion molecule 1: An inducible receptor for neutrophils related to complement regulatory proteins and lectins. *Science* 243:1160, 1989.

13. Lowe JB, Stoolman LM, Nair RP, et al: ELAM-1 dependent cell adhesion to vascular endothelium determined by a transfected human fucosyltransferase cDNA. *Cell* 63:475, 1990.

14. Picker LJ, Warnock RA, Burns AR, et al: The neutrophil selectin LECAM-1 presents carbohydrate ligands to the vascular selectins ELAM-1 and GMP-140. *Cell* 66:921, 1991.

15. Takagi J, Springer TA: Integrin activation and structural rearrangement. *Immunol Rev* 186:141, 2002.

16. Shimaoka M, Takagi J, Springer TA: Conformational regulation of integrin structure and function. *Annu Rev Biophys Biomol Struct* 31:485, 2002.

17. Hemler ME: VLA proteins in the integrin family: Structures, functions, and their role on leukocytes. *Annu Rev Immunol* 8:365, 1990.

18. Mulligan MS, Varani J, Warren JS, et al: Roles of β_2 integrins of rat neutrophils in complement- and oxygen radical-mediated acute inflammatory injury. *J Immunol* 148:1847, 1992.

19. Arfors KE, Lundberg C, Lindom L, et al: A monoclonal antibody to the membrane glycoprotein complex CD18 inhibits polymorphonuclear leukocyte accumulation and plasma leakage *in vivo*. *Blood* 69:338, 1987.

20. Doerschuk CM, Winn RK, Coxson HO, Harlan JM: CD18-dependent and -independent mechanisms of neutrophil emigration in the pulmonary and systemic microcirculation of rabbits. *J Immunol* 144:2327, 1990.

21. Foxman EF, Campbell JJ, Butcher EC: Multistep navigation and the combinatorial control of leukocyte chemotaxis. *J Cell Biol* 139:1349, 1997.

22. Faurschou M, Borregaard N: Neutrophil granules and secretory vesicles in inflammation. *Microbes Infect* 5:1317, 2003.

23. Klebanoff SJ: Oxygen metabolites from phagocytes, in *Inflammation: Basic Principles and Clinical Correlates*, 2d ed, edited by JJ Gallin, IM Goldstein, R Snyderman., p 541. Raven Press, New York, 1992.

24. Henson PM, et al: Phagocytosis, in *Inflammation: Basic Principles and Clinical Correlates*, 2d ed, edited by JJ Gallin, IM Goldstein, R Snyderman., p 511. Raven Press, New York, 1992.

25. Digstelbluem HM, Kallenberg CGM, Van de Winkel JGJ: Inflammation in autoimmunity: Receptors for IgG. *Trends Immunol* 22:510, 2001.

26. Furchgott RF, Zawadzki JV: The obligatory role of endothelial cells in the relaxation of arterial smooth muscle by acetylcholine. *Nature* 288:373, 1980.

27. MacMicking JD, Xie Q-w, Nathan C: Nitric oxide and macrophage function. *Annu Rev Immunol* 15:323, 1997.

28. Mulligan MS, Warren JS, Smith CW, et al: Lung injury after deposition of IgA immune complexes: Requirements for CD18 and L-arginine. *J Immunol* 148:3086, 1992.

29. Mulligan MS, Moncada S, Ward PA: Protective effects of inhibitors of nitric oxide synthase in immune complex-induced vasculitis. *Br J Pharmacol* 107:1159, 1992.

30. Abbas AK, Lichtman AH: *Cellular and Molecular Immunology*, 3rd ed, p 249. WB Saunders, Philadelphia, 1999.

31. Beutler B: TNF, immunity and inflammatory disease: Lessons of the past decade. *J Investig Med* 43:227, 1995.

32. Taub DD, Oppenheim JJ: Review of the chemokines. The Third International Meeting of Chemotactic Cytokines. *Cytokine* 5:175, 1993.

33. Adams DH, Lloyd AR: Chemokines: Leukocyte recruitment and activation cytokines. *Lancet* 349:490, 1997.

34. Kelvin DJ, Michiel DF, Johnston JAet al: Chemokines and serpentines. *J Leukoc Biol* 54:605, 1993.

35. Zurier RB: Prostaglandins, leukotrienes, and related compounds, in (eds.): *Kelley's Textbook of Rheumatology*, 6th ed, edited by ED Harris, Jr, RC Budd, GS Firestein, MC Genovese, JS, Sargent, S Ruddy., p 356. Saunders Elsevier, Philadelphia, 2005.

36. Zimmerman G, Golden M, Doherty K, et al: A fluid phase and cell-associated mediator of inflammation, in *Inflammation: Basic Principles and Clinical Correlates*, 2nd ed, edited by JJ Gallin, IM Goldstein, R Snyderman., p 149. Raven Press, New York, 1992.

37. Carmeliet P, Collen D: Molecular genetics of the fibrinolytic and coagulation systems in haemostasis, thrombogenesis, restenosis and atherosclerosis. *Curr Opin Lipidol* 8:118, 1997.

38. Busse W: Histamine mediator and modulator in inflammation, in *Chemical Messengers of the Inflammatory Process*, edited by JC Houck, p 1. Elsevier, Amsterdam, 1979.

39. Asghar SS, Pasch MC: Complement as a promiscuous signal transduction device. *Lab Invest* 78:1203, 1998.

40. Holers MV: Complement, in *Clinical Immunology: Principles and Practice*, 2nd ed, edited by RR Rich, TT Fleisher, WT Shearer, BL Kotizn, HW Schroeder Jr, p 21.1. Mosby, London, 2001.

41. McEver RP, Beckstead JH, Moore KL, et al: GMP-140, a platelet alpha-granule membrane protein, is also synthesized by vascular endothelial cells and is localized in Weibel-Palade bodies. *J Clin Invest* 84:92, 1989.

42. Argiles JM, Lopez-Soriano J, Busquets S, Lopez-Soriano FJ: Journey from cachexia to obesity by TNF. *FASEB J* 11:743, 1997.

43. Thomas R, Arend WP: Antigen-presenting cells, in *Kelley's Textbook of Rheumatology*, 6th ed, edited by ED Harris, Jr, RC Budd, GS Firestein, MC Genovese, JS, Sargent, S Ruddy, p 101. Elsevier Saunders, Philadelphia, 2005.

44. Teixeira MM, Wells TNC, Lukacs NW: Chemokine-induced eosinophil recruitment. Role for endogenous eotaxin. *J Clin Invest* 100:1657, 1997.

45. Boyce JA: The pathobiology of eosinophilic inflammation. *Allergy Asthma Proc* 18:253, 1997.

46. Jung U, Key K: Mice lacking two or all three selectins demonstrate overlapping and distinct functions for each selectin. *J Immunol* 162:6755, 1999.

47. Jung U, Ramos CL, Bullard DC, Ley K: Gene-targeted mice reveal importance of L-selectin-dependent rolling for neutrophil adhesion. *Am J Physiol Heart Circ Physiol* 274:H1785, 1998.

48. Lu B, Rutledge BJ, Gu L, et al: Abnormalities in monocyte recruitment and cytokine expression in monocyte chemoattractant protein 1-deficient mice. *J Exp Med* 187:601, 1998.

49. Kuziel WA, Morgan SJ, Dawson TC, et al: Severe reduction in leukocyte adhesion and monocyte extravasation in mice deficient in CC chemokine receptor 2. *Proc Natl Acad Sci U S A* 94:12053, 1997.

50. Low QE, Drugea IA, Duffner LA, et al: Wound healing in MIP-1α −/− and MCP-1 −/− mice. *Am J Pathol* 159:457, 2001.

INNATE IMMUNITY

BRUCE BEUTLER

The innate immune system provides immediate protection against infection and serves an essential antigen-presenting role that allows the adaptive immune response to occur during the days that follow. The key receptors that permit innate immune cells (macrophages and dendritic cells) to recognize specific molecules of microbial origin and respond to an infection have been identified, along with the central biochemical events that follow activation of these receptors. Susceptibility to infection in humans is strongly heritable, and among the many loci that influence it, those that encode proteins vital to the innate immune response are probably of central importance.

INNATE IMMUNITY VERSUS ADAPTIVE IMMUNITY

In humans, as in all mammals, resistance to microbial infection is based in part on lymphocytes, which yield highly specific responses to microbial antigens: either the production of antibodies, or the expansion of T cell clones that are directly cytotoxic to infected cells (see Chaps. 77 and 78). This, the *adaptive* immune response, is a recent fixture in evolution, witnessed only in vertebrates and traceable to the development of a mechanism for recombination of genomic DNA that arose approximately 450 million years ago. A more fundamental type of immunity, known as *innate* immunity, is represented in one form or another in all multicellular organisms. For this reason, a great deal of progress in the innate immunity field has come from the study of model animals, such as *Drosophila melanogaster*, and model plants, such as *Arabidopsis thaliana*. Despite the vast evolutionary distance that separates these organisms from *Homo sapiens*, both species use defensive proteins and signaling pathways that are ancestrally related to those represented in humans.

Like the adaptive immune system, the innate immune system is endowed with a means of detecting microbes, destroying microbes, and at the same time, exercising self-tolerance. These mechanisms are far older than the analogous adaptive mechanisms, and as a consequence, are more refined. While it is sometimes called the "primitive" immune system, the innate immune system actually shows remarkable sophistication. Moreover, adaptive immunity is entirely dependent on innate immunity in the sense that antigen presentation requires the participation of innate immune cells. The well-known adjuvant effect

of microbes (e.g., the ability of heat-killed mycobacteria in Freund adjuvant to augment the antibody response to a particular antigen) is also mediated by cells of the innate immune system.

Innate immunity, which acts immediately to protect the host in the event of microbial inoculation, fills a temporal gap that would otherwise exist in the global immune response. Days or weeks are required for an effective adaptive immune response to develop when the naive host encounters a new pathogen. During this time, innate immunity alone protects the host. Indeed, where host survival is concerned, innate immunity is more important than adaptive immunity, and prolonged survival would be impossible without it (Table 17-1).

TYPES OF INNATE IMMUNITY

Innate immunity embraces a large number of host resistance mechanisms. It is possible to divide the innate immune system into cellular and noncellular components, as well as into afferent and effector components. Noncellular components of innate immunity include antimicrobial peptides, which selectively disrupt microbial cell membranes, complement, components of which also disrupt cell membranes, and such proteins as hemopexin and haptoglobin, which deny iron to invasive microbes. Cellular components include cells of myeloid origin (*granulocytes, monocyte/macrophages, mast cells,* and *dendritic cells*) and lymphoid cells (*natural killer [NK] cells* and *natural killer T [NKT] cells*). As such, it can be seen that despite their recent evolutionary origin, some lymphoid cells have been co-opted to serve in the innate immune system rather than the adaptive immune system.

It is more difficult to cleanly divide innate immune responses into "afferent" and "effector" functions, because a response, once initiated, runs its course in a preprogrammed fashion, proceeding from microbial sensing all the way through to microbial killing. However, the proteins responsible for microbial recognition, signaling, and the development of a transcriptional response within innate immune cells are generally considered to be "afferent" components; the cytokines that mediate the response and the cellular weaponry that is used to destroy viruses and bacteria may be considered "effector" components.

The remainder of this chapter focuses on the afferent arm of cellular innate immunity, because the effector mechanisms (neutro-

Acronyms and abbreviations that appear in this chapter include: CMV, cytomegalovirus; CTLA, cytotoxic T lymphocyte antigen; dsRNA, double-stranded ribonucleic acid; G-CSF, granulocyte colony stimulating factor; GM-CSF, granulocyte-monocyte colony stimulating factor; IL, interleukin; IFN, interferon; IRAK, interleukin-1 receptor-associated kinase; IRF-3, interferon response factor-3; LPS, lipopolysaccharide; LRR, leucine-rich repeat; MCMV, mouse cytomegalovirus; MDP, muramyl dipeptide; NADPH, nicotinamide adenine dinucleotide phosphate; NBS, nucleotide binding sequence; NF-κB, nuclear factor-κB; NK, natural killer; PAMPs, pathogen-associated molecular patterns; PRRs, pattern recognition receptors; SOCS-1, suppressor of cytokine synthesis 1; TAK-1, transforming growth factor β activating kinase 1; TBK1, TANK-binding kinase 1; TIR, Toll/interleukin-1 receptor/resistance; TLRs, Toll-like receptors; TNF, tumor necrosis factor; UCM, up-regulation of costimulatory molecules.

TABLE 17-1   COMPARISONS BETWEEN INNATE AND ADAPTIVE IMMUNITY

	INNATE IMMUNITY	ADAPTIVE IMMUNITY
Sensing mechanism	TLRs, NK receptors; possibly NOD proteins, fMLP receptor	Immunoglobulins, T cell receptors
Cellular components	Macrophages, dendritic cells, granulocytes, mast cells, NK cells	T cells, B cells
Efferent mechanisms	Cytokine production, inflammatory response, phagocytosis, pathogen killing	Antibody production, cytokine production, cell killing
Purpose	Alert other innate and adaptive immune cells to pathogen presence; directly kill pathogen; encourage the development of an adaptive immune response	Assist in efficacy of innate immune response; produce highly specific ligands for pathogens
Time scale of response	Quick (maximal in minutes to hours)	Slow (maximal in days to weeks)
Specific memory	No	Yes
Phylogeny	Ancient (all multicellular organisms)	Recent (vertebrates only)

ABBREVIATIONS: fMLP, N-formyl-methyonyl-leucyl-phenylalanine; NK, natural killer; NOD, nondefinitive; TLRs, Toll-like receptors.

TABLE 17-2 TOLL-LIKE RECEPTORS, MICROBIAL SPECIFICITIES, AND TRANSDUCERS

TLR	KNOWN MACROMOLECULAR ASSOCIATIONS	LIGAND(S)	ADAPTER USE	REFERENCES
1	TLR2	Triacyl lipopeptides	MyD88, MAL	3–6
2	TLRs 1 or 6, or homodimer	Lipopeptides, lipoteichoic acid, glucans, protozoal GPI	MyD88, MAL	7
3	—	dsRNA	Trif	8–10
4	CD14, MD-2	LPS	MyD88, MAL, Trif, Tram	9–15
5	—	Flagellin	MyD88	16
6	TLR2	Diacyl lipopeptides, glucans, lipoteichoic acid	MyD88, MAL	17
7	—	ssRNA, imidazoquinolines	MyD88	18
8	—	ssRNA, imidazoquinolines	MyD88	19
9	—	Unmethylated CpG motifs	MyD88	20
10	—	Unknown	Unknown	21

ABBREVIATIONS: dsRNA, double-stranded ribonucleic acid, GPI, glycosylphoshoinositol; LPS, lipopolysaccanide; ssRNA, single-stranded ribonucleic acid.

philmediated killing, complement, and antimicrobial peptides) are discussed in other chapters (see Chaps. 16, 61, and 66). Our understanding of innate immune responses has improved dramatically as a result of using forward and reverse genetic methods to dissect the signaling pathways that permit host recognition of microbes.

MICROBIAL RECOGNITION AND THE TOLL-LIKE RECEPTORS

INNATE IMMUNE RECOGNITION IS BASED ON CONVENTIONAL RECEPTOR–LIGAND INTERACTIONS

Very regrettably, the microbial principles that are recognized by the innate immune system are often referred to as "danger signals" or "pathogen-associated molecular patterns" (so-called PAMPs), and the receptors for PAMPs are dubbed "pattern recognition receptors" (PRRs).[1] The use of these terms is unfortunate for two reasons. First, the notion that there are PAMPs or danger signals does not bespeak a new or correct principle in immunology. Rather, the existence, chemical structure, and properties of many immunostimulatory molecules of microbial origin were known long before the terms "danger signals" or "PAMPs" came into being. Second, the idea of immune activation by "patterns" or "danger" suggests a retreat from the long-held reductionist credo that definable *molecules* of microbial origin are targets for detection by specific receptors, which operate according the rules established for receptor–ligand interaction.[2] There is nothing "fuzzy" about innate immune detection, and one of the central goals of the science of innate immunity is to precisely define ligand–receptor interactions at the atomic level. The first steps have been taken with the molecular identification of many of the target ligands as well as the host receptors.

DISCOVERY OF THE MAMMALIAN TOLL-LIKE RECEPTORS AS THE PRIMARY SENSORS OF THE INNATE IMMUNE SYSTEM

The proteins chiefly responsible for microbial sensing are the Toll-like receptors (TLRs). These receptors collectively mediate the recognition of most, if not all, microbes. Ten TLRs are encoded in the human genome. The molecular specificity of nine of these TLRs has been established, at least in part. While publications may be found to sug-

gest that some of the TLRs (notably TLRs 2 and 4) detect dozens of molecules, the evidence favoring most of these interactions is slender, and a conservative viewpoint is preferred; hence, only those interactions that are deemed certain are presented in Table 17-2.

The microbial sensing function of the mammalian TLRs was discovered as a direct result of inquiry into the mechanism of endotoxin sensing. Endotoxin (later denoted as lipopolysaccharide [LPS]) was first described by Pfeiffer as a toxic component of *Vibrio cholerae* more than 100 years ago.[22] Its chemical structure was established many years later (reviewed in ref. 23), and a toxic "lipid A" moiety of LPS was synthesized artificially in 1985 and found to have full biologic activity.[24] The identity of the LPS receptor was established in 1998, through the positional cloning of *Lps*, a locus that was known to be required for all cellular responses to endotoxin, and for the effective clearance of gram-negative bacterial infections[25,26] in laboratory mice. In LPS-unresponsive mice, the *Tlr4* locus was shown to be mutationally inactivated.[13,14] It had previously been recognized that Toll, a *Drosophila* protein also known for its developmental effects,[27] was required for the innate immune response to fungal infection in flies.[28] Hence, the discovery of an LPS sensing function for TLR4, a homologue of Toll, made good evolutionary sense.

Other molecules of microbial origin (for example, di- and triacylated lipopeptides and lipoproteins, lipoteichoic acid, unmethylated DNA bearing CpG dinucleotides in a particular context, flagellin, and double-stranded ribonucleic acid [dsRNA]) were known to elicit responses qualitatively similar to those elicited by LPS. The other TLR paralogs seemed excellent candidate receptors for these molecules. Reverse genetic methods established that each of these molecules is indeed recognized by a particular TLR or heteromeric combination of TLRs.[3,7,8,16,20,29,30] Moreover, genetic complementation analyses have shown that at least some microbial ligands directly engage the TLRs to elicit a signal.[31–33] Conversely, other molecules enhance the signal, and also participate in ligand recognition. For example, CD14 binds LPS[11] and augments LPS responses.[34] CD36 augments responses to bacterial diacylglycerides. It is likely that these accessory molecules form complexes with the TLRs, which are responsible for transducing the signal across the cell membrane. TLR4, alone among the TLRs, is known to exist as a tight complex with MD-2, a small secreted protein that is required for TLR4 to reach the cell surface and is also required for LPS sensing.[12]

STRUCTURE OF THE TLRs

The TLRs are all single-spanning transmembrane proteins. All have leucine-rich repeat (LRR) motifs in their extracellular domains. All have a characteristic TIR (Toll/interleukin [IL]-1 receptor/resistance) motif in their cytoplasmic domains. This ancient protein fold[35] is evident in cytosolic plant disease resistance proteins (where it often is represented together with a nucleotide binding sequence [NBS] and/or LRR motifs), in proteins of the IL-1 and IL-18 receptor family, in the adapter proteins that carry signals from TLRs, and in the TLRs themselves. The function of the LRRs is uncertain. These motifs are known to create "horseshoe" shapes when repeated many times in close proximity, but are scattered at irregular intervals in some of the TLR ectodomains. It is believed that the TLRs are dimeric on the basis of *Drosophila* studies, which show that membrane-proximal cysteine mutations are hypermorphic,[36] and on the basis of transfection studies suggesting that enforced dimerization of TLR4 can yield a signal.[37] Some of the TLR ectodomains clearly form tight associations with other proteins. This is the case for TLR4, which is tightly complexed with MD-2[38] and in contact with CD14 as well.[39]

TLR2 is known to form heteromeric complexes with TLRs 1 or 6,[40] and is believed to exist and signal as a homodimer as well. TLR2:6 heteromers signal the presence of diacyl lipopeptides; TLR2:1 heteromers signal the presence of triacyl lipopeptides.[30] While it was once supposed that many different heteromeric complexes might form among the different TLRs and yield very broad specificity, no other examples of heteromeric interaction are presently known. The function of TLR10, while still unknown, may be similar to that of TLRs 1 and 6, given that it is more structurally similar to these proteins than to other TLRs.

TLRs 3, 7, 8, and 9 are believed to be intracellular because no surface expression can be detected, and tagged versions of the molecules are found to reside within the interior of transfected cells.[41] It is likely that these TLRs, as well as a fraction of the other TLRs, project into endocytic vesicles and detect foreign molecules there rather than within the extracellular space. It may be assumed, then, that other proteins of the cell are required as a conduit to bring microbial inducers into contact with these TLRs.

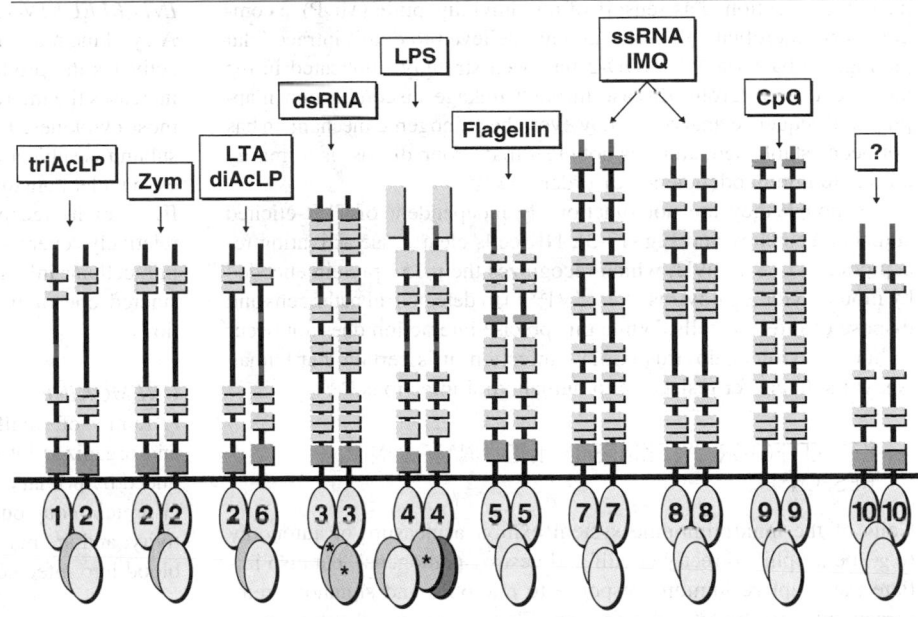

FIGURE 17-1   The human TLRs, their ligands, and their transducers. It is believed that all TLRs signal as homodimers or heterodimers. *Pale blue boxes*, leucine-rich repeats. *Dark blue boxes*, membrane-proximal leucine-rich repeats. *Pale blue vertical rectangle*, MD-2; *pale blue numbered ovals*, TIR domains. Other ovals: *pale blue*, MyD88; *four medium blue*, MAL/Tirap; *three asterisked ovals*, Trif; *dark blue*, Tram. CpG, unmethylated DNA; ds, double-stranded; IMQ, imidazoquinolines; LP, lipopeptide; LPS, lipopolysaccharide; LTA, lipoteichoic acid; ss, single-stranded; zym, zymosan.

TIR ADAPTER SIGNALING

A total of five TIR adapter proteins are encoded in the human genome. These adapters are MyD88, MAL (also known as Tirap), Trif (also known as Ticam-1 and first identified by a mutant allele known as *Lps2*), Tram, and Sarm. The function of Sarm is not presently known. However, the four remaining adapters have well-defined roles in signal transduction. All of these adapters are required for normal signaling from the LPS receptor TLR4. MyD88 and MAL act in concert with one another, and Trif and Tram act in concert with one another, so that two primary "branches" of the LPS signaling pathway diverge at the level of the receptor. Trif alone serves TLR3 signaling; MyD88 and MAL (but neither Trif nor Tram) serve TLR2; and MyD88 alone serves TLRs 7, 8, and 9 (Fig. 17-1). Mutational inactivation of MyD88 creates a severe immunodeficiency state in mice, and compound homozygosity for mutations at both MyD88 and Trif loci causes immunodeficiency that is still more severe, in which animals are essentially unable to sense the presence of most microbes.

It is probable that the adapter proteins exist as dimers in a total of five homomeric and heteromeric complexes with one another. Although this has not been established by rigorous methods, the existence of dimers would best explain the diversity of signals that are observed to emanate from the TLRs. MAL and Tram probably function as "bridges" joining MyD88 and Trif respectively to the TLR4 receptor. However, MyD88 can directly engage other receptors (TLRs 7, 8, and 9, for example), and Trif can directly engage TLR3.[42] MAL/MyD88 signaling is very different from Tram/Trif signaling in several respects.

MyD88, when activated, recruits interleukin-1 receptor-associated kinase 4 (IRAK4), a serine kinase, through an interaction involving death domains on each molecule. This, in turn, leads to the phosphorylation of IRAK (IRAK1), and to the recruitment of TRAF6, a cellular scaffold protein that coordinates the recruitment of several other protein kinases. Transforming growth factor β activating kinase 1 (TAK-1) is among these, and phosphorylates IκB, leading to its degradation and nuclear translocation of nuclear factor-κB (NF-κB), a transcription factor required for the expression of numerous cytokine genes.

When Trif is activated, it is capable of circumventing IRAK4 and directly activating TRAF6, thereby causing activation of NF-κB.[43] In addition, Trif activates a serine kinase (TANK-binding kinase 1 [TBK1]),[44,45] which, in turn, activates interferon response factor-3 (IRF-3), a transcription factor that initiates expression of the interferon beta (IFN-β) gene. INF-β mediates antiviral effects, and also is required for the up-regulation of costimulatory proteins (e.g., CD40, CD80, and CD86) that enhance the activation of an adaptive immune response. Hence, the adjuvant effects of LPS and dsRNA are dependent upon the type I interferon receptor.[46]

MyD88 homodimers, activated by TLRs 7, 8, and 9, are also able to activate INF-β gene expression. However, the heteromeric MyD88/MAL complex is incapable of doing so.

Countervailing Influences in TIR Adapter Signaling   IRAK-M, a homolog of IRAKs 1, 2, and 4, is an inhibitor of TIR domain signaling and may participate in feedback inhibition of signaling known as "endotoxin tolerance."[47] In addition, suppressor of cytokine synthesis 1 (SOCS-1) inhibits signal transduction from the JAK/STAT pathway, activated by type I interferon, one of the key cytokines elicited in the course of an innate immune response.[48] Still more distally, inhibition of signaling via antiinflammatory cytokines (such as IL-10 or TGF-β) may limit the response to infectious organisms.

OTHER SENSORS

Other molecules may represent entirely TLR-independent pathways for microbial sensing. Among these, the NOD-1 and NOD-2 proteins have been mentioned as sensors of muramyl dipeptide (MDP), a component of microbial cell walls, and are believed to detect intracellular pathogenic bacteria.[49–51] NOD-2 has been strongly implicated in the pathogenesis of Crohn disease through linkage disequilibrium mapping and sequence analysis[52]; however, the pathogenic mechanism has not been established, and it is not clear that Crohn disease is primarily an innate immunodeficiency disorder.

Although they are not functionally independent of TLR-elicited signals (see below and Fig. 17-3), NK cells clearly use activating receptors (such as Ly49H, which recognizes the m157 protein encoded by mouse cytomegalovirus [MCMV][53,54]) to detect viral pathogens and dispose of infected cells. While this precise interaction does not occur in human cytomegalovirus (CMV) infection, it is certain that human NK cells do confer resistance to human viral infections.[55,56]

KEY EFFECTOR CYTOKINES IN THE INNATE IMMUNE RESPONSE

Cells of the innate immune system exhibit a measure of autonomy (e.g., neutrophils directly engulf and destroy pathogens), but also initiate the adaptive immune response to microbes and summon "reinforcements" to the site of infection. These functions depend on the production of cytokines too numerous to describe in this chapter. However, a few of the key mediators are listed here.

TUMOR NECROSIS FACTOR ALPHA

A homotrimeric cytokine that is made by many cells, tumor necrosis factor (TNF) is synthesized in greatest amounts by mononuclear phagocytes that have been exposed to LPS or other TLR-activating stimuli. It was recognized as a key endogenous mediator of endotoxicity,[57] and later, as a mediator of other forms of inflammation (including sterile inflammation, as observed in rheumatoid arthritis, Crohn disease, ankylosing spondylitis, and psoriasis). The TNF signaling pathway depends upon two receptors, involves NF-κB activation, and is ancestrally related to the *Drosophila* IMD (immunodeficiency) pathway for recognition of gram-negative bacteria.[58] The ancient phylogenetic origins of TNF signaling, its large representation in distant species, the remarkable therapeutic efficacy of TNF neutralization in the diseases just mentioned, and the immunocompromising effects of TNF and TNF receptor mutations in animals suggest that TNF is one of the most important of the cytokines used by the innate immune system for effective containment of infection.

INTERLEUKIN-1

Once known as pleiotropic inflammatory cytokines, IL-1α and IL-1β, two distantly related ligands that share the same set of receptors, are produced in response to innate immune stimuli and evoke fever, swelling, and neutrophil adhesion in the region of an infectious nidus. The type I IL-1 receptor, responsible for most or all of the agonist activity of the IL-1 proteins, has two chains, each of which is endowed with a cytoplasmic TIR domain. The receptor complex signals via MyD88, and no other adapters are known to be required. IL-1 signaling may act as an amplification mechanism that augments the primary infectious signal, and transmits awareness of infection to cells that lack the innate immune sensors required for detection of microbes.

INTERLEUKIN-6

Signaling via a receptor that utilizes the JAK/STAT pathway, IL-6 activates many elements of the "acute phase response," that is, hepatic production of fibrinogen, serum amyloid A protein, and C-reactive protein. It also has thrombopoietic activity, which may assist in the generation of platelets, often consumed in the course of a serious infection.

INTERLEUKIN-12

A cytokine made in abundance in response to TLR stimulation, IL-12 activates the production of INF-γ by lymphoid cells, which, in turn, increases the microbicidal activity of mononuclear phagocytes. Unlike most cytokines, IL-12 is a heterodimeric protein, and the IL-12 p40 subunit is subject to induction, whereas the p35 subunit is synthesized even under nonstimulated conditions. Mutations of the genes encoding IL-12 or its receptor, or IFN-γ or its receptor, are known to cause relatively severe susceptibility to infection by mycobacteria and other intracellular infections. Hence the IL-12/IFN-γ feedback loop is considered one of the most important innate/adaptive immune interactions.

CHEMOKINES

A family of small proteins, highly redundant in receptor specificity and organized into CC and CXC subfamilies, the chemokines are induced by primary microbial stimuli and by TNF and IL-1. Binding to G-protein coupled receptors, they exhibit neutrophil chemotactic activity, and are believed to contribute to the egress of neutrophils from blood into infected tissue.

GRANULOCYTE COLONY STIMULATING FACTOR AND GRANULOCYTE-MONOCYTE COLONY STIMULATING FACTOR

The central hematopoietic response is attuned to events in the peripheral tissues, and granulocyte colony stimulating factor (G-CSF) and granulocyte-monocyte colony stimulating factor (GM-CSF) encourage the production and release of granulocytes and monocytes to cope with an infectious challenge. These cytokines are produced in direct response to TLR signaling, and also in response to secondary cytokines such as TNF. They signal via JAK/STAT-coupled receptors.

INTERFERONS

Type I interferons (IFN-α and IFN-β) are expressed immediately in response to LPS, dsRNA, or unmethylated DNA, and have broad activity in the containment of viral infections. LPS-induced type I interferon production depends upon TLR4 and the adapters Trif and Tram. dsRNA-induced type I interferon depends upon TLR3 and Trif (but not Tram). The stimulation of Type I interferon production by unmethylated CpG is dependent on MyD88. Although many cells are induced to an antiviral state as the result of interferon stimulation, NK cells, which are specialized for the elimination of virus-infected targets, are particularly dependent on type I interferon signaling,[59] and require it for the elimination of specific pathogens such as CMV.[60] The type I interferons may also be involved in protection against bacterial infection, and type I interferon signaling is important for the development of endotoxic shock.[61] Plasmacytoid dendritic cells are a particularly important source of type I interferon.[62]

Type II interferon (IFN-γ) has less antiviral activity than type I interferon, is produced by T cells in response to IL-12 receptor stimulation, and is crucial for the elimination of intracellular pathogens such as mycobacteria, which reside within macrophages of the infected host.

THE ACTIVATION OF ADAPTIVE IMMUNITY

The adjuvant effect of microbes has been known since the classic studies of Lewis and Loomis[63] who coined the term *allergic irritability* to describe the augmented production of antibodies against a protein antigen in guinea pigs infected with *Mycobacterium tuberculosis*. Freund and McDermott[64] demonstrated that heat-killed mycobacteria were also capable of eliciting an exaggerated antibody response when coadministered with a protein antigen: a fact that indicated that molecular components of microbes (rather than infection per se) were responsible for adjuvanticity. LPS was shown to be endowed with adjuvant activity by Condie et al. in 1955,[65] and by 1975 the *Lps* locus was shown to be required for this effect of LPS (as it was required for all other cellular effects of LPS).[66] By deduction, the positional cloning of *Lps* thus revealed the essential role of TLR4 in LPS adjuvanticity.[14]

Activation of an adaptive immune response to a specific antigen has long been known to depend on two signals that occur in the course of antigen presentation. First, the T cell receptor must be activated. In addition, costimulatory molecules up-regulated on the antigen-presenting cell (e.g., CD40, CD69, CD80, and CD86) are known to interact with receptors (or in some cases ligands) on the T cell. An exchange of signals occurs over a period of approximately 12 hours,[67] ultimately leading to autonomous expansion of the T cell clone, and, in turn, activation of specific B cells. Some of these signals are well characterized. For example, CD80 and CD86 both engage CD28 and cytotoxic T lymphocyte antigen (CTLA) on the T cell surface, and abrogation of signaling via these costimulatory receptors is known to substantially attenuate the adaptive immune response.[68]

Consequently, up-regulation of costimulatory molecules (UCM) is essential, although not by itself sufficient, for activation of the adaptive immune response. LPS depends upon Trif (and specifically on Trif-mediated type I interferon gene expression) to elicit UCM,[9,10,46] and absent Trif, LPS cannot exert an adjuvant effect. Tram is also required for UCM.[15] Although MyD88 does not elicit UCM, it does contribute to LPS-induced adjuvanticity in an experimental setting.[46] It is likely that IL-12, a cytokine that is largely MyD88 dependent, also contributes to the adjuvant effect, along with other proteins yet to be identified. As noted below, adaptive immune responses are at least grossly intact in human patients with IRAK4 deficiency, and normal levels of immunoglobulin are measured in the blood of such patients. This suggests that at least in response to some antigenic stimuli and some microbial adjuvants, adaptive immune responses can take place in vivo. As previously mentioned, dsRNA-induced NF-κB activation may proceed by way of Trif → TRAF6 interaction.[45]

dsRNA is partly Trif dependent. However, dsRNA-induced UCM also proceeds by way of a separate pathway that is neither TLR3 nor Trif dependent.[46] Unmethylated DNA can also induce UCM, and presumably, does so by way of MyD88 homodimers (whereas MyD88/MAL heteromers are incapable of eliciting UCM). In all instances, the final common pathway to UCM depends upon the induction of type I interferon (Fig. 17-2).

TLR-MEDIATED RESISTANCE TO VIRAL INFECTIONS

The clinical features of viral and bacterial infections are often similar to one another or indistinguishable. This similarity originates at the level of the TLRs and the adapters that serve them. Gram-negative bacterial LPS activates TLR4, whereas viral dsRNA activates TLR3. But both receptors signal via the adapter protein Trif; consequently, both bacterial and viral infections induce the production of a common set of cytokine mediators, which elicit a similar clinical syndrome.[9]

Although the importance of the *Lps* locus (now known to encode TLR4[13,14]) in the containment of bacterial infections has been known for decades,[25,26,69] the essential role of TLRs in viral sensing and in protection against viral infection was demonstrated only recently. In mice, TLR3 and TLR9 are both of key importance in the response to MCMV infection,[70] as are the corresponding adapter molecules Trif and MyD88.[9,70] The antiviral effect is mediated by type I interferon, produced in response to TLR3 and/or TLR9 signaling. Inter-

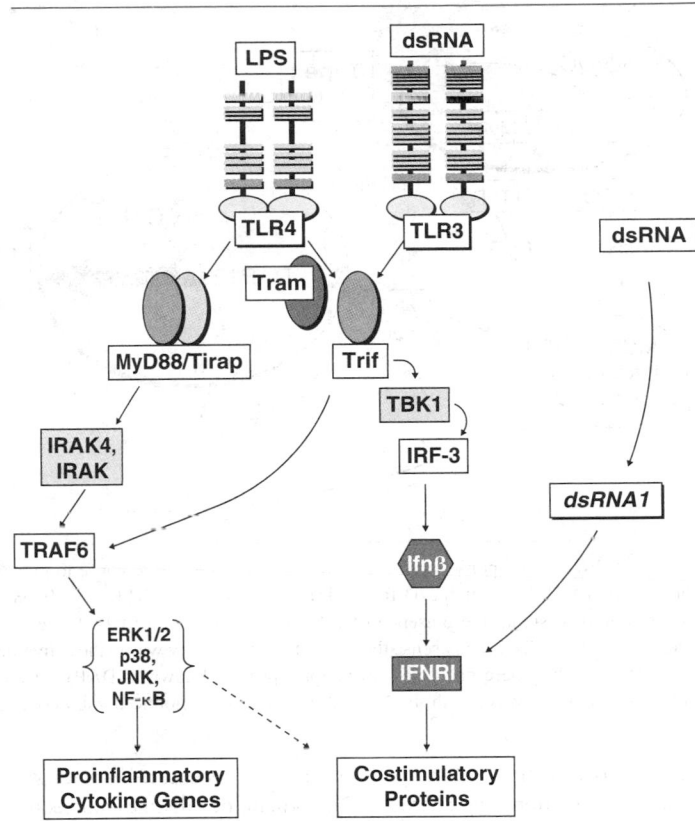

FIGURE 17-2 Separation of the up-regulation of inflammatory cytokine genes from the up-regulation of molecules involved in costimulation during antigen presentation. TLRs 3 and 4 both use Trif (TLR4 additionally requires Tram) to initiate the up-regulation of costimulatory molecules and, hence, to mediate adjuvant effects. Abbreviations are as used in the text.

estingly, although both pathways elicit interferon production, neither pathway alone is sufficient to provide full protection. This may suggest that other, nonredundant factors induced by each pathway are also important to the protective effect.

Because NK cells are known to be the final executors of the host response to MCMV,[71–73] and because type I interferons are also required for NK cell activation,[74] it is probable that combined input from both the Ly49H receptor and the type I interferon receptor is required for the NK cell to mount an effective response to a virally infected target cell (Fig. 17-3).

DISEASES CAUSED BY INNATE IMMUNE DEFECTS

Premature death from infection is strongly heritable in humans,[75] but the loci that confer this heritability remain uncertain. Defects of the innate immune sensing apparatus are expected to cause hypersusceptibility to infection in humans as they clearly do in mice, and specific examples of such mutations have recently come to light. Missense mutations of TLR4 that are very rare among the normal white population are quite common in patients with systemic meningococcal disease, and have been assigned a role in susceptibility on this basis.[76] A nonsense mutation of TLR5 was found to be overrepresented in patients who developed Legionnaires disease as compared to a comparably exposed population that remained disease-free.[77] Mutations of IRAK4 create susceptibility to suppurative gram-positive infections.[78]

On the effector side, examples of immunocompromise from innate immune defects are far better known, and include diseases caused by

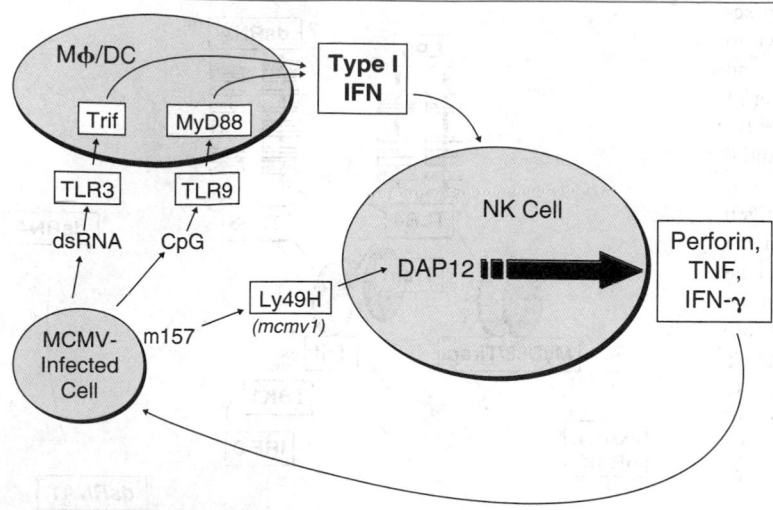

FIGURE 17-3   Response circuits required for an effective response to infection by the herpesvirus MCMV. Both the TLR3 → Trif pathway and the TLR4 → MyD88 pathways are required to signal the presence of infection via release of type I interferon. At the same time, NK cells directly sense the viral protein m157 by way of the activating receptor Ly49H. Signaling here occurs by an adapter protein known as DAP12. Defects in the TIR signaling pathways or in the NK pathway cause pronounced immunodeficiency.

mutations affecting IFN-γ,[79] IL-12[80] and its receptor,[81,82] defects of granule formation,[83] and defects of nicotinamide adenine dinucleotide phosphate (NADPH) oxidase.[84]

THE GENERAL STRATEGY OF INNATE IMMUNE RESPONSES AND THE CONCEPT OF "INNATE AUTOIMMUNITY"

Although the term *autoimmunity* is reserved for inappropriate adaptive immune responses that damage tissues of the host, the innate immune system may also cause injury or death, and typically does so when systemic activation occurs in the course of a serious infection. Innate immune responses, which entail cytokine-mediated inflammation and coagulation, evolved to contain small inoculates of microorganisms by encouraging the influx of granulocytes to engulf and destroy these pathogens, and by stimulating the development of an adaptive immune response. The mechanisms that are employed to these ends can be lethal if they are generalized rather than focal.

Beyond this, the innate immune system may, indeed, contribute to sterile inflammation, as witnessed in many human diseases that have so far eluded etiologic decipherment. A number of diseases in humans occur as the result of untoward elaboration and action of specific cytokines. Best known among the pathogenic cytokines is TNF-α, which has a well-established role in rheumatoid arthritis, Crohn disease, ankylosing spondylitis, and psoriasis; hence, TNF neutralization using antibodies or soluble receptor derivatives is very effective in the treatment of these diseases. The primary cause of TNF production in sterile inflammatory disorders is unknown. However, TNF production by myeloid cells is minimally dependent upon NF-κB activation,[85] and NF-κB is well known to be activated via TLR signaling pathways. The possibility that dysregulation of the TNF gene results from primary defects in the innate immune sensing pathways, or from untoward activation of these pathways by endogenous molecules, must therefore be considered. CD36, which binds endogenous lipids[86] and proteins[87,88] and also serves the recognition of microbial ligands, may be viewed as a possible conduit between endogenous mediators of inflammation and the host innate immune system.

In "classical" autoimmune diseases, the TLR signaling pathways may also be important. It has been reported, for example, that endogenous DNA, signaling via TLR9, is responsible for the generation and perpetuation of antinucleoprotein antibodies in a mouse model of systemic lupus erythematosus.[89] The involvement of other TLRs cannot be excluded.

REFERENCES

1. Janeway CA Jr: Approaching the asymptote? Evolution and revolution in immunology. *Cold Spring Harb Symp Quant Biol* 54(Pt 1):1, 1989.
2. Beutler B: Not "molecular patterns" but molecules. *Immunity* 19:155, 2003.
3. Takeuchi O, Sato S, Horiuchi T, et al: Cutting edge: role of Toll-like receptor 1 in mediating immune response to microbial lipoproteins. *J Immunol* 169:10, 2002.
4. Fitzgerald KA, Palsson-McDermott EM, Bowie AG, et al: Mal (MyD88-adapter-like) is required for Toll-like receptor-4 signal transduction. *Nature* 413:78, 2001.
5. Horng T, Barton GM, Medzhitov R: TIRAP: an adapter molecule in the Toll signaling pathway. *Nat Immunol* 2:835, 2001.
6. Yamamoto M, Sato S, Hemmi H, et al: Essential role for TIRAP in activation of the signalling cascade shared by TLR2 and TLR4. *Nature* 420:324, 2002.
7. Takeuchi O, Hoshino K, Kawai T, et al: Differential roles of TLR2 and TLR4 in recognition of gram-negative and gram-positive bacterial cell wall components. *Immunity* 11:443, 1999.
8. Alexopoulou L, Holt AC, Medzhitov R, Flavell RA: Recognition of double-stranded RNA and activation of NF-kappaB by Toll-like receptor 3. *Nature* 413:732, 2001.
9. Hoebe K, Du X, Georgel P, et al: Identification of Lps2 as a key transducer of MyD88-independent TIR signaling. *Nature* 424:743, 2003.
10. Yamamoto M, Sato S, Hemmi H, et al: Role of adapter TRIF in the MyD88-independent Toll-like receptor signaling pathway. *Science* 301:640, 2003.
11. Wright SD, Ramos RA, Tobias PS, et al: CD14, a receptor for complexes of lipopolysaccharide (LPS) and LPS binding protein. *Science* 249:1431, 1990.
12. Nagai Y, Akashi S, Nagafuku M, et al: Essential role of MD-2 in LPS responsiveness and TLR4 distribution. *Nat Immunol* 3:667, 2002.
13. Poltorak A, Smirnova I, He XL, et al: Genetic and physical mapping of the *Lps* locus—identification of the toll-4 receptor as a candidate gene in the critical region. *Blood Cells Mol Dis* 24:340, 1998.
14. Poltorak A, He X, Smirnova I, et al: Defective LPS signaling in C3H/HeJ and C57BL/10ScCr mice: mutations in *Tlr4* gene. *Science* 282:2085, 1998.
15. Yamamoto M, Sato S, Hemmi H, et al: TRAM is specifically involved in the Toll-like receptor 4-mediated MyD88-independent signaling pathway. *Nat Immunol* 4:1144, 2003.
16. Hayashi F, Smith KD, Ozinsky A, et al: The innate immune response to bacterial flagellin is mediated by Toll-like receptor 5. *Nature* 410:1099, 2001.
17. Takeuchi O, Kawai T, Muhlradt PF, et al: Discrimination of bacterial lipoproteins by Toll-like receptor 6. *Int Immunol* 13:933, 2001.
18. Hemmi H, Kaisho T, Takeuchi O, et al: Small anti-viral compounds activate immune cells via the TLR7 MyD88-dependent signaling pathway. *Nat Immunol* 3:196, 2002.
19. Jurk M, Heil F, Vollmer J, et al: Human TLR7 or TLR8 independently confer responsiveness to the antiviral compound R-848. *Nat Immunol* 3:499, 2002.

20. Hemmi H, Takeuchi O, Kawai T, et al: A Toll-like receptor recognizes bacterial DNA. *Nature* 408:740, 2000.
21. Chuang T, Ulevitch RJ: Identification of hTLR10: a novel human Toll-like receptor preferentially expressed in immune cells. *Biochim Biophys Acta* 1518:157, 2001.
22. Pfeiffer R: Untersuchungen über das Choleragift. *Z Hygiene* 11:393, 1892.
23. Raetz CR, Whitfield C: Lipopolysaccharide endotoxins. *Annu Rev Biochem* 71:635, 2002.
24. Galanos C, Luderitz O, Rietschel ET, et al: Synthetic and natural *Escherichia coli* free lipid A express identical endotoxic activities. *Eur J Biochem* 148:1, 1985.
25. O'Brien AD, Rosenstreich DL, Scher I, et al: Genetic control of susceptibility to *Salmonella typhimurium* in mice: role of the LPS gene. *J Immunol* 124:20, 1980.
26. Rosenstreich DL, Weinblatt AC, O'Brien AD: Genetic control of resistance to infection in mice. *CRC Crit Rev Immunol* 3:263, 1982.
27. Anderson KV, Bokla L, Nusslein-Volhard C: Establishment of dorsal-ventral polarity in the *Drosophila* embryo: the induction of polarity by the Toll gene product. *Cell* 42:791, 1985.
28. Lemaitre B, Nicolas E, Michaut L, et al: The dorsoventral regulatory gene cassette spatzle/Toll/cactus controls the potent antifungal response in *Drosophila* adults. *Cell* 86:973, 1996.
29. Takeuchi O, Kaufmann A, Grote K, et al: Preferentially the R-stereoisomer of the mycoplasmal lipopeptide macrophage-activating lipopeptide-2 activates immune cells through a Toll-like receptor 2- and MyD88-dependent signaling pathway. *J Immunol* 164:554, 2000.
30. Morr M, Takeuchi O, Akira S, et al: Differential recognition of structural details of bacterial lipopeptides by Toll-like receptors. *Eur J Immunol* 32:3337, 2002.
31. Poltorak A, Ricciardi-Castagnoli P, Citterio A, Beutler B: Physical contact between LPS and Tlr4 revealed by genetic complementation. *Proc Natl Acad Sci U S A* 97:2163, 2000.
32. Lien E, Means TK, Heine H, et al: Toll-like receptor 4 imparts ligand-specific recognition of bacterial lipopolysaccharide. *J Clin Invest* 105:497, 2000.
33. Bauer S, Kirschning CJ, Hacker H, et al: Human TLR9 confers responsiveness to bacterial DNA via species-specific CpG motif recognition. *Proc Natl Acad Sci U S A* 98:9237, 2001.
34. Haziot A, Ferrero E, Kontgen F, et al: Resistance to endotoxin shock and reduced dissemination of gram-negative bacteria in CD14-deficient mice. *Immunity* 4:407, 1996.
35. Xu Y, Tao X, Shen B, et al: Structural basis for signal transduction by the Toll/interleukin-1 receptor domains. *Nature* 408:111, 2000.
36. Schneider DS, Hudson KL, Lin TY, Anderson KV: Dominant and recessive mutations define functional domains of Toll, a transmembrane protein required for dorsal-ventral polarity in the *Drosophila* embryo. *Genes Dev* 5:797, 1991.
37. Medzhitov R, Preston-Hurlburt P, Janeway CA Jr: A human homologue of the *Drosophila* Toll protein signals activation of adaptive immunity. *Nature* 388:394, 1997.
38. Shimazu R, Akashi S, Ogata H, et al: MD-2, a molecule that confers lipopolysaccharide responsiveness on Toll-like receptor 4. *J Exp Med* 189:1777, 1999.
39. Da Silva CJ, Soldau K, Christen U, et al: Lipopolysaccharide is in close proximity to each of the proteins in its membrane receptor complex: transfer from CD14 to TLR4 and MD-2. *J Biol Chem* 276:21129, 2001.
40. Ozinsky A, Underhill DM, Fontenot JD, et al: The repertoire for pattern recognition of pathogens by the innate immune system is defined by cooperation between toll-like receptors. *Proc Natl Acad Sci U S A* 97:13766, 2000.
41. Ahmad-Nejad P, Hacker H, Rutz M, et al: Bacterial CpG-DNA and lipopolysaccharides activate Toll-like receptors at distinct cellular compartments. *Eur J Immunol* 32:1958, 2002.
42. Oshiumi H, Matsumoto M, Funami K, et al: TICAM-1, an adaptor molecule that participates in Toll-like receptor 3-mediated interferon-beta induction. *Nat Immunol* 4:161, 2003.
43. Jiang Z, Zamanian-Daryoush M, Nie H, et al: Poly(dI.dC)-induced Toll-like receptor 3 (TLR3)-mediated activation of NFkappa B and MAP kinase is through an interleukin-1 receptor-associated kinase (IRAK)-independent pathway employing the signaling components TLR3-TRAF6-TAK1-TAB2-PKR. *J Biol Chem* 278:16713, 2003.
44. Fitzgerald KA, McWhirter SM, Faia KL, et al: IKKepsilon and TBK1 are essential components of the IRF3 signaling pathway. *Nat Immunol* 4:491, 2003.
45. Sato S, Sugiyama M, Yamamoto M, et al: Toll/IL-1 receptor domain-containing adaptor inducing IFN-beta (TRIF) associates with TNF receptor-associated factor 6 and TANK-binding kinase 1, and activates two distinct transcription factors, NF-kappa B and IFN-regulatory factor-3, in the Toll-like receptor signaling. *J Immunol* 171:4304, 2003.
46. Hoebe K, Janssen EM, Kim SO, et al: Upregulation of costimulatory molecules induced by lipopolysaccharide and double-stranded RNA occurs by Trif-dependent and Trif-independent pathways. *Nat Immunol* 4:1223, 2003.
47. Kobayashi K, Hernandez LD, Galan JE, et al: IRAK-M is a negative regulator of Toll-like receptor signaling. *Cell* 110:191, 2002.
48. Kinjyo I, Hanada T, Inagaki-Ohara K, et al: SOCS1/JAB is a negative regulator of LPS-induced macrophage activation. *Immunity* 17:583, 2002.
49. Girardin SE, Boneca IG, Viala J, et al: Nod2 is a general sensor of peptidoglycan through muramyl dipeptide (MDP) detection. *J Biol Chem* 278:8869, 2003.
50. Girardin SE, Travassos LH, Herve M, et al: Peptidoglycan molecular requirements allowing detection by Nod1 and Nod2. *J Biol Chem* 278:41702, 2003.
51. Girardin SE, Boneca IG, Carneiro LA, et al: Nod1 detects a unique muropeptide from gram-negative bacterial peptidoglycan. *Science* 300:1584, 2003.
52. Hugot JP, Chamaillard M, Zouali H, et al: Association of NOD2 leucine-rich repeat variants with susceptibility to Crohn's disease. *Nature* 411:599, 2001.
53. Brown MG, Dokun AO, Heusel JW, et al: Vital involvement of a natural killer cell activation receptor in resistance to viral infection. *Science* 292:934, 2001.
54. Smith HR, Heusel JW, Mehta IK, et al: Recognition of a virus-encoded ligand by a natural killer cell activation receptor. *Proc Natl Acad Sci U S A* 99:8826, 2002.
55. Sayos J, Wu C, Morra M, et al: The X-linked lymphoproliferative-disease gene product SAP regulates signals induced through the co-receptor SLAM. *Nature* 395:462, 1998.
56. Benoit L, Wang X, Pabst HF, et al: Defective NK cell activation in X-linked lymphoproliferative disease. *J Immunol* 165:3549, 2000.
57. Beutler B, Milsark IW, Cerami A: Passive immunization against cachectin/tumor necrosis factor (TNF) protects mice from the lethal effect of endotoxin. *Science* 229:869, 1985.
58. Georgel P, Naitza S, Kappler C, et al: *Drosophila* immune deficiency (IMD) is a death domain protein that activates antibacterial defense and can promote apoptosis. *Dev Cell* 1:503, 2001.
59. Orange JS, Biron CA: Characterization of early IL-12, IFN-alpha beta, and TNF effects on antiviral state and NK cell responses during murine cytomegalovirus infection. *J Immunol* 156:4746, 1996.
60. Andrews DM, Scalzo AA, Yokoyama WM, et al: Functional interactions between dendritic cells and NK cells during viral infection. *Nat Immunol* 4:175, 2003.
61. Karaghiosoff M, Steinborn R, Kovarik P, et al: Central role for type I interferons and Tyk2 in lipopolysaccharide-induced endotoxin shock. *Nat Immunol* 4:471, 2003.

62. Cella M, Jarrossay D, Facchetti F, et al: Plasmacytoid monocytes migrate to inflamed lymph nodes and produce large amounts of type I interferon. *Nat Med* 5:919, 1999.

63. Lewis PA, Loomis D: The formation of anti-sheep hemolytic amboceptor in the normal and tuberculous guinea pig. *J Exp Med* 40:503, 1924.

64. Freund J, McDermott K: Sensitization to horse serum by means of adjuvants. *SEBM* 49:548, 1942.

65. Condie RM, Zak SJ, Good RA: Effect of meningococcal endotoxin on the immune response. *Proc Soc Exp Biol Med* 90:355, 1955.

66. Skidmore BJ, Chiller JM, Morrison DC, Weigle WO: Immunologic properties of bacterial lipopolysaccharide (LPS): correlation between the mitogenic, adjuvant, and immunogenic activities. *J Immunol* 114:770, 1975.

67. Germain RN, Jenkins MK: In vivo antigen presentation. *Curr Opin Immunol* 16:120, 2004.

68. Borriello F, Sethna MP, Boyd SD, et al: B7-1 and B7-2 have overlapping, critical roles in immunoglobulin class switching and germinal center formation. *Immunity* 6:303, 1997.

69. Hagberg L, Hull R, Hull S, et al: Difference in susceptibility to gramnegative urinary tract infection between C3H/HeJ and C3H/HeN mice. *Infect Immun* 46:839, 1984.

70. Tabeta K, Georgel P, Janssen E, et al: TLR9 and TLR3 as essential components of innate immune defense against mouse cytomegalovirus. *Proc Natl Acad Sci U S A* 101:3516, 2004.

71. Bukowski JF, Warner JF, Dennert G, Welsh RM: Adoptive transfer studies demonstrating the antiviral effect of natural killer cells in vivo. *J Exp Med* 161:40, 1985.

72. Bukowski JF, Woda BA, Welsh RM: Pathogenesis of murine cytomegalovirus infection in natural killer cell-depleted mice. *J Virol* 52:119, 1984.

73. Bukowski JF, Woda BA, Habu S, et al: Natural killer cell depletion enhances virus synthesis and virus-induced hepatitis in vivo. *J Immunol* 131:1531, 1983.

74. Salazar-Mather TP, Lewis CA, Biron CA: Type I interferons regulate inflammatory cell trafficking and macrophage inflammatory protein 1alpha delivery to the liver. *J Clin Invest* 110:321, 2002.

75. Sorensen TI, Nielsen GG, Andersen PK, Teasdale TW: Genetic and environmental influences on premature death in adult adoptees. *N Engl J Med* 318:727, 1988.

76. Smirnova I, Mann N, Dols A, et al: Assay of locus-specific genetic load implicates rare Toll-like receptor 4 mutations in meningococcal susceptibility. *Proc Natl Acad Sci U S A* 100:6075, 2003.

77. Hawn TR, Verbon A, Lettinga KD, et al: A common dominant TLR5 stop codon polymorphism abolishes flagellin signaling and is associated with susceptibility to legionnaires' disease. *J Exp Med* 198:1563, 2003.

78. Picard C, Puel A, Bonnet M, et al: Pyogenic bacterial infections in humans with IRAK-4 deficiency. *Science* 299:2076, 2003.

79. Jouanguy E, Altare F, Lamhamedi S, et al: Interferon-gamma-receptor deficiency in an infant with fatal bacille Calmette-Guérin infection. *N Engl J Med* 335:1956, 1996.

80. Picard C, Fieschi C, Altare F, et al: Inherited interleukin-12 deficiency: IL12B genotype and clinical phenotype of 13 patients from six kindreds. *Am J Hum Genet* 70:336, 2002.

81. Altare F, Durandy A, Lammas D, et al: Impairment of mycobacterial immunity in human interleukin-12 receptor deficiency. *Science* 280:1432, 1998.

82. De Jong R, Altare F, Haagen IA, et al: Severe mycobacterial and *Salmonella* infections in interleukin-12 receptor-deficient patients. *Science* 280:1435, 1998.

83. Barbosa MD, Nguyen QA, Tchernev VT, et al: Identification of the homologous beige and Chédiak-Higashi syndrome genes. *Nature* 382:262, 1996.

84. Royer-Pokora B, Kunkel LM, Monaco AP, et al: Cloning the gene for an inherited human disorder—chronic granulomatous disease—on the basis of its chromosomal location. *Nature* 322:32, 1986.

85. Shakhov AN, Collart MA, Vassalli P, et al: kappaB-type enhancers are involved in lipopolysaccharide-mediated transcriptional activation of the tumor necrosis factor α gene in primary macrophages. *J Exp Med* 171:35, 1990.

86. Ibrahimi A, Abumrad NA: Role of CD36 in membrane transport of long-chain fatty acids. *Curr Opin Clin Nutr Metab Care* 5:139, 2002.

87. Asch AS, Barnwell J, Silverstein RL, Nachman RL: Isolation of the thrombospondin membrane receptor. *J Clin Invest* 79:1054, 1987.

88. El Khoury JB, Moore KJ, Means TK, et al: CD36 mediates the innate host response to beta-amyloid. *J Exp Med* 197:1657, 2003.

89. Leadbetter EA, Rifkin IR, Hohlbaum AM, et al: Chromatin-IgG complexes activate B cells by dual engagement of IgM and Toll-like receptors. *Nature* 416:603, 2002.

DENDRITIC CELLS AND THE CONTROL OF INNATE AND ADAPTIVE IMMUNITY

MADHAV DHODAPKAR

RALPH M . STEINMAN

The term *dendritic cell* defines a diverse and multifunctional group of cells that serve as sentinels, adjuvants, and controllers of many immune functions. The cells play important roles in both the innate and adaptive immune response to invading pathogens. Dendritic cells have receptors for substances found in the environment, providing the cells with the capacity to respond rapidly to invading pathogens. In this capacity, they can play an important role in activation of innate immune effector mechanisms involved as the first-line defense against infection. In addition, these cells can serve as highly effective antigen-presenting cells that can induce T cell proliferation (activation) or lack of activation (anergy) in response to recognition of peptides presented by the dendritic cells' major histocompatibility complex antigens. As such, the cells help regulate the responses to antigen by the adaptive immune system involving T and B lymphocytes. This chapter describes the varied types and functions of this important class of cells.

FUNCTIONS OF DENDRITIC CELLS

Host defense against pathogens, both infectious and neoplastic, is mediated by innate and adaptive responses, often in concert. Innate immune mechanisms act quickly to resist pathogens but do not develop improved function or memory following an initial exposure (see Chap. 17). Adaptive responses by B and T lymphocytes are acquired over days to months and are capable of memory, that is, improved responses upon pathogen reexposure (see Chaps. 77 and 78). Dendritic cells (DCs) are important mediators of both innate and adaptive immunity and often are responsible for linking together these two forms of resistance.

DENDRITIC CELLS AND INNATE IMMUNITY

Among the many mechanisms of innate resistance (Table 18-1), DCs participate by producing large amounts of protective cytokines, including interleukin (IL)-12 and type I and II interferons, and by activating innate lymphocytes such as like natural killer (NK) cells, NK T cells, and $\gamma\delta$ T cells. The innate response of DCs, particularly cytokine and chemokine production, frequently is mediated by toll-like

Acronyms and abbreviations that appear in this chapter include: APRIL, a proliferation-induced ligand; BAFF, B cell activating factor belonging to the tumor necrosis factor family; BlyS, B lymphocyte stimulator; CD, cluster of differentiation; CMV, cytomegalovirus; DC, dendritic cell; GM-CSF, granulocyte-monocyte colony stimulating factor; HIV, human immunodeficiency virus; Ig, immunoglobulin; IL, interleukin; MHC, major histocompatibility complex; NK, natural killer; TLR, toll-like receptors; TNF, tumor necrosis factor.

TABLE 18-1   SOME INNATE MECHANISMS OF HOST RESISTANCE

Phagocytic cells: granulocytes and macrophages
Innate lymphocytes: NK cells, NK T cells, $\gamma\delta$T cells
Mast cells
Complement
Microbial-binding lectins and pentraxins
Cytokines, including interferons
Chemokines

receptors (TLRs), which recognize distinct microbial ligands.[1,2] TLRs do not have the exquisite specificity provided by the antigen receptors for adaptive immunity on B and T cells (see Chaps. 77 and 78). Nevertheless, TLRs recognize specific ligands such as oligonucleotides, lipopolysaccharides, and other microbial constituents. DCs express TLRs and respond quickly and vigorously to the corresponding microbial ligands. DCs also respond to noninfectious stimuli, but more research is required to determine the extent to which responses to infectious and noninfectious stimuli share signal transduction pathways, including the TLRs. Noninfectious stimuli, which include heat shock proteins and different types of lymphocytes involved in innate responses, may be important for activating DCs to initiate host responses following transplantation or in disease states such as cancer or allergy.

DENDRITIC CELLS AND CONTROL OF ADAPTIVE IMMUNITY

Adaptive immunity comprises several major activities of B and T lymphocytes (Table 18-2). DCs control many features of adaptive immunity, except for one, apparently, the generation of new immunocompetent lymphocytes in the marrow and thymus. These lymphocytes have exquisite diversity and specificity by virtue of antibody and immunoglobulin-like receptors for antigen on B cells and T cells, respectively. The receptor genes undergo rearrangements and other somatic diversification mechanisms to create an immense array of antigen receptors (see Chap. 77). An essential counterpart to adaptive immunity is adaptive tolerance, which is the silencing of cells with receptors that are reactive to self or harmless environmental antigens. DCs play a role here, especially with regard to T cells, which develop tolerance centrally in the thymus and peripherally in lymphoid organs (see Chaps. 76 and 78). During immunization, B and T cells undergo extensive clonal expansion, followed by several mechanisms that eventually remove most of the responding lymphocytes. DCs initiate the clonal expansion of T cells and may influence the growth of B cells. In addition, DCs can control the subsequent differentiation of lymphocytes, such that the properties of the lymphocytes are appropriate to the invading pathogen. For example, T cells, under the influence of DCs, can polarize themselves to produce either interferon gamma (Th1 cells) or IL-4, IL-5, and IL-13 (Th2 cells) (see Chap. 78). Th1 cells are valuable for activating the antimicrobial killing mechanisms of macrophages, which are important in combating infections such as tuberculosis. Th2 cells mobilize resistance to helminths and mediate many allergic responses. Finally, adaptive immunity imparts memory to the host. The memory can be induced by antigen-bearing DCs, but the mechanisms are obscure. Nevertheless, memory provides

TABLE 18-2   SOME FEATURES OF ADAPTIVE IMMUNITY BY B AND T LYMPHOCYTES

Diversity and specificity: somatically rearranged immunoglobulin receptors
Tolerance: specific silencing to self and harmless environmental antigens
Clonal expansion and its regulation: increased, then decreased, numbers of antigen-specific lymphocytes during an immune response
Appropriateness: pathogen-relevant, differentiation of lymphocytes
Memory: long-lived capacity for improved function upon reexposure to antigen

TABLE 18-3   SOME KEY CONSEQUENCES OF DENDRITIC CELL FUNCTION

Sensors: rapid and appropriate differentiation in response to pathogen-associated molecular patterns and other signals
Sentinels: positioned in peripheral tissues to optimize antigen capture and migrate to lymphoid tissues
Tolerance: deletion and anergy of self-reactive lymphocytes and induction of regulatory T cells
Innate resistance: activation of innate lymphocytes, including NK and NK T cells, secretion of protective cytokines
Adaptive immunity: differentiation of quiescent, naive T cells to form effectors, establishment of memory lymphocytes, antibody responses

a population of lymphocytes that allow the host to respond more rapidly and effectively to rechallenge with antigen. The frequency and function of antigen-specific lymphocytes are improved, leading to more rapid production of protective antibodies, cytokines, or killer molecules.

DENDRITIC CELL FUNCTION

DCs may function as sentinels of the immune system, conductors of the immune orchestra, and nature's adjuvants (Table 18-3).[3–8] As sentinels, DCs sense a variety of environmental stimuli, often more quickly than other leukocytes. They can produce cytokines, such as IL-12, that help stimulate immune responses.[9] DCs express most types of TLR.[8,10] DCs also can respond to a number of endogenous stimuli, ranging from inflammatory cytokines, including tumor necrosis factor alpha (TNF-α), IL-1, or interferons, to metabolites such as uric acid, or to heat sock proteins. DCs capture microbes and tumor cells, processing their component antigens for presentation to the adaptive immune system. In addition to antigen processing and presentation, sentinel DCs produce chemokines and cytokines. They migrate to lymphoid tissues, recruiting naive antigen-specific lymphocytes and instructing their subsequent development.

On the other hand, DCs can silence self-reactive T cells, either deleting or anergizing (paralyzing) the lymphocytes.[11] In addition, DCs can recruit antigen-specific regulatory lymphocytes that suppress immune responses by other so-called effector cells.

DCs can activate lymphocytes, such as NK and NK T cells. Such activation contributes to the expansion in numbers of such cells in response to virus infections. It also can enhance their killing activity and capacity to produce cytokines. Reciprocally, these cells act back on DCs, enhancing their capacity to mature into DCs that can help develop adaptive immune responses. Interaction of DCs with such lymphocytes is an example of cross-talk between cell types involving multiple cell surface molecules and cytokines.

Finally, DCs are a critical bridge between innate and adaptive immunity including memory. As part of the innate response, DCs differentiate or mature to become potent initiators of adaptive immunity. The type of mature DC varies according to the challenge, for example, some parasite products cause DCs to induce a Th2 type of T cell response, whereas some viruses and bacteria cause DCs to induce Th1 type of immunity. In short, the presence of antigen and lymphocytes often is not sufficient to induce many innate and adaptive responses. A third party, the DC system of antigen-presenting cells, typically is pivotal.

LIFE HISTORY AND HETEROGENEITY OF DENDRITIC CELLS

TISSUE DISTRIBUTION

DC progenitors in the marrow give rise to circulating precursors that home to lymphoid and nonlymphoid tissues. Most of the DCs in these tissues are considered "immature" because they are not yet able to act as potent initiators of immunity. Nevertheless, immature DCs are specialized cells. They express numerous receptors for environmental stimuli, such as TLRs and cytokine receptors, and endocytic receptors that can facilitate antigen uptake and processing. Immature DCs line body surfaces, such as the airway and intestine. They also are found in the interstitial spaces of most organs, including the heart and kidney, but they are not found in the brain parenchyma. Although immature DCs usually are nonproliferating, data indicate some populations, such as epidermal DCs (termed Langerhans cells), are capable of self-renewal.[12] Some DCs continually traffic through tissues in the steady state, typically moving via the afferent lymphatics to lymph nodes. The traffic can increase upon appropriate stimulation, as initially revealed by research on contact allergens. In the steady state, the migration of DCs, such as through the intestinal and airway epithelium, allows DCs to carry samples of self and environmental antigens to regional lymph nodes,[13–15] with the potential of tolerizing the T cell repertoire. In contrast, under maturation conditions, such as infection with influenza in the lung,[15] the migrating DCs are the critical link for initiating immunity in the draining lymphoid tissues. However, this general scheme of the life history of DCs must be placed in the context of DC heterogeneity, because many types of DCs exist (Table 18-4).

DENDRITIC CELL PRECURSORS IN MARROW AND BLOOD

At the progenitor level in the marrow, DCs are unique in that they can be derived from lymphoid (shared with B, T, NK cells) and myeloid (shared with macrophages and granulocytes) progenitors. The consequence of this dual origin is not known. Importantly, progenitors for DCs express flt3, a receptor tyrosine kinase that is activated upon binding to flt3 ligand.[16] Activation of flt3 induces DC proliferation.[17] At the precursor level in the blood, distinct subsets of DCs, termed myeloid DC and plasmacytoid DC, can be distinguished by their differential expression of several marker proteins and distinctive functions. The myeloid subset of DCs expresses the cluster of differentiation (CD)11c integrin and BDCA-1. The plasmacytoid subset of human DCs lacks CD11c and expresses the lectin BDCA-2. An important feature of plasmacytoid DCs is their ability to produce very high levels of type I interferons upon contact with enveloped viruses, including ultraviolet-inactivated viruses.[18,19] The process likely involves ligation of TLR-7 and TLR-9 by viral RNA,[20,21] and DNA, respectively.[22,23] The myeloid–plasmacytoid terminology can be confusing because plasmacytoid DCs can originate from so called myeloid progenitors. Nevertheless, most investigators agree that myeloid and plasmacytoid DCs in blood and tissues represent distinct states of differentiation with unique transcriptional controls.

Another DC population obtained from blood is monocyte-derived DCs. These cells are differentiated from blood monocytes in tissue culture, usually by applying a combination of granulocyte-monocyte colony stimulating factor (GM-CSF) and IL-4 or IL-13.[24,25] More work is required to identify the counterpart of monocyte-derived DCs *in situ*.

TABLE 18-4   DENDRITIC CELL HETEROGENEITY: ORIGIN, SUBSETS, AND NOMENCLATURE

Marrow: lymphoid and myeloid progenitors
Blood: plasmacytoid and myeloid subsets
Peripheral tissues: epidermal (epithelial) and dermal (interstitial) subsets
Lymphoid tissues: plasmacytoid and other subsets
Other: interdigitating cells, monocyte-derived dendritic cells

DENDRITIC CELLS IN PERIPHERAL TISSUES

As illustrated by the skin, distinct subsets of DCs are associated with epithelia (e.g., epidermal Langerhans cells) and interstitial spaces (dermal DCs).[26,27] These subsets have different markers, including molecules with a potential role in antigen presentation. Langerhans cells express a C-type lectin called Langerin/CD207, which can be internalized into special compartments called Birbeck granules, and the CD1a form of CD1 glycolipid-presenting molecules. Dermal DCs express abundant mannose receptor/CD206 and the CD1b and CD1c forms of glycolipid-presenting molecules.[28]

DENDRITIC CELLS IN LYMPHOID TISSUES, ESPECIALLY PERIPHERAL LYMPHOID ORGANS

Representatives of the Langerhans cells and plasmacytoid DCs and additional subsets of DCs that again exhibit differences in endocytic capacities are present in the lymphoid tissues. For example, in mouse spleen,[29] one subset of DCs lacks the integrin CD11b but selectively expresses an endocytic receptor termed DEC-205/CD205[30] and takes up dying cells, including targets killed by NK lymphocytes.[31] Another subset of DCs expresses CD11b and is capable of phagocytic and pinocytic activity, but it lacks DEC-205 and appears not to ingest many types of dying cells.

By electron microscopy, DCs in lymphoid tissues often are termed "interdigitating cells." These cells appear as large stellate cells with a lucent "empty"-appearing cytoplasm. Whether these interdigitating cells primarily represent the subset of DCs that also express high levels of DEC-205 remains to be determined.

DCs involved in induction of immune tolerance can be called "tolerogenic DCs." Tolerogenic DCs may represent a distinct subset, although all types of DCs may be capable of inducing tolerance. The type of tolerance depends on the state of DC maturation and the environments in which the DCs are located.

MEANING OF DENDRITIC CELL HETEROGENEITY

Investigators currently are studying the significance of the heterogeneity of DCs. In one view, DC subsets are precommitted to carry out select innate responses and in turn, perhaps, distinct types of adaptive immunity. Plasmacytoid DCs are a major source of type I interferons, particularly with inactivated viruses,[18,19] yet other DCs can be a rich source of interferon after certain live viral infections and signaling through protein kinase R.[32] Some evidence indicates different subsets of DCs polarize helper T cells to either the Th1- or Th2-type pathway of differentiation (see Chap. 78).[33] In contrast, other data indicate these same subsets are plastic, influenced by the pathogen to bring about different types of innate and adaptive immunity.[34] The field of DC subsets is perplexing at this time and is limited by the relative lack of direct analyses of DCs *in vivo*, as opposed to data on DCs studied *ex vivo* or following reinfusion.

ELEMENTS OF DENDRITIC CELL FUNCTION FOR INITIATION OF IMMUNITY

DCs are "antigen-presenting cells." An antigen-presenting cell is *any* cell that uses its major histocompatibility complex (MHC) products or other antigen-presenting molecules, such as the CD1 molecules that present glycolipids and lipoglycans, to bind and display (i.e., "present") fragments of antigen to lymphocytes (see Chaps. 78 and 129). DCs are much more specialized or professional than other antigen-presenting cells. When DCs mature in response to antigen, hundreds and even thousands of gene transcripts can be up-regulated or

down-regulated.[35,36] Most of the early attention on the function of DCs was on their ability to stimulate T cell immunity, but the significant roles of DCs in the induction of tolerance and in the regulation of other types of lymphocytes, such as NK, NK T cells, γδ T cells, and B cells, are increasingly evident (Table 18-5).

ANTIGEN CAPTURE

Many different endocytic receptors are expressed by DCs, where they enhance the efficiency of antigen capture, processing, and presentation.[37] One example, which has been pursued *in vivo* in mice, involves the engineering of antigens into antibodies that bind to the endocytic receptor DEC-205/CD205. The modified antibody then targets the antigen selectively to DCs in lymphoid tissues.[38,39] Antibody-mediated targeting to DCs in lymphoid tissues enhances presentation of the associated antigen more than 100-fold to CD8+ and CD4+ T cells.[40] In other words, although DCs are positioned to pick up antigens and process them for presentation in lymphoid organs, receptor-based pathways exist through which antigen capture (and in some cases, antigen processing) is enormously improved.

Many potential antigen uptake receptors are predicted to be C-type lectins,[41] but in many cases their natural ligands have not been identified. DCs also express Fcγ and Fcε receptors for immune complexes and several scavenger receptors for uptake of dying cells and microbes. Recognition of pathogens by DC receptors can have two outcomes. One outcome is antigen presentation. In the second outcome, the pathogen may use the receptor to exploit and evade the host. An example studied in tissue culture is the lectin DC-SIGN/CD209, which is expressed by monocyte derived DCs. DC-SIGN is commandeered by different agents, such as human immunodeficiency virus (HIV)-1 and cytomegalovirus (CMV), to be transmitted to T cells and endothelial cells, respectively[42,43]; by Dengue virus to replicate within DCs[44]; and by *Mycobacterium tuberculosis* to trigger production of the suppressive cytokine IL-10.[45,46]

ANTIGEN PROCESSING

Following uptake, efficient processing of antigen yields peptides that bind to MHC class II and class I products. The terminology can be confusing, but by definition, "exogenous" antigens are processed directly following uptake, whereas "endogenous" antigens are processed following biosynthesis in the antigen-presenting cell. The more classic or earliest defined routes involved processing of "exogenous" antigens for presentation of MHC II–peptide complexes to CD4+ T lymphocytes and "endogenous" antigens for presentation of MHC class I–peptide complexes to CD8+ T cells.

However, a more recently appreciated route leads to the presentation of exogenous antigens on MHC I products. This pathway often is termed "cross-presentation" and can be particularly well developed

TABLE 18-5   SOME IMPORTANT COMPONENTS OF DENDRITIC CELL FUNCTION

Antigen handling: specialized antigen uptake receptors and processing pathways for classic (MHC) and nonclassic (CD1 and others) presenting molecules

Environmental sensing: multiple receptors for microbial and nonmicrobial products and exaggerated responses to the products

Cytokine receptors, including hematopoietins (flt3L and GM-CSF, but not M-CSF, G-CSF)

Chemokine receptors, especially for homing to tissues (CCR6) and lymph nodes (CCR7)

Induction of peripheral tolerance via intrinsic and extrinsic pathways

Activation of innate lymphocytes

in DCs, especially those cells in lymphoid tissues *in vivo* where cross-presentation leads efficiently to either tolerance or immunity in CD8+ T lymphocytes, depending upon the DC maturation stimulus.[39,47] The exogenous pathways are particularly efficient in DCs, as illustrated by the uptake of dying cells,[47,48] which model the capture of cell-associated antigens from transplants, tumors, foci of infection, and self tissues. The pathway is called "cross-presentation" because antigens that are located in a dying cell "cross" over to the processing and presentation machinery of the DC. Nevertheless, cross-presentation of antigens onto MHC class I often involves the proteasome and transporters for antigenic peptides, which are used in the presentation of endogenous antigens. Cross-presentation has been proposed to occur in endocytic vacuoles that have fused with elements of the rough endoplasmic reticulum.[49,50] New evidence indicates a conserved tyrosine in the cytoplasmic tail of MHC class I products traffics these molecules to special cross-presenting compartments.[51]

DCs are a major cell type involved in cross-presentation, both proteins[52] and probably lipids.[53] Cross-presentation has been observed with nonreplicating microbes, dying cells, ligands for the DEC-205 receptor, and immune complexes including antibody-coated tumor cells. These examples allow DCs to induce tolerance or immunity to antigens that are not synthesized *de novo* in these cells. Fcγ receptors, in addition to mediating presentation, can influence DC maturation, either enhancing maturation through activating forms of the receptor or preventing maturation through inhibitory forms.[54] Such consequences of antibody binding to DC Fc receptors, with regard to DC maturation and cross-presentation, must be considered when trying to understand the use of antibodies as therapeutic agents in patients.

DCs are a major site for expression of the CD1 family of antigen-presenting molecules, although individual CD1 molecules can be restricted to subsets of DCs. For example, CD1a typically is found on epidermal Langerhans cells in skin, whereas CD1b and CD1c are expressed on dermal DCs. CD1 molecules present glycolipids, whereas microbial glycolipids are the best studied to date with regard to CD1a, CD1b, and CD1c.[55] In addition, CD1d molecules on DCs efficiently present the synthetic glycolipid α-galactosylceramide. This process leads to activation of distinct lymphocytes with a restricted T cell repertoire, the NK T cells.[56] NK T cells have significant potential as effector cells because they can produce large amounts of interferon gamma and lyse tumor targets.

REGULATION AND MATURATION OF DENDRITIC CELLS

Maturation refers to the stimulus-dependent differentiation of DCs that in turn allows differentiation of lymphocytes for immunity and memory. Immature DCs efficiently take up antigen but do not induce immunity, that is, the production of immune effectors and the establishment of memory. For immune induction to occur, DCs require additional stimuli that lead to an intricate differentiation process called maturation. Maturation comprises changes in the endocytic and antigen processing machineries, the production of chemokines and cytokines, and the expression of many cell surface molecules, including those of the B7, TNF, and Notch ligand families. Therefore, DCs can separate in time two of the vital components for initiating immunity: antigen uptake by immature DCs and expression of costimulatory functions for lymphocytes by mature cells.[57]

In the case of DCs derived from marrow and monocyte precursors, DC maturation is accompanied by exquisite changes in the endocytic system. Lysosomal processing is activated by assembly of an active proton pump.[58] This ATPase acidifies the lysosome so that processing of antigens and the MHC class II associated invariant chain can proceed. The MHC–peptide complexes form within the endocytic system of the maturing DCs,[59] which then traffic in distinct nonlysosomal

compartments to the cell surface.[60] DC maturation also increases presentation on MHC I. One change is the formation of an "immunoproteasome," a combinatorial form of proteasome that increases the spectrum of peptides destined to be presented on MHC I.[61] Another regulated process involves the uptake or endocytosis step itself. During maturation, uptake is dampened as a result of inactivation of a rho-GTPase termed cdc42.[62] Therefore, DCs have an endocytic system that is tightly regulated and devoted to presentation of captured antigens, rather than clearance and scavenging.

More research is needed to understand the mechanisms of DC maturation, but different stimuli, such as specific pathogens and cytokines, likely drive DCs along distinct pathways with distinct immune consequences. DCs expressing the notch ligand "delta" trigger Th1 type of immune responses, whereas DCs induced to express the other notch ligand "jagged" allow for Th2-type responses.[63] A hallmark of DC maturation in response to several stimuli is up-regulation of costimulatory molecules such as CD80 and CD86. The up-regulation seems to result from production of inflammatory cytokines, particularly TNF-α. Nonetheless, CD86 up-regulation should not be equated directly with immunogenicity, which requires other DC functions, such as those triggered by CD40 ligation.[56]

ACTIVATION OF INNATE LYMPHOCYTES

Increasing attention is now being paid to cross-talk between DCs and other innate effectors such as NK cells.[64] DCs can prime resting NK cells, which, after activation, might induce further maturation of DCs. NK-mediated killing of virus-infected cells or tumor cells may provide a source of antigens for generation of T cell responses via DCs, further linking innate and adaptive immunity. NK cells also negatively regulate DC function by killing immature DCs.[65] A significant proportion of NK cells reside in the T cell regions of lymphoid tissues, thereby providing an opportunity for direct interaction between DC and NK cells *in vivo*.[66]

GENERATION OF ANTIBODY-FORMING B CELLS

DCs enhance antibody formation by promoting formation of antigen-specific CD4+ helper T cells.[67] In addition, DCs can have direct effects on B cells[68] that greatly enhance immunoglobulin (Ig) secretion and isotype switching, including production of the IgA class of antibodies, which contribute to mucosal immunity.[69] DCs also can induce a B cell class switch in a CD40-independent manner, through production of ligands such as B lymphocyte stimulator (BlyS; B cell activating factor belonging to the tumor necrosis factor family [BAFF]) and a proliferation-induced ligand (APRIL), including T cell-independent induction of IgA antibodies to commensal organisms.[70] Data have shown an important role for plasmacytoid DCs in antibody responses to influenza virus in culture.[71] Production of antibodies by any of these mechanisms may lead to interaction with DC FcγR and thereby an adaptive response by T cells.

POSITIONING AND MIGRATION OF DENDRITIC CELLS

DCs are strategically positioned as immature cells along body surfaces (skin, airway, gut) and in the interstitial spaces of many organs, such as the heart and kidneys. In the steady state, DCs appear to migrate continuously from tissues into afferent lymphatics and probably blood. The precursors of these migrating DCs (originally called "veiled" cells because of their sheet-like processes or veils) seem to include a subset of monocytes and committed myeloid DCs in the blood. Steady-state traffic of DCs may allow the DCs to sample self and environmental antigens for purposes of tolerance. Interestingly, the "tolerogenic" DC may not be the migratory cell itself. Instead, the migrating DC may die in the lymph node and be processed by resident DCs in that organ,[48] or additional mechanisms may transfer antigen and MHC peptide complexes to more "resident" DCs. Most DCs in a lymph node often are assumed to represent immigrants from the tissues, but this situation may not always be true. Many DCs in the T cell areas also may be derived from blood progenitors of plasmacytoid and nonplasmacytoid DCs.

TOLEROGENIC PROPERTIES OF DENDRITIC CELLS

Much of the early focus on DCs was on their immunogenic properties, but increasing evidence indicates DCs *in situ* can mediate antigen-specific unresponsiveness or tolerance in the central lymphoid organs and in the periphery. In the thymus, DCs generate tolerance by deleting self-reactive T cells.[72] Other cells, particularly the specialized epithelium of the thymic medulla,[73] are important in deletional tolerance or negative selection.

DCs also induce tolerance in peripheral lymphoid organs. For example, DCs may induce tolerance to antigens present in dying self tissues. Uptake, especially when receptor mediated, leads to presentation of antigens on MHC class I and II products.[38,39,47] In mice, the targeting of antigens to receptors on resting DCs can lead to deletion of the corresponding T cells and unresponsiveness to antigenic challenge. However, if a stimulus for DC maturation is coadministered, the mice develop immunity. DCs also can contribute to the expansion and differentiation of T cells that can suppress or regulate other immune cells.[74,75] One possibility is that distinct developmental stages and subsets of DCs account for the different pathways, leading to peripheral tolerance, such as deletion or suppression of self-reactive T cells.

DENDRITIC CELLS IN IMMUNOTHERAPY

At this time, the principal hematologic field addressed from the perspective of DC biology is that of the host response to malignancy and associated strategies for immunotherapy of cancer. The features of DCs outlined in Table 18-5 explain their relevance to these fields. Malignant cells express a large number of alterations that are viewed as antigens by the immune system. Antibodies, T cells, and NK cells also can act against tumors. DCs can efficiently process antigens from a variety of different sources, such as tumor cells, and initiate responses by the different kinds of innate and adaptive lymphocytes. Therefore, harnessing DCs to manipulate the host response to tumors and to other hematologic antigens seems logical.

An interesting example is myeloma, in which both T cells and tumor cells from the marrow can be studied. In the premalignant state, termed essential monoclonal gammopathy, myeloma-reactive T cells are detected in the marrow.[76] Using DCs to present myeloma cells as antigens, the presence of both CD4+ helper T cells and CD8+ killer T cells in the marrow can be detected. In contrast, myeloma-reactive T cells cannot be detected in patients with advanced myeloma. Nonetheless, myeloma-reactive CD4+ and CD8+ T cells can be generated when the T cells are cultured for 1 to 2 weeks in the presence of DCs that have captured myeloma cells.[77] Interestingly, the presentation of myeloma cells is greatly enhanced when they are coated with antisyndecan antibodies.[77,78]

DCs have important potential roles in immunotherapy.[6,79] Several approaches are being used to generate DCs under clinical grade conditions, load them with tumor antigens *ex vivo*, and reinfuse the cells to actively immunize patients against cancer antigens or, more broadly, to study several aspects of the human immune response to cancer. This field of research is in its early stages. One approach to DC-based immunotherapy utilizes blood DCs that are differentiated and charged with tumor antigens. A second approach generates DCs *ex vivo* from proliferating progenitors within CD34+ populations. This process provides a composite of cells with properties of epidermal and dermal DCs. A third approach differentiates DCs from blood monocytes.

Ex vivo–derived and antigen-loaded DCs have been used to expand antigen-specific T cell responses in healthy volunteers,[80,81] and in cancer patients.[82–85] These early studies have yielded some evidence of clinical activity, with tumor regressions in patients with either solid tumors or hematologic malignancies.[82–85] An important advantage of the *ex vivo* approach to immunotherapy is that several key parameters of DC function can be controlled and researched, such as the loading of DCs with multiple antigens (from whole tumor cells or with RNA from whole tumor cells) and the control of the DC maturation state. Injection of immature DCs may lead to inhibition of T cell responses and induction of regulatory T cells.[80] Furthermore, DCs can boost innate lymphocytes such as NK cells[86] and glycolipid-reactive NK T cells.[87]

Another approach, still in the preclinical setting, targets antigens to DCs directly *in situ*. This objective can be achieved by incorporating the antigens into monoclonal antibodies specific for receptors expressed selectively or at much higher levels on DCs or DC subsets. Targeting via the DEC-205 receptor is an early example and stresses the need to simultaneously consider the maturation state of the antigen-capturing DCs. In the steady state, tolerance can ensue.[38,88] For immunity, a complex process of maturation must be induced, for example, by the actions of agonistic anti-CD40 antibodies[40] and by innate lymphocytes.[56]

REFERENCES

1. Beutler B: Inferences, questions, and possibilities in Toll-like receptor signaling. *Nature* 430:257, 2004.
2. Akira S, Takeda K: Toll-like receptor signaling. *Nat Rev Immunol* 4:499, 2004.
3. Kapsenberg ML: Dendritic-cell control of pathogen-driven T-cell polarization. *Nat Rev Immunol* 3:984, 2003.
4. Sher A, Pearce E, Kaye P: Shaping the immune response to parasites: Role of dendritic cells. *Curr Opin Immunol* 15:421, 2003.
5. Cerundolo V, Hermans IF, Salio M: Dendritic cells: A journey from laboratory to clinic. *Nat Immunol* 5:7, 2004.
6. Figdor CG, De Vries IJ, Lesterhuis WJ, Melief CJ: Dendritic cell immunotherapy: Mapping the way. *Nat Med* 10:475, 2004.
7. Hackstein H, Thomson AW: Dendritic cells: Emerging pharmacological targets of immunosuppressive drugs. *Nat Rev Immunol* 4:24, 2004.
8. Pulendran B: Modulating vaccine responses with dendritic cells and toll-like receptors. *Immunol Rev* 199:227, 2004.
9. Reis e Sousa C, Hieny S, Scharton-Kersten T, et al: In vivo microbial stimulation induces rapid CD40L-independent production of IL-12 by dendritic cells and their re-distribution to T cell areas. *J Exp Med* 186:1819, 1997.
10. Mazzoni A, Segal DM: Controlling the Toll road to dendritic cell polarization. *J Leukoc Biol* 75:721, 2004.
11. Steinman RM, Hawiger D, Nussenzweig MC: Tolerogenic dendritic cells. *Annu Rev Immunol* 21:685, 2003.
12. Merad M, Manz MG, Karsunky H, et al: Langerhans cells renew in the skin throughout life under steady-state conditions. *Nat Immunol* 3:1135, 2002.
13. Huang F-P, Platt N, Wykes M, et al: A discrete subpopulation of dendritic cells transports apoptotic intestinal epithelial cells to T cell areas of mesenteric lymph nodes. *J Exp Med* 191:435, 2000.
14. Vermaelen KY, Carro-Muino I, Lambrecht BN, Pauwels RA: Specific migratory dendritic cells rapidly transport antigen from the airways to the thoracic lymph nodes. *J Exp Med* 193:51, 2001.

15. Brimnes MK, Bonifaz L, Steinman RM, Moran TM: Influenza virus-induced dendritic cell maturation is associated with the induction of strong T cell immunity to a coadministered, normally nonimmunogenic protein. *J Exp Med* 198:133, 2003.

16. D'Amico A, Wu L: The early progenitors of mouse dendritic cells and plasmacytoid predendritic cells are within the bone marrow hemopoietic precursors expressing Flt3. *J Exp Med* 198:293, 2003.

17. Pulendran B, Banchereau J, Burkeholder S, et al: Flt3-ligand and granulocyte colony-stimulating factor mobilize distinct human dendritic cell subsets in vivo. *J Immunol* 165:566, 2000.

18. Siegal FP, Kadowaki N, Shodell M, et al: The nature of the principal type 1 interferon-producing cells in human blood. *Science* 284:1835, 1999.

19. Cella M, Jarrossay D, Facchetti F, et al: Plasmacytoid monocytes migrate to inflamed lymph nodes and produce large amounts of type I interferon. *Nat Med* 5:919, 1999.

20. Diebold SS, Kaisho T, Hemmi H, et al: Innate antiviral responses by means of TLR7-mediated recognition of single-stranded RNA. *Science* 303:1529, 2004.

21. Heil F, Hemmi H, Hochrein H, et al: Species-specific recognition of single-stranded RNA via toll-like receptor 7 and 8. *Science* 303:1526, 2004.

22. Lund J, Sato A, Akira S, et al: Toll-like receptor 9-mediated recognition of herpes simplex virus-2 by plasmacytoid dendritic cells. *J Exp Med* 198:513, 2003.

23. Tabeta K, Georgel P, Janssen E, et al: Toll-like receptors 9 and 3 as essential components of innate immune defense against mouse cytomegalovirus infection. *Proc Natl Acad Sci U S A* 101:3516, 2004.

24. Sallusto F, Lanzavecchia A: Efficient presentation of soluble antigen by cultured human dendritic cells is maintained by granulocyte/macrophage colony-stimulating factor plus interleukin 4 and downregulated by tumor necrosis factor α. *J Exp Med* 179:1109, 1994.

25. Romani N, Gruner S, Brang D, et al: Proliferating dendritic cell progenitors in human blood. *J Exp Med* 180:83, 1994.

26. Nestle FO, Turka LA, Nickoloff BJ: Characterization of dermal dendritic cells in psoriasis. Autostimulation of T lymphocytes and induction of Th1 type cytokines. *J Clin Invest* 94:202, 1994.

27. Caux C, Vanbervliet B, Massacrier C, et al: CD34+ hematopoietic progenitors from human cord blood differentiate along two independent dendritic cell pathways in response to GM-CSF+ TNF α. *J Exp Med* 184:695, 1996.

28. Ebner S, Ehammer Z, Holzmann S, et al: Expression of C-type lectin receptors by subsets of dendritic cells in human skin. *Int Immunol* 16:877, 2004.

29. Vremec D, Shortman K: Dendritic cells subtypes in mouse lymphoid organs. Cross-correlation of surface markers, changes with incubation, and differences among thymus, spleen, and lymph nodes. *J Immunol* 159:565, 1997.

30. Jiang W, Swiggard WJ, Heufler C, et al: The receptor DEC-205 expressed by dendritic cells and thymic epithelial cells is involved in antigen processing. *Nature* 375:151, 1995.

31. Iyoda T, Shimoyama S, Liu K, et al: The CD8+ dendritic cell subset selectively endocytoses dying cells in culture and in vivo. *J Exp Med* 195:1289, 2002.

32. Diebold SS, Montoya M, Unger H, et al: Viral infection switches nonplasmacytoid dendritic cells into high interferon producers. *Nature* 424:324, 2003.

33. Moser M, Murphy KM: Dendritic cell regulation of Th1-Th2 development. *Nat Immunol* 1:199, 2000.

34. Boonstra A, Asselin-Paturel C, Gilliet M, et al: Flexibility of mouse classical and plasmacytoid-derived dendritic cells in directing T helper type 1 and 2 cell development: Dependency on antigen dose and differential toll-like receptor ligation. *J Exp Med* 197:1, 2003.

35. Granucci F, Vizzardelli C, Pavelka N, et al: Inducible IL-2 production by dendritic cells revealed by global gene expression analysis. *Nat Immunol* 2:882, 2001.

36. Huang Q, Liu do N, Majewski P, et al: The plasticity of dendritic cell responses to pathogens and their components. *Science* 294:870, 2001.

37. Mellman I, Steinman RM: Dendritic cells: Specialized and regulated antigen processing machines. *Cell* 106:255, 2001.

38. Hawiger D, Inaba K, Dorsett Y, et al: Dendritic cells induce peripheral T cell unresponsiveness under steady state conditions in vivo. *J Exp Med* 194:769, 2001.

39. Bonifaz L, Bonnyay D, Mahnke K, et al: Efficient targeting of protein antigen to the dendritic cell receptor DEC-205 in the steady state leads to antigen presentation on major histocompatibility complex class I products and peripheral CD8+ T cell tolerance. *J Exp Med* 196:1627, 2002.

40. Bonifaz LC, Bonnyay DP, Charalambous A, et al: In vivo targeting of antigens to the DEC-205 receptor on maturing dendritic cells improves T cell vaccination. *J Exp Med* 199:815, 2004.

41. Figdor CG, Van Kooyk Y, Adema GJ: C-type lectin receptors on dendritic cells and Langerhans cells. *Nat Rev Immunol* 2:77, 2002.

42. Geijtenbeek TB, Kwon DS, Torensma R, et al: DC-SIGN, a dendritic cell specific HIV-1 binding protein that enhances trans-infection of T cells. *Cell* 100:587, 2000.

43. Halary F, Amara A, Lortat-Jacob H, et al: Human cytomegalovirus binding to DC-SIGN is required for dendritic cell infection and target cell trans-infection. *Immunity* 17:653, 2002.

44. Tassaneetrithep B, Burgess TH, Granelli-Piperno A, et al: DC-SIGN (CD209) mediates dengue virus infection of human dendritic cells. *J Exp Med* 197:823, 2003.

45. Van Kooyk Y, Geijtenbeek TB: DC-SIGN: Escape mechanism for pathogens. *Nat Rev Immunol* 3:697, 2003.

46. Tailleux L, Schwartz O, Herrmann J-L, et al: DC-SIGN is the major Mycobacterium tuberculosis receptor on human dendritic cells. *J Exp Med* 197:121, 2003.

47. Liu K, Iyoda T, Saternus M, et al: Immune tolerance after delivery of dying cells to dendritic cells in situ. *J Exp Med* 196:1091, 2002.

48. Inaba K, Turley S, Yamaide F, et al: Efficient presentation of phagocytosed cellular fragments on the MHC class II products of dendritic cells. *J Exp Med* 188:2163, 1998.

49. Houde M, Bertholet S, Gagnon E, et al: Phagosomes are competent organelles for antigen cross-presentation. *Nature* 425:402, 2003.

50. Guermonprez P, Saveanu L, Kleijmeer M, et al: ER-phagosome fusion defines an MHC class I cross-presentation compartment in dendritic cells. *Nature* 425:397, 2003.

51. Lizee G, Basha G, Tiong J, et al: Control of dendritic cell cross-presentation by the major histocompatibility complex class I cytoplasmic domain. *Nat Immunol* 4:1065, 2003.

52. Jung S, Unutmaz D, Wong P, et al: In vivo depletion of CD11c+ dendritic cells abrogation priming of CD8+ T cells by exogenous cell-associated antigens. *Immunity* 17:211, 2002.

53. Wu DY, Segal NH, Sidobre S, et al: Cross-presentation of disialoganglioside GD3 to natural killer T cells. *J Exp Med* 198:173, 2003.

54. Kalergis AM, Ravetch JV: Inducing tumor immunity through the selective engagement of activating Fcγ receptors on dendritic cells. *J Exp Med* 195:1653, 2002.

55. Vincent MS, Gumperz JE, Brenner MB: Understanding the function of CD1-restricted T cells. *Nat Immunol* 4:517, 2003.

56. Fujii S, Liu K, Smith C, et al: The linkage of innate to adaptive immunity via maturing dendritic cells in vivo requires CD40 ligation in addition to antigen presentation and CD80/86 costimulation. *J Exp Med* 199:1607, 2004.

57. Romani N, Koide S, Crowley M, et al: Presentation of exogenous protein antigens by dendritic cells to T cell clones: Intact protein is presented

best by immature, epidermal Langerhans cells. *J Exp Med* 169:1169, 1989.

58. Trombetta ES, Ebersold M, Garrett W, et al: Activation of lysosomal function during dendritic cell maturation. *Science* 299:1400, 2003.

59. Inaba K, Turley S, Iyoda T, et al: The formation of immunogenic MHC class II-peptide ligands in lysosomal compartments of dendritic cells is regulated by inflammatory stimuli. *J Exp Med* 191:927, 2000.

60. Chow A, Toomre D WG, Mellman I: Dendritic cell maturation triggers retrograde transport of MHC class II transport from lysosomes to the plasma membrane. *Nature* 418:988, 2002.

61. Morel S, Levy F, Burlet-Schiltz O, et al: Processing of some antigens by the standard proteasome but not by the immunoproteasome results in poor presentation by dendritic cells. *Immunity* 12:107, 2000.

62. Garrett WS, Chen LM, Kroschewski R, et al: Developmental control of endocytosis in dendritic cells by Cdc42. *Cell* 102:325, 2000.

63. Amsen D, Blander JM, Lee GR, et al: Instruction of distinct CD4 T helper cell fates by different notch ligands on antigen-presenting cells. *Cell* 117:515, 2004.

64. Zitvogel L: Dendritic and natural killer cells cooperate in the control/switch of innate immunity. *J Exp Med* 195:F9, 2002.

65. Ferlazzo G, Tsang ML, Moretta L, et al: Human dendritic cells activate resting NK cells and are recognized via the NKp30 receptor by activated NK cells. *J Exp Med* 195:343, 2002.

66. Ferlazzo G, Thomas D, Lin SL, et al: The abundant NK cells in human secondary lymphoid tissues require activation to express killer cell Ig-like receptors and become cytolytic. *J Immunol* 172:1455, 2004.

67. Inaba K, Steinman RM: Protein-specific helper T lymphocyte formation initiated by dendritic cells. *Science* 229:475, 1985.

68. Balazs M, Martin F, Zhou T, Kearney JF: Blood dendritic cells interact with splenic marginal zone B cells to initiate T-independent immune responses. *Immunity* 17:341, 2002.

69. Fayette J, Dubois B, Vandenabelle S, et al: Human dendritic cells skew isotype switching of CD40 activated naive B cells towards IgA1 and IgA2. *J Exp Med* 185:1909, 1997.

70. Macpherson AJ, Uhr T: Induction of protective IgA by intestinal dendritic cells carrying commensal bacteria. *Science* 303:1662, 2004.

71. Jego G, Palucka AK, Blanck JP, et al: Plasmacytoid dendritic cells induce plasma cell differentiation through type I interferon and interleukin 6. *Immunity* 19:225, 2003.

72. Zal T, Volkmann A, Stockinger B: Mechanisms of tolerance induction in major histocompatibility complex class II-restricted T cells specific for a blood-borne self-antigen. *J Exp Med* 180:2089, 1994.

73. Kyewski B, Derbinski J, Gotter J, Klein L: Promiscuous gene expression and central T-cell tolerance: More than meets the eye. *Trends Immunol* 23:364, 2002.

74. Yamazaki S, Iyoda T, Tarbell K, et al: Direct expansion of functional CD25+ CD4+ regulatory T cells by antigen processing dendritic cells. *J Exp Med* 198;235, 2003.

75. Tarbell KV, Yamazaki S, Olson K, et al: CD25+ CD4+ T cells, expanded with dendritic cells presenting a single autoantigenic peptide, suppress autoimmune diabetes. *J Exp Med* 199:1467, 2004.

76. Dhodapkar MV, Krasovsky J, Osman K, Geller MD: Vigorous premalignancy-specific effector T cell response in the bone marrow of patients with monoclonal gammopathy. *J Exp Med* 198:1753, 2003.

77. Dhodapkar MV, Krasovsky J, Olson K: T cells from the tumor microenvironment of patients with progressive myeloma can generate strong, tumor-specific cytolytic responses to autologous, tumor-loaded dendritic cells. *Proc Natl Acad Sci U S A* 99:13009, 2002.

78. Dhodapkar KM, Krasovsky J, Williamson B, Dhodapkar MV: Antitumor monoclonal antibodies enhance cross-presentation of cellular antigens and the generation of myeloma-specific killer T cells by dendritic cells. *J Exp Med* 195:125, 2002.

79. Steinman RM, Dhodapkar M: Active immunization against cancer with dendritic cells: The near future. *Int J Cancer* 94:459, 2001.

80. Dhodapkar MV, Steinman RM: Antigen-bearing, immature dendritic cells induce peptide-specific, CD8+ regulatory T cells in vivo in humans. *Blood* 100:174, 2002.

81. Dhodapkar MV, Steinman RM, Krasovsky J, et al: Antigen specific inhibition of effector T cell function in humans after injection of immature dendritic cells. *J Exp Med* 193:233, 2001.

82. Hsu FJ, Benike C, Fagnoni F, et al: Vaccination of patients with B-cell lymphoma using autologous antigen-pulsed dendritic cells. *Nat Med* 2:52, 1996.

83. Nestle FO, Alijagic S, Gilliet M, et al: Vaccination of melanoma patients with peptide- or tumor lysate-pulsed dendritic cells. *Nat Med* 4:328, 1998.

84. Thurner B, Haendle I, Röder C, et al: Vaccination with Mage-3A1 peptide-pulsed mature, monocyte-derived dendritic cells expands specific cytotoxic T cells and induces regression of some metastases in advanced stage IV melanoma. *J Exp Med* 190:1669, 1999.

85. Banchereau J, Palucka AK, Dhodapkar M, et al: Immune and clinical responses in patients with metastatic melanoma to CD34+ progenitor-derived dendritic cell vaccine. *Cancer Res* 61:6451, 2001.

86. Ferlazzo G, Munz C: NK cell compartments and their activation by dendritic cells. *J Immunol* 172:1333, 2004.

87. Fujii S, Shimizu K, Kronenberg M, Steinman RM: Prolonged interferon-γ producing NKT response induced with α-galactosylceramide-loaded dendritic cells. *Nat Immunol* 3:867, 2002.

88. Hawiger D, Masilamani RF, Bettelli E, et al: Immunological unresponsiveness characterized by increased expression of CD5 on peripheral T cells induced by dendritic cells in vivo. *Immunity* 20:695, 2004.

THERAPEUTIC PRINCIPLES

PHARMACOLOGY AND TOXICITY OF ANTINEOPLASTIC DRUGS

BRUCE A. CHABNER

WYNDHAM WILSON

JEFFREY SUPKO

The safe and effective use of anticancer drugs in the treatment of hematologic malignancies requires an in-depth knowledge of the pharmacology of these agents. In this field of medicine, the margin of safety is narrow and the potential for serious toxicity is real. At the same time, anticancer drugs cure many hematologic malignancies and provide palliation for others. The discovery and development of treatments for leukemia and lymphoma have provided a paradigm for approaches to the improved treatment of the more common solid tumors.

The intelligent use of these drugs begins with an understanding of their mechanism of action. Most anticancer drugs inhibit the synthesis of DNA or directly attack its integrity through the formation of DNA adducts or enzyme-mediated breaks. These DNA-directed actions are recognized by repair processes and by the checkpoints that monitor DNA integrity, including most prominently p53. If DNA damage cannot be repaired, and if the DNA damage reaches thresholds for activating programmed cell death, then DNA damage is translated into tumor regression. Attention has turned to the possibility of identifying molecular targets unique to tumor cells, or dramatically overexpressed in those cells, including molecules involved in cell signaling and cell cycle control, but the principles of drug action and resistance to these compounds remain the same. Resistance to drug action can arise from alterations in any one of the critical steps required for drug activity; these steps include drug uptake and distribution through the bloodstream or across the blood–brain barrier; transport across the cell membrane; transformation of the parent drug to its active form within the tumor cell or in the liver; interaction of the drug with its target protein or nucleic acid; enzymatic or chemical inactivation of the agent; drug transport out of the cell; and elimination of the agent from the body through the kidneys or through metabolic transformation. The underlying mutability of tumors leads to the spontaneous generation of cells with alterations in drug uptake, transformation, inactivation, and target binding. In the presence of the selective pressure of a cytotoxic drug, drug-resistant tumors grow out as the dominant tumor population. Combination chemotherapy evades resistance that carries specificity for single agents, but the expression of multidrug resistance (MDR) genes, as well as loss of the apoptotic response, can result in resistance even to combination drug therapy.

In addition to the molecular determinants of drug action, pharmacokinetics (the disposition of drugs in humans) plays a critical role in determining drug effectiveness and toxicity. Drug regimens are designed to achieve a maximally effective concentration in plasma and tumor cells for an effective duration of exposure. Because of the potential of these agents for toxicity, it is critical for oncologists to understand the pathways of drug clearance and to adjust dose in the presence of compromised organ function. Drugs such as methotrexate, hydroxyurea, and the newer purine antagonists (fludarabine and cladribine) are eliminated primarily by renal excretion and should not be used in full doses in patients with renal dysfunction. Similarly, hepatic dysfunction with elevated serum bilirubin concentrations should alert clinicians to decrease doses of the taxanes, vinca alkaloids, and (with less certainty) the anthracyclines. In addition, clinicians must be alert to the potential for drug interactions, particularly the ability of drugs that induce or inhibit cytochrome P450 (CYP) 3A4 and CYP 2B6 to alter the metabolism of taxanes.

A growing body of knowledge indicates inherited genetic variations in drug-metabolizing enzymes may lead to differences in drug toxicity and response. The most important of these familial syndromes affecting treatment of leukemia is the deficiency of thiopurine methyltransferase, which slows the elimination of 6-mercaptopurine and leads to unanticipated toxicity during maintenance chemotherapy for acute lymphocytic leukemia. Pharmacokinetic monitoring has a standard role in the use of certain therapies, particularly high-dose methotrexate, and in the evaluation of new drugs or new drug combinations. Major cancer centers must have the capability of performing pharmacokinetic studies in conjunction with their clinical research programs.

To assure appropriate dose reduction, regimen choice, and management of toxicity, there is no substitute for therapy based on standard protocols and peer-reviewed clinical trials. Adherence to protocols assures that the pharmacologic and pharmacogenetic variables affecting cancer chemotherapy can be recognized early in the course of treatment and that serious untoward events can be avoided while maintaining effective therapy.

Acronyms and abbreviations that appear in this chapter include: ABVD, Adriamycin (doxorubicin), bleomycin, vinblastine, and dacarbazine; ADCC, antibody-dependent cellular cytotoxicity; ADH, antidiuretic hormone; ALL, acute lymphocytic leukemia; AML, acute myelogenous leukemia; APL, acute promyelocytic leukemia; ara-C, cytarabine; ara-CTP, cytarabine triphosphate; ara-G, arabinosylguanine; ara-GTP, arabinosylguanine triphosphate; ara-U, arabinosyluracil; ATRA, all-*trans*-retinoic acid; BCNU, bischloroethylnitrosourea; CDA, chlorodeoxyadenosine; CHOP, cyclophosphamide, Adriamycin (hydroxydaunorubicin), vincristine (Oncovin), prednisone; CLL, chronic lymphocytic leukemia; CML, chronic myelogenous leukemia; CTP, cytosine triphosphate; CYP, cytochrome P450; DCF, deoxycoformycin; dCK, deoxycytidine kinase; dCTP, deoxycytidine triphosphate; DHFR, dihydrofolate reductase; EGFR, epidermal growth factor receptor; FGF, fibroblast growth factor; GIST, gastrointestinal stromal tumor; HAMA, human antimouse antibody; HDAC, histone deacetylase; HIT, heparin-induced thrombocytopenia; HPRT, hypoxanthine-guanine phosphoribosyl transferase; IC_{50}, inhibiting growth by concentration 50 percent; IL, interleukin; MDR, multidrug resistance; MP, mercaptopurine; MRP, multidrug resistance-associated protein; MTD, maximum tolerated dose; NF-κB, nuclear factor-κB; PDGFR, platelet-derived growth factor receptor; RARA, retinoic acid receptor-alpha; TG, thioguanine; 6-TG, 6-thioguanine; TGF, transforming growth factor; VEGF, vascular endothelial growth factor.

HISTORY

The leukemias and lymphomas have been the proving ground for chemotherapy. The first evidence for antitumor activity of a chemical agent came from experiments with nitrogen mustard in a patient with Hodgkin disease in 1942.[1] The even more startling discovery of remission induction by antifolates in acute lymphocytic leukemia 6 years later ushered in the modern era of chemotherapy.[2] Subsequent clinical experiments in these diseases established the basic principles of cyclic combination therapy and dose intensification,[3] developed effective strategies for high-dose therapy with marrow reconstitution,[4] and demonstrated the importance of specific mechanisms of drug resistance. The concept of molecularly targeted therapy achieved its first success with the development of imatinib mesylate for chronic myelogenous leukemia.[5] Other promising molecular targets in leukemic cells have been identified; the FLT3 tyrosine kinase receptor undergoes an activating mutation in approximately 30 percent of cases of acute myelogenous leukemia (AML), and confers a poor prognosis.[6] Drugs designed as inhibitors of this kinase induce apoptosis in cells carrying this mutation, and have entered clinical trial. It is likely that genetic profiles of lymphomas and leukemias will reveal distinct subsets of major classes of cancer, and will identify new targets and pathways for future therapies.

As an alternative to low molecular weight chemicals, antibodies have greater specificity, and may be directed against targets on the cell surface. The first successes of antibody-based therapy, either as antibody alone (rituximab) or antibody linked to toxins (gemtuzumab ozogamicin), were demonstrated in hematologic malignancy, and are described below. These clinical experiments in the hematologic malignancies have led to important new therapies while simultaneously proving the effectiveness of a new approach to therapy of cancer.

BASIC PRINCIPLES OF CANCER CHEMOTHERAPY

The safe and effective use of chemotherapy in clinical practice requires a thorough understanding of the basic aspects of drug action as well as knowledge of the important clinical toxicities, pharmacokinetics, and drug interactions. Antineoplastic chemotherapy is often complex, and there is the potential for serious or fatal side effects. Patients are best served if their treatment is based on evidence from clinical trials. Likewise, the modification of doses and schedules should be based on data, not empirical improvisation. The specific protocol chosen for treatment should be appropriate not only for the stage and histology of the tumor but should consider individual patient tolerance and susceptibility to specific potential toxicities. Thus, bleomycin is usually not an appropriate choice for a patient with serious underlying lung disease, nor is doxorubicin an appropriate drug for use in a patient with a history of congestive heart failure.

Changes in the dose and schedule of a drug may lead to a spectrum of unique toxicities. With the development of techniques for marrow or blood stem cell storage and reinfusion, previously fatal doses of chemotherapy can be administered in an attempt to cure malignancies refractory to standard chemotherapy. In general, these regimens produce a spectrum of organ toxicities not seen at conventional doses—including pulmonary dysfunction, cardiac failure, and hepatic and renal insufficiency—and are ordinarily reserved for patients of younger age and with normal baseline organ function (see Chap. 22).[4]

The greater susceptibility of malignant cells to drug toxicity, as reflected in the phenomenon of leukemia remission induction, cannot be explained at present but may result from the relative insensitivity of normal marrow stem cells to drug injury. These stem cells exist in a nonreplicating phase of the cell cycle, where they are less susceptible to damage by DNA-directed agents. In addition, there is growing evidence that cancer cells lack cell cycle checkpoints that recognize DNA damage and activate repair of DNA strand breaks, base deletions, or other lesions induced by chemotherapy.[7] This differential in repair capability may allow normal cells to escape with less intrinsic damage and favors their recovery from chemotherapy-induced injury.

COMBINATION CHEMOTHERAPY

Most leukemias and lymphomas are highly drug sensitive, but, with the exception of Burkitt lymphoma treated with cyclophosphamide and hairy cell leukemia treated with cladribine, are rarely cured with single-agent chemotherapy. Combination chemotherapy forestalls the emergence of drug-resistant cells and thus is curative in settings where individual agents are ineffective. Empirical principles have resulted from the clinical experience of the past 4 decades of combination therapy. In general, drugs selected for combination therapy should, with few exceptions (such as the rescue agent leucovorin), have demonstrable antineoplastic activity, or at least biologic effects, against the tumor in question. However, a significant body of preclinical and clinical evidence suggests that drugs that inhibit signal transduction, angiogenesis, or other molecular targets may have limited ability to cause tumor regression on their own, but may significantly augment the action of cytotoxics.[8] A basic principle of combination design states that individual agents in a combination should have different mechanisms of action and the agents should not share a common mechanism of resistance such as MDR. The dose-limiting toxicities of the agents chosen should not overlap; otherwise, they could not be used together at or near full doses. The clinical use of specific combinations should be based on preclinical evidence of synergistic interaction. Favorable drug interactions may be dependent on specific sequences and schedules of administration. For these reasons, clinical protocols should attempt to duplicate the most favorable preclinical regimens.

Another important consideration in designing clinical protocols is dose intensity, the dose administered per unit time, which should be maintained throughout a treatment regimen. Achieving this objective may require the use of hematopoietic growth factors to hasten marrow recovery, prevent repeated episodes of febrile neutropenia, and allow on-time administration of the next treatment cycle.

Interdigitation of chemotherapy with surgery and irradiation makes it possible to take advantage of favorable cytokinetic or radiosensitizing effects of chemotherapy, while avoiding enhancement of toxicity. Thus, 5-fluorouracil is used with radiation therapy to enhance local tumor control in malignancies of the head and neck,[9] esophagus,[10] rectum,[11] and anus.[12] Surgical reduction of tumor bulk increases the response rate of ovarian tumors to chemotherapy, perhaps by eliminating poorly perfused tumor masses.[13] In the treatment of lymphomas, the toxicity of radiation therapy to sensitive organs such as skin, lung, heart, and brain may be significantly increased by concurrent administration of anthracyclines, a consideration that has prompted the use of radiation therapy either before or after chemotherapy.

CELL KINETICS AND CANCER CHEMOTHERAPY

The cell-killing characteristics of cancer chemotherapeutic agents vary according to their mechanism of action. Many of the most effective agents in antileukemic therapy belong to the antimetabolite class, including cytosine arabinoside and methotrexate. These drugs kill cells most effectively during the DNA-synthetic phase (S phase) of the cell cycle. They have greatly diminished toxicity for nondividing cells. For these agents, a prolonged period of tumor exposure to drug is essential in order to maximize the number of cells exposed during the vulnerable period of the cell cycle. As would be predicted, the antimetabolite drugs are primarily active against rapidly dividing tumors such as acute leukemias and intermediate and high-grade lymphomas. High-dose regimens achieve a number of worthwhile objectives for these agents, including an enhancement of cross-membrane transport, saturation of anabolic pathways inside the cell, and prolongation of the period of effective drug concentration. However, achieving these objectives is realized at the cost of increased toxicity to normal proliferating marrow precursor cells and may produce significant and unexpected damage to normal organs, such as hepatic venoocclusive disease (alkylating agents), cerebellar toxicity (cytosine arabinoside), or pulmonary toxicity (nitrosoureas and alkylating agents). Because hematopoietic stem cells can be harvested, stored, and reinfused, dose-limiting toxicities of high-dose chemotherapy are generally those affecting nonhematologic organs.

A number of other anticancer drugs do not require cells to be exposed during a specific phase of the cell cycle, although like the antimetabolites, these drugs are generally more effective against actively proliferating cells as compared to resting cells. These agents include the anthracyclines, the epipodophyllotoxins, and certain alkylating agents such as cyclophosphamide. Still others, most notably the nitrosoureas and busulfan, are equally toxic to dividing and nondividing cells, and at the same time, deplete marrow stem cells. In general, the toxicity of alkylating agents is determined by the total dose of drug, while for the cell cycle-specific drugs (such as methotrexate and cytosine arabinoside), both drug concentration and duration of exposure determine cytocidal effect. However, for drugs that act through alternate mechanisms, such as the taxanes, myelosuppression correlates best with the duration of exposure above a threshold plasma concentration, which is approximately 50 to 100 nM for paclitaxel and 200 nM for docetaxel.[14]

The choice of an appropriate dose and schedule of drug administration depends on a number of factors: (1) the drug's cell cycle dependence; (2) the often empirically derived relationship between toxicity to marrow and other organs, and the drug dose and schedule; (3) pharmacokinetic behavior and the need to maintain a specific drug concentration for a given period of time; (4) potential interactions with other drugs; and (5) patient tolerance. The last factor will vary among individuals and will depend on physiologic parameters such as renal and hepatic functions (Table 19-1), which determine the patient's ability to eliminate drug. Tolerance may also depend on the patient's prior treatment experience, performance status, and age. Protocols for cancer chemotherapy must contain provisions for adjusting dose to accommodate these variables and should be followed diligently.

DRUG RESISTANCE

Inadequate treatment of a sensitive tumor tends to select for the outgrowth of drug-resistant clones of the original tumor. It has been proposed that the basis for drug resistance is the spontaneous generation of resistant mutants, with subsequent selection of the drug-resistant mutant under the pressure of chemotherapeutic drugs. The first formal proof of the clonal selection hypothesis has come from clinical observations in patients treated with imatinib mesylate, who often exhibit a small population of drug-resistant cells prior to treatment (see below). In addition, cancer drugs and irradiation are themselves intrinsically mutagenic and increase the rate of generation of drug-resistant mutants. To discourage the outgrowth of resistant cells, multiple agents with differing mechanisms of resistance should be used simultaneously, because the likelihood of there being a doubly or triply resistant cell is the product of the probabilities of the independent drug-resistant mutations occurring at the same time in a single cell. The probability of a cell division resulting in mutation at any given genetic locus is approximately 10^{-6} for somatic cells; thus the probability of multiple independent mutations arising in the same cell is 10^{-12} or lower. Mutation rates may be distinctly higher in tumor cells and may be further increased by exposure to alkylating agents and irradiation. Some mutations, such as those affecting apoptosis, may confer resistance to diverse agents. Thus, the probability of encountering multiply drug-resistant cells is much higher in reality.

In choosing drugs for combination therapy, one must bear in mind potential mechanisms of resistance. Classical MDR as a consequence,

TABLE 19-1 DOSE MODIFICATION IN PATIENTS WITH RENAL OR HEPATIC DYSFUNCTION

Renal dysfunction (creatinine clearance <60 ml/min)
- Reduce dose in proportion to reduction in creatinine clearance.

Drugs

1.	Methotrexate	6.	Hydroxyurea
2.	Cisplatin	7.	Deoxycoformycin
3.	Carboplatin	8.	Fludarabine phosphate
4.	Bleomycin	9.	Cladribine
5.	Etoposide	10.	Topotecan

Hepatic dysfunction
- For bilirubin >1.5 mg/dl reduce initial dose by 50%.
- For bilirubin >3.0 mg/dl reduce initial dose by 75%.

Drugs

1.	Amsacrine	5.	Vinblastine
2.	Doxorubicin	6.	Paclitaxel and docetaxel
3.	Daunorubicin	7.	Mitoxantrone
4.	Vincristine		

of increased expression of drug efflux pumps such as the P-glycoprotein or the multidrug resistance-associated proteins (MRPs)[15,16] confers resistance to a broad spectrum of agents derived from natural products, including taxanes, anthracyclines, vinca alkaloids, and epipodophyllotoxins. Other mechanisms, such as amplification of a target gene such as dihydrofolate reductase[17] or *BCR-ABL* kinase,[18] are highly specific for a single drug. Table 19-2 lists the common mechanisms of resistance. While none of these biochemical changes are routinely measured either prior to or following therapy, these mechanisms should be considered in developing new protocols and in choosing new therapy for patients who relapse from primary treatment.

In addition to drug-specific mechanisms of resistance, mutations that abolish recognition of DNA damage, such as those affecting the mismatch repair gene complex,[19] seem to block initiation of apoptosis by cisplatin, thiopurine, or alkylating agents. Other mutations that block the induction of apoptosis, such as loss of p53[20] or overexpression of the antiapoptotic factors such as BCL-2,[21] may render tumor cells insensitive to a broad array of drugs and modalities, including ionizing irradiation, alkylating agents, antimetabolites, and anthracyclines. Although the specific contribution of these factors to clinical resistance is still uncertain, emerging evidence suggests that mutations involving genes that control cell cycle and apoptosis, such as loss of p53 function, are strongly associated with clinically resistant and aggressive tumors and may be more relevant causes of drug resistance in the clinic than are the classical drug-specific mechanisms found in experimental tumors.

CELL CYCLE-ACTIVE AGENTS

METHOTREXATE

Farber and associates showed that the folate antagonist aminopterin induced a complete remission in children with acute lymphoblastic leukemia (ALL), thereby launching the modern era of chemotherapy. Unfortunately, these remissions were short-lived, and the leukemia invariably became resistant within months to further treatment. Subsequently, methotrexate, a 4-amino, N-10 methyl analogue of folic acid, supplanted aminopterin because it had a better therapeutic index. Methotrexate continues to be a key drug in maintenance therapy of ALL, in the intrathecal prophylaxis and treatment of central nervous system (CNS) leukemia, and in combination therapy of intermediate- and high-grade lymphomas.

MECHANISMS OF ACTION

Methotrexate enters cells through an active uptake process mediated in most tumor cells by the reduced folate transporter[22,23] and is actively

TABLE 19-2 MECHANISMS OF RESISTANCE TO ANTICANCER DRUGS

MECHANISMS	DRUGS AFFECTED	CLINICAL ROLE
1. Decreased drug uptake		
Reduced folate transporter	Methotrexate	ALL
Nucleoside transporter	Cytosine arabinoside	AML
2. Increased drug efflux		
MDR transporter (P-glycoprotein)	Anthracyclines, vinca alkaloids, taxanes, etoposide	Myeloma, AML, non-Hodgkin lymphoma
MRP transporter	Anthracyclines, vinca alkaloids, taxanes, etoposide	Uncertain
3. Decreased drug activation in tumor		
Deoxycytidine kinase deletion	Cytarabine (likely fludarabine and cladribine as well)	AML
Hypoxanthine phosphoribosyl transferase deletion	6-Mercaptopurine	Uncertain
Folylpolyglutamation	Methotrexate	Acute leukemias
4. Increased drug inactivation		
Thiopurine methyl transferase	6-Mercaptopurine	ALL
Bleomycin hydrolase	Bleomycin	Uncertain
Glutathione transferase	Alkylating agents	Uncertain
5. Decreased target enzyme		
Topoisomerase I	Camptothecins	Uncertain
Topoisomerase II	Anthracyclines, etoposide	Uncertain
6. Increased target enzyme		
Dihydrofolate reductase	Methotrexate	Acute leukemia, small cell lung cancer
Thymidylate synthase	5-Fluorouracil	Solid tumors
Adenosine deaminase	Deoxycoformycin	Uncertain
7. Altered intracellular target		
BCR-ABL kinase	Imatinib mesylate	CML
Tubulin	Vinca alkaloids, taxanes	Uncertain
Topoisomerase I	Camptothecins	Uncertain
Topoisomerase II	Anthracyclines, etoposide	Uncertain
8. Increase DNA repair		
Guanine-0–6-methyl transferase	Procarbazine, nitrosoureas temozolomide	Brain tumors
Nucleotide excision repair	Platinating drugs	Ovarian cancer
9. Decreased DNA damage recognition		
p53 mutation	Many cancer drugs, radiation	Leukemias, lymphomas
Mismatch DNA repair mutations	Platinating agents, thiopurines	Colon cancer

ALL, acute lymphocytic leukemia; AML, acute myelogenous leukemia; CML, chronic myelogenous leukemia. See text for references and explanation.

effluxed from cells by the MRP class of exporters.[23] A second uptake transporter, the membrane folate-binding protein, has lower affinity for methotrexate, but may contribute to uptake of other antifolates. By virtue of its 4-amino substitution, methotrexate potently inhibits the enzyme dihydrofolate reductase (DHFR), which recycles oxidized dihydrofolate to its active tetrahydrofolate state. Inhibition of DHFR leads to rapid depletion of the intracellular tetrahydrofolate coenzymes required for thymidylate and purine biosynthesis. As a result, DNA synthesis is blocked and cell replication stops. Methotrexate is retained in tumor cells for many hours as a consequence of an enzymatic process that adds up to six glutamate moieties to the γ-carboxyl group of the drug (see Chap. 39). Polyglutamation is an important determinant of methotrexate selectivity. Methotrexate polyglutamates, in addition to their long persistence in cells and their potent inhibition of DHFR, have greatly increased inhibitory effects on other folate-dependent enzymes, including thymidylate synthase and enzymes that synthesize purines. Cells that convert the drug to polyglutamates efficiently, such as leukemic myeloblasts and lymphoblasts, are more susceptible to the drug than are normal myeloid precursors, which have limited capability for polyglutamation.[24] Accumulation of polyglutamates correlates with increased cytotoxicity and treatment response in childhood lymphoblastic leukemia.[25] Hyperdiploid ALLs are particularly efficient in transporting methotrexate and in producing polyglutamated species—factors that may contribute to their good prognosis.[26] Other steps in methotrexate action may enhance drug sensitivity. Acquired resistance

to methotrexate in patients with leukemia is associated with increased levels of dihydrofolate reductase as a consequence of gene amplification,[17] defective polyglutamation,[27] and impaired drug uptake, or increased efflux by the MRP class of transporters.[28]

CLINICAL PHARMACOLOGY

Methotrexate is well absorbed when administered orally at low doses ($5-10$ mg/m^2), but when doses exceed 30 mg/m^2, absorption is variable. Consequently, doses greater than 25 mg/m^2 should be administered parenterally.

The concentration of methotrexate in plasma declines in a polyexponential manner. A very rapid initial disposition phase persists for only a few minutes after intravenous administration. The intermediate disposition phase has a 2- to 3-hour half-life and persists for 12 to 24 hours after dosing. The terminal phase of drug decay is considerably slower, with an 8- to 10-hour half-life. Methotrexate is primarily excreted unchanged by the kidney, although with large doses a minor fraction of the drug ($7-30\%$) is inactivated by hepatic hydroxylation at the 7 position. Thus, patients with renal impairment should not be treated with methotrexate, because the prolonged exposure to high blood levels may result in life-threatening hematologic and gastrointestinal toxicity.[29] High-dose methotrexate (>0.5 g/m^2) together with leucovorin rescue is used to treat patients with high-grade lymphoma, osteosarcoma, and ALL.[29] Dose adjustment of methotrexate to maintain a target area under the concentration $\times$ time ($C \times T$) curve improves treatment outcome.[30] In patients receiving high-dose methotrexate, urine should be maintained at an alkaline pH, because methotrexate is a weak acid and has limited solubility below pH 6. Leucovorin is administered in doses of 10 to 15 mg/m^2 at 6-hour intervals, starting 6 to 24 hours after the injection of methotrexate, and continuing until plasma concentrations of the drug fall below 1 μM. In patients receiving high-dose methotrexate, drug levels are routinely assayed 24 to 48 hours after dosing to determine the rate of drug elimination and the safety of discontinuing leucovorin. Both methotrexate and its hydroxylated metabolite are organic acids, which, like uric acid, are much more soluble in alkaline urine. In patients receiving such therapy, renal toxicity may result from intrarenal precipitation of the parent drug or its 7-OH metabolite, and is generally the cause of decreased drug clearance. Renal dysfunction can be prevented by alkalinizing the urine to pH 7.0 with intravenous sodium bicarbonate prior to and during therapy, and patients should be given intensive hydration. If drug concentrations in plasma at 48 hours after high-dose therapy exceed 1 μM, leucovorin should be continued at doses of 50 to 100 mg/m^2 every 6 hours until methotrexate concentrations fall below 0.1 μM. In cases of extreme renal failure, with stable drug levels in the 10 μM range, leucovorin will not be effective. In this setting, continuous flow hemodialysis may provide a sustained reduction in drug levels.[31] An alternative effective measure in this circumstance is the administration of carboxypeptidase G, a bacterial enzyme that degrades antifolates.[32] The enzyme can be obtained from the Cancer Therapy Evaluation Program of the National Cancer Institute (301-496-6138) and may be lifesaving.

ADVERSE EFFECTS

The dose-limiting toxicities of methotrexate are myelosuppression and gastrointestinal toxicity. Toxic doses of methotrexate can induce thrombocytopenia and/or leukopenia, although leukopenia is more common. An early indication of methotrexate toxicity to the gastrointestinal tract is oral mucositis, while more severe toxicity may be manifested as diarrhea and gastrointestinal bleeding. Less common toxic effects of methotrexate are skin rash (10%), pneumonitis, and chemical hepatitis. The latter is reversible in most patients, and without sequelae, but low-dose chronic administration may lead to fibrosis and cirrhosis of the liver in a small percentage of patients.

Methotrexate given intrathecally in doses of 12 mg every 4 days for children older than age 3 years and for adults is used to prevent or treat meningeal leukemia and lymphoma. Dose adjustment is required for children younger than age 3 years, and should be made according to established protocols. Because the drug distributes poorly into the ventricular system after spinal injection, patients with active meningeal leukemia are frequently treated through an indwelling ventricular reservoir. Toxicities caused by this route of administration include acute arachnoiditis with nuchal rigidity and headache, as well as more chronic CNS toxicities, such as dementia, motor deficits, seizures, and coma.[33] Rarely, these neurotoxicities develop hours after intrathecal drug administration, but more commonly they occur in the days or weeks after initiation of intrathecal treatment, and are more often seen in patients with active meningeal leukemia. Leucovorin is ineffective in reversing or preventing these toxicities. Patients exhibiting such signs should undergo evaluation to rule out progressive central nervous system leukemia or lymphoma, and if neither of these is present intrathecal cytosine arabinoside should be given instead of methotrexate.

Methotrexate is synergistic with inhibitors of purine biosynthesis, such as 6-mercaptopurine. L-Asparaginase, an inhibitor of protein synthesis, blocks cells from entering DNA synthesis and antagonizes the effects of methotrexate, when used before the antifolate. The two drugs are not used concurrently.

Nonsteroidal antiinflammatory drugs, which diminish renal blood flow, may reduce methotrexate clearance, as may nephrotoxic antibiotics and platinum derivatives, and should not be administered to patients during high-dose methotrexate therapy.

CYTARABINE (CYTOSINE ARABINOSIDE, ARABINOSYL CYTOSINE, ARA-C)

Cytarabine is an antimetabolite analogue of cytidine, differing in the configuration at the substituent on C_2' position of the sugar, with the C_2'-hydroxyl group being cis-oriented relative to the C_1'-N-glycosyl bond, in contrast to the trans configuration of the ribose nucleoside. Cytarabine is a mainstay in the induction of remission in patients with AML. When used with an anthracycline, remissions may be achieved in 60 to 80 percent of patients with this disease.

High doses (1–3 g/m^2) of cytarabine given at 12-hour intervals for 6 to 12 doses are more effective alone or in a combination with anthracyclines than conventional doses (100–150 mg/m^2 q 12 h) in consolidation therapy of AML, and they confer particular benefit in patients with cytogenetic abnormalities [t(8:21), inv[16], t(9:16), and del(16)] related to the core binding factor that regulates hematopoiesis.[34] Cytarabine has also been used to treat ALL, lymphoma, and both the chronic and the blast phases of chronic myelogenous leukemia (CML), but its exact role in the treatment of these malignancies is less well defined. In ALL, with rearrangement of the MLL gene (llq23), high sensitivity to cytarabine correlates with increased expression of the nucleoside transporter, hENTI.[35]

MECHANISM OF ACTION

Cytarabine is converted to the nucleoside triphosphate (ara-CTP) intracellularly. Ara-CTP is an inhibitor of DNA polymerase and is also incorporated into DNA, where it terminates strand elongation.[36] Cytarabine and its mononucleotide are deaminated and inactivated by two intracellular enzymes, cytidine deaminase and deoxycytidylate deaminase, respectively. The arabinosyluracil (ara-U) formed as a consequence of cytarabine deamination is more slowly cleared from plasma than is cytarabine and may inhibit subsequent inactivation of cytarabine in high-dose regimens.

Acquired cytarabine resistance in experimental leukemias consistently results from the loss of deoxycytidine kinase, the initial activating enzyme in the cytarabine pathway.[37] Other changes implicated in experimental tumors include decreased drug uptake because of decreased expression of the equilibrative nucleoside transporter, increased deamination, increased pool size of competitive deoxycytidine triphosphate, and inhibition of the apoptotic pathway. Some of these changes have been reported in studies of human leukemia, but these results have not been confirmed in definitive trials.[38]

CLINICAL PHARMACOLOGY

Cytarabine is administered intravenously either as a bolus injection or a continuous infusion. It is not orally bioavailable because of its degradation by cytidine deaminase, which is present in the gastrointestinal epithelium and liver. Cytarabine distributes rapidly throughout total-body water and is eliminated from plasma with a biologic half-life of 7 to 20 minutes. Most of the dose is excreted as ara-U, an inactive metabolite, which is formed in plasma, the liver, granulocytes, and other tissues. Inhibition of cytarabine deamination by ara-U may be responsible for the prolongation of the biologic half-life of the drug as larger doses are administered.[39] Single-bolus injections and short infusions (30-minute to 1-hour duration) at doses as high as 5 g/m^2 produce little myelotoxicity because of the drug's rapid clearance, whereas continuous intravenous infusion of only 1 g/m^2 over 48 hours produces severe marrow toxicity. Unlike most drugs, a relatively high concentration of cytarabine is achieved in the cerebrospinal fluid after intravenous administration, which may approach 50 percent of the corresponding concentration in plasma.

Cytarabine is also used intrathecally to treat meningeal leukemia. Doses of 50 to 70 mg in adults are usually employed and afford cerebrospinal fluid levels of the drug near 1.0 mM, which decline with a half-life of 2 hours. Cytarabine (50 mg, given every 2 weeks) has been impregnated into a gel matrix, in a formulation called DepoCyt, for sustained release into the cerebrospinal fluid, thus avoiding the need for repeated spinal taps. Initial clinical results in spinal lymphomatous meningitis indicate that it has efficacy equal to that of methotrexate.[40,41]

ADVERSE EFFECTS

The dose-limiting toxicity for conventional dosing regimens of cytarabine, 100 to 150 mg/m² per day for 5 to 10 days, is myelosuppression. Some nausea and vomiting also occur at these doses, the severity of which increases markedly when higher doses are employed, although repeated administration of the drug results in some tolerance. The nadir of the white count and platelet count occurs at about days 7 to 10 after the last dose of drug. Neurologic, gastrointestinal, and liver toxicity have also been observed when high-dose regimens are used. Hepatotoxicity ranges from abnormalities in serum transaminase levels to frank jaundice. The severity of these effects increases as the duration of therapy is prolonged; however, toxic effects rapidly subside upon discontinuation of treatment. Pulmonary infiltrates due to noncardiogenic pulmonary edema are frequently observed in leukemic patients receiving cytarabine, as are gastrointestinal ulcerations with bleeding and infrequently perforation. Cytarabine treatment is also reported to predispose to *Streptococcus viridans* pneumonia.[42]

In patients older than 60 years of age, high-dose cytarabine (3 g/m² q 12 h for 6 doses) causes cerebellar toxicity, manifested as ataxia and slurred speech.[43] Confusion and dementia may supervene, leading to a fatal outcome. Cerebellar toxicity is more frequent in patients with abnormal renal function because of slowed elimination of ara-U, with consequent inhibition of cytarabine deamination. Intrathecal cytarabine is usually well tolerated, but neurologic side effects have been reported (seizures, alterations in mental status).

GEMCITABINE

Although primarily used for solid tumors, gemcitabine, a 2′-2′-difluoro analogue of deoxycytidine, has significant activity against Hodgkin disease. Its mechanism of action is very similar to *cytarabine*, in that, as a nucleotide, it competes with deoxycytidine triphosphate (dCTP) for incorporation into the elongating DNA strand, where it terminates DNA synthesis. It is also self-potentiating in that at a second site of action, it reduces competitive pools of dCTP through inhibition of ribonucleotide reductase. It achieves higher nucleotide levels in tumor cells than does ara-CTP, and has a longer intracellular half-life. Its clinical pharmacokinetics are determined primarily by its rapid deamination by cytidine deaminase, yielding a short plasma $t_{1/2}$ of less than 1 hour.

Toxicities are mainly acute myelosuppression, mild hepatic enzyme elevations, uncommonly a reversible pneumonitis, and with prolonged usage, a progressive hemolytic uremic syndrome with capillary leak, leading to pleural effusions, ascites, and renal failure.[44]

5-AZACYTIDINE

Both 5-azacytidine and decitabine (5-aza-2′-deoxycytidine), its closely related deoxy analogue, exhibit cytotoxic activity and also induce differentiation of malignant cells at low doses. The latter action is believed to result from an inhibition of methylation of cytosine bases in DNA, leading to enhanced transcription of otherwise silent genes.[45]

The differentiating effects of 5-azacytidine are the basis for its experimental use in the induction of fetal hemoglobin synthesis in patients with sickle cell anemia and thalassemia[46] and in low-dose therapy of myelodysplastic syndromes. The usual doses of 5-azacytidine are 150 to 200 mg/m² per day for 5 days. Lower doses are used in treating myelodysplasia.

5-Azacytidine and decitabine are rapidly deaminated and converted to a chemically unstable metabolite that immediately degrades into inactive products. Pharmacologic activity results from phosphorylation of the parent compound by cytidine kinase or deoxycytidine kinase, with subsequent conversion to a triphosphate nucleotide that becomes incorporated into RNA and DNA. The precise mechanism of cytotoxicity has not been defined. The primary clinical toxicities of both 5-azacytidine and decitabine[47] include reversible myelosuppression, rather severe nausea and vomiting, hepatic dysfunction, myalgias, and fever and rash.

PURINE ANALOGUES

Purine analogues have won an important role in remission induction and maintenance for ALL, and in the past decade new analogues have shown remarkable activity in chronic leukemias and small cell lymphomas. With methotrexate, 6-mercaptopurine (6-MP) is a critical component in the maintenance phase of curative therapy of childhood ALL. Other clinically useful purine analogues include azathioprine, a 6-MP precursor and potent immunosuppressive agent; allopurinol, an inhibitor of xanthine oxidase, useful in the prevention of uric acid nephropathy; 2-chlorodeoxyadenosine, effective in the treatment of hairy cell leukemia and other lymphoid malignancies; 6-thioguanine (6-TG), an antileukemic agent; and fludarabine phosphate (2-fluoro-ara-adenosine monophosphate), an effective agent for chronic lymphocytic leukemia and follicular lymphomas, and for suppression of graft-versus-host disease in transplantation. A new purine analogue, nelarabine, is an a ara-guanine prodrug, with strong activity against T cell diseases, including lymphoblastic leukemias and lymphomas.[48] The basis for this T cell sensitivity appears to be the resistance of arabinosylguanine (ara-G) to degradation by the catabolic enzyme, purine nucleoside phosphorylase. High levels of arabinosylguanine triphosphate (ara-GTP) accumulate in T cell neoplasms, leading to Fasligand-mediated apoptosis. Deoxycoformycin, a potent inhibitor of adenosine deaminase, is also effective in the treatment of T cell malignancies and hairy cell leukemia.

MECHANISM OF ACTION OF 6-THIOPURINES

Both 6-MP and 6-TG have a thiol group substituted for the 6-oxo or 6-hydroxy group of hypoxanthine or guanine, respectively. Both compounds are converted to nucleotides by the enzyme hypoxanthine-guanine phosphoribosyl transferase (HPRT). The exact mechanism whereby these analogues exert their cytotoxic effects is unknown.[49] De novo purine synthesis is blocked by the 6-TG nucleotide, as is the conversion of inosine monophosphate to adenosine and guanosine monophosphates.[50] The nucleotides of both 6-MP and 6-TG are incorporated into DNA. Thiopurines incorporated into DNA are recognized by the mismatch repair system, triggering apoptosis. Cell death correlates with the extent of their incorporation into DNA.

In experimental tumor cells, resistance is most commonly caused by decreased activity of HPRT, but it is poorly understood in humans. Patients differ in their rates of metabolic clearance of 6-MP. Rapid clearance of the drug, as mediated by methylation of the thiol group by 5-thiopurine-methyl transferase,[50,51] is associated with a high leukemia recurrence rate in ALL maintenance therapy. Low levels of red blood cell thiopurine nucleotides correlate with a high risk of clinical relapse in patients with ALL,[52] while decreased activity of thiopurine methyl transferase, because of an inherited polymorphism, is associated with increased drug toxicity (see "Clinical Pharmacology of 6-Thiopurines" below).

Methotrexate and 6-MP are highly synergistic, possibly because methotrexate blocks the de novo synthesis of purines and enhances the use of preformed purines and purine analogues such as 6-MP.

CLINICAL PHARMACOLOGY OF 6-THIOPURINES

Both 6-TG and 6-MP are given orally at doses of 50 to 100 mg/m² per day. Oral absorption of 6-MP is erratic, as only 16 to 50 percent of an oral dose is systemically available.[53] Food and antibiotics may decrease absorption. Both 6-MP and 6-TG are inactivated by metabolism, and have half-lives of approximately 1 hour in plasma. During 6-TG treatment, 6-thioguanine nucleotides accumulate to much higher levels in leukemic cells, as compared to 6-MP treatment, but 6-thiomethyl nucleotides are almost thirtyfold higher after 6-MP, and do have reduced, but significant inhibitory activity.[54] 6-MP is inactivated by metabolism to 6-thiouric acid, a reaction catalyzed by xanthine oxidase. Allopurinol inhibits the metabolic inactivation of 6-MP, but not of 6-TG. Therefore, it is generally recommended that dosages of orally administered 6-MP must be reduced by 75 percent in patients receiving allopurinol. 6-TG is inactivated primarily by S-methylation, followed by oxidation and desulfuration. Dose reduction is not necessary when 6-TG and allopurinol are administered together.

ADVERSE EFFECTS OF 6-THIOPURINES

Both 6-TG and 6-MP are myelotoxic, producing nadirs of white blood cells and platelets at 7 to 10 days after treatment, although 6-TG appears to cause greater myelosuppression, especially thrombocytopenia, in maintenance therapy of childhood ALL.[55] Moderate nausea and vomiting may also be observed. Patients may experience mild but rapidly reversible hepatotoxicity after treatment with either compound. Cirrhosis has occurred in some children with leukemia who are receiving long-term therapy with 6-MP. Thiopurine methyl transferase, which inactivates 6-thiopurines, occurs in several polymorphic forms that fail to metabolize the analogues. Approximately 1 person in 10 of the white population is heterozygous for ineffective polymorphic forms of the enzyme and has increased sensitivity to thiopurines, whereas 1 patient in 300 is homozygous for the inactive forms and at risk for overwhelming toxicity.

FLUDARABINE PHOSPHATE

Originally synthesized as a deamination-resistant analogue of adenosine, fludarabine phosphate has outstanding activity in chronic lymphocytic leukemia (CLL).[56] It is strongly immunosuppressive, like the other purine analogues, and is frequently used in nonmyeloablative allogeneic bone marrow transplantation[57] and in the treatment of collagen vascular diseases.

The pharmacology of fludarabine phosphate requires removal of the phosphate group in plasma to allow cellular uptake by nucleoside transporters, and then intracellular rephosphorylation. Fludarabine is activated to the monophosphate level by deoxycytidine kinase. The triphosphate inhibits DNA polymerase and becomes incorporated into both DNA and RNA.[58] Its mechanism of cytotoxicity is believed to result from DNA chain termination and induction of apoptosis, although it also inhibits ribonucleotide reductase and becomes incorporated into RNA.[59] Its triphosphate has a long intracellular half-life of 15 hours in CLL cells.

The drug is available in the United States as an intravenous preparation, although in Europe it is approved for oral use. It has 60 to 80 percent bioavailability. Because it is resistant to adenosine deaminase, fludarabine is eliminated primarily by renal excretion

(60%), with a terminal $t_{1/2}$ of 10 hours. For patients treated with a standard dose of 25 mg/m² for 5 days, the time to treatment-limiting toxicity is a function of creatinine clearance.[60] In patients with renal impairment, a 20 percent dose reduction for a creatinine clearance of 17 to 40 ml/min/m², and a 40 percent dose reduction for a creatinine clearance less than 17 ml/min/m² yields an area under the curve (AUC) approximately equal to that seen in patients with normal renal function receiving full doses of fludarabine.[61]

In CLL, the recommended doses are 25 mg/m² per day for 5 days given as 2-hour infusions and repeated every 4 weeks. When administered at these doses, fludarabine causes only moderate myelosuppression. In CLL patients, its antileukemic effect will lead to a progressive, but relatively slow, improvement in marrow function over a period of two to three cycles of treatment, with a median time to disease progression of 31 months. However, the drug also exerts cytotoxic effects against both B and T lymphocytes, lowering CD4 T cell counts to 150 to 200 cells/μl and predisposing patients to opportunistic infection. In patients with a large tumor burden, rapid tumor lysis may rarely lead to hyperuricemia, renal failure, and hypocalcemia (tumor lysis syndrome).[62] Thus, patients should be well hydrated and their urine alkalinized prior to beginning therapy. The primary toxicity is acute and reversible myelosuppression. Peripheral sensory and motor neuropathy may occur during standard-dose therapy; rare episodes of hemolytic anemia with both warm and cold antibodies have been reported.[63] Approximately 10 percent of CLL patients receiving fludarabine may develop a hypersensitivity syndrome of pulmonary infiltrates, hypoxemia, and fever, responsive to corticosteroids.[64] At higher doses (125 mg/m² per day for 5 days) altered mental status, seizures, coma, and optic neuritis have been reported.

CLADRIBINE (2-CHLORODEOXYADENOSINE, 2-CDA)

The extreme sensitivity of normal and malignant lymphocytes to deamination-resistant purine analogues is further exemplified by the potent activity of cladribine in hairy cell leukemia, CLL, and low-grade lymphomas.[65,66] A single course of cladribine, typically 0.09 mg/kg per day for 7 days by continuous intravenous infusion, induces complete response in 80 percent of patients with hairy cell leukemia, and partial responses in the remainder. Administration by subcutaneous injection or by 2-hour intravenous infusions for 5 days to the same total dose achieves similar results. The drug has much the same intracellular fate as fludarabine, undergoing phosphorylation by deoxycytidine kinase (dCK) and further conversion to a triphosphate that becomes incorporated into DNA. The triphosphate of cladribine has a very long intracellular half-life of 9.7 hours in CLL cells isolated from patients treated with the drug.[67] The triphosphate also accumulates in mitochondria, disrupting oxidative phosphorylation, and inhibits ribonucleotide reductase and depletes nicotinamide adenine dinucleotide (NAD) levels in tumor cells. All of these actions might help explain the drug's toxicity to slowly dividing lymphoid malignancies such as hairy cell leukemia and CLL. The actual mechanisms by which cladribine induces DNA strand breaks are not completely understood. However, similar to fludarabine, it inhibits DNA chain extension and daughter strand synthesis.[68] Furthermore, the drug inhibits ribonucleotide reductase, thus lowering levels of the competitive nucleotide dCTP. The cumulative effects of cladribine induce apoptosis (programmed cell death).

Cladribine is eliminated primarily (>50%) by renal excretion, with a terminal plasma half-life of 20 hours. In a patient with renal failure, continuous flow hemodialysis effectively cleared the drug and prevented serious myelosuppression.[69] Cladribine retains effectiveness in at least a fraction of hairy cell leukemia patients resistant to deoxycoformycin or fludarabine, although clinical experience with sequential use of these drugs is limited. Toxicities of cladribine include transient myelosuppression, fever, and occasional opportunistic infections possibly related to immunosuppression. The development of cumulative thrombocytopenia during treatment with repeated courses of the drug may limit its use. Resistance develops in experimental tumors through loss of the activating enzyme dCK, by increased ribonucleotide reductase activity, or by induction of 5'-nucleotidase activity.[70]

PENTOSTATIN (2-DEOXYCOFORMYCIN)

Pentostatin contains a unique seven-carbon primary ring system that closely resembles the transition-state intermediate of the adenosine deaminase reaction. As such, pentostatin is a potent inhibitor of the enzyme, leading to accumulation of intracellular adenosine and deoxyadenosine nucleotides. In addition, the triphosphate of pentostatin is incorporated into DNA. The imbalance in purine nucleotide pools produced by pentostatin probably accounts for its cytotoxicity.

Although initial trials of pentostatin demonstrated striking renal and neurologic toxicities at doses of 10 mg/m^2 per day or greater, lower doses (4 mg/m^2 biweekly) are extremely effective in inducing pathologically confirmed complete responses in hairy cell leukemia. At this lower dose, severe depletion of normal T cells occurs and may predispose to opportunistic infection.[71] The optimal dose may be lower than 4 mg/m^2 biweekly. The drug is eliminated entirely by renal excretion, necessitating proportional dose reduction in patients with reduced creatinine clearance.

HYDROXYUREA

Hydroxyurea inhibits ribonucleotide reductase, the enzyme that converts ribonucleotide diphosphates to deoxyribonucleotides. Hydroxyurea is most commonly used in the treatment of polycythemia vera, essential thrombocythemia, and the chronic phase of CML and to lower the leukocyte count rapidly during blast crisis of CML. Resistance to hydroxyurea occurs in experimental tumors as a consequence of an increase in ribonucleotide reductase activity, or through mutations that produce an enzyme that binds the drug with decreased affinity.

CLINICAL PHARMACOLOGY

Hydroxyurea is usually administered orally and is well absorbed, even when large doses such as 50 to 75 mg/kg are given. Peak plasma levels following oral administration are achieved at about 1 hour and decline rapidly thereafter. Renal excretion is the major route of drug elimination.

ADVERSE EFFECTS

The major toxicities of hydroxyurea are leukopenia and the induction of megaloblastic changes. Except for nausea, drug fever, and maculopapular skin rash, little other toxicity has been observed with this drug, even when large doses are administered. Hydroxyurea, like cytosine arabinoside, is an S phase-specific agent. Accordingly, single large doses affect little toxicity other than myelosuppression. The nadir of the leukocyte count occurs 6 to 7 days after a single dose of drug, and the leukocyte count recovers rapidly. When hydroxyurea is used as therapy for essential thrombocythemia, there may be an increase in the incidence of acute myelogenous leukemia.[72] The agent is also used in nonmalignant disorders, notably sickle cell anemia (see Chap. 47).

ANTITUBULINS

THE VINCA ALKALOIDS

Among the three vinca alkaloids that have been extensively evaluated during the past 3 decades, vinblastine, vincristine, and vinorelbine (Navelbine), only the first two are used widely in the treatment of hema-

tologic neoplasms: vinblastine because of its excellent activity in the treatment of Hodgkin disease, and vincristine in lymphomas and childhood leukemia. Vinorelbine is used primarily for the treatment of breast and lung cancers.

MECHANISM OF ACTION

The vinca alkaloids exert their cytotoxic action by binding to tubulin, a protein found in the cytoplasm of cells. Microtubules, assembled through polymerization of tubulin dimers, form the spindle along which the chromosomes migrate during mitosis and maintain cell structure. Binding of the vinca alkaloids to tubulin leads to inhibition of the process of assembly of the mitotic spindle,[73] arresting cells in metaphase and inducing apoptosis. Resistance to the vinca alkaloids may be acquired through the expression of multidrug resistance, which causes increased efflux of the drugs from the resistant cells. Alternatively, resistant cells may contain mutant tubulin with decreased avidity of vinca binding.[74] The clinical significance of these resistance mechanisms, however, is still unproven.

CLINICAL PHARMACOLOGY

Vincristine and vinblastine are both administered by the intravenous route. The average single dose of vincristine is 1.4 mg/m^2 and that of vinblastine 8 to 9 mg/m^2. Sequential doses of the drugs are usually given at 2- to 4-week intervals. These doses provide peak plasma drug concentrations of approximately 1 μM. The plasma concentration-time profile of vincristine is characterized by a very rapid initial disposition phase followed by two slower phases of decay, with half-lives of 3 hours and 23 to 85 hours. In comparison, the intermediate and terminal disposition phases of vinblastine have half-lives of 1 hour and 20 hours, respectively. Almost 70 percent of a dose of vincristine is metabolized by the liver and excreted in the feces. Metabolism is also the major route of inactivation of vinblastine, but details are lacking with respect to the site of metabolism and the identity of metabolic products. Accordingly, the dose of vincristine or vinblastine should be reduced in patients with hepatic impairment. While specific guidelines for dose reduction have not been completely developed, a 50 percent decrease in dose is recommended for patients presenting with a bilirubin count of 1.5 to 3 mg/dl and a 75% reduction for levels greater than 3 mg/dl. Dose reduction is not necessary for patients with impaired renal function, as very little intact drug is excreted in urine.

ADVERSE EFFECTS

The dose-limiting side effect of vincristine is neurotoxicity, which usually occurs when the total dose received exceeds 6 mg/m^2. The initial signs of neurotoxicity are paresthesia of the fingers and lower extremities and loss of deep tendon reflexes. Continued administration may lead to profound loss of motor strength, such as weakness of dorsiflexion of the foot and extension of the wrists. Elderly patients are particularly susceptible to such toxicities. Occasionally, cranial nerve palsies may lead to vocal chord paralysis or diplopia, and severe jaw pain may result from vincristine administration. At high doses of vincristine (>3 mg total single dose), autonomic neuropathy may cause obstipation and paralytic ileus. Sensory changes and reflex abnormalities slowly improve when the drug is discontinued; however, motor impairment improves less rapidly and may be irreversible. Inappropriate antidiuretic hormone (ADH) release resulting in symptomatic dilutional hyponatremia is sometimes observed.

While marrow suppression is not common with vincristine administration, some marrow toxicity may be noted in patients with impaired marrow function as a consequence of prior treatment with other drugs.

The primary toxicity of vinblastine is leukopenia. The white count reaches a nadir at day 7 and reverses rapidly thereafter. Mucositis may result from higher doses (>8 mg/m^2) of vinblastine or when it is used in combination with other cytotoxic drugs. Neurotoxicity is rare, but ileus may occur at high doses.

Both drugs cause severe pain and local toxicity if extravasated. Neither drug should ever be given intrathecally. Vincristine administered inadvertently into the cerebrospinal fluid causes acute neurologic dysfunction, coma, and death.

TAXANES

The newest of the antimitotic drugs are the taxanes, paclitaxel (Taxol) and docetaxel (Taxotere). Paclitaxel was purified from an extract of the bark of *Taxus brevifolia*, whereas docetaxel is a closely related semisynthetic derivative. Neither drug has won an important role in the treatment of hematologic malignancies. Taxanes are highly active in a number of solid tumors, including breast, ovarian, and lung cancers. They bind to the β-tubulin subunit of microtubules and promote the polymerization of microtubules, leading to disordered mitotic spindle formation and a block in the progression through mitosis.[75] Both drugs induce apoptosis in tumor cells irrespective of p53 status of the cells and kill cells at 10-nM concentrations in cell culture in a time-dependent manner.[76] In experimental settings, resistance is related to increased drug efflux, mutations in β-tubulin, or increased expression of antiapoptic proteins such as survivin,[77] or of the mitosis-related aurora kinase.[78]

The taxanes are subject to MDR mediated by the *mdr* and *mrp* genes, as well as to β-tubulin mutations. Because they are highly insoluble in aqueous solution, both drugs are formulated in lipid-based solvents that cause occasional hypersensitivity reactions. Thus, paclitaxel is given after pretreatment with antihistamines (cimetidine and diphenhydramine hydrochloride [Benadryl]) and dexamethasone sodium phosphate (Decadron). Both drugs are cleared primarily by hepatic CYP metabolism, although by different isoenzymes (paclitaxel predominantly by CYP 2B6 and docetaxel by CYP 3A4) with terminal plasma half-lives of 10 to 13 hours. Their metabolism is stimulated by phenytoin (Dilantin) and other CYP-inducing drugs and inhibited by ketoconazole. Their major toxicities, aside from hypersensitivity, are a sharp but brief leukopenia, milder thrombocytopenia, and mucositis. High-dose or repeated cycles of the taxanes cause a sensory and motor peripheral neuropathy that is reversible with drug discontinuation. Occasional patients have experienced atrial conduction block or atrial or ventricular arrhythmias after paclitaxel administration, and the combination of paclitaxel with doxorubicin may produce a greater incidence of congestive heart failure than seen with doxorubicin alone.[79] A syndrome of progressive fluid retention and peripheral edema occurs in patients receiving multiple cycles of docetaxel and can be at least partially prevented by pretreatment with glucocorticoids.[80]

Although the taxanes have not found a valuable role in the treatment of hematologic malignancy, a number of analogues and new formulations are under development, and may find useful applications in these diseases. New classes of natural products, the epothilones, which have a similar mechanism of action but less sensitivity to MDR, have attracted particular interest in early trials.[81]

TOPOISOMERASE I INHIBITORS

CAMPTOTHECINS

This group of compounds includes synthetic derivatives of 20 (*S*)-camptothecin, a naturally occurring compound initially isolated from the *Camptotheca acuminata* bush. The campothecins interact with a unique target, topoisomerase I, stabilizing the enzyme's complex with DNA and preventing the resealing of DNA single-strand breaks induced by the enzyme. Resistance arises through mutation, deletion, or

decreased expression of the topoisomerase I gene. The primary agents in clinical use are irinotecan, which is approved for treatment of colon cancer, and topotecan, approved for use against ovarian cancer and small cell lung cancer. Irinotecan, most commonly administered intravenously at a dose of 125 mg/m^2 once each week for 4 weeks every 42 days, has shown promise against lymphomas in phase II trials performed in Japan.[82] Response rates of 42 percent in previously treated patients with non-Hodgkin lymphoma, and of 38 percent in patients with refractory or relapsed adult T cell leukemia-lymphoma, were reported. However, these encouraging results remain to be confirmed. In contrast, topotecan has some remission-inducing activity in patients with myelodysplasia and chronic myelomonocytic leukemia, both as a single agent (1.5 mg/m^2 per day for 5 days) and in combination with cytarabine.[83,84] Objective responses have also been observed in phase I clinical trials in patients with acute myelogenous leukemia.[85] The two drugs differ substantially in their profile of toxicities and pharmacokinetic behavior. Irinotecan is a water-soluble prodrug that converts to the active species, SN-38, by carboxyl esterase-mediated cleavage of the basic promoiety. SN-38 and its parent drug are eliminated by biliary excretion, either directly as in the case of the parent drug, or upon glucuronidation of the active metabolite SN-38. Therefore, irinotecan must be used with caution and at lower doses in patients with Gilbert disease or hepatic dysfunction.[86] Approximately two-thirds of the dose of topotecan is eliminated by renal excretion, with the remainder being cleared by biliary excretion. Dose adjustment proportional to creatinine clearance is indicated in patients with renal failure.[87] Topotecan toxicity consists mainly of myelosuppression and, to a lesser degree, mucositis, whereas irinotecan causes a profound diarrhea, which is responsive to loperamide, and a more modest myelosuppression. The maximum tolerated dose for the daily 30-minute IV infusion × 5 schedule in patients hematologic malignancies is 4.5 mg/m^2 per day.[88] This is considerably greater than the approved dose and gastrointestinal side effects, such as mucositis and diarrhea, become dose-limiting at these higher doses.

ANTHRACYCLINE ANTIBIOTICS

DOXORUBICIN, DAUNORUBICIN, IDARUBICIN

The anthracyclines in general clinical use are doxorubicin, daunorubicin, and idarubicin, and in Europe, epirubicin. Mitoxantrone (Novantrone), a closely related anthracenedione, has very similar pharmacologic properties. The anthracyclines are produced by a *Streptomyces* species, whereas mitoxantrone is a synthetic compound not containing a sugar moiety. Doxorubicin (Adriamycin) has a broad spectrum of activity against neoplastic disease; it is an important drug in the treatment of hematologic malignancies, especially Hodgkin disease and the other lymphomas. Daunorubicin (Daunomycin) and idarubicin are used almost exclusively in combination with cytarabine for the treatment of AML. Mitoxantrone is employed for the treatment of AML and breast cancer.

MECHANISM OF ACTION

These drugs exert their effects by forming a complex with DNA and topoisomerase II, leading to double-stranded DNA strand breaks. The various anthracycline analogues differ in their specificity for binding to DNA base sequences. To varying degrees they generate free radicals through oxidation-reduction cycling of their quinone groups, an action that may contribute to their cardiac toxicity. The anthracyclines enter cells through a passive transport process and are pumped out by both the MRP and the P-glycoprotein transport system.[16] Other mechanisms for anthracycline resistance include decreased or altered topoisomerase II activity.

CLINICAL PHARMACOLOGY

Doxorubicin and daunorubicin are converted to active hydroxyl metabolites, and thereafter to a spectrum of inactive products in the liver. Only a minor fraction of the dose is excreted in the urine as the parent drug or active metabolite. The pharmacokinetics of the clinically useful anthracyclines are predominantly influenced by their terminal disposition phases, which exceed 10 hours. While prolongation of the half-life of doxorubicin has been reported in studies of patients with compromised liver function, no clear correlations with toxicity have been established. Idarubicin is the only anthracycline that exhibits reasonable oral bioavailability, being 20 percent for the parent drug and 40 percent for parent plus idarubicinol, the primary active metabolite. Idarubicinol has a very prolonged biologic half-life, ranging from 50 to 60 hours, and is likely responsible for the antitumor activity of this drug. In contrast to doxorubicin and daunorubicin, it is eliminated significantly by renal excretion. Mitoxantrone has a brief initial plasma half-life of 1.1 hours and a considerably longer terminal half-life of 23 to 42 hours. Only a minor fraction of unchanged drug is excreted in the urine (<10%) or stool (<20%). The majority of the drug is probably metabolized or bound to tissues. Patients with impaired hepatic function may have a more prolonged elimination of mitoxantrone.

The usual dose of doxorubicin when administered as a single agent by bolus intravenous injection is 60 to 75 mg/m^2 every 3 to 4 weeks. Less cardiac toxicity may result from schedules that avoid high peak plasma concentrations, such as weekly doses (15–25 mg/m^2) or continuous intravenous infusion over 48 to 96 hours. When given in combination with other myelotoxic agents such as cyclophosphamide, the dose of doxorubicin is usually decreased by one-third to one-half. Although daunorubicin has been used as the anthracycline of choice in the treatment of AML, usually in combination with cytarabine, doxorubicin, mitoxantrone, and idarubicin may be equally effective.

ADVERSE EFFECTS

Myelosuppression is the primary acute toxicity of this class of drugs, with a nadir occurring 7 to 10 days after single-dose administration and recovery by 2 weeks. Mitoxantrone produces less nausea and vomiting than does either daunorubicin or doxorubicin. Doxorubicin may cause mucositis, especially when used in maximally tolerated divided doses given over 2 to 3 days or when used in combination with other drugs that cause mucositis. These drugs may also cause a reaction in previously irradiated tissues, especially when the drug is administered just prior to or in the weeks following irradiation. Alopecia often occurs. Extravasation of these drugs results in tissue necrosis. Like the epipodophyllotoxins, the anthracyclines have caused a low but clear incidence of AML 1 to 4 years after treatment. The characteristic cytogenetic feature of these cases is the translocation at 11q23 involving the *MLL* gene.

Cardiac toxicity is a major toxic effect of doxorubicin and daunorubicin.[89,90] In mice, it appears to be mediated by a carbonyl reductase that activates the quinone moiety on doxorubicin.[91] Cardiac toxicity appears to be mediated by free radical formation catalyzed by the quinone function of the anthracycline nucleus and can be averted by free radical-scavenging agents (sulfhydryl compounds) or by iron chelators such as dexrazoxane (ICRF-187).[90] It is not known whether these modulators affect antitumor activity. Both acute effects, manifested by arrhythmias, conduction abnormalities, and a "pericarditis-myocarditis syndrome," and chronic congestive heart failure may occur. Ejection fraction measurements have been helpful as a noninvasive technique to demonstrate a decline in myocardial function and a rising risk of myocardial failure with increasing doses. Anthracycline therapy should be discontinued when the ejection fraction falls below 40 percent. Most patients will tolerate total doses of 450 to 550 mg/m^2 dox-

orubicin or daunorubicin before the risk of cardiac damage exceeds 5 percent.[92] There is a high risk of cardiac damage at lower cumulative doses in patients receiving mantle irradiation. Once clinically overt cardiac toxicity occurs, usually manifested by congestive heart failure, the mortality rate is high. Congestive heart failure usually occurs during therapy or less than 1 month following cessation of treatment; rarely, heart failure may occur many months later, or may be elicited by a second drug, such as mitoxantrone or mitomycin C. Children treated with anthracyclines may show abnormal cardiac development and late congestive heart failure in their teenage years.[93] Those children who received greater than 300 mg/m^2 demonstrated decreased myocardial contractility and increased ventricular dimension when tested years later, thus leading to the recommendation that total anthracycline dose be limited to no more than 300 mg/m^2 in children. Low-dose schedules cause less cardiac toxicity. Treatment with idarubicin or mitoxantrone is associated with a lower risk of cardiac toxicity, but the data are less complete for these newer agents.

TOPOISOMERASE II INHIBITORS

EPIPODOPHYLLOTOXINS

Two semisynthetic derivatives of podophyllotoxin, VP-16 (etoposide) and VM-26 (teniposide), have significant clinical activity in hematologic malignancies. Etoposide has been incorporated into combination therapy regimens for Hodgkin disease, diffuse aggressive lymphomas, and leukemias and is frequently used as a component of high-dose chemotherapy regimens. Teniposide has been used investigationally to treat various forms of childhood acute leukemia and appears to be synergistic with cytarabine.[94]

These compounds induce double-stranded breaks in DNA through their sequence-specific binding to DNA in complex with topoisomerase II, a DNA repair enzyme.[95] One mechanism of resistance is increased expression of the MDR phenotype.[16] A second mechanism results from decreased topoisomerase II activity or mutation of the enzyme, resulting in decreased drug binding.[96,97]

CLINICAL PHARMACOLOGY

Etoposide has excellent oral bioavailability and may be administered either orally or intravenously. The usual intravenous dose schedule used for etoposide is 100 to 120 mg/m^2 per day for 3 days, either consecutively or every other day. When administered orally, the dose should be increased twofold over the intravenous dose, because 50 to 67 percent of the dose is absorbed. Approximately 30 to 40 percent of an intravenous dose of etoposide is excreted intact in the urine; thus, doses of etoposide require modification for patients with compromised renal function but not hepatic dysfunction.[98] The biologic half-life of etoposide is 15 hours. The clinical activity of etoposide is highly schedule dependent. Single conventional doses are essentially without antitumor effect as compared to consecutive daily doses for 3 to 5 days. The oral administration of 50 mg per day for 2 to 3 weeks is a commonly used regimen that takes advantage of that schedule dependency.

The pharmacokinetics of teniposide are very similar to those of etoposide, with a terminal plasma half-life of 20 to 48 hours. However, little parent drug appears intact in the urine, and dose modification for patients with renal dysfunction is unnecessary.

ADVERSE EFFECTS

When administered intravenously, both etoposide and teniposide should be infused over a 30-minute period to avoid hypotensive episodes. The major toxicity of both drugs is leukopenia, which is rapidly reversible. Thrombocytopenia is less common. Nausea and vomiting often follow etoposide administration. Alopecia may occur with both drugs. Other toxicities, such as fever, mild elevation of liver function tests, or peripheral neuropathy, are relatively uncommon. Because the major toxicity of etoposide is limited to the marrow, this drug is under intensive investigation as a component of high-dose regimens followed by marrow transplantation. In high-dose etoposide protocols (3 to 4 g/m^2 given over 3 to 5 days) oropharyngeal mucositis becomes a prominent toxicity. Less frequent high-dose toxicities include hepatocellular damage and, rarely, anaphylactic-like symptoms, probably related to the chromophore-based vehicle. Secondary acute myeloid leukemia associated with translocation at 11q23 may follow etoposide treatment in children with ALL[99] and in adults with solid tumors.[100]

BLEOMYCIN

Bleomycin is a mixture of peptides produced by the fungus *Streptomyces verticillis*.[101] Because it has antitumor effects with little or no marrow toxicity, it is commonly used as part of combination regimens (such as Adriamycin [doxorubicin], bleomycin, vinblastine, and dacarbazine [ABVD]) to treat Hodgkin disease, the aggressive lymphomas, and with cisplatin and vinblastine to treat germ cell tumors. Bleomycin acts by causing both single- and double-strand breaks in DNA. These breaks form as a consequence of a bleomycin:Fe (II) complex with DNA leading to proton abstraction from the deoxyribose and cleavage at the 4'-carbon.[102,103] In experimental tumors, resistance to bleomycin has been attributed to increased concentrations of an aminohydrolase that cleaves and inactivates the drug.[104] Some resistant cell lines exhibit enhanced capacity to repair strand breaks, and in others, resistance results from decreased drug accumulation. Additional factors, such as increased free radical detoxification may also influence toxicity. The tumor specificity of bleomycin and its lack of toxicity to marrow and the gastrointestinal tract may be a result of different levels of a bleomycin-inactivating enzyme in these tissues. The aminohydrolase is found in low concentrations in the lung and skin, a possible explanation for the susceptibility of these two normal organs to damage by this drug. Cell killing occurs throughout the cell cycle.

CLINICAL PHARMACOLOGY

Bleomycin may be administered intravenously or intramuscularly for systemic therapy, as well as intrapleurally or intraperitoneally for control of malignant effusions. The half-life of drug elimination from plasma is estimated to be 2 to 3 hours. After a single intravenous injection, more than half the dose is excreted, unchanged, in the urine within 24 hours.[105] Bleomycin elimination may be markedly impaired in patients with poor renal function; such patients are at risk of overwhelming skin and lung toxicity. Dose reduction proportional to creatinine clearance should be considered in these patients.

ADVERSE EFFECTS

Bleomycin has few or no effects on normal marrow; however, in patients given other myelosuppressive drugs or recovering from marrow toxicity from these agents, additional mild myelosuppression may be observed. The primary toxicities that result from bleomycin are pulmonary fibrosis and skin changes. In experimental settings, the drug induces the secretion of numerous cytokines, including interleukin (IL)-6 and transforming growth factor β (TGF-β), by alveolar macrophages, leading to collagen deposition.[106] The risk of pulmonary toxicity is related to the cumulative dose administered, increasing to 10 percent in patients given more than 450 mg. Risk is also greater in patients older than age 70 years, in patients with underlying lung disease, in patients receiving bleomycin who are given high oxygen concentrations, and in patients who have had previous radiotherapy to the lungs. Single doses of 25 mg/m^2 or more predispose to this toxic effect. Symptoms of pulmonary toxicity include cough and dyspnea. Chest

x-rays show nonspecific infiltrates, especially in the lower lobes. Open lung biopsy may be required to distinguish bleomycin pulmonary toxicity from infection or malignant disease. Findings of bleomycin toxicity include an inflammatory alveolar infiltrate with edema, pulmonary hyaline formation, and squamous metaplasia of the alveolar lining cells. These changes progress to intraalveolar and interstitial fibrosis over a period of months. Patients with bleomycin lung toxicity have a defect in carbon monoxide diffusing capacity, a test of possible value in predicting potential pulmonary toxicity.[107] Because there is no specific therapy for patients with bleomycin lung toxicity, close attention should be paid to early pulmonary symptoms and radiographic changes. In patients with bleomycin pulmonary toxicity, some improvement may be seen on discontinuation of the drug, but the pulmonary fibrosis is usually not reversible. Glucocorticoids may decrease inflammation, but are of no proven benefit once fibrosis has occurred.

The dermatologic toxicity of bleomycin is also dose related. Erythema, hyperpigmentation, hyperkeratosis, and even ulceration may occur when the drug is given in conventional daily doses for longer than 2 to 3 weeks. Areas of skin pressure, especially of the hands, fingers, and joints, are initially affected. Nail changes and alopecia may also occur with continued use of the drug. In combination regimens (e.g., ABVD) where bleomycin is used intermittently, skin toxicity usually does not occur.

Fever and malaise are common symptoms and may be alleviated with the use of acetaminophen. Hypersensitivity reactions have also been observed. Idiosyncratic cardiovascular collapse has been rarely noted. A 1- or 2-mg test dose administered to such susceptible patients may result in hypotension, tachycardia, pulmonary insufficiency, or anaphylactoid reactions within 30 to 60 minutes. Their occurrence precludes further treatment with bleomycin.

ASPARAGINASE

The enzyme L-asparaginase is used clinically in the treatment of lymphoid malignancies, in particular in poor-risk B cell ALL, T cell ALL, and the lymphomas.

MECHANISM OF ACTION

The cells causing these lymphoid malignancies require exogenous L-asparaginase for growth; they obtain this amino acid from the circulating pool of amino acids generated primarily by the liver. The enzyme L-asparaginase, which catalyzes the hydrolysis of asparagine to aspartic acid and ammonia, is capable of rapidly depleting the serum level of L-asparaginase. This induces an asparagine deficiency in lymphoid malignant cells. Resistant tumors are able to respond by rapid induction of asparagine synthetase,[108] thereby restoring intracellular pools of asparagine. For reasons not well understood, hyperdiploid ALL cells are particularly sensitive to L-asparaginase.[109] In vitro incubation of leukemic cells with drug appears to predict sensitivity,[110] but is unproven as a useful tool for choosing therapy.

Three L-asparaginase preparations are available in the United States.[111–113] The product purified from *Escherichia coli* is employed as a first-line agent, while a second preparation (pegaspargase), derived by attachment of polyethylene glycol to the *E. coli* enzyme, is primarily reserved for patients with hypersensitivity to the unmodified enzyme. A third preparation, purified from *Erwinia chrysanthemi*, can be obtained from the National Cancer Institute of the United States for patients hypersensitive to the *E. coli* enzyme, but is rarely used. The various preparations differ in their pharmacokinetics and recommended doses. The *E. coli* enzyme is usually given in doses of 6000 to 10,000 IU every third day for 3 to 4 weeks, although much higher doses have been used in ALL treatment. Levels are maintained continuously above 0.03 IU/ml serum, leading to total abolition of aspar-agine in the systemic circulation. The *E. coli* enzyme has an elimi-nation half-life of 14 to 24 hours. Polyethylene glycol (PEG) conjugated to the enzyme reduces its immunogenicity and extends its half-life to 6 days. PEG-asparaginase is used in patients hypersensitive to the unmodified enzyme, in doses of 2500 IU/m^2 every 2 weeks. Some patients remain hypersensitive to both preparations of *E. coli* enzyme; enzyme from *Erwinia* has a low incidence of hypersensitivity and approximately equal catalytic activity to the *E. coli* preparation, but a more rapid clearance. Additionally, *Erwinia* enzyme must be used in higher doses.

ADVERSE EFFECTS

Reactions to the first dose are uncommon, but after two or more doses of the drug, hypersensitivity may develop, varying from urticarial re-actions to hypotension, laryngospasm, and cardiac arrest. Skin testing to predict allergic reactions is helpful in some, but not all, cases, and should be performed to confirm a clinical suspicion of hypersensitiv-ity. Hypersensitive patients may have antibodies to L-asparaginase in their plasma. However, more than half the patients with such circu-lating antibodies will not display an overt allergic reaction to the drug, but these patients may have more rapid disappearance of drug from plasma and an inadequate clearance of asparagine from plasma and cells, leading to therapeutic failure. Patients who are treated with L-asparaginase should be observed carefully for several hours after dos-ing, and epinephrine should be available in case anaphylactic reactions occur. Anaphylaxis is less likely when L-asparaginase is given intra-muscularly than when it is administered intravenously.

The other major toxic effects of L-asparaginase are a consequence of the ability of this drug to inhibit protein synthesis in normal tissues. Inhibition of protein synthesis in the liver will result in hypoalbumi-nemia, a decrease in clotting factors, a decrease in serum lipoproteins, and a marked increase in plasma triglycerides. Inhibition of insulin production may lead to hyperglycemia. The clotting abnormalities that are regularly observed as a consequence of L-asparaginase treatment include initial decreases in the anticoagulant factors antithrombin III, protein C, and protein S, leading to either arterial or venous thrombosis in occasional patients.[114] With more prolonged therapy, bleeding se-quelae may result from inhibition of the synthesis of procoagulant proteins such as fibrinogen and factors II, VII, IX, and X. Conse-quently, monitoring of coagulation factors is recommended. High doses of L-asparaginase may cause cerebral dysfunction that manifests as confusion, stupor, or coma, and cortical sinus thrombosis has been documented by magnetic resonance imaging (MRI) scan in such pa-tients.[115] Clinical thromboembolic episodes may occur in up to 35 percent of children with ALL.[116] These events are mostly asympto-matic thrombi associated with central venous catheters; less frequently cortical sinus and atrial thrombi may occur. Preexisting clotting ab-normalities, such as antiphospholipid antibodies or factor V Leiden, may predispose to thromboembolic complications.[117]

Acute nonhemorrhagic pancreatitis occurs as a complication of L-asparaginase treatment, especially in patients who have extreme ele-vations of plasma triglycerides (>2 g/dl).[118]

Because L-asparaginase manifests little toxicity in marrow or gas-trointestinal mucosa, it has been used in combination with other drugs that do have such toxicities.

MOLECULARLY TARGETED SMALL MOLECULES

IMATINIB MESYLATE

The first molecularly targeted drug to make a major impact on cancer treatment was imatinib mesylate (Gleevec), an inhibitor of ABL ty-rosine kinase activity and notably the mutant ABL characteristic of the BCR-ABL fusion protein in chronic myelogenous leukemia. That this agent should prove uniformly effective, while others similarly directed at proliferation linked kinases, such as the epidermal growth factor receptor (EGFR), have produced only occasional responses in solid tumors, has been ascribed to the unique role of the 9:22 trans-location and the resultant BCR-ABL fusion protein in CML. This sin-gle molecular event produces growth factor independence and by itself is sufficient to cause and maintain malignant transformation in exper-imental settings.[119] The drug was selected for clinical study by scien-tists at Ciba-Geigy (later Novartis) based on a high throughput screen for kinase inhibition. Preclinical experiments established that contin-uous exposure to drug concentrations of 1 μM or higher could lead to apoptosis of cells carrying the activated kinase, but had little effect on normal hematopoietic cells, a conclusion borne out by subsequent clin-ical trials.

Imatinib mesylate potently inhibits BCR-ABL kinase (inhibitory concentration of 50 percent [IC_{50}] = 100 nM), as well as the c-KIT kinase[120] and the platelet-derived growth factor receptor (PDGFR) ki-nase. The latter two kinases are targets for imatinib mesylate in the treatment of gastrointestinal stromal tumors (GIST),[121] which ex-presses a mutated c-KIT, and in some cases of hypereosinophilia syn-drome,[122] chronic myelomonocytic leukemia,[123] and dermatofibrosar-coma protuberans,[124] each of which contain activating mutations of PDGFR. Crystallographic and mutagenesis studies indicate that ima-tinib mesylate binds to a segment of the BCR-ABL tyrosine kinase domain that fixes the enzyme in a closed, or nonfunctional state, in which the protein is unable to bind its substrate, adenosine triphosphate (ATP).[125] The contact points between imatinib mesylate and the en-zyme become sites of mutations in drug-resistant leukemic cells, pre-venting tight binding of the drug and locking the enzyme in its open configuration, in which it has access to substrate.

The drug is well absorbed by the oral route and subject to clearance by hepatic P450 (CYP 3A4) metabolism.[126] It has a terminal half-life of approximately 10 hours and therefore can be administered once per day. Doses of 400 mg produce a peak drug concentration in blood of 4 to 7 μM and trough levels at 24 hours of 1.5 to 2.0 μM in most patients. Clearance is delayed in patients with renal dysfunction, ap-parently as a result of decreased P450 activity in the presence of renal failure. Limited data indicate that imatinib mesylate penetrates poorly into the cerebrospinal fluid, achieving concentrations of 1 percent of simultaneous drug levels in the systemic circulation.[127]

The drug is more than 99 percent protein bound, largely by α_1-acid glycoprotein (AGP), a binding protein present in higher concen-trations in humans than in mice.[128] Thus therapeutic studies in mice may overpredict drug activity. AGP concentrations vary over a four-fold range in human subjects, and total drug concentrations in plasma appear to be a function of AGP levels. Clindamycin displaces imatinib mesylate from binding to AGP and, in mice, increases the concentra-tion of drug found in cells.

Preclinical studies suggest that conclusions regarding the adequacy of 1 μM imatinib mesylate may be premature, and that patients with higher levels of binding protein may demonstrate "pharmacokinetic" resistance, and may require higher doses of drug to maintain enzyme inhibition. Clinical experience suggests that a fraction (30%) of pa-tients with CML who demonstrate hematologic or cytogenetic pro-gression while on standard doses of imatinib may benefit from dose escalation to 600 to 800 mg/day.[129] Whether these responses result from overcoming pharmacokinetics resistance or from inhibition of mutated or amplified enzyme remains to be established.

Resistance in human malignancies arises from point mutations in three separate segments of the kinase domain.[130] The most relevant of these mutations are those that hold the enzyme in its open confirmation and maintain kinetic activity. The most common mutations associated with clinical resistance affect amino acids 255 and 315, both of which serve as contact points for the drug; these mutations confer high-level resistance to imatinib mesylate. Other mutations affect the phosphate-binding region and the "activation loop" of the domain with varying degrees of associated resistance. Some mutations, such as at amino acids 351 and 355, confer low levels of resistance and these tumor cells may remain sensitive to higher drug doses.[131] This theory may explain the clinical response of some resistant patients to dose escalation. Experimental studies of enzyme mutagenesis indicate that mutations in regions outside the kinase domain, and affecting interactions with proteins that dock with the kinase, can also confer resistance, but these have uncertain relevance to clinical resistance.[132]

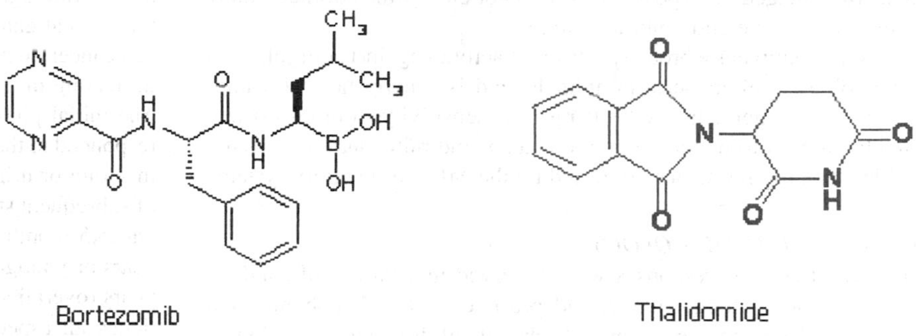

Bortezomib

Thalidomide

FIGURE 19-1   The planar chemical structure of thalidomide and bortezomib (Velcade).

Kinase mutations known to cause drug resistance may be detected in some patients prior to initiation of therapy, particularly in patients with Ph+ ALL[133,134] or CML and blastic crisis. This finding strongly supports the hypothesis that drug-resistant cells arise through spontaneous mutation, and are further selected by drug exposure. Among CML patients, mutations are readily detectable in patients receiving imatinib mesylate, including one-third of those undergoing treatment in the accelerated phase and in late (longer than 4 years from diagnosis) chronic phase CML.[135] Most patients with mutations demonstrate clinical resistance at the time a mutation is detected, or shortly thereafter. Mutations involving the phosphate binding loop are associated with rapid disease progression and death within a median of 4.5 months.

In addition to kinase mutation, amplification of the wild-type kinase gene, leading to overexpression of the enzyme, has been identified in tumor samples from a minority of patients with resistance to treatment.[136] The *MDR* gene, which codes for a drug efflux protein, confers resistance experimentally[137]; thus far this mechanism has not been implicated in clinical resistance.

Experimental studies suggest strategies to prevent or overcome *BCR-ABL* mutations. Alternative kinase inhibitors, such as PD180970 and related compounds, bind to the "open" confirmation of the enzyme, inhibit its catalytic activity,[138] and remain effective against some mutations involving the kinase domain. Combination therapy with drugs unrelated to imatinib might discourage outgrowth of resistant clones, although the poor response of blastic-phase CML to conventional agents suggests that new drugs are needed. Imatinib mesylate-resistant cells remain sensitive to histone deacetylase (HDAC)[139] or farnesyl transferase inhibition.[140] HDAC inhibitors and heat shock protein-binding drugs (such as geldanamycin) promote degradation of both wild-type and mutant kinase, and increase apoptosis in imatinib-resistant cells.[141] None of these strategies have reached clinical evaluation at this time.

Not all resistance is explained by kinase amplification or mutation, or by pharmacokinetic factors. There is a growing awareness of the appearance of mutant Ph− clones carrying the karyotype of myelodysplastic cells in patients receiving imatinib for CML, and a few cases of progression to myelodysplastic syndrome (MDS) and AML have been reported.[142,143]

At conventional doses of 400 mg/day, imatinib mesylate has modest toxicity. Periorbital edema occurs in 60 percent of patients, a maculopapular rash in 32 percent, and diarrhea, myalgia, fatigue, and headache in less than 33 percent. In less than 5 percent of patients are symptoms serious enough to warrant discontinuation of therapy.[144] A minor fraction of patients will develop myelosuppression necessitating dose reduction. In rare patients, pulmonary edema, pleural or pericar-

dial effusion, or severe peripheral edema will lead to drug discontinuation. Hepatic toxicity, associated with hepatocellular necrosis on biopsy, has been reported. Imatinib causes a spectrum of skin reactions,[145] including a common maculopapular drug eruption, erythema nodosum, Stevens-Johnson syndrome, or vasculitis. The typical maculopapular rash is dose related, and will respond to dose reduction or administration of concomitant glucocorticoids.

BORTEZOMIB (VELCADE)

After a brief, 3-year clinical trial, bortezomib has become an important new agent for treating myeloma. Its accelerated marketing approval was based on the results of two phase II trials in which it produced a 25 to 30 percent clinical response rate in patients who had progressed after primary therapy.[146,147] It inhibits a unique target, the proteasome, which is responsible for degradation of intracellular proteins, and is believed to alter the balance of signals for apoptosis and proliferation, leading to cell death.

MECHANISM OF ACTION
Bortezomib has a unique structure in which boron is covalently bound to a pyrazinyl-carbonyl side chain linked to a phenyl group (Fig. 19-1). It was discovered in a screen for inhibition of proteasome function, and found to be a potent (K_i = 0.6 nM) inhibitor of the serine protease component of the proteasome.[148] This action blocks the degradation of a number of cellular proteins. Although it is unclear which of these changes lead to cell death, a leading candidate is the effect of bortezomib on the nuclear factor-κB (NF-κB) pathway. NF-κB is an important regulatory protein that promotes the transcription of a variety of growth-promoting, angiogenic, and antiapoptotic genes, thereby protecting cells against hypoxia, DNA damage, and other "environmental" stress, including cellular damage caused by chemotherapy. In most normal cells it exists in an inactivated state, bound to an inhibitor, IkB. In tumor cells, either through increased synthesis of NF-κB or increased proteosomal degradation of IkB, the level of free NF-κB is increased and the program of stress response and angiogenesis is activated. The same pathway protects tumor cells from undergoing apoptosis after exposure to chemotherapy or radiation, both of which trigger IkB degradation. Bortezomib, through its inhibition of the proteasome, elevates IkB, which, in turn, inactivates NF-κB, promoting tumor cell apoptosis. Bortezomib has attracted great interest, not only in its own right, but also as an enhancer of cytotoxic chemotherapy or radiation therapy.[149]

In addition to its effects on IkB, bortezomib blocks production of IL-6, a key growth factor in myeloma proliferation, and inhibits angiogenesis. It promotes phosphorylation and proteolytic cleavage of the antiapoptotic factor Bcl-2. It also blocks proteolysis of p21 and p27, an action that inhibits cell cycle progression and promotes apoptosis of damaged or hypoxic cells. It is not clear which of these many effects contribute antitumor activity.[150]

Bortezomib has a broad spectrum of activity against both solid and hematologic malignancies in animals, and is synergistic with camptothecins and gemcitabine.[149] It restores sensitivity of drug-resistant myeloma cells to doxorubicin, melphalan, and mitoxantrone. It is not subject to drug resistance conferred by the MDR drug efflux system.

CLINICAL PHARMACOLOGY

In phase I studies, responses were observed in a variety of solid tumors, including lung, kidney, and prostate, and in lymphomas and myeloma. Using the now standard schedule of drug administration on days 1, 4, 8, and 11 (twice weekly for 2 weeks, with a 10-day rest period), the maximum tolerated dose is 1.3 mg/m^2. At this dose, proteasome function is inhibited by 60 to 80 percent, a level associated with acceptable toxicity in animal toxicology experiments and with therapeutic activity in mice.[151] Drug concentrations in plasma of 2 ng/ml or greater are associated with 50 percent or greater inhibition of proteasome function. Dose-limiting toxicities are thrombocytopenia, diarrhea, and fatigue, but myelosuppression at the maximal therapeutic dose (MTD) is usually modest and readily reversible. Approximately 10 percent of patients receiving multiple cycles of treatment may develop a painful sensory peripheral neuropathy, and some may choose to discontinue treatment.[152,153]

Bortezomib undergoes deboronation, followed by hydroxylation via CYP 3A4 and 2D6. The primary metabolites are inactive. Because the drug has a terminal $t_{1/2}$ of 5.45 hours, dose reduction is not necessary for patients with mild renal dysfunction. Its half-life tends to increase with subsequent cycles of therapy, although no consistent scheme for dose reduction is required in routine use in the absence of serious toxicity. Information is lacking regarding its pharmacokinetics in severe renal failure or hepatic dysfunction.

THALIDOMIDE

Thalidomide (α-phthalimidoglutarimide), approved in 1953 as a sedative, was withdrawn from clinical use because of its teratogenicity. It causes dysmelia (i.e., stunted limb growth) when used during early pregnancy. However, it has since resurfaced as an antibacterial and antitumor agent, with clear effectiveness against leprosy and myeloma.[154]

The mechanism of action of thalidomide in each of these indications is poorly understood, and indeed may differ, but there is considerable preclinical evidence for a prominent antiangiogenic effect against tumors,[155] for immune modulation, and for cytokine inhibition. It inhibits basic fibroblast growth factor (bFGF)- and vascular endothelial growth factor (VEGF)-induced neovascularization in the mouse cornea, blocks proliferation of endothelial cells in culture,[156] and inhibits secretions of VEGF and other angiogenic cytokines; antiangiogenic effects have also been ascribed to its metabolites and analogues, including CC 5013 (Revlimid), a related compound that has reached advanced stages of clinical testing.[157,158] Revlimid potently stimulates phosphorylation and activation of the CD28 costimulatory molecule.[159] Thalidomide has a broad range of effects on cytokine secretion, lowering levels of tumor necrosis factor alpha (TNF-α) and γ-interferon in leprosy patients, and stimulating T cell function.

Pharmacokinetics of thalidomide reveal a slow absorption with peak levels achieved in 2.9 to 4.3 hours[160,161] after doses ranging from 50 to 400 mg. There is no evidence for induction of metabolism on a daily dosing regimen. Drug concentrations in plasma decay with a half-life of 5 to 7 hours, the major pathways for elimination including spontaneous hydrolysis of the imide esters, and further metabolism by the liver. Less than 1 percent of the drug is excreted unchanged in the urine. Although thalidomide has been evaluated against a number of human malignancies, with occasional responses in brain tumors, renal cell cancer, hepatoma, and Kaposi sarcoma, it has an established value in treating multiple myeloma refractory to first-line chemotherapy.[162] The initial phase II trial in 84 patients demonstrated that 32 percent responded to thalidomide as defined by a 25 percent or greater decrease in serum or urine paraprotein, a response rate confirmed by a number of subsequent studies.[163] The median time for progression-free survival was 5.5 months in a recent Australian trial, although patients age 65 years or younger did significantly better than those older than age 65 years (overall survival: 26 months vs. 9.2 months). In responding patients, all aspects of the disease, including bone marrow infiltration with tumor cells, anemia, and performance status, improved with therapy. Thalidomide has synergistic myeloma-inhibiting activity with glucocorticoids, interferon alpha, and cytotoxic agents.[164] Clinical trials exploring its use in combination with glucocorticoids and cytotoxic drugs are presently being performed, with promising early results as initial therapy in combination with dexamethasone.[165]

Thalidomide is generally well tolerated in doses of 50 to 1200 mg daily. In treating myeloma, a 1-month trial is usually sufficient to observe a decline in paraprotein and an improvement in symptoms. Doses can usually be escalated 200 mg every 2 weeks until dose-limiting toxicity is reached at 600 to 800 mg/day. Patients older than age 65 years are less tolerant of side effects, particularly sedation, constipation, fatigue, and peripheral sensory neuropathy, and receive a median dose of 400 mg/day, while those younger may tolerate up to a median of 800 mg/day. At doses below 400 mg/day, the peripheral neuropathy usually improves with dose reduction or drug discontinuation, but may be irreversible in patients receiving higher doses of thalidomide. Other side effects include rash, dizziness and orthostatic hypotension, neutropenia, mood changes or depression, and nausea. Hypersensitivity and bradycardia have also been reported. Thalidomide in combination with doxorubicin or with prednisone is associated with an increased incidence of thromboembolism, a complication that can be prevented by concurrent treatment with low molecular weight heparin.[166] Because of its teratogenicity, patients of child-bearing age should take precautions to prevent pregnancy while on therapy. Because of the synergy with interferon alpha in preclinical experiments, this drug combination has been evaluated, with unclear benefit. Up to one third of patients who have achieved stable disease on thalidomide do reach a partial response with interferon.[163] However, in trials of this combination against renal cell carcinoma, in which high doses of interferon (9 million units subcutaneously 3 times per week) were used, 4 of 13 patients developed complex partial seizures and visual disturbances.[167] Two of 19 patients on low-dose interferon (1.5 to 3.0 units three times weekly) developed complex partial seizures in a trial against melanoma.[163]

In the United States, thalidomide is approved for use under a special restricted distribution program, the System for Thalidomide Education and Prescribing Safety (STEPS). The analogue, Revlimid, with significant activity against myeloma, causes significantly less sedation, constipation, and neurotoxicity, but greater myelosuppression. It seems most effective in doses of 25 mg/day for 20 doses every 28 days, and is progressing through phase III trials.[158,168]

AGENTS ACTIVE THROUGHOUT THE CELL CYCLE

THE ALKYLATING DRUGS

These drugs are important in the treatment of hematopoietic malignancies either as single agents or as components of combination regimens. Their role as treatment for both acute and chronic hematologic malignancies results from their lack of cell cycle specificity. In combination with cell cycle-specific agents, they may eradicate noncycling cells that escape cycle-active components of the treatment. Although these agents share the common property of forming covalent bonds with electron-rich sites on DNA (oxygen and nitrogen substituents), they exhibit important differences in their intrinsic reactivity, route of cellular uptake, favored sites of alkylation on DNA bases, and the specific mechanism of DNA repair that determines cell survival. These differences are borne out in experimental settings, where cross-resistance to alkylating agents is incomplete. Thus, protocols employing multiple alkylators, particularly in high-dose regimens, have a rational basis.[169] Alkylating agents differ as well in their patterns of toxicity. The majority of these drugs cause myelosuppression and mucositis as their primary acute toxicities, as well as delayed pulmonary fibrosis and late secondary leukemias. They also cause vascular endothelial damage in occasional patients when used in high doses. However, cyclophosphamide and bischloroethylnitrosourea (BCNU) cause less mucositis in high-dose regimens, although cyclophosphamide rarely produces a hemorrhagic myocarditis. 4-Hydroperoxycyclophosphamide, an activated analogue of cyclophosphamide, appears to spare marrow stem cells relative to tumor cells and is used for *in vitro* purging of marrow in autologous transplantation.[170]

Although platinum analogues are not true alkylating agents in that they form metal adducts rather than carbon adducts with DNA, RNA, and protein, their range of toxicities and mechanisms of resistance have much in common with the classical alkylators. They have limited use in hematologic malignancy, mainly finding a role in high-dose chemotherapy for lymphomas (see Chap. 96). Their intrastrand DNA adducts, the primary molecular lesion, is subject to repair by nucleotide excision repair, a process dependent on functional p53 activity.[171] Polymorphisms of the repair pathways, associated with decreased ability to repair adducts, may be associated with drug resistance.[172] This paradox may be related to the need for recognition of the platinum adduct by the repair machinery in order to create DNA strand breaks. It is unclear whether these polymorphisms in the nucleotide-excision repair (NER) pathway confer resistance in leukemic cells and whether this resistance extends to traditional alkylating agents.

MECHANISM OF ACTION

All alkylating agents have in common the generation of highly reactive carbonium intermediates that attack electron-rich sites on DNA, such as the N-7, O-2, and O-6 positions of guanine and the N-1, N-3, and N-7 positions of adenine. For many of these agents, the alkylating group must undergo a preliminary activation reaction mediated either by chemical rearrangement of the molecule, as in the case of nitrogen mustard and the nitrosoureas, or by metabolic activation followed by chemical rearrangement, as for cyclophosphamide, ifosfamide, and procarbazine. In some alkylating agents the reactive intermediate contains two reactive centers, usually chloroethyl groups, and therefore may cross-link opposing strands of DNA. Methylating agents produce only single-strand alkylation but may be highly carcinogenic, as, for example, procarbazine. In general, the most commonly used drugs of this class, including cyclophosphamide, ifosfamide, melphalan, and chlorambucil, produce the same spectrum of myelosuppressive, carcinogenic, and genotoxic actions.

Experimental systems have elucidated the mechanisms of resistance to alkylating agents that are unique to these compounds.[173] Some mechanisms are specific for certain alkylating agents (e.g., impaired uptake of nitrogen mustard as a consequence of an alteration in the membrane carrier for choline, or deletion of the amino acid carrier used by melphalan), while others appear to be less specific (e.g., drug inactivation associated with an increase in intracellular sulfhydryl compounds, and enhanced nucleotide-excision repair of DNA cross-links). The primary resistance mechanisms for various alkylating

drugs, as documented in experimental tumors, include increased degradation by aldehyde dehydrogenase (cyclophosphamide)[174]; increased conjugation of the reactive intermediates with glutathione or glutathione transferase (all chloroethylating agents and platinum analogues); increased repair of the O-6 guanine alkyl lesions by a specific alkyl transferase (nitrosoureas, procarbazine, dacarbazine)[175]; increased nucleotide excision repair (all platinum derivatives and chloroethylating agents, except nitrosoureas); decreased uptake (melphalan, nitrogen mustard); and decreased ability to recognize DNA damage (alkylating agents and platinum derivatives). The clinical basis of alkylating agent resistance is incompletely understood.

CLINICAL PHARMACOLOGY

In general, the alkylating agents and their reactive intermediates have short residence times in the systemic circulation and within cells. They are eliminated predominantly by hydrolysis, by chemical or biochemical conjugation to the sulfhydryl groups of glutathione or proteins, or by oxidative metabolism, therefore, dose reduction is not required in patients with diminished renal function. Cyclophosphamide and ifosfamide are closely related molecules that undergo hepatic activation. Their active metabolites generate a highly toxic metabolite, acrolein, which is excreted in the urine.[176] To counteract toxicity to kidneys and bladder, mercaptoethane sulfonate (MESNA) is administered simultaneously in equivalent doses to patients receiving ifosfamide or high-dose cyclophosphamide. Nitrogen mustard is a highly reactive compound that may be administered topically, intravenously, or intrapleurally. It is a potent vesicant, and care must be taken in the mixing and administration of the drug. Extravasation may lead to severe tissue injury. The second-generation alkylating agents, which include cyclophosphamide, melphalan, busulfan, and chlorambucil, are more chemically stable and absorbed reasonably well when given orally.

ADVERSE EFFECTS

Marrow toxicity, which is cumulative and a function of total dose, is the most important toxic effect of these compounds. Other toxicities, including lung, cardiac, and endothelial damage, have been described above. Because alkylating agents all react with DNA, mutations and secondary leukemias are major long-term effects of these agents. This hazard appears to be related to the total dose administered. The monofunctional methylating agents (e.g., procarbazine) are especially potent in this regard and may have a major role in the increased incidence of secondary malignancies noted in patients who have been treated with chemotherapy. The dose-limiting toxicity of one of these drugs, dacarbazine, is nausea and vomiting rather than marrow suppression.

Nitrosoureas produce a characteristic delayed myelosuppression that reaches a nadir 4 to 6 weeks after administration. Busulfan, like the nitrosoureas, depletes stem cells and can cause profound marrow hypoplasia or permanent aplasia when administered over prolonged periods of time and must be used with caution. All alkylating agents, but particularly busulfan and the nitrosoureas, may produce pulmonary fibrosis. The nitrosoureas also cause nephrotoxicity, particularly after total doses of 1200 mg/m^2 BCNU or methylcyclohexylchloroethylnitrosourea.[177]

HIGH-DOSE ALKYLATING AGENT THERAPY

The development of marrow stem cell rescue techniques has made it clinically possible to administer doses of chemotherapy that would otherwise produce life-threatening aplasia. To be of benefit, however, high-dose therapy must employ agents that have a relatively steep dose–response relationship and must not have lethal extramedullary toxicity at high doses. Among the classes of cytotoxics, alkylators have a particularly favorable linear relationship between dose and cytotoxicity in experimental systems. Their hematopoietic toxicity is generally

TABLE 19-3 DOSE-LIMITING EXTRAMEDULLARY TOXICITIES OF SINGLE-AGENT CHEMOTHERAPY

DRUG	MAXIMUM TOLERATED DOSE, MG/M²*	INCREASE OVER STANDARD DOSE†	MAJOR TOXICITIES‡
Cyclophosphamide	7000	7.0	Cardiac
Ifosfamide	16,000	2.7	Renal, CNS
Thiotepa§	1005	18.0	GI, CNS
Melphalan§	180	5.6	GI
Busulfan§	640	9.0	GI, hepatic
BCNU§	1050	5.3	Lung, hepatic
Cisplatin	200	2.0	Renal, neuropathy
Carboplatin§	2000	5.0	Hepatic, renal
Etoposide	3000	6.0	GI
Cytarabine	3000	10–30	Neurologic, mucositis

BCNU, bischloroethyl nitrosourea; CNS, central nervous system; GI, gastrointestinal.
* Independent of hematopoietic toxicity.[178–184]
† Fold increase: This is an approximation because standard doses may vary.
‡ All drugs listed in this table cause vascular endothelial damage and venoocclusive disease, as well as late secondary leukemias.
§ With stem cell support.

limiting within standard dose ranges, but other organ toxicities are infrequent until doses are increased manyfold, making them ideal candidates for high-dose regimens. When agents are administered with stem cell rescue, marrow toxicity ceases to be dose limiting and extramedullary toxic effects are seen. Depending on the agent and the toxicity profile, doses may only be escalated by as little as twofold, as seen with cisplatin because of renal toxicity, or to as high as 18-fold in the case of thiotepa (Table 19-3).[178–184] However, when agents are combined into a high-dose regimen, overlapping extramedullary tox-

icities of the agents must be considered in order to avoid serious new additive and/or synergistic toxicities (Table 19-4). Overlapping extramedullary toxicities (particularly the risk of pulmonary or hepatic dysfunction or secondary leukemia) cannot be completely avoided, but rational drug selection can minimize the dose reductions of the individual agents, compared to their single-agent maximum tolerated dose, that are required to make a combination regimen safe. This is illustrated in Table 19-4, which shows the fraction of the single-agent MTD that can be administered in combination with other drugs. As might be expected, this fraction is quite variable depending on the drug combinations, with the average fractional MTD used in combination ranging from 0.5 to 1. Depending on the regimen, significant gastrointestinal, pulmonary, hepatic, and/or renal toxicities are encountered and become dose limiting. For these reasons, high-dose regimens are safest in patients who are younger (<70 years) and who have had minimal prior chemotherapy and radiation therapy.

MATURING (TERMINAL DIFFERENTIATING) AGENTS

Certain chemical agents have the ability to cause maturation of malignant cells.[190,191] Although referred to as *differentiating* agents, they induce the maturation of a single lineage precursor to its terminal form. The most prominent among these are members of the vitamin A family (carotenes and retinoids), vitamin D and its analogues, phenylacetic acid, various cytotoxic agents used in low concentrations (such as hydroxyurea and 5-azacytidine), and inhibitors of histone deacetylase, exemplified by hexamethylene bisacetamide (HMBA), depsipeptide, and various benzamides.[192] In addition, biologic agents such as the interferons and interleukins induce terminal differentiation of both malignant and normal cells, but the role of terminal differentiation in the anticancer action of these drugs in humans is uncertain, as they have multiple biologic effects. Among the terminal differentiating agents,

TABLE 19-4 TOXICITIES AND DOSES OF HIGH-DOSE REGIMENS ADMINISTERED WITH STEM CELL SUPPORT

REGIMEN	DOSE, MG/M²	FRACTION OF MTD* (AVERAGE)	MAJOR TOXICITIES	TUMOR TARGETS	REFERENCES
Cyclophosphamide	6000	0.86	GI, cardiac	Breast	185
Thiotepa	500	0.5			
Carboplatin	800	0.4 (0.59)			
Cyclophosphamide	6000	0.86	Lung, GI	Lymphomas	186
BCNU	300	0.29			
Etoposide	750	0.25 (0.47)			
Busulfan	640	1.0	Lung, GI, hepatic	Leukemia	187
Cyclophosphamide	8000	1.0 (1.0)		Lymphomas	
Ifosfamide	16,000	1.0	Renal, hepatic, GI	Lymphomas	188
Carboplatin	1800	0.9		Breast	
Etoposide	1500	0.5 (0.8)		Testicular	
Cyclophosphamide	5625	0.8	Cardiac, hepatic, renal	Breast	169
BCNU	600	0.57			
Cisplatin	164	0.82 (0.73)			
Cyclophosphamide	5250	0.75	GI, renal	Breast	189
Etoposide	1200	0.4			
Cisplatin	180	0.9 (0.68)			

BCNU, bischloroethylnitrosourea; GI, gastrointestinal; MTD, maximum tolerated dose.
* This is the fraction of the single-agent MTD (See Table 19-3, Col. 2). Calculation based on Eder et al.[185]

the retinoids are the only drugs that have clearly identified therapeutic value in the treatment and prevention of cancer, although the benzamides and related drugs have produced interesting early results. Most notably, retinoids can drive leukemic promyelocytes to a cell akin to a segmented neutrophil. In so doing, apoptosis of these leukemic neutrophils, former leukemic promyelocytes, occurs, relieving the inhibition of polyclonal hematopoiesis and resulting in a remission in a very high proportion of patients with acute promyelocytic leukemia (APL).

RETINOIDS

As the first effective terminal differentiating agent in cancer therapy, all-*trans*-retinoic acid (ATRA) induces complete responses in a high percentage of patients with APL.[193] ATRA acts through binding to a nuclear receptor formed by the heterodimerization of the RARA receptor and the retinoid X receptor. In APL, an abnormal fusion protein, composed of portions of the RARA receptor and a unique transcription factor (the *PML* gene product) results from the characteristic 15;17 chromosomal translocation found in this disease.[194] The fusion protein has a lower affinity for retinoids than does the wild-type molecule. High concentrations of retinoids are required to displace a corepressor bound to the protein, and activate differentiation.[195] In experimental settings, resistance to ATRA differentiating activity results from mutation in the *PML-RARA* fusion gene, indicating that the fusion gene product plays a role in retinoid responsiveness, and sensitivity can be restored by transfection of a functional *RARA* gene.[196]

ATRA is administered to APL patients in doses of 45 mg/m² per day until complete remission is achieved and reaches peak serum levels of 300 ng/ml 1 to 2 hours after administration.[197] It disappears from serum with a half-life of less than 1 hour during the initial course of treatment, but its rate of clearance greatly accelerates with continued treatment, a factor that may contribute to resistance to ATRA therapy. Induction of CYP-mediated metabolism is suspected to underlie this accelerated clearance, and may account for the high rate of disease recurrence if ATRA is used as a single agent.[198] The primary toxicities of ATRA resemble those of other retinoids and vitamin A, specifically dry skin, cheilitis, mild and reversible hepatic dysfunction, bone tenderness and hyperostosis on x-ray, and occasional cases of pseudotumor cerebri; in addition, approximately 15 percent of patients with APL, particularly those with an initial leukemic cell count greater than 5000/μl, develop a syndrome of hyperleukocytosis, fever, altered mental status, and respiratory failure (the "retinoic acid syndrome").[199] Hyperleukocytosis results from a rapid increase in the number of mature leukemic cells in the blood and from the increased expression of integrins on the leukemic cell surface in response to ATRA. In patients with white blood cell counts above 20 × 10³ cells/μl (20 × 10⁹ cells/ liter), pleural and pericardial effusions and peripheral edema develop rapidly, and respiratory distress, cardiac failure, and renal insufficiency may lead to death. Anecdotal reports indicate that high-dose glucocorticoids reverse this syndrome, which is mediated by leukocyte adhesion and clogging of small vessels and/or by cytokine release.[200] The early introduction of cytotoxic chemotherapy during remission induction, or the use of dexamethasone sodium phosphate (10 mg twice daily for 3 or more days), drastically lowers the incidence of the syndrome and improves the safety of ATRA therapy.

ARSENIC TRIOXIDE

In the 1930s, arsenic was used to treat CML and other malignancies with little effect. Based on further clinical trials of arsenic trioxide (As_2O_3) in Shanghai in the 1990s, it resurfaced as an impressively effective treatment for relapsed promyelocytic leukemia, and appears to also be active against multiple myeloma and myelodysplasia.[201,202]

Its mechanism of action remains obscure.[203] It is readily converted to methylated derivatives, which have uncertain effects. Arsenic trioxide promotes free radical production. It induces maturation and promotes apoptosis in APL cells[203], accelerating degradation of the PML-RAR fusion protein. In addition it has antiangiogenic effects. In a general reactive mechanism, it binds to cysteine-rich sequences of numerous proteins. It alters many signal transduction pathways, up-regulating p53 and other gene products, including caspases, associated with apoptosis. It promotes degradation of NF-κB, a transcription factor that responds to cell damage. The sum of these actions is potent antitumor activity in some but not all tumor cells. In APL patients refractory to ATRA and conventional chemotherapy (see Chap. 87), it produces strikingly durable complete responses, and is therefore under study as a part of primary treatment regimens for this disease.[201]

Patients are treated with a 2-hour IV infusion of 10 mg per day for 60 days, or until bone marrow remission is achieved, with further consolidation therapy beginning 3 weeks after remission. Remissions appear in 2 to 3 months after beginning doses of 0.15 mg/kg/day for 25 days every 3 to 6 weeks, with evidence of leukemic cell differentiation and a progressive peripheral blood leukocytosis after 2 weeks of therapy.[204,205] Side effects of arsenic trioxide in APL may include hyperglycemia, elevated liver enzymes, and hypokalemia, none of which require discontinuation of therapy. Occasional patients complain of fatigue, dysesthesias, and lightheadedness. A pulmonary distress syndrome, similar to that encountered with APL cell maturation after ATRA therapy, occurs in approximately 10 percent of patients, and is managed with glucocorticoids, oxygen, and temporary withholding of arsenic trioxide. Arsenic trioxide prolongs the cardiac QT interval, and uncommonly produces atrial or ventricular arrhythmias; it is important to maintain serum K⁺ at normal concentrations during arsenic trioxide therapy.[206]

A maximum plasma concentration of 5.5 to 7.3 μM was achieved in the initial studies from China, and small amounts of drug are eliminated in the urine, the rest residing in tissues.[207]

THERAPEUTIC MONOCLONAL ANTIBODIES

Monoclonal antibodies are an important new class of agents for the treatment of lymphoid malignancies. As a group, lymphoid cells express a variety of antigens that are attractive targets for monoclonal-based therapy, as shown in Tables 19-5 and 19-6. Development of monoclonal antibodies against specific targets has been largely accomplished by the empiric method of immunizing mice against human tumor cells and screening the hybridomas for antibodies of interest. Because murine antibodies have a short half-life and induce a human antimouse antibody (HAMA) immune response, they are usually chimerized or humanized when used as therapeutic reagents. Presently, several monoclonal antibodies have received Food and Drug Administration approval for non-Hodgkin lymphoma and CLL, including rituximab and alemtuzumab. Although several mechanism(s) of action have been described for monoclonal antibodies, including direct induction of apoptosis, antibody-dependent cellular cytotoxicity (ADCC), and complement-dependent cytotoxicity (CDC), the clinically important mechanisms for most antibodies remain uncertain.[208,209]

Monoclonal antibodies may also be engineered to combine the antibody with a toxin (immunotoxin), or a radioactive isotope (radioimmunoconjugates), or to contain a second specificity (bispecific antibodies) (see Tables 19-5 and 19-6).[210–213] For example, it is possible to conjugate an antibody with specificity to B cell lymphomas with an antibody against CD3, which binds to and activates normal T cells, in order to enhance T-cell-mediated lysis of the lymphoma cell. One such example of a bispecific antibody contains anti-CD3 and anti-CD19 specificity. Monoclonal antibodies raised against the immuno-

TABLE 19-5 MONOCLONAL ANTIBODY-BASED DRUGS

TARGET ANTIGEN AND PRIMARY CELL TYPE	FUNCTION	UNLABELED	RADIOISOTOPE BASED	TOXIN BASED
CD20: B cells	Proliferation/differentiation	Rituximab (chimeric)	^{131}I-tositumomab ^{90}Y-ibritumomab tiuxetan	None
CD22: B cells	Activation	Epratuzumab (humanized)	LL2 [31]Iodine, LL2 [90]Yttrium	BL-22 (*Pseudomonas* toxin)
CD52: B and T cells	Unknown	Alemtuzumab (humanized)	None	None
Tac (CD25 α subunit): B and T cells	Activation	Daclizumab (humanized)	None	Denileukin difitox (diphtheria toxin)

globulin idiotype on a B cell lymphoma represent another therapeutic strategy, which was first reported in 1982 by Miller and associates.[214]

NAKED MONOCLONAL ANTIBODIES

RITUXIMAB

Rituximab is the first monoclonal antibody to receive Food and Drug Administration approval (see Tables 19-5 and 19-6). Rituximab is a chimeric antibody, containing the human immunoglobulin (Ig) G1 and κ constant and murine variable regions, which targets the CD20 B cell antigen.[215,216] CD20 is expressed on the surface of normal B cells and on more than 90 percent of B cell neoplasms, and is present from the pre-B cell stage through terminal differentiation to plasma cells.[217,218] To date, the biologic functions of CD20 remain uncertain, although incubation of B cells with anti-CD20 antibody has variable effects on cell cycle progression, depending on the monoclonal antibody type.[219,220] Mechanistically, monoclonal antibody binding to CD20 generates transmembrane signals that produce a number of events including autophosphorylation and activation of serine/tyrosine protein kinases, and induction of c-myc oncogene expression and major histocompatibility complex class II molecules.[221] Studies show that CD20 is also associated with transmembrane Ca^{2+} conductance through its possible function as a Ca^{2+} channel.[221] These studies demonstrate the importance of CD20 in B cell regulation, but do not in themselves indicate how ligation of the receptor produces cell death independent of ADCC or complement-mediated pathways.

Rituximab was initially approved for relapsed indolent lymphomas, but it has shown activity in a wide variety of clinical settings.[222,223] In the initial phase II study of rituximab in 37 patients with relapsed low-grade lymphoma, 46 percent responded with a median time to progression of 10 months.[216] Notably, rituximab was also shown to be effective in 40 percent of patients who had previously responded to rituximab, with a median time to progression of 18 months.[224] Studies also demonstrate significant activity of rituximab in mantle cell lymphoma, relapsed aggressive B cell lymphomas, and CLL.[215,222,223,225] The use of maintenance rituximab has gained increased acceptance, based on demonstration of delayed time to progression, but effects on survival have not been demonstrated.[226]

Increasingly evident are the synergistic effects of rituximab and chemotherapy, suggesting it sensitizes lymphoma cells to the apoptotic effects of chemotherapy by directly acting on tumor cells.[227,228] Based on *in vitro* studies showing synergistic effects of chemotherapy and rituximab, rituximab is being clinically combined with agents like fludarabine and combinations such as cyclophosphamide, doxorubicin, vincristine, and prednisone (CHOP).[229,230] In one study of 29 patients with indolent lymphoma or leukemia, rituximab and fludarabine produced an overall response rate of 83 percent, of which 35 percent were complete responses.[231] Excellent response rates have also been reported with CHOP plus rituximab, including long durations of remission.[230] Of great importance is the finding that the addition of rituximab to CHOP chemotherapy significantly improves the event-free survival of diffuse large B cell lymphoma patients.[232,233] Rituximab has a limited spectrum of toxicities which are mostly related to infusion reactions (see Table 19-2).[215] However, there are increasing reports of rituximab causing late-onset neutropenia, as well as rare reports of severe skin toxicity.[234]

ALEMTUZUMAB

Alemtuzumab (Campath) is a humanized monoclonal antibody targeted against the CD52 antigen present on the surface of normal neutrophils and lymphocytes as well as most B and T cell lymphomas (see Tables 19-1 and 19-2).[235] CD52 is expressed at reasonable levels and does not modulate with antibody binding, making it a good target for unconjugated monoclonal antibodies. Mechanistically, alemtuzumab can induce tumor cell death through ADCC and CDC (see Table 19-2).[236] Clinical activity has been demonstrated in low-grade lymphomas and CLL, including in patients with purine analogue refractory disease.[237] In refractory CLL, response rates from 33 percent to 59 percent have been described, with higher response rates in patients with untreated CLL.[238] The most concerning side effects are from acute infusion reactions and from depletion of normal neutrophils and T cells (see Table 19-6). Opportunistic infections are a serious side effect, particularly in patients who have received purine analogues, and have resulted in patient deaths.[239] The broad expression of CD52 in T cells has led to the testing of Campath in T cell lymphomas.

TABLE 19-6 DOSE AND TOXICITY OF FDA-APPROVED MONOCLONAL ANTIBODY-BASED DRUGS

DRUG	MECHANISM	DOSE AND SCHEDULE	MAJOR TOXICITY
Rituximab[215,228]	Antibody-dependent cytotoxicity, complement activation, induction of apoptosis	375 mg/m² IV infusion weekly × 4	Infusion related; late-onset neutropenia
Alemtuzumab[249]	Complement activation, antibody-dependent cytotoxicity, possible induction of apoptosis	Escalation 3, 10, 30 mg/m² IV TIW followed by 30 mg/m² TIW for 4 to 12 weeks	Infusion-related toxicity with fever, rash, and dyspnea; T cell depletion with increased infections
[90]Y-ibritumomab tiuxetan[250]	Targeted radiotherapy	0.4 mCi/kg IV	Hematologic toxicity, myelodysplasia
[131]I-tositumomab[247]	Targeted radiotherapy	Patient-specific dosimetry	Hematologic toxicity, myelodysplasia
Denileukin difitox[245]	Targeted diphtheria toxin with inhibition of protein synthesis	9–18 μg/kg/day IV × 5 every 21 days	Fever, arthralgia, asthenia, hypotension

Studies show a high response rate in mycosis fungoides, and investigators at the National Cancer Institute are testing the combination of Campath and dose-adjusted-EPOCH (etoposide, prednisone, vincristine [Oncovin], cyclophosphamide, doxorubicin [hydroxydaunorubicin]) chemotherapy in aggressive T cell lymphomas.[240]

IMMUNOTOXINS

Immunotoxins have been engineered using a variety of antigen and toxin combinations (see Tables 19-5 and 19-6). Traditionally, immunotoxins were developed from the intact monoclonal antibody or its deglycosylated form or the Fab fragment, with conjugation to either ricin A chain or *Pseudomonas* exotoxin. Bioengineered immunotoxins incorporating a single-chain variable-domain fragment, consisting of the antibody variable region, fused to a 38-Kd truncated form of *Pseudomonas* exotoxin A (PE38) have been made.

BL22

BL22 is an immunotoxin that targets the CD22 antigen found on normal B cells and B cell malignancies.[241] In a phase I study, this recombinant immunotoxin containing an anti-CD22 variable domain, fused to truncated pseudomonas exotoxin, was administered in a dose-escalation trial by intravenous infusion every other day for three doses each cycle. Among 16 cladribine-refractory patients with hairy cell leukemia, 11 achieved complete and 2 achieved partial responses.[242] Phase I and II studies are underway and planned to determine the optimal dose and schedule, and to assess its activity against a variety of lymphoid malignancies, including CLL. Of note, their unique spectrum of toxicities, which include vascular leak syndrome and hemolytic uremic syndrome, requires further investigation.

DENILEUKIN DIFTITOX

Denileukin diftitox (Ontak, DAB389 IL-2) is an immunotoxin made from the genetic recombination of IL-2 and the catalytically active fragment of diphtheria toxin.[243] The human IL-2 receptor consists of three discrete subunits, CD25 (α chain, Tac, p55), CD122 (β chain, p70), and CD132 (γ chain, p64), assembled as a trimolecular complex to generate the high-affinity IL-2R. CD25, the low-affinity IL-2R, is incapable of internalizing IL-2, whereas CD122, the β chain of the IL-2R, internalizes IL-2 and has an intermediate affinity. It is in a complex with CD25 that CD122 produces the high affinity IL-2R with a dissociation coefficient two logs higher than the intermediate affinity receptor. The high affinity IL-2R is not expressed on resting T cells but is up-regulated by antigen activation and is constitutively expressed on malignant lymphocytes of both T cell and B cell origin. The limited tissue expression of the high-affinity IL-2R makes this an attractive target for cancer treatments as cells that do not express the IL-2R or express only the intermediate or low affinity receptor are significantly less sensitive to this agent. Toxicities associated with denileukin diftitox are typically acute hypersensitivity reactions, a vascular leak syndrome, and constitutional toxicities; steroid premedication significantly decreases toxicity (Table 19-2).[244] Immunologic reactivity to denileukin diftitox can be detected in virtually all patients after treatment, but does not preclude clinical benefit with continued treatment. Denileukin diftitox clearance is accelerated in later cycles of treatment by two- to threefold as a result of development of antibodies, but serum levels are greater than that required to produce cell death in IL-2R-expressing cells lines (1 to 10 ng/ml for more than 90 minutes). Patients with a history of hypersensitivity reactions to diphtheria toxin or IL-2 should not be treated.

Clinically, denileukin diftitox produced an overall response rate of 30 percent in a phase I study in patients with cutaneous T-cell lymphoma, with a higher response rate at the higher dose levels.[245] In this study, the median duration of response was 6.9 months with a range of 2.7 to 46.1 months, and the median time to response was 6 weeks. Similar response rates were achieved in the phase I/II trials (13/35, 37%). A larger proportion of patients showed clinical benefit but did not meet the objective criteria for response. Denileukin diftitox is being evaluated in patients with CD25-negative tumors, and modulators of CD25 expression are being combined to in an attempt to increase response rates. This latter approach is attractive because it may allow higher levels of intracellular toxin to be delivered. Bexarotene increases the level of CD25 expression on malignant T cells and provides a rationale for combining these agents.[246]

RADIOIMMUNOCONJUGATES

Radioimmunoconjugates provide monoclonal antibody targeted delivery of radioactive particles to tumor cells (see Tables 19-5 and 19-6).[247,248] [131]Iodine (^{131}I) is a commonly used radioisotope because it is readily available, relatively inexpensive, and easily conjugated to a monoclonal antibody. The gamma particles emitted by ^{131}I can be used for both imaging and therapy, but have the drawbacks of releasing free ^{131}I and ^{131}I-tyrosine into the blood and of being a potential health hazard to caregivers. The beta-emitter [90]Yttrium (^{90}Y) has emerged as an attractive alternative to ^{131}I, based on its higher energy and longer path length, which may be more effective in tumors with larger diameters. It also has a short half-life and remains conjugated, even after endocytosis, providing a safer profile for outpatient use. However, its disadvantages include its inability to image, and it is less available and more expensive. Clinically, radioimmunoconjugates have been developed with murine monoclonal antibodies against CD20 conjugated with [131]I (tositumomab or Bexxar) and [90]Y (ibritumomab tiuxetan or Zevalin). Both drugs have shown responses rates in relapsed lymphoma of 65 to 80 percent.[247,248] These agents have been well tolerated with most toxicity attributable to bone marrow suppression. However, there have been worrisome reports of secondary leukemias (see Table 19-2).

Pretargeting has been used to increase the therapeutic index of radioimmunoconjugates by taking advantage of the high binding affinity of avidin and biotin. Patients are initially treated with avidin-labeled monoclonal antibody, followed 1 to 2 days later, after maximal binding of the monoclonal antibody to the target, by administration of yttrium-conjugated biotin. This technique may improve the specificity of radioisotope delivery to tumor cells, and increase the therapeutic index.

GEMTUZUMAB OZOGAMICIN

An alternative to unarmed antibody, or radiolabeled antibody, is the concept of linking a potent toxin, which would otherwise become lethal to the host, to the antibody, thereby limiting exposure to the specific tissue displaying the antigen. The success of this approach depends on stability of the antibody-toxin conjugate, the specificity of binding to tumor, and the ability of the bound antigen to internalize the complex and release the toxin. The most successful application of this approach has been gemtuzumab ozogamicin (Mylotarg), a humanized mouse antibody covalently linked to a chemical toxin. The antibody recognizes CD33, an antigen expressed by more than 90 percent of AML cells but not on normal marrow hematopoietic stem cells (although it is expressed on myeloid progenitor cells). The toxin calicheamicin dimethyl hydrazide is cleaved from the antibody inside the cell and binds to the minor groove of DNA, producing strand breaks and caspase-9-dependent apoptosis.[251] Activation of calicheamicin depends on reduction of an internal disulfide, producing a di-radical that links to deoxyribose sugars on opposing DNA strands.[252]

The antibody conjugate produced a 30 percent complete response rate in relapsed AML, when administered at a dose of 9 mg/m^2 for up to 3 doses at 2-week intervals. Most patients require two to three doses to achieve remission. Its primary toxicities include myelosuppression in all patients treated, and hepatocellular damage in 30 to 40 percent of patients, manifested by hyperbilirubinemia and enzyme elevations. It is also associated with the occurrence of a syndrome that resembles hepatic venoocclusive disease when patients subsequently undergo myeloablative therapy, or when gemtuzumab ozogamicin follows high-dose chemotherapy.[253] The cause of hepatic injury appears to be direct injury to hepatic sinusoids rather than venules. Defibrotide may have value in preventing severe or fatal hepatic injury in patients receiving a stem cell transplant following gemtuzumab ozogamicin.[254] Prolonged myelosuppression, particularly that affecting platelet recovery, has also been observed following remission induction with gemtuzumab ozogamicin.[255]

The pharmacokinetics of gemtuzumab ozogamicin are incompletely understood. Some free toxin is released in the bloodstream and undergoes hepatic degradation, perhaps accounting for the hepatic toxicity. Resistance to Mylotarg may be mediated by export of the calicheamicin by the MDR transporter in tumor cells, by modulation of CD33 expression,[256] or by failure to saturate a high density of CD33 antigen on tumor cells.[257]

REFERENCES

1. Goodman LS, Wintrobe MM, Dameshek W, et al: Nitrogen mustard therapy: Use of methylbis (B-chlorethyl) amino hydrochloride for Hodgkin's disease, lymphosarcoma, leukemia and certain allied and miscellaneous disorders. *JAMA* 132:126, 1946.
2. Farber S, Diamond LK, Mercer RD, et al: Temporary remissions in acute leukemia in children produced by folic acid antagonist, 4-aminopteroylglutamic acid (aminopterin). *N Engl J Med* 238:787, 1948.
3. Devita V, Serpick A, Carbone P: Combination chemotherapy in the treatment of advanced Hodgkin's disease. *Ann Intern Med* 73:881, 1970.
4. Doney K, Fisher LD, Appelbaum FR, et al: Treatment of adult acute lymphoblastic leukemia with allogeneic bone marrow transplantation. Multivariate analysis of factors affecting acute graft-versus-host disease, relapse and relapse-free survival. *Bone Marrow Transplant* 7:453, 1991.
5. Druker BJ, Tamura S, Buchdunger E, et al: Effects of a selective inhibitor of the ABL tyrosine kinase on the growth of BCR-ABL positive cells. *Nat Med* 2:561, 1996.
6. Tse KF, Mukherjee G, Small D: Constitutive activation of FLT3 stimulates multiple intracellular signal transducers and results in transformation. *Leukemia* 14:1766, 2000.
7. Hartwell L: Defects in a cell cycle checkpoint may be responsible for the genomic instability of cancer cells. *Cell* 71:543, 1992.
8. Slamon DJ, Leyland-Jones B, Shak S, et al: Use of chemotherapy plus a monoclonal antibody against HER2 for metastatic breast cancer that overexpresses HER2. *N Engl J Med* 344:783, 2001.
9. Vokes EE, Schilsky RL, Weichselbaum RR, et al: Induction chemotherapy with cisplatin, fluorouracil, and high-dose leucovorin for locally advanced head and neck cancer: A clinical and pharmacologic analysis. *J Clin Oncol* 8:241, 1990.
10. Seitz JF, Giovanni M, Padaut-Cesana J, Fuentes C: Inoperable nonmetastatic squamous cell carcinoma of the esophagus managed by concomitant chemotherapy (5-fluorouracil and cisplatin) and radiation therapy. *Cancer* 66:214, 1990.
11. Willett CG, Boucher Y, Di Tomaso E, et al: Direct evidence that the VEGF-specific antibody bevacizumab has antivascular effects in human rectal cancer. *Nat Med* 10:145, 2004.
12. Leichman L, Nigro N, Vaitkevicius VK, et al: Cancer of the anal canal: Model for preoperative adjuvant combined modality therapy. *Am J Med* 78:211, 1985.
13. Omura GA, Bundy BN, Berek JS, et al: Randomized trial of cyclophosphamide plus cisplatin with or without doxorubicin in ovarian carcinoma: A Gynecologic Oncology Group study. *J Clin Oncol* 7:457, 1989.
14. Bruno R, Hille D, Riva A, et al: Population pharmacokinetics/pharmacodynamics of docetaxel in phase II studies in patients with cancer. *J Clin Oncol* 16:187, 1998.
15. Kruh GD, Zeng H, Rea PA, et al: MRP subfamily transporters and resistance to anticancer agents. *J Bioenerg Biomembr* 33:493, 2001.
16. Boorst P, Oude Elferink R: Mammalian ABC transporters in health and disease. *Annu Rev Biochem* 71:537, 2002.
17. Goker E, Waltham M, Kheradpour A, et al: Amplification of the dihydrofolate reductase gene is a mechanism of acquired resistance to methotrexate in patients with acute lymphoblastic leukemia and is correlated with p53 gene mutations. *Blood* 86:677, 1995.
18. Nimmanapalli R, Bhalla K: Mechanisms of resistance to imatinib mesylate in Bcr-Abl-positive leukemias. *Curr Opin Oncol* 14:616, 2002.
19. Fink D, Aebi S, Howell S: The role of DNA mismatch repair in drug resistance. *Clin Cancer Res* 4:1, 1998.
20. Kirsch D, Kastan M: Tumor-suppressor p53: Implications for tumor development and prognosis. *J Clin Oncol* 16:3158, 1998.
21. Hannun Y: Apoptosis and the dilemma of cancer chemotherapy. *Blood* 89(6):1845, 1997.
22. Moscow JA, Connolly T, Myers TG, et al: Reduced folate carrier gene (RFC1) expression and anti-folate resistance in transfected and nonselected cell lines. *Int J Cancer* 72:184, 1997.
23. Barrado JC, Synold TW, Laver J, et al: Co-administration of probenecid, an inhibitor of a cMOAT/MRP-like plasma membrane ATPase, greatly enhanced the efficacy of a new 10-deazaaminopterin against human solid tumors *in vivo. Clin Cancer Res* 6:3705, 2000.
24. Galpin A, Schuetz J, Mason E, et al: Differences in folylpolyglutamate synthetase and dihydrofolate reductase expression in human B-lineage versus T-lineage leukemic lymphoblasts: Mechanisms for lineage differences in methotrexate polyglutamylation and cytotoxicity. *Mol Pharmacol* 52:155, 1997.
25. Masson E, Relling MV, Synold TW, et al: Accumulation of methotrexate polyglutamates in lymphoblasts is a determinant of antileukemic effects *in vivo*. A rationale for high-dose methotrexate. *J Clin Invest* 97:73, 1996.
26. Synold TW, Relling MV, Boyett JM, et al: Blast cell methotrexate polyglutamate accumulation *in vivo* differs by lineage, ploidy, and methotrexate dose in acute lymphoblastic leukemia. *J Clin Invest* 94:1996, 1994.
27. Longo GS, Gorlick R, Tong WP, et al: Gamma-glutamyl hydrolase and folylpolyglutamate synthetase activities predict polyglutamylation of methotrexate in acute leukemia. *Oncol Res* 9:259, 1997.
28. Assaraf YG, Rothem L, Hooijberg JH, et al: Loss of multidrug resistance protein 1 expression and folate efflux activity results in a highly concentrative folate transport in human leukemia cells. *J Biol Chem* 278:6680, 2003.
29. Stoller RG, Hande KR, Jacobs SA, et al: Use of plasma pharmacokinetics to predict and prevent methotrexate toxicity. *N Engl J Med* 297:630, 1977.
30. Evans W, Crom W, Abromowitch M, et al: Clinical pharmacodynamics of high-dose methotrexate in acute lymphocytic leukemia: Identification of a relation between concentration and effect. *N Engl J Med* 314:471, 1986.
31. Wall SM, Johansen MJ, Maloney DA, et al: Effective clearance of methotrexate using high-flux hemodialysis membranes. *Am J Kidney Dis* 28:846, 1996.

32. Widemann BC, Balis FM, Murphy RF, et al: Carboxypeptidase-G2, thymidine, and leucovorin rescue in cancer patients with methotrexate-induced renal dysfunction. *J Clin Oncol* 15:2125, 1997.

33. Shapiro WR, Allen JC, Horten BC: Chronic methotrexate toxicity to the central nervous system. *Clin Bull Memorial-Sloan Kettering* 10:49, 1980.

34. Bloomfield CD, Lawrence D, Byrd JC, et al: Frequency of prolonged remission duration after high-dose cytarabine intensification in acute myeloid leukemia varies by cytogenetic subtype. *Cancer Res* 58:4173, 1998.

35. Stam RW, Den Boer ML, Meijerink JPP, et al: Differential mRNA expression of Ara-C sensitivity in MLL gene-rearranged infant acute lymphoblastic leukemia. *Blood* 101(4):1270, 2003.

36. Kufe DW, Munroe D, Herrick D, et al: Effects of 1-β-D-arabinofuranosylcytosine incorporation on eukaryotic DNA template function. *Mol Pharmacol* 26:128, 1984.

37. Owens JK, Shewach DS, Ullman B, Mitchell RS: Resistance to 1-β-D-arabinofuranosylcytosine in human T-lymphoblasts mediated by mutations within the deoxycytidine kinase gene. *Cancer Res* 52:2389, 1992.

38. Flasshove M, Strumberg D, Ayscue L, et al: Structural analysis of the deoxycytidine kinase gene in patients with the acute myeloid leukemia and resistance to cytosine arabinoside. *Leukemia* 8:780, 1993.

39. Capizzi RL, Powell BL: Sequential high-dose ara-C and asparaginase versus high-dose ara-C alone in the treatment of patients with relapsed and refractory acute leukemias. *Semin Oncol* 14(Suppl 1):40, 1987.

40. Glantz MJ, Jaeckle KA, Chamberlain MC, et al: A Randomized controlled trial comparing intrathecal sustained-release cytarabine (DepoCyt) to intrathecal methotrexate in patients with neoplastic meningitis from solid tumors. *Clin Cancer Res* 5:3394, 1999.

41. Cole BF, Glantz MJ, Jaeckle KA, et al: Quality-of-life-adjusted survival comparison of sustained-release cytosine arabinoside versus intrathecal methotrexate for treatment of solid tumor neoplastic meningitis. *Cancer* 97:3053, 2003.

42. Kern W, Kurrle E, Schmeiser T: Streptococcal bacteremia in adult patients with leukemia undergoing aggressive chemotherapy. A review of 55 cases. *Infection* 18:138, 1990.

43. Herzig RH, Hines JD, Herzig GP, et al: Cerebellar toxicity with high-dose cytosine arabinoside. *J Clin Oncol* 5:927, 1987.

44. Walter RB, Joerger M, Pestalozzi BC: Gemcitabine-associated hemolytic-uremic syndrome. *Am J Kidney Dis* 40(4):E16, 2002.

45. Claus R, Lubbert M: Epigenetic targets in hematopoietic malignancies. *Oncogene* 22:6489, 2003.

46. Ley TJ, DeSimone J, Anagnon NP, et al: 5-Azacytidine selectively increases gamma chain synthesis in a patient with β-thalassemia. *N Engl J Med* 307:1469, 1982.

47. Kantarjian HM, O'Brien S, Cortes J, et al: Results of decitabine (5-aza-2'-deoxycytidine) therapy in 130 patients with chronic myelogenous leukemia. *Cancer* 98:522, 2003.

48. Rodriguez CO Jr, Stellrecht CM, Gandhi V: Mechanisms for T cell selective cytotoxicity of arabinosylguanine. *Blood* 102(5):1842, 2003.

49. Christie NT, Drake S, Meyn RE, et al: 6-Thiopurine-induced DNA damage as a determinant of cytotoxicity in cultured Chinese hamster ovary cells. *Cancer Res* 44:3665, 1984.

50. Lilleyman J, Lennard L: Mercaptopurine metabolism and risk of relapse in childhood lymphoblastic leukaemia. *Lancet* 343:1188, 1994.

51. Lennard L, Lillyman JS: Are children with lymphoblastic leukaemia given enough 6-mercaptopurine? *Lancet* 2:785, 1987.

52. Lennard L, Lilleyman JS, Van Loon J, Weinshilboum RM: Genetic variation in response to 6-mercaptopurine for childhood acute lymphoblastic leukaemia. *Lancet* 336:225, 1990.

53. Zimm S, Collins JM, Riccardi R, et al: Variable bioavailability of oral 6-mercaptopurine: Is maintenance chemotherapy in acute lymphoblastic leukemia being optimally delivered? *N Engl J Med* 308:1005, 1983.

54. Erb N, Janka-Schaub G: Pharmacokinetics and metabolism of thiopurines in children with acute lymphoblastic leukemia receiving 6-thioguanine versus 6 mercaptopurine. *Cancer Chemother Pharmacol* 42:266, 1998.

55. Harms DO, Gobel U, Spaar HJ, et al: Thioguanine offers no advantage over mercaptopurine in maintenance treatment of childhood ALL: Results of the randomized trial COALL-92. *Blood* 102(8):2736, 2003.

56. Keating MJ, O'Brien S, Lerner S, et al: Long-term follow-up of patients with chronic lymphocytic leukemia (CLL) receiving fludarabine regimens as initial therapy. *Blood* 92(4):1165, 1998.

57. Slavin S, Nagler A, Naparstek E, et al: Nonmyeloablative stem cell transplantation and cell therapy as an alternative to conventional bone marrow transplantation with lethal cytoreduction for the treatment of malignant and nonmalignant hematologic diseases. *Blood* 91(3):756, 1998.

58. Brockman RW, Cheng Y-C, Schabel FM Jr, et al: Metabolism and chemotherapeutic activity of 9-β-D-arabinofuranosyl-2-fluoroadenine against murine leukemia L1210 and evidence for its phosphorylation by deoxycytidine kinase. *Cancer Res* 40:3610, 1980.

59. Gandhi V, Plunkett W: Cellular and clinical pharmacology of fludarabine. *Clin Pharmacokinet* 41(2):93, 2002.

60. Martell RE, Peterson BL, Cohen HJ, et al: Analysis of age, estimated creatine clearance and pretreatment hematologic parameters as predictors of fludarabine toxicity in patients treated for chronic lymphocytic leukemia: A CALGB (9011) coordinated intergroup study. *Cancer Chemother Pharmacol* 50:37, 2002.

61. Lichtman SM, Etcubanas E, Budman DR, et al: The pharmacokinetics and pharmacodynamics of fludarabine phosphate in patients with renal impairment: A prospective dose adjustment study. *Cancer Invest* 20:904, 2002.

62. Cheson B, Frame J, Vena D, et al: Tumor lysis syndrome: an uncommon complication of fludarabine therapy of chronic lymphocytic leukemia. *J Clin Oncol* 16:2313, 1998.

63. Cheson BD: Immunologic and immunosuppressive complications of purine analogue therapy. *J Clin Oncol* 13:2431, 1995.

64. Helman DL Jr, Byrd JC, Ales NC, et al: Fludarabine-related pulmonary toxicity: A distinct clinical entity in chronic lymphoproliferative syndromes. *Chest* 122(3):785, 2002.

65. Estey EH, Kurzrock R, Kantarjin HM, et al: Treatment of hairy cell leukemia with 2-chlorodeoxyadenosine (2-CdA). *Blood* 79:882, 1992.

66. Kay AC, Saven A, Carrera CJ, et al: 2-Chlorodeoxyadenosine treatment of low-grade lymphomas. *J Clin Oncol* 10:371, 1992.

67. Albertoni F, Lindemalm S, Reichelova V, et al: Pharmacokinetics of cladribine in plasma and its 5-monophosphate and 5-triphosphate in leukemic cells of patients with chronic lymphocytic leukemia 1. *Clin Cancer Res* 4:653, 1998.

68. Beutler E: Cladribine (2-chlorodeoxyadenosine). *Lancet* 340:952, 1992.

69. Crews KR, Wimmer PS, Hudson JQ, et al: Pharmacokinetics of 2-chlorodeoxyadenosine in a child undergoing hemofiltration and hemodialysis for acute renal failure. *J Pediatr Hematol Oncol* 24(8):677, 2002.

70. Hunsucker SA, Spychala J, Mitchell BS: Human cytosolic 5'-nucleotidase I: Characterization and role in nucleoside analog resistance. *J Biol Chem* 276(13):10498, 2001.

71. Steis R, Urba WJ, Kopp WC, et al: Kinetics of recovery of CD4+ cells in peripheral blood of deoxycoformycin-treated patients. *J Natl Cancer Inst* 83:1678, 1992.

72. Sterkers Y, Preudhomme C, Lai J-L, et al: Acute myeloid leukemia and myelodysplastic syndromes following essential thrombocythemia treated with hydroxyurea: High proportion of cases with 17p deletion. *Blood* 91:616, 1998.

73. Madoc-Jones H, Mauro F: Interphase action of vinblastine and vincristine: Differences in their lethal action through the mitotic cycle of cultured mammalian cells. *J Cell Physiol* 72:185, 1968.

74. Cabral FR, Brady RC, Schiber MJ: A mechanism of cellular resistance to drugs that interfere with microtubule assembly. *Ann N Y Acad Sci* 46: 748, 1986.

75. Rowinsky EK, Donehower RC: Paclitaxel (Taxol). *N Engl J Med* 332: 1004, 1995.

76. Lopes NM, Adams EG, Pitts TW, et al: Cell kill kinetics and cell cycle effects of Taxol on human hamster ovarian cell lines. *Cancer Chemother Pharmacol* 32:235, 1993.

77. Zaffaroni N, Pennati M, Colella G, et al: Expression of the anti-apoptotic gene survivin correlates with Taxol resistance in human ovarian cancer. *Cell Mol Life Sci* 59:1406, 2002.

78. Anand S, Penrhyn-Lowe S, Venkitaraman AR: AURORA-A amplification overrides the mitotic spindle assembly checkpoint, inducing resistance to Taxol. *Cancer Cell* 3(1):51, 2003.

79. Gianni L, Vigano L, Locatelli A, et al: Human pharmacokinetic characterization and in vitro study of the interaction between doxorubicin and paclitaxel in patients with breast cancer. *J Clin Oncol* 15:1906, 1997.

80. Semb K, Aamdal S, Oian P: Capillary protein leak syndrome appears to explain fluid retention in cancer patients who receive docetaxel treatment. *J Clin Oncol* 16(10):3426, 1998.

81. Wartmann M, Altmann KH: Biology and medicinal chemistry of epothilones. *Curr Med Chem* 2:123, 2002.

82. Ohno R, Okada K, Masaoka T, et al: An early phase II study of CPT-11: A new derivative of camptothecin, for the treatment of leukemia and lymphoma. *J Clin Oncol* 8:1907, 1990.

83. Beran M, Kantarjian H, Obrien S, et al: Topotecan, a topoisomerase I inhibitor, is active in the treatment of myelodysplastic syndrome and chronic myelomonocytic leukemia. *Blood* 88:2473, 1996.

84. Beran M, Estey E, O'Brien S, et al: Topotecan and cytarabine is an active combination regimen in myelodysplastic syndromes and chronic myelomonocytic leukemia. *J Clin Oncol* 17:2819, 1999.

85. Kantarjian HM, Beran M, Ellis A, et al: Phase I study of topotecan, a new topoisomerase I inhibitor, in patients with refractory or relapsed acute leukemia. *Blood* 81:1146, 1993.

86. Iyer L, King C, Whitington P, et al: Genetic predisposition to the metabolism of irinotecan (CPT-11). Role of uridine glucuronosyltransferase isoform 1A1 in the glucuronidation of its active metabolite (SN-38) in human liver microsomes. *J Clin Invest* 101:847, 1998.

87. Grochow LB, Rowinski EK, Johnson R, et al: Pharmacokinetics and pharmacodynamics of topotecan in patients with advanced cancer. *Drug Metab Dispos* 20:706, 1992.

88. Rowinsky EK, Kaufmann SH, Baker, SD, et al: A phase I and pharmacological study of topotecan infused over 30 minutes for five days in patients with refractory acute leukemia. *Clin Cancer Res* 2:1921, 1996.

89. Moreb JS, Oblon DJ: Outcome of clinical congestive heart failure induced by anthracycline chemotherapy. *Cancer* 70:2637, 1992.

90. Speyer JL, Green MD, Kramer E, et al: Protective effect of the bispiperazinedione, ICRF-187, against doxorubicin-induced cardiac toxicity in women with advanced breast cancer. *N Engl J Med* 319:745, 1988.

91. Olson LE, Bedja D, Alvey SJ, et al: Protection from doxorubicin-induced cardiac toxicity in mice with a null allele of carbonyl reductase 1. *Cancer Res* 63(20):6602, 2003.

92. Lipschultz SE, Colan SD, Gelber RD, et al: Late cardiac effects of doxorubicin in therapy for acute lymphoblastic leukemia in childhood. *N Engl J Med* 324:808, 1991.

93. Nysom K, Holm K, Lipsita S: Relationship between cumulative anthracycline dose and late cardiotoxicity in childhood acute lymphoblastic leukemia. *J Clin Oncol* 16(2):545, 1998.

94. Odom LF, Gordon EM: Acute monoblastic leukemia in infancy and early childhood: Successful treatment with an epipodophyllotoxin. *Blood* 64:875, 1984.

95. Capranico G, Zunino F: Antitumor inhibitors of DNA topoisomerases. *Curr Pharm Des* 1:1, 1995.

96. Zwelling LA, Hinds M, Chan D, et al: Characterization of an amsacrine-resistant line of human leukemia cells. Evidence for a drug resistant form of topoisomerase II. *J Biol Chem* 264:16411, 1989.

97. Buggs BY, Danks MK, Beck WT, Suttle DP: Expression of a mutant topoisomerase II in CCRF-CEM human leukemia cells selected for resistance to teniposide. *Proc Natl Acad Sci U S A* 88:7654, 1991.

98. Stewart CF, Arbuck SG, Fleming RA, et al: Changes in the clearance of total and unbound etoposide in patients with liver dysfunction. *J Clin Oncol* 8:1874, 1990.

99. Winick N, McKenna R, Shuster JJ, et al: Secondary acute myeloid leukemia in children with B-lineage acute lymphoblastic leukemia treated with an epipodophyllotoxin. *J Clin Oncol* 11:209, 1993.

100. Ratain MJ, Kaminer LS, Bitran JD, et al: Acute nonlymphocytic leukemia following etoposide and cisplatin combination chemotherapy for advanced non-small-cell carcinoma of the lung. *Blood* 70:1412, 1987.

101. Umezawa H, Maeda K, Takeuchi T, et al: New antibiotics, bleomycin A and B. *J Antibiot (Tokyo)*; 19:200, 1966.

102. Petering DH, Byrnes RW, Antholine WE: The role of redox-active metals in the mechanism of action of bleomycin. *Chem Biol Interact* 73: 133, 1990.

103. Burger R: Cleavage of nucleic acids by bleomycin. *Chem Rev* 98:1153, 1998.

104. Sebti SM, Jani JP, Mistry JS, et al: Metabolic inactivation: A mechanism of human tumor resistance to bleomycin. *Cancer Res* 51:227, 1991.

105. Alberts DS, Chen HSG, Liu R, et al: Bleomycin pharmacokinetics in man: I. Intravenous administration. *Cancer Chemother Pharmacol* 1: 177, 1978.

106. Karmiol S, Remick DG, Kunkel SL, Phan SL: Regulation of rat pulmonary endothelial cell interleukin-6 production by bleomycin: Effects of cellular fatty acid composition. *Am J Respir Cell Mol Biol* 9:628, 1993.

107. Comis RL: Detecting bleomycin pulmonary toxicity: A continued conundrum. *J Clin Oncol* 8:765, 1990.

108. Hutson RG, Kitoh T, Moraga Amador DA: Amino acid control of asparagine synthetase: relation to asparaginase resistance in human leukemia cells. *Am J Physiol* 272:1691, 1997.

109. Kaspers GJ, Veerman AJ, Pieters R, et al: *In vitro* cellular drug resistance and prognosis in newly diagnosed childhood acute lymphoblastic leukemia. *Blood* 90:2723, 1997.

110. Den Boer ML, Harms DO, Pieters R, et al: Patient stratification based on prednisolone-vincristine-asparaginase resistance profiles in children with acute lymphoblastic leukemia. *J Clin Oncol* 21(17):3262, 2003.

111. Asselin BL, Whitin JC, Coppola DJ, et al: Comparative pharmacokinetic studies of three asparaginase preparations. *J Clin Oncol* 101(7):2743, 1993.

112. Holle LM: Pegaspargase: An alternative? *Ann Pharmacother* 31:616, 1997.

113. Asselin BL, Whitin JC, Coppola DJ, et al: Comparative pharmacokinetic studies of three asparaginase preparations. *J Clin Oncol* 11:1770, 1993.

114. Semeraro N, Montemurro P, Giordano P, et al: Unbalanced coagulation fibrinolysis potential during L-asparaginase therapy in children with acute lymphoblastic leukaemia. *Thromb Haemost* 64:38, 1990.

115. Bushara KO, Rust RS: Reversible MRI lesions due to pegaspargase treatment of non-Hodgkin's lymphoma. *Pediatr Neurol* 17:185, 1997.

116. Michell LG, PARKAA Group: A prospective cohort study determining the prevalence of thrombotic events in children with acute lymphoblastic leukemia and a central venous line who are treated with L-asparaginase. *Cancer* 97(2):508, 2003.

117. Nowak-Gottl U, Wermes C, Junker R, et al: Prospective evaluation of the thrombotic risk in children with acute lymphoblastic leukemia car-

rying the MTHFR TT 677 genotype, the prothrombin G20210A variant, and further prothrombotic risk factors. *Blood* 93:1595, 1999.

118. Parsons SK, Skapek SX, Neufeld EJ, et al: Asparaginase-associated lipid abnormalities in children with acute lymphoblastic leukemia. *Blood* 89:1886, 1997.

119. Druker B: Perspectives on the development of a molecularly targeted agent. *Cancer Cell* 1:31, 2002.

120. Heinrich MC, Griffith DJ, Drucker BJ, et al: Inhibition of c-kit receptor tyrosine kinase by STI 571, a selective tyrosine kinase inhibitor. *Blood* 96:925, 2000.

121. Demetri GD, von Mehren M, Blanke CD, et al: Efficacy and safety of imatinib mesylate in advanced gastrointestinal stromal tumors. *N Engl J Med* 347(7):472, 2002.

122. Cools J, DeAngelo D, Gotlib J, et al: A tyrosine kinase created by fusion of the PDGFRA and FIP1L1 genes as a therapeutic target of imatinib in idiopathic hypereosinophilic syndrome. *N Engl J Med* 348(13):1201, 2003.

123. Magnusson MK, Meade KE, Nakamura R, et al: Activity of STI571 in chronic myelomonocytic leukemia with a platelet-derived growth factor β receptor fusion oncogene. *Blood* 100(3):1088, 2002.

124. Sirvent N, Maire G, Pedeutour F: Genetics of dermatofibrosarcoma protuberans family of tumors: From ring chromosomes to tyrosine kinase inhibitor treatment. *Genes Chromosomes Cancer* 37:1, 2003.

125. Wisniewski D, Lambek CL, Liu C, et al: Characterization of potent inhibitors of the Bcr-Abl and the c-Kit receptor tyrosine kinases. *Cancer Res* 62:4244, 2002.

126. Gambacorti-Passerini C, Piazza R, D'Incalci M: Bcr-Abl mutations, resistance to imatinib, and imatinib plasma levels [letter]. *Blood* 102(5):1933, 2003.

127. Takayama N, Sato N, O'Brien SG, et al: Imatinib mesylate has limited activity against the central nervous system involvement of Philadelphia chromosome-positive acute lymphoblastic leukemia due to poor penetration into cerebrospinal fluid. *Br J Haematol* 119:106, 2002.

128. Gambacorti-Passerini C, Zucchetti M, Russo D, et al: α1 Acid glycoprotein binds to imatinib (STI571) and substantially alters its pharmacokinetics in chronic myeloid leukemia patients. *Clin Cancer Res* 9:625, 2003.

129. Kantarjian H, Talpaz M, O'Brien S, et al: Dose escalation of imatinib mesylate can overcome resistance to standard-dose therapy in patients with chronic myelogenous leukemia. *Blood* 101(2):473, 2003.

130. Shah NP, Nicoll JM, Nagar B, et al: Multiple BCR-ABL kinase domain mutations confer polyclonal resistance to the tyrosine kinase inhibitor imatinib (STI571) in chronic phase and blast crisis chronic myeloid leukemia. *Cancer Cell* 2:117, 2002.

131. Corbin AS, La Rosee P, Stoffregen EP, et al: Several Bcr-Abl kinase domain mutants associated with imatinib mesylate resistance remain sensitive to imatinib. *Blood* 101(11):4611, 2003.

132. Azam M, Latek RR, Daley GQ: Mechanisms of autoinhibition and STI571/imatinib resistance revealed by mutagenesis of BCR-ABL. *Cell* 112:831, 2003.

133. Roche-Lestienne C, Lai JL, Darre S, et al: A mutation conferring resistance to imatinib at the time of diagnosis of chronic myelogenous leukemia [letter]. *N Engl J Med* 348(22):2265, 2003.

134. Hofmann WK, Komor M, Wassmann B, et al: Presence of the BCR-ABL mutation Glu255Lys prior to STI571 (imatinib) treatment in patients with Ph+ acute lymphoblastic leukemia. *Blood* 102(2):659, 2003.

135. Banford S, Rudzki Z, Walsh S, et al: Detection of BCR-ABL mutations in patients with CML treated with imatinib is virtually always accompanied by clinical resistance, and mutations in the ATP phosphate-binding loop (P-loop) are associated with a poor prognosis. *Blood* 102(1):276, 2003.

136. Morel F, Bris MJ, Herry A, et al: Double minutes containing amplified bcr-abl fusion gene in a case of chronic myeloid leukemia treated by imatinib. *Eur J Haematol* 70:235, 2003.

137. Mahon FX, Belloc F, Lagarde V, et al: MDR1 gene overexpression confers resistance to imatinib mesylate in leukemia cell line models. *Blood* 101(6):2368, 2003.

138. La Rosee P, Corbin A, Stoffregen EP, et al: Activity of the Bcr-Abl kinase inhibitor PD180970 against clinically relevant Bcr-Abl isoforms that cause resistance to imatinib mesylate. *Cancer Res* 62:7149, 2002.

139. Nimmanapalli R, Fuino L, Bali P, et al: Histone deacetylase inhibitor LAQ824 both lowers expression and promotes proteasomal degradation of Bcr-Abl and induces apoptosis of imatinib mesylate-sensitive or -refractory chronic myelogenous leukemia-blast crisis cells. *Cancer Res* 63:5126, 2003.

140. Hoover RR, Mahon FX, Melo JV, Daley GQ: Overcoming STI571 resistance with the farnesyl transferase inhibitor SCH66336. *Blood* 100(3):1068, 2002.

141. Nimmanapalli R, O'Bryan E, Huang M, et al: Molecular characterization and sensitivity of STI-571 (imatinib mesylate, Gleevec)-resistant, Bcr-Abl-positive, human acute leukemia cells to SRC kinase inhibitor PD180970 and 17-allylamino-17-demethoxygeldanamycin. *Cancer Res* 62:5761, 2002.

142. Bumm T, Muller C, Al-Ali HK, et al: Emergence of clonal cytogenic abnormalities in Ph- cells in some CML patients in cytogenetic remission to imatinib but restoration of polyclonal hematopoiesis in the majority. *Blood* 101(5):1941, 2003.

143. Andersen MK, Pedersen-Bjergaard J, Kjeldsen L, et al: Clonal Ph-negative hematopoiesis in CML after therapy with imatinib mesylate is frequently characterized by trisomy 8 [letter]. *Leukemia* 16:1390, 2002.

144. Kantarjian H, Sawyers C, Hochhaus A, et al: Hematologic and cytogenetic responses to imatinib mesylate in chronic myelogenous leukemia. *N Engl J Med* 346(9):645, 2002.

145. Philip S, Bermon, S: A spectrum of skin reactions caused by the tyrosine kinase inhibitor imatinib mesylate (STI 571, Glivec). *Br J Haematol* 120:907, 2003.

146. Jagannath S, Barlogie B, Berenson J, et al: A phase II multicenter randomized study of the proteasome inhibitor bortezomib (Velcade, formerly PS-341) in multiple myeloma patients relapsed after front-line therapy. *Blood* 100:3027, 2002.

147. Richardson PG, Barlogie B, Berenson J, et al: A phase 2 study of bortezomib in relapsed, refractory myeloma, *N Engl J Med* 348:2609, 2003.

148. Adams J: Development of the proteasome inhibitor PS-341. *Oncologist* 7(1):9, 2002.

149. Ma MH, Yang HH, Parker K, et al: The proteasome inhibitor PS-341 markedly enhances sensitivity of multiple myeloma tumor cells to chemotherapeutic agents. *Clin Cancer Res* 9:1136, 2003.

150. Hideshima T, Mitsiades C, Akiyama M, et al: Molecular mechanisms mediating antimyeloma activity of proteasome inhibitor PS-341. *Blood* 101(4):1530, 2003.

151. Hideshima T, Richardson P, Chauhan D, et al: The proteasome inhibitor PS-341 inhibits growth, induces apoptosis, and overcomes drug resistance in human multiple myeloma cells. *Cancer Res* 61:3071, 2001.

152. Mitchell BS: The proteasome—An emerging therapeutic target in cancer. *N Engl J Med* 348(26):2597, 2003.

153. Kane RC, Bross PF, Farrell AT, Pazdur R: Velcade: U.S. FDA approval for the treatment of multiple myeloma progressing on prior therapy. *Oncologist* 8:508, 2003.

154. Calderon P, Anzilotti M, Phelps R: Thalidomide in dermatology. New indications for an old drug. *Int J Dermatol* 1997;36:881.

155. D'Amato RJ, Loughnan MS, Flynn E, et al: Thalidomide is an inhibitor of angiogenesis. *Proc Natl Acad Sci U S A* 91:4082, 1994.

156. Moreira AL, Friedlander DR, Shif B, et al: Thalidomide and a thalidomide analogue inhibit endothelial cell proliferation *in vitro*. *J Neurooncol* 43(2):109, 1999.

157. Mueller G, Chen R, Huang SY. et al: Amino-substituted thalidomide analogs: potent inhibitors of TNF-alpha production. *Bioorg Med Chem Lett* 9:1625, 1999.

158. Richardson PG, Schlossman RL, Weller E, et al: Immunomodulatory drug CC-5013 Overcomes drug resistance and is well tolerated in patients with relapsed multiple myeloma. *Blood* 100:3063, 2002.

159. LeBlanc R, Hideshia T, Catley L, et al: Immunomodulatory drug co-stimulates T- cells via B7-CD28 pathway. *Blood* 103:1787, 2004.

160. Teo SK, Scheffler MR, Kook KA, et al: Thalidomide dose proportionality assessment following single doses to healthy subjects. *J Clin Pharmacol* 41(6):662, 2001.

161. Piscitelli SC, Figg WD, Hahn B, et al: Single-dose pharmacokinetics of thalidomide in human immunodeficiency virus-infected patients. *Antimicrob Agents Chemother* 41(12):2797, 1997.

162. Singhal S, Mehta J, Desikan R, et al: Antitumor activity of thalidomide in refractory multiple myeloma. *N Engl J Med* 341:1565, 1999.

163. Mileshikin L, Biagi J, Underhil C, et al: Multicenter phase 2 trial of thalidomide in relapsed/refractory multiple myeloma: Adverse prognostic impact of advanced age. *Blood* 102:69, 2003.

164. Mitsiadis N, Mitsiadis CS, Poulaki V: Biologic sequelae of nuclear factor-kappa B blockade in multiple myeloma: Therapeutic applications. *Blood* 99:4079, 2002.

165. Rajkumar SV, Hayman S, Gertz M, et al: Combination therapy with thalidomide plus dexamethasone for newly diagnosed myeloma. *J Clin Oncol* 20:4319, 2002.

166. Barlogie B, Shaughnessey J, Tricot G, et al: Treatment of multiple myeloma. *Blood* 103:20, 2004.

167. Nathan PD, Gore ME, Eisen TG. Unexpected toxicity of combination thalidomide and interferon-alpha-2a treatment in metastatic renal cell carcinoma. *J Clin Oncol* 20:1429, 2002.

168. Mitsiades N, Mitsiadis CS, Poulaki V, et al: Apoptotic signaling induced by immunomodulatory thalidomide analogs in human multiple myeloma cells: Therapeutic implications. *Blood* 99:4525, 2002.

169. Peters WP, Shpall EJ, Jones RB, et al: High-dose combination alkylating agents with bone marrow support as initial treatment for metastatic breast cancer. *J Clin Oncol* 6:1368, 1988.

170. Yeager AM, Kaizer H, Santos GW, et al: Autologous bone marrow transplantation in patients with acute nonlymphocytic leukemia using ex vivo marrow treatment with 4-hydroperoxycyclophosphamide. *N Engl J Med* 315:141, 1986.

171. Reed E: Platinum-DNA adduct, nucleotide excision repair and platinum based anti-cancer chemotherapy. *Cancer Treat Rev* 24:331, 1998.

172. Gurubhagavatula S, Liu G, Park S, et al: XPD and XRCC1 genetic polymorphisms are prognostic factors in advanced non-small cell lung cancer patients treated with platinum chemotherapy. *J Clin Oncol* 22:2594, 2004.

173. Tew KD, Colvin M, Chabner BA: Alkylating agents, in *Cancer Chemotherapy and Biotherapy: Principles and Practice*, 3rd ed, edited by BA Chabner, DL Longo, p 297. Lippincott, Philadelphia, 2001.

174. Hilton J: Role of aldehyde dehydrogenase in cyclophosphamide-resistant L1210 leukemia. *Cancer Res* 44:5156, 1984.

175. Erickson L: The role of *O*-6 methylguanine DNA methyltransferase (MGMT) in drug resistance and strategies for its inhibition. *Sem Cancer Biol* 2:257, 1991.

176. Droller MJ, Saral R, Santos G: Prevention of cyclophosphamide-induced hemorrhagic cystitis. *Urology* 20:256, 1982.

177. Schacht RG, Baldwin DS: Chronic interstitial nephritis and renal failure due to nitrosourea (NU) therapy. *Kidney Int* 14:661, 1978.

178. Gianni AM, Bregni M, Siena S, et al: Recombinant human granulocyte-macrophage colony stimulating factor reduces hematologic toxicity and widens clinical applicability of high-dose cyclophosphamide treatment in breast cancer and non-Hodgkin's lymphoma. *J Clin Oncol* 8:768, 1990.

179. Elias AD, Eder JP, Shea T, et al: High-dose ifosfamide with mesna uroprotection: A phase I study. *J Clin Oncol* 8:170, 1990.

180. Lazarus HM, Reed MD, Spitzer TR, et al: High-dose IV thiotepa and cryopreserved autologous bone marrow transplantation for therapy of refractory cancer. *Cancer Treat Rep* 71:689, 1987.

181. Peters WP, Henner WD, Grochow LB, et al: Clinical and pharmacologic effects of high dose single agent busulfan with autologous bone marrow support in the treatment of solid tumors. *Cancer Res* 47:6402, 1987.

182. Phillips GL, Wolff SN, Fay JW, et al: Intensive 1,3-bis(2-chloroethyl)-1-nitrosourea (BCNU) monochemotherapy and autologous marrow transplantation for malignant glioma. *J Clin Oncol* 4:639, 1986.

183. Ozols RF, Corden BJ, Jacob J, et al: High dose cisplatin in hypertonic saline. *Ann Intern Med* 100:19, 1984.

184. Shea TC, Flaherty M, Elias A, et al: A phase I clinical and pharmacokinetic study of carboplatin and autologous bone marrow support. *J Clin Oncol* 7:651, 1989.

185. Eder JP, Elias A, Shea TC, et al: A phase I-II study of cyclophosphamide, thiotepa, and carboplatin with autologous bone marrow transplantation in solid tumor patients. *J Clin Oncol* 8:1239, 1990.

186. Kessinger A, Armitage JO, Smith DM, et al: High-dose therapy and autologous peripheral blood stem cell transplantation for patients with lymphoma. *Blood* 74:1260, 1989.

187. Jones RJ, Piantadosi S, Mann RB, et al: High-dose cytotoxic therapy and bone marrow transplantation for relapsed Hodgkin's disease. *J Clin Oncol* 8:527, 1990.

188. Wilson WH, Jain V, Bryant G, et al: Phase I and II study of high-dose ifosfamide, carboplatin, and etoposide with autologous bone marrow rescue in lymphomas and solid tumors. *J Clin Oncol* 10:1712, 1992.

189. Dunphy FR, Spitzer G, Buzdar AU, et al: Treatment of estrogen receptor-negative or hormonally refractory breast cancer with double high-dose chemotherapy intensification and bone marrow support. *J Clin Oncol* 8:1207, 1990.

190. Kizaki M, Nakazato T, Ito K, et al: A novel therapeutic approach for hematological malignancies based on cellular differentiation and apoptosis. *Int J Hematol* 1(Suppl 1):250, 2002.

191. Parkinson DR, Smith MA: Retinoid therapy for acute promyelocytic leukemia: A coming of age for the differentiation therapy of malignancy [editorial]. *Ann Intern Med* 117:338, 1992.

192. Sandor V, Bakke S, Robey RW, et al: Phase I trial of the histone deacetylase inhibitor, depsipeptide (FR901228, NSC 630176), in patients with refractory neoplasms. *Clin Cancer Res* 8:718, 2002.

193. Warrell RP Jr, Frankel SR, Miller WH Jr, et al: Differentiation therapy of acute promyelocytic leukemia with tretinoin (all-*trans*-retinoic acid). *N Engl J Med* 324:1385, 1991.

194. Kazizuka A, Miller WH Jr, Umesono K, et al: Chromosomal translocation t(15;17) in human acute promyelocytic leukemia fuses RARα with a novel putative transcription factor, PML. *Cell* 66:663, 1991.

195. Lin RJ, Nagy L, Inoue S, et al: Role of the histone deacetylase complex in acute promyelocytic leukemia. *Nature* 391:811, 1998.

196. Robertson KA, Emami B, Collins SJ: Retinoic acid-resistant HL-60R cells harbor a point mutation in the retinoic acid receptor ligand binding domain that confers dominant negative activity. *Blood* 80:1885, 1992.

197. Muindi JRF, Frankel SR, Huselton C, et al: Clinical pharmacology of oral all-*trans*-retinoic acid in patients with acute promyelocytic leukemia. *Cancer Res* 52:2138, 1992.

198. Muindi J, Frankel SR, Miller WH Jr, et al: Continuous treatment with all-*trans*-retinoic acid causes a progressive reduction in plasma drug concentrations: Implications for relapse and retinoid "resistance" in patients with acute promyelocytic leukemia. *Blood* 79:299, 1992.

199. Frankel SR, Eardley A, Lauwers G, et al: The "retinoic acid syndrome" in acute promyelocytic leukemia. *Ann Intern Med* 117:292, 1992.

200. De Botton S, Dombret H, Sanz M, et al: Incidence, clinical features, and outcome of all-*trans*-retinoic acid syndrome in 413 cases of newly diagnosed acute promyelocytic leukemia. *Blood* 92(8):2712, 1998.

201. Soignet SL, Maslak P, Wang Z-G, et al: Complete remission after treatment of acute promyelocytic leukemia with arsenic trioxide. *N Engl J Med* 339(19):1341, 1998.

202. List AF, Schiller GJ, Mason J, et al: Trisenox (arsenic trioxide) in patients with myelodysplastic syndromes (MDS): Preliminary findings in a phase 2 clinical study [abstract]. *Blood* 102(11):423a, 2003.

203. Miller WH Jr, Schipper HM, Lee JS, et al: Mechanisms of action of arsenic trioxide. *Cancer Res* 62:3893, 2002.

204. Mulford DA, Maslak PG, Weiss MA, et al: Reducing standard postremission chemotherapy in acute promyelocytic leukemia (APL) with risk-adapted therapy [abstract]. *Blood* 102(11):619a, 2003.

205. Chen G-Q, Shi X-G, Tang W, et al: Use of arsenic trioxide (As$_2$O$_3$) in the treatment of acute promyelocytic leukemia (APL): I. As$_2$O$_3$ exerts dose-dependent dual effects on APL cells. *Blood* 89:3345, 1997.

206. Shen Z-X, Chen G-Q, Ni J-H, et al: Use of arsenic trioxide (As$_2$O$_3$) in the treatment of acute promyelocytic leukemia (APL): II. Clinical efficacy and pharmacokinetics in relapsed patients. *Blood* 89(9):3354, 1997.

207. Shen ZX, Chen GQ, Ni JH, et al: Use of arsenic trioxide (As$_2$O$_3$) in the treatment of acute promyelocytic leukemia (APL): II. Clinical efficacy and pharmacokinetics in relapsed patients. *Blood* 89(9):3354, 1997.

208. Mathas SBK, Dorken B, Mapara MY: Anti-CD20 antibody mediated apoptosis is dependent on caspase 3 activation [abstract]. *Proc Am Soc Hematol* 92:1671, 1998.

209. Shan D, Ledbetter JA, Press OW: Apoptosis of malignant human B cells by ligation of CD20 with monoclonal antibodies. *Blood* 91:1644, 1998.

210. Onda M, Wang QC, Guo HF, et al: *In vitro* and *in vivo* cytotoxic activities of recombinant immunotoxin 8H9(Fv)-PE38 against breast cancer, osteosarcoma, and neuroblastoma. *Cancer Res* 64:1419, 2004.

211. Withoff S, Helfrich W, De Leij LF, Molema G: Bi-specific antibody therapy for the treatment of cancer. *Curr Opin Mol Ther* 3:53, 2001.

212. Withoff S, Bijman MN, Stel AJ, et al: Characterization of BIS20x3, a bi-specific antibody activating and retargeting T-cells to CD20-positive B-cells. *Br J Cancer* 84:1115, 2001.

213. Silverman DH, Delpassand ES, Torabi F, et al: Radiolabeled antibody therapy in non-Hodgkins lymphoma: radiation protection, isotope comparisons and quality of life issues. *Cancer Treat Rev* 30:165, 2004.

214. Miller RA, Maloney DG, Warnke R, Levy R. Treatment of B-cell lymphoma with monoclonal anti-idiotype antibody. *N Engl J Med* 306:517, 1982.

215. Maloney DG, Liles TM, Czerwinski DK, et al: Phase I clinical trial using escalating single-dose infusion of chimeric anti-CD20 monoclonal antibody (IDEC-C2B8) in patients with recurrent B-cell lymphoma. *Blood* 84:2457, 1994.

216. Maloney DG, Grillo-Lopez AJ, White CA, et al: IDEC-C2B8 (Rituximab) anti-CD20 monoclonal antibody therapy in patients with relapsed low-grade non-Hodgkin's lymphoma. *Blood* 90:2188, 1997.

217. Stashenko P, Nadler LM, Hardy R, Schlossman SF: Characterization of a human B lymphocyte-specific antigen. *J Immunol* 125:1678, 1980.

218. Bhan AK, Nadler LM, Stashenko P, et al: Stages of B cell differentiation in human lymphoid tissue. *J Exp Med* 154:737, 1981.

219. Tedder TF, Forsgren A, Boyd AW, et al: Antibodies reactive with the B1 molecule inhibit cell cycle progression but not activation of human B lymphocytes. *Eur J Immunol* 16:881, 1986.

220. Smeland E, Godal T, Ruud E, et al: The specific induction of myc protooncogene expression in normal human B cells is not a sufficient event for acquisition of competence to proliferate. *Proc Natl Acad Sci U S A* 82:6255, 1985.

221. Deans JP, Schieven GL, Shu GL, et al: Association of tyrosine and serine kinases with the B cell surface antigen CD20. Induction via CD20 of tyrosine phosphorylation and activation of phospholipase C-gamma 1 and PLC phospholipase C-gamma 2. *J Immunol* 151:4494, 1993.

222. Coiffier B, Haioun C, Ketterer N, et al: Rituximab (anti-CD20 monoclonal antibody) for the treatment of patients with relapsing or refractory aggressive lymphoma: A multicenter phase II study. *Blood* 92:1927, 1998.

223. Foran JM, Rohatiner AZ, Cunningham D, et al: European phase II study of rituximab (chimeric anti-CD20 monoclonal antibody) for patients with newly diagnosed mantle-cell lymphoma and previously treated mantle-cell lymphoma, immunocytoma, and small B-cell lymphocytic lymphoma. *J Clin Oncol* 18:317, 2000.

224. Davis TA, Grillo-Lopez AJ, White CA, et al: Rituximab anti-CD20 monoclonal antibody therapy in non-Hodgkin's lymphoma: safety and efficacy of re-treatment. *J Clin Oncol* 18:3135, 2000.

225. O'Brien SM, Kantarjian H, Thomas DA, et al: Rituximab dose-escalation trial in chronic lymphocytic leukemia. *J Clin Oncol* 19:2165, 2001.

226. Hainsworth JD: Prolonging remission with rituximab maintenance therapy. *Semin Oncol* 31:17, 2004.

227. Reed JC, Kitada S, Kim Y, Byrd J: Modulating apoptosis pathways in low-grade B-cell malignancies using biological response modifiers. *Semin Oncol* 29:10, 2002.

228. Maloney DG, Smith B, Rose A: Rituximab: Mechanism of action and resistance. *Semin Oncol* 29:2, 2002.

229. Alas S, Bonavida B, Emmanouilides C: Potentiation of fludarabine cytotoxicity on non-Hodgkin's lymphoma by pentoxifylline and rituximab. *Anticancer Res* 20:2961, 2000.

230. Czuczman MS, Fallon A, Mohr A, et al: Rituximab in combination with CHOP or fludarabine in low-grade lymphoma. *Semin Oncol* 29:36, 2002.

231. Savage DG, Cohen NS, Hesdorffer CS, et al: Combined fludarabine and rituximab for low grade lymphoma and chronic lymphocytic leukemia. *Leuk Lymphoma* 44:477, 2003.

232. Coiffier B, Lepage E, Briere J, et al: CHOP chemotherapy plus rituximab compared with CHOP alone in elderly patients with diffuse large-B-cell lymphoma. *N Engl J Med* 346:235, 2002.

233. Wilson WH PS, Pittaluga S, Gutierrez M, et al: Dose-adjusted EPOCH-rituximab in untreated diffuse large B-cell lymphoma: Benefit of rituximab appears restricted to tumors harboring anti-apoptotic mechanisms. *Proc Am Soc Hematol* 102:105a, 2003.

234. Lemieux B, Tartas S, Traulle C, et al: Rituximab-related late onset neutropenia after autologous stem cell transplantation for aggressive non-Hodgkin's lymphoma. *Bone Marrow Transplant* 33:921, 2004.

235. Kumar S, Kimlinger TK, Lust JA, et al: Expression of CD52 on plasma cells in plasma cell proliferative disorders. *Blood* 102:1075, 2003.

236. Villamor N, Montserrat E, Colomer D: Mechanism of action and resistance to monoclonal antibody therapy. *Semin Oncol* 30:424, 2003.

237. Rai KR, Freter CE, Mercier RJ, et al: Alemtuzumab in previously treated chronic lymphocytic leukemia patients who also had received fludarabine. *J Clin Oncol* 20:3891, 2002.

238. Osterborg A, Dyer MJ, Bunjes D, et al: Phase II multicenter study of human CD52 antibody in previously treated chronic lymphocytic leukemia. European Study Group of CAMPATH-1H Treatment in Chronic Lymphocytic Leukemia. *J Clin Oncol* 15:1567, 1997.

239. Tang SC, Hewitt K, Reis MD, Berinstein NL. Immunosuppressive toxicity of CAMPATH1H monoclonal antibody in the treatment of patients with recurrent low grade lymphoma. *Leuk Lymphoma* 24:93, 1996.

240. Kennedy GA, Seymour JF, Wolf M, et al: Treatment of patients with advanced mycosis fungoides and Sézary syndrome with alemtuzumab. *Eur J Haematol* 71:250, 2003.

241. Cesano A, Gayko U: CD22 as a target of passive immunotherapy. *Semin Oncol* 30:253, 2003.

242. Kreitman RJ, Wilson WH, Bergeron K, et al: Efficacy of the anti-CD22 recombinant immunotoxin BL22 in chemotherapy-resistant hairy-cell leukemia. *N Engl J Med* 345:241, 2001.

243. Foss FM. Interleukin-2 fusion toxin: targeted therapy for cutaneous T cell lymphoma. *Ann N Y Acad Sci* 941:166, 2001.

244. Foss FM, Bacha P, Osann KE, et al: Biological correlates of acute hypersensitivity events with DAB(389)IL-2 (denileukin diftitox, ONTAK) in cutaneous T-cell lymphoma: Decreased frequency and severity with steroid premedication. *Clin Lymphoma* 1:298, 2001.

245. Olsen E, Duvic M, Frankel A, et al: Pivotal phase III trial of two dose levels of denileukin diftitox for the treatment of cutaneous T-cell lymphoma. *J Clin Oncol* 19:376, 2001.

246. Gorgun G, Foss F: Immunomodulatory effects of RXR rexinoids: Modulation of high-affinity IL-2R expression enhances susceptibility to denileukin diftitox. *Blood* 100:1399, 2002.

247. Kaminski MS, Zelenetz AD, Press OW, et al: Pivotal study of iodine I 131 tositumomab for chemotherapy-refractory low-grade or transformed low-grade B-cell non-Hodgkin's lymphomas. *J Clin Oncol* 19:3918, 2001.

248. Gordon LI, Witzig TE, Wiseman GA, et al: Yttrium 90 ibritumomab tiuxetan radioimmunotherapy for relapsed or refractory low-grade non-Hodgkin's lymphoma. *Semin Oncol* 29:87, 2002.

249. Ferrajoli A, O'Brien SM, Cortes JE, et al: Phase II study of alemtuzumab in chronic lymphoproliferative disorders. *Cancer* 98:773, 2003.

250. Wiseman GA, Kornmehl E, Leigh B, et al: Radiation dosimetry results and safety correlations from 90Y-ibritumomab tiuxetan radioimmunotherapy for relapsed or refractory non-Hodgkin's lymphoma: Combined data from 4 clinical trials. *J Nucl Med* 44:465, 2003.

251. Prokop A, Wrasidlo W, Lode H, et al: Induction of apoptosis by enediyne antibiotic calicheamicin theta II proceeds through a caspase-mediated mitochondrial amplification loop in an entirely Bax-dependent manner. *Oncogene* 22(57):9107, 2003.

252. Zein N, Sinha AM, McGahren WJ, et al: Calicheamicin gamma 1: An antitumor antibiotic that cleaves double-stranded DNA site specifically. *Science* 240:1198, 1988.

253. Wadleigh M, Richardson P, Zahreieh D, et al: Prior gemtuzumab ozogamicin exposure significantly increases the risk of veno-occlusive disease in patients who undergo myeloablative allogenic stem cell transplantation. *Blood* 102:1578, 2003.

254. Versluys B, Bhattacharaya R, Steward C, et al: Prophylaxis with defibrotide prevents veno-occlusive disease in stem cell transplantation after gemtuzumab ozogamicin exposure. *Blood* 103(5):1968, 2004.

255. Tomblyn MR, Tallman MS: New developments in antibody therapy for acute myeloid leukemia. *Semin Oncol* 30(4):502, 2003.

256. Naito K, Takeshita A, Shigeno K, et al: Calicheamicin-conjugated humanized anti-CD33 monoclonal antibody (gemtuzumab zogamicin, CMA-676) shows cytocidal effect on CD33-positive leukemia cell lines, but is inactive on P-glycoprotein-expressing sublines. *Leukemia* 14: 1436, 2000.

257. Van der Velden VH, Boeckx N, Jedema I, et al: High CD33-antigen loads in peripheral blood limit the efficacy of gemtuzumab ozogamicin (Mylotarg) treatment in acute myeloid leukemia patients. *Leukemia* 18(5):983, 2004.

TREATMENT OF INFECTIONS IN THE IMMUNOCOMPROMISED HOST

STEVEN M. BEUTLER

Infection is a major cause of morbidity and mortality in patients receiving chemotherapy for treatment of hematologic neoplasms. Severe neutropenia and monocytopenia often result from the combined effects of replacement of marrow with malignant cells and superimposed intense chemotherapy. The severity and duration of the neutropenia determine the risk of infection. Bacterial infections may result in rapid clinical deterioration and, if not treated appropriately, death. Fungal, viral, and parasitic infections also may result in potentially lethal complications during and after chemotherapy. Methods of diagnosis of bacterial, fungal, viral, and protozoal infection are considered and treatment regimens described. The introduction of home antibiotic therapy is noted and may be appropriate for certain patients. Because prevention of infection during periods of neutropenia should reduce morbidity and improve outcome, attention is focused on various means of prophylaxis of bacterial, parasitic, viral, and fungal infections.

The profound pancytopenia that results from cytoreductive chemotherapy is a common and dramatic manifestation of hematopoietic suppression. During the periods of neutropenia that follow such chemotherapy, infection develops in most patients. Patients with neoplasms of the lymphoid system commonly manifest altered humoral and cellular immunity, resulting in an increased incidence of nonbacterial infection.

RISK FACTORS AND INFECTING ORGANISMS

SEVERITY OF NEUTROPENIA

Bacterial, fungal, viral, and parasitic organisms may cause infection in neutropenic patients. Bacterial infections are the most frequent and usually the most serious. The risk for bacterial infection increases when the neutrophil count falls to less than $500/\mu l$ (0.5×10^9/liter) and becomes especially pronounced at neutrophil counts less than 100 ml (0.1×10^9/liter; see Fig. 20-1).[1] The rate of decline and duration of granulocyte count are important in determining the risk of bacterial infection. Disruption of mucosal barriers, especially in the oral cavity, esophagus, and bowel, further favors the development of infection by providing portals of entry.

BACTERIAL PATHOGENS

Historically, gram-negative bacilli have been the most commonly isolated pathogens. These organisms include *Pseudomonas*, *Klebsiella*,

Escherichia coli, and *Proteus*. These bacteria are responsible for a variety of infections, including pneumonia, soft tissue infections, perirectal infections, and primary bacteremia. Urinary tract infections are infrequent unless a urinary catheter is present or urinary tract obstruction has developed. Meningitis is uncommon.

During the past 2 decades, the incidence of gram-positive infection has increased.[2] Staphylococcal species, enterococcus, and *Corynebacterium* are now the pathogens most frequently isolated from neutropenic patients. This finding may result, in part, from the popularity of semipermanent venous catheters and from the use of prophylactic regimens that are active against gram-negative rods. Several reports document the increasing frequency of *Streptococcus viridans* as a major pathogen in neutropenic patients,[3] especially in those receiving marrow transplant, perhaps because these patients have a higher incidence of mucositis. Septic shock may occur in these patients.[4] Anaerobic infections are less common unless periodontal or gastrointestinal pathology coexists.

Patients with Hodgkin lymphoma, other lymphomas, or chronic lymphocytic leukemia primarily suffer from impaired cell-mediated immunity and diminished antibody production.[5] Consequently, the spectrum of infections in these patients differs from that found in neutropenic patients. Bacterial infections, when they occur, tend to result from encapsulated organisms such as *Pneumococcus* or *Haemophilus*. *Listeria* and *Nocardia* infections also are seen more frequently in this group of patients.

FUNGAL PATHOGENS

Fungal infections are common during periods of prolonged neutropenia and in patients with lymphomas or chronic lymphocytic leukemia. *Candida* species are most frequently isolated, but *Aspergillus* and *Phycomycetes* also are found. The gastrointestinal tract serves as a reservoir for candidiasis (thrush), and erosive esophagitis may develop. *Candida* may enter the bloodstream via indwelling catheters. *Aspergillus* and *Phycomycetes* tend to colonize and infect the sinuses and bronchopulmonary tree. Because cell-mediated immunity is required for defense against fungal infections, infections with *Cryptococcus*, *Aspergillus*, *Coccidioides*, *Histoplasma*, and *Candida* are more common in patients with leukemia or lymphoma who have required chronic glucocorticoid treatment.

VIRAL PATHOGENS

Viral infections are especially frequent in patients with impaired cell-mediated immunity. Among viruses that cause infections in immunocompromised hosts, herpes simplex, varicella zoster, cytomegalovirus (CMV), and adenoviruses are the most important. Cutaneous lesions and mucositis often are caused by herpes simplex. Herpes zoster infections may be especially severe and have a propensity for dissemination. Left untreated, primary varicella infections are associated with a high mortality rate. CMV may cause febrile illnesses associated with pneumonia, hepatitis, and/or gastrointestinal tract ulcerations. This virus may be isolated by culture or demonstrated by the presence of viral antigens or viral DNA in clinical specimens.[6] Respiratory infections resulting from respiratory syncytial virus (RSV) have been documented in approximately 18 percent of marrow transplant recipients with pulmonary symptoms during the winter months.[7] Influenza virus, picornavirus, and other viruses have been isolated.

PROTOZOAL PATHOGENS

Pneumocystis carinii (now called *Pneumocystis jiroveci*), a ubiquitous, endogenous parasite, may cause pneumonia in neutropenic patients and in those with defective cell-mediated immunity. It often becomes clinically evident after glucocorticoids have been tapered or discontin-

---

Acronyms and abbreviations that appear in this chapter include: CMV, cytomegalovirus; MRSA, methicillin-resistant *Staphylococcus aureus*; RSV, respiratory syncytial virus; VRE, vancomycin-resistant enterococcus.

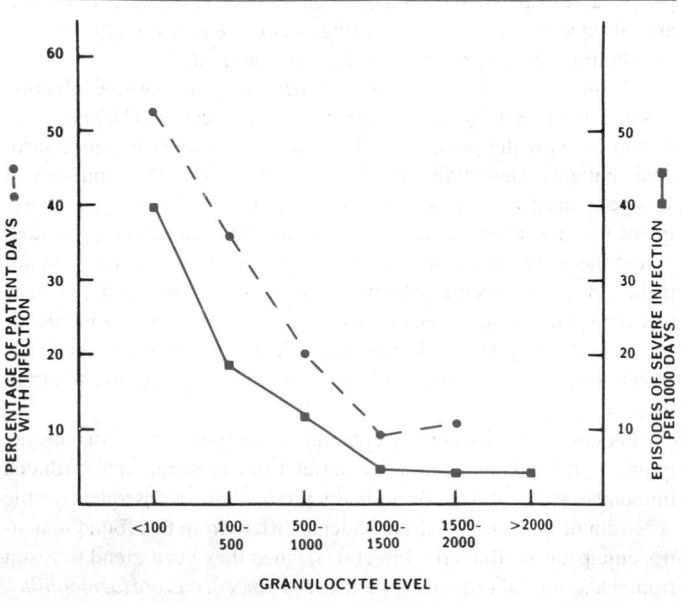

FIGURE 20-1   Relationship between granulocyte count and percentage of patient days with infection (●---●) and episodes of severe infections per 1000 days (■---■). (Based on data from Bodey et al.[1])

ued. *Toxoplasma gondii*, another protozoan parasite, may be responsible for brain abscesses in patients with lymphoma or chronic lymphocytic leukemia, especially in those treated with glucocorticoids. Glucocorticoid-treated patients also are at risk for *Strongyloides* hyperinfection.

MYCOBACTERIAL INFECTIONS

The association between lymphoid malignancies and tuberculosis has been recognized for more than a century and threatens to become a more frequent, serious problem with the resurgence of tuberculosis and the increased prevalence of drug-resistant strains.[8] Atypical mycobacterial infections are very common in HIV-positive patients but are fairly rare in patients receiving chemotherapy.

RECOGNITION AND DIAGNOSIS OF INFECTION

The development of an infection in a neutropenic patient may be accompanied by dramatic clinical manifestations or by none at all. Any fever that develops is very suggestive of infection. However, hypothermia, declining mental status, myalgias, or lethargy also may indicate infection in these patients. The usual local signs of infection may be absent or delayed because they are mediated by neutrophils.[9]

A careful physical examination should be performed when such a change in condition is observed. Special attention should be paid to the mouth and teeth for evidence of thrush or periodontal disease. The skin should be examined in detail. Innocuous-appearing skin lesions may be septic emboli. Trivial injuries inflicted by venipuncture or intravenous catheters may become infected and result in septicemia. An increased incidence of perianal and perirectal infection is observed in neutropenic patients.[10] Examination of the rectum may provide a clue to the source of fever in patients without other clinical findings. Although such examinations should not be performed unnecessarily on an immunocompromised patient, rectal or pelvic examination should not be deferred when searching for a cause of fever.

Chest x-ray films should be obtained initially and may need to be repeated, although this practice has been questioned in patients without respiratory complaints.[11] Chest computed tomography may reveal le-

sions not detected on routine radiograms.[12] Sinus x-ray films may be helpful if symptoms are present.

Blood cultures should be collected prior to institution of antibiotic therapy and periodically thereafter if fever persists. If an indwelling venous catheter is present, some of the cultures should be obtained from the catheter. The common practice of separating blood cultures by 10 to 15 minutes does not seem to have any physiologic or experimental basis. However, obtaining two to three cultures improves the likelihood of recovering fastidious organisms. To improve the likelihood of isolating fungal pathogens, the specimens should be retained by the laboratory for at least 10 days. Urine and sputum cultures may be helpful. Results of the latter, however, must be interpreted with caution, because the results may reflect the flora colonizing the oropharynx rather than the pathogens infecting the lung. Skin lesions of a suspicious nature should be biopsied and cultured. Stools should be examined for *Clostridium difficile* toxin in patients with diarrhea. Potentially infected intravenous lines should be cultured upon removal. Nasal cultures may be useful in predicting pulmonary aspergillosis.[13] Fungal and viral infections, which may be difficult to document using conventional culture techniques, may be diagnosed by polymerase chain reaction and antigen detection.[14,15]

Open lung biopsies once were advocated for further evaluation of neutropenic patients with pulmonary infiltrates.[16] However, this procedure should not be routinely performed in immunocompromised patients with pneumonia because the result rarely establishes a treatable diagnosis. The procedure may be useful under certain limited circumstances, for example, when further empiric therapy would be unacceptably toxic in a patient whose clinical condition is deteriorating.

Transbronchial lung biopsies are generally considered unsafe in patients with thrombocytopenia because of the high risk of uncontrolled bleeding. Obtaining material via bronchial brushing or lavage carries a lower risk and may yield useful information.[17]

TREATMENT

INITIAL TREATMENT

BACTERIAL INFECTIONS
The need for prompt, effective therapy is dramatized by the finding that mortality rates approach 100 percent in bacteremic neutropenic patients treated with regimens lacking activity against the organisms subsequently isolated.[18] In contrast, patients receiving appropriate therapy have much lower mortality rates.[19] Therefore, selection of potent, broad-spectrum agents when initiating empiric antimicrobial therapy in the neutropenic patient is critical.[20,21]

In general, antibiotics should be given at the maximum recommended doses (Table 20-1). Aminoglycoside and vancomycin levels should be measured to establish proper doses. High peak levels of aminoglycosides are desirable. The increasingly common practice of administering aminoglycosides as a single, daily dose seems to be effective in neutropenic patients.[22,23] Aminoglycoside selection depends on institutional sensitivity patterns. In the case of β-lactam drugs, frequent or continuous administration following a loading dose ensures constant therapeutic levels and may be advantageous.[24]

Many different regimens have been evaluated and found to be acceptable for empiric therapy in neutropenic patients. Table 20-2 lists several regimens. Generally, combinations of two or three drugs have been favored for initial empiric therapy, but single-drug therapy also may be efficacious. Imipenem,[25] meropenem,[26] cefepime,[27,28] and ceftazidime[24] each has been studied as a single agent. These drugs are active against most of the virulent pathogens infecting neutropenic patients, and subsequent modification of therapy can optimize treatment. Antibiotic toxicity is reduced by omitting the aminoglycoside

TABLE 20-1 MAXIMUM RECOMMENDED DOSES OF ANTIBIOTICS

DRUG CATEGORY	DRUG	BRAND NAME	DOSE	ADJUSTMENT FOR RENAL INSUFFICIENCY	ACTIVITY	TOXICITY
Anti-pseudomonal penicillins	Ticarcillin-clavulanic acid	Timentin	3.1 g q4h	++	Methicillin-sensitive *Staphylococcus*, *Streptococcus*, anaerobes, *Pseudomonas aeruginosa*	Hypokalemia, antiplatelet effect
	Piperacillin-tazobactam	Zosyn	4.5 g q6h	+		
Anti-pseudomonal cephalosporins	Ceftazidime	Fortaz	2 g q8h	+++	*Pseudomonas aeruginosa*, enteric gram-negative rods, methicillin-sensitive *Staphylococcus*	
	Cefepime	Maxipime	2 g q12h			
Aminoglycosides	Amikacin	Amikin	15 (mg/kg)/day[a]	+++	Enteric gram-negative rods, *Pseudomonas aeruginosa*	Nephrotoxicity, ototoxicity
	Tobramycin	Nebcin	4–5 (mg/kg)/day[a]			
	Gentamicin	Garamycin	4–5 (mg/kg)/day[a]			
Glycopeptide	Vancomycin	Vancocin	30 (mg/kg)/day in 2 doses[a]	+++	*Staphylococcus* (including MRSA), *Streptococcus*, *Corynebacterium*	Ototoxicity, red-man syndrome with rapid infusion
Carbapenem	Imipenem	Primaxin	0.5–1 g q6h	++–+++	Gram-negative rods, *Pseudomonas aeruginosa (except for ertapenem)*, methicillin sensitive, *Staphylococcus*, enterococcus, anaerobes	Nausea, seizures (Primaxin)
	Meropenem	Merrem	1 g q8h	+		
	Ertapenem	Invanz	1 g q24h			
Monobactam	Aztreonam	Azactam	2 g q6h	+	Gram-negative rods, *Pseudomonas aeruginosa*	
Sulfonamides	Trimethoprim-sulfamethoxazole	Bactrim; Septra	10–20 (mg/kg)/day (based on trimethoprim) in 2–4 doses/day	++	*Pneumocystis carinii*, gram-negative rods, *Haemophilus*, *Staphylococcus*	Sulfa allergy, increased creatinine, nausea, rash
Fluoroquinolones	Ciprofloxacin	Cipro	500–750 mg q12h PO or 200–400 mg IV q12h	+	Gram-negative rods, *Pseudomonas aeruginosa* (Cipro)	Nausea. Not for use in children
	Levofloxacin	Levaquin	500 mg PO or IV q24h	+++		
Nucleosides	Acyclovir	Zovirax	15 (mg/kg)/day IV [30 (mg/kg)/day IV for encephalitis or for herpes zoster] in 3 divided doses; comparable oral dose approximately twice as high	+–++	Herpes simplex and zoster	Crystalluria
	Valacyclovir	Valtrex	1000 mg bid (tid in herpes zoster) PO	++	Herpes simplex and zoster	
	Famciclovir	Famvir	250–500 mg tid PO	+++	CMV, herpes simplex	
	Ganciclovir	Cytovene	10 (mg/kg)/day in 2 divided doses IV or 1000 mg PO tid	++		Neutropenia
Phosphonoformate	Foscarnet	Foscavir	180 (mg/kg)/day in 3 doses	++	CMV	Renal failure, electrolyte abnormalities
Polyene antifungals	Amphotericin B	Fungizone	0.7–1.0 (mg/kg)/day in a single daily dose over 2–6 h	0	*Candida, Aspergillus, Torulopsis*, other fungus	Nausea, vomiting, chills, fever, renal failure, hypokalemia, hypomagnesemia
	Ampho B lipid complex	Abelcet	5 (mg/kg)/day		*Candida, Aspergillus, Torulopsis*, other fungus	Fever, chills, nausea, vomiting, increased creatinine
	Ampho B cholesteryl sulfate complex	Amphotec	4 (mg/kg)/day		*Candida, Aspergillus, Torulopsis*, other fungus	Fever, chills, nausea, vomiting, increased creatinine
	Ampho B liposomal ampho	AmBisome	5 (mg/kg)/day		*Candida, Aspergillus, Torulopsis*, other fungus	Fever, chills, nausea, vomiting, increased creatinine
	Ampho B colloidal dispersion	Amphocil	6 (mg/kg)/day		*Candida, Aspergillus, Torulopsis*, other fungus	Fever, chills, nausea, vomiting, increased creatinine
Azole	Fluconazole	Diflucan	400 mg/day PO/IV	++	*Candida albicans, Cryptococcus, Coccidioides immitis*, histoplasmosis	LFT abnormality
	Itraconazole	Sporanox	200 mg bid	0	*Aspergillus*	Nausea
	Voriconazole	VFend	300 mg bid			
Echinocandin	Caspofungin	Cancidas	70 mg × 1; then 50 mg qd	0	*Aspergillus*, candida	
Diamidine	Pentamidine	Pentam	4 mg/kg q24h IV	++(?)	*Pneumocystis carinii*	Renal failure, hypotension, hypoglycemia
Oxazolidinone	Linezolid	Zyvox	600 mg q12h PO or IV	0	MRSA, VRE	Thrombocytopenia, anemia
Lipopeptide	Daptomycin	Cubicin			MRSA	

[a] Adjust dose based on levels.

NOTE: 0 = no adjustment required; + = small adjustment for creatinine clearance <20; ++ = moderate adjustment required; +++ = nearly complete renal excretion; dose to be reduced proportionally to renal function.

bid = twice per day; CMV = cytomegalovirus; ESBL = extended-spectrum β-lactamase; IV = intravenous; LFT = liver function tests; MRSA = methicillin-resistant *Staphylococcus aureus*; tid = three times per day.

TABLE 20-2 REGIMENS FOR EMPIRIC THERAPY IN NEUTROPENIC
PATIENTS

Ceftazidime + aminoglycoside ± vancomycin
Imipenem (or meropenem) + aminoglycoside ± vancomycin
Piperacillin + aminoglycoside ± vancomycin
Cefepime + aminoglycoside ± vancomycin
Ciprofloxacin + aminoglycoside
Ciprofloxacin + ceftazidime
"Monotherapy" (imipenem, meropenem, ceftazidime, or cefepime)

from the regimen. However, development of resistant organisms during single-drug therapy is of concern. Aminoglycosides may provide synergy against gram-negative bacilli and further broaden the spectrum of antimicrobial activity. Note that none of these agents is active against methicillin-resistant *Staphylococcus aureus* (MRSA). More than half of the hospital-acquired strains of *Staphylococcus aureus* now are methicillin resistant. Cefepime and ceftazidime lack activity against enterococcus. In addition, over the past 5 years, an increasing prevalence of enteric pathogens, particularly *Klebsiella*, which produce extended-spectrum beta lactamases (ESBLs), has been observed.[29] These organisms are resistant to all cephalosporins and exhibit varying and unpredictable degrees of sensitivity to aminoglycosides and quinolones. The carbapenems (imipenem, meropenem, ertapenem) are active against these pathogens.

No good evidence supports the simultaneous use of two β-lactam drugs. Quinolones, usually in conjunction with another antibiotic, are effective in patients who have not received quinolone prophylaxis.[30]

Use of single-drug therapy cannot be recommended for all patients with stem cell failure. Single-drug therapy may be appropriate for patients with less profound neutropenia, those who are not overtly septic, and those who may have problems tolerating aminoglycosides. Differences in institutional sensitivity patterns influence antibiotic selection.

Vancomycin-resistant enterococcus (VRE) is being isolated with increasing frequency and presents a major challenge.[31] Synercid (quinupristin/dalfopristin),[32] linezolid (Zyvox),[33] and daptomycin are the only agents currently available for treatment of this pathogen. The latter has not received Food and Drug Administration (FDA) approval for this indication. All three agents are highly active against MRSA. Linezolid causes thrombocytopenia and therefore must be used with caution in patients who are receiving chemotherapy.

Therapeutic use of granulocytes is rarely necessary (see Chap. 25), may result in transmission of CMV disease, and may cause severe reactions.

FUNGAL INFECTIONS

Amphotericin B is the drug of choice for the majority of fungal infections that develop in neutropenic hosts, although its position has been challenged by the introduction of two other medications. The dose of amphotericin should be advanced rapidly so that the full therapeutic dose is given by the first or second day. Serum creatinine, potassium, and magnesium levels should be monitored. Fever and chills associated with administration of this drug may be treated or prevented with meperidine (Demerol) or diphenhydramine hydrochloride (Benadryl) and acetaminophen. This will not be necessary in all patients, and systemic reactions tend to decrease after several doses. Twenty-five to 50 mg of hydrocortisone added to the infusion may attenuate the reactions. Infusions should be given over 2 to 6 hours.

Flucytosine provides synergy against *Cryptococcus neoformans* and some strains of *Candida* but not against *Aspergillus*. The drug is myelotoxic and may cause hepatitis and colitis; therefore, it should not be used routinely for treatment of fungal infections in these patient groups.

Several preparations of liposomal amphotericin B are available.[34] They are more likely than nonliposomal amphotericin B to cause infusion-related symptoms[35] but are less nephrotoxic.[36,37] Higher doses are required to achieve a clinical response, and the cost is considerably greater than that of amphotericin B. Therefore, these formulations should be reserved for patients who have underlying renal insufficiency or who have experienced nephrotoxicity with amphotericin B.

Fluconazole, an azole drug that can be administered orally or intravenously, is approved for treatment of *Candida albicans, C. neoformans,* and *Coccidioides immitis*. It is less active against non-albicans *Candida* species and is completely inactive against *Candida krusei*. It can be used to treat patients with sensitive strains of fungus who cannot tolerate or do not respond to amphotericin B. It has been used as first-line therapy in hepatosplenic candidiasis and may be appropriate for patients with nonsystemic fungal infections.

Voriconazole, a newer azole drug, has consistent activity against *Aspergillus*.[38] It is less toxic than amphotericin and in initial studies led to improved survival rates. It is available in intravenous and oral forms. The intravenous preparation may result in the acute development of visual loss, which is generally temporary and reversible.

Caspofungin is highly active against aspergillus. In addition, it can be used to treat invasive candida infections,[39] including those caused by non-albicans *Candida* such as *C. krusei*.[40] It is available only for intravenous administration.

Itraconazole can be used for treatment of *Aspergillus* infection, although amphotericin, voriconazole, and caspofungin are more active.

VIRAL INFECTIONS

A limited number of options are available for treatment of viral infections. Acyclovir is active against herpes simplex and, at higher doses, against varicella zoster. It is not useful against CMV or Epstein-Barr virus. Newer agents (e.g., famciclovir and valacyclovir) may be administered less frequently but are not available for intravenous administration. Valacyclovir has been shown to be efficacious in the prevention of CMV in renal transplant patients,[41] but otherwise these agents are not well studied in immunosuppressed patients.

Ganciclovir and foscarnet have efficacy in treatment of CMV disease and are also active against herpes simplex. They are most effective when they are used early in the course of the infection. Hence, frequent screening for antigenemia in high-risk (e.g., marrow transplant) patients may allow for improved outcomes.[42] Both agents have been used successfully in conjunction with CMV immunoglobulin for treatment of CMV pneumonia in marrow transplant patients.[43] Ganciclovir results in neutropenia in a significant percentage of patients who receive it. Foscarnet therapy may be complicated by azotemia and electrolyte abnormalities. Ribavirin can be used to treat RSV. Rimantadine should be used if influenza A is suspected.

PARASITIC INFECTIONS

Pneumocystis carinii (now called *Pneumocystis jiroveci*) may be treated with trimethoprim-sulfamethoxazole or with pentamidine. Table 20-1 lists the recommended doses. Other regimens, including dapsone-trimethoprim, primaquine-clindamycin, and atovaquone, have proved efficacious in patients with AIDS but are largely untested in patients with chemotherapy-related immunosuppression.

ADJUSTING THERAPY

Adjustment or modification of the initial antimicrobial regimen may be necessary for several reasons. Results of cultures may suggest another regimen would be more active or less toxic. All cultures may remain negative while the patient fails to respond to the regimen. Fever may recur following an initial response to therapy, raising the possibility of a superinfection.

Adjusting therapy based on a culture report usually is straightforward, but the other two situations may pose dilemmas. In these circumstances, resistant organisms or noninfectious causes of fever must be considered. Repeat cultures and careful clinical reappraisal may prove helpful. Empiric modification of the antibiotic regimen to enhance the effect on gram-positive or fungal pathogens may be successful. Vancomycin is active against gram-positive organisms. Antifungal therapy should be strongly considered if a combination of antibacterial agents proves ineffective after 5 to 7 days of treatment.[21] Addition of a nonsteroidal antiinflammatory agent may eliminate fever caused by tumor or tumor lysis.

DURATION OF THERAPY

Antibiotics usually should be discontinued when the neutropenia resolves or clinical evidence of infection is no longer present. Often however, the fever resolves, while neutropenia is expected to continue for a prolonged period. Antibiotic therapy is commonly continued until the granulocyte count reaches $500/\mu l$ (0.5×10^9/liter). Although this therapy reduces the number of relapsing infections, it likely increases the risk of superinfection and antibiotic toxicity. Marrow recovery may be delayed by cephalosporins and sulfa drugs. Therefore, discontinuing antibiotics after an appropriate course in patients who have responded promptly and completely to therapy is reasonable.[44,45] If antibiotics are discontinued, close observation is required and therapy should be reinstituted at any suggestion of recurrent infection.

The duration of antifungal therapy varies considerably. Parasitic infection with Pneumocystis requires 2 to 3 weeks of therapy. Herpetic infections generally are treated for 7 days.

FEVER FOLLOWING RECOVERY FROM CHEMOTHERAPY

Fevers occasionally persist after the granulocyte count has returned to normal levels. Drug fever is a consideration in this setting, but more commonly a deep-seated infection is present.[46] Pulmonary and hepatic[47] fungal infections must be considered. Elevated serum alkaline phosphatase levels and a characteristic image on computed tomography are common with hepatic involvement.[48] Hepatic ultrasound[49] and magnetic resonance imaging[50] are diagnostically useful, but biopsy may be required to establish the diagnosis. Hepatosplenic candidiasis requires prolonged therapy. Several regimens have been proposed, including fluconazole[51] and liposomal amphotericin B.[52] Cure is difficult to achieve regardless of the regimen used.

Indwelling catheter infection should be considered when fevers continue after marrow recovery.

CATHETER-RELATED INFECTIONS

Minor exit site infections generally respond promptly to antibiotic therapy. Infection of indwelling catheters with Staphylococcus epidermidis and other avirulent pathogens often can be cured with a prolonged course (at least 2 weeks) of an appropriate antibiotic. If a tunnel infection is present, successful therapy is less likely. Gram-negative infections or fungal infections[53] of the catheter usually necessitate its removal. This may be followed, if necessary, by insertion of a new catheter at a different site. Catheters impregnated with antibiotics may resist infection but have not been widely studied in neutropenic patients. Chlorhexidine and silver-impregnated central venous catheters do not appear to prevent bloodstream infections in neutropenic patients.[54] Catheter infections and their management are reviewed elsewhere.[55,56]

OUTPATIENT THERAPY

Ten years ago, treatment of the febrile neutropenic patient outside of the hospital would have been unthinkable. Economic pressures, coupled with the widespread availability of home infusion services and more potent oral antibiotics, have made outpatient therapy an option for some of these patients.[57,58] Outcomes seem to be comparable to those observed in hospitalized patients, provided the patients are selected properly and appropriate monitoring can be ensured. Suitable candidates for home intravenous therapy include patients who are expected to have a short-duration neutropenia. Individuals who remain febrile, who require multiple antibiotics, or who are unreliable are not candidates for home intravenous therapy. Nurses must be experienced in the evaluation of chemotherapy patients and familiar with catheter care and maintenance. Rigorous family education is crucial for a successful outcome.

PREVENTION OF INFECTIONS

BACTERIAL INFECTIONS

In view of the high mortality rate associated with infections in neutropenic patients, preventive measures remain a priority. Instrumentation should be avoided whenever possible. Intravenous access sites should be carefully maintained. The earliest strategies included administration of nonabsorbable oral antibiotics usually consisting of gentamicin, vancomycin, and nystatin.[59] Unfortunately, this combination is poorly tolerated. Therefore, this practice has been abandoned in favor of systemic antibiotics. Trimethoprim-sulfamethoxazole has been especially well studied and is beneficial for some patients, particularly those with severe neutropenia expected to last more than 2 weeks. The therapy has the additional advantage of preventing Pneumocystis, but it causes a rash in 5 to 10 percent of individuals. Its use may be associated with infections with resistant organisms, and it may result in delayed marrow recovery.[60]

The fluorinated quinolones have received considerable attention for their ability to prevent gram-negative infections in neutropenic patients.[61,62] Unfortunately, indiscriminate use of these agents in the community has diminished their value as resistant bacteria have developed.[63] Infection with gram-positive organisms is more common in patients receiving quinolones prophylactically.[64,65] Prophylactic use also eliminates these agents from therapeutic use in the same patient. Quinolone prophylaxis has resulted in an increased incidence of bacteremia with quinolone-resistant S. viridans.[66] For these reasons, some centers have abandoned the use of prophylactic quinolones, at least in some patients.[67,68]

Isoniazid hydrazide therapy is recommended for all tuberculin-positive patients who require chemotherapy unless they have been treated previously.

Prophylactic antibiotics are beneficial for some patients with acute leukemia receiving induction chemotherapy. The best regimen remains to be determined and may vary among institutions. Perhaps equally important for preventing infection is careful attention to sterile technique and personal hygiene.[69]

The ability of granulocyte-macrophage colony stimulating factor and granulocyte colony stimulating factor to raise the granulocyte count in neutropenic patients may prevent bacterial infections in this group of patients. Some series show a small reduction in the infection rate in patients receiving these agents,[70] whereas others do not.[71–73] Although a subset of patients may benefit from this therapy,[74] definitive methods for selecting such patients are lacking.

Various forms of immunotherapy have been reviewed. Intravenous immunoglobulin has been advocated for prevention of bacterial infection in some patients with chronic severe hypogammaglobulinemia, as may occur in chronic lymphocytic leukemia and multiple myeloma, but its value has not been proved.[75] The value of special diets and reverse isolation has not been established. Granulocyte transfusions have no role in the prevention of infection.

PARASITIC INFECTIONS
Pneumocystis jiroveci pneumonia can be prevented with trimethoprim-sulfamethoxazole. Pentamidine administered monthly in aerosolized form also is effective.[76] Although *P. carinii* is a ubiquitous organism, institutional variability in the incidence of infection is observed; therefore, the need for prophylaxis varies.

VIRAL INFECTIONS
Acyclovir has proved useful for prevention of recurrent herpes simplex infections in patients receiving chemotherapy and marrow transplantation.[77,78] Such prophylaxis probably is unnecessary in patients who lack antibodies to herpes simplex virus. Varicella zoster immunoglobulin given to susceptible individuals reduces the incidence of varicella following exposure.

The incidence of CMV infection can be reduced by avoiding blood products from CMV-seropositive individuals.[79] Passive immunization has provided benefit in some studies. Acyclovir is ineffective in treating CMV infections but may reduce their incidence.[80] Ganciclovir[81] and foscarnet[82] have been used successfully to prevent CMV infections in marrow recipients, but these strategies have not been applied to patients receiving conventional chemotherapy.

Active immunizations with killed vaccines (e.g., influenza) are of some benefit. Attenuated vaccines (e.g., measles) should be avoided.

FUNGAL INFECTIONS
Studies on prevention of fungal infections in neutropenic patients are difficult to evaluate. Results of the various studies have been conflicting, partly because different definitions were applied, different doses of antifungal agents were administered, and the numbers of study patients were small.

Nystatin,[83] amphotericin B,[84] clotrimazole,[85] and ketoconazole[86] have been studied. Each has been effective in reducing colonization and mucositis, but none has been consistently effective in preventing systemic fungal infections and improving survival.

Several studies have documented a statistically significant reduction in superficial and invasive fungal infections when fluconazole is used prophylactically.[87,88] However, many failures have been reported, including breakthrough fungemia.[89] Not all studies have documented a benefit of using fluconazole prophylactically.[90,91] Superinfection with *Aspergillus*, *Torulopsis glabrata*, and *C. krusei* has occurred when fluconazole was used prophylactically.[92] Itraconazole may be effective in preventing *Aspergillus* infection.[93]

Thus, although antifungal prophylaxis appears to diminish the incidence of mucositis, close observation and early treatment of mucositis also provide a reasonable approach to this problem. The ability of antifungal agents to prevent systemic infection is not consistent. Prophylactic use of these agents may select more resistant strains of fungus and may not reduce mortality. Therefore, pending the results of additional studies, earlier and more aggressive empiric antifungal therapy may be preferable to prophylaxis.[94] Exceptions to this approach include patients undergoing marrow transplantation and patients in facilities having a high incidence of invasive *C. albicans* infections.

INFECTIONS IN MARROW TRANSPLANTATION RECIPIENTS

Patients receiving marrow transplants are at risk for the same infections occurring in patients rendered neutropenic by chemotherapy. Graft-versus-host disease and the immunosuppressive agents used to treat it result in a particularly high incidence of infection in this group of patients. Viral infections, especially CMV and varicella zoster virus, are especially troublesome. Infection in marrow transplant patients has been reviewed[95,96] and is discussed in Chap. 22.

REFERENCES

1. Bodey GP, Buckley M, Sathe YS, Freireich EJ: Quantitative relationships between circulating leukocytes and infection in patients with acute leukemia. *Ann Intern Med* 64:328, 1966.
2. Oppenheim BA: The changing pattern of infection in neutropenic patients. *J Antimicrob Chemother* 41(suppl D):7, 1998.
3. Tunkey AR, Sepkowitz KA: Infections caused by viridans streptococci in patients with neutropenia. *Clin Infect Dis* 34:1524, 2002.
4. Martino R, Manteiga R, Sanchez I, et al: *Viridans* streptococcal shock syndrome during bone marrow transplantation. *Acta Haematol* 94:69, 1995.
5. Morrison VA: The infectious complications of chronic lymphocytic leukemia. *Semin Oncol* 25:98, 1998.
6. Matsunaga T, Sakamaki S, Ishigaki S, et al: Use of PCR serum in diagnosing and monitoring cytomegalovirus reactivation in bone marrow transplant recipients. *Int J Hematol* 69:105, 1999.
7. Whimbey E, Champlin RE, Couch RB, et al: Community respiratory virus infections among hospitalized adult bone marrow transplant recipients. *Clin Infect Dis* 5:778, 1996.
8. Libshitz HI, Pannu HK, Elting LS, Cooksley CD: Tuberculosis in cancer patients: An update. *J Thorac Imaging* 12:41, 1997.
9. Sickles EA, Greene EA, Wiernik PH: Clinical presentation of infection in granulocytopenic patients. *Arch Intern Med* 135:715, 1975.
10. Cohen JS, Paz BI, O'Donnell MR: Treatment of perianal infection following bone marrow transplantation. *Dis Colon Rectum* 39:981, 1996.
11. Korones DN, Hussong MR, Gullace MA: Routine chest radiography of children with cancer hospitalized for fever and neutropenia. *Cancer* 80:1160, 1997.
12. Heussel CP, Kauczor HU, Heussel G, et al: Early detection of pneumonia in febrile neutropenic patients: Use of thin-section CT. *AJR Am J Roentgenol* 169:1347, 1997.
13. Aisner J, Murillo J, Schimpff SC, Steere AC: Invasive aspergillosis in acute leukemia: Correlation with nose cultures and antibiotic use. *Ann Intern Med* 90:4, 1979.
14. Einsele H, Hebart H, Roller C, et al: Detection and identification of fungal pathogens in blood by using molecular probe. *J Clin Microbiol* 35:1353, 1997.
15. Richardson MD, Kokki MH: Diagnosis and prevention of fungal infection in the immunocompromised patient. *Blood Rev* 12:24, 1998.
16. Toledo-Pereyra LH, DeMeester TR, Kinealey A, et al: The benefits of open lung biopsy in patients with previous nondiagnostic transbronchial lung biopsy. *Chest* 77:647, 1980.
17. Pagano L, Pagliari G, Busso A, et al: The role of bronchoalveolar lavage in the microbiological diagnosis of pneumonia in patients with haematological malignancies. *Ann Med* 29:535, 1997.
18. Love LJ, Schimpff SC, Schiffer CA, Wiernik PH: Improved prognosis for granulocytopenic patients with gram-negative bacteremia. *Am J Med* 68:643, 1980.
19. Elting LS: Outcomes of bacteremia in patients with cancer and neutropenia: Observations from two decades of epidemiological clinical trials. *Clin J Infect Dis* 25:247, 1997.
20. Dompeling EC, Donnelly JP, Deresinski SC, et al: Early identification of neutropenic patients at risk of gram-positive bacteraemia and the impact of empirical administration of vancomycin. *Eur J Cancer* 32:1332, 1996.
21. Link H, Bohme A, Cornely OA: Antimicrobial therapy of unexplained fever in neutropenic patients—Guidelines of the Infectious Diseases

Working Party (AGIHO) of the German Society of Hematology and Oncology (DGHO); Group Interventional Therapy of Unexplained Fever, Arbeitsgemeinschaft Supportivmassnahmen in der Onkologie (ASO) of the Deutsche Krebsgesellschaft (DKG-German Cancer Society). *Ann Hematol Suppl* Epub 2:S105, 2003.

22. Gerberding JL: Aminoglycoside dosing: Timing is of the essence. *Am J Med* 105:256, 1998.

23. Hatala R, Dinh TT, Cook DJ: Single daily dosing of aminoglycosides in immunocompromised adults: A systematic review. *Clin Infect Dis* 24: 810, 1997.

24. Egerer G, Goldschmidt H, Salwender H, et al: Efficacy of continuous infusion of ceftazidime for patients with neutropenic fever after high-dose chemotherapy and peripheral blood stem cell transplantation. *Int J Antimicrob Agents* 15:119, 2000.

25. Klastersky JA: Use of imipenem as empirical treatment of febrile neutropenia. *Int J Antimicrob Agents* 21:393, 2003.

26. Behre G, Link H, Maschmeger G, et al: Meropenem monotherapy versus combination therapy with ceftazidime and amikacin for empirical treatment of febrile neutropenic patients. *Ann Hematol* 76:73, 1998.

27. Raad II, Escalante C, Hachem RY, et al: Treatment of febrile neutropenic patients with cancer who require hospitalization: A prospective randomized study comparing imipenem and cefepime. *Cancer* 98:1039, 2003.

28. Yamamura D, Gucaip R, Carlisle P, et al: Open randomized study of cefepime versus piperacillin-gentamicin for treatment of febrile neutropenic cancer patients. *Antimicrob Agents Chemother* 41:1704, 1997.

29. Burgess DS, Hall RG, Lewis JS: Clinical and microbiologic analysis of a hospital's extended-spectrum-beta-lactamase-producing isolates over a 2-year period. *Pharmacotherapy* 23:1232, 2003.

30. Ghazal HH, Ghazal CD, Tabbara IA: Ceftazidime and ciprofloxacin as empiric therapy in febrile neutropenic patients undergoing hematopoietic stem cell transplantation. *Clin Ther* 19:520, 1997.

31. Moellering RO: Vancomycin-resistant enterococci. *Clin Infect Dis* 26: 1196, 1998.

32. Eliopoulos GM, Wennersten GB, Gold HS, et al: Characterization of vancomycin-resistant *Enterococcus faecium* isolates from the United States and their susceptibility in vitro to dalfopristin-quinupristin. *Antimicrob Agents Chemother* 42:1088, 1998

33. Birmingham MC, Rayner CR, Meagher AK, et al: Linezolid for the treatment of multidrug-resistant, gram-positive infections: Experience from a compassionate-use program. *Clin Infect Dis* 36:159, 2003.

34. Wong-Beringer A, Jacobs RA, Guglielmo BJ: Lipid formulations of amphotericin B: Clinical efficacy and toxicities. *Clin Infect Dis* 27:603, 1998.

35. White MH, Bowden RA, Sandier ES, et al: Randomized, double-blind clinical trial of amphotericin B colloidal dispersion vs. amphotericin B in the empirical treatment of fever and neutropenia. *Clin Infect Dis* 27: 296, 1998.

36. Lube RG, Boyle JA: Renal effects of amphotericin B lipid complex. *Am J Kidney Dis* 31:780, 1998.

37. Prentice HG, Hann IM, Herbrecht R, et al: A randomized comparison of liposomal versus conventional amphotericin B for the treatment of pyrexia of unknown origin in neutropenic patients. *Br J Haematol* 98: 711, 1997.

38. Herbrecht R, Denning DW, Patterson, TF, et al: Voriconazole versus Amphotericin B for primary therapy of invasive aspergillosis. *N Engl J Med* 347:408, 2002.

39. Mora-Duarte J, Betts R, Colombo AL, et al: Comparison of caspofungin and amphotericin B for invasive candidiasis. *N Engl J Med* 25:2020, 2002.

40. McGee WT, Tereso GJ: Successful treatment of Candida krusei infection with caspofungin acetate: A new antifungal agent. *Crit Care Med* 5:1577, 2003.

41. Lowance D, Neumayer HH, Legendre CM, et al: Valacyclovir for the prevention of cytomegalovirus disease after renal transplantation: International Valacyclovir Cytomegalovirus Prophylaxis Transplantation Study Group. *N Engl J Med* 340.1462, 1999.

42. Stocchi R, Ward KN, Fanin R, et al: Management of human cytomegalovirus infection and disease after allogeneic bone marrow transplantation. *Haematologica* 84:71, 1999.

43. Ljungman P: Cytomegalovirus pneumonia: Presentation, diagnosis, and treatment. *Semin Respir Infect* 10:209 1995.

44. Dinubile MJ: Stopping antibiotic therapy in neutropenic patients. *Ann Intern Med* 108:289,1988.

45. Cornelissen JJ, Rozenberg-Arska M, Dekker AW: Discontinuation of intravenous antibiotic therapy during persistent neutropenia patients receiving prophylaxis with oral ciprofloxacin. *Clin Infect Dis* 21:1300, 1995.

46. Barton TD, Schuster MG: The cause of fever following resolution of neutropenia in patients with acute leukemia. *Clin J Infect Dis* 22:1064, 1996.

47. Sallah S: Hepatosplenic candidiasis in patients with acute leukemia: Increasingly encountered complications. *Anticancer Res* 19:757, 1999.

48. Thaler M, Pastakia B, Shawker TH, et al: Hepatic candidiasis in cancer patients: The evolving picture of the syndrome. *Ann Intern Med* 108: 88, 1988.

49. Karthaus M, Huebner G, Elser C, et al: Early detection of chronic disseminated candida infection in leukemia patients with febrile neutropenia: Value of computer-assisted serial ultrasound documentation. *Ann Hematol* 77:41, 1998.

50. Sallah S, Semelka R, Kelekis N, et al: Diagnosis and monitoring response to treatment of hepatosplenic candidiasis in patients with acute leukemia using magnetic resonance imaging. *Acta Haematol* 100·77, 1998.

51. Torres-Valdivieso MJ, Lopes J, Melero O, et al: Hepatosplenic candidosis in an immunosuppressed patient responding to fluconazole. *Mycoses* 37:443, 1994.

52. Walsh TJ, Whitcomb P, Piscitelli S, et al: Safety, tolerance, and pharmacokinetics of amphotericin B lipid complex in children with hepatosplenic candidiasis. *Antimicrob Agents Chemother* 41:1944, 1997.

53. Klein NC, Gill MV, Cunha BA: Unusual organisms causing intravenous line infections in compromised hosts: II. Fungal infections. *Infect Dis Clin Pract* 5:303, 1996.

54. Logghe C, Van Ossel C, D'Hoore W, et al: Evaluation of chlorhexidine and silver-sulfadiazine impregnated central venous catheters for the prevention of bloodstream infection in leukaemic patients: A randomized controlled trial. *J Hosp Infect* 37:145, 1997.

55. Raad, II, Hanna, HA: Intravascular catheter-related infections: New horizons and recent advances. *Arch Int Med* 162:2253, 2002

56. Lane RK, Matthay MA: Central line infections. *Curr Opin Crit Care* 8: 441, 2002.

57. Escalante CP, Rubenstein KB, Roiston KV: Outpatient antibiotic therapy for febrile episodes in low-risk neutropenic patients with cancer. *Cancer Invest* 15:237, 1997.

58. Tice AD: Outpatient parenteral antibiotic therapy for fever and neutropenia. *Infect Dis Clin North Am* 12:963, 1998.

59. Schimpff SC, Greene WH, Young VM, et al: Infection prevention in acute nonlymphocytic leukemia. *Ann Intern Med* 82:351, 1975.

60. Kovatch AL, Wald ER, Albo VD, et al: Oral trimethoprim-sulfamethoxazole for prevention of bacterial infection during the induction phase of cancer chemotherapy in children. *Pediatrics* 76:754, 1985.

61. Engels BA, Lau J, Barza M: Efficacy of quinolone prophylaxis in neutropenic cancer patients: A meta-analysis. *J Clin Oncol* 16:1179, 1998.

62. Cruciani M, Rampazo R, Malena M, et al: Prophylaxis with fluoroquinolones for bacterial infections in neutropenic patients: A meta-analysis. *Clin Infect Dis* 23:795, 1996.

63. Neuhauser MM, Weinstein RA, Rydman R, et al: Antibiotic resistance among gram-negative bacilli in U.S. intensive care units: Implications for fluoroquinolone use. *JAMA* 289:885, 2003.

64. Bochud PY, Calandra T, Francioli P: Bacteremia due to *viridans* streptococci in neutropenic patients: A review. *Am J Med* 97:256, 1994.

65. Patrick CC: Use of fluoroquinolones as prophylactic agents in patients with neutropenia. *Pediatr Infect Dis J* 12:135, 1997.

66. Razonable RR, Litzow MR, Khaliq Y, et al: Bacteremia due to viridans group Streptococci with diminished susceptibility to Levofloxacin among neutropenic patients receiving levofloxacin prophylaxis. *Clin Infect Dis* 34:1469, 2002.

67. Gomez L, Garau J, Estrada C, et al: Ciprofloxacin prophylaxis in patients with acute leukemia and granulocytopenia in an area with a high prevalence of ciprofloxacin-resistant Escherichia coli. *Cancer* 97:419, 2003.

68. Baum HV, Franz U, Geiss HK: Prevalence of ciprofloxacin-resistant Escherichia coli in hematologic-oncologic patients. *Infection* 28:278, 2000.

69. Schimpff SC: Infection prevention during granulocytopenia, in *Current Clinical Topics in Infectious Disease*, vol 1, edited by JS Remington, MN Swartz, p 85. McGraw-Hill, New York, 1980.

70. Mitchell PLR, Morland B, Stevens MOG, et al: Granulocyte colony-stimulating factor in established febrile neutropenia: A randomized study of pediatric patients. *J Clin Oncol* 15:1163, 1997.

71. Pui OH, Boyett JM, Hughes WI, et al: Human granulocyte colony-stimulating factor after induction chemotherapy in children with acute lymphoblastic leukemia. *N Engl J Med* 336:1781, 1997.

72. Ohno R, Miyawaki S, Hatake K, et al: Human urinary macrophage colony-stimulating factor reduces the incidence and duration of febrile neutropenia and shortens the period required to finish three courses of intensive consolidation therapy in acute myeloid leukemia: A double-blind controlled study. *J Clin Oncol* 15:2954, 1997.

73. Hartmann LC, Tschetter LK, Habermann TM, et al: Granulocyte colony-stimulating factor in severe chemotherapy-induced afebrile neutropenia. *N Engl J Med* 336:1776, 1997.

74. Repetto L, Biganzoli L, Koehne CH, et al: EORTC Cancer in the Elderly Task Force guidelines for the use of colony-stimulating factors in elderly patients with cancer. *Eur J Cancer* 39:2264, 2003.

75. Siber GR, Snydman DR: Use of immune globulins in the prevention and treatment of infections. *Curr Clin Top Infect Dis* 12:208, 1992.

76. Weinthal J, Frost JD, Briones G, Cairo MS: Successful *Pneumocystis carinii* pneumonia prophylaxis using aerosolized pentamidine in children with acute leukemia. *J Clin Oncol* 12:136, 1994.

77. Saral R, Ambinder RF, Burns WH, et al: Acyclovir prophylaxis against herpes simplex virus infection in patients with leukemia: A randomized, double-blind placebo-controlled study. *Ann Intern Med* 99:773, 1983.

78. Wade JO, Newton B, Fluornoy N, Meyers JD: Oral acyclovir for prevention of herpes simplex virus reactivation after marrow transplantation. *Ann Intern Med* 100:823, 1984.

79. Bowden ERA, Sages M, Gleaves CA, et al: Cytomegalovirus. Seronegative blood components for the prevention of primary cytomegalovirus infection after marrow transplant. Considerations for blood banks. *Transfusion* 27:478, 1987.

80. Prentice HG, Gluckman E, Powles RL, et al: Long-term survival in allogeneic bone marrow transplant recipients following acyclovir pro-

phylaxis for CMV infections: The European Acyclovir for CMV Prophylaxis Study Group. *Bone Marrow Transplant* 19:129, 1997.

81. Verdonck LF, Dekker AW, Rozenberg-Arska M, Van den Hoek MR: A risk-adapted approach with a short course of ganciclovir to prevent cytomegalovirus (CMV) pneumonia in CMV-seropositive recipients of allogeneic bone marrow transplants. *Clin Infect Dis* 24:901, 1997.

82. Reusser P, Gambertoglio JG, Lilleby K, Meyers JD: Phase I-II trial of foscarnet for prevention of cytomegalovirus infection in autologous and allogeneic marrow transplant recipients. *J Infect Dis* 166:473, 1992.

83. Pizzuto J, Conte G, Aviles A, et al: Nystatin prophylaxis in leukemia and lymphoma [letter]. *N Engl J Med* 299:661, 1978.

84. Perfect JR, Klotman ME, Gilbert CC, et al: Prophylactic intravenous amphotericin B in neutropenic autologous bone marrow transplant recipients. *J Infect Dis* 156:891, 1992.

85. Cuttner J, Troy KM, Funaro L, et al: Clotrimazole treatment for prevention of oral candidiasis in patients with acute leukemia undergoing chemotherapy. *Am J Med* 61:771, 1986.

86. Hansen RM, Einerio N, Sohnle PG, et al: Ketoconazole in the prevention of candidiasis in patients with cancer: A prospective randomized, controlled, double-blind study. *Arch Intern Med* 147:710, 1987.

87. Goodman JL, Winston DJ, Green RA, et al: A controlled trial of fluconazole to prevent fungal infections in patients undergoing bone marrow transplantation. *N Engl J Med* 362:845, 1992.

88. Rotstein C, Bow EJ, Laverdiere M, et al: Randomized placebo-controlled trial of fluconazole prophylaxis for neutropenic cancer patients: Benefit based on purpose and intensity of cytotoxic therapy. The Canadian Fluconazole Prophylaxis Study Group. *Clin Infect Dis* 28:331, 1999.

89. Girmenia C, Martino P: Breakthrough candidemia during antifungal treatment with fluconazole in patients with hematologic malignancies. *Blood* 87:838, 1996.

90. Kern W, Behre G, Rudolf T, Kerkhoff A: Failure of fluconazole prophylaxis to reduce mortality or the requirement of systemic amphotericin B therapy during treatment for refractory acute myeloid leukemia: Results of a prospective randomized phase III study. German AML Cooperative Group. *Cancer* 83:291, 1998.

91. Schaffner A, Schaffner M: Effect of prophylactic fluconazole on the frequency of fungal infections, amphotericin B use, and health care costs in patients undergoing intensive chemotherapy for hematologic neoplasias. *J Infect Dis* 172:1035, 1995.

92. Wingard JR, Merz WG, Rinaldi MG, et al: Increase in *Candida krusei* infection among patients with bone marrow transplantation and neutropenia treated prophylactically with fluconazole. *N Engl J Med* 325:1274, 1991.

93. Lamy T, Bernard M, Courtois A, et al: Prophylactic use of itraconazole for the prevention of invasive pulmonary aspergillosis in high-risk neutropenic patients. *Leuk Lymphoma* 30:63, 1998.

94. De Pauw B: Preventive use of antifungal drugs in patients treated for cancer. *J Antimicrob Chemother* 53:130, 2004.

95. Nichols WG: Management of infectious complications in the hematopoietic stem cell transplant recipient. *J Intens Care Med* 18:295, 2003.

96. Blume KG, Forman SJ, Applebaum, FR(eds): *Thomas' Hematopoietic Cell Transplantation*, 3rd ed. Blackwell-Science, Boston, 2004.

PRINCIPLES OF ANTITHROMBOTIC THERAPY

CHARLES W. FRANCIS

KAREN L. KAPLAN

Antithrombotic drugs are among the most commonly used in medicine and are generally separated into anticoagulants, fibrinolytic agents, and platelet inhibitors based on their primary mechanism of action. Warfarin is the only currently available oral anticoagulant. It acts by inhibiting vitamin K action, has a prolonged effect, requires monitoring, and is widely used for prevention and treatment. Unfractionated heparin and the low molecular weight heparins are the most commonly used rapidly acting parenteral anticoagulants; they inhibit activated serine proteases through antithrombin. One synthetic agent in this class, fondaparinux, is specific for inhibition of factor Xa, and is effective for prevention and treatment of venous thromboembolism. Several direct thrombin inhibitors have excellent anticoagulant action and offer an alternative to heparins. Several fibrinolytic agents are available, all of which convert plasminogen to plasmin to accelerate clot lysis. Differences among them include their degree of fibrin specificity, half-life, and antigenicity. Antiplatelet agents play an important role in prevention and treatment of arterial thrombosis. Aspirin is a cyclooxgenase-1 inhibitor that is effective and widely used in the prevention of stroke and myocardial infarction. Drugs that modulate cyclic adenosine monophosphate (cAMP) levels include dipyridamole, pentoxifylline, and cilostazol, and are primarily used in treatment of peripheral vascular disease. Adenosine diphosphate (ADP) receptor blockers such as clopidogrel are effective in treatment of coronary and peripheral arterial disease. Examples of inhibitors of fibrinogen interaction with glycoprotein IIb-IIIa are abciximab, tirofiban, and eptifibutide. These drugs are highly effective in treatment of patients with acute coronary syndromes.

OVERVIEW

Antithrombotic agents are highly effective and are among the most commonly used drugs in medicine because thrombotic diseases are the leading cause of mortality and morbidity in Western countries. Antithrombotic agents are generally characterized separately as anticoagulants, antiplatelet agents, or fibrinolytic drugs, depending on their primary mechanism, although there is overlap in their activities (Table 21-1). Their greatest use is in prevention of thrombosis in patients at high risk, but they also have important applications for treating acute thrombosis. For many agents the risk-to-benefit ratio is narrow, with the result that bleeding complications occur, which are the most common adverse effects. Consequently, the clinician should carefully weigh the risks and benefits for each patient when selecting treatment. Generally, these drugs do not cause bleeding by themselves, but rather they exacerbate preexisting bleeding or predispose to bleeding from pathologic lesions that may be found in the gastrointestinal or genitourinary tracts or central nervous system. A careful review of comorbid conditions that may increase bleeding risk is important when deciding on therapy.

Anticoagulant therapy acts to decrease fibrin formation by inhibiting the formation and action of thrombin, and its most common use is in treating venous thrombosis and atrial fibrillation. Anticoagulant therapy is often monitored using coagulation testing because of marked biologic variation in effect. Antiplatelet agents act to inhibit platelet function, and their primary uses are in preventing thrombotic complications of cerebrovascular and coronary artery disease. They also have a role in treatment of acute myocardial infarction and some effect in preventing venous thrombosis. Fibrinolytic agents accelerate lysis of thrombi by increasing conversion of plasminogen to plasmin, and are primarily used in the acute management of myocardial infarction and also in selected patients with stroke or venous thromboembolism. Fibrinolytic therapy is associated with a higher risk of bleeding complications than treatment with either anticoagulants or antiplatelet agents. Treatment of acute thrombosis often involves combinations of agents with multiple actions for maximum effect.

Antithrombotic therapy is an area of intense research in new drug development with many promising agents in clinical trials. These efforts are based on scientific developments in recent years that have elucidated details of the biochemistry and cell and molecular biology of the hemostatic system. Newer agents are typically targeted toward specific enzymes, whereas older drugs affect multiple sites.

VITAMIN K ANTAGONISTS

The development of vitamin K antagonists as oral anticoagulants began in the 1920s with a hemorrhagic disease in cattle, the cause of which was eventually traced to moldy hay leading to hypoprothrombinemia.[1,2] A coumarin that inhibited vitamin K was purified and eventually introduced into clinical practice in the 1940s.[3-5] Several coumarin derivatives with differing pharmacologic properties are now available as anticoagulants worldwide, and are collectively referred to as vitamin K antagonists, but warfarin is nearly universally used in North America. These agents are widely used to prevent or treat common thrombotic diseases and represent the only oral anticoagulants currently available.[6,7]

PHARMACOLOGY

The coumarins are competitive inhibitors of vitamin K. They inhibit γ-carboxylation reactions required for synthesis of several coagulation proteins, including factors II, VII, IX, and X, as well as proteins C and S, which are involved in inhibitory regulation of hemostasis. The synthesis of these proteins requires a posttranslational modification of several glutamic acid residues, converting them to γ-carboxylated glutamic acid, which is required for proper membrane interaction and biologic activity (see Chap. 106).[8-11] The carboxylation reaction requires reduced vitamin K, which is converted to vitamin K epoxide in the reaction. Vitamin K epoxide subsequently undergoes reduction by an enzyme that is inhibited by warfarin.[12-14] Therefore, treatment with warfarin causes reduced γ-carboxylation, leading to synthesis of molecules with impaired activity of vitamin K proteins.[15-18]

TABLE 21-1 TYPES AND FUNCTION OF ANTITHROMBOTIC AGENTS

Anticoagulants—decrease fibrin formation by inhibiting thrombin or thrombin formation
  Agents
    Oral—warfarin and other vitamin K antagonists
    Parenteral—heparin, low molecular weight heparin, fondaparinux, direct thrombin inhibitors (argatroban, desirudin, bivalirudin)
  Narrow therapeutic margin
    Warfarin, heparin, and direct thrombin inhibitors; require monitoring for dose adjustment
Antiplatelet agents—inhibit platelet function
  Agents
    Aspirin, clopidogrel, dipyridamole, abciximab, integrilin, eptifibatide, tirofiban
    Primary use is in preventing and treating arterial thrombosis
Fibrinolytic agents—plasminogen activators that convert plasminogen to plasmin and accelerate clot lysis
  Agents
    Streptokinase, urokinase, alteplase, reteplase, tenecteplase
    Primary use is in treatment of acute myocardial infarction; also used in selected patients with stroke, pulmonary embolism, and deep vein thrombosis
    Bleeding complications are frequent

Warfarin preparations consist of a racemic mixture of S and R enantiomers in approximately equal proportion in an oral formulation with high bioavailability. Warfarin is water soluble and rapidly absorbed after oral administration, reaching a peak concentration after 60 to 90 minutes. An intravenous preparation is also available for patients who cannot take oral medications or who have malabsorption. It is tightly bound to plasma proteins with a half-life of 35 to 45 hours, with only the free, nonbound form having biologic activity.[6,19] Warfarin is metabolized through the cytochrome P450 system, the activity of which is influenced by environmental factors and also by genetic polymorphisms that alter the structure of common enzymes.[20–22] Other vitamin K antagonists have similar activities but exhibit differences in absorption and elimination.

Because warfarin is a vitamin K antagonist, its action is influenced by the vitamin K content of the diet. Naturally occurring vitamin K is found in a variety of vegetables, and changes in diet can affect the vitamin K availability and warfarin effect.[23] This may be seen particularly in patients receiving warfarin who are on strict weight reduction diets or in those with little oral intake because of illness. Also, diarrhea can affect vitamin K availability as can administration of broad-spectrum antibiotics leading to marked warfarin sensitivity in hospitalized patients. Ingestion of vitamin K in dietary supplements or vitamins also affects sensitivity to warfarin. Liver disease can increase sensitivity to warfarin because of impaired synthesis of coagulation factors, and hyper- or hypometabolic states may also alter sensitivity. Hereditary resistance to warfarin has been described.[24,25] Many drug interactions can influence the pharmacodynamics of warfarin by altering synthesis or clearance of vitamin K-dependent coagulation factors or interfering with warfarin metabolism, and patients should be advised to consult their physician or pharmacist about effects on anticoagulation when changing drug therapy or starting new medication (Table 21-2). Other commonly used drugs affecting hemostasis such as aspirin, nonsteroidal antiinflammatory agents, heparins, and other anticoagulants can potentiate the antihemostatic effects of warfarin and can lead to bleeding.

ADMINISTRATION AND MONITORING

The anticoagulant effect of warfarin is the result of decreased levels of vitamin K-dependent coagulation factors, and their concentration represents a balance of synthesis and metabolism. Warfarin administration impairs synthesis, and levels of vitamin K-dependent factors fall in relation to their metabolism. This is short for factor VII, with a half-life of approximately 5 hours, but longer for factors X and IX ($t_{1/2}$ = 24 hours) and longest for factor II (prothrombin) with a half-life of approximately 72 hours. The desired anticoagulant effect results from a balanced reduction of all factors and requires several days to achieve. Imbalances in reduction of coagulation factors may occur during initiation of therapy as factor VII level falls rapidly, whereas others, especially factor II, decline more slowly. The initial rapid fall in factor VII level may lead to an early elevation in the prothrombin time (PT) expressed as international normalized ratio (INR) without reflecting the desired anticoagulant effect. Because protein C, a natural inhibitor of coagulation, has a short half-life (approximately 8 hours), its level may fall rapidly, theoretically inducing a procoagulant state during initiation of therapy.

Because the anticoagulant effect of warfarin is delayed, therapy must be initiated with a rapidly acting agent such as heparin or low molecular weight heparin (LMWH) if immediate anticoagulation is needed. For example, patients with venous thromboembolism are typically given heparin or LMWH for rapid effect, and warfarin is also administered within the first 24 hours. After a period of 5 or more days, the necessary anticoagulant effect of warfarin is achieved, and the parenteral anticoagulant can be stopped. Anticoagulation should be initiated with a dose close to the expected daily maintenance requirement, which is usually between 5 and 10 mg.[26] There is, however, great variability in the doses required, and smaller amounts should be used for frail, elderly, or poorly nourished patients or those with an increased bleeding risk. "Loading doses" of warfarin were recom-

TABLE 21-2 EFFECT OF DRUGS ON WARFARIN RESPONSE

Potentiate Effect

α-Methyldopa	Isoniazid
Acetaminophen	Mefenamic acid
Acetohexamide	Methimazole
Allopurinol	Methotrexate
Androgenic and anabolic steroids	Methylphenidate
Antibiotics that disrupt intestinal flora (tetracyclines, streptomycin, erythromycin, kanamycin, nalidixic acid, neomycin)	Nalidixic acid
	Nortriptyline
	Oxyphenbutazone
	p-Aminosalicylic acid
Cephaloridine	Paromomycin
Chloramphenicol	Phenylbutazone
Chlorpromazine	Phenyramidol
Chlorpropamide	Phenytoin
Chloral hydrate	Propylthiouracil
Cimetidine	Quinidine
Clofibrate	Salicylate
Diazoxide	Sulfinpyrazone
Disulfiram	Sulfonamides
Ethacrynic acid	Thyroid hormone
Glucagon	Tolbutamide
Guanethidine	
Indomethacin	

Depress Effect

Antipyrine	Glutethimide
Barbiturates	Griseofulvin
Carbamazepine	Haloperidol
Chlorthalidone	Oral contraceptives
Digitalis	Phenobarbital
Ethanol	Prednisone
Ethchlorvynol	Vitamin preparations containing vitamin K

mended in the past, but these are inappropriate and may cause hemorrhage without shortening the time to achieve adequate anticoagulation. In patients with a low level of protein C or protein S as a result of an inherited deficiency, initiation of warfarin therapy without concomitant heparin or other immediately acting anticoagulant can lead to very low levels of these natural anticoagulants with ensuing thrombosis such as skin necrosis.

MONITORING

The anticoagulant effect is monitored using the PT, which is sensitive to decreases in vitamin K-dependent factors and is progressively lengthened as the vitamin K-dependent factors reach lower levels. A critical component of the PT is the thromboplastin reagent that is used, and variability in composition leads to variation in results. The INR has improved standardization of results.[27-29] Manufacturers determine the potency of thromboplastins by measuring the International Sensitivity Index (ISI), and this is used as a correction factor for the responsiveness of the thromboplastin in the PT. The INR represents the ratio of the patient PT to control PT corrected by the ISI. By this method, INR values obtained in different laboratories can be reliably compared for therapeutic monitoring.

During initiation of therapy, the INR should be checked every 2 to 3 days for 1 to 2 weeks until a stable therapeutic effect is achieved. The target INR for most indications is 2.5 with a desirable therapeutic range from 2 to 3 (Table 21-3). A higher INR is recommended for patients with mechanical heart valve replacement or for those who failed anticoagulant therapy despite well-documented INR values in the 2 to 3 range. During chronic therapy, the INR should be monitored every 2 to 3 weeks depending on stability of the response, and minor dose adjustments are frequently needed. Monitoring can also be performed using portable instruments that are suitable for home use.[30-32] Specialized clinics devoted to monitoring warfarin typically achieve better results in maintaining patients within the therapeutic range, resulting in fewer bleeding complications.[33,34] Problems with keeping patients within the therapeutic range often result from failure of compliance, changes in diet or medication, or intercurrent illnesses.

COMPLICATIONS

The most serious and common complication of oral anticoagulation is bleeding, and its risk is related primarily to patient characteristics, the intensity of the anticoagulation, and the length of therapy. Risk factors for bleeding include older age, recent surgery or trauma, a history of recent gastrointestinal bleeding, renal insufficiency, hypertension, cerebrovascular disease, and use of drugs with potentiating activity (see Table 21-2).[35,36] The intensity of anticoagulation as reflected by the INR is the most important predictor of bleeding risk, which is low in the therapeutic range but increases as the INR prolongs further. The cumulative risk of bleeding increases with a longer duration of treatment, whereas the absolute risk is greatest early, possibly caused by pathologic lesions present at the time therapy is started. Overall, the total risk of bleeding with a 6-month course of anticoagulation for venous thromboembolism is between 3 and 5 percent.[37] A rare complication of warfarin therapy is skin necrosis that usually occurs early in the course of anticoagulation.[38] Typical initial complaints are burning and tingling at the affected site, which usually involves a region with a large amount of subcutaneous tissue such as the breast, buttock, or thigh. Painful hemorrhagic full-thickness skin infarction develops and frequently requires skin grafting. Thrombosis in dermal and subdermal venules is the underlying cause, and this may be caused by disproportionately rapid reduction in proteins C and S.

Oral anticoagulation should be avoided in pregnancy because warfarin crosses the placenta, and exposure during organogenesis in the first trimester can lead to fetal embryopathy with significant cranial bone malformations.[39] Anticoagulation during pregnancy increases bleeding complications, especially later in pregnancy. Oral anticoagulants may be considered during the second trimester, but heparin or LMWH are preferable alternatives. Vitamin K antagonists are safe during lactation.[40]

REVERSAL OF ANTICOAGULATION

Anticoagulation must be reversed for episodes of bleeding, surgery, trauma, or overdosage. Appropriate interventions for patients with excessively prolonged INRs without bleeding include holding warfarin doses, administering low doses of vitamin K (0.5–1.0 mg), and increasing the frequency of monitoring[41,42] (Table 21-4). Serious bleeding or major warfarin overdosage requires factor replacement and/or larger vitamin K doses that may need to be given intravenously. Anticoagulated patients who need invasive procedures represent management problems, and decisions should be based on balancing the risk of thromboembolism with that of bleeding from the procedure.[43] The goal is to reduce the intensity of anticoagulation during and immediately after surgery, while avoiding thromboembolism caused by the underlying disease. Generally, the risk of recurrence is greatest in the period shortly after an episode of acute thrombosis and declines progressively over time. If possible, elective surgery and other invasive procedures associated with a high bleeding risk should be postponed during the first several months following acute thrombosis. Generally, the bleeding risk is highest during surgery and decreases rapidly to baseline after approximately 7 to 10 days. Most surgery can be done with a minimal bleeding risk in patients receiving warfarin and an INR of 1.5 or less. For patients at moderate or high risk of thrombotic recurrence, heparin or LMWH should be administered when the INR become subtherapeutic. Full anticoagulation can be resumed after the invasive procedure when the bleeding risk declines.

HEPARIN AND LOW MOLECULAR WEIGHT HEPARINS

PHARMACOLOGY

Heparin and the related LMWHs are the most widely used, rapidly acting, parenteral anticoagulants. Heparin derives its name from its

TABLE 21-3   RECOMMENDED INR VALUES DURING ORAL ANTICOAGULANT THERAPY

CONDITION	TARGET INR (RANGE)
Deep venous thrombosis treatment	2.5 (2.0–3.0)
Pulmonary embolism treatment	2.5 (2.0–3.0)
Deep venous thrombosis prophylaxis	2.5 (2.0–3.0)
Atrial fibrillation	2.5 (2.0–3.0)
Cardiac valve replacement	
Tissue valves	2.5 (2.0–3.0)
Mechanical valves	3.0 (2.5–3.5)
Acute myocardial infarction	2.5 (2.0–3.0)

TABLE 21-4   REVERSING WARFARIN THERAPY

INDICATION	ACTION
Excessively long INR	
INR <6	Lower dose
INR 6–10	Give vitamin K, 1–2 mg orally, or subcutaneously; recheck INR 12–24 h later
INR >10	Give vitamin K, 2–4 mg orally or subcutaneously; recheck INR 12–24 h later
Serious bleeding or major overdose	Give vitamin K, 5–10 mg intravenously, and consider fresh-frozen plasma or prothrombin complex concentrate

original description as an aqueous extract of liver (hepar) that exhibited anticoagulant activity *in vitro*.[44-46] It is a mixture of sulfated glycosaminoglycans composed of chains of alternating residues of D-glycosamine and iduronic acid. Heparin is very heterogeneous in composition and includes molecules varying in chain lengths and M_r from 5000 to 30,000 daltons with an average of approximately 15,000 daltons and a chain length of 50 saccharide units. It is extracted from lungs and intestinal tissue of cows and swine, and is assayed biologically by its ability to prolong blood clotting *in vitro*.[47] Heparin has no direct anticoagulant effect, but it acts through antithrombin (AT), a serine protease inhibitor. Only about one-third of heparin molecules contain the necessary unique pentasaccharide sequence required to interact with AT and have anticoagulant activity.[48-51]

AT inhibits thrombin, factor Xa, and other coagulation serine proteases in a reaction that is slow by itself, but is accelerated approximately 1000-fold in the presence of heparin.[52,53] To inhibit thrombin, heparin binds to both the enzyme and AT, forming a ternary complex.[54,55] The inhibition of factor Xa, however, occurs through binding to heparin/AT complex without the requirement for heparin binding directly also to factor Xa.[55] The requirement for a ternary heparin/AT/thrombin complex requires heparin molecules with 19 or more saccharide units, whereas smaller heparin molecules are effective in promoting factor Xa inactivation. Heparin also stimulates release of tissue factor pathway inhibitor from endothelial cells, and this may contribute to anticoagulant activity.[56,57] Thrombin and factor Xa are relatively protected from inhibition by heparin/AT complex when they are surface immobilized within thrombi or on cells.[58-60] Heparin also interacts with heparin cofactor II; high concentrations of heparin accelerate thrombin inhibition by heparin cofactor II.[61,62]

Heparin is not absorbed after oral ingestion, so it must be given either subcutaneously or intravenously. Following parenteral administration, heparin exerts an immediate anticoagulant effect. It interacts with proteins and cells in the blood, resulting in complex pharmacokinetics characterized by rapid equilibration and slower clearance.[63-66] The initial binding to cells is saturable within concentrations used clinically, resulting in a dose-dependent half-life that increases from approximately 1 hour at a dose of 100 U/kg to 2.5 hours at 400 U/kg. Pharmacodynamics vary among individuals and also depend on the method of administration. After subcutaneous injection, bioavailability may be less than 50 percent in low doses, but increases at higher, therapeutic doses.[66-68]

ADMINISTRATION AND MONITORING

To achieve a full anticoagulant effect rapidly, heparin is usually administered intravenously. A common protocol uses an initial intravenous bolus of 5000 units or 75 U/kg, followed by a maintenance infusion of 1250 to 1660 U/hour or 18 U/kg per hour. Clinical studies demonstrate a lower occurrence of bleeding complications with continuous intravenous rather than intermittent bolus therapy. The anticoagulant effect is immediate, but laboratory monitoring is needed because of the variability in response among patients. Monitoring is most convenient with the activated partial thromboplastin time (aPTT), which is sensitive to plasma heparin concentrations of 0.1 U/ml or higher. Because different reagents and measuring systems have differing sensitivities to heparin, it is recommended that the therapeutic range be established for each laboratory by calibrating the aPTT to a plasma heparin concentration of 0.2 to 0.4 units by protamine sulfate titration, or 0.3 to 0.7 U/ml using an antifactor Xa assay.[47] The usual aPTT range for heparin therapy is between 1.5 and 2.5 times the mean of the normal range. Clinically useful nomograms are available for adjusting heparin dose using either fixed- or weight-based dosing.[69,70] Alternatively, monitoring can be performed using anti-Xa levels,

which is a useful approach when the aPTT is unreliable, as in patients with baseline prolongation of the aPTT as a consequence of lupus anticoagulant. Rapid achievement of a therapeutic level as reflected by the aPTT or anti-Xa is important in ensuring an adequate anticoagulant effect.

Some patients appear to respond poorly to heparin, with inadequate prolongation of the aPTT despite apparently adequate or even high heparin dosage. This is often referred to as *heparin resistance* and is rarely caused by AT deficiency but more commonly is caused by the acute-phase response that results in high levels of procoagulant proteins, including factor VIII. The antithrombotic effect of heparin correlates best with plasma heparin levels, which may be adequate in these circumstances despite a subtherapeutic aPTT.[71] For patients who require heparin doses of greater than 35,000 U/day to increase the aPTT into the therapeutic range, consideration should be given to using heparin levels determined by an anti-Xa assay. Substitution of LMWH for unfractionated heparin is another consideration. Although AT deficiency may cause heparin resistance, most AT-deficient patients can be adequately anticoagulated with heparin in usual doses, although very low AT levels can cause heparin resistance. No monitoring is recommended when low doses of heparin are used for prophylaxis of venous thromboembolic disease, although minimal prolongation of the aPTT may occur.

REVERSAL

Heparin has a short half-life, and its anticoagulant effect disappears several hours after discontinuation of an intravenous infusion. Therefore, stopping the infusion and local measures are usually adequate to control bleeding. However, in major or life-threatening bleeding, the anticoagulant effect can be neutralized with protamine sulfate, which is a basic polypeptide that binds tightly to the acidic heparin molecule. The usual dose of protamine required is 1 mg to neutralize 100 units of heparin. The dose to be administered is based on the amount of heparin remaining in the circulation. Protamine is routinely used to neutralize heparin after cardiopulmonary bypass using standard formulas and activated clotting time monitoring.

ADVERSE EFFECTS

The most frequent complication of heparin administration is bleeding, which is related to the dose and intensity of treatment as well as to patient characteristics. Heparin-induced thrombocytopenia (HIT) is an immune-mediated platelet consumption caused by an antibody directed against a complex of heparin and platelet factor 4 (see Chap. 124). Despite thrombocytopenia, HIT is more commonly associated with thrombotic complications than bleeding, and it occurs in approximately 3 percent of patients when defined as a 50 percent reduction in baseline platelet count or development of a platelet count of less than $150,000/\mu l$ during therapy.[72,73] Platelet counts should be monitored during treatment and heparin discontinued if thrombocytopenia occurs. An alternative anticoagulant should be used instead. Long-term heparin therapy can also cause osteoporosis, and radiographic evidence of bone loss occurs in approximately 15 percent of women receiving prolonged treatment during pregnancy, with symptomatic vertebrae fractures in approximately 2 percent. The bone loss resolves after heparin is discontinued.[74,75]

LOW MOLECULAR WEIGHT HEPARIN

Limitations of unfractionated heparin led to studies correlating structural and functional relationships of heparin, and this eventually resulted in the development of LMWHs, several of which are now available. LMWH preparations are produced by treating heparin chemically or enzymatically to decrease the size of the polysaccharide chains, yield-

287

ing products with restricted molecular weight distributions with a mean of approximately 4000 to 5000 daltons.[76] Like heparin, LMWHs exert antithrombotic effects through interaction with AT. In the presence of LMWH, AT inactivates factor Xa in the same way as unfractionated heparin, but it is less able to inactivate thrombin because the shorter polysaccharide length does not allow formation of the necessary ternary complex with AT and thrombin. Consequently, LMWHs have a greater proportion of antifactor Xa than antithrombin activity.

LMWHs also have different pharmacokinetic properties than unfractionated heparin.[67,76-78] Following subcutaneous administration, LMWHs are nearly completely absorbed, a clear benefit over unfractionated heparin, which exhibits variable and dose-dependent absorption. LMWH also exhibits less binding to plasma proteins and cells than unfractionated heparin, resulting in more predictable blood levels and anticoagulant effects.[76] LMWHs have a longer plasma half-life than unfractionated heparins, allowing once or twice daily subcutaneous administration for many applications.

LMWHs have significant renal clearance, and high levels can accumulate in patients with renal insufficiency. Care must be taken in dosing LMWH in patients with reduced renal function, and monitoring with antifactor Xa levels may be needed. Similarly, monitoring may be necessary to achieve appropriate levels in very obese patients. Protamine sulfate does not completely reverse the anticoagulant effect of LMWH but is partially effective and can be useful in patients with serious hemorrhage.[79,80] Several LMWH preparations are available and approved for both prophylaxis and treatment of venous and arterial thrombotic diseases. Each preparation differs slightly and must be regarded as unique, although the results of clinical trials are very similar with this group of agents. Table 21-5 lists the doses used for common indications.

Similar to unfractionated heparin, the most common adverse effect is bleeding, which occurs at approximately the same frequency and severity when used in similar patient groups for the same indication. HIT is much less common than with unfractionated heparin, occurring only in 0.3 to 0.45 percent of patients.[72] However, cross-reactivity of the antibody occurs, and LMWH is not an acceptable choice for continued anticoagulation in patients with HIT. Animal studies suggest that osteoporosis may be less common with LMWH, but little clinical data is available.

CHOICE OF HEPARIN OR LOW MOLECULAR WEIGHT HEPARIN

The factors governing the choice of heparin or LMWH concern effectiveness, safety, convenience, and cost. Evidence suggests that heparin and LMWH are equally effective for prophylaxis of venous thromboembolism in most surgical and medical patients.[81] LMWH is more effective than heparin, however, in patients undergoing major orthopedic surgery. For treatment of venous thromboembolic disease, the safety and efficacy of heparin and LMWH are comparable, but LMWH offers better convenience because subcutaneous administration permits outpatient treatment, which is preferable for most patients. LMWH may be difficult to use in patients with renal insufficiency because of decreased clearance, and intravenous heparin may offer advantages in such patients. LMWH is incompletely reversed by protamine sulfate, making it more difficult to use for cardiac bypass surgery. Unfractionated heparin may be preferable in patients who require an invasive procedure on an urgent basis because of its shorter half-life. LMWH may offer some advantages for patients with acute coronary syndromes.

DANAPAROID

Danaparoid is a mixture of glycosaminoglycans and is composed of approximately 84 percent heparan sulfate, 12 percent dermatan sulfate,

TABLE 21-5 TREATMENT REGIMENS WITH LOW MOLECULAR WEIGHT HEPARIN

	DRUG*	REGIMEN
Prophylaxis		
General surgery		
Low risk	Dalteparin	2500 U, 1–2 h preoperation and qd
	Enoxaparin	20 mg, 1–2 h preoperation and qd
	Nadroparin	3100 U, 2 h preoperation and qd
	Tinzaparin	3500 U, 2 h preoperation and qd
High risk	Dalteparin	5000 U, 10–12 h preoperation and qd
	Enoxaparin	40 mg 10–12 h preoperation and qd
	Danaparoid†	750 U bid
Orthopedic surgery	Dalteparin	5000 U, 8–12 h preoperation and qd
	Enoxaparin	30 mg q 12 h starting 12–24 h postoperation or 40 mg qd starting 12 h preoperation
	Ardeparin	50 U/kg q 12 h starting 12–24 h postoperation
	Nadroparin	40 U/kg 2 h preoperation and qd; then 60 U/kg qd
	Tinzaparin	50 U/kg 2 h preoperation and qd or 75 U/kg qd starting 12–24 h postoperation
	Danaparoid†	750 U, 1–2 h preoperation and bid
	Fondaparinux	2.5 mg daily, starting 6–8 h postoperation
Spinal injury	Enoxaparin	30 mg q 12 h
Multiple trauma	Enoxaparin	30 mg q 12 h
Medical patients	Enoxaparin	20 mg qd (40 mg qd more effective in high-risk patients)
	Dalteparin	2500 U qd
	Danaparoid†	750 U bid
Treatment		
Venous thromboembolism	Enoxaparin	1 mg/kg q 12 h; or 1.5 mg/kg qd
	Dalteparin	100 U/kg q 12 h; or 200 U/kg qd
	Nadroparin	90 U/kg q 12 h
	Tinzaparin	175 U/kg qd
Unstable angina	Enoxaparin	1 mg/kg q 12 h
	Dalteparin	100 U/kg q 12 h

* Brand names: ardeparin, Normiflo; danaparoid, Orgaran; dalteparin, Fragmin; enoxaparin, Lovenox; fondaparinux, Arixtra; nadroparin, Fraxiparine; tinzaparin, Innohep.
† Danaparoid sodium is not an LMWH but a closely related glycosaminoglycan mixture composed of heparan sulfate, dermatan sulfate, and chondroitin sulfate.

and 4 percent chondroitin sulfate. It is an AT-dependent anticoagulant with predominant antifactor Xa activity.[82] The plasma half-life is approximately 24 hours with predominant renal clearance. Danaparoid is not reversed by protamine sulfate. Danaparoid differs structurally from heparin and it has been used successfully to treat patients with HIT.[83-85] Although there is in vitro cross-reactivity of 10 to 20 percent of heparin antibodies with danaparoid, this is of uncertain clinical relevance. Danaparoid is administered subcutaneously, and levels may be monitored with antifactor Xa assays.

FONDAPARINUX
Fondaparinux is a unique heparin-like anticoagulant with selective antifactor Xa activity.[86,87] It is a completely synthetic pentasaccharide whose structure is based on the heparin sequence that interacts with AT. It binds reversibly and with high affinity to AT, resulting in a conformational change that renders it effective in inhibiting factor Xa but not thrombin. Whereas unfractionated heparin and all LMWHs are derived from animal sources, fondaparinux is synthesized in a structurally homogenous form containing no animal products. Consequently, fondaparinux does not induce allergic responses. Because it inhibits factor Xa but has no direct action on thrombin, its mechanism of action depends on reducing thrombin generation.

TABLE 21-6   CLINICAL INDICATIONS AND USE OF DIRECT THROMBIN INHIBITORS

AGENT*	CLINICAL INDICATION	REGIMEN	MONITORING	HALF-LIFE
Lepirudin	HIT	0.4 mg/kg bolus 0.1–0.15 mg/kg/h	aPTT	2.8 h
Bivalirudin	Angioplasty	1 mg/kg bolus 2.5 mg/kg/h × 4 h 0.2 mg/kg/h to 20 h	aPTT	24–45 min
Argatroban	HIT HIT with PCI	2 µg/kg 350 µg/kg bolus, then 15–40 µg/kg/min	aPTT ACT	39–51 min
Ximelagatran	DVT prophylaxis[†] DVT/PE treatment[†] Atrial fibrillation[†]	24 or 36 mg twice daily 36 mg twice daily 36 mg twice daily	None	2.5–3.5 h

ACT, activated clotting time; aPTT, activated partial thromboplastin time; DVT, deep vein thrombosis; HIT, heparin-induced thrombocytopenia; PCI, percutaneous coronary intervention; PE, pulmonary embolism.
* Brand names: argatroban, Novastan; bivalirudin, Angiomaz; lepirudin, Refludan; ximelagatran, Exanta.
† Not FDA approved.

Pharmacologic studies show that maximum plasma levels are reached approximately 2 hours after subcutaneous administration with an elimination half-life of approximately 17 hours independent of the dose.[88] Bioavailability is nearly complete after subcutaneous or intravenous administration. There is a low intra- and intersubject variability with little accumulation after multiple daily doses. Elimination is primarily renal, and the agent is excreted unchanged in the urine. Fondaparinux plasma levels can be measured with the antifactor Xa assay, but there is no effect on other coagulation assays including the activated clotting time (ACT), aPTT, or thrombin clotting time.

Clinical studies have evaluated the use of fondaparinux in prevention and treatment of venous thromboembolism,[86,89] and it is approved by the FDA for prevention of venous thromboembolism in patients undergoing major orthopedic surgery. For this purpose it is administered subcutaneously in a dose of 2.5 mg once daily. Studies evaluating its use in treatment and prevention of venous thromboembolism at a dose of 7.5 mg administered subcutaneously daily show an effectiveness that is comparable with LMWH.[90]

The principal adverse effect is bleeding, and its frequency and severity have been comparable to those observed with LMWH. Elevated levels may occur in patients with renal insufficiency, and caution should be exercised in using fondaparinux in patients with renal compromise. Cross-reactivity with antibodies causing HIT does not occur,[91–93] and fondaparinux may be a good choice for an anticoagulant in patients with HIT, particularly those needing subcutaneous administration.[94]

DIRECT THROMBIN INHIBITORS

HIRUDIN

Hirudin, the anticoagulant present in the salivary glands of the medicinal leech, *Hirudo medicinalis*, is a highly specific direct inhibitor of thrombin. Hirudin forms a stable, noncovalent but very strong complex with thrombin with a dissociation constant of approximately 2×10^{-14} mol/liter.[95,96] The carboxyl-terminal end of the protein binds to exosite I of thrombin (the fibrinogen-binding site) via electrostatic, polar, and hydrophobic interactions, and the amino-terminal end binds to the active site via a hydrogen bond between Ile-1 of hirudin and Ser-525 of thrombin.[97] The closely related biosynthetic polypeptide called *lepirudin* is composed of 65 amino acids and is identical to natural hirudin except for substitution of leucine for isoleucine at the N-terminus of the molecule and the absence of a sulfate group on tyrosine 63. Lepirudin has bioavailability of approximately 88 percent after subcutaneous administration with peak plasma levels after a single dose in 1.3 to 2.5 hours. The half-life is 1 to 3 hours in normal volunteers with predominantly renal catabolism, but it may be as long as 2 days in

dialysis-dependent patients.[98–103] Lepirudin prolongs the aPTT in a concentration-dependent manner,[104] but the ecarin clotting time may be better as a measure of blood levels.[105]

Lepirudin is approved for use in treatment of HIT (Table 21-6) and has also been used successfully in clinical trials for prevention and treatment of deep vein thrombosis (DVT) and in patients with acute coronary syndromes. It has no structural homology with heparin and exhibits no cross-reactivity with HIT antibodies. The recommended dosing depends on renal function. For patients with normal function, treatment is initiated with a bolus of 0.4 mg/kg followed by an infusion of 0.1 to 0.15 mg/kg per hour to maintain the aPTT at 1.5 to 2.5 times normal. With renal insufficiency, both the bolus and infusion rate should be decreased.

The primary adverse effect is bleeding. Also, formation of anti-hirudin antibodies has been observed in approximately 40 percent of HIT patients treated with lepirudin, which may decrease drug clearance and thus increase the anticoagulant effect, possibly because of delayed renal elimination of lepirudin-antibody complexes, which retain anticoagulant properties.[106–109] There is no available agent to reverse the effects of lepirudin. The infusion should be discontinued in a case of bleeding complications or overdosage and aPTT and other coagulation parameters monitored as appropriate. Hemofiltration or hemodialysis may be useful with very high levels or renal compromise. Also, factor VIIa decreases bleeding in patients receiving lepirudin.

BIVALIRUDIN

Bivalirudin, a recombinant protein based on the structure of hirudin, is composed of a dodecapeptide analogue of the carboxy-terminal region of hirudin linked by a four-glycine residue to a structure directed to the active site of thrombin.[110] The glycine bridge permits easy cleavage of the molecule, providing a more reversible interaction with the catalytic site of thrombin than hirudin,[111] and this may result in fewer bleeding complications. Pharmacokinetic studies show that plasma clearance is rapid (4.6 ml/min/kg) in patients with normal renal function with a volume of distribution of 0.2 liter/kg and elimination of half-life of approximately 30 minutes.[112] There is dose-dependent prolongation of the ACT and aPTT that correlates with plasma concentrations. There are both renal and hepatic clearance,[113] and dose modification is recommended for patients with moderate-to-severe functional impairment or who are dialyzed.

Bivalirudin is effective when used with aspirin in patients with unstable angina or postinfarction angina undergoing angioplasty, and it is approved for this use (see Table 21-6). The recommended dose is an intravenous bolus of 1 mg/kg followed by a continuous infusion of 2.5 mg/kg per hour for 4 hours with an additional 0.2 mg/kg per hour for up to 20 hours if needed. Bivalirudin has also shown efficacy in preventing restenosis after coronary angioplasty, as an adjunct to streptokinase in acute myocardial infarction, and in preventing venous thrombosis after orthopedic surgery and in patients with HIT. The most common adverse effect is bleeding, and no specific antidote is available. The infusion should be discontinued in patients with bleeding complications and blood levels monitored with the aPTT or other coagulation parameters. Antibivalirudin antibodies have not been detected following therapy.

ARGATROBAN

Argatroban is a small molecule arginine derivative that reversibly inhibits thrombin by binding directly to the active catalytic site with a

K_i of 3.9×10^{-8} mol/liter.[114] Because of its small size, argatroban is an effective inhibitor of thrombin both bound to surfaces and in solution.[115] The anticoagulant effect can be assessed with either the aPTT or ACT, and both correlate with plasma concentrations of the drug.[116] Argatroban is approximately 50 percent protein bound and has a volume of distribution of 0.2 liter/kg and an elimination half-life of 39 to 51 minutes.[117,118] Metabolism is primarily hepatic, and the clearance and half-life are prolonged in patients with hepatic functional abnormalities requiring dose reduction. Renal function does not affect argatroban pharmacokinetics.

Argatroban is approved for treatment and prophylaxis of HIT and for percutaneous interventions in patients with HIT (see Table 21-6). It has also shown some benefit in patients with thrombotic stroke in clinical trials. For treatment of HIT, argatroban is administered at 2 μg/kg per hour and adjusted to maintain the aPTT at 1.5 to 3 times baseline. For patients with HIT undergoing percutaneous coronary interventions, the drug is administered as a bolus of 350 μg/kg followed by a continuous infusion of 15 to 400 μg/kg per minute for a target ACT of 300 to 450 seconds. As with other direct thrombin inhibitors, the main side effect is bleeding, and no specific agent is available to reverse its action. The anticoagulant effect may be prolonged in patients with hepatic impairment. If overdosage or excess bleeding occurs, the infusion should be discontinued and the aPTT and other coagulation parameters monitored.

The transition from argatroban to warfarin in patients requiring long-term anticoagulation is complicated because argatroban has a significant effect on both the PT and the aPTT.[119] Two possible methods for this transition have been used. The argatroban infusion can be discontinued 1 hour prior to checking the INR. Alternatively, a goal of an INR of 4 while the patient is on dual therapy indicates an effective warfarin therapeutic effect.

MELAGATRAN AND XIMELAGATRAN

Ximelagatran is an inactive prodrug formulation of melagatran, a potent direct thrombin inhibitor that is in late-phase clinical trials as a new oral anticoagulant.[120] Development of the novel prodrug approach was essential because melagatran and other active direct thrombin inhibitors exhibit poor intestinal absorption.[121,122] Following oral administration, ximelagatran is rapidly and nearly completely absorbed and then rapidly metabolized, with approximately 20 percent converted to the active form, melagatran,[122,123] with low interindividual variability in absorption and conversion. The peak melagatran concentration following oral ximelagatran occurs in approximately 2 hours.[120,122,123]

Melagatran, the active metabolite, is a competitive, reversible active site inhibitor of thrombin. It is a dipeptide whose structure mimics the sequence N-terminal to the cleavage site for thrombin on the fibrinogen Aα chain. It is effective in inhibiting both fluid phase and surface-immobilized thrombin, thrombin complexed with thrombomodulin, and platelet activation by cleavage of protease activator receptor-1.[124–126] Melagatran can be administered intravenously or subcutaneously but has poor oral bioavailability. More than 80 percent of melagatran is excreted unchanged in the urine, and thus plasma half-life and concentration increase with declining renal function.[127,128] Protein binding is less than 15 percent, and the plasma half-life in normal young subjects is approximately 3 hours. Melagatran prolongs coagulation tests, including the aPTT, thrombin time, and PT. The ecarin clotting time is probably the best coagulation test for assessing plasma levels.[126,129,130]

Ximelagatran is not approved for clinical use in the United States but has undergone extensive phase III clinical evaluation for prevention and treatment of venous thromboembolism[131–134] and prevention of stroke in patients with atrial fibrillation.[135] Also, a large phase II trial was conducted in patients with acute myocardial infarction.[136] These studies are promising, as efficacy and bleeding complications were similar to currently used drugs. Unexpectedly, elevations of liver function tests 4 to 6 weeks after administration are observed in 5 to 10 percent of patients and thus monitoring of serum transaminase levels during long-term administration is necessary. The significance of this finding is uncertain.

FIBRINOLYTIC THERAPY

Fibrinolytic therapy is administered by infusing high doses of a plasminogen activator to accelerate the conversion of plasminogen to the active fibrinolytic enzyme plasmin, which proteolytically degrades fibrin (see Chap. 127). The specific biochemical and pharmacologic properties of different agents are important determinants of the administration regimen, the efficacy of clot lysis, and the nature of adverse effects (Table 21-7). For example, some fibrinolytic drugs are bacterial products that are antigenic and can cause allergic responses, whereas others are recombinant human proteins. Some agents activate plasminogen prominently both in blood and at the clot surface and induce a systemic fibrinolytic state in addition to accelerating clot

TABLE 21-7 PROPERTIES OF FIBRINOLYTIC AGENTS

DRUG*	FDA APPROVAL	ORIGIN	FIBRIN SPECIFICITY	HALF-LIFE (MIN)	ANTI-GENICITY	NOTE
Streptokinase	Yes	Bacterial	No	20	Yes	Acts indirectly by forming 1:1 complex with plasminogen.
Urokinase	Yes	Cell culture	Low	15	No	Normally present in urine. Currently not available because of manufacturing problems.
Alteplase	Yes	Recombinant	Moderate	5	No	Naturally occurring activator synthesized in endothelium.
Anistreplase	Yes	Streptococci; plasminogen, plasma derived	Moderate	70	Yes	Complex of streptococci and plasmin-plasminogen with active site blocked. Activates after administration.
Reteplase	Yes	Recombinant	Moderate	15	No	Modified form of t-PA with longer half-life.
Tenecteplase	Yes	Recombinant	Enhanced	30–120	No	Bioengineered variant of t-PA with longer half-life, resistance to inactivation by PAI-1, and enhanced fibrin specificity.
Single chain urokinase plasminogen activator (scu-PA)	No	Recombinant	Enhanced	15	No	Single-chain form of t-PA.
Staphylokinase	No	Recombinant	Enhanced		Yes	Fibrinolytic protein from staphylococci.

PAI-1, plasminogen-activator inhibitor; t-PA, tissue-plasminogen activator.
* Brand names: alteplase, Activase; anistreplase, Eminase; reteplase, Retevase; scu-PA, Saruplase; streptokinase, Streptase; tenecteplase, Metalyse; urokinase, Abbokinase.

lysis, whereas the activity of other agents is more specifically limited to the clot surface with less systemic effects. Fibrinolytic therapy is used for treatment of both venous and arterial thrombosis and represents standard treatment for many patients presenting with acute myocardial infarction because it accelerates reperfusion, decreases mortality, and reduces morbidity (Chap. 126). Thrombolytic therapy has also become standard for many patients presenting with thrombosis of peripheral arteries and bypass grafts. It is used for treatment of selected patients with thrombotic stroke, resulting in decreased disability. Fibrinolytic therapy improves outcome in selected patients with large pulmonary emboli associated with hemodynamic compromise and in some patients with venous thrombosis (Chap. 125).

STREPTOKINASE

Streptokinase was the first clinically employed plasminogen activator. It is derived from β-hemolytic streptococci and has a unique indirect mechanism of action. By itself, streptokinase has no enzymatic activity, but it combines with plasminogen to form an equimolar streptokinase–plasminogen complex that can then convert another plasminogen molecule to plasmin.[137,138] Additionally, the streptokinase–plasminogen complex can undergo proteolytic cleavage itself, resulting in activation. When administered in therapeutic doses, streptokinase is an effective thrombolytic agent. The streptokinase–plasmin(ogen) complex can bind to fibrin through the "kringle" domains of plasmin and activate clot-bound plasminogen to accelerate clot lysis (see Chap. 127),[139,140] but can also act on plasminogen in the blood to produce plasmin, giving rise to systemic proteolysis termed the *lytic state*.[141,142] This results in consumption of plasminogen and α_2-antiplasmin, degradation of fibrinogen, factor V, and VIII, proteolysis of platelet membrane proteins by plasmin, and platelet activation. Streptokinase has a rapid plasma clearance with a half-life of approximately 20 minutes, but the duration of the proteolytic effect is more prolonged.

Streptokinase is typically administered intravenously and can be used to treat either venous or arterial thrombosis. For treatment of venous thromboembolic disease, streptokinase is usually administered as initial bolus of 250,000 units followed by a constant infusion of 100,000 units per hour for up to 3 days (Table 21-8). The purpose of the initial bolus is to overcome circulating neutralizing antibodies, which are common because of the frequency of streptococcal infec-

TABLE 21-8 SYSTEMIC THROMBOLYTIC THERAPY REGIMENS

DRUG	ADMINISTRATION
Deep vein thrombosis (DVT) and pulmonary embolism (PE)	
Streptokinase	250,000 U loading dose IV followed by 100,000 U/h; 24 h for PE; up to 3 days for DVT
Urokinase	2000 U/kg loading dose IV followed by 2000 U/kg/h 12–24 h for PE; up to 3 days for DVT
t-PA	100 mg over 2 h for PE
Thrombolytic therapy for acute myocardial infarction	
Streptokinase	1,500,000 U over 1 h IV
t-PA	15 mg bolus IV, then 0.75 mg/kg over 30 min (not to exceed 50 mg); then 0.75 mg/kg over 60 min (not to exceed 35 mg) *or* 100 mg total over 3 h; 60 mg in first hour (6–10 mg as a bolus), 20 mg over the second hour, and 20 mg over the third hour
APSAC	30 U over 5 min IV
Reteplase	10 U IV bolus; repeat once after 30 min
Thrombolytic therapy for stroke*	
t-PA	0.9 mg/kg (maximum 90 mg) IV, with 10% total dose as a bolus and the remainder over 60 min

* Strict attention to criteria for patient selection is required.

tions in the population.[143,144] Occasionally, individuals have a high titer of antibodies that neutralize this amount of streptokinase, resulting in resistance. Consequently, it is useful to ensure proteolytic activity of streptokinase in blood after 1 to 2 hours of administration by validating a decrease in fibrinogen concentration or prolongation of the thrombin clotting time. If these parameters do not become abnormal, a second bolus infusion may be needed to overcome inhibition. Streptokinase is antigenic, and high-titer antibodies develop 1 to 2 weeks after use, precluding retreatment until the titer declines. High titers can also cause febrile or hypotensive reactions. The regimen of streptokinase used to treat acute myocardial infarction differs from that recommended for venous thrombosis; a higher dose (1,500,000 U) over a shorter period of time (1 hour) is used to achieve a maximum effect.

ANISTREPLASE

Anisoylated plasminogen activator complex (anistreplase), a chemically modified streptokinase derivative with improved pharmacologic properties, in which streptokinase is complexed with plasminogen and the active site of plasminogen is protected by modification with a p-anisoyl group, has been developed.[145] This activator binds to fibrinogen through the plasminogen kringle domain and has a significantly prolonged half-life of approximately 40 minutes, allowing it to be administered for therapy in a bolus dose. The agent is enzymatically inactive until active-site deacylation occurs, either in the blood or after binding to a thrombus. The fibrin-binding properties result in a greater activity at the site of fibrin deposition, and systemic plasminemia and fibrinogen depletion are less than with streptokinase or urokinase but more than with tissue-plasminogen activator (t-PA). Because it contains a streptokinase moiety, anistreplase is immunogenic, and resistance to therapy or allergic reactions can occur in patients with high-titer antibodies. Anistreplase has been evaluated clinically primarily in the setting of acute myocardial infarction. Its particular advantage is that it can be administered as a single bolus injection with a high rate of coronary reperfusion.

UROKINASE

Urokinase is a naturally occurring plasminogen activator synthesized by the renal tubular epithelium that is normally present in the urine.[146–148] A single-chain urokinase-type plasminogen activator (scu-PA) is synthesized in endothelial cells and converted to a two-chain derivative by limited hydrolysis by plasmin or kallikrein.[149–151] This form and a smaller two-chain cleavage product are used clinically. For therapeutic use, urokinase can be prepared from embryonic kidney cell culture, but concern over possible viral contamination has recently limited commercial production and clinical use. Urokinase can also be produced by recombinant DNA technology. Two-chain urokinase is a direct plasminogen activator that proteolytically converts plasminogen to plasmin, whereas scu-PA has little activity until it is proteolytically converted to the active two-chain form.[152–154] Urokinase is cleared primarily by the liver and has a half-life of approximately 15 minutes. In usual doses it produces systemic plasminemia, with degradation of circulating fibrinogen reflecting the lytic state. Urokinase has been used effectively in treatment of DVT, pulmonary embolism (PE), myocardial infarction, arterial occlusion, and stroke. However, its primary use has been in treating venous thromboembolic disease and peripheral arterial occlusion. The same doses are used for treatment of DVT and PE, although a shorter duration of treatment of 12 hours is typical for PE, whereas a longer duration of up to several days may be used for DVT (see Table 21-8). For peripheral arterial occlusion, urokinase is typically administered through a catheter placed within the thrombus.

TISSUE-PLASMINOGEN ACTIVATOR

t-PA is a naturally occurring plasminogen activator that is structurally and immunologically distinct from urokinase.[155-157] t-PA is synthesized by endothelial cells as a single-chain polypeptide and was originally produced from cell culture for pharmacologic use, but is now synthesized by recombinant techniques (alteplase). t-PA directly converts plasminogen to plasmin in a reaction that is accelerated several hundred-fold in the presence of fibrin.[158-160] In the absence of fibrin, t-PA has much less activity, and this property accounts for the relative "fibrin specificity" of t-PA observed physiologically. However, when administered pharmacologically in a high dose, significant proteolysis of plasma fibrinogen often occurs, but this is typically less prominent than observed with treatment using either streptokinase or urokinase. The half-life of t-PA following intravenous administration is 4 to 5 minutes, which requires a constant infusion to maintain therapeutic plasma levels. t-PA is not antigenic because it is a physiologic enzyme.

t-PA has been evaluated in treatment of DVT, PE, myocardial infarction, stroke, and peripheral arterial occlusion. In patients with PE, a regimen of 100 mg intravenously over 2 hours results in a high rate of clot lysis and hemodynamic improvement (see Table 21-8). t-PA has been evaluated in many large studies for acute myocardial infarction and administration results in improved mortality and morbidity. t-PA has also been evaluated in treatment of stroke and results in significant benefit in highly selected patients who are treated within 3 hours of symptom onset (see Chap. 126).

RETEPLASE

Recombinant technology has been used to engineer many t-PA mutants in an attempt to improve pharmacologic properties. The structural modifications in reteplase result in reduced fibrin binding and a significantly longer half-life of 15 minutes compared to 4 minutes with t-PA, so it can be administered as an intravenous bolus rather than a continuous infusion.[161,162] Reteplase has been evaluated primarily for treatment of acute myocardial infarction and is administered in two bolus injections of 10 units each given 30 minutes apart.

TENECTEPLASE

Tenecteplase (TNK-tissue plasminogen activator) is another bioengineered variant of t-PA with a longer half-life, increased resistance to inactivation by plasminogen activator inhibitor-1, and improved fibrin specificity.[163] Advantages include a longer half-life, greater fibrin specificity, ease and rapidity of administration, and similar clinical efficacy as t-PA for treatment of acute myocardial infarction. It has a half-life of more than 30 minutes.

OTHER PLASMINOGEN ACTIVATORS

Many other plasminogen activators have been characterized, prepared for clinical use, and tested in limited trials. These include a variety of genetically engineered mutants of t-PA and urokinase-plasminogen activator (u-PA) as well as chimeric forms of t-PA and u-PA and bifunctional agents that include antiplatelet agents. These are of great research interest but are not approved for use. A particularly interesting plasminogen activator is staphylokinase, a 15.5-kDa protein produced by *Staphylococcus aureus* and known to have fibrinolytic properties for many years. Similar to streptokinase, it is an indirect activator and forms a 1:1 stoichiometric complex with plasminogen, which then forms plasmin. It is much more fibrin-specific than streptokinase, producing high rates of clot lysis without significant effects on the levels of fibrinogen, plasminogen, or α_2-antiplasmin.[164] It is, however, antigenic, and neutralizing antibodies develop following therapy. It has been evaluated in preliminary clinical trials and shows promise. Another novel but naturally occurring plasminogen activator is derived from the vampire bat, which secretes plasminogen activators in its saliva.[165,166] One form was developed for possible clinical use and shows high potency and fibrin specificity with very few systemic effects.

ANTIPLATELET DRUGS

Platelets play an important role in hemostasis and thrombosis (see Chaps. 105 and 126). Platelets adhere to exposed subendothelium, become activated, release contents of their dense and α granules, and form aggregates. Additional platelets from the circulating blood are then recruited by ADP, which is released from dense granules, and also by thromboxane A2 synthesized by activated platelets in the aggregate. Simultaneous with the initial platelet adhesion and aggregation, thrombin generation is initiated (see Chap. 106). The activated platelet phospholipid membrane is an effective surface for binding of coagulation factors to enhance the rate of thrombin generation. As thrombin is formed it activates additional platelets and also cleaves fibrinopeptides from fibrinogen to form fibrin in and around the platelet plug, consolidating it. The role of platelets in initiating thrombosis is greater in the arterial circulation than in the venous circulation because higher shear forces present in arteries activate platelets. Therefore, antiplatelet drugs are more effective in arterial than in venous thrombosis. The type of drugs, their use in clinical settings, their mechanism of action, and their dosages are summarized in Tables 21-9 and 21-10.

CYCLOOXYGENASE-1 INHIBITORS

Cyclooxygenase-1 (COX-1) is an enzyme that is present in most cells. It converts arachidonic acid released from phospholipids by phospholipase A_2 or phospholipase C and diacylglycerol[167] to prostaglandin G_2 (see Chap. 108). A peroxidase converts prostaglandin G_2 to prostaglandin H_2, which is then converted by thromboxane synthase in platelets to thromboxane A2.[168] Thromboxane A2 is a potent activator of platelets. In endothelial cells prostaglandin H_2 is converted to prostacyclin, a potent inhibitor of platelet function, through an increase in intraplatelet cAMP.

Aspirin (acetylsalicylic acid) was recognized as an inhibitor of platelet function in the 1960s, although the mechanism of its action was unknown at that time.[169-171] It prolonged the bleeding time in normal subjects slightly, although usually not out of the normal range, and its effect lasted for several days. If the bleeding time in a patient taking aspirin is very prolonged, it usually means that an underlying

TABLE 21-9   ANTIPLATELET AGENTS BY MECHANISM OF ACTION AND CLINICAL USE

Cyclooxygenase inhibitors	
Aspirin	Coronary and cerebrovascular disease
Agents that increase cAMP	
Dipyridamole	Coronary, cerebrovascular, peripheral arterial disease
Pentoxifylline	Peripheral arterial disease
Cilostazol	Peripheral arterial disease
ADP receptor blockers	
Ticlopidine	Cerebrovascular disease
Clopidogrel	Cerebrovascular disease, PCI
Glycoprotein IIb-IIIa inhibitors	
Abciximab	ACS, PCI
Eptifibatide	ACS, PCI
Tirofiban	ACS, PCI

ACS, acute coronary syndrome; cAMP, cyclic adenosine monophosphate; PCI, percutaneous coronary intervention.

TABLE 21-10 ANTIPLATELET AGENTS

AGENT	USUAL DOSE	DURATION OF EFFECT
Aspirin	75–650 mg daily	7–10 days (life of the platelet)
Dipyridamole	75–100 mg qid	$t_{1/2}$ 40 min
Pentoxifylline	400 mg bid	$t_{1/2}$ 1–1.6 h
Cilostazol	100 mg bid	$t_{1/2}$ 11–13 h
Ticlopidine	250 mg bid	7–10 days (life of the platelet)
Clopidogrel	75 mg daily	7–10 days (life of the platelet)
Abciximab	0.25 mg/kg, then 10 μg/kg/min	<10 min and 30 min
Eptifibatide	ACS 180 μg/kg, then 2 μg/kg/min PCI 180 μg/kg, then 2 μg/kg/min with 180 μg/kg at 10 min*	$t_{1/2}$ 2.5 h
Tirofiban	0.4 μg/kg/min × 30 min, then 0.1 μg/kg/min*	$t_{1/2}$ 2 h

ACS, acute coronary syndrome; PCI, percutaneous coronary intervention.
* Decrease infusion rate by 50 percent for renal dysfunction.

hemostatic defect is also present. It was demonstrated that acetylation of cyclooxygenase is important in platelet inhibition by aspirin.[172–174] Because platelets cannot synthesize new COX, irreversible enzyme inhibition by aspirin means that inhibition persists for the life span of the platelet. Most cells have two forms of COX, known as COX-1 and COX-2. COX-1 is synthesized constitutively, whereas COX-2 is only synthesized under stress conditions.[175] Both COX-1 and COX-2 are inhibited by aspirin and most nonsteroidal antiinflammatory drugs (NSAIDs), with aspirin acetylating both forms. The nonaspirin COX inhibitors are reversible inhibitors, so they are active only while in the circulation. It was thought initially that only COX-1 is found in platelets, but more recently COX-2 was found in platelets transiently, especially when there was a rapid platelet turnover.[176,177] Because COX-1 is the major COX in platelets, COX-2–specific inhibitors have minimal effect on platelet function.

Aspirin and several of the commonly used NSAIDs (e.g., indomethacin, ibuprofen, and naproxen) have similar *in vitro* effects on platelet function. Platelet aggregometry demonstrates that the second wave of aggregation induced by ADP or epinephrine in citrated platelet-rich plasma (PRP) is abolished after aspirin ingestion and that aggregation induced by low concentrations of collagen is markedly decreased.[169,170] Arachidonic acid-induced aggregation is abolished after aspirin ingestion.[177] Additionally, secretion of dense granule components (ADP, ATP, and serotonin)[178] and of α-granule proteins by ADP, epinephrine, collagen, and arachidonic acid is inhibited in citrated PRP after aspirin ingestion or with addition of indomethacin to citrated PRP.[179]

Because of these *in vitro* effects of aspirin, the drug has been used extensively as an inhibitor of platelet function *in vivo*,[180,181] with beneficial effects in primary and secondary prevention and in treatment of myocardial infarction (see Chap. 126). Aspirin is also beneficial in stroke prevention with carotid artery disease[182,183] and embolic stroke,[184–187] although anticoagulation with warfarin or its analogues is generally more effective than aspirin in embolic stroke in most patients with a cardiac embolic source.[184–189] Aspirin is rarely used to prevent venous thrombosis. Other drugs that inhibit COX-1 are not used to prevent either arterial or venous thrombosis.

DRUGS THAT MODULATE CYCLIC ADENOSINE MONOPHOSPHATE LEVELS

cAMP in platelets is formed from ATP by the action of adenylate cyclase[190] and degraded by cAMP phosphodiesterase.[191,192] Basal lev-

els of cAMP in platelets are low (approximately 0.04% of metabolic nucleotide, or 3–7 nmol/10^{11} platelets).[193] Elevated levels of intra-platelet cAMP are induced by inhibition of cAMP phosphodiesterase, or by stimulation of adenylate cyclase activity, resulting in inhibition of platelet activation[193–196] through several pathways: (1) modulation of phosphorylation of specific proteins; (2) inhibition of several steps in metabolism of phosphoinositol phosphates; and (3) lowering of preelevated levels of intracellular Ca^{2+}, and accumulation of Ca^{2+} by platelet microsomes.[197] Agents that inhibit the cAMP phosphodiesterase include theophylline, papaverine, and dipyridamole,[193] as well as pentoxifylline[198,199] and cilostazol.[200] Several prostaglandins stimulate adenylate cyclase, including prostaglandin E_1 (PGE$_1$),[193–195,201] PGD$_2$,[201,202] and PGI$_2$ (prostacyclin).[178,203,204]

Clinical use of drugs that elevate cAMP levels is confined to dipyridamole, pentoxifylline, and cilostazol. Dipyridamole is used alone or in combination with aspirin. A study of more than 6000 patients with previous stroke or transient ischemic attack showed a reduction in stroke with dipyridamole plus aspirin compared with aspirin alone,[81] but a review of randomized trials in 19,000 patients with nonembolic arterial vascular disease concluded that dipyridamole with or without aspirin was not better than other antiplatelet drugs (primarily aspirin) in preventing vascular death.[205] There was a slight benefit of aspirin plus dipyridamole in preventing vascular events, because of the results of the study referred to above.[81] The question of added benefit from dipyridamole is thus not completely resolved.

The other two phosphodiesterase inhibitors (pentoxifylline and cilostazol) are used primarily in patients with peripheral vascular disease. In addition to their inhibitory effect on platelets they exert a beneficial effect on blood rheology and the microcirculation by increasing red cell deformability, thereby reducing blood viscosity.[206] Cilostazol increases vascular endothelial growth factor levels, which may lead to an increase in collateral circulation.[207] Pentoxifylline inhibits vascular smooth-muscle cell proliferation and collagen synthesis,[208] which may enhance vasodilation.

Clinical studies in peripheral vascular disease have shown benefit in some patients with peripheral vascular disease for pentoxifylline[206,209,210] and for cilostazol.[210–212] Both cilostazol plus aspirin and ticlopidine plus aspirin after coronary stenting have an equivalent efficacy, but cilostazol is probably safer because of the potential for neutropenia with ticlopidine.[213–216] Cilostazol may also prevent restenosis.[216]

ADENOSINE DIPHOSPHATE RECEPTOR BLOCKERS

The third class of platelet inhibitors is the ADP receptor blockers, ticlopidine and clopidogrel.[217] These agents are thienopyridines and they selectively inhibit platelet activation induced by ADP.[217] The drugs are not active *in vitro*, indicating that they must be metabolized. Hepatic metabolism is necessary for clopidogrel activity[218] and the cytochrome P450 (CYP) 01A pathway is involved.[219] There are three ADP receptors on platelet membranes (see Chap. 105), with the thienopyridines inhibiting one of them, the P2Y12 receptor. The inhibition of binding of ADP to the P2Y12 receptor results in inhibition of adenylate cyclase.[220,221]

Ticlopidine was available for clinical use before clopidogrel. The Canadian American Ticlopidine Study was a randomized, placebo-controlled, double blind study of the efficacy and safety of ticlopidine in patients with recent stroke. The primary outcome efficacy variable was recurrent stroke, myocardial infarction, or vascular death. There was a risk reduction of 30.2 percent with ticlopidine. In terms of safety, there was a 1 percent incidence of severe neutropenia with ticlopidine and 2 percent incidence of skin rash and of diarrhea.[222] A review of four trials of ticlopidine plus aspirin versus oral anticoagulants[223] for coronary stenting showed benefit to the combination in terms of reduced risk of nonfatal myocardial infarction and revascularization at 30 days, combined negative events (mortality, myocardial infarction, revascularization at 30 days), and major bleeding, but increased the risk of thrombocytopenia and neutropenia. Ticlopidine plus aspirin also reduced the risk of stent thrombosis. Strict monitoring of blood cell counts was recommended. Drug reactions included thrombotic thrombocytopenia purpura, thrombocytopenia, marrow aplasia, anemia, pancytopenia, agranulocytosis, and neutropenia.[224] Two meta-analyses of aspirin with ticlopidine versus clopidogrel after coronary stenting showed superior efficacy and a significantly better safety profile for clopidogrel.[225,226] A systematic review of antiplatelet therapy with aspirin and clopidogrel concluded that dual treatment should be used for at least 12 months after stenting.[227]

The first clinical trial of clopidogrel was the Clopidogrel versus Aspirin in Patients at Risk of Ischemic Events (CAPRIE) trial, a large randomized, blinded trial of clopidogrel versus aspirin in 19,000 patients at risk of ischemic events.[228] Patients were enrolled after recent myocardial infarction or stroke or if they had symptomatic peripheral arterial disease. The primary outcome was the occurrence of ischemic stroke, myocardial infarction, or vascular death. With a mean follow-up of 1.91 years, there was a relative risk reduction of 8.7 percent in the clopidogrel group (p = 0.043). No major differences were noted in terms of safety. Neutropenia occurs rarely with clopidogrel.[229]

Clopidogrel is also used in acute coronary syndromes, based on the Clopidogrel in Unstable angina to prevent Recurrent Events (CURE) study.[227,230] The CREDO study also examined aspirin with and without clopidogrel in acute coronary syndromes and showed a consistent benefit of extended clopidogrel for each component of the composite end point of cardiovascular death, myocardial infarction, or stroke.[231] Another use of clopidogrel is for peripheral arterial disease, where it reduces the risk of atherothrombotic events.[228,232] Based on studies with ticlopidine, it may also be useful to increase the patency of arteriovenous fistulas.[233]

Clopidogrel use is increasing in patients after a first ischemic stroke.[234] Several studies of clopidogrel or aspirin, for prevention of stroke in patients after transient ischemic attacks are ongoing (FASTER and ATARI), and the combination of aspirin and clopidogrel is being evaluated in the MATCH, CHARISMA, ARCH, CARESS, and SPS3 studies in patients with ischemic brain syndromes.[235]

GPIIB-IIIA BLOCKERS

Fibrinogen binds specifically and saturably to the surface of activated platelets[236,237], and the glycoprotein (GP) IIb-IIIa complex is the fibrinogen receptor.[236] Platelets of patients with Glanzmann thrombasthenia[238] are unable to aggregate, but do respond to stimuli with shape change and secretion of their granular contents (see Chap. 112).[239–241] These patients lack the GPIIb-IIIa complex.[242] This complex mediates platelet aggregation induced by all physiologic agonists.[243–245] The critical amino acids on fibrinogen for binding to the GPIIb-IIIa complex are located in the C-terminal dodecapeptide of the γ chain and an arginine-glycine-aspartic acid (RGD) sequence of the α chain.[246–248] Of the monoclonal antibodies that have been developed that bind to the GPIIb-IIIa complex, some react with the complex on resting or activated platelets,[243,249–252]whereas others react better after platelets have been activated, for example, by ADP.[249,253,254] Fibrinogen binds only to the activated conformation of the receptor.[254]

Because monoclonal antibodies against the GPIIb-IIIa receptor block platelet aggregation by preventing ligand binding to the receptor, they were introduced as antiplatelet agents. The first two antibodies developed were 10E5 and 7E3, but the latter had better pharmacologic properties.[243,254] The clinical version of 7E3, called *abciximab*, is the Fab'$_2$ fragment of a chimeric mouse-human antibody.[255] Animal stud-

ies with abciximab showed that it prevented arterial thrombosis in animal models.[256,257] Initial human pharmacodynamic studies were performed in patients with unstable angina[258] and in patients undergoing high-risk coronary angioplasty,[259] and dose-related inhibition of platelet function was found. No spontaneous bleeding was observed, despite prolongation of the template bleeding time. Because of the mouse component of abciximab, it may induce antimouse antibodies, preventing repeated use in patients.[260]

The first large clinical trial of abciximab was the Evaluation of c7E3 for the Prevention of Ischemic Complications (EPIC) trial, published in 1994, in which the drug was used in patients with high-risk coronary angioplasty.[261] Abciximab reduced ischemic events after angioplasty when given together with heparin and aspirin, but it also increased the risk of bleeding.[262] A subsequent study of patients undergoing percutaneous coronary intervention, the Evaluation in PTCA to Improve Long-term Outcome with Abciximab GP IIb/IIIa Blockade (EPILOG) study, demonstrated efficacy in both low-risk and high-risk patients without any increase in major bleeding.[263]

Other types of inhibitors of fibrinogen binding to platelets have also been developed. Those in clinical use are eptifibatide, a cyclic heptapeptide based on a rattlesnake venom peptide,[264–266] and tirofiban, a nonpeptide derivative of tyrosine.[267] Animal studies of eptifibatide were performed in a canine model of coronary thrombosis, showing suppression of platelet-dependent flow reduction.[268] Pharmacokinetic and pharmacodynamic studies in animals and humans showed a rapid onset of action, short plasma half-life, and rapid reversibility of action.[265] The pharmacodynamics of eptifibatide are substantially altered by anticoagulants that chelate calcium,[269] and pharmacokinetic modeling suggests that optimal dosing is obtained by giving a second bolus 10 minutes after the first bolus.[269] Eptifibatide is not immunogenic.[270]

The first major clinical trial of eptifibatide was the Integrilin to Minimize Platelet Aggregation and Coronary Thrombosis (IMPACT) II trial in patients undergoing any kind of coronary intervention.[271] There was a highly significant reduction in the composite end point of death, myocardial infarction, coronary artery bypass grafting, repeat urgent or emergent coronary intervention, or stent placement for abrupt closure at 24 hours with both eptifibatide dosing arms. There was no increase in major bleeding. The effect was no longer significant at 30 days on intention-to-treat analysis.

Animal studies with tirofiban were performed in dogs.[267,272] Dose-dependent inhibition of *ex vivo* platelet aggregation was achieved, with rapid reversibility at the end of the infusion.[267] Electrically induced coronary artery thrombosis was markedly reduced by tirofiban infusion, without significant extension of the bleeding time.[272] Pharmacokinetic and pharmacodynamic studies in humans showed that tirofiban provided a well-tolerated reversible means of inhibiting platelet function.[273–275] Bleeding time was prolonged, and ADP-induced aggregation was blocked by at least 80 percent in normal volunteers.[274] The plasma half-life was 1.6 hours.[274] ADP- and collagen-induced platelet aggregation in normal volunteers returned to 55 percent and 89 percent of baseline by 3 hours after the end of infusion.[273] Similar results were found in a dose-ranging study in patients undergoing coronary angioplasty.[275]

The first major clinical trial of tirofiban was the Randomized Efficacy Study of Tirofiban for Outcomes and Restenosis (RESTORE) trial, in which tirofiban was compared with placebo in patients thought to be at increased risk for abrupt arterial occlusion closure because of unstable angina, recent myocardial infarction, or direct angioplasty during an acute myocardial infarction.[276] There was a highly significant difference in the composite end point at day 2 favoring tirofiban over placebo, with loss of significance at 30 days.

A meta-analysis is available on the effect of GPIIb-IIIa inhibitors on 30-day survival in percutaneous coronary interventions for acute coronary syndromes.[277] This analysis included 12 trials involving more than 20,000 patients. Overall, 30-day mortality was significantly reduced with GPIIb-IIIa inhibition (odds ratio 0.73 [0.55–0.96], p = 0.024). This translated into preventing approximately 1 of every 3 deaths that occur within 30 days after percutaneous coronary intervention, saving 2.8 lives per 1000 patients treated. Reduction of mortality approached significance at 6 months. Another meta-analysis of the effect of these inhibitors in medically managed patients with acute coronary syndromes showed that GPIIb-IIIa blockade was associated with a significant reduction (from 11.5% to 10.7%, p = 0.02) in death or nonfatal myocardial infarction at 30 days.[278]

REFERENCES

1. Schofield FW: A brief account of a disease in cattle simulating hemorrhagic septicaemia due to feeding sweet clover. *Can Vet Rec* 3:74, 1922.
2. Overman RS, Satahmann MA, Sullivan WR, et al: Studies on the haemorrhagic sweet clover disease. *J Biol Chem* 141:941, 1941.
3. Allen EV, Barker NW, Waugh JM: A preparation from spoiled sweet clover (3,3′-methylene-bis-(4-hydroxycoumarin)) which prolongs coagulation and prothrombin time of the blood. A clinical study. *JAMA* 120:1009, 1942.
4. Butsch WC, Stewart JD: Clinical experience with dicoumarin 3,3′-methylene-bis-(4-hydroxycoumarin). *JAMA* 120:10256, 1942.
5. Lehmann J: Hypoprothrombinaemia produced by methylene-bis-(hydroxycoumarin): Its use in thrombosis. *Lancet* 1:318, 1942.
6. Hirsh J, Dalen J, Anderson DR, et al: Oral anticoagulants: mechanism of action, clinical effectiveness, and optimal therapeutic range. *Chest* 119:8S, 2001.
7. Ansell J, Hirsh J, Dalen J, et al: Managing oral anticoagulant therapy. *Chest* 119:22S, 2001.
8. Nelsestuen GL, Zytkovicz TH, Howard JB: The mode of action of vitamin K. Identification of gamma-carboxyglutamic acid as a component of prothrombin. *J Biol Chem* 249:6347, 1974.
9. Stenflo I, Fernlund P, Egan W, et al: Vitamin K dependent modifications of glutamc acid residues in prothrombin. *Proc Natl Acad Sci U S A* 71:2730, 1974.
10. Freedman SJ, Blostein MD, Baleja JD, et al: Identification of the phospholipid binding site in the vitamin K-dependent blood coagulation protein factor IX. *J Biol Chem* 271:16227, 1996.
11. Magnusson S, Sottrup-Jensen L, Petersen TE, et al: Primary structure of the vitamin K-dependent part of prothrombin. *FEBS Lett* 44:189, 1974.
12. Whitlon DS, Sadowski JA, Suttie JW: Mechanism of coumarin action: significance of vitamin K epoxide reductase inhibition. *Biochemistry* 17:1371, 1978.
13. Fasco MJ, Hildebrandt EF, Suttie JW: Evidence that warfarin anticoagulant action involves two distinct reductase activities. *J Biol Chem* 257:11210, 1982.
14. Morris DP, Soute, BA, Vermeer C, et al: Characterization of the purified vitamin K-dependent gamma-glutamyl carboxylase. *J Biol Chem* 268:8735, 1993.
15. Paul B, Oxley A, Brigham K, et al: Factor II, VII, IX and X concentrations in patients receiving long-term warfarin. *J Clin Pathol* 40:94, 1987.
16. Malhotra OP: Dicoumarol-induced prothrombins containing 6, 7, and 8 gamma-carboxyglutamic acid residues: Isolation and characterization. *Biochem Cell Biol* 67:411, 1989.
17. Esnouf MP, Prowse CV: The gamma-carboxy glutamic acid content of human and bovine prothrombin following warfarin treatment. *Biochim Biophys Acta* 490:471, 1977.
18. Ratcliffe JV, Furie B, Furie BC: The importance of specific gamma-carboxyglutamic acid residues in prothrombin. Evaluation by site-specific mutagenesis. *J Biol Chem* 268:24339, 1993.

19. Wessler S, Gitel SN: Warfarin. From bedside to bench. *N Engl J Med* 311:645, 1984.
20. Taube J, Halsall D, Baglin T: Influence of cytochrome P-450 CYP2C9 polymorphisms on warfarin sensitivity and risk of over-anticoagulation in patients on long-term treatment. *Blood* 96:1816, 2000.
21. Margaglione M, Colaizzo D, D'Andrea G, et al: Genetic modulation of oral anticoagulation with warfarin. *Thromb Haemost* 84:775, 2000.
22. Alving BM, Strickler MP, Knight RD, et al: Hereditary warfarin resistance. Investigation of a rare phenomenon. *Arch Intern Med* 145:499, 1985.
23. Wells PS, Holbrook AM, Crowther NR, et al: Interactions of warfarin with drugs and food. *Ann Intern Med* 121:676, 1994.
24. O'Reilly RA, Pool JG, Aggeler PM: Hereditary resistance to coumarin anticoagulant drugs in man and rat. *Ann N Y Acad Sci* 151:913, 1968.
25. O'Reilly RA, Aggeler PM, Hoag MS, et al: Hereditary transmission of exceptional resistance to coumarin anticoagulant drugs. *N Engl J Med* 308:1229, 1983.
26. Harrison L, Johnston M, Massicotte MP, et al: Comparison of 5-mg and 10-mg loading doses in initiation of warfarin therapy. *Ann Intern Med* 126:133, 1997.
27. Loeliger EA, van den Besselaar AM, Lewis SM: Reliability and clinical impact of the normalization of the prothrombin times in oral anticoagulant control. *Thromb Haemost* 53:148, 1985.
28. Kovacs MJ, Wong A, MacKinnon K, et al: Assessment of the validity of the INR system for patients with liver impairment. *Thromb Haemost* 71:727, 1994.
29. Taberner DA, Poller L, Thomson JM, et al: Effect of international sensitivity index (ISI) of thromboplastins on precision of international normalised ratios (INR). *J Clin Pathol* 42:92, 1989.
30. Anderson DR, Harrison L, Hirsh J: Evaluation of a portable prothrombin time monitor for home use by patients who require long-term oral anticoagulant therapy. *Arch Intern Med* 153:1441, 1993.
31. Ansell JE, Patel N, Ostrovsky D, et al: Long-term patient self-management of oral anticoagulation. *Arch Intern Med* 155:2185, 1995.
32. Massicotte P, Marzinotto V, Vegh P, et al: Home monitoring of warfarin therapy in children with a whole blood prothrombin time monitor. *J Pediatr* 127:389, 1995.
33. Ansell JE, Hughes R: Evolving models of warfarin management: anticoagulation clinics, patient self-monitoring, and patient self-management. *Am Heart J* 132:1095, 1996.
34. Chiquette E, Amato MG, Bussey HI: Comparison of an anticoagulation clinic with usual medical care: anticoagulation control, patient outcomes, and health care costs. *Arch Intern Med* 158:1641, 1998.
35. Landefeld CS, McGuire E 3rd, Rosenblatt MW: A bleeding risk index for estimating the probability of major bleeding in hospitalized patients starting anticoagulant therapy. *Am J Med* 89:569, 1990.
36. Fihn SD, Callahan CM, Martin DC, et al: The risk for and severity of bleeding complications in elderly patients treated with warfarin. The National Consortium of Anticoagulation Clinics. *Ann Intern Med* 124:970, 1996.
37. Levine MN, Raskob G, Landefeld CS, et al: Hemorrhagic complications of anticoagulant treatment. *Chest* 119(Suppl):1085, 2001.
38. Sallah S, Thomas DP, Roberts HR: Warfarin and heparin-induced skin necrosis and the purple toe syndrome: Infrequent complications of anticoagulant treatment. *Thromb Haemost* 78:785, 1997.
39. Ginsberg JS, Greer I, Hirsh J: Use of antithrombotic agents during pregnancy. *Chest* 119(Suppl):1225, 2001.
40. Ito S: Drug therapy for breast-feeding women. *N Engl J Med* 343:118, 2000.
41. Shetty HG, Backhouse G, Bentley DP, et al: Effective reversal of warfarin-induced excessive anticoagulation with low dose vitamin K1. *Thromb Haemost* 67:13, 1992.
42. Crowther MA, Donovan D, Harrison L, et al: Low-dose oral vitamin K

reliably reverses over-anticoagulation due to warfarin. *Thromb Haemost* 79:1116, 1998.

43. Kearon C, Hirsh J: Management of anticoagulation before and after elective surgery. *N Engl J Med* 336:1506, 1997.

44. McLean J: The thromboplastic action of cephalin. *Am J Physiol* 41:250, 1916.

45. Brinkhous KM, Smith HP, Warner ED, et al: The inhibition of blood clotting: An unidentified substance which acts in conjunction with heparin to prevent the conversion of prothrombin into thrombin. *Am J Physiol* 125:683, 1939.

46. Howell WH: Heparin as an anticoagulant. *Am J Physiol* 63:434, 1923.

47. Hirsh J, Warkentin TE, Shaughnessy SG, et al: Heparin and low-molecular-weight heparin: Mechanisms of action, pharmacokinetics, dosing, monitoring, efficacy, and safety. *Chest* 119:64S, 2001.

48. Lam LH, Silbert JE, Rosenberg RD: The separation of active and inactive forms of heparin. *Biochem Biophys Res Commun* 69:570, 1976.

49. Lindahl U, Backstrom G, Hook M, et al: Structure of the antithrombin-binding site in heparin. *Proc Natl Acad Sci U S A* 76:3198, 1979.

50. Casu B, Oreste P, Torri G, et al: The structure of heparin oligosaccharide fragments with high anti-(factor Xa) activity containing the minimal antithrombin III-binding sequence. Chemical and 13C nuclear-magnetic-resonance studies. *Biochem J* 197:599, 1981.

51. Choay J, Lormeau JC, Petitou M, et al: Structural studies on a biologically active hexasaccharide obtained from heparin. *Ann N Y Acad Sci* 370:644, 1981.

52. Abildgaard U: Highly purified antithrombin 3 with heparin cofactor activity prepared by disc electrophoresis. *Scand J Clin Lab Invest* 21:89, 1968.

53. Rosenberg RD, Damus PS: The purification and mechanism of action of human antithrombin-heparin cofactor. *J Biol Chem* 248:6490, 1973.

54. Danielsson A, Raub E, Lindahl U, et al: Role of ternary complexes, in which heparin binds both antithrombin and proteinase, in the acceleration of the reactions between antithrombin and thrombin or factor Xa. *J Biol Chem* 261:15467, 1986.

55. Jordan RE, Oosta GM, Gardner WT, et al: The kinetics of hemostatic enzyme-antithrombin interactions in the presence of low molecular weight heparin. *J Biol Chem* 255:10081, 1980.

56. Lupu C, Poulsen E, Roquefeuil S, et al: Cellular effects of heparin on the production and release of tissue factor pathway inhibitor in human endothelial cells in culture. *Arterioscler Thromb Vasc Biol* 19:2251, 1999.

57. Gori AM, Pepe G, Attanasio M, et al: Tissue factor reduction and tissue factor pathway inhibitor release after heparin administration. *Thromb Haemost* 81:589, 1999.

58. Teitel JM, Rosenberg RD: Protection of factor Xa from neutralization by the heparin-antithrombin complex. *J Clin Invest* 71:1383, 1983.

59. Hogg PJ, Jackson CM: Fibrin monomer protects thrombin from inactivation by heparin-antithrombin III: implications for heparin efficacy. *Proc Natl Acad Sci U S A* 86:3619, 1989.

60. Weitz JI, Hudoba M, Massel D, et al: Clot-bound thrombin is protected from inhibition by heparin-antithrombin III but is susceptible to inactivation by antithrombin III-independent inhibitors. *J Clin Invest* 86:385, 1990.

61. Tollefsen DM, Majerus DW, Blank MK: Heparin cofactor II. Purification and properties of a heparin-dependent inhibitor of thrombin in human plasma. *J Biol Chem* 257:2162, 1982.

62. Blinder MA, Marasa JC, Reynolds CH, et al: Heparin cofactor II: cDNA sequence, chromosome localization, restriction fragment length polymorphism, and expression in *Escherichia coli*. *Biochemistry* 27:752, 1988.

63. Lane DA, Denton J, Flynn AM, et al: Anticoagulant activities of heparin oligosaccharides and their neutralization by platelet factor 4. *Biochem J* 218:725, 1984.

64. Young E, Prins M, Levine MN, et al: Heparin binding to plasma proteins, an important mechanism for heparin resistance. *Thromb Haemost* 67:639, 1992.

65. de Swart CA, Nijmeyer B, Roelofs JM, et al: Kinetics of intravenously administered heparin in normal humans. *Blood* 60:1251, 1982.

66. Olsson P, Lagergren H, Ek S: The elimination from plasma of intravenous heparin. An experimental study on dogs and humans. *Acta Med Scand* 173:619, 1963.

67. Bara L, Billaud E, Gramond G, et al: Comparative pharmacokinetics of a low molecular weight heparin (PK 10 169) and unfractionated heparin after intravenous and subcutaneous administration. *Thromb Res* 39:631, 1985.

68. Pini M, Pattachini C, Quintavalla R, et al: Subcutaneous vs intravenous heparin in the treatment of deep venous thrombosis—A randomized clinical trial. *Thromb Haemost* 64:222, 1990.

69. Cruickshank MK, Levine MN, Hirsh J, et al: A standard heparin nomogram for the management of heparin therapy. *Arch Intern Med* 151:333, 1991.

70. Raschke RA, Reilly BM, Guidry JR, et al: The weight-based heparin dosing nomogram compared with a "standard care" nomogram. A randomized controlled trial. *Ann Intern Med* 119:874, 1993.

71. Levine MN, Hirsh J, Gent M, et al: A randomized trial comparing activated thromboplastin time with heparin assay in patients with acute venous thromboembolism requiring large daily doses of heparin. *Arch Intern Med* 154:49, 1994.

72. Warkentin TE, Levine MN, Hirsh J, et al: Heparin-induced thrombocytopenia in patients treated with low-molecular-weight heparin or unfractionated heparin. *N Engl J Med* 332:1330, 1995.

73. Kaplan KL, Francis CW: Heparin-induced thrombocytopenia. *Blood Rev* 13:1, 1999.

74. Dahlman T, Lindvall N, Hellgren M: Osteopenia in pregnancy during long-term heparin treatment: a radiological study post partum. *Br J Obstet Gynaecol* 97:221, 1990.

75. Dahlman TC: Osteoporotic fractures and the recurrence of thromboembolism during pregnancy and the puerperium in 184 women undergoing thromboprophylaxis with heparin. *Am J Obstet Gynecol* 168:1265, 1993.

76. Weitz JI: Low-molecular-weight heparins. *N Engl J Med* 337:688, 1997.

77. Frydman AM, Bara L, Le Roux Y, et al: The antithrombotic activity and pharmacokinetics of enoxaparine, a low molecular weight heparin, in humans given single subcutaneous doses of 20 to 80 mg. *J Clin Pharmacol* 28:609, 1988.

78. Briant L, Caranobe C, Saivin S, et al: Unfractionated heparin and CY 216: pharmacokinetics and bioavailabilities of the antifactor Xa and IIa effects after intravenous and subcutaneous injection in the rabbit. *Thromb Haemost* 61:348, 1989.

79. Racanelli A, Fareed J, Walenga JM, et al: Biochemical and pharmacologic studies on the protamine interactions with heparin, its fractions and fragments. *Semin Thromb Hemost* 11:176, 1985.

80. Van Ryn-McKenna J, Cai L, Ofosu FA, et al: Neutralization of enoxaparine-induced bleeding by protamine sulfate. *Thromb Haemost* 63:271, 1990.

81. Nurmohamed MT, Rosendaal FR, Buller HR, et al: Low-molecular-weight heparin versus standard heparin in general and orthopaedic surgery: A meta-analysis. *Lancet* 340:152, 1992.

82. Wilde MI, Markham A: Danaparoid. A review of its pharmacology and clinical use in the management of heparin-induced thrombocytopenia. *Drugs* 54:903, 1997.

83. Chong BH: Heparin-induced thrombocytopenia. *J Thromb Haemost* 1:1471, 2003.

84. Ibbotson T, Perry CM: Danaparoid: a review of its use in thromboembolic and coagulation disorders. *Drugs* 62:2283, 2002.

85. Farner B, Eichler P, Kroll H, et al: A comparison of danaparoid and lepirudin in heparin-induced thrombocytopenia. *Thromb Haemost* 85: 950, 2001.

86. Turpie AG: Pentasaccharides. *Semin Hematol* 39:158, 2002.

87. Samama MM, Gerotziafas GT: Evaluation of the pharmacological properties and clinical results of the synthetic pentasaccharide (fondaparinux). *Thromb Res* 109:1, 2003.

88. Boneu B, Necciari J, Cariou R, et al: Pharmacokinetics and tolerance of the natural pentasaccharide (SR90107/Org31540) with high affinity to antithrombin III in man. *Thromb Haemost* 74:1468, 1995.

89. Turpie AG, Bauer KA, Eriksson BI, et al: Fondaparinux vs enoxaparin for the prevention of venous thromboembolism in major orthopedic surgery: A meta-analysis of 4 randomized double-blind studies. *Arch Intern Med* 162:1833, 2002.

90. Buller HR, Davidson BL, Decousus H, et al: Subcutaneous fondaparinux versus intravenous unfractionated heparin in the initial treatment of pulmonary embolism. *N Engl J Med* 349:1695, 2003.

91. Amiral J, Lormeau JC, Marfaing-Koka A, et al: Absence of cross-reactivity of SR90107A/ORG31540 pentasaccharide with antibodies to heparin-PF4 complexes developed in heparin-induced thrombocytopenia. *Blood Coagul Fibrinolysis* 8:114, 1997.

92. Ahmed S, Jeske WP, Walenga JM, et al: Synthetic pentasaccharides do not cause platelet activation by antiheparin-platelet factor 4 antibodies. *Clin Appl Thromb Haemost* 5:259, 1999.

93. Elalamy I, Lecrubier C, Potevin F, et al: Absence of in vitro cross-reaction of pentasaccharide with the plasma heparin-dependent factor of twenty-five patients with heparin-associated thrombocytopenia. *Thromb Haemost* 74:1384, 1995.

94. Parody R, Oliver A, Souto JC, et al: Fondaparinux (ARIXTRA) as an alternative anti-thrombotic prophylaxis when there is hypersensitivity to low molecular weight and unfractionated heparins. *Haematologica* 88: ECR32, 2003.

95. Stone SR, Braun PJ, Hofsteenge J: Identification of regions of alpha-thrombin involved in its interaction with hirudin. *Biochemistry* 26:4617, 1987.

96. Stone SR, Hofsteenge J: Kinetics of the inhibition of thrombin by hirudin. *Biochemistry* 25:4622, 1986.

97. Tulinsky A: Molecular interactions of thrombin. *Semin Thromb Hemost* 22:117, 1996.

98. Meiring SM, Lotter MG, Badenhorst PN, et al: Sites of elimination and pharmacokinetics of recombinant [131I]lepirudin in baboons. *J Pharm Sci* 88:523, 1999.

99. Meyer BH, Luus HG, Muller FO, et al: The pharmacology of recombinant hirudin, a new anticoagulant. *S Afr Med J* 78:268, 1990.

100. Cardot JM, Lefevre GY, Godbillon JA: Pharmacokinetics of rec-hirudin in healthy volunteers after intravenous administration. *J Pharmacokinet Biopharm* 22:147, 1994.

101. Zoldhelyi P, Webster MW, Fuster V, et al: Recombinant hirudin in patients with chronic, stable coronary artery disease. Safety, half-life, and effect on coagulation parameters. *Circulation* 88:2015, 1993.

102. Verstraete M, Nurmohamed M, Kienast J, et al: Biologic effects of recombinant hirudin (CGP 39393) in human volunteers. European Hirudin in Thrombosis Group. *J Am Coll Cardiol* 22:1080, 1993.

103. Esslinger HU, Haas S, Maurer R, et al: Pharmacodynamic and safety results of PEG-hirudin in healthy volunteers. *Thromb Haemost* 77:911, 1997.

104. Tripodi A, Chantarangkul V, Arbini AA, et al: Effects of hirudin on activated partial thromboplastin time determined with ten different reagents. *Thromb Haemost* 70:286, 1993.

105. Potzsch B, Hund S, Madlener K, et al: Monitoring of recombinant hirudin: assessment of a plasma-based ecarin clotting time assay. *Thromb Res* 86:373, 1997.

106. Huhle G, Hoffmann U, Song X, et al: Immunologic response to recombinant hirudin in HIT type II patients during long-term treatment. *Br J Haematol* 106:195, 1999.

107. Song X, Huhle G, Wang L, et al: Generation of anti-hirudin antibodies in heparin-induced thrombocytopenic patients treated with r-hirudin. *Circulation* 100:1528, 1999.

108. Huhle G, Liebe V, Hudek R, et al: Anti-r-hirudin antibodies reveal clinical relevance through direct functional inactivation of r-hirudin or prolongation of r-hirudin's plasma halflife. *Thromb Haemost* 85:936, 2001.

109. Eichler P, Friesen HJ, Lubenow N, et al: Antihirudin antibodies in patients with heparin-induced thrombocytopenia treated with lepirudin: incidence, effects on aPTT, and clinical relevance. *Blood* 96:2373, 2000.

110. Maraganore JM, Bourdon P, Jablonski J, et al: Design and characterization of hirulogs: a novel class of bivalent peptide inhibitors of thrombin. *Biochemistry* 29:7095, 1990.

111. Parry MA, Maraganore JM, Stone SR: Kinetic mechanism for the interaction of Hirulog with thrombin. *Biochemistry* 33:14807, 1994.

112. Fox I, Dawson A, Loynds P, et al: Anticoagulant activity of Hirulog, a direct thrombin inhibitor, in humans. *Thromb Haemost* 69:157, 1993.

113. Robson R: The use of bivalirudin in patients with renal impairment. *J Invasive Cardiol* 12 Suppl F:33F 2000.

114. Kikumoto R, Tamao Y, Tezuka T, et al: Selective inhibition of thrombin by (2R,4R)-4-methyl-1-[N2-[(3-methyl-1,2,3,4-tetrahydro-8-quinolinyl++ +) sulfonyl]-1-arginyl)]-2-piperidinecarboxylic acid. *Biochemistry* 23:85, 1984.

115. Berry CN, Girardot C, Lecoffre C, et al: Effects of the synthetic thrombin inhibitor argatroban on fibrin- or clot-incorporated thrombin: Comparison with heparin and recombinant Hirudin. *Thromb Haemost* 72: 381, 1994.

116. Hursting, MJ, Alford KL, Becker JC, et al: Novastan (brand of argatroban): A small-molecule, direct thrombin inhibitor. *Semin Thromb Hemost* 23:503, 1997.

117. McKeage K, Plosker GL: Argatroban. *Drugs* 61:515, 2001.

118. Swan SK, Hursting MJ: The pharmacokinetics and pharmacodynamics of argatroban: effects of age, gender, and hepatic or renal dysfunction. *Pharmacotherapy* 20:318, 2000.

119. Gosselin RC, Dager WE, King JH, et al: Effect of direct thrombin inhibitors, bivalirudin, lepirudin, and argatroban, on prothrombin time and INR values. *Am J Clin Pathol* 121:593, 2004.

120. Francis CW: Ximelagatran: A new oral anticoagulant *Best Prac Res Clin Haematol* 17:139,2004.

121. Gustafsson D, Nystrom J, Carlsson S, et al: The direct thrombin inhibitor melagatran and its oral prodrug H 376/95: Intestinal absorption properties, biochemical and pharmacodynamic effects. *Thromb Res* 101:171, 2001.

122. Eriksson UG, Bredberg U, Hoffmann KJ, et al: Absorption, distribution, metabolism, and excretion of ximelagatran, an oral direct thrombin inhibitor, in rats, dogs, and humans. *Drug Metab Dispos* 31:294, 2003.

123. Johansson LC, Frison L, Logren U, et al: Influence of age on the pharmacokinetics and pharmacodynamics of ximelagatran, an oral direct thrombin inhibitor. *Clin Pharmacokinet* 42:381, 2003.

124. Nylander S, Mattsson C: Thrombin-induced platelet activation and its inhibition by anticoagulants with different modes of action. *Blood Coagul Fibrinolysis* 14:159, 2003.

125. Sarich TC, Wolzt M, Eriksson UG, et al: Effects of ximelagatran, an oral direct thrombin inhibitor, r-hirudin and enoxaparin on thrombin generation and platelet activation in healthy male subjects. *J Am Coll Cardiol* 41:557, 2003.

126. Mattsson C, Menschik-Lundin A, Nylander S, et al: Effect of different types of thrombin inhibitors on thrombin/thrombomodulin modulated activation of protein C *in vitro. Thromb Res* 104:475, 2001.

127. Hauptmann J: Pharmacokinetics of an emerging new class of anticoagulant/antithrombotic drugs. A review of small-molecule thrombin inhibitors. *Eur J Clin Pharmacol* 57:751, 2002.

128. Eriksson H, Eriksson UG, Frison L, et al: Pharmacokinetics and pharmacodynamics of melagatran, a novel synthetic LMW thrombin inhibitor, in patients with acute DVT. *Thromb Haemost* 81:358, 1999.

129. Gustafsson D, Antonsson T, Bylund R, et al: Effects of melagatran, a new low-molecular-weight thrombin inhibitor, on thrombin and fibrinolytic enzymes. *Thromb Haemost* 79:110, 1998.

130. Hafner G, Roser M, Nauck M: Methods for the monitoring of direct thrombin inhibitors. *Semin Thromb Hemost* 28:425, 2002.

131. Francis CW, Davidson BL, Berkowitz SD, et al: Ximelagatran versus warfarin for the prevention of venous thromboembolism after total knee arthroplasty. A randomized, double-blind trial. *Ann Intern Med* 137:648, 2002.

132. Francis CW, Berkowitz SD, Comp PC, et al: Comparison of ximelagatran with warfarin for the prevention of venous thromboembolism after total knee replacement. *N Engl J Med* 349:1703, 2003.

133. Colwell CW Jr, Berkowitz SD, Davidson BL, et al: Comparison of ximelagatran, an oral direct thrombin inhibitor, with enoxaparin for the prevention of venous thromboembolism following total hip replacement. A randomized, double-blind study. *J Thromb Haemost* 1:2119, 2003.

134. Huisman M: Efficacy and safety of the oral direct thrombin inhibitor ximelagatran compared with current standard therapy for acute symptomatic deep vein thrombosis with or without pulmonary embolism, a double-blind, multinational trial. Abstracts of the XIX Congress of the ISTH, 2003.

135. Halperin JL: Ximelagatran compared with warfarin for prevention of thromboembolism in patients with nonvalvular atrial fibrillatiom: Rationale, objectivers and design of a pair of clinical studies and baseline patient characteristics (SPORTIF III and V). *Am Heart J* 146:431, 2003.

136. Wallentin L, Wilcox RG, Weaver WD, et al: Oral ximelagatran for secondary prophylaxis after myocardial infarction: the ESTEEM randomised controlled trial. *Lancet* 362:789, 2003.

137. Wohl RC, Summaria L, Arzadon L, et al: Steady state kinetics of activation of human and bovine plasminogens by streptokinase and its equimolar complexes with various activated forms of human plasminogen. *J Biol Chem* 253:1402, 1978.

138. Castellino FJ: A unique enzyme-protein substrate modifier reaction: plasmin/streptokinase interaction. *Trends Biochem Sci* 4:1, 1979.

139. Cederholm-Williams SA: The binding of plasmin-streptokinase complex to fibrin monomer-Sepharose. *Thromb Res* 17.573, 1980.

140. Cederholm-Williams SA, De Cock F, Lijnen HR, et al: Kinetics of the reactions between streptokinase, plasmin and alpha 2-antiplasmin. *Eur J Biochem* 100:125, 1979.

141. Marder VJ: The use of thrombolytic agents: Choice of patient, drug administration, laboratory monitoring. *Ann Intern Med* 90:802, 1979.

142. Marder VJ, Sherry S: Thrombolytic therapy: Current status (1). *N Engl J Med* 318:1512, 1988.

143. Buchalter MB: Is the development of antibodies to streptokinase clinically relevant? *Drugs* 48:133, 1994.

144. Ojalvo AG, Pozo L, Labarta V, et al: Prevalence of circulating antibodies against a streptokinase C-terminal peptide in normal blood donors. *Biochem Biophys Res Commun* 263:454, 1999.

145. Smith RAG, Dupe RJ, English PD, et al: Fibrinolysis with acyl enzymes: A new approach to thrombolytic therapy. *Nature* 290:505, 1981.

146. Holmes WE, Pernica D, Blaber M, et al: Cloning and expression of the gene for prourokinase in E. coli. *Biotechnology* 3:923, 1985.

147. Hussain S, Gurewich V, Lipinski B: Purification and characterization of a single-chain high-molecular-weight form of urokinase from human urine. *Arch Biochem Biophys* 220:31, 1983.

148. Wun TC, Schleuning WD, Reich E: Isolation and characterization of urokinase from human plasma. *J Biol Chem* 257:3276, 1982.

149. Ichinose A, Fujikawa K, Suyama T: The activation of pro-urokinase by plasma kallikrein and its inactivation by thrombin. *J Biol Chem* 261:3486, 1986.

150. List K, Jensen ON, Bugge TH, et al: Plasminogen-independent initiation of the pro-urokinase activation cascade in vivo. Activation of pro-urokinase by glandular kallikrein (mGK-6) in plasminogen-deficient mice. *Biochemistry* 39:508, 2000.

151. Lijnen HR, Van Hoef B, Collen D: Activation with plasmin of two-chain urokinase-type plasminogen activator derived from single-chain urokinase-type plasminogen activator by treatment with thrombin. *Eur J Biochem* 169:359, 1987.

152. Ellis V, Scully MF, Kakkar VV: Plasminogen activation by single-chain urokinase in functional isolation. A kinetic study. *J Biol Chem* 262:14998, 1987.

153. Pannell R, Gurewich V: Activation of plasminogen by single-chain urokinase or by two-chain urokinase—A demonstration that single-chain urokinase has a low catalytic activity (pro-urokinase). *Blood* 69:22, 1987.

154. Lijnen HR, Van Hoef B, De Cock F, et al: The mechanism of plasminogen activation and fibrin dissolution by single chain urokinase-type plasminogen activator in a plasma milieu in vitro. *Blood* 73:1864, 1989.

155. Pennica D, Holmes WE, Kohr WJ, et al: Cloning and expression of human tissue-type plasminogen activator cDNA in E. coli. *Nature* 301:214, 1983.

156. Edlund T, Ny T, Ranby M, et al: Isolation of cDNA sequences coding for a part of human tissue plasminogen activator. *Proc Natl Acad Sci U S A* 80:349, 1983.

157. Rijken DC, Collen D: Purification and characterization of the plasminogen activator secreted by human melanoma cells in culture. *J Biol Chem* 256:7035, 1981.

158. Nieuwenhuizen W, Voskuilen M, Vermond A, et al: The influence of fibrin(ogen) fragments on the kinetic parameters of the tissue-type plasminogen-activator-mediated activation of different forms of plasminogen. *Eur J Biochem* 174:163, 1988.

159. Suenson E, Bjerrum P, Holm A, et al: The role of fragment X polymers in the fibrin enhancement of tissue plasminogen activator-catalyzed plasmin formation. *J Biol Chem* 265:22228, 1990.

160. Suensen E, Petersen LD: Fibrin and plasminogen structures essential to stimulation to plasmin formation by tissue-type plasminogen activator. *Biochem Biophys Acta* 870:510, 1986.

161. Kohnert U, Rudolph R, Verheijen JH, et al: Biochemical properties of the kringle 2 and protease domains are maintained in the refolded t-PA deletion variant BM 06.022. *Protein Eng* 5:93, 1992.

162. Martin U, Von Mollendorff E, Akpan W, et al: Dose-ranging study of the novel recombinant plasminogen activator BM 06.022 in healthy volunteers. *Clin Pharmacol Ther* 50:429, 1991.

163. Keyt BA, Paoni NF, Refino CJ, et al: A faster-acting and more potent form of tissue plasminogen activator. *Proc Natl Acad Sci U S A* 91:3670, 1994.

164. Collen D: Staphylokinase: A potent, uniquely fibrin-selective thrombolytic agent. *Nat Med* 4:279, 1998.

165. Hawkey C: Plasminogen activator in saliva of the vampire bat *Desmodus rotundus. Nature* 211:434, 1966.

166. Gardell SJ, Duong LT, Diehl RE, et al: Isolation, characterization, and cDNA cloning of a vampire bat salivary plasminogen activator. *J Biol Chem* 264:17947, 1989.

167. Needleman P, Turk J, Jakschik BA, et al: Arachidonic acid metabolism. *Annu Rev Biochem* 55:69, 1986.

168. Hamberg M, Samuelsson B: Prostaglandin endoperoxides. Novel transformations of arachidonic acid in human platelets. *Proc Natl Acad Sci U S A* 71:3400, 1974.

169. Weiss, HJ, Aledort LM: Impaired platelet-connective-tissue reaction in man after aspirin ingestion. *Lancet* 2:495, 1967.

170. Zucker MB, Peterson J: Inhibition of adenosine diphosphate-induced secondary aggregation and other platelet functions by acetylsalicylic acid ingestion. *Proc Soc Exp Biol Med* 127:547, 1968.

171. Evans G, Packham MA, Nishizawa EE, et al: The effect of acetylsalicylic acid on platelet function. *J Exp Med* 128:877, 1968.

172. Mills DG, Hirst M, Philp RB: The effects of some salicylate analogues on human blood platelets. 2. The role of platelet acetylation in the inhibition of platelet aggregation. *Life Sci* 14:673, 1974.

173. Roth GJ, Majerus PW: The mechanism of the effect of aspirin on human platelets. I: Acetylation of a particulate fraction protein. *J Clin Invest* 56:624, 1975.

174. Roth GJ, Stanford N, Majerus PW: Acetylation of prostaglandin synthase by aspirin. *Proc Natl Acad Sci U S A* 72:3073, 1975.

175. Mitchell JA, Akarasereenont P, Thiemermann C, et al: Selectivity of nonsteroidal antiinflammatory drugs as inhibitors of constitutive and inducible cyclooxygenase. *Proc Natl Acad Sci U S A* 90:11693, 1993.

176. Rocca B, Secchiero P, Ciabattoni G, et al: Cyclooxygenase-2 expression is induced during human megakaryopoiesis and characterizes newly formed platelets. *Proc Natl Acad Sci U S A* 99:7634, 2002.

177. Silver MJ, Smith JB, Ingerman C, et al: Arachidonic acid-induced human platelet aggregation and prostaglandin formation. *Prostaglandins* 4:863, 1973.

178. Higgs GA, Moncada S, Vane JR: Prostacyclin (PGI2) inhibits the formation of platelet thrombi induced by adenosine diphosphate (ADP) in vivo [proceedings]. *Br J Pharmacol* 61:137P 1977.

179. Kaplan KL, Broekman MJ, Chernoff A, et al: Platelet alpha-granule proteins: studies on release and subcellular localization. *Blood* 53:604, 1979.

180. Hennekens CH: Update on aspirin in the treatment and prevention of cardiovascular disease. *Am Heart J* 137:S9, 1999.

181. Mehta P: Aspirin in the prophylaxis of coronary artery disease. *Curr Opin Cardiol* 17:552, 2002.

182. Gent M, Barnett HJ, Sackett DL, et al: A randomized trial of aspirin and sulfinpyrazone in patients with threatened stroke. Results and methodologic issues. *Circulation* 62:V97, 1980.

183. Barnett HJ: Therapy of carotid arteriosclerosis. *Annu Rev Med* 45:53, 1994.

184. Hull RD, Raskob GE, Pineo GF, et al: Subcutaneous low-molecular-weight heparin compared with continuous intravenous heparin in the treatment of proximal-vein thrombosis. *N Engl J Med* 326:975, 1992.

185. Chunilal SD, Ginsberg JS: Strategies for the diagnosis of deep vein thrombosis and pulmonary embolism. *Thromb Res* 97:V33, 2000.

186. Pini M, Aiello S, Manotti C, et al: Low molecular weight heparin versus warfarin in the prevention of recurrences after deep vein thrombosis. *Thromb Haemost* 72:191, 1994.

187. Colwell CW Jr, Collis DK, Paulson R, et al: Comparison of enoxaparin and warfarin for the prevention of venous thromboembolic disease after total hip arthroplasty. Evaluation during hospitalization and three months after discharge. *J Bone Joint Surg Am* 81:932, 1999.

188. Forgione MA, Leopold JA, Loscalzo J: Roles of endothelial dysfunction in coronary artery disease. *Curr Opin Cardiol* 15:409, 2000.

189. Hylek EM, Go AS, Chang Y, et al: Effect of intensity of oral anticoagulation on stroke severity and mortality in atrial fibrillation. *N Engl J Med* 349:1019, 2003.

190. Wolfe SM, Shulman NR: Adenyl cyclase activity in human platelets. *Biochem Biophys Res Commun* 35:265, 1969.

191. Ardlie NG, Glew G, Schultz BG, et al: Inhibition and reversal of platelet aggregation by methyl xanthines. *Thromb Diath Haemorrh* 18:670, 1967.

192. Song SY, Cheung WY: Cyclic 3′,5′-nucleotide phosphodiesterase properties of the enzyme of human blood platelets. *Biochim Biophys Acta* 242:593, 1971.

193. Mills DC, Smith JB: The influence on platelet aggregation of drugs that affect the accumulation of adenosine 3′:5′-cyclic monophosphate in platelets. *Biochem J* 121:185, 1971.

194. Marquis NR, Vigdahl RL, Tavormina PA: Platelet aggregation. I. Regulation by cyclic AMP and prostaglandin E1. *Biochem Biophys Res Commun* 36:965, 1969.

195. Vigdahl RL, Marquis NR, Tavormina PA: Platelet aggregation. II. Adenyl cyclase, prostaglandin E1, and calcium. *Biochem Biophys Res Commun* 37:409, 1969.

196. Salzman EW, Rubino EB, Sims RV: Cyclic 3,′5′-adenosine monophosphate in human blood platelets. 3. The role of cyclic AMP in platelet aggregation. *Ser Haematol* 3:100, 1970.

197. Holmsen H: *Cyclic AMP-Dependent Protein Kinases and Protein Kinase C in Platelet Responses and Metabolism*, p 51. CRC Press, Boca Raton, FL, 1987.

198. Weithmann KU: Reduced platelet aggregation by effects of pentoxifylline on vascular prostacyclin isomerase and platelet cyclic AMP. *Gen Pharmacol* 14:161, 1983.

199. Hammerschmidt DE, Kotasek D, McCarthy T, et al: Pentoxifylline inhibits granulocyte and platelet function, including granulocyte priming by platelet activating factor. *J Lab Clin Med* 112:254, 1988.

200. Sudo T, Tachibana K, Toga K, et al: Potent effects of novel anti-platelet aggregatory cilostamide analogues on recombinant cyclic nucleotide phosphodiesterase isozyme activity. *Biochem Pharmacol* 59:347, 2000.

201. Moncada S, Vane JR, Whittle BJ: Relative potency of prostacyclin, prostaglandin E1 and D2 as inhibitors of platelet aggregation in several species [proceedings]. *J Physiol* 273:2P, 1977.

202. Mills DC, Macfarlane DE: Stimulation of human platelet adenylate cyclase by prostaglandin D2. *Thromb Res* 5:401, 1974.

203. Moncada S, Higgs EA, Vane JR: Human arterial and venous tissues generate prostacyclin (prostaglandin x), a potent inhibitor of platelet aggregation. *Lancet* 1:18, 1977.

204. Gorman RR, Bunting S, Miller OV: Modulation of human platelet adenylate cyclase by prostacyclin (PGX). *Prostaglandins* 13:377, 1977.

205. Heit JA, Silverstein MD, Mohr DN, et al: Risk factors for deep vein thrombosis and pulmonary embolism: A population-based case-control study. *Arch Intern Med* 160:809, 2000.

206. Ward A, Clissold SP: Pentoxifylline. A review of its pharmacodynamic and pharmacokinetic properties, and its therapeutic efficacy. *Drugs* 34:50, 1987.

207. Lee TM, Su SF, Tsai CH, et al: Differential effects of cilostazol and pentoxifylline on vascular endothelial growth factor in patients with intermittent claudication. *Clin Sci (Lond)* 101:305, 2001.

208. Chen YM, Wu KD, Tsai TJ, et al: Pentoxifylline inhibits PDGF-induced proliferation of and TGF-beta-stimulated collagen synthesis by vascular smooth muscle cells. *J Mol Cell Cardiol* 31:773, 1999.

209. Hood SC, Moher D, Barber GG: Management of intermittent claudication with pentoxifylline: Meta-analysis of randomized controlled trials. *CMAJ* 155:1053, 1996.

210. Tjon JA, Riemann LE: Treatment of intermittent claudication with pentoxifylline and cilostazol. *Am J Health Syst Pharm* 58:485, 2001.

211. Money SR, Herd JA, Isaacsohn JL, et al: Effect of cilostazol on walking distances in patients with intermittent claudication caused by peripheral vascular disease. *J Vasc Surg* 27:267, 1998.

212. Dawson DL, Cutler BS, Meissner MH, et al: Cilostazol has beneficial effects in treatment of intermittent claudication: results from a multicenter, randomized, prospective, double-blind trial. *Circulation* 98:678, 1998.

213. Ochiai M, Isshiki T, Takeshita S, et al: Use of cilostazol, a novel antiplatelet agent, in a post-Palmaz-Schatz stenting regimen. *Am J Cardiol* 79:1471, 1997.

214. Yoon Y, Shim WH, Lee DH, et al: Usefulness of cilostazol versus ticlopidine in coronary artery stenting. *Am J Cardiol* 84:1375, 1999.

215. Tanigawa T, Nishikawa M, Kitai T, et al: Increased platelet aggregability in response to shear stress in acute myocardial infarction and its inhibition by combined therapy with aspirin and cilostazol after coronary intervention. *Am J Cardiol* 85:1054, 2000.

216. Kamishirado H, Inoue T, Mizoguchi K, et al: Randomized comparison of cilostazol versus ticlopidine hydrochloride for antiplatelet therapy after coronary stent implantation for prevention of late restenosis. *Am Heart J* 144:303, 2002.

217. Defreyn G, Gachet C, Savi P, et al: Ticlopidine and clopidogrel (SR 25990C) selectively neutralize ADP inhibition of PGE1-activated platelet adenylate cyclase in rats and rabbits. *Thromb Haemost* 65:186, 1991.

218. Savi P, Herbert JM, Pflieger AM, et al: Importance of hepatic metabolism in the antiaggregating activity of the thienopyridine clopidogrel. *Biochem Pharmacol* 44:527, 1992.

219. Savi P, Combalbert J, Gaich C, et al: The antiaggregating activity of clopidogrel is due to a metabolic activation by the hepatic cytochrome P450-1A. *Thromb Haemost* 72:313, 1994.

220. Mills DC, Puri R, Hu CJ, et al: Clopidogrel inhibits the binding of ADP analogues to the receptor mediating inhibition of platelet adenylate cyclase. *Arterioscler Thromb* 12:430, 1992.

221. Foster CJ, Prosser DM, Agans JM, et al: Molecular identification and characterization of the platelet ADP receptor targeted by thienopyridine antithrombotic drugs. *J Clin Invest* 107:1591, 2001.

222. Gent M, Blakely JA, Easton JD, et al: The Canadian American Ticlopidine Study (CATS) in thromboembolic stroke. *Lancet* 1:1215, 1989.

223. Cosmi B, Rubboli A, Castelvetri C, et al: Ticlopidine versus oral anticoagulation for coronary stenting. *Cochrane Database Syst Rev* CD002133, 2001.

224. Dunlop H, Siu K: Serious hematologic reactions associated with ticlopidine—update. *CMAJ* 161:867, 1999.

225. Casella G, Ottani F, Pavesi PC, et al: Safety and efficacy evaluation of clopidogrel compared to ticlopidine after stent implantation: An updated meta-analysis. *Ital Heart J* 4:677, 2003.

226. Bhatt DL, Bertrand ME, Berger PB, et al: Meta-analysis of randomized and registry comparisons of ticlopidine with clopidogrel after stenting. *J Am Coll Cardiol* 39:9, 2002.

227. Jneid H, Bhatt DL, Corti R, et al: Aspirin and clopidogrel in acute coronary syndromes: therapeutic insights from the CURE study. *Arch Intern Med* 163:1145, 2003.

228. Anonymous: A randomised, blinded, trial of clopidogrel versus aspirin in patients at risk of ischaemic events (CAPRIE). CAPRIE Steering Committee. *Lancet* 348:1329, 1996.

229. McCarthy MW, Kockler DR: Clopidogrel-associated leukopenia. *Ann Pharmacother* 37:216, 2003.

230. Peters RJ, Mehta SR, Fox KA, et al: Effects of aspirin dose when used alone or in combination with clopidogrel in patients with acute coronary syndromes: Observations from the Clopidogrel in Unstable angina to prevent Recurrent Events (CURE) study. *Circulation* 108:1682, 2003.

231. Teal PA: Recent clinical trial results with antiplatelet therapy: Implications in stroke prevention. *Cerebrovasc Dis* 17 Suppl 3:6, 2004.

232. Bradberry JC: Peripheral arterial disease: pathophysiology, risk factors, and role of antithrombotic therapy. *J Am Pharm Assoc (Wash DC)* 44: S37, 2004.

233. Da Silva AF, Escofet X, Rutherford PA: Medical adjuvant treatment to increase patency of arteriovenous fistulae and grafts. *Cochrane Database Syst Rev* CD002786, 2003.

234. Carswell JL, Beard KA, Chevrette MM, et al: Tracking trends in secondary stroke prevention strategies. *Ann Pharmacother* 38:215, 2004.

235. Hankey GJ: Ongoing and planned trials of antiplatelet therapy in the acute and long-term management of patients with ischaemic brain syndromes: Setting a new standard of care. *Cerebrovasc Dis* 17 Suppl 3: 11, 2004.

236. Bennett JS, Vilaire G: Exposure of platelet fibrinogen receptors by ADP and epinephrine. *J Clin Invest* 64:1393, 1979.

237. Marguerie GA, Plow EF, Edgington TS: Human platelets possess an inducible and saturable receptor specific for fibrinogen. *J Biol Chem* 254:5357, 1979.

238. Caen JP, Vainer H, Gautier A: Thrombasthenia. *Thromb Diath Haemorrh Suppl* 26:223, 1967.

239. Weiss HJ: Platelet aggregation, adhesion and adenosine diphosphate release in thrombopathia (platelet factor 3 deficiency). A comparison with Glanzmann's thrombasthenia and von Willebrand's disease. *Am J Med* 43:570, 1967.

240. Gartner TK, Gerrard JM, White JG, et al: The endogenous lectin of human platelets is an alpha-granule component. *Blood* 58:153, 1981.

241. Haverstick DM, Dixit VM, Grant GA, et al: Characterization of the platelet agglutinating activity of thrombospondin. *Biochemistry* 24: 3128, 1985.

242. Nachman RL: Thrombasthenia: Immunologic evidence of a platelet protein abnormality. *J Lab Clin Med* 67:411, 1966.

243. Coller BS, Peerschke EI, Scudder LE, et al: A murine monoclonal antibody that completely blocks the binding of fibrinogen to platelets produces a thrombasthenic-like state in normal platelets and binds to glycoproteins IIb and/or IIIa. *J Clin Invest* 72:325, 1983.

244. Bennett JS, Hoxic JA, Leitman SF, et al: Inhibition of fibrinogen binding to stimulated human platelets by a monoclonal antibody. *Proc Natl Acad Sci U S A* 80:2417, 1983.

245. Phillips DR, Charo IF, Parise LV, et al: The platelet membrane glycoprotein IIb-IIIa complex. *Blood* 71:831, 1988.

246. Kloczewiak M, Timmons S, Lukas TJ, et al: Platelet receptor recognition site on human fibrinogen. Synthesis and structure-function relationship of peptides corresponding to the carboxy-terminal segment of the gamma chain. *Biochemistry* 23:1767, 1984.

247. Lam SC, Plow EF, Smith MA, et al: Evidence that arginyl-glycyl-aspartate peptides and fibrinogen gamma chain peptides share a common binding site on platelets. *J Biol Chem* 262:947, 1987.

248. Pytela R, Pierschbacher MD, Ginsberg MH, et al: Platelet membrane glycoprotein IIb/IIIa: member of a family of Arg-Gly-Asp–specific adhesion receptors. *Science* 231:1559, 1986.

249. McEver RP, Bennett EM, Martin MN: Identification of two structurally and functionally distinct sites on human platelet membrane glycoprotein IIb-IIIa using monoclonal antibodies. *J Biol Chem* 258:5269, 1983.

250. Pidard D, Montgomery RR, Bennett JS, et al: Interaction of AP-2, a monoclonal antibody specific for the human platelet glycoprotein IIb-IIIa complex, with intact platelets. *J Biol Chem* 258:12582, 1983.

251. Vilella R, Lozano T, Mila J, et al: An antiplatelet monoclonal antibody that inhibits ADP and epinephrine-induced aggregation. *Thromb Haemost* 51:93, 1984.

252. Di Minno G, Thiagarajan P, Perussia B, et al: Exposure of platelet fibrinogen-binding sites by collagen, arachidonic acid, and ADP: Inhibition by a monoclonal antibody to the glycoprotein IIb-IIIa complex. *Blood* 61:140, 1983.

253. McEver RP, Martin MN: A monoclonal antibody to a membrane glycoprotein binds only to activated platelets. *J Biol Chem* 259:9799, 1984.

254. Coller BS: A new murine monoclonal antibody reports an activation-dependent change in the conformation and/or microenvironment of the platelet glycoprotein IIb/IIIa complex. *J Clin Invest* 76:101, 1985.

255. Coller BS, Scudder LE, Berger HJ, et al: Inhibition of human platelet function in vivo with a monoclonal antibody. With observations on the newly dead as experimental subjects. *Ann Intern Med* 109:635, 1988.

256. Coller BS, Folts JD, Scudder LE, et al: Antithrombotic effect of a monoclonal antibody to the platelet glycoprotein IIb/IIIa receptor in an experimental animal model. *Blood* 68:783, 1986.

257. Coller BS, Folts JD, Smith SR, et al: Abolition of *in vivo* platelet thrombus formation in primates with monoclonal antibodies to the platelet GPIIb/IIIa receptor. Correlation with bleeding time, platelet aggregation, and blockade of GPIIb/IIIa receptors. *Circulation* 80:1766, 1989.

258. Gold HK, Gimple LW, Yasuda T, et al: Pharmacodynamic study of F(ab')2 fragments of murine monoclonal antibody 7E3 directed against

human platelet glycoprotein IIb/IIIa in patients with unstable angina pectoris. *J Clin Invest* 86:651, 1990.

259. Tcheng JE, Ellis SG, George BS, et al: Pharmacodynamics of chimeric glycoprotein IIb/IIIa integrin antiplatelet antibody Fab 7E3 in high-risk coronary angioplasty. *Circulation* 90:1757, 1994.

260. Tcheng JE, Kereiakes DJ, Lincoff AM, et al: Abciximab readministration: Results of the ReoPro Readministration Registry. *Circulation* 104:870, 2001.

261. EPIC Investigators: Use of a monoclonal antibody directed against the platelet glycoprotein IIb/IIIa receptor in high-risk coronary angioplasty. *N Engl J Med* 330:956, 1994.

262. Aguirre FV, Topol EJ, Ferguson JJ, et al: Bleeding complications with the chimeric antibody to platelet glycoprotein IIb/IIIa integrin in patients undergoing percutaneous coronary intervention. EPIC Investigators. *Circulation* 91:2882, 1995.

263. Platelet glycoprotein IIb/IIIa receptor blockade and low-dose heparin during percutaneous coronary revascularization. The EPILOG investigators. *N Engl J Med* 336:1689, 1997.

264. Bednar RA, Gaul SL, Hamill TG, et al: Identification of low molecular weight GP IIb/IIIa antagonists that bind preferentially to activated platelets. *J Pharmacol Exp Ther* 285:1317, 1998.

265. Phillips DR, Scarborough RM: Clinical pharmacology of eptifibatide. *Am J Cardiol* 80:11B 1997.

266. Fisher MJ, Gunn B, Harms CS, et al: Non-peptide RGD surrogates which mimic a Gly-Asp beta-turn: Potent antagonists of platelet glycoprotein IIb-IIIa. *J Med Chem* 40:2085, 1997.

267. Egbertson MS, Chang CT, Duggan ME, et al: Non-peptide fibrinogen receptor antagonists. 2. Optimization of a tyrosine template as a mimic for Arg-Gly-Asp. *J Med Chem* 37:2537, 1994.

268. Ramjit DR, Lynch JJ Jr, Sitko GR, et al: Antithrombotic effects of MK-0852, a platelet fibrinogen receptor antagonist, in canine models of thrombosis. *J Pharmacol Exp Ther* 266:1501, 1993.

269. Gilchrist IC, O'Shea JC, Kosoglou T, et al: Pharmacodynamics and pharmacokinetics of higher-dose, double-bolus eptifibatide in percutaneous coronary intervention. *Circulation* 104:406, 2001.

270. Lorenz TJ, Macdonald F, Kitt MM: Nonimmunogenicity of eptifibatide, a cyclic heptapeptide inhibitor of platelet glycoprotein IIb-IIIa. *Clin Ther* 21:128, 1999.

271. Tcheng JE, Harrington RA, Kottke-Marchant K, et al: Multicenter, randomized, double-blind, placebo-controlled trial of the platelet integrin glycoprotein IIb/IIIa blocker Integrelin in elective coronary intervention. IMPACT Investigators. *Circulation* 91:2151, 1995.

272. Lynch JJ Jr, Cook JJ, Sitko GR, et al: Nonpeptide glycoprotein IIb/IIIa inhibitors. 5. Antithrombotic effects of MK-0383. *J Pharmacol Exp Ther* 272:20, 1995.

273. Peerlinck K, De Lepeleire I, Goldberg M, et al: MK-383 (L-700,462), a selective nonpeptide platelet glycoprotein IIb/IIIa antagonist, is active in man. *Circulation* 88:1512, 1993.

274. Barrett JS, Murphy G, Peerlinck K, et al: Pharmacokinetics and pharmacodynamics of MK-383, a selective non-peptide platelet glycoprotein-IIb/IIIa receptor antagonist, in healthy men. *Clin Pharmacol Ther* 56:377, 1994.

275. Kereiakes DJ, Kleiman NS, Ambrose J, et al: Randomized, double-blind, placebo-controlled dose-ranging study of tirofiban (MK-383) platelet IIb/IIIa blockade in high-risk patients undergoing coronary angioplasty. *J Am Coll Cardiol* 27:536, 1996.

276. Gibson CM, Goel M, Cohen DJ, et al: Six-month angiographic and clinical follow-up of patients prospectively randomized to receive either tirofiban or placebo during angioplasty in the RESTORE trial. Randomized Efficacy Study of Tirofiban for Outcomes and Restenosis. *J Am Coll Cardiol* 32:28, 1998.

277. Kong DF, Hasselblad V, Harrington RA, et al: Meta-analysis of survival with platelet glycoprotein IIb/IIIa antagonists for percutaneous coronary interventions. *Am J Cardiol* 92:651, 2003.

278. Roffi M, Chew DP, Mukherjee D, et al: Platelet glycoprotein IIb/IIIa inhibition in acute coronary syndromes. Gradient of benefit related to the revascularization strategy. *Eur Heart J* 23:1441, 2002.

PRINCIPLES OF HEMATOPOIETIC CELL TRANSPLANTATION

ROBERT S. NEGRIN

KARL G. BLUME

Hematopoietic cell transplantation has evolved from a treatment of last resort for patients with refractory leukemias to an effective, and in some instances front-line, therapy for a broad array of hematologic malignancies and genetic disorders of the marrow and selected solid tumors. In this chapter, the underlying biologic principles are discussed along with future goals and potential applications of this treatment modality. Mechanisms by which this form of therapy can offer curative potential are discussed, as well as complications of immunologic incompetence, graft-versus-host disease, and toxicity. Selected results demonstrating important principles are highlighted.

HISTORY

Transplantation of marrow to rescue patients from the lethal effects of radiation and chemotherapy or to correct abnormal hematopoiesis has evolved over the past four decades as an act of desperation administered only to patients with end-stage disease to a highly successful form of therapy employed in the course of a variety of malignant and nonmalignant disorders. Advances in transplantation biology and supportive care have made that evolution possible and have helped usher in the modern era of hematopoietic cell transplantation.

Table 22-1 lists key historical events leading to the successful application of hematopoietic cell transplantation (HCT). The first description of marrow as a blood-forming tissue was made in 1868 by German and Italian investigators nearly simultaneously. The first documented human marrow transplant was attempted in 1939, for a patient with gold-induced aplasia who was given marrow intravenously from a brother with identical blood group antigens. The transplant was not

successful and the patient died 5 days later.[1] In the early 1950s, in an effort to explain the lethal effects of radiation, laboratory experiments demonstrated that splenic shielding or the intravenous administration of marrow cells protected animals from an otherwise lethal dose of radiation.[2,3] These findings were explained first by the humeral hypothesis, followed later by the cellular hypothesis of marrow reconstitution. In 1955, Main and Prehn first described studies of lethally irradiated mice who were protected from the effects of radiation and were able to tolerate skin grafts following a marrow transplant.[4] Subsequent to these studies, patients with end-stage hematologic malignancies were treated with high doses of radiation or chemotherapy followed by marrow infusion. Although these early studies in the late 1950s and early 1960s were largely unsuccessful, they did demonstrate at least transient engraftment in some patients, which provided a reference for future studies.[5] Sustained engraftment was first documented in 1965 in a patient with acute lymphoblastic leukemia who received radiation and chemotherapy followed by intravenous infusion of marrow from six different related donors.[6] Unfortunately, the patient died of recurrent leukemia 20 months later.

Studies initially in the dog demonstrated the importance of immunologic matching for a successful outcome.[7] The discovery of the human leukocyte antigen (HLA) system and development of histocompatibility typing methods in the 1960s led to a new phase of marrow transplantation. The first successful marrow transplants were performed in 1968 in children with severe combined immunodeficiency,[8,9] and with Wiskott-Aldrich syndrome.[10] In the early 1970s, increasing numbers of patients with acute leukemia who had failed conventional therapy and a patient with advanced aplastic anemia underwent marrow transplantation from identical twin donors[11] and histocompatible siblings.[12,13] For the first time, a significant percentage of patients became long-term disease-free survivors and many of those patients are still surviving more than 30 years later.[14] In 1977 and 1980, the first successful HCT procedures from unrelated marrow donors were reported.[15,16] At the end of 1978, the first series of successful autologous HCTs for lymphoma were reported.[17,18] Based on these early studies, the Nobel Prize in Medicine/Physiology was award to Dr. E.D. Thomas in 1990. By the year 2000, more than 500,000 patients had been transplanted worldwide during the previous three decades.

STEM CELL MODEL OF HEMATOPOIESIS

The scientific basis for hematopoiesis has evolved over many decades. The stem cell model for hematopoiesis predicted the existence of a pluripotent hematopoietic stem cell. The first phenotypic description of a murine hematopoietic stem cell was reported in 1988.[19] These studies ushered in intense interest in the characterization of different hematopoietic stem and progenitor cell populations, as well as studies to determine the factors and genes that control and regulate hematopoiesis.

Hematopoietic stem cells are central to the biologic basis of HCT. The concept that all cellular populations of the hematopoietic and lymphoid systems are derived from a common hematopoietic stem cell population is firmly established. This concept predicts that following successful allogeneic HCT there is transfer not only of hematopoiesis and blood type, but also of immunity. A variety of early in vitro and in vivo assay systems were developed to identify the biologic activity of hematopoietic stem cells.[20,21] Through these studies it was determined that an immature population of cells capable of giving rise to all hematolymphoid cells was present in the bone marrow. Various antigen-presenting cells found in the liver, gastrointestinal tract, lung, and brain were also derived from hematopoietic stem cells.

In murine systems, the development of monoclonal antibodies that recognized specific cell surface antigens allowed for the isolation of

TABLE 22-1   HISTORICAL MARKERS IN HEMATOPOIETIC CELL
TRANSPLANTATION

YEARS	EVENTS/PERIODS
1868	First description of marrow as blood-forming tissue
1939	First documented clinical marrow transplant attempt
1949–1956	The humoral and cellular hypotheses of marrow reconstitution
1956–1959	Renewed efforts in marrow grafting in human diseases
1956–present	Advances in marrow grafting through animal studies
1968–1969	First successful allogeneic HCT in patients with SCID
1975	First large series of allogeneic HCT for leukemia
1977, 1980	Successful HCT procedures from unrelated marrow donors
1978	First series of successful autologous HCT for lymphoma
1988	Isolation of the murine hematopoietic stem cell
1990	Nobel Prize in Medicine/Physiology awarded to Dr. E.D. Thomas
2000	More than 500,000 patients transplanted worldwide during the past three decades

HCT, hematopoietic cell transplantation; SCID, severe combined immunodeficiency.

rare populations of hematopoietic cells capable of performing the functions defined for hematopoietic stem cells, namely, to rescue animals from lethal radiation and to be capable of reisolation and secondary transfer. Using fluorescence-activated cell sorting it has been possible to isolate highly purified marrow cells that can be identified as hematopoietic stem cells (HSCs) by virtue of being capable of rescuing lethally irradiated animals. The phenotypic characteristics of these cells included being positive for stem cell antigen 1 (SCA-1), Thy-1, and c-Kit ligand, yet not expressing various markers found on committed B, T, erythroid, and myeloid cells (Lin−).[19] In addition, HSCs pump out the vital dye rhodamine and express multidrug resistance. Cells of this phenotype are present in the marrow at a frequency of approximately 1×10^{-3} to 1×10^{-4} and morphologically appear similar to normal lymphocytes. More recently, multipotent progenitor cells that commit either to the myeloid lineage, forming common myeloid progenitors (CMPs), or to the lymphoid lineage, forming common lymphoid progenitors (CLPs), were isolated using a similar strategy.[22–25]

The search for HSCs in humans has been more difficult because of the lack of assays of stem cell function as described above. Nevertheless, the use of fluorescence-activated cell sorting has identified human cells that express CD34 and Thy-1 and that are negative for lineage markers that have in vitro and in vivo properties of stem cells.[26,27]

A significant debate following HCT concerns which cells are responsible for hematopoietic engraftment. Several possibilities exist, including that engraftment is initiated by committed progenitor cells followed by stem cell engraftment over a more delayed time frame. Alternatively, stem cells themselves may be solely responsible for hematopoietic engraftment. Murine studies using highly purified populations of HSCs that were transplanted into congenic mouse strains revealed that the time to engraftment, as measured by the return of white blood cells, platelets, and red cells in the blood, was nearly identical between HSC and unfractionated marrow, assuming sufficient numbers of HSCs were administered.[28] The time to hematopoietic cell engraftment was directly related to the dose of purified HSCs infused.[29] In syngeneic (similar to autologous transplantation) murine experiments, as few as 100 HSCs were capable of reconstituting lethally irradiated animals. Escalation of the dose of HSCs up to 5000 per animal reduced the time to engraftment to what is commonly seen in human transplantation of approximately 9 to 10 days. Assuming the average weight of a mouse of 25 g, the equivalent dose of purified

HSCs that would give rapid trilineage hematopoietic engraftment should be approximately 2 to 4×10^5 HSCs/kg.

Initial studies have been performed in humans by isolating CD34+Thy-1+ cells by high-speed cell sorting and performing autologous transplantation. These studies demonstrated that rapid trilineage hematopoietic reconstitution occurs in patients with multiple myeloma, non-Hodgkin lymphoma, and metastatic breast cancer even when cell doses as low as 5×10^5 CD34+Thy-1+ cells/kg were administered.[30–32] These studies indicate that highly purified populations of CD34+Thy-1+ HSCs alone were capable of multilineage engraftment with similar kinetics as observed with unfractionated blood progenitor cells. In addition, these highly purified cell populations were consistently free of malignant cell contamination. Interestingly, the kinetics predicted in murine models is very similar to that observed in patients.

SOURCES OF HEMATOPOIETIC STEM CELLS

A variety of sources have been used for the collection of HSCs for transplantation procedures. These include marrow, blood, and umbilical cord blood obtained at the time of delivery.

MARROW

Marrow has served as the traditional source for HSCs for both allogeneic and autologous transplantation. The marrow is typically aspirated from the posterior iliac crest under either regional or general anesthesia. The cell dose required for stable long-term engraftment has not been defined with certainty, however, a typical collection contains more than 2×10^8 nucleated cells/kg recipient body weight. Current guidelines indicate that collection of up to 20 mL/kg donor body weight are considered safe.

Marrow harvesting is considered a very safe procedure and complications generally involve anesthesia. In a report of 1270 allogeneic marrow harvests from normal donors there were 6 (0.5%) life-threatening complications.[33] Review of the National Marrow Donor experience of volunteer donors in 493 harvests showed that there was only 1 serious adverse event (apnea) and 3 patients (0.6%) required a blood transfusion. Patients typically required up to 16 days to recover and 10 percent of donors still had not completely recovered at the end of the first month following marrow harvest.[34]

PERIPHERAL BLOOD

HSCs are present in the blood at very low levels; however, a number of different stimuli, including chemotherapy, various hematopoietic growth factors, and inhibitors of certain chemokine receptors, result in the mobilization of HSCs into the blood. These cells can then be easily collected with apheresis and have been termed *peripheral blood progenitor cells* (PBPCs) to differentiate them from the terminology of blood stem cells, which should be reserved for instances where the stem cell population itself has been isolated. A variety of different mobilization agents have been used, including granulocyte colony stimulating factor (G-CSF), granulocyte-monocyte colony stimulating factor (GM-CSF), interleukin (IL)-3, thrombopoietin, and more recently the chemokine-related receptor (CXCR4) antagonist AMD3100.[35–38]

The measurement of the absolute number of CD34+ cells/kg recipient weight collected is a reliable and practical method for determining the adequacy of the stem cell product. Most laboratories measure CD34+ cell content by fluorescent-activated cell sorting (FACS). Significant variability exists from laboratory to laboratory, requiring that adequate quality control measures be in place for reliance on a particular value. Most transplantation centers have observed that stem cell products containing more than 2×10^6 CD34+ cells/kg result in rapid trilineage engraftment. Some studies suggest that higher stem cell doses may lead to more rapid platelet recovery.[39] Although the minimum cell dose required for hematopoietic engraftment has not been defined with certainty, most transplantation centers will accept cell doses of $>1\times10^6$ CD34+ cells/kg. Although inadequate mobilization of healthy donors is rare, patients with prior malignancies undergoing mobilization for autologous transplantation often have difficulty collecting adequate numbers of CD34+ cells. Approximately 10 to 20 percent of patients do not mobilize sufficient numbers of CD34+ cells using G-CSF alone or chemotherapy plus G-CSF. Unfortunately, it has been relatively difficult to prospectively identify these individuals. Efforts to add combinations of hematopoietic growth factors to improve mobilization efficiency have met with relatively limited success to date. Nevertheless, collection of blood progenitor cells has emerged as a far simpler, better tolerated procedure for collection of hematopoietic cell grafts for transplantation.

The use of mobilized PBPCs has had a major impact on autologous transplantation. In this clinical setting there is little debate that mobilized PBPCs are a superior product as compared with marrow. A number of phase II clinical trials have documented accelerated engraftment with PBPC products that contain $>2\times10^6$ CD34+ cells/kg. Randomized clinical trials have confirmed these results. In these studies, recovery of hematopoietic cells, such as absolute neutrophil count, platelet recovery, and red blood cell transfusion requirement, have all improved with the use of mobilized PBPCs. In a randomized trial of 58 patients with advanced Hodgkin disease or high-grade non-Hodgkin lymphoma who received either PBPCs (n = 27) or marrow (n = 31), the time to neutrophil recovery of absolute neutrophil count (ANC) $>5\times10^9$/liter was reduced from 14 days with marrow to 11 days with PBPCs (p = 0.005). In addition, time to platelet recovery of $>20\times10^9$/liter was 23 days for patients receiving marrow versus 16 days in the PBPC group (p = 0.02). Patients who received PBPC also required fewer red blood cell and platelet transfusions and spent less time in the hospital. Overall survival was similar in the two groups.[40] On the basis of these and other results, most transplant centers use mobilized PBPCs and have adopted a CD34 cell minimum of $>1\times10^6$ CD34+ cells/kg and a preferred content of $>2\times10^6$ CD34+ cells/kg.

In the allogeneic setting, the situation is considerably more complex. Here, because of the significantly greater numbers of T cells contained in PBPC grafts, the concern is that the higher number of T cells may result in an increased incidence and severity of graft-versus-host disease (GVHD). In the initial phase II studies, the incidence and severity of GVHD somewhat surprisingly were similar among patients who received G-CSF mobilized PBPCs as compared to historical cohorts of patients who received marrow. Table 22-2 summarizes a series of prospective randomized clinical trials that were performed. In the majority of these studies, no clear differences in the incidence of acute GVHD (grades II to IV) were observed.[41-45] The study by Schmitz et al. was an exception where an incidence of acute GVHD of 52% for patients receiving PBPCs versus 39% for patients who received marrow (p = 0.013) was reported.[46] In the studies that evaluated grades III and IV GVHD, no differences were noted. Similar to previous studies in the autologous setting, hematopoietic reconstitution was significantly faster in patients who received mobilized PBPCs as compared with marrow. These studies were largely performed with patients who had HLA-histocompatible siblings and there are relatively few data yet in the unrelated donor setting.

The risk of chronic GVHD (limited and extensive) is more controversial. Some studies have not shown a significant difference, including a randomized collaborative study from the Fred Hutchinson Cancer Research Center, the City of Hope National Medical Center,

TABLE 22-2 ACUTE AND CHRONIC GVHD AFTER TRANSPLANTATION OF HEMATOPOIETIC CELLS FROM BLOOD OR MARROW (PROSPECTIVE TRIALS)

AUTHORS (REFERENCE)	ACUTE GVHD (GRADES II–IV)			CHRONIC GVHD (LIMITED AND EXTENSIVE)		
	BLOOD (%)	MARROW (%)	P VALUE	BLOOD (%)	MARROW (%)	P VALUE
Bensinger et al. (41)	64	57	0.35	46	35	0.54
Blaise et al. (42)	44	42	N/A	50	28	<0.03
Couban et al. (43)	44	44	>0.9	85	69	0.62
Schmitz et al. (46)	52	39	0.013	67	54	0.0066
Powles et al. (44)	50	47	N/A	—	—	—
Vigorito et al. (45)	27	19	0.53	—	—	—

and Stanford University. In this study, the incidence of chronic GVHD for patients who received mobilized blood was 46% versus 35% in the patients receiving marrow (p = 0.54).[47] In other studies, there has been an increased risk of chronic GVHD, in particular, the studies by Blaise et al.[42] and Schmitz et al.[46] where a higher risk of chronic GVHD was noted for those patients who received PBPCs. Therefore, additional followup of these patients and other studies is important to resolve this issue. However, it has been found that chronic GVHD has also resulted in reduced relapse risk. In addition, in patients with high-risk disease, more rapid hematopoietic reconstitution could result in improved outcomes, which was observed in the study by Bensinger et al., where patients with high risk disease (beyond first complete remission [CR1] or after first chronic phase of chronic myelogenous leukemia [CML]) had improved overall survival if they received PBPCs as compared with those patients with advanced disease characteristics who received marrow.[41] Patients with standard risk (CR1 or first chronic phase of CML) had similar outcomes. Consequently, some centers have used an approach where patients with high-risk disease receive mobilized PBPCs, whereas those with standard-risk disease continue to receive marrow. In the unrelated donor setting, several randomized clinical trials are ongoing in an effort to address this important question.

UMBILICAL CORD BLOOD

Umbilical cord blood collected from the umbilical vessels in the placenta at the time of delivery is a rich source of HSCs. The relative immaturity of the cord blood cells allows for engraftment across immunologic barriers more easily than when other stem cell sources are used.[48] Registries have been established that can be searched for histocompatible cord blood units. A significant advantage of cord blood is that the cells are readily available, avoiding long search times. However, a major limitation has been the relatively small number of cells available in the cord blood, which has made transplantation feasible mainly for pediatric patients.[49-51] A limited number of studies have been performed in adults with relatively prolonged engraftment times.[52] Efforts have also been made to expand HSCs from cord blood or potentially use multiple cord blood samples for transplantation to accelerate hematopoietic immune reconstitution.[53]

DISEASES TREATED WITH HEMATOPOIETIC CELL TRANSPLANTATION

Table 22-3 lists disorders that have been successfully treated with HCT. Patients with malignancies of the hematopoietic lineage, including acute and chronic leukemias, non-Hodgkin lymphoma, Hodgkin disease, myelodysplastic syndromes, multiple myeloma, and myelo-

TABLE 22-3   CLINICAL USE OF HEMATOPOIETIC CELL
TRANSPLANTATION (HCT)

DISEASE/CONDITION	ALLOGENEIC HCT	AUTOLOGOUS HCT
Acute leukemia (myeloblastic; lymphoblastic)	+	+
Chronic myelogenous leukemia	+	–
Chronic lymphocytic leukemia	+	+
Myelodysplastic syndromes	+	–
Myeloproliferative syndromes	+	–
Non-Hodgkin lymphoma	+	+
Hodgkin disease	–	+
Multiple myeloma	+	+
Amyloidosis	–	+
Neuroblastoma	–	+
Selected solid tumors (testicular cancer, pediatric tumors)	–	+
Aplastic anemia	+	–
Fanconi anemia	+	–
Thalassemia	+	–
Sickle cell anemia	+	–
Congenital pure red cell aplasia	+	–
Paroxysmal nocturnal hemoglobinuria	+	–
Severe combined immunodeficiency	+	–
Wiskott-Aldrich syndrome	+	–
Congenital leukocyte dysfunction syndromes	+	–
Osteoporosis	+	–
Familial erythrophagocytic lymphohistiocytosis	+	–
Hereditary storage disorders	+	–
Glanzmann disease	+	–
Selected autoimmune disorders	+	+

proliferative disorders, have all benefited from transplantation. In addition, patients with selected solid tumors, such as testicular cancer, neuroblastoma, and other pediatric tumors, have had successful outcomes with HCT. Other chapters summarize the results obtained with transplantation in these various disease entities. In addition to hematopoietic malignancies, a variety of studies have been performed in patients with selected solid tumors, such as women with breast and ovarian carcinoma, and limited studies in renal cell carcinoma and small-cell lung cancer, as well as selected other solid tumors. These studies have been less convincing that there is a defined role for HCT in the treatment of these diseases. In patients with breast cancer, a number of randomized clinical trials are still ongoing to evaluate the potential role of HCT in this disease setting.

In addition to malignancies, HCT is an effective approach for the treatment of a variety of other acquired and congenital disorders. Most notable is HCT for patients with severe aplastic anemia where outstanding results have been achieved for those individuals who have an HLA-matched sibling donor; upwards of 80 to 90 percent of these patients enjoy long-term disease-free control and complete hematologic remissions.[54] In other studies, the treatment of patients with thalassemia has been very successful, especially in patients without significant liver disease.[55] Patients with amyloidosis who can tolerate autologous HCT also appear to benefit from this form of therapy.[56]

The choice of performing an autologous versus allogeneic HCT procedure is largely based on the disease being treated, as well as the availability of a histocompatible donor. For some diseases, such as patients with myelodysplastic syndromes, aplastic anemia, and various myeloproliferative disorders, as well as patients with congenital dis-

orders, only allogeneic transplants can be considered. In contrast, in those patients with malignancies, either autologous or allogeneic transplants have been performed. In general terms, the allogeneic transplant has been far more successful in controlling disease recurrence in virtually all of these settings, with a statistically significant reduction in disease relapse risk. However, the risk of the transplant, which includes GVHD, toxicity, and infections, has negatively impacted the overall survival of patients. Given the relative ease of an autologous as compared to an allogeneic transplant in situations where outcomes are similar, autologous transplantation is preferred. Examples include patients with non-Hodgkin lymphoma and Hodgkin disease. In contrast, in other disease settings where there is robust graft-versus-tumor (GVT) effect and significantly reduced risk of disease relapse, allogeneic transplantation is favored. Examples include patients with CML, acute myelogenous leukemia (AML), and acute lymphoblastic leukemia (ALL).

CONCEPTS OF CURATIVE THERAPY

AUTOLOGOUS HEMATOPOIETIC CELL TRANSPLANTATION

In pursuing autologous HCT, the concept whereby effective control of disease can be accomplished is largely through the effects of high-dose chemotherapy and/or radiation. Here the delivery of drugs at the maximally tolerated dose in an attempt to overcome drug resistance and improve tumor cell killing is the major basis of disease control. The choice of drugs in the preparative regimen includes those agents that can be significantly dose-escalated and have improved tumor cell killing at higher doses without unacceptable toxicities. In addition, regimens are constructed to use drugs that have nonoverlapping toxicities; for example, a commonly used regimen includes carmustine (BCNU), etoposide (VP-16), and cyclophosphamide. This regimen was chosen because of the ability to dose-escalate each of these drugs, which has significant impact on the disease,[57,58] yet these drugs have nonoverlapping toxicities. For example, the organ impacted at the maximally tolerated dose of BCNU is largely the lungs, VP-16 largely impacts the liver, and cyclophosphamide largely impacts the heart. Consequently, using these drugs below the maximally tolerated doses results in a regimen that has a relatively low risk of regimen-related mortality yet maximizes the possibility of tumor cell kill to overcome drug resistance. Significant problems following autologous transplantation that occur in the majority of patients include nausea, vomiting, alopecia, infection, bleeding, mucositis, and infertility. The use of mobilized PBPCs has significantly accelerated the rate of hematopoietic cell reconstitution, which has a positive impact on many of these potential problems. The introduction of mobilized PBPCs has reduced the transplant-related mortality from approximately 8 to 10 percent with marrow to 1-3 percent with mobilized PBPCs in most centers. In addition, the reduced risks and faster engraftment times have allowed many centers to pursue outpatient transplantation, further easing the difficulty of patients undergoing this procedure, as well as reducing costs.

A consistent concern in autologous transplantation has been the risk that tumor cells may be present in the stem cell products. The relative contributions of tumor cell contamination of the stem cell product and residual disease in the patient are difficult, if not impossible, to evaluate outside the setting of a prospective randomized clinical trial. In addition, the methodologies used to reduce tumor cell burden within the graft must be such that there is consistent and documented removal of tumor cells without damaging the HSCs in order for such a prospective randomized clinical trial to be of value. However, it seems reasonable to assume that both sources of tumor cells, namely, those within the stem cell product and residual cells within the patient, are capable of contributing to eventual relapse. Gene marking studies have definitively demonstrated that tumor cells can be transplanted within the graft and contribute to disease relapse.[59,60] In addition, as patient selection and treatment are optimized, tumor cell contamination of the graft is likely to be even more important to address in order to further improve outcomes following autologous transplantation.

A number of retrospective studies have suggested that the infusion of tumor cells within the graft is associated with higher rates of relapse. These studies include patients with AML whose marrow products have been treated with an activated form of cyclophosphamide (4-hydroperoxycyclophosphamide) or with mafosfamide, a related drug that is associated with a lower relapse rate than seen in historical control patients who received unmanipulated cells.[61,62] Although further followup of these patients continues to show positive outcomes, these drugs do impact the rapidity of hematopoietic cell engraftment, which has limited enthusiasm for this approach. Other strategies have been to attempt to remove potential malignant cells from the graft by using monoclonal antibody-mediated methods employing magnetic beads, complement, drugs, or toxins with or attached to the monoclonal antibodies. Generally a cocktail of monoclonal antibodies directed against determinants on the tumor cells is used, such as anti-B cell monoclonal antibodies for patients with B cell non-Hodgkin lymphoma. Sensitive polymerase chain reaction (PCR)-based methods have been used to evaluate the efficacy of tumor cell removal.[63,64] In one retrospective analysis, patients who had been successfully depleted of PCR-positive products were compared with patients who remained PCR-positive. This study demonstrated significantly improved outcomes for the patients who received a PCR-negative product.[65]

Another approach has been to positively select for HSCs, thereby depleting tumor cells from the cells to be infused. Positive stem cell selection has resulted in a significant reduction in tumor cell contamination through the use of sensitive immunohistochemical and molecular approaches. The most widely used strategy has been to select for CD34+ cells with immunomagnetic techniques. Clinical application of CD34 selected cells results in rapid multilineage engraftment. This approach is not without potential complications as some studies suggest that CD34 selected grafts in the setting of autologous HCT may result in an increased risk of infection.[66,67] However, no clinical trials have documented improved clinical outcome for patients who received CD34+ selected autografts as compared to those patients who received unmanipulated autografts. In a randomized prospective study in patients with multiple myeloma, the outcomes were similar with respect to disease-free and overall survival, as well as infectious risks.[68] Without a prospective randomized clinical trial, many centers have found it hard to justify additional manipulations and costs associated with CD34 selection of the stem cell product. However, given that disease relapse is the greatest risk of failure following autologous HCT, removal of tumor cells in the graft continues to be an important goal for future development.

Despite CD34 cell selection a number of positive selection studies have demonstrated that there continues to be contamination of tumor cells within the graft. To overcome this contamination, further purification of stem cells using high-speed cell sorting, for example, CD34+Thy-1+ isolation, has been pursued in patients with multiple myeloma, breast cancer, and non-Hodgkin lymphoma.[30–32] These studies consistently demonstrate that the purification of CD34+Thy-1+ cells results in grafts with undetectable tumor burden.

An alternative approach has been to attempt to use in vivo purging by collecting cells at a time when there is relatively low tumor burden. Two such strategies have been employed. The first uses combination chemotherapy, largely in patients with acute leukemias where cells are collected at a time of early recovery following induction chemotherapy. Several studies document that these collections appear to be relatively free of tumor burden.[69,70] An alternative approach has been to use rituximab, the anti-B cell monoclonal antibody that can be combined with mobilizing agents such as cyclophosphamide. In several relatively small studies, tumor cell contamination based on sensitive PCR-based methodologies revealed significant tumor reduction following rituximab-based mobilization strategies.[71,72]

Despite these various approaches to treat the graft, a consistent problem following HCT continues to be relapse of the underlying disease. Relapse often occurs at sites of previous disease, suggesting that residual cells within the patient are responsible for the recurrence. Strategies in the posttransplant setting to reduce disease recurrence have been explored. These strategies include the use of selected radiation therapy to sites of previous bulk and several studies suggest that this strategy might reduce disease recurrence.[73–75] However, because of the nature of many of the diseases treated with transplantation, radiation therapy is sometimes difficult to administer in many patients, making it extremely difficult to study in a prospective fashion. Other approaches include immunologic interventions in an effort to generate either a GVT response in the autologous setting or to use monoclonal antibody-based therapies directed at the tumor cells. Vaccination strategies, such as using idiotype pulsed dendritic cells or other vaccination approaches, have been explored in early phase clinical trials and have shown relative safety and immunologic responses in some patients.[76,77] Further studies are required to determine whether these immunologic responses predict or influence overall disease outcome.

An alternative approach has been to use monoclonal antibody-based therapies in an effort to reduce disease recurrence. This strategy is most feasible in patients with B cell non-Hodgkin lymphoma where rituximab is an effective therapy. In the autologous transplant setting, patients with chemotherapy-sensitive relapsed B cell lymphoma undergoing autologous HCT have been treated with rituximab in the posttransplant setting with excellent disease-free and overall survival in phase II clinical trials. Figure 22-1 shows the results of one such trial where 35 patients who underwent autologous transplantation followed by rituximab therapy at approximately 6 weeks and 6 months enjoyed excellent overall results.[78] Interestingly, in several studies patients treated with rituximab developed an isolated neutropenia through as yet unexplained mechanisms. The use of rituximab in the transplant setting in an effort to reduce disease relapse in patients with relapsed B cell non-Hodgkin lymphoma is being explored in a randomized prospective clinical trial in the United States.

ALLOGENEIC HEMATOPOIETIC CELL TRANSPLANTATION

The choice of pursuing allogeneic HCT is based on the type, prognosis, and remission status of the underlying disease being treated, the performance status of the patient, and the availability of an appropriate donor. Both HLA-matched sibling donors and unrelated donors obtained through national and international registries are frequently used for allogeneic HCT. Figure 22-2 illustrates the principles to consider in the successful application of allogeneic HCT. In the allogeneic setting, a major obstacle which must be overcome is the immune competence of the recipient. The potential for rejection by the recipient against infused donor cells is mediated predominantly through T and natural killer (NK) cells. Immunosuppressive strategies include high-dose chemotherapy, radiation, immunosuppressive drugs, and donor-derived T cells within the graft. Other strategies under investigation are the use of monoclonal antibodies directed against T cell determinants and antibodies conjugated with radioactive isotopes. To reestablish donor-derived hematopoiesis, there must be a source of HSCs that can be achieved with any of the sources described above, most com-

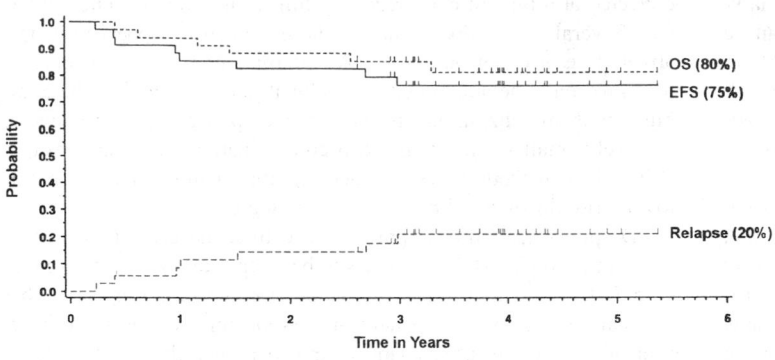

FIGURE 22-1   Outcome for 35 patients with relapsed non-Hodgkin lymphoma who then received a course of rituximab at approximately 6 weeks and 6 months following autologous transplantation.[78]

monly with marrow or G-CSF mobilized PBPCs. The beneficial effects of an allogeneic transplant are mediated through the impact of the preparative regimen and, more importantly, through an immunologic-mediated event termed the *GVT effect*. The GVT effect, which is discussed separately below, is mediated by T and NK cell populations. However, donor-derived T cells are also responsible for the major risk of allogeneic HCT, namely GVHD. Therefore, strategies to enhance GVT while minimizing GVHD remain at the forefront of research.

MYELOABLATIVE HEMATOPOIETIC CELL TRANSPLANTATION

The standard approach to prepare the patient for allogeneic transplantation has been to pursue high-dose chemotherapy with or without total body irradiation (TBI) in an effort to treat the underlying disease and overcome rejection by the recipient. The most commonly used preparative regimens for allogeneic HCT include the use of TBI in the range of 1200 to 1320 rads combined with cyclophosphamide (Cy), 60 mg/kg, on two successive days.[79] Radiation is typically fractionated (fractionated total body irradiation [FTBI]) to reduce complications. The FTBI/Cy regimen has been widely used in a variety of clinical settings and has been reasonably well tolerated, with the major complications being nausea, vomiting, alopecia, mucositis, and infertility. In addition, with radiation-based regimens there is a significant risk of cataracts; however, the use of FTBI has significantly reduced this risk and has also made the regimen more tolerable.[80] The maximally tolerated dose of FTBI is approximately 1500 cGy. In randomized studies of two different doses of TBI (1220 vs. 1575 cGy), a decreased relapse rate was noted with the higher radiation dose. However, this advantage was not associated with improved survival because of the increased incidence of regimen-related mortality.[81] Therefore, most groups have used FTBI in the dose range of 1200 to 1320 cGy. In addition, excellent results have been reported combining FTBI with VP-16 at the maximally tolerated dose of 60 mg/kg.[82] The combination of FTBI and VP-16 has resulted in particularly promising results in patients with acute lymphoblastic leukemia.[83]

A variety of different regimens that do not include radiation have also been developed for use in the autologous and allogeneic setting. The most widely used of these regimens combines busulfan at a dose of 16 mg/kg given over 4 days with cyclophosphamide at 120 mg/kg over 2 days.[84] A randomized comparison between FTBI/Cy and busulfan and cyclophosphamide (BuCy) demonstrated that the BuCy regimen was better tolerated; however, FTBI/Cy resulted in similar outcomes.[85] More recently, the development of intravenous busulfan has improved the tolerability of this regimen.[86] A retrospective analysis of cohorts of patients receiving oral versus IV busulfan revealed that

fewer patients treated with intravenous drug developed venoocclusive disease (VOD).[87] Pharmacologic monitoring has demonstrated that patients who receive doses of busulfan such that the mean dose is above 917 ng/ml have a decreased risk of relapse.[88] These findings have led to the concept of adjusted dose busulfan with cyclophosphamide, which is used in a variety of centers. Several other regimens have been developed for use in both the autologous and allogeneic transplant settings.

NONMYELOABLATIVE PREPARATIVE REGIMENS

The demonstration of the beneficial effects of immune-mediated mechanisms in controlling minimal residual disease has challenged the concept that relatively toxic myeloablative preparative regimens are required for cure. Regimens with reduced toxicity may be particularly useful in older patients or in those individuals who have comorbid medical conditions who may not be able to tolerate aggressive myeloablative preparative regimens. In addition, patients with relatively indolent disease who do not require the immediate cytoreductive capacity of these aggressive preparative regimens may be particularly suitable candidates for nonmyeloablative transplantation. Less toxic regimens could also be extremely useful in patients with genetic disorders or autoimmune diseases, or potentially for the induction of tolerance for solid-organ transplantation.

The goal of nonmyeloablative transplantation is to use the minimum amount of myelosuppressive and immunosuppressive therapy required to achieve durable engraftment of donor-derived hematopoiesis. A variety of regimens have been developed with differing dose intensities. One regimen includes six daily infusions of fludarabine at 30 mg/m², busulfan at 4 mg/kg/d for 2 consecutive days, and anti-T lymphocyte globulin at 10 mg/kg for 4 consecutive days. Patients then receive G-CSF mobilized PBPCs from an HLA-matched sibling donor. Hematopoietic toxicity is modest and overall survival in patients, for example, with CML, is quite favorable.[89,90]

Another approach has been to use fludarabine at doses between 90 and 150 mg/m² and cyclophosphamide at a dose of between 900 and

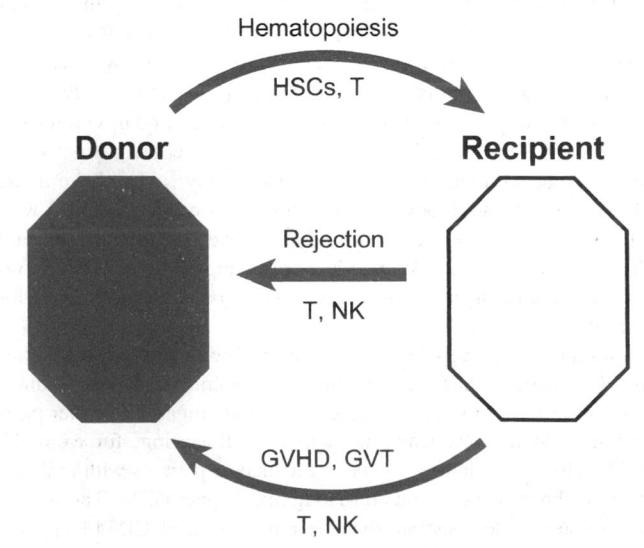

FIGURE 22-2   Theoretical considerations in performing allogeneic hematopoietic cell transplantation. HSCs, hematopoietic stem cells; GVHD, graft-versus-host disease; GVT, graft-versus-tumor effect; NK, natural killer cell; T, T cell.

2000 mg/m² followed by allogeneic hematopoietic cell infusion from an HLA-matched sibling donor. This approach, combined with rituximab, has been particularly favorable in patients with indolent lymphoma and potentially mantle cell lymphoma.[91]

An alternative approach is based on careful studies in a canine model and uses low-dose radiation of 200 cGy followed by immunosuppression with mycophenolate mofetil and cyclosporine in an attempt to suppress the recipient T cells from rejecting the graft.[92] Studies performed in patients with a variety of malignancies resulted in consistent hematopoietic engraftment, with chimerism achieved in all lineages.[93] In the initial study, approximately 20 percent of patients eventually rejected their grafts, following which fludarabine 30 mg/m² for 3 days was added. The addition of fludarabine to low-dose TBI successfully reduced the risk of rejection to less than 5 percent. This nonmyeloablative transplant approach may be particularly successful in patients with indolent hematologic malignancies such as chronic leukemias or multiple myeloma.[94]

Yet another approach has been to use a preparative regimen involving total lymphoid irradiation (TLI) and antithymocyte globulin (ATG) based on studies in rodent models that indicated that animals prepared in this fashion were resistant to GVHD induction by donor-derived T cells. In these rodent models, as many as 1000 times the number of donor-derived T cells could be infused without recipients developing significant acute lethal GVHD. The mechanism underlying this observation is related to a relative increase in IL-4 producing NK T cells that suppress the GVHD response.[95] This strategy has been successfully translated to the clinic where an initial study showed that patients treated with TLI and ATG experienced a very low incidence of acute GVHD sustained with donor-derived hematopoiesis (Lowsky, in preparation).

The development of nonmyeloablative allogeneic transplantation has been a major advance in the field. This transplant approach has resulted in the ability to offer allogeneic transplantation to patients who would otherwise be ineligible because of age or comorbid medical conditions. Sustained hematopoietic engraftment has been achieved in the majority of patients. Initial studies suggested that donor leukocyte infusions (DLIs) could be used to improve donor-derived engraftment and generate a more potent antitumor response. However, the use of DLIs has largely been reserved for patients with persistent or relapsed disease because of the risks of GVHD. In addition, the majority of patients eventually achieve either full donor chimerism or, more rarely, reject their graft, and relatively few patients continue to have mixed chimerism following these types of transplant procedures. The relative merits of nonmyeloablative allogeneic transplantation compared with alternative therapies such as autologous transplantation are currently under evaluation.

NOVEL PREPARATIVE REGIMENS

Because the preparative regimen clearly has a major impact on disease burden, alternative strategies have been developed in an effort to enhance clinical efficacy. As discussed earlier, although higher doses of radiation are associated with improved control of the underlying disease, they are also associated with increased mortality as a consequence of toxicity. These observations led to the concept of using targeted radiotherapy to augment the preparative regimen. Several different approaches have been used that conjugate monoclonal antibodies with radioactive isotopes with the goal of delivering an increased dose of radiation to sites of disease. For example, in one study, anti-CD33 antibodies were conjugated to radioactive iodine (^{131}I). In the initial study, the majority of patients had favorable biodistribution such that the marrow and spleen received more radiation than any nonhematopoietic organ.[96] Other studies with ^{131}I-labeled anti-CD45 mono-

clonal antibodies were used in combination with FTBI/Cy. The toxicity observed was not thought to be greater than that observed with FTBI/Cy alone.[97,98] These studies demonstrate that radiolabeled monoclonal antibodies can be combined with standard preparative regimens and higher doses of radiation can be successfully delivered. Other studies performed with ^{131}I-conjugated anti-CD20 monoclonal antibodies for the treatment of patients with B cell non-Hodgkin lymphoma appeared favorable as compared with a historical cohort of patients.[99] Additional studies are required to demonstrate improved disease-free and overall survival using this approach. Nonradioactive antibodies such as the anti-CD20 monoclonal antibody rituximab have also been incorporated into the preparative regimen with excellent results in patients with follicular lymphoma.[91]

GRAFT-VERSUS-TUMOR EFFECT

The concept that transfer of immunity from donor to recipient following successful allogeneic transplantation is capable of eradicating residual disease in the patient is one of the most significant biologic findings with implications well beyond the transplant setting. This concept, now beyond dispute, was developed from observations in a variety of clinical settings. The first major observation came from rare instances where patients with hematologic malignancies were transplanted with genetically identical (syngeneic) donors. The finding that such patients did not develop GVHD yet had a higher incidence of disease relapse was a striking and unexpected finding.[100] Larger numbers of patients revealed that the risk of relapse was not only dependent on the remission status of the patient, but also related to the underlying disease. Patients with CML had the greatest allogeneic effect and a significantly higher risk of relapse following syngeneic as compared with HLA-matched allogeneic transplantation. A significant impact, albeit to a lesser extent, was also observed for patients with AML, whereas patients with ALL had less of an allogeneic donor effect.[101] These observations led to the concept that not all diseases were immunologically identical and that some were well recognized whereas others were less well recognized.

Further support for the allogeneic effect came from studies of T cell depletion of the graft. The motivation to perform T cell depletion was based on the expectation that removal of donor-derived T cells would reduce the risk of GVHD. The finding that GVHD could be almost completely eliminated by successful T cell depletion even in the absence of immunosuppressive drugs was a major finding. The later observation that these patients had a much higher risk of disease recurrence as well as a higher incidence of graft rejection was sobering.[102] These results linked GVHD with GVT, further supporting the finding that patients who developed some degree of GVHD, especially chronic GVHD, had a significantly reduced risk of disease relapse, providing further evidence for the GVT effect.[103–105]

The final and definitive demonstration of a GVT effect came from the application of DLIs. The observation that patients who had undergone allogeneic HCT and later relapsed could be rendered back into remission, in some instances even a molecular remission, by the simple application of donor-derived lymphocytes was a thrilling finding.[106–111] The treatment of larger numbers of patients again demonstrated variable responses, with some diseases, such as CML, being very responsive, whereas others, such as ALL, were less responsive.[111,112] Long-term followup of patients successfully treated with DLI revealed that patients who respond, especially with a molecular response, have remarkably durable remissions and excellent outcomes.[113]

These observations have definitively established the GVT effect as a biologic entity capable of controlling an otherwise lethal condition such as acute leukemia. Despite these findings, the biologic basis for the GVT effect remains relatively obscure. The cells responsible for the GVT effect clearly include T cells and there is emerging evidence that NK cells are also responsible for tumor cell control, especially in some special situations such as following haploidentical transplantation.[114–116] A major question continues to be whether the T cells resulting in GVHD are the same populations of cells as those responsible for the GVT effect. The structures recognized by the immune effector cells have been proposed to be alloantigens, such as minor histocompatibility antigens, unique structures on the malignant cells, such as products of chromosomal translocations, or other specific markers of the malignant phenotype.

The demonstration of the GVT effect has led to the concept that perhaps GVHD may be separable from GVT. A variety of strategies have been proposed in an effort to enhance the GVT effect while minimizing GVHD. One approach has been to manipulate DLI to reduce the risk of GVHD inherent in its use. The depletion of CD8+ cells by immunomagnetic techniques has resulted in a relatively low incidence of GVHD.[117,118] The finding that some patients developed powerful disease responses without GVHD has provided support that these biologic reactions can be separated. An alternative approach has been to introduce a suicide gene into the donor lymphocytes such that they can be eradicated should GVHD develop.[119] To enhance specificity, others have attempted to clone T cells capable of recognizing the tumor cells but not normal host cells such as fibroblasts or lymphoblastoid cells.[120] Tumor-reactive T cells have been developed and even used clinically.[121–124] Although this approach is elegant, there are a number of technical limitations. An alternative strategy has been to use engineered populations of effector cells capable of expansion ex vivo, which have limited capacity for GVHD induction. One such population of cells derived from T cells which upon activation with the timed addition of interferon-γ, anti-CD3 monoclonal antibodies, and IL-2 result in the dramatic expansion of effector cells, which share phenotypic and functional properties of both T and NK cells. These cells, termed *cytokine-induced killer cells*, have biologic activity in a number of different animal models and have a limited capacity for GVHD induction partly because of the production of interferon-γ.[125,126] Other groups have used NK cells, which have GVT activity but a limited capacity for GVHD induction through as-yet-unexplained mechanisms.[116]

A variety of cytokines have been evaluated for their ability to impact GVHD without limiting GVT reactions. These studies are largely performed in animal model systems with defined end points that serve as preclinical models. Cytokines, such as IL-2, keratinocyte growth factor, and other interleukins such as IL-18, maintain or enhance GVT while reducing GVHD.[127–130] Another strategy has been to use phenotypically defined populations of T cells that have the capability to regulate immune responses. The best characterized population of such regulatory T (T_{reg}) cells are CD4+ T cells that coexpress the IL-2α receptor CD25. Adjusting the number of T_{reg} cells within the graft has resulted in the control of GVHD in murine models even across major histocompatibility barriers.[131–133] More recent studies indicate that the combination of defined numbers of conventional CD4+ and CD8+ T cells with T_{reg} cells resulted in control of GVHD with maintenance of GVT reactions.[134,135] These exciting observations suggest that manipulation of the graft could have a major impact on diverse biologic reactions such as GVHD and GVT, which will be explored in future clinical trials.

Yet another approach has been to attempt to manipulate the immune environment of the recipient to raise the barrier required for GVHD induction. Studies discussed above in murine models have demonstrated that the combination of total lymphoid irradiation with anti-T cell antiserum dramatically alters the immune environment of the recipient such that up to 1000 times the number of donor-derived T cells can be infused without induction of GVHD.[95,136] One possible

unifying mechanism to explain these experimental results is that for GVHD to develop, alloreactive T cells must be present capable of activation and proliferation in response to recipient alloantigens. Conversely, GVT also requires T cell activation yet may not require such profound T cell proliferation. These murine models have advanced a number of experimental concepts that are now being applied in the clinic in an effort to reduce the incidence and severity of GVHD while maintaining GVT, which could have a major impact on results of allogeneic HCT because GVHD remains the major obstacle to a successful outcome.

FACTORS INFLUENCING OUTCOME

A number of factors have been identified that consistently impact results obtained following treatment with HCT. These factors include disease status at transplantation, type of donor, recipient's age, and comorbid medical conditions. They must be considered when evaluating a patient for potential transplantation as they often significantly impact outcome.

DISEASE STATUS AT TIME OF TRANSPLANTATION

Disease status at the time of transplantation is the most powerful predictor of long-term disease-free survival. Early studies were largely performed on patients with advanced disease who had failed a variety of other treatment strategies. Although a small percentage of these patients were salvaged,[79] this strategy was unsuccessful in the majority of patients treated. Results following treatment of patients earlier in the course of disease have consistently been superior. An example is shown in Figure 22-3 for patients with leukemia who underwent allogeneic HCT at Stanford University. This analysis of 532 patients treated uniformly at a single institution included 277 patients in CR1 or first chronic phase (CP). Their overall outcome with followup beyond 10 years is approximately 65–70 percent. In contrast, patients who were beyond CR1 or first CP (N = 255) had an outcome of approximately 35 percent beyond 10 years (p <0.0001). Similar data have been obtained from a variety of sources, indicating that disease status has a major impact on disease-free and overall survival. Attempts at salvaging patients with advanced disease who have failed multiple therapies are rarely successful and if transplantation is to be considered a viable treatment strategy, it is best to consider this modality early in the course of therapy. Clearly these discussions are complex as earlier allogeneic transplantation carries risks of GVHD, toxicity, and opportunistic infections. When compared to the use of autologous transplantation or chemotherapy for diseases such as AML, virtually all studies demonstrate improved disease control and many studies demonstrate improved event-free and overall survival.[137–151] A number of other criteria are important in evaluating disease status, including the presence of cytogenetic abnormalities, immune phenotype, evidence of extramedullary disease, blood counts, and response to therapy.[152] It is hoped that advanced genetic techniques may provide even more insight into cohorts of patients likely to fare well versus poorly with standard therapies for whom allogeneic HCT should be performed earlier in the course of disease.

TYPE OF DONOR

A major limitation of allogeneic HCT is the requirement for a histocompatible donor. As discussed above, siblings are the most likely source of an appropriate donor. However, patients who do not have siblings, or who do not have a match following HLA analysis, should be considered for an unrelated donor search. Because finding a suitably matched donor may require 3 to 6 months, early searching is critical in avoiding unnecessary delays in pursuing an allogeneic transplant procedure.

An alternative approach in selected patients has been to perform transplantation with a half matched or haploidentical donor. These types of transplants have the advantage that virtually all patients have a haploidentical donor who can be a parent, child, sibling, or relative. GVHD and graft rejection have been significant problems which can be overcome by using intensive regimens capable of immunosuppressing the recipient with grafts containing high numbers of stem cells and extremely low T cell content. Encouraging results have been obtained, especially in patients with AML.[153] Here alloreactive NK cells which are not inhibited by HLA class I molecules of the recipient play a major role in disease control.[116] Similar circumstances may exist in some unrelated donor transplants and donor–recipient pairs mis matched at HLA-C. Improved outcomes have been found in some, but not all, studies.[154,155]

Cord blood transplantation is another potential option, especially for children who do not have HLA-matched sibling donors.[48,156] In this setting, it has been possible to use cord blood units that are not completely matched with a lower risk of GVHD than would be expected. A major advantage is that these cord blood units have already been collected and are available, thereby reducing the search time to find an acceptable graft.

PATIENT AGE

Another major factor impacting outcomes following HCT is the age of the patient at the time of transplantation. With better supportive care the ability to perform transplants successfully in older patients has steadily improved; however, age continues to have a significant impact. For example, patients with leukemia who undergo allogeneic HCT fared best if they were younger than 21 years of age, with approximately 60–80 percent achieving long-term disease-free survival. However, because most of the diseases treated with allogeneic HCT are more common in older patients, results were evaluated for older patients in the age groups of 21 to 36, 37 to 50, and older than 50 years. A worsening in outcome was observed with advancing age, which is most apparent for patients older than 50 years of age. The reasons for this effect are complex and include overall condition, comorbid medical issues, potential differences in disease characteristics, and ability to tolerate the rigors of allogeneic transplantation. For these reasons, patients older than 50 to 55 years of age are generally considered for nonmyeloablative allogeneic transplantation, which is better tolerated and possible to perform in patients in their seventh decade of life. Following autologous transplantation there is less impact of age and successful transplantations can be performed for patients even older than 70 years of age. Careful screening for other comorbid medical conditions, such as heart, lung, kidney, and liver disease, are critically important to avoid potential complications wherever possible.

COMORBID CONDITIONS

Comorbid medical conditions can have a major impact on outcomes following transplantation. Routine screening of heart and lung function to detect occult abnormalities is of critical importance, especially in older patients. Evaluation of liver and kidney function, as well as exposures to potential pathogens such as cytomegalovirus, hepatitis B and C, herpes viruses, and human immunodeficiency virus (HIV) are routine and should be performed in all patients. Another major factor impacting outcome following transplantation is the body weight of the

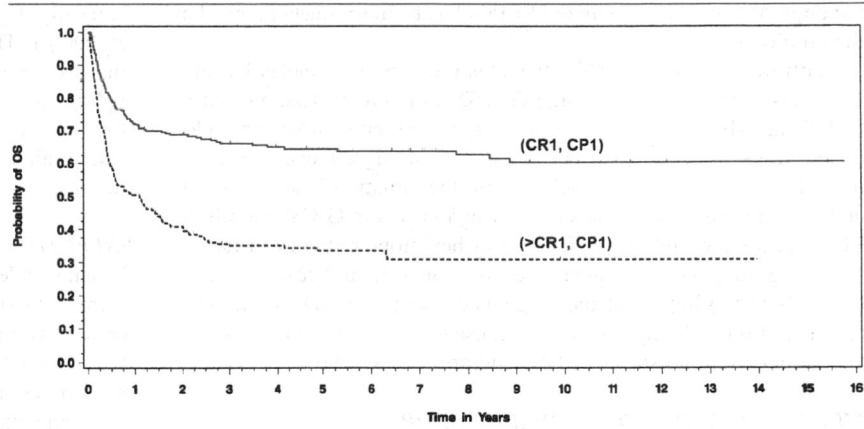

FIGURE 22-3   Long-term outcome of patients with acute leukemia treated at a single institution based on disease status at time of transplantation, of first complete remission or chronic phase (N = 277), or beyond first complete remission or first chronic phase (N = 255) (p <0.0001).

recipient. In one study, patients who weighed more than 30 percent over ideal body weight had increased transplant-related mortality and poorer outcomes.[157] Every effort should be made to encourage potential patients to maintain good health practices, including weight loss if sufficient time exists, discontinuation of alcohol and smoking, and avoiding illicit drug use permanently.

With improved transplantation techniques, outcomes continue to improve. HCT, especially allogeneic HCT, carries significant risks that must be considered and managed effectively. Improvements in eliminating or managing some of these complications continue to result in improved outcomes.

COMPLICATIONS OF HEMATOPOIETIC CELL TRANSPLANTATION

SHORT TERM (DAYS 0 TO 100)

The early transplant period is often the time of greatest risk following both autologous and allogeneic HCT. Care by physicians skilled in the management of patients undergoing these types of treatments is of critical importance. Progress in the supportive care of patients is critically important in improving overall outcomes. The development and use of PBPCs with more rapid hematologic engraftment also reduce risk such that many transplantation patients are routinely managed in the outpatient setting.

ENGRAFTMENT AND SUPPORTIVE CARE
Probably the single most important advance in reducing the morbidity and mortality of HCT has been the introduction of mobilized PBPCs. This advance has been most clearly observed in the autologous HCT setting. Grafts containing >2×10⁶ CD34+ cells/kg routinely result in hematopoietic engraftment within 10 to 15 days. The more rapid recovery observed following transplantation with mobilized PBPCs has reduced antibiotic requirements, use of total parenteral nutrition (TPN), transfusion requirements, and length of hospitalization. Hematopoietic growth factors such as G-CSF are often used following autologous transplantation, which appears to accelerate neutrophil recovery modestly.[158,159] Many centers begin G-CSF therapy 5 to 7 days after the transplant procedure, which appears to provide an adequate acceleration of neutrophil recovery. These advances have led to a reduction in mortality risk from 7 to 15 percent following marrow transplantation to 1–5 percent following PBPC transplantation, such that

the approach of using mobilized PBPCs has been routinely adopted in the autologous setting.

Following allogeneic HCT the situation is more complex because of the risks of acute and chronic GVHD. In many centers, mobilized PBPCs are also used on a routine basis for patients undergoing allogeneic transplantation with HLA-matched sibling donors. In the setting of unrelated donor transplantation, the situation is less resolved and randomized clinical trials comparing marrow to G-CSF mobilized PBPC grafts are underway. The use of hematopoietic growth factors following allogeneic transplantation is controversial because of concerns about the impact of these agents on acute GVHD and immune reconstitution.[160] Many centers do not use growth factors in this setting except under circumstances where engraftment is delayed.

MUCOSITIS AND NUTRITIONAL SUPPORT

The majority of patients who undergo HCT, especially patients who receive FTBI as part of the preparative regimen or methotrexate for GVHD prophylaxis, develop moderate to severe mucositis. Mucositis is often regarded as the most difficult issue from the patient's perspective. Current management is unsatisfactory and includes frequent rinsing with antimicrobial and antifungal medications, antiviral treatment for patients with history of herpes simplex virus (HSV) seropositivity, and pain control. Pain medications include topical numbing agents or, if these are not successful, parenteral narcotics. Newer therapeutics for either topical or systemic use are eagerly awaited. Novel strategies, including the use of growth factors such as keratinocyte growth factor, are under investigation.[161] In addition to impacting mucositis, this agent may also impact GVHD.[127,162]

Patients who develop mucositis often have significant issues with respect to pain control, frequently reactivate herpes virus infections, and have difficulty maintaining adequate oral nutritional support. Many such patients require TPN support. One randomized clinical trial performed prior to the routine use of mobilized PBPCs reported that use of TPN was associated with improved overall survival as compared with the use of dextrose alone.[163] A second randomized trial did not find an improvement in overall survival and instead suggested that TPN may suppress the appetite associated with a delay in resumption of oral intake.[164] One study reported that glutamine supplementation decreased the risk of opportunistic infection; however, this observation was not confirmed in a second randomized trial.[165,166] Therefore, TPN is frequently used, if necessary, but discontinued as soon as adequate oral intake of fluids can be accomplished.

HEMORRHAGE

Life-threatening bleeding complications are frequently worrisome but, fortunately, relatively rare following HCT. Although patients are at significant risk for hemorrhage caused by chronic thrombocytopenia and tissue injury, serious or life-threatening bleeding events are relatively uncommon. Minor hemorrhage such as petechiae, nose bleeds, and urinary and gastrointestinal bleeding are relatively common and stressful for patients. Fortunately, these events are usually time limited or relatively easy to control with simple measures, such as applying pressure or platelet transfusions. Severe bleeding events occurred at a frequency of 11 percent, which contributed to death in 2 percent of patients in a survey of 798 patients treated at marrow transplant programs in the United States and Canada.[167] Interestingly, these events did not occur with any greater frequency in patients with severe, as compared with moderate, thrombocytopenia. These and other results have called into question the rationale for routine platelet transfusions. A comparative study of routinely transfusing nonbleeding patients with a platelet count of $20,000/\mu l$ as compared to $10,000/\mu l$ did not reveal any significant differences in outcome measures.[168,169] Consequently, most centers perform platelet transfusions for patients with clinically significant hemorrhage or for platelet counts less than $10,000/\mu l$. The study of comparing the routine use of platelet transfusions at this level of thrombocytopenia as compared with only providing transfusions for patients with bleeding events has not been performed. Platelet transfusions are relatively safe, yet are costly and can lead to alloreactions that limit the effectiveness of subsequent transfusions.

INFECTIONS

Patients undergoing HCT, especially allogenic transplantation, are at increased risk for infection with bacterial, viral, fungal, and parasitic organisms. Immunoglobulin infusions have been used by some centers to reduce infections following allogeneic HCT. Early use of immunoglobulins reduced infections and other risks in the first 90 days following allogeneic HCT in a randomized clinical trial.[170] Little benefit was found when the immunoglobulin infusions were continued for 1 year.[171] As a result, many centers use infusions of intravenous immunoglobulins to allogeneic HCT recipients only until day 90.

Bacterial Bacterial infections are common during the early period of neutropenia. These are most typically caused by gram-positive organisms although gram-negative infections also occur. This increased risk is not only caused by neutropenia, but is also caused by the presence of indwelling catheters and tissue injury from the preparative regimen. Good hygiene by the patient, including frequent mouth and catheter care, may be helpful in reducing risks. Consideration of staff hygiene is also critically important to avoid nosocomial infection. Frequent handwashing is critical. Some centers also institute other measures such as gowning and masking, although there is less evidence that these actions reduce infection risk. Patients who develop signs or symptoms of infection must be evaluated immediately with a low threshold for the institution of antimicrobial medications. Removal of venous catheters is sometimes required for patients who do not respond promptly to treatment. Specific strategies and regimens for treating bacterial infections are considered in Chap. 20.

Fungal Fungal infections, especially invasive *Aspergillus* infections, are a particularly dreaded complication following allogeneic stem cell transplantation.[172–175] *Candida* and *Aspergillus* represent the most common fungal pathogens; however, other organisms can also cause life-threatening infections. The incidence of fungal infection varies considerably among transplant centers because of a variety of factors, including geographic location, nearby construction, and prophylactic regimen employed. The treatment and prophylaxis of fungal infections are discussed in Chap. 20.

Viral Viral infections are also discussed in Chap. 20.[176–186] Cytomegalovirus (CMV) represents a particular problem in HCT patients, however, and it is worth emphasizing that the best method of control of CMV is prevention. This can most easily be accomplished by using a seronegative donor if the patient is also seronegative. Following HCT, the transfusion of seronegative blood products effectively eliminates the risk of CMV transmission.[176] Although primary infection can occur, these events are rare. However, because many patients are either seropositive themselves or only have a seropositive donor, other strategies must be developed. The early use of anti-CMV therapy with ganciclovir or foscarnet in association with intravenous immunoglobulin (IVIg) is associated with a significant reduction in risk of CMV mortality.[177–179] Sensitive screening tests using CMV-specific antigenemia or PCR assays are now readily available and in routine use. The strategy of preemptively treating patients who develop positive results with these tests is established therapy. Major questions remain with respect to the duration of therapy, relative merits of oral preparations of ganciclovir, and effective treatment of late CMV disease, especially in the setting of gastrointestinal GVHD. Other approaches for prevention of CMV have also been pursued, including the use of anti-CMV cytotoxic T cells, which is elegant, although not practical in many centers.[180]

ACUTE GRAFT-VERSUS-HOST DISEASE

Acute graft-versus-host disease (AGVHD) remains one of the most serious and challenging complications following allogeneic HCT. GVHD is caused by immunologically competent donor-derived T cells that react with recipient tissue antigens. Billingham introduced the requirements for developing AGVHD, which include that the graft must contain immunologically competent cells, the recipient must express tissue antigens not found in the donor, and the recipient must be immunologically suppressed enough that an effective response against transplanted cells cannot be made.[187] There are a number of risk factors for developing AGVHD, which include the degree of HLA disparity between donor and recipient, age, gender disparity (in some studies, males receiving cells from female donors has increased the risk), and the type of immune prophylaxis used.

By definition, AGVHD occurs prior to day 100 and primarily affects skin, gastrointestinal tract, and liver. Severity is clinically based, although biopsies of affected organs are often helpful in making a definitive diagnosis and ranges between grades 0 and IV are defined by involvement of each organ system. An overall grade of between II and IV is generally considered clinically significant disease.

Clinically significant AGVHD occurs in 20 to 50 percent of patients who receive an allogeneic HCT from a histocompatible sibling donor. As discussed in "Sources of Hematopoietic Stem Cells," above, the donor source with respect to marrow versus PBPC does not seem to impact greatly the incidence of clinically significant AGVHD. Grade II AGVHD is not typically associated with poor outcome; however, severe (grades III and IV) AGVHD is associated with a high risk of mortality. Patients undergoing allogeneic HCT with T cell replete grafts require GVHD prophylaxis. The mainstay of prevention of AGVHD is prophylaxis with immunosuppressive drugs. The most commonly used regimen includes cyclosporine and methotrexate and despite multiple attempts at improvement, this regimen continues to be one of the most effective regimens to prevent AGVHD.[188,189] A randomized trial comparing cyclosporine and methotrexate to a combination of cyclosporine, prednisone, and methotrexate did not show any significant differences with respect to GVHD incidence, relapse risk, and overall outcomes.[190] Tacrolimus (FK506) has also been used to prevent GVHD. Randomized clinical trials in the setting of HLA-matched sibling and HLA-matched unrelated allogeneic HCT have shown a slight reduction in the incidence of AGVHD but no change in overall survival for those patients randomized to the FK506-methotrexate as compared with cyclosporine-methotrexate.[191-193] On the basis of these studies, primary prophylaxis using either cyclosporine-methotrexate or FK506-methotrexate has been the mainstay of prevention.

An alternative approach for the prevention of AGVHD has been to deplete donor T cells from the graft prior to infusion. A variety of techniques have been employed, including physical separation, density gradient centrifugation, monoclonal antibody-based depletion methods, and CD34 cell positive selection. Although extensive removal of donor-derived T cells is effective in eradicating AGVHD, it is associated with an unacceptably high risk of graft rejection and relapse.[102,194-197] The concept of less rigorous depletion of T cells has also been forwarded. One approach has been to use soybean agglutinin and erythrocyte-rosetting (E-rosetting), which has resulted in sufficient T cell depletion to reduce the risk of AGVHD to very low levels without immune prophylaxis and excellent outcomes in patients with acute leukemia.[198] Patients who receive T cell depleted grafts are at an increased risk of other opportunistic infections, including Epstein-Barr

virus-associated lymphoproliferative disease.[199] A randomized clinical trial comparing results obtained for patients receiving T cell depleted with T cell replete unrelated donor transplantation was performed.[200]

An alternative approach has been the use of Campath 1H antibody, which is an immunoglobulin (Ig) M antibody that binds to CD52, a molecule expressed on a variety of cells, including T cells. Campath 1H has been used for in vitro depletion of the graft, as well as in vivo depletion of recipients following graft infusion.[201,202] Although acute GVHD has been low, patients are at risk for opportunistic infections.

Established AGVHD can be difficult to treat. A variety of measures have been attempted. The first-line of therapy is glucocorticoids, which are the mainstay of treatment. Typically, glucocorticoids are begun at a dose of 1-2 mg/kg with subsequent tapering once disease activity resolves. A comparison of low-dose (2 mg/kg/d) to high-dose (10 mg/kg/d) regimens did not show differences in evolution to more advanced GVHD, CMV infection, or survival.[203] Individuals who develop steroid-refractory GVHD have an extremely poor outlook. A variety of other approaches have been explored in the treatment of AGVHD, including the use of other immunosuppressive agents, antibody-based therapies either to T cells or cytokines, and photopheresis. Although responses have been noted in many of these studies, it is difficult to determine whether these therapies improve overall survival in these patients.

VENOOCCLUSIVE DISEASE

VOD of the liver is one of the most feared complications of allogeneic and autologous HCT. The incidence of VOD varies significantly from center to center, depending on which criteria is used for diagnosis.[204,205] The typical signs and symptoms of VOD include unexplained weight gain, jaundice, abdominal pain, and ascites. Doppler ultrasonography demonstrating reversal of portal flow and elevated serum plasminogen activator inhibitor-1 is associated with patients who have clinically significant VOD.[206] Patients with a prior history of hepatitis B or C infection and liver function abnormalities or those with seropositive donors are at increased risk for developing VOD.[207,208] Although no individual preparative regimen has emerged as increasing the risk of patients developing VOD, those patients who received busulfan who had an area under the curve of greater than 1500 μmol/min per liter appeared to have a higher incidence of VOD.[209] Controlled studies have not shown any specific therapy for VOD to be effective and the treatment is largely supportive. Patients with mild to moderate VOD may spontaneously improve over time. Most patients who recover from VOD regain normal liver function and rarely develop sequelae of chronic liver disease. Attempts have been made to identify risk factors associated with disease progression and death in patients who develop clinical features of VOD. One study evaluated risk factors associated with the development of severe VOD at different time points following HCT in a cohort of 355 patients. This model was validated prospectively in a separate cohort of 392 patients. The logistic projection model identified serum bilirubin and percent weight gain within 1 to 2 weeks of HCT as the most important independent predictors of progression to severe disease.[205]

The treatment of established VOD has very limited effectiveness. A variety of approaches have been used and include recombinant tissue-plasminogen activator (t-PA) and heparin, which results in improvement in some patients, but is associated with a very high incidence of hemorrhage, especially in those patients with more severe disease.[210,211] Another approach has been to use defibrotide, which is a polydeoxyribonucleotide, rather than multiple antithrombotic and fibrinolytic agents.[212] Defibrotide has little anticoagulant activity and encouraging results have been observed in patients even with severe VOD and multiorgan dysfunction.[213] An experience of 88 patients

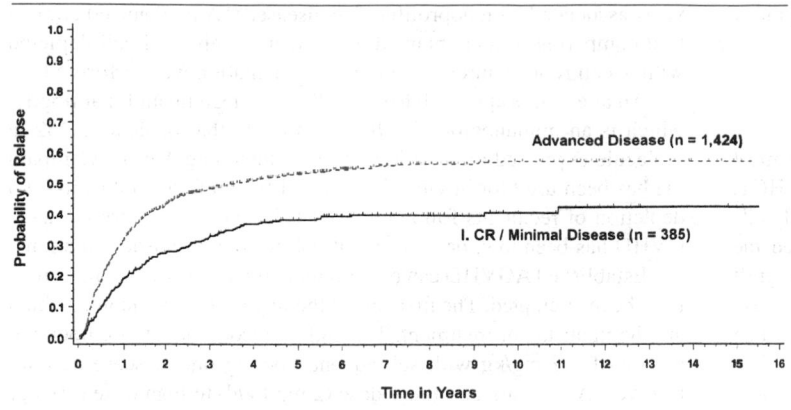

FIGURE 22-4 Relapse risk according to disease status prior to autologous transplantation.

with moderate to severe VOD treated with defibrotide resulted in complete resolution in 36 percent of patients with relatively low toxicity.[214] Antithrombin III concentrates have also been used in patients with VOD with some clinical improvement.[215]

In the absence of specific effective therapy, efforts have been made to develop prophylaxis strategies to reduce the incidence and severity of VOD. Heparin has been explored by low-dose continuous infusion in a prospective randomized clinical trial of 161 patients who underwent allogeneic or autologous HCT. Patients were randomized to either low-dose heparin (100 U/kg total dose per day) by continuous intravenous infusion or placebo. The heparin was initiated prior to the start of the preparative regimen and continued until 30 days after HCT. A significantly lower incidence of VOD was noted in the heparin-treated group of 2.5 percent versus 13.7 percent in the control group. There was no increased risk of bleeding or other toxicities in the patients treated with heparin.[216] The beneficial effect of heparin has not been observed in all studies, however, and the schedule of treatment was not used in an identical manner, which may be important. In another study where benefit was not observed, heparin was begun at the day of stem cell transplantation rather than at the beginning of high-dose therapy.[217] In addition, other respective analyses have not consistently found benefit with the prophylactic use of heparin.[218] A pilot study of 61 patients also suggested that prophylaxis with low molecular weight heparin resulted in a lower incidence of VOD.[219]

Another approach has been to use ursodeoxycholic acid for prophylactic use to reduce the incidence of VOD. In a prospective randomized clinical trial, prophylaxis with ursodeoxycholic acid resulted in a reduced risk of hepatic complications following allogeneic HCT.[220] The use of nonmyeloablative allogeneic transplantation is associated with a low risk of developing VOD. It is still unclear whether patients who are at high risk of developing VOD—for example, those patients with a history of hepatitis, infections, and/or liver function abnormalities—will also have a high risk of VOD following nonmyeloablative allogeneic transplantation. Caution clearly should be exercised in this area.

PULMONARY COMPLICATIONS

Lung toxicity is a relatively common problem following either autologous or allogeneic HCT. The causes of lung injury or interstitial pneumonitis can be infection (bacterial or viral), chemical (BCNU being the most common), bleeding, or idiopathic. Interstitial pneumonitis occurs in 10–15 percent of patients, the etiology of which can often be difficult to discern.[221] Risk factors for developing interstitial pneumonitis include increasing age and prior history of lung irradia-

tion.[222] Children with a prior history of atopy have a higher risk of interstitial pneumonitis.[223] Idiopathic interstitial pneumonitis is typically treated with glucocorticoids, generally at a dose of 1 mg/kg with a weekly taper.[224] Pulmonary function tests with carbon monoxide diffusion capacity measurements are generally required to confirm the presence of interstitial pneumonitis associated, for example, with the use of BCNU in the preparative regimen. This complication generally occurs between days 20 and 60 following transplantation. Idiopathic interstitial pneumonitis is often rapidly responsive to corticosteroids; it can recur in a small percentage of patients following steroid taper.

Diffuse alveolar hemorrhage (DAH) is a clinical syndrome that occurs generally within the first 40 days following HCT. It is characterized by dyspnea, hypoxia, diffuse pulmonary infiltrates on chest radiograph, and progressively bloody fluid return on a bronchoalveolar lavage. DAH has been reported in up to 20 percent of patients undergoing autologous HCT; however, this incidence varies among transplantation centers. Prompt treatment with high-dose glucocorticoids has been successful in this disorder, which otherwise carries a high risk of mortality.[225]

LONG-TERM COMPLICATIONS (BEYOND DAY 100)

DISEASE RELAPSE AND NONRELAPSE MORTALITY

Nonrelapse mortality and disease relapse are significant concerns following HCT. The reasons for late complications vary but often are associated with risks of chronic GVHD and infection in the allogeneic setting and occasionally organ toxicity in the autologous setting. The overall risk is clearly related to prior treatment history, comorbid medical conditions, and a history of prior AGVHD. Figure 22-4 is a retrospective analysis of 1809 patients treated with autologous HCT at Stanford University Medical Center. Of the 385 patients who underwent HCT while in complete remission or a minimal disease state approximately 30–40 percent eventually relapsed. Those patients with more advanced disease clearly carried a higher relapse rate of 50 to 60 percent. Relapse was most likely to occur within the first year of transplantation with roughly 75 percent of patients who eventually relapsed doing so in the first year. By year 3 the vast majority of relapses had occurred.

Relapse following transplantation is an ominous clinical event. Every effort should be made to carefully and completely document potential relapses as it is common for patients to have residual radiographic abnormalities following transplantation, especially in patients with lymphoma. GVT effects often take weeks and even months to develop with continued and ongoing clinical responses. For example, molecular evidence of CML may persist for up to 6 months following allogeneic HCT, which has no bearing on eventual clinical outcomes.[226] In patients with multiple myeloma, gradual reductions in paraprotein levels may take 6 to 12 months to reach maximal effect. Therefore, because patients are highly sensitized to the possibility of disease relapse, clear and unequivocal documentation is required prior to declaring that a patient has relapsed.

Treatment of relapse has generally been unsuccessful with the exception of patients who receive DLI, for example, for a cytogenetic relapse of CML. The use of further chemotherapy can result in disease responses; however, they are unlikely to be durable. Performing a second myeloablative transplant procedure has largely been unsuccessful because of excessive toxicity and nonrelapse transplant-related mortality, which can approach 50–80 percent.[227–229] One exception may be children or adolescents who relapse beyond 1 to 2 years from the original transplant; they may benefit from a second allogeneic transplant procedure.[230]

The development of nonmyeloablative allogeneic transplantation has brought new possibilities for selected patients who relapse following autologous HCT where reasonable tolerability has been observed.[231-234] The durability of remission following nonmyeloablative allogeneic transplant is an area of ongoing investigation. A variety of strategies are under investigation in an effort to reduce the risk of disease relapse following autologous HCT. The use of cytokines such as IL-2 with or without interferon-γ, monoclonal antibodies, cellular immunotherapy, and vaccination strategies are all areas of active research.[76-78,235,236]

Not only is the relapse rate significantly higher in patients who undergo transplantation for advanced disease, but so is the risk of nonrelapse mortality. In a cohort of 1809 patients undergoing autologous transplantation, those patients treated in CR1 had a nonrelapse mortality of less than 10 percent, whereas those patients with advanced disease had a nonrelapse mortality of approximately 20 percent (Fig. 22-5). Clearly, the introduction of mobilized PBPC has reduced the nonrelapse mortality risk significantly. The lower nonrelapse mortality for patients undergoing autologous HCT allows for consideration of treatment earlier in the course of disease. For example, patients with non-Hodgkin lymphoma at high risk of disease recurrence may benefit by performing autologous HCT while in CR1 rather than at first relapse in an effort to prevent rather than treat disease relapse.[237-240]

CHRONIC GVHD

Chronic graft-versus-host disease (cGVHD) is another significant complication following allogeneic HCT. By definition, cGVHD occurs beyond 100 days from the transplant with the clinical manifestations being broad and possibly resembling those of an autoimmune disorder such as scleroderma or dermatomyositis.[241,242] cGVHD has been broadly defined as either limited or extensive, although this definition is often not very useful and better, more predictive staging systems are needed. Patients with extensive cGVHD have an increased mortality rate, especially patients with platelet counts less than $100,000/\mu l$ on day +100 and those patients with low serum albumin. Treatment for cGVHD is complex and involves the use of immunosuppressive drugs.[243] The mainstay of treatment continues to be prednisone, which was found to be equally effective in combination with other immunosuppressive medications such as cyclosporine.[244] Because of the chronic nature of disease, long-term treatment is often required. Alternate-day dosing has been found to help reduce some of the toxicity of immunosuppressive medications such as corticosteroids.[245] Treatment of cGVHD is an art and the slow taper of immunosuppressive medications is a necessity, keeping careful watch for issues of immunosuppression, infection, and disease flares.[246,247] The immunosuppressive medications have significant toxicities along with the risk of infection. Many patients with cGVHD are at high risk of infections, primarily as a result of gram-positive organisms. The use of vaccinations, IVIg, and rotating antibiotics is sometimes helpful in patients with recurrent infections, especially those patients who are hypogammaglobulinemic as a result of cGVHD. A variety of newer agents are being explored for the treatment of cGVHD. Such drugs include thalidomide, which has resulted in encouraging responses in some patients.[248-250] An attempt to use thalidomide as prophylaxis for cGVHD was not successful.[251] A variety of other agents, including psoralen plus ultraviolet A (PUVA), have been used to treat cGVHD with some success, especially in some patients with sclerodermatous-like skin changes.[252] Rapamycin has efficacy in some patients with

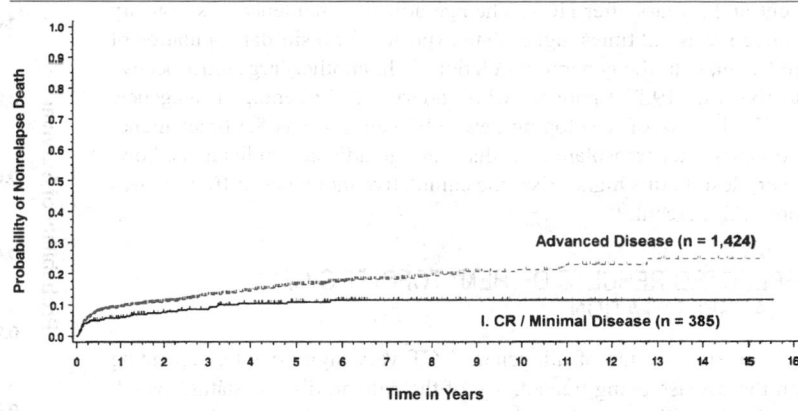

FIGURE 22-5 Nonrelapse mortality for patients undergoing autologous transplantation in CR1 or minimal residual disease as compared with patients with more advanced disease.

cGVHD.[253] cGVHD continues to be a significant clinical problem which requires new therapies.

INFERTILITY

A significant issue following both autologous and allogeneic HCT, when high-dose myeloablative regimens are used, is the risk of infertility.[254,255] This is of particular concern in those individuals, especially women, who are of childbearing age at the time of HCT. Sperm banking for men is an acceptable solution and should be offered to all interested patients.[256] The success rate using banked sperm is significant and represents an effective alternative for male patients. Successful pregnancies after allogeneic HCT using embryos collected prior to transplantation have been reported, especially in those individuals who have fertilized embryos stored.[257,258] Gynecologic abnormalities such as atrophic vaginitis and problems related to ovarian failure are common. If observed, these problems can be effectively reversed with estrogen administration, either systemically or locally.[259]

GROWTH AND DEVELOPMENT

Growth and development problems can occur in pediatric patients, especially in patients receiving TBI-based regimens.[260] Hypothyroidism is also occasionally observed and is readily correctable with thyroid replacement therapy.[261]

SECONDARY MALIGNANCIES

The success of both autologous and allogeneic HCT has led to the realization that some patients who are long-term survivors may be at increased risk for second malignancies. This is especially true in patients with severe aplastic anemia and Fanconi anemia, but it has also been observed following HCT for a variety of malignancies. A major risk is that of secondary myelodysplastic syndrome (MDS) and AML, which can occur 2 to 7 years following transplantation with accumulative risk of approximately 8 to 18 percent.[262-265] Careful analyses of marrow cells, including cytogenetic evaluation prior to autologous HCT, can help to identify patients at increased risk for these secondary malignancies.[266] The avoidance of alkylator-based regimens is associated with a decreased risk of developing this complication in the treatment of patients prior to consideration for HCT. For example, avoiding the use of melphalan in patients with multiple myeloma prior to autologous HCT has resulted in a much lower incidence of MDS.[267]

Secondary malignancies may also occur following allogeneic HCT. In one retrospective analysis of 557 patients, 9 patients developed secondary cancers for an accumulative actuarial risk of 12 percent at 11 years after HCT. The age-adjusted incidence of secondary cancers was 4.2 times higher than expected for a similar population of individuals in the general population.[268] In another large retrospective analysis of 19,229 patients who underwent allogeneic or syngeneic HCT, the risk of developing new solid cancers was 8.3 times higher 10 years after transplantation than for age-adjusted individuals; however, despite this higher risk, the cumulative incidence at 10 years was only 2.2 percent.[269]

SELECTED RESULTS OF HEMATOPOIETIC CELL TRANSPLANTATION

The overall results of allogeneic HCT vary significantly, depending on the disease being treated, age of the patient, disease status, overall medical condition, and a variety of other factors. Many of these issues are discussed in other chapters. As discussed, the overriding factor that most significantly impacts results is the disease stage at the time of HCT. Table 22-4 shows the expected overall survival for patients with acute AML, ALL, and CML who undergo allogeneic HCT. For patients treated while in CR1 or CP, between 60 and 80 percent achieve long-term disease-free survival. Recent results using adjusted dose BuCy for patients with CML in first CP who undergo allogeneic HCT within 1 year of diagnosis indicate that more than 80 percent achieve long-term disease-free survival and are PCR negative (Fig. 22-6).[270] Clearly, results following HCT continue to improve as various transplantation-related complications are controlled. Discussions with patients to determine which treatment options are most suitable requires careful consideration of a variety of different factors, including the availability and results of alternative therapies, as well as the risk associated with transplantation in that individual patient. Biologic assignment studies have been performed to analyze results of transplantation for patients with AML and ALL. In these studies, the trial design is to assign patients with HLA-matched sibling donors to allogeneic transplantation and those that do not to either chemotherapy or possibly randomization between chemotherapy and autologous transplantation. A series of studies with this general design have been performed for the treatment of patients with AML in CR1. In virtually all of the studies, the risk of disease relapse was significantly reduced following allogeneic HCT, as a result of GVT effects. In a number of studies the reduced risk of disease relapse resulted in improvements in overall survival, however, in other studies similar outcomes were observed as a consequence of transplantation-related complications. As improved strategies are developed to address and treat GVHD, accelerate immune reconstitution, and reduce toxicity, it is expected that overall results with allogeneic HCT will continue to improve. Clearly, it is preferable to pursue allogeneic HCT early in the course of therapy in appropriate patients.

In the autologous setting, a series of randomized prospective clinical trials have been performed documenting the value of autologous HCT in a variety of different clinical settings. These trials have utilized

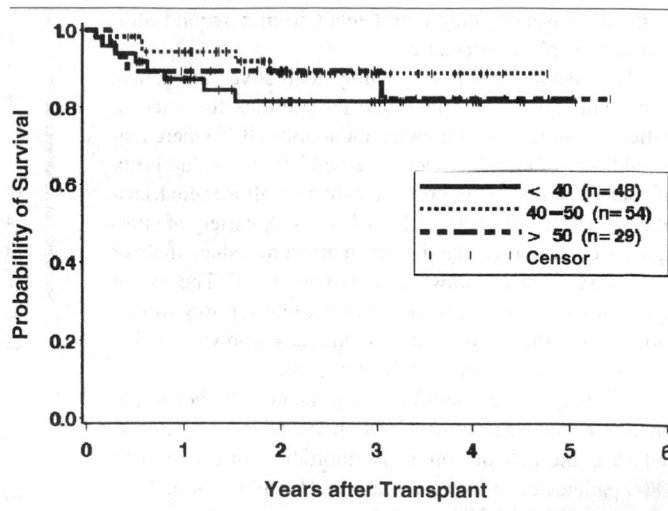

FIGURE 22-6   Allogeneic transplantation for patients with chronic myeloid leukemia transplanted with targeted-dose busulfan and cyclophosphamide using an HLA-matched sibling donor.[270]

an intention to treat analysis whereby patients assigned to transplantation are analyzed within that group irrespective of the treatment that was actually rendered. For example, two studies evaluated the role of autologous transplantation as compared with chemotherapy as first-line treatment for patients with advanced stage multiple myeloma.[271,272] In these studies, a statistically significant improvement in disease-free and overall survival was noted for the patients randomized to transplantation despite the fact that nearly 25 percent of patients did not receive the planned therapy. A more recent study compared the use of tandem autologous transplantation for patients with multiple myeloma as compared with a single transplant, demonstrating that at 7 years overall survival was improved in those patients who received a tandem transplant.[273,274] Consequently, the use of tandem transplants is currently being compared to autologous transplantation followed by nonmyeloablative allogeneic transplantation in patients with multiple myeloma through the US Clinical Trials Network.

In patients with relapsed non-Hodgkin lymphoma with chemotherapy-responsive disease, improved overall survival was demonstrated for patients treated with high-dose therapy and autologous transplantation as compared with continued chemotherapy.[275] Improvement of these results may be achieved with other immunologic therapies such as posttransplant rituximab, which is the subject of a phase III randomized clinical trial. Additional studies addressing the question of whether performing HCT in patients who have a high risk of disease prior to relapse based on the International Prognosis Scoring Index will improve outcomes are ongoing. A recent study compared standard chemotherapy with cyclophosphamide, doxorubicin, vincristine, and prednisone to chemotherapy followed by autologous HCT (Fig. 22-7). The estimated event-free survival at 5 years was significantly better for the patients randomized to autologous transplantation (55% vs. 37%; p = 0.037).[240] Therefore, as therapies evolve, results need to be continuously evaluated in an effort to more definitively determine the best therapeutic option.

FUTURE ROLE OF HEMATOPOIETIC CELL TRANSPLANTATION

HCT is the best example of the successful use of cell-based therapeutics currently practiced in clinical medicine. The concept of using cellular products to treat diseases as complex as malignancy is at the

TABLE 22-4   EXPECTED RESULTS WITH ALLOGENEIC HEMATOPOIETIC CELL TRANSPLANTATION FOR THE TREATMENT OF PATIENTS WITH LEUKEMIAS

	CR1 OR CP (%)	>CR1 OR AP (%)	RELAPSE OR BC (%)
AML	60–70	40–50	10–20
ALL	50–70	30–50	0–20
CML	60–80	30–50	10–20

Abbreviations: ALL, acute lymphoblastic leukemia; AML, acute myelogenous leukemia; AP, acute phase; BC, blast crisis; CML, chronic myelogenous leukemia; CR, complete remission; CP, chronic phase.

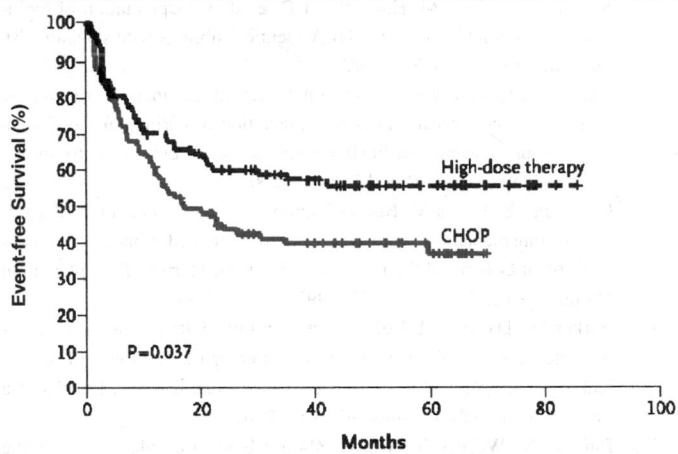

FIGURE 22-7 Event-free survival for patients with non-Hodgkin lymphoma comparing cyclophosphamide, doxorubicin, vincristine, and prednisone (CHOP) chemotherapy to high-dose therapy.[240]

forefront of clinical research. Understanding the mechanisms and targets of GVT reactions continues to be an area of intense interest. In addition, understanding the complexities of immunologic reactions has revealed that not only are T cell populations responsible for the effector phase, but also that other T cell populations may regulate these responses. The concept of using regulatory T cells to control such adverse effects such as GVHD has been successful in murine models and holds significant promise in its application to the treatment of patients. Other defined cellular populations, cytokines, and vaccination strategies show promise in reducing the risk of disease relapse following HCT. In addition, improved strategies to reduce the risk of acute and chronic GVHD could enable extension of allogeneic HCT beyond the treatment of patients with hematologic malignancies. For example, animal models of autoimmune diseases demonstrate that these disorders can be effectively treated with HCT and preliminary evidence in patients is supportive. In addition, a variety of different animal studies clearly demonstrate that following HCT tolerance develops to genetic determinants of the donor, which could lead to combined HCT with solid-organ transplantation to reduce the risk of graft rejection. Preliminary studies suggest that extension of allogeneic HCT to these and other disease settings could provide new therapeutic concepts to improve outcomes for patients with diverse clinical problems.

HCT has emerged from a treatment of last resort in patients with refractory malignancies to an effective therapy for patients with a broad range of disorders and, in some instances, to a first-line therapy. Elucidating the underlying biology is of primary importance to improve outcomes and reduce complications. HCT represents the best example of cellular-based therapeutics as commonly practiced in clinical medicine, which will likely become a mainstay of treatment for a variety of disorders in the future.

REFERENCES

1. Osgood EE, Riddle MC, Mathew TJ: Aplastic anemia treated with daily transfusions and intravenous marrow; case report. *Ann Intern Med* 13: 357, 1939.
2. Jacobson LO, Marks EK, Robson MJ, et al: Effect of spleen protection on mortality following X-irradiation. *J Lab Clin Med* 34:1538, 1949.
3. Lorenz E, Uphoff D, Reid TR, et al: Modification of irradiation injury in mice and guinea pigs by bone marrow injections. *J Natl Cancer Inst* 12:157, 1951.
4. Main JM, Prehn RT: Successful skin homografts after the administration of high dosage X radiation and homologous bone marrow. *J Natl Cancer Inst* 15:1023, 1955.
5. Thomas ED, Lochte HL, Lu WC, et al: Intravenous infusion of bone marrow in patients receiving radiation and chemotherapy. *N Engl J Med* 257:491, 1957.
6. Mathe G, Amiel JL, Schwarzenberg L, et al: Successful allogeneic bone marrow transplantation in man: chimerism, induced specific tolerance and possible anti-leukemic effects. *Blood* 25:179, 1965.
7. Storb R, Epstein RB, Graham TC, et al: Methotrexate regimens for control of graft-versus-host disease in dogs with allogeneic marrow grafts. *Transplantation* 9:240, 1970.
8. Gatti RA, Meuwissen HJ, Allen HD, et al: Immunological reconstitution of sex-linked lymphopenic immunological deficiency. *Lancet* 2:1366, 1968.
9. Hong R, Cooper MD, Allan MJ, et al: Immunological restitution in lymphopenic immunological deficiency syndrome. *Lancet* 1:503, 1968.
10. Bach FH, Albertini RJ, Joo P, et al: Bone-marrow transplantation in a patient with the Wiskott-Aldrich syndrome. *Lancet* 2:1364, 1968.
11. Fefer A, Cheever MA, Greenberg PD, et al: Treatment of chronic granulocytic leukemia with chemoradiotherapy and transplantation of marrow from identical twins. *N Engl J Med* 306:63, 1982.
12. Buckner CD, Epstein RB, Rudolph RH, et al: Allogeneic marrow engraftment following whole body irradiation in a patient with leukemia. *Blood* 35:741, 1970.
13. Santos GW, Sensenbrenner LL, Burke PJ, et al: Allogeneic marrow grafts in man using cyclophosphamide. *Transplant Proc* 6:345, 1974.
14. Thomas ED, Storb R, Clift RA, et al: Bone-marrow transplantation. *N Engl J Med* 292:832, 1975.
15. O'Reilly RJ, Dupont B, Pahwa S, et al: Reconstitution in severe combined immunodeficiency by transplantation of marrow from an unrelated donor. *N Engl J Med* 297:1311, 1977.
16. Hansen JA, Clift RA, Thomas ED, et al: Transplantation of marrow from an unrelated donor to a patient with acute leukemia. *N Engl J Med* 303: 565, 1980.
17. Abrams RA, Glaubiger D, Appelbaum FR, et al: Result of attempted hematopoietic reconstitution using isologous, peripheral blood mononuclear cells: a case report. *Blood* 56:516, 1980.
18. Netzel B, Haas RJ, Rodt H, et al: Immunological conditioning of bone marrow for autotransplantation in childhood acute lymphoblastic leukaemia. *Lancet* 1:1330, 1980.
19. Spangrude GJ, Heimfeld S, Weissman IL: Purification and characterization of mouse hematopoietic stem cells. *Science* 241:58, 1988.
20. Till JE, McCulloch EA: A direct measurement of the radiation sensitivity of normal mouse bone marrow cells. *Radiat Res* 14:213, 1961.
21. Whitlock CA, Witte ON: Long-term culture of B lymphocytes and their precursors from murine bone marrow. *Proc Natl Acad Sci U S A* 79: 3608, 1982.
22. Kondo M, Weissman IL, Akashi K: Identification of clonogenic common lymphoid progenitors in mouse bone marrow. *Cell* 91:661, 1997.
23. Akashi K, Traver D, Miyamoto T, et al: A clonogenic common myeloid progenitor that gives rise to all myeloid lineages. *Nature* 404:193, 2000.
24. Galy A, Travis M, Cen D, et al: Human T, B, natural killer, and dendritic cells arise from a common bone marrow progenitor cell subset. *Immunity* 3:459, 1995.
25. Shizuru JA, Negrin RS, Weissman IL: Hematopoietic stem and progenitor cells: clinical and preclinical regeneration of the hematolymphoid system. *Annu Rev Med.* 56:509, 2005.
26. Baum CM, Weissman IL, Tsukamoto AS, et al: Isolation of a candidate human hematopoietic stem-cell population. *Proc Natl Acad Sci U S A* 89:2804, 1992.
27. Craig W, Kay R, Cutler RL, et al: Expression of thy-1 on human hematopoietic progenitor cells. *J Exp Med* 177:1331, 1993.

28. Uchida N, Aguila HL, Fleming WH, et al: Rapid and sustained hematopoietic recovery in lethally irradiated mice transplanted with purified Thy-1.110 Lin-Sca-1+ hematopoietic stem cells. *Blood* 83:3758, 1994.

29. Uchida N, Tsukamoto A, He D, et al: High doses of purified stem cells cause early hematopoietic recovery in syngeneic and allogeneic hosts. *J Clin Invest* 101:961, 1998.

30. Michallet M, Philip T, Philip I, et al: Transplantation with selected autologous peripheral blood CD34+Thy1+ hematopoietic stem cells (HSCs) in multiple myeloma: Impact of HSC dose on engraftment, safety, and immune reconstitution. *Exp Hematol* 28:858, 2000.

31. Negrin RS, Atkinson K, Leemhuis T, et al: Transplantation of highly purified CD34+Thy-1+ hematopoietic stem cells in patients with metastatic breast cancer. *Biol Blood Marrow Transplant* 6:262, 2000.

32. Vose JM, Bierman PJ, Lynch JC, et al: Transplantation of highly purified CD34+Thy-1+ hematopoietic stem cells in patients with recurrent indolent non-Hodgkin's lymphoma. *Biol Blood Marrow Transplant* 7:680, 2001.

33. Buckner CD, Clift RA, Sanders JE, et al: Marrow harvesting from normal donors. *Blood* 64:630, 1984.

34. Stroncek DF, Holland PV, Bartch G, et al: Experiences of the first 493 unrelated marrow donors in the National Marrow Donor Program. *Blood* 81:1940, 1993.

35. Siena S, Bregni M, Brando B, et al: Circulation of CD34+ hematopoietic progenitor cells in the peripheral blood of high-dose cyclophosphamide-treated patients: Enhancement by intravenous human granulocyte-macrophage colony-stimulating factor. *Blood* 74:1905, 1989.

36. Chao NJ, Schriber JR, Grimes K, et al: Granulocyte colony-stimulating factor "mobilized" peripheral blood progenitor cells accelerate granulocyte and platelet recovery after high-dose chemotherapy. *Blood* 81:2031, 1993.

37. Glaspy JA, Shpall EJ, LeMaistre CF, et al: Peripheral blood progenitor cell mobilization using stem cell factor in combination with filgrastim in breast cancer patients. *Blood* 90:2939, 1997.

38. Liles WC, Broxmeyer HE, Rodger E, et al: Mobilization of hematopoietic progenitor cells in healthy volunteers by AMD3100, a CXCR4 antagonist. *Blood* 102:2728, 2003.

39. Shpall EJ, Champlin R, Glaspy JA: Effect of CD34+ peripheral blood progenitor cell dose on hematopoietic recovery. *Biol Blood Marrow Transplant* 4:84, 1998.

40. Schmitz N, Linch DC, Dreger P, et al: Randomized trial of filgrastim-mobilised peripheral blood progenitor cell transplantation versus autologous bone-marrow transplantation in lymphoma patients. *Lancet* 347:353, 1996.

41. Bensinger W, Martin P, Storer B, et al: A prospective, randomized trial of transplantation of marrow vs. peripheral blood cells from HLA-identical siblings in patients treated for hematologic malignancies. *N Engl J Med* 344:175, 2001.

42. Blaise D, Kuentz M, Fortanier C, et al: Randomized trial of bone marrow versus lenograstim-primed blood cell allogeneic transplantation in patients with early-stage leukemia: A report from the Societe Francaise de Greffe de Moelle. *J Clin Oncol* 18:537, 2000.

43. Couban S, Simpson DR, Barnett MJ, et al: A randomized multicenter comparison of bone marrow and peripheral blood in recipients of matched sibling allogeneic transplants for myeloid malignancies. *Blood* 100:1525, 2002.

44. Powles R, Mehta J, Kulkarni S, et al: Allogeneic blood and bone-marrow stem-cell transplantation in haematological malignant diseases: A randomised trial. *Lancet* 355:1231, 2000.

45. Vigorito AC, Marques Junior JF, Aranha FJ, et al: A randomized, prospective comparison of allogeneic bone marrow and peripheral blood progenitor cell transplantation in the treatment of hematologic malignancies: An update. *Haematologica* 86:665, 2001.

46. Schmitz N, Beksac M, Hasenclever D, et al: Transplantation of mobilized peripheral blood cells to HLA-identical siblings with standard-risk leukemia. *Blood* 100:761, 2002.

47. Flowers ME, Parker PM, Johnston LJ, et al: Comparison of chronic graft-versus-host disease after transplantation of peripheral blood stem cells versus bone marrow in allogeneic recipients: Long-term follow-up of a randomized trial. *Blood* 100:415, 2002.

48. Gluckman E, Rocha V, Boyer-Chammard A, et al: Outcome of cord-blood transplantation from related and unrelated donors. Eurocord Transplant Group and the European Blood and Marrow Transplantation Group. *N Engl J Med* 337:373, 1997.

49. Barker JN, Davies SM, DeFor T, et al: Survival after transplantation of unrelated donor umbilical cord blood is comparable to that of human leukocyte antigen-matched unrelated donor bone marrow: Results of a matched-pair analysis. *Blood* 97:2957, 2001.

50. Barker JN, Wagner JE: Umbilical-cord blood transplantation for the treatment of cancer. *Nat Rev Cancer* 3:526, 2003.

51. Wagner JE, Barker JN, DeFor TE, et al: Transplantation of unrelated donor umbilical cord blood in 102 patients with malignant and non-malignant diseases: influence of CD34 cell dose and HLA disparity on treatment-related mortality and survival. *Blood* 100:1611, 2002.

52. Long GD, Laughlin M, Madan B, et al: Unrelated umbilical cord blood transplantation in adult patients. *Biol Blood Marrow Transplant* 9:772, 2003.

53. Barker JN, Weisdorf DJ, Wagner JE: Creation of a double chimera after the transplantation of umbilical-cord blood from two partially matched unrelated donors. *N Engl J Med* 344:1870, 2001.

54. Deeg HJ, Leisenring W, Storb R, et al: Long-term outcome after marrow transplantation for severe aplastic anemia. *Blood* 91:3637, 1998.

55. Lucarelli G, Clift RA, Galimberti M, et al: Bone marrow transplantation in adult thalassemic patients. *Blood* 93:1164, 1999.

56. Skinner M, Sanchorawala V, Seldin DC, et al: High-dose melphalan and autologous stem-cell transplantation in patients with AL amyloidosis: An 8-year study. *Ann Intern Med* 140:85, 2004.

57. Horning SJ, Chao NJ, Negrin RS, et al: High-dose therapy and autologous hematopoietic progenitor cell transplantation for recurrent or refractory Hodgkin's disease: Analysis of the Stanford University results and prognostic indices. *Blood* 89:801, 1997.

58. Wheeler C, Eickhoff C, Elias A, et al: High-dose cyclophosphamide, carmustine, and etoposide with autologous transplantation in Hodgkin's disease: A prognostic model for treatment outcomes. *Biol Blood Marrow Transplant* 3:98, 1997.

59. Brenner MK, Rill DR, Moen RC, et al: Gene-marking to trace origin of relapse after autologous bone-marrow transplantation. *Lancet* 341:85, 1993.

60. Deisseroth AB, Zu Z, Claxton D, et al: Genetic marking shows that Ph+ cells present in autologous transplants of chronic myelogenous leukemia (CML) contribute to relapse after autologous bone marrow in CML. *Blood* 83:3068, 1994.

61. Yeager AM, Kaizer H, Santos GW, et al: Autologous bone marrow transplantation in patients with acute nonlymphocytic leukemia, using ex vivo marrow treatment with 4-hydroperoxycyclophosphamide. *N Engl J Med* 315:141, 1986.

62. Gorin NC, Aegerter P, Auvert B, et al: Autologous bone marrow transplantation for acute myelocytic leukemia in first remission: A European survey of the role of marrow purging. *Blood* 75:1606, 1990.

63. Negrin RS, Blume KG: The use of the polymerase chain reaction for the detection of minimal residual malignant disease. *Blood* 78:255, 1991.

64. Negrin RS, Pesando J: Detection of tumor cells in purged bone marrow and peripheral blood mononuclear cells by polymerase chain reaction amplification of bcl-2 translocations. *J Clin Oncol* 12:1021, 1994.

65. Gribben JG, Freedman AS, Neuberg D, et al: Immunologic purging of

marrow assessed by PCR before autologous bone marrow transplantation for B-cell lymphoma. *N Engl J Med* 325:1525, 1991.

66. Crippa F, Holmberg L, Carter RA, et al: Infectious complications after autologous CD34-selected peripheral blood stem cell transplantation. *Biol Blood Marrow Transplant* 8:281, 2002.

67. Holmberg LA, Boeckh M, Hooper H, et al: Increased incidence of cytomegalovirus disease after autologous CD34-selected peripheral blood stem cell transplantation. *Blood* 94:4029, 1999.

68. Vescio R, Schiller G, Stewart AK, et al: Multicenter phase III trial to evaluate CD34(+) selected versus unselected autologous peripheral blood progenitor cell transplantation in multiple myeloma. *Blood* 93:1858, 1999.

69. Carella AM, Congiu AM, Gaozza E, et al: High-dose chemotherapy with autologous bone marrow transplantation in 50 advanced resistant Hodgkin's disease patients: an Italian study group report. *J Clin Oncol* 6:1411, 1988.

70. Carella AM, Dejana A, Lerma E, et al: In vivo mobilization of karyotypically normal peripheral blood progenitor cells in high-risk MDS, secondary or therapy-related acute myelogenous leukaemia. *Br J Haematol* 95:127, 1996.

71. Flinn IW, O'Donnell PV, Goodrich A, et al: Immunotherapy with rituximab during peripheral blood stem cell transplantation for non-Hodgkin's lymphoma. *Biol Blood Marrow Transplant* 6:628, 2000.

72. Lazzarino M, Arcaini L, Bernasconi P, et al: A sequence of immunochemotherapy with Rituximab, mobilization of in vivo purged stem cells, high-dose chemotherapy and autotransplant is an effective and non-toxic treatment for advanced follicular and mantle cell lymphoma. *Br J Haematol* 116:229, 2002.

73. Pezner RD, Nademanee A, Forman SJ: High-dose therapy and autologous bone marrow transplantation for Hodgkin's disease patients with relapses potentially treatable by radical radiation therapy. *Int J Radiat Oncol Biol Phys* 33:189, 1995.

74. Mundt AJ, Sibley G, Williams S, et al: Patterns of failure following high-dose chemotherapy and autologous bone marrow transplantation with involved field radiotherapy for relapsed/refractory Hodgkin's disease. *Int J Radiat Oncol Biol Phys* 33:261, 1995.

75. Poen JC, Hoppe RT, Horning SJ: High-dose therapy and autologous bone marrow transplantation for relapsed/refractory Hodgkin's disease: the impact of involved field radiotherapy on patterns of failure and survival. *Int J Radiat Oncol Biol Phys* 36:3, 1996.

76. Reichardt VL, Okada CY, Liso A, et al: Idiotype vaccination using dendritic cells after autologous peripheral blood stem cell transplantation for multiple myeloma—a feasibility study. *Blood* 93:2411, 1999.

77. Davis TA, Hsu FJ, Caspar CB, et al: Idiotype vaccination following ABMT can stimulate specific anti-idiotype immune responses in patients with B-cell lymphoma. *Biol Blood Marrow Transplant* 7:517, 2001.

78. Horwitz SM, Negrin RS, Blume KG, et al: Rituximab as adjuvant to high-dose therapy and autologous hematopoietic cell transplantation for aggressive non-Hodgkin lymphoma. *Blood* 103:777, 2004.

79. Thomas ED, Buckner CD, Banaji M, et al: One hundred patients with acute leukemia treated by chemotherapy, total body irradiation, and allogeneic marrow transplantation. *Blood* 49:511, 1977.

80. Deeg HJ, Flournow N, Sullivan KM, et al: Cataracts after total body irradiation and marrow transplantation: a sparing effect of dose fractionation. *Int J Radiat Oncol Biol Phys* 10:957, 1984.

81. Clift RA, Buckner CD, Appelbaum FR, et al: Allogeneic marrow transplantation in patients with chronic myeloid leukemia in the chronic phase. A randomized trial of two irradiation regimens. *Blood* 77:1660, 1991.

82. Blume KG, Forman SJ: High-dose etoposide (VP-16)-containing preparatory regimens in allogeneic and autologous bone marrow transplantation for hematologic malignancies. *Semin Oncol* 19:63, 1992.

83. Jamieson CH, Amylon MD, Wong RM, et al: Allogeneic hematopoietic cell transplantation for patients with high-risk acute lymphoblastic leukemia in first or second complete remission using fractionated total-body irradiation and high-dose etoposide: A 15-year experience. *Exp Hematol* 31:981, 2003.

84. Tutschka PJ, Copelan EA, Klein JP: Bone marrow transplantation for leukemia following a new busulfan and cyclophosphamide regimen. *Blood* 70:1382, 1987.

85. Clift RA, Buckner CD, Thomas ED, et al: Marrow transplantation for chronic myeloid leukemia: a randomized study comparing cyclophosphamide and total body irradiation with busulfan and cyclophosphamide. *Blood* 84:2036, 1994.

86. Andersson BS, Kashyap A, Gian V, et al: Conditioning therapy with intravenous busulfan and cyclophosphamide (IV BuCy2) for hematologic malignancies prior to allogeneic stem cell transplantation: A phase II study. *Biol Blood Marrow Transplant* 8:145, 2002.

87. Kashyap A, Wingard J, Cagnoni P, et al: Intravenous versus oral busulfan as part of a busulfan/cyclophosphamide preparative regimen for allogeneic hematopoietic stem cell transplantation: decreased incidence of hepatic venoocclusive disease (HVOD), HVOD-related mortality, and overall 100-day mortality. *Biol Blood Marrow Transplant* 8:493, 2002.

88. Slattery JT, Clift RA, Buckner CD, et al: Marrow transplantation for chronic myeloid leukemia: the influence of plasma busulfan levels on the outcome of transplantation. *Blood* 89:3055, 1997.

89. Slavin S, Nagler A, Naparstek E, et al: Nonmyeloablative stem cell transplantation and cell therapy as an alternative to conventional bone marrow transplantation with lethal cytoreduction for the treatment of malignant and nonmalignant hematologic diseases. *Blood* 91:756, 1998.

90. Or R, Shapira MY, Resnick I, et al: Nonmyeloablative allogeneic stem cell transplantation for the treatment of chronic myeloid leukemia in first chronic phase. *Blood* 101:441, 2003.

91. Khouri IF, Saliba RM, Giralt SA, et al: Nonablative allogeneic hematopoietic transplantation as adoptive immunotherapy for indolent lymphoma: Low incidence of toxicity, acute graft-versus-host disease, and treatment-related mortality. *Blood* 98:3595, 2001.

92. Storb R, Yu C, Wagner JL, et al: Stable mixed hematopoietic chimerism in DLA-identical littermate dogs given sublethal total body irradiation before and pharmacological immunosuppression after marrow transplantation. *Blood* 89:3048, 1997.

93. Sandmaer BM, Maloney DG, Hegenbart U, et al: Non-myeloablative conditioning for HLA-identical related allografts for hematologic malignancies. *Blood* 96:479a, 2000.

94. Maloney DG, Molina AJ, Sahebi F, et al: Allografting with non-myeloablative conditioning following cytoreductive autografts for the treatment of patients with multiple myeloma. *Blood* 10:10, 2003.

95. Lan F, Zeng D, Higuchi M, et al: Host conditioning with total lymphoid irradiation and antithymocyte globulin prevents graft-versus-host disease: the role of CD1-reactive natural killer T cells. *Biol Blood Marrow Transplant* 9:355, 2003.

96. Matthews DC, Appelbaum FR, Eary JF, et al: Phase I study of (131)I-anti-CD45 antibody plus cyclophosphamide and total body irradiation for advanced acute leukemia and myelodysplastic syndrome. *Blood* 94:1237, 1999.

97. Appelbaum FR, Matthews DC, Eary JF, et al: The use of radiolabeled anti-CD33 antibody to augment marrow irradiation prior to marrow transplantation for acute myelogenous leukemia. *Transplantation* 54:829, 1992.

98. Matthews DC, Appelbaum FR, Eary JF, et al: Development of a marrow transplant regimen for acute leukemia using targeted hematopoietic irradiation delivered by ^{131}I-labeled anti-CD45 antibody, combined with cyclophosphamide and total body irradiation. *Blood* 85:1122, 1995.

99. Press OW, Eary JF, Gooley T, et al: A phase I/II trial of iodine-131-tositumomab (anti-CD20), etoposide, cyclophosphamide, and autolo-

gous stem cell transplantation for relapsed B-cell lymphomas. *Blood* 96: 2934, 2000.

100. Fefer A, Einstein AB, Thomas ED, et al: Bone-marrow transplantation for hematologic neoplasia in 16 patients with identical twins. *N Engl J Med* 290:1389, 1974.

101. Gale RP, Horowitz MM, Ash RC, et al: Identical-twin bone marrow transplants for leukemia. *Ann Intern Med* 120:646, 1994.

102. Martin PJ, Hansen JA, Buckner CD, et al: Effects of in vitro depletion of T cells in HLA-identical allogeneic marrow grafts. *Blood* 66:664, 1985.

103. Weiden PL, Flournoy N, Thomas ED, et al: Antileukemic effect of graft-versus-host disease in human recipients of allogeneic-marrow grafts. *N Engl J Med* 300:1068, 1979.

104. Weiden PL, Sullivan KM, Flournoy N, et al: Antileukemic effect of chronic graft versus host disease. Contribution of improved survival after allogeneic marrow transplantation. *N Engl J Med* 304:1529, 1981.

105. Sullivan KM, Weiden PL, Storb R, et al: Influence of acute and chronic graft-versus-host disease on relapse and survival after bone marrow transplantation from HLA-identical siblings as treatment of acute and chronic leukemia. *Blood* 73:1720, 1989.

106. Kolb HJ, Mittermuller J, Clemm CH, et al: Donor leukocyte transfusions for treatment of recurrent chronic myelogenous leukemia in marrow transplant patients. *Blood* 76:2462, 1990.

107. Drobyski WR, Keever CA, Roth MS, et al: Salvage immunotherapy using donor leukocyte infusions as treatment for relapsed chronic myelogenous leukemia after allogeneic bone marrow transplantation: efficacy and toxicity of a defined T-cell dose. *Blood* 82:2310, 1993.

108. Porter DL, Roth MS, McGarigle C, et al: Induction of graft-versus-host disease as immunotherapy for relapsed chronic myelogenous leukemia. *N Engl J Med* 330:100, 1994.

109. Collins RH Jr, Pineiro LA, Nemunaitis JJ, et al: Transfusion of donor buffy coat cells in the treatment of persistent or recurrent malignancy after allogeneic bone marrow transplantation. *Transfusion (Paris)* 35: 891, 1995.

110. Slavin S, Naparstek E, Nagler A, et al: Allogeneic cell therapy with donor peripheral blood cells and recombinant human interleukin-2 to treat leukemia relapse after allogeneic bone marrow transplantation. *Blood* 87:2195, 1996.

111. Collins RH, Shpilberg O, Drobyski WR, et al: Donor leukocyte infusions in 140 patients with relapsed malignancy after allogeneic bone marrow transplantation. *J Clin Oncol* 15:433, 1997.

112. Kolb HJ, Schattenberg A, Goldman JM, et al: Graft-versus-leukemia effect of donor lymphocyte transfusions in marrow grafted patients. *Blood* 86:2041, 1995.

113. Dazzi F, Szydlo RM, Cross NC, et al: Durability of responses following donor lymphocyte infusions for patients who relapse after allogeneic stem cell transplantation for chronic myeloid leukemia. *Blood* 96:2712, 2000.

114. Hauch M, Gazzola MV, Small T, et al: Anti-leukemia potential of interelukin-2 activated natural killer cells after bone marrow transplantation for chronic myelogenous leukemia. *Blood* 75:2250, 1990.

115. Ruggeri L, Capanni M, Casucci M, et al: Role of natural killer cell alloreactivity in HLA-mismatched hematopoietic stem cell transplantation. *Blood* 94:333, 1999.

116. Ruggeri L, Capanni M, Urbani E, et al: Effectiveness of donor natural killer cell alloreactivity in mismatched hematopoietic transplants. *Science* 295:2097, 2002.

117. Alyea EP, Soiffer RJ, Canning C, et al: Toxicity and efficacy of defined doses of CD4+ donor lymphocytes for treatment of relapse after allogeneic bone marrow transplant. *Blood* 91:3671, 1998.

118. Champlin R, Ho W, Gajewski J, et al: Selective depletion of CD8+ T lymphocytes for prevention of graft-versus-host disease after allogeneic bone marrow transplantation. *Blood* 76:418, 1990.

119. Bonini C, Ferrari G, Verzeletti S, et al: HSV-TK gene transfer into donor lymphocytes for control of allogeneic graft-versus-leukemia. *Science* 276:1719, 1997.

120. Warren EH, Tykodi SS, Murata M, et al: T-cell therapy targeting minor histocompatibility Ags for the treatment of leukemia and renal-cell carcinoma. *Cytotherapy* 4:441, 2002.

121. Smit WM, Rijnbeek M, Van Bergen CA, et al: T cells recognizing leukemic CD34(+) progenitor cells mediate the antileukemic effect of donor lymphocyte infusions for relapsed chronic myeloid leukemia after allogeneic stem cell transplantation. *Proc Natl Acad Sci U S A* 95:10152, 1998.

122. Yee C, Thompson JA, Byrd D, et al: Adoptive T cell therapy using antigen-specific CD8+ T cell clones for the treatment of patients with metastatic melanoma: In vivo persistence, migration, and antitumor effect of transferred T cells. *Proc Natl Acad Sci U S A* 99:16168, 2002.

123. Heslop H, Rooney C, Brenner M, et al: Administration of neomycin resistance gene-marked EBV-specific cytotoxic T-lymphocytes as therapy for patients receiving a bone marrow transplant for relapsed EBV-positive Hodgkin disease. *Hum Gene Ther* 11:1465, 2000.

124. Roskrow MA, Suzuki N, Gan Y, et al: Epstein-Barr virus (EBV)-specific cytotoxic T lymphocytes for the treatment of patients with EBV-positive relapsed Hodgkin's disease. *Blood* 91:2925, 1998.

125. Baker J, Verneris MR, Ito M, et al: Expansion of cytolytic CD8(+) natural killer T cells with limited capacity for graft-versus-host disease induction due to interferon gamma production. *Blood* 97:2923, 2001.

126. Verneris M, Ito M, Baker J, et al: Engineering hematopoietic grafts: purified allogeneic hematopoietic stem cells plus expanded CD8+ NK-T cells in the treatment of lymphoma. *Biol Blood Marrow Transplant* 7:532, 2001.

127. Clouthier SG, Cooke KR, Teshima T, et al: Repifermin (keratinocyte growth factor-2) reduces the severity of graft-versus-host disease while preserving a graft-versus-leukemia effect. *Biol Blood Marrow Transplant* 9:592, 2003.

128. Reddy P, Teshima T, Hildebrandt G, et al: Interleukin 18 preserves a perforin-dependent graft-versus-leukemia effect after allogeneic bone marrow transplantation. *Blood* 100:3429, 2002.

129. Reddy P, Teshima T, Kukuruga M, et al: Interleukin-18 regulates acute graft-versus-host disease by enhancing Fas-mediated donor T cell apoptosis. *J Exp Med* 194:1433, 2001.

130. Giralt S, O'Brien S, Talpaz M, et al: Interferon-alpha and interleukin-2 as treatment for leukemia relapse after allogeneic bone marrow transplantation. *Cytokines Mol Ther* 1:115, 1995.

131. Hoffmann P, Ermann J, Edinger M, et al: Donor type CD4+CD25+ regulatory T cells suppress lethal acute graft-versus-host disease after allogeneic bone marrow transplantation. *J Exp Med* 196:389, 2002.

132. Taylor PA, Lees CJ, Blazar BR: The infusion of ex vivo activated and expanded CD4(+)CD25(+) immune regulatory cells inhibits graft-versus-host disease lethality. *Blood* 99:3493, 2002.

133. Cohen JL, Trenado A, Vasey D, et al: CD4(+)CD25(+) immunoregulatory T cells: New therapeutics for graft-versus-host disease. *J Exp Med* 196:401, 2002.

134. Edinger M, Hoffmann P, Ermann J, et al: CD4(+)CD25(+) regulatory T cells preserve graft-versus-tumor activity while inhibiting graft-versus-host disease after bone marrow transplantation. *Nat Med* 9:1144, 2003.

135. Trenado A, Charlotte F, Fisson S, et al: Recipient-type specific CD4+CD25+ regulatory T cells favor immune reconstitution and control graft-versus-host disease while maintaining graft-versus-leukemia. *J Clin Invest* 112:1688, 2003.

136. Lan F, Zeng D, Higuchi M, et al: Predominance of NK1.1(+)TCRalphabeta(+) or DX5(+)TCRalphabeta(+) T cells in mice conditioned with fractionated lymphoid irradiation protects against graft-versus-host disease: "Natural suppressor" cells. *J Immunol* 167: 2087, 2001.

137. Powles RL, Watson JG, Morgenstern GR, et al: Bone-marrow transplantation in leukaemia remission [letter]. *Lancet* 1:336, 1982.

138. Appelbaum FR, Fisher LD, Thomas ED: Chemotherapy v marrow transplantation for adults with acute nonlymphocytic leukemia: A five-year follow-up. *Blood* 72:179, 1988.

139. Champlin RE, Ho WG, Gale RP, et al: Treatment of acute myelogenous leukemia. A prospective controlled trial of bone marrow transplantation versus consolidation chemotherapy. *Ann Intern Med* 102:285, 1985.

140. Marmot A, Bacigalupo A, Van Lint MT, et al: Bone marrow transplantation versus chemotherapy alone for acute nonlymphoblastic leukemia. *Exp Hematol* 13:40, 1985.

141. Zander AR, Keating M, Dicke K, et al: A comparison of marrow transplantation with chemotherapy for adults with acute leukemia of poor prognosis in first complete remission. *J Clin Oncol* 6:1548, 1988.

142. Conde E, Iriondo A, Rayon C, et al: Allogeneic bone marrow transplantation versus intensification chemotherapy for acute myelogenous leukaemia in first remission: A prospective controlled trial. *Br J Haematol* 68:219, 1988.

143. Reiffers J, Gaspard MH, Maraninchi D, et al: Comparison of allogeneic or autologous bone marrow transplantation and chemotherapy in patients with acute myeloid leukaemia in first remission: A prospective controlled trial. *Br J Haematol* 72:57, 1989.

144. Löwenberg B, Verdonck LJ, Dekker AW, et al: Autologous bone marrow transplantation in acute myeloid leukemia in first remission: Results of a Dutch prospective study. *J Clin Oncol* 8:287, 1990.

145. Schiller GJ, Nimer SD, Territo MC, et al: Bone marrow transplantation versus high-dose cytarabine-based consolidation chemotherapy for acute myelogenous leukemia in first remission. *J Clin Oncol* 10:41, 1992.

146. Cassileth PA, Lynch E, Hines JD, et al: Varying intensity of postremission therapy in acute myeloid leukemia. *Blood* 79:1924, 1992.

147. Archimbaud E, Thomas X, Michallet M, et al: Prospective genetically randomized comparison between intensive postinduction chemotherapy and bone marrow transplantation in adults with newly diagnosed acute myeloid leukemia. *J Clin Oncol* 12:262, 1994.

148. Mitus AJ, Miller KB, Schenkein DP, et al: Improved survival for patients with acute myelogenous leukemia. *J Clin Oncol* 13:560, 1995.

149. Hewlett J, Kopecky KJ, Head D, et al: A prospective evaluation of the roles of allogeneic marrow transplantation and low-dose monthly maintenance chemotherapy in the treatment of adult acute myelogenous leukemia (AML): A Southwest Oncology Group study. *Leukemia* 9:562, 1995.

150. Harousseau JL, Cahn JY, Pignon B, et al: Comparison of autologous bone marrow transplantation and intensive chemotherapy as postremission therapy in adult acute myeloid leukemia. The Groupe Ouest Est Leucémies Aiguës Myéloblastiques (GOELAM). *Blood* 90:2978, 1997.

151. Cassileth PA, Harrington DP, Appelbaum FR, et al: Chemotherapy compared with autologous or allogeneic bone marrow transplantation in the management of acute myeloid leukemia in first remission. *N Engl J Med* 339:1649, 1998.

152. Bloomfield CD, Lawrence D, Byrd JC, et al: Frequency of prolonged remission duration after high-dose cytarabine intensification in acute myeloid leukemia varies by cytogenetic subtype. *Cancer Res* 58:4173, 1998.

153. Aversa F, Tabilio A, Velardi A, et al: Transplantation for high-risk acute leukemia with high doses of T-cell-depleted hematopoietic stem cells from full-haplotype incompatible donors. *N Engl J Med* 339:1186, 1998.

154. Davies SM, Ruggieri L, DeFor T, et al: Evaluation of KIR ligand incompatibility in mismatched unrelated donor hematopoietic transplants. Killer immunoglobulin-like receptor. *Blood* 100:3825, 2002.

155. Giebel S, Locatelli FW, Lamparelli T, et al: Survival advantage with KIR ligand incompatibility in hematopoietic stem cell transplantation from unrelated donors. *Blood* 10:10, 2003.

156. Michel G, Rocha V, Chevret S, et al: Unrelated cord blood transplantation for childhood acute myeloid leukemia: A Eurocord Group analysis. *Blood* 102:4290, 2003.

157. Dickson TM, Kusnierz-Glaz CR, Blume KG, et al: Impact of admission body weight and chemotherapy dose adjustment on the outcome of autologous bone marrow transplantation. *Biol Blood Marrow Transplant* 5:299, 1999.

158. Linch DC, Milligan DW, Winfield DA, et al: G-CSF after peripheral blood stem cell transplantation in lymphoma patients significantly accelerated neutrophil recovery and shortened time in hospital: results of a randomized BNLI trial. *Br J Haematol* 99:933, 1997.

159. Spitzer G, Adkins DR, Spencer V, et al: Randomized study of growth factors post-peripheral-blood stem-cell transplant: Neutrophil recovery is improved with modest clinical benefit. *J Clin Oncol* 12:661, 1994.

160. Volpi I, Perruccio K, Tosti A, et al: Postgrafting administration of granulocyte colony-stimulating factor impairs functional immune recovery in recipients of human leukocyte antigen haplotype-mismatched hematopoietic transplants. *Blood* 97:2514, 2001.

161. Farrell CL, Bready JV, Rex KL, et al: Keratinocyte growth factor protects mice from chemotherapy and radiation-induced gastrointestinal injury and mortality. *Cancer Res* 58:933, 1998.

162. Hill GR, Ferrara JL: The primacy of the gastrointestinal tract as a target organ of acute graft-versus-host disease: rationale for the use of cytokine shields in allogeneic bone marrow transplantation. *Blood* 95:2754, 2000.

163. Weisdorf SA, Lysne J, Wind D, et al: Positive effect of prophylactic total parenteral nutrition on long-term outcome of bone marrow transplantation. *Transplantation* 43:833, 1987.

164. Charuhas P, Fosberg K, Bruemmer B, et al: A double-blind randomized trial comparing outpatient parenteral nutrition with intravenous hydration: effect on resumption of oral intake after marrow transplantation. *JPEN J Parenter Enteral Nutr* 21:157, 1997.

165. Ziegler TR, Young LS, Benfell K, et al: Clinical and metabolic efficacy of glutamine-supplemented parenteral nutrition after bone marrow transplantation. *Ann Intern Med* 116:821, 1992.

166. Coghlin-Dickson T, Wong R, Negrin R, et al: Effect of oral glutamine supplementation during bone marrow transplantation. *JPEN J Parenter Enteral Nutr* 24:61, 2000.

167. Bernstein SH, Nademanee AP, Vose JM, et al: A multicenter study of platelet recovery and utilization in patients after myeloablative therapy and hematopoietic stem cell transplantation. *Blood* 91:3509, 1998.

168. Rebulla R, Finazzi G, Marangoni F, et al: A multicenter randomized study of the threshold for prophylactic platelet transfusions in adults with acute myeloid leukemia. Gruppo Italiano Malattie Ematologiche Maligne dell'Adulto. *N Engl J Med* 337:1870, 1997.

169. Heckman KD, Weiner GJ, Davis CS, et al: Randomized study of prophylactic platelet transfusion threshold for adult acute leukemia: 10,000/microL versus 20,000/microL. *J Clin Oncol* 15:1143, 1997.

170. Sullivan KM, Kopecky KJ, Jocom J, et al: Immunomodulatory and antimicrobial efficacy of intravenous immunoglobulin in bone marrow transplantation. *N Engl J Med* 323:705, 1990.

171. Sullivan KM, Storek J, Kopecky KJ, et al: A controlled trial of long-term administration of intravenous immunoglobulin to prevent late infection and chronic graft-vs.-host disease after marrow transplantation: Clinical outcome and effect on subsequent immune recovery. *Biol Blood Marrow Transplant* 2:44, 1996.

172. Rousey SR, Russler S, Gottlieb M, et al: Low-dose amphotericin B prophylaxis against invasive *Aspergillus* infections in allogeneic marrow transplantation. *Am J Med* 91:484, 1991.

173. O'Donnell M, Schmidt GM, Tegtmeier BR, et al: Prediction of systemic fungal infection in allogeneic marrow recipients: Impact of amphotericin prophylaxis in high-risk patients. *J Clin Oncol* 12:827, 1994.

174. Goodman JL, Winston DJ, Greenfield RA, et al: A controlled trial of fluconazole to prevent fungal infections in patients undergoing bone marrow transplantation. *N Engl J Med* 326:845, 1992.

175. Bow EJ, Laverdiere M, Lussier N, et al: Antifungal prophylaxis for severely neutropenic chemotherapy recipients: A meta analysis of randomized-controlled clinical trials. *Cancer* 94:3230, 2002.

176. Bowden RA, Sayers M, Flournoy N, et al: Cytomegalovirus immune globulin and seronegative blood products to prevent primary cytomegalovirus infection after marrow transplantation. *N Engl J Med* 314:1006, 1986.

177. Schmidt GM, Horak DA, Niland JC, et al: A randomized, controlled trial of prophylactic ganciclovir for cytomegalovirus pulmonary infection in recipients of allogeneic bone marrow transplants. *N Engl J Med* 324:1005, 1991.

178. Goodrich JM, Mori M, Gleaves CA, et al: Early treatment with ganciclovir to prevent cytomegalovirus disease after allogeneic bone marrow transplantation. *N Engl J Med* 325:1601, 1991.

179. Winston DJ, Ho WG, Bartoni K, et al: Ganciclovir prophylaxis of cytomegalovirus infection and disease in allogeneic bone marrow transplant recipients. *Ann Intern Med* 118:179, 1993.

180. Walter EA, Greenberg PD, Gilbert MJ, et al: Reconstitution of cellular immunity against cytomegalovirus in recipients of allogeneic bone marrow by transfer of T-cell clones from the donor. *N Engl J Med* 333:1038, 1995.

181. Wade JC, Newton B, McLaren C, et al: Intravenous acyclovir to treat mucocutaneous herpes simplex virus infection after marrow transplantation: A double blind trial. *Ann Intern Med* 96:265, 1982.

182. Cone R, Hackman R, Huang M, et al: Human herpesvirus 6 in lung tissue from patients with pneumonitis after bone marrow transplantation. *N Engl J Med* 329:156, 1993.

183. Drobyski W, Knox K, Majewski D, et al: Brief report: Fatal encephalitis due to variant B human herpesvirus-6 infection in a bone marrow transplant recipient. *N Engl J Med* 330:1356, 1994.

184. Harrington R, Hooton T, Hackman R, et al: An outbreak of respiratory syncytial virus in a bone marrow transplant center. *J Infect Dis* 165:987, 1992.

185. Shields AF, Hackman RC, Fife KH, et al: Adenovirus infections in patients undergoing bone-marrow transplantation. *N Engl J Med* 312:529, 1985.

186. Arthur RR, Shah KV, Baust SJ, et al: Association of BK viruria with hemorrhagic cystitis in recipients of bone marrow transplants. *N Engl J Med* 315:230, 1986.

187. Billingham RE: The biology of graft-versus-host reactions, in *The Harvey Lectures*, p 62:21. Academic Press New York, 1966.

188. Storb R, Deeg HJ, Farewell V, et al: Marrow transplantation for severe aplastic anemia: methotrexate alone compared with a combination of methotrexate and cyclosporine for prevention of acute graft-versus-host disease. *Blood* 68:119, 1986.

189. Storb R, Deeg HJ, Whitehead J, et al: Methotrexate and cyclosporine compared with cyclosporine alone for prophylaxis of acute graft versus host disease after marrow transplantation for leukemia. *N Engl J Med* 314:729, 1986.

190. Chao NJ, Snyder DS, Jain M, et al: Equivalence of 2 effective graft-versus-host disease prophylaxis regimens: Results of a prospective double-blind randomized trial. *Biol Blood Marrow Transplant* 6:254, 2000.

191. Ratanatharathorn V, Nash RA, Przepiorka D, et al: Phase III study comparing methotrexate and tacrolimus (Prograf, FK506) with methotrexate and cyclosporine for graft-versus-host disease prophylaxis after HLA-identical sibling bone marrow transplantation. *Blood* 92:2303, 1998.

192. Nash RA, Piñeiro LA, Storb R, et al: FK506 in combination with methotrexate for the prevention of graft-versus-host disease after marrow transplantation from matched unrelated donors. *Blood* 88:3634, 1996.

193. Hiroka A: Results of a phase III study on prophylactic use of FK506 for acute GVHD compared with cyclosporin in allogeneic bone marrow transplantation. *Blood* 90(suppl 1):561a, 1997.

194. Goldman JM, Gale RP, Horowitz MM, et al: Bone marrow transplantation for chronic myelogenous leukemia in chronic phase. Increased risk for relapse associated with T-cell depletion. *Ann Intern Med* 108:806, 1988.

195. Filipovich AH, Vallera DA, Youle RJ, et al: Ex vivo treatment of donor bone marrow with anti-T-cell immunotoxins for prevention of graft-versus-host disease. *Lancet* 1:469, 1984.

196. Prentice HG, Blacklock HA, Janossy G, et al: Use of anti-T-cell monoclonal antibody OKT3 to prevent acute graft-versus-host disease in allogeneic bone-marrow transplantation for acute leukaemia. *Lancet* 1:700, 1982.

197. Kernan NA, Flomenberg N, Dupont B, et al: Graft rejection in recipients of T-cell-depleted HLA-nonidentical marrow transplants for leukemia. Identification of host-derived antidonor allocytotoxic T lymphocytes. *Transplantation* 43:842, 1987.

198. Papadopoulos EB, Carabasi MH, Castro-Malaspina H, et al: T-cell-depleted allogeneic bone marrow transplantation as postremission therapy for acute myelogenous leukemia: freedom from relapse in the absence of graft-versus-host disease. *Blood* 91:1083, 1998.

199. Small TN, Avigan D, Dupont B, et al: Immune reconstitution following T-cell depleted bone marrow transplantation: effect of age and posttransplant graft rejection prophylaxis. *Biol Blood Marrow Transplant* 3:65, 1997.

200. Wagner JE, Thompson JS, Carter S, et al: Impact of graft-versus-host disease (GVHD) prophylaxis on 3-year disease-free survival (DFS): Results of a multi-center, randomized phase II-III trial comparing T cell depletion/cyclosporine (TCD) and methotrexate/cyclosporine (M/C) in 410 recipients of unrelated donor bone marrow (BM). *Blood* 100:75a[abstract], 2002.

201. Novitzky N, Thomas V, Hale G, et al: Ex vivo depletion of T cells from bone marrow grafts with CAMPATH-1 in acute leukemia: graft-versus-host disease and graft-versus-leukemia effect. *Transplantation* 67:620, 1999.

202. Hale G, Zhang MJ, Bunjes D, et al: Improving the outcome of bone marrow transplantation by using CD52 monoclonal antibodies to prevent graft-versus-host disease and graft rejection. *Blood* 92:4581, 1998.

203. Van Lint MT, Uderzo C, Locasciulli A, et al: Early treatment of acute graft-versus-host disease with high- or low-dose 6-methylprednisolone: A multicenter randomized trial from the Italian Group for Bone Marrow Transplantation. *Blood* 92:2288, 1998.

204. McDonald GB, Hinds MS, Fisher LD: Veno-occlusive disease of the liver and multiorgan failure after bone marrow transplantation: A cohort study of 355 patients. *Ann Intern Med* 118:255, 1993.

205. Bearman SI, Anderson GL, Mori M, et al: Venoocclusive disease of the liver: Development of a model for predicting fatal outcome after marrow transplantation. *J Clin Oncol* 11:1729, 1993.

206. Salat C, Holler E, Kolb HJ, et al: Plasminogen activator inhibitor-1 confirms the diagnosis of hepatic veno-occlusive disease in patients with hyperbilirubinemia after bone marrow transplantation. *Blood* 89:2184, 1997.

207. Rozman C, Carreras E, Qian C, et al: Risk factors for hepatic veno-occlusive disease following HLA-identical sibling bone marrow transplants for leukemia. *Bone Marrow Transplant* 17:75, 1996.

208. Locasciulli A, Alberti A, Bandini G, et al: Allogeneic bone marrow transplantation from HBsAg+ donors: A multicenter study from the Gruppo Italiano Trapianto di Midollo Osseo (GITMO). *Blood* 86:3236, 1995.

209. Dix SP, Wingard JR, Mullins RE, et al: Association of busulfan area under the curve with veno-occlusive disease following BMT. *Bone Marrow Transplant* 17:225, 1996.

210. Bearman SI, Lee JL, Baron AE, et al: Treatment of hepatic venoocclusive disease with recombinant human tissue plasminogen activator and heparin in 42 marrow transplant patients. *Blood* 89:1501, 1997.

211. Haaglund H, Ringden O, Ericzon BG, et al: Treatment of hepatic

venoocclusive disease with recombinant human tissue plasminogen activator or orthotopic liver transplantation after allogeneic bone marrow transplantation. *Transplantation* 62:1076, 1996.

212. Bacher P, Kindel G, Walenga JM, et al: Modulation of endothelial and platelet function by a polydeoxyribonucleotide derived drug "defibrotide." A dual mechanism in the control of vascular pathology. *Thromb Res* 70:343, 1993.

213. Richardson PG, Elias AD, Krishnan A, et al: Treatment of severe veno-occlusive disease with defibrotide: compassionate use results in response without significant toxicity in a high-risk population. *Blood* 92:737, 1998.

214. Richardson PG, Murakami C, Jin Z, et al: Multi-institutional use of defibrotide in 88 patients after stem cell transplantation with severe veno-occlusive disease and multisystem organ failure: Response without significant toxicity in a high-risk population and factors predictive of outcome. *Blood* 100:4337, 2002.

215. Morris JD, Harris RE, Hashmi R, et al: Antithrombin-III for the treatment of chemotherapy-induced organ dysfunction following bone marrow transplantation. *Bone Marrow Transplant* 20:871, 1997.

216. Attal M, Hueguet F, Rubie H, et al: Prevention of hepatic veno-occlusive disease after bone marrow transplantation by continuous infusion of low-dose heparin: A prospective, randomized trial. *Blood* 79:2834, 1992.

217. Marsa-Vila L, Gorin NC, Laporte JP, et al: Prophylactic heparin does not prevent liver veno-occlusive disease following autologous bone marrow transplantation. *Eur J Haematol* 47:346, 1991.

218. Carreras E, Bertz H, Arcese W, et al: Incidence and outcome of hepatic veno-occlusive disease after blood or marrow transplantation: A prospective cohort study of the European Group for Blood and Marrow Transplantation. European Group for Blood and Marrow Transplantation Chronic Leukemia Working Party. *Blood* 92:3599, 1998.

219. Or R, Nagler A, Shpilberg O, et al: Low molecular weight heparin for the prevention of veno-occlusive disease of the liver in bone marrow transplantation patients. *Transplantation* 61:1067, 1996.

220. Ruutu T, Eriksson B, Remes K, et al: Ursodeoxycholic acid for the prevention of hepatic complications in allogeneic stem cell transplantation. *Blood* 100:1977, 2002.

221. Wingard JR, Sostrin MB, Vriesendorp HM, et al: Interstitial pneumonitis following autologous bone marrow transplantation. *Transplantation* 46:61, 1988.

222. Pecego R, Hill R, Appelbaum FR, et al: Interstitial pneumonitis following autologous bone marrow transplantation. *Transplantation* 42:515, 1986.

223. Frankovich J, Donaldson SS, Lee Y, et al: High-dose therapy and autologous hematopoietic cell transplantation in children with primary refractory and relapsed Hodgkin's disease: Atopy predicts idiopathic diffuse lung injury syndromes. *Biol Blood Marrow Transplant* 7:49, 2001.

224. Seiden MV, Elias A, Ayash L, et al: Pulmonary toxicity associated with high dose chemotherapy in the treatment of solid tumors with autologous marrow transplant: An analysis of four chemotherapy regimens. *Bone Marrow Transplant* 10:57, 1992.

225. Chao NJ, Duncan SR, Long GD, et al: Corticosteroid therapy for diffuse alveolar hemorrhage in autologous bone marrow transplant recipients. *Ann Intern Med* 114:145, 1991.

226. Radich JP, Gehly G, Gooley T, et al: Polymerase chain reaction of the BCR-ABL fusion transcript after allogeneic marrow transplantation for chronic myeloid leukemia: Results and implications in 346 patients. *Blood* 85:2632, 1995.

227. Tsai T, Goodman S, Saez R, et al: Allogeneic bone marrow transplantation in patients who relapse after autologous transplantation. *Bone Marrow Transplant* 20:859, 1997.

228. Di Grazia C, Raiola AM, Van Lint MT, et al: Conventional hematopoietic stem cell transplants from identical or alternative donors are feasible in recipients relapsing after an autograft. *Haematologica* 86:646, 2001.

229. Radich JP, Gooley T, Sanders JE, et al: Second allogeneic transplantation after failure of first autologous transplantation. *Biol Blood Marrow Transplant* 6:272, 2000.

230. Hale GA, Tong X, Benaim E, et al: Allogeneic bone marrow transplantation in children failing prior autologous bone marrow transplantation. *Bone Marrow Transplant* 27:155, 2001.

231. Nagler A, Or R, Naparstek E, et al: Second allogeneic stem cell transplantation using nonmyeloablative conditioning for patients who relapsed or developed secondary malignancies following autologous transplantation. *Exp Hematol* 28:1096, 2000.

232. Porter DL, Luger SM, Duffy KM, et al: Allogeneic cell therapy for patients who relapse after autologous stem cell transplantation. *Biol Blood Marrow Transplant* 7:230, 2001.

233. Dey BR, McAfee S, Sackstein R, et al: Successful allogeneic stem cell transplantation with nonmyeloablative conditioning in patients with relapsed hematologic malignancy following autologous stem cell transplantation. *Biol Blood Marrow Transplant* 7:604, 2001.

234. Corradini P, Tarella C, Olivieri A, et al: Reduced-intensity conditioning followed by allografting of hematopoietic cells can produce clinical and molecular remissions in patients with poor-risk hematologic malignancies. *Blood* 99:75, 2002.

235. Nagler A, Ackerstein A, Or R, et al: Immunotherapy with recombinant human interleukin-2 and recombinant interferon-alpha in lymphoma patients postautologous marrow or stem cell transplantation. *Blood* 89:3951, 1997.

236. Stein AS, O'Donnell MR, Slovak ML, et al: Interleukin-2 after autologous stem-cell transplantation for adult patients with acute myeloid leukemia in first complete remission. *J Clin Oncol* 21:615, 2003.

237. Haioun C, Lepage E, Gisselbrecht C, et al: Benefit of autologous bone marrow transplantation over sequential chemotherapy in poor-risk aggressive non-Hodgkin's lymphoma: Updated results of the prospective study LNH87-2. Groupe d'Etude des Lymphomes de l'Adulte. *J Clin Oncol* 15:1131, 1997.

238. Nademanee A, Molina A, O'Donnell MR, et al: Results of high-dose therapy and autologous bone marrow/stem cell transplantation during remission in poor-risk intermediate- and high-grade lymphoma: International index high and high-intermediate risk group. *Blood* 90:3844, 1997.

239. Gianni AM, Bregni M, Siena S, et al: High-dose chemotherapy and autologous bone marrow transplantation compared with MACOP-B in aggressive B-cell lymphoma. *N Engl J Med* 336:1290, 1997.

240. Milpied N, Deconinck E, Gaillard F, et al: Initial treatment of aggressive lymphoma with high-dose chemotherapy and autologous stem-cell support. *N Engl J Med* 350:1287, 2004.

241. Shulman HM, Sale GE, Lerner KG, et al: Chronic cutaneous graft-versus-host disease in man. *Am J Pathol* 91:545, 1978.

242. Shulman HM, Sullivan KM, Weiden PL, et al: Chronic graft-versus-host syndrome in man. A long-term clinicopathologic study of 20 Seattle patients. *Am J Med* 69:204, 1980.

243. Sullivan KM, Shulman HM, Storb R, et al: Chronic graft-versus-host disease in 52 patients: Adverse natural course and successful treatment with combination immunosuppression. *Blood* 57:267, 1981.

244. Koc S, Leisenring W, Flowers ME, et al: Therapy for chronic graft-versus-host disease: A randomized trial comparing cyclosporine plus prednisone versus prednisone alone. *Blood* 100:48, 2002.

245. Sullivan KM, Witherspoon RP, Storb R, et al: Alternating-day cyclosporine and prednisone for treatment of high-risk chronic graft-v-host disease. *Blood* 72:555, 1988.

246. Vogelsang GB: How I treat chronic graft-versus-host disease. *Blood* 97:1196, 2001.

247. Flowers ME, Lee S, Vogelsang G: An update on how to treat chronic GVHD. *Blood* 102:2312, 2003.

248. Vogelsang GB, Farmer ER, Hess AD, et al: Thalidomide for the treatment of chronic graft-versus-host disease. *N Engl J Med* 326:1055, 1992.

249. Parker PM, Chao N, Nademanee A, et al: Thalidomide as salvage ther-apy for chronic graft-versus-host disease. *Blood* 86:3604, 1995.

250. Koc S, Leisenring W, Flowers ME, et al: Thalidomide for treatment of patients with chronic graft-versus-host disease. *Blood* 96:3995, 2000.

251. Chao NJ, Parker PM, Niland JC, et al: Paradoxical effect of thalidomide prophylaxis on chronic graft-vs.-host disease. *Biol Blood Marrow Transplant* 2:86, 1996.

252. Kapoor N, Pelligrini AE, Copelan EA, et al: Psoralen plus ultraviolet A (PUVA) in the treatment of chronic graft versus host disease: Preliminary experience in standard treatment resistant patients. *Semin Hematol* 29:108, 1992.

253. Benito AI, Furlong T, Martin PJ, et al: Sirolimus (rapamycin) for the treatment of steroid-refractory acute graft-versus-host disease. *Transplantation* 72:1924, 2001.

254. Alston PK, Kuller JA, McMahon MJ: Pregnancy in transplant recipients. *Obstet Gynecol Surv* 56:289, 2001.

255. Watson M, Wheatley K, Harrison GA, et al: Severe adverse impact on sexual functioning and fertility of bone marrow transplantation, either allogeneic or autologous, compared with consolidation chemotherapy alone: analysis of the MRC AML 10 trial. *Cancer* 86:1231, 1999.

256. Apperley JF, Reddy N: Mechanism and management of treatment-related gonadal failure in recipients of high dose chemoradiotherapy. *Blood Rev* 9:93, 1995.

257. Lipton JH, Virro M, Solow H: Successful pregnancy after allogeneic bone marrow transplant with embryos isolated before transplant. *J Clin Oncol* 15:3347, 1997.

258. Demeestere I, Simon P, Englert Y, et al: Preliminary experience of ovarian tissue cryopreservation procedure: alternatives, perspectives and feasibility. *Reprod Biomed Online* 7:572, 2003.

259. Schubert MA, Sullivan KM, Schubert MM, et al: Gynecological abnormalities following allogeneic bone marrow transplantation. *Bone Marrow Transplant* 5:425, 1990.

260. Sanders JE, Pritchard S, Mahoney P, et al: Growth and development following marrow transplantation for leukemia. *Blood* 68:1129, 1986.

261. Sklar CA, Kim TH, Ramsay NK: Thyroid dysfunction among long-term survivors of bone marrow transplantation. *Am J Med* 73:688, 1982.

262. Miller JS, Arthur DC, Litz CE, et al: Myelodysplastic syndrome after autologous bone marrow transplantation: an additional late complication of curative cancer therapy. *Blood* 83:3780, 1994.

263. Stone RM, Neuberg D, Soiffer R, et al: Myelodysplastic syndrome as a late complication following autologous bone marrow transplantation for non-Hodgkin's lymphoma. *J Clin Oncol* 12:2535, 1994.

264. Bhatia S, Ramsay NK, Steinbuch M, et al: Malignant neoplasms following bone marrow transplantation. *Blood* 87:3633, 1996.

265. André M, Henry-Amar M, Blaise D, et al: Treatment-related deaths and second cancer risk after autologous stem-cell transplantation for Hodgkin's disease. *Blood* 92:1933, 1998.

266. Chao NJ, Nademanee AP, Long GD, et al: Importance of bone marrow cytogenetic evaluation before autologous bone marrow transplantation for Hodgkin's disease. *J Clin Oncol* 9:1575, 1991.

267. Govindarajan R, Jagannath S, Flick JT, et al: Preceding standard therapy is the likely cause of MDS after autotransplants for multiple myeloma. *Br J Haematol* 95:349, 1996.

268. Lowsky R, Lipton J, Fyles G, et al: Secondary malignancies after bone marrow transplantation in adults. *J Clin Oncol* 12:2187, 1994.

269. Curtis RE, Rowlings PA, Deeg HJ, et al: Solid cancers after bone marrow transplantation. *N Engl J Med* 336:897, 1997.

270. Radich JP, Gooley T, Bensinger W, et al: HLA-matched related hematopoetic cell transplantation for CML chronic phase using a targeted busulfan and cyclophosphamide preparative regimen. *Blood* 20:20, 2003.

271. Attal M, Harousseau JL, Stoppa AM, et al: A prospective, randomized trial of autologous bone marrow transplantation and chemotherapy in multiple myeloma. Intergroupe Francais du Myelome. *N Engl J Med* 335:91, 1996.

272. Child JA, Morgan GJ, Davies FE, et al: High-dose chemotherapy with hematopoietic stem-cell rescue for multiple myeloma. *N Engl J Med* 348:1875, 2003.

273. Barlogie B, Jagannath S, Vesole DH, et al: Superiority of tandem autologous transplantation over standard therapy for previously untreated multiple myeloma. *Blood* 89:789, 1997.

274. Attal M, Harousseau JL, Facon T, et al: Single versus double autologous stem-cell transplantation for multiple myeloma. *N Engl J Med* 349:2495, 2003.

275. Philip T, Guglielmi C, Hagenbeek A, et al: Autologous bone marrow transplantation as compared with salvage chemotherapy in relapses of chemotherapy-sensitive non-Hodgkin's lymphoma. *N Engl J Med* 333:1540, 1995.

PRINCIPLES OF IMMUNE CELL THERAPY

CAROLINA BERGER
STANLEY R. RIDDELL

Antigen-specific T cells, which recognize processed fragments of proteins presented in association with major histocompatibility complex (MHC) molecules, represent an important component of the host response to intracellular pathogens and tumors. Adoptive T cell immunotherapy, in which T cells are administered to augment or establish an immune response, is an emerging modality for the treatment of both infectious and malignant diseases. Studies in murine models have elucidated many of the principles for effective T cell therapy and provided valuable insights for applying this approach to the treatment of human disease. Over the past few years, advances in cellular and molecular immunology have resulted in the identification of candidate target antigens for immunotherapy and the development of efficient techniques for isolating and propagating T cells. Dendritic cells (DCs) have been identified as specialized antigen-presenting cells (APCs) that elicit and regulate antigen-specific CD4+ and CD8+ T cell immunity in vivo. Culture techniques that use DCs have been used to facilitate the in vitro isolation of antigen-reactive T cells for cell therapy and to generate cell-based vaccines to induce antitumor immunity in vivo. Clinical trials of cell-based immunotherapy have been performed and the results have provided insight into the obstacles to effectively using this modality in humans. It is expected that with further development, immune cell therapy will become an increasingly available and effective therapy.

ADOPTIVE CELLULAR THERAPY OF VIRAL DISEASES

Two subsets of antigen-specific T cells cooperate to terminate acute viral infections and control reactivation of latent viruses. CD8+ cytotoxic T lymphocytes (CTLs) recognize viral peptides presented by major histocompatibility complex (MHC) class I molecules, lyse the infected cell by perforin/granzyme release, and produce inflammatory cytokines. CD4+ T helper (Th) cells recognize viral peptides presented by class II MHC molecules and produce cytokines that amplify T cell responses or promote B cell proliferation and antibody production. A deficiency of CD8+ and CD4+ helper T cells occurs after allogeneic hematopoietic stem cell transplantation (HCT) as a consequence of the administration of intensive chemoradiotherapy, anti-T cell monoclonal antibodies (MAbs), and/or posttransplant immunosuppressive drugs, and these patients are at risk for life-threatening viral infection.[1] Studies in mouse models demonstrate that the adoptive transfer of virus-specific T cells can restore immunity, providing a rationale for developing T cell therapy in humans.[2,3] Clinical investigation of this approach for the treatment of cytomegalovirus (CMV) and Epstein-Barr virus (EBV) infection has focused on patients receiving allogeneic HCT, because the stem cell donor can serve as a source of T cells for therapy. T cell therapy for these viruses requires knowledge of the antigens presented by infected cells, strategies for propagating T cells of the appropriate phenotype, specificity, and function, modification of the host to improve cell transfer, and methods for monitoring the in vivo activity of transferred cells (Fig. 23-1).[4]

T CELL THERAPY OF CYTOMEGALOVIRUS INFECTION

CMV is a large DNA virus that infects several cell types in vivo, including hematopoietic progenitors, monocytes, and endothelium. CMV establishes latency in some cells, and expresses proteins that interfere with antigen presentation by class I and class II MHC molecules in cells that are replicating virus to evade complete elimination by host immunity.[5] CMV frequently reactivates after allogeneic HCT and contributes to morbidity and mortality. The administration of the antiviral drug ganciclovir at the onset of CMV reactivation reduces the incidence of CMV disease early after HCT,[6] but CMV disease continues to occur later when the antiviral drug is discontinued.[7]

Normal CMV+ individuals have approximately 5 to 10 percent of CD8+ T cells and 1 to 5 percent of CD4+ T cells in the blood that are specific for CMV antigens, and it is essential these responses be maintained for life to control infection.[8,9] The essential role of T cells in protection from CMV disease after allogeneic HCT is supported by several observations. Recovery of endogenous CMV-specific CD8+ and CD4+ T cell responses, but not CMV-specific antibodies, correlates with protection from CMV disease in the first 3 months after allogeneic HCT.[10] An absolute lymphocytopenia and deficiency of functional CMV-specific T cells persist for several months in many HCT recipients, and this deficiency correlates with the occurrence of late CMV disease.[7] Thus, suppression of CMV replication with antiviral drugs provides temporary control of reactivation, but restoration of immune function is essential to contain CMV infection.

TARGET ANTIGENS FOR CYTOMEGALOVIRUS-SPECIFIC T CELLS

Studies of the specificity of CMV-specific T cells isolated from immunocompetent CMV-infected individuals have provided insights into appropriate antigens to target in T cell therapy. CMV expresses approximately 190 viral proteins in permissively infected cells.[11] However, the majority of CD8+ CTLs cells elicited by in vitro stimulation with autologous CMV-infected cells are specific for virion proteins, including the pp65 and pp150 matrix proteins. These viral antigens are introduced into the cytoplasm of cells immediately following viral penetration of the plasma membrane and are rapidly processed and presented to CD8+ CTL cells. Thus, CTL cells specific for pp65 and pp150 are capable of lysing infected cells before class I MHC is downregulated by the viral immune evasion genes.[12] Recent studies have used stimulation with panels of CMV peptides or with cells infected with a CMV strain that is deleted of the viral immune evasion genes to further probe the specificity of CD8+ T cells in CMV+ donors.[13,14]

Acronyms and abbreviations that appear in this chapter include: ALL, acute lymphoblastic leukemia; AML, acute myeloid leukemia; APC, antigen-presenting cell; cDNA, complementary DNA; CDR3, complementarity-determining region 3; CEA, carcinoembryonic antigen; CML, chronic myeloid leukemia; CMV, cytomegalovirus; CTL, cytotoxic T lymphocyte; DC, dendritic cell; E, early; EBV, Epstein-Barr virus; gB, glycoprotein B; GVHD, graft-versus-host disease; GVL, graft-versus-leukemia; HCT, hematopoietic stem cell transplantation; HLA, human leukocyte antigen; HSV-TK, herpes simplex virus-thymidine kinase; H-Y antigen, minor histocompatibility antigen encoded by the Y chromosome; IE, immediate early; IFN-α, interferon alpha; IFN-γ, interferon gamma; IL, interleukin; L, late; LCL, lymphoblastoid cell line; LPD, lymphoproliferative disease; mHAg, minor histocompatibility antigen; MAb, monoclonal antibody; MHC, major histocompatibility complex; neo, neomycin phosphotransferase gene; NOD SCID, nonobese diabetic severe combined immune deficiency; PBMC, peripheral blood mononuclear cell; PCR, polymerase chain reaction; PET, positron emission tomography; PML-RARα, promyelocytic leukemia-retinoic acid receptor-α; PR-3, proteinase 3; TCR, T cell receptor; Th, T helper (cell); TIL, tumor-infiltrating lymphocyte; WT-1, Wilms tumor antigen 1.

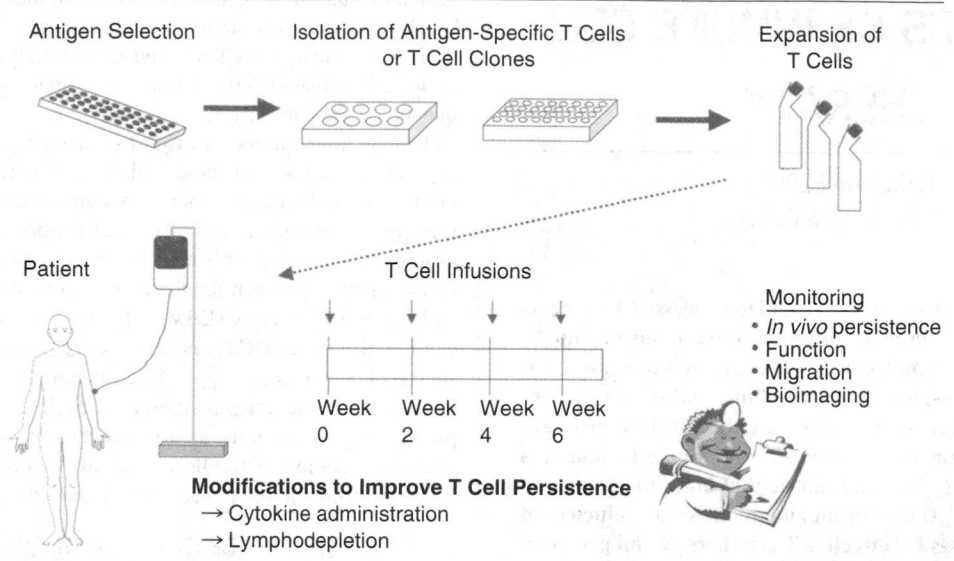

Antigen Selection

Isolation of Antigen-Specific T Cells
or T Cell Clones

Expansion of
T Cells

Patient

T Cell Infusions

Monitoring
• *In vivo* persistence
• Function
• Migration
• Bioimaging

Week 0   Week 2   Week 4   Week 6

Modifications to Improve T Cell Persistence
→ Cytokine administration
→ Lymphodepletion

FIGURE 23-1   Scheme for adoptive T cell therapy with antigen-specific T cells. T cells are selected based on antigen specificity, phenotype, and function, and expanded by *in vitro* culture. Patients receiving T cells are monitored after each cell infusion for toxicity, persistence, and migration of transferred cells and for efficacy.

A significant number of CD8+ T cells specific for intermediate early (IE) or early (E) viral proteins are also detected with these approaches, even though IE and E antigens are not efficiently presented to T cells *in vitro* by cells replicating wild-type CMV. This finding raises the question as to how these CTL cells might function to control CMV *in vivo*. One possibility is that IE- and E-specific T cells are capable of recognizing cells that are reactivating CMV from latency. Thus, reconstitution of responses both to virion and IE or E antigens may be necessary to restore to immunodeficient hosts the immunologic control possessed by normal individuals.

CD4+ Th cells are required for optimal CD8+ CTL cell responses and may eliminate CMV-infected cells that express class II MHC *in vivo*. The specificity of the CD4+ Th cell response to CMV has not been as well characterized as for CD8+ T cells. Studies using recombinant pp65, IE-1, or glycoprotein B (gB) proteins to stimulate peripheral blood mononuclear cells (PBMCs) from normal CMV+ donors have shown that CD4+ Th cells recognize one or more of these antigens.[15]

TECHNIQUES FOR ISOLATION AND ADOPTIVE TRANSFER OF CYTOMEGALOVIRUS-SPECIFIC T CELLS

In a murine model of T cell therapy for CMV, CD8+ CTL cells alone provided protection from lethal infection,[2,3] whereas CD4+ Th cells alone were not protective but provided antiviral activity in selected organs and improved the efficacy of CD8+ CTL.[16] Extending T cell therapy to human CMV in allogeneic HCT recipients required the development of approaches to reliably isolate CMV-specific T cells from the stem cell donor, and to remove potentially alloreactive T cells that could cause graft-versus-host disease (GVHD). The initial clinical study of T cell therapy employed CD8+ CMV-specific T cell clones that were isolated after *in vitro* culture of donor lymphocytes with autologous CMV-infected fibroblasts and expanded to several billion cells.[17] The T cell clones were screened to exclude reactivity with noninfected recipient cells prior to adoptive transfer making it unlikely that therapy would cause GVHD. In a phase I study, 14 allogeneic HCT recipients received four escalating weekly doses ($3.3 \times 10^7 - 1 \times 10^9/m^2$) of CD8+ CMV-specific CTL clones as prophylaxis for

CMV disease. The treatment did not cause serious toxicity or exacerbate GVHD. In 11 patients who were deficient in CTL responses immediately prior to infusion, CMV-specific cytolytic activity was increased after therapy to levels equivalent to those in the donor (Fig. 23-2A).[18] Transferred CTLs were detected for more than 12 weeks after infusion, but the magnitude of the response declined in the subset of patients who did not recover endogenous CD4+ CMV-specific Th cell responses, suggesting that CD4+ Th cells may be required for CD8+ T cell persistence.[18] None of the 14 patients developed CMV viremia or disease, which was expected to occur with a frequency of 50 percent and 40 percent, respectively, providing encouraging evidence for the antiviral activity of prophylactic CD8+ CTL infusions.[18]

The observation that maintenance of antiviral CD8+ T cells may depend on the presence of a functional CD4+ Th cell response provided a rationale for restoring both subsets of CMV-specific T cells by adoptive therapy. At the Fred Hutchinson Cancer Research Center, 35 allogeneic HCT recipients received infusions of both CD8+ and CD4+ CMV-specific T cell clones early after transplantation as prophylaxis for CMV disease. The infusion of CMV-specific CD4+ Th cell clones resulted in reconstitution of the CD4+ Th cell response in deficient patients and augmented CD8+ T cell responses in some patients (see Fig. 23-2B). However, the persistence of transferred T cell responses was diminished in the subset of patients receiving glucocorticoid therapy to treat preexisting GVHD.[12]

The results of T cell therapy trials for CMV suggest this approach is an attractive alternative to antiviral drugs for controlling CMV infection in HCT recipients. However, more efficient culture methods for isolating T cells for therapy are needed for broader application. Strategies that circumvent the use of live virus and the requirement for dermal fibroblasts as APCs have been developed for generating CMV-specific T cells. DCs pulsed with CMV peptides or CMV antigen, and EBV-lymphoblastoid cell lines (LCLs) modified by gene transfer to express one or more CMV antigens have been effective as alternative APCs to generate CMV-specific CD8+ and CD4+ T cells.[19,20] Clinical trials of T cell therapy with polyclonal CD4+ T cells or both CD4+ and CD8+ T cells generated using such alternative methods have been performed. CD4+ CMV-specific T cells obtained

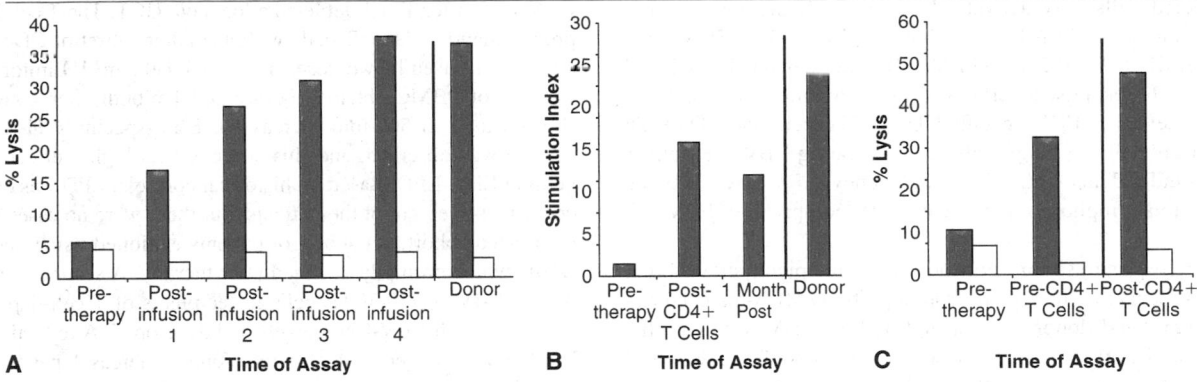

FIGURE 23-2   Adoptive transfer of CMV-specific T cell clones reconstitutes immunity in immunodeficient allogeneic HCT recipients. (A) CMV-specific cytotoxic T cell responses of PBMCs obtained from eleven recipients of CMV-specific CD8+ T cell clones prior to T cell therapy, and 2 days after each infusion. The T cell response of the donors is shown for comparison. Target cells are autologous CMV-infected (■) and mock-infected fibroblasts (□). (B) CMV-specific Th cell response of PBMC obtained from a recipient of CMV-specific CD4+ T cell clones prior to T cell therapy, 2 days after the CD4+ T cell infusion, and 1 month after the T cell infusion. The response present in the donor is shown for comparison. (C) CMV-specific CD8+ CTL responses in the same patient shown in (B), prior to and 1 week after the adoptive transfer of CD4+ T cell clones. Target cells are autologous CMV-infected (■) and mock-infected fibroblasts (□).

by sequential *in vitro* stimulation of donor PBMCs with CMV antigen were administered in a dose of $10^7/m^2$ to HCT recipients with persistent CMV infection. Treatment was accompanied by restoration of both CD4+ and CD8+ CMV-specific T cell responses, suggesting the CD4+ Th cells provided helper function for endogenous CD8+ CTL cells. Moreover, sustained viral clearance was achieved in 5 of 7 patients.[21] A second study infused even smaller doses (10^5/kg) of polyclonal CMV-specific CD4+ and CD8+ T cells to 16 patients with early CMV infection.[20] In this study, the infused T cells were not rigorously purified to remove potentially alloreactive T cells, and mild GVHD was observed after therapy in 3 of 16 patients. Importantly, a dramatic *in vivo* expansion of CMV-specific T cells was observed after the T cell infusions, and subsequent CMV reactivation was prevented in 14 of the 16 patients. Most patients in this study were severely lymphopenic at the time of T cell therapy because anti-T cell MAb was given prior to transplantation as part of the conditioning regimen.[20] Thus, the *in vivo* proliferation of CMV-specific T cells may have been induced in part by homeostatic mechanisms that operate in lymphopenia to restore T cell numbers.

MONITORING PERSISTENCE, FUNCTION, AND MIGRATION OF ADOPTIVELY TRANSFERRED CYTOMEGALOVIRUS-SPECIFIC T CELLS

Transferred T cells must persist as functional memory T cells and migrate to sites of virus persistence to be effective. Methods based on functional or structural properties of T cells have been developed for tracking transferred T cells. In the study of therapy with CD8+ CMV-specific T cell clones, assays of cytolytic activity provided a semi-quantitative analysis of T cell function.[18] New approaches such as intracellular staining of cytokines that are induced after antigen stimulation can now be employed to enumerate functional cells on a single cell level by flow cytometry.[22] The use of genetic markers in transferred T cells is a useful adjunct to functional studies. The unique DNA sequences of the rearranged T cell receptor (TCR) V_α or V_β genes of transferred T cells were used to evaluate cell survival in the first trial of CMV-specific T cell therapy.[18] Real-time polymerase chain reaction (PCR) with TCR-specific primers that flank the unique CDR3 sequence has been developed and can provide precise quantitation of transferred T cells in blood samples.

Monitoring the trafficking of CMV-specific T cells to tissue sites is a more formidable problem. Dynamic and sensitive measures to examine *in vivo* migration of adoptively transferred cells might contribute to understanding the basis for success or failure of cell therapy in a variety of settings. However, the available imaging modalities are useful only in small animals.[23] Positron emission tomography (PET) imaging is a noninvasive technique that has permitted repeated *in vivo* assessment of the migration of adoptively transferred T cells in murine studies.[24] This methodology may potentially be applicable to humans, but studies in large animal models have not yet been performed.

FUTURE DIRECTIONS IN CYTOMEGALOVIRUS-SPECIFIC T CELL THERAPY

Advances in our understanding of the immunobiology of CMV and techniques for isolating CMV-specific T cells promise to improve the feasibility and efficacy of T cell therapy for CMV infection in HCT recipients. Innovative methods have been developed for isolating antigen-specific T cells directly from the blood using bispecific MAbs to capture T cells that produce interferon gamma (IFN-γ) in response to antigen stimulation or using MHC/peptide tetramers that bind T cells based on TCR specificity.[25,26] These methods can shorten the time needed to generate CD4+ and CD8+ CMV-specific T cells to as little as 10 days.[27] Subsets of patients who are most likely to benefit from cell therapy such as those undergoing T cell-depleted HCT have been identified. These patients have delayed T cell reconstitution but require less posttransplant immunosuppressive drug therapy that interferes with the survival and function of transferred T cells. The introduction of genes that render transferred T cells resistant to immunosuppressive drugs may be necessary for optimal efficacy of T cell therapy after unmodified allogeneic HCT.

T CELL THERAPY OF EPSTEIN-BARR VIRUS INFECTION

EBV infection occurs in more than 90 percent of individuals and can cause an infectious mononucleosis syndrome (see Chap. 84), but is more commonly not clinically apparent as it is rapidly contained by the host immune system.[28] However, EBV is never completely cleared and persists in a latent form in B lymphocytes. Some latently infected B cells express only EBNA-1, which has glycine-alanine repeats that inhibit its translation and processing for presentation to CD8+ T cells.[29] Infected cells may activate the latency III program of viral genes that includes EBNA-1, EBNA-2, EBNA-3A, EBNA-3B, EBNA-3C, LMP-1, LMP-2A, and LMP-2B, and which induces B cell proliferation.[28] In response to EBV infection, immunocompetent hosts develop high levels of EBV-specific CD8+ CTL cells and CD4+ Th cells, which prevent the outgrowth of proliferating EBV+ B cells.[30] However, in individuals with a T cell deficiency, EBV may reactivate and progress to a lymphoproliferative disorder comprised of EBV+ B cells.

Retrospective analysis of allogeneic HCT recipients showed that patients who received a transplant from a partially HLA-matched relative or an unrelated donor were at high risk of EBV-lymphoproliferative disease (LPD) because of the severe immunodeficiency caused by T cell depletion to prevent GVHD, or intensive immunosuppression to treat GVHD.[31] Solid organ allograft recipients are also at risk for EBV-LPD, particularly those that require anti-T cell MAbs to treat graft rejection.[32] Historically, patients with EBV-LPD have had a grave prognosis, responding poorly to both antiviral drug therapy and chemotherapy. Thus, restoration of EBV-specific T cell immunity by adoptive T cell therapy represents an alternative strategy for prophylaxis of high-risk patients or to treat established EBV-LPD.

TARGET ANTIGENS FOR EPSTEIN-BARR VIRUS-SPECIFIC T CELLS

The CD8+ CTL response to EBV infection in normal hosts is mainly directed against lytic viral proteins and the EBNA-3A, -3B, and -3C latency proteins.[30,33] The CD4+ Th cell response to EBV is similarly directed against both lytic and latent EBV antigens, and may contribute to eliminating class II MHC+ EBV-infected cells in vivo.[34] A quantitative deficiency of EBV-specific CTLs frequently exists in the first 6 months after allogeneic HCT.[35] This deficiency of EBV-specific T cells allows the unimpeded lytic infection of memory B cells that can spread to additional B cells, some of which may activate the latency III program and undergo proliferation characteristic of LPD.[36]

TECHNIQUES FOR ISOLATION AND ADOPTIVE TRANSFER OF EPSTEIN-BARR VIRUS-SPECIFIC T CELLS

The efficacy of T cell therapy for EBV-LPD was demonstrated in a study in which unselected donor lymphocytes were administered to five patients with EBV-LPD after T cell-depleted allogeneic HCT. A dose of approximately 1×10^6 CD3+ T cells/kg was infused because of the concern that higher T cell doses would cause severe GVHD and resulted in complete resolution of EBV-LPD in all patients.[37] Unfortunately, therapy was complicated by fatal respiratory failure in two patients with EBV-LPD in the lungs, and all of the surviving patients developed GVHD, which suggested that future studies should focus on methods to select EBV-specific T cells for therapy.[37]

In vitro culture techniques have been developed to generate EBV-specific T cell lines from allogeneic HCT donors using autologous EBV-LCLs, which express the latency III viral genes as stimulator cells. The T cell lines become oligoclonal after repeated stimulations in vitro and are depleted of alloreactive T cells that cause GVHD. The adoptive transfer of such EBV-specific T cell lines was effective in 2 of 3 HCT recipients with established EBV-LPD without causing GVHD.[38] One patient had progressive LPD despite T cell infusions; analysis of this patient's tumor revealed a mutation in the EBNA-3B gene that eliminated the region encoding the epitopes targeted by the CTL cell line.[39] This finding illustrates the problem of targeting only a few antigenic epitopes, particularly when treating a large tumor burden that may contain escape variants.

Prophylactic infusion of EBV-specific T cells should diminish the probability that escape variants would emerge. A subsequent study administered donor EBV-specific T cell lines to 36 patients at risk for EBV-LPD after T cell-depleted allogeneic HCT. The T cell lines were predominantly CD8+ T cells with a smaller subset of CD4+ T cells, and were infused in two doses of 2×10^7 cells/m².[40] Limiting dilution analysis of PBMC obtained before and 1 month after T cell therapy showed a 2- to 500-fold increase in EBV-specific CTL cells.[40] No GVHD was observed, and this strategy was highly effective in preventing EBV-LPD. Based on historical controls, LPD was expected to occur in 14 percent of the patients, but there were no cases of LPD in the treated cohort.[40] A subset of patients exhibited rising plasma EBV DNA, which promptly declined after therapy. A second study administered EBV-specific CTL cells to recipients of T cell-depleted HCT only after high EBV-DNA levels had developed. A reduction of EBV DNA was observed in 4 of 5 recipients, whereas 1 patient, who received a T cell line that lacked an EBV-specific component, progressed to EBV-LPD.[41] Thus, transfer of EBV-specific T cells safely and rapidly reconstituted immunity, mediated antiviral activity, and protected the majority of patients from EBV-LPD.

MONITORING PERSISTENCE, FUNCTION, AND MIGRATION OF TRANSFERRED EPSTEIN-BARR VIRUS-SPECIFIC T CELLS

A retrovirus encoding the neomycin phosphotransferase gene (neo) was introduced into a subset of the infused EBV-specific T cells to provide a genetic marker for tracking persistence of the transferred cells. In one patient treated for established LPD, biopsy of the tumor after therapy revealed infiltration of T cells containing the marker gene. Moreover, neo+ T cells were detected in EBV-specific T cell lines generated from PBMCs 86 months after infusion, confirming the transferred T cells can persist as long-term memory cells.[42]

FUTURE DIRECTIONS IN EPSTEIN-BARR VIRUS-SPECIFIC T CELL THERAPY

T cell therapy is now established as an important modality for EBV-LPD in allogeneic HCT recipients at risk for this complication. Therapy with anti-CD20 MAbs can also induce a remission of EBV-LPD in a substantial fraction of patients, and be curative if accompanied by a reduction in immunosuppression and resolution of the T cell immunodeficiency.[43] However, in situations where anti-CD20 MAbs fail or where T cell recovery is likely to be delayed, T cell therapy provides an attractive alternative. The use of cellular therapy for EBV-LPD in solid-organ transplant recipients has been challenging because of the lack of a donor from whom to generate T cells for therapy, and the need to continue immunosuppression to prevent organ rejection. Efforts to isolate and expand rare EBV-reactive T cells from the patient or to use EBV-specific T cells from unrelated donors have met with limited success,[44] and novel strategies such as the use of TCR gene transfer to engineer autologous T cells to be specific for EBV may be beneficial.[45]

Other malignancies, such as Hodgkin disease or nasopharyngeal carcinoma, are associated with EBV. These tumors express a limited number of EBV proteins that are recognized by a low frequency of T cells in normal hosts. Preliminary studies demonstrate the feasibility of isolating and expanding these T cells; however, effective T cell therapy of sporadic EBV+ tumors will likely require strategies to overcome immune evasion mechanisms employed by these tumors.[46]

ADOPTIVE CELLULAR THERAPY OF MALIGNANCY

The identification of antigens expressed by tumor cells has renewed optimism that T cell therapy might be developed for nonviral malignant disease. Studies in animal models demonstrate that T cells, particularly CD8+ CTL cells, can eradicate disseminated tumors. Immunogenic proteins in human tumors have been identified by

TABLE 23-1   CATEGORIES OF TUMOR ANTIGENS

ANTIGEN	TUMOR	EXPRESSION IN NORMAL TISSUES
Antigens arising from mutations or gene rearrangements		
p21ras	Acute leukemia, others	—
p53	~50% of tumors	—
BCR/ABL	CML	
PML/RARα	APL	
Caspase-8	Head and neck cancer	—
CDK-4, MUM-1	Melanoma	—
β-Catenin	Melanoma, lung, others	—
Tissue-specific differentiation antigens		
Tyrosinase	Melanoma	Melanocytes
MART-1/Melan-A	Melanoma	Melanocytes
GP100	Melanoma	Melanocytes
Cancer-testis antigens		
MAGE-1, MAGE-2, MAGE-3	Melanoma	Testis, placenta
GAGE and others	Melanoma	Testis, placenta
NY-ESO-1	Melanoma, breast cancer	Testis, placenta
Nonmutated overexpressed proteins		
HER-2/neu	Breast cancer, ovarian cancer	Breast tissue, ovary
Telomerase catalytic protein	Colon cancer, others	Liver, others
CEA	Various tumors	
CD20, idiotype proteins	Immunoglobulin molecule of B cells	B lymphocytes
Oncofetal proteins		
CEA	Colon cancer, others	Liver, others
AFP	Liver cancer	—
Viral proteins		
HPV E6 and E7	Cervical cancer	—
EBV LMP-1 and EBNA-1 proteins	Hodgkin disease, nasopharyngeal lymphoma	—

screening of tumor complementary DNA (cDNA) libraries with tumor-specific T cells isolated from the blood or tumor microenvironment[47] or by screening of patient sera for antibody responses against tumor-associated proteins.[48] Distinct categories of tumor antigens have been uncovered, and several are being investigated as targets for T cell therapy or vaccination (Table 23-1). The development of immune cell therapy for malignancy has focused on melanoma because target antigens have been identified,[49] and on amplifying the graft-versus-leukemia (GVL) effect after allogeneic HCT because of the evidence that donor T cells mediate tumor eradication in this setting.[50]

CELLULAR THERAPY OF MELANOMA

The isolation and expansion of polyclonal populations of tumor-infiltrating lymphocytes (TILs) *in vitro* with high concentrations of interleukin (IL)-2, and their infusion with the administration of high-dose IL-2 in patients with melanoma, were associated with responses in 31 percent of patients.[51] Most of the responses were transient and the high-dose IL-2 caused severe toxicity. Nevertheless, the results encouraged efforts to define the antigens recognized by TILs in responding patients, and to develop cell therapy strategies to target potential tumor-rejection antigens using adoptive transfer of *in vitro* cultured tumor-reactive T cells or DCs engineered to express tumor-associated antigens.

TARGET ANTIGENS FOR MELANOMA-SPECIFIC T CELLS

Melanoma has served as a model for the discovery of human tumor antigens because T cells specific for melanoma cells can often be detected in the blood or tumor microenvironment. A landmark in cancer immunotherapy was the identification by cDNA expression cloning of MAGE-1, a tumor-specific gene product recognized by T cells derived from a melanoma patient.[47] Several additional melanoma antigens recognized by CD8+ and/or CD4+ T cells have been discovered, including proteins that function in normal melanocyte physiology such as tyrosinase, gp100, and MART-1, cancer testis antigens such as MAGE-1, and mutated proteins that arise as a consequence of the genetic instability of tumors.[47,49]

TECHNIQUES FOR ISOLATION AND ADOPTIVE TRANSFER OF MELANOMA-SPECIFIC T CELLS

Adoptive therapy with tumor-specific T cell clones or oligoclonal populations of T cells expanded *ex vivo* provides an alternative in which the magnitude and function of the T cell response can be more rigorously controlled. Methods have been developed for isolating melanoma-specific T cells *in vitro*.[52] If the tumor is easily accessible, T cells can be isolated directly from the tumor biopsies by culture in high dose IL-2.[52] Alternatively, autologous DCs pulsed with synthetic peptides corresponding to defined melanoma antigens can be used as stimulators to expand reactive T cells from the blood.[53] A problem with the latter approach is that T cells with low avidity for the antigen are often isolated.[54] T cells with higher avidity can be preferentially expanded using lower concentrations of peptide, by varying the cytokines used for T cell expansion, or by using APCs transfected with the genes encoding the antigen or pulsed with lysates of the tumor.[55,56]

Pilot clinical trials have evaluated the adoptive transfer of CD8+ T cell clones specific for MART-1 or gp100. In a study of 10 patients by Yee and associates, four infusions of autologous CD8+ T cell clones at a dose of $3.3 \times 10^9/m^2$ were safely administered at 14- to 21-day intervals.[57] A peak frequency of between 0.5 percent and 2.2 percent of all CD8+ T cells was achieved in the blood after the T cell infusions. Low-dose IL-2 ($0.25-1.0 \times 10^6$ U/m²) was administered for 14 days following some infusions and improved the persistence of transferred CTL cells without causing toxicity. The T cells localized to tumor sites and mediated an antitumor response in some patients with advanced disease.[57]

This study also identified several issues that may limit efficacy of T cell therapy. One issue is that tumors evade the immune response by loss of antigen expression, down-regulation of MHC, and production of immunosuppressive factors. The growth of tumor that had lost expression of the antigen targeted by the T cells was observed in 3 of 5 patients studied in detail,[57] suggesting that targeting multiple antigens may improve efficacy. A second issue is that transferred T cells may need to persist long term for optimal antitumor efficacy. The administration of IL-2 after T cell transfer resulted in only a modest improvement in the duration of T cell persistence from a median of approximately 7 to 17 days.[57] The lack of clonal persistence could be a result of a requirement for antigen-specific CD4+ Th cells, terminal differentiation of clones during expansion, or activation-induced T cell death at the tumor site. IL-2 is routinely employed *in vitro* to promote T cell growth, but excessive or prolonged exposure of T cells to IL-2 can increase susceptibility to cell death and inhibit the establishment of T cell memory.[58] Other cytokines, such as IL-7 and IL-15, are known to have a role in T cell memory and may be useful for propagating cells *in vitro* and supporting T cell survival *in vivo*.[59,60]

An alternative strategy that might enhance the persistence of transferred T cells and promote their *in vivo* expansion is to take advantage of host homeostatic responses to lymphopenia.[52,61,62] The transfer of gp100 or MART-1-specific CD4+ and CD8+ T cell lines into 13 patients with metastatic melanoma after lymphodepletion with cyclo-phosphamide and fludarabine, along with high-dose IL-2, resulted in proliferation of the transferred T cells in vivo.[62] The cells displayed functional activity and persisted in large numbers in the peripheral blood. Objective tumor responses were observed in 7 of 13 patients, and mixed responses were seen in 4 additional patients. Although the antitumor activity was encouraging, autoimmunity related to destruction of normal melanocytes and long-term abnormalities in the T cell repertoire were observed. Thus, additional evaluation is necessary to define the short- and long-term safety of T cell therapy after a lymphodepleting regimen.

DENDRITIC CELL VACCINATION

The identification of T cell defined antigens for melanoma and other tumors has also led to the investigation of cell-based vaccines to elicit T cell immunity in vivo. The use of DCs to present tumor antigens may have advantages over peptide vaccines, which may successfully elicit tumor-reactive T cells but rarely induce tumor regression, potentially because of a defect in frequency or function of CTL cells.[49,63] DCs have been identified as the most potent APCs that when appropriately activated and matured display a unique ability to initiate immune responses of both CD8+ and CD4+ T cells.[64,65] In murine models, DCs have been pulsed with tumor lysates or peptides, transfected with RNA- or DNA-encoding tumor antigens, or fused to tumor cells for use in vaccination, and have induced protective tumor-specific immunity.[65,66] These observations suggested that DC-based vaccination might serve to overcome tolerance to tumor antigens, many of which are self-proteins.

Clinical studies of DC-based vaccine strategies are now being actively pursued for therapy of a variety of tumors including melanoma. Immunization with ex vivo-generated DCs has proven feasible and safe and has resulted in the augmentation of tumor-specific T cell responses and the regression of disease in a subset of melanoma patients.[67-69] Fong and associates demonstrated that vaccination of colon and breast cancer patients with DCs displaying a carcinoembryonic antigen (CEA) peptide that is altered to promote more efficient engagement of TCR elicited high levels of CD8+ CTLs specific for the cognate antigen and tumor regression in a subset of patients.[70,71] In these studies, administration of Flt-3 ligand, which serves as a growth and differentiation factor for hematopoietic progenitors and expands DCs in vivo, assisted in obtaining large numbers of DCs by leukapheresis and minimized the ex vivo culture needed for vaccine generation. Although these data are encouraging, systematic studies are needed to define the most effective ways of employing DC as a vaccine vehicle.[69] Multiple strategies can be used for introducing antigens into DCs, and it is unclear which strategy will be most effective. Among the variables being evaluated for improving immunogenicity and clinical efficacy are the subsets of DCs used for vaccination, activation and maturation signals that are delivered, vaccine schedule, and strategies to direct migration of DCs to secondary lymphoid organs in vivo or to over-express costimulatory molecules.[69] Alternatively, vaccine strategies that obviate ex vivo culture of DCs by directing antigen to these cells in situ have been proposed.[69,72]

FUTURE DIRECTIONS IN MELANOMA-SPECIFIC T CELL THERAPY

Although significant progress has been made in cellular therapy for melanoma, the optimal and safest regimens for both effective immunotherapies that employ the adoptive transfer of tumor-reactive T cells and DC-based vaccines, respectively, remain to be defined. Advances in our understanding of the role of individual cytokines in T cell survival in vitro and in vivo, and of the regulation of T cell activation and homeostasis will surely provide new opportunities for improving the

persistence of in vitro-expanded T cells after transfer. Systematic studies in animal models that are predictive for clinical utility are likely to be important for defining approaches that best improve the persistence and function of transferred tumor-reactive T cells, and fully exploit the immune-stimulatory capacity of DCs to elicit antitumor immunity. Extending cellular therapy to other malignancies will require strategies to overcome the apparent lack of immunogenicity of many tumor cells, to define relevant tumor antigens, and to efficiently generate functional antigen-specific T cells in vitro. One novel approach for generating antigen-specific T cells from every patient involves transfer of the genes encoding the TCR for the antigen.[45]

CELLULAR THERAPY OF LEUKEMIA

It is well established that a GVL effect mediated by allogeneic donor T cells contained in or derived from the stem cell graft contributes to the eradication of malignancy after allogeneic HCT.[73] The potency of the GVL effect is illustrated by studies in which unselected donor lymphocytes were adoptively transferred to patients who relapsed after allogeneic HCT.[74] This treatment is very successful in patients with relapsed chronic myeloid leukemia (CML). Unfortunately, the administration of unselected donor lymphocytes is less effective in acute leukemias and is often complicated by acute and chronic GVHD.[74] Efforts are in progress to identify target antigens on leukemic cells that would allow separation of GVL from GVHD and the induction of a potent immune response to acute leukemia by T cell therapy.

TARGET ANTIGENS FOR LEUKEMIA-SPECIFIC T CELLS

GVHD and GVL effects are usually linked, but a GVL effect is observed after HCT in the absence of GVHD.[73] Thus, it is presumed there are antigens presented by leukemic cells but not by tissues that are targets of GVHD. Several categories of antigens that could be potential targets of selective GVL activity have been identified. These include (1) minor histocompatibility antigens (mHAgs) that are selectively expressed in hematopoietic cells including leukemic cells, (2) tumor-specific proteins resulting from chromosome translocations or mutations, and (3) normal proteins that are overexpressed in leukemic cells. Proteins in the latter two classes could be targets both in the transplant and nontransplant setting, whereas mHAgs are only relevant after allogeneic HCT.

Minor Histocompatibility Antigens   The increased potency of the GVL effect after allogeneic HCT compared with syngeneic HCT emphasizes the importance of disparity in mHAgs for immune-mediated eradication of malignancy.[73] mHAgs are peptides derived from proteins that differ between the donor and recipient as a result of genetic polymorphisms and are presented by class I and class II molecules on recipient cells.[75] In murine models, the adoptive transfer of T cells specific for a single mHAg eradicated leukemia without causing GVHD, illustrating the potential of this approach.[76] In humans, donor T cells reactive with recipient mHAgs can be isolated after transplantation from most allogeneic HCT recipients.[75,77] Analysis of the specificity of such T cell clones shows that many mHAgs are expressed preferentially in hematopoietic cells, including leukemic blasts, and might permit the separation of GVL from GVHD (Fig. 23-3).[77,78] Such mHAg-specific CD8+ CTLs prevent engraftment of human leukemia in nonobese diabetic (NOD)/severe combined immune deficiency (SCID) mice, providing evidence that the rare leukemic stem cell is susceptible to T cell recognition.[79]

The genes that encode mHAgs are now being identified using peptide elution and mass spectrometry, cDNA expression cloning, and genetic linkage analysis.[50] Both autosomal and Y-chromosome–encoded mHAgs that are attractive targets for therapy of leukemia after allogeneic HCT have been discovered. Two mHAgs (HA-1 and HA-

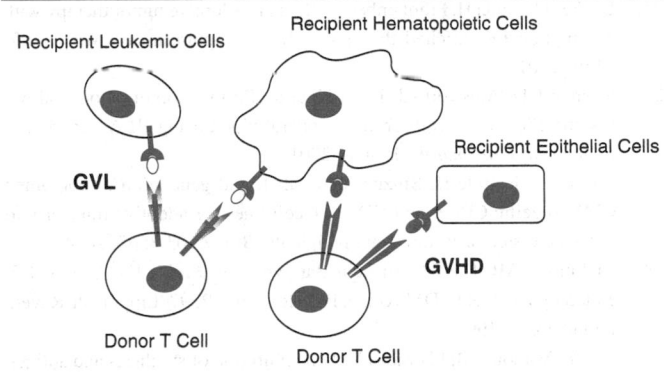

FIGURE 23-3   Tissue-specific expression of minor histocompatibility antigens may permit separation of GVHD from GVL effects. The genes that encode mHAgs may be ubiquitously expressed on recipient tissues and be targets for both GVHD and GVL effects or be selectively expressed on hematopoietic cells and be targets for a GVL effect without GVHD.

2) encoded by the autosomal genes KIAA0023 and MY01G, respectively, and presented by HLA-A2, are selectively transcribed in leukemic cells.[80–82] A study using HLA-A2/peptide tetramers to detect HA-1- and HA-2-reactive T cells demonstrated a dramatic expansion of these T cells in patients who responded to treatment with donor lymphocyte infusions for posttransplant relapse.[83]

Clinical and laboratory studies also support a potential role of Y-chromosome–encoded mHAgs in the GVL effect. Male recipients of allogeneic HCT from female donors have a higher risk of GVHD but exhibit a lower risk of leukemia relapse than do other donor/recipient gender combinations, even after controlling for GVHD.[84] Several H-Y antigens are ubiquitously expressed in tissues, providing an explanation for the increased GVHD. However, an mHAg encoded by the Y-chromosome gene UTY and presented by HLA-B8 is preferentially expressed in hematopoietic cells and is not associated with GVHD.[85] CD8+ CTL cells specific for B8/UTY lysed leukemic blasts and prevented engraftment of acute myeloid leukemia (AML) in NOD/SCID mice.[79] UTY is very polymorphic with its X-chromosome homologue and likely to encode peptides that bind to other HLA alleles,[86] suggesting that it may be a broadly applicable target for a GVL response in male recipients of HCT from female donors. The identification of genes that encode additional human mHAgs will facilitate the development of clinical trials of T cell therapy to augment the GVL effect after allogeneic HCT.

Leukemia-Associated Proteins Leukemia-associated proteins that could be targets for cellular therapy have been identified. These include mutated proteins such as p21/ras or chromosome translocations such as bcr/abl and promyelocytic leukemia-retinoic acid receptor alpha (PML-RARα), which can provide unique peptides that represent potential tumor-specific targets.[87–89] Nonpolymorphic normal proteins, such as proteinase 3 (PR-3)[90] and Wilms' tumor antigen-1 (WT-1),[91] which are overexpressed in some leukemias, also represent potential targets for T cell therapy. PR-3 is a serine protease normally expressed in promyelocytes, but it is overexpressed in myeloid leukemia. CD8+ T cells reactive with an epitope of PR-3 presented by HLA-A2 have been isolated from normal donors by stimulation of PBMCs with a synthetic peptide termed PR-1.[90] PR-1-specific CTL were of sufficient avidity to lyse CML cells and inhibit leukemic colony formation *in vitro*, but did not affect normal hematopoietic progenitors.[92] Expansion of functional PR-1-specific T cells was also observed in patients with CML who responded to interferon alpha (IFN-α) or allogeneic HCT, suggesting that these T cells may have participated in the response to therapy.[93] T cells specific for WT-1,

which is expressed at high levels in myeloid leukemias but at low levels in normal hematopoietic cells, have also been isolated from normal donors by *in vitro* stimulation of PBMCs with synthetic peptides.[94] WT-1–specific CTL selectively lysed leukemic blasts and prevented engraftment of leukemia in immunodeficient mice, suggesting that these T cells may mediate an antileukemic effect without affecting normal hematopoiesis *in vivo*.[91,95] Collectively, these findings suggest that monomorphic epitopes derived from both PR-3 and WT-1, respectively, could serve as attractive targets for T cell therapy.

An alternative or complementary approach to the adoptive transfer of leukemia-reactive T cells is to elicit antitumor responses *in vivo* by vaccination. Although this strategy may be easier to apply more broadly, it has limitations, including the potential for toxicity of targeting self-proteins. However, vaccination could assist in delineating the role of candidate antigens as potential targets for immunotherapy and may facilitate the isolation of high-avidity T cells specific for defined antigens that could be used for T cell therapy of leukemia. For example, patients who had relapsed with acute or chronic leukemia were vaccinated with PR-1 or WT-1 peptides, respectively. Following vaccination, peptide-specific CD8+ T cells were detected in the blood of a subset of patients and their presence correlated with an antileukemic effect.[96,97] It is conceivable that strategies that employ DCs as professional APCs might further enhance the benefit of this approach.

FUTURE DIRECTIONS FOR T CELL THERAPY OF LEUKEMIA

The feasibility of adoptive therapy using T cells reactive with mHAgs that are selectively or preferentially expressed on recipient hematopoietic cells has been demonstrated,[98] and trials of T cell therapy targeting leukemia-associated antigens are now being initiated. Leukemia patients have been vaccinated with PR-3 or WT-1 peptides with encouraging results.[96,97] However, adverse effects such as leukopenia and erythema have been reported in one patient after WT-1 vaccination,[99] and there is a risk of GVHD in trials of therapy targeting mHAgs. An approach that may improve safety of T cell therapy is to introduce a suicide gene into the T cells that could be activated if toxicity occurred. Introduction of the herpes simplex virus-thymidine kinase (HSV-TK) gene has been effective in reversing GVHD after donor lymphocyte infusion.[100] However, the viral thymidine kinase is immunogenic and can result in premature elimination of transferred T cells that do not cause toxicity.[101] A suicide gene based on inducing cell death through the Fas pathway using a chemical dimerizer to activate an engineered chimeric human Fas transgene product has been developed and evaluated in animal models, and may circumvent the problem of immunogenicity.[102,103] If T cell therapy for leukemia can be accomplished safely, this could provide a method for improving the GVL effect after low-intensity allogeneic HCT, or it could be used in conjunction with engineering of the stem cell graft to reduce GVHD without compromising the GVL effect.

REFERENCES

1. Einsele H, Hebart H: Cellular immunity to viral and fungal antigens after stem cell transplantation. *Curr Opin Hematol* 9:485, 2002.

2. Reddehase MJ, Weiland F, Münch K, et al: Intestinal murine cytomegalovirus pneumonia after irradiation: Characterization of cells that limit viral replication during established infection of the lungs. *J Virol* 55:264, 1985.

3. Reddehase MJ, Mutter W, Münch K, et al: CD8-positive T lymphocytes specific for murine cytomegalovirus immediate-early antigens mediate protective immunity. *J Virol* 61:3102, 1987.

4. Riddell SR, Greenberg PD: Principles for adoptive T cell therapy of human viral diseases. *Annu Rev Immunol* 13:545, 1995.

5. Mocarski ES Jr: Immunomodulation by cytomegaloviruses: Manipulative strategies beyond evasion. *Trends Microbiol* 10:332, 2002.

6. Boeckh M, Nichols WG, Papanicolaou G, et al: Cytomegalovirus in hematopoietic stem cell transplant recipients: Current status, known challenges, and future strategies. *Biol Blood Marrow Transplant* 9:543, 2003.

7. Boeckh M, Leisenring W, Riddell SR, et al: Late cytomegalovirus disease and mortality in recipients of allogeneic hematopoietic stem cell transplants: Importance of viral load and T-cell immunity. *Blood* 101:407, 2003.

8. Bitmansour AD, Waldrop SL, Pitcher CJ, et al: Clonotypic structure of the human CD4+ memory T cell response to cytomegalovirus. *J Immunol* 167:1151, 2001.

9. Gillespie GMA, Wills MR, Appay V, et al: Functional heterogeneity and high frequencies of cytomegalovirus-specific CD8+ T lymphocytes in healthy seropositive donors. *J Virol* 74:8140, 2000.

10. Li C-R, Greenberg PD, Gilbert MJ, et al: Recovery of HLA-restricted cytomegalovirus (CMV)-specific T-cell responses after allogeneic bone marrow transplant: Correlation with CMV disease and effect of ganciclovir prophylaxis. *Blood* 83:1971, 1994.

11. Murphy E, Rigoutsos I, Shibuya T, et al: Reevaluation of human cytomegalovirus coding potential. *Proc Natl Acad Sci U S A* 100:13585, 2003.

12. Riddell SR, Greenberg PD: T-cell therapy of cytomegalovirus and human immunodeficiency virus infection. *J Antimicrob Chemother* 45(suppl T3):35, 2000.

13. Kern F, Surel IP, Faulhaber N, et al: Target structures of the CD8+-T-cell response to human cytomegalovirus: The 72-kilodalton major immediate-early protein revisited. *J Virol* 73:8179, 1999.

14. Manley TJ, Luy L, Jones T, et al: Cytomegalovirus immune evasion genes do not prevent the induction of a diverse CD8+ CTL response in viral infection. *Blood* 104:1075, 2004.

15. Vaz-Santiago J, Lulé J, Rohrlich P, et al: *Ex vivo* stimulation and expansion of both CD4+ and CD8+ T cells from peripheral blood mononuclear cells of human cytomegalovirus-seropositive blood donors by using a soluble recombinant chimeric protein, IE1-pp65. *J Virol* 75:7840, 2001.

16. Lucin P, Pavic I, Polic B, et al: Gamma interferon-dependent clearance of cytomegalovirus infection in salivary glands. *J Virol* 66:1977, 1992.

17. Riddell SR, Watanabe KS, Goodrich JM, et al: Restoration of viral immunity in immunodeficient humans by the adoptive transfer of T cell clones. *Science* 257:238, 1992.

18. Walter EA, Greenberg PD, Gilbert MJ, et al: Reconstitution of cellular immunity against cytomegalovirus in recipients of allogeneic bone marrow by transfer of T-cell clones from the donor. *N Engl J Med* 333:1038, 1995.

19. Kleihauer A, Grigoleit U, Hebart H, et al: *Ex vivo* generation of human cytomegalovirus-specific cytotoxic T cells by peptide-pulsed dendritic cells. *Br J Haematol* 113:231, 2001.

20. Peggs KS, Verfuerth S, Pizzey A, et al: Adoptive cellular therapy for early cytomegalovirus infection after allogeneic stem-cell transplantation with virus-specific T-cell lines. *Lancet* 362:1375, 2003.

21. Einsele H, Roosnek E, Rufer N, et al: Infusion of cytomegalovirus (CMV)-specific T cells for the treatment of CMV infection not responding to antiviral chemotherapy. *Blood* 99:3916, 2002.

22. Waldrop SL, Pitcher CJ, Peterson DM, et al: Determination of antigen-specific memory/effector CD4+ T cell frequencies by flow cytometry. *J Clin Invest* 99:1739, 1999.

23. Dubey P, Su H, Adonai N, et al: Quantitative imaging of the T cell antitumor response by positron-emission tomography. *Proc Natl Acad Sci U S A* 100:1232, 2003.

24. Brentjens RJ, Latouche J-B, Santos E, et al: Eradication of systemic B-cell tumors by genetically targeted human T lymphocytes co-stimulated by CD80 and interleukin-15. *Nat Med* 9:279, 2003.

25. Becker C, Pohla H, Frankenberger B, et al: Adoptive tumor therapy with T lymphocytes enriched through an IFN-γ capture assay. *Nat Med* 7:1159, 2001.

26. Keenan RD, Ainsworth J, Khan N, et al: Purification of cytomegalovirus-specific CD8 T cells from peripheral blood using HLA-peptide tetramers. *Br J Haematol* 115:428, 2001.

27. Rauser G, Einsele H, Sinzger C, et al: Rapid generation of combined CMV-specific CD4+ and CD8+ T-cell lines for adoptive transfer into allogeneic stem cell transplant recipients. *Blood* 103:3565, 2004.

28. Rickinson AB, Kieff E. Epstein-Barr virus, in *Fields Virology*, vol 2, edited by BN Fields, DM Knipe, PM Howley, p 2397. Lippincott-Raven, Philadelphia, 1996.

29. Yin Y, Manoury B, Fåhraeus R: Self-inhibition of synthesis and antigen presentation by Epstein-Barr virus-encoded EBNA1. *Science* 301:1371, 2003.

30. Tan LC, Gudgeon N, Annels NE, et al: A re-evaluation of the frequency of CD8+ T cells specific for EBV in healthy virus carriers. *J Immunol* 162:1827, 1999.

31. Curtis RE, Travis LB, Rowlings PA, et al: Risk of lymphoproliferative disorders after bone marrow transplantation: A multi-institutional study. *Blood* 94:2208, 1999.

32. Nalesnik MA: Lymphoproliferative disease in organ transplant recipients. *Springer Semin Immunopathol* 13:199, 1991.

33. Annels NE, Callan MFC, Tan L, et al: Changing patterns of dominant TCR usage with maturation of an EBV-specific cytotoxic T cell response. *J Immunol* 165:4831, 2000.

34. Amyes E, Hatton C, Montamat-Sicotte D, et al: Characterization of the CD4+ T cell response to Epstein-Barr virus during primary and persistent infection. *J Exp Med* 198:903, 2003.

35. Lucas KG, Burton RL, Zimmerman SE, et al: Semiquantitative Epstein-Barr virus (EBV) polymerase chain reaction for the determination of patients at risk for EBV-induced lymphoproliferative disease after stem cell transplantation. *Blood* 91:3654, 1998.

36. Timms JM, Bell A, Flavell JR, et al: Target cells of Epstein-Barr-virus (EBV)-positive post-transplant lymphoproliferative disease: Similarities to EBV-positive Hodgkin's lymphoma. *Lancet* 361:217, 2003.

37. Papadopoulos EB, Ladanyi M, Emanuel D, et al: Infusions of donor leukocytes to treat Epstein-Barr-virus-associated lymphoproliferative disorders after allogeneic bone marrow transplantation. *N Engl J Med* 330:1185, 1994.

38. Rooney CM, Smith CA, Ng CYC, et al: Use of gene-modified virus-specific T lymphocytes to control Epstein-Barr-virus-related lymphoproliferation. *Lancet* 345:9, 1995.

39. Gottschalk S, Edwards OL, Sili U, et al: Generating CTLs against the subdominant Epstein-Barr virus LMP1 antigen for the adoptive immunotherapy of ABV-associated malignancies. *Blood* 101:1905, 2003.

40. Rooney CM, Smith CA, Ng CYC, et al: Infusion of cytotoxic T cells for the prevention and treatment of Epstein-Barr virus-induced lymphoma in allogeneic transplant recipients. *Blood* 92:1549, 1998.

41. Gustafsson A, Levitsky V, Zou JZ, et al: Epstein-Barr virus (EBV) load in bone marrow transplant recipients at risk to develop posttransplant lymphoproliferative disease: Prophylactic infusion of EBV-specific cytotoxic T cells. *Blood* 95:807, 2000.

42. Heslop HE, Stevenson FK, Molldrem JJ: Immunotherapy of hematologic malignancies. *Hematology (Am Soc Hematol Educ Program)* 331, 2003.

43. Kuehnle I, Huls MH, Liu Z, et al: CD20 monoclonal antibody (rituximab) for therapy of Epstein-Barr virus lymphoma after hemopoietic stem-cell transplantation. *Blood* 95:1502, 2000.

44. Haque T, Wilkie GM, Taylor C, et al: Treatment of Epstein-Barr-virus-positive post-transplantation lymphoproliferative disease with partly HLA-matched allogeneic cytotoxic T cells. *Lancet* 360:436, 2002.

45. Schumacher TNM: T-cell-receptor gene therapy. *Nat Rev Immunol* 2: 512, 2002.

46. Huls MII, Rooney CM, Heslop HF: Adoptive T-cell therapy for Epstein-Barr virus-positive Hodgkin's disease. *Acta Haematol* 110:149, 2003.

47. Van der Bruggen P, Traversari C, Chomez P, et al: A gene encoding an antigen recognized by cytolytic T lymphocytes on a human melanoma. *Science* 254:1643, 1991.

48. Chen Y-T, Scanlan MJ, Sahin U, et al: A testicular antigen aberrantly expressed in human cancers detected by autologous antibody screening. *Proc Natl Acad Sci U S A* 94:1914, 1997.

49. Rosenberg SA: Progress in human tumour immunology and immunotherapy. *Nature* 411:380, 2001.

50. Riddell SR, Berger C, Murata M, et al: The graft versus leukemia response after allogeneic hematopoietic stem cell transplantation. *Blood Rev* 17:153, 2003.

51. Rosenberg SA, Aebersold P, Cornetta K, et al: Gene transfer into humans—immunotherapy of patients with advanced melanoma, using tumor-infiltrating lymphocytes modified by retroviral gene transduction. *N Engl J Med* 323:570, 1990.

52. Dudley ME, Rosenberg SA: Adoptive-cell transfer: Therapy for the treatment of patients with cancer. *Nat Rev Cancer* 3:666, 2003.

53. Yee C, Savage PA, Lee PP, et al: Isolation of high avidity melanoma-reactive CTL from heterogeneous populations using peptide-MHC tetramers. *J Immunol* 162:2227, 1999.

54. Alexander-Miller MA, Leggatt GR, Berzofsky JA: Selective expansion of high- or low-avidity cytotoxic T lymphocytes and efficacy for adoptive immunotherapy. *Proc Natl Acad Sci U S A* 93:4102, 1996.

55. Meyer zum Büschenfelde C, Nicklisch N, Rose-John S, et al: Generation of tumor-reactive CTL against the tumor-associated antigen HER2 using retrovirally transduced dendritic cells derived from CD34+ hemopoietic progenitor cells. *J Immunol* 165:4133, 2000.

56. Parkhurst MR, DePan C, Riley JP, et al: Hybrids of dendritic cells and tumor cells generated by electrofusion simultaneously present immunodominant epitopes from multiple human tumor-associated antigens in the context of MHC class I and class II molecules. *J Immunol* 170:5317, 2003.

57. Yee C, Thompson JA, Byrd D, et al: Adoptive T cell therapy using antigen-specific CD8+ T cell clones for the treatment of patients with metastatic melanoma: *In vivo* persistence, migration, and antitumor effect of transferred cells. *Proc Natl Acad Sci U S A* 99:16168, 2002.

58. Van Parijs L, Refaeli Y, Lord JD, et al: Uncoupling IL-2 signals that regulate T cell proliferation, survival, and Fas-mediated activation-induced cell death. *Immunity* 11:281, 1999.

59. Ku CC, Murakami M, Sakamoto A, et al: Control of homeostasis of CD8+ memory T cells by opposing cytokines. *Science* 288:675, 2000.

60. Schluns KS, Lefrançois L: Cytokine control of memory T-cell development and survival. *Nat Rev Immunol* 3:269, 2003.

61. Dummer W, Niethammer AG, Baccala R, et al: T cell homeostatic proliferation elicits effective antitumor autoimmunity. *J Clin Invest* 110: 185, 2002.

62. Dudley ME, Wunderlich JR, Robbins PF, et al: Cancer regression and autoimmunity in patients after clonal repopulation with antitumor lymphocytes. *Science* 298:850, 2002.

63. Rosenberg SA, Yang JC, Schwartentruber DJ, et al: Immunologic and therapeutic evaluation of a synthetic peptide vaccine for the treatment of patients with metastatic melanoma. *Nat Med* 4:321, 1998.

64. Banchereau J, Steinman RM: Dendritic cells and the control of immunity. *Nature* 392:245, 1998.

65. Banchereau J, Briere F, Caux C, et al: Immunobiology of dendritic cells. *Annu Rev Immunol* 18:767, 2000.

66. Wang J, Saffold S, Cao X, et al: Eliciting T cell immunity against poorly immunogenic tumors by immunization with dendritic cell-tumor fusion vaccines. *J Immunol* 161:5516, 1998.

67. Banchereau J, Palucka K, Dhodapkar MV, et al: Immune and clinical responses in patients with metastatic melanoma to CD34+ progenitor-derived dendritic cell vaccine. *Cancer Res* 61:6458, 2001.

68. Nestle FO, Banchereau J, Hart D: Dendritic cells. On the move from bench to bedside. *Nat Med* 7:761, 2001.

69. Cerundolo V, Hermans IF, Salio M: Dendritic cells: A journey from laboratory to clinic. *Nat Immunol* 5:7, 2004.

70. Fong L, Hou Y, Rivas A, et al: Altered peptide ligand vaccination with Flt3 ligand expanded dendritic cells for tumor immunotherapy. *Proc Natl Acad Sci U S A* 98:8809, 2001.

71. Riddell SR: Progress in cancer vaccines by enhanced self-presentation. *Proc Natl Acad Sci U S A* 98:8933, 2001.

72. Merad M, Sugie T, Engleman EG, et al: *In vivo* manipulation of dendritic cells to induce therapeutic immunity. *Blood* 99:1676, 2002.

73. Horowitz MM, Gale RP, Sondel PM, et al: Graft-versus-leukemia reactions after bone marrow transplantation. *Blood* 75:555, 1990.

74. Kolb H-J, Schmid C, Barrett AJ, et al: Graft-versus-leukemia reactions in allogeneic chimeras. *Blood* 103:767, 2004.

75. Goulmy E: Human minor histocompatibility antigens: New concepts for marrow transplantation and adoptive immunotherapy. *Immunol Rev* 157: 125, 1997.

76. Fontaine P, Roy-Proulx G, Knafo L, et al: Adoptive transfer of minor histocompatibility antigen-specific T lymphocytes eradicates leukemia cells without causing graft-versus-host disease. *Nat Med* 7:789, 2001.

77. Warren EH, Greenberg PD, Riddell SR: Cytotoxic T-lymphocyte-defined human minor histocompatibility antigens with a restricted tissue distribution. *Blood* 91:2197, 1998.

78. Smit WM, Rijnbeek M, Van Bergen CAM, et al: T cells recognizing leukemic CD34+ progenitor cells mediate the antileukemic effect of donor lymphocyte infusions for relapsed chronic myeloid leukemia after allogeneic stem cell transplantation. *Proc Natl Acad Sci U S A* 95:10152, 1998.

79. Bonnet D, Warren EH, Greenberg PD, et al: CD8+ minor histocompatibility antigen-specific cytotoxic T lymphocyte clones eliminate human acute myeloid leukemia stem cells. *Proc Natl Acad Sci U S A* 96: 8639, 1999.

80. Den Haan JM, Meadows LM, Wang W, et al: The minor histocompatibility antigen HA-1: A diallelic gene with a single amino acid polymorphism. *Science* 279:1054, 1998.

81. Den Haan JMM, Sherman NE, Blokland E, et al: Identification of a graft versus host disease-associated human minor histocompatibility antigen. *Science* 268:1476, 1995.

82. Pierce RA, Field ED, Mutis T, et al: The HA-2 minor histocompatibility antigen is derived from a diallelic gene encoding a novel human class I myosin protein. *J Immunol* 167:3223, 2001.

83. Marijt WAE, Heemskerk MHM, Kloosterboer FM, et al: Hematopoiesis-restricted minor histocompatibility antigens HA-1- or HA-2-specific T cells can induce complete remissions of relapsed leukemia. *Proc Natl Acad Sci U S A* 100:2742, 2003.

84. Randolph SSB, Gooley TA, Warren EH, et al: Female donors contribute to a selective graft versus leukemia effect in male recipients of HLA matched related hematopoietic cell transplants. *Blood* 103:347, 2004.

85. Warren EH, Gavin MA, Simpson E, et al: The human UTY gene encodes a novel HLA-B8-restricted H-Y antigen. *J Immunol* 164:2807, 2000.

86. Vogt MHJ, Goulmy E, Kloosterboer FM, et al: UTY gene codes for an HLA-B60-restricted human male-specific minor histocompatibility antigen involved in stem cell graft rejection: Characterization of the critical polymorphic amino acid residues for T-cell recognition. *Blood* 96:3126, 2000.

87. Bocchia M, Korontsvit T, Xu Q, et al: Specific human cellular immunity to bcr-abl oncogene-derived peptides. *Blood* 87:3587, 1996.

88. Van Elsas A, Nijman HW, Van der Minne CE, et al: Induction and

characterization of cytotoxic T-lymphocytes recognizing a mutated p21ras peptide presented by HLA-A*0201. *Int J Cancer* 61:389, 1995.

89. Clark RE, Dodi A, Hill SC, et al: Direct evidence that leukemic cells present HLA-associated immunogenic peptides derived from the BCR-ABL b3a2 fusion protein. *Blood* 98:2887, 2001.

90. Molldrem JJ, Clave E, Jiang YZ, et al: Cytotoxic T lymphocytes specific for a nonpolymorphic proteinase 3 peptide preferentially inhibit chronic myeloid leukemia colony-forming units. *Blood* 90:2529, 1997.

91. Bellantuono I, Gao L, Parry S, et al: Two distinct HLA-A0201-presented epitopes of the Wilms tumor antigen 1 can function as targets for leukemia-reactive CTL. *Blood* 100:3835, 2002.

92. Molldrem J, Dermime S, Parker K, et al: Targeted T-cell therapy for human leukemia: Cytotoxic T lymphocytes specific for a peptide derived from proteinase 3 preferentially lyse human myeloid leukemia cells. *Blood* 88:2450, 1996.

93. Molldrem JJ, Lee PP, Wang C, et al: Evidence that specific T lymphocytes may participate in the elimination of chronic myelogenous leukemia. *Nat Med* 6:1018, 2000.

94. Menssen HD, Renkl HJ, Entezami M, et al: Wilms' tumor gene expression in human CD34+ hematopoietic progenitors during fetal development and early clonogenic growth. *Blood* 89:3486, 1997.

95. Gao L, Bellantuono I, Elsässer A, et al: Selective elimination of leukemic CD34+ progenitor cells by cytotoxic t lymphocytes specific for WT1. *Blood* 95:2198, 2000.

96. Molldrem JJ, Kant S, Lu S, et al: Peptide vaccination with PR1 elicits active T cell immunity that induces cytogenetic remission in acute myelogenous leukemia [abstract]. *Blood* 100:6a, 2002.

97. Mailänder V, Scheibenbogen C, Thiel E, et al: Complete remission in a patient with recurrent acute myeloid leukemia induced by vaccination with WT1 peptide in the absence of hematological or renal toxicity. *Leukemia* 18:165, 2004.

98. Falkenburg JHF, Wafelman AR, Joosten P, et al: Complete remission of accelerated phase chronic myeloid leukemia by treatment with leukemia-reactive cytotoxic T lymphocytes. *Blood* 94:1201, 1999.

99. Oka Y, Tsuboi A, Murakami M, et al: Wilms tumor gene peptide-based immunotherapy for patients with overt leukemia from myelodysplastic syndrome (MDS) or MDS with myelofibrosis. *Int J Hematol* 78:56, 2003.

100. Bonini C, Ferrari G, Verzeletti S, et al: HSV-TK gene transfer into donor lymphocytes for control of allogeneic graft-versus-leukemia. *Science* 276:1719, 1997.

101. Riddell SR, Elliott M, Lewinsohn DA, et al: T-cell mediated rejection of gene-modified HIV-specific cytotoxic T lymphocytes in HIV-infected patients. *Nat Med* 2:216, 1996.

102. Thomis DC, Marktel S, Bonini C, et al: A Fas-based suicide switch in human T cells for the treatment of graft-versus-host disease. *Blood* 97:1249, 2001.

103. Berger C, Blau CA, Huang ML, et al: Pharmacologically regulated Fas-mediated death of adoptively transferred T cells in a nonhuman primate model. *Blood* 103:1261, 2004.

PRINCIPLES OF VACCINE THERAPY

LARRY W. KWAK

Vaccines are biologic substances that are designed to stimulate the host immune system to elicit a neutralizing response against clinically relevant targets. Active immunotherapy with vaccines has been extremely effective as prevention against self-limiting infectious pathogens. However, effective vaccine therapy of chronic infectious diseases or cancer, in the therapeutic setting, remains a promising but largely unrealized goal. Hematologic malignancies are an excellent model system for vaccine therapies, in part because of accessibility and susceptibility to immune effector mechanisms and availability of tumor cells for studies of mechanism.

INTRODUCTION

ADVANTAGES OF A VACCINE

Immunity elicited by vaccines offers several advantages over passive immunotherapy using monoclonal antibodies. In active immune therapy, all components of the effector immune response are host-derived (without murine or xenogeneic components that could cause indirect toxicity). The lack of foreign components also suggests that the host immune response may be sustained. Also, if the vaccine contains more than a single determinant of the target antigen, the immune response could be broad in scope, recognizing more than a single epitope in the antigen (polyclonal). This feature might be of particular importance for cancer immunotherapy, as mutation of individual peptide epitopes is a possible mechanism of immune evasion by tumors. In addition to inducing antibodies, which can recognize intact proteins on the surface of tumor cells, vaccines induce T cells that can recognize peptide fragments derived from proteins, which may be endogenously processed and presented on the surface of tumor cells. Such T cells have various effector mechanisms capable of neutralizing tumor cells, including lysis of the tumor cell by cell-to-cell contact and local production of cytokines that might directly neutralize tumor cells (e.g., γ-interferon).

IMPEDIMENTS TO A VACCINE

Factors that potentially limit the success of active immunization, and strategies to overcome them, need to be identified.[1] Naturally operating regulatory mechanisms in the host, including (1) CD4+ CD25+, negative regulatory T cells, (2) negative costimulatory molecules on T cells (e.g., CTLA4 or CD152), (3) activation-induced cell death of T cells, and (4) the deletion of precursor T cells, could account for the failure to mount a protective immune response against tumor antigens.[2,3] In addition, tumor cell-associated mechanisms, such as loss of antigen or expression of human leukocyte antigen (HLA), the lack of immune costimulatory molecules, and the ability of tumor cells to produce suppressive soluble factors (e.g., transforming growth factor β [TGF-β]), also can account for the failure of the immune system to suppress tumors.[4,5]

ANTIGEN DISCOVERY

Conventional, as well as novel, technologies used to define cancer-associated antigens, such as serologic analysis by recombinant expression cloning (SEREX), serial analysis of gene expression (SAGE), screening tumor complementary DNA (cDNA) libraries with tumor-reactive T cells, and characterization of peptides eluted from tumor-derived HLA molecules, have resulted in a rapidly growing list of candidate tumor antigens for various hematologic malignancies (Table 24-1). The majority of these candidate antigens have been identified since 1998. Furthermore, the application of genomic and proteomic techniques, combined with the feasibility of isolating sufficient quantities of clonogenic tumor cells from individual patients, should identify additional targets.

Desirable characteristics for candidate target antigens for immune therapy include antigens that are selectively expressed by the tumor or that are required to maintain the malignant cell phenotype or cell survival. Host T cell recognition of such antigens requires that they are naturally processed and presented by tumor cells into peptides that bind host HLA molecules. Optimally, the candidate antigen should contain both CD4+ and CD8+ T cell epitopes. Antigens recognized by humoral immune responses must be expressed on the tumor cell surface, and the relevant epitopes must be accessible to antibody molecules. Candidate tumor antigens should be immunogenic (capable of being recognized by the host immune system).

Vaccine therapy does not necessarily require a completely defined tumor antigen. Vaccines can consist of whole tumor cells or subcellular components containing putative antigens. For example, autologous tumor cells engineered to overexpress cytokines such as granulocyte-macrophage colony stimulating factor (GM-CSF),[17,18] or activated ex vivo by CD40 receptor engagement,[19] can be effective at inducing tumor-specific T cells with as yet undefined antigen specificity. Similarly, transfer of the gene encoding CD40– ligand into chronic lymphocytic leukemia cells induced CD4+ and CD8+ T cell responses in human patients.[20] Vaccination with mixtures of heat shock proteins, which are intracellular chaperones for potential tumor peptides isolated from autologous human tumor cells, is also in clinical testing.[21]

VACCINE DELIVERY

Effective delivery of the target antigen to the immune system is critical for the successful induction of immunity. For most tumor antigens,

TABLE 24-1   EXAMPLES OF CANDIDATE HUMAN TUMOR ANTIGENS FOR HEMATOLOGIC CANCERS

ANTIGEN	REFERENCE
Minor histocompatibility antigens (HA-1, HA-2)	6
Proteinase-3	7
Wilms tumor antigen-1	8
B cell receptor (immunoglobin idiotype)	9
Anaplastic lymphoma kinase	10
Sperm protein 17	11
Sperm protein associated with the nucleus on X chromosome (SPAN-X)	12
CML-66	13
Survivin	14
HM1.24	15
Immature laminin receptor protein	16

Acronyms and abbreviations that appear in this chapter include: cDNA, complementary DNA; GM-CSF, granulocyte-monocyte colony stimulating factor; HLA, human leukocyte antigen; IL, interleukin; KLH, keyhole limpet hemocyanin; TGF, transforming growth factor.

this is a daunting challenge, as most antigens (with the exception of viral antigens associated with cancers) are weakly immunogenic, self, or tissue differentiation antigens.

Many vaccine-delivery strategies use dendritic cells. These key antigen-presenting cells are principally responsible for initiating a host immune response.[22] These cells, represented in minute quantities, have the powerful capacity to take up antigens, and once activated, to present processed peptides to T cells. Accordingly, optimizing the delivery of tumor antigens to these specialized antigen-presenting cells is critical. Such efforts have included isolation of dendritic cells from blood, followed by physical loading with protein or peptide antigens, or introducing the genes for candidate antigens by transfection with cDNA or messenger RNA (mRNA) or by fusion with whole tumor cells. Loaded dendritic cells have been administered to patients as vaccines.[23]

An alternative strategy is to target the delivery of antigens to dendritic cells in vivo. Traditional approaches focused on attempts to make the antigen look foreign to the host immune system; for example, by chemical linkage to larger, highly immunogenic proteins (carriers) or incorporation into liposomes. Rational approaches to increase the efficiency of antigen delivery to dendritic cells have included genetic fusion of the gene encoding the antigen to one encoding biologically active molecules that has the ability to target cell surface receptors on antigen-presenting cells. Such targeting molecules have included cytokines, chemokines, antibody Fc or Fab fragments, transferrin, CD40, and mannose, which serve as ligands for specific receptors on antigen-presenting cells.[24] Such molecular vaccines can be administered as naked DNA or as fusion proteins. Other promising approaches to target dendritic cells in vivo are represented by recombinant viral or bacterial vectors or virus-like particles.[25,26]

IMMUNOSTIMULANTS TO ENHANCE VACCINE EFFICACY

Traditionally, immunologic adjuvants, described by the late Charles Janeway as "immunology's dirty little secret," such as alum and oil-in-water emulsions (e.g., incomplete Freund adjuvant), provide a physical depot for slow release of antigen. Adjuvants also serve as general immune stimulants by providing a danger signal to activate antigen-presenting cells. This feature describes classical adjuvant components, such as bacterial cell wall extracts, as well as unmethylated CpG DNA sequences, which deliver maturation signals to dendritic cells through toll-like receptors.[27] The incorporation of either recombinant cytokines or their genes into vaccine formulations may increase vaccine potency by broadly enhancing the function of either antigen-presenting cells or T cells. Consequently, cytokines, such as γ-interferon, interleukin (IL)-2, and IL-15, may be useful as components of vaccines.[28] Such cytokines also can help direct the type of immune response elicited. For example, IL-12 elicits primarily T helper (Th) 1 cell responses, whereas the inclusion of IL-4 or IL-10 generally induces predominantly a Th2 cell response. Some cytokines, such as GM-CSF, which can induce dendritic cell differentiation, can also function as an adjuvant by recruiting antigen-presenting cells to local vaccination sites.[29] In the early 2000s, biologic agents or small molecules which block immunoregulatory signals (e.g., anti-CTLA4) were found to also enhance vaccine efficacy.[39]

CLINICAL TRIAL DESIGN

Cancer vaccine trials might not fit into the paradigm developed for chemotherapeutic agents, which have direct effects on tumor and normal host cells. For example, studies in heavily pretreated patients with terminal disease might be inappropriate for vaccines, which generally require an intact host immune system. For this reason, even safety

cannot be evaluated completely in patients who cannot make an immune response, because any toxicity will likely be indirect, resulting from the immune response elicited. In addition, animal models show that the immune system may be more effective at clearing minimal residual disease than at clearing advanced tumor cell burdens. Accordingly, several late stage clinical trials of cancer vaccines are testing this approach in the setting of clinical remission, after primary surgery or chemotherapy.

Although conventional clinical trials generally test one experimental agent at a time, vaccine formulations may contain several components. The simultaneous optimization of multiple variables (e.g., vaccine and adjuvant dose and schedule, and routes of administration) in a single clinical study often requires the application of novel, more flexible clinical trial designs.[30]

ASSAYS OF VACCINE EFFICACY

The development of surrogate measures of vaccine efficacy has potential value for answering the scientific question of whether it is even possible to vaccinate human patients against a candidate antigen. Traditional assays of immune response, including simple lymphoproliferation and cytotoxicity assays, requiring prolonged periods of prior stimulation, are being replaced by quantitative assays that can measure effector function of T cells directly sampled from blood (e.g., enzyme-linked immunospot assay [ELISPOT]) and by sensitive tetramer binding assays (Table 24-2).[31] In some cases, tetramer-binding assays have been combined with intracellular cytokine production to provide both quantitative and functional analyses of antigen-specific T cells.[32] An important aim of clinical trials is to determine which, if any, of these measures of immune response are valid surrogates for vaccine efficacy.

B CELL ANTIGEN RECEPTOR VACCINES AS SCIENTIFIC PROOF OF PRINCIPLE

B cells are clonally restricted to express surface Ig receptors that have unique epitopes present in the antibody variable region termed idiotypes. Idiotypes expressed by B cell malignancies are clonally distributed and thus can serve as tumor-specific target antigen for specific immunotherapy. Idiotypes were initially validated as tumor rejection antigens in mouse models of myeloma and lymphoma,[33,34] and the first clinical trial testing this approach in human patients with lymphoma was reported in 1992.[35,36] Customized idiotype proteins were isolated

TABLE 24-2 MONITORING OF HUMAN IMMUNE RESPONSES

TYPE OF RESPONSE	REPRESENTATIVE ASSAY
CD4+ T cells (Th1)	Cytokine induction
	Cytokine ELISPOT (IFN-γ)
	Intracellular cytokine
CD4+ T cells (Th2)	Proliferation
CD8+ T cells	Cytotoxicity
	Limiting dilution analysis
	Tetramer
Antibody	ELISA
	Flow cytometry
	ELISPOT
Multiple	Microarray
	Cytokine mRNA by RT-PCR
	T cell spectratyping

ELISA, enzyme-linked immunoabsorbent assay; ELISPOT, enzyme-linked immunospot assay, IFN, interferon; RT-PCR, reverse transcriptase polymerase chain reaction.

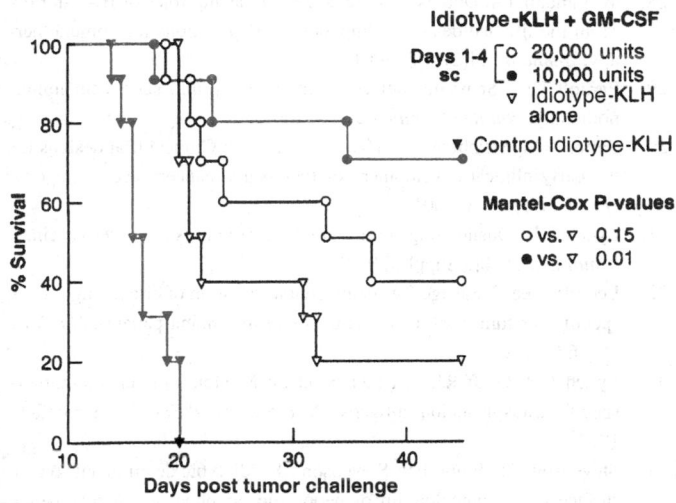

FIGURE 24-1 GM-CSF enhances lymphoma vaccine potency. Mice were vaccinated subcutaneously with idiotype KLH protein, together with or without various doses of GM-CSF and challenged with a lethal dose of syngeneic lymphoma cells. The use of 10,000 units of GM-CSF+ idiotype KLH conjugate on days 1 to 4 (*closed dots*) resulted in a significantly longer survival after tumor challenge than did idiotype KLH conjugate vaccination alone.

by heterohybridoma fusion, conjugated chemically to keyhole limpet hemocyanin (KLH), which functioned as a carrier, and emulsified in a simple oil-in-water emulsion. These vaccines elicited predominantly antibody responses.

Subsequently, guided by additional data from murine lymphoma models (Fig. 24-1), recombinant GM-CSF protein was substituted as the immunologic adjuvant. Soluble GM-CSF, initially mixed with the vaccine and then administered for three additional daily doses subcutaneously as close as possible to the original site of immunization, significantly enhanced vaccine potency, consistent with previous gene

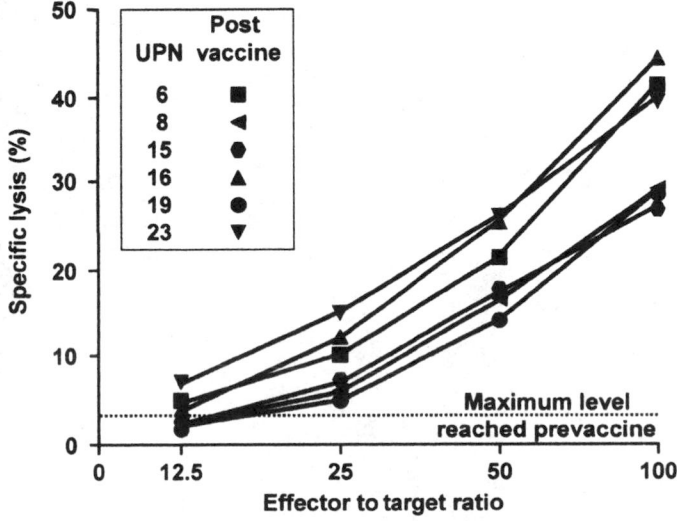

FIGURE 24-2 T cell-mediated lysis of human autologous lymphoma cells after vaccination with idiotype KLH protein plus GM-CSF. Representative results are shown from six individual patients, designated by unique patient number (UPN). (Adapted from M Bendandi, CD Gocke, CB Kobrin, et al.,[9] with permission.)

therapy studies.[37] The cellular mechanism of this effect required CD8+ and CD4+ T cells.[38]

A phase II study was designed to test these vaccines in the setting of minimal residual disease, defined as first remission after chemotherapy in follicular lymphoma patients.[9] Previously untreated patients first received treatment with uniform chemotherapy to achieve complete remission. After a 6-month break to allow for immune reconstitution, idiotype proteins conjugated with KLH plus GM-CSF vaccines were administered in five monthly doses. Surrogate assays for vaccine efficacy were developed that used autologous lymphoma cells as targets for both B and T cell responses. In 19 patients (86%), vaccination elicited CD8+ cytotoxic T lymphocyte cells reactive with the lymphoma cell (Fig. 24-2). More than half of the patients remain in continuous first complete remission, even after a median followup of more than 7 years. Controlled, randomized phase III trials are in progress, testing idiotype vaccines (produced by heterohybridoma fusion as originally described, or by newer recombinant technologies), also in combination with GM-CSF and administered in first remission.

REFERENCES

1. Waldmann T: Immunotherapy: Past, present and future. *Nat Med* 9(3): 269, 2003.
2. Chambers CA, Kuhns MS, Egen JG, Allison JP: CTLA-4 mediated inhibition in regulation of T-cell responses: Mechanisms and manipulation in tumor immunotherapy. *Annu Rev Immunol* 19:565, 2001.
3. Woo EY, Yeh H, Chu CS, et al: Cutting edge: Regulatory T cells from lung cancer patients directly inhibit autologous T cell proliferation. *J Immunol* 168(9):4272, 2002.
4. Rivoltini L, Carrabba M, Huber V, et al: Immunity to cancer: Attack and escape in T lymphocyte-tumor cell interaction. *Immunol Rev* 188: 97, 2002.
5. Phan GQ, Wang E, Marincola FM: T-cell-directed cancer vaccines: Mechanisms of immune escape and immune tolerance. *Expert Opin Biol Ther* 1(3):511, 2001.
6. Marijt WA, Heemskerk MH, Kloosterboer FM, et al: Hematopoiesis-restricted minor histocompatibility antigens HA-1- or HA-2-specific T cells can induce complete remissions of relapsed leukemia. *Proc Natl Acad Sci U S A* 100(5):2742, 2003.
7. Molldrem JJ, Komanduri K, Wieder E: Overexpressed differentiation antigens as targets of graft-versus-leukemia reactions. *Curr Opin Hematol* 9(6):503, 2002.
8. Bellantuono I, Gao L, Parry S, et al: Two distinct HLA-A0201-presented epitopes of the Wilms tumor antigen 1 can function as targets for leukemia-reactive CTL. *Blood* 100(10):3835, 2002.
9. Bendandi M, Gocke CD, Kobrin CB, et al: Complete molecular remissions induced by patient-specific vaccination plus granulocyte-monocyte colony-stimulating factor against lymphoma. *Nat Med* 5:1171, 1999.
10. Passoni L, Scardino A, Bertazzoli C, et al: ALK as a novel lymphoma-associated tumor antigen: Identification of 2 HLA-A2.1-restricted CD8+ T-cell epitopes. *Blood* 99(6):2100, 2002.
11. Lim SH, Wang Z, Chiriva-Internati M, et al: Sperm protein 17 is a novel cancer-testis antigen in multiple myeloma. *Blood* 97(5):1508, 2001.
12. Wang Z, Zhang Y, Liu H, et al: Gene expression and immunologic consequence of SPAN-Xb in myeloma and other hematologic malignancies. *Blood* 101(3):955, 2003.
13. Yang XF, Wu CJ, Mclaughlin S, et al: CML66, a broadly immunogenic tumor antigen, elicits a humoral immune response associated with remission of chronic myelogenous leukemia. *Proc Natl Acad Sci U S A* 98(13):7492, 2001.
14. Zeis M, Siegel S, Wagner A, et al: Generation of cytotoxic responses in mice and human individuals against hematological malignancies using

survivin-RNA-transfected dendritic cells. *J Immunol* 170(11):5391, 2003.

15. Chiriva-Internati M, Liu Y, Weidanz JA, et al: Testing recombinant adeno-associated virus-gene loading of dendritic cells for generating potent cytotoxic T lymphocytes against a prototype self-antigen, multiple myeloma HM1.24. *Blood* 102(9):3100, 2003.

16. Siegel S, Wagner A, Kabelitz D, et al: Induction of cytotoxic T-cell responses against the oncofetal antigen-immature laminin receptor for the treatment of hematologic malignancies. *Blood* 102(1):4416, 2003.

17. Levitsky HI, Montgomery J, Ahmadzadeh M, et al: Immunization with granulocyte-macrophage colony-stimulating factor-transduced, but not B7-1-transduced, lymphoma cells primes idiotype-specific T cells and generates potent systemic antitumor immunity. *J Immunol* 156(10): 3858, 1996.

18. Dranoff G: Cytokines in cancer pathogenesis and cancer therapy. *Nat Rev Cancer* 4(1):11, 2004.

19. von Bergwelt-Baildon MS, Vonderheide RH, Maecker B, et al: Human primary and memory cytotoxic T lymphocyte responses are efficiently induced by means of CD40-activated B cells as antigen-presenting cells: Potential for clinical application. *Blood* 99(9):3319, 2002.

20. Wierda WG, Cantwell MJ, Woods SJ: CD40-ligand (CD154) gene therapy for chronic lymphocytic leukemia. *Blood* 96(9):2917, 2000.

21. Srivastava, PK: Roles of heat-shock proteins in innate and adaptive immunity. *Nat Rev Immunol* 2:185, 2002.

22. Liu YJ: Dendritic cell subsets and lineages, and their functions in innate and adaptive immunity. *Cell* 106:259, 2001.

23. Cerundolo V, Hermans IF, Salio M: Dendritic cells: A journey from laboratory to clinic. *Nat Immunol* 5(1):7, 2004.

24. Biragyn A, Kwak LW: Designer cancer vaccines are still in fashion. *Nat Med* 6(9):966, 2000.

25. Tartour E, Benchetrit F, Haicheur N, et al: Synthetic and natural non-live vectors: Rationale for their clinical development in cancer vaccine protocols. *Vaccine* 20[Suppl 4]:A32, 2002.

26. Zhang L, Tang Y, Akbulut H, et al: An adenoviral vector cancer vaccine that delivers a tumor-associated antigen/CD40-ligand fusion protein to dendritic cells. *Proc Natl Acad Sci U S A* 100(25):15101, 2003.

27. Kreig AM: CpG motifs in bacterial DNA and their immune effects. *Annu Rev Immunol* 20:709, 2002.

28. Waldmann TA, Dubois S, Tagaya Y: Contrasting roles of IL-2 and IL-15 in the life and death of lymphocytes: Implications for immunotherapy. *Immunity* 14(2):105, 2001.

29. Pardoll DM: Spinning molecular immunology into successful immunotherapy. *Nat Rev Immunol* 2:227, 2002.

30. Simon RM, Steinberg SM, Hamilton M, et al: Clinical trial designs for the early clinical development of therapeutic cancer vaccines. *J Clin Oncol* 19(6):1848, 2001.

31. Lyerly HK: Quantitating cellular immune responses to cancer vaccines. *Semin Oncol* 30[3 Suppl 8]:9, 2003.

32. Lee PP, Yee C, Savage PA, et al: Characterization of circulating T cells specific for tumor-associated antigens in melanoma patients. *Nat Med* 5(6):677, 1999.

33. Lynch RG, Graff RJ, Sirisinha S, et al: Myeloma proteins as tumor-specific transplantation antigens. *Proc Natl Acad Sci U S A* 69:1540, 1972.

34. Stevenson GT, Elliott EV, Stevenson FK: Idiotypic determinants on the surface of immunoglobulin of neoplastic lymphocytes: A therapeutic target. *Fed Proc* 36:2268, 1977.

35. Kwak LW, Campbell MJ, Czerwinski DK, et al: Induction of immune responses in patients with B-cell lymphoma against the surface-immunoglobulin idiotype expressed by their tumors. *N Engl J Med* 327:1209, 1992.

36. Hsu FJ, Caspar CB, Czerwinski D, et al: Tumor-specific idiotype vaccines in the treatment of patients with B-cell lymphoma—Long-term results of a clinical trial. *Blood* 89:3129, 1997.

37. Dranoff G, Jaffee E, Lazenby A, et al: Vaccination with irradiated tumor cells engineered to secrete murine granulocyte-macrophage colony-stimulating factor stimulates potent, specific, and long-lasting anti-tumor immunity. *Proc Natl Acad Sci U S A* 90(8):3539, 1993.

38. Kwak LW, Young HA, Pennington RW, et al: Vaccination with syngeneic lymphoma-derive immunoglobulin idiotype combined with granulocyte/macrophage colony-stimulating factor primes mice for a protective T-cell response. *Proc Natl Acad Sci U S A* 93:10972, 1996.

39. Phan GQ, Yang JC, Sherry RM, et al: Cancer regression and autoimmunity induced by cytotoxic T lymphocyte-associated antigen 4 blockade in patients with metastatic melanoma. *Proc Natl Acad Sci U S A* 100:8372, 2003.

PRINCIPLES OF THERAPEUTIC APHERESIS: INDICATIONS, EFFICACY, AND COMPLICATIONS

BRUCE C. MCLEOD

Therapeutic apheresis provides a means to rapidly alter the composition of blood components. It can be a valuable and safe initial treatment of a number of illnesses associated with quantitative and/or qualitative abnormalities of blood cells or plasma. Cell depletions are useful in symptomatic thrombocythemia and hyperleukocytosis. They provide autologous or allogeneic stem and progenitor cells for hematopoietic reconstitution or immunocytes for immunomodulation. Plasma exchange is useful in certain paraproteinemias, antibody-mediated disorders, and toxin-mediated diseases. It also can be used to replace a deficient plasma constituent. Red cell exchange is used primarily for severe manifestations of sickle cell disease. Selective extraction techniques are available for immunoglobulin G and low-density lipoprotein, and modulation of certain immune responses is possible with photopheresis. Adverse effects with current techniques are infrequent and usually mild.

INTRODUCTION

Therapeutic apheresis comprises a set of related techniques in which the amount or composition of a blood component is manipulated for a therapeutic purpose, usually with a continuous-flow centrifugal blood separation instrument. Available techniques are divided into three main categories: blood cell depletion, blood component exchange, and blood component modification (Table 25-1). Cell depletion procedures usually target excess platelets or leukocytes. These procedures currently are undertaken almost exclusively for hematologic diseases. Similar techniques adapted for autologous or allogeneic leukocyte donation provide cells for transplantation and/or immunotherapy. Blood component exchanges target plasma or red cells. Plasma exchange is beneficial in a number of antibody-mediated conditions, many of which are not usually considered hematologic diseases. Specialized techniques have been developed for online selective extraction of certain individual constituents, such as immunoglobulin (Ig) G and low-density lipoproteins (LDLs) from plasma separated by

Acronyms and abbreviations that appear in this chapter include: ADAMTS13, von Willebrand cleaving metalloproteinase; ALL, acute lymphocytic leukemia; AML, acute myelogenous leukemia; CML, chronic myelogenous leukemia; CTCL, cutaneous T cell lymphoma; HPA, human platelet alloantigen; Ig, immunoglobulin; LDL, low-density lipoprotein; MNC, mononuclear cell; PBPC, peripheral blood progenitor cell; SPS, stiff person syndrome; TTP, thrombotic thrombocytopenic purpura.

TABLE 25-1   THERAPEUTIC APHERESIS TECHNIQUES

Cell depletion
  Plateletpheresis
  Leukapheresis
    Therapeutic white blood cell removal
    Peripheral blood progenitor cell collection
    Immunocyte collection
Blood component exchange
  Plasma exchange (plasmapheresis)
  Red cell exchange
Blood component modification
  Selective extraction of a plasma constituent
  Photopheresis

an apheresis instrument, and for photochemical modification of separated lymphocytes (photopheresis).

The goal of therapeutic apheresis usually is therapeutic depletion. Candidate entities for therapeutic depletion should be pathogenic and susceptible to depletion by apheresis. The latter provision implies that a substantial portion of the total body burden is intravascular and that the half-life is relatively long. In practice, this limits utility to blood cells and large, slowly catabolized plasma proteins such as immunoglobulins and low-density lipoproteins (LDLs).[1] Infusion of normal blood constituents in quantity may be important in some instances. Apheresis therapy depletes rapidly but does not decrease production of an abnormal blood constituent. Therefore, in most illnesses apheresis therapy is best used acutely to control symptoms until more definitive therapy takes effect. Chronic apheresis therapy is seldom appropriate unless more convenient treatments are ineffective or contraindicated.

Adverse effects of therapeutic apheresis with modern instruments occur infrequently and generally are mild. Symptomatic hypotension occurs in 1 to 2 percent of patients. Hypocalcemia as a result of citrate infusion can occur. Urticaria may be seen when donor plasma is infused in plasma exchange. Deaths are extremely rare. Most deaths are attributable to central venous catheter placement or to the progression of the disease rather than to apheresis therapy *per se*.[2-5] Table 25-2 lists the overall nonaccess-related adverse effect rates for common procedures observed in one large multicenter study.[3]

CELL DEPLETION

PLATELETPHERESIS

Thrombocythemia usually can be managed pharmacologically with hydroxyurea or anagrelide. However, therapeutic plateletpheresis can be valuable in patients with symptomatic thrombocythemia who require rapid reduction of platelet count or who cannot tolerate drug

TABLE 25-2   NONACCESS-RELATED ADVERSE EFFECT RATES FOR COMMON THERAPEUTIC APHERESIS PROCEDURES

PROCEDURE	ADVERSE EFFECT RATE, %
Plasma exchange	
Without plasma infusion	3.4
With plasma infusion	7.8
Leukapheresis	5.7
Plateletpheresis	0.0
Red cell exchange	10
Peripheral blood progenitor cell collection	1.7

Adapted from McLeod et al.[3]

therapy.[6] Platelet count usually can be lowered by approximately 50 percent with each procedure, although the decrement may be less if platelets are mobilized from an enlarged spleen during apheresis. Plateletpheresis can reverse clinical manifestations of myocardial or cerebral ischemia, pulmonary embolism, and gastrointestinal bleeding. Multiple procedures at intervals of a few days usually are needed until chemotherapy takes effect. Whether prophylactic plateletpheresis lowers the incidence of thrombosis or hemorrhage is not known; however, prophylactic plateletpheresis may prevent placental infarction and fetal death in pregnant patients with thrombocythemia.[7] Long-term plateletpheresis is logistically and financially burdensome and is seldom indicated as the sole therapy for thrombocythemia (see Chap. 111).

LEUKAPHERESIS

The most common therapeutic application of leukapheresis is removal of malignant leukocytes. Leukapheresis has been performed in acute and chronic leukemias and in the leukemic phase of lymphoma. The usual goal of leukapheresis is relieving or forestalling acute symptoms of hyperleukocytosis, but leukapheresis occasionally has been used as a primary method of disease control.[6] Immunomodulation by removal of nonmalignant lymphocytes also has been attempted[8,9] but has not become an accepted treatment of any illness.

The threshold white cell count for pulmonary and/or cerebral dysfunction (leukostasis) in patients with leukemia is not known. The count may depend on rheologic variables that differ among different leukemias and even among patients with the same type of leukemia. Clinical manifestations of hyperleukocytosis may occur in acute myelogenous leukemia (AML) when the white cell count is 75×10^9/liter[10,11] but more likely occur when the white cell count exceeds 200×10^9/liter.[12] Although controlled trials documenting benefit are lacking, therapeutic leukapheresis often is performed urgently in patients with AML if the white cell count is greater than 100×10^9/liter because this is a risk factor for early death.[13] Patients with acute lymphocytic leukemia (ALL) often are treated similarly, even though symptoms occur less frequently in this condition. In one study of ALL patients, leukapheresis led to a lower incidence of electrolyte abnormalities.[14]

White cell removal in chronic myelogenous leukemia (CML) was one of the earliest applications of apheresis instruments in patients.[15] Repeated leukapheresis as therapy for CML also provided leukocytes for transfusion to infected neutropenic patients with acute leukemia.[16] Some CML patients experienced reduced organomegaly and amelioration of constitutional symptoms, but chronic leukapheresis did not prolong life or delay onset of blast transformation.[17] Logistical and financial issues make this approach impractical except in unusual circumstances such as pregnancy,[18] in which delayed chemotherapy is desirable. Leukapheresis therapy for CML usually is reserved for patients who have white cell counts of 300 to 500×10^9/liter and signs of leukostasis. Even higher white cell counts are tolerated in chronic lymphocytic leukemia.[19]

In Sézary syndrome, a leukemic phase of cutaneous T cell lymphoma (CTCL), repeated leukapheresis reduces the number of circulating malignant (Sézary) cells and improves or resolves skin lesions.[20,21] Photopheresis (extracorporeal photochemotherapy) has been used to treat CTCL, especially in the erythrodermic phase.[22] In photopheresis, leukocytes removed by apheresis are exposed to ultraviolet A light in the presence of 8-methoxypsoralen and then returned to the patient. Photochemical damage to DNA is believed to render the malignant cells immunomodulatory, thereby stimulating host antitumor immunity.[23] Photopheresis has resulted in sustained remissions in CTCL.[24]

The extent to which the white cell count should be lowered is not known with certainty for any application of therapeutic leukapheresis. Processing at least two patient blood volumes has been recommended, with white cell count reductions of 15 to 86 percent reported in acute leukemias.[6] Predicting the outcome of a procedure is difficult because of mobilization of cells into the bloodstream, underestimation of patient blood volume by standard formulas, and patient-specific differences in the behavior of leukemic cells in a centrifugal instrument. In practice, monitoring the white cell count during a procedure and continuing until a 30 to 50 percent decline is achieved is worthwhile.

MONONUCLEAR CELL COLLECTION

Leukapheresis techniques optimized for mononuclear cell (MNC) depletion have been adapted for collection of stem and progenitor cells and various immunocytes from circulating blood. These techniques are described here, although the therapeutic effect derives from subsequent infusion (transplantation) of cells rather than from depletion, even in the autologous setting.

PERIPHERAL BLOOD PROGENITOR CELL COLLECTION

Stem and progenitor cells in quantities adequate to support hematopoietic reconstitution after myeloablative therapy can be obtained from most individuals by MNC collection. Prospective donors are pretreated with conventional chemotherapy (autologous only) and/or hematopoietic growth factors (autologous or allogeneic) to "mobilize" the desired cells from the marrow into the circulating blood. Unlike marrow harvest, peripheral blood progenitor cell (PBPC) collection does not require general anesthesia. Also, PBPC collection yields cells that engraft more rapidly after transplantation than marrow-derived cells. The latter two properties are significant advantages. As a result, PBPC collection has largely supplanted marrow harvest for allogeneic and autologous stem cell transplantation. PBPC transplants contain more T cells and may cause more frequent and/or more severe graft-versus-host disease in the allogeneic setting; however, this potential disadvantage does not offset the perceived advantages for donor and recipient[25] (see Chap. 20). PBPCs are a convenient substrate for some instances of gene insertion therapy[26] (see Chap. 26). Complications of PBPC collection occur infrequently (see Table 25-2)[3]; however, mobilization with granulocyte colony stimulating factor has led to splenic rupture in a healthy allogeneic donor[27] and fatal sickle cell crisis in an allogeneic donor with mild hemoglobin SC disease.[28]

IMMUNOCYTE COLLECTION

MNC collection from individuals who have not been "mobilized" still can serve as a source of T cells, natural killer cells, dendritic cells, or other cells having a role in the immune response to tumors or infectious agents. Deliberate infusion of T cells from a matched allogeneic stem cell donor (donor lymphocyte infusion) can enhance the graft-versus-tumor effect in preventing or combatting relapse[29] (see Chap. 23). Methods whereby autologous MNCs are manipulated *ex vivo* to boost a specific immune response to tumor or microbial antigens and then reinfused[30] are being explored (see Chap. 24).

BLOOD COMPONENT EXCHANGES

PHYSIOLOGY

Therapeutic blood component exchange reduces the concentration of a harmful blood constituent by removing patient material and simultaneously replacing the material with a substitute lacking the unwanted constituent. In a plasma exchange, the extent of depletion of an unwanted macromolecule X can be estimated at any point by the formula[31]:

$$X_n = X_0 e^{-n}$$

where X_0 = starting concentration of X; n = volume exchanged, expressed in patient plasma volumes; X_n = concentration of X after exchange of n plasma volumes; and e = base natural log.

This formula describes an asymptotic function that predicts (assuming equilibrium with extravascular substance is slow) exchange of one plasma volume lowers the intravascular concentration of a substance by about 65 percent, whereas exchange of a second plasma volume lowers the intravascular concentration only about 23 percent more. Removal is more efficient in the early portion of an exchange, so many exchanges are limited to a single plasma volume. For IgG antibodies, the existence of a substantial extravascular reservoir provides a further rationale for a series of single plasma volume exchanges separated by intervals adequate to allow reequilibration between intravascular and extravascular spaces. Applied in a reciprocal manner, the formula works equally well for predicting the outcome of a red cell exchange, although the final concentration of normal red cells can be increased efficiently beyond the predicted level by removing some red cells while infusing a plasma substitute at the beginning of a procedure and infusing red cells while removing plasma at the end of a procedure.[32]

A protein-containing replacement fluid must be given during plasma exchange. Usually either normal plasma or 5 percent albumin is chosen. For most applications, 5 percent albumin is preferred because it does not transmit viral infections or cause urticarial reactions, and it can be administered without regard to blood type. As expected, IgG levels fall by approximately 63 percent after a single plasma volume exchange for albumin and then take several weeks to recover. Coagulation factor levels also fall, with transient prolongation of the prothrombin time and partial thromboplastin time. However, clinical bleeding usually is not encountered, and all coagulant proteins except fibrinogen return to the normal range within 6 to 24 hours after an exchange.[31] Because most other plasma protein levels also recover quickly between exchanges, a series of thrice-weekly exchanges of patient plasma for 5 percent albumin produces selective depression in immunoglobulin levels.[33] Plasma replacement may be necessary in certain illnesses, such as thrombotic thrombocytopenic purpura (TTP), to achieve the desired therapeutic effect. Plasma may be given in the final portion of an exchange to replete coagulation factors when a patient has a preexisting bleeding diathesis.

PLASMA EXCHANGE

Therapeutic plasma exchange has been used to treat several types of plasma constituent abnormalities (Table 25-3). In most instances, the goal is removing a pathogenic immunoglobulin from the patient's blood. Cases can be subdivided based on whether the antigenic specificity of the immunoglobulin or an abnormal physical property imparted to the blood by its presence (e.g., hyperviscosity) mediates the disease process. In a few instances, plasma exchange can help by removing substances other than immunoglobulin (e.g., LDL). Plasma exchange can replete a deficient factor to a higher level than plasma infusion alone.

IMMUNOGLOBULINS WITH PATHOGENIC PHYSICAL PROPERTIES

Almost all of the conditions in this category are caused by monoclonal proteins. The hyperviscosity syndrome, which can be a feature of macroglobulinemia and rarely results from the effects of species of IgG or

TABLE 25-3 INDICATION CATEGORIES FOR PLASMA EXCHANGE

GOAL	EXAMPLE
Immunoglobulin removal	
Abnormal physical properties	Hyperviscosity syndrome
Specific antibody	Goodpasture syndrome
Nonimmunoglobulin constituent removal	Familial hypercholesterolemia
Factor replacement	Thrombotic thrombocytopenic purpura

IgA, probably is the oldest indication for therapeutic apheresis.[34,35] The hyperviscosity syndrome is particularly amenable to plasma exchange because IgM is distributed largely in the plasma and not in the extravascular fluid. Because the relationship between paraprotein concentration and viscosity is nonlinear, reduced viscosity sufficient to relieve both hemorrhagic and ischemic symptoms can be achieved with exchange of only 500- to 1000-ml plasma by manual bag techniques. Larger automated exchanges are even more effective. Plasma exchange can reverse clinical manifestations of cryoglobulinemia, such as vasculitis, glomerulonephritis, and Raynaud phenomenon.[36,37] In both instances, plasma exchange is best used as a temporizing strategy until more definitive therapy directed at the protein-producing cells take effect. However, long-term treatment can be effective in unusual circumstances.

Plasma exchange may be beneficial in renal failure associated with multiple myeloma.[38,39] In one prospective, randomized study of oliguric patients requiring dialysis, only patients treated with plasma exchange and chemotherapy recovered renal function.[39]

IMMUNOGLOBULINS WITH PATHOGENIC SPECIFICITY

A number of diseases are mediated by circulating antibody specific for a host tissue antigen. Although autoreactive, some of these antibodies probably are stimulated by exposure to alloantigens (e.g., anti-human platelet antigen [HPA]-1a in posttransfusion purpura). Plasma exchange therapy is useful in many such illnesses, including the examples listed in Table 25-4.

Hematologic Diseases In posttransfusion purpura, thrombocytopenia develops abruptly about 1 week after a blood transfusion, in association with an alloantibody response to a platelet-specific antigen. The mechanism by which the patient's antigen-negative platelets are

TABLE 25-4 EXAMPLES OF SPECIFIC ANTIBODIES IN DISEASES TREATED WITH PLASMA EXCHANGE

ANTIBODY SPECIFICITY	DISEASE
Autoantibodies	
Motor endplate acetylcholine receptor	Myasthenia gravis
Nerve ending calcium channel active zone	Lambert-Eaton myasthenic syndrome
Peripheral nerve myelin	Guillain-Barré syndrome, chronic inflammatory demyelinating polyneuropathy
Red cell I/i	Cold agglutinin disease
Factor VIII	Acquired hemophilia
$\alpha3$ Chain of type IV collagen	Goodpasture syndrome
Alloantibodies	
HPA-1a or other platelet antigen	Posttransfusion purpura
Anti-A, anti-B	ABO-incompatible transplant
Anti-D	Hydrops fetalis
Factor VIII	Hemophilia A inhibitor

destroyed is not clear.[40] Plasma exchange hastens recovery from this self-limited syndrome, as does IV γ-globulin infusion.[41]

Plasma exchange reportedly was beneficial in some trials of acute idiopathic thrombocytopenic purpura[42,43] but has since been superseded by IV γ-globulin.[44] In chronic idiopathic thrombocytopenic purpura associated with HIV infection or unresponsive to glucocorticoids and splenectomy, platelet count reportedly improves after infusions of autologous plasma that has passed through a protein A/silica affinity column.[45,46] The procedure can be performed offline on stored plasma or online in series with the plasma circuit of an apheresis device. Exposure to protein A apparently is immunomodulatory rather than subtractive, given that the amounts of immune complexes and platelet-associated antibodies removed by the column are insufficient to account for a salutary effect.[46]

Plasma exchange is not routinely recommended for warm autoimmune hemolytic anemia[47] but may be helpful in refractory cases when used in combination with IV γ-globulin[48] or pulse cyclophosphamide.[49] In cold agglutinin disease, significant but transient reductions in antibody titer and hemolysis severity have been reported.[50–53] In such cases, warming the extracorporeal circuit and replacement fluids is very important.

Coagulation factor inhibitors (autoantibodies and alloantibodies) can be removed by plasma exchange. Removal alone will not control bleeding caused by a high-titer inhibitor but may reduce the titer enough to allow replacement factor to circulate temporarily. The replacement fluid for such exchanges should be fresh-frozen plasma.[54,55] Repeated antibody removal by online immunoadsorption with a protein A/Sepharose affinity column, in combination with factor replacement and immunosuppression, may induce tolerance in alloimmunized hemophiliacs.[56–58]

Plasma exchange has been attempted in patients with disorders of blood cell production that can be linked to circulating antibody, including aplastic anemia and pure red cell aplasia.[58]

Removal of alloantibodies to red blood cells can be accomplished by therapeutic apheresis. Plasma exchange and isoagglutinin-specific immunoadsorption have been used to prepare patients for ABO-incompatible marrow transplants.[59–61] Apheresis instruments can also be used to remove red cells from the graft; this has become the preferred alternative because it involves a single manipulation that does not inconvenience the patient.[62] In sensitized Rh-negative women, removal of maternal IgG by plasma exchange during pregnancy to ameliorate destruction of fetal red cells has largely been supplanted by intrauterine transfusion of compatible cells.[63] Plasma exchange still may be attempted if therapy is needed prior to 18 to 20 weeks' gestation, when intrauterine transfusion is not technically feasible.[64,65]

Neurologic Diseases Neurologic diseases account for many plasma exchange treatments. The effectiveness of plasma exchange treatment complements other evidence supporting an autoimmune etiology for several neuropathic and neuromuscular disorders.

In Guillain-Barré syndrome, early treatment with plasma exchange clearly hastens recovery[66–68] from an illness in which antibodies to myelin frequently are found,[69] possibly in response to infection with *Campylobacter jejuni*.[70–72] Antimyelin antibodies may be found in chronic inflammatory demyelinating polyneuropathy.[73–75] A controlled trial in chronic inflammatory demyelinating polyneuropathy showed patients treated with plasma exchange improved significantly.[76,77] Chronic neuropathy in the context of a monoclonal gammopathy also may respond to plasma exchange.[78]

Myasthenia gravis and Lambert-Eaton syndrome are mediated by autoantibodies to structures in the neuromuscular junction.[79] In myasthenia gravis, the target is the acetylcholine receptor on the muscle cell. In Lambert-Eaton syndrome, antibodies are directed against structures in the nerve ending. Both illnesses respond to plasma exchange,[80,81] which has been most useful in severe myasthenia gravis.

Autoantibodies that may block central nervous system neurotransmission are implicated in other neurologic diseases. Many patients with stiff person syndrome (SPS) make an antibody to glutamic acid decarboxylase that may inhibit synthesis of the neurotransmitter γ-aminobutyric acid.[82] Paraneoplastic SPS may be caused by antibody to one of two synaptic proteins, amphiphysine[83] or gephyrin.[84] In Rasmussen encephalitis, antibodies to the Glu R3 receptor for the neurotransmitter glutamate are present.[85] Plasma exchange reportedly benefits individual patients with these antibodies.

Several other paraneoplastic syndromes with neurologic manifestations are associated with autoantibodies to neural antigens, such as encephalomyelitis with anti-Hu, cerebellar degeneration with anti-Yo, opsoclonus-myoclonus with anti-Ri, and retinal degeneration with anti-CAR. Results from plasma exchange have been disappointing.[86,87]

Renal and Rheumatic Diseases Goodpasture syndrome of glomerulonephritis and lung hemorrhage is caused by linear deposition of autoantibody to a collagen found in pulmonary and renal basement membranes.[88] Prompt intervention with plasma exchange and cyclophosphamide is the treatment of choice.[89] By contrast, controlled trials of nephritis associated with systemic lupus erythematosus have shown that oral cyclophosphamide and plasma exchange are no better than oral cyclophosphamide alone.[90,91] One study of pauciimmune rapidly progressive glomerulonephritis suggested benefit from plasma exchange in patients with dialysis-dependent renal failure[92]; however, no benefit has been observed in controlled trials of dialysis-independent patients.[93,94] Plasma exchange has been attempted in patients with several categories of severe vasculitis,[95–97] but studies of severe nonrenal lupus erythematosus reported excess deaths from infection when plasma exchange was added to pulse intravenous cyclophosphamide therapy.[98,99] Multiple controlled trials have shown that plasma exchange is ineffective in reversing renal transplant rejection.[100] However, favorable outcomes in uncontrolled series of patients with circulating donor-specific antibody have rekindled interest in this topic.[101,102] Pretransplant plasma exchange may allow successful transplantation despite HLA or ABO incompatibility.[103,104]

NONIMMUNOGLOBULIN CONSTITUENTS

Removal of LDLs by plasma exchange can lower cholesterol levels and promote resorption of xanthomas and atheromas in patients with familial hypercholesterolemia.[105,106] Online selective extraction of lipoproteins from patient plasma can be accomplished by chemical or immunological means.[107–109] Two methods —dextran sulfate absorption[109] and heparin-induced LDL precipitation[110]—have been approved by the FDA for patients with severe hypercholesterolemia resistant to dietary and drug therapy. Removal of phytanic acid by plasma exchange[111] or selective LDL extraction[112] can prevent or reverse neurologic manifestations in Refsum disease. Plasma exchange can remove excessive levels of low molecular weight drugs, toxins, and hormones bound to plasma proteins.[100]

NORMAL FACTOR REPLACEMENT

Conceptually, plasma exchange (normal plasma for the patient's deficient plasma) can be used to correct a deficiency of any plasma factor that is not available in a concentrated form. Plasma exchange can achieve higher levels (theoretically 65 percent of normal with a single plasma volume exchange) than simple plasma infusion, without inducing volume overload. Repletion of coagulation factors is part of the rationale for using plasma exchange to support patients with acute liver failure until recovery or liver transplantation.[113]

TTP was found empirically to respond to daily plasma exchange with normal plasma replacement.[114–116] Some patients respond to simple plasma infusion, but results of treatment are better with plasma exchange,[117] suggesting that replacement of a deficient plasma factor is an important element of the therapeutic effect. The success of plasma exchange in TTP led to its application in patients with thrombocytopenia and microangiopathy whose clinical features suggest hemolytic uremic syndrome or are difficult to classify.

Many patients with TTP have severe deficiency (<5% of normal activity) of the von Willebrand cleaving metalloproteinase ADAMTS13, which limits the size of circulating von Willebrand factor multimers.[118,119] In adult patients with "acquired" TTP, the deficiency is caused by an IgG autoantibody inhibitor,[118,119] which provides a basis for a variety of immunosuppressive therapies. Simultaneous depletion of inhibitor and infusion of enzyme provide an especially strong and satisfying rationale for plasma exchange (see Chap. 124). In other patients with thrombotic microangiopathy, many of whom have the clinical picture of hemolytic uremic syndrome, ADAMTS13 levels are not severely depressed.[118,120] The rationale for plasma exchange in such patients remains uncertain, and efficacy is doubtful.[121]

A rapid assay for ADAMTS13 might be useful to guide plasma exchange and other immunosuppressive measures in patients with thrombotic microangiopathy. In one retrospective report on a heterogenous group of 142 patients, ADAMTS13 levels did not seem predictive of response to plasma exchange; however, only 13 percent of the patients were severely deficient, and most did not receive initial corticosteroid therapy.[122] In another report from the same center, 27 percent of patients treated for thrombotic microangiopathy had serious therapy-related complications (2 percent fatal); 84 percent of the complications were attributed to central venous catheters placed for plasma exchange.[123] This degree of risk emphasizes the need for prospective studies addressing the efficacy of plasma exchange and other immunosuppressive treatments, especially in patients without severe ADAMTS13 deficiency, to refine future management practices.

RED CELL EXCHANGE

Most red cell exchanges are performed in patients with complications of sickle cell disease. The goal of exchanging patient cells for cells containing hemoglobin A is creating a red cell mixture that has far fewer hemoglobin SS cells. This change may interrupt the vicious cycle of sickling, stasis, vasoocclusion, and progressive ischemia.[124] The ratio of hemoglobin AA cells to hemoglobin SS cells needed to accomplish a salutary effect is not known, but red cell exchanges should aim for a posttreatment blood hemoglobin A level greater than 70 percent so that a level greater than 50 percent persists for several weeks. Exchange may be indicated in severe crises such as stroke,[125] chest syndrome,[126,127] cholestasis,[128,129] and priapism.[130,131] Exchange in priapism sometimes is associated with neurologic events occurring up to 11 days later.[132] Prophylactic exchange is not indicated for simple pain crisis[133] but may prevent future events in patients with frequent or overlapping crises. Prophylactic red cell exchange has been recommended for pregnant patients and prior to general anesthesia, but these two indications are controversial.[134] Long-term maintenance of a hemoglobin A level greater than 70 percent is recommended for patients who have sustained a stroke or have imaging evidence of brain ischemia.[134,135] Prophylactic red cell exchange can achieve this level with a far lower risk of iron overload than frequent simple transfusion but requires exposure to more red cell units.[136]

In other applications, red cell exchange can lower parasite load in severe falciparum malaria and babesiosis.[124] Exchange of red cells for a plasma substitute can lower hematocrit rapidly, without hypovolemia, in polycythemic states[137] and deplete iron more rapidly than simple phlebotomy in hemochromatosis.[138] Finally, exchange of plasma for red cells can rapidly raise hematocrit without producing hypervolemia.[139]

REFERENCES

1. McLeod BC: An approach to evidenced-based therapeutic apheresis. *J Clin Apheresis* 17:124, 2002.
2. Strauss RG, McLeod BC: Complications of therapeutic apheresis, in *Transfusion Reactions*, edited by MA Popovsky, p 281. AABB Press, Bethesda, MD, 1996.
3. McLeod BC, Price TH, Owen H, et al: Frequency of immediate adverse effects associated with therapeutic apheresis. *Transfusion* 39:282, 1999.
4. Bolan CD, Greer SE, Cecco SA, et al: Comprehensive analysis of citrate effects during plateletpheresis in normal donors. *Transfusion* 41:1165, 2001.
5. Bolan CD, Cecco SA, Wesley RA, et al: Controlled study of citrate effects and response to i.v. calcium administration during allogeneic peripheral blood progenitor cell donation. *Transfusion* 42:935, 2002.
6. Hester J: Therapeutic cell depletion, in *Apheresis: Principles and Practice*, 2nd ed, edited by BC McLeod, TH Price, R Weinstein, p 283. AABB Press, Bethesda, MD, 2003.
7. Mercer B, Drouin J, Jolly E, D'Anjou G: Primary thrombocythemia in pregnancy: A report of two cases. *Am J Obstet Gynecol* 159:127, 1988.
8. Klippel JH: Apheresis: Biotechnology and the rheumatic diseases. *Arthritis Rheum* 27:1081, 1984.
9. McFarland HF, Rose JW: Lymphocytapheresis in the treatment of multiple sclerosis. *Plasma Ther Transfus Technol* 3:411, 1982.
10. Fritz RD, Forkner GE, Freireich EJ, et al: The association of fatal intracranial hemorrhage and blastic "crisis" in patients with acute leukemia. *N Engl J Med* 261:59, 1959.
11. Freireich E, Thomas L, Rei E, et al: A distinctive type of intracerebral hemorrhage associated with "blastic crisis" in patients with leukemia. *Cancer* 13:146, 1960.
12. McKee LC, Collins RD: Intravascular leukocyte thrombi and aggregates as a cause of morbidity and mortality in leukemia. *Medicine* 53:463, 1974.
13. Ventura GJ, Hester JP, Smith TL, Keating MJ: Acute myeloblastic leukemia with hyperleukocytosis: Risk factors for early mortality in induction. *Am J Hematol* 27:34, 1988.
14. Maurer HS, Steinharz PG, Gaynon PS, et al: The effect of initial management of hyperleukocytosis on early complications and outcome of children with acute lymphoblastic leukemia. *J Clin Oncol* 6:1425, 1988.
15. Morse EE, Carbone PP, Freireich EJ, et al: Repeated leukapheresis of patients with chronic myelocytic leukemia. *Transfusion* 6:175, 1966.
16. Morse EE, Freireich EJ, Carbone PP, et al: The transfusion of leukocytes from donors with chronic myelocytic leukemia to patients with leukopenia. *Transfusion* 6:183, 1966.
17. Hester JP, McCredie KB, Freireich EJ: Response to chronic leukapheresis procedures and survival of chronic myelogenous leukemia patients. *Transfusion* 22:305, 1982.
18. Caplan SM, Coco FV, Berkman EM: Management of chronic myelocytic leukemia in pregnancy by cell pheresis. *Transfusion* 18:120, 1978.
19. Lichtman MA, Rowe JM: Hyperleukocytic leukemias: Rheological, clinical, and therapeutic considerations. *Blood* 60:279, 1982.
20. Edelson R, Factor M, Andrews A, et al: Successful management of the Sézary syndrome. *N Engl J Med* 291:293, 1974.
21. Belter SV, Knop J, Bruske K, Sorg C: Leukapheresis in the treatment of cutaneous T-cell lymphomas. *Br J Dermatol* 115:159, 1986.
22. Edelson RL, Berger C, Gasparro F, et al: Treatment of cutaneous T-cell lymphoma by extracorporeal photochemotherapy. *N Engl J Med* 316:297, 1987.

23. Marks DI, Rockman SP, Oziemski MA, Fox RM: Mechanisms of lymphocytotoxicity induced by extracorporeal photochemistry for cutaneous T cell lymphoma. *J Clin Invest* 86:2080, 1990.

24. Lim HW, Edelson RL: Photopheresis for the treatment of cutaneous T-cell lymphoma. *Hematol Oncol Clin North Am* 9:1117, 1995.

25. Mechanic SA, Krause D, Proytcheva MA, Snyder EL: Mobilization and collection of peripheral blood progenitor cells, in *Apheresis: Principles and Practice*, 2nd ed, edited by BC McLeod, TH Price, R Weinstein, p 503. AABB Press, Bethesda, MD, 2003.

26. Klein HG: Cellular gene therapy, in *Apheresis: Principles and Practice*, 2nd ed, edited by BC McLeod, TH Price, R Weinstein, p 643. AABB Press, Bethesda, MD, 2003.

27. Becker PS, Wagle M, Matous S, et al: Spontaneous splenic rupture following administration of granulocyte colony-stimulating factor (G-CSF): Occurrence in an allogeneic donor of peripheral blood stem cells. *Biol Blood Marrow Transplant* 3:45, 1997.

28. Adler BK, Salzman DE, Calabresi H, et al: Fatal sickle cell crisis after granulocyte colony-stimulating factor administration. *Blood* 97:3313, 2001.

29. Porter DL: The graft-vs-tumor potential of allogeneic cell therapy: An update on donor leukocyte infusions and nonmyeloablative allogeneic stem cell transplantation. *J Hematother Stem Cell Res* 10:465, 2001.

30. Ribas A, Butterfield LH, Glaspy JA, Economou JS: Current developments in cancer vaccines and cellular immunotherapy. *J Clin Oncol* 21:2415, 2003.

31. Weinstein R: Basic principles of therapeutic blood exchange, in *Apheresis: Principles and Practice*, 2nd ed, edited by BC McLeod, TH Price, R Weinstein, p 295. AABB Press, Bethesda, MD, 2003.

32. Rawal A, Anderson C, Rodgers ZR, et al: Isovolemic hemodilution followed by red cell exchange in patients with sickle cell disease [abstract]. *J Clin Apheresis* 17:153, 2002.

33. McLeod BC, Sassetti RJ, Stefoski D, Davis FA: Partial plasma protein replacement in therapeutic plasma exchange. *J Clin Apheresis* 1:115, 1983.

34. Schwab PJ, Fahey JL: Treatment of Waldenström's macroglobulinemia by plasmapheresis. *N Engl J Med* 263:574, 1960.

35. Solomon A, Fahey JL: Plasmapheresis therapy in macroglobulinemia. *Ann Intern Med* 58:789, 1963.

36. Berkman EM, Orlin JB: Use of plasmapheresis and partial plasma exchange in the management of patients with cryoglobulinemia. *Transfusion* 20:171, 1980.

37. McLeod BC, Sassetti RJ: Plasmapheresis with return of cryoglobulin-depleted autologous plasma (cryoglobulinpheresis) in cryoglobulinemia. *Blood* 55:866, 1980.

38. Wahlin A, Lofvenberg E, Holm J: Improved survival in multiple myeloma with renal failure. *Acta Med Scand* 221:205, 1987.

39. Johnson WJ, Kyle RA, Pineda AA, et al: Treatment of renal failure associated with multiple myeloma. *Arch Intern Med* 150:863, 1990.

40. McCrae KR, Herman JH: Posttransfusion purpura: Two unusual cases and a literature review. *Am J Hematol* 52:205, 1996.

41. Mueller-Eckhardt C, Kiefel V: High dose IgG for post-transfusion purpura revisited. *Blut* 57:163, 1988.

42. Marder VJ, Nusbacher J, Anderson FW: One-year follow-up of plasma exchange therapy in 14 patients with idiopathic thrombocytopenic purpura. *Transfusion* 21:291, 1981.

43. Blanchette VS, Hogan VA, McCombie NE, et al: Intensive plasma exchange therapy in ten patients with idiopathic thrombocytopenic purpura. *Transfusion* 24:388, 1984.

44. Bussel JB: Autoimmune thrombocytopenic purpura. *Hematol Oncol Clin North Am* 4:179, 1990.

45. Mittelman A, Bertram H, Henry DH, et al: Treatment of patients with HIV thrombocytopenia and hemolytic uremic syndrome with protein A

46. Snyder HW, Cochran SK, Balint JP, et al: Experience with Protein A-immunoadsorption in treatment resistant immune thrombocytopenic purpura. *Blood* 79:2237, 1992.

47. Koo AP: Therapeutic apheresis in autoimmune and rheumatic disorders. *J Clin Apheresis* 15:18, 2000.

48. Hughes P, Toogood A: Plasma exchange as a necessary prerequisite for the induction of remission by human immunoglobulin in auto-immune haemolytic anemia. *Acta Haematol* 91:166, 1994.

49. Silva VA, Seder RH, Weintraub LR: Synchronization of plasma exchange and cyclophosphamide in severe and refractory autoimmune hemolytic anemia. *J Clin Apheresis* 9:120, 1994.

50. Brooks BD, Steane EA, Sheehan RG, et al: Therapeutic plasma exchange in the immune hemolytic anemias and immunologic thrombocytopenic purpura. *Prog Clin Biol Res* 106:317, 1982.

51. Silberstein LE, Berkman EM: Plasma exchange in autoimmune hemolytic anemia (AIHA). *J Clin Apheresis* 1:238, 1983.

52. Valbonesi M, Guzzini D, Zerbi D, et al: Successful plasma exchange for a patient with chronic demyelinating polyneuropathy and cold agglutinin disease due to anti-Pr_a. *J Clin Apheresis* 3:109, 1986.

53. Geurs F, Ritter K, Mast A, Van Maele V: Successful plasmapheresis in corticosteroid-resistant hemolysis in infectious mononucleosis: Role of autoantibodies against triosephosphate isomerase. *Acta Haematol* 88:142, 1992.

54. Nilsson IM, Berntorp E, Freiburghaus C: Treatment of patients with factor VIII and IX inhibitors. *Thromb Haemost* 70:56, 1993.

55. Cohen AJ, Kessler CM: Acquired inhibitors. *Baillieres Clin Haematol* 9:331, 1996.

56. Nilsson IM, Berntorp E, Zettervoll O: Induction of immune tolerance in patients with hemophilia and antibodies to factor VIII by combined treatment with intravenous IgG, cyclophosphamide, and factor VIII. *N Engl J Med* 318:947, 1988.

57. Uehlinger J, Button GR, McCarthy JM, et al: Immunoadsorption for coagulation factor inhibitors. *Transfusion* 31:269, 1991.

58. Grima KM: Therapeutic apheresis in hematological and oncological diseases. *J Clin Apheresis* 15:28, 2000.

59. Berkman EM, Caplan W, Kim GS: ABO-incompatible bone marrow transplantation: Preparation by plasma exchange and in vivo antibody absorption. *Transfusion* 18:504, 1978.

60. Bensinger WL, Baker DA, Buckner CD, et al: Immunoadsorption for removal of A and B blood group antibodies. *N Engl J Med* 304:160, 1981.

61. Bensinger WL, Baker DA, Buckner CD, et al: In vitro and in vivo removal of anti-A erythrocyte antibody by adsorption to a synthetic immunoadsorbent. *Transfusion* 21:335, 1981.

62. Braine HG, Sensenbrenner LL, Wright SK, et al: Bone marrow transplantation with major ABO incompatibility using erythrocyte depletion of marrow prior to infusion. *Blood* 60:420, 1982.

63. Rock G, Lafreniere I, Chan L, McCombie N: Plasma exchange in the treatment of hemolytic disease of the newborn. *Transfusion* 21:546, 1981.

64. Filbey D, Berseus O, Lindeberg S, Wesstrom G: A management programme for Rh alloimmunization during pregnancy. *Early Hum Dev* 15:11, 1987.

65. Watson WJ, Katz VL, Bowes WA: Plasmapheresis during pregnancy. *Obstet Gynecol* 76:451, 1990.

66. The Guillain-Barré Syndrome Study Group: Plasmapheresis and acute Guillain-Barré syndrome. *Neurology* 35:1096, 1985.

67. Osterman PG, Lundemo G, Pirskanen R, et al: Beneficial effects of plasma exchange in acute inflammatory polyradiculoneuropathy. *Lancet* 2:1296, 1984.

68. French Cooperative Group on Plasma Exchange and Guillain-Barré Syndrome: Efficiency of plasma exchange in Guillain-Barré syndrome: Role of replacement fluids. *Ann Neurol* 22:753, 1987.

(Prosorba column) immunoadsorption. *Semin Hematol* 26(suppl 1):15, 1989.

69. Vriesendorp FJ, Mishu B, Blaser MJ, Koski CL: Serum antibodies to GM1, GD16, peripheral nerve myelin, and *Campylobacter jejuni* in patients with Guillain-Barré syndrome and controls. *Ann Neurol* 34:130, 1993.

70. Rees JH, Gregson NA, Hughes RA: Anti-ganglioside GM1 antibodies in Guillain-Barré syndrome and their relationship to *Campylobacter jejuni* infection. *Ann Neurol* 38:809, 1995.

71. Rees JH, Soudain SE, Gregson NA, Hughes RAC: *Campylobacter jejuni* infection and Guillain-Barré syndrome. *N Engl J Med* 333:1374, 1995.

72. Hadden RDM, Karch H, Hartung H-P, et al: Preceding infections, immune factors, and outcome in Guillain-Barré syndrome. *Neurology* 56:758, 2001.

73. Connolly AM, Pestronk A, Trotter JL, et al: High-titer selective anti-beta-tubulin antibodies in chronic demyelinating polyneuropathy. *Neurology* 43:557, 1993.

74. Simone IL, Annunziata P, Maimone D, et al: Serum and CSF anti-GM1 antibodies in patients with Guillain-Barré syndrome and chronic inflammatory demyelinating polyneuropathy. *J Neurol Sci* 114:49, 1993.

75. Khalili-Shirazi A, Atkinson P, Gregson N, Hughes RAC: Antibody response to P$_0$ and P$_2$ myelin proteins in Guillain-Barré syndrome and chronic inflammatory demyelinating polyradiculoneuropathy. *J Neuroimmunol* 46:245, 1993.

76. Dyck PJ, Daube J, O'Brien P, et al: Plasma exchange in chronic inflammatory demyelinating polyradiculoneuropathy. *N Engl J Med* 314:461, 1986.

77. Hahn AF, Bolton CF, Pillay N, et al: Plasma exchange therapy in chronic inflammatory demyelinating polyneuropathy. *Brain* 119:1055, 1996.

78. Dyck PJ, Low PA, Windebank AJ, et al: Plasma exchange in polyneuropathy associated with monoclonal gammopathy of undetermined significance. *N Engl J Med* 325:1482, 1991.

79. Masselli RA: Pathophysiology of myasthenia gravis and Lambert-Eaton syndrome. *Neurol Clin* 12:285, 1994.

80. Seybold ME: Plasmapheresis in myasthenia gravis. *Ann N Y Acad Sci* 505:584, 1987.

81. Lisak RP: Plasma exchange in neurologic disease. *Arch Neurol* 41:654, 1984.

82. Dalakas MC, Fujii M, Li M, McElroy B: The clinical spectrum of anti-GAD antibody-positive patients with stiff-person syndrome. *Neurology* 55:1531, 2000.

83. Moll JWB, Vecht CJ: Immune diagnoses of paraneoplastic neurologic disease. *Clin Neurol Neurosurg* 97:71, 1995.

84. Butler MH, Hayashi A, Ohkoshi N, et al: Autoimmunity to gephyrin in stiff-man syndrome. *Neuron* 26:307, 2000.

85. Rodgers SW, Andress PI, Gahring LC, et al: Autoantibodies to glutamate receptor Glu R3 in Rasmussen's encephalitis. *Science* 265:648, 1994.

86. Moll JWB, Vecht CJ: Immune diagnosis of paraneoplastic neurological disease. *Clin Neurol Neurosurg* 97:71, 1995.

87. Das A, Hochberg FH, McNelis S: A review of the therapy of paraneoplastic neurologic syndromes. *J Neurooncol* 41:181, 1999.

88. Kalluri R, Gunwar S, Reeders ST, et al: Goodpasture syndrome: Localization of the epitope for the autoantibodies to the carboxy terminal region of the alpha 3(IV) chain of basement membrane collagen. *J Biol Chem* 266:24018, 1991.

89. Levy JB, Turner AN, Rees AJ, Pusey CD: Long-term outcome of anti-glomerular basement membrane antibody disease treated with plasma exchange and immunosuppression. *Ann Intern Med* 134:1033, 2001.

90. Lewis EJ, Hunsicker LG, Lan S-P, et al: A controlled trial of plasmapheresis therapy in severe lupus nephritis. *N Engl J Med* 326:1373, 1992.

91. Doria A, Piccoli A, Vesco P, et al: Therapy of lupus nephritis. *Ann Med Interne (Paris)* 145:307, 1994.

92. Pusey CD, Rees AJ, Evans DJ, et al: Plasma exchange in focal necrotizing glomerulonephritis without anti-GBM antibodies. *Kidney Int* 40:757, 1991.

93. Glöckner WM, Sieberth HG, Wichmann HE, et al: Plasma exchange and immunosuppression in rapidly progressive glomerulonephritis: A controlled, multi-center study. *Clin Nephrol* 29:1, 1988.

94. Cole E, Cattran D, Magil A, et al: A prospective randomized trial of plasma exchange as additive therapy in idiopathic crescentic glomerulonephritis. *Am J Kidney Dis* 20:261, 1992.

95. Gerraty RP, McKelvie PA, Byrne E: Aseptic meningoencephalitis in primary Sjögren's syndrome. *Acta Neurol Scand* 88:309, 1993.

96. Jenkins HR, Jewkes F, Vujanic GM: Systemic vasculitis complicating infantile autoimmune enteropathy. *Arch Dis Child* 71:534, 1994.

97. Fauci AS, Leavitt RY: Systemic vasculitis, in *Current Therapy in Allergy, Immunology and Rheumatology*, edited by LM Liechtenstein, AS Fauci, p 149. Decker, Toronto, 1988.

98. Aringer M, Smolen J, Graninger W: Severe infections in plasmapheresis-treated systemic lupus erythematosus. *Arthritis Rheum* 41:414, 1998.

99. Schroeder JO, Schwab U, Zennet R, et al: Plasmapheresis and subsequent pulse cyclophosphamide in severe systemic lupus erythematosus. Preliminary results of the LPSG-Trial. *Arthritis Rheum* 40:S325, 1997.

100. Winters JL, Pineda A, McLeod BC, Grima K: Therapeutic apheresis in renal and metabolic diseases. *J Clin Apheresis* 15:53, 2000.

101. Crespo M, Pascual M, Tolkoff-Rubin N, et al: Acute humoral rejection in renal allograft recipients: I. Incidence, serology and clinical characteristics. *Transplantation* 71:652, 2001.

102. Montgomery RA, Zachary AA, Racusen LC, et al: Plasmapheresis and intravenous immune globulin provides effective rescue therapy for refractory humoral rejection and allows kidneys to be successfully transplanted into crossmatch-positive recipients. *Transplantation* 70:887, 2000.

103. Taube D, Palmer A, Welsh K, et al: Removal of anti-HLA antibodies prior to transplantation: An effective and successful strategy for highly sensitised renal allograft recipients. *Transplant Proc* 21:694, 1989

104. Montgomery R, Ratner L, Samaniego M, et al: Successful transplantation across HLA and ABO sensitization. *Hum Immunol* 63(suppl 10):S83, 2002.

105. Ginsberg HN: Update on the treatment of hypercholesterolemia, with a focus on HMG-CoA reductase inhibitors and combination regimens. *Clin Cardiol* 18:307, 1995.

106. Mabuchi H, Koizumi J, Michishita I, et al: Effects on coronary atherosclerosis of long-term treatment of familial hypercholesterolemia by LDL-apheresis. *Beitr Infusionther* 23:87, 1988.

107. Lane DM, McConathy WJ, Laughlin LO, et al: Weekly treatment of diet/drug-resistant hypercholesterolemia with the heparin-induced extracorporeal low-density lipoprotein precipitation (HELP) system by selective plasma low-density lipoprotein removal. *Am J Cardiol* 71:816, 1993.

108. Knisel W, Pfohl M, Müller M, et al: Comparative long-term experience with immunoadsorption and dextran sulfate cellulose adsorption for extracorporeal elimination of low-density lipoproteins. *Clin Invest* 72:660, 1994.

109. Gordon BR, Kelsey SF, Dan P, et al: Long-term effects of low-density lipoprotein apheresis using an automated dextran sulfate cellulose adsorption system. *Am J Cardiol* 81:407, 1998.

110. Lane DM, McConathy WJ, Laughlin LO, et al: Weekly treatment of diet/drug-resistant hypercholesterolemia with the heparin-induced extracorporeal low-density lipoprotein precipitation (HELP) system by selective plasma low-density lipoprotein removal. *Am J Cardiol* 71:816, 1993.

111. Gibberd FB: Plasma exchange for Refsum's disease. *Transfus Sci* 14:23, 1993.

112. Gutsche H-U, Siegmund JB, Hoppmann I: Lipapheresis: An immuno-globulin-sparing treatment for Refsum's disease. *Acta Neurol Scand* 94: 190, 1996.

113. Kondrup J, Almdal T, Vilstrup H, et al: High volume plasma exchange in fulminant hepatic failure. *Int J Artif Organs* 15:669, 1992.

114. Byrnes JJ, Moake JL, Periman P: Effectiveness of the cryosupernatant fraction of plasma in the treatment of refractory thrombotic thrombocytopenic purpura. *Am J Hematol* 34:169, 1990.

115. Welborn JL, Emrick P, Acevedo M: Rapid improvement of thrombotic thrombocytopenic purpura with vincristine and plasmapheresis. *Am J Hematol* 35:18, 1990.

116. Rock G, Shumak K, Kelton J, et al: Thrombotic thrombocytopenic purpura: Outcome in 24 patients with renal impairment treated with plasma exchange. *Transfusion* 32:710, 1992.

117. Rock GA, Shumak KH, Buskard NA, et al: Comparison of plasma exchange with plasma infusion in the treatment of thrombotic thrombocytopenic purpura. *N Engl J Med* 325:393, 1991.

118. Furlan M, Robles R, Galbusera M, et al: Von Willebrand factor-cleaving protease in thrombotic thrombocytopenic purpura and the hemolytic-uremic syndrome. *N Engl J Med* 339:1578, 1998.

119. Tsai H-M, Lian EC-Y: Antibodies to von Willebrand factor-cleaving protease in acute thrombotic thrombocytopenic purpura. *N Engl J Med* 339:1585, 1998.

120. Veyradier A, Obert B, Houllier A, et al: Specific von Willebrand factor-cleaving protease in thrombotic microangiopathies: A study of 111 cases. *Blood* 98:1765, 2001.

121. McLeod BC: Thrombotic microangiopathies in bone marrow and organ transplant patients. *J Clin Apheresis* 17:118, 2002.

122. Vesely SK, George JN, Lämmele B, et al: ADAMTS13 activity in thrombotic thrombocytopenic purpura-hemolytic uremic syndrome: Relation to presenting features and clinical outcomes in a prospective cohort. *Blood* 102:60, 2003.

123. McMinn JR Jr, Thomas IA, Terrell DR, et al: Complication of plasma exchange in thrombotic thrombocytopenic purpura-hemolytic uremic syndrome. A study of 78 additional patients. *Transfusion* 43:415, 2003.

124. Pepkowitz S: Red cell exchange and other therapeutic alterations of red cell mass, in *Apheresis: Principles and Practice*, 2nd ed, edited by BC McLeod, TH Price, R Weinstein, p 411. AABB Press, Bethesda, MD, 2003.

125. Adams RJ: Stroke prevention and treatment in sickle cell disease. *Arch Neurol* 58:565, 2001.

126. Vichinsky EP, Syles LA, Colangelo LH, et al: Acute chest syndrome in sickle cell disease: Clinical presentation and course. *Blood* 89:1787, 1997.

127. Emre U, Miller ST, Gutierez M, et al: Effect of transfusion in acute chest syndrome of sickle cell disease. *Pediatrics* 127:901, 1995.

128. Rossof AH, McLeod BC, Holmes AW, Fried W: Intrahepatic sickling crisis in hemoglobin SC disease: Management by partial exchange transfusion. *Plasma Ther* 2:7, 1981.

129. Sheehy TW, Law DE, Wade BH: Exchange transfusion for sickle cell intrahepatic cholestasis. *Arch Intern Med* 140:1364, 1980.

130. Hamre MR, Harmon EP, Kirkpatrick DV, et al: Priapism as a complication of sickle cell disease. *J Urol* 145:1, 1991.

131. Chakrabarty A, Upadhyay J, Dhabuwala CB, et al: Priapism associated with sickle cell hemoglobinopathy in children: Long-term effects on potency. *J Urol* 155:1419, 1996.

132. Rackoff WR, Ohene-Frempong K, Month S, et al: Neurologic events after partial exchange transfusion for priapism in sickle cell disease. *J Pediatr* 120:882, 1992.

133. Kleinman SH, Hurvitz CG, Goldfinger D: Use of erythrocytapheresis in the treatment of patients with sickle cell disease. *J Clin Apheresis* 2: 170, 1984.

134. Telen MJ: Principles and problems of transfusion in sickle cell disease. *Semin Hematol* 38:315, 2001.

135. Cohen AR, Martin MB, Silber JH, et al: A modified transfusion program for prevention of stroke in sickle cell disease. *Blood* 79:1657, 1992.

136. Vichinsky E: Consensus document for transfusion-related iron overload. *Semin Hematol* 38:2, 2001.

137. Kaboth U, Rumph KW, Liersch T, et al: Advantages of isovolemic large-volume erythrocytapheresis as a rapidly effective and long-lasting treatment modality for red blood cell depletion in patients with polycythemia vera. *Ther Apheresis* 1:131, 1997.

138. Cesana M, Mandelli C, Tiribelli C, et al: Concomitant primary hemochromatosis and β-thalassemia trait: Iron depletion by erythrocytapheresis and desferrioxamine. *Am J Gastroenterol* 84:150, 1989.

139. McLeod BC, Reed SR, Viernes AV, Valentino L: Rapid red cell transfusion by apheresis. *J Clin Apheresis* 9:142, 1994.

PRINCIPLES OF GENE TRANSFER FOR THERAPY

JANUARIO E. CASTRO

THOMAS J. KIPPS

The term "gene therapy" describes treatment resulting from insertion of a gene(s) into somatic cells. High-level expression of a transferred gene (or *transgene*) can be achieved in almost any type of mammalian cell. Once inside the cell, the transgene can direct synthesis of an intracellular cell surface or secreted protein that can complement a genetic deficiency or confer upon the cell a desired phenotype or function. Alternatively, the transferred genetic material can repress expression of genes encoding unwanted or mutated proteins through "gene interference" or gene complementation. Conceivably, transfer and expression of appropriate genes could correct genetic deficiencies or generate somatic cells with a desired characteristic(s) that can result in therapeutic benefit. Many clinical trials have involved gene therapy for patients with various hematologic diseases, such as leukemia, lymphoma, Gaucher disease, aplastic anemia, hemoglobinopathies, or coagulation factor deficiencies.[1] The full application of this technology in clinical practice has not yet been realized. Results from some clinical trials suggest gene therapy may be useful for treatment of a variety of genetic or acquired diseases, including hematologic disorders. This chapter reviews the basic principles of gene transfer and the results of selected preclinical and clinical studies.

MECHANISM OF GENE TRANSFER

VIRUS VECTORS

Vectors can be derived from viruses such as retroviruses or adenoviruses. Such vectors can transfer their genetic material into somatic cells with high efficiency. Virus entry can be accomplished by binding to cell surface receptors or through nonspecific attachment. Typically, such viruses bind and enter host cells via receptor-mediated endocytosis, allowing for efficient entry of the virus genetic material into the cell. Table 26-1 lists the cell receptors for specific virus vectors.

Virus vectors generally use viruses that are modified such that they are unable to generate progeny virus except in specific cell lines. The cell lines that can propagate such virus vectors generally have been genetically modified to complement the replication defect of the virus

Acronyms and abbreviations that appear in this chapter include: AAV, adeno-associated virus; ADA, adenosine deaminase; AIDS, acquired immunodeficiency syndrome; AML, acute myelogenous leukemia; CAR, coxsackie adenovirus receptor; cDNA, copy or complementary DNA; CLL, chronic lymphocytic leukemia; CMV, cytomegalovirus; CTL, cytotoxic T lymphocytes; dsDNA, double-stranded DNA; dsRNA, double-stranded RNA; FA, Fanconi anemia; GC, glucocerebrosidase; HIV, human immunodeficiency virus; HSV, herpes simplex virus; Hve-A, herpes virus entry mediator-A; IFN, interferon; IL, interleukin; *IL2RG*, interleukin-2 receptor gene; kb, kilobase; NPM-ALK, nucleophosmin-anaplastic lymphoma kinase; RNAi, RNA interference; SCID-Xl, X-linked severe combined immune deficiency disease; siRNA, small interfering RNA; TLR, Toll-like receptor; TNF, tumor necrosis factor.

vector. These so-called *"packaging cell lines"* express a gene(s) that is deleted or mutated in the virus vector that is essential for generating progeny virus capable of infecting other cells. Ordinary somatic cells that lack this gene(s) cannot complement the genetic defect of such virus vectors and therefore cannot produce infectious progeny virus.

Virus vectors also can be produced by packaging cells that are genetically modified to synthesize and replace the virus vector's envelope proteins with those of another virus, such as vesicular stomatitis virus-G.[2,3] These modified, virus particles are called *pseudotyped* viruses because they have the envelope protein(s) of virus that is distinct from that of the genetic material confined within the particle. Generally, the envelope protein(s) selected for generating pseudotyped viruses is derived from viruses that have a broader or more-desired tissue tropism and/or more resilient physical characteristics. Table 26-1 lists some examples of pseudotyped virus and their receptors.

Upon binding and entry into the target cell, the virus vector inserts its genetic material into the infected cell. The RNA of retroviruses must first be modified prior to its transport to the nucleus. For this purpose, retroviruses carry a reverse transcriptase that converts the virus single-stranded RNA into copy or complementary DNA (cDNA). DNA viruses, such as adenovirus or adeno-associated virus (AAV), on the other hand, do not require such modification. In any case, during productive infection, the virus genome or its cDNA is transported to the nucleus, where it usurps host cellular machinery to direct the synthesis of virus-specific proteins and assembly of new virus particles (Fig. 26-1).

TABLE 26-1   VECTORS USED IN GENE THERAPY AND THEIR RECEPTORS

VECTOR	CELLULAR RECEPTORS
Retroviruses	
Amphotropic retrovirus	Sodium-phosphate symporters (e.g., Ram-1)
Ecotropic retrovirus	Cationic amino acid transport proteins (e.g., CAT 1 or Rec-1)
Lentivirus (HIV-1)	CD4 and CCR5 or CXCR4
Viruses Used to Make *Pseudotyped* Vectors	
Vesicular stomatitis virus (VSV)	Phosphatidylserine
Gibbon ape leukemia virus (GALV)	Sodium-phosphate symporters (e.g., Glvr-1)
Adenovirus serotype 27 (Ad37)	(see Ad37 below)
Adeno-associated virus serotype 6 (AAV-6)	(see AAV-6 below)
Adenovirus	
Ad2, Ad4, Ad5, Ad17 serotypes	Coxsackievirus/adenovirus receptor (CAR) (1° receptor) and integrins $\alpha_\gamma\beta_3$ or $\alpha_\gamma\beta_5$ (2° receptors for internalization)
Ad11, Ad16, Ad21, Ad35 serotypes	Complement regulatory protein CD46 and/or receptors other than CAR
Ad37 serotype	Sialic acid residues or a 50-kDa membrane receptor protein that appears more broadly expressed than CAR
Adeno-associated Virus (AAV)	
AAV-2, AAV-3	Heparan sulfate (1° receptor) or fibroblast growth factor receptor-1 (alternative receptor for AAV-2) and integrin $\alpha_\gamma\beta_5$ (2° receptor for internalization)
AAV-6	Receptor other than that used by AAV-2 that is expressed at high level on skeletal muscle
Herpes Simplex Virus	
HSV-1	Herpesvirus entry mediator-A (Hve-A), nectin-1 (HveC/CD111), and/or 3-*O*-sulfated glucosamine residues
HSV-2	Nectin-2

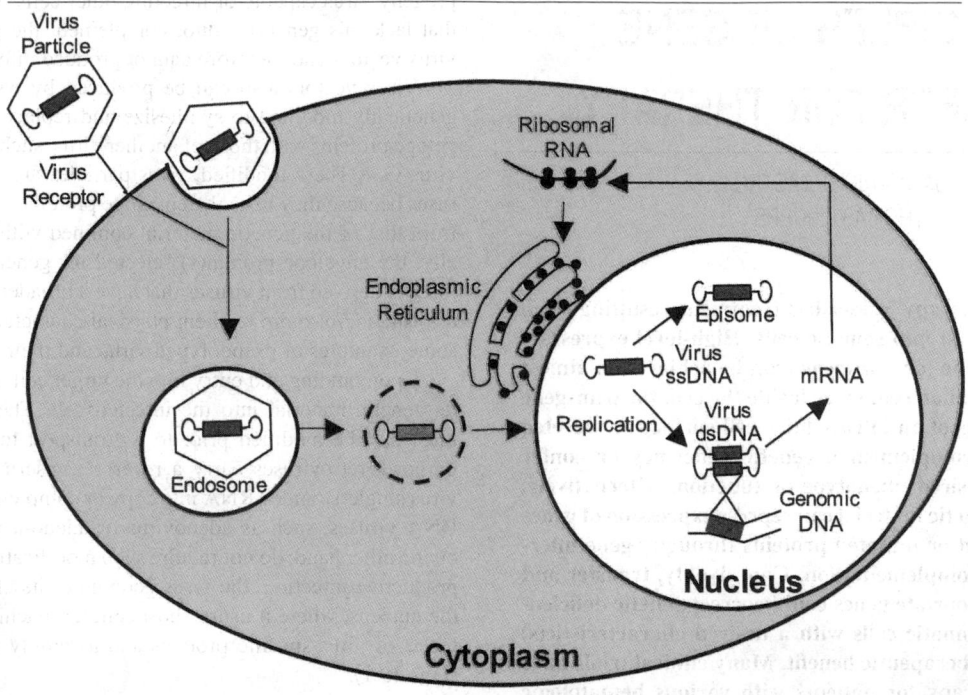

FIGURE 26-1   Interaction of vector with target cells. Virus vector binding to the target cell, its passage through the cell membrane, and subsequent release of the vector genome from the endosome are shown. Following trafficking of the vector genome to the nucleus, the genes within the episomal or integrated vector genome can be transcribed, allowing for production of transgene RNA, which then can be translated into protein. ssDNA, single stranded DNA; dsDNA, double-stranded DNA.

RETROVIRUS VECTORS

Retrovirus vectors are lipid-enveloped particles containing a positive-sense, single-stranded RNA that typically is 7 to 11 kilobases (kb) in length. These vectors produce stable, high-level transgene expression in the infected cell and its progeny.

The *Retroviridae* family includes several members that are used as vectors in gene therapy. The viruses initially evaluated were the mammalian and avian C-type retroviruses (oncoretroviruses). More recently, spumavirus and lentivirus, which includes the human immune deficiency virus (HIV), have been modified for use in gene transfer.

The preintegration nuclear protein complex of oncoretroviruses, such as murine leukemia virus, is relatively unstable and cannot be used for effecting transgene expression in nondividing cells. In contrast, the preintegration complex of lentiviruses is more stable and can transit through the intact nuclear membrane.[4] Therefore, lentivirus-derived vectors have an advantage over previously used retrovirus vectors in that their cDNA can enter into the nucleus of nondividing cells,[5] where it can integrate into the host cell's genome, a requirement for retrovirus transgene expression.

Both oncoretrovirus and lentivirus vectors integrate into the host cell genome, a requirement for expression of virus-encoded transgenes. Insertions in or near host cell genes can result in "insertional mutagenesis." Such insertional mutagenesis has been implicated in the development of leukemia in patients with X-linked severe combined immune deficiency (SCID-X1) who were treated with lentivirus-vectors encoding the interleukin (IL)-2 receptor gene *IL2RG*.[6,7]

Retrovirus vectors can be used for cell marking with genes encoding neomycin resistance or green fluorescent protein and for biologic tracking of transplanted hematopoietic cells during engraftment or at the time of clinical relapse.[8–10]

ADENOVIRUS VECTORS

Adenovirus vectors also are used for gene therapy. More than 50 different human adenovirus serotypes exist, but current vectors primarily are derived from serotypes 2 and 5.[11] In some cases, these vectors are modified by deleting important replication genes, rendering the virus replication incompetent and creating space for insertion of a desired transgene(s).[12] In contrast to retrovirus vectors, adenovirus vectors do not pose a risk for insertional mutagenesis because they do not integrate into the host cell's genome.[11]

Several qualities make adenoviruses good candidates for gene therapy. Adenoviruses can be produced and purified with high titers,[13] they can generate high levels of transgene expression in nonproliferating cells, and their double-stranded DNA (dsDNA) genome remains episomal, mitigating the problem of insertional mutagenesis.[14]

However, adenovirus vectors have some disadvantages, including low-level expression of the transgene without a suitable promoter/enhancer to direct gene expression, the inability to transfer the transgene to successive generations of progeny daughter cells, and the capacity to induce T cell–directed immune responses against virus-infected cells that often lead to clearance of transgene-expressing cells.[15,16] Furthermore, antibodies that develop against adenovirus proteins following the initial infection can neutralize the capacity of adenovirus vectors to infect cells *in vivo*.[17] On the other hand, the so-called *immunogenicity* of adenovirus-infected cells can be considered an advantage because immunogenicity may enhance development of antitumor immunity in response to adenovirus-infected tumor cells.[17,18]

The susceptibility to adenovirus type 5 infection generally correlates with the relative expression of coxsackie adenovirus receptor (CAR) protein.[19–21] Because CAR expression is low in many human cells, new adenovirus vectors capable of infecting cells via CAR-independent endocytosis are being developed and evaluated in clinical trials.[22–24]

ADENO-ASSOCIATED VIRUS

AAV is a human parvovirus that initially was discovered as a contaminant in adenovirus preparations. AAV requires a helper virus, such as adenovirus, to mediate a productive infection.[25] Of the 11 known human virus serotypes, AAV-2 is the best studied.[26] No known human disease is associated with AAV.

AAV vectors have a number of qualities that make them highly suitable for gene therapy. The viral dsDNA may remain episomal or integrate into the host cell's genome. This process permits persistent gene expression in nondividing cells and long-term transgene expression in successive generations of daughter cells after genome integration.[26–28] Finally, AAV vectors generally do not induce inflammatory responses or cytotoxic immune responses against infected cells.[29–31]

However, like adenovirus vectors, injection of AAV can elicit neutralizing antibodies that inhibit the capacity of AAV in subsequent injections to infect cells in vivo. Also, AAV can only accept transgenes of relatively small size (<5 kb). Large-scale production and purification of this vector are fraught with problems and require the development of improved packaging cell lines and chromatographic methods.[32,33]

HERPES SIMPLEX VIRUS

Herpes viruses are DNA viruses that can be modified for use as vehicles for gene transfer into somatic cells. Among this family of virus, herpes simplex virus type 1 (HSV-1) is the most extensively studied for potential use in human gene therapy. Its genome consists of 152 kb of linear dsDNA containing at least 84 contiguous genes, of which only 50 percent is essential for virus replication. For this reason, HSV-1 vectors can carry very large transgene inserts (approximately 30 kb), potentially allowing HSV-1 vectors to contain multiple transgenes that can be individually or coordinately expressed.[34]

After deletion of the immediate early gene region, HSV vectors can be grown only in specially engineered packaging cell lines. Such HSV vectors can infect a broad range of somatic cells that in turn cannot produce infectious virus particles.[35] Another attractive feature of HSV vectors is that they can effect high-level expression of a transgene in many different cell types.[36]

HSV can function as a recombinant vector that encodes the transgene of interest or as part of a plasmid-based delivery system or "amplicon," in which the transgene sequence is cloned into a eukaryotic expression plasmid that contains one HSV origin of replication and a packaging signal. This process enables the amplicon to replicate and undergo packaging with the HSV gene products encoded by a cotransfected helper HSV vector.[37,38] Use of such amplicons simplifies vector construction and minimizes the adverse effects caused by infection with live HSV particles.[39]

HSV offers advantages in cellular systems where other vectors are less effective. For example, chronic lymphocytic leukemia (CLL) B cells, which are relatively resistant to infection with retroviruses or adenovirus, are highly sensitive to infection with HSV-1 vectors.[40] The sensitivity results in part because CLL B cells and other lymphoid cells express high levels of the herpes virus entry mediator-A (Hve-A) protein, one of the known receptors for HSV-1.

NONVIRUS-MEDIATED GENE TRANSFER AND INTERFERENCE

Nonvirus vectors use different combinations of DNA or RNA. In general, these systems are easier to produce than are virus vectors.[23,41] Such nonvirus vectors generally lack the efficiency of virus vector–mediated gene delivery systems. However, multiple strategies are being developed to improve gene delivery of nonvirus vectors, including those using cationic lipids,[42] in vivo electroporation,[43] hydrodynamic injection of isotonic saline,[44] cell-penetrating peptides,[45] liposome encapsulation,[46] neoglycoproteins, or glycosylated plasmids.[47] Conceivably, any one or a combination of these techniques someday may improve the efficacy of nonvirus vector systems to levels approaching those of virus-based vector delivery systems.

PLASMID DNA EXPRESSION VECTORS

DNA plasmid expression vectors can be used for gene transfer.[48] Generally, the transgene is placed downstream of a strong promoter, such as the heterologous cytomegalovirus (CMV) promoter/enhancer region and upstream of a polyadenylation signal sequence to allow for appropriate RNA processing and transport from the nucleus.

The efficiency of gene expression following intravascular or intramuscular delivery of naked DNA generally is highest in muscle and liver. High-level transgene expression can be achieved in larger animals, including primates. Improved DNA expression vectors may allow for sustained transgene expression over prolonged periods.[49] Finally, DNA fusion vaccines containing immune-stimulatory sequences can augment the immune response to vector-encoded transgene antigens.[50–52]

OLIGONUCLEOTIDES

Oligonucleotides are short pieces of synthetic, generally single-stranded DNA. Oligonucleotides can be generated with a phosphorothioate backbone that resists degradation by nucleases that otherwise rapidly metabolize standard, single-stranded pieces of DNA and enhances the oligonucleotide half-life.

Oligonucleotides can produce "gene interference" or inhibition of expression of aberrant or undesired genes.[53] Gene interference involves oligonucleotide binding to complementary sequences in a target RNA sequence, thereby inhibiting its processing or expression. The first antisense oligonucleotide was approved in 1998 for treatment of patients with CMV retinitis.[54,55] Several other oligonucleotides with antisense sequences are being evaluated in clinical trials applied to solid tumors and hematologic malignancies.[56]

Certain oligonucleotides can directly stimulate cells, such as macrophages, dendritic cells, or B cells, by interacting with certain toll-like receptors (TLR), such as TLR-9[57] (see Chap. 17). This property is associated with nonmethylated CpG dinucleotides that may be present in the sequence of the oligonucleotide.[58,59]

Finally, oligonucleotides with certain G-rich DNA sequences form G-quartet structures that can specifically interact with and inhibit the function of a selected target protein(s), such as telomerase, thrombin, or signal transduction proteins.[60] Some of these G-quartet DNA oligonucleotides are being developed as potential anticancer agents.

DOUBLE-STRANDED RNA

Double-stranded RNA (dsRNA) can cause selective silencing of genes in multiple cell types.[61] The interference of gene expression that can be affected by dsRNA is termed RNA interference (RNAi).[62]

Several mechanisms have been proposed to account for the mechanism(s) underlying RNAi: (1) dsRNA-directed destruction of target RNA[63,64]; (2) dsRNA suppression of gene transcription by affecting the chromatin structure of the targeted genes[65,66]; (3) dsRNA-directed methylation and silencing of genomic regions that contain the target genes[65,67]; (4) dsRNA-directed inhibition of translation of target genes[68]; and (5) dsRNA-mediated chromosomal rearrangements.[69]

RNAi may have application in gene therapy. RNAi can suppress replication of HIV or other RNA viruses in human cells.[70,71] In addition, RNAi may be used to silence unwanted genes more efficiently than antisense oligonucleotide.[56,72]

dsRNA is an unstable molecule with a relatively short half-life. Several systems are being developed to overcome the problem of dsRNA's instability. For example, one system generates small interfering RNA (siRNA) by virus vectors that produce small stem-loop RNA,[73,74] which can be transcribed using either polymerase III or II promoters. The vector-encoded RNA can be processed inside the cells by the Dicer enzyme into siRNA, which in turn can regulate the expression of selected target genes.[74,75]

GENE THERAPY APPLICATIONS

HEMATOPOIETIC STEM CELLS

Hematopoietic stem cells can be modified with gene therapy protocols to treat a variety of diseases, including primary immune deficiency disease (see Chap. 82), hemoglobinopathies (see Chaps. 46 and 47), metabolic diseases, and various genetic disorders.[76] The main advantage of modifying hematopoietic stem cells is that these cells can undergo self-renewal and/or differentiate into mature cells of different lineages.[77–79]

GENE MARKING OF HEMATOPOIETIC STEM CELLS

The initial clinical trials on the application of hematopoietic stem cells used gene marking to investigate the origin of relapse of leukemia patients subjected to autologous hematopoietic cell transplantation. For this purpose, hematopoietic stem cells were transduced with retrovirus vectors encoding sequences of marker genes. The transduced hematopoietic stem cells were transplanted into the patients, and the marker gene was assessed in normal or neoplastic cells. These studies demonstrated that clinical relapse in patients with acute myelogenous leukemia (AML) and CML resulted from the presence of contaminating residual leukemia cells in the transplanted stem cell collection.[80,81]

INHERITED DISORDERS

ADENOSINE DEAMINASE DEFICIENCY

Adenosine deaminase (ADA) deficiency causes SCID in newborns (see Chap. 82). Currently, ADA-deficient patients who lack an appropriate hematopoietic stem cell donor are treated with pegylated ADA. This expensive treatment is required throughout life and cannot restore the capacity to generate protective immunity in all of these patients.

The genetic treatment of ADA-deficient patients was the first attempt to cure an inherited disease by a gene therapy approach. Retrovirus transduction of the normal ADA gene into blood T lymphocytes of affected patients corrected the deficiency *in vitro* and suggested the feasibility of a gene transfer approach *in vivo*.[82] Subsequently, clinical studies showed encouraging results after transfer of the ADA gene into blood lymphocytes of ADA-deficient patients[83] or when patients were treated with autologous ADA-transduced umbilical cord stem cells.[84]

A later protocol showed the relevance of nonmyeloablative conditioning as a procedure to facilitate engraftment of ADA-transduced CD34+ stem cells.[85] In this trial, investigators observed in treated patients a sustained engraftment of transduced hematopoietic stem cells, increased leukocyte counts, and improved immune function.

X-LINKED SEVERE COMBINED IMMUNE DEFICIENCY

SCID-Xl is caused by mutations in the *IL2RG* X-linked gene that encodes the common γ-chain (γc) of the lymphocyte receptors for IL-2 and other cytokines[86] (see Chap. 82). The only therapy available for this form of SCID is allogeneic hematopoietic cell transplantation,[87] which is predicated upon finding a suitable donor (see Chap. 22).

The initial work in humans used retrovirus-transduced CD34+ autologous hematopoietic stem cells. In treated patients, transgene expression was detectable for prolonged periods and was associated with normalization of immune repertoire of T cells, B cells, and NK cells.[88] These encouraging findings were confirmed in a followup study of six more patients treated under the same protocol. Nine of 11 treated children experienced sustained improvements in immune function.[89]

Some of the patients, however, experienced a late serious adverse effect of therapy. Two patients developed T cell acute lymphoblastic leukemia.[6,90] Both of these patients were found to have insertions of the vector genetic material near the *LMO2* gene in their leukemia T

cells, resulting in dysregulated *LMO2* gene expression.[89–91] This unexpected complication appears to be a complication of insertional mutagenesis.[92]

HEMOGLOBINOPATHIES

High-level regulated globin gene expression is required for therapy of severely affected patients with sickle cell disease (see Chap. 47) or β-thalassemia (see Chap. 46).[93]

Two research groups have achieved transfer and expression of curative levels of β-globin in the red cell progeny of murine stem cells in animal models of β-thalassemia and sickle cell disease.[94,95] Another study evaluated the use of lentivirus vectors encoding a β-globin transgene to transduced, human progenitor stem cells from patients lacking normal β-globin genes. After transfer to immunodeficient mice, the β-globin–transduced human stem cells were able to produce erythroid cells with stable levels of β-globin expression. These animals produced erythroid cells that expressed human β-globin at levels that should be therapeutic in patients with sickle cell anemia or β-thalassemia.[96]

GAUCHER DISEASE

Gaucher disease is a lysosomal storage disorder resulting from a deficiency of glucocerebrosidase (GC) (see Chap. 79). Transduction of murine hematopoietic stem cells has been achieved, with long-term expression of the GC gene in macrophages of transplanted mice.[97] Two clinical trials using Maloney-based retrovirus vectors targeted to human CD34+ cells yielded similar results with low transduction of blood cells.[98,99]

Using AAV- and HIV-1–derived lentivirus vectors, stable expression of human GC protein has been achieved in the blood and liver of experimental animals and in fibroblast derived from patients with Gaucher disease.[100,101]

FANCONI ANEMIA

Fanconi anemia (FA) is an inherited cancer susceptibility syndrome caused by mutations in a DNA repair pathway including at least six Fanconi anemia-complementing genes (see Chap. 33). The A and C genes (*FANCA* and *FANCC*) have been genetically engineered into retrovirus and AAV vectors.[102]

Recombinant lentivirus vectors have been tested in FANCA-/- and FANCC-/- mice.[103] For these particular experiments, long-term repopulating hematopoietic progenitors were transduced with lentivirus vectors encoding the normal gene. Following lentivirus transduction, resistance to DNA-damaging agents was restored, allowing for *in vivo* selection of the corrected cells with nonmyeloablative doses of cyclophosphamide. This approach requires validation using human cells.

HEMOPHILIA

Sustained therapeutic levels of clotting factors VIII and IX could significantly affect the clinical course of patients with hemophilia (see Chap. 115).

Patients with hemophilia B have received intramuscular injections of a recombinant AAV encoding factor IX. No evidence of local or systemic toxicity has been observed up to 40 months after the initial injection. Preexisting high-titer antibodies to AAV did not prevent gene transfer or expression. Despite evidence for gene transfer and expression, circulating levels of factor IX were less than 2 percent in all cases.[104] Another study evaluated the use of AAV encoding factor IX injected directly into the hepatic artery. One of the treated patients experienced significant improvement of the serum levels of factor IX, suggesting the route of administration may be a factor in the efficiency of this approach.[105]

Twelve patients with hemophilia A received intravenous infusion of retrovirus encoding factor VIII.[106] Plasma factor VIII levels increased in six of the treated patients and were associated with a reduced tendency for bleeding. An *ex vivo* approach using nonvirus plasmid transfection of autologous fibroblasts in culture also has been reported.[107] Four of 12 patients with hemophilia A had transient improvement in factor VIII plasma levels.

In general, the outcomes of human trials have been inferior to results observed in animals. Further development in gene delivery and expression systems is required to achieve serum levels of clotting factors that are clinically relevant.

ACQUIRED DISORDERS

ACQUIRED IMMUNODEFICIENCY SYNDROME

HIV/acquired immunodeficiency syndrome (AIDS) currently is best treated with pharmaceutical inhibitors of reverse transcriptase and virus proteases (see Chap. 83). Nevertheless, concerns exist over the long-term efficacy of such treatment, the need for chronic drug administration, the lack of compliance of some patients, and long-term toxicity of the medications. Alternative genetic therapies that could overcome such problems are the subject of much interest.

The potential for generation of a cytotoxic response to HIV-specific elements in HIV patients has provided the bases for vaccination protocols. One study evaluated the activity of autologous fibroblasts modified to express envelope proteins of HIV IIIB as artificial antigen-presenting cells.[108] The study demonstrated that HIV-specific cytotoxic T lymphocyte (CTL) responses could be generated by this protocol. No local or systemic side effects related to treatment were observed.[109]

Other investigators have studied the use of T lymphocytes transduced with vectors expressing the chimeric protein CD4/CD3ζ, which is assembled using the extracellular domain of CD4 and the intracellular domain of the ζ-chain of the T cell receptor. In theory, this chimeric molecule could bind to HIV and, after engagement of the receptor, generate signaling events similar to those elicited by specific antigen binding. In a phase II clinical trial, HIV patients infused with CD4/CD3ζ-transduced T lymphocytes experienced decreased virus load in reservoir sites, such as the rectal mucosa.[110,111]

In another trial using CD34+ hematopoietic stem cells derived from patients with HIV-associated lymphomas, the investigators transduced hematopoietic stem cells with a *trans*-dominant Rev protein.[112] These approaches generated relatively few transduced hematopoietic stem cells with short-term engraftment.

LEUKEMIA AND LYMPHOMA

GENE INTERFERENCE

Strategies using antisense oligonucleotides currently are under evaluation in clinical trials. For example, antisense oligonucleotides targeting the open reading frame of the *BCL-2* mRNA can down-regulate its expression, resulting in increased susceptibility to apoptosis.[113] A phase I clinical trial was performed in which nine lymphoma patients were given repeated daily subcutaneous injections of Genasense™, an 18-base phosphorothioate *BCL-2* antisense oligonucleotide. One patient reportedly had a complete response, and three had stable disease after therapy.[114] This oligonucleotide also has been evaluated in patients with CLL. Some of the patients treated with this oligonucleotide had reduced blood lymphocyte cell counts following therapy, including one patient who apparently experienced a "tumor lysis syndrome."[115] Current studies are evaluating whether such oligonucleotides can enhance the activity of anticancer drugs in patients with different types of malignancies.

Other antisense oligonucleotides targeting *BCR-ABL*, protein kinase C-α, and human telomerase reverse transcriptase have been evaluated in preclinical studies and in phase I and II clinical trials.[116–118] The results of these studies have shown the feasibility and safety of this approach and in some cases partial responses to the treatment modality.

Studies also have evaluated the activity of siRNA in leukemia and lymphoma cells. In one study, three different chemically synthesized siRNAs were used to target the nucleophosmin-anaplastic lymphoma kinase (NPM-ALK) fusion gene that is expressed in anaplastic large cell lymphomas. The siRNAs decreased expression of NPM-ALK protein and increased susceptibility to apoptosis.[119] Similar results were observed in a different study that evaluated siRNA targeting the multidrug resistance mediated by P-glycoprotein.[120]

GENE TRANSFER FOR DEVELOPMENT OF TUMOR VACCINES

Studies have evaluated the use of lymphoma or leukemia cells transduced with immune-stimulatory genes to generate enhanced antitumor responses. Some examples include the use of vectors encoding IL-2, IL-12, interferon gamma (IFN-γ), and granulocyte-macrophage colony stimulating factor, and genes for immune accessory molecules, including tumor necrosis factor alpha (TNF-α), CD80, and the ligand for CD40 (CD154).

Immune Costimulatory Surface Molecules Transduction of CLL B cells with an adenovirus encoding CD154 (Ad-CD154) can induce leukemia cells to express immune costimulatory molecules, thereby enhancing their capacity to present antigens to autologous T lymphocytes (CTL).[121] Eleven patients received a single infusion of autologous CLL cells transduced *ex vivo* with Ad-CD154.[122] Nearly all treated patients exhibited increased serum levels of IL-12 and IFN-γ, enhanced expression of immune costimulatory molecules on bystander leukemia cells, increased absolute numbers of blood T cells, and reduced blood leukemia cell counts and lymph node size. After additional infusions of Ad-CD154–transduced cells, patients showed disease stabilization, with delayed disease progression and the need for further treatment. Two of the treated patients did not require additional therapy 4 years after treatment.[123]

Immune Stimulatory Cytokines Human leukemia cells typically express negligible levels of CD80 and low levels of CD86, causing the cells to be ineffective at stimulating T cells in response to presented antigens.[124] Primary human leukemic cells from patients with AML can be transduced with retrovirus vectors to express CD80. *In vitro*, such transduced leukemia cells could stimulate proliferation of allogeneic T cells in mixed lymphocyte culture.[125] CLL B cells transduced with HSV-based amplicon vectors encoding CD80 can stimulate allogeneic T cells in mixed lymphocyte reactions and stimulate T cells to produce IL-2 and IFN-γ.[126] Studies performed in animal models using transduced leukemia cells with CD80 or CD86 have shown modest antitumor immunity.[127–129] To date, results of clinical trials using this approach have not been reported.

Murine B lymphoma cells transduced to express IL-2 and the lymphotactic chemokine lymphotactin are better able to induce antitumor immunity than nontransduced lymphoma cells or lymphoma cells transduced to express IL-2 alone.[130] Two clinical trials using transduction of IL-2 in prostate cancer have been reported.[131,132] Clinical trials of this approach for treatment of patients with leukemia or lymphoma are lacking.

Preclinical studies have shown that mouse lymphoma B cells (A20) transduced with a retrovirus encoding IL-12 could induce immunity against A20 cells in syngeneic mice more efficiently than A20 cells transduced with control vectors.[133] Additionally, dendritic cells transfected with a plasmid encoding IL-12 are an effective alternative for generating enhanced antigen presentation and antitumor immune responses in a murine model of lymphoma.[134]

Transduction of cells with TNF-α inhibits the development or progression of leukemia in experimental animals.[135,136] However, systemic administration of TNF-α induces serious toxicities that limit its clinical application.[137,138] Membrane-bound TNF molecules may lack the undesirable side effects of soluble TNF-α. Coincubation of CLL cells expressing a membrane-stabilized form of TNF-α induced bystander CLL cells to express immune accessory molecules, such as CD80 and CD54. Conceivably, such modified forms of active TNF-α that resist changes from the plasma membrane may be used in gene therapy of various hematologic cancers.

REFERENCES

1. National Institutes of Health-Office of Biotechnology Activities: Clinical Trials in Human Gene Transfer-Recombinant and Gene Transfer, vol 2004. Available at: http://www4.od.nih.gov/oba/rac/clinicaltrial.htm. Accessed January 2005.

2. Gene Therapy Clinical Trials Web Page, vol 2004. Available at: http://www.wiley.co.uk/wileychi/genmed/clinical. Accessed January 2005.

3. Abe A, Emi N, Kanie T, et al: Expression cloning of oligomerization-activated genes with cell-proliferating potency by pseudotype retrovirus vector. *Biochem Biophys Res Commun* 320:920, 2004.

4. Naldini L, Blomer U, Gage FH, et al: Efficient transfer, integration, and sustained long-term expression of the transgene in adult rat brains injected with a lentiviral vector. *Proc Natl Acad Sci U S A* 93:11382, 1996.

5. Kay MA, Glorioso JC, Naldini L: Viral vectors for gene therapy: The art of turning infectious agents into vehicles of therapeutics. *Nat Med* 7:33, 2001.

6. Hacein-Bey-Abina S, von Kalle C, Schmidt M, et al: A serious adverse event after successful gene therapy for X-linked severe combined immunodeficiency. *N Engl J Med* 348:255, 2003.

7. Dave UP, Jenkins NA, Copeland NG: Gene therapy insertional mutagenesis insights. *Science* 303:333, 2004.

8. Verhasselt B, De Smedt M, Verhelst R, et al: Retrovirally transduced CD34++ human cord blood cells generate T cells expressing high levels of the retroviral encoded green fluorescent protein marker in vitro. *Blood* 91:431, 1998.

9. Dunbar CE, Cottler-Fox M, O'Shaughnessy JA, et al: Retrovirally marked CD34-enriched peripheral blood and bone marrow cells contribute to long-term engraftment after autologous transplantation. *Blood* 85:3048, 1995.

10. Stewart AK, Sutherland DR, Nanji S, et al: Engraftment of gene-marked hematopoietic progenitors in myeloma patients after transplant of autologous long-term marrow cultures. *Hum Gene Ther* 10:1953, 1999.

11. Douglas JT: Adenovirus-mediated gene delivery: An overview. *Methods Mol Biol* 246:3, 2004.

12. Curiel DT: Strategies to adapt adenoviral vectors for targeted delivery. *Ann N Y Acad Sci* 886:158, 1999.

13. Kamen A, Henry O: Development and optimization of an adenovirus production process. *J Gene Med* 6(suppl 1):S184, 2004.

14. Nasz I, Adam E: Recombinant adenovirus vectors for gene therapy and clinical trials. *Acta Microbiol Immunol Hung* 48:323, 2001.

15. Yang Y, Ertl HC, Wilson JM: MHC class I-restricted cytotoxic T lymphocytes to viral antigens destroy hepatocytes in mice infected with E1-deleted recombinant adenoviruses. *Immunity* 1:433, 1994.

16. Yang Y, Wilson JM: Clearance of adenovirus-infected hepatocytes by MHC class I-restricted CD4+ CTLs in vivo. *J Immunol* 155:2564, 1995.

17. Sumida SM, Truitt DM, Kishko MG, et al: Neutralizing antibodies and CD8+ T lymphocytes both contribute to immunity to adenovirus serotype 5 vaccine vectors. *J Virol* 78:2666, 2004.

18. Borgland SL, Bowen GP, Wong NC, et al: Adenovirus vector-induced expression of the C-X-C chemokine IP-10 is mediated through capsid-dependent activation of NF-κB. *J Virol* 74:3941, 2000.

19. McDonald D, Stockwin L, Matzow T, et al: Coxsackie and adenovirus receptor (CAR)-dependent and major histocompatibility complex (MHC) class I-independent uptake of recombinant adenoviruses into human tumour cells. *Gene Ther* 6:1512, 1999.

20. Santis G, Legrand V, Hong SS, et al: Molecular determinants of adenovirus serotype 5 fibre binding to its cellular receptor CAR. *J Gen Virol* 80:1519, 1999.

21. Hidaka C, Milano E, Leopold PL, et al: CAR-dependent and CAR-independent pathways of adenovirus vector-mediated gene transfer and expression in human fibroblasts. *J Clin Invest* 103:579, 1999.

22. Krasnykh V, Dmitriev I, Navarro JG, et al: Advanced generation adenoviral vectors possess augmented gene transfer efficiency based upon coxsackie adenovirus receptor-independent cellular entry capacity. *Cancer Res* 60:6784, 2000.

23. Kouraklis G: Gene therapy for cancer: From the laboratory to the patient. *Dig Dis Sci* 45:1045, 2000.

24. Meier O, Greber UF: Adenovirus endocytosis. *J Gene Med* 6(suppl 1):S152, 2004.

25. Muzyczka N: Use of adeno-associated virus as a general transduction vector for mammalian cells. *Curr Top Microbiol Immunol* 158:97, 1992.

26. Flotte TR: Gene therapy progress and prospects: Recombinant adeno-associated virus (rAAV) vectors. *Gene Ther* 11:805, 2004.

27. Duan D, Sharma P, Yang J, et al: Circular intermediates of recombinant adeno-associated virus have defined structural characteristics responsible for long-term episomal persistence in muscle tissue. *J Virol* 72:8568, 1998.

28. Nakai H, Iwaki Y, Kay MA, Couto LB: Isolation of recombinant adeno-associated virus vector-cellular DNA junctions from mouse liver. *J Virol* 73:5438, 1999.

29. Russell DW, Kay MA: Adeno-associated virus vectors and hematology. *Blood* 94:864, 1999.

30. Monahan PE, Samulski RJ: Adeno-associated virus vectors for gene therapy: More pros than cons? *Mol Med Today* 6:433, 2000.

31. Tal J: Adeno-associated virus-based vectors in gene therapy. *J Biomed Sci* 7:279, 2000.

32. Brument N, Morenweiser R, Blouin V, et al: A versatile and scalable two-step ion-exchange chromatography process for the purification of recombinant adeno-associated virus serotypes-2 and -5. *Mol Ther* 6:678, 2002.

33. Davidoff AM, Ng CY, Sleep S, et al: Purification of recombinant adeno-associated virus type 8 vectors by ion exchange chromatography generates clinical grade vector stock. *J Virol Methods* 121:209, 2004.

34. Krisky DM, Marconi PC, Oligino TJ, et al: Development of herpes simplex virus replication-defective multigene vectors for combination gene therapy applications. *Gene Ther* 5:1517, 1998.

35. Wolfe D, Goins WF, Kaplan TJ, et al: Herpesvirus-mediated systemic delivery of nerve growth factor. *Mol Ther* 3:61, 2001.

36. Burton EA, Huang S, Goins WF, Glorioso JC: Use of the herpes simplex viral genome to construct gene therapy vectors. *Methods Mol Med* 76:1, 2003.

37. Frenkel N, Singer O, Kwong AD: Minireview: The herpes simplex virus amplicon—A versatile defective virus vector. *Gene Ther* 1:S40, 1994.

38. Latchman DS: Gene therapy with herpes simplex virus vectors: Progress and prospects for clinical neuroscience. *Neuroscientist* 7:528, 2001.

39. Calderwood MA, White RE, Whitehouse A: Development of herpes-virus-based episomally maintained gene delivery vectors. *Expert Opin Biol Ther* 4:493, 2004.

40. Eling DJ, Johnson PA, Sharma S, et al: Chronic lymphocytic leukemia B cells are highly sensitive to infection by herpes simplex virus-1 via herpesvirus-entry-mediator A. *Gene Ther* 7:1210, 2000.

41. Han S, Mahato RI, Sung YK, Kim SW: Development of biomaterials for gene therapy. *Mol Ther* 2:302, 2000.

42. Tranchant I, Thompson B, Nicolazzi C, et al: Physicochemical optimisation of plasmid delivery by cationic lipids. *J Gene Med* 6(suppl 1):S24, 2004.

43. Bloquel C, Fabre E, Bureau MF, Scherman D: Plasmid DNA electrotransfer for intracellular and secreted proteins expression: New methodological developments and applications. *J Gene Med* 6(suppl 1):S11, 2004.

44. Andrianaivo F, Lecocq M, Wattiaux-De Coninck S, et al: Hydrodynamics-based transfection of the liver: Entrance into hepatocytes of DNA that causes expression takes place very early after injection. *J Gene Med* 6:877, 2004.

45. Jarver P, Langel U: The use of cell-penetrating peptides as a tool for gene regulation. *Drug Discov Today* 9:395, 2004.

46. Luo D, Saltzman WM: Synthetic DNA delivery systems. *Nat Biotechnol* 18:33, 2000.

47. Monsigny M, Rondanino C, Duverger E, et al: Glyco-dependent nuclear import of glycoproteins, glycoplexes and glycosylated plasmids. *Biochim Biophys Acta* 1673:94, 2004.

48. Herweijer H, Wolff JA: Progress and prospects: Naked DNA gene transfer and therapy. *Gene Ther* 10:453, 2003.

49. Miao CH, Thompson AR, Loeb K, Ye X: Long-term and therapeutic-level hepatic gene expression of human factor IX after naked plasmid transfer in vivo. *Mol Ther* 3:947, 2001.

50. Zhu D, Rice J, Savelyeva N, Stevenson FK: DNA fusion vaccines against B-cell tumors. *Trends Mol Med* 7:566, 2001.

51. Rice J, Elliott T, Buchan S, Stevenson FK: DNA fusion vaccine designed to induce cytotoxic T cell responses against defined peptide motifs: Implications for cancer vaccines. *J Immunol* 167:1558, 2001.

52. Stevenson FK, Rosenberg W: DNA vaccination: A potential weapon against infection and cancer. *Vox Sang* 80:12, 2001.

53. Yuen AR, Sikic BI: Clinical studies of antisense therapy in cancer. *Front Biosci* 5:D588, 2000.

54. Henry SP, Miner RC, Drew WL, et al: Antiviral activity and ocular kinetics of antisense oligonucleotides designed to inhibit CMV replication. *Invest Ophthalmol Vis Sci* 42:2646, 2001.

55. Roehr B: Fomivirsen approved for CMV retinitis: First antisense drug. *J Int Assoc Physicians AIDS Care* 4:14, 1998.

56. Wright P: Antisense and siRNA Technologies—SMi's Second Annual Conference, 16–17 February 2003, London, U.K. *IDrugs* 7:233, 2004.

57. Hemmi H, Takeuchi O, Kawai T, et al: A Toll-like receptor recognizes bacterial DNA. *Nature* 408:740, 2000.

58. Wu CC, Castro JE, Motta M, et al: Selection of oligonucleotide aptamers with enhanced uptake and activation of human leukemia B cells. *Hum Gene Ther* 14:849, 2003.

59. Krieg AM: CpG motifs: The active ingredient in bacterial extracts? *Nat Med* 9:831, 2003.

60. Jing N, Li Y, Xiong W, et al: G-quartet oligonucleotides: A new class of signal transducer and activator of transcription 3 inhibitors that suppresses growth of prostate and breast tumors through induction of apoptosis. *Cancer Res* 64:6603, 2004.

61. Mello CC, Conte D Jr.: Revealing the world of RNA interference. *Nature* 431:338, 2004.

62. Rocheleau CE, Downs WD, Lin R, et al: Wnt signaling and an APC-related gene specify endoderm in early C. elegans embryos. *Cell* 90:707, 1997.

63. Parrish S, Fleenor J, Xu S, et al: Functional anatomy of a dsRNA trigger: Differential requirement for the two trigger strands in RNA interference. *Mol Cell* 6:1077, 2000.

64. Zamore PD, Tuschl T, Sharp PA, Bartel DP: RNAi: Double-stranded RNA directs the ATP-dependent cleavage of mRNA at 21 to 23 nucleotide intervals. *Cell* 101:25, 2000.

65. Tabara H, Sarkissian M, Kelly WG, et al: The rde-1 gene, RNA interference, and transposon silencing in C. elegans. *Cell* 99:123, 1999.

66. Pal-Bhadra M, Bhadra U, Birchler JA: Cosuppression in Drosophila: Gene silencing of alcohol dehydrogenase by white-Adh transgenes is polycomb dependent. *Cell* 90:479, 1997.

67. Mette MF, Aufsatz W, van der Winden J, et al: Transcriptional silencing and promoter methylation triggered by double-stranded RNA. *EMBO J* 19:5194, 2000.

68. Olsen PH, Ambros V: The lin-4 regulatory RNA controls developmental timing in Caenorhabditis elegans by blocking LIN-14 protein synthesis after the initiation of translation. *Dev Biol* 216:671, 1999.

69. Mochizuki K, Fine NA, Fujisawa T, Gorovsky MA: Analysis of a piwi-related gene implicates small RNAs in genome rearrangement in tetrahymena. *Cell* 110:689, 2002.

70. Gitlin L, Karelsky S, Andino R: Short interfering RNA confers intracellular antiviral immunity in human cells. *Nature* 418:430, 2002.

71. Novina CD, Murray MF, Dykxhoorn DM, et al: SiRNA-directed inhibition of HIV-1 infection. *Nat Med* 8:681, 2002.

72. Stephens AC, Rivers RP: Antisense oligonucleotide therapy in cancer. *Curr Opin Mol Ther* 5:118, 2003.

73. Brummelkamp TR, Bernards R, Agami R: A system for stable expression of short interfering RNAs in mammalian cells. *Science* 296:550, 2002.

74. Paddison PJ, Caudy AA, Bernstein E, et al: Short hairpin RNAs (shRNAs) induce sequence-specific silencing in mammalian cells. *Genes Dev* 16:948, 2002.

75. Devroe E, Silver PA: Retrovirus-delivered siRNA. *BMC Biotechnol* 2:15, 2002.

76. Bueren JA, Guenechea G, Casado JA, et al: Genetic modification of hematopoietic stem cells: Recent advances in the gene therapy of inherited diseases. *Arch Med Res* 34:589, 2003.

77. Mollah ZU, Aiba S, Manome H, et al: Cord blood CD34+ cells differentiate into dermal dendritic cells in co-culture with cutaneous fibroblasts or stromal cells. *J Invest Dermatol* 118:450, 2002.

78. Krivit W, Sung JH, Shapiro EG, Lockman LA: Microglia: The effector cell for reconstitution of the central nervous system following bone marrow transplantation for lysosomal and peroxisomal storage diseases. *Cell Transplant* 4:385, 1995.

79. Matayoshi A, Brown C, DiPersio JF, et al: Human blood-mobilized hematopoietic precursors differentiate into osteoclasts in the absence of stromal cells. *Proc Natl Acad Sci U S A* 93:10785, 1996.

80. Deisseroth AB, Zu Z, Claxton D, et al: Genetic marking shows that Ph+ cells present in autologous transplants of chronic myelogenous leukemia (CML) contribute to relapse after autologous bone marrow in CML. *Blood* 83:3068, 1994.

81. Brenner MK, Rill DR, Moen RC, et al: Gene-marking to trace origin of relapse after autologous bone-marrow transplantation. *Lancet* 341:85, 1993.

82. Kantoff PW, Kohn DB, Mitsuya H, et al: Correction of adenosine deaminase deficiency in cultured human T and B cells by retrovirus-mediated gene transfer. *Proc Natl Acad Sci U S A* 83:6563, 1986.

83. Blaese RM.: Development of gene therapy for immunodeficiency: Adenosine deaminase deficiency. *Pediatr Res* 33:S49, 1993.

84. Kohn DB, Hershfield MS, Carbonaro D, et al: T lymphocytes with a normal ADA gene accumulate after transplantation of transduced autologous umbilical cord blood CD34+ cells in ADA-deficient SCID neonates. *Nat Med* 4:775, 1998.

85. Aiuti A, Slavin S, Aker M, et al: Correction of ADA-SCID by stem cell gene therapy combined with nonmyeloablative conditioning. *Science* 296:2410, 2002.

86. Noguchi M, Yi H, Rosenblatt HM, et al: Interleukin-2 receptor gamma chain mutation results in X-linked severe combined immunodeficiency in humans. *Cell* 73:147, 1993.

87. Haddad E, Landais P, Friedrich W, et al: Long-term immune reconstitution and outcome after HLA-nonidentical T-cell-depleted bone mar-

row transplantation for severe combined immunodeficiency: A European retrospective study of 116 patients. *Blood* 91:3646, 1998.

88. Cavazzana-Calvo M, Hacein-Bey S, De Saint Basile G, et al: Gene therapy of human severe combined immunodeficiency (SCID)-X1 disease. *Science* 288:669, 2000.

89. Hacein-Bey-Abina S, Le Deist F, Carlier F, et al: Sustained correction of X-linked severe combined immunodeficiency by ex vivo gene therapy. *N Engl J Med* 346:1185, 2002.

90. Hacein-Bey-Abina S, Von Kalle C, Schmidt M, et al: LMO2-associated clonal T cell proliferation in two patients after gene therapy for SCID-X1. *Science* 302:415, 2003.

91. McCormack MP, Forster A, Drynan L, et al: The LMO2 T-cell oncogene is activated via chromosomal translocations or retroviral insertion during gene therapy but has no mandatory role in normal T-cell development. *Mol Cell Biol* 23:9003, 2003.

92. Stocking C, Bergholz U, Friel J, et al: Distinct classes of factor-independent mutants can be isolated after retroviral mutagenesis of a human myeloid stem cell line. *Growth Factors* 8:197, 1993.

93. von Kalle C, Baum C, Williams DA: Lenti in red: Progress in gene therapy for human hemoglobinopathies. *J Clin Invest* 114:889, 2004.

94. May C, Rivella S, Callegari J, et al: Therapeutic haemoglobin synthesis in beta-thalassaemic mice expressing lentivirus-encoded human beta-globin. *Nature* 406:82, 2000.

95. Pawliuk R, Westerman KA, Fabry ME, et al: Correction of sickle cell disease in transgenic mouse models by gene therapy. *Science* 294:2368, 2001.

96. Imren S, Fabry ME, Westerman KA, et al: High-level beta-globin expression and preferred intragenic integration after lentiviral transduction of human cord blood stem cells. *J Clin Invest* 114:953, 2004.

97. Nolta JA, Sender LS, Barranger JA, Kohn DB: Expression of human glucocerebrosidase in murine long-term bone marrow cultures after retroviral vector-mediated transfer. *Blood* 75:787, 1990.

98. Barranger JA, Rice EO, Swaney WP: Gene transfer approaches to the lysosomal storage disorders. *Neurochem Res* 24:601, 1999.

99. Dunbar CE, Kohn DB, Schiffmann R, et al: Retroviral transfer of the glucocerebrosidase gene into CD34+ cells from patients with Gaucher disease: In vivo detection of transduced cells without myeloablation. *Hum Gene Ther* 9:2629, 1998.

100. Kim EY, Hong YB, Lai Z, et al: Expression and secretion of human glucocerebrosidase mediated by recombinant lentivirus vectors in vitro and in vivo: Implications for gene therapy of Gaucher disease. *Biochem Biophys Res Commun* 318:381, 2004.

101. Hong YB, Kim EY, Yoo HW, Jung SC: Feasibility of gene therapy in Gaucher disease using an adeno-associated virus vector. *J Hum Genet* 2004.

102. Croop JM: Gene therapy for Fanconi anemia. *Curr Hematol Rep* 2:335, 2003.

103. Galimi F, Noll M, Kanazawa Y, et al: Gene therapy of Fanconi anemia: Preclinical efficacy using lentiviral vectors. *Blood* 100:2732, 2002.

104. Manno CS, Chew AJ, Hutchison S, et al: AAV-mediated factor IX gene transfer to skeletal muscle in patients with severe hemophilia B. *Blood* 101:2963, 2003.

105. Kay MA, High K, Glader B, et al: A phase I/II clinical trial for liver directed AAV-mediated gene transfer for hemophilia B. *Blood* 100:115a, 2002.

106. Powell JS, Ragni MV, White GC 2nd, et al: Phase 1 trial of FVIII gene transfer for severe hemophilia A using a retroviral construct administered by peripheral intravenous infusion. *Blood* 102:2038, 2003.

107. Roth DA, Tawa NE Jr, O'Brien JM, et al: Nonviral transfer of the gene encoding coagulation factor VIII in patients with severe hemophilia A. *N Engl J Med* 344:1735, 2001.

108. Galpin JE, Casciato DA, Richards SB: A phase I clinical trial to evaluate the safety and biological activity of HIV-IT (TAF) (HIV-1IIIBenv-trans-duced, autologous fibroblasts) in asymptomatic HIV-1 infected subjects. *Hum Gene Ther* 5:997, 1994.

109. Ziegner UH, Peters G, Jolly DJ, et al: Cytotoxic T-lymphocyte induction in asymptomatic HIV-1-infected patients immunized with retrovector-transduced autologous fibroblasts expressing HIV-1IIIB Env/Rev proteins. *AIDS* 9:43, 1995.

110. Deeks SG, Wagner B, Anton PA, et al: A phase II randomized study of HIV-specific T-cell gene therapy in subjects with undetectable plasma viremia on combination antiretroviral therapy. *Mol Ther* 5:788, 2002.

111. Walker RE, Bechtel CM, Natarajan V, et al: Long-term in vivo survival of receptor-modified syngeneic T cells in patients with human immunodeficiency virus infection. *Blood* 96:467, 2000.

112. Kang EM, de Witte M, Malech H, et al: Nonmyeloablative conditioning followed by transplantation of genetically modified HLA-matched peripheral blood progenitor cells for hematologic malignancies in patients with acquired immunodeficiency syndrome. *Blood* 99:698, 2002.

113. Cotter FE, Johnson P, Hall P, et al: Antisense oligonucleotides suppress B-cell lymphoma growth in a SCID-hu mouse model. *Oncogene* 9:3049, 1994.

114. Webb A, Cunningham D, Cotter F, et al: BCL-2 antisense therapy in patients with non-Hodgkin lymphoma. *Lancet* 349:1137, 1997.

115. Chanan-Khan A: Bcl-2 antisense therapy in hematologic malignancies. *Curr Opin Oncol* 16:581, 2004.

116. Skorski T, Nieborowska-Skorska M, Nicolaides NC, et al: Suppression of Philadelphia1 leukemia cell growth in mice by BCR-ABL antisense oligodeoxynucleotide. *Proc Natl Acad Sci U S A* 91:4504, 1994.

117. Rao S, Watkins D, Cunningham D, et al: Phase II study of ISIS 3521, an antisense oligodeoxynucleotide to protein kinase C alpha, in patients with previously treated low-grade non-Hodgkin's lymphoma. *Ann Oncol* 15:1413, 2004.

118. Yuan Z, Mei HD: Inhibition of telomerase activity with hTERT antisense increases the effect of CDDP-induced apoptosis in myeloid leukemia. *Hematol J* 3:201, 2002.

119. Ritter U, Damm-Welk C, Fuchs U, et al: Design and evaluation of chemically synthesized siRNA targeting the NPM-ALK fusion site in anaplastic large cell lymphoma (ALCL). *Oligonucleotides* 13:365, 2003.

120. Peng Z, Xiao Z, Wang Y, et al: Reversal of P-glycoprotein-mediated multidrug resistance with small interference RNA (siRNA) in leukemia cells. *Cancer Gene Ther* 2004.

121. Kato K, Cantwell MJ, Sharma S, Kipps TJ: Gene transfer of CD40-ligand induces autologous immune recognition of chronic lymphocytic leukemia B cells. *J Clin Invest* 101:1133, 1998.

122. Wierda WG, Cantwell MJ, Woods SJ, et al: CD40-ligand (CD154) gene therapy for chronic lymphocytic leukemia. *Blood* 96:2917, 2000.

123. Castro JE, Cantwell MJ, Prussak CE, et al: Long-term follow up of chronic lymphocytic leukemia patients treated with CD40-ligand (CD154) gene therapy. *Blood* 102:1790a, 2003.

124. Hirano N, Takahashi T, Ohtake S, et al: Expression of costimulatory molecules in human leukemias. *Leukemia* 10:1168, 1996.

125. Hirst WJ, Buggins A, Darling D, et al: Enhanced immune costimulatory activity of primary acute myeloid leukaemia blasts after retrovirus-mediated gene transfer of B7.1. *Gene Ther* 4:691, 1997.

126. Tolba KA, Bowers WJ, Hilchey SP, et al: Development of herpes simplex virus-1 amplicon-based immunotherapy for chronic lymphocytic leukemia. *Blood* 98:287, 2001.

127. Dunussi-Joannopoulos K, Weinstein HJ, Arceci RJ, Croop JM: Gene therapy with B7.1 and GM-CSF vaccines in a murine AML model. *J Pediatr Hematol Oncol* 19:536, 1997.

128. Hirano N, Takahashi T, Azuma M, et al: Protective and therapeutic immunity against leukemia induced by irradiated B7-1 (CD80)-transduced leukemic cells. *Hum Gene Ther* 8:1375, 1997.

129. Stripecke R, Cardoso AA, Pepper KA, et al: Lentiviral vectors for efficient delivery of CD80 and granulocyte-macrophage-colony-stimulating factor in human acute lymphoblastic leukemia and acute myeloid leukemia cells to induce antileukemic immune responses. *Blood* 96: 1317, 2000.

130. Dilloo D, Bacon K, Holden W, et al: Combined chemokine and cytokine gene transfer enhances antitumor immunity. *Nat Med* 2:1090, 1996.

131. Pantuck AJ, Van Ophoven A, Gitlitz BJ, et al: Phase I trial of antigen-specific gene therapy using a recombinant vaccinia virus encoding MUC-1 and IL-2 in MUC-1-positive patients with advanced prostate cancer. *J Immunother* 27:240, 2004.

132. Pantuck AJ, Belldegrun AS: Phase I clinical trial of interleukin 2 (IL-2) gene therapy for prostate cancer. *Curr Urol Rep* 2:33, 2001.

133. Nishimura T, Watanabe K, Yahata T, et al: The application of IL-12 to cytokine therapy and gene therapy for tumors. *Ann N Y Acad Sci* 795: 375, 1996.

134. Chen HW, Lee YP, Chung YF, et al: Inducing long-term survival with lasting anti-tumor immunity in treating B cell lymphoma by a combined dendritic cell-based and hydrodynamic plasmid-encoding IL-12 gene therapy. *Int Immunol* 15:427, 2003.

135. Gautam SC, Pindolia KR, Xu YX, et al: Antileukemic activity of TNF-alpha gene therapy with myeloid progenitor cells against minimal leukemia. *J Hematother* 7:115, 1998.

136. Gautam SC, Xu YX, Pindolia KR, et al: TNF-alpha gene therapy with myeloid progenitor cells lacks the toxicities of systemic TNF-alpha therapy. *J Hematother* 8:237, 1999.

137. Villani F, Galimberti M, Mazzola G, et al: Pulmonary toxicity of alpha tumor necrosis factor in patients treated by isolation perfusion. *J Chemother* 7:452, 1995.

138. Krigel RL, Padavic-Shaller KA, Rudolph AA, et al: Hemorrhagic gastritis as a new dose-limiting toxicity of recombinant tumor necrosis factor. *J Natl Cancer Inst* 83:129, 1991.

PAIN MANAGEMENT

WEONJEONG LIM
KAMALA S. THOMAS
JOEL E. DIMSDALE

The ancient Greeks said it well: "Call no mortal happy til he has passed the final limit of his life secure from pain" (Sophocles, *Oedipus the King*, trans. David Grene [University of Chicago Press, 1954]). Hematologists are singularly trained to appreciate the wisdom of this quote. Pain is a frequent visitor to the hematologist's waiting room. This chapter reviews the definition, measurement, and mechanisms of pain. The chapter discusses pharmacologic, surgical, behavioral, and complementary medicine approaches to pain treatment. The chapter's major focus is cancer-related pain, but the chapter also discusses pain states associated with sickle cell anemia because this illness is seen frequently in hematologic practice.

DEFINITION OF PAIN

According to the International Association for the Study of Pain (ISAP), pain is "an unpleasant sensory and emotional experience associated with actual or potential tissue damage or described in terms of such damage." The ISAP notes that "pain is always subjective" and that if individuals describe "their experience as pain and if they report it in the same ways as pain caused by tissue damage, it should be accepted as pain."[1] This broad definition recognizes that sensory fibers reflecting tissue damage and emotional factors reflecting suffering form an amalgam that is difficult to sort out.[2]

Cancer-related pain often is experienced throughout the course of the disease, thus placing a great burden on patients and their families. Cancer pain is associated with the disease process itself but also can result from treatment of the disease.[3] Unfortunately, cancer pain is undertreated, which is particularly disappointing because cancer pain can be controlled in up to 90 percent of cases.[4]

For treatment purposes, cancer-related pain is divided into five categories[5,6]:

1. *Cancer patients with acute pain*: Patients with acute pain respond well to treatment. However, they often develop tolerance to strong analgesics and require more medication to alleviate long-lasting pain. After the pain eases, patients wean themselves off medication easily and voluntarily.
2. *Cancer patients with chronic pain*: Patients have pain related to the disease process, chemotherapy, radiation therapy, and surgery. Cancer-related pain often worsens over time, unlike symptoms that may not change over many years in patients with nonmalignant chronic pain.
3. *Cancer patients with preexisting chronic pain*: Patients are at increased risk for drug addiction and escalating psychological prob-

lems. Some of these patients are cured of the cancer yet suffer from intractable pain.
4. *Cancer patients with drug abuse problems*: Patients with a prior history of drug abuse are at high risk for addiction. Physical dependence and tolerance may develop, but the clinician's primary obligation is easing the patient's discomfort. Patients who are actively abusing or taking opioids already are tolerant to the drug and must be given a larger amount of medication to achieve adequate pain control. The need for a large dose should not be regarded as drug abusing behavior. Patients require treatment, not a suspicious, withholding approach.
5. *Dying patients*: A poignant dilemma for dying patients is choosing between pain relief and alertness. If a large amount of opioid is needed for pain relief, wakefulness can be episodically increased using psychostimulants.

PAIN MECHANISMS

TYPES OF PAIN

Diverse types of pain frequently overlap and often require complex treatment regimens that address the multifaceted origins of the patient's pain.[5]

Pain can result from inflammation around nerves, injury to nerves, or physical irritation of nerves. This kind of pain, which can be directly linked to physical causes, is called nociceptive pain. Somatic pain results when nerve receptors in the skin, muscle, and deep tissue are stimulated.[7] Somatic pain is well localized and generally described as an "aching" or "gnawing" feeling in the affected area. Common causes of somatic pain in cancer patients include bone metastasis and postsurgical pain.[8] Visceral pain often is described as "squeezing," "colicky," and "crampy." The pain is poorly localized, deep, or pressure like. The pain frequently is associated with nausea, vomiting, and sweating.[7] Somatic and visceral pains respond to opiates.

Pain caused by neural tissue injury may result from either the cancer itself (e.g., tumor infiltration of a nerve, plexus, or the spinal cord) or the anticancer therapy (e.g., peripheral neuropathy caused by vinca alkaloids, postradiation neuritis, or fibrosis).[8] This type of pain, which is common among cancer patients with chronic pain, often is severe and constant. The pain typically is described as a dull ache or vice-like pressure accompanied by paroxysms of burning pain or electrical shock. Neuropathic pain is difficult to diagnose and treat effectively because the pain cannot be explained by a single etiology, mechanism, or anatomical lesion.[7] Hyperalgesia, a decreased threshold or exaggerated nociceptive response to a noxious stimulus, is closely tied to neuronal sensitization resulting from inflammatory processes. Allodynia, an exaggerated nociceptive response to innocuous stimuli, is the behavioral modality responsible for much of the debilitation caused by chronic neuropathic pain syndrome.[9]

Pain may have no apparent physical or biologic cause; rather, pain may be a way of coping with emotional distress. Individuals with "psychogenic pain" are not conscious of the psychological nature of their symptoms.[6] Although pure psychogenic pain is rare in cancer patients, psychological factors potently exacerbate or ameliorate all cancer-related pain.

PAIN-ELICITING NEUROCHEMICALS

Research has clarified the neuroanatomical circuits and cellular mechanisms underlying pain induction.[10] The role of inflammatory mediators in pain induction is widely appreciated, but investigators also are exploring novel mechanisms such as protons, adenosine triphosphate, neurotrophins (growth factors), nitric oxide (NO), dopamine, serotonin, norepinephrine, and histamine. Other work focuses on the role of N-methyl-D-aspartate (NMDA) receptor activation, which induces neuronal sensitization and pain. Pain is exacerbated when inhibitory interneuron tone in the dorsal horn is reduced. These sorts of diverse pain mediators imply different pharmacologic treatment strategies.

Different chemicals play major roles, depending on the pain state. Three pain states are defined according to the underlying spinal connectivity and biology. Treatment of pain resulting from acute stimuli, such as heat injury, is achieved by blocking the opening of voltage-sensitive Ca^{2+} channels or desensitization of the terminal. Receptors of μ- and δ-opioids, α_2-adrenoreceptors, and neuropeptide Y affect voltage-sensitive Ca^{2+} channels.[11] Capsaicin and nicotine desensitize the terminal.[12] Tissue injury leads to persistent afferent input in the spinal cord, which can augment neuronal responses to a given afferent input.[13] Substance P, Ca^{2+} channels, excitatory amino acid products and their receptors, NO synthetase, cyclooxygenase (COX)-2, protein kinase C, and tachykinin receptors are involved.[11] Peripheral nerve injury, commonly seen in patients with diabetes or postherpetic neuropathy or who are undergoing radiotherapy and chemotherapy, is associated with hyperalgesia and allodynia. The mechanisms responsible for these phenomena involve loss of dorsal horn γ-aminobutyric acid (GABA), increased sympathetic flow, spontaneous neuronal activity, and release of cytokines.[11,14] Accordingly, GABA receptor agonists, NMDA receptor blockades, adenosine A_1, N-type Ca^{2+} channel blockades, and α_2-adrenoreceptor agonists are important candidates of antiallodynic drugs.[11]

Animal models suggest cytokines play an important role in promoting pain and increasing pain severity, lethargy, anorexia, and nausea.[15] The hyperalgesic effects of proinflammatory agents such as endotoxin are mediated by interleukin (IL)-1, tumor necrosis factor (TNF), IL-6, and IL-8.[16] Cytokines may sensitize patients to the "flu-like" aches and generalized discomfort sometimes associated with allodynia or other pains occurring in patients dying of advanced cancer.[17] TNF can cause muscle soreness via an unknown mechanism.[18]

After nerve injury, the inducible prostaglandin-synthesizing enzyme COX is up-regulated in the spinal cord and peripheral nerve. The latter is positively associated with TNF,[19] suggesting that COX inhibitors are effective in reducing some types of neuropathic pain, although COX inhibitors are generally considered ineffective in neuropathic pain.[20] In a study that examined whether COX inhibitors attenuate pain behavior induced by chronic constrictive sciatic nerve injury or intraneural injection of TNF, mechanical allodynia was reduced by ibuprofen but not by celecoxib treatment 5 and 7 days after injection. Thus, monotherapy with COX inhibitors for treatment of neuropathic pain seems to be insufficient, but combined treatment regimens with other analgesic drugs may be useful.[21]

Endorphins lower pain perception by reducing signal transmission between nerve cells. Endorphins are produced by the pituitary gland and hypothalamus. The pharmacologic effects of these endogenous peptides mimic the effects of opium and its analogues.[22]

Opioid receptors modulate pain by binding to endogenous opioid peptides and exogenous opioids.[23] Five major categories of opioid receptors have been identified and cloned: mu (μ), kappa (κ), sigma (σ), delta (δ), and epsilon (ε).[22] Commercially available opiate analgesics act on κ-, δ-, and μ-receptor sites. In general, functional studies using selective agonists and antagonists revealed substantial parallels between μ- and δ-receptors and contrasts between μ-/δ- and κ-receptors.[6] μ-Receptors are of primary interest to clinicians because these receptors mediate the analgesic effects of opioids. μ-Receptor activation may produce euphoria, respiratory and physical depression, miosis, and reduced gastrointestinal motility. κ-Receptors mediate pentazocine-like analgesia at the spinal level. κ-Receptors also mediate the prominent sedating effect of opiates, respiratory depression, and dysphoria.[22]

The important role of the NMDA receptor in pain mechanisms is increasingly recognized,[10] but a narrow therapeutic window and side effect profiles limit the utility of NMDA antagonists for pain relief.[6] Drugs that act on specific NMDA receptor subtypes may be less likely to produce unwanted side effects. The antipain effect of some peptides derived from cone snail venom result from inhibition of the NR2B or NR2A NMDA receptor subtypes. These peptides suppress pain behavior and conantokin G–reversed mechanical allodynia in mice.[24]

PREVALENCE OF PAIN

Figure 27-1 demonstrates the complexity of cancer-related pain. Approximately 60 percent of cancer patients experience cancer-related pain. The likelihood of pain increases with advancing cancer stage.[25] Patients who experience pain have lower quality of life, greater

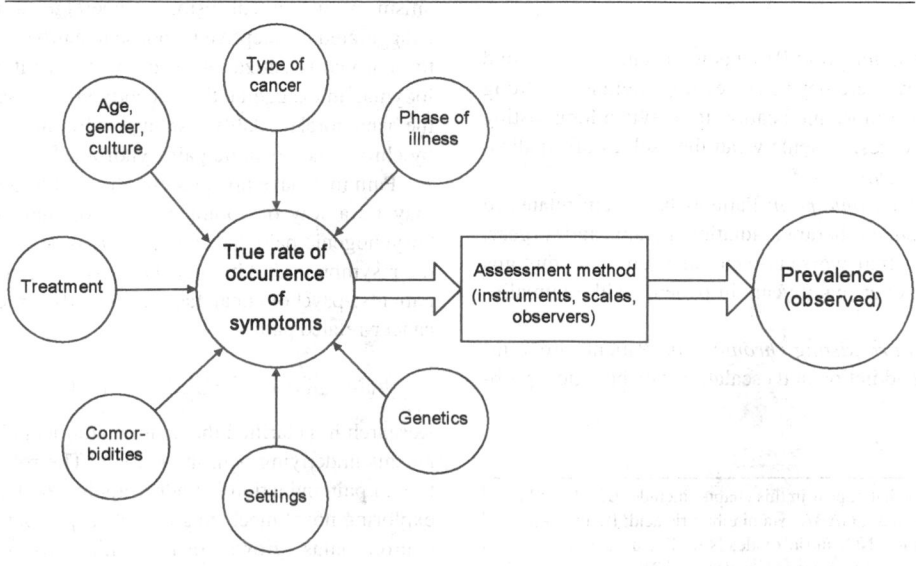

FIGURE 27-1 Factors contributing to the prevalence of pain symptoms. (Adapted from the Agency for Healthcare Research and Quality: Evidence Report/Technology Assessment No. 61.[139])

sleep disruption, impaired functionality, and more depressive symptoms.[26–28]

Individuals from minority populations, women, socioeconomically disadvantaged persons, and elderly individuals are at greater risk for undertreatment for cancer-related pain.[29–32] Poor communication between patients and physicians may be a major barrier to adequate pain management.[29,33] In a study examining physicians' attitudes toward their patients' pain management needs, physicians more likely underestimated the pain management needs of their female than their male patients.[29]

Another barrier to effective pain management in cancer patients is lack of availability of analgesics for severe cancer-related pain.[31] Data from a survey of 347 neighborhood pharmacies in diverse ethnic and social class neighborhoods in New York City reveal that pharmacies in nonwhite and low-income neighborhoods less likely carry opioid analgesics sufficient to treat patients in severe pain.[31]

ASSESSMENT OF PAIN

Pain is a complex, subjective experience that is not directly measurable in patients. Instead, pain must be operationally defined and estimated using patient self-report. Pain assessment conducted before and periodically after treatment allows the physician to increase pain medication dosage as needed.

Visual analogue scales consist of a straight line on which patients indicate their current level of pain by placing a mark on the side of the line that best represents their pain state.[34] Categorical pain descriptions (also known as word scales), such as "none," "mild," "moderate," and "severe," also are used to assess pain in cancer patients, who indicate the category that best describes their current pain.

Multidimensional scales for pain can be used to assess the intensity of pain and factors that aggravate pain. The Brief Pain Inventory (BPI)[35] is a multidimensional scale that assesses the severity of pain and the impact of pain on daily functions. An advantage of this scale is that the BPI provides a diagram in which patients shade-in the areas of their body where they feel pain. The BPI also assesses the effectiveness of current pain treatments. The BPI has been translated and validated for use in diverse populations, including Chinese,[36] Hindi,[37] Italian,[38] and Spanish[39] populations.

PSYCHOLOGICAL FACTORS AND CANCER PAIN

DEPRESSION AND CANCER PAIN

Prevalence rates for major depression are as high as 42 percent in cancer patients[40] compared to 7 percent in the general population.[41] Cancer patients experience emotional distress related to fear of death, dependency, disfigurement, disability, financial status, and disrupted relationships. Many of these individuals develop depressive symptoms as they learn to cope with major life changes caused by the cancer diagnosis itself, cancer-related pain, and cancer treatments.

Mood and behavior changes in cancer patients may be caused by physiologic changes in response to illness. Proinflammatory cytokines released by tissue damage can impact neurotransmitter and neuroendocrine function, leading to "sickness behavior."[42] Sickness behavior is characterized by anhedonia, cognitive dysfunction, anxiety, irritability, psychomotor retardation, fatigue, anorexia, sleep disruption, and increased sensitivity to pain.[43] Cytokines used to treat malignancies, such as IL-2 or interferon alpha-2B, often induce depressive symptoms.[44]

Depression typically is underdiagnosed in cancer patients. A major complication in diagnosing major depressive disorder in cancer patients is that the diagnostic criteria for major depression include several somatic symptoms that are commonly experienced by cancer patients.[45] Many widely used assessment tools for diagnosing depression include sleep disturbance, motor retardation, loss of energy, and change in appetite/weight as criteria.

Severe depression is associated with reports of increased pain intensity in cancer patients.[46] Depressed cancer patients tend to have more metastases and pain than do their nondepressed counterparts.[47] Chronic pain, whether a result of cancer or some other source, often leads to psychological symptoms, including depression, anger, and anxiety. These emotions can cause increased stress and muscle tension, which produce more pain. Depressed patients often have lower energy levels and engage in fewer physical activities. Decreased activity results in increased muscle weakness and, in turn, more pain.

FATIGUE AND CANCER PAIN

Fatigue often is comorbid with cancer pain[48] and is related to poor quality of life in cancer patients.[49] The greater fatigue reported by individuals who complain of pain may partially be a side effect of pain medications.[49] Analgesics used to treat cancer pain often cause sleep disturbance, leading to greater daytime fatigue.[49] Although use of analgesics for pain control is an independent contributor to fatigue, studies show that pain alone is a significant predictor of fatigue in cancer patients, regardless of analgesic use.[28]

Greater daytime fatigue among cancer patients can be explained by sleep disturbance resulting from pain. Studies reveal that greater than 50 percent of cancer patients report significant sleep problems.[29] Among chronically ill patients, sleep disturbances are related to poorer quality of life, diminished work productivity, and greater use of health care services.[50] Pain sensations at night may lead to sleep disruption and, in turn, cause daytime fatigue. However, the mechanisms underlying the relationship among pain, sleep, and fatigue are not completely understood.

TREATMENT OF PAIN

PHARMACOLOGIC INTERVENTIONS

When selecting treatment regimens that consider the patient's needs, clinicians must consider the nature and etiology of the pain. Patient well-being can be compromised not only by the pain itself but also by many of the therapeutic interventions involved in pain treatment. Some interventions may not be appropriate for certain types of pain.[51] For instance, neuropathic pain can be unresponsive to opiates. Consequently, morphine and other narcotic analgesics that are considered the "gold standard" of analgesics not only may fail to produce pain relief but may worsen other symptoms, such as nausea.[52]

The World Health Organization's three-step ladder for cancer pain control (Fig. 27-2) is a drug-treatment method with documented ef-

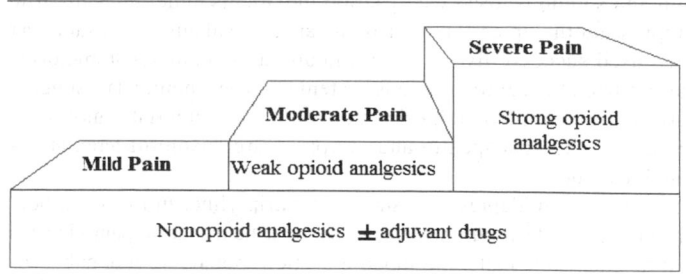

FIGURE 27-2 Analgesic steps. (Adapted from the World Health Organization analgesic ladder.[53])

fectiveness in many settings.[53] Treatment begins with the use of non-narcotic analgesics, moves to moderately strong opiates and then to strong opiates, and culminates in a continuous morphine drip if necessary. Nonnarcotic analgesics can play an important role in treatment as an adjuvant because they potentiate the effects of stronger analgesics.[54]

NONOPIOID AND ADJUVANT ANALGESIC DRUGS

The effectiveness of nonsteroidal antiinflammatory drugs (NSAIDs) is well established for initial treatment of mild to moderate pain and, when combined with an opioid, for treatment of moderate to severe cancer pain. NSAIDs may be particularly helpful in treating metastatic bone pain.

Acetaminophen has a less potent antiinflammatory effect[8] but is included in this group because it has analgesic potency and pharmacologic characteristics similar to other NSAIDs. Acetaminophen does not inhibit platelet function, so it is useful in thrombocytopenic patients. NSAIDs do not produce physical dependence or tolerance. However, they have a ceiling effect such that increasing the dose beyond a certain level does not increase the analgesic effect but may increase toxic side effects.[55] NSAIDs inhibit peripheral and central COX, which catalyzes conversion of arachidonic acid to prostaglandins and leukotrienes.[56] Because these substances are important inflammatory mediators that sensitize nociceptors to painful stimuli, inhibition of their synthesis can explain the analgesic properties of NSAIDs. NSAIDs have a central action at the brain or spinal cord level that also may play an important role in their analgesic effects.[57]

COX-1 and COX-2 are the two main forms of COX. COX-1 enzymes are necessary for normal physiologic function of stomach, kidney, and platelets. COX-2 enzymes are inducible and are involved in inflammation.[54] Nonselective COX inhibitors inhibit platelet function to a variable degree. The most serious side effects associated with conventional NSAIDs include bleeding and gastric ulceration, renal failure, and hepatic dysfunction.[58] Clinical studies suggest specific COX-2 inhibitors may provide an improved risk-to-benefit ratio in terms of gastrointestinal safety compared with conventional NSAIDs.[59] However, recent postmarketing studies have led to concerns over their adverse vascular effects, leading to the removal of rofecoxib from the market and an increased caution in the use of any agent in this class of analgesics.

Glucocorticoids provide a wide range of effects, including enhancement of analgesia, antiinflammatory activity, mood elevation, increased energy level, antiemetic activity, and appetite stimulation. They are useful for metastatic bone pain, pain related to nerve compression, and pain from spinal cord compression. Well-known side effects associated with steroid therapy include myopathy, hyperglycemia, weight gain, dysphoria, mood disruption, and oral candidiasis.[60]

Anticonvulsants such as phenytoin, carbamazepine, valproate, and clonazepam are useful for management of selected neuropathic pain syndromes (e.g., lancinating pain and paroxysmal stabbing pain), perhaps by reducing spontaneous discharges of neurons.[61] Carbamazepine can cause dose-related transient bone marrow suppression and should be used with caution in patients undergoing marrow suppressant therapies.[62] Lamotrigine, an atypical anticonvulsant, has been used successfully in cases of neuropathic pain syndrome originating from the central nervous system.[63] Experimental data suggest gabapentin is antihyperalgesic in animals and potentiates morphine analgesia when gabapentin and morphine are coadministered at subanalgesic doses.[64]

Tricyclic antidepressants such as amitriptyline, imipramine, nortriptyline, and desipramine effectively treat neuropathic pain via several mechanisms, including mood elevation, potentiation or enhancement of opioid analgesia,[65] and direct analgesic effects.[66] The analgesic effect of these drugs is not directly related to their antidepressant activity. Pain relief occurs about 1 to 2 weeks after initiation of therapy.

Selective serotonin reuptake inhibitors are a newer class of antidepressants with a more benign side effect profile; however, they are less effective analgesics than tricyclic antidepressants.[67]

Evidence suggests systemic local anesthetic drugs are effective for neuropathic pain.[68] Intraspinal administration with an opioid may provide additional analgesia and permit successful treatment of patients unresponsive to spinal morphine alone.[69] However, in most cases, chronic therapy is accomplished using oral local anesthetic drugs. Oral formulations of mexiletine, tocainide, and flecainide have analgesic efficacy and may be valuable in the treatment of neuropathic pain.[70]

The analgesic ability of clonidine and other α_2-agonists, which work through nonopioid mechanisms, suggests these agents offer an advantage over opioids for patients who are tolerant, nonresponsive, or allergic to opioids. Antinociceptive effects of clonidine may be mediated via inhibitory interactions with presynaptic and postsynaptic primary afferent nociceptive projections in the dorsal horn neurons and by inhibition of substance P release. Epidural administration of clonidine has been approved in the United States for use in cancer patients with intractable pain. No documented cases of toxicity in animal or human bolus dose studies have been reported to date.[71] Clonidine can be administered via the oral or transdermal route. Higher doses often are poorly tolerated because they lead to somnolence, dry mouth, and dizziness.[72]

NMDA receptor antagonists such as ketamine, memantine, and dextromethorphan may provide new tools for the broad range of adjuvant analgesics (Table 27-1). Intrathecal injection of the GABA$_A$ antagonist bicuculline elicits touch-evoked agitation and spinal release of amino acids. Allodynia from GABA$_A$ antagonism is blocked by NMDA receptor antagonism. The NMDA antagonist-sensitive allodynia may reflect loss of GABAergic inhibition and increased spinal glutamate release secondary to loss of inhibition.[73] Preclinical studies established that NMDA receptor is involved in the development of neuropathic pain and opioid tolerance.[11] New data confirm the substantial benefit resulting from addition of ketamine to opioid therapy in different chronic pain states. Ketamine in subanesthetic doses appears to be a safe and effective agent that can be recommended for terminally ill patients.[74]

WEAK OPIOIDS

Opioids produce analgesia by binding to specific opioid receptors in the brain and spinal cord.[22] Current thinking recognizes two classes of opioid drugs: "weak" and "strong." Codeine, dihydrocodeine, tramadol, and dextropropoxyphene are prime examples of the weak class. Morphine, methadone, oxycodone, buprenorphine, hydromorphone, fentanyl, and heroin are examples of the strong class.[6,51] Weak opioids often are marketed in combination with a nonopioid such as aspirin or an NSAID, with the latter component limiting the dose. Weak drugs often are expensive with respect to their potential benefits.[75]

The efficacy of codeine (200–400 mg/day) in moderate cancer-related pain has been confirmed. Codeine is a prodrug of morphine with a biotransformation of approximately 10 percent. The pharmacodynamic effects of codeine largely result from production of its active metabolite morphine.[76] Conversion of codeine to morphine is effected by the cytochrome P450 enzyme CYP2D6. Well-characterized genetic polymorphisms in CYP2D6 lead to the inability to convert codeine to morphine, thus making codeine ineffective as an analgesic for approximately 10 percent of the Caucasian population.[77] Metabolism varies among different ethnic groups. For example, Chinese patients produce less morphine from codeine than do Caucasians because Chinese patients produce less morphine-6-glucuronide.[78] Codeine can be used in combination with aspirin or acetaminophen. Oral doses greater than 200 mg are associated with significant side effects of nausea and vomiting.[79]

TABLE 27-1 ADJUNCTIVE ANALGESICS COMMONLY USED FOR CANCER PAIN

CLASS AND DRUGS	ORAL DOSAGE RANGE (MG/DAY)	MAIN USE OF THE CLASS	COMMENTS FOR THE CLASS
Nonsteroidal antiinflammatory drugs (NSAIDs)			
Acetaminophen	650–4000	Initial therapy for treatment of mild pain; adjuvant analgesics for severe pain	Relative contraindications include peptic ulcer disease, thrombocytopenia, and renal impairment; parenteral formulation of ketorolac is available in United States
Indomethacin	50–200		
Ibuprofen	900–2400		
Piroxicam	10–40		
Ketorolac	10–40		
Celecoxib	200–400		
Tricyclic antidepressants			
Amitriptyline	25–200	Adjunctive therapy for neuropathic pain (e.g., vincristine-induced, radiation plexopathy, tumor invasion, dysesthesia); helpful in treating insomnia and depression	Start with lowest dose and titrate to effect; patient monitoring includes regular electrocardiogram, measurement of blood pressure, and blood level of the drugs
Imipramine	10–200		
Desipramine	25–150		
Nortriptyline	10–150		
Anticonvulsants			
Carbamazepine	200–1200	Adjunctive therapy for neuropathic pain	Carbamazepine should be used with caution in patients undergoing other bone marrow suppressant therapies; monitor for hematologic, hepatic allergic reactions
Phenytoin	250–400		
Valproate	375–1000		
Clonazepam	1.5–8		
Gabapentin	300–1800		
Glucocorticoids			
Dexamethasone	0.75–10	Adjunctive therapy for neuropathic pain or metastatic bone pain; alleviate headache from raised intracranial pressure; improve appetite, mood, nausea, and malaise	Short-term administration of high doses recommended for epidural cord compression
Cortisone	25–300		
Methylprednisolone	4–30		
Local anesthetics			
Mexiletine	600–900	Adjunctive therapy for lancinating neuropathic pain; can be used in combination with long-acting corticosteroids	
Tocainide	600–1200		
α_2-Adrenergic agonist			
Clonidine	0.1–0.3	Adjunctive therapy for sympathetically mediated pain; sedative and anxiolytic action	Blood pressure and heart rate decrease dose dependently; rapid administration may cause increased blood pressure and reflex bradycardia
Psychostimulants			
Dextroamphetamine	10–60	Potentiate opioid analgesics; enhance alertness	Administer second dose in early afternoon to avoid sleep disturbances
Methylphenidate	5–40		

Adapted from Ahmedzai[140] with additional information from multiple references.[6,8,141]

The analgesic strength of propoxyphene is about half to two thirds that of codeine. Propoxyphene in high doses can cause cardiac conduction depression, convulsions, central nervous system depression, and respiratory depression.[79]

Tramadol administered with NSAIDs is useful for relieving spastic visceral pain. The maximum daily dose is 500 to 600 mg. The drug is contraindicated in patients taking monoamine oxidase inhibitors or serotonergic blocking agents.[80]

STRONG OPIOIDS

Morphine is the most commonly used strong opioid for treatment of moderate to severe pain (Table 27-2).[8] Use of strong opioids is associated with tolerance, physical dependence, and addiction. These terms have specific meanings. "Tolerance" refers to a decline in the effectiveness of an opioid with continued use, such that higher doses are required to maintain the same analgesic effect. Tolerance is rarely a major problem in patients with stable pain syndromes.[81] Worsening pain in the cancer patient usually results from disease progression and not tolerance. "Physical dependence" is a physiologic state characterized by a withdrawal syndrome when therapy is discontinued abruptly or dose is reduced substantially. The phenomenon is observed when repeated and substantial doses of opioids are administered for more than a few days. Withdrawal symptoms include anxiety, irritability,

chills, hot flashes, joint pain, lacrimation, rhinorrhea, diaphoresis, nausea, vomiting, abdominal cramps, and diarrhea. Neither tolerance nor physical dependence represents drug addiction. "Addiction" is a psychological and behavioral syndrome characterized by continued drug use despite harm to the individual.[82] Everyone worries about addiction, but addiction is seldom a problem with cancer patients. In fact, unwarranted fear of addiction is one of the main obstacles to adequate pain management.[8]

Common side effects associated with opioids include constipation and sedation.[8] Some patients experience dry mouth, nausea and vomiting, respiratory depression, skin flushing, pruritus, urinary retention, sweating, myoclonus, muscle rigidity, tremor, dysphoria, euphoria, confusion, delirium, hallucination, dizziness, disrupted cognition, hypertension or hypotension, headache, convulsion, sleep disturbances, sexual dysfunction, physiologic dependence, and inappropriate secretion of antidiuretic hormone.[6,8] Tolerance to most side effects occurs with chronic therapy, but tolerance to the constipating effects of opioids either does not occur or occurs very slowly.[8]

The route of opioid administration (oral, transdermal, or spinal) influences the dose at which side effects emerge. Pragmatic suggestions can be easily incorporated in oncology settings.[83] Guidelines advise oral administration with morphine every 4 hours and the same dose for breakthrough pain. The total daily dose of morphine should

TABLE 27-2   OPIOID ANALGESICS COMMONLY USED FOR SEVERE PAIN

NAME	EQUINANALGESIC INTRAMUSCULAR DOSE (MG)	STARTING ORAL DOSE RANGE (MG)	MAIN USE AND COMMENTS	PRECAUTIONS
Agonists				
Morphine	10	30–60	Standard of comparison for opioid analgesics; sustained-release preparations are available	Reduce doses for aged patients; compromised respiratory function; head injury or increased intracranial pressure; liver failure; renal disease; hypotension
Levorphanol	2	2–4	Less effective when given orally; long plasma half-life	Like morphine; less nausea and vomiting than morphine; repeated administration at short interval may lead to drug accumulation
Meperidine	75	Not recommended	Onset of analgesic effect is faster (within 10 min); not the drug of choice for treatment of severe or prolonged pain and should not be used for >48 hours or in doses >600 mg/24 h	Large doses repeated at short intervals produce central nervous system excitation (hallucination, convulsion, tremor); not for patients with impaired renal or hepatic function; not for patients taking monoamine oxidase inhibitors
Fentanyl	0.1	—	Sustained-release transdermal patches are effective for >48 h; used intravenously, epidurally, or intrathecally; anesthetic adjuvant; transmucosal fentanyl is not recommended in opioid-naive patients because of side effects	Respiratory depression is similar with morphine, but the onset is more rapid
Methadone	10	20	Good oral potency; long plasma half-life; treatment of opioid abstinence syndrome	Like morphine; delayed toxicity from accumulation
Oxymorphone	1	10 (rectal)	No oral form; available as a rectal suppository; rectal route is contraindicated in patients with neutropenia or lesions of anus	Like morphine
Mixed agonist-antagonists				
Pentazocine	30–60	100	Oral route should be used whenever possible to diminish possibility of abuse; patients who had been receiving morphine-like opioids require brief (1–2 days) drug-free interval	Higher doses (parenteral doses >60 mg) elicit dysphoric and psychotomimetic effects (weird thoughts, anxiety, nightmare, hallucination); may precipitate opioid withdrawal symptoms in opioid-dependent patients
Nalbuphine	10	Not available	Patients who had been receiving morphine-like opioids require brief (1–2 days) drug-free interval	Incidence of psychotomimetic effects is lower than pentazocine
Butorphanol	2–3	Not available	Better suited for relief of acute rather than chronic pain	Like nalbuphine; not for congestive heart failure or myocardial infarction
Partial agonist				
Buprenorphine	0.4	Not available	Sublingual preparation is not yet in United States. FDA approval for use in treatment of heroin addiction is pending	Precipitates opioid withdrawal symptoms in opioid-dependent patients; after discontinuation, delayed withdrawal symptoms develop 2 days to 2 weeks later

Adapted from Inturrisi[143] with additional information from multiple references.[5,6,8,141]

be reviewed daily. If rescue doses are required consistently, the regular dose should be increased. For patients receiving morphine immediate-release formulation every 4 hours, a double dose at bedtime helps prevent awakening because of pain. Morphine can be given subcutaneously, but intramuscular use for treatment of chronic cancer pain is less advisable to minimize pain on injection. Intravenous administration may be preferred for generalized edema, skin troubles, coagulation disorders, and poor peripheral circulation.[83]

Intravenous dosing has rapid onset of action. Oral or rectal medications require higher doses than parenteral medications because of hepatic metabolism. Morphine and oxycodone also are available in controlled-release forms. Patients should be cautioned not to crush or divide these formulations because such action alters drug bioavailability.[6,8,75]

Orally administered patient-controlled analgesia (PCA) is becoming standard practice in cancer pain management. The rescue dose of opioid can be calculated as approximately 5 to 10 percent of the total daily dose and administered every 2 to 3 hours.[84] If patients have an intravenous or subcutaneous access portal and report irregular and sud-denly exaggerating pain, intravenous or subcutaneous PCA is recommended. Immediate pain relief increases patient satisfaction and decreases patient anxiety.[85] This technique is contraindicated for confused and sedated patients.[86]

OPIOID WITHDRAWAL

Withdrawal likely will develop with continuous use of opioids at moderate to high doses for more than 1 week. Withdrawal is characterized by pervasive symptoms of gastrointestinal distress, myalgias, and dysphoria. Withdrawal can be minimized by careful tapering of opioids. Tapering regimens vary, but a reasonable approach is tapering opioids by 33 percent in the first 2 days and thereafter by approximately 10 to 20 percent per day.

NONPHARMACOLOGIC TREATMENT OF PAIN

Nonpharmacologic treatments are widely used to manage pain and cope with emotional distress. Treatments range from conventional techniques, such as behavioral and cognitive behavioral therapies, to complementary and alternative medicine interventions, which include food supplements and herbs, meditation, and energy therapies.

COGNITIVE BEHAVIORAL THERAPY

Cognitive behavioral therapy is based on the belief that a person's distressing physical and mental symptoms partially result from maladaptive thoughts, feelings, or behaviors. Thus, therapy focuses on recognizing and modifying thoughts, feelings, and behaviors that contribute to physical and emotional distress. When used as an adjunct to medical treatments, this approach is effective in reducing pain[87] and distress[88] and increasing quality of life in cancer patients.[89]

Relaxation Techniques Relaxation techniques involve repetitive focus on a word, sound, prayer, phrase, or muscular activity. Several studies demonstrated the effectiveness of relaxation training in reducing cancer-related pain, depression, anxiety, and tension. Guided imagery induces a relaxed state through use of a visual image, such as a peaceful scene that enhances the sense of relaxation.[90] This technique often is used in conjunction with muscle relaxation training and is effective in treating pain.[91]

Hypnosis Hypnosis is a widely used technique that involves induction of a deep state of relaxation or trance. Patients receive suggestions to alter sensations, behavior, feelings, or thoughts while they are in an hypnotic state.[90] Research supports use of hypnosis for relieving cancer-related pain in adults.[92,93] Results of studies examining the effectiveness of hypnosis in children are contradictory.[94-96]

Nutrition and Physical Activity Initial studies have examined the effects of nutritional and dietary approaches on cancer pain.[97,98] Although the findings are preliminary and have not been supported in cancer patients, evidence suggests increased intake of fruits and vegetables helps reduce the pain associated with inflammatory states.[98] Increasing physical activity can help improve quality of life in cancer patients.[99,100] Most studies examining the effect of exercise on chronic pain were conducted in noncancer patients; nonetheless, the results suggest exercise interventions help reduce chronic pain.[101-103]

COMPLEMENTARY AND ALTERNATIVE MEDICINE

These therapies and techniques are used as a complement or alternative to conventional care to prevent illness or promote health and well-being. Approximately 31 percent of cancer patients use these techniques,[90] which include dietary treatment, herbs, acupuncture, massage therapy, spiritual healing, and meditation. Complementary and alternative therapies are widely used, but few clinical trials have examined the effectiveness of these techniques in managing cancer-related pain.

Acupuncture Acupuncture is a technique based on traditional Chinese medical theory. According to Chinese medicine, a network of energy flows through the body, and an imbalance in this energy flow creates a disease process. Acupuncture is believed to restore balance in the body.[90] Many health professionals who currently practice this method believe acupuncture points correspond to peripheral nerve junctions.[90] Results of clinical trials do not yet support the use of acupuncture in managing cancer-related pain.

Meditation Meditation and spiritual healing were developed within a religious context and ultimately aim for spiritual growth, personal transformation, or a transcendental experience. Transcendental meditation consists of repeating a silent word or phrase (a mantra), with the goal of quieting mental dialogue. Mindfulness meditation consists of observing or attending to thoughts, emotions, or sensations as the patient becomes aware of them. Studies suggest meditation can be effective in managing cancer-related pain[104] and relieving stress in patients with cancer-related pain.[105]

ANESTHETIC AND SURGICAL APPROACHES

Local anesthetic blocks can have a diagnostic role in addition to a therapeutic role because they allow patients to experience the sensation of numbness. Some patients prefer pain to complete loss of sensation.[106] Clinicians must consider the onset, duration of action, degree of sensory and motor blockade, and side effects of the anesthetic drug. Central nervous system toxicity and cardiotoxicity, which can result from accidental intravascular or intrathecal injections, are the most serious adverse effects of local anesthetics.[107]

Neurosurgical anesthetic approaches for pain control consist of three main categories[108]:

1. *Neuropharmacologic procedures*: This technique delivers analgesic drugs directly to the central nervous system, usually via epidural, intracranial, or intraventricular spaces.
2. *Neuroablative techniques*: These techniques interrupt pain transmission by destroying nerves. Techniques include nerve avulsion, cordotomy, rhizotomy, myelotomy, spinothalamic tractotomies, cingulotomy, and dorsal root entry zone lesion.
3. *Neurostimulatory procedures*: These techniques modulate rostral nociceptive transmission by stimulating selected regions of the peripheral or central nervous system via implanted electrodes.

Epidural and intrathecal opioids are indicated if systemic analgesic treatments fail because of unacceptable side effects or inadequate pain relief. Less than 2 percent of patients with cancer pain are candidates for spinal opioids.[109] Although high efficacy of spinal opioids with much smaller doses of morphine has been reported,[110] failure rates up to 30 percent have been reported.[111] Lack of consensus exists regarding appropriate dose. Side effects such as infection, fibrosis around the catheter, cerebral spinal fluid leakage, mechanical pump failure, catheter kinking, obstruction, dislodgment, and neurologic complications pose problems.[112]

Clinicians should carefully select patients with severe intractable chronic pain for intraventricular morphine treatment. The technique should be used only after all other treatments have been attempted.[113]

Open cordotomy involves dividing the anterolateral quadrant of the spinal cord, which contains the spinothalamic tract. The procedure can lessen pain perception on the contralateral side, up to a level several segments below the lesion.[108] Cordotomy should be considered when all medical and minimally invasive methods have failed to adequately control pain, the severity of the pain warrants surgery, and no medical contraindications to the procedures exist. Cordotomy can be useful for unilateral and well-localized pain that is transmitted via spinal cord pathways.[114]

Neurostimulatory treatment may provide relief for patients with radiating pain, continued pain following back surgery, and ischemic pain from inoperable peripheral vascular diseases.[8] Electrical signals sent by spinal cord stimulation "confuse" the brain as to the modality being experienced. Consequently, patients feel a tingling sensation instead of pain.[115] Transcutaneous electrical nerve stimulation is a noninvasive and simple technique involving cutaneous application of electrical currents. Transcutaneous electrical nerve stimulation may mediate antihyperalgesia through activation of opiate systems. Transcutaneous electrical nerve stimulation combined with exogenous analgesics can enhance the analgesic effect and reduce side effects.[116]

SPECIAL CONSIDERATIONS

SICKLE CELL ANEMIA

In sickle cell anemia, red blood cells intermittently cause vasoocclusion that leads to episodes of ischemic pain. Sickle cell anemia affects large numbers of Americans[117] of African descent and individuals of Saudi-Arabian, Indian, and Mediterranean ancestry (see Chap. 47).

Pain is the most common and distressing symptom related to sickle cell disease (see Chap. 47). Sickle cell pain differs from other types of pain because it is unpredictable, recurrent, and persistent. Intense pain occurs in the joint or organ where sickled blood cells block oxygen flow to tissues, leading to tissue damage. Tissue damage, in turn, releases several inflammatory mediators that aggravate the pain. Pain usually occurs deep in the bones and muscles of the arms, legs, and back. The frequency of pain experienced by sickle cell patients ranges from one to 15 or more episodes per year. The episodes can last from only a few hours to several weeks. Environmental factors, including physical stress, trauma, dehydration, and infections, influence pain in sickle cell patients.[117]

Mild or moderate acute sickle cell pain usually can be treated at home using the World Health Organization's three-step analgesic ladder. Over-the-counter medications, such as acetaminophen and ibuprofen, usually are adequate to treat this type of pain. However, severe sickle cell pain often requires treatment at an emergency room or medical facility. Chronic sickle cell pain lasting longer than a few weeks can be caused by bone or nerve damage resulting from blocked blood flow. This type of pain can be treated with a combination of long-acting opioids and a short-acting opioid.[117]

Standard treatments for sickle cell disease include rest, rehydration, and analgesia. Pain management in sickle cell disease includes pharmacologic and nonpharmacologic treatments. Nonpharmacologic treatments for sickle cell pain include transcutaneous electrical nerve stimulation, heat, cold, vibration, distraction, relaxation, massage, music, guided imagery, self-hypnosis, acupuncture, and biofeedback. Self-hypnosis is among the most widely used behavioral treatments for coping with sickle pain. In one study, self-hypnosis was associated with a significantly reduced number of days during which sickle cell patients experienced pain, decreased pain medication doses, and improved sleep.[118] Although no controlled trials have examined the efficacy of these treatments for sickle cell pain management, several studies have demonstrated their effectiveness for treatment of other types of pain.

Pharmacologic treatments for sickle cell pain include use of nonopioids and opioids. Use of adjuvants such as hypnosis have been beneficial in some patients.[117] Use of opioids for managing sickle cell pain may be hindered by medical staff and patient concerns about drug addiction. Medical staff perceptions about dependence may lead to undertreatment of pain.[119] The incidence of drug dependence in sickle cell patients is not known. Wildly discrepant rates of drug dependence in the sickle cell population have been reported, with incidence rates ranging from 5 to 31 percent in different studies.[117,119] Factors such as sample characteristics influence discrepancies. However, evidence suggests the potential for drug dependence in sickle cell patients is no greater than in any other medical population.[117]

PCA has been used to treat sickle cell pain. Several studies demonstrated the effectiveness of PCA compared to traditional methods.[120] Some patients prefer PCA to traditional nurse-administered analgesia because PCA restores patient control over pain relief during hospitalization and provides quick pain relief and relative independence from staff.[120] More data are needed in this area, but some data suggest PCA is beneficial and safe for treatment of sickle cell pain in children and adolescents.[120]

PAIN OF CHILDHOOD CANCER

Pain is highly prevalent in children with cancer. However, assessment of pain in pediatric cancer patients is difficult.[121] In young children, pain evoked by cancer leads to depression-like reactions that correlate with pain intensity.[122] The prevalence of childhood cancer pain was studied in children aged 10 to 18 years treated at Memorial Sloan Kettering Cancer Center in New York. Pain was the most prevalent symptom in the inpatient group (84.4 percent). The pain was rated as moderate to severe by 87 percent of the children and highly distressing by 53 percent. Pain was experienced by 35 percent of the outpatient group. The pain was rated as moderate to severe by 75 percent of the outpatients.[121]

Pediatric cancer patients can experience multiple sources of pain. Distention or infiltrations of tissue or bone by tumor cause pain. Inflammations from infection, necrosis, or obstruction contribute to pain. Side effects from treatment, including massive infection, organ(s) failure, mucositis, neutropenic enterocolitis, and skin breakdown, are important settings for pain.[123] With more aggressive cancer treatment protocols, pain often is related to the treatment and procedure (e.g., bone marrow aspiration, needle puncture, lumbar puncture, removal of central venous line) rather than the cancer.[124] Neuropathic pain occurs when nerves are injured as a result of tumor infiltration or as a side effect from chemotherapy or radiation therapy.[125] Children with cancer may experience pain unrelated to the disease, just as any other child would. The pain may stem from mild trauma resulting from minor bumps and scrapes that occur during play, major injury, or coexisting illness with a pain component, such as otitis media or juvenile rheumatoid arthritis.[126]

Anxiety, poorly managed painful procedures, anticipatory fear of pain, fear of the unknown, loss of trust, and social and physical isolation are problematic aspects of disease and treatment for children and adults. Educating parents about pain management may help alleviate parental anxiety and distress, which often result from a lack of knowledge about the child's typical reaction to the pain.[127] Nonpharmacologic treatments can be used in conjunction with drug treatments to provide children with pain relief. Children can use distraction and relaxation techniques to control pain and anxiety. Medical play, singing, counting, pretending, and storytelling can help younger children to cope with pain. Teenagers may prefer using a technique such as rhythmic breathing or playing video games.[127]

Acetaminophen is one of the most common nonopioid analgesics used in children (Table 27-3). Acetaminophen has a potential to cause hepatic and renal injury,[128] but these side effects are uncommon in therapeutic doses. The antipyretic action of acetaminophen may be contraindicated in neutropenic patients in whom fever monitoring is important. Oral doses of 15 mg/kg every 4 hours is recommended, with a maximum daily dosage of 90 mg/kg per day in children and 60 mg/kg per day in younger children.[129] No data on the safety, efficacy, and tolerability of COX-2 inhibitors in children with cancer have been reported.[130]

Codeine usually is prescribed for moderate pain. Codeine often is administered in oral doses of 0.5 to 1.0 mg/kg every 4 hours for children older than 6 months. Oxycodone has a higher clearance and a shorter elimination half-life in children aged 2 to 20 years than in adults.[131] Oral morphine at a starting dosage of 1.5 to 2 mg/kg/day is recommended for children with pain unrelieved by mild- or moderate-strength analgesics.[132] Sustained-release oral preparations of morphine are available for children and usually are administered at twice-daily intervals.

BONE INVOLVEMENT

The clinical course of bone disease in myeloma is relatively long. Symptoms include bone pain, fractures, hypercalcemia, and spinal cord compression, all of which may profoundly impair a patient's quality of life.[133]

Bone pain may be poorly localized. The pain often has a deep boring quality that aches or burns and is accompanied by episodes of stabbing discomfort. The pain often is worse at night, is little helped by sleep, and is not necessarily relieved by lying down.[133]

TABLE 27-3   OPIOID ANALGESICS FOR CHILDREN

DRUG	USUAL IV STARTING DOSE (≤50 KG)	USUAL IV STARTING DOSE (≥50 KG)	USUAL PO STARTING DOSE (≤50 KG)	USUAL PO STARTING DOSE (≥50 KG)	EQUIANALGESIC DOSE (PARENTERAL)
Morphine	Bolus dose 0.1 mg/kg q3–4h; continuous infusion 0.03–0.05 mg/kg/h	5–10 mg q3–4h	0.3 mg/kg q3–4h	30 mg q3–4h	10 mg
Controlled-release morphine*	Not available	Not available	0.6 mg/kg q8h or 0.9 mg/kg q12h	30–60 mg q12h	—
Hydromorphone	0.015 mg/kg q3–4h	1–1.5 mg q3–4h	0.06 mg/kg q3–4h	4–8 mg q3–4h	1.5 mg
Codeine	Not available	Not available	0.5–1 mg/kg q3–4h	60 mg q3–4h	130 mg
Oxycodone	Not available	Not available	0.2 mg/kg q3–4h	10 mg q3–4h	—
Meperidine†	0.75 mg/kg q2–3h	75–100 mg q3h	Not recommended	Not recommended	75 mg
Fentanyl	Continuous infusion 0.5–1.5 μg/kg/h	25–75 μg q1–2h	Not available	Not available	100 μg
Methadone‡	0.1 mg/kg q4–8h	5–10 mg q4–8h	0.2 mg/kg q4–8h	10 mg q4–8h	10 mg

Doses are for opioid naive patients.
For infants <6 months, start at ¼ – ⅓ of the suggested dose and titrate to effect.
* Crushing sustained-released tablets produces immediate release of morphine.
† Meperidine is not generally recommended for children with chronic pain but is acceptable for short painful procedures.
‡ Methadone has a risk of delayed sedation and overdosage occurring several days after initiation of treatment. If patients become oversedated, stop dosing, if not, just reduce the dose.

Method of opioid administration:
1. Oral route is the first choice for majority of children.
2. Intramuscular administration should be avoided.
3. Rectal administration is discouraged because of concern regarding infection and the great variability of rectal absorption.
4. Rescue dose of opioid may be calculated as approximately 5–10% of the total daily requirement and administered every hour. If more than approximately six rescue doses are given in a 24-h period, the total daily dose should be increased. An alternative is to increase infusion by 50%.
5. Opioid switching: If changing between short half-life opioids, start new opioid at 50% of equianalgesic dose. If changing from short to long half-life opioid, start at 10–20% of equianalgesic dose and titrate to effect.
6. Opioid tapering. Anyone taking opioid for >1 week must be tapered to avoid withdrawal. Taper by 50% for 2 days and then decrease by 25% every 2 days. When dose is equianalgesic to an oral morphine dose of 0.6 mg/kg/day if <50 kg or 30 mg/day if >50 kg, dose can be stopped.

Adapted from McGrath[142] with additional information from multiple references.[129,130]

The most likely cause of bone pain is osteoclast-induced bone resorption by the tumor, which results in osteoporosis, hypercalcemia, microfractures, or pathologic fractures.[134] Pharmacologic agents that decrease bone resorption, such as bisphosphonates and calcitonin, are used in the management of hypercalcemia and pain caused by bony metastasis. A double-blind, randomized trial comparing salmon calcitonin to a placebo demonstrated that calcitonin 100 IU/day administered subcutaneously resulted in reduced analgesic consumption, shorter duration of pain, and subjective improvement.[135]

Biphosphonates are effective for treatment of myeloma and carcinoma of the breast when they are given to patients with asymptomatic disease or are given prophylactically to patients at high risk for bone involvement. Reductions in spinal fractures in myeloma and bone fractures in breast cancer have been demonstrated.[136]

Radiotherapy is well established as an effective treatment for pain secondary to bone metastasis. Local radiotherapy remains the treatment of choice for local metastatic bone pain in most situations. Underlying pathologic fractures for which surgical fixation may be required prior to radiotherapy must be excluded. A single dose of radiation reportedly alleviates pain within 4 to 6 weeks in 60 to 80 percent of patients, although higher re-treatment rates and pathologic fracture rates remain problems.[137]

Systemic isotopes are an alternative means of delivering radiation to the skeleton. Strontium 89 is the most widely used isotope, but alternatives include phosphorus, rhenium, and samarium.[138]

REFERENCES

1. International Association for the Study of Pain: Subcommittee on Taxonomy in Pain Terms: A list with definitions and notes on usage. *Pain* 6:249, 1979.

2. Suchdev PK: Pathophysiology of pain, in *Manual of Pain Management*, 2nd ed, edited by CA Warfield, HJ Fausett, p 6. Lippincott, Williams & Wilkins, Philadelphia, 2002.

3. Jacox AK, Carr DB, Payne R: Management of cancer pain: Clinical Practice Guideline number 9, edited by U.S. Dept. of Health and Human Services, Agency for Health Care Policy and Research, AHCPR publication number 94-0592, Rockville, MD, 1994.

4. Kochhar SC: Cancer pain, in *Manual of Pain Management*, 2nd ed, edited by CA Warfield, HJ Fausett, p 165. Lippincott, Williams & Wilkins, Philadelphia, 2002.

5. Lederberg MS, Holland JC: Psycho-Oncology, in *Comprehensive Textbook of Psychiatry*, 7th ed, edited by HI Kaplan, BJ Sadock, p 1860. Lippincott, Williams & Wilkins, Philadelphia, 2000.

6. Gustein HB, Akil H: Opioid analgesics, in *Goodman and Gilman's The Pharmacological Basis of Therapeutics*, 10th ed, edited by JG Hardman, LE Limbird, AG Gilman, p 569. McGraw-Hill, New York, 2001.

7. Koenig HG: Pain is a common problem, in *Chronic Pain, Biomedical and Spiritual Approaches*, edited by HG Koenig, p 15. Haworth Pastoral Press, New York, 2003.

8. Gordin V, Weaver MA, Hahn DM: Acute and chronic pain management in palliative care. *Best Pract Res Clin Obstet Gynaecol* 15:203, 2001.

9. Colburn RW, Munglani R: Central and peripheral components of neuropathic pain, in *Pain, Current Understanding, Emerging Therapies and Novel Approaches to Drug Discovery*, edited by C Bountra, R Munglani, WK Schmidt, p 45. Marcel Dekker, New York, 2003.

10. Millan MJ: The induction of pain: An integrative review. *Prog Neurobiol* 57:1, 1999.

11. Yaksh TL: Spinal systems and pain processing: Development of novel analgesic drugs which mechanically defined models. *Trends Pharmacol Sci* 20:329, 1999.

12. Jhamandas K, Yaksh TL, Harty G, et al: Action of intrathecal capsaicin and its structural analogues on the content and release of spinal substance P: Selectivity of action and relationship to analgesia. *Brain Res* 306:215, 1984.

13. Nozaki-Taguchi N, Yaksh TL: A novel model of primary and secondary hyperalgesia after mild thermal injury in the rat. *Neurosci Lett* 254:25, 1998.

14. Wagner R, Myers RR: Schwann cells produce tumor necrosis factor alpha: Expression in injured and non-injured nerves. *Neuroscience* 76:845, 1997.

15. Watkins LR, Maier SF, Goehler LE: Immune activation: The role of pro-inflammatory cytokines in inflammation, illness responses and pathological pain states. *Pain* 63:289, 1995.

16. Gadient RA, Otten UH: Postnatal expression of interleukin-6 (IL-6) and IL-6 receptor (IL-6R) mRNAs in rat sympathetic and sensory ganglia. *Brain Res* 724:41, 1995.

17. Luchter I, Hunt E: The last 48 hours of life. *J Palliat Care* 6:7, 1990.

18. Blick M, Sherwin M, Rosenblum M: Phase I trial of recombinant tumor necrosis factor in cancer patients. *Cancer Res* 47:2986, 1987.

19. Marziniak M, Sommer C: Upregulation of cyclooxygenase-2 is dependent on tumor necrosis factor receptor 1 and 2 after chronic constriction injury. *J Neurol* 247(III):125, 2000.

20. Weber H, Holme I, Amlie E: The natural course of acute sciatica with nerve root symptoms in a double-blind placebo-controlled trial evaluating the effect of piroxicam. *Spine* 18:1433, 1993.

21. Schafers M, Marziniak M, Sorkin LS, et al: Cyclooxygenase inhibition in nerve-injury- and TNF-induced hyperalgesia in the rat. *Exp Neurol* 185:160, 2004.

22. Stranc DS: Endogeneous opioids, in *Manual of Pain Management*, 2nd ed, edited by CA Warfield, HJ Fausett, p 13. Lippincott, Williams & Wilkins, Philadelphia, 2002.

23. Summers S: Evidence-based practice part 1: Pain definitions, pathophysiologic mechanisms and theories. *J Perinanesth Nursing* 14:357, 2000.

24. Malmberg AB, Gilbert H, McCabe RT, Basbaum AI: Powerful antinociceptive effects of the cone snail venom-derived subtype specific NMDA receptor antagonist conantokins G and T. *Pain* 101:109, 2003.

25. Daut RL, Cleeland CS: The prevalence and severity of pain in cancer. *Cancer* 50:615, 1982.

26. Blesch KS, Paice JA, Wickham R, et al: Correlates of fatigue in people with breast or lung cancer. *Oncol Nurs Forum* 18:81, 1991.

27. Dersch J, Polatin PB, Gatchel RJ: Chronic pain and psychopathology: Research findings and theoretical considerations. *Psychosom Med* 64:773, 2002.

28. Hwang SS, Chang VT, Rue M, Kasimis B: Multidimensional independent predictors of cancer-related fatigue. *J Pain Symptom Manage* 26:604, 2003.

29. Anderson KO, Mendoza TR, Valero V, et al: Minority cancer patients and their providers: Pain management attitudes and practice. *Cancer* 88:1929, 2000.

30. Ng B, Dimsdale JE, Shragg GP: Deutsch. Ethnic differences in analgesic consumption for postoperative pain. *Psychosom Med* 58:125, 1996.

31. Morrison RS, Wallenstein S, Natale DK, et al: "We don't carry that": Failure of pharmacies in predominantly nonwhite neighborhoods to stock opioid analgesics. *N Engl J Med* 342:1023, 2000.

32. Cleeland CS, Gonin R, Hatfield AK, et al: Pain and its treatment in outpatients with metastatic cancer. *N Engl J Med* 330:592, 1994.

33. Green CR, Anderson KO, Baker TA, et al: The unequal burden of pain: Confronting racial and ethnic disparities in pain. *Pain Med* 4:277, 2003.

34. McCormack HM, Horne DJL, Sheather S: Clinical application of visual analogue scales: A critical review. *Psychol Med* 18:1007, 1988.

35. Daut RL, Cleeland CS, Flanery RC: Development of the Wisconsin Brief Pain Questionnaire to assess pain in cancer and other diseases. *Pain* 17:197, 1983.

36. Ger LP, Ho ST, Sun WZ, et al: Validation of the Brief Pain Inventory in a Taiwanese population. *J Pain Symptom Manage* 18:316, 1999.

37. Saxena A, Mendoza T, Cleeland CS: The assessment of cancer pain in north India: The validation of the Hindi Brief Pain Inventory—BPI-H. *J Pain Symptom Manage* 17:27, 1999.

38. Caraceni A, Mendoza TR, Mencaglia E, et al: A validation study of an Italian version of the Brief Pain Inventory (Breve Questionario per la Valutazione del Dolore). *Pain* 65:87, 1996.

39. Badia X, Muriel C, Gracia A, et al: Validation of the Spanish version of the Brief Pain Inventory in patients with oncological pain. *Med Clin* 120:52, 2003.

40. National Institutes of Health State of the Science Panel, National Institutes of Health State of the Science Conference Statement: Symptom management in cancer: Pain, depression, and fatigue, July 15–17, 2002. *J Natl Cancer Inst* 95:1110, 2003.

41. Mental Health: A Surgeon General Report. Retrieved December 5, 2003 from http://www.surgeongeneral.gov/library/mentalhealth/chapter4/sec3.html.

42. Dunn AJ, Wang J, Ando T: Effects of cytokines on cerebral neurotransmission. Comparison with the effects of stress. *Adv Exp Med Biol* 461:117, 1999.

43. Kent S, Bluthe RM, Kelley KW, Dantzer R: Sickness behavior as a new target for drug development. *Trends Pharmacol Sci* 155:172, 1992.

44. Capuron L, Ravaud A, Dantzer R: Timing and specificity of the cognitive changes induced by interleukin-2 and interferon-alpha treatments in cancer patients. *Psychosom Med* 63:376, 2001.

45. Akechi T, Nakano T, Akizuki N, et al: Somatic symptoms for diagnosing major depression in cancer patients. *Psychosomatics* 44:244, 2003.

46. Spiegel D, Giese-Davis J: Depression and cancer: Mechanisms and disease progression. *Biol Psychiatry* 54:269, 2003.

47. Ciaramella A, Poli P: Assessment of depression among cancer patients: The role of pain, cancer type and treatment. *Psychooncology* 10:156, 2001.

48. Chang VT, Hwang SS, Feuerman M, Kasimis BS: Symptom and quality-of-life survey of medical oncology patients at a Veterans Affairs medical center: A role for symptom assessment. *Cancer* 88:1175, 2000.

49. Moore P, Dimsdale JE: Opioids, sleep, and cancer-related fatigue. *Med Hypotheses* 58:77, 2002.

50. Mannocchia M, Keller S, Ware JE: Sleep problems, health-related quality of life, work functioning and health care utilization among the chronically ill. *Qual Life Res* 10:331, 2001.

51. Ahmedzai S: New approaches to pain control in patients with cancer. *Eur J Cancer* 33:S8, 1997.

52. Fausett HJ, Warfield CA: Systemic analgesics: An overview, in *Manual of Pain Management*, 2nd ed, edited by CA Warfield, HJ Fausett, p 237. Lippincott, Williams & Wilkins, Philadelphia, 2002.

53. World Health Organization: *Cancer Pain Relief and Palliative Care*, 2nd ed, edited by World Health Organization, Geneva, 1990.

54. Portenoy RK: Current pharmacotherapy of chronic pain. *J Pain Symptom Manage* 19:S16, 2000.

55. Inturrisi CE: Management of cancer pain: Pharmacology and principles of management. *Cancer* 63:2308, 1989.

56. Sunshine A, Olson NZ: Non-narcotic analgesics, in *Textbook of Pain*, 2nd ed, edited by PD Wall, R Melzack, p 650. Churchill Livingstone, New York, 1989.

57. Malmberg AB, Yaksh TL: Hyperalgesia mediated by spinal glutamate or substance P receptor blocked by spinal cyclooxygenase inhibitor. *Science* 257:1276, 1992.

58. Eisenberg E, Berkey CS, Carr DB: Efficacy and safety of nonsteroidal anti-inflammatory drugs for cancer pain: A meta-analysis. *J Clin Oncol* 12:2756, 1994.

59. Bombardier C, Laine L, Reicin A: Comparison of upper gastrointestinal toxicity of rofecoxib and naproxen in patient with rheumatoid arthritis. VIGOR Study Group. *N Engl J Med* 343:1520, 2000.

60. Hanks GW, Trueman T, Twycross RG: Corticosteroid in terminal cancer: A prospective analysis of current practice. *Postgrad Med J* 59:702, 1983.

61. Swerdlow M: Anticonvulsant drugs and chronic pain. *Clin Neuropharmacol* 7:51, 1984.

62. Rosenberg JM, Harrell C, Ristic H: The effect of gabapentin on neuropathic pain. *Clin J Pain* 13:251, 1997.

63. Canavero S, Bonicalzi V: Lamotrigine control of central pain. *Pain* 68:179, 1996.

64. Shimoyama M, Shimoyama N, Inturrisi CE, Elliott KJ: Gabapentin enhances the antinociceptive effects of spinal morphine in the rat tail-flick test. *Pain* 72:375, 1997.

65. Ventafridda V, Bianchi M, Ripamonti C: Studies on the effects of antidepressant drugs on the antinociceptive action of morphine and on plasma morphine in rat and man. *Pain* 43:155, 1990.

66. Max MB, Schafer SC, Culnane M: Amitriptyline, but not lorazepam, relieves postherpetic neuralgia. *Neurology* 38:1427, 1988.

67. Sindrup SH, Gram LF, Brosen K, et al: The selective serotonin reuptake inhibitor paroxetine is effective in the treatment of diabetic neuropathy symptoms. *Pain* 42:135, 1990.

68. Chong SF, Bretscher ME, Mailliard JA: Pilot study evaluating local anesthetics administered systemically for treatment of pain in patients with advanced cancer. *J Pain Symptom Manage* 13:112, 1997.

69. Sjoberg M, Nitescu P, Appelgren L, Curelaru I: Long-term intrathecal morphine and bupivacaine in patients with refractory cancer pain. Results from a morphine:Bupivacaine dose regimen of 0.5:4.75 mg/ml. *Anesthesiology* 80:284, 1994.

70. Galer BS, Harle J, Rowbotham MC: Response to intravenous lidocaine infusion predicts subsequent response to oral mexiletine: A prospective study. *J Pain Symptom Manage* 12:161, 1996.

71. Stuart A, Dunbar MB: Alpha2-adrenoceptor agonists in the management of chronic pain. *Baillieres Clin Anaesthesiol* 14:471, 2000

72. Portenoy RK, Rowe G: Adjuvant analgesic drugs, in *Cancer Pain*, edited by ED Bruera, RK Portenoy, p 188. Cambridge University Press, New York, 2003.

73. Ishikawa T, Marsala M, Sakabe T, Yaksh TL: Characterization of spinal amino acid release and touch-evoked allodynia produced by spinal glycine or GABAA receptor antagonist. *Neuroscience* 95:781, 2000.

74. Luczak J, Dickenson AH, Kotlinska-Lemieszek A: The role of ketamine, an NMDA receptor antagonist, in the management of pain. *Prog Palliat Care* 3:127, 1995.

75. Ripamonti C: Pharmacology of opioid analgesia: Clinical principles, in *Cancer Pain*, edited by ED Bruera, RK Portenoy, p 125. Cambridge University Press, New York, 2003.

76. Caraco Y, Sheller J, Wood AJ: Pharmacogenetic determination of the effects of codeine and prediction of drug interactions. *J Pharmacol Exp Ther* 278:1165, 1996.

77. Eichelbaum M, Evert B: Influence of pharmacogenetics on drug disposition and response. *Clin Exp Pharmacol Physiol* 23:983, 1996.

78. Caraco Y, Sheller J, Wood AJ: Impact of ethnic origin and quinidine coadministration on codeine's disposition and pharmacokinetic effects. *J Pharmacol Exp Ther* 290:413, 1999.

79. Tran ML: Opioids, in *Manual of Pain Management*, 2nd ed, edited by CA Warfield, HJ Fausett, p 266. Lippincott, Williams & Wilkins, Philadelphia, 2002.

80. Camu F, Vanlersberghe C: Pharmacology of systemic analgesic. *Best Pract Res Clin Anaesthesiol* 16:475, 2002.

81. Twycross RG: Clinical experience with diamorphine in advanced malignant disease. *Int J Clin Pharmacol Ther* 9:184, 1974.

82. Portenoy RK, Payne R: Acute and chronic pain, in *Comprehensive Textbook of Substance Abuse*, edited by JH Lowinson, P Ruiz, R Millman, J Langrod, p 691. Williams & Wilkins, Baltimore, 1992.

83. Expert Working Group of the European Association for Palliative Care: Morphine in cancer pain: Modes of administration. *BMJ* 312:823, 1996.

84. Coluzzi PH: Oral patient-controlled analgesia. *Semin Oncol* 24(suppl 16):35, 1997.

85. Ripamonti C, Bruera E: Current status of patient-controlled analgesia in cancer patients. *Oncology* 11:373, 1997.

86. Ferrell BR, Cronin NC, Warfield C: The role of patient-controlled analgesia in the management of cancer pain. *J Pain Symptom Manage* 7:149, 1992

87. Devine EC. Meta-analysis of the effect of psychoeducational interventions on pain in adults with cancer. *Oncol Nurs Forum* 30:75, 2003.

88. Cruess DG, Antoni MH, McGregor BA, et al: Cognitive-behavioral stress management reduces serum cortisol by enhancing benefit finding among women being treated for early stage breast cancer. *Psychosom Med* 62:304, 2000.

89. Sandgren AK, McCaul KD, King B, et al: Telephone therapy for patients with breast cancer. *Oncol Nurs Forum* 27:683, 2000.

90. Vickers AJ, Cassileth BR: Unconventional therapies for cancer and cancer-related symptoms. *Oncology* 1:226, 2001.

91. Syrjala KL, Donaldson GW, Davis MW, et al: Relaxation and imagery cognitive-behavioral training reduce pain during cancer treatment: A controlled clinical trial. *Pain* 63:189, 1995.

92. Lynch DJ Jr: Empowering the patient: Hypnosis in the management of cancer, surgical disease and chronic pain. *Am J Clin Hypn* 42:122, 1999.

93. Trijsburg RW, Van Kippenberg FC, Rijpma SE: Effects of psychological treatment on cancer patients: A critical review. *Psychosom Med* 54:489, 1992.

94. Liossi C, Hatira P: Clinical hypnosis versus cognitive behavioral training for pain management with pediatric cancer patients undergoing bone marrow aspirations. *Int J Clin Exp Hypn* 47:104, 1999.

95. Ellenberg L, Kellerman J, Dash J, et al: Use of hypnosis for multiple symptoms in an adolescent girl with leukemia. *J Adolesc Health Care* 1:132, 1980.

96. Wall VJ, Womack W: Hypnotic versus active cognitive strategies for alleviation of procedural distress in pediatric oncology patients. *Am J Clin Hypn* 31:181, 1989.

97. Paillaud E, Bories PN, Aita SL, et al: Prognostic value of dietary intake and inflammation on survival in patients with advanced cancer: Relationship with performance status, pain, and digestive disorders. *Nutr Cancer* 45:30, 2003.

98. Seaman DR: The diet-induced proinflammatory state: A cause of chronic pain and other degenerative disease? *J Manipulative Physiol Ther* 25:168, 2002.

99. Segal R, Evans W, Johnson D, et al: Structured exercise improves physical functioning in women with stages I and II breast cancer: Results of a randomized controlled trial. *J Clin Oncol* 9:657, 2001.

100. Segal RJ, Reid RD, Courneya KS, et al: Resistance exercise in men receiving androgen deprivation therapy for prostate cancer. *J Clin Oncol* 21:1653, 2003.

101. Borman P, Keskin D, Bodur H: The efficacy of lumbar traction in the management of patients with low back pain. *Rheumatol Int* 23:82, 2003.

102. Heintjes E, Berger M, Bierma-Zeinstra S, et al: Exercise therapy for patellofemoral pain syndrome. *Cochrane Database Syst Rev* 4:CD003472, 2003.

103. Taylor NF, Evans OM, Goldie PA: The effect of walking faster on people with acute low back pain. *Eur Spine J* 12:166, 2003.

104. Speca M, Carlson LE, Goodey E, Angen M: A randomized, wait-list controlled clinical trail: The effect of a mindfulness meditation-based stress reduction program on mood and symptoms of stress in cancer outpatients. *Psychosom Med* 62:613, 2000.

105. Carlson LE, Speca M, Patel KD, Goodey E: Mindfulness-based stress reduction in relation to quality of life, mood, symptoms of stress, and immune parameters in breast and prostate cancer outpatients. *Psychosom Med* 65:571, 2003.

106. Loeser JD: Neurosurgical approaches in palliative care, in *Oxford Textbook of Palliative Medicine*, edited by D Doyle, G Hanks, N MacDonald, p 221. Oxford Medical Publications, Oxford, 1993.

107. Sabrine A, Lyons G: New local anesthetic analgesics, in *Pain*, edited by C Bountra, R Munglani, WK Schmodt, p 795. Marcel Dekker, New York, 2003

108. Jones B, Finlay I, Ray A, Simpson B: Is there still a role for open cordotomy in cancer pain management? *J Pain Symptom Manage* 25: 179, 2003.

109. Zech DFJ, Grond S, Lynch J, et al: A validation of World Health Organization guidelines for cancer pain relief: A 10 year prospective study. *Pain* 63:65, 1995.

110. Plummer JL, Cherry DA, Cousins MJ, et al: Long-term spinal administration of morphine in cancer and non-cancer pain: A retrospective study. *Pain* 44:215, 1991.

111. Chrubasik J, Chrubasik S, Martin E: Patient-controlled spinal opiate analgesia in terminal cancer. *Drugs* 43:799, 1992.

112. Mercadante S: Problems of long-term spinal opioid treatment in advanced cancer patients. *Pain* 79:1, 1999.

113. Meynadier J, Blond S, Willer JC, Le Bars D: Intraventricular morphine: When, how, and why?, in *Cancer Pain Management*, edited by WCV Parris, p 198. Butterworth-Heinemann, Newton, MA, 1997.

114. Sundaresan N, Digiacinto G, Hughes J: Neurosurgery in the treatment of cancer pain. *Cancer* 63(suppl 11):2365, 1989.

115. Brara HS: Neurosurgical procedures, in *Manual of Pain Management*, 2nd ed, edited by CA Warfield, HJ Fausett, p 345. Lippincott, Williams & Wilkins, Philadelphia, 2002.

116. Sluka KA, Chandran P: Enhanced reduction in hyperalgesia by combined administration of clonidine and TENS. *Pain* 100:183, 2002.

117. Platt A, Eckman JR, Beasley J, Miller G: Treating sickle cell pain: An update from the Georgia comprehensive sickle cell center. *J Emerg Nurs* 28:297, 2002.

118. Dinges DF, Whitehouse WG, Orne EC, et al: Self-hypnosis training as an adjunctive treatment in the management of pain associated with sickle cell disease. *Int J Clin Exp Hypn* 45:417, 1997.

119. Elander J, Lusher J, Bevan D, Telfer P: Pain management and symptoms of substance dependence among patients with sickle cell disease. *Soc Sci Med* 57:1683, 2003.

120. Trentadue NO, Kachoyeanos MK, Lea G: A comparison of two regimens of patient-controlled analgesia for children with sickle cell disease. *J Pediatr Nurs* 13:15, 1998.

121. Collins JJ, Byrnes ME, Dunkel I: The measurement symptoms in children with cancer. *J Pain Symptom Manage* 19:363, 2000.

122. Gauvain-Piquard A, Rodary C, Rezvani A, Lemerle J: Pain in children aged 2-6 years: A new observational rating scale elaborated in a pediatric oncology unit—Preliminary report. *Pain* 31:177, 1987.

123. Hooke C, Hellsten MB, Stutzer C, Forte K: Pain management for the child with cancer in end-of-life care: APON position paper. *J Pediatr Oncol Nurs* 19:43, 2002.

124. Elliott SC, Miser AW, Dose AM: Epidemiological features of pain in pediatric cancer patients: A co-operative community-based study. *Clin J Pain* 7:263, 1991.

125. World Health Organization: *Cancer Pain Relief and Palliative Care in Children*. World Health Organization, Geneva, 1998.

126. Bossert EA, Van Cleve L, Adlard K, Saverdra M: Pain and leukemia: The stories of three children. *J Pediatr Oncol Nurs* 19:2, 2002.

127. Chrstensen J, Fatchett D: Promoting parental use of distraction and relaxation in pediatric oncology patients during invasive procedures. *J Pediatr Oncol Nurs* 19:127, 2002.

128. Sandler DP, Smit JC, Weinberg CR: Analgesic use and chronic renal disease. *N Engl J Med* 320:1238, 1989.

129. Collins JH: Cancer management in children. *Eur J Pain* 5(suppl A):37, 2001.

130. Collins JH, Berde C: Cancer pain in children, in *Cancer Pain*, 2nd ed, edited by ED Bruera, RK Portenoy, p 346. Cambridge University Press, New York, 2003.

131. Poyhia R, Seppala T: Lipid solubility and protein binding of oxycodone in vitro. *Pharmacol Toxicol* 74:23, 1994.

132. Hunt A, Joel S, Dick G, Goldman A: Population pharmacokinetics of oral morphine and its glucuronides in children receiving morphine as immediate-release liquid or sustained release tablets. *J Pediatr* 135:47, 1999.

133. Coleman RE: Metastatic bone disease: Clinical features, pathophysiology and treatment strategies. *Cancer Treat Rev* 27:165, 2001.

134. Ascari E, Attardo-Parrinello G, Merlini G: Treatment of painful bone lesions and hypercalcemia. *Eur J Haematol* 43:135, 1989.

135. Roth A, Kolaric K: Analgesic activity of calcitonin in patients with painful osteolytic metastases of breast cancer. *Oncology* 43:283, 1986.

136. Bloomfield DJ: Should biphosphonates be part of the standard therapy of patients with multiple myeloma or bone metastases from other disease? An evidence-based review. *J Clin Oncol* 16:1218, 1998.

137. Sze WM, Shelley MD, Held I, et al: Palliation of metastatic bone pain: Single fraction versus multifraction radiotherapy—A systematic review of randomized trials. *Clin Oncol* 15:345, 2003.

138. Quilty PM, Kirk D, Bolger JJ, et al: A comparison of the palliative effects of strontium-89 and external beam radiotherapy in metastatic prostate cancer. *Radiother Oncol* 31:33, 1994.

139. Agency for Healthcare Research and Quality: Management of cancer symptoms: Pain, depression, and fatigue. Evidence Report/Technology Assessment 61:02, 2002.

140. Ahmedzai S: Pain control in patients with cancer. *Eur J Cancer* 33(suppl 4):855, 1997.

141. *Saunders Nursing Drug Handbook 2003*. Elsevier Science, Philadelphia, 2003.

142. McGrath PA: Development of WHO guidelines on cancer pain and palliative care in children. *J Pain Symptom Manage* 12:87, 1996.

143. Inturrisi CE: Pharmacology of analgesia in *Cancer Pain*, edited by ED Bruera, RK Portenoy, p 112. Cambridge University Press, New York, 2003.

THE ERYTHROCYTE

MORPHOLOGY OF THE ERYTHRON

BRIAN S. BULL

Collectively, the progenitor and adult red cells are termed the *erythron* to reinforce the idea that they function as an organ. The widely dispersed cells constituting this organ arise from undifferentiated, pluripotential stem cells. Following commitment, erythroid progenitors progress through several replicative stages, each having a characteristic ultrastructural morphology. As the cells mature, hemoglobin is synthesized with increasing intensity. The nucleus becomes more pyknotic and eventually is extruded. The mature erythrocyte adopts a variety of forms. Two sequences—from discocyte to echinocyte and from discocyte to stomatocyte—consist of a series of reversible stages through which a single erythrocyte can pass as a result of changes in pH, blood protein levels, and presence of amphipathic drugs. Other shapes, once acquired, are irreversible and not infrequently give evidence of a particular pathophysiologic process. Names derived from Greek terms have been attached to these erythrocyte shapes because there is significant benefit to standardized terminology.

ERYTHRON

Collectively, the progenitor and adult red cells are termed the *erythron* to reinforce the idea that they function as an organ. The widely dispersed cells constituting this organ arise from undifferentiated, pluripotential stem cells. Following commitment, erythroid progenitors progress through several replicative stages, becoming more functionally specialized with maturation. In the process, they acquire the human blood group antigens (Figure 28-1).[1] Eventually the reticulocyte and finally the mature circulating erythrocyte are produced.

ERYTHROID PROGENITORS AND STIMULATING FACTORS

BURST-FORMING UNIT–ERYTHROID

The earliest characterized progenitor committed to the erythroid lineage is the burst forming unit–erythroid (BFU-E). BFU-E is defined *in vitro* by its ability to create a "burst" on semisolid media, that is, a colony consisting of several hundred to thousand cells in 10 to 14 days. This progenitor requires interleukin-3, granulocyte-macrophage colony stimulating factor, erythropoietin, and other factors for proliferation, prevention of apoptosis, and differentiation to morphologically recognizable erythroid precursors.

COLONY-FORMING UNIT–ERYTHROID

As maturation progresses, a late progenitor, colony forming unit–erythroid (CFU-E) can be defined *in vitro*. CFU-E is very sensitive to erythropoietin (see Chap. 15) and can undergo only a few divisions. Thus, CFU-E forms a small colony of morphologically recognizable erythroid precursors in 2 to 5 days.

ERYTHROBLASTIC ISLAND

The anatomical unit of erythropoiesis in the normal adult is the *erythroblastic island*.[2] The erythroblastic island consists of one or two centrally located macrophages surrounded by maturing erythroid cells (Figure 28-2). Adhesion between erythroid cells and macrophages occurs at the CFU-E stage of maturation.[3] The ligand LW gp, a member of the intercellular adhesion molecule family that is virtually restricted in its expression to erythroid cells, appears at this stage and may help stabilize the erythroblastic island.[4] Phase-contrast microcinematography reveals the macrophage is far from passive or immobile. Its pseudopodium-like cytoplasmic extensions move rapidly over cell surfaces of the surrounding wreath of erythroblasts. On scanning electron micrographs, the central macrophage of the erythroblastic island appears sponge-like, with surface invaginations in which the erythroblasts lie. As the erythroblast matures, it moves along a cytoplasmic extension of the macrophage away from the main body. When the erythroblast is sufficiently mature for nuclear expulsion, the erythroblast makes contact with an endothelial cell, passes through a pore in the cytoplasm of the endothelial cell, and enters the circulation (see Chap. 4). The nucleus is ejected prior to egress from the marrow, phagocytized, and degraded by the marrow macrophages.

In addition to fibronectin,[5,6] a cell-to-cell recognition system almost certainly undergirds formation of the erythroblastic island. Maturing erythroid cells express adhesion molecules belonging to the immunoglobulin superfamily, integrins, selectins, sialomucins, and cadherins.[4] Marrow macrophages express hemagglutinin ligands, sialoadhesins, and erythroblast receptors.[7] The cell recognition system also is operative *in vitro*. Erythroblastic islands form in long-term marrow cultures with an adherent stromal cell layer. Likewise, erythroblasts grown from BFU–E in methylcellulose or in plasma clots form erythroid islands if the clots are lysed, permitting erythroblast–macrophage association.[8,9] Despite the central role of erythroid islands in erythropoiesis, morphologically normal development of erythroid cells occurs *in vitro* without these structures as long as developing cells are provided with appropriate cytokines and growth factors.[10]

The erythroblastic island is a fragile structure. It usually is disrupted in the process of obtaining a marrow specimen by needle aspiration. Maturing erythroblasts juxtaposed to a macrophage fragment are encountered only occasionally in stained films of marrow aspirates. Macrophage fragments typically are rich in iron and thus more easily seen in iron-stained preparations. Erythroblastic islands are commonly seen in marrow films only in clinical situations with accelerated erythroblastic activity, such as acute hemolytic anemia and erythroleukemia.

MARROW IRON METABOLISM

Details of iron metabolism are discussed in Chap. 40. In normal humans, the marrow macrophage plays a major role in iron conservation. Aged and damaged erythrocytes, identified and trapped within the marrow microcirculation, are phagocytosed by the macrophage. Lysosomes release their lytic enzymes into the primary phagosome of the macrophage. Digestion of the engulfed red cell is virtually complete within 60 minutes. The membrane is reduced to multiple myelin laminae, and erythrocyte iron is transformed into aggregates of ferritin (Figure 28-3).

Ferritin is a 440-kDa protein consisting of 24 subunits arranged to form a hollow sphere. The central cavity can store 4500 iron atoms[11] in the form of electron-dense particles of approximately 6 nm (60 Å) (see Figure 28-3). Microdiffraction techniques have shown that the

Acronyms and abbreviations that appear in this chapter include: BFU-E, burst forming unit–erythroid; CFU-E, colony forming unit–erythroid; DMT1, divalent metal transporter; MCHC, mean corpuscular hemoglobin concentration.

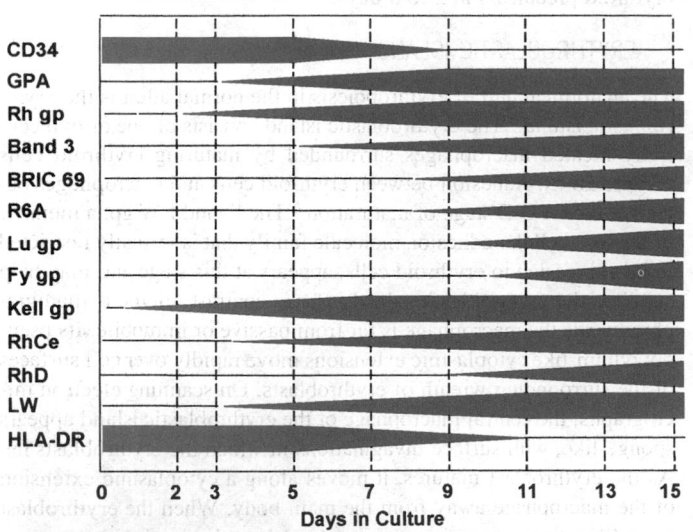

FIGURE 28-1 Sequence in which specific erythroid epitopes appear in *in vitro* cultures of placental cord blood cells. The thickness of the bar represents the percentage of positive cells expressing that marker; full thickness represents 100 percent. (From Southcott et al,[1] with permission.)

iron cores display a hexagonal structure.[12] Under the light microscope, hemosiderin is the intracellular yellowish iron-containing pigment in iron-loaded tissues. Under the electron microscope, hemosiderin is largely composed of dense clusters of ferritin, most of which are membrane enclosed.[13] Ferritin is converted into hemosiderin upon partial degradation of its protein shell by lysosomal enzymes.[14]

The outer membrane of erythroblasts possesses transferrin receptors on clathrin-coated pits. Adherence of transferrin to these portions of the cell membrane initiates a local membrane invagination, and intracytoplasmic vesicles are formed. The vesicles rapidly shed their clathrin coats and fuse with lysosomes, forming endosomes.[11,15] The acid pH in the endosome permits release of iron from transferrin.[11] DMT1 protein is present in the endosomal membrane, where it transports iron released from the transferrin complex into the cytoplasm for heme synthesis (see Chap. 40). Direct mitochondria–endosome interaction is involved[16] and may involve another protein mobilferrin.[17]

Apotransferrin and transferrin receptor molecules are cycled back to the cell membrane, where apotransferrin is released into the extracellular medium. Ferritin molecules also are endocytosed by coated pits on erythroblasts. This phenomenon was termed *rhopheocytosis*[18] before it became evident that this mechanism of acquiring iron was only one example of a more general cellular mechanism for recycling receptors. Immunocytochemical labeling of transferrin receptors has shown that the same pit can contain the transferrin receptors and ferritin molecules.[19] Calculations suggest the coated vesicle transfers 1000 times more iron via ferritin than via transferrin[15]; however, ferritin iron does not appear to be utilized for hemoglobin synthesis.

Despite the efficiency of this transfer mechanism, whether ferritin iron can support the biosynthesis of heme in mitochondria is not clear.[20,21] Possibly the cytosolic ferritin in early red cell precursors is utilized for hemoglobin synthesis, while the ferritin clusters in mature erythroblasts represent storage of excess iron. The H ferritin (see Chap. 40) mRNA accumulates specifically during early erythroid differentiation.[22]

Uncomplexed iron and superoxide form a lethal mixture containing reactive hydroxyl radicals. Hydroxyl radicals cause lipid peroxidation and DNA strand breakage, establishing a self-amplifying and self-propagating redox reaction capable of destroying the developing erythroid cell.[23] This disastrous outcome may not be realized because iron is kept in the safe, bound ferric form (extracellular transferrin, intracellular ferritin, membrane-encapsulated hemosiderin)[24] and the bound iron is transferred directly from endosomes to mitochondria.[23,24]

ERYTHROBLASTIC SERIES

EARLY PROGENITORS

Numerically, BFU−E and CFU−E represent only a minute proportion of human marrow. In mice, CFU−E can be generated in large numbers and then enriched by centrifugal elutriation and Percoll density gradient centrifugation. Under the electron microscope, these cells show large nucleoli, abundant polyribosomes, and large mitochondria (Figure 28-4).[25] Isolation of CD34+ cells from cord blood and marrow has replaced the laborious elutriation/density gradient centrifugation process. *In vitro* cultures using CD34+ cells as the starting material have identified the critical cytokines required for differentiation and maturation[1,10,26,27] and enabled identification and tracing of pure co-

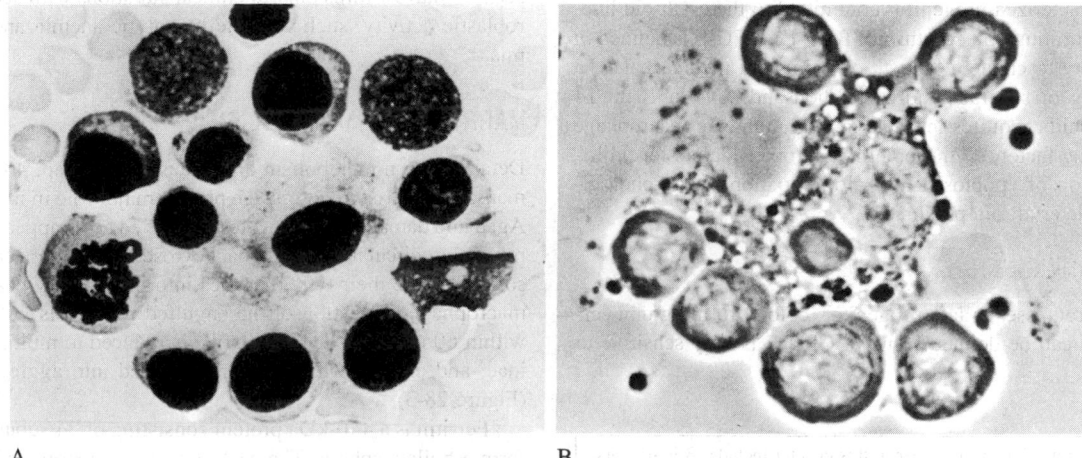

FIGURE 28-2 Erythroblastic island. (*A*) Erythroblastic island as seen in Giemsa-stained marrow. (*B*) Erythroblastic island in the living state examined by phase-contrast microscopy. The macrophage shows dynamic movement in relation to its surrounding erythroblasts.

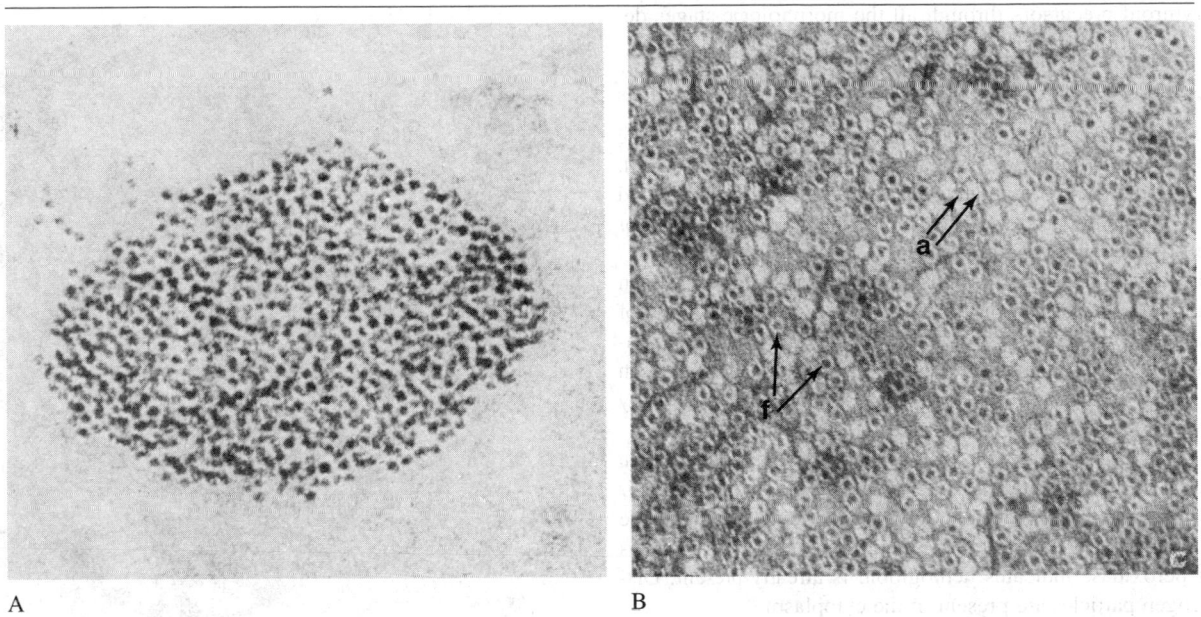

FIGURE 28-3   Ultrastructural aspects of ferritin. (A) Electron micrograph of a membrane-bound erythroblast siderosome showing that the siderosome is composed of individual ferritin molecules. (B) Electron micrograph of negatively stained ferritin and apoferritin mixture showing the ferritin molecule (f) with its protein coat and central dense iron core. Apoferritin molecules (a) lack the central iron cores. (From Bessis and Breton-Gorius[144] with permission.)

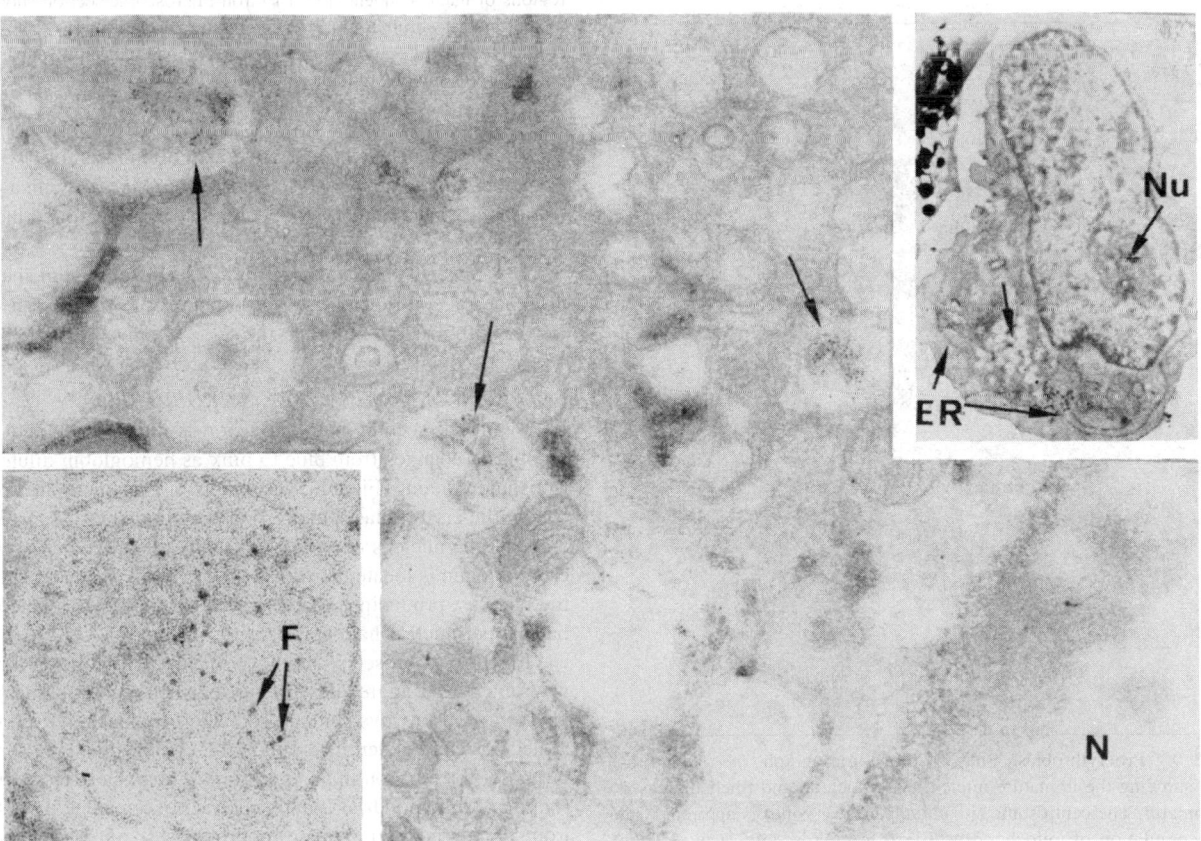

FIGURE 28-4   *Right inset*: Unstained section of a normal presumptive CFU-E that was enriched by panning from marrow, using the monoclonal antibody FA-152.[145] This blast has a large nucleolus (Nu). Incubation in diaminobenzidine medium reveals weak peroxidase activity in the endoplasmic reticulum (ER). In the Golgi zone, several granules appear as vacuoles (arrow). *Main figure*: On enlargement of the Golgi zone, a portion of the nucleus (N) is seen surrounded by a perinuclear cistern containing weak peroxidase activity. Several granules with a pale matrix contain ferritin molecules (arrows). *Left inset*: High magnification of a granule showing ferritin molecules (F) of characteristic structure and density. (Adapted from Breton-Gorius et al,[146] with permission.)

horts of erythroid precursors through all the morphologic stages described in the sections that immediately follow.[28]

PROERYTHROBLASTS

On stained films, the proerythroblast (Figure 28-5) appears as a large cell, 20 to 25 μm in diameter, irregularly rounded or slightly oval. The nucleus occupies approximately 80 percent of the cell area and contains fine chromatin delicately distributed in small clumps. One or several well-defined nucleoli are present.

Polyribosomes arranged in groups of two to six are numerous in the cytoplasm and are typical of this stage. The high concentration of polyribosomes gives the cytoplasm of these cells its characteristic intense basophilia. At high magnification, ferritin molecules are seen dispersed singly throughout the cytoplasm. Rhopheocytosis is easily observed at cell margins.

Three to 12 granules present in the Golgi zone contain ferritin molecules.[29] The granules stain for acid phosphatase, indicating their lysosomal nature, and differ from another class of small granules, the catalase-containing granules. Diffuse cytoplasmic density on sections stained for peroxidase indicates hemoglobin is already present. Dispersed glycogen particles are present in the cytoplasm.[30]

BASOPHILIC ERYTHROBLASTS

Basophilic erythroblasts are smaller than proerythroblasts, measuring 16 to 18 μm (Figure 28-6). The nucleus occupies three fourths of the cell area and is composed of characteristic dark violet heterochromatin interspersed with pink-staining clumps of euchromatin linked by ir-

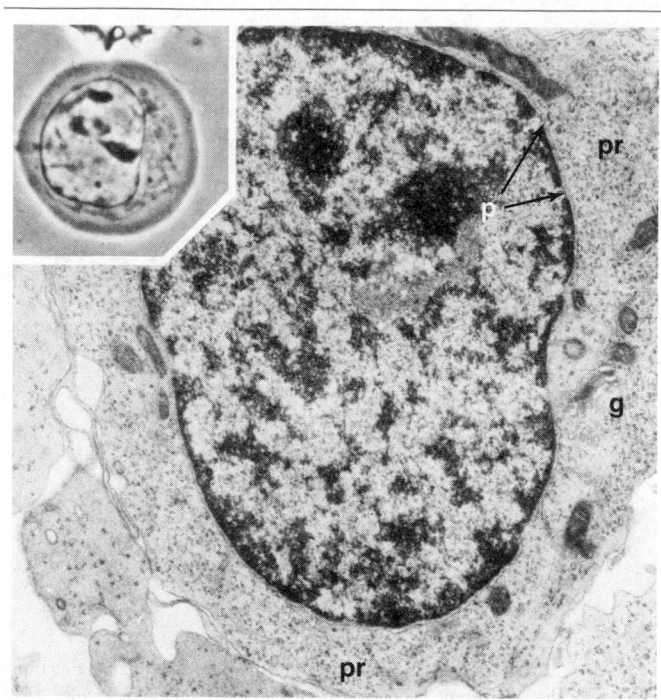

FIGURE 28-6   Basophilic erythroblast. Phase-contrast photomicrograph (*inset*) shows increased clumping of the nuclear chromatin and further rounding of the cell, with aggregation of the mitochondria and centrosome into the regions of nuclear indentation. Electron microscopic section shows clumping of the nuclear chromatin, nuclear pores (p), organization of the nucleoli, increased density of polyribosomes (pr), well-developed Golgi apparatus (g), and a decrease in smooth endoplasmic reticulum.

regular strands. The whole arrangement often resembles wheel spokes or a clock face. The cytoplasm stains deep blue, leaving a perinuclear halo that expands into a juxtanuclear clear zone around the Golgi apparatus.

Cytoplasmic basophilia at this stage results from the continued presence of polyribosomes. Microtubules are often seen connecting two erythroblasts in mitosis.

POLYCHROMATOPHILIC ERYTHROBLASTS

Following the second mitotic division of the erythropoietic series, the cytoplasm changes from blue to pink as hemoglobin dilutes the polyribosome content (Figure 28-7). Cells at this stage are smaller than basophilic erythroblasts, measuring approximately 12 to 15 μm in diameter. The nucleus occupies less than half of the cell area. The heterochromatin is located in well-defined clumps spaced regularly about the nucleus, producing a checkerboard pattern. The nucleolus is lost, but the perinuclear halo persists.

Electron microscopy of the polychromatophilic erythroblast reveals increased aggregation of nuclear heterochromatin. Active rhopheocytosis is always evident, and siderosomes and dispersed ferritin molecules can be identified within the cytoplasm.[2] This normal distribution of ferritin iron in the erythroblast characterizes the *normal sideroblast*. Mitochondrial iron usually is not apparent, even though the iron is incorporated into protoporphyrin in the mitochondria. The Golgi apparatus becomes quite small and may contain lysosomes.

ORTHOCHROMIC ERYTHROBLASTS

After the final mitotic division of the erythropoietic series, the concentration of hemoglobin increases within the erythroblast. More than

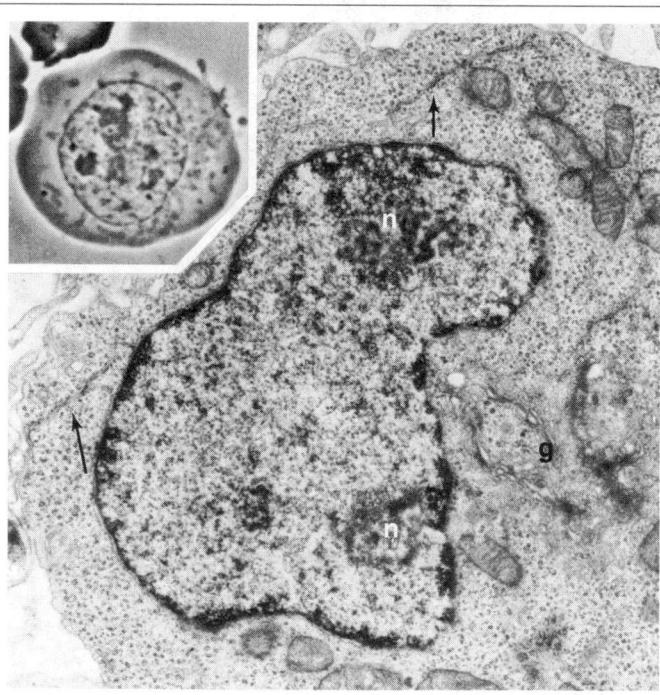

FIGURE 28-5   Proerythroblast. Phase-contrast micrograph (*inset*) of a proerythroblast showing the immature nucleus with nucleoli and finely dispersed nuclear chromatin. The centrosome (juxtanuclear clear zone) is apparent with its dense accumulation of mitochondria. Electron microscopic section of the proerythroblast shows nucleoli (n) in contact with the nuclear membrane. Chromatin is finely dispersed and forms small aggregates in the fixed nuclear membrane. The perinuclear canal is narrow but well defined. Polyribosome groups, many in helical configuration, are dispersed throughout the cytoplasm. The Golgi apparatus (g) is well developed, and regions of endoplasmic reticulum (arrows) are seen.

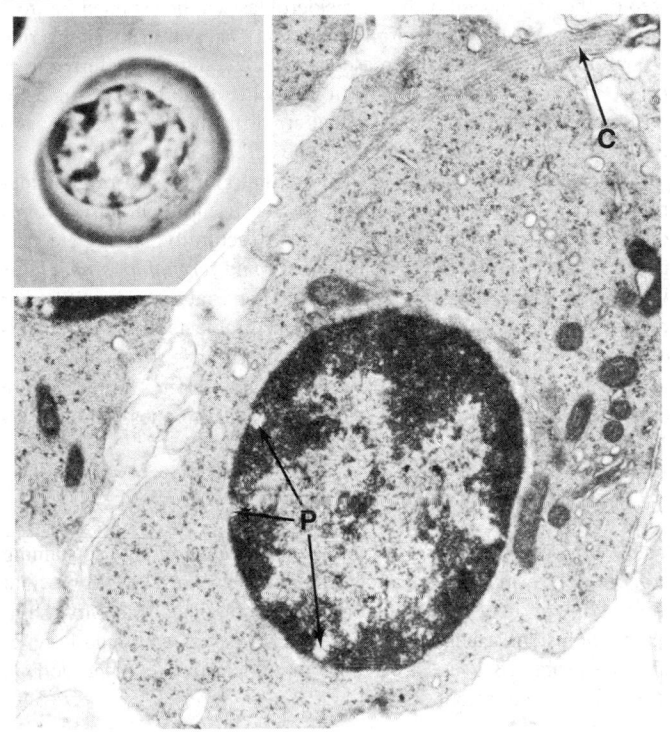

FIGURE 28-7   Polychromatophilic erythroblast. Phase-contrast micrograph (*inset*) demonstrates diminished size of this cell compared with its precursor. Further clumping of nuclear chromatin gives the nucleus a checkerboard appearance. The centrosome is condensed, and a perinuclear halo has developed. Electron microscopic section demonstrates relative reduction of the density of polyribosomes and dilution by the moderately osmiophilic hemoglobin in the cytoplasm. Nuclear chromatin shows a marked increase in clumping, and nuclear pores (P) are enlarged.

any of its predecessors, the orthochromic erythroblast stains like a mature erythrocyte (Figure 28-8); however, it is always somewhat polychromatophilic because of residual monoribosomes and polyribosomes.

Under the light microscope, the nucleus appears almost completely dense and featureless. It is measurably decreased in size. This cell is the smallest of the erythroblastic series, varying from 10 to 15 μm in diameter. The nucleus occupies approximately one fourth the cell area and is eccentric.

A surprising motility can be appreciated under the phase-contrast microscope. Round projections appear suddenly in different parts of the cell periphery and are just as quickly retracted. The movements probably are made in preparation for ejection of the nucleus.[2]

The cell ultrastructure is characterized by irregular borders, reflecting its motile state. The nucleus is eccentric; the heterochromatin forms large masses. The cytoplasmic ribosomes are further dispersed into diribosomes and monoribosomes. Mitochondria are reduced in number and size. Hemoglobin is present within the nucleus itself.[30,31]

RETICULOCYTE

BIRTH

Prior to enucleation, intermediate filaments and the marginal band of microtubules disappear. Tubulin and actin become concentrated at the point where the nucleus will exit.[32] These changes, accompanied by microtubular rearrangements, play a role in nuclear expulsion.[33,34]

Expulsion of the nucleus *in vitro* is not an instantaneous phenomenon; it requires a period of minutes.[2] The process begins with several vigorous contractions around the midportion of the cell, followed by a division of the cell into unequal portions. The smaller portion consists of the expelled nucleus accompanied by a thin rim of hemoglobinized cytoplasm. Loss of a "corona" of hemoglobin with the nucleus leads, in part, to an increase in the "early peak" of stercobilin when the rate of erythropoiesis is increased.[35]

In vivo, expulsion of the nucleus may occur while the erythroblast is still part of an erythroblastic island (Figure 28-9), or the nucleus may be lost during passage through the wall of a marrow sinus. The nucleus, which cannot traverse the small opening, remains in the marrow. In either case, the expelled nucleus is rapidly ingested by a macrophage.

Two proposals have been advanced to explain how the reticulocyte exits the marrow. The precise mechanism is unknown. The reticulocyte may actively traverse the sinus epithelium.[36] More likely, however, the reticulocyte may be driven across by a pressure differential because it appears incapable of directed amoeboid motion.[37,38]

MATURATION

The reticulocyte, as it enters the circulation, retains mitochondria, small numbers of ribosomes, the centriole, and remnants of the Golgi apparatus. The reticulocyte contains no endoplasmic reticulum. Supravital staining with brilliant cresyl blue or new methylene blue produces aggregates of ribosomes, mitochondria, and other cytoplasmic

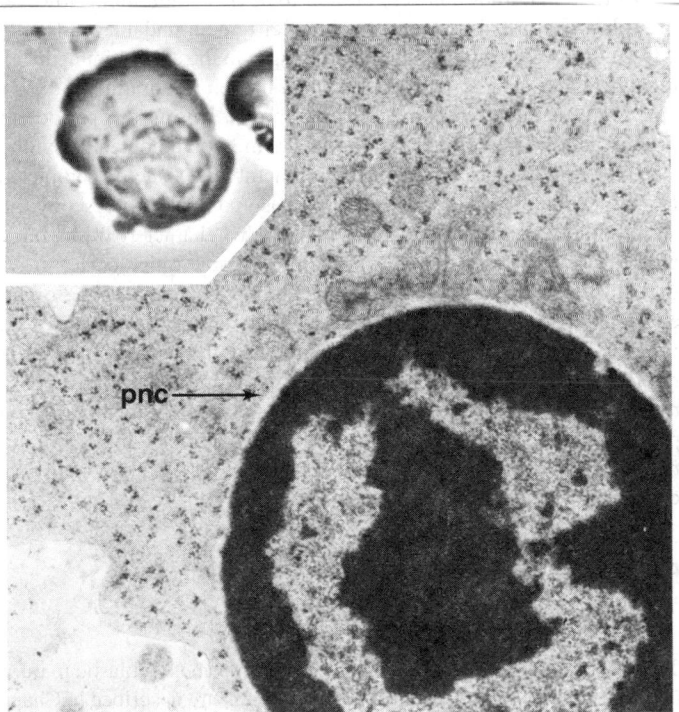

FIGURE 28-8   Orthochromic erythroblast. Phase-contrast appearance of this cell in the living state (*inset*) shows the irregular borders indicative of its characteristic motility, the eccentric nucleus making contact with the plasmalemma, further pyknosis of the nuclear chromatin, and condensation of the centrosome. Electron microscopic section shows further dilution of polyribosomes, some of which appear to be disintegrating into monoribosomes, by the increasing hemoglobin. The number of mitochondria is decreased, and some mitochondria are degenerating. Nuclear chromatin is clumped into large masses, and a perinuclear canal (pnc) is seen.

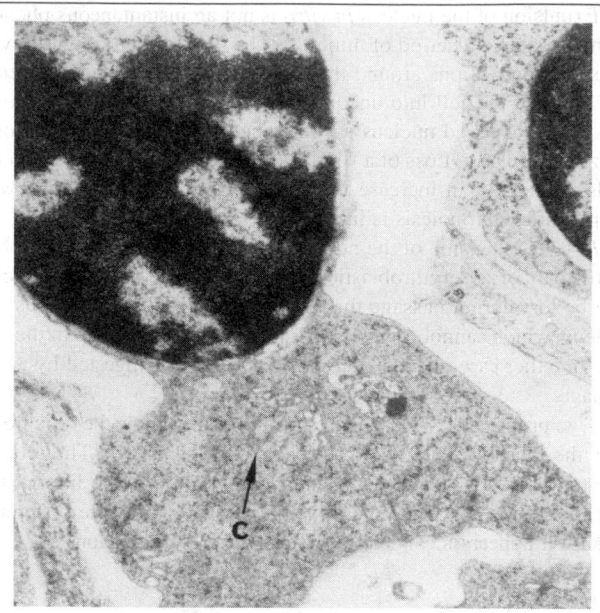

FIGURE 28-9   Orthochromic erythroblast ejecting its nucleus. A thin rim of cytoplasm surrounds the nucleus. In the cytoplasm, a single centriole (c) is partially encircled by some Golgi saccules.

organelles. These artifactual aggregates stain deep blue and, arranged in reticular strands, give the reticulocyte its name.

In vitro maturation is very similar to *in vivo* maturation. However, in a plasma clot culture the naked nuclei remain undamaged (Figure 28-10). If the clot is lysed, the macrophages in the culture immediately recognize and phagocytose the expelled nuclei. Maturation of the circulating reticulocyte requires 24 to 48 hours. During this period, approximately 20 percent of the ultimate hemoglobin content is synthesized and the final assembly of the submembrane skeleton completed. Living reticulocytes observed by phase-contrast microscopy are slightly motile, irregularly shaped cells with a characteristically puckered exterior. Examined by electron microscopy, reticulocytes are irregularly shaped and contain many remnant organelles. The organelles, small smooth vesicles, and an occasional centriole are grouped in the hilar region. In "young" reticulocytes, the vast majority of ribosomes dispersed throughout the cytoplasm are in the form of polyribosomes. As protein synthesis diminishes during maturation, the polyribosomes gradually transform into monoribosomes. Simultaneously, loss of transferrin receptors occurs,[39,40] and eventually the capacity for endocytosis disappears.[41]

PATHOLOGIC ERYTHROBLASTS

MEGALOBLASTS AND DYSERYTHROPOIESIS

The morphologic abnormalities characterizing megaloblastic maturation and polyclonal dyserythropoietic anemias are described in Chaps. 37 and 39.

PATHOLOGIC SIDEROBLASTS

A heterogeneous group of erythrocyte maturation disorders is accompanied by ineffective erythropoiesis and hyperferremia. Erythrocyte maturation disorders include acquired idiopathic sideroblastic anemia, pyridoxine-responsive anemia, alcohol-induced sideroblastic anemia, lead intoxication, dyserythropoietic anemia, and certain hemoglobinopathies (see Chaps. 37, 50, and 58). These conditions are character-

ized by the presence of pathologic sideroblasts. When stained for iron, these cells may show small iron-containing granules arranged in a ring around the nucleus. For this reason, they are commonly referred to as *ringed sideroblasts*.[42] Iron stains of normal erythroid precursors demonstrate a few very fine granules that are difficult to see without carefully focusing up and down through the cell.

Electron microscopic studies show that granules in ringed sideroblasts are iron-loaded mitochondria. Because mitochondrial iron is distinct from ferritin antigenically, ultrastructurally, and by electron probe analysis, mitochondrial iron is termed *ferruginous micelles*.[2] In hereditary sideroblastic anemia, mitochondrial iron deposits occur primarily in late, polychromatophilic erythroblasts. In acquired sideroblastic anemia, iron overload affects the early proerythroblast.[43] In cells with iron-loaded mitochondria, many ferritin molecules are deposited between adjacent erythroblast membranes (Figure 28-11).[44]

PATHOLOGY OF RETICULOCYTE AND ERYTHROCYTE

The reticulocyte may show pathologic alterations in size or staining properties. The reticulocyte may contain inclusions visible by light microscopy or identifiable only on ultrastructural analysis. Most pathologic inclusions usually attributed to erythrocytes are found in reticulocytes (Table 28-1) and are nuclear or cytoplasmic remnants derived from late-stage normoblasts.

HOWELL-JOLLY BODIES

Howell-Jolly bodies[45] are small nuclear remnants that have the color of a pyknotic nucleus on Wright-stained films and give a positive Feulgen reaction for DNA.[46] They are spherically shaped and usually no larger than 0.5 μm in diameter. Howell-Jolly bodies may be numerous, although generally only one is present. In pathologic situations, they appear to represent chromosomes that have separated from the mitotic spindle during abnormal mitosis.[47] More commonly, during normal maturation they arise from nuclear fragmentation (karyorrhexis) or incomplete expulsion of the nucleus.[48] Howell-Jolly bodies are pitted from the reticulocytes in their passage through the interendothelial slits of the splenic sinus. They are characteristically present in the blood of splenectomized persons and in patients suffering from hemolytic anemia, megaloblastic anemia, and hyposplenic states.

POCKED (OR PITTED) RED CELLS

When viewed by interference-phase microscopy, pocked red cells appear to have surface membrane "pits" or craters.[49] The vesicles or indentations characterizing these cells represent autophagic vacuoles adjacent to the cell membrane.[50] The vacuoles appear to be instrumental in disposal of cellular debris as the erythrocyte passes through the microcirculation of the spleen.[51] Within 1 week following splenectomy, pocked red cell counts begin to rise, reaching a plateau at 2 to 3 months.[52] Pocked red blood cell counts sometimes are used as a test for splenic function.

CABOT RINGS

The ring-like or figure-of-eight structures sometimes seen in megaloblastic anemia within reticulocytes and in an occasional, heavily stippled, late intermediate megaloblast[53] are designated *Cabot rings*. Their exact composition is questionable. Some investigators have suggested that Cabot rings originate from spindle material that was mishandled during abnormal mitosis.[54] Others have found no indication of DNA or spindle filaments but have shown the rings are associated with adherent granular material containing arginine-rich histone and nonhemoglobin iron.[55] Because histone biosynthesis and iron metabolism/

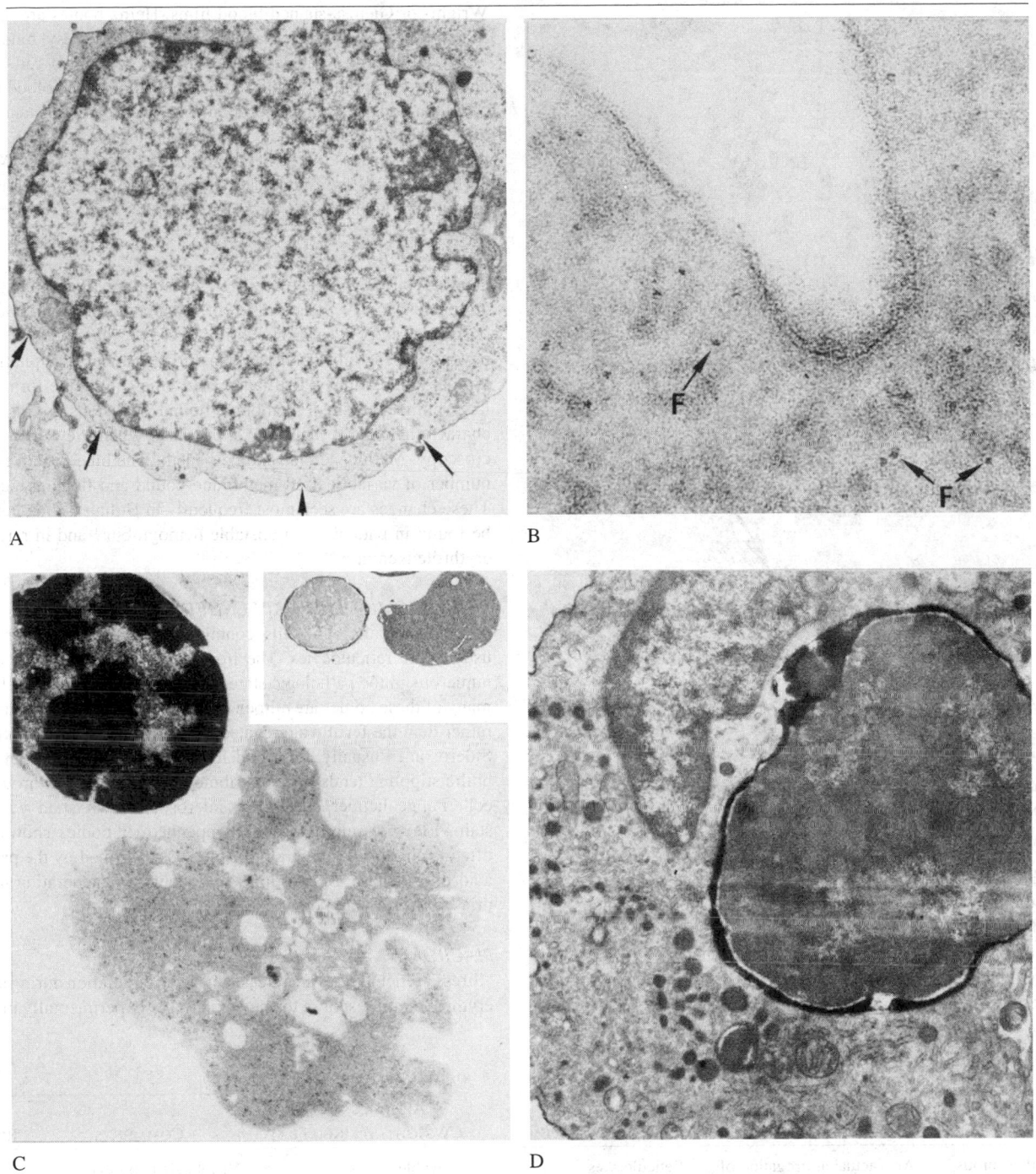

FIGURE 28-10   Erythroblast maturation in an *in vitro* plasma clot from BFU-E. (*A*) At day 9 of culture, a cell resembling the *in vivo* proerythroblast exhibits numerous rhopheocytotic invaginations (arrows). (*B*) One invagination seen at high magnification. Note the numerous ferritin molecules (F) dispersed in the cytoplasm. (*C*) At day 12 of culture, an extruded nucleus is seen close to a reticulocyte. *Inset*: When the hemoglobin is emphasized by cytochemical staining, the thin rim of cytoplasm surrounding the nucleus is clearly visible. (*D*) In the cell suspension produced by clot lysis, a macrophage phagocytoses a hemoglobin-rimmed erythroblast nucleus that was recently extruded. (Panels *C* and *D* adapted from Breton-Gorius et al,[9] with permission.)

mobilization are abnormal in pernicious anemia, Cabot rings may simply be markers of "cytoplasmic currents" within the cell.[2]

BASOPHILIC STIPPLING

Basophilic stippling consists of granulations of variable size and number that stain deep blue with Wright stain. Electron microscopic studies have shown that *punctate basophilia* represents aggregated ribo-

somes.[56] Clumps form during the course of drying and postvital staining of the cells, much as "reticulum" in reticulocytes precipitates from ribosomes during supravital staining. The clumped ribosomes may include degenerating mitochondria and siderosomes. In conditions such as lead intoxication and thalassemia, the altered reticulocyte ribosomes have a greater propensity to aggregate. As a result, basophilic granulation appears larger and is referred to as *coarse basophilic stippling*.

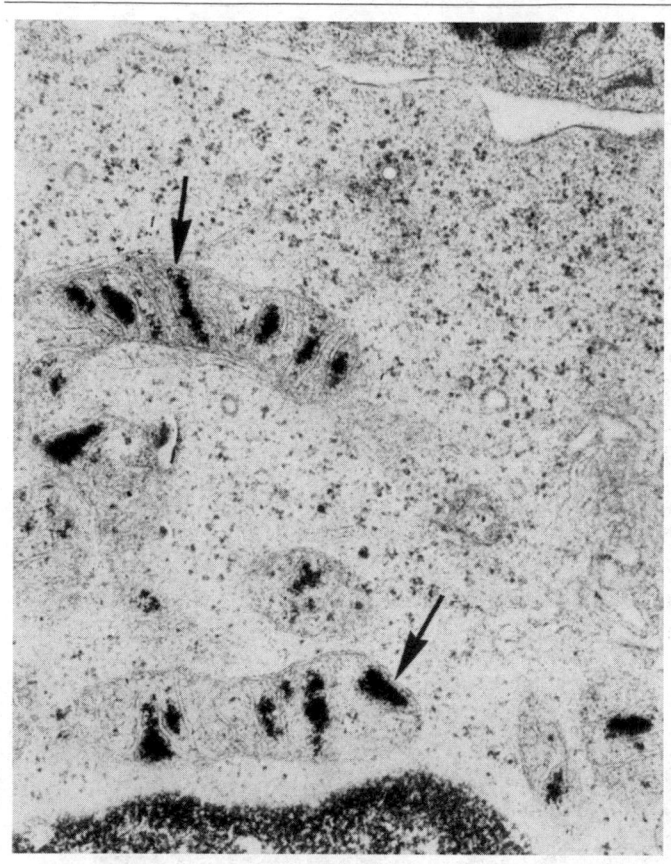

FIGURE 28-11 Pathologic sideroblast is an erythroblast characterized by the presence of mitochondrial deposits of iron-containing ferruginous micelles (arrows) between the cristae.

HEINZ BODIES

Heinz bodies are composed of denatured proteins, primarily hemoglobin, that form in red cells as a result of chemical insult (see Chap. 50); in hereditary defects of the hexose monophosphate shunt (see Chap. 45); in the thalassemias (see Chap. 46); and in unstable hemoglobin syndromes (see Chap. 47).[57] Heinz bodies are not seen on ordinary Wright- or Giemsa-stained blood films. Heinz bodies are readily visible in red cells stained supravitally with brilliant cresyl blue or crystal violet. They tend to adhere to the interior of the red cell membrane and protrude into the cytoplasm. On dried and stained blood films they characteristically are located about one third of the distance in from the edge of the disk, where membrane curvature is at a minimum, presumably because of the membrane stiffening they cause. Membrane stiffening likely is responsible for their removal as red cells traverse the interepithelial slits of the splenic sinus.[58]

HEMOGLOBIN H INCLUSIONS

Hemoglobin H is composed of β_4 tetramers, indicating that β chains are present in excess as a result of impaired α-chain production. Exposure to redox dyes such as brilliant cresyl blue, methylene blue, or new methylene blue results in denaturization and precipitation of abnormal hemoglobin.[59] Brilliant cresyl blue causes the formation of a large number of small membrane-bound inclusions, giving the cell a characteristic "golf ball-like" appearance when viewed by light microscopy. Methylene blue and new methylene blue generate a smaller number of variably sized membrane-bound and floating inclusions.[60] These changes are seen most frequently in β-thalassemia but also can be found in patients with unstable hemoglobin[61] and in rare cases of erythroleukemia.[62,63]

SIDEROSOMES AND PAPPENHEIMER BODIES

Normal or pathologic cells containing siderosomes ("iron bodies") usually are reticulocytes. The iron granulations are larger and more numerous in the pathologic state. Electron microscopy has shown that many of these bodies are mitochondria containing ferruginous micelles rather than the ferritin aggregates characterizing normal siderocytes.[64] Siderosomes usually are found in the cell periphery, whereas basophilic stippling tends to be distributed homogeneously throughout the cell. Pappenheimer bodies are siderosomes that stain with Wright stain. Electron microscopy of Pappenheimer bodies shows the iron often is contained within a lysosome, as confirmed by the presence of acid phosphatase. Siderosomes may contain degenerating mitochondria, ribosomes, and other cellular remnants.

MACRORETICULOCYTES

"Stress" reticulocytes are released into the circulation during an intense erythropoietin response to acute anemia or experimentally in response

TABLE 28-1 ERYTHROCYTE AND RETICULOCYTE INCLUSIONS

INCLUSIONS	COMPOSITION	CELL TYPE	APPEARANCE ON WRIGHT-STAINED FILM	COMMENTS	REFERENCE
"Reticulofilamentous substance"	Artifactual aggregation of ribosomes	Reticulocytes	Invisible	Visible after supravital staining	2
Howell-Jolly bodies	Nuclear fragment containing aberrant chromosomes	Reticulocytes; rarely erythrocytes	Dense blue spherical granule(s)	Visible in unstained cells	45–48
Cabot rings	Spindle remnant or histone-rich and iron-rich "cytoplasmic currents"	Reticulocytes; heavily stippled late intermediate megaloblasts	Ring or figure-of-eight strand stained purple	Visible in some hemolytic states	2, 53–55
Basophilic stippling	Pathologic precipitation of ribosomes	Reticulocytes	Dispersed blue granulations		56
Heinz bodies	Denatured hemoglobin	Erythrocytes; occasionally reticulocytes	Rarely visible	Refractile inclusions after staining with methylene or Nile blue dyes	57, 58
Hemoglobin H inclusions	Denatured hemoglobin (induced in vitro by exposure to brilliant cresyl blue, methylene blue, new methylene blue)	Erythrocytes; reticulocytes	Invisible	Gives "golf-ball" appearance to erythrocytes after incubation with appropriate supravital stains	59–63

to large doses of exogenously administered erythropoietin.[65] These cells may be twice the normal volume, with a corresponding increase in hemoglobin content. Whether the increase results from one less mitotic division during maturation or from some other process is not clear. In contrast, even under moderate erythropoietic stress, some reticulocytes in the marrow pool shift to the circulating pool. These "shift" reticulocytes contain a higher than normal RNA content and now can be quantified. Quantification is commonly performed by applying a fluorescent stain to the aggregated ribosomal material and then dividing reticulocytes into high-, medium-, and low-fluorescence categories using a fluorescence-sensitive flow cytometer. The "stress" reticulocytes of the older literature likely fall in the high- and medium-fluorescence categories.[65–68]

STRUCTURE AND SHAPE OF ERYTHROCYTES

The normal resting shape of the erythrocyte is a biconcave disk. Variations in the shape and dimensions of the red cell are useful in the differential diagnosis of anemias. Normal human red cells have a diameter of 7.5 to 8.7 μm, and the diameter decreases slightly with cell age. The size decrease likely results from removal of membrane and hemoglobin throughout the erythrocyte life span by spleen-facilitated vesiculation.[69] The cells have an average volume of 90 fl[70] and a surface area of approximately 136 μm[2].[71] The membrane is present in sufficient excess to allow the cell to swell to a sphere of approximately 150 fl or to enter a capillary with a diameter of 2.8 μm. The normal erythrocyte stains reddish-brown in Wright-stained blood films and pink with Giemsa stain. The central third of the cell appears relatively pale compared with the periphery, reflecting its biconcave shape. Red cells on dried blood films are 0.6 μm thick, having lost about two thirds of their normal thickness.[2] Many artifacts can be produced in the preparation of the blood film. They may result from contamination of the glass slide or coverslip with traces of fat, detergent, or other impurities.[72] Friction and surface tension involved in the preparation of the blood film produce fragmentation, "doughnut cells" or annulocytes, and crescent-shaped cells.[72] Observed under the phase-contrast or interference microscope, the red cell shows a characteristic internal scintillation known as red cell flicker.[73] The scintillation results from thermally excited undulations of the red cell membrane. Frequency analysis of the surface undulations has provided an estimate of the membrane curvature elastic constant and of changes in this constant resulting from alcohol, cholesterol loading, and exposure to cross-linking agents.[74]

RED CELL SHAPE AND SURVIVAL IN THE CIRCULATION

The red cell spends most of its circulatory life within the capillary channels of the microcirculation. During its 100- to 120-day life span, the red cell travels approximately 250 km. The long survival of the red cell is at least partially due to the unique capacity of its membrane to "tank tread," that is, to rotate around the red cell contents.[75] This arrangement transmits shocks from wall contact through the membrane to the viscous hemoglobin solution in the interior rather than concentrating the energy of contact in the membrane. The physical arrangement of membrane skeletal proteins in a uniform shell[76] of highly folded hexagonal/pentagonal units[77–79] permits this unusual behavior. The arrangement also is responsible for the characteristic biconcave shape of the resting cell.[80] Subtle differences in the discoid shape assumed by resting cells probably are related to variations in the elastic properties of the submembrane skeleton.[71] A deficiency in the amount of spectrin or the presence of mutant spectrin in the submembrane skeleton results in abnormal discoid cells in hereditary spherocytosis, elliptocytosis, and pyropoikilocytosis (see Chap. 44).[81] In regions of

circulatory standstill or very slow flow, red cells travel in aggregates of two to a dozen cells, forming rouleaux.[82] Within large vessels, aggregation is disrupted by increased shear forces.

NOMENCLATURE OF COMMON RED CELL SHAPES

An international terminology using uniform Greek word stems has been introduced to describe cells based on their three-dimensional morphology (Table 28-2).[83]

The discocyte is the form assumed by a red cell when it is not subjected to external deforming stress. It is a smooth, biconcave disk. A discocyte can be reversibly and rapidly transformed by a variety of environmental agents into two other forms: the stomatocyte, a uniconcave cup-shaped cell, and the echinocyte, covered by 10 to 30 short projections evenly spaced over the cell surface. In general, these changes can be superimposed on other red cell shapes, which suggests they represent membrane energy equilibrium states.[80]

The acanthocyte is irregularly shape, with two to 10 hemispherically tipped spicules of variable length and diameter. The bases of the spicules on the acanthocyte are of varying girth, unlike the spicules on echinocytes, which have remarkably uniform dimensions.

Notwithstanding the time-honored use of the word, the spherocyte is not a truly spherical cell. Its thickness is greatly increased so that the central concavity is significantly reduced and may be overlooked. On scanning electron microscopic examination, the spherocyte frequently bears a small dimple or irregular area suggesting derivation from a stomatocyte.

The schizocyte refers to a red cell fragment that characteristically assumes a half-disk shape with two or three pointed extremities. Because it is produced by the sealing of two opposing membrane surfaces followed by physical cleavage or fragmentation of a red cell, the schizocyte is smaller than the normal discocyte and may display one or more regions of stiffened and distorted membrane where the sealing and cleavage occurred.

The drepanocyte (sickle cell) describes the sickle cell and a variety of shapes induced by polymerization of sickle hemoglobin. Drepanocytes vary in shape, ranging from bipolar, spiculated forms to cells with long, irregular spicules and holly-leaf configurations.

The elliptocyte (ovalocyte) basically is an oval biconcave disk. It shows varying degrees of elliptical aberration, ranging from a slightly oval to an almost cylindrical, bipolar, elongated shape.

A relative excess of membrane in the codocyte (target cell) results in membrane recurvature in the center of the dimple. Hemoglobin accumulates where the upper and lower cell membranes separate when the cell is on a blood film, forming the central density, or "bull's eye," of the target.

The dacryocyte refers to a cell characterized by a single elongated or pointed extremity. This cell shape has been referred to as a teardrop, racket, or tail poikilocyte.

The leptocyte is a wafer-thin cell that has a generally large diameter, displays a thin rim of hemoglobin at the periphery, and has a large area of central pallor. Such a cell reflects an increased surface-to-volume ratio.

The keratocyte is a red cell with a relatively normal cell volume that was deformed by removal of a region of apposed and sealed membranes so that the cell presents with two or more points.

The "bite" cell is a red cell from which one or more semicircular portions were removed from the cell margin when Heinz bodies were pitted out by the splenic macrophages.[84]

If necessary, any shape variation of the red cell can be described precisely using compound terms such as spherostomatocyte. Addition of modifiers such as micro- to denote a changed volume may add to descriptive precision, as in microspherocyte or macroleptocyte.

TABLE 28-2 NOMENCLATURE OF RED CELL SHAPES AND ASSOCIATED DISEASE STATES

TERMINOLOGY (GREEK MEANING)	OLD TERMS, SYNONYMS	DESCRIPTION	MICROGRAPH	ASSOCIATED DISEASE STATES
Discocyte (disk)	Biconcave disk	Biconcave disk form of RBC		
Echinocyte (I–III) (sea urchin)	"Burr cell," crenated cell, "berry cell"	Spiculated RBC with short, equally spaced projections over entire surface; progressing from the "crenated disk" (echinocyte I) to the crenated sphere (echinocyte IV, not shown) with nearly complete loss of spicules		Uremia, liver disease Low-potassium red cells Immediately posttransfusion with aged or metabolically depleted blood Carcinoma of stomach and bleeding peptic ulcers
Acanthocyte (spike)	"Spur cell," acanthoid cell, acanthrocyte	Irregularly spiculated RBC with projections of varying length and position		Abetalipoproteinemia Alcoholic liver disease Postsplenectomy state Malabsorptive states
Stomatocyte (I–III) (mouth)	Mouth cell, cup form, mushroom cap, uniconcave disk, microspherocyte	Bowled-shaped RBC with single concavity; progressing from shallow bowl (I) to near sphere with small dimple (seen as mouth-shaped form in peripheral film)		Hereditary spherocytosis Hereditary stomatocytosis Alcoholism, cirrhosis, obstructive liver disease Erythrocyte sodium-pump defect
Spherostomatocyte (sphere)	Spherocyte, prelytic sphere, microspherocyte	Spherical RBC with dense hemoglobin content; scanning electron microscopy shows a persistent minimal dimple		Hereditary spherocytosis (cells actually spherostomatocytes) Immune hemolytic anemia Posttransfusion Heinz body hemolytic anemia Water-dilution hemolysis Fragmentation hemolysis
Schizocyte (cut)	Schistocyte, helmet cell, fragmented cell	Split RBC, often showing half-disk shape with two or three pointed extremities; may be small, irregular fragment		Microangiopathic hemolytic anemia (TTP, DIC, vasculitis, glomerulonephritis, renal graft rejection) Carcinomatosis Heart valve hemolysis (prosthetic or pathologic valves) Severe burns March hemoglobinuria

Variability in the size of red cells is designated *anisocytosis*. Any type of shape abnormality is designated as *poikilocytosis* (see Chap. 2).

NORMAL PHYSIOLOGY AND PATHOPHYSIOLOGY OF RED CELL SHAPES

BICONCAVE DISKS

A healthy red blood cell maintains its normal biconcave shape by minimizing bending energy in the membrane.[85] As the suspending medium becomes more hypotonic, red cells change from biconcave disks to spheres. This mathematically tractable transformation gave rise to the original hypothesis that the biconcave shape arose as a bending energy minimum. Developments in mathematical modeling of the various shapes assumed by a red cell have shown that, by in-cluding bending rigidity and stretch and shear elasticity contributed by the membrane skeleton,[86,87] the minimization-of-energy approach can reproduce, with surprising fidelity, all red cell shapes along the "main sequence" of shape transformation from stomatocyte to biconcave disk to echinocytes I, II, and III.[88,89] Additional evidence that the major mechanical forces are now reasonably well understood comes from "nonmain sequence" shapes such as *knizocytes* (three-dimpled cell) and triangular-mouthed stomatocytes, which also can be mathematically modeled by considering bending rigidity, stretch, and shear elasticity[88] (see Figure 28-12).

Does, however, the resistance to bending arise from changes in the relative surface area of the inner and outer leaflets of the bilaminar plasmamembranes, as the original "bilayer couple" hypothesis contemplates,[90] perhaps by incorporation of a cytoplasmic protein into the

TABLE 28-2 NOMENCLATURE OF RED CELL SHAPES AND ASSOCIATED DISEASE STATES (*Continued*)

TERMINOLOGY (GREEK MEANING)	OLD TERMS, SYNONYMS	DESCRIPTION	MICROGRAPH	ASSOCIATED DISEASE STATES
Elliptocyte (oval)	Ovalocyte	Oval to elongated ellipsoid RBC (with polarization of hemoglobin)		Hereditary elliptocytosis Thalassemia Iron deficiency Myelophthisic anemias Megaloblastic anemias
Drepanocyte (sickle)	Sickle cell	RBC containing polymerized hemoglobin S; showing varying shapes from bipolar, spiculated forms to holly-leaf and irregularly spiculated forms		Sickle cell disorders (SS, S trait, SC, SD, S thalassemia) Hemoglobin C-Harlem Hemoglobin Memphis/S
Codocyte (bell)	Target cell	Bell-shaped RBC that assumes a target shape on dried films of blood		Obstructive liver disease Hemoglobinopathies (S, C) Thalassemia Iron deficiency Postsplenectomy state Lecithin cholesterol acetyltransferase deficiency
Dacryocyte (tear)	Teardrop cell	RBC with a single elongated or pointed extremity		Myelofibrosis with mycloid metaplasia Myclophthisic anemias Thalassemia
Leptocyte (thin)	Thin cell, wafer cell	Thin, flat RBC with hemoglobin at periphery		Thalassemia Obstructive liver disease (±iron deficiency)
Keratocyte (horn)	Horn cell	RBC with spicules resulting from ruptured vacuole; cell appears half-moon shaped or spindle shaped		DIC or vascular prosthesis

DIC, disseminated intravascular coagulation; RBC, red blood cell; TTP, thrombotic thrombocytopenic purpura.

inner bilayer?[91] Or does the remarkable bending resistance of the membrane arise from interaction between the bilayer and the underlying spectrin cytoskeleton,[92–95] with the latter undergoing expansion or contraction as a result of a morphology change of the anion exchanger band 3?

STOMATOCYTE-ECHINOCYTE-DISCOCYTE EQUILIBRIUM

At physiologic pH and in the presence of normal plasma protein levels (particularly albumin), healthy red cells always are smooth, biconcave disks (Figure 28-13). As the pH is raised or the albumin concentration lowered, or in the presence of lysolecithin or anionic phenothiazine derivatives, the rim of the disk becomes bumpy. The bumps are low and widely spaced, and they involve only the membrane of the red cell rim. This form is an echinocyte I. Further environmental stress results in transformation to echinocytes II and III. These cells bear 10 to 30 projections of surprisingly uniform dimensions, equally spaced over the entire cell surface. If the environmental stress is sufficiently intense or is of sufficient duration so that the echinocyte III becomes a spheroechinocyte I or II, the process is irreversible.

Environmental stress caused by low pH, excess albumin, or cationic phenothiazine derivatives transforms the discocyte into an intermediate form having deeper biconcavities and then into a cup-shaped cell with only a single concavity: a stomatocyte. The changes are readily reversible, but if the single deep depression on the stomatocyte surface is obliterated by membrane loss, the transformation becomes irreversible and a spherostomatocyte results.

A wide array of agents in addition to pH and albumin cause stomatocytic-echinocytic changes in red cell shape. The agents include amphiphilic drugs and detergents, competitive transport inhibitors/affinity labels of band 3, and antibodies directed toward integral membrane constituents.[93]

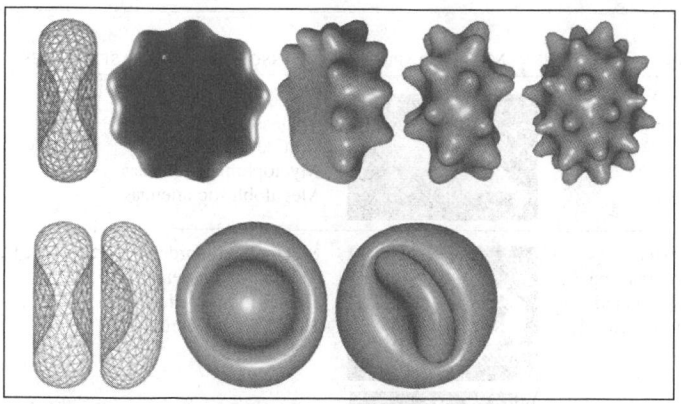

FIGURE 28-12 Discocyte-echinocyte and discocyte-stomatocyte transformation generated mathematically.[88,89] The match between real shapes depicted in Figure 28-13 and those generated mathematically is exceptionally good, even to the first appearance of the crenation spicules over the rim rather than in the dimple of the biconcave disk. (Adapted from Lim et al.,[88] with permission.)

AGED CELLS

The reticulocyte loses membrane as it matures into a discocyte. Membrane loss by vesiculation continues throughout the erythrocyte life span. The vesiculation process results in loss of up to 20 percent of the cell's hemoglobin with preferential loss of hemoglobin A_{1c} and hemoglobin A_{1e2}.[69] As erythrocytes age, the hemoglobin accumulates in endovesicles, which are removed by the spleen. These vesicles accumulate in asplenia. The notion that erythrocyte aging is synonymous with membrane loss, increasing mean corpuscular hemoglobin concentration (MCHC), and decreasing deformability largely results from studies on density-separated cells and the equating of dense cells with aged cells. Indeed, dense cells are dense because their MCHC is elevated, and an elevated MCHC exerts a profoundly depressant effect on red cell deformability. Thus, dense cells are always relatively nondeformable, but whether they are aged is not settled. One thing is clear: unlike the reticulocyte, the aged red cell is not easily distinguished morphologically. Red cell aging and senescence are discussed in Chapter 31.

CODOCYTES

In the circulation, the codocyte is a bell-shaped cell that assumes a target configuration when it is dried on a slide in preparation of a blood film.[72] On a flat surface, the codocyte tends to evert its concavity into a central projection into which hemoglobin redistributes. This action results in a central density (target) on the blood film. The codocyte is characterized by relative membrane excess due to either increased red cell surface area or decreased intracellular hemoglobin. In patients with obstructive liver disease, lecithin cholesterol acetyltransferase activity is depressed, which increases the cholesterol-to-phospholipid ratio[96] and produces an absolute increase in the surface area of the red cell membrane. In contrast, membrane excess is only relative in patients with iron-deficiency anemia and thalassemia because of the reduced quantity of intracellular hemoglobin.

ACANTHOCYTES

Acanthocytes are generated from normal red blood cells under conditions that alter their membrane lipid content, possibly by loss of glycerophospholipids resulting in a relative increase of sphingomyelin.[97] Once produced, the shape is irreversible except in the rare McLeod syndrome, where incubation of the acanthocytic cells with phosphatidylserine or chlorpromazine restores the discoid shape.[98] A

markedly increased membrane cholesterol-to-lecithin ratio is common in acanthocytes from patients with hepatocellular disease and abetalipoproteinemia.

DISCOCYTE-DREPANOCYTE TRANSFORMATION

The sickle cell, or drepanocyte, displays a characteristic variation of form on stained blood films. The fusiform cell in the crescent shape with two pointed extremities is encountered most commonly. Examination by phase-contrast microscopy of deoxygenated sickle cell blood reveals varied cell forms characterized by pointed extremities in holly-leaf and poikilocytic configurations, many with multiple spicules several micrometers long. The spicules are fragile and easily avulsed from the cell. If sickle cell formation is observed, the earliest change with deoxygenation is loss of flicker,[99] followed by slight deformation at the discocyte border with displacement of the hemoglobin to one region of the cell. The cell then elongates and becomes rigid as a result of polymerization of hemoglobin S in rods or filaments.[100] The rods are 15 to 18 nm (150–180 Å) in diameter and composed of monomolecular filaments 6 to 7 nm (60–70 Å) in diameter, intertwined into a six-stranded helix.[101] In partially sickled cells, the polymers display random orientation. As polymerization increases, the polymeric filaments undergo lateral reorientation into rods that are generally aligned with the long axis of the drepanocyte. Upon reoxygenation, the drepanocyte resumes the discocyte form and, in so doing, loses membrane by microspherulation and fragmentation during retraction of long spicules.[102] Evidence suggests more typical sickle-shaped cells form under slow deoxygenation. Thus, the cell membrane is maximally stressed, and more of the membrane is lost during the unsickling cycle after slow deoxygenation.[103] The unsickling process also leads to formation of micro-

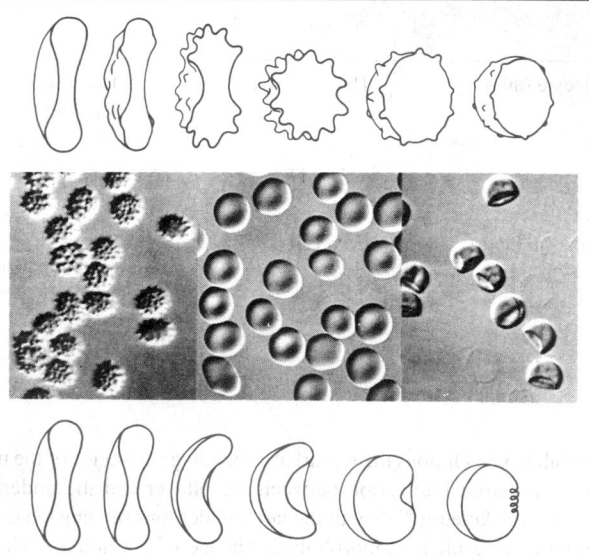

FIGURE 28-13 Discocyte-echinocyte and discocyte-stomatocyte transformation. *Upper panel* schematically depicts the echinocytic transformation as induced by a rise in pH, a lack of albumin in the suspension, or exposure to an anionic phenothiazine derivative. Note that the low protuberances heralding echinocytogenic transformation appear preferentially over the rim of the biconcave disk. *Lower panel* schematically depicts stomatocyte formation as induced by a cationic phenothiazine derivative, a lowering of pH, or an excess of albumin in the suspending medium. Note that the intermediate form between the disk and the early cup is not a bent disk but rather a bowtie form with very steep sides to the dimples.[147] *Center panel* shows the microscopic appearance in wet preparations of stomatocytes (*right*), discocytes (*middle*), and echinocytes (*left*).

Heinz bodies that adhere to the internal surface of the red cell membrane and contribute to increased membrane rigidity and cation leak.[57] With each sickle–unsickle cycle, membrane damage accumulates, as signaled by increasing amounts of an altered membrane protein β-actin. The alteration results from formation of a disulfide bond between [284]Cys and [373]Cys residues.[104] Eventually the cells become incapable of reversion to the biconcave disk shape, even when the cells are fully oxygenated. The cells become *irreversibly sickled cells*.[105] The cells have an increased hemoglobin concentration, increased cation permeability, decreased potassium, and increased sodium. Membrane deformability[105] and accumulation of irreversibly sickled cell β-actin are markedly decreased.[104] In addition to irreversibly sickled cells, the blood of patients with sickle cell anemia contains small numbers of another rigid, membrane-damaged cell: the sequestrocyte. Sequestrocytes are characterized by linear zones of membrane fusion that entrap lakes of hemoglobin. They appear massively vacuolated under the light microscope. Sequestrocytes presumably arise from a combination of physical damage from sickle–unsickle cycles and oxidative membrane damage that causes transcellular cross-bonding of the cell membrane.[106]

SCHIZOCYTES

Fibrin strands in damaged blood vessels can be arrayed so that they sieve the passing red cells. If a passing red cell folds over or otherwise attaches to the strand, the bloodstream pulls on the arrested cell, stretches it, and eventually fragments it.[107,108] If the two inner surfaces of the red cell membrane become approximated prior to rupture, the torn membranes seals[109] and the schizocyte contains hemoglobin. The more rigid schizocytes and those with a low relative surface area are rapidly removed by the spleen; the remainder may circulate for many days.

SPHEROCYTES AND STOMATOCYTES

Red cells sensitized with antibodies, complement, or immune complexes lose cholesterol and thus surface area, displaying the increased osmotic fragility of the spherocyte.[110] Heinz body formation leads to membrane depletion by fragmentation, with spherocyte formation.[111] A spherogenic mechanism common to Heinz body hemolytic anemias and immune hemolysis is partial phagocytosis of portions of the cell containing aggregates of denatured hemoglobin[111] and portions of the sensitized membrane,[112] respectively.

Stomatocytosis is a rare form of spherocytosis.[113] The anomaly is caused by abnormal permeability of the red cell membrane to the univalent cations Na^+ and K^+. The group of disorders is heterogenous and includes overhydrated and dehydrated hereditary stomatocytosis, cryohydrocytosis, and familial pseudohyperkalemia.[114] These disorders are discussed further in Chap. 44.

A spectrum of abnormal cells varying from normal discocytes to stomatocytes, spherostomatocytes, and dense microspherocytes is seen in hereditary spherocytosis.[115]

HEAT-INDUCED SHAPE CHANGES

Heating red cells to temperatures greater than 49°C depolymerizes spectrin. If the heating episode is brief and the inner surfaces of the biconcavities are in contact, the surfaces fuse upon cooling.[116] More vigorous heating causes marked spherulation of the entire cell. Microspherocytes bud from the cell surface, and the entire cell is transformed into small spherical fragments (*pyropoikilocytes*). The fragments can be recovered from the blood after severe burns.

ELLIPTOCYTES

In blood films of normal subjects, elliptical or oval cells usually constitute less than 1 percent of the erythrocytes. In various pathologic situations, with or without anemia (thalassemia trait, folate and iron deficiency), the number of elliptocytes can increase to 10 percent. Exceptionally, as in dyserythropoiesis, the proportion can be as high as 50 percent. In hereditary elliptocytosis (see Chap. 44), the number of elliptical erythrocytes varies greatly, from 0 to 98 percent.[117] Such fluctuations have forced hematologists to substitute a biochemical and functional (rheologic) definition of hereditary elliptocytosis for the original morphologic definition.[117] Qualitative and quantitative anomalies of spectrin, band 3,[81,118–120] and protein 4.1,[121,122] the major proteins of the membrane skeleton, are associated with hereditary elliptocytosis. As a consequence, rheologic membrane properties are impaired.[118,123] Severe hemolytic anemia is seen only in the homozygous form of the disease (hereditary pyropoikilocytosis) where *pyropoikilocytes* typically are present.

DACRYOCYTES

Dacryocytes typically are found in the bloodstream of patients with marrow fibrosis, often accompanied by extramedullary hemopoiesis. How these marrow changes give rise to dacryocytes is unknown. Aspiration of red cell membrane into a micropipette of appropriate dimensions produces a morphologically similar shape change; however, the cell usually recovers completely within minutes. Similar deformation in a reticulocyte can be permanent because the deformation occurred while the submembrane skeleton was being assembled. A delay during egress from the marrow or from extramedullary sites, such as in idiopathic myelofibrosis (see Chap. 89), provides such an opportunity.

KERATOCYTES ("HORN CELLS" OR "HELMET CELLS")

Keratocytes are erythrocytes from which one or more roughly circular bites were removed from the discocyte margin. They differ from schizocytes in that their hemoglobin content is normal or only slightly lower than normal. They are not formed by sectioning of a red cell. Rather, they appear to arise when all the hemoglobin is squeezed out of a portion near the edge of a discocytic red cell and the two opposite membrane surfaces fuse.[124] The process forms a pseudovacuole that soon ruptures, probably because of stiffening of the membrane skeleton in the fused portion. The result is a notch with bordering spicules or horns. Experimentally, membrane fusion with pseudovacuole formation can be produced by temperatures greater than 49°C[116] and by mechanical stress.[109] *In vitro* exposure to diamide and N-ethylmaleimide[125] produces this characteristic form.

"BITE" CELLS

"Bite" cells are formed when the Heinz bodies are pitted from the cells by splenic macrophages.[84] Emphasis on the missing portion rather than on the horns that remain led to the term *bite cell*.[126] *In vivo* exposure to sulfonamide drugs such as dapsone and sulfasalazine and the urinary tract antiseptic phenazopyridine results in "bite" cells in susceptible individuals.[127] Bite cells are a form of keratocyte. Bite cells should be distinguished from other keratocytes because bite cell formation involves removal of denatured hemoglobin (and membrane), whereas keratocytes in general appear to be formed by membrane apposition and subsequent removal of the apposed membranes.

CRYSTALS OF HEMOGLOBIN C DISEASE

In splenectomized patients with homozygous hemoglobin C disease, up to 10 percent of the circulating cells may contain tetrahedral crystals.[128] Crystal-containing cells are rare or absent in blood films from nonsplenectomized patients.[129] The efficiency in splenic removal may be a result of spherocyte formation from release of osmotically active particles as hemoglobin C crystals "melt" while undergoing deoxygenation in the spleen. "Melting" of hemoglobin C crystals upon deoxygenation occurs readily *in vitro*, behavior opposite to that of sickle hemoglobin crystals.[130] *In vitro* dehydration of hemoglobin C−containing cells for a 24-hour period between slide and coverslip[131] or hypertonic dehydration of red cells in 3% NaCl buffer for 4 to 12 hours readily produces crystals. In homozygous hemoglobin C disease, up to 75 percent of cells may show crystals. Lower percentages of crystals occur in hemoglobin SC and other hemoglobin C variants. Molecular subunits in a tetragonal or hexagonal arrangement may be identified within hemoglobin C crystals.[132] Hemoglobin Setif, like hemoglobin C, may precipitate as intracellular crystals when the tonicity of the suspending medium is raised.[133] The process occurs in oxygenated solutions and at osmolarities achieved in the renal medulla. No clinical symptoms among heterozygous carriers of the Setif gene have been reported.

OSMOTIC BEHAVIOR

The red cell behaves as an osmometer.[134] Red cells placed into a hypertonic solution shrink, and the inner surfaces of the biconcavities touch over a progressively larger central region. When red cells in hypotonic solutions reach their critical hemolytic volume, holes or pores greater than 10 nm (100 Å) in diameter appear[135] and the hemoglobin exits. The probability of pore formation is affected by elastic membrane properties and is delayed in thalassemic cells.[136] Following hemolysis (exit of the hemoglobin), the holes or tears close, and the cell resumes its original biconcave shape.

DEFORMABILITY

An important determinant of red cell survival in the circulation is the cell's deformability. The deformability of the intact cell consists of contributions from the intrinsic deformability of the membrane itself, the internal viscosity (for practical purposes, the MCHC), and the surface-to-volume ratio of the cell. The deformability of the intact cell can be measured by the time needed for a red cell suspension to traverse a filter of known pore size.[137] Alternatively, the cells can be suspended in a viscous medium and exposed to a shear force. The change in shape can be observed microscopically, as in the rheoscope,[138] or by laser diffraction, as in the ektacytometer.[139] Additional information can be obtained from ektacytometric analysis by varying the osmolarity of the suspending medium, which changes the surface-to-volume ratio and the internal viscosity of the cells during the analytical procedure.[140] Alternatively, the red cell can be folded over a spider web strand in the presence of rapidly flowing buffer. The deformability of the membrane can be estimated from the relationship between the flow rate of the buffer and the deformation of the red cell.[141]

A 20 percent increase in MCHC results in an approximately 600 percent increase in internal viscosity.[142] An increase of this magnitude still leaves the red cell with sufficient deformability to survive in the circulation, although such nondeformable cells probably experience a prolonged transit time through the spleen. This is not the case for erythrocytes from patients with xerocytosis or dessicocytosis. In such patients, the erythrocytes are always perilously close to the upper limits of internal viscosity, consistent with traversing the vasculature.[143]

In the circulation, the primary cause of decreased red cell deformability likely is insufficient membrane (spherocytosis) rather than stiffening of the membrane. The interendothelial slits of the splenic sinus stress cells with a normal surface-to-volume ratio, and splenic phagocytes remove cells with a lower than normal ratio. It is self-evident that a perfectly spherical red cell will be rigid no matter how low the MCHC or how flexible the isolated membrane.

REFERENCES

1. Southcott MJG, Tanner MJA, Anstee DJ: The expression of human blood group antigens during erythropoiesis in a cell culture system. *Blood* 93:4425, 1999.
2. Bessis M, Weed RI: *Living Blood Cells and Their Ultrastructure.* Springer-Verlag, New York, 1973.
3. Breton-Gorius J, Vuillet-Gaugler MH, Coulombel L, et al: Association between leukemic erythroid progenitors and bone marrow macrophages. *Blood Cells* 17:127, 1991.
4. Spring FA, Parsons SF: Erythroid cell adhesion molecules. *Transfus Med Rev* 14:351, 2000.
5. Wright SD, Meyer BC: Fibronectin receptor of human macrophages recognizes the sequence Arg-Gly-Asp-Ser. *J Exp Med* 162:762, 1985.
6. Patel VP, Lodish HF: The fibronectin receptor on mammalian erythroid precursor cells: Characterization and developmental regulation. *J Cell Biol* 102:449, 1986.
7. Fraser IP, Gordon S: Murine erythroleukemia (Mel) cells bear ligands for the sialoadhesin and erythroblast receptor macrophage hemagglutinins. *Eur J Cell Biol* 64:217, 1994.
8. Parmley RT, Ogawa M, Spicer SS, et al: Human marrow erythropoiesis in culture: III. Ultrastructural and cytochemical studies of cellular interactions. *Exp Hematol* 6:78, 1978.
9. Breton-Gorius J, Guichard J, Vainchenker W: Absence of erythroblastic islands in plasma clot culture and their possible reconstitution after clot lysis. *Blood Cells* 5:461, 1979.
10. Panzenbock B, Bartunek P, Mapara MY, et al: Growth and differentiation of human stem cell factor erythropoietin-dependent erythroid progenitor cells in vitro. *Blood* 92:3658, 1998.
11. Klausner RD, Harford JB, Rao K: Molecular aspects of the regulation of cellular iron metabolism, in *Proteins of Iron Storage and Transport*, edited by G Spik, J Montreuil, RR Crichton, J Mazurier, p 111. Elsevier Science Publishers, Amsterdam, 1985.
12. Quintana C, Bonnet N, Jeantet AY, et al: Crystallographic study of the ferritin molecule: New results obtained from natural crystals in situ (mollusk oocyte) and from isolated molecules (horse spleen). *Biol Cell* 59:247, 1987.
13. Iancu TC: Iron and neoplasia: Ferritin and hemosiderin in tumor cells. *Ultrastruct Pathol* 13:573, 1989.
14. Richter GW: Studies of iron overload: Rat liver siderosome ferritin. *Lab Invest* 50:26, 1984.
15. Pearse BMF: Coated vesicles from human placenta carry ferritin, transferrin, and immunoglobulin-G. *Proc Natl Acad Sci U S A* 79:451, 1982.
16. Ponka P, Sheftel AD, Zhang AS: Iron targeting to mitochondria in erythroid cells. *Biochem Soc Trans* 30:735, 2002.
17. Conrad ME, Umbreit JN, Moore EG, et al: Mobilferrin is an intermediate in iron transport between transferrin and hemoglobin in K562 cells. *J Clin Invest* 98:1449, 1996.
18. Policard A, Bessis M: Sur un mode d'incorporation des macromolecules par la cellule, visible au microscope électronique. *CR Hebd Seances Acad Sci* 246:3194, 1958.
19. Parmley RT, Hajdu I, Denys FR: Ultrastructural localization of the transferrin receptor and transferrin on marrow cell surfaces. *Br J Haematol* 54:633, 1983.
20. Speyer BE, Fielding J: Ferritin as a cytosol iron transport intermediate in human reticulocytes. *Br J Haematol* 42:255, 1979.
21. Grasso JA, Hillis TJ, Mooneyfrank JA: Ferritin is not a required intermediate for iron utilization in heme synthesis. *Biochim Biophys Acta* 797:247, 1984.
22. Drysdale J, Jain SK, Boyd D: Human ferritins: Genes and proteins, in *Proteins of Iron Storage and Transport*, edited by G Spik, J Montreuil, RR Crichton, J Mazurier, p 343. Elsevier Science Publishers, Amsterdam, 1985.

23. Scott MD, Eaton JW: Thalassemic erythrocytes: Cellular suicide arising from iron and glutathione-dependent oxidation reactions? *Br J Haematol* 91:811, 1995.

24. Harrison PM, Arosio P: Ferritins: Molecular properties, iron storage function and cellular regulation. *Biochim Biophys Acta* 1275:161, 1996.

25. Nijhof W, Wierenga PK: Isolation and characterization of the erythroid progenitor cell: CFU-E. *J Cell Biol* 96:386, 1983.

26. Malik P, Fisher TC, Barsky LLW, et al: An in vitro model of human red blood cell production from hematopoietic progenitor cells. *Blood* 91:2664, 1998.

27. Sato T, Maekawa T, Watanabe S, et al: Erythroid progenitors differentiate and mature in response to endogenous erythropoietin. *J Clin Invest* 106:263, 2000.

28. Kie JH, Jung YJ, Woo SY, et al: Ultrastructural and phenotypic analysis of in vitro erythropoiesis from human cord blood CD34(+) cells. *Ann Hematol* 82:278, 2003.

29. Bessis M, Breton-Gorius J: Ultrastructure du proerythroblaste. *Nouv Rev Fr Hematol* 1:529, 1961.

30. Breton-Gorius J, Reyes F: Ultrastructure of human bone marrow cell maturation. *Int Rev Cytol* 46:251, 1976.

31. Dvorak AM, Dvorak HF, Karnovsky MJ: Cytochemical localization of peroxidase activity in the developing erythrocyte. *Am J Pathol* 67:303, 1972.

32. Xue SP, Zhang SF, Du Q, et al: The role of cytoskeletal elements in the two-phase denucleation process of mammalian erythroblasts in vitro observed by laser confocal scanning microscope. *Cell Mol Biol* 43:851, 1997.

33. Lazarides E: From genes to structural morphogenesis: The genesis and epigenesis of a red blood cell. *Cell* 51:345, 1987.

34. Chasis JA, Prenant M, Leung A, et al: Membrane assembly and remodeling during reticulocyte maturation. *Blood* 74:1112, 1989.

35. Bessis M, Breton-Gorius J, Thiery JP: Role possible de l'hemoglobine accompagnant le noyau des erythroblastes dans l'origine de la stercobiline éliminée précocement. *CR Acad Sci III* 252:2300, 1961.

36. Wilson JG, Tavassoli M: Microenvironmental factors involved in the establishment of erythropoiesis in bone marrow. *Ann N Y Acad Sci* 718:271, 1994.

37. Lichtman MA, Santillo P: Red cell egress from the marrow: Vis-a-tergo. *Blood Cells* 12:11, 1986.

38. Waugh RE, Hsu LL, Clark P, et al: Analysis of cell egress in bone marrow, in *White Cell Mechanics: Basic Science and Clinical Aspects*, edited by HJ Meiselman, MA Lichtman, PL LaCelle, p 221. Alan R. Liss, New York, 1984.

39. Nunez MT, Glass J, Fischer S, et al: Transferrin receptors in developing murine erythroid cells. *Br J Haematol* 36:519, 1977.

40. Pan BT, Johnstone RM: Fate of the transferrin receptor during maturation of sheep reticulocytes in vitro: Selective externalization of the receptor. *Cell* 33:967, 1983.

41. Zweig S, Singer SJ: Concanavalin A-induced endocytosis in rabbit reticulocytes, and its decrease with reticulocyte maturation. *J Cell Biol* 80:487, 1979.

42. Bowman WD Jr: Abnormal ("ringed") sideroblasts in various hematologic and non-hematologic disorders. *Blood* 18:662, 1961.

43. Hines JD, Grasso JA: The sideroblastic anemias. *Semin Hematol* 7:86, 1970.

44. Flandrin G, Daniel MT, Breton-Gorius J, et al: Ilot érythroblastique anormal du au développement de jonctions intercellulaires (synartèse érythroblastique). Un nouveau mécanisme d'anémie. Problèmes posés par le diagnostic. *Nouv Rev Fr Hematol* 14:161, 1974.

45. Jolly J: Recherches sur la formation des globules rouges des mammifères. *Arch Anat Microsc* 9:133, 1907.

46. Discombe G: L'Origine des corps de Howell-Jolly et des anneaux de Cabot. *Sangre (Barc)* 29:262, 1948.

47. Rondanelli EG, Trenta A, Magliulo E, et al: Morphogenese des micronoyaux supplementaires (pseudo-corps de Jolly) dans les cellules erythropoietiques irradiées. *Acta Haematol* 35:232, 1966.

48. Koyama S: Studies on Howell-Jolly body. *Acta Haematol Jpn* 23:20, 1960.

49. Koyama S, Kihira H, Aoki S, et al: Postsplenectomy vacuole: A new erythrocytic inclusion body. *Mie Med J* 11:425, 1962.

50. Holroyde CP, Gardner FH: Acquisition of autophagic vacuoles by human erythrocytes. Physiological role of the spleen. *Blood* 36:566, 1970.

51. Ogrady JG, Harding B, Egan EL, et al: Pitted erythrocytes: Impaired formation in splenectomized subjects with congenital spherocytosis. *Br J Haematol* 57:441, 1984.

52. Buchanan GR, Holtkamp CA, Horton JA: formation and disappearance of pocked erythrocytes: Studies in human-subjects and laboratory animals. *Am J Hematol* 25:243, 1987.

53. Kass L: Origin and composition of Cabot rings in pernicious anemia. *Am J Clin Pathol* 64:53, 1975.

54. Van Oye E: L'Origine des anneaux de Cabot. *Rev Hematol* 9:173, 1954.

55. Kass L, Gray RH: Ultrastructural visualization of Cabot rings in pernicious anemia. *Experientia* 32:507, 1976.

56. Jensen WN, Moreno GD, Bessis MC: An electron microscopic description of basophilic stippling in red cells. *Blood* 25:933, 1965.

57. Lessin L, Wallas CP: Biochemical basis for membrane alterations in the irreversibly sickled cell. *Blood* 42:978, 1973.

58. Heinz R: Uber Blutdegeneration und Regeneration. *Beitr Pathol* 29:299, 1901.

59. Chinprasertsuk S, Piankijagum A, Wasi P: In vivo induction of intra-erythrocytic inclusion bodies in hemoglobin H disease: An electron microscopic study. *Birth Defects Orig Artic Ser* 23:317, 1987.

60. Wickramasinghe SN, Hughes M, Fucharoon S, et al: The morphology of redox-dye-treated Hb H-containing red cells: Differences between cells treated with brilliant cresyl blue, methylene blue and new methylene blue. *Clin Lab Haematol* 7:353, 1985.

61. Sansone G, Sciarratta GV, Ivaldi G, et al: Hb H-like inclusions in red cells of patients with unstable hemoglobin. *Haematologica* 72:481, 1987.

62. Wickramasinghe SN, Hughes M, Higgs DR, et al: Ultrastructure of red cells containing haemoglobin H inclusions induced by redox dyes. *Clin Lab Haematol* 3:51, 1981.

63. Beaven GH, Coleman PN, White JC: Occurrence of haemoglobin H in leukaemia: A further case of erythroleukaemia. *Acta Haematol* 59:37, 1978.

64. Bessis M, Breton-Gorius J: Iron particles in normal erythroblasts and pathological erythrocytes. *J Biophys Biochem Cytol* 3:503, 1957.

65. Brecher G, Haley JE, Prenant M, et al: Macronormoblasts, macroreticulocytes, and macrocytes. *Blood Cells* 1:547, 1975.

66. Major A, Bauer C, Breymann C, et al: Rh-erythropoietin stimulates immature reticulocyte release in man. *Br J Haematol* 87:605, 1994.

67. Davis BH, Dicorato M, Bigelow NC, et al: Proposal for standardization of flow cytometric reticulocyte maturity index (RMI) measurements. *Cytometry* 14:318, 1993.

68. Watanabe K, Kawai Y, Takeuchi K, et al: Reticulocyte maturity as an indicator for estimating qualitative abnormality of erythropoiesis. *J Clin Pathol* 47:736, 1994.

69. Willekens FLA, Roerdinkholder-Stoelwinder B, Groenen-Dopp YAM, et al: Hemoglobin loss from erythrocytes in vivo results from spleen-facilitated vesiculation. *Blood* 101:747, 2003.

70. Bull BS, Hay KL: Are red blood cell indexes international? *Arch Pathol Lab Med* 109:604, 1985.

71. Korpman RA, Dorrough DC, Brailsford JD, et al: The red cell shape as an indicator of membrane structure: Ponder's rule reexamined. *Blood Cells* 3:315, 1977.

72. Bessis M: *Blood Smears Reinterpreted*. Springer International, Berlin, 1977.

73. Burton AL, Anderson WL, Andrews RV: Quantitative studies on the flicker phenomenon in the erythrocytes. *Blood* 32:819, 1968.

74. Fricke K, Wirthensohn K, Laxhuber R, et al: Flicker spectroscopy of erythrocytes: A sensitive method to study subtle changes of membrane bending stiffness. *Eur Biophys J* 14:67, 1986.

75. Schmid-Schonbein H, Wells R: Tank treading of erythrocytes. *Science* 165:288, 1969.

76. Brailsford JD, Korpman RA, Bull BS: The red cell shape from discocyte to hypotonic spherocyte: A mathematical delineation based on a uniform shell hypothesis. *J Theor Biol* 60:131, 1976.

77. Byers TJ, Branton D: Visualization of the protein associations in the erythrocyte-membrane skeleton. *Proc Natl Acad Sci U S A* 82:6153, 1985.

78. Shen BW, Josephs R, Steck TL: Ultrastructure of the intact skeleton of the human-erythrocyte membrane. *J Cell Biol* 102:997, 1986.

79. Liu SC, Derick LH, Palek J: Visualization of the hexagonal lattice in the erythrocyte-membrane Skeleton. *J Cell Biol* 104:527, 1987.

80. Bull BS, Brailsford JD: Red blood cell shape, in *Red Blood Cell Membranes: Structure, Function, Clinical Implications*, edited by P Agre, JC Parker, p 401. Marcel Dekker, New York, 1989.

81. Liu SC, Derick LH, Agre P, et al: Alteration of the erythrocyte membrane skeletal ultrastructure in hereditary spherocytosis, hereditary elliptocytosis, and pyropoikilocytosis. *Blood* 76:198, 1990.

82. Branemark PI, Bagge U: Intravascular rheology of erythrocytes in man. *Blood Cells* 3:11, 1977.

83. Bessis M: Red cell shapes: An illustrated classification and its rationale, in *Red Cell Shape: Physiology, Pathology, Ultrastructure*, edited by M Bessis, R Weed, P LeBlond, p 1. Springer-Verlag, New York, 1973.

84. Prasad AS: Acquired hemolytic anemias, in *Hematology: Clinical and Laboratory Practice*, edited by RL Bick, p 391. Mosby Year Book, St. Louis, 1993.

85. Canham PB: The minimum energy of bending as a possible explanation of the biconcave shape of the human red blood cell. *J Theor Biol* 26:61, 1970.

86. Iglic A: A possible mechanism determining the stability of spiculated red blood cells. *J Biomech* 30:35, 1997.

87. Iglic A, Kralj-Iglic V, Hagerstrand H: Amphiphile induced echinocyte-spheroechinocyte transformation of red blood cell shape. *Eur Biophys J* 27:335, 1998.

88. Lim HWG, Wortis M, Mukhopadhyay R: Stomatocyte-discocyte-echinocyte sequence of the human red blood cell: Evidence for the bilayer-couple hypothesis from membrane mechanics. *Proc Natl Acad Sci U S A* 99:16766, 2002.

89. Lim GHW: A *Numerical Study of Morphologies and Morphological Transformations of Human Erythrocyte based on Membrane Mechanics* [PhD thesis]. Simon Fraser University, British Columbia, 2003.

90. Sheetz MP, Painter RG, Singer SJ: Biological membranes as bilayer couples: III. Compensatory shape changes induced in membranes. *J Cell Biol* 70:193, 1976.

91. Gedde MM, Yang EY, Huestis WH: Resolution of the paradox of red cell shape changes in low and high pH. *Biochim Biophys Acta* 1417:246, 1999.

92. Wong P: Mechanism of control of erythrocyte shape: A possible relationship to band-3. *J Theor Biol* 171:197, 1994.

93. Wong P: A basis of echinocytosis and stomatocytosis in the disc-sphere transformations of the erythrocyte. *J Theor Biol* 196:343, 1999.

94. Gimsa J, Ried C: Do band-3 protein conformational changes mediate shape changes of human erythrocytes. *Mol Membr Biol* 12:247, 1995.

95. Gimsa J: A possible molecular mechanism governing human erythrocyte shape. *Biophys J* 75:568, 1998.

96. Cooper RA, Jandl JH: Bile salts and cholesterol in the pathogenesis of target cells in obstructive jaundice. *J Clin Invest* 47:809, 1968.

97. Clark MR, Aminoff MJ, Chiu DT, et al: Red cell deformability and lipid composition in two forms of acanthocytosis: Enrichment of acanthocytic populations by density gradient centrifugation. *J Lab Clin Med* 113:469, 1989.

98. Redman CM, Huima T, Robbins E, et al: Effect of phosphatidylserine on the shape of McLeod red cell acanthocytes. *Blood* 74:1826, 1989.

99. Padilla F, Bromberg PA, Jensen WN: The sickle-unsickle cycle: A cause of cell fragmentation leading to permanently deformed cells. *Blood* 41:653, 1973.

100. Bessis M, Nomarski G, Thiery JP, et al: Étude sur la falciformation des globules rouges au microscope polarisant et microscope électronique. II L'Intérieur du globule; comparaison avec les cristaux intra-globulaires. *Rev Hematol* 13:249, 1958.

101. White JG: The fine structure of sickled hemoglobin in situ. *Blood* 31:561, 1968.

102. Jensen WN, Lessin LS: Membrane alterations associated with hemoglobinopathies. *Semin Hematol* 7:409, 1970.

103. Horiuchi K, Ballas SK, Asakura T: The effect of deoxygenation rate on the formation of irreversibly sickled cells. *Blood* 71:46, 1988.

104. Abraham A, Bencsath FA, Shartava A, et al: Preparation of irreversibly sickled cell beta-actin from normal red blood cell beta-actin. *Biochemistry (Mosc)* 41:292, 2002.

105. Bertles JF, Milner PF: Irreversibly sickled erythrocytes: A consequence of the heterogeneous distribution of hemoglobin types in sickle cell anemia. *J Clin Invest* 47:1731, 1968.

106. Weinstein RS, Warth JA, Near K, et al: Sequestrocytes: A manifestation of transcellular cross-bonding of the red cell membrane in sickle cell anemia. *J Cell Sci* 94:593, 1989.

107. Bull BS, Kuhn IN: The production of schistocytes by fibrin strands (a scanning electron microscope study). *Blood* 35:104, 1970.

108. Young TW, Keeney GL, Bull BS: Red cell fragmentation in human disease (a light and scanning electron microscope study). *Blood Cells* 10:493, 1984.

109. Bull BS, Weinstein RS, Korpman RA: On the thickness of the red cell membrane skeleton: Quantitative electron microscopy of maximally narrowed isthmus regions of intact cells. *Blood Cells* 12:25, 1986.

110. Cooper RA: Loss of membrane components in the pathogenesis of antibody-induced spherocytosis. *J Clin Invest* 51:16, 1972.

111. Rifkind RA, Danon D: Heinz body anemia: An ultrastructural study: I. Heinz body formation. *Blood* 25:885, 1965.

112. Rabinovitch M: Phagocytosis: The engulfment stage. *Semin Hematol* 5:134, 1968.

113. Lock SP, Smith RS, Hardisty RM: Stomatocytosis: A hereditary red cell anomaly associated with haemolytic anaemia. *Br J Haematol* 7:303, 1961.

114. Delaunay J, Stewart G, Iolascon A: Hereditary dehydrated and overhydrated stomatocytosis: Recent advances. *Curr Opin Hematol* 6:110, 1999.

115. Leblond PF, de Boisfleury A, Bessis M: La forme des erythrocytes dans la sphèrocytose héréditaire. *Nouv Rev Fr Hematol* 13:873, 1973.

116. Bull B: Holey red cells: A brief note. A commentary. *Blood Cells* 9:173, 1983.

117. Dhermy D, Feo C, Garbarz M, et al: Prenatal diagnosis of hereditary elliptocytosis with molecular defect of spectrin. *Prenat Diagn* 7:471, 1987.

118. Dhermy D, Garbarz M, Lecomte MC, et al: Hereditary elliptocytosis: Clinical, morphological and biochemical studies of 38 cases. *Nouv Rev Fr Hematol* 28:129, 1986.

119. Coetzer T, Palek J, Lawler J, et al: Structural and functional heterogeneity of alpha spectrin mutations involving the spectrin heterodimer self association site: Relationships to hematologic expression of homozy-

gous hereditary elliptocytosis and hereditary pyropoikilocytosis. *Blood* 75:2235, 1990.

120. Marchesi SL, Knowles WJ, Morrow JS, et al: Abnormal spectrin in hereditary elliptocytosis. *Blood* 67:141, 1986.

121. Agre P, Zinkham WH, Casella JF, et al: Spectrin deficiency is common to all forms of hereditary spherocytosis (HS): The degree of deficiency correlates with osmotic fragility. *Blood* 62(suppl 1):42a, 1983.

122. Marchesi SL, Conboy J, Agre P, et al: Molecular analysis of insertion deletion mutations in protein-4.1 in elliptocytosis: 1. Biochemical identification of rearrangements in the spectrin actin binding domain and functional characterizations. *J Clin Invest* 86:516, 1990.

123. Bull B, Feo C, Bessis M: Behavior of elliptocytes under shear stress in the rheoscope and ektacytometer. *Cytometry* 3:300, 1983.

124. Santillo PA, Lichtman MA: Holey red cells: A brief note. *Blood Cells* 9:169, 1983.

125. Fischer TM: Role of spectrin in cross bonding of the red cell membrane. *Blood Cells* 13:377, 1988.

126. Greenberg MS: Heinz body hemolytic anmea. "Bite cells"—A clue to diagnosis. *Arch Intern Med* 136:153, 1976.

127. Yoo D, Lessin LS: Drug-associated bite cell hemolytic anemia. *Am J Med* 92:243, 1992.

128. Diggs LW, Kraus AP, Morrison DB, et al: Intraerythrocytic crystals in a white patient with hemoglobin C in the absence of other types of hemoglobin. *Blood* 9:1172, 1954.

129. Fabry ME, Kaul DK, Raventos C, et al: Some aspects of the pathophysiology of homozygous Hb CC erythrocytes. *J Clin Invest* 67:1284, 1981.

130. Hirsch RE, Raventossuarez C, Olson JA, et al: Ligand state of intraerythrocytic circulating HbC crystals in homozygote CC patients. *Blood* 66:775, 1985.

131. Charache S, Conley CL, Waugh DF, et al: Pathogenesis of hemolytic anemia in homozygous hemoglobin C disease. *J Clin Invest* 46:1795, 1967.

132. Lessin LS, Jensen WN, Ponder E: Molecular mechanism of hemolytic anemia in homozygous hemoglobin C disease. Electron microscopic study by the freeze-etching technique. *J Exp Med* 130:443, 1969.

133. Charache S, Raik E, Holtzclaw D, et al: Pseudosickling of hemoglobin Setif. *Blood* 70:237, 1987.

134. Ponder E: *Hemolysis and Related Phenomena.* Grune & Stratton, New York, 1948.

135. Seeman P: Transient holes in the erythrocyte membrane during hypotonic hemolysis and stable holes in the membrane after lysis by saponin and lysolecithin. *J Cell Biol* 32:55, 1967.

136. Pribush A, Hatskelzon L, Kapelushnik J, et al: Osmotic swelling and hole formation in membranes of thalassemic and spherocytic erythrocytes. *Blood Cells Mol Dis* 31:43, 2003.

137. Stuart J, Bull BS, Juhan-Vague I: Microrheological techniques for the measurement of erythrocyte deformability, in *Investigative Microtechniques in Medicine and Biology*, edited by J Chayen, L Bitensky, p 297. Marcel Dekker, New York, 1984.

138. Schmid-Schonbein H, von Gosen J, Heinich L, et al: A counter-rotating "rheoscope chamber" for the study of the microrheology of blood cell aggregation by microscopic observation and microphotometry. *Microvasc Res* 6:366, 1973.

139. Bessis M, Mohandas N, Feo C: Automated ektacytometry: A new method of measuring red cell deformability and red cell indices. *Blood Cells* 6:315, 1980.

140. Mohandas N, Clark MR, Jacobs MS, et al: Analysis of factors regulating erythrocyte deformability. *J Clin Invest* 66:563, 1980.

141. Bull BS, Brailsford JD: A new method of measuring the deformability of the red cell membrane. *Blood* 45:581, 1975.

142. Williams AR, Morris DR: The internal viscosity of the human erythrocyte may determine its lifespan in vivo. *Scand J Haematol* 24:57, 1980.

143. Clark MR, Mohandas N, Caggiano V, et al: Effects of abnormal cation transport on deformability of desiccytes. *J Supramol Struct* 8:521, 1978.

144. Bessis MC, Breton-Gorius J: Iron metabolism in the bone marrow as seen by electron microscopy: A critical review. *Blood* 19:635, 1962.

145. Edelman P, Vinci G, Villeval JL, et al: A monoclonal antibody against an erythrocyte ontogenic antigen identifies fetal and adult erythroid progenitors. *Blood* 67:56, 1986.

146. Breton-Gorius J, Villeval JL, Mitjavila MT, et al: Ultrastructural and cytochemical characterization of blasts from early erythroblastic leukemias. *Leukemia* 1:173, 1987.

147. Jay AW: Geometry of the human erythrocyte: I. Effect of albumin on cell geometry. *Biophys J* 15:205, 1975.

C H A P T E R   2 9

COMPOSITION OF THE ERYTHROCYTE

ERNEST BEUTLER

Quantitative data have been published about many of the components of the red cell, including minerals, carbohydrates, enzymes and other proteins, vitamins, and lipids. Some of these are marred by the failure to rigorously remove white cells from the red cell pellet, but this chapter provides access to some of the large amount of data that is available.

The erythrocyte is a complex cell. The membrane is composed of lipids and proteins. The interior of the cell contains metabolic machinery designed to sustain the cell through its 120-day life span and maintain the integrity of hemoglobin function. Each component of red blood cells can be expressed as a function of red cell volume, grams of hemoglobin, or square centimeters of cell surface. These expressions are usually interchangeable, but under certain circumstances each may have specific advantages. However, because disease can produce changes in the average red cell size, hemoglobin content, or surface area, the use of any of these measurements individually may, at times, be misleading.

For convenience and uniformity, the data in the accompanying tables (Tables 29-1 through 29-9) are expressed in terms of cell constituent per milliliter of red cell and per gram of hemoglobin. In many instances, this process required recalculation of published data. These recalculations assume a hematocrit value of 45 percent and 33 g of hemoglobin per deciliter of red cells. To obtain concentration per gram of hemoglobin, the concentration per milliliter red blood cell (RBC) can be multiplied by 3.03. The tables list only some of the most commonly referred to constituents of the erythrocyte. The reference on which each value is based is the first number presented in the last column of each table. Where applicable, additional confirmatory references are given. Additional data and references can be found elsewhere.[1,2] In some instances, only the percentage of the total of the type of constituent present is given. Data regarding activities of red cell enzymes are presented in Chap. 45.

TABLE 29-1 HUMAN ERYTHROCYTE PROTEIN AND WATER CONTENT

COMPONENT	MG/ML RBC	REFERENCE
Water	721±17.3	3, 4
Total protein	371	4–7
Nonhemoglobin protein	9.2	4, 5
Insoluble stroma protein	6.3	5
Protein from enzymes	2.9	5

Acronyms and abbreviations that appear in this chapter include: RBC, red blood cell.

TABLE 29-2 HUMAN ERYTHROCYTE LIPIDS

FATTY ACIDS AS PERCENT OF TOTAL FATTY ACID		REFERENCE
Lauric (n-C_{17})	0.3	8
Myristic (n-C_{14})	0.8	8
Pentoenoic (n-C_{15})	0.3	8
Palmitoleic (16:1)	1.1	8
Palmitic (n-C_{16})	41.0	8
(n-C_{17}) branched	0.3	8
(n-C_{17})	0.3	8
Linoleic	15.3	8
Oleic	18.9	8
Oleic isomer	Trace	8
Stearic (n-C_{18})	7.9	8
Arachidonic (20:4)	7.9	8
C_{22} unsaturated (a)	2.5	8
C_{22} unsaturated (b)	2.0	8
Unknown C_{19}	2.9	8
Unknown C_{20}	3.1	8
Unknown C_{21}	5.6	8

LONG-CHAIN ALDEHYDES AS PERCENT OF TOTAL ALDEHYDES		REFERENCE
n-C_{14}	Trace	8
Branched C_{15}	0.8	8
n-C_{15}	0.6	8
Highly branched C_{16}	Trace	8
C_{16} monoene	0.4	8
n-C_{16}	24.2	8
Highly branched C_{17}	1.7	8
Branched C_{17}	7.5	8
n-C_{17}	1.3	8
C_{18} monoene	6.0	8
Isomeric C_{18} monoene	2.8	8
n-C_{18}	42.5	8

FATTY ACIDS AS PERCENT OF TOTAL NEUTRAL LIPIDS FATTY ACIDS		REFERENCE
n-C_{10}	0.0–0.6	9
n-C_{12}	1.1–2.2	9
n-C_{14}	5.9–17.3	9
16:1	3.2–6.0	9
n-C_{16}	15.2–22.6	9
18:2 and 3	11.4–21.1	9
18:1	28.8–29.1	9
n-C_{18}	5.7–10.7	9
Unsaturated C_{19}A	Trace	9
Arachidonic	7.4–8.3	9
Polyunsaturated C_{20}	Trace	9

TABLE 29-3 HUMAN ERYTHROCYTE PHOSPHOLIPIDS

LIPID	AMOUNT	REFERENCE
Total phospholipids	2.98 ± 0.20 mg/ml RBC	10
Cephalin	1.17 (0.38–1.91) mg/ml RBC	10
Ethanolamine phosphoglyceride	29% of total phospholipid	10
Mean plasmalogen content	67% of ethanolamine phosphoglyceride	10
Serine phosphoglyceride	10% of total phospholipid	10
Mean plasmalogen content	8% of serine phosphoglyceride	10
Lecithin	0.32 (0.03–0.95) mg/ml	11
Sphingomyelin	0.12–1.13 mg/ml	11
Lysolecithin	1.82% of total phospholipids	12

NOTE: Some results are given as mean ± standard deviation.

TABLE 29-4   FATTY ACID COMPOSITIONS OF ERYTHROCYTE PHOSPHOLIPIDS[6,7] (MOL %)

SHORTHAND DESIGNATION	MIXED PHOSPHOLIPIDS (METHANOL FRACTION)	ETHANOL-AMINE	SERINE	CHOLINE
12:0	0.1	—	—	0.1
14:0	0.5	0.2	Trace	0.5
14:0	0.3	0.2	Trace	0.3
16:0	28.8	18.9	7.1	33.0
cis 16:1[9]	0.7	0.6	0.4	0.1
17:0	0.4	Trace	0.3	0.5
18:0	15.1	8.0	41.6	11.7
cis 18:1[9]	18.3	21.6	7.9	17.9
trans 18:1[9]	2.9	3.6	5.1	2.7
cis,cis 18:2[9,12]	10.6	7.0	2.8	18.2
cis,cis,cis 18:3[9,12,15]	—	Trace	—	—
19:0 iso or ante-iso	Trace	0.2	—	—
20:0	0.1	—	Trace	0.2
20:1[11]	0.2	0.3	Trace	0.2
20:2[8,11]	—	Trace	—	—
20:2[11,14]	0.1	0.1	—	0.2
20:3[5,8,11]	1.6	1.0	2.1	1.6
20:4[5,8,11,14]	10.8	21.9	19.7	5.0
20:5[5,8,11,14,17]	0.8	1.4	0.3	0.5
(22:unsat.?)	1.7	4.7	2.2	0.3
22:5	0.7	0.8	0.9	1.7
22:5	2.3	2.3	2.0	2.7
22:5[7,10,13,16,19]	1.0	—	—	1.0
22:6[4,7,10,13,16,19]	2.1	3.9	4.2	1.1
14:0	Trace	—	—	0.8
Branched 15:0	2.8	2.6	5.5	—
15:0 iso or ante-iso	0.1	—	0.4	—
15:0	0.2	0.3	—	—
Unknown	0.1	—	1.6	1.0
cis 16:1[9]	Trace	—	—	0.2
16:0	18.2	15.9	17.1	49.8
Branched 17:0 unsat.?	0.9	1.5	—	—
Branched 17:unsat.?	2.4	3.0	—	—
Branched 17:0	5.8	5.5	11.3	6.9
17:0 iso or ante-iso	1.1	0.8	0.7	2.9
cis,cis 18:2[9,12]	Trace	—	1.4	—
cis 18:1[9]	6.8	7.0	5.4	5.3
18:1 isomer	13.2	18.8	10.5	7.7
18:0	37.1	40.4	32.3	19.2
Unknown	1.3	2.1	—	—

TABLE 29-5   NUCLEOTIDES

COMPOUND	μMOL/ML RBC	REFERENCE
Adenosine monophosphate	0.021 ± 0.003	13–19
Adenosine diphosphate	0.216 ± 0.036	13–18
Adenosine triphosphate	1.35 ± 0.035	15–17, 19–22
Cyclic adenosine monophosphate	0.015 ± .0024	23
Cyclic guanosine monophosphate	0.013 ± .0042	23
Guanosine diphosphate	0.018 ± 0.005	15
Guanosine triphosphate	0.052 ± 0.012	14, 15
Inosine monophosphate	0.031 ± 0.005	15–19
Nicotinamide adenine dinucleotide		
Reduced	0.0018 ± 0.001	24, 25
Oxidized	0.049 ± 0.006	24, 25
Nicotinamide adenine dinucleotide phosphate		
Reduced	0.032 ± 0.002	24, 25
Oxidized	0.0014 ± 0.0011	24, 25
S-adenosylmethionine	0.005	26
Total nucleotide	1.534 ± 0.033	27
Uridine diphosphoglucose	0.031 ± 0.005	15, 28
Uridine diphosphate N-acetyl glucosamine	0.018	28

NOTE: Some results are given as mean ± standard deviation.

TABLE 29-6   AMINO ACIDS AND OTHER NITROGEN-CONTAINING COMPOUNDS

COMPOUND	μMOL/ML RBC	REFERENCE
Alanine	0.275 ± 0.060	28–32
α-Amino butyrate	0.016 ± 0.009	29–31
Arginine	0.040 ± 0.013	29–31, 33, 34
Asparagine	0.121 ± 0.041	29, 30
Aspartate	0.306 ± 0.081*	29
Carnitine	0.23	35, 36
Citrulline	0.036 ± 0.005*	29
Glutamate	0.265 ± 0.089	29, 31, 37
Glutamine	0.624 ± 0.136	31, 38, 39
Glycine	0.347 ± 0.070	29, 30
Histidine	0.086 ± 0.013	29, 31, 34, 40
Isoleucine	0.058 ± 0.013	29, 30
Leucine	0.110 ± 0.009	29, 30
Lysine	0.139 ± 0.032	29, 31, 34
Methionine	0.015 ± 0.006	29, 31, 34
Ornithine	0.120 ± 0.028	29, 31
Phenylalanine	0.049 ± 0.006	29–31, 34
Proline	0.137 ± 0.035	29–31
Serine	0.149 ± 0.032	29–30
Taurine	0.349 ± 0.057	29
Threonine	0.116 ± 0.022	29–31
Tyrosine	0.059 ± 0.009	29–31, 34
Valine	0.171 ± 0.028	29–31, 34
Creatine	0.33 ± 0.11	41
Creatinine	0.159	42
Cystine	0.016 ± 0.002	34
Ergothioneine	0.355 ± 0.112	31
Ethanolamine	0.007	31
Glutathione		
Oxidized	0.0036 ± 0.0014	43
Reduced	2.234 ± 0.354	13
Tryptophan	0.024 ± 0.004	31, 33, 34, 44
Uric acid	0.113	31, 42
Urea	4.121 ± 0.420	31

* Measured in samples treated with sodium sulfite before analysis.
NOTE: Some results are given as mean ± standard deviation.

TABLE 29-7 HUMAN ERYTHROCYTE COENZYME AND VITAMINS

COMPOUND	μMOL/ML RBC	REFERENCE
Ascorbic acid	0.0199 ± 0.0023	45–47
Choline (free)	Trace	48
Cocarboxylase	0.00021	49
Coenzyme A	0.0027	50
Nicotinic acid	0.105	51
Pantothenic acid	0.001 ± 0.00028	52
Pyridoxine (pyridoxal, pyridoxamine)	1×10^{-5}	53
Riboflavin	0.00059 ± 0.00021	54
Flavin adenine dinucleotide	0.000398 ± 0.000042	55
Thiamine	0.00027	56

NOTE: Some results are given as mean ± standard deviation.

TABLE 29-8 HUMAN ERYTHROCYTE CARBOHYDRATES, ORGANIC ACIDS, AND METABOLITES

COMPOUND	μMOL/ML RBC	REFERENCE
Deoxyribonucleic acid	Trace	57
Dihydroxyacetone phosphate	0.0094 + 0.0028	13
2,3 Diphosphoglycerate	4.171 ± 0.636	13, 17, 21, 22
Fructose 6-P	0.0093 ± 0.002	13, 16, 21, 58
Fructose 3-P	0.013 ± 0.001	59, 60
Fructose 2,6-bisphosphate	48 ± 13*	61
Fructose 1,6-diphosphate	0.0019 ± 0.0006	13, 16, 17, 21, 58
Glucuronic acid	Trace	62
Glucose	In equilibrium with plasma	63, 64
Glucose 6-P	0.0278 ± 0.0075	13, 16, 21, 58
Glucose 1,6-diphosphate	0.18–0.30	16, 65
Glyceraldehyde 3-P	Not detectable	13
Lactic acid	0.932 ± 0.211	5, 13, 66
Mannose 1,6-diphosphate	0.150	65
Octulose 1,8-diphosphate	Trace	67
Pyruvate	0.0533 ± 0.0215	13
3-Phosphoglycerate	0.0449 ± 0.0051	13, 21
2-Phosphoglycerate	0.0073 ± 0.0025	13, 21
Phosphoenol pyruvate	0.0122 ± 0.0022	13
Ribonucleic acid	1.355 mg	68
Ribose 1,5-diphosphate	<0.02	69, 70
Ribulose 5-P	Trace	71
Sedoheptulose 7-P	Trace	71
Sedoheptulose diphosphate	Trace	72
Sialic acid	0.825 ± 0.028	69
Sorbitol	31.1 ± 5.3	59, 73
Sorbitol 3-P	0.013 ± 0.001	60

* Values are given in picomole.
NOTE: Some results are given as mean ± standard deviation.

TABLE 29-9 HUMAN ERYTHROCYTE ELECTROLYTES

ELECTROLYTE	μMOL/ML RBC	REFERENCE
Aluminum	0.0026	74
Bromide	0.1225	75, 76
Calcium	0.0089 ± 0.0030	76–78
Chloride	78	76, 79
Chromium	0.0004	80
Cobalt	0.0002	76, 81
Copper	0.018	82, 80, 83
Fluoride	0.0131	84
Iodine, protein-bound	0.0013	85
Lead	0.0082	74, 76, 82, 86
Magnesium	3.06	80, 87–89
Manganese	0.0034	74, 90
Nickel	0.0009	80
Phosphorus (acid soluble)		
Total P	13.2	91
Inorganic P	0.466	91
Lipid P	3.840	92
Unidentified P	0.955	91
Potassium	102.4 ± 3.9	87, 93–97
Rubidium	0.054	76
Silicon	Trace	49
Silver	Trace	74
Sodium	6.2 ± 0.8	93–95
Sulfur	0.0044	98
Tin	0.0022	74
Zinc	0.153	80, 99, 100

NOTE: Some results are given as mean ± standard deviation.

REFERENCES

1. Friedemann H, Rapoport SM: Enzymes of the red cell; a critical catalogue, in: *Cellular and Molecular Biology of Erythrocytes*, edited by H Yoshikawa, SM Rapoport, p 181. University Park Press, Baltimore, 1974.

2. Pennell RB: Comparison of normal human red cells, in: *The Red Blood Cell*, edited by DM Surgenor, p 98. Academic Press, New York, 1974.

3. Nichols G, Nichols N: Electrolyte equilibrium in erythrocytes during diabetic acidosis. *J Clin Invest* 32:113, 1953.

4. Ponder E: *Hemolysis and Related Phenomena*. Grune & Stratton, New York, 1948.

5. Behrendt H: *Chemistry of Erythrocytes*. Charles C. Thomas, Springfield, 1957.

6. Guidotti G: The protein of human erythrocyte membranes. I. Preparation, solubilization and partial characterization. *J Biol Chem* 243:1985, 1968.

7. Silverman L, Glick D: Measurement of protein concentration by quantitative electron microscopy. *J Cell Biol* 40:773, 1969.

8. Kates M, Allison AC, James AT: Phosphatides of human blood cells and their role in spherocytosis. *Biochim Biophys Acta* 48:571, 1961.

9. James AT, Lovelock JE, Webb JPW: The lipids of whole blood. I. Lipid biosynthesis in human blood in vitro. *Biochem J* 73:106, 1959.

10. Farquhar JW: Human erythrocytes phosphoglycerides. I. Quantification of plasmalogens, fatty acids and fatty aldehydes. *Biochim Biophys Acta* 60:80, 1962.

11. Kirk E: The concentration of lecithin, cephalin, ether-insoluble phosphatide, and cerebrosides in plasma and red blood cells of normal adults. *J Biol Chem* 123:637, 1938.

12. Phillips GB, Roome NS: Quantitative chromatographic analysis of the phospholipids of abnormal human red blood cells. *Proc Soc Exp Biol Med* 109:360, 1962.

13. Beutler E: *Red Cell Metabolism: A Manual of Biochemical Methods.* Grune & Stratton, New York, 1984.

14. Bishop C, Rankine D, Talbott JH: The nucleotides in normal human blood. *J Biol Chem* 234:1233, 1959.

15. Mandel P, Chambon P, Karon H, et al: Nucleotides libres des globules rouges et des reticulocytes. *Folia Haematol (Leipz)* 78:525, 1962.

16. Bartlett GR: Human red cell glycolytic intermediates. *J Biol Chem* 234:449, 1959.

17. Gerlach E, Fleckenstein A, Gross E: Der Intermediaere Phosphat-Stoffwechsel des Menschen-Erythrocyten. *Pflugers Arch* 266:528, 1958.

18. Löhr GW, Waller HD: The biochemistry of erythrocyte aging. *Folia Haematol (Leipz)* 78:384, 1961.

19. Yoshikawa H, Nakano M, Miyamoto K, Tatibana M: Phosphorus metabolism in human erythrocyte. II. Separation of acid-soluble phosphorus compounds incorporating p32 by column chromatography with ion exchange resin. *J Biochem (Tokyo)* 47:635, 1960.

20. Beutler E, Mathai CK: A comparison of normal red cell ATP levels as measured by the firefly system and the hexokinase system. *Blood* 30:311, 1967.

21. Minakami S, Suzuki C, Saito T, Yoshikawa H: Studies on erythrocyte glycolysis I, determination of the glycolytic intermediates in human erythrocytes. *J Biochem (Tokyo)* 58:543, 1965.

22. Ramos JLA, Nonoyama K, Quintal VS, Barretto OCDO: Red cell enzymes and intermediates in AGA term newborns, AGA preterm newborns and SGA term newborns. *Acta Paediatr Scand* 79:32, 1990.

23. Patterson WD, Hardman JG, Sutherland EW: A comparison of cyclic nucleotide levels in plasma and cells of rat and human blood. *Endocrinology* 95:325, 1974.

24. Canepa L, Ferraris AM, Miglino M, Gaetani GF: Bound and unbound pyridine dinucleotides in normal and glucose-6-phosphate dehydrogenase-deficient erythrocytes. *Biochim Biophys Acta* 1074:101, 1991.

25. Micheli V, Simmonds HA, Bari M, Pompucci G: HPLC determination of oxidized and reduced pyridine coenzymes in human erythrocytes. *Clin Chim Acta* 220:1, 1993.

26. Lagendijk J, Ubbink JB, Vermaak WJH: Quantification of erythrocyte S-adenosyl-L-methionine levels and its application in enzyme studies. *J Chromatogr Biomed Appl* 576:95, 1992.

27. Overgard-Hansen K, Jorgensen S: Determination and concentration of adenine nucleotides in human blood. *Scand J Clin Lab Invest* 12:10, 1960.

28. Mills GC: Uridine diphosphate glucose and uridine diphosphate N-acetylglucosamine in erythrocytes. *Tex Rep Biol Med* 18:446, 1960.

29. Hagenfeldt L, Arvidsson A: A distribution of amino acids between plasma and erythrocytes. *Clin Chim Acta* 100:133, 1980.

30. Leighton WP, Rosenblatt S, Chanley JD: Determination of erythrocyte amino acids by gas chromatography. *J Chromatogr* 164:427, 1979.

31. McMenamy RH, Lund CC, Neville GJ, Wallach DFH: Studies of unbound amino acid distributions in plasma, erythrocytes, leukocytes and urine of normal human subjects. *J Clin Invest* 39:1675, 1960.

32. Wiss O, Kruger R: Der Einfluss Enteral und Parenteral Verabreichter Glucose auf den Alaningehalt des Blutes. *Helv Chim Acta* 31:1774, 1948.

33. Hier SW, Bergeim O: The microbiological determination of certain free amino acids in human and dog plasma. *J Biol Chem* 163:129, 1946.

34. Johnson CA, Bergeim O: The distribution of free amino acids between erythrocytes and plasma in man. *J Biol Chem* 188:833, 1951.

35. Borum PR, York CM, Bennett SG: Carnitine concentration of red blood cells. *Am J Clin Nutr* 41:653, 1985.

36. Reichmann HV, Lindeneiner N: Carnitine analysis in normal human red blood cells, plasma, and muscle tissue. *Eur Neurol* 34:40, 1994.

37. Divino Filho JC, Hazel SJ, Furst P, et al: Glutamate concentration in plasma, erythrocyte and muscle in relation to plasma levels of insulin-like growth factor (IGF)-I, IGF binding protein-1 and insulin in patients on haemodialysis. *J Endocrinol* 156:519, 1998.

38. Preisler H, Browman G, Henderson E, et al: Treatment of acute myelocytic leukemia: Effects of early intensive consolidation. *ASCO Abstracts* 443, 1980.

39. Iyer GYN: Distribution of glutamine, glutamic acids, and aspartic acid between erythrocytes and plasma. *Indian J Med Res* 44:201, 1956.

40. von Euler H, Heller L: Free histidine in the blood serum of normal and Jensen sarcoma-bearing rats. *Arch Miner Geol* 24A:23, 1947.

41. Griffiths WJ, Fitzpatrick M: The effect of age on the creatine in red cells. *Br J Haematol* 13:175, 1967.

42. Jellinek EM, Looney JM: Statistics of some biochemical variables on healthy men in the age range of twenty to forty-five years. *J Biol Chem* 128:621, 1939.

43. Srivastava SK, Beutler E: Oxidized glutathione levels in erythrocytes of glucose-6-phosphate dehydrogenase-deficient subjects. *Lancet* 2:23, 1968.

44. Steele BF, Reynolds MS, Baumann CA: Amino acids in the blood and urine of human subjects ingesting different amounts of the same proteins. *J Nutr* 40:145, 1950.

45. Barkhan P, Howard AN: Distribution of ascorbic acid in normal and leukaemic human blood. *Biochem J* 70:163, 1958.

46. Butler AM, Cushman M: Distribution of ascorbic acid in the blood and its nutritional significance. *J Clin Invest* 19:459, 1940.

47. Sargent F: A study of the normal distribution of ascorbic acid between the red cells and plasma of human blood. *J Biol Chem* 171: 1947.

48. Luecke R, Pearson PB: The microbiological determination of free choline in plasma and urine. *J Biol Chem* 153:259, 1944.

49. Beerstecher E, Spangler S, Granick S, et al: Blood vitamins, hormones, enzymes. Blood coenzymes: Vertebrates, in: *Blood and Other Body Fluids*, edited by PL Altman, DS Dittmer, p 108. Federation of American Societies for Experimental Biology, Washington, DC, 1961.

50. Kaplan NO, Lipmann F: The assay of distribution of coenzyme A. *J Biol Chem* 174:37, 1948.

51. Klein JR, Perlzweig WA, Handler P: Determination of nicotinic acid in blood cells and plasma. *J Biol Chem* 145:27, 1942.

52. Pearson PB: The pantothenic acid content of the blood of mammalia. *J Biol Chem* 140:423, 1941.

53. Marsch ME, Greenberg LD, Rinehart JF: The relationship between pyridoxine ingestion and transaminase activity. *J Nutr* 56:115, 1955.

54. Burch HB, Bessey OA, Lowry OH: Fluorometric measurements of riboflavin and its natural derivatives in small quantities of blood serum and cells. *J Biol Chem* 175:457, 1948.

55. Beutler E: Glutathione reductase: Stimulation in normal subjects by riboflavin supplementation. *Science* 165:613, 1969.

56. Burch HB, Bessey OA, Love RH, Lowry OH: The determination of thiamine and thiamine phosphates in small quantities of blood and blood cells. *J Biol Chem* 198:477, 1952.

57. Metais P, Mandel P: Teneur en acide desoxypentosenucleique des leucocytes chez l'homme normal et a l'etat pathologique. *C R Acad Sci (Paris)* 144:277, 1950.

58. Lionetti FJ, McLellan WL, Fortier NL, Foster JM: Phosphate esters produced from inosine in human erythrocyte ghosts. *Arch Biochem* 94:7, 1961.

59. Kawaguchi M, Fujii T, Kamiya Y, et al: Effects of fructose ingestion on sorbitol and fructose 3-phosphate contents of erythrocytes from healthy men. *Acta Diabetol* 33:100, 1996.

60. Petersen A, Szwergold BS, Kappler F, et al: Identification of sorbitol 3-phosphate and fructose 3-phosphate in normal and diabetic human erythrocytes. *J Biol Chem* 265:17424, 1990.

61. Colomer D, Pujades A, Carballo E, Vives Corrons JL: Erythrocyte fructose 2,6-bisphosphate content in congenital hemolytic anemias. *Hemoglobin* 15:517, 1991.

62. Deichmann WB, Dierker M: The spectrophotometric estimation of hexuronates (expressed as glucuronic acid) in plasma or serum. *J Biol Chem* 163:753, 1946.

63. Jung CY: Carrier-mediated glucose transport across human red cell membranes, in: *The Red Blood Cell*, edited by DM Surgenor, p 705. Academic Press, New York, 1975.

64. Lacko L, Wittke B, Geck P: The temperature dependence of the exchange transport of glucose in human erythrocytes. *J Cell Physiol* 82:213, 1973.

65. Bartlett GR: Glucose and mannose diphosphates in the red blood cell. *Biochim Biophys Acta* 156:231, 1968.

66. Johnson RE, Edward HT, Dill DB, Wilson JW: Blood as a physicochemical system. XIII. The distribution of lactate. *J Biol Chem* 157:461, 1945.

67. Bartlett GR, Bucolo G: Octulose phosphates from the human red blood cell. *Biochem Biophys Res Commun* 3:474, 1960.

68. Mandel P, Métals P: Les acides nucléiques du plasma sanguin chez l'homme. *C R Acad Sci (Paris)* 142:241, 1948.

69. Aminoff D, Anderson J, Dabich L, Gathmann WD: Sialic acid content of erythrocytes in normal individuals and patients with certain hematologic disorders. *Am J Hematol* 9:381, 1980.

70. Vanderheiden BS: Ribosediphosphate in the human erythrocyte. *Biochem Biophys Res Commun* 6:117, 1961.

71. Bruns FH, Noltmann E, Vahlhaus E: Über den Stoffwechsel von Ribose-5-phosphat in Hämolysaten. I. Aktivitäts-messung und Eigenschaften der Phosphoribose-isomerase. II. Der Pentosephosphate-Cyclus in roten Blutzellen. *Biochem Z* 330:483, 1958.

72. Bucolo G, Bartlett GR: Sedoheptulose diphosphate formation by the human red blood cell. *Biochem Biophys Res Commun* 3:620, 1960.

73. Inoue S, Lin SL, Chang T, et al: Identification of free deaminated sialic acid (2-keto-3-deoxy-D-glycero-D-galacto-nononic acid) in human red blood cells and its elevated expression in fetal cord red blood cells and ovarian cancer cells. *J Biol Chem* 273:27199, 1998.

74. Kehoe RA, Cholak J, Story RV: A spectrochemical study of the normal ranges of concentration of certain trace metals in biological materials. *J Nutr* 19:579, 1940.

75. Hunter G: Micro-determination of bromide in body fluids. *Biochem J* 60:261, 1955.

76. Ojo JO, Oluwole AF, Durosinmi MA, et al: Baseline levels of elemental concentrations in whole blood, plasma, and erythrocytes of Nigerian subjects. *Biol Trace Elem Res* 43-44:461, 1994.

77. Bernard J-F, Bournier O, Boivin P: Human erythrocytic calcium concentration in hemolytic anemia. *Biomedicine* 23:431, 1975.

78. Shoji S, Komiyama A, Nakamura M, Nomoto S: Calcium content of healthy human erythrocytes. *Clin Chem* 35:1264, 1989.

79. Bernstein RE: Potassium and sodium balance in mammalian red cells. *Science* 120:459, 1954.

80. Herring WB, Leavell BS, Paizao LM, Yoe JH: Trace metals in human plasma and red blood cells: A study of magnesium, chromium, nickel, copper and zinc. I. Observations of normal subjects. *Am J Clin Nutr* 8:846, 1960.

81. Heyrovsky A: The biochemistry of cobalt. III. Amounts of cobalt in plasma, erythrocytes, urine, and feces of normal subjects. *Cas Lek Cesk* 91:680, 1952.

82. Mahalingam TR, Vijayalakshmi S, Prabhu RK, et al: Studies on some trace and minor elements in blood: A survey of the Kalpakkam (India) population. 2. Reference values for plasma and red cells, and correlation with coronary risk index. *Biol Trace Elem Res* 57:207, 1997.

83. Lahey ME, Gubler CJ, Cartwright GE, Wintrobe MM: Studies on copper metabolism. VI. Blood copper in normal human subjects. *J Clin Invest* 32:322, 1953.

84. Largent EJ, Cholak J: Blood electrolytes. Man, in: *Blood and Other Body Fluids*, edited by PL Altman, DS Dittmer, p 21. Federation of American Societies for Experimental Biology, Washington, DC, 1961.

85. McClendon JF, Foster WC: Protein-bound iodine in erythrocytes and plasma and elsewhere. *Am J Med Sci* 207:549, 1944.

86. Jensovsky L, Roth Z: Der normale Bleigehalt im menschlichen Blute. *Naturwissenschaften* 48:382, 1961.

87. McCance RA, Widdowson EM: The effect of development, anaemia, and undernutrition on the composition of the erythrocyte. *Clin Sci* 15:409, 1956.

88. Huijgen HJ, Sanders R, Van Olden RW, et al: Intracellular and extracellular blood magnesium fractions in hemodialysis patients; is the ionized fraction a measure of magnesium excess? *Clin Chem* 44:639, 1998.

89. Martin BJ, Lyon TD, Fell GS, McKay P: Erythrocyte magnesium in elderly patients: not a reliable guide to magnesium status. *J Trace Elem Med Biol* 11:44, 1997.

90. Miller DO, Yoe JH: Spectrophotometric determination of manganese in human plasma and red cells with benzohydroxamic acid. *Anal Chim Acta* 26:224, 1962.

91. Bartlett GR, Savage E, Hughes L, Marlow AA: Carbohydrate intermediates and related cofactors with benzohydroxamic acid. *J Appl Physiol* 6:51, 1953.

92. Ferranti F, Giannetti O: The microdetermination of phosphorus (inorganic, acid-soluble, lipoid and total) in the blood and excretions. *Diagn Tec Lab Napoli Riv Mens* 4:664, 1933.

93. Overman RR, Davis AK: The application of flame photometry to sodium and potassium determinations in biological fluids. *J Biol Chem* 168:641, 1947.

94. Mayer KDF, Starkey BJ: Simpler flame photometric determination of erythrocyte sodium and potassium: The reference range for apparently healthy adults. *Clin Chem* 23:275, 1977.

95. Bernard JF, Bournier O, Renoux M, et al: Unclassified haemolytic anaemia with splenomegaly and erythrocyte cation abnormalities: A disease of the spleen? *Scand J Haematol* 17:231, 1976.

96. Hald PM: Notes on the determination and distribution of sodium and potassium in cells and serum of normal human blood. *J Biol Chem* 163:429, 1946.

97. Streef GM: Sodium and calcium content of erythrocytes. *J Biol Chem* 129:661, 1939.

98. Reed L, Denis W: On the distribution of the non-protein sulfur of the blood between serum and corpuscles. *J Biol Chem* 73:623, 1927.

99. Vallee BL, Gibson JG: The zinc content of normal human whole blood, plasma, leucocytes, and erythrocytes. *J Biol Chem* 176:445, 1948.

100. Zak B, Nalbandian RM, Williams LA, Cohen J: Determination of human erythrocyte zinc: hemoglobin ratios. *Clin Chim Acta* 7:634, 1962.

PRODUCTION OF ERYTHROCYTES

JOSEF T. PRCHAL

Production of red cells—*erythropoiesis*—is a tightly regulated process. When one of the progeny of the multipotential hematopoietic stem becomes committed to the erythroid lineage, the early erythroid progenitor undergoes a series of divisions that eventually result in morphologically recognizable erythroblasts. After expulsion of the nucleus, the enucleated erythroid cell—the reticulocyte—leaves the bone marrow. Reticulocytes lose their mitochondria (which produce energy by oxidative phosphorylation) and ribosomes (with their protein synthesizing machinery), and the mature erythrocytes, which account for the vast majority of circulating blood cells, start their life span. Erythropoiesis is controlled by transcription factors and cytokines, principally GATA-1 and erythropoietin, which influence the rate of lineage commitment, proliferation, apoptosis, differentiation, and number of divisions from the earliest progenitor to late erythroblasts. The number of red cells produced varies in response to tissue oxygenation, which determines the level of the transcription factor hypoxia inducible factor-1 (HIF-1), the principal regulator of hypoxia response. HIF-1 modulates respiration, energy metabolism, vasculogenesis, and other physiologic processes. It is a crucial regulator of erythropoiesis, which synchronizes cellular responses, hemoglobin and iron metabolism, and other metabolic pathways, assuring optimal red cell production to satisfy body needs.

HISTORY

The red cell mass evolved largely for the purpose of transporting oxygen to tissues. Thus, the size of the red cell mass and the rate of red cell production must be closely related to supply and demand for oxygen in the tissues. Toward the end of the 19th century, French mountaineers and physiologists established that a low tissue tension of oxygen stimulates the rate of red cell production.[1] However, the mode of stimulation was hotly debated. In 1906, Dr. Paul Carnot, the Sorbonne professor, and Mademoiselle DeFlandre, his associate, suggested that hypoxia generates a humoral factor capable of stimulating red cell

*This chapter is based in part on Chapter 29 in the previous edition of this text by Dr. Ernest Beutler.

Acronyms and abbreviations that appear in this chapter include: ACEI, angiotensin converting-enzyme inhibitor; Ang-II, angiotensin II; Bcl-x$_L$, antiapoptotic factor; BFU-E, burst forming unit—erythroid; CFU-E, colony forming unit—erythroid; CIS, signal transduction protein that down-regulates activity of erythropoietin receptor; CPM, counts per minute; Epo, erythropoietin (protein); *EPO*, erythropoietin (gene); EpoR, erythropoietin receptor (protein); *EPOR*, erythropoietin receptor (gene); FOG, friend of GATA; GATA-1, transcription factor; HCP, hematopoietic cell phosphatase; Hct, hematocrit; HIF-1, hypoxia inducible factor-1; ICSH, International Committee on Standardization in Hematology; IGF, insulin-like growth factor; JAK2, janus kinase 2, a tyrosine kinase that interacts with erythropoietin receptor; PU.1, transcription factor; RAS, renin–angiotensin system; STAT-5, signal transduction protein that transduces activity of erythropoietin receptor.

---

production.[2] On the other hand, the biochemist Friederich Miescher[3] erroneously proposed that marrow hypoxia directly stimulates red cell production. Unfortunately, both hypotheses were based on highly questionable experimental data, and subsequent attempts to clarify the picture generated more heat than light. Finally, in 1950, in an ingenious study on parabiotic rats, Kurt Reissmann[4] provided strong support for the existence of an indirect humoral mechanism. A few years later, Erslev and colleagues[5,6] demonstrated convincingly that the plasma from anemic rabbits and primates contains a red cell stimulating factor. The factor was appropriately named erythropoietin (Epo). Epo generally became accepted as being involved in regulation of red cell production. In 1957, Jacobson and coworkers[7] reported that Epo was produced by the kidney, a finding that raised the possibility that Epo isolated in adequate amounts might be of therapeutic benefit to uremic patients. After *EPO* cloning and production of recombinant Epo in industrial quantities, Epo has proved to have much broader applicability. Widespread clinical use of Epo has surpassed original expectations.

PHYLOGENY OF RED CELL PRODUCTION

Hemoglobin is present in the most primitive animal forms, such as *Paramecium* and *Tetrahymena*. Some crustaceans, such as *Daphnia*, were capable of developing a fairly sophisticated oxygen transport system without circulating red cells.[8] An erythroid cell that can synthesize, carry, and protect hemoglobin from oxidation was found only with the development of a circulatory system. Circulating nucleated erythrocytes first appear in the worms of the phylum Nemertina and in the sessile marine creatures of the phylum Phoronida. Erythropoiesis in these primitive invertebrates takes place near or on the peritoneal surface, derived from endothelial cells.[9] Nonnucleated red cells are observed for the first time in the more advanced phylum Annelida. However, the evolutionary advantage derived from enucleation appears to be slight. Nucleated red cells are observed in much further advanced animals, such as reptiles and birds.[10] All mammalian erythrocytes are nonnucleated.[11] The emergence of red cells appears to be related to the protective and regulatory effect of intracellular compounds on hemoglobin and its oxygen affinity.

In premammalian species, the spleen is the fundamental erythropoietic organ. However, in some fish, the kidneys also are involved in red cell production.[12,13] In the vertebrates, an evolutionary shift occurred from the spleen to the liver and from the liver to the hollow bones. Any organ with a relatively stagnant sinusoidal vascular system may serve as a site for red cell production, and the sinusoidal structure of the bone cavities in mammals is particularly suited.[14] The homeostatic regulation of blood or hemoglobin production has been studied in Daphnia,[8] where a balance exists between oxygen need and hemoglobin production. In the higher animals, this relationship is maintained by adjusting red cell production. Studies of birds,[15] fish,[16] and mammals[17] indicate red cell production is controlled by Epo, which is capable of adjusting red cell production to the demands for oxygen in the tissues. Epo of mammals has a considerable biologic similarity and genetic homology.[18]

ONTOGENY OF RED CELL PRODUCTION

EMBRYONIC AND FETAL ERYTHROPOIESIS

The environment inside the bone apparently is optimal for cellular proliferation and maturation. However, bone cavities do not develop until the fifth fetal month. Other, presumably less favorable, sites are responsible for red cell production during early embryonic life (see Chap. 6). In the human, large nucleated blood cells are first formed in the yolk sac.[19] During the second gestational month, erythropoiesis moves to fetal liver, wherein smaller, but still macrocytic, nonnucleated cells are produced.[20,21] At birth, the hepatic phase of blood cell production ceases, and erythropoiesis moves to the marrow (see Chap. 6).

During the neonatal period, the volume of available marrow space is almost the same as the total volume of hematopoietic cells.[22] This process continues for a few years until the growth of bones and bone cavities exceeds the growth of hematopoietic mass. However, whenever the demand on erythropoiesis increases (blood loss, hypoxia, thalassemia, or hemolysis), the lack of reserve space in neonates and small children reactivates extramedullary erythropoiesis in the liver and spleen.[23] In adults, expansion of marrow space continues, and the amount of fatty tissue gradually increases in all bone cavities. Because of the abundant marrow space, compensatory reactivation of extramedullary sites rarely occurs in later life, even during periods of prolonged and intense demand for additional blood cell formation. Extramedullary hematopoiesis during these years usually indicates pathologic rather than compensatory blood formation.[24] During fetal life, Epo production is primarily hepatic.[25] At birth, a gradual switch to renal production of Epo occurs. In the adult, the kidney is responsible for 90 to 95 percent of total production.[26,27]

CELLULAR COMPONENTS OF ERYTHROPOIESIS

PROGENITOR CELLS

Our ability to evaluate early erythropoiesis rests on functional assays of hematopoietic progenitors. The earliest defined erythroid progenitor is the burst forming unit–erythroid (BFU-E). It is called a burst because it contains cells still capable of migration. These cells form smaller clusters around a larger central colony, giving the appearance of a sunburst, although all the cells in the colony are clonal. BFU-E takes longer to generate erythroblasts (~10–14 days) and forms a large BFU-E colony (~2000 cells). BFU-E expresses Epo receptors (EpoR). BFU-E then differentiates into colony forming unit–erythroid (CFU-E), the more restricted erythroid progenitor. CFU-E is the later, more differentiated erythroid progenitor that is identified *in vitro* by smaller colonies (50–200 cells) that grow in 3 to 5 days. However, EpoR density and Epo dependency increase gradually as progenitor cells mature, culminating at the level of the CFU-E.[28] BFU-E and CFU-E cannot be identified by microscopy (see Chap. 28), but they can be studied *in vitro* by their ability to generate microscopically recognizable hemoglobinized precursors (i.e., erythroblasts) by so-called clonogenic assays on semisolid media.

PRECURSOR CELLS

In contrast, the later stages of erythropoiesis can be identified by microscopy (see Chap. 28). The number of erythroid precursor cells determines to a great extent the number of red cells produced. The proerythroblasts also contain EpoRs that, in the presence of high levels of Epo, may accelerate their entry into the first mitotic division. This process may lead to a shortened marrow transit time of erythroblasts[29] and result in release of still immature reticulocytes, so-called stress reticulocytes.[30] Creation of a normal red cell is the end result of an orderly transformation of a proerythroblast with a large nucleus and a volume of approximately 900 fl to a hemoglobinized anucleated disc with a volume of approximately 90 fl. Although cytoplasmic maturation is continuous, the interposed mitotic divisions cause a stepwise reduction in cytoplasmic and nuclear volumes, enabling recognition of proerythroblasts, erythroblasts, and polychromatophilic red cell (reticulocytes) with light microscopy. Direct measurements of the number of marrow erythroblasts and reticulocytes have shown approxi-

TABLE 30-1   ERYTHROID POOLS

	CELL NUMBER $\times 10^8$ PER KG/BODY WEIGHT	
CELL TYPE	OBSERVED*	THEORETIC MODEL (FIG. 30-1)
Proerythroblasts	1	1
Erythroblasts	49	58
Marrow reticulocytes	82	64
Blood reticulocytes	31	32
Mature red cells	3300	3800

* Adapted from Donohue et al[31] and Finch et al.[32]

mately 50 erythroblasts and 113 reticulocytes for each proerythroblast (Table 30-1).[31,32] This distribution conforms to the number of cells in a theoretic erythroid pyramid (Table 30-1, Fig. 30-1). In the pyramid, each proerythroblast undergoes five mitotic divisions over 5 days before the proerythroblast loses its nucleus and enters a 2- to 3-day period of maturation before its release from the marrow. The size and shape of these erythroid pyramids undoubtedly vary, but the question is whether such variations are random or play a role in the physiologic control of red cell production. When production is suppressed, as in anemia of chronic renal disease, the distribution of erythroblasts appears normal, with no morphologic or ferrokinetic evidence of ineffective erythropoiesis or abnormal erythroblast apoptosis.[29] When production is increased, as in severe hemolytic anemia, the erythroblastic pyramids also appear normal, with no evidence of additional mitotic divisions. Consequently, the rate of red cell production likely depends on the number of erythroid pyramids (progenitors) formed and not on their shape.

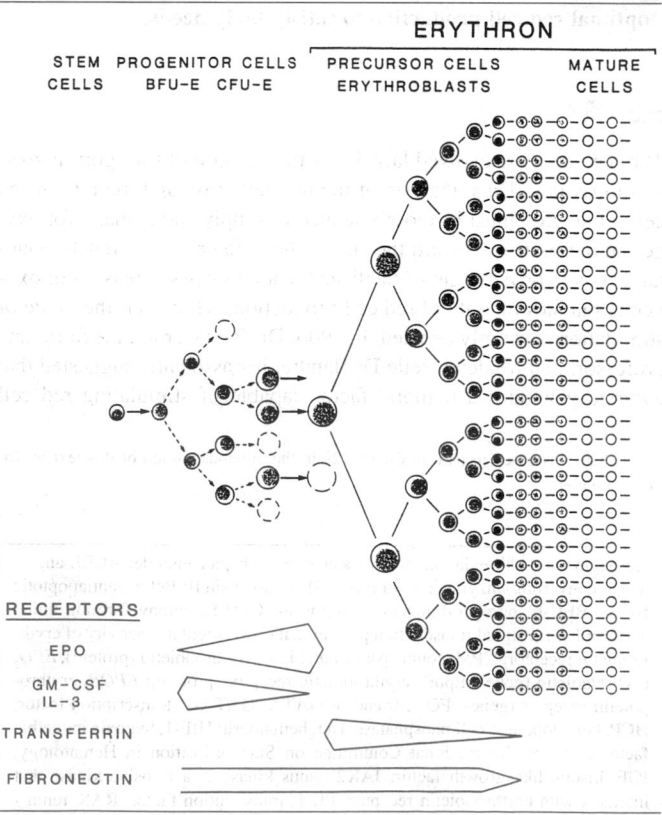

FIGURE 30-1   Theoretical model of proliferation of erythroid-committed marrow cells, including their most important receptors.

As the erythroblast matures, its synthetic activities increase rapidly, producing all proteins characteristic of mature red blood cells, particularly globin. Eventually 95 percent of all protein in the red cell is hemoglobin, almost all hemoglobin A ($\alpha_2\beta_2$) in adults, with only small amounts of hemoglobin F ($\alpha_2\gamma_2$) and hemoglobin A_2 ($\alpha_2\delta_2$). Hemoglobin F is unequally distributed and is present only in some erythrocytes, designated as F cells (see Chap. 46).

EpoR density declines sharply on early erythroblasts, and EpoRs are absent from the more mature erythroblast forms. On the other hand, the number of receptors for transferrin increases sharply, reflecting the increased demands for iron for heme synthesis. The microenvironment may be important for proliferation and maturation of erythroblasts. However, *in situ* secreted or circulating growth factors and cytokines appear to be less important for precursor cells than for progenitor cells. Intercellular adhesion molecules secure the structural integrity of the marrow, and fibronectin is of special importance for erythroblasts.[33] Loss of fibronectin receptors heralds the migration of reticulocytes into blood, but some reticulocytes remain sticky even after release and are temporarily sequestered by the spleen (see Chap. 5). Because erythroid colonies developed *in vitro* consist mainly of nucleated red cells, enucleation may primarily be induced by marrow stromal or endothelial cells (see Chap. 28).

Microscopic determination of marrow cellularity and proportion of erythroblasts permits reasonably semiquantitative evaluation of erythropoiesis. However, in disease states the presence of ineffective erythropoiesis, as seen in iron deficiency, anemia of chronic disease, megaloblastic anemias, and thalassemias, makes the morphologic approach misleading (see Chaps. 39, 40, 43, and 46). Red cell production can be accurately estimated by ferrokinetic studies using radioactive [59]Fe. Similarly, the amount of final erythropoiesis product, red cell mass, also can be accurately measured. Unfortunately, the ever-increasing regulation of even minute amounts of radioisotopes used *in vivo* makes these methods available in few specialized centers.

Chapters 6, 29, 46 and 128 discuss developmental control of erythropoiesis, differential use of globin genes, and the crucial differences between embryonic yolk sac and fetal/adult definite erythropoiesis. This chapter concentrates mainly on adult erythropoiesis.

REGULATION OF ERYTHROPOIESIS

GATA-1, BCL-x_L, FOG-1, AND PU.1

Erythropoiesis is influenced by a number of hormones/cytokines, receptors, and transcription factors. The lineage-specific transcription factor GATA-1 plays essential roles in normal erythropoiesis and activates many erythroid specific genes including globins and cytoskeletal red cell proteins (see Chaps. 44 and 47). GATA-1, along with Epo, induces expression of the antiapoptotic protein Bcl-x_L[34] and interacts with multiple proteins, including FOG-1[35] and PU.1.[36] Direct physical interaction between GATA-1 and FOG-1 is essential for normal human erythroid and megakaryocyte maturation *in vivo*.[37] In contrast, GATA-1 interaction with PU.1 appears to counteract erythropoiesis by inducing differentiation of pluripotent stem cell to myeloid and B lymphopoiesis and inhibition of erythropoiesis.[36,38,39] Whereas PU.1 absence appears to be required for completion of terminal erythroid differentiation, low levels of PU.1 expression are essential for fetal erythropoiesis and for proper augmentation of adult erythropoiesis at times of stress.[40]

Multipotent progenitor (see Chap. 15) and primitive erythroid progenitor BFU-E require stem cell factor, interleukin-3, granulocyte-macrophage colony stimulating factor, and/or thrombopoietin for growth and survival (Fig. 30-2).

ERYTHROPOIETIN, OXYGEN SENSING, AND HYPOXIA-INDUCIBLE FACTOR

ERYTHROPOIETIN

The principal hormone regulating erythropoiesis is kidney-produced Epo.[7] Erythroid progenitors express their own Epo.[41] Different levels of kidney-produced Epo are optimal for various stages of erythroid maturation.[42] Purification of Epo provided a partial protein sequence that led to cloning of the gene and permitted mass production of the recombinant protein.[43] The *EPO* gene contains five exons, four introns, and functionally important 5′ and 3′ untranslated sequences.[44,45] From 80 to 90 percent homology exists between the human gene and genes for mouse and monkey EPO. The cDNA also encodes a 27-amino-acid leader peptide. The mature circulating Epo has 165 amino acids. Epo and its recombinant form are heavily glycosylated α-globulins with a molecular mass of 34,000 daltons and a specific activity of approximately 200,000 IU/mg.[44,45] Sixty percent of the molecular weight is contributed by amino acids; the other 40 percent is made up of carbohydrate. The classic study by Jacobson and coworkers[7] in 1957 suggested strongly that the kidney was the organ of production. Using molecular probes for EPO mRNA enabled the pinpointing of synthesis to cortical interstitial cells[46,47] of endothelial or fibroblastic lineage. The cells appear to function in an all-or-none fashion, with the overall production of mRNA dependent on the number of cells activated.[48]

Certain 5′ sequences located 6000 to 12,000 bp upstream also affect gene transcription. These sequences are not hypoxia-sensitive

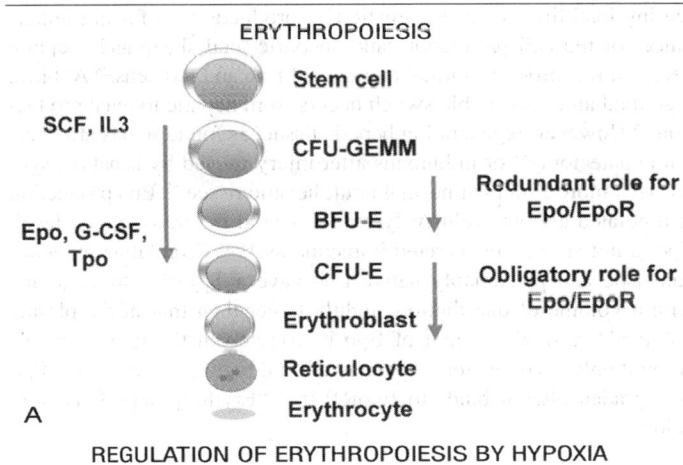

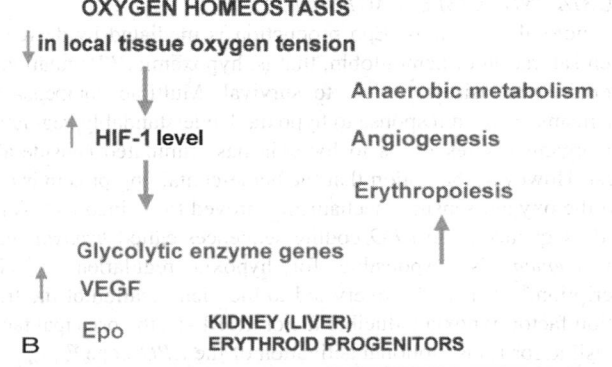

FIGURE 30-2   *A.* Cytokine influence on hematopoiesis. CFU-GEMM, colony forming unit–growing granulocyte, erythrocyte, megakaryocyte, and macrophage precursors; SCF, stem cell factor; IL3, interleukin-3; G-CSF, granulocyte colony stimulating factor; Tpo, thrombopoietin. *B.* Regulation of erythropoiesis by hypoxia HIF-1 hypoxia inducible factor; VEGF, vascular endothelial growth factor I; Epo, erythropoietin.

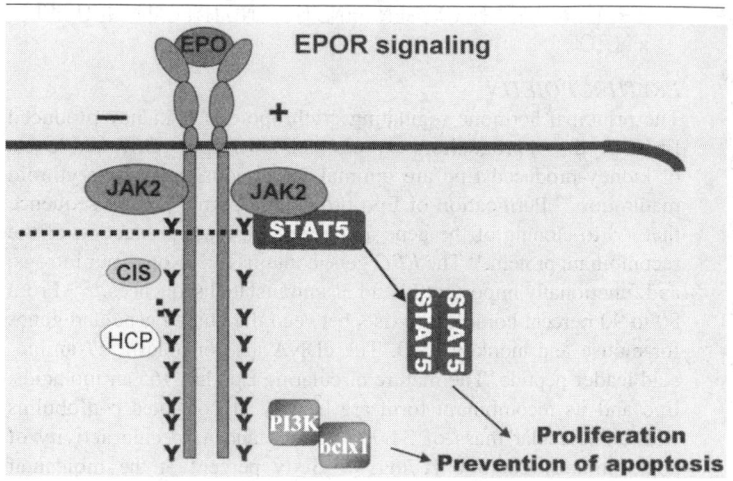

FIGURE 30-3   Outline of erythropoietin–erythropoietin receptor (Epo–EpoR) signaling. Activation of JAK2 and STAT5 represents erythropoiesis-promoting signals. Interaction of CIS and HCT inhibit erythropoiesis. PI3 kinase (PI3K) activation of Bcl-x_L inhibits apoptosis of erythroid progenitors.

but appear necessary for tissue and cellular specificity.[49] Hepatic production is contributed primarily by hepatocytes but is much less than renal production.[50] Hepatic production in rodents may contribute 10 to 15 percent of total Epo circulating in plasma, but less in humans. During fetal life, however, hepatic Epo production is of major importance for red cell production, and anephric fetal sheep and anephric neonatal rats produce normal amounts of Epo and red cells.[25] At birth, a gradual and irreversible switch occurs from hepatic to renal production.[26] However, regenerating hepatic tissue, as found in rats after partial hepatectomy[51] or in humans after injury caused by hepatitis, synthesizes more Epo than normal adult hepatic tissue.[52] Epo production is regulated almost exclusively by hypoxia at the transcription level. Epo is not stored but secreted immediately.[46–48] Circulating recombinant Epo and presumably native Epo have a $T_{1/2}$ of 4 to 12 hours, with a volume of distribution slightly larger than that of the plasma volume.[53] A small amount of Epo is excreted in the urine, but this amount only accounts for 10 percent of total body Epo turnover.[54] Epo is degraded after it binds to EpoR[55] (see "Erythropoietin Receptor" below).

HYPOXIA INDUCIBLE FACTOR-1

Under normal conditions, Epo production is mediated by decreased oxygen saturation of hemoglobin, that is, hypoxemia.[42] Regulation of oxygen homeostasis is critical to survival. Multiple compensatory mechanisms occur in response to hypoxia. Understandably, regulation of an organism's responses to hypoxia has stimulated considerable interest. However, the notion that the heme-containing protein is central to the oxygen-sensing mechanism[56] proved to be incorrect. A nucleotide sequence 3′ to *EPO* coding sequences called *hypoxia regulatory element* is responsible for hypoxia regulation of EPO transcription.[57–60] This discovery led to the identification of the transcription factor hypoxia inducible factor-1 (HIF-1), the principal factor responsible for transcriptional activation of the *EPO* gene.[57]

HIF-1 is part of a widespread oxygen-sensing mechanism. It also is found in cells that do not express Epo.[60–62] HIF-1 regulates genes that promote cell survival under ischemic conditions. HIF-1 also regulates vasculogenesis, is required for embryonic development, elevates glucose uptake by cells, augments production of glycolytic enzymes, and plays an important role in carcinogenesis.[60–65] Thus, stimulation of Epo production by hypoxia is only one of many phenotypic mani-

festations of augmented hypoxia response. HIF-1 is composed of two subunits, HIF-1α and HIF-1β, which form the HIF-1 heterodimer.[66] Only HIF-1α is regulated by hypoxia. HIF-1α mRNA and protein levels are induced by hypoxia, and HIF-1α protein decays rapidly with return to normoxia. Posttranslational regulation of HIF-1α protein accounts for the majority of the hypoxic regulation of this gene.[67] Normoxia-induced, ubiquitin-mediated degradation of the HIF-1α protein regulates HIF-1α protein levels.[67,68] In the presence of oxygen, one of the proline residues of HIF-1α is hydroxylated by an iron-containing proline hydroxylase enzyme.[69,70] Three different genes encoding proline hydroxylase manifest tissue-specific expression.[71] Thus, oxygen allows generation of proline hydroxylated HIF-1α, which becomes a target for interaction with von Hippel–Lindau protein that initiates subsequent polyubiquitination and rapid destruction of HIF-1α in the proteasome complex. This complex (see Chaps. 32 and 56 and Fig. 32-1) constitutes the oxygen sensor.[69–71]

ERYTHROPOIETIN RECEPTOR

Interaction of Epo with its receptor EpoR results in (1) stimulation of erythroid cell division, (2) erythroid differentiation by induction of erythroid-specific protein expression, and (3) prevention of erythroid progenitor apoptosis (reviewed in ref. 72). Earlier models of this interaction were based on the ligand (Epo)-induced homodimerization of EpoR. EpoR already is present as a homodimer that changes its transmembrane orientation after Epo binding,[73] which initiates the Epo-specific erythroid signal transduction cascade (Fig. 30-3). The cytoplasmic portion of EpoR contains a positive regulatory domain that interacts with janus kinase 2 (JAK2).[74] Immediately after Epo binding, JAK2 phosphorylates itself, EpoR, and other proteins such as STAT-5, thus initiating a cascade of erythroid-specific signaling.[75] JAK2/STAT-5 signaling plays an essential role in Epo–EpoR-mediated regulation of erythropoiesis (Fig. 30-3).[76] Deficiency of Epo–EpoR is lethal by abrogating fetal liver erythropoiesis (but not the "primitive" yolk sac erythropoiesis). However, in these *EPO* or *EPOR* knockout mouse, differentiation of early pluripotent hematopoietic stem cell to BFU-E occurs, but not the subsequent erythroid differentiation. This occurrence demonstrates the crucial role of Epo in terminal erythroid maturation and differentiation.[77–79] The C-terminal cytoplasmic portion of EpoR also possesses a domain essential for prevention of apoptosis (Fig. 30-3) by inducing expression of Bcl-x_L via PI3 kinase.[34] However, the cytoplasmic portion of EpoR also contains a negative regulatory domain[80] that interacts with hematopoietic cell phosphatase (HCP, also known as SHP1) and down-modulates signal transduction.[81] Once recruited by EpoR tyrosine Y429, HCP attaches to the cytoplasmic EpoR domain and dephosphorylates JAK2. Inactivation of the HCP binding site leads to prolonged phosphorylation of JAK2/STAT-5.[81,82] CIS, another negative regulator of erythropoiesis, binds to the cytoplasmic portion of the EpoR tyrosine Y401 and suppresses Epo-dependent JAK2/STAT-5 signaling.[83,84] Thus, deletion of the distal C-terminal cytoplasmic portion of EpoR results in a truncated EpoR, abolishes negative regulatory elements, and results in increased proliferation of erythroid progenitor cells. Gain-of-function mutations resulting from deletion of the negative regulatory domain of the *EPOR* gene (see Chap. 56) have been demonstrated in a small proportion of patients with primary familial and congenital polycythemia but are rarely found in erythroleukemia.

Because the activation signal after Epo binding to its receptor is rapidly down-regulated and Epo rapidly disappears after binding to EpoR, Epo–EpoR internalization was proposed as one mechanism of down-regulation of Epo signaling.[55] This mechanism is indeed true. After Epo binds to the receptor, Epo–EpoR complexes are ubiquinated, rapidly internalized, and targeted for degradation. This process involves two proteolytic systems, the proteasomes that remove part of the intracellular domain of EpoR at the cell surface and the lysosomes that degrade the Epo–EpoR complex in the cytoplasm.[85]

Another yet incompletely understood mechanism of erythropoiesis regulation is the presence of several EpoR isoforms, some of which may have an inhibitory function on erythropoiesis.[86–88]

INSULIN-LIKE GROWTH FACTOR-1 AND RECEPTOR CROSS-TALK

Although *in vitro* studies of erythropoiesis have provided crucial information about erythropoiesis regulation, the experiments were performed in the presence of serum and serum-component proteins capable of stimulating and inhibiting erythropoiesis.[89,90] Using serum-free conditions, insulin-like growth factor-1 (IGF-1) can partially substitute for Epo in BFU-E cultures. Furthermore, anephric nonanemic patients with no detectable Epo have elevated levels of IGF-1.[91]

RENIN–ANGIOTENSIN SYSTEM AND HEMATOPOIESIS

The renin–angiotensin system (RAS) regulates fluid and electrolyte homeostasis and blood pressure.[92] The primary function of angiotensin during development is modulation of tissue growth and differentiation.[93] Angiotensin II (Ang-II) is a ligand for two distinct receptors, type 1 (AT1) and type 2. AT1 appears to have a major role in modulating cell proliferation.[94] The role of the RAS in regulating erythropoiesis has been long suspected, although the controlling mechanisms are complex and not fully elucidated. The RAS was first postulated to regulate erythropoiesis in the 1980s after the discovery that use of angiotensin-converting enzyme inhibitors (ACEI) for treatment of hypertension could cause anemia.[95] This hypothesis is based on the presumption that reduced oxygen pressure in the kidneys triggers HIF-1α to induce Epo release.[96] However, Ang-II significantly modulates erythropoiesis directly. Whereas Ang-II directly stimulated proliferation of hematopoietic progenitors *in vitro*,[97] inhibition of its effects using ACEI induced apoptosis of erythroid progenitors in renal transplant patients.[98] In an *in vivo* laboratory model, mice with ACE gene knockout developed normocytic anemia that was fully reversed with AngII infusion.[99]

MEASUREMENTS OF RED CELL MASS

The red cell mass is maintained and regulated by the marrow, which under steady-state conditions precisely replaces cells lost by senescence. Red cell mass defines anemia and polycythemia. The kinetics of red cell production and destruction helps establish their pathogenesis. A number of tests have been developed to measure the three main components of red cell kinetics: red cell mass, rate of red cell production, and rate of red cell destruction. Some of these tests are simple but indirect, such as hematocrit, reticulocyte count, haptoglobin, lactic dehydrogenase, and unconjugated bilirubin concentration. Examination of the marrow allows assessment of total cellularity and relative erythroid contribution but is limited in that the kinetics of cell production cannot be inferred from a single static image, obtained from a very small fraction of the whole marrow. These tests are very useful in the aggregate but can be supplemented by more complex but direct quantitation made possible by use of radioisotopes.

HEMATOCRIT

Packed red cell volume is commonly referred as the *hematocrit*. It can be measured as volume of blood composed of erythrocytes in 1 ml of blood. Total body hematocrit is the volume of red cells in the body divided by the total blood volume. Blood hematocrit is the simplest and most widely used test for estimating the size of red cell mass. In most anemic patients, blood hematocrit gives an excellent approximation of total red cell mass and a functional estimation of the oxygen-carrying capacity and whole blood viscosity. Its main drawback is that it is an indirect measure that is influenced by changes in plasma volume and may not reflect the size of the red cell mass in dehydrated or polycythemic patients. Dehydration usually is clinically apparent and in most cases can be taken into account when evaluating the significance of a specific hematocrit determination. A hematocrit that is moderately elevated may not reflect the total red cell mass. Only direct measurement of red cell mass can differentiate between relative and absolute polycythemia. However, when the hematocrit is greater than 60 percent, almost all patients have an increase in total red cell mass.[100] The extent of the increase cannot be estimated accurately from a hematocrit measurement alone (Fig. 30-4).

RED CELL MASS AND PLASMA VOLUME

A more direct and accurate estimate of the size of the red cell mass is obtained from labeling a known volume of red cells and determining the dilution of this label in blood. Radioactive iron is an excellent label of red cells because it is biosynthetically incorporated into hemoglobin *in vivo*. In experimental animals, radioactive iron can be given to a donor animal and the donor's cells transfused into the animal whose red cell volume is being assessed. However, the radiation exposure to the donor and the hazards of transfusing allogeneic cells preclude its use in humans. Thus, almost all current clinical methods use labeling of autologous red cells *in vitro* by any one of a number of isotopes. If studies must be performed in radio-sensitive individuals, such as pregnant women, red cell labeling can be performed by nonradioactive chromium[101] or by biotin, which is detected with streptavidin coupled to a fluorochrome.[102] Among the isotopes available, chromium-51 (^{51}Cr) is the most widely used label, although technetium-99m (^{99m}Tc) is convenient and accurate.[103] Chromium in the form of the chromate ion (CrO_2^-) readily enters the red cell and binds to globin chains. Excess isotope in the incubation mixture can be removed by washing or by using ascorbic acid to reduce the chromate ion to a nonpermeant chromic ion. Approximately 15 minutes after injection of a known amount of labeled cells, a sample of blood is obtained; its volume, hematocrit, and

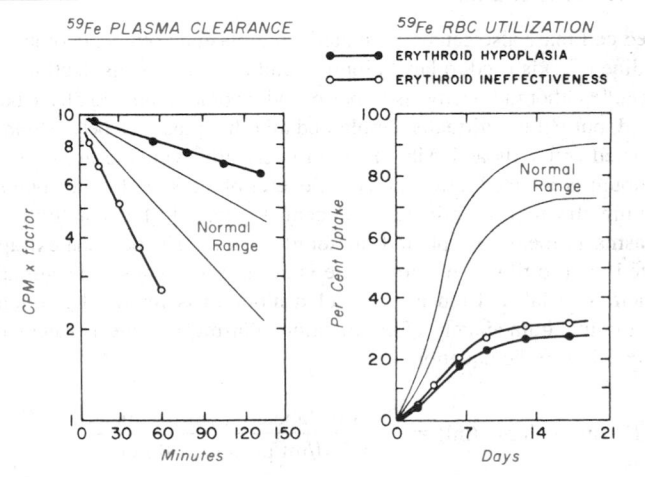

FIGURE 30-4   Iron clearance and iron utilization in normal subjects, patients with decreased effective red cell production (erythroid hypoplasia), and patients with ineffective red cell production.

radioactivity are determined; and the total red cell volume is calculated from the equation:

$$\text{Red cell mass (ml)} = \frac{\text{CPM of isotope injected}}{\text{CPM of red cells in sample}}$$

Sampling time is generally 15 minutes. Because ^{51}Cr also may label white cells, centrifuge and remove the buffy coat before labeling if the white cell count is elevated ($>25 \times 10^9$/liter).

No theoretical objection exists to measuring the red cell mass using labeled cells. It is independent of the hematocrit of the blood utilized to measure radioactivity, and replicate determination can be made with a coefficient of variation of approximately 1.5 percent.[104] The principal problem lies in reporting the measured red cell mass. The total red cell mass can be expressed as a volume related to body surface (ml/m^2) or as a volume related to body weight (ml/kg). A committee of the International Committee on Standardization in Hematology (ICSH) has extensively examined existing data and concluded that the most reproducible expressions of red cell mass are related to body surface area estimated from height and weight[105]:

$$\text{RCM}_{\text{Males}} = (1486 \times S) - 285$$

$$\text{RCM}_{\text{Females}} = (822 \times S) + (1.06 \times \text{Age})$$

where RCM = red cell mass, S = body surface area in square meters, and age = age in years.

The calculated values ± 25 percent included 98 percent of the measured male values and 99 percent of the measured female values.[9]

Despite the ICSH recommendation, the most common method is to report red cell mass values in terms of milliliters per kilogram. However, this method of expression gives erroneously low values in obese individuals because fat is hypovascular. A better method might be to express the red cell mass in terms of lean weight. In general, lean weight is 20 percent less than actual weight in normal males and 25 percent less in normal females.[103] However, estimation of lean weight in obese individuals is most inaccurate. From a practical point of view, red cell mass probably is best reported in terms of actual weight, with mental adjustments made based on body configuration. In general, the red cell mass of normal females ranges from 23 to 29 ml/kg body weight and of normal males ranges from 26 to 32 ml/kg.[105]

PLASMA LABELS

Red cell mass also can be estimated from plasma volume. Radioactive iodine (^{125}I) is used to label albumin and measure its distribution volume.[106] Other radioactive isotopes of iodine other than ^{99m}Tc have been used, but ^{125}I has virtually supplanted all other plasma labels. Albumin labeled with radioactive iodine is commercially available, and a known amount is injected intravenously. Several blood samples are obtained within the first 15 minutes and centrifuged. CPM per milliliter of plasma is measured, plotted on semilogarithmic paper, and extrapolated to zero time. This procedure is necessary because, in contradistinction to labeled red cells, labeled albumin is removed gradually, beginning immediately after injection. Plasma volume is calculated according to the equation:

$$\text{Plasma volume (ml)} = \frac{\text{CPM of labeled albumin injected}}{\text{CPM/ml plasma at 0 hour}}$$

The continuous exchange of intravascular with extravascular albumin is the major problem encountered when plasma volume is measured with labeled albumin. Even with extrapolation to 0 hour, plasma volume is somewhat larger than that measured with a strictly intravascular protein such as fibrinogen.[107] Consequently, if measurement of the plasma volume is used to calculate the size of the total red cell mass, it is a less reliable measure than determining red cell mass directly with tagged red cells. This inaccuracy is further aggravated by the fact that the venous hematocrit used to calculate red cell mass from measured plasma volume does not reflect accurately the distribution of plasma and red cells in the body. However, from a practical point of view, the results of estimating red cell mass from plasma volume are surprisingly accurate and have been advocated based on simplicity and low cost.[106,108]

TOTAL BODY HEMATOCRIT

When total red cell mass is measured with labeled red cells, the value is approximately 10 percent lower than that calculated from plasma volume and the hematocrit of peripheral blood. In fact, the mean hematocrit of blood in all of the vessels (total body hematocrit) clearly is somewhat lower than the hematocrit determined from blood obtained from large vessels.

Generally the ratio of total body hematocrit as estimated by direct measurements of red cell volume and plasma volume to the large-vessel hematocrit ranges from 0.89 to 0.92.[109] Consequently, when using the determined plasma volume to calculate red cell mass and total blood volume, a correction factor is necessary, and a value of 0.90 is generally used:

$$\text{Corrected red cell mass} = \frac{\text{Hct} \times \text{plasma volume} \times 0.90}{100 - \text{Hct}}$$

where Hct = hematocrit.

Recommended procedures for determination and evaluation of blood volume are outlined by the ICSH.[110]

MEASUREMENTS OF RED CELL PRODUCTION

Under normal circumstances, most human red cells produced in the marrow live, or have the potential to live, a normal life span. Under certain conditions, however, a fraction of red cell production is ineffective, with destruction of nonviable red cells either within the marrow or shortly after the cells reach the blood.[29]

EFFECTIVE RED CELL PRODUCTION

Effective erythropoiesis is most simply estimated by determining the reticulocyte count. This count usually is expressed as the percentage of red cells that are reticulocytes, but it also can be expressed as the total number of circulating reticulocytes per unit of blood (absolute reticulocyte count).

$$\text{Absolute reticulocyte count} = \frac{\% \text{ reticulocytes} \times \text{red cell count}}{100}$$

A simple clinical method to estimate effective erythropoiesis uses the reticulocyte count to calculate the reticulocyte index.[111] This measurement depends on several assumptions: (1) the human red cell life span is approximately 100 days (actually approximately 115); (2) the life span is finite and, thus, the oldest one of 100 or 1 percent of red cells is removed (and replaced) each day; (3) the reticulocyte is identifiable as such in the blood for 1 day using supravital stain; and (4) the reticulocyte count of 1 percent in a person with a normal hematocrit represents normal red cell production and thus "1" is the basal reticulocyte index.

$$\text{Corrected reticulocyte\%} = \text{reticulocyte\%} \times \frac{\text{actual hematocrit}}{\text{normal hematocrit}}$$

In anemic patients, two calculations are needed to measure the reticulocyte index and compare it to the normal of 1 in the basal state. To correct the reticulocyte percentage for the lower red cell count in anemic subjects, the reticulocyte percent is multiplied by the ratio of the patient's hematocrit over the normal mean hematocrit, providing a corrected reticulocyte index.

$$\text{Reticulocyte index} = \frac{\text{absolute reticulocyte count}}{\text{correction factor (usually 2)}}$$

Conversion of the corrected reticulocyte count to the reticulocyte index is achieved by taking into account the estimated life span of reticulocytes. The life span of reticulocytes in blood in a normal individual is approximately 1 day. However, when red cell production is increased under conditions of erythropoietic stress, for example, in anemia, reticulocytes are released prematurely and circulate as reticulocytes for 2 to 4 days, except in situations with low Epo levels, as in renal insufficiency. Accordingly, the elevated reticulocyte count may give an erroneous impression of the actual rate of daily red cell production. To take this situation into account when estimating the rate of red cell production in anemic patients with high reticulocyte counts, dividing the absolute reticulocyte count by a factor may provide a more accurate estimate of red cell production.[111] For simplicity, an average factor of 2 often is used; however, the factor depends on the degree of anemia: 1.5 in mild cases, 2.5 in moderate cases, and 3.0 in severe cases.

An example follows. A patient with autoimmune hemolytic anemia has a hematocrit of 10 and reticulocyte count of 70 percent. The marrow cannot increase production by 70-fold. To measure the approximate true increase, we calculate the reticulocyte index as follows: corrected reticulocyte count = 70 × 10/45 = 15, and reticulocyte index = 15/3 = 5 × basal. Thus, marrow erythroid production in response to this severe anemia has increased fivefold, a plausible response to this degree of severity of hemolytic anemia.

INEFFECTIVE RED CELL PRODUCTION

Ineffective erythropoiesis is suspected when the reticulocyte count is normal or only slightly increased despite erythroid hyperplasia of the marrow. Ineffective erythropoiesis was first recognized as an entity from the study of isotope incorporation into fecal urobilin following administration of labeled glycine, a precursor of heme.[112] Two peaks were observed: an early peak at 3 to 5 days and a late peak at 100 to 120 days. One of the sources of the early-labeled peak was suggested to be the hemoglobin of red cells that had never completed their development, having been destroyed either in the marrow or shortly after reaching the blood. Subsequent studies revealed that in certain disorders, such as pernicious anemia, thalassemia, and sideroblastic anemia, ineffective erythropoiesis is a major component of total erythropoiesis. This component can be quantitated by measuring ^{15}N-labeled glycine incorporation into the early bilirubin peaks.[112,113] or ferrokinetics.[29] Calculated from bilirubin peaks and turnover, ineffective erythropoiesis under normal conditions amounts to approximately 4 to 12 percent of total erythropoiesis. Using ferrokinetic methods, ineffective erythropoiesis is calculated as the difference between total plasma iron turnover and erythrocyte iron turnover plus storage iron turnover (see below "Ferrokinetics"). The values estimated from such studies in normal subjects are higher, ranging from 14 to 34 percent.[29] However, the results, both high and low, probably are misleading because none of the methods actually measures cell death but only the turnover of

heme and iron. It is possible that little premature death of cells occurs in normal subjects, but much of the early release of bilirubin and iron is derived from the rim of hemoglobin extruded during enucleation of erythroblasts (see Chap. 28).

TOTAL ERYTHROPOIESIS

Total erythropoiesis, which is the sum of effective and ineffective red cell production, can be estimated from a marrow examination. Films or sections from marrow aspirates and biopsies are first examined for relative content of fat and hematopoietic tissue. This examination gives an estimate of overall hematopoietic activity within the marrow space. A differential count then is performed, determining the ratio between granulocytic and erythroid precursors (M/E ratio). In a normal adult, the ratio is approximately 3:1 to 5:1. The ratio can be used to estimate whether erythropoiesis is normal, increased, or decreased (see Chap. 3). The ratio is only an approximation of total erythroid activity because the ratio can be altered by changing the myeloid and erythroid components, and an aspirate or biopsy of a small segment of the marrow may not always reflect total marrow activity. However, when used in conjunction with determination of red blood cell count and reticulocyte count, under most circumstances the ratio provides qualitative information about the rate and effectiveness of red blood cell production. A more accurate quantitation of total erythropoiesis can be made by measuring the rate of production of red cells (ferrokinetics) or, in steady-state conditions, the rate of destruction of red cells (red cell life span, bilirubin production, carbon monoxide excretion).

FERROKINETICS

In 1950, Huff and associates[114] first described a method for measuring the rate of red cell production utilizing a simple model of iron metabolism (Fig. 30-5; see Chap. 40). In this method, radioactive iron is complexed to transferrin *in vitro* and injected intravenously. Alternatively, ^{59}Fe can be injected directly intravenously as the gluconate without preincubation with the patient's own plasma, providing enough unbound transferrin is available, because binding is almost instantaneous. The rate of clearance of the transferrin-bound iron from the plasma (^{59}Fe plasma $T_{1/2}$) and the subsequent uptake in the red cells are measured. From these two values and from determinations of plasma iron concentration and plasma volume, the rate of formation of red cells can be calculated.[29]

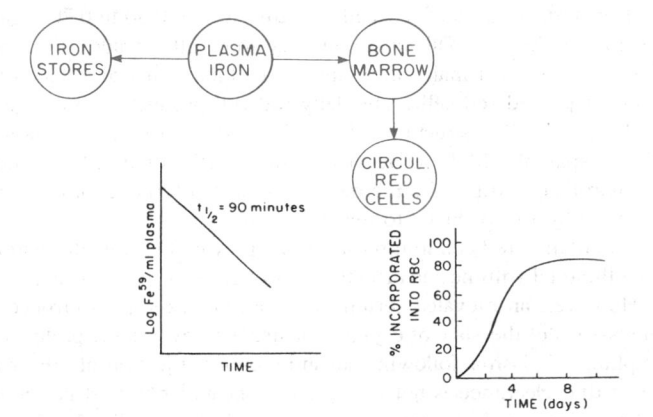

FIGURE 30-5 Single dynamic pool model of iron metabolism. Radioactive iron injected into the plasma iron pool is cleared from the plasma as a single exponential, and approximately 80 percent is incorporated into circulating blood cells.

The initial clearance of iron is exponential, and sampling during this period can be used to calculate $T_{1/2}$. In normal individuals, initial clearance averages approximately 90 minutes. Initial clearance is shorter in patients with hyperplasia of the erythropoietic tissue and longer in patients with marrow hypoplasia (Fig. 30-4). However, the clearance rate is not a direct measurement of erythropoietic activity because it depends on the size of the pool of unlabeled, circulating iron. Consequently, calculation of the plasma iron turnover rate must include the plasma iron concentration. Clearance is expressed in milligrams of iron. The point of reference can be hemoglobin mass, blood volume, or weight, but a commonly used expression is micrograms of iron per deciliters of whole blood per day.

$$\text{Plasma iron turnover rate (mg iron/dl blood/24 h)}$$
$$= \frac{\text{plasma iron (mg/dl) } \times (100 - \text{Hct})}{T_{1/2}(\text{min}) \times 100}$$

Under normal conditions, radioactive iron is incorporated into newly formed red cells after a few days and reaches a maximum approximately 10 to 14 days after injection (see Fig. 30-4). Normal utilization is 70 to 90 percent on day 10 to 14, a value that is so high that further increases have little significance. However, decreased utilization is an important finding and suggests immature red cells are destroyed in the marrow before they are released to the circulation (ineffective erythropoiesis) or that serum iron is diverted to nonerythropoietic tissues (marrow hypoplasia) because of slow marrow uptake. The shape of the red cell utilization curve also is important. An early and steep rise (rapid marrow transit time) suggests a high Epo level. Finally, an early rise in utilization with a subsequent fall off suggests hemolysis.

When calculating utilization, the blood volume must be known:

$$\text{Red cell iron utilization (\%)}$$
$$= \frac{\text{CPM of 1 ml blood} \times \text{blood volume} \times 100}{\text{CPM of } ^{59}\text{Fe injected}}$$

Using the plasma iron clearance and utilization of iron, the red cell turnover in milligrams per deciliter blood for 24 hours is calculated as follows:

$$\text{Red cell iron turnover (mg iron/dl blood/24h)}$$
$$= \text{plasma iron turnover} \times \text{maximal red cell iron utilization}$$

The normal value of red cell iron turnover is 0.30 to 0.70 mg/dl blood for 24 hours.[29] This range fits very well with a crude estimation of the iron used for maintaining the red cell mass in 1 dl of blood or 45 ml of packed red cells. The daily red cell production must equal the daily red cell destruction (45 ml/120 = 0.38 ml), assuming a red cell life span of 120 days. Because 1 ml of packed red cells contains approximately 1 mg of iron, a daily plasma iron turnover of 0.38 mg is needed by 1 dl of blood to maintain homeostasis.

Calculating red cell iron turnover has provided useful information about the total volume and effectiveness of erythroid tissue (Table 30-2). However, an elevated serum iron concentration gives erroneous impressions of the state of erythropoiesis. Moreover, more prolonged sampling of plasma following an intravenous injection of ^{59}Fe has shown that clearance is not a single exponential but must be represented by several exponential components.[115] This finding has led to the introduction of more complex models of iron kinetics with a single pool of plasma iron exchanging with a number of extravascular erythroid and nonerythroid pools. Careful analysis of such models has generated computer-supported methods calculating the degree and ef-

TABLE 30-2   PLASMA RADIOACTIVE IRON CLEARANCE AND RED BLOOD CELL UPTAKE

CONDITION	PLASMA ^{59}FE $T_{1/2}$	RED BLOOD CELL UPTAKE (%)
Normal	90 min	80–90
Increased erythropoiesis	Rapid (10–40 min)	80–90
Hemolytic anemia	Rapid	20–90*
Ineffective erythropoiesis	Normal to rapid	10–30
Iron deficiency anemia	Normal to rapid	100
Decreased erythropoiesis	Slow (≥180 min)	0–20

* Variability a result of variability in intensity of hemolysis and size of iron stores.

fectiveness of erythroid activity.[116] Although possibly more accurate than the conventional method of calculating iron turnover, the models appear to be too cumbersome for clinical use. Moreover, even these sophisticated methods may not give an accurate account of the state of erythropoiesis. Despite a constant rate of red cell production, the plasma iron turnover was found to increase with increasing plasma iron and transferrin saturation. This finding first was thought to result from increased nonerythroid iron uptake and led to the introduction of various correction factors in the calculation of red cell iron turnover.[115] However, the iron in plasma is present in two pools, a diferric and a monoferric transferrin pool, and the erythroid and nonerythroid receptors have a four times greater avidity for diferric transferrin than for monoferric transferrin. Consequently, total plasma iron turnover depends on the degree of saturation and does not necessarily reflect the number of transferrin receptors, presumably a critical measure of erythropoietic capacity.[117] To measure the number of transferrin receptors, adjusting the plasma iron turnover equations for both nonerythroid uptake and degree of transferrin saturation and expressing the plasma turnover in terms of transferrin rather than iron have been proposed.[118] Normal erythroid uptake of transferrin is 60 ± 12 μmol per liter of blood per day, a value that has appropriately decreased and increased in patients with hypoplastic and hyperplastic marrow.

REFERENCES

1. Erslev AJ: Blood and mountains, in *Blood, Pure, and Eloquent*, edited by MM Wintrobe, p 257. McGraw-Hill, New York, 1980.
2. Carnot P, Deflandre C: Sur l'activité hématopoiétique des serum au cours de la régénération du sang. *Acad Sci Med* 3:384, 1906.
3. Miescher F: Über die Beziehungen Zwischen Meereshohe und Beschaffenheit des Blutes. *Koresp Bltt Schweitz Aerzte* 24:809, 1893.
4. Reissmann KR: Studies on the mechanism of erythropoietic stimulation in parabiotic rats during hypoxia. *Blood* 5:372, 1950.
5. Erslev AJ: Humoral regulation of red cell production. *Blood* 8:349, 1953.
6. Erslev AJ, Lavietes PH, Van Wagenen G: Erythropoietic stimulation induced by "anemia" serum. *Proc Soc Exp Biol Med* 83:548, 1953.
7. Jacobson LO, Goldwasser E, Fried W, Plzak L: Role of the kidney in erythropoiesis. *Nature* 179:633, 1957.
8. Fox HM: The hemoglobin of Daphnia. *Proc R Soc Lond (Biol)* 135:195, 1948.
9. Scott RB: Comparative hematology: The phylogeny of the erythrocyte. *Blut* 12:340, 1966.
10. Andrew W: *Comparative Hematology*. Grune & Stratton, New York, 1965.
11. Bolliger A: Observations on the blood of a monotreme Tachyglossus aculeatus. *Aust J Sci* 22:257, 1959.
12. Jordan HE: Comparative hematology, in *Handbook of Hematology*, edited by H. Downey, p 703. Hoeber-Harper, New York, 1938.

13. Iorio RJ: Some morphologic and kinetic studies of the developing ery-throid cells of the common gold fish Carassius auratus. *Cell Tissue Kinet* 2:319, 1969.

14. Robb-Smith AHT: *The Growth of Knowledge of the Functions of the Blood*, edited by RG Macfarlane, AHT Robb-Smith. Academic Press, New York, 1961.

15. Rosse WF, Waldmann TA: Factors controlling erythropoiesis in birds. *Blood* 27:654, 1966.

16. Zanjani ED: Humoral factors influencing erythropoiesis in the fish (Blue Gourami-Trichogaster trichopteras). *Blood* 33:573, 1969.

17. Erslev AJ: Control of red cell production. *Annu Rev Med* 11:315, 1959.

18. Shoemaker C, Mitsock LD: Murine erythropoietin gene: Cloning, expression and human gene homology. *Mol Cell Biol* 6:849, 1986.

19. Le Douarin NM: Cell migrations in embryos. *Cell* 38:353, 1984.

20. Hoyes AD, Riches DJ, Martin BGH: The fine structure of haemato-poiesis in the human fetal liver. *J Anat* 115:99, 1973.

21. Palis J, Robertson S, Kennedy M, et al: Development of erythroid and myeloid progenitors in the yolk sac and embryo proper of the mouse. *Development* 126:5073, 1999.

22. Hudson G: Bone marrow volume in the human foetus and newborn. *Br J Haematol* 11:446, 1965.

23. Brannon D: Extramedullary hematopoiesis in anemia. *Bull Johns Hopkins Hosp* 41:104, 1927.

24. Erslev A: Medullary and extramedullary blood formation. *Clin Orthop* 52:25, 1967.

25. Zanjani ED, Poster J, Burlington H, et al: Liver as the primary site of erythropoietin formation in the fetus. *J Lab Clin Med* 89:640, 1977.

26. Zanjani ED, Ascensao JL, McGlare PG, et al: Studies on the liver to kidney switch of erythropoietin production. *J Clin Invest* 67:1183, 1981.

27. Flake AW, Harrison MR, Adzick NS, Zanjani ED: Erythropoietin production by the fetal liver in an adult environment. *Blood* 70:542, 1987.

28. Sawyer ST, Penta K: Erythropoietin cell biology. *Hematol Oncol Clin North Am* 8:895, 1994.

29. Finch CA, Deubelbeiss K, Cook JD, et al: Ferrokinetics in man. *Medicine (Baltimore)* 49:17, 1970.

30. Noble NA, Xu Q-P, Hoge LL: Reticulocytes: II. Reexamination of the in vivo survival of stress reticulocytes. *Blood* 75:1877, 1990.

31. Donohue DM, Reiff RH, Hanson ML, et al: Quantitation measurement of the erythrocytic and granulocytic cells of marrow and blood. *J Clin Invest* 37:1571, 1958.

32. Finch CA, Harker LA, Cook JD: Kinetics of the formed elements of human blood. *Blood* 50:699, 1977.

33. Goltry KL, Patel VP: Specific domains of fibronectin mediate adhesion and migration of early murine erythroid progenitors. *Blood* 90:138, 1997.

34. Gregory T, Yu C, Ma A, et al: GATA-1 and erythropoietin cooperate to promote erythroid cell survival by regulating bcl-xL expression. *Blood* 94:87, 1999.

35. Tsang AP, Visvader JE, Turner CA, et al: FOG, a multitype zinc finger protein, acts as a cofactor for transcription factor GATA-1 in erythroid and megakaryocytic differentiation. *Cell* 90:109, 1997.

36. Nerlov C, Querfurth E, Kulessa H, Graf T: GATA-1 interacts with the myeloid PU.1 transcription factor and represses PU.1-dependent transcription. *Blood* 95:2543, 2000.

37. Ohneda K, Yamamoto M: Roles of hematopoietic transcription factors GATA-1 and GATA-2 in the development of red blood cell lineage. *Acta Haematol* 108:237, 2002.

38. Xie H, Ye M, Feng R, Graf T: Stepwise reprogramming of B cells into macrophages. *Cell* 117:663, 2004.

39. Cantor AB, Orkin SH: Transcriptional regulation of erythropoiesis: An affair involving multiple partners. *Oncogene* 213:368, 2002.

40. Back J, Dierich A, Bronn C, et al: PU.1 determines the self-renewal capacity of erythroid progenitor cells. *Blood* 103:3615, 2004.

41. Stopka T, Zivny JH, Stopkova P, et al: Human hematopoietic progenitors express erythropoietin. *Blood* 91:3766, 1998.

42. Krantz SB: Erythropoietin. *Blood* 77:419, 1991.

43. Lappin TR, Rich IN: Erythropoietin—the first 90 years. *Clin Lab Haematol* 18:137, 1996.

44. Jelkmann W: Erythropoietin: Structure, control of production, and function. *Physiol Rev* 72:449, 1992.

45. Jelkmann W, Metzen E: Erythropoietin in the control of red cell production. *Anat Anz* 178:391, 1996.

46. Koury ST, Boudurant MC, Koury MJ: Localization of erythropoietic synthesizing cells in murine kidneys by in situ hybridization. *Blood* 71:524, 1988.

47. Lacombe C, Da Silva J-L, Bruneval P, Fournier J-G: Peritubular cells are the site of erythropoietin synthesis in the murine hypoxic kidney. *J Clin Invest* 81:620, 1988.

48. Koury ST, Koury MJ, Bondurant MC, et al: Quantitation of erythro-poietic-producing cells in kidneys of mice by in situ hybridization: Correlation with hematocrit, renal erythropoietin mRNA, and serum erythropoietin concentration. *Blood* 71:645, 1989.

49. Semenza GL, Dureza RC, Traystman MD, et al: Human erythropoietin gene expression in transgenic mice: Multiple transcription initiation sites and cis-acting regulatory elements. *Mol Cell Biol* 10:930, 1990.

50. Schuster SJ, Koury ST, Bohrer M, et al: Cellular sites of extrarenal and renal erythropoietin production in anaemic rats. *Br J Haematol* 81:153, 1992.

51. Naughton BA, Kaplan SM, Roy M, et al: Hepatic regeneration and erythropoietin production in the rat. *Science* 196:301, 1977.

52. Brown S, Caro J, Erslev AJ, Murray T: Spontaneous increase in erythropoietin and hematocrit value associated with transient liver enzyme abnormalities in an anephric patient undergoing hemodialysis. *Am J Med* 68:280, 1980.

53. Flaharty KK, Caro J, Erslev A, et al: Pharmacokinetics and erythropoietic response to human recombinant erythropoietin in healthy men. *Clin Pharmacol Ther* 47:557, 1990.

54. Sytkowski AJ, Lunn ED, Davis KL, et al: Human erythropoietin dimers with markedly enhanced in vivo activity. *Proc Natl Acad Sci U S A* 95:1184, 1998.

55. Sawyer ST, Krantz SB, Goldwasser E: Binding and receptor-mediated endocytosis of erythropoietin in Friend virus-infected erythroid cells. *J Biol Chem* 262:5554, 1987.

56. Goldberg MA, Dunning SP, Bunn HF: Regulation of the erythropoietin gene: Evidence that the oxygen sensor is a heme protein. *Science* 242:1412, 1988.

57. Semenza GL, Wang GL: A nuclear factor induced by hypoxia via de novo protein synthesis binds to the human erythropoietin gene enhancer at a site required for transcriptional activation. *Mol Cell Biol* 12:5447, 1992.

58. Semenza GL, Agani F, Booth G, et al: Structural and functional analysis of hypoxia-inducible factor 1. *Kidney Int* 51:553, 1997.

59. Maxwell PH, Pugh CW, Ratcliffe PJ: Inducible operation of the erythropoietin 3′ enhancer in multiple cell lines: Evidence for a widespread oxygen-sensing mechanism. *Proc Natl Acad Sci U S A* 90:2423, 1993.

60. Beck I, Weinmann R, Caro J: Characterization of hypoxia-responsive enhancer in the human erythropoietin gene shows presence of hypoxia-inducible 120-Kd nuclear DNA-binding protein in erythropoietin-producing and nonproducing cells. *Blood* 82:704, 1993.

61. Semenza GL, Roth PH, Fang HM, Wang GL: Transcriptional regulation of genes encoding glycolytic enzymes by hypoxia-inducible factor 1. *J Biol Chem* 269:23757, 1994.

62. Wiener CM, Booth G, Semenza GL: In vivo expression of mRNAs encoding hypoxia-inducible factor 1. *Biochem Biophys Res Commun* 225:485, 1996.

63. Carmeliet P, Dor Y, Herbert JM, et al: Role of HIF-1 alpha in hypoxia-mediated apoptosis, cell proliferation and tumour angiogenesis. *Nature* 394:485, 1998.

64. Iyer NV, Kotch LE, Agani F, et al: Cellular and developmental control of O_2 homeostasis by hypoxia-inducible factor 1 alpha. *Genes Dev* 12: 149, 1998.

65. Ryan HE, Lo J, Johnson RS: HIF-1 alpha is required for solid tumor formation and embryonic vascularization. *EMBO J* 17:3005, 1998.

66. Wang GL, Semenza GL: General involvement of hypoxia-inducible factor 1 in transcriptional response to hypoxia. *Proc Natl Acad Sci U S A* 90:4304, 1993.

67. Maxwell PH, Wiesener MS, Chang GW, et al: The tumour suppressor protein VHL targets hypoxia-inducible factors for oxygen-dependent proteolysis. *Nature* 399:271, 1999.

68. Sutter CH, Laughner E, Semenza GL: Hypoxia-inducible factor 1α protein expression is controlled by oxygen-regulated ubiquitination that is disrupted by deletions and missense mutations. *Proc Natl Acad Sci U S A* 97:4748, 2000.

69. Ivan M, Kondo K, Yang H, et al: HIF alpha targeted for VHL-mediated destruction by proline hydroxylation: Implications for O_2 sensing. *Science* 292:464, 2001.

70. Jaakkola P, Mole DR, Tian YM, et al: Targeting of HIF-alpha to the von Hippel-Lindau ubiquitylation complex by O_2-regulated prolyl hydroxylation. *Science* 292:449, 2001.

71. Epstein AC, Gleadle JM, McNeill LA, et al: C. elegans EGL-9 and mammalian homologs define a family of dioxygenases that regulate HIF by prolyl hydroxylation. *Cell* 107:43, 2001.

72. Ebert BL, Bunn HF: Regulation of the erythropoietin gene. *Blood* 94: 1864, 1999.

73. Constantinescu SN, Keren T, Socolovsky M, et al: Ligand-independent oligomerization of cell-surface erythropoietin receptor is mediated by the transmembrane domain. *Proc Natl Acad Sci U S A* 984:379, 2001.

74. Witthuhn B, Quelle FW, Silvennoinen O, et al: JAK2 associates with the erythropoietin receptor and is tyrosine phosphorylated and activated following stimulation with erythropoietin. *Cell* 74:227, 1993.

75. Damen JE, Wakao H, Miyajima A, et al: Tyrosine 343 in the erythropoietin receptor positively regulates erythropoietin-induced cell proliferation and STAT5 activation. *EMBO J* 14:5557, 1995.

76. Parganas E, Wang D, Stravopodis D, et al: JAK2 is essential for signaling through a variety of cytokine receptors. *Cell* 93:385, 1998.

77. Lin CS, Lim SK, D'Agati V, et al: Differential effects of an erythropoietin receptor gene disruption on primitive and definitive erythropoiesis. *Genes Dev* 10:154, 1996.

78. Wu H, Liu X, Jaenisch R, et al: Generation of committed erythroid BFU-E and CFU-E progenitors does not require erythropoietin or the erythropoietin receptor. *Cell* 83:59, 1995.

79. Divoky V, Prchal JT: Mouse surviving solely on human erythropoietin receptor (EPOR): Model of human EPOR-linked disease. *Blood* 99: 3873, 2002.

80. D'Andrea AD, Yoshimura A, Youssoufian H, et al: The cytoplasmic region of the erythropoietin receptor contains non-overlapping positive and negative growth-regulatory domains. *Mol Cell Biol* 11:1980, 1991.

81. Klingmuller U, Lorenz U, Cantley, LC, et al: Specific recruitment of SH-PTP1 to the erythropoietin receptor causes inactivation of JAK2 and termination of proliferative signals. *Cell* 80:729, 1995.

82. Arcasoy MO, Harris KW, Forget BG: A human erythropoietin receptor gene mutant causing familial erythrocytosis is associated with deregulation of the rates of Jak2 and Stat5 inactivation. *Exp Hematol* 27:63, 1999.

83. Marine JC, McKay C, Wang D, et al: SOCS3 is essential in the regulation of fetal liver erythropoiesis. *Cell* 98:617, 1999.

84. Sasaki A, Yasukoawa H, Shouda T, et al: Cis3/SOCS3 suppresses erythropoietin signaling by binding to EPOR and JAK2. *J Biol Chem* 275: 29338, 2000.

85. Walrafen P, Verdier F, Zahra Kadri Z, et al: Both proteasomes and lysosomes degrade the activated erythropoietin receptor. *Blood* 105:600, 2005.

86. Nakamura Y, Nakauchi H: A truncated erythropoietin receptor and cell death: A reanalysis. *Science* 264:588, 1994.

87. Barron C, Migliaccio AR, Migliaccio G, et al: Alternatively spliced mRNAs encoding soluble isoforms of the erythropoietin receptor in murine cell lines and bone marrow. *Gene* 147:263, 1994.

88. Arcasoy MO, Jiang X, Haroon ZA: Expression of erythropoietin receptor splice variants in human cancer. *Biochem Biophys Res Commun* 307: 999, 2003.

89. Mirza AM, Ezzat S, Axelrad A: Insulin-like growth factor binding protein-1 is elevated in patients with polycythemia vera and stimulates erythroid burst formation in vitro. *Blood* 89:1862, 1997.

90. Correa PN, Eskinazi D, Axelrad AA: Circulating erythroid progenitors in polycythemia vera are hypersensitive to insulin-like growth factor I in vitro: Studies in an improved serum-free medium. *Blood* 83:99, 1994.

91. Brox AG, Congote LF, Fafard J, Fauser AA: Identification and characterization of an 8-kd peptide stimulating late erythropoiesis. *Exp Hematol* 17:769, 1989.

92. Gomez AR, Norwood VF: Developmental consequences of the renin-angiotensin system. *Am J Kidney Dis* 26:409, 1995.

93. Ray PE, Aguilera G, Kopp JB, et al: Angiotensin II receptor-mediated proliferation of cultured human fetal mesangial cells. *Kidney Int* 40:764, 1991.

94. Tufro-Meddie A, Gomer RA: Ontogeny of the renin-angiotensin system. *Semin Nephrol* 13:519, 1993.

95. Verhaaren HA, Vande Walle J, Devloo-Blancquaert A: Captopril in severe childhood hypertension--reversible anaemia with high dosage. *Eur J Pediatr* 144:554, 1986.

96. Wang AY, Yu AW, Lam CW, et al: Effects of losartan or enalapril on hemoglobin, circulating erythropoietin, and insulin-like growth factor-1 in patients with and without posttransplant erythrocytosis. *Am J Kidney Dis* 39:600, 2002.

97. Mrug M, Stopka T, Julian BA, et al: Angiotensin II facilitates erythropoietin mediated proliferation of normal early erythroid progenitors. *J Clin Invest* 115:508,1997.

98. Glezerman I, Patel H, Glicklich D, et al: Angiotensin-converting enzyme inhibition induces death receptor apoptotic pathways in erythroid precursors following renal transplantation. *Am J Nephrol* 23:195, 2003.

99. Cole J, Ertoy D, Lin H, et al: Lack of angiotensin II-facilitated erythropoiesis causes anemia in angiotensin-converting enzyme-deficient mice. *J Clin Invest* 106:1391, 2000.

100. Pearson TC, Botterill CA, Glass UH, Wetherley-Mein G: Interpretation of measured red cell mass and plasma volume in males with elevated venous PCV values. *Scand J Haematol* 33:68, 1984.

101. Sioufi HA, Button LN, Jacobson MS, Kevy SV: Nonradioactive chromium technique for red cell labeling. *Vox Sang* 58:204, 1990.

102. Cavill I, Trevett D, Fisher J, Hoy T: The measurement of the total volume of red cells in man: A non-radioactive approach using biotin. *Br J Haematol* 70:491, 1988.

103. Jones J, Mollison PL: A simple and efficient method of labeling red cells with 99m Tc for determination of red cell volume. *Br J Haematol* 38: 141, 1978.

104. Chaplin H Jr: Precision of red cell volume measurement using P^{32} labeled cells. *J Physiol* 123:22, 1954.

105. Pearson TC, Guthrie DL, Simpson J, et al: Interpretation of measured red cell mass and plasma volume in adults: Expert Panel on Radionuclides of the International Council for Standardization in Haematology. *Br J Haematol* 89:748, 1995.

106. Fairbanks VF, Klee GG, Wiseman GA, et al: Measurement of blood volume and red cell mass: Re-examination of ^{51}Cr and ^{125}I methods. *Blood Cells Mol Dis* 22:169, 1996.

107. Larson RA: Studies of the body hematocrit phenomenon: Dynamic hematocrit of large vessel and initial distribution space of albumin and fibrinogen in the whole body. *Scand J Clin Lab Invest* 22:189, 1998.

108. Fairbanks VF: Measurement of blood volume and red cell mass: Re-examination of ^{51}Cr and ^{125}I methods [commentary]. *Blood Cells Mol Dis* 22:186C, 1996.

109. Button LN, Gibson JG II, Walter CW: Simultaneous determination of the volume of red cells and plasma for survival studies of stored blood. *Transfusion* 5:143, 1965.

110. International Committee for Standardization in Haematology: Recommended methods for measurement of red-cell and plasma volume. *J Nucl Med* 21:793, 1980.

111. Hillman RS, Finch CA: Erythropoiesis: Normal and abnormal. *Semin Hematol* 4:327, 1967.

112. Samson D, Halliday D, Nicholson DC, Chanarin I: Quantitation of in effective erythropoiesis from the incorporation of [^{15}N] delta-aminolae-vulinic acid and [^{15}N] glycine into early labeled bilirubin: I. Normal subjects. *Br J Haematol* 34:33, 1976.

113. Samson D, Halliday D, Nicholson DC, Chanarin I: Quantitation of in-effective erythropoiesis from the incorporation of [^{15}N] delta-aminolae-vulinic acid and [^{15}N] glycine into early labeled bilirubin: II. Anaemic patients. *Br J Haematol* 34:45, 1976.

114. Huff RI, Hennessey TG, Austin RE: Plasma and red cell iron turnover in normal subjects and in patients having various hematopoietic disorders. *J Clin Invest* 29:1041, 1950.

115. Cook JD, Marsaglia G, Eschbach JW, et al: Ferrokinetics: A biologic model for plasma iron exchange in man. *J Clin Invest* 49:197, 1970.

116. Ricketts C, Cavill I, Napier JA, Jacobs A: Ferrokinetics and erythropoiesis in man: An evaluation of ferrokinetic measurements. *Br J Haematol* 35:41, 1977.

117. Bauer W, Stray S, Huebers H, Finch C: The relationship between plasma iron and plasma iron turnover in the rat. *Blood* 57:239, 1981.

118. Beguin Y: The soluble transferrin receptor: Biological aspects and clinical usefulness as quantitative measure of erythropoiesis. *Haematologica* 77:1, 1992.

COLOR PLATES

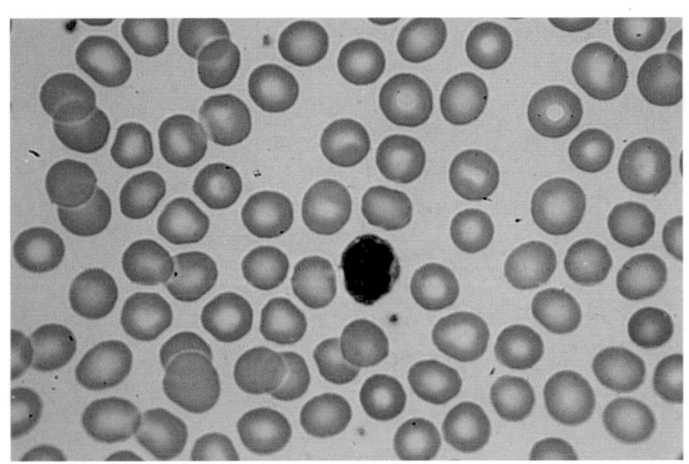

PLATE I-1   Normal erythrocytes. Small lymphocyte in center of field.

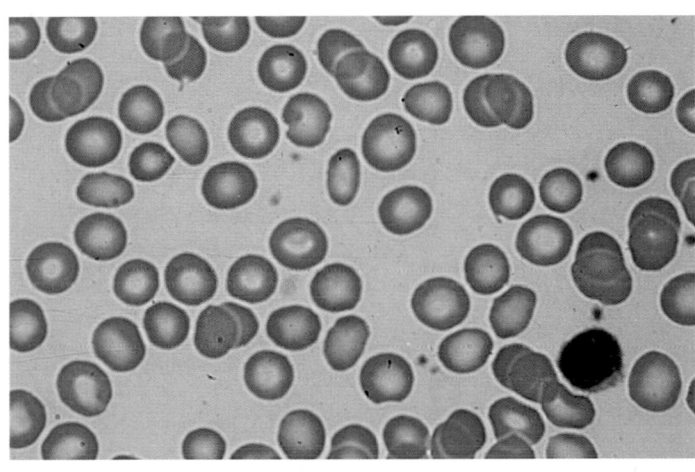

PLATE I-2   Slight hypochromia and microcytosis in early iron deficiency anemia. Small lymphocyte right lower corner.

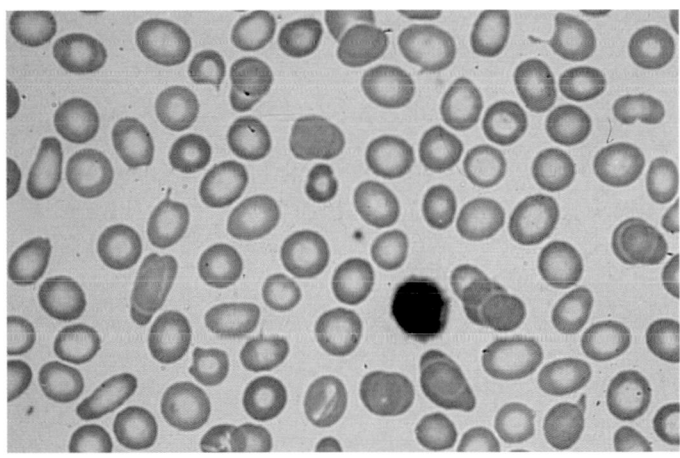

PLATE I-3   Severe hypochromia and microcytosis in iron deficiency anemia. Small lymphocyte in field.

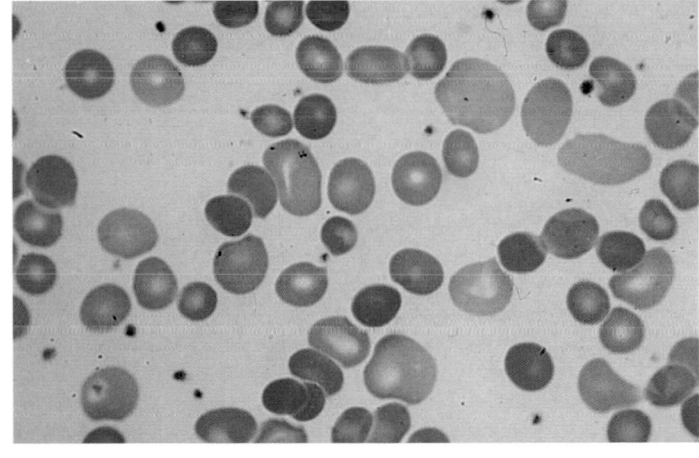

PLATE I-4   Polychromatophilia. Note large red cells with light purple coloring.

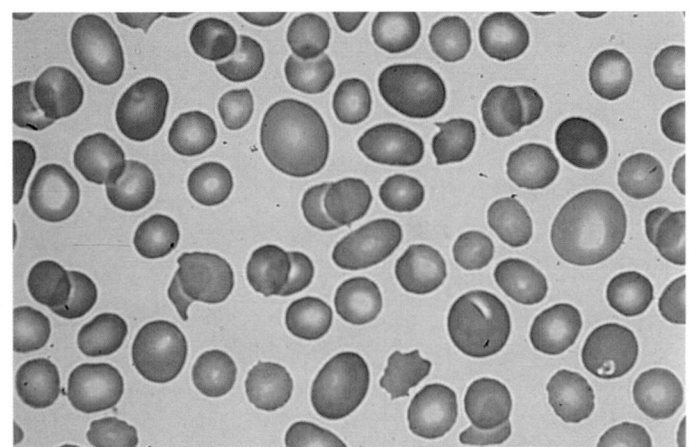

PLATE I-5   Macrocytosis.

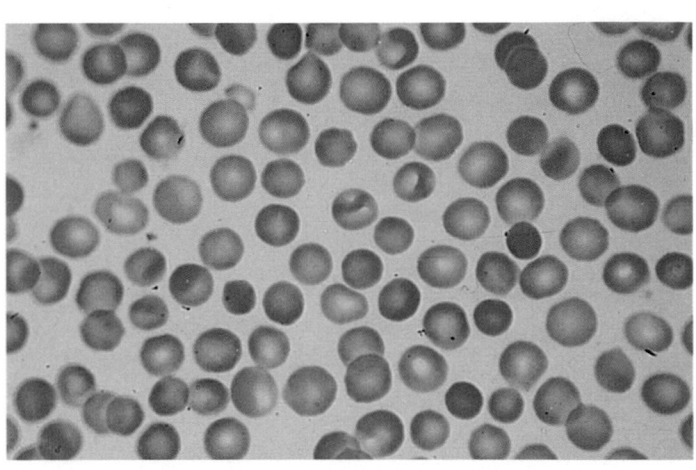

PLATE I-6   Spherocytosis. Note small hyperchromatic cells.

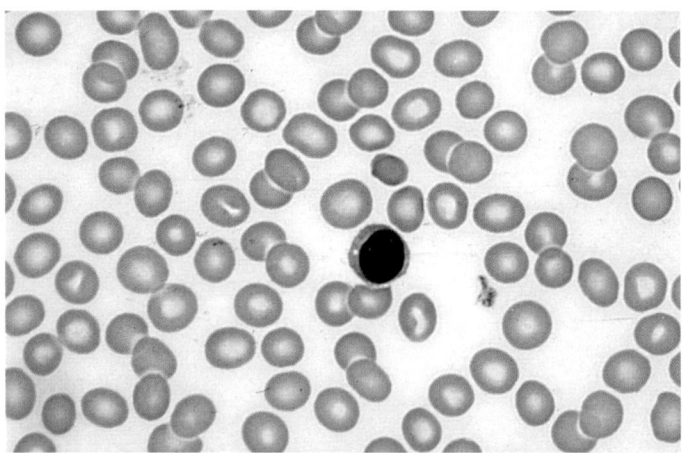

PLATE I-7   Normal red cells distribution. Small lymphocyte in center of field.

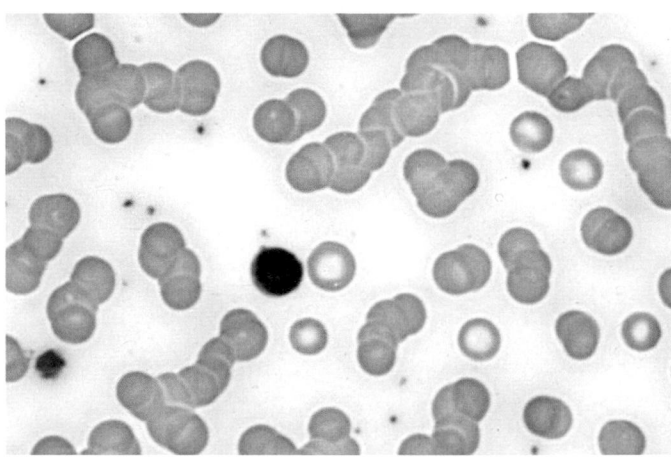

PLATE I-8   Rouleaux formation. Small lymphocyte in center of field.

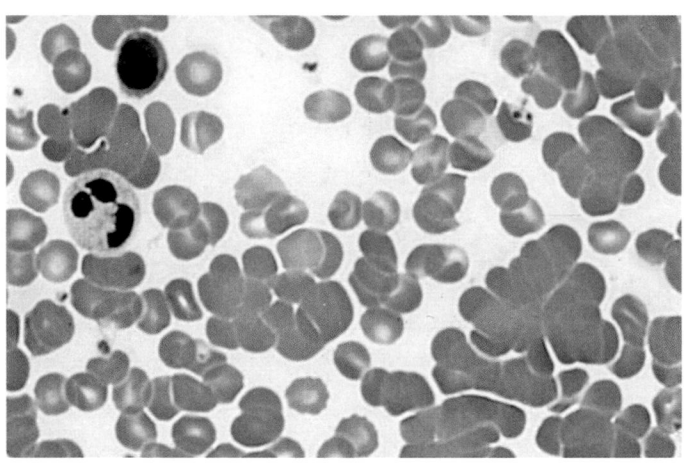

PLATE I-9   Erythrocyte agglutination. Small lymphocyte and segmented neutrophil upper left corner.

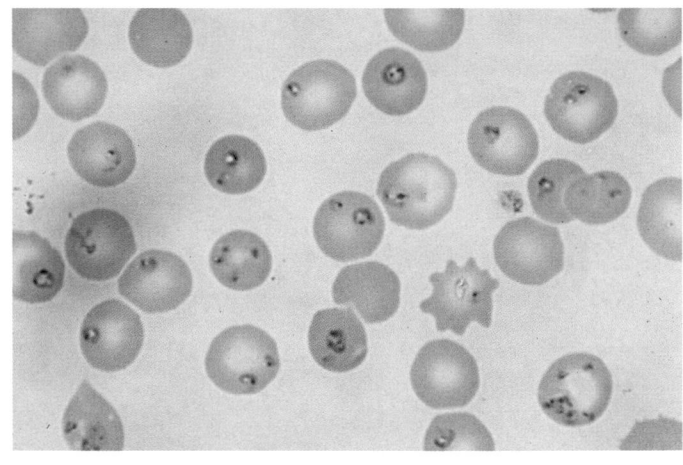

PLATE I-10   Red cell containing *Babesia microti*.

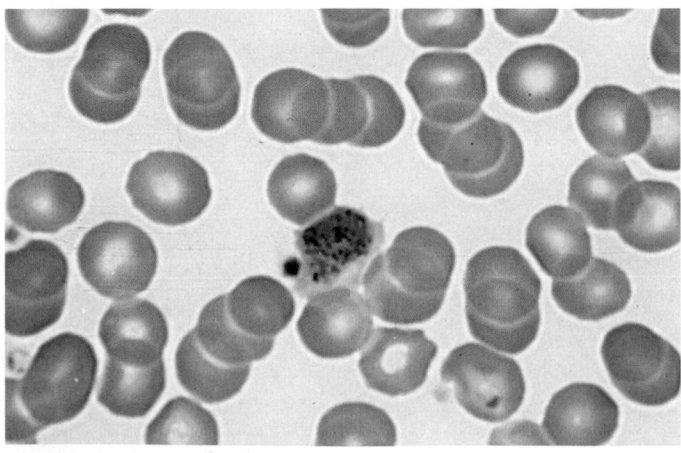

PLATE I-11   A red cell containing a trophozoite of *Plasmodium vivax*.

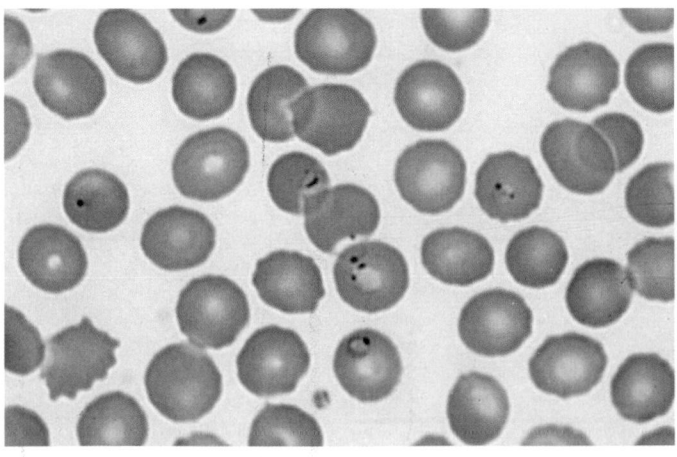

PLATE I-12   Red cells containing *Plasmodium falciparum* ring forms.

(I-1 through I-12 are blood films.)

P L A T E I I
RED CELL MORPHOLOGY

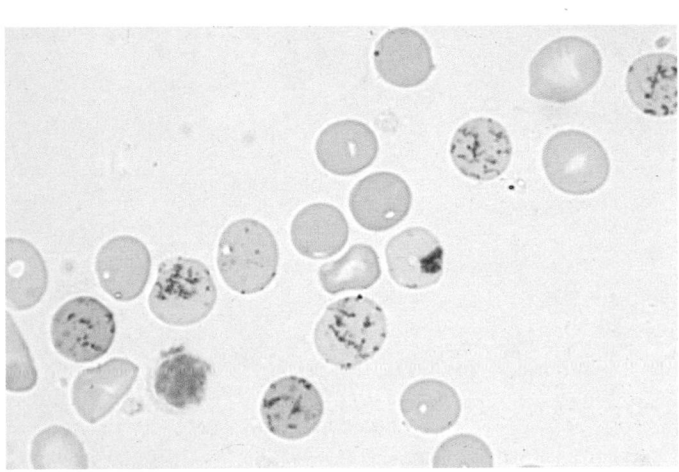

PLATE II-1   Red cells stained supravitally with new methylene blue. Reticulocytes retain intracellular stained precipitates of ribosomal RNA.

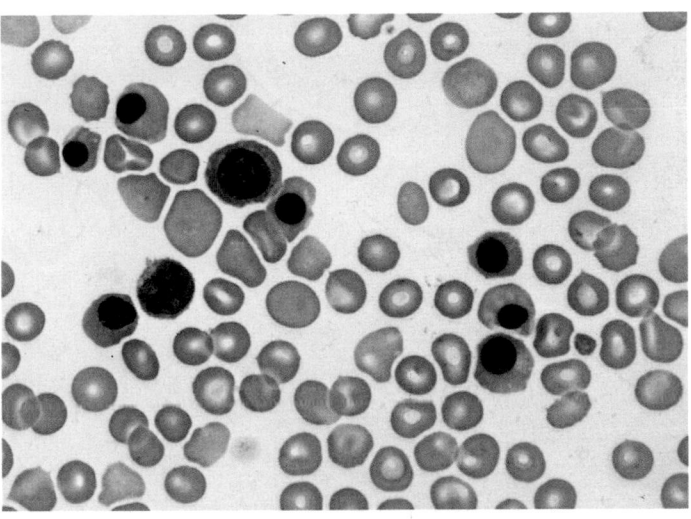

PLATE II-2   Hemolytic disease of the newborn (erythroblastosis fetalis). Polychromatophilic cells, spherocytes, and circulating erythroblasts.

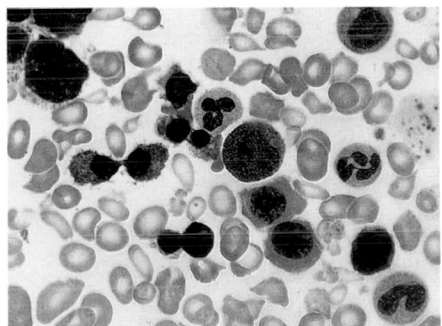

PLATE II-3   Marrow film. Congenital dyserythropoietic anemia. Red cell shape abnormalities and nuclear anomalies of the erythroblasts (bridging).

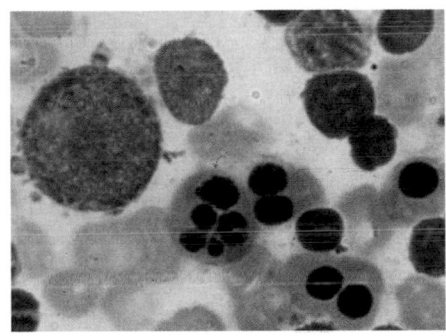

PLATE II-4   Marrow film. Erythroblastic multinuclearity.

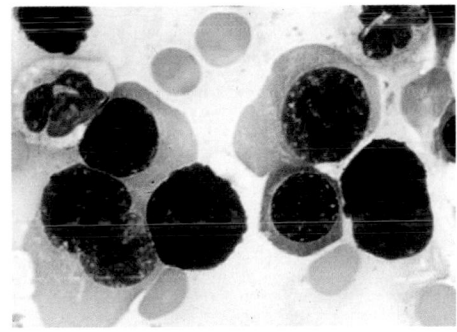

PLATE II-5   Marrow film. Congenital dyserythropoietic anemia. Note giant erythroblasts and binucleated erythroblast.

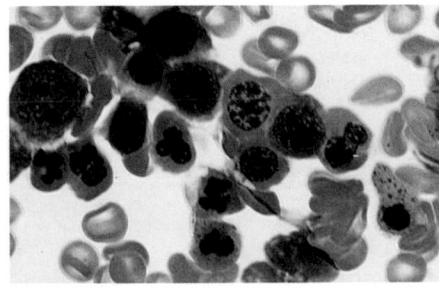

PLATE II-6   Chronic arsenic poisoning. Marrow film. Marked dyserythropoiesis.

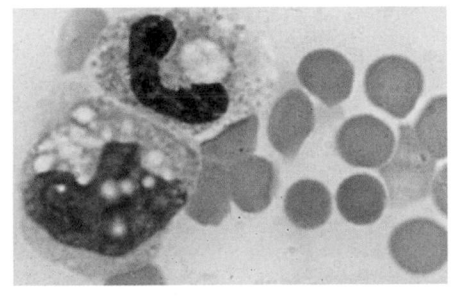

PLATE II-7   Clostridium septicemia. Erythrophagocytosis by a macrophage and neutrophil. Microspherocytes and profound decrease in red cells.

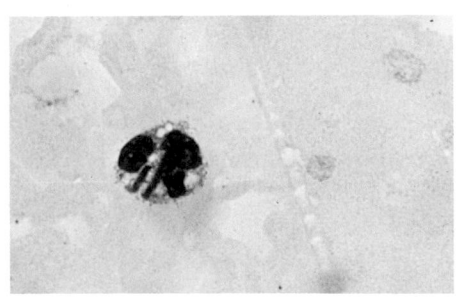

PLATE II-8   Clostridial septicemia. *Clostridium* bacilli in a neutrophil.

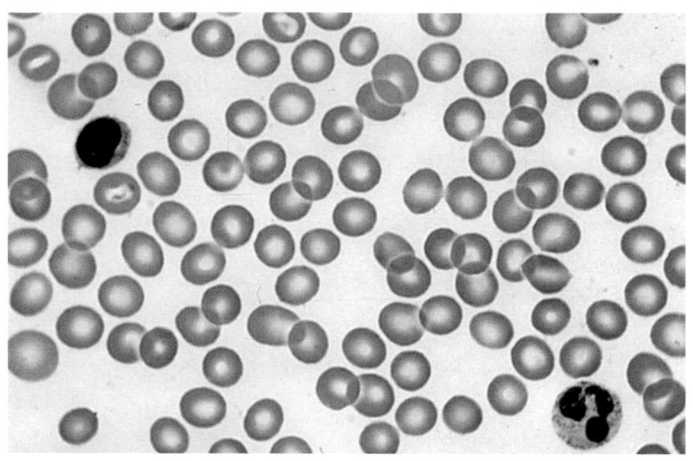

PLATE III-1   Normal blood film. Small lymphocyte and segmented neutrophil in field.

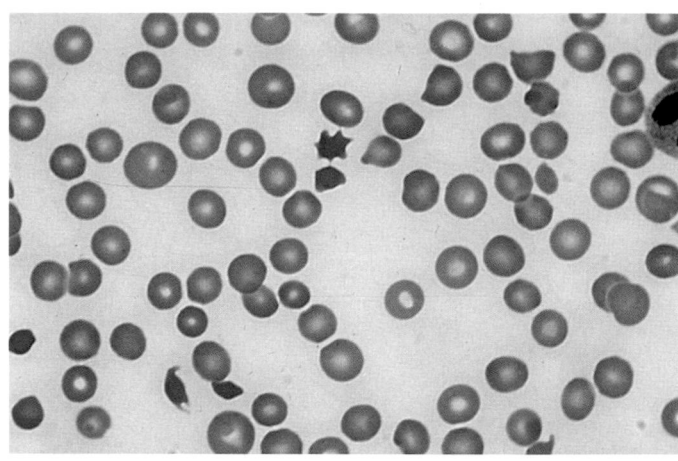

PLATE III-2   Fragmented red cells: Disseminated intravascular coagulation.

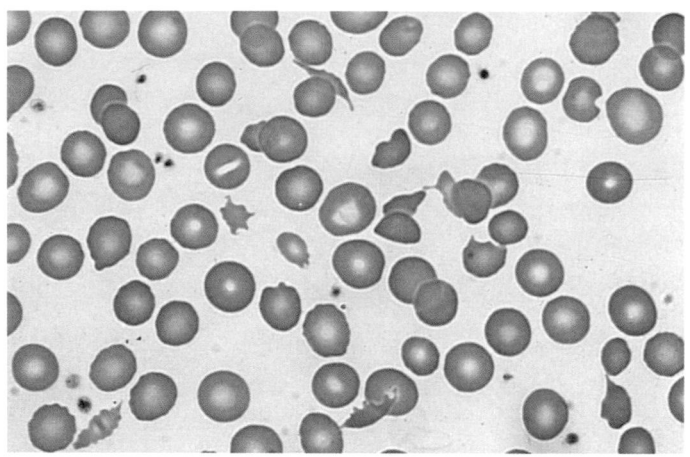

PLATE III-3   Fragmented red cells: Heart valve hemolysis.

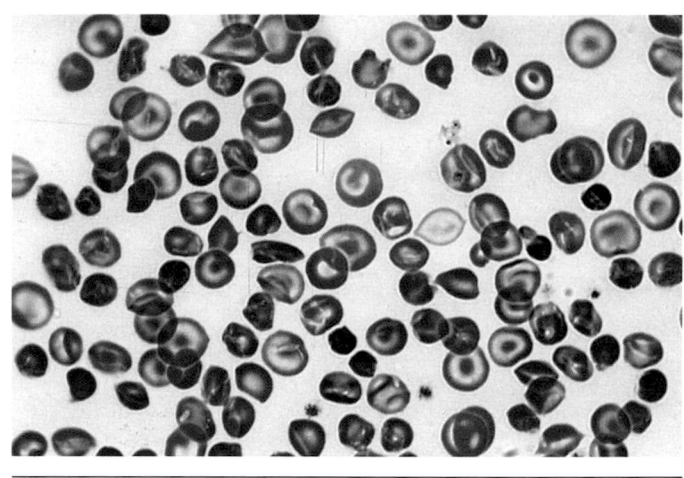

PLATE III-4   Target cells and microspherocytes. Hemoglobin C disease.

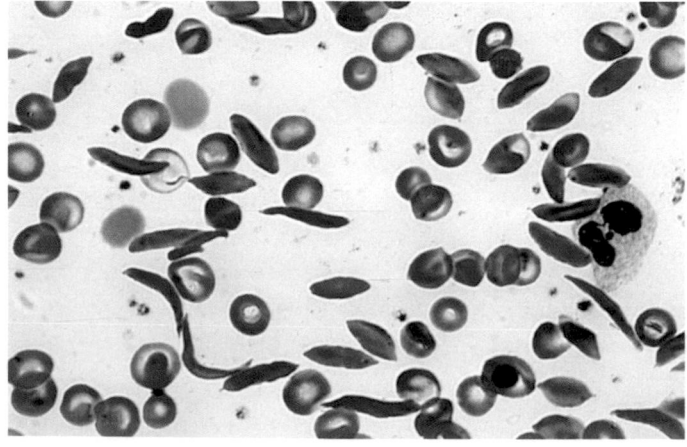

PLATE III-5   Sickle cells. Homozygous sickle cell disease. Nucleated red cell and segmented neutrophil in field.

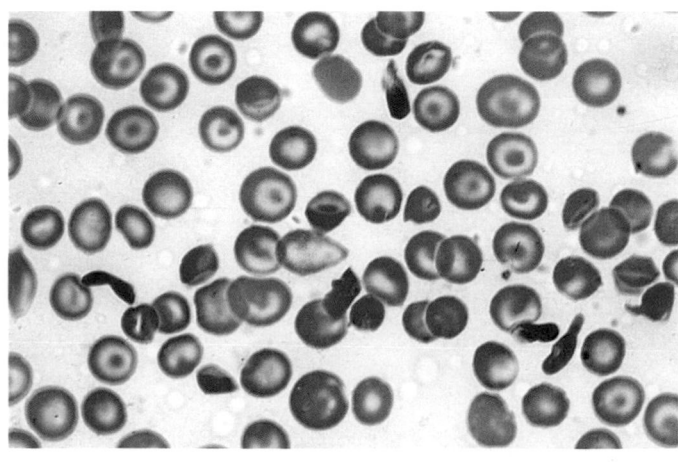

PLATE III-6   Target cells and sickle cells: Hemoglobin SC disease.

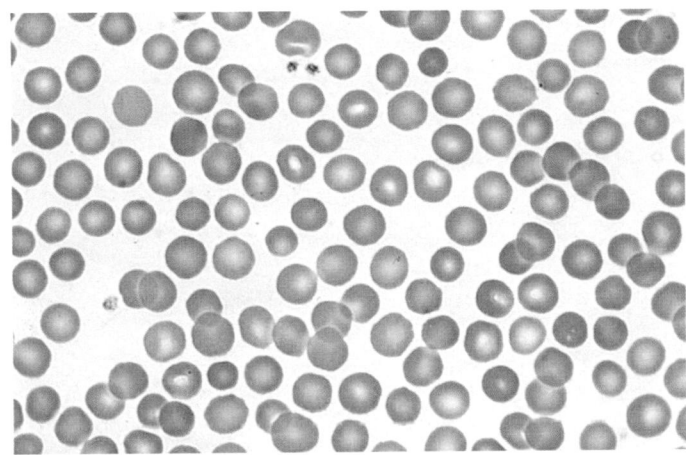

PLATE III-7   Spherocytes: Hereditary spherocytosis.

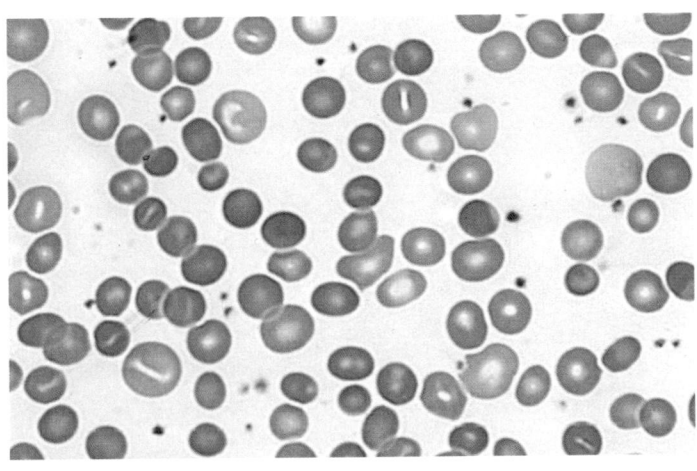

PLATE III-8   Spherocytes: Autoimmune hemolytic anemia.

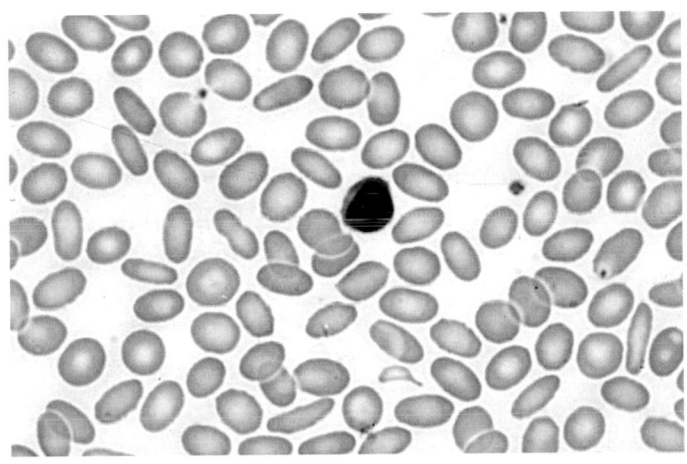

PLATE III-9   Elliptocytes. Hereditary elliptocytosis. Small lymphocyte in center of field.

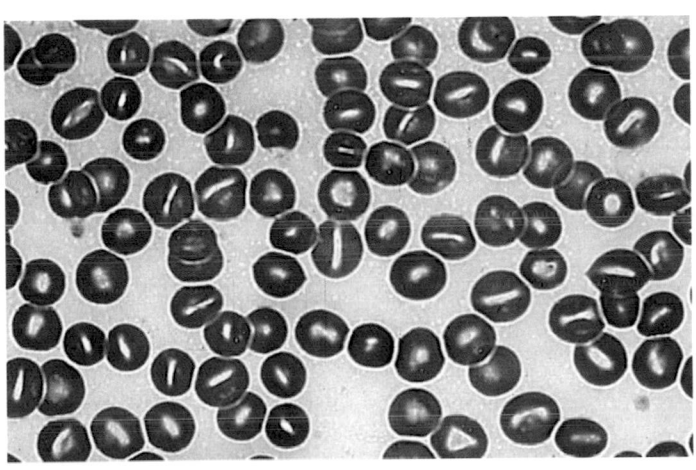

PLATE III-10   Stomatocytosis.

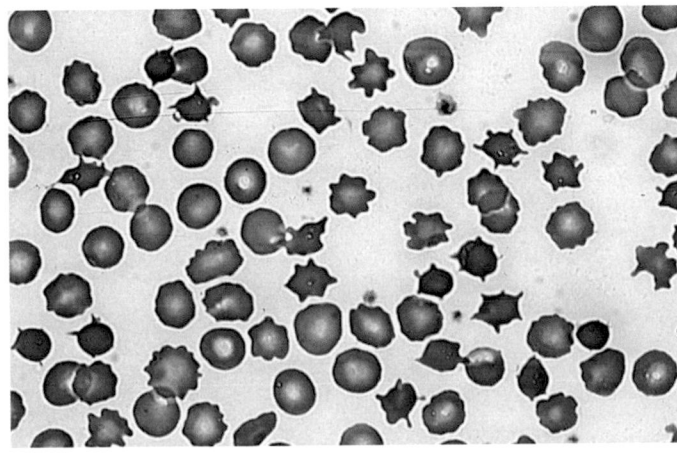

PLATE III-11   Acanthocytosis.

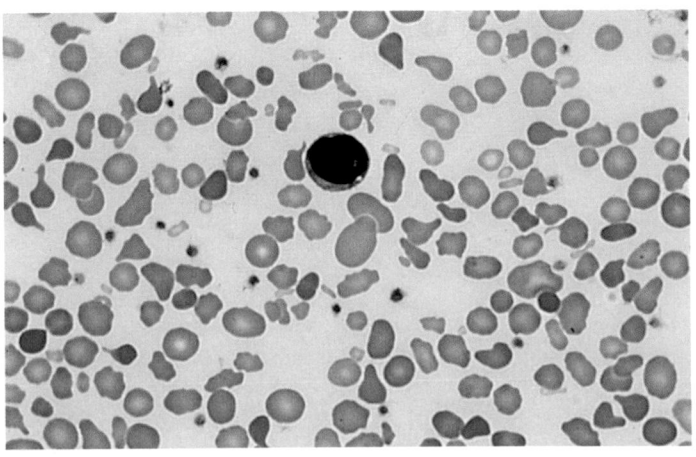

PLATE III-12   Poikilocytosis. Hereditary pyropoikilocytosis. Small lymphocyte in field.

(III-1 through III-12 are blood films.)

P L A T E   I V
RED CELL MORPHOLOGY

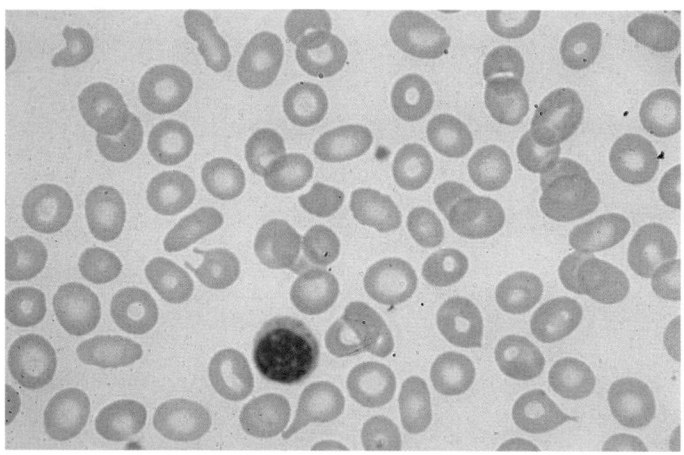

PLATE IV-1   Thalassemia minor. Mild hypochromia, poikilocytosis, and stippled red cell. Small lymphocyte in field.

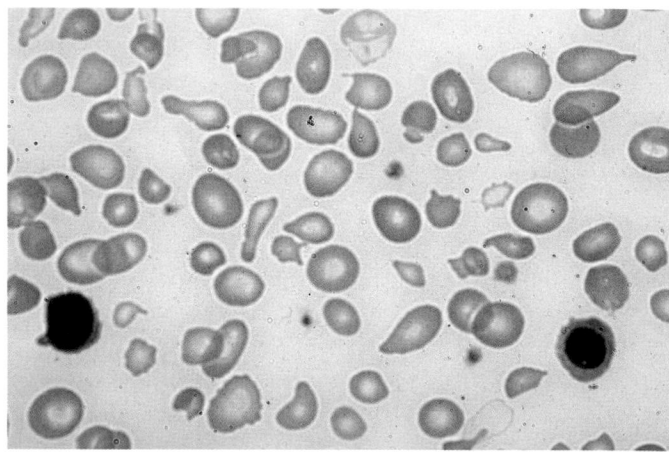

PLATE IV-2   Thalassemia major. Severe poikilocytosis, mild hypochromia, nucleated red cell. Small lymphocyte on left. Nucleated red cell on right.

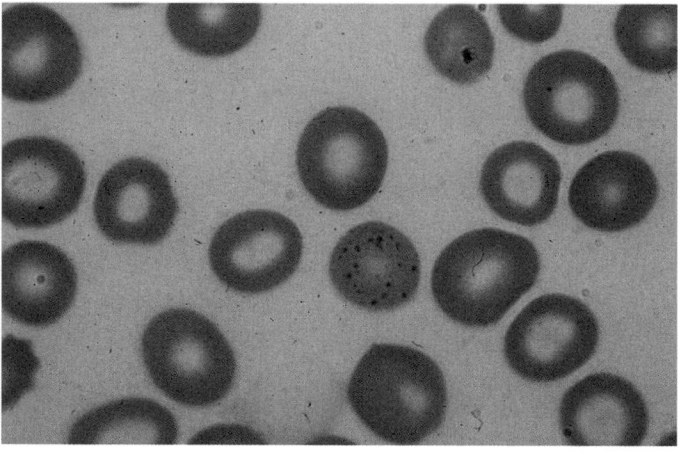

PLATE IV-3   Lead poisoning. Mild hypochromia. Coarsely stippled red cell.

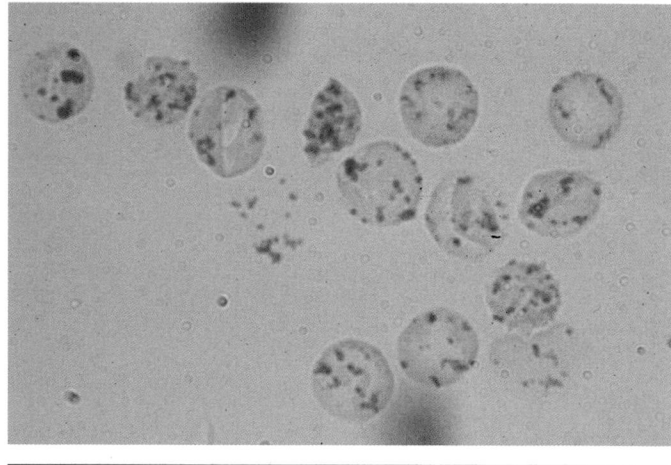

PLATE IV-4   Heinz bodies. Blood mixed with hypotonic solution of crystal violet. Precipitates of denatured hemoglobin within the cells.

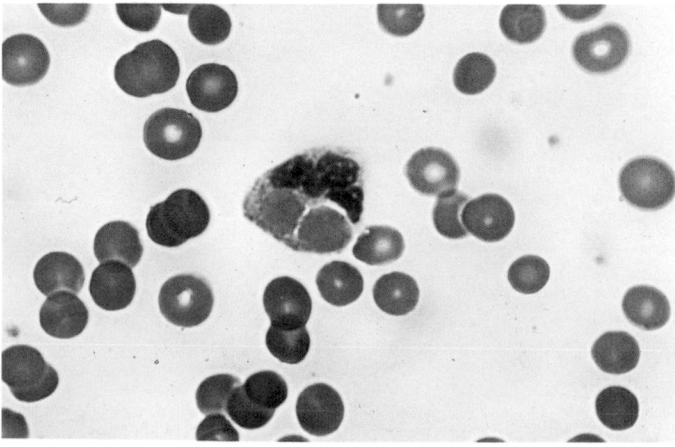

PLATE IV-5   Severe autoimmune hemolytic anemia. Scant red cells on film, frequent microspherocytes, erythrophagocytosis by blood monocyte.

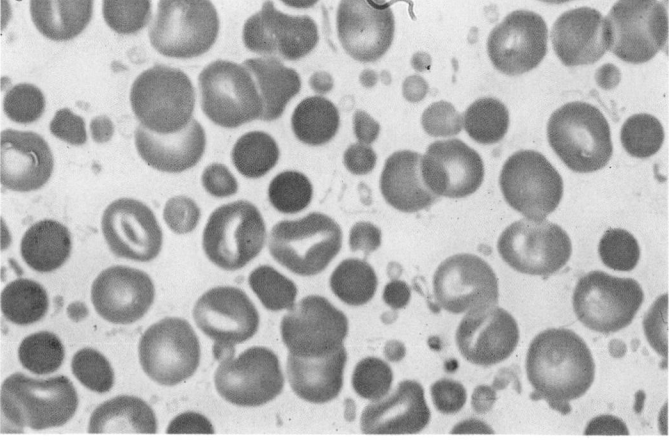

PLATE IV-6   Extensive third degree burns. Spherocytosis, including extremely small spherical "cells."

(IV-1 through IV-3, IV-5, and IV-6 are blood films.)

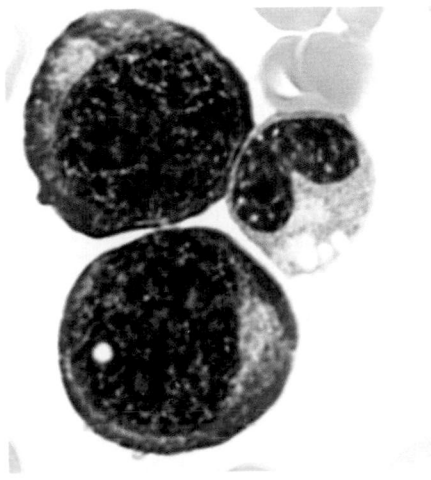

PLATE V-1   Two proerythroblasts and a neutrophilic metamyelocyte.

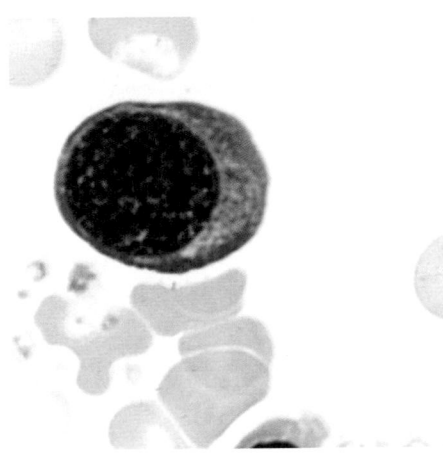

PLATE V-2   Basophilic erythroblasts.

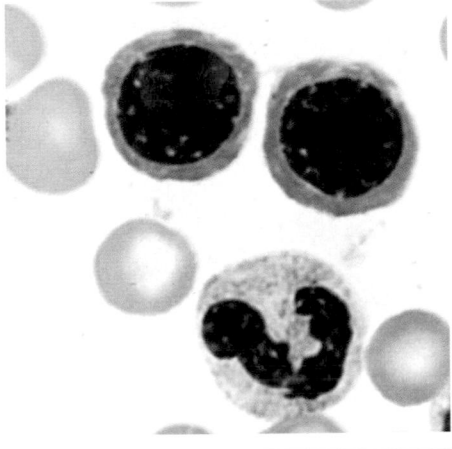

PLATE V-3   Polychromatophilic erythroblasts and segmented neutrophil.

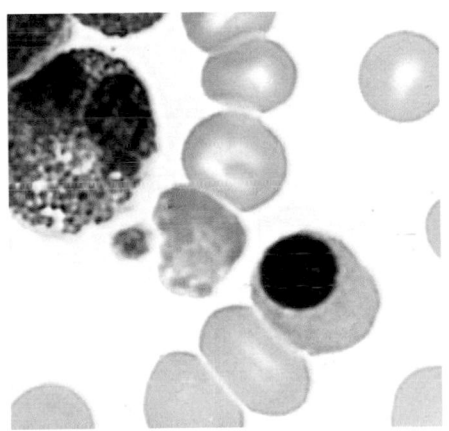

PLATE V-4   Orthochromatic erythroblast and eosinophil.

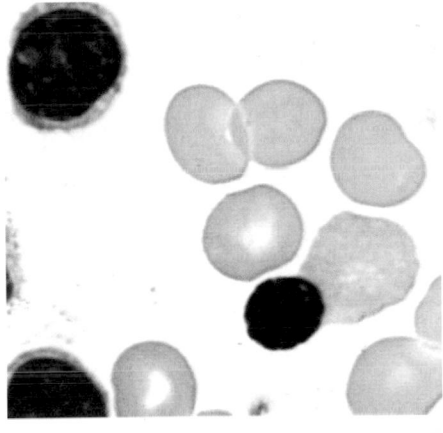

PLATE V-5   Enucleation of orthochromatic erythroblast,

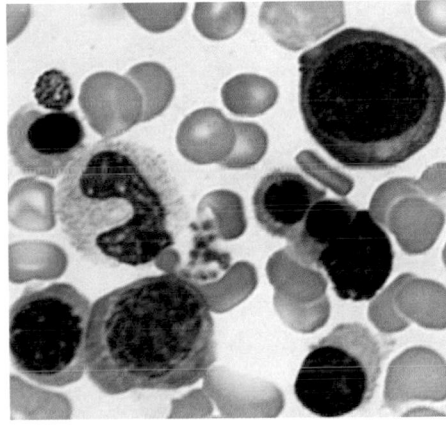

PLATE V-7   Proerythroblast, basophilic erythroblast, polychromatophilic erythroblast, orthochromatic erythroblasts (also, note small plasma cell).

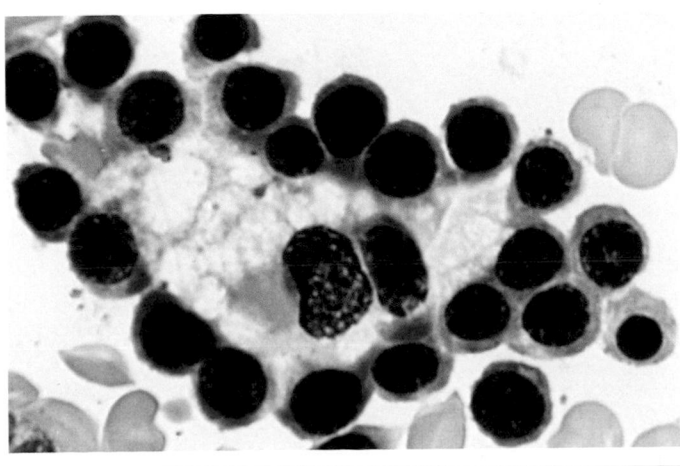

PLATE V-6   Erythroid islet: Central macrophage with surrounding erythroblasts.

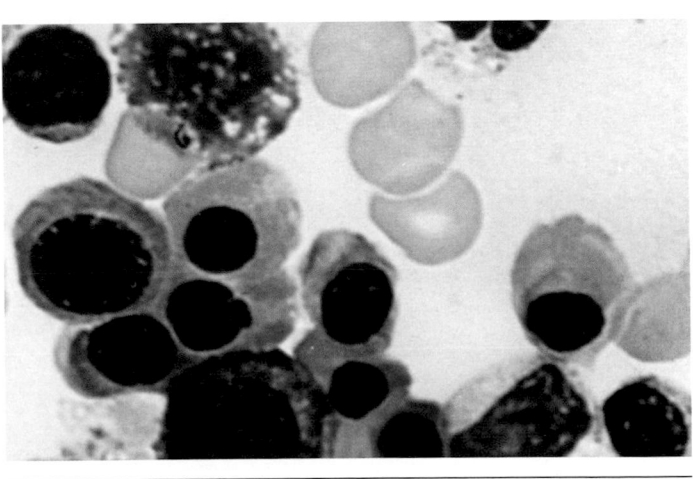

PLATE V-8   Basophilic, polychromatophilic, and orthochromatic erythroblasts.

(V-1 through V-8 are marrow cells.)

P L A T E   V I
MEGALOBLASTIC ERYTHROPOIESIS

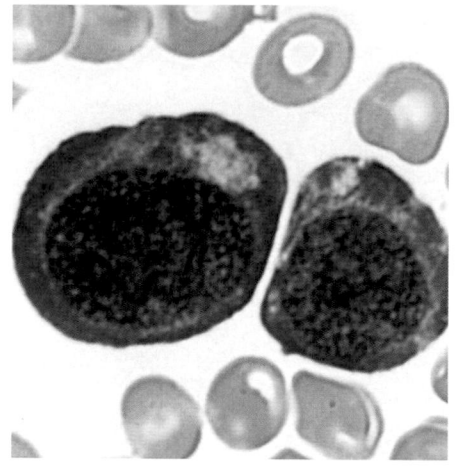

PLATE VI-1   Promegaloblasts.

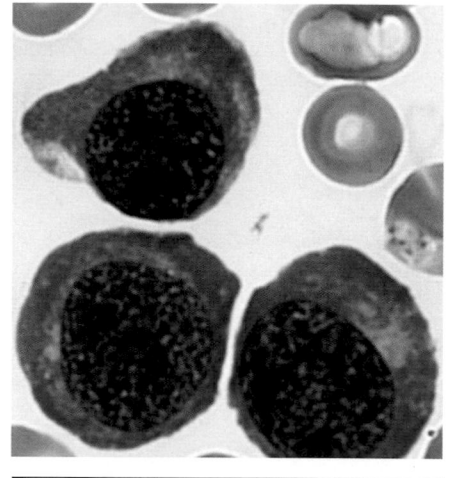

PLATE VI-2   Basophilic megaloblasts.

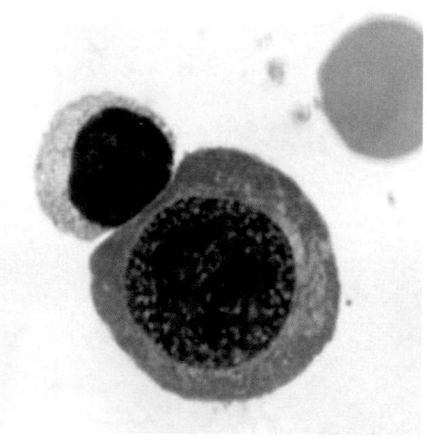

PLATE VI-3   Polychromatophilic megaloblasts.

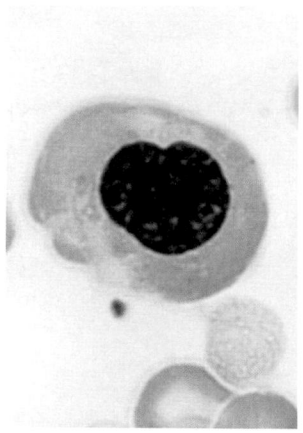

PLATE VI-4   Orthochromatic megaloblast.

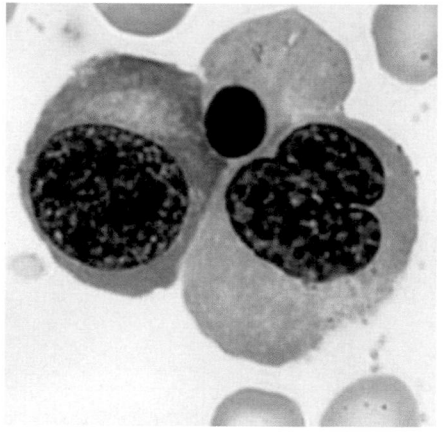

PLATE VI-5   Basophilic, polychromatophilic, and enucleating orthochromatic megaloblasts.

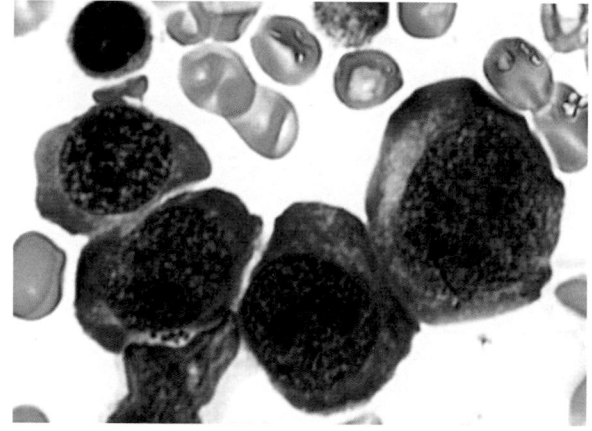

PLATE VI-6   Promegaloblast, basophilic megaloblast, and polychromatophilic megaloblast.

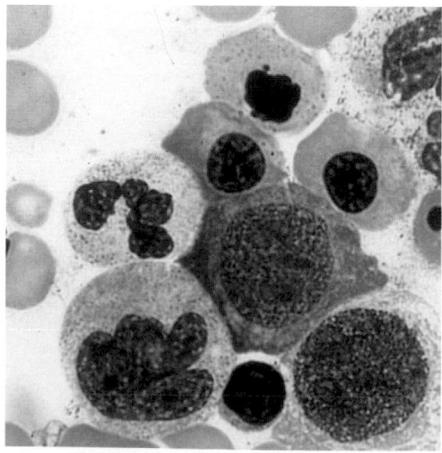

PLATE VI-7   Giant band, basophilic and several orthochromatic megaloblasts with one pyknotic nucleus.

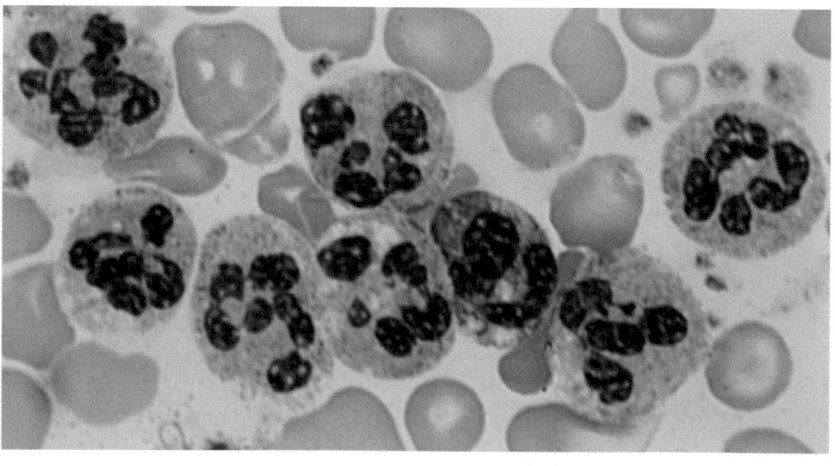

PLATE VI-8   Hypersegmented neutrophils in the buffy coat of a patient with pernicious anemia. An eosinophil is in the field also.

(VI-1 through VI-8 are marrow films.)

PLATE VII
GRANULOCYTE AND MONOCYTE MORPHOLOGY

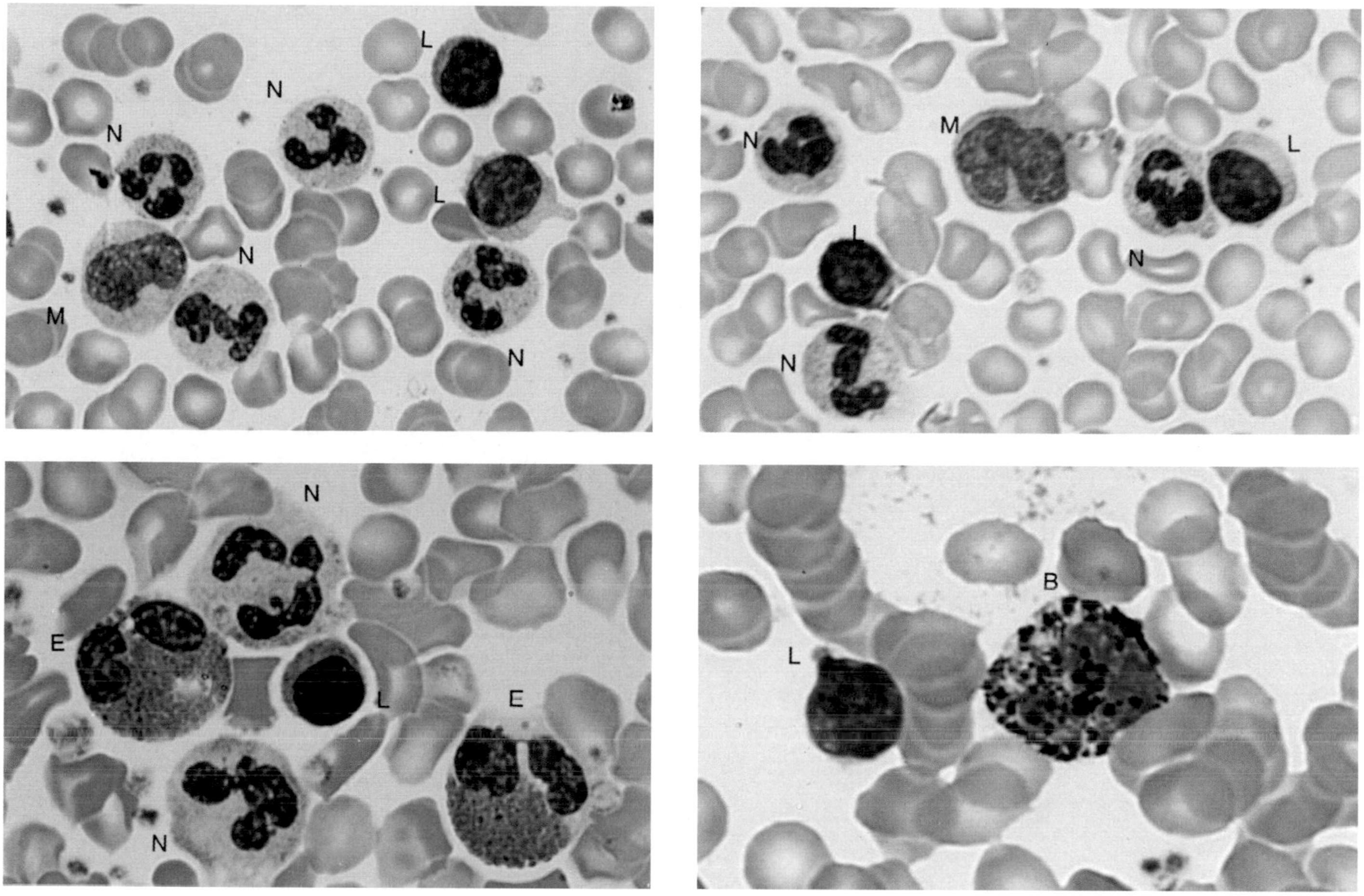

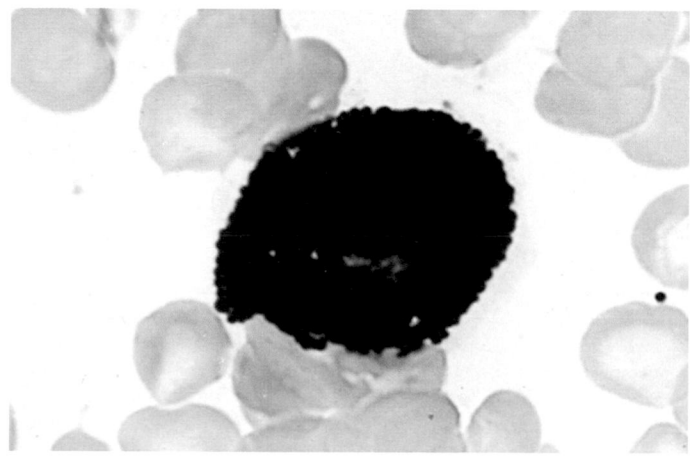

PLATE VII-1, 2, 3, 4 The film was prepared from the buffy coat of the blood from a normal donor. L, lymphocyte; M, monocyte; N, neutrophil; E, eosinophil; B, basophil.

PLATE VII-5 Marrow mast cell.

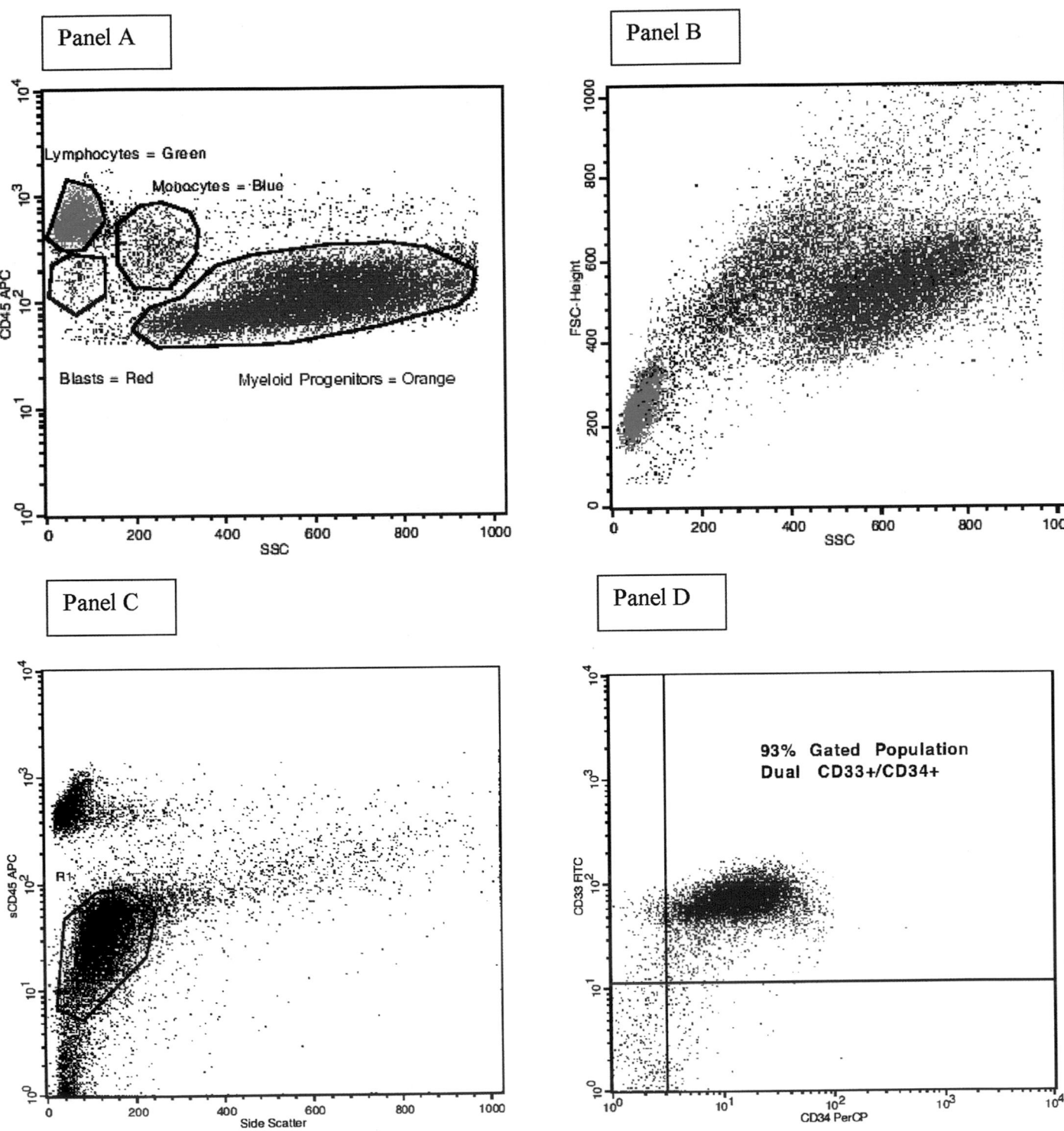

PLATE VII-6   Panels *A* and *B* illustrate the distribution of normal marrow progenitors on CD45 vs side-scatter (SSC) and forward angle (FSC) vs SSC histograms. Identical populations are illustrated in the same colors. Note that many of the populations distinguished as single populations on CD45 vs SSC show considerable overlap when displayed on light scatter alone. This is particularly true for the immature precursor ("blast") population, shown in red. Panels *C* and *D* illustrate the utility of CD45 based gating in isolating the blast population in a myeloid leukemia. Panel *C* shows the ungated data on CD45 vs side-scatter, indicating the population to be gated in for phenotypic analysis ("R1"). Panel *D* illustrates the staining pattern for the gated R1 population (red) when examined for expression of the myeloid marker CD33 and the early progenitor marker CD34. The phenotype is clearly CD34+/CD33+, consistent with myeloid leukemia. Additional markers would be studied to confirm this conclusion. (See Chap. 3, "Examination of the Marrow.")

PLATE VIII
GRANULOCYTE MORPHOLOGY

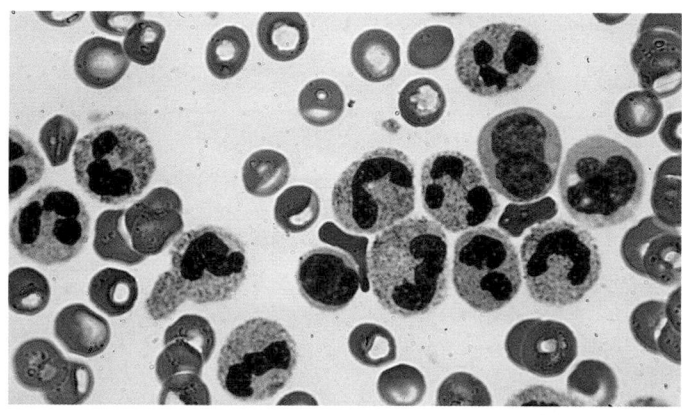

PLATE VIII-1   Extreme neutrophilia (leukemoid reaction). Most cells are band and segmented neutrophils. Two monocytes and a lymphocyte are also in the field.

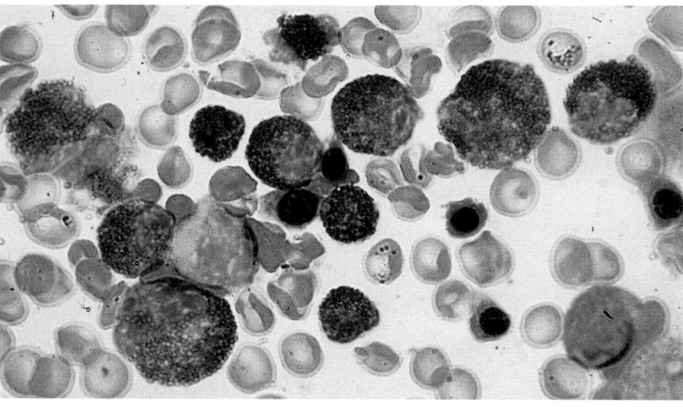

PLATE VIII-2   Hypereosinophilic syndrome. Intense marrow eosinophilia. Eosinophilic myelocytes and segmented forms.

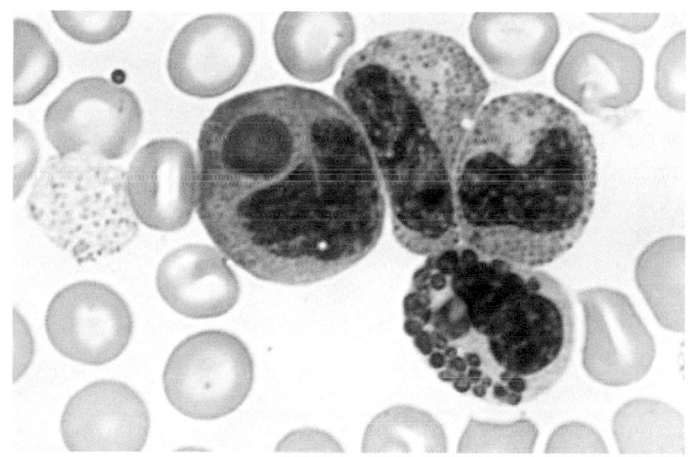

PLATE VIII-3   Chédiak-Higashi disease. Note monstrous granule in monocyte and giant granules in band neutrophil.

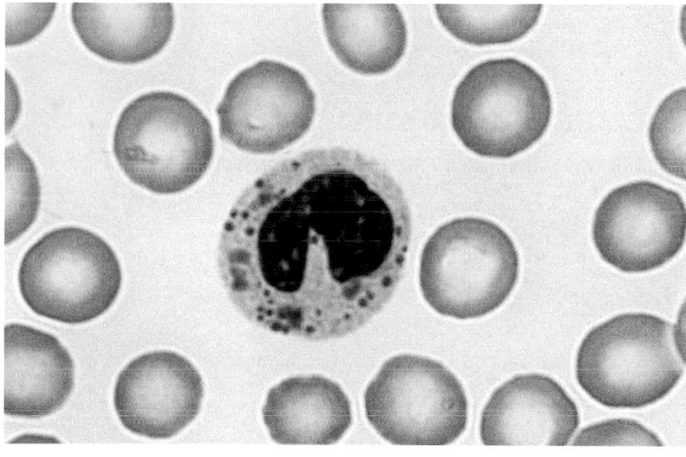

PLATE VIII-4   Chédiak-Higashi disease. Note giant granules in neutrophil.

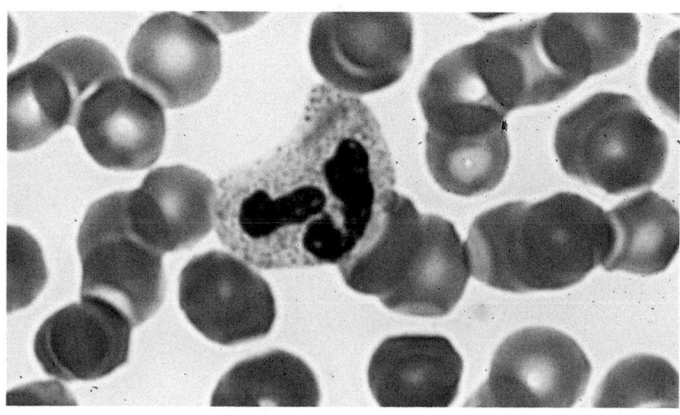

PLATE VIII-5   May-Hegglin anomaly. Note violaceous Döhle-body-like inclusion.

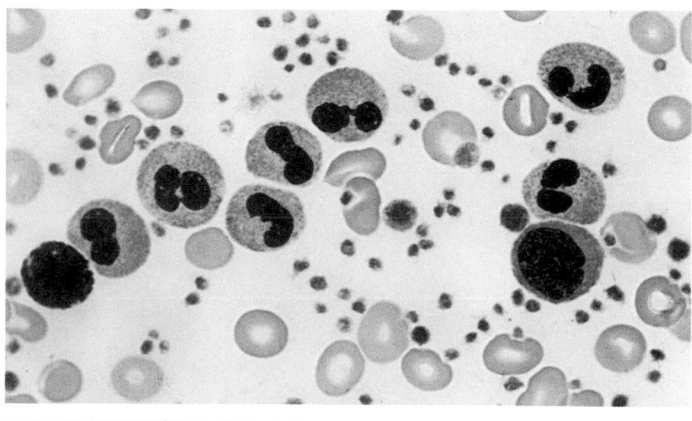

PLATE VIII-6   Heterozygote for the Pelger-Huët anomaly of leukocyte nuclei. Bilobed (pince-nez shape) nuclei (buffy coat).

(VIII-1, VIII-3 through VIII-6 are blood films.)

PLATE IX
MACROPHAGES

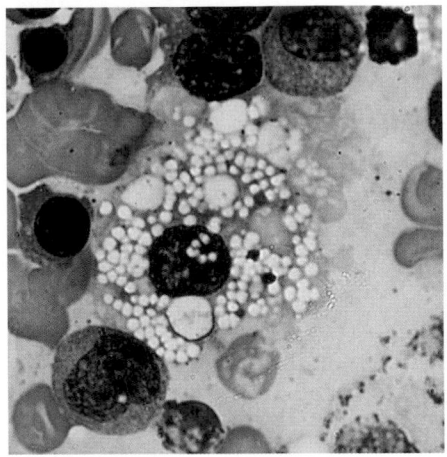

PLATE IX-1   Active macrophage.

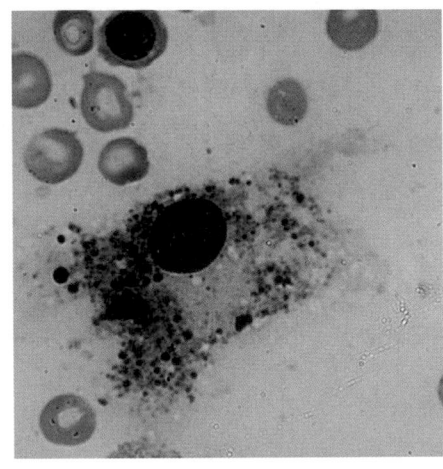

PLATE IX-2   Macrophage with iron particles. Wright stain.

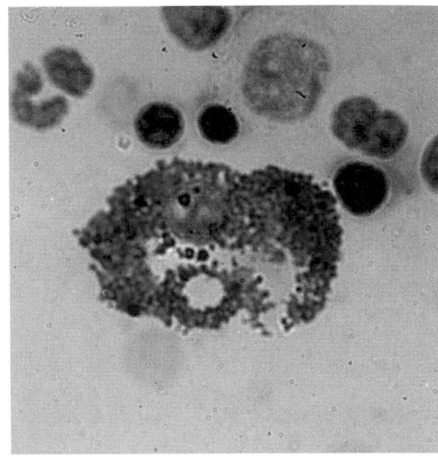

PLATE IX-3   Macrophage with iron particles. Prussian blue stain.

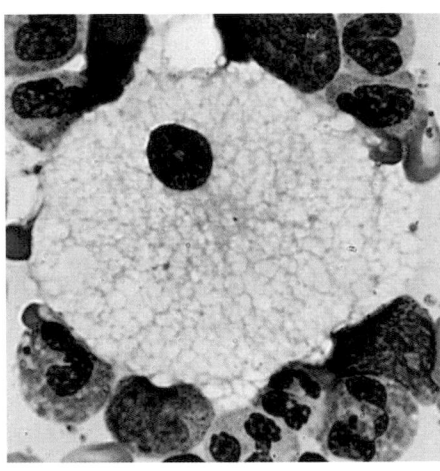

PLATE IX-4   Niemann-Pick cell.

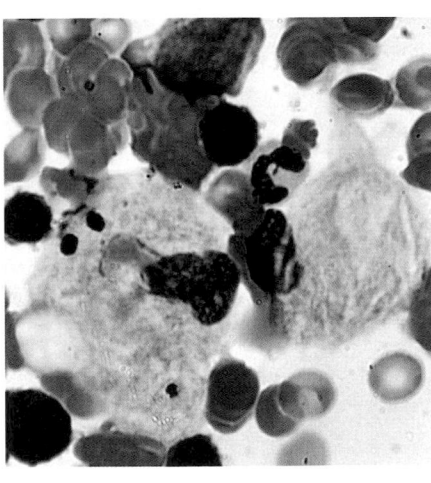

PLATE IX-5   Gaucher cells in the adult form of the disease.

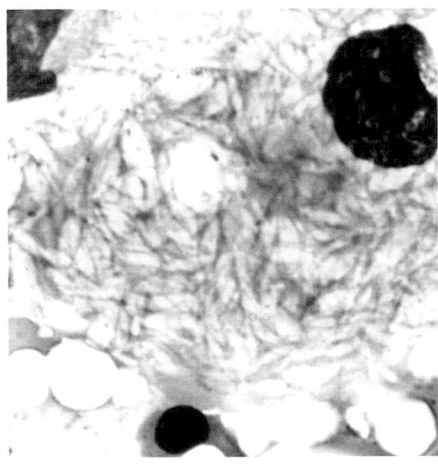

PLATE IX-6   Pseudo-Gaucher cells in a patient with chronic myelogenous leukemia.

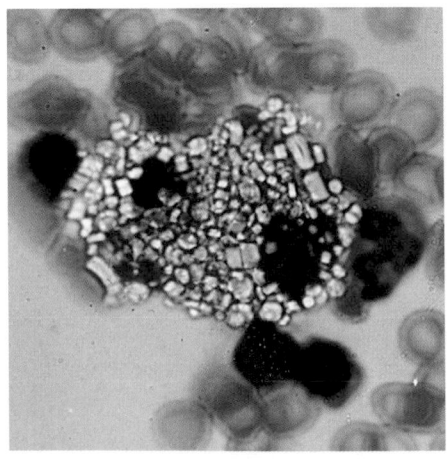

PLATE IX-7   Macrophage engorged with cystine crystals.

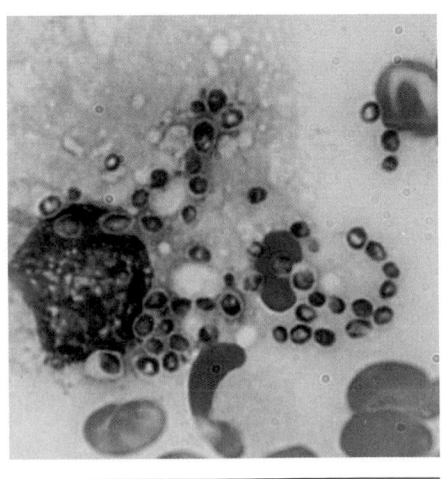

PLATE IX-8   Macrophage containing *Histoplasma capsulatum*.

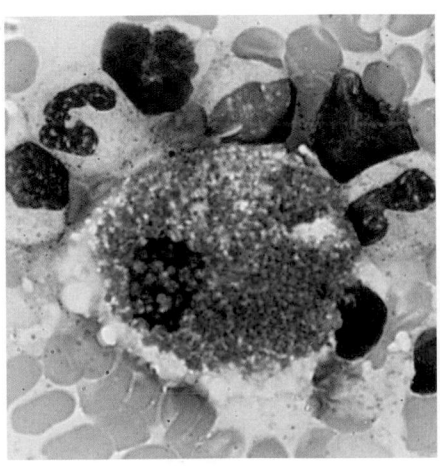

PLATE IX-9   Macrophage in sea blue histiocytosis.

(IX-1 through IX-9 are marrow macrophages.)

P L A T E   X
NORMAL NEUTROPHILOPOIESIS

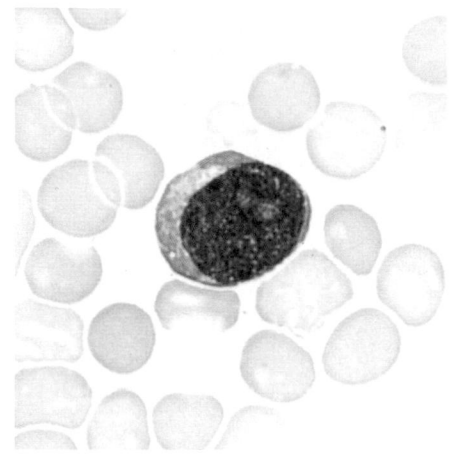

PLATE X-1   Myeloblast.

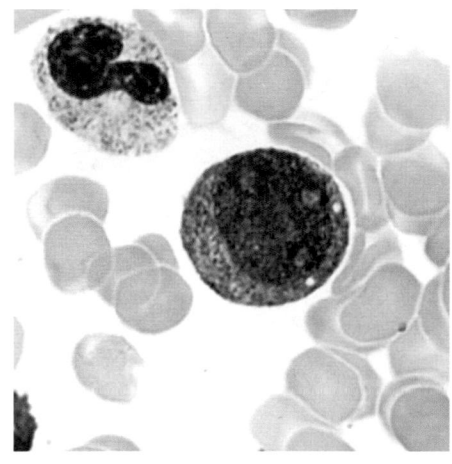

PLATE X-2   Promyelocyte.

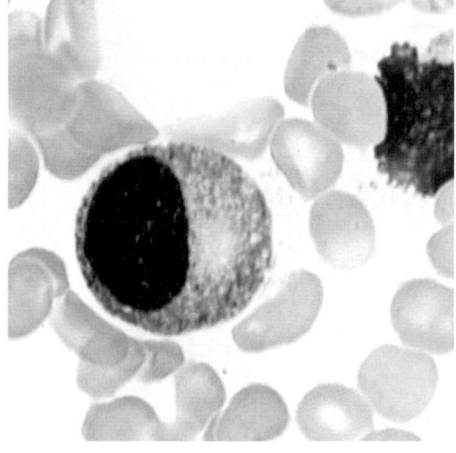

PLATE X-3   Early neutrophilic myelocyte.

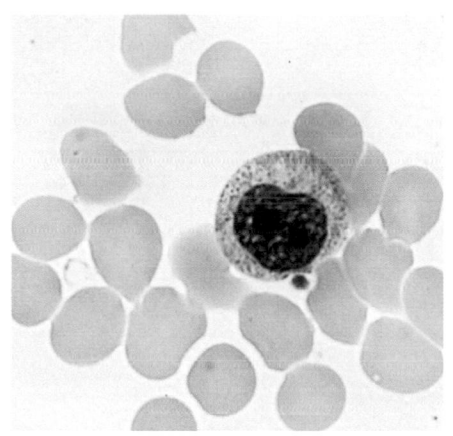

PLATE X-4   Late neutrophilic myelocyte.

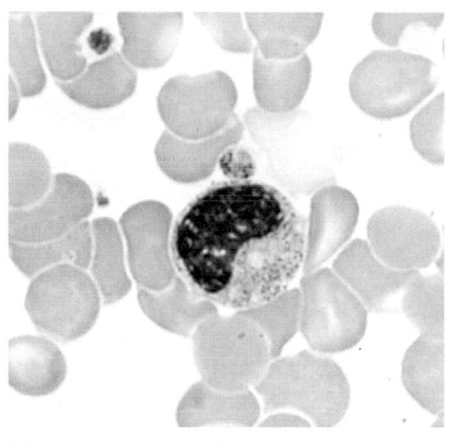

PLATE X-5   Neutrophilic metamyelocyte.

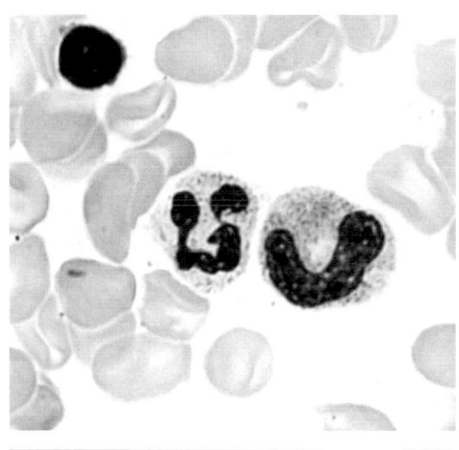

PLATE X-6   Band and segmented neutrophils.

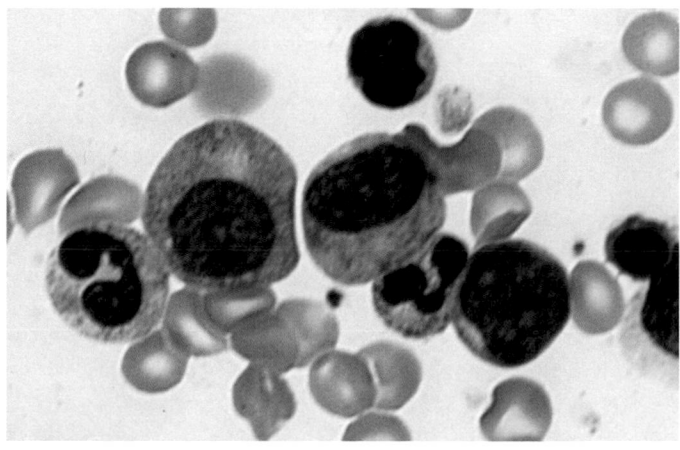

PLATE X-7   Myeloblast, early myelocytes, band and segmented neutrophils.

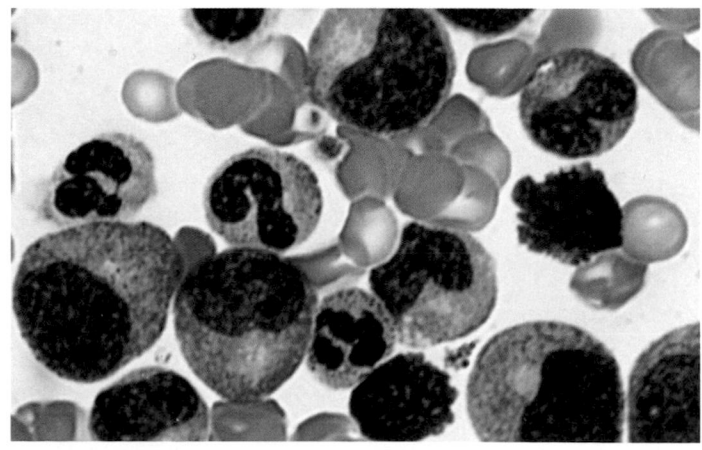

PLATE X-8   Promyelocyte, early myelocytes, metamyelocytes, band and segmented neutrophils.

(X-1 through X-8 are marrow films.)

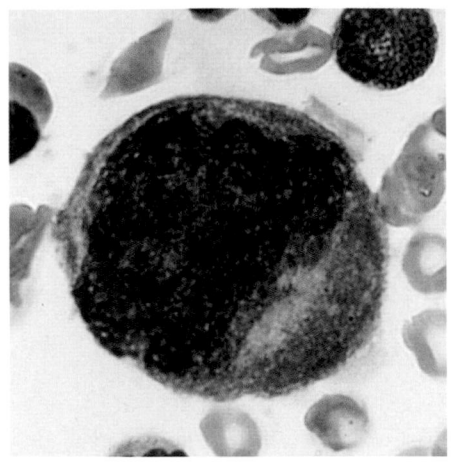

PLATE XI-1   Immature megakaryocyte.

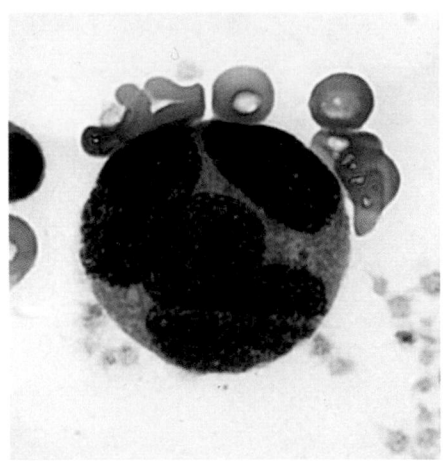

PLATE XI-2   Immature megakaryocyte.

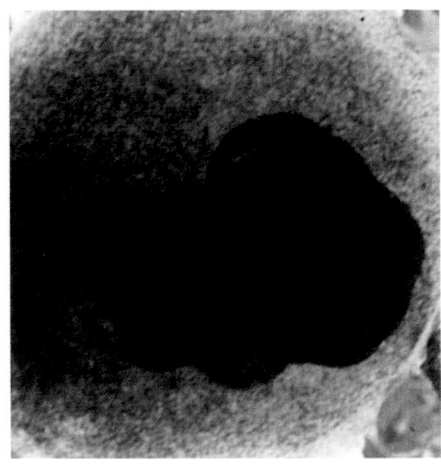

PLATE XI-3   Mature megakaryocyte.

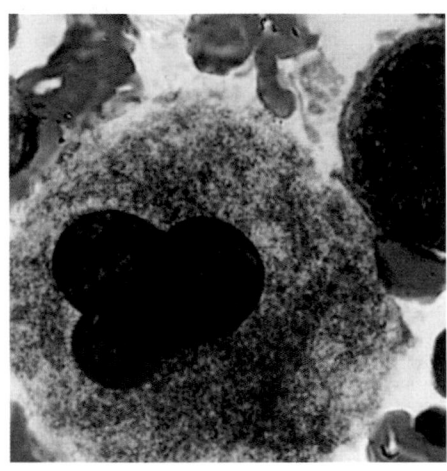

PLATE XI-4   Mature megakaryocyte.

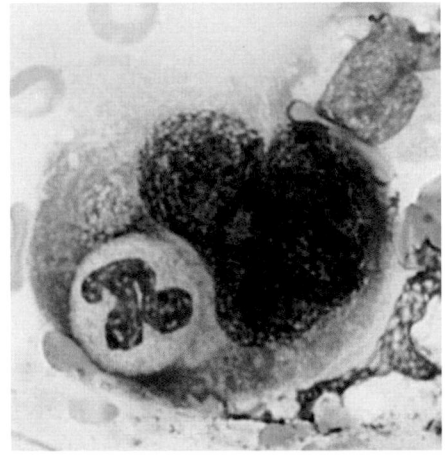

PLATE XI-5   Emperipolesis, the migration of a neutrophil into the canalicular system of megakaryocyte cytoplasm.

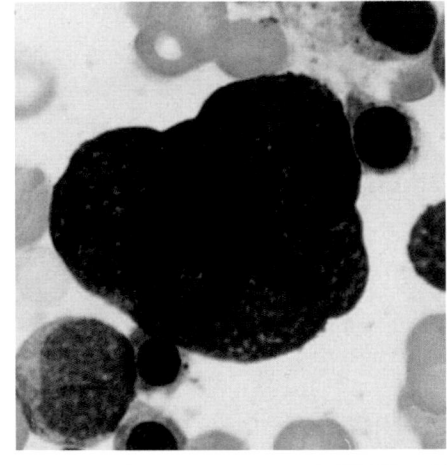

PLATE XI-6   The residue of a megakaryocyte nucleus.

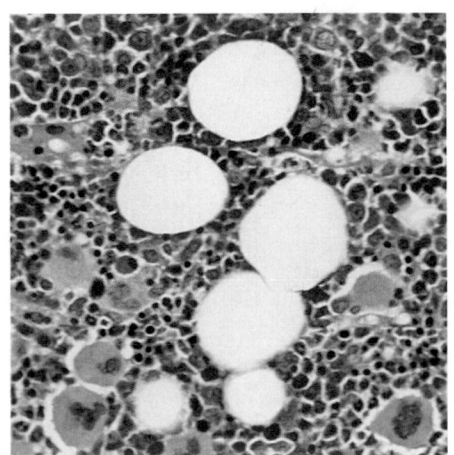

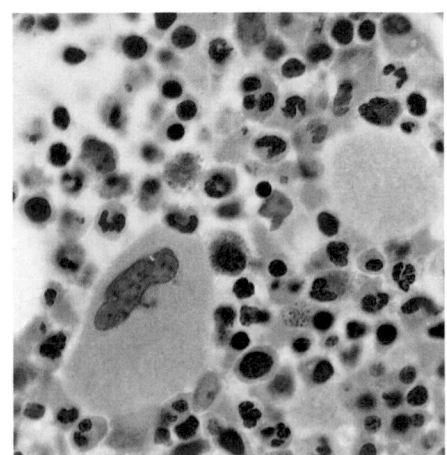

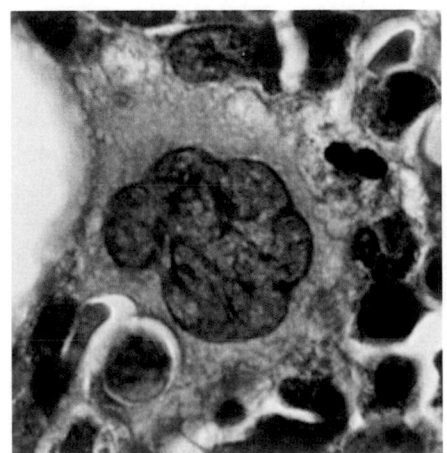

PLATE XI-7, 8, 9   Marrow biopsies demonstrating megakaryocytes.

(XI-1 through XI-6 are marrow films.)

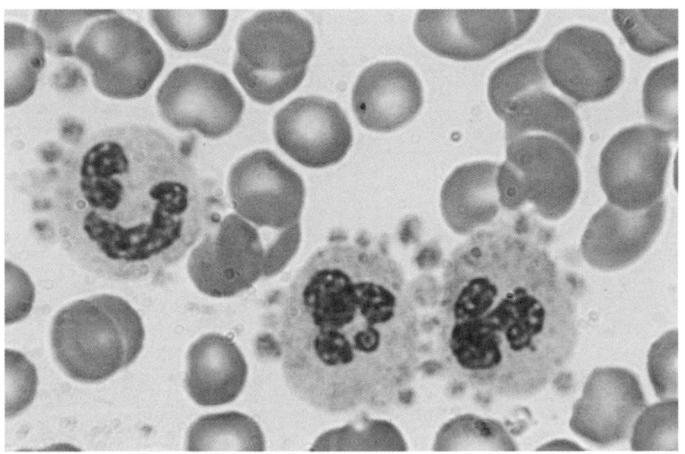

PLATE XII-1   Platelet satellitism.

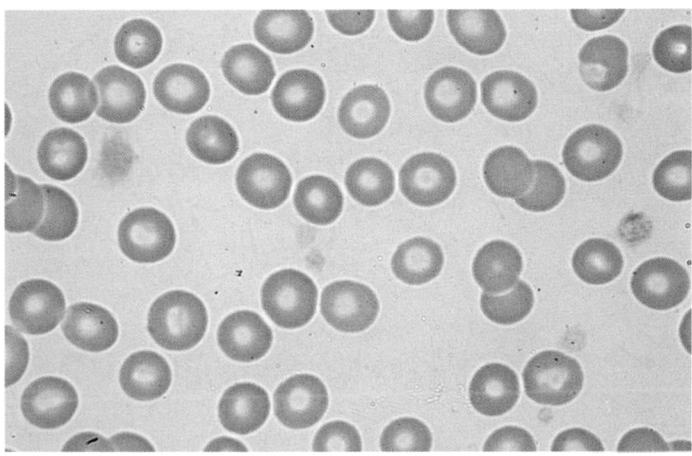

PLATE XII-2   Gray platelet syndrome.

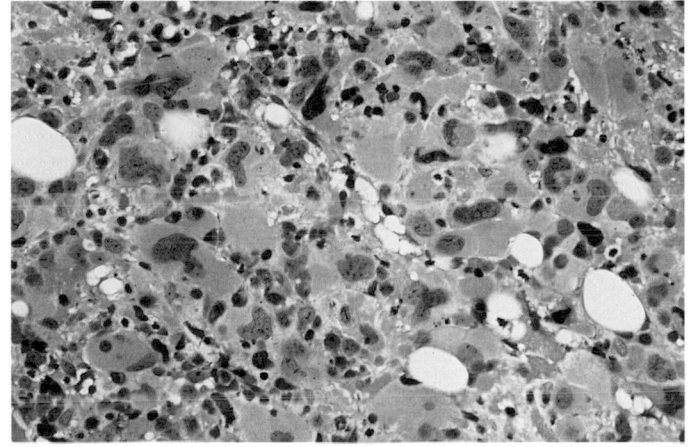

PLATE XII-3   Acute megakaryocytic leukemia. Marrow section.

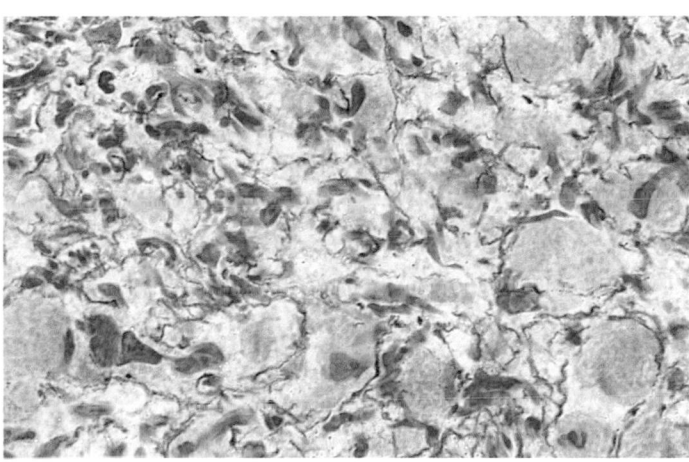

PLATE XII-4   Acute megakaryocytic leukemia. Marrow section. Silver stain demonstrating increased reticulin fibers.

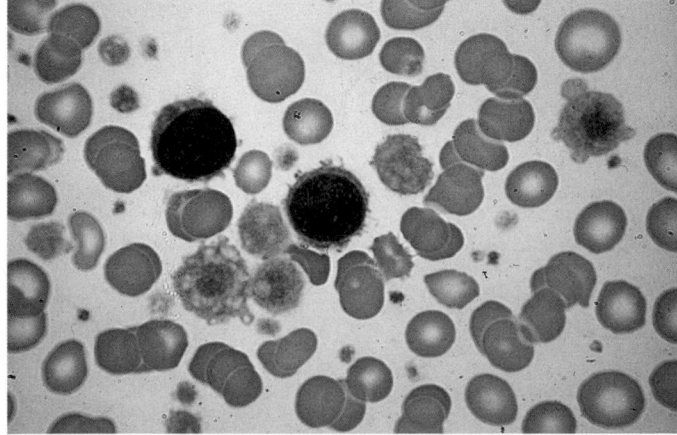

PLATE XII-5   Idiopathic myelofibrosis (agnogenic myeloid metaplasia) and probable megakaryocytic leukemic conversion. Dwarfed megakaryocyte and enormous platelets (megakaryocytic cytoplasmic fragments). Post-splenectomy.

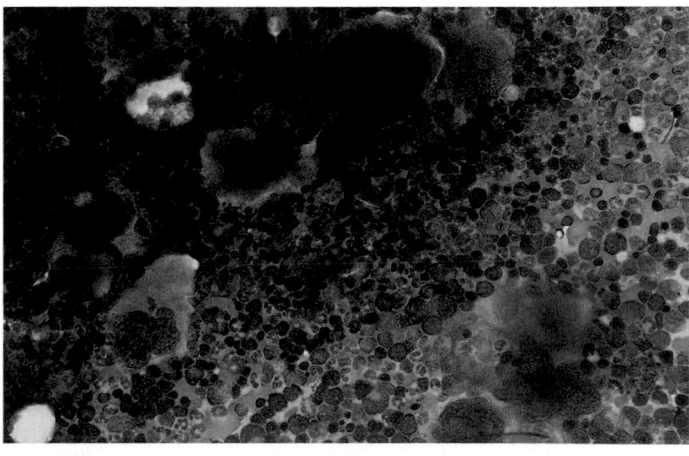

PLATE XII-6   Essential thrombocythemia. Marrow film. Marked increase in megakaryocytes.

(XII-1, XII-2, and XII-5 are blood films.)

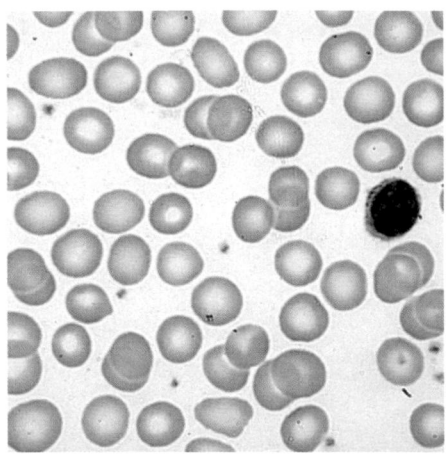

PLATE XIII-1   Normal platelets.

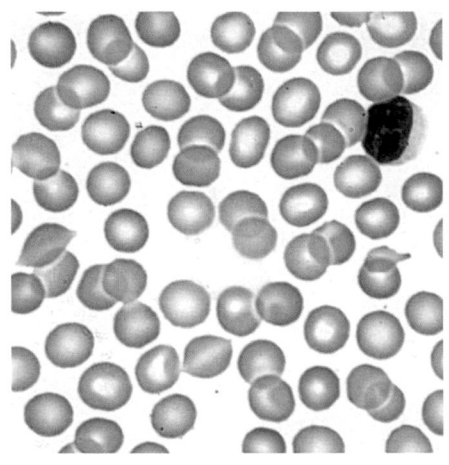

PLATE XIII-2   Severe thrombocytopenia. Absence of platelets in this field.

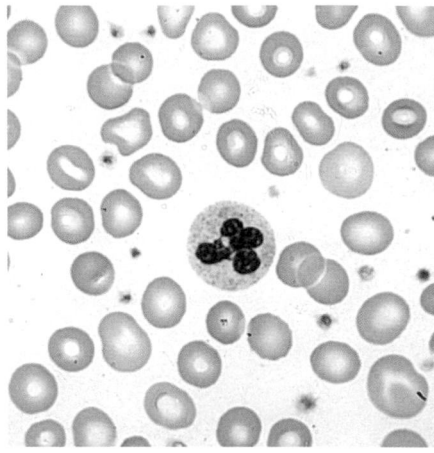

PLATE XIII-3   Marked increase in platelets. Some increase in platelet size. (Compare to normal platelets).

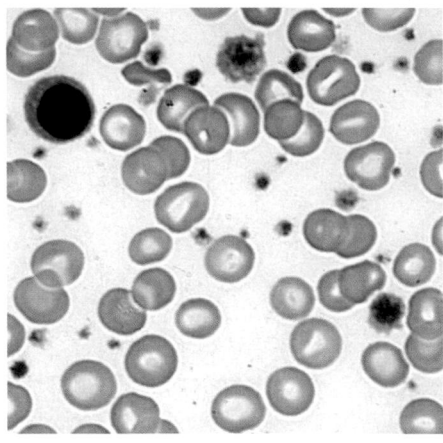

PLATE XIII-4   Thrombocythemia. Increased number and size of platelets. Two are approximately the area of red cells. A lymphocyte is also in the field.

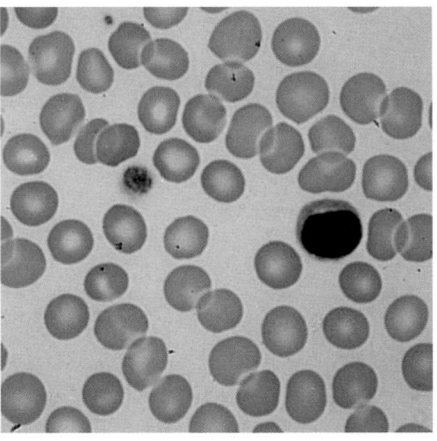

PLATE XIII-5   Giant platelets (megathrombocyte).

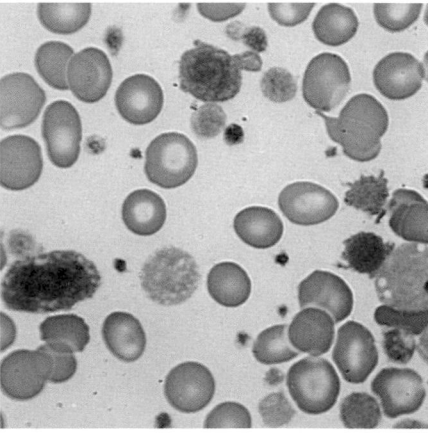

PLATE XIII-6   Giant platelets as large or larger than red cells (megakaryocyte cytoplasmic fragments). All of the blue- and gray-staining elements in the field are platelets.

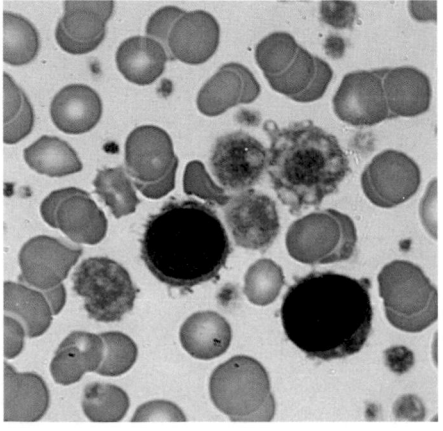

PLATE XIII-7   Two dwarf megakaryocytes with cytoplasmic blebs. Megakaryocyte cytoplasmic fragments and giant platelets.

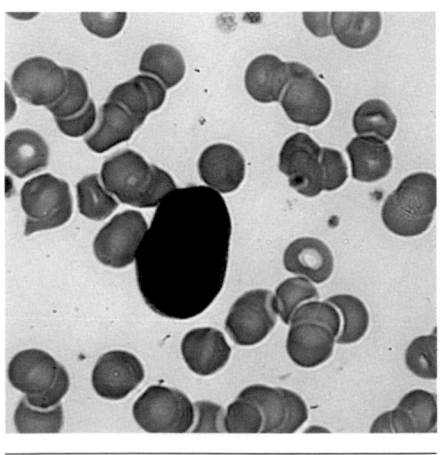

PLATE XIII-8   Megakaryocyte nucleus.

(XIII-1 through XIII-8 are blood films.)

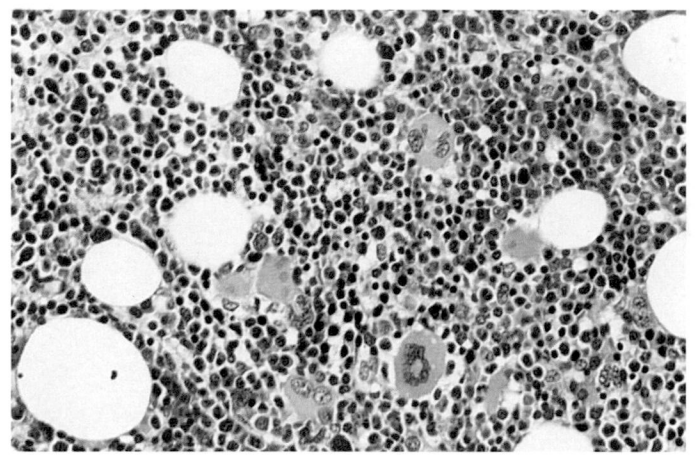

PLATE XIV-1   Normal.

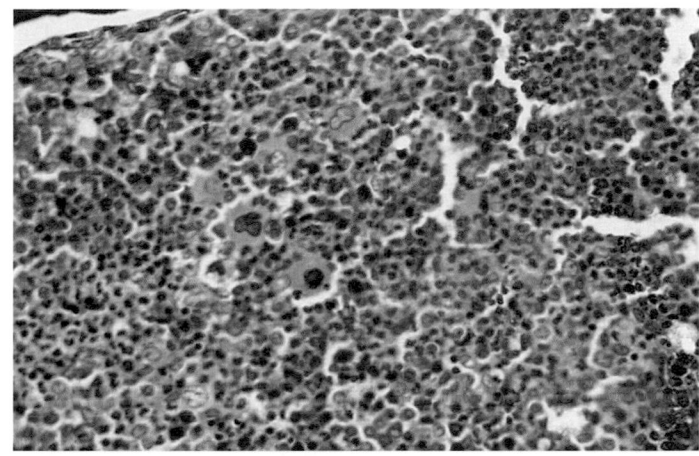

PLATE XIV-2   Hypercellular.

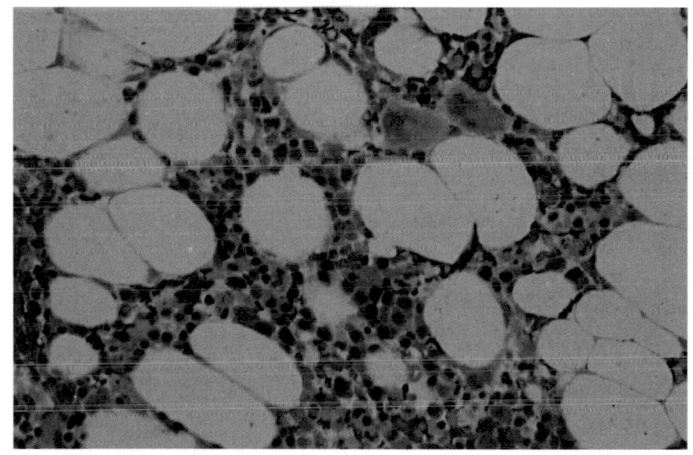

PLATE XIV-3   Hypocellular.

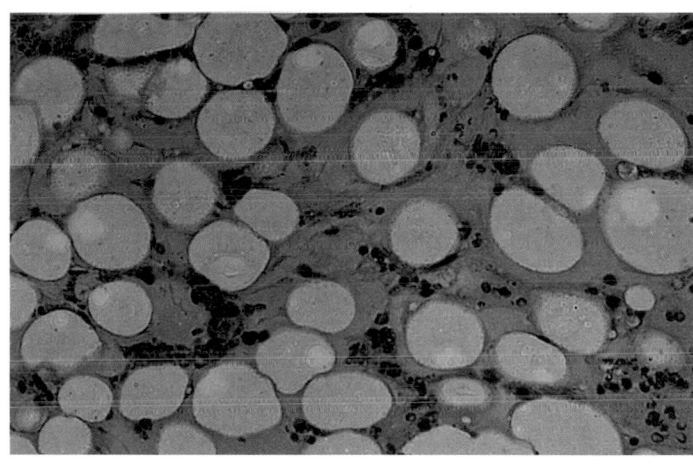

PLATE XIV-4   Aplasia.

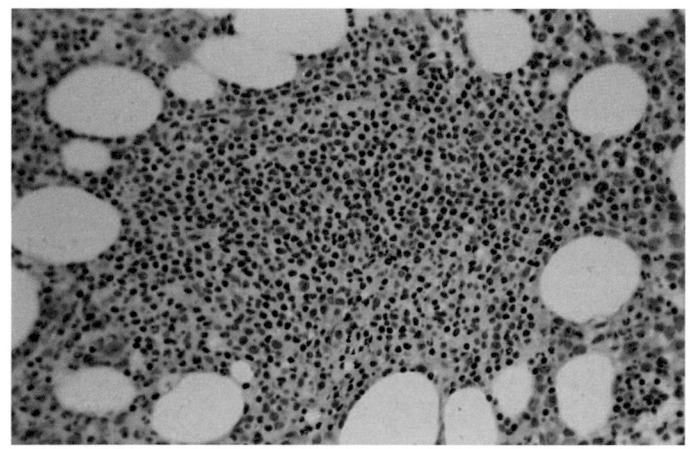

PLATE XIV-5   Lymphoid aggregate: Uncertain significance.

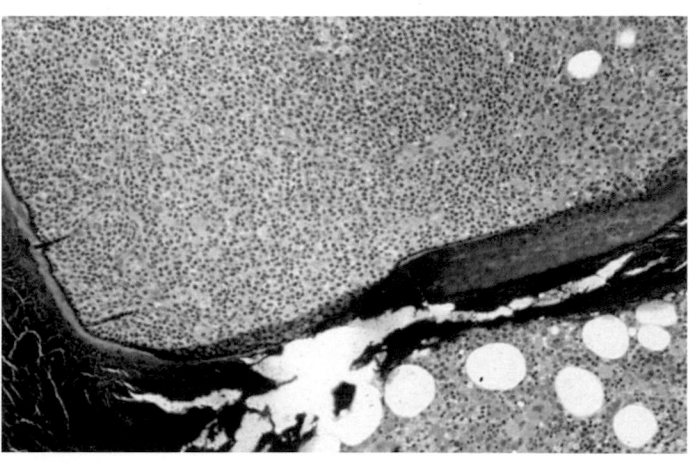

PLATE XIV-6   Lymphoma in marrow: Note paratrabecular location.

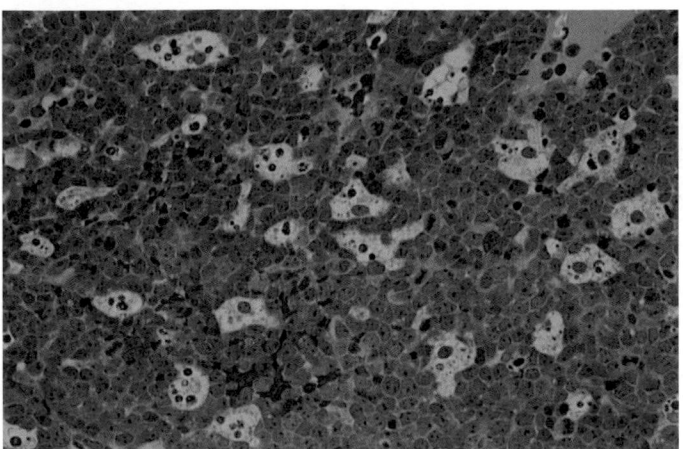

PLATE XIV-7   Burkitt lymphoma: Note the starry sky appearance as a result of the interspersed macrophages.

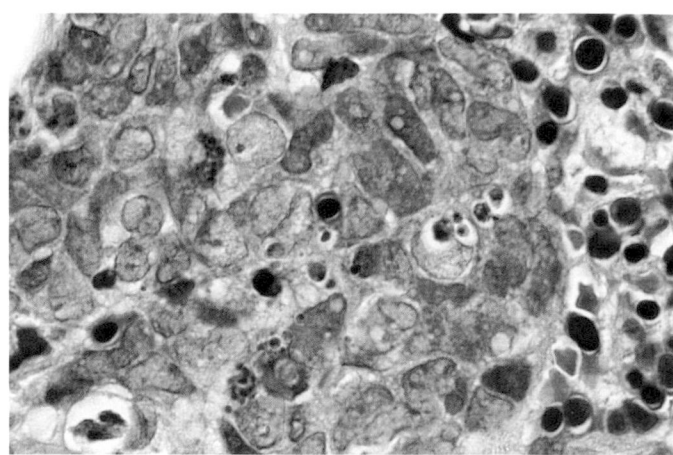

PLATE XIV-8   Metastatic carcinoma.

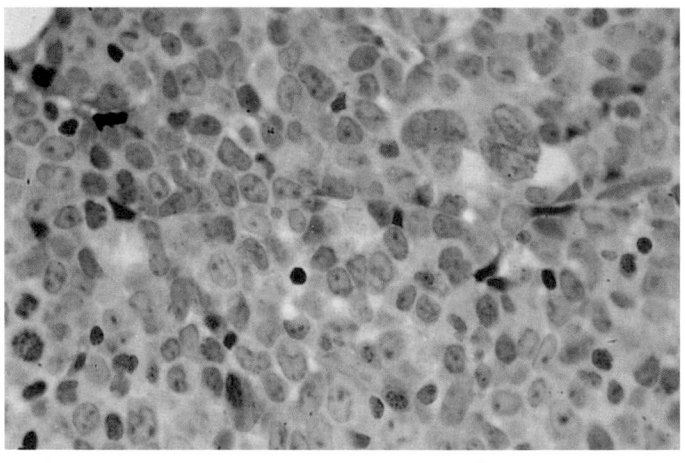

PLATE XIV-9   Acute myelogenous leukemia.

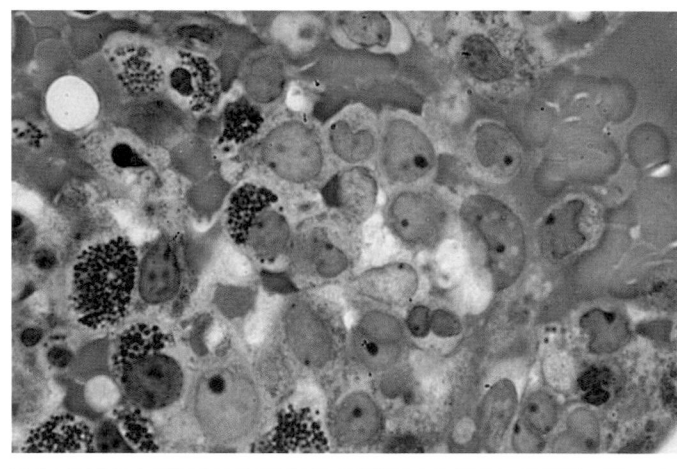

PLATE XIV-10   Acute myelogenous leukemia with marked increase in eosinophils.

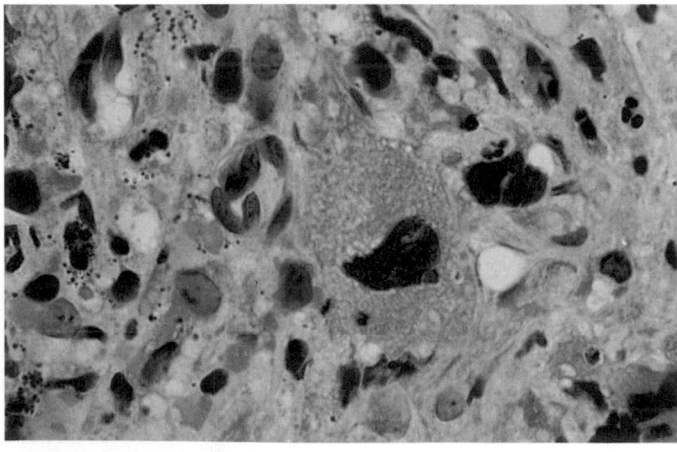

PLATE XIV-11   Myelofibrosis: Increased numbers of megakaryocytes and decreased marrow cellularity.

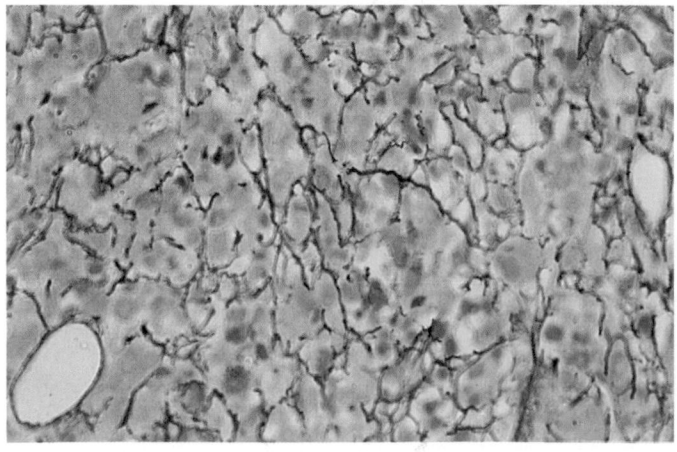

PLATE XIV-12   Myelofibrosis: Silver stain showing increased reticulin.

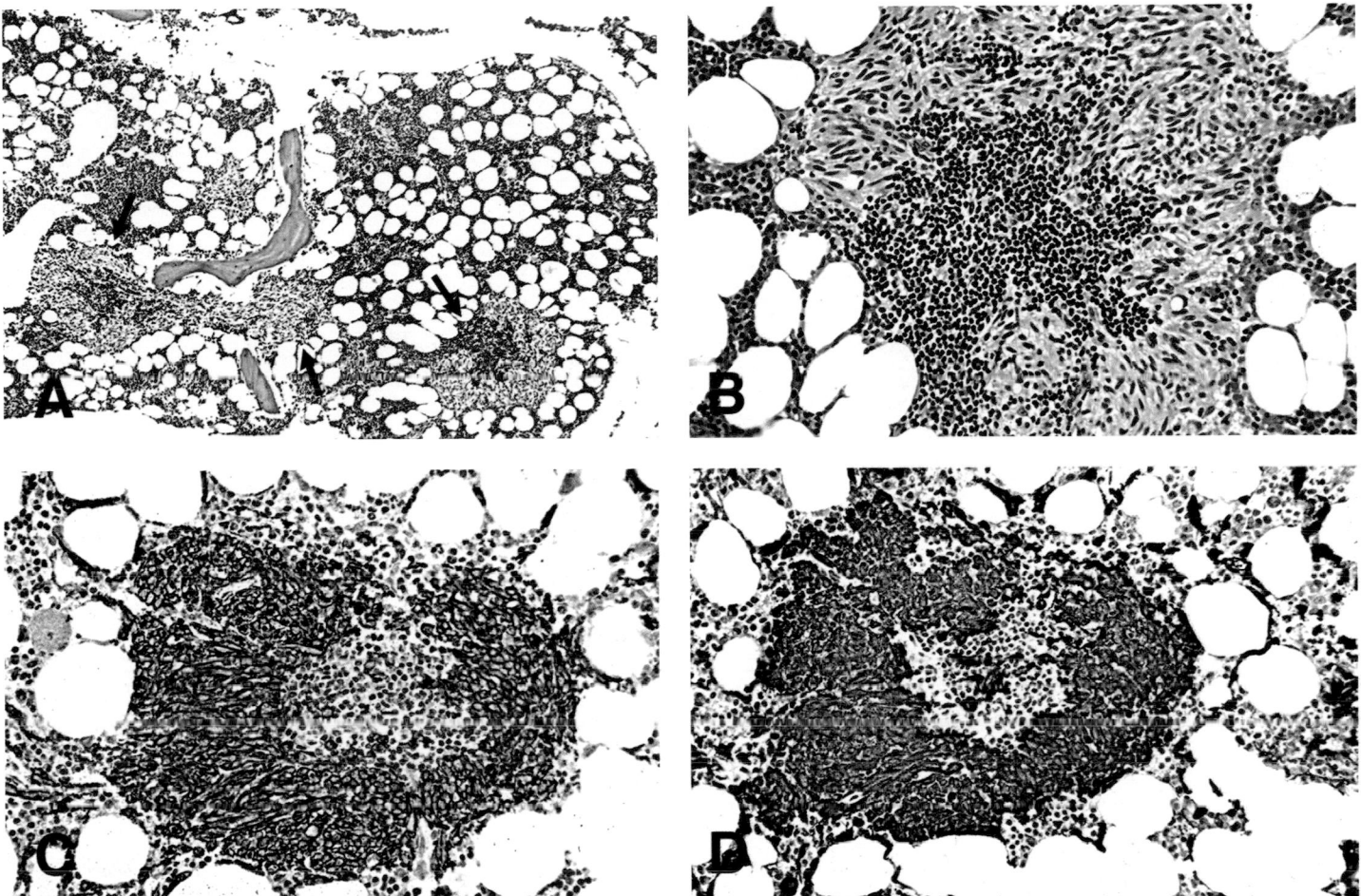

PLATE XIV-13   Bone marrow biopsy from an adult with indolent systemic mastocytosis showing characteristic focal aggregates of mast cells, some of which are spindle-shaped, with admixed eosinophils and numerous small lymphocytes; different areas of the specimen were stained by H&E (A, B; 40× and 200×, respectively) or with an antibody to human CD117 (C; 200×) or tryptase (D; 200×). Areas that contain many mast cells are depicted with arrows in A. (See Chapter 63, "Basophils and Mast Cells and Their Disorders.")

(XIV-1 through XIV-13 are marrow biopsies.)

PLATE XV
NON-HEMATOPOIETIC CELLS IN MARROW

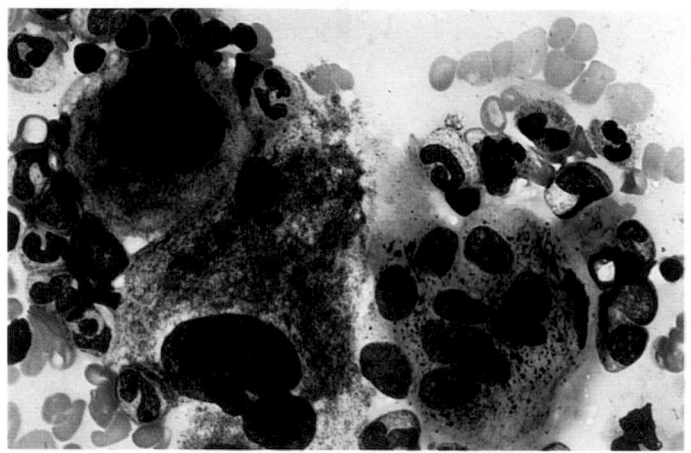

PLATE XV-1   Osteoclast. Note non-overlapping of multiple nuclei.

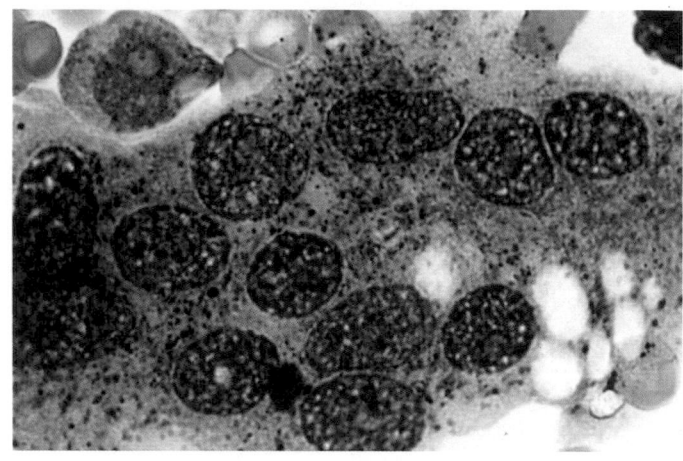

PLATE XV-2   Higher magnification of an osteoclast.

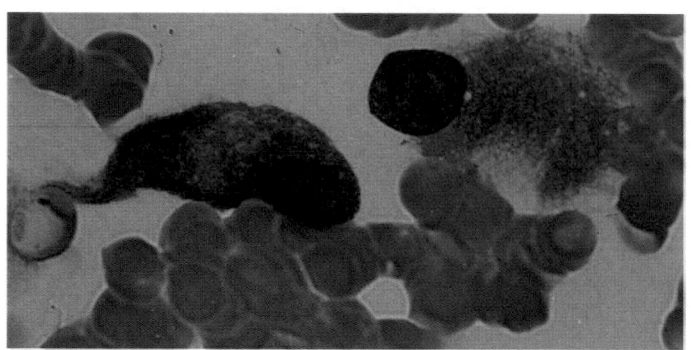

PLATE XV-3   Osteoblasts with typical elongated oval cell shape and extremely eccentric single nucleus.

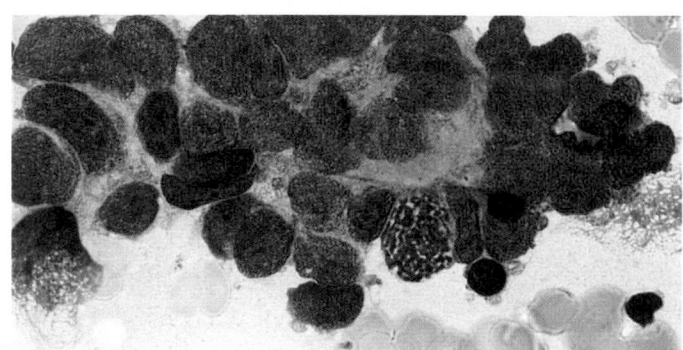

PLATE XV-4   Aggregate of metastatic lung carcinoma cells.

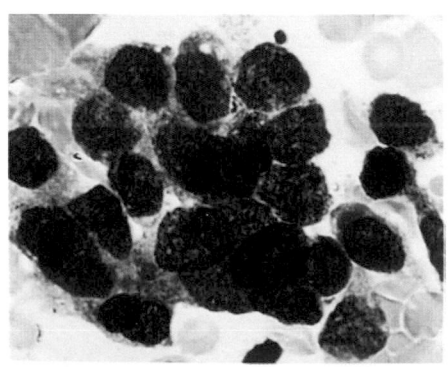

PLATE XV-5   Aggregate of metastatic prostate carcinoma cells.

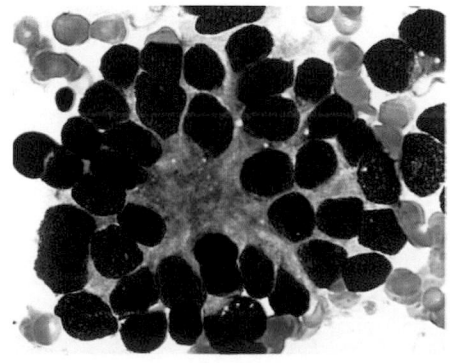

PLATE XV-6   Metastatic neuroblastoma cells: Note the characteristic rosette appearance.

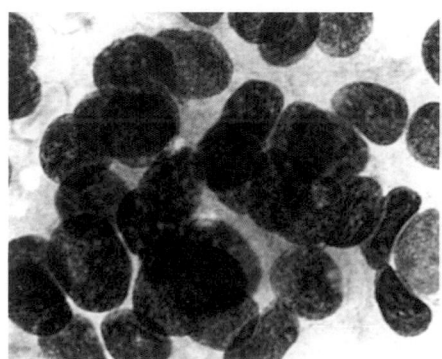

PLATE XV-7   Metastatic breast carcinoma cells.

(XV-1 through XV-7 are marrow films.)

P L A T E   X V I
ACUTE MYELOGENOUS LEUKEMIA

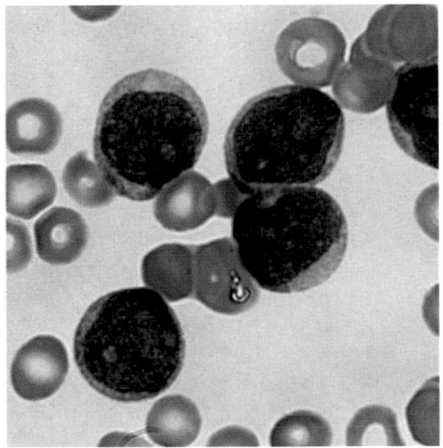

PLATE XVI-1   Leukemic myeloblasts.

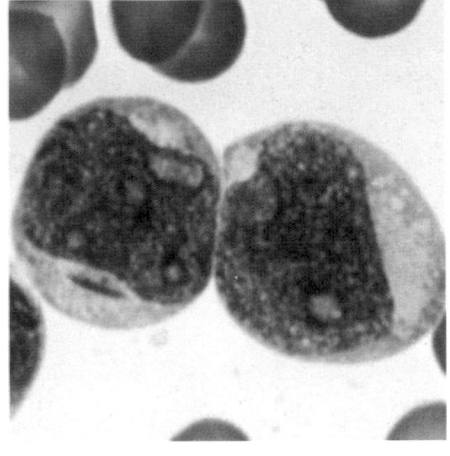

PLATE XVI-2   Leukemic myeloblast with an Auer rod. Note two to four large, prominent nucleoli in each cell.

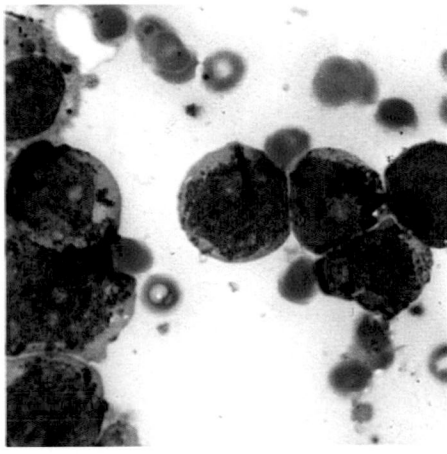

PLATE XVI-3   Leukemic myeloblasts stained with peroxidase: Note the staining of an Auer rod.

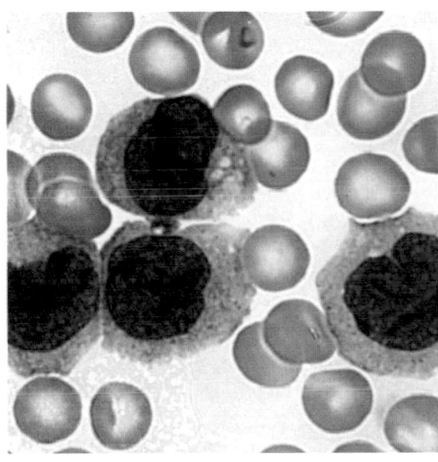

PLATE XVI-4   Leukemic monocytes.

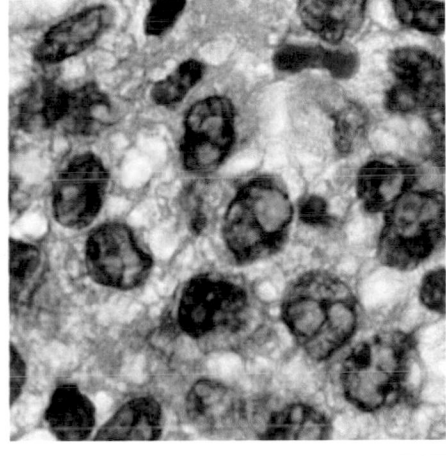

PLATE XVI-5   A skin biopsy showing infiltration of leukemic monocytes.

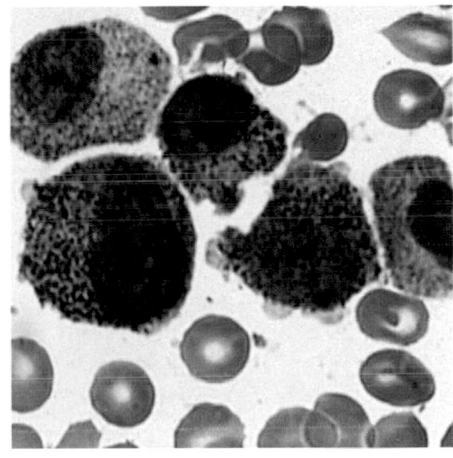

PLATE XVI-6   Leukemic promyelocytes.

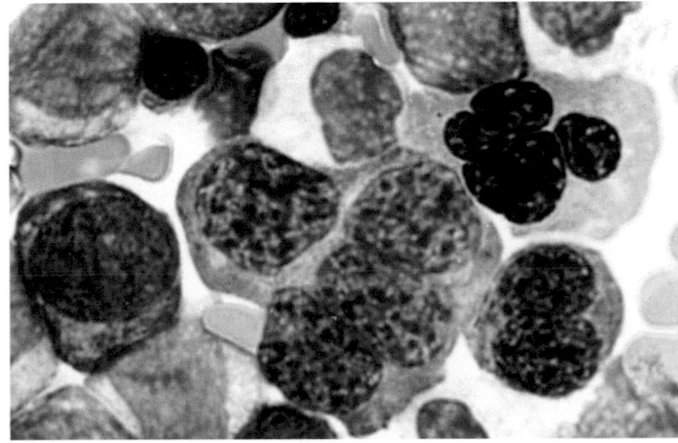

PLATE XVI-7   Erythroleukemia cells. Note giant dysmorphic erythroblasts, two are binucleate and one is multinucleate.

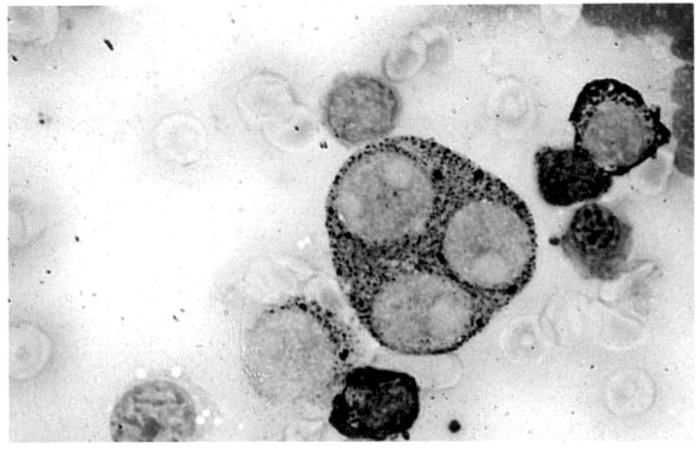

PLATE XVI-8   Erythroleukemia cells stained with periodic acid-Schiff.

(XVI-1 through XVI-8 are marrow films.)

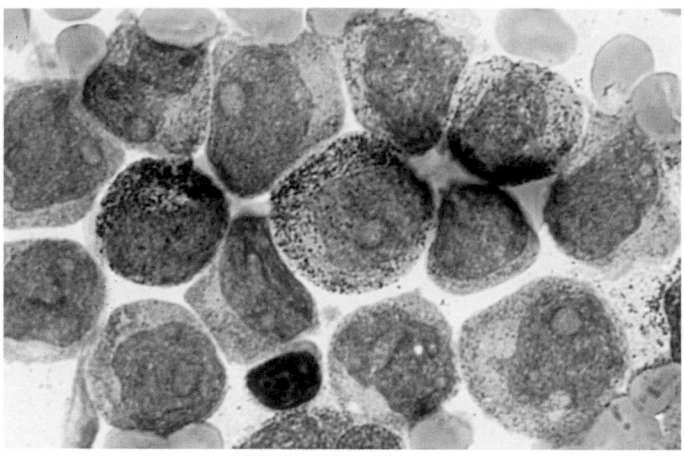

PLATE XVII-1   Acute promyelocytic leukemia. Marrow film. Predominance of promyelocytes, many with large nucleoli.

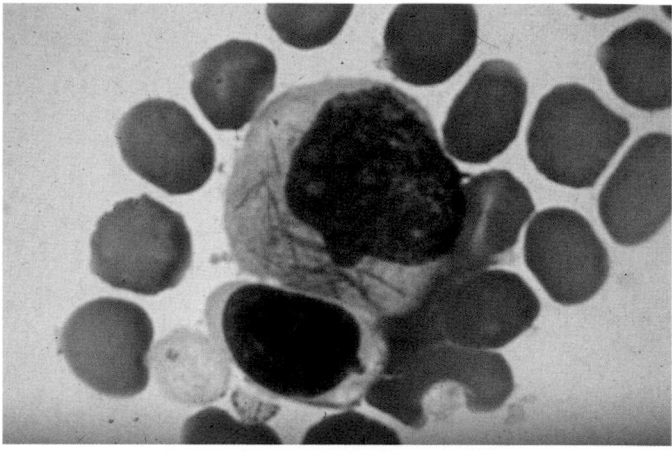

PLATE XVII-2   Acute promyelocytic leukemia. Marrow film. Multiple Auer rods in leukemic cell.

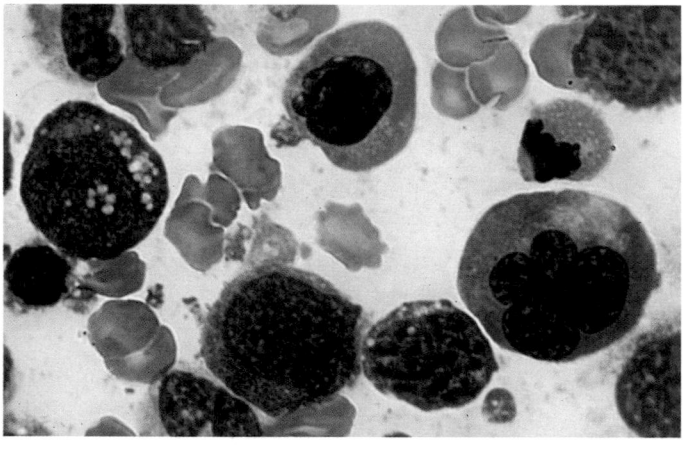

PLATE XVII-3   Acute erythroid leukemia. Marrow film. Large erythroblasts with bizarre nuclear morphology.

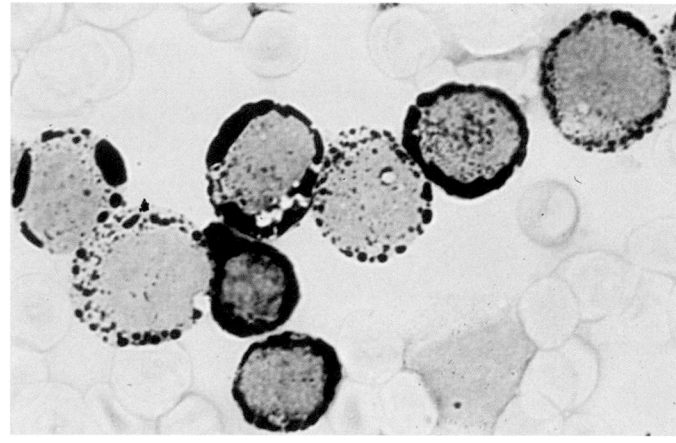

PLATE XVII-4   Acute erythroid leukemia. Marrow film stained with periodic acid Schiff reagent. Intense PAS-positive staining of leukemic erythroblasts.

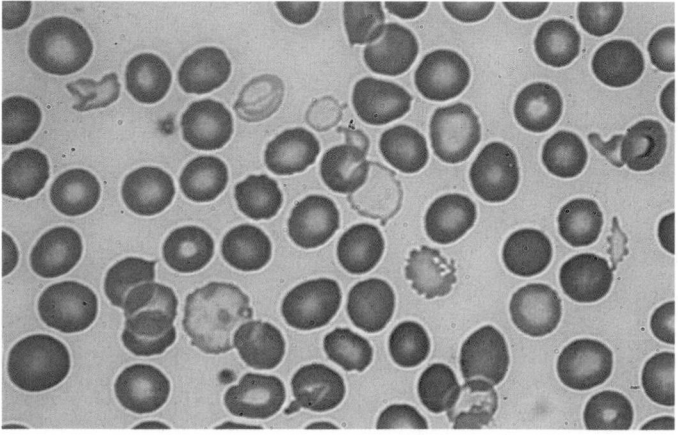

PLATE XVII-5   Acute erythroid leukemia. Blood film. Striking anisochromia and poikilocytosis. Some red cells are so poorly hemoglobinized that they mimic red cell ghosts.

MYELODYSPLASIA

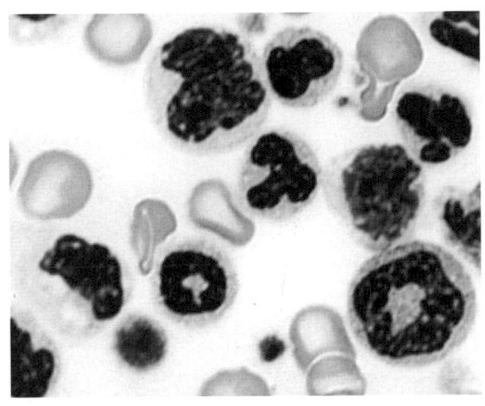

PLATE XVIII-1   Erythrocyte abnormalities: Anisocytosis, poikilocytosis, anisochromia.

PLATE XVIII-2   Buffy coat showing neutrophil abnormalities including ringed nuclei, hyperdense nuclear pattern, and decreased nuclear segmentation.

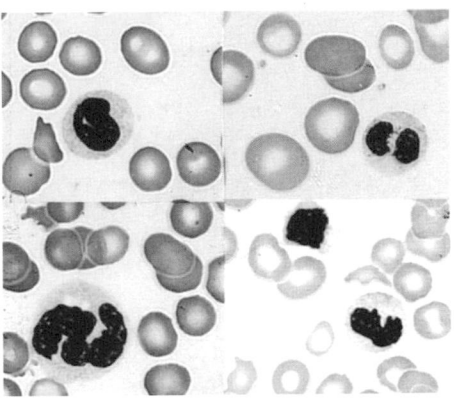

PLATE XVIII-3   Hyposegmented neutrophil nuclei (acquired Pelger-Hüet abnormality). Note pince-nez shape in upper right image.

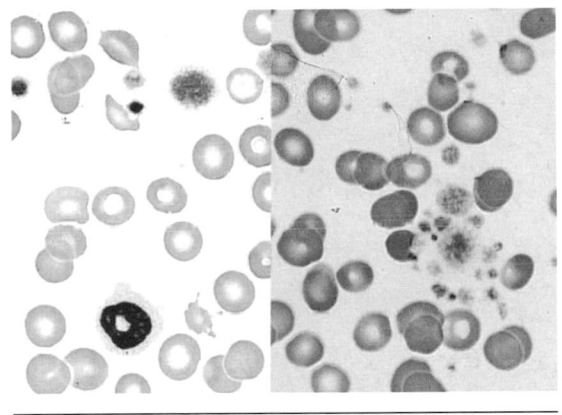

PLATE XVIII-4   Giant platelets, red cell abnormalities, and neutrophil with ringed nucleus.

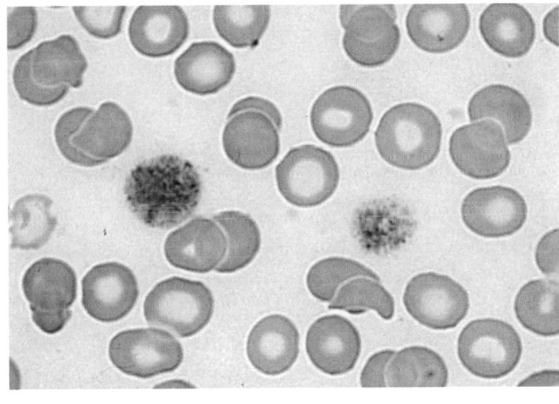

PLATE XVIII-5   Giant, dysmorphic platelets.

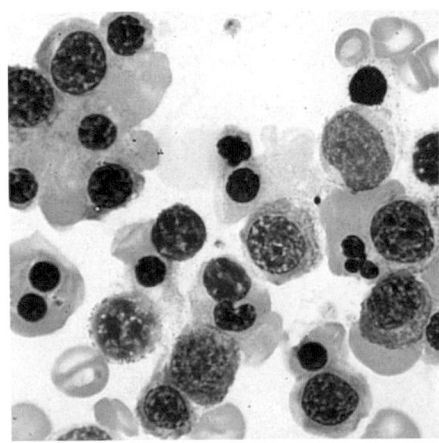

PLATE XVIII-6   Dyserythropoiesis with binucleate and fragmented erythroblastic nuclei, and ineffective erythropoiesis.

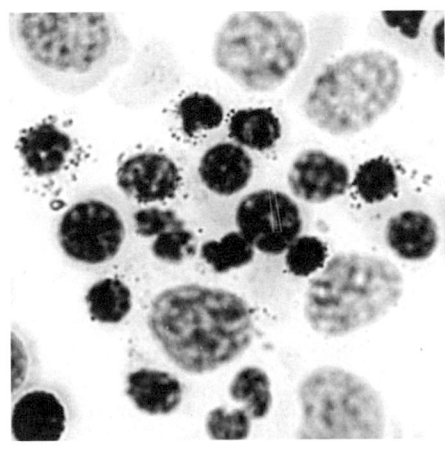

PLATE XVIII-7   Marrow stained with Prussian blue. Pathological sideroblasts showing marked increase in number and size of siderotic granules in erythroblast cytoplasm. Most have siderotic granules in a circumferential pattern around the nucleus (ringed sideroblasts).

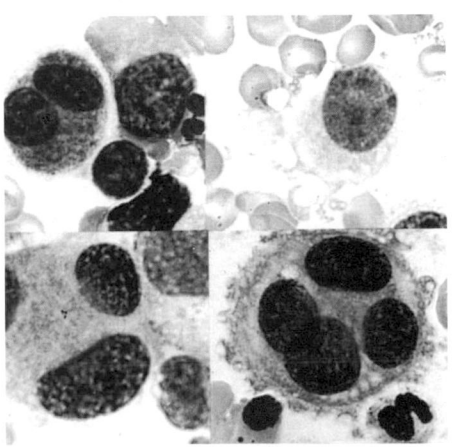

PLATE XVIII-8   Abnormal megakaryocytes.

(XVIII-1, XVII-3 through XVIII-5 are blood films; XVIII-6 through XVIII-8 are marrow films.)

CHRONIC MYELOGENOUS LEUKEMIA

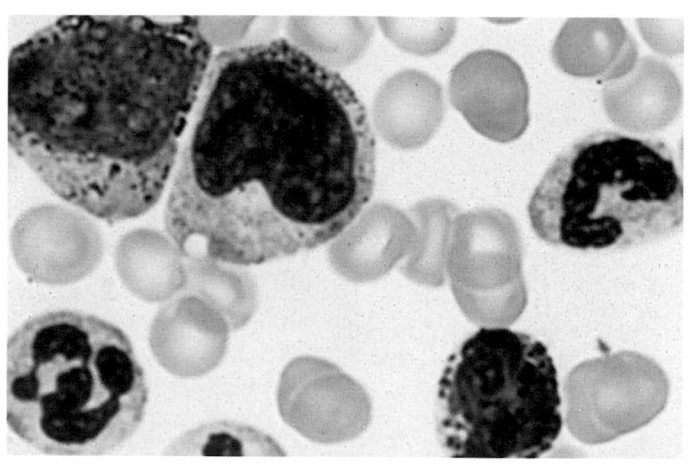

PLATE XIX-1   Myelocytes, neutrophils, and a basophil.

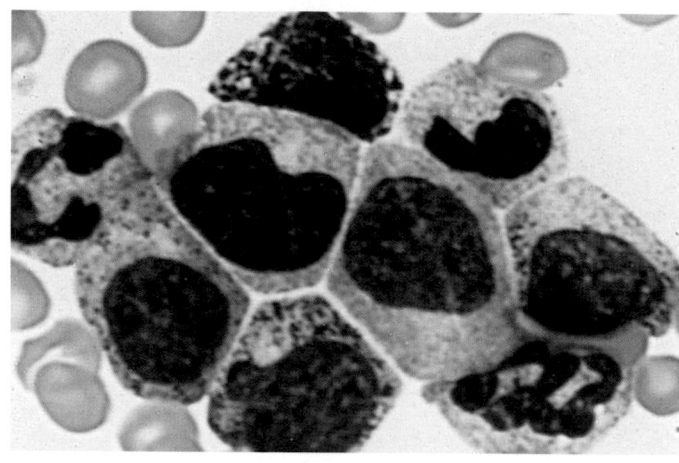

PLATE XIX-2   Myelocytes, neutrophils, and a basophil.

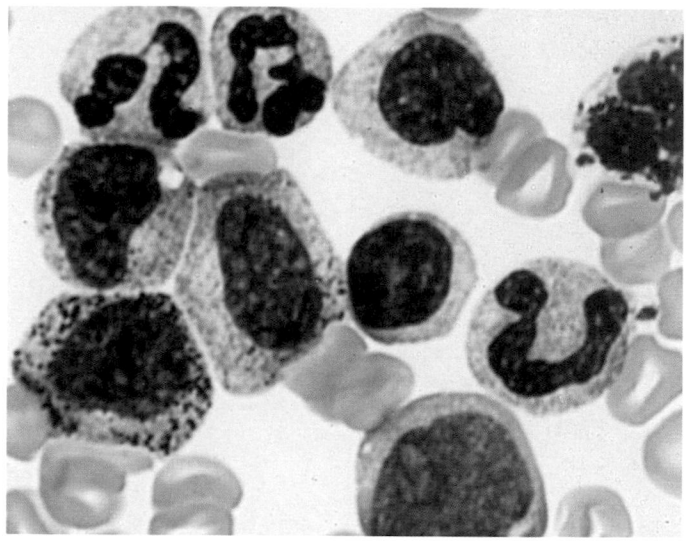

PLATE XIX-3   Myeloblast, myelocytes, and neutrophils.

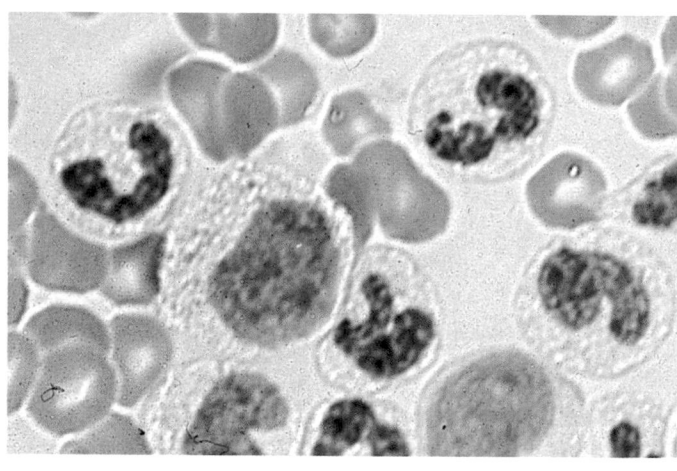

PLATE XIX-4   Absence of leukocyte alkaline phosphatase staining of the neutrophils.

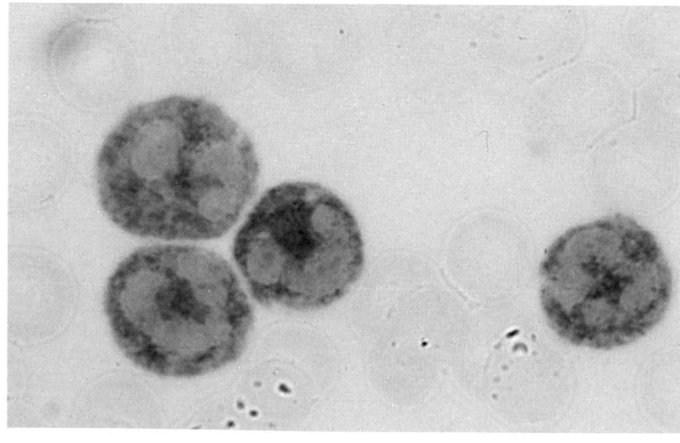

PLATE XIX-5   Leukocyte alkaline phosphatase staining of inflammatory neutrophils.

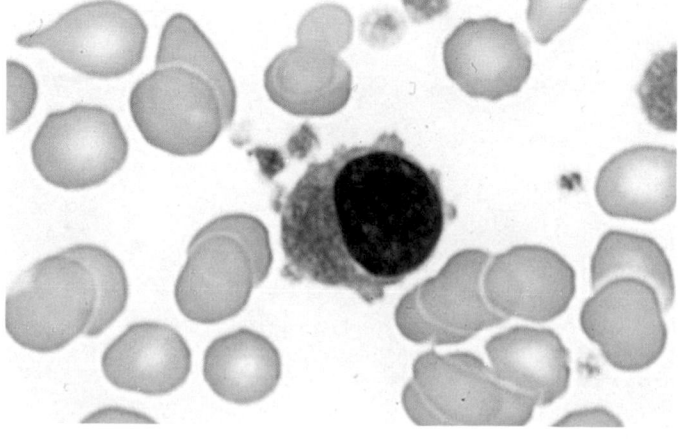

PLATE XIX-6   Micromegakaryocyte in a patient undergoing acute transformation.

(XIX-1 through XIX-6 are blood films.)

PLATE XX
LYMPHOCYTES AND ACUTE AND CHRONIC LYMPHOCYTIC LEUKEMIA

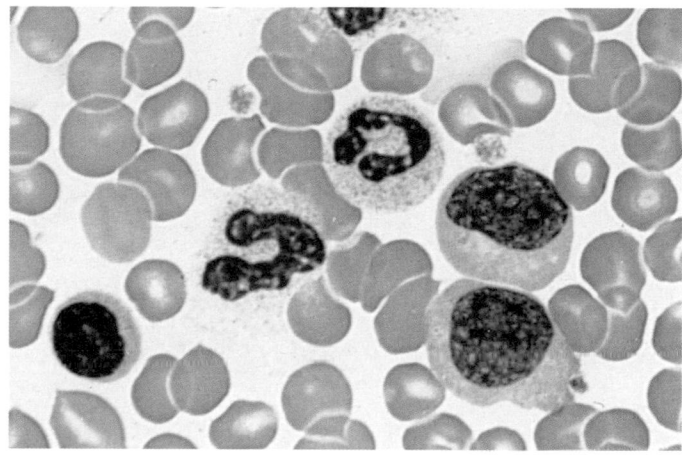

PLATE XX-1   Buffy coat from patient with infectious mononucleosis: Two large reactive lymphocytes.

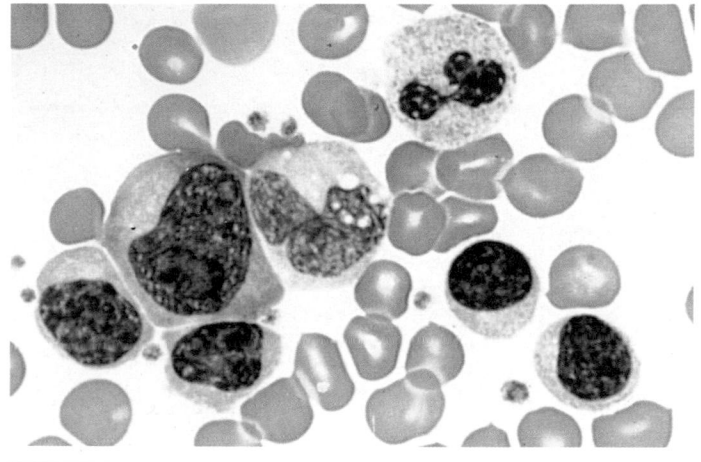

PLATE XX-2   Buffy coat from patient with infectious mononucleosis: Reactive lymphocytes, plasmacytoid lymphocytes, and monocyte.

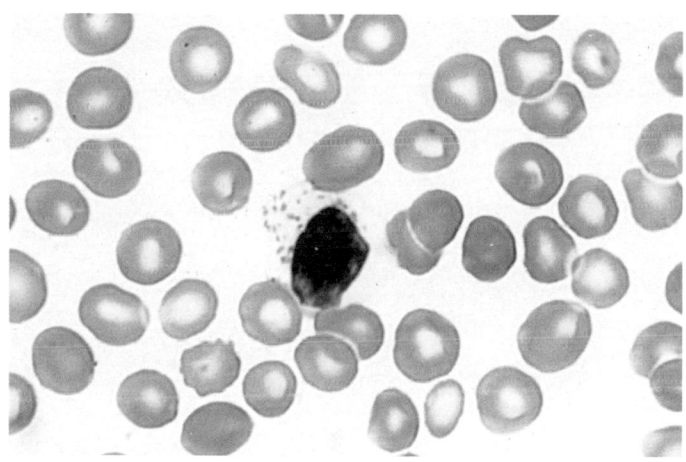

PLATE XX-3   Large granular lymphocyte.

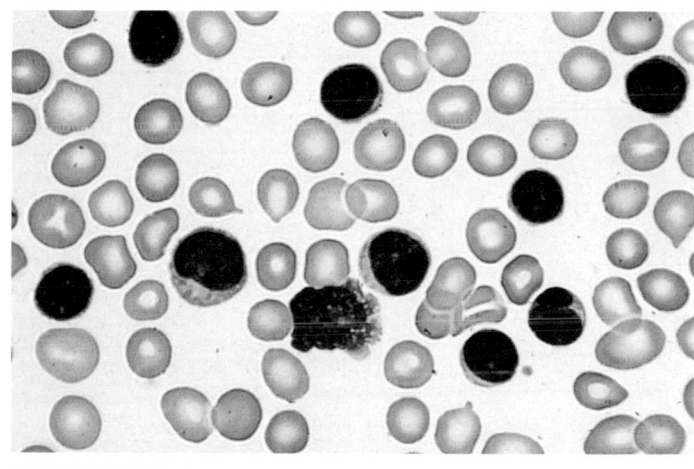

PLATE XX-4   Chronic lymphocytic leukemia.

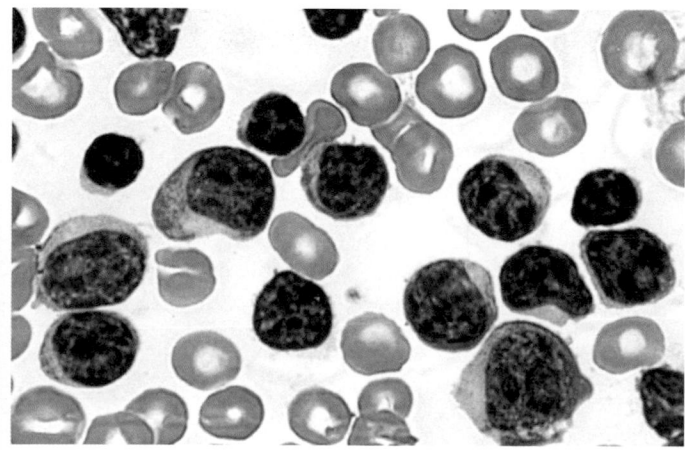

PLATE XX-5   Chronic lymphocytic leukemia.

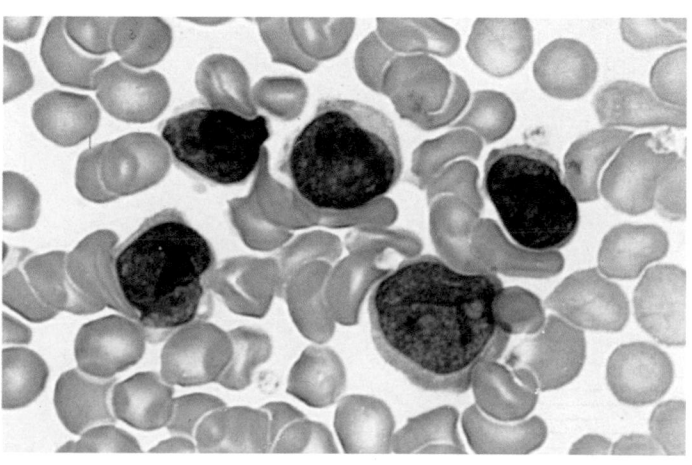

PLATE XX-6   Sézary cell leukemia. Note clefts and folds in nuclei.

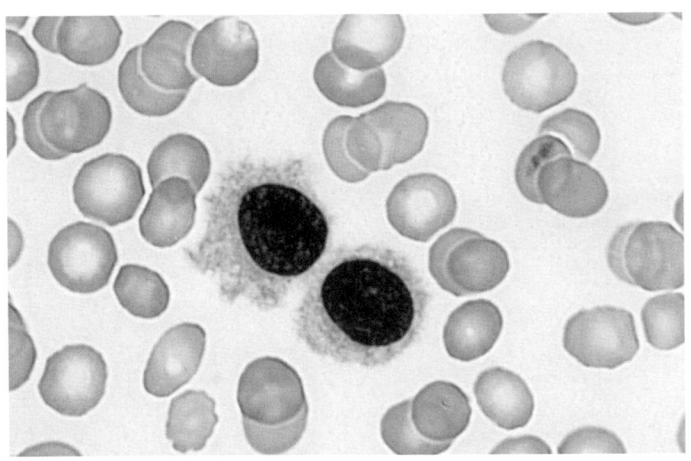

PLATE XX-7   Hairy cell leukemia.

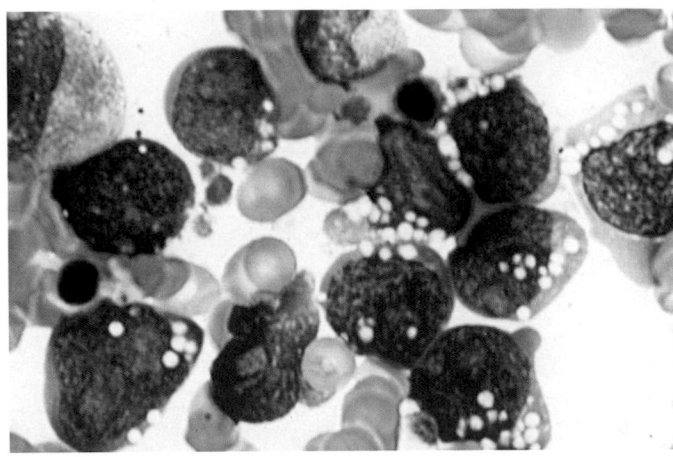

PLATE XX-8   Burkitt cell leukemia.

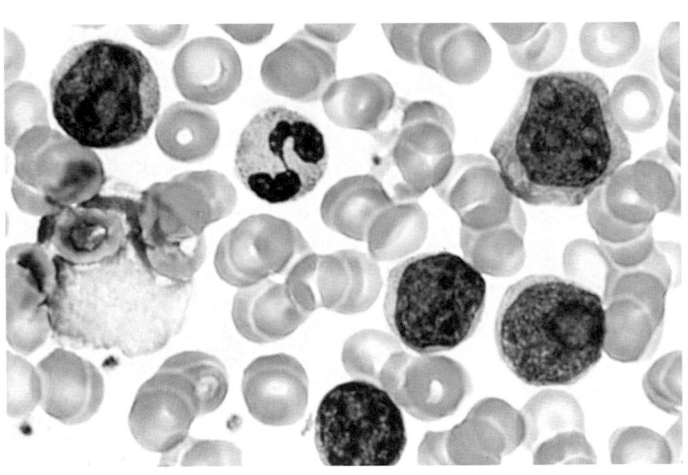

PLATE XX-9   Acute prolymphocytic leukemia.

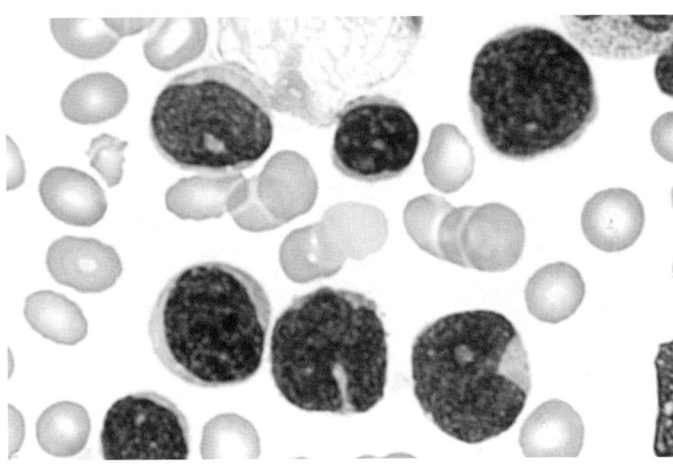

PLATE XX-10   Leukemic phase of small cell, cleaved follicular lymphoma.

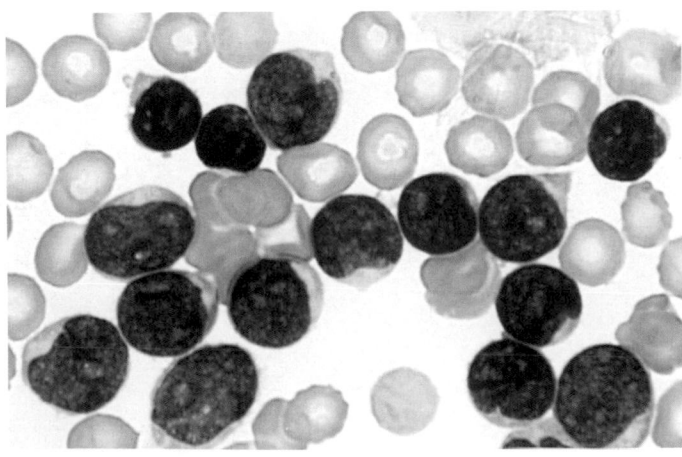

PLATE XX-11   Acute lymphocytic leukemia.

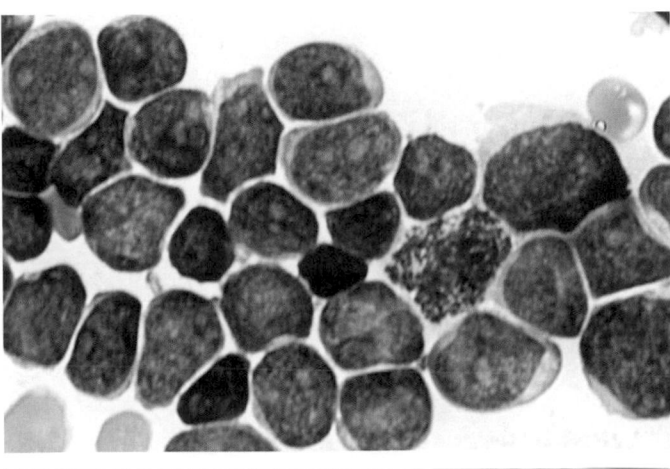

PLATE XX-12   Acute lymphocytic leukemia stained with peroxidase: Note that the blast cells are unreactive and the neutrophil is stained.

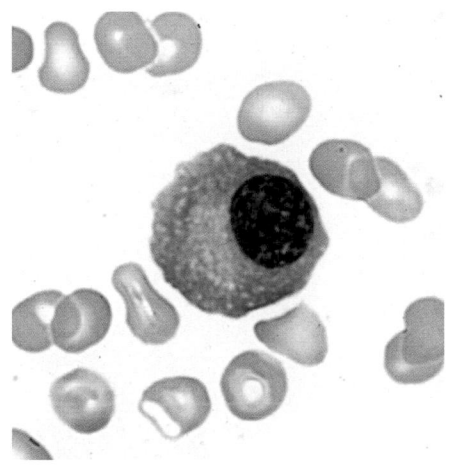

PLATE XXI-1   Plasma cell.

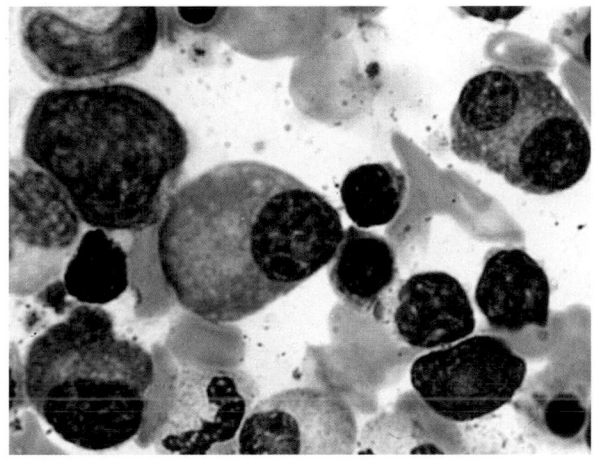

PLATE XXI-2   Plasma cells.

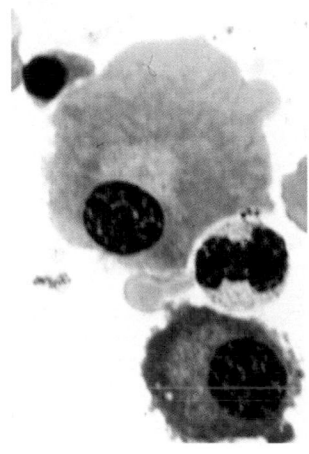

PLATE XXI-3   Plasma cells.

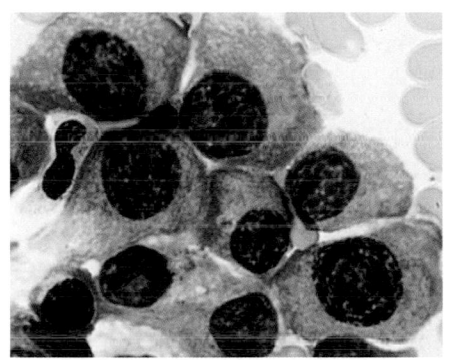

PLATE XXI-4   Myeloma cells.

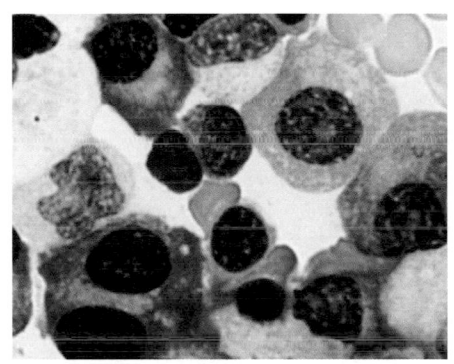

PLATE XXI-5   Myeloma cells.

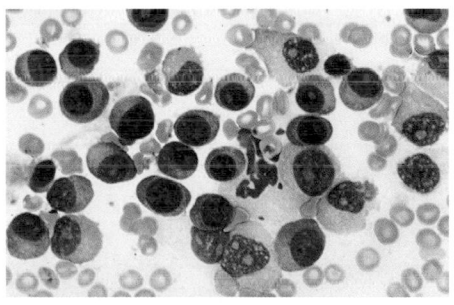

PLATE XXI-6   Blood film of patient with plasma cell leukemia.

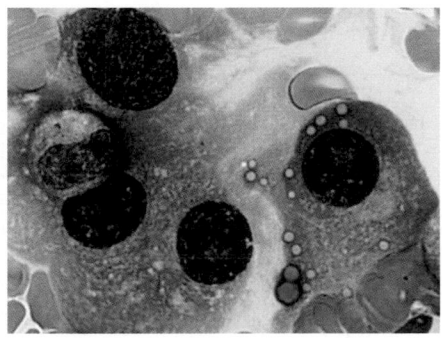

PLATE XXI-7   Myeloma cells.

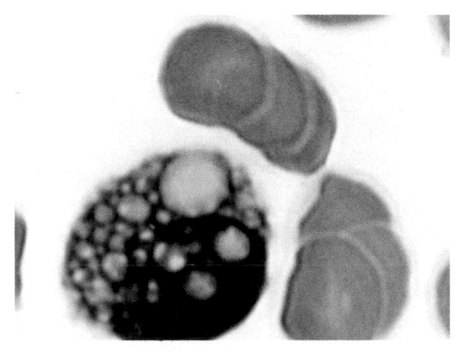

PLATE XXI-8   Mott cells.

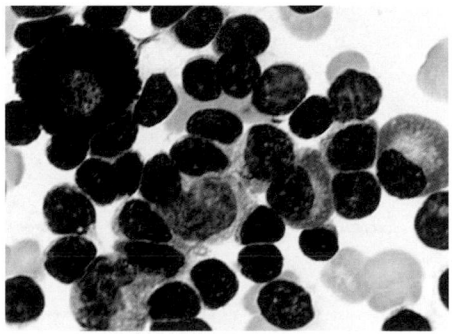

PLATE XXI-9   Waldenström macroglobuline-mia: Increased lymphocytes, occasional plasma cells, and a mast cell.

(XXI-1 through XXI-9 are marrow films.)

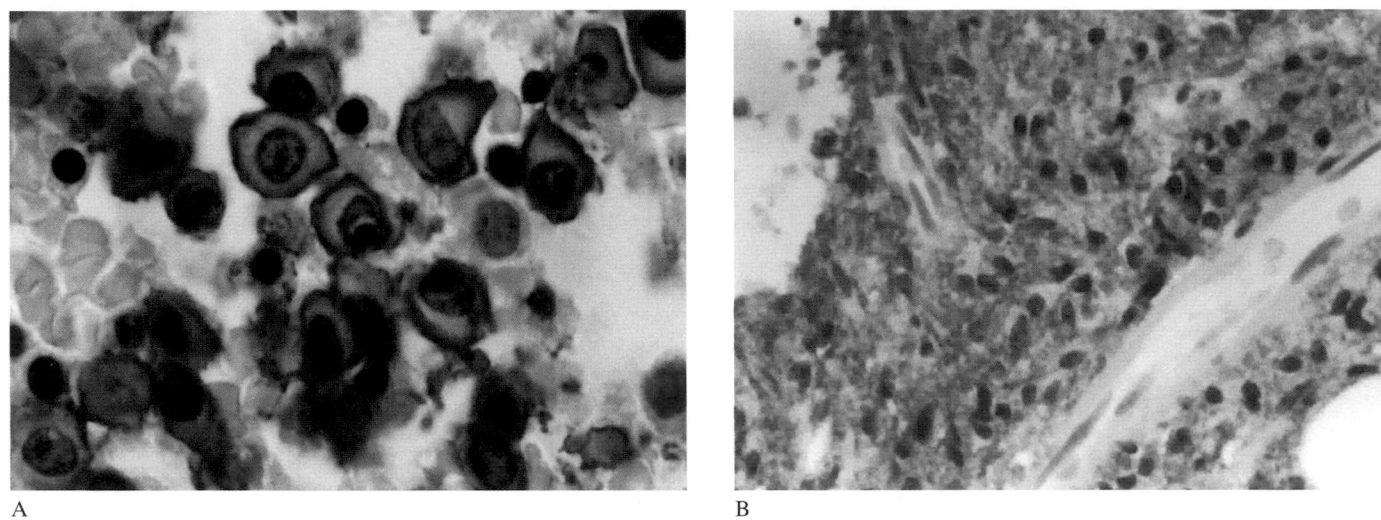

A

B

PLATE XXI-10 Staining of patient marrow biopsies with antibody against the syndecan-1 core protein. Syndecan-1 accumulates in fibrotic marrow. *A.* Syndecan-1 is expressed on the surface of myeloma cells. *B.* When shed, Syndecan-1 accumulates within the fibrotic extracellular matrix. Most cells present are marrow stromal cells. (From Sanderson RD, Yang Y, Suva LJ, Kelly T. Heparan sulfate proteoglycans and heparanase—partners in osteolytic tumor growth and metastasis. *Matrix Biol* 2004; 23:341–352, with permission.)

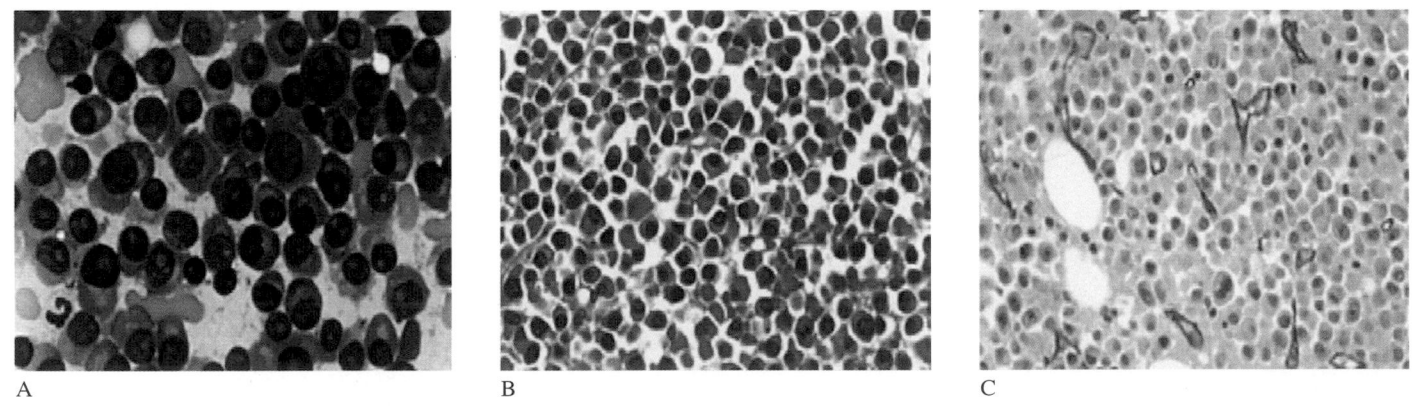

A

B

C

PLATE XXI-11 Marrow biopsy in myeloma. *A.* Hemotoxalin and eosin stain of marrow aspirate showing polymorphic plasma cells with nuclear prominence. *B.* Marrow biopsy. *C.* Increased microvessel density (anti-CD34 staining).

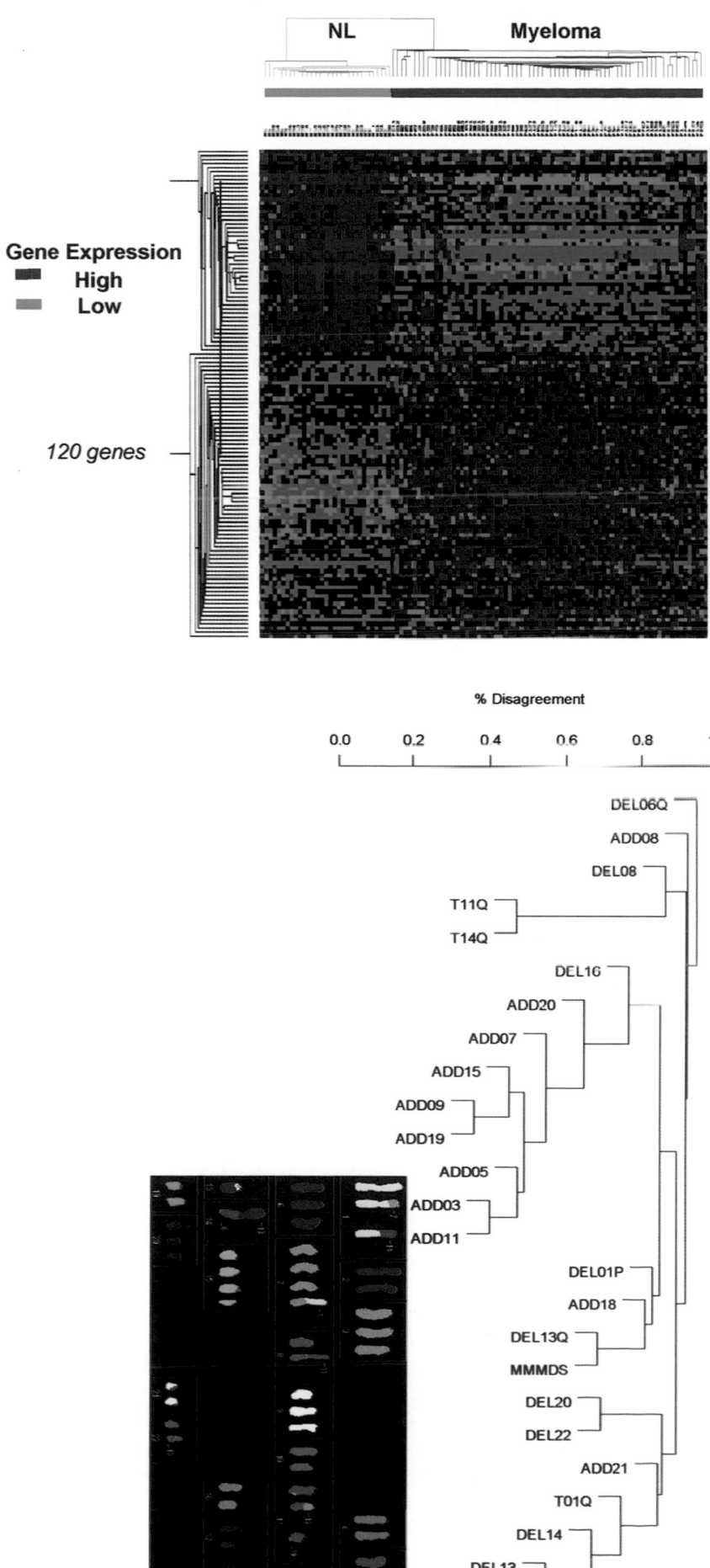

PLATE XXI-12 Myeloma and normal plasma cells distinguished by DNA microarray analysis. (See Chap. 100, "Disease Evolution and Genetic Alterations.")

PLATE XXI-13 Genomic chaos in myeloma: Cluster tree of chromosomal abnormalities. (See Chap. 100, "Disease Evolution and Genetic Alterations.")

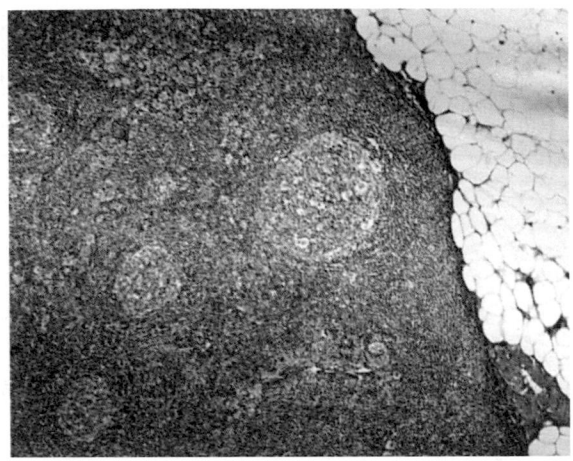

PLATE XXII-1   Normal lymph node.

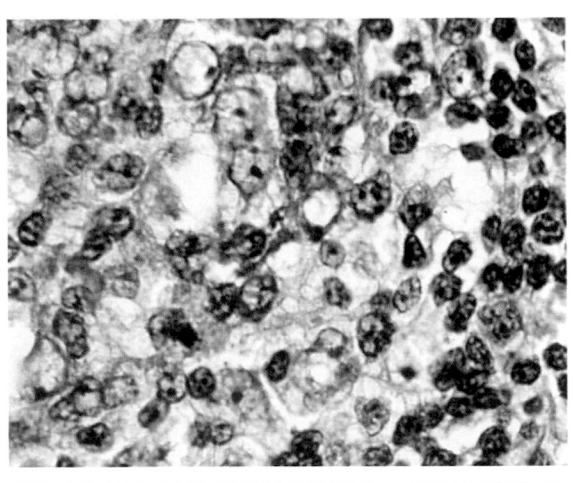

PLATE XXII-2   Normal lymph node.

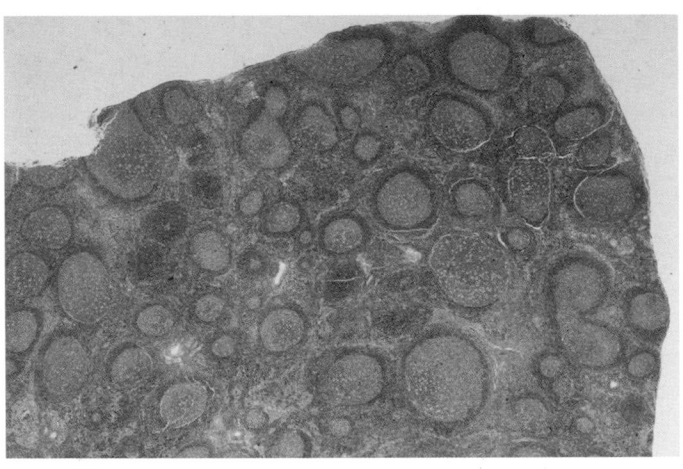

PLATE XXII-3   Reactive lymph node with follicular hyperplasia.

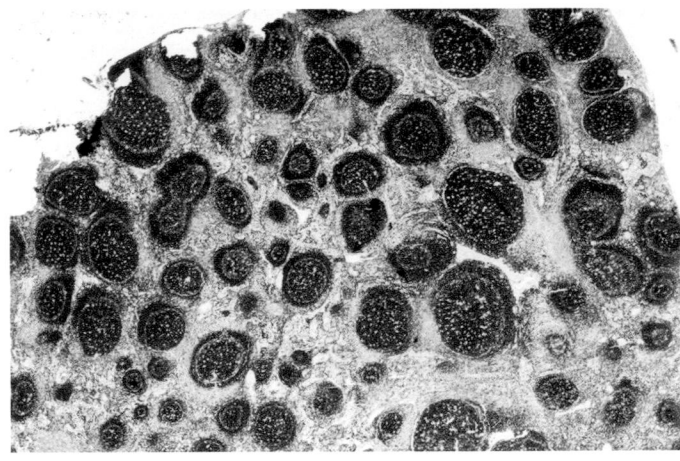

PLATE XXII-4   Same reactive lymph node stained with an antibody to CD20 (B cell marker).

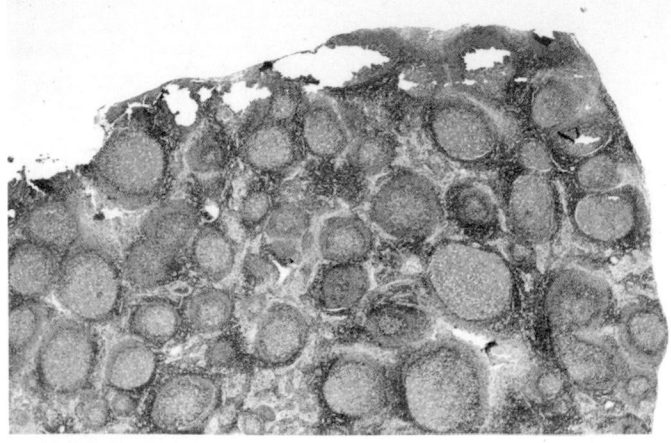

PLATE XXII-5   Same reactive lymph node stained with an antibody to CD3 (T cell marker).

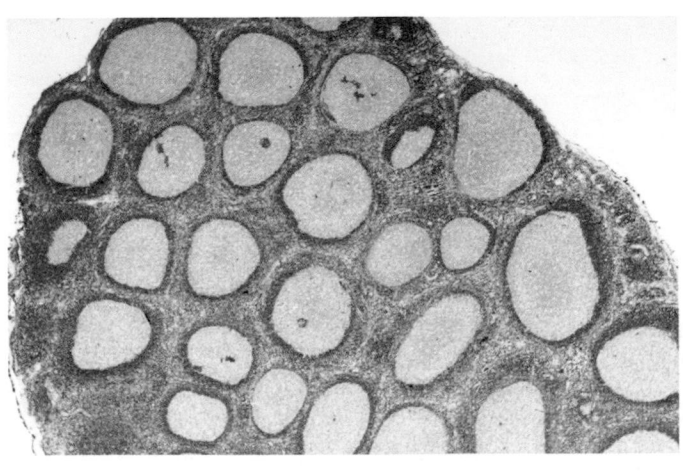

PLATE XXII-6   Same reactive lymph node stained with an antibody to the anti-apoptotic protein Bc1-2. Note the negative staining of the germinal centers where most of the cells will die during the maturation process.

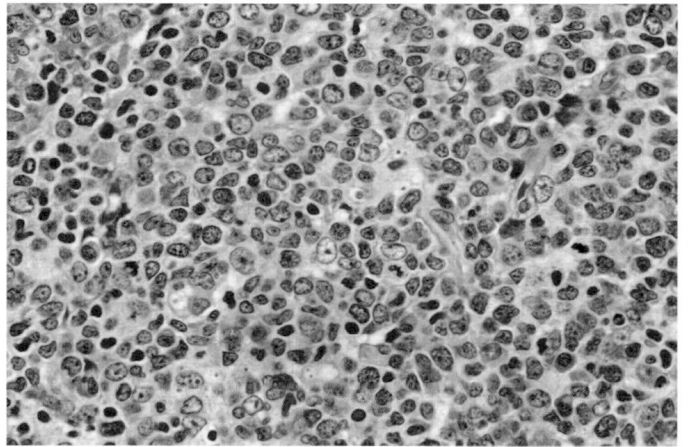

PLATE XXII-7   The typical cellular appearance of a benign germinal center.

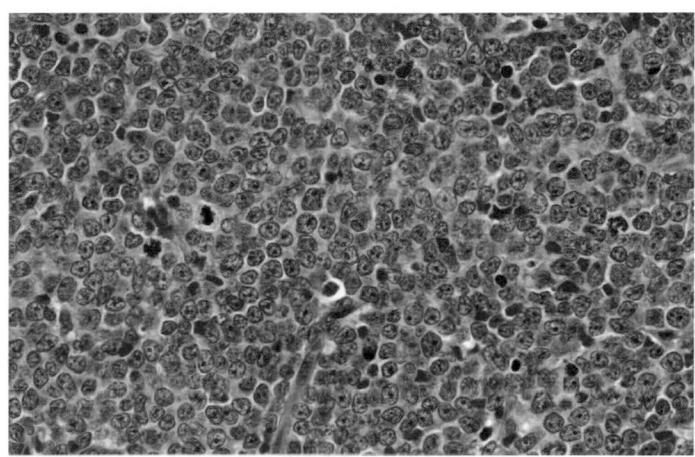

PLATE XXII-8   Lymphoblastic lymphoma of T cell type.

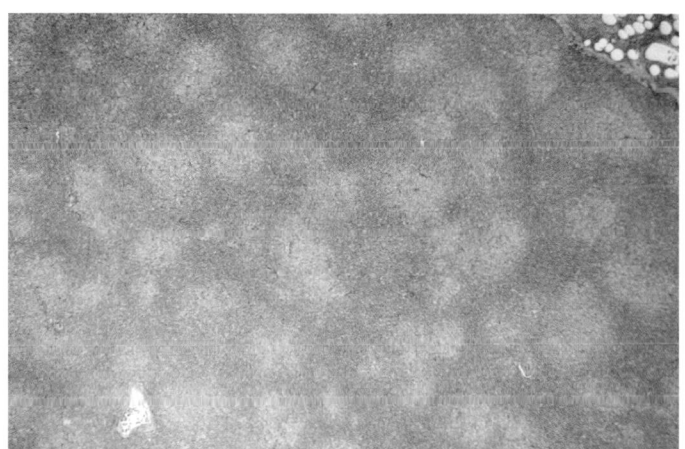

PLATE XXII-9   Small lymphocytic lymphoma with vague nodular appearance (pseudo-follicular pattern).

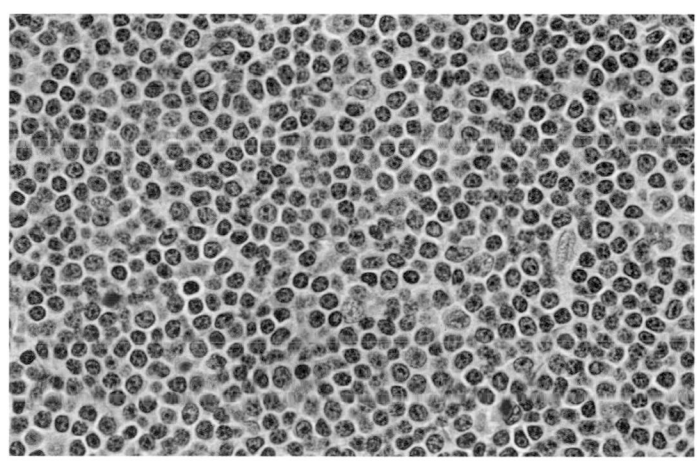

PLATE XXII-10   Characteristic nuclear features of small lymphocytic lymphoma.

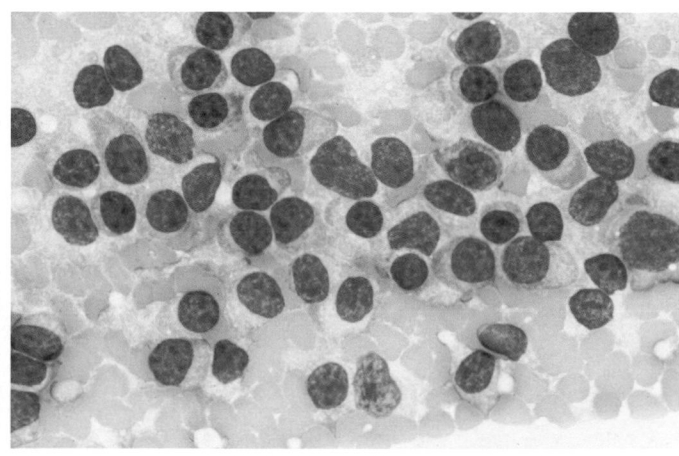

PLATE XXII-11   Imprint preparation of lymphoplasmacytic lymphoma.

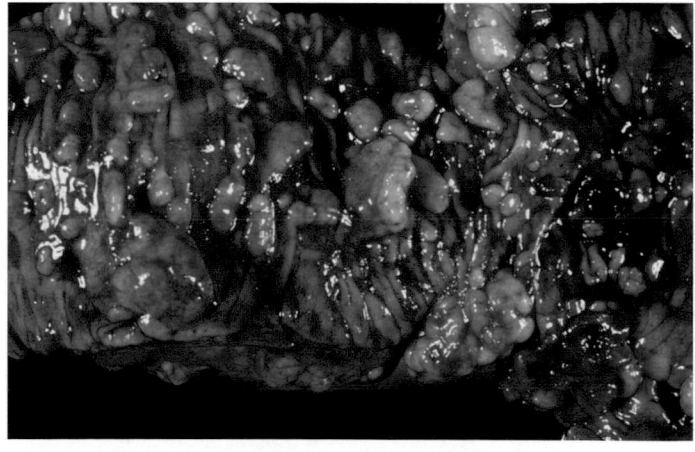

PLATE XXII-12   Large bowel involved with MCL (multiple lymphomatous polyposis).

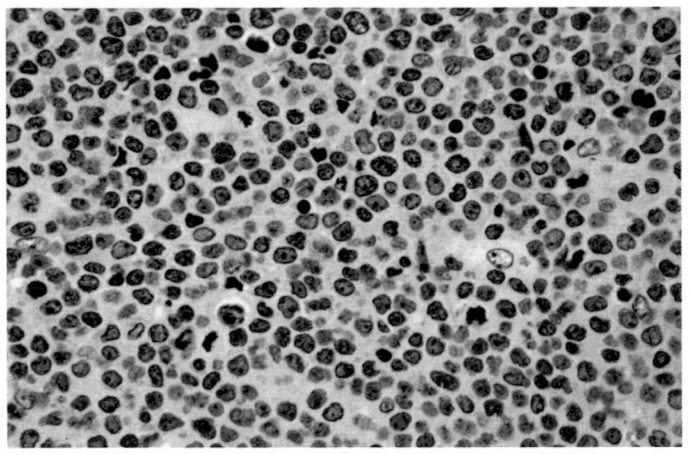

PLATE XXII-13   Mantle cell lymphoma (MCL) with a diffuse pattern.

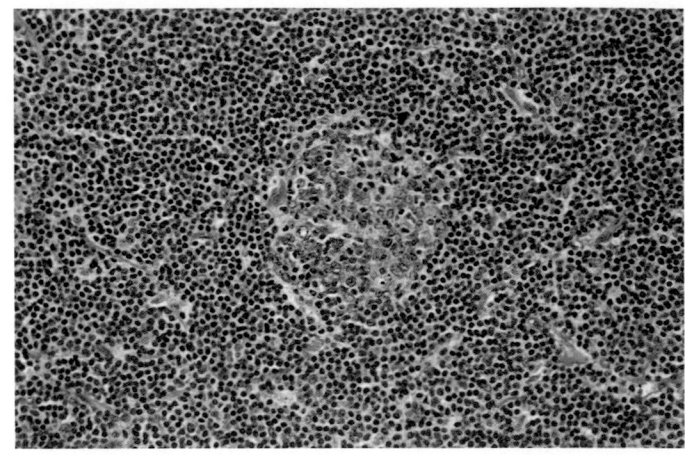

PLATE XXII-14   Mantle cell lymphoma with a mantle-zone pattern.

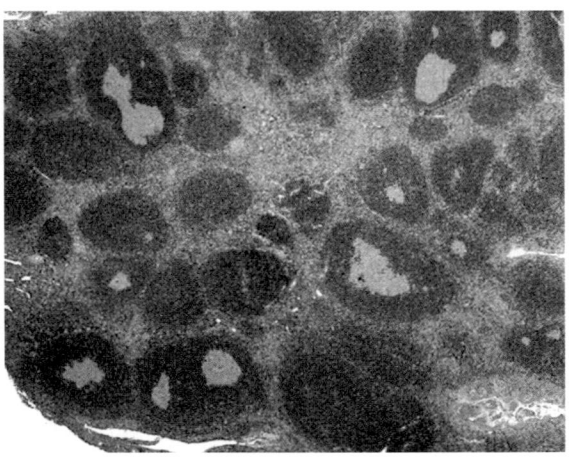

PLATE XXII-15   MCL with mantle-zone pattern stained with antibody to cyclin D1.

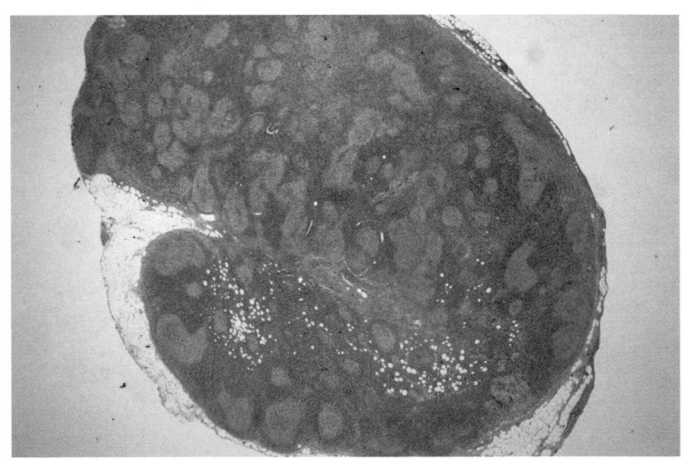

PLATE XXII-16   Grade 2 follicular lymphoma (low-power magnification).

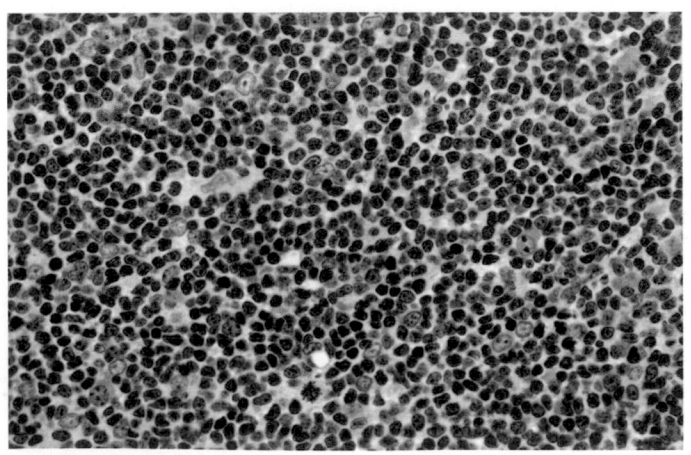

PLATE XXII-17   Center of a neoplastic follicle in grade 1 follicular lymphoma with almost exclusively small centrocytes.

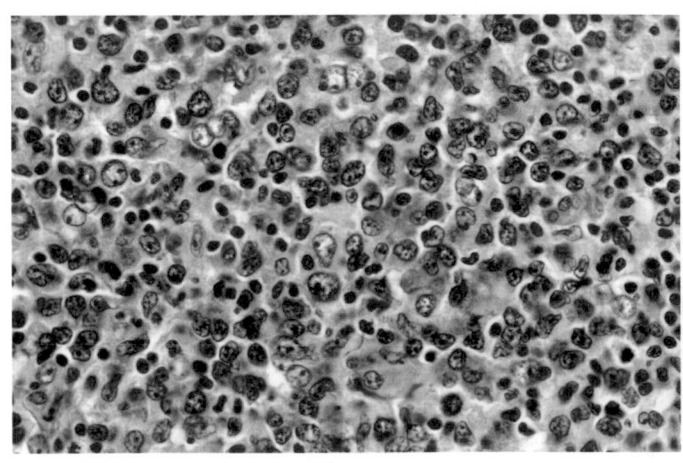

PLATE XXII-18   Grade 3A follicular lymphoma with <15 centroblasts per high-power field.

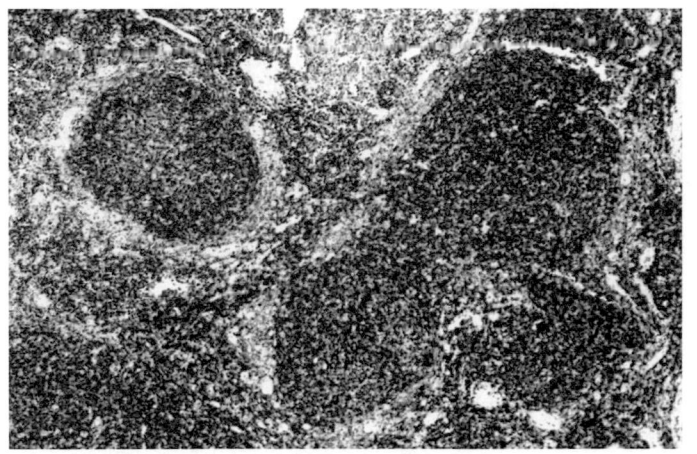

PLATE XXII-19 BCL-2 immunostain of a follicular lymphoma (contrast with Plate XXII-6).

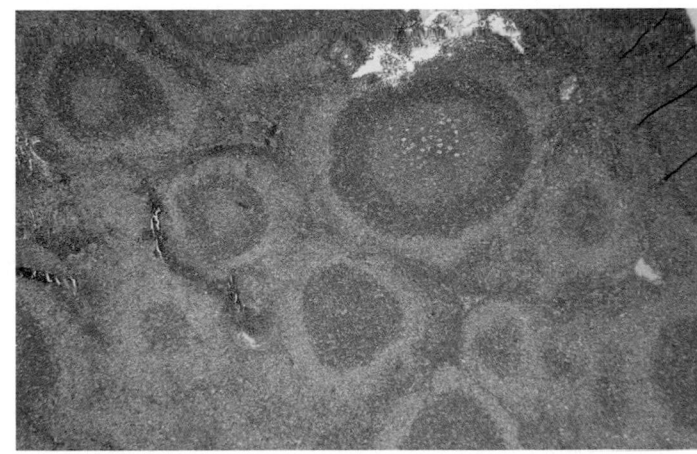

PLATE XXII-20 Lymph node involved by marginal zone B cell lymphoma.

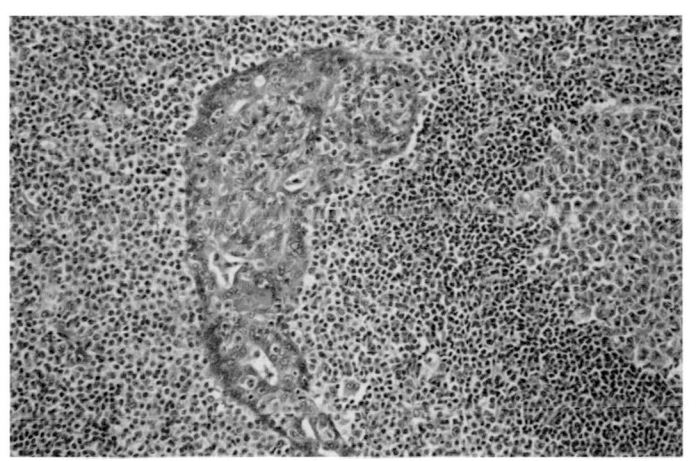

PLATE XXII-21 Salivary gland involved by MALT lymphoma.

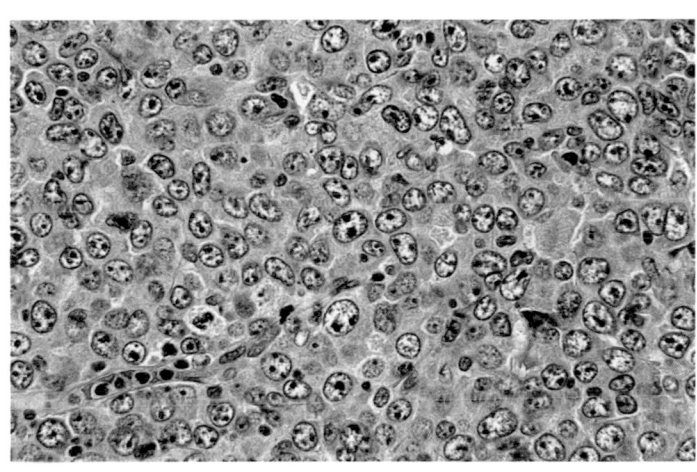

PLATE XXII-22 Diffuse large B cell lymphoma.

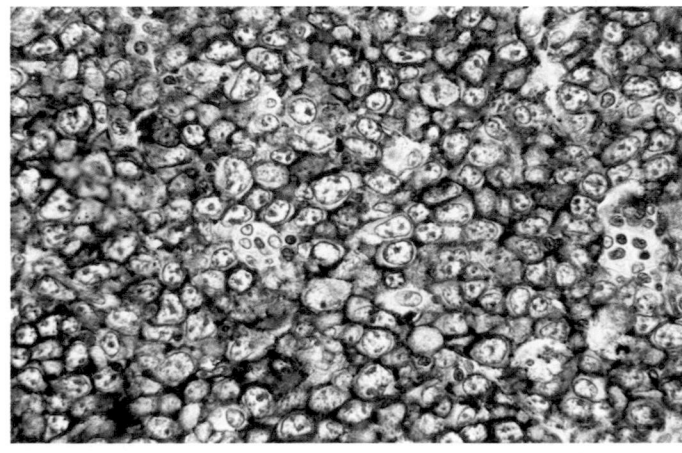

PLATE XXII-23 Diffuse large B cell lymphoma stained with antibody to CD20.

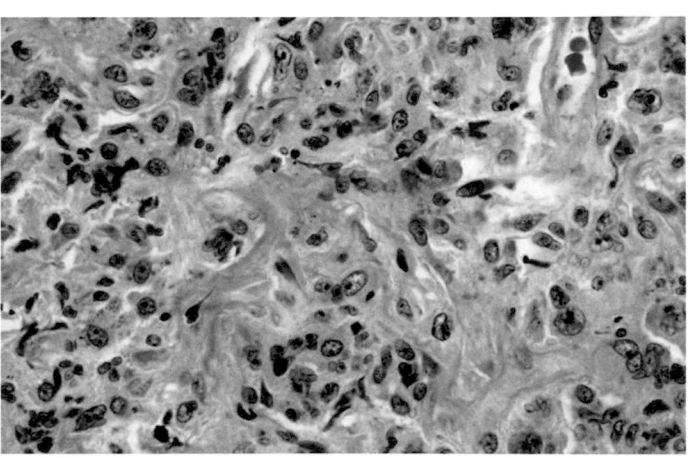

PLATE XXII-24 Primary mediastinal large B cell lymphoma with sclerosis.

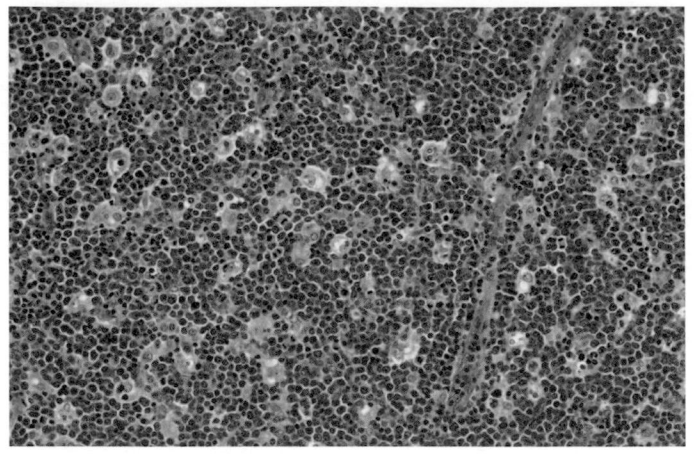

PLATE XXII-25   Burkitt lymphoma with starry-sky appearance.

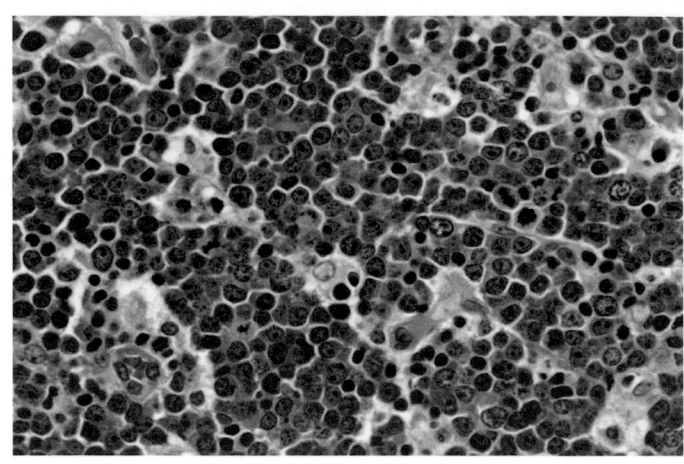

PLATE XXII-26   Burkitt lymphoma.

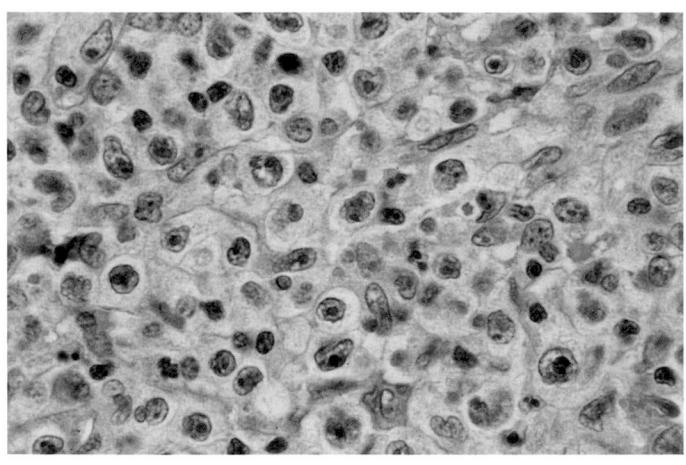

PLATE XXII-27   Peripheral T cell lymphoma, unspecified.

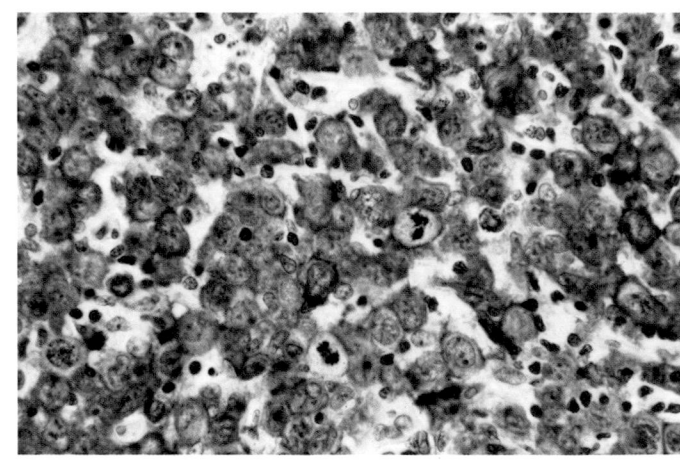

PLATE XXII-28   Peripheral T cell lymphoma stained with antibody to CD3.

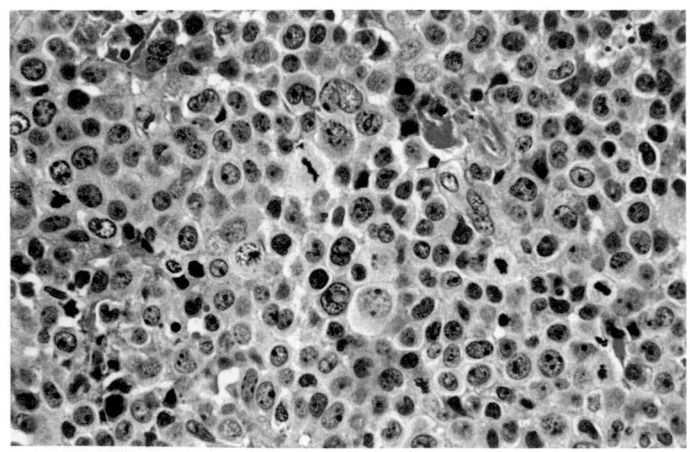

PLATE XXII-29   Anaplastic large cell lymphoma, T cell type.

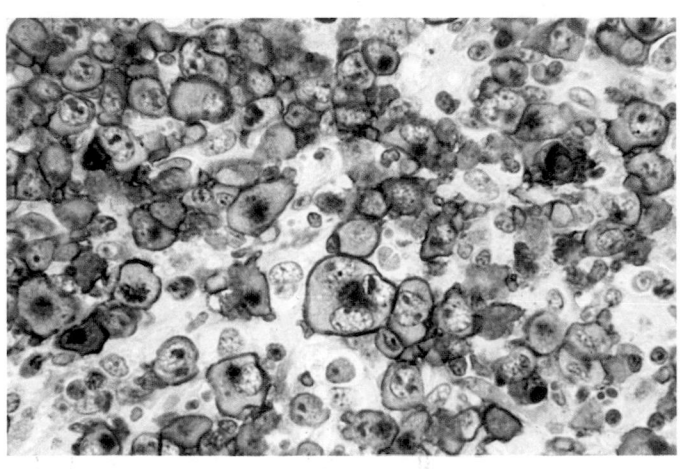

PLATE XXII-30   Anaplastic large cell lymphoma stained with antibody to CD30.

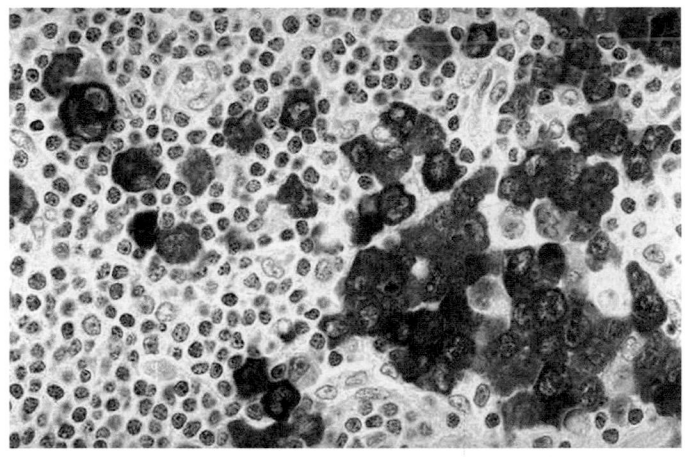

PLATE XXII-31   Anaplastic large cell lymphoma stained with antibody to ALK (anaplastic lymphoma kinase).

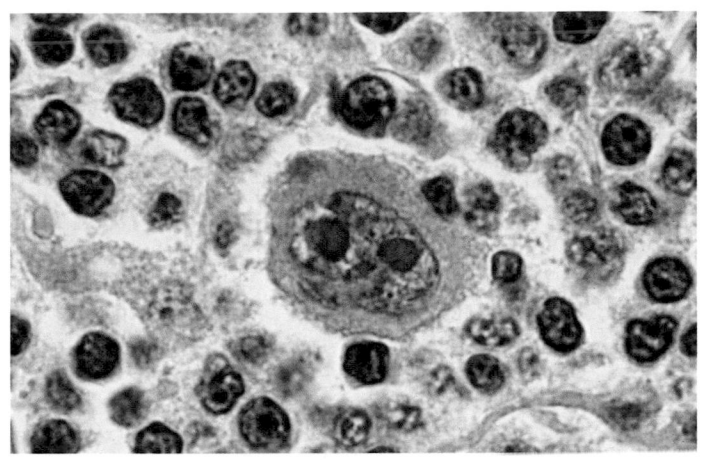

PLATE XXII-32   Diagnostic Reed-Sternberg cell in Hodgkin lymphoma.

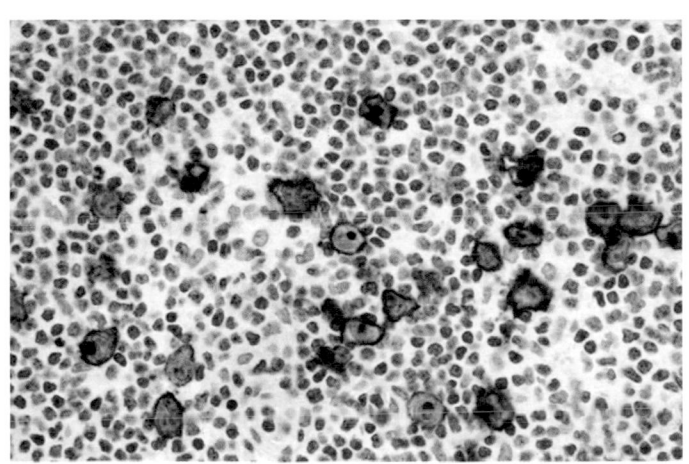

PLATE XXII-33   Classical Hodgkin lymphoma stained with antibody to CD30.

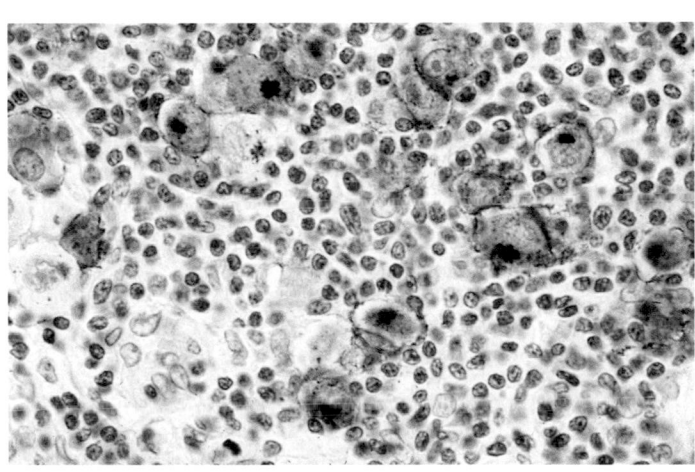

PLATE XXII-34   Classical Hodgkin lymphoma with Reed-Sternberg cells clearly identified with antibody to CD15.

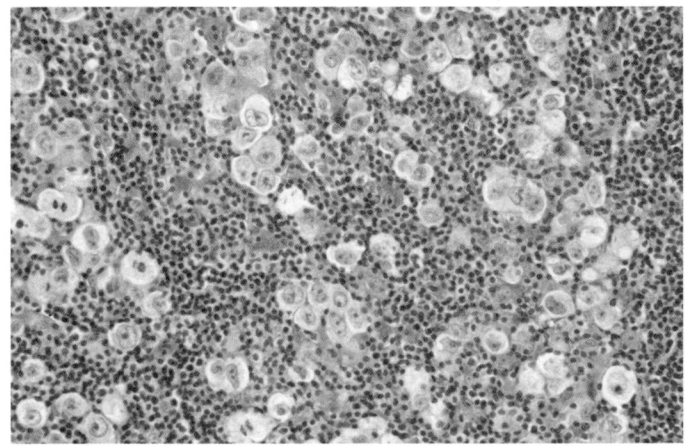

PLATE XXII-35   Classical Hodgkin lymphoma, nodular sclerosis type with characteristic lacunar cells.

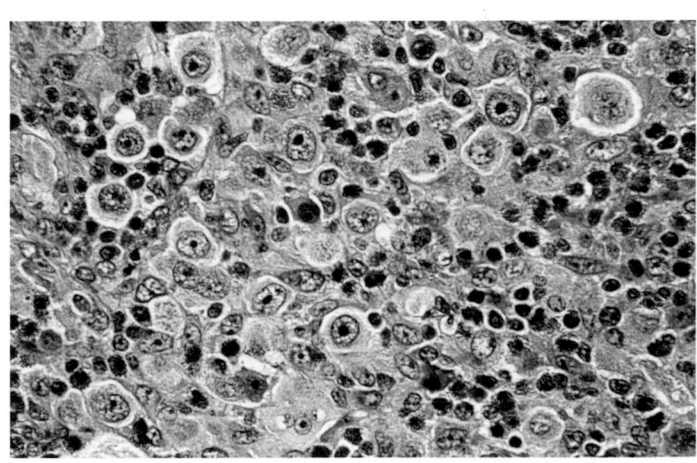

PLATE XXII-36   Mixed cellularity Hodgkin lymphoma.

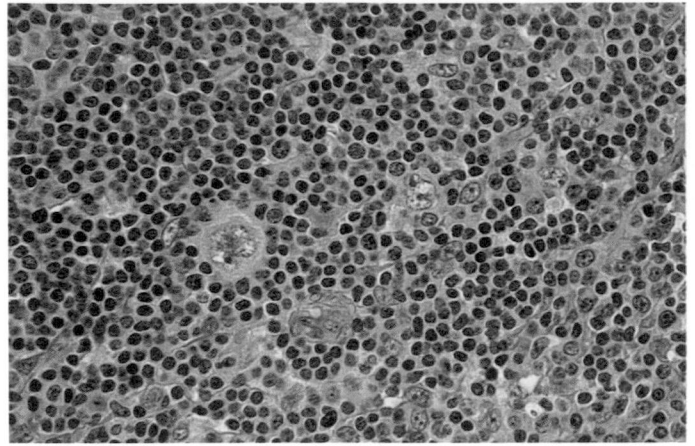

PLATE XXII-37 Nodular lymphocyte predominance Hodgkin lymphoma showing characteristic "L&H cells" (popcorn cells).

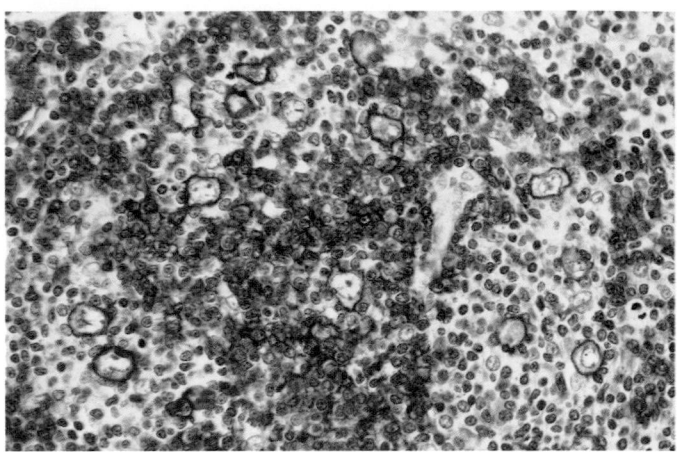

PLATE XXII-38 Nodular lymphocyte predominance Hodgkin lymphoma stained with antibody to CD20. Note the positive staining of the L & H cells (popcorn cells).

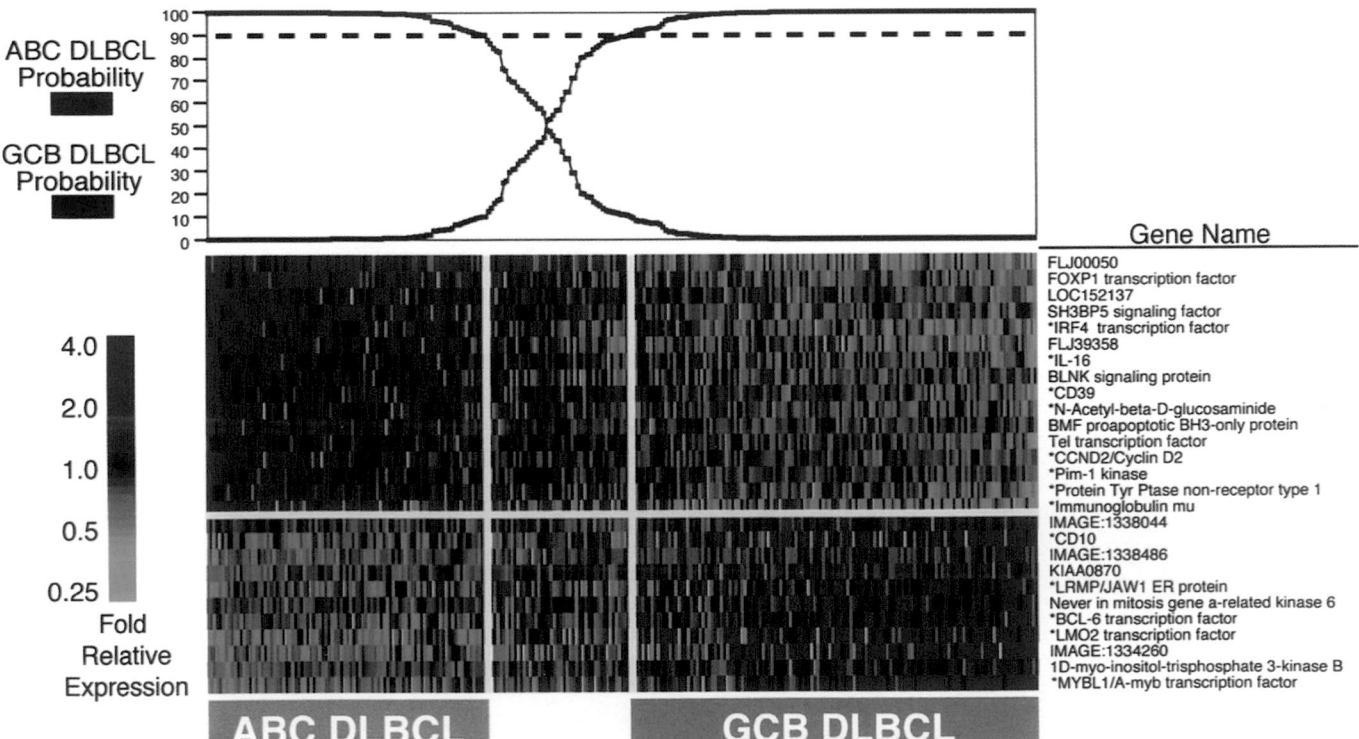

PLATE XXII-39 Gene expression profiling of diffuse large B cell lymphoma, showing the subgroup discriminator used to divide cases into germinal center B cell-like (GCB) and activated B cell-like (ABC). Each vertical column represents an individual patient and each horizontal row a unique gene. Red is relative over-expression of a gene and green relative under-expression. Using a probability of subgroup assignment of 90%, approximately 15% of cases are left unclassified (cases between the vertical yellow bars that are neither GCB or ABC). This approach allows one to analyze thousands of genes from a single patient in one experiment, and forms the basis of the new molecular classification of lymphomas. (Reproduced from Proceedings of the National Academy of Sciences, USA, 2003, 100: pp 9991–9996, by copyright permission of the National Academy of Sciences, USA.) (See Chap. 95, "Pathology of Malignant Lymphomas.")

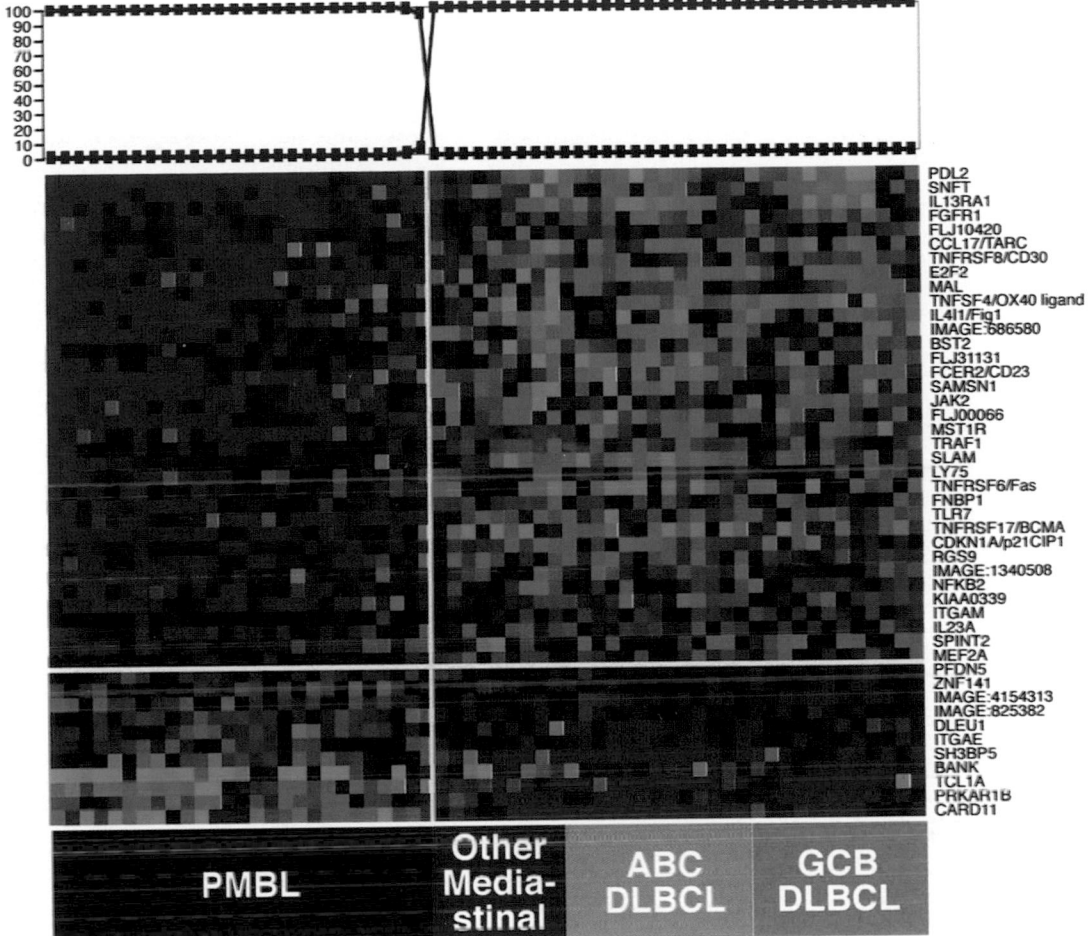

PLATE XXII-40 Gene expression profiling of primary mediastinal large B cell lymphoma (PMBCL), contrasting the expression profile with nodal diffuse large B cell lymphomas (DLBCL). This figure shows numerous genes that are over-expressed in PMBCL (red). Many of these genes are shared with classical Hodgkin lymphoma, suggesting a biological overlap between these two diseases. Cases listed as "Other Mediastinal" refer to those cases of DLBCL with mediastinal involvement, but not felt to be typical of PMBCL. This is borne out by the gene expression data, showing that these cases are more closely related to DLBCL rather than PMBCL. (Reproduced from the *Journal of Experimental Medicine*, 2003, 198: pp 851–862, by copyright permission of The Rockefeller University Press.) (See Chap. 95, "Pathology of Malignant Lymphomas.")

FLUORESCENCE *IN SITU* HYBRIDIZATION (FISH) FOR CYTOGENETIC ANALYSIS

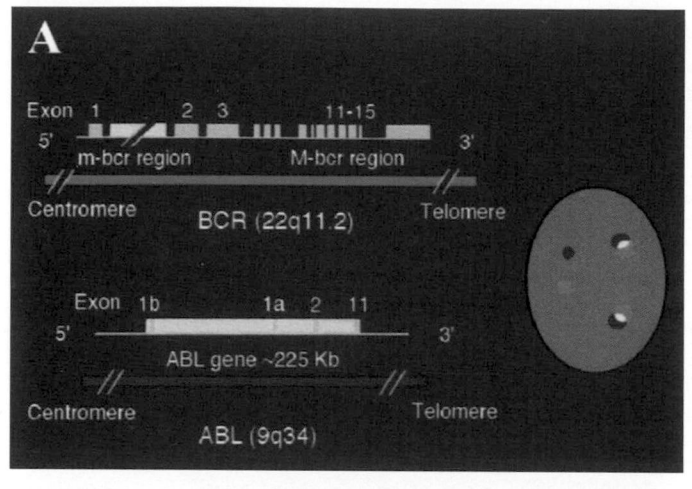

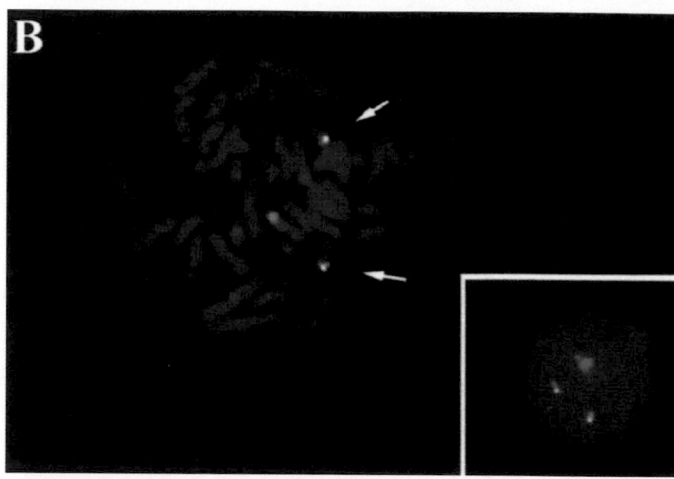

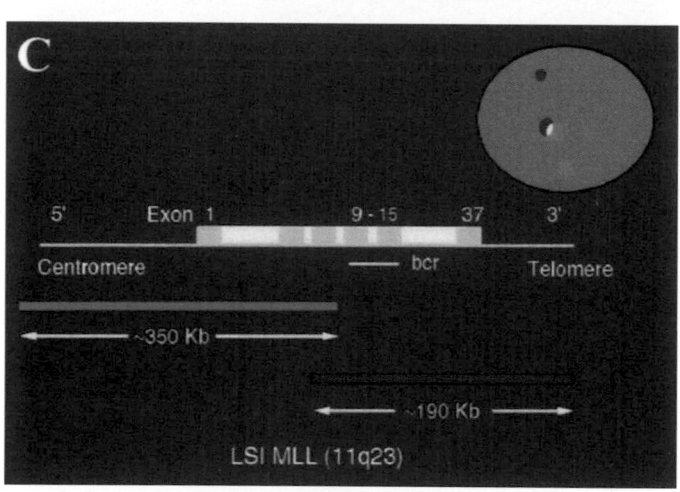

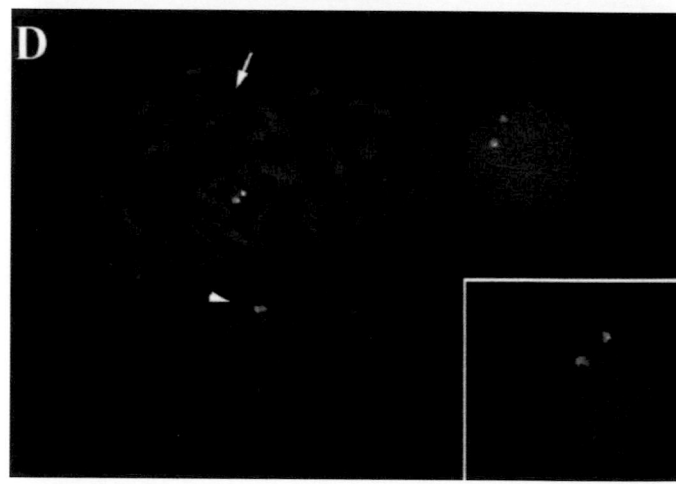

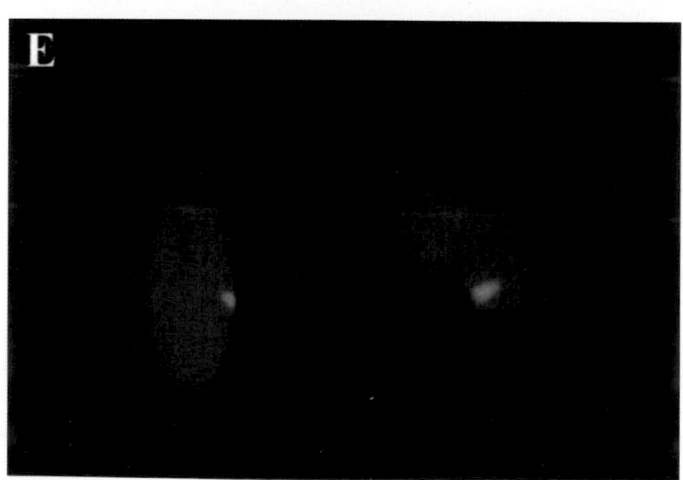

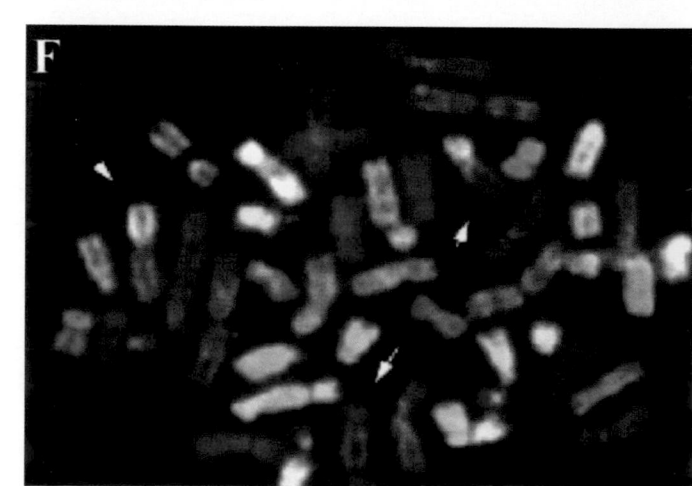

PLATE XXIII Fluorescence *in situ* hybridization and spectral karyotyping analysis of hematologic malignant diseases. Panels B, D, and E illustrate images of metaphase and interphase cells following FISH; the cells are counterstained with 4,6-diamidino-2-phenylindole-dihydrochloride (DAPI). (*A*) Schematic diagram of the *BCR* and *ABL* loci, location of the *BCR* and *ABL* dual fusion probe (Vysis, Inc), and configuration of signals in interphase cells. (*B*) Hybridization of the *BCR-ABL* dual fusion probe to metaphase and interphase cells with the t(9;22). In cells with the t(9;22), only one green and one red signal is observed on the normal 9 and 22 homologs, and two yellow fusion signals (arrows) are observed on the der(9) and the der(22) (Ph chromosome) chromosomes as a result of the juxtaposition of the *ABL* and *BCR* sequences. (*C*) Schematic diagram of the *MLL* gene, location of the *MLL* break-apart probe (Vysis Inc.), and configuration of signals in interphase cells. (*D*) Hybridization of the *MLL* break-apart probe to metaphase and interphase cells with a t(11q23). In cells with *MLL* translocation, a yellow fusion signal is observed for the germline configuration on the normal chromosome 11 homologue, a green signal is observed in the der(11) chromosome, and a red signal is observed on the partner chromosome. (*E*) Hybridization of directly-labeled centromere-specific probes for the X (CEPX Spectrum Orange, Vysis Inc.) and Y (CEPX Spectrum Green, Vysis Inc.) chromosomes to interphase cells from a marrow aspirate of a female patient with AML who received a marrow transplant from a male donor. Centromere-specific probes hybridize to the repetitive DNA sequences that are present at the centromeres of human chromosomes. (*F*) Spectral karyotyping analysis of a metaphase cell from an AML-M7. Twenty-four differentially labeled probes representing each human chromosome are co-hybridized, and imaging analysis software assigns a unique color to each. A complex karyotype was identified by conventional cytogenetic analysis, including a derivative chromosome 1 with additional material of unknown origin on 1p, a deletion of 8p, a derivative chromosome 11 resulting from an unbalanced translocation involving 1 and 11, and a derivative chromosome 12, consisting of 11q and 12q. The results of spectral karyotyping confirmed the identity of the rearranged chromosome 12 (arrowhead), but clarified the other abnormalities. The additional material on 1p was derived from chromosome 8 (long arrow, blue signal), and the der(11) actually consisted of material from chromsomes 1, 11, and 12 (short arrow, 11p white signal, chromosome 12 brown signal; 1p blue-pink signal).

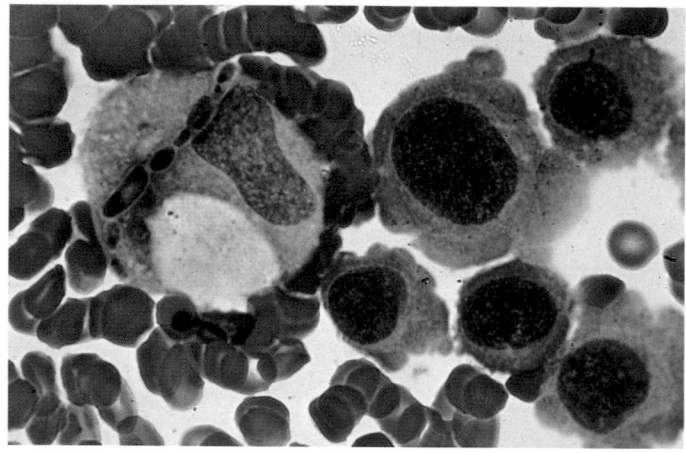

PLATE XXIV-1   Candidiasis. Pleural fluid film. Macrophage with ingested Candida. Adjacent mesothelial cells.

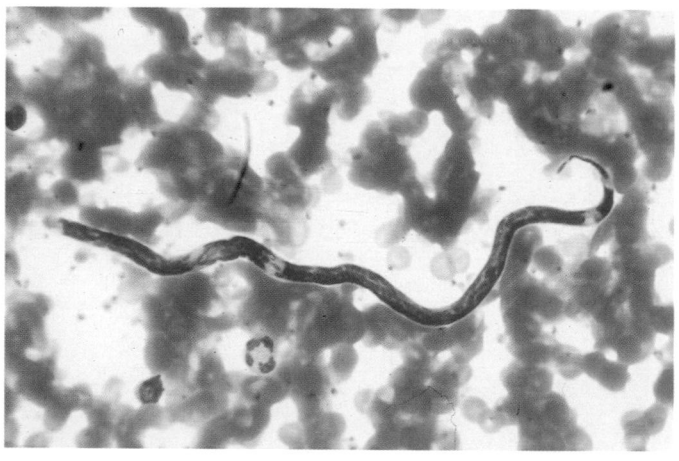

PLATE XXIV-2   Microfilaria of *Loa loa*. Blood film.

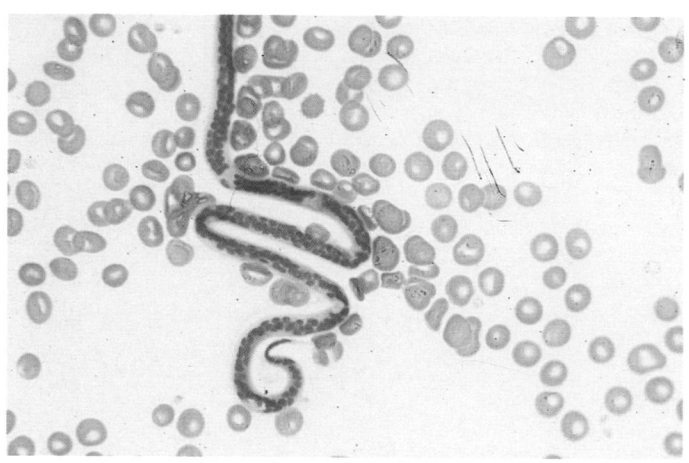

PLATE XXIV-3   Microfilaria of *Wuchereria bancrofti*. Blood film.

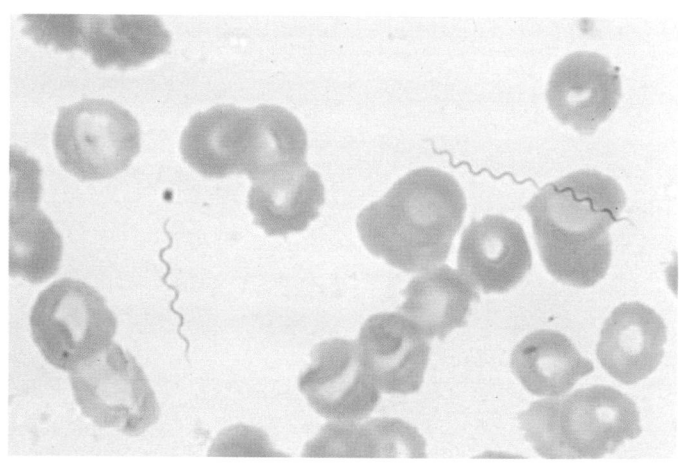

PLATE XXIV-4   Spirochetes of *Borrelia* species. Blood film.

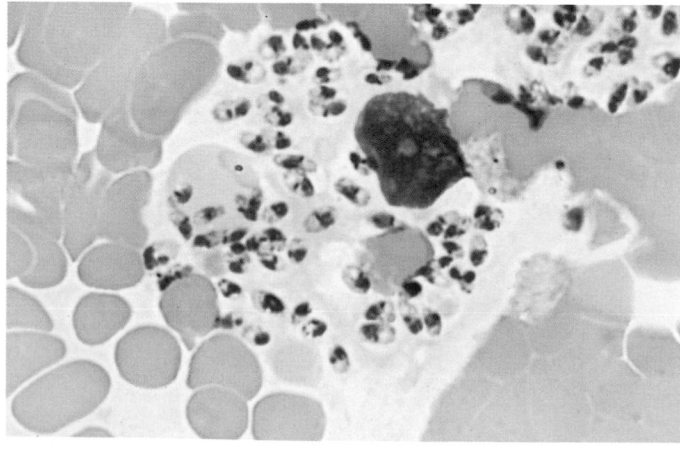

PLATE XXIV-5   Macrophages loaded with the amastiogotes of *Leishmania* species. Pleural fluid film. The "T" shapes are in contrast to those of *Histoplasma capsulatum* (see Plate IX-8).

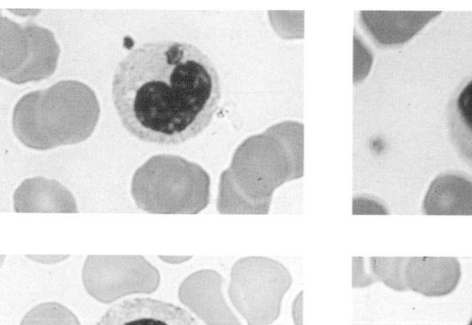
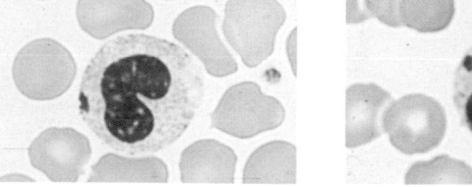

PLATE XXIV-6   Ehrlichiosis. Blood film. The intracellular *Ehrlichia* are evident.

PLATE XXV
CUTANEOUS LESIONS

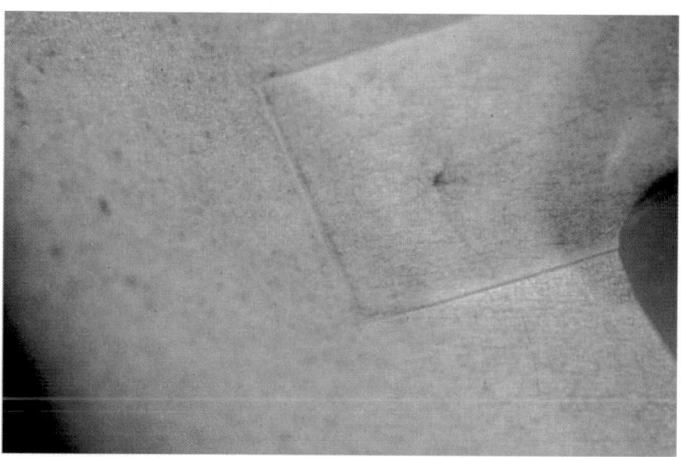

PLATE XXV-1   Spider telangiectasia.

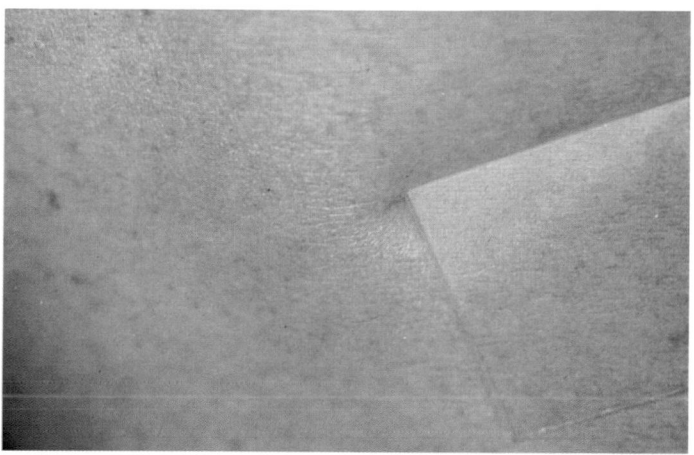

PLATE XXV-2   Blanching of spider telangiectasia. Note that spider telangiectasia blanches with diascopy.

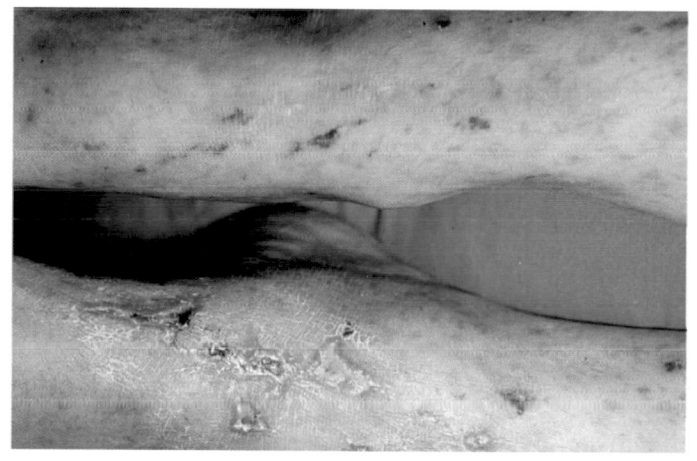

PLATE XXV-3   Cryoglobulinemia: Peripheral purpura.

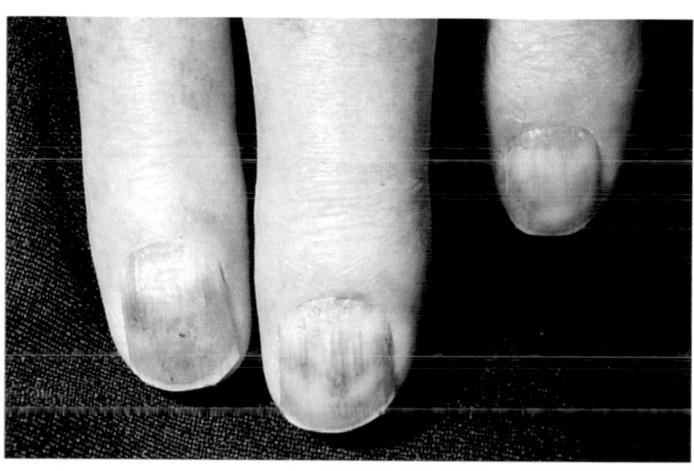

PLATE XXV-4   Cryoglobulinemia: Subungual purpura.

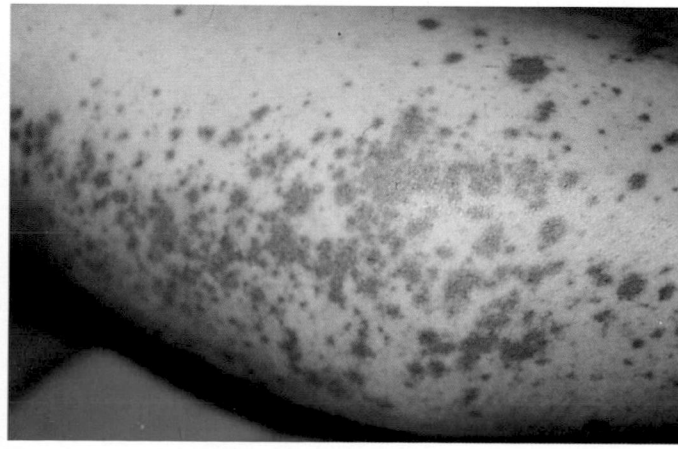

PLATE XXV-5   Waldenström hyperglobulinemic purpura. Note discrete and coalescing petechiae on lower limb.

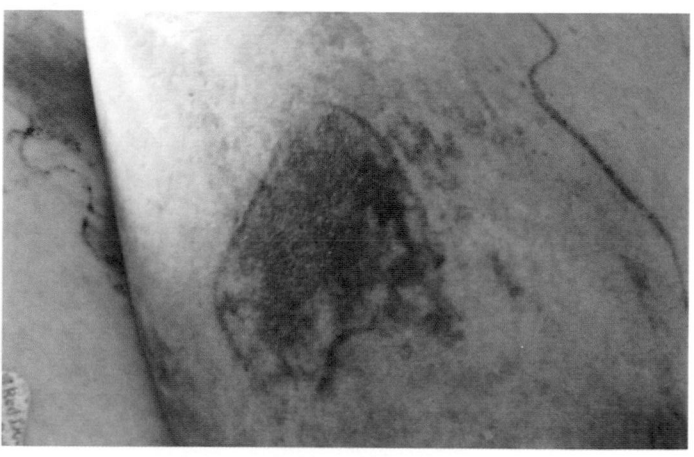

PLATE XXV-6   Coumadin necrosis. Develops in acral areas and areas of fat deposition such as buttocks or breast (as shown here).

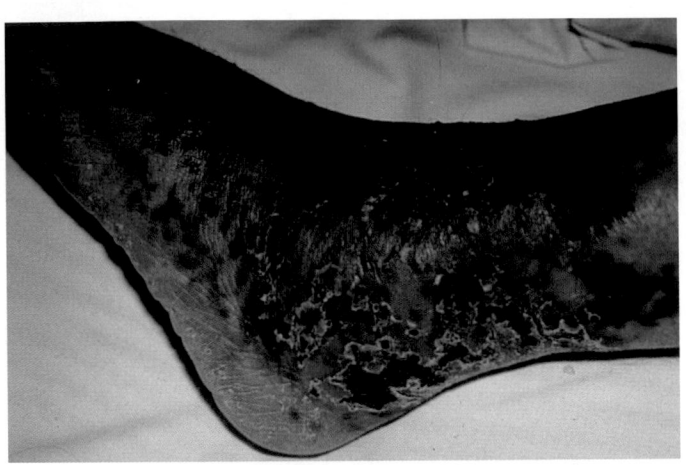

PLATE XXV-7   Antiphospholipid antibody syndrome. Anticardiolipin antibody.

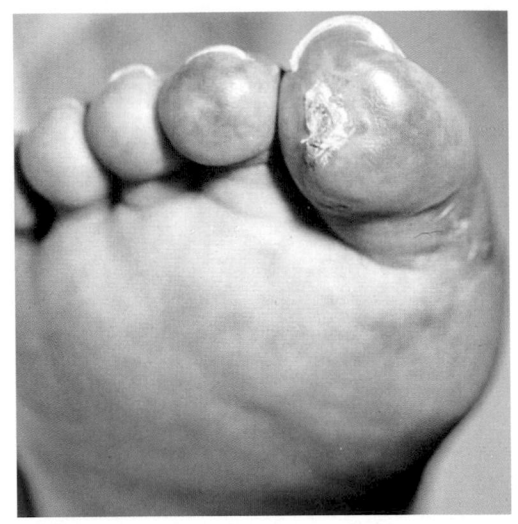

PLATE XXV-8   Antiphospholipid antibody syndrome: Lupus anticoagulant.

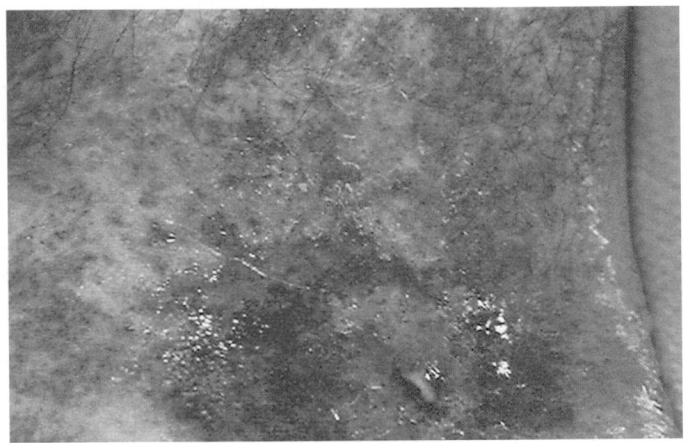

PLATE XXV-9   Livedoid vasculitis.

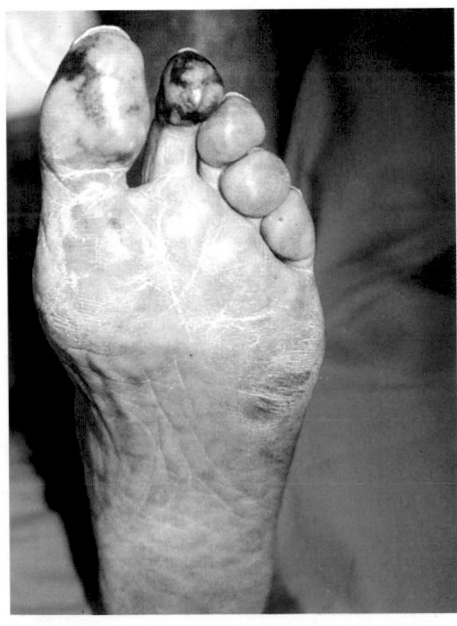

PLATE XXV-10   Cholesterol emboli.

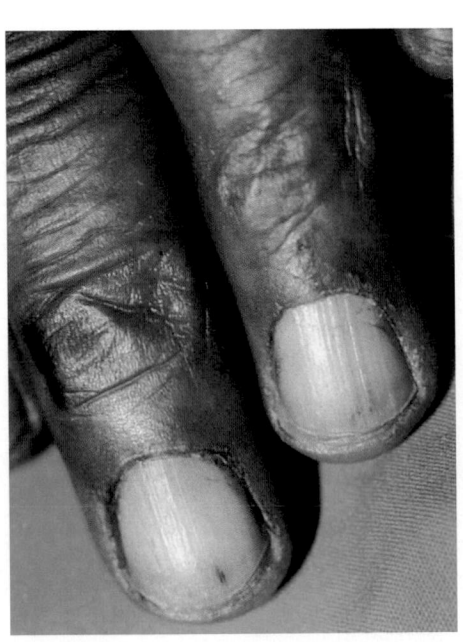

PLATE XXV-11   Cholesterol emboli: Splinter hemorrhages.

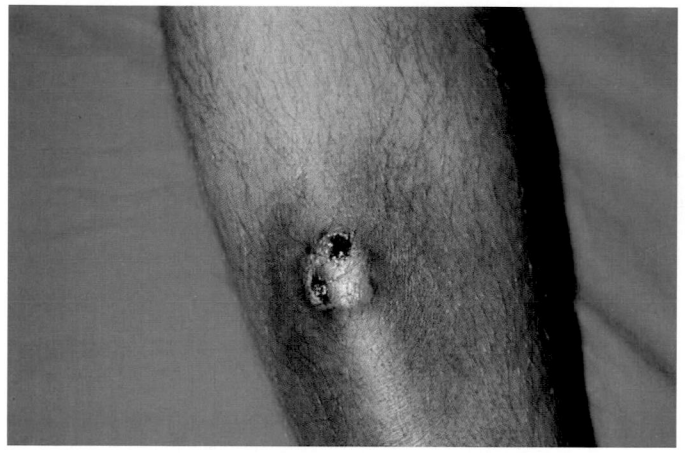

PLATE XXV-12   Pyoderma gangrenosum: Central purpuraa.

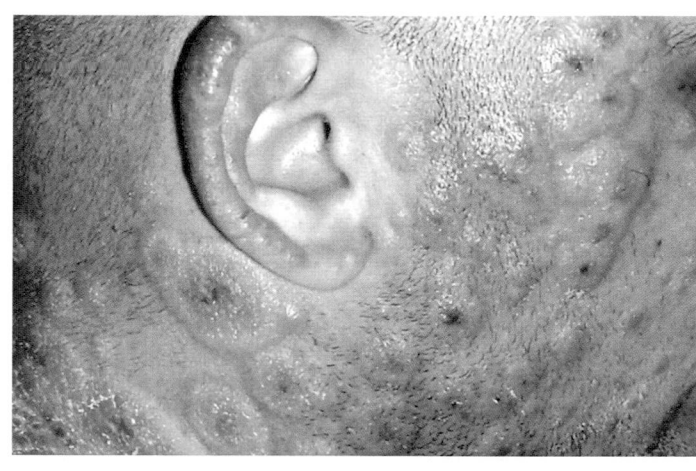

PLATE XXV-13   Sweet syndrome.

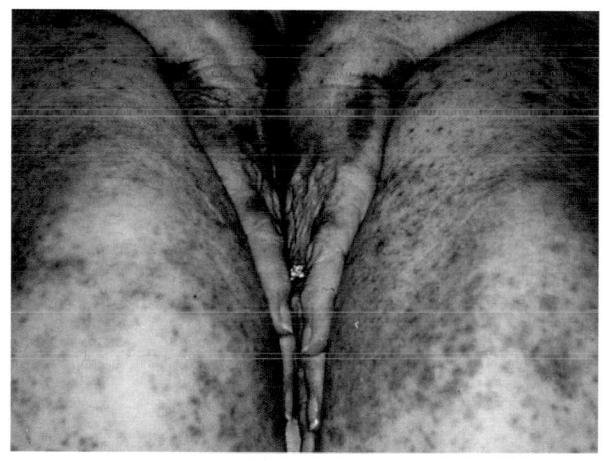

PLATE XXV-14   Serum sickness due to antithymocyte globulin.

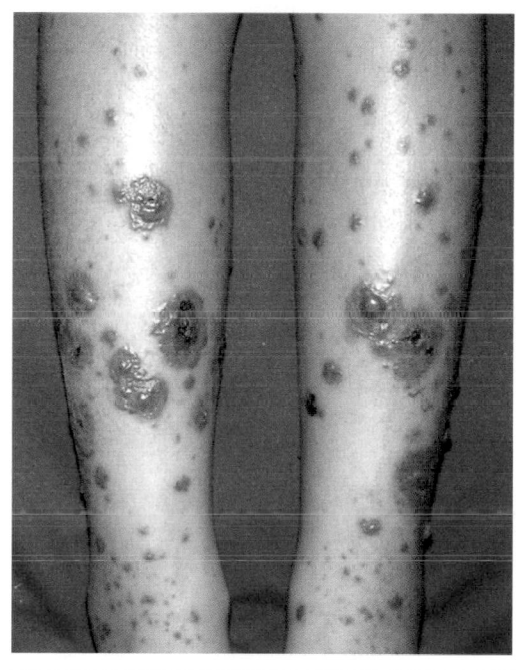

PLATE XXV-15   Henoch-Schönlein purpura. Urticarial papules and plaques can evolve into palpable purpura.

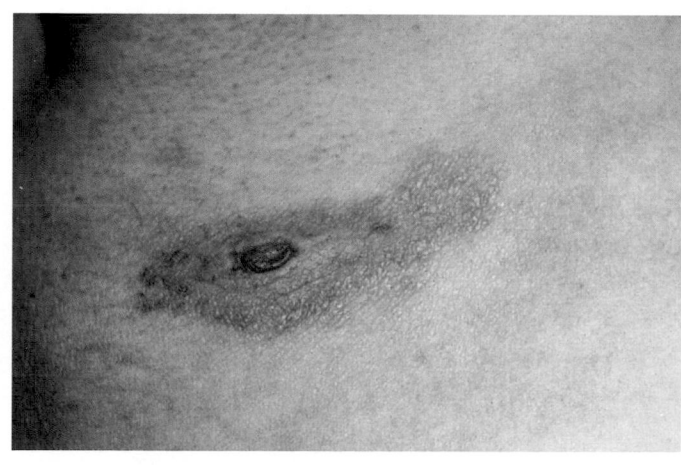

PLATE XXV-16   Ecthyma gangrenosum.

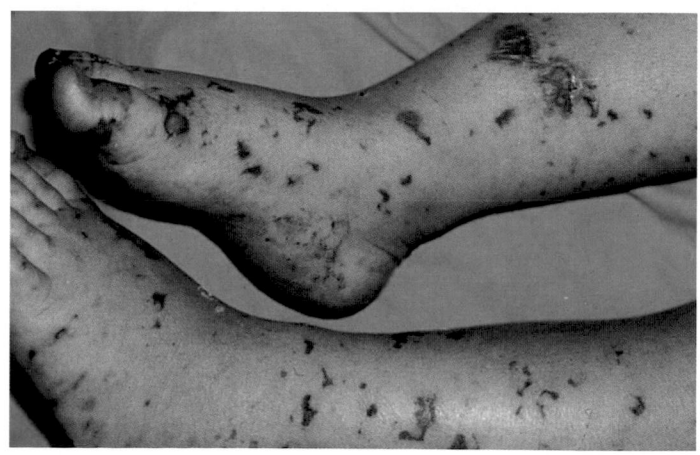

PLATE XXV-17   Meningococcemia: Stellate purpura.

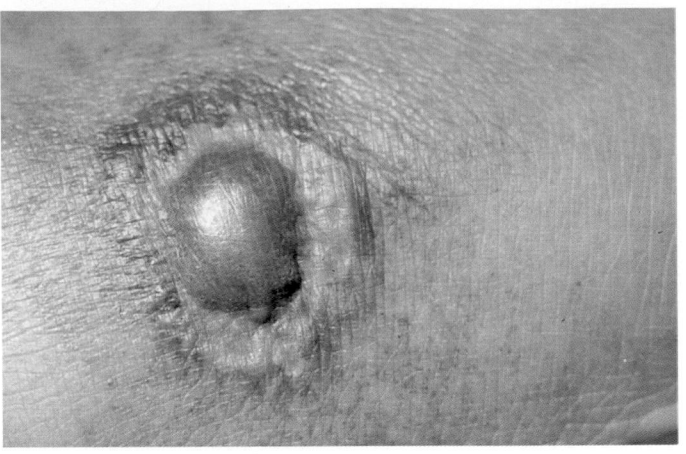

PLATE XXV-18   Lyme disease. Erythema migrans with a central hemorrhagic bulla.

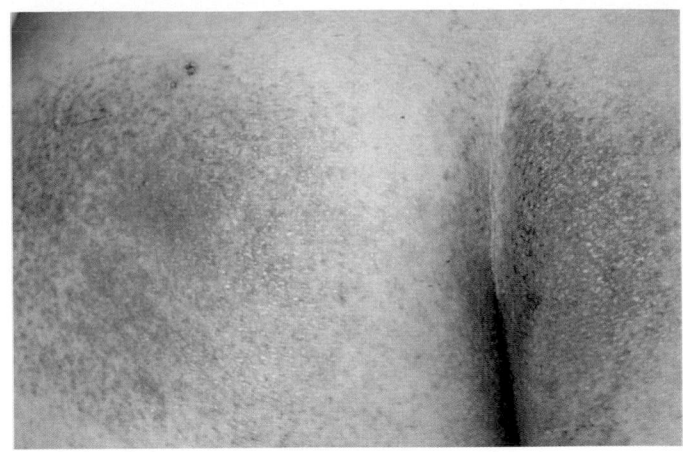

PLATE XXV-19   Parvovirus B-19.

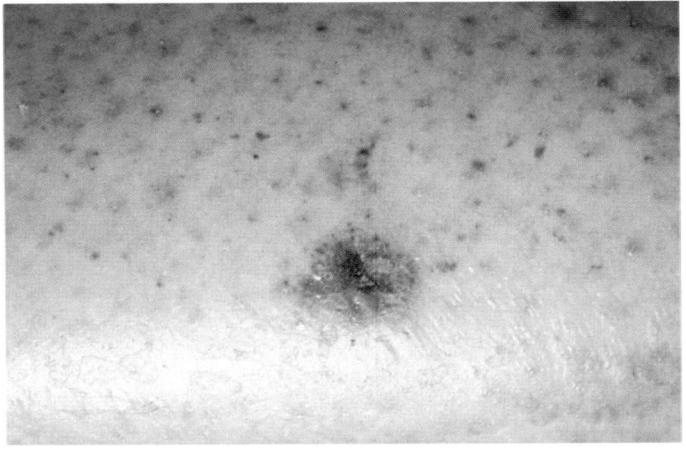

PLATE XXV-20   Disseminated candidiasis. Purpuric nodule in a patient with acute myelogenous leukemia.

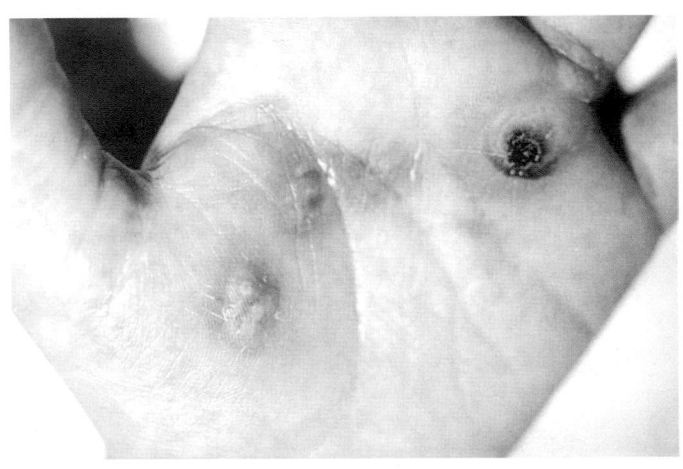

PLATE XXV-21   Aspergillosis: Primary cutaneous inoculation from contaminated armboard.

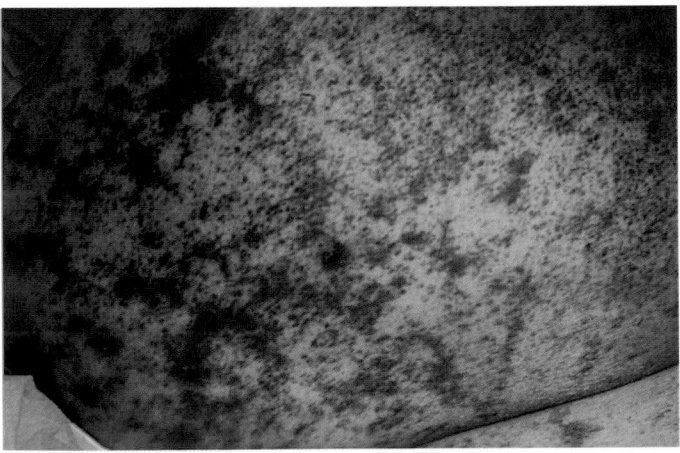

PLATE XXV-22   Disseminated strongyloidiasis.

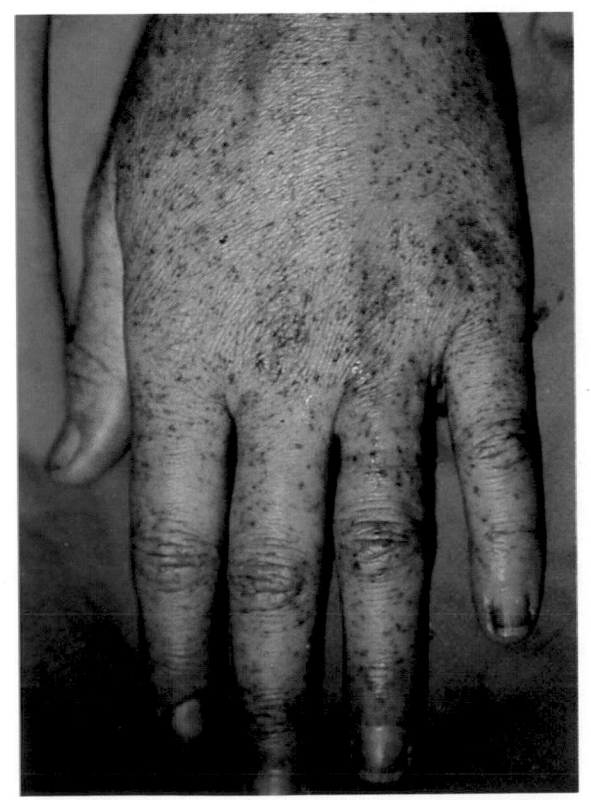

PLATE XXV-23   Rocky Mountain spotted fever. Petechiae on the dorsum of the hand.

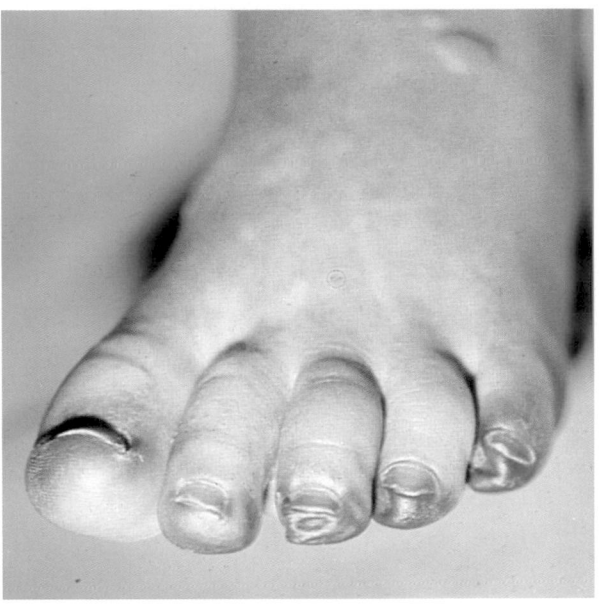

PLATE XXV-24   Rocky Mountain spotted fever. Peripheral purpuric gangrene.

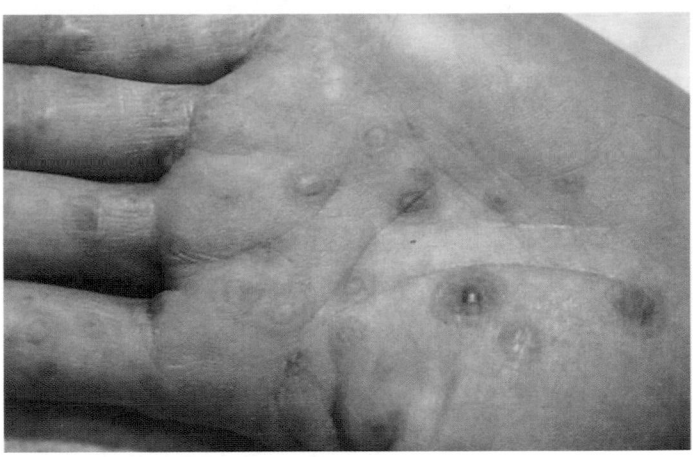

PLATE XXV-25   Erythema multiforme. Note characteristic targetoid lesions.

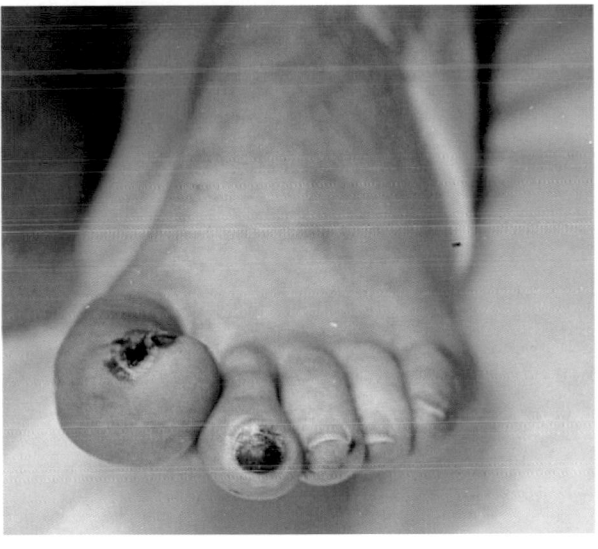

PLATE XXV-26   Polyarteritis nodosa. Acral purpura accompanying tender erythematous nodules.

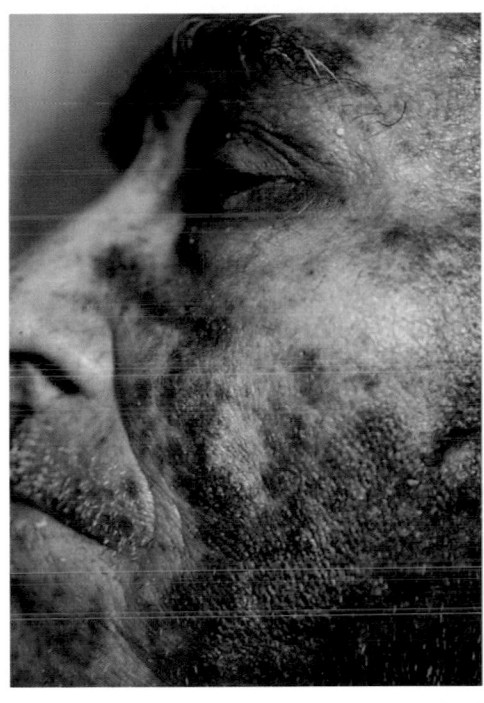

PLATE XXV-27   Paraneoplastic vasculitis. Acute myelogenous leukemia blast cells infiltrating the skin.

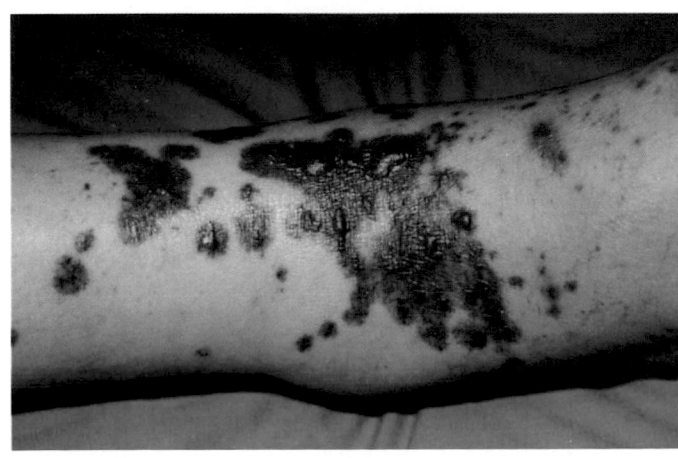

PLATE XXV-28   Leukocytoclastic vasculitis secondary to furosemide.

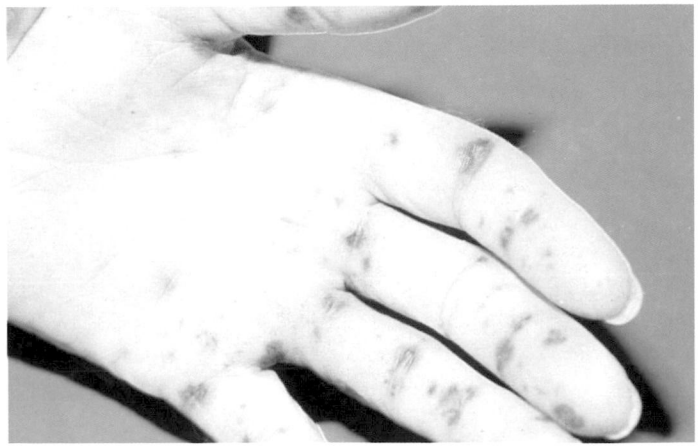

PLATE XXV-29   Wegener granulomatosis.

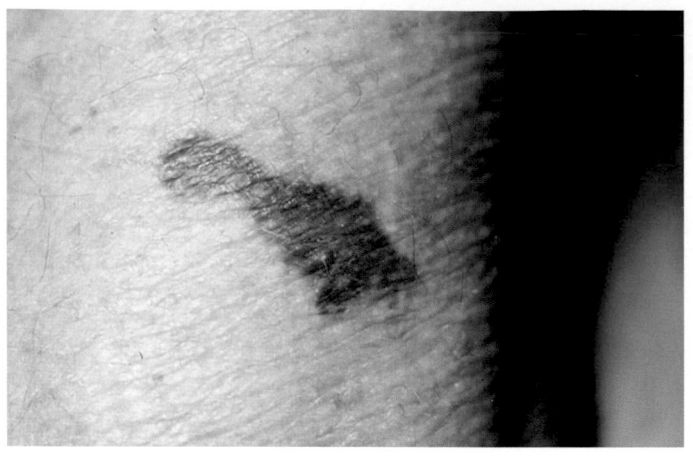

PLATE XXV-30   Senile purpura.

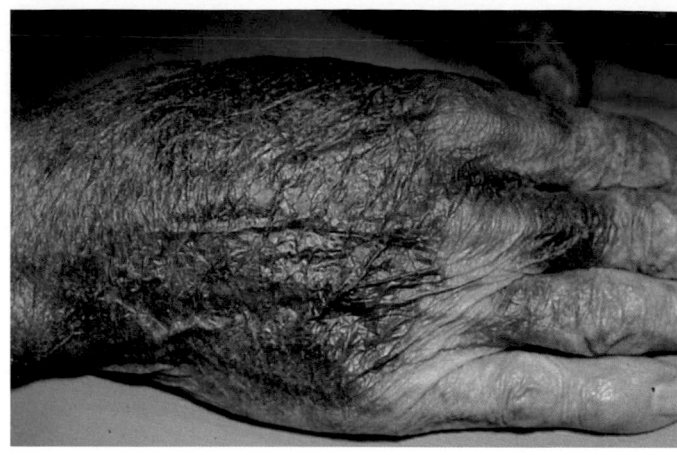

PLATE XXV-31   Senile purpura. Note accompanying skin atrophy.

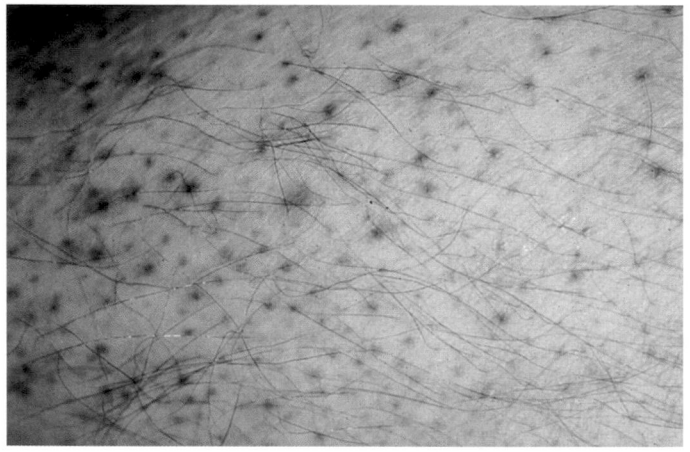

PLATE XXV-32   Scurvy. Note parafollicular petechiae.

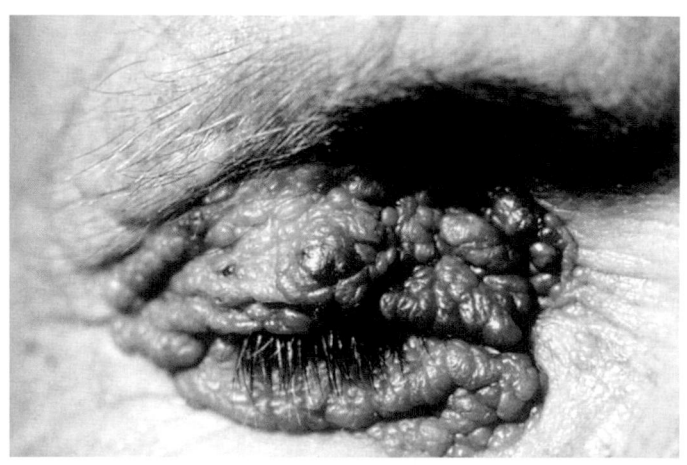

PLATE XXV-33   Amyloidosis of inferior palpebrum. Note waxy surface.

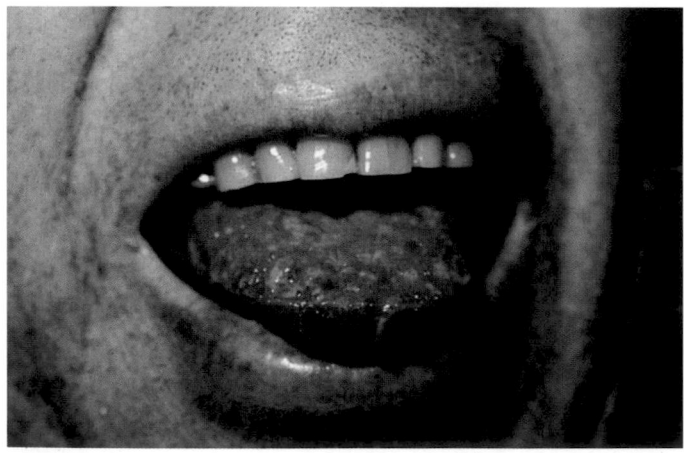

PLATE XXV-34   Amyloidoses of tongue.

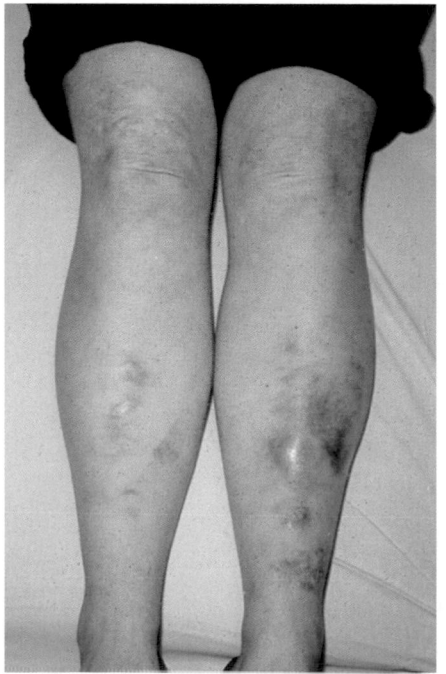

PLATE XXV-35   Ehlers-Danlos Syndrome. Purpura on lower extremities.

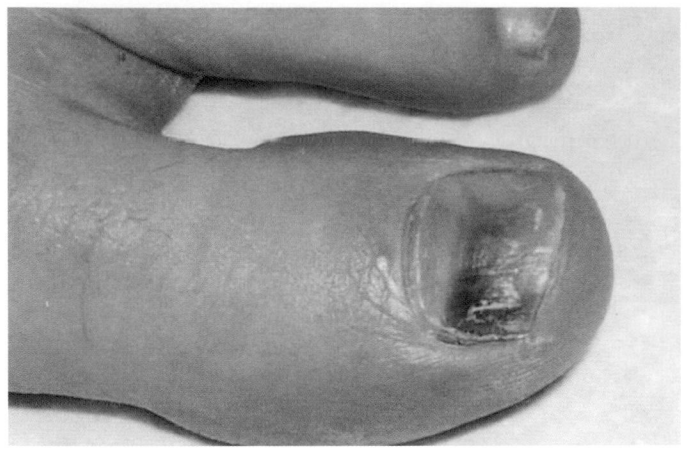

PLATE XXV-36 Subungual hematoma. Can be confused with subungual melanoma. A proximal nail fold clear of pigmentation favors the diagnosis of hematoma.

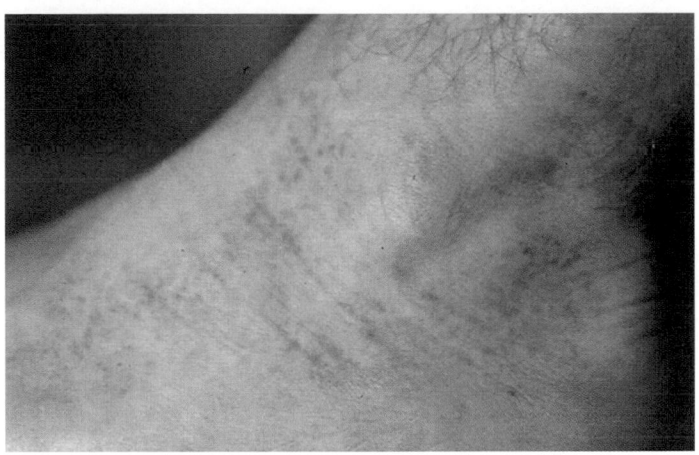

PLATE XXV-37 Schamberg disease. Note characteristic "cayenne pepper petechiae."

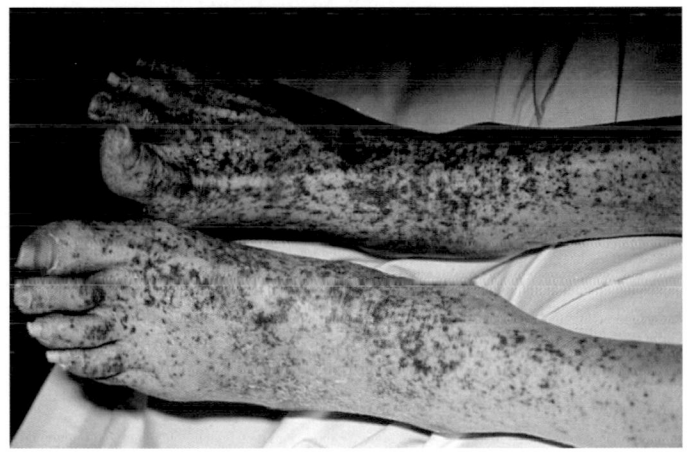

PLATE XXV-38 Quinidine purpura.

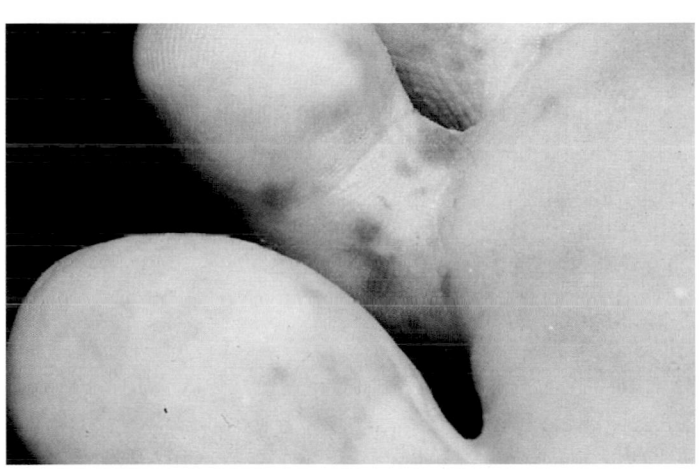

PLATE XXV-39 Systemic lupus erythematosus vasculitis.

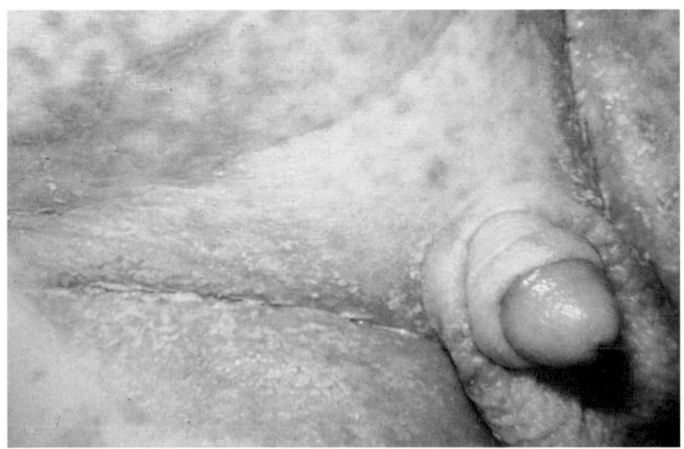

PLATE XXV-40 Langerhans cell histiocytosis.

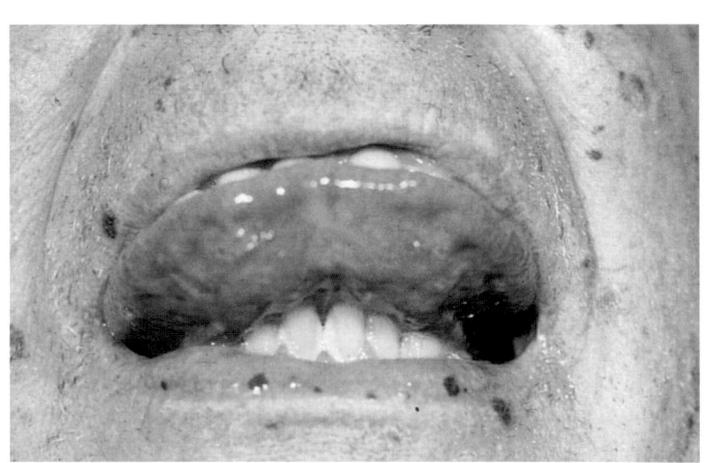

PLATE XXV-41 Hereditary hemorrhagic telangiectasia: Sublingual and labial telangiectasia.

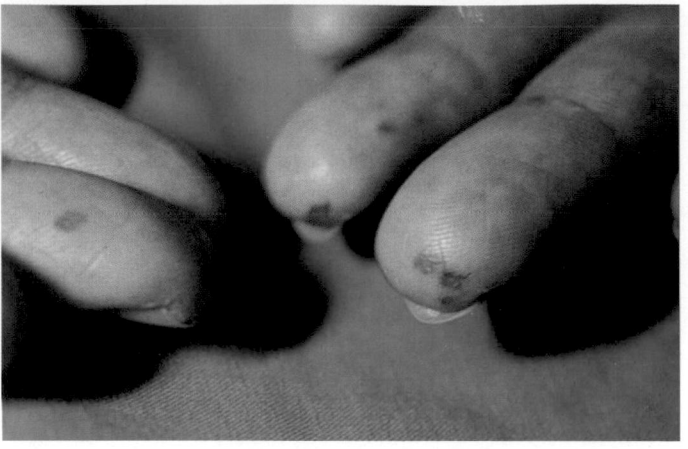

PLATE XXV-42   Hereditary hemorrhagic telangiectasia: Acral telangiectasias.

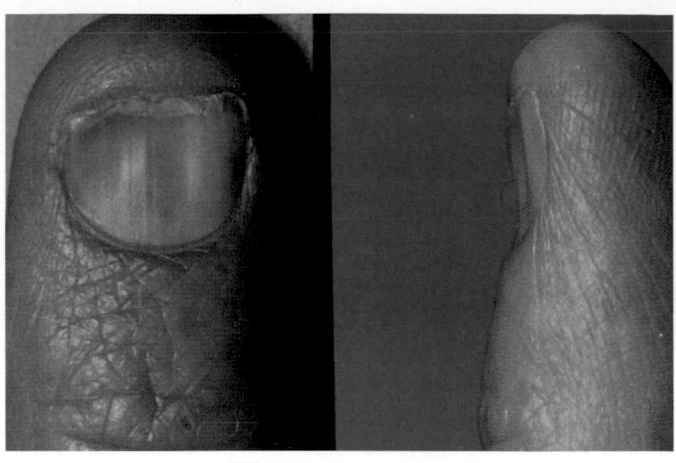

PLATE XXV-43   Koilonychia in severe iron deficiency.

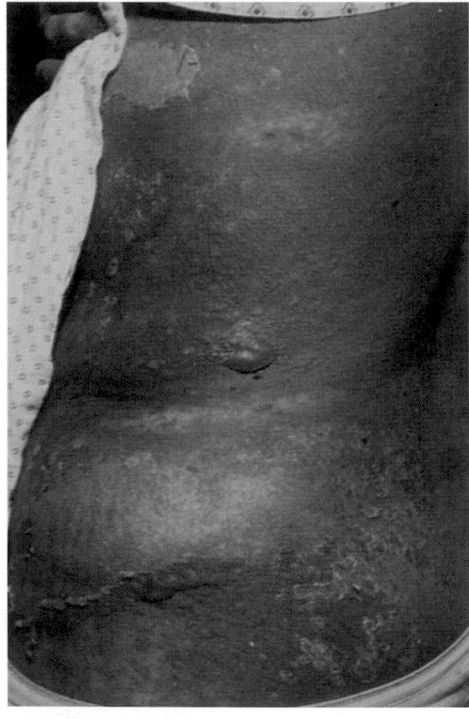

PLATE XXV-44   Grade IV graft-versus-host disease of the skin with diffuse erythroderma and bullous formation.

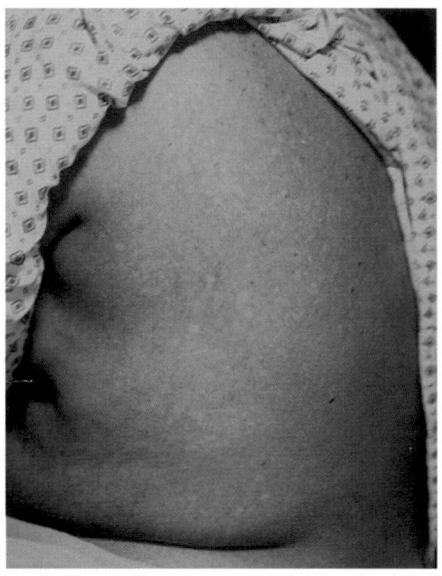

PLATE XXV-45   Complete resolution of grade IV graft-versus-host disease after therapy with high-dose glucocorticoids and antithymocyte globulin.

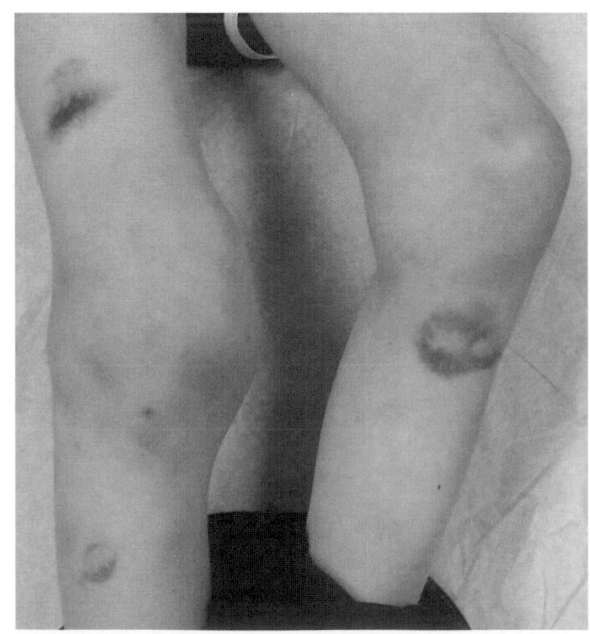

PLATE XXV-46   Hemophilia A. Swelling from recurrent knee joint bleeding. Cutaneous ecchymoses.

DESTRUCTION OF ERYTHROCYTES

ERNEST BEUTLER

The survival of red cells in the circulation can be measured in a variety of ways: (1) by labeling with isotopes, particularly ^{51}Cr, and assessing the disappearance of the tag from the circulation over time; (2) by labeling the erythrocytes with biotin or fluorescent dye and measuring this marker over time; (3) by determining the disappearance of transfused allogeneic erythrocytes using immunologic markers; and (4) by measuring the excretion of CO, a product of heme catabolism.

Such studies show that normal human red cells have a finite life span averaging 120 days, with very little random destruction. During maturation of the reticulocyte, cell density increases, but after a few days of intravascular life span there is little further increase in density or other changes in the physical property of the red cells. This has made the senescent changes in the red cell that mark it for destruction difficult to study, but the exposure of phosphatidylserine on the membrane appears to be of major importance.

MEASUREMENT OF RED CELL DESTRUCTION

RED CELL LIFE SPAN

The original method for the measurement of the red cell life span consisted of the transfusion of cells that were compatible but identifiable immunologically—the Ashby technique; type O red cells were infused into individuals with type A or B cells and the recipients' own cells were removed using anti-A or anti-B serum.[1] During World War II and shortly after, this method was used extensively, but in recent years, because of the hazards associated with the administration of allogeneic erythrocytes, it has been completely replaced by techniques based on labeling of autologous blood.

In 1946, Shemin and Rittenberg demonstrated that the incorporation of ^{15}N-labeled glycine into heme could be used to measure the life span of the red cells.[2] Since then a number of other isotopic methods have been developed. These can be divided into three groups: (1) those that label a cohort of cells; (2) those that label cells randomly; and (3) those that use indirect measurements such as the rate of production of red cells or the rate of heme breakdown. The first two classes yield information about the nature of the shortening of the red cell life span, age-dependent or random. The last group yields only mean life span.

COHORT METHODS

Cohort methods depend on the biosynthetic incorporation of the label into the developing red cells. In these methods a group of cells of approximately the same age is labeled. The labels used are glycine-containing labeled nitrogen (^{15}N),[2] radioactive carbon (^{14}C),[3] or radioactive iron, either ^{55}Fe or ^{59}Fe.[4–6] The main disadvantage of cohort labeling is the need for prolonged periods of sampling, especially if the life span is only moderately reduced (Fig. 31-1). In addition, radioiron from destroyed red cells may be reutilized making it difficult to interpret results.

RANDOM-LABEL METHODS

The random-label methods are the Ashby differential agglutination technique,[1] which uses an immunologic marker, and/or the use of various red cell labels such as chromium (^{50}Cr, ^{51}Cr, or ^{53}Cr),[7,8] diisopropylfluorophosphate (DFP) labeled with ^{32}P,[9] ^{3}H[10] or ^{14}C,[11] ^{14}C cyanate,[12] a lipophilic dye,[13,14] or biotin.[15–17]

By far the most commonly used radioactive isotope for the measurement of the red cell life span is ^{51}Cr, which as the chromate ion penetrates the red cell membrane and binds to the β and γ chains of globin. Unfortunately, these bonds are not covalent and there is a continuous elution of the isotope, varying from 0.5 to 2.9 percent per day.[18] DFP, on the other hand, is irreversibly bound to red cell cholinesterase. There is some elution of unbound DFP during the first 2 to 3 days of study, but after that DFP disappearance closely matches red cell destruction.[19,20] Nevertheless, because sample preparation is somewhat complicated this label is not commonly used.

To accurately calculate red cell life span using a random label method requires steady-state conditions or that correction can be made for concurrent blood loss or blood transfusion. Fortunately, it is usually possible to gain an accurate estimate of red cell half-life by sampling three times a week for 1 to 2 weeks.

In the normal human the red cell life span is finite, with an average of about 120 days, with very little random destruction, that is, loss irrespective of cell age (0.06% to 0.4% per day). In some mammalian species the amount of random destruction is much greater.[21] The survival curve of randomly labeled human red cells should be nearly linear from day 0 to day 120 with a half life of 60 days. When ^{51}Cr is used as the label, approximately 1 percent of label elutes per day and the survival curve becomes exponential with a half-life of about 30 days (see Fig. 31-1). For clinical use the red cell life span is usually expressed as chromium $t_{1/2}$ and compared to the normal of 30 days.

Because merely expressing the red cell life span measured by chromium as chromium $t_{1/2}$ will not give information as to the character of destruction, senescence versus random, it has been recommended that in addition a correction factor for chromium elution be used and the data recorded using linear coordinates.[22] If the data lie on a straight line, the destruction is by senescence and the life span can be calculated as twice the half-life. If the data indicate exponential disappearance and it is necessary to use semilogarithmic paper in order to depict the data on a straight line, the destruction is random and the life span is 1.44 times the half-life. One objection to this method is that the degree of chromium elution is not a constant but varies from day to day and from disease to disease.[18] Furthermore, the best fit of data is rarely linear or exponential but somewhere in between. Computer-assisted methods can resolve ambiguities, but the inherent biologic and technical variations in measuring red cell life span are such that it is better to rely on chromium $t_{1/2}$ with intuitive adjustments based on clinical findings.

INDIRECT METHODS

There are two approaches to the calculation of the red cell life span by indirect methods: from a measurement of the rate of production of red cells using radioactive iron or from a measurement of the rate of breakdown of heme to bilirubin[23] and or the release of carbon monoxide from catabolized heme.[24] Both of these compounds are derived

Acronyms and abbreviations that appear in this chapter include: AMP, adenosine monophosphate; C3, third component of complement; DFP, diisopropylfluorophosphate; Ig, immunoglobulin.

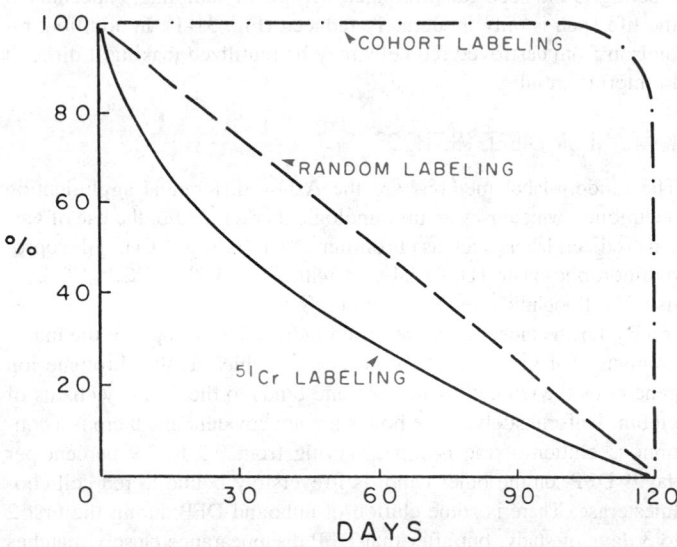

FIGURE 31-1   Red cell life span measured by cohort labeling or random labeling. When red cells are labeled randomly with ^{51}Cr there is a daily 1 percent elution that needs to be corrected for in the calculation of total red cell life span.

almost exclusively from catabolized hemoglobin and measurements of their rate of production have provided useful information about the red cell life span. There are probably too many variables that affect the serum bilirubin level to make it a reliable, quantitative measurement of red cell destruction. The measurement of CO production was formerly very tedious, requiring elaborate rebreathing apparatus. With the development of newer technologies,[25,26] measuring CO levels has become more practical. An advantage of the measurement of blood CO as an indication of the rate of red cell destruction is that it gives the rate of destruction at a single point in time.

IN SITU LOCALIZATION OF RED CELL PRODUCTION AND DESTRUCTION

As part of routine erythrokinetic studies both radioactive iron and radioactive chromium may be used to localize red cell production and red cell destruction. This is accomplished by positioning probes for external counting over the sacrum, liver, spleen, and heart and measuring the distribution of radioactivity in the body.[27]

In a normal subject, ^{59}Fe injected intravenously is cleared rapidly from the plasma, and within 24 hours approximately 85 percent of the radioactivity can be accounted for in the marrow. The liver and the spleen divide the remaining 15 percent. Over the next 10 days, the marrow radioactivity decreases gradually as a result of the release into circulating blood of red cells labeled with radioactive hemoglobin. Patterns showing different uptake and distribution of the radioactive iron have been found for various hematologic disorders.[28] In hypersplenism, the trapping and destruction of iron-labeled cells in the spleen will increase splenic radioactivity rapidly, and in patients with erythroid hypoplasia the distribution of radioactive iron between liver and marrow is reversed (Fig. 31-2).

More effective methods demonstrating in situ erythropoiesis involve imaging marrow, liver, and spleen with a ^{99m}Tc sulfur colloid or ^{111}In.[29] Although these isotopes label primarily the monocyte–macrophage system, their uptake is similar to that of ^{59}Fe and they can be used as surrogate markers to estimate the distribution of erythroid tissue.

Surface counting for ^{51}Cr-labeled red cells provides a characteristic organ distribution of radioactivity and has been used to demonstrate the degree of red cell sequestration and destruction in an enlarged spleen[30] (Fig. 31-3). This approach has been used to predict the results of elective splenectomy, but the utility of this method has been challenged.[31] The in situ localization of red cell sequestration or destruction can also be determined by following the tissue distribution of ^{59}Fe-labeled red cells, especially if the red cell life span is very short.

MECHANISMS OF DESTRUCTION

INTRAVASCULAR DESTRUCTION

If the red cell membrane is breached in the circulation the red cell is destroyed. This mode of demise of the erythrocyte occurs at a low frequency normally but may be the predominant mode of destruction in some hemolytic disorders, for example, ABO-incompatible transfusions (Chap. 52) and paroxysmal nocturnal hemoglobinuria (Chap. 38) where the complement complex creates holes in the red cell membrane, and in cardiac valve hemolysis (Chap. 49) and microangiopathic hemolytic anemia (Chap. 121) where the shear stress may be so strong as to break open the membrane.

EXTRAVASCULAR DESTRUCTION

Most commonly the life of the red cell comes to an end when it is ingested by a macrophage. Clearly, signals that allow the macrophage to distinguish the younger normal red cell from a damaged or senescent

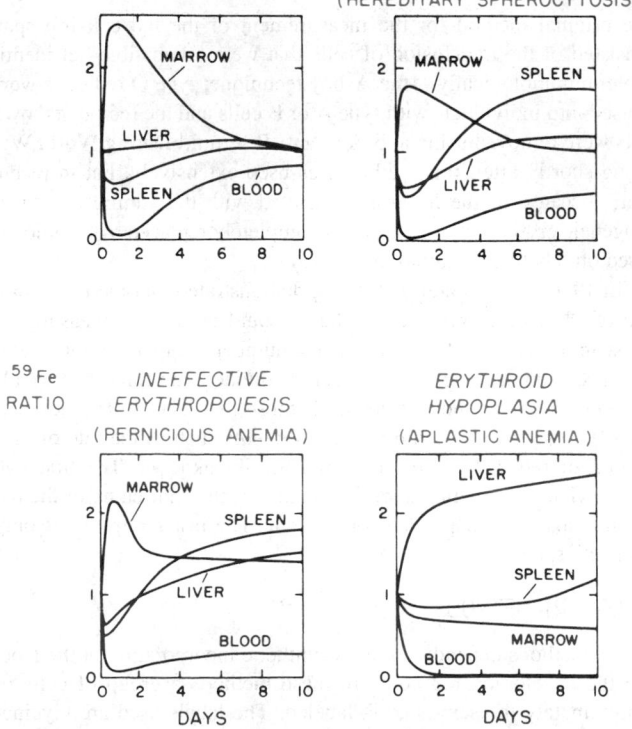

FIGURE 31-2   Tissue distribution of ^{59}Fe in normal subjects, hypersplenic patients, and anemic patients with ineffective and effective erythropoiesis. The radioactivity is expressed on the ordinate as a ratio relative to the radioactivity measured in the same organ 15 minutes after the intravenous administration of the isotope. (Redrawn from RS Hillman, CA Finch,[28] with permission.)

cell must exist. Such signals consist of decreased deformability and/or altered surface properties.

DECREASED DEFORMABILITY

The red cell does not circulate as the biconcave disc that we are accustomed to observing under the microscope. Instead, it is normally greatly distorted by the shear stresses in the circulation and such distortion is an absolute requirement for the red cell to be able to negotiate the narrow slits that separate the splenic pulp from the sinuses (Chap. 5). The deformability of the erythrocyte can be measured clinically using the ektacytometer, an instrument that displays the diffraction pattern of a red cell suspension under shear stress.[32-34] The red cell membrane, a lipid bilayer, bends readily but has very little capacity to stretch. Thus, deformability is a largely a function of the excess red cell membrane intrinsic to the biconcave disc shape of the cell and to some extent of the viscosity of the hemoglobin solution within the cell. As the red cell loses membrane it assumes a spherical shape and loses its ability to deform. Hereditary spherocytosis and hereditary elliptocytosis are prototypic of hemolytic anemias in which decreased deformability as a result of a decreased surface/volume ratio plays a key role in red cell destruction (Chap. 44). However, loss of membrane plays a role in many types of pathologic hemolysis, including autoimmune hemolytic anemia (Chap. 52). In sickle cell disease and hemoglobin C disease (Chap. 47) the internal viscosity of the cell is increased. Loss of water from the red cell, as may occur when the membrane is damaged and leaks potassium as in hereditary xerocytosis (Chap. 44), also markedly impairs the deformability of the cell.

Altered Surface Properties The surface of the red cell membrane can be altered by binding of antibodies to surface antigens, by binding of complement components, and by chemical alterations, particularly oxidation of membrane components. Immunoglobulin (Ig) G-coated red cells[35] and red cells coated by C3[36,37] are bound by Fc receptors on macrophages and undergo partial phagocytosis. This results in the formation of a spherocyte. The same process occurs in the mononuclear phagocyte system of patients with autoimmune hemolytic anemia (Chap. 52). *In vitro* oxidation of red cells with phenylhydrazine or ADP plus iron causes clustering of band 3 protein in the membrane. Although the physiologic significance of this is far from clear, it has been suggested that the clustered proteins serve as a recognition site for the binding of IgG.[38,39] Oxidative damage to the membrane may play a role in the removal of sickle cells (Chap. 47) and thalassemic cells from the circulation (Chap. 46).

SENESCENCE OF NORMAL ERYTHROCYTES

The classic 1949 studies of London and associates,[40] in which the heme in erythrocytes was labeled with ^{15}N glycine, established that most red cells have a finite life span of between 100 and 140 days.[41]

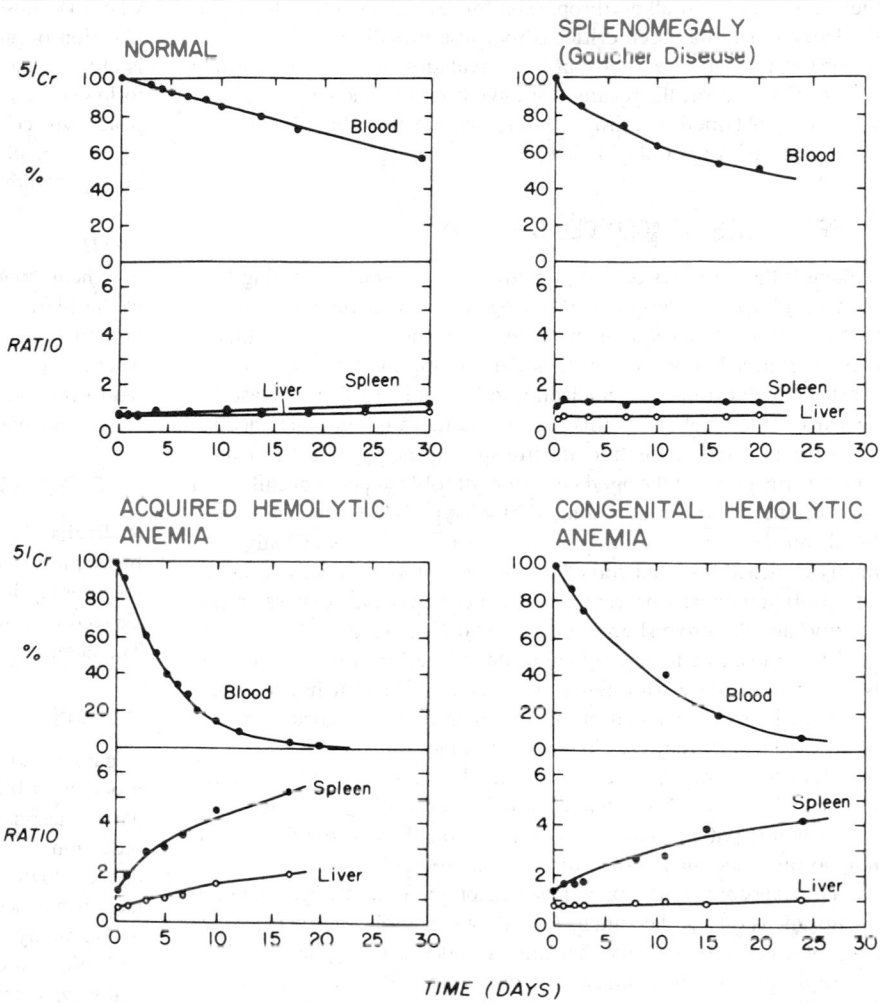

FIGURE 31-3 Tissue distribution of red cells labeled with ^{51}Cr in normal subjects and in patients with hypersplenism. The radioactivity of blood is given on the ordinate in percent of the radioactivity found 15 minutes after injection. The radioactivity of the spleen and liver is expressed as a ratio relative to the radioactivity determined simultaneously over the precordium. (Redrawn from JH Jandl, MS Greenberg, RH Yonemoto, WB Castle,[30] with permission.)

METHODOLOGIC CONSIDERATIONS

Labeling a cohort of human erythrocytes with ^{59}Fe and centrifuging the cells in a density gradient demonstrates that reticulocytes and young red cells are less dense than mature red cells.[42,43] However, at the end of the life span of the labeled cohort, radioactivity is fairly evenly distributed throughout red cells of all densities with only a slight tendency of the radioactivity to be concentrated in the more dense cells. Unfortunately, many studies of the properties of senescent cells in the past have been based upon the characteristics of the most dense fraction of erythrocytes, using various fractionating techniques. In fact, the most dense fraction of red cells is only slightly enriched with old erythrocytes.[44-46]

There are two animal models and one human disease model that provide cells that are truly aged. In mice, *in vivo* aged cells have been produced by serially transfusing mice, maintaining polycythemia to suppress virtually all erythropoiesis.[47] In other species, particularly the rabbit, red cells have been labeled with traces of biotin, which enables them to be recovered from the circulation.[48] The human model is transient erythroblastopenia of childhood (Chap. 34), a disorder in which there is cessation of all erythropoiesis for several months. The use of the latter model has been criticized because this disorder is not fully understood and the red cells in the circulation may not be entirely normal.[49] However, the results that have been obtained are consistent with those obtained in animal models and are probably reliable (see "Properties of Aged Cells" below).

PROPERTIES OF AGED CELLS

Although the activities of a large number of enzymes, including hexokinase, glucose-6-phosphate dehydrogenase, and pyruvate kinase, are higher in reticulocytes than in mature erythrocytes, the activities of these enzymes do not continue to decline during the aging of the erythrocyte.[48,50] Pyrimidine-5'-nucleotidase[51,52] and AMP-deaminase[53–55] appear to be exceptions to this rule in that there is continuing decline of enzyme activity throughout the life span of the red cell. The density and deformability of the aged cells in erythroblastopenia of childhood are normal.[44] Fluorescent sorting of blood type NN erythrocytes transfused into humans shows that the most dense fractions are only minimally enriched with old cells,[56] and biotinylated aged cells of rabbits have only a modestly decreased surface area, volume, cell water, and density, and therefore slightly decreased deformability.[45,57]

The amount of immunoglobulin on red cell membranes has been reported to increase with aging of the cells,[58,59] and it has been proposed that such accumulation of immunoglobulin mediates removal of senescent erythrocytes. However, immunoglobulin levels on aged, biotinylated rabbit cells are not increased,[60] and the fact that red cell life span has never been demonstrated to be prolonged in agammaglobulinemic patients casts serious doubt on the concept that immunoglobulins mediate removal of senescent red cells.

The exposure of phosphatidylserine on the outer leaflet of the cell membrane is one of the signals that allows macrophages to recognize apoptotic cells. It is likely that this is, indeed, the signal by which macrophages recognize senescent erythrocytes.[17,61,62] A model that has been developed suggests that the average time during which phosphatidylserine is exposed is only 0.3 to 0.5 days, so that few cells with increased exposure of the phospholipid are in the circulation at any time. It is not yet clear whether this is the only, or even the primary, signal that indicates that a cell has reached the end of its life span, but it is the only major difference between senescent and nonsenescent erythrocytes that has been documented clearly.

FATE OF DESTROYED RED CELLS

INTRAVASCULAR DESTRUCTION

HEMOGLOBIN

When red cells are destroyed in the vascular compartment the hemoglobin escaping into the plasma is bound to haptoglobin. A dimeric glycoprotein, each molecule of haptoglobin can bind two hemoglobin dimers.[63] The haptoglobin–hemoglobin complex is cleared from the plasma with a $t_{1/2}$ of 10 to 30 minutes.[64] After the complex is carried to the liver parenchyma,[65] the heme of the hemoglobin is converted to iron and biliverdin by heme oxygenase and the biliverdin is further catabolized to bilirubin. CO is released in the course of cleavage of heme by heme oxygenase.

Free haptoglobin, in contrast to the hemoglobin–haptoglobin complex has a $t_{1/2}$ of 5 days, and when large amounts of the rapidly turned over haptoglobin–hemoglobin complex are formed, the haptoglobin content of the plasma is depleted. The haptoglobin content of the plasma is diminished not only in the plasma of patients undergoing frank intravascular hemolysis, but also from the plasma of patients

who, like those with sickle cell disease, have accelerated red cell destruction occurring primarily within macrophages. Presumably there is either enough intravascular hemolysis in such hemolytic disorders to lower the plasma haptoglobin level or sufficient leakage from the phagocytic cells into the plasma to bind to haptoglobin. Thus the measurement of plasma haptoglobin levels has some usefulness in diagnosing the presence of hemolysis.

HEME

Free heme that is released into the circulation is bound in a 1:1 ratio to the plasma glycoprotein hemopexin,[66] which is cleared from the plasma with a $t_{1/2}$ of 7 to 8 hours.[67,68] The heme is delivered to the liver where it is converted to bilirubin. When the capacity of hemopexin to bind heme has been saturated, excess heme may bind to albumin to form methemalbumin.[69]

EXTRAVASCULAR DESTRUCTION

Red cells that are engulfed by phagocytic cells are degraded within lysosomes into lipids, protein, and heme. The proteins and lipids are reprocessed in their respective catabolic pathways and the heme is cleaved by a microsomal heme oxygenase[70] into iron and biliverdin. The latter is catabolized to bilirubin.

BILIRUBIN EXCRETION

Regardless of the site of destruction of hemoglobin one of the final products is bilirubin, and this is excreted through the bile into the gastrointestinal tract where it is converted to urobilinogens by bacterial reduction.[71] A small fraction of urobilinogen is reabsorbed and excreted into the urine. Thus, the fecal and urinary urobilinogen excretion have been used as an indicator of the rate of hemolysis, but are only uncommonly used for this purpose in modern practice because the collections are cumbersome and because alternatively degradative pathways detract severely from the accuracy of the estimates of the rate of heme catabolism.

REFERENCES

1. Ashby W: The determination of the length of life of transfused blood corpuscles in man. *J Exp Med* 29:267, 1919.
2. Shemin D, Rittenberg D: Life span of human red blood cell. *J Biol Chem* 166:627, 1946.
3. Berlin NI, Meyer LM, Lazarus M: Life span of the rat red blood cell as determined by glycine-2-C[14]. *Am J Physiol* 165:565, 1951.
4. Beutler E, Dern RJ, Alving AS: The hemolytic effect of primaquine: IV. The relationship of cell age to hemolysis. *J Lab Clin Med* 44:439, 1954.
5. Birgens HS, Hansen OP, Henriksen JH, Wantzin P: Quantitation of erythropoiesis in myelomatosis. *Scand J Haematol* 22:357, 1979.
6. Weinstein IM, Beutler E: The use of Cr-51 and Fe-59 in a combined procedure to study erythrocyte production and destruction in normal human subjects and in patients with hemolytic or aplastic anemia. *J Lab Clin Med* 45:616, 1955.
7. Heaton WA: Evaluation of posttransfusion recovery and survival of transfused red cells. *Transfus Med Rev* 6:153, 1992.
8. Silver HM, Seebeck MA, Cowett RM, et al: Red cell volume determination using a stable isotope of chromium. *J Soc Gynecol Investig* 4:254, 1997.
9. Cohen JA, Warringa MGPJ: The fate of P[32] labeled diisopropyl fluorophosphonate in the human body and its use as a labeling agent in study of turnover of blood plasma and red cells. *J Clin Invest* 33:459, 1954.

10. Cline MJ, Berlin NI: Measurement of red cell survival with tritiated diisopropyl flurophosphate. *J Lab Clin Med* 60:826, 1962.

11. Milner PF, Charache S: Life span of carbamylated red cells in sickle cell anemia. *J Clin Invest* 52:3161, 1973.

12. Eschbach JW, Korn D, Finch CA: ^{14}C cyanate as a tag for red cell survival in normal and uremic man. *J Lab Clin Med* 89:823, 1977.

13. Horan PK, Slezak SE: Stable cell membrane labeling. *Nature* 340:167, 1989.

14. Slezak SE, Horan PK: Fluorescent *in vivo* tracking of hematopoietic cells. Part I. Technical considerations. *Blood* 74:2172, 1989.

15. Suzuki T, Dale GL: Biotinylated erythrocytes: *In vivo* survival and *in vitro* recovery. *Blood* 70:791, 1987.

16. Wardrop KJ, Tucker RL, Anderson EP: Use of an *in vitro* biotinylation technique for determination of posttransfusion viability of stored canine packed red blood cells. *Am J Vet Res* 59:397, 1998.

17. Boas FE, Forman L, Beutler E: Phosphatidyl serine exposure and red cell viability in red cell ageing and in hemolytic anemia. *Proc Natl Acad Sci U S A* 95:3077, 1998.

18. Bentley SA, Glass HI, Lewis SM, Szur L: Elution correction in ^{51}Cr red cell survival studies. *Br J Haematol* 26:179, 1974.

19. Cline MJ, Berlin NI: Simultaneous measurement of the survival of two populations of erythrocytes with the use of labeled diisopropyl fluorophosphate. *J Lab Clin Med* 61:249, 1963.

20. McCurdy PR, Sherman AS: Irreversibly sickled cells and red cell survival in sickle cell anemia: A study with both DF32P and 51CR. *Am J Med* 64:253, 1978.

21. Eadie GS, Brown IW Jr: Red blood cell survival studies. *Blood* 8:1110, 1953.

22. International Committee for Standardization in Haematology: Recommended method for radioisotope red-cell survival studies. *Br J Haematol* 45:659, 1980.

23. Berlin NI, Berk PD: Quantitative aspects of bilirubin metabolism for hematologists. *Blood* 57:983, 1981.

24. Doyle J, Vreman HJ, Stevenson DK, et al: Does vitamin C cause hemolysis in premature newborn infants? Results of a multicenter double-blind, randomized, controlled trial. *J Pediatr* 130:103, 1997.

25. Furne JK, Springfield JR, Ho SB, Levitt MD: Simplification of the end-alveolar carbon monoxide technique to assess erythrocyte survival. *J Lab Clin Med* 142:52, 2003.

26. Vreman HJ, Stevenson DK: Carboxyhemoglobin determined in neonatal blood with a CO-oximeter unaffected by fetal oxyhemoglobin. *Clin Chem* 40:1522, 1994.

27. ICSH Panel on Diagnostic Applications of Radioisotopes in Hematology: Recommended methods for surface counting to determine sites of red cell destruction. *Br J Haematol* 30:249, 1975.

28. Hillman RS, Finch CA: Erythropoiesis: Normal and abnormal. *Semin Hematol* 4:327, 1967.

29. Datz FL, Taylor AJ: The clinical use of radionuclide bone marrow imaging. *Semin Nucl Med* 15:239, 1985.

30. Jandl JH, Greenberg MS, Yonemoto RH, Castle WB: Clinical determination of the sites of red cell sequestration in hemolytic anemias. *J Clin Invest* 35:842, 1956.

31. Ferrant A, Cauwe F, Michaux JL, et al: Assessment of the sites of red cell destruction using quantitative measurements of splenic and hepatic red cell destruction. *Br J Haematol* 50:591, 1982.

32. Rigal CS: The place of instruments in the scientific work of Marcel Bessis (1917–1994): The electron microscope and the ektactometer. *Hematol Cell Ther* 42:250, 2000.

33. Johnson RM, Ravindranath Y: Osmotic scan ektacytometry in clinical diagnosis. *J Pediatr Hematol Oncol* 18:122, 1996.

34. Kuypers FA, Scott MD, Schott MA, et al: Use of ektacytometry to determine red cell susceptibility to oxidative stress. *J Lab Clin Med* 116:535, 1990.

35. Lo Buglio AF, Cotran RS, Jandl JH: Red cells coated with immunoglobulin G: Binding and sphering by mononuclear cells in man. *Science* 158:1582, 1967.

36. Jandl JH, Tomlinson AS: The destruction of red cells by antibodies in man: II. Pyrogenic, leukocytic and dermal responses to immune hemolysis. *J Clin Invest* 37:1202, 1958.

37. Lutz HU, Stammler P, Kock D, et al: Opsonic potential of C3b-antiband 3 complexes when generated on senescent and oxidatively stressed red cells or in fluid phase, in *Red Blood Cell Aging*, edited by M Magnani, A DeFlora, p 367. Plenum Press, New York, 1991.

38. Low PS, Waugh SM, Zinke K, Drenckhahn D: The role of hemoglobin denaturation and band 3 clustering in red blood cell aging. *Science* 227:531, 1985.

39. Beppu M, Mizukami A, Nagoya M, Kikugawa K: Binding of anti-band 3 autoantibody to oxidatively damaged erythrocytes. Formation of senescent antigen on erythrocyte surface by an oxidative mechanism. *J Biol Chem* 265:3226, 1990.

40. London IM, Shemin D, West R, Rittenberg D: Heme synthesis and red blood cell dynamics in normal humans and in subjects with polycythemia vera, sickle-cell anemias, and pernicious anemia. *J Biol Chem* 179:463, 1949.

41. Bratosin D, Mazurier J, Tissier JP, et al: Cellular and molecular mechanisms of senescent erythrocyte phagocytosis by macrophages. A review. *Biochimie* 80:173, 1998.

42. Borun ER, Figueroa WG, Perry SM: The distribution of Fe59 tagged human erythrocytes in centrifuged specimens as a function of cell age. *J Clin Invest* 36:676, 1957.

43. Luthra MG, Friedman JM, Sears DA: Studies of density fractions of normal human erythrocytes labeled with iron-59 in vivo. *J Lab Clin Med* 94:879, 1979.

44. Linderkamp O, Friederichs E, Boehler T, Ludwig A: Age dependency of red blood cell deformability and density: Studies in transient erythroblastopenia of childhood. *Br J Haematol* 83:125, 1993.

45. Dale GL, Norenberg SL: Density fractionation of erythrocytes by Percoll/Hypaque results in only a slight enrichment for aged cells. *Biochim Biophys Acta* 1036:183, 1990.

46. Beutler E: Isolation of the aged. *Blood Cells* 14:1, 1988.

47. Ganzoni AM, Oakes R, Hillman RS: Red cell aging in vivo. *J Clin Invest* 50:1373, 1971.

48. Suzuki T, Dale GL: Senescent erythrocytes: Isolation of in vivo aged cells and their biochemical characteristics. *Proc Natl Acad Sci U S A* 85:1647, 1988.

49. Haram S, Carriero D, Seaman C, Piomelli S: The mechanism of decline of age-dependent enzymes in the red blood cell. *Enzyme* 45:47, 1991.

50. Zimran A, Forman L, Suzuki T, et al: In vivo aging of red cell enzymes: Study of biotinylated red blood cells in rabbits. *Am J Hematol* 33:249, 1990.

51. Beutler E, Hartman G: Age-related red cell enzymes in children with transient erythroblastopenia of childhood and hemolytic anemia. *Pediatr Res* 19:44, 1985.

52. Beutler E: The relationship of red cell enzymes to red cell life-span. *Blood Cells* 14:69, 1988.

53. Dale GL, Norenberg SL: Time-dependent loss of adenosine 5′-monophosphate deaminase activity may explain elevated adenosine 5′-triphosphate levels in senescent erythrocytes. *Blood* 74:2157, 1989.

54. Paglia DE, Valentine WN, Nakatani M, Brockway RA: AMP deaminase as a cell-age marker in transient erythroblastopenia of childhood and its role in the adenylate economy of erythrocytes. *Blood* 74:2161, 1989.

55. Dale GL, Norenberg SL, Suzuki T, Forman L: Altered adenine nucleotide metabolism in senescent erythrocytes from the rabbit. *Prog Clin Biol Res* 319:259, 1989.

56. Clark MR, Corash L, Jensen RH: Density distribution of aging, transfused human red cells. *Blood* 74[Suppl 1]:217a, 1989.

57. Waugh RE, Narla M, Jackson CW, et al: Rheologic properties of senescent erythrocytes: Loss of surface area and volume with red blood cell age. *Blood* 79:1351, 1992.

58. Kay MMB, Marchalonis JJ, Schluter SF, Bosman G: Human erythrocyte aging: Cellular and molecular biology. *Transfus Med Rev* 5:173, 1991.

59. Sheiban E, Gershon H: Recognition and sequestration of young and old erythrocytes from young and elderly human donors: *In vitro* studies. *J Lab Clin Med* 121:493, 1993.

60. Dale GL: Does surface bound immunoglobulin mediate erythrocyte death? Commentary. *Blood Cells* 14:36, 1988.

61. Connor J, Pak CC, Schroit AJ: Exposure of phosphatidylserine in the outer leaflet of human red blood cells. Relationship to cell density, cell age, and clearance by mononuclear cells. *J Biol Chem* 269:2399, 1994.

62. Kuypers FA, De J: The role of phosphatidylserine in recognition and removal of erythrocytes. *Cell Mol Biol* 50:147, 2004.

63. Nagel RL, Gibson QH: The binding of hemoglobin to haptoglobin and its relation to subunit dissociation of hemoglobin. *J Biol Chem* 246:69, 1971.

64. Garby L, Noyes WD: Studies on hemoglobin metabolism: I. The kinetic properties of the plasma hemoglobin pool in normal man. *J Clin Invest* 38:1479, 1959.

65. Hershko C: The fate of circulating hemoglobins. *Br J Haematol* 29:199, 1975.

66. Baker HM, Anderson BF, Baker EN: Dealing with iron: Common structural principles in proteins that transport iron and heme. *Proc Natl Acad Sci U S A* 100:3579, 2003.

67. Sears DA: Disposal of plasma heme in normal man and patients with intravascular hemolysis. *J Clin Invest* 49:5, 1970.

68. Wochner RD, Spilberg I, Iio A, et al: Hemopexin metabolism in sickle-cell disease, porphyrias and control subjects—Effects of heme injection. *N Engl J Med* 290:822, 1974.

69. Rosen H, Sears DA: Spectral properties of hemopexin-heme: The Schumm test. *J Lab Clin Med* 74:941, 1969.

70. Maines MD: The heme oxygenase system: A regulator of second messenger gases. *Annu Rev Pharmacol Toxicol* 37:517, 1997.

71. Elder G, Gray CH, Nicholson DG: Bile pigment fate in gastrointestinal tract. *Semin Hematol* 9:71, 1972.

CLINICAL MANIFESTATIONS AND CLASSIFICATION OF ERYTHROCYTE DISORDERS

JOSEF T. PRCHAL

Anemias are characterized by a decrease and polycythemias by an increase in red cell mass. The anemias typically but not always are associated with a decrease in the oxygen-carrying capacity of blood, so they usually are expressed in terms of hemoglobin concentration. The anemias may cause symptoms resulting from tissue hypoxia (e.g., fatigue, dyspnea on exertion). Manifestations also are caused by compensatory attempts to ameliorate hypoxia (e.g., hyperventilation, tachycardia, increased cardiac output). Tissue hypoxia sensing is ubiquitous and is mediated by an increased level of a transcription factor, hypoxia-inducible transcription factor 1 (HIF-1). HIF-1 upregulates the transcription of many genes that are involved in angiogenesis, energy metabolism, iron balance, and erythropoiesis, including erythropoietin, the principal erythropoietic factor. Classification of anemia is evolving because the classification should take into account new kinetic and molecular findings. The polycythemias are best expressed in terms of the packed red cell volume (hematocrit) because their clinical manifestations are primarily related to the expanded red cell mass and resulting increased viscosity of blood and to specific features related to the pathophysiology stemming from the molecular causative defect (e.g., thrombosis in polycythemia vera, cyanosis in congenital methemoglobinemia). The polycythemias result from (1) aberrant growth of hematopoietic progenitors—primary polycythemias (e.g., a monoclonal expansion of a multipotential hematopoietic cell; polycythemia vera), (2) gain-of-function mutations of an erythropoietin progenitor, or (3) increased levels of circulating erythropoiesis stimulating factors, usually erythropoietin-secondary polycythemias (e.g., chronic pulmonary disease, cobalt poisoning, Chuvash polycythemia). Spurious polycythemia designates an elevated hematocrit resulting from normal red cell mass but a contracted plasma volume.

ANEMIA

PATHOPHYSIOLOGY AND MANIFESTATIONS

EFFECT ON OXYGEN TRANSPORT

The clinical manifestations of anemia are a function of the degree of tissue hypoxia and the etiology and pathogenesis of the specific anemia (e.g., splenomegaly characteristic of hereditary spherocytosis, mucosal tongue atrophy of pernicious anemia). Reduced oxygen-carrying capacity mobilizes compensatory mechanisms designed to prevent or

---

Acronyms and abbreviations that appear in this chapter include: HIF-1, hypoxia-inducible transcription factor.

---

ameliorate tissue anoxia. The red cells also carry carbon dioxide from the tissues to the lungs and help distribute nitric oxide throughout the body, but transport of these gases does not appear to be dependent on the number of red cells available and remains normal in anemic patients. Tissue hypoxia occurs when the pressure of oxygen in the capillaries is too low to provide cells with enough oxygen for the cells' metabolic needs. In an average person, the red cell mass must provide the total body tissues with about 250 ml/min of oxygen to support life. Because the oxygen-carrying capacity of normal blood is 1.34 ml per gram of hemoglobin (approximately 200 ml per liter of normal blood) and cardiac output is approximately 5000 ml/min, 1000 ml/min of oxygen is available at the tissue level. Extraction of one fourth of this amount reduces the oxygen tension of 100 torr in the arterial end of the capillary to 40 torr in the venous end. This partial extraction ensures the presence of sufficient diffusion pressure throughout the capillaries to provide all cells with enough oxygen for the cells' metabolic needs (Fig. 32-1). In anemia, extraction of the same amount of oxygen leads to greater hemoglobin desaturation and lower oxygen tension at the venous end of the capillary. The resulting anoxia in the immediate vicinity initiates a number of compensatory and frequently symptomatic adjustments in the supply of blood and oxygen.

Hypoxia-Inducible Transcription Factor 1 Hypoxia-inducible transcription factor 1 (HIF-1) plays a central role in the body's response to hypoxia (see Chaps. 30 and 56). HIF-1 was first identified as a factor regulating the transcriptional activity of erythropoietin gene[1] (see Chap. 30). The essential role of this transcriptional factor in global regulation of protection against hypoxia soon became clear. Its actions include respiratory control, transcriptional regulation of glycolytic enzyme genes, angiogenesis, and energy metabolism.[2–4] The prediction that hypoxia-regulated subunit of HIF-1 (HIF 1α) degradation is controlled by an enzyme sensitive to the presence or absence of oxygen[5] proved to be prescient. The current knowledge of hypoxia sensing is described in greater detail in Chap. 30. Tissue-specific and known and unknown factors are responsible for tissue-specific mobilization of the compensatory mechanisms listed below that permit survival under hypoxic conditions. Figure 32-2 outlines the regulation of some physiologic processes by hypoxia.

DECREASED OXYGEN CONSUMPTION

Energy metabolism at the optimal oxygen supply is generated by efficient oxidative phosphorylation. In hypoxia, energy is produced by less efficient glycolysis accomplished by up-regulation of transcription of glycolytic enzyme genes[4] and increased glucose transport, a process known as the Pasteur effect. Pasteur and its cancer exception, i.e., the Warburg effect, are explained at the molecular level by changes in HIF-1 levels.[4,6–8]

DECREASED OXYGEN AFFINITY

Efficient increase of tissue oxygen delivery is accomplished by decreasing the affinity of hemoglobin for oxygen (right-shifted hemoglobin oxygen dissociation curve). This action permits increased oxygen extraction from the same amount of hemoglobin[9] (see Chap. 47). Acutely, a very small shift in pH produces a large effect on the dissociation curve because of the Bohr effect. In chronic anemia, increased oxygen tissue delivery is accomplished by increased amounts of 2,3-bisphosphoglycerate[9] (see Chap. 45). The increased synthesis of 2,3-bisphosphoglycerate in anemia is accomplished by increasing the intracellular pH of red cells (see Chap. 45) by respiratory alkalosis resulting from increased respiration. This effect is clearly demonstrated in individuals with high-altitude hypoxemia.[10]

INCREASED TISSUE PERFUSION

The effect of decreased oxygen-carrying capacity on the tissue tension of oxygen can be compensated by increasing tissue perfusion by

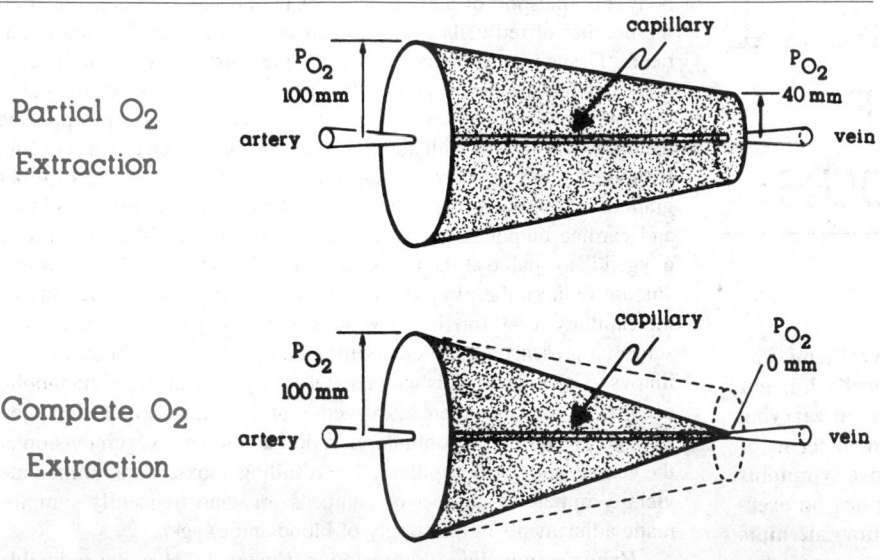

Partial O₂ Extraction

Complete O₂ Extraction

FIGURE 32-1   Theoretical tissue segment provided with oxygen from one capillary. With an arterial diffusion pressure of oxygen of 100 torr and partial oxygen extraction resulting in a venous oxygen pressure of 40 torr, one capillary can provide oxygen to cells within a truncated cone segment. With complete oxygen extraction, however, oxygen cannot be supplied to cells within a rim of tissue around the apex of the cone.

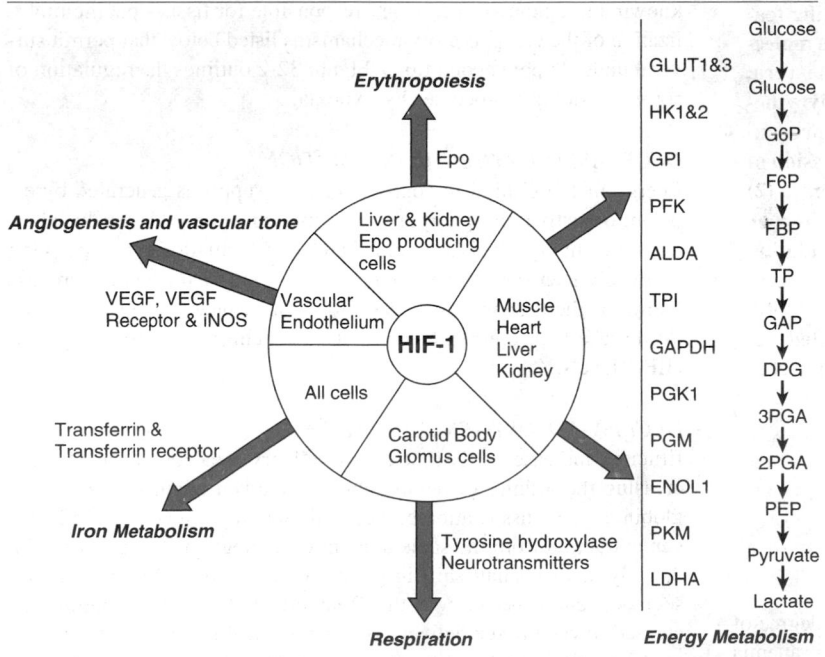

FIGURE 32-2   Regulation of erythropoiesis, angiogenesis, iron metabolism, respiration, and energy metabolism by HIF-1 are examples of physiologic processes regulated by hypoxia. iNOS, inducible nitrous oxide synthase; VEGF, vascular endothelial growth factor. *Right panel, left column*: GLUT1&3, glucose transporter 1 and 3. Glycolytic enzymes: HK1&2, hexokinase 1 and 2; GPI, glucose phosphate isomerase; PFK, phosphofructokinase; ALDA, aldolase A; TPI, triosophosphate isomerase; GAPDH, glycerol phosphate dehydrogenase; PGK1, phosphoglycerate kinase; PGM, phosphoglycerate mutase; ENOL1, enolase 1; PKM, pyruvate kinase M isoform; LDHA, lactic dehydrogenase A isoform. *Right column*: Metabolic intermediates generated by the depicted enzymes.

changing vasomotor activity and angiogenesis.[2] Because in most anemias the blood volume is not changed (Fig. 32-3),[11] increased tissue perfusion is organ selective, accomplished by shunting the blood from nonvital donor areas to oxygen-sensitive essential recipient organs. In acute anemia, the major donor areas for redistribution of blood are the mesenteric and iliac beds.[12] In chronic anemia in humans, the donor areas are the cutaneous tissue[13] and the kidneys.[14] Vasoconstriction and oxygen deprivation in the skin causes characteristic pallor of anemia. In the kidneys, the oxygen supply under normal conditions exceeds oxygen demands. The arteriovenous oxygen difference in the kidney is as low as 1.4 ml/dl (compared with the myocardium, where the difference can be as high as 20 ml/dl), indicating that even a severe reduction in kidney perfusion can be tolerated. Nevertheless, enough renal hypoxia must be present to activate HIF-1 and stimulate increased erythropoietin production and erythropoiesis (see Chap. 30). The effect on renal excretory mechanisms is slight because the reduction in renal blood flow is offset by high plasmacrit. Even in severe anemia where renal blood flow reduced by almost 50 percent, the total renal plasma flow is only moderately reduced. Severe anemia can cause retinal hemorrhages.[15] Thus, organs with the most pressing need for oxygen, such as myocardium, brain, and muscles, are largely unimpeded by a moderate reduction in oxygen-carrying capacity.

INCREASED CARDIAC OUTPUT

Increased cardiac output is an excellent but metabolically expensive compensatory device.[16] It decreases the fraction of oxygen that must be extracted during each circulation, thereby maintaining high oxygen pressure. Because the viscosity of blood in anemia is decreased and selective vascular dilatation decreases peripheral resistance, high cardiac output can be maintained without any increase in blood pressure.[17] In an otherwise healthy person, a measurable increase in resting cardiac output does not occur until hemoglobin concentration is less than 7 g/dl, and clinical signs of cardiac hyperactivity usually are not present until hemoglobin concentration reaches even lower levels.[18]

Signs of cardiac hyperactivity include tachycardia, increased arterial and capillary pulsation, and hemodynamic "flow" murmurs.[19] The murmurs usually are heard during systole at the apex, over the pulmonary valve area, or at the pulmonary valve area. Murmurs and bruits have been described in many regions, such as over the jugular vein, the closed eye, and the parietal region of the skull, and may be sensed by the patient as roaring in the ears (tinnitus), especially at night. They disappear promptly after the hemoglobin concentration is restored to normal.[19] The myocardium tolerates a prolonged period of sustained hyperactivity. However, angina pectoris and high-output failure may supervene if anemia is so extreme that it exceeds myocardial oxygen demands or if the patient has coronary artery disease. Cardiomegaly, pulmonary congestion, ascites, and edema have been observed, and they require prompt treatment with oxygen and transfusion of packed red cells.

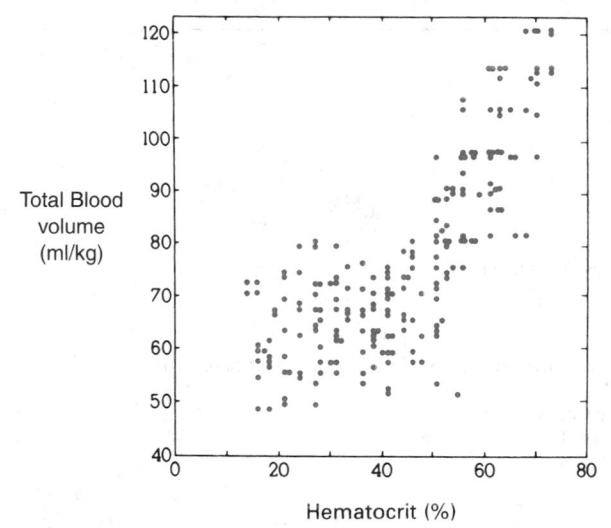

FIGURE 32-3   Relationship between hematocrit and total blood volume in normal individuals and in patients with anemia and polycythemia. (Reproduced from Huber et al.[11])

INCREASED PULMONARY FUNCTION

Significant anemia leads to compensatory increase in respiratory rate that decreases the oxygen gradient from ambient air to alveolar air and increases the amount of oxygen available to oxygenate a greater than normal cardiac output. Consequently, exertional dyspnea and orthopnea are characteristic clinical manifestations of severe anemia.[18–21]

INCREASED RED CELL PRODUCTION

The most appropriate response to anemia is a compensatory increase of red cell production, which may increase about twofold to threefold acutely and fourfold to sixfold chronically, and occasionally as much as 10-fold in the latter case. The increase is mediated by increased production of erythropoietin. The rate of erythropoietin synthesis is inversely and logarithmically related to hemoglobin concentration (see Chap. 30). Erythropoietin concentration can increase from approximately 10 mU/ml at normal hemoglobin concentrations to 10,000 mU/ml in severe anemia (Fig. 32-4).[22,23] The change in erythropoietin levels ensures red cell production fully balances red cell destruction (compensated hemolysis) or chronic moderate blood loss. Augmented erythroid activity expands marrow space, which can cause sternal tenderness and diffuse bone pains. The number and proportion of reticulocytes increase. Because erythroid transit time through the marrow is shortened, "stress reticulocytes" having increased cell volume and surface area appear. Nucleated red cells may be observed in severe anemia.[24]

Administration of human recombinant erythropoietin augments or replaces endogenous synthesis. At pharmacologic amounts, the effect on hemoglobin concentration is most noticeable if endogenous production is subnormal as a result of renal failure or systemic illnesses (see Chaps. 35 and 43). In severe anemia where endogenous erythropoietin production (providing production is not impaired) has already increased red cell production maximally, administration of erythropoietin generally does not help, and the patients require transfusion.[23]

UNCORRECTED TISSUE HYPOXIA

A certain residual degree of tissue hypoxia remains despite mobilization of compensatory mechanisms. Hypoxia is essential for initiation of adequate cardiovascular and erythropoietic compensation mechanisms, but severe tissue hypoxia can cause the following symptoms:

dyspnea on exertion or even at rest, angina, intermittent claudication, muscle cramps typically at night, headache, light-headedness, and fatigue. A number of diffuse gastrointestinal and genitourinary symptoms are associated with anemia (e.g., abdominal cramps, nausea), but whether the symptoms should be attributed to tissue hypoxia, compensatory redistribution of blood, or the underlying cause of anemia is uncertain.

CLASSIFICATION

Based on determination of the red cell mass, anemia and polycythemia can be classified as (1) *relative* or (2) *absolute*. Relative anemia and relative polycythemia are characterized by a normal total red cell mass. The conditions usually are not thought of as hematologic disorders but rather as disturbances in plasma volume regulation. However, dilution anemia and dehydration polycythemia are of clinical and differential diagnostic importance for the hematologist.

Classification of the *absolute anemias* with decreased red cell mass is difficult because the classification has to consider kinetic, morphologic, and pathophysiologic interacting criteria. Initially, all anemias should be divided into anemias caused by decreased production and anemias caused by increased destruction of red cells. The differentiation is based largely on the reticulocyte count. Subsequent diagnostic breakdown can be based on either morphologic or pathophysiologic criteria.

Morphologic classification subdivides anemia into (1) macrocytic anemia, (2) normocytic anemia, and (3) microcytic hypochromic anemia. The main advantages of this classification are that the classification is simple, is based on readily available red cell indices (MCV and MCHC), and forces the physician to consider the most important types of curable anemia: vitamin B_{12}, folic acid, and iron-deficiency anemias. Such practical considerations have led to wide acceptance of this classification. *Pathophysiologic classification* (Table 32-1) is best suited for relating disease processes to potential treatment. In addition, anemia resulting from deficiency states occurs in a significant proportion of patients with normal indices.

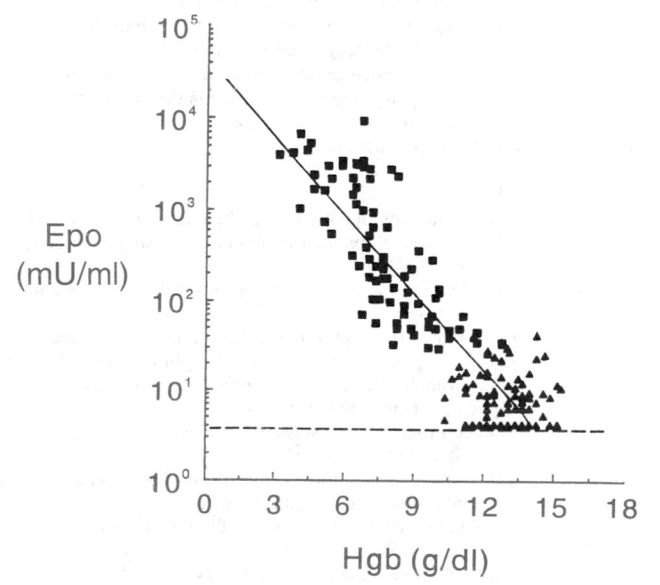

FIGURE 32-4   Erythropoietin levels in plasma of normal individuals and patients with anemia uncomplicated by renal or inflammatory disease. The lower limit of accuracy of the erythropoietin assay is 3 mU/ml and is indicated by the broken line. ■, anemias; ▲, normals.

TABLE 32-1 CLASSIFICATION OF ANEMIA

I. Absolute anemia (decreased red cell volume)
   A. Decreased red cell production
      1. Acquired
         a. Pluripotential stem cell failure
            (1) Aplastic anemia (see Chap. 33)
                (a) Radiation induced
                (b) Drugs and chemicals (chloramphenicol, benzene, etc.)
                (c) Viruses (hepatitis, Epstein-Barr virus, etc.)
                (d) Idiopathic
            (2) Anemia of leukemia and of myelodysplastic syndromes (see Chaps. 86, 87, and 91)
            (3) Anemia associated with marrow infiltration (see Chap. 42)
            (4) Postchemotherapy (see Chap. 19)
         b. Erythroid progenitor cell failure
            (1) Pure red cell aplasia parvovirus B19 infection, drugs, associated with thymoma, autoantibodies, etc. [see Chap. 34])
            (2) Endocrine disorders (see Chap. 36)
            (3) Acquired sideroblastic anemia (drugs, copper deficiency, etc. [see Chaps. 58 and 86])
         c. Functional impairment of erythroid and other progenitors due to nutritional and other causes
            (1) Megaloblastic anemias (see Chap. 39)
                (a) B_{12} deficiency
                (b) Folate deficiency
                (c) Acute megaloblastic anemia due to nitrous oxide (N_2O)
                (d) Drug-induced megaloblastic anemia (pemetrexed, methotrexate, phenytoin toxicity, etc.)
            (2) Iron-deficiency anemia (see Chap. 40)
            (3) Anemia resulting from other nutritional deficiencies (see Chap. 41)
            (4) Anemia of chronic disease and inflammation (see Chap. 43)
            (5) Anemia of renal failure (see Chap. 35)
            (6) Anemia due to chemical agents (lead toxicity [see Chap. 50])
            (7) Acquired thalassemias (seen in some clonal hematopoietic disorders [see Chaps. 46, 86, and 89])
            (8) Erythropoietin antibodies (see Chap. 35)
      2. Hereditary
         a. Pluripotential stem-cell failure (see Chap. 33)
            (1) Fanconi anemia
            (2) Shwachman syndrome
            (3) Dyskeratosis congenita
         b. Erythroid progenitor cell failure
            (1) Diamond-Blackfan syndrome (see Chap. 34)
            (2) Congenital dyserythropoietic syndromes (see Chap. 37)
         c. Functional impairment of erythroid and other progenitors due to nutritional and other causes
            (1) Megaloblastic anemias (see Chap. 39)
                (a) Selective malabsorption of vitamin B_{12} (Imerslund-Gräsbeck disease)
                (b) Congenital intrinsic factor deficiency
                (c) Transcobalamin II deficiency
                (d) Inborn errors of cobalamin metabolism (methylmalonic aciduria, homocystinuria, etc.)
                (e) Inborn errors of folate metabolism (congenital folate malabsorption, dihydrofolate deficiency, methyltransferase deficiency, etc.)
            (2) Inborn purine and pyrimidine metabolism defects (Lesch-Nyhan syndrome, hereditary orotic aciduria, etc.)
            (3) Disorders of iron metabolism (see Chap. 40)
                (a) Hereditary atransferrinemia
                (b) Hypochromic anemia due to DMT1 mutation
            (4) Hereditary sideroblastic anemia (see Chap. 58)
            (5) Thalassemias (see Chap. 46)
   B. Increased red cell destruction
      1. Acquired
         a. Mechanical
            (1) Macroangiopathic (march hemoglobinuria, artificial heart valves [see Chap. 49])
            (2) Microangiopathic (disseminated intravascular coagulation, DIC; thrombotic thrombocytopenic purpura, TTP; vasculitis [see Chaps. 49, 121, and 124])
            (3) Parasites and microorganisms (malaria, bartonellosis, babesiosis, *Clostridium welchii*, etc. [see Chap. 51])
         b. Antibody-mediated
            (1) Warm-type autoimmune hemolytic anemia (see Chap. 52)
            (2) Cryopathic syndromes (cold agglutinin disease, paroxysmal cold hemoglobinuria, cryoglobulinemia [see Chaps. 38 and 52])
            (3) Transfusion reactions (immediate and delayed [see Chaps. 53 and 128])
         c. Hypersplenism (see Chap. 55)
         d. Red cell membrane disorders (see Chap. 44)
            (1) Spur cell hemolysis
            (2) Acquired acanthocytosis and acquired stomatocytosis, etc.
         e. Chemical injury and complex chemicals (arsenic, copper, chlorate, spider, scorpion, and snake venoms, etc. [see Chap. 50])
         f. Physical injury (heat, oxygen, radiation [see Chap. 50])
      2. Hereditary
         a. Hemoglobinopathies (see Chap. 47)
            (1) Sickle cell disease
            (2) Unstable hemoglobins
          b. Red cell membrane disorders (see Chap. 44)
            (1) Cytoskeletal membrane disorders (hereditary spherocytosis, elliptocytosis, pyropoikilocytosis)
            (2) Lipid membrane disorders (hereditary abetalipoproteinemia, hereditary stomatocytosis, etc.)
            (3) Membrane disorders associated with abnormalities of erythrocyte antigens (McLeod syndrome, Rh deficiency syndromes, etc.)

TABLE 32-1   CLASSIFICATION OF ANEMIA (*Continued*)

      (4) Membrane disorders associated with abnormal transport (hereditary xerocytosis)
    c. Red cell enzyme defects (pyruvate kinase, $5'$ nucleotidase, glucose-6-phosphate dehydrogenase deficiencies, other red cell membrane disorders [see Chap. 45])
    d. Porphyrias (congenital erythropoietic and hepatoerythropoietic porphyrias, rarely congenital erythropoietic protoporphyria [see Chap. 57])
  C. Blood loss and blood redistribution
    1. Acute blood loss (see Chap. 54)
    2. Splenic sequestration crisis (see Chap. 47)
II. Relative (increased plasma volume)
  A. Macroglobulinemia (see Chap. 102)
  B. Pregnancy (see Chap. 7)
  C. Athletes (see Chap. 31)
  D. Postflight astronauts (see Chap. 31)

This chapter presents a classification based on our present concepts of normal red cell production and red cell destruction. Figure 32-5 outlines the cascade of proliferation, differentiation, and maturation underlying the transformation of a multipotential stem cell, first to erythroid progenitor cells, then to erythroid precursor cells, and finally to mature red cells. Each of these steps can become impaired and cause anemia. Therapeutic intervention depends on identifying the defective step and instituting the specific therapy. The limitation of such a classification is that, in most anemias, the pathogenesis involves several steps. For example, a decreased rate of production most often results in production of defective red cells with a shortened life span. Thus,

the outline provided is a conceptual guide to our present understanding of the processes underlying the production and destruction of red cells.

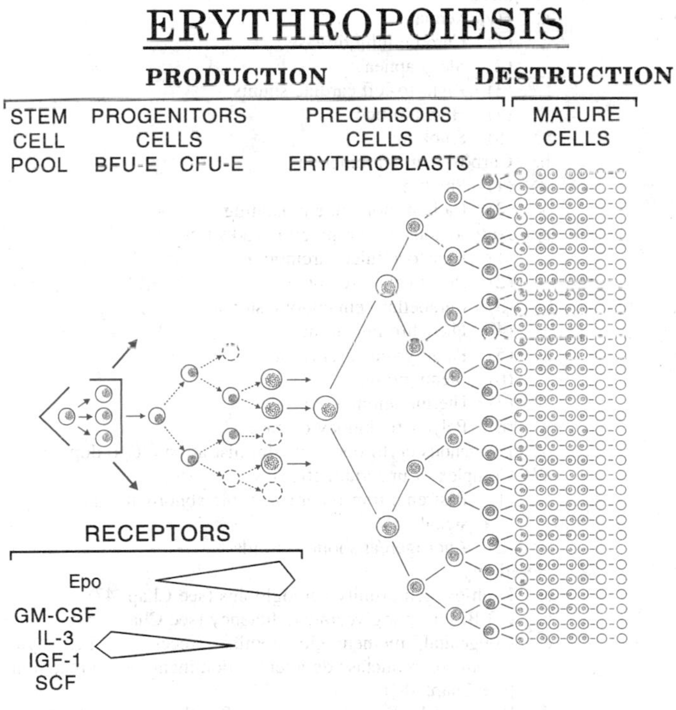

POLYCYTHEMIA (ERYTHROCYTOSIS)

PATHOPHYSIOLOGY AND MANIFESTATIONS

The production and presence of an increased number of red cells are associated with general and specific effects generated by changes in blood viscosity and blood volume.

At hematocrit readings greater than 50 percent, the viscosity of blood increases steeply (Fig. 32-6). The resulting decrease in blood flow reduces the transport of oxygen, with optimal values at hematocrit readings between 40 and 45 percent.[25,26] In a study of red cells from a number of animal species, the optimal value of oxygen transport corresponded closely to their normal hematocrits[27] and may explain the evolutionary choice of certain hematocrit levels as optimal.[28] However, before concluding that polycythemia always is a suboptimal condition, realize that it may be premature to translate viscosity readings, derived from blood tested in a rigid glass viscosimeter (Ostwald) or

ERYTHROPOIESIS

PRODUCTION **DESTRUCTION**

STEM CELL POOL	PROGENITORS CELLS BFU-E CFU-E	PRECURSORS CELLS ERYTHROBLASTS	MATURE CELLS

RECEPTORS

Epo

GM-CSF
IL-3
IGF-1
SCF

FIGURE 32-5   Outline of the process of differentiation, proliferation, and maturation underlying the production and destruction of red blood cells. Multipotential stem cells responding to a number of growth factors, including granulocyte-monocyte colony stimulating factors (GM-CSF), interleukin 3 (IL-3), insulin growth factor 1 (IGF-1), and stem cell factor (SCF), differentiate to progenitor cells committed to erythroid development. Progenitor cells, burst forming unit–erythroid (BFU-E), and colony forming unit–erythroid (CFU-E) proliferate under the control of erythropoietin (Epo) and finally differentiate to precursor cells (erythroblasts). In the presence of adequate amounts of nutrients, such as vitamin B_{12}, folic acid, and iron, precursor cells proliferate and mature into nucleated red cells, reticulocytes, and mature red blood cells. After a 120-day life span, these cells age and are destroyed.

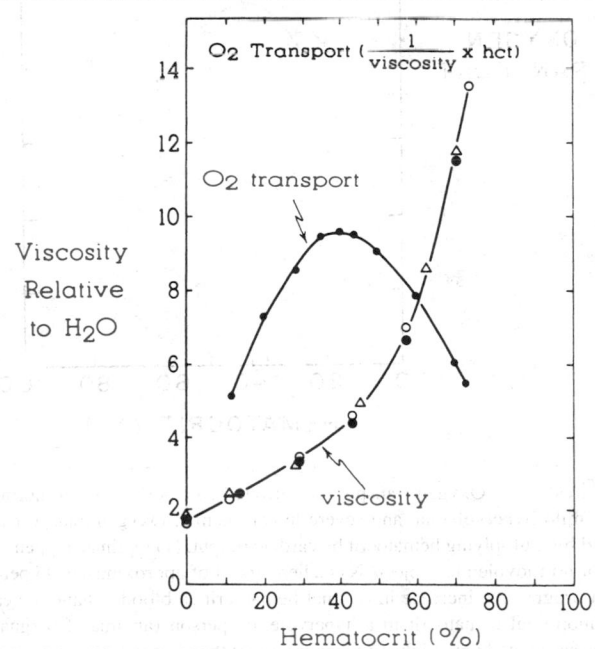

FIGURE 32-6   Viscosity of heparinized normal human blood related to hematocrit (hct). Viscosity is measured with an Ostwald viscosimeter at 37°C and expressed in relation to viscosity of saline solution. Oxygen transport is computed from hct and O_2 flow (1/viscosity) and is recorded in arbitrary units.

even in a cone-plate viscosimeter, into blood flow through tiny distensible vessels *in vivo*.[29] First, the flow through these narrow channels is rapid (high shear rate), which in a non-newtonian fluid such as blood causes a marked decrease in viscosity. Second, blood flowing through narrow channels *in vivo* is axial, with a central core of packed red cells sliding over a peripheral layer of lubricating low-viscosity plasma. Finally, and most important, absolute polycythemia is not normovolemic but is accompanied by increased blood volume, which, in turn, enlarges the vascular bed and decreases peripheral resistance. Because blood pressure remains stable, the increased blood volume must be associated with increased cardiac output and increased oxygen transport (cardiac output times hematocrit). Using measurements of cardiac output in dogs[30] and tissue oxygen tension in rats and mice,[29] construction of curves (Fig. 32-7) that relate oxygen transport to hematocrit in normovolemic and hypervolemic states is possible. The curves show that hypervolemia *per se* increases oxygen transport and that the optimum oxygen transport in these conditions occurs at higher hematocrit values than in normovolemic states. Consequently, despite the increased viscosity, a moderate increase in hematocrit is beneficial. The same may not be true of a more pronounced increase in hematocrit. Observations in humans[31] and experimental animals[30] indicate high viscosity causes reduced blood flow to most tissues and may be responsible for the cerebral and cardiovascular impairment experienced occasionally by high-altitude dwellers,[32] patients with severe polycy-

themia,[33,34] and athletes self-administering overdoses of erythropoietin (see Chap. 56).

The rate of red cell production is increased in true polycythemias, but changes in marrow morphology can be unimpressive, although marrow is hypercellular in a typical patient with polycythemia vera. Under normal conditions, the rate of red cell production is adjusted to maintain the red cell mass at about 30 ml per kilogram of body weight. Because the life span of red cells in polycythemia is normal, a mere doubling of the daily rate of red cell production is adequate to maintain a polycythemic red cell mass of 60 ml/kg. Consequently, the morphology and volume of the marrow are only moderately altered in polycythemia compared with the changes observed in some types of hemolytic anemia, in which the rate of red cell production can be six to 10 times normal. In erythrocytosis, the number of red cells destroyed daily merely causes a slight increase in bilirubin levels. The presence of secondary gout and splenomegaly usually are signs of a myelopro-

TABLE 32-2   CLASSIFICATION OF POLYCYTHEMIA

I. Absolute (true) polycythemia (increased red cell volume)
  A. Primary polycythemia
    1. Acquired
      a. Polycythemia vera
    2. Hereditary
      a. Primary familial and congenital polycythemia
        (1) Erythropoietin receptor mutations
        (2) Unknown gene mutations
  B. Secondary polycythemia
    1. Acquired
      a. Hypoxemia
        (1) Chronic lung disease
        (2) Sleep apnea
        (3) Right-to-left cardiac shunts
        (4) High altitude
        (5) Smoking
      b. Carboxyhemoglobinemia
        (1) Smoking
        (2) Carbon monoxide poisoning
      c. Autonomous erythropoietin production
        (1) Hepatocellular carcinoma
        (2) Renal cell carcinoma
        (3) Cerebellar hemangioblastoma
        (4) Pheochromocytoma
        (5) Parathyroid carcinoma
        (6) Meningioma
        (7) Uterine leiomyoma
        (8) Polycystic kidney disease
      d. Exogenous erythropoietin administration ("Epo doping")
      e. Complex or uncertain etiology
        (1) Postrenal transplant (probable abnormal angiotensin II signaling)
        (2) Androgen/anabolic steroids
    2. Hereditary
      a. High-oxygen affinity hemoglobins (see Chap. 47)
      b. 2,3-Bisphosphoglycerate deficiency (see Chap. 45)
      c. Congenital methemoglobinemias (recessive, i.e., cytochrome b5 reductase deficiency, dominant globin mutations [see Chap. 48])
      d. Recessive high erythropoietin polycythemias not due to von Hippel-Lindau gene mutations
      e. Autosomal dominant high erythropoietin polycythemias not due to von Hippel-Lindau gene mutations
  C. Mixed primary and secondary polycythemia
    1. Proven or suspected congenital disorders of hypoxia sensing
      a. Chuvash polycythemia
      b. High erythropoietin polycythemias due to mutations of von Hippel-Lindau gene other than Chuvash mutation
II. Relative (spurious) polycythemia (normal red cell volume)
  A. Dehydration
  B. Diuretics
  C. Smoking
  D. Gaisböck syndrome

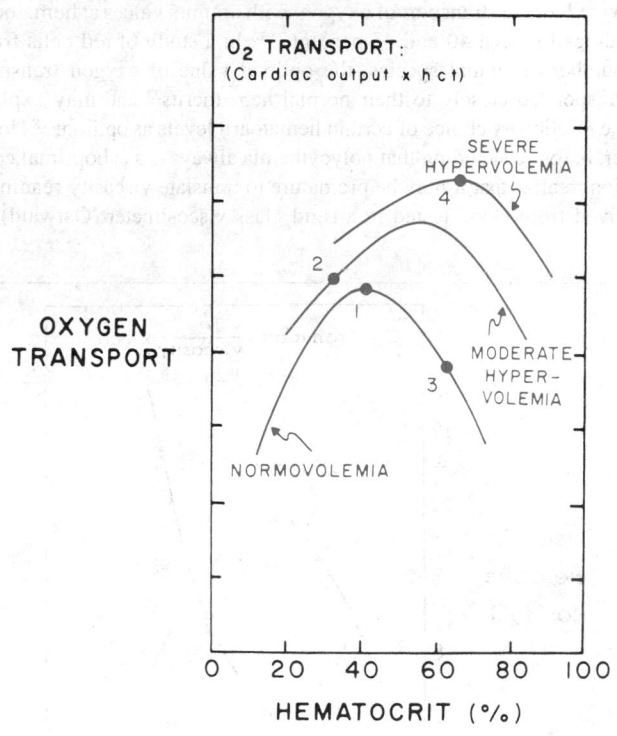

FIGURE 32-7   Oxygen transport at various hematocrit levels in normovolemia, mild hypervolemia, and severe hypervolemia. Oxygen transport is estimated by multiplying hematocrit by cardiac output. (1) Optimal oxygen transport for normovolemic subjects is at a hematocrit of approximately 45 percent, with a progressive increase in optimal hematocrit as blood volume increases. (2) Suboptimal hematocrit in a hypervolemic person (anemia of pregnancy) may be associated with higher oxygen transport than in a normovolemic person with normal hematocrit. (3) High hematocrit without an increase in blood volume may be associated with an absolute reduction in oxygen transport and tissue hypoxia. (4) Only high hematocrit coupled with high blood volume enhances oxygen transport to the tissues. (Adapted from Murray et al.[28] and Thorling and Erslev.[29])

liferative disorder rather than of erythrocytosis alone. Although considerable homology exists between erythropoietin and thrombopoietin,[35] erythropoietin-driven erythrocytosis is not associated with increased platelet production.

The increased viscosity and vascular space are responsible for many of the signs and symptoms of polycythemia. The characteristic *rubor* in patients with polycythemia vera is caused by excessive deoxygenation of blood flowing sluggishly through dilated cutaneous vessels. Nonspecific symptoms such as headaches, dizziness, tinnitus, and a feeling of fullness of the face and head probably are caused by a combination of increased viscosity and vascular dilatation. In extreme polycythemia and some specific types of polycythemia (e.g., methemoglobinemia, see Chap. 48), *cyanosis* can result from greater than 4 gm/dl of deoxygenated hemoglobin (accomplished more easily at higher hemoglobin concentrations [see "blue bloaters" and "pink puffers" in Chap. 56]) or greater than 1.5 gm/dl of methemoglobin.

Hemorrhages from the nose or stomach in patients with normal platelets and coagulation proteins can be attributed to capillary distention. However, circulatory stagnation causing ischemia and necrosis may contribute. Thromboses are common in polycythemia vera but are not seen at similar frequencies in other types of polycythemias (see Chap. 56). Coronary blood flow is decreased in polycythemia,[33] so the risk of coronary thrombosis in patients with a high hematocrit is assumed to be increased; however, statistical analyses have yielded equivocal results.[34,36,37] Polycythemia reportedly does not pose a risk in surgical patients.[38] Although cerebral blood flow is materially reduced in patients with moderately elevated hematocrit,[31,39] such reductions may have little practical significance.

CLASSIFICATION

Polycythemia, or *erythrocytosis,* is a condition in which the hematocrit percentage is above the upper limit of normal: greater than 51 percent in men and greater than 48 percent in women. Polycythemia can be classified as relative, in which the red cell mass is normal but the plasma volume is decreased, or absolute, in which the red cell mass is increased above normal (see Chap. 56). Table 32-2 outlines the polycythemic states.

Differentiation of absolute from relative polycythemia can be difficult at hematocrits less than 60 percent. Designation of a measured red cell mass as normal is imprecise because the red cell mass depends on the patient's age, sex, weight, height, and body frame and because only increases above the mean greater than 25 percent are considered abnormal.

PRIMARY POLYCYTHEMIAS

Primary polycythemias are caused by either acquired (polycythemia vera) or congenital mutations (such as gain-of-function erythropoietin receptor causing primary familial and congenital polycythemia) expressed within hematopoietic progenitors leading to increased production of red cells.

SECONDARY POLYCYTHEMIAS

Secondary polycythemias are caused by augmentation of erythropoiesis by circulating stimulatory factors such as erythropoietin (polycythemia of high altitude), cobalt, or insulin-like growth factor 1 (see Chap. 56).

CHUVASH POLYCYTHEMIA

Chuvash polycythemia has features of primary and secondary polycythemia (see Chap. 56).

REFERENCES

1. Semenza GL, Nejfelt MK, Chi SM, Antonarakis SE: Hypoxia-inducible nuclear factors bind to an enhancer element located 3′ to the human erythropoietin gene. *Proc Natl Acad Sci U S A* 88:5680, 1991.
2. Guillemin K, Krasnow MA: The hypoxic response: Huffing and HIFing. *Cell* 89:9, 1997.
3. Hochachka PW, Buck LT, Doll CJ, Land SC: Unifying theory of hypoxia tolerance: Molecular/metabolic defense and rescue mechanisms for surviving oxygen lack. *Proc Natl Acad Sci U S A* 93:9493, 1996.
4. Semenza GL: O_2-regulated gene expression: Transcriptional control of cardiorespiratory physiology by HIF-1. *J Appl Physiol* 96:1173, 2004.
5. Srinivas V, Zhu X, Salceda S, et al: Hypoxia-inducible factor 1α (HIF-1α) is a non-heme iron protein. *J Biol Chem* 273:18019, 1998.
6. Ivan M, Kondo K, Yang H, et al: HIF-alpha targeted for VHL-mediated destruction by proline hydroxylation: Implications for O_2 sensing. *Science* 292:464, 2001.
7. Jaakkola P, Mole DR, Tian Y, et al: Targeting of HIF alpha to the von Hippel-Lindau ubiquitylation complex by O_2-regulated prolyl hydroxylation. *Science* 292,468, 2001.
8. Epstein AC, Gleadle JM, McNeill LA, et al: *C. elegans* EGL-9 and mammalian homologs define a family of dioxygenases that regulate HIF by propyl hydroxylation. *Cell* 107:43, 2001.
9. Edwards MJ, Novy MJ, Walters CL, Metcalfe J: Improved oxygen release: An adaptation of mature red cells to hypoxia. *J Clin Invest* 47:1851, 1968.
10. Moore LG, Brewer GJ: Beneficial effect of rightward hemoglobin-oxygen dissociation curve shift for short-term high-altitude adaptation. *J Lab Clin Med* 98:145, 1981.
11. Huber H, Lewis SM, Szur L: The influence of anaemia, polycythaemia and splenomegaly on the relationship between venous haematocrit and red-cell volume. *Br J Haematol* 10:567, 1964.
12. Vatner SF: Effects of hemorrhage on regional blood flow distribution in dogs and primates. *J Clin Invest* 54:225, 1974.
13. Abramson DJ, Fierst SM, Flachs K: Resting peripheral blood flow in the anemic state. *Am Heart J* 25:609, 1954.
14. Bradley SE, Bradley GP: Renal function during chronic anemia in man. *Blood* 2:192, 1947.
15. Merin S, Freund M: Retinopathy in severe anemia. *Am J Ophthalmol* 66:1102, 1968.
16. Duke M, Abelman WH: The hemodynamic response to chronic anemia. *Circulation* 39:503, 1969.
17. Sharpey-Schafer EP: Cardiac output in severe anemia. *Clin Sci* 5:125, 1944.
18. Wintrobe MM: The cardiovascular system in anemia. *Blood* 1:121, 1946.
19. Wales RT, Martin EA: Arterial bruits in anemia. *BMJ* 2:1444, 1963.
20. Blumgart HL, Altschule MD: Clinical significance of cardiac and respiratory adjustments in chronic anemia. *Blood* 3:329, 1948.
21. Fatemian M, Gamboa A, Leon-Velarde F, et al: Selected contribution: Ventilatory response to CO_2 in high-altitude natives and patients with chronic mountain sickness. *J Appl Physiol* 94:1279, 2003.
22. Adamson JW: The erythropoietin/hematocrit relationship in normal and polycythemic man: Implications of marrow regulation. *Blood* 32:597, 1968.
23. Erslev AJ: Erythropoietin. *N Engl J Med* 324:1339, 1991.
24. Ward HP, Halman J: The association of nucleated red cells in the peripheral smear with hypoxemia. *Ann Intern Med* 67:1190, 1967.
25. Dintenfass I: A preliminary outline of the blood high viscosity syndromes. *Arch Intern Med* 118:427, 1966.
26. Stone HO, Thompson HK Jr, Schmidt-Nielson K: Influence of erythrocytes on blood viscosity. *Am J Physiol* 221:913, 1968.
27. Erslev AJ, Caro J, Schuster SJ: Is there an optimal hemoglobin level? *Transfus Med Rev* 3:237, 1989.

28. Murray JF, Gold P, Johnson BL Jr: The circulatory effects of hematocrit variations in normovolemic and hypervolemic dogs. *J Clin Invest* 42: 1150, 1963.

29. Thorling EB, Erslev AJ: The "tissue" tension of oxygen and its relation to hematocrit and erythropoiesis. *Blood* 31:332, 1968.

30. Fan FC, Chen RYZ, Schuessler GB, Chien S: Effects of hematocrit variations on regional hemodynamics and oxygen transport in the dog. *Am J Physiol* 238:H545, 1980.

31. Pearson TC, Humphrey PRD, Thomas DJ, et al: Hematocrit, blood viscosity, cerebral blood flow, and vascular occlusion, in *Clinical Aspects of Blood Viscosity and Cell Deformability*, edited by GDO Lowe, p 97. Springer-Verlag, New York, 1981.

32. Monge CM, Monge CC: *High Altitude Diseases: Mechanism and Management*, p 34. Thomas, Springfield, IL, 1966.

33. Kershenovich S, Modiano M, Ewy GA: Markedly decreased coronary blood flow in secondary polycythemia. *Am Heart J* 123:521, 1992.

34. Conley CL, Russell RP, Thomas CB, Tumulty PA: Hematocrit values in coronary artery disease. *Arch Intern Med* 113:170, 1969.

35. Kaushansky K: Thrombopoietin. *N Engl J Med* 339:749, 1998.

36. Mayer GA: Hematocrit and coronary heart disease. *CMAJ* 93:1151, 1965.

37. Hershberg PJ, Wells RE, McGandy RB: Hematocrit and prognosis in patients with acute myocardial infarction. *JAMA* 219:855, 1972.

38. Lubarsky DA, Gallagher CJ, Berend JL: Secondary polycythemia does not increase the risk of perioperative hemorrhagic or thrombotic complications. *J Clin Anesth* 3:99, 1991.

39. Thomas DJ, Marshall J, Russell RWR, et al: Cerebral blood flow in polycythemia. *Lancet* 2:161, 1977

APLASTIC ANEMIA

GEORGE B. SEGEL
MARSHALL A. LICHTMAN

Aplastic anemia **is a clinical syndrome manifested as a deficiency of red cells, neutrophils, monocytes, and platelets in the blood, and fatty replacement of the marrow with a near absence of hematopoietic precursor cells. Reticulocytopenia, neutropenia, monocytopenia, and thrombocytopenia, when severe, are life-threatening because of the risk of infection and bleeding, complicated by severe anemia. Most cases occur without an evident precipitating cause and result from expression of autoreactive T lymphocytes that suppress or destroy primitive hematopoietic cells. The disorder also can occur (1) after prolonged high-dose exposure to certain toxic chemicals (e.g., benzene), (2) after specific viral infections (e.g., Epstein-Barr virus), (3) as an idiosyncratic response to certain pharmaceuticals (e.g., ticlopidine), (4) as a feature of a connective tissue or autoimmune disorder (e.g., lupus erythematosus), or (5) rarely in association with pregnancy. Aplastic hematopoiesis is the primary manifestation of several uncommon inherited disorders (e.g., Fanconi anemia). Differential diagnosis includes other causes of a hypoplastic marrow, which can occur in paroxysmal nocturnal hemoglobinuria or hypoplastic myelogenous leukemia. Allogeneic stem cell transplantation is curative in approximately 80 percent of younger patients with a suitable donor, although the posttransplant period may be marred by graft-versus-host disease. The disease can be significantly ameliorated or rarely cured by anti–T cell therapy, especially with antithymocyte globulin and cyclosporine. After successful treatment with immunosuppressive agents, the disease has a propensity to evolve into a clonal hematopoietic disorder, such as paroxysmal nocturnal hemoglobinuria, a clonal cytopenia, or oligoblastic or polyblastic myelogenous leukemia.**

DEFINITION AND HISTORY

Aplastic anemia is a clinical syndrome that results from marked diminution of marrow blood cell production. The decreased production results in reticulocytopenia, anemia, granulocytopenia, monocytopenia, and thrombocytopenia. Severe aplastic anemia is defined as pancytopenia accompanied by a markedly hypocellular marrow and two of the following three features: (1) a corrected reticulocyte count less than 1 percent, (2) fewer than $500/\mu l$ granulocytes, or (3) fewer than $20,000/\mu l$ platelets. Most cases of aplastic anemia are acquired. Fewer cases are the result of an inherited disorder, such as Fanconi anemia.

Acronyms and abbreviations that appear in this chapter include: ALG, antilymphocyte globulin; ATG, antithymocyte globulin; BFU-E, burst forming unit–erythroid; CFU-GM, colony forming unit–granulocyte-macrophage; CMV, cytomegalovirus; DDT, dichlorodiphenyltrichloroethane; EBV, Epstein-Barr virus; G-CSF, granulocyte colony stimulating factor; GM-CSF, granulocyte-macrophage colony stimulating factor; HLA, human leukocyte antigen; IFN-γ, interferon gamma; IL, interleukin; MRI, magnetic resonance imaging; PCP, pentachlorophenol; PNH, paroxysmal nocturnal hemoglobinuria; SCF, stem cell factor; TNT, trinitrotoluene.

Aplastic anemia was first recognized by Ehrlich[1] in 1888. He described a young pregnant woman who died of severe anemia and neutropenia. Autopsy examination revealed a fatty marrow with essentially no hematopoiesis. The name *aplastic anemia* subsequently was applied to this disease by the French hematologist Chauffard[2] in 1904. Although the term is anachronistic because morbidity is the result of pancytopenia, the designation is entrenched in medical usage. For the following 30 years, many conditions that caused pancytopenia were confused with aplastic anemia based on incomplete or inadequate histologic study of the patient's marrow.[3] The development of improved instruments for percutaneous marrow biopsy in the last half of the 20th century improved diagnostic precision. The disease initially was thought to result from atrophy of primitive marrow hematopoietic cells. The unexpected recovery of marrow recipients who were given immunosuppressive conditioning but who did not engraft with donor stem cells raised the possibility that the disease was not intrinsic to primitive hematopoietic cells but resulted from suppression of hematopoietic cells by immune cells.[4] This supposition was confirmed by a clinical trial that established antilymphocyte globulin (ALG) alone as effective therapy for aplastic anemia.[5]

EPIDEMIOLOGY

Retrospective analysis in the United States estimated the incidence of aplastic anemia at two to five cases per 1,000,000 population per year.[6] The International Aplastic Anemia and Agranulocytosis Study and a French study brought the number closer to two per 1,000,000 persons per year.[7,8] The highest frequency of aplastic anemia occurs in persons aged 15 to 25 years; a second peak occurs at age 65 to 69 years.[9] Aplastic anemia is more prevalent in the Far East, where the incidence is approximately seven per 1,000,000 in China,[10] approximately four per 1,000,000 in Thailand,[11] and approximately five per 1,000,000 in Malaysia.[12] The explanation for the twofold or greater incidence in the Orient compared to the Occident is unclear. A study showing that the incidence of aplastic anemia in Hawaiians of Japanese ancestry is similar to that observed in the West does not support a genetic basis.[13] Use of chloramphenicol in Asia probably is not an explanation given that the occurrence of aplastic anemia remained high even after decreased use of the agent.[14,15] Poorly regulated exposure of workers to benzene may be a factor.[16]

ETIOLOGY AND PATHOGENESIS

Table 33-1 lists potential causes of aplastic anemia. The final common pathway to the clinical disease is decreased blood cell formation. The numbers of marrow colony forming unit–granulocyte-macrophage (CFU-GM) and burst forming unit–erythroid (BFU-E) are reduced markedly in patients with aplastic anemia.[17–22] The number of long-term culture-initiating cells is reduced to approximately 1 percent of normal values.[23] CD34+ hematopoietic cells, the fraction in which hematopoietic stem cells may reside, are correspondingly low.[24,25] Potential mechanisms responsible for acquired marrow cell failure include (1) direct toxicity to hematopoietic stem cells, (2) a defect in the stromal microenvironment of the marrow required for hematopoietic cell development, (3) impaired production or release of essential hematopoietic growth factors, and (4) cellular or humoral immune suppression of marrow progenitor cells. Little experimental evidence for a stromal microenvironmental defect or a deficit of critical hematopoietic growth factors exists. Thus, reduced hematopoiesis appears to represent an acquired toxic injury to primitive hematopoietic cells or, alternatively, immune suppression of hematopoietic progenitor cells. The accumulated evidence points primarily to suppression of hematopoiesis by autoreactive T lymphocytes.[26,27] The inheritance of mutations in genes such as *TERC* or *TERT* results in impaired mainte-

TABLE 33-1   ETIOLOGIC CLASSIFICATION OF APLASTIC ANEMIA

Acquired
  Idiopathic (autoimmune)
    TERC, TERT, TERF 1 & 2, *TIN2* susceptibility mutations
  Drugs (see Table 33-2)
  Toxins
    Benzene
    Chlorinated hydrocarbons
    Organophosphates
  Viruses
    Epstein-Barr virus
    Non-A, non-B, non-C, non-D, non-E, and non-G hepatitis virus
    Human immunodeficiency virus
  Paroxysmal nocturnal hemoglobinuria
  Autoimmune/connective tissue disorders
    Eosinophilic fasciitis
    Immune thyroid disease (Graves disease, Hashimoto thyroiditis)
    Rheumatoid arthritis
    Systemic lupus erythematosus
    Thymoma
  Pregnancy
  Iatrogenic
    Radiation
    Cytotoxic drug therapy
Hereditary
  Fanconi anemia
  Dyskeratosis congenita
  Shwachman-Diamond syndrome
  Other rare syndromes (see Table 33-4)

nance of telomere length. Shortened telomere length in the hematopoietic cells may heighten susceptibility to immune or other injury. These mutations may, therefore, predispose to the development of aplastic anemia.[278,279]

AUTOREACTIVE T LYMPHOCYTES ("IDIOPATHIC" APLASTIC ANEMIA)

Early studies showed that marrow lymphocytes or blood or marrow mononuclear cells from patients with aplastic anemia inhibited colony growth when the cells were cocultured with normal marrow.[17,20,28–30] Inhibition could have resulted from transfusion sensitization rather than autoimmunity.[31,32] However, culture studies in patients with aplastic anemia prior to transfusion[33] or before and after successful treatment[34,35] were highly suggestive of T cell–mediated suppression of marrow cell development. Furthermore, some marrow transplant recipients recovered from marrow aplasia without engraftment after the initial immunosuppressive preparative treatment, a finding compatible with successful treatment of a suppressor cell population.[36] Also, transplantation of a patient with aplastic anemia from an identical twin often resulted in engraftment failure unless a conditioning regimen (immunosuppression) was administered prior to transplantation.[37,38] Because the latter treatment is not required to prevent graft rejection between identical twins, the requirement also supported the need to eradicate in the recipient a cell population that interfered with restitution of normal hematopoiesis. Taken together, these *in vitro* and clinical observations support a T cell–mediated mechanism for genesis of idiopathic aplastic anemia.[39] Immune injury to the marrow after drug-, viral-, or toxin-induced marrow aplasia could result from induction of neoantigens that provoke a secondary T cell–mediated attack on hematopoietic cells. This mechanism could explain the response to immunosuppressive treatment after exposure to an ex-

ogenous agent. Levels of cytokines with inhibitory effects on hematopoiesis increase in the marrow of patients with severe aplastic anemia. Spontaneous or mitogen-induced increases in mononuclear cell production of interferon gamma (IFN-γ),[40,41] interleukin (IL) 2,[42] and tumor necrosis factor alpha[43,44] occur. Elevated serum levels of IFN-γ have been found in 30 percent of patients with aplastic anemia, and IFN-γ expression has been detected in the marrow of most patients with acquired aplastic anemia.[45] Addition of antibodies to IFN enhances *in vitro* colony growth of marrow cells from affected patients.[40] This indicates a role for IFN-γ in either the initiation or propagation of the aplastic anemia defect. Aplastic anemia now is considered to result from immune inhibition of primitive hematopoietic progenitors, mediated in part by inhibitory cytokines released by cytotoxic T lymphocytes. Several putative target antigens on affected hematopoietic cells have been identified. Autoantibodies to kinectin, one putative antigen, have been found in patients with aplastic anemia. T cells, which are responsive to kinectin-derived peptides, suppress granulocyte-monocyte colony growth *in vitro*. However, in these studies cytotoxic T lymphocytes with that specificity were not isolated from patients.[273]

DRUGS

Chloramphenicol is the most notorious drug documented to cause aplastic anemia. Although this drug is directly myelosuppressive at very high dose because of mitochondrial toxicity, the occurrence of aplastic anemia appears to be idiosyncratic, perhaps related to an inherited sensitivity to a nitroso-containing toxic intermediate.[46] This sensitivity may produce immunologic marrow suppression, given the substantial numbers of affected patients who respond to immunosuppressive therapy.[47] The risk of developing aplastic anemia in patients treated with chloramphenicol is approximately one in 20,000, or 10 to 50 times that of the general population.[6,48,49] Unfortunately, fatal aplastic anemia with topical or systemic drug use still is reported.[50,51]

Epidemiologic evidence established that quinacrine (Atabrine) increased the risk of aplastic anemia.[52] This drug was administered to all US troops in the South Pacific and Asiatic theaters of operations as prophylaxis for malaria during 1943 and 1944. The incidence of aplastic anemia was seven to 28 cases per 1,000,000 personnel per year in the prophylaxis zones, whereas untreated soldiers had one to two cases per 1,000,000 personnel per year. The aplasia occurred during administration of the offending agent and was preceded by a characteristic rash in nearly half the cases. Many other drugs reportedly increase the risk of aplastic anemia, but the spectrum of drug-induced aplastic anemia may not be fully appreciated because of incomplete reporting of information and the infrequency of the association. Table 33-2 lists the drugs that have been associated with aplastic anemia.

Many of the drugs induce selective cytopenias, such as agranulocytosis, which usually are reversible after the offending agent is discontinued. These reversible reactions are not correlated with the risk of aplastic anemia, which casts doubt on the effectiveness of routine monitoring of blood counts as a strategy to avoid aplastic anemia.

Aplastic anemia remains a rare event that can occur because of an underlying genetic, metabolic, or immunologic predisposition in susceptible individuals. Delayed oxidation and clearance of acetanilide, a related compound, occur in patients with phenylbutazone-associated marrow aplasia compared to either normal controls or patients with aplastic anemia resulting from other causes.[53] This finding suggests excess accumulation of the drug as a potential mechanism for the aplasia. Drug interactions or synergy may be required to induce marrow aplasia in some cases. Cimetidine, a histamine H_2-receptor antagonist, occasionally is implicated in the onset of cytopenias and aplastic anemia, perhaps because of a direct effect on hematopoietic stem cells.[54,55]

TABLE 33-2 DRUGS ASSOCIATED WITH APLASTIC ANEMIA

Category	High Risk	Intermediate Risk	Low Risk
Analgesic			Phenacetin, aspirin, salicylamide
Antiarrhythmic			Quinidine, tocainide
Antiarthritics		Gold salts	Colchicine
Anticonvulsant		Carbamazepine, hydantoins, felbamate	Ethosuximide, phenacemide, primidone, trimethadione, sodium valproate
Antihistamine			Chlorpheniramine, pyrilamine, tripelennamine
Antihypertensive			Captopril, methyldopa
Antiinflammatory		Penicillamine, phenylbutazone, oxyphenbutazone	Diclofenac, ibuprofen, indomethacin, naproxen, sulindac
Antimicrobial			
Antibacterial		Chloramphenicol	Dapsone, methicillin, penicillin, streptomycin, β-lactam antibiotics
Antifungal			Amphotericin, flucytosine
Antiprotozoal		Quinacrine	Chloroquine, mepacrine, pyrimethamine
Antineoplastic drugs			
Alkylating agents	Busulfan, cyclophosphamide, melphalan, nitrogen mustard		
Antimetabolites	Fluorouracil, mercaptopurine, methotrexate		
Cytotoxic antibiotics	Daunorubicin, doxorubicin, mitoxantrone		
Antiplatelet			Ticlopidine
Antithyroid			Carbimazole, methimazole, methylthiouracil, potassium perchlorate, propylthiouracil, sodium thiocyanate
Sedative and tranquilizer			Chlordiazepoxide, chlorpromazine (and other phenothiazines), lithium, meprobamate, methyprylon
Sulfonamides and derivatives			
Antibacterial			Numerous sulfonamides
Diuretic		Acetazolamide	Chlorothiazide, furosemide
Hypoglycemic			Chlorpropamide, tolbutamide
Miscellaneous			Allopurinol, interferon, pentoxifylline

NOTE: Drugs that invariably cause marrow aplasia with high doses are termed *high risk*; drugs with at least 30 reported cases are listed as *moderate risk*; others are less often associated with aplastic anemia (*low risk*).

SOURCES: This list was compiled from the AMA Registry,[125] publications of the International Agranulocytosis and Aplastic Anemia Study,[126–130] other reviews and studies,[87,131–133,183] previous compilations of offending agents,[134,135] and selected reports. An additional comprehensive source for potentially offending drugs can be found in reference 272.

This drug accentuates the marrow-suppressive effects of the chemotherapy drug carmustine.[56] In several instances, cimetidine reportedly was a possible cause of marrow aplasia when cimetidine was given with chloramphenicol.[51]

TOXIC CHEMICALS

Benzene was the first chemical linked to aplastic anemia, based on studies of factory workers before the 20th century.[57] Benzene is used as a solvent in the manufacture of chemicals, drugs, dyes, and explosives. It has been a vital chemical in the manufacture of rubber and leather goods and has been used widely in the shoe industry, leading to an increased risk for aplastic anemia and leukemia in workers in these industries.[58,59] In China, toxic effects of benzene were found in 0.5 percent of exposed workers; occurrence of aplastic anemia among workers was sixfold higher than in the general population.[16]

The US Occupational Safety and Health Administration has lowered the permissible exposure limit to benzene to 1 ppm,[60] after exposure to 100 ppm was shown to be associated with leukopenia in about one third of workers.[61] Other hematologic abnormalities, such as hemolytic anemia, marrow hyperplasia, myeloid metaplasia, and acute myelogenous leukemia, have been observed in patients exposed to benzene.[16,58,59,62]

Chlorinated hydrocarbons and organophosphate compounds have been implicated in the onset of aplastic anemia.[63] Chlorophenothane (dichlorodiphenyltrichloroethane [DDT]), lindane, and chlordane are the most common insecticides involved. Aplastic anemia was reported following use of lindane in home vaporizers for disinfection. This practice continued until the 1970s, when more than 30 case reports of aplastic anemia led to curtailment of chlorophenothane use.[64] Cases still occur occasionally after heavy exposure at industrial plants or after its use as a pesticide.[65] Lindane is metabolized in part to pentachlorophenol (PCP), another potentially toxic chlorinated hydrocarbon that is manufactured for use as a wood preservative. Many cases of aplastic anemia and related blood disorders have been attributed to PCP over the past 25 years.[64–67] Prolonged exposures to petroleum distillates in the form of Stoddard solvent[68] and acute exposure to toluene through glue sniffing[69] reportedly cause marrow aplasia. Trinitrotoluene (TNT), an explosive used extensively during World Wars I and II, is absorbed readily by inhalation and through the skin. Fatal cases of aplastic anemia were observed in munitions workers exposed to TNT in Great Britain from 1940 to 1946.[70]

VIRUSES

NON-A, NON-B, NON-C, NON-D, NON-E, AND NON-G HEPATITIS VIRUSES

A number of case reports have studied the relationship between hepatitis and subsequent development of aplastic anemia. The association was emphasized by two major reviews in the 1970s.[71,72] In aggregate, the reports summarized findings in more than 200 cases. In many instances, the hepatitis was improving or had resolved when the aplastic anemia was noted 4 to 12 weeks later. Approximately 10 percent of cases occurred more than 1 year after the initial diagnosis of hepatitis. Most patients were young (aged 18–20 years), two thirds were male, and their survival was short (10 weeks). Although hepatitis A and B have been implicated in aplastic anemia in a small number of cases, most cases are related to non-A, non-B, and non-C hepatitis.[73,74] Severe aplastic anemia developed in nine of 31 patients who underwent liver transplantation for non-A, non-B, or non-C hepatitis but in none of 1463 patients transplanted for other indications.[75] Several lines of evidence indicate no association with hepatitis C virus, which suggests an unknown viral agent is involved.[76–78] No evidence of hepatitis A, B, C, D, E, or G, transfusion-transmitted virus, or parvovirus B19 was found in 15 patients with posthepatitic aplastic anemia.[79]

EPSTEIN-BARR VIRUS

EBV has been implicated in the pathogenesis of aplastic anemia.[80] Onset usually occurs within 4 to 6 weeks of infection. Infectious mononucleosis is subclinical in some cases. Reactive lymphocytes are noted on the blood film, and serologic results are consistent with a recent infection. EBV has been detected in marrow cells,[81] but whether marrow aplasia results from a direct effect or is an immunologic response by the host is uncertain. Some patients have recovered after antithymocyte globulin therapy.[76,81]

OTHER VIRUSES

Human immunodeficiency virus infection frequently is associated with varying degrees of cytopenia. The marrow often is cellular, but occasional cases of aplastic anemia have been noted.[82–84] In these patients, marrow hypoplasia may result from viral suppression and from the drugs used to control viral replication in this disorder.

A number of other viruses have been implicated in the pathogenesis of marrow failure. B19 parvovirus, the cause of fifth disease, leads to transient erythroid aplasia but is not known to induce aplastic anemia.[76,85] Human herpes virus 6 has caused severe marrow aplasia subsequent to bone marrow transplantation for other disorders.[86]

AUTOIMMUNE/CONNECTIVE TISSUE DISEASES

The incidence of severe aplastic anemia was sevenfold greater than expected in patients with rheumatoid arthritis.[87] Whether the aplastic anemia is related directly to rheumatoid arthritis or to the various drugs used to treat the condition (gold salts, D-penicillamine, nonsteroidal agents) is uncertain. Occasional cases of aplastic anemia are seen in conjunction with systemic lupus erythematosus.[88] In vitro studies found either an antibody[89] or a suppressor cell[90,91] directed against hematopoietic progenitor cells. Patients have recovered after plasmapheresis,[89] glucocorticoids,[91] or cyclophosphamide therapy,[90,92] suggesting an immune etiology.

Eosinophilic fasciitis is an uncommon connective tissue disorder with painful swelling and induration of the skin and subcutaneous tissue associated with aplastic anemia.[93,94] The disorder is antibody mediated in some cases but is largely unresponsive to therapy.[93] Stem cell transplantation, immunosuppressive therapy using cyclosporine,[93] antithymocyte globulin (ATG), or ATG and cyclosporine has cured or significantly ameliorated the disease in a few patients.[94]

Severe aplastic anemia has been reported in association with immune thyroid disease[95,96] and thymoma.[97,98]

PREGNANCY

Cases of pregnancy-associated aplastic anemia have been reported, but the relationship between the two conditions is not clear.[99–101] In some patients, pregnancy exacerbates preexisting aplastic anemia, which improves after the pregnancy is terminated.[99,100] In other cases, the aplasia develops during pregnancy, with recurrences during subsequent pregnancies.[100,101] Termination of pregnancy or delivery may improve marrow function, but the disease may progress to a fatal outcome even after delivery.[99–101] Therapy can include elective termination of early pregnancy, supportive care, immunosuppressive therapy, or marrow transplantation after delivery. Pregnancy in women previously treated with immunosuppression for aplastic anemia can result in the birth of a normal newborn.[102] In a series of 36 pregnancies, 22 were uncomplicated, 7 were complicated by a relapse of the marrow aplasia, and 5 without aplasia required red cell transfusion during delivery.[102] One death as a result of cerebral thrombosis occurred in a patient with paroxysmal nocturnal hemoglobinuria (PNH) and aplasia.

IATROGENIC CAUSES

Although marrow toxicity from cytotoxic chemotherapy or radiation directly damages stem cells and more mature cells and results in marrow aplasia, most patients with acquired aplastic anemia cannot relate an exposure that would be responsible for marrow damage.

Chronic exposure to low doses of radiation or use of spinal radiation for ankylosing spondylitis is associated with an increased, but delayed, risk of developing aplastic anemia and acute leukemia.[103,104] Patients who were given thorium dioxide (Thorotrast) as an intravenous contrast medium suffered numerous late complications, including malignant liver tumors, acute leukemia, and aplastic anemia.[105] Chronic radium poisoning with osteitis of the jaw, osteogenic sarcoma, and aplastic anemia was seen in workers who painted watch dials with luminous paint when the workers moistened the brushes orally.[106]

Acute exposures to large doses of radiation are associated with development of marrow aplasia and a gastrointestinal syndrome.[107,108] Total body exposure between 1 and 2.5 Gy leads to gastrointestinal symptoms and depression of leukocyte counts, but most patients recover. A 4.5-Gy dose leads to death in half of individuals (LD_{50}) as a result of marrow failure. Higher doses of approximately 10 Gy are universally fatal unless the patient receives extensive supportive care followed by marrow transplantation. Aplastic anemia associated with nuclear accidents was seen after the Chernobyl nuclear power station disaster in the Ukraine in 1986.[109]

Antineoplastic drugs such as alkylating agents, antimetabolites, and certain cytotoxic antibiotics have the potential to produce marrow aplasia. In general, the effect is transient, is an extension of the drugs' pharmacologic action, and resolves within several weeks of completing chemotherapy. Severe hypoplasia, although unusual, can follow use of the alkylating agent busulfan and persist for extended intervals. Patients may develop marrow aplasia 2 to 5 years after discontinuing alkylating agent therapy. These cases often evolve into hypoplastic myelodysplastic syndromes.

STROMAL MICROENVIRONMENT AND GROWTH FACTORS

Short-term clonal assays for marrow stromal cells show variable defects in stromal cell function. Serum levels of stem cell factor (SCF) were either moderately low or normal in several studies of aplastic anemia.[110–112] Although SCF augments the growth of hematopoietic colonies from aplastic marrows,[113] its use in patients has not led to clinical remissions. Flt-3 ligand, another early-acting growth factor, is 30- to 100-fold elevated in the serum of patients with aplastic anemia.[114] Fibroblasts grown from patients with severe aplastic anemia have subnormal cytokine production. However, serum levels of granulocyte colony stimulating factor (G-CSF),[115] erythropoietin,[116] and thrombopoietin[117] usually are high. Synthesis of IL-1, an early stimulator of hematopoiesis, is decreased in mononuclear cells from patients with aplastic anemia.[118] Studies of the microenvironment have shown relatively normal stromal cell proliferation and growth factor production.[119–121] These findings, coupled with the limited response of patients with aplastic anemia to growth factors, suggest cytokine deficiency is not the etiologic problem in most cases. The most compelling argument is that most patients transplanted for aplastic anemia are cured with allogeneic donor stem cells and autologous stroma.[37,122–124]

HEREDITARY APLASTIC ANEMIA

FANCONI ANEMIA

DEFINITION AND HISTORY

Fanconi anemia, the most common form of constitutional aplastic anemia, was described in three brothers by Fanconi[136] in 1927. It is inherited as an autosomal recessive condition that results from defects in genes that modulate DNA stability.

EPIDEMIOLOGY

Since its initial description, more than 1300 cases of Fanconi anemia have been recorded through reports in the literature or from an International Fanconi Anemia Registry.[137] Fanconi anemia is estimated to be present in one in 1,000,000 individuals, although it occurs more frequently in Afrikaners of European descent and in southern Italy.

ETIOLOGY AND PATHOGENESIS

Eleven complementation groups, defined by somatic cell hybridization, are associated with development of Fanconi anemia.[138] The complementation groups are designated FANCA, B, C, D1, D2, E, F, G, I, J, and L. Table 33-3 lists the gene mutations corresponding to eight complementation groups. The great majority of patients have mutations of FANCA, C, or G.[139] The A and C gene products, which are cytoplasmic proteins, have been proposed to form a complex with the products of genes B, E, F, and G, which are adaptors or phosphorylators. The complex translocates to the nucleus, where it protects the cell from DNA cross-linking and likely participates in DNA repair by interacting with BRCA2, Rad51, and possibly BRCA1.[139] Normal function is disturbed in the presence of a mutant gene product, leading to damaging effects in sensitive tissues, including hematopoietic cells. Mutation of the D product appears to affect tissue cells through a different mechanism, perhaps downstream from the complex.[140,141] An eighth gene, FANCL, has been identified. The gene product is necessary for FANCD2 monoubiquitination, and its mutation can lead to Fanconi anemia.[274] Two additional genes, FANCI and FANCJ, have been described in a group of patients with Fanconi anemia.[275] FANCI anemia also involves a defect in monoubiquitination of FANCD2.

In addition to the genetic defects leading to DNA instability and an inability to repair DNA, tumor necrosis factor (TNF) alpha and TNF gamma are overexpressed in the marrow of Fanconi anemia patients.[276] The excess TNF-α may play a role in suppression of erythropoiesis in these patients.

CLINICAL FEATURES

The onset of marrow failure, usually during the last half of the first decade of life, is gradual. Anemia, weakness, fatigue, dyspnea on exertion, thrombocytopenia, epistaxis, purpura, or other unexpected bleeding are the principal findings. Hepatosplenomegaly is not a feature of the disease. Café au lait spots, an abnormal skin pigmentation consisting of flat, light brown lesions ranging from 1 to 12 cm in diameter, may be evident. Growth retardation results in short stature. Skeletal anomalies, especially dysplastic radii and thumbs, occur in half the patients. Heart, kidney, and eye defects may be present. Microcephaly and mental retardation may be a feature. Hypogonadism may be evident. Hematologic and visceral manifestations are combined in more than one third of patients, but some may have cytopenias and inconspicuous somatic changes, whereas others may have somatic anomalies with no or a nominal disorder of blood cell formation. Some who carry the gene may be virtually unaffected.[140,142] In a review of the more than 1300 patients reported in the literature, 100 patients (14%) without anomalies were identified by chromosome breakage studies (see "Laboratory Features," below) as a result of affected siblings.[143] In the past, children in Fanconi families with onset of aplastic anemia without congenital abnormalities were thought to have a different disorder termed Estren-Dameshek syndrome.[144] However, children whose lymphocytes show sensitivity to diepoxybutane are considered to have Fanconi anemia without skeletal abnormalities.

LABORATORY FEATURES

Blood counts and marrow cellularity often are normal until the patient is 5 to 10 years old, when pancytopenia develops over an extended interval. Macrocytosis with anisocytosis and poikilocytosis may be present before cytopenia occurs. Thrombocytopenia may precede the development of granulocytopenia and anemia. The marrow becomes hypocellular, and in vitro colony assays reveal decreased CFU-GM and BFU-E.[142]

Random chromatid breaks are present in myeloid cells, lymphocytes, and chorionic villus biopsy samples. This chromosome damage is intensified after exposure to DNA cross-linking agents such as mitomycin C or diepoxybutane. The hypersensitivity of the chromosomes of marrow cells or lymphocytes to the latter agent is used as a diagnostic test for the condition. Cell cycle progression is prolonged at the G_2 to M transition, and the cells are more susceptible to oxygen toxicity when cultured in vitro.[145] It is important to test the lymphocytes from pediatric patients with aplastic anemia for sensitivity to diepoxybutane, since therapy for Fanconi anemia differs from that used for aplastic anemia.

In the near future, clinical laboratories will be able to genotype suspected patients. Determining the specific gene mutation responsible in a patient (see Table 33-3) is important because it confirms the diagnosis, identifies the genotype linked to BRCA2 which may predispose to a cancer (breast, ovary), and permits carrier detection.[146]

TABLE 33-3 FANCONI ANEMIA GENES

GENE	APPROXIMATE INCIDENCE AMONG FANCONI ANEMIA PATIENTS (%)	CHROMOSOMAL LOCATION	EXON NUMBER	AMINO ACID RESIDUES
FANCA	70*	16q24.3	43	1455
FANCC	10	9q22.3	14	558
BRCA2†	1	13q12.3	27	3418
FANCD2	1	3p25.3	44	1451
FANCE	5	6p21.3	10	536
FANCF	2	11p15	1	374
FANCG	10	9p13	14	622
FANCL	1	2p16.1	?	373

* There are more than 100 mutant FANCA alleles, approximately 40 percent of which are large intragenic deletions. Whereas FA alleles of BRCA2 are found in FA-D1 cells, a sufficient number of FANCB cells have not been tested at this time to conclude that BRCA2 mutations account for both FA-B and FA-D1.
† Although a BRCA2 null genotype is an embryonic lethal phenotype, certain homozygous BRCA2 mutations that lead to C-terminal truncations lead to FA of the D1 complementation group.
Reproduced with permission from reference 139.

DIFFERENTIAL DIAGNOSIS

Differential diagnosis of Fanconi anemia includes other causes of aplastic anemia, particularly familial syndromes associated with skeletal anomalies and other dysmorphic features. Other familial types of aplastic anemia have been reported with or without associated anomalies. In instances in which no sensitivity to DNA damaging agents is observed, the syndrome does not represent Fanconi anemia. Several uncommon syndromes of this type are described below and in Table 33-4.

THERAPY AND PROGNOSIS

Most patients with Fanconi anemia do not respond to ATG or cyclosporine. Patients improve with androgen preparations, often for as long as several years. Cytokines can improve blood counts, but studies in a mouse model suggest the effects will not be sustained.[162] Relapses occur gradually. Death from progressive marrow failure or conversion to myelodysplastic syndrome, acute myelogenous leukemia (approximately 10 percent of patients), or development of a variety of other cancers occurs eventually by age 10 to 20 years.[137] The presence of a clonal cytogenetic abnormality or marrow morphology consistent with myelodysplasia markedly reduces the 5-year survival rate.[163] Allogeneic stem cell transplantation is curative for Fanconi anemia.[164,165] A marked reduction in dosage of the marrow-conditioning regimen of cyclophosphamide and radiation is necessary because of the undue sensitivity of the tissues to alkylating agents.[164] Early studies of gene therapy that introduce normal cDNA into cells from patients may restore resistance to DNA-damaging agents.[166,167] Difficulties in this approach include the paucity of stem cells in these patients and the toxicity of the gene transfer methodology.

DYSKERATOSIS CONGENITA, SHWACHMAN-DIAMOND SYNDROME, AND OTHER INHERITED SYNDROMES

Dyskeratosis congenita and Shwachman-Diamond syndrome (pancreatic insufficiency with neutropenia) are two rare disorders that may evolve into aplastic anemia. Dyskeratosis usually is inherited as a re-cessive X chromosome–linked disorder, although rare cases are autosomal dominant or recessive. Mutations of the *DKC1* gene are responsible for the X-linked form and mutations of the *TERC* gene for the autosomal dominant form.[151,153,154] *DKC1* encodes dyskerin, which is a protein component of the telomerase complex, and hTR is the RNA component of telomerase. Dyskeratosis congenita likely results from defective telomerase activity resulting from mutations in these two genes.[151,153,154] The disease is reflected in reticulate skin pigmentation, leukoplakia, and dystrophic nails. A variety of noncutaneous anomalies are observed. Skin and mucosal lesions appear in adolescence, and aplastic anemia usually develops in early adulthood.[168]

Shwachman-Diamond syndrome results from a mutation in the *SBDS* gene and is manifest by pancreatic insufficiency and steatorrhea.[158] Neutropenia is present in virtually all patients and neutropenia and thrombocytopenia in about one third to one half of patients. Thus, a substantial plurality of patients has bicytopenia or tricytopenia with hypoplastic marrows. A significant risk of progression to myelogenous leukemia exists.[169,170] Severe hematopoietic dysfunction can be treated successfully with allogeneic stem cell transplantation.

Table 33-4 lists other rare syndromes associated with aplastic anemia. Reticular dysgenesis appears to result from a stem cell defect, given that lymphoid and myeloid precursors are affected. Seckel syndrome involves the *ATR* gene, and marrow cells exhibit heightened sister chromatid exchange.[156,171] The genetic bases of marrow failure in the other syndromes are unknown.

CLINICAL FEATURES

The onset of symptoms of aplastic anemia may be gradual. Pallor, weakness, dyspnea, and fatigue result from the decrease in red cells. Dependent petechiae, bruising, epistaxis, vaginal bleeding, and unexpected bleeding at other sites secondary to thrombocytopenia are frequent presenting signs of the underlying marrow disorder. Rarely, the symptoms are more dramatic. Fever, chills, and pharyngitis or other sites of infection result from neutropenia. Physical examination generally is unrevealing, except for evidence of anemia (e.g., conjunctival

TABLE 33-4   RARE SYNDROMES ASSOCIATED WITH APLASTIC ANEMIA

DISORDER	FINDINGS	INHERITANCE	GENE	REFERENCES
Ataxia-pancytopenia	Cerebellar atrophy Pancytopenia	Autosomal dominant	Unknown	146–148
Dubowitz syndrome	Growth failure Microcephaly Abnormal facies Pancytopenia, AML, ALL	Autosomal recessive	Unknown	149,150
Dyskeratosis congenita	Skin pigmentation Leukoplakia Dystrophic nails Pancytopenia	X-linked recessive Rarely: Autosomal dominant Autosomal recessive	*DKC1* *TERC* Unknown	151–154
Reticular dysgenesis	Lymphopenia Granulocytopenia (mostly seen in males) Often anemia	X-linked recessive	Unknown	155
Seckel syndrome	Growth failure Microcephaly Abnormal facies Occasional pancytopenia AML (1 case)	Autosomal recessive	*ATR* (and *RAD3* related gene)	156,157
Shwachman-Diamond	Pancreatic insufficiency and neutropenia Pancytopenia in 1/3 to 1/2 AML	Autosomal recessive	*SBDS*	158–160
WT syndrome	Radial/ulnar abnormalities Pancytopenia, AML	Autosomal dominant	Unknown	161

A number of other isolated cases of familial aplastic anemia with or without associated anomalies that are not consistent with Fanconi anemia have been reported (see reference 143).
AML, acute myelogenous leukemia; ALL, acute lymphoblastic leukemia.

History and physical examination

Initial laboratory studies

   Complete blood counts, reticulocyte count, and examination of blood film

   Marrow aspiration and biopsy

   Marrow cytogenetics to evaluate clonal myeloid disease

   Red cell hemoglobin F content and DNA stability test as markers of Fanconi anemia

   Immunophenotyping of red and white cells, especially for CD59 to exclude paroxysmal nocturnal hemoglobinuria

   Direct and indirect Coombs test to rule out immune cytopenia

   Serum lactate dehydrogenase and uric acid that may reflect neoplastic cell turnover

   Liver function tests to assess evidence of recent hepatitis virus exposure

   Screening tests for hepatitis viruses A, B, and C

   Screening tests for cytomegalovirus, Epstein-Barr virus, and human immunodeficiency virus

   Serum B_{12} and red cell folic acid levels to rule out megaloblastic pancytopenia

   Serum iron, iron-binding capacity, and ferritin as a baseline prior to chronic transfusion therapy

and cutaneous pallor, resting tachycardia), cutaneous bleeding (e.g., ecchymoses and petechiae), or gingival bleeding and intraoral purpura. Lymphadenopathy and splenomegaly are not features of aplastic anemia; such findings suggest an alternative diagnosis such as leukemia or lymphoma.

LABORATORY FEATURES

BLOOD FINDINGS

Patients with aplastic anemia have varying degrees of pancytopenia. Anemia is associated with a low reticulocyte index. The reticulocyte count usually is less than 1.0 percent and may be zero despite the high levels of erythropoietin.[172] Macrocytes may be present. The total leukocyte count and platelet counts are low. The differential white cell count reveals a decrease in neutrophils and monocytes. An absolute neutrophil count less than 500×10^6/liter and a platelet count less than $20,000 \times 10^6$/liter are indicative of severe disease. A neutrophil count less than 200×10^6/liter indicates very severe disease. Lymphocyte production is thought to be normal, but patients may have mild lymphopenia. Platelets are reduced but function normally. Significant

qualitative changes of red cell, leukocyte, or platelet morphology are not features of classic acquired aplastic anemia. On occasion, only one cell line is depressed initially, which may lead to an early diagnosis of red cell aplasia or amegakaryocytic thrombocytopenia. In such patients, other cell lines fail shortly thereafter (days to weeks) and permit a definitive diagnosis (Table 33-5).

PLASMA FINDINGS

Plasma contains high levels of hematopoietic growth factors, including erythropoietin, thrombopoietin, and myeloid colony stimulating factors.[115–117] Serum iron values usually are high, and ^{59}Fe clearance is prolonged, with decreased incorporation into circulating red cells.[173]

MARROW FINDINGS

MORPHOLOGY

Marrow aspirate typically contains numerous spicules with empty, fat-filled spaces and relatively few hematopoietic cells. Lymphocytes, plasma cells, macrophages, and mast cells may be prominent, reflecting a lack of other cells rather than an increase in these elements. On occasion, some spicules are cellular or even hypercellular ("hot spots"), but megakaryocytes usually are reduced. These focal areas of residual hematopoiesis do not appear to be of prognostic significance. Residual granulocytic cells generally appear normal, but mild macronormoblastic erythropoiesis, presumably because of high levels of erythropoietin, is not unusual. Marrow biopsy is essential to confirm the overall hypocellularity (Fig. 33-1) because a poor yield of cells occasionally is obtained from marrow aspirates from patients with other disorders, especially if fibrosis is present.

In severe aplastic anemia as defined by the International Aplastic Anemia Study Group,[174] less than 25 percent cellularity or less than 50 percent cellularity with less than 30 percent hematopoietic cells is seen in the marrow.

If lymphocytosis is noted in the marrow or blood, an atypical case of hairy cell leukemia[175] or the occasional hypoplastic presentation of acute lymphocytic leukemia should be considered (see "Differential Diagnosis," below).[176]

PROGENITOR CELL GROWTH

In vitro CFU-GM and BFU-E colony assays reveal a marked reduction in progenitor cells.[17–22,28–34] Improvement in colony growth after incubation with anti–T cell monoclonal antibodies may predict improvement after immunosuppressive therapy[177]; however, this has not been a universal finding.

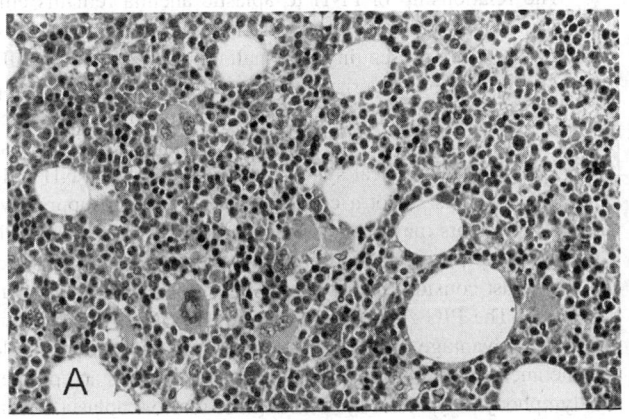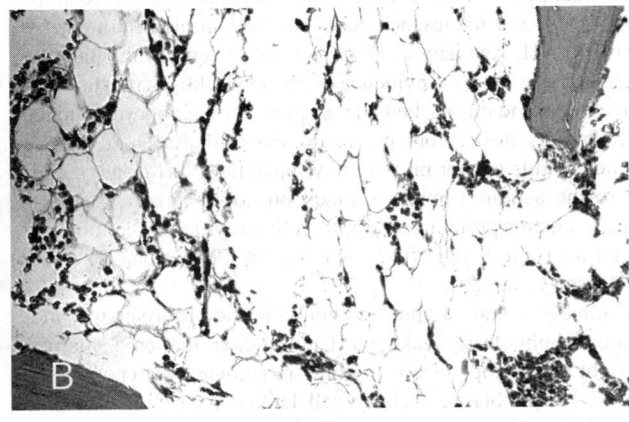

FIGURE 33-1 Marrow biopsy in aplastic anemia. (A) Normal marrow biopsy. (B) Marrow in aplastic anemia is devoid of hematopoietic cells and contains only scattered lymphocytes and stromal cells.

CYTOGENETIC STUDIES

Cytogenetic analysis may be difficult because of low cellularity; thus, multiple aspirates may be required to provide sufficient cells for study. The results of analysis are normal in aplastic anemia. Clonal cytogenetic abnormalities in otherwise apparent aplastic anemia are indicative of an underlying hypoproliferative clonal myeloid disease.[178]

IMAGING STUDIES

Magnetic resonance imaging (MRI) can be used to distinguish between marrow fat and hematopoietic cells.[179] This may be a more useful overall estimate of marrow hematopoietic cell density than morphologic techniques and may help differentiate hypoplastic myelogenous leukemia from aplastic anemia.[180,181]

DIFFERENTIAL DIAGNOSIS

Any disease that can present with pancytopenia may mimic aplastic anemia if only the blood counts are considered. Measurement of reticulocyte count and examination of the blood film and marrow biopsy are essential early steps to arrive at a diagnosis. A reticulocyte percentage of 0.5 to zero is strongly indicative of aplastic erythropoiesis and, coupled with leukopenia and thrombocytopenia, points to aplastic anemia. Absence of qualitative abnormalities of cells on the blood film and a markedly hypocellular marrow are characteristic of acquired aplastic anemia. The disorders most commonly confused with severe aplastic anemia include the myelodysplastic syndromes in the approximately 5 to 10 percent of patients who present with a hypoplastic rather than a hypercellular marrow. Myelodysplasia should be considered if abnormal blood film morphology consistent with myelodysplasia (e.g., poikilocytosis, basophilic stippling, granulocytes with the pseudo-Pelger-Hüet anomaly) is observed. Marrow erythroid precursors in myelodysplasia may have dysmorphic features. Pathologic sideroblasts are inconsistent with aplastic anemia and are a frequent feature of myelodysplasia. Granulocyte precursors may have reduced or abnormal granulation. Megakaryocytes may have abnormal nuclear lobulation (e.g., unilobular micromegakaryocytes) (see Chap. 86). A clonal myeloid disorder, especially myelodysplastic syndrome or hypocellular myelogenous leukemia, is likely if clonal cytogenetic abnormalities are found. MRI studies of bone may be useful in differentiating severe aplastic anemia from clonal myeloid syndromes. The former gives a fatty signal and the latter a diffuse cellular pattern.[179–181]

A hypocellular marrow frequently is associated with PNH. PNH is characterized by an acquired mutation in the PIG-A gene that encodes a glycosyl-phosphatidylinositol anchor protein (CD59). This protein anchors protein inhibitors of the complement pathway to blood cell membranes, and its absence accounts for complement-mediated hemolysis in PNH. As many as 50 percent of patients with otherwise typical aplastic anemia have evidence of glycosyl-phosphatidylinositol molecule defects and diminished anchor protein on leukocytes and red cells as judged by flow cytometry, analogous to that seen in PNH.[182] The absence of this anchor protein may make the PNH clone of cells resistant to the acquired immune attack on normal marrow components, or the anchor protein on normal cells provides an epitope that initiates an aberrant T cell attack, leaving the PNH clone relatively resistant[183] (see Chap. 38).

Occasionally, apparent aplastic anemia is the prodrome to childhood acute lymphoblastic leukemia. Careful examination of marrow cells by light microscopy or flow cytometry can uncover a population of leukemic lymphoblasts.[176] Hairy cell leukemia rarely is preceded by a period of marrow hypoplasia.[175] Use of tartrate-resistant acid phosphatase or immunophenotyping by flow cytometry for CD25 may uncover the presence of hairy cells. Other clinical features may be distinctive (see Chap. 93). Organomegalies such as lymphadenopathy, hepatomegaly, or splenomegaly are inconsistent with the atrophic (hypoproliferative) features of aplastic anemia.

RELATIONSHIP AMONG APLASTIC ANEMIA, PAROXYSMAL NOCTURNAL HEMOGLOBINURIA, AND CLONAL MYELOID DISEASES

In addition to the diagnostic difficulties occasionally presented by patients with hypoplastic myelodysplastic syndromes, hypoplastic acute myelogenous leukemia (AML), or PNH and hypocellular marrows, a more fundamental relationship may exist among these three diseases and aplastic anemia. The development of clonal cytogenetic abnormalities such as monosomy 7 or trisomy 8 in a patient with aplastic anemia portends the evolution of a myelodysplastic syndrome or acute leukemia. Occasionally, these cytogenetic markers are transient. Hematologic improvement has occurred in cases with disappearance of monosomy 7.[184] Persistent monosomy 7 carries a poor prognosis compared to trisomy 8.[185,186]

As many as 15 to 20 percent of patients with aplastic anemia have a 5-year probability of developing myelodysplasia.[184] If any transformation to a clonal myeloid disorder that occurs up to 6 months after treatment is excluded, to avoid misdiagnosis among the hypoplastic myeloid diseases, the frequency of a clonal disorder was nearly 15 times greater in patients treated with immunosuppression compared to patients treated with marrow transplantation after 39 months of observation.[187] This finding suggests that immune suppression by anti–T cell therapy enhances the evolution of a neoplastic clone or that the therapy does not suppress the intrinsic tendency of aplastic anemia to evolve to a clonal disease but provides the increased longevity of the patient required to express that potential. The latter interpretation is more likely given that patients successfully treated solely with androgens develop clonal disease as frequently as patients treated with immunosuppression.[188] Transplantation may reduce the potential to clonal evolution in patients with aplastic anemia by reestablishing robust hematolymphopoiesis.

Telomere shortening may play a pathogenetic role in the evolution of aplastic anemia into myelodysplasia. Patients with aplastic anemia had shorter telomere lengths than matched controls, and patients with aplastic anemia with persistent cytopenias had greater telomere shortening over time than matched controls. Three of five patients with telomere lengths less than 5 kb developed clonal cytogenetic changes, whereas patients with longer telomeres did not develop such diseases.[189]

The relationship of PNH to aplastic anemia remains enigmatic. Because hematopoietic stem cells lacking the phosphatidylinositol anchor proteins are present in very small numbers in many or all normal persons,[190] it is not surprising that more than 50 percent of patients with aplastic anemia may have a PNH cell population as detected by immunophenotyping.[182] The probability of patients with aplastic anemia developing a clinical syndrome consistent with PNH is 10 to 20 percent, and this is not a consequence of immunosuppressive treatment.[184] Patients may present with the hemolytic anemia of PNH and later develop progressive marrow failure, so any pathogenetic explanation must consider both types of development of aplastic marrows in PNH. The PIG-A mutation may confer either a proliferative or a survival advantage to PNH cells.[191] A survival advantage could result if the anchor protein or one of its ligands served as an epitope for the T lymphocyte cytotoxicity inducing the marrow aplasia. In this case, the presenting event could reflect either cytopenias or the sensitivity of red cells to complement lysis and hemolysis, depending on the intrinsic proliferative potential of the PNH clone.

Within our current state of knowledge, aplastic anemia is an autoimmune process. Any residual hematopoiesis presumably is polyclonal. This is a critical distinction from hypoplastic leukemia and PNH, which are clonal (neoplastic) diseases. The environment of the aplastic marrow, however, may favor the eventual evolution of a mutant (malignant) clone.

TREATMENT

APPROACH TO THERAPY

Severe anemia, bleeding from thrombocytopenia, and, rarely at the time of diagnosis, infection secondary to granulocytopenia and monocytopenia require prompt attention to remove potential life-threatening conditions and improve patient comfort (Table 33-6). More specific treatment of marrow aplasia involves three principal options: (1) allogeneic stem cell transplantation, (2) combination immunosuppressive therapy, or (3) high-dose cyclophosphamide. Selection of the specific mode of treatment depends on several factors, including the patient's age and condition and the availability of a suitable stem cell donor. In general, transplantation is the preferred treatment for children and most otherwise healthy adults. Histocompatibility testing is of particular importance because it establishes whether a sibling donor is available to the patient for transplantation. The preferred stem cell source is a histocompatible sibling matched at the human leukocyte antigen (HLA)-A, B, and DR loci. The outcome is compromised if there is a mismatch at one or more loci, and immunosuppression with combined therapy is the preferred treatment.

SUPPORTIVE CARE

USE OF BLOOD PRODUCTS

Sparing use of red cell and platelet transfusions in potential transplant recipients has been recommended to minimize sensitization to histocompatibility antigens. However, this recommendation has become less important since ATG and cyclophosphamide have been used as the preparative regimen for transplantation in aplastic anemia because the combination markedly reduces the problem of graft rejection.[192]

Cytomegalovirus (CMV)-negative blood products should be given to potential transplant recipients to minimize problems with CMV infections after transplantation. This restriction is no longer necessary once a patient is CMV positive. Leukocyte-depletion filters decrease the risk of CMV transmittal.

RED CELL TRANSFUSION

Packed red cells given to alleviate symptoms of anemia are indicated when hemoglobin values are less than 7 to 8 g/dl unless comorbid medical conditions require a higher hemoglobin concentration. These

TABLE 33-6 INITIAL MANAGEMENT OF APLASTIC ANEMIA

- Discontinue any potential offending drug and use an alternative class of agents if essential
- Anemia: transfusion of leukocyte-depleted red cells as required for severe anemia
- Severe thrombocytopenia or thrombocytopenic bleeding: use ε-aminocaproic acid; transfusion of platelets as required
- Infectious precautions if severe neutropenia
- Infection: cultures, broad-spectrum antibiotics if specific organism not identified, G-CSF in dire cases; if low body weight and profound infection (e.g., gram-negative bacteria, fungus) are present, consider granulocyte transfusion from a G-CSF–pretreated donor
- Assessment for allogeneic stem cell transplantation: histocompatibility testing of patient, parents, and siblings

G-CSF, granulocyte colony stimulating factor.

products should be leukocyte depleted to lessen leukocyte and platelet sensitization and to reduce subsequent transfusion reactions. Blood products should be irradiated in those patients requiring immunosuppression. It is important not to transfuse patients with red cells (or platelets) from family members if transplantation is remotely possible, because this approach may sensitize patients to minor histocompatibility antigens, increasing the risk of graft rejection after marrow transplantation. Following a marrow transplant or in individuals in whom transplantation is not a consideration, family members may be ideal donors for platelet products. Because each unit of red cells adds approximately 200 to 250 mg of iron to the total body iron, transfusion-induced iron overload may occur over the long term. This is not a major problem in patients who respond to transplantation or immunosuppressive therapy but is an issue in nonresponders who require continued transfusion support. In the latter case, consideration should be given to iron chelation therapy with deferoxamine (see Chap. 46).

PLATELET TRANSFUSION

Assessment of the risk of bleeding in each patient is important. Most patients tolerate platelet counts of 8 to 10×10^9/liter without undue bruising or bleeding, unless a systemic infection is present.[193,194] Administration of ε-aminocaproic acid, 100 mg/kg per dose every 4 hours (maximum dose 5 g) orally or intravenously, may reduce the bleeding tendency.[195] Pooled random-donor platelets can be used until sensitization ensues, although use of single-donor platelets from the onset to minimize sensitization to HLA or platelet antigens is preferable. Single-donor apheresis products or HLA-matched platelets may be required later.

Platelet refractoriness is a major problem with long-term transfusion support. The refractoriness may occur transiently, with fever or infection, or as a chronic problem secondary to HLA sensitization. In the past, the problem occurred in approximately 50 percent of patients after 8 to 10 weeks of transfusion support. Filtration of blood and platelet concentrates to remove leukocytes reduces this problem to approximately 15 to 20 percent of patients receiving chronic transfusions.[196] In some patients refractory to platelets, this problem can be overcome by administering high-dose intravenous γ-globulin[197,198] or by immunoabsorbent pheresis, using a column to remove circulating immunoglobulin G complexes.[199]

MANAGEMENT OF NEUTROPENIA

Neutropenic precautions should be applied to hospitalized patients with a severely depressed neutrophil count. The level of neutrophils requiring precautions is debated but is approximately less than 0.75×10^9/liter. One approach is use of private rooms, with requirements for face masks and hand washing with antiseptic soap. Unwashed fresh fruits and vegetables should be avoided because they are sources of bacterial contamination. Patients with aplastic anemia uncommonly present with significant infection. When patients with aplastic anemia become febrile, cultures should be obtained from the throat, sputum (if any), blood, urine, and any suspicious lesions. Broad-spectrum antibiotics should be initiated promptly, without awaiting culture results (see Chap. 20). The choice of antibiotics depends on the prevalence of organisms and their antibiotic sensitivity in the local setting. Organisms of concern usually include *Staphylococcus aureus, S. epidermidis* (in patients with venous access devices), and gram-negative organisms. Patients with persistent culture-negative fevers should be considered for antifungal treatment (see Chap. 20).

In the past, leukocyte transfusions were used on a daily basis to reduce the short-term mortality from infections. Detection of more than 100 to 200 neutrophils per microliter for more than a few hours after transfusion was unusual. Neutrophil yield can be increased by administering granulocyte-macrophage colony stimulating factor

(GM-CSF) or G-CSF to the donor,[200] but most physicians avoid using white cell products because present-day antibiotics usually are sufficient to treat an episode of sepsis. Notable exceptions include documented invasive aspergillosis unresponsive to amphotericin (particularly in the posttransplant setting), infections with organisms resistant to all known antibiotics, and disorders in which blood cultures remain positive despite antibiotic treatment.

HEMATOPOIETIC STEM CELL TRANSPLANTATION

Prompt therapy usually is indicated for patients with severe disease. The major curative approach is hematopoietic stem cell transplantation from a histocompatible sibling.[37,122] This treatment modality is described in Chap. 22. Only approximately 30 percent of patients in the United States have compatible sibling donors. The outcome is compromised if there is a mismatch at one or more loci, and immunosuppression with combined therapy is preferred. Transplants have been performed using stem cells from partially matched siblings or from unrelated histocompatible donors recruited through the National Marrow Donor Program or similar organizations in other countries.[201] Umbilical cord blood is an alternative source of stem cells from unrelated donors (or rarely siblings) for transplantation in children.[202] Use of high-resolution DNA-based HLA typing of a matched unrelated donor markedly improves the prognosis for transplantation from an unrelated donor.[203] This may be the preferred treatment for patients who no longer respond to immunotherapy rather than repeated courses of immunosuppression.[203]

COMPONENTS OF ANTI-T LYMPHOCYTE (IMMUNOSUPPRESSIVE) THERAPY

ANTILYMPHOCYTE GLOBULIN AND ANTITHYMOCYTE GLOBULIN

ATG and ALG act principally by reducing cytotoxic T cells. The process involves ATG-induced apoptosis through both Fas and TNF pathways.[204] Cathepsin B also plays a role in T cell cytotoxicity at clinical concentrations of ATG but may involve an independent apoptosis pathway.[271] ATG and ALG also release hematopoietic growth factors from T cells.[205,206] Horse and rabbit ATGs are licensed in the United States. Skin tests against horse serum should be performed prior to administration.[207] If the result is positive, the patient may be desensitized. ATG therapy with doses of 15 to 40 mg/kg is given daily for 4 to 10 days. Fever and chills are common during the first day of treatment. Concomitant treatment with glucocorticoids, such as methylprednisolone (1 mg/kg/day), lessens the reaction to ATG.

ATG treatment may accelerate platelet destruction, reduce the absolute neutrophil count, and cause a positive direct antiglobulin test. This effect may increase transfusion requirements during the 4- to 10-day treatment interval. Serum sickness, characterized by spiking fevers, skin rashes, and arthralgias, occurs commonly 7 to 10 days from the first dose. The clinical manifestations of serum sickness can be diminished by increasing the glucocorticoid dose from day 10 to day 17 after treatment. Approximately one third of patients no longer require transfusion support after treatment with ATG alone.[208–210]

Of 358 patients responding to immunosuppressive therapy, principally ATG alone, 74 (21 percent) relapsed after a mean of 2.1 years. The actuarial incidence of relapse was 35 percent at 10 years.[211] Similar results were observed when 227 patients were treated with immunosuppression, primarily ATG alone.[212] The actuarial survival at 15 years was 38 percent following immunosuppression.[211] However, a combination of immunosuppressive agents provides more effective therapy than ATG alone (see "Combination Immunotherapy," below).

Twenty-two percent of 129 patients treated with ALG developed myelodysplasia, leukemia, paroxysmal nocturnal hemoglobinuria, or combined disorders.[213] The tendency to relapse and develop clonal hematologic disorders was reviewed by the European Cooperative Group for Bone Marrow Transplantation in 468 patients, most of whom received ATG.[214] The risk of a hematologic complication increased continuously and reached 57 percent at 8 years after immunosuppressive therapy. A further survey found 42 (5 percent) malignancies in 860 patients treated with immunosuppression, whereas only 9 (1 percent) malignancies were seen in 748 patients who received marrow transplants.[215]

CYCLOSPORINE

Administration of cyclosporine, a cyclic polypeptide that inhibits IL-2 production by T lymphocytes and prevents expansion of cytotoxic T cells in response to IL-2, is another approach to immunotherapy. After the initial report of its ability to induce remission in 1984,[216] several groups have utilized cyclosporine (1) as primary treatment,[217–220] (2) in patients refractory to ATG or glucocorticoids,[218–223] (3) in combination with G-CSFs,[224,225] or (4) in varying combinations with other modes of therapy.[226] Cyclosporine is administered orally at 10 to 12 mg/kg/day for at least 4 to 6 months. Dosage adjustments may be required to maintain trough blood levels of 200 to 400 ng/ml. Renal impairment is common and may require increased hydration or dose adjustments to keep creatinine values less than 2 mg/dl. Cyclosporine may cause moderate hypertension, a variety of neurologic manifestations, and other side effects. Several drug classes interact with cyclosporine to either increase (e.g., some antibiotics and antifungals) or decrease (e.g., some anticonvulsants) blood levels. Responses usually are seen by 3 months and range from achieving transfusion independence to complete remission. Approximately 25 percent of patients respond to this agent used alone, but the reported response rate ranges from 0 to 80 percent.[226]

Although immunosuppression with ALG or ATG has been used the longest and has a seemingly better response rate, cyclosporine has certain advantages. The drug does not require hospitalization or use of central venous catheters. Fewer platelet transfusions are required during the first few weeks of therapy compared to treatment with ALG or ATG. A French cooperative trial showed equal effectiveness of ATG plus prednisone compared to cyclosporine.[227] In this crossover study of newly diagnosed patients, survival of approximately 65 percent was observed 12 months after diagnosis. Improved *in vitro* tests for predicting responsiveness may help tailor specific therapy for each patient in the future.[222]

HIGH-DOSE GLUCOCORTICOIDS

Marrow recovery can occur after very high doses of glucocorticoids.[228,229] Methylprednisolone in the range from 500 to 1000 mg daily for 3 to 14 days has been successful, but the side effects can be severe. Side effects include marked hyperglycemia and glycosuria, electrolyte disturbances, gastric irritation, psychosis, increased infections, and aseptic necrosis of the hips. Glucocorticoids at lower doses commonly are used only as a component of combination therapy for aplastic anemia. In this role, they are useful in modulating the adverse reactions to ATG and in providing additional lymphocyte suppression.

COMBINATION IMMUNOTHERAPY

Combination treatment of severe aplastic anemia usually includes ATG 40 mg/kg/day for 4 days, cyclosporine 10 to 12 mg/kg/day for 6 months, and methylprednisolone 1 mg/kg/day for 2 weeks.[230] The cyclosporine dose is adjusted to maintain a trough level of 200 to 400 ng/ml. Prophylaxis for *Pneumocystis carinii* with daily trimethoprim-sulfamethoxazole (160/800 mg qd orally) or with monthly pentamidine inhalations should be considered for these patients as they receive immunosuppressive therapy.

Addition of cyclosporine to the combination of ALG and glucocorticoids improves response rates to approximately 70 percent.[231,232] Although G-CSF used alone in patients with aplastic anemia may be detrimental,[233] G-CSF added to ALG, glucocorticoids, and cyclosporine appeared to permit 5-year actuarial survival of greater than 80 percent in 100 patients with very severe aplastic anemia.[234] Response usually is defined as a significant improvement in red cells, white cells, and platelets to eliminate risk of infection and bleeding and the requirement for red cell transfusions.

Five-year survival after completion of combination immunosuppressive therapy may approximate that after stem cell transplantation.[235] Forty-eight children treated between 1983 and 1992 had a 10-year survival of approximately 75 percent after marrow transplantation and approximately 75 percent after combined immunosuppressive therapy, although there were only half the number of severely affected patients in the immunosuppressive therapy group.[236] Thus, immunosuppression may be preferable for patients who are older than 30 years and for patients who experience a delay in finding a suitable donor. Marrow transplants are curative for aplastic anemia, whereas more frequent sequelae occur after immunosuppressive therapy,[237–239] notably a substantial rate of evolution to a myelodysplastic syndrome or acute myelogenous leukemia.

A recent National Institutes of Health protocol was designed to increase immune tolerance by specific deletion of activated T lymphocytes that target primitive hematopoietic progenitor cells.[240] Concurrent administration of cyclosporine with ATG may diminish the ATG tolerizing effect so that, in this program, cyclosporine is introduced at a later time. Addition of new immunosuppressive agents, such as mycophenolate mofetil, rapamycin, or monoclonal antibodies to the IL-2 receptor, may provide more effective induction of tolerance so that the activated lymphocytes spare the targeted hematopoietic stem cells.[240]

HIGH-DOSE CYCLOPHOSPHAMIDE

High-dose cyclophosphamide has been used as a form of immunosuppression.[241] Although it seems inappropriate to administer high doses of chemotherapy to patients with severe marrow aplasia, this approach was based on observations of autologous recovery after preparative therapy for allogeneic transplants.[241] Ten patients received cyclophosphamide at 45 mg/kg/day intravenously for 4 days with or without cyclosporine for an additional 100 days. Gradual neutrophil and platelet recovery ensued over 3 months. Seven patients responded completely and remain in remission 11 years after treatment. Interest in high-dose cyclophosphamide treatment has been renewed because hematopoietic stem cells have high levels of aldehyde dehydrogenase and are relatively resistant to cyclophosphamide.[242,243] Thus, cyclophosphamide in this situation is more immunosuppressive than it is myelotoxic. The most extensive trial of high-dose cyclophosphamide resulted in complete response by 65 percent of patients at 50 months.[244] However, the role of this regimen as initial therapy is not clear because early toxicity may exceed that of the ATG and cyclosporine combination.[245] The probability of a durable remission may be superior, but insufficient data exist to allow conclusion on whether ATG and cyclosporine or high-dose cyclophosphamide provides better long-term results. Cyclophosphamide, also, is effective in inducing marrow recovery in some patients who have not responded to immunosuppressive therapy.[280]

ANDROGENS

Randomized trials have not shown efficacy when androgens were used as primary therapy for severe or moderately severe aplastic ane-

mia.[174,246] These agents have been replaced by immunosuppression or stem cell transplantation.

Androgens stimulate the production of erythropoietin, and their metabolites stimulate erythropoiesis when they are added to marrow cultures in vitro.[247] High doses of androgens were beneficial in some patients with moderately severe aplasia.[248] Large series of patients in whom survival seemed improved compared with historical controls have been reported, but this finding could have resulted from improved supportive care.[188]

Androgens, if used, should be continued for at least 3 to 6 months because responses may require prolonged treatment. Nandrolone decanoate administered at 400 mg intramuscularly per week is one approach. Local hematomas can be minimized by firm local pressure for 30 minutes after the injection. Long-term survivors after androgen therapy have essentially the same progression to clonal hematologic disorders as patients treated with immunosuppressive agents.[188]

CYTOKINES

Despite their effectiveness in accelerating recovery from chemotherapy, cytokines have been far less effective in achieving long-term benefits in patients with severe aplastic anemia. Daily treatment with GM-CSF[249–251] or G-CSF[252] has improved marrow cellularity and increased neutrophil counts approximately 1.5- to 10-fold. Unfortunately, the blood counts return to baseline within several days of cessation of therapy in nearly all patients. Although occasional patients show evidence of trilineage marrow recovery with long-term therapy,[252–254] the vast majority of patients do not respond. In fact, physicians have been cautioned not to use hematopoietic growth factors as primary therapy.[233] Therapy with myeloid growth factors probably is best reserved for episodes of severe infection or as a preventive measure prior to dental work or other procedures that can compromise mucosal barriers. Prophylactic use of growth factors is not warranted. G-CSF at a dose of 5 μg/kg by subcutaneous injection is easiest to administer and seems to be associated with the fewest side effects. The drug can be given daily or fewer times per week, depending on the response. Newer pegylated preparations have greater longevity and usually are administered at less frequent, every-other-week intervals.

IL-1, a potent stimulator of marrow stromal cell production of other cytokines, and IL-3 have been ineffective in small numbers of patients with severe aplastic anemia.[255,256] These disappointing results with cytokines are not unexpected, given that previous work has found high serum levels of growth factors in patients with aplastic anemia. Moreover, the majority of patients have suppression of very primitive progenitors, which may be unresponsive to factors that act on more mature progenitor cells.

SPLENECTOMY

Removal of the spleen does not increase hematopoiesis but may increase neutrophil and platelet counts twofold to threefold and improve survival of transfused red cells or platelets in highly sensitized individuals.[257] Surgical morbidity and mortality in patients with few platelets and white cells makes splenectomy a questionable therapeutic procedure. Because more successful methods of therapy that attack the fundamental problem are available, splenectomy is rarely used today.

OTHER THERAPY

High doses of intravenous γ-globulin have been given to small numbers of patients with severe aplastic anemia[258,259] because of its success in treating certain cases of antibody-mediated pure red cell aplasia. Some improvement was noted in four of six patients treated. Another treatment that occasionally is successful is lymphocytapheresis administered to deplete T cells.[260,261]

COURSE AND PROGNOSIS

At diagnosis, the prognosis is largely related to the absolute neutrophil count and the platelet count. The absolute neutrophil count is the most important prognostic feature. A count of less than $500/\mu l$ ($0.5 \times 10^9/$ liter) is considered severe aplastic anemia, and a count less than $200/\mu l$ ($0.2 \times 10^9/$liter) is associated with a poor response to immunotherapy and a dire prognosis if early successful allogeneic transplant is not available. In the past, the prognosis appeared worse when the disease occurred after hepatitis.[71,72] Results with immunosuppression[262] or marrow transplant[263] are equivalent to results seen in idiopathic or drug-induced cases. Children appear to respond better than adults.[264] Constitutional aplastic anemia responds temporarily to androgens and glucocorticoids but usually is fatal unless it is treated by transplantation.[142,164]

Before marrow transplantation and immunosuppressive therapy, greater than 25 percent of patients with severe aplastic anemia died within 4 months of diagnosis; half died within 1 year.[265,266] Marrow transplantation is curative for approximately 80 percent of patients younger than 20 years, approximately 70 percent of patients aged 20 to 40 years, and approximately 50 percent of patients older than 40 years.[267] Unfortunately, as many as 40 percent of transplant survivors suffer the deleterious consequences of chronic graft-versus-host disease,[212] and the risk of subsequent cancer can be as high as 11 percent in older patients or after cyclosporine therapy prior to stem cell transplantation.[277] The best outcomes occur in patients who have not been exposed to immunosuppressive therapy prior to transplantation, not exposed and sensitized to blood cell products, and not subjected to irradiation in the conditioning regimen for transplantation.[277]

Combined immunosuppressive therapy with ATG and cyclosporine leads to marked improvement in at least 70 percent of patients.[268] Although some patients have normal blood counts, many continue having moderate anemia or thrombocytopenia. The disease may progress over 10 years to paroxysmal nocturnal hemoglobinuria, a myelodysplastic syndrome, or acute myelogenous leukemia in as many as 40 percent of patients who initially responded to immunosuppressive therapy.[211,213–215,237–239] In 168 transplanted patients, actuarial survival at 15 years was 69 percent, and in 227 patients receiving immunosuppressive therapy survival was only 38 percent.[269]

Treatment with high-dose cyclophosphamide produces early results similar to the results seen with the combination of ATG and cyclosporine.[245,270] However, cyclophosphamide has greater early toxicity and slower hematologic recovery but may generate more durable remissions.[245]

REFERENCES

1. Ehrlich P: Über einen Fall von Anämie mit Bemerkungen über regenerative Veränderungen des Knochenmarks. *Charite Ann* 13:300, 1888.

2. Chauffard M: Un cas d'anémie pernicieuse aplastique. *Bull Soc Med Hop Paris* 21:313, 1904.

3. Scott JL, Cartwright GE, Wintrobe MM: Acquired aplastic anemia: An analysis of thirty-nine cases and review of the pertinent literature. *Medicine* 38:119, 1959.

4. Thomas ED, Storb R, Giblett B, et al: Recovery from aplastic anemia following attempted marrow transplantation. *Exp Hematol* 4:97, 1976.

5. Speck B, Gluckman E: Treatment of aplastic anemia by antilymphocyte globulin with and without allogeneic bone marrow infusions. *Lancet* II: 1145, 1977.

6. Wallerstein RO, Condit PK, Kasper PK, et al: Statewide study of chloramphenicol therapy and fatal aplastic anemia. *JAMA* 208:2045, 1969.

7. Kaufman DW, Kelly JP, Levy M, et al: *The Drug Etiology of Agranulocytosis and Aplastic Anemia.* Oxford University Press, New York, 1991.

8. Mary JY, Baumelou E, Guiguet M: Epidemiology of aplastic anemia in France: A prospective multicenter study. *Blood* 75:1646, 1990.

9. Young NS, Alter BP: *Aplastic Anemia: Acquired and Inherited*, p 26. WB Saunders, New York, 1994.

10. Chongli Y, Ziaobo Z: Incidence survey of aplastic anemia in China. *Chin Med Sci J* 6:203, 1991.

11. Issaragrisil S: Epidemiology of aplastic anemia in Thailand. Thai Aplastic Anemia Study Group. *Int J Hematol* 70:137, 1999.

12. Yong AS, Goh AS, Rahman M, et al: Epidemiology of aplastic anemia in the state of Sabah, Malaysia. *Med J Malaysia* 53:59, 1998.

13. Aoki K, Fujiki N, Shimizu H, et al: Geographic and ethnic differences of aplastic anemia in humans, in *Medullary Aplasia*, edited by Y Najean, p 79. Masson, New York, 1980.

14. Shimizu H, Kuroishi T, Tominaga S, et al: Production amount of chloramphenicol and mortality rate of aplastic anemia in Japan. *Acta Haematol Jpn* 42:689, 1979.

15. Mizuno S, Aoki K, Ohno Y, et al: Time series analysis of age-sex specific death rates from aplastic anemia and the trend in the production of chloramphenicol. *Nagoya J Med Sci* 44:103, 1982.

16. Yin SN, Li GL, Tain FD, et al: Leukaemia in benzene workers: A retrospective cohort study. *Br J Indust Med* 44:124, 1987.

17. Kagan WA, Ascensao J, Pahwa R, et al: Aplastic anemia: Presence in human bone marrow of cells that suppress myelopoiesis. *Proc Natl Acad Sci U S A* 73:2890, 1976.

18. Kern P, Heimpel H, Heit W, et al: Granulocytic progenitor cells in aplastic anaemia. *Br J Haematol* 35:613, 1977.

19. Haak HL, Goselink HM, Veenhof W, et al: Acquired aplastic anaemia in adults: IV. Histological and CFU studies in transplanted and nontransplanted patients. *Scand J Haematol* 19:159, 1977.

20. Hoffman R, Zanjani ED, Lutton JD, et al: Suppression of erythroid-colony formation by lymphocytes from patients with aplastic anemia. *N Engl J Med* 296:10, 1977.

21. Hansi W, Rich I, Heimpel H, et al: Erythroid colony forming cells in aplastic anaemia. *Br J Haematol* 37:483, 1977.

22. Moriyama Y, Sato M, Kinoshita Y: Studies of hematopoietic stem cells: XI. Lack of erythroid burst-forming units (BFU-E) in patients with aplastic anemia. *Am J Hematol* 6:11, 1979.

23. Maciejewski JP, Selleri C, Sato T, et al: A severe and consistent deficit in marrow and circulating primitive hematopoietic cells (long-term culture-initiating cells) in acquired aplastic anemia. *Blood* 88:1983, 1996.

24. Maciejewski JP, Anderson S, Katevas P, Young NS: Phenotypic and functional analysis of bone marrow progenitor cell compartment in bone marrow failure. *Br J Haematol* 87:227, 1994.

25. Scopes J, Bagnara M, Gordon-Smith EC, et al: Haemopoietic progenitor cells are reduced in aplastic anaemia. *Br J Haematol* 86:427, 1994.

26. Young NS: Immune pathophysiology of acquired aplastic anaemia. *Eur J Haematol* 57(suppl):55, 1996.

27. Young NS, Maciejewski J: The pathophysiology of acquired aplastic anemia. *N Engl J Med* 336:1365, 1997.

28. Ascensao J, Kagan W, Moore M, et al: Aplastic anemia: Evidence for an immunological mechanism. *Lancet* 1:669, 1976.

29. Nissen C, Cornu P, Gratwohl A, Speck B: Peripheral blood cells from patients with aplastic anaemia in partial remission suppress growth of their own bone marrow precursors in culture. *Br J Haematol* 45:233, 1980.

30. Bacigalupo A, Podesta M, VanLint MT, et al: Severe aplastic anaemia: Correlation of in vitro tests with clinical response to immunosuppression in twenty patients. *Br J Haematol* 47:423, 1981.

31. Singer JW, Brown JE, James MC, et al: Effect of peripheral blood lymphocytes from patients with aplastic anemia on granulocyte colony growth from HLA-matched and mismatched marrows: Effect of transfusion sensitization. *Blood* 52:37, 1978.

32. Torok-Storb B, Sieff C, Storb R, et al: In vitro tests for distinguishing possible immune-mediated aplastic anemia from transfusion-induced sensitization. *Blood* 55:211, 1980.

33. Singer JW, Doney KC, Thomas ED: Co-culture studies of 16 untransfused patients with aplastic anemia. *Blood* 54:180, 1979.

34. Mangan KF, Mullaney MT, Rosenfeld CS, Shadduck RK: In vitro evidence for disappearance of erythroid progenitor T suppressor cells following allogeneic bone marrow transplantation for severe aplastic anemia. *Blood* 71:144, 1988.

35. Teramura M, Kobayashi S, Iwabe K, et al: Mechanism of action of antithymocyte globulin in the treatment of aplastic anaemia: In vitro evidence for the presence of immunosuppressive mechanism. *Br J Haematol* 96:80, 1997.

36. Mathé G, Amiel JL, Schwarzenberg L, et al: Bone marrow graft in man after conditioning by antilymphocytic serum. *Br Med J* 2:131, 1970.

37. Storb R, Longton G, Anasetti C, et al: Changing trends in marrow transplantation for aplastic anemia. *Bone Marrow Transplant* 10(suppl 1):45, 1992.

38. Champlin RE, Feig SA, Sparkes RS, Gale RP: Bone marrow transplantation from identical twins in the treatment of aplastic anaemia: Implication for the pathogenesis of the disease. *Br J Haematol* 56:455, 1984.

39. Young NS, Maciejewski J: Mechanisms of disease: The pathophysiology of acquired aplastic anemia. *N Engl J Med* 336:1365, 1997.

40. Zoumbos N, Gascon P, Djeu J, Young NS: Interferon is a mediator of hematopoietic suppression in aplastic anemia in vitro and possibly in vivo. *Proc Natl Acad Sci U S A* 82:188, 1985.

41. Laver J, Castro-Malaspina H, Kernan NA, et al: In vitro interferon-gamma production by cultured T-cells in severe aplastic anaemia: Correlation with granulomonopoietic inhibition in patients who respond to anti-thymocyte globulin. *Br J Haematol* 69:545, 1988.

42. Gascon P, Zoumbos NC, Scala G, et al: Lymphokine abnormalities in aplastic anemia: Implications for the mechanism of action of antithymocyte globulin. *Blood* 65:407, 1985.

43. Hinterberger W, Adolf G, Bettelheim P, et al: Lymphokine overproduction in severe aplastic anemia is not related to blood transfusions. *Blood* 74:2713, 1989.

44. Shinohara K, Ayame H, Tanaka M, et al: Increased production of tumor necrosis factor alpha by peripheral blood mononuclear cells in the patients with aplastic anemia. *Am J Hematol* 37:75, 1991.

45. Nistico, A, Young, NS: Gamma-interferon gene expression in the bone marrow of patients with aplastic anemia. *Ann Intern Med* 120:463, 1994.

46. Yunis AA: Chloramphenicol toxicity: 25 years of research. *Am J Med* 87:44N, 1989.

47. Young NS: Acquired aplastic anemia. Available at http://aplasticcentral.com/Aplastic_Facts/NIH_Young.htm. Last accessed October 2004.

48. Modan B, Segal S, Shani M, Sheba C: Aplastic anemia in Israel: Evaluation of the etiological role of chloramphenicol on a community-wide basis. *Am J Med Sci* 270:441, 1975.

49. Smick K, Condit PK, Proctor RL, Sutcher V: Fatal aplastic anemia: An epidemiological study of its relationship to the drug chloramphenicol. *J Chronic Dis* 17:899, 1964.

50. Brodsky E, Zeidan Z, Biger Y, Schneider M: Topical application of chloramphenicol eye ointment followed by fatal bone marrow aplasia. *Isr J Med Sci* 25:54, 1989.

51. West BC, DeVault GA Jr, Clement JC, Williams DM: Aplastic anemia associated with parenteral chloramphenicol: Review of 10 cases, including the second case of possible increased risk with cimetidine. *Rev Infect Dis* 10:1048, 1988.

52. Custer RP: Aplastic anemia in soldiers treated with Atabrine (quinacrine). *Am J Med Sci* 212:211, 1946.

53. Cunningham JL, Leyland MJ, Delamore IW, Price-Evans DA: Acetanilide oxidation in phenylbutazone-associated hypoplastic anaemia. *Br Med J* 3:313, 1974.

54. Chang HK, Morrison SL: Bone marrow suppression associated with cimetidine. *Ann Intern Med* 91:580, 1979.

55. Tonkonow B, Hoffman R: Aplastic anemia and cimetidine. *Arch Intern Med* 140:1123, 1980.

56. Volkin RL, Shadduck RK, Winkelstein A, et al: Potentiation of carmustine-cranial-irradiation-induced myelosuppression by cimetidine. *Arch Intern Med* 142:243, 1982.

57. Santesson GG: Über chronische Vergiftungen mit Steinkohlenteerbenzin. vier Todesfälle. *Arch Hyg Berl* 31:336, 1897.

58. Rangau U, Snyder R: Scientific update on benzene. *Ann N Y Acad Sci* 837:105, 1997.

59. Snyder R: Benzene and Leukemia. *Crit Rev Toxicol* 32:155, 2002.

60. Yardley-Jones A, Anderson D, Parke DV: The toxicity of benzene and its metabolism and molecular pathology in human risk assessment. *Br J Ind Med* 48:437, 1991.

61. Hamilton A: The lessening menace of benzol poisoning in American industry. *J Ind Hyg* 10:227, 1928.

62. Aksoy M, Dincol K, Akgun T, et al: Hematological effects of chronic benzene poisoning in 217 workers. *Br J Indust Med* 28:296, 1971.

63. Fleming LE, Timmeny MA: Aplastic anemia and pesticides. *J Occup Med* 35:1106, 1993.

64. Rugman FP, Cosstick R: Aplastic anaemia associated with organochlorine pesticide: Case reports and review of evidence. *J Clin Pathol* 43:98, 1990.

65. Rauch AE, Kowalsky SF, Lesar TS, et al: Lindane (Kwell)-induced aplastic anemia. *Arch Intern Med* 150:2393, 1990.

66. Sanchez-Medal L, Castanedo JP, Garcia-Rojas F: Insecticides and aplastic anemia. *N Engl J Med* 269:1365, 1963.

67. Roberts HJ: Pentachlorophenol-associated aplastic anemia, red cell aplasia, leukemia and other blood disorders. *J Fla Med Assoc* 77:86, 1990.

68. Prager D, Peters C: Development of aplastic anemia and the exposure to Stoddard solvent. *Blood* 35:286, 1970.

69. Powers D: Aplastic anemia secondary to glue sniffing. *N Engl J Med* 273:700, 1965.

70. Crawford MAD: Aplastic anaemia due to trinitrotoluene intoxication. *Br Med J* 2:430, 1954.

71. Ajlouni K, Doeblin TD: The syndrome of hepatitis and aplastic anaemia. *Br J Haematol* 27:345, 1974.

72. Hagler L, Pastore RA, Bergin JJ: Aplastic anemia following viral hepatitis: Report of 2 fatal cases and literature review. *Medicine (Baltimore)* 54:139, 1975.

73. Pol S, Driss F, Devergie A, et al: Is hepatitis C virus involved in hepatitis-associated aplastic anemia? *Ann Intern Med* 113:435, 1990.

74. Hibbs JR, Frickhofen N, Rosenfeld SJ, et al: Aplastic anemia and viral hepatitis: Non-A, non-B, non-C? *JAMA* 267:2051, 1992.

75. Tzakis AG, Arditi M, Whitington PF, et al: Aplastic anemia complicating orthotopic liver transplantation for non-A, non-B hepatitis. *N Engl J Med* 319:393, 1988.

76. Kurtzman G, Young N: Viruses and bone marrow failure. *Baillieres Clin Haematol* 2:51, 1989.

77. Hibbs JR, Issaragrisl S, Young NS: High prevalence of hepatitis C viremia among aplastic anemia patients and controls from Thailand. *Am J Trop Med Hyg* 46:564, 1992.

78. Brown KE, Tisdale J, Barrett AJ, et al: Hepatitis-associated aplastic anemia. *N Engl J Med* 336:1059, 1997.

79. Safadi R, Or R, Ilan Y, et al: Lack of known hepatitis virus in hepatitis-associated aplastic anemia and outcome after bone marrow transplantation. *Bone Marrow Transplant* 27:183, 2001.

80. Lazarus KH, Baehner RL: Aplastic anemia complicating infectious mononucleosis: A case report and review of the literature. *Pediatrics* 67:907, 1981.

81. Baranski B, Armstrong G, Truman JT, et al: Epstein-Barr virus in the bone marrow of patients with aplastic anemia. *Ann Intern Med* 109:695, 1988.

82. Vinters HV, Mah V, Mohrmann R, Wiley CA: Evidence for human immunodeficiency virus (HIV) infection of the brain in a patient with aplastic anemia. *Acta Neuropathol* 76:311, 1988.

83. Samuel D, Castaing D, Adam R, et al: Fatal acute HIV infection with aplastic anaemia, transmitted by liver graft. *Lancet* 1:1221, 1988.

84. Morales CE, Sriram I, Baumann MA: Myelodysplastic syndrome occurring as possible first manifestation of human immunodeficiency virus infection with subsequent progression to aplastic anaemia. *Int J STD AIDS* 1:55, 1990.

85. Young N: Hematologic and hematopoietic consequences of B-19 parvovirus infection. *Semin Hematol* 25:159, 1988.

86. Rosenfeld CS, Rybka WB, Weinbaum D, et al: Late graft failure due to dual bone marrow infection with variants A and B of human Herpesvirus-6. *Exp Hematol* 23:626, 1995.

87. Baumelou E, Guiguet M, Mary JY, et al: Epidemiology of aplastic anemia in France: A case control study: I. Medical history and medication use. *Blood* 81:1471, 1993.

88. Pavithran K, Raji NL, Thomas M: Aplastic anemia complicating lupus erythematosus–Report of a case and review of the literature. *Rheumatol Int* 22:253, 2002.

89. Bailey FA, Lilly M, Bertoli LF, Ball GV: An antibody that inhibits in vitro bone marrow proliferation in a patient with systemic lupus erythematosus and aplastic anemia. *Arthritis Rheum* 31:901, 1989.

90. Roffe C, Cahill MR, Samanta A, et al: Aplastic anaemia in systemic lupus erythematosus: A cellular immune mechanism? *Br J Rheumatol* 30:301, 1991.

91. Sumimoto S, Kawai M, Kasajima Y, Hamamoto T: Aplastic anemia associated with systemic lupus erythematosus. *Am J Hematol* 38:329, 1991.

92. Winkler A, Jackson RW, Kay DS, et al: High-dose intravenous cyclophosphamide treatment of systemic lupus erythematosus-associated aplastic anemia [letter]. *Arthritis Rheum* 31:693, 1988.

93. Kim SW, Rice L, Champlin R, Udden MM: Aplastic Anemia in eosinophilic fasciitis: Responses to immunosuppression and marrow transplantation. *Haematologica* 28:131, 1997.

94. Debusscher L, Bitar N, DeMaubeuge J, et al: Eosinophilic fasciitis and severe aplastic anemia: Favorable response to either antithymocyte globulin or cyclosporin A in blood and skin disorders. *Transplant Proc* 20:310, 1988.

95. Kumar M, Goldman J: Severe aplastic anemia and Grave's disease in a paediatric patient. *Br J Haematol* 118:327, 2002.

96. Tomonari A, Tojo A, Iseki T, et al: Severe aplastic anemia with autoimmune thyroiditis showing no hematological response to intensive immunosuppressive therapy. *Acta Haematol* 109:90, 2003.

97. Dincol G, Saka B, Aktan M, et al: Very severe aplastic anemia following resection of lymphocytic thymoma: Effectiveness of antilymphocyte globulin, cyclosporin A and granulocyte-colony stimulating factor. *Am J Hematol* 64:78, 2000.

98. Ritchie DS, Underhill C, Grigg AP: Aplastic anemia as a late complication of thymoma in remission. *Eur J Haematol* 68:389, 2002.

99. Aitchison RGM, Marsh JCW, Hows JM, et al: Pregnancy associated aplastic anaemia: A report of 5 cases and review of current management. *Br J Haematol* 73:541, 1989.

100. Pajor A, Kelemen E, Szak'acs Z, Lehoczky D: Pregnancy in idiopathic aplastic anemia (report of 10 patients). *Eur J Obstet Gynecol Reprod Biol* 45:19, 1992.

101. Bourantas K, Makrydimas G, Georgiou I, et al: Aplastic anemia: Report of a case with recurrent episodes in consecutive pregnancies. *J Reprod Med* 42:672, 1997.

102. Tichelli A, Socie G, Marsh J, et al: Outcome of pregnancy and disease course among women with aplastic anemia treated with immunosuppression. *Ann Intern Med* 137:164, 2002.

103. Court-Brown WM, Doll R: Mortality from cancer and other causes after radiotherapy for ankylosing spondylitis. *Br Med J* 2:1317, 1965.

104. Darby SC, Doll R, Gill SK, Smith PG: Long term mortality after a single treatment course with x-rays in patients treated with ankylosing spondylitis. *Br J Cancer* 55:179, 1987.

105. Johnson SAN, Bateman CJT, Beard MEJ, et al: Long-term haematological complications of Thorotrast. *Q J Med* 182:259, 1977.

106. Martland HS: The occurrence of malignancy in radioactive persons: A general review of data gathered in the study of the radium dial painters, with special reference to the occurrence of osteogeneic sarcoma and the inter-relationship of certain blood diseases. *Am J Cancer* 15:2435, 1931.

107. Cronkite EP, Haley TJ: Clinical aspects of acute radiation injury, in *Manual on Radiation Haematology*, p 169. International Atomic Energy Agency, Vienna, 1971.

108. Mettler FA Jr, Moseley RD Jr: *Medical Effects of Ionizing Irradiation*, p 1. Grune & Stratton, New York, 1985.

109. Gale RP: USSR: Follow-up after Chernobyl. *Lancet* 1:401, 1990.

110. Wodnar-Filipowicz A, Yancik S, Moser Y, et al: Levels of soluble stem cell factor in serum of patients with aplastic anemia. *Blood* 81:3159, 1993.

111. Nimer SD, Leung DHY, Wolin MJ, Golde DW: Serum stem cell factor levels in patients with aplastic anemia. *Int J Hematol* 60:185, 1994.

112. Kojima S, Matsuyama T, Kodera Y: Plasma levels and production of soluble stem cell factor by marrow stromal cells in patients with aplastic anaemia. *Br J Haematol* 99:440, 1997.

113. Wodnar-Filipowicz A, Tichelli A, Zsebo KM, et al: Stem cell factor stimulates the in vitro growth of bone marrow cells from aplastic anemia patients. *Blood* 79:3196, 1992.

114. Lyman SD, Seaberg M, Hanna R, et al: Plasma/serum levels of flt3 ligand are low in normal individuals and highly elevated in patients with Fanconi anemia and acquired aplastic anemia. *Blood* 86:4091, 1995.

115. Kojima S, Matsuyama T, Kodera Y, et al: Measurement of endogenous plasma granulocyte colony-stimulating factor in patients with acquired aplastic anemia by a sensitive chemiluminescent immunoassay. *Blood* 87:1303, 1996.

116. Kojima S, Matsuyama T, Kodera Y: Circulating erythropoietin in patients with acquired aplastic anaemia. *Acta Haematol* 94:117, 1995.

117. Emmons RVD, Reid DM, Cohen RL, et al: Human thrombopoietin levels are high when thrombocytopenia is due to megakaryocyte deficiency and low when due to increased platelet destruction. *Blood* 87:4068, 1996.

118. Nakao S, Matsushima K, Young N: Deficient interleukin I production by aplastic anaemia monocytes. *Br J Haematol* 71:431, 1989.

119. Marsh JC, Chang J, Testa NG, et al: In vitro assessment of marrow "stem cell" and stromal cell function in aplastic anaemia. *Br J Haematol* 78:258, 1991.

120. Kojima S, Matsuyama T, Kodera Y: Hematopoietic growth factors released by marrow stromal cells from patients with aplastic anemia. *Blood* 79:2256, 1992.

121. Holmberg LA, Seidel K, Leisenring W, Torok-Storb B: Aplastic anemia: Analysis of stromal cell function in long-term marrow cultures. *Blood* 84:3685, 1994.

122. Margolis DA, Cammita BM: Hematopoietic stem cell transplantation for severe aplastic anemia. *Curr Opin Hematol* 5:441, 1998.

123. Georges GE, Storb R: Stem cell transplantation for aplastic anemia. *Int J Hematol* 75:141, 2002.

124. Stute N, Fehse B, Schroder J, et al: Human mesenchymal stem cells are not of donor origin in patients with severe aplastic anemia who underwent sex-mismatched allogeneic bone marrow transplant. *J Hematother Stem Cell Res* 11:977, 2002.

125. Best WR: Drug-associated blood dyscrasias. *JAMA* 185:286, 1963.

126. The International Agranulocytosis and Aplastic Anemia Study: Risks of agranulocytosis and aplastic anemia: A first report of their relation to drug use with special reference to analgesics. *JAMA* 256:1749, 1986.

127. Retsagi G, Kelly JP, Kaufman DW: Risk of agranulocytosis and aplastic

anaemia in relation to use of antithyroid drugs: International Agranulocytosis and Aplastic Anaemia Study. *Br Med J* 297:262, 1988.

128. International Agranulocytosis and Aplastic Anemia Study: Anti-infec-
tive drug use in relation to the risk of agranulocytosis and aplastic anemia. *Arch Intern Med* 149:1036, 1989.

129. Kelly JP, Kaufman DW, Shapiro S: Risks of agranulocytosis and aplastic
anemia in relation to the use of cardiovascular drugs: The International
Agranulocytosis and Aplastic Anemia Study. *Clin Pharmacol Ther* 49:
330, 1991.

130. Kaufmann DW, Kelly JP, Jurgelon JM, et al: Drugs in the aetiology of
agranulocytosis and aplastic anaemia. *Eur J Haematolo* 57(suppl):23, 1996.

131. Bithell TC, Wintrobe MM: Drug-induced aplastic anemia. *Semin Hematol* 4:194, 1967.

132. Williams DM, Lynch RE, Cartwright GE: Drug-induced aplastic anemia. *Semin Hematol* 10:195, 1973.

133. Heimpel H, Heit W: Drug-induced aplastic anaemia. *Clin Haematol* 9:
641, 1980.

134. Williams DM: Pancytopenia, aplastic anemia and pure red cell aplasia,
in *Wintrobe's Clinical Hematology*, 10th ed, edited by GR Lee, J Foers-
ter, J Lukens, p 1452. Williams & Wilkins, Baltimore, 1999.

135. Adamson JW, Erslev AJ: Aplastic anemia, in *Hematology*, 4th ed, edited
by WJ Williams, E Beutler, AJ Erslev, MA Lichtman, p 158. McGraw-
Hill, New York, 1990.

136. Fanconi G: Familiäre infantile perniziosaartige anämie (perniziöses blut-
bild und konstitution). *Jahrbuch Kinderheil* 117:257, 1927.

137. Alter BP: Cancer in Fanconi anemia. *Cancer* 97:425, 2003.

138. Rosenberg PS, Huang Y, Alter BP: Individualized risks of first adverse
events in patients with Fanconi anemia. *Blood* 104:350, 2004.

139. Bagby GC: Genetic basis of Fanconi anemia. *Curr Opin Hematol* 10:
68, 2003.

140. D'Apolito M, Zelante L, Savoia A: Molecular basis of Fanconi anemia.
Hematologica 83:533, 1998.

141. Garcia-Higuera I, Kuang Y, D'Andrea AD: The molecular and cellular
biology of Fanconi anemia. *Curr Opin Hematol* 6:83, 1999.

142. Alter BP: Fanconi's anemia: Current concepts. *Am J Pediatr Hematol
Oncol* 14:170, 1992.

143. Young NA, Alter BP: *Aplastic Anemia: Acquired and Inherited*. WB
Saunders, Philadelphia, 1994.

144. Estren S, Damshek W: Familial hypoplastic anemia of childhood: Report
of 8 cases in 2 families with beneficial effects of splenectomy in 1 case.
Am J Dis Child 73:671, 1947.

145. Gonzalez-del AA, Cervera M, Gomez L, et al: Ataxia-pancytopenia syndrome. *Am J Med Genet* 90:252, 2000.

146. Swhimamura A, D'Andrea AD: Subtyping of Fanconi anemia patients:
Implications for clinical management. *Blood* 102:3459, 2003.

147. Mahmood F, King MD, Smyth OO, et al: Familial cerebellar hypoplasia
and pancytopenia without chromosomal breakages. *Neuropediatrics* 29:
302, 1998.

148. Li FP, Hecht F, Kaiser-McCaw B, et al: Ataxia-pancytopenia: Syndrome
of cerebellar ataxia, hypoplastic anemia, monosomy 7 and acute myelogenous leukemia. *Cancer Genet Cytogenet* 4:189, 1981.

149. Berthold F, Fuhrmann W, Lampert F: Fatal aplastic anemia in a patient
with Dubowitz syndrome. *Eur J Pediatr* 146:605, 1987.

150. Walters TR, Desposito F: Aplastic anemia in Dubowitz syndrome. *J
Pediatr* 106:622, 1985.

151. Dokal I, Vulliamy T: Dyskeratosis congenita: Its link to telomerase and
aplastic anemia. *Blood Rev* 17:217, 2003.

152. Drachman RA, Alter BP: Dyskeratosis congenita. *Dermatol Clin* 13:33,
1995.

153. Mason PJ: Stem cells, telomerase and dyskeratosis congenita. *Bioessays*
25:126, 2003.

154. Bessler M, Wilson DB, Mason PJ: Dyskeratosis congenita and telomerase. *Curr Opin Pediatr* 16:23, 2004.

155. Revesz T, Kardos G, Schuler D: Rare congenital forms of bone marrow
deficiency. *Orv Hetil* 134:1147, 1993.

156. Esperou-Bourdeau H, Leblanc T, Schaison G, et al: Aplastic anemia
associated with "bird-headed" dwarfism (Seckel syndrome). *Nouv Rev
Fr Hematol* 35:99, 1993.

157. O'Driscoll M, Ruiz-Perez VL, Woods CG, et al: A splicing mutation
affecting expression of ataxia-telangiectasia and RAD3-related protein
(ATR) results in Seckel syndrome. *Nature Genet* 33:497, 2003.

158. Boocock GR, Morrison JA, Popovic M, et al: Mutations in SBDS are
associated with Shwachman-Diamond syndrome. *Nature Genet* 33:97,
2003.

159. Dror Y, Freedman MH: Shwachman-Diamond syndrome. *Br J Haematol* 118:701, 2002.

160. Smith OP: Shwachman-Diamond syndrome. *Semin Hematol* 39:95,
2002.

161. Gonzalez CH, Durkin-Stamm MV, Geimer NF, et al: The WT syndrome—A "new" autosomal dominant pleiotropic trait of radial/ulnar
hypoplasia with high risk of bone marrow failure and/or leukemia. *Birth
Defects Orig Artic Ser* 13:31, 1977.

162. Carreau M, Liu L, Gan OI, et al: Short-term granulocyte colony-stimulating factor and erythropoietin treatment enhances hematopoiesis and
survival in the mitomycin C-conditioned Fancc(-/-) mouse model, while
long-term treatment is ineffective. *Blood* 100:1499, 2002.

163. Alter BP, Caruso JP, Drachman RA, et al: Fanconi anemia: Myelodysplasia as a predictor of outcome. *Cancer Genet Cytogenet* 117:125,
2000.

164. Gluckman E, Auerbach A, Horowitz MM, et al: Bone marrow transplantation for Fanconi anemia. *Blood* 86:2856, 1995.

165. Guardiola Ph, Pasquini R, Dokal I, et al: Outcome of 69 allogeneic stem
cell transplantations for Fanconi anemia using HLA-matched unrelated
donors. *Blood* 95:422, 2000.

166. Croop JM: Gene therapy for Fanconi anemia. *Curr Hematol Rep* 1:335,
2003.

167. Galimi F, Noll M, Kanazawa Y, et al: Gene therapy of Fanconi anemia:
Preclinical efficacy of lentiviral vectors. *Blood* 100:2732, 2002.

168. Dokal I: Dyskeratosis congenita: An inherited bone marrow failure syndrome. *Br J Haematol* 92:775, 1996.

169. Ginzberg H, Shin J, Ellis L, et al: Shwachman syndrome: Phenotypic
manifestations of sibling sets and isolated cases in a large patient cohort
are similar. *J Pediatr* 135:81, 1999.

170. Dror Y, Freedman MH: Shwachman-Diamond syndrome. *Blood* 94:
3048, 1999.

171. Hayani A, Suarez CR, Molnar Z, et al: Acute myeloid leukemia in a
patient with Seckel syndrome. *J Med Genet* 31:148, 1994.

172. Alexanian R: Erythropoietin excretion in bone marrow failure and hemolytic anemia. *J Lab Clin Med* 82:438, 1973.

173. Finch CA, Duebelbeiss K, Cook JD, et al: Ferrokinetics in man. *Medicine (Baltimore)* 49:17, 1970.

174. Camitta BM, Thomas ED, Nathan DG, et al: A prospective study of
androgens and bone marrow transplantation for treatment of severe
aplastic anemia. *Blood* 53:504, 1979.

175. Krause JR: Aplastic anemia terminating in hairy cell leukemia. A report
of 2 cases. *Cancer* 53:1533, 1984.

176. Reid MM, Summerfield GP: Distinction between a leukaemic prodrome
of childhood acute lymphoblastic leukaemia and aplastic anaemia. *J Clin
Pathol* 45:697, 1992.

177. Torok-Storb B, Doney K, Brown SL, Prentice RL: Correlation of two
in vitro tests with clinical response to immunosuppressive therapy in 54
patients with severe aplastic anemia. *Blood* 63:349, 1984.

178. Applebaum FR, Barrall J, Storb R, et al: Clonal cytogenetic abnormalities in patients with otherwise typical aplastic anemia. *Exp Hematol* 15:
1134, 1987.

179. Olson DO, Shields AF, Scheurich CJ, et al: Magnetic resonance imaging

of the bone marrow in patients with leukemia, aplastic anemia, and lymphoma. *Invest Radiol* 21:540, 1986.

180. Steiner RM, Mitchell DG, Rao VM, et al: Magnetic resonance imaging of bone marrow: Diagnostic value in diffuse hematologic disorders. *Magn Reson Q* 6:17, 1990.

181. Negendank W, Weissman D, Bey TM, et al: Evidence for clonal disease by magnetic resonance imaging in patients with hypoplastic marrow disorders. *Blood* 78:2872, 1991.

182. Schrezenmeier H, Hertenstein B, Wagner B, et al: A pathogenetic link between aplastic anemia and paroxysmal nocturnal hemoglobinuria is suggested by a high frequency of aplastic anemia patients with a deficiency of phosphatidylinositol glycan anchored proteins. *Exp Hematol* 23:81, 1995.

183. Young N: Acquired aplastic anemia. *Ann Intern Med* 136:534, 2002.

184. Socie G, Rosenfeld S, Frickhofen N, et al: Late clonal diseases of aplastic anemia. *Semin Hematol* 37:91, 2000.

185. Gordon-Smith EC, Marsh JC, Gibson FM: Views on the pathophysiology of aplastic anemia. *Int J Hematol* 76(suppl 2):163, 2002.

186. Maciejewski JP, Risitano A, Sloand EM, et al: Distinct clinical outcomes for cytogenetic abnormalities evolving from aplastic anemia. *Blood* 99:3129, 2002.

187. Socie G, Henryamar M, Bacigalupo A, et al: Malignant tumors occurring after treatment of aplastic anemia. *N Engl J Med* 329:1152, 1993.

188. Najean Y, Haguenauer O, the Cooperative Group for the Study of Aplastic and Refractory Anemias: Long-term (5–20 years) evolution of nongrafted aplastic anemias. *Blood* 76:2222, 1990.

189. Ball SE, Gibson FM, Rizzo S: Progressive telomere shortening in aplastic anemia. *Blood* 91:3582, 1998.

190. Rosse WF: New insights into paroxysmal nocturnal hemoglobinuria. *Curr Opin Hematol* 8:61, 2001.

191. Nakakuma H, Kawaguchi T: Pathogenesis of selective expansion of PNH clones. *Int J Hematol* 77:121, 2003.

192. Storb R, Blume KG, O'Donnell MR, et al: Cyclophosphamide and antithymocyte globulin to condition patients with aplastic anemia for allogeneic marrow transplantation: The experience in four centers. *Biol Blood Transplant* 7:39, 2001.

193. Sagmeister M, Oec L, Gmur J: A restrictive platelet transfusion policy allowing long-term support of outpatients with severe aplastic anemia. *Blood* 93:3124, 1999.

194. Lawrence JB, Yomtovian RA, Hammons T, et al: Lowering the prophylactic platelet transfusion threshold: A prospective analysis. *Leuk Lymphoma* 41:67, 2001.

195. Zeigler ZR: Effects of epsilon aminocaproic acid on primary haemostasis. *Haemostasis* 21:313, 1991.

196. Sniecinski I, O'Donnell MR, Nowicki B, Hill LR: Prevention of refractoriness and HLA-alloimmunization using filtered blood products. *Blood* 71:1402, 1988.

197. Zeigler ZR, Shadduck RK, Rosenfeld CS, et al: High-dose intravenous gamma globulin improves responses to single-donor platelets in patients refractory to platelet transfusion. *Blood* 70:1433, 1987.

198. Zeigler ZR, Shadduck RK, Rosenfeld CS, et al: Intravenous gamma globulin decreases platelet associated IgG and improves transfusion responses in platelet refractory states. *Am J Hematol* 38:15, 1991.

199. Christie DJ, Howe RB, Lennon SS, Sauro SC: Treatment of refractoriness to platelet transfusion by protein A column therapy. *Transfusion* 33:234, 1993.

200. Caspar CB, Seger RA, Burger J, Gmür J: Effective stimulation of donors for granulocyte transfusions with recombinant methionyl granulocyte colony-stimulating factor. *Blood* 81:2866, 1993.

201. Davies SM, Kollman C, Anasetti C, et al: Engraftment and survival after unrelated-donor bone marrow transplantation: A report from the national marrow donor program. *Blood* 96:4096, 2000.

202. Wagner JE, Rosenthal J, Sweetman R, et al: Successful transplantation of HLA-matched and HLA-mismatched umbilical cord blood from unrelated donors: Analysis of engraftment and acute graft-versus-host disease. *Blood* 88:795, 1996.

203. Georges GE, Storb R: Stem cell transplantation for aplastic anemia. *Int J Hematol* 75:141, 2002.

204. Dubey S, Nityanand S: Involvement of Fas and TNF pathways in the induction of apoptosis of T cells by antithymocyte globulin. *Ann Hematol* 82:496, 2003.

205. Mangan KF, D'Alessandro L, Mullaney MT: Action of antithymocyte globulin on normal human erythroid progenitor cell proliferation in vitro: Erythropoietic growth-enhancing factors are released from marrow accessory cells. *J Lab Clin Med* 107:353, 1986.

206. Kawano Y, Nissen C, Gratwohl A, Speck B: Immunostimulatory effects of different antilymphocyte globulin preparations: A possible clue to their clinical effect. *Br J Haematol* 68:115, 1988.

207. Bielory L, Wright R, Nienhuis AW, et al: Antithymocyte globulin hypersensitivity in bone marrow failure patients. *JAMA* 260:3164, 1988.

208. Camitta B, O'Reilly RJ, Sensenbrenner L: Antithoracic duct lymphocyte globulin therapy of severe aplastic anemia. *Blood* 62:883, 1983.

209. Champlin R, Ho W, Gale RP: Antithymocyte globulin treatment in patients with aplastic anemia: A prospective randomized trial. *N Engl J Med* 308:113, 1983.

210. Young N, Griffin P, Brittain E, et al: A multicenter trial of antithymocyte globulin in aplastic anemia and related diseases. *Blood* 72:1861, 1988.

211. Schrezenmeier H, Marin P, Raghavachar A, et al: Relapse of aplastic anaemia after immunosuppressive treatment: A report from the European Bone Marrow Transplantation Group SAA Working Party. *Br J Haematol* 85:371, 1993.

212. Doney K, Leisenring W, Storb R, Appelbaum FR: Primary treatment of acquired aplastic anemia: Outcomes with bone marrow transplantation and immunosuppressive therapy. *Ann Intern Med* 126:107, 1997.

213. Tichelli A, Gratwohl A, Nissen C, Speck B: Late clonal complications in severe aplastic anemia. *Leuk Lymphoma* 12:167, 1994.

214. De Planque MM, Bacigalupo A, Würsch A, et al: Long-term follow-up of severe aplastic anaemia patients treated with antithymocyte globulin. *Br J Haematol* 73:121, 1989.

215. Socié G, Henry-Amar M, Bacigalupo A, et al: Malignant tumors occurring after treatment of aplastic anemia. *N Engl J Med* 319:1152, 1993.

216. Stryckmans PA, Dumont JP, Velu T, Debusscher L: Cyclosporine in refractory severe aplastic anemia [letter]. *N Engl J Med* 310:655, 1984.

217. Lazzarino M, Morra E, Canevari A, et al: Cyclosporine in the treatment of aplastic anaemia and pure red-cell aplasia. *Bone Marrow Transplant* 4(suppl 4):165, 1989.

218. Hinterberger-Fischer M, Höcker P, Lechner K, et al: Oral cyclosporin-A is effective treatment for untreated and also for previously immunosuppressed patients with severe bone marrow failure. *Eur J Haematol* 43:136, 1989.

219. Tötterman TH, Höglund M, Bengtsson M, et al: Treatment of pure red-cell aplasia and aplastic anaemia with cyclosporin: Long-term clinical effects. *Eur J Haematol* 42:126, 1989.

220. Leeksma OC, Thomas LLM, van der Lelie J, et al: Effectiveness of low dose cyclosporine in acquired aplastic anaemia with severe neutropenia. *Neth J Med* 41:143, 1992.

221. Leonard EM, Raefsky E, Griffith P, et al: Cyclosporine therapy of aplastic anaemia, congenital and acquired red-cell aplasia. *Br J Haematol* 72:278, 1989.

222. Tong J, Bacigalupo A, Piaggio G, et al: Severe aplastic anemia (SAA): Response to cyclosporin A (CyA) in vivo and in vitro. *Eur J Haematol* 46:212, 1991.

223. Nakao S, Yamaguchi M, Shiobara S, et al: Interferon-g gene expression in unstimulated bone marrow mononuclear cells predicts a good response to cyclosporine therapy in aplastic anemia. *Blood* 79:2531, 1992.

224. Kojima S, Fukada M, Miyajima Y, Matsuyama T: Cyclosporine and

recombinant granulocyte colony-stimulating factor in severe aplastic anemia [letter]. *N Engl J Med* 313:920, 1990.

225. Bertrand Y, Amri F, Capdeville R, et al: The successful treatment of two cases of severe aplastic anaemia with granulocyte colony-stimulating factor and cyclosporine A (case report). *Br J Haematol* 79:648, 1991.

226. Schrezenmeier H, Schlander M, Raghavachar A: Cyclosporin A in aplastic anemia—Report of a workshop. *Ann Hematol* 65:33, 1992.

227. Gluckman E, Esperou-Bourdeau H, Baruchel A, et al: Multicenter randomized study comparing cyclosporine-A alone and antithymocyte globulin with prednisone for treatment of severe aplastic anemia. *Blood* 79:2540, 1992.

228. Bacigalupo A, Van Lint MT, Cerri R, et al: Treatment of severe aplastic anemia with bolus 6-methylprednisolone and antilymphocyte globulin. *Blut* 41:168, 1980.

229. Issaragrisil S, Tangnai-Trisorana Y, Siriseriwan T, et al: Methylprednisolone therapy in aplastic anaemia: Correlation of in vitro tests and lymphocyte subsets with clinical response. *Eur J Haematol* 40:343, 1988.

230. Rosenfeld S, Follmann D, Nunez O, et al: Antithymocyte globulin and cyclosporine for severe aplastic anemia: Association between hematologic response and long-term outcome. *JAMA* 289:1130, 2003.

231. Rosenfeld SJ, Kimball J, Vining D, Young NS: Intensive immunosuppression with antithymocyte globulin and cyclosporine as treatment for severe acquired aplastic anemia. *Blood* 85:3058, 1995.

232. Marsh J, Schrezenmeier H, Marin P, et al: Prospective randomized multicenter study comparing cyclosporine alone versus the combination of antithymocyte globulin and cyclosporine for treatment of patients with nonsevere aplastic anemia: A report from the European blood and marrow transplant (EBMT) severe aplastic anemia working party. *Blood* 93:2191, 1999.

233. Marsh JCW, Socie G, Schrezenmeier H, et al: Haemopoietic growth factors in aplastic anaemia: A cautionary note. *Lancet* 344:172, 1994.

234. Bacigalupo A, Bruno B, Saracco P, et al: Antilymphocyte globulin, cyclosporine, prednisolone and granulocyte colony-stimulating factor for severe aplastic anemia: An update of the GITMO/EBMT study on 100 patients. *Blood* 95:1931, 2000.

235. Bacigalupo A, Brand R, Oneto R, et al: Treatment of acquired severe aplastic anemia: Bone marrow transplantation compared with immunosuppressive therapy—The European group for blood and marrow transplantation experience. *Semin Hematol* 37:69, 2000.

236. Gillio AP, Boulad F, Small TN, et al: Comparison of long-term outcome of children with severe aplastic anemia treated with immunosuppression versus bone marrow transplantation. *Biol Blood Marrow Transplant* 3:18, 1997.

237. De Planque MM, Kluin-Nelemans HC, Van Krieken HJM, et al: Evolution of acquired severe aplastic anaemia to myelodysplasia and subsequent leukaemia in adults. *Br J Haematol* 70:55, 1988.

238. Tichelli A, Gratwohl A, Würsch A, et al: Late haematological complications in severe aplastic anaemia. *Br J Haematol* 69:413, 1988.

239. Moore MAS, Castro-Malaspina H: Immunosuppression in aplastic anemia—Postponing the inevitable? *N Engl J Med* 314:1358, 1991.

240. Young NS: Acquired aplastic anemia. *Ann Intern Med* 136:534, 2002.

241. Brodsky RA, Sensenbrenner LL, Jones RJ: Complete remission in severe aplastic anemia after high-dose cyclophosphamide without bone marrow transplantation. *Blood* 87:491, 1996.

242. Jones RJ, Barber JP, Vala MS, et al: Assessment of aldehyde dehydrogenase in viable cells. *Blood* 85:2742, 1995.

243. Kastan MB, Schlaffer I, Russo JE, et al: Direct demonstration of aldehyde dehydrogenase in human hematopoietic progenitor cells. *Blood* 75:1947, 1990.

244. Brodsky RA, Sensenbrenner LL, Smith BD, et al: Durable treatment-free remission following high-dose cyclophosphamide for previously untreated severe aplastic anemia. *Ann Intern Med* 135:477, 2001.

245. Brodsky RA: High-dose cyclophosphamide for aplastic anemia and autoimmunity. *Curr Opin Oncol* 14:143, 2002.

246. Champlin RE, Ho WG, Feig SA, et al: Do androgens enhance the response to antithymocyte globulin in patients with aplastic anemia? A prospective randomized trial. *Blood* 66:184, 1985.

247. Shahidi NT: Androgens and erythropoiesis. *N Engl J Med* 289:72, 1973.

248. French Cooperative Group for the Study of Aplastic and Refractory Anemias: Androgen therapy in aplastic anemia: A comparative study of high and low doses of 4 different androgens. *Scand J Haematol* 36:346, 1986.

249. Antin JH, Smith BR, Holmes W, Rosenthal DS: Phase I/II study of recombinant human granulocyte-macrophage colony-stimulating factor in aplastic anemia and myelodysplastic syndrome. *Blood* 72:705, 1988.

250. Vadhan-Raj S, Buescher S, Broxmeyer HE, et al: Stimulation of myelopoiesis in patients with aplastic anemia by recombinant human granulocyte-macrophage colony-stimulating factor. *N Engl J Med* 319:1628, 1988.

251. Guinan EC, Sieff CA, Oette DH, Nathan DG: A phase I/II trial of recombinant granulocyte-macrophage colony-stimulating factor for children with aplastic anemia. *Blood* 76:1077, 1990.

252. Sonoda Y, Ohno Y, Fujii H, et al: Multilineage response in aplastic anemia patients following long-term administration of filgrastim (recombinant human granulocyte colony stimulating factor). *Stem Cells* 11:543, 1993.

253. Bessho M, Jinnai I, Hirashima K, et al: Trilineage recovery by combination therapy with recombinant human granulocyte colony-stimulating factor and erythropoietin in patients with aplastic anemia and refractory anemia. *Stem Cells* 12:604, 1994.

254. Imamura M, Kobayashi M, Kobayashi S, et al: Combination therapy with recombinant human granulocyte colony stimulating factor and erythropoietin in aplastic anemia. *Am J Hematol* 48:29, 1995.

255. Ganser A, Lindemann A, Siepelt G, et al: Effects of recombinant human interleukin-3 in aplastic anemia. *Blood* 76:1287, 1990.

256. Walsh CE, Liu JM, Anderson SM, et al: A trial of recombinant human interleukin-1 in patients with severe refractory aplastic anaemia. *Br J Haematol* 80:106, 1992.

257. Speck B, Tichelli A, Widmer E, et al: Splenectomy as an adjuvant measure in the treatment of severe aplastic anaemia. *Br J Haematol* 92:818, 1996.

258. Sadowitz PD, Dubowy RL: Intravenous immunoglobulin in the treatment of aplastic anemia. *Am J Pediatr Hematol Oncol* 12:198, 1990.

259. Bodenstein H: Successful treatment of aplastic anemia with high-dose immunoglobulin [letter]. *N Engl J Med* 314:1368, 1991.

260. Ito T, Haraiwa M, Ishikawa Y, et al: Lymphocytapheresis in a patient with severe aplastic anaemia. *Acta Haematol* 80:167, 1988.

261. Morales-Polanco MR, Sanchez-Valle E, Guerrero-Rivera S, et al: Treatment results of 23 cases of severe aplastic anemia with lymphocytapheresis. *Arch Med Res* 28:85, 1997.

262. Bacigalupo A: Aetiology of severe aplastic anaemia and outcome after allogeneic bone marrow transplantation or immunosuppression therapy. *Eur J Haematol* 57(suppl):16, 1996.

263. Kiem HP, McDonald GB, Myerson D, et al: Marrow transplantation for hepatitis-associated aplastic anemia: A follow-up of long-term survivors. *Biol Blood Marrow Transplant* 2:93, 1996.

264. Locasciulli A: Acquired aplastic anemia in children: Incidence, prognosis and treatment options. *Paediatr Drugs* 4:761, 2002.

265. Lewis SM: Course and prognosis in aplastic anemia. *Br Med J* 1:1027, 1965.

266. Lynch RE, Williams DM, Reading JC, Cartwright GE: The prognosis in aplastic anemia. *Blood* 45:517, 1975.

267. Horowitz MM: Current status of allogeneic bone marrow transplantation in acquired aplastic anemia. *Semin Hematol* 37:30, 2000.

268. Bacigalupo A, Frickhofen N, Rosenfeld S: Immunosuppressive treat-

ment of aplastic anemia with antithymocyte globulin and cyclosporine. *Semin Hematol* 37:56, 2000.

269. Doney K, Leisenring W, Storb R, et al: Primary treatment of acquired aplastic anemia: Outcomes with bone marrow transplantation and immunosuppressive therapy. *Ann Intern Med* 126:107, 1997.

270. Tisdale JF, Dunn DE, Maciejewski J: Cyclophosphamide and other new agents for the treatment of severe aplastic anemia. *Semin Hematol* 37: 102, 2000.

271. Michallet M-C, Saltel F, Preville X, et al: Cathepsin-B-dependent apoptosis triggered by antithymocyte globulins: A novel mechanism of T-cell depletion. *Blood* 102:3719, 2003.

272. Kaufman DW, Kelly JP, Levy M, Shapiro S: *The Drug Etiology of Agranulocytosis and Aplastic Anemia.* Oxford University Press, United Kingdom, 1991.

273. Hirano N, Butler MO, Von Bergwelt-Baildon MS, et al: Autoantibodies frequently detected in patients with aplastic anemia. *Blood* 102:4567, 2003.

274. Meetei AR, De Winter JP, Medhurst AL, et al: A novel ubiquitin ligase is deficient in Fanconi anemia. *Nat Genet* 35:165, 2003.

275. Levitus M, Rooimans MA, Steltenpool J, et al: Heterogeneity in Fanconi anemia: Evidence for 2 new genetic subtypes. *Blood* 103:2498, 2004.

276. Dufour C, Corcione A, Svahn J, et al: TNF-α and TNF-γ are overexpressed in the bone marrow of Fanconi anemia patients and TNF-α suppresses erythropoiesis in vitro. *Blood* 102:2053, 2003.

277. Ades L, Mary J-Y, Robin M, et al: Long-term outcome after bone marrow transplantation for severe aplastic anemia. *Blood* 103:2490, 2004.

278. Calado RT, Hinh L, Yamaguchi H, et al: Mutations in *TERT*, the gene encoding telomerase reverse transcriptase, in "acquired" aplastic anemia inhibit enzymatic function by a dominant negative mechanism of action. *Blood* 104:5a, 2004.

279. Calado RT, Savage SA, Lansdorp PM, et al: Genes encoding telomere-binding proteins TERF1, TERF2 and TIN2 are mutated in patients with acquired aplastic anemia. *Blood* 104:53a, 2004.

280. Brodsky RA, Chen AR, Brodsky I, Jones RJ: High-dose cyclophosphamide as salvage therapy for severe aplastic anemia. *Exp Hematol* 32: 435, 2004.

PURE RED CELL APLASIA

NEAL S. YOUNG

Pure red cell aplasia results in an anemia associated with severe reticulocytopenia and absence of marrow erythroid precursor cells. Thus, this aregenerative anemia is caused by the selective failure of erythropoiesis. A correct diagnosis is important because most patients can be treated successfully. Like other marrow failure syndromes, pure red cell aplasia can be inherited or acquired, and its pathophysiology is heterogeneous. Inherited pure red cell aplasia, Diamond-Blackfan anemia, appears in early life and frequently is responsive to glucocorticoids, often at low doses. Mutations in a few genes have been mapped in some families with Diamond-Blackfan anemia, but the mechanism of this form of erythropoietic failure is not understood. Acquired pure red cell aplasia is a disease of older persons. It can be a solitary diagnosis or appear in association with immunologic diseases, especially chronic lymphocytic leukemia (CLL) or thymoma. Occasionally, pure red cell aplasia results from an idiosyncratic drug reaction. Immunosuppressive therapies often are effective in the treatment of acquired pure red cell aplasia. Approximately 15 percent of acquired pure red cell aplasia is caused by persistent parvovirus B19 infection, almost always in a host (1) with an inherited immunodeficiency disorder, (2) undergoing immunosuppressive therapy, or (3) infected with the human immunodeficiency virus. Parvovirus is cytotoxic to human erythroid progenitor cells, and immunoglobulin therapy can neutralize the viral infection and resolve its hematologic manifestation. Acute parvovirus infection suppresses erythropoiesis in all infected individuals but causes transient aplastic crisis (a sudden decline in hemoglobin to dangerously low levels) in individuals with underlying hemolysis, such as sickle cell disease or hereditary spherocytosis. Transient erythroblastopenia of childhood occurs in the setting of a nonspecific viral infection and is a short-lived suppression of erythropoiesis.

Pure red cell aplasia is the term now widely applied to isolated anemia secondary to failure of erythropoiesis. The cardinal findings are a low hemoglobin level, reticulocytopenia, and absent or extremely infrequent erythroid precursor cells in the marrow. Historical names for pure red cell aplasia include *erythroblast hypoplasia, erythroblastopenia, red cell agenesis, hypoplastic anemia,* and *aregenerative anemia*. *Aplastic anemia* confers the same meaning, of course, but is applied to pancytopenia and an empty bone marrow (see Chap. 33). Pure red cell aplasia was first separated from aplastic anemia by Kaznelson in 1922. The association of red cell aplasia and thymoma interested physicians in the 1930s and ultimately led to laboratory studies linking pure red cell aplasia to immune mechanisms, including the early identification of antierythroid precursor cell antibodies by Krantz and later characterization of T cells that

inhibited erythropoiesis. Red cell aplasia as an acute and life-threatening complication of sickle cell disease and other hemolytic anemias was recognized in the 1940s, presaging the role of a specific virus in the etiology of both acute and chronic erythropoietic failure. Despite its infrequency, pure red cell aplasia has been a subject of much laboratory research because of its link to an immune mechanism of erythropoietic failure and as a manifestation of parvovirus B19 infection and destruction of marrow red cell progenitors. However, because of its infrequency, pure red cell aplasia has not been the subject of large or controlled clinical trials; as a result, therapeutic recommendations are based on single cases or small series. Table 34-1 lists a pragmatic classification of pure red cell aplasia.

INHERITED PURE RED CELL APLASIA (DIAMOND-BLACKFAN ANEMIA)

DEFINITION AND HISTORY

Anemia in infancy and early childhood associated with absent reticulocytes in the blood and erythroid precursor cells in the marrow was described by Joseph[1] in 1936 as a "failure of erythropoiesis" and by Diamond and Blackfan[2] in 1938 as "congenital hypoplastic anemia." Gasser[3] first reported a response of a patient to glucocorticoids in 1951, and Diamond and associates[4] presented a series of treated patients. Genetic linkage studies have identified a causative mutated gene in a subset of patients with inherited red cell aplasia.[5] Hundreds of cases have been reported, and many excellent reviews have been published.[6–15] Although Josephs was the first to describe the disorder, the anemia invariably is referred to as either *Blackfan-Diamond* or *Diamond-Blackfan anemia*.

ETIOLOGY AND PATHOGENESIS

An annual incidence of five cases per million live births has been estimated from registry data.[16] Well-characterized pedigrees are consistent with an autosomal dominant or, less often, recessive inheritance pattern. Sporadic cases are seen most frequently. Retrospective studies may reveal subtle hematologic or biochemical lesions, or an abnormal gene, in an affected parent or another relative without clinical ane-

TABLE 34-1   CLASSIFICATION OF PURE RED CELL APLASIA

Fetal red cell aplasia (nonimmune hydrops fetalis)
    Parvovirus B19 *in utero*
Inherited (Diamond-Blackfan anemia)
    RPS19 mutations (~25% cases)
Acquired
    Transient PRCA
        Acute B19 parvovirus infection in hemolytic disease (transient aplastic crisis; ~100%)
        Transient erythroblastopenia of childhood
    Chronic PRCA
        Idiopathic
        Large granular lymphocytic leukemia
        Chronic lymphocytic leukemia
        Clonal myeloid diseases (especially 5q-syndrome)
        Persistent B19 parvovirus infection in immunodeficient host (~15% cases)
        Thymoma
        Collagen vascular diseases
        Post stem cell transplant
            Anti-ABO antibodies
        Drug-induced
        Antierythropoietin antibodies
        Pregnancy

mia.[17] Linkage analyses of several dozen European families mapped to a site on chromosome 19q13[18] and the finding of a translocation in one individual allowed cloning of the *RPS19* gene, which encodes a protein involved in ribosome assembly.[5] *RPS19* behaves as a dominant gene; it requires disruption of both copies of the gene in the mouse to prevent implantation.[19] *RPS19* is expressed ubiquitously. The apparently specific role of *RSP19* in red cell development has not been elucidated.[20] In tissue culture experiments, silencing of *RPS19* profoundly affects erythropoietic differentiation and, to lesser degrees, myelopoiesis.[21,22] Considerable phenotypic heterogeneity must exist, because mutations in this gene were found in only approximately 25 percent of patients with inherited red cell aplasia.[23] Other genes have been implicated in positional cloning studies.[24] Mutated c-kit receptor (cytokine receptor on hematopoietic stem cells) and the gene *SCF* for its ligand (stem cell factor) produce animal models of disordered erythropoiesis, but these genes and the erythropoietin receptor are normal in human patients.[25]

Diminished erythroid progenitor cell numbers (colony forming unit–erythroid [CFU-E] and burst forming unit–erythroid [BFU-E]) are characteristic; decreased sensitivity to erythropoietin and interleukin 3 (IL-3)[26,27] have been improved by stem cell factor[28] or the addition of a glucocorticoid *in vitro*.[29] In cell culture systems, early, erythropoietin-independent erythropoiesis is relatively normal; consistent defect in the late stage of erythropoietin-dependent erythroid cell expansion and maturation is present; and late-stage erythroid colonies are small.[30] A defect in late erythroid differentiation is compatible with the classic findings of macrocytosis and increased hemoglobin F expression in inherited red cell aplasia. Granulopoiesis in the colony forming unit–granulocyte-macrophage assay and the earlier hematopoietic progenitors as measured *in vitro* by long-term culture-initiating cell assay (an assay for an early multipotential hematopoietic progenitor) frequently are abnormal but to a lesser degree than CFU-E and BFU-E.[31]

Despite responsiveness of patients to glucocorticoids, there is little evidence of an immune mechanism, cellular or humoral, underlying inherited red cell aplasia.

CLINICAL FEATURES

About one third of patients are diagnosed at birth or within a few weeks of delivery, and almost all are identified within the first year of life.[7] Considerable variations are noted with regard to severity of phenotype, ranging from hydrops fetalis[32,33] to presentation in adulthood, when diagnosis is inferred from associated physical anomalies.[34] No sex predominance exists. Increased rates of prematurity in patients and of miscarriages in families have been inferred from collected cases.[9] Symptoms of anemia in early childhood include pallor, apathy, poor appetite, and "failure to thrive." Physical anomalies include craniofacial dysmorphism, which occurs in approximately 20 percent of cases. The classic appearance described by Cathie[35] is "tow-colored hair, snub nose, wide set eyes, thick upper lips, and an intelligent expression." Malformations of the thumbs and short stature are frequent, followed by abnormalities of the urogenital system, web neck, and skeletal and cardiac defects.[7,12,16] These physical anomalies are less prevalent than the abnormalities seen in Fanconi anemia.

LABORATORY FEATURES

The degree of anemia is highly variable at diagnosis. Erythrocytes may be macrocytic or normocytic. Reticulocytopenia is profound. The marrow, which usually is devoid of erythroid precursors, may show small numbers of megaloblastoid early erythroid cells with apparent "mat-

uration arrest." Platelets are normal or elevated. Leukocytes may be normal or slightly decreased at presentation. Neutrophils often decline with age, and in adult survivors neutropenia occasionally is severe enough to predispose to fatal infection.[36]

Erythrocyte adenosine deaminase level is elevated high in approximately 75 percent of patients but also may be increased in other aregenerative anemias of childhood.[37] Serum erythropoietin level, serum iron level, and total iron-binding capacity are high. Ferritin level increases as patients receive multiple transfusions and develop iron overload if they are not treated with chelation therapy.

DIFFERENTIAL DIAGNOSIS

The characteristic triad consists of the clinical diagnostic features of anemia, reticulocytopenia, and a paucity or absence of erythroid precursors in the marrow. These findings may by supplemented by increased activity of red cell adenosine deaminase and mutation in the *RPS19* gene sequence. Fanconi anemia can be excluded by cytogenetic analyses under clastogenic stress and determination of FA gene mutations (see Chap. 33). Transient erythroblastopenia of childhood, which unusually occurs in the first year of life, is established by spontaneous recovery. When presentation occurs at older ages, the distinction between inherited and acquired aplastic anemia is somewhat arbitrary[11] because the hematologic features are similar. A positive family history, physical anomalies, and characteristic cytogenetic enzymatic, or genetic findings strongly indicate an inherited disorder.

THERAPY, COURSE, AND PROGNOSIS

Untreated inherited pure red cell aplasia is fatal; death results from severe anemia and congestive heart failure. Transfusions, glucocorticoids, and allogeneic stem cell transplantation are of proven efficacy. With better survival, the risk of late development of leukemia has become apparent. Four of 76 patients followed at Children's Hospital in Boston died of acute myelogenous leukemia, with a calculated relative risk of greater than 200 times expected.[8] Predictors of a response to glucocorticoids include older age at presentation, a family history, and a normal platelet count. Younger age at presentation and premature birth correlate with continued red cell transfusion dependence.[38] Supportive care consists of red cell transfusions. To avoid transfusional hemosiderosis, chelation with desferrioxamine should be initiated early. Injury to visceral organs from iron overload has been a major cause of death in the past and can be prevented by an adequate iron chelation program (see Chap. 40). The inconvenience and discomfort of desferrioxamine administration are impediments to patient compliance, especially when children enter adolescence. The anticipated approval of effective oral iron chelators[39] should improve an often frustrating feature of medical management of this disease.

Red cell transfusions should be leukocyte depleted to avoid alloimmunization (see Chap. 131). Erythrocytes are administered with the goal of eliminating symptoms and permitting normal growth and sexual development, usually achieved by maintaining hemoglobin levels between 7 and 9 g/dl (70–90 g/liter). Glucocorticoids are effective in many patients. Although the mechanism of action of glucocorticoids in this disease is not understood, their toxicities are substantial, and a response is not predictable. Once the diagnosis is established, prednisone is administered at 2 mg/kg daily in three or four divided doses.[8–10] A reticulocyte response is seen in the majority of patients 1 to 4 weeks later, followed by a rise in hemoglobin level. Once the hemoglobin level reaches 9 to 10 g/dl (90–100 g/liter), very slow reduction of the glucocorticoid dose is undertaken by decreasing the number of daily doses. When a single daily dose is achieved, an alternate-day schedule is adopted. In general, severe anemia can be avoided with continued glucocorticoid administration. The maintenance dose may be low (1–2 mg/day). Some patients may tolerate complete withdrawal of prednisone, but relapse is frequent and most responders become glucocorticoid dependent. A variety of patterns of response have been described, ranging from prompt recovery and apparent cure to refractoriness after years of responsiveness.[9] Conversely, a second trial of glucocorticoids years after an apparent therapeutic failure may be successful. In a series of 76 patients followed for the long term, 59 were treated with prednisone; 31 initially responded, and 2 of the 25 who initially failed later responded.[8] Glucocorticoid responsiveness is strongly associated with better survival, and patients who require low doses of prednisone, or those few who spontaneously remit, may have normal life expectancies. Long-term use of high-dose prednisone results in significant toxicity, including some combination of growth retardation, cushingoid facies, buffalo hump, osteoporosis, aseptic necrosis of the hip and fractures, diabetes, hypertension, and cataracts. Red cell transfusions with iron chelation may be preferable to such an outcome.

Allogeneic stem cell marrow transplantation, when successful, is curative (see Chap. 22), but the procedure has not been widely applied to children responding to medical measures. The median life expectancy of patients requiring transfusions and iron chelation is 30 to 40 years. A less favorable outcome is related to poor compliance and cardiac and hepatic disease from iron overload.[8] Because of the morbidity and mortality associated with allogeneic stem cell transplant, most patients have been transplanted late in their disease course, after large numbers of transfusions, accumulation of heavy iron loads, and alloimmunization. Despite the poor predictive factors, 15 of 19 patients of the first published series of cases survived 5 months to many years posttransplant.[12] Comparable survival rates have been reported from European[40] and Japanese registries.[41] Stem cell transplantation from unrelated stem cell donors or use of cord blood stem cells[40,41] has been less successful; most patients die of treatment-related complications. Recurrent red cell aplasia despite full engraftment was reported in one child after allogeneic stem cell transplant.[42]

Other therapies have not gained wide acceptance despite promising pilot studies, including IL-3,[43] high-dose methylprednisolone,[44] cyclosporine and other immunosuppressive agents,[45,46] and prolactin induction by metoclopropamide.[47]

Gene transfer *in vitro* has functionally corrected cells defective in *RSP19* (gene encoding ribosomal protein),[48] offering the possibility of gene therapy for *RSP19* mutant patients.

TRANSIENT APLASTIC CRISIS AND TRANSIENT ERYTHROBLASTOPENIA OF CHILDHOOD

DEFINITION AND HISTORY

Temporary failure of erythropoiesis is clinically identical to pure red cell aplasia except for spontaneous resolution of symptoms and of the laboratory findings of normocytic and normochromic anemia and marrow erythroid hypoplasia, usually over the course of a few weeks. Erythrocyte production is halted (1) by acute B19 parvovirus infection, typically in the context of underlying hemolytic disease (called transient aplastic crisis); (2) in normal children, usually after an infection by another [unknown] childhood virus (transient erythroblastopenia of childhood); or (3) as a transient reaction to a drug.

An anemic crisis was described in the 1940s first by Lyngar[49] and then by Owren,[50] Gasser,[3] and Dameshek and Bloom[51] in kindreds with hereditary spherocytosis. Several children within a family suffered anemic crises and exhibited low, rather than the usually high, reticulocyte numbers. Transient aplastic crisis also was noted as a complication of sickle cell disease.[52,53] Marrow examination showed decrease or absence of erythroid precursor cells, and often giant erythroblasts.[50,51] An infectious etiology was suspected from the history of a preceding febrile illness in families and its simultaneous occurrence in siblings. After the serendipitous discovery of B19 parvovirus in a normal blood donor, Pattison and colleagues screened large numbers of stored sera for evidence of recent infection. Immunoglobulin (Ig) M antibody or viral antigen was found in the blood of Jamaican children in London, all of whom had transient aplastic crisis of sickle cell disease.[54] B19 parvovirus later was established as the agent also responsible for fifth disease.[55] In the large cohort of sickle cell patients in Jamaica reported by Serjeant and colleagues,[56,57] virtually all episodes of transient aplastic crisis could be linked to B19 parvovirus. In retrospect, red cell aplasias blamed on kwashiorkor, vitamin deficiency, bacterial infections, and chemical exposures represented parvovirus infection.

Gasser (cited in reference 50) described erythroblastopenia in normal children who ultimately recovered[50]; the disease was recognized as an entity by Wranne[58] in the 1970s. Transient erythroblastopenia of childhood has an unclear etiology but may represent a postviral immune-mediated syndrome.

ETIOLOGY AND PATHOGENESIS

B19 parvovirus, a small DNA virus, commonly infects humans. Most of the adult population has IgG antibodies specific to B19.[55] The virus is tropic for erythroid progenitor cells,[59] mainly due to their P antigen or globoside, the receptor for entry of B19 into the cell.[60,61] Infection lyses the target cell and abrogates erythropoiesis *in vitro* and *in vivo*. Reticulocytopenia probably accompanies B19 parvovirus infection in all infected persons.[62] Anemia only manifests if red cell survival is decreased. Infection ordinarily is terminated by production of neutralizing antibodies to the virus (when such antibodies are absent, persistence of the virus produces chronic pure red cell aplasia). B19 parvovirus may appear in epidemics of fifth disease in the normal population and of transient aplastic crisis, for example, in hematology clinics specializing in sickle cell disease.[63,64] In fifth disease, IgM antibody is present in the blood, and virus levels are low or not detectable. Symptoms and signs of a typical "slapped cheek" cutaneous eruption and arthralgia or arthritis are secondary to antibody–virus immune complex deposition.

In contrast, in transient aplastic crisis, high concentrations of virus are present in the circulation, and patients do not develop fifth disease. In children with sickle cell disease, the incidence of B19 parvovirus infection was estimated at approximately 11 percent, and 75 percent of patients were infected by age 20 years.[65] In this setting, parvovirus infection was associated with transient aplastic crisis, a higher frequency of fever, pain, acute chest syndrome, and acute splenic sequestration syndrome.[65] As in normal individuals, parvovirus infection can be asymptomatic in sickle cell disease.[66]

The origins of transient erythroblastopenia of childhood are poorly understood. An apparent viral prodrome is typical,[67] and temporal and seasonal clustering of cases may occur.[68–70] B19 parvovirus is not the etiology,[71,72] and no other virus has been consistently implicated.[67] Erythroid colony numbers (see Chap. 28) usually are low.[73] An immune pathophysiology has been inferred from *in vitro* experiments in which IgG from sera of patients inhibited erythropoiesis[74] in the majority of cases.[75] Cell-mediated mechanisms also may play a causal role. In one report, T cell depletion led to a dramatic increase in CFU-

E formation.[76] A possible relationship between transient erythroblastopenia of childhood and inherited red cell aplasia has been suggested by the clustering of polymorphic alleles in familial transient erythroblastopenia.[77]

The same drugs implicated in chronic pure red cell aplasia apply to transient erythropoietic failure.[78] Laboratory investigations of red cell aplasia secondary to diphenylhydantoin[79] and rifampicin[80] are consistent with a hapten mechanism, in which serum antibody affects erythroid progenitor cells only in the presence of drug.

CLINICAL FEATURES

Transient aplastic crisis typically occurs in younger patients who are chronically anemic as a result of hereditary spherocytosis, sickle cell disease, or another hemolytic anemia. The decrease in erythropoiesis results in more evident pallor, fatigue on exertion or at rest, lassitude, and dyspnea on exertion. Gastrointestinal complaints or headache may be associated.[81] Parvovirus infection can unmask previously undiagnosed underlying hemolytic anemia. Physical examination may reveal signs of anemia, such as pallor, tachycardia, and a flow murmur. No rash or joint swelling is seen. Elevated serum bilirubin or overt icterus may be a clue to underlying hemolysis. In contrast, transient erythroblastopenia of childhood presents as an acute anemia in a previously well child. The syndrome has an estimated incidence rate of four to five cases per million children.[82–84] Transient erythroblastopenia is a frequent diagnosis in children with severe anemia,[83,85] and is the most common cause of acquired red cell aplasia in pediatric patients.[6,82] Most patients are 1 to 3 years old,[6,85] but transient erythroblastopenia of childhood can occur in the first year of life and through adolescence. Rare complications include seizures and transient neurologic abnormalities.[86–88]

LABORATORY EVALUATION

In both syndromes, anemia is the hallmark, and hemoglobin levels may be markedly depressed. Reticulocytes usually are absent from the blood, and erythroid precursor cells are not present or markedly decreased in the marrow. Red cell indices are normal. White blood cell and platelet counts are normal or elevated. Occasionally, neutropenia and thrombocytopenia of mild or moderate degree are present (especially if splenic function is intact, as in hereditary spherocytosis and in transient erythroblastopenia of childhood).[85] If the episode is brief and diagnosed during marrow recovery, patients may present with reticulocytosis, and nucleated red blood cells may be seen on the blood film.

DIFFERENTIAL DIAGNOSIS

The reticulocyte count readily distinguishes the cause of increasing anemia in a patient with hemolytic disease as transient aplastic crisis. The most important differential diagnosis for transient erythroblastopenia of childhood is inherited pure red cell aplasia. For the former, the age at presentation is older, the patient usually has no family history (but transient erythroblastopenia of childhood may be familial and can occur simultaneously in siblings[89]), physical anomalies are absent, and the syndrome resolves spontaneously. In transient erythroblastopenia of childhood (in contrast to inherited red cell aplasia), erythrocyte adenosine deaminase levels are normal, and red cells do not show "stress" patterns of fetal hemoglobin and i antigen (red cell antigen expressed primarily on feral erythrocytes) expression. The patient's medical history, the red cell indices, and appropriate serum assays should allow prompt exclusion of more common causes of anemia in children, such as iron deficiency or other nutritional deficiencies. When transient erythroblastopenia is associated with neutropenia, acute lymphoblastic leukemia and aplastic anemia may be suspected: marrow examination clarifies the diagnosis.[90] A record of current medications, more important in adults, may provide the basis for a tentative diagnosis of drug-induced rather than idiopathic disease.

THERAPY, COURSE, AND PROGNOSIS

Transient aplastic crisis resolves as neutralizing antibodies to B19 parvovirus are made, usually within 1 to 2 weeks of infection. Ensuing reticulocytosis may be brisk, and the hemoglobin may transiently rise to higher than normal values. White cell and platelet numbers may "rebound," and some bone pain from marrow expansion may be present. Severe anemia may require transfusion of red blood cells (see Chap. 131). No established role for administration of immunoglobulins exists.

Transient erythroblastopenia of childhood typically terminates after a few weeks, but anemia may persist occasionally for months.[6] Transfusions may be required during that interval.

For drug-associated transient failure of erythropoiesis, the suspected offending drug is discontinued and the diagnosis established from subsequent clinical improvement.

ACQUIRED PURE RED CELL APLASIA

DEFINITION AND HISTORY

Acquired pure red cell aplasia is an uncommon cause of anemia that occurs principally in older adults. The blood counts and marrow appearance are indistinguishable from the picture of Diamond-Blackfan anemia, that is, anemia, severe reticulocytopenia, and absent marrow erythroid precursor cells. The nosologic origins of acquired pure red cell aplasia are obscure. Early descriptions are intermixed with those of aplastic anemia (in retrospect, a poor term for generalized marrow failure). Kaznelson[91] is credited with the first case report in 1922. Early distinction of the two syndromes was stimulated by the relationship of red cell aplasia to thymoma. Although red cell aplasia shares with aplastic anemia an immune pathophysiology and responsiveness to immunosuppressive therapies, the absence of involvement of neutrophils, monocytes, and platelets makes the diagnostic distinction evident. Many of the diverse clinical associations (Table 34-1) are consistent with an immune-mediated pathophysiology. The mechanism of red cell failure is best understood for T cell–mediated autoimmune destruction and persistent B19 parvovirus infection.

ETIOLOGY AND PATHOGENESIS

IMMUNE-MEDIATED ERYTHROPOIETIC FAILURE
Clinical and laboratory evidence supports both antibody and cellular mechanisms of inhibition of erythropoiesis. Red cell aplasia is associated with autoimmune diseases, such as rheumatoid arthritis, systemic lupus erythematosus, myasthenia gravis, autoimmune hemolytic anemia, acquired hypoimmunoglobulinemia, and thymoma, and with lymphoproliferative processes, such as CLL and Hodgkin disease, in which immune dysregulation is common. Serum inhibitors can be detected in the laboratory. Krantz and colleagues showed that immunoglobulin fractions from the patient's blood inhibited heme synthesis and red cell progenitor assays *in vitro*.[75] Antibodies that inhibit BFU-E and CFU-E colony formation are present frequently in patients with red cell aplasia. A pathophysiologic role can be inferred, first from the response of patients to specific treatments directed at antibodies, such as plasmapheresis and monoclonal antibody to CD20 (an antigen

present on B cells), and second from decreased or absent plasma antibody in recovered patients. Antibodies may be involved in the red cell aplasia of pregnancy.[92]

Autoantibodies to erythropoietin rarely have caused this disease.[93,94] More frequently, red cell aplasia secondary to antibodies is elicited by administration of recombinant erythropoietin to patients undergoing renal dialysis (see Chap. 35).[95–97] Anemia can be profound, and some patients remain transfusion dependent despite discontinuation of hormone therapy. Glycosylation of recombinant erythropoietin is different from the native molecule, but antibodies are directed against conformational epitopes of the protein and not to the sugar moieties. The second example of antibodies of known specificity causing red cell aplasia occurs after hematopoietic stem cell transplantation using donors mismatched at a major ABO locus, which can lead to delayed donor erythroid engraftment or late erythropoietic failure.[98–100] In most instances, however, the target antigen(s) responsible for this outcome is(are) not known.

Suppression of erythropoiesis by T cells may be more common than antibody inhibition as a mechanism of erythropoietic failure.[101] Suggestive clinical observations include the frequent association of red cell aplasia with CLL (approximately 6 percent of cases)[102] and with large granular lymphocytic leukemia (approximately 7 percent of cases).[103] In a series of 47 red cell aplasia patients, four had CLL and nine had large granular lymphocytic leukemia (LGL).[104] More sensitive flow cytometric and molecular methods may detect clonal T cell expansion in patients with normal numbers of circulating lymphocytes.[105] Lymphocytes from patients with idiopathic pure red cell aplasia[106–109] or red cell aplasia associated with CLL,[110,111] LGL,[112–114] thymoma,[115] other lymphoid malignancies,[116,117] Epstein-Barr virus infection,[118] and human T cell leukemia virus 1 infection[119] suppressed erythropoiesis in colony assays. Several mechanisms of cell killing have been suggested.[14,103] When effector cells show histocompatibility locus A class I–restricted killing, recognition of a specific antigen peptide is implied by a T cell with an $\alpha\beta$-T cell receptor.[120] In one man with red cell aplasia and LGL, erythropoiesis was inhibited by non–MHC (major histocompatibility antigen) restricted $\gamma\delta$–T cells that lysed CFU-E. T cells downregulated class I histocompatibility antigens and thus were unable to engage the natural killer cell's inhibitory receptors.[114]

PERSISTENT B19 PARVOVIRUS INFECTION

B19 parvovirus specifically infects and is toxic to erythroid progenitor cells. Parvovirus infection normally is terminated by the humoral immune response within 1 to 2 weeks of infection. Linear neutralizing epitopes are localized to a relatively small region of the capsid protein.[121] In the absence of an effective antibody response, infection persists and causes pure red cell aplasia.[55,121] Erythropoietic failure may be the only evidence of parvoviral infection. Persistence of B19 parvovirus infection may occur in the setting of immunodeficiency, most commonly caused by chemotherapeutic and immunosuppressive drugs,[122] human immunodeficiency virus 1 infection,[123] and occasionally with Nezelof syndrome's subtle immunologic abnormalities.[124] Parvovirus at one time may have accounted for approximately 15 percent of severe anemia in patients with acquired immunodeficiency syndrome,[125] but highly effective antiretroviral drug regimens have reduced its role.[126] Persistent B19 parvovirus infection can occur in the fetus exposed during the midtrimester of pregnancy. The infection can cause hydrops fetalis as a result of viral cytotoxicity for erythroid progenitors in the fetal liver and death of the newborn as a result of severe anemia and congestive heart failure.[55] In rare instances, parvovirus-infected or hydropic infants res-

cued by red cell transfusion show congenital red cell aplasia or dyserythropoietic anemia.[33]

INTRINSIC CELLULAR DEFECTS LEADING TO FAILED RED BLOOD CELL PRODUCTION

Red cell aplasia can be the first or the major manifestation of myelodysplasia.[127] Discrete genetic defects can lead to failure of erythropoiesis. Acquired somatic mutations similar to those in some patients with Diamond-Blackfan anemia have not been described in acquired red cell aplasia. Activating point mutations in *N-RAS* (oncogene in RAS group) occur in some cases of myelodysplastic syndrome.[128,129] Mutant *N-RAS in vitro* can induce a proliferative defect in erythroid progenitor cells.[130]

MEDICATIONS

Idiosyncratic drug reactions account for a far smaller proportion of red cell aplasia than of agranulocytosis (see Chap. 65). Case reports have implicated various agents, such as diphenylhydantoin,[79,131,132] sulfa and sulfonamide drugs,[133–136] azathioprine,[137] allopurinol,[138] isoniazid,[139,140] procainamide,[141] ticlopidine,[142] ribavirin,[143] and penicillamine. Causality is impossible to assign from case reports. As with nonsteroidal antiinflammatory drugs, gold, and colchicine, the underlying rheumatic syndrome may be the etiologic link.

CLINICAL FEATURES

Symptomatic anemia in the older patient may manifest as pallor, fatigue, lassitude, pulsatile tinnitus, and anginal chest pain. Iatrogenic Cushing syndrome and the physical stigmata of secondary hemochromatosis are seen in patients after prolonged glucocorticoid administration and long-term red cell transfusion therapy. Concomitant diseases include CLL and lymphomas, collagen vascular disorders, myasthenia gravis, especially in the setting of thymoma, and some cancers. Red cell aplasia also occurs with pregnancy. Persistent B19 parvovirus infection should be suspected in the anemic cancer patient after stem cell transplantation, in patients treated with immunosuppressive drugs, in patients with AIDS, and in patients with a family or personal history suggestive of inherited immune disorder. Other viral infections have been implicated in pure red cell aplasia, including infectious mononucleosis and, in some patients, hepatitis (an unknown agent in seronegative hepatitis).

LABORATORY FEATURES

Anemia is either normocytic or macrocytic, reticulocytopenia is profound, and white cell and platelet counts are generally normal. The marrow shows absent or very few erythroid precursor cells but normal granulopoiesis and megakaryocytopoiesis. Iron saturation and ferritin level frequently are elevated and rise further after repeated red cell transfusions. Erythroid colony assays may predict responsiveness to immunosuppressive treatment. The presence of marrow or blood BFU-E and CFU-E correlates with hematologic improvement,[106,144,145] but these tests may not be generally available.

A thymoma should be sought by chest imaging, including computed tomographic scan. The association of thymoma and pure red cell aplasia has been emphasized but is uncommon. One experienced investigator found thymoma in only two of 37 patients,[146] and other series reported a low incidence.[101,104] The thymomas usually are encapsulated and have a spindle cell histology. In one series, 10 of 56 cases were considered malignant because of their locally infiltrating character[147]; therefore, the tumors should be surgically excised, if feasible.

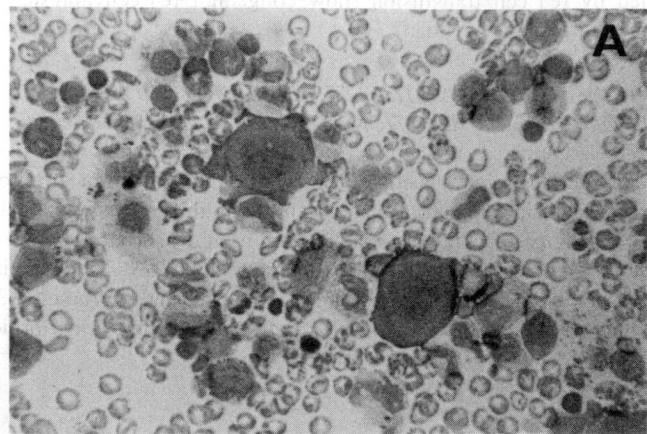

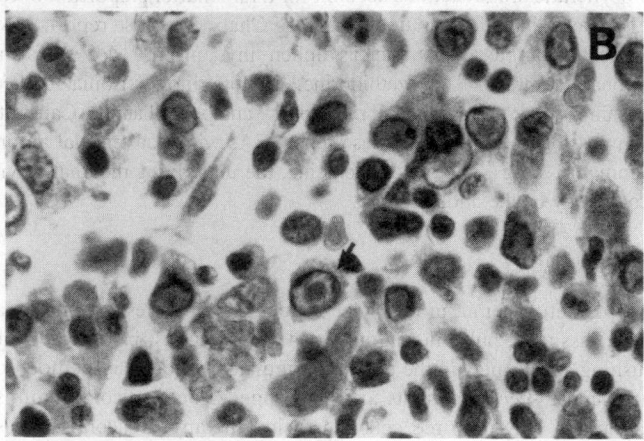

FIGURE 34-1   (A and B) Giant pronormoblasts in the marrow aspirate of a patient with chronic pure red cell aplasia secondary to persistent B19 parvovirus infection.

Chronic lymphocyte leukemia should be evident based on elevated lymphocyte count and immunophenotyping for monoclonality. Large granular lymphocytosis (see Chap. 94), which frequently underlies red cell aplasia, may be more subtle. Diagnosis requires careful examination of the blood film for typical lymphocytic forms, flow cytometry for cell surface markers characteristic of natural killer and cytotoxic lymphocytes, and demonstration of monoclonal T cell proliferation by molecular studies.

Persistent parvovirus infection can be difficult to diagnose. Giant pronormoblasts scattered on the marrow film are the most characteristic of the condition (Fig. 34-1), but such typical cells may not be observed. Marrow morphologies that are dysplastic or suggestive of leukemia also have been described. Serum antibodies specific to the virus are absent or only IgM is positive. Parvovirus DNA should be present in high concentrations in the blood and readily measured by molecular techniques.

DIFFERENTIAL DIAGNOSIS

The distinction between inherited and acquired red cell aplasia may be impossible to make in the younger patient. Rarely, pure red cell aplasia is difficult to distinguish from more generalized marrow failure if other blood counts are borderline. A dysmorphic marrow smear and abnormal chromosomes point to myelodysplasia as responsible for isolated anemia and reticulocytopenia. B19 parvovirus infection should always be suspected and searched for in any immunosup-

pressed individual who is anemic because the infection can be treated.

THERAPY, COURSE, AND PROGNOSIS

TREATMENT

Transfusion Therapy   As with inherited red cell aplasia, transfusions and iron chelation are basic to management. In an adult, one unit of packed erythrocytes per week can replace marrow erythropoiesis, which for convenience usually is transfused as two units every 2 weeks. The goal of preventing symptoms of anemia is achievable in most patients if the nadir hemoglobin is greater than 7 g/dl (70 g/liter). A goal greater than 9 g/dl (90 g/liter) may be preferable in patients with cardiac or pulmonary disease and in older patients. Even refractory pure red cell aplasia is consistent with a prolonged and perhaps even normal life expectancy, and desferrioxamine therapy can be initiated based on the ferritin level (see Chap. 40).

Immunosuppression   Immunosuppressive agents are used to treat disease with suspected immune origin. Response is likely in the majority of patients, but sequential treatment with a variety of agents often is required. Some patients, however, remain refractory to treatment.[101,148,149] Typically, prednisone 1 to 2 mg/kg/day is given first, and about half of patients improve. A 1- to 2-month trial can be associated with significant toxicity and evidence of Cushing syndrome. Higher response rates have been cited for cyclosporine, and some investigators advocate using this drug first.[45,150–153] Cytotoxic agents, especially azathioprine and cyclophosphamide,[154] can be beneficial but are not first-choice because of their mutagenic and leukemogenic properties. These drugs may be preferred for red cell aplasia associated with large granular lymphocytic leukemia, in which cytoreduction is required.[105,155] Acquired pure red cell aplasia often responds to antithymocyte globulin.[106,156,157] More specific monoclonal antibodies have less toxicity than does antilymphocyte globulin and can be administered without hospitalization.[158] Success has been reported in a few otherwise refractory cases using rituximab (anti-CD20 monoclonal antibody)[159,160] and alemtuzumab (anti-CD52 [antigen on B lymphocytes]).[161,162] Some patients with resistant disease also respond to fludarabine and cladribine.[163,164] Plasmapheresis[165,166] has produced long-lasting improvement in a few patients, presumably by removing pathogenic antibodies.[165]

A thymoma should be excised to prevent local spread of a malignant tumor, but thymectomy does not necessarily improve marrow function.[147] Red cell aplasia is rarely an indication for stem cell transplantation because the aplasia usually can be managed with other approaches. Unresponsive patients have been cured by infusion of allogeneic stem cells after cyclophosphamide conditioning.[167,168]

Other Therapies   Despite early favorable case reports, androgens, erythropoietin, and splenectomy are not routinely used to treat pure red cell aplasia.

Immunoglobulins for Persistent B19 Parvovirus Infection   Persistent parvovirus infection results from the inability of the host to mount an effective humoral immune response. It can be effectively treated in almost all cases by administration of commercial immunoglobulins, an excellent source of neutralizing antibodies present in a large proportion of the normal population. Infusion of immunoglobulins at 0.4 g/kg/day for 5 to 10 days should produce brisk reticulocytosis and restore a hemoglobin level appropriate for the patient. A single course may be adequate to cure long-standing red cell aplasia resulting from an underlying inherited immunodeficiency syndrome,[169] but patients with acquired immunodeficiency syndrome may not show complete clearance of parvovirus from the circulation and may relapse, requiring retreatment[123] or maintenance immunoglobulin injections (Figure 34-2).[123,170] Patients suffering from per-

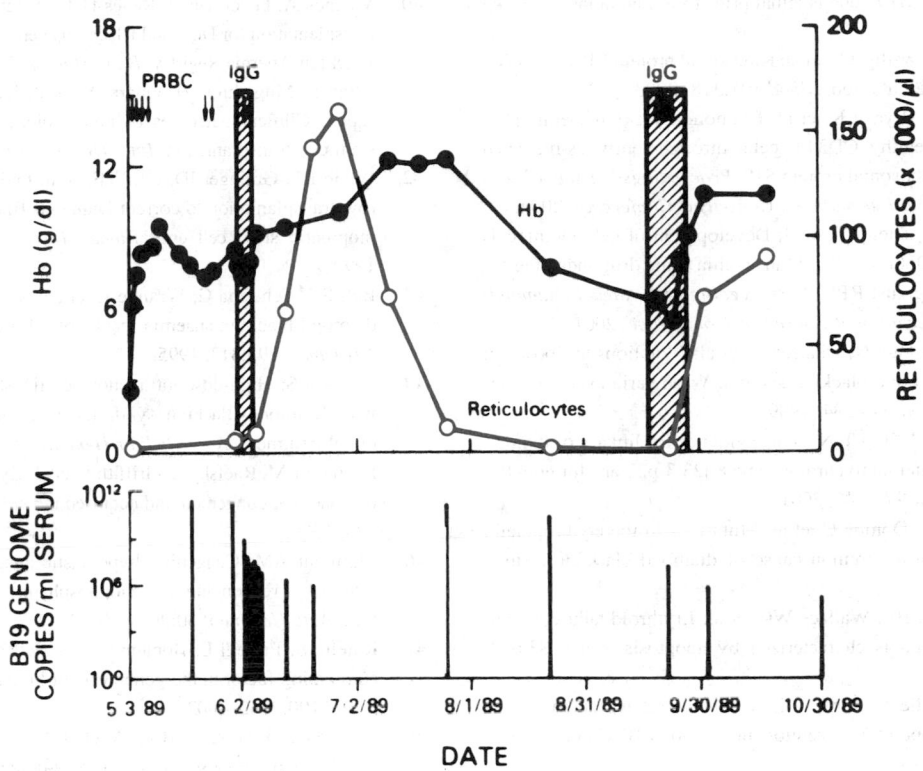

FIGURE 34-2   Diagram of the clinical course of a human immunodeficiency virus 1–infected patient with red cell aplasia due to B19 persistent parvovirus.[123] Note the increase of the reticulocyte count (*open circles*) to the first infusion of immunoglobulin (*hatched bar*) and the subsequent decline in parvovirus titers. Thereafter, the reticulocyte count and the hemoglobin concentration (*closed circles*) decrease, reflecting the return of the anemia. A second immunoglobulin treatment increases the reticulocyte count and hemoglobin concentration and decreases the parvovirus titers.

sistent B19 parvovirus infection do not have typical manifestations of a viral infection, such as fever. In these patients, immunoglobulin infusions can induce fifth disease symptoms of variable severity, including cutaneous eruptions and arthritis. Older case reports of red cell aplasia responsive to immunoglobulin infusions likely represent treatment of patients with previously unrecognized parvovirus infection.

REFERENCES

1. Joseph WH: Anemia of infancy and early childhood. *Medicine* 15:307, 1936.
2. Diamond LK, Blackfan KD: Hypoplastic anemia. *Am J Dis Child* 56:464, 1938.
3. Gasser C: Aplasia of erythropoiesis. *Pediatr Clin North Am* 4:445, 1957.
4. Diamond LK, Wang WC, Alter BP: Congenital hypoplastic anemia. *Adv Pediatr* 22:349, 1976.
5. Draptchinskaia N, Gustavsson P, Anderson B, et al: The gene encoding ribosomal protein S19 is mutated in Diamond-Blackfan anaemia. *Nat Genet* 21:169, 1999.
6. Glader BE: Diagnosis and management of red cell aplasia in children. *Hematol Oncol Clin North Am* 1:431, 1987.
7. Halperin SD, Freedman HM: Diamond-Blackfan anemia: Etiology, pathophysiology, and treatment. *Am J Pediatr Hematol Oncol* 11:380, 1989.
8. Janov A, Leong T, Nathan D, et al: Diamond-Blackfan anemia, natural history and sequelae of treatment. *Medicine* 75:77, 1996.
9. Alter BP. Diamond-Blackfan anemia, in *Aplastic Anemia, Acquired and Inherited*, edited by NS Young, BP Alter, p 361. WB Saunders, Philadelphia, 1994.
10. Willig TN, Gazda H, Sieff CA: Diamond-Blackfan anemia. *Curr Opin Hematol* 7:85, 2000.
11. Freedman MH: Pure red cell aplasia in childhood and adolescence: Pathogenesis and approaches to diagnosis (clinical annotations). *Br J Haematol* 85:246, 1993.
12. Tisdale J, Dunbar CE: Pure red cell aplasia, in *The Bone Marrow Failure Syndromes* edited by NS Young. WB Saunders, Philadelphia, pp 135–155, 2000.
13. Dessypris EN: Aplastic anemia and pure red cell aplasia. *Curr Opin Hematol* 1:157, 1994.
14. Fisch P: Pure red cell aplasia. *Br J Haematol* 111:1010, 2000.
15. Croisille L, Tchernia G, Casadevall N: Autoimmune disorders of erythropoiesis. *Curr Opin Hematol* 8:68, 2001.
16. Ball SE, McGuckin CP, Jenkins G, et al: Diamond-Blackfan anaemia in the U.K.: Analysis of 80 cases from a 20-year birth cohort. *Br J Haematol* 94:645, 1996.
17. Ball S, DBA Study Group: Normal parental results should not be taken as evidence of sporadic de novo DBA: Results of family studies from the U.K. DBA Registry. *Proceedings 5th Annual Diamond-Blackfan Anemia International Consensus Conference*, 2004.
18. Gustavsson P, Willig TN, Van Haederingen A: Diamond-Blackfan anaemia: Genetic homogeneity for a gene on chromosome 19q13 restricted to 1.8 Mb. *Nat Genet* 16:368, 1997.
19. Matsson H, Davey EJ, Draptchinskaia N, et al: Targeted disruption of

the ribosomal protein S19 gene is lethal prior to implantation. *Mol Cell Biol* 24:4032, 2004.

20. Da Costa L, Narla G, Willig TN, et al: Ribosomal protein S19 expression during erythroid differentiation. *Blood* 101:318, 2003.

21. Flygare J, Kiefer T, Miyake K, et al: Diamond-Blackfan anemia phenotype created in healthy CD34+ cells through lentivirus-mediated siRNA silencing of ribosomal protein S19. *Proceedings 5th Annual Diamond-Blackfan Anemia International Consensus Conference*, 2004.

22. Miyake K, Flygare J, Kiefer T, et al: Development of cell line models for RPS19 deficient Diamond-Blackfan anemia using drug-inducible expression of siRNA against RPS19. *Proceedings 5th Annual Diamond-Blackfan Anemia International Consensus Conference*, 2004

23. Wilig TN, Draptchinskaia N, Dianzani I, et al: Mutations in ribosomal protein S19 gene diamond blackfan anemia: Wide variations in phenotypic expression. *Blood* 94:4294, 1999.

24. Gazda H, Lipton JM, Willig T-N, et al: Evidence for linkage of familial Diamond-Blackfan anemia to chromosome 8p23.3-p22 and for non-19q non-8p disease. *Blood* 97:2145, 2001.

25. Dianzani I, Garelli E, Dompè C, et al: Mutations in the erythropoietin receptor gene are not a common cause of diamond-blackfan anemia. *Blood* 87:2568, 1996.

26. Perdahl EB, Naprstek BL, Wallace WC, et al: Erythroid failure in Diamond-Blackfan anemia is characterized by apoptosis. *Blood* 83:645, 1994.

27. Casadevall N, Croisille L, Auffray I, et al: Age-related alterations in erythroid and granulopoietic progenitors in Diamond-Blackfan anaemia. *Brit J Haem* 87:369, 1994.

28. Alter BP, Knoblock ME, He L, et al: Effect of stem cell factor on in vitro erythropoiesis in patients with bone marrow failure syndromes. *Blood* 80:3000, 1992.

29. Chan HSL, Saunders EF, Freedman MH: Diamond-Blackfan syndrome: I. In vitro corticosteroid effect on erythropoiesis. *Pediatr Res* 16:477, 1982.

30. Ball S, DBA Study Group: Further definition of the erythroid defect in DBA, and the modulatory effect of steroids and prolactin. *Proceedings 5th Annual Diamond Blackfan Anemia International Consensus Conference*, 2004.

31. Giri N, Kang E, Tisdale JF, Follman D, et al: Clinical and laboratory evidence for a trilineage haematopoietic defect in patients with refractory Diamond-Blackfan anaemia. *Br J Haematol* 108:167, 2000.

32. Scimeca PG, Weinblatt ME, Slepowitz G, et al: Diamond-Blackfan syndrome: An unusual cause of hydrops fetalis. *Am J Pediatr Hematol Oncol* 10:241, 1988.

33. Brown KE, Green SW, Antunez-de-Mayolo J, et al: Congenital anemia following transplacental B19 parvovirus infection. *Lancet* 343:895, 1994.

34. Balaban EP, Buchanan GR, Graham M, et al: Diamond-Blackfan syndrome in adult patients. *Am J Med* 78:533, 1985.

35. Cathie IA: Erythrogenesis imperfecta. *Arch Dis Child* 25:313, 1950.

36. Schofield KP, Evans DIK: Diamond-Blackfan syndrome and neutropenia. *J Clin Pathol* 44:742, 1991.

37. Glader BE, Backer K: Elevated red cell adenosine deaminase activity: A marker of disordered erythropoiesis in Diamond-Blackfan anaemia and other haematologic diseases. *Brit J Haematol* 68:165, 1988.

38. Willig TN, Niemeyer CM, Leblanc T, et al: Identification of new prognosis factors from the clinical and epidemiologic analysis of a registry of 229 Diamond-Blackfan anemia patients: DBA group of Societé d'Hematologic et d'Immunologie Pediatrique, Gesellschaft fur Padiatrische Onkologie und Hamatologie, and the European Society for Pediatric Hematology and Immunology (ESPHI). *Pediatr Res* 46:553, 1999.

39. Nich H, Acklin P, Lattmann R, et al: Development of tridentate iron chelators: From desferrithiocin to ICL670. *Curr Med Chem* 10:1065, 2003.

40. Vlachos A, Federman N, Reyes-Haley C, et al: Hematopoietic stem cell transplantation for Diamond Blackfan anemia: A report from the Diamond Blackfan Anemia Registry. *Bone Marrow Transplant* 27:381, 2001.

41. Ohga S, Mugishima H, Ohara A, et al: Diamond-Blackfan anemia in Japan: Clinical outcomes of prednisolone therapy and hematopoietic stem cell transplantation. *Int J Hematol* 79:22, 2004.

42. Wynn RF, Grainger JD, Carr TF, et al: Failure of allogeneic bone marrow transplantation to correct Diamond-Blackfan anaemia despite haemopoietic stem cell engraftment. *Bone Marrow Transplant* 24:803, 1999.

43. Ball SE, Tchernia G, Wranne L, et al: Is there a role for interleukin-3 diamond-blackfan anaemia results of a European multicentre study. *Br J Haematol* 91:313, 1995.

44. Ozsoylu S: High-dose intravenous corticosteroid treatment for patients with Diamond-Blackfan syndrome resistant or refractory to conventional treatment. *Am J Pediatr Hematol Oncol* 10:217, 1988.

45. Leonard EM, Raefsky E, Griffith P, et al: Cyclosporine therapy of aplastic anaemia, congenital and acquired red cell aplasia. *Br J Haematol* 72:278, 1989.

46. Marmont AM: Congenital hypoplastic anaemia refractory to corticosteriods but responding to cyclophosphamide and antilymphocytic globulin. *Acta Haematol* 60:90, 1978.

47. Rutella S, Pierelli L, Bonanno G, et al: Role for granulocyte colony-stimulating factor in the generation of human T regulatory type 1 cells. *Blood* 100:2562, 2002.

48. Hamaguchi I, Ooka A, Brun A, et al: Gene transfer improves erythroid development in ribosomal protein S19-deficient Diamond-Blackfan anemia. *Blood* 100:2724, 2002.

49. Lyngar E: Samtidig optreden av anemisk kriser hos 3 barn i en familie med hemolytisk ikterus. *Nord Med* 14:1246, 1942.

50. Owren PA: Congenital hemolytic jaundice: The pathogenesis of the "hemolytic crisis". *Blood* 3:231, 1948.

51. Dameshek W, Bloom ML: The events in the hemolytic crisis of hereditary spherocytosis, with particular reference to the reticulocytopenia, pancytopenia and an abnormal splenic mechanism. *Blood* 3:1381, 1948.

52. Chernoff AI, Josephson AM: Acute erythroblastopenia in sickle-cell anemia and infectious mononucleosis. *Am J Dis Child* 82:310, 1951.

53. Singer K, Motulsky AG, Wile SA: Aplastic crisis in sickle cell anemia. A study of its mechanism and its relationship to other types of hemolytic crises. *J Lab Clin Med* 35:721, 1950.

54. Pattison JR, Jones SE, Hodgson J, et al: Parvovirus infections and hypoplastic crisis in sickle cell anemia. *Lancet* 1:664, 1981.

55. Young NS, Brown KE: Parvovirus B19. *N Eng J Med* 350:586, 2003.

56. Serjeant GR, Topley JM, Mason K, et al: Outbreak of aplastic crises in sickle cell anaemia associated with parvovirus-like agent. *Lancet* 2:595, 1981.

57. Serjeant GR, Serjeant BE, Thomas PW, et al: Human parvovirus infection in homozygous sickle cell disease. *Lancet* 341:1237, 1993.

58. Wranne L: Transient erythroblastopenia in infancy and childhood. *Scand J Haematol* 7:76, 1970.

59. Young NS, Harrison M, Moore JG, et al: Direct demonstration of the human parvovirus in erythroid progenitor cells infected in vitro. *J Clin Invest* 74:2024, 1984.

60. Brown KE, Anderson SM, Young NS: Erythrocyte P antigen: Cellular receptor for B19 parvovirus. *Science* 262:114, 1993.

61. Brown KE, Hibbs JR, Gallinella G, et al: Resistance to parvovirus B19 due to lack of virus receptor (erythrocyte P antigen). *N Engl J Med* 330:1192, 1994.

62. Anderson MJ, Higgins PG, Davis LR, et al: Experimental parvoviral infection in humans. *J Infect Dis* 152:257, 1985.

63. Saarinen UM, Chorba TL, Tattersall P, et al: Human parvovirus B19-induced epidemic acute red cell aplasia in patients with hereditary hemolytic anemia. *Blood* 67:1411, 1986.

64. Chorba TL, Coccia P, Holman RC, et al: Role of parvovirus B19 in aplastic crisis and erythema infectiosum (fifth disease). *J Infect Dis* 154: 383, 1986.

65. Smith-Whitley K, Zhao H, Hodinka RL, et al: The epidemiology of human parvovirus B19 in children with sickle cell disease. *Blood* 103: 422, 2004.

66. Serjeant BE, Hambleton RR, Kerr S, et al: Haematological response to parvovirus B19 infection in homozygous sickle-cell disease. *Lancet* 341: 1237, 1993.

67. Skeppner G, Kreuger A, Elinder G: Transient erythroblastopenia of childhood: Prospective study of 10 patients with special reference to viral infections. *J Pediatr Hematol Oncol* 24:294, 2002.

68. Beresford CH, MacFarlane SD: Temporal clustering of transient erythroblastopenia (cytopenia) of childhood. *Aust Paediatr J* 23:351, 1987.

69. Bhambhani K, Inoue S, Sarnaik SA: Seasonal clustering of transient erythroblastopenia of childhood. *Am J Dis Child* 142:175, 1988.

70. Hays T, Lane PA, Shafer F: Transient erythroblastopenia of childhood. A review of 26 cases and reassessment of indications for bone marrow aspirate. *Am J Dis Child* 143:605, 1989.

71. Young NS, Mortimer PP, Moore JG, et al: Characterization of a virus that causes transient aplastic crisis. *J Clin Invest* 73:224, 1984.

72. Rogers BB, Rogers ZR, Timmons CF: Polymerase chain reaction amplification of acrchival material for parvovirus B19 in children with transient erythroblastopenia of childhood. *Pediatr Pathol Lab Med* 16:471, 1996.

73. Gussetis ES, Peristeri J, Kitra V, et al: Clinical value of bone marrow cultures in childhood pure red cell aplasia. *J Pediatr Hematol Oncol* 20: 120, 1998.

74. Koenig HM, Lightsey AL, Nelson DP, et al. Immune suppression of erythropoiesis in transient erythroblastopenia of childhood. *Blood* 54: 742, 1979.

75. Dessypris EN, Krantz SB, Roloff JS, et al: Mode of action of the IgG inhibitor of erythropoiesis in transient erythroblastopenia of childhood. *Blood* 59:114, 1982.

76. Tamary H, Kaplinsky C, Shvartzmayer S, et al: Transient erythroblastopenia of childhood: Evidence for cell-mediated suppression of erythropoiesis. *Am J Pediatr Hematol* 15:386, 1993.

77. Gustavsson P, Klar J, Matsson H, et al: Familiar transient erythroblastopenia of childhood is associated with the chromosome 19q13.2 region but not caused by mutations in coding sequences of the ribosomal protein S19 (RPS19) gene. *Br J Haematol* 119:261, 2002.

78. Thompson DF, Gales MA: Drug-induced pure red cell aplasia. *Pharmacotherapy* 16:1002, 1996.

79. Dessypris EN, Redline S, Harris JW, et al: Diphenylhydantoin-induced pure red cell aplasia. *Blood* 65:789, 1985.

80. Mariette Y, Mitjavila MT, Moulinie PR, et al: Rifampicin-induced pure red cell aplasia. *Am J Med* 87:459, 1989.

81. Smith JC, Megason GC, Iyer RV, et al: Clinical characteristics of children with hereditary hemolytic anemias and aplastic crisis: A 7-year review. *South Med J* 87:702, 1994.

82. Kynaston JA, West NC, Reid MM: A regional experience of red cell aplasia. *Eur J Pediatr* 152:306, 1993.

83. Farhi DC, Leubbers E, Rosenthal N: Bone marrow biopsy findings in childhood anemia - prevalence of transient erythroblastopenia of childhood. *Arch Pathol Lab Med* 122:638, 1998.

84. Skeppner G, Wranne L: Transient erythroblastopenia of childhood in Sweden: Incidence and findings at the time of diagnosis. *Acta Paediatr* 82:574, 1993.

85. Cherrick I, Karayalcin G, Lanzkowsky P: Transient erythroblastopenia of childhood: Prospective study of fifty patients. *Am J Pediatr Hematol* 16:320, 1994.

86. Michelson AD, Marshall PC: Transient neurological disorder associated with transient erythroblastopenia of childhood. *Am J Pediatr Hematol* 9:161, 1987.

87. Young RSK, Rannels E, Hilmi A, et al: Severe anemia in childhood presenting as transient ischemic attacks. *Stroke* 14:622, 1983.

88. Chan GCF, Kanwar VS, Wilimas J: Transient erythroblastopenia of childhood associated with transient neurologic deficity: Report of a case and review of the literature. *J Paediatr Child Health* 34:299, 1998.

89. Skeppner G, Forestier E, Henter JI, et al: Transient red cell aplasia in siblings: A common environmental or a common hereditary factor? *Acta Paediatr* 87:43, 1998.

90. Leuschner S, Bödewaldt-Radzun S, Rister M: Increase of CALLA-positive stimulated lymphoid cells in transient erythroblastopenia of childhood. *Eur J Pediatr* 149:551, 1990.

91. Kaznelson P: Zur Enstehung der Blut Plattchen. *Verh Dtsch Ges Inn Med* 34:557, 1922.

92. Baker RI, Manoharan A, De Luca E, Begley CG: Pure red cell aplasia of pregnancy: A distinct clinical entity. *Br J Haematol* 85:619, 1993.

93. Peschle C, Marmont AM, Marone G, et al: Pure red cell aplasia: Studies on an IgG serum inhibitor neutralizing erythropoietin. *Br J Haematol* 30:411, 1975.

94. Casadevall N, Dupuy E, Molho-Sabatier P, et al: Autoantibodies against erythropoietin in a patient with pure red-cell aplasia. *N Engl J Med* 334: 630, 1996.

95. Prabhakar SS, Muhlfelder T: Antibodies to recombinant human erythropoietin causing pure red cell aplasia. *Clin Nephrol* 47:331, 1997.

96. Casadevall N, Nataf J, Viron BP, et al: Pure red-cell aplasia and anti-erythropoietin antibodies in patients treated with recombinant erythropoietin. *N Eng J Med* 346:469, 2002.

97. Locatelli F, Del Vecchio L: Pure red cell aplasia secondary to treatment with erythropoietin. *J Nephrol* 16:461, 2003.

98. Bolan CD, Leitman SF, Griffith LM, et al: Delayed donor red cell chimerism and pure red cell aplasia following major ABO-incompatible nonmyeloablative hematopoietic stem cell transplantation. *Blood* 98: 1687, 2001.

99. Grigg AP, Juneja SK: Pure red cell aplasia with the onset of graft versus host disease. *Bone Marrow Transplant* 32:1099, 2003.

100. Hayden PJ, Gardiner N, Molloy K, et al: Pure red cell aplasia after a major ABO-mismatched bone marrow transplant for chronic myeloid leukaemia: Response to re-introduction of cyclosporin. *Bone Marrow Transplant* 34:545, 2004.

101. Charles RJ, Sabo KM, Kidd PG, et al: The pathophysiology of pure red cell aplasia: Implications for therapy. *Blood* 87:4831, 1996.

102. Chikkappa G, Zarrabi MH, Tsan MF: Pure red-cell aplasia in patients with chronic lymphocytic leukemia. *Medicine* 65:339, 1986.

103. Go RS, Lust JA, Phyliky RL: Aplastic anemia and pure red cell aplasia associated with large granular lymphocyte leukemia. *Semin Hematol* 40: 196, 2003.

104. Lacy MQ, Kurtin PJ, Tefferi A: Pure red cell aplasia: Association with large granular lymphocyte leukemia and the prognostic value of cytogenetic abnormalities. *Blood* 87:3000, 1996.

105. Yamada O: Clonal T cell proliferation in patients with pure red cell aplasia. *Leuk Lymphoma* 35:69, 1999.

106. Abkowitz JL, Powell JS, Nakamura JM, et al: Pure red cell aplasia: Response to therapy with anti-thymocyte globulin. *Am J Hematol* 23: 363, 1986.

107. Abkowitz JL, Kadin ME, Powell JS, et al: Pure red cell aplasia: Lymphocyte inhibition of erythropoiesis. *Br J Haematol* 63:59, 1986.

108. Hanada T, Abe T, Nakamura H, Aoki Y: Pure red cell aplasia: Relationship between inhibitory activity of T cells to CFU-E and erythropoiesis. *Br J Haematol* 58:107, 1984.

109. Linch DC, Cawley JC, MacDonald SM, et al: Acquired pure red-cell aplasia associated with an increase of T cells bearing receptors for the Fc of IgG. *Acta Haematol* 65:270, 1981.

110. Mangan KF, D'Alessandro L: Hypoplastic anemia in B cell chronic lymphocytic leukemia: Evolution of T cell-mediated suppression of erythropoiesis in early-stage and late-stage disease. *Blood* 66:533, 1985.

111. Mangan KF, Chikkappa G, Farley PC: T gamma cells suppress growth of erythroid colony-forming units in vitro in the pure red cell aplasia of B-cell chronic lymphocytic leukemia. *J Clin Invest* 70:1148, 1982.

112. Hoffman R, Kopel S, Hsu SD, et al: T cell chronic lymphocytic leukemia: Presence in bone marrow and peripheral blood of cells that suppress erythropoiesis in vitro. *Blood* 52:255, 1978.

113. Nagasawa T, Abe T, Nakagawa T: Pure red cell aplasia and hypogammaglobulinemia associated with T-cell chronic lymphocytic leukemia. *Blood* 57:1025, 1981.

114. Handgretinger R, Geiselhart A, Moris A: Pure red cell aplasia associated with clonal expansion of granular lymphocytes expressing killer-cell inhibitory receptors. *N Engl J Med* 340:278, 1999.

115. Mangan KF, Volkin R, Winkelstein A: Autoreactive erythroid progenitor-T suppressor cells in the pure red cell aplasia associated with thymoma and panhypogammaglobulinemia. *Am J Hematol* 23:167, 1986.

116. Akard LP, Brandt J, Lu Li, et al: Chronic T cell lymphoproliferative disorder and pure red cell aplasia. *Am J Med* 83:1069, 1987.

117. Reid TJI, Mullancy M, Burrell LM, et al: Pure red cell aplasia after chemotherapy for Hodgkin's lymphoma: In vitro evidence for T cell mediated suppression of erythropoiesis and response to sequential cyclosporin and erythropoietin. *Am J Hematol* 46:48, 1994.

118. Socinksi MA, Ershler WB, Tosato G, et al: Pure red blood cell aplasia associated with chronic Epstein-Barr virus infection: Evidence for T cell-mediated suppression of erythroid colony forming units. *J Lab Clin Med* 104:995, 1984.

119. Levitt LJ, Reyes GR, Moonka DK, et al: Human T cell leukemia virus-I-associated T-suppressor cell inhibition of erythropoiesis in a patient with pure red cell aplasia and chronic T-gamma-lymphoproliferative disease. *J Clin Invest* 81:538, 1988.

120. Lipton JM, Nadler LM, Canellos GP, et al: Evidence for genetic restriction in the suppression of erythropoiesis by a unique subset of T lymphocytes in man. *J Clin Invest* 72:694, 1983.

121. Kurtzman G, Cohen R, Field AM, et al: The immune response to B19 parvovirus infection and an antibody defect in persistent viral infection. *J Clin Invest* 84:1114, 1989.

122. Geetha D, Zachary JB, Baldado HM, et al: Pure red cell aplasia caused by Parvovirus B19 infection in solid organ transplant recipients: A case report and review of literature. *Clin Transplant* 14:586, 2000.

123. Frickhofen N, Abkowitz J, Safford M, et al: Persistent parvovirus infection in patients infected with human immunodeficiency virus type 1 (HIV-1): A treatable cause of anemia in AIDS. *Ann Intern Med* 113:926, 1990.

124. Kurtzman G, Frickhofen N, Kimball J, et al: Pure red-cell aplasia of 10 years' duration due to persistent parvovirus B19 infection and its cure with immunoglobulin therapy. *N Engl J Med* 321:519, 1989.

125. Abkowitz JL, Brown KE, Wood RW, et al: Clinical relevance of parvovirus B19 as a cause of anemia in patients with human immunodeficiency virus infection. *J Infect Dis* 176:269, 1997.

126. Mylonakis E, Dickinson BP, Mileno MD, et al: Persistent parvovirus B19 related anemia of seven year's duration in an HIV-infected patient: Complete remission associated with highly active antiretroviral therapy. *Am J Hematol* 60:164, 1999.

127. Garcia-Suárez J, Pascual T, Muñoz MA, et al: Myelodysplastic syndrome with erythroid hypoplasia/aplasia: A case report and review of the literature. *Am J Hematol* 58:319, 1998.

128. Hirai H: Molecular pathogenesis of MDS. *Int J Hematol* 76:213, 2002.

129. Pellagatti A, Esoof N, Watkins F, et al: Gene expression profiling in the myelodysplastic syndromes using cDNA microarray technology. *Br J Haematol* 125:576, 2004.

130. Darley RL, Hoy TG, Baines P, et al: Mutant N-RAS induces erythroid lineage dysplasia in human CD34+ cells. *J Exp Med* 185:1337, 1997.

131. Brittingham TE, Lutcher CL, Murphy DI: Reversible erythroid aplasia induced by diphenylhydantoin. *Arch Intern Med* 113:764, 1964.

132. Yunis AA, Arimura GK, Lutcher CL, et al: Biochemical lesion in dilantin-induced erythroid aplasia. *Blood* 30:587, 1967.

133. Strauss AM: Erythrocyte aplasia following sulfathiazole. *Am J Clin Pathol* 13:249, 1943.

134. Stephens ME: Transient erythroid hypoplasia in a patient on long-term co-trimoxazole therapy. *Postgrad Med J* 50:235, 1974.

135. Planas AT, Kranwinkel RN, Soletsky HB, et al: Chlorpropamide-induced pure RBC aplasia. *Arch Intern Med* 140:707, 1980.

136. Krivoy N, Ben-Arieh Y, Carter A, et al, Methazolamide-induced hepatitis and pure RBC aplasia. *Arch Intern Med* 141:1229, 1981.

137. McGrath BP, Ibels LS, Raik E, et al: Erythroid toxicity of azathioprine: Macrocytosis and selective marrow hypoplasia. *Q J Med* 44:57, 1975.

138. Lin YW, Okazaki S, Hamahata K, et al: Acute pure red cell aplasia associated with allopurinol therapy. *Am J Hematol* 61:209, 1999.

139. Hoffman R, McPhedran P, Benz EJ, et al: Isoniazid-induced pure red cell aplasia. *Am J Med Sci* 286:2, 1983.

140. Marseglia GL, Locatelli F: Isoniazid-induced pure red cell aplasia in two siblings. *J Pediatr* 132:898, 1998.

141. Agudelo CA, Wise CM, Lyles MF: Pure red cell aplasia in procainamide induced systemic lupus erythematosus. Report and review of the literature. *J Rheumatol* 15:1431, 1988.

142. Kawakita T, Okano H, Sugimoto K, et al: Ticlopidine induced acute cholestatic hepatitis complicated with pure red cell aplasia. *J Clin Gastroenterol* 38:84, 2004.

143. Tanaka N, Ishida F, Tanaka E: Ribavirin-induced pure red-cell aplasia during treatment of chronic hepatitis C. *N Eng J Med* 350:1264, 2004.

144. Lacombe C, Casadevall N, Muller O, et al: Erythroid progenitors in adult chronic pure red cell aplasia: Relationship of in vitro erythroid colonies to therapeutic response. *Blood* 64:71, 1984.

145. Mangan KF, Shadduck RK: Successful treatment of chronic refractory pure red cell aplasia with antithymocyte globulin: Correlation with in vitro erythroid culture studies. *Am J Hematol* 17:417, 1984.

146. Clark DA, Dessypris EN, Krantz SB: Studies on pure red cell aplasia: XI. Results of immunosuppressive treatment of 37 patients. *Blood* 63:277, 1984.

147. Hirst E, Robertson TI: The syndrome of thymoma and erythroblastopenic anemia. *Medicine* 46:225, 1967.

148. Firkin FC, Maher D: Cytotoxic immunosuppressive drug treatment strategy in pure red cell aplasia. *Eur J Haematol* 41:212, 1988.

149. Kwong YL, Wong KF, Liang RHS, et al: Pure red cell aplasia: Clinical features and treatment results in 16 cases. *Ann Hematol* 72:137, 1996.

150. Mamiya S, Itoh T, Miura AB: Acquired pure red cell aplasia in Japan. *Eur J Haematol* 59:199, 1997.

151. Yamada O, Motoji T, Mizoguchi H: Selective effect of cyclosporine monotherapy for pure red cell aplasia not associated with granular lymphocyte-proliferative disorders. *Br J Haematol* 106:371, 1999.

152. Raghavachar A: Pure red cell aplasia: Review of treatment and proposal for a treatment strategy. *Blut* 61:47, 1990.

153. Tötterman TH, Höglund M, Bengtsson M, et al: Treatment of pure red-cell aplasia and aplastic anaemia with ciclosporin: Long-term clinical effects. *Eur J Haematol* 42:126, 1989.

154. Yamada O, Mizoguchi H, Oshimi K: Cyclophosphamide therapy for pure red cell aplasia associated with granular lymphocyte-proliferative disorders. *Br J Haematol* 97:392, 1997.

155. Go RS, Li C-Y, Tefferi A, et al: Acquired pure red cell aplasia associated with lymphoproliferative disease of granular T lymphocytes. *Blood* 98:483, 2001.

156. Harris SI, Weinberg JB: Treatment of red cell aplasia with antithymo-cyte globulin: Repeated inductions of complete remissions in two patients. *Am J Hematol* 20:183, 1985.

157. Mangan KF, Shadduck RK: Successful treatment of chronic refractory pure red cell aplasia with antithymocyte globulin: Correlation with in vitro erythroid culture studies. *Am J Hematol* 17:417, 1984.

158. Robak T: Monoclonal antibodies in the treatment of autoimmune cytopenias. *Eur J Haematol* 72:79, 2004.

159. Ghazal H: Successful treatment of pure red cell aplasia with rituximab in patients with chronic lymphocytic leukemia. *Blood* 9:1092, 2002.

160. Auner HW, Wolfler A, Beham-Schmid C, et al: Restoration of erythropoiesis by rituximab in an adult patient with primary acquired pure red cell aplasia refractory to conventional treatment. *Br J Haematol* 116: 725, 2002.

161. Willis F, Marsh JCW, Bevan DH, et al: The effect of treatment with Campath-1H in patients with autoimmune cytopenias. *Br J Haematol* 114:891, 2001.

162. Ru X, Liebman HA: Successful treatment of refractory pure red cell aplasia associated with lymphoproliferative disorders with the anti-CD52 monoclonal antibody alemtuzumab (Campath-1H). *Br J Haematol* 123:278, 2004.

163. Ahn JH, Lee KH, Lee JH, et al: A case of refractory idiopathic pure red cell aplasia responsive to fludarabine treatment. *Br J Haematol* 112:527, 2001.

164. Robak T, Kaszn M, Blo KI, et al: Pure red cell aplasia in patients with chronic lymphocytic leukaemia treated with cladribine. *Br J Haematol* 112:1083, 2001

165. Messner HA, Fauser AA, Curtis JE, et al; Control of antibodymediated pure red-cell aplasia by plasmapheresis. *N Engl J Med* 304:1334, 1981.

166. Freund LG, Hippe E, Strandgaard S, et al: Complete remission in pure red cell aplasia after plasmapheresis. *Scand J Haematol* 35:315, 1985.

167. Müller BU, Tichelli A, Passweg JR, et al: Successful treatment of refractory acquired pure red cell aplasia (PRCAP) by allogeneic bone marrow transplantation. *Bone Marrow Transplant* 23:1205, 1999.

168. Tseng SB, Lin SF, Chang CS, et al: Successful treatment of acquired pure red cell aplasia (PRCA) by allogeneic peripheral blood stem cell transplantation. *Am J Hematol* 74:273, 2003.

169. Kurtzman GJ, Ozawa K, Cohen B, et al: Chronic bone marrow failure due to persistent B19 parvovirus infection. *N Engl J Med* 317:287, 1987.

170. Ramratnam B, Schiffman FJ, Rintels P, et al: Management of persistent B19 parvovirus infection in AIDS. *Br J Haematol* 91:90, 1995.

ANEMIA OF CHRONIC RENAL FAILURE

JAIME CARO

Anemia is an almost constant complication of chronic renal failure that significantly contributes to the symptoms and complications of the disease. The anemia of chronic renal disease is caused by failure of renal excretory and endocrine function. Accumulation of toxic metabolic end products plays a secondary role in the pathogenesis of the anemia; however, the effects of these end products largely can be overcome by exogenous erythropoietin (Epo) treatment. Use of recombinant human Epo to ameliorate the anemia in patients with chronic renal disease has been successful and has confirmed deficiency in the renal production and secretion of the hormone as the primary cause of the anemia. Failure of renal excretory function causes a moderate reduction of red cell life span, impairment of blood platelet function, and suppression of marrow activity. Intensive dialysis is the most effective treatment for the metabolic effects resulting from inadequate renal excretory function. Failure of renal endocrine function (decreased Epo production) is managed by replacement treatment with recombinant human Epo. If adequate iron sources are available, a hematocrit of approximately 35 percent can be maintained by subcutaneous or intravenous Epo injections. Approximately 95 percent of patients respond to the hormone without significant side effects.

HISTORY AND DEFINITION

Anemia is one of the most characteristic and visible manifestations of chronic renal failure. In 1836, Richard Bright[1] first commented on the pallor of patients with renal disease. Since that time, numerous observers have described and attempted to explain the underlying anemia. Untreated anemia can, depending on its severity, be associated with a number of abnormalities, including decreased oxygen delivery to the tissues, increased cardiac output and cardiomegaly, decreased cognition and mental acuity, and overall decrease in patient welfare. The degree of anemia appears to be roughly proportional to the severity of renal failure,[2] but a strict linear relationship between hematocrit and creatinine clearance does not exist. At creatinine clearances of less than 20 ml/min, however, the hematocrit almost always is less than 30 percent (Fig. 35-1). Infectious, neoplastic, immunologic, or metabolic disorders that can accompany renal disease may affect the degree of anemia and its response to treatment.[3]

ETIOLOGY AND PATHOGENESIS

Experimental and clinical observations on the effect of intensive dialysis, bilateral nephrectomy, and treatment with Epo have clarified some of the pathophysiologic mechanisms responsible for the anemia

Acronyms and abbreviations that appear in this chapter include: Epo, erythropoietin; HIF, hypoxia-inducible factor; Na+-K+, sodium-potassium; PRCA, pure red cell aplasia; VHL, von Hippel-Lindau.

of chronic renal disease. The primary cause of the anemia is decreased production of Epo by the failing kidneys.[2,4] A diminished capacity to excrete potentially toxic metabolic end products may contribute to the anemia by shortening the red cell life span and causing blood loss and marrow suppression.[5,6] Concomitant inflammatory conditions and/or malnutrition may aggravate the anemia and impair its response to therapy.[3]

RENAL EXCRETORY FAILURE

The life span of red cells in patients with chronic renal disease usually is shorter than normal. Because the red cells survive normally when they are injected into healthy recipients and normal red cells may have a shortened life span in uremic recipients,[5,6] the metabolic or mechanical environment in uremic patients is unfavorable for normal survival of red cells. However, the mildly shortened red cell life span can be compensated in the presence of a normal erythropoietic response.

METABOLIC RED CELL DYSFUNCTION

The inverse relationship between blood urea nitrogen and red cell life span[5-7] and the occasional normalization of the red cell life span after intensive dialysis[7] suggest the presence of an erythrocyte metabolic defect. However, most red cell enzymes show normal or increased activity in uremia, and the intracellular level of adenosine triphosphate is high, possibly as a result of a high serum phosphate concentration.[8]

The intracellular concentration of 2,3-bisphosphoglycerate is appropriately increased in response to anemia and hyperphosphatemia,[9] with a moderate decrease in the affinity of hemoglobin for oxygen.[10] In the presence of uremic acidosis, the decrease in oxygen is augmented by a rightward shift of the oxygen dissociation curve, that is, Bohr effect affinity (see Chap. 47). However, acidosis also tends to decrease the concentration of intracellular organic phosphates, establishing a condition of opposing effects on the oxygen affinity of hemoglobin.[11] Intensive dialysis may initially reduce the concentration of intracellular organic phosphate compounds, possibly because of hypophosphatemia.[12] The result is increased oxygen affinity of hemoglobin and temporary aggravation of tissue hypoxia, which may play a role in the so-called dialysis disequilibrium syndrome.[13]

Only the activities of transketolase, a hexose monophosphate shunt enzyme (see Chap. 45),[14] and adenosine triphosphatase, which powers the sodium-potassium (Na+-K+) membrane pumps,[15] are decreased in uremia. The decreased response of the hexose monophosphate shunt renders the hemoglobin and red cell membrane excessively sensitive to oxidant drugs or chemicals.[16,17] For example, tap water used for hemodialysis and purified with chloramine can cause the formation of Heinz bodies and hemolytic anemia.[18] The decreased activity of the Na+-K+ pumps can cause changes in red cell shape and rigidity and, in turn, life span. The toxic substances responsible for these metabolic impairments presumably are dialyzable but have not been identified. Other exogenous toxins introduced by dialysis fluids, such as copper, nitrates, and formaldehyde, can contribute to hemolysis and occasionally produce severe, even fatal, hemolytic episodes.[19] Parathyroid hormone, often increased in renal failure, can contribute to hemolysis by increasing red cell osmotic fragility.[20,21]

MECHANICAL RED CELL DESTRUCTION

Despite the data supporting a metabolic basis for hemolysis, a considerable number of investigators have failed to find a clear-cut correlation between red cell life span and degree of renal failure.[2] Red cell injury and premature destruction may be caused by mechanical trauma rather than metabolic alterations.[22] Normal red cells exposed to strong shearing stress, especially at a fibrin interphase, become deformed and vulnerable to monocyte-macrophage sequestration. In some cases of malignant hypertension, extensive red cell fragmentation occurs with

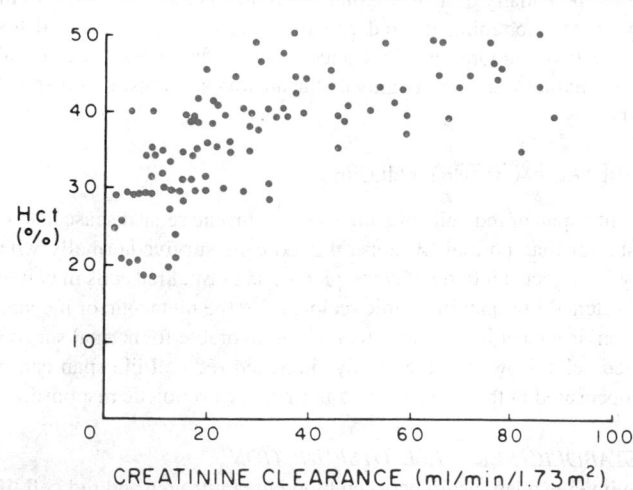

FIGURE 35-1 Relationship between hematocrit and creatinine clearance in patients with chronic renal disease. Anemia is inversely related to the degree of renal impairment in most patients with chronic renal disease. (Redrawn from Radtke et al.[2])

severe hemolytic anemia,[23] but in most cases of chronic renal disease the hemolysis and morphologic changes are only moderate. Current reasoning relates premature destruction of red cells in uremia with mechanical disruption of metabolically impaired cells.

HEMOLYTIC UREMIC SYNDROME

Hemolytic uremic syndrome is a distinct entity[24] that usually is acute. The hemolysis is not secondary to the uremia, and its manifestations are similar to those found in other microangiopathic disorders (see Chap. 49) or disseminated intravascular coagulation (see Chap. 121). The syndrome was first described in 1955 by Gasser and coworkers,[25] who found hemolysis and uremia in infants and young children subsequent to episodes of gastrointestinal or upper respiratory infections. Since that time, the syndrome has been recognized in patients of all ages and associated with a variety of exogenous agents.[26] The syndrome is initiated by damage to the endothelium of glomerular capillaries and renal arterioles.[27] The damage leads to local platelet deposition, intravascular coagulation, and ischemic renal cortical necrosis.[27] Clinical manifestations are pallor, purpura, jaundice, and oliguria. Laboratory tests reveal anemia. Blood film displays many deformed and fragmented red cells (Fig. 35-2), increased number of reticulocytes, and occasional nucleated red cells.[26,28] Epo levels usually are increased despite an elevated serum creatinine concentration.[29] Thrombocytopenia and a compensatory increase in marrow megakaryocytes are noted. Distinguishing hemolytic uremic syndrome from the syndrome of thrombotic thrombocytopenic purpura can be difficult in many cases (see Chaps. 49 and 124). Normal cleaving of von Willebrand multimers is impaired in thrombotic thrombocytopenic purpura because of either a congenital absence of a multimer-cleaving protease or immunologic inactivation of the protease.[30,31] Most cases of this syndrome clear spontaneously, but severe cases may cause life-threatening renal failure. Drug-induced hemolytic uremic syndrome/TTP (thrombotic thrombocytopenic purpura) is becoming an increasingly described entity, especially associated with the use of chemotherapeutic or immunosuppressive agents.[32]

BLOOD LOSS

Purpura and gastrointestinal and gynecologic bleeding occur in one third to one half of all patients with chronic renal failure.[33] In addition,

blood is lost during laboratory testing and in discarded dialysis tubing. All of these occurrences constitute a significant loss of iron and may contribute to the development of anemia and its response to therapy. The pathogenesis of the bleeding tendency is poorly understood. Thrombocytopenia, when present, is rarely of sufficient magnitude to explain spontaneous blood loss. However, platelet or vascular function, as judged from bleeding time, platelet adhesiveness and aggregation, clot retraction, thromboxane formation, or prostacyclin production by vessel walls, is abnormal in the majority of cases and may, alone or in combination, account for the bleeding tendency[33] (see Chaps. 105 and 110). Dialysis corrects or ameliorates both the laboratory and clinical manifestations of abnormal platelet function, but the dialyzable agent responsible has not been identified. Urea or creatinine probably is not involved, but certain guanidine compounds are suspected.[34]

MARROW SUPPRESSION

Although Epo deficiency in itself could explain the development of anemia, uremic toxins also may impair erythroid activity and be partly responsible for the development of anemia.[35] Earlier studies have suggested that such uremic toxins exist, but all attempts to identify and isolate the toxins have been unsuccessful.[36] Spermine, an attractive candidate,[37] suppresses all cellular elements, not only the erythroid tissue, when administered in toxic doses. Parathyroid hormone,[38] another contender, causes general marrow suppression by inducing marrow fibrosis.[39] Exogenous Epo is equally effective when administered to patients before and after successful kidney transplantation.[40] These observations indicate that uremia per se does not affect normal erythroid metabolism in vivo. Nevertheless, the response to Epo in stable,

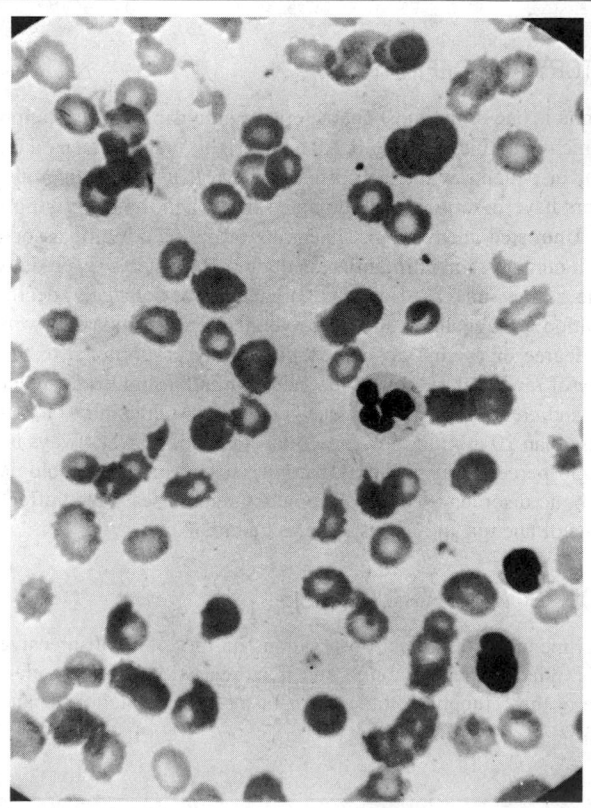

FIGURE 35-2 Microangiopathic hemolytic anemia in renal disease. Blood film from a patient with hemolytic-uremic syndrome shows fragmentation and distortion of red blood cells.

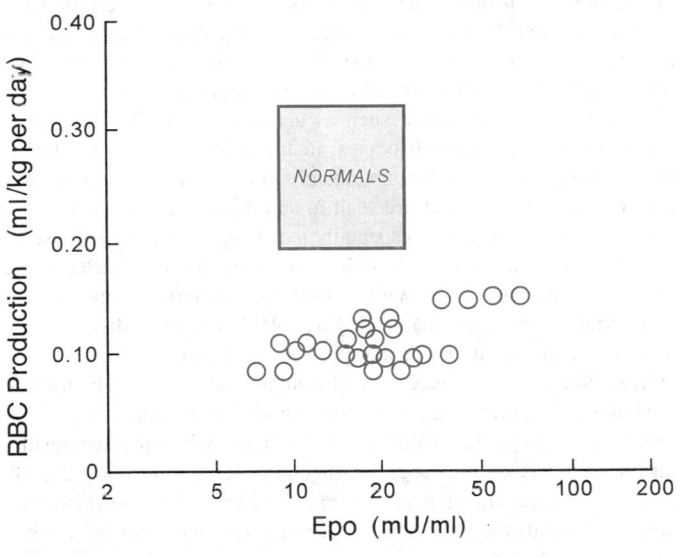

FIGURE 35-3 Relationship between red cell production and Epo levels in uremic patients. Given their stable hematocrits, the rate of red cell production must equal the rate of red cell destruction, which was calculated by dividing red cell mass by red cell life span. The *square* denotes the rate of red cell production in normal individuals at normal Epo levels. Results indicate that uremic patients have decreased red cell production for equivalent serum Epo concentrations compared to normal individuals.[41]

well-dialyzed patients is about half the response in normal individuals[41] (Fig. 35-3). Whether the decreased erythroid responsiveness is the result of uremic toxins, associated inflammatory conditions, or relative iron deficiency is not clear.

Iron may be in short supply because of excessive blood loss in most patients with renal failure[42]; therefore, iron supplementation in uremic patients receiving Epo may be necessary (see Chap. 40) for their response to therapy. Aluminum in dialysis water may interfere with iron incorporation in erythroid cells and cause microcytic anemia and occasionally osteomalacia and encephalopathy.[43] In the rare case of nephrotic syndrome, urinary loss of transferrin reportedly causes low iron-binding capacity, with impairment in metabolic cycling of iron.[44] Folic acid deficiency should be treated with folic acid replacement in patients undergoing intensive dialysis because folic acid is dialyzable and may be lost in the dialysis bath.[45]

FAILURE OF RENAL ENDOCRINE FUNCTION

ERYTHROPOIETIN

Epo is a 34-kDa glycoprotein hematopoietic growth factor that can control the rate of red cell production by acting on erythroid precursors in the bone marrow[46] (see Chap. 30). In 1957, Jacobson and coworkers[47] reported that nephrectomized and uremic rats failed to respond to blood loss by releasing Epo, whereas ureter-ligated and equally uremic rats responded in an almost normal manner. This important observation led to the hypothesis that the kidney produces Epo. In the 1970s, studies on isolated perfused kidneys supported the kidney's direct role in Epo production.[48] However, the kidney was not established as an Epo-producing organ until *EPO* mRNA was demonstrated in renal tissue.[49–51]

In situ hybridization studies have localized the Epo-producing cells to the cortical interstitium of mouse and rat kidneys.[52,53] Immunoelectron microscopic techniques showed that Epo-expressing cells also express the surface enzyme ecto-5′-nucleotidase,[54,55] a marker restricted to fibroblastic cells. A number of Epo-producing cells are re-

cruited to express the gene in an all-or-none fashion, with recruitment spreading outward from the corticomedullary boundary.[53]

Hypoxia is followed within 1 hour by a measurable accumulation of *EPO* mRNA in the kidneys and shortly afterward by an increase in circulating Epo.[56] The molecular mechanisms by which hypoxia-anemia controls production of Epo and other hypoxia-responsive genes are an area of active research (see Chap. 30). A hypoxia-responsive enhancer sequence element that controls the hypoxia response was identified in the 3′-flanking sequence of the human *EPO* gene.[57] This sequence acts as the DNA-binding site for a hypoxia-inducible transcription factor 1 (HIF-1) complex, which activates transcription of the *EPO* gene. The HIF-1 complex is formed by two subunits: HIF-1β, which is constitutively expressed, and HIF-1α, which is expressed only under hypoxic conditions.[58] The HIF-1α subunit normally is ubiquinated and degraded by the proteasomal system in a process that requires the von Hippel-Lindau (VHL) protein, which acts as an ubiquitin ligase.[59–61] During normoxic conditions, HIF-1α is hydroxylated in specific prolyl-residues by prolyl-hydroxylase enzymes in an oxygen-dependent reaction.[62–64] Hydroxylation of HIF-1α facilitates its interaction with the VHL protein and its degradation by the proteasome system. Thus, under hypoxic or anemic conditions, HIF-1α is not degraded and interacts with HIF-1β to activate transcription of the *EPO* gene (Fig. 35-4). Of interest, patients with VHL mutations overexpress HIF and may develop erythrocytosis secondary to increased Epo production.[65]

Extrarenal sites of Epo production exist and account for approximately 15 to 20 percent of total Epo secretion in adult rodents.[66] In humans, very low but still detectable levels of Epo are found in severely anemic anephric individuals (see Fig. 35-4)[4], consistent with extrarenal sites of Epo synthesis. During fetal life, extrarenal production of Epo by the liver predominates, with a gradual change to renal production at birth. In the liver, two types of cells express the *EPO* gene, hepatocytes and the nonparenchymal Ito cells,[67–69] which are morphologically and functionally similar to the interstitial fibroblasts in the kidneys. The genomic *EPO* determinants of expression in kidney

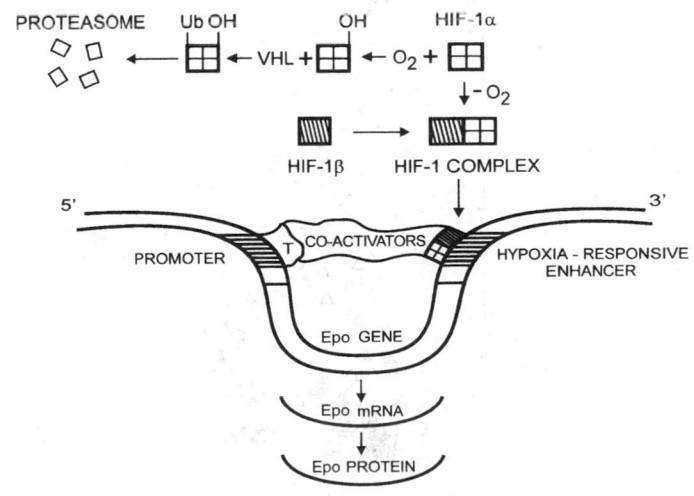

FIGURE 35-4 Molecular control of the *EPO* gene. Schematic representation of the transcriptional control of the *EPO* gene by the hypoxia-inducible factor 1 (HIF-1) complex. Under normoxic conditions, HIF-1α is hydroxylated (OH) by oxygen- and iron-dependent prolyl-hydroxylase enzymes. Hydroxylated HIF is ubiquinated (Ub) by the von Hippel-Lindau protein (VHL) and degraded by the proteasomal system. During hypoxic or anemic conditions, HIF-1α is not degraded and interacts with HIF-1β to form an active HIF-1 complex that stimulates transcription of the *EPO* gene (Epo mRNA).

and liver are different. The kidney requires a 14-kb upstream fragment that is not needed by the liver.[70] Inappropriate production of Epo by renal and extrarenal tumors appears to be accomplished by cells different from those responsible for normal, regulated Epo synthesis.

In patients with renal disease, the reduction in Epo production is roughly proportional to the degree of excretory impairment. However, even nonfunctioning kidneys produce some Epo and can maintain hemoglobin levels higher than those found in anephric patients (see Fig. 35-5).[4] The remaining capacity of remnant kidneys to produce Epo is at least partly responsible for the polycythemia (see Chap. 56) that occurs in 10 to 15 percent of patients following kidney transplantation.[71] It also is responsible for the brief but significant increase in Epo levels seen in end-stage uremic patients following episodes of acute hypoxia or blood loss.[72,73]

CLINICAL AND LABORATORY FEATURES

The symptoms and physical manifestations of renal failure depend primarily on the underlying disorder. However, anemia almost invariably is present and is of major clinical concern.

BLOOD

The anemia is characteristically normocytic and normochromic and is associated with a normal or slightly decreased number of reticulocytes. A few red cells appear deformed on blood films. Some cells have multiple tiny spicules; others have grossly abnormal contour and loss

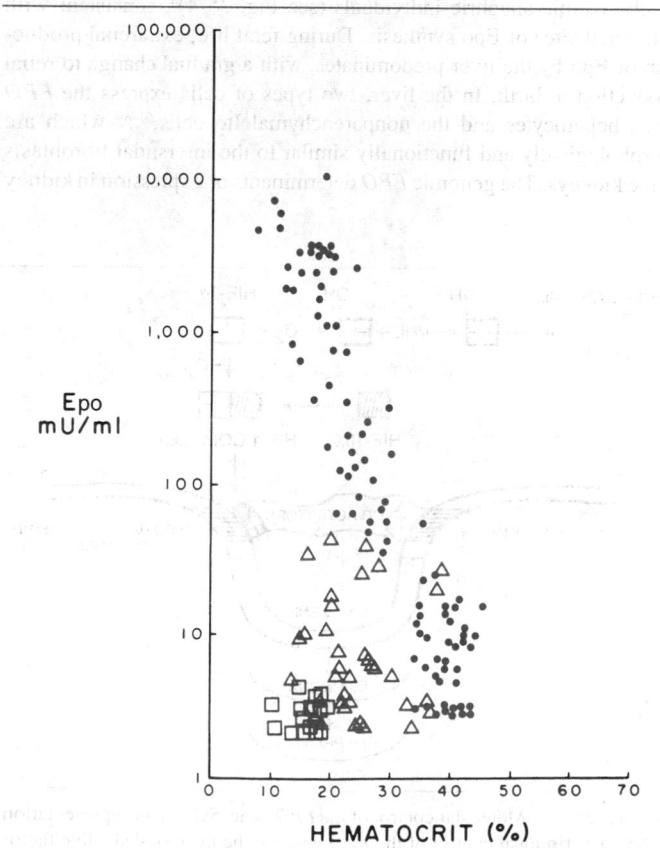

FIGURE 35-5   Circulating Epo levels are decreased in uremic patients. Epo levels in nephric and anephric uremic patients are compared to levels in individuals with intact kidneys. •, Normal subjects and patients with simple anemia; □, anephric patients; △, and uremic-nephric patients. All determinations were made by bioassay of plasma concentrates in hypertransfused mice.

of volume. The former cells, echinocytes or burr cells, were thought to be characteristic of chronic renal failure.[74] However, even normal cells undergo a reversible transformation to burr cell-like echinocytes when exposed to a glass surface or incubated uremic plasma.[75]

Grossly deformed cells, such as acanthocytes with a few large spicules or fragmented schistocytes, are formed in the microcirculation *in vivo*. They are found most abundantly in the hemolytic uremic syndrome (see Fig. 35-2) but are seen in small numbers on blood films from most uremic patients, especially in the presence of hypertension.

The total and differential leukocyte count and the platelet count usually are normal, but, as with all other hematologic parameters, the underlying disorder plays a modifying role. Uremia and dialysis may have an effect on leukocytes and platelets. The phagocytic activity of granulocytes may be reduced,[76] and complement activation by the hemodialysis membrane may cause pulmonary leukostasis with temporary granulocytopenia.[77] Cell-mediated immunity is depressed, resulting in an increased incidence of infections but also prolonged graft survival. Platelet function is abnormal and related to the degree of uremia and dialysis. The resulting bleeding tendency may be another anemia contributor.

MARROW

The marrow usually appears normal and is in the maturation sequence of all cellular elements, including the nucleated red cells. Normal marrow morphology is inappropriate in the context of reduced hemoglobin concentration because a compensatory increase in erythroid activity is expected.[78] However, the marrow may be hypoplastic, and severe erythroid hypoplasia in acute renal failure has been described.

PLASMA

The level of circulating Epo and the iron turnover are within the "normal range," which also is inappropriate for the degree of anemia.[4] Iron utilization is regularly decreased in renal insufficiency. Again, these "normal" levels contrast with the increased levels found at similar degrees of anemia but with normal kidney function (see Fig. 35-4). In many cases, the underlying disease causes specific changes in iron kinetics and in the serum concentrations of folic acid, iron, and transferrin. These changes modify and aggravate the relative marrow failure characterizing the anemia of chronic renal disease.[79]

THERAPY, COURSE, AND PROGNOSIS

In the past, anemia was often considered a relatively minor problem for patients suffering from the many metabolic consequences of failing kidneys. The development of efficient hospital and home dialysis provided partial relief for many of the metabolic problems but left the anemia unchanged until the availability of Epo.

DIALYSIS

Dialysis per se typically has little effect with regard to correcting the anemia, although a mild increase in hemoglobin concentration may result from the decrease in bleeding tendency. However, for still unexplained reasons, ambulatory peritoneal dialysis may ameliorate and, on occasions, completely correct the anemia.[80]

IRON AND FOLATE SUPPLEMENTATION

Although overt folic acid or iron deficiency may not be evident, these compounds are given routinely to most patients with renal disease. A serum ferritin level of 100 ng/ml must be maintained because effective treatment requires an adequate iron supply to the erythroid cells.

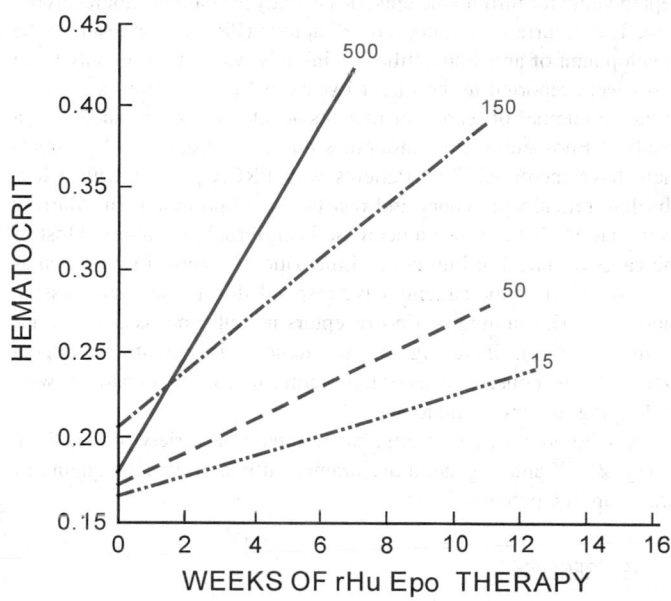

FIGURE 35-6   Erythropoietic response to recombinant human (rHu) Epo therapy in patients with renal disease. The slopes of hematocrit increase in uremic patients after weekly administration of various doses of recombinant Epo. —, 500 units/kg; — . —, 150 units/kg; – – –, 50 units/kg; — ·· —, 15 units/kg. (From Eschbach et al.,[84] with permission.)

ANDROGEN USE

Androgens have been widely used to stimulate Epo production and action. Even with the advent of appropriate Epo treatment, androgens occasionally are used in apparently resistant patients. Of the many preparations available, nandrolone decanoate[81] and fluoxymesterone[82] usually are effective. However, minor and major side effects occur, and androgen use is now rarely justified given the availability of Epo.

TRANSFUSION THERAPY

Transfusions with packed red cells are necessary to counteract the effects of acute blood loss. Transfusions occasionally are needed to maintain acceptable hemoglobin concentrations in patients who do not respond adequately to Epo.

RECOMBINANT ERYTHROPOIETIN ADMINISTRATION

Replacement therapy with Epo, the most rational approach to treatment of the anemia of renal disease, became a reality in 1987 with the introduction of mass-produced recombinant human Epo.[83,84] The recombinant product has the same amino acid composition as natural human Epo[85] and an almost identical carbohydrate composition[86]; thus, antibodies against the recombinant product are rarely found in Epo-treated patients. Epo administration can ameliorate the anemia in almost all patients treated, irrespective of the underlying cause of the renal disorder (Fig. 35-6).

The National Kidney Foundation has published detailed guidelines for Epo administration to patients with the anemia of chronic renal diseases.[87] In short, the presence of an anemia with hematocrits of less than 33 percent or hemoglobins of less than 11 g/dl should initiate a thorough search for conditions unrelated to decreased Epo production or action. Measurements of folic acid and B_{12} levels should be carried out, with special attention to iron, iron-binding capacity, and ferritin levels. Determination of Epo levels is not necessary. Complicating chronic illnesses that can aggravate the anemia should be ruled out

(see Chap. 43). Although the anemia of renal disease is roughly proportional to the severity of renal failure, anemia can occur with serum creatinine levels as low as 2 mg/dl.

Because of the availability of venous access in dialysis patients, Epo has been given primarily by the intravenous route. However, pharmacokinetic studies of normal volunteers and patients with chronic renal disease have shown that subcutaneous administration may be equally or more effective.[88,89] The half-life of intravenous Epo is between 6 and 9 hours, with a volume of distribution slightly larger than that of the plasma volume (Fig. 35-7a).[90,91] When the subcutaneous route is used, no peaks are observed, and plasma levels are lower but more sustained throughout the course (Fig. 35-7b).[90] However, bioavailability after subcutaneous injections appears to be less predictable, possibly because of erratic tissue absorption. Subcutaneous Epo administration can maintain a target hematocrit value of 30 to 33 percent, with use of approximately 30 percent lower doses of Epo.[92,93]

Based on the initial clinical trials, the US Food and Drug Administration approved the clinical use of Epo in June 1989, setting the target hematocrit at 30 to 33 percent. In its 1997 guidelines,[87] the National Kidney Foundation recommended an increase in the target hematocrit to 33 to 36 percent and target hemoglobin to 11 to 12 g/dl. In addition, the National Kidney Foundation recommended subcutaneous Epo administration as the preferred route and intravenous, rather than oral, routine iron supplementation to optimize the response. Some

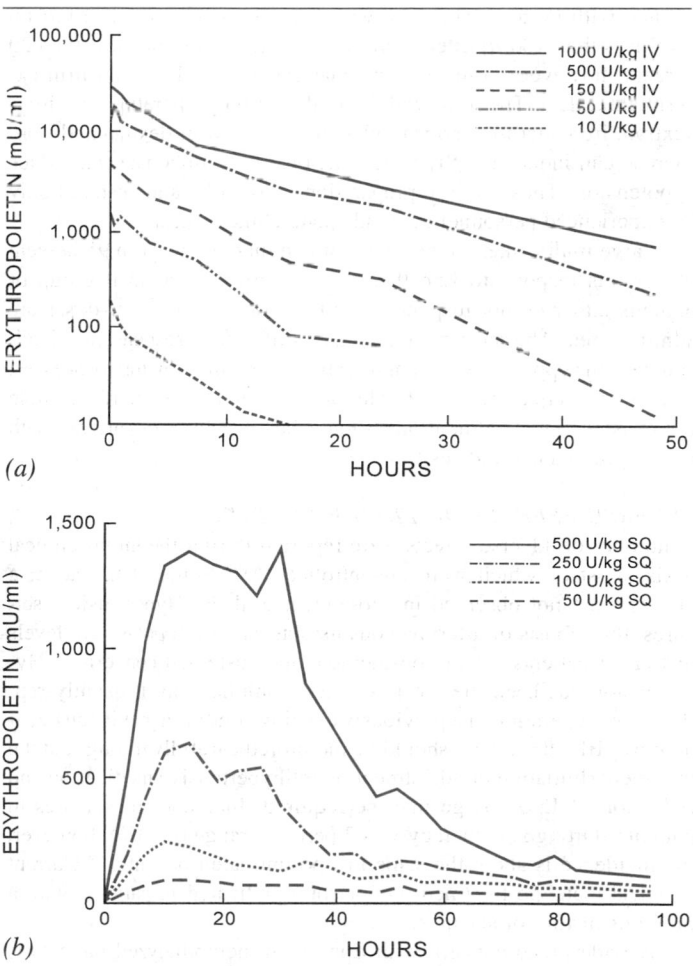

FIGURE 35-7   Pharmacokinetics of plasma Epo in normal volunteers. Plasma concentrations were measured after (a) intravenous administration and (b) subcutaneous administration.

physicians have advocated higher target hematocrits, close to the normal range, but a disappointing number of complications can occur in the near-normal hematocrit group.[94,95]

To achieve the target hematocrit within 3 to 4 months of therapy, the initial Epo dose in adult patients should be 80 to 120 units/kg/week divided into two or three subcutaneous injections or 120 to 180 units/kg/week given as three intravenous injections. The response should be monitored by measuring hematocrit and hemoglobin at least once every 2 weeks. Once the target hematocrit is reached, most adult patients can be maintained by a total Epo administration of approximately 50 to 100 units/kg/week.[96] Pediatric patients (younger than 5 years) usually require higher initial and maintenance doses. Newer Epo preparations with a more prolonged plasma half-life have been developed by modifying the sialic content of the Epo molecule (Darbepoetin).[97] Darbepoetin allows for prolongation of the periods between injections, which can now be extended to every 2 weeks. Other longer half-life Epo preparations (e.g., pegylated Epo) are being clinically evaluated. Anemia in predialysis patients can be corrected with exogenous Epo. Such corrections will not jeopardize renal function[98–100] and may prevent the development of cardiac hypertrophy.

Adequate iron supplies must be maintained for erythropoiesis. Although the National Kidney Foundation expresses a preference for intravenous iron, many physicians, especially those who administer Epo subcutaneously, prefer an oral iron preparation that provides at least 100 mg of elemental iron per day.[101] A diagnosis of absolute or functional iron deficiency should be made before patients are supplemented with IV iron. The most widely used criteria include a ferritin level less than 100 μg/liter and/or a transferrin saturation less than 20 percent; however, these recommendations are not based on firm experimental data. The most widely used IV iron preparations are iron-dextran, iron-sucrose, and iron-gluconate.[102,103] Iron-dextran and iron-sucrose can induce anaphylactic reactions; iron-gluconate can induce hypotension. Thus, IV iron preparations should be administered only by experienced personnel in an adequate clinical setting.

Large multicenter studies have shown that greater than 95 percent of patients respond to Epo therapy. Nevertheless, a small group of patients either do not respond or first respond when larger doses are administered. The most common causes of a poor response are inadequate iron supply, intercurrent infections and inflammatory processes, and splenic sequestration.[3,104] Aluminum toxicity may be responsible for resistance to treatment and should be suspected in patients with microcytic red cell indices.[105]

ADVERSE EFFECTS OF ERYTHROPOIETIN

A number of adverse effects were reported during the initial clinical trials, most of which were uncontrolled.[106,107] Some of the adverse effects were not observed in subsequent trials.[108] Hypertension, seizures, thrombosis of arteriovenous fistulas, and high potassium levels in treated patients are of considerable and sustained concern.[106] Hypertension has been the most common complication. It usually represents exaggeration of a previously existing condition, but it can occur de novo. Blood pressure should be monitored carefully throughout the treatment. Initiation or adjustment of antihypertensive medication and reduction of Epo dosage may be required. Incidence of seizures in patients starting Epo therapy was 3 percent (range 0–13%); however, the incidence is about the same in Epo-untreated patients.[108] Current belief is that Epo treatment is not contraindicated in patients with a previous history of seizures.

A widespread concern with Epo use in hemodialyzed patients is the possible effect of higher hematocrits on the native fistulas or synthetic shunts. In a review of 26 studies that enrolled 4100 patients, the average incidence of thrombosis of the access routes in patients receiving Epo was 7.5 percent.[109] This number is well within the accepted value for thrombotic episodes in dialyzed patients not receiving Epo. The occurrence of pure red cell aplasia (PRCA) as a result of the development of anti-Epo antibodies initially was very low; only three cases were reported in the first 10 years of Epo use. However, since 1998 the number of reports of patients developing severe anemia as a result of Epo-neutralizing antibodies during the course of Epo treatment have increased.[110,111] Patients with PRCA present with a low absolute reticulocyte count and resistance to Epo treatment. Marrow examinations have shown a decrease in erythroid precursors. Most of the cases occurred in Europe, and the patients received Epo subcutaneously. Most of the patients have responded to immunosuppressive therapy.[111] The finding of Epo receptors in cells and tissues of nonerythroid origin, including several tumors, is potentially important.[112,113] The consequences of long-term Epo therapy in patients with underlying tumors is unknown.

Amelioration of the anemia has resulted in a variety of beneficial changes[114–116] and in general has dramatically improved the quality of life of uremic patients.[116–118]

REFERENCES

1. Bright R: Cases and observations, illustrative of renal disease accompanied with the secretion of albuminous urine. *Guys Hosp Rep* 1:340, 1836.
2. Radtke HW, Claussner A, Erbes PM, et al: Serum erythropoietin concentration in chronic renal failure: Relationship to degree of anemia and excretory function. *Blood* 54:877, 1979.
3. Kalantar-Zadeh K, McAllister CJ, Lehn RS, et al: Effect of malnutrition-inflammation complex syndrome on EPO hyporesponsiveness in maintenance hemodialysis patients. *Am J Kidney Dis* 42:761, 2003.
4. Caro J, Brown S, Miller O, et al: Erythropoietin levels in uremic nephric and anephric patients. *J Lab Clin Med* 93:449, 1979.
5. Ragen PA, Hagedorn AB, Owen CA: Radioisotope study of anemia in chronic renal disease. *Arch Intern Med* 105:518, 1960.
6. Adamson JW, Eschbach J, Finch CA: The kidney and erythropoiesis. *Am J Med* 44:725, 1968.
7. Berry ER, Rambach WA, Alt HL, Del Greco G: Effect of peritoneal dialysis on erythrokinetics and ferrokinetics of azotemic anemia. *Trans Am Soc Artif Intern Organs* 10:415, 1965.
8. Mansell M, Grimes AJ: Red and white cell abnormalities in chronic renal failure. *Br J Haematol* 42:168, 1979.
9. Chillar RK, Desforges JF: Red cell organic phosphates in patients with chronic renal failure on maintenance haemodialysis. *Br J Haematol* 26:549, 1974.
10. Mitchell TR, Pegrum GD: The oxygen affinity of haemoglobin in chronic renal failure. *Br J Haematol* 21:463, 1971.
11. Lichtman MA, Murphy MS, Whitbeck AA, Kearney EA: Oxygen binding to haemoglobin in subjects with hypoproliferative anaemia, with and without chronic renal disease: Role of pH. *Br J Haematol* 27:439, 1974.
12. Lichtman MA, Miller OR, Freeman RB: Erythrocyte adenosine triphosphate depletion during hypophosphatemia in a uremic subject. *N Engl J Med* 280:240, 1969.
13. Torrance JD, Milne FJ, Hurwitz S, et al: Changes in oxygen delivery during hemodialysis. *Clin Nephrol* 3:53, 1975.
14. Lonergan ET, Semar M, Sterzel RB, et al: Erythrocyte transketolase activity in dialyzed patients: A reversible metabolic lesion of uremia. *N Engl J Med* 284:1399, 1971.
15. Cole CH: Decreased ouabain-sensitive adenine triphosphatase activity in the erythrocyte membrane of patients with chronic renal disease. *Clin Sci* 45:775, 1973.
16. Yawata Y, Howe R, Jacob HS: Abnormal red cell metabolism causing hemolysis in uremia: A defect potentiated by tap water hemodialysis. *Ann Intern Med* 79:362, 1973.

17. Rosenwund A, Binswanger U, Straub PW: Oxidative injury to erythrocytes, cell rigidity, and splenic hemolysis in hemodialyzed uremic patients. *Ann Intern Med* 82:460, 1975.

18. Eaton JW, Kolpin CF, Swofford HS, et al: Chlorinated urban water: A cause of dialysis-induced hemolytic anemia. *Science* 181:463, 1973.

19. Orringer EP, Mattern WDL: Formaldehyde-induced hemolysis in chronic hemodialysis. *N Engl J Med* 294:416, 1976.

20. Rao DS, Shih M, Mohini R: Effect of serum PTH and bone marrow fibrosis on the response to erythropoietin in uremia. *N Engl J Med* 328:171, 1993.

21. Okmai M, Telfer N, Ansani A, et al: Erythrocyte survival in chronic renal failure: Role of secondary hyperparathyroidism. *J Clin Invest* 76:1695, 1985.

22. Brain MC: The haemolytic-uremic syndrome. *Semin Hematol* 6:162, 1969.

23. Capelli JP, Wesson LG, Erslev AJ: Malignant hypertension and red cell fragmentation syndrome. *Ann Intern Med* 64:128, 1966.

24. Hosler GA, Cusumano AM, Hutchins GM: Thrombotic thrombocytopenic purpura and hemolytic uremic syndrome are distinct pathologic entities. *Arch Pathol Lab Med* 127:834, 2003.

25. Gasser C, Gautier E, Steck A, et al: Hämolytisch-urämische Syndrome: Bilaterale Nierenrindennekrosen bei akuten erworbenen hämolytischen Anämien. *Schweiz Med Wochenschr* 85:906, 1955.

26. Lieberman E, Heuser E, Donnell GN, et al: Hemolytic-uremic syndrome: Clinical and pathological considerations. *N Engl J Med* 275:277, 1966.

27. Mitra D, Jaffe EA, Weksler B, et al: Thrombotic thrombocytopenic purpura and sporadic hemolytic-uremic syndrome plasmas induce apoptosis in restricted lineages of human microvascular endothelial cells. *Blood* 89:1224, 1997.

28. Moake JL: Haemolytic-uraemic syndrome. Basic science. *Lancet* 343:393, 1994.

29. Miller RP, Denny WF: Hemolytic anemia during acute renal failure: Observations on plasma erythropoietin levels. *South Med J* 61:29, 1968.

30. Furlan M, Robles R, Galbusera M, et al: Von Willebrand factor–cleaving protease in thrombotic thrombocytopenic purpura and the hemolytic-uremic syndrome. *N Engl J Med* 339:1578, 1998.

31. Tsai HM, Lian EC: Antibodies to von Willebrand factor–cleaving protease in acute thrombotic thrombocytopenic purpura. *N Engl J Med* 339:1585, 1998.

32. Lin CC, King KL, Chao YW, et al: Tacrolimus-associated hemolytic uremic syndrome: A case analysis. *J Nephrol* 16:580, 2003.

33. Castaldi PA, Gorman DJ: Disordered platelet function in renal disease, in *Hemostasis and Thrombosis*, edited by RW Colman, J Hirsch, VJ Marder, EW Salzman, p 750. Lippincott, Philadelphia, 1987.

34. Horowitz HJ, Stein JM, Cohen BD, White JM: Further studies on the platelet inhibitory effect of guanidinosuccinic acid and its role in uremic bleeding. *Am J Med* 49:336, 1970.

35. Fisher JW: Mechanism of the anemia of chronic renal failure. *Nephron* 25:106, 1980.

36. Bozzini CE, Devoto FCH, Tomio JM: Decreased responsiveness of hematopoietic tissue to erythropoietin in acutely uremic rats. *J Lab Clin Med* 68:411, 1966.

37. Radtke HW, Rege AB, La Mouche MB, et al: Identification of spermine as an inhibitor of erythropoiesis in patients with chronic renal failure. *J Clin Invest* 67:1623, 1981.

38. Caro J, Erslev AJ: Uremic inhibitors of erythropoiesis. *Semin Nephrol* 5:128, 1985.

39. Brancaccio D, Cozzolino M, Gallieni M: Hyperparathyroidism and anemia in uremic subjects: A combined therapeutic approach. *J Am Soc Nephrol* 15:S21, 2004.

40. Eschbach JW, Haley NR, Egrie JC, Adamson JW: A comparison of the responses to rHEpo in normal and uremic subjects. *Kidney Int* 42:407, 1992.

41. Erslev AJ, Besarab A: Erythropoietin in the pathogenesis and treatment of the anemia of chronic renal disease. *Kidney Int* 51:622, 1997.

42. Eschbach JW, Cook JD, Scribner BH, Finch CA: Iron balance in hemodialysis patients. *Ann Intern Med* 87:710, 1977.

43. Wills MR, Savory J: Aluminum poisoning: Dialysis encephalopathy, osteomalacia, and anaemia. *Lancet* 1:29, 1983.

44. Rifkind D, Kravetz HM, Knight V, Schade AL: Urinary excretion of iron binding protein in the nephrotic syndrome. *N Engl J Med* 265:115, 1961.

45. Hampers CL, Streiff R, Nathan DK, et al: Megaloblastic hematopoiesis in uremia and in patients on long-term hemodialysis. *N Engl J Med* 276:551, 1967.

46. Erslev AJ: Humoral regulation of red cell production. *Blood* 8:349, 1953.

47. Jacobson LO, Goldwasser E, Fried W, Plazak L: Role of the kidney in erythropoiesis. *Nature* 179:633, 1957.

48. Erslev AJ: In vitro production of erythropoietin by kidneys perfused with a serum-free solution. *Blood* 44:77, 1974.

49. Bondurant MC, Koury M: Anemia induces accumulation of erythropoietin mRNA in the kidney and liver. *Mol Cell Biol* 6:2731, 1986.

50. Beru N, McDonald J, Lacombe C, Goldwasser E: Expression of the erythropoietin gene. *Mol Cell Biol* 6:2571, 1986.

51. Schuster SJ, Wilson J, Erslev AJ, Caro J: Physiologic regulation and tissue localization of renal erythropoietin mRNA. *Blood* 70:316, 1987.

52. Lacombe C, DaSilva J-L, Bruneval P, et al: Peritubular cells are the site of erythropoietin synthesis in the murine hypoxic kidney. *J Clin Invest* 81:620, 1988.

53. Koury ST, Bondurant MC, Koury MJ: Localization of erythropoietin-synthesizing cells in murine kidneys by in situ hybridization. *Blood* 71:524, 1988.

54. Maxwell PH, Ferguson DJP, Nicholls LG, et al: Sites of erythropoietin production. *Kidney Int* 51:393, 1997.

55. Maxwell PH, Ratcliffe PJ: The erythropoietin-producing cells. *Exp Nephrol* 4:309, 1996.

56. Schuster SJ, Badiavas E, Costa-Giomi P, et al: Stimulation of erythropoietin gene transcription during hypoxia and cobalt exposure. *Blood* 73:13, 1989.

57. Beck I, Ramirez S, Weinmann R, Caro J: Enhancer element at the 3'-flanking region controls transcriptional response to hypoxia in the human erythropoietin gene. *J Biol Chem* 266:15563, 1991.

58. Semenza GL: Hypoxia-inducible factor 1: Master regulator of O_2 homeostasis. *Curr Opin Genet Dev* 8:588, 1998.

59. Salceda S, Caro J: Hypoxia-inducible factor 1alpha (HIF-1alpha) protein is rapidly degraded by the ubiquitin-proteasome system under normoxic conditions. Its stabilization by hypoxia depends on redox-induced changes. *J Biol Chem* 272:22642, 1997.

60. Huang LE, Gu J, Schau M, Bunn HF: Regulation of hypoxia-inducible factor 1alpha is mediated by an O_2-dependent domain via the ubiquitin-proteasome pathway. *Proc Natl Acad Sci U S A* 95:7987, 1998.

61. Maxwell PH, Wiesener MS, Chang GW, et al: The tumour suppressor protein VHL targets hypoxia-inducible factors for oxygen-dependent proteolysis. *Nature* 399:271, 1999.

62. Jaakkola P, Mole DR, Tian YM, et al: Targeting of HIF-alpha to the von Hippel-Lindau ubiquitylation complex by O_2-regulated prolyl hydroxylation. *Science* 292:468, 2001.

63. Ivan M, Kondo K, Yang H, et al: HIF-alpha targeted for VHL-mediated destruction by proline hydroxylation: Implications for O_2 sensing. *Science* 292:464, 2001.

64. Epstein AC, Gleadle JM, McNeill LA, et al: C. elegans EGL-9 and mammalian homologs define a family of dioxygenases that regulate HIF by prolyl hydroxylation. *Cell* 107:43, 2001.

65. Pastore Y, Jedlickova K, Guan Y, et al: Mutations of von Hippel-Lindau tumor-suppressor gene and congenital polycythemia. *Am J Hum Genet* 73:412, 2003.

66. Erslev AJ, Caro J, Kansu E, Silver R: Renal and extrarenal erythropoietin production in anemic rats. *Br J Haematol* 45:65, 1980.

67. Koury JT, Bondurant MC, Koury MJ, Semenza GL: Localization of cells producing erythropoietin in murine liver by in situ hybridization. *Blood* 77:2497, 1991.

68. Schuster SJ, Koury S, Borher M, et al: Cellular sites of extrarenal and renal erythropoietin production in anemic rats. *Br J Haematol* 81:153, 1992.

69. Maxwell PH, Ferguson DJ, Osmond MK, et al: Expression of a homologously recombined erythropoietin-SV40 T antigen fusion gene in mouse liver: Evidence for erythropoietin production by Ito cells. *Blood* 84:1823, 1994.

70. Köchling J, Curtis PT, Madan A: Regulation of human erythropoietin gene induction by upstream flanking sequences in transgenic mice. *Br J Haematol* 103:960, 1998.

71. Dagher FJ, Ramos E, Erslev AJ, et al: Are the native kidneys responsible for erythrocytosis in renal allorecipients? *Transplantation* 28:496, 1979.

72. Walle AJ, Wong GY, Clemons GK, et al: Erythropoietin-hematocrit feedback circuit in the anemia of end-stage renal disease. *Kidney Int* 31:1205, 1987.

73. Eckardt K-U, Druecke T, Leski M, Kurtz A: Unutilized reserves: The production capacity for erythropoietin appears to be conserved in chronic renal disease. *Contrib Nephrol* 88:18, 1991.

74. Schwartz SO, Motto SA: The diagnostic significance of "burr" red blood cells. *Am J Med Sci* 218:563, 1949.

75. Brecher G, Bessis M: Present status of spiculed red cells and their relationship to the discocyte-echinocyte transformation: A critical review. *Blood* 40:333, 1972.

76. Goldblum SE, Reed WP: Host defenses and immunologic alterations associated with chronic hemodialysis. *Ann Intern Med* 93:597, 1980.

77. Craddock PR, Fehr J, Brigham KL, et al: Complement and leukocyte-mediated pulmonary dysfunction in hemodialysis. *N Engl J Med* 296:769, 1977.

78. Pasternack A, Wahlberg P: Bone marrow in acute renal failure. *Acta Med Scand* 181:505, 1967.

79. Eschbach JW, Funk D, Adamson JW, et al: Erythropoiesis in patients with renal failure undergoing chronic dialysis. *N Engl J Med* 276:653, 1967.

80. Zappacosta AR, Caro J, Erslev A: The normalization of hematocrit in end-stage renal disease patients on continuous ambulatory peritoneal dialysis: The role of erythropoietin. *Am J Med* 72:53, 1982.

81. Eschbach JW, Adamson JW: Improvement in the anemia of chronic renal failure with fluoxymesterone. *Ann Intern Med* 78:527, 1973.

82. Neff MS, Goldberg J, Slifkin RF, et al: A comparison of androgens for anemia in patients on hemodialysis. *N Engl J Med* 304:871, 1981.

83. Winearls CG, Oliver DO, Pippard MJ, et al: Effect of human erythropoietin derived from recombinant DNA on the anemia of patients maintained by chronic haemodialysis. *Lancet* 2:1175, 1986.

84. Eschbach JW, Egrie JC, Downing MR, et al: Correction of the anemia of end-stage renal disease with recombinant human erythropoietin. *N Engl J Med* 316:73, 1987.

85. Recny MA, Scoble HA, Kim Y: Structural characterization of natural human urinary and recombinant DNA-derived erythropoietin. *J Biol Chem* 262:17156, 1987.

86. Tsuda E, Kawanishi G, Ueda M, et al: The role of carbohydrate in recombinant human erythropoietin. *Eur J Biochem* 188:405, 1990.

87. NKF-DOA: Anemia work group: Guidelines. *Am J Kidney Dis* 30:8196, 1997.

88. Besarab A, Flaharty KK, Erslev A, et al: Clinical pharmacology and economics of recombinant human erythropoietin in end stage renal disease: The case for subcutaneous administration. *J Am Soc Nephrol* 2:1405, 1992.

89. Watson A, Gimenez L, Cotton J, et al: Treatment of anemia of chronic renal failure with subcutaneous rHEpo. *Am J Med* 89:432, 1990.

90. Flaharty KK, Caro J, Erslev A, et al: Pharmacokinetics and erythropoietic response to human recombinant erythropoietin in healthy men. *Clin Pharmacol Ther* 47:557, 1990.

91. Spivak J, Cotes M: Pharmacokinetics of erythropoietin, in *Erythropoietin: Molecular, Cellular, and Clinical Biology*, edited by AJ Erslev, JW Adamson, JW Eschbach, CG Winearls, p 62. Johns Hopkins University Press, Baltimore, 1992.

92. Newmayer H, Brockmoller J, Fritscka E, et al: Pharmacokinetics of rHEpo after sc administration and in long-term IV treatment in patients on hemodialysis. *Contrib Nephrol* 76:131, 1989.

93. Kaufman JS, Reda DJ, Fye CL, et al: Subcutaneous compared with intravenous epoietin in patients receiving hemodialysis. *N Engl J Med* 339:578, 1998.

94. Eschbach J, Adamson J: Guidelines for rHEpo therapy. *Am J Kidney Dis* 14(suppl 1):2, 1989.

95. Besarab A, Bolton WK, Browne JK, et al: The effects of normal as compared with low hematocrit values in patients with cardiac disease who are receiving hemodialysis and epoietin. *N Engl J Med* 389:584, 1998.

96. Cazzola M: How and when to use erythropoietin. *Curr Opin Hematol* 5:103, 1998.

97. Egrie JC, Dwyer E, Browne JK, et al: Darbepoetin alfa has a longer circulating half-life and greater in vivo potency than recombinant human erythropoietin. *Exp Hematol* 31:290, 2003.

98. Koene R, Frenken LA: Renal function of pre-dialysis patients during treatment with rHEpo. *Contrib Nephrol* 80:192, 1991.

99. Kuriyama H, Tomonari H, Yoshida H, et al: Reversal of anemia by erythropoietin therapy retards the progression of chronic renal failure, especially in non-diabetic patients. *Nephron* 77:176, 1997.

100. Rossert J, Fouqueray B, Boffa JJ: Anemia management and the delay of chronic renal failure progression. *J Am Soc Nephrol* 14:S173, 2003.

101. Sunder-Plassmann G, Horl WH: Erythropoietin and iron. *Clin Nephrol* 47:141, 1997.

102. Fishbane S: Safety in iron management. *Am J Kidney Dis* 41:18, 2003.

103. Yee J, Besarab A: Iron sucrose: The oldest iron therapy becomes new. *Am J Kidney Dis* 40:1111, 2002.

104. Drueke T: Modulating factors in the hemopoietic response to erythropoietin. *Am J Kidney Dis* 18(suppl 1):87, 1991.

105. Rosenlof K, Fyhrquist F, Tenfunen R: Erythropoietin, aluminum and anemia in patients on hemodialysis. *Lancet* 335:247, 1990.

106. Casati S, Passerini P, Campise MR, et al: Benefits and risks of protracted treatment with human recombinant erythropoietin in patients having haemodialysis. *Br Med J* 295:1017, 1987.

107. Eschbach J: The anemia of chronic renal failure: Pathophysiology and the effects of rHEpo. *Kidney Int* 25:134, 1989.

108. Buccianti G, Colombi L, Battistel V: Use of recombinant human erythropoietin (rh-EPO) in the treatment of anemia in hemodialysis patients: A multicenter Italian experience. *Haematologica* 78:111, 1993.

109. Laupacis A: Changes in quality of life and functional capacity in hemodialysis patients treated with recombinant human erythropoietin. *Semin Nephrol* 10:11, 1990.

110. Casadevall N, Nataf J, Viron B, et al: Pure red-cell aplasia and anti-erythropoietin antibodies in patients treated with recombinant erythropoietin. *N Engl J Med* 348:469, 2002.

111. Eckardt K-U, Casadevall N: Pure red-cell aplasia due to anti-erythropoietin antibodies. *Nephrol Dial Transplant* 18:865, 2003.

112. Arcasoy MO, Karayal AK, Chou SC, et al: Functional significance of erythropoietin receptor expression in breast cancer. *Lab Invest* 82:911, 2002.

113. Loprinzi C: Epoetin for cancer patients: A boon or a danger? *J Natl Cancer Inst* 95:1820, 2003.

114. Moia M, Vizotto L, Cattaneo M, et al: Improvement in the haemostatic defect of uraemia after treatment with recombinant human erythropoietin. *Lancet* 2:1227, 1987.

115. Schaefer R, Kokot F, Heidland A: Improvement of rHEpo on sexual function on hemodialyzed patients. *Contrib Nephrol* 76:273, 1989.

116. Silberberg J, Racine N, Barre P, Sniderman AD: Regression of left ventricular hypertrophy in dialysis patients following correction of anemia with recombinant human erythropoietin. *Can J Cardiol* 6:1, 1990.

117. Evans RW, Rader B, Manninen DL: The quality of life of hemodialysis recipients treated with recombinant human erythropoietin. *JAMA* 263: 825, 1990.

118. Adamson JW, Eschbach JW: Erythropoietin for end-stage renal disease [editorial]. *N Engl J Med* 339:625, 1998.

ANEMIA OF ENDOCRINE DISORDERS

XYLINA T. GREGG

JOSEF T. PRCHAL

Anemia may be the first recognized manifestation of an endo-crine disorder. Anemia resulting from endocrine disease gen-erally is mild to moderate; however, a decreased plasma vol-ume in some of these disorders may mask the severity of anemia. Anemia in endocrine deficiency states may be physio-logic as a result of decreased oxygen requirements, but a direct influence of hormones on erythropoiesis may contribute to ane-mia. The pathophysiologic basis of the anemia seen in endo-crine disorders is not well understood.

THYROID DYSFUNCTION

HYPOTHYROIDISM

Since the 1880s, anemia has been a recognized complication of thy-roidectomy[1] or other causes of hypothyroidism.[2] The anemia usually is mild to moderate, with hemoglobin concentrations rarely less than 8 to 9 g/dl (80–90 g/liter). A concomitant decrease in plasma volume[3] makes the hemoglobin concentration an unreliable indicator of the red cell mass.[4] Dogs subjected to thyroidectomy have a normocytic, nor-mochromic anemia that is associated with reticulocytopenia and marrow erythroid hypoplasia.[5] In humans with hypothyroidism, the associated anemia has been described variably as normocytic, mac-rocytic, or microcytic.[6] Coexisting deficiencies of iron, B_{12}, and folate may explain some of the heterogeneity. Hypothyroidism may contrib-ute to the development of iron deficiency as a result of increased pre-disposition to menorrhagia.[7] Males with hypothyroidism may be iron deficient, possibly because of an associated achlorhydria[8] or because thyroid hormone augments iron absorption.[9,10] Conversely, iron defi-ciency impairs thyroid hormone synthesis by reducing the activity of heme-dependent thyroid peroxidase.[11] Although macrocytosis may be seen in uncomplicated anemia of hypothyroidism,[12] significant ele-vations in mean corpuscular volume usually result from accompanying B_{12} or folate deficiency.[13] Nevertheless, macrocytosis is not a sensitive means of identifying patients with hypothyroidism complicated by B_{12} deficiency.[12] An association between hypothyroidism and pernicious anemia is established,[14–16] but the underlying mechanism is unknown. When these confounding causes of anemia are excluded, it is evident that anemia also is a direct consequence of thyroid hormone defi-ciency.[13,17]

In hypothyroid humans and thyroidectomized animals, the red cell life span is normal, and results of ferrokinetic studies are compatible with hypoproliferative erythropoiesis.[5,18,19] Administration of thyroid hormones increases the rate of red cell production in experimental animals,[20,21] whereas thyroidectomy decreases red cell production.[22,23] Because thyroid hormones affect the cellular needs for oxygen, these

responses are compatible with an appropriate physiologic adjustment. Evidence of a direct effect of thyroid hormones on erythropoiesis ex-ists. *In vitro* studies have shown that triiodothyronine (T_3), thyroxine (T_4), and noncalorigenic resin triiodothyronine (rT_3) all potentiate the effect of erythropoietin on erythroid colony formation.[24] Thyroid hor-mones increase hypoxia-induced production of erythropoietin in the rat kidney and a human hepatoma cell line.[25] Other *in vitro* studies have shown an inhibitory effect of T_3 on erythroid colony formation, particularly in combination with all-*trans*-retinoic acid.[26]

The response to thyroid hormone therapy is gradual. Slow im-provement in hemoglobin concentration is seen over a several-month period.[12,13] White blood cell and platelet counts usually are unaffected in hypothyroidism. However, pancytopenia in association with mar-row hypoplasia has been reported in a patient with myxedema coma; the hematologic abnormalities in this patient resolved with thyroid hormone replacement.[27]

HYPERTHYROIDISM

Although thyroid hormone administration increases red cell produc-tion in animals,[20,21] humans with hyperthyroidism generally do not have polycythemia. Anemia is present in 10 to 25 percent of these patients.[28–30] This finding may be the result of increased plasma vol-ume[3]; however, decreased red cell survival[31] and ineffective erythro-poiesis[32] also have been described in patients with hyperthyroidism. Treatment with [131]I (radioactive iodine)[30] or methimazole[33] has ame-liorated the anemia. A patient with autoimmune hemolytic anemia and hyperthyroidism has been described; the hemolysis in this patient abated with treatment of the hyperthyroidism.[34]

ADRENAL INSUFFICIENCY

A normocytic normochromic anemia may be seen in primary adrenal insufficiency (Addison disease),[35,36] but the anemia may be masked by the concomitant reduction in plasma volume that is common in this disease. In a series of patients with Addison disease, untreated patients had normal hemoglobin levels but developed transient anemia after initiation of hormone replacement therapy (presumably secondary to an increased plasma volume).[37]

In experimental animals, adrenalectomy causes a mild anemia that responds to glucocorticoids or erythropoietin.[23,35,38] The pathophysi-ologic basis of the anemia and any influence of adrenal cortical hor-mones on erythropoiesis are not well defined. Glucocorticoids interact with erythropoietin *in vitro* to enhance erythroid colony prolifera-tion.[39,40] Glucocorticoid receptors, activated by their cognate ligand, initiate Janus kinase 2 phosphorylation-mediated cytoplasmic signal transduction, which may stimulate erythropoiesis by a mechanism shared with erythropoietin (see Chap. 30). Polycythemia has been re-ported in Cushing syndrome,[41,42] primary aldosteronism,[43] and Bartter syndrome.[44] Pheochromocytomas are rarely associated with polycy-themia. This finding is believed to be the result of autonomous eryth-ropoietin production by the tumor,[45] often mediated by von Hippel-Lindau mutations that cause or contribute to pheochromocytoma development (see Chap. 56).

Pernicious anemia occurs in patients with autoimmune adrenal in-sufficiency but is seen primarily in patients with type I polyglandular autoimmune syndrome, whose other manifestations include mucocu-taneous candidiasis and hypoparathyroidism.[46,47] Up to 15 percent of these patients develop pernicious anemia, often at a young age.[46] Ane-mia as a result of primary erythropoietin deficiency has been reported in one patient with this syndrome.[48]

ANDROGEN DEFICIENCY

Sexually mature males have higher hemoglobin levels than prepubertal males, older males, and females.[49] The difference is attributed to androgen production. Orchiectomy results in a median decrease in hemoglobin concentration of 1.2 g/dl (12 g/liter).[50] "Medical" castration with combined androgen blockade by gonadotropin-releasing agonists and antiandrogens also causes anemia.[51]

The erythropoietic effects of androgens are well documented[52,53] and have been widely exploited for the treatment of various anemias, especially before the development of recombinant erythropoietin. Androgen therapy reverses anemia and may even cause polycythemia.[53] Testosterone therapy in hypogonadal men increased the mean hematocrit from 38.0 to 43.1 percent within 3 months.[54] The mechanism of androgen action appears to be complex, with evidence for stimulation of erythropoietin secretion[55] and a direct effect on the marrow.[56] Androgen receptors have been identified in the marrow cells of human males and females. The cells expressing the receptors include stromal cells, endothelial cells, macrophages, and myeloid precursors but not erythroid cells.[57]

Estrogens may have a suppressive effect on erythropoiesis. Exogenous administration of large doses of estrogen led to moderately severe anemia,[58,59] and castration of female rats resulted in an increase in hemoglobin.[60]

PITUITARY INSUFFICIENCY

The most common cause of pituitary insufficiency is pituitary tumors or consequences of their therapy.[61] Other etiologies include hypothalamic tumors or dysfunction, sarcoidosis or other infiltrative diseases, pituitary hemorrhage or infarct, genetic causes, or idiopathic pituitary failure. Regardless of the cause, hypopituitarism results in a moderately severe normochromic normocytic anemia, with an average hemoglobin of 10 g/dl (100 g/liter).[35,62,63] Anemia and erythroid hypoplasia have been described in hypophysectomized animals.[64-66]

In rats, removal of the posterior lobe of the pituitary, which secretes vasopressin and oxytocin, does not result in anemia.[67] Thus, the anemia of hypopituitarism presumably results from the absence of the anterior lobe hormones, adrenocorticotropic hormone, thyroid-stimulating hormone, follicle-stimulating hormone, luteinizing hormone, growth hormone, and prolactin, although the exact role of each of these hormones in the pathogenesis of anemia is unknown. The resulting deficiencies of thyroid hormones, adrenal hormones, and androgens are likely the major contributors to anemia. Combined adrenalectomy and thyroidectomy in animals results in an anemia that is similar but not identical to that seen after hypophysectomy.[68] A correlation between low testosterone levels and anemia has been observed in human males with hypopituitarism resulting from nonfunctioning pituitary adenomas.[69] The data regarding the role of growth hormone are conflicting. Growth hormone stimulates erythropoietin-induced erythropoiesis in vitro,[70,71] but whether this is of physiologic significance is unclear.[72] Children with isolated growth hormone deficiency become anemic.[73] Growth hormone replacement therapy in adults with growth hormone deficiency increased hemoglobin levels in one study but not in another.[74,75] Limited information about the influence of prolactin is available.[76] Prolactin administration in mice increased the number of erythroid and myeloid progenitor cells and partially corrected anemia induced by azidothymidine.[77] Metoclopramide, which stimulates prolactin secretion, improved hemoglobin levels or reduced transfusions in three of nine patients with Diamond-Blackfan anemia.[78] The prolactin receptor can substitute for the erythropoietin receptor in in vitro studies of erythroid differentiation.[79,80]

Red cell survival is normal in hypopituitarism, but the marrow is hypoplastic. The results of ferrokinetic studies are consistent with decreased erythropoiesis.[35,66,81] In addition to anemia, leukopenia and even pancytopenia can occur.[82,83] Replacement therapy with a combination of thyroid, adrenal, and gonadal hormones usually effectively corrects anemia and other cytopenias.[83,84] Erythropoietin therapy also was effective in one case of postoperative hypopituitarism refractory to hormone replacement therapy.[85]

HYPERPARATHYROIDISM

Anemia not attributable to other causes is present in 3 to 5 percent of patients with primary hyperparathyroidism; these patients usually have severe hyperthyroidism.[86,87] The anemia is normochromic and normocytic and resolves or improves after parathyroidectomy.[86,87] The cause of the anemia is unknown; marrow fibrosis has been described in a few patients.[86]

Studies using crude bovine extracts described an inhibitory effect of parathyroid hormone (PTH) on murine erythroid colony formation.[88] However, studies using purified PTH did not demonstrate an inhibitory effect on human or mouse erythroid progenitors.[89,90]

Although anemia in patients with renal failure is multifactorial, secondary hyperparathyroidism may contribute to refractoriness to erythropoietin therapy. Parathyroidectomy or medical treatment of hyperparathyroidism may improve anemia in some patients.[91-93]

REFERENCES

1. Kocher T: Ueber Kropfexstirpation und Ihre Folgen. *Arch Klin Chir* 29: 254, 1883.
2. Charcot M: Myxedéme, cachexie pachydermique ou état cretinoide. *Gaz Hop Paris* 54:73, 1881.
3. Muldowney F, Crooks J, Wayne E: The total red cell mass in thyrotoxicosis and myxoedema. *Clin Sci* 16:309, 1957.
4. Das K, Mukherjee M, Sarkar T, et al: Erythropoiesis and erythropoietin in hypo- and hyperthyroidism. *J Clin Endocrinol Metab* 40:211, 1975.
5. Cline M, Berlin N: Erythropoiesis and red cell survival in the hypothyroid dog. *Am J Physiol* 204:415, 1963.
6. Bomford R: Anemia in myxedema and the role of the thyroid gland in erythropoiesis. *Q J Med* 7:495, 1938.
7. Goldsmith R: The menstrual pattern in thyroid disease. *J Clin Endocrinol Metab* 12:846, 1952.
8. Lerman J, Means J: The gastric secretion in exophthalmic goiter and myxoedema. *J Clin Invest* 11:167, 1932.
9. Pirzio-Biroli G, Bothwell T, Finch C: Iron absorption: II. The absorption of radio iron administered with standard meal. *J Lab Clin Med* 51:37, 1958.
10. Donati RM, Fletcher JW, Warnecke MA, Gallagher NI: Erythropoiesis in hypothyroidism. *Proc Soc Exp Biol Med* 144:78, 1973.
11. Zimmermann M, Kohrle J: The impact of iron and selenium deficiencies on iodine and thyroid metabolism: Biochemistry and relevance to public health. *Thyroid* 12:867, 2002.
12. Horton L, Coburn R, England J, Himsworth R: The haematology of hypothyroidism. *Q J Med* 45:101, 1976.
13. Tudhope GR, Wilson GM: Anaemia in hypothyroidism. Incidence, pathogenesis, and response to treatment. *Q J Med* 29:513, 1960.
14. Green ST, Ng JP, Chan-Lam D: Insulin-dependent diabetes mellitus, myasthenia gravis, pernicious anaemia, autoimmune thyroiditis and autoimmune adrenalitis in a single patient. *Scott Med J* 33:213, 1988.
15. Carmel R, Spencer CA: Clinical and subclinical thyroid disorders associated with pernicious anemia. Observations on abnormal thyroid-stimulating hormone levels and on a possible association of blood group O with hyperthyroidism. *Arch Intern Med* 142:1465, 1982.
16. Petite J, Rosset N, Chapuis B, Jeannet M: Genetic factors predisposing to autoimmune diseases. Study of HLA antigens in a family with pernicious anemia and thyroid diseases. *Schweiz Med Wochenschr* 117: 2032, 1987.

17. Hines JD, Halsted CH, Griggs RC, Harris JW: Megaloblastic anemia secondary to folate deficiency associated with hypothyroidism. *Ann Intern Med* 68:792, 1968.

18. Kiely JM, Purnell DC, Owen CA Jr: Erythrokinetics in myxedema. *Ann Intern Med* 67:533, 1967.

19. Axelrod AR, Berman L: The bone marrow in hyperthyroidism and hypothyroidism. *Blood* 6:436, 1951.

20. Donati RM, Warnecke MA, Gallagher NI: Effect of Triiodothyronine administration on erythrocyte radioiron incorporation in rats. *Proc Soc Exp Biol Med* 115:405, 1964.

21. Shalet M, Coe D, Reissmann KR: Mechanism of erythropoietic action of thyroid hormone. *Proc Soc Exp Biol Med* 123:443, 1966.

22. Gordon A, Kadow P, Finkelstein G, Charipper H: The thyroid and blood regeneration in the rat. *Am J Med Sci* 212:385, 1946.

23. Crafts RC: The effect of endocrines on the formed elements of the blood: I. The effects of hypophysectomy, thyroidectomy and adrenalectomy on the blood of the adult female rat. *Endocrinology* 29:596, 1941.

24. Golde D, Bersch N, Chopra I, Cline M: Thyroid hormones stimulate erythropoiesis in vitro. *Br J Haematol* 37:173, 1977.

25. Fandrey J, Pagel H, Frede S, et al: Thyroid hormones enhance hypoxia-induced erythropoietin production in vitro. *Exp Hematol* 22:272, 1994.

26. Perrin M, Blanchet J, Mouchiroud G: Modulation of human and mouse erythropoiesis by thyroid hormone and retinoic acid: Evidence for specific effects at different steps of the erythroid pathway. *Hematol Cell Ther* 39:19, 1997.

27. Song S, McCallum C, Campbell I: Hypoplastic anaemia complicating myxoedema coma. *Scott Med J* 43:149, 1998.

28. Rivlin RS, Wagner HN Jr: Anemia in hyperthyroidism. *Ann Intern Med* 70:507, 1969.

29. Nightingale S, Vitek PJ, Himsworth RL: The haematology of hyperthyroidism. *Q J Med* 47:35, 1978.

30. Perlman J, Sternthal P: Effect of ^{131}I on the anemia of hyperthyroidism. *J Chronic Dis* 36:405, 1983.

31. McClellan J, Donegan C, Thorup OA, Leavell BS: Survival time of the erythrocyte in myxedema and hyperthyroidism. *J Lab Clin Med* 51:91, 1958.

32. Donati RM, Warnecke MA, Gallagher NI: Ferrokinetics in hyperthyroidism. *Ann Intern Med* 63:945, 1965.

33. Jyo-Oshiro Y, Nomura S, Fukushima T, et al: Primary hyperthyroidism induced erythropoietin-resistant anemia? *Intern Med* 36:903, 1997.

34. Ogihara T, Katoh H, Yoshitake H, et al: Hyperthyroidism associated with autoimmune hemolytic anemia and periodic paralysis: A report of a case in which antihyperthyroid therapy alone was effective against hemolysis. *Jpn J Med* 26:401, 1987.

35. Daughaday W, Williams R, Daland G: The effect of endocrinopathies on the blood. *Blood* 3:1342, 1948.

36. Baez-Villasenor J, Rath C, Finch C: The blood picture in Addison's disease. *Blood* 3:769, 1958.

37. Irvine WJ, Stewart AG, Scarth L: A clinical and immunological study of adrenocortical insufficiency (Addison's disease). *Clin Exp Immunol* 2:31, 1967.

38. Van Dyke DC, Contopoulos AN, Williams BS, et al: Hormonal factors influencing erythropoiesis. *Acta Haematol* 11:203, 1954.

39. von Lindern M, Zauner W, Mellitzer G, et al: The glucocorticoid receptor cooperates with the erythropoietin receptor and c-kit to enhance and sustain proliferation of erythroid progenitors in vitro. *Blood* 94:550, 1999.

40. Golde DW, Bersch N, Cline MJ: Potentiation of erythropoiesis in vitro by dexamethasone. *J Clin Invest* 57:57, 1976.

41. Plotz CM, Knowlton AI, Ragan C: The natural history of Cushing's syndrome. *Am J Med* 13:597, 1952.

42. Ross EJ, Marshall-Jones P, Friedman M: Cushing's syndrome: Diagnostic criteria. *Q J Med* 35:149, 1966.

43. Mann DL, Gallagher NI, Donati RM: Erythrocytosis and primary aldosteronism. *Ann Intern Med* 66:335, 1967.

44. Erkelens DW, Statius van Eps LW: Bartter's syndrome and erythrocytosis. *Am J Med* 55:711, 1973.

45. Drenou B, Le Tulzo Y, Caulet-Maugendre S, et al: Pheochromocytoma and secondary erythrocytosis: Role of tumour erythropoietin secretion. *Nouv Rev Fr Hematol* 37:197, 1995.

46. Neufeld M, Maclaren NK, Blizzard RM: Two types of autoimmune Addison's disease associated with different polyglandular autoimmune (PGA) syndromes. *Medicine (Baltimore)* 60:355, 1981.

47. Eisenbarth GS, Gottlieb PA: Autoimmune polyendocrine syndromes. *N Engl J Med* 350:2068, 2004.

48. Toonkel R, Levine M, Gardner L: Erythropoietin-deficient anemia associated with autoimmune polyglandular syndrome type I. *Am J Hematol* 75:84, 2004.

49. Hawkins WW, Speck E, Leonard VG: Variation of the hemoglobin level with age and sex. *Blood* 9:999, 1954.

50. Fonseca R, Rajkumar SV, White WL, et al: Anemia after orchiectomy. *Am J Hematol* 59:230, 1998.

51. Bogdanos J, Karamanolakis D, Milathianakis C, et al: Combined androgen blockade-induced anemia in prostate cancer patients without bone involvement. *Anticancer Res* 23:1757, 2003.

52. Kennedy BJ, Gilbertsen AS: Increased erythropoiesis induced by androgenic-hormone therapy. *N Engl J Med* 256:719, 1957.

53. Shahidi NT: Androgens and erythropoiesis. *N Engl J Med* 289:72, 1973.

54. Snyder P, Peachey H, Berlin J, et al: Effects of testosterone replacement in hypogonadal men. *J Clin Endocrinol Metab* 85:2670, 2000.

55. Alexanian R: Erythropoietin and erythropoiesis in anemic man following androgens. *Blood* 33:564, 1969.

56. Beran M, Spitzer G, Verma D: Testosterone and synthetic androgens improve the in vitro survival of human marrow progenitor cells in serum-free suspension cultures. *J Lab Clin Med* 99:247, 1982.

57. Mantalaris A, Panoskaltsis N, Sakai Y, et al: Localization of androgen receptor expression in human bone marrow. *J Pathol* 193:361, 2001.

58. Dukes PP, Goldwasser E: Inhibition of erythropoiesis by estrogens. *Endocrinology* 69:21, 1961.

59. Piliero SJ, Medici PT, Haber C: The interrelationships of the endocrine and erythropoietic systems in the rat with special reference to the mechanism of action of estradiol and testosterone. *Ann N Y Acad Sci* 149:336, 1968.

60. Gemzell CA, Sjostrand T: The effect of the gonads on the total amount of haemoglobin and blood volume in rats. *Acta Endocrinol (Copenh)* 21:86, 1956.

61. Bates A, Van't Hoff W, Jones P, Clayton R: The effect of hypopituitarism on life expectancy. *J Clin Endocrinol Metab* 81:1169, 1996.

62. Escamilla R, Lasser H: Simmonds' disease. *J Clin Endocrinol* 2:65, 1948.

63. Grieg H, Metz J, Sunn L: Anemia in hypopituitarism. Treatment with testosterone and cortisone. *S Afr J Lab Clin Med* 2:52, 1956.

64. Crafts RC, Meineke HA: The anemia of hypophysectomized animals. *Ann N Y Acad Sci* 77:501, 1959.

65. Berlin NI, Van Dyke DC, Siri WE, Williams CP: The effect of hypophysectomy on the total circulating red cell volume of the rat. *Endocrinology* 47:429, 1950.

66. Bozzini CE: Decrease in the number of erythrogenic elements in the blood-forming tissues as the cause of anemia in hypophysectomized rats. *Endocrinology* 77:977, 1965.

67. Van Dyke DC, Garcia JF, Simpson ME, et al: Maintenance of circulating red cell volume in rats after removal of the posterior and intermediate lobes of the pituitary. *Blood* 7:1005, 1952.

68. Crafts RC: The similarity between anemia induced by hypophysectomy and that induced by a combined thyroidectomy and adrenalectomy in adult female rats. *Endocrinology* 53:465, 1953.

69. Ellegala D, Alden T, Couture D, et al: Anemia, testosterone, and pituitary adenoma in men. *J Neurosurg* 98:974, 2003.

70. Merchav S, Tatarsky I, Hochberg Z: Enhancement of erythropoiesis in vitro by human growth hormone is mediated by insulin-like growth factor I. *Br J Haematol* 70:267, 1988.

71. Golde DW, Bersch N, Li CH: Growth hormone: Species-specific stimulation of erythropoiesis in vitro. *Science* 196:1112, 1977.

72. Jepson JH, McGarry EE: Hemopoiesis in pituitary dwarfs treated with human growth hormone and testosterone. *Blood* 39:229, 1972.

73. Eugster E, Fisch M, Walvoord E, et al: Low hemoglobin levels in children with an idiopathic growth hormone deficiency. *Endocrine* 18:135, 2002.

74. Kotzmann H, Riedl M, Clodi M, et al: The influence of growth hormone substitution therapy on erythroid and myeloid progenitor cells and on peripheral blood cells in adult patients with growth hormone deficiency. *Eur J Clin Invest* 26:1175, 1996.

75. Ten Have SM, van der Lely AJ, Lamberts SW: Increase in haemoglobin concentrations in growth hormone deficient adults during human recombinant growth hormone replacement therapy. *Clin Endocrinol (Oxf)* 47: 565, 1997.

76. Jepson JH, Lowenstein L: Effect of prolactin on erythropoiesis in the mouse. *Blood* 24:726, 1964.

77. Woody M, Welniak L, Sun R, et al: Prolactin exerts hematopoietic growth-promoting effects in vivo and partially counteracts myelosuppression by azidothymidine. *Exp Hematol* 27:811, 1999.

78. Abkowitz JL, Schaison G, Boulad F, et al: Response of Diamond-Blackfan anemia to metoclopramide: Evidence for a role for prolactin in erythropoiesis. *Blood* 100:2687, 2002.

79. Socolovsky M, Fallon A, Lodish H: The prolactin receptor rescues EpoR−/− erythroid progenitors and replaces EpoR in a synergistic interaction with c-kit. *Blood* 92:1491, 1998.

80. Socolovsky M, Dusanter-Fourt I, Lodish H: The prolactin receptor and severely truncated erythropoietin receptors support differentiation of erythroid progenitors. *J Biol Chem* 272:14009, 1997.

81. Degrossi O, Houssay A, Varela J, Capalbo E: Erythrokinetic studies in the anemia of thyroid and pituitary insufficiency, in *Advances in Thyroid Research*, edited by R Pitt-Rivers, p 410. Pergamon, New York, 1961.

82. Rudzki Z, Matynia A, Przybylik-Mazurek E, et al: Hypopituitarism and hematological abnormalities mimicking myelodysplastic syndrome. Report of four cases. *Pol Arch Med Wewn* 110:1003, 2003.

83. Kim D, Kim J, Park Y, et al: Case of complete recovery of pancytopenia after treatment of hypopituitarism. *Ann Hematol* 83:309, 2004.

84. Ferrari E, Ascari E, Bossolo PA, Barosi G: Sheehan's syndrome with complete bone marrow aplasia: Long-term results of substitution therapy with hormones. *Br J Haematol* 33:575, 1976.

85. Nomiyama J, Shinohara K, Inoue H: Improvement of anemia by recombinant erythropoietin in a patient with postoperative hypopituitarism. *Am J Hematol* 47:249, 1994.

86. Boxer M, Ellman L, Geller R, Wang CA: Anemia in primary hyperparathyroidism. *Arch Intern Med* 137:588, 1977.

87. Abarca J, Trigonis C, Hamberger B, Granberg PO: Anaemia in primary hyperparathyroidism—Fantasy or reality. *Ann Chir Gynaecol* 74:74, 1985.

88. Meytes D, Bogin E, Ma A, et al: Effect of parathyroid hormone on erythropoiesis. *J Clin Invest* 67:1263, 1981.

89. Delwiche F, Garrity MJ, Powell JS, et al: High levels of the circulating form of parathyroid hormone do not inhibit in vitro erythropoiesis. *J Lab Clin Med* 102:613, 1983.

90. Komatsuda A, Hirokawa M, Haseyama T, et al: Human parathyroid hormone does not influence human erythropoiesis in vitro. *Nephrol Dial Transplant* 13:2088, 1998.

91. Barbour GL: Effect of parathyroidectomy on anemia in chronic renal failure. *Arch Intern Med* 139:889, 1979.

92. Urena P, Eckardt K, Sarfati E, et al: Serum erythropoietin and erythropoiesis in primary and secondary hyperparathyroidism: Effect of parathyroidectomy. *Nephron* 59:384, 1991.

93. Argiles A, Mourad G, Lorho R, et al: Medical treatment of severe hyperparathyroidism and its influence on anaemia in end-stage renal failure. *Nephrol Dial Transplant* 9:1809, 1994.

THE CONGENITAL DYSERYTHROPOIETIC ANEMIAS

ERNEST BEUTLER

The congenital dyserythropoietic anemias are a heterogenous group of uncommon disorders characterized by anemia, the presence of multinuclear erythroid precursors in the marrow, ineffective erythropoiesis, and iron overload. Patients have been classified as type I, II, and III, but some patients who appear to fit into the general category of congenital dyserythropoietic anemia do not fit into any of these three groups. Types I and II congenital dyserythropoietic anemia are inherited as autosomal recessive disorders, and type III disease is dominant. Type I disease is caused by mutations of the codanin-1 gene, the function of which is unknown. Type II congenital dyserythropoietic anemia is also known by the acronym HEMPAS, which describes serologic findings that are characteristic of this form of the disorder. Abnormal complex carbohydrates are present in patients with the type II disease. The gene causing this disease has been mapped to 20q11.2, but remains unidentified. Type III disease is clinically milder than the other two forms of congenital dyserythropoietic anemia. There is no specific treatment, and management has included transfusions, removal of excess storage iron, splenectomy, and marrow transplantation.

The term *congenital dyserythropoietic anemia* applies to a group of hereditary refractory anemias characterized by ineffective erythropoiesis, erythroid multinuclearity, and accumulation of tissue iron. Anemia is usually first noted in infancy or childhood. The life span of circulating erythrocytes may be normal to moderately shortened, but dyserythropoiesis with a large component of intramedullary cell death is the dominant factor in pathogenesis. Ineffective erythropoiesis results in increased plasma iron turnover, diminished incorporation of tracer iron into circulating red cells, mild increases in the level of indirect-reacting bilirubin, elevated fecal stercobilin level, increased endogenous carbon monoxide production (presumably derived from heme catabolism), intense marrow erythroid hyperplasia, and normal, or at most slightly elevated, absolute reticulocyte counts. Splenomegaly, variably severe anemia, and mild increases in indirect-reacting serum bilirubin are present. Congenital dyserythropoietic anemias have been classified into three types[1] (Table 37-1). In addition, a number of cases that do not fit clearly into any of these three categories have been described.

EPIDEMIOLOGY

The congenital dyserythropoietic anemias are quite uncommon. In a survey of the United Kingdom between 1994 and 1996, 47 cases were identified. Twelve had type I, 13 type II, 2 type III, and 20 had types that did not fit into this classification.[2] All three major types are inherited; I and II as autosomal recessive disorder, and type III disease

in a dominant manner. The geographic distribution of affected patients suggests a higher frequency of type II disease in northwest Europe, Italy, and North Africa.[3] It seems to be particularly prevalent in southern Italy, and a founder effect has been suggested.[4]

CONGENITAL DYSERYTHROPOIETIC ANEMIA TYPE I

Type I dyserythropoietic anemia generally first becomes manifest in infancy, childhood, or adolescence, and is characterized by slight hyperbilirubinemia, moderate anemia (hematocrit usually 25–36%), and, commonly, splenomegaly.[5–14] The mode of genetic transmission is autosomal recessive, and the disorder has been documented in identical twins.[15] Linkage analysis narrowed localization of the gene responsible for this disorder to a 0.5-centimorgan interval in the q15.1 to q15.3 region.[16] The mutations responsible have been identified in a gene designated *CDAN1*, which encodes codanin-1, a putative o-glycosylated protein of 1226 amino acids, with no obvious transmembrane domains.[17] How these mutations result in the clinical phenotype of congenital dyserythropoietic anemia is unknown.

The level of serum haptoglobin is low; that of serum iron is normal or high. The red cell morphologic picture is characterized by well-marked anisocytosis and poikilocytosis and slight to moderate macrocytosis. The intensely cellular erythroid marrow shows megaloblastoid features.[5,6,18] The majority of erythroblasts have varying degrees of abnormality by light microscopy. In particular, three morphologic aberrations are regarded as typical: (1) very large cells containing an irregularly shaped nuclear mass with two nuclear segments suggesting incomplete nuclear division (1–2% of erythroblasts), (2) double nucleated cells in which the two nuclei differ in size, structure, and stainability (0.3–0.8% of erythroblasts), and (3) pairs of erythroblasts connected by thin chromatin bridges of different lengths (0.8–2.3% of erythroblasts) (see Color Plate II-5).[6] Only the erythroid series shows significant abnormalities by electron and light microscopy. The pores of the nuclear envelope of the erythroid cells become abnormally numerous and wide, with progressive maturation. Later the cytoplasm has invaded between the nuclear chromatin strands of many cells, and there is intense clumping of the dense chromatin. In even more severely affected cells, the cytoplasm separates the chromatin fragments and gives the nucleus a spongy appearance.[6,7,9,10,19] The persistence of cytoplasmic microtubules has also been demonstrated.[9] Some mitochondria show deposition of ferruginous micelles, causing a loss of normal structure, but these changes are quantitatively much less severe than in the sideroblastic anemias (see Chap. 58). In other studies, hypertetraploid DNA values were found in a high proportion of erythroblasts, and RNA synthesis was markedly reduced, leading to impaired hemoglobin synthesis.[12,20] Serologic abnormalities, such as occur in congenital dyserythropoietic anemia type II, have usually not been present. An increase in the α-/β-globin chain synthetic ratio has been reported. An animal model of the disease has been described.[21]

No effective treatment is available. Most subjects do not require transfusions, which are to be avoided if at all possible because iron overload is often present.[22–24] The cautious use of phlebotomy or administration of iron-chelating agents to help prevent tissue siderosis has been suggested by some studies[25] but not by two others.[13,22] Although co-inheritance of hereditary hemochromatosis and type I congenital dyserythropoietic anemia has been reported,[26] the association seems to have been an unusual coincidence. Most iron-loaded patients with the disorder do not have *HFE* mutations.[14,27] Successful hematopoietic stem cell transplantation has been documented.[28]

CONGENITAL DYSERYTHROPOIETIC ANEMIA TYPE II (HEMPAS)

Most commonly known as HEMPAS, a somewhat whimsical acronym for *H*ereditary *E*rythroblastic *M*ultinuclearity associated with a *P*osi-

TABLE 37-1 CONGENITAL DYSERYTHROPOIETIC ANEMIA TYPES I, II, AND III: MARROW AND SEROLOGIC FEATURES

	MARROW			
CDA TYPE	LIGHT MICROSCOPY	ELECTRON MICROSCOPY	SEROLOGY	INHERITANCE
I	Most erythroid cells abnormal: megaloblastoid changes; large cells with incompletely divided nuclear segments; double nuclei, internuclear chromatin bridges	Widened nuclear pores, cytoplasmic invasion of nucleus, disaggregation of ribosomes, presence of cytoplasmic microtubules	No serologic abnormalities	Autosomal recessive
II "HEMPAS"	Late polychromatophilic and orthochromic erythroblasts often contain 2–7 normal-appearing nuclei	Excess endoplasmic reticulum appearing as a double cell membrane	Cells possess unique "HEMPAS" antigen and are lysed by 30% of acidified normal sera; increased agglutination by anti-I; increased lysis by anti-I	Autosomal recessive
III	Giant erythroblasts, up to 50 μm in diameter, with up to 12 nuclei; prominent basophilic stippling	Clefts and blebs within nuclear region, autolytic areas in cytoplasm, some iron-filled mitochondria, myelin figures	Data inadequate; a single case showed increased agglutination by anti-i and increased lysis by anti-I, but a negative acidified serum test	Autosomal dominant

tive Acidified Serum test, type II congenital dyserythropoietic anemia was first described in 1962.[29,30] The unusual serologic abnormalities characterizing this disorder were defined in the late 1960s.[31] By 1975, the clinical and hematologic features of 84 patients in 55 families had been described and reviewed.[32] A considerable number of additional patients with HEMPAS have since been reported.[11,33-44] Both sexes are affected. The mode of genetic transmission is autosomal recessive,[45] although abnormalities in the levels of some glycoconjugates have been found in carriers.[46] The mean age at presentation is 5.2 years and at correct diagnosis was 15.9 years.[44] In one study, two thirds of patients were anemic; in another all were anemic.[47] The degree of anemia varies from mild to very severe.[48] Jaundice is present in over half of affected individuals and is most severe in patients who also have inherited the UDPGT1 mutation of Gilbert disease.[49] Secondary hemochromatosis is the most serious complication of the disorder.[33,35,37,40,47,49,50] It has been suggested that cirrhosis is common in this disorder, even in the absence of frank iron overload. Priapism has been documented in one patient.[51]

The red cell membrane of HEMPAS patients characteristically contains abnormal complex carbohydrate patterns[52] (Fig. 37-1). Presumably as a consequence of the abnormality in glycosylation, the electrophoretic mobilities of membrane proteins of the red cells from patients with HEMPAS deviate markedly from normal,[48] and this could occur as a result of either a genetic defect in N-acetylglucosaminyltransferase II[53] or α-mannosidase II.[21,54,55] The putative gene responsible for this disorder has been mapped to the long arm of chromosome 20 (20q11.2),[56] and a number of candidate genes have been excluded.[57,58] Its identity remains unknown.

A characteristic feature of HEMPAS is the behavior of the patient's cells in serologic tests. HEMPAS cells are lysed by certain group-compatible sera at pH 6.8, resembling in this respect cells of paroxysmal nocturnal hemoglobinuria (PNH) (see Chap. 38).[31,45,59] However, HEMPAS cells differ from those in PNH in several important respects.[45,59] The sucrose hemolysis test (see Chap. 38) is negative[45] (although an exception has been noted[60]), and the cells are not lysed by their own acidified serum. Only about 30 percent of group-compatible sera lyse HEMPAS cells. Unlike PNH cells, HEMPAS cells behave as a single population in quantitative lysis tests. The lysis of HEMPAS cells appears to be caused by a naturally occurring immunoglobulin M complement-binding antibody that can be removed by absorption with HEMPAS but not with normal or PNH cells. The antigen recognized by antibody is unknown. A constant finding in HEMPAS is the strong reactivity of the red cells with anti-i autoantibodies. In this respect, the red cells resemble those of newborn infants.[31,45,59] HEMPAS cells are agglutinated and lysed more readily

than normal cells by cold-reacting agglutinins (anti-I and anti-i). It appears that this is largely explained by increased antibody binding rather than by increased sensitivity to complement.[61]

Multinuclearity and karyorrhexis are present in 15 to 20 percent of late erythroblasts from patients with HEMPAS, and autoradiography indicates that these cells are no longer synthesizing DNA (see Color Plates II-3 and 4).

The circulating red cells exhibit moderate to marked anisocytosis and poikilocytosis and anisochromia. There are also a few irregularly contracted spherocytes. Ferrokinetic studies document the ineffective erythropoiesis.[31,45] Reticulocyte counts are normal or slightly elevated. Body iron stores and serum iron levels are usually increased, and the occurrence of frank hemochromatosis has been observed.[35] From 10 to 30 percent of the erythroblasts, chiefly the more mature stages, have two or more nuclei or lobulated nuclei (Fig. 37-2). Gaucher-like cells may develop as a result of phagocytosis of erythroblasts by macrophages. Ringed sideroblasts are not conspicuous. No satisfactory treatment is available, but partial benefit has been reported with splenectomy.[43-45,47] Hematopoietic stem cell transplantation was reported in one patient with possible type II disease.[62] One patient was successfully phlebotomized, removing 1.2 g of iron, in spite of an initial hemoglobin of 7 g/dl, a level that improved in the course of phlebotomy.[42,63]

CONGENITAL DYSERYTHROPOIETIC ANEMIA TYPE III

A third type of congenital dyserythropoietic anemia was first described in a woman and all three of her children, in whom 16 to 22.7 percent of marrow erythroblasts were multinucleated.[64] Giant-sized erythrocytes were present in the blood, and giant erythroblasts with coarse basophilic stippling and up to 12 nuclei were present in the marrow. All patients were asymptomatic, with absent or minimal anemia. The reticulocyte count was less than 3 percent. A similar, dominantly transmitted disorder was described in 15 members of a large Swedish family[65] under the name of hereditary benign erythroreticulosis, and other cases have been reported subsequently.[66,67]

Precipitation of β-chains has been observed within the abnormal erythroblasts.[68,69] The defect in the erythrocyte precursors is intrinsic to the stem cell; it can be reproduced in tissue culture, in which both morphologically normal and giant multinuclear erythroblasts are found.[70,71]

OTHER FORMS OF CONGENITAL DYSERYTHROPOIETIC ANEMIA AND SIMILAR DISORDERS

A number of cases of congenital dyserythropoietic anemia that do not have the features of types I, II, and III have been reported,[72-85]

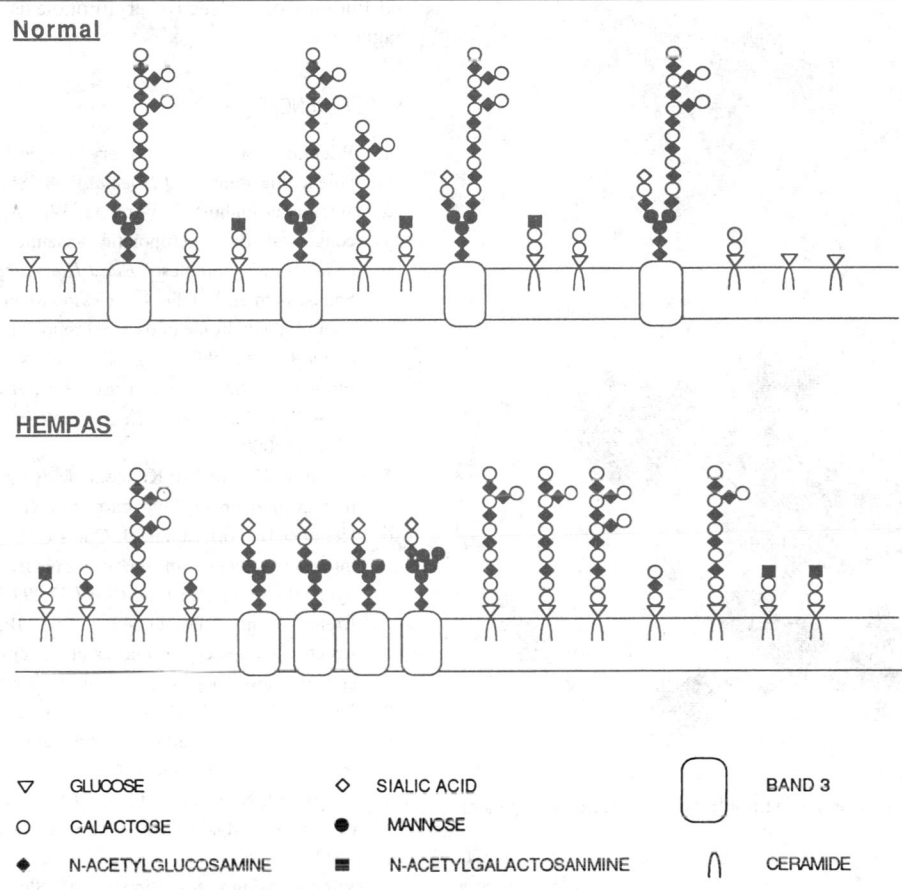

Normal

HEMPAS

▽	GLUCOSE	◇	SIALIC ACID	▢	BAND 3
○	GALACTOSE	●	MANNOSE		
◆	N-ACETYLGLUCOSAMINE	▆	N-ACETYLGALACTOSANMINE	∩	CERAMIDE

FIGURE 37-1   Schematic models for erythrocyte glycoproteins and glycolipids of normal, HEMPAS, and variant G.K. Band 3 glycoproteins in normal erythrocyte membranes are glycosylated by large carbohydrate chains — the polyactosaminoglycans. Most glycolipids have short carbohydrate chains but have small amounts of polyactosaminylceramide. In HEMPAS erythrocytes, band 3 has truncated hybrid-type oligosaccharides, and most polylactosamines shift to lipid acceptors. In variant G.K., band 3 has high mannose-type oligosaccharides, and polyactosamines are not present in glycolipids. Incompletely glycosylated band 3s in HEMPAS and variant G.K. appear to be clustered in the membranes. (Reprinted from Fukuda MN: Congenital dyserythropoietic anaemia type II (HEMPAS) and its molecular basis. *Bailliere's Clinical Hematology*, Vol, 6, pp 493–511, 1993. By permission of the publisher, WB Saunders Company Limited, London.[54])

and it has been suggested that one of these be designated as type IV.[78] The salient features of some of the earlier cases of atypical congenital dyserythropoietic anemia have been reviewed.[75] In two kindreds, congenital dyserythropoietic anemia was inherited in a dominant fashion. In some patients, marrow erythroid multinuclearity resembled that of HEMPAS, but the acidified serum lysis test was negative.[77,78] Long-lasting erythroblastosis occurring after splenectomy of such patients has been attributed to impaired denucleation of erythroblasts.[77] Unbalanced globin-chain synthesis with excess production of α chains was documented in several patients. In one such kindred, a disorder with features of both thalassemia and hereditary erythroid multinuclearity was dominantly transmitted.[74] In variant syndromes, there were also differences in the degree of agglutination by anti-i antibodies and in the concentrations of hemoglobins F and A₂. In one case of congenital dyserythropoietic anemia, the acidified serum lysis test was positive, but erythroid multinuclearity was absent.

Still other ill-defined forms of congenital dyserythropoietic anemia undoubtedly exist. Several cases of apparently lifelong anemia, thought to be hereditary, have been described.[76] These are characterized by marked aniso- and poikilocytosis and occasional teardrop and fragmented erythrocytes in the blood. Hyperplastic marrows showed megaloblastoid features without multinuclearity or ringed sideroblasts,[76] but a case with prominent ringed sideroblasts has also been described.[81] Neutropenia is commonly present, and thrombocytopenia has been observed in some patients. Cytogenetic studies of marrow revealed no chromosomal abnormalities. The reticulocyte response to anemia was absent or inappropriately low in all patients. In most cases, studies of parents failed to reveal abnormalities, suggesting an autosomal recessive mode of transmission. High-dose androgen therapy appeared partially to benefit two subjects.[76]

An X-linked form of the dyserythropoiesis and thrombocytopenia was associated with a *GATA-1* mutation.[43]

ERYTHROCYTE ENZYME ABNORMALITIES IN CONGENITAL DYSERYTHROPOIETIC ANEMIA

In both congenital dyserythropoietic anemia types I and II, as well as in certain less well-defined but apparently hereditary dyserythropoietic anemias, a diversity of abnormalities of individual red cell enzyme and findings of ineffective erythropoiesis should point to the correct diagnosis.

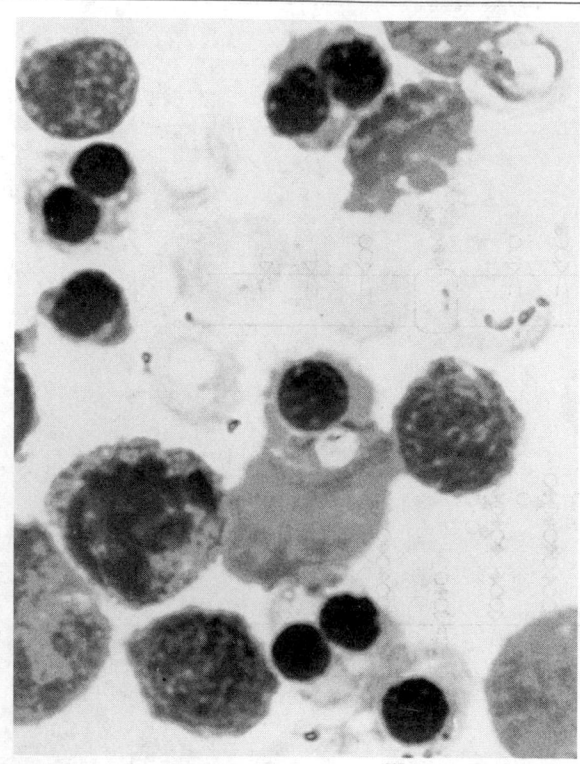

FIGURE 37-2 Multinuclearity of the erythroblasts in the marrow of a patient with HEMPAS.

activities and of activity ratios have been identified.[76,86] Enzyme patterns differ strikingly from those of either normal red cells or reticulocyte-rich blood. They resemble closely, however, patterns observed in a variety of disorders characterized by ineffective erythropoiesis, including certain acquired and congenital sideroblastic anemias, certain preleukemic states, and certain refractory, nonsideroblastic anemias with cellular marrow.[76]

DIFFERENTIAL DIAGNOSIS

Congenital dyserythropoietic anemia may be confused with the thalassemic syndromes because of the frequent presence of marked anisocytosis and poikilocytosis, hypochromia, and evidence of ineffective erythropoiesis. The readily evident erythroid multinuclearity of congenital dyserythropoietic anemia type II and the marrow gigantocytes of the rarer congenital dyserythropoietic anemia type III point toward the correct diagnosis in these conditions. The marrow changes in congenital dyserythropoietic anemia type I are, however, more subtle and more easily missed.[10,11] In one patient, parvovirus B19 simulated the marrow appearance of congenital dyserythropoietic anemia.[87] Family studies and evaluation of hemoglobin A_2 levels indicate that thalassemia is not present. The megaloblastoid marrow structure may cause some confusion with other disorders associated with abnormalities of vitamin B_{12}, folic acid, and nucleic acid metabolism. Some forms of congenital dyserythropoietic anemia also resemble some of the acquired or hereditary sideroblastic anemias, but sideroblastosis is usually not prominent and the other marrow features described earlier point to the correct diagnosis. The abnormal serologic tests observed with HEMPAS are of obvious major diagnostic importance. Otherwise, indirect hyperbilirubinemia and splenomegaly may suggest a hemolytic process, but low reticulocyte counts, the marrow features,

REFERENCES

1. Wickramasinghe SN: Dyserythropoiesis and congenital dyserythropoietic anaemias. *Br J Haematol* 98:785, 1997.
2. Wickramasinghe SN, Vora AJ, Will A, et al: Transfusion-dependent congenital dyserythropoietic anaemia with non-specific dysplastic changes in erythroblasts. *Eur J Haematol* 60:140, 1998.
3. Sandstroem H, Wahlin A, Eriksson M, et al: Angioid streaks are part of a familial syndrome of dyserythropoietic anaemia (CDA III). *Br J Haematol* 98:845, 1997.
4. Iolascon A, Servedio V, Carbone R, et al: Geographic distribution of CDA-II: Did a founder effect operate in Southern Italy? *Haematologica* 85:470, 2000.
5. Wendt F, Heimpel H: Kongenitale dyserythropoietische Anämie bei einem zweieiigen Zwillingsparr. *Med Klin* 62:172, 1967.
6. Heimpel H, Forteza-Vila J, Queisser W, Spiertz E: Electron and light microscopic study of the erythroblasts of patients with congenital dyserythropoietic anemia. *Blood* 37:299, 1971.
7. Breton-Gorius J, Daniel MT, Clauvel JP, Dreyfus B: Anomalies ultrastructurales des érythroblastes et des érythrocytes dan six cas de dysérythropoïése congénitale. *Nouv Rev Fr Hematol* 13:23, 1973.
8. Faille A, Najean Y, Dresch C: Cinétique de l'érythropoïése dans 14 cas "d'erythropoïése inéfficase" avec anomalies morphologiques des érythroblastes et polynucléarité. *Nouv Rev Fr Hematol* 12:113, 1972.
9. Lewis SM, Nelson DA, Pitcher CS: Clinical and ultrastructural aspects of congenital dyserythropoietic anaemia Type I. *Br J Haematol* 23:113, 1972.
10. Wickramasinghe SN, Pippard MJ: Studies of erythroblast function in congenital dyserythropoietic anaemia, type I: Evidence of impaired DNA, RNA, and protein synthesis and unbalanced globin chain synthesis in ultrastructurally abnormal cells. *J Clin Pathol* 39:881, 1986.
11. Alloisio N, Jaccoud P, Dorleac E, et al: Alterations of globin chain synthesis and of red cell membrane proteins in congenital dyserythropoietic anemia I and II. *Pediatr Res* 16:1016, 1982.
12. Meuret G, Tschan P, Schlüter G, et al: DNA-, histone-, RNA-, hemoglobin-content and DNA synthesis in erythroblasts in a case of congenital dyserythropoietic anemia type I. *Blut* 24:32, 1972.
13. Maeda K, Saeed SM, Rebuck JW, Monto RW: Type I dyserythropoietic anemia. A 30-year follow-up. *Am J Clin Pathol* 73:433, 1980.
14. Shalev H, Kapleushnik Y, Haeskelzon L, et al: Clinical and laboratory manifestations of congenital dyserythropoietic anemia type I in young adults. *Eur J Haematol* 68:170, 2002.
15. Facon T, Mannessier L, Lepelley P, et al: Congenital diserythropoietic anemia type I. Report on monozygotic twins with associated hemochromatosis and short stature. *Blut* 61:248, 1990.
16. Tamary H, Shalmon L, Shalev H, et al: Localization of the gene for congenital dyserythropoietic anemia type I to a <1-cM interval on chromosome 15q15.1-15.3. *Am J Hum Genet* 62:1062, 1998.
17. Dgany O, Avidan N, Delaunay J, et al: Congenital dyserythropoietic anemia type I is caused by mutations in codanin-1. *Am J Hum Genet* 71:1467, 2002.
18. Heimpel H, Wendt F, Klemm D, et al: Kongenitale dyserythropoietische Anämie. *Arch Klin Med* 215:174, 1968.
19. Woessner S, Pardo P, Lafuente R, et al: Congenital dyserythropoietic anemia type I. Report of a case. *Blut* 42:47, 1981.
20. Meuret VG, Boll I, Keyserlingk DG, Heissmeyer H: Morphologische und kinetische Befinde bei einer kongenitalen dyserythropoietischen Anämie. *Blut* 21:341, 1970.
21. Steffen DJ, Elliott GS, Leipold HW, Smith JE: Congenital dyserythropoiesis and progressive alopecia in Polled Hereford calves: Hemato-

logic, biochemical, bone marrow cytologic, electrophoretic, and flow cytometric findings. *J Vet Diagn Invest* 4:31, 1992.

22. Hanna WT, Machado EA, Montgomery RN, Lange RD. Variant of congenital dyserythropoietic anemia. *South Med J* 78:616, 1985.

23. Smithson WA, Perrault J: Use of subcutaneous deferoxamine in a child with hemochromatosis associated with congenital dyserythropoietic anemia, type I. *Mayo Clin Proc* 57:322, 1982.

24. Cazzola M, Barosi G, Bergamaschi G, et al: Iron loading in congenital dyserythropoietic anaemias and congenital sideroblastic anaemias. *Br J Haematol* 54:649, 1983.

25. Choudhry VP, Saraya AK, Kasturi J, Rath PK: Congenital dyserythropoietic anaemias: Splenectomy as a mode of therapy. *Acta Haematol (Basel)* 66:195, 1981.

26. Fargion S, Valenti L, Fracanzani AL, et al: Hereditary hemochromatosis in a patient with congenital dyserythropoietic anemia. *Blood* 96:3653, 2000.

27. Wickramasinghe SN, Thein SL, Srichairatanakool S, Porter JB: Determinants of iron status and bilirubin levels in congenital dyserythropoietic anaemia type I. *Br J Haematol* 107:522, 1999.

28. Ayas M, al Jefri A, Baothman A, et al: Transfusion-dependent congenital dyserythropoietic anemia type I successfully treated with allogeneic stem cell transplantation. *Bone Marrow Transplant* 29:681, 2002.

29. DeLozzio CB, Valencia JI, Accame E: Chromosomal study in erythroblastic endopolyploidy. *Lancet* 1:1004, 1962.

30. Roberts PD, Wallis PG, Jackson ADM: Haemolytic anaemia with multinucleated normoblasts in the marrow [letter]. *Lancet* 1:1186, 1962.

31. Crookston JH, Crookston MC, Burnie KL, et al: Hereditary erythroblastic multinuclearity associated with a positive acidified-serum test: A test of congenital dyserythropoietic anaemia. *Br J Haematol* 17:11, 1969.

32. Verwilghen RL: Congenital dyserythropoietic anaemia, type II (HEMPAS), in *Congenital Disorders of Erythropoiesis, Ciba Foundation Symposium 37 (new series)*, p 151. Elsevier/Excerpta Medica, North Holland, Amsterdam, 1976.

33. Bird AR, Jacobs P, Moores P: Congenital dyserythropoietic anaemia (type II) presenting with haemosiderosis. *Acta Haematol (Basel)* 78:33, 1987.

34. Zdebska E, Anselstetter V, Pacuszka T, et al: Glycolipids and glycopeptides of red cell membranes in congenital dyserythropoietic anaemia type II (CDA II). *Br J Haematol* 66:385, 1987.

35. Halpern Z, Rahmani R, Levo Y: Severe hemochromatosis: The predominant clinical manifestation of congenital dyserythropoietic anemia type 2. *Acta Haematol (Basel)* 74:178, 1985.

36. Ventura A, Panizon F, Soranzo MR, et al: Congenital dyserythropoietic anaemia type II associated with a new type of G6PD deficiency (G6PD Gabrovizza). *Acta Haematol (Basel)* 71:227, 1984.

37. Faruqui S, Abraham A, Berenfeld MR, Gabuzda TG: Normal serum ferritin levels in a patient with HEMPAS syndrome and iron overload. *Am J Clin Pathol* 78:97, 1982.

38. Chrobak L, Radochova D, Smetana K, et al: Congenital dyserythropoietic anemia, type II (HEMPAS) in three siblings. *Folia Haematol (Leipz)*, 107:628, 1980.

39. McCann SR, Firth R, Murray N, Temperley IJ: Congenital dyserythropoietic anaemia type II (HEMPAS): A family study. *J Clin Pathol* 33:1197, 1980.

40. Greiner TC, Burns CP, Dick FR, et al: Congenital dyserythropoietic anemia type II diagnosed in a 69-year-old patient with iron overload. *Am J Clin Pathol* 98:522, 1992.

41. Gangarossa S, Romano V, Del Giudice EM, et al: Congenital dyserythropoietic anemia type II associated with G6PD Seattle in a Sicilian child. *Acta Haematol (Basel)* 93:36, 1995.

42. Hofmann WK, Kaltwasser JP, Hoelzer D, et al: Successful treatment of iron overload by phlebotomies in a patient with severe congenital dyserythropoietic anemia type II. *Blood* 89:3068, 1997.

43. Nichols KE, Crispino JD, Poncz M, et al: Familial dyserythropoietic anaemia and thrombocytopenia due to an inherited mutation in GATA1. *Nat Genet* 24:266, 2000.

44. Iolascon A, Delaunay J, Wickramasinghe SN, et al: Natural history of congenital dyserythropoietic anemia type II. *Blood* 98:1258, 2001.

45. Crookston MC: HEMPAS: Congenital dyserythropoietic anemia (type II). *Q J Med* 66:257, 1973.

46. Zdebska E, Mendek-Czajkowska E, Ploski R, et al: Heterozygosity of CDAN II (HEMPAS) gene may be detected by the analysis of erythrocyte membrane glycoconjugates from healthy carriers. *Haematologica* 87:126, 2002.

47. Heimpel H, Anselstetter V, Chrobak L, et al: Congenital dyserythropoietic anemia type II: Epidemiology, clinical appearance, and prognosis based on long-term observation. *Blood* 102:4576, 2003.

48. Iolascon A, D'Agostaro G, Perrotta S, et al: Congenital dyserythropoietic anemia type II: Molecular basis and clinical aspects. *Haematologica* 81:543, 1996.

49. Perrotta S, Del Giudice EM, Carbone R, et al: Gilbert's syndrome accounts for the phenotypic variability of congenital dyserythropoietic anemia type II (CDA-II). *J Pediatr* 136:556, 2000.

50. Hovinga JA, Solenthaler M, Dufour JF: Congenital dyserythropoietic anaemia type II (HEMPAS) and haemochromatosis: A report of two cases. *Eur J Gastroenterol Hepatol* 15:1141, 2003.

51. Edney MT, Schned AR, Cendron M, et al: Priapism in a 15-year-old boy with congenital dyserythropoietic anemia type II (hereditary erythroblastic multinuclearity with positive acidified serum lysis test). *J Urol* 167:309, 2002.

52. Fukuda MN: HEMPAS. *Biochim Biophys Acta* 1455:231, 1999.

53. Fukuda MN, Dell A, Scartezzini P: Primary defect of congenital dyserythropoietic anemia type II. Failure in glycosylation of erythrocyte lactosaminoglycan proteins caused by lowered N-acetylglucosaminyltransferase II. *J Biol Chem* 262:7195, 1987.

54. Fukuda MN: Congenital dyserythropoietic anaemia type II (HEMPAS) and its molecular basis. *Baillieres Clin Haematol* 6:493, 1993.

55. Chui D, Oh-Eda M, Liao YF, et al: Alpha-mannosidase-II deficiency results in dyserythropoiesis and unveils an alternate pathway in oligosaccharide biosynthesis. *Cell* 90:157, 1997.

56. Gasparini P, Del Giudice EM, Delaunay J, et al: Localization of the congenital dyserythropoietic anemia II locus to chromosome 20q11.2 by genomewide search. *Am J Hum Genet* 61:1112, 1997.

57. Iolascon A, Miraglia del Giudice E, Perrotta S, et al: Exclusion of three candidate genes as determinants of congenital dyserythropoietic anemia type II (CDA-II). *Blood* 90:4197, 1997.

58. Lanzara C, Ficarella R, Totaro A, et al: Congenital dyserythropoietic anemia type II: Exclusion of seven candidate genes. *Blood Cells Mol Dis* 30:22, 2003.

59. Crookston JH, Crookston MC: Hereditary anemia with multinuclear erythroblasts ("HEMPAS"), in *Birth Defects, Original Article Series, Clinical Delineation of Birth Defects*, vol. 8, edited by D Bergsma, p 15. Williams & Wilkins, Baltimore, 1972.

60. Koduri PR, Gowrishankar S: Congenital dyserythropoietic anemia type II with a positive sucrose hemolysis test. *Am J Hematol* 71:64, 2002.

61. Lewis SM, Grammaticos P, Dacie JV: Lysis by anti-I in dyserythropoietic anaemias: Role of increased uptake of antibody. *Br J Haematol* 18:465, 1970.

62. Remacha AF, Badell I, Pujol-Moix N, et al: Hydrops fetalis-associated congenital dyserythropoietic anemia treated with intrauterine transfusions and bone marrow transplantation. *Blood* 100:356, 2002.

63. Mager J, Glaser G, Razin A, et al: Metabolic effects of pyrimidines derived from fava bean glycosides on human erythrocytes deficient in glucose-6-phosphate dehydrogenase. *Biochem Biophys Res Commun* 20:235, 1965.

64. Wolff JA, von Hofe FH: Familial erythroid multinuclearity. *Blood* 6: 1274, 1951.

65. Bergström I, Jacobsson L: Hereditary benign erythroreticulosis. *Blood* 19:296, 1962.

66. Lind L, Sandstrom H, Wahlin A, et al: Localization of the gene for congenital dyserythropoietic anemia type III, CDAN3, to chromosome 15q21-q25. *Hum Mol Genet* 4:109, 1995.

67. Soderquist AM, Carpenter G: Developments in the mechanism of growth factor action: Activation of protein kinase by epidermal growth factor. *Fed Proc* 42:2615, 1983.

68. Villegas A, Gonzalez L, Furio V, et al: Congenital dyserythropoietic anemia type III with unbalanced globin chain synthesis. *Eur J Haematol* 52:251, 1994.

69. Waller HD, Schlegel B, Mueller AA, Löhr GW: Der Hemiglobingehalt in alternden Erythrocyten. *Klin Wochenschr* 37:898, 1959.

70. McCluggage WG, Hull D, Mayne E, et al: Malignant lymphoma in congenital dyserythropoietic anaemia type III. *J Clin Pathol* 49:599, 1996.

71. Desforges JF, Kalaw E, Gilchrist P: Inhibition of glucose-6-phosphate dehydrogenase by hemolysis inducing drugs. *J Lab Clin Med* 55:757, 1960.

72. McBride JA, Wilson WE, Baille N: Congenital dyserythropoietic anaemia-type IV. *Blood* 38:837, 1971.

73. Hruby MA, Mason RG, Honig GR: Unbalanced globin chain synthesis in congenital dyserythropoietic anemia. *Blood* 42:843, 1973.

74. Weatherall DJ, Clegg JB, Knox-Macaulay HHM, et al: A genetically determined disorder with features both of thalassemia and congenital dyserythropoietic anemia. *Br J Haematol* 24:681, 1973.

75. David G, Van Dorpe A: Aberrant congenital dyserythropoietic anaemias, in *Dyserythropoiesis*, edited by SM Lewis, RL Verwilghen, p 93. Academic Press, London, 1977.

76. Valentine WN, Konrad PN, Paglia DE: Dyserythropoiesis, refractory anemia, and "preleukemia": Metabolic features of the erythrocytes. *Blood* 41:857, 1973.

77. Bethlenfalvay NC, Hadnagy C, Heimpel H: Unclassified type of congenital dyserythropoietic anaemia (CDA) with prominent peripheral erythroblastosis. *Br J Haematol* 60:541, 1985.

78. Bird AR, Karabus CD, Hartley PS: Type IV congenital dyserythropoietic anemia with an unusual response to splenectomy. *Am J Pediatr Hematol Oncol* 7:196, 1985.

79. Ohisalo JJ, Viitala J, Lintula R, Ruutu T: A new congenital dyserythropoietic anaemia. *Br J Haematol* 68:111, 1988.

80. Pothier B, Morle L, Alloisio N, et al: Aberrant pattern of red cell membrane and cytosolic proteins in a case of congenital dyserythropoietic anaemia. *Br J Haematol* 66:393, 1987.

81. Brien WF, Mant MJ, Etches WS: Variant congenital dyserythropoietic anaemia with ringed sideroblasts. *Clin Lab Haematol* 7:231, 1985.

82. Wickramasinghe SN, Illum N, Wimberley PD: Congenital dyserythropoietic anaemia with novel intra-erythroblastic and intra-erythrocytic inclusions. *Br J Haematol* 79:322, 1991.

83. Sansone G, Masera G, Cantù-Rajnoldi A, Terzoli S: An unclassified case of congenital dyserythropoietic anaemia with a severe neonatal onset. *Acta Haematol (Basel)* 88:41, 1992.

84. Agre P, Smith BL, Baumgarten R, et al: Human red cell aquaporin CHIP: II. Expression during normal fetal development and in a novel form of congenital dyserythropoietic anemia. *J Clin Invest* 94:1050, 1994.

85. Woessner S, Trujillo M, Florensa L, et al: Congenital dyserythropoietic anaemia other than type I to III with a peculiar erythroblastic morphology. *Eur J Haematol* 71:211, 2003.

86. Valentine WN, Crookston JH, Paglia DE, Conrad P: Erythrocyte enzymatic abnormalities in HEMPAS (hereditary erythroblastic multinuclearity with a positive acidified-serum test). *Br J Haematol* 23:107, 1972.

87. Carpenter SL, Zimmerman SA, Ware RE: Acute parvovirus B19 infection mimicking congenital dyserythropoietic anemia. *J Pediatr Hematol Oncol* 26:133, 2004.

PAROXYSMAL NOCTURNAL HEMOGLOBINURIA

ERNEST BEUTLER

Paroxysmal nocturnal hemoglobinuria (PNH) is an acquired hematopoietic stem cell disease characterized by chronic hemolytic anemia, thrombotic episodes, and often pancytopenia. It is a clonal disorder caused by a somatic mutation of the X-linked gene phosphatidylinositol glycan class A (PIG-A), which is required for formation of the phosphatidylinositol anchor. As a result, many membrane proteins, including some inhibitors of the complement cascade, are missing from the cell surface, and the erythrocytes are usually sensitive to the hemolytic effect of complement. The abnormal clone seems to arise in the context of marrow damage, and many patients have an antecedent history of marrow failure before the existence of PNH becomes apparent. The disease is diagnosed provisionally with the sucrose hemolysis test and definitively by flow cytometry. Treatment with glucocorticoids and/or androgenic steroids is sometimes helpful. The median survival is approximately 10 years. Hematopoietic stem cell transplantation can be curative.

DEFINITION AND HISTORY

Although commonly regarded as a type of hemolytic anemia, paroxysmal nocturnal hemoglobinuria (PNH) actually is in reality a hematopoietic stem cell disorder characterized by the formation of defective platelets, granulocytes, and possibly lymphocytes as well as abnormal erythrocytes. The abnormality of the red cells predisposes them to intravascular complement-mediated lysis that waxes and wanes in severity. The name suggests that cyclic variation in hemoglobinuria is an important feature of this disease. However, in many patients, hemoglobinuria is quite irregular or occult. The classic diagnostic feature of PNH is the increased sensitivity of the red blood cells to the hemolytic action of complement.

In a scholarly historical review of PNH, Crosby[1] attributed the first definitive account of this disease to Strübing,[2] who in 1882 described a patient with hemoglobinuria after sleep. The patient's plasma was red, and Strübing suggested that the erythrocytes were being destroyed within the bloodstream. He also detected a fine-grained yellowish-brown material in the urine, presumably hemosiderin. Hijmans van den Bergh[3] demonstrated that erythrocytes from a similar patient were lysed in normal serum as well as in the patient's serum if the mixture was acidified with carbon dioxide. Marchiafava and Micheli also were early students of the disease, and for a time the disease was designated Marchiafava-Micheli syndrome, an appellation that has fallen into disuse.

Acronyms and abbreviations that appear in this chapter include: DAF, decay accelerating factor; FACS, fluorescent-activated cell sorting; GPI, glycosylphosphatidylinositol; HRF, homologous restriction factor; LFA, lymphocyte function-associated antigen; MIRL, membrane inhibitor of reactive lysis; PIG-A, phosphatidylinositol glycan class A; PNH, paroxysmal nocturnal hemoglobinuria.

Many different proteins that have in common attachment to a phosphatidylinositol anchor are missing from the surface of blood cells in PNH, and it was recognized that the underlying defect in PNH would be likely to affect this structure. The detection of the defect in an X-linked gene designated PIG-A (for phosphatidylinositol glycan class A)[4] was the culmination of more than 100 years of research into this once mysterious disorder.

ETIOLOGY AND PATHOGENESIS

CLONAL ORIGIN OF PNH

In contrast to all the other intrinsic abnormalities of the erythrocyte, PNH is an acquired disorder; in a number of cases, only one of a pair of identical twins was affected.[5–7] Before the basic lesion had been discovered, the expression of glucose-6-phosphate dehydrogenase alleles,[8] methylation of polymorphic restriction sites,[9] and cytogenetic studies[10] had all demonstrated the clonal nature of PNH. Thus, PNH arises, like a neoplasm, from the transformation of a single cell.

THE PIG-A MUTATION

The underlying defect in PNH is one or several of many different mutations in the PIG-A gene, an X-linked gene that plays a major role in the formation of the phosphatidylinositol anchor. Many different mutations have been documented in PNH patients,[11] most of them nonsense mutations or insertions or deletions producing frame shifts. It is no accident that the gene that is mutated is X-linked. In this way a single somatic mutation is enough to affect formation of the anchor. If an autosomal gene were to cause the disease, damage to both copies of the gene would be required, a statistically unlikely event. The abnormal clone appears to arise most commonly in a damaged marrow; many patients with PNH have a prior history of aplastic anemia,[12] either idiopathic or drug induced. Although it is been known for many years[13] that complement-sensitive cells are present in the circulation of many patients with aplastic anemia,[14] myelodysplastic syndromes,[15–17] and even normal subjects,[16,18] it is apparent that mutations in the phosphatidylinositol anchor arise sporadically in hematopoietic precursors, and that the environment provided by the abnormal marrow allows mutant clone(s) to be selected. Cells with PIG-A mutations do not appear to have a proliferative advantage in vitro or in hybrid animal models made with PIG-A knockouts,[19] but they have been found to be relatively resistant to apoptosis in some studies,[20–23] but not in others.[24,25] Some patients have multiple clones, each with a distinct mutation.[26,27] This implies that mutations of the PIG-A gene may not be altogether rare, and when the conditions are such that a PNH clone has a selective advantage, several independent mutational events may come to light.[28]

FUNCTION OF PIG-A

The PIG-A gene plays a vital role in a very early step in the conversion of N-acetylglucosamine and glucosamine-phosphoinositol into mature mannolipids.[29] Transformed lymphoblasts are unable to incorporate labeled mannose into glycosylphosphatidylinositol (GPI) anchor precursors, and when provided with uridine diphospho-N-acetyl[³H] glucosamine there is marked reduction in the production of anchor phospholipids. Transfection with the PIG-A cDNA corrects the defect in GPI anchor synthesis.[4]

MEMBRANE ABNORMALITIES IN PNH

A large number of membrane protein deficiencies have been observed in PNH. These include deficiencies of acetylcholinesterase,[30] leukocyte alkaline phosphatase,[31] "decay accelerating factor" ([DAF] CD55),[32] CD59 antigen (membrane inhibitor of reactive lysis

[MIRL]), homologous restriction factor ([HRF] C8 binding protein),[33] CD58 (lymphocyte function-associated antigen-3 [LAF-3]),[34] 5'-ectonucleotidase,[35] CD16 (the low-affinity Fc receptor of granulocytes),[36] urokinase-type plasminogen activator,[37] and CD14 antigen.[38] The common denominator is that all of these proteins are attached to the GPI anchor (see Chap. 44).

COMPLEMENT SENSITIVITY

The classic abnormality of PNH erythrocytes is their increased sensitivity to complement-mediated lysis, whether the complement is activated by the classic or the alternative pathway (see Chap. 16). Activation of complement may be achieved by a variety of means:[39] lowering of pH, as in the acid hemolysis test; reducing ionic strength, as in the sucrose hemolysis test; treating the plasma with cobra venom; increasing the magnesium concentration; or coating the cells with antibodies such as anti-A. Using graded amounts of complement, it is possible to identify several populations of cells, that have been designated PNH I, PNH II, PNH IIIa, and PNH IIIb, manifesting progressively increasing sensitivity to complement lysis and deposition of increasing amounts of C3 on the PNH membranes.[12] The existence of multiple populations, once difficult to explain in a clonal disorder, presumably results from the coexistence of several different clones with different mutations.[26,27]

Although several of the abnormalities involve proteins that modulate complement function, a variety of findings suggest that the absence of the CD59 antigen plays the most critical role in the complement sensitivity of PNH erythrocytes. Inherited deficiency of DAF is not associated with clinical hemolysis, although a weakly positive acid hemolysis test may be present,[40,41] whereas a hereditary deficiency of CD59 is associated with PNH.[42] CD59 knockout mice show some of the hematologic manifestations of PNH.[43,44] Restoration *in vitro* of CD59 corrects the complement sensitivity of red cells more completely than restoration of DAF,[45] and PNH may occur in the absence of DAF deficiency.[46] The trimodal distribution of complement sensitivity of the red cells of some patients with PNH[30] appears to be related to the degree of deficiency of CD59 and DAF among the erythrocytes of such patients.[47,48]

DISTRIBUTION OF THE DEFECT AMONG BLOOD CELLS

Granulocytes and platelets, like red cells, show increased sensitivity to complement-mediated lysis[49] and are deficient in DAF.[50] Chemotactic responses of PNH granulocytes are also impaired.[51] Even blood lymphocytes[52] and lymphoblastoid cell lines from some patients with PNH show abnormalities in CD59 and DAF.[53]

CLINICAL FEATURES

HEMOGLOBINURIA

The nocturnal hemoglobinuria from which PNH derives its name, that is, the passage of red or brownish urine in the morning on rising, occurs in only a small proportion of patients. When it does follow the classical cyclic pattern, the hemoglobinuria occurs during sleep regardless of the time of day.[54] It was originally believed that nocturnal hemoglobinuria was a function of a lowered blood pH during sleep, but this is not the case.[55] Hemoglobinuria may be the result of the production of increased numbers of abnormal cells rather than of an increase in hemolytic processes.

In most patients with PNH, hemoglobinuria occurs irregularly. Bouts of hemolysis may be initiated by infections, surgery, and possibly even strenuous exercise. The injection of contrast dyes, as in intravenous pyelography or myelography, may precipitate hemolysis by activating complement.[56]

CHRONIC HEMOLYSIS

Patients with PNH manifest all the clinical and laboratory signs of chronic hemolytic anemia. Weakness, dyspnea, and pallor are common, particularly when the anemia is quite severe. Splenomegaly is present in some patients, but the enlargement of the spleen is usually quite modest.

IRON DEFICIENCY

Iron deficiency is often a manifestation of PNH because of urinary loss of iron as hemosiderin and hemoglobin. The administration of iron to iron-deficient patients sometimes results in overt signs of hemolysis manifested by the appearance of frank hemoglobinuria. Although this effect of iron has sometimes been attributed to its peroxidatic effect increasing damage to the red cell membrane,[57] it seems more likely that it results from increased production of both normal and abnormal red cells by the marrow, the newly formed abnormal cells undergoing hemolysis.[58]

BLEEDING

Thrombocytopenia varies greatly in severity. It may be very mild and persist for years, or be very severe. In the latter instance extensive hemorrhagic complications may be a prominent part of the clinical presentation of patients with PNH.

THROMBOSIS

Although thrombotic complications occur in other forms of hemolytic anemia as well, they are particularly prominent and severe in PNH. The 10-year risk for thrombosis was 44 percent in patients in whom more than 50 percent of granulocytes were PNH cells but was only 5.8 percent among patients with smaller clones. The reason for the high prevalence of thrombosis is not entirely clear, but it may be related to activation of platelets by complement,[12] the procoagulant activity of red cell membranes, or the intravascular release of ADP from red cells, leading to platelet aggregation. The prevalence of factor V Leiden is not increased in PNH.[59] Venous thromboses represent one of the most frequent clinical manifestations of PNH. The Budd-Chiari syndrome, which results from hepatic vein thrombosis, has been observed repeatedly. In one study of 40 patients with Budd-Chiari syndrome, five had PNH.[60] Thus, PNH should be a serious consideration in any patient with hepatic vein thrombosis. Budd-Chiari syndrome has an ominous prognosis when fully developed.[61,62] It may also occur in a milder, subclinical form detectable by ultrasonography,[63] and early therapy has been recommended.[60] Pain in the abdomen or in the lower part of the back also appears to be more common in patients with PNH than in those with other types of hemolytic anemia. The abdominal pain is often colicky in nature and the abdomen is tender on palpitation. Frank intestinal infarction or bleeding into the intestinal wall has sometimes been found.[64,65] Esophageal spasm has been observed in patients who are undergoing hemolysis and has been likened to the symptoms that have occurred in patients who are receiving hemoglobin solutions as a blood substitute, symptoms that are probably related to removal of ambient nitric oxide.[12] Pulmonary hypertension has occurred and has been attributed to widespread thromboses in the pulmonary microvasculature.[66] Arterial as well as venous thrombosis has been documented.[67]

PREGNANCY

Pregnancy has been associated with abortion and venous thromboembolism, but the outcome is sometimes normal.[68–71] In a study of 38 pregnant patients with PNH, pregnancy was uncomplicated in one third of the cases, and life-threatening complications in mothers were found to be uncommon.[70] There were no maternal deaths, but 11 of the pregnancies ended in miscarriage, six were terminated, and three were born preterm. The other 18 mothers delivered normal infants.

RENAL MANIFESTATIONS

A variety of abnormalities of renal function is observed. Included are hyposthenuria, abnormal tubular function, and declining creatinine clearance. Hypertension was observed in eight of a series of 21 patients who had been followed for a long period of time. Radiologic findings included enlarged kidneys and cortical infarcts, cortical thinning, and papillary necrosis. Most patients have some episodes of hematuria and proteinuria distinct from hemoglobinuria.[56] Acute and chronic renal failure may occur.[56,72–75]

NEUROLOGIC MANIFESTATIONS

Severe headaches or pains in the eyes occur in patients with PNH without any objectively demonstrable neurologic abnormalities. These complications may result from small venous occlusions. Frank cerebral venous thrombosis is a grave and fortunately uncommon complication of PNH.[76]

LABORATORY FEATURES

BLOOD

Anemia may be very severe, with hemoglobin levels below 5 g/dl, but in some cases the hemoglobin concentration of the blood is normal. A mild to moderate reticulocytosis is usually present; the reticulocyte count tends to be lower than in other patients with chronic hemolysis who manifest the same degree of anemia. A modest degree of macrocytosis commensurate with the increased reticulocyte count is usually present. However, if the patient has become iron deficient, the red cells may be microcytic and hypochromic. In this case, the plasma iron and ferritin levels are usually low and the iron binding capacity elevated.

The leukocyte count is characteristically low, principally because of a diminution of the number of granulocytes. The leukocyte alkaline phosphatase activity[31] may be diminished and surface urokinase receptors absent.[77] The platelet count is often low, but may be 150,000/μL or more in about 20 to 50 percent of patients.[78] Platelet survival is usually normal.[49]

MARROW

Erythroid hyperplasia is usually present but the overall marrow cellularity is generally not greatly increased, and the marrow may even be aplastic. Stainable iron is often absent.

URINE

Hemoglobin is sometimes but by no means always present in the urine. Hemoglobin casts may be present. Hemosiderinuria is one of the most constant features of the disease and is of considerable diagnostic importance.

DIFFERENTIAL DIAGNOSIS

The diagnosis of PNH should be entertained in any patient with pancytopenia of unknown origin, particularly when accompanied by reticulocytosis. Isolated defects in a single lineage, such as thrombocytopenia, may also be the presenting finding. PNH arises within the context of marrow failure states such as aplastic anemia. When such patients manifest moderate numbers of reticulocytes in the blood, tests for PNH may demonstrate that a complement-sensitive clone has appeared. A search for PNH may also occasionally prove rewarding in the case of patients with repeated unexplained thrombotic episodes.

The most convenient screening tests for PNH are the sucrose hemolysis test[79] and the examination of urine for hemosiderin. Occasionally, the characteristically complement-sensitive red cells cannot be demonstrated in patients with well-established PNH. This probably occurs when the production of PNH cells is relatively low and most of the PNH cells that have been made have already been destroyed either in the marrow or in the circulation. Thus a single normal sucrose hemolysis test cannot be considered to be strong evidence that a patient does not have PNH. Hemosiderinuria is a more constant feature of the disease and is helpful in identifying patients who may have PNH with a transiently normal sucrose hemolysis test. The diagnosis can be definitively established using fluorescent-activated cell sorting (FACS) of granulocytes using either anti-CD55 or anti-CD59 antibodies[43,80,81] or the fluorescently labeled inactive variant of the anchor-binding protein aerolysin.[82] It has been suggested that both CD59 and CD55 should be measured in erythrocytes and that when granulocytes are studied two anchor-linked antigens (e.g., CD55/CD16 or CD59/CD16) and one non–anchor-linked antigen (CD15 or CD33) should be measured.[83] Older methods for establishing the diagnosis, such as the Ham acid hemolysis test, have been replaced by FACS analysis as the definitive diagnostic test.

Thrombocytopenia and leukopenia are features of PNH that help to differentiate this disorder from other types of hemolytic anemia. Hemosiderinuria, a constant feature of PNH, does not usually occur in other forms of hemolytic anemia, except for those in which there is considerable intravascular destruction of erythrocytes, such as in the hemolytic anemia associated with prosthetic cardiac valves. Although HEMPAS (herediary erythroblastic multinuclearity with a positive acidified serum lysis test) is characterized, as its name implies, by a positive acidified lysis test, there should be no difficulty in distinguishing this disorder from PNH (see Chap. 37). Lysis of HEMPAS cells results from the presence in normal serum of antibodies to unusual antigens on the surface of HEMPAS cells. The serum of patients lacks the required alloantibody, and HEMPAS cells do not lyse in their own serum. Moreover, HEMPAS is a hereditary disorder and is not associated with leukopenia or thrombocytopenia.

THERAPY, COURSE, AND PROGNOSIS

TREATMENT

Treatment of PNH consists chiefly of supportive measures such as transfusion, antibiotics, and anticoagulants as may be required. Suitable patients may be cured by marrow transplantation.

TRANSFUSIONS

Transfusions with red cells are often necessary in the management of patients with severe PNH. Although washed red cells are usually recommended so as to avoid transfusing the complement contained in plasma, analysis of a large number of transfusions given to PNH patients suggests that packed red cells are equally safe.[84,85]

IRON THERAPY

The iron deficiency that often occurs in patients with PNH because of the urinary loss of iron should be treated. The oral administration of iron is usually entirely satisfactory (see Chap. 40). Although an increase in hemoglobinuria may occur during iron therapy because of increased production of PNH cells by the marrow, the net positive effect of the administration of iron may lessen the requirements for blood transfusion.

STEROIDS

Both androgens and glucocorticoids have been used in the treatment of PNH. Fluoxymestrone (Halotestin) in doses of 20 to 30 mg/day usually produces some increase in the hemoglobin concentration of the blood.[86] The administration of danazol has given mixed results.[87–89] The administration of glucocorticoids has also been reported to be useful both in the treatment of hemolysis and thrombotic episodes.[12] Doses ranging from 20 to 60 mg of prednisone on alternate days may be tried. In view of the potential side effects, particularly when these drugs are administered chronically, steroid therapy should be limited to those patients whose transfusion requirement is significantly decreased at well-tolerated doses.

ANTICOAGULANTS

The principal role of anticoagulants in the management of PNH is in the treatment of thrombotic complications such as the Budd-Chiari syndrome,[90] but prophylactic anticoagulation with warfarin has been advocated for patients with large (>50% of granulocyte) clones.[91] Thrombolytic therapy with streptokinase and urokinase was considered safe and effective in two patients with PNH,[92] as was fibrinolytic therapy with recombinant tissue plasminogen activator given intravenously in another patient.[93]

The anticomplementary effect of heparin or low molecular weight heparin may exert a beneficial effect on the disease.[94] Sometimes a trial of anticoagulation therapy is used with patients who have repeated episodes of abdominal and back pain, but the usefulness of this approach remains to be established. The administration of drugs associated with an increased incidence of thrombosis, particularly oral contraceptives, should be avoided.

SPLENECTOMY

Generally, splenectomy is not indicated, although favorable responses have been reported in occasional patients.[78] Because of the considerable risk of thromboembolic complications in patients with PNH, elective surgery of any type, including splenectomy, is best avoided.

STEM CELL TRANSPLANTATION

As in other stem cell disorders, stem cell transplantation is an effective, albeit high-risk, method for treatment of PNH.[95–97] As might be expected, the abnormalities in the phosphoinositol-anchored proteins are corrected by this procedure. A large study from 1978 suggested that transplantation restores normal marrow function in about 50 percent of patients. The outlook may be somewhat more favorable with modern transplantation techniques (see Chap. 22). The experience with stem cell transplantation is not sufficient to provide clear guidelines for indications for the procedure. In general, however, it should be reserved for patients with life-threatening complications, such as venous thrombosis, and those who have a good match for allogeneic transplantation.[68]

OTHER TREATMENTS

Erythropoietin therapy seemed to have a beneficial effect in some patients but not in others.[98,99] Hemolysis may be diminished temporarily by the infusion of a dextran solution,[100,101] but this measure does not seem to have a role in the clinical management of PNH. Some selective suppression of PNH cells was documented with 6-mercaptopurine treatment, but this did not prove to be of any clinical value.[102] Cyclosporine, sometimes in combination with granulocyte colony stimulat-

ing factor, has seemed helpful in some patients.[103,104] A C5-blocking monoclonal antibody was found useful in controlling hemolysis.[105]

COURSE

The clinical course of PNH is enormously variable. In rare instances, the patient may succumb to this disease within a few months of the first onset of symptoms. Other patients experience a chronic course in which the severity of the disease waxes and wanes as the normal cells and the PNH clone alternately appear to gain ascendancy. Sometimes the abnormal clone disappears altogether, and the patient appears to be cured. It has been suggested that the course is more severe in children and adolescents with PNH.[106]

It has been suggested that 5 to 15 percent of patients with PNH ultimately develop acute leukemia.[107] Myelodysplastic syndrome also occurs in patients with PNH.[108–110] Not surprisingly, the defect seems to arise in the PNH clone.[111]

PROGNOSIS

As with so many other diseases, initial reports on PNH tended to emphasize the more severely affected patients, so the prognosis was generally deemed to be very grave. As physicians developed a higher index of suspicion concerning this disorder, and as simplified methods for diagnosis became available, milder cases were diagnosed, and these tend to have the better long-term outlook. Nonetheless, even today the disease must be considered a very serious one, and most patients eventually succumb to its complications. The most commonly lethal of these are probably thrombotic episodes such as the Budd-Chiari syndrome, but the various complications of pancytopenia also may lead to death, and in a few patients the terminal episode has been the development of acute leukemia.[112] In a study of 220 patients with PNH followed for up to 46 years, the Kaplan-Meier survival estimate was 65 percent at 10 years and 48 percent at 15 years after diagnosis.[113] In another study of 80 consecutive patients the outlook was similar: the median survival after diagnosis was 10 years, with 28 percent of patients surviving for 25 years.[114] Eight-year cumulative incidence rates of the main complications of pancytopenia, thrombosis, and myelodysplastic syndrome were 15 percent, 28 percent, and 5 percent, respectively. Poor survival was associated with age over 55 years at the time of diagnosis, the occurrence of thrombosis as a complication, evolution to pancytopenia, a myelodysplastic syndrome or acute leukemia, and thrombocytopenia at diagnosis. The prognosis of patients in whom aplastic anemia antedated PNH was better than in those in whom it did not.[113]

REFERENCES

1. Crosby WH: Paroxysmal nocturnal hemoglobinuria. A classic description by Paul Strübing in 1882, and a bibliography of the disease. *Blood* 6:270, 1951.
2. Strübing P: Paroxysmale Haemoglobinurie. *Dtsch Med Wochenschr* 8:1, 1882.
3. Hijmans Van Den Bergh AA: Ictère hémolytique avec crises hémoglobinuriques fragilité globulaire. *Rev Med* 31:63, 1911.
4. Takeda J, Miyata T, Kawagoe K, et al: Deficiency of the GPI anchor caused by a somatic mutation of the PIG-A gene in paroxysmal nocturnal hemoglobinuria. *Cell* 73:703, 1993.
5. Freeman H, Hill R, Edwards AM, Wolowyk MW: Paroxysmal nocturnal hemoglobinuria in an identical twin. *CMAJ* 109:1002, 1973.
6. Endo M, Beatty PG, Vreeke TM, et al: Syngeneic bone marrow transplantation without conditioning in a patient with paroxysmal nocturnal hemoglobinuria: In vivo evidence that the mutant stem cells have a survival advantage. *Blood* 88:742, 1996.

7. Kolb HJ, Holler E, Bender-Gotze C, et al: Myeloablative conditioning for marrow transplantation in myelodysplastic syndromes and paroxysmal nocturnal haemoglobinuria. *Bone Marrow Transplant* 4:29, 1989.

8. Oni SB, Osunkoya BO, Luzzatto L: Paroxysmal nocturnal hemoglobinuria: Evidence for monoclonal origin of abnormal red cells. *Blood* 36:145, 1970.

9. Josten KM, Tooze JA, Borthwick-Clarke C, et al: Acquired aplastic anemia and paroxysmal nocturnal hemoglobinuria: Studies on clonality. *Blood* 78:3162, 1991.

10. Parlier V, Tiainen M, Beris P, et al: Trisomy 8 detection in granulo-monocytic, erythrocytic and megakaryocytic lineages by chromosomal in situ suppression hybridization in a case of refractory anaemia with ringed sideroblasts complicating the course of paroxysmal nocturnal haemoglobinuria. *Br J Haematol* 81:296, 1992.

11. Luzzatto L, Bessler M: The dual pathogenesis of paroxysmal nocturnal hemoglobinuria. *Curr Opin Hematol* 3:101, 1996.

12. Rosse WF: Paroxysmal nocturnal hemoglobinuria as a molecular disease. *Medicine* 76:63, 1997.

13. Ben-Bassat I, Brok-Simoni F, Ramot B: Complement-sensitive red cells in aplastic anemia. *Blood* 46:357, 1975.

14. Mortazavi Y, Merk B, McIntosh J, et al: The spectrum of PIG-A gene mutations in aplastic anemia/paroxysmal nocturnal hemoglobinuria (AA/PNH): A high incidence of multiple mutations and evidence of a mutational hot spot. *Blood* 101:2833, 2003.

15. Iwanaga M, Furukawa K, Amenomori T, et al: Paroxysmal nocturnal haemoglobinuria clones in patients with myelodysplastic syndromes. *Br J Haematol* 102:465, 1998.

16. Ware RE, Pickens CV, DeCastro CM, Howard TA: Circulating PIG-A mutant T lymphocytes in healthy adults and patients with bone marrow failure syndromes. *Exp Hematol* 29:1403, 2001.

17. Wang HB, Chuhjo T, Yasue S, et al: Clinical significance of a minor population of paroxysmal nocturnal hemoglobinuria-type cells in bone marrow failure syndrome. *Blood* 100:3897, 2002.

18. Araten DJ, Nafa K, Pakdeesuwan K, Luzzatto L: Clonal populations of hematopoietic cells with paroxysmal nocturnal hemoglobinuria genotype and phenotype are present in normal individuals. *Proc Natl Acad Sci U S A* 96:5209, 1999.

19. Rosti V, Tremml G, Soares V, et al: Murine embryonic stem cells without PIG-A gene activity are competent for hematopoiesis with the PNH phenotype but not for clonal expansion. *J Clin Invest* 100:1028, 1997.

20. Brodsky RA, Vala MS, Barber JP, et al: Resistance to apoptosis caused by PIG-A gene mutations in paroxysmal nocturnal hemoglobinuria. *Proc Natl Acad Sci U S A* 94:8756, 1997.

21. Horikawa K, Nakakuma H, Kawaguchi T, et al: Apoptosis resistance of blood cells from patients with paroxysmal nocturnal hemoglobinuria, aplastic anemia, and myelodysplastic syndrome. *Blood* 90:2716, 1997.

22. Chen TG, Nagarajan S, Prince GM, et al: Impaired growth and elevated fas receptor expression in PIGA(+) stem cells in primary paroxysmal nocturnal hemoglobinuria. *J Clin Invest* 106:689, 2000.

23. Heeney MM, Ormsbee SM, Anthony MM, et al: Increased expression of anti-apoptosis genes in peripheral blood cells from patients with paroxysmal nocturnal hemoglobinuria. *Mol Genet Metab* 78:291, 2003.

24. Ware RE, Nishimura J, Moody MA, et al: The PIG-A mutation and absence of glycosylphosphatidylinositol-linked proteins do not confer resistance to apoptosis in paroxysmal nocturnal hemoglobinuria. *Blood* 92:2541, 1998.

25. Yamamoto T, Shichishima T, Shikama Y, et al: Granulocytes from patients with paroxysmal nocturnal hemoglobinuria and normal individuals have the same sensitivity to spontaneous apoptosis. *Exp Hematol* 30:187, 2002.

26. Bessler M, Mason P, Hillmen P, Luzzatto L: Somatic mutations and cellular selection in paroxysmal nocturnal haemoglobinuria. *Lancet* 343:951, 1994.

27. Nishimura J, Inoue N, Wada H, et al: A patient with paroxysmal nocturnal hemoglobinuria bearing four independent PIG-A mutant clones. *Blood* 89:3470, 1997.

28. Johnson RJ, Hillmen P: Paroxysmal nocturnal haemoglobinuria: Nature's gene therapy? *Mol Pathol* 55:145, 2002.

29. Hirose S, Ravi L, Prince GM, et al: Synthesis of mannosylglucosaminylinositol phospholipids in normal but not paroxysmal nocturnal hemoglobinuria cells. *Proc Natl Acad Sci U S A* 89:6025, 1992.

30. Chow FL, Hall SE, Rosse WF, Telen MJ: Separation of the acetylcholinesterase-deficient red cells in paroxysmal nocturnal hemoglobinuria. *Blood* 67:893, 1986.

31. Beck WS, Valentine WN: Biochemical studies on leucocytes: II. Phosphatase activity in chronic lymphatic leukemia, acute leukemia, and miscellaneous hematologic conditions. *J Lab Clin Med* 38:245, 1951.

32. Pangburn MK, Schreiber RD, Muller-Eberhard HJ: Dysfunction of two erythrocyte membrane proteins in paroxysmal nocturnal hemoglobinuria. *Proc Natl Acad Sci U S A* 80:5430, 1983.

33. Zalman LS, Wood LM, Frank MM, Muller-Eberhard HJ: Deficiency of the homologous restriction factor in paroxysmal nocturnal hemoglobinuria. *J Exp Med* 165:572, 1987.

34. Selvaraj P, Dustin ML, Silber R, et al: Deficiency of lymphocyte function-associated antigen 3 (LFA-3) in paroxysmal nocturnal hemoglobinuria. Functional correlates and evidence for a phosphatidylinositol membrane anchor. *J Exp Med* 166:1011, 1987.

35. Rosse WF: Paroxysmal nocturnal hemoglobinuria and decay-accelerating factor. *Annu Rev Med* 41:431, 1990.

36. Selvaraj P, Rosse WF, Silber R, Springer TA: The major Fc receptor in blood has a phosphatidylinositol anchor and is deficient in paroxysmal nocturnal haemoglobinuria. *Nature* 333:565, 1988.

37. Ploug M, Plesner T, Ronne E, et al: The receptor for urokinase-type plasminogen activator is deficient on peripheral blood leukocytes in patients with paroxysmal nocturnal hemoglobinuria. *Blood* 79:1447, 1992.

38. Simmons DL, Tan S, Tenen DG, et al: Monocyte antigen CD14 is a phospholipid anchored membrane protein. *Blood* 73:284, 1989.

39. Rosse WF: Paroxysmal nocturnal hemoglobinuria. *Curr Top Microbiol Immunol* 178:163, 1992.

40. Merry AH, Rawlinson VI, Uchikawa M, et al: Studies on the sensitivity to complement-mediated lysis of erythrocytes (Inab phenotype) with a deficiency of DAF (decay accelerating factor). *Br J Haematol* 73:248, 1989.

41. Telen MJ, Green AM: The Inab phenotype: Characterization of the membrane protein and complement regulatory defect. *Blood* 74:437, 1989.

42. Yamashina M, Ueda E, Kinoshita T, et al: Inherited complete deficiency of 20-kilodalton homologous restriction factor (CD59) as a cause of paroxysmal nocturnal hemoglobinuria. *N Engl J Med* 323:1184, 1990.

43. Richards SJ, Rawstron AC, Hillmen P: Application of flow cytometry to the diagnosis of paroxysmal nocturnal hemoglobinuria. *Cytometry* 42:223, 2000.

44. Holt DS, Botto M, Bygrave AE, et al: Targeted deletion of the CD59 gene causes spontaneous intravascular hemolysis and hemoglobinuria. *Blood* 98:442, 2001.

45. Wilcox LA, Ezzell JL, Bernshaw NJ, Parker CJ: Molecular basis of the enhanced susceptibility of the erythrocytes of paroxysmal nocturnal hemoglobinuria to hemolysis in acidified serum. *Blood* 78:820, 1991.

46. Ono H, Kuno Y, Tanaka H, et al: A case of paroxysmal nocturnal hemoglobinuria without deficiency of decay-accelerating factor on erythrocytes. *Blood* 75:1746, 1990.

47. Shichishima T, Terasawa T, Hashimoto C, et al: Heterogenous expression of decay accelerating factor and CD59/membrane attack complex inhibition factor on paroxysmal nocturnal haemoglobinuria (PNH) erythrocytes. *Br J Haematol* 78:545, 1991.

48. Hillmen P, Hows JM, Luzzatto L: Two distinct patterns of glycosyl-phosphatidylinositol (GPI) linked protein deficiency in the red cells of patients with paroxysmal nocturnal haemoglobinuria. *Br J Haematol* 80: 399, 1992.

49. Devine DV, Siegel RS, Rosse WF: Interactions of the platelets in paroxysmal nocturnal hemoglobinuria with complement. Relationship to defects in the regulation of complement and to platelet survival in vivo. *J Clin Invest* 79:131, 1987.

50. Okuda K, Kanamaru A, Ueda E, et al: Membrane expression of decay-accelerating factor on neutrophils from normal individuals and patients with paroxysmal nocturnal hemoglobinuria. *Blood* 75:1186, 1990.

51. Craddock PR, Fehr J, Jacob HS: Complement-mediated granulocyte dysfunction in paroxysmal nocturnal hemoglobinuria. *Blood* 47:931, 1976.

52. Alfinito F, Del Vecchio L, Rocco S, et al: Blood cell flow cytometry in paroxysmal nocturnal hemoglobinuria: A tool for measuring the extent of the PNH clone. *Leukemia* 10:1326, 1996.

53. Hillmen P, Bessler M, Crawford DH, Luzzatto L: Production and characterization of lymphoblastoid cell lines with the paroxysmal nocturnal hemoglobinuria phenotype. *Blood* 81:193, 1993.

54. Ham TH: Studies on destruction of red blood cells: I. Chronic hemolytic anemia with paroxysmal nocturnal hemoglobinuria: An investigation of the mechanism of hemolysis, with observations on five cases. *Arch Intern Med* 64:1271, 1939.

55. Crosby WH: Paroxysmal nocturnal hemoglobinuria. Relation of the clinical manifestations to underlying pathogenic mechanisms. *Blood* 8:769, 1953.

56. Clark DA, Butler SA, Braren V, et al: The kidneys in paroxysmal nocturnal hemoglobinuria. *Blood* 57:83, 1981.

57. Mengel CE, Kann HE Jr, O'Malley BW: Increased hemolysis after intramuscular iron administration in patients with paroxysmal nocturnal hemoglobinuria: Report of six occurrences in four patients, and speculations on a possible mechanism. *Blood* 26:74, 1965.

58. Rosse WF, Gutterman LG: The effect of iron therapy in paroxysmal nocturnal hemoglobinuria. *Blood* 36:559, 1970.

59. Nafa K, Bessler M, Mason P, et al: Factor V Leiden mutation investigated by amplification created restriction enzyme site (ACRES) in PNH patients with and without thrombosis. *Haematologica* 81:540, 1996.

60. Valla D, Dhumeaux D, Babany G, et al: Hepatic vein thrombosis in paroxysmal nocturnal hemoglobinuria. A spectrum from asymptomatic occlusion of hepatic venules to fatal Budd-Chiari syndrome. *Gastroenterology* 93:569, 1987.

61. Leibowitz AI, Hartmann RC: Annotation: The Budd-Chiari syndrome and paroxysmal nocturnal haemoglobinuria. *Br J Haematol* 48:1, 1981.

62. Wyatt HA, Mowat AP, Layton M: Paroxysmal nocturnal haemoglobinuria and Budd-Chiari syndrome. *Arch Dis Child* 72:241, 1995.

63. Birgens HS, Hancke S, Rosenklint A, Hansen NE: Ultrasonic demonstration of clinical and subclinical hepatic venous thrombosis in paroxysmal nocturnal haemoglobinuria. *Br J Haematol* 64:737, 1986.

64. Blum SF, Gardner FH: Intestinal infarction in paroxysmal nocturnal hemoglobinuria. *N Engl J Med* 274:1137, 1966.

65. Doukas MA, DiLorenzo PE, Mohler DN: Intestinal infarction caused by paroxysmal nocturnal hemoglobinuria. *Am J Hematol* 16:75, 1984.

66. Heller PG, Grinberg AR, Lencioni M, et al: Pulmonary hypertension in paroxysmal nocturnal hemoglobinuria. *Chest* 102:642, 1992.

67. Klein KL, Hartmann RC: Acute coronary artery thrombosis in paroxysmal nocturnal hemoglobinuria. *South Med J* 82:1169, 1989.

68. Meyers G, Parker CJ: Management issues in paroxysmal nocturnal hemoglobinuria. *Int J Hematol* 77:125, 2003.

69. Jacobs P, Wood L: Paroxysmal nocturnal haemoglobinuria and pregnancy. *Lancet* 2:1099, 1986.

70. De Gramont A, Krulik M, Debray J: Paroxysmal nocturnal haemoglobinuria and pregnancy. *Lancet* 1:868, 1987.

71. Beresford CH, Gudex DJ, Symmans WA: Paroxysmal nocturnal haemoglobinuria and pregnancy. *Lancet* 2:1396, 1986.

72. Blaisdell RK, Priest RE, Beutler E: Paroxysmal nocturnal hemoglobinuria: A case report with a negative Ham presumptive test associated with serum properdin deficiency. *Blood* 13:1074, 1958.

73. Jose MD, Lynn KL: Acute renal failure in a patient with paroxysmal nocturnal hemoglobinuria. *Clin Nephrol* 56:172, 2001.

74. Chow KM, Lai FM, Wang AY, et al: Reversible renal failure in paroxysmal nocturnal hemoglobinuria. *Am J Kidney Dis* 37:E17, 2001.

75. Zachée P, Henckens M, Van Damme B, et al: Chronic renal failure due to renal hemosiderosis in a patient with paroxysmal nocturnal hemoglobinuria. *Clin Nephrol* 39:28, 1993.

76. Hauser D, Barzilai N, Zalish M, et al: Bilateral papilledema with retinal hemorrhages in association with cerebral venous sinus thrombosis and paroxysmal nocturnal hemoglobinuria. *Am J Ophthalmol* 122:592, 1996.

77. Olson D, Hillmen P, Luzzatto L, Blasi F: Absence of a cell surface urokinase receptor in the white blood cells of three patients with paroxysmal nocturnal hemoglobinuria. *Blood Coagul Fibrinolysis* 6(Suppl 4):89, 1992.

78. Dacie JV: *The Haemolytic Anaemias*. Grune & Stratton, New York, 1967.

79. Hartmann RC, Jenkins DE Jr: The "sugar-water" test for paroxysmal nocturnal hemoglobinuria. *N Engl J Med* 275:155, 1965.

80. Guimbretière L, Bernard D, Maisonneuve H, et al: Paroxysmal nocturnal haemoglobinuria. Diagnosis aided by a monoclonal antibody directed against the decay accelerating factor glycoprotein. *Presse Med* 22:467, 1993.

81. Meletis J, Michali E, Samarkos M, et al: Detection of "PNH red cell" populations in hematological disorders using the sephacryl gel test micro typing system. *Leuk Lymphoma* 28:177, 1997.

82. Brodsky RA, Mukhina GL, Li S, et al: Improved detection and characterization of paroxysmal nocturnal hemoglobinuria using fluorescent aerolysin. *Am J Clin Pathol* 114:459, 2000.

83. Hillmen P, Richards SJ: Implications of recent insights into the pathophysiology of paroxysmal nocturnal hemoglobinuria. *Br J Haematol* 108:470, 2000.

84. Brecher ME, Taswell HF: Paroxysmal nocturnal hemoglobinuria and the transfusion of washed red cells: A myth revisited. *Transfusion* 29:681, 1989.

85. Rosse WF: Transfusion in paroxysmal nocturnal hemoglobinuria: To wash or not to wash. *Transfusion* 29:663, 1989.

86. Hartmann RC, Jenkins DE Jr, McKee LC, Heyssel RM: Paroxysmal nocturnal hemoglobinuria: Clinical and laboratory studies relating to iron metabolism and therapy with androgen and iron. *Medicine* 45:331, 1966.

87. Harrington WJS, Kolodny L, Horstman LL, et al: Danazol for paroxysmal nocturnal hemoglobinuria. *Am J Hematol* 54:149, 1997.

88. Katayama Y, Hiramatsu Y, Kohriyama K: Monitoring of CD59 expression in paroxysmal nocturnal hemoglobinuria treated with danazol. *Am J Hematol* 68:280, 2001.

89. Lippman SM, Durie BG, Garewal HS, et al: Efficacy of danazol in pure red cell aplasia. *Am J Hematol* 23:373, 1986.

90. Hartmann RC, Luther AB, Jenkins DE Jr, et al: Fulminant hepatic venous thrombosis (Budd-Chiari syndrome) in paroxysmal nocturnal hemoglobinuria: Definition of a medical emergency. *Johns Hopkins Med J* 146:247, 1980.

91. Hall CJ, Richards SJ, Hillmen P: Primary prophylaxis with warfarin prevents thrombosis in paroxysmal nocturnal hemoglobinuria (PNH). *Blood* 102:3587, 2003.

92. Sholar PW, Bell WR: Thrombolytic therapy for inferior vena cava thrombosis in paroxysmal nocturnal hemoglobinuria. *Ann Intern Med* 103:539, 1985.

93. Hauser AC, Brichta A, Pabinger-Fasching I, Jager U: Fibrinolytic therapy with rt-PA in a patient with paroxysmal nocturnal hemoglobinuria and Budd-Chiari syndrome. *Ann Hematol* 82:299, 2003.

94. Ninomiya H, Kawashima Y, Nagasawa T: Inhibition of complement-mediated haemolysis in paroxysmal nocturnal haemoglobinuria by heparin or low-molecular weight heparin. *Br J Haematol* 109:875, 2000.

95. Lee JL, Lee JH, Choi SJ, et al: Allogeneic hematopoietic cell transplantation for paroxysmal nocturnal hemoglobinuria. *Eur J Haematol* 71: 114, 2003.

96. Flotho C, Strahm B, Kontny U, et al: Stem cell transplantation for paroxysmal nocturnal haemoglobinuria in childhood. *Br J Haematol* 118: 124, 2002.

97. Ditschkowski M, Trenschel R, Kummer G, et al: Allogeneic CD34-enriched peripheral blood stem cell transplantation in a patient with paroxysmal nocturnal haemoglobinuria. *Bone Marrow Transplant* 32:633, 2003.

98. Astori C, Bonfichi M, Pagnucco G, et al: Treatment with recombinant human erythropoietin (rHuEpo) in a patient with paroxysmal nocturnal haemoglobinuria: Evaluation of membrane proteins CD55 and CD59 with cytofluorometric assay. *Br J Haematol* 97:586, 1997.

99. Stebler C, Tichelli A, Dazzi H, et al: High-dose recombinant human erythropoietin for treatment of anemia in myelodysplastic syndromes and paroxysmal nocturnal hemoglobinuria: A pilot study. *Exp Hematol* 18:1204, 1990.

100. Stratton F, Wilkinson JF, Israels MCG: Clinical dextran for acute episodes in paroxysmal nocturnal hemoglobinuria. *Lancet* 1:831, 1958.

101. Gardner FH, Laforet MT: The use of clinical dextran in patients with paroxysmal nocturnal hemoglobinuria. *J Lab Clin Med* 55:946, 1960.

102. Beutler E, Collins Z: The effect of 6-mercaptopurine (6-MP) administration in paroxysmal nocturnal hemoglobinuria (PNH). Proceedings of the 10th Congress of the International Society of Hematology, Stockholm, Sweden, August 30–September 4, 1964.

103. Schubert J, Scholz C, Geissler RG, et al: G-CSF and cyclosporin induce an increase of normal cells in hypoplastic paroxysmal nocturnal hemoglobinuria. *Ann Hematol* 74:225, 1997.

104. Van Kamp H, Van Imhoff GW, de Wolf JT, et al: The effect of cyclosporine on haematological parameters in patients with paroxysmal nocturnal haemoglobinuria. *Br J Haematol* 89:79, 1995.

105. Hillmen P, Hall C, Marsh JC, et al: Effect of eculizumab on hemolysis and transfusion requirements in patients with paroxysmal nocturnal hemoglobinuria. *N Engl J Med* 350:552, 2004.

106. Ware RE, Hall SE, Rosse WF: Paroxysmal nocturnal hemoglobinuria with onset in childhood and adolescence. *N Engl J Med* 325:991, 1991.

107. Harris JW, Koscick R, Lazarus HM, et al: Leukemia arising out of paroxysmal nocturnal hemoglobinuria. *Leuk Lymphoma* 32:401, 1999.

108. Aymard JP, Buisine J, Gregoire MJ, et al: Refractory anaemia with excess of blasts as a terminal evolution of paroxysmal nocturnal haemoglobinuria. *Acta Haematol (Basel)* 74:181, 1985.

109. Ko W-S, Chen L-M, Chao T-Y, Hwang W-S: Myeloblastic leukemoid reaction in paroxysmal nocturnal hemoglobinuria associated with myelodysplasia. *Acta Haematol (Basel)* 87:75, 1992.

110. Graham DL, Gastineau DA: Paroxysmal nocturnal hemoglobinuria as a marker for clonal myelopathy. *Am J Med* 93:671, 1992.

111. Devine DV, Gluck WL, Rosse WF, Weinberg JB: Acute myeloblastic leukemia in paroxysmal nocturnal hemoglobinuria: Evidence of evolution from the abnormal paroxysmal nocturnal hemoglobinuria clone. *J Clin Invest* 79:314, 1987.

112. Zittoun R, Bernadou A, James IM, et al: Acute myelo-monocytic leukaemia: A terminal complication of paroxysmal nocturnal haemoglobinuria. *Acta Haematol (Basel)* 53:241, 1975.

113. Socie G, Mary JY, De Gramont A, et al: Paroxysmal nocturnal haemoglobinuria: Long-term follow-up and prognostic factors. *Lancet* 348: 573, 1996.

114. Hillmen P, Lewis SM, Bessler M, et al: Natural history of paroxysmal nocturnal hemoglobinuria. *N Engl J Med* 333:1253, 1995.

FOLATE, COBALAMIN, AND MEGALOBLASTIC ANEMIAS

BERNARD M. BABIOR*

Folate in its tetrahydro form is a transporter of one-carbon fragments, which it can carry at any of three oxidation levels: methanol, formaldehyde, and formic acid. The oxidation levels of the folate-bound one-carbon fragments can be altered by oxidation and reduction reactions that require nicotinamide adenine dinucleotide phosphate and nicotinamide adenine dinucleotide phosphate (reduced form), respectively. The chief source of the folate-bound one-carbon fragments is serine, which is converted to glycine as it passes its terminal carbon to folate. The one-carbon fragments are used for biosynthesis of purines, thymidine, and methionine. During biosynthesis of purines and methionine, free folate is released in its tetrahydro form. During biosynthesis of thymidine, tetrahydrofolate is oxidized to the dihydro form and must be re-reduced by dihydrofolate reductase in order to continue functioning in one-carbon metabolism. Methotrexate acts as an anticancer agent because it is an exceedingly powerful inhibitor of dihydrofolate reductase.

In the cell, folates are conjugated by the addition of a chain of seven or eight glutamic acid residues. These residues prevent the folates from leaking out of the cell. When folates are absorbed from the intestine, a process that occurs chiefly in the duodenum and proximal jejunum, all but one of the glutamates are removed by the enzyme conjugase. Folates travel in the bloodstream and are taken up by the cells, mainly in the form of unconjugated methyltetrahydrofolate. The newly absorbed folates are rapidly reconjugated in the cell. If reconjugation is prevented, the folates leak back out of the cell, resulting in an intracellular folate deficiency.

Cobalamin is required for two reactions: conversion of methylmalonyl coenzyme A (CoA) a product of catabolism of branched-chain amino acids, to succinyl CoA, a Krebs cycle intermediate, and conversion of homocysteine to methionine, a reaction in which the methyl group of methyltetrahydrofolate is donated to the sulfur atom of homocysteine. In cobalamin deficiency, methyltetrahydrofolate accumulates because, for practical purposes, donation of the methyl group to homocysteine is the only method of generating free tetrahydrofolate from methyltetrahydrofolate. Free tetrahydrofolate is an excellent substrate for the conjugase; methyltetrahydrofolate is a poor substrate. Consequently, much of the methyltetrahydrofolate taken up by a cobalamin-deficient cell leaks out of the cell before it can be conjugated. The megaloblastic anemia of cobalamin deficiency results from an intracellular folate deficiency that arises because of the cell's limited ability to conjugate methyltetrahydrofolate.

Absorption of cobalamin is a highly complex process. Upon arriving in the stomach, cobalamin is taken up by R binder (also called *haptocorrin* or *cobalophilin*), a glycoprotein found in virtually all secretions. When the cobalamin–R binder complex enters the duodenum, the R binder is digested and the cobalamin is released into the intestinal lumen, where it is taken up by intrinsic factor, a protein secreted by the gastric parietal cells. The cobalamin–intrinsic factor complex is absorbed by cells in the ileum, where the cobalamin is released and transported to the bloodstream. Here the vitamin binds to transcobalamin (TC) II, which delivers its cargo of cobalamin to cells throughout the body. Folic acid (pteroylglutamic acid) and cobalamin (vitamin B_{12}) play key roles in the metabolic economy of proliferating cells.

Megaloblastic anemia most commonly results from folate or cobalamin (vitamin B_{12}) deficiency. Folate deficiency usually is nutritional in origin. It may be seen in alcoholics and the elderly poor but also is seen in patients on hyperalimentation or hemodialysis. In pregnancy, even a mild folate deficiency is associated with defects in neural tube closure in the fetus, so pregnant women should always be given folate supplements. Diagnosis is based on measurements of folate in serum, which furnishes information about the current level of folate, and in red cells, which provides data on folate levels over the preceding 6 weeks. Nutritional folate deficiency is treated with folic acid by mouth.

Folate deficiency as a result of malabsorption occurs in tropical and nontropical sprue. Folate deficiency as a result of tropical sprue is treated with folate supplements and antibiotics. In nontropical sprue, the treatment is folate plus a gluten-free diet.

The most common cause of cobalamin deficiency is pernicious anemia (PA), a condition in which the portion of gastric mucosa that contains the parietal cells is destroyed through an autoimmune mechanism. The parietal cells secrete intrinsic factor, which is essential for cobalamin absorption. Without intrinsic factor, a state of cobalamin deficiency develops over the course of years. Cobalamin deficiency leads not only to megaloblastic anemia but also to a demyelinating disease that manifests itself as peripheral neuropathy, spastic paralysis with ataxia (so-called combined system disease of the spinal cord), dementia, psychosis, or a combination of the foregoing. "Subtle" cobalamin deficiency, manifested as neurologic symptoms without anemia, appears to be relatively widespread among the elderly. The incidence of gastric cancer is increased by a factor of two to three in patients with PA. Other causes of cobalamin deficiency are gastric resection; stasis of the small intestinal contents as a result of blind loops, strictures, or hypomotility (e.g., as seen in amyloid); and disease or resection of the terminal ileum. Patients on a vegan diet become cobalamin deficient. Cobalamin deficiency is diagnosed by measuring the level of the vitamin in the blood or by measuring serum methylmalonic acid, which accumulates in the bloodstream in patients

*Deceased 6/29/04.

Acronyms and abbreviations that appear in this chapter include: AdoCbl, adenosylcobalamin; AICAR, 5-amino-4-imidazole carboxamide ribotide; ATP, adenosine 5′-triphosphate; ATPase, adenosine triphosphatase; AZT, azidothymidine; BFU-E, burst forming unit–erythroid; CnCbl, cyanocobalamin; CNS, central nervous system; CoA, coenzyme A; dTMP, deoxythymidine monophosphate; dU, deoxyuridine; dUMP, deoxyuridine monophosphate; FH$_4$, tetrahydrofolate; FIGlu, formiminoglutamic acid; [³H]Thd, [³H]thymidine; HCl, hydrochloric acid; HIV, human immunodeficiency virus; IM, intramuscular; LDH, lactate dehydrogenase; MCV, mean corpuscular volume; MeCbl, methylcobalamin; MRI, magnetic resonance imaging; MTHFR, methylenetetrahydrofolate reductase; NAD, nicotinamide adenine dinucleotide; NADH, nicotinamide adenine dinucleotide (reduced form); NADP, nicotinamide adenine dinucleotide phosphate; NADPH, nicotinamide adenine dinucleotide phosphate (reduced form); N$_2$O, nitrous oxide; OHCbl, hydroxycobalamin; PA, pernicious anemia; SAH, S-adenosylhomocysteine; SAM, S-adenosylmethionine; TC, transcobalamin; UTP, uridine triphosphate.

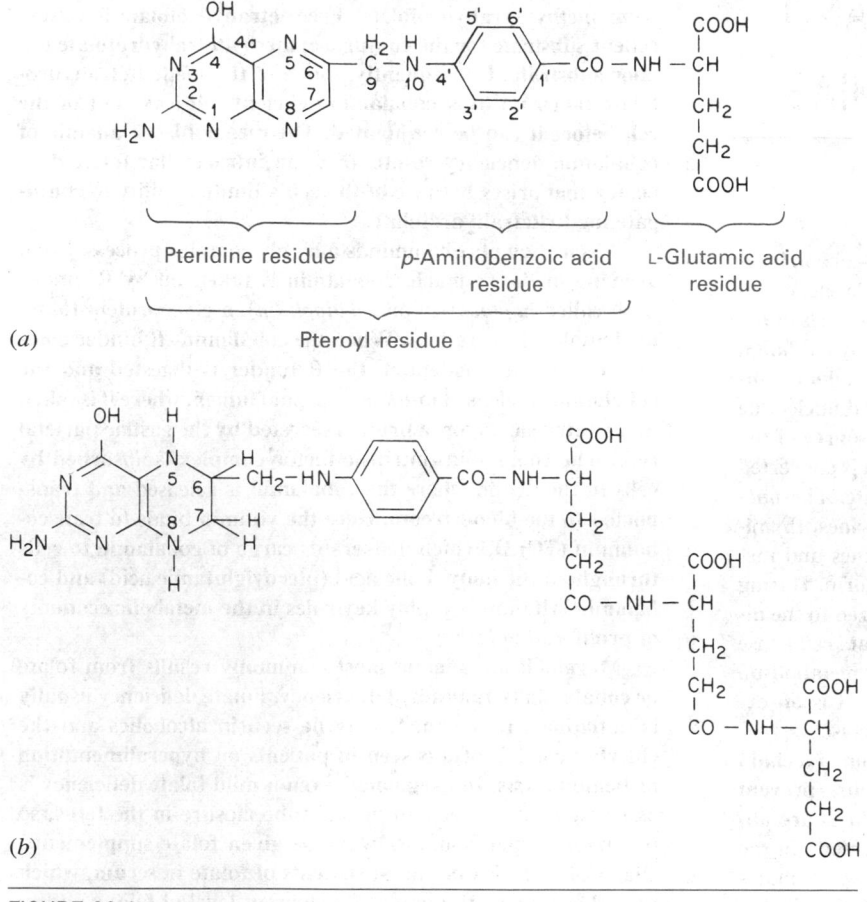

(a)

(b)

FIGURE 39-1 Folic acid. (*a*) Folic acid (pteroylglutamic acid) and its components. (*b*) Tetrahydrofolate triglutamate.

with cobalamin deficiency. The cause of cobalamin deficiency often can be determined by the Schilling test, a measure of cobalamin absorption. In patients with nutritional megaloblastic anemia, folate or cobalamin deficiency as the cause of the anemia must be determined. If a patient with cobalamin deficiency is treated with folic acid, the anemia is corrected but the neurologic abnormalities progress. Patients with cobalamin deficiency usually are treated with parenteral cobalamin.

Megaloblastic anemia can develop as an acute disorder with rapid development of leukopenia and/or thrombocytopenia. Nitrous oxide anesthesia is responsible for some cases of acute megaloblastic anemia. The anemia is seen in patients with a marginal folate status in intensive care units. The condition resembles an immune cytopenia but can be ruled out by examining the bone marrow, which exhibits a floridly megaloblastic picture.

Other causes of megaloblastic anemia include drugs (e.g., hydroxyurea, nucleoside analogues), hemolytic anemia causing folate deficiency by increasing folate demand for augmented erythropoiesis, and certain inborn errors of metabolism. Of the inherited conditions, TCII deficiency is singled out because it causes a severe megaloblastic anemia in infants who respond completely to high-dose cobalamin. Irreversible neurologic complications supervene if the deficiency is not detected in time. Megaloblastic anemia is seen in refractory megaloblastic anemia, a form of the myelodysplastic syndrome, and in early stages of acute myeloblastic leukemia of the M6 type (Di Guglielmo syndrome). The anemia of refractory megaloblastic anemia sometimes responds to very high doses of pyridoxine.

METABOLIC ASPECTS OF FOLATE AND COBALAMIN

Folic acid (pteroylglutamic acid) and cobalamin (vitamin B_{12}) play key roles in the metabolism of proliferating cells.

FOLIC ACID

CHEMISTRY

Folic acid (pteroylglutamic acid) is composed of a pteridine derivative, a *p*-aminobenzoate residue, and an L-glutamic acid residue (Fig. 39-1*a*). The first two together are called *pteroic acid*.[1] In nature, folic acid occurs largely as conjugates in which multiple glutamic acids are linked by peptide bonds involving their γ-carboxyl groups (Fig. 39-1*b*). Conjugates are named according to the length of the glutamate chain (e.g., pteroylglutamate, pteroyldiglutamate, pteroylhexaglutamate). Therapeutic folic acid (abbreviated PteGlu, or F) has one glutamic acid.

To form a functional compound, folate must be reduced to tetrahydrofolate (FH_4) (see Fig. 39-1*b*). In this reduction, dihydrofolate (FH_2) is an intermediate. A single enzyme, *dihydrofolate reductase*, catalyzes both F→FH_2 and FH_2→FH_4.

The folate family consists largely of FH_4 derivatives bearing a one-carbon substituent (symbolized as FH_4-C). The varieties of FH_4-C differ with regard to the identity of the one-carbon unit and the site of its attachment to FH_4 (Fig. 39-2). One-carbon substituents of biochemical significance include the following:

formyl	$-CH=O$
formimino	$-CH=NH_2$
hydroxymethyl	$-CH_2OH$
methenyl	$=CH-$
methylene	$=CH_2$
methyl	$-CH_3$

These substituents are attached to FH_4 through N^5, N^{10}, or both (see Fig. 39-2). Specific enzymes interconvert these various FH_4 derivatives through oxidations that require nicotinamide adenine dinucleotide (NAD) and reductions that utilize nicotinamide adenine dinucleotide phosphate [reduced form (NADPH)].

Reduced derivatives of folic acid usually are sensitive to air oxidation. A clinically important exception is N^5-formyl FH_4, also called *citrovorum factor, leucovorin,* or *folinic acid.*

NUTRITION

SOURCES

Folic acid comes from many sources. The richest vegetable sources are asparagus, broccoli, endive, spinach, lettuce, and lima beans. Each vegetable contains more than 1 mg of folate per 100 g dry weight. The best fruit sources are lemons, bananas, and melons. Folates also are abundant in liver, kidney, yeast, and mushrooms. An average daily American diet contains 400 to 600 μg of folate.[2] Foods are readily depleted of folate by excessive cooking, especially with large amounts of water.

DAILY REQUIREMENTS

In the normal adult, the minimum daily requirement for folic acid is approximately 50 μg. The average diet contains many times this amount, but some of the folic acid may be unavailable. Accordingly, the officially recommended daily allowance of *food* folate for an adult is 0.4 mg.[3] The body is thought to contain approximately 5 mg of folate.[4] When folate intake is reduced to 5 μg/day, megaloblastic anemia develops in approximately 4 months.[5]

Folic acid requirements increase in hemolytic anemia, leukemia, and other malignant diseases, in alcoholism,[6] during growth, and in pregnancy and lactation. Requirements increase threefold to sixfold.[7] Adequate folate supplies are particularly important in pregnant women, in whom the recommended intake is 400 μg/day.[8]

FOLATE METABOLISM

FOLATE-DEPENDENT ENZYMES

FH_4 is an intermediate in reactions involving the transfer of one-carbon units from a donor X—C to an acceptor Y:

$$X-C + FH_4 \rightarrow FH_4-C + X$$
$$\underline{FH_4-C + Y \rightarrow Y-C + FH_4}$$
$$\text{Sum: } X-C + Y \rightarrow Y-C + X$$

Table 39-1 summarizes and reference 9 reviews the metabolic systems of animal tissues known to require folic acid coenzymes.

One-carbon units enter the folate pool principally via the serine hydroxymethyltransfcrase reaction.[10]

$$\text{Serine} + FH_4 \leftrightarrow \text{glycine}$$
$$+ N^5, N^{10}\text{-methylene } FH_4 + H_2O$$

which requires pyridoxal phosphate as cofactor.

Conversion of methionine to polyamines is accompanied by the production of one-carbon fragments that combine with folate at the oxidation level of formate[11] (Fig. 39-3). Less important sources of one-carbon units are the catabolism of histidine[12] and the adenosine 5'-triphosphate (ATP)-dependent formation of N^5-formyl FH_4 (folinic acid) from formic acid and FH_4.[13]

Among the one-carbon transfers mediated by folic acid, the transfer that appears to be clinically the most important is the methylation of deoxyuridylate to thymidylate, catalyzed by the enzyme thymidylate synthase.[14] This reaction is an essential step in the synthesis of DNA (Fig. 39-4). In carrying out this reaction, N^5, N^{10}-methylene FH_4 simultaneously transfers and reduces a one-carbon group, itself serving as the hydrogen donor for the reduction.[15] The reaction generates FH_2 (Fig. 39-5), which must be reduced again to FH_4 by dihydrofolate reductase and NADPH before it can again be utilized as a coenzyme:

$$dUMP + N^5, N^{10}\text{-methylene } FH_4 \rightarrow FH_2 + dTMP$$
$$FH_2 + NADPH + H^+ \rightarrow FH_4 + NADP^+$$

Limitation of thymidylate synthesis in folic acid deficiency causes incorporation of uracil instead thymine into DNA.[16]

Folate deficiency diminishes purine biosynthesis by slowing (1) the folate-dependent formylation of glycinamide ribotide to N-formylglycinamide ribotide, the reaction that places the C-8 in the purine ring, and (2) the folate-dependent conversion of 5-amino-4-imidazole carboxamide ribotide (AICAR) to 5-formamido-4-imidazole carbox-

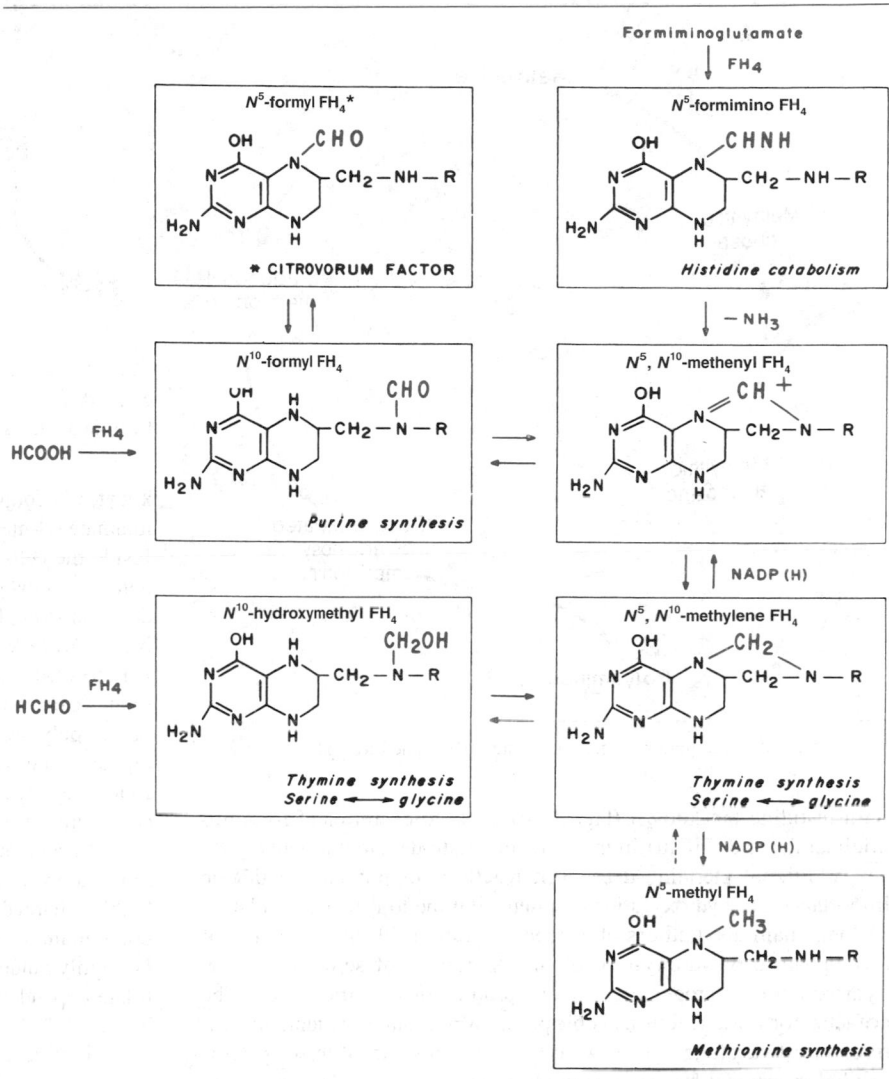

FIGURE 39-2 Derivatives of tetrahydrofolic acid (FH_4), their interconversions, and the metabolic pathways in which they participate. One-carbon substituents are shown in *blue*.

amide ribotide, the reaction that places the C-2 in the purine ring.[17] The decrease in purine synthesis, however, is offset by the ability of AICAR to slow purine degradation by inhibiting adenosine deaminase and adenylate deaminase.[1] This may explain why no clinical manifestations have been traced to the block in purine synthesis. Interference

TABLE 39-1 METABOLIC SYSTEMS REQUIRING FOLIC ACID COENZYMES IN ANIMAL CELLS

SYSTEM	RELATED TRANSFORMATIONS OF FOLIC ACID COENZYMES
Serine $\rightleftharpoons$ glycine	Serine + FH_4 $\rightleftharpoons$ N^5,N^{10}-methylene FH_4 + glycine
Thymidylate synthesis	Deoxyuridylate (dUMP) + N^5,N^{10}-methylene FH_4 $\rightarrow$ FH_2 + thymidylate (dTMP)
Histidine catabolism	Formiminoglutamate + FH_4 $\rightarrow$ N^5-formimino FH_4 + glutamate
Methionine synthesis	Homocysteine + N^5-methyl FH_4 $\rightarrow$ FH_4 + methionine
Purine synthesis	Glycinamide ribotide + N^{10}-formyl FH_4 $\rightarrow$ FH_4 + formylglycinamide ribotide
Purine synthesis	5-Amino-4-imidazole carboxamide ribotide + N^{10}-formyl FH_4 $\rightarrow$ FH_4 + 5-formamido-4-imidazole carboxamide ribotide

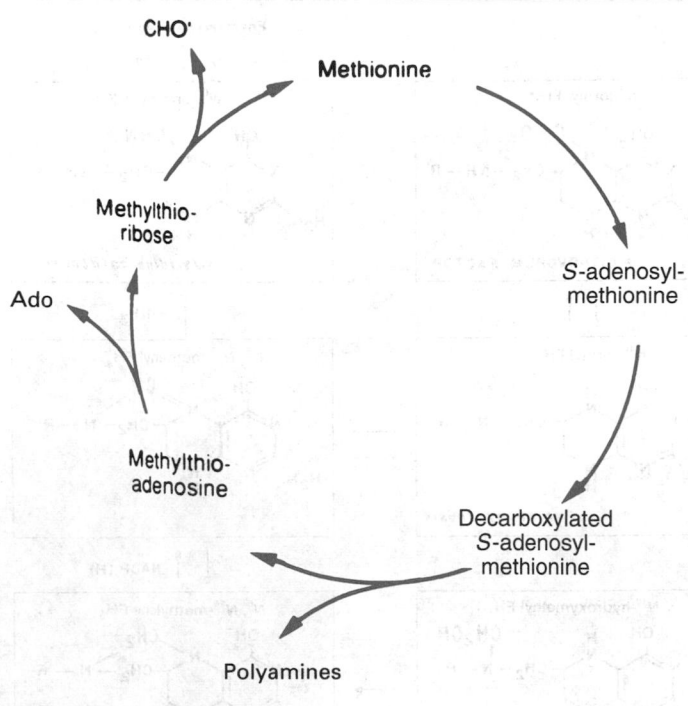

FIGURE 39-3   Formate production during polyamine biosynthesis.

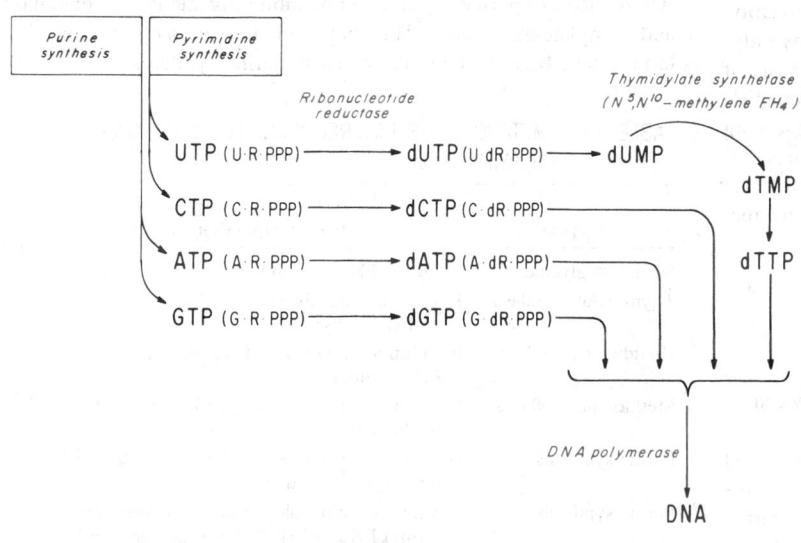

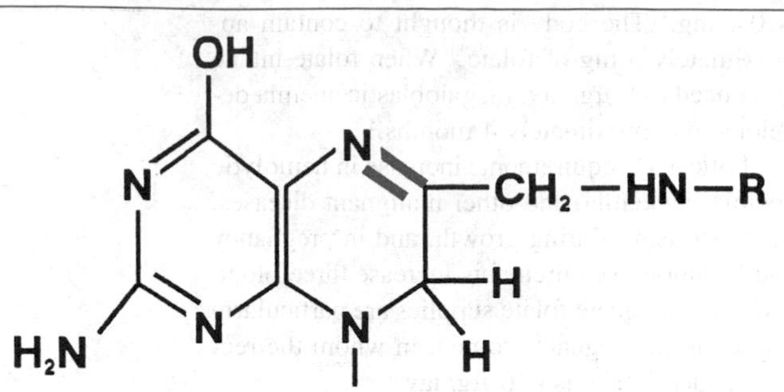

FIGURE 39-5   Dihydrofolate (FH_2). The double bond formed when tetrahydrofolate loses two hydrogens is shown in *blue*.

with histidine breakdown (Fig. 39-6) leads to excretion of formiminoglutamic acid (FIGlu) in the urine of folate-deficient patients.

Additional pteridine-dependent reactions of potential metabolic importance are hydroxylation of phenylalanine to tyrosine, oxidation of long-chain alkyl ethers of glycerol to fatty acid, hydroxylation of tryptophan to 6-hydroxytryptophan (a precursor of serotonin), 17-α-hydroxylation of progesterone,[18] and production of nitric oxide.[19] The cofactor for these reactions is biopterin, a nonfolate pteridine derivative. Tetrahydrofolic acid is weakly active in some of these systems *in vitro*[20]; whether it plays any such role *in vivo* is not known.

SIGNIFICANCE OF FOLYLPOLYGLUTAMATES

Intracellular folates exist primarily as polyglutamate conjugates.[9] Approximately 75 percent of the folate in human erythrocytes and leukocytes is conjugated.[21] Plasma folate consists largely of the monoglutamate N^5-methyl FH_4 and is transported into the cells in this form.[22] Inside the cells, the polyglutamate chain is added by an ATP-dependent *folylpoly-γ-glutamyl synthase*.[23] The activity of human synthase depends strongly on the form of the folate substrate, declining in the order $FH_4 > N^{10}$-formyl $FH_4 > FH_4 = N^{10}$-formyl THF $> N^5$-methyl FH_4, toward which the enzyme is almost inert.[24] In humans, conjugated folates carry on average seven to eight glutamyl residues.[25] The length of the polyglutamate chain can be determined by the ability of the higher folate polyglutamates to inhibit folylpolyglutamyl synthase.[26] Evidence suggests folylpolyglutamyl synthase is regulated within cells, with its activity closely paralleling rates of DNA synthesis.[27]

Intracellular folylmonoglutamates leak out of the cells at a fairly rapid rate whereas polyglutamates do not, presumably because of the highly charged polyglutamate tail.[28] Therefore, attachment of the polyglutamylate chain is essential for retaining folates within cells. Folylpolyglutamates are superior to monoglutamates as substrates for folate-dependent enzyme reactions.[29]

PHYSIOLOGY

INTESTINAL ABSORPTION

The proximal jejunum is the principal site of folate absorption. Absorption of a dose of either unconjugated or conjugated folate begins within minutes. Peak levels are reached in 1 to 2 hours. Because only folylmonoglutamate appears in plasma, all folylpolyglutamates are deconjugated during absorption across the intestine.[30] Deconjugating enzymes ("conjugases") play an important but poorly understood role in the intestinal absorption of folate.[31] Folylpolyglutamate may be hydrolyzed within the lumen of the intestine, and the monoglutamate product may be absorbed subsequently.[32] Alternatively, hydrolysis may occur at the brush border of the intestinal cell (Fig. 39-7). A brush border conjugase purified from human jejunum catalyzes the Zn^{2+}-dependent deconjugation of folate polyglutamates ranging from $PteGlu_2$ to at least $PteGlu_7$ ($K_m = 0.6$ μM for both substrates).[33] It is an exopeptidase that successively removes single glutamate residues from the end of the polyglutamate chain, yielding the folylmonoglutamate.

Conjugases are found not only in the intestine. For example, human plasma contains sufficient conjugase to convert polyglutamates containing more than three glutamyl residues to monoglutamates.[34] Other conjugases appear to be lysosomal carboxypeptidases[35] that are not involved in absorption of folates from the intestine.

Once deconjugated, the folates are actively transported across the intestinal epithelium[36] by a carrier-

FIGURE 39-4   Pathways of deoxynucleotide and DNA synthesis.

mediated mechanism (K_m = 1–2 μM) that is independent of Na^+, K^+, and transmembrane potential.[37] The mechanism uses the pH gradient between the jejunal lumen (pH ~ 6) and the interior of the epithelial cell to drive folate into the cell against a concentration gradient.[38] Passive transport also may occur.[39] In the intestinal cell, the absorbed folate monoglutamates are reduced if necessary, and then converted to N^5-methyl FH_4 (some N^{10}-formyl FH_4 also is made) and transported into the bloodstream without further change.[40]

Folate undergoes an enterohepatic cycle in which it is first secreted against a concentration gradient into the bile, appearing there chiefly as N^5-methyl FH_4 monoglutamate, and then is reabsorbed from the small intestine.[41] Bile contains approximately two to 10 times the folate concentration of normal serum,[41] with biliary excretion accounting for up to 0.1 mg of folate per day. This quantity is sufficiently large that interruption of the enterohepatic cycle by biliary diversion causes serum folate levels to fall by more than 50 percent in less than 1 day.[42] The enterohepatic cycle has been proposed to redistribute folate between hepatic stores and peripheral tissues according to the state of the exogenous folate supplies[43]; however, this view is disputed.[44]

METABOLISM

Tritiated folylmonoglutamate (³H-F) administered intravenously is almost completely removed from the bloodstream in a few minutes.[45] Uptake involves two classes of folate-binding proteins[46]: *high-affinity folate receptors*[47] that concentrate folate in intracellular vesicles and a *membrane folate transporter* that transports folate from the vesicles into the cytosol. The high-affinity receptors, which are attached to the outer surface of the cell membrane by glycosyl-phosphatidylinositol linkages,[48] bind very tightly (K_d in the nanomolar range) to most physiologic folate monoglutamates,[49] particularly N^5-methyl FH_4, the major circulating folate.[50] Their very high affinity enables the receptors to take up N^5-methyl FH_4 from the plasma, even at its ambient concentration of approximately 10 nM. The membrane folate transporter is a probenecid-inhibitable organic anion carrier that, among other functions, carries reduced folates and methotrexate (but not oxidized folate itself) in and out of the cytoplasm.[46] Its K_m for folate is in the micromolar range. These two classes of receptors cooperate in the following way to transport N^5-methyl FH_4 into the cell[51]: (1) A region of membrane containing a group of folate-loaded high-affinity receptors is internalized as a vesicle (the *caveola*); (2) the caveola is acidified, releasing the folate into the vesicle lumen; (3) the folate is passed from the caveola to the cytoplasm by the membrane folate transporter; and finally, (4) the caveola recycles to the cell surface, where its high-affinity receptors take on another load of N^5-methyl FH_4. Once internalized, the folates are retained by the cells partly through polyglutamylation[52] but also through tight association with a set of intracellular folate-binding proteins.[53] Three of these proteins are enzymes involved in methyl group metabolism: sarcosine dehydrogenase and dimethylglycine dehydrogenase (mitochondrial)[54] and glycine N-methyl transferase (cytosolic).[55] Why these enzymes bind folate so avidly or whether this binding affects overall methyl group metabolism is not known, although glycine N-methyl transferase is speculated to regulate methyl group metabolism by controlling the tissue concentration of S-adenosylhomocysteine (SAH), one of its reaction products and a potent inhibitor of most methyltransferases.

Folates have been found in all body tissues that have been analyzed. The principal form of the vitamin in tissues and in blood appears

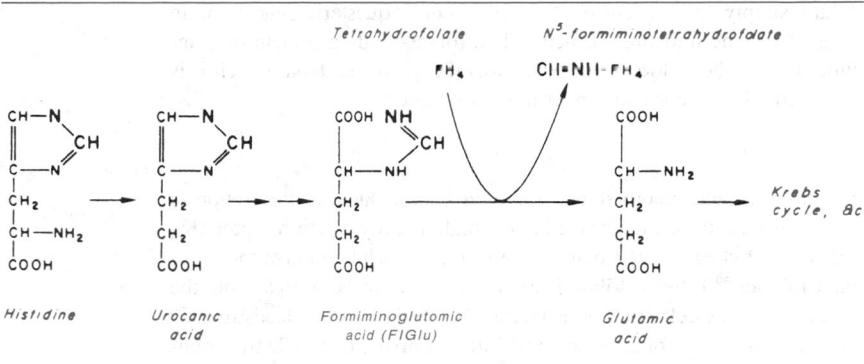

FIGURE 39-6 Catabolism of histidine.

to be the N^5-methyl form.[56] Human liver contains 0.7 to 17 μg of folate per gram.[57]

The total folate pool turns over very slowly.[58] Degradation accounts for a portion of this turnover. p-Aminobenzoylglutamate has been identified as a breakdown product. The fate of the pteridine moiety is unknown.

FOLATE-BINDING PROTEINS OF SERUM AND MILK

The soluble folate-binding proteins of serum and milk are high-affinity folate receptors that are released from cell membranes by proteolysis.[59] These proteins can be detected in approximately 15 percent of normal individuals[60] and are found at increased levels in some pregnant women, women taking oral contraceptives, folate-deficient alcoholics (but not patients with cobalamin deficiency),[61] and patients with uremia, hepatic cirrhosis, and chronic myelogenous leukemia.[62] In normal subjects, the proteins are about two thirds saturated and have a total folate-binding capacity of approximately 175 pg/ml of serum.[63] The proteins may not be detected in some subjects because of prior saturation of the proteins with unlabeled folate.[64] Serum protein has an M_r of 40,000 and prefers oxidized to reduced folates.[64]

Folate-binding proteins have been found in milk and in normal granulocytes.[65] Folate bound to the milk folate binder is absorbed chiefly in the ileum[66] rather than the jejunum, the principal site of absorption of free folate. The milk folate binder, a glycoprotein, also promotes folate transport into the liver via the asialoglycoprotein receptor.[67] The milk folate binder is speculated to protect an infant's

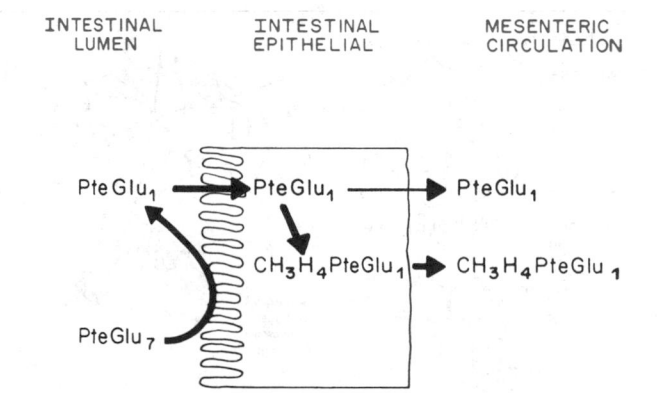

FIGURE 39-7 Digestion and absorption of folate polyglutamate by the intestine. The polyglutamate (in this case, $PteGlu_7$) is hydrolyzed in the intestinal lumen or at the brush border. The resulting pteroylglutamate (PteGlu) is transported into the intestinal cell, where it is reduced and methylated, appearing in the circulation chiefly as N^5-methyl FH_4.

folate supply by preventing bacteria from sequestering the vitamin away from the intestinal lumen.[44] The folate-binding protein in granulocytes has been localized to the specific granules, from which it is released when the granulocytes are stimulated.[68]

EXCRETION

Folates are both resorbed and secreted by the kidney. Resorption is accomplished by a membrane-bound high-affinity folate receptor (K_m for N^5-methyl $FH_4 = 0.4$ nM) located in the brush borders of the proximal tubules.[69] Filtered folate is carried rapidly by the receptor into the proximal tubule cell, from which it travels slowly into the bloodstream.[70] At the same time, folate is secreted into the proximal tubule by a nonspecific probenecid-sensitive organic anion carrier that is closely related or identical to the membrane folate transporter and is responsible for renal secretion of p-aminohippuric acid (which blocks renal folate secretion), penicillin, and uric acid.[70] The net result of these two processes is resorption of most, but not all, of the filtered folate.

In humans, intact folates and their cleavage products are excreted by the kidney at a rate of 2 to 5 μg/day.[71] Folates given in doses less than 15 μg/kg are excreted in the urine in reduced forms, particularly as N^{10}-formyl FH_4.[72] When folate doses greater than 15 μg/kg are given, large amounts of folate are excreted unchanged.

A small percentage of parenterally administered ³H-F is recoverable in the feces and mainly represents overflow from the enterohepatic cycle.

ASSAY OF SERUM FOLATE

Folates are measured by isotopic methods using various folate binders. Isotopic folate assays are identical in principle to radioimmunoassays.

COBALAMIN

CHEMISTRY

STRUCTURE AND NOMENCLATURE

The cobalamin molecule has two major portions: a porphyrinlike near-planar macrocycle known as corrin, and a nucleotide that lies almost perpendicular to the corrin ring (Fig. 39-8). The corrin moiety contains four reduced pyrrole rings[73] that bind a central cobalt atom whose two remaining coordination positions are occupied by a 5,6-dimethylbenzimidazolyl group (below the ring) and various ligands (above the ring; in this case, —N).

Compounds containing the corrin ring are known as *corrinoids*. The cobalamins are corrinoids whose nucleotide contains 5,6-dime-

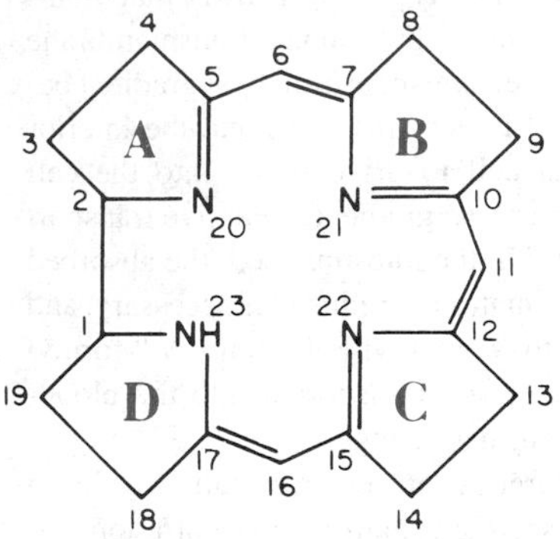

FIGURE 39-9   Corrin ring showing ring designations and standard numbering of the atoms.

thylbenzimidazole. Two connections exist between the corrin and the nucleotide: (1) a bond between the nucleotide phosphate and a side chain in ring D, and (2) a bond between cobalt and a nitrogen atom of benzimidazole. Figure 39-9 summarizes the numbering and ring designations of the corrin system.

The term *vitamin B₁₂* is sometimes used as a generic term for the corrinoids. The term probably is best reserved, however, as an alternative name for cyanocobalamin, the usual therapeutic corrinoid.

Four cobalamins are important in animal cell metabolism. Two are *cyanocobalamin* (CnCbl; vitamin B_{12}) and *hydroxycobalamin* (OHCbl). The other two cobalamins are alkyl derivatives that are synthesized from OHCbl and serve as coenzymes. In one, *adenosylcobalamin* (AdoCbl), a 5′-deoxyadenosyl replaces OH as the cobalt ligand above the ring (Fig. 39-10).[74] In the second, *methylcobalamin* (MeCbl), the upper lig-

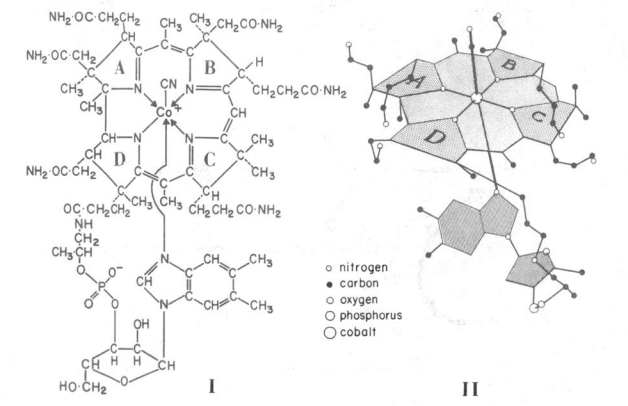

FIGURE 39-8   (*I*) Structure of cyanocobalamin (CnCbl; vitamin B_{12}). (*II*) Partial structure of CnCbl showing the relationship between the corrin ring and the nucleotide.

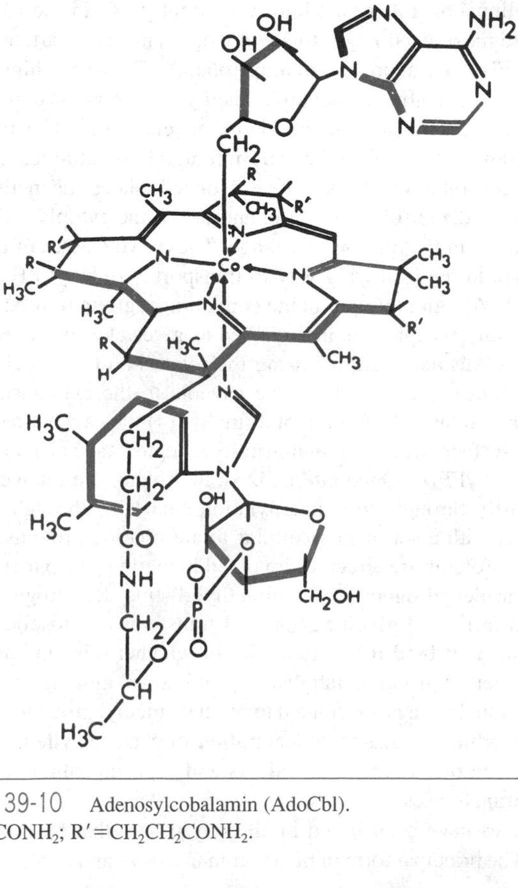

FIGURE 39-10   Adenosylcobalamin (AdoCbl).
R=CH_2CONH_2; R′=$CH_2CH_2CONH_2$.

and is a methyl group. MeCbl is the major form of cobalamin in human blood plasma.[75]

NUTRITION

SOURCES

Cobalamin is synthesized only by certain microorganisms; animals ultimately depend on microbial synthesis for their cobalamin supply. Foods that contain cobalamin are of animal origin: meat, liver, seafood, and dairy products. Cobalamin has not been found in plants.

DAILY REQUIREMENTS

The average daily diet in Western countries contains 5 to 30 μg of cobalamin. Of this, 1 to 5 μg is absorbed.[76] Less than 250 ng appears in the urine; the unabsorbed remainder appears in the feces. Total body content is 2 to 5 mg in an adult,[77] with approximately 1 mg in the liver. The kidneys also are rich in cobalamin.[78] Relative to the daily requirement, body reserves of cobalamin are much larger than those of folate.

Cobalamin has a daily rate of obligatory loss of approximately 0.1 percent of the total body pool, irrespective of the pool size. For this reason, a deficiency state does not develop for several years after cessation of cobalamin intake. The officially recommended daily allowance for adults[3] is 5 μg; growth, hypermetabolic states, and pregnancy increase daily requirements. The recommended daily allowance for infants during the first year is 1 to 2 μg. In cobalamin-deficient subjects, a normal diet containing approximately 15 μg/day replenishes depleted body stores.[79]

ROLE IN METABOLISM

The only two recognized cobalamin-dependent enzymes in human cells are AdoCbl-dependent *methylmalonyl CoA mutase* and MeCbl-dependent *methyltetrahydrofolate-homocysteine methyltransferase*. The presence in humans of a third cobalamin-dependent enzyme, leucine 2,3-aminomutase, is controversial.[80]

METHYLMALONYL COENZYME A MUTASE

Methylmalonyl CoA mutase is a mitochondrial enzyme that participates in the disposal of the propionate formed during breakdown of valine and isoleucine. The enzyme is a homodimer of a 78-kDa subunit that is encoded by a gene on chromosome 6.[81] In the reaction catalyzed by methylmalonyl CoA mutase, methylmalonyl CoA, which is produced during catabolism of propionate,[82] is converted to succinyl CoA, a Krebs cycle intermediate. In the course of this reaction, a hydrogen on the methyl carbon of the substrate exchanges places with the —COSCoA group (Fig. 39-11).

The coenzyme serves as an intermediate hydrogen carrier, accepting the hydrogen from the substrate in the initial phase of the reaction and returning it to the product after migration of —COSCoA. The place for the migrating hydrogen is created by cleavage of the carbon-

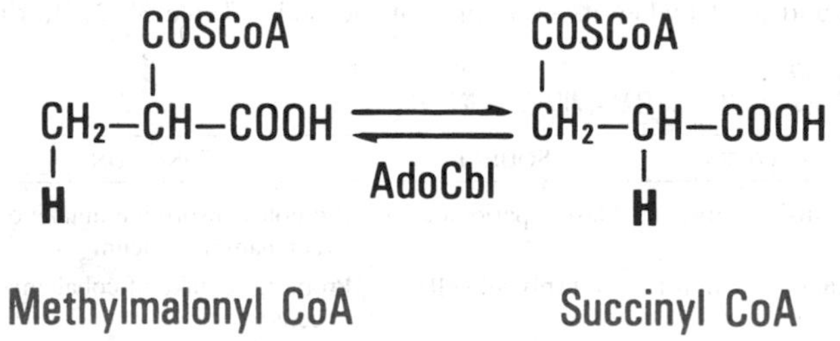

FIGURE 39-11   Methylmalonyl coenzyme A (CoA) mutase reaction.

cobalt bond to form cob(II)alamin and the 5′-deoxyadenos-5′-yl radical at the active site of the enzyme. This is an example of an enzyme-catalyzed reaction mediated by an active-site free radical situated on an unactivated carbon.

N^5-METHYLTETRAHYDROFOLATE-HOMOCYSTEINE METHYLTRANSFERASE

MeCbl participates in cobalamin-dependent synthesis of methionine.[83] S-adenosylmethionine (SAM) and methionine synthase reductase are required for methyltransferase activity, probably to reactivate enzyme molecules whose coenzyme is inactivated by oxidation of the cobalt.[84] The reductase converts the oxidized cobalt to the readily alkylatable Co^{1+}, which then accepts a methyl group from SAM, a powerful biologic methylating agent, thereby restoring activity of the methyltransferase. In humans, this pathway also serves as a mechanism for converting N^5-methyltetrahydrofolate to tetrahydrofolate. The demethylation of N^5-methyl FH_4 is a prerequisite for attachment of the polyglutamate chain to newly acquired folate, which is largely taken up by the cell in the form of N^5-methyl FH_4 monoglutamate.[22] Nitrous oxide (N_2O) impairs methyltransferase by oxidizing cob(I)alamin (a catalytic intermediate in the methyltransferase reaction) to cob(II)alamin.[85] This reaction depletes MeCbl and produces a cobalamin deficiency-like state.[86]

A mutant form of methylenetetrahydrofolate reductase (MTHFR), MTHFR 677C→T, is of some clinical importance. This designation refers to the mutation in the DNA; the amino acid does not change.[87] Despite the lack of change in the amino acid, the mutation affects the levels of homocysteine, an amino acid whose rate of production depends on both folate and cobalamin. These effects are discussed further below in "Folate-Cobalamin Relationship."

NONENZYMATIC METABOLISM

Cobalamin has the capacity to bind cyanide; therefore, cobalamin may participate in the metabolism of this toxin in humans. Tobacco and certain foods (fruits, beans, and nuts) contain cyanide. Although the evidence is inconclusive, cobalamin is believed to play a role in neutralizing cyanide taken in via these substances.[88]

FOLATE-COBALAMIN RELATIONSHIP

In both folate deficiency and cobalamin deficiency, the megaloblastic anemias are fully corrected by treatment with the appropriate vitamin. The megaloblastic anemia of cobalamin deficiency also is largely corrected by folic acid supplementation even if no cobalamin is given. Conversely, the anemia of folate deficiency is not helped at all by cobalamin. These clinical observations indicate that the megaloblastic anemia in cobalamin deficiency actually results from an abnormality in folate metabolism.[28] The observation that urinary excretion of FIGlu and AICAR, normally regarded as a sign of folate deficiency, is seen occasionally in pure cobalamin deficiency[89] provides further evidence that folate metabolism is deranged by cobalamin deficiency. Two explanations have been proposed to account for the folate responsiveness of cobalamin-deficient megaloblastic anemia: (1) the *methylfolate trap* hypothesis, which is accepted by the majority of authorities, and (2) the *formate starvation* hypothesis (Fig. 39-12).

METHYLFOLATE TRAP HYPOTHESIS

The methylfolate trap hypothesis[90] is based on the fact that the folate-requiring enzyme N^5-methyl FH_4—homocysteine methyltransferase is also dependent on cobalamin. The hypothesis states that in cobalamin deficiency tissue folates are gradually diverted into the N^5-methyl FH_4 pool because of slowing of the methyltransferase reaction,[91] the only route out of that pool for folate. As N^5-methyl FH_4 levels increase, the

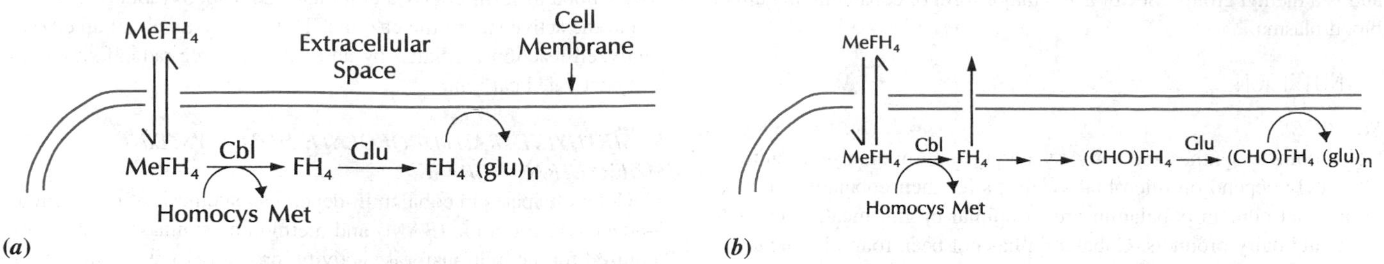

FIGURE 39-12   Methods by which cobalamin deficiency decreases intracellular folate levels. Methyltetrahydrofolate (MeFH$_4$), the principal form of folate in the bloodstream, circulates in the unconjugated form (i.e., it has no polyglutamate side chain). This and other forms of unconjugated FH$_4$ can be taken into cells but leak out again unless they are conjugated. Methyl FH$_4$ is not a substrate for the conjugating enzyme, so conjugation cannot occur until the methyl FH$_4$ is converted to another form of folate. Cobalamin is necessary for this process because it is the cofactor for the reaction that converts methyl FH$_4$ to FH$_4$. In cobalamin deficiency, the conversion of methyl FH$_4$ to FH$_4$ is defective. Newly transported folate remains in the form of methyl FH$_4$, which cannot be conjugated and leaks back out of the cell. According to the *methylfolate trap hypothesis (a)*, all forms of FH$_4$ other than methyl FH$_4$ can be conjugated, so methyl FH$_4$ is the only folate species that leaks out of the cell. The *formate starvation hypothesis (b)* differs from the methylfolate trap hypothesis solely in assuming that only the formylated folates (N^{10}-formyl FH$_4$ and/or N^5,N^{10}-methenyl FH$_4$) can be conjugated, so newly transported methyl FH$_4$, N^5,N^{10}-methylene FH$_4$ and free FH$_4$ leak out of the cell. (CH$_2$) FH$_4$=N^5,N^{10}-methylene FH$_4$; (CHO) FH$_4$=N^{10}-formyl FH$_4$ or N^5,N^{10}-methenyl FH$_4$.

levels of other forms of folate decline, with a consequent fall in the rates of reactions in which those forms participate. In particular, the synthesis of deoxythymidine monophosphate (dTMP) is slowed, and megaloblastic anemia ensues.

In its simplest form, the hypothesis predicts that in cobalamin deficiency tissue levels of N^5-methyl FH$_4$ are abnormally high and those of other forms of folate are abnormally low. Although serum N^5-methyl FH$_4$ levels are elevated in cobalamin deficiency,[92] tissue folate levels actually decline, whereas increases in the fraction of tissue folates in the form of N^5-methyl FH$_4$ may[93] or may not[94] occur. The polyglutamates are the folates whose relative levels consistently fall as total folate levels decline.[95] The decreased level appears to be related to the substrate specificity of the folate-conjugating enzyme. This enzyme works very poorly with N^5-methyl FH$_4$; therefore, it is unable to carry out normal γ-glutamylation of newly internalized N^5-methyl FH$_4$ monoglutamate in cobalamin-deficient cells because the freshly acquired folate cannot be converted into a suitable substrate (i.e., free FH$_4$ or formyl FH$_4$). Thus, although sequestration of tissue folates in an expanded N^5-methyl FH$_4$ pool may account for some of the effects of the blockade in methyltransferase activity, the major problem seems to be a failure to convert newly acquired folate into a form that can be retained by the cell. The upshot is development of tissue folate deficiency as the unconjugated folate leaks out (Fig. 39-13). The whole process is aggravated by a drop in tissue levels of SAM as the methionine supply is curtailed because of the diminished activity of the methyltransferase.[96] SAM, which is necessary for methyltransferase activity, is also a powerful inhibitor of N^5,N^{10}-methylene FH$_4$ reductase,[97] the enzyme responsible for production of N^5-methyl FH$_4$. The relief of this inhibition as SAM levels fall accelerates the flow of folates toward N^5-methyl FH$_4$, further aggravating the metabolic imbalance resulting from impairment in methyltransferase activity.

This problem could be overcome if N^5-methyl FH$_4$ were converted into a substrate for the conjugating enzyme by another route. In theory, this could be accomplished by reversal of the N^5,N^{10}-methylene FH$_4$ reductase reaction or by catabolism of N^5-methyl FH$_4$ via the methylation of biogenic amines.[98] For practical purposes, however, the N^5,N^{10}-methylene FH$_4$ reductase reaction is irreversible *in vivo*,[99] and the methylation of biogenic amines by N^5-methyl FH$_4$ is too slow to provide much relief.

FORMATE STARVATION HYPOTHESIS

This hypothesis holds that formate starvation is the basis for folate-responsive megaloblastic anemia of cobalamin deficiency.[100] This theory is based on the diminished capacity of cobalamin-deficient lymphoblasts to incorporate formaldehyde into purine and methionine[96] and on experiments showing that N^5-formyl FH$_4$ is more effective than FH$_4$ at correcting some of the abnormalities in folate metabolism seen in cobalamin deficiency.[101] The hypothesis states that with the decrease in methionine production in cobalamin-deficient conditions, the generation of formate is depressed (because normally the methyl group of excess methionine is rapidly oxidized to formate[102]), leading to a decline in the production of N^5-formyl FH$_4$. If N^5-formyl FH$_4$ but not FH$_4$ is a substrate for the conjugating enzyme,[103] then the low tissue folate levels seen in cobalamin deficiency cannot result merely from impaired demethylation of N^5-methyl FH$_4$ by a cobalamin-deficient homocysteine methyltransferase but must reflect a decreased production of methionine, the source of the formate needed to produce the conjugable substrate N^5-formyl FH$_4$.

INTESTINAL ABSORPTION

INTRINSIC FACTOR

Intrinsic factor is one of a number of proteins to which cobalamin is bound as it makes its way through the body (Table 39-2). Intrinsic

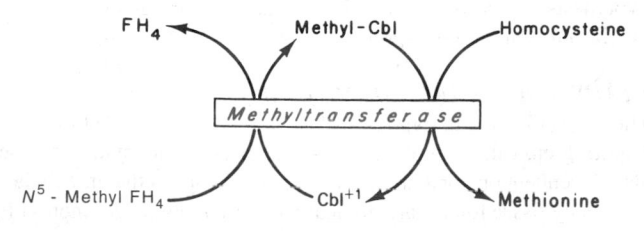

FIGURE 39-13 N^5-methyl FH$_4$–homocysteine methyltransferase reaction.

TABLE 39-2   COBALAMIN-BINDING PROTEINS

PROTEIN	SOURCE	FUNCTION
Intrinsic factor	Gastric parietal cells	Promotes absorption uptake of cobalamin by ileum
Transcobalamin II	Probably all cells	Promotes uptake of cobalamin by cells
R proteins	Exocrine glands, phagocytes	Helps dispose of cobalamin analogues (?)

factor is needed for the absorption of cobalamins given orally at physiologic dosage levels. Human intrinsic factor is a glycoprotein (M_r approximately 44,000) encoded by a gene on chromosome 11.[104] It has binding sites for cobalamin and a specific ileal receptor, the former situated near the carboxy terminus and the latter near the amino terminus of the intrinsic factor molecule.[105] Binding to cobalamin is very tight.[106] Table 39-3 summarizes the properties of intrinsic factor. Bound vitamin alters the conformation of intrinsic factor, producing a more compact form that is resistant to proteolytic digestion.

In humans, intrinsic factor is synthesized and secreted by the parietal cells of the cardiac and fundic mucosa.[107] Secretion of intrinsic factor usually parallels that of hydrochloric acid (HCl). It is enhanced by the presence of food in the stomach,[108] vagal stimulation,[109] and histamine and gastrin.[110] Gastric juice also contains other cobalamin-binding proteins.[111] These proteins are known as the *R proteins* because of their rapid electrophoretic mobility compared with intrinsic factor.

ABSORPTION OF COBALAMIN: CUBULIN

Cobalamins in foods are liberated in the stomach by peptic digestion.[112] They are then bound not to intrinsic factor but to R proteins because cobalamin binds much more tightly to R proteins than to intrinsic factor at the acid pH of the stomach.[113] Upon entering the duodenum, cobalamin is released from the cobalamin–R protein complex by digestion with pancreatic proteases, which in normal subjects act by selectively degrading R proteins and the cobalamin–R protein complex while sparing intrinsic factor.[113] At this point, cobalamin finally reaches the intrinsic factor to form the intrinsic factor–cobalamin complex.

The intrinsic factor–cobalamin complex, which is very resistant to digestion,[114] journeys down the intestine until it reaches the intrinsic factor receptor *cubulin*,[115] a 460-kDa peripheral membrane protein located in the microvillus pits of the ileal mucosa.[116] (The same receptor is found in the brush border of renal proximal tubule cells,[117] but its purpose there is unknown.) The ileal mucosa occupies the distal half of the small intestine, and the cubulin is found all along this portion of the intestine. Its concentration rises progressively until a maximum is reached near the terminal ileum.[118] A specific site on the intrinsic factor molecule avidly attaches to a receptor in a binding reaction that requires a pH of 5.4 or greater and Ca^{2+} (or other divalent cations) but no energy.[119]

Following attachment of the intrinsic factor–cobalamin complex to the receptor, the vitamin is taken into the ileal mucosal cells over 30 to 60 minutes by endocytosis.[120] The vitamin then is passed by the mucosal cells into the portal blood over many hours, while the receptors recycle to the surfaces of the microvilli for another load of intrinsic factor–cobalamin complex.[120] During its sojourn in the ileal enterocyte, the vitamin first appears in the lysosomes, but by 4 hours most of the vitamin is located in the cytosol.[121] During absorption, the entire intrinsic factor–cobalamin complex appears to be taken into the cell, where the cobalamin is released while the intrinsic factor is degraded.[122]

Cobalamin from a small oral dose (10–20 μg) starts to appear in the blood after 3 to 4 hours, and the vitamin reaches a peak level in 8 to 12 hours. In the portal blood, the cobalamin is complexed with a cobalamin-transporting protein known as *transcobalamin (TC) II*.[123] The cobalamin—TCII complex probably is formed in the ileal enterocyte, one of a variety of cells that synthesize TC.[124] Large oral doses (1 mg) of cobalamin are absorbed by simple diffusion that is not mediated by intrinsic factor. In these instances, vitamin appears in blood within minutes, again as the cobalamin–TCII complex.

Like the folates, the cobalamins participate in an enterohepatic cycle. In humans, between 0.5 and 9 μg/day of cobalamins is secreted into the bile, where the cobalamins bind to an R protein and enter the intestine.[125] In the intestine, the cobalamin–R protein complexes of biliary origin are treated exactly like those delivered from the stomach. The cobalamin is released by digestion of the R protein by pancreatic proteases, and then is taken up by intrinsic factor and reabsorbed. From 65 to 75 percent of biliary cobalamin is estimated to be reabsorbed by this mechanism.[126] Because of the size of the cobalamin storage pool and the existence of this enterohepatic circulation, a very long time—sometimes 20 years—is required for a clinically significant cobalamin deficiency to develop from a diet providing insufficient cobalamin (e.g., a strictly vegetarian diet).[127] Patients who fail to absorb the vitamin, however, become clinically deficient in only 3 to 6 years because biliary and dietary cobalamin are lost.[128]

COBALAMIN IN THE CELL: TRANSCOBALAMIN II

UPTAKE OF COBALAMIN BY CELLS

TCII is the plasma protein that mediates the transport of cobalamin into the tissues.[129] A simple protein of $M_r = 43,000$, TCII binds cobalamin with exceedingly high affinity ($K_a = 10^{-11}$ M).[130,131] Unlike intrinsic factor, whose binding is relatively specific for cobalamins, TCII also can bind certain corrins that are chemically related to the cobalamins but have no function in mammalian systems and are known as cobalamin "analogues."[132] TCII is synthesized by many types of cells, including enterocytes, hepatocytes, mononuclear phagocytes, fibroblasts, and hematopoietic precursors in the marrow.[124] Although circulating TCII carries only a minor fraction of the cobalamin in the plasma, it is the protein to which newly acquired cobalamin is first bound. Cobalamin given parenterally associates almost immediately with unsaturated TCII,[133] whereas cobalamin absorbed through the intestine probably is carried into the portal blood as the preformed cobalamin–TCII complex. These cobalamin–TCII complexes are transported into the tissues within minutes of appearing in the bloodstream.[134] The transport process begins with binding of the cobalamin–TCII complex to a membrane receptor that is present on a wide variety of cells.[135] The receptor-bound complex is internalized by pinocytosis and delivered to a lysosome, where the TCII is digested and the cobalamin is freed.[136] The cobalamin is actively exported from the lysosome into the cytosol by a specific Mg^{2+}-dependent carrier (K_m for CnCbl = 3.5 μM) that uses a proton gradient as the energy source.[137]

FORMATION OF ADENOSYLCOBALAMIN AND METHYLCOBALAMIN

To be useful to the cell, CnCbl and OHCbl must be converted to AdoCbl and MeCbl, the coenzymatically active cobalamins. The conversion is accomplished by reduction and alkylation. CnCbl and OHCbl are first reduced to the Co^{2+} form [cob(II)alamin] by NADPH- and nicotinamide adenine dinucleotide ([reduced form] NADH)-dependent reductases that are present in mitochondria and microsomes.[138] (NADPH–cobalamin reductase activity may be identical to

TABLE 39-3 PROPERTIES OF HUMAN INTRINSIC FACTOR

PROPERTY	VALUE	REFERENCE
M_r (approximate)	44,000	80
Cyanocobalamin-binding capacity (μg/mg)	30.1	80
Association constant for cyanocobalamin (M^{-1})	1.5×10^{10}	80
Composition:		
Carbohydrate content (%)	15.0	80
Hexoses, including fucose (%)	6.9	81
Hexosamine (residues/mol)	4.1	81
Sialic acid (residues/mol)	1.7	81

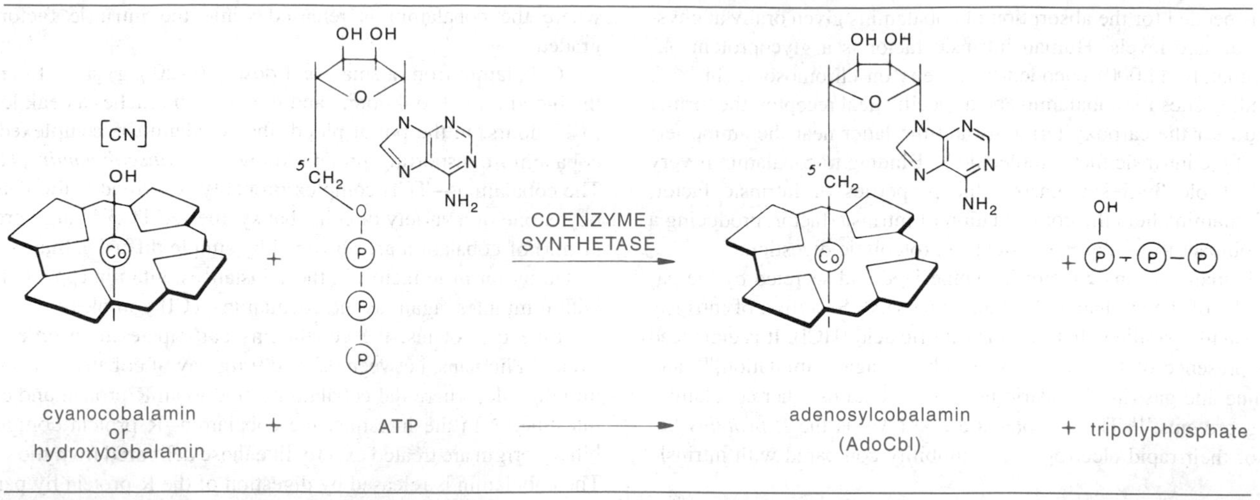

FIGURE 39-14   Biosynthesis of adenosylcobalamin (AdoCbl).

that of NADPH–cytochrome c reductase[139] and NADH–cobalamin reductase in the cytochrome b_5/cytochrome b_5 reductase system[140]). CN^- and OH^- are displaced from the metal during reduction. Some of the cob(II)alamin in the mitochondria is reduced further to the intensely nucleophilic Co^+ form [cob(I)alamin]. This is then alkylated by ATP to form AdoCbl in a reaction in which the 5′-deoxyadenosyl moiety of ATP is transferred to the cobalamin and the three phosphates of ATP are released as inorganic triphosphate (Fig. 39-14). The rest of the cobalamin binds to cytosolic N^5-methyltetrahydrofolate-homocysteine methyltransferase, where it is converted to MeCbl.[142]

PLASMA "R" PROTEINS: TRANSCOBALAMINS I AND III

The R proteins are a group of immunologically related proteins of apparent M_r approximately 60,000 consisting of a single polypeptide species variably substituted with oligosaccharides that terminate with different quantities of sialic acid.[143] They are found in milk, plasma, saliva, gastric juice, and numerous other body fluids. They appear to be synthesized by mucosal cells of the organs that secrete them [144] and by phagocytes.[145] Although the R proteins bind cobalamin, they lack intrinsic factor activity, that is, they are unable to promote the intestinal absorption of the vitamin.

TCI is the principal R protein of plasma and carries most of the circulating cobalamin. It contains nine potential glycosylation sites[146] and is encoded by a gene on chromosome 11, the same chromosome that carries the intrinsic factor gene.[147] In contrast to TCII, TCI clearance from the plasma is very slow ($T_{1/2}$ 9–10 days).[148] The asialyglycoprotein receptor carries the cobalamin–TCI complexes into the hepatocytes, where they are chiefly eliminated. The complexes are degraded, and their load of cobalamins is excreted in the bile.[149] TCI binds its ligands more tightly than does either intrinsic factor or TCII. TCI is less restrictive than either intrinsic factor or TCII with respect to ligand specificity; it avidly takes up corrinoids of widely varying structure.[150] The ligand-binding properties of TCI and its mode of clearance by the liver suggest that TCI helps clear the system of nonphysiologic cobalamin analogues that may be accidentally acquired in the normal course of events.[151] As the liver metabolizes analogue–TCI complexes, it secretes the analogues into the bile. Because these analogues are bound poorly by intrinsic factor,[131] they are poorly reabsorbed from the intestine and instead are eliminated in the feces. An alternative proposal is that TCI is a storage protein for cobalamins.[152] In reality, the physiologic role of TCI is unknown.

A second circulating R protein is TCIII.[153] This protein is found in the plasma and in granulocytes,[154] where it constitutes the cobala-

min-binding protein of the specific granules and from which it is released into the serum when blood clots.[155] Structurally, TCI is richer in sialic acid than is TCIII. The plasma R proteins likely consist of half a dozen or more species whose pI values range from 2.9 to 4.0, with "TCI" and "TCIII" representing the arbitrary division of these R proteins into a group with a lower average isoelectric point and a group with a higher average isoelectric point, respectively.

ASSAY OF SERUM COBALAMIN AND THE TRANSCOBALAMINS

As with folate, cobalamin is measured with a radioisotope assay using a cobalamin-binding protein.[156] The misleading results previously provided by this assay were explained by the discovery in serum and tissue of a class of cobalamin analogues that are detected by the radioisotope assay when R protein is used as the binder but not when intrinsic factor is the binder.[157] Current assays use intrinsic factor as the binder and give accurate values for serum cobalamin. The chemical nature and biologic significance of the analogues are unknown.[158]

TCI and TCII are present in plasma in trace quantities (approximately 7 and 20 μg/liter, respectively). TCIII often is undetectable. In fasting plasma, at least 70 percent of the circulating cobalamin is bound to TCI.[159] Nevertheless, TCI has substantial unsaturated binding capacity.[160] TCII binds only 10 to 25 percent of the total plasma cobalamin[161] but provides the majority (approximately 75 percent) of the total unsaturated cobalamin-binding capacity of plasma.[160] Less than 2 percent of the TCII in plasma is saturated at any given moment. Table 39-4 lists alterations in unsaturated cobalamin-binding capacity and in TCI and TCII levels in various disease states.

MEGALOBLASTIC ANEMIAS

GENERAL CONSIDERATIONS

DEFINITION

Megaloblastic anemias are disorders caused by impaired DNA synthesis. The presence of megaloblastic cells is the morphologic hallmark of this group of anemias. Megaloblastic red cell precursors are larger than normal and have more cytoplasm relative to the size of the nucleus. Promegaloblasts show a blue granule-free cytoplasm and a granular chromatin that contrasts with the ground-glass texture of its normal counterpart (see Color Plate VI-1). As the cell differentiates, the chromatin condenses more slowly than normal into dark aggregates that coalesce, giving the nucleus a characteristic fenestrated appearance. Condensation of chromatin to a homogeneous mass either fails

TABLE 39-4 LEVELS AND BINDING CAPACITY OF COBALAMIN-BINDING PROTEINS IN DISEASE

BINDER	DISEASE
Increased TCI (R protein)	Myeloproliferative disorders
	Polycythemia vera
	Myelofibrosis
	Benign neutrophilia
	Chronic myelocytic leukemia
	Hepatoma (occasionally)
	Metastatic cancer
Increased TCII	Myeloproliferative disorders
	Liver disease
	Inflammatory disorders
	Gaucher disease
	Anti–TCII antibodies
Unsaturated cobalamin binders	
Increased	Transient neutropenia
	Elevated TCI
Decreased	Liver disease
	Elevated serum cobalamin

From reference 156.

or is delayed. The growing maturity of the cytoplasm as it acquires hemoglobin contrasts with the immature-looking nucleus, a feature termed *nuclear-cytoplasmic asynchrony*.

Megaloblastic granulocyte precursors are larger than normal. They show nuclear-cytoplasmic asynchrony, with cytoplasm that looks less mature than the cytoplasm of their normal counterparts. A characteristic cell is the *giant metamyelocyte*, which has a large horseshoe-shaped nucleus, sometimes irregularly shaped, containing ragged chromatin.

Megaloblastic megakaryocytes may be abnormally large, with deficient granulation of the cytoplasm. In severe megaloblastosis, the nucleus may show unattached lobes.

ETIOLOGY AND PATHOGENESIS

Table 39-5 lists the causes of megaloblastic anemia. By far the most common causes are folate deficiency and cobalamin deficiency. Megaloblastic cells have much more cytoplasm and RNA than do their normal counterparts, but they have a relatively normal amount of DNA,[162] suggesting that cytoplasmic constituents (RNA and protein) are synthesized faster than is DNA. Evidence that maturation is retarded in megaloblastic precursors supports this conclusion.[163] DNA synthesis is impaired,[164] migration of the DNA replication fork and the joining of DNA fragments synthesized from the lagging strand (Okazaki fragments) are delayed,[165] and S phase is prolonged.[164]

Slowing of DNA replication in the megaloblastic anemias of folate and cobalamin deficiency appears to arise from failure of the folate-dependent conversion of deoxyuridine monophosphate (dUMP) to deoxythymidine monophosphate (dTMP). Because of this failure and the fact that DNA polymerase has difficulty distinguishing deoxyuridine triphosphate (dUTP) from deoxythymidine triphosphate (dTTP), dUTP instead of dTTP is incorporated into the DNA of folate-deficient cells.[166] Recognizing the mistake, the cells try to repair the DNA by replacing uridine with thymidine, but these repair attempts tend to fail for the same reason that uridine triphosphate (UTP) was incorporated into the DNA in the first place. The result is a frustrated effort at DNA repair that ultimately leads to DNA fragmentation followed by cell death.

Deoxyuridine (dU) normally inhibits the incorporation of tritiated thymidine into DNA, probably because it is converted via dUMP→dTMP to unlabeled dTTP, which competes with the tritiated thymidine. In megaloblastic cells, this effect of dU is greatly diminished. This finding is consistent with impairment in the dUMP→dTMP reaction in the megaloblastic cells and is the basis for the *dU suppression test*. This model also explains the chromosome breaks and other abnormalities that occur in megaloblastic cells.[167]

A curious group of findings suggests that the megaloblastic line arises from a more "primitive" precursor than is the case for the normoblastic line. Megaloblasts contain high concentrations of fetal hemoglobin[168] and the fetal isozyme of thymidine kinase.[169] Like megaloblasts, burst forming unit–erythroid (BFU-E) (see Chaps. 15 and 30) grown with monocyte-conditioned medium are rich in γ-globin chains and appear megaloblastic. BFU-E from the same source but grown with T lymphocytes appear normal and contain the usual proportion of γ-globin chains.[170] The relationship between these observations and the pathogenesis of the nutritional megaloblastic anemias remains to be determined.

CLINICAL FEATURES

All megaloblastic anemias share certain general clinical features. Because the anemia develops slowly, it produces few symptoms until the hematocrit is severely depressed. Symptoms, when they appear, are those of anemia: weakness, palpitation, fatigue, light-headedness, and shortness of breath. Severe pallor and slight jaundice combine to produce a telltale lemon-yellow skin. Leukocyte and platelet counts may

TABLE 39-5 CAUSES OF MEGALOBLASTIC ANEMIAS

Folate deficiency
  Decreased intake
  Poor nutrition
  Old age, poverty, alcoholism
  Hyperalimentation
  Hemodialysis
  Premature infants
  Spinal cord injury
  Children on synthetic diets
  Goat's milk anemia
  Impaired absorption
  Nontropical sprue
  Tropical sprue
  Other disease of the small
    intestine
Increased requirements
  Pregnancy
  Increased cell turnover
  Chronic hemolytic anemia
  Exfoliative dermatitis
  Cobalamin deficiency
Impaired absorption
  Gastric causes
  Pernicious anemia
  Gastrectomy
  Zollinger-Ellison syndrome
  Intestinal causes
    Ileal resection or disease
    Blind loop syndrome
    Fish tapeworm
  Pancreatic insufficiency
Decreased intake
  Vegans

Acute megaloblastic anemia
  Nitrous oxide exposure
  Severe illness with
    Extensive transfusion
    Dialysis
    Total parenteral nutrition
    Exposure to weak folate antagonists
      (e.g., trimethoprim or low-dose
      methotrexate)
Drugs
  Dihydrofolate reductase inhibitors
  Antimetabolites
  Inhibitors of deoxynucleotide synthesis
  Anticonvulsants
  Oral contraceptives
  Others
Inborn errors
  Cobalamin deficiency
    Imerslund-Gräsbeck disease
    Congenital deficiency of intrinsic
      factor
    Transcobalamin II deficiency
  Errors of folate metabolism
    Congenital folate malabsorption
    Dihydrofolate reductase deficiency
    N^5-methyl FH$_4$ homocysteine–
      methyltransferase deficiency
  Errors of cobalamin metabolism
    "Cobalamin mutant" syndromes with
      homocystinuria
  Other errors
    Hereditary orotic aciduria
    Lesch-Nyhan syndrome
    Thiamine-responsive megaloblastic
      anemia
  Unexplained
    Congenital dyserythropoietic anemia
    Refractory megaloblastic anemia
    Erythroleukemia

be low but rarely cause clinical problems. Details of the clinical manifestations are given in the sections on the specific forms of megaloblastic anemia later in this chapter.

LABORATORY FEATURES

BLOOD CELLS

All cell lines are affected. Erythrocytes vary markedly in size and shape, often are large and oval, and in severe cases can show basophilic stippling and nuclear remnants (Cabot rings, and Howell-Jolly bodies). Erythroid activity in the marrow is enhanced, although the megaloblastic cells usually die before they are released, accounting for the reduced reticulocyte count. The more severe the anemia, the more pronounced the morphologic changes in the red cells. When the hematocrit is less than 20 percent, erythroblasts with megaloblastic nuclei, including an occasional promegaloblast, may appear in the blood. The anemia is macrocytic (mean corpuscular volume [MCV] = 100–150 fl or more), although coexisting iron deficiency, thalassemia trait, or inflammation can prevent macrocytosis.[171] Slight macrocytosis often is the earliest sign of megaloblastic anemia.

Neutrophil nuclei often have more than the usual three to five lobes[172] (Fig. 39-15). Typically, more than 5 percent of the neutrophils have five lobes. Cells may contain six or more lobes, a morphology never seen in normal neutrophils. In nutritional megaloblastic anemias, hypersegmented neutrophils are an early sign of megaloblastosis[172,173] and persist in the blood for many days after treatment.[174] Chromosomes are elongated and broken.[175] Specific therapy corrects these abnormalities, usually within 2 days, although some abnormalities do not disappear for months.[167] Platelets are slightly smaller than normal and vary more widely in size (increased platelet distribution width).[176]

MARROW

Aspirated marrow is cellular and shows striking megaloblastic changes, especially in the erythroid series. The high apoptosis rate of erythroid precursor cells in the marrow creates more globin lysis and, thus, jaundice. Sideroblasts are increased in number and contain increased numbers of iron granules. The ratio of myeloid to erythroid precursors falls to 1:1 or lower, and granulocyte reserves may be decreased.[177] In severe cases, promegaloblasts containing an unusually large number of mitotic figures are plentiful. Macrophage iron content often is increased.

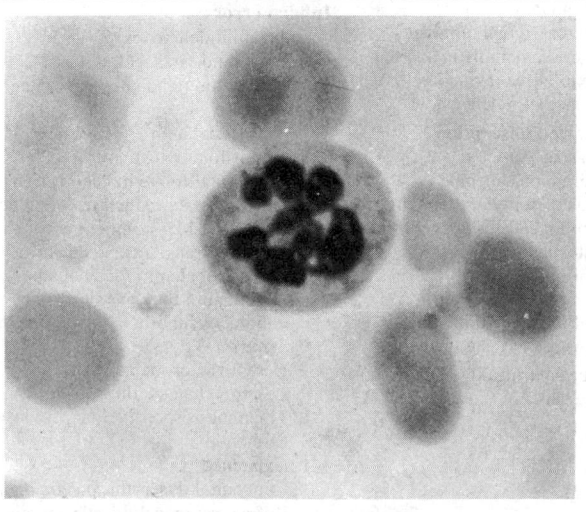

FIGURE 39-15   Megaloblastic hypersegmented neutrophil (×1500).

ATYPICAL MORPHOLOGY IN MEGALOBLASTIC ANEMIA

Under certain circumstances, megaloblastic anemia may be overlooked because its characteristic morphology is imperfectly expressed. For example, a measurable proportion of patients with cobalamin deficiency do not have an MCV above the normal limit.

COEXISTING MICROCYTIC ANEMIA

Many features of megaloblastic anemia may be masked when megaloblastic anemia is combined with a microcytic anemia.[178] The anemia can be normocytic or even microcytic, whereas the blood film may show both microcytes and macro-ovalocytes (a "dimorphic anemia") or microcytes alone if the microcytic component is sufficiently severe. The marrow may contain "intermediate" megaloblasts[179] that are smaller and look less "megaloblastic" than usual. In this kind of mixed anemia, the microcytic component usually is iron-deficiency anemia.[171] but it may be thalassemia minor or the anemia of chronic disease.[180] Even megaloblastic anemia masked by a severe microcytic anemia usually shows hypersegmented neutrophils in the blood and giant metamyelocytes and bands in the marrow. Neutrophil myeloperoxidase levels are high.[181]

The megaloblastic component of a mixed iron-deficiency anemia can be overlooked, and the patient may be treated only with iron. In this case, the anemia responds only partly to therapy, and megaloblastic features emerge as iron stores fill.

INCOMPLETE MEGALOBLASTIC ANEMIA

If a patient with a full-blown megaloblastic anemia receives cobalamin or folate before marrow aspiration, the anemia persists but the megaloblastic changes may be obscured. Attenuated megaloblastic changes also are seen in patients with early megaloblastic anemia, in patients with coexisting infection, or in patients after transfusion.

MEGALOBLASTIC ANEMIA MISDIAGNOSED AS ACUTE LEUKEMIA

Occasionally, very severe megaloblastic anemia produces marrow morphology so bizarre as to be mistaken for acute leukemia. The mistaken identification occurs especially if the marrow lacks classic megaloblasts and displays as its principal cell type the bizarre megaloblastic white cell precursors that, in a more typical morphologic background, supports the diagnosis of a megaloblastic anemia. In some cases, the erythroid series does not mature, and the megaloblastic pronormoblast dominates the marrow, raising the possibility of erythroid leukemia.

MEGALOBLASTIC CHANGES IN OTHER CELLS

In most forms of megaloblastic anemia, cytologic abnormalities resembling megaloblastosis may appear in other proliferating cells. Epithelial cells from the mouth, stomach, small intestine, and cervix uteri may look megaloblastic, appearing larger than their normal counterparts and containing atypical immature-looking nuclei.[182] Distinguishing these "megaloblastic" changes from the changes of malignancy can be difficult.

CHEMICAL CHANGES IN BODY FLUIDS

Plasma bilirubin, iron, and ferritin levels are increased.[183] Serum lactate dehydrogenase-1 (LDH-1) and LDH-2, both found in red cells, are markedly elevated as a result of rapid intramedullary erythroblast turnover and increase with the severity of the anemia.[184] In megaloblastic anemia LDH-1 is greater than LDH-2, whereas in other anemias LDH-2 is greater than LDH-1.[185] Serum muramidase (lysozyme) levels are high,[186] whereas serum glutamic oxaloacetic transaminase is normal.[187] Erythropoietin levels rise, but less than in other anemias of similar severity.[188] Surprisingly, the elevated erythropoietin levels fall sharply within 1 day of beginning treatment, an interval too short to affect the hematocrit.

CYTOKINETICS

Megaloblastic anemia is associated with two pathophysiologic abnormalities: *ineffective erythropoiesis* and *hemolysis*. Ineffective erythropoiesis increases the red cell precursor to reticulocyte ratio, plasma iron turnover,[189] LDH-1 and LDH-2 levels,[190] and "early-labeled" bilirubin.[191] Extramedullary hemolysis occurs in megaloblastic anemia, with red cell life span decreased by 30 to 50 percent.[192]

Increased serum muramidase in megaloblastic anemia can be caused by increased granulocyte turnover,[186] possibly induced by disintegration of granulocyte precursors in the marrow (ineffective granulopoiesis). In cobalamin deficiency, platelet production is only 10 percent of that expected from the megakaryocyte mass,[193] perhaps reflecting ineffective thrombopoiesis. Platelets in severe cobalamin deficiency are functionally abnormal.[194]

FOLIC ACID DEFICIENCY

ETIOLOGY AND PATHOGENESIS

Folate deficiency is caused by (1) dietary deficiency, (2) impaired absorption, and (3) increased requirements (see Table 39-5).

DECREASED INTAKE CAUSED BY POOR NUTRITION

An inadequate diet is the major cause of folate deficiency. Because folate reserves are small, deficiency develops rapidly in malnourished persons, typically the old, the poor, and the alcoholic. Folate deficiency can occur during *hyperalimentation*[195] or during *hemodialysis*, where folate is lost in the dialysis fluid.[196] Subclinical folate deficiency has been reported in subtotal gastrectomy.[197] Folate deficiency can occur in *premature infants*, especially with infection, diarrhea, or hemolytic anemia[198]; in children on a *synthetic diet* because of inborn errors[199]; and in infants raised on *goat's milk*, which is poor in folate.[200] Destruction of folate through excessive cooking can aggravate folate deficiency.

In alcoholic cirrhosis, megaloblastic anemia usually is caused by folate deficiency.[174] Alcohol may acutely depress serum folate, even if folate stores are full,[201] and accelerates the development of megaloblastic anemia in persons with early folate deficiency.[202] Alcohol causes acute marrow suppression, decreases in reticulocyte, platelet, and granulocyte levels[203]; reversible vacuolation of erythroid and myeloid precursors[204]; and dysfunction of granulocytes.[204] These changes occur even if large doses of folate are given with the alcohol.[205]

DECREASED INTAKE CAUSED BY IMPAIRED ABSORPTION

Nontropical Sprue Nontropical sprue (*celiac disease* in children) is related to ingestion of wheat gluten.[206] Pathologically, nontropical sprue shows atrophy and chronic inflammation of the small intestinal mucosa that is most severe proximally. Findings include weight loss, glossitis (typical of folate deficiency), other signs of a generalized vitamin deficiency, diarrhea, and passage of light-colored, bulky stools with an unusually foul odor. Iron deficiency, hypocalcemia, osteoporosis, and osteomalacia may occur.

Folate malabsorption occurs in most patients with this disorder.[207] Serum folate levels are low,[208] and megaloblastic anemia occurs frequently.

Tropical Sprue Tropical sprue is endemic in the West Indies, southern India, parts of southern Africa, and Southeast Asia. It can be acquired by travelers to those regions and persists for many years after the travelers return.[209] Tropical sprue is rapidly corrected by folate therapy, even though folate deficiency does not cause the disease. The

etiology of tropical sprue is unknown, although the response of the disease to antibiotics suggests infection.[210]

Clinically and pathologically, tropical sprue is like nontropical sprue, except that tropical sprue is more severe in the distal small intestine.[211] Therefore, tropical sprue usually leads to cobalamin deficiency[212] and should be strongly considered as a cause of cobalamin deficiency in former residents of the tropics, even though they have been away from the tropics for 20 years or more. Folate malabsorption may occur,[213] possibly because the diseased intestine fails to deconjugate folate polyglutamates.[214] Therefore, megaloblastic anemia is very common in patients with this disease[215] and may result from both folate and cobalamin deficiency.

Other Intestinal Disorders Malabsorption of folic acid commonly occurs in regional enteritis,[215] after extensive resections of the small intestine,[216] and in conditions such as lymphomatous or leukemic infiltration of the small intestine,[217] Whipple disease,[217] scleroderma and amyloidosis,[218] and diabetes mellitus.[219] Systemic bacterial infections impair folate absorption.[220]

INCREASED FOLATE REQUIREMENTS

Pregnancy During pregnancy (see Chap. 7),[221] folate requirements increase fivefold to tenfold because of transfer of folate to the growing fetus,[222] which draws down maternal folate stores even in the face of severe maternal folate deficiency.[223] Further increases may result from the presence of multiple fetuses, a poor diet, infection, coexisting hemolytic anemia, or anticonvulsant medication. Lactation aggravates folate deficiency.[224] Consequently, folate deficiency is very common in pregnancy[225] and is the major cause of the megaloblastic anemia of pregnancy.[226]

Folate deficiency is difficult to diagnose in pregnancy because the signs of deficiency are obscured by the normal hematologic changes of pregnancy. During pregnancy, a physiologic "anemia" develops because of increased plasma volume that is only partly offset by an accompanying increase in red cell mass (Fig. 39-16). Hemoglobin levels may fall to 10 g/dl. The anemia is associated with a physiologic macrocytosis; MCV increases to 120 fl, although the average at term is 104 fl.[227] Serum and red cell folate levels fall steadily during pregnancy, even in well-nourished women.[228] All these changes are false clues suggesting folate deficiency even when folate levels are normal. Conversely, hypersegmented neutrophils, usually a reliable clue to early megaloblastic anemia, are missing in early megaloblastic anemia of pregnancy.[229] In many cases, the only finding that reliably distinguishes the physiologic anemia of pregnancy from folate deficiency is a megaloblastic marrow.

Increased Cell Turnover Because of increased marrow cell turnover, the folate requirement rises sharply in chronic *hemolytic anemia*.[230] During bouts of acute hemolysis that can occur in these anemias, the marrow may become megaloblastic within days.

Folic acid deficiency may arise in chronic *exfoliative dermatitis*, in which folate losses of 5 to 20 μg/day may occur.[231] Patients with psoriasis who are treated with methotrexate have an added reason for developing signs of folate deficiency. Pretreating such patients with folate may prevent these signs without impairing the therapeutic effect of methotrexate.[231]

CLINICAL FEATURES

The clinical picture of folate deficiency includes all the nonspecific manifestations of megaloblastic anemia *plus* the following specific features: (1) a history and laboratory studies indicating folate deficiency, (2) absence of the neurologic signs of cobalamin deficiency (see "Cobalamin Deficiency" below), and (3) a full response to *physiologic* doses of folate.

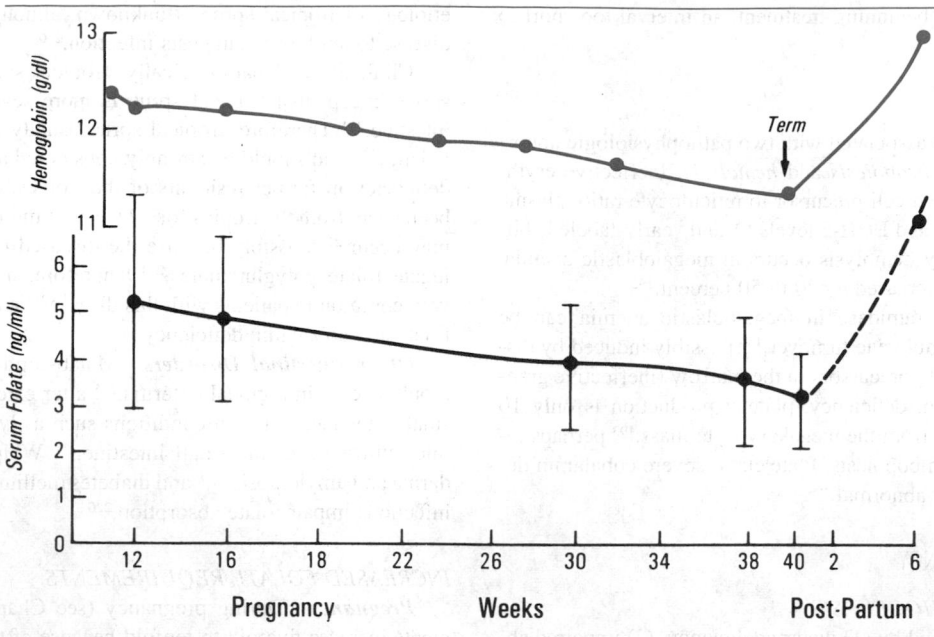

FIGURE 39-16   Hemoglobin and serum folate levels during pregnancy and the postpartum period. (Adapted from Shojania.[221])

LABORATORY FEATURES

The earliest indicator of folate deficiency is a *low serum folate*. Serum folate follows folate intake closely, so a low serum folate (less than approximately 3 ng/ml) may indicate only a drop in folate intake over the preceding few days.[173] Similarly, a low serum folate rises quickly on refeeding.

A better indicator of the tissue folate status is the *red cell folate*,[232] which remains relatively unchanged while a red cell is circulating and thus reflects folate turnover over the preceding 2 to 3 months. Red cell folate usually is quite low in folate-deficient megaloblastic anemia. However, red cell folate also is low in more than 50 percent of patients with cobalamin-deficient megaloblastic anemia[233]; therefore, it cannot be used to distinguish between these two deficiencies. Conversely, red cell folate may be normal in the megaloblastic state that occurs, often with little accompanying anemia, in rapidly developing folate deficiency (see "Acute Megaloblastic Anemia" below).[234]

The dU suppression test is used in research on pathogenetic mechanisms in megaloblastic states. It adds little to the clinical evaluation of a megaloblastic anemia. The test is discussed in full in "Deoxyuridine Suppression Test" below.

DIFFERENTIAL DIAGNOSIS

Macrocytosis occurs in alcoholism without megaloblastic anemia, liver disease, hypothyroidism, aplastic anemia, certain forms of myelodysplasia, pregnancy, and any condition associated with reticulocytosis (e.g., autoimmune hemolytic anemia). However, MCV rarely exceeds 110 fl in these conditions. A full hematologic response to physiologic doses of folate (i.e., 200 μg daily) distinguishes folate deficiency from cobalamin deficiency, in which a response occurs only at *pharmacologic* doses of folate (e.g., 5 mg daily).[182] This is *not* recommended as a diagnostic test because neurologic problems may develop in cobalamin-deficient patients treated with folate alone. Cobalamin may produce a partial response in folate deficiency.[235]

The diagnosis of nontropical sprue rests on (1) the demonstration of malabsorption, (2) a jejunal biopsy showing villus atrophy, and (3) the response to a gluten-free diet. In 80 percent of patients, a gluten-

free diet gradually reverses the functional disorder by correcting folate malabsorption.[236]

NONHEMATOLOGIC EFFECTS OF FOLATE DEFICIENCY

The hematologic problems associated with folate deficiency have been recognized for decades. However, folate deficiency is related to a number of serious disorders not involving the hematopoietic system. Moreover, these disorders occur at folate levels usually regarded as low to normal. They include congenital anomalies, fragile site syndromes, and, most common of all, atherosclerosis.

ABNORMALITIES OF NEURAL TUBE CLOSURE

A close association exists between mild folate deficiency and congenital anomalies of the fetus, most notably defects in neural tube closure, but also abnormalities involving the heart, urinary tract, limbs, and other sites.[237] A portion of the neural tube closure defects appear to be associated with antibodies against folate receptors that may be overcome by higher folate intake.[237a] Mutations affecting enzymes of folate metabolism, especially the common 677C→T mutation of the *MTHFR* gene (also designated as *MTHFR* 677C→T),[238] also predispose to congenital anomalies.

Levels of TCII in normal pregnant women correlate with their likelihood of bearing an infant with a defect in neural tube closure. Patients in the lowest quintile of TCII concentration are five times more likely to give birth to a defective infant as patients in the highest quintile.[239]

Poorly defined neuropsychiatric abnormalities that respond to folate therapy have been reported in patients with folate deficiency.[235]

VASCULAR DISEASE

A mildly elevated homocysteine level is a major risk factor for atherosclerosis and venous thrombosis, possibly because of an effect on the vascular endothelium.[240] Homocysteine levels can decrease with folate, cobalamin, and pyridoxine supplements, possibly reducing the risk of vascular disease.[241] The *MTHFR* polymorphism *MTHFR* 677C→T leads to increased homocysteine levels in subjects with low folate or cobalamin levels,[242] although controversy exists as to whether MTHFR 677C→T causes an increased incidence of vascular disease.[243] Like folate, cobalamin seems to be important in decreasing the risk of vascular disease, further reducing serum homocysteine levels in subjects supplemented with folic acid.[244] A 1561C→T polymorphism in the gene for glutamate carboxypeptidase-II increases serum folate and decreases serum homocysteine in the homozygote, presumably protecting against vascular disease.[245]

HELLP SYNDROME

Severe folate deficiency reportedly mimics the hemolysis, elevated liver enzymes, low platelets (HELLP) syndrome (preeclampsia with liver swelling and abnormal liver function studies in pregnant women) (see Chap. 7).[246] In these patients, the diagnosis of severe folate deficiency can be made based on the presence of anemia and a megaloblastic blood film and marrow. Serum and red cell folate, serum cobalamin, homocysteine, and methylmalonic acid levels all should be assayed before treatment is started. The patient should immediately be given high doses of folate plus cobalamin, the latter in case the megaloblastic anemia actually results from cobalamin deficiency. A major goal of treatment is preventing preterm delivery of the fetus.

COLON CANCER

A large study of nurses in the United States indicated that supplementation with more than 400 μg of folate per day reduces the incidence of colon cancer by 31 percent.[247] This finding has important implications for public health. Preliminary evidence suggests individuals who are homozygous for the 677C→T MTHFR mutation also have a decreased incidence for colon cancer compared with 677C→T heterozygotes and normal controls.[248]

THERAPY, COURSE, AND PROGNOSIS

Folate 1 to 5 mg/day is given orally, although 1 mg usually is sufficient. At this dose, anemia usually is corrected even in patients with malabsorption. A parenteral preparation containing 5 mg/ml of folate also is available.

Treatment for *tropical sprue* consists of the usual doses of folate, plus cobalamin if indicated. To prevent relapse, treatment should be maintained for at least 2 years. Broad-spectrum antibiotics are helpful adjuncts, although antibiotics alone fail to correct the condition.

Pregnant women must given at least 400 μg of folate per day.[249] As to the possibility of overlooking cobalamin deficiency resulting from folate administration, PA in pregnancy is rare.[250] In pregnant women at risk for cobalamin deficiency (e.g., vegans or patients with malabsorption), the deficiency is easily prevented with vitamin B_{12}, 1 mg given parenterally every 3 months during the pregnancy.

Therapeutic doses of folate partly correct the hematologic abnormalities in cobalamin deficiency, but the neurologic manifestations can progress, with disastrous results.[251] Therefore, both folate status and cobalamin status must be evaluated early in the workup of a megaloblastic anemia. If treatment is urgent and the nature of the deficiency is unclear, both folate and cobalamin can be given after samples have been obtained for assay.

Patients who receive low-dose methotrexate therapy as an immunosuppressant may develop side effects, the worst of which is hepatotoxicity. The incidence of side effects, including hepatotoxicity, has been correlated with reduced folate levels.[252] Administration of folic or folinic acid can prevent side effects without reducing the therapeutic effect of low-dose methotrexate.

COBALAMIN DEFICIENCY

ETIOLOGY AND PATHOGENESIS

Table 39-5 lists disorders that lead to cobalamin deficiency.

DECREASED UPTAKE CAUSED BY IMPAIRED ABSORPTION

Cobalamin deficiency most often results from defective absorption, most commonly PA, a condition characterized by failure of intrinsic factor production. Many other causes of defective cobalamin absorption involve the stomach, pancreas, or small intestine.

GASTRIC DISORDERS

PERNICIOUS ANEMIA*

PA is a disease of insidious onset that generally begins in middle age or later (usually after age 40 years).[253] In this condition, intrinsic factor secretion fails because of gastric mucosal atrophy. PA is an autoimmune disease. The gastric atrophy of PA probably results from immune destruction of the acid- and pepsin-secreting portion of the gastric mucosa.

In patients with PA, antibodies occur that recognize the H^+/K^+-adenosine triphosphatase (ATPase), which resides in the secretory membrane of the parietal cell and is responsible for acidifying the stomach contents. These antiparietal cell antibodies occur in approximately 60 percent of patients with simple atrophic gastritis and in 90 percent of patients with PA, but in only 5 percent of a random 30- to 60-year-old population.[254] Antiparietal cell antibodies also occur in a significant percentage of patients with thyroid disease.[255] Conversely, patients with PA have a higher than expected incidence of antibodies against thyroid epithelium, lymphocytes, and renal collecting duct cells.[256]

Antiparietal cell antibodies are not thought to be responsible for the pathogenesis of PA. Rather, studies in mice suggest the gastric atrophy in PA anemia is caused by CD4+ T cells whose receptors recognize the H^+/K^+-ATPase. Thus, thymectomized BALB/c mice develop an autoimmune atrophic gastritis similar to that seen in PA patients. CD4+ T cells from these mice produce atrophic gastritis when injected into nude mice.[257]

Antibodies to intrinsic factor ("type I," or "blocking," antibodies) or the intrinsic factor–Cbl complex ("type II," or "binding," antibodies) are highly specific to PA patients.[256] Blocking antibodies, which prevent formation of the intrinsic factor–Cbl complex, are found in 70 percent of PA sera.[258] Binding antibodies, which prevent the intrinsic factor–Cbl complex from binding to its ileal receptors, are found in about half the sera that contain blocking antibody. In the second part of the Schilling test, these antibodies may produce a false-positive result by interfering with the action of exogenous intrinsic factor.[259]

Some findings in humans support the idea that T cells are responsible for the gastric atrophy in PA. First, lymphocytes from patients with PA are hyperresponsive to gastric antigens.[260] Second, the correlation between antiparietal cell antibodies and PA is not perfect.[261] Finally, the incidence of PA is higher than expected in patients with agammaglobulinemia, even though their sera contain none of the antibodies typical of PA.[262]

OTHER AUTOIMMUNE DISEASES

Antiparietal cell antibodies and PA are unexpectedly frequent in patients with other autoimmune diseases,[263] including autoimmune thyroid disorders (thyrotoxicosis, hypothyroidism, and Hashimoto thyroiditis),[264] type I diabetes mellitus, hypoparathyroidism,[265] Addison disease, postpartum hypophysitis,[266] ulcerative colitis,[267] vitiligo,[268] acquired agammaglobulinemia,[262] infertility in female patients younger than 40 years,[269] and hypospermia and infertility in males.[270]

---

*The term *pernicious anemia* sometimes is used as a synonym for cobalamin deficiency, but it should be reserved for the condition resulting from defective secretion of intrinsic factor by an atrophic gastric mucosa.

The coexistence of these diseases and PA is further evidence that PA is an autoimmune disease.

INHERITED PREDISPOSITION TO PERNICIOUS ANEMIA

Predisposition to PA can be inherited. The disease is associated with human leukocyte antigen types A2, A3, B7, and B12[271] and with blood group A.[272] PA and antiparietal cell antibodies occur more frequently than expected in the families of PA patients.[273] In one study, gastric atrophy was found in more than 30 percent of the relatives of patients with PA; of these relatives, 65 percent had antiparietal cell antibodies and 22 percent had anti-intrinsic factor antibodies.[274] PA occurs relatively frequently in northern Europeans (especially Scandinavians)[274] and African Americans[275] but is uncommon in Asians. In African Americans, the disease tends to begin early, occurs with high frequency in women, and often is severe.[275]

STOMACH AND INTESTINE IN PERNICIOUS ANEMIA

Gastric manifestations of PA include achlorhydria, acquired intrinsic factor deficiency demonstrable by the Schilling test, and an increased incidence of certain malignancies: an approximately twofold increase in the incidence of gastric cancer, similar increases in the incidence of certain hematologic malignancies, and an increase in the incidence of gastric carcinoid.[276] Achlorhydria may precede by many years the loss of intrinsic factor secretion and the development of PA.[277] Achlorhydria is present if the pH of gastric juice after stimulation with pentagastrin (6 μg/kg subcutaneously) remains greater than 3.5 and does not decrease by more than 1 pH unit. The absence of achlorhydria excludes the diagnosis of PA. Measurement of gastric acid secretion has been supplanted by serum cobalamin and methylmalonic acid levels and the Schilling test.[278]

Helicobacter pylori, a microorganism that infects the gastric mucosa, is a major cause of gastritis and peptic ulcers. Evidence is conflicting regarding the role of *H. pylori* in PA. In two studies, cultures of gastric biopsies showed a very low incidence of *H. pylori* infection in PA patients.[279] One study reported that anti–*H. pylori* antibodies were found in only a small fraction of the sera from these patients. The other study reported that these antibodies were present in most of the PA sera, indicating that most of the patients described in the study had been infected previously. Whether *H. pylori* participates in the pathogenesis of PA is an open question.

Fasting plasma gastrin levels are high in most patients with PA, whereas somatostatin levels are low.[280] In biopsies from PA stomachs, however, fundal gastrin and somatostatin levels were high, correlating with increases in argyrophilic cells in the basal crypts; antral gastrin and somatostatin were normal. Gastrin levels are high in simple achlorhydria without PA.[281]

The stomach shows characteristic histologic abnormalities in PA (Fig. 39-17). The mucosa of the cardia and fundus is atrophic, containing few chief (i.e., pepsin-secreting) or parietal cells. The withered mucosa is infiltrated with lymphocytes[282] and plasma cells. In contrast, the antral and pyloric mucosa are normal. Gastric atrophy is partly reversible by glucocorticoid treatment, with some regeneration and return of intrinsic factor secretion, further evidence for the autoimmune nature of PA.[283]

Megaloblastic changes reversible by cobalamin are seen in the gastrointestinal epithelium. Cells recovered by lavage are large[142] and show atypical nuclei resembling early malignant change.[284] Small intestinal biopsy shows decreased mitoses in crypts, shortening of villi, megaloblastic changes in epithelial cells, and infiltration in the lamina propria.[285] These changes may account for the occasional malabsorption of D-xylose and carotene in PA.[286]

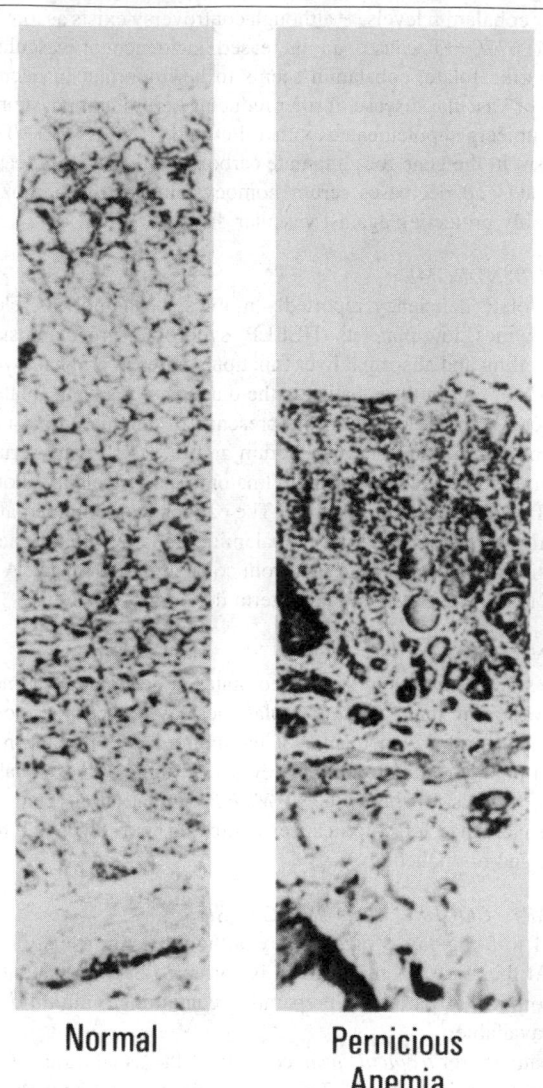

Normal **Pernicious Anemia**

FIGURE 39-17 Gastric histology in pernicious anemia. (*Left*) Normal fundus. The thick mucosa is packed with gastric glands composed mostly of chief cells and parietal cells. The mucus-secreting cells are concentrated in the necks of the glands. (*Right*) Fundus in pernicious anemia. Gastric glands in the atrophic mucosa are sparse and consist mainly of mucus-secreting cells. The mucosa is densely infiltrated by lymphocytes.

RECOGNIZING PERNICIOUS ANEMIA MAY BE DIFFICULT

PA combines the general features of megaloblastic anemia and features specific for cobalamin deficiency with unique clinical features related to its (probable) autoimmune etiology and gastric pathology. The disease is easily missed because of its (1) insidious onset, (2) tendency to be masked by the use of multivitamin preparations containing folic acid,[287] and (3) many atypical presentations,[288] including its presentation as a neurologic disease without hematologic findings and its tendency to be overlooked in patients with another autoimmune disease.

Antiparietal cell and anti-intrinsic factor antibodies are rarely measured, even though anti-intrinsic factor antibodies in particular could be of considerable diagnostic value.[234] Anti-intrinsic factor antibody is highly specific for PA (although its sensitivity is only modest), and its presence in a megaloblastic anemia makes the diagnosis of PA almost certain.

GASTRECTOMY SYNDROMES

Gastric surgery often leads to anemia. Iron-deficiency anemia is most common, but cobalamin deficiency with megaloblastic anemia can occur. After *total gastrectomy*, cobalamin deficiency develops within 5 or 6 years because the operation removes the source of intrinsic factor.[289] The delay between surgery and the onset of cobalamin deficiency reflects the time needed to exhaust cobalamin stores after cobalamin absorption ceases.

After *partial gastrectomy*, few patients show frank cobalamin deficiency, but approximately 5 percent have intermediate megaloblastosis, approximately 25 to 50 percent have low serum cobalamin levels, and many have decreased intrinsic factor secretion (Schilling test).[290] Achlorhydria not present before surgery often develops some years after gastrectomy. Postgastrectomy patients with low serum cobalamin levels usually have low serum iron levels,[291] in contrast to the high iron levels typical of cobalamin deficiency.

Cobalamin deficiency after partial gastrectomy can be caused by mucosal atrophy in the unresected remnant of the stomach[292] or, if a gastrojejunostomy was performed, by bacterial overgrowth in the afferent loop (see "Blind Loop Syndrome" below). Postgastrectomy folate deficiency from malabsorption or reduced dietary intake accounts for more cases of postgastrectomy megaloblastic anemia than does cobalamin deficiency. The two deficiencies often occur together.

ZOLLINGER-ELLISON SYNDROME

In Zollinger-Ellison syndrome, a gastrin-producing tumor, usually in the pancreas, stimulates the gastric mucosa to secrete immense amounts of HCl. The major clinical problem is a severe ulcer diathesis. Malabsorption of cobalamin occurs when the vast quantities of HCl secreted by the overactive gastric mucosa cannot be completely neutralized by the pancreatic secretions. The resulting acidification of the duodenal contents inactivates pancreatic proteases, preventing transfer of Cbl from R binder to intrinsic factor.[293]

INTESTINAL DISEASES

A number of intestinal disorders can lead to cobalamin deficiency. They include (1) extensive resection of the ileum,[294] (2) regional ileitis[295] or other disease affecting the ileum (e.g., lymphoma, radiation damage[296]), (3) cobalamin malabsorption associated with hypothyroidism,[297] or certain drugs, (4) the effects of cobalamin deficiency itself,[298] and (5) sprue, either tropical or, less often, nontropical.[212] In each of these disorders, exogenous intrinsic factor fails to correct an abnormal Schilling test.

COMPETING INTESTINAL FLORA AND FAUNA: "BLIND LOOP SYNDROME"

The *blind loop syndrome* is a state of cobalamin malabsorption with megaloblastic anemia caused by intestinal stasis from anatomic lesions (strictures, diverticula, anastomoses, surgical blind loops) or impaired motility (scleroderma, amyloid).[299] Serum cobalamin is low, but intrinsic factor secretion is normal. Cobalamin malabsorption is not corrected by exogenous intrinsic factor. The defect in cobalamin absorption is caused by colonization of the diseased small intestine by bacteria that take up ingested cobalamin before it can be absorbed from the intestine.[300] Steatorrhea is also seen in the blind loop syndrome.

Another cause of cobalamin deficiency is infestation with the fish tapeworm *Diphyllobothrium latum*. Prevalence is highest near the Baltic Sea, Canada, and Alaska. Figure 39-18 illustrates the life cycle of the worm. Humans are infected by eating undercooked fish or fish roe. Once ingested, the sparganum larva becomes an adult in 5 to 6 weeks and may live for years.

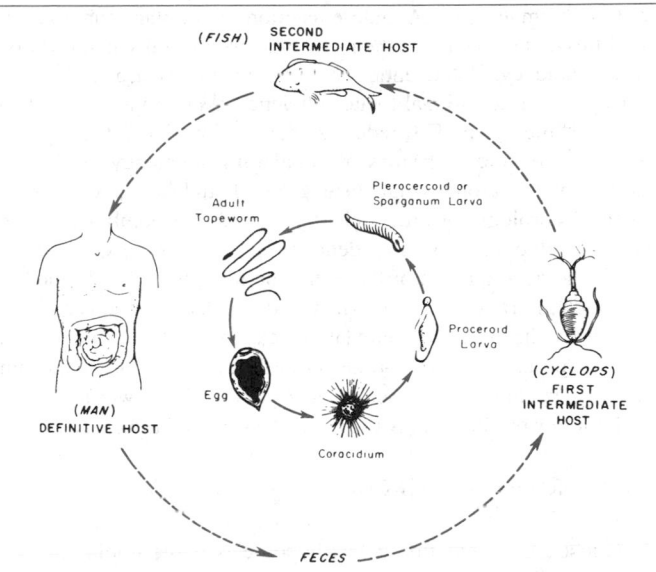

FIGURE 39-18   Life cycle of *Diphyllobothrium latum. Inner circle* represents developmental stages of parasite: (1) adult worm, (2) eggs, (3) embryonated egg (coracidium), (4) procercoid larva, (5) plerocercoid larva. *Outside circle* shows first intermediate host (*Cyclops*), second intermediate host (fish), and definitive host (man). (Adapted from Wirth WA, Farrow CC: Human sparganosis. *JAMA* 177:76, 1961.)

Cobalamin deficiency results from competition between the worm and the host for ingested cobalamin.[301] The clinical picture of *D. latum* infestation ranges from no symptoms to a full-blown megaloblastic anemia with neurologic changes. Only approximately 3 percent of persons harboring the parasite become anemic.[302] The infestation is diagnosed by finding tapeworm ova in the feces.

PANCREATIC DISEASE

Cobalamin malabsorption can be demonstrated by the Schilling test in 50 to 70 percent of patients with exocrine pancreatic insufficiency.[303] Cobalamin malabsorption in pancreatic insufficiency is caused by a deficiency in pancreatic proteases, resulting in a partial failure to destroy R binder–Cbl complexes whose destruction is a prerequisite for the transfer of cobalamin to intrinsic factor. The defect in cobalamin absorption in chronic pancreatitis is corrected by oral trypsin or by presaturating the R binder with cobinamide, a cobalamin analogue that is taken up by R binder but not by intrinsic factor.[304] Despite the high incidence of abnormal Schilling tests in pancreatic insufficiency, this disorder almost never causes clinically significant cobalamin deficiency.[305]

DIETARY COBALAMIN DEFICIENCY

Dietary cobalamin deficiency is very unusual. It occurs mainly in vegetarians who also do not consume dairy products and eggs (vegans).[306] Low serum cobalamin levels occur in 50 to 60 percent of individuals in this group.[307] Breast-fed infants of vegan mothers also may develop cobalamin deficiency.[308] Cobalamin deficiency in vegans presents with mild megaloblastic anemia, glossitis, and neurologic disturbances.

Cobalamin deficiency may occur in severe general malnutrition. A megaloblastic anemia not related to cobalamin deficiency may accompany kwashiorkor or marasmus.[309]

NEUROLOGIC EFFECTS OF COBALAMIN DEFICIENCY

Formerly, the neurologic abnormalities of cobalamin deficiency were attributed to disordered metabolism of myelin lipids caused by an impaired methylmalonyl CoA mutase reaction.[310] Similar neurologic abnormalities do not occur in patients with inherited methylmalonyl CoA mutase deficiency.[254] Authentic combined system disease has occurred in a patient with nutritional folate deficiency[311] and in another patient with N^5,N^{10}-methylene FH$_4$ reductase deficiency.[312] The latter reports suggest the neurologic lesions of cobalamin deficiency result from deranged methyl group metabolism. Animal studies support this hypothesis. Neurologic disorders closely resembling combined system disease develop in cobalamin-deficient pigs, fruit bats, and monkeys.[313] The development of these disorders is prevented by methionine, which is produced in a cobalamin-dependent reaction and is the precursor of the biologic methylating reagent SAM. A finding that further supports a methylation defect is that brains from cobalamin-deficient pigs contain increased levels of SAH,[314] a powerful methylation inhibitor produced in SAM-dependent methylation reactions:

$$SAM + RH \rightarrow SAH + RCH_3$$

Against the methylation defect hypothesis is the finding that cobalamin deficiency had no effect on SAM, SAH, or methylation of phospholipids or myelin basic protein[315] in the brains of fruit bats. Are humans more like pigs or fruit bats? Draw your own conclusions.[316]

CLINICAL FEATURES

The clinical picture of cobalamin deficiency includes the nonspecific manifestations of megaloblastosis, which include anemia, thrombocytopenia, neutropenia, smooth tongue, cardiomyopathy, pale yellow skin and/or weight loss, plus specific features caused by the lack of cobalamin, chiefly neurologic abnormalities. Because cobalamin reserves are large, years may pass between the cessation of cobalamin absorption and the appearance of deficiency symptoms. This interval is shortened in patients whose enterohepatic cobalamin cycle is interrupted.

NEUROLOGIC ABNORMALITIES

Cobalamin deficiency causes a neurologic syndrome that is particularly dangerous because the syndrome can develop in isolation,[317] with no megaloblastic anemia suggesting a lack of cobalamin,[318] and because the syndrome cannot be reversed by treatment when it is sufficiently far advanced. The syndrome usually begins with paresthesias in feet and fingers as a result of early peripheral neuropathy and disturbances of vibratory sense and proprioception. The earliest signs, which precede other neurologic findings by months, are loss of position sense in the second toe and loss of vibration sense for a 256-Hz but not a 128-Hz tuning fork.[319] Left untreated, the neurologic disorder progresses to spastic ataxia resulting from demyelination of the dorsal and lateral columns of the spinal cord, so-called *combined system disease* (Fig. 39-19).[320]

The peripheral nerves, the spinal cord, and the brain are affected by cobalamin deficiency. Somnolence and perversion of taste, smell, and vision with occasional optic atrophy are accompanied by slow waves on the electroencephalogram. A dementia mimicking Alzheimer disease can develop.[321] Psychological derangements, including psychotic depression and paranoid schizophrenia, can occur.[322] Frank psychosis in cobalamin deficiency has been termed "megaloblastic madness."[323]

The neurologic lesions of cobalamin deficiency can be detected by magnetic resonance imaging (MRI). Demyelination appears as T2-weighted hyperintensity of the white matter. MRI is particularly useful for confirming the diagnosis of a neurologic disorder resulting from cobalamin deficiency. MRI also has been used to follow the progress of neurologic abnormalities during treatment of cobalamin-deficient patients.[324]

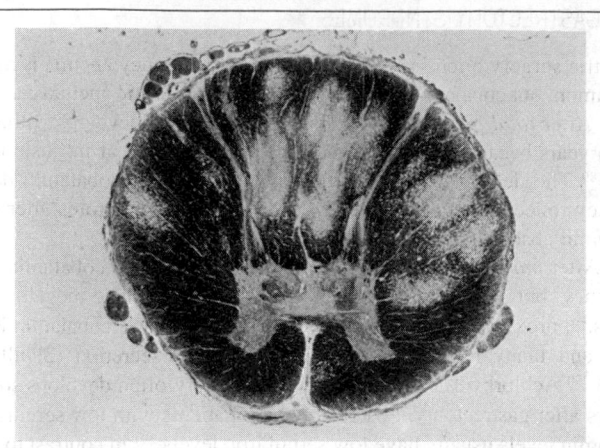

FIGURE 39-19   Degeneration of spinal cord in combined system disease. (From Harris JW, Kellermeyer RW: *The Red Cell: Production, Metabolism, Destruction: Normal and Abnormal*, rev ed, Harvard University Press, Cambridge, 1970.)

SUBTLE COBALAMIN DEFICIENCY

Some observations suggest the existence of a large group of patients who are hematologically normal, with a normal hematocrit and MCV, but have cobalamin-responsive neuropsychiatric disease.[325] The views are conflicting.[102] Neuropsychiatric findings include peripheral neuropathy, gait disturbance, memory loss, and psychiatric symptoms, often with abnormal evoked potentials. Serum cobalamin may be normal, borderline, or low, but tissue cobalamin deficiency is suggested by consistently high levels of serum methylmalonic acid and/or homocysteine,[326] very high levels of methylmalonic acid in the cerebrospinal fluid, and an abnormal dU suppression test. Most of the neuropsychiatric abnormalities appear to respond to cobalamin therapy.

LABORATORY FEATURES

SERUM COBALAMIN LEVELS

Serum cobalamin is low in most but not all patients with cobalamin deficiency.[326] Cobalamin levels are normal in cobalamin deficiency resulting from N_2O, TCII deficiency, and inborn errors of cobalamin metabolism. Levels also may be normal in cobalamin-deficient patients with high TCI levels resulting from myeloproliferative diseases.[327] Conversely, serum cobalamin levels may be low in the presence of normal tissue cobalamins in vegetarians, in subjects taking megadoses of ascorbic acid,[328] in pregnancy (25 percent), in the presence of TCI deficiency,[329] and in megaloblastic anemia resulting from folate deficiency (30 percent).[327] Serum folate may be higher than expected in cobalamin deficiency. Patients deficient in both cobalamin and folate may show normal serum folate levels.

METHYLMALONIC ACIDURIA

Except when caused by an inborn error, methylmalonic aciduria is a reliable indicator of cobalamin deficiency.[330] Normal subjects excrete only traces of methylmalonate (0–3.4 mg/day). In cobalamin deficiency, urine methylmalonate usually is elevated. Cobalamin therapy restores excretion to normal in a few days.

SERUM METHYLMALONIC ACID AND HOMOCYSTEINE

Elevated serum methylmalonic acid and homocysteine levels are indicators of *tissue* cobalamin deficiency. Their levels are high in more than 90 percent of cobalamin-deficient patients and rise before serum cobalamin falls to subnormal levels.[331] Elevated serum methylmalonic acid and/or elevated homocysteine probably are the most reliable indicators of cobalamin deficiency in patients without a congenital disorder in their metabolism.

Spinal fluid methylmalonic acid levels are markedly elevated in cobalamin deficiency.[332]

SCHILLING TEST: ASSAYS OF COBALAMIN ABSORPTION AND INTRINSIC FACTOR

The Schilling test assays cobalamin absorption by measuring urinary radioactivity after an oral dose of radioactive cobalamin. The test can be performed even after cobalamin deficiency has been treated. After voiding, a fasting patient drinks 0.5 μCi (0.5–2.0 μg) of radioactive CnCbl in water. A 24-hour urine collection is started. At 2 hours, 1 mg of unlabeled CnCbl is given intramuscularly (IM) to saturate the circulating cobalamin-binding proteins, after which the patient may eat. The amount of radioactivity in the 24-hour urine collection is measured. Normal subjects excrete at least 7 percent of the administered radioactivity in the first 24 hours.

If excretion of radioactivity is low, the second part of the Schilling test is performed after a 5-day delay. The interval allows the unlabeled cobalamin given in the first part of the test to correct intestinal megaloblastosis.[333] The procedure is the same except that 60 mg of *active* hog intrinsic factor (equivalent of 1 national formulary unit) is given orally with the radioactive cobalamin. If poor excretion in the first part resulted from intrinsic factor deficiency, excretion in the second part will be normal. Intrinsic factor will not correct cobalamin malabsorption resulting from other causes.

The Schilling test gives a false-negative result in patients who absorb free cobalamin but fail to release the vitamin from food (e.g., after partial gastrectomy[334] and vagotomy,[335] in a gastric ulcer,[336] and during treatment with agents that block the gastric H^+/K^+-ATPase (e.g., omeprazole[337]). Failure to absorb food cobalamin can be established by a modified Schilling test in which the source of labeled vitamin is an omelet of eggs obtained from a chicken fed on radioactive cobalamin.[331] Cobalamin deficiency occasionally results from malabsorption of protein-bound cobalamin only.[338]

The major source of error in the Schilling test is incomplete urine collection. Completeness of collection can be assessed by measuring the creatinine in the specimen (normal >15 mg/kg/day). Renal disease may delay excretion of radioactivity, giving a false-positive Schilling test.[339] Whole-body counting can be used to measure cobalamin absorption in severe renal insufficiency.[340] Other causes of a false-positive result are inadequate saturation of cobalamin-binding proteins by unlabeled cobalamin (first part of test), inactive intrinsic factor or neutralization of intrinsic factor by anti-intrinsic factor antibodies in the stomach[259] (second part), and malabsorption as a result of megaloblastic changes in the ileum[341] (second part). A false-negative result can be caused by isotope given with an earlier Schilling or other test.

DEOXYURIDINE SUPPRESSION TEST

The dU suppression test is based on the finding that unlabeled dU can suppress the uptake of [³H]thymidine ([³H]Thd) into the DNA of cultured lymphocytes or marrow cells.[342] Thymidine enters DNA through the dTMP pool, into which it is fed by thymidine kinase (Fig. 39-20). Deoxyuridine also enters DNA through the dTMP pool. It first is phosphorylated to dUMP by thymidine kinase and then is methylated to dTMP by thymidylate synthetase. The theory of the dU suppression test is that treating normal cells with dU loads them with *unlabeled* dTMP, which competes for uptake into DNA with the *labeled* dTMP formed during a later incubation with [³H]Thd. Thus, dU suppresses the uptake of [³H]Thd into DNA. If thymidylate synthetase activity is low, conversion of dU into dTMP is slowed, and the suppressive effect of dU on [³H]Thd uptake into DNA is diminished. Because thymidylate synthetase uses N^5,N^{10}-methylene FH_4 as a methylating agent,

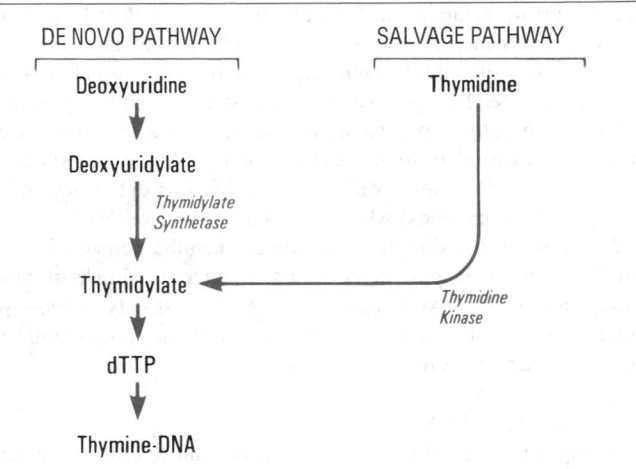

FIGURE 39-20   Incorporation of thymidine into DNA via the *de novo* and salvage pathways. (Adapted from Metz.[342])

its activity depends directly on folate and indirectly on cobalamin. Failure of dU suppression becomes an indication of cellular folate or cobalamin deficiency. The foregoing theory is highly oversimplified,[343] but experience indicates the dU suppression test can answer questions about cellular folate and cobalamin.

To perform the assay, cultured lymphocytes or marrow cells from a patient and control are incubated for 1 hour at 37°C with and without 0.1 μM dU. [³H]Thd is added, and the cells are incubated for another 0.5 to 3.0 hours. Incorporation of [³H]Thd is determined, and dU suppression is calculated as $100 \times$ (³H incorporation in dU-treated cells/ ³H incorporation by control cells), expressed as a percentage. Normally, dU depresses the uptake of [³H]Thd into DNA to less than 10 percent of control values. Deoxyuridine suppression is relieved in megaloblastic anemias of nutritional origin and in certain inherited disorders of folate or cobalamin metabolism[343] but not in other megaloblastic states.[344] In the nutritional anemias, dU suppression can be restored with folate or cobalamin according to a pattern that depends on the nature of the deficiency (Table 39-6).[343] The dU suppression test even can detect subclinical deficiency states.[345]

The dU suppression test is chiefly a research tool. It can help diagnose certain special clinical problems,[342] but these problems also can be diagnosed using other laboratory tests, therapeutic trials with vitamins or iron, or watchful waiting. Furthermore, in more than 30 years of use, the test has not moved from the research laboratory into the clinic. The dU suppression test seems unlikely to enjoy more widespread clinical use in the future.

THERAPY, COURSE, AND PROGNOSIS

Treatment consists of parenteral CnCbl (vitamin B_{12}) or OHCbl to replace daily losses and refill storage pools, which normally contain 2 to 5 mg of cobalamin.[346] Toxicity is unusual, although severe hypokalemia leading to cardiac arrhythmias can be seen.[346a,346b] Doses ex-

TABLE 39-6   CORRECTION OF THE DEOXYURIDINE SUPPRESSION TEST IN NUTRITIONAL MEGALOBLASTIC ANEMIA

	CORRECTED BY			
DEFICIENCY	CNCBL	FOLATE	N^5-FORMYL FH_4	N^5-METHYL FH_4
Folate	−	+	+	+
Cobalamin	+	+	+	−

CnCbl, cyanocobalamin (vitamin B_{12}); FH_4, tetrahydrofolic acid.

ceeding 100 μg saturate the TCs, and the excess is lost in the urine. A typical treatment schedule consists of 1000 μg cobalamin IM daily for 2 weeks, then weekly until the hematocrit is normal, and then monthly for life. For neurologic manifestations, 1000 μg every 2 weeks for 6 months is recommended. Higher doses are given for certain inherited disorders (e.g., TCII deficiency). Cobalamin should be given by mouth to patients with dietary cobalamin deficiency and patients (e.g., hemophiliacs) who cannot take IM injections.

Transfusion occasionally is required when the hematocrit is less than 15 percent or the patient is debilitated, infected, or in heart failure. In such instances, packed cells should be given slowly to avoid pulmonary edema. Infections can impair the response to cobalamin and must be treated vigorously.

RESPONSE TO TREATMENT

Following parenteral administration of cobalamin to deficient patients, elevated plasma bilirubin, iron, and LDH levels fall rapidly (Fig. 39-21).[347] Decreasing plasma iron turnover and fecal urobilinogen reflect cessation of ineffective erythropoiesis. Within 12 hours, the marrow begins to change from megaloblastic to normoblastic, a process that is complete in 2 to 3 days. Reticulocytosis begins on days 3 to 5 and peaks on days 4 to 10.[348] The new red cells come from new normoblasts, not from the old megaloblasts, most of which die before leaving the marrow. Blood hemoglobin concentration becomes normal within 1 to 2 months. If normal values are not achieved by 2 months, another cause of anemia should be sought.

Other changes include the following: (1) prompt improvement in the sense of well-being; (2) normalization of leukocyte and platelet counts, although neutrophil hypersegmentation persists for 10 to 14 days; (3) rise in serum cobalamin and folate; and (4) drop in serum potassium.[349] Cobalamin deficiency does not respond to a physiologic dose of folate (100–400 μg/day), although this dose produces a maximal response in folate deficiency. Larger doses of folate (5–15 mg/day) can produce a reticulocytosis and partially correct the anemia in cobalamin deficiency.

SPECIAL CIRCUMSTANCES

After Gastrectomy   Cobalamin should always be given after total gastrectomy. Cobalamin administration is not necessary after partial gastrectomy, but patients need to be watched for megaloblastic anemia, bearing in mind that this anemia can be masked by postgastrectomy iron deficiency.

Blind Loop Syndrome   The anemia of the blind loop syndrome can be treated by parenteral cobalamin therapy. It also responds after approximately 1 week to oral broad-spectrum antibiotics [cephalexin monohydrate (Keflex) 250 mg qid plus metronidazole 250 mg tid for 10 days],[350] and the Schilling test becomes normal. Successful surgical correction of an anatomic lesion cures the syndrome.

Fish Tapeworm   Treatment consists of a single 2 g dose of niclosamide.

USE OF ORAL COBALAMIN

Much interest has been kindled regarding the possibility of treating cobalamin deficiency with oral cobalamin.[351] Oral cobalamin can be used not only for treatment of dietary cobalamin deficiency that occurs in vegans and in patients with very severe general malnutrition but also for patients with food cobalamin malabsorption[352] and for patients with PA, provided the patients are followed carefully.[353] In patients lacking intrinsic factor, approximately 1 percent of an oral dose of the vitamin is forced across the intestinal epithelium by mass action. Therefore, 1000 to 2000 μg/day of oral cobalamin supplies most PA patients with their daily cobalamin requirement without the need for injections and their accompanying pain and expense.

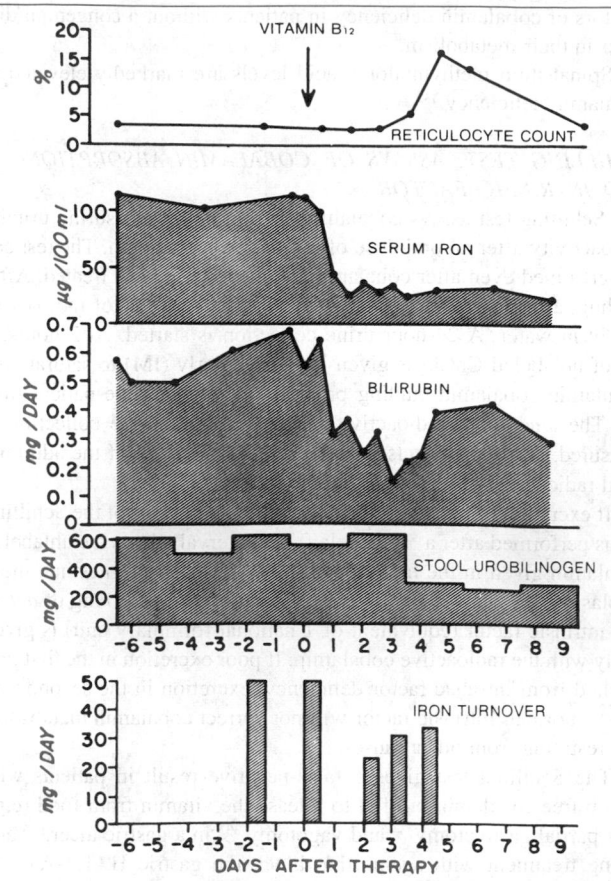

FIGURE 39-21   Effect of cyanocobalamin on reticulocyte count, serum iron, serum bilirubin, stool urobilinogen, and plasma iron turnover. (Adapted from Finch et al.[347])

ACUTE MEGALOBLASTIC ANEMIA

Megaloblastic anemia usually is a chronic condition that requires weeks or months to develop, but a potentially fatal megaloblastic state resulting from acute tissue folate or cobalamin deficiency can arise over the course of only a few days. Patients with acute megaloblastic anemia present with rapidly developing thrombocytopenia and/or leukopenia and counts that sometimes fall to very low levels, but little change in red cell levels unless another cause of anemia is present. The clinical picture can suggest an immune cytopenia. The diagnosis is made from the marrow aspirate, which is floridly megaloblastic, and confirmed by the rapid response to appropriate replacement therapy.

The most common cause of acute megaloblastic anemia is N_2O anesthesia. N_2O rapidly destroys MeCbl,[354] leading quickly to a megaloblastic state. AdoCbl eventually is lost, SAM and total folate levels decline, and the proportion of folate in the form of N^5-methyl FH_4 increases.[355]

Clinical findings develop quickly. Impairment of dU suppression with a cobalamin-deficiency pattern (see Table 39-6) appears after 6 hours of exposure. Grossly megaloblastic changes are seen in the marrow after 12 to 24 hours.[356] Hypersegmented neutrophils do not appear until 5 days after exposure but then persist for several days.[357] Some investigators report that the hematologic effects of N_2O can be prevented by folinic acid (30 mg at surgery and 12 hours later).[358] The effects of N_2O disappear spontaneously after a few days; disappearance can be hastened by folinic acid or cobalamin.[359]

Fatalities resulting from N_2O-induced megaloblastosis have occurred in tetanus patients given N_2O for weeks.[360] Long-term recreational use of N_2O has led to psychosis[361] and to a neurologic disorder similar to combined system disease.[362] Operating room personnel are not at risk for N_2O-induced megaloblastic anemia.[363]

Acute megaloblastic anemia occurs in other clinical settings. A rapidly developing megaloblastic state with acute thrombocytopenia has occurred in seriously ill patients, often in intensive care units.[364] Especially at risk are patients transfused extensively at surgery,[365] those on dialysis or total parenteral nutrition, and those receiving weak folate antagonists such as trimethoprim.[366] Morphologic clues to the diagnosis (e.g., hypersegmented neutrophils) often are absent from the blood film. Both red cell folate and serum cobalamin levels may be normal, but the marrow is always megaloblastic. A rapid response to therapeutic doses of parenteral folate (5 mg/day) and cobalamin (1 mg) is the rule.

MEGALOBLASTIC ANEMIA CAUSED BY DRUGS

Table 39-7 lists the drugs that cause megaloblastic anemia. *Aminopterin* and *methotrexate* are almost structurally identical to folic acid. After they enter cells via the folate carrier[367] and acquire a polyglutamate chain,[368] they act as very powerful inhibitors of dihydrofolate reductase.[369] By blocking the $FH_2 \rightarrow FH_4$ reaction and perhaps inhibiting other enzymes of folate metabolism, they effect the rapid withdrawal of folates from the 1-carbon fragment carrier pool, causing a fall in nucleotide (especially thymidine) biosynthesis that leads to a major derangement in DNA replication (see Chap. 9).[370]

Toxic effects include necrotic mouth lesions; ulcerations of the esophagus, small intestine, and colon, with abdominal pain, vomiting, and diarrhea; megaloblastic anemia; alopecia; and hyperpigmentation. The drug is excreted by the kidney, so effects and toxicity are prolonged and enhanced if renal function is impaired. Toxicity caused by

TABLE 39-7 DRUGS THAT CAUSE MEGALOBLASTIC ANEMIA

AGENTS	COMMENTS	REFERENCE
Antifolates		
Methotrexate	Very potent inhibitor of dihydrofolate reductase	421
Aminopterin	Treat overdose with folinic acid	370
Pyrimethamine	Much weaker than methotrexate and aminopterin	366
Trimethoprim	Treat with folinic acid or by withdrawing the drug	422
Sulfasalazine	Can cause acute megaloblastic anemia in susceptible patients, especially those with low folate stores	423
Chlorguanide (Proguanil)		424
Triamterene		
Pemetrexed (Alimta)	Use of folate and cobalamin during pemetrexed treatment reduces toxicity	
Purine analogues		
6-Mercaptopurine	Megaloblastosis precedes hypoplasia, usually mild	425
6-Thioguanine	Responds to folinic acid but not folate	426
Azathioprine		427
Acyclovir	Megaloblastosis at high doses	428
Pyrimidine analogues		
5-Fluorouracil	Mild megaloblastosis	429
Floxuridine (5-fluorodeoxyuridine)		429
6-Azauridine	Blocks uridine monophosphate production by inhibiting orotidyl decarboxylase; occasional megaloblastosis with orotic acid and orotidine in urine	430
Zidovudine (AZT)	Severe megaloblastic anemia is the major side effect	373
Ribonucleotide reductase inhibitors		
Hydroxyurea	Marked megaloblastosis within 1–2 days of starting therapy; quickly reversed by withdrawing drug	431
Cytarabine (cytosine arabinoside)	Early megaloblastosis is routine	432
Anticonvulsants		
Phenytoin (diphenylhydantoin)	Occasional megaloblastosis, associated with low folate levels; responds to high-dose folate (1–5 mg/day);	433
Phenobarbital	how anticonvulsants cause low folate is not understood, but may be related to a drug-induced rise in	434
Primidone	cytochrome P450	435
Carbamazepine		436
Other drugs that depress folates		
Oral contraceptives	Occasional megaloblastosis; sometimes dysplasia of uterine cervix, corrected with folate	437
Glutethimide		438
Cycloserine		438
H^+/K^+-ATPase inhibitors		
Omeprazole	Long-term use causes decreased serum cobalamin levels	337
Lansoprazole		
Miscellaneous		
N_2O	See "Acute Megaloblastic Anemia"	
p-Aminosalicylic acid	Causes cobalamin malabsorption with occasional mild megaloblastic anemia	438
Metformin		439
Phenformin	Causes cobalamin malabsorption but not anemia	
Colchicine		440
Neomycin		441
Arsenic	Causes myelodysplastic hematopoiesis, sometimes with megaloblastic changes	442

these folate antagonists is treated with folinic acid (N^5-formyl FH$_4$). Folate itself is useless because the blocked reductase cannot convert folate to the active tetrahydro form. Folinic acid is already in the tetrahydro form, so folinic acid is effective despite reductase blockade. The usual dose of folinic acid is 3 to 6 mg/day IM. Larger doses are given in chemotherapy protocols that use folinic acid to rescue patients deliberately treated with otherwise fatal doses of methotrexate. Folinic acid was used intrathecally in a patient in whom a large overdose of methotrexate was accidentally delivered into the subarachnoid space.[371]

Zidovudine (azidothymidine [AZT]) is used for human immunodeficiency virus (HIV) infections (AIDS) (see Chap. 83).[372] Its principal toxic effect is severe megaloblastic anemia. Anemia or neutropenia produced by zidovudine may limit use of this drug.[373]

HIV infection itself suppresses hematopoiesis, leading to pancytopenia with myelodysplastic features (see Chaps. 83 and 86). The blood film shows vacuolated monocytes. Megaloblastosis in HIV infection may result from folate or cobalamin deficiency[374] or AZT or trimethoprim toxicity.

Hydroxyurea is used at high doses to treat chronic myelogenous leukemia, polycythemia vera, and essential thrombocythemia and at lower doses to treat psoriasis (see Chap. 19). It inhibits conversion of ribonucleotides to deoxyribonucleotides.[375] Marked megaloblastic changes are routinely found in the marrow 1 to 2 days after initiating hydroxyurea therapy.[376] These changes are rapidly reversed after the drug is withdrawn. Megaloblastosis as a result of N$_2$O is discussed in "Acute Megaloblastic Anemia" above.

Long-term use of *omeprazole* and presumably other H$^+$/K$^+$-ATPase inhibitors is associated with reduced serum cobalamin levels, presumably because of the ability of these drugs to inhibit parietal cell function.[337] Reduced serum cobalamin levels are not a problem when these drugs are used for short intervals.[377]

Pemetrexed (Alimta; Eli Lilly) is an antifolate approved for use in mesothelioma. It also has been used for treatment of non-small cell lung cancer. Like other antifolate agents, pemetrexed can result in a megaloblastic anemia that is treated with cobalamin and folate.

MEGALOBLASTIC ANEMIA IN CHILDHOOD

MALABSORPTION OF COBALAMIN
Cobalamin malabsorption occurs in five childhood conditions: (1) cobalamin malabsorption in the presence of normal intrinsic factor secretion, (2) congenital abnormality of intrinsic factor, (3) TCII deficiency, (4) congenital R-binder deficiency, and (5) true PA of childhood. The management of cobalamin deficiency in childhood has been thoughtfully reviewed.[378]

Selective Malabsorption of Cobalamin, Imerslund-Gräsbeck Disease Imerslund-Gräsbeck disease[379] is an inherited failure of transport of the intrinsic factor–Cbl complex by the ileum, usually accompanied by proteinuria (mostly albumin).[380] It may be the most common cause of cobalamin deficiency in infancy.[381] Cobalamin deficiency usually is seen before age 2 years but may appear later.[382] Both parts of the Schilling test are abnormal, but intrinsic factor and HCl secretion, TCI and TCII levels, and gastric and intestinal histology are normal. Intrinsic factor antibodies are absent.[383] Intrinsic factor–Cbl receptors are present in some but not all patients.[384] The molecular defect responsible for this disease is unknown.

Patients are treated with IM cobalamin. The anemia is corrected, but proteinuria persists.

Congenital Intrinsic Factor Deficiency Congenital intrinsic factor deficiency is an autosomal recessive disease in which parietal cells fail to produce functionally normal intrinsic factor.[385] Patients present with irritability and megaloblastic anemia when cobalamin stores (<25 μg at birth) are exhausted. The disease usually presents at age

6 to 24 months. HCl secretion and gastric histology are normal, proteinuria is not present, and anti-intrinsic factor antibodies are absent.[382] The abnormal Schilling test is corrected by oral intrinsic factor.[386] Treatment consists of standard doses of IM cobalamin.

Transcobalamin II Deficiency Transcobalamin deficiency[387] is an autosomal recessive disorder causing a flagrant megaloblastic anemia that generally presents in early infancy.[388] The disease is dangerously deceptive because it results from a very severe deficiency of tissue cobalamin, usually with normal serum cobalamin levels. Undiagnosed transcobalamin deficiency causes irreversible central nervous system (CNS) damage.[389] Patients are healthy at birth but over the next few weeks develop signs and symptoms of cobalamin deficiency, such as rapidly progressive pancytopenia, mouth ulcers, vomiting, and diarrhea. Recurrent bacterial infections may occur.[390] Neurologic findings are not prominent in the early stages of the disease.[389]

Serum folate and cobalamin are normal (the latter because most cobalamin is carried by TCI, not TCII). Little homocysteine or methylmalonic acid is found in the urine.[391] The marrow is megaloblastic (a few patients showed severe erythroid hypoplasia[392]). The Schilling test usually[387] but not always[393] is abnormal and is never corrected by intrinsic factor. The diagnosis is made by measuring serum TCII.[394] Prenatal diagnosis may be possible.[395] Serum should be obtained prior to treatment because TCII levels in normal individuals drop sharply after cobalamin is given.[387] TCII deficiency is treated with cobalamin doses sufficiently large to force enough vitamin into the cells to allow normal function. Initial therapy can consist of oral vitamin B$_{12}$ or OHCbl 500 to 1000 μg twice a week, or IM OHCbl 1000 μg/week. Blood counts and symptoms should be monitored and doses adjusted upward if necessary.

R-Binder Deficiency Congenital R-binder deficiency has been reported in six patients.[329] None of the patients clinically manifested cobalamin deficiency, although the patients' serum cobalamin levels were well below normal. R binders were deficient in leukocytes, saliva, and plasma. These patients show that the R binders are not essential for health.

True Juvenile Pernicious Anemia True PA, with gastric atrophy and a defect in intrinsic factor secretion, is exceedingly rare in childhood.[396] Patients usually present in their teens with cobalamin deficiency. Serum anti-intrinsic factor antibodies usually are present.[260] The diagnosis and treatment are the same as for PA in adults.

INBORN ERRORS OF COBALAMIN METABOLISM

Cobalamin is converted to AdoCbl and MeCbl by a complex series of transformations involving several steps.[397] Seven disorders affecting this cobalamin transformation pathway have been described, one for each of the steps. Because the molecular causes of these disorders have not yet been fully characterized, the disorders themselves are not named for a defective protein but instead are designated by letter, as in "cobalamin mutant class 'cobalamin A'" or "CblA." The disorders can be grouped into three clinical syndromes based on the abnormal metabolites in the patient's urine (Table 39-8).

METHYLMALONIC ACIDURIA ONLY (CblA, CblB, AND CblF)
In CblA and CblB,[398] AdoCbl production is impaired[399] but MeCbl production is normal. In CblF, cobalamin export from lysosomes to cytosol is defective. Patients present in infancy with acidosis because they cannot catabolize methylmalonic acid. Symptoms include lethargy and failure to thrive, vomiting, and neurologic problems. Mental retardation is not prominent, and megaloblastic anemia is absent. Most patients respond to 1000 μg/day of OHCbl or CnCbl.[399]

TABLE 39-8 COBALAMIN MUTANT CLASS SYNDROMES

SYNDROME	METHYLMALONIC ACIDURIA	HOMOCYSTINURIA	MEGALOBLASTIC ANEMIA
CblA, CblB, CblF	+	−	−
CblE, CblG	−	+	+
CblC, CblD	+	+	±

HOMOCYSTINURIA ONLY (CblE AND CblG)

In these disorders, N^5-methyltetrahydrofolate-homocysteine methyltransferase can produce methionine but has difficulty making MeCbl.[400] In patients with CblG, methionine synthase is missing or defective.[401] CblE results from failure to reactivate methionine synthase that was inactivated by oxidation of its bound cobalamin.[402] Patients present in infancy with vomiting, mental retardation, and megaloblastic anemia. They respond well to CnCbl 1000 μg/day or 1000 μg/week. Infants diagnosed prenatally and treated from birth usually show normal development.

METHYLMALONIC ACIDURIA AND HOMOCYSTINURIA (CblC AND CblD)

In these disorders, the defect in Cbl transformation affects AdoCbl and MeCbl, probably because reduction of cobalt from Co^{2+} to Co^{1+} is defective.[403] The age at initial presentation ranges from early infancy to adolescence. In addition to lethargy and failure to thrive, affected infants present with serious neurologic difficulties. Older patients present with psychological problems, progressive dementia, and motor signs and symptoms. In one fetus at risk for CblC, the diagnosis was excluded prenatally by chorionic villus sampling.[403] Megaloblastic anemia occurs in about half the cases. Patients respond partially to 1000 μg/day of OHCbl or CnCbl.

A tentative diagnosis of a cobalamin mutation can be made by demonstrating methylmalonic aciduria and/or homocystinuria in a patient with the clinical findings described above in "Methylmalonic Aciduria Only," or "Homocystinuria Only," respectively. Establishing a diagnosis requires a specialized laboratory. In a patient suspected of having a cobalamin mutation, treatment should be started pending the test results because early high-dose cobalamin treatment is risk-free and may reduce the chance of damage to the CNS. Fetuses with these diseases have been successfully treated *in utero* with very large doses of CnCbl given parenterally to the mother.[404]

INBORN ERRORS OF FOLATE METABOLISM

Megaloblastic anemia in infancy has been described in three inherited disorders of folate metabolism.[405]

CONGENTIAL FOLATE MALABSORPTION

Patients cannot absorb folate from the gastrointestinal tract or transport it into the cerebrospinal fluid.[406] Patients present with severe megaloblastic anemia, seizures, mental retardation, and other CNS findings. Folate levels are low in the serum and nil in the cerebrospinal fluid. Folate given parenterally has corrected the anemia and seizures in some patients but has had no effect on other CNS symptoms or on the cerebrospinal fluid folate level.

DIHYDROFOLATE REDUCTASE DEFICIENCY

A patient postulated to have dihydrofolate reductase deficiency presented with isolated megaloblastic anemia at age 6 weeks. His anemia responded to folinic acid but not to folic acid.[407]

N^5-METHYL FH_4–HOMOCYSTEINE METHYLTRANSFERASE DEFICIENCY

Decreased methyltransferase activity was found in a liver biopsy from a child with megaloblastic anemia and mental retardation. The anemia failed to respond to folate, cobalamin, or pyridoxal phosphate.[408]

OTHER INBORN ERRORS

HEREDITARY OROTIC ACIDURIA

Hereditary orotic aciduria is an autosomal recessive disorder of pyrimidine metabolism[409] characterized by megaloblastic anemia, growth impairment, and excretion of orotic acid in the urine. Cobalamin and folate levels are normal.

LESCH-NYHAN SYNDROME

The Lesch-Nyhan syndrome is an X-linked disorder of purine metabolism characterized by hyperuricemia, hyperuricosuria, and a neurologic disease with self-mutilation. It is caused by a hypoxanthine-guanine phosphoribosyltransferase deficiency. One patient had megaloblastic anemia.[410]

THIAMINE-RESPONSIVE MEGALOBLASTIC ANEMIA

Seven children with severe megaloblastic anemia, sensorineural deafness, and diabetes mellitus, all beginning in infancy, have been reported.[411] The anemia responded to thiamine (25–100 mg/day). The marrow was reported as myelodysplastic in two patients with the disorder.[412] The gene for this puzzling disorder has been mapped to the long arm of chromosome 1,[413] but the biochemical defect is completely unknown.

OTHER CAUSES OF MEGALOBLASTIC ANEMIA

CONGENITAL DYSERYTHROPOIETIC ANEMIA

The congenital dyserythropoietic anemias are lifelong anemias. They often are mild, showing dysplastic changes affecting the red cell line only, most typically multinuclearity of the normoblasts. They appear to result from defects in glycosylation of polylactosaminoglycans linked to membrane proteins and ceramides.[414] They present as iron storage disorders. Of the three types, two (type I usually[415] and type III occasionally[416]) show megaloblastic red cell precursors (see Chap. 37).

REFRACTORY MEGALOBLASTIC ANEMIA

Refractory megaloblastic anemia is regarded as a manifestation of myelodysplastic and sideroblastic syndromes (see Chaps. 86 and 58). The megaloblastic changes are atypical. Dysplastic features are confined to the erythroid series. Giant metamyelocytes and bands are absent from the marrow. The combination of a myeloproliferative disorder and true cobalamin deficiency can create a confusing picture.[417] A few patients with refractory megaloblastic anemia respond to pharmacologic doses of pyridoxine (200 mg/day),[418] perhaps because of an effect on serine transformylase, which requires both pyridoxine and folate.

ACUTE MYELOID LEUKEMIA TYPE M6 (ERYTHROLEUKEMIA; DI GUGLIELMO SYNDROME)

Erythroleukemia is the earliest stage of M6 acute myelogenous leukemia (see Chap. 87).[419] Nucleated red cells appear on the blood film, and the marrow shows hyperplasia involving very bizarre-looking megaloblastic red cell precursors, often containing multiple nuclei or nuclear fragments. The disease usually evolves fairly quickly into classic acute myelogenous leukemia.

USE OF HYDROXYCOBALAMIN IN CYANIDE POISONING

The symptoms of cyanide poisoning are quite general: rapidly developing coma, respiratory arrest, and cardiovascular collapse. Severe lactic acidosis (>8 mmol/liter of plasma) is a specific and sensitive indicator of cyanide poisoning, but plasma lactate must be obtained immediately because cyanide kills quickly.

Because cobalamin has such a high affinity for cyanide ($K_d \sim 10^{-13}$ M), it can be used for treatment of cyanide poisoning.[420] For this purpose, OHCbl, *not CnCbl (i.e., not "vitamin B$_{12}$"),* must be used, and it should be given rapidly and as soon as possible. The cyanide in 1 mmol of NaCN (49 mg, a near-lethal to lethal dose) requires approximately 1.5 g of OHCbl for complete neutralization. Other than temporarily turning the skin and urine red, OHCbl is completely harmless, so it can be given in this and even larger doses. It also can be given before the lactate value is available if cyanide poisoning is suspected. Because of the doses required, however, OHCbl use in patients exposed to large amounts of cyanide is impractical. For these patients, OHCbl in maximum doses can be given but must be supplemented with methylene blue and continuous sodium thiosulfate infusions.

REFERENCES

1. Baggott JE, Vaughn WH, Hudson BB: Inhibition of 5-aminoimidazole-4-carboxamide ribotide transformylase, adenosine deaminase and 5'-adenylate deaminase by polyglutamates of methotrexate and oxidized folates and by 5-aminoimidazole-4-carboxamide riboside and ribotide. *Biochem J* 236:193, 1986.
2. Butterworth CE Jr, Santini R Jr, Frommeyer WB Jr: The pteroylglutamate components of American diets as determined by chromatographic fractionation. *J Clin Invest* 42:1929, 1963.
3. Food and Nutrition Board: *National Research Council: Recommended Dietary Allowances.* Washington, 1968.
4. von der Porten AE, Gregory JF III, Toth JP, et al: In vivo folate kinetics during chronic supplementation of human subjects with deuterium-labeled folic acid. *J Nutr* 122:1293, 1992.
5. Herbert V: Minimal daily adult folate requirement. *Arch Intern Med* 110:649, 1962.
6. Halsted CH: Folate deficiency in alcoholism. *Am J Clin Nutr* 33:2736, 1980.
7. Alperin JB, Hutchinson HT, Levin WC: Studies of folic acid requirements in megaloblastic anemia of pregnancy. *Arch Intern Med* 117:681, 1966.
8. Schwarz RH, Johnston RB Jr: Folic acid supplementation: When and now. *Obstet Gynecol* 88:886, 1996.
9. Bird OD, McGlohom VM, Vaitkus JW: Naturally occurring folates in the blood and liver of rats. *Anal Biochem* 12:18, 1965.
10. Ulevitch R, Kallen RG: Purification and characterization of pyridoxal 5'-phosphate dependent serine hydroxymethylase from lamb liver and its action upon b-phenylserines. *Biochemistry* 16:5342, 1977.
11. Johnson FB, Sinclair DA, Guarente L: Molecular biology of aging. *Cell* 96:291, 1999.
12. Tabor H, Wyngaarden L: The enzymatic formation of formiminotetrahydrofolic acid, 5,10-methyltetrahydrofolic acid and 10-formiminohydrofolic acid in the metabolism of formiminoglutamic acid. *J Biol Chem* 234:1830, 1959.
13. Himes RH, Harmony JA: Formyltetrahydrofolate synthetase. *CRC Crit Rev Biochem* 1:501, 1973.
14. Deacon R, Chanarin I, Perry J, Lumb M: Marrow cells from patients with untreated pernicious anaemia cannot use tetrahydrofolate normally. *Br J Haematol* 46:523, 1980.
15. Wahba AJ, Friedkin M: The enzymatic synthesis of thymidylate: I. Early steps in the purification of thymidylate synthetase of *Escherichia coli. J Biol Chem* 237:3794, 1962.
16. Fenech M: The role of folic acid and vitamin B$_{12}$ in genomic stability of human cells. *Mutat Res* 475:57, 2001.
17. Huennekens FM: Folic acid coenzymes in the biosynthesis of purines and pyrimidines. *Vitam Horm* 26:375, 1968.
18. Kaufman S: The phenylalanine hydroxylating system from mammalian liver. *Adv Enzymol* 35:245, 1971.
19. Kwon NS, Nathan CF, Stuehr DJ: Reduced biopterin as a cofactor in the generation of nitrogen oxides by murine macrophages. *J Biol Chem* 264:20496, 1989.
20. Banerjee SP, Snyder SH: Methyltetrahydrofolic acid mediates N- and O-methylation of biogenic amines. *Science* 182:74, 1973.
21. Chanarin I, Perry J, Lumb M: The biochemical lesion in vitamin B$_{12}$ deficiency in man. *Lancet* 1:1251, 1974.
22. Pratt RF, Cooper BA: Folates in plasma and bile in man after feeding folic acid-^{3}H and 5-formyltetrahydrofolate (folinic acid). *J Clin Invest* 50:455, 1971.
23. Kisliuk RL: Pteroylpolyglutamates. *Mol Cell Biochem* 39:331, 1979.
24. Atkinson I, Garrow T, Brenner A, Shane B: Human cytosolic folylpoly-gamma-glutamate synthase. *Methods Enzymol* 281:134, 1997.
25. Sussman DJ, Milman G, Shane B: Characterization of human folylpolyglutamate synthetase expressed in chinese hamster ovary cells. *Somatic Cell Mol Genet* 12:531, 1986.
26. Cook JD, Cichowicz DJ, George S, et al: Mammalian folylpoly-γ-glutamate synthetase: IV. In vitro and in vivo metabolism of folates and analogues and regulation of folate homeostasis. *Biochemistry* 26:530, 1987.
27. Siddarth R, Beck WS: Evidence that folylpolyglutamate synthetase is under regulatory control. *Clin Res* 29:552A, 1981.
28. Shane B, Stokstad EL: Vitamin B$_{12}$-folate interrelationships. *Annu Rev Nutr* 5:115, 1985.
29. Coward JK, Chello PL, Cashmore AR, et al: 5-Methyl-5,6,7,8-tetrahydropteroliogo-γ-L-glutamates: Synthesis and kinetic studies with methionine synthetase from bovine brain. *Biochemistry* 14:1548, 1975.
30. Butterworth CE Jr, Baught CM, Krumdieck C: A study of folate absorption and metabolism in man utilizing carbon-14-labeled polyglutamates synthesized by the solid phase method. *J Clin Invest* 48:1131, 1969.
31. Rosenberg IH, Godwin HA: The digestion and absorption of dietary folate. *Gastroenterology* 60:445, 1999.
32. Kesavan V, Noronha JM: Folate malabsorption in aged rats related to low levels of pancreatic folyl conjugase. *Am J Clin Nutr* 37:262, 1983.
33. Chandler CJ, Wang TTY, Halsted CH: Pteroylpolyglutamate hydrolase from human jejunal brush borders: Purification and characterization. *J Biol Chem* 261:928, 1986.
34. Wolff R, Drouet PL, Karlin R: Recherches sur la vitamin-B$_c$-conjugase: Action de quelques effecteurs sur l'activité conjugasique du plasma. *Bull Soc Chim Biol* 31:1439, 1949.
35. Elsenhans B, Ahmad O, Rosenberg IH: Isolation and characterization of pteroylpolyglutamate hydrolase from rat intestinal mucosa. *J Biol Chem* 259:6364, 1984.
36. Cohen N: Differential microbiological assay in study of folic acid absorption in vitro by everted intestinal sacs. *Clin Res* 13:252, 1965.
37. Schron CM: PH Modulation of the kinetics of rabbit jejunal, brush-border folate transport. *J Membr Biol* 120:192, 1991.
38. Schron CM, Washington C, Jr, Blitzer BL: The transmembrane pH gradient drives uphill folate transport in rabbit jejunum: Direct evidence for folate/hydroxyl exchange in brush border membrane vesicles. *J Clin Invest* 76:2030, 1985.
39. Zimmerman J, Selhub J, Rosenberg IH: Role of sodium ion in transport of folic acid in the small intestine. *Am J Physiol* 251:G218, 1986.
40. Perry J, Chanarin I: Intestinal absorption of reduced folate compounds in man. *Br J Haematol* 18:329, 1970.
41. Herbert V: Excretion of folic acid in bile. *Lancet* 1:913, 1965.

42. Steinberg SE, Campbell CL, Hillman RS: Kinetics of the normal folate enterohepatic cycle. *J Clin Invest* 64:83, 1979.

43. Steinberg SE: Mechanisms of folate homeostasis. *Am J Physiol* 246: G319, 1984.

44. Henderson GB: Folate-binding proteins. *Annu Rev Nutr* 10:319, 1990.

45. Johns DG, Sperti S, Burgen ASV: The metabolism of tritiated folic acid in man. *J Clin Invest* 40:1684, 1961.

46. Antony AC: The biological chemistry of folate receptors. *Blood* 79: 2807, 1992.

47. Weitman SD, Weinberg AG, Coney LR, et al: Cellular localization of the folate receptor: Potential role in drug toxicity and folate homeostasis. *Cancer Res* 52:6708, 1992.

48. Luhrs CA, Slomiany BL: A human membrane-associated folate binding protein is anchored by a glycosyl-phosphatidylinositol tail. *J Biol Chem* 264:21446, 1989.

49. Green T, Ford HC: Human placental microvilli contain high-affinity binding sites for folate. *Biochem J* 218:75, 1984.

50. Rothberg KG, Ying Y, Kolhouse JF, et al: The glycophospholipid-linked folate receptor internalizes folate without entering the clathrin-coated pit endocytic pathway. *J Cell Biol* 110:637, 1990.

51. Matsue H, Rothberg KG, Takashima A, et al: Folate receptor allows cells to grow in low concentrations of 5-methyltetrahydrofolate. *Proc Natl Acad Sci U S A* 89:6006, 1992.

52. Hilton JG, Cooper BA, Rosenblatt DS: Folate glutamate synthesis and turnover in cultured human fibroblasts. *J Biol Chem* 254:8498, 1979.

53. Zamierowski MM, Wagner C: High molecular weight complexes of folic acid in mammalian tissues. *Biochem Biophys Res Commun* 60:81, 1974.

54. Duch DS, Bowers SW, Nichols CA: Analysis of folate cofactor levels in tissues using high-performance liquid chromatography. *Anal Biochem* 130:385, 1983.

55. Cook RJ, Wagner C: Glycine N-methyltransferase is a folate binding protein of rat liver cytosol. *Proc Natl Acad Sci U S A* 81:3631, 1984.

56. Rosenblatt DS, Cooper BA, Lue-Shing S, et al: Folate distribution in cultured human cells: Studies on 5,10-CH$_2$-H$_4$ Pte Glu reductase deficiency. *J Clin Invest* 63:1019, 1979.

57. Chanarin I, Hutchinson M, McLean A, Moule M: Hepatic folate in man. *Br Med J* 1:396, 1966.

58. Stites TE, Bailey LB, Scott KC, et al: Kinetic modeling of folate metabolism through use of chronic administration of deuterium-labeled folic acid in men. *Am J Clin Nutr* 65:53, 1997.

59. Elwood PC, Deutsch JC, Kolhouse JF: The conversion of the human membrane-associated folate binding protein (folate receptor) to the soluble folate binding protein by a membrane-associated metalloprotease. *J Biol Chem* 266:2346, 1991.

60. Colman N, Herbert V: Total folate binding capacity of normal human plasma and variations in uremia, cirrhosis, and pregnancy. *Blood* 48: 911, 1976.

61. Waxman S: Folate binding proteins. *Br J Haematol* 29:23, 1975.

62. Waxman S, Schreiber C: Measurement of serum folate binding factor in some leukemic cells. *Blood* 42:281, 1973.

63. Colman N, Herbert V: Folate-binding proteins. *Annu Rev Med* 31:433, 1980.

64. Waxman S, Schreiber C: Characteristics of folate acid-binding protein in folate deficient serum. *Blood* 42:291, 1973.

65. Rothenberg SP: A macromolecular factor in some leukemic cells which binds folic acid. *Proc Soc Exp Biol Med* 133:428, 1970.

66. Mason JB, Selhub J: Folate binding protein and the absorption of folic acid in the small intestine of the suckling rat. *Am J Clin Nutr* 48:620, 1988.

67. Rubinoff M, Abramson R, Schreiber C, Waxman S: Effect of a folate-binding protein on the plasma transport and tissue distribution of folic acid. *Acta Haematol (Basel)* 65:145, 1981.

68. Colman N, Herbert V: Studies using the calcium ionophore A23187 suggest localization of the human granulocyte folate binder in specific (secondary) granules. *Clin Res* 27:291A, 1979.

69. Selhub J, Emmanouel D, Stavropoulos T, Arnold R: Renal folate absorption and the kidney folate binding protein: I. Urinary clearance studies. *Am J Physiol* 252:F750, 1987.

70. Williams WM, Huang KC: Renal tubular transport of folic acid and methotrexate in the monkey. *Am J Physiol* 242:F484, 1982.

71. O'Brien JS: Urinary excretion of folic acid and folinic acids in normal adults. *Proc Soc Exp Biol Med* 104:354, 1960.

72. McLean A, Chanarin I: Urinary excretion of 5-methyltetrahydro-folate in man. *Blood* 27:386, 1966.

73. Blount BC, Mack MM, Wehr CM, et al: Folate deficiency causes uracil misincorporation into human DNA and chromosome breakage: Implications for cancer and neuronal damage. *Proc Natl Acad Sci U S A* 94: 3290, 1997.

74. Lenhert PG, Hodgkin DC: Structure of the 5,6-dimethyl-benzimidazo-lylcobamide coenzyme. *Nature* 192:937, 1961.

75. Stahlberg KG: Studies on methyl-B$_{12}$ in man. *Scand J Haemat* 4(suppl 1):1, 1967.

76. Heyssel RM, Bozian RC, Darby WC, Bell MC: Vitamin B$_{12}$ turnover in man: The assimilation of vitamin B$_{12}$ from natural foodstuff by man and estimates of minimal daily dietary requirements. *Am J Clin Nutr* 18:176, 1966.

77. Gräsbeck R: Calculations on vitamin B$_{12}$ turnover in man. *Scand J Clin Lab Invest* 11:250, 1959.

78. Hsu JM, Kawin B, Minor P, Mitchell JA: Vitamin B$_{12}$ concentrations in human tissues. *Nature* 210:1264, 1966.

79. Poston JM: Cobalamin-dependent formation of leucine and b-leucine by rat and human tissue. Changes in pernicious anemia. *J Biol Chem* 255: 10067, 1980.

80. Stabler SP, Lindenbaum J, Allen RH: Failure to detect beta-leucine in human blood or leucine 2,3-aminomutase in rat liver using capillary gas chromatography-mass spectrometry. *J Biol Chem* 263:5581, 1988.

81. Nham SU, Wilkemeyer MF, Ledley FD: Structure of the human methylmalonyl-CoA mutase (MUT) locus. *Genomics* 8:710, 1990.

82. Beck WS, Flavin M, Ochoa S: Metabolism of propionic acid in animal tissues: III. Formation of succinate. *J Biol Chem* 229:997, 1957.

83. Peytremann R, Thorndike J, Beck WS: Studies on N^5-methyltetrahydro-folate-homocysteine methyltransferase in normal and leukemic leukocytes. *J Clin Invest* 56:1293, 1975.

84. Taylor RT, Weissbach H: Enzymatic synthesis of methionine: Formation of a radioactive cobamide enzyme with N^5-methyl-^{14}C-tetrahydrofolate. *Arch Biochem Biophys* 119:572, 1967.

85. Banks RGS, Henderson RJ, Pratt JM: Reactions of gases in solution: III. Some reactions of nitrous oxide with transition-metal complexes. *J Chem Soc* (A):2886, 1968.

86. Chanarin I: Cobalamins and nitrous oxide: A review. *J Clin Pathol* 33: 909, 1980.

87. Sunder-Plassmann G, Fodinger M: Genetic determinants of the homocysteine level. *Kidney Int Suppl* S141, 2003.

88. Matthews DM, Wilson J: Cobalamins and cyanide metabolism in neurological diseases, in *The Cobalamins: A Glaxo symposium*, edited by HRV Arnstein, RJ Wrighton, p 115. Williams & Wilkins, Baltimore, 1971.

89. Knowles JP, Prankerd TA: Abnormal folic acid metabolism in vitamin B$_{12}$ deficiency. *Clin Sci* 22:233, 1962.

90. Herbert V, Zalusky R: Interrelations of vitamin B$_{12}$ and folic acid metabolism: Folic acid clearance studies. *J Clin Invest* 41:1263, 1962.

91. Kano Y, Sakamoto S, Hida K, et al: 5-Methyltetrahydrofolate related enzymes and DNA polymerase a activities in bone marrow cells from patients with vitamin B$_{12}$ deficient megaloblastic anemia. *Blood* 59:832, 1982.

92. Waters AH, Mollin DL: Observations on the metabolism of folic acid in pernicious anaemia. *Br J Haematol* 9:319, 1963.

93. Wilson SD, Horne DW: Effect of nitrous oxide inactivation of vitamin B_{12} on the levels of folate coenzymes in rat bone marrow, kidney, brain, and liver. *Arch Biochem Biophys* 244:248, 1986.

94. Smith RM, Osborne-White WS: Folic acid metabolism in vitamin B_{12}-deficient sheep: Depletion of liver folates. *Biochem J* 136:279, 1973.

95. Jeejeebhoy KN, Pathare SM, Noronha JM: Observations on conjugated and unconjugated blood folate levels in megaloblastic anemia and the effects of vitamin B_{12}. *Blood* 26:354, 1965.

96. Boss GR: Cobalamin inactivation decreases purine and methionine synthesis in cultured lymphoblasts. *J Clin Invest* 76:213, 1985.

97. Chanarin I: The methyl-folate trap and the supply of S-adenosylmethionine. *Lancet* 2:755, 1965.

98. Taylor RT, Hanna ML: 5-Methyltetrahydrofolate aromatic alkylamine N-methyltransferase: An artefact of 5,10-methylene-tetrahydrofolate reductase activity. *Life Sci* 17:111, 1975.

99. Katzen HM, Buchanan JM: Enzymatic synthesis of the methyl group of methionine: VIII. Repression-derepression, purification and properties of 5,10-methylenetetrahydrofolate reductase from *E. coli*. *J Biol Chem* 240:825, 1980.

100. Chanarin I, Deacon R, Lumb M, Perry J: Vitamin B_{12} regulates folate metabolism by the supply of formate. *Lancet* 2:505, 1980.

101. Taheri MR, Wickremasinghe RG, Jackson BF, Hoffbrand AV: The effect of folate analogues and vitamin B_{12} on provision of thymine nucleotides for DNA synthesis in megaloblastic anemia. *Blood* 59:634, 1982.

102. Chanarin I, Deacon R, Lumb M, et al: Cobalamin and folate: Recent developments. *J Clin Pathol* 45:277, 1992.

103. Perry J, Chanarin I, Deacon R, Lumb M: The substrate for folate polyglutamate biosynthesis in the vitamin B_{12}-inactivated rat. *Biochem Biophys Res Commun* 91:678, 1979.

104. Hewitt JE, Gordon MM, Taggart RT, et al: Human gastric intrinsic factor: Characterization of cDNA and genomic clones and localization to human chromosome 11. *Genomics* 10:432, 1991.

105. Tang LH, Chokshi H, Hu CB, et al: The intrinsic factor (IF)-cobalamin receptor binding site is located in the amino-terminal portion of IF. *J Biol Chem* 267:22982, 1992.

106. Visuri K, Gräsbeck R: Human intrinsic factor: Isolation by improved conventional methods and properties of the preparation. *Biochim Biophys Acta* 303:319, 1973.

107. Levine JS, Nakane PK, Allen RH: Immunocytochemical localization of human intrinsic factor: The nonstimulated stomach. *Gastroenterology* 79:493, 1980.

108. Deller DJ, Germar H, Witts LJ: Effect of food on absorption of radioactive vitamin B_{12}. *Lancet* 1:574, 1961.

109. Meikle DD, Bull J, Callendar ST, Truelove SC: Intrinsic factor secretion after vagotomy. *Br J Surg* 96:795, 1977.

110. Lawrie JH, Anderson NM: Secretion of gastric intrinsic factor. *Lancet* 1:68, 1967.

111. Stenman UH: Vitamin B_{12}-binding proteins of R-type cobalophilin: Characterization and comparison of cobalophilin from different sources. *Scand J Haematol* 14:91, 1975.

112. Cooper BA, Castle WB: Sequential mechanisms in the enhanced absorption of vitamin B_{12} by intrinsic factor in the rat. *J Clin Invest* 39:199, 1966.

113. Allen RH, Seetharam B, Podell ER, Alpers DH: Effect of proteolytic enzymes on the binding of cobalamin to R protein and intrinsic factor: In vitro evidence that a failure to partially degrade R protein is responsible for cobalamin malabsorption in pancreatic insufficiency. *J Clin Invest* 61:47, 1978.

114. Abels J, Schilling RF: Protection of intrinsic factor by vitamin B_{12}. *J Lab Clin Med* 64:375, 1964.

115. Titenko-Holland N, Jacob RA, Shang N, et al: Micronuclei in lymphocytes and exfoliated buccal cells of postmenopausal women with dietary changes in folate. *Mutat Res* 417:101, 1998.

116. Levine JS, Allen RH, Alpers DH: Immunocytochemical localization of the intrinsic factor-cobalamin receptor in dog ileum: Distribution of intracellular receptor during cell maturation. *J Cell Biol* 98:1111, 1984.

117. Seetharam S, Ramanujam KS, Seetharam B: Synthesis and brush border expression of intrinsic factor-cobalamin receptor from rat renal cortex. *J Biol Chem* 267:7421, 1992.

118. Hagedorn CH, Alpers DH: Distribution of intrinsic factor-vitamin B_{12} receptors inhuman intestine. *Gastroenterology* 73:1019, 1977.

119. Kapadia CR, Serfilippi D, Voloshin K, Donaldson RM Jr: Intrinsic factor-mediated absorption of cobalamin by guinea pig ileal cells. *J Clin Invest* 71:440, 1983.

120. Robertson JA, Gallagher MD: In vivo evidence that cobalamin is absorbed by receptor-mediated endocytosis in the mouse. *Gastroenterology* 88:908, 1985.

121. Horadagoda NU, Batt RM: Lysosomal localization of cobalamin during absorption by the ileum of the dog. *Biochim Biophys Acta* 838:206, 1985.

122. Rothenberg SP, Weisberg H, Ficarra A: Evidence for the absorption of immunoreactive intrinsic factor into the intestinal epithelial cell during vitamin B_{12} absorption. *J Lab Clin Med* 79:578, 1972.

123. Hall CA: Transcobalamins I and II as natural transport proteins of vitamin B_{12}. *J Clin Invest* 56:1125, 1975.

124. Savage CR, Green PD: Biosynthesis of transcobalamin II by adult rat liver parenchymal cells in culture. *Arch Biochem Biophys* 173:691, 1976.

125. Gräsbeck R, Nyberg W, Reizenstein P: Biliary and fecal vitamin B_{12} excretion in man: An isotope study. *Proc Soc Exp Biol Med* 97:780, 1958.

126. Booth MA, Spray GH: Vitamin B_{12} activity in the serum and liver of rats after total gastrectomy. *Br J Haematol* 6:288, 1960.

127. Antony AC: Vegetarianism and vitamin B_{12} (cobalamin) deficiency. *Am J Clin Nutr* 78:3, 2003.

128. Dorscherholmen A, Hagen PS, Liu M: A dual mechanism of vitamin B_{12} plasma absorption. *J Clin Invest* 36:1551, 1957.

129. Seetharam B, Alpers DH: Cellular uptake of cobalamin. *Nutr Rev* 43:97, 1985.

130. Seetharam S, Dahms N, Li N, Seetharam B: Functional expression of transcobalamin II cDNA in Xenopus laevis oocytes. *Biochem Biophys Res Commun* 181:1151, 1991.

131. Hippe E, Olesen H: Nature of vitamin B_{12} binding: III. Thermodynamics of binding to human intrinsic factor and transcobalamins. *Biochim Biophys Acta* 243:83, 1999.

132. Kolhouse JF, Allen RH: Absorption, plasma transport and cellular retention of cobalamin analogues in the rabbit. *J Clin Invest* 60:1381, 1977.

133. Donaldson RM, Brand M, Serfilippi D: Changes in circulating transcobalamin II after injection of cyanocobalamin. *N Engl J Med* 296:1427, 1977.

134. Schneider RJ, Burger RL, Hehlman CS, Allen RH: The role and fate of rabbit and human transcobalamin II in the plasma transport of vitamin B_{12} in the rabbit. *J Clin Invest* 57:27, 1978.

135. Youngdahl-Turner P, Rosenberg LE, Allen RH: Binding and uptake of transcobalamin II by human fibroblasts. *J Clin Invest* 61:133, 1978.

136. Pletsch QA, Coffey JW: Properties of the proteins that bind vitamin B_{12} in subcellular fractions of rat liver. *Arch Biochem Biophys* 151:157, 1972.

137. Idriss J-M, Jonas AJ: Vitamin B_{12} transport by rat liver lysosomal membrane vesicles. *J Biol Chem* 266:9438, 1991.

138. Watanabe F, Nakano Y: Comparative biochemistry of vitamin B_{12} (cobalamin) metabolism: Biochemistry diversity in the systems for intra-

cellular cobalamin transfer and synthesis of the coenzymes. *Int J Biochem* 23:1353, 1991.

139. Watanabe F, Nakano Y, Saido H, et al: NADPH-cytochrome c (P 450) reductase has the activity of NADPH-linked aquacobalamin reductase in rat liver microsomes. *Biochim Biophys Acta* 119:175, 1992.

140. Watanabe F, Nakano Y, Saido H, et al: Cytochrome b_5/cytochrome b_5 reductase complex in rat liver microsomes has NADH-linked aquacobalamin reductase activity. *J Nutr* 122:940, 1992.

141. Van Scott EJ, Auerback R, Weinstein GD: Parental methotrexate in psoriasis. *Arch Dermatol* 89:550, 1964.

142. Boddington MM, Spriggs AI: The epithelial cells in megaloblastic anaemias. *J Clin Pathol* 12:228, 1969.

143. Burger RL, Allen RH: Characterization of vitamin B_{12}-binding proteins isolated from human milk and saliva by affinity chromatography. *J Biol Chem* 249:7220, 1974.

144. Hurlimann J, Zuber C: Vitamin B_{12} binders in human body fluids: II. Synthesis in vitro. *Clin Exp Immunol* 4:141, 1974.

145. Simons K, Weber T: The vitamin B_{12} binding protein in human leukocytes. *Biochim Biophys Acta* 117:201, 1966.

146. Johnston J, Bollekens J, Allen RH, Berliner N: Structure of the cDNA encoding transcobalamin I, a neutrophil granule protein. *J Biol Chem* 264:15754, 1989.

147. Johnston J, Yang-Feng T, Berliner N: Genomic structure and mapping of the chromosomal gene for transcobalamin I (TCN1): Comparison to human intrinsic factor. *Genomics* 12:459, 1992.

148. Burger RL, Schneider RJ, Mehlman CS, Allen RH: Human plasma R-type vitamin B_{12}-binding proteins: II. The role of transcobalamin I, transcobalamin III, and the normal granulocyte vitamin B12-binding protein in the plasma transport of vitamin B_{12}. *J Biol Chem* 250:7707, 1975.

149. Gueant JL, Monin B, Boissel P, et al: Biliary excretion of cobalamin and cobalamin analogues in man. *Digestion* 30:151, 1984.

150. Gottlieb C, Retief FP, Herbert V: Blockage of vitamin B_{12}-binding sites in the gastric juice, serum and saliva by analogues and derivatives of vitamin B_{12} and by antibody to intrinsic factor. *Biochim Biophys Acta* 141:560, 1967.

151. Allen RH: Human vitamin B_{12} transport proteins. *Prog Hematol* 9:57, 1975.

152. Retief FP, Gottlieb CW, Herbert V: Delivery of Co^{57} B_{12} by human and mouse tumour cells. *Nature* 191:393, 1961.

153. Carmel R: Vitamin B_{12} binding abnormality in subjects without myeloproliferative disease: I. Elevated serum vitamin B_{12} binding capacity in patients with leucocytosis. *Br J Haematol* 22:43, 1972.

154. Stenman UH, Simons K, Gräsbeck R: Vitamin B_{12} binding proteins in normal and leukemic leukocytes and sera. *Scand J Clin Invest* 21(suppl 101):103, 1974.

155. Carmel R, Herbert V: Vitamin B_{12}-binding protein of leukocytes as a possible major source of the third vitamin B_{12}-binding protein of serum. *Blood* 40:452, 1972.

156. Kelly A, Herbert V: Coated charcoal assay of erythrocyte vitamin B_{12}. *Blood* 29:139, 1967.

157. Kolhouse JF, Kondo H, Allen NC, et al: Cobalamin analogues are present in human plasma and can mask cobalamin deficiency because current radioisotope dilution assays are not specific for true cobalamin. *N Engl J Med* 299:785, 1978.

158. Kondo H, Kolhouse JF, Allen RH: Presence of cobalamin analogues in animal tissues. *Proc Natl Acad Sci U S A* 77:817, 1980.

159. Hom BL: Plasma turnover of ^{57}cobalt-vitamin B_{12} bound to transcobalamin I and II. *Scand J Haematol* 4:321, 1967.

160. Hom BL, Ahluwalia BK: The vitamin B_{12} binding capacity of transcobalamin I and II on normal serum. *Scand J Haematol* 5:64, 1967.

161. Carmel R: The distribution of endogenous cobalamin among cobalamin-binding proteins in the blood of normal and abnormal states. *Am J Clin Nutr* 41:713, 1985.

162. Bertaux O, Mederic C, Valencia R: Amplification of ribosomal DNA in the nucleolus of vitamin B_{12}-deficient Euglena cells. *Exp Cell Res* 195:119, 1991.

163. Rondanelli EG, Gorini P, Magliulo E, Fiori GP: Differences in proliferative activity between normoblasts and pernicious anemia megaloblasts. *Blood* 24:542, 1964.

164. Steinberg SE, Fonda S, Campbell CL, Hillman RS: Cellular abnormalities of folate deficiency. *Br J Haematol* 54:605, 1983.

165. Wickremasinghe RG, Hoffbrand AV: Reduce rate of DNA replication fork movement in megaloblastic anemia. *J Clin Invest* 65:26, 1980.

166. Duthie SJ, McMillan P: Uracil misincorporation in human DNA detected using single cell gel electrophoresis. *Carcinogenesis* 18:1709, 1997.

167. Das KC, Mohanty D, Garewell G: Cytogenetics in nutritional megaloblastic anaemia: Prolonged persistence of chromosomal abnormalities in lymphocytes after remission. *Acta Haematol (Basel)* 76:146, 1986.

168. Forni M, Meyer PR, Levy NB, et al: An immunohistochemical study of hemoglobin A, hemoglobin F, muramidase, and transferrin in erythroid hyperplasia and neoplasia. *J Clin Pathol* 80:145, 1983.

169. Ellims PH, Hayman RJ, Van Der Weyden MB: Plasma thymidine kinase in megaloblastic anemia. *Br J Haematol* 44:167, 1980.

170. Reid CD, Baptista LC, Deacon R, Chanarin I: Megaloblastic change is a feature of colonies derived from an early erythroid progenitor (BFU-E) stimulated by monocytes in culture. *Br J Haematol* 49:551, 1981.

171. Spivak JL: Masked megaloblastic anemia. *Arch Intern Med* 142:2111, 1982.

172. Lindenbaum J, Nath BJ: Megaloblastic anaemia and neutrophil hypersegmentation. *Br J Haematol* 44:511, 1980.

173. Herbert V: Experimental nutritional folate deficiency in man. *Trans Assoc Am Physicians* 75:307, 1962.

174. Savage D, Lindenbaum J: Anemia in alcoholics. *Medicine (Baltimore)* 65:322, 1986.

175. Lawler SD, Roberts PD, Hoffbrand AV: Chromosome studies in megaloblastic anemia before and after treatment. *Scand J Haematol* 8:309, 1971.

176. Bessman JD, Williams LJ, Gilmer PR: Platelet size in health and hematologic disease. *Am J Clin Pathol* 78:150, 1982.

177. Liu YK, Sullivan LW: Marrow granulocyte reserve in pernicious anemia. *Clin Res* 14:321, 1966.

178. Sue-A-Quan AK, Fialkow L, Vlahos CJ, et al: Inhibition of neutrophil oxidative burst and granule secretion by Wortmannin: Potential role of MAP kinase and renaturable kinases. *J Cell Physiol* 172:94, 1997.

179. Fudenberg H, Estren S: The intermediate megaloblasts in the differential diagnosis of pernicious and related anemias. *Am J Med* 25:198, 1958.

180. Green R, Kuhl W, Jacobson R, et al: Masking of macrocytosis by alpha-globin chain deletions in Blacks with pernicious anemia. *N Engl J Med* 307:1322, 1982.

181. Gulley ML, Bentley SA, Ross DW: Neutrophil myeloperoxidase measurement uncovers masked megaloblastic anemia. *Blood* 76:1004, 1990.

182. Marshall RA, Jandl HH: Responses to "physiologic" doses of folic acid in the megaloblastic anemias. *Arch Intern Med* 105:353, 1960.

183. Hussein S, Laulicht M, Hoffbrand AV: Serum ferritin in megaloblastic anemia. *Scand J Haematol* 20:241, 1978.

184. Emerson PM, Wilkinson JH: Lactate dehydrogenase in the diagnosis and assessment of response to treatment of megaloblastic anemia. *Br J Haematol* 12:678, 1966.

185. Winston RM, Warburton FG, Scott A: Enzymatic diagnosis of megaloblastic anaemia. *Br J Haematol* 19:587, 1970.

186. Hansen NE, Karle H: Blood and bone marrow lysozyme in neutropenia: An attempt towards pathogenetic classification. *Br J Haematol* 21:261, 1971.

187. Heller P, Weinstein HG, West M, Zimmerman HJ: Glycolytic, citric acid cycle, and hexose monophosphate shunt enzymes of plasma in megaloblastic anemia. *J Lab Clin Med* 55:425, 1960.

188. De Klerk G, Rosengarten PC, Vet RJ, Goudsmit R: Serum erythropoietin (EST) titers in anemia. *Blood* 58:1164, 1981.

189. Myhre E: Studies on the erythrokinetics in pernicious anemia. *Scand J Clin Lab Invest* 16:391, 1964.

190. Heller P, Weinstein HG, Zimmerman HJ: Enzymes in anemia: A study of abnormalities of several enzymes of carbohydrate metabolism in the plasma and erythrocytes in patients with anemia, with preliminary observations of bone marrow enzymes. *Ann Intern Med* 53:898, 1960.

191. Lindahl J: Quantification of ineffective erythropoiesis in megaloblastic anaemia by determination of endogenous production of ^{14}CO after administration of glycine-2-^{14}C. *Scand J Haematol* 24:281, 1980.

192. Hamilton HE, Sheets RF, DeGowin EL: Studies with inagglutinable erythrocyte counts: VII. Further investigation of the hemolytic mechanism in untreated pernicious anemia and the demonstration of a hemolytic property in the plasma. *J Lab Clin Med* 51:942, 1958.

193. Harker LA, Finch CA: Thrombokinetics in man. *J Clin Invest* 48:963, 1969.

194. Aikawa R, Komuro I, Yamazaki T, et al: Oxidative stress activates extracellular signal-regulated kinases through Src and Ras in cultured cardiac myocytes of neonatal rats. *J Clin Invest* 100:1813, 1997.

195. Ballard HS, Lindenbaum J: Megaloblastic anemia complicating hyperalimentation therapy. *Am J Med* 56:740, 1974.

196. Whitehead VM, Comty CH, Posen GA, Kay M: Homeostasis of folic acid in patients undergoing maintenance hemodialysis. *N Engl J Med* 279:970, 1968.

197. Mollin DL, Hines JD: Observations on the nature and pathogenesis of anemia following partial gastrectomy. *Proc R Soc Med* 57:575, 1964.

198. Hoffbrand AV: Folate deficiency in premature infants. *Arch Dis Child* 45:441, 1970.

199. Royston NJW, Parry TE: Megaloblastic anaemia complicating dietary treatment of phenylketonuria in infancy. *Arch Dis Child* 37:430, 1962.

200. Ford JD, Scott KJ: The folic acid activity of some milk foods for babies. *J Dairy Res* 35:85, 1968.

201. Eichner ER, Hillman RS: Effect of alcohol on serum folate level. *J Clin Invest* 52:584, 1973.

202. Lieber CS: Metabolism and metabolic effects of alcohol. *Semin Hematol* 17:85, 1980.

203. Post RM, Desforges JF: Thrombocytopenia and alcoholism. *Ann Intern Med* 68:1230, 1963.

204. Liu YK: Effects of alcohol on granulocyte and lymphocytes. *Semin Hematol* 17:130, 1980.

205. Lindenbaum J, Lieber CS: Hematological effects of alcohol in man in the absence of nutritional deficiency. *N Engl J Med* 281:333, 1969.

206. Trier JS: Celiac sprue. *N Engl J Med* 325:1709, 1991.

207. Halsted CH, Reisenauer AM, Romero JJ, et al: Jejunal perfusion of simple and conjugated folates in celiac sprue. *J Clin Invest* 59:933, 1977.

208. Hjelt K, Krasilnikoff PA: The impact of gluten on haematological status, dietary intakes of haemopoietic nutrients and vitamin B_{12} and folic acid absorption in children with coeliac disease. *Acta Paediatr Scand* 79:911, 1990.

209. Klipstein FA: Tropical sprue in New York City. *Gastroenterology* 47:457, 1964.

210. Klipstein FA, Schenck EA, Samloff IM: Folate repletion associated with oral tetracycline therapy in tropical sprue. *Gastroenterology* 51:317, 1966.

211. Klipstein FA: Progress in gastroenterology: Tropical sprue. *Gastroenterology* 54:275, 1968.

212. Sheehy TW, Perez-Santiago E, Rubini ME: Tropical sprue and vitamin B_{12}. *N Engl J Med* 265:1232, 1961.

213. Klipstein FA: Folate in tropical sprue. *Br J Haematol* 23:119, 1972.

214. Corcino JJ, Coll G, Klipstein FA: Pteroylglutamic acid malabsorption in tropical sprue. *Blood* 45:577, 1975.

215. Chanarin I, Bennett MC: Absorption of folic acid and D-xylose as tests of small intestinal function. *Br Med J* 1:985, 1962.

216. Booth CC: Metabolic effects of intestinal resection in man. *Postgrad Med J* 37:725, 1961.

217. Pitney WR, Joske RA, Mackinnon NL: Folic acid and other absorption tests in lymphosarcoma, chronic lymphocytic leukemia and some related conditions. *J Clin Pathol* 13:440, 1960.

218. Hoskins LC, Norris TH, Gottlieb LS, Zamcheck N: Functional and morphologic alterations of the gastrointestinal tract in progressive systemic sclerosis (scleroderma). *Am J Med* 33:459, 1962.

219. Vinnik IE, Kern F, Struthers JE: Malabsorption and the diarrhea of diabetes mellitus. *Gastroenterology* 43:507, 1962.

220. Cook GC, Morgan JO, Hoffbrand AV: Impairment of folate absorption by systemic bacterial infections. *Lancet* 2:1417, 1974.

221. Shojania M: Folic acid and vitamin B_{12} deficiency in pregnancy and in the neonatal period. *Clin Perinatol* 11:2, 1984.

222. Landon MJ, Eyre DH, Hytten FE: Transfer of folate to the fetus. *Br J Obstet Gynaecol* 82:12, 1975.

223. Pritchard JA, Scott DE, Whalley PJ: Infants of mothers with megaloblastic anemia due to folate deficiency. *JAMA* 211:1982, 1970.

224. Shapiro J, Alperts HW, Welch P, Metz J: Folate and vitamin B_{12} deficiency associated with lactation. *Br J Haematol* 11:498, 1965.

225. Blot I, Papierhik F, Kaltwasser JP, et al: Influence of routine administration of folic acid and iron during pregnancy. *Gynecol Obstet Invest* 12:294, 1981.

226. Strieff RR, Little AB: Folic acid deficiency in pregnancy. *N Engl J Med* 276:776, 1967.

227. Chanarin I, McFadyen IR, Kyle R: The physiological macrocytosis of pregnancy. *Br J Obstet Gynaecol* 84:504, 1977.

228. Avery B, Ledger WJ: Folic acid metabolism in well-nourished pregnant women. *Obstet Gynecol* 35:616, 1970.

229. Giles C: An account of 335 cases of megaloblastic anemia of pregnancy. *J Clin Pathol* 19:1, 1966.

230. Lindenbaum J, Klipstein FA: Folic acid deficiency in sickle cell anemia. *N Engl J Med* 269:875, 1963.

231. Hild D: Folate losses from the skin in exfoliative dermatitis. *Arch Intern Med* 123:51, 1969.

232. Hoffbrand AV, Newcombe BFA, Mollin DL: Method of assay of red cell folate activity and the value of the assay as a test for folate deficiency. *J Clin Pathol* 19:17, 1999.

233. Chanarin I: Folate in blood, cerebrospinal fluid and tissues, in *The Megaloblastic Anemias*, 3rd ed, p 187. Blackwell, Oxford, 1990.

234. Lindenbaum J: Status of laboratory testing in the diagnosis of megaloblastic anemia. *Blood* 61:624, 1983.

235. Zalusky R, Herbert V, Castle AB: Cyanocobalamin therapy effect in folic acid deficiency. *Arch Intern Med* 109:545, 1962.

236. Kinnear DG, Johns DG, McIntosh PC: Intestinal absorption of tritium-labeled folic acid in idiopathic steatorrhea: Effect of a gluten-free diet. *CMAJ* 89:957, 1963.

237. MRC Vitamin Study Research Group: Prevention of neural tube defects: Results of the medical research council vitamin study. *Lancet* 338:131, 1991.

237a. Rothenberg SP, da Costa MP, Sequeira JM, et al: Autoantibodies against folate receptors in women with a pregnancy complicated by a neural-tube defect. *N Engl J Med* 350:134, 2004.

238. Van der Put NM, Gabreels F, Stevens EM, et al: A second common mutation in the methylenetetrahydrofolate reductase gene: An additional risk factor for neural-tube defects. *Am J Hum Genet* 62:1044, 1998.

239. Afman LA, Van der Put NM, Thomas CM, et al: Reduced vitamin B_{12} binding by transcobalamin II increases the risk of neural tube defects. *Q J Med* 94:159, 2001.

240. Schnyder G, Roffi M, Pin R, et al: Decreased rate of coronary restenosis after lowering of plasma homocysteine levels. *N Engl J Med* 345:1593, 2001.

241. Nilsson K, Gustafson L, Hultberg B: Folate and cobalamin levels as determinants of plasma homocysteine in different age groups of healthy controls and psychogeriatric patients. *Clin Chem Lab Med* 41:681, 2003.

242. Kluijtmans LA, Young IS, Boreham CA, et al: Genetic and nutritional factors contributing to hyperhomocysteinemia in young adults. *Blood* 101:2483, 2003.

243. Ward M, McNulty H, McPartlin J, et al: Plasma homocysteine, a risk factor for cardiovascular disease, is lowered by physiological doses of folic acid. *Q J Med* 90:519, 1997.

244. Quinlivan EP, McPartlin J, McNulty H, et al: Importance of both folic acid and vitamin B_{12} in reduction of risk of vascular disease. *Lancet* 359:227, 2002.

245. Lievers KJ, Kluijtmans LA, Boers GH, et al: Influence of a glutamate carboxypeptidase II (GCPII) polymorphism (1561C→T) on plasma homocysteine, folate and vitamin B(12) levels and its relationship to cardiovascular disease risk. *Atherosclerosis* 164:269, 2002.

246. Walker SP, Wein P, Ihle BU: Severe folate deficiency masquerading as the syndrome of hemolysis, elevated liver enzymes, and low platelets. *Obstet Gynecol* 90:655, 1997.

247. Giovannucci E, Stampfer MJ, Colditz GA, et al: Multivitamin use, folate, and colon cancer in women in the nurses' health study. *Ann Intern Med* 129:517, 1998.

248. Fenech M, Aitken C, Rinaldi J: Folate, vitamin B_{12}, homocysteine status and DNA damage in young Australian adults. *Carcinogenesis* 19:1163, 1998.

249. Rosenberg IH: Folic acid and neural-tube defects—Time for action. *N Engl J Med* 327:1875, 1992.

250. Hibbard ED, Spencer WS: Low serum B_{12} levels and latent Addisonian anaemia in pregnancy. *J Obstet Gynaecol Br Commonw* 77:52, 1970.

251. Vilter CF, Vilter RW, Spies TD: The treatment of pernicious and related anemias with synthetic folic acid: I. Observations on the maintenance of a normal hematologic status and on the occurrence of combined system disease at the end of one year. *J Lab Clin Med* 32:262, 1947.

252. Andersen LS, Hansen EL, Knudsen JB, et al: Prospectively measured red cell folate levels in methotrexate treated patients with rheumatoid arthritis: Relation to withdrawal and side effects. *J Rheumatol* 24:830, 1997.

253. Toh BH, Van Driel IR, Gleeson PA: Pernicious anemia. *N Engl J Med* 337:1441, 1997.

254. Kano K, Sakamoto S, Miura Y, Takaku F: Disorders of cobalamin metabolism. *CRC Crit Rev Oncol Hematol* 3:1, 1985.

255. Irvine WJ, Davies SH, Teitelbaum S: The clinical and pathological significance of gastric parietal cell antibody. *Ann N Y Acad Sci* 124:657, 1965.

256. Gardner PI, Heier HE: A human autoantibody to renal collecting duct cells associated with thyroid and gastric autoimmunity and possibly renal tubular acidosis. *Clin Exp Immunol* 51:19, 1983.

257. Suri-Payer E, Kehn PJ, Cheever AW, Shevach EM: Pathogenesis of post-thymectomy autoimmune gastritis. Identification of the anti-H/K adenosine triphosphatase-reactive T cells. *J Immunol* 157:1799, 1996.

258. Kapadia CR, Donaldson RM: Disorders of cobalamin (vitamin B_{12}) absorption and transport. *Annu Rev Med* 36:93, 1985.

259. Rose MS, Chanarin I: Intrinsic-factor antibody and absorption of vitamin B_{12} in pernicious anaemia. *Br Med J* 1:25, 1971.

260. Chanarin I, James D: Humoral and cell-mediated intrinsic factor antibody in pernicious anaemia. *Lancet* 1:1078, 1974.

261. Carmel R, Johnson CS: Racial patterns in pernicious anemia. *N Engl J Med* 298:647, 1978.

262. Conn HO, Binder H, Burns B: Pernicious anemia and immunologic deficiency. *Ann Intern Med* 68:603, 1968.

263. Sharpstone P, James DG: Pernicious anemia and immunologic deficiency. *Ann Intern Med* 68:603, 1968.

264. Ardeman S, Chanarin I, Krafchik B, Singer W: Addisonian pernicious anaemia and intrinsic factor antibodies in thyroid disorders. *Q J Med* 35:421, 1966.

265. Comin DB, Hines JD, Wieland RG: Coexistent pernicious anemia and idiopathic hypoparathyroidism in a women. *JAMA* 207:1147, 1969.

266. Mazzone T, Kelly W, Ensinck J: Lymphocytic hypophysitis associated with antiparietal cell antibodies and vitamin B_{12} deficiency. *Arch Intern Med* 143:1794, 1983.

267. Perillie PE, Nagler R: Development of pernicious anemia in a young patient with chronic ulcerative colitis. *N Engl J Med* 261:1175, 1959.

268. Howitz J, Schwartz M: Vitiligo, achlorhydria, and pernicious anemia. *Lancet* 1:1331, 1971.

269. Jackson I, Doig WB, McDonald G: Pernicious anemia as a cause of infertility. *Lancet* 2:1159, 1967.

270. Watson AA: Seminal vitamin B_{12} and sterility. *Lancet* 2:644, 1962.

271. Ungar B, Matthews JD, Tait BD, Cowling DC: HLA-DR patterns in pernicious anaemia. *Br Med J* 282:768, 1981.

272. Hoskins LC, Loux HA, Britten A, Zamcheck N: Distribution of ABO blood groups in patients with pernicious anemia, gastric carcinoma and gastric carcinoma associated with pernicious anemia. *N Engl J Med* 273:633, 1965.

273. Wangel AG, Callender ST, Spray GH, Wright R: A family study of pernicious anaemia: I. Autoantibodies, achlorhydria, serum pepsinogen and vitamin B_{12}. *N Engl J Med* 273:633, 1968.

274. Varis K, Ihamaki T, Harkonen M, et al: Gastric morphology, function, and immunology in first-degree relatives of probands with pernicious anemia and controls. *Scand J Gastroenterol* 14:129, 1979.

275. Solanki DL, Jacobson RJ, Green R, et al: Pernicious anemia in Blacks. *Am J Clin Pathol* 75:96, 1981.

276. Eriksson S, Clas L, Moquist-Olsson I: Pernicious anemia at risk factor in gastric cancer: The extent of the problem. *Acta Med Scand* 210:481, 1981.

277. Wilkinson JF: Gastric secretions in pernicious anemia. *Q J Med* 1:361, 1932.

278. Shojania AM: Problems in the diagnosis and investigation of megaloblastic anemia. *CMAJ* 122:999, 1980.

279. Karnes WE Jr, Samloff IM, Siurala M: Positive scrum antibody and negative tissue staining for *Helicobacter pylori* in subjects with atrophic body gastritis. *Gastroenterology* 101:167, 1991.

280. Slingerland DW, Cardarelli JA, Burrows BA, Miller A: The utility of serum gastrin levels in assessing the significance of low serum B_{12} levels. *Arch Intern Med* 144:1167, 1984.

281. Ganguli PC, Cullen DR, Irvine WJ: Radioimmunoassay of plasma-gastrin in pernicious anemia, achlorhydria without pernicious anemia, hypochlorhydria, and in controls. *Lancet* 1:155, 1971.

282. Kaye MD, Whorwell PJ, Wright R: Gastric mucosal lymphocyte subpopulations in pernicious anemia and in normal stomach. *Clin Immunol Immunopathol* 28:431, 1983.

283. Rodbro P, Dige-Petersen H, Schwartz M, Dalggard OZ: Effect of steroids on gastric mucosal structure and function in pernicious anemia. *Acta Med Scand* 181:445, 1967.

284. Neiburgs HE, Glass GBJ: Gastric-cell maturation disorders in atrophic gastritis, pernicious anemia, and carcinoma. *Am J Dig Dis* 8:135, 1963.

285. Foroozan P, Trier JS: Mucosa of the small intestine in pernicious anemia. *N Engl J Med* 277:553, 1967.

286. Bezman A, Kinnear DG, Zamcheck N: D-xylose and potassium iodide absorption and serum carotene in pernicious anemia. *J Lab Clin Med* 53:226, 1959.

287. Ellison AB: Pernicious anemia masked by multivitamins containing folic acid. *JAMA* 173:240, 1960.

288. Stefanini M, Karaca M: Acquired thrombocytopathy in patients with pernicious anemia. *Lancet* 1:400, 1966.

289. MacLean LD, Sunberg RD: Incidence of megaloblastic anemia after total gastrectomy. *N Engl J Med* 254:885, 1956.

290. Gozzard DI, Dawson DW, Lewis MJ: Experiences with dual protein bound aqueous vitamin B$_{12}$ absorption test in subjects with low serum vitamin B$_{12}$ concentrations. *J Clin Pathol* 40:633, 1987.

291. Van Der Weyden MB, Rother M, Firkin BG: Megaloblastic maturation masked by iron deficiency: A biochemical basis. *Br J Haematol* 22:299, 1973.

292. Lees F, Ganjean LC: The gastric and jejunal mucosae in healthy patients with partial gastrectomy. *Arch Intern Med* 101:943, 1958.

293. Shimoda SS, Saunders DR, Rubin CF: The Zollinger-Ellison syndrome with steatorrhea: II. The mechanism of fat and vitamin B$_{12}$ malabsorption. *Gastroenterology* 55:705, 1968.

294. Kennedy HJ, Callender ST, Truelove SC, Warner GT: Haematological aspects of life on an ileostomy. *Br J Haematol* 52:445, 1982.

295. Steinberg F: The megaloblastic anemia of regional ileitis. *N Engl J Med* 264:186, 1961.

296. Anderson CG, Walton KR, Chanarin I: Megaloblastic anaemia after pelvic radiotherapy for carcinoma of the cervix. *J Clin Pathol* 34:151, 1981.

297. Tudhope GR, Wilson GM: Deficiency of vitamin B$_{12}$ in hypothyroidism. *Lancet* 1:703, 1962.

298. McLean LD: Incidence of megaloblastic anemia after subtotal gastrectomy. *N Engl J Med* 257:262, 1957.

299. Cameron DG, Watson GM, Witts LJ: The clinical association of macrocytic anemia with intestinal stricture and anastomosis. *Blood* 4:793, 1949.

300. Murphy MF, Sourial NA, Burman JF, et al: Megaloblastic anaemia due to vitamin B$_{12}$ deficiency caused by small intestinal bacterial overgrowth: Possible role of vitamin B$_{12}$ analogues. *Br J Haematol* 62:7, 1986.

301. Nyberg W: The influence of *Diphyllobothrium latum* on the vitamin B$_{12}$-intrinsic factor complex: I. In vivo studies with Schilling test technique. *Acta Med Scand* 167:185, 1960.

302. Nyberg W: *Diphyllobothrium latum* and human nutrition with particular reference to vitamin B$_{12}$ deficiency. *Proc Nutr Soc* 22:8, 1963.

303. Guéant JL, Champigneulle B, Gaucher P, Nicolas J-P: Malabsorption of vitamin B$_{12}$ in pancreatic insufficiency of the adult and of the child. *Pancreas* 5:559, 1999.

304. Toskes PP, Deren JJ, Conrad ME: Trypsin-like nature of the pancreatic factor that corrects vitamin B$_{12}$ malabsorption associated with pancreatic dysfunction. *J Clin Invest* 52:1660, 1973.

305. Henderson JT, Simpson JD, Warwick RRG, Shearman DJC: Does malabsorption of vitamin B$_{12}$ occur in chronic pancreatitis? *Lancet* 2:241, 1972.

306. Gilois C, Wierzbicki AS, Hirani N: The hematological and electrophysiological effects of cobalamin: Deficiency secondary to vegetarian diets. *Ann N Y Acad Sci* 669:345, 1992.

307. Ford MJ: Megaloblastic anaemia in a vegetarian. *Br J Clin Pract* 34:222, 1980.

308. Michaud JL, Lemieux B, Ogier H, Lambert MA: Nutritional vitamin B$_{12}$ deficiency: Two cases detected by routine newborn urinary screening. *Eur J Pediatr* 151:218, 1992.

309. Wickramasinghe SN, Akinyanju OÒ, Grange A, Litwinczuk RA: Folate levels and deoxyuridine suppression tests in protein-energy malnutrition. *Br J Haematol* 53:135, 1983.

310. Frenkel EP: Abnormal fatty acid metabolism in peripheral nerves of patients with pernicious anemia. *J Clin Invest* 52:1237, 1973.

311. Lever EG, Elwes RD, Williams A, Reynolds EH: Subacute combined degeneration of the cord due to folate deficiency: Response to methyl folate treatment. *J Neurol Neurosurg Psychiatry* 49:1203, 1986.

312. Clayton PT, Smith I, Harding B, et al: Subacute combined degradation of the cord, dementia and Parkinsonism due to an inborn error of folate metabolism. *J Neurol Neurosurg Psychiatry* 49:920, 1986.

313. Green R, Van Tonder SV, Oettle GJ, et al: Neurologic changes in fruit bats deficient in vitamin B$_{12}$. *Nature* 254:148, 1975.

314. Weir DG, Keating S, Molloy A, et al: Methylation deficiency causes vitamin B$_{12}$-deficient monkeys with combined system disease: I. B$_{12}$-deficient patterns in bone marrow deoxyuridine suppression tests without morphologic or functional abnormalities. *J Neurochem* 51:1949, 1988.

315. Deacon R, Purkiss P, Green R, et al: Vitamin B$_{12}$ neuropathy is not due to failure to methylate myelin basic protein. *J Neurol Sci* 72:113, 1986.

316. Surtees R, Leonard J, Austin S: Association of demyelination with deficiency of cerebrospinal-fluid S-adenosylmethionine in inborn errors of methyl transfer pathway. *Lancet* 388:15504, 1991.

317. Beck WS: Neuropsychiatric consequences of cobalamin deficiency. *Adv Intern Med* 36:33, 1991.

318. Victor M, Lear A: Subacute combined degeneration of the spinal cord: Current concepts of the disease: Value of serum vitamin B$_{12}$ determinations in clarifying some of the common clinical problems. *Am J Med* 20:896, 1956.

319. Herbert V: Biology of disease: Megaloblastic anemias. *Lab Invest* 52:3, 1985.

320. DiLazzaro V, Restuccia D, Fogli D, et al: Central sensory and motor conduction in vitamin B$_{12}$ deficiency. *Electroencephalogr Clin Neurophysiol* 84:433, 1992.

321. Fraser TN: Cerebral manifestations of Addisonian pernicious anemia. *Lancet* 2:258, 1960.

322. Shulman R: Psychiatric aspects of pernicious anaemia. *Br Med J* 3:266, 1967.

323. Smith ADM: Megaloblastic madness. *Br Med J* 2:1840, 1960.

324. Stojsavljevic N, Levic Z, Drulovic J, Dragutinovic G: A 44-month clinical-brain MRI follow-up in a patient with B$_{12}$ deficiency. *Neurology* 49:878, 1997.

325. Lindenbaum J, Healton EB, Savage DG, et al: Neuropsychiatric disorders caused by cobalamin deficiency in the absence of anemia or macrocytosis. *N Engl J Med* 318:1720, 1988.

326. Rasmussen K, Vyberg B, Pedersen KO, Brochner-Mortensen J: Methylmalonic acid in renal insufficiency: Evidence of accumulation and implications for diagnosis of cobalamin deficiency. *Clin Chem* 36:1523, 1990.

327. Malleson P: Isolated gastroduodenal Crohn disease in a ten-year-old girl. *Postgrad Med J* 56:294, 1980.

328. Shojania AM: Physician's management of suspected vitamin B$_{12}$ deficiency. *CMAJ* 123:1127, 1999.

329. Carmel R: R-binder deficiency: A clinically benign cause of cobalamin pseudodeficiency. *JAMA* 250:1886, 1983.

330. Kahn SB, Williams WS, Barness LA, et al: Methylmalonic acid excretion: A sensitive indicator of vitamin B$_{12}$ deficiency. *J Lab Clin Med* 66:75, 1965.

331. Lindenbaum J, Savage DG, Stabler SP, Allen RH: Diagnosis of cobalamin deficiency: II. Relative sensitivities of serum cobalamin, methylmalonic acid and total homocysteine concentrations. *Am J Hematol* 34:99, 1990.

332. Stabler SP, Allen RH, Barrett RE: Cerebrospinal fluid methylmalonic acid levels in normal subjects and patients with cobalamin deficiency. *Neurology* 41:1627, 1991.

333. Fairbanks VF, Wahner HW, Phyliky RL: Tests for pernicious anemia: The Schilling test. *Mayo Clin Proc* 63:480, 1983.

334. Nelp WB, Wagner HN Jr, Reba RC: Renal excretion of vitamin B$_{12}$ and its use in measurements of glomerular filtration rate in man. *J Lab Clin Med* 63:480, 1964.

335. Rath CE, McCurdy PR, Duffy BJ: Effect of renal disease on the Schilling test. *N Engl J Med* 256:111, 1956.

336. Akun SN, Miller IF, Meyer LM: Vitamin B$_{12}$ absorption tests. *Acta Haematol (Basel)* 41:341, 1969.

337. Termanini B, Gibril F, Sutliff VE, et al: Effect of long-term gastric acid suppressive therapy on serum vitamin B_{12} levels inpatients with Zollinger-Ellison syndrome. *Am J Med* 104:422, 1998.

338. Miller A, Furlong D, Burrows BA, Slingerland DW: Bound vitamin B_{12} absorption in patients with low serum B_{12} levels. *Am J Hematol* 40:163, 1992.

339. Streeter AM, Duncombe VM, Boyle R, Pheils MT: A simple method of measuring the absorption of protein-bound vitamin B_{12}. *Aust N Z J Med* 5:382, 1975.

340. Steinberg WM, King CE, Toskes PP: Malabsorption of protein-bound cobalamin but not unbound cobalamin during cimetidine administration. *Dig Dis Sci* 25:188, 1980.

341. Forshaw J: Effect of vitamin B_{12} and folic acid deficiency in small intestinal absorption. *J Clin Pathol* 22:551, 1969.

342. Metz J: The deoxyuridine suppression test. *CRC Crit Rev Clin Lab Sci* 20:205, 1984.

343. Das KC, Manusselis C, Herbert V: In vitro DNA synthesis by bone marrow cells and PHA-stimulated lymphocytes: Suppression by nonradioactive thymidine of the incorporation of ^{3}H-deoxyuridine into DNA: Enhancement of incorporation when inadequate vitamin B_{12} or folate is corrected. *Br J Haematol* 44:51, 1980.

344. Das D, Garawal G, Mohanty D: Derangement of DNA synthesis in erythroleukaemia: Normal deoxyuridine suppression and impaired thymidine incorporation in bone marrow culture. *Acta Haematol (Basel)* 64:121, 1980.

345. Carmel R, Karnaze DS: The deoxyuridine suppression test identifies subtle cobalamin deficiency in patients without typical megaloblastic anemia. *JAMA* 253:1284, 1985.

346. Boddy K, King P, Mervyn L, et al: Retention of cyanocobalamin hydroxocobalamin and coenzyme B_{12} after parenteral administration. *Lancet* 2:710, 1968.

346a. Lawson DH, Murray RM, Parker JL. Early mortality in the megaloblastic anaemias. *Q J Med* 41:1, 1972,

346b. Omboni E, Checchini M, Longoni F: Hypopotassemia and megaloblastic anemia. Presentation of a case. *Minerva Med* 78:1255, 1987.

347. Finch CA, Coleman DH, Motulsky AG, et al: Erythrokinetics in pernicious anemia. *Blood* 11:807, 1956.

348. Hillman RS, Adamson J, Burka E: Characteristics of vitamin B_{12} correction of the abnormal erythropoiesis of pernicious anemia. *Blood* 31:419, 1968.

349. Lawson DH, Murray RM, Parker JLW, Hay G: Hypokalemia in megaloblastic anaemias. *Lancet* 2:558, 1970.

350. Paalk EA Jr, Farrar WE Jr: Diverticulosis of the small intestine and megaloblastic anemia: Intestinal flora and absorption before and after tetracycline administration. *Am J Med* 37:473, 1964.

351. Kuzminski AM, Del Giacco EJ, Allen RH, et al: Effective treatment of cobalamin deficiency with oral cobalamin. *Blood* 92:1191, 1998.

352. Andres E, Kurtz JE, Perrin AE, et al: Oral cobalamin therapy for the treatment of patients with food-cobalamin malabsorption. *Am J Med* 111:126, 2001.

353. Lederle FA: Oral cobalamin for pernicious anemia: Medicine's best kept secret. *JAMA* 265:94, 1999.

354. Kondo H, Osborne ML, Kolhouse JF: Nitrous oxide has multiple deleterious effects on cobalamin metabolism and causes decreases in activities of both mammalian cobalamin-dependent enzymes in rats. *J Clin Invest* 67:1270, 1981.

355. Lumb M, Sharer N, Deacon R, et al: Effects of nitrous oxide-induced inactivation of cobalamin on methionine and S-adenosylmethionine metabolism in the rat. *Biochim Biophys Acta* 756:354, 1983.

356. O'Sullivan H, Jennings F, Ward K, et al: Human bone marrow biochemical function and megaloblastic hematopoiesis after nitrous oxide anesthesia. *Anesthesiology* 55:645, 1981.

357. Skacel PO, Hewlett AM, Lewis JD, et al: Studies on the haemopoietic toxicity of nitrous oxide in man. *Br J Haematol* 53:189, 1983.

358. Skacel PO, Chanarin I, Hewlett A, Nunn JF: Failure to correct nitrous oxide toxicity with folinic acid. *Anesthesiology* 57:557, 1982.

359. Kano Y, Sakamoto S, Sakuraya K, et al: Effects of leucovorin and methylcobalamin with N_2O anesthesia. *J Lab Clin Med* 104:711, 1984.

360. Amess JAL, Burman JR, Rees GM: Megaloblastic haemopoiesis in patients receiving nitrous oxide. *Lancet* 2:339, 1978.

361. Brodsky L, Zuniga J: Nitrous oxide: A psychotogenic agent. *Comp Psychiatry* 16:185, 1975.

362. Layzer RB, Fishman RA, Schafer JA: Neuropathy following abuse of nitrous oxide. *Neurology* 28:504, 1978.

363. Salo M, Rajamaki A, Nikoskelainen J: Absence of signs of vitamin B_{12}–nitrous oxide interaction in operating theatre personnel. *Acta Anaesthesiol Scand* 28:106, 1984.

364. Easton DJ: Severe thrombocytopenia associated with acute folic acid deficiency and severe hemorrhage in two patients. *CMAJ* 130:418, 1984.

365. Beard ME, Hatipov CS, Hamer JW: Acute onset of folate deficiency in patients under intensive care. *Crit Care Med* 8:500, 1980.

366. Chan MK, Beale D, Moorhead JF: Acute megaloblastosis due to cotrimoxazole. *Br J Clin Pract* 34:187, 1980.

367. Henderson GB, Suresh MR, Vitols KS, Huennekens FM: Transport of folate compounds in L1210 cells: Kinetic evidence that folate influx proceeds via the high-affinity transport system for 5-methyltetrahydrofolate and methotrexate. *Cancer Res* 46:1639, 1986.

368. Schoo MM, Pristupa ZB, Vickers PJ, Scrimgeour KG: Folate analogues as substrates of mammalian folylpolyglutamate synthetase. *Cancer Res* 46:1639, 1985.

369. Huennekens FM, Duffy TH, Pope LE: Biochemistry of methotrexate: Teaching an old drug new tricks, in *Cancer Biology and Therapeutics*, edited by JG Corry, A Szentivanyi, p 45. Plenum, New York, 1987.

370. Kesavan V, Sur P, Doig MT: Effect of methotrexate on folates in Krebs ascites and L1210 murine leukemia cells. *Cancer Lett* 30:55, 1986.

371. Spiegel RJ, Cooper PR, Blum RH, et al: Treatment of massive intrathecal methotrexate overdose by ventriculolumbar perfusion. *N Engl J Med* 311:386, 1984.

372. Yarchoan R, Broder S: Development of antiretroviral therapy for the acquired immunodeficiency syndrome and related disorders. *N Engl J Med* 316:557, 1987.

373. Richman DD, Fischl MA, the AZT Collaborative Working Group, et al: The toxicity of azidothymidine (AZT) in the treatment of patients with AIDS and AIDS-related complex. A double-blind, placebo-controlled trial. *N Engl J Med* 317:192, 1987.

374. Boudes P, Zittoun J, Sober A: Folate, vitamin B_{12}, and HIV infection. *Lancet* 335:1401, 1990.

375. Krakoff IH, Brown NC, Reichard P: Inhibition of ribonucleoside diphosphate reductase by hydroxyurea. *Cancer Res* 28:1559, 1968.

376. Krakoff JH: Clinical and physiologic effects of hydroxyurea, in *Antineoplastic and Immunosuppressive Agents*, edited by AC Sartorelli, DG Johus, p 780. Springer-Verlag, Berlin, 1975.

377. Koop H, Bachem MG: Serum iron, ferritin, and vitamin B_{12} during prolonged omeprazole therapy. *J Clin Gastroenterol* 14:288, 1992.

378. Parry TE: The diagnosis of megaloblastic anaemia. *Clin Lab Haematol* 2:89, 1980.

379. Gräsbeck R, Gordin R, Kantero I, Kuhlback B: Selective vitamin B_{12} malabsorption and proteinuria in young people: A syndrome. *Acta Med Scand* 167:289, 1960.

380. Goldenberg LS, Fudenberg HH: Familial selective malabsorption of vitamin B_{12}: Re-evaluation of an in vitro intrinsic factor inhibitor. *N Engl J Med* 279:405, 1968.

381. Zimram A, Hershko C: The changing pattern of megaloblastic anemia: Megaloblastic anemia in Israel. *Am J Clin Nutr* 37:855, 1983.

382. Cooper BA, Rosenblatt DS: Inherited defects of vitamin B$_{12}$ metabolism. *Annu Rev Nutr* 7:291, 1987.

383. Chisolm JC: Selective malabsorption of vitamin B$_{12}$ and vitamin B$_{12}$-intrinsic factor complex with megaloblastic anemia in an adult. *JAMA* 77:835, 1985.

384. Burman JF, Jenkins WJ, Walker-Smith JA, et al: Absent ileal uptake of IF-bound-vitamin B$_{12}$ in the Imerslund-Gräsbeck syndrome (familial B$_{12}$ malabsorption with proteinuria). *Gut* 26:311, 1985.

385. Carmel R: Gastric juice in congenital pernicious anemia contains no immunoreactive intrinsic factor molecule: Study of three kindreds with variable ages at presentation, including a patient first diagnosed in adulthood. *Am J Hum Genet* 35:66, 1983.

386. Miller DR, Bloom GE, Streiff RR, et al: Juvenile "congenital" pernicious anemia: Clinical and immunologic studies. *N Engl J Med* 275:978, 1966.

387. Hall CA: Congenital disorders of vitamin B$_{12}$ transport and their contributions to concepts: II. *Yale J Biol Med* 54:485, 1981.

388. Frater-Schröder M, Luthy R, Haurani FI, Hitzig WH: Transcobalamin II polymorphisms: Biochemische und klinische Aspekven Seltener Variaten. *Schweiz Med Wochenschr* 109:1373, 1982.

389. Thomas PK, Hoffbrand AV, Smith IS: Neurological involvement in hereditary transcobalamin II deficiency. *J Neurol Neurosurg Psychiatry* 45:74, 1982.

390. Frater-Schröder M, Sacher M, Hitzig WH: Inheritance of transcobalamin II (TC II) in two families with TC II deficiency and related immunodeficiency. *J Inherit Metab Dis* 4:165, 1981.

391. Carmel R, Ravindranath Y: Congenital transcobalamin II deficiency presenting atypically with a low serum cobalamin level: Studies demonstrating the coexistence of a circulating transcobalamin I (R binder) complex. *Blood* 63:598, 1984.

392. Rana SR, Colman N, Goh KO, et al: Transcobalamin II deficiency associated with usual bone marrow findings and chromosomal abnormalities. *Am J Hematol* 14:89, 1983.

393. Haurani FI, Hall CA, Rubin R: Megaloblastic anemia as a result of an abnormal transcobalamin II. *J Clin Invest* 64:1253, 1979.

394. Fernandes-Costa F, Metz J: Vitamin B$_{12}$ binders (transcobalamins) in serum. *CRC Crit Rev Clin Lab Sci* 18:1, 1983.

395. Rosenblatt DS, Hosack A, Matiaszuk N: Expression of transcobalamin II by amniocytes. *Prenat Diagn* 7:35, 1987.

396. McIntyre OR, Sullivan LW, Jeffries GH, Silver RH: Pernicious anemia in childhood. *N Engl J Med* 272:981, 1965.

397. Fowler B: Genetic defects of folate and cobalamin metabolism. *Eur J Pediatr* 157:S60, 1998.

398. Rosenblatt DS, Hosack A, Matiaszuk NV: Defect in vitamin B$_{12}$ release from lysosomes: Newly described inborn error of vitamin B$_{12}$ metabolism. *Science* 228:1219, 1985.

399. Chalmers RA, Bain MD, Mistry J, et al: Enzymologic studies on patients with methylmalonic aciduria: Basis for a clinical trial of deoxyadenosylcobalamin in a hydroxocobalamin-unresponsive patient. *Pediatr Res* 30:560, 1991.

400. Rosenblatt DS, Cooper BA, Pottier A: Altered vitamin B$_{12}$ metabolism in fibroblasts from a patient with megaloblastic anemia and homocystinuria due to a new defect in methionine biosynthesis. *J Clin Invest* 74:2149, 1984.

401. Leclerc D, Campeau E, Goyette P, et al: Human methionine synthase: CDNA cloning and identification of mutations in patients of the *cblG* complementation group of folate/cobalamin disorders. *Hum Mol Genet* 5:1867, 1996.

402. Gulati S, Chen Z, Brody LC, et al: Defects in auxiliary redox proteins lead to functional methionine synthase deficiency. *J Biol Chem* 272:19171, 1997.

403. Zammarchi E, Lippi A, Falorni S, et al: Case report and monitoring of a pregnancy at risk by chorionic villus sampling. *Clin Invest Med* 13:139, 1980.

404. Van der Meer SB, Spaapen LJM, Fowler B, et al: Prenatal treatment of a patient with vitamin B$_{12}$-responsive methylmalonic acidemia. *J Pediatr* 117:923, 1990.

405. Erbe RW: Inborn errors of folate metabolism: II. *N Engl J Med* 293:807, 1975.

406. Lanzkowsky P: Congenital malabsorption of folate. *Am J Med* 48:580, 1970.

407. Walters T: Congenital megaloblastic anemia responsive to N^5-formyl tetrahydrofolic acid administration. *J Pediatr* 70:686, 1967.

408. Arakawa T, Narisawa K, Tanno K, et al: Megaloblastic anemia and mental retardation associated with hyperfolic-acidemia: Probably due to N^5-methyltetrahydrofolate transferase deficiency. *Tohoku J Exp Med* 93:1, 1967.

409. Fox RM, Wood MH, Royse-Smith D, O'Sullivan WJ: Hereditary orotic aciduria: Types I and II. *Am J Med* 55:791, 1973.

410. van der Zee SPM: Megaloblastic anemia in the Lesch-Nyhan syndrome. *Lancet* 1:1427, 1968.

411. Thiamine-responsive megaloblastic anemia. *Nutr Res* 38:374, 1980.

412. Bazarbachi A, Muakkit S, Ayas M, et al: Thiamine-responsive myelodysplasia. *Br J Haematol* 102:1098, 1998.

413. Neufeld EJ, Mandel H, Raz T, et al: Localization of the gene for thiamine-responsive megaloblastic anemia syndrome, on the long arm of chromosome 1, by homozygosity mapping. *Am J Hum Genet* 61:1335, 1997.

414. Zdebska E, Mendek-Czajkowska E, Ploski R, et al: Heterozygosity of CDAN II (HEMPAS) gene may be detected by the analysis of erythrocyte membrane glycoconjugates from healthy carriers. *Haematologica* 87:126, 2002.

415. Maeda K, Saeed SM, Rebuck JW: Type I dyserythropoietic anemia. A 30-year follow-up. *Am J Clin Pathol* 73:433, 1980.

416. Wickramasinghe SN, Parry TE, Williams C: A new case of congenital dyserythropoietic anaemia, type III: Studies of the cell cycle distribution and ultrastructure of erythroblasts and of nucleic acid synthesis in marrow cells. *J Clin Pathol* 35:1103, 1982.

417. Ahmann FR, Durie BG: Acute myelogenous leukaemia modulated by B$_{12}$ deficiency: A case with bone marrow blast cell assay corroboration. *Br J Haematol* 58:91, 1984.

418. Najfeld V, McArthur J, Shashty GG: Monosomy 7 in a patient with pancytopenia and abnormal erythropoiesis. *Acta Haematol (Basel)* 66:12, 1981.

419. Roggli VL, Saleem A: Erythroleukemia: A study of 15 cases and literature review. *Cancer* 49:101, 1982.

420. Megarbane B, Delahaye A, Goldgran-Toledano D, Baud FJ: Antidotal treatment of cyanide poisoning. *J Chin Med Assoc* 66:193, 2003.

421. Matherly LH, Barlowe CK, Phillips VM, Goldman ID: The effect of 4-aminoantifolates on 5-formyltetrahydrofolate metabolism. *J Biol Chem* 262:710, 1987.

422. Magee F, O'Sullivan H, McCann SR: Megaloblastosis and low-dose trimethoprim sulfamethoxazole [letter]. *Ann Intern Med* 95:657, 1981.

423. Swinson CM, Perry J, Lumb M, Levi AJ: Role of sulphasalazine in the aetiology of folate deficiency in ulcerative colitis. *Gut* 22:456, 1981.

424. Boots M, Phillips M, Curtis JR: Megaloblastic anemia and pancytopenia due to proguanil in patients with chronic renal failure. *Clin Nephrol* 18:106, 1981.

424a. Fossella FV: Pemetrexed for treatment of advanced non-small cell lung cancer. *Semin Oncol* 31:100, 2004.

425. Bethell FH, Thompson DS: Treatment of leukemia and related disorders with 6-mercaptopurine. *Ann N Y Acad Sci* 60:436, 1954.

426. Cristoph R, Pisnay D, Hartl W: Megaloblastic anaemia following treatment of rheumatoid arthritis with Imuran. *Med Welt* 46:1824, 1971.

427. Klippel JH, Decker JL: Relative macrocytosis in cyclophosphamide and azathioprine therapy. *JAMA* 229:180, 1974.

428. Amos RJ, Amess JA: Megaloblastic haemopoiesis due to acyclovir [letter]. *Lancet* 1:242, 1983.

429. Reyes P, Heidelberger C: Fluorinated pyrimidines. *Mol Pharmacol* 1: 14, 1963.

430. Cornell RC, Milstein HG, Fox CM: Anemia of azaribine in the treatment of psoriasis. *Arch Dermatol* 112:1717, 1976.

431. Frenkel EP, Arthur C: Induced ribotide reductive conversion by hydroxyurea and its relationship to megaloblastosis. *Cancer Res* 27:1016, 1967.

432. Papac RJ: Clinical and hematologic studies with 1-b-D-arabinosylcytosine. *J Natl Cancer Inst* 40:997, 1968.

433. Druskin MS, Wallen MH, Bonagura L: Anticonvulsant-associated anemia. *N Engl J Med* 267:483, 1962.

434. Gerson CD, Hepner GW, Brown N, et al: Inhibition of diphenylhydantoin of folic acid absorption in man. *Gastroenterology* 63:246, 1972.

435. Carl GF, Smith ML, Furman GM, et al: Phenytoin treatment and folate supplementation affect folate concentrations and methylation capacity in rats. *J Nutr* 121:1214, 1991.

436. Isojarvi FI, Pakarinen AJ, Myllyla VV: Basic haematological parameters, serum gamma-glutamyl-transferase activity, and erythrocyte folate and serum vitamin B_{12} levels during carbamazepine and oxcarbazepine therapy. *Seizure* 6:207, 1997.

437. Lindenbaum J, Whitehead N, Reyner F: Oral contraceptive hormones, folate metabolism and cervical epithelium. *Am J Clin Nutr* 28:346, 1975.

438. Hainivaara O, Palva IP: Malabsorption and deficiency of vitamin B_{12} caused by treatment with para-aminosalicylic acid. *Acta Med Scand* 177: 337, 1965.

439. Callaghan TS, Hadden DR, Tomkin GH: Megaloblastic anaemia due to vitamin B_{12} malabsorption associated with long-term metformin treatment. *Br Med J* 280:1214, 1980.

440. Webb DI, Chodos RB, Mahar CQ, Faloon WW: Mechanism of vitamin B_{12} malabsorption in patients receiving colchicine. *N Engl J Med* 279: 845, 1968.

441. Dobbins WO, Herrero BA, Mansbach CM: Morphological alterations associated with neomycin induced malabsorption. *Am J Med Sci* 255: 63, 1968.

442. Lerman BB, Ali N, Green D: Megaloblastic, dyserythropoietic anemia following arsenic ingestion. *Ann Clin Lab Sci* 10:515, 1980.

DISORDERS OF IRON METABOLISM

ERNEST BEUTLER

Iron is a component of all living organisms. It plays an important metabolic role, particularly in electron transfer reactions. Much of the iron in the human body is in circulating red cells, which contain 1 mg of iron per 1 ml of packed cells. Iron is stored in the form of ferritin or hemosiderin. Smaller amounts of iron are present in myoglobin and in many enzymes. Because little iron is lost from the body, the iron content of the body is regulated by modulating iron absorption. Separate pathways exist for the absorption of heme and inorganic iron. The precise mechanism by which iron passes across the intestinal mucosa into the plasma has not yet been elucidated. The process appears to involve a ferrireductase, an integrin, a divalent iron transporter DMT-1, hephaestin, and ferroportin-1. Iron absorption is increased in the presence of iron deficiency and it decreases when there is iron overload. The main regulator of iron homeostasis seems to be the antimicrobial peptide hepcidin.

Once ferric iron enters the plasma, it is bound by transferrin, which, after forming a complex with the transferrin receptor, transports the metal into cells. The transferrin receptor is internalized together with bound transferrin and iron, and the iron is released inside the cell into an acidified vacuole. The transferrin receptor then moves back to the cell surface.

Many of the proteins involved in iron homeostasis are regulated by the amount of available iron through binding of one of the iron regulatory proteins (IRPs) with iron-responsive elements (IREs), which exist as stem-loop structures in RNA. IRP-1 is cytoplasmic aconitase that binds to the IRE when it is not complexed with iron and does not bind when iron is present. IRP-2, a closely related protein, is destabilized by the presence of iron. When IRPs bind to IREs at the $5'$ end of the mRNA they prevent translation; when they bind at the $3'$ end they stabilize the message.

Iron deficiency and iron-deficiency anemia are common nutritional and hematologic disorders in North America and world-wide. In infants and young children iron deficiency is most commonly due to insufficient dietary iron. In young women it is most often the result of blood loss in menstruation or as a result of pregnancy. In older adults bleeding may be from the gastrointestinal tract, as from hemorrhoids, bleeding peptic ulcer, hiatus hernia, colon cancer or angiodysplasia. It may result from uterine leiomyomas or carcinoma, or a renal tumor. Pulmonary blood loss is usually evidenced by chronic hemoptysis due to infection, malignancy, or as a result of idiopathic pulmonary hemosiderosis. However, bloody sputum may be swallowed, and pulmonary bleeding may be mistaken for gastrointestinal bleeding. Iron deficiency has adverse effects on activity of numerous enzymes, and in infants can result in impairment of growth and intellectual development. The hematologic features of iron deficiency are non-specific and too often confused with other causes of microcytic anemia such as thalassemias, chronic disease, renal neoplasms, and other disorders. A low serum ferritin concentration is a good indicator of iron deficiency, but is elevated by inflammation, which lessens its sensitivity for the detection of iron deficiency coexisting with the anemia of chronic disease. The plasma iron is decreased and the iron binding capacity increased in severe iron deficiency, but these alterations are not uniformly present in mild iron deficiency, and low plasma iron levels are also characteristic of the anemia of chronic disease. Erythrocyte zinc protoporphyrin assay is a useful screening test but lacks specificity. Other laboratory tests that are useful include assays for serum transferrin receptor, erythrocyte ferritin concentration, and reticulocyte hemoglobin content. Diagnosis of iron deficiency, particularly in an adult, obliges the clinician to determine the site and cause of blood loss, and to rectify it whenever possible. Treatment of iron deficiency with ferrous salts, in doses of 100–200 mg of elemental iron daily, is superior to, much safer, and far less costly than parenteral therapy. Enteric-coated and prolonged-release preparations should be avoided. Complete correction of anemia is expected in 8–12 weeks, depending on patient's age. If this response is not achieved, the patient and the diagnosis require re-evaluation. Administration of iron should be continued for 8 months after correction of anemia, or as long as bleeding continues. Parenteral iron is used in patients with gastrointestinal disease, noncompliant patients, and patients undergoing renal dialysis. Iron sucrose and iron gluconate complexes are preferred to iron dextran because they are less likely to cause anaphylactic reactions.

Increased body iron stores have the capacity to produce tissue damage. Iron storage disease (hemochromatosis) can be the result of mutations of genes that are involved in regulation of iron homeostasis or transport. These genes include HFE, ferroportin-1 (SCL40A1), hepcidin, and hemojuvelin. Alternatively, hemochromatosis can be the result of iron given in the form of red blood cell transfusions, particularly in individuals with ineffective erythropoiesis, a disorder that seems to facilitate iron absorption. Among the most common causes of secondary hemochromatosis are thalassemia major, myelodysplastic anemias, dyserythropoietic anemias, and pyruvate kinase deficiency.

The diagnosis of hemochromatosis depends, in large part, upon increased serum ferritin levels, which tend to reflect increased iron stores. However, ferritin levels are also increased in patients with chronic inflammation or neoplasia or with the hyperferritinemia cataract syndrome, a disorder due to mutations in the IRE of the ferritin light chain. The transferrin saturation is usually increased in patients with hereditary hemochromatosis, even when the ferritin level is normal.

Full-blown hemochromatosis is characterized by cirrhosis of the liver, darkening of the skin, diabetes, cardiomyopathies, and possibly by arthropathies. Iron deposition is primarily in hepatocytes, with macrophages and intestinal mucosal cells being relatively iron-poor. The most common causes of genetic hemochromatosis are mutations of the HFE gene. Two muta-

Acronyms and abbreviations that appear in this chapter include: dcytb, duodenal cytochrome b; DMT, divalent metal transporter; GRACILE syndrome, Growth Retardation, Aminoaciduria, Cholestasis, Iron overload, Lactic acidosis, and Early death syndrome; HLA, human leukocyte antigen; IRE, iron-responsive element; IRP, iron regulatory protein; MAO, monoamine oxidase; MCHC, mean corpuscular hemoglobin concentration; MCV, mean corpuscular volume; MRI, magnetic resonance imaging; RDA, recommended daily allowance; RDW, red cell distribution width; TfR, transferrin receptor; TIBC, total iron-binding capacity; TS, transferrin saturation; UIBC, unsaturated iron-binding capacity.

tions are involved, the c.854G→A (C282Y), and c.187C→G (H63D) substitutions. Increased transferrin saturation values, serum ferritin levels, and iron stores were found in a majority of homozygotes for the C282Y mutation and in many compound heterozygotes for C282Y/H63D or homozygotes for H63D. However, clinical manifestations, even among homozygotes for the C282Y mutation, are rare, in contrast to biochemical and/or histological manifestations of the increased iron levels, which are common. The penetrance of the C282Y homozygous state with respect to clinical manifestations is approximately 1 percent, and that of the other HFE genotypes is probably on the order of 0.01 percent. An earlier onset and a more severe type of hemochromatosis with high penetrance, juvenile hemochromatosis, is the result of mutations of the hemojuvelin or the hepcidin gene. Ferroportin-1 deficiency produces an autosomal dominant form of iron overload in which the iron is deposited chiefly in macrophages.

Iron can be removed from patients with hereditary hemochromatosis by serial phlebotomy but in patients with impaired erythropoiesis iron chelation therapy with either desferrioxamine or deferiprone is required.

Iron is a key element in the metabolism of all living organisms. In plants, ferredoxins are essential for an early step of photosynthesis. DNA synthesis requires the enzyme ribonucleotide reductase to convert ribonucleotides to deoxyribonucleotides. Neither bacteria nor nucleated cells proliferate when the supply of iron is insufficient. Iron is a part of heme, which is the active site of electron transport in cytochromes and cytochrome oxygenase, essential coenzymes in the Krebs cycle. Heme is also the site of O_2 uptake by myoglobin and hemoglobin, providing the means of O_2 transport to tissues. In the root nodules of legumes hemoglobin catalyzes the fixation of atmospheric N_2 by symbiotic bacteria. This is an important natural means of fertilization of soil and for synthesis of plant proteins. Heme is also the active site of peroxidases that protect cells from oxidative injury by reducing peroxides to water.

DISTRIBUTION OF IRON

The most important iron compartments are summarized in Table 40-1.

HEMOGLOBIN

Hemoglobin, which is 0.34 percent iron by weight, contains approximately 2 g of body iron in men and 1.5 g in women. One milliliter of packed erythrocytes contains approximately 1 mg of iron.

TABLE 40-1   IRON COMPARTMENTS IN NORMAL MAN*

COMPARTMENT	IRON CONTENT (MG)	TOTAL BODY IRON (%)
Hemoglobin iron	2000	67
Storage iron (ferritin, hemosiderin)	1000	27
Myoglobin iron	130	3.5
Labile pool	80	2.2
Other tissue iron	8	0.2
Transport iron	3	0.08

* Values represent estimates for an "average" person, that is, weight 70 kg, height 177 cm (70 inches). The values are derived from data in several sources.

STORAGE COMPARTMENT

Iron is stored either as ferritin or as hemosiderin. The former is water soluble; the latter is water insoluble. The protein shell apoferritin is composed of 24 similar or identical subunits arranged as 12 dimers forming a dodecahedron that approximates a hollow sphere (Fig. 40-1). The apoferritin monomers are of H (heavy) or L (light) type. L-monomers have 15 hydrophilic residues that may bind iron, thereby promoting its retention and serving as sites for ferrihydrite crystal growth. H-monomers have fewer hydrophilic residues but contribute an iron-binding histidyl to the intermonomeric pore (where iron atoms enter or exit). H-monomers have ferroxidase activity, thereby enabling apoferritin to take up or release iron quite rapidly. Apoferritin that is rich in H-monomers takes up iron more readily but retains it less avidly than does ferritin composed predominantly of L-monomers. Much of the storage iron in liver and spleen is in ferritin containing mostly L-monomers.

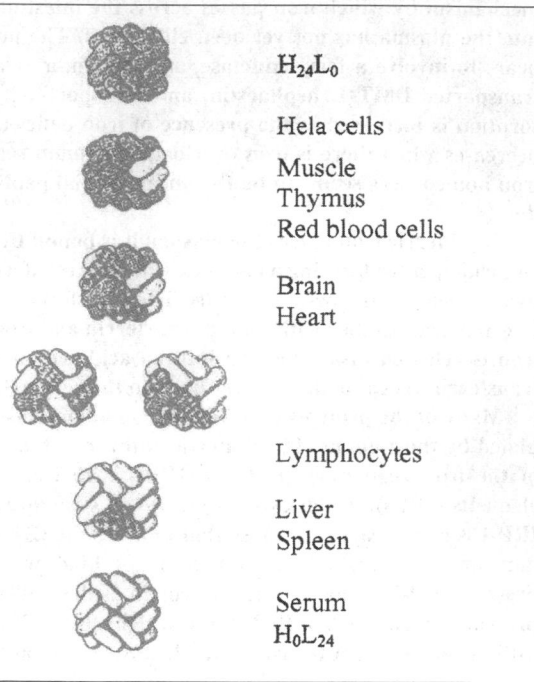

$H_{24}L_0$

Hela cells

Muscle
Thymus
Red blood cells

Brain
Heart

Lymphocytes

Liver
Spleen

Serum
H_0L_{24}

FIGURE 40-1   Schematic diagram of human "isoferritins" of different subunit compositions. Each ferritin subunit is depicted as a "sausage" and subunits are packed in a symmetrical shell. Twelve of the 24 subunits are visible. Mammalian ferritins are composed of two subunits of different primary structures, known as H and L. In the diagram, *stippled* subunits represent human H-chains, and *unstippled* subunits represent L-chains. H-chain and L-chain homopolymers are shown at the *top* and *bottom* of the figure, respectively. Heteropolymers of descending H content are placed between the homopolymers. Coassembly of the two subunit types is possible because many of the intersubunit contact residues are conserved. The sources of various ferritins are listed in the *right-hand column*, such that their average subunit compositions are indicated (e.g., muscle ferritin about 20 H 4 L, liver ferritin about 2–3 H: 22–21 L). Most of the data were obtained by immunoassay using H- or L-chain specific antisera. The composition of human brain ferritin was measured after subunit separation by gel electrophoresis. The pair of molecules in the *fourth position* indicates that subunits may be clustered differently in molecules of the same composition. *In vitro* assembly experiments indicate that dimers are a first assembly intermediate, and it is likely that these dimers are antiparallel pairs formed by association of subunits along their axes as shown here. It may be supposed that H-chains (or L-chains) forming on their polysomes would associate into homodimers before co-assembly into heteropolymers, although there is no evidence for this. (From PM Harrison, P Arosio,[670] with permission from Elsevier.)

Ferritin is found in virtually all cells of the body and also in tissue fluids. In blood plasma ferritin is present in minute concentration. It is glycosylated and largely composed of H subunits. The plasma (serum) ferritin concentration usually correlates roughly with total-body iron stores, making measurement of serum ferritin levels important in the diagnosis of disorders of iron metabolism. It has been suggested that the iron content of ferritin may vary with the size of iron stores,[1] but the value of this approach could not be confirmed.[2]

The size of the storage compartment is quite variable. Normally in adult men it amounts to 800 to 1000 mg; in adult women it is a few hundred milligrams. The mobilization of storage iron involves the reduction of Fe^{+++} to Fe^{++}, its release from the core crystal, and its diffusion out of the apoferritin shell. As it passes from cytosol to plasma, it must be reoxidized, either by hephaestin in the cell membrane or by ceruloplasmin in plasma, before it binds to transferrin.

Hemosiderin is found predominantly in macrophages. Microscopically, in unstained tissue sections or marrow films it appears as clumps or granules of golden refractile pigment. Hemosiderin contains approximately 25 to 30 percent iron by weight. Under pathologic conditions, it may accumulate in large quantities in almost every tissue of the body. Hemosiderin is heterogeneous and is structurally related to the mineral ferrihydrite.[3]

MYOGLOBIN

Myoglobin is structurally similar to hemoglobin, but it is monomeric: each myoglobin molecule consists of a heme group nearly surrounded by loops of a long polypeptide chain containing approximately 150 amino acid residues. It is present in small amounts in all skeletal and cardiac muscle cells, where it may serve as an oxygen reservoir to protect against cellular injury during periods of oxygen deprivation.

LABILE IRON POOL

The existence of a labile iron pool was postulated from studies of the rate of clearance of injected ^{59}Fe from plasma.[4,5] Iron leaves the plasma and enters the interstitial and intracellular fluid compartments for a brief time before it is incorporated into heme or storage compounds. Some of the iron reenters plasma, causing a biphasic curve of ^{59}Fe clearance 1 to 2 days after injection. The change in slope defines the size of the labile pool, normally 80 to 90 mg of iron. It is now sometimes considered to be equivalent to the chelatable iron pool.[6]

TISSUE IRON COMPARTMENT

Tissue iron normally amounts to 6 to 8 mg. This includes cytochromes and iron-containing enzymes. Although a small compartment, it is an extremely vital one that is sensitive to iron deficiency.[7–9]

TRANSPORT COMPARTMENT

From the standpoint of its total iron content, normally about 3 mg, the transport compartment of plasma is the smallest but the most active of the iron compartments: its iron normally turns over at least 10 times each day. This is a common pathway for interchange of iron between compartments.

Transferrins and lactoferrins comprise a group of glycoproteins that transport iron in plasma and in milk, respectively. They are single polypeptide chains with an M_r of approximately 80 kDa. Each molecule has two binding sites for Fe^{+++}. Each is bilobed, and within each lobe the iron-binding site is in a cleft between two domains that are designated N and C (for amino-terminal and carboxy-terminal). Thus, each complete transferrin or lactoferrin molecule has two N domains and two C domains. Within each lobe, Fe^{+++} is bound to both the N and C domains, which fold over and enclose the Fe^{+++}.[10,11] Normally,

approximately one third of the transferrin iron-binding sites are occupied by iron. About 200 mg (2.5 μmol) of transferrin, carrying about 100 μg (1.8 μmol) of iron per deciliter, is normally present in human plasma. Apotransferrin (transferrin devoid of iron) is synthesized by hepatocytes and by cells of the monocyte-macrophage system.[12,13] At least 30 genetically determined molecular variants of transferrin have been described in humans.[14] In most cases, their properties are normal, but there are exceptions,[15] and one relatively common transferrin variant has been found to be a risk factor for iron-deficiency anemia,[16] although its kinetic properties seem to be normal.[17]

DIETARY IRON

CONTENT

An average American male ingests 10 to 20 mg of iron daily[18,19] Table 40-2 shows daily requirements that are age and sex specific. The amount of iron absorbed by a normal adult male need only balance the small amount that is excreted, mostly in the stool, approximately 1 mg per day.[20] A higher iron requirement exists during growth periods or when there is blood loss. In women, iron absorbed must be sufficient to replace that lost through menstruation or diverted to the fetus during pregnancy.

The iron gained by food during cooking or other food processing is in the form of simple inorganic salts iron-amino acid complexes. Heme, as from hemoglobin and myoglobin, normally comprises about one-third of dietary iron.

BIOAVAILABILITY

Oxalates, phytates, and phosphates complex with iron and retard iron absorption, while simple reducing substances, among these hydroquinone, ascorbate, lactate, pyruvate, succinate, fructose, cysteine, and sorbitol,[21–23] increase iron absorption. The effect of ethanol on iron absorption seems to be relatively minor.[26,27] Red wine, contrary to popular belief, inhibits iron absorption,[28,29] probably because of the presence of polyphenols. Gastric secretion, the transit time, and mucus secretion all play roles in iron absorption.[30]

IRON ABSORPTION

Iron normally enters the body through the gastrointestinal tract, mostly through the duodenum. The amount of iron absorbed is normally tightly regulated according to body needs. Active erythropoiesis and/or iron deficiency up-regulates absorption; iron overload down-regulates absorption. The regulatory role that the intestine plays in iron homeostasis has been recognized since 1937,[31] but the mechanism of regulation has remained elusive.

TABLE 40-2 MINIMAL DAILY IRON REQUIREMENTS

	AMOUNTS THAT MUST BE ABSORBED DAILY FOR HEMOGLOBIN SYNTHESIS (MG)	MINIMAL AMOUNT THAT SHOULD BE INGESTED DAILY (MG)
Infants	1	10
Children	0.5	5
Young nonpregnant women	2	20
Pregnant women	3	30
Men and postmenopausal women	1	10

Gastric juice stabilizes dietary ferric ion, preventing its precipitation as insoluble ferric hydroxide.[32] This may result, in part, from chelation of Fe^{+++} by small molecules in the gastric juice, such as amino acids and keto sugars,[33,34] and by mucin.[35]

MECHANISM OF TRANSPORT ACROSS THE INTESTINAL MUCOSA

Understanding of the mechanism of iron absorption has been made more difficult by the fact that the pathways for the absorption of inorganic iron and for heme are different. These pathways do seem to merge within the intestinal cell, however, since the feeding of heme is not followed by the appearance of heme in the plasma.[36] The existence of a heme receptor on intestinal cells has been described,[37] but neither the putative receptor nor its function has been well characterized. The entry of iron into intestinal cells has been studied by the use of pulse-chase experiments, and the existence of a pathway in which a β_3-integrin and a protein designated mobilferrin are involved in transporting iron into the cell.[38] The partial amino acid sequence of the latter has been found to be that of calreticulin. These proteins are believed to form a complex that has been designated paraferritin (although it contains no ferritin) and which also contains the divalent metal transporter-1 (DMT-1). Paraferritin appears to have ferrireductase activity.[38] However, another protein, duodenal cytochrome b (dcytb) reductase,[39,40] that seems to reduce ferric iron to ferrous iron, has been characterized. Figure 40-2 illustrates some of the steps that are thought to be involved in iron transport across the mucosal cell.

MAINTENANCE OF IRON HOMEOSTASIS

The mechanism by which body iron content is regulated by modulation of iron absorption has been a subject of intense interest for the past 60 years, but the manner in which regulation is achieved has continued to be elusive. The concept of the existence of a "mucosal block", the notion that the administration of a dose of iron prevents any further absorption for a considerable period of time, was introduced in 1943,

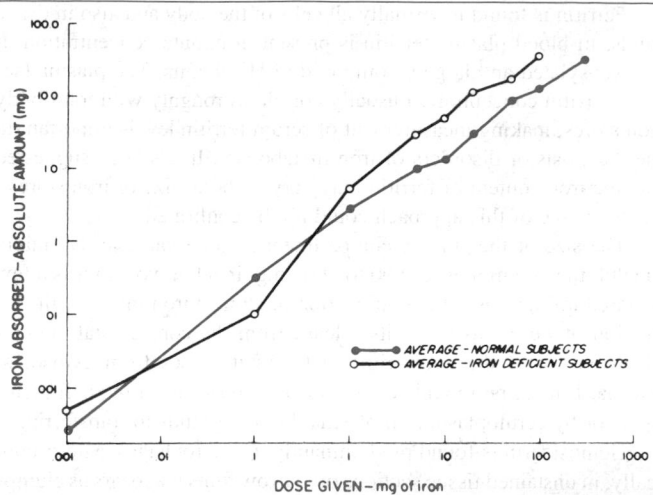

FIGURE 40-3   The relationship between oral iron dosage and amount of iron absorbed in humans. When the logarithm of the dose is plotted against the logarithm of the amount of iron absorbed, a rectilinear relationship is observed. Thus, at all levels, the greater the dose of iron, the more that it is absorbed, although the percent of the dose absorbed progressively declines. (Drawn from data of Smith and Pannacciuli.[43])

but was based on faulty experimental evidence.[41] In reality, no such block exists; for each increment in dose of an inorganic iron compound, there is a corresponding increment in the amount of iron absorbed (Fig. 40-3).[42,43] However, it is clear that there is a close relationship between iron need and iron dose, on the one hand and the amount of iron absorbed on the other[41] and the fact that this relationship exists is probably best designated as *mucosal intelligence*.

A number of genes that encode proteins with demonstrated effects on iron homeostasis have been identified (Table 40-3). To some extent, their role can be deduced from the effect of their deletion in human mutations or knockout mice or from their overproduction. Several different models incorporating these proteins in schemes of iron absorption and regulation of absorption have been proposed,[68,69] but their exact role has not yet been definitively assigned. It is postulated that iron is reduced by the duodenal cytochrome b5 and the ferrous iron is then transported into the cell by means of DMT-1. To exit into the plasma from the abluminal surface of the cell, the iron is reoxidized by hephaestin and transported from the cell by ferroportin.

How the rate and quantity of iron absorbed by the body through the gastrointestinal tract is regulated remains unclear. Because mutations of the *HFE* gene in man and its targeted disruption in the mouse results in iron accumulation, it was thought that hfe (the protein product of the *HFE* gene) might be the primary regulator of iron homeostasis. Its interaction with the transferrin receptor (TfR) may be a key to the function of the HFE molecule, but how this interaction functions to limit iron absorption from the small bowel remains unclear, in spite of several hypotheses that have been put forward. It has been proposed that the signal for iron absorption is built into the crypt cells of the intestinal mucosa[69,70] but the fact that the up-regulation of iron absorption as a response to hypoxia or anemia is more rapid than the lifespan of the enterocytes makes it unlikely that this is the only mechanism.[71]

The primary regulator of iron homeostasis may be hepcidin, an antimicrobial peptide that is only 20 to 25 amino acids in length and has four disulfide bonds.[72] Interdicting function of the gene encoding this peptide results in severe iron overload,[65] and mutations in humans result in juvenile hemochromatosis. A regulatory role for this peptide

INTESTINAL LUMEN

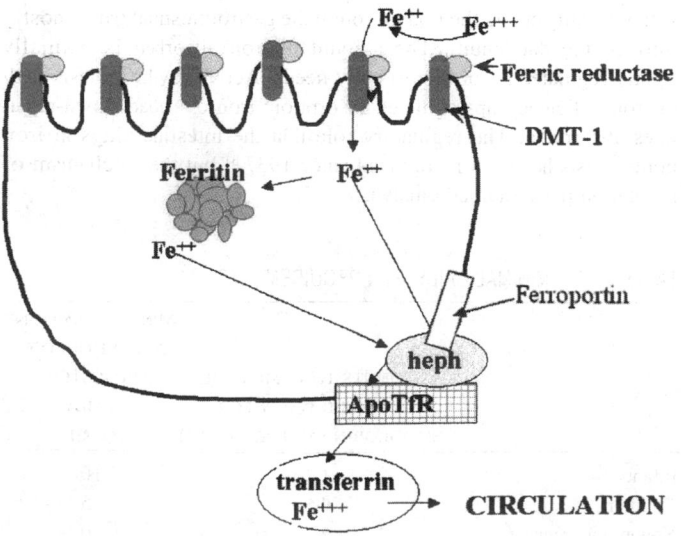

FIGURE 40-2   Schematic representation of iron uptake from the intestine and transfer to the plasma by an intestinal villus cell. The existence of an apotransferrin receptor has not been clearly demonstrated; it may be identical to the transferrin receptor. ApoTfR, apotransferrin receptor; heph, hephaestin.

TABLE 40-3   PROTEINS THAT PLAY A ROLE IN IRON HOMEOSTASIS

PROTEINS THAT AFFECT IRON HOMEOSTASIS IN MAN AND MOUSE	EFFECT OF DEFICIENCY	HUMAN DATA	MURINE DATA	COMMENTS
HFE	Fe Increased	44	45–47	Most patients with hereditary hemochromatosis are homozygous for the 845 A→G (C282Y) mutation of this gene
Ferroportin (SLC11A3)	Macrophage Fe increased	48		Autosomal dominant
β_2-microglobulin	Fe Increased		49,50	Believed to function by facilitating transport of hfe to membrane
Transferrin	Fe Increased	51,52	53	
Transferrin receptor-1	Lethal, central nervous system Fe increased	Unknown	45	
Transferrin receptor-2	Fe increased	54	55	
Hephaestin	Fe deficiency	Unknown	56	Sex-linked gene, deletion of exons is cause of *sla* mouse
Iron-regulatory protein-2 (IRP-2)	Fe increased	Unknown	57	Brain deposition
Ferritin H-chain	Fe increased	58		Dominant IRE mutation
Duodenal cytochrome B (dcytb)	Unknown		39	
Nramp1 (SLC11A1)	Alters iron distribution in macrophages	Unknown	59	Deficiency increases susceptibility to infection in mice
Nramp2 (DMT-1)	Fe deficiency	Unknown	60, 61	Same naturally occurring mutations found in the *mk* mouse and the Belgrade rat
Ceruloplasmin	Fe increased	62	63	Brain accumulation and neurologic disease
Hepcidin	Fe increased	64	65,66	May be the ultimate regulator of iron homeostasis, with respect to both total body iron and iron in infection
Hemojuvelin	Fe increased	67	Unknown	May be part of signaling pathway to hepcidin

is implied by the fact that it is markedly up-regulated in iron-loaded mice[66] and in humans with iron storage disease.[64] Overexpression of hepcidin results in marked iron-deficiency anemia in mice[73] and a refractory anemia resembling the anemia of chronic disease in humans,[74] and injection of synthetic hepcidin down-regulates iron absorption.[75] However, merely exposing hepatocytes to increased concentrations of iron does not up-regulate hepcidin,[76] it actually decreases the amount of hepcidin message.[66,77] Hepcidin mRNA expression is stimulated by erythropoietin, hypoxia, and inflammation.[77–79] An important exception to the rule that iron storage up-regulates hepcidin is the iron storage that occurs in *HFE* defects.[77,80,81] This implies that hfe may be a part of the signaling pathway to hepcidin. IL-1 and IL-6 stimulate hepcidin production by liver cells,[77,676] but it seems likely that this may be a property of the acute antimicrobial function of the peptide, serving to deprive bacteria of iron. It may be that in this way hepcidin plays an important role in the anemia of chronic infection (see Chap. 43). Ferroportin serves as the receptor for hepcidin. When hepcidin binds to ferroportin the latter transport molecule is internalized and undergoes proteolysis. As a result the capacity of cells to export iron is decreased.[677]

Hemojuvelin encoded by transcript LOC148738 on chromosome 1 may well be another protein in the signaling pathway to hepcidin; patients with juvenile hemochromatosis who have mutations of hemojuvelin manifest low hepcidin levels.[67]

TRANSPORT OF IRON

Once an atom of iron enters the body, it is virtually in a closed system (Fig. 40-4) in which it cycles almost endlessly from the plasma to the developing erythroblast (where it is utilized in hemoglobin synthesis), thence into the circulating blood for about 4 months, and then to phagocytic macrophages. Here it is removed from heme by heme oxygenase and released back into the plasma to repeat the cycle.

The major function of the transport protein transferrin is to move iron from wherever it enters the plasma (intestinal villi, splenic sinusoids) to the erythroblasts of the marrow and to other sites of utilization.

ENDOCYTOSIS OF TRANSFERRIN

Diferric transferrin binds to the transferrin receptor (TfR) on the cell surface, and the transferrin–TfR complex forms clusters in pits on the cell membrane.[82] The complex is then internalized by endocytosis (Fig. 40-5). Within the cytosol, the transferrin-TfR complex is in a clathrin coated vesicle. The vesicles fuse with endosomes, in which occur acidification and release of iron from transferrin. Transformation into lysosomes does not occur. Neither transferrin nor TfR is degraded in the process. Within the vesicle, a low pH (approximately pH 5) causes the release of one iron atom. The apotransferrin-TfR complex then returns to the cell membrane, where, at neutral pH, apotransferrin is released to the interstitial fluid to reenter plasma and take up more iron.[83]

The transferrin receptor is a protein consisting of two subunits that are linked by disulfide bonds.[84] It is a group II transmembrane protein: its amino-terminus is on the cytoplasmic side of the membrane and its carboxy-terminus, on the outer surface.[85] Because of the role of TfR in the binding and endocytosis of diferric transferrin, control of TfR biosynthesis is a major mechanism for regulation of iron metabolism. Synthesis of TfR is induced by iron deficiency or, experimentally, by incubation with an iron-chelating agent such as desferrioxamine. Conversely, synthesis of TfR is inhibited by heme.[86] The transferrin receptor binds to hfe,[87–89] the product of the *HFE* gene involved in hereditary hemochromatosis, but the functional consequences of this interaction are unclear.

IRON IN THE ERYTHROBLAST

Once within the developing erythroblast, iron must be transported to mitochondria to be incorporated into heme or taken up by ferritin within siderosomes. Within the vesicle, another protein (DMT-1; Nramp2) effects the release of Fe^{+++} into the cytosol, where it is taken up by mitochondria for heme synthesis.

Within mitochondria, iron is inserted into protoporphyrin by heme synthetase (ferrochelatase). When heme synthesis is impaired, as in lead poisoning or in the sideroblastic anemias (see Chap. 58), the mitochondria accumulate excessive amounts of amorphous iron aggregates.

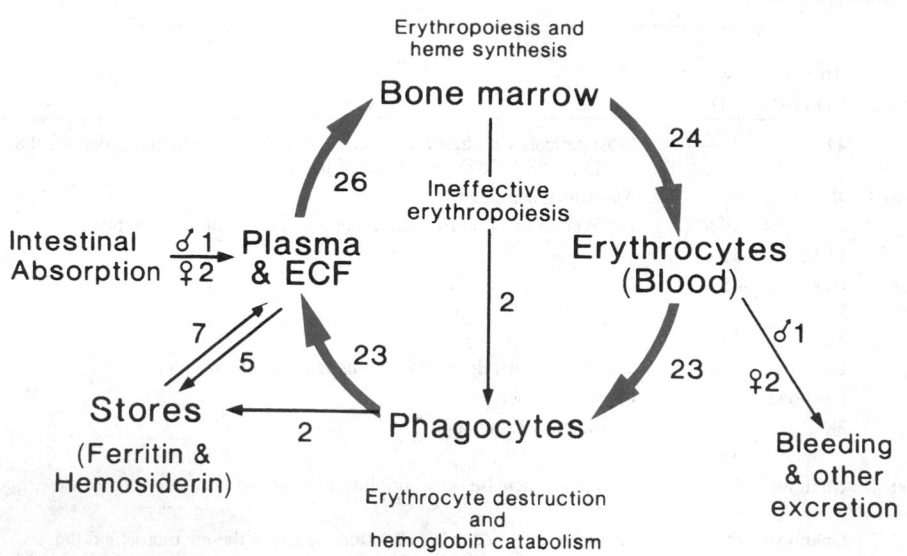

FIGURE 40-4   Iron cycle in humans. Iron is tightly conserved in a nearly closed system in which each iron atom cycles repeatedly from plasma and extracellular fluid (ECF) to the marrow, where it is incorporated into hemoglobin. Then it moves into the blood within erythrocytes and circulates for 4 months. It then travels to phagocytes of the reticuloendothelial system, where senescent erythrocytes are engulfed and destroyed, hemoglobin is digested, and iron is released to plasma, where the cycle continues. With each cycle, a small proportion of iron is transferred to storage sites, where it is incorporated into ferritin or hemosiderin, a small proportion of storage iron is released to plasma, a small proportion is lost in urine, sweat, feces, or blood, and an equivalent small amount of iron is absorbed from the intestinal tract. In addition, a small proportion (about 10%) of newly formed erythrocytes normally is destroyed within the bone marrow and its iron released, bypassing the circulating blood part of the cycle (ineffective erythropoiesis). The numbers indicate the approximate amount of iron (in milligrams) that enters and leaves each of these iron compartments every day in healthy adults who do not have bleeding and other blood disorders.

The mitochondria can then be stained by the Prussian blue reaction and are seen by light microscopy as a ring of large blue siderotic granules encircling the erythroblast nucleus (ringed sideroblast). In normal marrow, siderotic granules are also demonstrable in erythroblast cytoplasm. However, these are very small, usually only one to three in number, and randomly distributed in the cytoplasm. These normal siderotic granules are ferritin aggregates located in lysosomal organelles designated siderosomes.[90] Erythroblasts containing these siderotic granules, *sideroblasts*, normally represent 20 to 50 percent of the erythrocyte precursors of the marrow and are visualized by light microscopy. In iron deficiency and in the anemia that accompanies chronic disorders, sideroblasts almost disappear from the marrow. Conversely, in some states of iron overload characterized by dyserythropoiesis, they may become more numerous and contain more siderotic granules than normal.

INTRACELLULAR REGULATION OF IRON METABOLISM

The synthesis of apoferritin, TfR, δ-aminolevulinic acid (ALA) synthase, apotransferrin, aconitase, DMT-1 and ferroportin is regulated posttranscriptionally. The mRNA for each of these proteins contains one or several iron-responsive elements, or IREs. If the IRE is located at the 5′ end of the mRNA it serves to regulate translation; 3′ IREs regulate the stability of the mRNA. Each IRE consists of a stem and loop structure, in which the loop is the nucleotide sequence CAGUGC (Fig. 40-6). The apoferritin mRNA has, as its IRE, a single stem-loop structure in the 5′ (upstream) untranslated region. In contrast to the apoferritin IRE, there are as many as five stem-loops present in the 3′ (downstream) untranslated portion of TfR mRNA.[91] The IREs exert their effect by binding one of the two iron regulatory proteins (IRPs).

IRP-1 is cytoplasmic aconitase with four iron–sulfur clusters and the ability to bind iron, which is required for its aconitase activity. IRP-2 is highly homologous to IRP-1 but differs by the presence of a 73-amino-acid insertion in the N-terminus and a lack of aconitase activity. In the absence of iron, IRP-1 binds to IREs, but in its presence becomes a cytoplasmic aconitase. IRP-2, on the other hand, is proteolyzed in the presence of iron. Nitric oxide has an effect on the IRE/IRP system. It increases binding of IRP-1 to IREs and enhances degradation of IRP-2, therefore exerting contradictory effects on the regulation of protein synthesis. Moreover, nitric oxide may also destabilize IRP-2.[92–94]

Although the first-discovered IRP-1 has received the most attention, the importance of IRP-2 is emphasized by the fact that targeted disruption of the gene that encodes this protein causes a severe adult-onset neurologic disorder, whereas disruption of IRP-1 causes no obvious phenotype.[95] The effect of binding of IRPs to 3′ IREs is to increase the stability of the mRNA and thus to enhance the synthesis of the gene product; conversely, when the iron content of cytosol is high, the displacement of IRPs from these IREs leads to decreased synthesis of these proteins. Figure 40-7 illustrates these relationships for the regulation of synthesis of apoferritin and TfR.

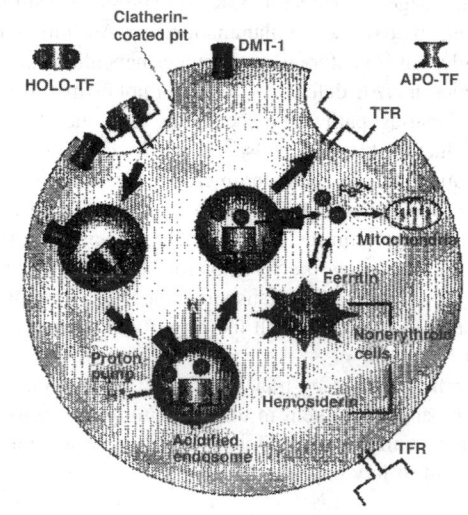

FIGURE 40-5   The transferrin cycle. Holotransferrin (HOLO-TF) binds to transferrin receptors (TfR) on the cell surface. The complexes localize to clathrin-coated pits, which invaginate to initiate endocytosis. Specialized endosomes form and become acidified through the action of a proton pump. Acidification leads to protein conformational changes that release iron from transferrin. Acidification also enables proton-coupled iron transport out of the endosomes through the activity of the divalent metal transporter-1 protein (DMT-1). Subsequently, apotransferrin (APO-TF) and the transferrin receptor both return to the cell surface, where they dissociate at neutral pH. Both proteins participate in further rounds of iron delivery. In nonerythroid cells, iron is stored as ferritin and hemosiderin. (From NC Andrews,[671] with permission from Nature Reviews Drug Discovery, 2000, Macmillan Magazines Ltd.)

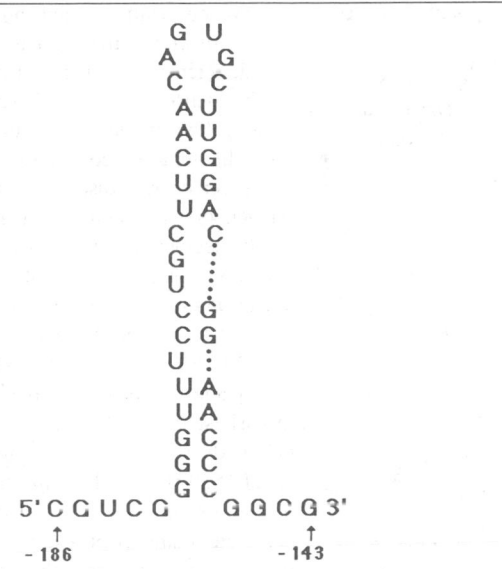

```
        G U
      A     G
      C     C
      A     U
      A     U
      C     G
      U     G
      U     A
      C     C
      G     :
      U     C     G
      C     G
      U     A
      U     A
      G     C
      G     C
      G C
5'CGUCG     GGCG3'
      ↑           ↑
    -186        -143
```

FIGURE 40-6   Stem-loop structure that is the iron-responsive element of apoferritin mRNA. (From MW Hentze, SW Canylunan, JL Casey, et al.,[672] with permission.)

In addition to mechanisms for regulation of iron metabolism at the mRNA level, the expression of some genes is regulated at the transcriptional level. Although the mechanism of transcriptional regulation is not well understood, it may operate, in some cases, by virtue of the ability of iron to generate oxygen free radicals.[96]

ROLE OF THE MONOCYTE-MACROPHAGE SYSTEM

Destruction of aged erythrocytes and hemoglobin degradation occur within macrophages (see Chap. 31). This proceeds at a rate sufficient to release from the cell to the plasma compartment approximately 20 percent of the hemoglobin iron within a few hours. Approximately 80 percent of this iron is rapidly reincorporated into hemoglobin. Thus, 19 to 69 percent of the hemoglobin iron of nonviable erythrocytes reappears in circulating red cells in 12 days. The remainder of the iron enters the storage pool as ferritin or hemosiderin and then turns over very slowly. In normal subjects, approximately 40 percent of this iron remains in storage after 140 days. When there is an increased iron demand for hemoglobin synthesis, however, storage iron may be mobilized more rapidly.[97] Conversely, in the presence of infection, other inflammatory process, or malignancy, iron is much more slowly reutilized in hemoglobin synthesis.[97-100]

IRON EXCRETION

The body conserves iron with remarkable efficiency. Most iron loss occurs by way of desquamated intestinal cells in the feces and it normally amounts to about 1 mg per day, less than one thousandth of total body iron. Exfoliation of skin and dermal appendages and perspiration result in much smaller losses. Even in tropical climates, the loss of iron in sweat is minimal.[101] Very small amounts of iron are lost in the urine. Lactation may cause excretion of about 1 mg iron daily, thus doubling the overall rate of iron loss. Blood loss by normal menstruation contributes to negative iron balance.

Although total daily iron loss is normally about 1 mg for males,[20] it averages about 2 mg for menstruating women. Persons with marked

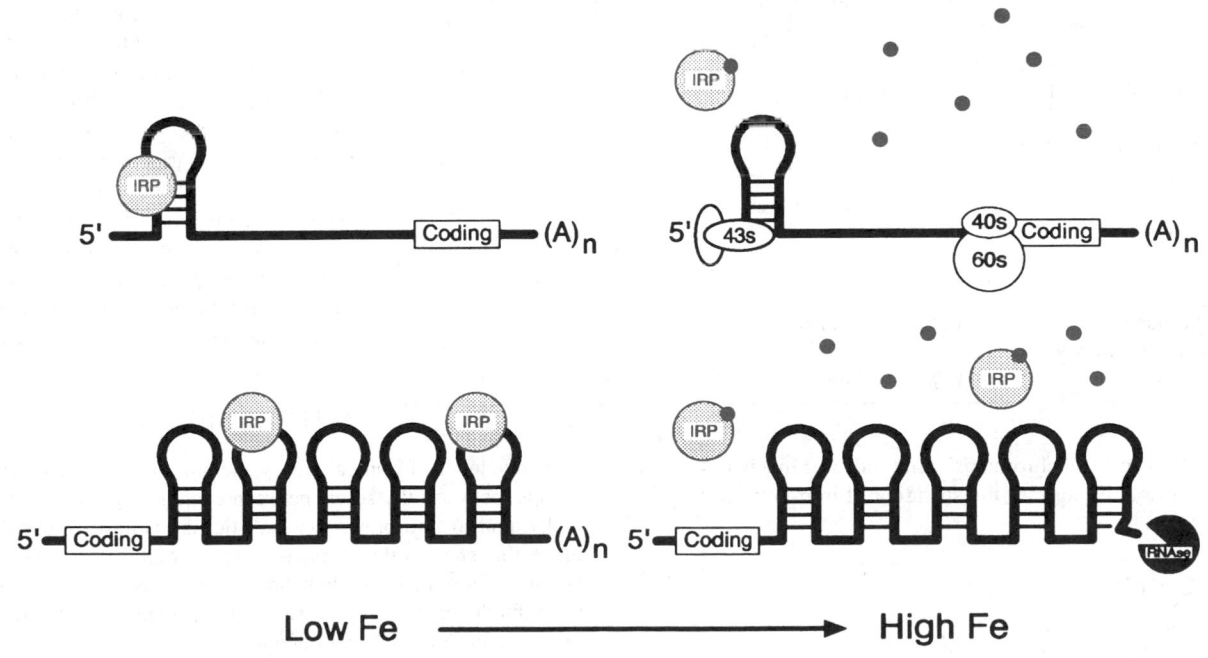

Low Fe ⟶ High Fe

FIGURE 40-7   Regulation of iron metabolism at the cytoplasmic mRNA level by interaction of iron regulatory protein (IRP-1) and the iron responsive elements (IREs) to apoferritin mRNA (top) and transferrin receptor (TfR) mRNA (bottom). When the cytoplasmic iron concentration is low (left side of illustration), IRP-1 binds to the IREs of both mRNAs. This represses the translation of apoferritin mRNA, where the IRE is at the 5' end of the mRNA, thereby reducing the amount of apoferritin formed. It stabilizes and increases the translation of TfR mRNA, where the IRE is at the 3' end of the mRNA, thereby increasing the amount of TfR formed. Conversely, when there is an abundance of iron in the cytoplasm (right side of illustration), IRP-1 is displaced from both species of mRNA. This results in derepression of apoferritin synthesis and destabilization and degradation of TfR mRNA. (Modified from AS Knisely,[673] with permission from Mosby/Year Book.)

TABLE 40-4   PREVALENCE OF IRON DEFICIENCY AND IRON DEFICIENCY ANEMIA IN SOME SELECTED POPULATIONS

POPULATION	SEX	AGE GROUP	IRON DEFICIENCY	IRON DEFICIENCY ANEMIA
Chile[106]		Full-term infants	30.7	22.6
Inner City, USA[107]		Third and fourth graders	2.9	1
Sweden[108]	F	15–16 years	40	
	M		15	
USA (1999–2000)[109]		1–2	7	2
		2–4	5	
		6–11	4	
	M	12–15	5	
	M	16–69	2	
	M	>70	3	
	F	12–49	12	3
	F	50–69	9	3
	F	>70	6	1
Canada[110]		Infants		4.3
Southern California HFE wt/wt[111]	F	26–49	12.4	3.2
	M	26–95	0.7	0.4
USA (1988–1994)[112]		1–2		
		3–5		<1
		6–11		<1
	F	12–15		2
		16–19		3
		20–49		
		50–69		
		>70		
	M	12–15		<1
		16–19	<1	<1
		20–49	<1	<1
		50–69		1
		>70		2
Columbia school children and adolescents[113]	F, M	6–18	4.9	0.6
Mexican pregnant and adolescents[114]	F	11–17		80
Ethiopian lactating women[115]	F	28.4 ± 6.12		22.3
Iranian children[116]	F, M	6 months–5 years		19.7
Belgian pregnant women[117]	F	15–44		
Trimester 1				1.5
Trimester 3				23
New Zealand children[118]	F, M	6–24 months	5.6	4.3
South African factory workers[119]	F	18–55	40	27.4
Urban New Zealand[118]	F, M	6–24 months	18.6	5.6

uration, but without frank anemia. *Iron-deficiency anemia* is the most advanced stage of iron deficiency. It is characterized by decreased or absent iron stores, low serum iron concentration, low transferrin saturation, and low blood hemoglobin concentration.

In certain rare disorders, such as idiopathic pulmonary hemosiderosis or paroxysmal nocturnal hemoglobinuria (see Chap. 38), iron-deficiency anemia may occur without iron depletion as a result of redistribution of body iron, and thus its inaccessibility for hemoglobin synthesis.

The clinical manifestations of iron-deficiency anemia appear to have been recognized in earliest times. A disease characterized by pallor, dyspnea, and edema was described in about 1500 B.C. in the *Papyrus Ebers*, a manual of therapeutics believed to be the oldest complete manuscript extant.[102] This ancient disease may have been due to chronic blood loss from hookworm infestation. Chlorosis, or "green sickness," was well known to European physicians after the middle of the 16th century. In France, by the middle of the 17th century, iron salts and other remedies (including, oddly enough, phlebotomy) were used in its treatment. Not long thereafter, iron was recommended by Sydenham as a specific remedy for chlorosis. For the 100 years preceding 1930, iron was used in the treatment of chlorosis, often in ineffective doses, although the mechanism of action of iron and the appropriateness of its use were highly controversial.

By the beginning of the 20th century, it had been established that chlorosis was characterized by a decrease in the iron content of the blood and by the presence of hypochromic erythrocytes, but it was not until the classic 1932 studies by Heath, Strauss, and Castle[103] that it was shown that the response of anemia to iron was stoichometrically related to the amount of iron given and that chlorosis was, indeed, iron deficiency. The history of iron deficiency has been reviewed in greater detail elsewhere.[41,104]

EPIDEMIOLOGY

The prevalence of iron-deficiency anemia varies so much between age groups, between the sexes, between economic groups, and by geography, that overall prevalence statistics are almost meaningless. Estimates that suggest that as many as three fourths of the world's population is iron deficient have been made, but these estimates are undoubtedly extravagant.[105] Table 40-4 provides some data regarding the prevalence in different populations.

iron overload, as in hemochromatosis, may lose as much as 4 mg of iron daily, probably because of the shedding of iron-laden cells, principally macrophages.

IRON DEFICIENCY

DEFINITION AND HISTORY

Iron deficiency is the state in which the content of iron in the body is less than normal. It occurs in varying degrees of severity that merge imperceptibly into one another. Iron depletion is the earliest stage of iron deficiency, in which storage iron is decreased or absent but serum iron concentration, transferrin saturation and blood hemoglobin levels are normal. Iron deficiency without anemia is a somewhat more advanced stage of iron deficiency, characterized by decreased or absent storage iron, usually low serum iron concentration and transferrin sat-

ETIOLOGY AND PATHOGENESIS

ETIOLOGY

Iron deficiency may occur as a result of chronic blood loss, inadequate dietary iron intake, malabsorption of iron, diversion of iron to fetal and infant erythropoiesis during pregnancy and lactation, intravascular hemolysis with hemoglobinuria, or a combination of these factors. Genetic factors seem to be important, also, based upon twin studies.[120]

With the exception of a transferrin polymorphism that increases the risk of developing iron-deficiency anemia[16] and a platelet collagen receptor polymorphism,[121] the nature of the putative genetic factors that influence iron deficiency remains unknown.

Bleeding   Gastrointestinal. In men and in postmenopausal women. iron deficiency is most commonly caused by chronic bleeding from the gastrointestinal tract. A list of causes of such blood loss is presented in Table 40-5. In the adult the most common causes of gastrointestinal bleeding are peptic ulcer, hiatal hernia, gastritis (including that due to alcohol or aspirin ingestion), hemorrhoids, vascular anomalies (such as angiodysplasia), and neoplasms. In one study of 114 outpatients referred to gastroenterologists for investigation of iron deficiency, 45 had upper gastrointestinal and 18 colonic sources of bleeding.[122] In 100 other patients in whom the site of bleeding could not be established by any means short of laparotomy, a malignancy was found to be the cause in 10 percent.[123] Enteritis after therapeutic irradiation of abdominal viscera may also be a cause of gastrointestinal bleeding leading to iron-deficiency anemia.[173] Colon cancer, colonic diverticula, periampullary tumors, leiomyomas, adenomas, and other malignant or benign neoplasms of the intestine are among the causes of chronic blood loss.[124–128]

TABLE 40 5   SOURCES OF BLOOD LOSS

Respiratory tract
  Carcinoma
  Epistaxis
  Idiopathic pulmonary hemosiderosis
  Infections
  Telangiectases
Alimentary tract
  Esophagus
    Varices
  Stomach
    Angiodysplasia
    Antral vascular ectasia
    Carcinoma
    Gastritis
    Hemangioma
    Hiatus hernia
    Hypergastrinemia
    Leiomyoma (Ménétrier disease)
    Mucosal hypertrophy
    Ulcer
    Varices
    "Watermelon stomach"
  Colon
    Amebiasis
    Angiodysplasia
    Carcinoma
    Diverticulum
    Hemangioma
    Polyps
    Telangiectasia
    Ulcerative colitis
Biliary tract
  Aberrant pancreas
  Carcinoma
  Cholelithiasis
  Intrahepatic bleeding
  Ruptured aneurysm
  Trauma

Diaphragmatic Hernia. Diaphragmatic (hiatal) hernia frequently is associated with gastrointestinal bleeding. The frequency of anemia ranges from 8 to 38 percent.[129–132] Bleeding is much more likely to occur in patients with paraesophageal or large hernias than in those with sliding hernias or small ones.[129,130,133] It is likely that hemorrhage follows mucosal injury at the neck of the sac, where the herniated stomach rides to and fro over the crus of the diaphragm during respiration.[129,130,132] Mucosal changes cannot always be demonstrated by esophagoscopy or gastroscopy in patients who have had blood loss from hiatus hernia. However, a linear gastric erosion, also called a "Cameron ulcer," commonly occurs on the crests of mucosal folds at the level of the diaphragm and appears to be the site of bleeding. In a series of 109 cases of large diaphragmatic hernias, one third had linear erosions, and most of these patients were anemic.[133]

Gastritis. Gastritis resulting from drug ingestion is another common cause of bleeding. Aspirin ingestion is as likely to cause bleeding in patients without preexisting ulcer as in those with peptic ulcer.[134] Other medications (e.g., glucocorticoids, indomethacin, ibuprofen, other nonsteroidal antiinflammatory drugs) may also cause bleeding by inducing gastric or duodenal ulcers or colitis.[135] Gastritis resulting from alcohol ingestion may also cause significant blood loss.

Varices. Chronic blood loss from esophageal or gastric varices may lead to iron-deficiency anemia. Chronic blood loss is often the cause of anemia in rheumatoid arthritis (perhaps a result of the aspirin or glucocorticoid therapy), ulcerative colitis, and regional enteritis.[136] Hemorrhoidal bleeding may lead to severe iron-deficiency anemia. Chronic blood loss may result from diffuse gastric mucosal hypertrophy (Ménétrier disease).[137]

Gastric and Duodenal Ulcers. Peptic ulcers of the stomach or duodenum are common causes of iron deficiency, and an association between infection with *Helicobacter pylori* and iron-deficiency anemia has been documented in numerous studies.[138] Surprisingly, it has been found in some studies, one of them controlled,[139] that putative iron-deficient patients infected with *H. pylori* do not respond to oral iron alone but do respond to eradication of *H. pylori*. This has been interpreted as suggesting that the organism itself may sequester iron and render it unavailable for absorption.[138] This would require sequestration of an enormous amount of iron, and an alternative explanation may be that response to this particular organism results in laboratory findings that simulate iron deficiency, but that this represents a subset of anemia of chronic infection. Indeed, some have considered the evidence of a causal association between *H. Pylo*ri and iron deficiency unproven.[140]

Gastric ulceration and bleeding may also occur in disorders of hypergastrinemia, as in Zollinger-Ellison syndrome and pseudo–Zollinger-Ellison syndrome.[141] Intestinal parasitism, particularly by hookworms, is a major cause of gastrointestinal blood loss in many parts of the world.[142] Achlorhydria seems common in such patients[143] and may play a role.

Anemia that follows subtotal gastrectomy has usually been attributed to reduced absorption of dietary iron[144] (see "Malabsorption" below), but occult intermittent gastrointestinal bleeding may also be a contributory factor. Of eight patients whose erythrocytes were labeled with $Na_2^{51}CrO_4$ to permit precise quantitation of daily fecal blood loss,[145] seven were shown to lose from 3.2 to 6.5 ml of blood per day. This is a very slight but significant increase in daily fecal blood loss that over a span of several years could well lead to iron-deficiency anemia. Chemical tests for fecal blood loss are usually insensitive to a daily loss of less than 5 to 10 ml of blood, although the sensitivity of the test depends to some extent on the site of bleeding within the gastrointestinal tract.

Vascular Anomalies. The lesions of angiodysplasia may occur in any part of the gastrointestinal tract but are most frequent in the cecum or ascending colon.[146] These tiny vascular anomalies may be the cause of significant blood loss. Endoscopy is usually required for diagnosis.[146] Gastric antral vascular ectasia exhibits a characteristic endoscopic appearance ("watermelon stomach") and is another cause of blood loss.[147,148] Hemorrhage into the gallbladder is a rare cause of chronic iron-deficiency anemia.[126]

Tortuous, dilated sublingual venous structures, the cherry hemangiomas commonly seen in the elderly, and the spider telangiectases of chronic liver disease are usually easily distinguished from the lesions of hereditary hemorrhagic telangiectasia. Bleeding from intestinal telangiectases has also been observed in scleroderma[149] and Turner syndrome[150] as a manifestation of bleeding from abnormal blood vessels. Cutaneous hemangiomas (blue rubber bleb nevus) may be associated with hemorrhage from intestinal hemangiomas.[151–153]

In hereditary hemorrhagic telangiectasia (see Chap. 114 and Color Plates XXV-41 and 42), characteristic lesions commonly occur on fingertips, nasal septum, tongue, lips, margins (helices) of ears, oral and pharyngeal mucosa, palms and soles, and other epithelial and cutaneous surfaces throughout the body. Those lesions that occur in the gastrointestinal tract are particularly likely to bleed and to cause iron deficiency.

Bleeding Disorders. Hemostatic defects, particularly those related to abnormal platelet function or number, may lead to gastrointestinal bleeding. Gastrointestinal bleeding is common in von Willebrand disease (see Chap. 118). Polycythemia vera is typically associated with iron deficiency as a result either of spontaneous gastrointestinal hemorrhage that commonly occurs in this disorder, or phlebotomy therapy, or both mechanisms (see Chap. 56).

When a patient with a disorder of hemostasis suffers from gastrointestinal bleeding, one must consider the possibility that the bleeding may not be caused by a hemostatic defect alone, but that an anatomic lesion of the gastrointestinal tract may also be present.

Cow's Milk Anemia. Ingestion of whole cow's milk may induce protein-losing enteropathy and gastrointestinal bleeding in infants,[154,155] probably on the basis of hypersensitivity or allergy. In four such cases observed endoscopically, erosive gastritis or gastroduodenitis was demonstrated as the probable source of bleeding.[156] At least during the first year of life, children should not be given whole bovine milk, either raw or pasteurized.[154,155,157] More protracted heating, as in preparation of infant formulas, eliminates this problem. Intrinsic lesions of the gastrointestinal tract, such as those listed above, may cause bleeding in infants and in older children as well. In infants or small children, peptic ulcer is an uncommon cause of gastrointestinal bleeding. Because Meckel diverticulum is usually not demonstrated by gastrointestinal x-ray examination, it is easily overlooked as a cause of gastrointestinal hemorrhage.

Respiratory Tract. Recurrent hemoptysis may lead to iron-deficiency anemia. It may be caused by congenital anomalies of the respiratory tract, endobronchial vascular anomalies, chronic infections, neoplasms, or valvular heart disease. Severe iron-deficiency anemia is a manifestation of idiopathic pulmonary hemosiderosis and Goodpasture syndrome (progressive glomerulonephritis with intrapulmonary hemorrhage).[158] In some of these disorders, hemoptysis may not be observed, but sufficient amounts of blood-laden sputum may be swallowed to result in positive tests for occult blood in the stools. Iron deficiency occurs in a large proportion of patients with cystic fibrosis, and is related to the volume of sputum but not to the degree of pancreatic insufficiency, suggesting that iron loss in sputum may play an important role.[159]

Genitourinary Tract. Menstrual bleeding is a very common cause of iron deficiency.[160] The amount of blood lost with menstruation varies markedly from one woman to another and is often difficult to evaluate by questioning the patient. The average menstrual blood loss is about 40 ml per cycle. Blood loss exceeds 80 ml (equivalent to about 30 mg of iron) per cycle in only 10 percent of women.[161] The volume of blood lost in the course of one menstrual cycle may be as high as 495 ml in apparently healthy, nonanemic women who do not regard their menstrual flow to be excessive. The amount of menstrual blood lost does not seem to vary markedly from one cycle to another for any given individual.[162] Oral contraceptives reduce menstrual blood loss,[163,164] but the uUse of an intrauterine coil for contraception increases menstrual blood loss,[165] especially during the first year of use. Because absorption of 1 mg of iron per day requires a dietary intake of between 10 and 20 mg of iron, it is easy to understand why, with an average dietary iron intake of approximately 10 mg per day, iron balance in many menstruating women is precarious.

Excessive bleeding may be caused by uterine fibroids and malignant neoplasms. Neoplasms, stones, or inflammatory disease of the kidney, ureter, or bladder may cause enough chronic blood loss to produce iron deficiency. In one unusual case, urinary iron loss was documented after red cell transfusions.[166]

Factitious Anemia. Factitious anemia resulting from self-inflicted bleeding may present a formidable diagnostic and therapeutic problem. This rare condition has also been called, in literary allusion to a fictitious character, "Lasthénie de Ferjol syndrome." (In Barbey d'Aurevilly's gloomy novel, *Une Histoire Sans Nom,* Lasthénie de Ferjol was a young woman noted for extreme pallor and languor, who habitually and secretly practiced auto-desanguination by thrusting needles into her heart.) Most patients are women. There is often a history of numerous blood transfusions. The anemia is chronic and may be severe, with blood hemoglobin concentration persistently as low as 5 to 6 g/dl. The site of induced blood loss is obscure. Hence, patients are subjected to numerous radiographic and endoscopic examinations, usually to no avail. The patients are usually refractory to medical advice and therapy.[167,168] The patients may be depressed and suicidal; some also suffer anorexia nervosa. Psychiatric care is needed, but often is unsuccessful. Rarely the outcome of self-bleeding may be fatal.[168]

Nosocomial (Iatrogenic) Anemia. During the course of medical care, repetitive blood sampling may result in removal of a large amount of blood,[169,170] and this iatrogenic phlebotomy can result in iron-deficiency anemia.

Anemia Incident to Blood Donation. Each whole blood donation removes about 200 mg of iron from the body. Lesser amounts of iron are removed in the course of donating platelets or leukocytes. Potential donors are screened in blood banks, so that those with frank anemia are not phlebotomized. Yet by the time they are excluded from donation, some blood donors are iron depleted and may readily develop iron-deficiency anemia with relatively small additional blood loss.[171,172]

Pregnancy and Parturition In pregnancy, the average iron loss resulting from diversion of iron to the fetus, blood loss at delivery (equivalent to an average of 150–200 mg of iron), and lactation is altogether about 900 mg; in terms of iron content, this is equivalent to the loss of over 2 liters of blood. Approximately 30 mg of iron may be expended monthly in lactation. Because most women begin pregnancy with low iron reserves, these additional demands frequently result in iron deficiency anemia. Iron depletion has been reported in 85 to 100 percent of pregnant women. The incidence is lower in women who take oral iron supplementation.[173–175] Iron-deficient mothers are likely to have smaller babies with low iron reserves.[176–179] Although some groups have suggested that routine iron supplementation of pregnant women is not indicated,[180] most experts seem to agree that iron supplementation during pregnancy is desirable, but it is often neglected.[181]

Dietary Iron Deficiency In infants, iron deficiency is most often a result of the use of unsupplemented milk diets, which contain an inadequate amount of iron. During the first year of life, the full-term infant requires approximately 160 mg and the premature infant about 240 mg of iron to meet the needs of an expanding red cell mass. About 50 mg of this need is met by the destruction of erythrocytes, which occurs physiologically during the first week of life. The rest must come from the diet. Milk products are very poor sources of iron, and prolonged breast-feeding or bottle feeding of infants frequently leads to iron-deficiency anemia unless there is iron supplementation. This is especially true of premature infants. Table 40-6 lists the iron content of several widely used infant foods. In recognition of the high prevalence of iron deficiency and its adverse effects, when infant formula is not iron supplemented, the American Academy of Pediatrics[182] has urged that all infant formulas be iron fortified; unfortunately, this practice is not universal in North America. In older children, an iron-poor diet may also contribute to the development of iron-deficiency anemia, particularly during rapid growth periods.

Estimates of average daily iron intake for various segments of the U.S. population are shown in Table 40-7. These estimates used surveys based on 24-hour recall of the food intake of participants and then estimated the iron intake from the known content of the foods consumed. For most persons in the United States, iron intake is approximately 5 to 7 mg/1000 cal. Children and young women are usually in precarious iron balance, their iron intake being less than 80 percent of the recommended daily allowance (RDA).[183] Fortification of bread and cereals with ferrous sulfate or metallic iron[184] has become commonplace. When this practice has been suspended because of concern for the possibility of increasing iron storage in patients with the hemochromatosis genotype, the result has been an increased incidence of iron-deficiency anemia.[185]

The scant iron supply of the American diet places young women and children at particular risk of negative iron balance (see Table 40-7). Among men in the 18- to 20-year age range, iron deficiency may be found without bleeding, presumably because of the iron demands imposed by the recent growth spurt.[186] Because the adult male needs to absorb only about 1 mg iron daily from his diet in order to maintain

TABLE 40-6   IRON CONTENT OF INFANT FOODS

LIQUID FOOD	IRON CONTENT (MG/LITER)*
Breast milk	1.1
Evaporated milk	1.8
Evaporated milk, diluted 13:19	0.7
Whole cow's milk	0.7
Similac™, "low iron"	1.3
Similac™, "with iron"	11.5
Enfamil™, "low iron"	0.45
Enfamil™, "with iron"	11.5

SEMISOLID FOOD	IRON CONTENT (MG/SERVING)†
Cereal, various (Gerber)	6.75
Purees	
Vegetables	0–0.60
Meat and vegetable mixes	0.30–1.20

* For commercially prepared infant formulas, iron content is as stated by manufacturer in 1999. The brand-name products listed are examples only and do not imply endorsement by the authors.

† For cereal and puree preparations, iron content was calculated from statement of the manufacturer, ambiguously expressed as "percent of daily amount." Communication with Gerber Products, Inc., indicated that the "daily amount" is 15 mg, i.e., the old RDA, which is 2.5-fold greater than the current RDA for infants. Thus, the many (Gerber) cereal products examined, whether wheat, rice, or mixed grains, all contain (according to the manufacturer) 6.75 mg of reduced iron per 15 g of dry powder (500 ppm), which is intended to be mixed with water, milk, or formula in volume up to 250 ml, for each serving.

TABLE 40-7   DAILY DIETARY IRON INTAKE IN THE UNITED STATES (MEAN VALUES FOR SELECTED GROUPS)*

AGE/SEX	ESTIMATED FE INTAKE/ (MG/DAY)	RECOMMENDED DAILY ALLOWANCE (MG)	% OF RECOMMENDED ALLOWANCE
Infant, 6–11 months	11.9	6	200
Child, 1–2 years	8.4	10	84
Female, 14–30 years	10.5	15	70
Female, pregnant	14	30	47
Female, lactating	14	15	93
Female, 60–65 years	10.2	10	102
Male, ≥12 years	>12	12	>100

* Modified from data obtained from 1982–1984 and published in "Mineral Contents of Foods and Total Diets: The Selected Minerals in Foods Survey, 1982 to 1984"[19], and from data collected from 1989–1990 in the Third National Health and Nutrition Examination Survey, NHANES-III. The data obtained in these two large surveys, which were undertaken 7 years apart, provided nearly identical results. Hence, they have been combined in this table. Note that, in the latter survey, RDAs for iron were based on the RDAs recommended in 1989, following substantial reduction in the estimated dietary iron requirements for infants, children, and young females. Differences between ethnic groups were negligible. To simplify the table, results for all males age 12 years and older were combined because of only minimal differences between the age groups. A similar simplification was made by combining data for all females in the age range 14–30 years, exclusive of those who were pregnant or lactating.

normal iron balance, iron deficiency in older men is only very rarely caused by insufficient dietary intake alone. Exceptions to this rule are known, such as the case of a man who remained on a nearly iron-free diet for 27 years.[187]

Malabsorption of Iron   Gastric secretion of hydrochloric acid is often reduced in iron deficiency.[188–191] Histamine-fast achlorhydria has been found in as many as 43 percent of patients with iron deficiency.[149,191] Gastric function may improve after correction of the iron deficiency, so that iron deficiency may be both a cause and a result of impairment of gastric iron secretion. However, in persons over the age of 30 the achlorhydria is usually irreversible.[192] Furthermore, when atrophic gastritis coexists with iron deficiency, no improvement in gastric secretory function has followed iron therapy.[193]

Intestinal malabsorption of iron is quite an uncommon cause of iron deficiency except after gastrointestinal surgery and in malabsorption syndromes. From 10 to 34 percent of patients who have undergone subtotal gastric resection develop iron-deficiency anemia years later.[144] Many such patients have impaired absorption of food iron, caused in part by more rapid gastrojejunal transit and in part by partially digested food bypassing some of the duodenum because of the location of the anastomosis. Fortunately, medicinal iron is well absorbed in post–partial gastrectomy patients. Moreover, gastrointestinal blood loss may also play an important role in anemia following gastric resection (see "Bleeding, gastrointestinal" above). In malabsorption syndromes, absorption of iron may be so limited that iron-deficiency anemia develops over a period of years. Celiac disease, whether overt or occult, may be associated with iron-deficiency anemia.[144,194]

Intravascular Hemolysis and Hemoglobinuria   Iron-deficiency anemia may occur in paroxysmal nocturnal hemoglobinuria (see Chap. 38) and in hemolysis resulting from mechanical erythrocyte trauma from intracardiac myxomas,[195] valvular prostheses, or patches[196–198] (see Chap. 50). In these disorders, iron is lost in the urine as hemosiderin and ferritin in desquamated tubular cells, and as hemoglobin.[198]

Iron deficiency occurs frequently in athletes engaged in a variety of sports (see Chap. 49). There may be mild anemia. Increased intravascular hemolysis[199] presumably with some renal loss of iron may play a role, but gastrointestinal blood loss has been demonstrated in persons engaged in strenuous athletic pursuits, and this is presumably the major cause of the iron deficiency.[200–203]

Dialysis Treatment of Chronic Renal Disease The use of extracorporeal dialysis for treatment of chronic renal disease may cause iron deficiency, often superimposed upon the anemia of chronic renal disease. The retention of blood in the dialyzing equipment is a major cause, along with gastrointestinal bleeding, blood sampling, and bleeding incident to vascular access.[204]

PATHOGENESIS

As iron deficiency develops, different compartments are depleted in iron in a sequential, overlapping fashion, as illustrated schematically in Fig. 40-8.

Erythrocyte Survival and Ferrokinetics Slight to moderate shortening of erythrocyte survival is characteristic of iron-deficiency anemia, particularly when it is severe.[205,206] A study of the movement of iron between various iron compartments (e.g., plasma pool, labile pool, hemoglobin compartment) may be performed by intravenous injection of radioactive iron, (^{59}Fe) followed by measurement of the rate of clearance of ^{59}Fe from plasma and of its incorporation into the hemoglobin of circulating erythrocytes. The principles underlying such "ferrokinetic" studies are discussed in Chap. 30.

In iron deficiency, plasma iron clearance is rapid and is closely inversely correlated with the serum iron concentration. The plasma iron transport rate may be normal or increased. The percentage of iron utilized in hemoglobin synthesis is normal or increased.[206] There is usually little or no evidence of ineffective erythropoiesis.

Iron-Containing Proteins As the body becomes depleted of iron, changes occur in many tissues. Hemosiderin and ferritin virtually disappear from marrow and other storage sites. There is a decreased activity of many other important iron proteins, such as cytochrome c, cytochrome oxidase, succinic dehydrogenase, aconitase,[7,8,207] xanthine oxidase,[208] and myoglobin.[209] Reduced activity has also been reported for some enzymes that do not contain or require iron. Phosphocreatine content is decreased and inorganic phosphorus is increased in skeletal muscle of iron-deficient rats.[210] Many of the affected enzymes are in the oxidative glycolysis (Krebs) cycle of mitochondria. On the other

hand, the activities of several mitochondrial matrix enzymes are increased in skeletal muscle of iron-deficient animals.[210,211]

In iron deficiency, the levels of some of the proteins involved in iron homeostasis, such as dcytb, hephaestin, DMT-1, and ferroportin, are up-regulated.[212]

Muscular Function and Exercise Tolerance Iron-deficient rats have impaired exercise tolerance and are prone to lactic acidosis when exercised. The activity of α-glycerophosphate dehydrogenase was diminished in the skeletal muscle of iron-deficient rats, and this finding might explain the greater proclivity of iron-deficient rats to lactic acidosis upon exercise.[213] However, in skeletal muscle of iron deficient guinea pigs, the activity of this enzyme is normal.[214] The brown fat of iron-deficient rats has lower than normal activities of NADH and of succinate and α-glycerophosphate oxidases.[215]

Besides these metabolic aberrations of muscle cells in iron-deficient rodents, ultrastructural studies show swollen mitochondria with distorted cristae, and there is evidence of mtDNA damage.[216] Despite these changes, mitochondrial cytochrome c increases adaptively on repetitive electrical stimulus of muscle.[217]

A study of energy transport pathways of submitochondrial particles of rat liver and skeletal muscle showed the latter to be less sensitive to iron depletion than the former.[218] ^{31}Phosphorus magnetic resonance spectroscopy studies demonstrated increased breakdown of phosphocreatine in muscles of iron-deficient rats,[219] but mitochondrial abnormalities could not be demonstrated in humans.[220]

Neurologic Changes Monoamine oxidase (MAO) activity is low in the liver and platelets of patients with iron deficiency.[221–224] MAO is involved in the synthesis and catabolism of important neurotransmitters such as dopamine, norepinephrine, and serotonin. Furthermore, iron-deficient children and iron-deficient rats excrete substantially more urinary norepinephrine than do iron-replete children or rats, an anomaly that is corrected within a few days of inception of iron therapy.[223,224] The brains of iron-deficient rats exhibit reduction in the number of dopamine D2 receptors that are also important in neurotransmission.[225]

Weanling rats given iron-deficient diets showed poor feeding efficiency, growth retardation, decrease in concentration, and greater than normal rates of turnover of norepinephrine in brown fat and heart, hypertrophy of brown fat and heart, reduction in plasma thyroxine and triiodothyronine, low hepatic content of carnitine, and impaired ketogenesis.[226,227] Prolonged iron deficiency in rats also caused abnormal formation of teeth[228] and cochlea[229] and hearing loss.[230] However, these effects have not been described in humans.

Host Defenses Iron deficiency affects immune function and the susceptibility to infection.[231,232] Some studies found that iron depletion prevents growth of microorganisms and therefore protects against infections; others observed that iron deficiency impairs host defenses. Iron-deficient mice fail to develop autoimmune encephalomyelitis, an animal model of human multiple sclerosis.[233]

Growth and Metabolism Iron-deficiency anemia is associated with reduction in children's height[234,235] and treatment promotes growth.[236] Together with zinc deficiency it has been held responsible for dwarfism.[237] The larger birth weight of infants from iron-supplemented mothers is discussed above (see "Pregnancy"). Impaired thermoregulation has also been demonstrated.[238]

Histologic Findings Iron deficiency may lead to histologic changes in various organs. The rapidly proliferating cells of the upper part of the alimentary tract seem particularly susceptible to the effects of iron deficiency. There may be atrophy of the mucosa of the tongue and esophagus,[239] stomach,[240,241] and small intestine.[242,243] The epithelium of the lateral margins of the tongue is reduced in thickness despite increase in the progenitor compartment. This thinning presumably reflects accelerated exfoliation of epithelial cells.[244] Buccal mucosa has shown thinning and keratinization of epithelium and increased mitotic

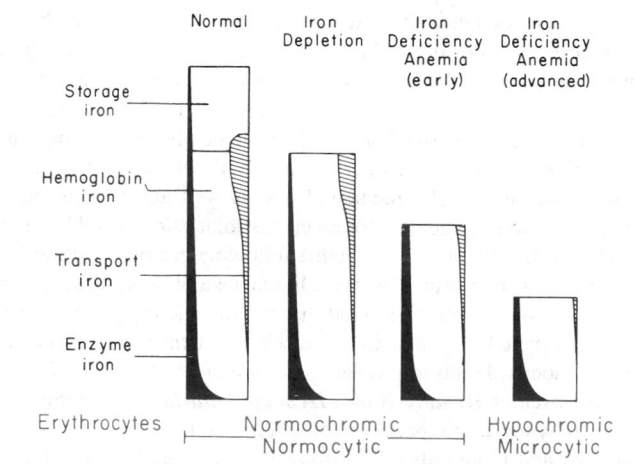

FIGURE 40-8 Stages in the development of iron deficiency. Early iron deficiency (iron depletion) is usually not accompanied by any abnormalities in blood; at this stage, serum iron concentration is occasionally below normal values and storage iron is markedly depleted. As iron deficiency progresses, development of anemia precedes appearance of morphologic changes in blood, although some cells may be smaller and paler than normal; serum iron concentration is usually low at this time, but it may be normal. With advanced iron depletion, classic changes of hypochromic, microcytic, hypoferremic anemia become manifest.

activity.[245,246] However, light microscopic and electron microscopic examination of exfoliated oral mucosal cells showed no aberrations in morphology of nuclei or cytoplasm of the cells of patients with iron-deficiency anemia.[247]

In iron-deficiency anemia resulting from idiopathic pulmonary hemosiderosis, characteristic pathologic changes are found in the lungs, including intense deposition of iron in the littoral cells of the alveoli and interstitial fibrosis.[248]

Widening of diploic spaces of bones, particularly those of the skull and hands,[249,250] may be a consequence of chronic iron deficiency beginning in infancy. In the skull, this is of the same character as in thalassemia, except that in β-thalassemia major there is maxillary hypertrophy, whereas in severe iron-deficiency anemia maxillary growth and pneumatization are normal. The sella turcica may be abnormally small in iron-deficient children, and it has been suggested that this implies reduction in pituitary hormonal secretion in long-standing iron-deficiency anemia.[251]

CLINICAL FEATURES

CLINICAL MANIFESTATIONS OF ANEMIA

The anemia in iron-deficient patients can be very severe, with blood hemoglobin levels less than 4 g/dl being encountered in some patients. Severe iron-deficiency anemia is associated with all of the various symptoms of anemia, resulting from hypoxia and the body's response to hypoxia as described in Chapter 32. Thus, tachycardia with palpitations and pounding in the ears, headache, light-headedness, and even angina pectoris may all occur in patients who are severely anemic.

CLINICAL MANIFESTATIONS THAT MAY BE UNRELATED TO ANEMIA

The clinical features of iron deficiency encompass those caused by a deficiency of an element essential for life, viz, iron, and symptoms caused by the anemia itself. The question of whether these can, at least in some patients, be dissociated is one that is difficult to approach experimentally, and the question of whether "iron deficiency without anemia" can cause symptoms cannot be considered definitively settled. Nonetheless, the idea that clinical chlorosis could occur without anemia has been observed clinically for more than a century (for reviews see refs. 41 and 252), and a number of controlled studies seemed to show that various manifestations of iron-deficiency anemia can occur in individuals whose hemoglobin is within the accepted normal range,[253–258] but there have also been a few studies in which no effect could be discerned.[259] In one randomized, double-blind study, patients with iron deficiency had greater symptomatic improvement with iron medication than with placebos[252]; in other studies with a somewhat different experimental design, this was not true.[260,261]

Decreased Work Performance Objective measurements of work performance and studies using O_2 consumption as an index of work performance have given contradictory results, but a comprehensive review led to the conclusion that severe iron deficiency (Hb >8 g/dl) and mild iron deficiency (Hb between 8 and 12 g/dl) led to decreased work performance, primarily as estimated by VO_{2max} measurements,[262] but the evidence that nonanemic iron deficiency had such an effect was less convincing.[262] However, in athletes with low ferritin levels but normal hemoglobin levels, iron-supplemented subjects showed an increased VO_{2max} without a change in their red cell mass,[254] and in other studies, nonanemic subjects treated with iron showed improved performance and/or VO_{2max}.[255–258,263]

Headache Iron-deficient patients frequently complain of headache,[264–266] but headache is a common symptom, and the data that have been presented are all anecdotal.

Paresthesias and Other Neurologic Symptoms Paresthesias are thought to be common in iron deficiency,[264] but there are no controlled studies to support this impression. Our investigations show that numbness in the extremities is no more common in iron-deficient than in iron-sufficient patients. (Table 40-8). In children, breath-holding spells have been attributed to iron deficiency.[267] Anecdotal reports of intracranial hypertension with papilledema are buttressed by apparent response to iron therapy.[265,267–270] Stroke in children has been associated with iron-deficiency anemia.[267]

Oral and Nasopharyngeal Symptoms Burning of the tongue[271,272] has also been described anecdotally in many accounts of iron deficiency, and although this symptom has been observed to diminish with treatment, no controlled studies have been performed. Indeed, it has been suggested that the tongue symptoms might be due to concurrent pyridoxine deficiency.[273] We have had the opportunity of comparing the frequencies of these symptoms in a large population of women attending a health appraisal clinic, and found that none of these symptoms occurred at a higher frequency in an iron deficient group of women (transferrin receptor [TS] <16%; serum ferritin <20 ng/ml) when compared with a group of iron-sufficient women (TS >20%; serum ferritin >60 ng/ml) (see Table 40-8). Iron deficiency has been proposed as a cause of atrophic rhinitis.[274,275] The evidence for this is equivocal; perhaps it is a contributory factor.

Dysphagia In the laryngopharynx, mucosal atrophy may lead to web formation in the postcricoid region, thereby giving rise to dysphagia (Paterson-Kelly/Plummer-Vinson syndrome).[276] If these alterations are of long duration, they may lead to pharyngeal carcinoma. Although it has been generally thought that these changes are secondary to long-standing iron deficiency, this mechanism is not universally accepted.[272] Although the frequency of the condition is considered to have decreased considerably[276] and its very existence has sometimes been doubted, cases with the features of this disorder continue to be reported.[194,277–279] Abnormal motility of the esophagus has also been documented in iron-deficient patients.[280]

Menstrual Bleeding An increase in the volume of menstrual blood loss has been considered to be a result as well as a cause of iron deficiency,[281,282] but this observation has been disputed.[283]

Pica The craving to eat unusual substances, such as dirt, clay, ice, laundry starch, salt, cardboard, or hair, is a classic manifestation of iron deficiency and is usually cured promptly by iron therapy.[284–286]

Restless Legs Restless legs is a common nocturnal problem, especially in the elderly, and has been associated with iron deficiency.[287–290]

Hair Loss It has been suggested that hair loss may be a consequence of iron deficiency,[291] and in one study there were significantly lowered ferritin levels in women with androgenetic alopecia and alopecia areata but not in those with telogen effluvium or alopecia areata totalis/universalis,[292] but the validity of a cause-and-effect relationship has been challenged.[293]

TABLE 40-8   FREQUENCY OF SOME SYMPTOMS COMMONLY ASCRIBED TO IRON DEFICIENCY IN WHITE WOMEN AGED 20–49 YEARS ATTENDING A HEALTH APPRAISAL CLINIC

SYMPTOM	IRON DEFICIENT (n*)	NON–IRON DEFICIENT (n)	IRON DEFICIENT, HEMOGLOBIN <10 G/DL
Frequent headaches	30.8% (452)	30.7% (685)	40.0% (15)
Mouth, tongue, or jaw problem	18.5% (470)	17.4% (688)	12.5% (16)
Numbness in hands or feet	38.8% (469)	36.6% (687)	62.5% (16)
Tired or decreased energy	41.2% (461)	38.9% (684)	43.8% (16)
Severe fatigue, tiredness, or exhaustion	19.1% (450)	19.7% (678)	33.3% (15)

* n = number of women who responded to the question on the questionnaire.

Infant and Childhood Development   In infants, iron deficiency is associated with poor attention span, poor response to sensory stimuli, and retarded behavioral and developmental achievement, even in the absence of anemia.[267,294] Although a considerable number of studies with a positive outcome have been reported,[295] many of these have been criticized because of a lack of controls, and the possibility that socio-economic factors may have a confounding effect.[296]

PHYSICAL FINDINGS

The physical findings in iron-deficiency anemia include pallor, glossitis (smooth, red tongue), stomatitis, and angular cheilitis. Koilonychia, once a common finding, is now encountered rarely (Fig. 40-9). Retinal hemorrhages and exudates may be seen in severely anemic patients (e.g., hemoglobin concentration ≤5 g/dl). Splenomegaly has occasionally been attributed to iron-deficiency anemia,[186] but when it occurs it is probably due to other causes.[297]

LABORATORY FEATURES

In severe uncomplicated iron-deficiency anemia, the erythrocytes are hypochromic and microcytic, the plasma iron concentration is diminished, the iron-binding capacity increased, the serum ferritin concentration is low, the serum transferrin receptor and erythrocyte zinc protoporphyrin concentrations are increased, and the marrow is depleted of stainable iron. Unfortunately, the classic combination of laboratory findings occurs consistently only when iron-deficiency anemia is far advanced, when there are no complicating factors such as infection or malignant neoplasms, and when there has not been previous therapy with transfusions or parenteral iron.

BLOOD CELLS

Erythrocytes   Anisocytosis is the earliest recognizable morphologic change of erythrocytes in iron-deficiency anemia (Fig. 40-10).[298,299] The anisocytosis is typically accompanied by mild ovalocytosis. As the iron deficiency worsens, a mild normochromic, normocytic anemia often develops.[298–302] With further progression, hemoglobin concentration, erythrocyte count, mean corpuscular volume (MCV), and mean erythrocyte hemoglobin (MCH) all decline together.

In infants and children, hypochromia may occur earlier in the course of iron deficiency, and erythrocyte counts greater than 5×10^{12}/liter (5,000,000/μl) encountered.[303] As the indices change, the erythrocytes appear microcytic and hypochromic on stained blood films. Target cells may sometimes be present. Elongated hypochromic elliptocytes may be seen, in which the long sides are nearly parallel. Such

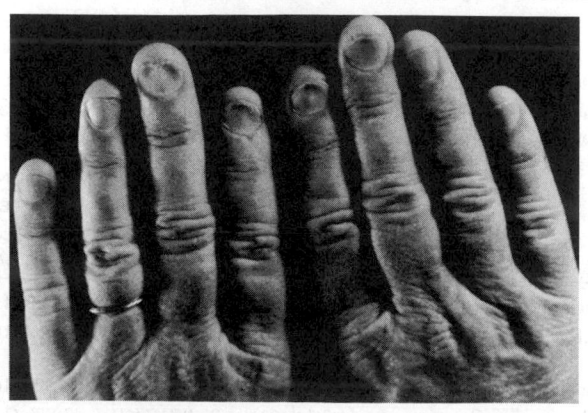

FIGURE 40-9   Koilonychia. Note the ridging, thinning, splitting, and spoonlike concavity of the fingernails.

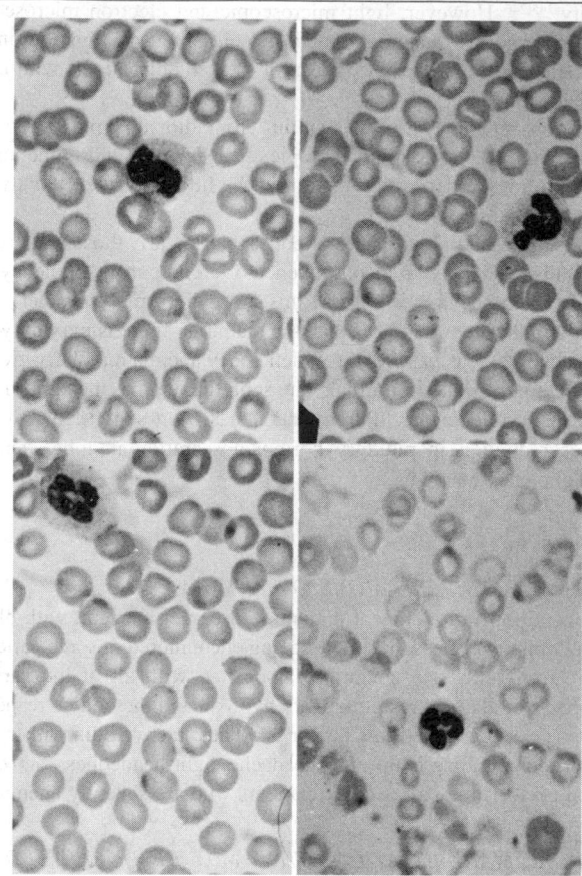

FIGURE 40-10   Variability in morphologic diagnosis of iron-deficiency anemia from blood film. Interpret and compare them with those of nine experienced hematologists who reviewed the original slides. The slides were part of a coded series that contained blood films from normal subjects and from iron-deficiency anemia patients in random order. The fields reproduced here were typical for each slide (×600). (From VF Fairbanks,[299] with permission from the J.B. Lippincott Company.) *(Top left)* From a young woman with iron-deficiency anemia due to excessive menstrual bleeding. Hemoglobin 10.1 g/dl, serum iron 36 μg/dl (6.4 μmol/liter). After treatment with ferrous gluconate, hemoglobin concentration increased to 13.1 g/dl. On 13 examinations of this slide by nine hematologists, 11 opinions were that there was no evidence to suggest iron deficiency. *(Top right)* From a normal woman. Hemoglobin 14.6 g/dl, mean corpuscular hemoglobin concentration (MCHC) 34 percent, serum iron 77 μg/dl (13.8 μmol/liter), total iron-binding capacity 300 μg/dl (53.7 μmol/liter). Three of nine hematologists who reviewed this film thought the erythrocytes were morphologically abnormal and consistent with iron-deficiency anemia. *(Bottom left)* From a normal young man. Hemoglobin 15.8 g/dl, MCHC 34 percent, serum iron 141 μg/dl (25.2 μmol/liter), total iron-binding capacity 278 μg/dl (49.8 μmol/liter). Nine hematologists made a total of 13 examinations of this slide; one examiner reported the slide showed evidence of iron deficiency. *(Bottom right)* From a 56-year-old man with anemia due to bleeding from paraesophageal hiatus hernia. Hemoglobin 4.0 g/dl, erythrocyte count 2.24 × 10^{12}/liter, reticulocyte count 2.5 percent, serum iron 2 μg/dl (0.4 μmol/liter). Hypochromia was marked, and all observers agreed that morphologically the cells suggested iron-deficiency anemia.

cells have been called *pencil cells*, although they more nearly resemble cigars in shape.

The red cell indices are consistently abnormal in adults only when iron-deficiency anemia is moderate or severe (e.g., in males with hemoglobin concentrations <12 g/dl or in women with hemoglobin concentrations <10 g/dl) (Fig. 40-11). Measurement of the distribution of erythrocyte volume (e.g., red cell distribution width [RDW]) is made

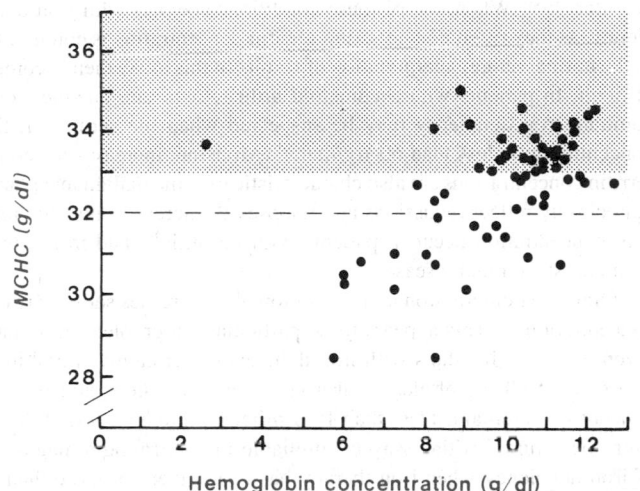

MCHC VALUES IN IRON DEFICIENCY ANEMIA

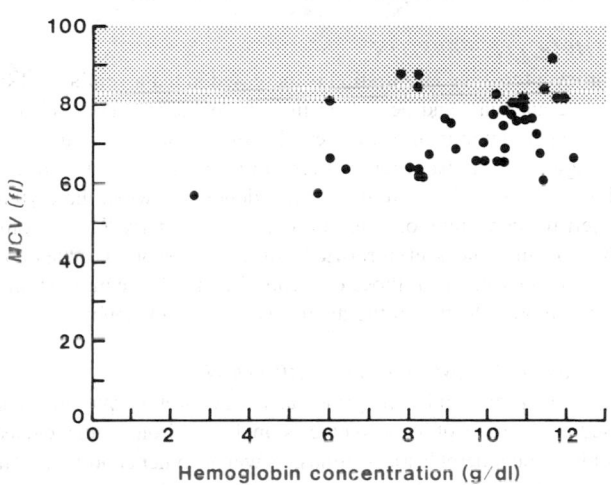

MCV VALUES IN IRON DEFICIENCY ANEMIA

FIGURE 40-11   Erythrocyte indices in iron-deficiency anemia of adults (data obtained with Coulter Counter, Model S). Normal ranges of indices observed in approximately 500 healthy adults[348] using the same instrument are indicated by *stippling*. The *dashed line* in the *top panel* indicates the more widely accepted lower normal limit of mean corpuscular hemoglobin concentration (MCHC) stated in this text. *(Top)* Correlation between venous blood hemoglobin concentration and MCHC. More than half of the 62 patients with iron-deficiency anemia had MCHC values clearly in the normal range. *(Bottom)* Correlation between venous blood hemoglobin concentrations and mean corpuscular volume (MCV). Nearly 70 percent of cases exhibited distinct microcytosis. Thus, when indices are determined by automated cell-counting methods, the MCV is much more sensitive than is the MCHC in detecting changes of iron deficiency. However, at least 30 percent of cases of iron-deficiency anemia will be misdiagnosed if physicians rely on the erythrocyte indices. (From E Beutler, VF Fairbanks,[674] with permission from Academic Press.)

easy by modern cell counters. With some of these instruments the RDW is reported as the coefficient of variation (in percent) of erythrocyte volume (see "Differential Diagnosis" below) The sensitivity and specificity of erythrocyte indices for iron deficiency may be increased by use of formulae that incorporate MCV, RDW, serum ferritin concentration, and serum transferrin saturation to produce an iron index[304] or combinations of other functions.[305–307]

Leukocytes   Leukopenia has been found in some patients with iron-deficiency anemia,[191] but the overall distribution of leukocyte counts in iron-deficient patients seems to be approximately normal.[300]

Platelets   Thrombocytopenia and thrombocytosis have both been attributed to iron deficiency. Thrombocytosis has been reported in 50 to 75 percent of adults with classic iron-deficiency anemia due to chronic blood loss.[300,308] However, thrombocytosis usually occurs only in those patients who are actively bleeding.[309] In infants and children, thrombocytopenia occurs almost as frequently (28%) as does thrombocytosis (35%); thrombocytopenia is associated with more severe anemia.[310,311] Marked thrombocytopenia may also occur in iron-deficient adults, either as the presenting hematologic problem or early during the response to iron therapy for anemia.[312–314]

Reticulocytes   It is sometimes stated that the reticulocyte count is normal or decreased in iron deficiency,[186,271] but in series of patients in which the number of reticulocytes is reported the number is often mildly increased,[243,300,315,316] a finding consistent with the increased erythroid activity of the marrow (see "Marrow" below).

MARROW

Both the degree of cellularity of the marrow and the relative proportion of erythroid to myeloid cells are variable.[317] In severe iron deficiency, erythroblasts of the marrow may be smaller than normal, with narrow, ragged rims of cytoplasm containing little hemoglobin. However, the morphologic changes in the marrow are not sufficiently distinctive to be of diagnostic value.

Decreased or absent hemosiderin in the marrow is characteristic of iron deficiency. Hemosiderin appears in the unstained marrow film as golden refractile granules, but the hemosiderin content of the marrow film is more readily and more reliably evaluated after staining by the simple Prussian blue method. Stored iron in the macrophages of the marrow can be seen in marrow spicules in marrow sections or in marrow aspirate films. Iron granules, normally found in the cytoplasm of 10 percent or more of erythroblasts, become rare but may not be entirely absent.

Because most body iron is divided between stores and the red cell mass and iron is not excreted, most anemias are characterized by increased storage iron. Iron-deficiency anemia is the exception, because iron stores are depleted before the red cell mass is compromised. Thus, evaluation of iron stores should be a sensitive and usually reliable means for differentiation between iron-deficiency anemia and all other anemias. Clinically, this is most directly achieved by evaluating the amount of iron in marrow macrophages, and this direct assessment of iron stores has long been considered the "gold standard" for the diagnosis of iron deficiency.[318,319] There are, however, technical barriers to the accurate histochemical determination of marrow iron. First of all, an invasive procedure, marrow aspiration, is required. Secondly, the differentiation of iron within macrophages from artifacts is no trivial matter, and it takes considerable experience and skill to obtain accurate results. In one study only 74 of 108 cases had been accurately reported.[320] Moreover, misleading results may be obtained in patients who have been transfused or who have been treated with parenteral iron.[319] The marrow of such patients may contain normal, or even increased, quantities of stainable iron in the face of typical iron-responsive iron-deficiency anemia. In such patients, iron that is seen on marrow examination is not readily available for erythropoiesis. Further, the ability of marrow to store iron seems to be impaired in some patients with chronic myelogenous leukemia[321] and possibly in those with myelofibrosis. In such patients, absence of marrow iron is often observed without other evidence of iron deficiency, and such patients do not respond to iron therapy. For such reasons, the primacy of marrow iron estimation has been questioned.[322]

SERUM IRON CONCENTRATION

The serum iron concentration is usually low in untreated iron-deficiency anemia; however, it may be normal.[302,323,324] The serum iron concentration also is influenced by many pathologic and physiologic states. Physiologically, the serum iron concentration has a diurnal rhythm; it decreases in late afternoon and evening, reaching a nadir near 9 PM, and increases to its maximum between 7 and 10 AM. Although numerous studies have shown that diurnal variation occurs,[325–327] it is doubtful whether this is of sufficient clinical importance to require all serum iron values to be drawn in the morning.[328] Serum iron levels decrease at about the time of menstrual bleeding, either when menses are under normal hormonal control[329,330] or when bleeding occurs after withdrawal of oral contraceptive agents.[163,331] The serum iron concentration is reduced in the presence of either acute or chronic inflammatory processes[332,333] or malignancy[334] and following acute myocardial infarction.[335,336] The serum iron concentration under these circumstances may be decreased sufficiently to suggest iron deficiency. On the other hand, during chemotherapy of malignancy, the serum iron concentration may be quite elevated. This effect is observed from the third to the seventh day after inception of chemotherapy of a variety of tumors.[337]

Normal or high concentrations of serum iron are commonly observed even in patients with iron-deficiency anemia if such patients receive iron medication before blood is drawn for these measurements. Even multiple vitamin preparations, which commonly contain about 18 mg of elemental iron per tablet, can result in this effect. Oral iron medication should be withheld for 24 hours. Parenteral injection of iron dextran may result in a very high serum iron concentration (e.g., 500–1000 μg/dl), at least with some methods,[338] for several weeks.

IRON-BINDING CAPACITY AND TRANSFERRIN SATURATION

The iron-binding capacity is a measure of the amount of transferrin in circulating blood. Normally, there is enough transferrin present in 100 mL serum to bind 4.4 to 8.0 μmol (250–450 μg) of iron; because the normal serum iron concentration is about 1.8 μmol/dl (100 μg/dl), transferrin may be found to be about one third saturated with iron. The unsaturated or latent iron-binding capacity (UIBC) is easily measured with radioactive iron or by spectrophotometric techniques. The sum of the UIBC and the plasma iron represents total iron-binding capacity (TIBC). TIBC may also be measured directly. In iron-deficiency anemia, UIBC and TIBC are often increased; a transferrin saturation of 15 percent or less is usually found. However, exceptions are so common as to detract considerably from the diagnostic value of measuring transferrin saturation in the diagnosis of iron deficiency.[319] A normal value for transferrin saturation often accompanies a low serum iron concentration in the anemia of chronic disease.

SERUM FERRITIN

The serum ferritin concentration correlates with total-body iron stores,[339,340] although the correlation is not as strong as has sometimes been suggested.[341–343] Serum ferritin concentrations of 10 μg/liter or less are characteristic of iron-deficiency anemia. In iron deficiency without anemia, serum ferritin concentration typically ranges from 10 to 20 μg/liter. In one series of 73 patients, marrow iron was depleted whenever the serum ferritin level was less than 70 μg/liter.[344] In another study in which patients with iron-deficiency anemia were compared with those with anemia of chronic disease, a cutoff point of 32 μg/liter provided a sensitivity of 79.2 percent and a specificity of 96.9 percent.[345] As noted earlier (see "Storage Compartment" above), serum ferritin predominantly consists of H-monomers, which contain less iron than do L-monomers; hence, serum ferritin contains relatively little iron. Moderate increase in serum ferritin concentration occurs in inflammatory disorders, such as rheumatoid arthritis, in chronic renal disease, and in malignancies.[346] In Gaucher disease, the serum ferritin concentration is commonly in the range of thousands of micrograms per liter.[347,348] When one of these conditions coexists with iron deficiency, as they often do, the serum ferritin concentration is commonly in the normal range; interpretation of results of this assay then becomes difficult. In patients with rheumatoid arthritis who are anemic, concomitant iron deficiency may be suspected when the serum ferritin concentration is less than 60 μg/liter.[349] Moderate increases in serum ferritin concentrations are also characteristic of some malignancies and may closely reflect remissions and relapses.[350] Increases in serum ferritin concentration occur in patients with hepatitis[351] and in patients with end-stage renal disease.[352]

Oral or parenteral iron administration also increases serum ferritin concentration.[353] This appears to be particularly a problem in infants given oral iron. In adults with iron-deficiency anemia given oral iron in a dose of 60 mg of elemental iron thrice daily, the serum ferritin concentration remained less than 10 μg/liter for 2 to 3 weeks.[353] However, the serum ferritin assay is unreliable in confirming a diagnosis of iron deficiency when iron therapy has been given for more than 3 weeks. Parenteral administration of iron dextran results in a rise in serum ferritin concentration to normal or supranormal values within 24 hours, and this effect persists for at least 1 month.[353]

ERYTHROCYTE FERRITIN

Erythrocyte ferritin concentration is increased in thalassemias and sideroblastic anemias, and decreased in iron deficiency. These changes appear to parallel those of serum ferritin concentration, although it has been suggested that basic red cell ferritin is not influenced by inflammation, and could therefore detect iron deficiency when the erythrocyte ferritin concentration was normal in the elderly.[354] In another study of anemic males, erythrocyte ferritin determinations appeared to have no more value than those of serum ferritin. The combination of both was more effective in the diagnosis of iron deficiency.[355]

ERYTHROCYTE ZINC PROTOPORPHYRIN

Erythrocyte protoporphyrin, principally zinc protoporphyrin, is increased in disorders of heme synthesis, including iron deficiency, lead poisoning, and sideroblastic anemias, as well as other conditions. This procedure requires small blood samples. It is quite sensitive in the diagnosis of iron deficiency and practical for large-scale screening programs designed to identify children with either iron deficiency or lead poisoning.[356] It does not differentiate between iron deficiency and chronic lead poisoning[357] or the anemia that accompanies inflammatory or malignant processes.[358]

SERUM TRANSFERRIN RECEPTOR

The role of transferrin receptor in transporting transferrin iron into cells was described earlier (see "Transport of Iron" above). The circulating receptor is a truncated form of the cellular receptor, lacking the transmembrane and cytoplasmic domains of the cellular receptor. It circulates bound to transferrin. Sensitive immunologic methods can detect about 5 mg/liter of receptor in serum. The levels of circulating transferrin receptor apparently mirror the amount of cellular receptor, and because receptor synthesis is greatly increased when cells lack iron, the amount of the circulating receptor increases in iron deficiency but not in the anemia of chronic disease.[359–361] This test for iron deficiency has gradually come into clinical use, but the methodology has not yet been standardized, making laboratory-to-laboratory comparisons difficult. Like the serum ferritin and serum iron, serum transferrin receptor assay results may be confounded by poorly understood variations in patients with malignancies, in whom the serum transferrin receptor concentration is reduced, and in patients with rheumatoid arthritis or thalassemia trait, in whom, in the absence of iron deficiency, it is increased. Thus, to be clinically useful, separate normal ranges need to be defined for serum transferrin receptor in these common conditions.[362-365] The ratio of serum transferrin receptor to serum ferritin seems to be a particularly accurate reflection of body iron stores.[366,367]

RETICULOCYTE HEMOGLOBIN CONTENT

Automated hematology instruments may offer, as a new method for diagnosis of iron deficiency, an assay of hemoglobin content within reticulocytes. This parameter seems to be an early indicator of iron deficiency, but does not otherwise seem to have any major advantages over other methods of establishing a diagnosis of iron deficiency.[368-370]

IRON TOLERANCE TESTS

In an iron tolerance test, the patient receives an oral dose of an inorganic iron compound, and the subsequent change in the serum iron concentration is measured. In iron deficiency, there is an increased rate of absorption of the test dose, and this is sometimes reflected in a more rapid increase and a higher plateau than in normal subjects. This procedure was espoused for the diagnosis of iron deficiency more than 50 years ago.[371] However it is not reliable,[319] presumably because the plasma iron levels represent the balance between absorption rate, which is increased in iron deficiency, and iron clearance, which is also increased. Although attempts have been made from time-to-time to reintroduce this method,[372] it is rarely used today.

DIFFERENTIAL DIAGNOSIS

Iron deficiency anemia is characterized by many abnormal laboratory features. Because none of these are unique, a small deviation from normal will detect most cases of iron deficiency (high sensitivity), but also falsely identify non-iron deficient subjects as being iron deficient (low specificity). On the other hand, a large deviation from normal will exclude most non–iron-deficient patients (high specificity), but miss many iron-deficient subjects (low sensitivity). This tradeoff is shown graphically in so-called *receiver operator characteristic curves*. These curves are constructed by plotting the sensitivity against the false-positive rate (1 – specificity) at various values of the analyte. Figure 40-12 shows receiver operator characteristic curves for some tests for iron deficiency. The situation is complicated in the case of iron deficiency by the fact that the diagnostic problem faced by the physician is not one of differentiating a patient with iron-deficiency anemia from a normal person, but rather from a patient who has an anemia with a different etiology. It is partly for this reason that a simple algorithm for the diagnosis of iron deficiency does not exist. In a severely anemic patient microcytosis would have very high specificity and high sensitivity compared to normal, but compared to a patient with thalassemia the specificity would be very low, indeed. Similarly, a low serum ferritin level is an excellent test in the general population, but it is a relatively little value in patients with chronic renal disease. Another problem that is inherent in evaluating diagnostic tests for iron deficiency is the standard that is applied to decide who is iron deficient and who is not. Marrow iron has served as one "gold standard" but has limitations, as discussed earlier (see "Marrow" above). Alternatively, the response to iron therapy serves as a powerful indicator of whose anemia is actually due to deficiency of iron. Here, too, there are limitations, in that some iron deficient patients may fail to respond adequately because of factors such as infection. Lacking an absolute test for iron deficiency, the ability of the physician to use judgment relevant to the particular patient's circumstances is of paramount importance.

The forms of anemia that must be distinguished from iron-deficiency anemia most frequently include those of thalassemia minor,

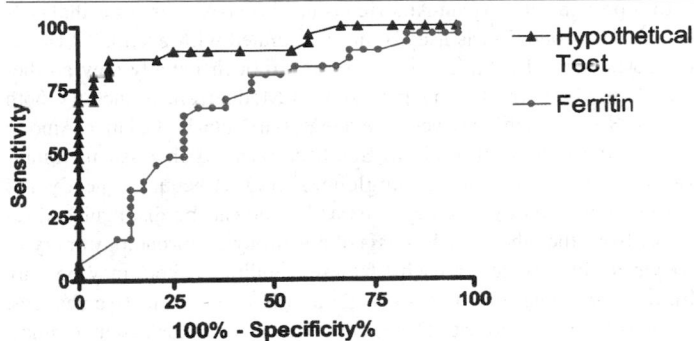

FIGURE 40-12 Two receiver operator characteristic curves. As the specificity increases, the sensitivity decreases. The receiver-operator properties of serum ferritin are far from ideal. When the specificity is high (to the *left on the abscissa*), the sensitivity is low; only when the specificity is low is the sensitivity adequate. The curve that would be obtained with a nearly ideal test for iron deficiency gives high specificity and high sensitivity. In the curve shown, a cutoff value could be found that allows one to identify 75 percent of patients with iron deficiency with a specificity greater than 90 percent. Unfortunately, no such test exists.

chronic inflammatory disease, malignancy, chronic liver disease, chronic renal disease, hemolytic anemia, and aplastic anemia. It is the microcytic anemias that are most likely to be confused with iron deficiency. Such anemias are summarized in Table 40-9, and each is discussed elsewhere in this volume. Attention will be directed here primarily to laboratory aids for differentiating iron-deficiency anemia from the frequently occurring disorders that may have similar manifestations.

THALASSEMIA MINOR

In many parts of the world and in many communities of North America, the frequency of β-thalassemia minor is second only to that of iron deficiency as a cause of hypochromic microcytic anemia (see Chap. 46). In African Americans, homozygosity for α-thalassemia 2, that is, the state in which only a single α-globin gene is present on each chromosome, is a common cause of microcytosis. Approximately

TABLE 40-9 MICROCYTIC DISORDERS THAT MAY BE CONFUSED WITH IRON DEFICIENCY

Thalassemias and hemoglobinopathies (see Chap. 46)
  β-thalassemia major
  β-thalassemia minor
  δβ-thalassemia minor
  α-thalassemia minor
  Hemoglobin Lepore trait
  Hemoglobin E trait
  Homozygous hemoglobin E disease
  Hemoglobin H disease
  Combination of above (compound heterozygotes)
Blockade of heme synthesis caused by chemicals (see Chap. 58)
  Lead
  Pyrazinamide
  Isoniazid
Other disorders
  Sideroblastic anemias (see Chap. 58)
    Hereditary sex-linked
    Idiopathic acquired
  Anemia of chronic disease (see Chap. 43)

1 to 3 percent of African-Americans are homozygous for α-thalassemia 2. The condition is usually not associated with anemia.[373] Heterozygotes may also have microcytosis, although usually they are hematologically normal. Among persons of Mediterranean ancestry, both α- and β-thalassemia are very prevalent, particularly the latter. Among Asians, particularly those from Southeast Asia, α-thalassemia minor, β-thalassemia minor, and hemoglobin E trait all occur frequently. All are characterized by microcytosis, and none can be distinguished reliably from the others on the basis of erythrocyte morphology or erythrocyte indices alone. In each of these conditions there may be only mild to moderate microcytosis without any other distinctive changes. However, in the majority of patients with α- or β-thalassemia minor, hemoglobin Lepore trait, and hemoglobin E trait, the erythrocyte count is greater than 5×10^{12}/liter (5,000,000/μl), despite low hemoglobin concentration.[374,375] Homozygous hemoglobin E is also characterized by marked hypochromia, microcytosis, abundant target cells, and elevated erythrocyte count but usually not by more than minimal anemia[376] (see Chap. 47).

In contrast to the findings in these hemoglobinopathies, erythrocyte counts of 5×10^{12}/liter (5,000,000/μl) or higher are relatively uncommon among adults with iron-deficiency anemia.[377] However, erythrocytosis may be seen in children with iron-deficiency anemia or in polycythemia vera patients who have become iron deficient following hemorrhage or therapeutic phlebotomy.[303] Consequently, although MCV is almost always reduced in α- or β-thalassemia minor and in homozygous hemoglobin E, with values of 60 to 70 fl being the rule, values this low are seen only in severe iron-deficiency anemia. In hemoglobin Lepore trait and hemoglobin E trait, only minimal microcytosis is observed.[374–376] The widespread adoption of the routine measurement of MCV has led to proposals that criteria for differentiation of iron deficiency from thalassemia minor might be based, in part, on the values of the erythrocyte count and MCV.[378] Some proposed rules could separate iron deficiency from thalassemia minor, with 90 percent reliability when groups of iron deficiency and thalassemic patients were of nearly equal numbers.[379] However, in a population in which iron deficiency is more prevalent than thalassemia minor, use of these criteria would result in an excessive number of diagnostic errors. None of these and other proposed rules seems completely reliable for distinguishing iron deficiency from thalassemia.[307,380,381]

Because anisocytosis is an early morphologic feature of iron deficiency, it has been suggested that measurements of variation in erythrocyte size permit discrimination between iron-deficiency anemia and other microcytic anemias.[380,382] However, hemoglobinopathies and thalassemias[382–384] commonly exhibit increased RDW values, as do some anemias that are due to chronic disease.[312,385,386] Hence, these conditions cannot be differentiated reliably by such measurements.

Mild reticulocytosis, polychromatophilia, and basophilic stippling are more likely to be encountered in β-thalassemia minor, $\delta\beta$-thalassemia minor, and hemoglobin Lepore trait than in iron-deficiency anemia but may be absent in these disorders. The serum iron concentration is usually normal or increased in thalassemic syndromes and is usually low in iron-deficiency anemia. Similarly, examination of marrow iron stores helps to differentiate these disorders. The presence of thalassemia is substantiated by the demonstration of increased proportions of hemoglobin A_2 or F or by the presence on electrophoresis of hemoglobin H or Lepore (see Chap. 46). At present the diagnosis of α-thalassemia minor is usually made on the basis of exclusion of other causes of microcytosis but it can be confirmed by measuring globin chain synthetic rates or by direct demonstration of mutations by DNA-based techniques.

Iron deficiency may mask concurrent thalassemia. The amounts of both hemoglobin A_2 and hemoglobin H are diminished disproportionately to the reduction in hemoglobin A in the presence of iron deficiency (see Chap. 46).[387] Thus, when a patient with proven iron deficiency and normal hemoglobin studies continues to exhibit microcytosis and hypochromia after adequate therapy, the concentration of hemoglobin A_2 should be measured again and electrophoresis performed to determine whether hemoglobin H is present.

ANEMIA OF CHRONIC DISEASE

The anemia of chronic disease (see Chap. 43) is usually normochromic and normocytic, but hypochromic microcytic anemia occurs in 20 to 30 percent of patients with chronic infections or malignancies.[332,333] Thus, these disorders cannot be distinguished from iron-deficiency anemia by examination of the blood film. Furthermore, the serum iron concentration is usually decreased in these disorders,[332,333,388] sometimes severely. However, while in iron deficiency, the TIBC is usually increased, whereas in inflammatory and neoplastic diseases it is commonly decreased, there is considerable overlap among TIBC values of normal subjects, those with iron-deficiency anemia, and those with chronic inflammatory diseases.

In iron-deficiency anemia, the transferrin saturation is usually less than 16 percent, whereas in chronic diseases it is usually greater than 16 percent.[333] However, this widely used criterion is actually quite unreliable. Transferrin saturation may be normal in iron-deficiency anemia, and conversely, low saturation is sometimes observed in chronic disease.[333] However, circulating transferrin receptors increase in iron deficiency but not in the anemia of chronic disease.[346,359–361,389] The serum ferritin level is usually diminished in iron deficiency but it is generally increased in chronic inflammatory and neoplastic disorders.[344,390] Measurement of the ratio of soluble transferrin receptor to ferritin has been found to be very useful in distinguishing the anemia of chronic disease from that of iron deficiency.[389] Examination of the marrow for stainable iron is particularly helpful. The latter is greatly decreased in amount or absent in iron deficiency anemia and normal or increased in the other disorders.

ANEMIA OF CHRONIC LIVER DISEASE

The erythrocytes on the blood film from patients with chronic liver disease may be normochromic and normocytic, macrocytic, or hypochromic. Target cells are frequently present in large numbers. Because the blood film in iron-deficiency anemia may also display these features, differential diagnosis must be based on other observations. Serum ferritin levels are useful in detecting iron deficiency in the setting of cirrhosis.[391,392] The serum iron concentration, however, does not seem to correlate well with iron stores.[392]

ANEMIA OF CHRONIC RENAL DISEASE

Iron deficiency is frequent in patients with chronic renal disease (see "Dialysis Treatment of Chronic Renal Disease" above). Iron-deficiency anemia is particularly difficult to diagnose in patients with chronic renal disease (see Chap. 35). Because the problem is fairly common and perhaps because of commercial interest in identifying those patients who can benefit from iron therapy, a large number of studies have been done to determine the best way to diagnose iron deficiency in patients undergoing extracorporeal dialysis. The serum iron concentration may be normal or decreased, depending on the cause of the renal disease. In one study,[393] the percentage of hypochromic erythrocytes was the most efficient, with other tests ranking as follows: reticulocyte hemoglobin > soluble transferrin receptor > erythrocyte zinc protoporphyrin > transferrin saturation > ferritin. But in another study,[394] the area under the receiver operator characteristic curve was largest for serum ferritin but less for transferrin receptor and erythrocyte ferritin. Other measurements, including the total iron-binding capacity, transferrin saturation and serum transferrin receptor had even less predictive value. Another comparison showed erythrocyte ferritin to be somewhat less efficient in the diagnosis of iron deficiency than serum ferritin.[394] Still another study averred that the reticulocyte hemoglobin content and reticulocytes in a high fluorescent intensity region, a measure of reticulocyte immaturity, were the best methods, particularly if the results of the two tests were combined.[395] Reticulocyte hemoglobin levels have become quite popular in the management of patients in renal failure[395,396] and may have the advantage of giving results that reflect the current iron status in patients who are being treated.[397]

ANEMIA OF HEMOLYTIC DISEASE

Hemolytic disease can usually be distinguished from iron-deficiency anemia based on the blood film. The marked poikilocytosis, polychromatophilia, and other morphologic features characteristic of hemolysis usually are not seen in iron-deficiency anemia. Furthermore, reticulocytosis is usually marked in hemolytic disorders but minimal or absent in iron deficiency anemia. However, there are some outstanding exceptions to these generally valid principles.

In unstable hemoglobin disorders, such as hemoglobin H disease or hemoglobin Köln disease, erythrocytic hypochromia may be pronounced. In these disorders, there is moderate reticulocytosis, which helps to differentiate them from iron-deficiency anemia. The serum iron concentration is normal or increased. The detection of unstable hemoglobins is discussed in Chapter 48.

When there is chronic intravascular hemolysis, erythrocytes in the blood film may display marked morphologic abnormalities, such as burr cells and schizocytes. Yet, because of loss of iron in the urine, iron deficiency may be the dominant cause of the resulting anemia. Evaluation of iron content marrow aspirates or measurement of serum iron concentration and TIBC may clarify the diagnosis in this form of anemia.

HYPOPLASTIC AND APLASTIC ANEMIA

In their early phases, these disorders cannot reliably be differentiated from mild iron-deficiency anemia on the basis of erythrocyte morphology alone (see Chap. 33. The reticulocyte count is generally less than in 0.5 percent in hypoplastic or aplastic anemia. The presence of neutropenia and thrombocytopenia suggests a diagnosis of aplastic anemia, but mild neutropenia may also occur in iron-deficiency anemia. The serum iron concentration is usually increased in aplastic anemia; the percentage transferrin saturation may be high. Marrow aspiration may produce scant material for cytologic study, and marrow biopsy may be necessary. Iron stain usually reveals increased amounts of hemosiderin in aplastic or hypoplastic anemia. However, if chronic bleeding has occurred, for example, because of thrombocytopenia, iron stores may be depleted.

MYELOPROLIFERATIVE DISEASES

In polycythemia vera, erythrocytes may be small and hypochromic (see Chap. 56). Even in the absence of distinctive morphologic changes in erythrocytes, the serum iron concentration is usually decreased, the TIBC is normal or increased, and marrow aspirates show little or no hemosiderin. Ferrokinetic studies show accelerated plasma iron incorporated into the hemoglobin of circulating erythrocytes.[398] These findings simply reflect iron deficiency, which is almost always present in this disease, as a result of marked expansion in total hemoglobin mass, increased gastrointestinal blood loss, or therapeutic phlebotomy. The marrow hemosiderin content is often decreased in other myeloproliferative disorders,[321] possibly because of a defect in macrophage storage of iron.

SIDEROBLASTIC ANEMIA

In this heterogeneous group of disorders (see Chap. 58), the blood findings often simulate those of iron-deficiency anemia. Reticulocytosis is usually absent, and the serum iron and serum ferritin levels are generally normal or increased. Marrow examination shows increased amounts of both are present.

CONGENITAL DYSERYTHROPOIETIC ANEMIA

In the rare congenital dyserythropoietic anemias, erythrocyte morphologic abnormalities may resemble those of iron deficiency or thalassemia (see Chap. 37). In general, in congenital dyserythropoietic anemias, poikilocytosis is very striking and occurs with less reduction in MCV than in iron deficiency or thalassemias. Often, however, such cases are believed to be thalassemic until the marrow is examined.

MEGALOBLASTIC ANEMIA

In pernicious anemia and other types of megaloblastic anemia (see Chap. 39), the blood film usually shows changes sufficiently distinctive that there is little difficulty in differential diagnosis. One potential source of error is the change in serum iron concentration that occurs after therapy. In the untreated patient with pernicious anemia or folic acid deficiency, the serum iron concentration decreases markedly as iron is utilized rapidly for hemoglobin synthesis.[399] Thus, the finding of a low serum iron concentration in such circumstances should not be taken as evidence of iron deficiency. Iron-deficiency anemia and anemia due to folic acid or vitamin B_{12} deficiency may coexist. During the course of treatment, with the rapid increase in the number of red cells, the typical manifestations of severe iron deficiency may develop.[400]

ANEMIA OF MYXEDEMA

The anemia of myxedema (see Chap. 36) is usually normochromic and normocytic and may be accompanied by mild to moderate depression of serum iron concentration. Ferrokinetic studies may show a decreased rate of plasma iron transport but normal iron utilization. Marrow examination may be required to determine whether iron deficiency is present, especially because iron deficiency often complicates myxedema because of menorrhagia, which is common in this disorder.

THERAPEUTIC TRIAL

In the final analysis, the response to iron therapy is the proof of correctness of diagnosis of iron-deficiency anemia. Furthermore, some physicians or patients may not have access to all the techniques described for diagnosis of iron-deficiency anemia. In this event, the patient's response to therapy may become a primary diagnostic measure. Iron administration in such a therapeutic trial should usually be by the oral route only. A therapeutic trial under any circumstance should be followed carefully. If the cause of anemia is iron deficiency, adequate iron therapy should result in reticulocytosis with a peak occurring after 1 to 2 weeks of therapy, although if anemia is mild, the reticulocyte response may be minimal. A significant increase in the hemoglobin concentration of the blood should be evident 3 to 4 weeks later, and the hemoglobin concentration should attain a normal value within 2 to 4 months. Unless there is evidence of continued, substantial blood loss, a malabsorption syndrome, or evidence of H. pylori infection, the absence of these changes must be taken as evidence that iron deficiency is not the cause of anemia. Iron therapy should be discontinued and another mechanism sought.

SPECIAL STUDIES TO DELINEATE THE CAUSE OF IRON DEFICIENCY

The physician who establishes a diagnosis of iron deficiency resulting from blood loss has the obligation to determine the site and cause of hemorrhage. Examination of the stools for the presence of blood is particularly helpful in determining what additional studies should be carried out. Specimens should be examined on several days because bleeding may be intermittent. Occasionally, it is helpful to label the patient's erythrocytes with ^{51}Cr sodium chromate and to determine quantitatively the amount of blood lost daily. When there is reason to believe that bleeding is from the gastrointestinal tract, roentgenographic and other imaging studies and endoscopic investigation are indicated. The latter often include gastroscopy, esophagoscopy, and colonoscopy. Numerous clinical studies indicate that intensive investigation of patients, particularly men and postmenopausal women, reveals unexpected bleeding lesions, many of which are curable or treatable.[128,401–404]

Percutaneous retrograde angiography of celiac or mesenteric arteries has proved valuable in localizing sites of active gastrointestinal bleeding, when rate of blood flow into the intestinal lumen is 0.5 ml/min or greater.[124,405] This procedure should be considered for any patient actively bleeding from the gastrointestinal tract, in whom the site of blood loss has not been established by other methods, including endoscopy, and for whom surgery is contemplated. Angiography should be carried out prior to barium contrast studies. The rate of bleeding may be increased following angiography.[405] The diverticula often contain ectopic gastric mucosa, which concentrate pertechnetate following intravenous injection for scintigraphic study; such scintigrams have been useful in identifying Meckel diverticulum as the cause of gastrointestinal blood loss.[406,407] H. pylori infection should be sought, particularly in patients who are iron deficient but do not seem to respond to therapy.

In some cases, small bowel endoscopy by laparoscopy may detect bleeding lesions when less invasive methods have failed.[408,409] Rarely, exploratory laparotomy may be warranted, because some adults with unexplained occult bleeding have gastrointestinal malignancies.

An iron stain of sputum may reveal hemosiderin-laden macrophages when there is intrapulmonary bleeding.

THERAPY

Once it has been established that a patient is deficient in iron, replacement therapy should be instituted without further delay.

Iron may be administered in one of several forms—orally, as simple iron salts; parenterally, as an iron–carbohydrate complex; or as a blood transfusion. In general, the oral route is preferred. In most patients, iron-deficiency anemia is a disorder of long duration and slow progression. Precipitous measures to restore a normal hemoglobin concentration by transfusing the patient are never warranted and are, indeed, hazardous. There is usually time to wait for normal mechanisms of erythropoiesis to respond to the body's needs and for gradual adjustment of the cardiovascular system to reexpansion of the total circulating erythrocyte volume.

ORAL IRON THERAPY

Dietary Therapy The patient should be encouraged to eat a diversified diet supplying all nutritional requirements. Nonetheless, it must be emphasized that neither meat nor any other dietary article contains enough iron to be useful therapeutically. Meat contains small amounts of myoglobin and hemoglobin (blood trapped in capillaries) and insignificant amounts of iron in other proteins. Although heme iron is better absorbed than inorganic iron, the quantity of heme iron in meat is actually quite small. In fact, an average (3-ounce) serving of steak provides only about 3 mg of iron. Provision of sufficient dietary iron to permit a maximal rate of recovery from iron-deficiency anemia might require a daily intake of at least 10 pounds of steak. For these and other reasons, medicinal iron is much superior to dietary iron in the therapy of iron deficiency.

Iron Preparations The pharmaceutical market is glutted with iron preparations in nearly every conceivable form; each promoted to appeal to physician or patient for one reason or another. The following simple principles may help the physician to find a way through this chaos.

1. Each dose of an inorganic iron preparation for an adult should contain between 30 and 100 mg of elemental iron. Doses of this magnitude cause unpleasant side effects relatively infrequently.[410,411] Smaller doses have been popular in the past, but these may result in a slower recovery of the patient, or no recovery at all. Small doses of iron preparations containing some heme have been reported to be effective in correcting iron deficiency in pregnancy.[412,413]

2. The iron should be readily released in acidic or neutral gastric juice or duodenal juice (usually pH 5–6), because maximal absorption occurs when iron is presented to the duodenal mucosa. Enteric-coated and prolonged-release preparations dissolve slowly in any of these fluids. Thus with such preparations the iron that eventually is released may be presented to a portion of the intestinal mucosa in which absorption is least efficient. Some patients who have been treated unsuccessfully with enteric-coated or prolonged-release iron preparations respond promptly to the administration of nonenteric-coated ferrous salts (Fig. 40-13).

3. The iron, once released, should be readily absorbed. Iron is absorbed in the ferrous form; consequently, only ferrous salts should be used.

4. Side effects should be infrequent. This seems not to be a particular problem for any of the common commercially available iron compounds. Despite the claims of pharmaceutical companies, there is no convincing evidence that any one effective preparation is superior in this respect to any other.

5. The cost to the patient should be small.

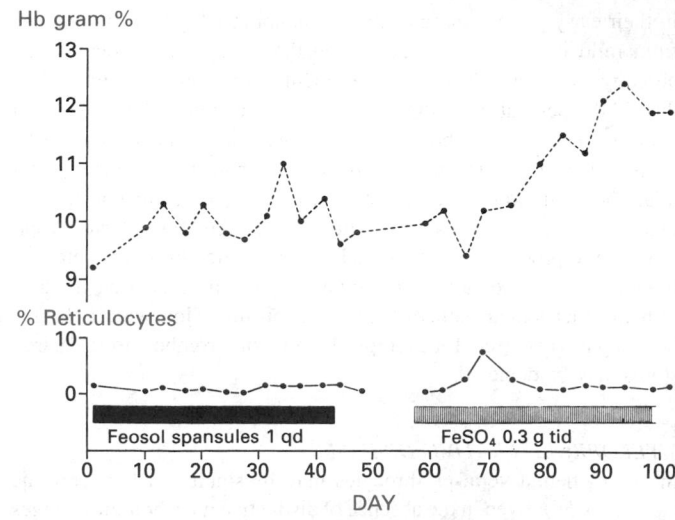

FIGURE 40-13 Rate of response of patient with iron-deficiency anemia to 43 days of treatment with prolonged-release Feosol Spansules (containing 225 mg ferrous sulfate), one capsule daily, the dosage recommended by the manufacturer, followed by 43 days of treatment with nonenteric ferrous sulfate (0.3 g three times daily). Clearly, 225 mg of ferrous sulfate daily in prolonged-release form failed to elicit any significant hematopoietic response in this case. The rapid response subsequently elicited with conventional ferrous sulfate may be taken as a typical response to effect therapy in adequate dosage, whether by oral or parenteral route. (From E Beutler, G Meerkreebs,[675] with permission from the Massachusetts Medical Society.)

CHAPTER 40 DISORDERS OF IRON METABOLISM

531

6. The use of preparations containing several therapeutic agents is to be condemned.

Physicians should be aware that if ferrous sulfate is prescribed generically, the choice of preparation is left to the pharmacist, who may dispense enteric-coated tablets. It is advisable to specify "nonenteric" or to prescribe by brand name a product that is not enteric coated.

Although substances such as ascorbic acid, succinate, and fructose have been shown to enhance iron absorption, the gain is offset to a large extent by the increase in frequency of side effects or cost of therapy, or both. There is no convincing evidence to support the use of chelated forms of iron or of iron in combination with wetting agents.

Dosage. For the therapy of iron deficiency in adults, the dosage should be sufficient to provide between 150 and 200 mg elemental iron daily. The iron may be taken orally in three or four doses 1 hour before meals. Infants may be given 6 mg/kg [414] daily in divided doses for therapy or a daily dose of 12.5 mg daily for prophylaxis of iron deficiency (Table 40-10).[415]

Side Effects. Mild gastrointestinal side effects occur occasionally in the form of nausea, heartburn, constipation, or looseness of stools. A metallic taste may be experienced. In some patients these side effects may be psychological in origin.[410] The majority of patients tolerate the usual therapeutic doses of iron without the least side effect. However, there is no doubt that some patients, perhaps one or two of 10, experience symptoms that may be ascribed to the iron preparation and may be related in part to the size of the dose.[411,416] In such cases, reduction of the frequency of administration to one tablet a day for a few days may alleviate the symptoms; later, the patient may be able to tolerate treatment in full dosage. It may also be useful to change to another iron preparation, especially one with a different external appearance.

Carbonyl iron has been proposed as an alternative to iron salts, on the assertion that it can be given in large doses with minimal side effects. This substance is actually metallic iron powder, with a particle size less than 5 μm. Because it is insoluble, it is not absorbed until converted to the ionic form. The bioavailability of carbonyl iron has been estimated to be about 70 percent of that of an equivalent amount of ferrous sulfate,[417] but oral doses of 1 to 3 g/day may be required for optimal therapy. Oral doses as high as 600 mg three times daily did not produce toxic effects.[418]

There has been speculation in the medical literature[419] and some data[420] suggesting that iron might be a risk factor for cardiovascular disease. However, the bulk of evidence suggests that no such effect exists,[421–427] nor does it seem that iron supplementation causes an increased frequency of infections.[428] Similarly, it has been claimed that there is association between elevated ferritin levels and diabetes,[429,430] but this has not been the case in most investigations.[431]

Acute Iron Poisoning. Acute iron poisoning is usually a consequence of the accidental ingestion by infants or small children of iron-containing medications intended for use by adults. Any potent oral preparation may cause acute iron poisoning, and this serious disorder is not at all rare. For example, in the Los Angeles area alone there were five deaths from iron poisoning among children 11 to 18 months of age in the 7-month period following June 1992.

The earliest manifestation of iron poisoning is vomiting, usually within 1 hour of the ingestion. There may be hematemesis or melena. Restlessness, hypotension, tachypnea, and cyanosis may develop soon thereafter and may be followed within a few hours by coma and death. So inexorable a course is not the rule, however, and only about 1 percent of such poisonings have a fatal outcome.[432] Usually, medical aid is sought early, and, with proper treatment, most iron-poisoned children should survive. The initial treatment is prompt evacuation of the stomach. In the home this may be induced by digital stimulation of the pharyngeal gag reflex. Oral administration of a tepid solution of baking soda serves two useful purposes: it may provoke emesis, and the bicarbonate ion complexes with the iron and retards absorption. If a child has ingested more than 60 mg of iron per kg body weight, hospital treatment is indicated.[433] In the emergency room, gastric intubation and lavage should be performed promptly, preferably with a solution containing 4 g sodium bicarbonate (or 3.6 g disodium phosphate and 0.8 g monosodium phosphate) per deciliter. Before the tube is withdrawn, a solution containing 5 to 10 g desferrioxamine, or approximately 60 ml of the bicarbonate or phosphate solution, should be introduced into the stomach. Supportive measures should be used as needed for shock or for metabolic acidosis should these develop. Desferrioxamine is the agent of choice for specific therapy of hyperferremia. It usually should be administered intramuscularly at an initial dose of 1 g, followed by 0.5 g intramuscularly 4 and 8 hours later, and thereafter at 12-hour intervals as the clinical status warrants. If the child is hypotensive, the dose may be administered intravenously at a rate not exceeding 15 mg/kg/hour for a total initial dose of 1 g, with repetition of this dosage started every 4 to 12 hours as the clinical status of the patient seems to warrant.[434] Improvement often appears several hours to a few days after onset of iron poisoning. This improvement may be permanent, but it may also be misleading, because pneumonitis or severe hepatic or neurologic decompensation may soon supervene. There may be seizures, coma, hyperreflexia, jaundice, and bilirubinemia. Children who survive for 3 or 4 days usually recover without sequelae. However, gastric strictures and fibrosis or intestinal stenosis may occur as late complications. These have been reported as early as 6 weeks after acute iron poisoning.[433,435–437]

PARENTERAL IRON THERAPY

Indications In view of the significantly greater hazards and cost of parenteral therapy, the choice of this mode of administration must be carefully considered, but occasionally it becomes necessary to administer iron by the parenteral route. The indications are malabsorption, intolerance to iron taken orally, iron need in excess of an amount that can be taken orally, and non-compliance of the patient. Parenteral iron administration, together with erythropoietin, appears to alleviate the anemia that otherwise may complicate long-term dialysis treatment of patients with chronic renal disease. For reasons that are not well understood, these patients do not appear to respond adequately to oral iron therapy.[438,439]

Calculating Dosage It is easy to estimate the amount of iron that need be given by merely remembering that 1 mL of red cells contain about 1 mg of iron. However, various formulas have been used for estimating total dose required for treatment. Because total blood volume is approximately 65 ml/kg and the iron content of hemoglobin is 0.34 percent by weight, the simplest formula for estimating the total dose required for correction of anemia only is as follows:

TABLE 40-10 IRON PREPARATIONS FOR PEDIATRIC USE

CHEMICAL DESIGNATION	IRON CONTENT (MG/ML)	COMMERCIAL (PROPRIETARY) DESIGNATION	THERAPEUTIC DOSAGE
Ferrous sulfate solution, USP	8		1, 2 or 3 times per day
Ferrous sulfate solution, concentrated	25	Fer-In-Sol	1 ml, 3 or 4 times per day
Ferrous sulfate elixir (5% ethanol)	9	Feosol elixir	1 tsp, 2 or 3 times per day

Dose of iron (mg) = Whole blood hemoglobin deficit (g/dl)

$$\times \text{ Body weight (lb).}$$

Assuming a normal mean hemoglobin concentration of 16 g/dl, a male weighing 170 pounds whose hemoglobin concentration is 7 g/dl would require (16 − 7) × 170 = 1530 mg of iron to correct the anemia. To this amount should be added a sufficient quantity of iron to replete iron stores, approximately 1000 mg for men and approximately 600 mg for women. Thus, a 170-pound male with a hemoglobin concentration of 7 g/dl should receive 2530 mg of iron.

Preparations   *Iron Sucrose.*   Known under a variety of generic names, iron sucrose (Eisenzucker; ferric hydroxide sucrose; ferric oxide, saccharated; ferrum oxydatum saccharatum; iron (III) hydroxide–sucrose complex; Oxyde de Fer Sucre; saccharated iron oxide; XI-921) is the oldest of the intravenous iron preparations, having been first used in humans in 1947.[440] For many years it was largely replaced by iron dextran, but iron sucrose complexes have enjoyed a renaissance in recent years, the newer complexes having the advantage of greater safety.

Iron sucrose is a complex of polynuclear iron ferric hydroxide in sucrose. It has a molecular mass of approximately 34,000 to 60,000 daltons.[441] Sold in the United States as Venofer®, it contains 20 mg of iron per milliliter. After intravenous injection, iron is cleared from the plasma with an initial half-life of about 30 minutes,[441] after which it is removed with a half-life of about 6 hours. It is taken up by macrophages, where the iron is released.

The dose recommended by the manufacturer is 5 ml (100 mg of elemental iron), administered no more frequently than three times weekly. However, iron sucrose has been administered to patients with chronic kidney disease at a dosage of 500 mg infused over 3 hours on 2 consecutive days, and considered to be safe and effective[442]; it has also been suggested that high doses may depress neutrophils' intracellular killing function.[443]

Adverse events reported by more than 5 percent of treated patients included hypotension (36%), cramps (23%), nausea, headache, vomiting, and diarrhea. It is not certain to what extent these are actually due to the iron preparation. Less common adverse effects have included headache, fever, chest pain, hypertension, dizziness, dyspnea, cough, pleuritis, and pain at the site of reaction. It has been estimated that 20 million doses of iron sucrose administered to more than one million patients worldwide resulted in 52 anaphylactoid reactions, of which 22 were considered serious. There were no deaths. [441] Iron sucrose has been administered without adverse event to patients who manifest sensitivity reactions to iron dextran or sodium ferric gluconate.[444,445]

Iron Dextran.   Iron dextran is a complex of iron and dextran with an average mass equivalent to 165,000 g/mole with a range of approximately ±10 percent daltons. The commercial preparation (INFeD Injection®; Watson in the United States) is marketed as a stable, dark brown, slightly acidic (pH 6) solution containing 50 mg of elemental iron per milliliter. The manufacturer recommends intravenous test doses of 0.5 ml before therapy is started and that each dose consist of only 2 ml or less. Much larger doses ("total dose infusion") have also been employed very widely and are generally considered more convenient, safe, and cost effective,[179,446–451] although an increase in minor reactions has been noted.[452] It may even be argued that a single infusion is less likely to elicit an immune response than multiple injections given over a period of several weeks. If any adverse effect is noted, injection must be terminated at once and appropriate countermeasures taken. A syringe containing a solution of epinephrine should be immediately accessible for treatment of anaphylaxis should this occur.

After intramuscular injection, iron dextran is slowly absorbed; approximately 72 hours are required for 50 percent of the dose to move

out of the injection site.[453,454] It is slowly cleared from plasma. Peak plasma concentrations of thousands of micrograms of iron per deciliter are found even 10 days after intramuscular injection; the plasma iron concentration decreases slowly, reaching normal values after 3 to 4 weeks.[455] Iron dextran is cleared from plasma by the macrophages, and ultimately the iron is used in hemoglobin synthesis. Mobilization of iron dextran from an intramuscular site is relatively slow and incomplete; 20 to 35 percent of the dose may remain at the injection site 1 month later.[456,457] Furthermore, the rate of incorporation of iron dextran into hemoglobin is somewhat slower than that for simpler ferric hydroxide colloids.[457,458] It appears that the iron dextran complex is only slowly dissociated in macrophages, and iron granules may be seen in marrow macrophages in iron dextran-treated patients even after iron-deficiency anemia has recurred.

Intramuscular administration of iron dextran causes a moderate degree of pain at the injection site and a dark stain in the skin that may remain for as long as 1 to 2 years. "Z-track" and other techniques of injection recommended by the manufacturer reduce, but do not eliminate, the discoloration of the skin. Intravenous administration also may cause local side effects, in the form of thrombophlebitis. This occurs most commonly when iron dextran is diluted with 5 percent glucose solution, less frequently when diluted with isotonic saline solution, and infrequently when iron dextran is injected undiluted. Thrombophlebitis at the injection site appears to be unusual with the technique of total-dose infusion, and other adverse effects appear to be no more frequent than with the intramuscular route.

The frequency of systemic reactions of iron dextran therapy has been markedly variable in different series, ranging from less than 2 percent to more than 25 percent of patients.[459] Dextran is a biologic product, the exact structure of which is apparently difficult to control, and the frequency of adverse effects varies, probably due to variations in manufacturing techniques. Arthralgias and fever may be experienced by as many as one third of patients. Other systemic reactions are infrequent and include hypotension, myalgia, headache, abdominal pain, nausea and vomiting, dizziness, lymphadenopathy, pleural effusion, pruritus, urticaria, seizures, flushing, chills, and phlebitis. Lymphadenopathy[460,461] and allergic purpura[462] have been noted. Several cases have been observed in which iron dextran infusion was followed by an acute febrile illness accompanied by tender lymphadenopathy and splenomegaly lasting 10 to 14 days.[451,463] Pleocytosis of the cerebrospinal fluid has been observed during a febrile reaction to iron dextran[464]; in this case there was also a blood leukocyte count of 88×10^9/liter (88,000/μL). In another patient, meningismus without increased leukocytes in the spinal fluid but a high spinal fluid iron concentration was documented.[465] Pancytopenia may follow iron dextran therapy.[466] Acute, severe exacerbation of arthritis has been observed following iron dextran therapy in patients with rheumatoid arthritis[459] or ankylosing spondylitis.[467] Intramuscular deposition of iron dextran has led to malignancy in some experimental animals.[468,469] Fibrosarcoma and undifferentiated pleomorphic sarcoma have developed at the site of injection in several human subjects following repeated or protracted iron dextran therapy.[470–472] This appears to be an extremely rare phenomenon and may in some cases have been coincidental rather than causally related.

The most dangerous complication of iron dextran therapy is anaphylactic reaction. This occurs in fewer than 1 percent of patients treated by either the intramuscular or intravenous route. It is not dose dependent and may follow the infusion of only a few drops of diluted iron dextran solution or a fraction of a milliliter of intramuscularly injected iron dextran. This calls into question the usefulness of giving a test dose, and it is doubtful whether such a test dose serves any useful purpose. Characteristically, during the first few minutes of infusion, the patient complains of difficulty breathing, or a choking or smothering sensation, becomes sweaty and anxious, may complain of nausea, and may vomit. Respiratory stridor may be observed, followed by apnea. The blood pressure may drop abruptly; stupor and coma may quickly supervene. At the first evidence of this reaction, the infusion must be terminated, and epinephrine should immediately be injected subcutaneously (0.5 ml of 1:1000 aqueous epinephrine). Other measures to combat shock and anaphylaxis are appropriate. Most patients survive, but 31 fatalities were reported in the United States between 1976 and 1996.[473] Stroke or myocardial infarction may follow anaphylactic shock induced by iron dextran.[474]

Freshly opened vials of iron dextran may contain as much as 100 mg of divalent iron per deciliter. Iron dextran causes hypotension when administered intravenously to cats, and the hypotensive effect correlates to some extent with the amount of divalent iron in the solution.[475] Successful administration of iron dextran after pretreatment with methylprednisolone, diphenhydramine, ephedrine, and Promit (very low molecular weight dextran) has been reported in a patient with a previous anaphylactic response,[476] and the use of glucocorticoids to prevent delayed reactions had been advocated,[451] but circumstances would need to be very unusual to justify readministration of iron dextran to a patient who had experienced a severe reaction.

Sodium Ferric Gluconate Complex in Sucrose Injection. Sodium ferric gluconate complex, sold in the United States as Ferrlecit®, is a stable macromolecular complex of innate and ferric iron with a molecular weight approximating 289,000 to 440,000 daltons. Each milliliter contains 12.5 mg of elemental iron. The manufacturer recommends administration of doses of 125 mg of elemental iron with the preparation eluted in 100 ml of 0.9 percent sodium chloride and given intravenously over a period of 1 hour.[477] However, doses as high as 500 mg have been given with apparent safety.[478,479] Adverse reactions include hypotension (29%), cramps (25%), dizziness (13%), dyspnea (11%), paresthesias (6%), coughing (6%), nausea, vomiting, and/or diarrhea (2%), hypertension (0.6%), allergic reaction (0.5%), chest pain (0.5%), pleuritis (0.5%), and back pain (0.4).[477] It is by no means clear that all of these symptoms were actually related to the drug. Injection site reactions have been reported by 33 percent of the subjects. Severe life-threatening hypersensitivity reactions are rare but do occur.[473] In contrast to those occurring with iron dextran, such episodes have not been reported to have a fatal outcome with sodium ferric gluconate. Although the number of reactions to these two iron preparations seem to be similar, the more severe reactions, leading to death, seem to be more common with iron dextran.[473,480]

COURSE AND PROGNOSIS

COURSE

If therapy is adequate, the correction of iron deficiency anemia is usually gratifying. Symptoms such as headache, fatigue, pica, paresthesias, and burning sensation of the oropharyngeal mucosa may abate within a few days. In the blood, the reticulocyte count begins to increase after a few days, usually reaches a maximum at about 7 to 12 days, and thereafter decreases. When anemia is mild, little or no reticulocytosis may be observed. Little change in hemoglobin concentration or hematocrit value is to be expected for the first 2 weeks, but then the anemia is corrected rapidly. The hemoglobin concentration in the blood may be halfway back to normal after 4 to 5 weeks of therapy. By the end of 2 months of therapy, and often much sooner, the hemoglobin concentration should have reached a normal level. There is little difference in the rate of response whether iron is administered by the oral or the parenteral route,[481] except in patients with intestinal malabsorption.[482] Differences that have been encountered may well be due to noncompliance of patients given oral iron.[483] If the diagnosis of iron-deficiency anemia is correct, anemia and other manifestations

of iron deficiency will respond to adequate therapy. However, the physician is occasionally disappointed in the results of treatment of patients who seem to have iron-deficiency anemia. In some cases this apparent failure of therapy is a result of treatment of patients with iron preparations that are virtually insoluble, enteric-coated, or contain iron in only minute amounts. Careful inquiry into the nature, duration, and regularity of iron therapy may reveal a reason for the failure of therapy and permit a gratifying response to be elicited with adequate therapy. Other questions that should be asked in evaluation of such a case are these: (1) Has bleeding been controlled? (2) Has the patient been on iron therapy long enough to show a response? (3) Has the dose of iron been adequate? (4) Are there other factors, such as inflammatory disease, neoplastic disease, hepatic or renal disease, concomitant deficiencies (vitamin B_{12}, folic acid, thyroid), that might retard response? It has been suggested that ingestion of large amounts of black tea[484–486] and *H. pylori*[138,139,144] may prevent the response of an iron-deficient patient to what would otherwise be adequate therapy. (5) Is the diagnosis correct?

PROGNOSIS

When the cause of the iron deficiency is a benign disorder, the prognosis is excellent, provided bleeding is controlled or can be compensated for by continual iron therapy. Too often, therapy is interrupted as soon as anemia has been corrected, and iron stores are not replenished. Such inadequately treated patients are likely to have recurrent anemia.[487,488] For this reason, and because iron therapy brings about replenishment of iron stores very slowly, oral therapy should be continued for at least 12 months after anemia has been corrected. If there is a benign cause of recurrent bleeding that is corrected, such as hiatal hernia, menorrhagia, or hereditary hemorrhagic telangiectasia, oral iron therapy may be continued indefinitely; if the bleeding is especially brisk, supplementation with parenterally administered iron or, rarely, with transfusion may be needed. Continuous iron administration may also be required in patients with iron deficiency secondary to intravascular hemolysis with hemoglobinuria.

IRON STORAGE DISEASE

DEFINITION AND HISTORY

The terms *iron storage disease* and *hemochromatosis* are used to designate an increase of tissue iron resulting in a disease state. *Hemosiderosis*, on the other hand denotes an increase of tissue iron stores with or without tissue damage. Classically, hemochromatosis has been characterized by bronzing of the skin, cirrhosis, and diabetes, and was once called *bronzed diabetes*. Since the 1970s, usage of the term hemochromatosis has expanded well beyond its original meaning. This diagnosis is now commonly applied to persons who have increased body iron as suggested by increased serum ferritin levels, and even to those who merely have the hemochromatosis *HFE* genotype, regardless of the level of their iron stores.

Hemochromatosis may be divided into genetic forms and acquired forms. The former have sometimes been designated as *primary* and the latter as *secondary* forms. The disorder—once designated as *idiopathic hemochromatosis* and more recently as *hereditary hemochromatosis*—usually is the most common genetic form of the disorder. It is found principally in those of northern European ancestry and is caused by mutations in the *HFE* gene. This form of the disease has also been called *type I hemochromatosis*, and we prefer to designate it as *classical hemochromatosis*. But there are other forms of hereditary hemochromatosis as well. *Juvenile hemochromatosis*, hemochromatosis due to ferroportin mutations, and *African iron overload* are among these. *Neonatal hemochromatosis* is a term that has been ap-

TABLE 40-11   CLASSIFICATION OF HEMOCHROMATOSIS

I. Hereditary hemochromatosis
  A. Classical hemochromatosis (hereditary hemochromatosis; *HFE* hemochromatosis) (type 1)
  B. Juvenile hemochromatosis (type 2)
    1. Abnormality in hemojuvelin
    2. Abnormality of hepcidin
  C. Transferrin receptor-2 deficiency (type 3)
  D. Ferroportin deficiency (includes some cases of African iron overload[490–492] (type 4)
  E. Ferritin H-chain IRE mutation[58]
  F. African iron overload
  G. Neonatal hemochromatosis (?)
II. Secondary hemochromatosis

plied to what is probably a heterogeneous group of disorders of the newborn in whom there is congenital cirrhosis or fulminant hepatitis with hepatic and extrahepatic iron deposits. It is not clear that this is a disorder of iron homeostasis[489] and will be discussed further here. A classification of hereditary hemochromatosis is presented in Table 40-11. *Secondary hemochromatosis* occurs in patients who receive multiple blood transfusions, particularly when they have ineffective erythropoiesis.

Iron accumulation in localized sites, particularly the brain, occurs in disorders other than hemochromatosis. One of these is termed *neonatal hemochromatosis*. It is of unknown origin and is characterized by hepatic and extrahepatic iron deposition and fulminant hepatitis.[489] The GRACILE (Growth Retardation, Aminoaciduria, Cholestasis, Iron overload, Lactic acidosis, and Early death) syndrome is an autosomal recessive disorder that is found mostly among Finns and a mutation in the *BCS1L* gene.[493] Neuroferritinopathy is a neurologic disorder that results from a structural mutation near the carboxy end of the ferritin light chain. Clinical features include a dystonic dysarthria with chorea, dystonia, and parkinsonian manifestations found in some patients.[494] Increased iron deposition also is characteristic of atransferrinemia.[51,52] Increased quantities of brain iron are characteristic of aeruloplasminemia[62,495] and are found in Alzheimer disease, parkinsonism, Friedreich ataxia, Hallervorden Spatz syndrome, and multiple system atrophy.[496] Because none of these disorders is primarily hematologic and in most the role of iron deposition is secondary to another underlying pathology, they are not discussed further here.

Hemochromatosis was first described by Trousseau in 1865 (cited in ref. 497). The massive accumulation of iron that occurred in this disease was recognized as its hallmark, but other metals also accumulate. Some investigators thought the toxic metal might be copper.[498] The ingenious development by Davis and Arrowsmith[499] in 1952 of serial phlebotomy used for treatment of the disease made clear that iron accumulation was the most important pathogenetic factor. In 1935, Sheldon[500] helped to focus attention on the disease in a classic monograph. He suggested that the disease might be hereditary, and he addressed the prevalence of hemochromatosis. Sheldon proposed that although hemochromatosis was not as rare as had been thought, it was a relatively uncommon disorder. Sheldon's view that hemochromatosis might have a genetic basis was strongly contested by MacDonald,[501,502] who considered the disorder to be caused by increased iron intake, particularly the iron in wine. However, the existence of a hereditary factor was firmly established when Simon and colleagues[503] showed that the disease was tightly linked to the human leukocyte antigen (HLA) locus. These investigators demonstrated both linkage within families and linkage disequilibrium in populations.[504] They realized that the HLA-A or HLA-B gene products themselves were not involved in the pathogenesis of the disease; rather the gene that did cause hemochromatosis was located nearby. A quarter of a century

passed before one of the many attempts succeeded in cloning the gene responsible for the disease. Surprisingly, the gene proved to be *HFE*, one of the many HLA-like genes on chromosome 6.[44] This finding, and the availability of new, powerful animal models for the study of iron homeostasis, resulted in the discovery of many new genes involved in the regulation of body iron content (see Table 40-3).

The identification of the *HFE* gene made possible, for the first time, accurate assessment of the gene frequency and penetrance of the *HFE* mutations. This assessment brought about a fusion of the apparently contrasting views of MacDonald and Simon. The penetrance of the homozygous state is so low that it could be considered a risk factor rather than the major cause of the disease.[505]

EPIDEMIOLOGY

At one time, all forms of hemochromatosis were considered rare. The male to female ratio was 18:1.[264,500] With the widespread availability in the 1970s of means for measuring serum iron, transferrin saturation, and ferritin levels, hereditary hemochromatosis grew to be regarded as a very common disorder with a sex ratio of about 1.5:1.[506] As discussed later (see "Genetics" below), the prevalence of *HFE* gene mutations is very high. The most significant is the c.845 A→G (C282Y) mutation. With a gene frequency of approximately 0.07 in the northern European population, approximately five in 1000 northern Europeans are homozygous for the mutation. The C282Y and S65C mutations are almost entirely confined to individuals of European ancestry. The H63D mutation is more widespread geographically but also is most common in Europeans. Within Europe, the highest gene frequencies are encountered in the southern British Isles and northern France.[507] Table 40-12 summarizes the prevalence of these polymorphic mutations. In addition to the relatively common mutations, many sporadic mutations confined to single families have been documented.[517–522] Not all patients with hereditary hemochromatosis have mutations of the *HFE* gene. Whereas in northern Europe almost all patients with hemochromatosis have *HFE* gene mutations, iron storage disease in southern Europe much more likely results from mutations in other, mostly unidentified gene.[523,524]

Although earlier studies attributed nonspecific symptoms in patients to hemochromatosis,[525–527] large controlled series showed that the symptoms were not present in homozygotes for the C282Y mutation at a higher frequency than in controls.[528–530] These findings are consistent with the very low prevalence of hemochromatosis reported

TABLE 40-12   PREVALENCE OF COMMON HEMOCHROMATOSIS ALLELES IN DIFFERENT POPULATION

POPULATION	NO. OF SUBJECTS	C282Y	S65C	H63D	REFERENCE
African-American	1373	0.016		0.032	508
98.6% White	1001	0.066		0.151	509
New Zealand	1064	0.079		0.130	510
Brittany	1000	0.065		ND	511
Europe	1450	0.038		0.136	512
California White	31,227	0.062	0.016*	0.149	513
California Black	1501	0.019	0.0068†	0.045	513
California Asian	1815	0.001	0‡	0.036	513
England	6261	0.068		0.141	514
Northern Italy	1132	0.032	0.013	0.134	515
Southeastern Italy	500	0.015	0.005	0.14	516

* Only 7739 tested.
† Only 369 tested.
‡ Only 450 tested.
ND = not done.

in autopsy series[531–533] and hospital surveys.[534,535] The probable prevalence of symptomatic clinical hemochromatosis in northern European populations probably is only approximately five in 100,000 individuals. If patients with abnormal liver function tests and/or fibrosis on liver biopsy are included, the number of affected patients may be several-fold higher. The factors that determine whether a patient with the C282Y homozygous genotype develops disease are not well understood. The patient's sex clearly is a modifying factor, with more severe manifestations observed in males.[536] Pregnancy and menstrual losses tend to ameliorate the disease in women. A high proportion of severely affected patients have a large alcohol intake. Other genetic factors that might interact with the C282Y homozygous genotype in producing clinically significant iron storage disease have been sought but have not been found,[537] except for rare instances in which co-inheritance of mutations of the hepcidin gene may be responsible.[538,539]

The widespread perception that classical hereditary hemochromatosis frequently led to clinical disease resulted in widespread enthusiasm for population-based screening.[540–543] However, the cost to benefit analysis used was based upon the assumption that life-threatening disease manifestations occur in 43 percent of males and 28 percent of females,[540] estimates that were based upon the prevalence of the disease in patients of whom most had been diagnosed clinically with hemochromatosis. With the realization that the clinical penetrance is much lower, interest in screening the general population for hemochromatosis has largely disappeared, and efforts have been made to find high-risk groups in which screening could be justified (Fig. 40-14).[544]

The prevalences of other forms of hemochromatosis, including juvenile hemochromatosis, hemochromatosis due to ferroportin deficiency, and atransferrinemia, are much lower than the prevalence of classical hereditary hemochromatosis. These forms of hemochromatosis appear to be truly rare diseases.

ETIOLOGY AND PATHOGENESIS

TOXICITY OF IRON

Accepting and releasing electrons is the main basis of the importance of iron to living organisms. The same capacity to undergo reversible oxidation-reduction reactions appears to be the basis of the harm caused by excessive amounts of iron. One of the pathways considered to be of greatest importance is the Haber-Weiss reaction:

$$Fe^{++} + H_2O_2 \rightarrow Fe^{+++} + OH^- + \cdot HO$$
$$O_2^{\cdot -} + Fe^{+++} \rightarrow O_2 + Fe^{++}$$

The sum of these two reactions is the Fenton reaction:

$$O_2^{\cdot -} + H_2O_2 \rightarrow O_2 + OH^- + \cdot HO$$

The hydroxyl radical ($\cdot OH$) is second in reactivity only to atomic oxygen and has been implicated in damaging polysaccharides, DNA, and enzymes and causing lipid peroxidation.[545] Although no direct evidence exists that hydroxyl radical generation is the main pathway of tissue damage in hemochromatosis, this common conjecture seems reasonable. A possible role of ferryl ions (FeO_2^+) in mediating tissue damage also has been suggested.[546]

Demonstrating a damaging affect of iron alone on experimental animals has been difficult. Although subtle biochemical defects have been documented in some studies,[547–549] frank cirrhotic changes have not been found. In iron-loaded gerbils, cirrhosis did not occur if the diet was enriched in vitamin E.[550] Memory and motor behavior deficits were found in rats treated with large amounts of iron as pups.[551] In rats, iron alone does not cause fibrosis, and alcohol alone causes only

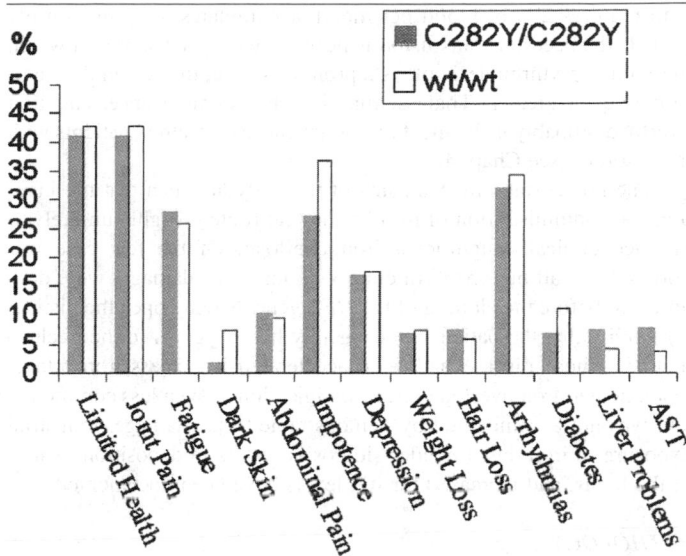

FIGURE 40-14 Penetrance of hemochromatosis in a large outpatient population. Patients were assessed by questionnaire, laboratory studies, and physical examination before the patient or physician was aware of the results of genotyping for the C282Y or H63D *HFE* mutation. There were 156 homozygotes for the C282Y mutation and more than 19,000 wild-type (wt/wt) controls. The only significant difference was in the aspartate amino transferase (AST). Only one patient had atypical symptoms and findings of hemochromatosis.

minor liver abnormalities. However, administration of both excess iron and alcohol results in fibrosis.[552] These findings in rats are consistent with the strong association demonstrated between alcohol ingestion and cirrhosis in patients with the hemochromatosis genotype.[553,554]

CAUSES OF IRON OVERLOAD

Because body iron content is maintained by regulating absorption, excess body iron can accumulate only when absorption is dysregulated or when iron is injected into the body, either in the form of medicinal iron or as transfused erythrocytes.

Dysregulation of Iron Absorption A variety of mutations cause increased iron absorption in experimental animals and in man (Table 40-3). Mutations of the genes encoding *HFE*, transferrin receptor-2, ferroportin-1, and hepcidin all have been associated with iron overload. Although a number of different models of systems through which such mutations dysregulate iron absorption have been proposed,[68,555–558] the actual mechanism remains unknown. In the case of hemochromatosis resulting from *HFE* mutations, a link with expression of hepcidin has been established. Normally, hepcidin is up-regulated when body iron increases. However, this process does not occur in *HFE* knockout mice[80,81] or in human disease.[76] A likely interpretation is that HFE is part of the signaling pathway that regulates hepcidin expression.

Ineffective Erythropoiesis A strong relationship between ineffective erythropoiesis and total body iron burden exists.[559] The amount of body iron may greatly exceed the quantity that can be accounted for through blood transfusion.[560] The mechanism by which active erythropoiesis and destruction of red cell precursors in the marrow stimulate iron absorption is unknown. However, of note, iron storage disease is particularly common in disorders such as thalassemia, hereditary dyserythropoietic anemia, and pyruvate kinase deficiency.

Transfusion or Iron Therapy Iron overload can be iatrogenic in origin. Because erythrocytes contain 1 mg of iron per milliliter, transfusion of 450 ml of whole blood or 200 ml of red cells add 200 mg of total iron to the body, iron that will not be excreted. Thus, a patient who requires 2 U of blood per month accumulates 4.8 g of iron per year. If the need for transfusion is necessitated by a disorder in which ineffective erythropoiesis plays a prominent role, the accumulation of iron is even greater. Thalassemia is such a circumstance, and iron overload probably is the most important cause of death in patients with the disorder (see Chap. 46).

The homeostatic mechanisms of the body are such that the inappropriate administration of iron by the oral route is highly unlikely to produce clinically significant iron overload. Of the few cases reported,[561–565] all but one[563] (a child without tissue damage) were documented before the cloning of the *HFE* gene, leaving open the distinct possibility that the patients were merely homozygotes for hemochromatosis whose disease had been accelerated by excess iron intake. Documented iron overload after iron injection is even less common[566] and was not accompanied by demonstrable tissue damage. Industrial exposure to iron dust (Welder siderosis) results in deposition of iron in the lungs, and increased ferritin levels have been documented.[567]

PATHOLOGY

Affected tissues and organs exhibit a deep brown color. Histologic examination reveals prominent hemosiderin deposition in many tissues and organs.

Liver   The liver often is enlarged. After cirrhosis develops, the liver becomes granular or coarsely nodular. In the liver of patients with classical hemochromatosis, transferrin receptor-2 mutations, and in juvenile hemochromatosis, hemosiderin, is found primarily in hepatocytes, bile duct epithelium, and, to a lesser degree, Kupffer cells and other mesenchymal cells. Prior to the development of cirrhosis, the hemosiderin accumulates primarily in periportal hepatocytes and is less toward the central veins. The iron of cirrhotic livers is mostly in the periphery of regenerative nodules. Fibrosis begins periportally, then fibrous septa traverse the lobules. Usually, the distortion of the architecture is not as severe or as uniform as in alcoholic cirrhosis.[568] The cirrhosis of hemochromatosis usually has a micronodular appearance. Iron in bile duct epithelium has sometimes been considered a specific marker for hemochromatosis but is not reliable. The amount of iron in the liver is always greatly increased. This is apparent on inspection of sections stained for iron with the Prussian Blue reaction and can be quantitated on liver biopsy specimens. An iron concentration greater than 300 μmol/g dry weight is considered strong evidence for hemochromatosis when factors such as transfusions are eliminated as the cause.

In the original description of African iron overload, the liver pathology was deemed to be indistinguishable from that of classical hemochromatosis,[569] but in more recent studies[570] it seems that only some of the affected patients manifest iron storage primarily in the hepatocytes; some have storage primarily in Kupffer cells. In ferroportin deficiency storage of iron takes place mostly in the Kupffer cells,[490,571,572] and fibrosis seems to be absent.

Marrow   The quantity of iron in the marrow of patients with classical hereditary hemochromatosis is only modestly increased, if at all. The iron is characteristically distributed into small equal-size granules,[573] and these have been found to be located in endothelial lining cells rather than in macrophages.[574] Indeed, in classical hereditary hemochromatosis, both macrophages[575] and intestinal mucosal cells are relatively iron-poor.

Other Tissues   Although more iron than normal is found in intestinal mucosal cells,[576] in relationship to total iron burden as indicated by the serum ferritin level, the amount of iron is strikingly decreased.[577] The same relationship has been noted in *HFE* knockout mice.[578] In contrast, in patients with transfusional iron overload, macrophages are heavily laden with iron, presumably derived from transfused red cells.

The myocardium is thickened and the heart is often enlarged. Testes are often atrophic.

GENETICS

Genetic factors play a central role in the etiology of iron storage disease. This is true not only in the primary forms of the disorder but also in secondary hemochromatosis, where genetic disorders of erythropoiesis are the most common causes. The genetics of these disorders, including the thalassemias, dyserythropoietic anemias, and red cell enzymopathies, are described elsewhere in this text (Chapters 37, 45, and 46). Mutations of several genes that play an important role in iron homeostasis have been found to lead to iron storage disease.[579]

HFE **Mutations**   The most common cause of hereditary hemochromatosis is a mutation of the *HFE* gene. This HLA-like gene resides on chromosome 6. Three polymorphic mutations have been identified. These are located at nucleotides 187, 193, and 845 of the cDNA and encode the H63D, S65C, and C282Y mutations, respectively. The phenotypic effect of these mutations on iron homeostasis are manifested in the following order: C282Y > H63D > S65C. Hereditary hemochromatosis is essentially an autosomal recessive disorder. About two thirds of homozygotes for the C282Y and a slightly lower percentage of compound heterozygotes for the C282Y and H63D mutations manifest increased serum transferrin saturations and serum ferritin levels. Individuals heterozygous for either the C282Y or the H63D mutation have, on the average, significantly higher transferrin saturations and serum ferritin levels than do wild-type homozygotes. However, the magnitude of this increase is very low. For example, the average transferrin saturation of man with the wild-type genotype is 26.69 percent, and heterozygotes for the C282Y mutation have a transferrin saturation averaging 30.63 percent. The increase in the geometric mean of the serum ferritin is even less, from 118 to 122 ng/ml.[528] The effect of the H63D mutation is even less, and that of the S65C mutation barely perceptible.[580]

In spite of the minimal effect of the heterozygous state for *HFE* mutations on iron homeostasis it has been proposed by a number of investigators that heterozygotes are at increased risk for a variety of disorders. It has been suggested that heterozygosity for the C282Y mutation is associated with more fibrosis in chronic hepatitis[581–584] but not in alcoholic liver disease.[585–587] It has also been claimed that the prevalence of the heterozygous state is significantly higher in patients with autoimmune hepatitis.[588] In other studies, an association between the heterozygous state and hepatocellular carcinoma[589] or breast cancer[590] were found. What has not been taken into account in the studies is the fact that the *HFE* gene is in linkage disequilibrium with many immune response genes on chromosome 6; it is therefore not possible to distinguish the minor effects that *HFE* mutations may have on iron homeostasis from variation in the immune response. The suggestion that increased iron levels are a risk factor for cardiovascular disease has been made repeatedly,[591,592] but a number of well-conducted negative studies cast serious doubt on this premise.[422–424,426,593,594]

HAMP **(Hepcidin) Mutations**   Mutations of hepcidin are exceedingly rare. Three mutations, 93delG, 166C→T, and 208T→C, have been found in patients with severe juvenile hemochromatosis.[595,596]

SCL40A1 **(Ferroportin-1) Mutations**   Mutations of the gene encoding ferroportin-1 cause an autosomal dominant iron storage disease characterized by storage in macrophages.[48,572,597–600] A triplet deletion that causes loss of a valine has been encountered repeatedly. A common polymorphism c.744G→T (Gln284His) shows an association with African iron overload but is clearly not present in all patients who manifest this syndrome.[491,492]

TfR-2 Mutations   Mutations of transferrin receptor 2 cause an autosomal recessive disorder that is indistinguishable clinically from hereditary hemochromatosis.[54,601–604]

Hemojuvelin Mutations Several different mutations of a gene of unknown function that has variously been designated as *HFE2* and *HJV* cause juvenile hemochromatosis.[67]

ANIMAL MODELS

Naturally Occurring Models In nature, a number of animal species have been found to be iron loaded. Included are myna birds,[605,606] the toco toucan,[607,608] Salers cattle,[609] a pony,[610] horses,[611] lemurs,[612] and the browsing rhinoceros.[613] The latter two species may represent an interesting paradigm for iron storage in captive species. While browsing rhinoceros species become iron loaded, grazing species are not. It seems likely that because iron is not readily available in the leaves eaten by the browsing species, it has evolved to more efficiently take up iron from its diet, more efficiently than needed when fed a zoo diet. Comparison of the *HFE* gene of browsing and grazing rhinoceros species showed numerous differences, but it is not clear whether any of these are related to the hyperabsorption of iron that is observed.[614] Similarly, lemurs subsist on a diet rich in leaves in the wild state, but are fed an iron-rich diet in captivity.[612]

Models Produced by Iron Loading Numerous efforts have been made to create models of hemochromatosis by loading laboratory animals with iron, either by the oral or parenteral route.[615–620] Some of these appear to simulate the human disease in one respect or another. For example, the iron-loaded gerbil develops heart disease, features of which resemble the human disease.[620,621] Moreover, such models have been used for the study of potential chelating agents.

Targeted Disruption Models Targeted disruption of the *HFE* gene produces a mouse with increased iron stores.[47] The effect of various combinations of knockouts, including *HFE*, β_2-microglobulin, hephaestin, and transferrin receptor have been documented.

CLINICAL FEATURES

CLASSICAL HEREDITARY HEMOCHROMATOSIS

Onset The clinical features of the most common form of hereditary hemochromatosis are cirrhosis of the liver, darkening of the skin, cardiomyopathies, and diabetes. In contrast to the juvenile form of the disease, in which onset is usually in the second or third decade of life, classical hereditary hemochromatosis associated with mutations of the *HFE* gene generally is diagnosed in the fifth or six decade of life.

General Symptomatology Many symptoms have been attributed to hereditary hemochromatosis. These include abdominal pain, weakness, lethargy, fatigue, loss of libido, impotence, and arthropathies. However, all of these symptoms are common in an aging population, and epidemiologic studies have shown that none of them are more common in patients with the hemochromatosis genotype, even those with the biochemical phenotype, than they are in the general population.[528–530,622,623]

Arthropathies The arthralgia of patients with hemochromatosis is claimed to have characteristic features.[624] It is said to tend to begin at the small joints in the hands, especially the second and third metacarpal joints, and that in some cases episodes of acute synovitis may occur as in calcium pyrophosphosphate dehydrate deposition arthopathy (pseudogout; chondrocalcinosis). Radiologically the arthropathy resembles that of osteoarthritis with joint space loss, subchondral cysts, sclerosis and osteophytosis. The features that have been considered distinctive include the joint distribution, the presence of sharp osteophytes emerging from the radial sides of the metacarpal distal epiphysis, and the presence of radiolucent zones in the subchondral area of the femoral head. In one investigation using historical controls, a borderline statistically significant increase in the number of patients with chondrocalcinosis who were homozygous for the C282Y mutation was documented.[625] However, properly blinded, controlled studies have not shown that any form of arthritis is more common in hereditary hemochromatosis than in the general population.[140,530] It is interesting, from this point of view, that arthritis was not mentioned by Sheldon as one of the clinical manifestations of hemochromatosis in his detailed monograph.[500] Moreover, it is generally recognized that arthritis does not respond to phlebotomy therapy; in one study, 9.2 percent of patients reported improvement of joint pain with treatment and 34 percent said that it was worse.[626] In fact, in a large survey virtually none of the nonspecific findings reported by patients improved significantly with therapy.[626] The possibility that excess iron does produce joint symptoms does remain open but unproven.[627]

Liver When cirrhosis is present there is a greatly increased risk of the patient developing a hepatoma.[628,629]

Porphyria Cutanea Tarda Porphyria cutanea tarda is a disease that is well known to be associated with mild overload and that responds to phlebotomy treatment (see Chap. 57). Numerous studies document that the prevalence of patients with this disorder who also have mutations of the *HFE* gene is considerably increased. Some of these patients are homozygotes; others heterozygotes.[630–634]

JUVENILE HEMOCHROMATOSIS

The penetrance of the rare juvenile form of the disease seems to be high, and cardiomyopathies and endocrine deficiencies seem to be the major clinical features.[489,635] Joint manifestations were found to be relatively common in patients with juvenile hemochromatosis.[636]

AFRICAN IRON OVERLOAD

It is not clear to what extent African iron overload is symptomatic. Among the Bantu, where the disorder was originally described, there are many complicating factors including malnutrition and high alcohol intake. Among African-Americans various associated disorders have been noted, but a cause-and-effect relationship is not clear. In one series of 23 patients, five had arthropathy, two had diabetes mellitus, and two had hypogonadism, and there were no instances of cirrhosis.[570]

SECONDARY HEMOCHROMATOSIS

The clinical findings in patients with hemochromatosis secondary to blood transfusion and/or disorders of erythropoiesis are, in general, indistinguishable from those found in patients with primary hemochromatosis.[559]

LABORATORY FEATURES

The main laboratory features of hereditary hemochromatosis are an increased transferrin saturation and increased serum ferritin level. Five to 10 percent of patients with classical hemochromatosis manifest increased liver enzyme levels in the serum. In secondary hemochromatosis, anemia and the other manifestations of the underlying disorder are found. Macrocytosis of the erythrocytes is a common feature[637,638]; this finding seems unrelated to liver disease, and its cause is unknown.

DIFFERENTIAL DIAGNOSIS

A large number of methods have been introduced that allow the amount of storage iron to be estimated.[639] The suspicion that a patient may have primary hemochromatosis is generally raised by an increased serum transferrin saturation, particularly when it is found together with an elevated serum ferritin level. An increased transferrin saturation commonly occurs in patients with chronic liver disease who have no mutations in the *HFE* gene.[640] Ferritin is an acute phase protein, and levels are elevated in a variety of disorders. Particularly high levels are encountered in patients with Gaucher disease,[348] in some malignancies,[390,641] and in patients with the hyperferritinemia-cataract syndrome. The latter disorder is an uncommon autosomal dominant defect in which a mutation in the 5′ IRE of the ferritin light chain prevents binding of the IRPs, resulting in unrestrained constitutive production of the ferritin chains.[642,643]

Many clinicians have considered a liver biopsy the "gold standard" for the diagnosis of iron overload. The material obtained at biopsy not only provides the opportunity to assess the histopathology of the liver of the patient, but also to quantitate the amount of non-heme iron in the specimen. Dividing the iron content by the patient's age provides an iron index; a value greater than 2 implies the presence of hemochromatosis.[644] Although in some situations liver biopsy may provide useful information, it is an invasive procedure that, although low risk, cannot be considered to be free of risk. Enthusiasm for subjecting every patient with potential hemochromatosis to liver biopsy has diminished with the ready availability of genetic analysis. Moreover, a simple way to determine whether a patient is iron overloaded is to institute a program of phlebotomies. This is an essentially harmless way to determine how much storage iron the body contains. Other noninvasive, but less readily available methods, for determining whether excess iron is present in the liver are the superconducting quantum interference device (SQUID)[645] and magnetic resonance imaging (MRI).[639,646–649] MRI is able to detected increased amounts of iron in the liver, but generally special techniques are required, and accuracy is satisfactory only at relatively high iron levels.[639,646,648]

THERAPY

The treatment of hemochromatosis consists of removing the accumulated iron. In the case of patients who mount an erythropoietin response to phlebotomy, removal of blood is generally the treatment of choice. When the patient has marked impairment of erythropoiesis, as in thalassemia and dyserythropoietic anemia, it is necessary to employ chelating agents to remove iron, although occasionally serial phlebotomy will stimulate sufficient erythropoiesis to make it a viable therapy.[650]

PHLEBOTOMY

Each milliliter of packed red cells contains approximately 1 mg of iron. Thus, the removal of 500 ml of blood with a hematocrit of 40 percent removes approximately 200 mg of iron. As the red cell mass is restored to its prephlebotomy size, iron is mobilized from the stores. When the stores have been exhausted, the signs of iron deficiency develop, and this is the endpoint of the initial part of the phlebotomy program. The patient is then followed and a schedule of maintenance phlebotomies is established with the frequency of phlebotomies tailored to maintain the serum ferritin level, the best indicator of body stores, less than 100 ng/ml.

The actual volume of blood removed by each phlebotomy depends on the patient's size. 500 ml is well-tolerated by most average-sized patients, but patients who weigh 50 kg or less are better treated by the removal of correspondingly smaller volumes of blood. Many patients may complain of symptoms following the first few phlebotomies. Better compliance is achieved if such symptoms are minimized by performing phlebotomies only every 14 days initially, increasing the frequency to weekly phlebotomies once the patient has become accustomed to the procedure and the activity of the marrow has been stimulated so as to replace the lost erythrocytes rapidly. The hematocrit or hemoglobin and the MCV of the red cells should be measured before each phlebotomy is undertaken. If there has been a substantial decrease in the hematocrit or hemoglobin the phlebotomy should be deferred. The MCV may rise early in the treatment program, but as iron deficiency develops it will fall, signaling that the endpoint has been reached or is near. The transferrin saturation and serum ferritin level should be measured every 2 or 3 months. When the transferrin

saturation is less than 10 percent and the serum ferritin less than 10 ng/ml, phlebotomy should be discontinued and the patient monitored every 4 to 8 weeks. When the serum ferritin is in the 50 to 100 ng/ml range, the maintenance phase should be initiated. Some patients may require phlebotomies monthly to maintain a normal ferritin value, whereas others may only require two or three phlebotomies per year.

CHELATION THERAPY

Chelation therapy instituted in a timely manner can decrease the potential morbidity caused by iron overload and prolong the life of patients with hereditary chronic iron-loading disorders such as thalassemia major. It also has a place in the management of some patients with acquired marrow dysplasias provided that the prognosis of the underlying disorder, and the patient's psychological state, justifies the somewhat cumbersome implementation of parenteral chelation. As oral chelating agents become more readily available, the application of chelation therapy to myelodysplastic states may broaden.

DESFERRIOXAMINE

Desferrioxamine is a naturally occurring iron-chelating compound elaborated by the microorganism *Streptomyces pilosus*, having evolved to enable the microbe to obtain iron from its environment. One molecule of this chelator binds one atom of iron. Its molecular weight is 560 daltons. The iron complex is excreted into the urine and feces. Urine iron is derived primarily from red cells broken down by macrophages whereas fecal iron is believed to be from iron chelated in the liver.[651]

Desferrioxamine is poorly absorbed from the gastrointestinal tract and must therefore be given parenterally, either by the subcutaneous or intravenous route. Rapid intravenous or intramuscular injection results in the relatively little iron mobilization; instead, it is necessary to administer desferrioxamine by slow intravenous or subcutaneous infusion over a period of 8 to 10 hours. An alternate method is twice daily subcutaneous injection,[652] but this is not well tolerated by all patients.[653] Increasing doses of desferrioxamine results in increased iron excretion,[654] and the usual recommended dose is 30 to 50 mg/kg.[651] The administration of 200 mg of ascorbic acid *after* the infusion of desferrioxamine has been started increases the amount of iron excreted, and is therefore recommended. However, it is considered potentially hazardous to administer ascorbic acid to iron overloaded patients in the absence of a powerful chelating agent because the mobilization of iron from tissues has been thought to produce acute cardiac damage.[655] The amount of iron excreted will vary from patient to patient and depends to a large extent on the iron burden. Since the treatment is cumbersome and costly it is well to be reasonably certain that sufficient good is being accomplished to justify the effort. This can be achieved by measuring urine output of iron after a test desferrioxamine infusion, bearing in mind that urinary excretion may account for only one third of the iron excreted, with fecal excretion accounting for the rest.[656]

Desferrioxamine is usually well-tolerated. Minor local reactions such as local pruritus, induration, or pain at the site of infusion are not uncommon. Large doses have been associated with hearing loss, night blindness and other visual abnormalities, growth retardation, and the skeletal changes. At very high doses occasional cases of kidney and lung abnormalities have been reported.[651]

ORAL CHELATING AGENTS

The inconvenience and high cost of therapy with desferrioxamine has stimulated an intensive search for safe, orally active chelating agents. Deferiprone (L-1) is the only orally effective agent currently available. At the end of 2003, it was licensed in 27 countries (not including the United States). It is a bidentate chelating agent; three molecules of deferiprone bind one iron atom. Its molecular weight is only 139 daltons, and it is excreted almost entirely in the urine. The usual dose is 75 mg/kg/day divided into three doses. Deferiprone administration has been associated with a number of toxic effects. Included are gastrointestinal disturbances, transient increases in the serum levels of liver enzymes, and zinc deficiency. The main concern has centered on the propensity of the drug to produce neutropenia and agranulocytosis. The latter complication occurs in about 1 percent of patients. It appears to be idiosyncratic, is more common in females, and appears to be reversible. Neutropenia with a granulocyte level between 500 and 1500 per microliter recurs in an additional 5 percent of patients. Treatment should be stopped at the first sign of a fall in the leukocyte count.[366,651] It has been suggested that deferiprone may be more effective in removing iron from the heart and desferrioxamine more effective with respect to liver iron accumulations.[366] Preliminary investigations suggest that a combination of desferrioxamine and deferiprone may be more effective than either alone.[657,658]

COURSE AND PROGNOSIS

A century ago when classical hereditary hemochromatosis was first recognized as a disease entity, the average survival after diagnosis was only 18.5 months,[500] most of the deaths being due to diabetic coma in the pre-insulin era. The outlook in this disease has changed in the current century to one in which the life span of patients with hemochromatosis is normal or nearly so. This is largely due to the change in the definition of the disorder. In the early 20th century, the diagnosis was reserved for the rare patient with full-blown bronzed diabetes. Today, the diagnosis is applied to any person found to be homozygous for the C282Y mutation or, indeed, anyone with an increased transferrin saturation and elevated serum ferritin level. In reality, patients with a diagnosis of hemochromatosis based on genetic and/or biochemical criteria have a normal life span. Although this finding has erroneously been attributed to the institution of therapy,[629,659] it applies equally to untreated patients discovered in population surveys. If such untreated patients suffered an early demise in the absence of treatment one would expect their number to diminish in cohorts of increasing age, but this does not appear to be the case even in very large series.[660] Surprisingly, long-term followup of patients not treated by phlebotomy shows little or no increase of serum ferritin levels, even after a followup as long as 23 years.[622,661] This is not to suggest that patients do not die of hereditary hemochromatosis. It is simply that the penetrance of the disorder as detected on genetic or biochemical bases is so low that the few deaths that do occur cannot be detected even in very sizable series.

For those patients with classical hereditary hemochromatosis who are clinically affected, it is likely that removal of iron by phlebotomy prevents further complications and prolongs life span. Although controlled studies of the effect of phlebotomy are not ethically feasible, serial observations in patients undergoing phlebotomy suggest that cirrhosis is either stabilized[662] or may, at least in some patients, improve.[499,662–666] Platelet counts improved in a large proportion of patients with cirrhosis undergoing phlebotomy.[667]

The course of untreated juvenile hemochromatosis seems less benign. Cardiac deaths seem to be particularly common,[668] and in a few cases cardiac transplantation has been performed successfully,[489] but there are insufficient data concerning this rare disorder to allow one to provide more precise information about the outlook.

The prognosis in thalassemia major and similar disorders is grim when iron chelation is not performed (see Chap. 46).[669] Death is most frequently due to cardiac failure. It has been estimated that two to 4000 thalassemia patients die each year as a result of iron overload.[366]

REFERENCES

1. Herbert V, Jayatilleke E, Shaw S, et al: Serum ferritin iron, a new test, measures human body iron stores unconfounded by inflammation. *Stem Cells* 15:291, 1997.
2. Nielsen P, Gunther U, Durken M, et al: Serum ferritin iron in iron overload and liver damage: Correlation to body iron stores and diagnostic relevance. *J Lab Clin Med* 135:413, 2000.
3. Ward RJ, Legssyer R, Henry C, Crichton RR: Does the haemosiderin iron core determine its potential for chelation and the development of iron-induced tissue damage? *J Inorg Biochem* 79:311, 2000.
4. Pollycove M, Mortimer R: The quantitative determination of iron kinetics and hemoglobin synthesis in human subjects. *J Clin Invest* 40: 753, 1961.
5. Hosain F, Marsaglia G, Finch CA: Blood ferrokinetics in normal man. *J Clin Invest* 46:1, 1967.
6. Petrat F, de Groot H, Sustmann R, Rauen U: The chelatable iron pool in living cells. A methodically defined quantity. *Biol Chem* 383:489, 2002.
7. Beutler E: Tissue effects of iron deficiency, in: *Iron Metabolism*, edited by F Gross, SR Naegeli, HD Philps, p 256. Springer-Verlag, Berlin, 1963.
8. Dallman PR, Beutler E, Finch CA: Effects of iron deficiency exclusive of anaemia. *Br J Haematol* 40:179, 1978.
9. Lozoff B: Perinatal iron deficiency and the developing brain. *Pediatr Res* 48:137, 2000.
10. Bailey S, Evans RW, Garratt RC, et al: Molecular structure of serum transferrin at 3.3 Å resolution. *Biochemistry* 27:5804, 1988.
11. van Haeringen B, de Lange F, van Stokkum IHM, et al: Dynamic structure of human serum transferrin from transient electric birefringence experiments. *Proteins* 23:233, 1998.
12. Haurani FI, Meyer A, O'Brien R: Production of transferrin by the macrophage. *J Reticuloendothel Soc* 14:309, 1973.
13. Thorbecke GJ, Liem HH, Knight S, et al: Sites of formation of the serum proteins transferrin and hemopexin. *J Clin Invest* 52:725, 1973.
14. Welch S, Langmead L: A comparison of the structure and properties of normal human transferrin and a genetic variant of human transferrin. *Int J Biochem* 22:275, 1990.
15. Young SP, Bomford A, Madden AD, et al: Abnormal in vitro function of a variant human transferrin. *Br J Haematol* 56:581, 1984.
16. Lee PL, Halloran C, Trevino R, et al: Human transferrin G277S mutation: A risk factor for iron deficiency anaemia. *Br J Haematol* 115:329, 2001.
17. Aisen P: The G277S mutation in transferrin does not disturb function. *Br J Haematol* 121:674, 2003.
18. Moore CV: Iron nutrition and requirements. *Ser Haematol* 6:1, 1965.
19. Pennington JA, Young BE, Wilson DB, et al: Mineral content of foods and total diets: The Selected Minerals in Foods Survey, 1982 to 1984. *J Am Diet Assoc* 86:876, 1986.
20. Dubach R, Moore CV, Callender S: Studies in iron transportation and metabolism IX. The excretion of iron as measured by the isotope technique. *J Lab Clin Med* 45:599, 1955.
21. Herndon JF, Rice EG, Tucker RG, et al: Iron absorption and metabolism: III. The enhancement of iron absorption in rats by D-sorbitol. *J Nutr* 64: 615, 1958.
22. Hallberg L, Sölvell L: Iron absorption studies: [1] Determination of the absorption rate of iron in man. [2] Absorption of a single dose of iron in man. [3] Iron absorption during constant intragastric infusion of iron in man. [4] Effect of iron and transferrin intravenously on iron absorption and turnover in man (Sölvell alone). *Acta Med Scand Suppl* 358:1, 1960.
23. Pollack S, Kaufman RM, Crosby WH: Iron absorption: Effects of sugars and reducing agents. *Blood* 24:577, 1964.

24. Slatkavitz CA, Clydesdale FM: Solubility of inorganic iron as affected by proteolytic digestion. *Am J Clin Nutr* 47:487, 1988.

25. Taylor PG, Martinez-Torres C, Romano EL, Layrisse M: The effect of cysteine-containing peptides released during meat digestion on iron absorption in humans. *Am J Clin Nutr* 43:68, 1986.

26. Charlton RW, Jacobs P, Seftel H, Bothwell TH: Effect of alcohol on iron absorption. *BMJ* 2:1427, 1964.

27. Celada A, Rudolf H, Donath A: Effect of a single ingestion of alcohol on iron absorption. *Am J Hematol* 5:225, 1978.

28. Bezwoda WR, Torrance JD, Bothwell TH, et al: Iron absorption from red and white wines. *Scand J Haematol* 34:121, 1985.

29. Cook JD, Reddy MB, Hurrell RF: The effect of red and white wines on nonheme-iron absorption in humans. *Am J Clin Nutr* 61:800, 1995.

30. Hankes LV, Jansen CR, Schmaeler M: Ascorbic acid catabolism in Bantu with hemosiderosis (scurvy). *Biochem Med* 9:244, 1974.

31. McCance RA, Widdowson EM: Absorption and excretion of iron. *Lancet* 2:680, 1937.

32. Beutler E, Fairbanks VF, Fahey JL: *Clinical Disorders of Iron Metabolism.* Grune & Stratton, New York, 1963.

33. Conrad ME, Umbreit JN: Iron absorption—The mucin-mobilferrin-integrin pathway. A competitive pathway for metal absorption. *Am J Hematol* 42:67, 1993.

34. Van Campen D: Enhancement of iron absorption from ligated segments of rat intestine by histidine, cysteine, and lysine: Effects of removing ionizing groups and of stereoisomerism. *J Nutr* 103:139, 1973.

35. Conrad ME, Umbreit JN, Moore EG: A role for mucin in the absorption of inorganic iron and other metal cations. A study in rats. *Gastroenterology* 100:129, 1991.

36. Weintraub LR, Weinstein MB, Huser H, Rafal S: Absorption of hemoglobin iron: The role of a heme-splitting substance in the intestinal mucosa. *J Clin Invest* 47:531, 1968.

37. Worthington MT, Cohn SM, Miller SK, et al: Characterization of a human plasma membrane heme transporter in intestinal and hepatocyte cell lines. *Am J Physiol Gastrointest Liver Physiol* 280:G1172, 2001.

38. Conrad ME, Umbreit JN: Pathways of iron absorption. *Blood Cells Mol Dis* 29:336, 2002.

39. Latunde-Dada GO, Van der Westhuizen J, Vulpe CD, et al: Molecular and functional roles of duodenal cytochrome B (dcytb) in iron metabolism. *Blood Cells Mol Dis* 29:356, 2002.

40. McKie AT, Barrow D, Latunde-Dada GO, et al: An iron-regulated ferric reductase associated with the absorption of dietary iron. *Science* 291:1755, 2001.

41. Beutler E: History of iron in Medicine. *Blood Cells Mol Dis* 29:297, 2002.

42. Beutler E, Kelly BM, Beutler F: The regulation of iron absorption: II. Relationship between iron dosage and iron absorption. *Am J Clin Nutr* 11:559, 1962.

43. Smith MD, Pannacciulli IM: Absorption of inorganic iron from graded doses: Its significance in relation to iron absorption tests and the "mucosal block" theory. *Br J Haematol* 4:428, 1958.

44. Feder JN, Gnirke A, Thomas W, et al: A novel MHC class I-like gene is mutated in patients with hereditary haemochromatosis. *Nat Genet* 13:399, 1996.

45. Levy JE, Montross LK, Andrews NC: Genes that modify the hemochromatosis phenotype in mice. *J Clin Invest* 105:1209, 2000.

46. Beutler E: Commentary. Targeted disruption of the HFE gene. *Proc Natl Acad Sci U S A* 95:2033, 1998.

47. Zhou XY, Tomatsu S, Fleming RE, et al: HFE gene knockout produces mouse model of hereditary hemochromatosis. *Proc Natl Acad Sci U S A* 95:2492, 1998.

48. Njajou OT, Vaessen N, Joosse M, et al: A mutation in SLC11A3 is associated with autosomal dominant hemochromatosis. *Nat Genet* 28:213, 2001.

49. de Sousa M, Reimao R, Lacerda R, et al: Iron overload in beta 2-microglobulin-deficient mice. *Immunol Lett* 39:105, 1994.

50. Rothenberg BE, Voland JR: B₂ Knockout mice develop parenchymal iron overload: A putative role for class I genes of the major histocompatibility complex in iron metabolism. *Proc Natl Acad Sci U S A* 93:1529, 1996.

51. Asada-Senju M, Maeda T, Sakata T, et al: Molecular analysis of the transferrin gene in a patient with hereditary hypotransferrinemia. *J Hum Genet* 47:355, 2002.

52. Beutler E, Gelbart T, Lee P, et al: Molecular characterization of a case of atransferrinemia. *Blood* 96:4071, 2000.

53. Trenor CC, Campagna DR, Sellers VM, et al: The molecular defect in hypotransferrinemic mice. *Blood* 96:1113, 2000.

54. Camaschella C, Roetto A, Cali A, et al: The gene TFR2 is mutated in a new type of haemochromatosis mapping to 7q22. *Nat Genet* 25:14, 2000.

55. Fleming RE, Ahmann JR, Migas MC, et al: Targeted mutagenesis of the murine transferrin receptor-2 gene produces hemochromatosis. *Proc Natl Acad Sci U S A* 2002.

56. Vulpe CD, Kuo YM, Murphy TL, et al: Hephaestin, a ceruloplasmin homologue implicated in intestinal iron transport, is defective in the sla mouse. *Nat Genet* 21:195, 1999.

57. LaVaute T, Smith S, Cooperman S, et al: Targeted deletion of the gene encoding iron regulatory protein-2 causes misregulation of iron metabolism and neurodegenerative disease in mice. *Nat Genet* 27:209, 2001.

58. Kato J, Fujikawa K, Kanda M, et al: A mutation, in the iron-responsive element of H ferritin mRNA, causing autosomal dominant iron overload. *Am J Hum Genet* 69:191, 2001.

59. Wyllie S, Seu P, Goss JA: The natural resistance-associated macrophage protein 1 Slc11a1 (formerly Nramp1) and iron metabolism in macrophages. *Microbes Infect* 4:351, 2002.

60. Fleming MD, Trenor CC3, Su MA, et al: Microcytic anaemia mice have a mutation in Nramp2, a candidate iron transporter gene. *Nat Genet* 16:383, 1997.

61. Fleming MD, Romano MA, Su MA, et al: Nramp2 is mutated in the anemic Belgrade (b) rat: Evidence of a role for nramp2 in endosomal iron transport. *Proc Natl Acad Sci U S A* 95:1148, 1998.

62. Nittis T, Gitlin JD: The copper-iron connection: Hereditary aceruloplasminemia. *Semin Hematol* 39:282, 2002.

63. Harris ZL, Durley AP, Man TK, Gitlin JD: Targeted gene disruption reveals an essential role for ceruloplasmin in cellular iron efflux. *Proc Natl Acad Sci U S A* 96:10812, 1999.

64. Roetto A, Papanikolaou G, Politou M, et al: Mutant antimicrobial peptide hepcidin is associated with severe juvenile hemochromatosis. *Nat Genet* 33:21, 2003.

65. Nicolas G, Bennoun M, Devaux I, et al: Lack of hepcidin gene expression and severe tissue iron overload in upstream stimulatory factor 2 (USF2) knockout mice. *Proc Natl Acad Sci U S A* 98:8780, 2001.

66. Pigeon C, Ilyin G, Courselaud B, et al: A new mouse liver-specific gene, encoding a protein homologous to human antimicrobial peptide hepcidin, is overexpressed during iron overload. *J Biol Chem* 276:7811, 2001.

67. Papanikolaou G, Samuels ME, Ludwig EH, et al: Mutations in HFE2 cause iron overload in chromosome 1q-linked juvenile hemochromatosis. *Nat Genet* 36:77, 2004.

68. Fleming RE, Sly WS: Mechanisms of iron accumulation in hereditary hemochromatosis. *Annu Rev Physiol* 64:663, 2002.

69. Roy CN, Enns CA: Iron homeostasis: New tales from the crypt. *Blood* 96:4020, 2000.

70. Townsend A, Drakesmith H: Role of HFE in iron metabolism, hereditary haemochromatosis, anaemia of chronic disease, and secondary iron overload. *Lancet* 359:786, 2002.

71. Frazer DM, Anderson GJ: The orchestration of body iron intake: How and where do enterocytes receive their cues? *Blood Cells Mol Dis* 30:288, 2003.

72. Park CH, Valore EV, Waring AJ, Ganz T: Hepcidin, a urinary antimicrobial peptide synthesized in the liver. *J Biol Chem* 276:7806, 2001.

73. Nicolas G, Bennoun M, Porteu A, et al: Severe iron deficiency anemia in transgenic mice expressing liver hepcidin. *Proc Natl Acad Sci U S A* 99:4596, 2002.

74. Weinstein DA, Roy CN, Fleming MD, et al: Inappropriate expression of hepcidin is associated with iron refractory anemia: Implications for the anemia of chronic disease. *Blood* 100:3776, 2002.

75. Laftah AH, Ramesh B, Simpson RJ, et al: Effect of hepcidin on intestinal iron absorption in mice. *Blood* 103: 3940, 2004.

76. Ganz T: Hepcidin, a key regulator of iron metabolism and mediator of anemia of inflammation. *Blood* 102:783, 2003.

77. Nemeth E, Valore EV, Territo M, et al: Hepcidin, a putative mediator of anemia of inflammation, is a type II acute-phase protein. *Blood* 101: 2461, 2003.

78. Nicolas G, Viatte L, Bennoun M, et al: Hepcidin, a new iron regulatory peptide. *Blood Cells Mol Dis* 29:327, 2002.

79. Nicolas G, Chauvet C, Viatte L, et al: The gene encoding the iron regulatory peptide hepcidin is regulated by anemia, hypoxia, and inflammation. *J Clin Invest* 110:1037, 2002.

80. Ahmad KA, Ahmann JR, Migas MC, et al: Decreased liver hepcidin expression in the HFE knockout mouse. *Blood Cells Mol Dis* 29:361, 2002.

81. Nicolas G, Viatte L, Lou DQ, et al: Constitutive hepcidin expression prevents iron overload in a mouse model of hemochromatosis. *Nat Genet* 34.97, 2003.

82. Dautry-Varsat A: Receptor-mediated endocytosis: The intracellular journey of transferrin and its receptor. *Biochimie* 68:375, 1986.

83. Kaplan J: Mechanisms of cellular iron acquisition: Another iron in the fire. *Cell* 111:603, 2002.

84. Schneider C, Williams JG: Molecular dissection of the human transferrin receptor. *J Cell Sci* 3(suppl):139, 1985.

85. Zerial M, Melancon P, Schneider C, Garoff H: The transmembrane segment of the human transferrin receptor functions as a signal peptide. *EMBO J* 5:1543, 1986.

86. Zimmerman RA, Gill F, Goldberg HI, et al: MRI of sickle cell cerebral infarction. *Neuroradiology* 29:232, 1987.

87. Lebrón JA, Bennett MJ, Vaughn DE, et al: Crystal structure of the hemochromatosis protein HFE and characterization of its interaction with transferrin receptor. *Cell* 93:111, 1998.

88. West AP, Giannetti AM, Herr AB, et al: Mutational analysis of the transferrin receptor reveals overlapping HFE and transferrin binding sites. *J Mol Biol* 313:385, 2001.

89. Fergelot P, Orhant M, Thenie A, et al: Over-expression of wild-type and mutant HFE in a human melanocytic cell line reveals an intracellular bridge between MHC class I pathway and transferrin iron uptake. *Biol Cell* 95:243, 2003.

90. Cartwright GE, Deiss A: Sideroblasts, siderocytes, and sideroblastic anemia. *N Engl J Med* 292:185, 1975.

91. Cairo G, Pietrangelo A: Iron regulatory proteins in pathobiology. *Biochem J* 352(pt 2):241, 2000.

92. Bouton C, Drapier JC: Iron regulatory proteins as NO signal transducers. *Sci STKE* 2003:e17, 2003.

93. Kim S, Ponka P: Nitric oxide-mediated modulation of iron regulatory proteins: Implication for cellular iron homeostasis. *Blood Cells Mol Dis* 29:400, 2002.

94. Kim S, Wing SS, Ponka P: S-Nitrosylation of IRP2 regulates its stability via the ubiquitin-proteasome pathway. *Mol Cell Biol* 24:330, 2004.

95. Rouault TA: Post-transcriptional regulation of human iron metabolism by iron regulatory proteins. *Blood Cells Mol Dis* 29:309, 2002.

96. Templeton DM, Liu Y: Genetic regulation of cell function in response to iron overload or chelation. *Biochim Biophys Acta* 1619:113, 2003.

97. Noyes WD, Bothwell TH, Finch CA: The role of the reticulo-endothelial cell in iron metabolism. *Br J Haematol* 6:43, 1960.

98. Haurani FI, Burke W, Martinez EJ: Defective reutilization of iron in the anemia of inflammation. *J Lab Clin Med* 65:560, 1965.

99. Haurani FI, Young K, Tocantins LM: Reutilization of iron in anemia complicating malignant neoplasms. *Blood* 22:73, 1963.

100. O'Shea MJ, Kershenobich D, Tavill AS: Effects of inflammation on iron and transferrin metabolism. *Br J Haematol* 25:707, 1973.

101. Green R, Charlton R, Seftel H, et al: Body iron excretion in man: A collaborative study. *Am J Med* 45:336, 1968.

102. Bryan CP: *The Papyrus Ebers*. Appleton-Century-Crofts, New York, 1931.

103. Heath CW, Strauss MB, Castle WB: Quantitative aspects of iron deficiency in hypochromic anemia. *J Clin Invest* 11:1293, 1932.

104. Poskitt EME: Early history of iron deficiency. *Br J Haematol* 122:554, 2003.

105. Stoltzfus R: Defining iron-deficiency anemia in public health terms: A time for reflection. *J Nutr* 131:565S, 2001.

106. Lozoff B, De A, I, Castillo M, et al: Behavioral and developmental effects of preventing iron-deficiency anemia in healthy full-term infants. *Pediatrics* 112:846, 2003.

107. Tershakovec AM, Weller SC: Iron status of inner-city elementary school children: Lack of correlation between anemia and iron deficiency. *Am J Clin Nutr* 54:1071, 1991.

108. Hallberg L, Hultén L, Lindstedt G, et al: Prevalence of iron deficiency in Swedish adolescents. *Pediatr Res* 34:680, 1993.

109. Centers for Disease Control and Prevention: Iron deficiency—United States, 1999-2000. *MMWR Morb Mortal Wkly Rep* 51:897, 2002.

110. Zlotkin SH, Ste-Marie M, Kopelman H, et al: The prevalence of iron depletion and iron-deficiency anaemia in a randomly selected group of infants from four Canadian cities. *Nutr Res* 16:729, 1996.

111. Beutler E, Felitti V, Gelbart T, Waalen J: Haematological effects of the C282Y HFE mutation in homozygous and heterozygous states among subjects of northern and southern European ancestry. *Br J Haematol* 120:887, 2003.

112. Looker AC, Dallman PR, Carroll MD, et al: Prevalence of iron deficiency in the United States. *JAMA* 277:973, 1997.

113. Agudelo GM, Cardona OL, Posada M, et al: Prevalence of iron-deficiency anemia in schoolchildren and adolescents, Medellin, Colombia, 1999. *Rev Panam Salud Publica* 13:376, 2003.

114. Casanueva E, Jimenez J, Meza-Camacho C, et al: Prevalence of nutritional deficiencies in Mexican adolescent women with early and late prenatal care. *Arch Latinoam Nutr* 53:35, 2003.

115. Haidar J, Muroki NM, Omwega AM, Ayana G: Malnutrition and iron deficiency in lactating women in urban slum communities from Addis Ababa, Ethiopia. *East Afr Med J* 80:191, 2003.

116. Kadivar MR, Yarmohammadi H, Mirahmadizadeh AR, et al: Prevalence of iron deficiency anemia in 6 months to 5 years old children in Fars, Southern Iran. *Med Sci Monit* 9:CR100, 2003.

117. Massot C, Vanderpas J: A survey of iron deficiency anaemia during pregnancy in Belgium: Analysis of routine hospital laboratory data in Mons. *Acta Clin Belg* 58:169, 2003.

118. Soh P, Ferguson EL, McKenzie JE, et al: Iron deficiency and risk factors for lower iron stores in 6–24-month-old New Zealanders. *Eur J Clin Nutr* 58:71, 2004.

119. Wolmarans P, Dhansay MA, Mansvelt EP, et al: Iron status of South African women working in a fruit-packing factory. *Public Health Nutr* 6:439, 2003.

120. Whitfield JB, Treloar S, Zhu G, et al: Relative importance of female-specific and non-female-specific effects on variation in iron stores between women. *Br J Haematol* 120:860, 2003.

121. Carlsson LE, Hempel S, Greinacher A: Iron deficiency anaemia in young women—A hypothesis on the impact of the platelet collagen receptor GPIaIIa polymorphism GPIa-C807T. *Eur J Haematol* 68:341, 2002.

122. McIntyre AS, Long RG: Prospective survey of investigations in outpatients referred with iron deficiency anaemia. *Gut* 34:1102, 1993.

123. Retzlaff JA, Hagedorn AB, Bartholomew LG: Abdominal exploration for gastrointestinal bleeding of obscure origin. *JAMA* 177:104, 1961.

124. Baum S, Nusbaum M, Blakemore WS, Finkelstein AK: The preoperative radiographic demonstration of intra-abdominal bleeding from undetermined sites by percutaneous selective celiac and superior mesenteric arteriography. *Surgery* 58:797, 1965.

125. Prichard PJ, Tjandra JJ: Colorectal cancer. *Med J Aust* 169:493, 1998.

126. Fitzpatrick J: Hemocholecyst: A neglected cause of gastrointestinal hemorrhage. *Ann Intern Med* 55:1008, 1961.

127. Kaminski N, Shaham D, Eliakim R: Primary tumours of the duodenum. *Postgrad Med J* 69:136, 1993.

128. Coban E, Timuragaoglu A, Meric M: Iron deficiency anemia in the elderly: Prevalence and endoscopic evaluation of the gastrointestinal tract in outpatients. *Acta Haematol (Basel)* 110:25, 2003.

129. Windsor CW, Collis JL: Anaemia and hiatus hernia: Experience in 450 patients. *Thorax* 22:73, 1967.

130. Holt JM, Mayet FG, Warner GT, et al: Iron absorption and blood loss in patients with hiatus hernia. *BMJ* 3:22, 1968.

131. Moskovitz M, Fadden R, Min T, et al: Large hiatal hernias, anemia, and linear gastric erosion: Studies of etiology and medical therapy. *Am J Gastroenterol* 87:622, 1992.

132. Weston AP: Hiatal hernia with cameron ulcers and erosions. *Gastrointest Endosc Clin N Am* 6:671, 1996.

133. Cameron AJ, Higgins JA: Linear gastric erosion. A lesion associated with large diaphragmatic hernia and chronic blood loss anemia. *Gastroenterology* 91:338, 1986.

134. Roth WL, Valdes-Dapena A, Pieses P, Buchman E: Topical action of salicylates in gastrointestinal erosion and hemorrhage. *Gastroenterology* 44:146, 1963.

135. Faucheron JL, Parc R: Non-steroidal anti-inflammatory drug-induced colitis. *Int J Colorectal Dis* 11:99, 1996.

136. Oldenburg B, Koningsberger JC, Henegouwen GPV, et al: Review article: Iron and inflammatory bowel disease. *Aliment Pharmacol Ther* 15:429, 2001.

137. Singh AK, Cumaraswamy RC, Corrin B: Diffuse hypertrophy of gastric mucosa (Menetrier's disease) and iron-deficiency anaemia. *Gut* 10:735, 1969.

138. Barabino A: Helicobacter pylori-related iron deficiency anemia: A review. *Helicobacter* 7:71, 2002.

139. Choe YH, Kim SK, Son BK, et al: Randomized placebo-controlled trial of Helicobacter pylori eradication for iron-deficiency anemia in preadolescent children and adolescents. *Helicobacter* 4:135, 1999.

140. Bini EJ: Helicobacter pylori and iron deficiency anemia: Guilty as charged? *Am J Med* 111:495, 2001.

141. Zaatar R, Younoszai MK, Mitros F: Pseudo-Zollinger-Ellison syndrome in a child presenting with anemia. *Gastroenterology* 92:508, 1987.

142. Crompton DW, Nesheim MC: Nutritional impact of intestinal helminthiasis during the human life cycle. *Annu Rev Nutr* 22:35, 2002.

143. Annibale B, Capurso G, Lahner E, et al: Concomitant alterations in intragastric pH and ascorbic acid concentration in patients with Helicobacter pylori gastritis and associated iron deficiency anaemia. *Gut* 52:496, 2003.

144. Annibale B, Capurso G, Delle FG: The stomach and iron deficiency anaemia: A forgotten link. *Dig Liver Dis* 35:288, 2003.

145. Kimber C, Patterson JF, Weintraub LR: The pathogenesis of iron deficiency anemia following partial gastrectomy. A study of iron balance. *JAMA* 202:935, 1967.

146. Sorbi D, Conio M, Gostout CJ: Vascular disorders of the small bowel. *Gastrointest Endosc Clin N Am* 9:71, 1999.

147. Toyota M, Hinoda Y, Nakagawa N, et al: Gastric antral vascular ectasia causing severe anemia. *J Gastroenterol* 31:710, 1996.

148. Blanc P, Phelip JM, Bertolino JG, et al: Watermelon stomach: A rare cause of iron deficiency anemia, surgically treatable; a new case with review of the literature. *Ann Chir* 128:462, 2003.

149. Holt JM, Wright R: Anaemia due to blood loss from the telangiectases of scleroderma. *BMJ* 3:537, 1967.

150. Reinhart WH, Mordasini C, Staubli M, Scheurer U: Abnormalities of gut vessels in Turner's syndrome. *Postgrad Med J* 59:122, 1983.

151. Hagood MF, Gathright JB Jr: Hemangiomatosis of the skin and gastrointestinal tract: Report of a case. *Dis Colon Rectum* 18:141, 1975.

152. Ohishi M, Tanaka Y, Higuchi Y, et al: Multiple facial hemangiomas and iron-deficiency anemia: Blue rubber-bleb nevus syndrome. *Head Neck Surg* 7:249, 1985.

153. Morris SJ, Kaplan SR, Ballan K, Tedesco FJ: Blue rubber-bleb nevus syndrome. *JAMA* 239:1887, 1978.

154. Male C, Persson LA, Freeman V, et al: Prevalence of iron deficiency in 12-month-old infants from 11 European areas and influence of dietary factors on iron status (Euro-Growth study). *Acta Paediatr* 90:492, 2001.

155. Oski FA: Is bovine milk a health hazard? *Pediatrics* 75:182, 1985.

156. Coello-Ramirez P, Larrosa-Haro A: Gastrointestinal occult hemorrhage and gastroduodenitis in cow's milk protein intolerance. *J Pediatr Gastroenterol Nutr* 3:215, 1984.

157. Karr MA, Mira M, Alperstein G, et al: Iron deficiency in Australian-born children of Arabic background in central Sydney. *Med J Aust* 174:165, 2001.

158. Hudson BG, Tryggvason K, Sundaramoorthy M, Neilson EG: Alport's syndrome, Goodpasture's syndrome, and type IV collagen. *N Engl J Med* 348:2543, 2003.

159. Reid DW, Withers NJ, Francis L, et al: Iron deficiency in cystic fibrosis: Relationship to lung disease severity and chronic Pseudomonas aeruginosa infection. *Chest* 121:48, 2002.

160. Hallberg L, Hulthen L, Bengtsson C, et al: Iron balance in menstruating women. *Eur J Clin Nutr* 49:200, 1995.

161. Hallberg L, Hogdahl AM, Nilsson L, Rybo G: Menstrual blood loss— A population study. Variation at different ages and attempts to define normality. *Acta Obstet Gynecol Scand* 45:320, 1966.

162. Hallberg L, Nilsson L: Constancy of individual menstrual blood loss. *Acta Obstet Gynecol Scand* 43:352, 1964.

163. Burton JL: Effect of oral contraceptives on haemoglobin, packed-cell volume, serum-iron, and total iron-binding capacity in healthy women. *Lancet* 1:978, 1967.

164. Escobedo L, Lee NC: Beyond contraception: The health benefits and risks of the pill. *IPPF Med Bull* 22:1, 1988.

165. Kivijarvi A, Timonen H, Rajamaki A, Gronroos M: Iron deficiency in women using modern copper intrauterine devices. *Obstet Gynecol* 67:95, 1986.

166. Kildahl-Andersen O, Dahl IM, Thorstensen K, Sagen E: Iron deficiency anemia in a patient with excessive urinary iron loss. *Eur J Haematol* 64:204, 2000.

167. Fey MF, Radvila A: Long term follow-up of factitious anaemia. *BMJ* 296:1504, 1988.

168. Hirayama Y, Sakamaki S, Tsuji Y, et al: Fatality caused by self-bloodletting in a patient with factitious anemia. *Int J Hematol* 78:146, 2003.

169. Henry ML, Garner WL, Fabri PJ: Iatrogenic anemia. *Am J Surg* 151:362, 1986.

170. Dale JC, Ruby SG: Specimen collection volumes for laboratory tests. *Arch Pathol Lab Med* 127:162, 2003.

171. Boulton F, Collis D, Inskip H, et al: A study of the iron and HFE status of blood donors, including a group who failed the initial screen for anaemia. *Br J Haematol* 108:434, 2000.

172. Milman N, Byg KE, Ovesen L, et al: Iron status in Danish men 1984–1994: A cohort comparison of changes in iron stores and the prevalence of iron deficiency and iron overload. *Eur J Haematol* 68:332, 2002.

173. Makrides M, Crowther CA, Gibson RA, et al: Efficacy and tolerability

of low-dose iron supplements during pregnancy: A randomized controlled trial. *Am J Clin Nutr* 78:145, 2003.

174. Bashiri A, Burstein E, Sheiner E, Mazor M: Anemia during pregnancy and treatment with intravenous iron: Review of the literature. *Eur J Obstet Gynecol Reprod Biol* 110:2, 2003.

175. Bayoumeu F, Subiran-Buisset C, Baka NE, et al: Iron therapy in iron deficiency anemia in pregnancy: Intravenous route versus oral route. *Am J Obstet Gynecol* 186:518, 2002.

176. Hercberg S, Galan P, Preziosi P, Aissa M: Consequences of iron deficiency in pregnant women—Current issues. *Clin Drug Invest* 19:1, 2000.

177. Villar J, Merialdi M, Gulmezoglu AM, et al: Nutritional interventions during pregnancy for the prevention or treatment of maternal morbidity and preterm delivery: An overview of randomized controlled trials. *J Nutr* 133:1606S, 2003.

178. Rasmussen KM, Stoltzfus RJ: New evidence that iron supplementation during pregnancy improves birth weight: New scientific questions. *Am J Clin Nutr* 78:673, 2003.

179. Mamula P, Piccoli DA, Peck SN, et al: Total dose intravenous infusion of iron dextran for iron-deficiency anemia in children with inflammatory bowel disease. *J Pediatr Gastroenterol Nutr* 34:286, 2002.

180. Cook JD: Iron-deficiency anaemia. *Baillieres Clin Haematol* 7:787, 1994.

181. Cogswell ME, Kettel-Khan L, Ramakrishnan U: Iron supplement use among women in the United States: Science, policy and practice. *J Nutr* 133:1974S, 2003.

182. Anonymous: Iron fortification of infant formulas. American Academy of Pediatrics. Committee on Nutrition. *Pediatrics* 104:119, 1999.

183. Federation of American Societies for Experimental Biology LSRO: Third Report on Nutritional Monitoring in the U.S. Executive Summary. U.S. Government Printing Office, Washington, DC, 1995.

184. Hurrell R, Bothwell T, Cook JD, et al: The usefulness of elemental iron for cereal flour fortification: A SUSTAIN Task Force report. Sharing United States Technology to Aid in the Improvement of Nutrition. *Nutr Rev* 60:391, 2002.

185. Hallberg L, Hulthen L: Perspectives on iron absorption. *Blood Cells Mol Dis* 29:562, 2002.

186. Leonard BJ: Hypochromic anaemia in R.A.F. recruits. *Lancet* 1:899, 1954.

187. Rosenbaum E, Leonard JW: Nutritional iron deficiency anemia in an adult male. Report of a case. *Ann Intern Med* 60:683, 1964.

188. Shearman DJ, Delamore IW, Gardner DL: Gastric function and structure in iron deficiency. *Lancet* 1:845, 1966.

189. Dagg JH, Goldberg A, Gibbs WN, Anderson JR: Detection of latent pernicious anaemia in iron-deficiency anaemia. *BMJ* 2:619, 1966.

190. Voigt D, Bruschke G: Gastric mucosa and iron deficiency. *Dtsch Med Wochenschr* 92:1082, 1967.

191. Voigt D, Dieterich WR, Brushke G, Herrmann H: On blood concentrations of leukocytes and thrombocytes in iron deficiency. *Blut* 14:267, 1967.

192. Stone WD: Gastric secretory response to iron therapy. *Gut* 9:99, 1968.

193. Davidson WM, Markson JL: The gastric mucosa in iron-deficiency anaemia. *Lancet* 269:639, 1955.

194. Dickey W, McConnell B: Celiac disease presenting as the Paterson-Brown Kelly (Plummer-Vinson) syndrome. *Am J Gastroenterol* 94:527, 1999.

195. Vuopio P, Nikkilä EA: Hemolytic anemia and thrombocytopenia in a case of left atrial myxoma associated with mitral stenosis. *Am J Cardiol* 17:585, 1966.

196. Eyster E, Mayer K, McKenzie S: Traumatic hemolysis with iron deficiency anemia in patients with aortic valve lesions. *Ann Intern Med* 68:995, 1968.

197. Reynolds RD, Coltman CA Jr, Beller BM: Iron treatment in sideropenic

intravascular hemolysis due to insufficiency of Starr-Edwards valve prostheses. *Ann Intern Med* 66:659, 1967.

198. Sears DA, Anderson PR, Foy AL, et al: Urinary iron excretion and renal metabolism of hemoglobin in hemolytic diseases. *Blood* 28:708, 1966.

199. Deitrick RW: Intravascular haemolysis in the recreational runner. *Br J Sports Med* 25:183, 1991.

200. Eliakim A, Nemet D, Constantini N: Screening blood tests in members of the Israeli National Olympic team. *J Sports Med Phys Fitness* 42:250, 2002.

201. Wilkinson JG, Martin DT, Adams AA, Liebman M: Iron status in cyclists during high-intensity interval training and recovery. *Int J Sports Med* 23:544, 2002.

202. Nielsen P, Nachtigall D: Iron supplementation in athletes. Current recommendations. *Sports Med* 26:207, 1998.

203. Mechrefe A, Wexler B, Feller E: Sports anemia and gastrointestinal bleeding in endurance athletes. *Med Health R I* 80:216, 1997.

204. Nissenson AR, Strobos J: Iron deficiency in patients with renal failure. *Kidney Int Suppl* 69:S18, 1999.

205. Loría A, Sanchez-Medal L, Lisker R, et al: Red cell life span in iron deficiency anaemia. *Br J Haematol* 13:294, 1967.

206. Pollycove M: Iron metabolism and kinetics. *Semin Hematol* 3:235, 1966.

207. Beutler E: Iron enzymes in iron deficiency. *Blut* 6:130, 1960.

208. Srivastava SK, Sanwal GG, Tewari KK: Biochemical alterations in rat tissue in iron deficiency anaemia & repletion with iron. *Indian J Biochem* 2:257, 1965.

209. Celsing F, Ekblom B, Sylvén C, et al: Effects of chronic iron deficiency anaemia on myoglobin content, enzyme activity, and capillary density in the human skeletal muscle. *Acta Med Scand* 223:451, 1988.

210. Ohira Y, Cartier LJ, Chen M, Holloszy JO: Induction of an increase in mitochondrial matrix enzymes in muscle of iron-deficient rats. *Am J Physiol* 253:C639, 1987.

211. Cartier LJ, Ohira Y, Chen M. et al: Perturbation of mitochondrial composition in muscle by iron deficiency. Implications regarding regulation of mitochondrial assembly. *J Biol Chem* 261:13827, 1986.

212. Zoller H, Theurl I, Koch RO, et al: Duodenal cytochrome B and hephaestin expression in patients with iron deficiency and hemochromatosis. *Gastroenterology* 125:746, 2003.

213. Finch CA, Gollnick PD, Hlastala MP, et al: Lactic acidosis as a result of iron deficiency. *J Clin Invest* 64:129, 1979.

214. MacDonald VW, Charache S, Hathaway PJ: Iron deficiency anemia: Mitochondrial alpha-glycerophosphate dehydrogenase in guinea pig skeletal muscle. *J Lab Clin Med* 105:11, 1985.

215. Mackler B, Person R, Grace R: Iron deficiency in the rat: Effects on energy metabolism in brown adipose tissue. *Pediatr Res* 19:989, 1985.

216. Walter PB, Knutson MD, Paler-Martinez A, et al: Iron deficiency and iron excess damage mitochondria and mitochondrial DNA in rats. *Proc Natl Acad Sci U S A* 99:2264, 2002.

217. Harlan WR, Williams RS: Activity-induced adaptations in skeletal muscles of iron-deficient rabbits. *J Appl Physiol* 65:782, 1988.

218. Evans TC, Mackler B: Effect of iron deficiency on energy conservation in rat liver and skeletal muscle submitochondrial particles. *Biochem Med* 34:93, 1985.

219. Thompson CH, Green YS, Ledingham JG, et al: The effect of iron deficiency on skeletal muscle metabolism of the rat. *Acta Physiol Scand* 147:85, 1993.

220. Thompson CH, Kemp GJ, Taylor DJ, et al: No evidence of mitochondrial abnormality in skeletal muscle of patients with iron-deficient anaemia. *J Intern Med* 234:149, 1993.

221. Youdim MBH, Green AR: Biogenic monoamine metabolism and functional activity in iron-deficient rats: Behavioural correlates. *Ciba Found Symp* 51:201, 1977.

222. Youdim MB, Green AR: Iron deficiency and neurotransmitter synthesis and function. *Proc Nutr Soc* 37:173, 1978.

223. Beard J, Tobin B, Smith SM: Norepinephrine turnover in iron deficiency at three environmental temperatures. *Am J Physiol* 255:R90, 1988.

224. Webb TE, Krill CE Jr, Oski FA, Tsou KC: Relationship of iron status to urinary norepinephrine excretion in children 7-12 years of age. *J Pediatr Gastroenterol Nutr* 1:207, 1982.

225. Youdim MB, Ben Shachar D: Minimal brain damage induced by early iron deficiency: Modified dopaminergic neurotransmission. *Isr J Med Sci* 23:19, 1987.

226. Bartholmey SJ, Sherman AR: Impaired ketogenesis in iron-deficient rat pups. *J Nutr* 116:2180, 1986.

227. Beard J: Feed efficiency and norepinephrine turnover in iron deficiency. *Proc Soc Exp Biol Med* 184:337, 1987.

228. Prime SS, MacDonald DG, Noble HW, Rennie JS: Effect of prolonged iron deficiency on enamel pigmentation and tooth structure in rat incisors. *Arch Oral Biol* 29:905, 1984.

229. Sun AH, Xiao SZ, Li BS, et al: Iron deficiency and hearing loss. Experimental study in growing rats. *ORL J Otorhinolaryngol Relat Spec* 49:118, 1987.

230. Sun AH, Xiao SZ, Zheng Z, et al: A scanning electron microscopic study of cochlear changes in iron-deficient rats. *Acta Otolaryngol* 104:211, 1987.

231. Beard JL: Iron biology in immune function, muscle metabolism and neuronal functioning. *J Nutr* 131:568S, 2001.

232. Ahluwalia N, Sun J, Krause D, et al: Immune function is impaired in iron-deficient, homebound, older women. *Am J Clin Nutr* 79:516, 2004.

233. Grant SM, Wiesinger JA, Beard JL, Cantorna MT: Iron-deficient mice fail to develop autoimmune encephalomyelitis. *J Nutr* 133:2635, 2003.

234. Chwang LC, Soemantri AG, Pollitt E: Iron supplementation and physical growth of rural Indonesian children. *Am J Clin Nutr* 47:496, 1988.

235. Pizarro F, Olivares M, Hertrampf E, Walter T: Growth in terms of length of Chilean infants of low socioeconomic status: 1978-1992. *Arch Latinoam Nutr* 46:107, 1996.

236. Bandhu R, Shankar N, Tandon OP: Effect of iron on growth in iron deficient anemic school going children. *Indian J Physiol Pharmacol* 47:59, 2003.

237. Prasad AS, Halsted JA, Nadimi M: Syndrome of iron deficiency anemia, hepatosplenomegaly, hypogonadism, dwarfism and geophagia. *Am J Med* 31:532, 1961.

238. Rosenzweig PH, Volpe SL: Iron, thermoregulation, and metabolic rate. *Crit Rev Food Sci Nutr* 39:131, 1999.

239. Baird IM, Dodge OG, Palmer FJ, Wawman RJ: The tongue and esophagus in iron-deficiency anaemia and the effect of iron therapy. *J Clin Pathol* 14:603, 1961.

240. Cheli R, Dodero M, Celle G, Vasalotti M: Gastric biopsy and secretory findings in hypochromic anaemias. *Acta Haematol (Basel)* 22:1, 1959.

241. Lees F, Rosenthal FD: Gastric mucosal lesions before and after treatment in iron deficiency anaemia. *Q J Med* 27:19, 1958.

242. Beutler E: Iron enzymes in iron deficiency: VI. Aconitase activity and citrate metabolism. *J Clin Invest* 38:1605, 1959.

243. Naiman JL, Oski FA, Diamond LK, et al: The gastrointestinal effects of iron deficiency anemia. *Pediatrics* 33:83, 1964.

244. Scott J, Valentine JA, St Hill CA, West CR: Morphometric analysis of atrophic changes in human lingual epithelium in iron deficiency anaemia. *J Clin Pathol* 38:1025, 1985.

245. Boddington MM: Changes in buccal cells in the anaemias. *J Clin Pathol* 12:222, 1959.

246. Jacobs A: The buccal mucosa in anaemia. *J Clin Pathol* 13:463, 1960.

247. Macleod RI, Hamilton PJ, Soames JV: Quantitative exfoliative oral cytology in iron-deficiency and megaloblastic anemia. *Anal Quant Cytol Histol* 10:176, 1988.

248. Milman N, Pedersen FM: Idiopathic pulmonary haemosiderosis. Epidemiology, pathogenic aspects and diagnosis. *Respir Med* 92:902, 1998.

249. Shahidi NT, Diamond LK: Skull changes in infants with chronic iron-deficiency anemia. *N Engl J Med* 262:137, 1960.

250. Moseley JE: Skeletal changes in the anemias. *Semin Roentgenol* 9:169, 1974.

251. Reimann F, Berker F, Gokmen E, Kucukcakirlar T: Behaviour of the sella turcica in juveniles with severe iron deficiency. *Rofo Fortschr Geb Rontgenstr Nuklearmed* 129:598, 1978.

252. Beutler E, Larsh SE, Gurney CW: Iron therapy in chronically fatigued, non-anemic women: A double-blind study. *Ann Intern Med* 52:378, 1960.

253. Halterman JS, Kaczorowski JM, Aligne CA, et al: Iron deficiency and cognitive achievement among school-aged children and adolescents in the United States. *Pediatrics* 107:1381, 2001.

254. Friedmann B, Weller E, Mairbaurl H, Bartsch P: Effects of iron repletion on blood volume and performance capacity in young athletes. *Med Sci Sports Exerc* 33:741, 2001.

255. Hinton PS, Giordano C, Brownlie T, Haas JD: Iron supplementation improves endurance after training in iron-depleted, nonanemic women. *J Appl Physiol* 88:1103, 2000.

256. Zhu YI, Haas JD: Altered metabolic response of iron-depleted nonanemic women during a 15-km time trial. *J Appl Physiol* 84:1768, 1998.

257. Zhu YI, Haas JD: Iron depletion without anemia and physical performance in young women. *Am J Clin Nutr* 66:334, 1997.

258. Rowland TW, Deisroth MB, Green GM, Kelleher JF: The effect of iron therapy on the exercise capacity of nonanemic iron-deficient adolescent runners. *Sports Med* 142:165, 1988.

259. Duport N, Preziosi P, Boutron-Ruault MC, et al: Consequences of iron depletion on health in menstruating women. *Eur J Clin Nutr* 57:1169, 2003.

260. Cochrane AL, Elwood PC: Iron deficiency without anaemia. *Lancet* 1:591, 1968.

261. Cusack RP, Brown WD: Iron deficiency in rats: Changes in body and organ weights, plasma proteins, hemoglobins, myoglobins, and catalase. *J Nutr* 86:383, 1965.

262. Haas JD, Brownlie T: Iron deficiency and reduced work capacity: A critical review of the research to determine a causal relationship. *J Nutr* 131:676S, 2001.

263. Brownlie T, Utermohlen V, Hinton PS, Haas JD: Tissue iron deficiency without anemia impairs adaptation in endurance capacity after aerobic training in previously untrained women. *Am J Clin Nutr* 79:437, 2004.

264. De Mulder R: Iron metabolism, biochemistry, and clinical physiology—Review of recent literature. *Arch Intern Med* 102:254, 1958.

265. Ikkala E, Laitinen L: Papilloedema due to iron deficiency anaemia. *Acta Haematol (Basel)* 29:368, 1963.

266. Morrow JJ, Dagg JH, Goldberg A: A controlled trial of iron therapy in sideropenia. *Scott Med J* 13:78, 1968.

267. Yager JY, Hartfield DS: Neurologic manifestations of iron deficiency in childhood. *Pediatr Neurol* 27:85, 2002.

268. Lubeck MJ: Papilledema caused by iron-deficiency anemia. *Trans Am Acad Ophthalmol Otolaryngol* 306, 1959.

269. Capriles LF: Intracranial hypertension and iron-deficiency anemia: Report of four cases. *Arch Neurol* 9:147, 1963.

270. Biousse V, Rucker JC, Vignal C, et al: Anemia and papilledema. *Am J Ophthalmol* 135:437, 2003.

271. Stevens AR Jr: The mechanism and treatment of iron-deficiency anemia. *Arch Intern Med* 96:550, 1956.

272. Jacobs A, Kilpatrick GS: The Paterson-Kelly syndrome. *BMJ* 2:79, 1964.

273. Jacobs A, Cavill I: The oral lesions of iron deficiency anaemia: Pyridoxine and riboflavin status. *Br J Haematol* 24:291, 1968.

274. Bernát I, Valló J: Ozaena: The causes of its familial occurrence. *Acta Med Acad Sci Hung* 20:89, 1964.

275. Akhnoukh S, Saad EF: Iron-deficiency in atrophic rhinitis & scleroma. *Indian J Med Res* 85:576, 1987.

276. Chen TS, Chen PS: Rise and fall of the Plummer-Vinson syndrome. *J Gastroenterol Hepatol* 9:654, 1994.

277. Yukselen V, Karaoglu AO, Yasa MH: Plummer-Vinson syndrome: A report of three cases. *Int J Clin Pract* 57:646, 2003.

278. Makharia GK, Nandi B, Garg PK, Tandon RK: Plummer Vinson syndrome: Unusual features. *Indian J Gastroenterol* 21:74, 2002.

279. Jani PG: Plummer Vinson syndrome: Case report. *East Afr Med J* 78:332, 2001.

280. Miranda AL, Dantas RO: Esophageal contractions and oropharyngeal and esophageal transits in patients with iron deficiency anemia. *Am J Gastroenterol* 98:1000, 2003.

281. Taymor ML, Sturgis SH, Yahia C: The etiological role of chronic iron deficiency in production of menorrhagia. *JAMA* 187:323, 1964.

282. Samuels AJ: Studies in patients with functional menorrhagia. The antihemorrhagic effect of the adequate repletion of iron stores. *Isr J Med Sci* 1:851, 1965.

283. Jacobs A, Butler EB: Menstrual blood-loss in iron-deficiency anaemia. *Lancet* 2:407, 1965.

284. Callinan V, O'Hare JA: Cardboard chewing: Cause and effect of iron-deficiency anemia. *Am J Med* 85:449, 1988.

285. Menge H, Lang A, Cuntze H: Pica in Germany—Amylophagia as the etiology of iron deficiency anemia. *Z Gastroenterol* 36:635, 1998.

286. Phillips MR, Zaheer S, Drugas GT: Gastric trichobezoar: Case report and literature review. *Mayo Clin Proc* 73:653, 1998.

287. Patel S: Restless legs syndrome and periodic limb movements of sleep: Fact, fad, and fiction. *Curr Opin Pulm Med* 8:498, 2002.

288. Earley CJ: Restless legs syndrome. *N Engl J Med* 348:2103, 2003.

289. Silber MH, Richardson JW: Multiple blood donations associated with iron deficiency in patients with restless legs syndrome. *Mayo Clin Proc* 78:52, 2003.

290. Sloand JA, Shelly MA, Feigin A, et al: A double-blind, placebo-controlled trial of intravenous iron dextran therapy in patients with ESRD and restless legs syndrome. *Am J Kidney Dis* 43:663, 2004.

291. Rushton DH. Nutritional factors and hair loss. *Clin Exp Dermatol* 27:400, 2002.

292. Kantor J, Kessler LJ, Brooks DG, Cotsarelis G: Decreased serum ferritin is associated with alopecia in women. *J Invest Dermatol* 121:985, 2003.

293. Chamberlain AJ, Dawber RPR: Significance of iron status in hair loss in women. *Br J Dermatol* 149:428, 2003.

294. Gordon N: Iron deficiency and the intellect. *Brain Dev* 25:3, 2003.

295. Dallman PR: Iron deficiency: Does it matter. *J Intern Med* 226:367, 1989.

296. Grantham-McGregor S, Ani C: A review of studies on the effect of iron deficiency on cognitive development in children. *J Nutr* 131:649S, 2001.

297. Aksoy M, Erdem S, Baserer G: On the pathogenesis of the hepatosplenomegaly in chronic iron deficiency anaemia. A study of five patients with a syndrome of chronic iron deficiency anaemia, hepatosplenomegaly, hypogonadism and dwarfism. *Acta Hepato-Splenologica* 15:241, 1968.

298. Bessman JD, Feinstein DI: Quantitative anisocytosis as a discriminant between iron deficiency and thalassemia minor. *Blood* 53:288, 1979.

299. Fairbanks VF: Is the peripheral blood film reliable for the diagnosis of iron deficiency anemia. *Am J Clin Pathol* 55:447, 1971.

300. Kasper CK, Whissell DYE, Wallerstein RO: Clinical aspects of iron deficiency. *JAMA* 191:359, 1965.

301. Conrad ME, Crosby WH: The natural history of iron deficiency induced by phlebotomy. *Blood* 20:173, 1962.

302. Beutler E: The red cell indices in the diagnosis of iron-deficiency anemia. *Ann Intern Med* 50:313, 1959.

303. Aslan D, Altay C: Incidence of high erythrocyte count in infants and young children with iron deficiency anemia: Re-evaluation of an old parameter. *J Pediatr Hematol Oncol* 25:303, 2003.

304. Charache S, Gittlelsohn AM, Allen H, et al: Noninvasive assessment of tissue iron stores. *Am J Clin Pathol* 88:333, 1987.

305. Witte DL, Kraemer DF, Johnson GF, et al: Prediction of bone marrow iron findings from tests performed on peripheral blood. *Am J Clin Pathol* 85:202, 1986.

306. Beck JR, Cornwell GG, Rawnsley HM: Multivariate approach to predictive diagnosis of bone-marrow iron stores. *Am J Clin Pathol* 70:665, 1978.

307. Junca J, Flores A, Roy C, et al: Red cell distribution width, free erythrocyte protoporphyrin, and England-Fraser index in the differential diagnosis of microcytosis due to iron deficiency or beta-thalassemia trait. A study of 200 cases of microcytic anemia. *Hematol Pathol* 5:33, 1991.

308. Kokkinos J, Levine SR: Thrombocytosis secondary to iron deficiency and recurrent cerebral ischemia possibly improved by plateletpheresis. *Cerebrovasc Dis* 3:177, 1993.

309. Dincol K, Aksoy M: On the platelet levels in chronic iron deficiency anemia. *Acta Haematol (Basel) 41*:135, 1969.

310. Gross S, Keefer V, Newman AJ: The platelets in iron-deficiency anemia: I. The response to oral and parenteral iron. *Pediatrics* 34:315, 1964.

311. Perlman MK, Schwab JG, Nachman JB, Rubin CM: Thrombocytopenia in children with severe iron deficiency. *J Pediatr Hematol Oncol* 24:380, 2002.

312. Marsh WL Jr, Bishop JW, Darcy TP: Evaluation of red cell volume distribution width (RDW). *Hematol Pathol* 1:117, 1987.

313. Soff GA, Levin J: Thrombocytopenia associated with repletion of iron in iron-deficiency anemia. *Am J Med Sci* 295:35, 1988.

314. Berger M, Brass LF: Severe thrombocytopenia in iron deficiency anemia. *Am J Hematol* 24:425, 1987.

315. de Lima GA, Grotto HZ: Soluble transferrin receptor and immature reticulocytes are not useful for distinguishing iron-deficiency anemia from heterozygous beta-thalassemia. *Sao Paulo Med J* 121:90, 2003.

316. Valentine WN, Tanaka KR: The glyoxalase content of human erythrocytes and leukocytes. *Acta Haematol (Basel)* 26:303, 1961.

317. Beutler E, Drennan W, Block M: The bone marrow and liver in iron deficiency anemia: A histopathologic study of sections with special reference to the stainable iron content. *J Lab Clin Med* 43:427, 1954.

318. Rath CE, Finch CA: Sternal marrow hemosiderin: A method for the determination of available iron stores in man. *J Lab Clin Med* 33:81, 1948.

319. Beutler E, Robson M, Buttenwieser E: A comparison of the serum iron, iron-binding capacity, sternal marrow iron and other methods in the clinical evaluation of iron stores. *Ann Intern Med* 48:60, 1958.

320. Barron BA, Hoyer JD, Tefferi A: A bone marrow report of absent stainable iron is not diagnostic of iron deficiency. *Ann Hematol* 80:166, 2001.

321. Cervantes F, Rozman C, Piera C, Fernandez M-R: Decreased bone marrow iron in chronic granulocytic leukaemia: A consistent finding not reflecting iron deficiency. *Blut* 53:305, 1986.

322. Cavill IA: Iron status indicators: Hello new, goodbye old? *Blood* 101:372, 2003.

323. Ellis LD, Jensen WN, Westerman MP: Marrow iron. An evaluation of depleted stores in a series of 1,332 needle biopsies. *Ann Intern Med* 61:44, 1964.

324. Garby L, Irnell L, Werner I: Iron deficiency in women of fertile age in a Swedish community: II. Efficiency of several laboratory tests to predict the response of iron supplementation. *Acta Med Scand* 185:107, 1969.

325. Hamilton LD, Gubler CJ, Cartwright GE, Wintrobe MM: Diurnal variation in the plasma iron level of man. *Proc Soc Exp Biol Med* 61:44, 1964.

326. Hoyer K: Physiologic variations in the iron content of human blood serum: I. The variations from week to week, from day to day, and through twenty-four hours: II. Further studies of the intra diem variations. *Acta Med Scand* 119:562, 1944.

327. Speck B: Diurnal variation of serum iron and the latent iron-binding in normal adults. *Helv Med Acta* 34:231, 1968.

328. Dale JC, Burritt MF, Zinsmeister AR: Diurnal variation of serum iron, iron-binding capacity, transferrin saturation, and ferritin levels. *Am J Clin Pathol* 117:802, 2002.

329. Zilva JF, Patston VJ: Variations in serum-iron in healthy women. *Lancet* 1:459, 1966.

330. Fujino M, Dawson EB, Holeman T, McGanity WJ: Interrelationships between estrogenic activity, serum iron and ascorbic acid levels during the menstrual cycle. *Am J Clin Nutr* 18:256, 1966.

331. Mardell M, Zilva JF: Effect of oral contraceptives on the variations in serum-iron during the menstrual cycle. *Lancet* 2:1323, 1967.

332. Cartwright GE: The anemia of chronic disorders. *Semin Hematol* 3:351, 1966.

333. Bainton DF, Finch CA: The diagnosis of iron deficiency anemia. *Am J Med* 37:62, 1964.

334. Banerjee RN, Narang RM: Haematological changes in malignancy. *Br J Haematol* 13:829, 1967.

335. Handjani AM, Banihashemi A, Rafiee R, Tolou H: Serum iron in acute myocardial infarction. *Blut* 23:363, 1971.

336. Syrkis I, Machtey I: Hypoferremia in acute myocardial infarction. *J Am Geriatr Soc* 21:28, 1973.

337. Follezou JY, Bizon M: Cancer chemotherapy induces a transient increase of serum-iron level. *Neoplasma* 33:225, 1986.

338. Seligman PA, Schleicher RB: Comparison of methods used to measure serum iron in the presence of iron gluconate or iron dextran. *Clin Chem* 45:898, 1999.

339. Lipschitz DA, Cook JD, Finch CA: A clinical evaluation of serum ferritin as an index of iron stores. *N Engl J Med* 290:1213, 1974.

340. Mazza P, Giua R, De Marco S, et al: Iron overload in thalassemia: Comparative analysis of magnetic resonance imaging, serum ferritin and iron content of the liver. *Haematologica* 80:398, 1995.

341. Beutler E, Felitti V, Ho N, Gelbart T: Relationship of body iron stores to levels of serum ferritin, serum iron, unsaturated iron binding capacity and transferrin saturation in patients with iron storage disease. *Acta Haematol (Basel)* 107:145, 2002.

342. Bonkovsky HL, Slaker DP, Bills EB, Wolf DC: Usefulness and limitations of laboratory and hepatic imaging studies in iron-storage disease. *Gastroenterology* 99:1079, 1990.

343. Hallberg L, Hulthen L: High serum ferritin is not identical to high iron stores. *Am J Clin Nutr* 78:1225, 2003.

344. Coenen JLLM, Van Dieijen-Visser MP, Van Pelt J, et al: Measurements of serum ferritin used to predict concentrations of iron in bone marrow in anemia of chronic disease. *Clin Chem* 37:560, 1991.

345. van Tellingen A, Kuenen JC, de Kieviet W, et al: Iron deficiency anaemia in hospitalized patients: Value of various laboratory parameters. Differentiation between IDA and ACD. *Neth J Med* 59:270, 2001.

346. Sears DA: Anemia of chronic disease. *Med Clin North Am* 76:567, 1992.

347. Zimran A, Kay AC, Gelbart T, et al: Gaucher disease: Clinical, laboratory, radiologic and genetic features of 53 patients. *Medicine* 71:337, 1992.

348. Morgan MAM, Hoffbrand AV, Laulicht M, et al: Serum ferritin concentration in Gaucher's disease. *BMJ* 286:1864, 1983.

349. Hansen TM, Hansen NE: Serum ferritin as indicator of iron responsive anaemia in patients with rheumatoid arthritis. *Ann Rheum Dis* 45:596, 1986.

350. Matzner Y, Konijn AM, Hershko C: Serum ferritin in hematologic malignancies. *Am J Hematol* 9:13, 1980.

351. Ioannou GN, Tung BY, Kowdley KV: Iron in hepatitis C: Villain or innocent bystander? *Semin Gastrointest Dis* 13:95, 2002.

352. Dennison HA: Limitations of ferritin as a marker of anemia in end stage renal disease. *ANNA J* 26:409, 1999.

353. Wheby MS: Effect of iron therapy on serum ferritin levels in iron-deficiency anemia. *Blood* 56:138, 1980.

354. Galfn P, Sangaré N, Preziosi P, et al: Is basic red cell ferritin a more specific indicator than serum ferritin in the assessment of iron stores in the elderly. *Clin Chim Acta* 189:159, 1990.

355. Balaban EP, Sheehan RG, Demian SE, et al: Evaluation of bone marrow iron stores in anemia associated with chronic disease: A comparative study of serum and red cell ferritin. *Am J Hematol* 42:177, 1993.

356. Mei Z, Parvanta I, Cogswell ME, et al: Erythrocyte protoporphyrin or hemoglobin: Which is a better screening test for iron deficiency in children and women? *Am J Clin Nutr* 77:1229, 2003.

357. Fischer AB, Georgieva R, Nikolova V, et al: Health risk for children from lead and cadmium near a non-ferrous smelter in Bulgaria. *Int J Hyg Environ Health* 206:25, 2003.

358. Houston T, Moore M, Porter D, et al: Abnormal haem biosynthesis in the chronic anaemia of rheumatoid arthritis. *Ann Rheum Dis* 53:167, 1994.

359. Cook JD, Skikne BS, Baynes RD: Serum transferrin receptor. *Annu Rev Med* 44:63, 1993.

360. Ahluwalia N: Diagnostic utility of serum transferrin receptors measurement in assessing iron status. *Nutr Rev* 56:133, 1998.

361. Provan D: Mechanisms and management of iron deficiency anaemia. *Br J Haematol* 105 (suppl 1):19, 1999.

362. Juncf J, Fernández-Avilés F, Oriol A, et al: The usefulness of the serum transferrin receptor in detecting iron deficiency in the anemia of chronic disorders. *Haematologica* 83:676, 1998.

363. Gimferrer F, Ubeda J, Remacha AF: Serum transferrin receptor levels are "physiologically" high in heterozygous beta-thalassemia. *Haematologica* 82:728, 1997.

364. North M, Dallalio G, Donath AS, et al: Serum transferrin receptor levels in patients undergoing evaluation of iron stores: Correlation with other parameters and observed versus predicted results. *Clin Lab Haematol* 19:93, 1997.

365. Pettersson T, Kivivuori SM, Siimes MA: Is serum transferrin receptor useful for detecting iron-deficiency in anaemic patients with chronic inflammatory diseases? *Br J Rheumatol* 33:740, 1994.

366. Beutler E, Hoffbrand AV, Cook JD: Iron deficiency and overload. *Hematology (Am Soc Hematol Educ Program)* 40, 2003.

367. Cook JD, Flowers CH, Skikne BS: The quantitative assessment of body iron. *Blood* 101:3359, 2003.

368. Brugnara C, Zurakowski D, DiCanzio J, et al: Reticulocyte hemoglobin content to diagnose iron deficiency in children. *JAMA* 281:2225, 1999.

369. Kaneko Y, Miyazaki S, Hirasawa Y, et al: Transferrin saturation versus reticulocyte hemoglobin content for iron deficiency in Japanese hemodialysis patients. *Kidney Int* 63:1086, 2003.

370. Mast AE, Blinder MA, Lu Q, et al: Clinical utility of the reticulocyte hemoglobin content in the diagnosis of iron deficiency. *Blood* 99:1489, 2002.

371. Jasinski B: Eisenresorptionsversuche für die Diagnose und Differentialdiagnose der Eisenmangelanämien insbesondere für die Erkennung der Eisenmangel-zustande ohne Anämie. *Schweiz Med Wochenschr* 79:291, 1949.

372. Crosby WH, O'Neil-Cutting MA: A small-dose iron tolerance test as an indicator of mild iron deficiency. *JAMA* 251:1986, 1984.

373. Johnson CS, Tegos C, Beutler E: Alpha-thalassemia. Prevalence and hematologic findings in American Blacks. *Arch Intern Med* 142:1280, 1982.

374. Duma H, Efremov G, Sadikario A, et al: Study of nine families with haemoglobin-Lepore. *Br J Haematol* 15:161, 1968.

375. Fairbanks VF, Gilchrist GS, Brimhall B, et al: Hemoglobin E trait reexamined: A cause of microcytosis and erythrocytosis. *Blood* 52:109, 1979.

376. Fairbanks VF, Oliveros R, Brandabur JH, et al: Homozygous hemoglo-

bin E mimics beta-thalassemia minor without anemia or hemolysis: Hematologic, functional, and biosynthetic studies of first North American cases. *Am J Hematol* 8:109, 1980.

377. Johnson C, Tegos C, Beutler E: Thalassemia minor: Routine erythrocyte measurements and differentiation from iron deficiency. *Am J Clin Pathol* 80:31, 1983.

378. England JM, Walford DM, Waters DA: Re-assessment of the reliability of the haematocrit. *Br J Haematol* 23:247, 1972.

379. Rose MS: Epitaph for the M.C.H.C. *BMJ* 4:169, 1971.

380. Han P, Fung KP: Discriminant analysis of iron deficiency anaemia and heterozygous thalassaemia traits: A 3-dimensional selection of red cell indices. *Clin Lab Haematol* 13:351, 1991.

381. Lin CK, Lin JS, Chen SY, et al: Comparison of hemoglobin and red blood cell distribution width in the differential diagnosis of microcytic anemia. *Arch Pathol Lab Med* 116:1030, 1992.

382. McClure S, Custer E, Bessman JD: Improved detection of early iron deficiency in nonanemic subjects. *JAMA* 253:1021, 1985.

383. Aslan D, Gumruk F, Gurgey A, Altay C: Importance of RDW value in differential diagnosis of hypochrome anemias. *Am J Hematol* 69:31, 2002.

384. Flynn MM, Reppun TS, Bhagavan NV: Limitations of red blood cell distribution width (RDW) in evaluation of microcytosis. *Am J Clin Pathol* 85:445, 1986.

385. Wians FH Jr, Urban JE, Keffer JH, Kroft SH: Discriminating between iron deficiency anemia and anemia of chronic disease using traditional indices of iron status vs transferrin receptor concentration. *Am J Clin Pathol* 115:112, 2001.

386. Thompson WG, Meola T, Lipkin M, Freedman ML: Red cell distribution width, mean corpuscular volume, and transferrin saturation in the diagnosis of iron deficiency. *Arch Intern Med* 148:2128, 1988.

387. Cartei G, Chisesi T, Cazzavillan M, et al: Relationship between Hb and HbA2 concentrations in beta-thalassemia trait and effect of iron deficiency anaemia. *Biomedicine* 25:282, 1976.

388. Meyer CT, Troncale FJ, Galloway S, Sheahan DG: Arteriovenous malformations of the bowel: An analysis of 22 cases and a review of the literature. *Medicine* 60:36, 1981.

389. Kohgo Y, Torimoto Y, Kato J: Transferrin receptor in tissue and serum: Updated clinical significance of soluble receptor. *Int J Hematol* 76:213, 2002.

390. Matthay KK, Villablanca JG, Seeger RC, et al: Treatment of high-risk neuroblastoma with intensive chemotherapy, radiotherapy, autologous bone marrow transplantation, and 13-*cis*-retinoic acid. *N Engl J Med* 341:1165, 1999.

391. Intragumtornchai T, Rojnukkarin P, Swasdikul D, Israsena S: The role of serum ferritin in the diagnosis of iron deficiency anaemia in patients with liver cirrhosis. *J Intern Med* 243:233, 1998.

392. Prieto J, Barry M, Sherlock S: Serum ferritin in patients with iron overload and with acute and chronic liver diseases. *Gastroenterology* 68:525, 1975.

393. Tessitore N, Solero GP, Lippi G, et al: The role of iron status markers in predicting response to intravenous iron in haemodialysis patients on maintenance erythropoietin. *Nephrol Dial Transplant* 16:1416, 2001.

394. Fernandez-Rodriguez AM, Guindeo-Casasus MC, Molero-Labarta T, et al: Diagnosis of iron deficiency in chronic renal failure. *Am J Kidney Dis* 34:508, 1999.

395. Chuang CL, Liu RS, Wei YH, et al: Early prediction of response to intravenous iron supplementation by reticulocyte haemoglobin content and high-fluorescence reticulocyte count in haemodialysis patients. *Nephrol Dial Transplant* 18:370, 2003.

396. Saito M, Tsuchiya K, Ando M, et al: Measuring the content of reticulocyte hemoglobin (CHr) in predialysis chronic renal failure (CRF) patients. *Nippon Jinzo Gakkai Shi* 45:430, 2003.

397. Fishbane S, Shapiro W, Dutka P, et al: A randomized trial of iron deficiency testing strategies in hemodialysis patients. *Kidney Int* 60:2406, 2001.

398. Ellis LD, Westerman MP, Balcerzak SP: The effect of iron stores on ferrokinetics in polycythaemia. *Br J Haematol* 13:892, 1967.

399. Hilal H, McCurdy PR: A pitfall in the interpretation of serum iron values. *Ann Intern Med* 66:983, 1967.

400. Demiroglu H, Dundar S: Pernicious anaemia patients should be screened for iron deficiency during follow up. *N Z Med J* 110:147, 1997.

401. Annibale B, Capurso G, Chistolini A, et al: Gastrointestinal causes of refractory iron deficiency anemia in patients without gastrointestinal symptoms. *Am J Med* 111:439, 2001.

402. Bampton PA, Holloway RH: A prospective study of the gastroenterological causes of iron deficiency anaemia in a General Hospital. *Aust N Z J Med* 26:793, 1996.

403. Kepczyk T, Cremins JE, Long BD, et al: A prospective, multidisciplinary evaluation of premenopausal women with iron-deficiency anemia. *Am J Gastroenterol* 94:109, 1999.

404. Rockey DC, Cello JP: Evaluation of the gastrointestinal tract in patients with iron-deficiency anemia. *N Engl J Med* 329:1691, 1993.

405. Chait A, Dann RH: G-I bleed after angiography. *N Engl J Med* 286:1418, 1972.

406. Al Onaizi I, Al Awadi F, Al Dawood AL: Iron deficiency anaemia: An unusual complication of Meckel's diverticulum. *Med Princ Pract* 11:214, 2002.

407. Berquist TH, Nolan NG, Adson MA, Schutt AJ: Diagnosis of Meckel's diverticulum by radioisotope scanning. *Mayo Clin Proc* 48:98, 1973.

408. Lu CC, Huang FC, Lee SY, Huang HY: Laparoscopy diagnosis and treatment excision of bleeding Meckel's diverticulum in a child: Report of one case. *Acta Paediatr Taiwan* 44:41, 2003.

409. Annibale B, Capurso G, Baccini F, et al: Role of small bowel investigation in iron deficiency anaemia after negative endoscopic/histologic evaluation of the upper and lower gastrointestinal tract. *Dig Liver Dis* 35:784, 2003.

410. Kerr DN, Davidson S: Gastrointestinal intolerance to oral iron preparations. *Lancet* 2:489, 1958.

411. Hallberg L, Ryttinger L, Sölvell L: Side-effects of oral iron therapy. A double-blind study of different iron compounds in tablet form. *Acta Med Scand* 459:3, 1966.

412. Eskeland B, Malterud K, Ulvik RJ, Hunskaar S: Iron supplementation in pregnancy: Is less enough? A randomized, placebo controlled trial of low dose iron supplementation with and without heme iron. *Acta Obstet Gynecol Scand* 76:822, 1997.

413. Fogelholm M, Suominen M, Rita H: Effects of low-dose iron supplementation in women with low serum ferritin concentration. *Eur J Clin Nutr* 48:753, 1994.

414. Leung AK, Chan KW: Iron deficiency anemia. *Adv Pediatr* 48:385, 2001.

415. Allen LH: Iron supplements: Scientific issues concerning efficacy and implications for research and programs. *J Nutr* 132:813S, 2002.

416. O'Sullivan DJ, Higgins PG, Wilkinson JF: Oral iron compounds: A therapeutic comparison. *Lancet* 269:482, 1955.

417. Gordeuk VR, Brittenham GM, Hughes M, et al: High-dose carbonyl iron for iron deficiency anemia: A randomized double-blind trial. *Am J Clin Nutr* 46:1029, 1987.

418. Brittenham GM, Klein HG, Kushner JP, Ajioka RS: Preserving the national blood supply. *Hematology (Am Soc Hematol Educ Program)* 422, 2001.

419. Sullivan JL: Iron and coronary heart disease. Iron makes myocardium vulnerable to ischaemia. *BMJ* 307:1066, 1993.

420. Tuomainen TP, Kontula K, Nyyssonen K, et al: Increased risk of acute myocardial infarction in carriers of the hemochromatosis gene

Cys282Tyr mutation—A prospective cohort study in men in eastern Finland. *Circulation* 100:1274, 1999.

421. Sempos CT, Looker AC, Gillum RF: Iron and heart disease: The epidemiologic data. *Nutr Rev* 54:73, 1996.

422. Waalen J, Felitti V, Gelbart T, et al: Prevalence of coronary heart disease associated with HFE mutations in adults attending a health appraisal center. *Am J Med* 113:472, 2002.

423. Knuiman MW, Divitini ML, Olynyk JK, et al: Serum ferritin and cardiovascular disease: A 17-year follow-up study in Busselton, Western Australia. *Am J Epidemiol* 158:144, 2003.

424. Auer J, Rammer M, Berent R, et al: Body iron stores and coronary atherosclerosis assessed by coronary angiography. *Nutr Metab Cardiovasc Dis* 12:285, 2002.

425. Bozzini C, Girelli D, Tinazzi E, et al: Biochemical and genetic markers of iron status and the risk of coronary artery disease: An angiography-based study. *Clin Chem* 48:622, 2002.

426. Claeys D, Walting M, Julmy F, et al: Haemochromatosis mutations and ferritin in myocardial infarction: A case-control study. *Eur J Clin Invest* 32(suppl 1):3, 2002.

427. Gunn IR, Maxwell FK, Gaffney D, et al: Haemochromatosis gene mutations and risk of coronary heart disease: A west of Scotland coronary prevention study (WOSCOPS) substudy. *Heart* 90:304, 2004.

428. Gera T, Sachdev HP: Effect of iron supplementation on incidence of infectious illness in children: Systematic review. *BMJ* 325:1142, 2002.

429. Jiang R, Manson JE, Meigs JB, et al: Body iron stores in relation to risk of type 2 diabetes in apparently healthy women. *JAMA* 291:711, 2004.

430. Moczulski DK, Grzeszczak W, Gawlik B: Role of hemochromatosis C282Y and H63D mutations in HFE gene in development of type 2 diabetes and diabetic nephropathy. *Diabetes Care* 24:1187, 2001.

431. Halsall DJ, McFarlane I, Luan J, et al: Typical type 2 diabetes mellitus and HFE gene mutations: A population-based case-control study. *Hum Mol Genet* 12:1361, 2003.

432. Klein-Schwartz W, Oderda GM, Gorman RL, et al: Assessment of management guidelines. Acute iron ingestion. *Clin Pediatr (Phila)* 29:316, 1990.

433. Walter T, Olivares M, Pizarro F, Munoz C: Iron, anemia, and infection. *Nutr Rev* 55:111, 1997.

434. Westlin WF: Deferoxamine in the treatment of acute iron poisoning. Clinical experiences with 172 children. *Clin Pediatr (Phila)* 5:531, 1966.

435. Greengard J, McEnery JT: Iron poisoning in children. *GP* 37:88, 1968.

436. Whitten CF, Brough AJ: The pathophysiology of acute iron poisoning. *Clin Toxicol* 4:585, 1971.

437. McEnery JT: Hospital management of acute iron ingestion. *Clin Toxicol* 4:603, 1971.

438. Silverberg DS, Iaina A, Peer G, et al: Intravenous iron supplementation for the treatment of the anemia of moderate to severe chronic renal failure patients not receiving dialysis. *Am J Kidney Dis* 27:234, 1996.

439. Nissenson AR, Berns JS, Sakiewicz P, et al: Clinical evaluation of heme iron polypeptide: Sustaining a response to rHuEPO in hemodialysis patients. *Am J Kidney Dis* 42:325, 2003.

440. Nissim JA: Intravenous administration of iron. *Lancet* 2:49, 1947.

441. Yee J, Besarab A: Iron sucrose: The oldest iron therapy becomes new. *Am J Kidney Dis* 40:1111, 2002.

442. Blaustein DA, Schwenk MH, Chattopadhyay J, et al: The safety and efficacy of an accelerated iron sucrose dosing regimen in patients with chronic kidney disease. *Kidney Int Suppl* 72, 2003.

443. Deicher R, Ziai F, Cohen G, et al: High-dose parenteral iron sucrose depresses neutrophil intracellular killing capacity. *Kidney Int* 64:728, 2003.

444. Van Wyck DB, Cavallo G, Spinowitz BS, et al: Safety and efficacy of iron sucrose in patients sensitive to iron dextran: North American clinical trial. *Am J Kidney Dis* 36:88, 2000.

445. Charytan C, Schwenk MH, Al Saloum MM, Spinowitz BS: Safety of iron sucrose in hemodialysis patients intolerant to other parenteral iron products. *Nephron Clin Pract* 96:C63, 2004.

446. Bhowmik D, Modi G, Ray D, et al: Total dose iron infusion: Safety and efficacy in predialysis patients. *Ren Fail* 22:39, 2000.

447. Sloand JA, Shelly MA, Erenstone AL, et al: Safety and efficacy of total dose iron dextran administration in patients on home renal replacement therapies. *Perit Dial Int* 18:522, 1998.

448. Ahsan N: Infusion of total dose iron versus oral iron supplementation in ambulatory peritoneal dialysis patients: A prospective, cross-over trial. *Adv Perit Dial* 16:80, 2000.

449. Auerbach M, Winchester J, Wahab A, et al: A randomized trial of three iron dextran infusion methods for anemia in EPO-treated dialysis patients. *Am J Kidney Dis* 31:81, 1998.

450. Reynoso-Gomez E, Salinas-Rojas V, Lazo-Langner A: Safety and efficacy of total dose intravenous iron infusion in the treatment of iron-deficiency anemia in adult non-pregnant patients. *Rev Invest Clin* 54:12, 2002.

451. Auerbach M, Witt D, Toler W, et al: Clinical use of the total dose intravenous infusion of iron dextran. *J Lab Clin Med* 111:566, 1988.

452. Khaodhiar L, Keane-Ellison M, Tawa NE, et al: Iron deficiency anemia in patients receiving home total parenteral nutrition. *JPEN J Parenter Enteral Nutr* 26:114, 2002.

453. Muranda M, Rivera H, Ortega F, et al: Experience with the use of iron-dextran labeled with ^{59}Fe. *Rev Med Chil* 93:134, 1965.

454. Will G: The absorption, distribution and utilization of intramuscularly administered iron-dextran: A radio-isotope study. *Br J Haematol* 14:395, 1968.

455. Marchasin S, Wallerstein RO: The treatment of iron-deficiency anemia with intravenous iron dextran. *Blood* 23:354, 1964.

456. Grimes AJ, Hutt MS: Metabolism of ^{59}Fe-dextran complex in human subjects. *BMJ* 33:1074, 1957.

457. Garby L, Sjolin S: Some observations on the distribution kinetics of radioactive colloidal iron (Imferon and ferric hydroxide). *Acta Med Scand* 157:319, 1957.

458. Henderson PA, Hillman RS: Characteristics of iron dextran utilization in man. *Blood* 34:357, 1969.

459. Burns DL, Pomposelli JJ: Toxicity of parenteral iron dextran therapy. *Kidney Int Suppl* 69:S119, 1999.

460. Theodoropoulos G, Makkous A, Constantoulakis M: Lymph node enlargement after a single massive infusion of iron dextran. *J Clin Pathol* 21:492, 1968.

461. Solanki SV, Kabrawala VN: Lymphadenopathy due to parenteral iron therapy. *J Indian Med Assoc* 51:22, 1968.

462. Amitai A, Acker M: Adverse effects of intramuscular iron injection. *Acta Haematol (Basel)* 68:341, 1982.

463. Hamstra RD, Block MH, Schocket AL: Intravenous iron dextran in clinical medicine. *JAMA* 243:1726, 1980.

464. Forristal T, Witt M: Pleocytosis after iron dextran injection. *Lancet* 1:1428, 1968.

465. Wallerstein RO: Intravenous iron-dextran complex. *Blood* 32:690, 1968.

466. Hurvitz H, Kerem E, Gross-Kieselstein E, et al: Pancytopenia caused by iron-dextran. *Arch Dis Child* 61:194, 1986.

467. Cantor RI, Downs GE, Abruzzo JL: Acute exacerbation of ankylosing spondylitis after an iron dextran infusion. *Ann Intern Med* 77:933, 1972.

468. Richmond HG: Induction of sarcoma in the rat by iron-dextran complex. *BMJ* 46:947, 1959.

469. Carter RL, Mitchley BC, Roe FJ: Induction of tumours in mice and rats with ferric sodium gluconate and iron dextran glycerol glycoside. *Br J Cancer* 22:521, 1968.

470. Greenberg G: Sarcoma after intramuscular iron injection. *BMJ* 1:1508, 1976.

471. MacKinnon AE, Bancewicz J: Sarcoma after injection of intramuscular iron. *BMJ* 2:277, 1973.

472. Robertson AG, Dick WC: Intramuscular iron and local oncogenesis. *BMJ* 1:946, 1977.

473. Faich G, Strobos J: Sodium ferric gluconate complex in sucrose: Safer intravenous iron therapy than iron dextrans. *Am J Kidney Dis* 33:464, 1999.

474. Mitchell ABS, Morton GA: Choice of iron therapy. *Practitioner* 213:370, 1974.

475. Cox JS, King RE, Reynolds GF: Valency investigations of iron dextran ("Imferon"). *Nature* 207:1202, 1965.

476. Altman LC, Petersen PE: Successful prevention of an anaphylactoid reaction to iron dextran. *Ann Intern Med* 109:346, 1988.

477. *Physicians' Desk Reference: PDR*. Medical Economics, Oradell, 2003.

478. Folkert VW, Michael B, Agarwal R, et al: Chronic use of sodium ferric gluconate complex in hemodialysis patients: Safety of higher-dose (> or =250 mg) administration. *Am J Kidney Dis* 41:651, 2003.

479. Jain AK, Bastani B: Safety profile of a high dose ferric gluconate in patients with severe chronic renal insufficiency. *J Nephrol* 15:681, 2002.

480. Eichbaum Q, Foran S, Dzik S: Is iron gluconate really safer than iron dextran? *Blood* 101:3756, 2003.

481. Pritchard JA, Hunt CF: A comparison of the hematologic responses following the routine prenatal administration of intramuscular and oral iron. *Surg Gynecol Obstet* 106:516, 1958.

482. McCurdy PR: Oral and parenteral iron therapy: A comparison. *JAMA* 191:859, 1965.

483. Komolafe JO, Kuti O, Ijadunola KT, Ogunniyi SO: A comparative study between intramuscular iron dextran and oral ferrous sulphate in the treatment of iron deficiency anaemia in pregnancy. *J Obstet Gynaecol* 23:628, 2003.

484. Gabrielli GB, De Sandre G: Excessive tea consumption can inhibit the efficacy of oral iron treatment in iron-deficiency anemia. *Haematologica* 80:518, 1995.

485. Hurrell RF, Reddy M, Cook JD: Inhibition of non-haem iron absorption in man by polyphenolic-containing beverages. *Br J Nutr* 81:289, 1999.

486. Mahlknecht U, Weidmann E, Seipelt G: The irreplaceable image: Black tea delays recovery from iron-deficiency anemia. *Haematologica* 86:559, 2001.

487. Fry J: Clinical patterns and course of anaemias in general practice. *BMJ* 2:1732, 1961.

488. Beveridge BR, Bannerman RM, Evanson JM, Witts LJ: Hypochromic anaemia. *Q J Med* 34:145, 1965.

489. Cox TM, Halsall DJ: Hemochromatosis-neonatal and young subjects. *Blood Cells Mol Dis* 29:411, 2002.

490. Pietrangelo A: The ferroportin disease. *Blood Cells Mol Dis* 32:131, 2004.

491. Beutler E, Barton JC, Felitti VJ et al: Ferroportin (*SCL40A1*) variant associated with iron overload in African-Americans. *Blood Cells Mol Dis* 31:305, 2003.

492. Gordeuk VR, Caleffi A, Corradini E, et al: Iron overload in Africans and African-Americans and a common mutation in the *SCL40A1* (ferroportin 1) gene. *Blood Cells Mol Dis* 31:299, 2003.

493. Fellman V: The GRACILE Syndrome, a neonatal lethal metabolic disorder with iron overload. *Blood Cells Mol Dis* 29:444, 2002.

494. Crompton DE, Chinnery PF, Fey C, et al: Neuroferritinopathy: A window on the role of iron in neurodegeneration. *Blood Cells Mol Dis* 29:522, 2002.

495. Loreal O, Turlin B, Pigeon C, et al: Aceruloplasminemia: New clinical, pathophysiological and therapeutic insights. *J Hepatol* 36:851, 2002.

496. Sipe JC, Lee P, Beutler E: Brain iron metabolism and neurodegenerative disorders. *Dev Neurosci* 24:188, 2002.

497. Fairbanks VF, Fahey JL, Beutler E: *Clinical Disorders of Iron Metabolism*. Grune & Stratton, New York, 1971.

498. Mallory FB: Hemochromatosis and chronic poisoning with copper. *Arch Intern Med* 37:336, 1926.

499. Davis WD, Arrowsmith WR: The effect of repeated phlebotomies in hemochromatosis. *J Lab Clin Med* 39:526, 1952.

500. Sheldon JH: *Haemochromatosis*. Oxford University Press, London, 1935.

501. MacDonald RA: Idiopathic hemochromatosis. Genetic or acquired? *Arch Intern Med* 112:82, 1963.

502. MacDonald RA: Primary hemochromatosis: Inherited or adquired? *Prog Hematol* 5:324, 1966.

503. Simon M, Pawlotsky Y, Bourel M, et al: Hémochromatose idiopathique: Maladie associée f l'antigène tissulaire. *Nouv Presse Med* 4:1432, 1975.

504. Simon M, Bourel R, Fauchet R, Genetet B: Association of HLA-A3 and HLA-B14 antigens with idiopathic hemochromatosis. *Gut* 17:332, 1976.

505. Beutler E: The HFE Cys282Tyr mutation as a necessary but not sufficient cause of hereditary hemochromatosis. *Blood* 101:3347, 2003.

506. Beutler E, Gelbart T, West C, et al: Mutation analysis in hereditary hemochromatosis. *Blood Cells Mol Dis* 22:187, 1996.

507. Lucotte G, Dieterlen F: A European allele map of the C282Y mutation of hemochromatosis: Celtic versus Viking origin of the mutation? *Blood Cells Mol Dis* 31:262, 2003.

508. Barton JC, Acton RT: Inheritance of two HFE mutations in African-Americans: Cases with hemochromatosis phenotypes and estimates of hemochromatosis phenotype frequency. *Genet Med* 3:294, 2001.

509. Bradley LA, Johnson DD, Palomaki GE, et al: Hereditary haemochromatosis mutation frequencies in the general population. *J Med Screen* 5:34, 1998.

510. Burt MJ, George PM, Upton JD, et al: The significance of haemochromatosis gene mutations in the general population: Implications for screening. *Gut* 43:830, 1998.

511. Jouanolle AM, Fergelot P, Raoul ML, et al: Prevalence of the C282Y mutation in Brittany: Penetrance of genetic hemochromatosis? *Ann Genet* 41:195, 1998.

512. Merryweather-Clarke AT, Pointon JJ, Shearman JD, Robson KJH: Global prevalence of putative haemochromatosis mutations. *J Med Genet* 34:275, 1997.

513. Beutler E, Felitti VJ, Waalen J, et al: Unpublished. 2003.

514. Chambers V, Sutherland L, Palmer K, et al: Haemochromatosis-associated HFE genotypes in English blood donors: Age-related frequency and biochemical expression. *J Hepatol* 39:925, 2003.

515. Mariani R, Salvioni A, Corengia C, et al: Prevalence of HFE mutations in upper Northern Italy: Study of 1132 unrelated blood donors. *Dig Liver Dis* 35:479, 2003.

516. Pietrapertosa A, Vitucci A, Campanale D, et al: HFE gene mutations an Apulian population: Allele frequencies. *Eur J Epidemiol* 18:685, 2003.

517. Barton JC, Sawada-Hirai R, Rothenberg BE, Acton RT: Two novel missense mutations of the HFE gene (I105T and G93R) and identification of the S65C mutation in Alabama hemochromatosis probands. *Blood Cells Mol Dis* 25:146, 1999.

518. Pointon JJ, Wallace D, Merryweather-Clarke AT, Robson KJH: Uncommon mutations and polymorphisms in the hemochromatosis gene. *Genet Test* 4:151, 2000.

519. Imanishi H, Liu W, Cheng J, et al: Idiopathic hemochromatosis with the mutation of Ala176Val heterozygous for HFE gene. *Intern Med* 40:479, 2001.

520. Beutler E, Griffin MJ, Gelbart T, West C: A previously undescribed nonsense mutation of the HFE gene. *Clin Genet* 61:40, 2002.

521. Steiner M, Ocran K, Genschel J, et al: A homozygous HFE gene splice site mutation (IVS5+1 G/A) in a hereditary hemochromatosis patient of Vietnamese origin. *Gastroenterology* 122:789, 2002.

522. Biasiotto G, Belloli S, Ruggeri G, et al: Identification of new mutations of the HFE, hepcidin, and transferrin receptor 2 genes by denaturing HPLC analysis of individuals with biochemical indications of iron overload. *Clin Chem* 49:1981, 2003.

523. De Marco F, Liguori R, Giardina MG, et al: High prevalence of non-

HFE gene-associated haemochromatosis in patients from southern Italy. *Clin Chem Lab Med* 42:17, 2004.

524. Camaschella C, Fargion S, Sampietro M, et al: Inherited HFE-unrelated hemochromatosis in Italian families. *Hepatology* 29:1563, 1999.

525. Adams P, Brissot P, Powell L: EASL International Consensus Conference on Haemochromatosis—Part II. Expert document. *J Hepatol* 33: 487, 2000.

526. Bulaj ZJ, Ajioka RS, Phillips JD, et al: Disease-related conditions in relatives of patients with hemochromatosis. *N Engl J Med* 343:1529, 2000.

527. Olynyk JK, Cullen DJ, Aquilia S, et al: A population-based study of the clinical expression of the hemochromatosis gene. *N Engl J Med* 341: 718, 1999.

528. Beutler E, Felitti VJ, Koziol JA, et al: Penetrance of the 845G6A (C282Y) HFE hereditary haemochromatosis mutation in the U.S.A. *Lancet* 359:211, 2002.

529. Waalen J, Felitti V, Gelbart T, et al: Prevalence of hemochromatosis-related symptoms in homozygotes for the C282Y mutation of the HFE gene. *Mayo Clin Proc* 77:522, 2002.

530. Lsberg A, Hveem K, Kruger O, Bjerve KS: Persons with screening-detected haemochromatosis: As healthy as the general population? *Scand J Gastroenterol* 37:719, 2002.

531. MacDonald RA: Hemochromatosis and cirrhosis in different geographic areas. *Am J Med Sci* 249:36, 1965.

532. MacSween RNM, Scott AR: Hepatic cirrhosis: A clinicopathological review of 520 cases. *J Clin Pathol* 26:936, 1972.

533. Yang Q, McDonnell SM, Khoury MJ, et al: Hemochromatosis-associated mortality in the United States from 1979 to 1992: An analysis of multiple-cause mortality data. *Ann Intern Med* 129:946, 1998.

534. McCune CA, Al Jader LN, May A, et al: Hereditary haemochromatosis: Only 1% of adult HFE C282Y homozygotes in South Wales have a clinical diagnosis of iron overload. *Hum Genet* 111:538, 2002.

535. Finch SC, Finch CA: Idiopathic hemochromatosis, an iron storage disease: A. Iron metabolism in hemochromatosis. *Medicine* 34:381, 1955.

536. Moirand R, Adams PC, Bicheler V, et al: Clinical features of genetic hemochromatosis in women compared with men. *Ann Intern Med* 127: 105, 1997.

537. Lee PL, Gelbart T, West C, et al: Seeking candidate mutations that affect iron homeostasis. *Blood Cells Mol Dis* 29:471, 2002.

538. Merryweather-Clarke AT, Cadet E, Bomford A, et al: Digenic inheritance of mutations in HAMP and HFE results in different types of haemochromatosis. *Hum Mol Genet* 12:2241, 2003.

539. Jacolot S, Le Gac G, Scotet V, et al: HAMP as a modifier gene that increase the phenotypic expression of the HFE p.C282Y homozygous genotype. *Blood* 103:2835, 2004.

540. Adams PC, Gregor JC, Kertesz AE, Valberg LS: Screening blood donors for hereditary hemochromatosis: Decision analysis model based on a 30-year database. *Gastroenterology* 109:177, 1995.

541. Kushner JP: Screening for hemochromatosis. *Gastroenterology* 109: 315, 1995.

542. Niederau C, Niederau CM, Lange S, et al: Screening for hemochromatosis and iron deficiency in employees and primary care patients in western Germany. *Ann Intern Med* 128:337, 1998.

543. Allen K, Williamson R: Screening for hereditary haemochromatosis should be implemented now. *BMJ* 320:183, 2000.

544. Pinsky LE, Imperatore G, Burke W: Diabetes and HFE mutations: Cause or coincidence? *West J Med* 176:114, 2002.

545. McCord JM: Iron, free radicals, and oxidative injury. *Semin Hematol* 35:5, 1998.

546. Gutteridge JM: Iron and oxygen: A biologically damaging mixture. *Acta Paediatr Scand Suppl* 361:78, 1989.

547. Brown EB Jr, Durbach R, Smith D, et al: Studies on iron transportation and metabolism: X. Long-term iron overload in dogs. *J Lab Clin Med* 50:862, 1957.

548. Bacon BR, Park CH, Brittenham GM, et al: Hepatic mitochondrial oxidative metabolism in rats with chronic dietary iron overload. *Hepatology* 5:789, 1985.

549. Houglum K, Filip M, Witztum JL, Chojkier M: Malondialdehyde and 4-hydroxynonenal protein adducts in plasma and liver of rats with iron overload. *J Clin Invest* 86:1991, 1990.

550. Pietrangelo A, Gualdi R, Casalgrandi G, et al: Molecular and cellular aspects of iron-induced hepatic cirrhosis in rodents. *J Clin Invest* 95: 1824, 1995.

551. Schroder N, Fredriksson A, Vianna MRM, et al: Memory deficits in adult rats following postnatal iron administration. *Behav Brain Res* 124: 77, 2001.

552. Tsukamoto H, Horne W, Kamimura S, et al: Experimental liver cirrhosis induced by alcohol and iron. *J Clin Invest* 96:620, 1995.

553. Fletcher LM, Powell LW: Hemochromatosis and alcoholic liver disease. *Alcohol* 30:131, 2003.

554. Scotet V, Merour MC, Mercier AY, et al: Hereditary hemochromatosis: Effect of excessive alcohol consumption on disease expression in patients homozygous for the C282Y mutation. *Am J Epidemiol* 158:129, 2003.

555. Waheed A, Parkkila S, Saarnio J, et al: Association of HFE protein with transferrin receptor in crypt enterocytes of human duodenum. *Proc Natl Acad Sci U S A* 96:1579, 1999.

556. Bomford A: Genetics of haemochromatosis. *Lancet* 360:1673, 2002.

557. West AP Jr, Bennett MJ, Sellers VM, et al: Comparison of the interactions of transferrin receptor and transferrin receptor 2 with transferrin and the hereditary hemochromatosis protein HFE. *J Biol Chem* 275: 38135, 2000.

558. Feder JN, Penny DM, Irrinki A, et al: The hemochromatosis gene product complexes with the transferrin receptor and lowers its affinity for ligand binding. *Proc Natl Acad Sci U S A* 95:1472, 1998.

559. Bottomley SS: Secondary iron overload disorders. *Semin Hematol* 35: 77, 1998.

560. Pippard MJ, Weatherall DJ: Iron absorption in non-transfused iron loading anaemias: Prediction of risk for iron loading, and response to iron chelation treatment, in beta thalassaemia intermedia and congenital sideroblastic anaemias. *Haematologia (Budap)* 17:17, 1984.

561. Castleman B, Towne VW: Case records of the massachusetts general hospital. Case 38512. *N Engl J Med* 247:992, 1952.

562. Johnson BF: Hemochromatosis resulting from prolonged oral iron therapy. *N Engl J Med* 278:1100, 1968.

563. Pearson HA, Ehrenkranz RA, Rinder HM, Riely CA: Hemosiderosis in a normal child secondary to oral iron medication. *Pediatrics* 105:429, 2000.

564. Turnberg LA: Excessive oral iron therapy causing haemochromatosis. *BMJ* 1:1360, 1965.

565. Wallerstein RO, Robbins SL: Hemochromatosis after prolonged oral iron therapy in a patient with chronic hemolytic anemia. *Am J Med* 14: 256, 1953.

566. Saven A, Beutler E: Iron overload after prolonged intramuscular iron therapy. *N Engl J Med* 321:331, 1989.

567. Doherty MJ, Healy M, Richardson SG, Fisher NC: Total body iron overload in welder's siderosis. *Occup Environ Med* 61:82, 2004.

568. Witte DL, Crosby WH, Edwards CQ, et al: Hereditary hemochromatosis. *Clin Chim Acta* 245:139, 1996.

569. Isaacson C, Seftel HC, Keeley KJ, Bothwell TH: Siderosis in the Bantu: The relationship between iron overload and cirrhosis. *J Lab Clin Med* 58:845, 1961.

570. Barton JC, Acton RT, Rivers CA, et al: Genetic and phenotypic heterogeneity of primary iron overload in African-Americans. *Blood Cells Mol Dis* 31:310, 2003.

571. Jouanolle AM, Douabin-Gicquel V, Halimi C, et al: Novel mutation in ferroportin 1 gene is associated with autosomal dominant iron overload. *J Hepatol* 39:286, 2003.

572. Devalia V, Carter K, Walker AP, et al: Autosomal dominant reticuloendothelial iron overload associated with a 3-base pair deletion in the ferroportin 1 gene *(SLC11A3)*. *Blood* 100:695, 2002.

573. Beutler E: The clinical evaluation of iron stores. *N Engl J Med* 256:692, 1957.

574. Düllmann J, Wulfhekel U: The diagnostic significance of bone-marrow iron in hereditary hemochromatosis. *Ann N Y Acad Sci* 526:357, 1988.

575. Ross CE, Muir WA, Ng ABP, et al: Hemochromatosis. Pathophysiologic and genetic considerations. *Am J Clin Pathol* 63:179, 1975.

576. Astaldi G, Meardi G, Lisino T: The iron content of jejunal mucosa obtained by Crosby's biopsy in hemochromatosis and hemosiderosis. *Blood* 28:70, 1966.

577. Whittaker P, Skikne BS, Covell AM, et al: Duodenal iron proteins in idiopathic hemochromatosis. *J Clin Invest* 83:261, 1989.

578. Simpson RJ, Debnam ES, Laftah AH, et al. Duodenal non-heme iron content correlates with iron stores in mice, but the relationship is altered by HFE gene knock-out. *Blood* 101:3316, 2003.

579. Beutler L, Beutler E: Hematologically important mutations: Hemochromatosis. *Blood Cells Mol Dis* 33: 40, 2004.

580. Beutler E, Felitti VJ, Ho NJ, Gelbart T: An *HFE* S65C variant is not associated with increased transferrin saturation in voluntary blood donors. Commentary by N Arya, S Chakrabrati, RA Hegele, PC Adams. *Blood Cells Mol Dis* 25:358, 1999.

581. Smith BC, Grove J, Guzail MA, et al: Heterozygosity for hereditary hemochromatosis is associated with more fibrosis in chronic hepatitis C. *Hepatology* 27:1695, 1998.

582. Bonkovsky HL, Troy N, McNeal K, et al: Iron and HFE or TfR1 mutations as comorbid factors for development and progression of chronic hepatitis C. *J Hepatol* 37:848, 2002.

583. Gehrke SG, Stremmel W, Mathes I, et al: Hemochromatosis and transferrin receptor gene polymorphisms in chronic hepatitis C: Impact on iron status, liver injury and HCV genotype. *J Mol Med* 81:780, 2003.

584. Martinelli ALC, Franco RF, Villanova MG, et al: Are haemochromatosis mutations related to the severity of liver disease in hepatitis C virus infection? *Acta Haematol (Basel)* 102:152, 1999.

585. Frenzer A, Rudzki Z, Norton ID, Butler WJ: Heterozygosity of the haemochromatosis mutation, C282Y, does not influence susceptibility to alcoholic cirrhosis. *Scand J Gastroenterol* 33:1324, 1998.

586. Grove J, Daly AK, Burt AD, et al: Heterozygotes for HFE mutations have no increased risk of advanced alcoholic liver disease. *Gut* 43:262, 1998.

587. Aldersley MA, Howdle PD, Wyatt JI, et al: Haemochromatosis gene mutation in liver disease patients. *Lancet* 349:1025, 1997.

588. Hohler T, Leininger S, Kohler HH, et al: Heterozygosity for the hemochromatosis gene in liver diseases—Prevalence and effects on liver histology. *Liver* 20:482, 2000.

589. Fargion S, Stazi MA, Fracanzani AL, et al: Mutations in the HFE gene and their interaction with exogenous risk factors in hepatocellular carcinoma. *Blood Cells Mol Dis* 27:505, 2001.

590. Kallianpur AR, Hall LD, Yadav M, et al: Increased prevalence of the HFE C282Y hemochromatosis allele in women with breast cancer. *Cancer Epidemiology, Biomarkers & Prevention* 13:205, 2004.

591. Yuan XM, Li W: The iron hypothesis of atherosclerosis and its clinical impact. *Ann Med* 35:578, 2003.

592. Wolff B, Volzke H, Ludemann J, et al: Association between high serum ferritin levels and carotid atherosclerosis in the Study of Health in Pomerania (SHIP). *Stroke* 35:453, 2004.

593. Candore G, Balistreri CR, Lio D, et al: Association between HFE mutations and acute myocardial infarction: A study in patients from Northern and Southern Italy. *Blood Cells Mol Dis* 31:57, 2003.

594. Heath ALM, Fairweather-Tait SJ: Health implications of iron overload: The role of diet and genotype. *Nutr Rev* 61:45, 2003.

595. Roetto A, Daraio F, Porporato P, et al: Screening hepcidin for mutations in juvenile hemochromatosis: Identification of a new mutation (C70r). *Blood* 103:2407, 2004.

596. Delatycki M, Allen K, Gow P, et al: A homozygous HAMP mutation in a multiply consanguineous family with pseudo-dominant juvenile hemochromatosis. *Clin Genet* 65:378, 2004.

597. Montosi G, Donovan A, Totaro A, et al: Autosomal-dominant hemochromatosis is associated with a mutation in the ferroportin *(SLC11A3)* gene. *J Clin Invest* 108:619, 2001.

598. Cazzola M, Cremonesi L, Papaioannou M, et al: Genetic hyperferritinaemia and reticuloendothelial iron overload associated with a three base pair deletion in the coding region of the ferroportin gene *(SLC11A3)*. *Br J Haematol* 119:539, 2002.

599. Roetto A, Merryweather-Clarke AT, Daraio F, et al: A valine deletion of ferroportin 1: A common mutation in hemochromatosis type 4? *Blood* 100:733, 2002.

600. Wallace DF, Clark RM, Harley HA, Subramaniam VN: Autosomal dominant iron overload due to a novel mutation of ferroportin1 associated with parenchymal iron loading and cirrhosis. *J Hepatol* 40:710, 2004.

601. Girelli D, Bozzini C, Roetto A, et al: Clinical and pathologic findings in hemochromatosis type 3 due to a novel mutation in transferrin receptor 2 gene. *Gastroenterology* 122:1295, 2002.

602. Mattman A, Huntsman D, Lockitch G, et al: Transferrin receptor 2 (TfR2) and HFE mutational analysis in non-C282Y iron overload: Identification of a novel TfR2 mutation. *Blood* 100:1075, 2002.

603. Roetto A, Totaro A, Piperno A, et al: New mutations inactivating transferrin receptor 2 in hemochromatosis type 3. *Blood* 97:2555, 2001.

604. Piperno A, Roetto A, Mariani R, et al: Homozygosity for transferrin receptor-2 Y250X mutation induces early iron overload. *Haematologica* 89:359, 2004.

605. Randell MG, Patnaik AK, Gould WJ: Hepatopathy associated with excessive iron storage in mynah birds. *J Am Vet Med Assoc* 179:1214, 1981.

606. Gosselin SJ, Kramer LW: Pathophysiology of excessive iron storage in mynah birds. *J Am Vet Med Assoc* 183:1238, 1983.

607. Spalding MG, Kollias GV, Mays MB, et al: Hepatic encephalopathy associated with hemochromatosis in a toco toucan. *J Am Vet Med Assoc* 189:1122, 1986.

608. Cornelissen H, Ducatelle R, Roels S: Successful treatment of a channel-billed Toucan (*Ramphastos vitellinus*) with iron storage disease by chelation therapy: Sequential monitoring of the iron content of the liver during the treatment period by quantitative chemical and image analyses. *J Avian Med Surg* 9:131, 1995.

609. House JK, Smith BP, Maas J, et al: Hemochromatosis in Salers cattle. *J Vet Intern Med* 8:105, 1994.

610. Lavoie JP, Teuscher E: Massive iron overload and liver fibrosis resembling haemochromatosis in a racing pony. *Equine Vet J* 25:552, 1993.

611. Pearson EG, Hedstrom OR, Poppenga RH: Hepatic cirrhosis and hemochromatosis in three horses. *J Am Vet Med Assoc* 204:1053, 1994.

612. Spelman LH, Osborn KG, Anderson MP: Pathogenesis of hemosiderosis in lemurs: Role of dietary iron, tannin, and ascorbic acid. *Zoo Biology* 8:239, 1989.

613. Paglia DE: Dietary iron overloads in browsing rhinoceroses. *Newsletter Zoo Nutrition Center Wildlife Conservation Society*, Bronx, February 3, 1999.

614. Beutler E, West C, Speir JA, et al: The HFE gene of browsing and grazing rhinoceroses: A possible site of adaptation to a low-iron diet. *Blood Cells Mol Dis* 27:342, 2001.

615. Awai M, Narasaki M, Yamanoi Y, Seno S: Induction of diabetes in animals by parenteral administration of ferric nitrilotriacetate. A model of experimental hemochromatosis. *Am J Pathol* 95:663, 1979.

616. Brighton CT, Bigley EJ, Smolenski BI: Iron-induced arthritis in immature rabbits. *Arthritis Rheum* 13:849, 1970.

617. Carthew P, Dorman BM, Edwards RE, et al: A unique rodent model for both the cardiotoxic and hepatotoxic effects of prolonged iron overload. *Lab Invest* 69:217, 1993.

618. Iancu TC, Ward RJ, Peters TJ: Ultrastructural observations in the carbonyl iron-fed rat, an animal model for hemochromatosis. *Virchows Arch B Cell Pathol Incl Mol Pathol* 53:208, 1987.

619. MacDonald RA, Pechet GS: Experimental hemochromatosis in rats. *Am J Pathol* 46:85, 1965.

620. Yang T, Dong WQ, Kuryshev YA, et al: Bimodal cardiac dysfunction in an animal model of iron overload. *J Lab Clin Med* 140:263, 2002.

621. Hershko C, Link G, Konijn AM, et al: The iron-loaded gerbil model revisited: Effects of deferoxamine and deferiprone treatment. *J Lab Clin Med* 139:50, 2002.

622. Andersen RV, Tybjaerg-Hansen A, Appleyard M, et al: Hemochromatosis mutations in the general population: Iron overload progression rate. *Blood* 103:2914, 2004.

623. Waalen J, Felitti VJ, Gelbart T, et al: Penetrance of hemochromatosis. *Blood Cells Mol Dis* 29:418, 2002.

624. Ines LS, Da Silva JAP, Malcata AB, Porto AL: Arthropathy of genetic hemochromatosis: A major and distinctive manifestation of the disease. *Clin Exp Rheumatol* 19:98, 2001.

625. Timms AE, Sathananthan R, Bradbury L, et al: Genetic testing for haemochromatosis in patients with chondrocalcinosis. *Ann Rheum Dis* 61:745, 2002.

626. McDonnell SM, Preston BL, Jewell SA, et al: A survey of 2,851 patients with hemochromatosis: Symptoms and response to treatment. *Am J Med* 106:619, 1999.

627. Jordan JM: Arthritis in hemochromatosis or iron storage disease. *Curr Opin Rheumatol* 16:62, 2004.

628. Milman N, Pedersen P, Steig T, et al: Clinically overt hereditary hemochromatosis in Denmark 1948-1985: Epidemiology, factors of significance for long-term survival, and causes of death in 179 patients. *Ann Hematol* 80:737, 2001.

629. Niederau C, Fischer R, Puerschel A, et al: Long-term survival in patients with hereditary hemochromatosis. *Gastroenterology* 110:1107, 1996.

630. Roberts AG, Whatley SD, Morgan R, et al: Increased frequency of the haemochromatosis Cys282Tyr mutation in sporadic porphyria cutanea tarda. *Lancet* 349:321, 1997.

631. Bulaj ZJ, Phillips JD, Ajioka RS, et al: Hemochromatosis genes and other factors contributing to the pathogenesis of porphyria cutanea tarda. *Blood* 95:1565, 2000.

632. Tannapfel A, Stolzel U, Kostler E, et al: C282Y and H63D mutation of the hemochromatosis gene in German porphyria cutanea tarda patients. *Virchows Arch* 439:1, 2001.

633. Chiaverini C, Halimi G, Ouzan D, et al: Porphyria cutanea tarda, C282Y, H63D and S65C HFE gene mutations and hepatitis C infection: A study from Southern France. *Dermatology* 206:212, 2003.

634. Stolzel U, Kostler E, Schuppan D, et al: Hemochromatosis (HFE) gene mutations and response to chloroquine in porphyria cutanea tarda. *Arch Dermatol* 139:309, 2003.

635. Camaschella C, Roetto A, De Gobbi M: Juvenile hemochromatosis. *Semin Hematol* 39:242, 2002.

636. Vaiopoulos G, Papanikolaou G, Politou M, et al: Arthropathy in juvenile hemochromatosis. *Arthritis Rheum* 48:227, 2003.

637. Barton JC, Bertoli LF, Rothenberg BE: Peripheral blood erythrocyte parameters in hemochromatosis: Evidence for increased erythrocyte hemoglobin content. *J Lab Clin Med* 135:96, 2000.

638. Beutler E, Felitti V, Gelbart T, Ho N: The effect of HFE genotypes in patients attending a health appraisal clinic. *Ann Intern Med* 133:329, 2000.

639. Jensen PD: Evaluation of iron overload. *Br J Haematol* 124:697, 2004.

640. Poullis A, Moodie SJ, Ang L, et al: Routine transferrin saturation measurement in liver clinic patients increases detection of hereditary haemochromatosis. *Ann Clin Biochem* 40:521, 2003.

641. Jacobs A: Serum ferritin and malignant tumours. *Med Oncol Tumor Pharmacother* 1:149, 1984.

642. Cazzola M, Skoda RC: Translational pathophysiology: A novel molecular mechanism of human disease. *Blood* 95:3280, 2000.

643. Craig JE, Clark JB, McLeod JL, et al: Hereditary hyperferritinemia-cataract syndrome: Prevalence, lens morphology, spectrum of mutations, and clinical presentations. *Arch Ophthalmol* 121:1753, 2003.

644. Bothwell TH, MacPhail AP: Hereditary hemochromatosis: Etiologic, pathologic, and clinical aspects. *Semin Hematol* 35:55, 1998.

645. Brittenham GM, Sheth S, Allen CJ, Farrell DE: Noninvasive methods for quantitative assessment of transfusional iron overload in sickle cell disease. *Semin Hematol* 38:37, 2001.

646. Wang ZJ, Haselgrove JC, Martin MB, et al: Evaluation of iron overload by single voxel MRS measurement of liver T2. *J Magn Reson Imaging* 15:395, 2002.

647. Pomerantz S, Siegelman ES: MR imaging of iron depositional disease. *Magn Reson Imaging Clin N Am* 10:105, 2002.

648. Bonkovsky HL, Rubin RB, Cable EE, et al: Hepatic iron concentration: Noninvasive estimation by means of MR imaging techniques. *Radiology* 212:227, 1999.

649. Alustiza JM, Artetxe J, Castiella A, et al: MR quantification of hepatic iron concentration. *Radiology* 230:479, 2004.

650. Hofmann WK, Kaltwasser JP, Hoelzer D, et al: Successful treatment of iron overload by phlebotomies in a patient with severe congenital dyserythropoietic anemia type II. *Blood* 89:3068, 1997.

651. Porter JB: Practical management of iron overload. *Br J Haematol* 115:239, 2001.

652. Borgna-Pignatti C, Cohen A: Evaluation of a new method of administration of the iron chelating agent deferoxamine. *J Pediatr* 130:86, 1997.

653. Franchini M, Gandini G, Veneri D, Aprili G: Safety and efficacy of subcutaneous bolus injection of deferoxamine in adult patients with iron overload: An update. *Blood* 103:747, 2004.

654. Blume KG, Beutler E, Chillar RK, et al: Continuous intravenous deferoxamine infusion treatment of secondary hemochromatosis in adults. *JAMA* 239:2149, 1978.

655. Nienhuis AW: Vitamin C and iron. *N Engl J Med* 304:170, 1981.

656. Kruger N, Kijewski H, Konig R, et al: Deferoxamine in hemosiderosis. Fecal iron excretion during continuous subcutaneous infusion. *Dtsch Med Wochenschr* 109:1682, 1984.

657. Gomber S, Saxena R, Madan N: Comparative efficacy of desferrioxamine, deferiprone and in combination on iron chelation in thalassemic children. *Indian Pediatr* 41:21, 2004.

658. Kattamis A, Kassou C, Berdousi H, et al: Combined therapy with desferrioxamine and deferiprone in thalassemic patients: Effect on urinary iron excretion. *Haematologica* 88:1423, 2003.

659. Niederau C, Fischer R, Sonnenberg A, et al: Survival and causes of death in cirrhotic and in noncirrhotic patients with primary hemochromatosis. *N Engl J Med* 313:1256, 1985.

660. Waalen J, Nordestgaard BG, Beutler E: Meta-analysis of survival of homozygotes for the HFE C282Y mutation. *JAMA* 2003.

661. Olynyk JK, Hagan SE, Cullen DJ, et al: Evolution of untreated hereditary hemochromatosis in the Busselton population: A 17-year study. *Mayo Clin Proc* 79:309, 2004.

662. Block M, Moore G, Wasi P, Haiby G: Histogenesis of the hepatic lesion in primary hemochromatosis: With consideration of the pseudo-iron deficient state produced by phlebotomies. *Am J Pathol* 47:89, 1965.

663. Blumberg RS, Chopra S, Ibrahim R, et al: Primary hepatocellular carcinoma in idiopathic hemochromatosis after reversal of cirrhosis. *Gastroenterology* 95:1399, 1988.

664. Knauer CM, Gamble CN, Monroe LS: The reversal of hemochromatotic

cirrhosis by multiple phlebotomies. Report of a case. *Gastroenterology* 49:667, 1965.

665. Powell LW, Kerr JF: Reversal of "cirrhosis" in idiopathic haemochromatosis following long-term intensive venesection therapy. *Australas Ann Med* 19:54, 1970.

666. Weintraub LR, Conrad ME, Crosby WH: The treatment of hemochromatosis by phlebotomy. *Med Clin North Am* 50:1579, 1966.

667. Franchini M: Platelet count increase following phlebotomy in iron overloaded patients with liver cirrhosis. *Hematology* 8:259, 2003.

668. De Gobbi M, Roetto A, Piperno A, et al: Natural history of juvenile haemochromatosis. *Br J Haematol* 117:973, 2002.

669. Borgna-Rignatti C, Zurlo MG, DeStefano P, et al: Survival in thalassemia with conventional treatment. *Prog Clin Biol Res* 309:27, 1989.

670. Harrison PM, Arosio P: The ferritins: Molecular properties, iron storage function and cellular regulation. *Biochim Biophys Acta* 1275:161, 1996.

671. Andrews NC: Iron homeostasis: Insights from genetics and animal models. *Nat Rev Genet* 1:208, 2000.

672. Hentze MW, Rouault TA, Caughman SW, et al: A cis-acting element is necessary and sufficient for translational regulation of human ferritin expression in response to iron. *Proc Natl Acad Sci U S A* 84:6730, 1987.

673. Knisely AS: Neonatal hemochromatosis. *Adv Pediatr* 39:383, 1992.

674. Beutler E, Fairbanks VF: The effects of iron deficiency, in: *Iron in Biochemistry and Medicine II*, edited by A Jacobs, M Worwood, p 393. Academic Press, New York, 1980.

675. Beutler E, Meerkreebs G: Letter to the editor. *N Engl J Med* 274:1152, 1966.

676. Lee P, Peng H, Gelbart T, Wang L, et al:. Regulation of hepcidin transcription by interleukin-1 and interleukin-6. *Proc. Natl. Acad. Sci. USA* 102: 1906, 2005.

677. Nemeth E, Tuttle MS, Powelson J, et al: Hepcidin Regulates Iron Efflux by Binding to Ferroportin and Inducing Its Internalization. *Science* 306: 2090, 2004.

ANEMIA RESULTING FROM OTHER NUTRITIONAL DEFICIENCIES

ERNEST BEUTLER

Anemia can result from nutritional deficiencies of a variety of vitamins and trace minerals. Vitamin deficiencies implicated as causes of anemia in humans, in addition to folic acid and vitamin B_{12}, include vitamins A, C, and E, and pyridoxine and riboflavin, members of the B group. In most instances, the relationship between the hematologic abnormality and a vitamin deficiency has been difficult to document in humans because multiple defects usually are present in a clinical setting. Copper and iron are recognized as minerals essential for optimal erythropoiesis. A number of different enzymes essential for iron metabolism are the cuproenzymes. Complex nutritional disturbances, such as those observed in starvation, protein-deficiency malnutrition, and alcoholism, are associated with anemia.

The anemias that result from deficiencies of vitamin B_{12}, folic acid (see Chap. 39), or iron (see Chap. 40) are clearly defined. They are relatively common and exist in pure states. In contrast, the characteristics of anemias that may occur with deficiencies of micronutrients, such as some of the other vitamins, are poorly defined. Many of these deficiencies are relatively rare in humans. When present, they exist not as isolated deficiencies of one vitamin or one mineral but rather as a combination of deficiencies. In this context, it is impossible to deduce which abnormalities are due to which deficiency. Studies in experimental animals, on the other hand, may not accurately reflect the role of micronutrients in humans. Accordingly, our knowledge of the effect of many micronutrients on hematopoiesis is fragmentary and based on clinical observations and interpretations that may be flawed. The daily requirements of some of the micronutrients are available at *www.nal.usda.gov/fnic/dga/rda.pdf* and the levels normally found in the serum, red cell, and leukocytes in Table 41-1.

VITAMIN-DEFICIENCY ANEMIAS

VITAMIN A DEFICIENCY

Chronic deprivation of vitamin A results in anemia similar to that observed in iron deficiency.[1-4] Mean corpuscular volume (MCV) and mean corpuscular hemoglobin concentration (MCHC) are reduced. Anisocytosis and poikilocytosis may be present, and serum iron levels are low. Unlike iron-deficiency anemia but similar to the anemia of chronic disease, the iron stores in the liver and marrow are increased, the serum transferrin concentration usually is normal or decreased, and administration of medicinal iron does not correct the anemia. The suggestion that vitamin A may facilitate iron absorption[5] could not be confirmed.[6]

Surveys conducted in developing countries have suggested vitamin A deficiency represents a public health problem among school children.[7,8] Although vitamin A deficiency is recognized to occur in the United States, the relationship between it and anemia is not known.

DEFICIENCIES OF MEMBERS OF THE VITAMIN B GROUP

Isolated nutritional deficiencies of members of the vitamin B group, with the exception of folic acid and vitamin B_{12}, apparently are very uncommon in humans. Evidence linking isolated nutritional deficiencies of pyridoxine, riboflavin, pantothenic acid, and niacin to anemia in patients is inconclusive. Deficiency states experimentally induced in animals are more commonly associated with hematologic abnormalities.

VITAMIN B_6 DEFICIENCY

Vitamin B_6 includes pyridoxal, pyridoxine, and pyridoxamine. These components are converted to pyridoxal 5-phosphate, which acts as a coenzyme in the decarboxylation and transamination of amino acids and in the synthesis of aminolevulinic acid, the porphyrin precursor. Vitamin B_6 deficiency induced in infants is associated with a hypochromic microcytic anemia.[9] A malnourished patient with a hypochromic anemia who failed to respond to iron therapy but subsequently responded to administration of vitamin B_6 has been described.[10] Occasionally, patients receiving therapy with antituberculosis agents, such as isoniazid, which interfere with vitamin B_6 metabolism, develop a microcytic anemia that can be corrected with large doses of pyridoxine.[11,12] Some patients with sideroblastic anemias (see Chap. 58) respond to the administration of pyridoxine, but these patients are not deficient in this vitamin.

RIBOFLAVIN DEFICIENCY

Riboflavin deficiency results in a decrease in red cell glutathione reductase activity since this enzyme requires flavin adenine dinucleotide for activation. The glutathione reductase deficiency induced by riboflavin deficiency is not associated with a hemolytic anemia or increased susceptibility to oxidant-induced injury.[13] Human volunteers maintained on a semisynthetic riboflavin-deficient diet and fed the riboflavin antagonist galactoflavin develop pure red cell aplasia.[14] Vacuolated erythroid precursors are evident prior to the development of aplasia. This anemia is reversed specifically by administration of riboflavin. Although it has been suggested that riboflavin deficiency causes anemia,[15] possibly by interfering with iron release from ferritin,[16] the relationship between dietary riboflavin deficiency and anemia is not at all clear.

PANTOTHENIC ACID DEFICIENCY

Pantothenic acid deficiency, when artificially induced in humans, is not associated with anemia.[17]

NIACIN DEFICIENCY

Pellagra (niacin deficiency) is associated with anemia, which responds to treatment with niacin.[18] However, it is not clear whether the anemia is a direct or an indirect effect of niacin deficiency.

VITAMIN C (ASCORBIC ACID) DEFICIENCY

Although approximately 80 percent of patients with scurvy[19] are anemic, attempts to induce anemia in human volunteers by severely restricting dietary ascorbic acid have been unsuccessful.[20] It seems that the anemia observed in subjects with scurvy is not due directly to a deficiency of ascorbic acid but rather due to bleeding or a deficiency of folic acid.[19] Human subjects with scurvy and megaloblastic anemia

---

This chapter is based upon the chapter contributed by the late Frank Oski, M.D., to the 5th edition of the book.

Acronyms and abbreviations that appear in this chapter include: MCHC, mean corpuscular hemoglobin concentration; MCV, mean corpuscular volume.

TABLE 41-1 BLOOD VITAMIN AND MINERAL LEVELS (ADULT VALUES)

VITAMIN OR MINERAL	SERUM LEVEL	PLASMA LEVEL	RED CELL LEVEL	WHITE CELL LEVEL
Copper	$11-24\ \mu mol/l$		$14-24\ \mu mol/l$	
Folate	$7-45$ nmol/l		>320 nmol/l	
Riboflavin (B$_2$)	$110-640$ nmol/l		$265-1350$ nmol/l	
Vitamin A	$1-3\ \mu mol/l$			
Vitamin B$_6$		$20-122$ nmol/l		
Vitamin C		$25-85\ \mu mol/l$		$11-30$ attomol/cell
Vitamin E	$12-40\ \mu mol/l$			
Selenium	$1200-2000$ nmol/l			
Zinc	$11-18\ \mu mol/l$			

SOURCE: Modified from Milne D: Trace Elements, Chapter 30, page 1029 and McCormick DB, Greene HL: Vitamins, Chapter 29, page 999, in: *Tietz Textbook of Clinical Chemistry*, 3rd ed, edited by CA Burtis, EF Ashwood. Philadelphia, WB Saunders, 1999.

fail to respond hematologically to vitamin C if they are maintained on a folic acid–deficient diet. When folic acid is given to these subjects in a dose of 50 μg/day, a prompt hematologic response is observed.[21]

Ascorbic acid is required for the maintenance of folic acid reductase in its reduced, or active, form. Impaired folic acid reductase activity results in an inability to form tetrahydrofolic acid, the metabolically active form of folic acid. Patients with scurvy and megaloblastic anemia excrete 10-formylfolic acid as the major urinary folate metabolite. Following ascorbic acid therapy, 5-methyltetrahydrofolic acid becomes the major urinary folate metabolite. This observation has led to the suggestion that ascorbic acid prevents the irreversible oxidation of methyltetrahydrofolic acid to formylfolic acid.[22] Failure to synthesize tetrahydrofolic acid or protect it from oxidation ultimately results in megaloblastic anemia. Under these circumstances, ascorbic acid therapy will produce a hematologic response only if enough folic acid is present to interact with the ascorbic acid.[23] Dietary iron deficiency in children often occurs in association with dietary ascorbic acid deficiency. Scurvy itself may cause iron deficiency as a consequence of external bleeding. Iron balance may be further compromised by the ascorbic acid deficiency because this vitamin serves to facilitate intestinal iron absorption. Patients with scurvy, particularly children, may require both iron and vitamin C to correct a hypochromic microcytic anemia.[24]

In patients with iron overload from repeated blood transfusions, the level of vitamin C in leukocytes is often decreased because of rapid conversion of ascorbate to oxalate.[25] Deferoxamine (desferrioxamine)-induced iron excretion is diminished when stores of vitamin C are reduced, but excretion returns to expected values with vitamin C supplementation.[26,27] It has been suggested, however, that large doses of ascorbic acid may be harmful in patients with iron overload and should be given only after an infusion of Desferal (deferoxamine mesylate) has been initiated (see Chap. 40). The presence of scurvy in patients with iron overload may protect them from tissue damage.[28] Both in scorbutic guinea pigs and in Bantu subjects with nutritional vitamin C deficiency and dietary hemosiderosis, iron accumulates in the monocyte-macrophage system rather than in the parenchymal cells of the liver.[29,30]

VITAMIN E DEFICIENCY

Vitamin E, α-tocopherol, is a fat-soluble vitamin that appears to be an antioxidant in humans. It is not as an essential cofactor in any recognized reactions. Nutritional deficiency of vitamin E in humans is extremely uncommon because of the widespread occurrence of α-tocopherol in food. The daily requirement of d-α-tocopherol for adults ranges from 5 to 7 mg, but the requirement varies with the polyun-

saturated fatty acid content of the diet and the content of peroxidizable lipids in tissues. Hematologic manifestations of vitamin E deficiency in humans are limited to the neonatal period and to pathologic states associated with chronic fat malabsorption.

Low-birth-weight infants are born with low serum and tissue concentrations of vitamin E. When these infants are fed a diet unusually rich in polyunsaturated fatty acids and inadequate in vitamin E, a hemolytic anemia will develop by 4 to 6 weeks of age, particularly if iron is also present in the diet.[31] The anemia often is associated with morphologic alterations of the erythrocytes,[32] thrombocytosis, and edema of the dorsum of the feet and pretibial area.[33] Treatment with vitamin E produces a prompt increase in hemoglobin level, a decrease in the elevated reticulocyte count, normalization of the red cell life span, and disappearance of thrombocytosis and edema. Modifications of infant formulas have all but eliminated vitamin E deficiency in preterm infants.[34]

Vitamin E deficiency is common in patients with cystic fibrosis if the patients are not receiving daily supplements of the water-soluble form of the vitamin.[35] Red cell life span in such patients is shortened to an average ^{51}Cr half-life of 19 days. After vitamin E therapy the red cell half-life increases to 27.5 days.[36] Severe anemia may be present.[35]

Pharmacologic doses of vitamin E have been employed with apparent success in the absence of vitamin deficiency to compensate for genetic defects that limit the erythrocytes' defense against oxidant injury. Chronic administration of vitamin E 400 to 800 U/day lengthened the red cell life span in some[37,38] but not all[39] studies of patients with hereditary hemolytic anemias associated with glutathione synthetase deficiency or glucose-6-phosphate dehydrogenase deficiency.

Administration of vitamin E 450 U/day for 6 to 36 weeks to patients with sickle cell anemia significantly reduced the number of irreversibly sickled erythrocytes.[40] Adult patients with sickle cell anemia have been reported to have significantly lower serum tocopherol values compared with normal controls,[41] and in children with sickle cell anemia, those with vitamin E deficiency have significantly more irreversibly sickled cells than did children without vitamin E deficiency.[42]

TRACE METAL DEFICIENCY

COPPER DEFICIENCY

Copper is present in a number of metalloproteins. Among the cuproenzymes are cytochrome *c* oxidase, dopamine β-hydroxylase, urate oxidase, tyrosine and lysyl oxidase, ascorbic acid oxidase, and superoxide dismutase (erythrocuprein). More than 90 percent of the copper in the blood is carried bound to ceruloplasmin, an α_2-globulin with ferro-oxidase activity. Copper appears to be required for the absorption and utilization of iron. Copper, in the form of hephaestin,[43] converts iron to the Fe^{+++} state for its transport by transferrin.

Copper deficiency has been described in malnourished children[44] and in both infants and adults[45–47] receiving parenteral alimentation. Copper deficiency is characterized by a microcytic anemia that is unresponsive to iron therapy, hypoferremia, neutropenia, and usually the presence of vacuolated erythroid precursors in the marrow.[45,46] Radiologic abnormalities generally are present in infants and young children with copper deficiency. These abnormalities include osteoporosis, flaring of the anterior ribs with spontaneous rib fractures, cupping and flaring of long-bone metaphyses with spur formation and submetaphyseal fractures, and epiphyseal separation. These changes have frequently been misinterpreted as signs of scurvy. Copper deficiency with a resultant microcytic anemia can be produced by chronic ingestion of massive quantities of zinc. Dietary zinc in large doses leads to copper deficiency by impairing copper absorption.[48,49]

The diagnosis of copper deficiency can be established by demonstrating a low serum ceruloplasmin or serum copper level, but the copper level is thought to be more reliable because ceruloplasmin behaves as an acute phase protein.[45] Adequate normal values for the first 2 to 3 months have not been well defined and normally are lower than the levels observed later in life. Despite these limitations, a serum copper level less than 40 μg/dl or a ceruloplasmin level less than 15 mg/dl after age 1 or 2 months can be regarded as evidence of copper deficiency. In later infancy, childhood, and adulthood, serum copper values should normally exceed 70 μg/dl. Low serum copper values may be observed in hypoproteinemic states, such as exudative enteropathies and nephrosis, and in Wilson disease. In these circumstances, a diagnosis of copper deficiency cannot be established by serum measurements alone but requires analysis of liver copper content or clinical response after a therapeutic trial of copper supplementation.

The anemia and neutropenia are quickly corrected by administration of copper. Treatment of copper-deficient infants consists of administration of approximately 2.5 mg of copper ($\sim$80 μg/kg/day) oral supplementation as a copper sulfate solution.[50] Intravenous bolus injection of copper chloride also has been used.[46]

ZINC DEFICIENCY

Zinc is required for a large number of zinc metalloenzymes, zinc-activated enzymes, and "zinc finger" transcription factors. Zinc deficiency occurs in a variety of pathologic states in humans, including hemolytic anemias such as thalassemia[51] and sickle cell anemia.[52] Zinc deficiency with or without an associated copper deficiency has been described in a patient receiving intensive desferrioxamine therapy[53] and in patients with decreased renal reabsorption of trace minerals.[54]

Although human zinc deficiency may produce growth retardation, impaired wound healing, impaired taste perception, immunologic abnormalities, and acrodermatitis enteropathica, at present there is no evidence that isolated zinc deficiency produces anemia.

SELENIUM DEFICIENCY

Selenium deficiency occurs in patients who live in areas where the selenium content of the soil is very low[55] and has been observed in patients receiving total parenteral nutrition.[56,57] Although this results in a striking decrease in the level of red cell glutathione peroxidase, there do not appear to be any adverse hematologic consequences.

ANEMIA OF STARVATION

Studies conducted during World War II among prisoners of war and conscientious objectors demonstrated that semistarvation for 24 weeks can result in a mild to moderate normocytic normochromic anemia.[58] Marrow cellularity is usually reduced and is accompanied by a decreased erythroid/myeloid ratio. Measurements of red cell volume and plasma volume suggest that dilution is a major factor responsible for the reduction in hemoglobin concentration.

In persons subjected to complete starvation either for experimental purposes or as treatment of severe obesity, anemia was not observed during the first 2 to 9 weeks of fasting.[59] Starvation for 9 to 17 weeks produced a decrease in hemoglobin and marrow hypocellularity.[60] Resumption of a normal diet was accompanied by reticulocytosis and disappearance of anemia. It has been suggested that the anemia of starvation is a response to a hypometabolic state with its attendant decrease in oxygen requirements.[61]

ANEMIA OF PROTEIN DEFICIENCY (KWASHIORKOR)

Even strict vegetarians do not seem to develop hematologic problems related to the absence of animal proteins,[62] except for some vegans who were reported to suffer from B$_{12}$ deficiency.[63] Kwashiorkor is largely a disease of the underdeveloped world but occasionally is seen even among the children of educated and well-to-do parents when the children are fed an inappropriate diet.[64,65]

In infants and children with protein-calorie malnutrition, the hemoglobin concentration may fall to 8 g/dl of blood,[65,66] but some children with kwashiorkor have normal hemoglobin levels, probably because of a decreased plasma volume. The anemia is normocytic and normochromic, but the size and shape of red cells on the blood film vary considerably. The white blood cells and the platelets usually are normal. The marrow is most often normally cellular or slightly hypocellular, with a reduced erythroid to myeloid ratio. Erythroblastopenia, reticulocytopenia, and a marrow containing a few giant pronormoblasts may be found, particularly if the children have an infection. With treatment of the infection, erythroid precursors may appear in the marrow and the reticulocyte count may rise. When nutrition is improved by giving high-protein diets (powdered milk or essential amino acids), reticulocytosis, a slight fall in hematocrit due to hemodilution, and then a rise in hemoglobin level, hematocrit, and red blood cell count occur. Improvement is very slow, however, and during the third or fourth week, when the children are clinically improved and serum protein levels are approaching normal, another episode of erythroid marrow aplasia may develop. The relapse is not associated with infection, does not respond to antibiotics, and does not remit spontaneously. It does respond to either riboflavin or prednisone. Children who develop this complication may die suddenly unless they are treated with riboflavin or prednisone. It has been suggested that the erythroblastic aplasia is a manifestation of riboflavin deficiency.[67]

Although the plasma volume is reduced to a variable degree in children with kwashiorkor, the total circulating red cell volume decreases in proportion to the decrease in lean body mass as protein deprivation reduces metabolic demands. During repletion, an increase in plasma volume may occur before an increase in red cell volume, and the anemia may seem to become more severe despite reticulocytosis.

From the study of the anemia of protein deficiency in rats, it was deduced that oxygen consumption and therefore erythropoietin production are reduced.[68] Other studies confirmed this observation but related the reduction to calorie deprivation with its associated decrease in the blood levels of triiodothyronine (T$_3$) and thyroxine (T$_4$).[61] As a result, erythropoiesis decreases and the reticulocyte count falls. The plasma iron turnover and red cell uptake of radioactive iron are markedly reduced, and the red cell volume gradually declines.[68] Protein deficiency also produces a maturation block at the erythroblast level and a slight decrease in the erythropoietin-sensitive progenitor cell pool.[69] If exogenous erythropoietin is provided, normal erythropoiesis is restored despite protein depletion,[70] an observation that explains the successful use of starved rats in the bioassay for erythropoietin.

ALCOHOLISM

Chronic alcohol ingestion often is associated with anemia. The anemia may result from nutritional deficiencies, chronic gastrointestinal bleeding, hepatic dysfunction, or direct toxic effects of alcohol on erythropoiesis. Quite commonly all these factors work in concert to produce the anemia. Pyridoxal phosphate and folate deficiency are common in alcoholics.[71] Alcohol affects not only the red cells, as described here, but also the platelets (see Chap. 110).[72,73]

Macrocytosis is common in chronic alcoholics[74] and is often associated with a megaloblastic anemia. Among hospitalized malnourished alcoholics it is the most common type of anemia,, occurring alone or in combination with ringed sideroblasts in approximately 40 percent of patients.[75,76] In contrast, megaloblastic anemia is rarely observed in nonhospitalized chronic alcoholics or relatively well-nourished subjects admitted to the hospital for alcohol withdrawal.[77] Anemia, when associated with megaloblastic marrow changes in alcoholics, almost always results from folate deficiency. Iron deficiency often is associated with folate deficiency in alcoholics.[77] In patients with both nutritional deficiencies, the blood film is "dimorphic," with macrocytes, hypersegmented neutrophils, and hypochromic microcytes. Although liver disease is frequently present in alcoholics with megaloblastic anemia, it is not responsible for the folate deficiency. Megaloblastic anemia occurs almost exclusively in alcoholics who have been eating poorly. It is seen more commonly in heavy drinkers of wine and whiskey, which contain little or no folate, than in drinkers of beer, which is a rich source of the vitamin. Although decreased dietary folate intake appears to be a necessary factor in the etiology of the megaloblastic anemia, ethanol itself interferes with folate metabolism (see Chap. 39).[78,79]

However, macrocytosis does not always indicate the presence of a megaloblastic anemia,[74] reticulocytosis secondary to hemolysis or bleeding, or liver disease. A so-called macrocytosis of alcoholism is found in as many as 82 to 96 percent of alcoholics.[80] In these patients, the macrocytosis usually is mild, with MCV in the range of 100 to 110 fl, and anemia is usually absent. In the blood film, the macrocytes are typically round rather than oval, and neutrophil hypersegmentation is not present. The macrocytosis persists until the patient abstains from alcohol. Even then, MCV does not become completely normal for periods of 2 to 4 months.[79]

Alcohol ingestion for 5 to 7 days produces vacuolization of early red cell precursors, and formation of vacuoles can be observed in *in vitro* marrow cell cultures.[76,81] These changes disappear promptly when alcohol ingestion is discontinued. Vacuolization of a similar appearance occurs in subjects who are fed a phenylalanine-deficient diet, patients treated with chloramphenicol or pyrazinamide, patients in hyperosmolar coma, and individuals deficient in copper or riboflavin.[80]

A relatively rare hematologic complication of alcoholism is Zieve syndrome,[82] consisting of transient hemolytic anemia, jaundice, hyperlipidemia, and alcohol-induced liver disease.

REFERENCES

1. Blackfan KD, Wolbach SB: Vitamin A deficiency in infants, a clinical and pathological study. *J Pediatr* 3:679, 1933.
2. Vitamin A and iron deficiency. *Nutr Rev* 47:1989.
3. Majia LA, Hodges RE, Arroyave G, et al: Vitamin A deficiency and anemia in Central American children. *Am J Clin Nutr* 30:1175, 1977.
4. Hodges RE, Sauberlich HE, Canham JE, et al: Hematopoietic studies in vitamin A deficiency. *Am J Clin Nutr* 31:876, 1978.
5. Kolsteren P, Rahman SR, Hilderbrand K, Diniz A: Treatment for iron deficiency anaemia with a combined supplementation of iron, vitamin A and zinc in women of Dinajpur, Bangladesh. *Eur J Clin Nutr* 53:102, 1999.
6. Walczyk T, Davidsson L, Rossander-Hulthen L, et al: No enhancing effect of vitamin A on iron absorption in humans. *Am J Clin Nutr* 77: 144, 2003.
7. Khatib IM: High prevalence of subclinical vitamin A deficiency in Jordan: A forgotten risk. *Food Nutr Bull* 23:228, 2002.
8. Palafox NA, Gamble MV, Dancheck B, et al: Vitamin A deficiency, iron deficiency, and anemia among preschool children in the Republic of the Marshall Islands. *Nutrition* 19:405, 2003.
9. Snyderman SE, Holt LE Jr, Carretero R, Jacobs KG: Pyridoxine deficiency in the human infant. *Am J Clin Nutr* 1:200, 1953.
10. Foy H, Kondi A: Hypochromic anemias of the tropics associated with pyridoxine and nicotinic acid deficiencies. *Blood* 13:1054, 1999.
11. McCurdy PR, Donohoe RF, Magovern M: Reversible sideroblastic anemia caused by pyrazinoic acid (Pyrazinamide). *Ann Intern Med* 64:1280, 1966.
12. Frimpter GW: Pyridoxine (B6) dependency syndromes. *Ann Intern Med* 68:1131, 1968.
13. Beutler E, Srivastava SK: Relationship between glutathione reductase activity and drug-induced haemolytic anaemia. *Nature* 226:759, 1970.
14. Lane M, Alfrey CP: The anemia of human riboflavin deficiency. *Blood* 22:811, 1963.
15. Foy H, Kondi A: A case of true red cell aplastic anaemia successfully treated with riboflavin. *J Pathol Bacteriol* 65:559, 1953.
16. Powers HJ: Riboflavin (vitamin B-2) and health. *Am J Clin Nutr* 77: 1352, 2003.
17. Hodges RE, Bean WB, Ohlson MA, Bleiler RE: Human pantothenic acid deficiency produced by omegamethylpantothenic acid. *J Clin Invest* 38:1421, 1959.
18. Spivak JL, Jackson DL: Pellagra: An analysis of 18 patients and a review of the literature. *Johns Hopkins Med J* 140:295, 1977.
19. Reuler JB, Broudy VC, Cooney TG: Adult scurvy. *JAMA* 253:805, 1985.
20. Hodges RE, Baker EM, Hood J, et al: Experimental scurvy in man. *Am J Clin Nutr* 22:535, 1969.
21. Zalusky R, Herbert V: Megaloblastic anemia in scurvy with response to 50 micrograms of folic acid daily. *N Engl J Med* 265:1033, 1961.
22. Stokes PL, Melikian V, Leeming RL, et al: Folate metabolism in scurvy. *Am J Clin Nutr* 28:126, 1975.
23. Cox EV, Meynell MJ, Northam BE, Cooke WT: The anaemia of scurvy. *Am J Med* 42:220, 1967.
24. Clark NG, Sheard NF, Kelleher JF: Treatment of iron-deficiency anemia complicated by scurvy and folic acid deficiency. *Nutr Rev* 50:134, 1992.
25. Wapnick AA, Lynch SR, Krawitz P, et al: Effects of iron overload on ascorbic acid metabolism. *BMJ* 3:704, 1968.
26. Wapnick AA, Lynch SR, Charlton RW, et al: The effect of ascorbic acid deficiency on desferrioxamine-induced urinary iron excretion. *Br J Haematol* 17:563, 1969.
27. Chapman RW, Hussain MA, Gorman A, et al: Effect of ascorbic acid deficiency on serum ferritin concentration in patients with beta-thalassaemia major and iron overload. *J Clin Pathol* 35:487, 1982.
28. Cohen A, Cohen IJ, Schwartz E: Scurvy and altered iron stores in thalassemia major. *N Engl J Med* 304:158, 1981.
29. Lipschitz DA, Bothwell TH, Seftel HC, et al: The role of ascorbic acid in the metabolism of storage iron. *Br J Haematol* 20:155, 1971.
30. Bothwell TH, Abrahams C, Bradlow BA, Charlton RW: Idiopathic and Bantu hemochromatosis. *Arch Pathol (Chicago)* 79:163, 1965.
31. Williams ML, Shoot RJ, O'Neal PL, Oski FA: Role of dietary iron and fat on vitamin E deficiency anemia of infancy. *N Engl J Med* 292:887, 1975.
32. Oski FA, Barness LA: Hemolytic anemia in vitamin E deficiency. *Am J Clin Nutr* 21:45, 1968.
33. Ritchie JH, Fish MB, McMasters V, Grossman M: Edema and hemolytic anemia in premature infants. A vitamin E deficiency syndrome. *N Engl J Med* 279:1185, 1968.
34. Zipursky A: Vitamin E deficiency anemia in newborn infants. *Clin Perinatol* 11:393, 1984.
35. Wilfond BS, Farrell PM, Laxova A, Mischler E: Severe hemolytic anemia associated with vitamin E deficiency in infants with cystic fibrosis. Implications for neonatal screening. *Clin Pediatr (Phila)* 33:2, 1994.
36. Farrell PM, Bieri JG, Fratantoni JF, et al: The occurrence and effects of human vitamin E deficiency. A study in patients with cystic fibrosis. *J Clin Invest* 60:233, 1977.

37. Corash L, Spielberg S, Bartsocas C, et al: Reduced chronic hemolysis during high-dose vitamin E administration in Mediterranean-type glucose-6-phosphate dehydrogenase deficiency. *N Engl J Med* 303:416, 1980.

38. Eldamhougy S, Elhelw Z, Yamamah G, et al: The vitamin E status among glucose-6 phosphate dehydrogenase deficient patients and effectiveness of oral vitamin E. *Int J Vitam Nutr Res* 58:184, 1988.

39. Johnson GJ, Vatassery GT, Finkel B, Allen DW: High-dose vitamin E does not decrease the rate of chronic hemolysis in glucose-6-phosphate dehydrogenase deficiency. *N Engl J Med* 308:1014, 1983.

40. Natta CL, Machlin LJ, Brin M: A decrease in irreversibly sickled erythrocytes in sickle cell anemia patients given vitamin E. *Am J Clin Nutr* 33:968, 1980.

41. Tangney CC, Phillips G, Bell RA, et al: Selected indices of micronutrient status in adult patients with sickle cell anemia (SCA). *Am J Hematol* 32:161, 1989.

42. Ndombi IO, Kinoti SN: Serum vitamin E and the sickling status in children with sickle cell anaemia. *East Afr Med J* 67:720, 1990.

43. Anderson GJ, Frazer DM, McKie AT, Vulpe CD: The ceruloplasmin homolog hephaestin and the control of intestinal iron absorption. *Blood Cells Mol Dis* 29:367, 2002.

44. Graham GG, Cordano A: Copper depletion and deficiency in the malnourished infant. *Johns Hopkins Med J* 124:139, 1969.

45. Spiegel JE, Willenbucher RF: Rapid development of severe copper deficiency in a patient with Crohn's disease receiving parenteral nutrition. *J Parenter Enteral Nutr* 23:169, 1999.

46. Hirase N, Abe Y, Sadamura S, et al: Anemia and neutropenia in a case of copper deficiency: Role of copper in normal hematopoiesis. *Acta Haematol (Basel)* 87:195, 1992.

47. Fuhrman MP, Herrmann V, Masidonski P, Eby C: Pancytopenia after removal of copper from total parenteral nutrition. *J Parenter Enteral Nutr* 24:361, 2000.

48. Hein MS: Copper deficiency anemia and nephrosis in zinc-toxicity: A case report. *S D J Med* 56:143, 2003.

49. Igic PG, Lee E, Harper W, Roach KW: Toxic effects associated with consumption of zinc. *Mayo Clin Proc* 77:713, 2002.

50. Cordano A: Clinical manifestations of nutritional copper deficiency in infants and children. *Am J Clin Nutr* 67:1012S, 1998.

51. Fuchs GJ, Tienboon P, Linpisarn S, et al: Nutritional factors and thalassaemia major. *Arch Dis Child* 74:224, 1996.

52. Prasad AS: Zinc deficiency in patients with sickle cell disease. *Am J Clin Nutr* 75:181, 2002.

53. Yuzbasiyan-Gurkan VA, Brewer GJ, Vander AJ, et al: Net renal tubular reabsorption of zinc in healthy man and impaired handling in sickle cell anemia. *Am J Hematol* 31:87, 1989.

54. De Virgiliis S, Congia M, Turco MP, et al: Depletion of trace elements and acute ocular toxicity induced by desferrioxamine in patients with thalassaemia. *Arch Dis Child* 63:250, 1988.

55. Thomson CD, Rea HM, Doesburg VM, Robinson MF: Selenium concentrations and glutathione peroxidase activities in whole blood of New Zealand residents. *Br J Nutr* 37:457, 1977.

56. Kien CL, Ganther HE: Manifestations of chronic selenium deficiency in a child receiving total parenteral nutrition. *Am J Clin Nutr* 37:319, 1983.

57. Cohen HJ, Brown MR, Hamilton D, et al: Glutathione peroxidase and selenium deficiency in patients receiving home parenteral nutrition: Time course for development of deficiency and repletion of enzyme activity in plasma and blood cells. *Am J Clin Nutr* 49:132, 1989.

58. Keys A, Brozek J, Henschel A, et al: *The Biology of Semistarvation.* University of Minnesota Press, Minneapolis, 1950.

59. Thomson TJ, Runcie J, Miller V: Treatment of obesity by total fasting for up to 249 days. *Lancet* 2:992, 1966.

60. Drenick EJ, Swendseid ME, Blahd WH, Tuttle SG: Prolonged starvation as treatment for severe obesity. *JAMA* 187:100, 1964.

61. Caro J, Silver R, Erslev AJ, et al: Erythropoietin production in fasted rats. Effects of thyroid hormones and glucose supplementation. *J Lab Clin Med* 98:860, 1981.

62. Lowik MR, Schrijver J, Odink J, et al: Long-term effects of a vegetarian diet on the nutritional status of elderly people (Dutch Nutrition Surveillance System). *J Am Coll Nutr* 9:600, 1990.

63. Chanarin I, Malkowska V, O'Hea AM, et al: Megaloblastic anaemia in a vegetarian Hindu community. *Lancet* 2:1168, 1985.

64. Carvalho NF, Kenney RD, Carrington PH, Hall DE: Severe nutritional deficiencies in toddlers resulting from health food milk alternatives. *Pediatrics* 107:E46, 2001.

65. Lunn PG, Morley CJ, Neale G: A case of kwashiorkor in the U.K. *Clin Nutr* 17:131, 1998.

66. Adams EB, Scragg JN, Naidoo BT, et al.: Observations on the aetiology and treatment of anaemia in kwashiorkor. *BMJ* 3:451, 1967.

67. Foy H, Kondi A: Comparison between erythroid aplasia in marasmus and kwashiorkor and the experimentally induced erythroid aplasia in baboons by riboflavin deficiency. *Vitam Horm* 26:653, 1968.

68. Delmonte L, Aschenasy A, Eyquem A: Studies on the hemolytic nature of protein-deficiency anemia in the rat. *Blood* 24:49, 1964.

69. Naets JP, Wittek M: Effect of starvation on the response to erythropoietin in the rat. *Acta Haematol (Basel)* 52:141, 1974.

70. Ito K, Reissmann KR: Quantitative and qualitative aspects of steady state erythropoiesis induced in protein starved rats by long-term erythropoietin injection. *Blood* 27:343, 1966.

71. Gloria L, Cravo M, Camilo ME, et al: Nutritional deficiencies in chronic alcoholics: Relation to dietary intake and alcohol consumption. *Am J Gastroenterol* 92:485, 1997.

72. Savage D, Lindenbaum J: Anemia in alcoholics. *Medicine* 65:322, 1986.

73. Girard DE, Kumar KL, McAfee JH: Hematologic effects of acute and chronic alcohol abuse. *Hematol Oncol Clin North Am* 1:321, 1987.

74. Fernando OV, Grimsley EW: Prevalence of folate deficiency and macrocytosis in patients with and without alcohol-related illness. *South Med J* 91:721, 1998.

75. Colman N, Herbert V: Hematologic complications of alcoholism: Overview. *Semin Hematol* 17:164, 1980.

76. Sullivan LW, Herbert V: Suppression of hematopoiesis by ethanol. *J Clin Invest* 43:2048, 1964.

77. Eichner ER, Hillman RS: Effect of alcohol on serum folate level. *J Clin Invest* 52:584, 1973.

78. Lindenbaum J: Folate and vitamin B₁₂ deficiencies in alcoholism. *Semin Hematol* 17:119, 1980.

79. Seppa K, Laippala P, Saarni M: Macrocytosis as a consequence of alcohol abuse among patients in general practice. *Alcohol Clin Exp Res* 15:871, 1991.

80. McCurdy PR, Rath CE: Vacuolated nucleated bone marrow cells in alcoholism. *Semin Hematol* 17:100, 1980.

81. Yeung KY, Klug PP, Lessin LS: Alcohol-induced vacuolization in bone marrow cells: Ultrastructure and mechanism of formation. *Blood Cells* 13:487, 1988.

82. Pilcher CR, Underwood RG, Smith HR: Zieve's syndrome a potential surgical pitfall? *J R Army Med Corps* 142:84, 1996.

ANEMIA ASSOCIATED WITH MARROW INFILTRATION

JOSEF T. PRCHAL

Myelophthisic anemia **is an anemia that results from marrow infiltration, typically by tumor but also by any nonhematopoietic tissue. It can present with overt myelocytes and nucleated red cells in the blood (leukoerythroblastic reaction) or with only a few teardrop-shaped red cells on a blood film. These changes may result from early spread of the tumor (or other nonhematopoietic tissue) to the marrow or may indicate massive replacement of the marrow space. Diagnosis can be made by standard marrow biopsy. The condition also can be diagnosed and quantified by radioisotope or by magnetic resonance imaging.**

DEFINITION AND HISTORY

Myelophthisic anemia is the term that has been used to describe diverse pathologic processes including Fanconi anemia[1] but currently refers to anemia resulting from the presence of spotty to massive marrow infiltration with abnormal cells or tissue components. Strictly speaking, the blasts of acute leukemia, plasma cells of myeloma, and cells of lymphoma, chronic leukemia, and myeloproliferative disorders fit this definition. However, the term *myelophthisic anemia*[2] is best reserved for marrow replacement by nonhematologic tumors and nonhematopoietic tissue. Minimal to moderate involvement usually does not cause symptoms or hematologic changes. However, such infiltration is clinically significant because in patients with an established diagnosis of cancer, it indicates metastatic dissemination of the tumor and usually an incurable disorder. Extensive infiltration may lead to anemia or even pancytopenia; however, anemia can be frequently accompanied by an elevated leukocyte count, often with immature myeloid cells in the blood. Platelets can be increased, decreased, or normal (megakaryocytic fragments are seen occasionally in the blood). The condition accompanied by teardrop-shaped red cells, prematurely released nucleated red cells, and immature myeloid cells is referred to as *leukoerythroblastic reaction*.[3]

ETIOLOGY AND PATHOGENESIS

Table 42-1 lists the most common causes of extensive cellular infiltration of marrow. In myelofibrotic disorders of both idiopathic and secondary origin, the malignant clone releases fibroblastic growth factors. The resultant fibrosis restricts the available bone marrow space and disrupts bone marrow architecture (see Chap. 89). The disruption may cause cytopenias with production of deformed red cells, especially poikilocytes and teardrop-shaped cells, and premature release of erythroblasts, myelocytes, and giant platelets. Circulating leukocytes also may be frequently elevated. Similar abnormalities in marrow replacement by calcium oxalate crystals have been reported.[4]

Anemia seen in metastatic cancer most frequently results from cytokine release leading to anemia of inflammation (see Chap. 43), iron deficiency (see Chap. 40), or other nutritional deficiencies (see Chaps. 39 and 41). However, marrow replacement causing a myelophthisic anemia as the sole cause of anemia also exists.[5] The marrow microenvironment is susceptible to implantation of bloodborne malignant cells. Almost all cancers can metastasize to the marrow,[6] but the most common are cancers of the lung, breast, and prostate. Metastatic foci in the marrow can be found in 20 to 30 percent of patients with small cell carcinoma of the lung at the time of diagnosis and in more than 50 percent at autopsy.[7] Development of a frank leukoerythroblastic blood picture occurs much less frequently,[5,6] and its absence should not be relied upon to indicate the marrow is not involved.

The characteristic abnormalities in hematopoiesis observed in patients with myelophthisic anemia may result partly from compensatory extramedullary blood formation.

A similar picture can be seen when the marrow is replaced by numerous granulomas and by macrophages containing indigestible lipids, as in Gaucher (see Chap. 73) and Niemann-Pick disease.[8]

Marrow necrosis can be an underlying cause of myelophthisic anemia. The morphologic picture, best observed in hematoxylin and eosin–stained biopsy of marrow,[9] consists of cell debris and occasional necrotic cells in a background of marrow fibrosis. Marrow necrosis is generally considered to be very rare, accounting for less than 1 percent of marrow biopsies. Tumors and septicemia are generally the underlying cause,[10] but sickle cell disease[11] and arsenic therapy in acute promyelocytic leukemia are other causes.[12] The frequency of the diagnosis of marrow necrosis is a function of the area of marrow that must be involved to draw such a conclusion. It is more common if a small area of necrotic marrow is considered sufficient to make the diagnosis.[13]

Because myelophthisic anemia is so rare, only a few rigorous studies of the pathogenesis of anemia in this entity have been conducted. *In vitro* study of hematopoietic progenitors reveals only a moderate decrease of their proportion and proliferative capacity.[14] Similar reports of erythropoiesis quantitation by ferrokinetic studies reveal only a moderate defect.[15] This finding suggests that when other confounding factors contributing to anemia, such as elevated hepcidin (see Chap. 43) and other factors, such as folate deficiency, are excluded, only massive bone marrow replacement leads to anemia.

CLINICAL FEATURES

Symptoms and signs associated with infiltrative marrow disorders usually are related to the underlying disease. Other symptoms, such as fatigue resulting from anemia, are related to cytopenias. Some patients are asymptomatic, and the incidental discovery of cytopenias and leukoerythroblastic blood morphology leads to diagnosis of an underlying disorder.

LABORATORY FEATURES

The anemia usually is mild to moderate, but it can be severe. White cell and platelet counts may vary, but the most characteristic feature is the morphologic appearance of red cells on the blood film. These cells may show anisocytosis and poikilocytosis, but the presence of teardrop forms and nucleated red cells is particularly suggestive of marrow infiltration (Fig. 42-1). The combination of nucleated red cells and immature myeloid precursors constitutes the leukoerythroblastic picture that is characteristic of marrow infiltration. The presence of cancer cells on the blood film occurs occasionally and always indicates marrow invasion.[16] Marrow biopsy is the most reliable procedure used to diagnose marrow-infiltrative disease and should be performed in all patients with suspected metastatic carcinoma or hematologic features of myelophthisic anemia.[5–7] Marrow aspiration[17] does not provide the

Acronyms and abbreviations that appear in this chapter include: MRI, magnetic resonance imaging; ^{99m}Tc, a radioisotope of technetium.

TABLE 42-1   CAUSES OF MARROW INFILTRATION

I. Fibroblasts and collagen
   A. Idiopathic myelofibrosis
   B. Fibrosis of other myeloproliferative disorders
   C. Fibrosis of hairy cell leukemia
   D. Metastatic malignancies
   E. Sarcoidosis
   F. Secondary myelofibrosis with pulmonary hypertension
II. Other noncellular material
   A. Oxalosis
III. Tumor cells
   A. Carcinoma (lung, breast, prostate)
   B. Sarcoma
IV. Granulomas (inflammatory cells)
   A. Miliary tuberculosis
   B. Fungal infections
   C. Sarcoidosis
V. Macrophages
   A. Gaucher disease
   B. Niemann-Pick disease
VI. Marrow necrosis
   A. Sickle cell anemia
   B. Septicemia
   C. Tumors
   D. Arsenic therapy

same yield of tumor cells and is particularly difficult in idiopathic or secondary myelofibrosis.[18] The inability to aspirate marrow (dry tap) leads to a high degree of suspicion of marrow replacement. Because the diagnostic marrow yield from biopsies depends on the amount of tissue examined, bilateral posterior iliac crest bone marrow biopsies may be necessary.

Technetium-99m (^{99m}Tc) sestamibi uptake reliably identifies marrow infiltration by Gaucher cells. Magnetic resonance imaging (MRI) also is helpful for defining the severity of marrow replacement and is being used with increasing frequency. This imaging approach is especially useful to follow resolution of marrow infiltration in patients with type 1 Gaucher disease treated with enzyme replacement therapy.[19] An isotopic bone scan or MRI study showing focal accumulation of radioactive tracers can be helpful in locating a suitable site for biopsy,[20] but a negative study of the area does not exclude the possibility of marrow involvement.

DIFFERENTIAL DIAGNOSIS

A myelophthisic blood picture ranging from a few teardrop-shaped red cells on the blood film to a full-blown leukoerythroblastic picture demands close attention. At times, this marrow biopsy reveals unsuspected malignancy, but typically an underlying disease causing marrow infiltration already has been diagnosed. In patients treated for a neoplastic disorder, careful marrow examination, even in the absence of red cell changes, may reveal neoplastic cells. Such an attempt today can be augmented by immunologic flow cytometric study using appropriate antibodies. Idiopathic myelofibrosis, a common cause of myelophthisic anemia among older subjects, may be difficult to distinguish from metastatic disease with focal reactive fibrosis[18] and should be considered in the differential diagnosis (see Chap. 89).

Nucleated red cells and leukocytosis can be seen in acute conditions, including overwhelming sepsis, acute severe hypoxia, postcardiac arrest, and chronic conditions such as thalassemia major and severe hemolytic anemia.

THERAPY, COURSE, AND PROGNOSIS

In general, the goal of treatment is managing the underlying disease. Patients with marrow infiltration caused by cancer should be treated

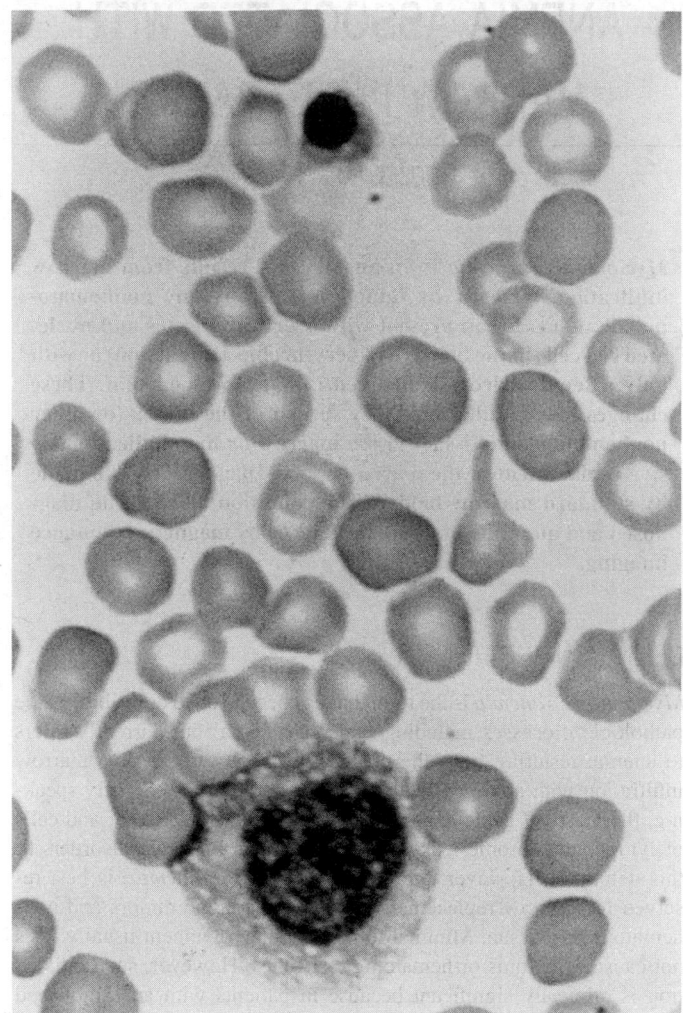

FIGURE 42-1   Blood film of a patient with prostatic adenocarcinoma metastatic to the marrow. The film shows an early myeloid cell, a nucleated red cell, and a classic teardrop-shaped red cell.

appropriately; however, in some instances the presence of marrow infiltration may not adversely affect the outcome. If treatment is successful, not only the malignant cells but also the reactive fibrosis surrounding metastatic foci may completely disappear. In hormone-refractory prostate cancer, the presence of a leukoerythroblastic picture does not seem to influence survival.[21] However, in most patients with cancers metastatic to the marrow, the prognosis is for only short-term survival.

REFERENCES

1. Baumann T: Constitutional general myelophthisis with multiple degeneration (Fanconi syndrome). *Ann Paediatr*177:65, 1951.

2. Rundles RW, Jousson U: Metastases in the bone marrow and myelophthisic anemia from carcinoma of the prostate. *Am J Med Sci* 218: 240, 1949.

3. Vaughan JM: Leuco-erythroblastic anaemia. *J Pathol Bacteriol* 42:541, 1936.

4. Hricik DE, Hussain R: Pancytopenia and hepatosplenomegaly in oxalosis. *Arch Intern Med* 144:167, 1984.

5. Laszlo J: Hematologic effects of cancer, in *Cancer Medicine*, 2nd ed, edited by JF Holland, E Frei, p 1275. Lea & Febiger, Philadelphia, 1982.

6. Makoni SN, Laber DA: Clinical spectrum of myelophthisis in cancer patients. Am *J Hematol* 76:92, 2004.

7. Hirsch FR, Hansen HH: Bone marrow involvement in small cell anaplastic carcinoma of the lung: Prognostic and therapeutic aspects. *Cancer* 46:206, 1980.

8. Hsu YS, Hwu WL, Huang SF, et al: Niemann-Pick disease type C (a cellular cholesterol lipidosis) treated by bone marrow transplantation. *Bone Marrow Transplant* 24:103, 1999.

9. Norgard MJ, Carpenter JT Jr, Conrad ME: Bone marrow necrosis and degeneration. *Arch Intern Med* 139:905, 1979.

10. Paydas S, Ergin M, Baslamisli F, et al: Bone marrow necrosis: Clinicopathologic analysis of 20 cases and review of the literature. *Am J Hematol* 70:300, 2002.

11. Conrad ME, Studdard H, Anderson LJ. Aplastic crisis in sickle cell disorders: Bone marrow necrosis and human parvovirus infection. *Am J Med Sci* 295:212, 1988.

12. Chim CS, Lam CC, Wong KF, et al: Atypical blasts and bone marrow necrosis associated with near-triploid relapse of acute promyelocytic leukemia after arsenic trioxide treatment. *Hum Pathol* 33:849, 2002.

13. Conrad ME: Bone marrow necrosis. Review. *J Intens Care Med* 10:171, 1995.

14. Dainiak N, Kulkarni V, Howard D, et al: Mechanisms of abnormal erythropoiesis in malignancy. *Cancer* 51:1101, 1983.

15. Cazzola M, Bergamaschi G, Huebers HA, Finch CA: Pathophysiological classification of acquired bone marrow failure based on quantitative assessment of erythroid function. *Eur J Haematol* 38:426, 1987.

16. Gallivan MVE, Lokich JJ: Carcinocythemia (carcinoma cell leukemia): Report of two cases with English literature review. *Cancer* 53:1100, 1984.

17. Garrett TJ, Gee TS, Lieberman PH, et al: The role of bone marrow aspiration and biopsy in detecting marrow involvement by nonhematologic malignancies. *Cancer* 38:2401, 1976.

18. Kiely JM, Silverstein MN: Metastatic carcinoma simulating agnogenic myeloid metaplasia and myelofibrosis. *Cancer* 24:1041, 1969.

19. Mariani G, Filocamo M, Giona F, et al: Severity of bone marrow involvement in patients with Gaucher's disease evaluated by scintigraphy with 99mTc-sestamibi. *J Nucl Med* 44:1253, 2003.

20. Terk MR, Dardashti S, Liebman HA: Bone marrow response in treated patients with Gaucher disease: Evaluation by T1-weighted magnetic resonance images and correlation with reduction in liver and spleen volume. *Skeletal Radiol* 29:563, 2000.

21. Shamdas GJ, Ahmann FR, Matzner MB, Ritchie JM: Leukoerythroblastic anemia in metastatic prostate cancer: Clinical and prognostic significance in patients with hormone-refractory disease. *Cancer* 71:3594, 1993.

ANEMIA OF CHRONIC DISEASE

TOMAS GANZ

Most patients who suffer from chronic infection, chronic inflammation, or some malignancies develop mild to moderate anemia. This anemia, designated *anemia of chronic disease* or *anemia of inflammation*, is characterized by a low serum iron level, low to normal transferrin level, and normal to elevated ferritin level. The anemia is caused by the inhibitory effects of inflammatory cytokines on erythrocyte production. Among the cytokines, interleukin-6 has a central role. Interleukin-6 increases the production of the iron regulatory hormone hepcidin by hepatocytes. Hepcidin blocks the release of iron from macrophages and hepatocytes, causing the characteristic hypoferremia associated with this anemia and limiting the availability of iron to the developing erythrocytes. Effective treatment of the underlying disease restores normal erythropoiesis. When the underlying disease cannot be alleviated but treatment of anemia is necessary, therapeutic trials have revealed that the anemia often responds to pharmacologic doses of erythropoietin.

DEFINITION AND HISTORY

The terms *anemia of chronic disease* or *anemia of chronic disorders* refer to mild to moderately severe anemias (hemoglobin [Hg] 7–12 g/dl) associated with chronic infections and inflammatory disorders and some malignancies.[1] The newer name, *anemia of inflammation* (AI), not only is more reflective of the pathophysiology of the disorders but also includes *anemia of critical illness*,[2] a condition that presents similarly to *anemia of chronic disease* but develops within days of the onset of illness. An anemia similar to AI is seen in some elderly patients in the absence of identifiable chronic disease.[3]

AI is characterized by inadequate erythrocyte production in the setting of low serum iron and low iron-binding capacity (i.e., low transferrin) despite preserved or even increased macrophage iron stores in the marrow. The erythrocytes usually are normocytic and normochromic but can be mildly hypochromic and microcytic. Anemia of critical illness[2] can develop acutely (within days) in intensive care settings where the effects of infection or inflammation are exacerbated by disease-related or iatrogenic blood loss or red cell destruction, which by themselves are not sufficiently severe to cause anemia. Anemia of aging[3] is diagnosed in the elderly when a normocytic normochromic anemia with low iron and preserved iron stores develops without an identified underlying disease. Elderly patients in this defined subset typically have an elevated sedimentation rate and/or elevated C-reactive protein (CRP), a high plasma interleukin-6 (IL-6) concentration, and frailty.

Physicians have known about the pale appearance of patients with chronic infections for hundreds of years. In 19th-century Europe, tuberculosis was the major killer, and the pallor associated with this disease was romanticized in the art literature of the time. The first

measurements of red cell mass revealed the association between inflammation and anemia. Discussing "the alterations in the condition of the Blood in Inflammation" in Section 372 of the 1859 edition of the *Principles of Human Physiology*, William B. Carpenter[4] described the connection between inflammation and anemia (author's parentheses): "With this increase in the proportion of fibrin and colorless corpuscles (leukocytes), separately or in combination, there is a diminution in the proportion of the red corpuscles, albumen and the salts of the blood." In 1961, 100 hundred years later, Maxwell Wintrobe,[5] in the fifth edition of *Clinical Hematology*, used the term "simple chronic anemia" for the normocytic anemia associated with the majority of infections and chronic systemic diseases. He described anemia associated with inflammation as a common subtype. Wintrobe proposed "profound alterations in iron and porphyrin metabolism" as the likely cause and referred to his own experiments that showed a decrease in erythrocyte survival of only 27 percent, which "could easily be met by increased erythropoiesis if the marrow functional capacity were not impaired." Despite advances in our understanding of the pathophysiology of this very common form of anemia, our knowledge is incomplete.

EPIDEMIOLOGY

The high prevalence of infectious diseases worldwide and the high prevalence of inflammatory and malignant disorders in industrialized countries suggest that AI is the second or third most common form of anemia after iron-deficiency anemia (IDA) and thalassemia.[6] Although the prevalence of iron deficiency in industrialized countries is rapidly decreasing,[6,7] AI is expected to increase as the proportion of the elderly in the population increases. Table 43-1 lists the most common diseases associated with AI.

ETIOLOGY AND PATHOGENESIS

In the chronic setting, AI predominantly results from the body's inability to increase erythrocyte production to compensate for relatively small decrements in erythrocyte survival (reviewed in reference 1). In the steady state, erythrocyte production is sufficiently high so that the resulting anemia is mild to moderate. The anemia associated with acute critical illness has the same pathogenesis as other forms of AI but develops more rapidly, perhaps because of the more extensive erythrocyte destruction and intensive diagnostic phlebotomy common in this setting. The key questions about the pathogenesis of AI, still only partially answered, are as follows: (1) What accounts for the inability of the AI marrow to increase erythropoiesis; and (2) How is this deficit connected to the characteristic hypoferremia and sequestration of iron in macrophages and hepatocytes.

RED CELL DESTRUCTION

Human studies indicate that transfused AI erythrocytes have a normal life span in normal recipients, but transfused normal erythrocytes have a decreased life span in AI recipients.[1] This finding suggests that increased erythrocyte destruction results from activation of host factors such as macrophages that prematurely remove aging erythrocytes from the bloodstream. The explanation is consistent with the predominance of young erythrocytes in AI. Whether extrinsic factors, such as bacterial toxins and medications, or host-derived antibodies or complement contribute to this process is unknown.

INADEQUATE ERYTHROPOIETIN SECRETION AND RESISTANCE TO ERYTHROPOIETIN

The normal response to increased destruction of erythrocytes is transient anemia followed by an increase in erythropoietin (Epo) produc-

TABLE 43-1   COMMON CONDITIONS ASSOCIATED WITH ANEMIA OF
INFLAMMATION

CATEGORY	DISEASES ASSOCIATED WITH AI
Infection	AIDS/HIV, tuberculosis, malaria (contributory), osteomyelitis, chronic abscesses, sepsis
Inflammation	Rheumatoid arthritis, other rheumatologic disorders, inflammatory bowel diseases, systemic inflammatory response syndrome
Malignancy	Carcinomas, multiple myeloma, lymphomas
Cytokine dysregulation	Anemia of aging

tion and subsequent compensatory increase in erythropoiesis. One proposed explanation for the inadequate marrow response in AI is less Epo production than expected in other types of anemia. Studies of patients with rheumatoid arthritis and AI indicated that Epo levels are increased but less so than in IDA.[8–13] The findings were similar in patients with anemias associated with solid tumors or hematologic malignancies.[14,15] However, these comparisons did not take into account the potentiating effect of iron deficiency on hypoxia sensing.[16] This effect could increase Epo production in IDA above that in other types of anemia and make Epo production in AI appear low in comparison. In support of the Epo suppression hypothesis are experiments with Epo-producing cell lines indicating that production of the hormone is inhibited by the inflammatory cytokines tumor necrosis factor alpha (TNF-α) and IL-1. The inhibition is mediated by the effects of the transcription factor GATA-1 on the Epo promoter, and the suppression of Epo production can be reversed by a GATA inhibitor.[17] Moreover, both baseline and hypoxia-induced Epo gene expression are suppressed in rats treated with bacterial lipopolysaccharide or IL-1β to mimic a septic state.[18] However, suppression of Epo production is not the major mechanism of AI. If it were, administration of relatively small amounts of Epo would be sufficient to reverse AI. Patients who had renal disease with inflammation, as measured by increased serum CRP greater than 20 mg/liter, required on the average 80 percent higher doses of Epo than patients with simple primary Epo deficiency resulting from renal disease.[19] In another study, patients with CRP greater than 50 mg/liter reached lower concentrations of Hg than patients with CRP less than 50, despite higher doses of Epo.[20] Inflammation thus induces a state of relative resistance to Epo.

ERYTHROPOIESIS RESTRICTION AS A RESULT OF IRON UNAVAILABILITY

INTERLEUKIN-6, HEPCIDIN, AND HYPOFERREMIA

Hypoferremia, one of the defining features of AI, develops within hours of the onset of inflammation.[1] Although previous studies of cytokine mediators of hypoferremia of inflammation were inconclusive, subsequent work[62] indicates the response is dependent on IL-6, which induces the newly discovered iron regulatory hormone hepcidin.[21] Unlike wild-type mice, mice deficient in either hepcidin[22] or IL-6[62] do not become hypoferremic during turpentine-induced inflammation. In hepatocyte cell cultures, IL-6 is a potent inducer of hepcidin. Neither IL-1 nor TNF-α shares this activity. The central role of IL-6 is further indicated by the observation that IL-6–deficient mice do not induce hepcidin in response to turpentine inflammation.[62] Infusion of IL-6 into human volunteers induces hepcidin release within hours and causes concomitant hypoferremia.[62] The IL-6–hepcidin axis now appears responsible for induction of hypoferremia during inflammation.

SERUM IRON CONCENTRATIONS ARE DEPENDENT ON IRON RELEASED FROM MACROPHAGES AND HEPATOCYTES

In the steady state, almost all of the approximately 20 to 25 mg of iron that daily enters the plasma iron/transferrin pool comes from macrophage recycling of senescent erythrocytes and from hepatocyte iron stores; only about 1 to 2 mg comes from dietary iron. Only about 2 to 4 mg of iron is bound to transferrin, but the entire daily iron flow transits through this compartment; thus, the iron in this pool turns over every few hours. During inflammation, release of iron from macrophages and probably also from liver stores is markedly inhibited.[23–29] Studies in transgenic mice lacking hepcidin and mice overexpressing hepcidin indicate the peptide is a negative regulator of iron release from macrophages and of intestinal iron uptake.[30,31] During inflammation, IL-6 induces hepcidin production, which in turn inhibits iron release from macrophages (and probably from hepatocytes), leading to hypoferremia (Fig. 43-1). Hepcidin acts by binding to cell membrane-associated ferroportin molecules that are the only conduits for iron export, and inducing ferroportin internalization and degradation.[61] As hepcidin concentrations increase, less and less ferroportin is available for iron export and the iron release into plasma from macrophages, hepatocytes and enterocytes decreases.

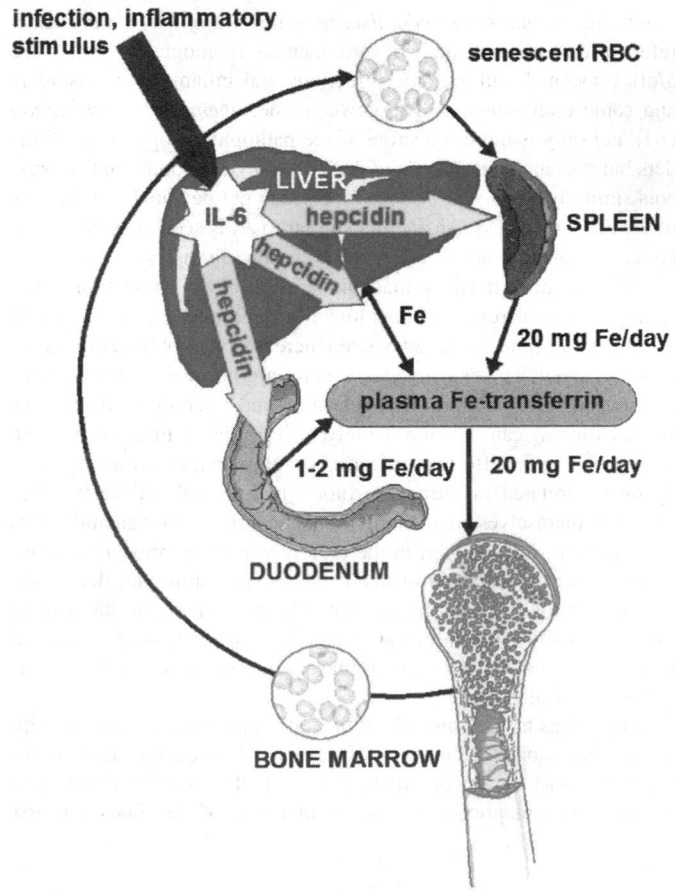

FIGURE 43-1   Effect of inflammation on iron concentrations in plasma. *Large blue open arrows* indicate control points where hepcidin inhibits iron flow into the plasma transferrin compartment.

ERYTHROPOIESIS IN ANEMIA OF INFLAMMATION IS LIMITED BY IRON

As an intermediate step during the synthesis of heme, iron becomes incorporated into protoporphyrin IX. However, zinc is an alternative protoporphyrin ligand. In iron deficiency, an increased amount of zinc is incorporated into protoporphyrin. In AI, zinc protoporphyrin also is increased.[32] Insufficient iron reaches the sites of heme synthesis in the developing erythrocytes, leading to the substitution of zinc. Moreover, the number of sideroblasts, nucleated erythrocyte precursors that stain for iron with Prussian blue, is decreased in AI.[1] A further indication of the limiting role of iron in patients with AI but no evidence of iron deficiency is that coadministration of parenteral iron can resolve the resistance of AI to Epo,[33,34] although higher doses of oral iron therapy also can overcome the problem. Attempts to treat AI with iron alone generally have been unsuccessful, as iron becomes rapidly trapped in the macrophage compartment.[1,35,36]

INHIBITION OF INTESTINAL ABSORPTION OF IRON

In long-standing AI, the erythrocytes can become hypochromic and microcytic, partly because progressive depletion of iron stores worsens the iron restriction. Intestinal absorption of iron is inhibited during inflammation,[37-39] presumably by an IL-6– and hepcidin-mediated mechanism.[22,31,40] Only 1 to 2 mg of the daily iron needed for erythropoiesis comes from the diet, and most adults have 400 to 1000 mg of iron stores; therefore, a considerable amount of time is needed to deplete the stored iron. True iron deficiency can eventually develop in chronic inflammatory diseases, especially in children who have limited iron stores or in conditions where IL-6 levels are particularly high, such as systemic-onset juvenile chronic arthritis.[41] The anemia in these children was accompanied by an appropriate Epo increase but was unresponsive to oral iron replacement. The anemia was corrected, at least partially, by parenteral iron.

Thus, AI is primarily the result of slightly decreased red cell survival and of macrophage iron sequestration leading to iron-restricted erythropoiesis. In some cases, the condition is compounded by inadequate Epo production, or depletion of iron stores.

CLINICAL FEATURES

The clinical manifestations of AI usually are obscured by the signs and symptoms of the underlying disease. Moderate anemia (Hg <10) can exacerbate the symptoms of preexisting ischemic heart disease or respiratory disease, or contribute to fatigue and exertional intolerance. The diagnosis is based on clinical features found in conjunction with typical laboratory abnormalities.

LABORATORY FEATURES

The erythrocytes in AI usually are normocytic and normochromic but, with increasing severity or duration, can become hypochromic and eventually microcytic.[1] The absolute reticulocyte count is normal or slightly elevated.

HYPOFERREMIA AND DECREASED SERUM TRANSFERRIN

Hypoferremia, a decrease in serum iron concentration, is a defining feature of AI. It develops within hours of the onset of infection or severe inflammation. The concentration of transferrin (measured as total iron-binding capacity) is moderately decreased in AI, unlike IDA in which transferrin concentration is increased. The decrease in transferrin concentrations develops more slowly than the decrease in serum

iron levels because of the longer half-life of transferrin (8–12 days)[42] compared to the half-life of iron (approximately 90 minutes).

INCREASED SERUM FERRITIN

Serum ferritin concentrations, which reflect iron stores, are increased in AI but decreased in iron deficiency. Thus, serum ferritin is useful in the differential diagnosis of patients with low serum iron concentrations.[43] Depleted iron stores in patients with coexisting inflammation may result in intermediate ferritin levels (Table 43-2 and Fig. 43-2) because ferritin is an acute-phase protein, and inflammatory cytokines increase ferritin synthesis. In this situation, iron deficiency should be suspected if ferritin concentrations are less than 60 μg/liter. If the etiology of the anemia remains unclear, the serum transferrin receptor assay[44] may clarify the diagnosis (Table 43-2). Soluble transferrin receptor levels are increased in iron deficiency but, unlike ferritin, are decreased during infection or inflammation.[44]

MARROW IRON STAIN

Marrow aspiration or biopsy is rarely required for diagnosis of AI. In general, the marrow morphology and stainable iron are normal, unless the underlying disease alters the picture. The most important information obtained from marrow examination is the content and distribution of iron. Iron in a marrow preparation can be found as storage iron in the cytoplasm of macrophages or as functional iron in nucleated red cells. In normal individuals, a few Prussian blue–staining particles can be found inside or adjacent to many macrophages. Approximately one third of nucleated red cells contain one to four fine blue inclusion bodies, and such cells are called *sideroblasts*. Both sideroblasts and macrophage iron are absent in iron deficiency. In contrast, sideroblasts are decreased or absent but macrophage iron is increased in AI. The increase in storage iron in association with a decreased level of circulating iron and a decreased number of sideroblasts is characteristic of AI. Although marrow stain could be considered the gold standard for differential diagnosis of AI and iron deficiency, the discomfort to the patient associated this procedure and the wide availability of the

TABLE 43-2   LABORATORY STUDIES OF IRON METABOLISM IN IRON DEFICIENCY ANEMIA AND ANEMIA OF INFLAMMATION

	IDA (N = 48)	AI (N = 58)	COMBI (N = 17)
Hemoglobin (g/liter)	93 ± 16 (96)	102 ± 12 (103)	88 ± 20 (90)
MCV (fl)	75 ± 9 (75)	90 ± 7 (91)	78 ± 9 (79)
Iron (μmol/L) [10–40]	8 ± 11 (4)	10 ± 6 (9)	6 ± 3 (6)
Transferrin (g/liter) [2.1–3.4m, 2.0–3.1f]	3.3 ± 0.4 (3.3)	1.9 ± 0.5 (1.8)	2.6 ± 0.6 (2.4)
Transferrin saturation (%)	12 ± 17 (5.7)	23 ± 13 (21)	12 ± 7 (8)
Ferritin (μg/L) [15–306m, 5–103f]	21 ± 55 (11)	342 ± 385 (195)	87 ± 167 (23)
TfR (mg/L) [0.85–3.05]	6.2 ± 3.5 (5.0)	1.8 ± 0.6 (1.8)	5.1 ± 2.0 (4.7)
TfR/log ferritin	6.8 ± 6.5 (5.4)	0.8 ± 0.3 (0.8)	3.8 ± 1.9 (3.2)

IDA, iron deficiency anemia; AI, anemia of inflammation; TfR, transferrin receptor (soluble form).
Diagnosis was defined by bone marrow iron stain and appropriate coexisting disease. Patients with a combination of no stainable marrow iron and either coexisting disease or elevated CRP were classified as "COMBI." Normal ranges for this laboratory for males (m) and females (f) are indicated in brackets. Measurements are presented as mean ± SD (median).
Modified from reference 44, with permission.

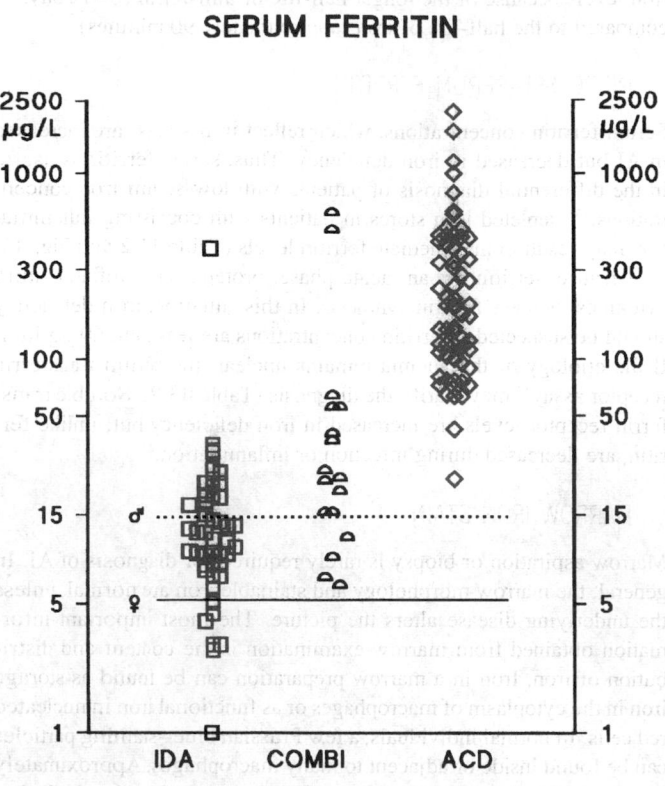

FIGURE 43-2 Distribution of serum ferritin measurements in patients with iron-deficiency anemia (IDA), anemia of chronic disease (ACD = anemia of inflammation), and combined IDA and ACD (COMBI). *Horizontal lines* indicate lower normal values for healthy men and women. (Used with permission from ref. 44.)

serum ferritin assay have decreased the use of marrow stain in this setting.

DIFFERENTIAL DIAGNOSIS

Most patients with chronic infections, inflammatory diseases, or neoplastic disorders are anemic. The diagnosis of AI should be made only if the anemia is mild to moderate, the serum iron and iron-binding capacity are low, and the serum ferritin is elevated. Underlying diseases and their treatments can cause many types of anemia, so other potential causes should be considered.

1. *Drug-induced marrow suppression or drug-induced hemolysis* can complicate infections, inflammatory disorders, and cancer. When the marrow is suppressed by cytotoxic drugs or idiopathic toxic reaction, serum iron tends to be high and reticulocyte count low. In hemolysis, reticulocyte counts, haptoglobin, bilirubin, and lactate dehydrogenase levels often are elevated.
2. *Chronic blood loss* depletes iron stores and decreases serum iron and serum ferritin but increases transferrin (see Chap. 40). When AI and chronic blood loss coexist, serum ferritin usually indicates the predominant disorder, although the level can increase as a result of the inflammation itself. Testing stool for occult blood and looking for other sources of overlooked blood loss, including phlebotomy and menorrhagia, often identify the source of bleeding. Once this issue is addressed, a successful trial of iron repletion with oral or parenteral iron confirms the diagnosis of combined AI and iron deficiency.

3. *Renal impairment* causes a deficiency of Epo with resulting decrease of erythropoiesis and a shortened red cell life span (see Chap. 35). Although the serum iron level is either normal or high in the anemia of uremia, the diagnosis rests on the finding of increased serum creatinine. AI can coexist with renal failure and should be suspected in the presence of an underlying inflammatory disorder, resistance to Epo therapy, and elevated markers of inflammation such as erythrocyte sedimentation rate or CRP.
4. *Endocrine disorders*, including hypothyroidism, hyperthyroidism, testicular failure, and diabetes mellitus, can be associated with a chronic normocytic, normochromic anemia (see Chap. 36). Unless inflammation or associated iron deficiency is present, serum iron should be normal in these disorders.
5. *Anemia resulting from metastatic invasion of the bone marrow* by tumors can be the presenting symptom of malignancy. The anemia can develop in the setting of a previous diagnosis of carcinoma or lymphoma and by itself is accompanied by normal or increased serum iron (see Chap. 42). It often develops in the setting of preexisting malignancy-related AI. The blood smear often is abnormal, with poikilocytes, teardrop-shaped red cells, normoblasts, or immature myeloid cells. Direct marrow examination often is necessary to establish the diagnosis.
6. *Thalassemia minor* is a common cause of anemia in many parts of the world. It can be confused with the anemia of chronic disease (see Chap. 46). Microcytosis is a lifelong condition and usually is more severe in this group of disorders than in the anemia of chronic disease.
7. *Dilution anemia* is seen in pregnancy and in patients with severely increased plasma protein levels as a result of multiple myeloma or macroglobulinemia.

THERAPY, COURSE, AND PROGNOSIS

Anemia that presents in the setting of infection, inflammation, or malignancy requires sufficient diagnostic studies to rule out reversible and potentially more threatening causes, such as occult hemorrhage; iron, B12, and folate deficiency; hemolysis; and drug reaction. If the anemia can be designated as AI after such studies, effective treatment of the underlying disease resolves the anemia. If treatment of the underlying disease is not effective and the patient has symptoms or medical complications attributable to anemia, one or more of the available anemia-specific treatment modalities should be considered (Table 43-3).

Acutely, transfusion of erythrocytes is indicated when anemia is moderate to severe and the patient is symptomatic. Epo therapy for treatment of AI has been tested in the setting of various cancers,[45,46] multiple myeloma and other hematologic malignancies,[15,47,48] rheumatoid arthritis,[49–52] and inflammatory bowel diseases.[53,54] In most reports, more than 50 percent of patients experienced Hg increases greater than 2 g/dl. Guidelines for Epo use in anemia associated with hematologic and nonhematologic malignancy were published in 2002 and form a reasonable guide for Epo treatment of AI.[55] The guidelines (used here with permission) recommend treating patients with Hg less than 10 g/dl in whom treatment of the underlying condition did not alleviate the anemia. The recommendations are based on evidence from trials in which Epo was administered subcutaneously three times per week. The recommended starting dose is 150 U/kg three times per week for a minimum of 4 weeks, with consideration given to dose escalation to 300 U/kg three times per week for an additional 4 to 8 weeks in patients who do not respond to the initial dose. An alternative weekly dosing regimen (40,000 U/week) can be considered. Dose escalation of weekly regimens should be considered under similar circumstances to the three-times-per-week regimens. Continuing Epo therapy beyond 6 to 8 weeks in the absence of response (i.e., 1–2 g/

TABLE 43-3 TREATMENT OF ANEMIA OF INFLAMMATION

MODALITY	INDICATIONS	TYPICAL SETTING	RISKS AND SIDE EFFECTS	BENEFITS
Transfusion	Cardiac ischemia Lack of response to other modalities	Hg <10 g/dl Chest pain and electrocardiographic changes	Infections Volume overload Transfusion reaction	Rapid correction of anemia
Erythropoietin[55]	Fatigue, exertional intolerance	Hg <10 g/dl Discretionary in Hg 10–12 g/dl Anemia symptoms	Response takes several weeks Rare red cell aplasia with some forms of erythropoietin[59] May worsen outcome in some cancers[60] Expensive	Usually well tolerated, relatively safe
Iron (oral or parenteral)[34]	Coexisting iron deficiency Resistance to erythropoietin (investigational)	Suspected or documented iron deficiency	Gastrointestinal side effects (oral) Systemic and local reactions (parenteral) May decrease resistance to infections	Inexpensive, relatively safe

dl rise in Hg), assuming appropriate dose increase was attempted in nonresponders, does not appear to be beneficial. Patients who do not respond should be investigated for underlying iron deficiency. As with other failed individual therapeutic trials, consideration should be given to discontinuing the medication. Hg levels can be raised to (or near) a concentration of 12 g/dl, at which time the dosage of Epo should be titrated to maintain that level or restarted when the level falls to near 10 g/dl. Insufficient evidence supports the "normalization" of Hg levels to greater than 12 g/dl. Baseline and periodic monitoring of iron, total iron-binding capacity, transferrin saturation, or ferritin levels and instituting iron repletion when indicated may be valuable in limiting the need for Epo, maximizing symptomatic improvement in patients, and determining why patients did not respond adequately to Epo.

The availability of darbepoietin, an Epo modified to have a longer half-life, should permit less frequent dosing of every 2 to 4 weeks.[46,48] Other Epo preparations, such as pegylated Epo, are being evaluated.

Coadministration of iron with Epo is a therapeutic strategy based on the idea that iron becomes limiting when marrow production of erythrocytes is stimulated. In some cases, occult iron deficiency coexists with AI.[44,54] In other situations, limited iron stores become depleted when Epo is initiated. How additional iron can be utilized if iron stores are present is uncertain. Existing iron therapies deliver most of the iron to macrophages; only a small percentage of the iron is delivered directly to transferrin.[56] Further studies are needed to determine whether the net effect on the transferrin iron pool is therapeutically important. Pending additional studies, coadministration of iron with Epo in AI in the absence of demonstrated iron deficiency remains investigational.[34] Concerns exist that iron supplementation in AI increases susceptibility to infections.[57,58]

REFERENCES

1. Cartwright GE: The anemia of chronic disorders. *Semin Hematol* 3:351, 1966.
2. Corwin HL, Krantz SB: Anemia of the critically ill: "Acute" anemia of chronic disease. *Crit Care Med* 28:3098, 2000.
3. Ershler WB: Biological interactions of aging and anemia: A focus on cytokines. *J Am Geriatr Soc* 51:S18, 2003.
4. Carpenter WB: *Principles of Human Physiology*, edited by FG Smith. Blanchard and Lea, Philadelphia, 1859.
5. Wintrobe MM: *Clinical Hematology*, 5th ed. Lea & Febiger, Philadelphia, 1961.
6. Dallman PR, Yip R, Johnson C: Prevalence and causes of anemia in the United States, 1976 to 1980. *Am J Clin Nutr* 39:437, 1984.
7. Ramakrishnan U, Yip R: Experiences and challenges in industrialized countries: Control of iron deficiency in industrialized countries. *J Nutr* 132:820S, 2002.
8. Baer AN, Dessypris EN, Goldwasser E, et al: Blunted erythropoietin response to anaemia in rheumatoid arthritis. *Br J Haematol* 66:559, 1987.
9. Hochberg MC, Arnold CM, Hogans BB, et al: Serum immunoreactive erythropoietin in rheumatoid arthritis: Impaired response to anemia. *Arthritis Rheum* 31:1318, 1988.
10. Vreugdenhil G, Wognum AW, Van Eijk HG, et al: Anaemia in rheumatoid arthritis: The role of iron, vitamin B_{12}, and folic acid deficiency, and erythropoietin responsiveness. *Ann Rheum Dis* 49:93, 1990.
11. Kendall R, Wasti A, Harvey A, et al: The relationship of haemoglobin to serum erythropoietin concentrations in the anaemia of rheumatoid arthritis: The effect of oral prednisolone. *Br J Rheumatol* 32:204, 1993.
12. Noe G, Augustin J, Hausdorf S, et al: Serum erythropoietin and transferrin receptor levels in patients with rheumatoid arthritis. *Clin Exp Rheumatol* 13:445, 1995.
13. Remacha AF, Rodriguez-de la Serna A, Garcia-Die F, et al: Erythroid abnormalities in rheumatoid arthritis: The role of erythropoietin. *J Rheumatol* 19:1687, 1992.
14. Miller CB, Jones RJ, Piantadosi S, et al: Decreased erythropoietin response in patients with the anemia of cancer. *N Engl J Med* 322:1689, 1990.
15. Cazzola M, Messinger D, Battistel V, et al: Recombinant human erythropoietin in the anemia associated with multiple myeloma or non-Hodgkins lymphoma: Dose finding and identification of predictors of response. *Blood* 86:4446, 1995.
16. Safran M, Kaelin WG Jr: HIF hydroxylation and the mammalian oxygen-sensing pathway. *J Clin Invest* 111:779, 2003.
17. Imagawa S, Nakano Y, Obara N, et al: A GATA-specific inhibitor (K-7174) rescues anemia induced by IL-1β, TNF-α, or L-NMMA. *FASEB J* 17:1742, 2003.
18. Frede S, Fandrey J, Pagel H, et al: Erythropoietin gene expression is suppressed after lipopolysaccharide or interleukin-1 beta injections in rats. *Am J Physiol* 273:R1067, 1997.
19. Barany P: Inflammation, serum C-reactive protein, and erythropoietin resistance. *Nephrol Dial Transplant* 16:224, 2001.
20. Macdougall IC, Cooper AC: Erythropoietin resistance: The role of inflammation and pro-inflammatory cytokines. *Nephrol Dial Transplant* 17:39, 2002.
21. Ganz T: Hepcidin, a key regulator of iron metabolism and mediator of anemia of inflammation. *Blood* 102:783, 2003.

22. Nicolas G, Chauvet C, Viatte L, et al: The gene encoding the iron regulatory peptide hepcidin is regulated by anemia, hypoxia, and inflammation. *J Clin Invest* 110:1037, 2002.

23. Freireich EM, Miller A, Emerson CP, et al: The effect of inflammation on the utilization of erythrocyte and transferrin-bound radio-iron for red cell production. *Blood* 12:972, 1957.

24. Haurani FI, Burke W, Martinez EJ: Defective reutilization of iron in the anemia of inflammation. *J Lab Clin Med* 65:560, 1965.

25. O'Shea MJ, Kershenobich D, Tavill AS: Effects of inflammation on iron and transferrin metabolism. *Br J Haematol* 25:707, 1973.

26. Hershko C, Cook JD, Finch CA: Storage iron kinetics: VI. The effect of inflammation on iron exchange in the rat. *Br J Haematol* 28:67, 1974.

27. Zarrabi MH, Lysik R, DiStefano J, et al: The anaemia of chronic disorders: Studies of iron reutilization in the anaemia of experimental malignancy and chronic inflammation. *Br J Haematol* 35:647, 1977.

28. Feldman BF, Kaneko JJ, Farver TB: Anemia of inflammatory disease in the dog: Ferrokinetics of adjuvant-induced anemia. *Am J Vet Res* 42:583, 1981.

29. Fillet G, Beguin Y, Baldelli L: Model of reticuloendothelial iron metabolism in humans: Abnormal behavior in idiopathic hemochromatosis and in inflammation. *Blood* 74:844, 1989.

30. Nicolas G, Bennoun M, Devaux I, et al: Lack of hepcidin gene expression and severe tissue iron overload in upstream stimulatory factor 2 (USF2) knockout mice. *Proc Natl Acad Sci U S A* 98:8780, 2001.

31. Nicolas G, Bennoun M, Porteu A, et al: Severe iron deficiency anemia in transgenic mice expressing liver hepcidin. *Proc Natl Acad Sci U S A* 99:4596, 2002.

32. Hastka J, Lasserre JJ, Schwarzbeck A, et al: Zinc protoporphyrin in anemia of chronic disorders. *Blood* 81:1200, 1993.

33. Taylor JE, Peat N, Porter C, et al: Regular low-dose intravenous iron therapy improves response to erythropoietin in haemodialysis patients. *Nephrol Dial Transplant* 11:1079, 1996.

34. Goodnough LT, Skikne B, Brugnara C: Erythropoietin, iron, and erythropoiesis. *Blood* 96:823, 2000.

35. Hume R, Currie WJ, Tennant M: Anaemia of rheumatoid arthritis and iron therapy. *Ann Rheum Dis* 24:451, 1965.

36. Beamish MR, Davies AG, Eakins JD, et al: The measurement of reticuloendothelial iron release using iron-dextran. *Br J Haematol* 21:617, 1971.

37. Gubler CJ, Cartwright GE, Wintrobe MM: The anemia of infection: X. The effect of infection on the absorption and storage of iron by the rat. *J Biol Chem* 184:563, 1950.

38. Weber J, Werre JM, Julius HW, et al: Decreased iron absorption in patients with active rheumatoid arthritis, with and without iron deficiency. *Ann Rheum Dis* 47:404, 1988.

39. Weber J, Julius HW, Verhoef CW, et al: Absorption and retention of iron in rheumatoid arthritis. *Ann Rheum Dis* 32:83, 1973.

40. Anderson GJ, Frazer DM, Wilkins SJ, et al: Relationship between intestinal iron-transporter expression, hepatic hepcidin levels and the control of iron absorption. *Biochem Soc Trans* 30:724, 2002.

41. Cazzola M, Ponchio L, De Benedetti F, et al: Defective iron supply for erythropoiesis and adequate endogenous erythropoietin production in the anemia associated with systemic-onset juvenile chronic arthritis. *Blood* 87:4824, 1996.

42. Awai M, Brown EB: Studies of the metabolism of I-131-labeled human transferrin. *J Lab Clin Med* 61:363, 1963.

43. Jacobs A, Worwood M: Ferritin in serum. Clinical and biochemical implications. *N Engl J Med* 292:951, 1975.

44. Punnonen K, Irjala K, Rajamaki A: Serum transferrin receptor and its ratio to serum ferritin in the diagnosis of iron deficiency. *Blood* 89:1052, 1997.

45. Ludwig H, Fritz E, Leitgeb C, et al: Prediction of response to erythropoietin treatment in chronic anemia of cancer. *Blood* 84:1056, 1994.

46. Smith RE, Tchekmedyian NS, Chan D, et al: A dose- and schedule-finding study of darbepoetin alpha for the treatment of chronic anaemia of cancer. *Br J Cancer* 88:1851, 2003.

47. Dammacco F, Castoldi G, Rodjer S: Efficacy of epoetin alfa in the treatment of anaemia of multiple myeloma. *Br J Haematol* 113:172, 2001.

48. Hedenus M, Adriansson M, San Miguel J, et al: Efficacy and safety of darbepoetin alfa in anaemic patients with lymphoproliferative malignancies: A randomized, double-blind, placebo-controlled study. *Br J Haematol* 122:394, 2003.

49. Peeters HR, Jongen-Lavrencic M, Bakker CH, et al: Recombinant human erythropoietin improves health-related quality of life in patients with rheumatoid arthritis and anaemia of chronic disease; utility measures correlate strongly with disease activity measures. *Rheumatol Int* 18:201, 1999.

50. Peeters HR, Jongen-Lavrencic M, Vreugdenhil G, et al: Effect of recombinant human erythropoietin on anaemia and disease activity in patients with rheumatoid arthritis and anaemia of chronic disease: A randomized placebo controlled double blind 52 weeks clinical trial. *Ann Rheum Dis* 55:739, 1996.

51. Goodnough LT, Marcus RE: The erythropoietic response to erythropoietin in patients with rheumatoid arthritis. *J Lab Clin Med* 130:381, 1997.

52. Kaltwasser JP, Kessler U, Gottschalk R, et al: Effect of recombinant human erythropoietin and intravenous iron on anemia and disease activity in rheumatoid arthritis. *J Rheumatol* 28:2430, 2001.

53. Schreiber S, Howaldt S, Schnoor M, et al: Recombinant erythropoietin for the treatment of anemia in inflammatory bowel disease. *N Engl J Med* 334:619, 1996.

54. Gasche C, Dejaco C, Reinisch W, et al: Sequential treatment of anemia in ulcerative colitis with intravenous iron and erythropoietin. *Digestion* 60:262, 1999.

55. Rizzo JD, Lichtin AE, Woolf SH, et al: Use of epoetin in patients with cancer: Evidence-based clinical practice guidelines of the American Society of Clinical Oncology and the American Society of Hematology. *J Clin Oncol* 20:4083, 2002.

56. Szilagyi G, Erslev AJ: Effect of organic iron compounds on the iron uptake of reticulocytes in vitro. *J Lab Clin Med* 75:275, 1970.

57. Jurado RL: Iron, infections, and anemia of inflammation. *Clin Infect Dis* 25:888, 1997.

58. Oppenheimer SJ: Iron and its relation to immunity and infectious disease. *J Nutr* 131:616S, 2001.

59. Rossert J, Casadevall N, Eckardt KU: Anti-erythropoietin antibodies and pure red cell aplasia. *J Am Soc Nephrol* 15:398, 2004.

60. Epoetin: For better or for worse? *Lancet Oncol* 5:1, 2004.

61. Nemeth E, Tuttle MS, Powelson J, Vaughn MB, Donovan A, Ward DM, Ganz T, Kaplan J: Hepcidin regulates cellular iron efflux by binding to ferroportin and inducing its internalization. *Science* 306:2090, 2004.

62. Nemeth E, Rivera S, Gabayan V, et al: Interleukin-6 mediates hypoferremia of inflammation by inducing the synthesis of the iron-regulatory hormone hepcidin. *J Clin Invest* 113:1271, 2004.

CHAPTER 44

DISORDERS OF THE RED BLOOD CELL MEMBRANE: HEREDITARY SPHEROCYTOSIS, ELLIPTOCYTOSIS, AND RELATED DISORDERS

PATRICK G. GALLAGHER

Hereditary spherocytosis is an inherited hemolytic anemia characterized by spherically shaped erythrocytes on the blood film, reticulocytosis, and splenomegaly. The principal cellular defect is the propensity to lose membrane surface area during passage through the splenic circulation, leading to spherical shape and decreased deformability. Splenic destruction of nondeformable spherocytes leads to anemia. Membrane loss results from defects in several membrane proteins, including ankyrin, band 3, α spectrin, β spectrin, or protein 4.2. Significant clinical, laboratory, biochemical, and genetic heterogeneities exist among patients with hereditary spherocytosis. *Hereditary elliptocytosis* is characterized by the presence of elliptical erythrocytes on the blood film, often with no or very slight shortening of red cell survival. The principal defect in the erythrocyte is a mechanical weakness caused by abnormalities in the proteins involved in membrane skeleton, including α spectrin, β spectrin, protein 4.1, or glycophorin C. The majority of patients are asymptomatic, and therapy is rarely necessary. *Hereditary pyropoikilocytosis* is a rare cause of severe hemolytic anemia characterized by erythrocyte morphology similar to that seen in thermal burns. *Acanthocytosis* is characterized by the presence of contracted, dense erythrocytes with irregular projections on blood films, which may be seen in patients with severe liver disease, abetalipoproteinemia, after splenectomy, various neurologic disorders, and as a correlate of certain aberrant red cell antigens. Acanthocytes have abnormal red cell membrane lipid composition. The associated hemolysis is mild and rarely requires therapy. *Stomatocytosis* is characterized by a wide transverse slit (or stoma) in the erythrocytes of patients with a variety of acquired and inherited red cell disorders. Stomatocytosis frequently is associated with abnormal red cell cation content, hydration, and membrane lipids. Great heterogeneity in the laboratory manifestations and clinical course of the stomatocytosis syndromes is observed. The specific membrane abnormality in these disorders of cation permeability is unknown.

THE RED CELL MEMBRANE

The erythrocyte membrane accounts for 1 percent of total weight of the red cell, yet it plays an integral role in the maintenance of erythrocyte integrity. The red cell membrane and its skeleton provide the erythrocyte the flexibility, durability, and tensile strength to undergo large deformations during repeated passages through narrow microcirculatory channels. The red cell membrane maintains a slippery exterior so that erythrocytes do not adhere to endothelial cells or aggregate and occlude the microcirculation. The membrane plays an important role in metabolism by selectively and reversibly binding and inactivating glycolytic enzymes. The membrane retains organic phosphates and other vital compounds and permits efflux of metabolic waste. The membrane sequesters the reductants required to prevent damage by oxygen. During erythropoiesis, the membrane responds to erythropoietin and imports the iron required for hemoglobin synthesis. At the level of the organism, the membrane participates in the maintenance of pH homeostasis by participating in the exchange of chloride and bicarbonate.

The easy accessibility of the human erythrocyte has resulted in the erythrocyte membrane being the most thoroughly studied. Erythrocytes are the cells about which the most detailed information is available concerning the normal structure and function of their membrane and the molecular pathology of disorders caused primarily by abnormal membrane or cytoskeletal structure. The erythrocyte membrane remains the paradigm for ongoing studies of other cell types. Although the primary structure (Fig. 44-1) and a number of the important functions of the red cell membrane are known, its study continues to yield important insights into our understanding of membrane structure and function. Genetic investigation of disorders of the erythrocyte membrane has advanced our understanding of the normal structure–function relationships of the membrane and has provided us with an understanding of the inheritance and expression of these disorders.

COMPOSITION OF THE ERYTHROCYTE MEMBRANE

The erythrocyte membrane is composed of three major structural elements: a lipid bilayer primarily composed of phospholipids and cholesterol that provides a permeability barrier between the external environment and the red cell cytoplasm; integral proteins embedded in the lipid bilayer that span the membrane; and a membrane skeleton on the internal side of the red cell membrane that provides structural integrity to the cell.

MEMBRANE LIPIDS

Composition Lipids compose 50 to 60 percent of red cell membrane mass. The principal membrane lipids are phospholipids and cholesterol, which are present in nearly equal amounts.[1] Small amounts of glycolipids, primarily globoside, are present. The primary phospholipids are phosphatidylcholine (28 percent of total phospholipids), phosphatidylethanolamine ([PE] 27 percent), sphingomyelin (26 percent), phosphatidylserine ([PS] 13 percent), and phosphatidylinositol.

Membrane phosphoinositides are phospholipids that contain phosphatidylinositol (PI) or its phosphorylated forms PI-4-monophosphate (PIP) and PI-4,5-biphosphate (PIP_2). In nucleated cells, phosphoinositides are precursors of important intracellular second messengers such

Acronyms and abbreviations that appear in this chapter include: AE1, anion exchanger-1; $α^{LELY}$, low-expression Lyon α spectrin; $α^{LEPRA}$, low-expression Prague α spectrin; AQP1, aquaphorin-1; ATP, adenosine triphosphate; BPG, bisphosphoglycerate; FP, familial pseudohyperkalemia; GPC, glycophorin C; GPD, glycophorin D; GSSG, oxidized glutathione; HAc, hereditary acanthocytosis; HE, hereditary elliptocytosis; HPP, hereditary pyropoikilocytosis; HS, hereditary spherocytosis; HSt, hereditary stomatocytosis; LCAT, lecithin-cholesterol acetyltransferase; MAGUK, membrane-associated guanylate kinase; MARCKS, myristoylated alanine-rich C kinase substrate; MCHC, mean corpuscular hemoglobin concentration; MCV, mean corpuscular volume; MRP1, multidrug resistance protein-1; PE, phosphatidylethanolamine; PI, phosphatidylinositol; PS, phosphatidylserine; RhAG, Rh-associated glycoproteins; SDS, sodium dodecyl sulfate; UDPGT1, uridine diphosphoglucuronate glucuronosyltransferase.

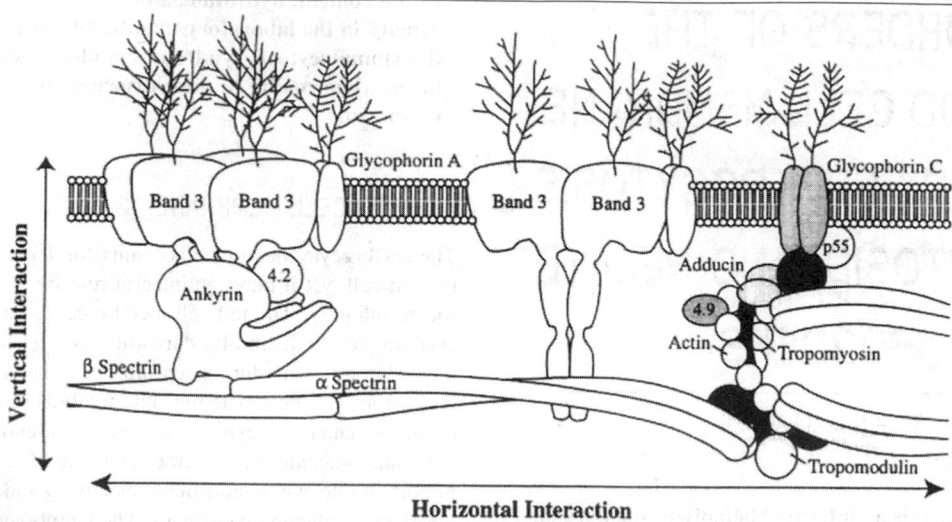

FIGURE 44-1   Schematic diagram illustrating the molecular assembly of the major erythrocyte membrane proteins and a model of the principal molecular defect in hereditary spherocytosis (HS), elliptocytosis (HE), and pyropoikilocytosis (HPP). Membrane protein–protein and protein–lipid associations can be divided into two categories: (1) *vertical interactions*, which are perpendicular to the plane of the membrane and involve spectrin–ankyrin–band 3 interaction, spectrin–protein 4.1–glycophorin C connection, and weak interactions between spectrin and the negatively charged lipids of the inner half of the membrane lipid bilayer; and (2) *horizontal interactions*, which are parallel to the plane of the membrane, and include α spectrin–β spectrin and β spectrin–protein 4.1 interactions. (From WT Tse and SE Lux, *Br J Haematol* 104:2, 1999, with permission.)

as inositol-1,4,5-triphosphate and diacylglycerol that participate in regulation of many cellular processes. In mature erythrocytes, phosphoinositides represent 2 to 5 percent of total phospholipids, residing largely at the inner membrane surface and undergoing rapid phosphorylation and dephosphorylation. In red cells, they are involved in regulation of calcium transport and interaction of transmembrane and skeletal proteins (e.g., glycophorin C and protein 4.1). They have been proposed to participate in the control of the discocyte-echinocyte shape transformation.[2]

In the erythrocyte, cholesterol is present in a free, unesterified form. It is almost entirely hydrophobic. Its primary role appears to be controlling membrane fluidity even under conditions that might lead to phospholipid crystallization and rigidification of the bilayer.

Membrane Lipid Distribution   Phospholipids are asymmetrically distributed in the red cell membrane with PS and PE primarily in the inner hemileaflet; sphingomyelin and phosphatidylcholine are outwardly oriented. This asymmetric distribution of phospholipids is a dynamic system involving a constant exchange ("flip-flop")[3] between the phospholipids of the two-bilayer leaflets. Maintenance of this asymmetry appears to be important in the regulation of hemostasis, as PS on the outer leaflet provides a site for prothrombinase binding, causing the red cell surface to become prothrombotic. Phospholipid flipping may contribute to the occurrence of thromboses in a variety of disorders, including sickle cell disease, thalassemia, and diabetes, because exposed phospholipids trigger conversion of prothrombin to thrombin and activate the coagulation cascade.[4] The presence of PS on the outer surface of the red cell is one of the earliest changes in apoptosis. It has been correlated with complement activation and red cell clearance by macrophages and liposomes.

Enzymes called *flippases* actively translocate PS and PE to the inner leaflet. *Floppases* catalyze translocation to the outer leaflet. Asymmetry seems to depend on the fact that flipping occurs at a higher rate than flopping. Flippase activity is mediated, at least in part, by a 130-kDa integral membrane protein that is a member of the Mg2+-dependent, P-glycoprotein ATPases family.[5] Floppase activity in red cell membranes appears to be mediated by the multidrug resistance protein-1 (MRP1).[6]

A *scramblase* activated by elevated intracellular calcium that promotes randomization and loss of asymmetry has been isolated and cloned.[7] Scramblase mediates redistribution of membrane phospholipids in activated, injured, or apoptotic cells.[8] Derangements within the red cell often raise intracellular calcium by direct or indirect damage to ion channels and pumps. Scott syndrome is a congenital bleeding disorder in which red cells and platelets expose subnormal amounts of PS on the outer surface in response to calcium, but the situation does not appear to result from scramblase deficiency.[9,10]

Glycolipids and cholesterol are intercalated between the phospholipids in the bilayer, with their long axes perpendicular to the bilayer plane. Red cell glycolipids are located entirely in the external half of the bilayer, with their carbohydrate moieties extending into the aqueous phase. They carry several important red cell antigens, including A, B, H, and P, and they may serve other important functions. The location of membrane cholesterol is less certain, but cholesterol appears to be present in about equal proportions on both sides of the bilayer.

Detergent-resistant membrane domains or lipid rafts are present in erythrocytes.[11] These membrane microdomains contain stomatin, flotillin-1 and flotillin-2, the Duffy receptor, heterotrimeric Gαs, CD55, CD58, and CD59. Alterations in erythrocyte calcium lead to shedding of rafts as large vesicles containing stomatin and small vesicles containing synexin and sorcin.[12] Neither of these vesicles contains flotillin. Lipid rafts play an important role in protein recruitment to the malarial parasite vacuole during erythrocyte invasion.[13]

Lipid Synthesis and Renewal   Synthesis and assembly of red cell membrane lipids occurs during erythropoiesis. Mature erythrocytes are unable to synthesize fatty acids, phospholipids, or cholesterol *de novo*. They depend on lipid exchange and fatty acid acylation for phospholipid repair and renewal. These renewal pathways, although limited, permit slow replacement of membrane lipid components.[14]

Lipid exchange rates vary considerably. Exchange of unesterified cholesterol occurs in several hours. Outer bilayer phospholipid phosphatidylcholine and sphingomyelin exchange with the phospholipids of plasma lipoproteins occurs over a period of days.[15,16] Because of their inaccessibility, the inner bilayer phospholipids PS and PE are unable to participate in lipid exchange.[15] Unesterified membrane cholesterol exchanges readily with the unesterified cholesterol in plasma lipoproteins, where the unesterified membrane cholesterol is partially converted to esterified cholesterol by lecithin-cholesterol acyltransferase (LCAT). Because the newly formed cholesteryl ester cannot return to the red cell membrane, LCAT catalyzes a unidirectional pathway that depletes the membrane of cholesterol and decreases its surface area. Virtually no esterified cholesterol is present in the membrane. The process is reversed when LCAT is absent or inactive, leading to a net accumulation of free cholesterol in the cells.

In addition to passive exchange, free fatty acids can be incorporated into red cell phospholipids in a two-step reaction requiring lysophospholipid, ATP, magnesium, and coenzyme A.[17] Following acyl-coenzyme A formation, the fatty acid is incorporated into the lysophospholipid at the inner bilayer leaflet. This pathway also participates in maintenance of phospholipid asymmetry, as evidenced by rapid outward translocation of the newly synthesized phosphatidylcholine.[18] Although this pathway consumes a small amount of energy, it may be important for detoxification of naturally formed lysophosphatides in the cells, as evidenced by their gradual accumulation during ATP depletion.

Lipid Bilayer Fluidity Under physiologic conditions, the lipid bilayer is in a liquid state, allowing transmembrane proteins and cell surface molecules (such as surface antigens) to move in the plane of the membrane. Lipid bilayer fluidity is influenced by several factors, including (1) temperature, which determines the phase transition between a liquid state and gel state; (2) free cholesterol content, as the rigid sterol ring of cholesterol decreases lipid bilayer fluidity; and (3) the length and degree of phospholipid fatty acid saturation. Saturated fatty acids with a relatively rigid backbone resist motion, whereas unsaturated fatty acids have relatively unrestricted movements, thereby increasing the fluidity of the lipid bilayer. Because of the differences in the composition of phospholipids between the two-bilayer halves, the bilayer is asymmetric in terms of the fluidity of the two hemileaflets.[17,18]

MEMBRANE PROTEINS

Several general observations can be made about erythrocyte membrane proteins. Most of these proteins also are present in nonerythroid cells, where they fulfill similar functions. Many of the proteins are members of superfamilies of proteins that are structurally related but genetically distinct. This genetic diversity explains why the clinical expression of many (but not all) red cell membrane protein mutations is confined to the erythroid lineage. Tissue- and developmental stage-specific alternative splicing or use of alternate initiation codons or alternate promoters creates multiple isoforms of many of these proteins. Finally, many are large, multifunctional proteins. As a result, mutations within a given region of the protein may lead to distinct differences in abnormalities of function and clinical phenotype.

Membrane proteins are classified according to the ease with which they can be removed from whole red cell membrane preparations in the laboratory. Integral proteins are firmly embedded into or through the lipid bilayer by hydrophobic domains within their amino acid sequences; only harsh reagents such as detergents can extract them. Peripheral proteins are more loosely associated; they are extractable by high or low salt or by high pH. Peripheral proteins are attached indirectly to the lipid bilayer by covalent or noncovalent binding to the (usually) cytoplasmic domains of embedded or anchored proteins. Peripheral proteins typically are associated with the interior or cytoplasmic face, whereas many integral proteins often protrude into both spaces. The affinity with which proteins associate with the membrane is not a static property. Rather, proteins can become more or less tightly bound according to their state of phosphorylation, methylation, glycosylation, or lipid modification (myristylation, palmitoylation, or farnesylation).[2]

Fairbanks and colleagues[19] assigned names to the proteins extracted from red cell membranes (see Fig. 44-1 and Table 44-1).[19] These designations were based on protein mobility in a sodium dodecyl sulfate (SDS)-acrylamide gel system. The slowest migrating band was band (or protein) 1, the next slowest band was band 2, and so on. Subbands were designated with decimals. After further analysis, some of these proteins, such as bands 1 and 2, were renamed α and β spectrin. Other proteins, such as protein 4.1, were never renamed.

INTEGRAL MEMBRANE PROTEINS

Band 3 This protein (*syn.* anion exchanger-1 [AE1]) is an abundant (10^6 copies per cell) transmembrane glycoprotein with a molecular mass of approximately 100 kDa. It serves as a regulator of ion content, red cell deformability, intermediary metabolism, and possibly red cell senescence.[20] The NH_2-terminus of the protein encodes a 43-kDa cytoplasmic domain with COOH-terminus of the protein folded into helices and β sheets to form the membrane-spanning domain. The region between the NH_2-terminus and the first membrane-spanning segment forms an interhinge domain.

Band 3 is the major anion (chloride–bicarbonate) exchanger of the red cell. It regulates metabolic pathways by sequestering key pathway enzymes, such as the glycolytic enzymes glyceraldehyde-3-phosphate dehydrogenase, phosphoglycerate kinase, and aldolase, and carbonic anhydrase II and IV. Band 3 contains important binding sites for interaction with other membrane proteins, including ankyrin, protein 4.1, protein 4.2, and the Rh–Rh-associated glycoproteins (RhAG) complex.[21,22] Binding of the cytoplasmic domain to ankyrin is one of the critical mechanisms for attachment of the membrane skeleton to the plasma membrane. The interdomain hinge at this attachment point may be a crucial determinant of the flexibility or rigidity of the erythrocyte.[23]

Extracellular domain polymorphisms of band 3 are the antigens for several blood groups, including the Diego and Wright blood groups, and several other low-incidence antigens.

Glycophorins Glycophorins are the most abundant integral membrane glycoproteins in erythrocytes. Because of their high sialic acid content, they account for more than 95 percent of the periodic acid–Schiff (PAS)-staining capacity of erythrocytes.[24] The glycophorins are O-glycosylated. They are composed of a single extracellular hydrophilic NH_2-terminal domain, a single membrane-spanning domain, and a COOH-terminal cytoplasmic tail. Characterization of cDNA and genomic clones encoding the glycophorins has revealed they fall into two distinct subgroups. Glycophorins A and B are homologous to each other and are encoded by two closely linked genes. Glycophorin C (GPC) and glycophorin D (GPD) arise from a single locus bearing no particular homology to the genes for glycophorins A and B. GPD differs from GPC by use of an alternate translation start site created by alternative splicing.

Glycophorins constitute more than 60 percent of the net negative surface charge of red cells; thus, they may modulate red cell–red cell and red cell–endothelial cell interactions. GPC, which interacts in a complex with protein 4.1 and p55, plays a critical role in regulating the stability, deformability, and shape of the membrane. GPC deficiency leads to elliptocytic erythrocytes that are less stable and

TABLE 44-1 MAJOR RED CELL MEMBRANE PROTEINS

BAND	PROTEIN	M_r (GEL)	M_r (CALC)	COPIES PER CELL ($\times 10^3$)	PERCENTAGE OF TOTAL[a]	GENE SYMBOL	CHROMOSOMAL LOCALIZATION	AMINO ACIDS	GENE SIZE (KB)	NO. OF EXONS	INVOLVEMENT IN HEMOLYTIC ANEMIAS
1	α Spectrin	240	280	240	16	SPTA1	1q22-q23	2429	80	52	HE, HS
2	β Spectrin	220	246	240	14	SPTB	14q23-q24.2	2137	>100	32	HE, HS
2.1	Ankyrin[b]	210	206	120	4.5	ANK1	8p11.2	1881	>100	40	HS
2.9	α Adducin[c]	103	81	30	2	ADDA	4p16.3	737	85	16	N
2.9	β Adducin[c]	97	80	30	2	ADDB	2p13-2p14	726	~100	17	N
3	Anion exchanger-1	90–100	102	1200	27	EPB3	17q21-qter	911	17	20	HS, SAO, HAc
4.1	Protein 4.1	80	66	200	5	EL11	1p33-p34.2	588[d]	>100	23	HE
4.2	Protein 4.2	72	77	200	5	EB42	15q15-q21	691	20	13	HS
4.9	Dematin[e]	48 + 52	43	40[f]	1	EPB49	8p21.1	383	—	—	N
4.9	p55[e]		55	53	80	—	MPP1	Xq28	466	—	—	N
5	β-Actin	43	42	400–500	5.5	ACTB	7pter-q22	375	>4	6	N
5	Tropomodulin	43	41	30	—	TMOD	9q22	359	—	—	N
6	G-3P-D[g]	35	37	500	3.5[g]	GAPD	12p13.31-p13.1	335	5	9	N
7	Stomatin	31	32	—	2.5	EPB72	9q33-q34	288	12	7	HSt
7	Tropomyosin	27 + 29	28	80	1	TPM3	1q31	239	—	—	N
PAS-1	Glycophorin A[h]	36	—	500–1000	85	GYPA	4q28-q31	131	>40	7	HE
PAS-2	Glycophorin C[h]	32	14	50–100	4	GYPC	2q14-q21	128	14	4	HE
PAS-3	Glycophorin B[h]	20	—	100–300	10	GYPB	4q28-q31	72	>30	5	N
	Glycophorin D[h]	23	—	20	1	GYPD	2q14-q21	107	14	4	N
	Glycophorin E	—	—	—	—	GYPE	4q28-q31	59	>30	4	N

[a] Quantitation based on scanning of SDS-PAGE gels of red cell membranes prepared from healthy blood donors. For glycophorins, values indicate the fraction of PAS-positive material.

[b] Bands 2.1, 2.2, 2.3, and 2.6 are protein isoforms of erythroid ankyrin, at least some of which are produced by alternative splicing of ankyrin mRNA.

[c] Because adducin comigrates with band 3, no numerical band designation is available.

[d] Numerous erythroid and nonerythroid isoforms of protein 4.1 produced by alternative splicing have been described. Values correspond to the major erythroid protein 4.1 isoform.

[e] Both dematin and p55 migrate within the 4.9 band.

[f] 40,000 of dematin trimers are present in one red cell.

[g] Variable amounts of band 6 are detected in red cell membranes.

[h] Detectable on PAS-stained gels only.

G-3-PD-glyceraldehyde, 3-phosphate dehydrogenase; HAc, hereditary acanthocytosis; HE, hereditary elliptocytosis; HPP, hereditary pyropoikilocytosis; HS, hereditary spherocytosis; HSt, hereditary stomatocytosis; N, no hematologic abnormalities reported; SAO, Southeast Asian ovalocytosis.

less deformable than normal red cells. Glycophorins serve as receptors for several infectious agents, including *Plasmodium falciparum*. The glycophorins carry a number of blood group antigens, including MN, Ss, Miltenberger V, En(a-), $M^K M^k$, and Gerbich (see Chap. 128).

Other Integral Membrane Proteins The red cell membrane contains other integral membrane proteins, including a number involved in clinical immunohematology, such as the Rh proteins (see Chap. 128), the Xk and Kell glycoprotein, and the Kidd, Duffy, and Lutheran glycoproteins. Rh proteins are part of a macromolecular complex composed of two Rh proteins, two RhAGs, CD47, LW glycoprotein, glycophorin B, and protein 4.2.[25,26] The Rh–RhAG complex interacts with ankyrin to link the membrane skeleton to the lipid bilayer. Evidence demonstrates Rh–RhAG complex linkage to band 3.[22]

Additional integral membrane proteins include stomatin, the LW protein, which may be involved in macrophage–erythroblast interactions during erythropoiesis, and various ion pumps and channels (see "Function of the Erythrocyte Membrane" below).

PERIPHERAL MEMBRANE PROTEINS

The major proteins of the erythrocyte membrane skeleton are spectrin, ankyrin, actin, proteins 4.1, 4.2, and 4.9, p55, and the adducins. These proteins form an interlocking network that attaches to the inner face of the membrane, primarily by binding to the cytoplasmic domains of band 3 and the glycophorins.

Spectrin This protein is the most abundant and largest in the erythrocyte membrane skeleton, constituting 75 percent of erythrocyte mass and present at a concentration of approximately 200,000 molecules per cell.[27] Spectrin is composed of two subunits, α and β, which, despite many similarities, are structurally distinct and encoded by separate genes (Fig. 44-2).[28] Both α and β spectrin contain homologous 106-amino-acid repeats that are folded into α-helical segments containing three antiparallel helices connected by short nonhelical segments. The presence of spectrin repeats suggests spectrin evolved from duplication of a single ancestral gene.[29]

The fundamental structure of the spectrin molecule is that of $\alpha\beta$ heterodimers that align and intertwine with each other in antiparallel fashion with respect to their NH_2-termini to form flexible, rod-like molecules (see Fig. 44-2).[27] These dimers further self-associate to form tetramers and higher-order oligomers. These tetramers, composed of multiple repeats, provide a strong, elastic, rod-like filament that associates into multimolecular complexes capable of lending shape and resiliency to the overlying plasma membrane via formation of a lattice-like meshwork linked to integral membrane proteins.[30] Direct interactions of a weaker nature also may occur between spectrin filaments and the lipid bilayer itself. The side-to-side assembly of α- and β-spectrin chains in a zipper-like fashion begins at a defined nucleation site composed of four repeats from each chain, α19 to α22 and β1 to β4, respectively.[31] After tight association of complementary nucleation sites, a conformational change is initiated that promotes pairing of the remainder of the two chains. A common α-spectrin variant, α^{LELY} (low-expression Lyon), interferes with normal nucleation and decreases the synthesis of functionally competent spectrin chains and may influence clinical expression of spectrin mutations (see "Membrane Biogenesis and Aging" below).[32]

The NH_2-terminus of α spectrin and the COOH-terminus of β spectrin are the regions involved in $\alpha\beta$ heterodimer self-association.[27]

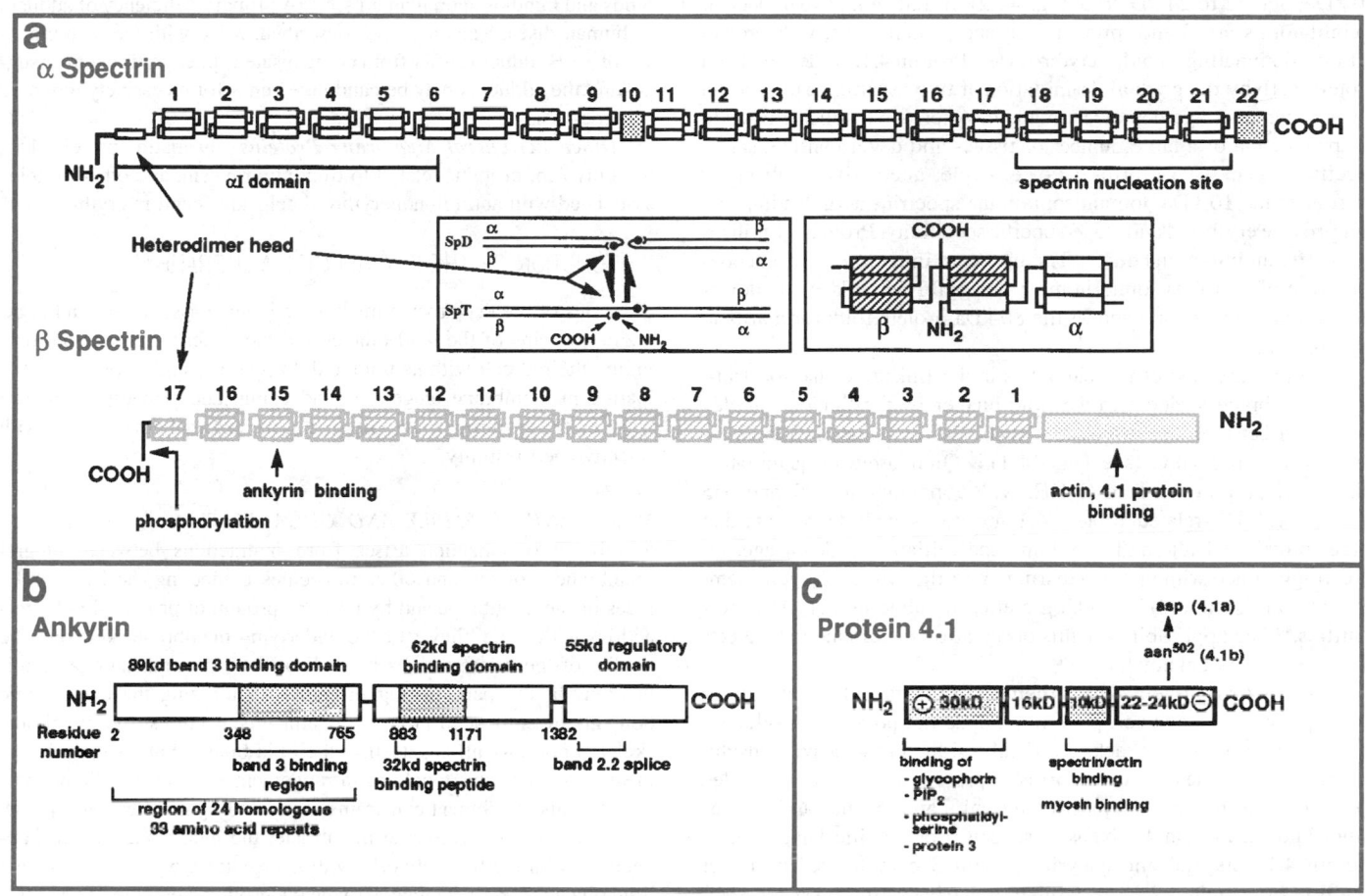

FIGURE 44-2   Spectrin, ankyrin, and protein 4.1. (a) α spectrin and β spectrin. Both proteins are composed of multiple homologous triple helical repetitive segments, numbered starting from the NH₂-terminus. α spectrin and β spectrin are shown in antiparallel orientation, their configuration in the spectrin heterodimer. *Stippled regions* represent nonhomologous segments. The αI domain (a tryptic peptide of α spectrin involved in spectrin self association), the spectrin nucleation site, and the ankyrin, actin, and protein 4.1 protein-binding sites are shown. In the head region of spectrin, α and β spectrin interact, forming either a heterodimer (SpD) or tetramer (SpT). The contact site between the α and β chains of a spectrin heterodimer or the opposed α and β chains of the tetramer is formed by a combined αβ triple helical segment (*inset*). (b) Ankyrin. The three major functional and structural domains, as defined by limited proteolytic digestion, are shown. The band 3 and spectrin-binding regions are *shaded*. The regulatory domain is subject to extensive alternative splicing, including the band 2.2 splice, which produces an activated form of ankyrin. (c) Protein 4.1. The four major functional and structural domains, as defined by limited proteolytic digestion, are shown. The regions where the 4.1 protein binds to other membrane proteins are *shaded*. The protein 4.1a isoform is derived from the 4.1b isoform by deamidation asparagine 508.

Spectrin also binds to actin and protein 4.1 via the NH₂-terminus of β spectrin and ankyrin via sites in repeats β15 and β16 near the COOH-terminus, respectively.[33,34] Other nonrepeat sequences in spectrin provide the recognition sites for binding to other modifiers, including kinases and calmodulin.

The functions of spectrin are to maintain cellular shape, regulate the lateral mobility of integral membrane proteins, and provide structural support for the lipid bilayer. Defects in the αβ self-association site are associated with hereditary elliptocytosis (HE) and hereditary pyropoikilocytosis (HPP). Compound heterozygosity or homozygosity for defects outside the αβ self-association site is associated with severe, recessively inherited spherocytosis.

Ankyrin   This asymmetric polar protein can be separated into three functional domains by mild proteolysis: an NH₂-terminal membrane-binding domain that contains sites for band 3 and other ligands, a central domain that contains sites for spectrin binding, and a COOH-terminal "regulatory" domain that influences ankyrin–protein interactions (see Fig. 44-2).[27,35] The membrane-binding domain contains 24 tandem repeats called *cdc10/ankyrin repeats*, which contain mul-

tiple protein-binding sites.[36] Ankyrin repeats are highly conserved, L-shaped structures composed of a pair of α-helices that form an antiparallel coiled-coil, followed by an extended loop perpendicular to the helices and a β hairpin.[37] These repeats have been found in proteins with a wide variety of functions. The regulatory domain consists of multiple isoforms generated by alternative splicing.[36] One of these isoforms (ankyrin 2.2) enhances ankyrin binding to band 3 and spectrin.

Ankyrin provides the primary linkage between the membrane skeleton via spectrin binding and the lipid bilayer via band 3 binding and interaction with the Rh–RhAG complex. Disruption of any of these linkages significantly decreases membrane stability. Ankyrin also appears to be involved in local segregation of integral membrane proteins within functional domains on the plasma membrane. The importance of ankyrin in the maintenance of membrane stability is underscored by the observation that abnormalities of ankyrin are the most common cause of typical hereditary spherocytosis (HS).

Protein 4.1   This phosphoprotein can be separated by mild chymotryptic digestion into four proteolytic domains: 30 kDa, 16 kD,

10 kDa, and 22 to 24 kDa (see Fig. 44-2). In red cells, two molecular weight forms are found, protein 4.1a and protein 4.1b, with protein 4.1a predominating in older erythrocytes. Protein 4.1a is derived from protein 4.1b by the gradual deamidation of two asparagine residues in a nonenzymatic, age-dependent manner. Alternative splicing leads to the production of a large number of tissue- and developmental stage-specific protein 4.1 isoforms.[38] For example, alternatively spliced isoforms of the 10 kDa domain contain the spectrin–actin binding site and provide erythroid and stage-specific specificity. Protein 4.1 utilizes two different initiation codons. The upstream initiation codon encodes a protein of 135 kDa found in most nonerythroid cells.[38] The downstream initiation codon encodes the 80-kDa protein found primarily in erythrocytes.

The primary role of protein 4.1 is in the linkage of the spectrin–actin membrane skeleton to the lipid bilayer by facilitating complex formation between spectrin–actin fibers, the cytoplasmic domain of band 3, and p55/GPC (see Fig. 44-1).[27] Qualitative or quantitative defects of protein 4.1 lead to HE, with concomitant GPC and p55 deficiency.[39] HE-related protein 4.1 mutations include variants that affect protein 4.1 alternative splicing and initiation codon usage. Interestingly, mice with targeted disruption of the protein 4.1 gene demonstrate, in addition to hematologic effects, subtle neurologic abnormalities.[40] The applicability of this observation to humans with defects of protein 4.1 is unknown.

Protein 4.2   Protein 4.2 is a member of the transglutaminase family of proteins.[41] However, protein 4.2 does not possess transglutaminase activity because it lacks a critical residue in the active transglutaminase site. At least four isoforms of protein 4.2 have been created by alternative splicing; the functional significance of the four isoforms is not known. Protein 4.2 binds to several proteins, including band 3, protein 4.1, ankyrin, and ankyrin–protein 3 complexes. The major function of protein 4.2 is to stabilize spectrin–actin–ankyrin association with band 3. It also may protect the membrane skeleton from premature aging by binding calcium and other cofactors that normally activate red cell transglutaminases, as these transglutaminases otherwise would cross-link proteins and lead to their inactivation. Deficiency of protein 4.2 has been associated with recessively inherited HS. Erythrocytes from mice with targeted inactivation of the protein 4.2 gene are dehydrated spherocytes with altered cation content (increased K^+/decreased Na^+).[42]

p55   This molecule is a phosphoprotein member of the membrane-associated guanylate kinase (MAGUK) family of proteins.[43] Homologues of p55 include signal transduction proteins, tumor suppressor genes, and proteins important in cell–cell interactions. The p55 molecule binds to protein 4.1 through a binding motif in the COOH-terminal MAGUK domain and to GPC via a PDZ motif.[43] A primary deficiency state for p55 has not been described, possibly because it is a widely expressed protein. p55 may play a critical role in protein–protein interactions in other tissues. Deficiency of protein 4.1 or GPC leads to concomitant p55 deficiency. Studies of this interesting protein may shed important light on mechanisms whereby the erythrocyte membrane influences other cellular processes.

Actin   The erythrocyte contains β-type actin assembled into short F-actin protofilaments of 12 to 18 monomers. Actin protofilaments are capped at the pointed end by tropomodulin and at the barbed end by adducin.

Adducin   Adducin, a calcium/calmodulin-binding phosphoprotein located at the spectrin–actin junctional complex, is composed of αβ adducin heterodimers. α and β adducin are structurally similar proteins encoded by separate genes. Adducin contains a myristoylated alanine-rich C kinase substrate (MARCKS) phosphorylation domain that regulates calcium/calmodulin-regulated capping and bundling of actin filaments. Adducin promotes interaction of spectrin and actin and

binds and bundles actin filaments.[44,45] A primary deficiency of adducin in human disease has not been described. Mice with targeted inactivation of β adducin suffer from compensated spherocytic anemia, suggesting the adducins may be candidate genes for recessively inherited spherocytosis.[46]

Other Peripheral Membrane Proteins   Dematin (protein 4.9), tropomyosin, proteins related to troponin, myosin, and other proteins associated with actin in nonerythroid cells are found in erythrocytes.

FUNCTION OF THE ERYTHROCYTE MEMBRANE

The roles of the erythrocyte membrane include assembling and organizing proteins of the lipid bilayer and the underlying skeleton, providing the red cell with its unique deformability and stability, participating in membrane biogenesis and aging, and providing a barrier between the erythrocyte cytoplasm and the external environment with selective permeability.

MEMBRANE ASSEMBLY AND ORGANIZATION

Membrane organization arises from interactions between integral membrane proteins and other molecules contacting the hydrophilic faces of the membrane and by protein–protein or protein–lipid interactions within the bilayer or the underlying membrane skeleton. The avidity of these interactions is modulated by posttranslational modifications of the participating proteins. By utilizing the cytoplasmic domains of embedded proteins as attachment points, the membrane skeleton not only affixes itself to the lipid bilayer but also provides a means to order the topologic arrangement of transmembrane proteins.[47] This attachment constrains motion along the transverse plane.

In the intact erythrocyte membrane, the membrane skeleton appears as a lattice-like network, with approximately 60 percent of the lipid bilayer directly laminated to the underlying membrane skeleton.[48] When skeletal preparations are stretched, the individual skeletal proteins can be visualized as a highly ordered lattice of hexagons. The corners of each hexagon are globular structures called the *junctional complex*, composed of complexes of F-actin, dematin, adducin, and protein 4.1.[49] Spectrin tetramers form the arms of the hexagons, cross-bridging individual junctional complexes. Spectrin cross-bridges are largely formed by spectrin tetramers, with occasional double tetramers or hexamers. Each spectrin tetramer is composed of two αβ heterodimers assembled at their "head" regions into tetramers. At their tails, the tetramers bind to junctional complexes of actin, with the aid of protein 4.1 and adducin. The *horizontal* protein contacts are important in the maintenance of the structural integrity of the cell, accounting for the high tensile strength of the erythrocyte (see Fig. 44-1).

The skeleton is affixed to the integral proteins of the membrane by several protein–protein interactions.[27] Spectrin tetramers are connected to ankyrin, the major skeleton/membrane linkage protein via an interaction site in β spectrin. Ankyrin links the underlying spectrin skeleton to tetramers of band 3, the major transmembrane protein of the red cell, and the Rh–RhAG complex. At the distal ends of spectrin tetramers, spectrin binds to the membrane via linkage to protein 4.1, which binds GPC and protein p55. In addition, both spectrin and protein 4.1 bind weakly to PS, which preferentially is located at the inner leaflet of the lipid bilayer. These *vertical* protein–protein and protein–lipid interactions are critical in the stabilization of the lipid bilayer, precluding its loss from the cells (see Fig. 44-1).

Hereditary spherocytosis is characterized by defects of *vertical* interactions, which lead to uncoupling of the lipid bilayer from the skeleton and a release of membrane microvesicles. In contrast, the principal defects in HE and pyropoikilocytosis involve *horizontal* interactions of membrane skeletal proteins, for example, interactions between α spectrin and spectrin that maintain the two-dimensional integrity of the skeleton. Overall, membrane protein interactions are more complex than this model but are a good starting point for understanding the pathophysiologic effects of membrane protein mutations. For instance, spectrin mutations that cause hemolytic anemia and do not directly destabilize spectrin self-association or spectrin–ankyrin binding have been described. These mutations disrupt cooperative interactions between proteins of the membrane skeleton, linkage adaptor proteins, and/or proteins of the lipid bilayer.[50]

Red cell membrane proteins are subject to a variety of posttranslational modifications or other regulatory effects, including phosphorylation, fatty acid acylation, methylation, glycosylation, deamidation, oxidation, and limited proteolytic cleavage.[2] With the exception of membrane protein phosphorylation, such modifications are relatively static and irreversible. In contrast, membrane protein phosphorylation represents a highly dynamic system of multiple protein kinases and phosphatases that constantly phosphorylate and dephosphorylate serine, threonine, and tyrosine residues, often in a manner that is amino acid and protein site specific, thereby tightly regulating association of membrane proteins. Additionally, membrane protein associations are influenced by a variety of intracellular factors, including calcium, calmodulin, phosphoinositides, and polyanions such as 2,3-bisphosphoglycerate (BPG).

The red cell surface is negatively charged, primarily because of a high concentration of neuraminic acid residues. Ninety percent of the residues reside on glycophorin A; the remainder are shared by the other glycophorins and band 3. Alterations in erythrocyte surface charge appear to have deleterious effects on the cell. For example, in sickle red cells, surface charge clustering may play a role in the adhesion of these cells to the surface of endothelial cells.

CELLULAR DEFORMABILITY AND MEMBRANE STABILITY

The most important property of red cells required for normal survival is cellular deformability.[51] *Deformability* refers to the ability of the erythrocyte to undergo distortions and deformations and then to resume its normal shape without fragmentation or loss of integrity. This situation is best exemplified in the wall of the splenic sinus, where red cells squeeze through narrow slits among the endothelial cells lining the splenic sinus wall. The cellular deformability of erythrocytes is determined by three factors: (1) cell geometry (biconcave disc shape); (2) cytoplasmic viscosity, principally determined by the properties and the concentration of hemoglobin in the cells; and (3) intrinsic viscoelastic properties of the red cell membrane (or membrane deformability). Among the three factors, cell geometry as determined by the contribution of the surface to volume ratio is the most important, as exemplified by the cellular lesion of hereditary spherocytes. On the other hand, the intrinsic viscoelastic properties of the red cell likely have a relatively small effect on red cell survival. Southeast Asian ovalocytes are very rigid, yet they have a normal survival *in vivo*.

The cellular geometry, that is, the biconcave disc shape of red cells, is critical for the cells' survival. This cell surface shape provides a high ratio of surface area to cellular volume. The normal volume of the erythrocyte is approximately 90 μm^3. The minimum surface area that could encase this volume is a sphere of approximately 98 μm^3. The surface area of a biconcave disc enclosing this volume is approximately 140 μm^3. Thus, shape alone provides the red cell with a considerable amount of redundant membrane and cytoskeleton. This feature provides the extra membrane surface area needed when red cells swell. More importantly, this geometric arrangement allows red cells to stretch as they undergo deformation and distortion in response to the mechanical stress of the circulation. Loss of membrane by partial phagocytosis in immune hemolytic anemias or by fragmentation of bits of membrane from the cell in patients with cytoskeletal defects leads to elliptocytic or spherocytic shapes having greatly reduced sur-

face area and, therefore, much less deformability.[52] The consequent reduction in tolerance of these cells to osmotic stress explains why anemias resulting from membrane defects often are accompanied by osmotic fragility, the basis for the clinical laboratory test. Similarly, if erythrocytes are engorged with water, they become macrospherocytic and less deformable.

Thus, the organization of the membrane skeleton and its attachment to the plasma membrane influence the stability and deformability of the red cell. In the resting state, the folded helical segments of spectrin are highly coiled. Membrane deformation is accompanied by a rearrangement of the spectrin–actin-based membrane skeleton network. Some spectrin molecules become uncoiled and extended, whereas others become more compressed and folded, resulting in no net change in surface area. Thus, shape changes but surface area does not. The extent to which stretching and compression are possible determines the extent of deformability. Mutations or acquired alterations in membrane proteins that influence the spectrin–actin-based lattice of proteins leads to membrane loss with a concomitant decrease in surface area and a change in cell geometry.

Red cell viscosity is largely determined by hemoglobin content.[52] At normal intracellular concentrations (27–35g/dl), viscosity contributes very little to cellular deformability. When erythrocytes become dehydrated, the effective intracellular hemoglobin concentration rises, and viscosity increases exponentially. Membrane pumps and channels normally maintain intracellular volumes that hold hemoglobin concentrations below the level at which cytoplasmic viscosity has an impact on deformability. Inherited anomalies of pumps or channels (e.g., hereditary xerocytosis) or derangements caused by polymerized or crystallized hemoglobin (e.g., sickle cell anemia or hemoglobin C disease), lead to cellular dehydration and greatly increased red cell viscosity.

MEMBRANE MATERIAL PROPERTIES

The material properties of the membrane reflect the properties of the lipid bilayer and the skeleton. During deformation, the membrane undergoes bending, which is restricted by the incompressibility of the lipid bilayer. Such bending has been proposed to be facilitated by rapid translocation of cholesterol from the inner to the outer hemileaflet (Fig. 44-3). Red cells that are suspended in hypotonic solutions, as during osmotic fragility testing (see "Laboratory Features" below), swell. They reach a nearly spherical shape because the bilayer membrane cannot expand its surface area more than 3 to 4 percent. Further lowering of osmotic pressure results in membrane rupture, and intracellular hemoglobin is discharged into the supernatant.

The membrane skeleton determines both the solid and semisolid properties of the membrane. The solid properties are exemplified by an elastic extension of cells that completely restores their normal shape after the applied force is removed. An example is a cell that was deformed when it passed through fenestrations of the splenic sinus wall. The elastic recovery of normal shape is facilitated by the unique molecular anatomy of the skeletal lattice. Here the individual hexagons are in a compact, unextended configuration, with the junctional complexes close to each other and the cross-linking arms of spectrin tetramers folded between them, thus allowing large unidirectional extensions without disruption of the lattice (see Fig. 44-3). The skeleton remains unperturbed during such deformation. On the other hand, application of large or prolonged forces allows the skeletal elements to reorganize into a new configuration, producing a permanent plastic deformation. When the force is excessive, membrane fragmentation ensues. An example is when red cells are trapped by fibrin strands in damaged vessels (see Chap. 49). After release from this site, the erythrocytes either are permanently deformed or are fragmented.

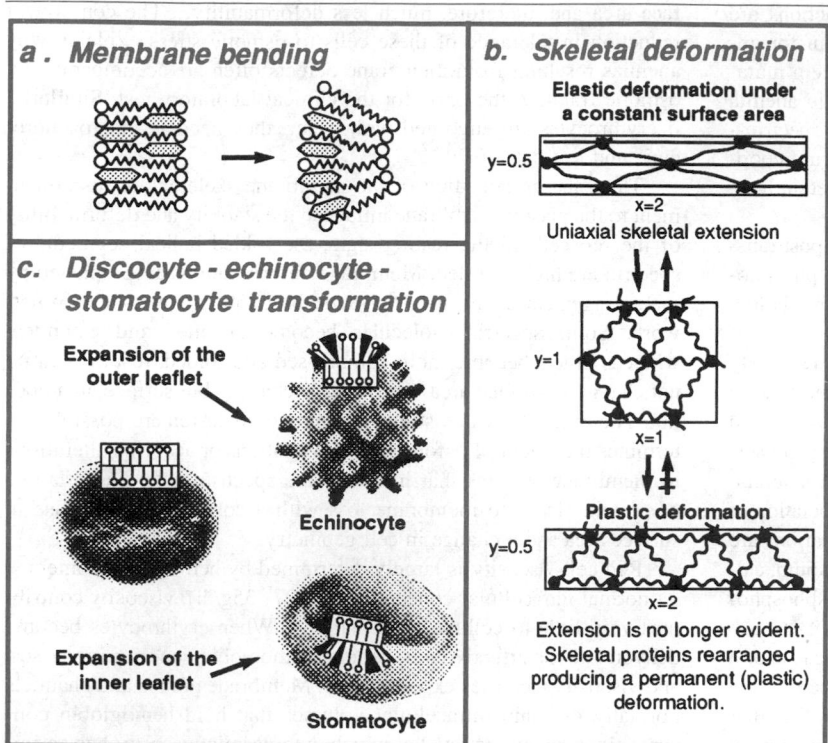

FIGURE 44-3   Material properties of the red cell membrane. (*a*) Membrane bending. The degree of membrane bending is restricted by the limited compressibility of the lipid bilayer. Rapid translocation of cholesterol (*shaded diamonds*) from the inner to the outer leaflet reduces compression of the inner bilayer leaflet, thereby facilitating bending. (*b*) Skeletal deformation. Although hydrophobicity of the red cell membrane lipid bilayer precludes the increase in its surface area without rupture, the membrane can undergo a large deformation under a constant surface area because of the viscoelastic properties of the membrane skeleton. During uniaxial extension, the skeleton undergoes stretching (*top rectangle*). After cessation of an external force, a square surface area is resumed because the protein connections within this elastic skeletal network remain intact. Extensive or prolonged uniaxial extension leads to rearrangement of the skeletal network because of disruption of existing skeletal protein connections and formation of new protein contacts. This process leads to a permanent plastic deformation (*bottom rectangle*). (*c*) Bilayer couple hypothesis and stomatocyte–discocyte–echinocyte transformation. Red cell shape reflects the ratio of the surface areas of the two hemileaflets of the lipid bilayer. The compounds (*black triangles*) that preferentially intercalate into the outer hemileaflet of the lipid bilayer produce its expansion, followed by red cell crenation (echinocytosis or acanthocytosis). In contrast, expansion of the inner lipid bilayer leaflet produces a cup shape (stomatocytosis) and surface invaginations.

MEMBRANE BIOGENESIS AND AGING

Membrane protein biosynthesis occurs asynchronously during erythropoiesis. Early in erythroid development, the major proteins of the membrane skeleton (spectrin, ankyrin, and protein 4.1) are synthesized.[53] However, they turn over rapidly and do not assemble into a permanent network. At the proerythroblast stage, synthesis of band 3 is initiated and, with synthesis of protein 4.1, increases up to the late erythroblast stage. During this time, mRNA levels and synthesis of spectrin and ankyrin protein decline. In contrast, the fraction of newly assembled spectrin and ankyrin protein on the membrane progressively increases, and the turnover of these proteins on the membrane declines.

Increased recruitment and stabilization of spectrin and ankyrin on the membrane despite declining synthesis of these proteins is temporally related to a progressive increase in the synthesis of band 3 and protein 4.1, the principal bilayer anchors of the membrane skeleton.[53] Early studies suggested the early steps of red cell membrane assembly were controlled by band 3 production where, after insertion into the

membrane, band 3 directed the assembly of stable macromolecular complexes from presynthesized pools of other proteins. The role of band 3 in membrane assembly has been questioned by the following findings: (1) the organization of preformed pools of cytoskeletal elements induced by band 3 synthesis is not seen in nontransformed cells; and (2) band 3 knockout mice exhibit normal membrane biogenesis even though their red cell membranes are unstable in the circulation.[54]

Biosynthesis and assembly of spectrin subunits is complex. β-spectrin biosynthesis exceeds α-spectrin biosynthesis in early erythroblasts derived from both embryonic (yolk sac) and fetal/adult (liver/spleen) origins. This ratio is preserved during later stages of erythropoiesis in embryonic cells, but not in fetal/adult-derived late erythroblasts and reticulocytes. In the latter cells, α-spectrin gene expression increases, whereas β-spectrin gene expression remains constant, resulting in a predominance of α-spectrin mRNA and protein during the late stages, when active assembly of the actual membrane occurs most rapidly. $\alpha\beta$-spectrin subunits are incorporated into the membrane in a 1:1 stoichiometric ratio, regardless of their synthesis rates.[55] This point is important in the analysis of inherited hemolytic anemias. Human α-spectrin synthesis exceeds that of β-spectrin by 2:1 to 4:1 during the later stages of erythropoiesis, when membrane assembly presumably proceeds rapidly. Therefore, the availability of β-spectrin subunits determines the maximum rate and amount of stable spectrin assembly. Thus, mutations reducing steady-state levels of newly synthesized β spectrin should have a far greater phenotypic impact than mutations causing comparable decreases in α-spectrin biosynthesis. Analyses of patients with hereditary hemolytic anemias support this prediction.

At the stage of orthochromatic erythroblast, when membrane biogenesis is nearly completed, the cell membrane undergoes a series of critical remodeling steps.[56,57] The membrane surrounding the nucleus contains an actin ring that likely participates in expulsion of the nucleus from the erythroblast. At the same time, the spectrin skeleton segregates into the region of the incipient reticulocyte, while some surface receptors cluster in membrane regions surrounding the extruded nucleus.

Some synthesis of spectrin, band 3, protein 4.1, and GPC continues in the newly enucleated reticulocyte, but most membrane remodeling occurs after translation. The reticulocyte is multilobular and motile. It possesses mitochondria, polyribosomes, and numerous membrane proteins that are either absent or much less abundant in mature red cells. In addition, phospholipid composition and inside–outside lipid distribution are different. Reticulocytes are far less deformable and considerably more unstable mechanically than are mature erythrocytes. Maturation begins in the bone marrow and lasts for 2 or 3 days. It is completed in the circulation and perhaps in the spleen, where it has been termed *splenic polishing*. Reticulocytes first become cup shaped before they acquire their final biconcave disc shape. This process involves major reorganization of membrane phospholipids and cytoskeletal and embedded proteins, and loss of lipids and proteins, including receptors for transferrin, insulin, and fibronectin.

RED CELL AGING

Chapter 31 discusses the mechanism of red cell aging.

FETAL RED CELLS

Fetal erythrocytes differ in a number of respects from adult cells, including activity of glycolytic and nonglycolytic enzymes, altered ATP and phosphate metabolism, differences in methemoglobin content and oxygen affinity, and altered storage characteristics.[58] These erythrocytes exhibit increased rigidity, increased mechanical fragility, and decreased life span (average 45–70 days) compared to adult red cells.

Membranes of fetal and adult erythrocytes differ. ABO and I antigens and the receptors for the adsorbed serum antigens of the Lewis system are incompletely expressed. Fetal membranes are more permeable to monovalent cations and contain less Na$^+$-K$^+$ ATPase activity. They contain more phospholipid and cholesterol per cell and, as a consequence, have a larger surface to volume ratio and are slightly more osmotically resistant than adult cells. The ratio of sphingomyelin to phosphatidylcholine is increased in fetal membranes, and differences in fatty acid composition exist. However, the changes likely balance each other, as membrane fluidity is normal. The protein composition of fetal red cell membrane is quantitatively normal.

MEMBRANE PERMEABILITY

The normal red cell membrane is nearly impermeable to monovalent and divalent cations, thereby maintaining a high potassium, low sodium, and very low calcium content. In contrast, the red cell is highly permeable to water and anions, which are readily exchanged. As a result, erythrocytes behave as nearly perfect osmometers. Water and ion transport pathways in the red cell membrane (Fig. 44-4) include energy-driven membrane pumps, gradient-driven systems, and various channels.[59] An important feature of the normal red cell is its ability to maintain a constant volume. The mechanisms by which red cells "sense" changes in cell volume and activate appropriate volume regulatory pathways are unknown. Glucose is transported without expenditure of energy utilizing a transporter. Larger charged molecules, such as ATP and related compounds, do not cross the normal red cell membrane, although phosphoenolpyruvate is an exception to this rule.[59]

The effects of disruption of the red cell permeability barrier are illustrated by complement-mediated hemolysis. Complement activation on the red cell surface leads to formation of the membrane attack complex, which is composed of terminal complement components embedded in the lipid bilayer. This multimolecular complex acts as a cation channel, allowing passive movements of sodium, potassium, and calcium across the membrane according to their concentration gradients. Attracted by fixed anions, such as hemoglobin, ATP, and 2,3-BPG, sodium accumulates in the cell in excess of potassium loss and of the compensatory efforts of the Na$^+$-K$^+$ pump. The resulting increase in intracellular monovalent cations and water is followed by cell swelling and ultimately colloid osmotic hemolysis.

ENERGY-DRIVEN MEMBRANE PUMPS

In the red cell, two ion-motive ATPase-dependent cation pumps maintain low intracellular sodium and calcium and high potassium.[59] The ouabain- inhibitable Na$^+$-K$^+$ ATPase (the sodium pump) extrudes sodium in exchange for potassium in a 3:2 stoichiometry. Ca^{2+} ATPase is a calmodulin-activated pump that extrudes calcium from the red cell and maintains a very low intracellular calcium concentration, thus protecting cells from multiple deleterious effects of calcium. Examples of deleterious effects include echinocytosis, membrane vesiculation, calpain activation, membrane proteolysis, and cellular dehydration. Elevated intracellular calcium plays an important role in the pathophysiology of sickle cell disease, as increased levels of intracellular calcium observed during sickling result from increased Ca^{2+} flux and reduced activity of Ca^{2+} ATPase. The membrane also contains an ATP-driven oxidized glutathione (GSSG) transporter and amino acid transport systems.[59]

GRADIENT-DRIVEN SYSTEMS

The Na$^+$-K$^+$ gradient established by the sodium pump is used by several passive, gradient-driven systems to move ions across the red cell membrane.[59] The systems include the K$^+$-Cl$^-$ cotransporter, band 3, the Na$^+$-K$^+$-Cl cotransporter, and the Na$^+$-H$^+$ exchanger. The Na$^+$-K$^+$-Cl$^-$ cotransporter plays only a minor role in the red cell. The Na$^+$-H$^+$ exchanger appears to play a role primarily in early erythrocyte maturation. The K$^+$-Cl$^-$ cotransporter is a typical carrier-mediated cotransporter, which is particularly active in reticulocytes.[60] It is activated by cell swelling, acidification, depletion of intracellular magnesium, and thiol oxidation.

CHANNELS

Channels of the red cell include voltage-gated channels (mediated via Na$^+$-K$^+$ ATPase), water channels (the aquaporins), and the Ca^{2+}-activated K$^+$ channel.[59] The Ca^{2+}-activated K$^+$ channel, also called the *Gardos channel* after its discoverer Dr. George Gardos, causes selective loss of K$^+$ in response to increased intracellular Ca^{2+}. In sickle cells, increased activity of the Gardos channel and the K$^+$-Cl$^-$ cotransporter leads to net loss of K$^+$ and water, leading to cellular dehydration and formation of intermediate and hyperdense erythrocytes.[61] These proteins have been manipulated pharmacologically in attempts to improve cellular hydration of the red cell and ameliorate the clinical course of patients with sickle cell disease.

The aquaporins are membrane channel proteins that serve as selective pores through which water crosses the plasma membrane.[62] Aquaporin-1 (AQP1), which is expressed in many tissues including erythrocytes, contributes to the ability of the red cell to adjust rapidly to changes in osmolality. AQP1 contains the epitope for the Colton blood group system. The genetic basis of the rare Colton null phenotype has been identified as a mutation of the highly conserved NPA (asparagine-proline-alanine) motif of AQP1 essential for channel function.[63] Colton null individuals exhibit no obvious clinical phenotype, although mice with targeted inactivation of AQP1 become hyperosmolar after fluid restriction.[63]

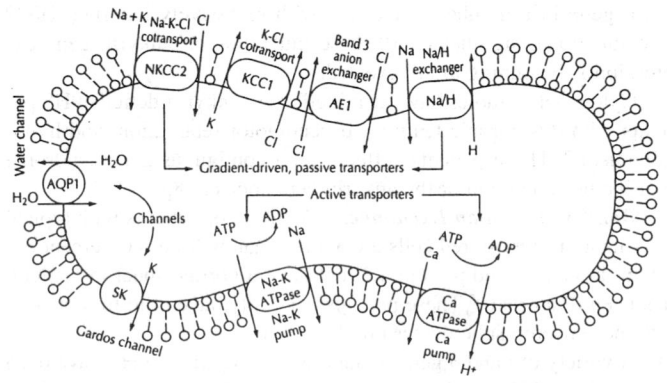

FIGURE 44-4 Principal ion transport pathways of the human erythrocyte. AE-1, band 3 anion exchanger; AQP1, water channel aquaporin 1; KCC1, KCl cotransport system of the family of chloride–cation cotransporters; NKCC2, basolateral molecular form of Na-K-Cl cotransport; SK, small conductance potassium channel. (From C Brugnara,[59] with permission.)

HEREDITARY SPHEROCYTOSIS, ELLIPTOCYTOSIS, AND RELATED DISORDERS

Hemolytic anemias resulting from defects in the erythrocyte membrane comprise an important group of hereditary anemias. HS, HE, and HPP are the most common disorders among this group. Originally classified by their morphologic presentation, detailed studies have demonstrated considerable overlap among these disorders and significant heterogeneity in their clinical, morphologic, laboratory, and molecular characteristics (Table 44-2). Advances in molecular biology have allowed further characterization of these disorders and, in many cases, detection of the precise genetic defect. These molecular analyses have provided additional information on the pathogenesis of these disorders and important insights into the structure–function relationships of erythrocyte membrane proteins.

HEREDITARY SPHEROCYTOSIS

DEFINITION AND HISTORY

Hereditary spherocytosis refers to a group of disorders characterized by spherical, doughnut-shaped erythrocytes with increased osmotic fragility. HS was first described more than 100 years ago by the two Belgian physicians Vanlair and Masius. Twenty years later, the disease was rediscovered by Wilson and Minkowsky, who reported eight cases of HS in three generations of one family. The description of increased erythrocyte osmotic fragility by Chauffard, reports of correction of anemia and hemolysis by splenectomy, and the studies of Ham and Castle implicating the spleen in the conditioning of hereditary spherocytes followed. Dacie[64] elegantly reviews the early history of HS.

A defect of the erythrocyte membrane was implicated when HS membranes were found to be leaky to sodium and to exhibit a loss of lipids, leading to surface area deficiency. Subsequently, abnormalities of proteins of the erythrocyte membrane were identified as the etiology of the HS defect.

EPIDEMIOLOGY

HS occurs in all racial and ethnic groups. It is the most common inherited anemia in individuals of northern European ancestry, affecting approximately one in 2500 individuals in the United States and England. Males and females are affected equally. Clinical, laboratory,

biochemical, and genetic heterogeneity characterize the spherocytosis syndromes.

ETIOLOGY AND PATHOGENESIS

The hallmark of HS erythrocytes is loss of membrane surface area relative to intracellular volume, accounting for the spheroidal shape and decreased deformability of the red cell.[65] The loss of surface area results from increased membrane fragility caused by defects in proteins of the erythrocyte membrane, including ankyrin, band 3, β spectrin, α spectrin, and protein 4.2. Increased fragility leads to membrane vesiculation and surface area loss (Fig. 44-5). Splenic trapping of nondeformable spherocytes, followed by conditioning and destruction of these abnormal erythrocytes, causes the hemolysis experienced by HS patients. Thus, the spleen plays an important role in hemolysis, secondary to the basic defect of the erythrocyte membrane.

RED CELL MEMBRANE PROTEIN DEFECTS

Study of erythrocyte membranes has revealed quantitative abnormalities of several membrane proteins.[65] Combined spectrin and ankyrin deficiency is most commonly observed, followed in frequency by band 3 deficiency, isolated spectrin deficiency, and protein 4.2 deficiency. Multiple genetic loci are involved. Except for rare exceptions, HS mutations are private, that is, each kindred has a unique mutation, implying no selective advantage to mutations.

Ankyrin Concomitant spectrin and ankyrin deficiency is the most common finding in HS erythrocyte membranes (Fig. 44-6). Several mechanisms, including decreased synthesis of ankyrin, decreased ankyrin assembly on the membrane, or assembly of an abnormal ankyrin, could lead to decreased assembly of spectrin on the membrane when spectrin-binding sites on ankyrin are decreased, absent, or defective.

Genetic screening has identified a number of ankyrin gene mutations in patients and has demonstrated that ankyrin defects are the most common cause of typical, dominant HS.[66,67] The majority of ankyrin mutations are either frameshift or nonsense mutations that lead to a defective ankyrin molecule, ankyrin deficiency, or both. Missense mutations may disrupt normal ankyrin–protein interactions. One such variant, ankyrin[Walsrode], identified in a kindred whose erythrocyte membranes were deficient in band 3, ankyrin, and spectrin, resulted from a mutation in the band 3 binding domain of ankyrin that decreased its affinity for band 3.[68] With one exception, all ankyrin mutations described to date have been private. The exception, ankyrin[Florianopolis], is a recurrent frameshift mutation associated with severe dominantly inherited HS.

Genetic variants have been identified in the promoter of the ankyrin gene in a number of patients with recessively inherited HS.[66] The functional significance of these mutations on ankyrin gene expression is beginning to be revealed.[69]

Cytogenetic studies have identified a few ankyrin-deficient HS patients with dysmorphic features, psychomotor retardation, and hypogonadism.[70] These patients suffer from a contiguous gene syndrome that includes deletion of the ankyrin gene locus at 8p11.2.

Band 3, the Anion Exchanger A subset of patients with typical dominant HS whose red cells are approximately 20 to 40 percent deficient in band 3 and protein 4.2, but have a normal spectrin content, has been described.[65] These patients generally have mild to moderate HS and pincered spherocytes on blood films.

A variety of band 3 gene mutations associated with HS have been identified, including missense, nonsense, duplication, insertion, deletion, and RNA-processing mutations.[71] The missense mutations include a group of mutations that replace highly conserved arginine residues in the transmembrane domain. The mutant proteins do not fold and fail to insert into the endoplasmic reticulum and, ultimately, into the erythrocyte membrane. Nonsense mutations lead to decreased band

TABLE 44-2   ERYTHROCYTE MEMBRANE PROTEIN DEFECTS IN INHERITED DISORDERS OF RED CELL SHAPE

PROTEIN	DISORDER	COMMENT
Ankyrin	HS	Most common cause of typical dominant HS
Band 3	HS, SAO, NIHF, HAc	"Pincered" HS spherocytes seen on blood film presplenectomy; SAO results from 9 amino acid deletion
β Spectrin	HS, HE, HPP, NIHF	"Acanthocytic" spherocytes seen on blood film presplenectomy; location of mutation in β spectrin determines clinical phenotype
α Spectrin	HS, HE, HPP, NIHF	Location of mutation in α spectrin determines clinical phenotype; α spectrin mutations most common cause of typical HE
Protein 4.2	HS	Primarily found in Japanese patients
Protein 4.1	HE	Found in certain European and Arab populations
GPC	HE	Concomitant protein 4.1 deficiency is basis of HE in GPC defects

GPC, glycophorin C; HAc, Hereditary acanthocytosis; HE, hereditary elliptocytosis; HPP, hereditary pyropoikilocytosis; HS, hereditary spherocytosis; NIHF, nonimmune hydrops fetalis; SAO, Southeast Asian ovalocytosis.

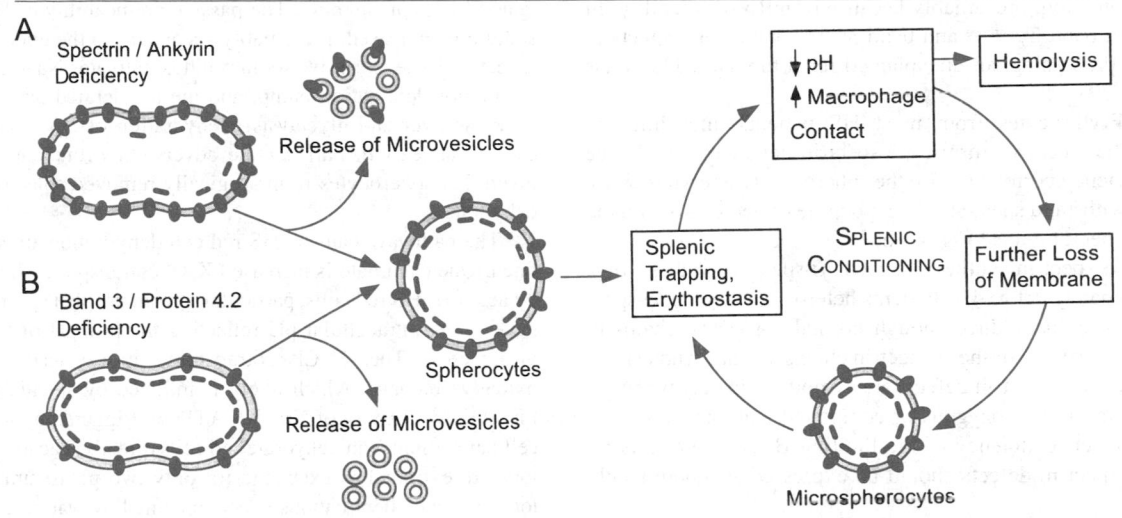

FIGURE 44-5   Pathobiology of HS. The primary defect in HS is a deficiency of membrane surface area, leading to spherocyte formation. Decreased surface area may be produced by two different mechanisms: (A) defects of spectrin and ankyrin lead to reduced density of the membrane skeleton, destabilizing the overlying lipid bilayer and releasing band 3-containing microvesicles; or (B) defects of band 3 or protein 4.2 lead to band 3 deficiency and loss of its lipid-stabilizing effect, resulting in loss of band 3 free microvesicles. Both pathways result in membrane loss, decreased surface area, and spherocyte formation with decreased deformability. The deformed erythrocytes become trapped in the hostile environment of the spleen, where splenic conditioning inflicts further membrane damage, amplifying the cycle of red cell membrane injury. (From PG Gallagher and P Jarolim: Red cell membrane disorders, in *Hematology: Basis Principles and Practice*, edited by R Hoffman, EJ Benz Jr, SJ Shattil, et al, p 576, WB Saunders, Philadelphia, with permission.)

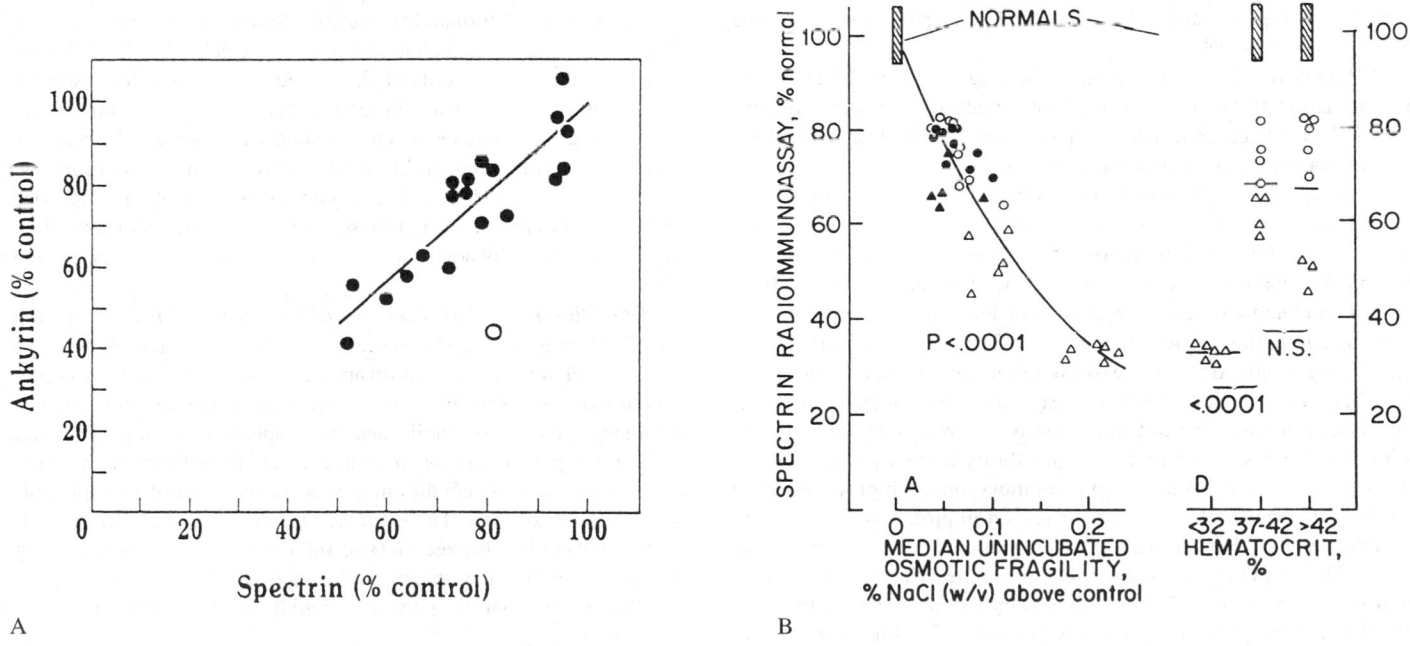

FIGURE 44-6   Role of ankyrin and spectrin in HS. (A) Correlation of spectrin and ankyrin deficiencies in 20 dominant HS kindreds. Each point, expressed as a percentage of the control (100%), represents the mean value for a kindred for both red cell spectrin and ankyrin levels. Within experimental error, the degree of spectrin and ankyrin deficiencies is essentially identical in these families with one exception *(open circle)*, an otherwise typical family in which red cells are primarily ankyrin deficient. (From S Eber and SE Lux,[65] with permission.) (B) Correlation between red cell spectrin deficiency and unincubated osmotic fragility (a measure of spheroidicity) in HS. Spectrin content, as measured by radioimmunoassay, is shown on the *vertical axis*. Osmotic fragility, as measured by NaCl concentration producing 50 percent hemolysis of erythrocytes, is shown on the *horizontal axis*. Circles represent patients with typical autosomal dominant HS. *Triangles* represent patients with atypical, nondominant HS. *Open symbols* represent patients who have undergone splenectomy. *(Right panel)* Hematocrit of every patient at least 4 months after splenectomy. Note that markedly spectrin-deficient patients have more spherical red cells and incomplete response to splenectomy. (From P Agre, A Asimos, JF Casella, et al,[75] with permission.)

3 mRNA accumulation, presumably because of mRNA instability. In HS patients with band 3[Campinas] and band 3[Pribram], which are defects in band 3 mRNA processing, an unexplained renal tubular acidosis has been observed.[72,73]

Spectrin Erythrocytes from most HS patients, including the dominant and the recessive forms, are spectrin deficient. The degree of spectrin deficiency correlates with the spheroidicity of erythrocytes, their ability to withstand shear stress, the degree of hemolysis, and the response to splenectomy (see Fig. 44-6).[74,75]

In humans, α-spectrin synthesis exceeds β-spectrin synthesis by a ratio of approximately 2:1 to 4:1. Patients heterozygous for an α-spectrin defect still should produce enough normal α-spectrin chains to pair with all, or nearly all, of the β-spectrin chains that are synthesized. Thus, patients with α-spectrin defects are symptomatic only when the defect is found in the homozygous or compound heterozygous state. In a similar manner, deficiency of the limiting β-spectrin chains resulting from β-spectrin defects should be expressed as a dominantly inherited trait.

α Spectrin The mechanisms of spectrin deficiency in most HS patients with recessively inherited HS are unknown. A number of patients with severe recessively inherited HS and marked spectrin deficiency have a mutant allele, α^{LEPRA} (low-expression Prague). α^{LEPRA} produces approximately one sixth the correctly spliced α-spectrin transcript as the normal allele because of aberrant mRNA processing. In one patient, the combination of the LEPRA allele with another defect of α spectrin *in trans*, a truncated α-spectrin chain, α^{Prague}, led to severe spectrin deficiency and severe spherocytic anemia.[76] Whether α^{LEPRA} is the etiology of many cases of α-spectrin-linked HS has not been determined. An amino acid substitution in the αII domain of spectrin, $\alpha^{Bug\ Hill}$, has been identified in many patients with spectrin-deficient, recessive HS.[77] Studies suggest $\alpha^{Bug\ Hill}$ is not itself responsible for HS but likely is a polymorphic variant that in some, but not all, cases is in linkage disequilibrium with another uncharacterized α-spectrin gene defect that causes HS.

β Spectrin A group of patients heterozygous for defects in the limiting β-spectrin chain associated with spectrin deficiency and dominant HS have been described.[65] These patients suffer from typical HS with a subpopulation of acanthocytes.

The majority of β-spectrin mutations have been associated with null alleles, including frameshift, nonsense, and initiator codon mutations. One frameshift mutation of β spectrin, caused by a single nucleotide deletion, spectrin[Houston], has been found in patients from several unrelated kindreds, suggesting the deletion might be a common β-spectrin mutation associated with HS.[78] Truncated β-spectrin chains caused by genomic deletions, exon skipping, and frameshift mutations have been described. A few missense mutations associated with HS have been reported. One of these missense mutations, spectrin[Kissimmee], is an unstable β spectrin that lacks the ability to bind protein 4.1 and binds poorly to actin because of a point mutation in a highly conserved region of β spectrin thought to be involved in protein 4.1 binding.[79]

Protein 4.2 Protein 4.2−deficient patients with recessively inherited HS, primarily from Japan, have been described.[71,80] One common variant, protein 4.2[Nippon], is caused by a point mutation that presumably affects protein 4.2 mRNA processing.[80] Other variants are caused by homozygosity or compound heterozygosity for frameshift, missense, or mRNA processing mutations of the protein 4.2 gene. Deficiency of protein 4.2 has been observed in patients with mutations in the cytoplasmic domain of band 3.[81,82] These mutations presumably involve the region of band 3−protein 4.2 interactions.

SECONDARY MEMBRANE DEFECTS

Cation Content and Membrane Permeability Potassium and water content are diminished in HS red cells, particularly those ob-

tained from splenic pulp. The passive permeability of HS red cells to sodium is increased, presumably secondary to the underlying skeletal defect.[55,83] The excessive sodium influx activates Na+-K+ ATPase and the monovalent cation pump, and the accelerated pumping increases ATP turnover and glycolysis. Dehydration of HS red cells likely is caused, at least in part, by the adverse environment of the spleen, given that spherocytes from surgically removed spleens are the most dehydrated.

The pathways causing HS red cell dehydration are not clearly defined. One candidate is increased K-Cl cotransport, which is activated by acid pH. HS red cells, particularly from unsplenectomized subjects, have a low intracellular pH reflecting the low pH of the splenic environment. . The K+-Cl− cotransport pathway also is activated by oxidative damage, which likely is inflicted by splenic macrophages. Finally, overactivity of Na+-K+ ATPase, triggered by increased intracellular sodium, can dehydrate red cells directly, because three sodium ions are extruded in exchange for only two potassium ions, and the loss of monovalent cations is accompanied by water.

Membrane Lipids The principal lipid abnormality of hereditary spherocytes is a symmetrical loss of each species of membrane lipid as part of the overall loss of membrane surface, the hallmark of HS pathobiology. The relative proportions of cholesterol and the various phospholipids are normal, and the phospholipids show the usual transmembrane asymmetry, even in severe cases.

ROLE OF THE SPLEEN

The spleen plays a secondary but important role in the pathophysiology of HS. Splenic destruction of abnormal erythrocytes with decreased deformability is the primary cause of hemolysis. Physical entrapment of spherocytes in the splenic microcirculation and ingestion by phagocytes are proposed mechanisms of destruction.

Splenic Trapping of Nondeformable Spherocytes Because of their diminished deformability, spherocytes are unable to traverse the slits between the endothelial and adventitial cells that form a wall separating the splenic cords of the red pulp from the splenic sinuses (see Chap. 5). The decrease in red cell deformability is primarily related to decreased surface area and secondarily to greater internal viscosity that results from mild cellular dehydration. In addition, the splenic environment is hostile to erythrocytes. Low pH, low glucose and ATP concentrations, and high local concentrations of toxic free radicals produced by adjacent phagocytes all contribute to membrane damage.

Conditioning and Destruction of Spherocytes in the Spleen Impeded spherocyte passage through the sinus wall fenestrations leads to a markedly engorged red pulp and pulp cords with relatively empty venous sinuses.[84] Red cells are "conditioned" in this location, becoming more osmotically fragile and more spherical, with a lower net sodium and potassium content than cells obtained from the systemic circulation.[85] Splenic conditioning is a consequence of multiple episodes of splenic stasis. The estimated residence time of HS erythrocytes in the cords is between 10 and 100 minutes. Only 1 to 10 percent of blood entering the spleen is detained by the congested cords, whereas greater than 90 percent is rapidly shunted into the venous circulation.

Macrophage phagocytosis in the spleen is the final step in the cycle of spherocyte destruction. The stimulus for phagocytosis by the macrophage is unknown.

INHERITANCE

The genes responsible for HS include ankyrin, β spectrin, band 3 protein, α spectrin, and protein 4.2. In approximately two thirds to three fourths of HS patients, inheritance is autosomal dominant. In the remaining patients, dominant inheritance cannot be demonstrated. Inheritance may be autosomal recessive or result from a *de novo* mutation. Cases with autosomal recessive inheritance result from defects in either α spectrin or protein 4.2. A surprising number of *de novo* mutations have been reported in the HS genes.[79,86,87] A few cases of HS resulting from homozygous or compound heterozygous defects in band 3 or spectrin that result in fetal death or severe hemolytic anemia presenting in the neonatal period have been reported.[88,89] In general, affected individuals of the same kindred experience similar degrees of hemolysis. Rarely, members of the same kindred experience varying degrees of hemolysis. When HS is identified in one or more siblings whose parents have no identifiable abnormalities or great variability exists in the clinical severity of affected HS family members, a number of explanations can be sought. Possible explanations include inheritance of a modifier allele that influences the expression of a membrane protein, leading to the variability in clinical expression; variable penetrance of the genetic defect; a *de novo* mutation; a mild form of recessively inherited HS; or tissue-specific mosaicism of the defect.[90]

CLINICAL FEATURES

The clinical manifestations of the spherocytosis syndromes vary widely. The typical clinical picture of HS combines evidence of hemolysis (anemia, jaundice, reticulocytosis, gallstones, splenomegaly) with spherocytosis (spherocytes on the blood film and increased osmotic fragility) and a positive family history. Mild, moderate, and severe forms of HS have been defined according to differences in hemoglobin, bilirubin, and reticulocyte counts (Table 44-3), which can be correlated with the degree of compensation for hemolysis. Initial assessment of a patient with suspected HS should include a family history and questions about history of anemia, jaundice, gallstones, and splenectomy. Physical examination should seek signs such as scleral icterus, jaundice, and splenomegaly.

TYPICAL HEREDITARY SPHEROCYTOSIS

Hereditary spherocytosis typically presents in infancy or childhood but may present at any age. In children, anemia is the most frequent finding (50%), followed by splenomegaly, jaundice, or a positive family history.[65] No comparable data exist for adults. Two thirds to three fourths of HS patients have incompletely compensated hemolysis and mild to moderate anemia. The anemia often is asymptomatic, except for fatigue and mild pallor or, with children, nonspecific parental complaints, such as irritability. Jaundice is seen at some time in about half of patients, usually in association with viral infections. When present, jaundice is acholuric, that is, unconjugated hyperbilirubinemia without detectable bilirubinuria. Palpable splenomegaly is detectable in most (75–95%) older children and adults. Typically the spleen is modestly enlarged (2–6 cm), but it may be massive. No proven correlation exists between the spleen size and the severity of HS. However, given the pathophysiology and response of the disease to splenectomy, such a correlation probably exists. Typical HS is associated with both dominant and recessive inheritance. Although the recessively inherited forms tend to be more severe, considerable overlap exists.

COMPENSATED HEREDITARY SPHEROCYTOSIS

Approximately 20 to 30 percent of HS patients have "compensated hemolysis," that is, production and destruction are balanced, and the hemoglobin concentration of the blood is normal.[65,90] Although the erythrocyte life span may only be approximately 20 to 30 days, patients adequately compensate for hemolysis with increased marrow erythropoiesis. Because they patients are not anemic, they usually are asymptomatic. In some cases, diagnosis may be difficult because hemolysis, splenomegaly, and spherocytosis are unusually mild. For example, in this group of patients, reticulocyte counts are generally less than 6 percent, and spherocytes are present on blood film in only approximately 60 percent of patients. Many of these individuals escape detection until adulthood when they are being evaluated for unrelated disorders or when complications related to anemia or chronic hemolysis occur. Hemolysis may become severe with illnesses that cause further splenomegaly, such as infectious mononucleosis, or may be exacerbated by other factors, such as pregnancy or sustained, vigorous exercise. Because of the asymptomatic course of HS in these patients, diagnosis of HS should be considered during evaluation of incidentally noted splenomegaly, gallstones at a young age, or anemia resulting from parvovirus B19 infection or other viral infections.

MODERATELY SEVERE AND SEVERE HEREDITARY SPHEROCYTOSIS

Approximately 5 to 10 percent of HS patients have moderately severe to severe anemia. Patients with "moderately severe" disease typically have a hemoglobin level of 6 to 8 g/dl, reticulocytes approximately bout 10 percent, bilirubin 2 to 3 mg/dl, and 40 to 80 percent of the normal red cell spectrin content. The category includes patients with both dominant and recessive HS and a variety of molecular defects. Patients with "severe" disease, by definition, have life-threatening anemia and are transfusion dependent. They almost always have recessive HS. Most have isolated, severe spectrin deficiency (<40%), which is thought to result from a defect in α spectrin.[74,75] Patients with severe

TABLE 44-3 CLASSIFICATION OF HEREDITARY SPHEROCYTOSIS

LABORATORY FINDINGS	HS TRAIT OR CARRIER	MILD SPHEROCYTOSIS	MODERATE SPHEROCYTOSIS	MODERATELY SEVERE SPHEROCYTOSIS[a]	SEVERE SPHEROCYTOSIS[b]
Hemoglobin (g/dl)	Normal	11–15	8–12	6–8	<6
Reticulocytes (%)	1–3	3–8	± 8	≥10	≥10
Bilirubin (mg/dl)	0–1	1–2	± 2	2–3	≥3
Spectrin content (% of normal)[c]	100	80–100	50–80	40–80[d]	20–50
Blood film	Normal	Mild spherocytosis	Spherocytosis	Spherocytosis	Spherocytosis and poikilocytosis
Osmotic fragility					
Fresh blood	Normal	Normal or slightly increased	Distinctly increased	Distinctly increased	Distinctly increased
Incubated blood	Slightly increased	Distinctly increased	Distinctly increased	Distinctly increased	Markedly increased

[a] Values in untransfused patients.
[b] By definition, patients with severe spherocytosis are transfusion dependent. Values were obtained immediately prior to transfusion.
[c] Normal, 245 ± 27 × 10³ spectrin dimers per erythrocyte.
[d] Spectrin content is variable in this group of patients, presumably reflecting heterogeneity of the underlying pathophysiology.
SOURCE: Compiled from S Eber et al.[90] and PG Gallagher and SE Lux.[168]

HS often have some irregularly contoured or budding spherocytes or bizarre poikilocytes in addition to typical spherocytes on blood film. Such cells are rare prior to splenectomy in patients with moderately severe disease, but some may be seen postsplenectomy. In addition to the risks of recurrent transfusions, patients often suffer from hemolytic and aplastic crises and may develop complications of severe uncompensated anemia, including growth retardation, delayed sexual maturation, and aspects of thalassemic facies.

ASYMPTOMATIC CARRIERS

Parents of patients with recessive HS are clinically asymptomatic and do not have anemia, splenomegaly, hyperbilirubinemia, or spherocytosis on the blood films. However, most have subtle laboratory signs of HS, including slight reticulocytosis (~2%), diminished haptoglobin levels, and slightly elevated osmotic fragility. The incubated osmotic fragility test probably is the most sensitive measure of this condition, particularly the 100 percent lysis point, which is significantly elevated in carriers (0.43 ± 0.05 g NaCl/dl) compared to normal subjects (0.23 ± 0.07).[90] However, no single test is sufficient. Carriers can be detected reliably only by considering the results of a battery of tests. At least 1.4 percent of the population is estimated to be silent carriers.

PREGNANCY AND HEREDITARY SPHEROCYTOSIS

Most patients do well during pregnancy.[91] Some patients experience anemia beyond that expected from expanded plasma volume resulting from increased hemolysis. A few patients are symptomatic only during pregnancy. Episodes of hemolytic crisis requiring transfusion and cases of folic acid deficiency have been described in pregnant HS patients.

HEREDITARY SPHEROCYTOSIS IN INFANCY

Anemia is the most common finding in neonates with HS, present in approximately 90 percent of cases.[54] Some infants have required blood transfusion to treat their anemia. Of interest, the degree of anemia seen in the neonatal period does not predict the severity of anemia seen in later life. Jaundice occurs in about half of HS neonates and may be severe enough to require phototherapy or exchange transfusion. Jaundice in neonates with HS may be accentuated by co-inheritance of Gilbert syndrome.[92] Because kernicterus is a risk, exchange transfusions may be necessary, but in most cases the jaundice can be controlled with phototherapy.

Rarely, patients suffer from severe hemolytic anemia presenting *in utero* or shortly after birth, continuing through the first year of life. Patients may require regular blood transfusions and, in some cases, early splenectomy. These severe HS patients usually suffer from significant spectrin deficiency resulting from presumed homozygosity or compound heterozygosity for α-spectrin gene defects. Several cases of hydrops fetalis in HS patients requiring intrauterine transfusion because of severe anemia associated with band 3 or spectrin defects have been reported.

COMPLICATIONS

Gallbladder Disease Chronic hemolysis leads to formation of bilirubinate gallstones, the most frequently reported complication in up to half of HS patients. Co-inheritance of Gilbert syndrome uridine diphosphoglucuronate glucuronosyltransferase (UDPGT1) gene polymorphism markedly increases the risk of gallstone formation.[93] Although gallstones have been detected in infants, most gallstones occur in adolescents, children, and young adults.[65,93] Routine management should include interval ultrasonography to detect gallstones because many patients with cholelithiasis and HS are asymptomatic. Interval ultrasonography allows prompt diagnosis and treatment and prevents complications of symptomatic biliary tract disease, including biliary obstruction, cholecystitis, and cholangitis.

Hemolytic, Aplastic and Megaloblastic Crises Hemolytic crises usually are associated with viral illnesses and typically occur in childhood. They generally are mild and characterized by jaundice, increased spleen size, decreased hematocrit, and reticulocytosis. Medical intervention rarely is necessary. During severe hemolytic crises, marked jaundice, anemia, lethargy, abdominal pain, and tender splenomegaly occur. Hospitalization and erythrocyte transfusion may be required.

Aplastic crises following virally induced bone marrow suppression are uncommon but may result in severe anemia with serious complications, including congestive heart failure or even death. The most common etiologic agent in these cases is parvovirus B19, which causes erythema infectiosum. Parvovirus infection typically presents with fever, chills, lethargy, vomiting, diarrhea, myalgias, and a maculopapular rash on the face (slapped cheek syndrome), trunk, and extremities.

Parvovirus B19 selectively infects erythropoietic progenitor cells and inhibits their growth (see Chap. 34).[94] Parvovirus infections frequently are associated with mild neutropenia, thrombocytopenia, or pancytopenia. During the aplastic phase, hematocrit level and reticulocyte count fall, marrow erythroblasts disappear, and, as the plasma iron turnover decreases, plasma iron level increases. Giant pronormoblasts, a hallmark of the cytopathic effects of parvovirus B19, often appear in the marrow. As production of new red cells declines, the remaining cells age, and microspherocytosis and osmotic fragility increase. Bilirubin levels may decrease as the number of abnormal red cells that can be destroyed declines. Return of marrow function is heralded by a fall in serum iron concentration and emergence of granulocytes, platelets, and, finally, reticulocytes.

Virally induced aplastic crisis brings many patients to medical attention, particularly asymptomatic HS patients with normally compensated hemolysis.[95] As expected, because parvovirus may simultaneously infect multiple members of a family, leading to aplastic crises, "epidemics" or "outbreaks" of HS have been reported.[96] Diagnostic confusion may arise during reemergence of marrow function, when the physician may mistake an aplastic crisis for a hemolytic crisis. Because aplastic crises usually last 10 to 14 days (about half the life span of typical HS red cells), the hemoglobin value usually falls to about half its usual level before recovery occurs. In patients with severe HS, the anemia may be profound, requiring hospitalization and transfusion.

Megaloblastic crisis occurs in HS patients with increased folate demands, such as pregnant patients, growing children, or patients recovering from an aplastic crisis. This complication is preventable with appropriate folate supplementation.

Other Complications Dermatologic manifestations of HS, including skin ulceration, gouty tophi, and chronic leg dermatitis, are uncommon.[97] These dermatologic manifestations usually heal rapidly after splenectomy. The pathogenesis of these manifestations is unknown but are proposed to be related to alterations in erythrocyte deformability, as suggested in patients with sickle cell anemia.

Findings attributable to extramedullary hematopoiesis have been described in some HS patients. The findings include poor growth and deformities of the hand and skull. Extramedullary tumors, particularly along the thoracic and lumbar spine or in the kidney hila, have been described in HS patients, including patients with untreated mild to moderate HS.[98,99] Biopsy may be performed because the masses may be mistaken for a malignant tumor. However, the biopsy procedure may be complicated by significant hemorrhage because of the composition of the masses. Magnetic resonance imaging appears to be a reliable and safer alternative diagnostic modality. Postsplenectomy, the masses involute and undergo fatty metamorphosis. However, they do not decrease in size.

HS has been suggested to predispose patients to hematologic malignancies, including myeloproliferative disorders, particularly multiple myeloma.[100] Chronic reticuloendothelial stimulation via splenic clearance of abnormal erythrocytes inducing proliferation of lymphocytes, plasma cells, and macrophages has been suggested as a possible pathogenic mechanism. Thrombosis has been reported in several HS patients, usually postsplenectomy.

Iron overload has been described in untreated HS patients with co-inherited hemochromatosis.[101] Untreated HS may aggravate underlying heart disease, particularly in the elderly. Progressive anemia resulting from loss of marrow reserve may gradually worsen underlying heart failure.

Angioid streaks have been described in the optic fundi of several adult HS patients.

NONERYTHROID MANIFESTATIONS

Clinical manifestations are confined to the erythroid lineage in most patients with HS, But a few exceptions have been observed. Several HS kindreds have been reported with cosegregating nonerythroid manifestations, particularly neuromuscular abnormalities including cardiomyopathy, slowly progressive spinocerebellar degenerative disease, spinal cord dysfunction, and movement disorders.

The observation that erythrocyte ankyrin and β spectrin are also expressed in muscle, brain, and spinal cord raises the possibility that these HS patients suffer from defects of one of these proteins.[22,65] The hypothesis is further supported by studies of ankyrin-deficient *nb/nb* mice.[102] These mice have almost no detectable ankyrin and suffer from

a severe, spherocytic hemolytic anemia and late-onset cerebellar ataxia that parallels a gradual loss of Purkinje cells. A further possibility is that another, yet to be described gene locus is causative. For example, mice that do not express the junctional complex membrane protein β adducin suffer from a spherocytic anemia and neurologic manifestations.[103]

Heterozygous defects of band 3 have been described in patients with inherited distal renal tubular acidosis and normal erythrocytes. This finding is in contrast to most patients with heterozygous mutations of band 3, who have normal renal acidification and abnormal erythrocytes. Two kindreds with co-inherited HS *and* renal acidification defects resulting from band 3 mRNA processing mutations, band 3[Pribram], and band 3[Campinas] have been described.[72,73]

LABORATORY FEATURES

Like the clinical presentation of HS, laboratory findings in HS are heterogeneous.

Blood Film   Erythrocyte morphology in HS is variable. Typical HS patients have blood films with easily identifiable spherocytes lacking central pallor (Fig. 44-7). Less commonly, patients present with only a few spherocytes on the film or, at the other end of the spectrum, with numerous small, dense spherocytes and bizarre erythrocyte morphology with anisocytosis and poikilocytosis. Rarely, spherostomatocytes are seen. Specific morphologic findings have been identified in patients with certain membrane protein defects, such as pincered erythrocytes (band 3) or spherocytic acanthocytes (β spectrin). When examining blood from a patient with suspected spherocytosis, a high-

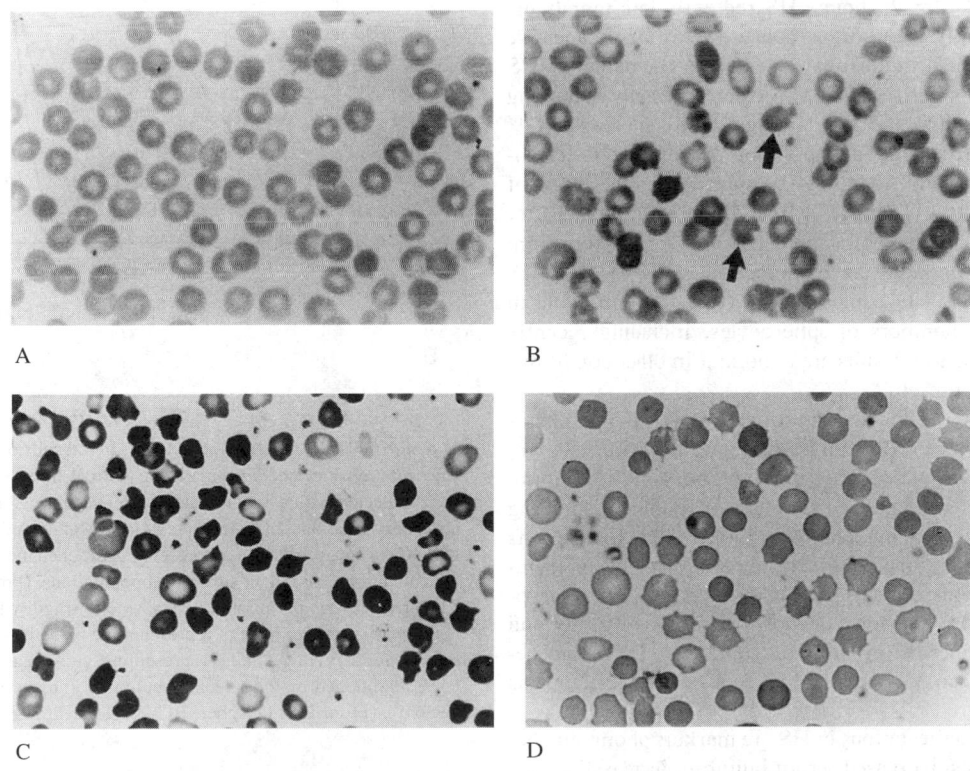

A

B

C

D

FIGURE 44-7   Blood films from patients with HS of varying severity. (*A*) Typical HS with mild deficiency of red cell spectrin and ankyrin. Although many cells have spheroidal shape, some cells retain a central concavity. (*B*) HS with pincered red cells (*arrows*), as typically seen in HS associated with band 3 deficiency. Occasionally, spiculated red cells also are present. (*C*) Severe atypical HS resulting from severe combined spectrin and ankyrin deficiency. In addition to spherocytes, many cells with irregular contour are present. (*D*) HS with isolated spectrin deficiency resulting from β-spectrin mutation. Some spherocytes have prominent surface projections resembling spheroacanthocytes (Blood film *D* courtesy of DL Wolfe.).

quality film with the erythrocytes well separated and some cells with central pallor in the field of examination is important because spherocytes are a common artifact.

Erythrocyte Indices   Most patients have mild to moderate anemia with hemoglobin in the 9 to 12g/dl range (see Table 44-3). Mean corpuscular hemoglobin concentration (MCHC) is increased (between 35 and 38%) because of relative cellular dehydration in approximately 50 percent of patients, but all HS patients have some dehydrated cells. The Technicon H1 blood counter and its successors (Technicon, Tarrytown, NY, USA) provide a histogram of MCHC that has been claimed to be sufficiently accurate to identify nearly all HS patients (Fig. 44-8A).[104] Finally, mean corpuscular volume (MCV) usually is normal except in cases of severe HS, when MCV is slightly decreased. Typically, MCV is relatively low for the age of the cells in most HS patients, reflecting the dehydrated state of the HS erythrocytes.

Osmotic Fragility   In the normal erythrocyte, a redundancy of cell membrane gives the cell its characteristic discoid shape and provides it with abundant surface area. Spherocytes have a decreased surface area relative to cell volume, resulting in their abnormal shape. This change is reflected in the increased osmotic fragility found in these cells (see Fig. 44-8B). Osmotic fragility is tested by adding increasingly hypotonic concentrations of saline solution to red cells. The normal erythrocyte is able to increase its volume by swelling, but spherocytes, which already are at maximum volume for surface area, burst at higher than normal saline concentrations. Some HS individuals have a normal osmotic fragility on freshly drawn red blood cells, with the osmotic fragility curve approximating the number of spherocytes seen on the blood film.[105] However, after incubation at 37°C (98.6°F) for 24 hours, HS red cells lose membrane surface area more readily than normal because their membranes are leaky and unstable. Thus, incubation accentuates the defect in HS erythrocytes and brings out the defect in osmotic fragility, making incubated osmotic fragility the standard test in diagnosing HS.[105] When the spleen is present, a subpopulation of very fragile erythrocytes that have been conditioned by the spleen form the "tail" of the osmotic fragility curve (see Fig. 44-8B). The tail disappears after splenectomy. Unfortunately, the osmotic fragility test suffers from poor sensitivity, with as many as 20 percent of mild cases of HS missed after incubation. The osmotic fragility test is unreliable in patients having small numbers of spherocytes, including recently transfused patients. The test results are abnormal in other conditions where spherocytes are present.

Additional Testing   Other investigations, such as the autohemolysis test, the hypertonic cryohemolysis test, and the acidified glycerol test, suffer from lack of specificity, are cumbersome to perform, and are not widely used. Specialized testing is available for studying difficult cases or cases requiring additional information. Useful tests for these purposes include structural and functional studies of erythrocyte membrane proteins, such as protein quantitation, limited tryptic digestion of spectrin, and ion transport. Membrane rigidity and fragility can be examined using an ektacytometer. cDNA and genomic DNA analyses can be performed when a molecular diagnosis is desired.

Other laboratory manifestations in HS are markers of ongoing hemolysis. Reticulocytosis, increased serum bilirubin, increased lactate dehydrogenase, increased urinary and fecal urobilinogen, and decreased serum haptoglobin reflect increased erythrocyte production or destruction and variable proportions of intravascular and extravascular hemolysis components. In many cases of HS, the reticulocyte count appears to be elevated disproportionately relative to the degree of anemia. This finding has been observed even in HS patients with normal hemoglobin levels.

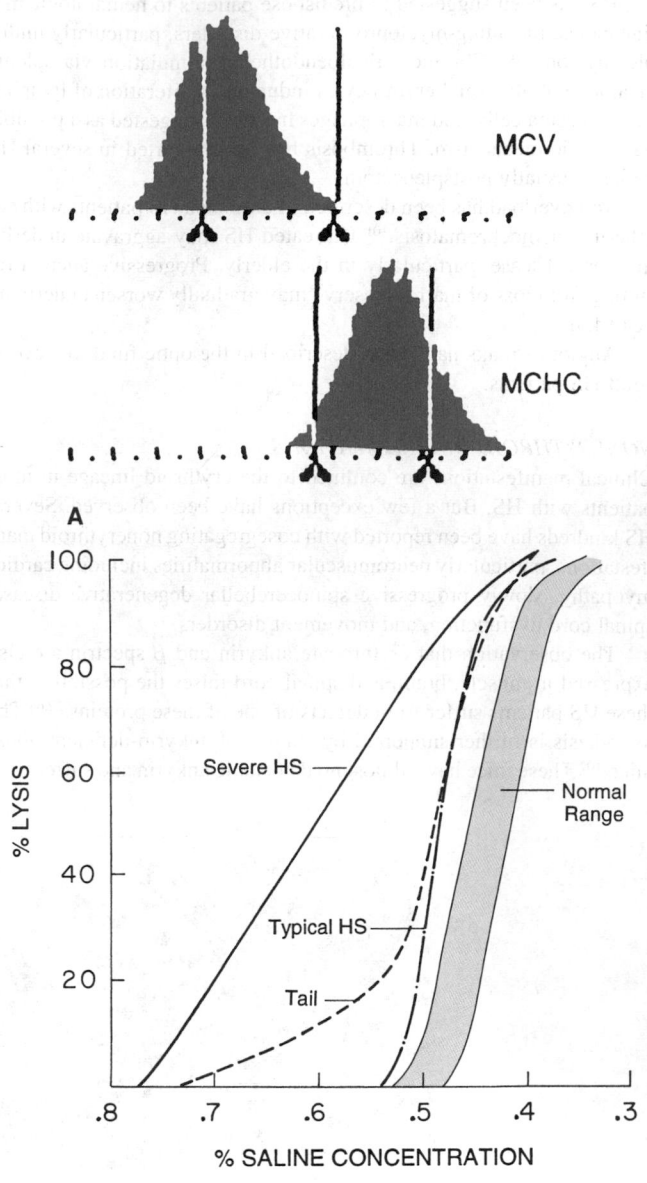

FIGURE 44-8   Laboratory diagnosis of HS. (*A*) Histograms of the distribution of (*top*) MCV and (*bottom*) MCHC in red cells of a patient with HS before splenectomy. *Vertical lines* mark the normal limits of the distributions. Data were collected with a Technicon H1 laser scattering blood counter. The patient has subpopulations of microcytes (low MCV) and dehydrated cells (high MCHC), which presumably represent conditioned microspherocytes. All 21 HS patients in one study had similar subpopulations. (From AR Pati, WN Patton, EI Harris,[104] with permission.) (*B*) Osmotic fragility testing. The *shaded area* is the normal range. Results representative of both typical and severe spherocytosis are shown. A "tail," representing very fragile erythrocytes that have been conditioned by the spleen, is common in many HS patients prior to splenectomy. (From PG Gallagher, BG Forget, SE Lux,[168] with permission.)

DIFFERENTIAL DIAGNOSIS

Initial laboratory investigation should include a complete blood count with a blood film, reticulocyte count, direct antiglobulin test (Coombs test), and serum bilirubin. An incubated osmotic fragility should be obtained. Rarely, additional specialized testing is required to confirm the diagnosis. In neonates, ABO incompatibility should be considered, but its differentiation from HS becomes clear several months after birth. Other causes of spherocytic hemolytic anemia, such as autoimmune hemolysis, clostridial sepsis, transfusion reactions, severe burns, and bites from snakes, spiders, bees, and wasps, should be viewed in the appropriate clinical context. Occasional spherocytes are seen in patients with a large spleen (e.g., in cirrhosis or myelofibrosis) or in patients with microangiopathic anemias (see Chap. 49), but differentiation of these conditions from HS does not usually present diagnostic difficulties.

HS may be obscured in disorders that increase the surface to volume ratio of erythrocytes, such as obstructive jaundice, iron deficiency, β-thalassemia trait or hemoglobin SC disease, and vitamin B_{12} or folate deficiency. In obstructive jaundice, spherocytosis can be obscured by accumulation of cholesterol and phospholipids in the membrane that characteristically accompanies this condition. In normal subjects, this process leads to target cell formation. Hereditary spherocytes acquire a discoidal appearance, and their survival in the circulation is improved. Iron deficiency corrects the abnormal shape but does not improve survival of HS erythrocytes.

THERAPY AND PROGNOSIS

Splenectomy Splenic sequestration is the primary determinant of erythrocyte survival in HS patients. Thus, splenectomy cures or alleviates the anemia in the overwhelming majority of patients, reducing or eliminating the need for red cell transfusions. Elimination of the need for chronic blood transfusions has obvious implications for future iron overload and risk of end-organ damage. The incidence of cholelithiasis is decreased. Postsplenectomy, spherocytosis, and altered osmotic fragility persist, but the "tail" of the osmotic fragility curve, created by conditioning of a subpopulation of spherocytes by the spleen, disappears. Erythrocyte life span nearly normalizes, and reticulocyte counts fall to normal or near-normal levels. Changes typical of the postsplenectomy state, including Howell-Jolly bodies, target cells, siderocytes, and acanthocytes, become evident on the blood film. Postsplenectomy, patients with the most severe forms of HS still suffer from shortened erythrocyte survival and hemolysis, but their clinical improvement is striking.[74,75] HS patients with spectrin/ankyrin-deficient erythrocytes may benefit more from splenectomy than patients with band 3–deficient cells.[106] Splenectomy prevents an early loss of young cells in both types of deficiencies. It also prolongs survival of mature spectrin/ankyrin-deficient cells because they escape the opsonization by band 3–containing vesicles.[106]

Complications of Splenectomy. Early complications of splenectomy include local infection or bleeding and pancreatitis, presumably resulting from injury to the tail of the pancreas incurred during spleen removal. In general, the morbidity of splenectomy for HS is lower than the morbidity of other hematologic disorders. Chapter 5 discusses the complications of splenectomy.

Indications for Splenectomy. In the past, splenectomy, which has a low operative mortality, was considered routine in HS patients. However, the risk of overwhelming postsplenectomy infection and the emergence of penicillin-resistant pneumococci have led to reevaluation of the role of splenectomy in the treatment of HS. Considering the risks and benefits, a reasonable approach is to splenectomize all patients with severe spherocytosis and all patients suffering from significant signs or symptoms of anemia, including growth failure, skeletal changes, leg ulcers, and extramedullary hematopoietic tumors. Other candidates for splenectomy are older HS patients suffering from vascular compromise of vital organs.

Whether patients with moderate HS and compensated, asymptomatic anemia should undergo splenectomy is controversial. Patients with mild HS and compensated hemolysis can be followed and referred for splenectomy if clinically indicated. Treatment of patients with mild

to moderate HS and gallstones is debatable, particularly because new treatments for cholelithiasis, including laparoscopic cholecystectomy, and endoscopic sphincterotomy, lower the risk of this complication. If such patients have symptomatic gallstones, a combined cholecystectomy and splenectomy can be performed, particularly if acute cholecystitis or biliary obstruction has occurred. No evidence indicates any benefit to performing cholecystectomy and splenectomy separately, as performed in the past.

Because the risk of postsplenectomy sepsis is very high during infancy and early childhood, splenectomy should be delayed until age 5 to 9 years if possible and to at least 3 years if feasible, even if chronic transfusions are required in the interim. No evidence indicates further delay is useful. In fact, further delay may be harmful because the risk of cholelithiasis increases dramatically in children older than 10 years.

When splenectomy is warranted, laparoscopic splenectomy has become the method of choice in centers with surgeons experienced in the technique.[107] If desired, the procedure can be combined with laparoscopic cholecystectomy. Laparoscopic splenectomy results in less postoperative discomfort, a quicker return to preoperative diet and activities, shorter hospitalization, decreased costs, and smaller scars. The risk of bleeding increases during the operation, and approximately 10 percent of laparoscopic operations (for all causes) must be converted to standard splenectomies. Even enormous spleens (>600 g) can be removed laparoscopically because the spleen is placed in a large bag, diced, and eliminated via suction catheters.

Partial splenectomy via laparotomy has been advocated for infants and young children with significant anemia associated with erythrocyte membrane disorders.[108] The goals of this procedure are to allow for palliation of hemolysis and anemia while maintaining some residual splenic immune function. Long-term follow-up data for this procedure have been variable.[109,110]

Prior to splenectomy, patients should be immunized with vaccines against pneumococcus, *Haemophilus influenzae* type B, and meningococcus, preferably several weeks preoperatively. Use of prophylactic antibiotics postsplenectomy for prevention of pneumococcal sepsis is controversial. Postsplenectomy, prophylactic antibiotics (penicillin V 125 mg orally twice daily for patients younger than 7 years or 250 mg orally twice daily for those older than 7 years, including adults), have been recommended for at least 5 years postsplenectomy by some and for life by others. The optimal duration of prophylactic antibiotic therapy postsplenectomy is unknown. Presplenectomy and, in severe cases, postsplenectomy, HS patients should take folic acid (1 mg/day orally) to prevent folate deficiency.

Splenectomy Failure. Splenectomy failure is uncommon. Failure may result from an accessory spleen missed during splenectomy, from development of splenunculi as a consequence of autotransplantation of splenic tissue during surgery, or from another intrinsic red cell defect, such as pyruvate kinase deficiency. Accessory spleens occur in 15 to 40 percent of patients and must always be sought. Recurrence of hemolytic anemia years or even decades following splenectomy should raise suspicion of an accessory spleen, particularly if Howell-Jolly bodies are no longer found on blood film. Definitive confirmation of ectopic splenic tissue can be achieved by a radiocolloid liver–spleen scan or a scan using ^{51}Cr-labeled, heat-damaged red cells.

GENETIC COUNSELING

After a patient is diagnosed with HS, family members should be examined for the presence of HS. A history, physical examination for splenomegaly, complete blood count, examination of the blood film for spherocytes, and a reticulocyte count should be obtained for parents, children, and siblings, if available.

HEREDITARY ELLIPTOCYTOSIS, PYROPOIKILOCYTOSIS, AND RELATED DISORDERS

DEFINITION AND HISTORY

HE is characterized by the presence of elliptical or oval erythrocytes on the blood films of affected individuals.[34,111,112] In 1904, Dresbach, a physiologist at Ohio State University in Columbus, Ohio, reported the first description of HE. Dresbach discovered the condition in a medical student during a laboratory exercise in which the students were examining their own blood.[113] The report elicited some controversy because the student died soon thereafter, leading to speculation that the student actually suffered from pernicious anemia. The demonstration of the disease in three generations of one family by Hunter and Adams[114] clearly established the hereditary nature of this disorder. Dacie[111] has reviewed the history of HE.

HPP is a rare cause of anemia first described in three children with severe neonatal anemia with erythrocyte morphology similar to that seen in patients suffering severe burns.[115] The erythrocytes from these patients also exhibited increased thermal sensitivity. Subsequently, other patients, mostly of African descent, with similar clinical and laboratory findings have been described.[116–118] A strong relationship exists between HE and HPP. Approximately one third of parents or siblings of patients with HPP have typical HE, and many of these family members share identical mutations in erythrocyte spectrin. In addition, many patients with HPP proceed to develop typical mild to moderate HE. Patients with HPP tend to experience severe hemolysis and anemia in infancy that gradually improves but then evolves toward typical hemolytic HE later in life. The blood film remains striking.

EPIDEMIOLOGY

The worldwide incidence of HE is estimated to be one in 2000 to one in 4000 individuals. The true incidence of HE is unknown because its clinical severity is heterogeneous and many patients are asymptomatic. It is common in individuals of African and Mediterranean descent, presumably because elliptocytes confer some resistance to malaria. The incidence of HE is 6 percent in Benin, Africa.[112] Genetic haplotyping studies suggest one HE mutation common in Africa has a "founder effect" with origins in central Africa similar to that attributed to hemoglobin S, Benin-type.

ETIOLOGY AND PATHOGENESIS

The principal defect in HE and HPP erythrocytes is mechanical weakness or fragility of the erythrocyte membrane skeleton. As in HS, study of erythrocyte membrane proteins in these disorders has identified abnormalities of various erythrocyte membrane proteins, including α and β spectrin, protein 4.1, and GPC. The majority of defects occur in spectrin, the principal structural protein of the erythrocyte membrane

skeleton. Most spectrin defects in HE and HPP impair the ability of spectrin dimers to self-associate into tetramers and oligomers, thereby disrupting the membrane skeleton.[34,119] Structural and functional defects of protein 4.1 lead to disruption of spectrin–actin attachment to the membrane via GPC, causing changes in cell shape and membrane stability similar to those found in abnormalities of spectrin. The mechanical instability in GPC variants appears to result from secondary protein 4.1 deficiency. In all of these defects, disruption of the membrane skeleton leads to mechanical instability sufficient to cause red cell fragmentation with hemolytic anemia under conditions of normal circulatory shear stress.[120]

The pathobiology of elliptocytic shape is less clear. Red cell precursors in common HE are round. The cells become progressively more elliptical as they age *in vivo*. Elliptocytes and poikilocytes may become permanently stabilized in shape because weakened spectrin heterodimer contacts facilitate skeletal reorganization following axial deformation of cells from prolonged or excessive shear stress. The reorganization likely involves breakage of the unidirectionally stretched protein connections, followed by formation of new protein contacts that preclude recovery of the normal biconcave shape. This process accounts for the permanent deformation of irreversibly sickled cells.

Spectrin in Hereditary Elliptocytosis and Pyropoikilocytosis The abnormalities of either α or β spectrin associated with the majority of cases of HE and HPP result from mutations in the spectrin heterodimer self-association site.[34,119] Figure 44-9 shows diagrammatically the repeats of spectrin involved in self-association and the locations of reported mutations. Most of the mutations are missense mutations at or very near highly conserved residues of α spectrin. The missense mutations are primarily either α helix-breaking mutations that replace the normal residue with a proline or glycine, or charge-shift mutations. In contrast to HS, the elliptocytosis and pyropoikilocytosis syndromes, while also quite heterogeneous, are associated with distinct spectrin mutations in persons of similar genetic backgrounds, suggesting a "founder effect" for the mutations.

HE or HPP phenotype–spectrin mutation genotype correlations are difficult to establish. Great clinical phenotypic heterogeneity exists among individuals with the same spectrin mutation. The heterogeneity exists even among individuals from the same kindred. A few general phenotype–genotype correlations can be made. Mutations at the contact sites of α and β spectrin in the spectrin self-association site tend to be more severe.[116,117] For example, mutations of codon 28, which is located in this contact site region, are generally associated with phenotypically severe HE or HPP. On the other hand, a common mutation in blacks from West and Central Africa, a leucine insertion at codon 154, is phenotypically very mild, even in the homozygous state.[121] Because of the great phenotypic variability, the presence of

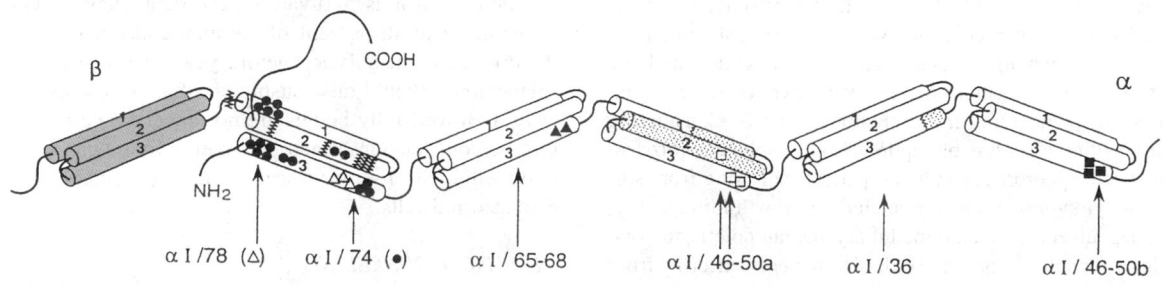

FIGURE 44-9 Defects of the spectrin self-association site in HE and HPP. A triple helical model of the spectrin repeats that constitute the spectrin self-association site is shown. *Symbols* denote positions of various genetic defects identified in patients with HE or HPP. Limited tryptic digestion of spectrin, followed by two-dimensional gel electrophoresis, identifies abnormal cleavage sites *(arrows)* in spectrin associated with various mutations. (Modified from PG Gallagher, BG Forget, SE Lux,[168] with permission.)

low-expression modifier alleles of spectrin has been postulated (see "Molecular Determinants of Clinical Severity" below).

In contrast to α spectrin mutations, a variety of β spectrin mutations have been identified in HE and HPP patients, including frameshift and splicing mutations that lead to truncated β-spectrin chains lacking the spectrin self-association site.[34] Three β-spectrin mutations, spectrin[Providence], spectrin[Cagliari], and spectrin[Buffalo],[122–124] lead to severe fetal or neonatal anemia and nonimmune hydrops fetalis when inherited in the homozygous state. Five of six homozygotes died; the one survivor remains transfusion dependent.

Protein 4.1 Protein 4.1 defects associated with HE are much less common than spectrin defects. Protein 4.1 is a multifunctional protein that undergoes complex patterns of tissue- and stage-specific alternative splicing. It contains several important functional sites, including a spectrin–actin binding domain and a GPC binding domain. Partial deficiency of protein 4.1 is associated with asymptomatic HE, whereas complete deficiency leads to hemolytic anemia.[34] Homozygous 4.1 (−/−) erythrocytes fragment more rapidly than normal at moderate shear stress, an indication of the intrinsic instability of the erythrocytes (Fig. 44-10). Membrane mechanical stability can be restored by reconstituting the deficient red cells with protein 4.1 or the protein 4.1–spectrin–actin binding site.[125] Homozygous protein 4.1 (−) erythrocytes also lack p55 and have only 30 percent of the normal content of GPC. The 4.1 (−) erythrocytes and GPC (−) Leach erythrocytes (see "Epidemiology" above) demonstrate decreased invasion and growth of *P. falciparum in vitro.*[126]

Most patients with protein 4.1–associated elliptocytosis are from certain European and Arab populations. Protein 4.1 utilizes tissue-specific translation start sites. Several HE mutations involve the downstream initiator codon.[34] In one HE mutant lacking the downstream initiator codon, an erythroid stage-specific switch occurs from the upstream initiator codon to the downstream initiator codon. In affected patients, HE phenotype does not develop until after the developmentally regulated switch has occurred.[127] HE-related protein 4.1 variants as a result of deletion or duplication of the exons involved in spectrin, actin, and protein 4.1 binding have been described.[34]

Glycophorin C Elliptocytes are present on the blood films of patients whose erythrocytes carry the Leach phenotype (i.e., lacking the Gerbich antigens Ge-1, Ge-2, Ge-3, and Ge-4) and lack both GPC and glycophorin D (GPD).[19] The Leach phenotype usually results from a 7-kb deletion of genomic DNA that removes exons 3 and 4 from the GPC/GPD locus.[128] A frameshift mutation resulting from a nucleotide deletion has been described as the cause of this phenotype. GPC-deficient subjects also are partially deficient in protein 4.1 and lack p55, presumably because these proteins form a complex and recruit or stabilize each other on the membrane. Protein 4.1 deficiency in Leach erythrocytes is speculated to be the cause of the elliptocytic shape. In contrast to other forms of HE, which are dominantly inherited, heterozygous carriers are asymptomatic, with normal red blood cell morphology, whereas homozygous subjects have no anemia, with only mild elliptocytosis seen on blood film.

MOLECULAR DETERMINANTS OF CLINICAL SEVERITY

The severity of hemolysis in common HE often varies not only among different kindreds but also within a given family. Erythrocyte spectrin content and the percentage of dimeric spectrin in crude spectrin extracts are the principal determinants of hemolysis severity. The percentage of dimeric spectrin in crude spectrin extracts depends on the degree of dysfunction of the mutant spectrin and the gene dose (i.e., heterozygote vs. homozygote or compound heterozygote) or the presence of other genetic defects *in trans.* Mutations in the spectrin self-association contact site produce a more severe defect of spectrin function and clinical phenotype than do other elliptocytogenic mutations.

The low-expression α-spectrin allele α^{LELY} is the best characterized abnormality affecting spectrin content and clinical severity. The allele is characterized by an amino acid substitution, Leu1857Val, and partial skipping of exon 46.[129] The abnormalities are located in the spectrin heterodimer nucleation site (i.e., where spectrin monomers assemble into heterodimers). The α-spectrin chains lacking exon 46 are poorly assembled into $\alpha\beta$ heterodimers and are rapidly degraded.[130] Alone, the α^{LELY} allele is clinically silent, even when inherited in the homozygous state, because α spectrin normally is synthesized in threefold to fourfold excess.[48] When the α^{LELY} allele is present *in trans* to an elliptocytogenic α-spectrin mutation, it increases the mutant spectrin concentration and worsens the disease severity. Conversely, when the α^{LELY} allele is *in cis* to an α-spectrin mutation, it mutes the elliptocytic phenotype.

Certain acquired factors may affect the clinical severity of HE. In neonatal red cells, the weak binding of 2,3-BPG by fetal hemoglobin leads to an increase in free 2,3-BPG, which in turn induces a superimposed destabilization of spectrin–actin–protein 4.1 interaction.[131] Finally, hemolytic anemia can be worsened by several acquired conditions, including those that alter microcirculatory stress to the cells.

INHERITANCE

HE is inherited as an autosomal dominant disorder in most patients. Clinical severity is highly variable among different kindreds, reflecting heterogeneous molecular lesions, and, to a lesser extent, in a given kindred, presumably because of other genetic or acquired defects that modify disease expression. Rare cases of *de novo* mutation have been described,[132] as has an HE kindred with a contiguous gene deletion syndrome inherited in an X-linked pattern.[133]

CLINICAL FEATURES

The clinical presentation of HE is heterogenous, ranging from asymptomatic carriers to patients with severe, life-threatening anemia.[34] The overwhelming majority of patients with HE are asymptomatic and are diagnosed incidentally during testing for unrelated conditions.

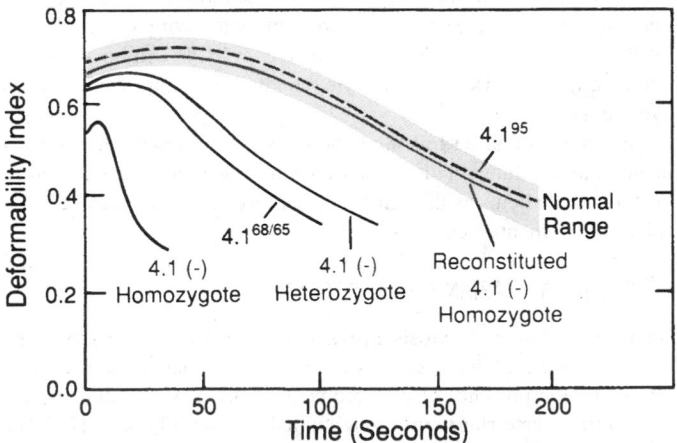

FIGURE 44-10 Erythrocyte membrane stability in defects of protein 4.1. Red cell membranes were subjected to shear stress in an ektacytometer, and deformability was measured as a function of time. A fall in deformability occurred as the membranes fragmented. Cells completely lacking protein 4.1 (−/−) have very fragile membranes, and normal fragility can be restored by reconstitution with normal protein 4.1. Heterozygous protein 4.1 mutant cells (+/− and the variant 65/68) have intermediate stability. (From N Mohandas and JA Chasis,[51] with permission.)

Asymptomatic carriers who possess the same molecular defect as an affected HE relative but who have normal or near normal blood films have been identified. The erythrocyte life span is normal, and the patients are not anemic. Asymptomatic HE patients may experience hemolysis in association with infections, hypersplenism, vitamin B_{12} deficiency, or microangiopathic hemolysis such as disseminated intravascular coagulation or thrombotic thrombocytopenic purpura. In the latter two conditions, worsening hemolysis may result from microcirculatory damage superimposed on the underlying mechanical instability of red cells.

HE patients with chronic hemolysis experience moderate to severe hemolytic anemia with elliptocytes and poikilocytes on blood film. Red cell life span is decreased, and patients may develop complications of chronic hemolysis, such as gallbladder disease. In some kindreds, the hemolytic HE has been transmitted through several generations. In other kindreds, not all HE subjects have chronic hemolysis; some have only mild hemolysis, presumably because another genetic factor modifies disease expression. The blood films of the most severe HE patients with chronic hemolysis exhibit elliptocytes, poikilocytes, and very small microspherocytes. Thus, their clinical presentation is indistinguishable from HPP.

HPP represents a subtype of common HE, as evidenced by the coexistence of HE and HPP in the same family and the presence of the same molecular defect of spectrin. Unlike HE subjects carrying the spectrin mutation, red cells of HPP subjects are partially deficient in spectrin. Typically, one parent of the HPP offspring carries an elliptocytogenic α-spectrin mutation, while the other parent is fully asymptomatic and has no detectable biochemical abnormality. In many patients, the asymptomatic parent carries a silent "thalassemia-like" defect of spectrin synthesis, enhancing the expression of the spectrin mutant and leading to a superimposed spectrin deficiency in HPP offspring. Some HPP subjects inherit two structural variants of α spectrin. In these HPP patients, spectrin deficiency may result from instability of the mutant spectrin. HPP is seen predominantly in subjects of African descent, but HPP also has been diagnosed in subjects of Arabic and European descent.

HEREDITARY ELLIPTOCYTOSIS AND PYROPOIKILOCYTOSIS IN INFANCY

Clinical symptoms of elliptocytosis are uncommon in the neonatal period. Typically, elliptocytes do not appear on the blood film until the patient is 4 to 6 months old. Occasionally, severe forms of HE present in the neonatal period with severe, hemolytic anemia with marked poikilocytosis and jaundice. These patients may require red cell transfusion, phototherapy, or exchange transfusion. Usually, even in severely affected patients, the hemolysis abates between 6 and 12 months of age, and the patient progresses to typical HE with mild anemia. Infrequently, patients remain transfusion dependent beyond the first year of life and require early splenectomy. In cases of suspected neonatal HE or HPP, review of family history and analysis of blood films from the parents usually are of greater diagnostic benefit than other available studies.

A few cases of hydrops fetalis accompanied by fetal or early neonatal death as a result of unusually severe forms of HE have been described.[122,123] One severely affected hydropic infant salvaged by intrauterine transfusions and early exchange transfusion has remained transfusion dependent for more than 2 years.

LABORATORY FEATURES

The hallmark of HE is the presence of cigar-shaped elliptocytes on blood film (Fig. 44-11). These normochromic, normocytic elliptocytes may number from a few to 100 percent. The degree of hemolysis does not correlate with the number of elliptocytes present. Spherocytes,

stomatocytes, and fragmented cells may be seen. Osmotic fragility is abnormal in severe HE and in HPP. The reticulocyte count generally is less than 5 percent but may be higher when hemolysis is severe. Other laboratory findings in HE are similar to those of other hemolytic anemias and are nonspecific markers of increased erythrocyte production and destruction. For example, increased serum bilirubin, increased urinary urobilinogen, and decreased serum haptoglobin reflect increased erythrocyte destruction.

In HPP, in addition to the blood film findings seen in HE, many HPP erythrocytes are bizarrely shaped, with fragmentation or budding. Microspherocytosis is common, and MCV usually is low (50–70 fl). Pyknocytes are prominent on blood films of neonates with HPP. The thermal instability of erythrocytes, originally reported as diagnostic of HPP, is not unique to this disorder; it is also commonly found in HE erythrocytes.

Specialized testing has been used in difficult cases or cases requiring a molecular diagnosis. Specialized tests include analysis of membrane proteins by one-dimensional gel electrophoresis, limited tryptic digestion of membrane spectrin followed by one- or two-dimensional gel electrophoresis, spectrin dimer self-association assays, ektacytometry, and cDNA and genomic DNA analyses.

DIFFERENTIAL DIAGNOSIS

Elliptocytes may be seen in association with several disorders, including megaloblastic anemias, hypochromic microcytic anemias (iron deficiency anemia and thalassemia), myelodysplastic syndromes, and myelofibrosis. In these conditions, elliptocytosis is acquired and generally represents less than one fourth of red cells seen on blood film. History and additional laboratory testing usually clarify the diagnosis of these disorders. Pseudoelliptocytosis is an artifact of blood film preparation. Pseudoelliptocytes are found only in certain areas of the film, usually near its tail. The long axes of pseudoelliptocytes are parallel, whereas the axes of true elliptocytes are distributed randomly.

THERAPY AND PROGNOSIS

Therapy is rarely needed in patients with HE. In rare cases, occasional red blood cell transfusions may be required. In cases of severe HE and HPP, splenectomy has been palliative, as the spleen is the site of erythrocyte sequestration and destruction. The same indications for splenectomy in HS can be applied to patients with symptomatic HE or HPP. Postsplenectomy, patients with HE or HPP exhibit increased hematocrit, decreased reticulocyte counts, and improved clinical symptoms.

Patients should be followed for signs of decompensation during acute illnesses. Interval ultrasonography to detect gallstones should be performed. Patients with significant hemolysis should receive daily folate supplementation.

SOUTHEAST ASIAN OVALOCYTOSIS

Southeast Asian ovalocytosis, also known as *Melanesian elliptocytosis* or *stomatocytic elliptocytosis*, is a dominantly inherited trait characterized by the presence of oval red cells, many of which contain one or two transverse ridges or a longitudinal slit (see Fig. 44-11D). The condition is widespread in certain ethnic groups of Malaysia, Papua New Guinea, the Philippines, and Indonesia.[34] Numerous abnormalities of Southeast Asian ovalocytosis erythrocytes have been reported, including increased red cell rigidity, decreased osmotic fragility, increased thermal stability, resistance to shape change by echinocytic agents, and reduced expression of many red cell antigens.[34] Thus, Southeast Asian ovalocytosis red cells are unique among the elliptocytes in that they are rigid and hyperstable rather than unstable.[134] A remarkable feature of Southeast Asian ovalocytosis erythrocytes is

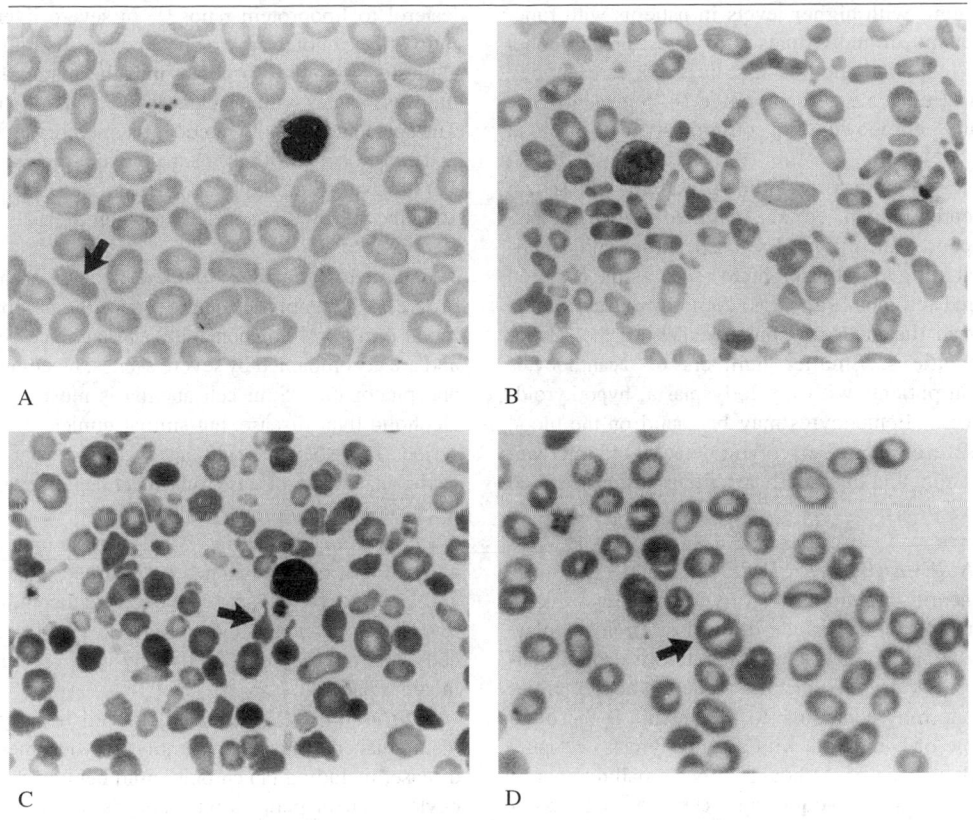

FIGURE 44-11   Blood films from patients with various forms of HE. (A) Simple heterozygote with mild common HE associated with an elliptocytogenic spectrin mutation. Note the predominant elliptocytosis, with some rod-shaped cells *(arrow)* and the virtual absence of poikilocytes. (B) Compound heterozygosity for common HE resulting from a double heterozygous state for two spectrin mutations. Both parents have mild HE. Many elliptocytes and numerous fragments and poikilocytes are present. (C) HPP. The patient is a compound heterozygote for an α-spectrin self-association site mutation and a defect characterized by reduced synthesis of the protein. Note prominent microspherocytosis, micropoikilocytosis, and fragmentation. Only a few elliptocytes are present. Some poikilocytes are in the process of budding *(arrow)*. (D) Southeast Asian (Melanesian) ovalocytosis. The majority of cells are oval. Some cells contain either a longitudinal slit or a transverse ridge *(arrow)*.

their resistance to *in vitro* invasion by several strains of malaria parasites, including *P. falciparum* and *Plasmodium knowlesi*.[135]

The Southeast Asian ovalocytosis phenotype is the result of heterozygosity for two band 3 mutations *in cis*: the deletion of 27 bp encoding amino acids 400 to 408 located at the boundary of the cytoplasmic and membrane domains of band 3 and the amino acid substitution Lys56Glu.[136] The latter is an asymptomatic polymorphism. Homozygosity for Southeast Asian ovalocytosis is hypothesized to lead to embryonic lethality.[137] Southeast Asian ovalocytosis erythrocytes exhibit increased binding of band 3 to ankyrin, increased tyrosine phosphorylation of band 3, inability to transport sulfate anions, and markedly restricted lateral and rotational mobility of the band 3 protein in the membrane.

Clinically, the finding on blood film of at least 30 percent oval-shaped red cells, some containing a central slit or a transverse ridge, and the notable absence of clinical and laboratory evidence of hemolysis in a patient from the above-noted ethnic groups are highly suggestive of the diagnosis. A useful screening test is the demonstration of resistance of ovalocytes or their ghosts to changes in shape resulting from treatments that produce spiculation in normal cells, such as overnight incubation of red cells or exposure of ghosts to salt solutions. Rapid genetic diagnosis can be made by amplifying the region containing the 27-bp deletion from genomic DNA or reticulocyte cDNA

and demonstrating a smaller band compared to control after electrophoresis.

In vivo, evidence indicates Southeast Asian ovalocytosis provides some protection against all forms of malaria, particularly against heavy infections and cerebral malaria.[138] The prevalence of Southeast Asian ovalocytosis increases with age in populations challenged by malaria, suggesting a selective advantage. The mechanism of malaria resistance of Southeast Asian ovalocytosis cells is speculative. Band 3 serves as one of the malaria receptors, as evidenced by inhibition of invasion *in vitro* by band 3–specific peptides.[139]

ACANTHOCYTOSIS

Spiculated red cells are classified into two types: acanthocytes and echinocytes. *Acanthocytes* are contracted, dense cells with irregular projections from the red cell surface that vary in width and length. *Echinocytes* have small, uniform projections spread evenly over the circumference of the red cell. The differences are clearly seen on scanning electron micrographs[140] but may be difficult to ascertain on blood films. Acanthocytes almost always are accompanied by echinocytes, but echinocytes may be present alone. Diagnostically, the distinction is not critical, and disorders of spiculated red cells generally are classified together. Normal adults may have up to 3 percent spiculated erythrocytes on blood film, with higher levels in patients with functional or actual splenectomy, in individuals after ingestion of alcohol or certain medications (e.g., indomethacin, salicylates, furosemide), and in premature infants (mean 5.5 percent, range 1–25 percent). Spiculated cells, particularly echinocytes, are common artifacts of blood film preparation.

Acanthocytes are present on the blood films of patients with severe liver disease, abetalipoproteinemia, certain inherited neurologic disorders without abetalipoproteinemia, and in association with inheritance of certain red cell antigen polymorphisms such as the McLeod phenotype. Abnormal red cell membrane lipid composition and altered lipid distribution between the inner and outer leaflets of the bilayer characterize these conditions. Smaller numbers of acanthocytes (<10%) may be seen in patients with myelodysplasia, hypothyroidism, and anorexia nervosa. Echinocytes may be found on the blood films of patients with severe uremia, glycolytic defects, and microangiopathic hemolytic anemia, and transiently after transfusion of stored red cells.

ACANTHOCYTOSIS IN SEVERE LIVER DISEASE

Definition The anemia in patients with liver disease is of complex etiology.[141] Common causes include blood loss, iron or folate deficiency, hypersplenism, and marrow suppression from alcohol, malnutrition, hepatitis infection, or other factors. Acquired abnormalities of the red cell membrane may contribute to the anemia in these patients; one is a syndrome of hemolysis with acanthocytosis or "spur" cells, so-called spur cell anemia.[142] Although only a small number of patients with end-stage liver disease acquire spur cell anemia, the prevalence of liver disease is so high that these individuals account for the majority of cases of acanthocytosis seen in clinical practice.

Etiology and Pathogenesis Acanthocyte formation *in vivo* is a two-step process involving accumulation of free (nonesterified) cholesterol in the red cell membrane and remodeling of abnormally shaped red cells by the spleen.[143,144] Acanthocytes result from increased acquisition of free cholesterol from the plasma because of abnormal cho-

lesterol to lipoprotein ratios.[143] In severe liver disease, a very high ratio of free cholesterol to phospholipids is found in lipoproteins. Free cholesterol readily partitions into the membrane, where it preferentially associates with the outer leaflet, making the membrane less fluid. The spleen attempts to remodel the membrane, leading to rigid, spherical erythrocytes with the characteristic spiculated projections (Fig. 44-12).[144] Over time, the poorly deformable cells have difficulty negotiating the narrow sinusoids of the splenic circulation and are hemolyzed (see Chap. 5).

Clinical Features Spur cell anemia is characterized by rapidly progressive hemolytic anemia with large numbers of acanthocytes on blood film.[143,145] Splenomegaly and jaundice become more prominent and are accompanied by severe ascites, bleeding diatheses, and hepatic encephalopathy. Spur cell anemia is most common in patients with alcoholic liver disease, but similar clinical syndromes have been described in association with advanced metastatic liver disease, cardiac cirrhosis, Wilson disease, fulminant hepatitis, and infantile cholestatic liver disease.

Laboratory Features Most patients have moderate anemia with a hematocrit of 20 to 30 percent, marked indirect hyperbilirubinemia, and laboratory evidence of severe hepatocellular disease. Blood films reveal significant acanthocytosis (see Fig. 44-12). Echinocytes, target cells, and microspherocytes, many with very fine spicules, are found in some patients.

Differential Diagnosis Spur cell hemolytic anemia should be distinguished from other hemolytic syndromes associated with liver disease, including (1) chronic, mild hemolysis with occasional spherocytes seen in patients with congestive splenomegaly, (2) transient hemolysis associated with fatty metamorphosis of the liver and hypertriglyceridemia (which does not appear to have a causal relationship to hemolysis), (3) transient hemolytic anemia with stomatocytosis, and (4) hemolytic anemia with rigid and occasionally spiculated red cells (echinocytes), which has been reported in malnourished alcoholics with severe hypophosphatemia. Spur cell anemia appears to differ from Zieve syndrome, a poorly defined syndrome of hyperlipoprotei-

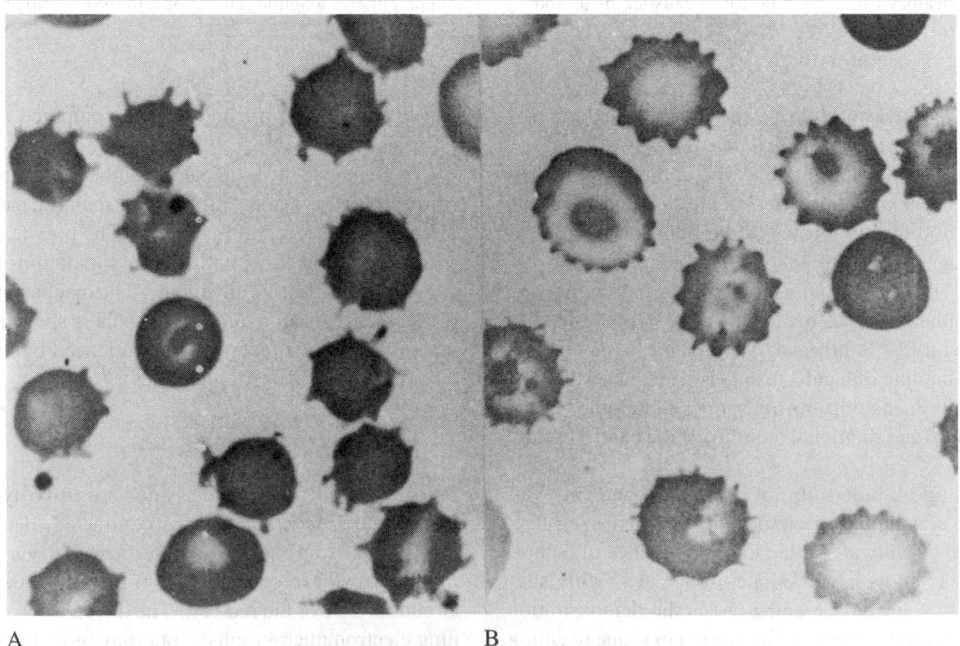

A   B

FIGURE 44-12   Panel A: Blood film from a patient with liver cirrhosis and spur cell anemia. Panel B: The conditioning effect of the spleen is evidenced by the spheroidal shape of the cells and the remodeling of the spicules. (From RA Cooper, DB Kimball, JR Durocher,[144] with permission.)

nemia, jaundice, and spherocytic hemolytic anemia that occurs in alcoholic patients with liver disease.[146]

Therapy, Course, and Prognosis The anemia of spur cell anemia usually is not a significant clinical problem, but it can aggravate pre-existing anemias, for example, resulting from gastrointestinal bleeding, to the point that erythrocyte transfusion is required. The life span of spur cells is markedly decreased because of splenic sequestration, and, as expected, hemolysis abates after splenectomy. However, splenectomy is a dangerous and potentially fatal procedure in these critically ill patients and is generally not recommended. Spur cell anemia is an ominous clinical marker of the terminal stages of liver disease. Prior to the availability of liver transplantation, patients who reached this stage rarely lived for more than a few weeks.

ABETALIPOPROTEINEMIA (BASSEN-KORNZWEIG SYNDROME)

Definition Abetalipoproteinemia is an autosomal recessive disorder characterized by progressive ataxic neurologic disease, celiac disease, retinitis pigmentosa, and acanthocytosis found in people of diverse ethnic backgrounds.[147]

Etiology and Pathogenesis The primary molecular defect in this disorder is a failure to synthesize or secrete lipoproteins containing products of the apolipoprotein B gene.[147] In some patients, the inability results from lack of microsomal transfer protein, which catalyzes the transport of triglyceride, cholesterol ester, and phospholipid from phospholipid surfaces.[148] Microsomal transfer protein, a heterodimer of protein disulfide isomerase and a large 88-kDa subunit, is located in the lumen of hepatic microsomes and intestinal epithelia, the sites of lipoprotein synthesis. Other than apolipoprotein B, microsomal transfer protein is the only tissue-specific component required for secretion of apoprotein B−containing lipoproteins. All lipoproteins that contain apolipoprotein B are absent in plasma. Consequently, preformed triglycerides are not transported from the intestinal mucosa, and plasma triglycerides are nearly absent. Plasma cholesterol and phospholipid levels are markedly decreased, with a relative increase of sphingomyelin at the expense of lecithin.

In this condition, marrow red cell precursors, nucleated red cells, and reticulocytes have normal shape. Acanthocytosis becomes apparent as the red cells mature in the circulation, worsening with increasing red cell age.[149] Incubating normal red cells in abetalipoproteinemic serum does not produce acanthocytes, but normal red cells acquire acanthocytic changes when transfused into an abetalipoproteinemic recipient. Erythrocyte membrane proteins are normal, but lipids are not.[150] The cholesterol to phospholipid ratio is normal or slightly increased, reflecting changes in the distribution of plasma phospholipids and a decrease in LCAT activity. The phosphatidylcholine concentration is decreased, and sphingomyelin is correspondingly increased. In abetalipoproteinemic acanthocytes, excess sphingomyelin is suggested to be preferentially confined to the outer membrane bilayer leaflet, causing an expansion of its surface area that may be responsible for the irregularities in cell surface contour.

Clinical Features The disorder manifests in the first month of life by steatorrhea. Intestinal biopsy typically reveals engorgement of mucosal cells with lipid droplets. Retinitis pigmentosa, which often results in blindness, and progressive neurologic abnormalities characterized by ataxia and intention tremors develop between 5 and 10 years of age and progress to death in the second or third decade.[147]

Laboratory Features Patients usually have mild anemia with normal red cell indices and normal or slightly increased reticulocyte counts.[147,149] Acanthocytosis is prominent, ranging from approximately 50 to 90 percent of red cells. Despite the lipid abnormalities and frequent concomitant vitamin E deficiency, the hemolysis is mild, especially compared to the hemolysis that occurs with spur cell anemia

(see "Acanthocytosis in Severe Liver Disease" above). The enlarged, congested spleen in patients with portal hypertension and spur cell anemia has been suggested to worsen the hemolysis, whereas the spleen is normal in patients with abetalipoproteinemia.

Differential Diagnosis The related disorders hypobetalipoproteinemia, normotriglyceridemic abetalipoproteinemia, and chylomicron retention disease are associated with partial production of apolipoprotein B−containing lipoproteins or with secretion of lipoproteins containing truncated forms of apolipoprotein B. Patients with these disorders may experience neurologic disease and acanthocytosis, depending on the severity of the underlying defect. Even patients with heterozygous hypobetalipoproteinemia may have acanthocytosis, but typically they do not.[151]

Therapy, Course, and Prognosis Treatment includes dietary restriction of triglycerides and supplementation of vitamins A, K, D, and E.[147] Water-soluble forms of vitamin E, such as D-α-tocopherol polyethylene glycol succinate, are available for use. The role of vitamin E in the pathophysiology and clinical symptomatology of abetalipoproteinemia is unknown. Vitamin E deficiency is suggested to be the primary stimulus for secondary manifestations of the disease, such as neuropathy. This hypothesis is based on the observations that vitamin E may stabilize or even improve neuromuscular and retinal abnormalities in these patients and because a similar neuropathy has been observed in patients with chronic cholestasis. Clinically evident vitamin A or D deficiencies are rarely observed.

ACANTHOCYTOSIS WITH NEUROLOGIC DISEASE AND NORMAL LIPOPROTEINS

Chorea-Acanthocytosis Syndrome Chorea-acanthocytosis is a rare autosomal recessive disorder characterized by normolipoproteinemic acanthocytosis and progressive neurodegenerative disease with onset in adolescence or adult life.[152] Chorea-acanthocytosis is characterized by progressive orofacial dyskineses with tics, limb chorea, lip and tongue biting; neurogenic muscle hypotonia and atrophy; absent or diminished reflexes; and increased serum creatine phosphokinase. Neuroimaging demonstrates abnormalities of the putamen and the head of the caudate.

Patients are not anemic, and red cell survival is only slightly decreased. In some patients, the acanthocytosis may precede the onset of neurologic symptoms. The mechanism of acanthocytosis in chorea-acanthocytosis is unknown. Plasma and erythrocyte membrane lipids and membrane fatty acid composition are normal except for a high content of saturated fatty acids.[153] Red cell membrane fluidity is decreased, and intramembrane particles are unevenly distributed, presumably because of altered lipid fluidity. Increased proteolysis of ankyrin, band 3, and protein 4.2 and increased membrane protein phosphorylation, especially of band 3, may contribute to the cell shape change. A point mutation near the COOH-terminus of band 3 has been identified in one unusual kindred with chorea-acanthocytosis.[154] The chorein gene has been cloned and mutations identified in chorea-acanthocytosis families from diverse ethnic backgrounds.[155–157] Chorein does not belong to any gene family, and no known structural motifs or domains have been identified.

Inherited neuroacanthocytosis syndromes other than chorea-acanthocytosis have been described. The syndromes include (1) a recessively inherited syndrome with acanthocytosis, tics, parkinsonism, and occasional motor neuron disease; (2) mitochondrial myopathy with encephalopathy, lactic acidosis, strokelike symptoms, and acanthocytosis; (3) Hallervorden-Spatz disease (progressive dementia, dystonia, spasticity, pallidal and retinal degeneration) with acanthocytosis; and (4) HARP syndrome (*h*ypoprebetalipoproteinemia, *a*canthocytosis, *r*etinitis pigmentosa, and *p*allidal degeneration with iron deposition).

ERYTHROCYTE DISORDERS ASSOCIATED WITH ABNORMALITIES OF KELL AND LUTHERAN BLOOD GROUPS

McLeod Syndrome The McLeod syndrome is an X-linked anomaly of the Kell blood group system characterized by mild compensated hemolytic anemia with variable acanthocytosis and, in some patients, late-onset myopathy or chorea.[158,159] The Kell antigen consists of two major protein components: a 37-kDa protein that carries the Kx antigen, a precursor molecule necessary for the Kell antigen expression, and a 93-kDa protein that carries the Kell blood group antigen. Red cells with the McLeod phenotype have no detectable Kx antigen, and they have a marked deficiency of the 93-kDa protein that carries the Kell antigen. The *XK* gene encodes a novel 444-amino-acid integral membrane transporter. Mutations of the *XK* gene have been identified in McLeod patients.[160] Male hemizygotes who lack Kx have 80 to 85 percent acanthocytes on the blood film and mild, compensated hemolysis. Because of red cell mosaicism—produced X inactivation, female heterozygote carriers may have occasional acanthocytes on blood film,[159] and women with markedly skewed X inactivation may have more severe symptoms.

McLeod red cells should be distinguished from Kell null (K$_o$) red cells, which have a normal shape. In K$_o$ cells, only the Kell antigen carrying 93-kDa glycoprotein is absent; the cells have twice the amount of the Kx antigen.[161] Patients with McLeod syndrome must be identified because they may develop antibodies that are compatible only with McLeod syndrome red cells if they receive transfusions.

The McLeod phenotype has been described in association with chronic granulomatous disease of childhood, retinitis pigmentosa, and Duchenne muscular dystrophy. These variable manifestations may result from contiguous gene deletion syndromes, as the genetic locus for these disorders is Xp21.[162] This situation may explain the occasional findings of either echinocytes or stomatocytes in Duchenne dystrophy or a choreiform disorder in some subjects with McLeod phenotype. Furthermore, some subjects with the McLeod phenotype exhibit laboratory features of myopathy and, later in life, a neurologic disorder that is first manifested by areflexia and, after the fifth decade, progresses to dystonia and choreiform movements.

Lutheran Blood Group Approximately one in 3000 to 5000 people inherit the dominantly acting inhibitor *In(Lu)*, which suppresses expression of Lu^a and Lu^b, the major antigens of the Lutheran blood group system. Patients with the *In(Lu)* Lu(a-b-) phenotype may have abnormally shaped red cells, including poikilocytes and acanthocytes, without evidence of anemia or hemolysis.[163] The osmotic fragility of fresh *In(Lu)* Lu(a-b-) erythrocytes is normal. However, after incubation, the cells lose potassium and become osmotically resistant.[164] The identity of the inhibitor has not been ascertained.

ACANTHOCYTOSIS IN OTHER CONDITIONS

A small number of acanthocytes are observed in malnutrition resulting from diverse causes, including anorexia nervosa and cystic fibrosis. The red cell shape normalizes after adequate nutritional status is restored. Very mild acanthocytosis (0.5−2%) is common in 20 to 65 percent of patients with hypothyroidism.[165] Because hypothyroidism is much more common than the other disorders that cause spiculated red cells, the finding of acanthocytes on the blood film should prompt consideration of the patient's thyroid function. This association may unmask undiagnosed cases of hypothyroidism.

STOMATOCYTOSIS AND RELATED DISORDERS

Stomatocytes are erythrocytes characterized by a wide transverse slit or stoma (thus *stomatocytes*) (Fig. 44-13).[166] No unifying theory explains this morphologic abnormality, which is an artifact resulting from folding of the cells during blood film preparation. Stomatocytes

are seen in a variety of acquired and inherited disorders. The latter often are associated with inherited abnormalities in red cell cation permeability that may be associated with abnormal red cell hydration or membrane lipids.[167] Disturbances of erythrocyte hydration range from the extremes of dehydration and overhydration. These variants have been divided into provisional categories based on clinical severity, morphology, cation content, lipid and protein composition, genetics, and response to splenectomy (Table 44-4).[168]

DEHYDRATED STOMATOCYTOSIS/HEREDITARY XEROCYTOSIS

Definition Dehydrated hereditary stomatocytosis (HSt), also known as *hereditary xerocytosis* or *dessicocytosis*, is the most common form of the HSt syndromes.[166–168] The predominant phenotype associated with this disorder is an autosomal dominant hemolytic anemia with red cell dehydration and decreased osmotic fragility. This phenotype has been extended to include recurrent fetal loss, hydrops fetalis, and pseudohyperkalemia (see "Therapy, Course, and Prognosis" below).

Etiology and Pathogenesis The underlying permeability defect is complex and involves a net loss of potassium from the red cells (typically approximately 20%) that is not accompanied by a proportional gain of sodium.[167,169] Consequently, the net intracellular cation content and cell water content are decreased. In some cases, erythrocytes have increased membrane lipids, particularly phosphatidylcholine, and reduced 2,3-BPG content.[170] No quantitative abnormalities of membrane lipids and proteins have been noted, except for increased membrane-associated glyceraldehyde-3-phosphate dehydrogenase.

The precise genetic basis of this disorder remains unknown. The dehydrated HSt locus has been mapped to 16q23-qter.[171]

Clinical Features Patients may present with compensated hemolytic anemia, jaundice, splenomegaly, and gallstones. This syndrome has been extended to include recurrent fetal loss, hydrops fetalis, neonatal hepatitis, and familial pseudohyperkalemia (FP).[167] Individuals with FP present with asymptomatic hyperkalemia attributable to an altered passive leak of potassium across the red cell membrane *in vitro*, similar to the mechanism considered defective in xerocytosis.[172] Pseudohyperkalemia is observed in approximately one third of xerocytosis patients. Xerocytosis, hydrops fetalis, and pseudohyperkalemia are linked in several kindreds.[173,174] Variable penetrance appears to present in this disorder, with significant disparity in clinical symptomatology between affected individuals in the same kindred. Genetic linkage analyses have mapped the FP locus to the same location as xerocytosis, supporting the hypothesis that the syndromes are allelic.[175]

Laboratory Features The hematologic picture is that of mild to moderate hemolytic anemia (see Table 44-4) with increased MCHC, a reflection of cellular dehydration. Frequently, MCV is mildly increased, an artifact of Coulter-type electronic counters. In these counters, conversion of pulse height (from the resistance of a cell passing through an electric field) to a cellular volume is dependent on cell shape. Xerocytes do not deform to the same degree as normal cells, which causes the MCV to be approximately 10 percent too high. The hematocrit level also is affected because the level is calculated from the MCV. Blood films do not always reveal stomatocytes, which are more prominent on wet films, but frequently target cells, dessicocytes, and spiculated cells are seen (see Fig. 44-13A). In some of the cells, hemoglobin is concentrated ("puddled") in discrete areas on the cell periphery. Erythrocyte osmotic fragility is decreased.

Therapy, Course, and Prognosis Most patients experience only mild anemia, and therapy is not required. The patients should receive folate supplementation and be monitored for complications of hemolysis.

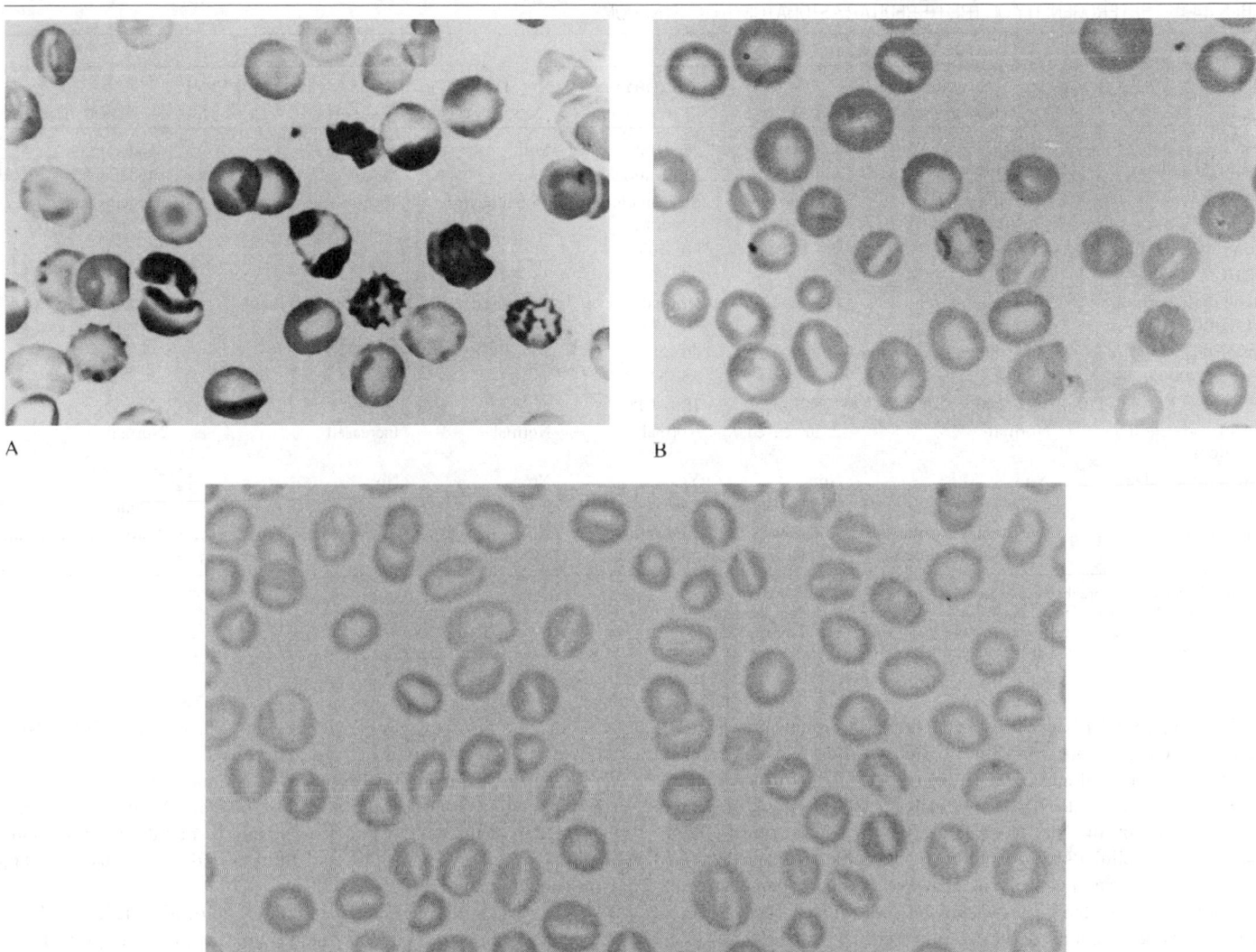

FIGURE 44-13   Stomatocytosis and variants. Blood film from patients with (A) hereditary xerocytosis (dessicocytosis), (B) stomatocytosis (hydrocytosis), and (C) acquired stomatocytosis as a result of alcoholic liver disease. (Panels A and B from WM Lande and WC Mentzer,[166] with permission.)

The effects of splenectomy have been variable, with many xerocytosis patients experiencing little or no improvement in anemia. Xerocytes have been suggested to be so functionally compromised that they are detected and eliminated in other areas of the macrophage-monocyte system. Splenectomy should be carefully considered in patients with hereditary xerocytosis. Several patients have developed hypercoagulability after splenectomy, leading to life-threatening thrombotic episodes.[176] Note that all cases of thrombosis have occurred after splenectomy. *In vitro*, stomatocytic erythrocytes from a splenectomized xerocytosis individual demonstrated increased endothelial adherence compared to stomatocytic erythrocytes from unsplenectomized family members without hypercoagulability.[177] In one hypercoagulable xerocytosis patient, pentoxifylline decreased red cell adherence.[177] Fortunately, the majority of HSt patients can maintain an adequate hemoglobin level so that splenectomy is not required. Results of treatment of splenectomized patients with long-term warfarin (Coumadin) have been variable. In a few severe cases, erythrocyte hypertransfusion has been beneficial. Un-

fortunately, the procedure is complicated by iron overload, a significant problem even in the absence of transfusion.

Neonates with xerocytosis have required phototherapy, red cell transfusion, and, in some cases, exchange transfusion, for treatment of anemia and hyperbilirubinemia. In a few cases, *in utero* transfusion has been required. The presence of hydrops fetalis is not a predictor of the severity of anemia later in life. Some infants experience little or no anemia later in childhood.

HEREDITARY STOMATOCYTOSIS-HYDROCYTOSIS

Definition and History   The overhydrated HSt syndromes, also known as *hereditary hydrocytosis*, are characterized by a dominantly inherited hemolytic anemia with red cell overhydration and macrocytosis. The syndrome was first described by Lock and coworkers[178] in a girl with dominantly inherited hemolytic anemia whose blood film contained red cells with a wide transverse slit, stomatocytes. Later, abnormal cation transport and cellular overhydration—hallmarks of this disorder—were discovered.[179]

TABLE 44-4 HETEROGENEITY OF THE HEREDITARY STOMATOCYTOSIS SYNDROMES

| | STOMATOCYTOSIS (HYDROCYTOSIS) | | INTERMEDIATE SYNDROMES | | | |
	SEVERE HEMOLYSIS	MILD HEMOLYSIS	CRYOHYDRO-CYTOSIS	STOMATOCYTIC XEROCYTOSIS	XEROCYTOSIS WITH HIGH PHOSPHATIDYLCHOLINE	XEROCYTOSIS
Hemolysis	Severe	Mild–moderate	Moderate	Mild	Moderate	Moderate
Anemia	Severe	Mild–moderate	Mild–moderate	None	Mild	Moderate
Blood film	Stomatocytes	Stomatocytes	Stomatocytes or normal	Stomatocytes	Targets	Targets, echinocytes
MCV (80–100 fl)[a]	110–150	95–130	90–105	91–98	84–92	100–110
MCHC (32–36%)	24–30	26–29	34–40	33–39	34–38	34–38
Unincubated osmotic fragility	Markedly increased	Increased	Normal	Decreased	Markedly decreased	Markedly decreased
RBC Na$^+$ (5–12)[b]	60–100	30–60	40–50	10–20	10–15	10–20
RBC K$^+$ (90–103)	20–55	40–85	55–65	75–85	75–90	60–80
RBC Na$^+$+K$^+$ (95–110)	110–140	115–145	100–105	87–103	93–99	75–90
Phosphatidylcholine content	Normal	± Increased	Normal	Normal	Increased	Normal
Cold autohemolysis	No	No	Yes	No	No	?
Effect of splenectomy[c]	Good	Good	Fair	?	?	? Poor
Inheritance	Autosomal dominant?, autosomal recessive	Autosomal dominant	Autosomal dominant	Autosomal dominant	Autosomal dominant	Autosomal dominant

[a] Values in parentheses are the normal range.
[b] Values for sodium, potassium, and sodium + potassium are mEq per liter RBC.
[c] Splenectomy may be contraindicated in these syndromes; see text for details.
SOURCE: From PG Gallagher et al,[168] with permission.

Etiology and Pathogenesis The principal lesion involves a sodium leak leading to increased intracellular sodium and water content and mildly decreased intracellular potassium.[167,169] This action is followed by a compensatory increase in the active transport of sodium and potassium by the Na$^+$-K$^+$ ATPase pump, which normally maintains low intracellular sodium and high potassium concentrations, and an ensuing increase in glycolysis. However, pump hyperactivity cannot compensate for the vastly increased sodium leak. The molecular basis of this permeability defect is unknown.

The osmotic fragility of hydrocytes is markedly increased because many of the swollen red cells approach their critical hemolytic volume. For unexplained reasons, red cell membrane lipids and, consequently, membrane surface area also are increased, but the increased area is insufficient to correct the osmotic fragility. Red cell deformability is decreased.

The red cells of some patients with overhydrated HSt lack a 31-kDa integral membrane protein called *band 7.2b* or *stomatin*.[180] Varying degrees of stomatin deficiency were subsequently described in most but not all patients with HSt, with younger erythroid cells demonstrating less deficiency.[181] However, the stomatin cDNA from several HSt patients was normal.[181] Mice lacking stomatin exhibit no hemolytic anemia, and the morphology, cell indices, cation content, and hydration status of their erythrocytes are normal.[182] The results suggest a stomatin defect is not the primary defect in HSt, but it may be involved in an as yet undiscovered volume regulatory pathway in the red cell.

Clinical Features The hydrocytosis syndromes are much less common than the xerocytosis disorders. Moderate to severe anemia is present.[167] Jaundice and splenomegaly are common, as are complications of chronic hemolysis such as cholelithiasis. A tendency for iron overload, independent of transfusion status or splenectomy, has been described. No other organ system abnormalities have been described. Neonatal anemia and hyperbilirubinemia have been reported.

Laboratory Features The blood film reveals striking stomatocytosis (see Fig. 44-13B). In addition to the anemia, red cell indices show decreased MCHC and elevated MCV (see Table 44-4). In some

patients, the macrocytosis is extreme, with MCV up to 150 fl. Erythrocyte osmotic fragility is markedly increased.

Therapy, Course, and Prognosis The majority of hydrocytosis patients suffer from significant lifelong anemia. Similar to patients with HS, patients with hydrocytosis should be monitored for complications of hemolysis, such as cholelithiasis and parvovirus infection, and should receive folate supplementation.

The results of splenectomy in this group of disorders have been variable.[168] In some patients, hemolytic anemia is improved, although often not fully corrected, by splenectomy. In other patients, the severity of hemolysis is unchanged. Splenectomy should be carefully considered in patients with the disorder. Like patients with xerocytosis, several patients with hydrocytosis have developed hypercoagulability after splenectomy, leading to catastrophic thrombotic episodes.[176] *In vivo*, venous thromboemboli predominate, sometimes with complicating pulmonary or portal hypertension. The thrombotic risk is independent of postsplenectomy thrombosis, and all cases of thrombosis have occurred in splenectomized patients. Results of treatment of splenectomized patients with long-term warfarin have been variable. In severe cases, erythrocyte hypertransfusion has been beneficial. Unfortunately, the procedure is complicated by iron overload, a significant problem even in the absence of transfusion.

Neonates with hydrocytosis have required phototherapy, red cell transfusion, and, in some cases, exchange transfusion for treatment of anemia and hyperbilirubinemia.

INTERMEDIATE SYNDROMES

Some reported cases of HSt share features of hereditary xerocytosis and hereditary hydrocytosis. These disorders have been characterized as *intermediate syndromes* (see Table 44-4).[168] Characteristically, patients have stomatocytes and/or target cells on blood film. Erythrocyte osmotic fragility is either normal or decreased. Red cell sodium and potassium permeabilities are increased, but the intracellular cation concentration and the red cell volume are either normal or slightly reduced. In a few patients, red cells undergo spontaneous *in vitro* hemolysis after storage at 5°C (41°F), hence the designation *cryohydrocytosis.*[183]

A dominantly inherited hemolytic anemia with stomatocytosis, occasional target cells, spherocytes, and decreased osmotic fragility, in which the main red cell membrane abnormality involved an almost 50 percent increase in phosphatidylcholine and a corresponding decrease in PE, has been described.[184,185] In wet preparations, approximately 30 percent of the cells were stomatocytes. The molecular basis of the syndrome is unclear. Because abnormalities in membrane phospholipid composition have not been systematically investigated, whether the disorder represents a distinct disease entity is unclear.

Rh Deficiency Syndrome Rh deficiency syndrome designates rare individuals who have either absent (Rh_{null}) or markedly reduced (Rh_{mod}) Rh antigen expression and reduced or absent proteins of the Rh–RhAG complex, including Rh, RhAG, LW, glycophorin B, CD47, and protein 4.2. Mild to moderate hemolytic anemia associated with the presence of stomatocytes and occasional spherocytes on blood film are observed.[186,187] Chapter 128 reviews the structure, localization, and functions of the Rh antigens.

Although the clinical syndromes are similar, the genetic bases of the Rh deficiency syndrome are heterogeneous, and at least two groups can be defined. The *amorph type* results from mutations of Rh30, the RhD and RhE polypeptides. The *regulatory type* results from mutations of Rh50, a modulator of Rh gene expression. Studies of these rare patients have provided evidence that both the Rh locus and Rh50 are required for the expression and function of Rh as a multimeric complex in the red cell membrane.

Red cells of some Rh_{null} patients have increased osmotic fragility reflecting a markedly reduced membrane surface area. The cells also are dehydrated, as indicated by decreased cell cation and water content and increased cell density. Potassium transport and Na+-K+ pump activity are increased, possibly because of reticulocytosis. Hemolytic anemia is improved by splenectomy.

FAMILIAL DEFICIENCY OF HIGH-DENSITY LIPOPROTEINS

Severe deficiency or absence of high-density lipoproteins leads to accumulation of cholesteryl esters in many tissues, leading to clinical findings of large orange tonsils and hepatosplenomegaly. Reported hematologic manifestations include moderately severe hemolytic anemia with stomatocytosis.[188] Membrane lipid analyses have shown a low cholesterol content leading to a decreased ratio of cholesterol to phospholipid and a relative increase in phosphatidylcholine at the expense of sphingomyelin.

ACQUIRED STOMATOCYTOSIS

Few stomatocytes (3–5%) are commonly found on blood films of normal subjects. Prospective analysis of films from a large number of hospitalized patients revealed an overall incidence of stomatocytosis (>5% of stomatocytes) of 2.3 percent.[189] Fifty-nine percent of the patients had 5 to 20 percent stomatocytes, 35 percent had 20 to 50 percent stomatocytes, and 6 percent had more than 50 percent stomatocytes. A wide variety of medications and diagnoses, including malignant neoplasms, cardiovascular disease, hepatobiliary disease, and alcoholism, were associated with stomatocytosis. Additional studies are required to determine which associations are specific and reproducible. For instance, acquired stomatocytosis is common in alcoholics, particularly those with acute alcoholism (see Fig. 44-13C).[190] Vinca alkaloids, such as vincristine and vinblastine, may induce hemolysis, with increased sodium permeability and stomatocytosis at the doses used for chemotherapy of leukemias and lymphomas.[191,192] The molecular basis of stomatocytosis in these conditions is unknown. Stomatocytosis is rarely associated with clinically significant hematologic abnormalities.

REFERENCES

1. Ways P, Hanahan DJ: Characterization and quantitation of red cell lipids in normal man. *J Lipid Res* 5:318, 1964.
2. Cohen CM, Gascard P: Regulation and post-translational modification of erythrocyte membrane and membrane-skeletal proteins. *Semin Hematol* 29:244, 1992.
3. Bevers EM, Comfurius P, Dekkers DW, Zwaal RF: Lipid translocation across the plasma membrane of mammalian cells. *Biochim Biophys Acta* 1439:317, 1999.
4. Andrews DA, Low PS: Role of red blood cells in thrombosis. *Curr Opin Hematol* 6:76, 1999.
5. Tang X, Halleck MS, Schlegel RA, Williamson P: A subfamily of P-type ATPases with aminophospholipid transporting activity. *Science* 272:1495, 1996.
6. Dekkers DW, Comfurius P, Schroit AJ, et al: Transbilayer movement of NBD-labeled phospholipids in red blood cell membranes: Outward-directed transport by the multidrug resistance protein 1 (MRP1). *Biochemistry* 37:14833, 1998.
7. Zhou Q, Zhao J, Stout JG, et al: Molecular cloning of human plasma membrane phospholipid scramblase. A protein mediating transbilayer movement of plasma membrane phospholipids. *J Biol Chem* 272:18240, 1997.
8. Zhao J, Zhou Q, Wiedmer T, Sims PJ: Level of expression of phospholipid scramblase regulates induced movement of phosphatidylserine to the cell surface. *J Biol Chem* 273:6603, 1998.
9. Dekkers DW, Comfurius P, Vuist WM, et al: Impaired Ca^{2+}-induced tyrosine phosphorylation and defective lipid scrambling in erythrocytes from a patient with Scott syndrome: A study using an inhibitor for scramblase that mimics the defect in Scott syndrome. *Blood* 91:2133, 1998.
10. Stout JG, Basse F, Luhm RA, et al: Scott syndrome erythrocytes contain a membrane protein capable of mediating Ca^{2+}-dependent transbilayer migration of membrane phospholipids. *J Clin Invest* 99.2232, 1997.
11. Salzer U, Prohaska R: Stomatin, flotillin-1, and flotillin-2 are major integral proteins of erythrocyte lipid rafts. *Blood* 97:1141, 2001.
12. Salzer U, Hinterdorfer P, Hunger U, et al: Ca++-dependent vesicle release from erythrocytes involves stomatin-specific lipid rafts, synexin (annexin VII), and sorcin. *Blood* 99:2569, 2002.
13. Murphy SC, Samuel BU, Harrison T, et al: Erythrocyte detergent-resistant membrane proteins: Their characterization and selective uptake during malarial infection. *Blood* 103:1920, 2004.
14. Mulder E, van Deenen LL: Metabolism of red-cell lipids. I. Incorporation in vitro of fatty acids into phospholipids from mature erythrocytes. *Biochim Biophys Acta* 106:106, 1965.
15. Reed CF: Incorporation of orthophosphate-^{32}P into erythrocyte phospholipids in normal subjects and in patients with hereditary spherocytosis. *J Clin Invest* 49:1668, 1968.
16. Shohet SB, Nathan DG, Karnovsky ML: Stages in the incorporation of fatty acids into red blood cells. *J Clin Invest* 47:1096, 1968.
17. Renooij W, Van Golde LM: Asymmetry in the renewal of molecular classes of phosphatidylcholine in the rat-erythrocyte membrane. *Biochim Biophys Acta* 558:314, 1979.
18. Shohet SB, Haley JE: Red cell membrane shape and stability: Relation to cell lipid renewal pathways and cell ATP. *Nouv Rev Fr Hematol* 12:761, 1972.
19. Fairbanks G, Steck TL, Wallach DFH: Electrophoretic analysis of the major polypeptides of the human erythrocyte membrane. *Biochemistry* 10:2606, 1971.
20. Tanner MJ: Band 3 anion exchanger and its involvement in erythrocyte and kidney disorders. *Curr Opin Hematol* 9:133, 2002.
21. Zhang D, Kiyatkin A, Bolin JT, Low PS: Crystallographic structure and functional interpretation of the cytoplasmic domain of erythrocyte membrane band 3. *Blood* 96:2925, 2000.

22. Bruce LJ, Beckmann R, Ribeiro ML, et al: A band 3-based macrocomplex of integral and peripheral proteins in the RBC membrane. *Blood* 101:4180, 2003.

23. Mohandas N, Winardi R, Knowles D, et al: Molecular basis for membrane rigidity of hereditary ovalocytosis. A novel mechanism involving the cytoplasmic domain of band 3. *J Clin Invest* 89:686, 1992.

24. Reid ME, Mohandas N: Red blood cell blood group antigens: Structure and function. *Semin Hematol* 41:93, 2004.

25. Nicolas V, Le Van Kim C, Gane P, et al: Rh-RhAG/ankyrin-R, a new interaction site between the membrane bilayer and the red cell skeleton, is impaired by Rh(null)-associated mutation. *J Biol Chem* 278:25526, 2003.

26. Dahl KN, Parthasarathy R, Westhoff CM, et al: Protein 4.2 is critical to CD47-membrane skeleton attachment in human red cells. *Blood* 103:1131, 2004.

27. Morrow JS, Rimm DL, Kennedy SP, et al: Of membrane stability and mosaics: The spectrin cytoskeleton, in *Handbook of Physiology*, edited by J Hoffman, J Jamieson, p 485. Oxford, London, 1997.

28. Gallagher PG, Forget BG: Spectrin genes in health and disease. *Semin Hematol* 30:4, 1993.

29. Thomas GH, Newbern EC, Korte CC, et al: Intragenic duplication and divergence in the spectrin superfamily of proteins. *Mol Biol Evol* 14:1285, 1997.

30. Grum VL, Li DN, MacDonald RI, Mondragon A: Structures of two repeats of spectrin suggest models of flexibility. *Cell* 98:523, 1999.

31. Ursitti JA, Kotula L, DeSilva TM, et al: Mapping the human erythrocyte beta-spectrin dimer initiation site using recombinant peptides and correlation of its phasing with the alpha-actinin dimer site. *J Biol Chem* 271:6636, 1996.

32. Alloisio N, Morle L, Marechal J, et al: Sp alpha V/41: A common spectrin polymorphism at the alpha IV-alpha V domain junction. Relevance to the expression level of hereditary elliptocytosis due to alpha-spectrin variants located in trans. *J Clin Invest* 87:2169, 1991.

33. Becker PS, Schwartz MA, Morrow JS, Lux SE: Radiolabel-transfer cross-linking demonstrates that protein 4.1 binds to the N-terminal region of beta spectrin and to actin in binary interactions. *Eur J Biochem* 193:827, 1990.

34. Kennedy SP, Warren SL, Forget BG, Morrow JS: Ankyrin binds to the 15th repetitive unit of erythroid and nonerythroid β spectrin. *J Cell Biol* 115:267, 1991.

35. Bennett V, Baines AJ: Spectrin and ankyrin-based pathways: Metazoan inventions for integrating cells into tissues. *Physiol Rev* 81:1353, 2001.

36. Gallagher PG, Tse WT, Scarpa AL, et al: Structure and organization of the human ankyrin-1 gene: Basis for complexity of pre-mRNA processing. *J Biol Chem* 272:19220, 1997.

37. Michaely P, Tomchick DR, Machius M, Anderson RG: Crystal structure of a 12 ANK repeat stack from human ankyrinR. *EMBO J* 21:6387, 2002.

38. Hou VC, Conboy JG: Regulation of alternative pre-mRNA splicing during erythroid differentiation. *Curr Opin Hematol* 8:74, 2001.

39. Gallagher PG: Hereditary elliptocytosis: Spectrin and protein 4.1R. *Semin Hematol* 41:142, 2004.

40. Shi ZT, Afzal V, Coller B, et al: Protein 4.1R-deficient mice are viable but have erythroid membrane skeleton abnormalities. *J Clin Invest* 103:331, 1999.

41. Yawata Y: Red cell membrane protein band 4.2: Phenotypic, genetic and electron microscopic aspects. *Biochim Biophys Acta* 1204:131, 1994.

42. Peters LL, Jindel HK, Gwynn B, et al: Mild spherocytosis and altered red cell ion transport in protein 4.2-null mice. *J Clin Invest* 103:1527, 1999.

43. Chishti AH: Function of p55 and its nonerythroid homologues. *Curr Opin Hematol* 5:116, 1998.

44. Li X, Matsuoka Y, Bennett V: Adducin preferentially recruits spectrin to the fast growing ends of actin filaments in a complex requiring the MARCKS-related domain and a newly defined oligomerization domain. *J Biol Chem* 273:19329, 1998.

45. Matsuoka Y, Li X, Bennett V: Adducin is an in vivo substrate for protein kinase C: Phosphorylation in the MARCKS-related domain inhibits activity in promoting spectrin-actin complexes and occurs in many cells, including dendritic spines of neurons. *J Cell Biol* 142:485, 1998.

46. Gilligan DM, Lozovatsky L, Gwynn B, et al: Targeted disruption of the beta-adducin gene (Add2) causes red blood cell spherocytosis in mice. *Proc Natl Acad Sci U S A* 96:10717, 1999.

47. De Matteis MA, Morrow JS: The role of ankyrin and spectrin in membrane transport and domain formation. *Curr Opin Cell Biol* 10:542, 1998.

48. Liu SC, Derick LH, Palek J: Visualization of the hexagonal lattice in the erythrocyte membrane skeleton. *J Cell Biol* 104:527, 1987.

49. Gilligan DM, Bennett V: The junctional complex of the membrane skeleton. *Semin Hematol* 30:74, 1993.

50. Giorgi M, Cianci CD, Gallagher PG, Morrow JS: Spectrin oligomerization is cooperatively coupled to membrane assembly: A linkage targeted by many hereditary hemolytic anemias? *Exp Mol Pathol* 70:215, 2001.

51. Mohandas N, Chasis JA: Red blood cell deformability, membrane material properties and shape: Regulation by transmembrane, skeletal and cytosolic proteins and lipids. *Semin Hematol* 30:171, 1993.

52. Narla M, Chasis JA, Shohet SB: The influence of membrane skeleton on red cell deformability, membrane material properties, and shape. *Semin Hematol* 20:225, 1983.

53. Hanspal M, Palek J: Biogenesis of normal and abnormal red blood cell membrane skeleton. *Semin Hematol* 29:305, 1992.

54. Peters LL, Shivdasani RA, Liu SC, et al: Anion exchanger 1 (band 3) is required to prevent erythrocyte membrane surface loss but not to form the membrane skeleton. *Cell* 86:917, 1996.

55. Peters LL, White RA, Birkenmeier CS, et al: Changing in cytoskeletal mRNA expression and protein synthesis patterns during murine erythropoiesis in vivo. *Proc Natl Acad Sci U S A* 89:5749, 1992.

56. Koury MJ, Bondurant MC, Rana SS: Changes in erythroid membrane proteins during erythropoietin-mediated terminal differentiation. *J Cell Physiol* 133:438, 1987.

57. Chasis JA, Prenant M, Leung A, Mohandas N: Membrane assembly and remodeling during reticulocyte maturation. *Blood* 74:1112, 1989.

58. Gallagher PG: Disorders of erythrocyte metabolism and shape, in *Hematologic Problems in the Neonate*, edited by RD Christensen, p 209. WB Saunders, Philadelphia, 1999.

59. Brugnara C: Erythrocyte membrane transport physiology. *Curr Opin Hematol* 4:122, 1997.

60. Lauf PK, Adragna NC: K-Cl cotransport: Properties and molecular mechanism. *Cell Physiol Biochem* 10:341, 2000.

61. Brugnara C: Sickle cell disease: From membrane pathophysiology to novel therapies for prevention of erythrocyte dehydration. *J Pediatr Hematol Oncol* 25:927, 2003.

62. Agre P, Kozono D: Aquaporin water channels: Molecular mechanisms for human diseases. *FEBS Lett* 555:72, 2003.

63. Chretien S, Cartron JP: A single mutation inside the NPA motif of aquaporin 1 found in a Colton-null phenotype. *Blood* 93:4021, 1999.

64. Dacie J: The life span of the red blood cell and circumstances of its premature death, in *Blood, Pure, and Eloquent*, edited by M Wintrobe, p 211. McGraw-Hill, New York, 1980.

65. Eber S, Lux SE: Hereditary spherocytosis—Defects in proteins that connect the membrane skeleton to the lipid bilayer. *Semin Hematol* 41:118, 2004.

66. Eber SW, Gonzalez JM, Lux ML, et al: Ankyrin-1 mutations are a major cause of dominant and recessive hereditary spherocytosis. *Nat Genet* 13:214, 1996.

67. Gallagher PG, Forget BG: Hematologically important mutations: Spectrin and ankyrin variants in hereditary spherocytosis. *Blood Cell Mol Dis* 24:539, 1998.

68. Eber SW, Pekrun A, Reinhardt D, et al: Hereditary spherocytosis with ankyrin Walsrode, a variant ankyrin with decreased affinity for band 3. *Blood* 84:362a, 1994.

69. Gallagher PG, Sabatino DE, Basseres DS, et al: Erythrocyte ankyrin promoter mutations associated with recessive hereditary spherocytosis cause significant abnormalities in ankyrin expression. *J Biol Chem* 276:41683, 2001.

70. Lux SE, Tse WT, Menninger JC, et al: Hereditary spherocytosis associated with deletion of human erythrocyte ankyrin gene on chromosome 8. *Nature* 345:736, 1990.

71. Gallagher PG, Forget BG: Hematologically important mutations: Band 3 and protein 4.2 variants in hereditary spherocytosis. *Blood Cell Mol Dis* 23:417, 1997.

72. Rysava R, Tesar V, Jirsa M Jr, et al: Incomplete distal renal tubular acidosis coinherited with a mutation in the band 3 (AE1) gene. *Nephrol Dial Transplant* 12:1869, 1997.

73. Lima PRM, Gontijo JAR, Lopes de Faria JB, et al: Band 3 Campinas: A novel splicing mutation in the band 3 gene (AE1) associated with hereditary spherocytosis, hyperactivity of Na⁺/Li⁺ countertransport and an abnormal renal bicarbonate handling. *Blood* 90:2810, 1997.

74. Agre P, Casella JF, Zinkham WH, et al: Partial deficiency of erythrocyte spectrin in hereditary spherocytosis. *Nature* 314:380, 1985.

75. Agre P, Asimos A, Casella JF, McMillan C: Inheritance pattern and clinical response to splenectomy as a reflection of erythrocyte spectrin deficiency in hereditary spherocytosis. *N Engl J Med* 315:1579, 1986.

76. Wichterle H, Hanspal M, Palek J, Jarolim P: Combination of two mutant alpha spectrin alleles underlies a severe spherocytic hemolytic anemia. *J Clin Invest* 98:2300, 1996.

77. Tse WT, Gallagher PG, Jenkins PB, et al: Amino acid substitution in α-spectrin commonly coinherited with nondominant hereditary spherocytosis. *Am J Hematol* 54:233, 1997.

78. Hassoun H, Vassiliadis JN, Murray J, et al: Characterization of the underlying molecular defect in hereditary spherocytosis associated with spectrin deficiency. *Blood* 90:398, 1997.

79. Becker PS, Tse WT, Lux SE, Forget BG: Beta spectrin Kissimmee: A spectrin variant associated with autosomal dominant hereditary spherocytosis and defective binding to protein 4.1. *J Clin Invest* 92:612, 1993.

80. Bouhassira EE, Schwartz RS, Yawata Y, et al: An alanine-to-threonine substitution in protein 4.2 cDNA is associated with a Japanese form of hereditary hemolytic anemia (protein 4.2^NIPPON). *Blood* 79:1846, 1992.

81. Rybicki AC, Qiu JJ, Musto S, et al: Human erythrocyte protein 4.2 deficiency associated with hemolytic anemia and a homozygous 40 glutamic acid→lysine substitution in the cytoplasmic domain of band 3 (band 3^Montefiore). *Blood* 81:2155, 1993.

82. Jarolim P, Palek J, Rubin HL, Prchal JT: Band 3 Tuscaloosa: Pro327-Arg327 substitution in the cytoplasmic domain of erythrocyte band 3 protein associated with spherocytic hemolytic anemia and partial deficiency of protein 4.2. *Blood* 80:523, 1992.

83. De Franceschi L, Olivieri O, Miraglia del Giudice E, et al: Membrane cation and anion transport activities in erythrocytes of hereditary spherocytosis: Effects of different membrane protein defects. *Am J Hematol* 55:121, 1997.

84. Young LE, Platzer RI, Ervin DM, Izzo MJ: Hereditary spherocytosis: II. Observations on the role of the spleen. *Blood* 6:1099, 1951.

85. Emerson CJ, Shen S, Ham T, et al: Studies on the destruction of red blood cells: IX. Quantitative methods for determining the osmotic and mechanical fragility of red cells in the peripheral blood and splenic pulp: The mechanism of increased hemolysis in hereditary spherocytosis (congenital hemolytic jaundice) as related to the function of the spleen. *Arch Intern Med* 97:1, 1956.

86. Miraglia del Giudice E, Francese M, Nobili B, et al: High frequency of de novo mutations in ankyrin gene (ANK1) in children with hereditary spherocytosis. *J Pediatr* 132:117, 1998.

87. Miraglia del Giudice E, Lombardi C, Francese M, et al: Frequent de novo monoallelic expression of β-spectrin gene (SPTB) in children with hereditary spherocytosis and isolated spectrin deficiency. *Br J Haematol* 101:251, 1998.

88. Ribeiro ML, Alloisio N, Almeida H, et al: Severe hereditary spherocytosis and distal renal tubular acidosis associated with the total absence of band 3. *Blood* 96:1602, 2000.

89. Perrotta S, Nigro V, Iolascon A, et al: Dominant hereditary spherocytosis due to band 3 Neapolis produces a life-threatening anemia at the homozygous state. *Blood* 92:9a, 1998.

90. Eber SW, Armbrust R, Schröter W: Variable clinical severity of hereditary spherocytosis: Relation to erythrocytic spectrin concentration, osmotic fragility, and autohemolysis. *J Pediatr* 117:409, 1990.

91. Pajor A, Lehoczky D, Szakacs Z: Pregnancy and hereditary spherocytosis: Report of 8 patients and a review. *Arch Gynecol Obstet* 253:37, 1993.

92. Iolascon A, Faienza MF, Moretti A, et al: UGT1 promoter polymorphism accounts for increased neonatal appearance of hereditary spherocytosis. *Blood* 91:1093, 1998.

93. Tamary H, Aviner S, Freud E, et al: High incidence of early cholelithiasis detected by ultrasonography in children and young adults with hereditary spherocytosis. *J Pediatr Hematol Oncol* 25:952, 2003.

94. Young NS, Brown KE: Parvovirus B19. *N Engl J Med* 350:586, 2004.

95. Lefrere JJ, Courouce AM, Girot R, et al: Six cases of hereditary spherocytosis revealed by human parvovirus infection. *Br J Haematol* 62:653, 1986.

96. McLellan NJ, Rutter N: Hereditary spherocytosis in sisters unmasked by parvovirus infection. *Postgrad Med J* 63:49, 1987.

97. Lawrence P, Aronson I, Saxe N, Jacobs P: Leg ulcers in hereditary spherocytosis. *Clin Exp Dermatol* 16:28, 1991.

98. Pulsoni A, Ferrazza G, Malagnino F, et al: Mediastinal extramedullary hematopoiesis as first manifestation of hereditary spherocytosis. *Ann Hematol* 65:196, 1992.

99. Sutton CD, Garcea G, Marshall LJ, et al: Pelvic extramedullary haematopoiesis associated with hereditary spherocytosis. *Eur J Haematol* 70:326, 2003.

100. Conti JA, Howard LM: Hereditary spherocytosis and hematologic malignancy. *N Engl J Med* 91:95, 1994.

101. Brandenberg JB, Demarmels BF, Lutz HU, et al: Hereditary spherocytosis and hemochromatosis. *Ann Hematol* 81:202, 2002.

102. Peters LL, Barker JE: Spontaneous and targeted mutations in erythrocyte membrane skeleton genes: Mouse models of hereditary spherocytosis, in *Hematopoiesis*, edited by L Zon. Oxford University Press, New York, 2001, pp 582–608.

103. Gilligan DM, Lozovatsky L, Gwynn B, et al: Targeted disruption of the beta-adducin gene (Add2) causes red blood cell spherocytosis in mice. *Proc Natl Acad Sci U S A* 96:10717, 1999.

104. Pati AR, Patton WN, Harris RI: The use of the Technicon H1 in the diagnosis of hereditary spherocytosis. *Clin Lab Haematol* 11:27, 1989.

105. Young LE, Izzo MJ, Platzer RF: Hereditary spherocytosis: I. Clinical, hematologic, and genetic features in 28 cases, with particular reference to the osmotic and mechanical fragility of incubated erythrocytes. *Blood* 6:1073, 1951.

106. Reliene R, Mariani M, Zanella A, et al: Splenectomy prolongs survival of erythrocytes differently in spectrin/ankyrin- and band 3-deficient hereditary spherocytosis. *Blood* 100:2208, 2002.

107. Rescorla FJ, Engum SA, West KW, et al: Laparoscopic splenectomy has become the gold standard in children. *Am Surg* 68:297, 2002.

108. Tchernia G, Gauthier F, Mielot F, et al: Initial assessment of the beneficial effect of partial splenectomy in hereditary spherocytosis. *Blood* 81:2014, 1993.

109. Bader-Meunier B, Gauthier F, Archambaud F, et al: Long-term evaluation of the beneficial effect of subtotal splenectomy for management of hereditary spherocytosis. *Blood* 97:399, 2001.

110. de Buys Roessingh AS, de Lagausie P, Rohrlich P, et al: Follow-up of partial splenectomy in children with hereditary spherocytosis. *J Pediatr Surg*; 37:1459, 2002.

111. Dacie J: Hereditary elliptocytosis, in *The Haemolytic Anaemias*, p 216. Churchill Livingstone, Edinburgh, 1985.

112. Glele-Kakai C, Garbarz M, Lecomte M-C, et al: Epidemiological studies of spectrin mutations related to hereditary elliptocytosis and spectrin polymorphisms in Benin. *Br J Haematol* 95:57, 1996.

113. Dresbach M: Elliptical human red corpuscles. *Science* 19:469, 1904.

114. Hunter WC, Adams RB: Hematologic study of three generations of a white family showing elliptical erythrocytes. *Ann Intern Med* 2:1162, 1929.

115. Zarkowsky HS, Mohandas N, Speaker CB, Shohet SB: A congenital haemolytic anaemia with thermal sensitivity of the erythrocyte membrane. *Br J Haematol* 29:537, 1975.

116. Coetzer T, Palek J, Lawler J, et al: Structural and functional heterogeneity of alpha spectrin mutations involving the spectrin heterodimer self-association site: Relationships to hematologic expression of homozygous hereditary elliptocytosis and hereditary pyropoikilocytosis. *Blood* 75:2235, 1990.

117. Coetzer TL, Sahr K, Prchal J, et al: Four different mutations in codon 28 of alpha spectrin are associated with structurally and functionally abnormal spectrin alpha I/74 in hereditary elliptocytosis. *J Clin Invest* 88:743, 1991.

118. Marchesi SL, Letsinger JT, Speicher DW, et al: Mutant forms of spectrin alpha-subunits in hereditary elliptocytosis. *J Clin Invest* 80:191, 1987.

119. Delaunay J: Genetic disorders of the red cell membrane. *Crit Rev Oncol Hematol* 19:79, 1995.

120. Mohandas N, Chasis JA: Red blood cell deformability, membrane material properties and shape: Regulation by transmembrane, skeletal and cytosolic proteins and lipids. *Semin Hematol* 30:171, 1993.

121. Roux AF, Morle F, Guetarni D, et al: Molecular basis of Spα$^{1/65}$ hereditary elliptocytosis in North Africa: Insertion of a TTG triplet between codons 147 and 149 in the alpha-spectrin gene from five unrelated families. *Blood* 73:2196, 1989.

122. Gallagher PG, Weed SA, Tse WT, et al: Recurrent fatal hydrops fetalis associated with a nucleotide substitution in the erythrocyte β-spectrin gene. *J Clin Invest* 95:1174, 1995.

123. Sahr KE, Coetzer TL, Moy LS, et al: Spectrin Cagliari. An Ala→Gly substitution in helix 1 of β spectrin repeat 17 that severely disrupts the structure and self-association of the erythrocyte spectrin heterodimer. *J Biol Chem* 268:22656, 1993.

124. Gallagher PG, Petruzzi MJ, Weed SA, et al: Mutation of a highly conserved residue of βI spectrin associated with fatal and near-fatal neonatal hemolytic anemia. *J Clin Invest* 99:267, 1997.

125. Takakuwa Y, Tchernia G, Rossi M, et al: Restoration of normal membrane stability to unstable protein 4.1-deficient erythrocyte membranes by incorporation of purified protein 4.1. *J Clin Invest* 78:80, 1986.

126. Chishti AH, Palek J, Fisher D, et al: Reduced invasion and growth of *Plasmodium falciparum* into elliptocytic red blood cells with a combined deficiency of protein 4.1, glycophorin C, and p55. *Blood* 87:3462, 1996.

127. Conboy JG, Chasis JA, Winardi R, et al: An isoform-specific mutation in the protein 4.1 gene results in hereditary elliptocytosis and complete deficiency of protein 4.1 in erythrocytes but not in nonerythroid cells. *J Clin Invest* 91:77, 1993.

128. Winardi R, Reid M, Conboy J, Mohandas N: Molecular analysis of glycophorin C deficiency in human erythrocytes. *Blood* 81:2799, 1993.

129. Wilmotte R, Marechal J, Morle L, et al: Low expression allele α^{LELY} of red cell spectrin is associated with mutations in exon 40 (α$^{V/41}$ polymorphism) and intron 45 and with partial skipping of exon 46. *J Clin Invest* 91:2091, 1993.

130. Wilmotte R, Harper SL, Ursitti JA, et al: The exon 46 encoded sequence is essential for stability of human erythroid α-spectrin and heterodimer formation. *Blood* 90:4188, 1996.

131. Mentzer WC Jr, Iarocci TA, Mohandas N, et al: Modulation of erythrocyte membrane mechanical stability by 2,3-diphosphoglycerate in the neonatal poikilocytosis/elliptocytosis syndrome. *J Clin Invest* 79:943, 1987.

132. Lorenzo F, Miraglia del Giudice E, Alloisio N, et al: Severe poikilocytosis associated with a de novo α 28 Arg→Cys mutation in spectrin. *Br J Haematol* 83:152, 1993.

133. Jonsson JJ, Renieri A, Gallagher PG, et al: Alport syndrome, mental retardation, midface hypoplasia, and elliptocytosis: A new X-linked contiguous gene deletion syndrome. *Am J Med Genet* 35:273, 1997.

134. Mohandas N, Lie-Injo LE, Friedman M, Mak JW: Rigid membranes of Malayan ovalocytes: A likely genetic barrier against malaria. *Blood* 63:1385, 1984.

135. Hadley T, Saul A, Lamont G, et al: Resistance of Melanesian elliptocytes (ovalocytes) to invasion *by Plasmodium knowlesi* and *Plasmodium falciparum* malaria parasites in vitro. *J Clin Invest* 71:780, 1983.

136. Jarolim P, Palek J, Amato D, et al: Deletion in erythrocyte band 3 gene in malaria-resistant Southeast Asian ovalocytosis. *Proc Natl Acad Sci U S A* 88:11022, 1991.

137. Liu SC, Jarolim P, Rubin HL, et al: The homozygous state for the band 3 protein mutation in Southeast Asian ovalocytosis may be lethal. *Blood* 84:3590, 1994.

138. Genton B, Al-Yaman F, Mgone CS, et al: Ovalocytosis and cerebral malaria. *Nature* 378:564, 1995.

139. Li X, Chen H, Oo TH, et al: A co-ligand complex anchors Plasmodium falciparum merozoites to the erythrocyte invasion receptor band 3. *J Biol Chem* 279:5765, 2004.

140. Bessis FA: Red cell shapes: An illustrated classification and its rationale, in *Red Cell Shape: Physiology, Pathology and Ultrastructure*, edited by M Bessis, RI Weed, PF Leblond, p 1. Springer-Verlag, New York, 1973.

141. Colman N, Herbert V: Hematologic complications of alcoholism: Overview. *Semin Hematol* 17:164, 1980.

142. Cooper RA: Hemolytic syndromes and red cell membrane abnormalities in liver disease. *Semin Hematol* 17:103, 1980.

143. Cooper RA, Diloy Puray M, Lando P, Greenverg MS: An analysis of lipoproteins, bile acids, and red cell membranes associated with target cells and spur cells in patients with liver disease. *J Clin Invest* 51:3182, 1972.

144. Cooper RA, Kimball DB, Durocher JR: Role of the spleen in membrane conditioning and hemolysis of spur cells in liver disease. *N Engl J Med* 290:1279, 1974.

145. Silber R, Amorosi E, Lhowe J, Kayden HJ: Spur-shaped erythrocytes in Laennec's cirrhosis. *N Engl J Med* 275:639, 1966.

146. Zieve L: Jaundice, hyperlipemia and hemolytic anemia: A heretofore unrecognized syndrome associated with alcoholic fatty liver and cirrhosis. *Ann Intern Med* 48:471, 1958.

147. Kane J, Havel R: Disorders of the biogenesis and secretion of lipoproteins containing the B apolipoproteins, in *The Metabolic and Molecular Bases of Inherited Disease*, edited by C Scriver, A Beaudet, W Sly, et al, p 2717. McGraw-Hill, New York, 2001.

148. Narcisi TM, Shoulders CC, Chester SA, et al: Mutations of the microsomal triglyceride-transfer-protein gene in abetalipoproteinemia. *Am J Hum Genet* 57:1298, 1995.

149. Simon E, Ways P: Incubation hemolysis and red cell metabolism in acanthocytosis. *J Clin Invest* 43:1311, 1964.

150. Jones JW, Ways P: Abnormalities of high density lipoproteins in abetalipoproteinemia. *J Clin Invest* 46:1151, 1967.

151. Ross RS, Gregg RE, Law SW, et al: Homozygous hypobetalipoproteinemia: A disease distinct from abetalipoproteinemia at the molecular level. *J Clin Invest* 81:590, 1988.

152. Hardie RJ, Pullon HW, Harding AE, et al: Neuroacanthocytosis. A clinical, haematological and pathological study of 19 cases. *Brain* 114:13, 1991.

153. Critchley EM, Clark DB, Wikler A: Acanthocytosis and neurological disorder without abetalipoproteinemia. *Arch Neurol* 18:134, 1968.

154. Bruce LJ, Kay MM, Lawrence C, Tanner MJ: Band 3 HT, a human red-cell variant associated with acanthocytosis and increased anion transport, carries the mutation Pro-868→Leu in the membrane domain of band 3. *Biochem J* 293:317, 1993.

155. Ueno S, Maruki Y, Nakamura M, et al: The gene encoding a newly discovered protein, chorein, is mutated in chorea-acanthocytosis. *Nat Genet* 28:121, 2001.

156. Rampoldi L, Dobson-Stone C, Rubio JP, et al: A conserved sorting-associated protein is mutant in chorea-acanthocytosis. *Nat Genet* 28:119, 2001.

157. Dobson-Stone C, Danek A, Rampoldi L, et al: Mutational spectrum of the CHAC gene in patients with chorea-acanthocytosis. *Eur J Hum Genet* 10:773, 2002.

158. Ballas SK, Bator SM, Aubuchon JP, et al: Abnormal membrane physical properties of red cells in McLeod syndrome. *Transfusion* 30:722, 1990.

159. Wimer BM, Marsh WL, Taswell HF, Galey WR: Haematological changes associated with the McLeod phenotype of the Kell blood group system. *Br J Haematol* 36:219, 1977.

160. Redman CM, Russo D, Lee S: Kell, Kx and the McLeod syndrome. *Baillieres Best Pract Res Clin Haematol* 12:621, 1999.

161. Redman CM, Marsh WL, Scarborough A, et al: Biochemical studies on McLeod phenotype red cells and isolation of Kx antigen. *Br J Haematol* 68:131, 1988.

162. Francke U, Ochs HD, De Martinville B, et al: Minor Xp21 chromosome deletion in a male associated with expression of Duchenne muscular dystrophy, chronic granulomatous disease, retinitis pigmentosa, and McLeod syndrome. *Am J Hum Genet* 37:250, 1985.

163. Udden MM, Umeda M, Hirano Y, Marcus DM: New abnormalities in the morphology, cell surface receptors, and electrolyte metabolism of In(Lu) erythrocytes. *Blood* 69:52, 1987.

164. Ballas SK, Marcolina MJ, Crawford MN: In vitro storage and in vivo survival studies of red cells from persons with the In(Lu) gene. *Transfusion* 32:607, 1992.

165. Wardrop C, Hutchison HE: Red-cell shape in hypothyroidism. *Lancet* 1:1243, 1969.

166. Lande WM, Mentzer WC: Haemolytic anaemia associated with increased cation permeability. *Clin Haematol* 14:89, 1985.

167. Delaunay J: The hereditary stomatocytoses: Genetic disorders of the red cell membrane permeability to monovalent cations. *Semin Hematol* 41:165, 2004.

168. Gallagher PG, Forget BG, Lux SE: Disorders of the erythrocyte membrane, in *Hematology of Infancy and Childhood*, edited by DG Nathan, SH Orkin, p 544. WB Saunders, Philadelphia, 1998.

169. Ellory JC, Gibson JS, Stewart GW: Pathophysiology of abnormal cell volume in human red cells. *Contrib Nephrol* 123:220, 1998.

170. Clark MR, Shohet SB, Gottfried EL: Hereditary hemolytic disease with increased red blood cell phosphatidylcholine and dehydration: One, two, or many disorders? *Am J Hematol* 42:25, 1993.

171. Carella M, Stewart G, Ajetunmobi JF, et al: Genomewide search for dehydrated hereditary stomatocytosis (hereditary xerocytosis): Mapping of locus to chromosome 16(16q23-qter). *Am J Hum Genet* 63:810, 1998.

172. Stewart GW, Corrall RJ, Fyffe JA, et al: Familial pseudohyperkalaemia. A new syndrome. *Lancet* 2:175, 1979.

173. Grootenboer S, Schischmanoff PO, Cynober T, et al: A genetic syndrome associating dehydrated hereditary stomatocytosis, pseudohyperkalaemia and perinatal oedema. *Br J Haematol* 103:383, 1998.

174. Grootenboer S, Schischmanoff PO, Laurendeau I, et al: Pleiotropic syndrome of dehydrated hereditary stomatocytosis, pseudohyperkalemia, and perinatal edema map to 16q23-q24. *Blood* 189a, 1999.

175. Iolascon A, Stewart GW, Ajetunmobi JF, et al: Familial pseudohyperkalemia maps to the same locus as dehydrated hereditary stomatocytosis (hereditary xerocytosis). *Blood* 93:3120, 1999.

176. Stewart GW, Amess JA, Eber SW, et al: Thrombo-embolic disease after splenectomy for hereditary stomatocytosis. *Br J Haematol* 93:303, 1996.

177. Smith BD, Segel GB: Abnormal erythrocyte endothelial adherence in hereditary stomatocytosis. *Blood* 89:3451, 1997.

178. Lock SP, Smith RS, Hardisty RM: Stomatocytosis: A hereditary red cell anomaly associated with haemolytic anaemia. *Br J Haematol* 7:303, 1961.

179. Zarkowsky HS, Oski FA, Sha'afi R, et al: Congenital hemolytic anemia with high sodium, low potassium red cells: I. Studies of membrane permeability *N Engl J Med* 278:573, 1968.

180. Lande WM, Thiemann PV, Mentzer WC Jr: Missing band 7 membrane protein in two patients with high Na, low K erythrocytes. *J Clin Invest* 70:1273, 1982.

181. Fricke B, Argent AC, Chetty MC, et al: The "stomatin" gene and protein in overhydrated hereditary stomatocytosis. *Blood* 102:2268, 2003.

182. Zhu Y, Paszty C, Turetsky T, et al: Stomatocytosis is absent in "stomatin"-deficient murine red cells. *Blood* 93:2404, 1999.

183. Fricke B, Jarvis HG, Reid CD, et al: Four new cases of stomatin-deficient hereditary stomatocytosis syndrome: Association of the stomatin-deficient cryohydrocytosis variant with neurological dysfunction. *Br J Haematol* 125:796, 2004.

184. Jaffe ER, Gottfried EL: Hereditary nonspherocytic hemolytic disease associated with an altered phospholipid composition of the erythrocytes. *J Clin Invest* 47:1375, 1968.

185. Lane PA, Kuypers FA, Clark MR, et al: Excess of red cell membrane proteins in hereditary high-phosphatidylcholine hemolytic anemia. *Am J Hematol* 34:186, 1990.

186. Nash R, Shojania AM: Hematological aspect of Rh deficiency syndrome: A case report and a review of the literature. *Am J Hematol* 24:267, 1987.

187. Avent ND, Reid ME: The Rh blood group system: A review. *Blood* 95:375, 2000.

188. Tall R, Breslow JL, Rubin EM: Genetic disorders affecting plasma high-density lipoproteins, in *The Metabolic and Molecular Bases of Inherited Disease*, edited by CR Scriver, AL Beaudet, WS Sly, et al, p 2915. McGraw-Hill, New York, 2001.

189. Davidson RJ, How J, Lessels S: Acquired stomatocytosis: Its prevalence and significance in routine haematology. *Scand J Haematol* 19:47, 1977.

190. Wisloff F, Boman D: Acquired stomatocytosis in alcoholic liver disease. *Scand J Haematol* 23:43, 1979.

191. Ohsaka A, Kano Y, Sakamoto S, et al: A transient hemolytic reaction and stomatocytosis following vinca alkaloid administration. *Nippon Ketsueki Gakkai Zasshi* 52:7, 1989.

192. Neville AJ, Rand CA, Barr RD, Mohan Pai KR: Drug-induced stomatocytosis and anemia during consolidation chemotherapy of childhood acute leukemia. *Am J Med Sci* 287:3, 1984.

DISORDERS OF RED CELLS RESULTING FROM ENZYME ABNORMALITIES

ERNEST BEUTLER

Red cells possess an active metabolic machinery that provides energy to pump ions against electrochemical gradients, to maintain red cell shape, to keep hemoglobin iron in the reduced form, and to maintain enzyme and hemoglobin sulfhydryl groups. The main source of metabolic energy comes from glucose. Glucose is metabolized through the glycolytic pathway and through the hexose monophosphate shunt. Glycolysis catabolizes glucose to pyruvate and lactate, which represent the end products of glucose metabolism in the erythrocyte, because it lacks the mitochondria required for further oxidation of pyruvate. Adenosine diphosphate (ADP) is phosphorylated to adenosine triphosphate (ATP), and nicotinamide adenine dinucleotide (NAD)$^+$ is reduced to NADH in glycolysis. 2,3-Bisphosphoglycerate, an important regulator of the oxygen affinity of hemoglobin, is generated during glycolysis. The hexose monophosphate shunt oxidizes glucose-6-phosphate, reducing NADP$^+$ to reduced nicotinamide adenine dinucleotide phosphate (NADPH). In addition to glucose, the red cell has the capacity to utilize some other sugars and nucleosides as a source of energy. The red cell lacks the capacity for *de novo* purine synthesis but has a salvage pathway that permits synthesis of purine nucleotides from purine bases. The red cell contains high concentrations of glutathione, which is maintained almost entirely in the reduced state by NADPH through the catalytic activity of glutathione reductase. Glutathione is synthesized from glycine, cysteine, and glutamic acid in a two-step process that requires ATP as a source of energy. Catalase and glutathione peroxidase serve to protect the red cell from oxidative damage. The maturation of reticulocytes into erythrocytes is associated with a rapid decrease in the activity of several enzymes. However, the decrease in activities of enzymes occurs much more slowly or not at all with aging.

Erythrocyte enzyme deficiencies may lead to hemolytic anemia; expression of the defect in other cell lines may lead to pathologic changes such as neuromuscular abnormalities. Glucose-6-phosphate dehydrogenase (G-6-PD) deficiency is the most common erythrocyte enzyme defect. In some populations, more than 20 percent of the population may be affected by this enzyme deficiency. In the common polymorphic forms, such as G-6-PD A−, G-6-PD Mediterranean, or G-6-PD Canton, hemolysis occurs only during the stress imposed by infection or administration of "oxidative" drugs and in some individuals upon ingestion of fava beans. Neonatal icterus, which appears largely to result from a defect in bilirubin conjugation, is the clinically most serious complication of G-6-PD deficiency. Patients with less common, functionally very severe, genetic variants of G-6-PD experience chronic hemolysis, a disorder designated hereditary nonspherocytic hemolytic anemia.

Hereditary nonspherocytic hemolytic anemia also occurs as a consequence of other enzyme deficiencies, the most common of which is pyruvate kinase deficiency. Glucosephosphate isomerase, triosephosphate isomerase, and pyrimidine 5′-nucleotidase deficiency are included among the relatively rare causes of hereditary nonspherocytic hemolytic anemia. In the case of some deficiencies, notably those of glutathione synthetase, triosephosphate isomerase, and phosphoglycerate kinase, the defect is expressed throughout the body, and neurologic defects may be a prominent part of the clinical syndrome.

Diagnosis is best achieved by determining red cell enzyme activity either with a quantitative assay or a screening test. Except for the stippling of erythrocytes that is characteristic of pyrimidine 5′ nucleotidase deficiency, red cell morphology is of little or no help in differentiation of red cell enzyme deficiencies from one another. A variety of molecular lesions have been defined in most of these enzyme deficiencies. Accurate diagnosis is necessary for genetic counseling and is helpful in recommendations for treatment, since patients with some enzyme deficiencies (e.g., glucosephosphate isomerase deficiency) tend to respond more favorably to splenectomy than do others (e.g., G-6-PD deficiency). It is also essential for genetic counseling, because some of the defects, such as pyruvate kinase and glucosephosphate isomerase deficiencies, are transmitted as autosomal recessive disorders, while G-6-PD and phosphoglycerate kinase deficiencies are X linked.

DEFINITION AND HISTORY

Deficiencies in the activities of a number of erythrocyte enzymes may lead to shortening of the red cell life span. Glucose-6-phosphate dehydrogenase (G-6-PD) deficiency was the first of these to be recognized and is the most common.

The recognition of G-6-PD deficiency was the result of investigations of the hemolytic effect of the antimalarial drug primaquine, carried out in the 1950s and described in detail elsewhere.[1-3] These early studies defined G-6-PD deficiency as a hereditary sex-linked enzyme deficiency that affected primarily the erythrocytes, older cells being more severely affected than newly formed ones. They showed that this enzyme deficiency was very prevalent in individuals of African, Mediterranean, and Oriental ethnic origins, but that it could be found in virtually any population. The common (polymorphic) forms of G-6-PD deficiency were found to be associated with anemia only under conditions of stress, such as the administration of oxidative drugs, infection, or the neonatal period.

Chronic hemolysis in the absence of a stress occurs in uncommon, functionally severe forms of G-6-PD deficiency and in patients with a variety of other red cell enzyme deficiencies. Such patients have one type of *hereditary nonspherocytic hemolytic anemia*. Although patients fitting the description of hereditary nonspherocytic hemolytic anemia had been documented earlier, the designation was first introduced by Crosby[4] in 1950. Dacie and colleagues[5] subsequently reported several families in which affected members manifested hemo-

Acronyms and abbreviations that appear in this chapter include: ADA, adenosine deaminase; ADP, adenosine diphosphate; ATP, adenosine triphosphate; BPG, bisphosphoglycerate; DPG, diphosphoglycerate; EDTA, ethylenediaminetetraacetic acid; G-6-PD, glucose-6-phosphate dehydrogenase; GSH, reduced glutathione; GSSG, oxidized glutathione; LDH, lactate dehydrogenase; NAD, nicotinamide adenine dinucleotide; NADPH, reduced nicotinamide adenine dinucleotide phosphate; PEP, phosphoenolpyruvate; PGM, phosphoglucomutase; PK, pyruvate kinase; TPI, triosephosphate isomerase; UDPG, uridine diphosphoglucose; UDPGT, uridine diphosphoglucuronate glucuronosyltransferase.

604

lytic anemia from an early age and in whom the osmotic fragility of the red cells was normal. The latter finding, and the fact that most of the affected individuals failed to benefit from splenectomy, distinguished this disorder from hereditary spherocytosis. Thus, defined essentially by exclusion as a hereditary hemolytic anemia that is not hereditary spherocytosis, it is not at all surprising that hereditary nonspherocytic hemolytic anemia has proven to be extremely heterogeneous both in etiology and in clinical manifestations. Sometimes this disorder is also designated *congenital nonspherocytic hemolytic anemia*, but the name hereditary is more accurate and is therefore preferable. While hereditary ovalocytosis, pyropoikilocytosis, stomatocytosis, and even sickle cell disease and thalassemia major are hereditary hemolytic anemias that are not spherocytic, they are not included in this category. Rather, the diagnosis of hereditary nonspherocytic hemolytic anemia is reserved for those patients who have no major aberration of red cell morphology.

Although a deficiency of G-6-PD was found to be responsible for hemolysis in a few patients with hereditary nonspherocytic hemolytic anemia,[6] in the overwhelming majority of cases the cause remained obscure. In 1954, Selwyn and Dacie[7] studied autohemolysis (spontaneous lysis of red cells after sterile incubation for 24–48 hours at 37°C) in four patients with hereditary nonspherocytic hemolytic anemia and found that in two of them lysis was only slightly increased and was prevented by glucose; these patients were designated as type 1 while the others, in whom glucose failed to correct autohemolysis, were classified as type 2. Autohemolysis of the erythrocytes of type 2 patients was modified by the addition of ATP, a substance that we now recognize does not penetrate the red cell membrane. Instead, its modifying influence was probably exerted chiefly by virtue of its effect on the osmolarity and pH of the suspending solution. However, the findings suggested to DeGruchy et al.[8,9] that patients with type 2 autohemolysis suffered from a defect in ATP generation. This proposal, born of a misunderstanding of red cell biochemistry, turned out to be correct: for one of the major causes of hereditary nonspherocytic hemolytic anemia proved to be a deficiency of the ATP-generating enzyme pyruvate kinase (PK),[10] but this was only the first of a large number of enzyme defects that have been shown to account for this heterogeneous syndrome.[11,12]

EPIDEMIOLOGY

The prevalence of G-6-PD deficiency among Caucasian populations ranges from less than one in 1000 among northern European populations to 50 percent of the males among Kurdish Jews. G-6-PD deficiency is also found among certain Chinese populations and in Southeast Asia, but it is rare in Japan. G-6-PD deficiency of the A– type is very common in West Africa, and the prevalence among African-American males is approximately 11 percent.[13] Some 16 percent of African-American males carry the nondeficient G-6-PD A+ gene. The distribution of G-6-PD deficiency among various population groups has been presented in detail elsewhere.[12,14,15]

The high frequency of G-6-PD–deficient genes in many populations implies that G-6-PD deficiency confers a selective advantage. The suggestion[16] that resistance to malaria could account for the frequency of G-6-PD deficiency was supported by studies in heterozygotes for G-6-PD A– that showed a higher degree of infestation of G-6-PD sufficient cells than of G-6-PD–deficient cells.[17] It has been suggested that deficient cells infested with malaria parasites may be phagocytosed more efficiently than normal cells.[18]

It has been suggested that a higher prevalence of G-6-PD deficiency in individuals with sickle cell disease than in the general African population reflects a favorable effect of the enzyme deficiency on the clinical course of the sickling disorders.[19,20] However, it seems that the increased prevalence of G-6-PD deficiency in patients with sickle disease may merely result from the markedly heterogeneous genetic composition of African-Americans; those with more African genes are more likely to inherit sickle hemoglobin and G-6-PD A–.[21–23] Similar factors may be responsible for the slight excess of G-6-PD deficiency observed among patients with SS hemoglobin in Arab populations.[24]

Pyruvate kinase (PK) deficiency is the most common cause of hereditary nonspherocytic hemolytic anemia. Estimates of heterozygote frequency have ranged from 0.24 percent[25] to 3.1 percent,[26] using screening techniques. More quantitative studies performed on a large number of cord blood samples have provided estimates of 1 percent in the white population and 2.4 percent in African-Americans.[27] Based on large-scale mutation analysis it has been estimated that the population prevalence of pyruvate kinase deficiency among whites is approximately 50 cases per million population.[490] Estimates of other deficiency alleles, such as those for adenylate kinase, diphosphoglycerate mutase, enolase, triosephosphate isomerase (TPI), and phosphoglycerate kinase, have also been made on large numbers of cord bloods.[27] A particularly high incidence of heterozygous TPI deficiency of greater than 4 percent in African-Americans is supported by family studies.[28] Since it is not reflected in a correspondingly high birth incidence, the allele might be lethal in the homozygous state. It was suggested that a promoter mutation at the -5 and -8 positions created such a lethal gene,[29] but the finding of normal adult homozygotes for these mutations shows that this is not the case.[30]

In addition to the common G-6-PD mutations, there are mutations in other enzymes that are repeatedly encountered in the population. Included are the 1529A mutation of PK,[31,32] the deletion of exon 11 found among gypsies,[33] and the 1591 C mutation of TPI.[34] In each of these instances, the existence of each mutation in the context of the same haplotype implies that there has been a *founder effect*, that is, the mutation occurred only once, and all individuals now carrying it are descendants of the person who sustained the original mutation. The expansion of the mutation could represent a selective advantage for heterozygotes but also may result from random factors or from a selective advantage provided by one or more tightly linked genes.

ETIOLOGY AND PATHOGENESIS

RED CELL METABOLISM

Although the binding, transport, and delivery of oxygen do not require the expenditure of metabolic energy by the red blood cell, a source of energy is required if the red cell is to perform its function efficiently and to survive in the circulation for its full life span of approximately 120 days. This energy is needed to maintain (1) the iron of hemoglobin in the divalent form, (2) the high potassium and low calcium and sodium levels within the cell against a gradient imposed by the high plasma calcium and sodium and low plasma potassium levels, (3) the sulfhydryl groups of red cell enzymes, hemoglobin, and membranes in the active, reduced form, and (4) the biconcave shape of the cell. If the red cell is deprived of a source of energy, it becomes sodium and calcium logged and potassium depleted, and the red cell shape changes from a biconcave disc to a sphere. Such a cell is quickly removed from the circulation by the filtering action of the spleen and by a perceptive monocyte-macrophage system. Even if it survived, such an energy-deprived cell would gradually turn brown as hemoglobin is oxidized to methemoglobin by the very high concentrations of oxygen within the erythrocyte. The cell would then be unable to perform its function of transporting oxygen and carbon dioxide.

The process of extracting energy from a substrate, such as glucose, and of utilizing this energy is carried out by a large number of enzymes (Table 45-1). Since the red cell loses its nucleus before it enters the

TABLE 45-1 ACTIVITIES OF SOME RED CELL ENZYMES

ENZYME	ACTIVITY AT 37°C IU/G HB (MEAN±SD)	REFERENCE
Acetylcholinesterase	36.93±3.83	1
Adenosine deaminase	1.11±0.23	1
Adenylate kinase	258±29.3	1
Aldolase	3.19±0.86	1
ATPase (Na$^+$-K$^+$)*	0.121±0.031	1
ATPase (Mg^{2+})	0.278±0.066	2
Bisphosphoglyceromutase	4.78±0.65	1
Catalase	153,117±2390	1
Enolase	5.39±0.83	1
Galactokinase	0.0291±0.004	1
Galactose-4-epimerase	0.231±0.061	1
Glucose phosphate isomerase	60.8±11.0	1
Glucose-6-phosphate dehydrogenase	8.34±1.59	1
γ-Glutamyl cysteine synthetase	1.05±0.19	3
Glutathione peroxidase*	30.82±4.65	1
Glutathione reductase without FAD	7.18±1.09	1
Glutathione reductase with FAD	10.4±1.50	1
Glutathione-S-transferase	6.66±1.81	1
Glutathione synthetase	0.34±0.06	3
Glyceraldehyde phosphate dehydrogenase	226±41.9	1
GOT without pyridoxal phosphate	3.02±0.67	1
GOT with pyridoxal phosphate	5.04±0.90	1
Hexokinase	1.78±0.38	1
Lactate dehydrogenase	200±26.5	1
Monophosphoglyceromutase	37.71±5.56	1
NADH-methemoglobin reductase	19.2±3.85(30°)	1
NADPH diaphorase	2.26±0.16	1
Nucleoside phosphorylase	359±32	4
Phosphofructokinase	11.01±2.33	1
Phosphoglucomutase	5.50±0.62	1
Phosphoglycerate kinase	320±36.1	1
Phosphoglycolate phosphatase	1.23±0.10	1
Phosphomannose isomerase	0.054+0.026	5
Pyrimidine 5′-nucleotidase	0.138±0.018	1
Pyruvate kinase	15.0±1.99	1
6-Phosphogluconate dehydrogenase	8.78±0.78	1
6-Phosphogluconolactonase	50.6±5.9	6
Ribosephosphate isomerase	200	1
Superoxide dismutase	2225±303	1
Transaldolase	1.21±0.24	7
Transketolase	0.725±0.17	7
Triose phosphate isomerase	2111±397	1

* For US–European subjects.

FAD = flavin adenine dinucleotide; GOT = glutamic oxaloacetic transaminase.

circulation and most of its RNA within 1 or 2 days of its release into the circulation, it does not have the capacity to synthesize new enzyme molecules to replace those that may become degraded during its life span. The enzymes present in the red cells were formed largely by the nucleated marrow cell and, to a lesser extent, the reticulocyte.

GLUCOSE METABOLISM

Glucose is the normal energy source of the red cell.[35] It is metabolized by the erythrocyte along two major routes, the glycolytic pathway and the hexose monophosphate shunt. The steps in these pathways are essentially the same as those found in other tissues and in other organisms, including even relatively simple ones such as *Escherichia*

coli and yeast. Unlike most other cells, however, the red cell lacks a citric acid cycle. Only the reticulocytes maintain some capacity for the breakdown of pyruvate to CO_2, with the attendant highly efficient production of ATP. The mature red cell must content itself with extracting energy from glucose almost solely by anaerobic glycolysis. Before glucose can be metabolized by the red cell, it must pass through the membrane. The membrane contains a carrier[36] that can combine with glucose and other sugars at the cell surface and release them at the interior surface of the membrane. The red cell membrane contains insulin receptors,[37] but the transport of glucose into red cells is independent of insulin.[38]

Pathways of Glucose Metabolism *Direct glycolytic pathway.* In the Embden-Meyerhof direct glycolytic pathway (Fig. 45-1), glucose is catabolized anaerobically to pyruvate or lactate. Although 2 moles of high-energy phosphate in the form of adenosine triphosphate (ATP) are utilized in preparing glucose for its further metabolism, up to 4 moles of adenosine diphosphate (ADP) may be phosphorylated to ATP during the metabolism of each mole of glucose, giving a net yield of 2 moles of ATP per mole of glucose metabolized. The rate of glucose utilization is limited largely by the hexokinase and phosphofructokinase reactions. Both of the enzymes catalyzing these reactions have a relatively high pH optimum; they have very little activity at pH levels lower than 7. For this reason, red cell glycolysis is very pH sensitive, being stimulated by a rise in pH. However, at higher than physiologic pH levels, the stimulation of hexokinase and phospho-

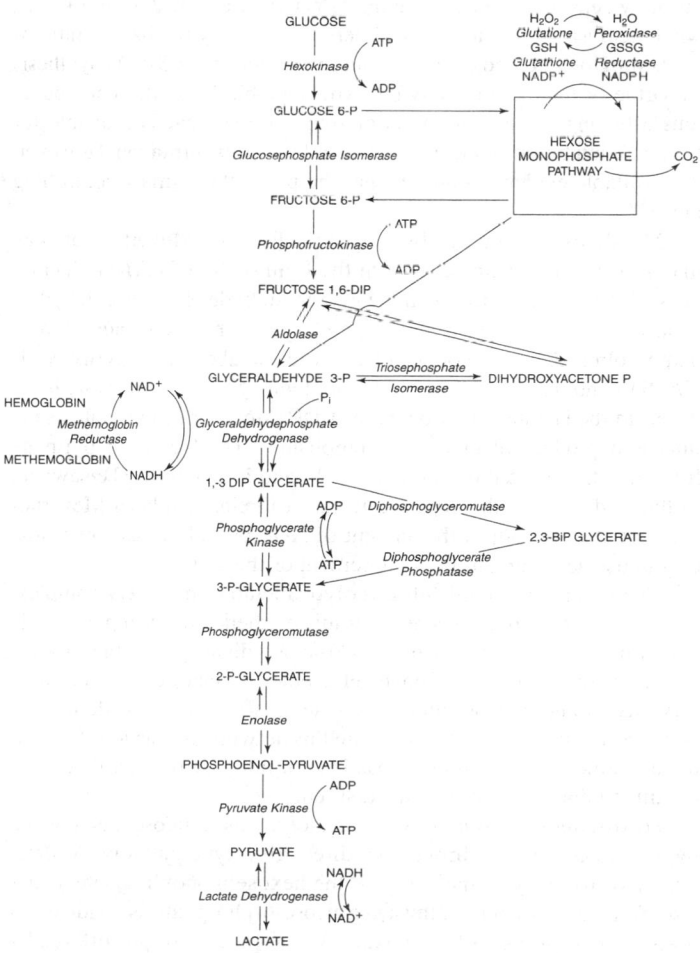

FIGURE 45-1 Glucose metabolism of the erythrocyte. The details of the hexose monophosphate pathway are shown in Fig. 45-2.

fructokinase activity merely results in the accumulation of fructose diphosphate and triose phosphates, because the availability of nicotinamide adenine dinucleotide (NAD)$^+$ for the glyceraldehyde phosphate dehydrogenase reaction becomes a limiting factor.

Branching of the metabolic stream after the formation of 1,3-bisphosphoglycerate (1,3-BPG) provides the red cell with flexibility in regard to the amount of ATP formed in the metabolism of each mole of glucose. 1,3-BPG may be metabolized to 2,3-bisphosphoglycerate (2,3-BPG) also known as 2,3-diphosphoglycerate (2,3-DPG), thus "wasting" the high-energy phosphate bond in position 1 of the glycerate. Removing the phosphate group at position 2 by bisphosphoglycerate phosphatase results in the formation of 3-phosphoglycerate. Alternatively, 3-phosphoglycerate may be formed directly from 1,3-BPG through the phosphoglycerate kinase step, resulting in phosphorylation of 1 mole of ADP to ATP. While metabolism of glucose through the 2,3-BPG step occurs without any net gain of high-energy phosphate bonds in the form of ATP, metabolism through the phosphoglycerate kinase step results in the formation of two such bonds per mole of glucose metabolized. This portion of the direct glycolytic pathway has been called the *energy clutch*.[39] Regulation of metabolism at this branch point determines not only the rate of ADP phosphorylation to ATP but also the concentration of 2,3-BPG, an important regulator of the oxygen affinity of hemoglobin (see Chap. 47). The concentration of 2,3-BPG depends on the balance between its rate of formation from 1,3-BPG by bisphosphoglycerate mutase and its degradation by bisphosphoglycerate phosphatase. Hydrogen ions inhibit the bisphosphoglycerate mutase reaction and stimulate the phosphatase reaction. Thus, red cell 2,3-BPG levels are exquisitely sensitive to pH: a rise in pH causes a rise in 2,3-BPG levels, while acidosis results in 2,3-BPG depletion. It may be that the ratio of oxyhemoglobin to deoxyhemoglobin also influences 2,3-BPG synthesis by virtue of the fact that only deoxyhemoglobin binds this compound, thus affecting the concentration of free 2,3-BPG that is available for feedback inhibition of the enzymes that lead to its formation. However, the available evidence suggests that the pH is the primary controlling factor.[40]

Metabolism of glucose by way of the Embden-Meyerhof pathway may also yield reducing energy in the form of NADH. The reduction of NAD$^+$ to NADH occurs in the glyceraldehyde phosphate dehydrogenase step. If NADH is reoxidized in reducing methemoglobin to hemoglobin, the end product of glucose metabolism is pyruvate. If NADH is not reoxidized by methemoglobin, however, pyruvate is reduced in the lactate dehydrogenase (LDH) step, forming lactate as the final end product of glucose metabolism.[35] The lactate or pyruvate formed is transported from the red cell[41] and is metabolized elsewhere in the body. Thus, the erythrocyte has a flexible Embden-Meyerhof pathway that can adjust the amount of ADP phosphorylated per mole of glucose according to the requirement of the cell.

The regulation of red cell glycolytic metabolism is very complex. Products of some reactions may stimulate others. For example, the PK reaction is exquisitely sensitive to fructose diphosphate, the product of phosphofructokinase. Conversely, other metabolic products may serve as strong enzyme inhibitors. Attempts have been made to construct computer models that simulate this network of reactions,[42–45] but the usefulness of such models has been limited by the fact that all of the interactions are not well understood.

Hexose monophosphate shunt.   Not all the glucose metabolized by the red cell passes through the direct glycolytic pathway. A direct oxidative pathway of metabolism, the hexose monophosphate shunt, also functions. In this pathway, glucose-6-phosphate is oxidized at position 1, yielding carbon dioxide. In the process of glucose oxidation, NADP$^+$ is reduced to NADPH (reduced nicotinamide adenine dinucleotide phosphate). The pentose phosphate formed when glucose is decarboxylated undergoes a series of molecular rearrangements,

eventuating in the formation of a triose, glyceraldehyde-3-phosphate, and a hexose, fructose-6-phosphate (Fig. 45-2). These are normal intermediates in anaerobic glycolysis and thus can rejoin that metabolic stream. Because the glucose phosphate isomerase reaction is freely reversible, allowing fructose-6-phosphate to be converted to glucose-6-phosphate, recycling through the hexose monophosphate pathway is also possible. Unlike the anaerobic glycolytic pathway, the hexose monophosphate pathway does not generate any high-energy phosphate bonds. Its primary function appears to be the reduction of NADP$^+$, and, indeed, the amount of glucose passing through this pathway appears to be regulated by the amount of NADP$^+$ that has been made available by the oxidation of NADPH. NADPH appears to function primarily as a substrate for the reduction of glutathione-containing disulfides in the erythrocyte through mediation of the enzyme glutathione reductase, which catalyzes the conversion of oxidized glutathione (GSSG) to reduced glutathione (GSH) and the reduction of mixed disulfides of hemoglobin and GSH.[46] NADP$^+$ also strongly binds to catalase and may affect its activity.[47,48]

As in the case of anaerobic glycolysis, efforts have been made to construct a computer model of the hexose monophosphate pathway of red cells.[49–51]

Enzymes of Glucose Metabolism   *Hexokinase.*   Hexokinase catalyzes the phosphorylation of glucose in position 6 by ATP (see Fig. 45-1). It thus serves as the first step in the utilization of glucose, whether by the anaerobic or the hexose monophosphate pathway. Mannose or fructose may also serve as a substrate for this enzyme.[52] Red cell hexokinase does not phosphorylate galactose.[53] The average normal activity of the hexokinase reaction is approximately five times the rate of glucose utilization by intact cells. Reticulocytes have much higher levels of hexokinase activity than do mature red cells.[54–56]

Hexokinase has an absolute requirement for magnesium. It is strongly inhibited by its product, glucose-6-phosphate, and is apparently released from this inhibition by the inorganic phosphate ion[57] and by high concentrations of glucose.[58] Inorganic phosphate enhances

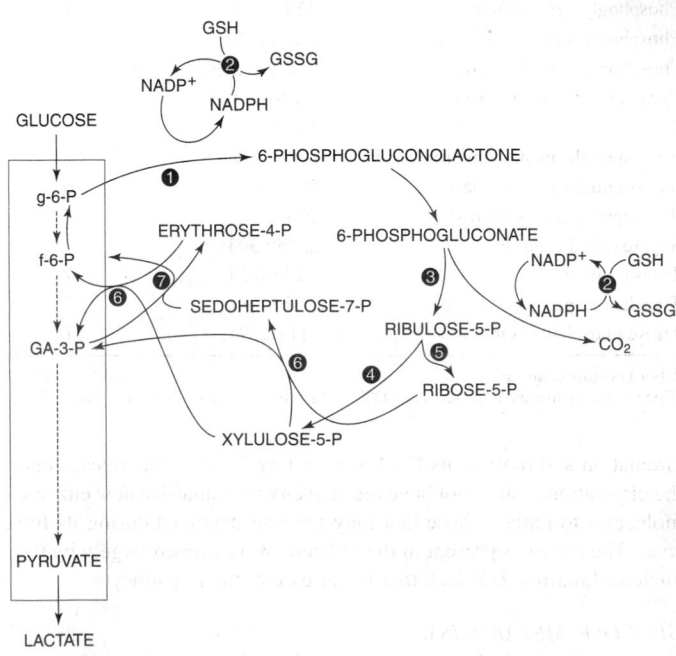

FIGURE 45-2   Hexose monophosphate pathway of the erythrocyte: (1) glucose-6-phosphate dehydrogenase, (2) glutathione reductase, (3) phosphogluconate dehydrogenase, (4) ribulosephosphate epimerase, (5) ribosephosphate isomerase, (6) transketolase, and (7) transaldolase.

the rate of glucose utilization by red cells. It has been suggested that this effect is not exerted through hexokinase but rather through stimulation of the phosphofructokinase reaction, resulting in a lowered glucose-6-phosphate concentration within the cell and thus releasing hexokinase from inhibition.[59] GSSG[60] and other disulfides and 2,3-BPG[61,62] inhibit hexokinase.

The human enzyme resolves into two major bands by electrophoresis.[63,64] Designated types I_A and I_F, both bands actually correspond to type I liver enzyme. Separated chromatographically, the two major fractions of red cell hexokinase have been designated HK and HK_R; the latter fraction being unique to erythrocytes and particularly to reticulocytes.[65] The hexokinase I gene has been cloned and its structure determined.[66] Evidence of an alternative red blood cell-specific exon 1 located upstream of the 5′ flanking region of the gene has been obtained,[66] and a hexokinase cDNA that appears to be unique to erythrocytes has been isolated.[67]

Rabbit reticulocytes appear to contain hexokinase fractions that are membrane bound and free.[68,69] It has been proposed that the ubiquitin-ATP proteolytic system selectively degrades the membrane-bound form of the enzyme, but the physiologic significance of such a process is not clear.[70] A small amount of type III hexokinase is also present in erythrocytes.

Hexokinase deficiency is a rare cause of hereditary nonspherocytic hemolytic anemia.

Glucose phosphate isomerase. Glucose-6-phosphate isomerase catalyzes the interconversion of glucose-6-phosphate and fructose-6-phosphate.[35] Electrophoresis resolves the normal enzyme into three bands, all of which are products of the same gene[71]; mutations that affect electrophoretic mobility are known.[71] Glucose phosphate isomerase deficiency is one of the causes of hereditary nonspherocytic hemolytic anemia.

Phosphofructokinase. Red cells contain two distinct types of phosphofructokinase. The classic (or type I) form of the enzyme catalyzes the phosphorylation of the 1-carbon of fructose-6-phosphate by ATP. The type II enzyme, fructose-6-phosphate 2-kinase, phosphorylates the second carbon of fructose-6-phosphate.[72] The product of this reaction, fructose-2,6-diphosphate, is a potent allosteric activator of type I phosphofructokinase. The type I enzyme requires magnesium for activity and is stimulated by ADP, inorganic phosphate, ammonia, and fructose-2,6-diphosphate.[73] The existence of the latter effector has been demonstrated in red cells.[72]

Red cell type I phosphofructokinase exists as a series of tetramers comprised of muscle (M) and liver (L) subunits. A platelet (P) subunit has also been identified.[74] Deficiency of type I phosphofructokinase may be associated with mild hemolytic anemia and with type VII glycogen storage disease.

Aldolase. Aldolase reversibly cleaves fructose-1,6-diphosphate into two trioses. The "upper" half of the fructose-1,6-diphosphate molecule becomes dihydroxyacetone phosphate and the "lower" half glyceraldehyde-3-phosphate. Red cells contain aldolase A, as is found in muscle, and no aldolase B (liver aldolase). On isoelectric focusing of hemolysates, however, five isoenzymes can be resolved, as is the case with other tissues.[75] The isoenzymes presumably represent mixed tetramers of native α polypeptide chains and chains that have undergone posttranscriptional deamidation, α′ chains. Young red cells contain more of the nondeamidated isoenzymes. Aldolase deficiency is a rare cause of hereditary nonspherocytic hemolytic anemia.

Triosephosphate isomerase. TPI is the enzyme of the anaerobic glycolytic pathway that has the highest activity. Its metabolic role is to catalyze interconversion of the two trioses formed by the action of aldolase: dihydroxyacetone phosphate and glyceraldehyde-3-phosphate.[35] Although equilibrium is in favor of dihydroxyacetone phosphate, glyceraldehyde-3-phosphate undergoes continued oxidation

through the action of glyceraldehyde phosphate dehydrogenase and is thus removed from the equilibrium. The gene encoding TPI has been cloned and sequenced.[76] A polymorphism in the promotor region[29] of uncertain significance has been identified.[77] A deficiency of TPI has been found in patients with hereditary nonspherocytic hemolytic anemia associated with a severe neuromuscular disorder.

Glyceraldehyde phosphate dehydrogenase. Glyceraldehyde phosphate dehydrogenase performs the dual functions of oxidizing and phosphorylating glyceraldehyde-3-phosphate, producing 1,3-BPG. In the process, NAD^+ is reduced to NADH. This enzyme is closely associated with the red cell membrane.[78] It interacts with and is stimulated by oxyhemoglobin, an interaction that could have a regulatory role.[79]

Phosphoglycerate kinase. Phosphoglycerate kinase effects the transfer to ADP of the high-energy phosphate from the 1-carbon of 1,3-DPG to form ATP. The reaction is readily reversible. Electrophoretically detectable mutations of the enzyme have been described,[80,81] and their transmission in families confirms that the structural gene for phosphoglycerate kinase is sex linked. Deficiency of phosphoglycerate kinase is a cause of nonspherocytic hemolytic anemia, often associated with neuromuscular abnormalities.

Bisphosphoglyceromutase-bisphosphoglycerate phosphatase. The same protein molecule is responsible for both bisphosphoglycerate mutase and bisphosphoglycerate phosphatase activities in the erythrocyte.[82,83] This enzyme is particularly important because it regulates the concentration of 2,3-BPG of erythrocytes. In its role as a bisphosphoglyceromutase, the enzyme competes with phosphoglycerate kinase for 1,3-BPG as a substrate. It changes 1,3-BPG to 2,3-BPG, thereby dissipating the energy of the high-energy acylphosphate bond.[84] It is inhibited by its product 2,3-BPG and by inorganic phosphate, and it is activated by 2-phosphoglycerate and by increased pH levels. It requires 3-phosphoglycerate for activity. Bisphosphoglycerate phosphatase catalyzes the removal of the phosphate group from carbon 2 of 2,3-BPG.[84] It is inhibited by its product 3-phosphoglycerate and by sulfhydryl reagents. It is most active at a slightly acid pH and is strongly stimulated by bisulfite and phosphoglycolate.

A deficiency of bisphosphoglyceromutase-bisphosphoglycerate phosphatase results in a marked decrease in red cell 2,3-BPG levels. The consequent left shift of the oxygen dissociation curve leads to polycythemia (see Chap. 56).

Phosphoglycolate, the most potent activator of phosphatase activity, is present in erythrocytes at very low concentrations,[85,86] but the source of this substance in red cells is a mystery.[87–89] Phosphoglycolate phosphatase, the enzyme that hydrolyzes phosphoglycolate, has also been identified in erythrocytes.[90,91]

Monophosphoglyceromutase. An equilibrium is established between 3-phosphoglycerate and 2-phosphoglycerate by phosphoglyceromutase.[92,93] 2,3-BPG acts as an essential cofactor for the transformation.

Enolase. Enolase establishes an equilibrium between 2-phosphoglycerate and phosphoenolpyruvate (PEP).[94] Electrophoresis of red cell enolase gives three bands, supporting the suggestion that it is composed of two different subunits that associate randomly into dimers.[95]

Pyruvate kinase. The transfer of phosphate from PEP to ADP, forming ATP and pyruvate, is catalyzed by PK.[96] This is one of the energy-yielding steps of glycolysis. There are two major types of PK. Four PK isoenzymes are present in mammalian tissues: M1 (in skeletal muscle), M2 (in leukocytes, kidney, adipose tissue, and lungs), L (in liver), and R (in red blood cells). The four PK isoenzymes are products of only two PK genes (*PKLR* and *PKM*). The PKM1 and PKM2 enzymes are formed from the *PKM* gene by alternative splicing. PKL (the liver enzyme) and PKR (the erythrocyte enzyme) are products of the other PK gene (*PKLR*), transcribed by two different, tissue-specific promoters. Exon 2 but not exon 1 is present in the processed liver transcript; in the red cell enzyme exon 1, but not exon 2, is represented.[97] Red cell PK is an allosteric enzyme, manifesting sigmoid kinetics with respect to PEP in the absence of fructose diphosphate. Hyperbolic kinetics are observed in the presence of even minute amounts of fructose diphosphate,[98,99] so that at low concentrations of PEP the enzyme activity is greatly increased by fructose diphosphate. PK deficiency is the most common cause of nonspherocytic hemolytic anemia.

Lactate dehydrogenase. LDH catalyzes the reversible reduction of pyruvate to lactate by NADH. The enzyme is composed of H (heart) and M (muscle) subunits. In red cells, the predominant subunit is LDH-H.[100] However, hereditary absence of the H subunit seems to be a benign condition, usually without clinical manifestations,[100–103] although one case with hemolysis has been reported.[104] Absence of the M subunit has been reported as well[100] and was unaccompanied by hematologic manifestations. Judging from the origin of the reports, LDH deficiency appears to be most common in Japan, where population surveys show a gene frequency of approximately 0.05 for each deficiency,[105,106] and several frameshift mutations have been identified.[106]

Glucose-6-phosphate dehydrogenase. G-6-PD is the most extensively studied erythrocyte enzyme.[105,107] It catalyzes the oxidation of glucose-6-phosphate to 6-phosphogluconolactone, which is rapidly hydrolyzed to 6-phosphogluconic acid. NADP$^+$ is reduced to NADPH in the reaction. The structure of the human enzyme has been deduced from its crystal structure.[108]

Much information is available regarding substrate specificity, Michaelis constants, and pH optimum curves. The M_r of the highly purified enzyme has been reported to be 240,000 daltons,[109] but in its natural state the M_r probably is approximately 105,000 daltons.[110,111] In the absence of NADP$^+$, G-6-PD dissociates into inactive subunits. The computed subunit M_r is 59,256 daltons. The enzyme is strongly inhibited by physiologic amounts of NADPH[112] and, to a lesser extent, by physiologic concentrations of ATP.[113,114] It is much more active in reticulocytes than mature red cells.[55,56] Many electrophoretic mutations are known, as are others involving the activity, stability, and kinetic properties of the enzyme.

Phosphogluconolactonase. Although 6-phosphogluconolactone, the direct product of the oxidation of glucose-6-phosphate by G-6-PD, hydrolyzes spontaneously at a relatively rapid rate at a physiologic pH, enzymatic hydrolysis is much more rapid and is required for normal metabolic flow through the stimulated hexose monophosphate pathway.[115,116] Partial deficiency of the enzyme has been observed[117] and is probably benign.[118]

Phosphogluconate dehydrogenase. Phosphogluconate dehydrogenase catalyzes the oxidation of phosphogluconate to ribulose-5-phosphate and CO$_2$ and the reduction of NADP$^+$ to NADPH. Variability of electrophoretic mobility of the enzyme is common in humans and in several animal species.[119] Deficiency of the enzyme has been observed only rarely and appears to be essentially innocuous.[120]

Ribosephosphate isomerase. Ribosephosphate isomerase catalyzes the interconversion of ribulose-5-phosphate and ribose-5-phosphate.[61,121]

Ribulosephosphate epimerase. Ribulosephosphate epimerase converts ribulose-5-phosphate to xylulose-5-phosphate.[61] The exact activity of this enzyme in human hemolysates has not been reported but seems to be less than that of ribosephosphate isomerase.

Transketolase. Transketolase effects the transfer of two carbon atoms from xylulose-5-phosphate to ribose-5-phosphate, resulting in the formation of the 7-carbon sugar sedoheptulose-7-phosphate and the 3-carbon sugar glyceraldehyde-3-phosphate.[61,122] It can also catalyze the reaction between xylulose-5-phosphate and erythrose-4-phosphate, producing fructose-6-phosphate and glyceraldehyde-3-phosphate. Thiamine pyrophosphate is a coenzyme for transketolase, and

the activity of erythrocyte transketolase has been used as an index of the adequacy of thiamine nutrition.[123,124]

Transaldolase. The conversion of seduheptulose-7-phosphate and glyceraldehyde-3-phosphate into erythrose-4-phosphate and fructose-6-phosphate is catalyzed by transaldolase.[122] This is another one in the series of molecular rearrangements that eventuate in the conversion of the 5-carbon sugar formed in the phosphogluconate dehydrogenase step to metabolic intermediates of the Embden-Meyerhof pathway.

L-Hexonate dehydrogenase. Red cells contain L-hexonate dehydrogenase, an enzyme that has the capacity to reduce aldoses such as glucose, galactose, or glyceraldehyde to their corresponding polyol (i.e., glucose to sorbitol, galactose to dulcitol, and glyceraldehyde to glycerol). NADPH serves as a hydrogen donor for this reaction.[125] Aldose reductase,[126] another enzyme that can catalyze this reaction, may also be present in red cells.

UTILIZATION OF SUBSTRATES OTHER THAN GLUCOSE AS ENERGY SOURCES

The red cell has the capacity to utilize several other substrates in addition to glucose as a source of energy. Among these are adenosine, inosine, fructose, mannose, galactose, dihydroxyacetone, and lactate. Although in the circulation red cells normally rely on glucose as their energy source, the utilization of other substrates, particularly during blood storage (see Chap. 131) and in certain experimental situations, is of interest.

Adenosine and Inosine Adenosine has been used as an experimental blood preservative, and it has been suggested that it may also be metabolized by human red cells *in vivo*.[127] Adenosine is deaminated to inosine by the enzyme adenosine deaminase (ADA)[128]:

$$\text{Adenosine} \xrightarrow{\text{ADA}} \text{Inosine} + \text{NH}_3$$

It apparently plays a regulatory role in the concentration of purine nucleotides in the red cell. Deficiency of ADA is associated with severe combined immunodeficiency (SCID) (see Chap. 82).[129,130] In this disorder, large quantities of deoxyadenine nucleotides, not normally present in erythrocytes, accumulate. Hereditary increase in activity of erythrocyte ADA results in the depletion of red cell ATP and nonspherocytic hemolytic anemia.[131] For reasons that are not understood, ADA activity also increases in the red cells of AIDS patients[132,133] and of those with Diamond-Blackfan anemia.[134]

Inosine formed in the ADA reaction or added directly to red cells may enter the erythrocyte and undergo phosphorolysis to form hypoxanthine and ribose-1-phosphate:

$$\text{Inosine} + \text{Pi} \xrightarrow{\text{Nucleoside phosphorylase}} \text{R-1-P} + \text{Hypoxanthine}$$

This reaction is of particular interest because it results in the introduction of a phosphorylated sugar, R-1-P, into the erythrocyte without the utilization of ATP.[128,135] The R-1-P may then be further metabolized to yield high-energy phosphate. The nucleoside phosphorylase reaction appears to be the only practical means by which ATP may be formed in the cell without first expending ATP to prepare an unphosphorylated substrate for further metabolism. The use of inosine has therefore received much attention in the field of blood banking (see Chap. 131). A deficiency of nucleoside phosphorylase has been associated with immunodeficiency.[130]

Fructose Fructose is readily utilized by the erythrocyte, although at a rate somewhat slower than that of glucose.[136] Fructose undergoes phosphorylation at position 6 in the hexokinase reaction:

$$\text{Fructose} + \text{ATP} \xrightarrow[\text{Mg}^{2+}]{\text{Hexokinase}} \text{Fructose-6-P} + \text{ADP}$$

Fructose-6-phosphate is a normal metabolic intermediate in the anaerobic glycolytic pathway. Thus, the result of fructose phosphorylation is exactly the same as the result of the phosphorylation of glucose.

Fructose may also be metabolized by another red cell enzyme, sorbitol dehydrogenase.[137,138] This enzyme reduces fructose to its corresponding polyol, sorbitol, with NADH serving as a hydrogen donor. The reaction is reversible, and a pathway therefore exists for the formation of fructose from glucose through L-hexonate dehydrogenase and sorbitol dehydrogenase.

Mannose Mannose is also phosphorylated in the hexokinase reaction[52]:

$$\text{Mannose} + \text{ATP} \xrightarrow[\text{Mg}^{2+}]{\text{Hexokinase}} \text{Mannose-6-P} + \text{ADP}$$

Mannose-6-phosphate must be isomerized to fructose-6-phosphate before it is further metabolized by erythrocytes. This is accomplished by phosphomannose isomerase[139,140]:

$$\text{Mannose-6-P} \xrightarrow[]{\text{PMI}} \text{Fructose-6-P}$$

Phosphomannose isomerase of red cells has very low activity, even at its pH optimum of 5.9.[52] The rate of mannose utilization is therefore limited by the activity of phosphomannose isomerase. Young red cells have enhanced phosphomannose isomerase activity and can therefore utilize mannose at a more rapid rate than can mature red cells.

Galactose The utilization of galactose by erythrocytes is more complex than that of most other substrates. At low concentrations of galactose, metabolism occurs by way of galactokinase, galactose-1-phosphate uridyltransferase, and phosphoglucomutase (PGM).[141] Unlike fructose, mannose, and glucose, galactose is phosphorylated at position 1:

$$\alpha\text{-Galactose} + \text{ATP} \xrightarrow[\text{Mg}^{2+}]{\text{Galactokinase}} \alpha\text{-Galactose-1-P} + \text{ADP}$$

The galactose-1-phosphate formed in the galactokinase reaction exchanges with the glucose-1-phosphate moiety of uridine diphosphoglucose (UDPG) in the galactose-1-phosphate uridyltransferase reaction:

$$\alpha\text{-Galactose-1-P} + \text{UDPG} \xrightarrow[]{\text{Transferase}} \alpha\text{-Glucose-1-P} + \text{UDPgalactose}$$

The uridine diphosphogalactose (UDPgalactose) formed in this reaction is epimerized to UDPG:

$$\text{UDPgalactose} \xrightarrow[\text{NAD}^+]{\text{Epimerase}} \text{UDPG}$$

The α-glucose-1-phosphate in the transferase reaction is transformed to α-glucose-6-phosphate in the PGM reaction[142] with glucose-1,6-diphosphate acting as coenzyme:

$$\alpha\text{-Glucose-1-P} \xrightarrow[\text{Glucose-1,6-diP}]{\text{PGM}} \alpha\text{-Glucose-6-P}$$

The α-glucose-6-phosphate formed may join the direct metabolic stream after conversion by phosphoglucose isomerase to fructose-6-phosphate. It may also undergo anomerization to β-glucose-6-phosphate and enter the hexose monophosphate pathway if $NADP^+$ is available. Very high concentrations of galactose appear to be metabolized by way of another pathway, as yet poorly delineated. This pathway is known not to involve galactose-1-phosphate uridyltransferase or to have the capacity to reduce NAD^+.[53]

Dihydroxyacetone and Glyceraldehyde As indicated earlier, glyceraldehyde can be reduced in erythrocytes to glycerol in the L-hexonate dehydrogenase reaction. In addition, glyceraldehyde and dihydroxyacetone can each be phosphorylated by ATP in the presence of the enzyme triokinase.[143] Like other kinases, this enzyme has a requirement for magnesium. A remarkable feature of this enzyme is its extraordinarily low K_m for dihydroxyacetone. It is half-saturated with this substrate at a concentration of only 0.5 μM. The products of the triokinase reaction, dihydroxyacetone phosphate or glyceraldehyde-3-phosphate, are normal metabolic intermediates and can be metabolized in the usual fashion. Because of its capacity to act as an alternate substrate for red cell energy metabolism and 2,3-BPG formation, dihydroxyacetone has been studied as an experimental additive for blood storage.[144,145]

GLYCOGEN METABOLISM

Red cells have the capacity to form and to break down glycogen. They contain the enzymes UDPG-glycogen glucosyltransferase, α-1,4-glucan: α-1,4-glucan-6-glycosyltransferase (the brancher enzyme) for the formation of glycogen from glucose-1-phosphate. They contain the enzymes phosphorylase and amylo-1,6-glucosidase (the debrancher enzyme) for the breakdown of glycogen.[146] Only very little glycogen is present in normal red cells,[147] and most of what was thought to be in red cells may actually be platelet and leukocyte glycogen.[148] The function of glycogen in red cell metabolism is not understood.

GLUTATHIONE METABOLISM OF THE ERYTHROCYTE

The red cell contains a high concentration (approximately 2 mM) of the sulfhydryl-containing tripeptide GSH.[35] Red cell GSH appears to undergo a rapid turnover, with a $T_{1/2}$ of approximately 4 days.[149] Synthesis occurs in two steps:

$$\text{Glutamate} + \text{Cysteine} + \text{ATP} \rightarrow \gamma\text{-Glutamyl cysteine} + \text{ADP} + P_i$$

$$\gamma\text{-Glutamyl cysteine} + \text{Glycine} + \text{ATP} \rightarrow \text{GSH} + \text{ADP} + P_i$$

Both steps are catalyzed by red cell hemolysates.[150] The red cell requires a system for the synthesis of GSH because of the active transport of GSSG from the erythrocyte.[151] It has also been suggested that a requirement for GSH synthesis comes from the amino acid-transporting function of the γ-glutamyl cycle.[152] However, this pathway is not present in red cells.[153–155]

One important function of GSH in the erythrocyte appears to be the detoxification of low levels of hydrogen peroxide that may form spontaneously or as a result of drug administration. In either event, the superoxide radical may be formed first and then be converted to H_2O_2 by the action of the copper-containing enzyme superoxide dismutase.[156] Hydrogen peroxide is reduced to water through the mediation of the enzyme glutathione peroxidase.[157,158] Glutathione peroxidase is a selenium-containing enzyme.[159] In New Zealand, dietary selenium intake is extremely low, and glutathione peroxidase activities are much lower than are observed elsewhere.[160] A polymorphism affecting the activity of the enzyme, which is most common in persons of Mediterranean descent,[161] has also been described. The consequent decreases in enzyme activity are without clinical effect. The genes for

TABLE 45-2   RED CELL ENZYME ABNORMALITIES LEADING TO HEMATOLOGIC DISEASE

ENZYME	CLINICAL FEATURES	INHERITANCE*	RED CELL MORPHOLOGY
Hexokinase	HNSHA	AR	Unremarkable
Glucose phosphate isomerase	HNSHA; neurologic abnormalities(?)	AR	Unremarkable
Phosphofructokinase	HNSHA and/or muscle glycogen storage disease	AR	Unremarkable
Aldolase	HNSHA and mild liver glycogen storage; ? mental retardation	AR	Unremarkable
Triosephosphate isomerase	HNSHA and severe neuromuscular disease	AR	Unremarkable
Phosphoglycerate kinase	HNSHA; myoglobinuria; behavioral disturbances	SL	Unremarkable
Bisphosphoglycerate mutase	HNSHA; polycythemia	AR	Unremarkable
Pyruvate kinase	HNSHA	AR	Usually unremarkable; occasionally contracted echinocytes
Glucose-6-phosphate dehydrogenase	HNSHA; drug- or infection-induced hemolysis; favism	SL	Usually unremarkable; rarely "bite cells"
Glutathione reductase (complete)	Drug-sensitive hemolytic anemia and favism	AR	Unremarkable
γ-Glutamyl cysteine synthetase	HNSHA; drug- or infection-induced hemolysis; spinocerebellar degeneration (?)	AR	Unremarkable
Glutathione synthetase	HNSHA; drug- or infection-induced hemolysis; neurologic defect and 5-oxoprolinuria in some cases	AR	Usually unremarkable
Pyrimidine 5'-nucleotidase	HNSHA; ? mental retardation in some cases	AR	Prominent stippling
Adenylate kinase	HNSHA	AR	Unremarkable
Adenosine deaminase (increased activity)	HNSHA	AD	Unremarkable
Adenosine deaminase (decreased activity)	Immunodeficiency	AR	Unremarkable
NADH-diaphorase (cytochrome b_5 reductase)	Methemoglobinemia; sometimes with mental retardation	AR	Unremarkable

* AR = autosomal recessive; AD = autosomal dominant; SL = sex linked.
† On a scale of 0 to 4+, where 4+ is a complete response. In many cases, data are meager.
‡ Very common if incidence is >5%. Unusual if >100 cases reported. Rare if 10–100 cases reported. Very rare if <10 cases reported.
¶ Recent reports. Comprehensive reviews[211] may be consulted for original descriptions and other reports.
HNSHA = hereditary nonspherocytic hemolytic anemia.

several glutathione peroxidases, including that of the erythrocyte, have been cloned.[162] The triplet UGA usually acts as a stop codon in this particular message and inserts selenocysteine in the proper location.[163] A unique tRNA that has complementary UCA anticodons is aminoacylated with serine. The seryl-tRNA is then converted to selenocysteyl-tRNA and is delivered to the ribosome.[164] Recognition elements within the mRNAs are essential for translation of UGA as selenocysteine rather than the usual stop codon.[164]

GSH also functions in maintaining integrity of the erythrocyte by reducing sulfhydryl groups of hemoglobin membrane.[165] In the process of reducing peroxides or oxidized protein sulfhydryl groups, GSH is converted to GSSG, or may form mixed disulfides. GSSG, like certain other disulfides, has the capacity to inhibit red cell hexokinase,[60,166] although greater than physiologic levels appear to be needed for this effect. It may also complex with hemoglobin A to form hemoglobin A3.[167] Glutathione reductase provides an efficient mechanism for the reduction of GSSG to GSH in the red cell. It is a flavin enzyme, and either NADPH or NADH may serve as a hydrogen donor.[168,169] In the intact cell, only the NADPH system appears to function.[170] The same enzyme system appears to have the capacity to reduce mixed disulfides of GSH and proteins.[46] Although inherited deficiencies of this enzyme exist,[171] the activity of red cell glutathione reductase is strongly influenced by the riboflavin content of the diet.[172] Red cells also contain thioltransferase that can catalyze GSH-dependent reduction of some disulfides.[173]

Oxidized glutathione is actively extruded from the erythrocyte[151,174,175] by a system consisting of at least two GSSG-activated ATPases that serve as an enzymatic basis for this transport process.[176] In addition to transporting GSSG, the system appears to have the capacity to transport thioether conjugates of GSH and electrophiles formed by the action of glutathione-S-transferase.[177,178] Blood cells, specifically including erythrocytes, contain a glutathione-S-transferase that is distinct from the predominant liver forms of the enzyme. This enzyme, designated type III or ρ to distinguish it from the liver enzymes, catalyzes the formation of a thioether bond between GSH and a variety of xenobiotics. The role of glutathione-S-transferase in the erythrocyte has not been established. It may be that it serves to cleanse the blood of xenobiotics to which the red cell membrane is permeable. Glutathione-S-transferase could conjugate such substances to glutathione, and the detoxified product of conjugation would be transported out of the red cell for subsequent disposal. The enzyme has the capacity to reversibly bind heme, and a possible role in heme transport has been postulated.[179]

EXAMPLES OF MUTATIONS CHARACTERIZED AT THE DNA LEVEL	DIAGNOSIS (REFERENCE)		RESPONSE TO SPLENECTOMY†	APPROXIMATE FREQUENCY‡	(REFERENCE)¶
	SCREENING TEST	ASSAY			
(185)	—	(186)	++	Rare	185
(187)	(186)	(186)	+++	Unusual	187
(188)	—	(186)	0	Rare	189
(190, 191)	—	(186)	?	Very rare	191
(192)	(186)	(186)		Rare	193
(194)	—	(186)	++	Rare	195
(196)	—	(186)		Rare	197
(198)	(186)	(186)	+|	Unusual	198
(199)	(186)	(186)	±	Very common	
	(186)	(186)	?	Very rare	171
(200)	(201)	(150)	?	Very rare	200
(202)	(201)	(150)	0	Rare	202
(203)	(204)	(205)	0	Rare	203
(206)	—	(186)		Rare	
	—	(186)		Rare	207
(208)	—	(186)		Rare	129
(209)	(210)	(186)		Unusual	See Chap. 48

Fairly severe deficiency of this enzyme has been associated with hemolytic anemia, but a cause and effect relationship has not been established.[180]

GENETICS

The great majority of red cell enzyme deficiencies that cause hemolytic anemia are hereditary. Most are inherited as autosomal recessive disorders, but G-6-PD deficiency and phosphoglycerate kinase deficiency are X linked. Occasionally, acquired forms of enzyme deficiencies, particularly PK deficiency, have been encountered, usually in patients with hematologic neoplasia.[181–184]

ENZYME DEFICIENCIES

Table 45-2 lists the erythrocyte enzyme deficiencies that have been shown to cause hemolytic anemia and other hematologic diseases.

Other red cell enzyme deficiencies (Table 45-3) do not appear to cause a functional abnormality of the erythrocyte.[237] For example, acatalasemia, the state in which there is a virtually total absence of red cell catalase, is devoid of hematologic manifestations. Similarly, red cells without cholinesterase[214] seem to survive normally in most cases. The lack of clinical manifestations is not always clear-cut. In some instances, hemolytic anemia is reported in some individuals with a given deficiency but not in others. For example, most subjects with LDH deficiency have had no anemia, but cases with hemolysis have been reported.[104] Aden-

ylate kinase deficiency has been associated with hemolysis in some kindreds[238,239] but not in others.[240] Such ambiguity could result from differences in environmental and genetic factors but also from bias of ascertainment. Erythrocyte enzyme assays are usually carried out on patients with hemolytic anemia. Thus, a benign enzyme defect may be thought, mistakenly, to cause hemolysis because it is found in a patient with hemolytic anemia. Deficiencies of phosphoglycerate kinase and of glutathione synthetase are usually associated with hereditary nonspherocytic hemolytic anemia, but cases have been reported in which these deficiencies were unassociated with any hematologic manifestations.[241,242] It has at times been suggested that moderate decreases in the activity of glutathione reductase and of glutathione peroxidase caused hemolytic anemia, but the best available evidence indicates that these enzymes are not ordinarily rate limiting in erythrocyte metabolism and are not associated with hemolytic anemia.[12] Even the total absence of glutathione reductase in the red cells of members of one family was associated with only rare episodes of hemolysis, possibly caused by fava beans, in otherwise hematologically normal individuals.[171] Table 45-3 includes deficiencies that may cause hemolytic anemia but for which a cause and effect relationship has not been clearly established, such as those of phosphogluconolactonase,[117] enolase,[225] glutathione-S-transferase,[180] and adenylate kinase.[240]

Patients with unstable hemoglobins (see Chap. 47) may present with the clinical picture of hereditary nonspherocytic hemolytic anemia. Hemolytic anemia resulting from abnormalities in the lipid com-

TABLE 45-3   RED CELL ENZYME ABNORMALITIES NOT LEADING TO HEMATOLOGIC DISEASE

ENZYME	CLINICAL FEATURES	INHERITANCE*	DIAGNOSIS, REFERENCE ASSAY	ESTIMATED FREQUENCY†	REFERENCE
6-Phosphogluconate dehydrogenase (complete deficiency)	None	AR	(186)	Unusual	120
6-Phosphogluconolactonase (partial defect)	Probably none	AD	(212)	Unusual	117, 118
δ-ALA dehydrase	None	AD	(213)		
Acetylcholinesterase	None	AR	(186)	Very rare	214
Adenine phosphoribosyl transferase	Kidney stones	AR	(215)	Rare	216, 217
AMP deaminase	None	AR	(218)	Unusual	219
Carbonic anhydrase I	None	AR	(220)	Rare	221
Carbonic anhydrase II	Osteoporosis	AR		Rare	222
Catalase	Oral ulcers in some types	AR	(186)	Rare	223, 224
Enolase	HNSHA?	AD?	(186)	Rare	225
Galactokinase	Cataracts	AR	(186)	Rare	226
Galactose-1-P-uridyltransferase	Cataracts; mental retardation; liver disease	AR	(186)	Rare	141
Glutathione peroxidase (partial deficiency)	None	AR and AD[186]	(186)	Very common	
Glutathione reductase (partial deficiency)	None	Usually not inherited[186]	(186)	Very common	12, 227
Glutathione-S-transferase	HNSHA	?	(186)	Very rare	180
Glyceraldehyde phosphate dehydrogenase (partial defect)	None	AD	(186)	Unusual	228
Glyoxalase I	None	AR		Rare	229
Hypoxanthine-guanine phosphoribosyl transferase (HGPRT)	Lesch-Nyhan syndrome (neurologic symptoms and gout)	SL	(230)	Rare	231
ITPase	None	AR	(221)	Rare	232
Lactate dehydrogenase	None	AR	(186)	Rare	102
NADPH diaphorase	None	AR	(186)	Rare	233
Phosphoglucomutase	None	AR	(186)	Rare	234
Uroporphyrinogen 1 synthase	Acute intermittent porphyria	AD	(235)	Unusual (common in selected populations)	236

* Very common if incidence is >5%, common if 1–5%, unusual if 0.01–1%, rare if <0.01%.
† See Table 45-2 for definition of inheritance abbreviations.
ALA = aminolevulinic acid; AMP = adenosine monophosphate; HNSHA = hereditary nonspherocytic hemolytic anemia; ITP = inosine triphosphate.

position of the red cell membrane, particularly increased phosphatidyl choline, occur rarely (see Chap. 44).[243–246]

MECHANISM OF HEMOLYSIS

G-6-PD DEFICIENCY AND OTHER DEFICIENCIES OF HEXOSE MONOPHOSPHATE SHUNT ENZYMES

The life span of G-6-PD–deficient red cells is shortened under many circumstances, particularly during drug administration and infection. The exact reason for this is not known.

Drug-Induced Hemolysis Drug-induced hemolysis in G-6-PD–deficient cells is generally accompanied by the formation of Heinz bodies, particles of denatured hemoglobin, and stromal protein (see Chap. 28), formed only in the presence of oxygen.[247] The mechanism by which Heinz bodies are formed and become attached to red cell stroma has been the subject of considerable investigation and speculation. Exposure of red cells to certain drugs results in the formation of low levels of hydrogen peroxide as the drug interacts with hemoglobin.[248] In addition, some drugs may form free radicals that oxidize GSH without the formation of peroxide as an intermediate.[249] The formation of free radicals of GSH through the action of peroxide or by the direct action of drugs may be followed either by oxidation of GSH to the disulfide form (GSSG) or complexing of the glutathione with hemoglobin to form a mixed disulfide. Such mixed disulfides are believed to form initially with the sulfhydryl group of the β-93 position of hemoglobin.[250] The mixed disulfide of GSH and hemoglobin is probably unstable and undergoes conformational changes exposing interior sulfhydryl groups to oxidation and mixed disulfide formation. Globin chain separation into free α- and β-chains also occurs.[251] Phenylhydrazine-like drugs also have been shown to form a hemochromogen directly with hemoglobin, a complex forming between the iron of ferriheme and the nitrogen bound to the benzene ring of the drug.[252] Once such oxidation has occurred, hemoglobin is denatured irreversibly and will precipitate as Heinz bodies. Normal red cells can defend themselves to a considerable extent against such changes by reducing GSSG to GSH and by reducing the mixed disulfides of GSH and hemoglobin through the glutathione reductase reaction.[46] However, the reduction of these disulfide bonds requires a source of NADPH. Since G-6-PD–deficient red cells are unable to reduce NADP+ to NADPH at a normal rate, they are unable to reduce hydrogen peroxide or the mixed disulfides of hemoglobin and GSH. Moreover, because catalase apparently contains tightly bound NADPH[253] that is required for activity, the lack of NADPH generation may impede an alternate pathway for the disposal of hydrogen peroxide.[254] When such cells are challenged by drugs, they form Heinz bodies more readily than do normal cells. Cells containing Heinz bodies encounter difficulty in traversing the splenic pulp[255] and are eliminated relatively rapidly from the circulation. The metabolic events that may lead to red cell damage and eventually destruction are summarized in Figure 45-3.

The formation of methemoglobin frequently accompanies the administration of drugs that have the capacity to produce hemolysis of G-6-PD–deficient cells.[256] The heme groups of methemoglobin become detached from the globin more readily than do the heme groups of oxyhemoglobin.[257] It is not clear whether methemoglobin formation plays an important role in the oxidative degradation of hemoglobin to Heinz bodies or whether formation of methemoglobin is merely an incidental side effect of oxidative drugs.[258,259]

Infection-Induced Hemolysis The mechanism of hemolysis induced by infection or occurring spontaneously in G-6-PD–deficient subjects is not well understood. The generation of hydrogen peroxide by phagocytizing leukocytes may play a role in this type of hemolytic reaction.[259]

Favism Substances capable of destroying red cell GSH have been isolated from fava beans.[260] Favism occurs only in G-6-PD–deficient subjects, but not all individuals in a particular family may be sensitive to the hemolytic effect of the beans. Nonetheless, some tendency toward familial occurrence has suggested the possibility that an additional genetic factor may be important.[261] The observation of increased excretion of glucaric acid[262] led to the suggestion that a defect in glucuronide formation might be present. An excess of individuals with the acid phosphatase ACP_1 A/C genotype has been found and attributed to a decrease in the *f* isoform of this tyrosine phosphatase.[263] Immunologic factors do not seem to play a role in favism.[264] Increased levels of red cell calcium[265,266] and consequent "cross-bonding" of membranes may occur. Such bonding of the facing inner membrane surfaces[267] may play a role in the destruction of red cells.

Neonatal Jaundice Icterus neonatorum in G-6-PD deficiency probably results principally from inadequate processing of bilirubin by the immature liver of G-6-PD–deficient infants, although shortening of red cell life span may play a role. Anemia does not appear to be present in these infants, and there is only a slight increase in carbon monoxide production, signifying a minimal decrease in red cell life span.[268,269] Severe jaundice resulting from G-6-PD deficiency seems to be limited to infants who have also inherited a mutation of the uridine diphosphoglucuronate glucuronosyltransferase-1 (UDPGT1) gene promoter[270] or, in Asia, the nt211 G→A coding mutation.[271] In adults, these mutations are associated with Gilbert syndrome. The limited data available on liver G-6-PD in deficient adults[272] suggest that a considerable degree of deficiency may be present. If such a deficiency also is present in infants, it may play a role in impairing the borderline ability of infant livers with the UDPGT1 promoter defect to catabolize bilirubin. While an increased incidence of neonatal icterus has been observed in Mediterranean infants with G-6-PD deficiency and among the Chinese,[273] jaundice seems to be less common among neonates with the A– type of enzyme deficiency, although some cases have been reported in G-6-PD–deficient infants, particularly in Africa[274–276] but also in the United States.[277] The cause of the relatively low incidence of neonatal jaundice in infants with G-6-PD A– mutation is not clear. It could result from the higher residual enzyme activity but does not appear to be related to the incidence of the UDPGT1 promoter mutation, which is actually more common in Africans and less common in Asians than it is in Europeans.[278]

DEFICIENCIES OF OTHER ENZYMES OF THE HEXOSE MONOPHOSPHATE SHUNT AND OF GLUTATHIONE METABOLISM

Deficiencies of γ-glutamyl synthetase[279,280] and of glutathione synthetase[280,281] are associated with a decrease in red cell GSH levels, and the mild hemolysis that occurs in these disorders probably has a pathogenesis similar to the hemolysis that occurs in G-6-PD deficiency. The same is probably true of the single case of glutathione reductase deficiency that has been documented.[171] Other defects of the hexose monophosphate and associated metabolic pathways, such as 6-phosphogluconolactone deficiency[117] and 6-phosphogluconate dehydrogenase deficiency,[120] are not associated with hemolysis.

Other Enzyme Deficiencies How deficiencies of enzymes other than those of the hexose monophosphate pathway result in shortening of red cell life span remains unknown, although it has been the object of much experimental work and of speculation. It is often believed that ATP depletion is a common pathway in producing damage to the cell leading to its destruction,[282] but the evidence that this is the case is not always compelling.[283] It is possible that, at least in some cases, alteration of the levels of red cell intermediate metabolites interferes with synthesis of cell components in early stages of development of the cell.

Animal Models G-6-PD deficiency has been encountered in the rat,[284] dog,[285] mouse,[286–288] and horse.[289,290] Targeted deletion in the mouse causes embryonic lethality.[291] PK deficiency is polymorphic in the Basenji dog[292] and has been found in mice.[293–295] Phosphofructokinase deficiency causes hemolytic anemia in dogs,[296] and glucosephosphate isomerase deficiency has been detected in the mouse.[297] Hexokinase deficiency is responsible for the Downeast anemia of mice.[298] Targeted disruption of the Manganese superoxide dismutase-2 gene causes hemolytic anemia in mice.[299] Mice with a red cell peroxiredoxin II deficiency have been found to have hemolytic anemia,[300,301] but a corresponding defect has not been identified in man.

BIOCHEMICAL GENETICS AND MOLECULAR BIOLOGY

GLUCOSE-6-PHOSPHATE DEHYDROGENASE

Biochemical Genetics The "normal" enzyme is designated as G-6-PD B. It represents the most common type of enzyme encountered in all the population groups that have been studied. Many variants of G-6-PD have been detected all over the world. Before it became pos-

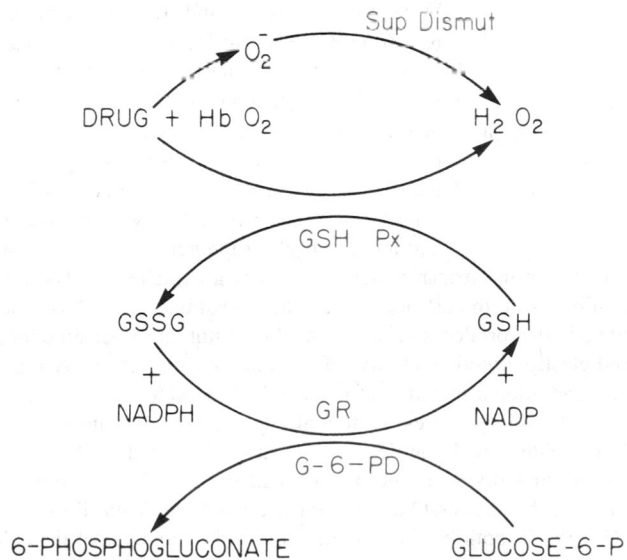

FIGURE 45-3 Reactions through which hydrogen peroxide is generated and detoxified in the erythrocyte. In G-6-PD deficiency, inadequate generation of NADPH results in accumulation of GSSG and probably of H_2O_2. The accumulation of these substances leads to hemoglobin denaturation, Heinz body formation, and consequently to decreased red cell survival. GR, glutathione reductase; GSH Px, glutathione peroxide; GSSG, glutathione disulfide (oxidized glutathione); Sup Dismut, superoxide dismutase.

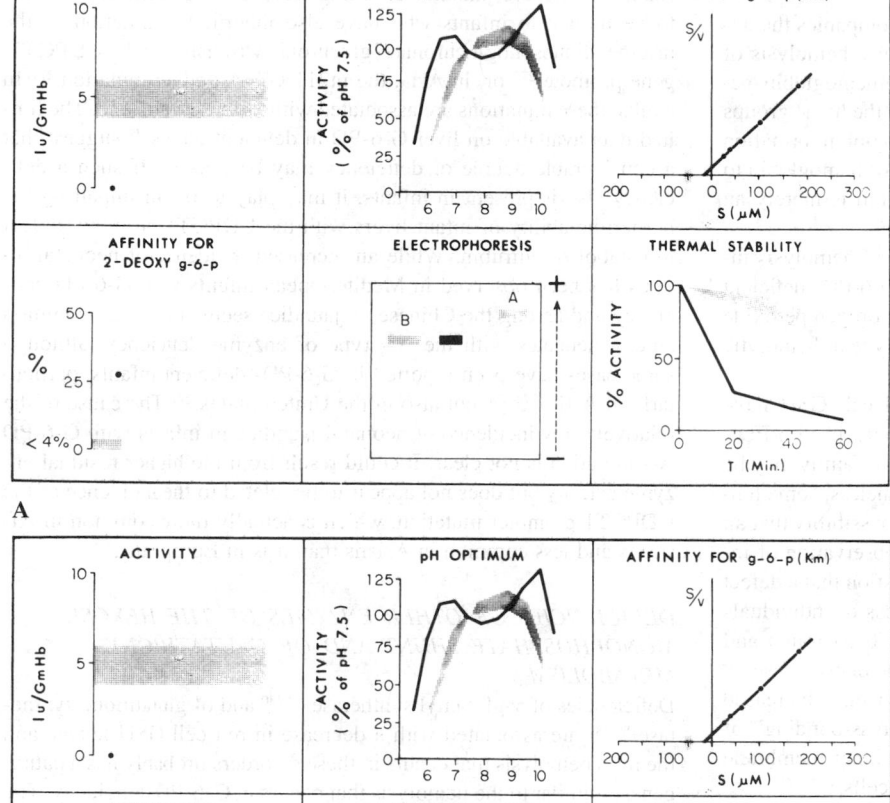

FIGURE 45-4 Biochemical properties of two common variants of G-6-PD. *(A)* The biochemical characteristics of G-6-PD A−. *(B)* The biochemical characteristics of G-6-PD Mediterranean. In each panel, the characteristics of the normal enzyme (types A and B) are indicated by the *shaded areas.*

sensitive to the inhibitory effect of NADPH. Detailed biochemical characteristics of some 400 putatively distinct G-6-PD variants have been tabulated.[308] Figure 45-4 shows a semischematic representation of the biochemical properties of two of the more common variants.

Molecular Biology The gene for G-6-PD is more than 20 kB in length, containing 13 exons. The coding sequence begins in exon 2. The intron between exons 2 and 3 is extraordinarily long, spanning 9857 base pairs.[309] Methylation of certain cytidines at the 3′ end is believed to have a regulatory function.[310] The enzyme is composed of 515 amino acids with a calculated molecular weight of 59,256 daltons. Aggregation of the inactive monomers into catalytically active dimers and higher forms requires the presence of NADP.[111] Thus, NADP appears to be bound to the enzyme both as a structural component and as one of the substrates of the reaction.[311–313] The glucose-6-phosphate binding site has been identified at amino acid 205 by locating a lysine that is reactive in competition with glucose-6-phosphate at this position.[314,315] Examination of mutants suggested that amino acids 386 and 387 bind one of the phosphates of NADP.[316] This seems to be borne out by crystallographic studies, which show this region to be close to the intersubunit interface where structural NADP is bound.[108]

African Variants Among persons of African descent, a mutant enzyme with normal activity is very prevalent. Designated G-6-PD A+, it migrates electrophoretically more rapidly than the normal B enzyme. A single amino acid substitution of Asn126Asp has been identified both by peptide analysis[317] and by DNA sequencing (c.376 A→G).[318] G-6-PD A− is the principal deficient variant found among people of African origin. The red cells contain only 5 to 15 percent of the normal amount of enzyme activity. The mobility of the enzyme present is rapid and is indistinguishable from that of the A+ variant in conventional electrophoretic systems. The fact that these two electrophoretically rapid variants are common in African populations is not a coincidence. These two mutations have in common a nucleotide substitution at cDNA nucleotide 376 that produces the amino acid substitution responsible for the rapid electrophoretic mobility. Most samples with G-6-PD A− manifest an additional mutation at nucleotide 202, which accounts for its *in vivo* instability.[319] Less commonly, the additional mutation is at a different site (see Table 45-4). Thus, it is evident that G-6-PD A− arose in an individual who already had the G-6-PD A+ mutation. However, the ancestral human sequence has been deduced to be that of G-6-PD B, both by showing that this is the sequence of the chimpanzee,[323] our nearest relative, and by analysis of linkage dysequilibrium.[339] Although it has been suggested that only interaction of the nt376 and nt202 mutations results in G-6-PD deficiency,[340] the nt202 mutation has been found in a patient to cause deficiency without the presence of the nt376 mutation.[341]

Variants in the Mediterranean Region Among Caucasian populations, G-6-PD deficiency is most common in Mediterranean countries. The most common enzyme variant in this region is G-6-PD Med-

sible to characterize these variants at the DNA level, they were distinguished from each other on the basis of biochemical characteristics, such as electrophoretic mobility, K_m for NADP and glucose-6-P, ability to utilize substrate analogues, pH activity profile, and thermal stability. To facilitate comparison of variants characterized in different laboratories, international standards for the methodology were established.[302] In the case of the common G-6-PD A− and G-6-PD Mediterranean mutations, the abnormal enzyme may be synthesized at normal or near-normal rates but has decreased stability *in vivo*.[303] The amount of enzyme antigen in the red cells declines concurrently with enzyme activity.[109,304] This suggests that the mutant protein in these variants is rendered unusually sensitive to proteolysis in the environment of the erythrocyte.[305] Other mutations also result in the formation of enzyme molecules with decreased enzyme activity[304] and with altered kinetic properties,[306] some of which may render them functionally inadequate. For example, G-6-PD Oklahoma[307] manifests a marked decrease in its affinity for the substrates glucose-6-phosphate and NADP, and G-6-PD Manchester and Tripler[112] are abnormally iterranean.[306] The enzyme activity of the red cells of individuals who have inherited this abnormal gene is barely detectable. Other variants are also prevalent in the Mediterranean region, including G-6-PD A– and G-6-PD Seattle (see Table 45-4).

Variants in Asia A great many different variants have been described in Asian populations. Some of these proved to be identical at a molecular level (e.g., G-6-PD Gifu, Agrigento, Canton, and Taiwan-Hakka all have the same mutation at cDNA nt1376), but DNA analysis has shown that more than 10 different mutations are found in various Asian populations.[334,342–344]

Variants Producing Hereditary Nonspherocytic Hemolytic Anemia Some mutations of G-6-PD result in chronic hemolysis without precipitating causes. From a functional point of view, these mutations are more severe than the more commonly occurring polymorphic forms of the enzyme, such as G-6-PD Mediterranean and G-6-PD A–, but the *in vitro* enzyme activity may actually be greater in such variants. It has been suggested that specific biochemical characteristics, such as susceptibility to inhibition by NADPH, might explain the chronic hemolysis that occurs in patients with such variants,[112] but no unifying principle that accounts for the clinical effects of variants has been found. On a molecular level, such variants usually are located in exon 10[316] or in the region of the glucose-6-phosphate binding site.[345] There are, however, exceptions to this rule. For example, deletion of a triplet near the 5′ end of the coding region[346] and a mutation very near the carboxy-terminus of the enzyme also have been found to result in hemolysis.[338]

PYRUVATE KINASE

PK deficiency, like G-6-PD deficiency, is genetically heterogeneous, with different mutations causing different kinetic and electrophoretic changes in the enzyme that is formed. Abnormalities include altered affinity for the substrate PEP and the allosteric activator fructose-1,6-diphosphate.[347–349] There are even cases in which the activity of PK as measured *in vitro* is higher than normal, but a kinetically abnormal enzyme is responsible for the occurrence of hemolytic anemia.[350] Kinetic characterization and analysis of PK mutants is considerably more complex, however, than analysis of G-6-PD mutants. Since two alleles are expressed in each cell, five different tetramers will be formed if the mutations are different: the two homotetramers and mixed tetramers containing different proportions of different subunits. There has been international agreement on standard methods for characterizing PK variants,[351] but because of the complexities mentioned above, the biochemical information is even less robust than that obtained

TABLE 45-4 SOME OF THE MORE IMPORTANT G-6-PD VARIANTS THAT HAVE BEEN CHARACTERIZED AT THE DNA LEVEL*

VARIANT	NUCLEOTIDE SUBSTITUTION	WHO CLASS†	AMINO ACID SUBSTITUTION	REFERENCE
Aures	143 T→C	2	48 Ile→Thr	320
A–	202 G→A	3	68 Val→Met	319
Distrito Federal				321
Matera				322
Castilla				321
Betica				323
Tepic				321
Ferrara				324
A	376 A→G	4	126 Asn→Asp	318
Santamaria	542 A→T	2	181 Asp→Val	325
	376 A→G		– 126 Asn→Asp	
Mediterranean	563 C→T	2	188 Ser→Phe	322
Dallas				326
Birmingham				326
Sassari				327
Cagliari				327
Panama				E Beutler (unpublished)
Minnesota	637 G→T	1	213 Val→Leu	328
Marion				
Gastonia				
A–	680 G→T	3	227 Arg→Lue	319
	376 A→G		126 Asn→Asp	
Seattle	844 G→C	2	282 Asp→His	327
Lodi				329
Modena				324
Viangchan	871 G→A	2	291 Val→Met	330
Jammu				
A–	968 T→C	3	323 Leu→Pro	319
Betica	376 A→G		126 Asn→Asp	
Selma				
Chatham	1003 G→A	3	335 Ala→Thr	322
Iowa	1156 A→G	1	386 Lys→Glu	316
Walter Reed				
Iowa City				
Springfield				
Guadalajara	1159 C→T		387 Arg→Cys	331
Mt. Sinai	1159 C→T	1	387 Arg→Cys	332
	376 A→G		126 Asn→Asp	
Beverly Hills	1160 G→A	1	387 Arg→His	316
Genova				A Argusti et al (personal communication)
Worcester				E Beutler (unpublished)
Nashville	1178 G→A	1	393 Arg→His	328
Anaheim				333
Calgary				
Portici				
Alhambra	1180 G→C	1	394 Val→Leu	331
Georgia	1284 C→A	1	428 Tyr→End	334
Taiwan-Hakka	1376 G→T	2	459 Arg→Leu	335
Gifu-like				
Agrigento-like				336
Canton				
Cosenza	1376 G→C	2	459 Arg→Pro	337
Kaiping	1388 G→A	2	463 Arg→His	335
Anant				
Dhon				
Petrich				
Sapporo				
Campinas	1463 G→T	1	488 Gly→Val	338

* See ref. 199 for a complete tabulation.
† Class 1 = nonspherocytic hemolytic anemia; class 2 = severe deficiency; class 3 = moderate deficiency; class 4 = not deficient.

TABLE 45-5   SOME PYRUVATE KINASE MUTATIONS

DESIGNATION	cDNA NT	SUBSTITUTION	AMINO ACID NO.	SUBSTITUTION	REFERENCE
	391-392 del	—	131	Ile→del	31
Linz	394	C→T	132	Arg→Cys	353
Beirut	946	C→T	353	Thr→Met	353–355
Tokyo					
Nagasaki					
Fukushima	1261	C→A	421	Gln→Gly	355
Maebashi					
Common European	1529	G→A	510	Arg→Gln	31
Gypsy	Exon 11 deleted				33

See ref. 352 for a more complete tabulation.

with G-6-PD variants. Mutations of the *PKLR* gene encoding the red cell PK have been identified in many deficient patients (see Table 45-5).[352] The same mutations are encountered repeatedly in apparently unrelated individuals; the existence of a common haplotype in such persons indicates that they are presumably offspring of a common ancestor.[32,33] The 1529A mutation, in particular, is encountered repeatedly in unrelated individuals, even in the homozygous state.[31] Deletion of exon 11 is characteristic of the mutation found among gypsies.[33] The nature of the mutation has relatively little predictive value with respect to the severity of the clinical course.[32,356] With the solution of the crystal structure of the human red cell enzyme, the functional effect of some of the mutants has been deduced to affect domain interfaces and catalytic and allosteric sites.[357] Previous efforts to deduce the structural effect of mutants had been based upon analogies drawn with the M type enzyme.[356]

OTHER ENZYME DEFICIENCIES

The mutations that cause other enzyme deficiencies have been identified in many instances. Table 45-3 provides references to some of the more recent studies in which the abnormalities in DNA sequence have been documented.

CLINICAL FEATURES

COMMON FORMS OF G-6-PD DEFICIENCY

Individuals who inherit the common (polymorphic) forms of G-6-PD deficiency, such as G-6-PD A− or G-6-PD Mediterranean, usually have no clinical manifestations. The major clinical consequence of G-6-PD deficiency is hemolytic anemia in adults and neonatal icterus in infants. Usually the anemia is episodic, but some of the unusual variants of G-6-PD may cause nonspherocytic congenital hemolytic disease (see "Variants Producing Hereditary Nonspherocytic Hemolytic Anemia" below). In general, hemolysis is associated with stress, most notably drug administration, infection, and, in certain individuals, exposure to fava beans.

DRUG-INDUCED HEMOLYTIC ANEMIA

A large number of drugs and other chemicals that may have the capacity to precipitate hemolytic reactions in G-6-PD–deficient individuals are listed in Table 45-6. Some drugs, such as chloramphenicol, may induce mild hemolysis in a person with severe, Mediterranean-type G-6-PD deficiency[376] but not in those with the milder A− or Canton[377] types of deficiency. Drugs that are innocuous when given in normal doses (Table 45-6) may be hemolytic when given in excessive doses. A case in point is ascorbic acid, which does not cause hemolytic anemia in normal doses but which can produce severe, even

fatal, hemolysis at doses of 80 g or more intravenously.[378–380] There appears, furthermore, to be a difference in the severity of the reaction to the same drug of different individuals with the same G-6-PD variant. For example, red cells from a single G-6-PD–deficient individual were hemolyzed in the circulation of some recipients who were given thiazolsulfone, but their survival was normal in the circulation of others.[247] Sulfamethoxazole, which was clearly hemolytic in experimental studies, does not appear to be a common cause of hemolysis in a clinical setting.[381] Undoubtedly, individual differences in the metabolism and excretion of drugs influence the extent to which G-6-PD–deficient red cells are destroyed.[382,383]

Typically, an episode of drug-induced hemolysis in G-6-PD–deficient individuals begins 1 to 3 days after drug administration is initiated.[384] Heinz bodies appear in the red cells, and the hemoglobin concentration begins to decline rapidly.[385] As hemolysis progresses, Heinz bodies disappear from the circulation, presumably as they or the erythrocytes that contain them are removed by the spleen. In severe cases, abdominal or back pain may occur. The urine may turn dark or even black. Within 4 to 6 days, there is generally an increase in the reticulocyte count, except in instances in which the patient has received the offending drug for treatment of an active infection. Because of the tendency of infections and certain other stressful situations to precipitate hemolysis in G-6-PD–deficient individuals, many drugs have been incorrectly implicated as a cause. Other drugs, such as aspirin, have appeared on many lists of proscribed medications because very large doses could slightly reduce the red cell life span. It is important to recognize that such drugs (Table 45-7) do not produce clinically significant hemolytic anemia. Advising patients not to ingest these drugs may not only deprive patients of potentially helpful medications, but will also weaken their confidence in the advice that they have received. Most G-6-PD–deficient patients, after all, have taken aspirin without untoward

TABLE 45-6   DRUGS AND CHEMICALS THAT SHOULD BE AVOIDED BY PERSONS WITH G-6-PD DEFICIENCY*

Acetanilid[247]
Dimercaptosuccinic acid[358]†
Furazolidone (Furoxone)[359,360]
Glibenclamide[362]†
Isobutyl nitrite[363,364]
Methylene blue[365]
Nalidixic acid (NeGram)[366,367]†
Naphthalene[369,370]
Niridazole (Ambilhar)[372,373]
Nitrofurantoin (Furadantin)[374]
Phenazopyridine (Pyridium)[375]
Phenylhydrazine[247]
Primaquine[247]
Sulfacetamide[247]
Toluidine blue[361]†
Sulfanilamide[247]
Sulfapyridine[247]
Thiazolesulfone[247]
Trinitrotoluene (TNT)[368]
Urate oxidase[371]

* Further details may be found in ref. 12.
† Single case reports. Cause and effect not certain.

TABLE 45-7   DRUGS THAT CAN PROBABLY SAFELY BE GIVEN IN NORMAL THERAPEUTIC DOSES TO G-6-PD–DEFICIENT SUBJECTS WITHOUT NONSPHEROCYTIC HEMOLYTIC ANEMIA*

Acetaminophen (paracetamol, Tylenol, Tralgon, hydroxyacetanilide)[247,386]

Acetophenetidin (phenacetin)[247]

Acetylsalicylic acid (aspirin)[1,386]

Aminopyrine (Pyramidon, aminopyrine)[387]

Antazoline (Antistine)[1]

Antipyrine[386]

Ascorbic acid (vitamin C)[1]

Benzhexol (Artane)[386]

Chloramphenicol[376,377,386]

Chlorguanidine (Proguanil, Paludrine)[386]

Chloroquine[1,386,388]

Colchicine[386]

Diphenyldramine (Benadryl)[1]

Isoniazid[386,389]

L-Dopa[386,390]

Menadione sodium bisulfite (Hykinone)[391]

p-Aminobenzoic acid[1]

p-Aminosalicylic acid[389]

Phenylbutazone[386]

Phenytoin[386]

Probenecid (Benemid)[386,391]

Procainamide hydrochloride (Pronestyl)[1]

Pyrimethamine (Daraprim)[1,386]

Quinine[391]

Streptomycin[386]

Sulfacytine[392]

Sulfadiazine[1,393]

Sulfaguanidine[393]

Sulfamerazine[1]

Sulfamethoxazole (Gantanol)[381]

Sulfamethoxypyridazine (Kynex)[394,395]

Sulfisoxazole (Gantrisin)[391,392]

Tiaprofenic acid[396]

Trimethoprim[386]

Tripelennamine (Pyribenzamine)[1]

Vitamin K[56]

* Further details may be found in ref. 12.

effect and are likely to distrust an advisor who counsels them that the ingestion of aspirin would have catastrophic effects.

In the A– type of G-6-PD deficiency, the hemolytic anemia is self-limited[384] because the young red cells produced in response to hemolysis have nearly normal G-6-PD levels and are relatively resistant to hemolysis.[397] The hemoglobin level may return to normal even while the same dose of drug that initially precipitated hemolysis is administered. In contrast, hemolysis is not self-limited in the more severe Mediterranean type of deficiency.[398]

HEMOLYTIC ANEMIA OCCURRING DURING INFECTION

Anemia often develops rather suddenly in G-6-PD–deficient individuals within a few days of onset of a febrile illness. The anemia is usually relatively mild, with a decline in the hemoglobin concentration of 3 or 4 g/dl. Hemolysis has been noted particularly in patients suffering from pneumonia and in those with typhoid fever. The fulminating form of the disease occurs particularly frequently among G-6-PD–deficient patients who are infected with Rocky Mountain spotted fever.[399] Jaundice is not a prominent part of the clinical picture, except where hemolysis occurs in association with infectious hepatitis.[400,401] In that case, it can be quite intense. Presumably because of the effect of the infection, reticulocytosis is usually absent, and recovery from the anemia is generally delayed until after the active infection has abated.

DIABETIC KETOACIDOSIS

Diabetic ketoacidosis has usually been considered a cause of hemolysis in G-6-PD–deficient individuals, but a review of 36 episodes of diabetic ketoacidosis in G-6-PD–deficient subjects yielded only 10 in whom hemolysis occurred and these all were associated with infection or drug ingestion.[402] It has been suggested that hypoglycemia may precipitate hemolysis.[403]

FAVISM

Favism is potentially one of the gravest clinical consequences of G-6-PD deficiency. It occurs much more commonly in children than in adults and occurs almost exclusively in persons who have inherited variants of G-6-PD that cause severe deficiency, but rarely the disorder has been noted in patients with G-6-PD A–.[404] The onset of hemolysis may be quite sudden, having been reported to occur within the first hours after exposure to fava beans. More commonly, the onset is gradual, hemolysis being noticed 1 to 2 days after ingestion of the beans.[405] The urine becomes red or quite dark, and in severe cases shock may develop within a short time. Sometimes the patient or parent does not realize that fava beans have been ingested, since they may be incorporated into foods such as Yewdow, eaten by the Chinese,[406] or falafel, eaten in the Middle East. Occasionally ingestion of other foodstuffs, such as unripe peaches[407] or a spiced Nigerian barbecued meat known as red suya,[408] has been reported to precipitate hemolysis.

NEONATAL ICTERUS

Icterus neonatorum without evidence of immunologic incompatibility occurs in some infants with G-6-PD deficiency.[409] The jaundice may be quite severe and, if untreated, may result in kernicterus. Thus, G-6-PD deficiency is a preventable cause of mental retardation,[410,411] and this aspect of the disorder has considerable public health significance.

EFFECTS ON OTHER TISSUES

In the common variants of G-6-PD, such as G-6-PD A– and Mediterranean, and even in most of the severely deficient variants, there is usually no demonstrated defect in leukocyte number or function.[412] However, there have been reports of isolated instances of leukocyte dysfunction associated with rare, severely deficient variants of G-6-PD.[413–418] In one patient, the apparently coincidental occurrence of Kostmann syndrome and G-6-PD deficiency was documented.[419] Patients with G-6-PD deficiency do not have a bleeding tendency, and studies of platelet function have yielded conflicting results.[420,421] Occasionally, cataracts have been observed in patients with variants of G-6-PD that produce nonspherocytic hemolytic anemia.[422–424] The incidence of senile cataracts may be increased in G-6-PD deficiency,[425,426] but this remains controversial.[427] Although claims have been made that an association exists between various kinds of G-6-PD deficiency and cancer,[428,429] the data are not convincing, and a detailed investigation of hematologic malignancies in patients with G-6-PD Mediterranean shows no effect.[430] Decrease in insulin release[431] and in cortisol levels after adrenocorticotropic hormone stimulation[432] have been reported to occur in G-6-PD–deficient men.

HEREDITARY NONSPHEROCYTIC HEMOLYTIC ANEMIA

Most patients with hereditary nonspherocytic hemolytic anemia manifest only the usual clinical signs and symptoms of chronic hemolysis.

The degree of anemia in this group of disorders varies widely. In some cases of very severe PK deficiency, scarcely any deficient cells survive in the circulation, and only transfused cells are found or steady-state hemoglobin levels as low as 5 g/dl may be encountered. Other patients with hereditary nonspherocytic hemolytic anemia may manifest compensated hemolysis with a normal steady-state hemoglobin concentration. Chronic jaundice is a common finding, and splenomegaly is often present. Gallstones are common. As in other forms of chronic hemolytic anemia, ankle ulcers may be present.[433,434] Pregnancy has been thought to precipitate hemolysis in patients with PK deficiency, perhaps even in heterozygotes.[435,436]

In the case of some enzyme defects, characteristic nonhematologic systemic manifestations may be present, and these may be the only sign of the enzyme deficiency. For example, patients with phosphofructokinase deficiency may have type VII muscle glycogen storage disease. In some with this defect, hemolysis is present without muscle manifestations, but in others both muscle abnormalities and hemolysis occur.[74] Glutathione synthetase deficiency may be associated with 5-oxoprolinuria and neuromuscular disturbances, and such abnormalities may occur either with[437] or without hematologic abnormalities.[242] On the other hand, some patients with glutathione synthetase deficiency manifest only the hematologic abnormalities.[280] Spinocerebellar degeneration was documented in the first case of γ-glutamylcysteine synthetase described[438,439] but was not present in subsequently investigated patients.[280,440] Patients with TPI deficiency nearly always manifest serious neuromuscular disease, and most of the patients who inherit this abnormality die in the first decade of life,[441–443] but there are exceptions, since only one of two brothers with the same genotype manifested neurologic disease.[193,444] Neurologic symptoms have also been noted in a patient with glucosephosphate isomerase deficiency.[445] This enzyme seems to be identical to neuroleukin, which could explain the existence of neurologic manifestations. Myoglobinuria has been encountered in patients with phosphoglycerate kinase,[241,446] aldolase,[191] and G-6-PD deficiency.[447] The clinical features of enzyme deficiencies causing nonspherocytic hemolytic anemia are summarized in Table 45-2.

LABORATORY FEATURES

In the absence of hemolysis, the light microscopic morphology of G-6-PD–deficient red cells appears to be normal. Differences in the texture of the membrane of the cells have, however, been observed under electron microscopy.[448]

Varying degrees of anemia and reticulocytosis are the main routine hematologic laboratory features of patients with hereditary nonspherocytic hemolytic anemia. Heinz bodies often are found in the erythrocytes of G-6-PD–deficient patients undergoing drug-induced hemolysis and in splenectomized but not unsplenectomized patients with unstable hemoglobins. When a hemolytic drug is administered to a G-6-PD–deficient patient, Heinz bodies (see Chap. 28) develop in the erythrocytes immediately preceding and in the early phases of the hemolytic episode. If the hemolytic anemia is very severe, spherocytosis and red cell fragmentation may be seen in the stained film. Although "bite cells" have been noted in the blood of a G-6-PD–deficient patient undergoing drug-induced hemolysis,[364] such cells have also been noted in nondeficient patients.[449,450]

The presence of small, densely staining cells has often been noted in the blood films of patients with hereditary nonspherocytic hemolytic anemia with defects other than G-6-PD deficiency. Particularly when manifesting an echinocytic appearance, such cells have been thought to be common in PK deficiency. In one reported case,[451] spectacular numbers of such cells were observed. However, cells of this type are seen in many blood films both from patients with gly-

colytic enzyme deficiencies and from those with other disorders and it is hazardous to attempt to make an enzymatic diagnosis on the basis of such findings. Basophilic stippling of the erythrocytes is prominent in most patients with pyrimidine 5′-nucleotidase deficiency but may not be apparent in blood that has been collected in ethylenediaminetetraacetic acid (EDTA) anticoagulant. Leukopenia occasionally is observed in patients with hereditary nonspherocytic hemolytic anemia, possibly secondary to splenic enlargement. Other laboratory stigmata of increased hemolysis may include increased levels of serum bilirubin, decreased haptoglobin levels, and increased serum lactic dehydrogenase activity.

Diagnosis of red cell enzyme deficiencies usually depends on the demonstration of decreased enzyme activity either through a quantitative assay or a screening test.[35,351,452,453] Assay of most of the enzymes generally is carried out by measuring the rate of reduction or oxidation of nicotinamide adenine nucleotides in an ultraviolet spectrophotometer, and a number of screening tests that depend upon the development or loss of fluorescence have been devised.[35] However, difficulties arise when the patient has been transfused so that the blood drawn represents a mixture of the patient's own cells and those obtained from the blood bank. Under the circumstances, DNA analysis may prove invaluable, since the DNA is extracted from blood leukocytes and transfused leukocytes do not persist in the circulation.

Although detection of G-6-PD deficiency in the healthy, fully affected (hemizygous) male can be achieved readily through either assay or screening tests, difficulties arise when a patient with G-6-PD deficiency of the A− type has undergone a hemolytic episode. As the older, more enzyme-deficient cells are removed from the circulation and are replaced by young cells, the level of the enzyme begins to increase toward normal. Under such circumstances, suspicion that the patient may be G-6-PD deficient should be raised by the fact that enzyme activity is not increased, even though the reticulocyte count is elevated. Centrifugation of the blood followed by testing of the most dense, reticulocyte depleted red cells has been employed as a means for the detection of G-6-PD deficiency in persons with the A− defect who recently have undergone hemolysis.[454,455] It is helpful to carry out family studies or to wait until the circulating red cells have aged sufficiently to betray their lack of enzyme.

Even greater difficulties are encountered in attempting to diagnose heterozygotes for G-6-PD deficiency.[456] Because the gene is X linked, a population of normal red cells coexists with the deficient cells (see Chap. 9). This may mask the enzyme deficiency when screening tests are used. Even enzyme assays carried out on erythrocytes of heterozygous females frequently may be in the normal range. Here methods that depend upon histochemical demonstration of individual red cell enzyme activity may be useful.[457,458] In addition, the ascorbate cyanide test,[459] in which screening is carried out on a whole cell population rather than on a lysate, may be more sensitive than the other screening procedures. However, when the nucleotide substitution is known, heterozygotes are easily detected by polymerase chain reaction-based analysis of the mutation.[328] Prenatal diagnosis of G-6-PD deficiency is also possible using this approach.[460]

Identifying specific G-6-PD variants on the basis of biochemical variations requires the use of relatively sophisticated techniques. The enzyme must be partially purified, and then its K_m for NADP+ and glucose-6-phosphate, utilization of substrate analogues, pH optima, and electrophoretic mobility must be determined in standard systems.[302] At best, there is often uncertainty regarding minor differences in the characteristics of enzymes studied in this way. Detailed biochemical characterization of G-6-PD variants largely has therefore been replaced by DNA sequence analysis.[461,462]

DIFFERENTIAL DIAGNOSIS

Drug-induced hemolytic anemia resulting from G-6-PD deficiency is similar in its clinical features and in certain laboratory features to drug-induced hemolytic anemia associated with unstable hemoglobins (see Chap. 47). Other enzyme defects affecting the pentose-phosphate shunt, such as a deficiency of GSH synthetase, also may mimic G-6-PD deficiency. The diagnosis of hemoglobinopathies can be excluded by performing a stability test and hemoglobin electrophoresis. Both of these are normal in G-6-PD deficiency. Some of the screening tests, particularly the ascorbate cyanide test,[459] may give positive results in the above-named disorders, but a G-6-PD assay or the fluorescent screening test will be positive only in G-6-PD deficiency.

Physicians often attempt to establish the cause of hereditary nonspherocytic hemolytic anemia on the basis of the appearance of red cells on a blood film and the results of the autohemolysis test. In reality, red cell morphology is helpful only in the diagnosis of pyrimidine 5'-nucleotidase deficiency because of the characteristic stippling of the red cells that is observed in that disorder. After splenectomy, the appearance of Heinz bodies suggests the possible presence of an unstable hemoglobin. Autohemolysis tests provide no diagnostic information of value, except occasionally in the confirmation of the presence of hereditary spherocytosis.[463]

Since the laboratory diagnosis of these disorders may entail considerable expenditure of time and effort, it is prudent to perform the simplest tests for the most common causes of hereditary nonspherocytic hemolytic anemia first. Accordingly, it is useful to carry out screening tests[35,452] for G-6-PD and PK activity and an isopropanol stability test[464] to detect an unstable hemoglobin. The characteristically elevated red cell 2,3-BPG level and the concentration of 3-phosphoglyceric acid[465] are also helpful in the diagnosis of PK deficiency. If the levels of these intermediates are normal, it is extremely unlikely that the patient has PK deficiency. If prominent stippling of erythrocytes is present, examination of the ultraviolet spectrum of a perchloric acid extract of the erythrocytes may help to establish the diagnosis of pyrimidine 5'-nucleotidase deficiency.[466] Beyond these relatively simple procedures it is probably rarely profitable to pick and choose individual enzyme assays on the basis of family history or clinical manifestations. Rather, it is usually appropriate to submit a blood sample to a reference laboratory that has the capability of performing all the enzyme assays listed in Table 45-2. The estimation of the red cell membrane lipid composition and the study of membrane proteins usually are carried out only in research laboratories.

Prenatal diagnosis of some of the defects causing hereditary nonspherocytic hemolytic anemia has been achieved.[467–469] For this purpose, DNA-based diagnosis is usually preferable because it can be carried out earlier in the pregnancy, and although the levels of red cell enzymes in fetal blood have been documented,[470] there is relatively little experience in prenatal diagnosis and little knowledge of what variables, such as leukocyte contamination, may affect the results.

THERAPY

G-6-PD DEFICIENCY

G-6-PD–deficient individuals should avoid drugs that might induce hemolytic episodes (see Table 45-6). However, it is important to realize that such patients are able to tolerate most drugs. Unfortunately, in the 1950s and 1960s, a number of case reports incorrectly suggested that some drugs had hemolytic potential that subsequently were shown to be safe. Table 45-7 lists such drugs. While it is possible that some of these may be hemolytic in some patients or under some circumstances, this is unlikely, and G-6-PD–deficient patients should not be deprived of the possible benefit of these drugs.

If hemolysis occurs as a result of drug ingestion or infection, particularly in the milder A– type of deficiency, transfusion usually is not required. If, however, the rate of hemolysis is very rapid, as may occur, for example, in favism, transfusions of whole blood or packed cells may be useful. Good urine flow should be maintained in patients with hemoglobinuria to avert renal damage. Infants with neonatal jaundice resulting from G-6-PD deficiency may require phototherapy or exchange transfusion; in areas in which G-6-PD deficiency is prevalent, care must be taken not to give G-6-PD–deficient blood to such newborns.[471] A single dose of Sn-mesoporphyrin, a potent inhibitor of heme oxygenase, has been advocated to eliminate the need for phototherapy.[472]

Patients with hereditary nonspherocytic hemolytic anemia resulting from G-6-PD deficiency usually do not require any therapy. Splenectomy is often ineffective, although some improvement has been reported in a number of cases following removal of the spleen.[12,491] In most cases, the anemia is not very severe, but in some instances frequent transfusions have been necessary.[338,473] The antioxidant properties of vitamin E have been tested in G-6-PD–deficient subjects, and a slight but statistically significant reduction in hemolysis was observed.[474,475] These results could not be confirmed in other studies.[476,477] It has been suggested that desferrioxamine decreases hemolysis.[478–480]

OTHER ENZYME DEFICIENCIES

Most patients with hereditary nonspherocytic hemolytic anemia secondary to red cell enzymopathies do not require therapy, but there are some patients with PK deficiency who need to be transfused continually. Patients with TPI deficiency generally die as children, not because of the severity of the anemia but rather because of the severe neuromuscular effects of the enzyme deficiency. PK deficiency has been treated successfully by stem cell transplantation,[481] and it has been proposed that the exogenous replacement of TPI might be useful for the treatment of this deficiency,[482] but no clinical trials have been carried out. The jaundice of glucosephosphate isomerase deficiency has been treated by the administration of phenobarbital.[483]

The principal decision that the physician must make regarding patients with hereditary nonspherocytic hemolytic anemia is whether or not they require a splenectomy. This decision is not made easily since the response is not predictable, and some patients who fail to respond may develop serious thrombotic complications resulting from postsplenectomy thrombocytosis that is often exaggerated when splenectomy does not ameliorate the hemolysis. The recommendation that is made should be based upon the following considerations: (1) severity of the disease, (2) family history of response to splenectomy, (3) the underlying defect, and (4) perhaps the need for cholecystectomy. Since it is unusual to obtain more than a partial response to splenectomy, this procedure should probably be reserved for patients whose quality of life is impaired by their anemia. The operation needs to be particularly considered for patients who need frequent transfusion and for those who require gallbladder surgery, in which splenectomy might be carried out as part of the same procedure. The best guide to the likely efficacy of splenectomy is probably the response to splenectomy of other affected family members. Unfortunately, such information is only occasionally available. The physician must therefore rely upon the experience of other patients with hereditary nonspherocytic hemolytic anemia of similar etiology to serve as a guide. However, even as the large group of patients with hereditary nonspherocytic hemolytic anemia represents a heterogeneous population, so individuals with a single enzymatic lesion, such as PK deficiency, are heterogeneous. Each family is likely to be afflicted with a distinct mutant enzyme, and the various mutants may differ both with respect to clinical manifestations and with respect to response to splenectomy. Some of the available information regarding response to splenectomy of patients with hereditary nonspherocytic hemolytic anemia has been reviewed[12] and is summarized in Table 45-2. Relatively little is known of the response of patients with unstable hemoglobins to splenectomy (see Chap. 47).

Glucocorticoids are of no known value in this group of disorders. Folic acid is often given, as in other patients with increased bone marrow activity, but without proven hematologic benefit. In the absence of iron deficiency, iron is contraindicated. Iron overload is not a frequent complication in this group of disorders but has been reported to occur, particularly in connection with PK deficiency.[484]

COURSE AND PROGNOSIS

Hemolytic episodes in the A– type of deficiency are usually self-limited, even if drug administration is continued. This is not the case in the more severe Mediterranean type of deficiency.[485] In patients with hereditary nonspherocytic hemolytic anemia resulting from G-6-PD deficiency, gallstones may occur, and the incidence of cholelithiasis may even be increased in patients with polymorphic forms of G-6-PD deficiency in Sardinia.[486] During periods of infections or drug administration, anemia may increase in severity. Otherwise, the hemoglobin level of affected subjects remains relatively stable.

Nearly all patients with drug- or infection-induced hemolysis recover uneventfully. Favism must be considered, by comparison, a relatively dangerous disease. Prior to the institution of modern hospital therapy, fatalities from favism were not uncommon. The other very serious complication of G-6-PD deficiency is neonatal icterus. If not recognized early and properly treated, it can lead to kernicterus. With the shortened period of hospitalization attending parturition, the incidence of this grave complication has increased.[487]

In one large population study, a decreasing incidence of G-6-PD deficiency was noted with increasing age of the population,[488] but no such change was observed in another.[23] While age stratification might represent evidence of a shorter life span for individuals with the A– deficiency, other factors are more likely explanations. Examination of the health records of more than 65,000 US Veterans Administration males failed to reveal any higher frequency of any illness in G-6-PD–deficient compared to nondeficient subjects.[13] In view of the benign nature of the common types of G-6-PD deficiency, community-based population screening is not recommended. However, screening for G-6-PD deficiency of all patients admitted to the hospital may be useful in anticipating hemolytic reactions and in understanding them if they occur. This is particularly prudent if a drug such as dapsone, known to cause hemolysis in G-6-PD–deficient individuals, is to be given. Study of family members of patients with this X-linked enzyme deficiency can be helpful in providing appropriate counseling to affected individuals.

The diagnosis of hereditary nonspherocytic hemolytic anemia has been made as late as the seventh decade,[237] and the disease can be fatal in the first few years of life. TPI deficiency appears to have the worst prognosis of all of the known defects that cause this disorder. With few exceptions, patients with this deficiency have died by the fifth or sixth year of life, usually of cardiopulmonary failure. PK deficiency, too, can be fatal in early childhood; the gene prevalent among the Amish of Pennsylvania produces particularly severe disease.[489] Unless the affected homozygous children have their spleens removed, the disorder is commonly lethal. In general, however, hereditary nonspherocytic hemolytic anemia is a relatively mild disease and most affected individuals lead a relatively normal life, apparently without much compromise of life span.

REFERENCES

1. Beutler E: The hemolytic effect of primaquine and related compounds. A review. *Blood* 14:103, 1959.
2. Beutler E: G6PD deficiency. *Blood* 84:3613, 1994.
3. Beutler E: The study of glucose-6-phosphate dehydrogenase: History and molecular biology. *Am J Hematol* 42:53, 1993.
4. Crosby WH: Hereditary nonspherocytic hemolytic anemia. *Blood* 5:233, 1950.
5. Dacie JV: The congenital anaemias, in *The Haemolytic Anaemias*, p 171. Grune & Stratton, New York, 1960.
6. Newton WA Jr, Bass JC: Glutathione sensitive chronic non-spherocytic hemolytic anemia. *Am J Dis Child* 96:501, 1958.
7. Selwyn JG, Dacie JV: Autohemolysis and other changes resulting from the incubation in vitro of red cells from patients with congenital hemolytic anemia. *Blood* 9:414, 1954.
8. Robinson MA, Loder PB, DeGruchy GC: Red-cell metabolism in non-spherocytic congenital haemolytic anaemia. *Br J Haematol* 7:327, 1961.
9. DeGruchy GC, Santamaria JN, Parsons IC, Crawford H: Nonspherocytic congenital hemolytic anemia. *Blood* 16:1371, 1960.
10. Valentine WN, Tanaka KR, Miwa S: A specific erythrocyte glycolytic enzyme defect (pyruvate kinase) in three subjects with congenital nonspherocytic hemolytic anemia. *Trans Assoc Am Phys* 74:100, 1961.
11. Dacie JV: Life and death of the red cell, in *Blood Pure and Eloquent*, edited by MM Wintrobe, p 211. McGraw-Hill, New York, 1980.
12. Beutler E: *Hemolytic Anemia in Disorders of Red Cell Metabolism*. Plenum Press, New York, 1978.
13. Heller P, Best WR, Nelson RB, Becktel J: Clinical implications of sickle-cell trait and glucose-6-phosphate dehydrogenase deficiency in hospitalized Black male patients. *N Engl J Med* 300:1001, 1979.
14. Luzzatto L, Battistuzzi G: Glucose-6-phosphate dehydrogenase, in *Advances in Human Genetics*, edited by H Harris, K Hirschhorn, p 217. Plenum Press, New York, 1985.
15. Luzzatto L, Mehta A: Glucose 6-phosphate dehydrogenase deficiency, in *The Metabolic and Molecular Bases of Inherited Disease*, edited by CR Scriver, AL Beaudet, WS Sly, D Valle, p 3367. McGraw-Hill, New York, 1995.
16. Motulsky AG: Metabolic metamorphisms and the role of infectious diseases in human evolution. *Hum Biol* 32:28, 1960.
17. Luzzatto L, Usanga EA, Reddy S: Glucose 6-phosphate dehydrogenase deficient red cells: Resistance to infection by malarial parasites. *Science* 164:839, 1969.
18. Cappadoro M, Giribaldi G, O'Brien E, et al: Early phagocytosis of glucose-6-phosphate dehydrogenase (G6PD)-deficient erythrocytes parasitized by plasmodium falciparum may explain malaria protection in G6PD deficiency. *Blood* 92:2527, 1998.
19. Piomelli S, Reindorf CA, Arzanian MT, Corash LM: Clinical and biochemical interactions of glucose-6-phosphate dehydrogenase deficiency and sickle-cell anemia. *N Engl J Med* 287:213, 1972.
20. Lewis RA, Hathorn M: Correlation of S hemoglobin with glucose-6-phosphate dehydrogenase deficiency and its significance. *Blood* 26:176, 1965.
21. Steinberg MH, Dreiling BJ: Glucose-6-phosphate dehydrogenase deficiency in sickle cell anemia. *Ann Intern Med* 80:217, 1974.
22. Beutler E, Johnson C, Powars D, West C: Prevalence of glucose-6-phosphate dehydrogenase deficiency in sickle cell disease. *N Engl J Med* 290:826, 1974.
23. Steinberg MH, West MS, Gallagher D, et al: Effects of glucose-6-phosphate dehydrogenase deficiency upon sickle cell anemia. *Blood* 71:748, 1988.
24. Warsy AS: Frequency of glucose-6-phosphate dehydrogenase deficiency in sickle-cell disease. *Hum Hered* 35:143, 1985.

25. Garcia SC, Moragon AC, Lopez-Fernandez ME: Frequency of glutathione reductase, pyruvate kinase and glucose-6-phosphate dehydrogenase deficiency in a Spanish population. *Hum Hered* 29:310, 1979.

26. Abu-Melha AM, Ahmed MAM, Knox-Macaulay H, et al: Erythrocyte pyruvate kinase deficiency in newborns of Eastern Saudi Arabia. *Acta Haematol (Basel)* 85:192, 1991.

27. Mohrenweiser HW: Functional hemizygosity in the human genome: Direct estimate from twelve erythrocyte enzyme loci. *Hum Genet* 77:241, 1987.

28. Mohrenweiser HW, Fielek S: Elevated frequency of carriers for triosephosphate isomerase deficiency in newborn infants. *Pediatr Res* 16:960, 1982.

29. Watanabe M, Zingg BC, Mohrenweiser HW: Molecular analysis of a series of alleles in humans with reduced activity at the triosephosphate isomerase locus. *Am J Hum Genet* 58:308, 1996.

30. Schneider A, Forman L, Westwood B, et al: The relationship of the -5, -8, and -24 mutations in African-Americans to triosephosphate isomerase (TPI) enzyme activity and to TPI deficiency. *Blood* 92:2959, 1998.

31. Baronciani L, Beutler E: Analysis of pyruvate kinase-deficiency mutations that produce nonspherocytic hemolytic anemia. *Proc Natl Acad Sci U S A* 90:4324, 1993.

32. Lenzner C, Nürnberg P, Jacobasch G, et al: Molecular analysis of 29 pyruvate kinase-deficient patients from Central Europe with hereditary hemolytic anemia. *Blood* 89:1793, 1997.

33. Baronciani L, Beutler E: Molecular study of pyruvate kinase deficient patients with hereditary nonspherocytic hemolytic anemia. *J Clin Invest* 95:1702, 1995.

34. Schneider A, Westwood B, Yim C, et al: The 1591C mutation in triosephosphate isomerase (TPI) deficiency. Tightly linked polymorphisms and a common haplotype in all known families. *Blood Cells Mol Dis* 22:115, 1996.

35. Beutler E: *Red Cell Metabolism: A Manual of Biochemical Methods.* Grune & Stratton, New York, 1984.

36. Baldwin SA, Lienhard GE: Purification and reconstitution of glucose transporter from human erythrocytes. *Methods Enzymol* 174:39, 1989.

37. Corry DB, Joolhar FS, Hori MT, Tuck ML: Decreased erythrocyte insulin binding in hypertensive subjects with hyperinsulinemia. *Am J Hypertens* 15:296, 2002.

38. Eadie GS, MacLeod JJR, Noble EC: Insulin and glycolysis. *Am J Physiol* 65:462, 1923.

39. Keitt AS, Bennett DC: Pyruvate kinase deficiency and related disorders of red cell glycolysis. *Am J Med* 41:762, 1966.

40. Gerlach E, Duhm J, Deuticke B: Metabolism of 2,3-diphosphoglycerate in red blood cells under various experimental conditions, in *Red Cell Metabolism and Function,* edited by GJ Brewer, p 155. Plenum Press, New York, 1970.

41. Poole RC, Halestrap AP: Identification and partial purification of the erythrocyte L-lactate transporter. *Biochem J* 283:855, 1992.

42. Heinrich R, Rapoport SM: The utility of mathematical models for the understanding of metabolic systems. *Biochem Soc Trans* 11:31, 1983.

43. Wiback SJ, Palsson BO: Extreme pathway analysis of human red blood cell metabolism. *Biophys J* 83:808, 2002.

44. Reddy VN, Liebman MN, Mavrovouniotis ML: Qualitative analysis of biochemical reaction systems. *Comput Biol Med* 26:9, 1996.

45. Mulquiney PJ, Kuchel PW: Model of the pH-dependence of the concentrations of complexes involving metabolites, haemoglobin and magnesium ions in the human erythrocyte. *Eur J Biochem* 245:71, 1997.

46. Srivastava SK, Beutler E: Glutathione metabolism of the erythrocyte. The enzymic cleavage of glutathione-haemoglobin preparations by glutathione reductase. *Biochem J* 119:353, 1970.

47. Scott MD, Wagner TC, Chiu DTY: Decreased catalase activity is the underlying mechanism of oxidant susceptibility in glucose-6-phosphate dehydrogenase-deficient erythrocytes. *Biochim Biophys Acta* 1181:163, 1993.

48. Gaetani GF, Ferraris AM, Rolfo M, et al: Predominant role of catalase in the disposal of hydrogen peroxide within human erythrocytes. *Blood* 87:1595, 1996.

49. Thorburn DR, Kuchel PW: Regulation of the human-erythrocyte hexose-monophosphate shunt under conditions of oxidative stress. *Eur J Biochem* 150:371, 1985.

50. Ni TC, Savageau MA: Application of biochemical systems theory to metabolism in human red blood cells: Signal propagation and accuracy of representation. *J Biol Chem* 271:7927, 1996.

51. Schuster R, Jacobasch G, Holzhütter HG: Mathematical modeling of metabolic pathways affected by an enzyme deficiency—Energy and redox metabolism of glucose-6-phosphate-dehydrogenase-deficient erythrocytes. *Eur J Biochem* 182:605, 1989.

52. Beutler E, Teeple L: Mannose metabolism in the human erythrocyte. *J Clin Invest* 48:461, 1969.

53. Beutler E, Mathai CK: Genetic variation in red cell galactose-1-phosphate uridyl transferase, in *Hereditary Disorders of Erythrocyte Metabolism,* edited by E Beutler, p 66. Grune & Stratton, New York, 1968.

54. Magnani M, Stocchi V, Chiarantini L, et al: Rabbit red blood cell hexokinase. Decay mechanism during reticulocyte maturation. *J Biol Chem* 261:8327, 1986.

55. Jansen G, Koenderman L, Rijksen G, et al: Age dependent behaviour of red cell glycolytic enzymes in haematological disorders. *Br J Haematol* 61:51, 1985.

56. Zimran A, Torem S, Beutler E: The in vivo ageing of red cell enzymes: Direct evidence of biphasic decay from polycythemic rabbits with reticulocytosis. *Br J Haematol* 69:67, 1988.

57. Rose IA, Warms JVB, O'Connell EL: Role of inorganic phosphate in stimulating the glucose utilization of human red blood cells *Biochem Biophys Res Commun* 15:33, 1964.

58. Fujii S, Beutler E: High glucose concentrations partially release hexokinase from inhibition by glucose-6-phosphate. *Proc Natl Acad Sci U S A* 82:1552, 1985.

59. Gerber G, Kloppick E, Rapoport S: Über den Einfluss des Anorganischen Phosphats auf die Glykolyse; seine Unwirksamkeit auf die Hexokinase des Menschenerythrozyten. *Acta Biol Med Ger* 18:305, 1967.

60. Beutler E, Teeple L: The effect of oxidized glutathione (GSSG) on human erythrocyte hexokinase activity. *Acta Biol Med Ger* 22:707, 1969.

61. Dische Z: The pentose phosphate metabolism in red cells, in *The Red Blood Cell,* edited by C Bishop, DM Surgenor, p 189. Academic Press, New York, 1964.

62. Beutler E: 2,3-Diphosphoglycerate affects enzymes of glucose metabolism in red blood cells. *Nat New Biol* 232:20, 1971.

63. Kaplan JC, Beutler E: Hexokinase isoenzymes in human erythrocytes. *Science* 159:215, 1968.

64. Altay C, Alper CA, Nathan DG: Normal and variant isoenzymes of human blood cell hexokinase and the isoenzyme patterns in hemolytic anemia. *Blood* 36:219, 1970.

65. Murakami K, Blei F, Tilton W, et al: An isozyme of hexokinase specific for the human red blood cell (HK$_R$). *Blood* 75:770, 1990.

66. Ruzzo A, Andreoni F, Magnani M: Structure of the human hexokinase type I gene and nucleotide sequence of the 5' flanking region. *Biochem J* 331:607, 1998.

67. Murakami K, Piomelli S: Identification of the cDNA for human red blood cell-specific hexokinase isozyme. *Blood* 89:762, 1997.

68. Magnani M, Stocchi V, Dacha M, Fornaini G: Rabbit red blood cell hexokinase: Intracellular distribution during reticulocytes maturation. *Mol Cell Biochem* 63:59, 1984.

69. Stocchi V, Magnani M, Piccoli G, Fornaini G: Hexokinase microheterogeneity in rabbit red blood cells and its behaviour during reticulocytes maturation. *Mol Cell Biochem* 79:133, 1988.

70. Thorburn DR, Beutler E: Decay of hexokinase during reticulocyte maturation: Is oxidative damage a signal for destruction? *Biochem Biophys Res Commun* 162:612, 1989.

71. Detter JC, Ways PO, Giblett ER, et al: Inherited variations in human phosphohexose isomerase. *Ann Hum Genet* 31:329, 1968.

72. Fujii S, Matsuda M, Okuya S, et al: Fructose-6-phosphate, 2-kinase activity in human erythrocytes. *Blood* 70:1211, 1987.

73. Boscá L, Aragón JJ, Sols A: Modulation of muscle phosphofructokinase at physiological concentration of enzyme. *J Biol Chem* 260:2100, 1985.

74. Vora S: Isozymes of human phosphofructokinase: Biochemical and genetic aspects, in *Isozymes: Current Topics in Biological and Medical Research*, edited by MC Rattazzi, JG Scandalios, GS Whitt, p 3. Alan R. Liss, New York, 1983.

75. Beutler E, Scott S, Bishop A, et al: Red cell aldolase deficiency and hemolytic anemia: A new syndrome. *Trans Assoc Am Phys* 86:154, 1974.

76. Maquat LE, Chilcote R, Ryan PM: Human triosephosphate isomerase cDNA and protein structure. *J Biol Chem* 260:3748, 1989.

77. Schneider A, Forman L, Westwood B, et al: New insights into the interrelationships of the -5, -8, and -24 mutations with triosephosphate isomerase (TPI) deficiency. *Blood* 90(suppl 1):273a, 1997.

78. Schrier SL: Organization of enzymes in human erythrocyte membranes. *Am J Physiol* 210:139, 1966.

79. Brookes PS, Land JM, Clark JB, Heales SJR: Stimulation of glyceraldehyde-3-phosphate dehydrogenase by oxyhemoglobin. *FEBS Lett* 416:90, 1997.

80. Chen S-H, Malcolm LA, Yoshida A, Giblett ER: Phosphoglycerate kinase: An X-linked polymorphism in man. *Am J Hum Genet* 23:87, 1971.

81. Yoshida A, Watanabe S, Chen S-H, et al: Human phosphoglycerate kinase II. Structure of a variant enzyme. *J Biol Chem* 247:446, 1972.

82. Rosa R, Gaillardon J, Rosa J: Diphosphoglycerate mutase and 2,3-diphosphoglycerate phosphatase activities of red cells: Comparative electrophoretic study. *Biochem Biophys Res Commun* 51:536, 1973.

83. Ikura K, Sasaki R, Narita H, et al: Multifunctional enzyme, bisphosphoglyceromutase/2,3-bisphosphoglycerate phosphatase/phosphoglyceromutase from human erythrocytes. *Eur J Biochem* 66:515, 1976.

84. Rose ZB: The enzymology of 2,3-bisphosphoglycerate. *Adv Enzymol* 51:211, 1980.

85. Rose ZB, Salon J: The identification of glycolate-2-P as a constituent of normal red blood cells. *Biochem Biophys Res Commun* 87:869, 1979.

86. Vora S, Spear D: Demonstration and quantitation of phosphoglycolate in human red cells. *Clin Res* 34:664A, 1986.

87. Fujii S, Beutler E: Glycolate kinase activity in human red cells. *Blood* 65:480, 1985.

88. Fujii S, Beutler E: Where does phosphoglycolate come from in red cells? *Acta Haematol (Basel)* 73:26, 1985.

89. Sasaki H, Fujii S, Yoshizaki Y, et al: Phosphoglycolate synthesis by human erythrocyte pyruvate kinase. *Acta Haematol (Basel)* 77:83, 1987.

90. Badwey JA: Phosphoglycolate phosphatase in human erythrocytes. *J Biol Chem* 252:2441, 1977.

91. Beutler E, West C: An improved assay and some properties of phosphoglycolate phosphatase. *Anal Biochem* 106:163, 1980.

92. Hass LF, Kappel WK, Muller KB, Engle RL: Evidence for structural homology between human red cell phosphoglycerate mutase and 2,3-bisphosphoglycerate synthase. *J Biol Chem* 253:77, 1978.

93. Chen S-H, Anderson JE, Giblett ER: Human red cell 2,3-diphosphoglycerate mutase and monophosphoglycerate mutase: Genetic evidence for two separate loci. *Am J Hum Genet* 29:405, 1977.

94. Hoorn RKJ, Filkweert JP, Staal GEJ: Purification and properties of enolase of human erythrocytes. *Int J Biochem* 5:845, 1974.

95. Chen S-H, Giblett ER: Enolase: Human tissue distribution and evidence for three different loci. *Ann Hum Genet* 39:277, 1976.

96. Valentine WN, Tanaka KR, Paglia DE: Hemolytic anemias and erythrocyte enzymopathies. *Ann Intern Med* 103:245, 1985.

97. Noguchi T, Yamada K, Inoue H, et al: The L- and R-type isozymes of rat pyruvate kinase are produced from a single gene by use of different promoters. *J Biol Chem* 262:14366, 1987.

98. Blume KG, Hoffbauer RW, Busch D, et al: Purification and properties of pyruvate kinase in normal and in pyruvate kinase deficient human red blood cells. *Biochim Biophys Acta* 227:364, 1971.

99. Kahn A, Marie J, Garreau H, Sprengers ED: The genetic system of the L-type pyruvate kinase forms in man. Subunit structure, interrelation and kinetic characteristics of the pyruvate kinase enzymes from erythrocytes and liver. *Biochim Biophys Acta* 523:59, 1978.

100. Takayasu S, Fujiwara S, Waki T: Hereditary lactate dehydrogenase M-subunit deficiency: Lactate dehydrogenase activity in skin lesions and in hair follicles. *J Am Acad Dermatol* 24:339, 1991.

101. Kitamura M, Iijima N, Hashimoto F, Hiratsuka A: Hereditary deficiency of subunit H of lactate dehydrogenase. *Clin Chim Acta* 34:419, 1971.

102. Miwa S, Nishina T, Kakehashi Y, et al: Studies on erythrocyte metabolism in a case with hereditary deficiency of H-subunit of lactate dehydrogenase. *Acta Haematol Jpn* 34:2, 1971.

103. Joukyuu R, Mizuno S, Amakawa T, et al: Hereditary complete deficiency of lactate dehydrogenase H-subunit. *Clin Chem* 35:687, 1989.

104. Wakabayashi H, Tsuchiya M, Yoshino K, et al: Hereditary deficiency of lactate dehydrogenase H-subunit. *Intern Med* 35:550, 1996.

105. Beutler E: G6PD: Population genetics and clinical manifestations. *Blood Rev* 10:45, 1996.

106. Maekawa M, Sudo K, Nagura K, et al: Population screening of lactate dehydrogenase deficiencies in Fukuoka Prefecture in Japan and molecular characterization of three independent mutations in the lactate dehydrogenase-B(H) gene. *Hum Genet* 93:74, 1994.

107. Yoshida A, Beutler E: *Glucose-6-Phosphate Dehydrogenase*. Academic Press, Orlando, FL, 1986.

108. Au SWN, Gover S, Lam VMS, Adams MJ: Human glucose-6-phosphate dehydrogenase: The crystal structure reveals a structural NADP(+) molecule and provides insights into enzyme deficiency. *Struct Fold Des* 8:293, 2000.

109. Yoshida A, Stamatoyannopoulos G, Motulsky A: Negro variant of glucose-6-phosphate dehydrogenase deficiency (A-) in man. *Science* 155:97, 1967.

110. Rattazzi MC: Glucose-6-phosphate dehydrogenase from human erythrocytes: Molecular weight determination by gel filtration. *Biochem Biophys Res Commun* 31:16, 1968.

111. Kirkman HN, Hendrickson EM: Glucose-6-phosphate dehydrogenase from human erythrocytes: II. Subactive states of the enzyme from normal persons. *J Biol Chem* 237:2371, 1962.

112. Yoshida A: Hemolytic anemia and G-6-PD deficiency. *Science* 179:532, 1973.

113. Avigad G: Inhibition of glucose-6-phosphate dehydrogenase by adenosine-5-triphosphate. *Proc Natl Acad Sci U S A* 56:1543, 1966.

114. Ben-Bassat I, Beutler E: Inhibition by ATP of erythrocyte glucose-6-phosphate dehydrogenase variants. *Proc Soc Exp Biol Med* 142:410, 1973.

115. Beutler E, Kuhl W: Limiting role of 6-phosphogluconolactonase in erythrocyte hexose monophosphate pathway metabolism. *J Lab Clin Med* 106:573, 1985.

116. Rakitzis ET, Papandreou P: Kinetic analysis of 6-phosphogluconolactone hydrolysis in hemolysates. *Biochem Mol Biol Int* 37:747, 1995.

117. Beutler E, Kuhl W, Gelbart T: 6-Phosphogluconolactonase deficiency, a hereditary erythrocyte enzyme deficiency: Possible interaction with glucose-6-phosphate dehydrogenase deficiency. *Proc Natl Acad Sci U S A* 82:3876, 1985.

118. Thorburn DR, Kuchel PW: Computer simulation of the metabolic consequences of the combined deficiency of 6-phosphogluconolactonase

and glucose-6-phosphate dehydrogenase in human erythrocytes. *J Lab Clin Med* 110:70, 1987.

119. Shih L, Justice P, Hsia DY: Purification and characterization of genetic variants of 6-phosphogluconate dehydrogenase. *Biochem Genet* 1:359, 1968.

120. Parr CW, Fitch LI: Inherited quantitative variations of human phosphogluconate dehydrogenase. *Ann Hum Genet* 30:339, 1967.

121. Bruns FH, Noltmann E, Vahlhaus E: Über den Stoffwechsel von Ribose-5-phosphat in Hämolysaten. I. Aktivitäts-messung und Eigenschaften der Phosphoribose-isomerase. II. Der Pentosephosphate-Cyclus in roten Blutzellen. *Biochem Z* 330:483, 1958.

122. Brownstone YS, Denstedt OF: The pentose phosphate metabolic pathway in the human erythrocyte: II. The transketolase and transaldolase activity of the human erythrocyte. *Can J Biochem* 39:533, 1961.

123. Nakasaki H, Ohta M, Soeda J, et al: Clinical and biochemical aspects of thiamine treatment for metabolic acidosis during total parenteral nutrition. *Nutrition* 13:110, 1997.

124. Wolfe SJ, Brin M, Davidson CS. The effect of thiamine deficiency on human erythrocyte metabolism. *J Clin Invest* 37:1476, 1958.

125. Beutler E, Guinto E: The reduction of glyceraldehyde by human erythrocytes. L-hexonate dehydrogenase activity. *J Clin Invest* 53:1258, 1974.

126. Das B, Srivastava SK: Purification and properties of aldose reductase and aldehyde reductase II from human erythrocyte. *Arch Biochem Biophys* 238:670, 1985.

127. Kim HD: Is adenosine a second metabolic substrate for human red blood cells. *Biochim Biophys Acta* 1036:113, 1990.

128. Gabrio BW, Finch CA, Huennekens FM: Erythrocyte preservation: A topic in molecular biochemistry. *Blood* 11:103, 1956.

129. Resta R, Thompson LF: SCID: The role of adenosine deaminase deficiency. *Immunol Today* 18:371, 1997.

130. Mitchell BS, Kelley WN: Purinogenic immunodeficiency diseases: Clinical features and molecular mechanisms. *Ann Intern Med* 92:826, 1980.

131. Valentine WN, Paglia DE, Tartaglia AP, Gilsanz F: Hereditary hemolytic anemia with increased red cell adenosine deaminase (45- to 70-fold) and decreased adenosine triphosphate. *Science* 195:783, 1977.

132. Casoli C, Lisa A, Magnani G, et al: Prognostic value of adenosine deaminase compared to other markers for progression to acquired immunodeficiency syndrome among intravenous drug users. *J Med Virol* 45:203, 1995.

133. Palomba E, David O, Boltri A, et al: Increased erythrocyte adenosine deaminase activity in children with perinatal human immunodeficiency virus infection. *Pediatr Infect Dis J* 8:862, 1989.

134. Glader BE, Backer K, Diamond LK: Elevated erythrocyte adenosine deaminase activity in congenital hypoplastic anemia. *N Engl J Med* 309:1486, 1983.

135. Accorsi A, Piacentini MP, Piatti E, Fazi A: Purine nucleoside phosphorylase from human erythrocytes: A kinetic study of the fully separated isoenzymes. *Biochem Int* 24:23, 1991.

136. Valentine WN, Oski FA, Paglia DE, et al: Erythrocyte hexokinase and hereditary hemolytic anemia, in *Hereditary Disorders of Erythrocyte Metabolism*, edited by E Beutler, p 288. Grune & Stratton, New York, 1968.

137. Morsches B, Holzmann H, Bettingen C: Zum Nachweis der Sorbit-dehydrogenase in menschlichen Erythrocyten. *Klin Wochenschr* 47:672, 1969.

138. Barretto OCO, Beutler E: The sorbitol oxidizing enzyme of red blood cells. *J Lab Clin Med* 85:645, 1975.

139. Bruns FH, Noltmann E: Phosphomannoisomerase, an SH-dependent metal-enzyme complex. *Nature* 181:1467, 1958.

140. Bruns FH, Noltmann E, Willemsen A: Phosphomannose-isomerase: I. Über die Aktivitätsmessung und die Sulfhydryl-sowie die Metallabhängigkeit der Enzymwirkung in einigen tierischen Geweben. *Biochem Z* 330:411, 1958.

141. Beutler E: Galactosemia: Screening and diagnosis. *Clin Biochem* 24:293, 1991.

142. Noltmann E, Bruns FH: Über die Phosphoglucomutase der Erythrocyten und des Serums. *Hoppe-Seyler's Z Physiol Chem* 313:194, 1959.

143. Beutler E, Guinto E: Dihydroxyacetone metabolism by human erythrocytes: Demonstration of triokinase activity and its characterization. *Blood* 41:559, 1973.

144. Brake JM, Deindoerfer FH: Preservation of red blood cell 2,3-diphosphoglycerate in stored blood containing dihydroxyacetone. *Transfusion* 13:84, 1973.

145. Wood L, Beutler E: The effect of ascorbate and dihydroxyacetone on the 2,3-diphosphoglycerate and ATP levels of stored human red cells. *Transfusion* 14:272, 1974.

146. Moses SW, Chayoth R, Levin S, et al: Glucose and glycogen metabolism in erythrocytes from normal and glycogen storage disease type III subjects. *J Clin Invest* 47:1343, 1968.

147. Sidbury JB Jr, Cornblath M, Fisher J, House E: Glycogen in erythrocytes of patients with glycogen storage disease. *Pediatrics* 27:103, 1961.

148. Bartels H: Untersuchungen zur Frage des Glykogen-Gehaltes von Erythrocyten, in *Metabolism and Membrane Permeability of Erythrocytes and Thrombocytes*, edited by E Deutsch, E Gerlach, K Moser, p 132. Georg Thieme Verlag, Stuttgart, 1968.

149. Dimant E, Landberg E, London IM: The metabolic behavior of reduced glutathione in human and avian erythrocytes. *J Biol Chem* 213:769, 1955.

150. Beutler E, Gelbart T: Improved assay of the enzymes of glutathione synthesis: Gamma-glutamylcysteine synthetase and glutathione synthetase. *Clin Chim Acta* 158:115, 1986.

151. Lunn G, Dale GL, Beutler E: Transport accounts for glutathione turnover in human erythrocytes. *Blood* 54:238, 1979.

152. Viña JR, Palacin M, Puertes IR, et al: Role of the gamma-glutamyl cycle in the regulation of amino acid translocation. *Am J Physiol* 257:E916, 1989.

153. Board PG, Smith JE: Erythrocyte gamma-glutamyl transpeptidase. *Blood* 49:667, 1977.

154. Srivastava SK, Awasthi YC, Miller SP, et al: Studies on gamma-glutamyl transpeptidase in human and rabbit erythrocytes. *Blood* 47:645, 1976.

155. Young JD, Ellory JC, Wright PC: Evidence against the participation of the gamma-glutamyltransferase-gamma-glutamylcyclotransferase pathway in amino acid transport by rabbit erythrocytes. *Biochem J* 152:713, 1975.

156. Winterbourn CC, Hawkins RE, Brian M, Carrell RW: The estimation of red cell superoxide dismutase activity. *J Lab Clin Med* 85:337, 1975.

157. Mills GC, Randall HP: Hemoglobin catabolism: II. The protection of hemoglobin from oxidative breakdown in the intact erythrocyte. *J Biol Chem* 232:589, 1958.

158. Cohen G, Hochstein P: Glutathione peroxidase: The primary agent for the elimination of hydrogen peroxide in erythrocytes. *Biochemistry* 2:1420, 1963.

159. Rotruck JT, Pope AL, Ganther HE, et al: Selenium: Biochemical role as a component of glutathione peroxidase. *Science* 179:588, 1973.

160. Thomson CD, Rea HM, Doesburg VM, Robinson MF: Selenium concentrations and glutathione peroxidase activities in whole blood of New Zealand residents. *Br J Nutr* 37:457, 1977.

161. Beutler E, Matsumoto F: Ethnic variation in red cell glutathione peroxidase activity. *Blood* 46:103, 1975.

162. Burk RF: Molecular biology of selenium with implications for its metabolism. *FASEB J* 5:2274, 1991.

163. Chambers I, Harrison PR: A new puzzle in selenoprotein biosynthesis: Selenocysteine seems to be encoded by the "stop" codon, UGA. *TIBS Rev* 12:255, 1987.

164. Stadtman TC: Selenocysteine. *Annu Rev Biochem* 65:83, 1996.

165. Jacob HS, Jandl JH: Effects of sulfhydryl inhibition on red blood cells: I. Mechanism of hemolysis. *J Clin Invest* 41:779, 1962.

166. Magnani M, Stocchi V, Ninfali P, et al: Action of oxidized and reduced glutathione on rabbit red blood cell hexokinase. *Biochim Biophys Acta* 615:113, 1980.

167. Huisman THJ, Dozy AM: Studies on the heterogeneity of hemoglobin: V. Binding of hemoglobin with oxidized glutathione. *J Lab Clin Med* 60:302, 1962.

168. Wong KK, Blanchard JS: Human erythrocyte glutathione reductase: pH dependence of kinetic parameters. *Biochemistry* 28:3586, 1989.

169. Icen A: Glutathione reductase of human erythrocytes. Purification and properties. *Scand J Clin Lab Invest* 96:1, 1967.

170. Beutler E, Yeh MKY: Erythrocyte glutathione reductase. *Blood* 21:573, 1963.

171. Loos H, Roos D, Weening R, Houwerzijl J: Familial deficiency of glutathione reductase in human blood cells. *Blood* 48:53, 1976.

172. Beutler E: Glutathione reductase: Stimulation in normal subjects by riboflavin supplementation. *Science* 165:613, 1969.

173. Mieyal JJ, Starke DW, Gravina SA, Hocevar BA: Thioltransferase in human red blood cells: Kinetics and equilibrium. *Biochemistry* 30:8883, 1991.

174. Srivastava SK, Beutler E: The transport of oxidized glutathione from human erythrocytes. *J Biol Chem* 244:9, 1969.

175. Kondo T, Dale GL, Beutler E: Glutathione transport by inside-out vesicles from human erythrocytes. *Proc Natl Acad Sci U S A* 77:6359, 1980.

176. Kondo T, Kawakami Y, Taniguchi N, Beutler E: Glutathione disulfide-stimulated Mg^{2+}-ATPase of human erythrocyte membranes. *Proc Natl Acad Sci U S A* 84:7373, 1987.

177. Board PG: Transport of glutathione S-conjugate from human erythrocytes. *FEBS Lett* 124:163, 1981.

178. Kondo T, Murao M, Taniguchi N: Glutathione S-conjugate transport using inside-out vesicles from human erythrocytes. *Eur J Biochem* 125:551, 1982.

179. Harvey JW, Beutler E: Binding of heme by glutathione S-transferase: A possible role of the erythrocyte enzyme. *Blood* 60:1227, 1982.

180. Beutler E, Dunning D, Dabe IB, Forman L: Erythrocyte glutathione S-transferase deficiency and hemolytic anemia. *Blood* 72:73, 1988.

181. Boivin P, Galand C, Dreyfus B: Activités enzymatiques erythrocytaires au cours des anemies refractaires. *Nouv Rev Fr Hematol* 9:105, 1969.

182. Abe S: Secondary red cell pyruvate kinase deficiency: I. Study of 30 subjects of malignant hematological disorders. *Acta Haematol Jpn* 39:247, 1976.

183. Kahn A, Cottreau D, Boyer C, et al: Causal mechanisms of multiple acquired red cell enzyme defects in a patient with acquired dyserythropoiesis. *Blood* 48:653, 1976.

184. Kornberg A, Goldfarb A: Preleukemia manifested by hemolytic anemia with pyruvate-kinase deficiency. *Arch Intern Med* 146:785, 1986.

185. Van Wijk R, Rijksen G, Huizinga EG, et al: HK Utrecht: Missense mutation in the active site of human hexokinase associated with hexokinase deficiency and severe nonspherocytic hemolytic anemia. *Blood* 101:345, 2003.

186. Beutler E: *Red Cell Metabolism: A Manual of Biochemical Methods*. Grune & Stratton, New York, 1975.

187. Clarke JL, Vulliamy TJ, Roper D, et al: Combined glucose-6-phosphate dehydrogenase and glucosephosphate isomerase deficiency can alter clinical outcome. *Blood Cells Mol Dis* 30:258, 2003.

188. Bruno C, Minetti C, Shanske S, et al: Combined defects of muscle phosphofructokinase and AMP deaminase in a child with myoglobinuria. *Neurology* 50:296, 1998.

189. Ronquist G, Rudolphi O, Engstrom I, Waldenstrom A: Familial phosphofructokinase deficiency is associated with a disturbed calcium homeostasis in erythrocytes. *J Intern Med* 249:85, 2001.

190. Kishi H, Mukai T, Hirono A, et al: Human aldolase A deficiency associated with a hemolytic anemia: Thermolabile aldolase due to a single base mutation. *Proc Natl Acad Sci U S A* 84:8623, 1987.

191. Kreuder J, Borkhardt A, Repp R, et al: Brief report: Inherited metabolic myopathy and hemolysis due to a mutation in aldolase A. *N Engl J Med* 334:1100, 1996.

192. Valentin C, Pissard S, Martin J, et al: Triose phosphate isomerase deficiency in 3 French families: Two novel null alleles, a frameshift mutation (TPI Alfortville) and an alteration in the initiation codon (TPI Paris). *Blood* 96:1130, 2000.

193. Hollan S, Magocsi M, Fodor E, et al: Search for the pathogenesis of the differing phenotype in two compound heterozygote Hungarian brothers with the same genotypic triosephosphate isomerase deficiency. *Proc Natl Acad Sci U S A* 94:10362, 1997.

194. Hamano T, Mutoh T, Sugie H, et al: Phosphoglycerate kinase deficiency: An adult myopathic form with a novel mutation. *Neurology* 54:1188, 2000.

195. Turner G, Fletcher J, Elber J, et al: Molecular defect of a phosphoglycerate kinase variant associated with haemolytic anaemia and neurological disorders in a large kindred. *Br J Haematol* 91:60, 1995.

196. Hoyer JD, Allen SL, Beutler E, et al: Erythrocytosis due to biphosphoglycerate mutase deficiency with concurrent glucose-6-phosphate dehydrogenase (G-6-PD) deficiency. *Am J Hematol* 75:205, 2004.

197. Lemarchandel V, Joulin V, Valentin C, et al: Compound heterozygosity in a complete erythrocyte bisphosphoglycerate mutase deficiency. *Blood* 80:2643, 1992.

198. Van Wijk R, Van Solinge WW, Nerlov C, et al: Disruption of a novel regulatory element in the erythroid-specific promoter of the human PKLR gene causes severe pyruvate kinase deficiency. *Blood* 101:1596, 2003.

199. Beutler E, Vulliamy TJ: Hematologically important mutations: Glucose-6-phosphate dehydrogenase. *Blood Cells Mol Dis* 28:93, 2002.

200. Hamilton D, Wu JH, Alaoui-Jamali M, Batist G: A novel missense mutation in the gamma-glutamylcysteine synthetase catalytic subunit gene causes both decreased enzymatic activity and glutathione production. *Blood* 102:725, 2003.

201. Beutler E, Duron O, Kelly BM: Improved method for the determination of blood glutathione. *J Lab Clin Med* 61:882, 1963.

202. Corrons JL, Alvarez R, Pujades A, et al: Hereditary non-spherocytic haemolytic anaemia due to red blood cell glutathione synthetase deficiency in four unrelated patients from Spain: Clinical and molecular studies. *Br J Haematol* 112:475, 2001.

203. Balta G, Gumruk F, Akarsu N, et al: Molecular characterization of Turkish patients with pyrimidine 5'-nucleotidase-I deficiency. *Blood* 102:1900, 2003.

204. Valentine WN, Fink K, Paglia DE, et al: Hereditary hemolytic anemia with human erythrocyte pyrimidine 5'-nucleotidase deficiency. *J Clin Invest* 54:866, 1974.

205. Torrance J, West C, Beutler E: A simple rapid radiometric assay for pyrimidine-5'-nucleotidase. *J Lab Clin Med* 90:563, 1977.

206. Vives-Corrons J-L, Varughese KI, Gelbart T, Beutler E: Red cell adenylate kinase deficiency. Molecular study of three new mutations (118G→A, 190G→A and GAC deletion) associated with hereditary nonspherocytic hemolytic anemia. *Blood* 102:353, 2003.

207. Chen EH, Tartaglia AP, Mitchell BS: Hereditary overexpression of adenosine deaminase in erythrocytes: Evidence for a *cis*-acting mutation. *Am J Hum Genet* 53:889, 1993.

208. Markert ML: Molecular basis of adenosine deaminase deficiency. *Immunodeficiency* 5:141, 1994.

209. Grabowska D, Plochocka D, Jablonska-Skwiecinska E, et al: Compound heterozygosity of two missense mutations in the NADH-cytochrome b5 reductase gene of a Polish patient with type I recessive congenital methaemoglobinaemia. *Eur J Haematol* 70:404, 2003.

210. Kaplan J-C, Nicolas A, Hanlickova-Leroux A, Beutler E: A simple spot screening test for fast detection of red cell NADH-diaphorase deficiency. *Blood* 36:330, 1970.

211. Jacobasch G, Rapoport SM: Hemolytic anemias due to erythrocyte enzyme deficiencies. *Mol Aspects Med* 17:143, 1996.

212. Beutler E, Kuhl W, Gelbart T: Blood cell phosphogluconolactonase: Assay and properties. *Br J Haematol* 62:577, 1986.

213. Bird TD, Hamernyik P, Nutter JY, Labbe RF: Inherited deficiency of delta-aminolevulinic acid dehydratase. *Am J Hum Genet* 31:662, 1979.

214. Shinohara K, Tanaka KR: Hereditary deficiency of erythrocyte acetylcholinesterase. *Am J Hematol* 7:313, 1979.

215. Kamatani N, Hakoda M, Otsuka S, et al: Only three mutations account for almost all defective alleles causing adenine phosphoribosyltransferase deficiency in Japanese patients. *J Clin Invest* 90:130, 1992.

216. Cartier P, Hamet M: Une nouvelle maladie metabolique: Le deficit complet en adenine-phosphoribosyltransferase avec lithiase de 2,8-dihydroxyadenine. *C R Acad Sci (Paris)* 279:883, 1974.

217. Hidaka Y, Palella TD, O'Toole TE, et al: Human adenine phosphoribosyltransferase. Identification of allelic mutations at the nucleotide level as a cause of complete deficiency of the enzyme. *J Clin Invest* 80:1409, 1987.

218. Ogasawara N, Goto H, Yamada Y, Watanabe T: Distribution of AMP-deaminase isozymes in rat tissues. *Eur J Biochem* 87:297, 1978.

219. Yamada Y, Makarewicz W, Goto H, et al: Gene mutations responsible for human erythrocyte AMP deaminase deficiency in Poles. *Adv Exp Med Biol* 431:347, 1998.

220. Armstrong JM, Myers DV, Verpoorte JA, Edsall JT: Purification and properties of human erythrocyte carbonic anhydrases. *J Biol Chem* 241:5137, 1966.

221. Kendall AG, Tashian RE: Erythrocyte carbonic anhydrase I: Inherited deficiency in humans. *Science* 197:471, 1977.

222. Roth DE, Venta PJ, Tashian RE, Sly WS: Molecular basis of human carbonic anhydrase II deficiency. *Proc Natl Acad Sci U S A* 89:1804, 1992.

223. Takahara S: Acatalasemia and hypocatalasemia in the Orient. *Semin Hematol* 8:397, 1971.

224. Aebi H, Bossi E, Cantz M, et al: Acatalas(em)ia in Switzerland, in *Hereditary Disorders of Erythrocyte Metabolism*, edited by E Beutler, p 41. Grune & Stratton, New York, 1968.

225. Boulard-Heitzmann P, Boulard M, Tallineau C, et al: Decreased red cell enolase activity in a 40-year-old woman with compensated haemolysis. *Scand J Haematol* 33:401, 1984.

226. Gitzelmann R: Hereditary galactokinase deficiency, a newly recognized cause of juvenile cataracts. *Pediatr Res* 1:14, 1967.

227. Beutler E: Effect of flavin compounds on glutathione reductase activity: In vivo and in vitro studies. *J Clin Invest* 48:1957, 1969.

228. McCann SR, Finkel B, Cadman S, Allen DW: Study of a kindred with hereditary spherocytosis and glyceraldehyde-3-phosphate dehydrogenase deficiency. *Blood* 47:171, 1976.

229. Valentine WN, Paglia DE, Neerhout RC, Konrad PN: Erythrocyte glyoxalase II deficiency with coincidental hereditary elliptocytosis. *Blood* 36:797, 1970.

230. Johnson LA, Gordon RB, Emmerson BT: Hypoxanthine-guanine phosphoribosyltransferase: A simple spectrophotometric assay. *Clin Chim Acta* 80:203, 1977.

231. Davidson BL, Tarle SA, Palella TD, Kelley WN: Molecular basis of hypoxanthine-guanine phosphoribosyltransferase deficiency in ten subjects determined by direct sequencing of amplified transcripts. *J Clin Invest* 84:342, 1989.

232. Vanderheiden BS: Genetic studies of human erythrocyte inosine triphosphatase. *Biochem Genet* 3:289, 1969.

233. Sass MD, Caruso CJ, Farhangi M: TPNH-methemoglobin reductase deficiency: A new red-cell enzyme defect. *J Lab Clin Med* 70:760, 1967.

234. Kaplan J-C, Alexandre Y, Dreyfus J-C: Deficit selectif d'un des loci genetiques de la phosphoglucomutase dans les globules rouges. *C R Acad Sci (Paris)* 270:1060, 1970.

235. Chamberlain BR, Buttery JE: Reappraisal of the uroporphyrinogen I synthase assay, and a proposed modified method. *Clin Chem* 26:1346, 1980.

236. Strand LJ, Meyer UA, Felsher BF, et al: Decreased red cell uroporphyrinogen I synthetase activity in intermittent acute porphyria. *J Clin Invest* 51:2530, 1972.

237. Beutler E: Red cell enzyme defects as non-diseases and as diseases. *Blood* 54:1, 1979.

238. Bianchi P, Zappa M, Bredi E, et al: A case of complete adenylate kinase deficiency due to a nonsense mutation in AK-1 gene (Arg 107→Stop, CGA→TGA) associated with chronic haemolytic anaemia. *Br J Haematol* 105:75, 1999.

239. Szeinberg A, Kahana D, Gavendo S, et al: Hereditary deficiency of adenylate kinase in red blood cells. *Acta Haematol (Basel)* 42:111, 1969.

240. Beutler E, Carson D, Dannawi H, et al: Metabolic compensation for profound erythrocyte adenylate kinase deficiency. *J Clin Invest* 72:648, 1983.

241. Rosa R, George C, Fardeau M, et al: A new case of phosphoglycerate kinase deficiency: PGK Creteil associated with rhabdomyolysis and lacking hemolytic anemia. *Blood* 60:84, 1982.

242. Marstein S, Jellum E, Halpern B, et al: Biochemical studies of erythrocytes in a patient with pyroglutamic acidemia (5-oxoprolinemia). *N Engl J Med* 295:406, 1976.

243. Shohet SB, Livermore BM, Nathan DG, Jaffe ER: Hereditary hemolytic anemia associated with abnormal membrane lipids: Mechanism of accumulation of phosphatidyl choline. *Blood* 38:445, 1971.

244. Lane PA, Kuypers FA, Clark MR, et al: Excess of red cell membrane proteins in hereditary high-phosphatidylcholine hemolytic anemia. *Am J Hematol* 34:186, 1990.

245. Shojania AM, Godin DV, Frohlich J: Hereditary high phosphatidylcholine hemolytic anemia: Report of a new family and review of the literature. *Clin Invest Med* 13:313, 1990.

246. Clark MR, Shohet SB, Gottfried EL: Hereditary hemolytic disease with increased red blood cell phosphatidylcholine and dehydration: One, two, or many disorders. *Am J Hematol* 42:25, 1993.

247. Dern RJ, Beutler E, Alving AS: The hemolytic effect of primaquine: V. Primaquine sensitivity as a manifestation of a multiple drug sensitivity. *J Lab Clin Med* 45:30, 1955.

248. Cohen G, Hochstein P: Generation of hydrogen peroxide in erythrocytes by hemolytic agents. *Biochemistry* 3:895, 1964.

249. Kosower NS, Song KR, Kosower EM, Correa W: Glutathione: II. Chemical aspects of azoester procedure for oxidation to disulfide. *Biochim Biophys Acta* 192:8, 1969.

250. Birchmeier W, Tuchschmid PE, Winterhalter H: Comparison of human hemoglobin A carrying glutathione as a mixed disulfide with the naturally occurring human hemoglobin A3. *Biochemistry* 12:3667, 1973.

251. Rachmilewitz EA, Harari E, Winterhalter KH: Separation of alpha- and beta-chains of hemoglobin A by acetylphenylhydrazine. *Biochim Biophys Acta* 371:402, 1974.

252. Itano HA, Hosokawa K, Hirota K: Induction of haemolytic anaemia by substituted phenylhydrazines. *Br J Haematol* 32:99, 1976.

253. Kirkman HN, Gaetani GF: Catalase: A tetrameric enzyme with four tightly bound molecules of NADPH. *Proc Natl Acad Sci U S A* 81:4343, 1984.

254. Gaetani GF, Rolfo M, Arena S, et al: Active involvement of catalase during hemolytic crises of favism. *Blood* 88:1084, 1996.

255. Rifkind RA: Heinz body anemia: An ultrastructural study: II. Red cell sequestration and destruction. *Blood* 26:433, 1965.

256. Bunn HEF, Jandl JH: Exchange of heme among hemoglobin molecules. *Proc Natl Acad Sci U S A* 56:974, 1966.

257. Jandl JH: The Heinz body hemolytic anemias. *Ann Intern Med* 58:702, 1963.

258. Beutler E: Abnormalities of glycolysis (HMP shunt). *Bibl Haematol* 29:146, 1968.

259. Baehner RL, Nathan DG, Castle WB: Oxidant injury of Caucasian glucose-6-phosphate dehydrogenase-deficient red blood cells by phagocytosing leukocytes during infection. *J Clin Invest* 50:2466, 1971.

260. Arese P, De Flora A: Denaturation of normal and abnormal erythrocytes: II. Pathophysiology of hemolysis in glucose-6-phosphate dehydrogenase deficiency. *Semin Hematol* 27:1, 1990.

261. Stamatoyannopoulos G, Fraser GR, Motulsky AG, et al: On the familial predisposition to favism. *Am J Hum Genet* 18:253, 1966.

262. Cassimos CHR, Malaka-Zafiriu K, Tsiures J: Urinary d-glucaric acid excretion in normal and G-6-PD deficient children with favism. *J Pediatr* 84:871, 1974.

263. Bottini E, Bottini FG, Borgiani P, Businco L: Association between ACP1 and favism: A possible biochemical mechanism. *Blood* 89:2613, 1997.

264. Fiorelli G, Podda M, Corrias A, Fargion S: The relevance of immune reactions in acute favism. *Acta Haematol (Basel)* 51:211, 1974.

265. Turrini F, Naitana A, Mannuzzu L, et al: Increased red cell calcium, decreased calcium adenosine triphosphatase, and altered membrane proteins during fava bean hemolysis in glucose-6-phosphate dehydrogenase-deficient (Mediterranean variant) individuals. *Blood* 66:302, 1985.

266. De Flora A, Benatti U, Guida L, et al: Favism: Disordered erythrocyte calcium homeostasis. *Blood* 66:294, 1985.

267. Fischer TM, Meloni T, Pescarmona GP, Arese P: Membrane cross bonding in red cells in favic crisis: A missing link in the mechanism of extravascular haemolysis. *Br J Haematol* 59:159, 1985.

268. Kaplan M, Vreman HJ, Hammerman C, et al: Contribution of haemolysis to jaundice in Sephardic Jewish glucose-6-phosphate dehydrogenase deficient neonates. *Br J Haematol* 93:822, 1996.

269. Kaplan M, Muraca M, Hammerman C, et al: Imbalance between production and conjugation of bilirubin: A fundamental concept in the mechanism of neonatal jaundice. *Pediatrics* 110:e47, 2002.

270. Kaplan M, Renbaum P, Levy-Lahad E, et al: Gilbert syndrome and glucose-6-phosphate dehydrogenase deficiency: A dose-dependent genetic interaction crucial to neonatal hyperbilirubinemia. *Proc Natl Acad Sci U S A* 94:12128, 1997.

271. Huang CS, Chang PF, Huang MJ, et al: Glucose-6-phosphate dehydrogenase deficiency, the UDP-glucuronosyl transferase 1A1 gene, and neonatal hyperbilirubinemia. *Gastroenterology* 123:127, 2002.

272. Oluboyede OA, Esan GJF, Francis TI, Luzzatto L: Genetically determined deficiency of glucose 6-phosphate dehydrogenase (type A-) is expressed in the liver. *J Lab Clin Med* 93:783, 1979.

273. Piomelli S: G6PD-related neonatal jaundice, in *Glucose-6-Phosphate Dehydrogenase*, edited by A Yoshida, E Beutler, p 95. Academic Press, Orlando, FL, 1986.

274. Ifekwunigwe AE, Luzzatto L: Kernicterus in G-6-PD-deficiency. *Lancet* 1:667, 1966.

275. Eshaghpour E, Oski FA, Williams M: The relationship of erythrocyte glucose-6-phosphate dehydrogenase deficiency to hyperbilirubinemia in Negro premature infants. *J Pediatr* 70:595, 1967.

276. Lopez R, Cooperman JM: Glucose-6-phosphate dehydrogenase deficiency and hyperbilirubinemia in the newborn. *Am J Dis Child* 122:66, 1971.

277. Herschel M, Ryan M, Gelbart T, Kaplan M: Hemolysis and hyperbilirubinemia in an African-American neonate heterozygous for glucose-6-phosphate dehydrogenase deficiency. *J Perinatol* 22:577, 2002.

278. Beutler E, Gelbart T, Demina A: Racial variability in the UDP-glucuronosyltransferase 1 (*UGT1A1*) promoter: A balanced polymorphism for regulation of bilirubin metabolism? *Proc Natl Acad Sci U S A* 95:8170, 1998.

279. Dahl N, Pigg M, Ristoff E, et al: Missense mutations in the human glutathione synthetase gene result in severe metabolic acidosis, 5-oxoprolinuria, hemolytic anemia and neurological dysfunction. *Hum Mol Genet* 6:1147, 1997.

280. Hirono A, Iyori H, Sekine I, et al: Three cases of hereditary nonspherocytic hemolytic anemia associated with red cell glutathione deficiency. *Blood* 87:2071, 1996.

281. Beutler E, Gelbart T, Pegelow C: Erythrocyte glutathione synthetase deficiency leads not only to glutathione but also to glutathione-S-transferase deficiency. *J Clin Invest* 77:38, 1986.

282. Valentine WN, Paglia DE: The primary cause of hemolysis in enzymopathies of anaerobic glycolysis: A viewpoint. *Blood Cells* 6:819, 1980.

283. Beutler E: The primary cause of hemolysis in enzymopathies of anaerobic glycolysis: A viewpoint. A commentary. *Blood Cells* 6:827, 1980.

284. Werth G, Mueller G: Vererbbarer Glucose-6-phosphatdehydrogenase-mangel in den Erythrocyten von Ratten. *Klin Wochenschr* 45:265, 1967.

285. Smith JE, Ryer K, Wallace L: Glucose-6-phosphate dehydrogenase deficiency in a dog. *Enzyme* 21:379, 1976.

286. Pretsch W, Charles DJ, Merkle S: X-linked glucose-6-phosphate dehydrogenase deficiency in Mus musculus. *Biochem Genet* 26:89, 1988.

287. Sanders S, Smith DP, Thomas GA, Williams ED: A glucose-6-phosphate dehydrogenase (G6PD) splice site consensus sequence mutation associated with G6PD enzyme deficiency. *Mutat Res* 374:79, 1997.

288. Felix K, Rockwood LD, Pretsch W, et al: Redox imbalance and mutagenesis in spleens of mice harboring a hypomorphic allele of Gpdx(a) encoding glucose 6-phosphate dehydrogenase. *Free Radic Biol Med* 34:226, 2003.

289. Nonneman D, Stockham SL, Shibuya H, et al: A missense mutation in the glucose-6-phosphate dehydrogenase gene associated with hemolytic anemia in an American saddlebred horse. *Blood* 82(suppl 1):466a, 1993.

290. Stockham SL, Harvey JW, Kinden DA: Equine glucose-6-phosphate dehydrogenase deficiency. *Vet Pathol* 31:518, 1994.

291. Longo L, Vanegas OC, Patel M, et al: Maternally transmitted severe glucose 6-phosphate dehydrogenase deficiency is an embryonic lethal. *EMBO J* 21:4229, 2002.

292. Whitney KM, Goodman SA, Bailey EM, Lothrop CD Jr: The molecular basis of canine pyruvate kinase deficiency. *Exp Hematol* 22:866, 1994.

293. Kanno H, Morimoto M, Fujii H, et al: Primary structure of murine red blood cell-type pyruvate kinase (PK) and molecular characterization of PK deficiency identified in the CBA strain. *Blood* 86:3205, 1995.

294. Morimoto M, Kanno H, Asai H, et al: Pyruvate kinase deficiency of mice associated with nonspherocytic hemolytic anemia and cure of the anemia by marrow transplantation without host irradiation. *Blood* 86:4323, 1995.

295. Tsujino K, Kanno H, Hashimoto K, et al: Delayed onset of hemolytic anemia in CBA-*Pk-1^slc/Pk-1^slc* mice with a point mutation of the gene encoding red blood cell type pyruvate kinase. *Blood* 91:2169, 1998.

296. Harvey JW, Pate MG, Mhaskar Y, Dunaway GA: Characterization of phosphofructokinase-deficient canine erythrocytes. *J Inherited Metab Dis* 15:747, 1992.

297. Merkle S, Pretsch W: Glucose-6-phosphate isomerase deficiency associated with nonspherocytic hemolytic anemia in the mouse: An animal model for the human disease. *Blood* 81:206, 1993.

298. Peters LL, Lane PW, Andersen SG, et al: Downeast anemia (dea), a new mouse model of severe nonspherocytic hemolytic anemia caused by hexokinase (HKI) deficiency. Importance of RDW value in differential diagnosis of hypochrome anemias. *Blood Cells Mol Dis* 27:850, 2001.

299. Friedman JS, Rebel VI, Derby R, et al: Absence of mitochondrial superoxide dismutase results in a murine hemolytic anemia responsive to therapy with a catalytic antioxidant. *J Exp Med* 193:925, 2001.

300. Lee T-H, Kim S-U, Yu S-L, et al: Peroxiredoxin II is essential for sustaining life span of erythrocytes in mice. *Blood* 101:5033, 2003.

301. Neumann CA, Krause DS, Carman CV, et al: Essential role for the peroxiredoxin *Prdx1* in erythrocyte antioxidant defense and tumour suppression. *Nature* 424:561, 2003.

302. Betke K, Beutler E, Brewer GJ, et al: Standardization of procedures for the study of glucose-6-phosphate dehydrogenase. Report of a WHO scientific group. *WHO Tech Rep Ser* 366, 1967.

303. Piomelli S, Corash LM, Davenport DD, et al: In vivo lability of glucose-6-phosphate dehydrogenase in GdA- and Gd Mediterranean deficiency. *J Clin Invest* 47:940, 1968.

304. Kahn A, Cottreau D, Boivin P: Molecular mechanism of glucose-6-phosphate dehydrogenase deficiency. *Humangenetik* 25:101, 1974.

305. Beutler E: Selectivity of proteases as a basis for tissue distribution of enzymes in hereditary deficiencies. *Proc Natl Acad Sci U S A* 80:3767, 1983.

306. Kirkman HN, Schettini F, Pickard BM: Mediterranean variant of glucose-6-phosphate dehydrogenase. *J Lab Clin Med* 63:726, 1964.

307. Kirkman HN, Riley HD Jr: Congenital nonspherocytic hemolytic anemia. *Am J Dis Child* 102:313, 1961.

308. Beutler E: Genetics of glucose-6-phosphate dehydrogenase deficiency. *Semin Hematol* 27:137, 1990.

309. Chen EY, Cheng A, Lee A, et al: Sequence of human glucose-6-phosphate dehydrogenase cloned in plasmids and a yeast artificial chromosome (YAC). *Genomics* 10:792, 1991.

310. Battistuzzi G, D'Urso M, Toniolo D, et al: Tissue-specific levels of human glucose-6-phosphate dehydrogenase correlate with methylation of specific sites at the 3' end of the gene. *Proc Natl Acad Sci U S A* 82:1465, 1985.

311. De Flora A, Morelli A, Giuliano F: Human erythrocyte glucose 6-phosphate dehydrogenase. Content of bound coenzyme. *Biochem Biophys Res Commun* 59:406, 1974.

312. De Flora A, Morelli A, Benatti U, et al: Human erythrocyte glucose 6-phosphate dehydrogenase. Interaction with oxidized and reduced coenzyme. *Biochem Biophys Res Commun* 60:999, 1974.

313. Canepa L, Ferraris AM, Miglino M, Gaetani GF: Bound and unbound pyridine dinucleotides in normal and glucose-6-phosphate dehydrogenase-deficient erythrocytes. *Biochim Biophys Acta* 1074:101, 1991.

314. Camardella L, Caruso C, Rutigliano B, et al: Human erythrocyte glucose-6-phosphate dehydrogenase: Identification of a reactive lysyl residue labeled with pyridoxal 5'-phosphate. *Eur J Biochem* 171:485, 1988.

315. Jeffery J, Wood I, Macleod A, et al: Glucose-6-phosphate dehydrogenase. Characterization of a reactive lysine residue in the *Pichia jadinii* enzyme reveals a limited structural variation in a functionally significant segment. *Biochem Biophys Res Commun* 160:1290, 1989.

316. Hirono A, Kuhl W, Gelbart T, et al: Identification of the binding domain for NADP+ of human glucose-6-phosphate dehydrogenase by sequence analysis of mutants. *Proc Natl Acad Sci U S A* 86:10015, 1989.

317. Yoshida A: A single amino acid substitution (asparagine to aspartic acid) between normal (B+) and the common Negro variant (A+) of human glucose-6-phosphate dehydrogenase. *Proc Natl Acad Sci U S A* 57:835, 1967.

318. Takizawa T, Yoneyama Y, Miwa S, Yoshida A: A single nucleotide base transition is the basis of the common human glucose-6-phosphate dehydrogenase variant A(+). *Genomics* 1:228, 1987.

319. Hirono A, Beutler E: Molecular cloning and nucleotide sequence of cDNA for human glucose-6-phosphate dehydrogenase variant A(-). *Proc Natl Acad Sci U S A* 85:3951, 1988.

320. Nafa K, Reghis A, Osmani N, et al: G6PD Aures: A new mutation (48 Ile→Thr) causing mild G6PD deficiency is associated with favism. *Hum Mol Genet* 2:81, 1993.

321. Beutler E, Kuhl W, Ramirez E, Lisker R: Some Mexican glucose-6-phosphate dehydrogenase (G6PD) variants revisited. *Hum Genet* 86:371, 1991.

322. Vulliamy TJ, D'Urso M, Battistuzzi G, et al: Diverse point mutations in the human glucose 6-phosphate dehydrogenase gene cause enzyme deficiency and mild or severe hemolytic anemia. *Proc Natl Acad Sci U S A* 85:5171, 1988.

323. Beutler E, Kuhl W, Vives-Corrons J-L, Prchal JT: Molecular heterogeneity of G6PD A-. *Blood* 74:2550, 1989.

324. Fiorelli G, Anghinelli L, Carandina G, et al: Point mutations in two G6PD variants previously described in Italy. *Blood* 76(suppl):7a, 1990.

325. Beutler E, Kuhl W, Sáenz GF, Rodriguez W: Mutation analysis of G6PD variants in Costa Rica. *Hum Genet* 87:462, 1991.

326. Beutler E, Kuhl W: The NT 1311 polymorphism of G6PD: G6PD Mediterranean mutation may have originated independently in Europe and Asia. *Am J Hum Genet* 47:1008, 1990.

327. De Vita G, Alcalay M, Sampietro M, et al: Two point mutations are responsible for G6PD polymorphism in Sardinia. *Am J Hum Genet* 44:233, 1989.

328. Beutler E, Kuhl W, Gelbart T, Forman L: DNA sequence abnormalities of human glucose-6-phosphate dehydrogenase variants. *J Biol Chem* 266:4145, 1991.

329. Ninfali P, Bresolin N, Baronciani L, et al: Glucose-6-phosphate dehydrogenase Lodi844C: A study on its expression in blood cells and muscle. *Enzyme* 45:180, 1991.

330. Beutler E, Prchal JT, Westwood B, Kuhl W: Definition of the mutations of G6PD Wayne, G6PD Viangchan, G6PD Jammu and G6PD "Le-Jeune." *Acta Haematol (Basel)* 86:179, 1991.

331. Beutler E, Westwood B, Prchal J et al: New glucose-6-phosphate dehydrogenase mutations from various ethnic groups. *Blood* 80:255, 1992.

332. Vlachos A, Westwood B, Lipton JM, Beutler E: G6PD Mt. Sinai: A new severe hemolytic variant characterized by dual mutations at nucleotides 376G and 1159T (N126D). *Hum Mutat Suppl* 1(6):S154, 1998.

333. Filosa S, Calabrò V, Vallone D, et al: Molecular basis of chronic nonspherocytic haemolytic anaemia: A new G6PD variant (393 Arg→His) with abnormal K_m^{GPD} and marked instability. *Br J Haematol* 80:111, 1992.

334. Xu W, Westwood B, Bartsocas CS, et al: Glucose-6 phosphate dehydrogenase mutations and haplotypes in various ethnic groups. *Blood* 85:257, 1995.

335. Zuo L, Chen E, Du CS, et al: Genetic study of Chinese G6PD variants by direct PCR sequencing. *Blood* 76(suppl):51a, 1990.

336. Stevens DJ, Wanachiwanawin W, Mason PJ, et al: G6PD Canton a common deficient variant in South East Asia caused by a 459 Arg→Leu mutation. *Nucleic Acids Res* 18:7190, 1990.

337. Calabrò V, Mason PJ, Filosa S, et al: Genetic heterogeneity of glucose-6-phosphate dehydrogenase deficiency revealed by single-strand conformation and sequence analysis. *Am J Hum Genet* 52:527, 1993.

338. Baronciani L, Tricta F, Beutler E: G6PD "Campinas": A deficient enzyme with a mutation at the far 3' end of the gene. *Hum Mutat* 2:77, 1993.

339. Vulliamy TJ, Othman A, Town M, et al: Polymorphic sites in the African population detected by sequence analysis of the glucose-6-phosphate dehydrogenase gene outline the evolution of the variants A and A-. *Proc Natl Acad Sci U S A* 88:8568, 1991.

340. Town M, Bautista JM, Mason PJ, Luzzatto L: Both mutations in G6PD A- are necessary to produce the G6PD deficient phenotype. *Hum Mol Genet* 1:171, 1992.

341. Hirono A, Kawate K, Honda A, et al: A single mutation 202G→A in the human glucose-6-phosphate dehydrogenase gene (G6PD) can cause acute hemolysis by itself. *Blood* 99:1498, 2002.

342. Huang C-S, Hung KL, Huang MJ, et al: Neonatal jaundice and molecular mutations in glucose-6-phosphate dehydrogenase deficient newborn infants. *Am J Hematol* 51:19, 1996.

343. Saha S, Saha N, Tay JSH, et al: Molecular characterisation of red cell glucose-6-phosphate dehydrogenase deficiency in Singapore Chinese. *Am J Hematol* 47:273, 1994.

344. Tang TK, Huang C-S, Huang M-J, et al: Diverse point mutations result in glucose-6-phosphate dehydrogenase (G6PD) polymorphism in Taiwan. *Blood* 79:2135, 1992.

345. Vulliamy T, Luzzatto L, Hirono A, Beutler E: Hematologically important mutations: Glucose-6-phosphate dehydrogenase. *Blood Cells Mol Dis* 23:302, 1997.

346. MacDonald D, Town M, Mason P, et al: Deficiency in red blood cells. *Nature* 350:115, 1991.

347. Miwa S: Pyruvate kinase deficiency. *Acta Haematol Jpn* 50:1445, 1987.

348. Kahn A, Kaplan J-C, Dreyfus J-C: Advances in hereditary red cell enzyme anomalies. *Hum Genet* 50:1, 1979.

349. Johnson ML, Jones DP, Freeman JM, Wang W: Biochemical and molecular characterization of variant pyruvate kinase enzymes and genes from three patients with red blood cell pyruvate kinase deficiency. *Acta Haematol (Basel)* 86:79, 1991.

350. Beutler E, Forman L, Rios-Larrain E: Elevated pyruvate kinase activity in patients with hemolytic anemia due to red cell pyruvate kinase "deficiency." *Am J Med* 83:899, 1987.

351. Miwa S, Boivin P, Blume KG, et al: Recommended methods for the characterization of red cell pyruvate kinase variants. *Br J Haematol* 43:275, 1979.

352. Bianchi P, Zanella A: Hematologically important mutations: Red cell pyruvate kinase (third update). *Blood Cells Mol Dis* 26:47, 2000.

353. Neubauer B, Lakomek M, Winkler H, et al: Point mutations in the L-type pyruvate kinase gene of two children with hemolytic anemia caused by pyruvate kinase deficiency. *Blood* 77:1871, 1991.

354. Kanno H, Fujii H, Hirono A, Miwa S: cDNA cloning of human R-type pyruvate kinase and identification of a single amino acid substitution (Thr[384]→Met) affecting enzymatic stability in a pyruvate kinase variant (PK Tokyo) associated with hereditary hemolytic anemia. *Proc Natl Acad Sci U S A* 88:8218, 1991.

355. Kanno H, Fujii H, Hirono A, et al: Identical point mutations of the R-type pyruvate kinase (PK) cDNA found in unrelated PK variants associated with hereditary hemolytic anemia. *Blood* 79:1347, 1992.

356. Demina A, Varughese KI, Barbot J, et al: Six previously undescribed pyruvate kinase mutations causing enzyme deficiency. *Blood* 92:647, 1998.

357. Valentini G, Chiarelli LR, Fortin R, et al: Structure and function of human erythrocyte pyruvate kinase—Molecular basis of nonspherocytic hemolytic anemia. *J Biol Chem* 277:23807, 2002.

358. Gerr F, Frumkin H, Hodgins P: Hemolytic anemia following succimer administration in a glucose-6-phosphate dehydrogenase deficient patient. *J Toxicol Clin Toxicol* 32:569, 1994.

359. Rajkondawar VL, Modi TH, Mishra SN: Drug induced acute haemolytic anaemia in glucose-6-phosphate dehydrogenase deficiency subjects. *J Assoc Physicians (India)* 16:589, 1968.

360. Omar MES, Wahab MFA: Treatment of typhoid and paratyphoid fever with furazolidone. *J Trop Med Hyg* 70:43, 1967.

361. Teunis BS, Leftwich EI, Pierce LE: Acute methemoglobinemia and hemolytic anemia due to toluidine blue. *Arch Surg* 101:527, 1970.

362. Meloni G, Meloni T: Glyburide-induced acute haemolysis in a G6PD-deficient patient with NIDDM. *Br J Haematol* 92:159, 1996.

363. Little C, Schacter B: Hemolytic anemia following isobutyl nitrate (IBN) inhalation in a patient with glucose-6-phosphate dehydrogenase (G6PD) deficiency. *Blood* 54(suppl 1):34A, 1979.

364. Beaupre SR, Schiffman FJ: Rush hemolysis. A "bite-cell" hemolytic anemia associated with volatile liquid nitrite use. *Arch Fam Med* 3:545, 1994.

365. Rosen PJ, Johnson C, McGehee WG, Beutler E: Failure of methylene blue treatment in toxic methemoglobinemia. Association with glucose-6-phosphate dehydrogenase deficiency. *Ann Intern Med* 75:83, 1971.

366. Belton EM, Jones RV: Haemolytic anaemia due to nalidixic acid. *Lancet* 2:691, 1965.

367. Mandal BK, Stevenson J: Haemolytic crisis produced by nalidixic acid (letter). *Lancet* 1:614, 1970.

368. Djerassi LS, Vitany L: Haemolytic episode in G6PD deficient workers exposed to TNT. *Br J Ind Med* 32:54, 1975.

369. Melzer-Lange M, Walsh-Kelly C: Naphthalene-induced hemolysis in a black female toddler deficient in glucose-6-phosphate dehydrogenase. *Pediatr Emerg Care* 5:24, 1989.

370. Todisco V, Lamour J, Finberg L: Hemolysis from exposure to naphthalene mothballs. *N Engl J Med* 325:1660, 1991.

371. Ducros J, Saingra S, Rampal M, et al: Hemolytic anemia due to G6PD deficiency and urate oxidase in a kidney-transplant patient. *Clin Nephrol* 35:89, 1991.

372. Lapierre J, Holler C, Tourte-Schaefer C, et al: Anémie hemolitque après traitment antibilharzien par le niridazole chez une antillaise deficiente en g6P.D. *Nouv Presse Med* 5:147, 1976.

373. Thomas M, Agnus D, Poirot JL, Golvan YJ: Hemolysis induced by niridazole in two patients with deficiency of G6PD. *Nouv Presse Med* 5:1537, 1976.

374. Chan TK, Todd D, Tso SC: Drug-induced haemolysis in glucose-6-phosphate dehydrogenase deficiency. *BMJ* 2:1227, 1976.

375. Tishler M: Phenazopyridine-induced hemolytic anemia in a patient with G6PD deficiency. *Acta Haematol (Basel)* 70:208, 1983.

376. McCaffrey RP, Halsted CH, Wahab MFA, Robertson RP: Chloramphenicol-induced hemolysis in Caucasian glucose-6-phosphate dehydrogenase deficiency. *Ann Intern Med* 74:722, 1971.

377. Chan TK, Chesterman CN, McFadzean AJS, Todd D: The survival of glucose-6-phosphate dehydrogenase-deficient erythrocytes in patients with typhoid fever on chloramphenicol therapy. *J Lab Clin Med* 77:177, 1971.

378. Mehta JB, Singhal SB, Mehta BC: Ascorbic-acid-induced haemolysis in G6PD deficiency. *Lancet* 336:944, 1990.

379. Campbell GD Jr, Steinberg MH, Bower JD: Ascorbic acid-induced hemolysis in G6PD deficiency. *Ann Intern Med* 82:810, 1975.

380. Rees DC, Kelsey H, Richards JDM: Acute haemolysis induced by high dose ascorbic acid in glucose-6-phosphate dehydrogenase deficiency. *BMJ* 306:841, 1993.

381. Markowitz N, Saravolatz LD: Use of trimethoprim-sulfamethoxazole in a glucose-6-phosphate dehydrogenase-deficient population. *Rev Infect Dis* 9(suppl 2):S218, 1987.

382. Magon AM, Leipzig RM, Zannoni VG, Brewer GJ: Interactions of glucose-6-phosphate dehydrogenase deficiency with drug acetylation and hydroxylation reactions. *J Lab Clin Med* 97:764, 1981.

383. Woolhouse NM, Atu-Taylor LC: Influence of double genetic polymorphism on response to sulfamethazine. *Clin Pharmacol Ther* 31:377, 1982.

384. Dern RJ, Beutler E, Alving AS: The hemolytic effect of primaquine: II. The natural course of the hemolytic anemia and the mechanism of its self-limited character. *J Lab Clin Med* 44:171, 1954.

385. Beutler E, Dern RJ, Alving AS: The hemolytic effect of primaquine: III. A study of primaquine-sensitive erythrocytes. *J Lab Clin Med* 44:177, 1954.

386. Chan TK, Todd D, Tso SC: Red cell survival studies in glucose-6-phosphate dehydrogenase deficiency. *Bull Hong Kong Med Assoc* 26:41, 1974.

387. Herman J, Ben-Meir S: Overt hemolysis in patients with glucose-6-phosphate dehydrogenase deficiency. *Isr J Med Sci* 2:340, 1975.

388. Gaetani GD, Mareni C, Ravazzolo R, Salvidio E: Haemolytic effect of two sulphonamides evaluated by a new method. *Br J Haematol* 32:183, 1976.

389. McCurdy PR, Donohoe RF: Pyridoxine-responsive anemia conditioned by isonicotinic acid hydrazide. *Blood* 27:352, 1966.

390. Gaetani G, Salvidio E, Pannacciulli I, et al: Absence of haemolytic effects of L-DOPA on transfused G6PD-deficient erythrocytes. *Experientia* 26:785, 1970.

391. Zail SS, Charlton RW, Bothwell TH: The haemolytic effect of certain drugs in Bantu subjects with a deficiency of glucose-6-phosphate dehydrogenase. S Afr J Med Sci 27:95, 1962.

392. Heinrich RA, Smith TC, Buchanan RA: A pharmacological study of a new sulfonamide in glucose-6-phosphate dehydrogenase deficient subjects. J Clin Pharmacol 11:428, 1971.

393. Szeinberg A, Pras M, Sheba C, et al: The hemolytic effect of various sulfonamides on subjects with a deficiency of glucose-6-phosphate dehydrogenase of erythrocytes. Isr J Med Sci 18:176, 1959.

394. Kellermeyer RW, Tarlov AR, Schrier SL, Alving AS: Hemolytic effect of commonly used drugs on erythrocytes deficient in glucose-6-phosphate dehydrogenase. J Lab Clin Med 52:827, 1958.

395. Kellermeyer RW, Tarlov AR, Brewer GJ, et al: Hemolytic effect of therapeutic drugs. Clinical considerations of the primaquine-type hemolysis. JAMA 180:388, 1962.

396. Mela Q, Perpignano G, Ruggiero V, Longatti S: Tolerability of tiaprofenic acid in patients with glucose-6-phosphate dehydrogenase (G6PD) deficiency. Drugs 35:107, 1988.

397. Beutler E, Dern RJ, Alving AS: The hemolytic effect of primaquine: IV. The relationship of cell age to hemolysis. J Lab Clin Med 44:439, 1954.

398. George JN, Sears DA, McCurdy P, Conrad ME: Primaquine sensitivity in Caucasians: Hemolytic reactions induced by primaquine in G6PD deficient subjects. J Lab Clin Med 70:80, 1967.

399. Walker DH, Hawkins HK, Hudson P: Fulminant Rocky Mountain spotted fever. Arch Pathol Lab Med 107:121, 1983.

400. Chau TN, Lai ST, Lai JY, Yuen H: Haemolysis complicating acute viral hepatitis in patients with normal or deficient glucose-6-phosphate dehydrogenase activity. Scand J Infect Dis 29:551, 1997.

401. Huo TI, Wu JC, Chiu CF, Lee SD: Severe hyperbilirubinemia due to acute hepatitis A superimposed on a chronic hepatitis B carrier with glucose-6-phosphate dehydrogenase deficiency. Am J Gastroenterol 91:158, 1996.

402. Shalev O, Wollner A, Menczel J: Diabetic ketoacidosis does not precipitate haemolysis in patients with the Mediterranean variant of glucose-6-phosphate dehydrogenase deficiency. BMJ 288:179, 1984.

403. Shalev O, Eliakim R, Lugassy GZ, Menczel J: Hypoglycemia induced hemolysis in glucose-6-phosphate dehydrogenase deficiency. Acta Haematol (Basel) 74:227, 1985.

404. Pietrapertosa A, Palma A, Campanale D, et al: Genotype and phenotype correlation in glucose-6-phosphate dehydrogenase deficiency. Haematologica 86:30, 2001.

405. Kattamis CA, Kyriazakou M, Chaidas S: Favism. Clinical and biochemical data. J Med Genet 6:34, 1969.

406. Wong WY, Powars D, Williams WD: "Yewdow"-induced anemia. West J Med 151:459, 1989.

407. Globerman H, Novak T, Chevion M: Haemolysis in a G6PD-deficient child induced by eating unripe peaches. Scand J Haematol 33:337, 1984.

408. Williams CKO, Osotimehin BO, Ogunmola GB, Awotedu AA: Haemolytic anaemia associated with Nigerian barbecued meat (red suya). Afr J Med Med Sci 17:71, 1988.

409. Kaplan M, Hammerman C: Severe neonatal hyperbilirubinemia. Clin Perinatol 25:575, 1998.

410. Fok T-F, Lau S-P: Glucose-6-phosphate dehydrogenase deficiency: A preventable cause of mental retardation. BMJ 292:829, 1986.

411. Singh H: Glucose-6-phosphate dehydrogenase deficiency: A preventable cause of mental retardation. BMJ 292:397, 1986.

412. Ardati KO, Bajakian KM, Tabbara KS: Effect of glucose-6-phosphate dehydrogenase deficiency on neutrophil function. Acta Haematol (Basel) 97:211, 1997.

413. Vives-Corrons JL, Feliu E, Pujades MA, et al: Severe glucose-6-phosphate dehydrogenase (G6PD) deficiency associated with chronic hemolytic anemia, granulocyte dysfunction and increased susceptibility to infections. Description of a new molecular variant (G6PD Barcelona). Blood 59:428, 1982.

414. Gray GR, Klebanoff SJ, Stamatoyannopoulos G, et al: Neutrophil dysfunction, chronic granulomatous disease, and nonspherocytic haemolytic anaemia caused by complete deficiency of glucose-6-phosphate dehydrogenase. Lancet 2:530, 1973.

415. Cooper MR, DeChatelet LR, McCall CE, et al: Complete deficiency of leukocyte glucose-6-phosphate dehydrogenase with defective bactericidal activity. J Clin Invest 51:769, 1972.

416. Van Bruggen R, Bautista JM, Petropoulou T, et al: Deletion of leucine 61 in glucose-6-phosphate dehydrogenase leads to chronic nonspherocytic anemia, granulocyte dysfunction, and increased susceptibility to infections. Blood 100:1026, 2002.

417. Roos D, van Zwieten R, Wijnen JT, et al: Molecular basis and enzymatic properties of glucose 6-phosphate dehydrogenase Volendam, leading to chronic nonspherocytic anemia, granulocyte dysfunction, and increased susceptibility to infections. Blood 94:2955, 1999.

418. Rosa-Borges A, Sampaio MG, Condino-Neto A, et al: Glucose-6-phosphate dehydrogenase deficiency with recurrent infections: Case report. J Pediatr (Rio J) 77:331, 2001.

419. Iancovici-Kidon M, Sthoger D, Abrahamov A, et al: A new exon 9 glucose-6-phosphate dehydrogenase mutation (G6PD "Rehovot") in a Jewish Ethiopian family, with variable phenotypes. Blood Cells Mol Dis 26:567, 2000.

420. Schwartz JP, Cooperberg AA, Rosenberg A: Platelet-function studies in patients with glucose-6-phosphate dehydrogenase deficiency. Br J Haematol 27:273, 1974.

421. Gray GR, Naiman SC, Robinson GCF: Platelet function and G6PD deficiency. Lancet 1:997, 1974.

422. Harley JD, Agar NS, Yoshida A: Glucose-6-phosphate dehydrogenase variants: Gd (+) Alexandra associated with neonatal jaundice and Gd (-) Camperdown in a young man with lamellar cataracts. J Lab Clin Med 91:295, 1978.

423. Harley JD, Agar NS, Gruca MA, et al: Cataracts with a glucose-6-phosphate dehydrogenase variant. BMJ 2:86, 1975.

424. Westring DW, Pisciotta AV: Anemia, cataracts, and seizures in patient with glucose-6-phosphate dehydrogenase deficiency. Arch Intern Med 118.385, 1966.

425. Panich V, Na-Nakorn S: G6PD deficiency in senile cataracts. Hum Genet 55:123, 1980.

426. Orzalesi N, Sorcinelli R, Guiso G: Increased incidence of cataract in male subjects deficient in glucose-6-phosphate dehydrogenase. Arch Ophthalmol 99:69, 1981.

427. Bhatia RPS, Patel R, Dubey B: Senile cataract and glucose-6-phosphate dehydrogenase deficiency in Indians. Trop Geogr Med 42:349, 1990.

428. Zampella EJ, Bradley EL, Pretlow TG: Glucose-6-phosphate dehydrogenase: A possible clinical indicator for prostatic carcinoma. Cancer 49:384, 1982.

429. Sulis E: G6PD deficiency and cancer. Lancet 1:1185, 1972.

430. Ferraris AM, Broccia G, Meloni T, et al: Glucose-6-phosphate dehydrogenase deficiency and incidence of hematologic malignancy. Am J Hum Genet 42:516, 1988.

431. Monte Alegre S, Saad STO, Delatre E, Saad MJA: Insulin secretion in patients deficient in glucose-6-phosphate dehydrogenase. Horm Metab Res 23:171, 1991.

432. Saad MJA, Monte-Alegre S, Saad STO: Cortisol levels in glucose-6-phosphate dehydrogenase deficiency. Horm Res 35:1, 1991.

433. Mueller-Soyano A, De Roura ET, Duke PR, et al: Pyruvate kinase deficiency and leg ulcers. Blood 47:807, 1976.

434. Curiel CD, Velasquez GA, Papa R: Hemolytic anemia and leg ulcers due to pyruvate kinase deficiency. Report of the second Venezuelan family. Sangre (Barc) 22:64, 1977.

435. Amankwah KS, Dick BW, Dodge S: Hemolytic anemia and pyruvate kinase deficiency in pregnancy. *Obstet Gynecol* 55(suppl):42S, 1980.

436. Vives Corrons J-L, García AM, Sosa AM, et al: Heterozygous pyruvate kinase deficiency and severe hemolytic anemia in a pregnant woman with concomitant, glucose-6-phosphate dehydrogenase deficiency. *Blut* 62:190, 1991.

437. Wellner VP, Sekura R, Meister A, Larsson A: Glutathione synthetase deficiency, an inborn error of metabolism involving the gamma-glutamyl cycle in patients with 5-oxoprolinuria (pyroglutamic aciduria). *Proc Natl Acad Sci U S A* 71:2505, 1974.

438. Konrad PN, Richards FI, Valentine WN, Paglia DE: Gamma-glutamylcysteine synthetase deficiency. *N Engl J Med* 286:557, 1972.

439. Richards FI, Cooper MR, Pearce LA, et al: Familial spinocerebellar degeneration, hemolytic anemia, and glutathione deficiency. *Arch Intern Med* 134:534, 1974.

440. Beutler E, Moroose R, Kramer L, et al: Gamma-glutamylcysteine synthetase deficiency and hemolytic anemia. *Blood* 75:271, 1990.

441. Skala H, Dreyfus JC, Vives-Corrons JL, et al: Triose phosphate isomerase deficiency. *Biochem Med* 18:226, 1977.

442. Valentine WN, Schneider AS, Baughan MA, et al: Hereditary hemolytic anemia with triosephosphate isomerase deficiency. *Am J Med* 41:27, 1966.

443. Schneider AS, Valentine WN, Baughan MA, et al: Triosephosphate isomerase deficiency. A multi-system inherited enzyme disorder: Clinical and genetic aspects, in *Hereditary Disorders of Erythrocyte Metabolism*, edited by E Beutler, p 265. Grune & Stratton, New York, 1968.

444. Hollan S, Fujii H, Hirono A, et al: Hereditary triosephosphate isomerase (TPI) deficiency: Two severely affected brothers one with and one without neurological symptoms. *Hum Genet* 92:486, 1993.

445. Kugler W, Breme K, Laspe P, et al: Molecular basis of neurological dysfunction coupled with haemolytic anaemia in human glucose-6-phosphate isomerase (GPI) deficiency. *Hum Genet* 103:450, 1998.

446. DiMauro S, Dalakas M, Miranda AF: Phosphoglycerate kinase deficiency: Another cause of recurrent myoglobinuria. *Ann Neurol* 13:11, 1983.

447. Bresolin N, Bet L, Moggio M, et al: Muscle glucose-6-phosphate dehydrogenase deficiency. *J Neurol* 236:193, 1989.

448. Danon D, Sheba C, Ramot B: The morphology of glucose-6-phosphate dehydrogenase deficient erythrocytes: Electron-microscopic studies. *Blood* 17:229, 1961.

449. Greenberg MS: Heinz body hemolytic anemia. *Arch Intern Med* 136:153, 1976.

450. Nathan DM, Siegel AJ, Bunn HF: Acute methemoglobinemia and hemolytic anemia with phenazopyridine. *Arch Intern Med* 137:1636, 1977.

451. Oski FA, Nathan DG, Sidel VW, Diamond LK: Extreme hemolysis and red-cell distortion in erythrocyte pyruvate kinase deficiency. *N Engl J Med* 270:1023, 1964.

452. Beutler E, Blume KG, Kaplan JC, et al: International committee for standardization in haematology: Recommended methods for red-cell enzyme analysis. *Br J Haematol* 35:331, 1977.

453. Beutler E, Blume KG, Kaplan JC, et al: International committee for standardization in haematology: Recommended screening test for glucose-6-phosphate dehydrogenase (G6PD) deficiency. *Br J Haematol* 43:465, 1979.

454. Herz F, Kaplan E, Scheye ES: Diagnosis of erythrocyte glucose-6-phosphate dehydrogenase deficiency in the Negro male despite hemolytic crisis. *Blood* 35:90, 1970.

455. Ringelhahn B: A simple laboratory procedure for the recognition of A- (African type) G6PD deficiency in acute haemolytic crisis. *Clin Chim Acta* 36:272, 1972.

456. Beutler E: X-inactivation in heterozygous G6PD variant females, in *Glucose-6-Phosphate Dehydrogenase*, edited by A Yoshida, E Beutler, p 405. Academic Press, Orlando, FL, 1986.

457. Beutler E: G6PD activity of individual erythrocytes and X-chromosomal inactivation, in *Biochemical Methods in Red Cell Genetics*, edited by JJ Yunis, p 95. Academic Press, New York, 1969.

458. Vogels IMC, Van Noorden CJF, Wolf BHM, et al: Cytochemical determination of heterozygous glucose-6-phosphate dehydrogenase deficiency in erythrocytes. *Br J Haematol* 63:402, 1986.

459. Jacob H, Jandl JH: A simple visual screening test for G6PD deficiency employing ascorbate and cyanide. *N Engl J Med* 274:1162, 1966.

460. Beutler E, Kuhl W, Fox M, et al: Prenatal diagnosis of glucose-6-P dehydrogenase (G6PD) deficiency. *Acta Haematol (Basel)* 87:103, 1992.

461. Luzzatto L, Mehta A: Glucose 6-phosphate dehydrogenase deficiency, in *The Metabolic and Molecular Bases of Inherited Disease*, edited by CR Scriver, AL Beaudet, WS Sly, D Valle, vol. III, p 3367. McGraw-Hill, New York, 1995.

462. Beutler E: Molecular biology of G6PD variants and other red cell enzyme defects. *Ann Rev Med* 43:47, 1992.

463. Beutler E: Why has the autohemolysis test not gone the way of the cephalin flocculation test? *Blood* 51:109, 1978.

464. Carrell RW, Kay R: A simple method for the detection of unstable haemoglobins. *Br J Haematol* 23:615, 1972.

465. Lestas AN, Kay LA, Bellingham AJ: Red cell 3-phosphoglycerate level as a diagnostic aid in pyruvate kinase deficiency. *Br J Haematol* 67:485, 1987.

466. Valentine WN, Paglia DE, Fink K, Madokoro G: Lead poisoning. Association with hemolytic anemia, basophilic stippling, erythrocyte pyrimidine 5'-nucleotidase deficiency, and intraerythrocytic accumulation of pyrimidines. *J Clin Invest* 58:926, 1976.

467. Pekrun A, Neubauer BA, Eber SW, et al: Triosephosphate isomerase deficiency: Biochemical and molecular genetic analysis for prenatal diagnosis. *Clin Genet* 47:175, 1995.

468. Beutler E: Red blood enzyme disorders, in *Hematologic Disorders in Maternal—Fetal Medicine*, edited by MM Bern, FD Frigoletto Jr, p 199. Wiley-Liss, New York, 1990.

469. Baronciani L, Beutler E: Prenatal diagnosis of pyruvate kinase deficiency. *Blood* 84:2354, 1994.

470. Lestas AN, Rodeck CH, White JM: Normal activities of glycolytic enzymes in the fetal erythrocytes. *Br J Haematol* 50:439, 1982.

471. Mimouni F, Shohat S, Reisner SH: G6PD-deficiency donor blood as a cause of hemolysis in two preterm infants. *Isr J Med Sci* 22:120, 1986.

472. Kappas A, Drummond GS, Valaes T: A single dose of Sn-mesoporphyrin prevents development of severe hyperbilirubinemia in glucose-6-phosphate dehydrogenase-deficient newborns. *Pediatrics* 108:25, 2001.

473. Beutler E, Mathai CK, Smith JE: Biochemical variants of glucose-6-phosphate dehydrogenase giving rise to congenital nonspherocytic hemolytic disease. *Blood* 31:131, 1968.

474. Spielberg SP, Boxer LA, Corash LM, Schulman JD: Improved erythrocyte survival with high dose vitamin E in chronic hemolyzing G6PD and glutathione synthetase deficiencies. *Ann Intern Med* 90:53, 1978.

475. Corash L, Spielberg S, Bartsocas C, et al: Reduced chronic hemolysis during high-dose vitamin E administration in Mediterranean-type glucose-6-phosphate dehydrogenase deficiency. *N Engl J Med* 303:416, 1980.

476. Johnson GJ, Vatassery GT, Finkel B, Allen DW: High-dose vitamin E does not decrease the rate of chronic hemolysis in glucose-6-phosphate dehydrogenase deficiency. *N Engl J Med* 308:1014, 1983.

477. Newman JG, Newman TB, Bowie LJ, Mendelsohn J: An examination of the role of vitamin E in glucose-6-phosphate dehydrogenase deficiency. *Clin Biochem* 12:149, 1979.

478. Ekert H, Rawlinson I: Deferoxamine and favism. *N Engl J Med* 312:1260, 1985.

479. Khalifa AS, El-Alfy MS, Mokhtar G, et al: Effect of desferrioxamine B on hemolysis in glucose-6-phosphate dehydrogenase deficiency. *Acta Haematol (Basel)* 82:113, 1989.

480. Al Rimawi HS, Al Sheyyab M, Batieha A, et al: Effect of desferrioxamine in acute haemolytic anaemia of glucose-6-phosphate dehydrogenase deficiency. *Acta Haematol (Basel)* 101:145, 1999.

481. Tanphaichitr VS, Suvatte V, Issaragrisil S, et al: Successful bone marrow transplantation in a child with red blood cell pyruvate kinase deficiency. *Bone Marrow Transplant* 26:689, 2000.

482. Ationu A, Humphries A, Lalloz MRA, et al: Reversal of metabolic block in glycolysis by enzyme replacement in triosephosphate isomerase-deficient cells. *Blood* 94:3193, 1999.

483. Schröter W: Successful long-term phenobarbital therapy of hyperbilirubinemia in congenital hemolytic anemia due to glucose phosphate isomerase deficiency. *Eur J Pediatr* 135:41, 1980.

484. Zanella A, Bianchi P, Iurlo A, et al: Iron status and HFE genotype in erythrocyte pyruvate kinase deficiency: Study of Italian cases. *Blood Cells Mol Dis* 27:653, 2001.

485. Pannacciulli I, Tizianello A, Ajmar F, Salvidio E: The course of experimentally-induced hemolytic anemia in a primaquine-sensitive Caucasian. A case study. *Blood* 25:92, 1965.

486. Meloni T, Forteleoni G, Noja G, et al: Increased prevalence of glucose-6-phosphate dehydrogenase deficiency in patients with cholelithiasis. *Acta Haematol (Basel)* 85:76, 1991.

487. Johnson LH, Bhutani VK, Brown AK: System-based approach to management of neonatal jaundice and prevention of kernicterus. *J Pediatr* 140:396, 2002.

488. Petrakis NL, Wiesenfeld SL, Sams BJ, et al: Prevalence of sickle-cell trait and glucose-6-phosphate dehydrogenase deficiency. *N Engl J Med* 282:767, 1970.

489. Bowman HS, McKusick VA, Dronamraju KR: Pyruvate kinase deficient hemolytic anemia in an Amish isolate. *Am J Hum Genet* 17:1, 1965.

490. Beutler E, Gelbart T: Estimating the prevalence of pyruvate kinase deficiency from the gene frequency in the general white population. *Blood* 95:3585, 2000.

491. Hamilton JW, Jones FG, McMullin MF: Glucose-6-phosphate dehydrogenase Guadalajara—a case of chronic non-spherocytic haemolytic anaemia responding to splenectomy and the role of splenectomy in this disorder. *Hematology* 9:307, 2004.

DISORDERS OF GLOBIN SYNTHESIS: THE THALASSEMIAS

DAVID J. WEATHERALL

The thalassemias are the most common monogenic diseases in man. They occur at a high gene frequency throughout the Mediterranean populations, the Middle East, the Indian subcontinent, Myanmar, and in a line stretching from southern China through Thailand and the Malay peninsula into the island populations of the Pacific. They are seen commonly in countries to which these high-frequency populations immigrate.

Thalassemia consists of two main classes, α and β, in which the α- and β-globin genes are involved. Rarer forms of thalassemia result from abnormalities of other globin genes. The conditions have in common an imbalanced rate of production of the globin chains of adult hemoglobin: excessive α chains in β-thalassemia and β chains in α-thalassemia. Several hundred different mutations at the α- and β-globin loci have been defined as the cause of the reduced or absent output of α or β chains. The high frequency and genetic diversity of the thalassemias are related to past or present heterozygote resistance to malaria.

The pathophysiology of the thalassemias can be traced to the deleterious effects of the excessively produced globin-chain subunits. In β-thalassemia, excess α chains damage the red cell precursors and red cells, leading to profound anemia. The result is extensive expansion of erythropoietic marrow, which is ineffective in producing mature red cells but impinges on developing bones, severely affecting development, bone formation, and growth. The major cause of morbidity and mortality is the effect of iron deposition on the endocrine organs, liver, and heart, which results from increased intestinal absorption and the effects of blood transfusion. The pathophysiology of the α-thalassemias is different because the excess β chains resulting from defective α-chain production form β_4 molecules, or hemoglobin H, which is soluble. However, hemoglobin H is unstable and precipitates in older red cells. Hence, the anemia of α-thalassemia is hemolytic rather than dyserythropoietic.

The clinical pictures of α- and β-thalassemia vary widely. Knowledge is gradually accumulating about the genetic and environmental factors that modify these phenotypes.

Because the carrier states for the thalassemias can be identified and affected fetuses can be diagnosed by DNA analysis after gestational weeks 9 to 10, these conditions are widely amenable to prenatal diagnosis. Marrow transplantation currently is the only cure for the thalassemias. Symptomatic management is based on regular blood transfusion, iron chelation therapy, and judicious use of splenectomy. Experimental approaches to their management include stimulation of fetal hemoglobin synthesis and attempts at somatic cell gene therapy.

Acronyms and abbreviations that appear in this chapter include: bp, base pairs; HPFH, hereditary persistence of fetal hemoglobin; LCR, locus control region; MCH, mean corpuscular hemoglobin; MCV, mean corpuscular volume; PCR, polymerase chain reaction; RFLP, restriction fragment length polymorphism.

DEFINITIONS AND HISTORY

In 1925, Cooley and Lee[1] first described a form of severe anemia that occurred early in life and was associated with splenomegaly and bone changes. In 1932, George H. Whipple and William L. Bradford[2] published a comprehensive account of the pathologic findings in this disease. Whipple coined the phrase *thalassic anemia*[3,4] and condensed it to *thalassemia*, from $\theta\alpha\lambda\alpha\sigma\sigma\alpha$, "the sea," because early patients were all of Mediterranean background. The true genetic character of the disorder became fully appreciated after 1940. The disease described by Cooley and Lee is the homozygous state of an autosomal gene for which the heterozygous state is associated with much milder hematologic changes. The severe homozygous condition became known as *thalassemia major*. The heterozygous states, thalassemia trait, were designated according to their severity as *thalassemia minor* or *minima*.[3,5–7] Later, the term *thalassemia intermedia* was used to describe disorders that were milder than the major form but more severe than the traits.

Thalassemia is not a single disease but a group of disorders, each resulting from an inherited abnormality of globin production.[7] The conditions form part of the spectrum of diseases known collectively as the *hemoglobinopathies*, which can be classified broadly into two types. The first subdivision consists of conditions, such as sickle cell anemia, that result from an inherited structural alteration in one of the globin chains. Although such abnormal hemoglobins may be synthesized less efficiently or broken down more rapidly than normal adult hemoglobin, the associated clinical abnormalities result from the physical properties of the abnormal hemoglobin (see Chap. 47). The second major subdivision of the hemoglobinopathies, the thalassemias, consists of inherited defects in the rate of synthesis of one or more of the globin chains. The result is imbalanced globin chain production, ineffective erythropoiesis, hemolysis, and a variable degree of anemia.

Several monographs describe the historical aspects of thalassemia in greater detail.[3,5,7]

DIFFERENT FORMS OF THALASSEMIA

Thalassemia can be defined as a condition in which a reduced rate of synthesis of one or more of the globin chains leads to imbalanced globin-chain synthesis, defective hemoglobin production, and damage to the red cells or their precursors from the effects of the globin subunits that are produced in relative excess.[7,8] Table 46-1 summarizes the main varieties of thalassemia that have been defined with certainty.

The β-thalassemias are divided into two main varieties. In one form, β^0-thalassemia, there is no β-chain production. In the other form, β^+-thalassemia, there is a partial deficiency of β-chain production. The hallmark of the common forms of β-thalassemia is an elevated level of hemoglobin A_2 in heterozygotes. In a less common class of β-thalassemias, heterozygotes have normal hemoglobin A_2 levels. Other rare forms include varieties of β-thalassemia intermedia that are inherited in a dominant fashion, that is, heterozygotes are severely affected, and there is a variety in which the genetic determinants are not linked to the β-globin gene cluster.[7,9,10]

The $\delta\beta$-thalassemias are heterogeneous. In some cases, no δ or β chains are synthesized. Originally, these disorders were classified according to the structure of the hemoglobin F produced, that is, $^G\gamma^A\gamma(\delta\beta)^0$- and $^G\gamma(\delta\beta)^0$-thalassemia. This classification is illogical. The conditions are best described by the globin chains that are defectively synthesized, that is, simply $(\delta\beta)^+$, $(\delta\beta)^0$, and $(^A\gamma\delta\beta)^0$-thalassemia.[7,10] In the $(\delta\beta)^+$-thalassemias, an abnormal hemoglobin is produced that has normal α chains combined with non-α chains consisting of the N-terminal residues of the δ chain fused to the C-terminal residues of the β chain. These fusion variants, called the *Lepore hemoglobins*, show structural heterogeneity.

TABLE 46-1 THALASSEMIAS AND RELATED DISORDERS

α-Thalassemia
    α^0
    α^+
    Deletion ($-\alpha$)
    Nondeletion (α^T)
β-Thalassemia
    β^0
    β^+
    Normal Hb A_2
    Dominant
    Unlinked to β-globin genes
$\delta\beta$-Thalassemia
    $(\delta\beta)^+$
    $(\delta\beta)^0$
    $(^A\gamma\delta\beta)^0$
γ-Thalassemia
δ-Thalassemia
    δ^0
    δ^+
$\varepsilon\gamma\delta\beta$-Thalassemia
HPFH
    Deletion
        $(\delta\beta)^0$, $(^A\gamma\delta\beta)^0$
    Nondeletion
        Linked to β-globin genes
            $^G\gamma\,\beta^+$, $^A\gamma\,\beta^+$
        Unlinked to β-globin genes

The δ-thalassemias[7,10] are characterized by reduced output of δ chains and hence reduced hemoglobin A_2 levels in heterozygotes and an absence of hemoglobin A_2 in homozygotes. They are of no clinical significance except that, when inherited with β-thalassemia trait, the level of hemoglobin A_2 is reduced to the normal range.

A disorder characterized by defective ε-, γ-, δ-, and β-chain synthesis has been defined at the clinical and molecular level.[7,10] The homozygous state for this condition, $\varepsilon\gamma\delta\beta$-thalassemia, presumably is not compatible with fetal survival. It has been observed only in heterozygotes.

Hereditary persistence of fetal hemoglobin (HPFH) is a heterogeneous condition characterized by persistent fetal hemoglobin.[7,9,10] It is classified into deletion and nondeletion forms. The deletion forms of HPFH can be classified, like $\delta\beta$-thalassemia, as $(\delta\beta)^0$ HPFH and then subdivided according to the particular population in which this occurs and its associated molecular defect. In effect, the deletion forms of HPFH are very similar to $\delta\beta$-thalassemia except for more efficient γ-chain synthesis and therefore less chain imbalance and a milder phenotype. The homozygous state is associated with mild thalassemic changes. In fact, the $\delta\beta$-thalassemias and deletion forms of HPFH form a clinical continuum. The nondeletion forms of HPFH also are heterogeneous. In some cases, they are associated with mutations that involve the β-globin gene cluster and in which there is β-chain synthesis cis to the HPFH determinant. These conditions are subdivided into $^G\gamma\beta^+$ HPFH and $^A\gamma\beta^+$ HPFH. Again, they often are subclassified according to the population in which they occur, for example, Greek HPFH, British HPFH, and so on. Finally, a heterogeneous group of HPFH determinants is associated with very low levels of persistent fetal hemoglobin, the genetic loci of which, at least in some cases, are not linked to the β-globin gene cluster.

Because α chains are present in both fetal and adult hemoglobins, a deficiency of α-chain production affects hemoglobin synthesis in fetal and in adult life. A reduced rate of α-chain synthesis in fetal life results in an excess of γ chains, which form γ_4 tetramers, or hemoglobin Bart's. In adult life, a deficiency of α chains results in an excess of β chains, which form β_4 tetramers, or hemoglobin H. Because there are two α-globin genes per haploid genome, the genetics of α-thalassemia is more complicated than that of β-thalassemia. There are two main groups of α-thalassemia determinants.[7,10] First, in the α^0-thalassemias (formerly called α-thalassemia 1), no α chains are produced from an affected chromosome, that is, both linked α-globin genes are inactivated. Second, in the α^+-thalassemias (formerly called α-thalassemia 2), the output of one of the linked pair of α-globin genes is defective. The α^+-thalassemias are subdivided into deletion and nondeletion types. Both the α^0-thalassemias and deletion and nondeletion forms of α^+-thalassemia are extremely heterogeneous at the molecular level. There are two major clinical phenotypes of α-thalassemia: the hemoglobin Bart's hydrops syndrome, which usually reflects the homozygous state for α^0-thalassemia, and hemoglobin H disease, which usually results from the compound heterozygous state for α^0- and α^+-thalassemia.

Because the structural hemoglobin variants and the thalassemias occur at a high frequency in some populations, the two types of genetic defect can be found in the same individual. The different genetic varieties of thalassemia and their combinations with the genes for abnormal hemoglobins produce a series of disorders known collectively as the *thalassemia syndromes*.[7]

EPIDEMIOLOGY AND POPULATION GENETICS

The β-thalassemias are distributed widely in Mediterranean populations, the Middle East, parts of India and Pakistan, and throughout Southeast Asia (Fig. 46-1).[7,11,12] The disease is common in the southern parts of the former Union of Soviet Socialist Republics and in the People's Republic of China. The β-thalassemias are rare in Africa, except for isolated pockets in West Africa, notably Liberia, and in parts of North Africa. However, β-thalassemia occurs sporadically in all racial groups and has been observed in the homozygous state in persons of pure Anglo-Saxon heritage. Thus, a patient's racial background does not preclude the diagnosis.

The $\delta\beta$-thalassemias have been observed sporadically in many racial groups, although no high-frequency populations have been defined. Similarly, the hemoglobin Lepore syndromes have been found in many populations, but, with the possible exceptions of central Italy, Western Europe, and parts of Spain and Portugal, these disorders have not been found to occur at a high frequency in any particular region.

The α-thalassemias occur widely throughout Africa, the Mediterranean countries, the Middle East, and Southeast Asia (Fig. 46-2).[7,11,12] The α^0-thalassemias are found most commonly in Mediterranean and Oriental populations but are extremely rare in African and the Middle Eastern populations. However, the deletion forms of α^+-thalassemia occur at a high frequency throughout West Africa, the Mediterranean, the Middle East, and Southeast Asia. Up to 80 percent of the population of some parts of Papua New Guinea are carriers for the deletion form of α^+-thalassemia. How common the nondeletion forms of α^+-thalassemia are in any particular populations is uncertain, but they have been reported quite frequently in some of the Mediterranean island populations and in the Middle Eastern and Southeast Asian populations. Because the hemoglobin Bart's hydrops syndrome and hemoglobin H disease require the action of an α^0-thalassemia determinant, these disorders are found at a high frequency only in Southeast Asia and in parts of the Mediterranean region. The α-chain termination mutants, such as hemoglobin Constant Spring, seem to be particularly common in Southeast Asia. Approximately 4 percent of the population in Thailand are carriers.

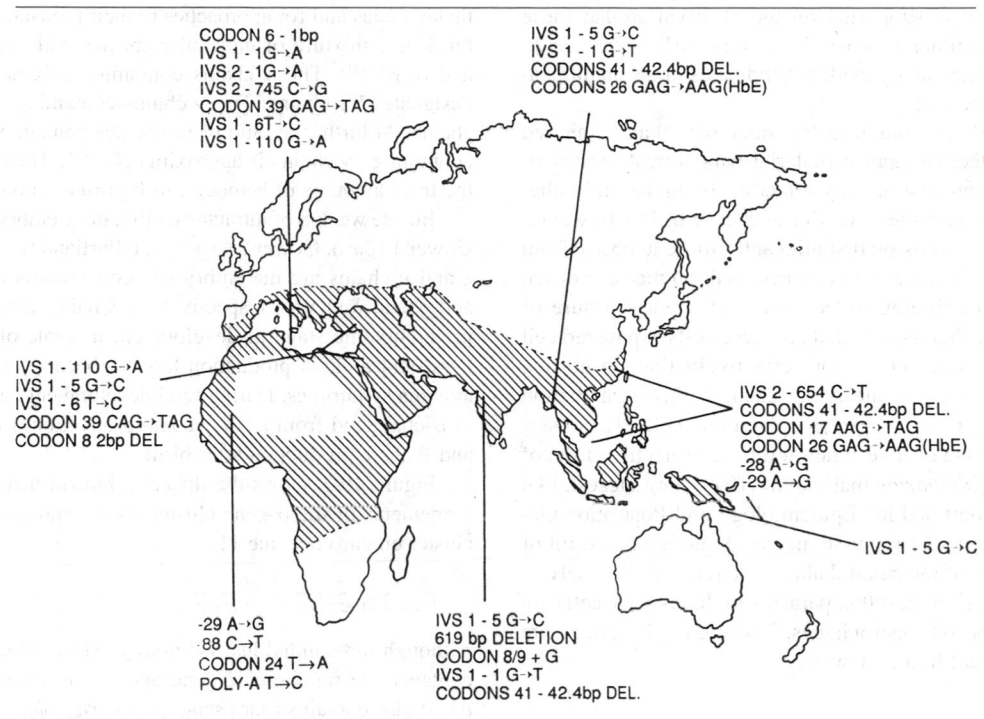

CODON 6 - 1bp
IVS 1 - 1G→A
IVS 2 - 1G→A
IVS 2 - 745 C→G
CODON 39 CAG→TAG
IVS 1 - 6T→C
IVS 1 - 110 G→A

IVS 1 - 5 G→C
IVS 1 - 1 G→T
CODONS 41 - 42.4bp DEL.
CODONS 26 GAG→AAG(HbE)

IVS 1 - 110 G→A
IVS 1 - 5 G→C
IVS 1 - 6 T→C
CODON 39 CAG→TAG
CODON 8 2bp DEL

IVS 2 - 654 C→T
CODONS 41 - 42.4bp DEL.
CODON 17 AAG→TAG
CODON 26 GAG→AAG(HbE)
-28 A→G
-29 A→G

IVS 1 - 5 G→C

-29 A→G
-88 C→T
CODON 24 T→A
POLY-A T→C

IVS 1 - 5 G→C
619 bp DELETION
CODON 8/9 + G
IVS 1 - 1 G→T
CODONS 41 - 42.4bp DEL.

FIGURE 46-1   World distribution of β-thalassemia.

In 1949, J.B.S. Haldane[13] suggested that thalassemia had reached its high frequency in tropical regions because heterozygotes are protected against malaria.[13] Although many population studies have tested this hypothesis, elucidation of some of the extremely complex population genetics underlying polymorphic systems such as the thalassemias has been possible only with the advent of recombinant DNA technology.

In each of the high-frequency areas for the β-thalassemias, a few common mutations and varying numbers of rare mutations are seen (see Fig. 46-1). Furthermore, in each of these regions the pattern of mutations is different, usually found in the context of different haplotypes in the associated β-globin gene cluster.[11,14,15] Similar observations have been made in the α-thalassemias (Fig. 46-2).[7,11] These studies suggest the thalassemias arose independently in different populations and then achieved their high frequency by selection. Although some movement of the thalassemia genes may have resulted from drift, independent mutation and selection undoubtedly provide the overall basis for their world distribution. Early studies in Sardinia showing that β-thalassemia is less common in the mountainous regions where malarial transmission is low supported Haldane's suggestion that β-thalassemia reached its high frequency because of protection against malarial infections. For many years these data remained the only convincing evidence for a protective effect.[11,16,17] However, later studies using malaria endemicity data and globin-gene mapping showed a clear altitude-related effect on the frequency of α-thalassemia in Papua New Guinea. In addition, a sharp cline in the frequency of α-thalassemia has been found in the region stretching south from Papua New Guinea through the island populations of Melanesia to New Caledonia. This is mirrored by a similar gradient in the distribution of malaria.[12] The effect of drift and founder effect in these island populations has been largely excluded by showing that other DNA polymorphisms have a random distribution through the region, with no evidence of a cline similar to that characterizing the distribution of α-thalassemia and malaria.

Firm evidence for protection of individuals with mild forms of α⁺-thalassemia against *Plasmodium falciparum* malaria has been provided. In a case control study performed in Papua New Guinea, the homozygous state for α⁺-thalassemia offered approximately 60 percent protection against hospital admittance because of serious complications of malaria, notably coma or profound anemia.[18] Long-term followup studies of cohorts of babies in the Vanuatan Islands showed surprisingly that, in the first years of life, patients homozygous for α⁺-thalassemia are more prone to both *Plasmodium vivax* and *P. falciparum* malaria.[19] This finding is of particular interest from the mechanistic viewpoint. The finding suggests α-thalassemic babies are more prone to infection at a time when they are less likely to die of malaria because they are protected by other mechanisms. The state of being more prone may induce an early immunization that results in later

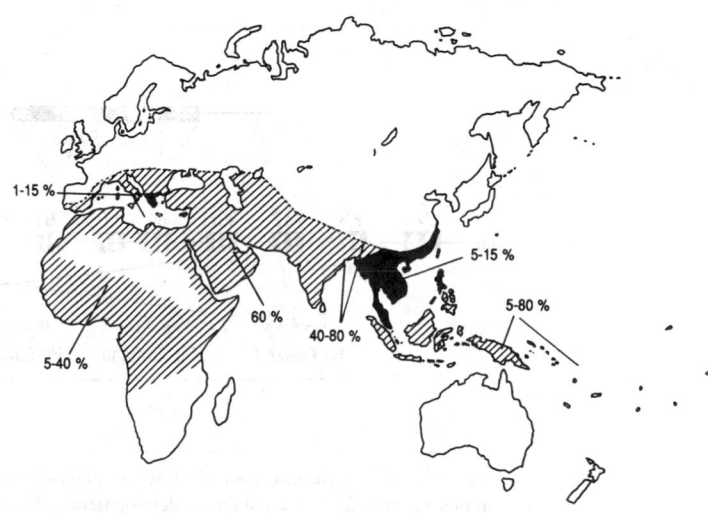

1-15 %

5-15 %

5-80 %

60 %

40-80 %

5-40 %

FIGURE 46-2   World distribution of α⁺- and α⁰-thalassemia.

protection. This concept is supported by the observation that these babies tend to get the milder *P. vivax* infections earlier than the *P. falciparum* infections. Increasing evidence indicates cross-immunization between the two species.

A great deal of work has sought to determine why thalassemic red cells appear to be protective against malarial parasites. A variety of studies have failed to demonstrate any effect of the thalassemia phenotype on the rates of parasite invasion and growth.[20,21] However, parasitized α-thalassemic cells bind significantly more antibody from the serum of patients with acute *P. falciparum* malaria than do normal red cells.[22] Whether this finding reflects more efficient exposure of malarial antigens by the thalassemic cells or these cells expose red cell neoantigens related to senescence more effectively than do normal cells when invaded by the parasite is not clear.[23] This phenomenon also has been observed in parasitized β-thalassemic cells. The observations raise a new avenue of investigation for the protective effect of thalassemia against *P. falciparum* malaria. In effect, they suggest, like the population studies outlined in "Epidemiology and Population Genetics," that the effect may be immune mediated and not the result of the particular properties of the small thalassemic red cells themselves. Several lines of evidence suggest that parasitized thalassemic cells are more prone to ingestion by macrophages. These complex issues are discussed in greater detail in a review article.[24]

ETIOLOGY AND PATHOGENESIS

GENETIC CONTROL AND SYNTHESIS OF HEMOGLOBIN

The structure and ontogeny of the hemoglobins are reviewed in Chaps. 6 and 47, respectively.[7,9,10] Only those aspects with particular relevance to the thalassemia problem are restated here.

Human adult hemoglobin is a heterogeneous mixture of proteins consisting of the major component hemoglobin A and the minor component hemoglobin A_2, which constitutes approximately 2.5 percent of the total. In intrauterine life, the main hemoglobin is hemoglobin F. The structure of these hemoglobins is similar. Each consists of two separate pairs of identical globin chains. Except for some of the embryonic hemoglobins (see below), all normal human hemoglobins have one pair of α chains. In hemoglobin A, the α chains are combined with β chains ($\alpha_2\beta_2$), in hemoglobin A_2 with δ chains ($\alpha_2\delta_2$), and in hemoglobin F with γ chains ($\alpha_2\gamma_2$).

Human hemoglobin shows further heterogeneity, particularly in fetal life, and this has important implications for understanding the

thalassemias and for approaches to their prenatal diagnosis. Hemoglobin F is a mixture of molecular species with the formulas $\alpha_2\gamma_2^{136Gly}$ and $\alpha_2\gamma_2^{136Ala}$. The γ chains containing glycine at position 136 are designated $^G\gamma$ chains. The γ chains containing alanine are called $^A\gamma$ chains. At birth, the ratio of molecules containing $^G\gamma$ chains to those containing $^A\gamma$ chains is approximately 3:1. The ratio varies widely in the trace amounts of hemoglobin F present in normal adults.

Before week 8 of intrauterine life, three embryonic hemoglobins—Gower 1 ($\zeta_2\varepsilon_2$), Gower 2 ($\alpha_2\varepsilon_2$), and Portland ($\zeta_2\gamma_2$)—are present. The ζ and ε chains are the embryonic counterparts of the adult α and β and γ and δ chains, respectively. ζ-Chain synthesis persists beyond the embryonic stage of development in some of the α-thalassemias. Persistent ε-chain production has not been found in any of the thalassemia syndromes. During fetal development, orderly switch from ζ- to α-chain and from ε- to γ-chain production occurs, followed by β- and δ-chain production after birth.

Figure 46-3 shows the different human hemoglobins and the arrangements of the α-gene cluster on chromosome 16 and the β-gene cluster on chromosome 11.

GLOBIN GENE CLUSTERS

Although some individual variability exists, the α-gene cluster usually contains one functional ζ gene and two α genes, designated $\alpha2$ and $\alpha1$. It also contains four pseudogenes: $\psi\zeta1$, $\psi\alpha1$, $\psi\alpha2$, and $\theta1$.[9,10] The latter is remarkably conserved among different species. Although it appears to be expressed early in fetal life, its function is unknown. It likely does not produce a viable globin chain. Each α gene is located in a region of homology approximately 4 kb long, interrupted by two small nonhomologous regions.[25–27] The homologous regions are believed to result from gene duplication, and the nonhomologous segments are believed to arise subsequently by insertion of DNA into the noncoding regions around one of the two genes. The exons of the two α-globin genes have identical sequences. The first intron in each gene is identical. The second intron of $\alpha1$ is nine bases longer and differs by three bases from that in the $\alpha2$ gene.[27–29] Despite their high degree of homology, the sequences of the two α-globin genes diverge in their 3' untranslated regions 13 bases beyond the TAA stop codon. These differences provide an opportunity to assess the relative output of the genes, an important part of the analysis of the α-thalassemias.[30,31] Production of $\alpha2$ messenger RNA appears to exceed that of $\alpha1$ by a factor of 1.5 to 3. $\psi\zeta1$ and $\zeta2$ genes also are highly homologous. The introns are much larger than those of α-globin genes. In contrast to the latter,

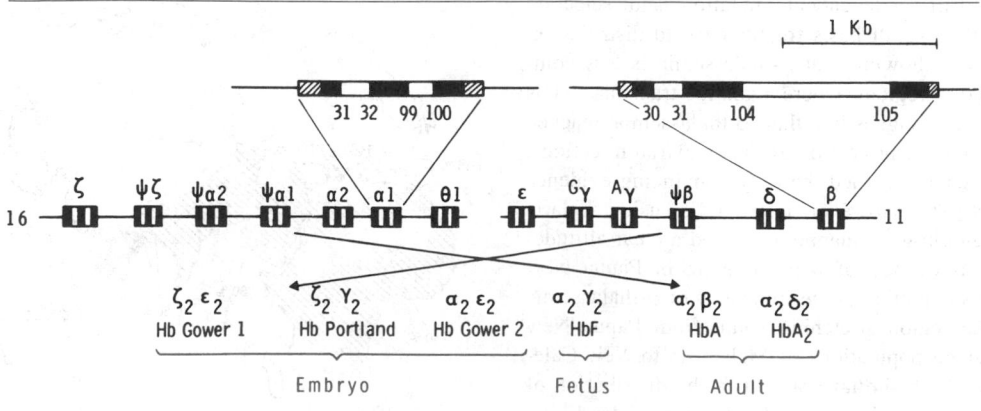

FIGURE 46-3 Genetic control of human hemoglobin. The main globin gene clusters are located on chromosomes 11 and 16. At each stage of development, different genes in these clusters are activated or repressed. The different globin chains directed by individual genes are synthesized independently and combine in random fashion as indicated by the *arrows*.

IVS-1 is larger than IVS-2. In each ξ gene, IVS-1 contains several copies of a simple repeated 14-base pair (bp) sequence that is similar to sequences located between the two ξ genes and near the human insulin gene. The coding sequence of the first exon of $\xi 1$ contains three base changes, one of which gives rise to a premature stop codon, thus making $\xi 1$ an inactive pseudogene.

The regions separating and surrounding the α-like structural genes have been analyzed in detail. Of particular relevance to thalassemia is the polymorphic nature of this gene cluster.[32] The cluster contains five hypervariable regions: one downstream from the $\alpha 1$ gene, one between the ξ and $\psi\xi$ genes, one in the first intron of both the ξ genes, and one 5' to the cluster. These regions consist of varying numbers of tandem repeats of nucleotide sequences. Taken together with single-base restriction fragment length polymorphisms (RFLPs), the variability of the α-globin gene cluster reaches a heterozygosity level of approximately 0.95. Thus, each parental α-globin gene cluster can be identified in the majority of persons. This heterogeneity has important implications for tracing the history of the thalassemia mutations.

Figure 46-3 shows the arrangement of the β-globin gene cluster on the short arm of chromosome 11. Each of the individual genes and their flanking regions have been sequenced.[33-36] Like the $\alpha 1$ and $\alpha 2$ gene pairs, the $^G\gamma$ and $^A\gamma$ genes share a similar sequence. In fact, the $^G\gamma$ and $^A\gamma$ genes on one chromosome are identical in the region 5' to the center of the large intron yet show some divergence 3' to that position. At the boundary between the conserved and divergent regions, a block of simple sequence may be a "hot spot" for initiation of recombination events that lead to unidirectional gene conversion.

Like the α-globin genes, the β-gene cluster contains a series of single point RFLPs, although in this case no hypervariable regions have been identified.[37,38] The arrangement of RFLPs, or haplotypes, in the β-globin gene cluster falls into two domains. The 5' side of the β gene, spanning about 32 kb from the ε gene to the 3' end of the $\psi\beta$ gene, contains three common patterns of RFLPs. The region encompassing about 18 kb to the 3' side of the β-globin gene also contains three common patterns in different populations. Between these regions is a sequence of about 11 kb in which there is randomization of the 5' and 3' domains; hence, a relatively higher frequency of recombination can occur.[38] The β-globin gene haplotypes are similar in most populations but differ markedly in individuals of African origin. These findings suggest the haplotype arrangements were laid down very early during evolution. The findings are consistent with data obtained from mitochondrial DNA polymorphisms pointing to the early emergence of a relatively small population from Africa with subsequent divergence into other racial groups.[39] Again, they are extremely useful for analyzing the population genetics and history of the thalassemia mutations.

The regions flanking the coding regions of the globin genes contain a number of conserved sequences essential for their expression.[7,40] The first conserved sequence is the TATA box, which serves accurately to locate the site of transcription initiation at the CAP site, usually about 30 bases downstream. It also appears to influence the rate of transcription. In addition, two so-called upstream promoter elements are present. A second conserved sequence, the CCAAT box, is located 70 or 80 bp upstream. The third conserved sequence, the CACCC homology box, is located further 5', approximately 80 to 100 bp from the CAP site. It can be either inverted or duplicated. These promoter sequences also are required for optimal transcription. Mutations in this region of the β-globin gene cause its defective expression. The globin

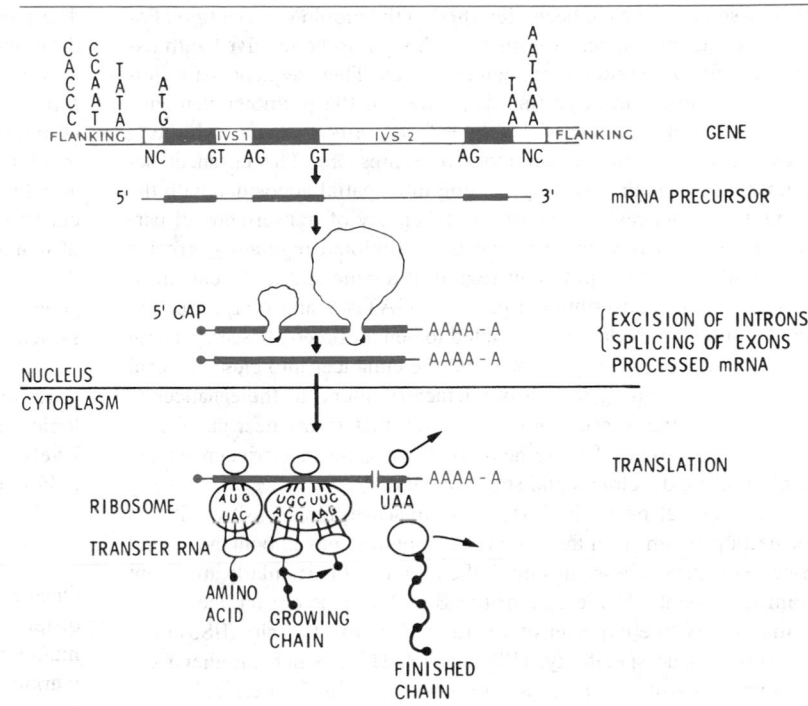

FIGURE 46-4   Expression of a human globin gene.

genes also have conserved sequences in their 3' flanking regions, notably AATAAA, which is the polyadenylation signal site.

REGULATION OF GLOBIN GENE CLUSTERS

Figure 46-4 summarizes the mechanism of globin gene expression. The primary transcript is an mRNA precursor containing both intron and exon sequences. During its stay in the nucleus, it undergoes a good deal of processing that entails capping the 5' end and polyadenylation of the 3' end, both of which probably serve to stabilize the transcript (see Chap. 9). The intervening sequences are removed from the mRNA precursor in a complex two-stage process that relies on certain critical sequences at the intron-exon junctions.

The method by which globin gene clusters are regulated is important to understanding the pathogenesis of the thalassemias. Many details remain to be determined, but studies performed over the last few years have provided at least an outline of some of the major mechanisms of globin gene regulation.[7,10,40,41]

Most of the DNA within cells that is not involved in gene transcription is packaged into a compact form that is inaccessible to transcription factors and RNA polymerase. Transcriptional activity is characterized by a major change in the structure of the chromatin surrounding a particular gene. These alterations in chromatin structure can be identified by enhanced sensitivity to exogenous nucleases. Erythroid lineage-specific nuclease-hypersensitive sites are found at several locations in the β-globin gene cluster, which vary during different stages of development. In fetal life, these sites are associated with the promoter regions of all four globin genes. In adult erythroid cells, the sites associated with the γ genes are absent. The methylation state of the genes plays an important role in their ability to be expressed. In human and other animal tissues, the globin genes are extensively methylated in nonerythroid organs and are relatively undermethylated in hematopoietic tissues. Changes in chromatin configuration around the globin genes at different stages of development are reflected by alterations in their methylation state.

In addition to the promoter elements, several other important regulatory sequences have been identified in the globin gene clusters. For example, several enhancer sequences thought to be involved with tissue-specific expression have been identified. Their sequences are similar to the upstream activating sequences of the promoter elements. Both consist of a number of "modules," or motifs, that contain binding sites for transcriptional activators or repressors. The enhancer sequences are thought to act by coming into spatial apposition with the promoter sequences to increase the efficiency of transcription of particular genes. It now is clear that transcriptional regulatory proteins may bind to both the promoter region of a gene and to the enhancer. Some of these transcriptional proteins, GATA-1 and NFE-2, for example, appear to be largely restricted to hematopoietic tissues.[41] These proteins may bring the promoter and the enhancer into close physical proximity, permitting transcription factors bound to the enhancer to interact with the transcriptional complex that forms near the TATA box. At least some of these hematopoietic gene transcription factors likely will be developmental stage specific.

Another set of erythroid-specific nuclease-hypersensitive sites is located upstream from the embryonic globin genes in both the α- and β-gene clusters. These sites mark the regions of particularly important control elements. In the case of the β-globin gene cluster, the region is marked by five hypersensitive sites.[40] The most 5' site (HS5) does not show tissue specificity. HS1 through HS4, which together form the locus control region (LCR), are largely erythroid specific. Each of the regions of the LCR contains a variety of binding sites for erythroid transcription factors. The precise function of the LCR is not known, but it is undoubtedly required to establish a transcriptionally active domain spanning the entire globin gene cluster. The α-globin gene cluster also has a major regulatory element of this kind, in this case HS40.[42] Its structure closely resembles HS2 of the β-globin gene cluster LCR. A 350-bp core fragment retains most of the activity and contains a duplicated NF-E2 binding site flanked by GATA-1 sites. Although deletions of this region inactivate the entire α-globin gene cluster, its action must be fundamentally different from that of the β-globin LCR because the chromatin structure of the α-gene cluster is in an open conformation in all tissues.

Some forms of thalassemia result from deletions involving these regulatory regions. In addition, the phenotypic effects of deletions of these gene clusters are strongly positional, which may reflect the relative distance of particular genes from the LCR and HS40.

DEVELOPMENTAL CHANGES IN GLOBIN GENE EXPRESSION

One particularly important aspect of human globin genes is regulation of the switch from fetal to adult hemoglobin. Because many of the thalassemias and related disorders of the β-globin gene cluster are associated with persistent γ-chain synthesis, a full understanding of their pathophysiology must include an explanation for this important phenomenon, which plays a considerable role in modifying their phenotypic expression.

The complex topic of hemoglobin switching has been the subject of several extensive reviews.[7,26,40] β-Globin synthesis commences early during fetal life, at approximately 8 to 10 weeks' gestation. β-Globin synthesis continues at a low level, approximately 10 percent of the total non–α-globin chain production, up to approximately 36 weeks' gestation, after which it is considerably augmented. At the same time, γ-globin chain synthesis starts to decline so that, at birth, approximately equal amounts of γ- and β-globin chains are produced. Over the first year of life, γ-chain synthesis gradually declines. By the end of the first year, γ-chain synthesis amounts to less than 1 percent of the total non–α-globin chain output. In, adults the small amount of hemoglobin F is confined to an erythrocyte population called F cells.

How this series of developmental switches is regulated is not clear.

The process is not organ specific but is synchronized throughout the developing hematopoietic tissues. Although environmental factors may be involved, the bulk of experimental evidence suggests some form of "time clock" is built into the hematopoietic stem cell. At the chromosomal level, regulation appears to occur in a complex manner involving both developmental stage-specific trans-activating factors and the relative proximity of the different genes of the β-globin gene cluster to LCR. The elements involved in the stage-specific regulation of human globin genes have not been identified, except for EKLF, a developmental stage-enriched protein that activates human β-globin gene expression and is involved in human γ- to β-globin gene switching.[43]

Fetal hemoglobin synthesis can be reactivated at low levels in states of hematopoietic stress and at higher levels in certain hematologic malignancies, notably juvenile myeloid leukemia. However, high levels of hemoglobin F production are seen consistently in adult life only in the hemoglobinopathies.

MOLECULAR BASIS OF THE THALASSEMIAS

Once cloning and sequencing of globin genes from patients with many different forms of thalassemia were possible, the wide spectrum of mutations underlying these conditions became clear. A picture of remarkable heterogeneity has emerged. For more extensive coverage of this topic, the reader is referred to several monographs and reviews.[7,9,10,44–46]

β-THALASSEMIA

β-Thalassemia is extremely heterogeneous at the molecular level.[7] More than 200 different mutations have been found in association with the β-thalassemia phenotype.[7] Broadly, they fall into deletions of the β-globin gene and nondeletional mutations that may affect the transcription, processing, or translation of β-globin messenger (see Table 46-4 and Fig. 46-5). Each major population group has a different set of β-thalassemia mutations, usually consisting of two or three mutations forming the bulk and large numbers of rare mutations. Because of this distribution pattern, only about 20 alleles account for the majority of all β-thalassemia determinants.

Gene Deletions At least 17 different deletions affecting only the β genes have been described. With one exception, the deletions are rare and appear to be isolated, single events. The 619-bp deletion at the 3' end of the β gene is more common,[47] but even that is restricted to the Sind and Gujarati populations of Pakistan and India, where it accounts for approximately 50 percent of β-thalassemia alleles.[48] The Indian 619-bp deletion removes the 3' end of the β gene but leaves the 5' end intact. Many of the other deletions remove the 5' end of the gene and leave the δ gene intact.[49–53] Homozygotes for these deletions have β^0-thalassemia. Heterozygotes for the Indian deletion have increased hemoglobin A_2 and F levels identical to those seen in heterozygotes for the other common forms of β-thalassemia. Heterozygotes for the other deletions all have unusually high hemoglobin A_2 levels.[46] Increased δ-chain production results from increased δ-gene transcription in cis to the deletion, possibly as a result of reduced competition from the deleted 5' β gene for transcription factors.

Other Transcriptional Mutations Several different base substitutions involve the conserved sequences upstream from the β-globin gene.[7,30] In every case, the phenotype is β^+-thalassemia, although considerable variability exists in the clinical severity associated with different mutations of this type. Several mutations, at positions −88 and −87 relative to the mRNA CAP site, for example,[54,55] are close to the CCAAT box, whereas others lie within the ATA box homology.[56–59]

Some mutations upstream from the β-globin gene are associated with even more subtle alterations in phenotype. For example, a C→T

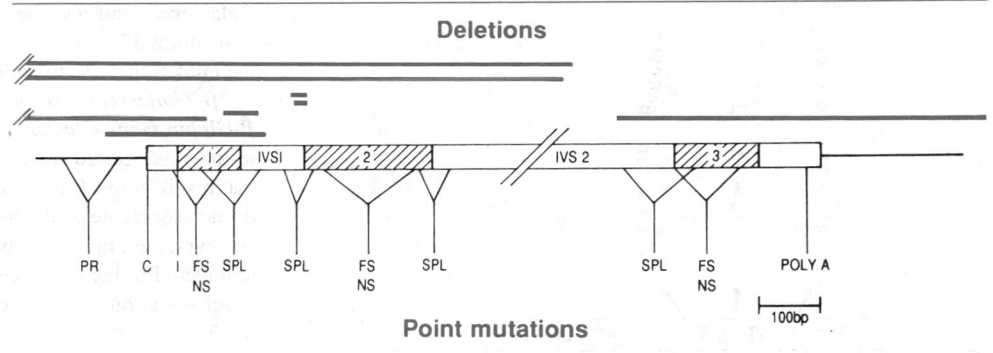

FIGURE 46-5 Classes of mutations that underlie β-thalassemia. PR, promoter; C, CAP site; I, initiation site; FS, frameshift; NS, nonsense mutation; SPL, splicing mutation; POLY A, polyA addition site mutation.

substitution at position −101, which involves one of the upstream promoter elements, is associated with "silent" β-thalassemia, that is, a completely normal ("silent") phenotype that can be identified only by its interaction with more severe forms of β-thalassemia in compound heterozygotes.[60] A single example of an A→C substitution at the CAP site (+1) was described in an Asian Indian who, despite being homozygous for the mutation, appeared to have the phenotype of the β-thalassemia trait.[61]

Upstream regulatory mutations confirm the importance of the role of conserved sequences in this region as regulators of the transcription of the β-globin genes and provide the basis for some of the mildest forms of β-thalassemia, particularly those in African populations, and for some varieties of "silent" β-thalassemia.

RNA-Processing Mutations One surprise about β-thalassemia has been the remarkable diversity of the single-base mutations that can interfere with the intranuclear processing of mRNA.

The boundaries of exons and introns are marked by invariant dinucleotides, GT at the 5′ (donor) and AG at the 3′ (receptor) sites. Single-base changes that involve either of these splice junctions totally abolish normal RNA splicing and result in the β⁰-thalassemia phenotype.[7,43,48,62–66]

Highly conserved sequences involved in mRNA processing surround the invariant dinucleotides at the splice junctions. Different varieties of β-thalassemia involve single-base substitutions within the consensus sequence of the IVS-1 donor site.[55,58,63,67–69] These mutations are particularly interesting because of the remarkable variability in their associated phenotypes. For example, substitution of the G in position 5 of IVS-1 by C or T results in severe β⁺-thalassemia.[55] On the other hand, a T→C change at position 6, found commonly in the Mediterranean region,[70] results in a very mild form of β⁺-thalassemia. The G→C change at position 5 has also been found in Melanesia and appears to be the most common cause of β-thalassemia in Papua New Guinea.[71]

RNA processing is affected by mutations that create new splice sites within either introns or exons. Again, these lesions are remarkably variable in their phenotypic effect, depending on the degree to which the new site is utilized compared with the normal splice site. For example, the G→A substitution at position 110 of IVS-1, which is one of the most common forms of β-thalassemia in the Mediterranean region, leads to only approximately 10 percent splicing at the normal site and hence results in a severe β⁺-thalassemia phenotype.[72,73] Similarly, a mutation that produces a new acceptor site at position 116 in IVS-1 results in little or no β-globin mRNA production and the β⁰-thalassemia phenotype.[74] Several mutations that generate new donor sites within IVS-2 of the β-globin gene have been described.[55,68]

Another interesting mechanism for abnormal splicing is activation of donor sites within exons (Fig. 46-6). For example, within exon 1 is a cryptic donor site in the region of codons 24 through 27. This site contains a GT dinucleotide. An adjacent substitution that alters the site so that it more closely resembles the consensus donor splice site results in its activation, even though the normal site is active. Several mutations in this region can activate this site so that it is utilized during RNA processing, with the production of abnormal mRNAs.[75–78] Three of the substitutions, A→G in codon 19, G→A in codon 26, and G→T in codon 27, result in reduced production of β-globin mRNA and an amino acid substitution so that the mRNA that is spliced normally is translated into protein. The abnormal hemoglobins produced are hemoglobins Malay, E, and Knossos, respectively, all of which are associated with a β-thalassemia phenotype, presumably as a result of reduced overall output of normal mRNA. A variety of other cryptic splice mutations within introns and exons have been described.[26,45]

Another class of processing mutations involves the polyadenylation signal site AAUAAA in the 3′ untranslated region of β-globin mRNA.[79–81] For example, a T→C substitution in this sequence leads to only one tenth the normal amount of β-globin mRNA and hence the severe β⁺-thalassemia phenotype.[79]

Mutations Causing Abnormal Translation of Messenger RNA Base substitutions that change an amino acid codon into a chain termination codon, that is, nonsense mutations, prevent translation of the mRNA and result in β⁰-thalassemia. Many substitutions of this type have been described.[7,45] For example, a codon 17 mutation is common in Southeast Asia,[82,83] and a codon 39 mutation occurs at a high frequency in the Mediterranean region.[84,85]

The insertion or deletion of one, two, or four nucleotides in the coding region of the β-globin gene disrupts the normal reading frame and results, upon translation of the mRNA, in the addition of anomalous amino acids until a termination codon is reached in the new reading frame. Several frameshift mutations of this type have been described.[7,45] Two mutations—the insertion of one nucleotide between codons 8 and 9 and a deletion of four nucleotides in codons 41 and 42—are common in Asian Indians.[63] The latter deletions are found frequently in different populations in Southeast Asia.[83]

An unusual β⁺-thalassemia was described in a patient from a Czech Republic in whom a full-length L1 transposon was inserted into the second intron of β-globin, creating a β⁺-thalassemia phenotype by an undefined molecular mechanism.[86]

Dominantly Inherited β-Thalassemia Families in which a picture indistinguishable from moderately severe β-thalassemia has segregated in Mendelian dominant fashion have been reported sporadically.[87,88] Because this condition often is characterized by the presence of inclusion bodies in the red cell precursors, it has been called *inclu-*

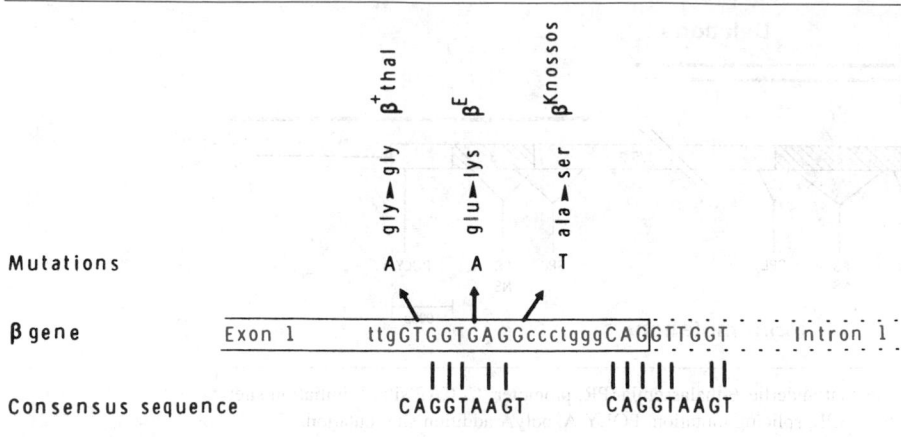

FIGURE 46-6 Activation of cryptic splice sites in exon 1 as the cause of β⁺-thalassemia, hemoglobin E, and hemoglobin Knossos. The similarities between the 5' splice region of intron 1 and the cryptic splice region in exon 1 are shown in *capitals*.

sion body β-thalassemia (hyperunstable hemoglobins). However, because all severe forms of β-thalassemia have inclusions in the red cell precursors, the term *dominantly inherited β-thalassemia* is preferred.[7,89] Sequence analysis has shown that these conditions are heterogeneous at the molecular level, but that many involve mutations of exon 3 of the β-globin gene. The mutations include frameshifts, premature chain termination mutations, and complex rearrangements that lead to synthesis of truncated or elongated and highly unstable β-globin gene products.[7,89–93] The most common mutation of this type is a GAA→TAA change at codon 121 that leads to synthesis of a truncated β-globin chain.[94] Although an abnormal β-chain product from loci affected by mutations of this type is unusual, many of these conditions are designated as hemoglobin variants.

The reason why mutations occurring in exons I and II produce the classic form of recessive β-thalassemia whereas the bulk of the dominant thalassemias result from mutations in exon III has become clearer. In the former case, very little abnormal β-globin mRNA is found in the cytoplasm of the red cell precursors, whereas exon III mutations are associated with full-length but abnormal mRNA accumulation. The different phenotypes of these premature termination codons have been suggested to reflect a phenomenon called *nonsense-mediated RNA decay*, a surveillance system to prevent transport of mRNA coding for truncated peptides. Presumably this process is active in the case of exon I or II mutations, in which affected mRNAs are degraded, but is not active in the case of exon III mutations.[95–97] A complete list of the mutations that underlie the dominant β-thalassemias is given in reference [7].

Unstable β-Globin Variants Some β-globin chain variants are highly unstable but are capable of forming a viable tetramer. The resulting unstable hemoglobins may precipitate in the red cell precursors or in the blood, giving rise to a spectrum of conditions ranging from dominantly inherited β-thalassemia to a hemolytic anemia similar to the anemia associated with other unstable hemoglobins. The first unstable hemoglobin to be described was hemoglobin Indianapolis.[98] Its structure was characterized by DNA analysis performed on stored autopsy material; however, the original description proved to be incorrect.[99]

Silent β-Thalassemia A number of extremely mild β-thalassemia alleles are either silent or almost unidentifiable in heterozygotes (Table 46-2). Some alleles are in the region of the promoter boxes of the β-globin gene, but others involve the CAP sites or the 5' or 3' untranslated regions.[7,45] These alleles usually are identified by finding a form of β-thalassemia intermedia in which one parent has a typical

thalassemia trait and the other parent appears to be normal but, in fact, is a carrier of one of the mild β-thalassemia alleles.

β-Thalassemia Mutations Unlinked to the β-Globin Gene Cluster Several family studies have suggested the existence of mutations that result in the β-thalassemia phenotype but do not segregate with the β-globin genes[100]; however, their molecular basis has not been determined. Further evidence for the existence of novel mutations of this type can be found in ref. [7].

Variant Forms of β-Thalassemia In several forms of β-thalassemia, the hemoglobin A₂ level is normal in heterozygotes. Some cases result from "silent" β-thalassemia alleles, whereas others reflect the co-inheritance of β- and δ-thalassemia.[7]

δβ-THALASSEMIA

The δβ-thalassemias are classified into the (δβ)⁺- and (δβ)⁰-thalassemias (Table 46-3). The (δβ)⁰-thalassemias are further divided into (δβ)⁰-thalassemia, in which both the δ- and β-globin genes are deleted, and (ᴬγδβ)⁰-thalassemia, in which the ᴳγ, δ, and β genes are deleted. Because many different deletion forms of δβ-thalassemia have been described, they are further classified according to the country in which they were first identified (Table 46-3).

(δβ)⁰- and (ᴬγδβ)⁰-Thalassemia Nearly all these conditions result from deletions involving varying lengths of the β-globin gene cluster. Many different varieties have been described in different pop-

TABLE 46-2 MOLECULAR PATHOLOGY OF THE β-THALASSEMIAS

β⁰- or β⁺-Thalassemia
  Transcription
    Deletions
    Insertions
    Promoter
    5' UTR
  Processing of mRNA
    Junctional
    Consensus splicing sequences
    Cryptic splice sites in introns
    Cryptic splice sites in exons
    Poly (A) addition site
  Translation
    Initiation
    Nonsense
    Frameshift
  Posttranslational stability
    Unstable β-chain variants
Normal Hb A₂ β-Thalassemia
  β-thalassemia and δ-thalassemia, *cis* or *trans*
  "Silent" β-thalassemia
    Some promoter mutations
    CAP +1, CAP +3, etc.
    5' UTR
    Some splice mutations
Dominant β-thalassemia
  Mainly point mutations or rearrangements in exon 3
  Other unstable variants

NOTE: A full list of mutations is given in refs. 7 and 45.

TABLE 46-3   δβ THALASSEMIAS

(δβ)⁺-Thalassemia
    Hb Lepore thalassemia
    Hb Lepore Washington-Boston
    Hb Lepore Hollandia
    Hb Lepore Baltimore
    Phenocopies of (δβ)⁺-thalassemia
        Sardinian δβ-thalassemia
        Corfu δβ-thalassemia
        Chinese δβ-thalassemia
        β-Thalassemia with δ-thalassemia

(δβ)⁰-Thalassemia
    Sicilian
    Indian
    Japanese
    Spanish
    Black
    Eastern European
    Macedonian
    Turkish
    Laotian
    Thai

(ᴬγδβ)⁰-Thalassemia
    Indian
    German
    Cantonese
    Turkish
    Malay 2
    Belgian
    Black
    Chinese
    Yunnanese
    Thai
    Italian

NOTE: Details of the molecular pathology of these conditions are given in refs. 7 and 45.

ulations (see Table 46-3), although their heterozygous and homozygous phenotypes are very similar.[7] Rare forms of these conditions result from more complex gene rearrangements. For example, one form of (ᴬγδβ)⁰-thalassemia, found in Indian populations, does not result from a simple linear deletion but rather from a complex rearrangement with two deletions, one affecting the ᴬγ gene and the other the δ and β genes. The intervening region is intact but inverted.[101] Figure 46-6 illustrates some of these conditions.

(δβ)⁺-Thalassemia   The (δβ)⁺-thalassemias usually are associated with the production of structural hemoglobin variants called Lepore.[7,9,10] Hemoglobin Lepore contains normal α chains and non-α chains that consist of the first 50 to 80 amino acid residues of the δ chains and the last 60 to 90 residues of the normal C-terminal amino acid sequence of the β chains. Thus, the Lepore non-α chain is a δβ fusion chain. Several different varieties of hemoglobin Lepore have been described—Washington-Boston, Baltimore, and Hollandia—in which the transition from δ to β sequences occurs at different points.[7] The fusion chains probably arose by nonhomologous crossing over between part of the δ locus on one chromosome and part of the β locus on the complementary chromosome (Fig. 46-7). This event results from misalignment of chromosome pairing during meiosis so that a δ-chain gene pairs with a β-chain gene instead of with its homologous partner.[102] Figure 46-8 shows such a mechanism should give rise to two abnormal chromosomes: the first, the Lepore chromosome, will have no normal δ or β loci but simply a δβ fusion

gene. Opposite the homologous pairs of chromosomes should be an anti-Lepore (βδ) fusion gene and normal δ and β loci. A variety of anti-Lepore–like hemoglobins have been discovered, including hemoglobins Miyada, P-Congo, Lincoln Park, and P-Nilotic.[7] All the hemoglobin Lepore disorders are characterized by a severe form of δβ-thalassemia. The output of the γ-globin genes on the chromosome with the δβ fusion gene is not increased sufficiently to compensate for the low output of the δβ fusion product. The reduced rate of production of the δβ fusion chains of hemoglobin Lepore presumably reflects the fact that its genetic determinant has the δ gene promoter region, which is structurally different from the β-globin gene promoter and is associated with a reduced rate of transcription of its gene product.

δβ-Thalassemia–like Disorders Resulting from Two Mutations in the β-Globin Gene Cluster   A heterogeneous group of nondeletion δβ-thalassemias has been described, most resulting from two mutations in the εγδβ-globin gene cluster (Table 46-4). Strictly speaking, they are not all δβ-thalassemias, but they often appear in the literature under this title because their phenotypes resemble the deletion forms of (δβ)⁰-thalassemia. In the Sardinian form of δβ-thalassemia, the β-globin gene has the common Mediterranean codon 39 nonsense mutation that leads to an absence of β-globin synthesis. The relatively high expression of the ᴬγ gene in cis gives this condition the δβ-thalassemia phenotype because of a point mutation at position −196 upstream from the ᴬγ gene (see "Hereditary Persistence of Fetal Hemoglobin" below). The phenotypic picture, in which heterozygotes have 15 to 20 percent hemoglobin F and normal hemoglobin A₂ levels, is identical to that of δβ-thalassemia.[103] Another condition having the δβ-thalassemia phenotype, with greater than 20 percent hemoglobin F in heterozygotes, has been described in a Chinese patient in whom defective β-globin chain synthesis appears to result from an A→G change in the ATA sequence in the promoter region of the β-globin gene.[104] The increased γ-chain synthesis, which appears to involve both ᴳγ and ᴬγ cis to this mutation, remains unexplained. A disorder originally called δβ-thalassemia has been described in the Corfu population.[105,106] The condition results from two mutations in the β-globin gene cluster: first, a 7201-bp deletion that starts in the δ-globin gene, IVS-2, position 818−822, and extends upstream to a 5′ breakpoint located 1719 to 1722 bp 3′ to the ψβ-gene termination codon; and second, a G→A mutation at position 5 in the donor site consensus region of IVS-1 of the β-globin gene. The output from this chromosome consists of relatively high levels of γ chains with very low levels of β chains. The condition resembles δβ-thalassemia in the homozygous state, with almost 100 percent hemoglobin F, traces of hemoglobin A, but no hemoglobin A₂. Heterozygotes have only slightly elevated hemoglobin F levels, with a phenotype similar to "normal A₂β-thalassemia."

εγδβ-THALASSEMIA

These rare conditions[107–113] result from long deletions that begin upstream from the β-gene complex 55 kb or more 5′ to the ε gene and terminate within the cluster (see Fig. 46-6). In two cases, designated Dutch[110,111] and English,[112] the deletions leave the β-globin gene intact, but no β-chain production occurs even though the gene is expressed in heterologous systems.

The molecular basis for inactivation of the β-globin gene cis to these deletions was clarified by the discovery of the LCR about 50 kb upstream from the εγδβ-globin gene cluster (see "Genetic Control and Synthesis of Hemoglobin," above). Removal of this critical regulatory region seems to completely inactivate the downstream globin gene complex. The Hispanic form of εγδβ-thalassemia[113] results from a deletion that includes most of the LCR, including four of the five DNase-1–hypersensitive sites. These lesions appear to close

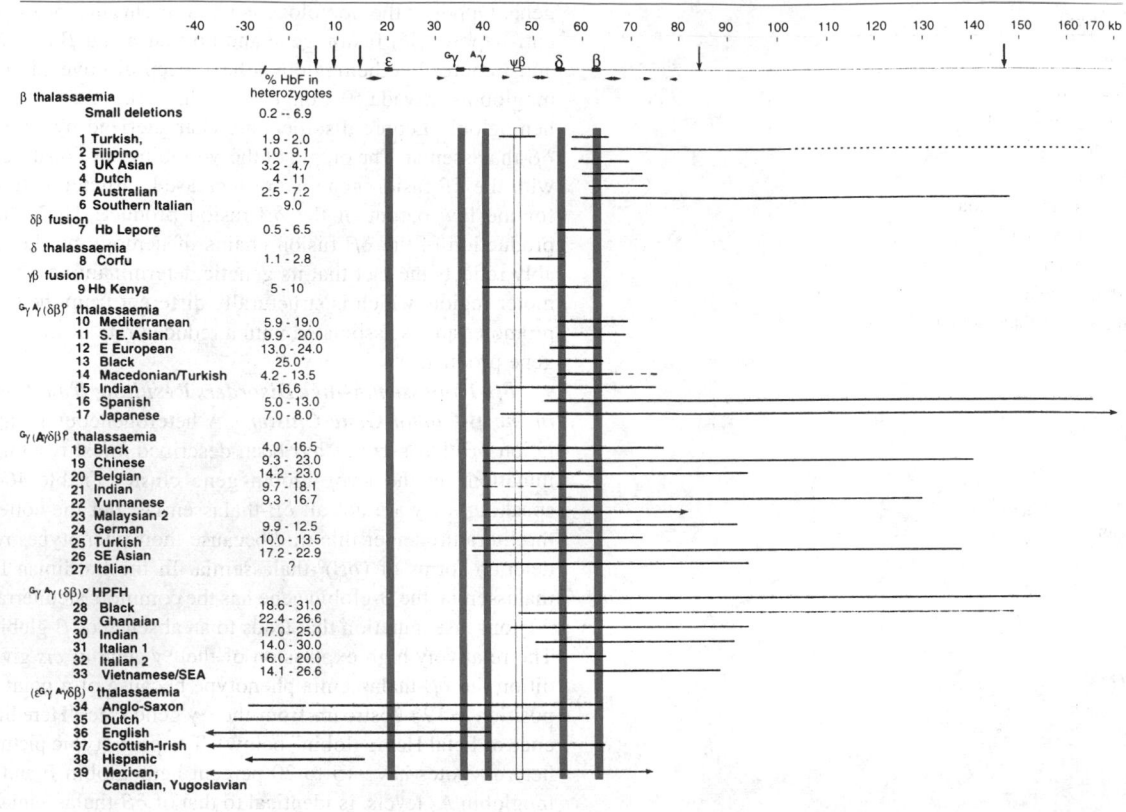

FIGURE 46-7   Some deletions responsible for the β- and (δβ)-thalassemias and hereditary persistence of fetal hemoglobin.

down the chromatin domain that usually is open in erythroid tissues and delay replication of the β-globin genes in the cell cycle. Thus, although they are rare, the lesions have been of considerable importance because analysis of the Dutch deletion first pointed to the possibility of a major control region upstream from the β-like–globin gene cluster and ultimately led to the discovery of the β-globin LCR.

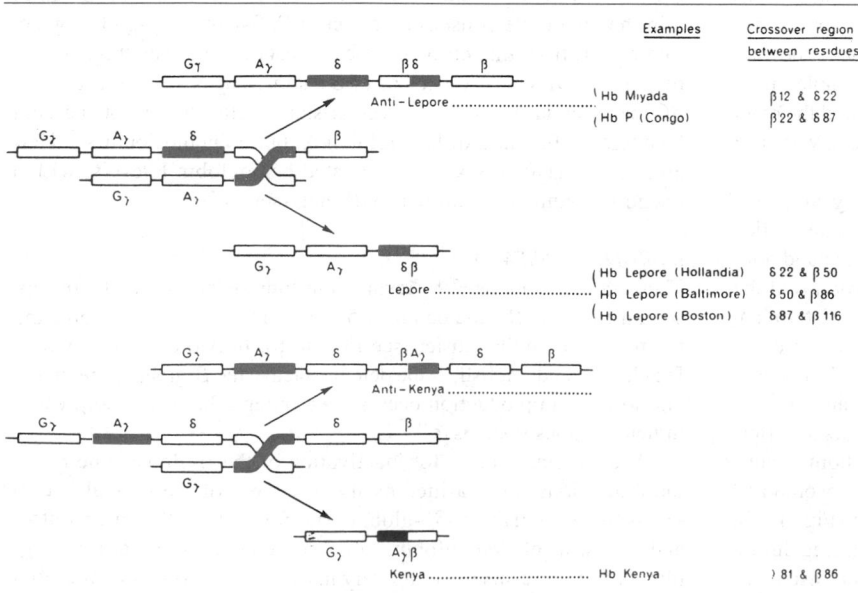

FIGURE 46-8   Mechanisms of production of the Lepore and anti-Lepore hemoglobins and hemoglobin Kenya.

HEREDITARY PERSISTENCE OF FETAL HEMOGLOBIN

This heterogeneous group of conditions produces phenotypes very similar to those of the δβ-thalassemias, except that defective β-chain production appears to be almost, but in some forms not completely, compensated by persistent γ-chain production. These conditions are best classified into deletion and nondeletion forms (see Table 46-4). In the past, the conditions were classified into pancellular and heterocellular varieties, depending on the intercellular distribution of fetal hemoglobin. However, this subdivision now appears to bear little relevance to their molecular basis and probably relates more to the particular level of fetal hemoglobin and how its cellular distribution is determined.[7]

The deletion forms of HPFH are heterogeneous (see Fig. 46-5). The two African varieties result from extensive deletions of similar length (<70 kb) but with staggered ends, differing phenotypically only in the proportions of Gγ and Aγ chains produced.[114] Another type of HPFH results from misalignment during crossing over between the Aγ- and β-globin genes, resulting in production of Aγβ fusion genes (see Fig. 46-8). The latter give rise to γβ fusion products that combine with α chains to form the hemoglobin variant called hemoglobin Kenya.[115,116] Hemoglobin Kenya is associated with an increased output of hemoglobin F, although at a lower level than in the deletion forms of HPFH. A theory that adequately explains the phenotypic differences between δβ-thalassemia and the deletion forms of HPFH has not been developed.[7]

The nondeletion determinants of HPFH can be classified into those that map within the β-globin

TABLE 46-4   HEREDITARY PERSISTENCE OF FETAL HEMOGLOBIN

Deletion (Pancellular*)

$(\delta\beta)^0$

  Black (HPFH 1)

  Ghanaian (HPFH 2)

  Indian (HPFH 3)

  Italian (HPFH 4 and 5)

  Vietnamese (HPFH 6)

$^G\gamma\,(^A\gamma\,\beta)^+$ (Hb Kenya)

Nondeletion

  Linked to β-globin gene cluster (pancellular*)

    $^G\gamma\,\beta^+$

      Black $^G\gamma$-202 C→G

      Tunisian $^G\gamma$-200+C

      Black/Sardinian $^G\gamma$-175 T→C

      Japanese $^G\gamma$-114 C→T

      Australian $^G\gamma$-114 C→G

    $^A\gamma\,\beta^+$

      Greek/Sardinian/Black $^A\gamma$-117 G→A

      British $^A\gamma$-198 T→C

      Black $^A\gamma$-202 C→T

      Italian/Chinese $^A\gamma$-196 C→T

      Brazilian $^A\gamma$-195 C→G

      Black $^A\gamma$-175 T→C

      Black $^A\gamma$-114 to −102 (del)

      Georgia $^A\gamma$-114 C→T

    $^G\gamma\,^A\gamma\,\beta^+$

  Linked to β-globin gene cluster (heterocellular*)

    Atlanta

    Czech

    Seattle

    Others (including some cases of $^G\gamma$-158 T→C)

  Unlinked to β-globin gene cluster (heterocellular*)

    Chromosome 6

    Others

* The intercellular distribution of Hb F is not always reported, and some inconsistencies are present within groups. Complete details are given in ref. 7.

gene cluster and those that segregate independently. The former are subdivided into $^G\gamma^+$ and $^A\gamma^+$ varieties, indicating persistent $^G\gamma$- or $^A\gamma$-chain synthesis in association with β-globin production directed by the β gene *cis* (on the same chromosome) to the HPFH determinant. Analysis of the overexpressed γ genes revealed in each case a single-base substitution in the region immediately upstream from the transcription start site.[7,117–120] Clustering of these substitutions and lack of

similar changes in normal γ genes suggest they are responsible for persistent hemoglobin F production (Fig. 46-9). This region of DNA likely is involved in binding of *trans*-acting proteins involved in the normal developmental repression of γ-gene expression, either by decreasing the affinity for an inhibitory factor normally present in adult life or by increasing the affinity for a factor promoting gene expression. The most common of these conditions are Greek $^A\gamma\beta^+$ HPFH and a form of $^G\gamma\beta^+$ HPFH, which has been found in several different African populations. If the upstream point mutations associated with persistent γ-chain production occur on the same chromosome as β-globin genes that carry β^0-thalassemia mutations, the clinical phenotype is converted from HPFH to $\delta\beta$-thalassemia, albeit with different hemoglobin A_2 levels.

In some cases, other nondeletional forms of HPFH have been related to small structural changes in the β-globin gene cluster (see Table 46-4). Although strictly speaking not a true form of HPFH, because even in homozygotes it may not be associated with increased hemoglobin F levels, the T→C polymorphism at position −158 to the $^G\gamma$-globin gene[121] may be associated with an increased output of hemoglobin F under conditions of erythropoietic stress.

Other forms of HPFH are characterized by the persistence of low levels of fetal hemoglobin production distributed in a heterocellular manner. In all populations studied, a small proportion of individuals have an increased amount of hemoglobin F and F cells, that is, red cells that can be detected when blood films are treated with antibodies against hemoglobin F. Although this condition originally was called the Swiss form of HPFH because it was first recognized in Swiss army recruits,[122] it is observed in every racial group. Some evidence suggests at least one genetic determinant responsible for determining the number of F cells is X linked, and a putative locus has been located at Xp22.2.[123,124] However, not all forms of hereditary persistence of low hemoglobin F levels are encoded by the X chromosome.[125–128] In studies of a large pedigree in which a form of HPFH segregated independently from β-thalassemia, the genetic determinant was localized to chromosome 6q23.[128] However, further studies indicated similar forms of HPFH were not linked to chromosome 6.[129] The different forms of HPFH that are unlinked to the β-globin gene cluster likely reflect mutations of transcription factors involved in the switch from fetal to adult hemoglobin production. The importance of these conditions lies in the fact that, when they are inherited together with the sickle-cell or β-thalassemia genes, they may increase the output of hemoglobin F to such an extent that they modify the phenotype of the associated disorders.

δ-THALASSEMIA

Several point mutations and deletions that reduce δ-globin synthesis have been described. They are summarized in ref. 7.

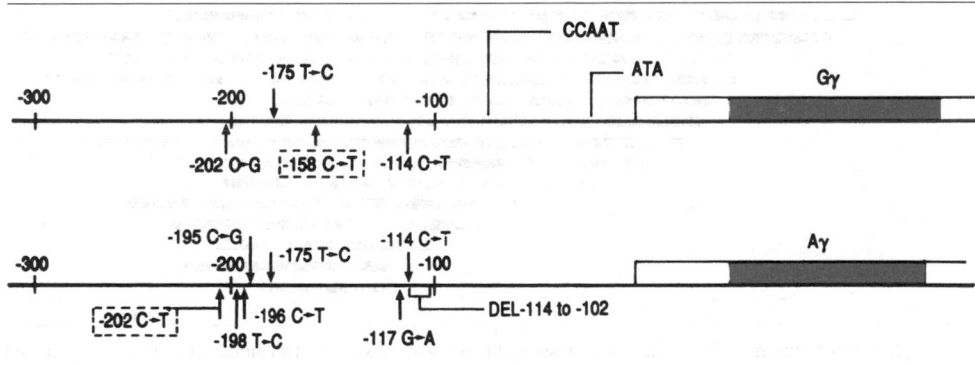

FIGURE 46-9   Some upstream point mutations associated with hereditary persistence of fetal hemoglobin.

TABLE 46-5   CLASSES OF MUTATIONS THAT CAUSE α-THALASSEMIA

α^0-Thalassemia
  Deletions involving both α-globin genes
  Deletions downstream from $\alpha2$ gene
  Truncations of telomeric region of 16p
  Deletions of HS40 region

α^+-Thalassemia
  Deletions involving $\alpha2$ or $\alpha1$ genes
  Point mutations involving $\alpha2$ or $\alpha1$ genes
    mRNA processing
      Splice site
      Poly(A) signal
    mRNA translation
    Initiation
    Nonsense, frameshift
    Termination
    Posttranslational
    Unstable α-globin variants

α-Thalassemia Mental Retardation
  ATR-16
    Deletions or telomeric truncations of 16p
    Translocations
  ATR-X
    Mutations of *ATR-X*
      Deletions
      Splice site
      Missense
      Nonsense

NOTE: Complete lists of individual mutations are found in refs. 7, 10, and 51.

α-THALASSEMIA

Table 46-5 summarizes the different classes of α-thalassemia. The α-globin gene haplotype can be written $\alpha\alpha$, indicating the $\alpha2$ and $\alpha1$ genes, respectively. A normal individual has the genotype $\alpha\alpha/\alpha\alpha$. A deletion involving one ($-\alpha$) or both ($-$ $-$) α genes can be further classified based on its size, written as a superscript; thus, $-\alpha^{3.7}$ indicates a deletion of 3.7 kb including one α gene. When the sizes of the deletions are not established, a superscript describing their geographic or family origin is useful; thus, $-$ $-^{MED}$ describes a deletion of both α genes first identified in individuals of Mediterranean origin. In thalassemia haplotypes in which both genes are intact, that is, nondeletion lesions, the nomenclature $\alpha^T\alpha$ is given, with the superscript T indicating the gene is thalassemic. However, when the precise molecular defect is known, as in hemoglobin Constant Spring, for example, $\alpha^T\alpha$ can be replaced by the more informative $\alpha^{CS}\alpha$. The molecular pathology and population genetics of the α-thalassemias have been the subject of several extensive reviews.[7,9,130,131]

α^0-Thalassemia   To date, 29 deletions that involve both α genes, and therefore abolish α-chain production from the affected chromosome, have been described (Fig. 46-10).[7] Several of the 3' breakpoints fall within a 6- to 8-kb region at the 3' end of the α-globin complex, suggesting this represents a breakpoint cluster region with a high level of recombination.[132] In at least five of the deletions, the 5' breakpoints also appear to cluster. This gives rise to a situation in which the 5' breakpoints are located approximately the same distance apart and in the same order along a chromosome as their respective 3' breakpoints. It is possible that such staggered deletions arise from illegitimate recombination events that delete an integral number of chromatin loops as they pass through their nuclear attachment points during replication. This mechanism has also been suggested to underlie some of the deletion forms of HPFH. One of these deletions ($-$ $-^{MED}$) involves a more complex rearrangement that introduces a new piece of DNA bridging the two breakpoints in the α-gene cluster. This new sequence originates upstream from the α cluster and appears to have been replicated into the junction in a manner suggesting that the upstream segment of DNA also lies at the base of a replication loop. At least some of these deletions seem to have arisen by recombination events between Alu repeat sequences.

Several other mechanisms for the generation of α^0-thalassemia have been identified. In one case of unusual genetic interest, a long (>18 kb) deletion that removes the $\alpha1$ gene and the region downstream was identified in which the $\alpha2$ gene remains intact but is completely inactivated, giving the α^0-thalassemia phenotype. Although the inactive $\alpha2$ gene retains all its local and remote *cis*-regulatory elements, its expression is completely silenced and its CpG island is completely methylated as a result of transcription of antisense RNA

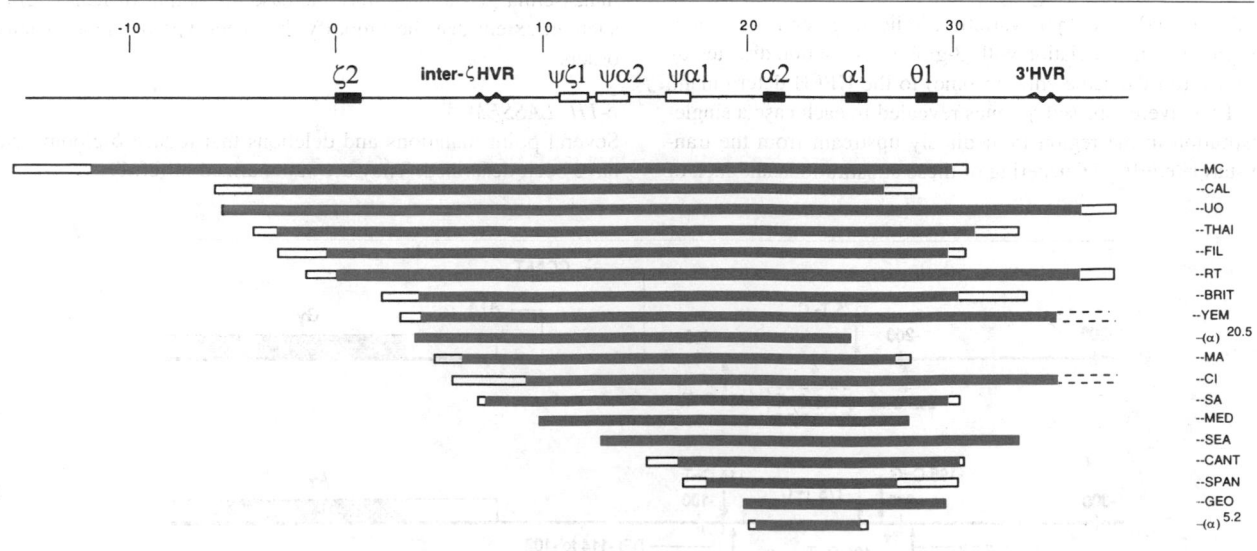

FIGURE 46-10   Some deletions of the α-globin gene cluster responsible for α^0-thalassemia. Deletions: MC, initials of patient; CAL, initials of patient; THAI, Thai; FIL, Filipino; CI, Conway Islands; BRIT, United Kingdom; SA, South Africa; MED, Mediterranean; SEA, Southeast Asian; SPAN, Spanish.

(A)

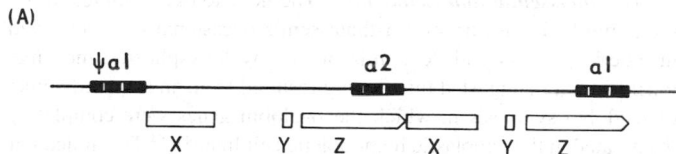

(B)   RIGHTWARD CROSSOVER

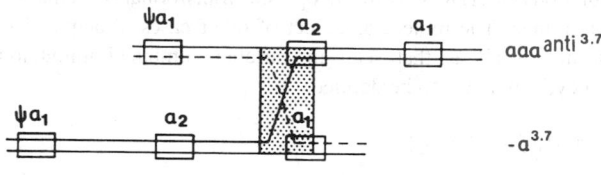

(C)   LEFTWARD CROSSOVER

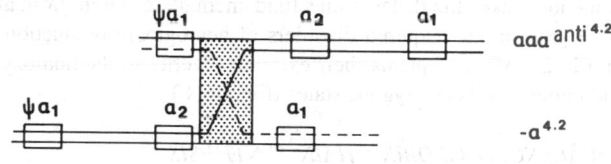

FIGURE 46-11   Mechanisms for production of the common deletion forms of α^+-thalassemia. (A) Normal α-globin gene cluster showing the homology boxes X, Y, and Z. (B) Rightward crossover through the Z bones, giving rise to the 3.7-kb deletion and a chromosome with three α-globin genes. (C) Leftward crossover through the Z boxes, giving rise to a 4.2 kb deletion and a chromosome containing three α genes.

expressed from a locus that had been juxtaposed to the $\alpha2$ gene because of the large deletion.[133,134] In some cases, this condition results from a terminal truncation of the short arm of chromosome 16 to a site 50 kb distal to the α-globin genes.[135] It is interesting that the telomeric consensus sequence (TTAGGGG)n has been added directly to the site of the break. Because this mutation is stably inherited, telomeric DNA alone appears sufficient to stabilize the broken chromosome end. This observation raises the possibility that other genetic diseases result from chromosomal truncations.

Several deletions have been identified that appear to down-regulate α-globin genes by removing the α-globin LCR (HS40).[7,136,137] In each case, the α-globin genes are left intact, although in one the 3' breakpoint is found between the ξ and $\psi\xi$ genes, thus removing the ξ gene.[138] These deletions appear to completely inactivate the α-globin gene complex, just as deletions of the β-globin LCR inactivate the entire β-gene complex. Such deletions have not been observed in the homozygous state, presumably because they would be lethal.

α^+-Thalassemia Gene Deletions   The most common forms of α^+-thalassemia ($-\alpha^{3.7}$ and $-\alpha^{4.2}$) involve deletion of one or the other of the duplicated α-globin genes (Figs. 46-10 and 46-11).

Each α gene is located within a region of homology approximately 4 kb long, interrupted by two nonhomologous regions. The homologous regions are believed to have resulted from an ancient duplication event and to have subsequently subdivided, presumably by insertions and deletions, to give three homologous subsegments referred to as X, Y, and Z (see Fig. 46-9). The duplicated Z boxes are 3.7 kb apart, and the X boxes are 4.2 kb apart. Misalignment and reciprocal crossover between these segments at meiosis can give rise to chromosomes with either single ($-\alpha$) or triplicated ($\alpha\alpha\alpha$) α-globin genes. Such an occurrence between homologous Z boxes deletes 3.7 kb of DNA (rightward deletion). A similar crossover between the two X blocks deletes 4.2 kb of DNA (leftward deletion $-\alpha^{4.2}$).[138] The corresponding

triplicated α-gene arrangements are referred to as $\alpha\alpha\alpha^{anti-3.7}$ and $\alpha^{anti-4.2}$.[139–141] More detailed analysis of these crossover events indicates they occur more commonly in the Z box. At least three different $-\alpha^{3.7}$ deletions have been found, depending on exactly where the crossover occurred.[142] These deletions are designated $-\alpha^{3.7I}$, $-\alpha^{3.7II}$, and $-\alpha^{3.7III}$, respectively. Other, rarer deletions of a single α gene are observed.[7]

Nondeletion α-Thalassemia   Because expression of the α_2 gene is two to three times greater than expression of the $\alpha1$ gene, the finding that most of the nondeletion mutants discovered to date affect predominantly $\alpha2$ gene expression is not surprising. Presumably this is ascertainment bias because of the greater phenotypic effect of these lesions. It also is possible that defective expression of the $\alpha2$ gene has come under greater selective pressure.

Like the β-thalassemia mutations, α-thalassemia mutations[7] can be classified according to the level of gene expression they affect (see Table 46-5). Several processing mutations have been identified. For example, a pentanucleotide deletion includes the 5' splice site of IVS-1 of the $\alpha2$-globin gene. This mutation involves the invariant GT donor splicing sequence and thus completely inactivates the $\alpha2$ gene.[143] A second mutant of this type, found commonly in the Middle East, involves the poly-A addition signal site (AATAAA→AATAAG) and down-regulates the $\alpha2$ gene by interfering with 3' end processing.[144,145]

A second group of nondeletion α-thalassemias results from mutations that interfere with translation of mRNA.[7] Several mutations involve the initiation codon.[146–149] In one case, for example, the initiation codon is inactivated by a T→C transition.[146] In another case, efficiency of initiation is reduced by a dinucleotide deletion in the consensus sequence around the start signal.[149] Five mutations that affect termination of translation and give rise to elongated α chains have been identified: hemoglobins Constant Spring, Icaria, Koya Dora, Seal Rock, and Pakse.[7] Each mutation specifically changes the termination codon TAA so that an amino acid is inserted instead of the chain terminating (Fig. 46-12). This process is followed by read-through of mRNA that is not normally translated until another "in-phase" stop codon is reached. Thus, each of these variants has an elongated α chain. The "read-through" of α-globin mRNA that usually is not utilized likely reduces its stability.[150] Several nonsense mutations are present, for example, one in exon 3 of the $\alpha2$ globin gene.[151] Finally, several mutations are present that cause α-thalassemia by producing highly unstable α-globin chains, including hemoglobins Quong Sze,[152] Suan Doc,[153] Petah Tikvah,[154] and Evanston.[155] A complete list of nondeletion α-thalassemia alleles is given in ref. 7.

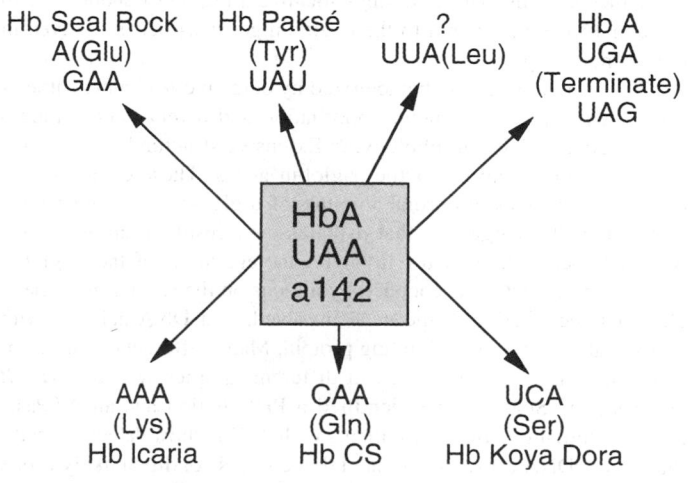

FIGURE 46-12   Point mutations in the α-globin gene termination codon.

Interactions of α-Thalassemia Haplotypes Many α-thalassemia haplotypes have been described, and potentially more than 500 interactions are possible![7] Phenotypically, these phenotypes result in four broad categories: (1) normal, (2) conditions characterized by mild hematologic changes but no clinical abnormality, (3) hemoglobin H disease, and (4) hemoglobin Bart's hydrops fetalis syndrome. The heterozygous states for deletion or nondeletion forms of α^+-thalassemia either cause extremely mild hematologic abnormalities or are completely silent. In populations where α-thalassemia is common, the homozygous state for α^+-thalassemia ($-\alpha/-\alpha$) can produce a hematologic phenotype identical to that of the heterozygous state for α^0-thalassemia ($--/\alpha\alpha$), that is, mild anemia with reduced mean cell hemoglobin and mean cell volume values.

Hemoglobin H disease usually results from the compound heterozygous state for α^0-thalassemia and either deletion or nondeletion α^+-thalassemia. It occurs most frequently in Southeast Asia ($--^{SEA}/-\alpha^{3.7}$) and the Mediterranean region (usually $--^{MED}/-\alpha^{3.7}$).

The hemoglobin Bart's hydrops fetalis syndrome usually results from the homozygous state for α^0-thalassemia, most commonly $--^{SEA}/--^{SEA}$ or $--^{MED}/--^{MED}$. A few infants with this syndrome who synthesized very low levels of α chains at birth have been reported. Gene-mapping studies suggest these cases result from interaction of α^0-thalassemia with nondeletion mutations $(\alpha\alpha^T)$.

Unusual Forms of α-Thalassemia Some unusual forms of α-thalassemia are completely unrelated to the common forms of the disease that occur in tropical populations. These conditions, which can occur in any racial groups, include α-thalassemia associated with mental retardation or leukemia. Their importance lies with the diagnostic problems they may present and, more importantly, the light that elucidation of the α-thalassemia pathology may shed on broader disease mechanisms.

Molecular Pathology of the α-Thalassemia–Mental Retardation Syndrome The first descriptions of noninherited forms of α-thalassemia associated with mental retardation suggested the lesions involving the α-globin gene locus were acquired in the paternal germ cells and that their molecular pathology might help elucidate the associated developmental changes.[156] Two separate syndromes of this type now are evident. In one group of patients, long deletions involve the α-globin gene cluster and remove at least one megabase.[157] This condition can arise in several ways, including unbalanced translocation involving chromosome 16, truncation of the tip of chromosome 16, and loss of the α-globin gene cluster and parts of its flanking regions by other mechanisms. These findings localize a region of about 1.7 Mb in band 16p13.3 proximal to the α-globin genes as being involved in mental handicap.[7]

The second group is characterized by defective α-globin synthesis associated with severe mental retardation and a relatively homogeneous pattern of dysmorphology.[158] Extensive structural studies have shown no abnormalities of the α-globin genes. These chromosomes direct the synthesis of normal amounts of α globin in mouse erythroleukemia cells, suggesting that α-thalassemia results from deficiency of a *trans*-activating factor involved in regulation of the α-globin genes. This condition is encoded by a locus on the short arm of the X chromosome.[159] ATX-R, the gene involved, is a DNA helicase with many features of a DNA-binding protein. Many different mutations of this gene have been identified in different families with the ATX-R syndrome.[160] Studies have identified a PHD region and an ATPase/helicase domain.[161] Because patients with ATX-R show defective methylation of rDNA arrays and related defects, this condition likely is one of a growing list of disorders that result from disordered chromatin remodeling.[162,163]

α-Thalassemia and Leukemia The hematologic findings of hemoglobin H disease or mild α-thalassemia occasionally are observed in elderly patients with leukemia or the myelodysplastic syndrome. Earlier studies suggested this finding resulted from an acquired defect of α-globin synthesis in which the α-globin genes were completely inactivated in the neoplastic hemopoietic cell line.[148,164] The molecular basis for this observation now is known to reside in a variety of different mutations involving ATR-X.[165] The relationship of these somatic mutations of ATR-X to the neoplastic transformation remains to be determined. The molecular defect of other cases of acquired α-thalassemia, such as that seen in variable combined immuniodeficiency,[166] remains to be defined.

PATHOPHYSIOLOGY

Almost all the pathophysiologic features of the thalassemias can be related to a primary imbalance of globin-chain synthesis. This phenomenon makes the thalassemias fundamentally different from all the other genetic and acquired disorders of hemoglobin production and, to a large extent, explains their extreme severity in the homozygous and compound heterozygous states (Fig. 46-13).

IMBALANCED GLOBIN-CHAIN SYNTHESIS

Measurements of *in vitro* globin-chain synthesis in the blood or marrow of patients with different types of thalassemia[167,168] and family studies that allow examination of the action of thalassemia genes in patients who also inherited α- or β-globin structural variants[7,8] provide a clear picture of the action of the thalassemia determinants. In homozygous β-thalassemia, β-globin synthesis is either absent or markedly reduced. The result is excessive production of α-globin chains. α-Globin chains are incapable of forming a viable hemoglobin tetra-

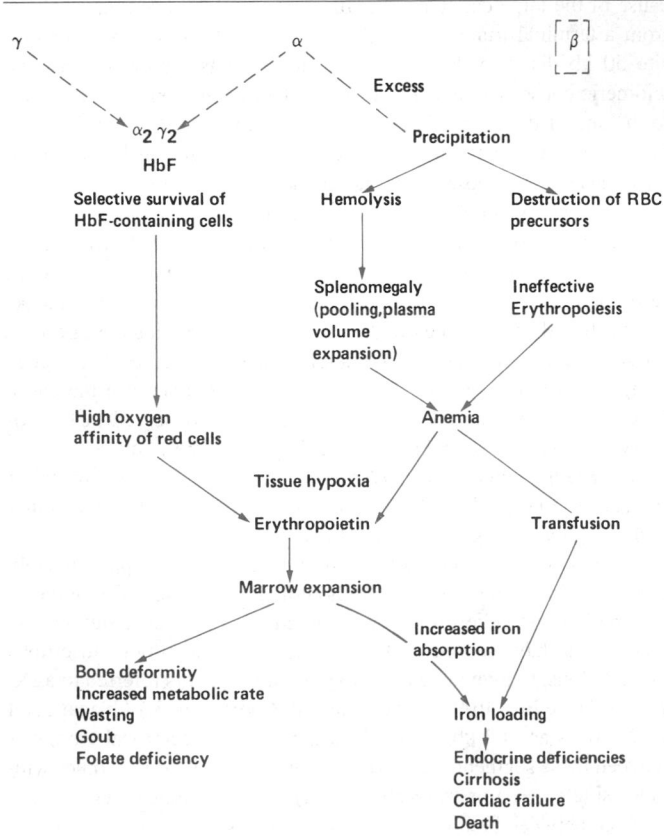

FIGURE 46-13 Pathophysiology of β-thalassemia.

mer, so the chains precipitate in red cell precursors. The resulting inclusion bodies can be demonstrated by both light and electron microscopy.[169,170] In the marrow, precipitation can be seen in the earliest hemoglobinized precursors and through the erythroid maturation pathway.[171] These large inclusions are responsible for intramedullary destruction of red cell precursors and hence for the ineffective erythropoiesis characterizing all the β-thalassemias. A large proportion of the developing erythroblasts are destroyed within the marrow in severe cases.[172] Any red cells that are released are prematurely destroyed by mechanisms that are considered below in "Mechanisms of Erythroid Precursor and Red Cell Damage." β-Thalassemia heterozygotes also have imbalanced globin-chain synthesis, but the magnitude of α-chain excess is much less and presumably can be resolved by the proteolytic enzymes of the red cell precursors.[173] Notwithstanding, a mild degree of ineffective erythropoiesis occurs.

MECHANISMS OF ERYTHROID PRECURSOR AND RED CELL DAMAGE

Damage to the red cell membrane by the globin-chain precipitation process occurs by two major routes: generation of hemichromes from excess α chains with subsequent structural damage to the red cell membrane, and similar damage mediated through the degradation products of excess α chains.[7,174–176] The degradation products of free α chains—globin, heme, hemin (oxidized heme), and free iron—also play a role in damaging red cell membranes. Excess globin chains bind to different membrane proteins and alter their structure and function. Excess iron, by generating oxygen free radicals, damages several red cell membrane components (including lipids and protein) and intracellular organelles. Heme and its products can catalyze the formation of a variety of reactive oxygen species that can damage the red cell membrane. These changes are reflected in an increased rate of apoptosis of red cell precursors.[177] The red cells are rigid and underhydrated, leak potassium, and have increased levels of calcium and low, unstable levels of ATP. Damage to the red cells can be mediated by the presence of rigid inclusion bodies during passage of the red cells through the spleen.

The anemia of β-thalassemia has three major components. First and most important is ineffective erythropoiesis with intramedullary destruction of a variable proportion of the developing red cell precursors. Second is hemolysis resulting from destruction of mature red cells containing α-chain inclusions. Third are hypochromic and microcytic red cells resulting from the overall reduction in hemoglobin synthesis.

Because the primary defect in β-thalassemia involves β-chain production, synthesis of hemoglobins F and A_2 should be unaffected. Fetal hemoglobin production *in utero* is normal. The clinical manifestations of thalassemia appear only when the neonatal switch from γ- to β-chain production occurs. However, fetal hemoglobin synthesis persists beyond the neonatal period in nearly all forms of β-thalassemia (see "Persistent Fetal Hemoglobin Production and Cellular Heterogeneity," below). β-Thalassemia heterozygotes have an elevated level of hemoglobin A_2. The elevated level appears to reflect not only a relative decrease in hemoglobin A as a result of defective β-chain synthesis but also an absolute increase in the output of δ chains both *cis* and *trans* to the mutant β-globin gene.[7]

The consequences of excess non–α-chain production in the α-thalassemias are quite different. Because α chains are shared by both fetal and adult hemoglobin (see Chaps. 6 and 47), defective α-chain production is manifest in both fetal and adult life. In the fetus, it leads to excess γ-chain production; in the adult, to an excess of β chains. Excess γ chains form γ_4 homotetramers or hemoglobin Bart's[178]; excess β chains form β_4 homotetramers or hemoglobin H.[179] The fact that γ and β chains form homotetramers is the reason for the funda-

mental difference in the pathophysiology of α- and β-thalassemia. Because γ_4 and β_4 tetramers are soluble, they do not precipitate to any significant degree in the marrow, and therefore the α-thalassemias are not characterized by severe ineffective erythropoiesis. However, β_4 tetramers precipitate as red cells age, with the formation of inclusion bodies. Thus, the anemia of the more severe forms of α-thalassemia in the adult results from a shortened survival of red cells consequent to their damage in the microvasculature of the spleen as a result of the presence of the inclusions. In addition, because of the defect in hemoglobin synthesis, the cells are hypochromic and microcytic. Hemoglobin Bart's is more stable than hemoglobin H and does not form large inclusions.

Although, as is the case in β-thalassemia, excess globin chains cause damage to the red cell membrane, the mechanisms are different in the two forms of the disease. As we saw in "Etiology and Pathogenesis," in β-thalassemia, excess α chains result in mechanical instability and oxidative damage to a variety of membrane proteins, notably protein 4.1. However, in α-thalassemia, the membranes are hyperstable, and no evidence of oxidation or dysfunction of this protein is present. Furthermore, the state of red cell hydration is different in α-thalassemia. Accumulation of excess β chains results in increased hydration. These differences in the pathophysiology of membrane damage between α- and β-thalassemia are discussed in detail in refs. 4 and 174–176.

Another factor exacerbates the tissue hypoxia of the anemia of the α-thalassemias. Both hemoglobin Bart's and hemoglobin H show no heme–heme interaction and have almost hyperbolic oxygen dissociation curves with very high oxygen affinities. Thus, they are not able to liberate oxygen at physiologic tissue tensions; in effect, they are useless as oxygen carriers.[7]

As a consequence, infants with high levels of hemoglobin Bart's have severe intrauterine hypoxia. This is the major basis for the clinical picture of homozygous α^0-thalassemia, which results in the stillbirth of hydropic infants late in pregnancy or at term. Oxygen deprivation is reflected by the grossly hydropic state of the infant, presumably as a result of increased capillary permeability, and by severe erythroblastosis. Deficient fetal oxygenation probably is responsible for the enormously hypertrophied placentas and possibly for the associated developmental abnormalities that occur with the severe forms of intrauterine α-thalassemia.[7]

PERSISTENT FETAL HEMOGLOBIN PRODUCTION AND CELLULAR HETEROGENEITY

Children with severe thalassemia have an increased level of hemoglobin F that persists into childhood and later.[7,10] In the β^0-thalassemias, hemoglobin F is the only hemoglobin produced, except for small amounts of hemoglobin A_2. Examination of the blood using staining methods specific for hemoglobin F shows that it is heterogeneously distributed among the red cells.[7] Persistent hemoglobin F production is not a major feature of the more severe forms of α-thalassemia.

The mechanism of persistent γ-chain synthesis in the thalassemias is incompletely understood. Normal adults have small quantities of hemoglobin F that are heterogeneously distributed among the red cells. Cells with demonstrable hemoglobin F are called *F cells*. One important mechanism for high hemoglobin F levels in the blood of patients with β-thalassemia is cell selection.[7,180–184] The major cause of ineffective erythropoiesis and shortened red cell survival in β-thalassemia is the deleterious effect of excess α chains on erythroid maturation in the marrow and on the survival of red cells in the blood. Therefore, red cell precursors that produce γ chains are at a selective advantage. Excess α chains combine with γ chains to produce hemoglobin F; therefore, the magnitude of α-chain precipitation is less. Differential centrifugation experiments[164] and *in vivo* labeling studies[180] have shown that populations of red cells with relatively large amounts of hemoglobin F are more efficiently produced and survive longer in the blood. The blood of patients with homozygous β-thalassemia shows remarkable cellular heterogeneity with respect to red cell survival, such as populations of cells containing predominantly hemoglobin F that are destroyed very rapidly in the spleen and elsewhere, cells with a much longer survival that contain relatively more hemoglobin F, and populations of intermediate age and hemoglobin constitution.[7,182]

Although cell selection of this type is the main mechanism for persistent γ-chain production in β-thalassemia,[183,184] an absolute increase in hemoglobin F production is possible in some cases. This process is seen in some milder forms of homozygous β^0-thalassemia, but in these cases other genetic factors are responsible for the relatively high level of γ-chain synthesis (see above in "Mechanisms of Eythroid Precursor and Red Cell Damage"). However, biosynthesis studies indicate that marrow expansion and the selective survival of F-cell precursors and their progeny are the major factors in hemoglobin F production in hemoglobin E/β-thalassemia.[183]

Because a reciprocal relation exists between γ- and δ-chain synthesis, the red cells of β-thalassemia homozygotes containing large amounts of hemoglobin F have relatively low hemoglobin A_2 levels.[7] Thus, the measured percent hemoglobin A_2 in these individuals is the average of a very heterogeneous cell population. This finding probably accounts for the extreme variability in hemoglobin A_2 levels found in homozygotes for this disorder. A further consequence of the persistence of hemoglobin F in β-thalassemia is the high oxygen affinity of the red cells.

CONSEQUENCES OF COMPENSATORY MECHANISMS FOR THE ANEMIA OF THALASSEMIA

The profound anemia of homozygous β-thalassemia and the high oxygen affinity of the blood produced combine to cause severe tissue hypoxia. Because of the high oxygen affinity of hemoglobins Bart's and H, a similar defect in tissue oxygenation occurs in the more severe forms of α-thalassemia. The major response is erythropoietin production and expansion of the dyserythropoietic marrow. The results are deformities of the skull and face and porosity of the long bones.[7] Extramedullary hematopoietic tumors may develop in extreme cases. Apart from the production of severe skeletal deformities, marrow expansion may cause pathologic fractures and sinus and middle ear infection as a result of ineffective drainage.

Another important effect of the enormous expansion of the marrow mass is the diversion of calories required for normal development to the ineffective red cell precursors. Thus, patients severely affected by thalassemia show poor development and wasting. The massive turnover of erythroid precursors may result in secondary hyperuricemia and gout and severe folate deficiency.

The effects of gross intrauterine hypoxia in homozygous α^0-thalassemia have been described. In the symptomatic forms of α-thalassemia (e.g., hemoglobin H disease) that are compatible with survival into adult life, bone changes and other consequences of erythroid expansion are seen, although less commonly than in β-thalassemia.

SPLENOMEGALY: DILUTIONAL ANEMIA

Constant exposure of the spleen to red cells with inclusions consisting of precipitated globin chains gives rise to the phenomenon of "work hypertrophy." Progressive splenomegaly occurs in both α- and β-thalassemia and may worsen the anemia.[7,10,185] A large spleen acts as a sump for red cells, sequestering a considerable proportion of the red cell mass. Furthermore, splenomegaly may cause plasma volume expansion, a complication that can be exacerbated by massive expansion of the erythroid marrow. The combination of pooling of the red cells in the spleen and plasma volume expansion can exacerbate the anemia

in both α- and β-thalassemia. The same process can occur in an enlarged liver, particularly after splenectomy.

ABNORMAL IRON METABOLISM

β-Thalassemia homozygotes who are anemic manifest increased intestinal iron absorption that is related to the degree of expansion of the red cell precursor population. Iron absorption is decreased by blood transfusion.[10,185] Increased absorption causes a steady accumulation of iron, first in the Kupffer cells of the liver and the macrophages of the spleen and later in the parenchymal cells of the liver (see Chap. 40). Most patients homozygous for β-thalassemia require regular blood transfusion; thus, transfusional siderosis adds to the iron accumulation. Iron accumulates in the endocrine glands,[7,186,187] particularly in the parathyroids, pituitary, pancreas, liver, and, most important, in the myocardium.[7,188] Iron accumulation in the myocardium leads to death by involving the conducting tissues or by causing intractable cardiac failure. Other consequences of iron loading include diabetes, hypoparathyroidism, hypothyroidism, and abnormalities of hypothalamic-pituitary function leading to growth retardation and hypogonadism.[7,186,187]

More accurate information now is available regarding the levels of body iron, as reflected by hepatic iron, at which patients are at risk for serious complications of iron overload.[7,189] These studies, which extrapolate data obtained from patients with genetic hemochromatosis, suggest that patients with hepatic iron levels of approximately 80 μmol of iron per gram of liver, wet weight ($\approx$15 mg of iron per gram of liver, dry weight), are at increased risk for hepatic disease and endocrine organ damage. Patients with higher body iron burdens are at particular risk for cardiac disease and early death.

Disordered iron metabolism is less common in the adult forms of α-thalassemia. The reason is not clear, but the milder degree of anemia, fewer transfusions, and the less marked erythroid expansion of the marrow are likely explanations.

All forms of severe thalassemia appear to be associated with an increased susceptibility to bacterial infection.[7,186,190] The reason is not known. The relatively high serum iron levels may favor bacterial growth. Another possible mechanism is blockade of the monocyte-macrophage system as a result of the increased rate of destruction of red cells. No consistent defects in white cell or immune function have been reported, and high serum iron levels as an important factor remain to be unequivocally demonstrated. The one exception is infection with *Yersinia enterocolitica*, a normally nonvirulent pathogen that can produce its own siderophore and hence can thrive in iron excess.

COAGULATION DEFECTS

The increasing knowledge about the potential hypercoagulable state in some forms of thalassemia has been reviewed in detail.[174–176] Evidence indicates that patients, particularly after splenectomy and with high platelet counts, may develop progressive pulmonary arterial disease as a result of platelet aggregation in the pulmonary circulation. Furthermore, using thalassemic red cells as a source of phospholipids, enhanced thrombin generation has been demonstrated in a thrombinase assay. The procoagulant effect of thalassemia cells appears to result from increased expression of anionic phospholipids on the red cell surface. Normally, neutral or negatively charged phospholipids are confined to the inner leaflet of the red cell membrane, an effect that is mediated by the action of aminophospholipid translocase, an enzyme sometimes known as flipase. In effect, this enzyme flips aminophospholipids that are diffused to the outer leaflet back to the inner leaflet (see Chap. 44). The current belief is that these aminophospholipids in thalassemic red cells are moved to the outer leaflet, thus providing a surface on which coagulation can be activated. Other nonspecific changes in the coagulation pathway and its antagonists have been observed in patients with different forms of thalassemia.

CLINICAL HETEROGENEITY

The pathophysiologic mechanisms described above provide the basis for the remarkably diverse clinical findings in the thalassemia syndromes.[7,191] All the manifestations of β-thalassemia can be related to excess α-chain production. Thus, any mechanism that reduces the excess of α chains should reduce the clinical severity of the disease. Several elegant "experiments of nature" have shown that this reasoning is true and, incidentally, have confirmed that globin-chain imbalance is the major factor determining the severity of the thalassemias.

Co-inheritance of α-thalassemia can reduce the severity of the more severe forms of β-thalassemia.[192–194] The effect is much more marked in individuals who are homozygotes or compound heterozygotes for different forms of β^+-thalassemia. β^0-thalassemia homozygotes who have inherited α-thalassemia seem to be protected little, if at all.

Severe β-thalassemia can be modified by the co-inheritance of genetic determinants for enhanced production of γ chains. Interaction of the heterocellular HPFH in the amelioration of homozygous β-thalassemia has been mentioned. Other determinants also may be involved. For example, inheritance of a particular RFLP haplotype in the region 5' to the β-globin gene may be an important factor.[184,195,196] This particular β-globin gene haplotype is associated with a single base change, C→T, at position −158 relative to the $^G\gamma$-globin gene, an alteration that creates a cleavage site for the restriction enzyme Xmn I.[121] An excess of individuals homozygous for T (XmnI++) with the phenotype of thalassemia intermedia exist compared with thalassemia major in different populations.[196,197] Whether this polymorphism is the only factor that increases hemoglobin F production in these cases is not absolutely clear. However, the association certainly points to an effect *cis* to the affected β gene as the basis for elevated fetal hemoglobin levels in these forms of thalassemia intermedia. Several varieties of heterocellular HPFH also can be co-inherited with β-thalassemia, leading to milder phenotypes.[4,125–127]

Some mutations that cause β-thalassemia are associated with a mild phenotype because they result in only modest reduction of β-chain production.[7] For example, mutations at positions −29 and −88 are associated with mild β^+-thalassemia in Africans. Similarly, particularly mild phenotypes are commonly found with a base substitution at position 6 in IVS-1 and at position −87 in the 5'-flanking region of the β-globin gene in Mediterranean populations. The homozygous state for the IVS-1 position 6 mutation usually produces an extremely mild form of β-thalassemia. When these "mild" mutations are co-inherited with more severe β-thalassemia determinants, the compound heterozygous states are characterized by a more severe form of thalassemia intermedia. Other forms of thalassemia intermedia are associated with the homozygous state for $\delta\beta$-thalassemia, the various interactions of $\delta\beta$-thalassemia with β-thalassemia, and heterozygous β-thalassemia of the severe variety or in association with triplicated α-gene loci.[7,10,198] These complex interactions are the subject of several extensive reviews.[198–200]

These mechanisms for the phenotypic variability of the β-thalassemias represent only the tip of the iceberg of the genetic diversity of these conditions. Hence, defining a series of genetic modifiers that act at different levels is useful. Primary modifiers represent the diversity of mutations at the β-globin gene locus. Secondary modifiers are those, such as α-thalassemia and increased hemoglobin F production, that directly modify the relative degree of the imbalanced globin chain output. However, an increasing number of tertiary modifiers, that is, genetic diversity, have an important effect on the complications of the disease. These include loci involved in iron, bone, and bilirubin metabolism and in determining resistance of susceptibility to infection. Furthermore, phenotypic diversity may reflect different degrees of adaptation to anemia and the effect of the environment. These complex

issues have been reviewed[191] and are illustrated in Fig. 46-14. Several more extensive reviews of the pathophysiology of the intermediate forms of β-thalassemia in different populations are available.[199,200]

The α-thalassemias, particularly hemoglobin H disease, show considerable clinical diversity. Some of this variability can be related to particular genotypes,[7,130,131] but the reasons for the heterogeneity of these disorders is not clear.

CLINICAL FEATURES

β- AND $\delta\beta$-THALASSEMIAS

The most clinically severe form of β-thalassemia is thalassemia major. A milder clinical picture, characterized by a later onset and either no transfusion requirement or at least fewer transfusions than are required to treat the major form of the illnesses, is designated β-*thalassemia intermedia*. β-*Thalassemia minor* is the term used to describe the heterozygous carrier state for β-thalassemia. More extensive accounts of the clinical features of these conditions are given in two monographs.[7,9]

β-THALASSEMIA MAJOR

The homozygous or compound heterozygous state for β-thalassemia, thalassemia major, produces the clinical picture first described by Cooley and Lee[1] in 1925. Affected infants are well at birth. Anemia usually develops during the first few months of life and becomes progressively more severe. The infants fail to thrive and may have feeding problems, bouts of fever, diarrhea, and other gastrointestinal symptoms. The majority of infants who develop transfusion-dependent homozygous β-thalassemia present with these symptoms within the first year of life. A later onset suggests the condition will develop into one of the intermediate forms of β-thalassemia (see "Pathophysiology," above).

The course of the disease in childhood depends almost entirely on whether the child is maintained on an adequate transfusion program.[7,9]

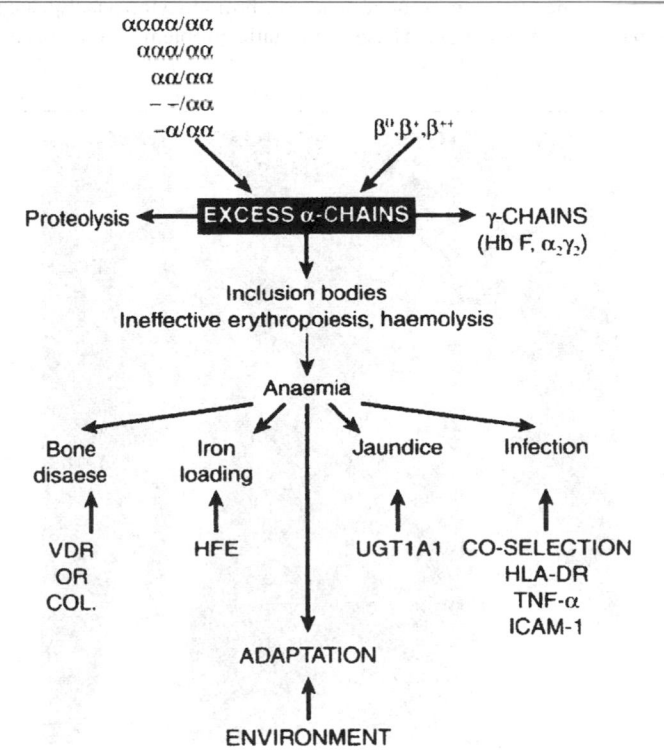

FIGURE 46-14 Different levels of modification of the β-thalassemia phenotype. (Adapted from refs. 7 and 191.)

The classic textbook picture of Cooley's anemia describes the disease as it was seen before these children could be maintained with relatively normal hemoglobin levels by regular blood transfusions. If adequate transfusion is possible, children grow and develop normally and have no abnormal physical signs. Few of the complications of the disorder occur during childhood. The disease presents a problem only when the effects of iron loading resulting from ineffective erythropoiesis and from repeated blood transfusions become apparent at the end of the first decade. Children who are treated with an adequate iron chelation regimen develop normally, although some of them remain short in height.

An inadequately transfused child develops the typical features of Cooley's anemia. Growth is stunted. With bossing of the skull and overgrowth of the maxillary region, the face gradually assumes a "mongoloid" appearance. These changes are associated with a characteristic radiologic appearance of the skull, long bones, and hands (Fig. 46-15). The diploe widens, with a "hair on end" or "sun ray" appearance and a lacy trabeculation of the long bones and phalanges. Gross skeletal deformities can occur. The liver and spleen are enlarged, and the pigmentation of the skin increases. Many features of a hypermetabolic state, as evidence by fever, wasting, and hyperuricemia, may develop.

The clinical course is characterized by severe anemia with frequent complications. These children are particularly prone to infection, which is a common cause of death. Spontaneous fractures occur commonly as a result of the expansion of the marrow cavities with thinning of the long bones and skull. Maxillary deformities often lead to dental problems from malocclusion. Formation of massive deposits of extramedullary hematopoietic tissue may cause neurologic complications. With the gross splenomegaly that may occur, secondary thrombocytopenia and leukopenia frequently develop, leading to a further tendency to infection and bleeding. Splenectomy is frequently performed to reduce transfusion frequency and severe thrombocytopenia; however, postsplenectomy infections are particularly common.[7] Bleeding tendency may be seen in the absence of thrombocytopenia. Epistaxis is particularly common. These hemostatic problems are associated

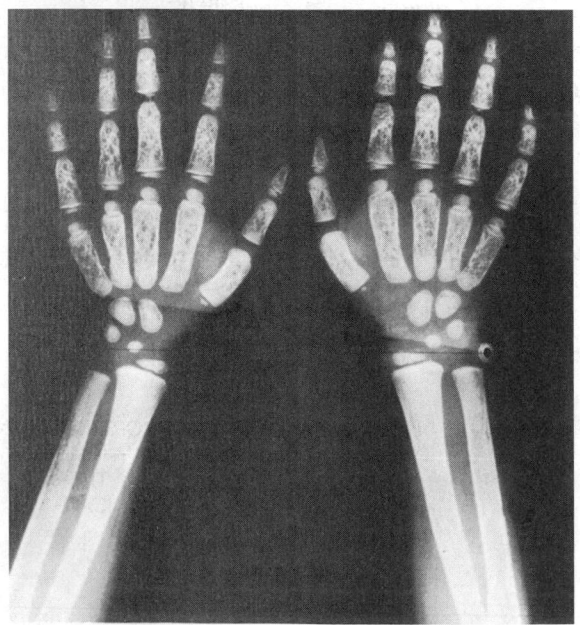

FIGURE 46-15 Radiologic appearances of the hands in homozygous β-thalassemia.

with poor liver function in some cases. Chronic leg ulceration may occur but is more common in thalassemia intermedia.

Children who have grown and developed normally throughout the first 10 years of life as a result of regular blood transfusion begin to develop the symptoms of iron loading as they enter puberty, particularly if they have not received adequate iron chelation.[167] The first indication of iron loading usually is the absence of the pubertal growth spurt and failure of the menarche. Over the succeeding years, a variety of endocrine disturbances may develop, particularly diabetes mellitus, hypogonadotrophic hypogonadism, and growth hormone deficiency. Hypothyroidism and adrenal insufficiency also occur but are less common.[4,185] Toward the end of the second decade, cardiac complications arise, and death usually occurs in the second or third decade as a result of cardiac siderosis.[4,186] Cardiac siderosis may cause an acute cardiac death with arrhythmia, or intractable cardiac failure. Both of these complications can be precipitated by intercurrent infection.

Even the adequately transfused child who has received chelation therapy may suffer a number of complications. Bloodborne infection, notably with hepatitis C[201] or HIV,[202] or malaria[203] is extremely common in some populations, although the frequency is decreasing with the use of widespread blood-donor screening programs. Delayed puberty and growth retardation are common and probably reflect hypogonadotrophic hypogonadism and damage to the pituitary gland.[201,204] Osteoporosis is being recognized increasingly and may, at least in part, be a reflection of hypogonadism.[201]

β-THALASSEMIA INTERMEDIA

The clinical phenotype of patients designated as having thalassemia intermedia is more severe than the usual asymptomatic thalassemia trait but milder than transfusion-dependent thalassemia major.[7,199,200] The syndrome encompasses disorders with a wide spectrum of disability. At the severe end, patients present with anemia later than patients with the transfusion-dependent forms of homozygous β-thalassemia and are just able to maintain a hemoglobin level of approximately 6 g/dl without transfusion. However, their growth and development are retarded. The patients become seriously disabled, with marked skeletal deformities, arthritis, and bone pain; progressive splenomegaly; growth retardation; and chronic ulcerations above the ankles. At the other end of the spectrum, patients remain completely asymptomatic until adult life and are transfusion independent, with hemoglobin levels as high as 10 to 12 g/dl. All varieties of intermediate severity are observed. Some patients become disabled simply from the effects of hypersplenism. Intensive studies of the molecular pathology of this condition have provided some guidelines about genotype–phenotype relationships that are useful for genetic counseling (Table 46-6).

Overall, the clinical features of the intermediate forms of β-thalassemia are similar to the features of β-thalassemia major. At the severe end of the spectrum, particularly in cases of growth retardation, patients should be treated with regular transfusion. However, a number of important complications, including progressive hypersplenism, occur in patients with milder forms. Clinically significant iron loading as a result of increased absorption is seen even in patients with infrequent transfusions (see Chap. 40). Iron overload results in frequent diabetes and endocrine disturbances, typically by fourth decade of life. A high incidence of pigment gallstones, skeletal deformities, bone and joint disease, leg ulcers, and thrombotic tendency, particularly after splenectomy, is observed.[7]

Hematologists should be aware that in patients heterozygous for rare forms of β-thalassemia, a phenotype of thalassemia intermedia that results in the clinical constellation of autosomal dominant thalassemia (discussed above in "Pathophysiology") is encountered on rare occasions.

TABLE 46-6   GENOTYPES OF PATIENTS WITH β-THALASSEMIA INTERMEDIA

Mild forms of β-thalassemia

  Homozygosity for mild β^+-thalassemia alleles

  Compound heterozygosity for two mild β^+-thalassemia alleles

  Compound heterozygosity for a "silent" or mild and more severe β-thalassemia allele

Inheritance of α- and β-thalassemia

  β^+-Thalassemia with α^0-thalassemia ($- -/\alpha\alpha$) or α^+-thalassemia($-\alpha/\alpha\alpha$ or $-\alpha/-\alpha$)

  β^+-Thalassemia with genotype of Hb H disease ($- -/-\alpha$)

β-Thalassemia with elevated γ-chain synthesis

  Homozygous β-thalassemia with heterocellular HPFH

  Homozygous β-thalassemia with homozygous $^G\gamma$ 158 T$\rightarrow$C change (some cases)

  Compound heterozygosity for β-thalassemia and deletion forms of HPFH

Compound heterozygosity for β-thalassemia and β-chain variants

  Hb E/β-thalassemia

  Other interactions with rare β-chain variants

Heterozygous β-thalassemia with triplicated or quadruplicated α-chain genes ($\alpha\alpha\alpha$ or $\alpha\alpha\alpha\alpha$)

Dominant forms of β-thalassemia

Interactions of β- and $(\delta\beta)^+$- or $(\delta\beta)^0$-thalassemia

---

β-THALASSEMIA MINOR

The heterozygous state for β-thalassemia is asymptomatic and not usually associated with any clinical disability. The abnormality is discovered only when blood examination is performed or during family studies of more severely affected relatives. The abnormality is most commonly discovered during periods of unrelated clinical situations, such as pregnancy or during severe infection, or on routine laboratory testing when a moderate degree of anemia with microcytosis may be found. Some patients with thalassemia minor have increased iron stores, but often this condition results from injudicious iron therapy initiated because of misdiagnosed microcytic anemia. Accurate diagnosis by an experienced physician will preclude unnecessary tests, expense, inconvenience, and erroneous diagnosis of this essentially laboratory abnormality.

α-THALASSEMIAS

HEMOGLOBIN BART'S HYDROPS FETALIS SYNDROME

This disorder is a frequent cause of stillbirth in Southeast Asia. Infants either are stillborn between 34 and 40 weeks' gestation or are born alive but die within the first few hours.[205,206] Pallor, edema, and hepatosplenomegaly are seen. The clinical picture resembles hydrops fetalis as a result of Rh blood group incompatibility. Massive extramedullary hemopoiesis and enlargement of the placenta are noted at autopsy. A variety of congenital anomalies have been observed.

The rescue of a few infants with this syndrome by prenatal detection and exchange transfusion has been reported. These babies have grown and developed normally, although they are blood transfusion dependent.[207,208]

This condition is associated with a high incidence of maternal toxemia of pregnancy and difficulties at the time of delivery because of the massive placenta.[205,206] The reason for placental hypertrophy is unknown, although severe intrauterine hypoxia is suspected because a similar phenomenon is observed in hydrops infants with Rh incompatibility.

HEMOGLOBIN H DISEASE

Hemoglobin H disease was described independently in the United States and in Greece in 1956.[209,210] The clinical findings are variable.

A few patients are affected almost as severely as patients with β-thalassemia major, but most patients have a much milder course.[7,211] Lifelong anemia with variable splenomegaly occurs; bone changes are unusual.

As discussed earlier in "Etiology and Pathogenesis," a few attempts have been made to correlate the genotype with the phenotype of hemoglobin H disease. In general, as expected, patients with a nondeletion form of α-thalassemia affecting the predominant $\alpha2$ gene interacting with an α^0-thalassemia determinant ($- -/\alpha^T\alpha$), $- -/\alpha^{\text{Constant Spring}}\alpha$, for example, have higher hemoglobin H levels, a greater degree of anemia, and, anecdotally, a more severe clinical course than patients with the $- -/-\alpha$ genotype.[212–215]

MILDER FORMS OF α-THALASSEMIA, INCLUDING THE TRAITS

Because two α-globin genes exist per haploid genome, a wide spectrum of different conditions with overlapping phenotypes result from their various interactions.[7] The carrier states for the deletion and nondeletion forms of α-thalassemia, $-\alpha/\alpha\alpha$ and $\alpha^T/\alpha/\alpha\alpha$, are symptomless. Similarly, the homozygous states for the deletion forms of α^+-thalassemia, $-\alpha/-\alpha$, and the heterozygous state for α^0-thalassemia, $- -/\alpha\alpha$, are symptomless, although they are associated with mild anemia and red cell changes. On the other hand, the homozygous states for the nondeletion forms of α-thalassemia, $\alpha^T\alpha/\alpha^T\alpha$, are associated with an extremely diverse series of phenotypes. As mentioned in "Interactions of α-Thalassemia Haplotypes" above in "Etiology and Pathogenesis," they sometimes result in the clinical picture of hemoglobin H disease. In other patients, they are associated with only mild hypochromic anemia.[7] The homozygous states for the chain termination mutants, notably hemoglobin Constant Spring, constitute a special case because they produce a particularly characteristic phenotype. In this case, moderate hemolytic anemia with splenomegaly and characteristic hematologic findings are seen.[7,216,217]

α-THALASSEMIA AND MENTAL RETARDATION

The clinical phenotype of these conditions associated with an intact α-globin locus is heterogeneous. In cases associated with chromosomal deletion (tip of chromosome 16; ATR-16), the clinical defects vary with the extent of chromosomal defect; only α-thalassemia and mental retardation are constant.

The clinical phenotype in the second group of these disorders, which are caused by mutations of ATR-X, includes skeletal abnormalities, dysmorphic face, neonatal hypotonus, genital abnormalities, and a variety of less constant features, in addition to mental retardation and α-thalassemia.

$\epsilon\gamma\delta\beta$-THALASSEMIA

The clinical picture varies with the stage of development. Neonates may be significantly anemic and require transfusions. In contrast, children and adults with this condition are asymptomatic. They have the clinical and laboratory picture of heterozygous β-thalassemia, with the exception of a normal hemoglobin A_2 level. The reason for this discrepancy of developmental differences of the clinical phenotype has not been identified.

LABORATORY FEATURES

β-THALASSEMIA MAJOR

Hemoglobin levels at presentation may range from 2 to 3 g/dl or even lower.[7,9] The red cells show marked anisopoikilocytosis, with hypochromia, target cell formation, and a variable degree of basophilic stippling (Fig. 46-16). The appearance of the blood film varies, depending on whether the spleen is intact. In nonsplenectomized patients, large poikilocytes are common. After splenectomy, large, flat macrocytes and small, deformed microcytes are frequently seen. The reticulocyte count is moderately elevated, and nucleated red cells nearly always are present in the blood. These red cell forms may reach very high levels after splenectomy. The white cell and platelet counts are slightly elevated unless secondary hypersplenism occurs. Staining of the blood with methyl violet, particularly in splenectomized subjects, reveals stippling or ragged inclusion bodies in the red cells.[169] These inclusions can nearly always be found in the red cell precursors in the marrow (Fig. 46-17). The marrow usually shows erythroid hyperplasia with morphologic abnormalities of the erythroblasts, such as striking basophilic stippling and increased iron deposition. Iron kinetic studies indicate markedly ineffective erythropoiesis, and red cell survival usually is shortened. Populations of cells with very short survival and longer-lived populations of cells are seen. The latter contain relatively more fetal hemoglobin. An increased level of fetal hemoglobin, ranging from less than 10 percent to greater than 90 percent, is characteristic of homozygous β-thalassemia. No hemoglobin A is produced in β^0-thalassemia. The acid elution test shows that fetal hemoglobin is heterogeneously distributed among the red cells. Hemoglobin A_2 levels in homozygous β-thalassemia may be low, normal, or high. However, expressed as a proportion of hemoglobin A, the hemoglobin A_2 level almost invariably is elevated. Differential centrifugation studies indicate some heterogeneity of hemoglobin F and A_2 distribution among thalassemic red cells, but their level in whole blood gives little indication of their total rates of synthesis.

In vitro hemoglobin synthesis studies using marrow or blood show a marked degree of globin-chain imbalance. Marked excess of α-chain over β- and γ-chain production is always observed. Other aspects of

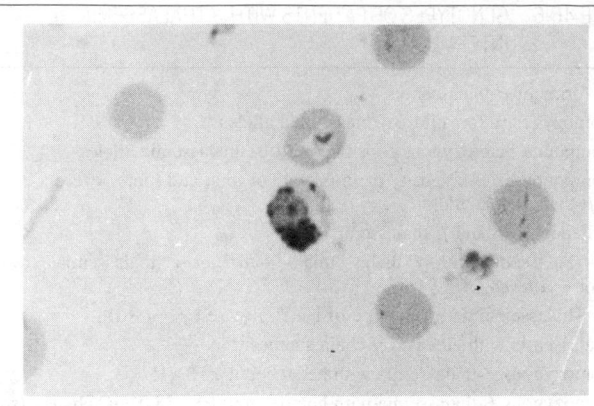

FIGURE 46-17   Red cell inclusions in peripheral blood of a homozygous β-thalassemia patient (postsplenectomy).

the laboratory findings in this condition, including red cell survival, iron absorption, ferrokinetics, erythrokinetics, and the consequences of iron loading, were discussed earlier (see "Etiology and Pathogenesis," above).

β-THALASSEMIA MINOR[7]

Hemoglobin values of patients with β-thalassemia minor usually range from 9 to 11 g/dl. The most consistent finding is small, poorly hemoglobinized red cells, resulting in MCH values of 20 to 22 pg and MCV values of 50 to 70 fl. The red cell indices are particularly useful in screening for heterozygous carriers of thalassemia in population surveys. The marrow in heterozygous β-thalassemia shows slight erythroid hyperplasia with rare red cell inclusions. Megaloblastic transformation as a result of folic acid deficiency occurs occasionally, particularly during pregnancy. A mild degree of ineffective erythropoiesis is noted, but red cell survival is normal or nearly normal. The hemoglobin A_2 level is increased to 3.5 to 7 percent. The level of fetal hemoglobin is elevated in approximately 50 percent of cases, usually to 1 to 3 percent and rarely to greater than 5 percent.

α-THALASSEMIAS[7]

HEMOGLOBIN BART'S HYDROPS FETALIS SYNDROME
In infants with the hydrops fetalis syndrome, the blood film shows severe thalassemic changes with many nucleated red cells. The hemoglobin consists mainly of hemoglobin Bart's, with approximately 10 to 20 percent hemoglobin Portland. Usually no hemoglobin A or F is present, although rare cases that seem to result from interaction of α^0-thalassemia with a severe nondeletion form of α^+-thalassemia show small amounts of hemoglobin A.

HEMOGLOBIN H DISEASE
The blood film shows hypochromia and anisopoikilocytosis. The reticulocyte count usually is approximately 5 percent. Incubation of the red cells with brilliant cresyl blue results in ragged inclusion bodies in almost all cells. These bodies form because of precipitation of hemoglobin H *in vitro* as a result of redox action of the dye. After splenectomy, large, single Heinz bodies are observed in some cells (Fig. 46-18). These bodies are formed by *in vitro* precipitation of the unstable hemoglobin H molecule and are seen only after splenectomy. Hemoglobin H constitutes between 5 and 40 percent of the total hemoglobin. Traces of hemoglobin Bart's may be present, and the hemoglobin A_2 level usually is slightly subnormal.

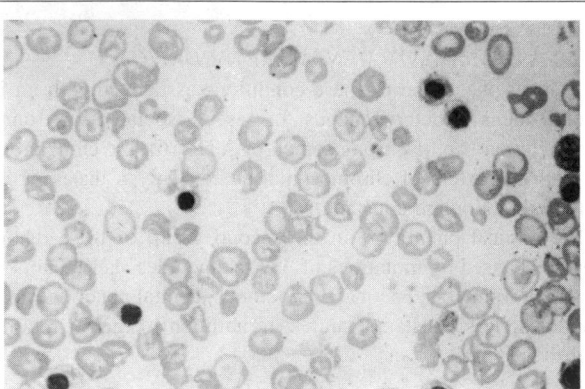

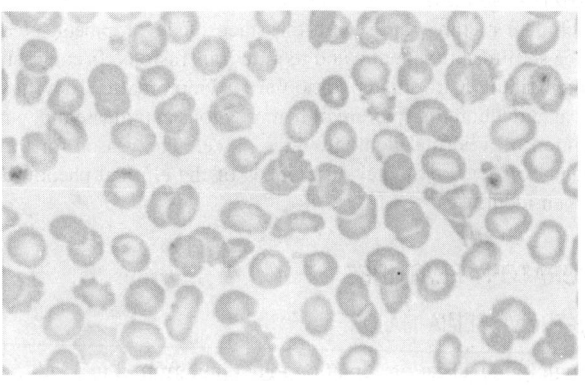

FIGURE 46-16   Blood film in homozygous β-thalassemia.

α^0-THALASSEMIA AND α^+-THALASSEMIA TRAITS

The α^0-thalassemia trait is characterized by the presence of 5 to 15 percent hemoglobin Bart's at birth.[7] This hemoglobin disappears during maturation and is not replaced by a similar amount of hemoglobin H. An occasional cell with hemoglobin H inclusion bodies may appear after incubation with brilliant cresyl blue. This phenomenon is often used as a diagnostic test for the α-thalassemia trait. However, the test is difficult to standardize and requires much experience to be useful. In adult life, the red cells of heterozygotes have morphologic changes of heterozygous thalassemia with low MCH and MCV values. The electrophoretic pattern is normal. Globin-synthesis studies show a deficit of α-chain production, with an α-/β-chain production ratio of approximately 0.7.

The α^+-thalassemia trait ($\alpha\alpha/\alpha-$) is characterized by no or minimal hematologic changes, 1 to 2 percent of hemoglobin Bart's at birth in some but not all cases, and a slightly reduced α-/β-chain production ratio of approximately 0.8; thus, this genotype often is referred to as *silent carrier*. Approximately 30 percent of African Americans carry one or two chromosomes with $-\alpha^{3.7}$ deletion,[218] so hematologists should be aware of the range of hematologic values associated with this genotype. Unfortunately, few firm data are available. However, in one study of African-American neonates, a large number of newborns with the $\alpha^{3.7}$ deletion had nondetectable hemoglobin Bart's. Globin-gene synthetic ratios can be distinguished from normal only by studying relatively large numbers of samples and comparing the mean α/β ratio with that of normal control subjects. This approach is not reliable for diagnosing individual cases of the α^+-thalassemia trait, and unfortunately no truly reliable method of diagnosis in adults is available except for DNA analysis.

Studies using DNA analysis indicate a marked overlap between the different α-thalassemia carrier states with regard to the hematologic and globin-synthesis findings (reviewed in ref. 7). In addition, the studies show that many α^+-thalassemia carriers do not have elevated levels of hemoglobin Bart's at birth. These studies confirm that, short of gene-mapping analysis, no method identifies specific α-thalassemia carrier states with certainty.

HOMOZYGOUS STATE FOR NONDELETION TYPES OF α-THALASSEMIA

The homozygous state for nondeletion forms of α-thalassemia involving the dominant ($\alpha2$) globin gene causes a more severe deficit of α chains than do the deletion forms of α^+-thalassemia. In some cases, the homozygous state produces hemoglobin H disease. The homozygous state for hemoglobin Constant Spring or other chain-termination mutations is associated with moderately severe hemolytic anemia in which, for reasons not explained, no hemoglobin H is present but small amounts of hemoglobin Bart's persist into adult life. The homozygous states for the other nondeletion forms of α^+-thalassemia are associated with hemoglobin H disease.

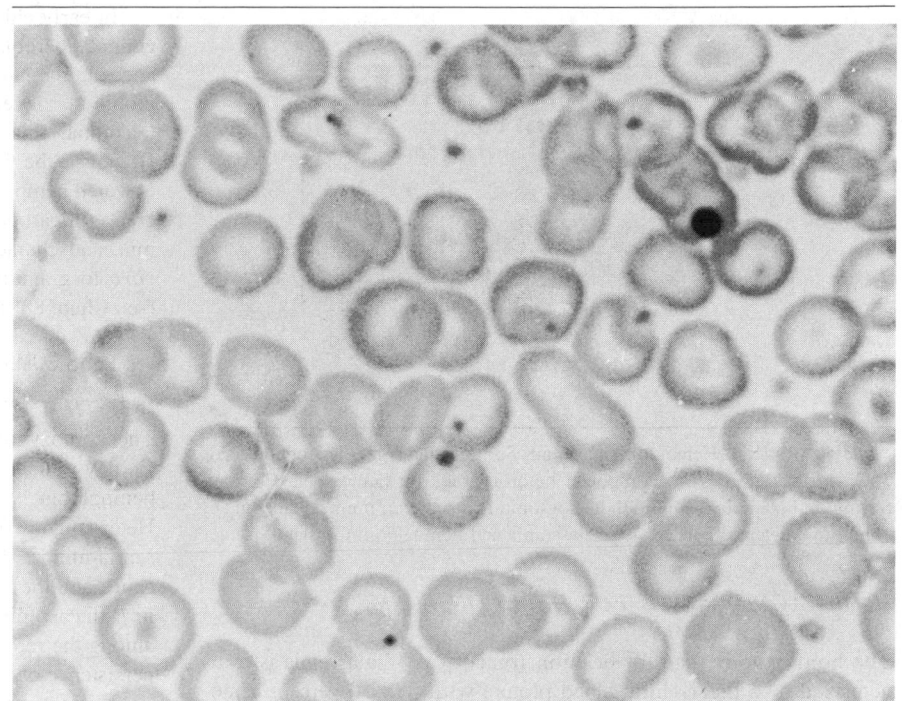

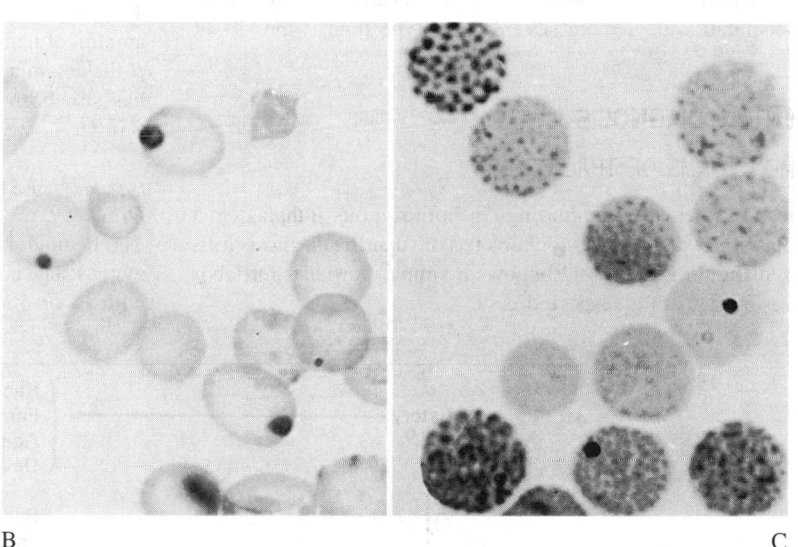

FIGURE 46-18   Hemoglobin H disease. *(A)* Blood film. *(B)* Preformed inclusions postsplenectomy. *(C)* Inclusions generated by brilliant cresyl blue.

In the homozygous state for hemoglobin Constant Spring, the blood picture shows mild thalassemic changes with normal-size red cells.[216,217] The hemoglobin consists of approximately 5 to 6 percent hemoglobin Constant Spring, normal hemoglobin A_2 levels, and trace amounts of hemoglobin Bart's. The remainder is hemoglobin A.

The heterozygous state for hemoglobin Constant Spring shows no hematologic abnormality. The hemoglobin pattern is normal except for the presence of approximately 0.5 percent hemoglobin Constant Spring. The latter can be observed on alkaline starch-gel electrophoresis as a faint band migrating between hemoglobin A_2 and the origin. It is best seen on heavily loaded starch gels and is easily missed if other electrophoretic techniques are used (Fig. 46-19). In the newborn, usually 1 to 3 percent hemoglobin Bart's is present in the cord blood.

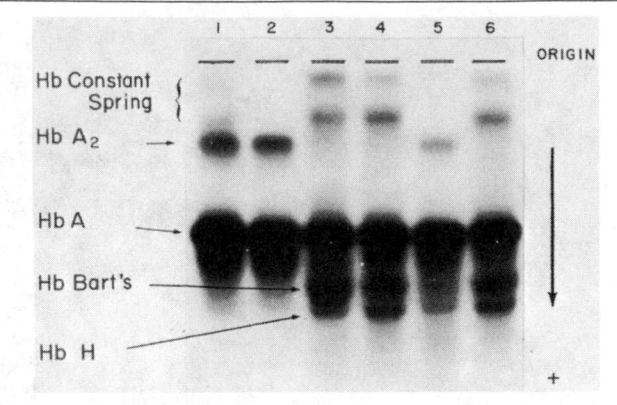

FIGURE 46-19   Hemoglobin Constant Spring. Starch gel electrophoresis of *1, 2,* normal adult; *3, 4,* compound heterozygotes for hemoglobin Constant Spring and α^0-thalassemia with hemoglobin H disease; *5,* normal adult; and *6,* compound heterozygote for α^0-thalassemia and hemoglobin Constant Spring.

HOMOZYGOUS STATE FOR DELETION FORMS OF α^+-THALASSEMIA

The homozygous state for deletion forms of α^+-thalassemia is characterized by a thalassemic blood picture with 5 to 10 percent hemoglobin Bart's at birth and hematologic findings similar to those in α^0-thalassemia heterozygotes in adult life.[141] In general, the $-\alpha^{4.2}$ deletion is associated with a more severe phenotype than is the $--^{3.7}$ deletion.[219]

DIFFERENTIAL DIAGNOSIS

COMMON FORMS OF THALASSEMIA

The clinical and hematologic findings in homozygous β-thalassemia and hemoglobin H disease are so characteristic that the diagnosis usually is not difficult. Figure 46-20 shows a simple flowchart for laboratory investigations of a suspected case.

In early childhood, distinguishing the thalassemias from the congenital sideroblastic anemias may be difficult, but the marrow appearances in the latter are quite characteristic. Because of the high hemoglobin F levels encountered in juvenile chronic myelogenous leukemia, this disorder may superficially resemble β-thalassemia. However, the finding of primitive cells in the marrow, the absence of elevated hemoglobin A_2 levels on hemoglobin electrophoresis, the decrease in carbonic anhydrase in juvenile chronic myelogenous leukemia, and characteristic *in vitro* responses of myeloid progenitors *in vitro* to granulocyte-monocyte colony stimulating factor (GM-CSF) (see Chap. 88) readily differentiate this disorder from β-thalassemia.

LESS COMMON FORMS OF THALASSEMIA

($\delta\beta)^0$-THALASSEMIA

The homozygous state for $\delta\beta$-thalassemia is clinically milder than Cooley's anemia and is one form of thalassemia intermedia.[220–222] Only hemoglobin F is present; hemoglobins A and A_2 are not produced. Heterozygous $\delta\beta$-thalassemia is hematologically similar to β-thalassemia minor.[7] The fetal hemoglobin level is higher (range 5–20 percent), and the hemoglobin A_2 value is normal or slightly reduced. As in β-thalassemia, the fetal hemoglobin is heterogeneously distributed among the red cells, thus distinguishing this disorder from hereditary persistence of fetal hemoglobin (Fig. 46-21).

Heterozygosity for both β-thalassemia and $\delta\beta$-thalassemia results in a condition clinically similar to but milder than Cooley's anemia. The hemoglobin consists largely of hemoglobin F, with a small amount of hemoglobin A_2. This finding is seen because the associated β-thalassemia gene has usually been the β^0 variety. $\delta\beta$-Thalassemia has also been observed in individuals heterozygous for hemoglobin S or C.[7]

($\delta\beta)^+$-THALASSEMIA AND HEMOGLOBIN LEPORE DISORDERS

The hemoglobin Lepore disorders have been described in the homozygous state and in the heterozygous state either alone or in association with β- or $\delta\beta$-thalassemia, hemoglobin S, or hemoglobin C.[7,9,223] In

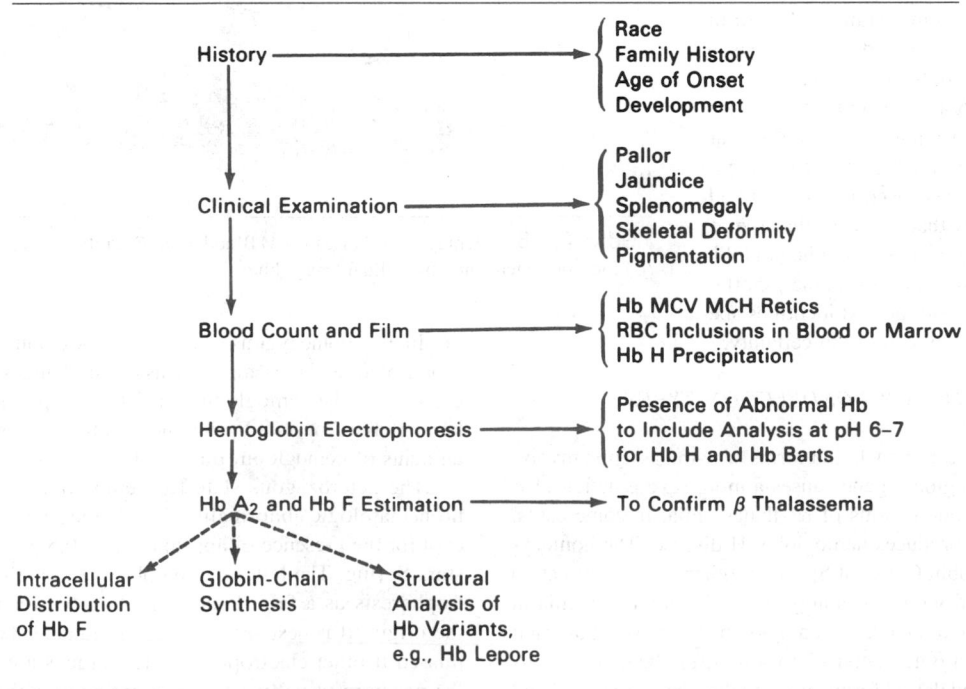

FIGURE 46-20   Flowchart showing an approach to diagnosis of the thalassemia syndromes.

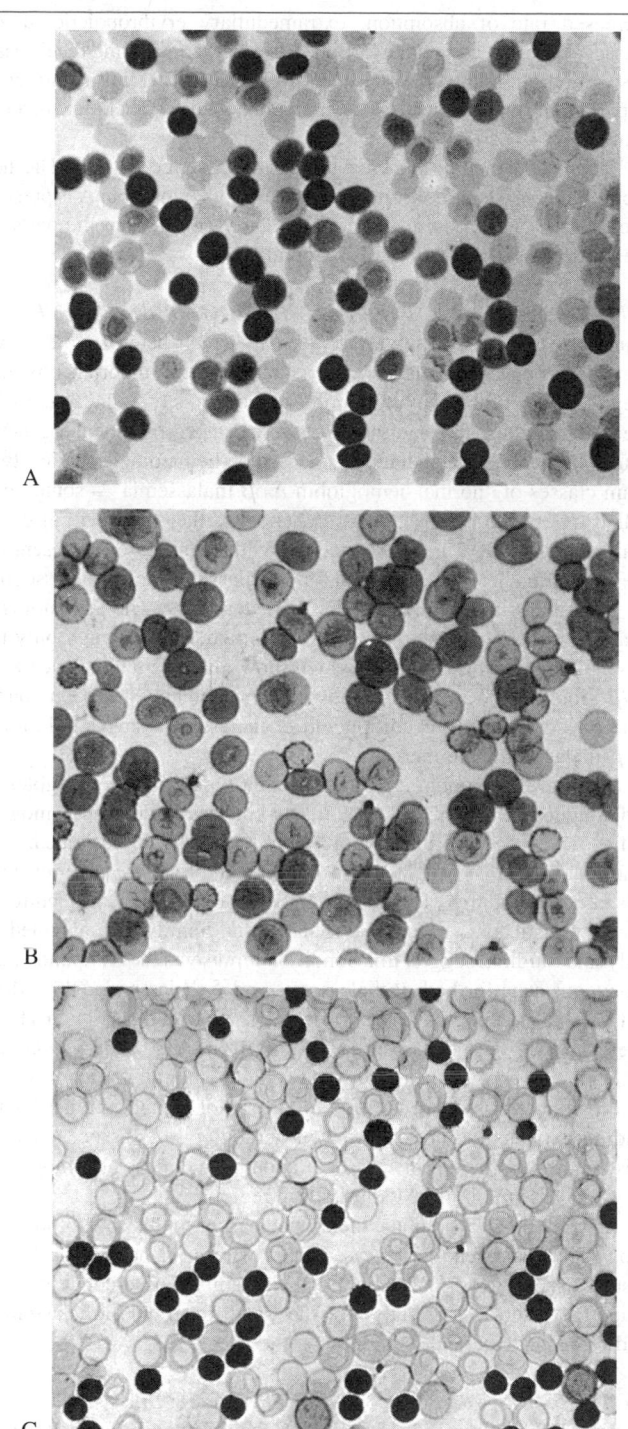

FIGURE 46-21   Acid elution preparations of blood films from *(A)* δβ-thalassemia, *(B)* hereditary persistence of fetal hemoglobin, and *(C)* artificial mixture of fetal and adult red cells.

the homozygous state, approximately 20 percent of the hemoglobin is of the Lepore type and 80 percent is fetal hemoglobin. Hemoglobins A and A_2 are absent. The clinical picture is variable. Some cases are identical to transfusion-dependent homozygous β-thalassemia; others are associated with the clinical picture of thalassemia intermedia. In the heterozygous state, the findings are similar to those of β-thalassemia minor. The hemoglobin consists of approximately 8 percent hemoglobin Lepore, with a reduced level of hemoglobin A_2 and a

slight but consistent increase in fetal hemoglobin level. The Lepore hemoglobins have been found sporadically in most racial groups. In the majority of cases, chemical analysis has shown that these hemoglobins are identical to hemoglobin Lepore Washington-Boston. Hemoglobin Lepore Hollandia and Lepore Baltimore have been observed in only a few patients.[7,223]

HEREDITARY PERSISTENCE OF FETAL HEMOGLOBIN

The current knowledge about the molecular pathology of HPFH was described earlier in "Etiology and Pathogenesis." Table 46-4 summarizes the currently accepted classification and nomenclature of this complex group of conditions. The different forms of HPFH are of very little clinical importance except that they may interact with thalassemia or the structural hemoglobin variants.

(δβ)⁰ HPFH   Homozygotes for $(\delta\beta)^0$ HPFH have 100 percent hemoglobin F. Their blood shows mild thalassemic changes with reduced MCH and MCV values very similar to those observed in heterozygous β-thalassemia. Similarly, they have imbalanced globin-chain production, with ratios in the range of those observed in β-thalassemia heterozygotes.[224] Heterozygotes have approximately 20 to 30 percent hemoglobin F, slightly reduced hemoglobin A_2 values, and completely normal blood pictures. Thus, this condition appears to be an extremely well-compensated form of δβ-thalassemia in which the output of γ chains almost but not entirely compensates for the complete absence of β and δ chains. The different molecular forms of this condition show no difference in phenotype except in the proportion of $^G\gamma$ chains. The African forms of $(\delta\beta)^0$ HPFH have been found in association with hemoglobins S and C or with β-thalassemia. These compound heterozygous states are associated with little clinical disability.[7]

Nondeletion Types of HPFH   Many nondeletion forms of HPFH associated with point mutations upstream from the γ-globin genes have been described (see Table 46-4). $^G\gamma\,\beta^+$ HPFH has been found in the heterozygous and compound heterozygous states with β-globin chain variants in African populations. No associated clinical or hematologic findings have been reported. Compound heterozygotes for $^G\gamma\,\beta^+$ HPFH and hemoglobins S or C produce 45 percent of the abnormal hemoglobin, 30 percent hemoglobin A, and 20 percent hemoglobin F containing only $^G\gamma$ chains.[225,226]

The most common form of nondeletion HPFH, $^A\gamma\,\beta^+$ HPFH, is found in Greeks.[227–229] In the homozygous state, no clinical or hematologic abnormalities are noted. The hemoglobin findings are characterized by approximately 25 percent fetal hemoglobin and reduced hemoglobin A_2 levels of approximately 0.8 percent.[230] Heterozygotes, who also are hematologically normal, have 10 to 15 percent hemoglobin F, almost all of the $^A\gamma$ variety. Compound heterozygotes with β-thalassemia have high hemoglobin F levels and a clinical picture that is only slightly more severe than the β-thalassemia trait.

In the British form of $^A\gamma\,\beta^+$ HPFH,[231] heterozygotes have approximately 5 to 12 percent hemoglobin F, whereas homozygotes have approximately 20 percent. No associated hematologic abnormalities are seen, although surprisingly in this form of nondeletion HPFH the hemoglobin F seems to be unevenly distributed among the red cells.

A heterogeneous group of conditions is associated with persistent production of small amounts of hemoglobin F in adult life. They are categorized under the general heading of *heterocellular HPFH*. Their clinical importance is that, when they are co-inherited with different forms of β-thalassemia, they may lead to greater output of hemoglobin F and hence a milder phenotype. This type of interaction should be suspected when one parent of a patient with β-thalassemia intermedia has an unusually high level of hemoglobin F for the β-thalassemia trait. Similarly, unaffected lateral relatives or other family members with slightly elevated hemoglobin F levels may be found. However, until the gene loci involved in these conditions are determined, identifying the loci with certainty is not possible.

β-THALASSEMIA ASSOCIATED WITH β-CHAIN STRUCTURAL HEMOGLOBIN VARIANTS

The most clinically important associations of β-thalassemia with β structural hemoglobin variants are sickle cell thalassemia, hemoglobin C thalassemia, and hemoglobin E thalassemia. In addition, many interactions of β-thalassemia with rare structural variants have been reported.[7,9,10]

Sickle cell thalassemia[7,232,233] occurs in parts of Africa and in the Mediterranean, particularly Greece and Italy. It also has been observed in the Middle East and parts of India. The clinical consequences of carrying one gene for hemoglobin S and one gene for β-thalassemia depend entirely on the type of β-thalassemia mutation. The interaction between the sickle cell gene and β⁰-thalassemia is characterized by a clinical disorder that is very similar to sickle cell anemia. Similarly, the interaction of the sickle cell gene with the more severe forms of β⁺-thalassemia associated with marked reduction in β-globin synthesis yields a similar clinical phenotype. On the other hand, the interaction of the sickle cell gene with very mild forms of β⁺-thalassemia may be quite innocuous.[234] The latter disorder is characterized by mild anemia associated with splenomegaly and a hemoglobin composition of approximately 60–70 percent hemoglobin S, 25 percent hemoglobin A, and an elevated level of hemoglobin A_2. In all these interactions, one parent shows the sickle cell trait, and the other parent shows the β-thalassemia trait.

Hemoglobin C thalassemia is a mild hemolytic disorder associated with splenomegaly.[7,9,10] Again, the hemoglobin pattern varies depending on whether the thalassemia gene is the β⁺ or β⁰ type. This relatively innocuous condition has been recorded mainly in North Africa, but it also is found in West Africa. It is characterized by a mild hemolytic anemia and splenomegaly with a blood picture showing the numerous target cells characteristic of all the hemoglobin C disorders.

Hemoglobin E thalassemia, which occurs at a high frequency in the eastern half of the Indian subcontinent and throughout Southeast Asia, is one of the most important hemoglobinopathies in the world population.[7,9,10,234–239] As mentioned earlier in "Etiology and Pathogenesis," hemoglobin E is synthesized at a reduced rate and hence produces the clinical phenotype of a mild form of β-thalassemia. Hence, when hemoglobin E is inherited with β-thalassemia—and most often this is a β⁰ or severe β⁺ thalassemia mutation in Southeast Asia and India—a marked deficit of β-chain production results, with the clinical picture of severe β-thalassemia. Hemoglobin E thalassemia shows a remarkable variability in clinical expression,[234,235,239] ranging from a mild form of thalassemia intermedia to a transfusion-dependent condition clinically indistinguishable from homozygous β-thalassemia. The reasons for this variability of expression are not understood, although some of the factors involved are identical to those that modify other forms of β-thalassemia.[240]

In more severe cases of hemoglobin E thalassemia, severe anemia with growth retardation, leg ulcers, bone deformity, marked tendency to infection, iron loading, and variable splenomegaly and hypersplenism are seen. Large tumor masses composed of extramedullary erythropoietic tissue may cause a variety of compression syndromes, including a clinical picture that closely mimics a cerebral tumor. Another curious picture that seems to be restricted to splenectomized patients is an obliterative occlusion of the pulmonary vasculature that is believed to result from an extremely high platelet count.[241]

The clinical course and complications in transfusion-dependent patients are similar to those observed in homozygous β-thalassemia. In the milder forms, the main complications are progressive hypersplenism, organ damage as a result of progressive iron loading from an increased rate of absorption, extramedullary erythropoietic tumor masses, bone disease, and infection. However, considering the disease is so common, relatively little is known about its natural history and, in particular, the reasons for its remarkable phenotypic clinical heterogeneity.

The blood picture shows a typical thalassemic pattern. The hemoglobin consists of E, F, and A_2. Usually no hemoglobin A is present because the β⁰-thalassemias are particularly common in the parts of the world where hemoglobin E is found.

β-THALASSEMIA WITH NORMAL HEMOGLOBIN A_2 LEVEL

Rare forms of β-thalassemia are seen in which heterozygotes have normal hemoglobin A_2 levels. Their main clinical importance is that they can be confused with the more severe forms of α-thalassemia in the heterozygous state and therefore may cause difficulties in genetic counseling and prenatal diagnosis. Based on hematologic studies, two main classes of "normal hemoglobin A_2 β-thalassemia"—sometimes called types 1 and 2—are seen.[242] Type 1 is the "silent" form of β-thalassemia. Type 2 is heterogeneous, with many cases representing the compound heterozygous state for β-thalassemia and δ-thalassemia.

"Silent" β-thalassemia[7,243] is characterized by no hematologic changes in heterozygotes. It can be identified with certainty only by globin-chain synthesis studies, which show mild chain imbalance with α-/β-globin chain synthesis ratios of approximately 1.3. Compound heterozygotes for this condition and β⁰-thalassemia have a mild form of β-thalassemia intermedia.

Normal hemoglobin A_2 β-thalassemia type 2 in heterozygotes is indistinguishable from typical β-thalassemia with elevated hemoglobin A_2 levels.[242] The homozygous state has not been described. The compound heterozygous state for this gene and for β-thalassemia with raised hemoglobin A_2 levels is characterized by a clinical picture of severe transfusion-dependent β-thalassemia. Family data obtained in Italy and Sardinia suggest this condition represents the compound heterozygous state for both β-thalassemia and δ-thalassemia.[244,245] Most of the δ-thalassemias have been observed *trans* to β-thalassemia. However, the form of δ-thalassemia resulting from loss of an A in codon 59 occurs on the same chromosome as the hemoglobin Knossos mutation, which is associated with a mild form of β-thalassemia.[246] This finding explains the normal level of hemoglobin A_2 associated with this condition, which is the most common form of normal hemoglobin A_2 β-thalassemia in the Mediterranean region.

Several other conditions, mentioned earlier in this chapter in "Etiology and Pathogenesis," are associated with a phenotype that is indistinguishable from normal A_2 β-thalassemia. These conditions include the heterozygous states for the Corfu form of δβ-thalassemia, and εγδβ-thalassemia.

OTHER UNUSUAL FORMS OF β-THALASSEMIA

The clinical features of the dominant β-thalassemias resemble the features of thalassemia intermedia.[7] Moderate anemia and splenomegaly are seen, with a blood picture showing thalassemic red cell changes. The marrow shows erythroid hyperplasia with well-marked inclusion bodies in the red cell precursors. The latter may be seen in the peripheral blood after splenectomy. Hemoglobin analysis shows hemoglobins A and A_2 are present, and the hemoglobin F level is not usually elevated much higher than that seen in β-thalassemia trait. Hemoglobin A_2 levels are always raised.

Other unusual varieties of β-thalassemia include those categorized by unusually high hemoglobin F or A_2 levels. Most of these conditions result from deletions involving the β-globin gene and its promoter region. For example, the so-called Dutch[247] form of β-thalassemia is associated with unusually high hemoglobin F levels in heterozygotes and high hemoglobin A_2 levels. Several other conditions of this type, which result from different-size deletions, have been reported (see ref. 7).

δ^0-THALASSEMIA

δ^0-Thalassemia causes a complete absence of hemoglobin A_2 in homozygotes and a reduced hemoglobin A_2 level in heterozygotes.[248] It is of no clinical significance except for its effect of reducing hemoglobin A_2 levels in β-thalassemia heterozygotes.

$\varepsilon\gamma\delta\beta$-THALASSEMIA

This heterogeneous condition has been observed only in the heterozygous state in a few families.[7,108,109] It is characterized by neonatal hemolysis and, in adult life, by the hematologic picture of heterozygous β-thalassemia with normal hemoglobin A_2 levels.

α-THALASSEMIA IN ASSOCIATION WITH α- AND β-CHAIN HEMOGLOBIN VARIANTS

Several α-globin structural variants are caused by single amino acid substitutions at α-chain loci on chromosomes that carry only a single α-chain gene. Individuals who inherit variants of this type and an α^0-thalassemia determinant have a form of hemoglobin H disease in which the hemoglobin consists of the α-chain variant hemoglobin and hemoglobin H. Well-documented examples include hemoglobin QH disease $(-\ -/-\alpha^Q)$,[249,250] hemoglobin G Philadelphia H disease $(-\ -/-\alpha^G)$,[251,252] and hemoglobin Hasharon H disease $(-\ -/-\alpha^{Hash})$.[253] Many examples of the coexistence of the homozygous or heterozygous states for β-chain hemoglobin variants and different α-thalassemia determinants have been reported.[7,9,10] Particularly well-characterized disorders include the various interactions of α^0- and α^+-thalassemia with hemoglobin E[7,237] and hemoglobin S.[254,255] Carriers for these hemoglobin variants who also have the α^0- or α^+-thalassemia traits have thalassemic red cell indices and unusually low levels of the abnormal hemoglobin. Individuals with sickle cell anemia who have α-thalassemia show thalassemic red cell changes, more persistent splenomegaly, and lower hemoglobin F values than do patients without the thalassemia genes.

THERAPY, COURSE, AND PROGNOSIS

The only forms of treatment available for thalassemic children are regular blood transfusions, iron chelation therapy in an attempt to prevent iron overload, judicious use of splenectomy in cases complicated by hypersplenism, and a good standard of general pediatric care.[7,9,256] Marrow transplantation has an important role in selected cases (see Chap. 22).

TRANSFUSION

Children with β-thalassemia who are maintained at a hemoglobin level of 9.5 to 14 g/dl grow and develop normally. They do not develop the distressing skeletal complications of thalassemia.[7,251] Maintaining a lower hemoglobin level than this range without any deleterious effects on development and with the added advantage of reducing the level of iron loading may be possible. This regimen maintains a mean pretransfusion level that does not exceed 9.5 g/dl.[257] A transfusion program should not be started too early, and it should be initiated only when the hemoglobin level is too low to be compatible with normal development. If transfusion is started too soon, thalassemia intermedia may be missed, and the child may be transfused unnecessarily. Usually blood transfusions are given every 4 weeks on an outpatient basis. To avoid transfusion reactions, washed, filtered, or frozen red cells should be used so that the majority of the white cells and plasma-protein components are removed (see Chap. 131).

IRON CHELATION

Every child who is maintained on a high-transfusion regimen ultimately develops iron overload and dies of siderosis of the myocardium. Therefore, such children must be started on a program of iron chelation within the first 2 to 3 years of life.[256] Despite extensive searches for an oral chelating agent, deferoxamine (desferrioxamine) is currently the only drug of proven long-term value for treatment of thalassemia. It is best administered by an 8- to 12-hour overnight pump-driven infusion in the subcutaneous tissues of the anterior abdominal wall.[258,259] Chelation therapy should commence by the time the serum ferritin level reaches approximately 1000 μg/dl. In practice, this level usually is seen after the 12th to 15th transfusion. Infants must not be overchelated when the iron burden is still low in order to prevent toxicity. The initial dose usually is 20 mg/kg 5 nights per week, with 100 mg of oral vitamin C (200 mg in older children and adults) on the day of infusion, after the infusion has been initiated.[260] Some evidence and a widespread opinion indicate ascorbate precipitates myocardiopathy in these patients if ascorbate is given before deferoxamine infusion is started.[261] In patients who are heavily iron loaded, particularly those patients with cardiac or endocrine complications, the body iron stores can be effectively lowered by continuous intravenous infusion of deferoxamine at a dose of up to 50 mg/kg body weight. The procedure usually entails insertion of an intravenous delivery system.

Monitoring the degree of iron loading using serial serum ferritin estimations is standard. However, the relationship between hepatic iron concentration and serum ferritin is not reliable, and all patients on regular transfusion should be monitored with hepatic iron studies (see "Abnormal Iron Metabolism" above and refs. 188 and 256). If such studies are not possible, serum ferritin levels should be maintained at less than 1500 μg/liter. Several noninvasive techniques are being developed for assessing iron stores, both in the liver and myocardium. Superconducting quantum interference device (SQUID) magnetometry is reliable but very expensive. Techniques based on computed tomography or magnetic resonance imaging require further evaluation.

Extensive experience with the use of deferoxamine and its toxic effects has been reported.[262] No serious complications occur other than local erythema and painful subcutaneous nodules at the site of infusions and extremely rare severe allergic reactions. These reactions can be controlled, at least in part, by including 5 to 10 mg hydrocortisone in the infusion. Probably of greatest concern is neurosensory toxicity, which has been documented in up to 30 percent of cases. Toxicity causes high-frequency hearing loss that may become symptomatic.[262,263] In a few cases, the toxicity did not respond to discontinuation of the drug, and permanent hearing loss resulted. Ocular toxicity has been reported.[262] Symptoms include visual failure, night and color blindness, and field loss. Reversal of symptoms after discontinuation of the drug has been reported. Deferoxamine may cause bone changes and growth retardation, sometimes associated with bone pain. Body measurements characteristically show a reduced crown-pubis/pubis-heel ratio.[264] These changes may be associated with radiological abnormalities of the vertebral column. These complications can be prevented by exercising extreme care in monitoring patients receiving long-term desferrioxamine therapy. Young children or individuals from whom most of the iron has been removed by chelation are at particularly high risk. Formal audiometry and ophthalmologic examinations at 6-month intervals are recommended.

The only oral iron chelating agent that has been studied extensively is 1,2-dimethyl-3-hydroxypyridin-4-one (deferiprone, L1). The current status of this drug has been reviewed.[265–266] Early studies were promising, but it now is apparent that some patients do not maintain iron balance at the dose currently used. Approximately 5 percent of patients develop severe neutropenia. Deaths from agranulocytosis have been reported. A disabling form of arthritis also has been reported. Given the early reports that this agent could potentiate liver fibrosis, the main problem in assessing the drug's role, at least as an alternate chelating agent, is the lack of long-term, carefully controlled trials of its efficacy and toxicity over a long period compared to that of deferoxamine. Preliminary studies indicate a new oral chelating agent, ICL670, may be effective in controlling iron accumulation, but further work on its efficacy and toxicity is required.[267]

Because of the extremely well-documented data showing long-term survival free of cardiac disease in patients adequately treated with deferoxamine,[268–270] this agent is recommended as the first-line choice for management of transfusion-dependent thalassemia. Patient compliance is the major problem with the drug's use, but every effort must be made to overcome this difficulty in view of the uncertainties regarding currently available oral chelating agents. In mice, L-type Ca^{2+} channels[272] are a major pathway for iron entry into cardiac myocytes, and cardiac (but not the liver) iron accumulation can be prevented by calcium channel blockers. However, in humans the efficacy of calcium channel blockers for cardiac iron overload must be proved in clinical trials.

Increasing evidence indicates children maintained at a high hemoglobin level do not develop hypersplenism.[7] However, enlargement of the spleen with increased transfusion requirements occurs commonly in patients maintained at a lower hemoglobin level. Splenectomy should be performed if transfusion requirements increase dramatically or pain develops because of the size of the spleen. Because of the risk of overwhelming pneumococcal infections,[271] splenectomy should not be performed in children younger than 5 years. These children should receive a pneumococcal vaccine prior to the procedure. They then should be placed on prophylactic oral penicillin after the operation. *Haemophilus influenzae* type B and meningococcal vaccines also are recommended.

Children with severe thalassemia are still prone to other infections. Presentation with abdominal pain, diarrhea, and vomiting should always suggest an infection with a member of the Yersinia class of bacteria. Empirical treatment should start immediately with either an aminoglycoside or a co-trimoxazole. Transfusion-transmitted virus infection is common in some populations. All chronically transfused patients should be tested annually for hepatitis C, hepatitis B, and HIV. Patients with serologic evidence of chronic active hepatitis should be considered for treatment with interferon alpha and/or ribavirin. As mentioned earlier in "Abnormal Iron Metabolism," subtle endocrine deficiencies are increasingly recognized, particularly those associated with growth retardation and hypogonadism. These patients require expert endocrinologic assessment and replacement therapy when appropriate.

MARROW TRANSPLANTATION

By 1997, more than 1000 marrow transplants had been performed at three centers in Italy.[273–276] Based on this experience and on later data,[7] the prognosis evidently depended on the adequacy of iron chelation up to the time of transplantation. Hence, patients were divided into three classes: class I patients have a history of adequate iron chelation and neither liver fibrosis nor hepatomegaly; class II patients have one or two of these characteristics; and class III have all three characteristics. Among children in class I who had undergone transplantation early in the course of the disease, disease-free survival was assessed at 90 to 93 percent at 5 years, with a 4 percent risk of mortality related to the procedure. For class II patients, who constitute the intermediate-

risk group, the survival and disease-free survival rates were 86 percent and 82 percent, respectively. For class III, the high-risk group, the survival and disease-free survival rates were 62 percent and 51 percent, respectively. Apart from the immediate complications of severe infection in the posttransplant period, most of the problems were related to development of acute or chronic graft-versus-host disease. The overall frequency of mild to severe grades ranges from 27 to 30 percent.[277] Modification of preparative drug regimens has reduced the frequency of drug toxicity. The occurrence of mixed chimerism may be a risk factor for graft-versus-host disease. No case of hematologic malignancy has been observed in the longest followup of patients between 15 and 20 years after transplantation. Removing excess body iron accumulated before transplantation by venesection appears to be more effective than chelation therapy.[278]

In experienced centers, marrow transplantation offers a genuine option for management of different forms of thalassemia. This topic and the current status of *in utero* and peripheral blood stem cell therapy are considered in Chap. 22.

GENERAL CARE

Management of thalassemia requires a high standard of general pediatric care. Infection should be treated early. If the diet is deficient in folate, supplements should be given. Supplementation probably is unnecessary in children maintained on a high-transfusion regimen. Particular attention should be paid to the ear, nose, and throat because of chronic sinus infection and middle-ear diseases resulting from bone deformity of the skull. Similarly, regular dental surveillance is essential because poorly transfused thalassemic children have a variety of deformities of the maxilla and poorly developed teeth. In the later stages of the illness, when iron loading becomes the major feature, endocrine replacement therapy may be necessary. Symptomatic treatment for metabolic bone disease and cardiac failure also may be needed.

THERAPIES OF SPECIAL TYPES OF THALASSEMIA

Hemoglobin H disease usually requires no specific therapy, although splenectomy may be of value in cases associated with severe anemia and splenomegaly.[7,9,10] Splenectomy may be followed by a higher incidence of thromboembolic disease than occurs in splenectomized children with β-thalassemia[7]; therefore, the spleen should be removed only in cases of extreme anemia and splenomegaly. Oxidant drugs should not be given to patients with hemoglobin H disease. The management of symptomatic sickle cell thalassemia follows the lines described for sickle cell anemia (see Chap. 47).

Thalassemia intermedia presents a particularly complex therapeutic problem. Whether a child with a steady-state hemoglobin level of 6 to 7 g/dl should be transfused is difficult to determine with certainty. Probably the best compromise is to watch such children very closely during the first years of life. If they grow and develop normally and no signs of bone changes are evident, they should be maintained without transfusion. If, however, their early growth pattern is retarded or their activity is limited because of their anemia, they should be placed on a regular transfusion regimen. If hypersplenism plays a role in their anemia as the children grow older, splenectomy should be performed. Because many of these patients have significant iron loading from the gastrointestinal tract, regular estimations of serum iron and ferritin should be obtained and chelation therapy instituted when appropriate.

EXPERIMENTAL APPROACHES TO TREATMENT

Two main experimental approaches are being pursued in the search for more effective therapy of the thalassemias: reactivation or augmentation of fetal hemoglobin production, and somatic gene therapy.

The main rationale for employing agents that have been used in attempts to increase hemoglobin F production is based on the observation that patients recovering from cytotoxic drug therapy or during other periods of erythroid expansion may reactivate hemoglobin F synthesis. In addition, the observation that butyrate analogues might have a stimulating effect on hemoglobin F production has led to a number of studies of their potential for management of thalassemia. A number of clinical trials have been performed.[279–282] Agents that have been used include various cytotoxic drugs, erythropoietin, and several different butyrate analogues. Overall, these agents, used alone or in combination, have produced some small effects on fetal hemoglobin production, but the results of these trials have been disappointing. Some notable exceptions were seen, however, particularly several cases of homozygosity or compound heterozygosity for hemoglobin Lepore in which use of either a combination of sodium phenylbutyrate and hydroxyurea or hydroxyurea alone produced a spectacular rise in hemoglobin F production. In the case of two homozygotes for hemoglobin Lepore, the necessity for further transfusion was eliminated.[283] This finding raises the intriguing possibility that certain mutations, possibly deletions of the β-globin gene cluster, are more susceptible to this type of approach. Appropriate combination therapy may improve the results in other forms of thalassemia.

The other experimental approach involves somatic gene therapy. Currently the therapy is mainly directed at gene transfer into potential hematopoietic stem cells using retroviral vectors.[284] Other approaches also are being taken, including attempts at the restoration of normal splicing in cases of splicing mutations[285] and use of trans-splicing ribozymes to correct β-globin gene transcripts.[286,287] However, studies using murine models with recombinant lentiviral vectors suggest that sustained, high-level globin gene expression may be possible, at least in this experimental system.[288,289] This approach likely will be applied toward correction of some of the β-globinopathies in the near future.

PROGNOSIS

The prognosis for patients with severe forms of β-thalassemia who are adequately treated by transfusion and chelation has improved dramatically over the years. Two large studies have investigated the influence of effective long-term desferrioxamine use on the development of cardiac disease.[269,270] In one study, patients who had maintained sustained reduction of body iron, as estimated by a serum ferritin level less than 2500 μg/liter over 12 years of followup, had an estimated cardiac disease–free survival rate of 91 percent. This finding is in contrast to patients in whom most determinations of serum ferritin level exceeded this value, in whom the estimated cardiac disease–free survival rate was less than 20 percent. In a second study, the relationship between survival and total body iron burden was measured directly using hepatic storage iron values. Patients who had maintained hepatic iron concentrations of at least 15 mg of iron per gram of liver, dry weight, had a 32 percent probability of survival to age 25 years. No cardiac disease developed in patients who maintained hepatic iron levels below this threshold. These studies provide unequivocal evidence that adequate transfusion and chelation are associated with longevity and good quality of life. On the other hand, poor compliance or unavailability of chelating agents still is associated with a poor prospect of survival much beyond the second decade.

PREVENTION

In parts of the world where the incidence of thalassemia is high, the disease places an immense economic burden on society. For example, if all the thalassemic children born in Cyprus were treated by regular blood transfusions and iron chelating therapy, it is estimated that within 15 years the total medical budget of the island would be required to treat this single disease.[290] Clearly, this approach is not always feasible, so considerable effort is directed toward developing programs for prevention of the different forms of thalassemia.

The goal of prevention can be achieved in two ways. The first is prospective genetic counseling, that is, screening total populations while the children still are at school and warning carriers about the potential risks of marriage to another carrier. Few data are available about the value of programs of this type; a pilot study in Greece was unsuccessful.[291] Because it is believed this approach likely will not be successful in many populations, considerable effort has been directed toward developing prenatal diagnosis programs.

Prenatal diagnosis for prevention of thalassemia entails screening mothers at the first prenatal visit, screening the father in cases in which the mother is a thalassemia carrier, and offering the couple the possibility of prenatal diagnosis and termination of pregnancy if both mother and father are carriers of a gene for a severe form of thalassemia. Currently, these programs are devoted mainly to prenatal diagnosis of the severe transfusion-dependent forms of homozygous β^+ or β^0-thalassemia. Considerable experience has been gained in prenatal diagnosis of mothers at risk for having a fetus with the hemoglobin Bart's hydrops syndrome, considering the distress caused by a long and difficult pregnancy and the obstetric problems resulting from the birth of a hydropic infant with a massive placenta.

The first efforts at prenatal detection of β-thalassemia utilized fetal blood sampling and globin-chain synthesis analysis carried out at about week 18 of pregnancy. Despite the technical difficulties involved, the method was applied successfully in many countries and has resulted in a reduced birth rate of infants with β-thalassemia.[292] The technique is associated with a low maternal morbidity rate, a fetal mortality rate of approximately 3 to 4 percent, and an error rate of 1 to 2 percent. Its main disadvantage is that it must be carried out relatively late in pregnancy. For this reason, efforts have turned to first-trimester prenatal diagnosis.

DNA technology has enabled diagnosis of important hemoglobin disorders in utero by fetal DNA analysis. Although analysis can be carried out on DNA derived from amniotic fluid, the approach has drawbacks because, again, it must be done relatively late in pregnancy, and often amniotic fluid cells must be grown in culture to obtain a sufficient amount of DNA.[288] However, DNA can be obtained as early as week 9 of pregnancy by chorionic villus sampling. Although the safety of this technique remains to be fully evaluated and limb reduction deformities may occur when the procedure is carried out very early in pregnancy (9 or 10 weeks), chorionic villus sampling has become the major method for prenatal diagnosis of the thalassemias based on subsequent experience with the technique.[7,293–297]

Identification of thalassemia in the fetus requires different approaches, depending on the nature of the molecular pathology involved.[298] Major deletions, such as those that cause α^0-thalassemia and some of the β^0-thalassemias, can be identified directly by Southern blotting analysis of fetal DNA. Approximately one third of the point mutations that produce β-thalassemia alter restriction enzyme sites; therefore, they also can be identified by gene mapping. If the mutation is known, oligonucleotide probes can be constructed to identify it directly. In families in which the mutation is not known, the affected parental chromosomes often can be defined by RFLP linkage analysis and determination made of whether the fetus has received both of the affected chromosomes from its parents. Experience with many hundred first-trimester prenatal diagnoses suggests determination of whether the fetus is affected can be made in approximately 80 percent of cases.[298] The main difficulties arise because many potentially affected fetuses are compound heterozygotes for a common and a rare β-thalassemia mutation or because the thalassemia chromosome cannot be defined by RFLP analysis.

Now that the mutations in so many different forms of α- and β-thalassemia have been determined, direct detection of these mutations can be the first-line approach to prenatal diagnosis. Because most racial groups have only a few common β-thalassemia mutations, determination of the mutations in the parents and then analysis of fetal DNA for the presence of these mutations are possible. The development of polymerase chain reaction (PCR), combined with the use of oligonucleotide probes to detect individual mutations, offers a wide variety of new approaches for facilitating the speed and accuracy of carrier detection and prenatal diagnosis.[297–300] For example, diagnoses can be made using hybridization of specific ^{32}P end-labeled oligonucleotides to an amplified region of the β-globin gene dotted onto a nylon membrane. Because the β-globin gene sequence can be amplified more than 10^6-fold, hybridization time can be limited to 1 hour, and the entire procedure can be carried out in 2 hours. Amplification refractory mutation systems (see Chap. 9) allow the diagnosis to be made in approximately 2 hours.[301,302] Other modifications of PCR involve the use of nonradioactively labeled probes.[302,303]

The error rate using these different approaches varies, depending on a number of factors, particularly the experience of the laboratory. Low rates of less than 1 percent have been reported from most laboratories using fetal DNA analysis. Potential sources of error include maternal contamination of fetal DNA, nonpaternity, genetic recombination in cases where RFLP linkage analysis is used, and other technical quirks.

The application of these approaches has caused a major reduction in the birth rate of infants with thalassemia in some populations, notably in the Mediterranean islands. A number of methods are being explored in an attempt to increase the options for prenatal detection of thalassemia. Harvesting of fetal cells from the maternal circulation is being explored, and a variety of ways are being investigated to isolate fetal cells by micromanipulation methods.[304,305] Because of the trauma of termination of pregnancy experienced by many women, preimplantation approaches are being explored. A few preimplantation diagnoses of β-thalassemia by polar body analysis have been successful.[306–308]

REFERENCES

1. Cooley TB, Lee P: A series of cases of splenomegaly in children with anemia and peculiar bone changes. *Trans Am Pediatr Soc* 37:29, 1925.
2. Whipple GH, Bradford WL: Racial or familial anemia of children associated with fundamental disturbances of bone and pigment metabolism (Cooley von Jaksch). *Am J Dis Child* 44:336, 1932.
3. Whipple CH, Bradford WL: Mediterranean disease—Thalassemia (erythroblastic anemia of Cooley): Associated pigment abnormalities simulating hemochromatosis. *J Pediatr* 9:279, 1936.
4. Weatherall DJ: Toward an understanding of the molecular biology of some common inherited anemias: The story of thalassemia, in *Blood, Pure and Eloquent*, edited by MM Wintrobe, p 373. McGraw-Hill, New York, 1980.
5. Bannerman RM: *Thalassemia: A Survey of Some Aspects.* Grune & Stratton, New York, 1961.
6. Chernoff AI: The distribution of the thalassemia gene: A historical review. *Blood* 14:899, 1959.
7. Weatherall DJ, Clegg JB: *The Thalassaemia Syndromes*, 4th ed. Blackwell, Oxford, 2001.
8. Ingram VM, Stretton AOW: Genetic basis of the thalassemia diseases. *Nature* 184:1903, 1959.
9. Steinberg MH, Forget BG, Higgs DR, Nagel RL: *Disorders of Hemoglobin.* Cambridge University Press, Cambridge, 2001.
10. Weatherall DJ, Clegg JB, Higgs DR, Wood WG: The hemoglobinopathies, in *The Metabolic and Molecular Bases of Inherited Disease*, 8th

ed, edited by CR Scriver, AL Beauder, WS Sly, D Valle, p 4571. McGraw-Hill, New York, 2001.
11. Flint J, Harding RM, Boyce AJ, Clegg JB: The population genetics of the haemoglobinopathies. *Clin Haematol* 11:1, 1998.
12. Weatherall DJ, Clegg JB: Inherited haemoglobin disorders: An increasing global health problem. *Bull World Health Organ* 79:704, 2001.
13. Haldane JBS: The rate of mutation of human genes. *Hereditas* 35(suppl): 267, 1949.
14. Orkin SH, Kazazian HH: The mutation and polymorphism of the human β-globin gene and its surrounding DNA. *Annu Rev Genet* 18:131, 1984.
15. Orkin SH, Antonarakis SE, Kazazian HH: Polymorphisms and molecular pathology of the human β-globin gene. *Prog Hematol* 13:49, 1983.
16. Siniscalco M, Bernini L, Filippi G, et al: Population genetics of haemoglobin variants, thalassemia and glucose-6-phosphate dehydrogenase deficiency, with particular reference to malaria hypothesis. *Bull World Health Organ* 34:379, 1966.
17. Flint J, Hill AVS, Bowden DK, et al: High frequencies of α thalassemia are the result of natural selection by malaria. *Nature* 321:744, 1986.
18. Allen SJ, O'Donnell A, Alexander NDE, et al: A$^+$-Thalassemia protects children against disease due to malaria and other infections. *Proc Natl Acad Sci U S A* 94:14736, 1997.
19. Williams TN, Maitland K, Bennett S, et al: High incidence of malaria in α-thalassemic children. *Nature* 383:522, 1996.
20. Pasvol G, Wilson RJM: The interaction of malaria parasites with red blood cells. *Br Med Bull* 38:133, 1982.
21. Luzzatto L: Malaria and the red cell, in *Recent Advances in Haematology*, edited by AV Hoffbrand, p 109. Churchill Livingstone, Edinburgh, 1985.
22. Luzzi GA, Merry AH, Newbold CI, et al: Surface antigen expression on *Plasmodium falciparum*–infected erythrocytes is modified in α- and β-thalassemia. *J Exp Med* 173:785, 1991.
23. Williams TN, Weatherall DJ, Newbold CI: The membrane characteristics of *Plasmodium falciparum*-infected and -uninfected heterozygous α^o thalassaemic erythrocytes. *Br J Haematol* 118:663, 2002.
24. Weatherall DJ, Clegg JB: Genetic variability in response to infection: Malaria and after. *Genes Immun* 3:331, 2002.
25. Orkin SH: The duplicated human α globin genes lie close together in cellular DNA. *Proc Natl Acad Sci U S A* 75:5950, 1978.
26. Lauer J, Shen C-KJ, Maniatis T: The chromosomal arrangement of human α-like globin genes: Sequence homology and α-globin gene deletions. *Cell* 20:119, 1980.
27. Liebhaber SA, Goossens N, Kan YW: Homology and concerted evolution at the α_1 and α_2 loci of human α-globin. *Nature* 290:26, 1981.
28. Liebhaber SA, Goossens MJ, Kan YW: Cloning and complete nucleotide sequence of human 5'-α-globin gene. *Proc Natl Acad Sci U S A* 77:7054, 1980.
29. Proudfoot NJ, Maniatis T: The structure of a human α-globin pseudogene and its relationship to α-globin duplication. *Cell* 21:537, 1980.
30. Liebhaber SA, Kan YW: Differentiation of the mRNA transcripts originating from the α_1- and α_2-globin loci in normals and α-thalassemics. *J Clin Invest* 68:439, 1981.
31. Orkin SH, Goff SC: The duplicated human α-globin genes: Their relative expression as measured by RNA analysis. *Cell* 24:345, 1981.
32. Higgs DR, Wainscoat JS, Flint J, et al: Analysis of the human α globin gene cluster reveals a highly informative genetic locus. *Proc Natl Acad Sci U S A* 83:5156, 1986.
33. Fritsch EF, Lawn RM, Maniatis T: Molecular cloning and characterization of the human β-like globin gene cluster. *Cell* 19:959, 1980.
34. Spritz RA, DeRiel JK, Forget BG, Weissman SM: Complete nucleotide sequence of the human δ-globin gene. *Cell* 21:639, 1980.
35. Baralle FE, Shoulders CC, Proudfoot NJ: The primary structure of the human ϵ globin gene. *Cell* 21:621, 1980.

36. Slightom JL, Blechl AE, Smithies O: Human $^G\gamma$- and $^A\gamma$-globin genes: Complete nucleotide sequences suggest that DNA can be exchanged between these duplicated genes. *Cell* 21:627, 1980.

37. Jeffrey AJ: DNA sequences in the $^G\gamma$-, $^A\gamma$-, δ-, and β-globin genes of man. *Cell* 18:1, 1979.

38. Antonarakis SE, Boehm CD, Giardina PVJ, Kazazian HH: Nonrandom association of polymorphic restriction sites in the β-globin gene complex. *Proc Natl Acad Sci U S A* 79:137, 1982.

39. Wainscoat JS, Hill AVV, Boyce A, et al: Evolutionary relationships of human populations from an analysis of nuclear DNA polymorphisms. *Nature* 319:491, 1982.

40. Stamatoyannopoulos G, Grosveld F: Hemoglobin switching, in *The Molecular Basis of Blood Disease*, 3rd ed, edited by G Stamatoyannopoulos, PW Majerus, RM Perlmutter, H Varmus, p 135. Saunders, Philadelphia, 1994.

41. Orkin SH: Transcription factors that regulate lineage decisions, in *The Molecular Basis of Blood Disease*, 3rd ed, edited by G Stamatoyannopoulos, PW Majerus, RM Perlmutter, H Varmus, p 80. Saunders, Philadelphia, 1994.

42. Jarman AP, Wood WG, Sharpe JA, et al: Characterization of the major regulatory element upstream of the human α globin gene cluster. *Mol Cell Biol* 11:4679, 1991.

43. Donze D, Townes TM, Bieker JJ. Role of erythroid Kruppel-like factor in human gamma- to beta-globin gene switching. *J Biol Chem* 270:1955, 1995.

44. Weatherall DJ: Thalassemia, in *The Molecular Basis of Blood Diseases*, 3rd ed, edited by G Stamatoyannopoulos, PW Majerus, RM Perlmutter, H Varmus, p 183. Saunders, Philadelphia, 2001.

45. Huisman THJ, Carver MFM, Baysal E: *A Syllabus of Thalassemia Mutations*. Sickle Cell Anemia Foundation, Augusta, 1997.

46. Thein SL: B-Thalassaemia, in *Bailliére's Clinical Haematology, International Practice and Research: Sickle Cell Disease and Thalassaemia*, edited by GP Rodgers, p 91. Bailliére Tindall, London 1998.

47. Orkin SH, Old JM, Weatherall DJ, Nathan DG: Partial deletion of β-globin gene DNA in certain patients with β^0-thalassemia. *Proc Natl Acad Sci U S A* 76:2400, 1979.

48. Thein SL, Old JM, Wainscoat JS, Weatherall DJ: Population and genetic studies suggest a single origin for the Indian deletion β^0 thalassaemia. *Br J Haematol* 57:271, 1984.

49. Anand R, Boehm CD, Kazazian HH, Vanin EF: Molecular characterization of a β^0-thalassemia resulting from a 1.4 kb deletion. *Blood* 72:636, 1988.

50. Padanilam BJ, Felice AE, Huisman THJ: Partial deletion of the 5' β globin gene region causes β^0 thalassemia in members of an American Black family. *Blood* 64:941, 1984.

51. Popovich BW, Rosenblatt DS, Kendall AG, Nishioka Y: Molecular characterization of an atypical β thalassemia caused by a large deletion in the 5' β-globin gene region. *Am J Hum Genet* 39:797, 1986.

52. Diaz-Chico JC, Yang KG, Kutlar A, et al: A 300 bp deletion involving part of the 5' β-globin gene region is observed in members of a Turkish family with β-thalassemia. *Blood* 70:583, 1987.

53. Aulehla-Scholtz C, Spielberg R, Horst J: A β-thalassemia mutant caused by a 300 bp deletion in the human β-globin gene. *Hum Genet* 81:298, 1989.

54. Orkin SH, Antonarakis SE, Kazazian HH: Base substitution at position -88 in a β-thalassemic globin gene: Further evidence for the role of the distal promoter element ACACCC. *J Biol Chem* 259:8679, 1984.

55. Orkin SH, Kazazian HH, Antonarakis SE, et al: Linkage of β-thalassemia mutations and β-globin gene polymorphisms with DNA polymorphisms in human globin gene cluster. *Nature* 296:267, 1982.

56. Poncz M, Ballantine M, Solowiejczyk D, et al: β-Thalassemia in a Kurdish Jew. *J Biol Chem* 257:5994, 1983.

57. Orkin SH, Sexton JP, Cheng TC, et al: ATA box transcription mutation in β-thalassemia. *Nucleic Acids Res* 11:4727, 1983.

58. Antonarakis SE, Orkin SH, Cheng T-C, et al: B-Thalassemia in American Blacks: Novel mutations in the TATA box and IVS-2 acceptor splice site. *Proc Natl Acad Sci U S A* 81:1154, 1984.

59. Surrey S, Delgrosso K, Malladi P, Schwartz E: Functional analysis of a β-globin gene containing a TATA box mutation from a Kurdish Jew with β-thalassemia. *J Biol Chem* 260:6507, 1985.

60. Gonzalez-Redondo JH, Stoming TA, Kutlar A, et al: A C→T substitution at nt -101 in a conserved DNA sequence of the promoter region of the β-globin gene is associated with "silent" β-thalassemia. *Blood* 73:1705, 1989.

61. Wong C, Dowling CE, Saiki RK, et al: Characterization of beta-thalassemia mutations using direct genomic sequencing of amplified single copy DNA. *Nature* 330:384, 1987.

62. Treisman R, Orkin SH, Maniatis T: Specific transcription and RNA splicing defects in five cloned β-thalassemia genes. *Nature* 302:591, 1983.

63. Kazazian HH, Orkin SH, Antonarakis SE, et al: Molecular characterization of seven β-thalassaemia mutations in Asian Indians. *EMBO J* 3:593, 1984.

64. Padanilam BJ, Huisman THJ: The β^0-thalassemia in an American Black family is due to a single nucleotide substitution in the acceptor splice junction of the second intervening sequence. *Am J Hematol* 22:259, 1986.

65. Atweh GF, Anagnou NP, Shearin J, et al: B-Thalassemia resulting from a single nucleotide substitution in an acceptor splice site. *Nucleic Acids Res* 13:777, 1985.

66. Orkin SH, Sexton JP, Goff SC, Kazazian HH: Inactivation of an acceptor splice site by a short deletion in β-thalassemia. *J Biol Chem* 258:7249, 1983.

67. Atweh GF, Wong C, Reed R, et al: A new mutation in IVS-1 of the human β globin gene causing β thalassemia due to abnormal splicing. *Blood* 70:147, 1987.

68. Cheng T, Orkin SH, Antonarakis SE, et al: B-Thalassemia in Chinese: Use of in vivo RNA analysis and oligonucleotide hybridization in systematic characterization of molecular defects. *Proc Natl Acad Sci U S A* 81:2821, 1984.

69. Gonzalez-Redondo JH, Stoming TA, Lanclos KD, et al: Clinical and genetic heterogeneity in Black patients with homozygous β-thalassemia from the southeastern United States. *Blood* 72:1007, 1988.

70. Tamagnini GP, Lopes MC, Castanheira ME, et al: B' thalassaemia—Portuguese type: Clinical, haematological and molecular studies of a newly defined form of β thalassaemia. *Br J Haematol* 54:189, 1983.

71. Hill AVS, Bowden DK, O'Shaughnessy DF, et al: B-Thalassemia in Melanesia: Association with malaria and characterization of a common variant. *Blood* 72:9, 1988.

72. Spritz RA, Jagadeeswaran P, Choudary PV, et al: Base substitution in an intervening sequence of a β^+ thalassemic human globin gene. *Proc Natl Acad Sci U S A* 78:2455, 1981.

73. Busslinger M, Moschanas N, Flavell RA: B$^+$ thalassemia: Aberrant splicing results from a single point mutation in an intron. *Cell* 27:289, 1981.

74. Metherall JE, Collins RS, Pan J, et al: B^0 thalassaemia caused by a base substitution that creates an alternative splice acceptor site in an intron. *EMBO J* 5:2551, 1986.

75. Orkin SH, Kazazian HH, Antonarakis SE, et al: Abnormal RNA processing due to the exon mutation of β^E-globin gene. *Nature* 300:768, 1982.

76. Goldsmith ME, Humphries RK, Bey T, et al: "Silent" nucleotide substitution in β^+ thalassemia globin gene activated splice site in coding sequence RNA. *Proc Natl Acad Sci U S A* 88:2318, 1983.

77. Orkin SH, Antonarakis SE, Loukopoulos D: Abnormal processing of β Knossos RNA. *Blood* 64:311, 1984.

78. Yang KG, Kutlar F, George E, et al: Molecular characterization of β-globin gene mutations in Malay patients with Hb E–β-thalassaemia major. *Br J Haematol* 72:73, 1989.

79. Orkin SH, Cheng T-C, Antonarakis SE, Kazazian HH: Thalassaemia due to a mutation in the cleavage-polyadenylation signal of the human β-globin gene. *EMBO J* 4:453, 1985.

80. Jankovic L, Efremov GD, Petkov G, et al: Three novel mutations leading to β thalassaemia. *Blood* 74:226, 1989.

81. Rund D, Filon D, Rachmilewitz EA, et al: Molecular analysis of β-thalassemia in Kurdish Jews: Novel mutations and expression studies. *Blood* 74:821, 1989.

82. Chang JC, Kan YW: β-Thalassemia: A nonsense mutation in man. *Proc Natl Acad Sci U S A* 76:2886, 1979.

83. Kazazian HH, Dowling CE, Waber PG, et al: The spectrum of β-thalassemia genes in China and Southeast Asia. *Blood* 68:964, 1986.

84. Trecartin RF, Liebhaber SA, Chang JC, et al: B Thalassemia in Sardinia is caused by a nonsense mutation. *J Clin Invest* 68:1012, 1981.

85. Rosatelli C, Leoni GB, Tuveri T, et al: B Thalassaemia mutations in Sardinians: Implications for prenatal diagnosis. *J Med Genet* 24:97, 1987.

86. Kimberland ML, Divoky V, Prchal J, et al: Full-length human L1 insertions retain the capacity for high frequency retrotransposition in cultured cells. *Hum Mol Genet* 8:1557, 1999.

87. Weatherall DJ, Clegg JB, Knox-Macaulay HHM, et al: A genetically determined disorder with features both of thalassaemia and congenital dyserythropoietic anaemia. *Br J Haematol* 24:681, 1973.

88. Stamatoyannopoulos G, Woodson R, Papayannopoulou T, et al: Inclusion-body β-thalassemia trait: A form of β thalassemia producing clinical manifestations in simple heterozygotes. *N Engl J Med* 290:939, 1974.

89. Thein SL: Dominant β thalassaemia: Molecular basis and pathophysiology. *Br J Haematol* 80:273, 1992.

90. Thein SL, Hesketh C, Taylor P, et al: Molecular basis for dominantly inherited inclusion body β thalassaemia. *Proc Natl Acad Sci U S A* 87:3924, 1990.

91. Beris RP, Miescher PA, Diaz-Chico JC, et al: Inclusion body β-thalassemia trait in a Swiss family is caused by an abnormal hemoglobin (Geneva) with an altered and extended β chain carboxy-terminus due to a modification in codon 114. *Blood* 72:801, 1988.

92. Kazazian HH, Dowling CE, Hurwitz RL, et al: Thalassemia mutations in exon 3 of the β-globin gene often cause a dominant form of thalassemia and show no predilection for malarial-endemic regions of the world. *Am J Hum Genet* 45:A242, 1989.

93. Fei YJ, Stoming TA, Kutlar A, et al: One form of inclusion body β thalassemia is due to a GAA→TAA mutation at codon 121 of the β chain. *Blood* 73:1075, 1989.

94. Kazazian HH, Orkin SH, Boehm CD, et al: Characterization of a spontaneous mutation to a β-thalassemia allele. *Am J Hum Genet* 38:860, 1986.

95. Sachs AB: Messenger RNA degradation in eukaryotes. *Cell* 74:413, 1993

96. Thermann R, Neu-Yilkins J, Deters A, et al: Binary specification of nonsense codons by splicing and cytoplasmic translation. *EMBO J* 17:3484, 1998.

97. Thein SL: Is it dominantly inherited β thalassaemia or just a β-chain variant that is highly unstable? *Br J Haematol* 107:12, 1999.

98. Adams JG, Steinberg MH, Boxer LA, et al: The structure of hemoglobin Indianapolis [(β112 (G14) arginine]: An unstable variant detectable only by isotopic labeling. *J Biol Chem* 254:3479, 1979.

99. Coleman MB, Steinberg MH, Adams JGI: Hemoglobin Terre Haute [β106 (G8) Arginine]: A posthumous correction to the original structure of Hb Indianapolis. *Blood* 76:57, 1990.

100. Thein SL, Wood WG, Wickramasinghe SN, Galvin MC: B-Thalassemia unlinked to the β-globin gene in an English family. *Blood* 82:961, 1993.

101. Jones RW, Old JM, Trent RJ, et al: Major rearrangement in the human β-globin gene cluster. *Nature* 291:39, 1981.

102. Baglioni C: The fusion of two peptide chains in hemoglobin Lepore and its interpretation as a genetic deletion. *Proc Natl Acad Sci U S A* 48:1880, 1962.

103. Ottolenghi S, Giglioni B, Pulazzini A, et al: Sardinian δβ⁰-thalassemia: A further example of a C to T substitution at position −196 of the ᴬγ globin gene promoter. *Blood* 69:1058, 1987.

104. Atweh GF, Zhu X-X, Brickner HW, et al: The β-globin gene on the Chinese δβ-thalassemia chromosome carries a promoter mutation. *Blood* 70:1470, 1987.

105. Wainscoat JS, Thein SL, Wood WG, et al: A novel deletion in the β globin gene complex. *Ann N Y Acad Sci* 445:20, 1985.

106. Kulozik A, Yarwood N, Jones RW: The Corfu δβ⁰ thalassemia: A small deletion acts at a distance to selectively β globin gene expression. *Blood* 71:457, 1988.

107. Fritsch EF, Lawn RM, Maniatis T: Characterization of deletions which affect the expression of fetal globin genes in man. *Nature* 279:598, 1979.

108. Orkin SH, Goff SC, Nathan DG: Heterogeneity of DNA deletion in γδβ-thalassemia. *J Clin Invest* 67:878, 1981.

109. Pirastu M, Kan YW, Lin CC, et al: Hemolytic disease of the newborn caused by a new deletion of the entire β-globin cluster. *J Clin Invest* 72:602, 1983.

110. Fearon EF, Kazazian HH, Waber PG, et al: The entire β-globin gene cluster is deleted in a form of γδβ-thalassemia. *Blood* 61:1269, 1983.

111. Van Der Ploeg LHT, Konings A, Cort M, et al: γβ-Thalassaemia studies showing that deletion of the γ- and δ-genes influence β-globin gene expression in man. *Nature* 283:637, 1980.

112. Curtin P, Pirastu M, Kan YW, et al: A distant gene deletion affects β-globin gene function in an γδβ-thalassemia. *J Clin Invest* 76:1554, 1985.

113. Driscoll MC, Dobkin CS, Alter BP: γδβ-Thalassemia due to a de novo mutation deleting the 5′ β-globin gene activation-region hypersensitive sites. *Proc Natl Acad Sci U S A* 86:7470, 1989.

114. Tuan D, Feingold E, Newman M, et al: Different 3′ end points of deletions causing δβ-thalassemia and hereditary persistence of fetal hemoglobin: Implications for the control of γ-globin gene expression in man. *Proc Natl Acad Sci U S A* 80:6937, 1983.

115. Kendall AG, Ojwang PJ, Schroeder WA, Huisman THJ: Hemoglobin Kenya, the product of a γ β fusion gene: Studies of the family. *Am J Hum Genet* 25:548, 1973.

116. Smith DH, Clegg JB, Weatherall DJ, Gilles HM: Hereditary persistence of foetal haemoglobin associated with a γ β fusion variant, haemoglobin Kenya. *Nat New Biol* 246:184, 1973.

117. Collins FS, Stoeckert CJ, Serjeant GR, et al: ᴳγβ⁺ hereditary persistence of fetal hemoglobin: Cosmid cloning and identification of a specific mutation 5′ to the ᴳγ gene. *Proc Natl Acad Sci U S A* 81:4894, 1984.

118. Giglioni B, Casini C, Mantovani R, et al: A molecular study of a family with Greek hereditary persistence of fetal hemoglobin and β-thalassemia. *EMBO J* 3:2641, 1984.

119. Gelinas R, Endlich B, Pfeiffer C, et al: G to A substitution in the distal CCAAT box of the ᴬγ-globin gene in Greek hereditary persistence of fetal haemoglobin. *Nature* 313:323, 1985.

120. Tate VE, Wood WG, Weatherall DJ: The British form of hereditary persistence of fetal haemoglobin results from a single base mutation adjacent to an S1 hypersensitive site 5′ to the ᴬγ globin gene. *Blood* 68:1389, 1986.

121. Gilman JG, Huisman THJ: DNA sequence variation associated with elevated fetal ᴳγ globin production. *Blood* 66:783, 1985.

122. Marti HR: *Normale und Abnormale Menschliche Haemoglobin*. Springer-Verlag, Berlin, 1963.

123. Miyoshi K, Kaneto Y, Kawai H, Huisman THJ: X-linked dominant control of F-cells in normal adult life. *Blood* 72:1854, 1988.

124. Dover GJ, Smith KD, Chang YC, et al: Fetal hemoglobin levels in sickle cell disease and normal individuals are partially controlled by an X-linked gene located at Xp22.2. *Blood* 80:816, 1992.

125. Wood WG, Weatherall DJ, Clegg JB: Interaction of heterocellular hereditary persistence of foetal haemoglobin with β thalassaemia and sickle cell anaemia. *Nature* 264:247, 1976.

126. Cappellini MD, Fiorelli G, Bernini LF: Interaction between homozygous β⁰ thalassaemia and the Swiss type of hereditary persistence of fetal haemoglobin. *Br J Haematol* 48:561, 1981.

127. Thein SL, Weatherall DJ: A non-deletion hereditary persistence of fetal hemoglobin (HPFH) determinant not linked to the β-globin gene complex, in *Hemoglobin Switching, Part B, Cellular and Molecular Mechanisms*, edited by G Stamatoyannopoulos, AW Nienhuis, p 97. Alan R. Liss, New York, 1989.

128. Craig JE, Rochette J, Fisher CA, et al: Dissecting the loci controlling fetal haemoglobin production on chromosomes 11p and 6q by the regressive approach. *Nat Genet* 12:58,1996.

129. Craig JE, Rochette J, Sampietro M, et al: Genetic heterogeneity in heterocellular hereditary persistence of fetal hemoglobin. *Blood* 90:428, 1997.

130. Higgs DR: A-Thalassaemia, in *Bailliére's Clinical Haematology. International Practice and Research: The Haemoglobinopathies*, edited by DR Higgs, DJ Weatherall, p 117. Bailliére Tindall, London, 1993.

131. Bernini LF, Harteveld CL: A-Thalassaemia, in *Bailliére's Clinical Haematology. International Practice and Research: The Haemoglobinopathies*, edited by GF Rogers, p 53. Bailliére Tindall, London, 1998.

132. Nicholls RB, Fischel-Ghodsian N, Higgs DR: Recombination at the human α globin gene cluster: Sequence features and topological constraints. *Cell* 49:369, 1987.

133. Barbour VM, Tufarelli C, Sharpe JA, et al: α-thalassemia resulting from a negative chromosomal position effect. *Blood* 96:800, 2000.

134. Tufarelli C, Stanley JA, Garrick D, et al: Transcription of antisense RNA leading to gene silencing and methylation as a novel cause of human genetic disease. *Nat Genet* 34:157, 2003.

135. Wilkie AOM, Lamb J, Harris PC, et al: A truncated human chromosome 16 associated with α thalassaemia is stabilized by addition of telomeric repeat (TTAGGG). *Nature* 346:868, 1990.

136. Hatton CSR, Wilkie AOM, Drysdale HC, et al: Alpha thalassemia caused by a large (62 kb) deletion upstream of the human α globin gene cluster. *Blood* 76:221, 1990.

137. Liebhaber SA, Griese E-U, Cash FE, et al: Inactivation of human α-globin gene expression by a de novo deletion located upstream of the α-globin gene cluster. *Proc Natl Acad Sci U S A* 81:9431, 1990.

138. Embury SH, Miller JA, Dozy AM, et al: Two different molecular organizations account for the single α-globin gene of the α-thalassemia-2 genotype. *J Clin Invest* 66:1319, 1980.

139. Higgs DR, Old JM, Pressley L, et al: A novel α-globin gene arrangement in man. *Nature* 284:632, 1980.

140. Goossens M, Dozy AM, Embury SH, et al: Triplicated α-globin loci in humans. *Proc Natl Acad Sci U S A* 77:518, 1980.

141. Trent RJ, Higgs DR, Clegg JB, Weatherall DJ: A new triplicated α-globin gene arrangement in man. *Br J Haematol* 49:149, 1981.

142. Higgs DR, Hill AVS, Bowden DK, Weatherall DJ: Independent recombination events between duplicated human α globin genes: Implications for their concerted evolution. *Nucleic Acids Res* 12:6965, 1984.

143. Orkin SH, Goff SC, Hechtman RL: Mutation in an intervening sequence splice junction in man. *Proc Natl Acad Sci U S A* 78:5041, 1981.

144. Higgs DR, Goodbourn SEY, Lamb J, et al: A-Thalassaemia caused by a polyadenylation signal mutation. *Nature* 306:398, 1983.

145. Thein SL, Wallace RB, Pressley L, et al: The polyadenylation site mutation in the α-globin gene cluster. *Blood* 71:313, 1988.

146. Pirastu M, Saglio G, Chang JC, et al: Initiation codon mutation as a cause of α thalassemia. *J Biol Chem* 259:12315, 1984.

147. Olivieri NF, Chang LS, Poon AO, et al: An α-globin gene initiation codon mutation in a Black family with Hb H disease. *Blood* 70:729, 1987.

148. Paglietti E, Galanello R, Moi P, et al: Molecular pathology of haemoglobin H disease in Sardinians. *Br J Haematol* 63:485, 1986.

149. Morle F, Lopez B, Henni T, Godet J: A-Thalassaemia associated with the deletion of two nucleotides at position −2 and −3 preceding the AUG codon. *EBMO J* 4:1245, 1985.

150. Weatherall DJ, Clegg JB: The α-chain termination mutants and their relationship to the α thalassaemias. *Philos Trans R Soc London B Biol Sci* 271:411, 1975.

151. Liebhaber SA, Coleman MB, Adams JG, et al: Molecular basis for non-deletion α thalassemia in American Blacks α₂¹¹⁶GAG→UAG. *J Clin Invest* 80:154, 1987.

152. Liebhaber SA, Kan YW: A Thalassemia caused by an unstable α-globin mutant. *J Clin Invest* 71:461, 1983.

153. Sanguansermsri T, Matrogoon S, Changlosh L, Fletz G: Hemoglobin Suan-Dok(α₂¹⁰⁹(G16)LEU→ARG β₂): An unstable variant associated with α thalassemia. *Hemoglobin* 3:161, 1979.

154. Honig GR, Shamsuddin M, Zaizov R, et al: Hemoglobin Petah Tikvah (α110 Ala→Asp): A new unstable variant with α-thalassemia-like expression. *Blood* 57:705, 1981.

155. Honig GR, Shamsuddin M, Vida LN, et al: Hemoglobin Evanston (α14 Trp→Arg): An unstable α-chain variant expressed as α-thalassemia. *J Clin Invest* 73:1740, 1984.

156. Weatherall DJ, Higgs DR, Bunch C, et al: Hemoglobin H disease and mental retardation: A new syndrome or a remarkable coincidence? *N Engl J Med* 305:607, 1981.

157. Wilkie AOM, Buckle VJ, Harris PC, et al: Clinical features and molecular analysis of the α thalassemia/mental retardation syndromes: I. Cases due to deletions involving chromosome band 16p13.3. *Am J Hum Genet* 46:1112, 1990.

158. Wilkie AOM, Zeitlin HC, Lindenbaum RH, et al: Clinical features and molecular analysis of the α-thalassemia/mental retardation syndromes: II. Cases without detectable abnormality of the α globin complex. *Am J Hum Genet* 46:1127, 1990.

159. Gibbons RJ, Suthers GK, Wilkie AOM, et al: X-linked α thalassemia/mental retardation (ATR-X) syndrome: Localization to Xq12-21.31 by X-inactivation and linkage analysis. *Am J Hum Genet* 51:1136, 1992.

160. Gibbons RJ, Picketts DJ, Villard L, Higgs DR: Mutations in a putative global transcriptional regulator cause X-linked mental retardation with α-thalassemia (ATR-X syndrome). *Cell* 80:837, 1995.

161. Gibbons RJ, Bachoo S, Picketts DJ, et al: Mutations in transcriptional regulator *ATRX* establish the functional significance of a PHD-like domain. *Nat Genet* 17:146, 1997.

162. Ausió J, Levin, DB, De Amorim GV, et al: Syndromes of disordered chromatin remodeling. *Clin Genet* 64:83, 2003.

163. Gibbons RJ, McDowell TL, Raman S, et al: Mutations in ATRX, encoding a SWI/SNF-like protein, cause diverse changes in the pattern of DNA methylation. *Nat Genet* 24:368, 2000.

164. Weatherall DJ, Old J, Longley J, et al: Acquired haemoglobin H disease in leukaemia: Pathophysiology and molecular basis. *Br J Haematol* 38:305, 1978.

165. Gibbons RJ, Pellagatti A, Garrick D, et al: Identification of acquired somatic mutations in the gene encoding chromatin-remodeling factor ATRX in the alpha-thalassemia myelodysplasia syndrome (ATMDS). *Nat Genet* 34:446, 2003.

166. Belickova M, Schroeder HW, Guan YL, et al: Clonal hematopoiesis and acquired thalassemia in common variable immunodeficiency: *Mol Med* 1:56, 1995.

167. Weatherall DJ, Clegg JB, Naughton MA: Globin synthesis in thalassemia: An in vitro study. *Nature* 208:1061, 1965.

168. Weatherall DJ, Clegg JB, Na-Nakorn S, Wasi P: The pattern of disordered haemoglobin synthesis in homozygous and heterozygous β-thalassaemia. *Br J Haematol* 16:251, 1969.

169. Fessas P: Inclusions of hemoglobin in erythroblasts and erythrocytes of thalassemia. *Blood* 21:21, 1963.

170. Wickramasinghe SN, Hughes M: Some features of bone marrow macrophages in patients with β-thalassaemia. *Br J Haematol* 38:23, 1978.

171. Yataganas X, Fessas P: The pattern of hemoglobin precipitation in thalassemia and its significance. *Ann N Y Acad Sci* 165:270, 1969.

172. Finch CA, Deubelbeiss K, Cook JD, et al: Ferrokinetics in man. *Medicine (Baltimore)* 49:17, 1970.

173. Chalavelakis G, Clegg JB, Weatherall DJ: Imbalanced globin chain synthesis in heterozygous β-thalassemic bone marrow. *Proc Natl Acad Sci U S A* 72:3853, 1975.

174. Rund D, Rachmilewitz E: Advances in the pathophysiology and treatment of thalassemia. *Crit Rev Oncol Hematol* 20:237, 1995.

175. Schrier SL: Pathobiology of thalassemic erythrocytes. *Curr Opin Haematol* 4:75, 1997.

176. Weatherall DJ: Pathophysiology of β-thalassaemia. *Clin Haematol* 11:127, 1998.

177. Yuan J, Angelucci E, Lucarelli G, et al: Accelerated programmed cell death (apoptosis) in erythroid precursors of patients with severe beta-thalassemia (Cooley's anemia). *Blood* 82:374, 1993.

178. Ager JAM, Lehmann H: Observations in some "fast" haemoglobins: K, J, N, and "Bart's." *Br Med J* 1:929, 1958.

179. Rigas DA, Kohler RD, Osgood EE: New hemoglobin possessing a higher electrophoretic mobility than normal adult hemoglobin. *Science* 121:372, 1955.

180. Gabuzda TG, Nathan DG, Gardner FH: The turnover of hemoglobins A F and A₂ in the peripheral blood of three patients with thalassemia. *J Clin Invest* 42:1678, 1963.

181. Loukopoulos D, Fessas P: The distribution of hemoglobin types in thalassemic erythrocyte. *J Clin Invest* 44:231, 1965.

182. Nathan DG, Gunn RB: Thalassemia: The consequences of unbalanced hemoglobin synthesis. *Am J Med* 41:815, 1966.

183. Rees DC, Porter JB, Clegg JB, Weatherall DJ: Why are hemoglobin F levels increased in Hb E/β thalassemia? *Blood* 94:3199, 1999.

184. Divoky V, Mrug M, Thornley-Brown D, et al: Non-anemic homozygous beta(o) thalassemia in an African-American family: Association of high fetal hemoglobin levels with beta thalassemia alleles. *Am J Hematol* 68:43, 2001.

185. Modell CB, Berdoukas VA: *The Clinical Approach to Thalassemia.* Grune & Stratton, New York, 1984.

186. Italian Working Group on Endocrine Complications in Non-endocrine Diseases: Multi-centre study on prevalence of endocrine complications in thalassemia major. *Clin Endocrinol* 42:581, 1995.

187. Wonke B, Hoffbrand AV, Pouloux P, et al: New approaches to the management of hepatitis and endocrine disorders in Cooley's anemia. *Ann N Y Acad Sci* 850:232, 1998.

188. Jessup M, Manno CS: Diagnosis and management of iron-induced heart disease in Cooley's anemia. *Ann N Y Acad Sci* 850:242, 1998.

189. Olivieri NF, Brittenham GM: Iron-chelating therapy and the treatment of thalassemia. *Blood* 89:739, 1997.

190. Hershko C, Peto TEA, Weatherall DJ: Iron and infection. *Br Med J* 296:660, 1988.

191. Weatherall DJ: Phenotype-genotype relationships in monogenic disease: Lessons from the thalassaemias. *Nat Rev Genet* 2:245, 2001.

192. Kan YW, Nathan DG: Mild thalassemia: The result of interactions of alpha and beta thalassemia genes. *J Clin Invest* 49:635, 1970.

193. Weatherall DJ, Pressley L, Wood WG, et al: The molecular basis for mild forms of homozygous β thalassaemia. *Lancet* 1:527, 1981.

194. Wainscoat JS, Old JM, Weatherall DJ, Orkin SH: The molecular basis for the clinical diversity of β thalassaemia in Cypriots. *Lancet* 1:1235, 1983.

195. Labie D, Pagnier J, Lapoumeroulie C, et al: Common haplotype dependency of high ᴳγ-globin gene expression and high Hb F levels in β-thalassemia and sickle cell anemia patients. *Proc Natl Acad Sci U S A* 82:2111, 1985.

196. Thein SL, Sampietro M, Old JM, et al: Association of thalassaemia intermedia with a beta-globin gene haplotype. *Br J Haematol* 65:370, 1987.

197. Thein SL, Hesketh C, Wallace RB, Weatherall DJ: The molecular basis of thalassaemia major and thalassaemia intermedia in Asian Indians: Application to prenatal diagnosis. *Br J Haematol* 70:225, 1988.

198. Ho PJ, Hall GW, Luo LY, et al: Beta thalassaemia intermedia: Is it possible to predict phenotype from genotype? *Br J Haematol* 100:70, 1998.

199. Camaschella C, Cappellini MD: Thalassemia intermedia. *Haematologica* 80:58, 1995.

200. Rund D, Oron-Karni V, Filon D, et al: Genetic analysis of β-thalassemia intermedia in Israel: Diversity of mechanisms and unpredictability of phenotype. *Am J Hematol* 54:16, 1997.

201. Wonke B, Hoffbrand AV, Bouloux P, et al: New approaches to the management of hepatitis and endocrine disorders in Cooley's anemia. *Ann N Y Acad Sci* 850:232, 1998.

202. Girot R, Lefrére JJ, Schettini F, et al: HIV infection and AIDS in thalassemia, in *Thalassemia 1990: 5th Annual Meeting of the COOLEY-CARE Group*, edited by P Rebulla, P Fessas, p 69. Centro Trasfusionale Ospedale Maggiore Policlinico Dio Milano, Athens, 1991.

203. Choudhury NV, Dubey ML, Jolly JG, et al: Post-transfusion malaria in thalassaemia patients. *Blut* 61:314, 1990.

204. Chatterjee R, Katz M, Cox TF, Porter JB: Prospective study of the hypothalmic-pituitary axis in thalassaemic patients who developed secondary amenorrhoea. *Clin Endocrinol* 39:287, 1993.

205. Liang ST, Wong VCW, So WWK, et al: Homozygous α-thalassaemia: Clinical presentation, diagnosis and management: A review of 46 cases. *Br J Obstet Gynaecol* 92:680, 1985.

206. Chui DHK, Waye JS: Hydrops fetalis caused by α-thalassaemia: An emerging health care problem. *Blood* 91:2213, 1998.

207. Beaudry MA, Ferguson DJ, Pearse K, et al: Survival of a hydropic infant with homozygous α-thalassaemia-1. *J Pediatr* 108:713, 1986.

208. Bianchi DW, Beyer EC, Stark AR, et al: Normal long-term survival with α thalassaemia. *J Pediatr* 108:716, 1986.

209. Gouttas A, Fessas P, Tsevrenis H, Xefteri E: Description d'une nouvelle variete d'anemie hemolytique congenitale. *Sang* 26:911, 1955.

210. Rigas DA, Koler RD, Osgood EE: Hemoglobin H: Clinical, laboratory, and genetic studies of a family with a previously undescribed hemoglobin. *J Lab Clin Med* 47:51, 1956.

211. Wasi P: Hemoglobinopathies in Southeast Asia, in *Distribution and Evolution of the Hemoglobin and Globin Loci*, edited by JE Bowman, p 179. Elsevier, New York 1983.

212. Kattamis C, Tzotzos S, Kanavakis E, et al: Correlation of clinical phenotype to genotype in haemoglobin H disease. *Lancet* 1:442, 1988.

213. Galanello R, Pirastu M, Melis MA, et al: Phenotype-genotype correlation in haemoglobin H disease in childhood. *J Med Genet* 20:425, 1983.

214. Fuchareon S, Winichagoon P, Pootrakul P, et al: Differences between two types of Hb H disease, α-thalassemia 1/α-thalassemia 2 and α-thalassemia 1/Hb Constant Spring. *Birth Defects Orig Artic Ser* 23:309, 1988.

215. Styles L, Foote DH, Kleman KM, et al: Hemoglobin H-Constant Spring disease: An under recognized, severe form of α thalassemia. *Int J Pediatr Hematol Oncol* 4:69, 1997.

216. Lie-Injo LE, Ganesan J, Clegg JB, Weatherall DJ: Homozygous state for Hb Constant Spring (slow-moving Hb X components). *Blood* 43:251, 1974.

217. Derry S, Wood WG, Pippard MJ, et al: Hematologic and biosynthetic studies in homozygous hemoglobin Constant Spring. *J Clin Invest* 73:1673, 1984.

218. Fei YJ, Kutlar F, Harris HF 2nd, et al: A search for anomalies in the zeta, alpha, beta, and gamma globin gene arrangements in normal Black, Italian, Turkish, and Spanish newborns. *Hemoglobin* 13:45, 1989.

219. Bowden DK, Hill AVS, Higgs DR, et al: Different hematologic phenotypes are associated with leftward ($-\alpha^{4.2}$) and rightward ($-\alpha^{3.7}$) α^+-thalassemia deletions. *J Clin Invest* 79:39, 1987.

220. Silvestroni E, Bianco L, Reitano G: Three cases of homozygous $\delta\beta$-thalassemia (or microcythemia) with high haemoglobin F in a Sicilian family. *Acta Hematol (Basel)* 40:220, 1968.

221. Ramot BN, Ben-Bassat I, Gafni D, Zaanoon R: A family with three $\delta\beta$-thalassemia homozygotes. *Blood* 35:158, 1970.

222. Tsistrakis GA, Amarantos SP, Konkouris LL: Homozygous $\beta\delta$-thalassaemia. *Acta Hematol (Basel)* 51:185, 1974.

223. Efremov GD: Hemoglobins Lepore and anti-Lepore. *Hemoglobin* 2:197, 1978.

224. Charache S, Clegg JB, Weatherall DJ: The Negro variety of hereditary persistence of fetal haemoglobin is a mild form of thalassaemia. *Br J Haematol* 34:527, 1976.

225. Huisman THJ, Miller A, Schroeder WA: A $^G\gamma$ type of hereditary persistence of fetal hemoglobin with β chain production in cis. *Am J Hum Genet* 27:765, 1975.

226. Higgs DR, Clegg JB, Wood WG, Weatherall DJ: $^G\gamma\delta\beta^+$-Type of hereditary persistence of fetal haemoglobin in association with Hb C. *J Med Genet* 16:288, 1979.

227. Fessas P, Stamatoyannopoulos G: Hereditary persistence of fetal hemoglobin in Greece: A study and a comparison. *Blood* 24:223, 1964.

228. Sofroniadou K, Wood WG, Nute PE, Stamatoyannopoulos G: Globin chain synthesis in Greek type ($^A\gamma$) of hereditary persistence of fetal haemoglobin. *Br J Haematol* 29:137, 1975.

229. Clegg JB, Metaxatou-Mavromati A, Kattamis C, et al: Occurrence of $^G\gamma$ Hb F in Greek HPFH: Analysis of heterozygotes and compound heterozygotes with β thalassaemia. *Br J Haematol* 43:521, 1979.

230. Camaschella C, Oggiano L, Sampietro M, et al: The homozygous state of G to A—117 $^A\gamma$ hereditary persistence of fetal hemoglobin. *Blood* 73:1999, 1989.

231. Weatherall DJ, Cartner R, Clegg JB, et al: A form of hereditary persistence of fetal haemoglobin characterized by uneven cellular distribution of haemoglobin F and the production of haemoglobins A and A$_2$ in homozygotes. *Br J Haematol* 29:205, 1975.

232. Silvestroni E, Bianco I: *La Malattia Microdrepanocitica*. Il Pensiero Scientifico, Rome, 1955.

233. Serjeant GR: *Sickle Cell Disease*, 2nd ed. Oxford University Press, New York, 1992.

234. Wasi P, Na-Nakorn S, Pootrakul S, et al: Alpha- and beta-thalassemia in Thailand. *Ann N Y Acad Sci* 165:60, 1969.

235. Rees DS, Styles J, Vichinsky EP, et al: The hemoglobin E syndromes. *Ann N Y Acad Sci* 850:334, 1998.

236. Agarwal S, Gulati R, Singh K: Hemoglobin E-beta thalassemia in Uttar Pradesh. *Indian Pediatr* 34:287, 1997.

237. Khanh NC, Thu LT, Truc DB, et al: Beta-thalassemia/hemoglobin E disease in Vietnam. *J Trop Pediatr* 36:43, 1990.

238. De Silva S, Fisher CA, Members of the Sri Lanka Thalassaemia Study, et al: Thalassaemia in Sri Lanka: Implications for the future health burden of Asian populations. *Lancet* 355:786, 2000.

239. Fucharoen S, Winichagoon P, Pootrakul P, et al: Variable severity of Southeast Asian β^0-thalassemia/Hb E disease, in *Thalassemia: Pathophysiology and Management*, Part A, edited by S Fucharoen, PT Rowley, NW Paul, p 241. Alan R. Liss, New York, 1988.

240. Fisher CA, Premawardhena A, De Silva S, et al: The molecular basis for the thalassaemias in Sri Lanka. *Br J Haematol* 121:1, 2003.

241. Sonakul D, Suwanagool P, Sirivaidyapong P, Fucharoen S: Distribution of pulmonary thromboembolic lesions in thalassemic patients, in *Thalassemia: Pathophysiology and Management*, Part A, edited by

S Fucharoen, PT Rowley, NW Paul, p 375. Alan R. Liss, New York, 1988.

242. Kattamis C, Metaxatou-Mavromati A, Wood WG, et al: The heterogeneity of normal Hb A$_2$-β thalassaemia in Greece. *Br J Haematol* 42:109, 1979.

243. Schwartz E: The silent carrier of beta thalassemia. *N Engl J Med* 281:1327, 1969.

244. Bianco I, Graziani B, Carboni C: Genetic patterns in thalassemia intermedia (constitutional microcytic anemia): Familial, hematologic and biosynthetic studies. *Hum Hered* 27:257, 1977.

245. Pirastu M, Ristaldi MS, Loudianos G, et al: Molecular analysis of atypical β-thalassemia heterozygotes. *Ann N Y Acad Sci* 612:90, 1990.

246. Olds RJ, Sura T, Jackson B, et al: A novel δ^0 mutation in cis with Hb Knossos: A study of different interactions in three Egyptian families. *Br J Haematol* 78:430, 1991.

247. Schokker RC, Went LN, Bok J: A new genetic variant of β-thalassaemia. *Nature* 209:44, 1966.

248. Ohta Y, Yamaoka K, Sumida I, et al: Homozygous delta-thalassemia first discovered in Japanese family with hereditary persistence of fetal hemoglobin. *Blood* 37:706, 1971.

249. Vella F, Wells RMC, Ager JAM: A haemoglobinopathy involving haemoglobin H and a new (Q) haemoglobin. *Br J Haematol* 1:752, 1958.

250. Lie-Injo LE, Pillay RP, Thuraisingham V: Further cases of Hb-Q-H disease (Hb Q-α-thalassemia). *Blood* 28:830, 1966.

251. Milner PF, Huisman THJ: Studies on the proportion and synthesis of haemoglobin G Philadelphia in red cells of heterozygotes, a homozygote, and a heterozygote for both haemoglobin G and α thalassemia. *Br J Haematol* 34:207, 1976.

252. Rieder RF, Woodbury DH, Rucknagel DL: The interaction of α-thalassaemia and haemoglobin G Philadelphia. *Br J Haematol* 32:159, 1976.

253. Pich P, Saglio G, Camaschella C, et al: Interaction between Hb Hasharon and α thalassemia: An approach to the problem of the number of human α loci. *Blood* 51:339, 1978.

254. Higgs DR, Aldridge BE, Lamb J, et al: The interaction of alpha-thalassemia and homozygous sickle cell disease. *N Engl J Med* 306:1441, 1982.

255. Embury SH, Dozy AM, Miller J, et al: Concurrent sickle-cell anemia and α-thalassemia. *N Engl J Med* 306:270, 1982.

256. Olivieri N: Thalassaemia: Clinical management. *Clin Haematol* 11:147, 1998.

257. Cazzola M, Borgna-Pignatti C, Locatelli F, et al: A moderate transfusion regimen may reduce iron loading in β-thalassemia major without producing excessive expansion of erythropoiesis. *Transfusion* 37:135, 1997.

258. Propper RD, Cooper B, Rufo RR, et al: Continuous subcutaneous administration of deferoxamine in patients with iron overload. *N Engl J Med* 297:418, 1977.

259. Pippard MJ, Callender ST, Letsky EA, Weatherall DJ: Prevention of iron loading in transfusion-dependent thalassaemia. *Lancet* 1:1178, 1978.

260. Pippard MJ, Callender ST, Finch CA: Ferrioxamine excretion in iron-loaded man. *Blood* 60:288, 1982.

261. Nienhuis AW: Safety of intensive chelation therapy. *N Engl J Med* 296:114, 1977.

262. Olivieri NF, Bunic JR, Chew E, et al: Visual and auditory neurotoxicity in patients receiving subcutaneous deferoxamine infusions. *N Engl J Med* 314:869, 1986.

263. Porter JB, Jawson MS, Huehns ER, et al: Desferrioxamine ototoxicity: Evaluation of risk factors in thalassaemia patients and guidelines for safe dosage. *Br J Haematol* 73:403, 1989.

264. Olivieri NF, Basran RK, Talbot AL, et al: Abnormal growth in thalassemia major associated with deferoxamine-induced destruction of spinal cartilage and compromise of sitting height. *Blood* 86:482a, 1995.

265. Pippard MJ, Weatherall DJ: Oral iron chelation therapy for thalassaemia: An uncertain scene. *Br J Haematol* 111:2, 2000.

266. Porter JB: Practical management of iron overload. *Br J Haematol* 115: 239, 2001.

267. Nisbet-Brown E, Olivieri NF, Giardina PJ, et al: Effectiveness and safety of ICL670 in iron-loaded patients with thalassaemia: A randomized, double-blind, placebo-controlled dose-escalation trial. *Lancet* 361:1597, 2003.

268. Wolfe L, Olivieri NF, Sallan D, et al: Prevention of cardiac disease by subcutaneous deferoxamine in patients with thalassemia major. *N Engl J Med* 312:1600, 1985.

269. Olivieri NF, Nathan DG, MacMillan JH, et al: Survival in medically treated patients with homozygous β-thalassemia. *N Engl J Med* 331: 574, 1994.

270. Brittenham GM, Griffith PM, Nienhuis AW, et al: Efficacy of deferoxamine in preventing complications of iron overload in patients with thalassemia major *N Engl J Med* 331:567, 1994.

271. Smith CH, Erlandson ME, Stern G, Hilgartner MW: Postsplenectomy infection in Cooley's anemia. *Ann N Y Acad Sci* 119:748, 1964.

272. Oudit GY, Sun H, Trivieri MG, et al: L-type Ca2+ channels provide a major pathway for iron entry into cardiomyocytes in iron-overload cardiomyopathy. *Nat Med* 9:1187, 2003.

273. Lucarelli G, Giardini C, Baronciani D: Bone marrow transplantation in β-thalassaemia. *Semin Hematol* 32:297, 1995.

274. Galimberti M, Angelucci M, Baronciani D, et al: Bone marrow transplantation in thalassemia: The experience of Pesaro. *Bone Marrow Transplant* 19(suppl 2):45, 1997.

275. Di Bartolomeo P, Di Girolamo G, Olioso P, et al: The Pescara experience of allogenic bone marrow transplantation in thalassemia. *Bone Marrow Transplant* 19(suppl 2):48, 1997.

276. Argiolu F, Sanna MA, Addari MC, et al: Bone marrow transplantation in thalassemia: The experience of Cagliari. *Bone Marrow Transplant* 19(suppl 2):65, 1997.

277. Gaziev D, Polchi P, Galimberti M, et al: Graft-versus-host disease following bone marrow transplantation for thalassemia: An analysis of incidence and risk factors. *Transplantation* 63:854, 1997.

278. Angelucci E, Ripalti M, Baronciani D, et al: Phlebotomy to reduce iron overload in patients cured of thalassemia by marrow transplantation. *Bone Marrow Transplant* 19(suppl 2):123, 1997.

279. Olivieri NF: Reactivation of fetal hemoglobin in patients with β thalassemia. *Semin Hematol* 33:24, 1996.

280. Olivieri NF, Weatherall DJ: The therapeutic reactivation of fetal haemoglobin. *Hum Mol Genet* 7:1655, 1998.

281. Swank RA, Stamatoyannopoulos G: Fetal gene reactivation. *Curr Opin Genet Dev* 8:366, 1998.

282. Weatherall DJ: Pharmacological treatment of monogenic disease. *Pharmacogenomics J* 3:264, 2003.

283. Olivieri NF, Rees DC, Ginder GD, et al: Treatment of thalassaemia major with phenylbutyrate and hydroxyurea. *Lancet* 350:491, 1997.

284. Sadelain M: Genetic treatment of the haemoglobinopathies: Recombinations and new combinations. *Br J Haematol* 98:247, 1997.

285. Dominski Z, Kole R: Restoration of correct splicing in thalassemic pre-mRNA by antisense oligonucleotides. *Proc Natl Acad Sci U S A* 90: 8673, 1993.

286. Lan N, Howrey RP, Lee S-W, et al: Ribozyme-mediated repair of sickle β-globin mRNAs in erythrocyte precursors. *Science* 280:1593, 1998.

287. Weatherall DJ: Gene therapy: Repairing haemoglobin disorders with ribozymes. *Curr Biol* 8:R696, 1998.

288. Rivella S, Sadelain M: Therapeutic globin gene delivery using lentiviral vectors. *Curr Opin Mol Ther* 4:505, 2002.

289. Persons DA, Nienhuis AW: Gene therapy for the hemoglobin disorders. *Curr Hematol Rep* 2:348, 2003.

290. WHO Working Group: Hereditary anemias: Genetic basis, clinical features, diagnosis and treatment. *Bull World Health Organ* 60:543, 1982.

291. Stamatoyannopoulos G: Problems of screening and counseling in the hemoglobinopathies, in *Proceedings of the IV International Conference on Birth Defects*, p. 268. Exerpta Medica, Vienna, 1974.

292. Alter BP: Antenatal diagnosis: Summary of results. *Ann N Y Acad Sci* 612:237, 1990.

293. Kazazian HH, Phillips JAI, Boehm CD, et al: Prenatal diagnosis of β-thalassemia by amniocentesis: Linkage analysis of multiple polymorphic restriction endonuclease sites. *Blood* 56:926, 1980.

294. Old JM, Ward RHT, Petrou M, et al: First trimester diagnosis for haemoglobinopathies: A report of 3 cases. *Lancet* 2:1413, 1982.

295. Old JM, Fitches A, Heath C, et al: First trimester fetal diagnosis for haemoglobinopathies: Report on 200 cases. *Lancet* 2:763, 1986.

296. Higgs DR, Lamb J, Aldridge BE, et al: Inadequacy of Hb Barts as an indicator of α-thalassaemia. *Br J Haematol* 51:177, 1982.

297. Pirastu M, Kan YW, Cao A, et al: Prenatal diagnosis of β-thalassemia: Detection of a single nucleotide mutation in DNA. *N Engl J Med* 309: 284, 1983.

298. Kogan SC, Doherty M, Gitschier J: An improved method for prenatal diagnosis of genetic diseases by analysis of amplified DNA sequences: Application to hemophilia. *N Engl J Med* 317:985, 1987.

299. Chehab F, Doherty M, Cai S, et al: Detection of sickle cell anaemia and thalassaemia. *Nature* 329:293, 1987.

300. Saiki RK, Chang C-A, Levenson CH, et al: Diagnosis of sickle cell anemia and β-thalassemia with enzymatically amplified DNA and non-radioactive allele-specific oligonucleotide probes. *N Engl J Med* 319: 537, 1988.

301. Old JM, Varawalla NY, Weatherall DJ: The rapid detection and prenatal diagnosis of β-thalassaemia in the Asian Indian and Cypriot populations in the U.K. *Lancet* 336:834, 1990.

302. Tan JAMA, Tay JSH, Lin LI, et al: The amplification refractory mutation system (ARMS): A rapid and direct prenatal diagnostic technique for β-thalassaemia in Singapore. *Prenatal Diagn* 14:1077, 1994.

303. Cai SP, Chang CA, Zhang JZ, et al: Rapid prenatal diagnosis of β-thalassemia using DNA amplification and nonradioactive probes. *Blood* 73:372, 1989.

304. Saiki RK, Walsh PS, Levenson CH, Erlich HA: Genetic analysis of amplified DNA with immobilized sequence-specific oligonucleotide probes. *Proc Natl Acad Sci U S A* 86:6230, 1989.

305. Takabayashi H, Kuwabara S, Ukita T, et al: Development of non-invasive fetal DNA diagnosis from maternal blood. *Prenatal Diagn* 15:74, 1995.

306. Cheung M-C, Goldberg JD, Kan YW: Prenatal diagnosis of sickle cell anemia and thalassemia by analysis of fetal cells in maternal blood. *Nat Genet* 14:264, 1996.

307. Kuliev A, Rechitsky S, Verlinsky O, et al: Preimplantation diagnosis of thalassemias. *J Assist Reprod Genet* 15:219, 1998.

308. Kuliev A, Rechitsky S, Verlinsky O, et al: Birth of healthy children after preimplantation diagnosis of thalassemia. *J Assist Reprod Genet* 16:201, 1999.

CHAPTER 47

DISORDERS OF HEMOGLOBIN STRUCTURE: SICKLE CELL ANEMIA AND RELATED ABNORMALITIES

ERNEST BEUTLER

Sickle hemoglobin is a mutant hemoglobin in which valine has been substituted for the glutamic acid normally at the sixth amino acid of the β-globin chain. This hemoglobin becomes polymerized and becomes poorly soluble when the oxygen tension is lowered and red cells that contain this hemoglobin become distorted and rigid. Sickle cell disease occurs when an individual is homozygous for the sickle cell mutation or is a compound heterozygote for sickle hemoglobin and β-thalassemia, hemoglobin C, and some less common β-globin mutations. Diagnosis depends upon demonstrating the presence of the abnormal hemoglobin(s) in the red cells. The disease is characterized by hemolytic anemia and by three types of crises: painful (vasoocclusive), sequestration, and aplastic. Complications include splenic infarction and autosplenectomy, stroke, bone infarcts and aseptic necrosis of the femoral head, leg ulcers, priapism, pulmonary hypertension, and renal failure. The severity of clinical manifestations varies greatly from patient to patient, and the aggressiveness of treatment needs to be modified accordingly. Early diagnosis, immunization against pneumococcal infection, and prompt treatment of infections that do occur have contributed to greatly improved survival of those born with these disorders. Stem cell transplantation, when successful, cures the disease. Treatment with hydroxyurea results in amelioration of crises. The original rationale for administration of hydroxyurea was its effect of increasing hemoglobin F levels, but there are probably other reasons for the success of this treatment, possibly including lowering of the white blood count, changes in red cell rheology, and indirect vascular affects. Sickle trait, the heterozygous state for sickle hemoglobin, affects approximately 8 percent of African-Americans and, with rare exceptions, is entirely benign. Hemoglobin C disease is associated with splenomegaly, but minimal hematologic changes, and the rare hemoglobin D disease is essentially asymptomatic. Hemoglobin E is very common in some parts of Asia. Hemoglobin E is greatly underproduced, and the homozygous state or compound heterozygous state with β-thalassemia resembles thalassemia.

Acronyms and abbreviations that appear in this chapter include: BPG, bisphosphoglycerate; CO, carbon monoxide; DPG, diphosphoglycerate; eNOS, endothelial nitric oxide synthase; G-6-PD, glucose-6-phosphate dehydrogenase; Hb, hemoglobin; HLA, human leukocyte antigen; Ig, immunoglobulin; MCHC, mean corpuscular hemoglobin concentration; NAD, nicotinamide adenine dinucleotide; NADH, nicotinamide adenine dinucleotide (reduced form); NO, nitric oxide.

Mutations that cause destabilization of the hemoglobin tetramer are an uncommon cause of hemolytic anemia. In contrast to the hemolytic anemias caused by enzyme deficiencies, a dominant mode of inheritance characterizes the unstable hemoglobins. Heinz bodies are a characteristic feature of the red cells in the blood when splenectomy has been performed. Hemolytic anemia may be precipitated by ingestion of "oxidative" drugs. The diagnosis is established by precipitating the unstable hemoglobin in a system in which the hemolysate is heated or incubated in a mixture of isopropanol and buffer. Although splenectomy has occasionally ameliorated the anemia, it should be avoided in most cases, because it has sometimes been followed by fatal thromboembolic complications.

DEFINITION AND HISTORY

James Herrick,[1] the astute Chicago physician who is also credited with description of the clinical syndrome of coronary thrombosis, was the first to observe sickled cells in the blood of an anemic African graduate student (Fig. 47-1). Emmel[2] demonstrated that red cells sickled when blood from such patients was sealed under glass and allowed to stand at room temperature for several days, but the fact that the transformation to sickled cells occurs in response to a fall in oxygen tension was not recognized until the classic studies of Hahn and Gillespie[3] in 1927. In 1923, the sickling phenomenon was shown to be inherited as an autosomal dominant trait.[4] Much later, Neel[5] and Beet[6] clarified the genetic basis of sickle cell anemia by demonstrating that heterozygosity for the sickle cell gene resulted in sickle cell trait without significant clinical symptoms, whereas homozygosity resulted in sickle cell anemia.

In 1949, Pauling and his colleagues[7] found that all the hemoglobin in patients with sickle cell anemia showed an abnormally slow rate of migration on electrophoresis, whereas the parents of these patients had normal as well as abnormal hemoglobin. Soon after, other abnormal hemoglobins were discovered by subjecting hemoglobin to electrophoresis. The biochemical nature of the defect in sickle cell anemia was elucidated by Ingram,[8] who digested hemoglobin with trypsin and separated the resulting peptides on paper by electrophoresis in one direction and chromatography in the other direction. This technique ("fingerprinting") demonstrated that one of the digestion products of sickle hemoglobin migrated differently from that of normal hemoglobin. Determination of the amino acid composition of this peptide indicated that sickle cell anemia was the result of the replacement of a glutamic acid residue by valine. This discovery established that the substitution of a single amino acid in a polypeptide chain can alter the function of the gene product sufficiently to produce widespread clinical effects. Conley[9] has chronicled the fascinating history of sickle cell disease.

NOMENCLATURE

STRUCTURAL AND MUTATION NOMENCLATURE

After the discovery that sickle hemoglobin, or hemoglobin S (Hb S), was electrophoretically altered, additional variants were assigned letters of the alphabet: C, D, E, etc. The letters of the alphabet were rapidly exhausted, however, and subsequent abnormal hemoglobins were named after the geographic location in which they were found (e.g., hemoglobin Memphis, hemoglobin Mexico). If the hemoglobin had the electrophoretic characteristics of a hemoglobin previously described by a letter, the geographic designation was added as a subscript (e.g., hemoglobin $M_{Saskatoon}$). In this case, M indicates an amino acid substitution resulting in a methemoglobin. In a fully characterized hemoglobin, the amino acid substitution has traditionally been designated by a superscript to the globin chain involved, for example, he-

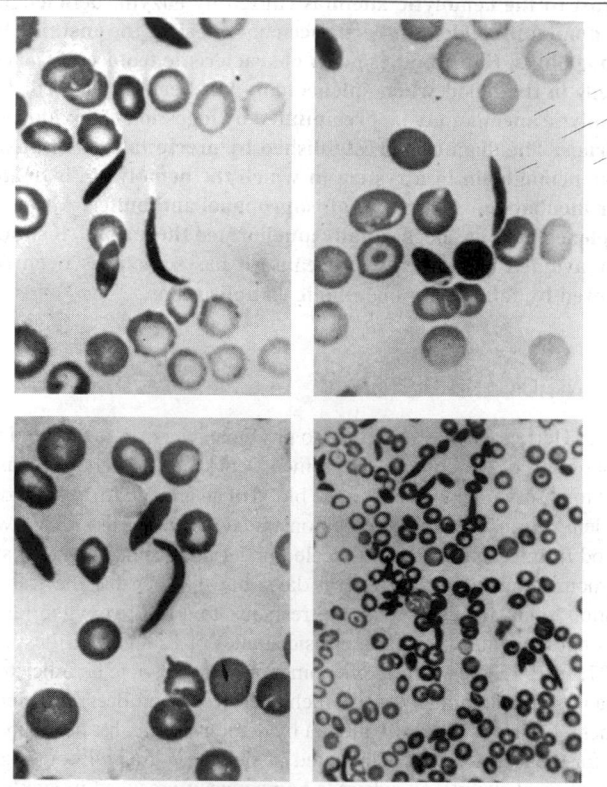

FIGURE 47-1   Peculiar elongated and sickle shaped red corpuscles in a case of severe anemia. (From JB Herrick,[1] with permission.)

moglobin S $\alpha_2\beta_2^{6Glu\rightarrow Val}$ and hemoglobin G$_{Norfolk}$ $\alpha_2^{35Asp\rightarrow Asn}\beta_2$. Thus, this notation indicates that hemoglobin S has a substitution of valine for glutamic acid in the sixth position of the β-chain and that hemoglobin G$_{Norfolk}$ is a substitution of asparagine for aspartic acid in the 35th position of the α-chain. These amino acid positions represent an aberration from the usual practice of naming the initiator methionine as amino acid number 1, because mutations in hemoglobin were numbered based on the processed, circulating protein. Moreover, because subscripts and superscripts do not lend themselves well to computerized databases, it has now been suggested that all capital letters be used and that the name and amino acid substitution not be subscripted.[10,11]

In another type of hemoglobin nomenclature, amino acids within helices (see "Structure and Function of the Hemoglobin Molecule") are designated by the amino acid number and the helix letter, whereas amino acids between helices bear the number of the amino acid and the letters of the two helices. Thus, residue EF3 is the third residue of the segment connecting the E and F helices, whereas residue F8 is the eighth residue of the F helix. Alignment according to helical designation makes homology evident: residue F8 is the proximal heme-linked histidine, and the histidine on the distal side of the heme is E7.

CLINICAL NOMENCLATURE

The term *sickle cell disorder* refers to states in which the red cell undergoes sickling when it is deoxygenated. The sickle cell diseases are disorders in which sickling produces prominent clinical manifestations. Included are sickle cell hemoglobin C disease (hemoglobin SC disease), sickle cell hemoglobin D disease (hemoglobin SD disease), sickle cell β-thalassemia, and sickle cell anemia. The latter term is reserved for the homozygous state for the sickle cell gene.

EPIDEMIOLOGY

Hemoglobin S occurs with greatest prevalence in tropical Africa. The heterozygote frequency usually is approximately 20 percent but in some areas reaches 40 percent. The sickle cell trait has a frequency of approximately 8 percent in African-American populations. The sickle cell gene is found to a lesser extent in the Middle East, in Greece, and in aboriginal tribes in India (Fig. 47-2). On occasion, sickle cell disease is found in Caucasians, especially where racial admixture has occurred over the centuries.[12]

The high prevalence of the gene for sickle hemoglobin in areas of the world where malaria has been common suggests that persons with sickle cell trait have a selective advantage over normal individuals when they contract this disease.[13] This advantage seems to be restricted to young children with sickle trait and *Plasmodium falciparum* infection. Although children with sickle cell trait are readily infected by *P. falciparum*, the parasite counts remain low. It may be that the infected red cell is preferentially sickled and destroyed, probably in the vascular system of the liver or spleen, where oxygen tensions are low and phagocytic cells abound. Whatever the mechanism, the result is that the infection is of short duration and the incidence of cerebral malaria and death is low.

At one time, one could only speculate as to whether the sickle cell mutation had arisen only once and had gradually gained a worldwide distribution or whether the same mutation had arisen independently in various populations and then had been the subject of selection, presumably through a protective effect against malaria. The ability to detect mutations in nontranscribed portions of DNA adjacent to the globin gene (see Chap. 9) has now provided insight into this problem. Such mutations are so close to the globin gene that the probability of a crossover (see Chap. 9) is vanishingly small. Thus, the relationship of the two mutations to one another will persist through hundreds of generations, permitting one to trace population movements. When the β-globin gene cluster is digested with restriction endonucleases, five distinct patterns are found in association with the sickle mutation. Four of these occur in Africa and have been designated the Senegal, Benin, Bantu, and Cameroon types.[14] An additional haplotype is typical of the Indian subcontinent.[15] These findings suggest that the sickle mutation arose independently at least five times.

The β-globin gene haplotypes have been a very useful tool for the study of gene flow.[16]

Hemoglobin C is found in 17 to 28 percent of West Africans, particularly east of the Niger River in the vicinity of North Ghana.[17,18] The selective factors that account for this high prevalence are unknown at present. The prevalence among African-Americans is 2 to 3 percent.[19,20] Sporadic cases also have been reported in other populations, including Italians[21] and Afrikaners.[12] Hemoglobin C probably confers some resistance to infection with malaria.[22]

Hemoglobin D Punjab, now recognized to be identical with hemoglobin D Los Angeles because both have the structure $\alpha_2\beta_2$121Glu$\rightarrow$Gln, also interacts with hemoglobin S in forming aggregates in the deoxy conformation. Hemoglobins D have been found in many parts of the world, including Africa, Northern Europe, and India.[23]

Hemoglobin E is so prevalent that it may be the most common abnormal hemoglobin[24] or second in prevalence only to hemoglobin S. Hemoglobin E is found principally in Burma, Thailand, Laos, Cambodia, Malaysia, and Indonesia. In some areas, hemoglobin E is found with an carrier rate of 30 percent.[25] On the other hand, it is not prevalent among the Chinese. Studies of restriction length polymorphisms in the β-globin cluster indicate the hemoglobin E mutation has arisen several times independently.[26] It, too, probably confers some resistance to infection with malaria.[27]

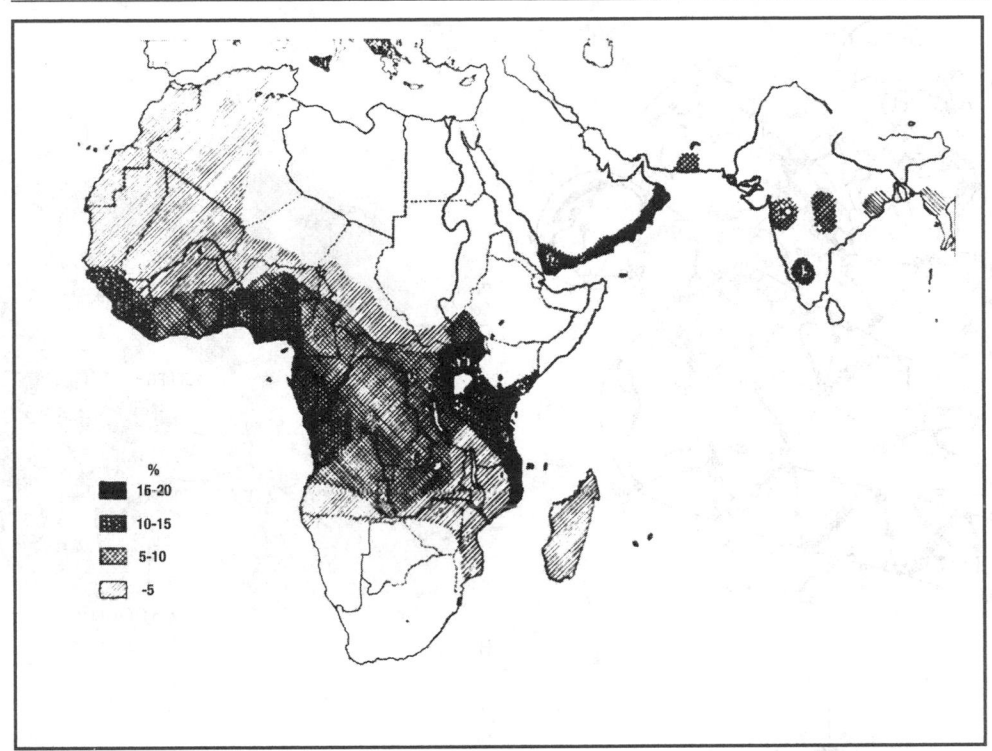

FIGURE 47 2   Distribution of sickle cell gene in Africa and Asia. (From AC Allison,[541] with permission.)

THE SICKLE CELL DISEASES

Sickle cell anemia (SS disease) may be considered the prototype of the sickle cell diseases. In general, the clinical features and treatment of all these disorders are the same and are therefore considered together here. The homozygous state, sickle cell anemia, is the most severe of these disorders. Hemoglobin SC disease and sickle cell β-thalassemia tend to be milder, and hemoglobin SD disease is the mildest of the group. However, there is a great deal of overlap in the severity of the clinical manifestations of these disorders; therefore, they are described together here. Some patients with sickle cell thalassemia or hemoglobin SC disease may be more anemic and have more severe and frequent crises than some mildly affected patients with sickle cell anemia. A major difference among these diseases is in their laboratory diagnosis.

ETIOLOGY AND PATHOGENESIS

STRUCTURE AND FUNCTION OF THE HEMOGLOBIN MOLECULE*

The red protein hemoglobin serves to transport oxygen from the lungs to the tissues and CO_2 from the tissues back to the lungs. Hemoglobin also destroys the physiologically important nitric oxide (NO) molecule. It has evolved to perform its transport functions in a highly efficient manner. The oxygen affinity of hemoglobin permits nearly complete saturation with oxygen in the lungs, as well as efficient oxygen unloading in the tissues because of its sigmoid oxygen dissociation curve. This curve results from the fact that hemoglobin is an allosteric molecule; its conformation, and hence the oxygen affinity, changes as each successive molecule of oxygen is bound. Hemoglobin also plays an important role in acid–base balance: deoxyhemoglobin binds protons and oxyhemoglobin releases protons.

*This section is based upon Chapter 28 by H.M. Ranney and V. Sharma in the sixth edition of this book.

Regulation of the oxygen dissociation curve to meet the needs of the body is remarkable. Hypoxic tissues become acidotic acutely, and the protons released produce a shift in the oxygen dissociation curve that enables more oxygen to be delivered to the tissue. However, longer-term acidosis or alkalosis (as occurs at high altitudes) is counteracted by modulation of red cell 2,3-diphosphoglycerate ([2,3-DPG]; 2,3 bisphosphoglycerate [2,3-BPG]) serving to decrease hemoglobin oxygen affinity (see Chap. 45).

Normal mammalian hemoglobins contain two pairs of unlike polypeptide chains: one chain of each pair is α or α-like and the other is non-α (β, γ, or δ). The α-chains of all human hemoglobins encountered after early embryogenesis are the same. The non-α-chains include the β-chain of normal adult hemoglobin [hemoglobin A ($\alpha_2\beta_2$)], the γ-chain of fetal hemoglobin [hemoglobin F ($\alpha_2\gamma_2$)], and the δ-chain of hemoglobin A_2 [hemoglobin A_2 ($\alpha_2\delta_2$)], the minor component of which accounts for 2.5 percent of the hemoglobin of normal adults. The regulation of production of the globin chains is discussed in Chapter 46.

Certain residues in the amino acid sequence of each polypeptide chain appear to be critical to stability and function. Such residues are usually the same (invariant) in α- or β-chains. The NH_2-terminal valines of the β-chains are important in 2,3-BPG interactions. The C-terminal residues are important in the salt bridges that characterize the unliganded molecules. Areas of contact between chains and between heme and globin tend to contain invariant residues.

The non-α- (β, γ, δ, or ε) chains are all 146 amino acids in length; the β-chain begins with valine and histidine. The C-terminal residues are Tyr β145 and His β146. The δ-chain (of hemoglobin A_2) differs from the β-chain (of hemoglobin A) in only 10 residues. The first eight residues and the C-terminal residues (127–146) are the same in δ- and β-chains.

The γ-chain of fetal hemoglobin (hemoglobin F) differs from the β-chain by 39 residues. The N-terminal residues of the γ-chain and β-

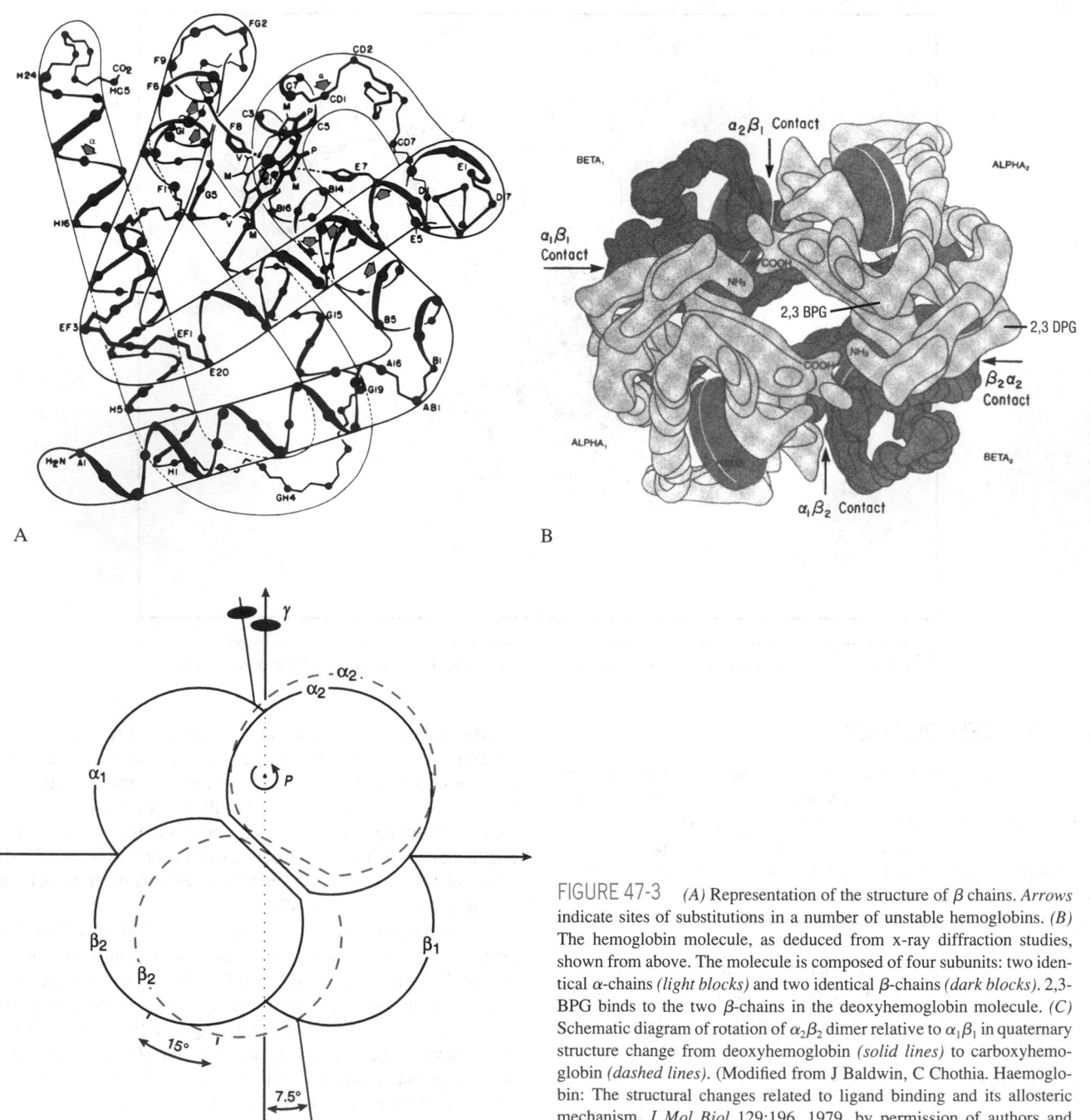

FIGURE 47-3   *(A)* Representation of the structure of β chains. *Arrows* indicate sites of substitutions in a number of unstable hemoglobins. *(B)* The hemoglobin molecule, as deduced from x-ray diffraction studies, shown from above. The molecule is composed of four subunits: two identical α-chains *(light blocks)* and two identical β-chains *(dark blocks)*. 2,3-BPG binds to the two β-chains in the deoxyhemoglobin molecule. *(C)* Schematic diagram of rotation of $\alpha_2\beta_2$ dimer relative to $\alpha_1\beta_1$ in quaternary structure change from deoxyhemoglobin *(solid lines)* to carboxyhemoglobin *(dashed lines)*. (Modified from J Baldwin, C Chothia. Haemoglobin: The structural changes related to ligand binding and its allosteric mechanism. *J Mol Biol* 129:196, 1979, by permission of authors and publisher, Academic Press Ltd., London.)

chain are glycine and valine, respectively, whereas the C-terminal residues Tyr145 and His146 are the same as in γ- and β-chains. In addition to the different N-terminal residues, several other differences in primary structure between the γ- and β-chains are noteworthy. The γ chain contains isoleucine, whereas the β-chains do not. The γ-genes are duplicated: one codes for glycine (Gγ) and the other for alanine (Aγ)[7] at residue 176, giving rise to two kinds of γ-chains. In addition, a common polymorphism, the substitution of threonine for isoleucine, is frequently found at residue 75 of the Aγ-chain.

Approximately 75 percent of the amino acids in α- or β-chains are in a helical arrangement. All hemoglobins studied have a similar helical content (Fig. 47-3A). Eight helical areas, lettered A to H, occur in

the β-chains. Hemoglobin nomenclature specifies that amino acids within helices are designated by the amino acid number and the helix letter, whereas amino acids between helices bear the number of the amino acid and the letters of the two helices. Thus, residue EF3 is the third residue of the segment connecting the E and F helices, whereas residue F8 is the eighth residue of the F helix. Alignment according to helical designation makes homology evident: residue F8 is the proximal heme-linked histidine, and the histidine on the distal side of the heme is E7.

Figure 47-3B and C shows the tertiary structure of the α- and β-chains. The prosthetic group of hemoglobin is ferroprotoporphyrin IX. Its structure is shown in Figure 47-4A. The heme group is located in

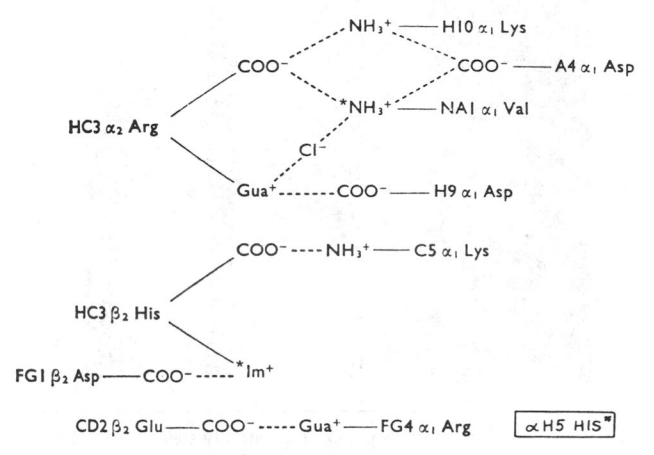

A   B

FIGURE 47-4 *(A)* Structure of heme (ferroprotoporphyrin IX). *(B)* Heme group and its environment in the unliganded α-chain. Only selected side chains are shown: the heme 4-propionate is omitted. (From BR Gelin, AW Lee, M Karplus,[542] with permission.)

a crevice between the E and F helices in each chain (Fig. 47-4B). The highly polar propionate side chains of the heme are on the surface of the molecule and are ionized at physiologic pH. The rest of the heme is inside the molecule, surrounded by nonpolar residues except for two histidines. The iron atom is linked by a coordinate bond to the imidazole nitrogen (N) of histidine F8. The E7 *distal* histidine, on the other side of the heme plane, is not bonded to the iron atom but is very close to the ligand-binding site.

The sigmoid oxygen dissociation curve is a function of the change of the conformation of the molecule from the liganded to the unliganded state (Table 47-1). In the deoxy state, the hemoglobin tetramer is held together by intersubunit salt bonds (Fig. 47-5) and intersubunit hydrophobic contacts (see Fig. 47-3B), in addition to a certain number of hydrogen bonds. In deoxyhemoglobin, 2,3-BPG is situated in the central cavity between the two β-chains (see Fig. 47-3B). The change in conformation of the hemoglobin molecule is brought about by a complex, coordinated series of changes in the structure of the molecule as heme binds oxygen.[20] The oxygen dissociation curve can be linearized by a transformation known as the Hill plot:

$$\log[y/(1-y)] = \log K + n \log Po_2,$$

where K is an empiric overall constant without physicochemical basis.

The slope n is taken as a convenient measure of cooperativity. Values of n in noninteracting hemoglobins that exhibit hyperbolic, not sigmoid, oxygen dissociation curves (e.g., myoglobin and hemoglobin H) are about 1. In a normal tetrameric hemoglobin with four oxygen-reactive sites, the maximum value for n is 4.0; however, n values of 2.7 to 3.0 are found in normal hemoglobin.

The point at which the hemoglobin is one-half saturated with oxygen (P_{50}) is the usual measurement of oxygen affinity. It depends upon pH (the Bohr effect), temperature, and 2,3-BPG concentration. In common practice, P_{50} is standardized at 37°C and pH 7.20. P_{50} of freshly drawn blood is about 26.7 torr under standard conditions, but the Po_2 of hemoglobin from which 2,3-BPG has been removed is only about 13 torr.[29] Although fetal and newborn red cells have 2,3-BPG levels similar to those of adults, their oxygen dissociation curve is left shifted (increased oxygen affinity) with a P_{50} of about 23 torr because fetal hemoglobin does not react as strongly with 2,3-BPG as does adult hemoglobin.

Although oxygen is the major physiologic ligand of the heme group of hemoglobin, the binding of carbon monoxide (CO) and NO by heme is of great importance. CO binds to hemoglobin with about 400 times the affinity of oxygen. As a result, relatively low ambient concentrations of CO may result in displacement of a large proportion of the oxygen from hemoglobin. To make matters worse, from a clinical point of view, CO has a pronounced effect of the oxygen dissociation curve, shifting it to the left. Thus, the clinical effect of CO poisoning is appreciably greater than that which can be accounted for on the basis of displacement of oxygen alone. When NO is bound by hemoglobin, the hemoglobin is oxidized to methemoglobin in the reaction:

TABLE 47-1 NOMENCLATURE OF HEMOGLOBIN QUATERNARY STRUCTURES

LIGANDED (OXYGEN BOUND)	UNLIGANDED (REDUCED)
Oxy	Deoxy
R-state	T-state
Relaxed	Tense
High-affinity	Low-affinity

FIGURE 47-5 Salt bridges in deoxyhemoglobin (* = ionizable group less protonated at pH 9.0 than at pH 7.0). These groups account for 60 percent of the alkaline Bohr effect. The remainder is due to αH5 His. (From MF Perutz, AJ Wilkinson, M Paoli, GG Dodson,[543] with permission.)

$$HbO_2 + NO \rightarrow MetHb + NO_3^-$$

Removal of NO by hemoglobin may play an important physiologic role and account for the esophageal pain sometimes encountered in paroxysmal nocturnal hemoglobinuria (see Chap. 38) and for the hypertension occurring after infusion of some experimental hemoglobin solutions.[30]

BIOCHEMICAL BASIS OF SICKLING

Sickle cell anemia results from the substitution of thymine for adenine in the glutamic acid DNA codon (GAG→GTG), which in turn results in substitution of valine for the sixth amino acid glutamic acid. Molecules of hemoglobin S that are in the deoxy conformation have a strong tendency to aggregate. Such aggregation requires the substitution of valine for glutamic acid in the sixth position, because only those hemoglobin variants with this substitution (e.g., S and Harlem) undergo sickling. Certain other structural features of the molecule also are important.[31,32]

Electron micrographs of deoxygenated sickle hemoglobin show the presence of multiple microtubules consisting of hemoglobin molecules stacked on top of each other (Fig. 47-6). The molecules do not

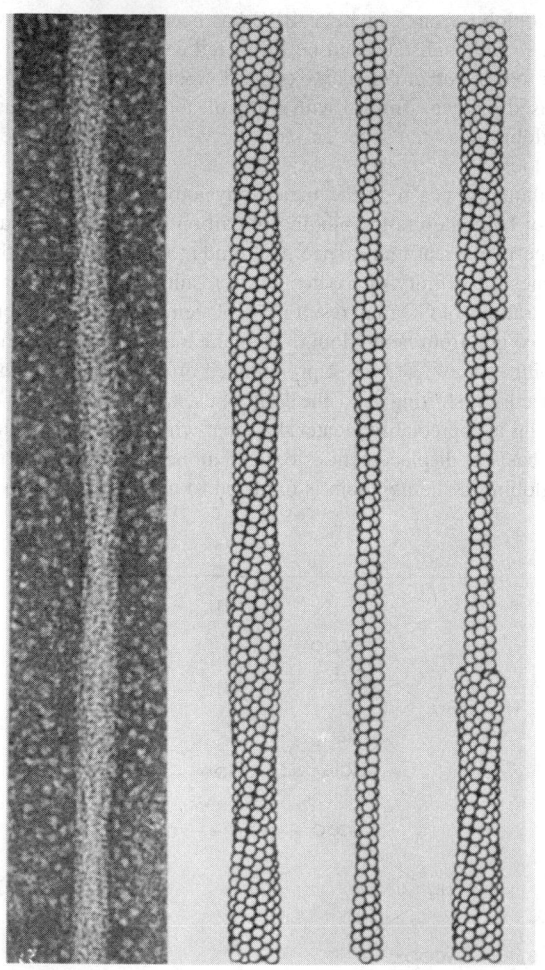

FIGURE 47-6　Electron micrograph of negatively stained fiber of hemoglobin S and the structure deduced by three-dimensional image reconstruction. The reconstructed fiber is presented as ball models, with each ball representing a hemoglobin S tetramer. The models are presented as the outer sheath (left), the inner core (center), and a combination of both inner and outer filaments (right). (From SJ Edelstein,[544] with permission.)

lie directly over one another, so a helical structure is formed. Fourteen strands of the fiber are organized into pairs,[33] giving rise to a fiber that is 21 nm in diameter. Most of the intermolecular contacts that give rise to this structure have been elucidated.[33,34]

The deoxygenated hemoglobin solution turns into a firm gel. The distorted sickled red cell is the visible end result of this molecular aggregation. The process is time dependent.[35] Initially, there is a rate-limiting nucleation process; a few molecules of sickle hemoglobin must aggregate, forming a "seed" on which aggregation of further molecules occurs rapidly. Thus, the sickling process is characterized by a long delay that is strongly dependent on temperature and concentration.[36] The delay is inversely proportional to approximately the 30th power of the hemoglobin concentration.[37] This delay is quite important in protecting the patient from even more dire consequences than might otherwise be anticipated. Even though the oxygen concentration of venous blood is sufficiently low so that at equilibrium about 85 percent of the red cells would contain sickle hemoglobin polymer, kinetic data suggest that about 80 percent of cells are prevented from sickling during their round trip through the circulation because they reach the lungs and become reoxygenated before significant polymerization has occurred.[35]

When a cell sickles and unsickles repeatedly, the membrane is affected and the cell becomes irreversibly sickled; it remains so even when the oxygen pressure is increased.[38] These are the sickled forms seen on air-dried films. An irreversibly sickled cell has a high hemoglobin concentration, high calcium and low potassium content, and it may be ATP-depleted.[39] These cells appear to be derived directly from reticulocytes[40] but have a short intravascular life span. The severity of the hemolytic process is directly related to the number of these cells in a patient's circulation.[41] However, the relationship between the number of irreversibly sickled cells and the number and severity of painful crises is an inverse one.[42,43]

MEMBRANE CHANGES IN SICKLE CELLS

Although the primary defect in sickle cell disease is clearly in the hemoglobin, secondary alterations in red cell metabolism and membrane structure and function have also been described. Rapid potassium loss occurs early in the sickling process.[44] Abnormalities of sickle cell membrane phosphorylation have been documented.[45–47] The calcium pump is abnormal.[48] Although the calcium content of sickle cell membranes, particularly of those cells that are irreversibly sickled, has been found to be increased,[45–50] the location of the excess calcium appears to be in endocytic vacuoles; therefore, from a functional point of view, its location is extracellular.[51,52] Increased generation of free radicals may occur in sickle cells,[53–55] and there is abnormal oxidation of thiols in sickle cells.[56] Superoxide dismutase activity of sickle cells is slightly reduced,[57] and the amount of nicotinamide adenine dinucleotide (NAD)+ and the ratio of NAD+ + NADH [nicotinamide adenine dinucleotide (reduced form)] to NADH are increased.[58] Binding of glyceraldehyde phosphate dehydrogenase to the membrane is decreased by 35 to 50 percent,[59] and the lipid bilayer appears to uncouple from the submembrane skeleton.[60] Macrophages seem to ingest sickle cells more readily than normal cells and this could be a result of excessive auto-oxidation of membrane components with the acquisition of immunoglobulins on the cell surface[61] or to loss of membrane phospholipid asymmetry, which is a constant finding in sickle cells[62,63] and may play an important role in their clearance from the circulation as well as activation of coagulation.[64]

Sickled erythrocytes lose some of their membrane phospholipid asymmetry exposing phosphatidylserine on the outside of the cell,[65,66] and this may result in activation of complement and/or coagulation. Co-inheritance of factor V Leiden does not appear to have an appreciable affect on the clinical manifestations of sickle cell disease,[67] although an anecdotal report of homozygous factor V Leiden in sickle cell disease suggested that such an interaction might be present.[68]

FACTORS THAT INFLUENCE THE SEVERITY OF SICKLE CELL DISEASE

Because a large number of inherited and acquired factors influence the pathogenesis of clinical symptoms, the sickle cell disorders vary in clinical severity from the virtually symptomless sickle cell trait to the potentially lethal state characteristic of sickle cell anemia. Wide variation in the severity of clinical manifestations also occurs within the group of patients with sickle cell anemia. Some die in the first few years of life, while others have been discovered late in life as a result of a chance survey.

Both intracellular and extracellular factors influence sickling. Included are the types of hemoglobin in the cell and their concentration, the level of 2,3-BPG (2,3-DPG), and the hydrogen ion concentration. Some of these factors are determined predominantly by genetic factors; others are environmentally modified. The variability of these factors as well as many others that are not understood probably accounts for the natural pattern of this group of diseases—periods of comparative well-being interspersed with periods of clinical deterioration (crises). Longitudinal studies of patients have suggested an increase in the number of dense and poorly deformable cells precedes the development of a crisis.[69] However, calculation of the mean polymer fraction from the 2,3-BPG concentration, mean corpuscular hemoglobin concentration (MCHC), internal pH, and percent non-sickle hemoglobin did not make possible prediction of the clinical course.[70] The precipitating circumstances responsible for the development of crises often are not clear. Of the events that seem to be associated with the appearance of crises, infections are probably among the most common. Since NO has been used for the therapy of the acute chest syndrome in patients with sickle cell disease, polymorphisms in the endothelial nitric oxide synthase (eNOS) have been examined and it has been claimed that female, but not male, subjects with the 786 T→C polymorphisms were more likely to develop pulmonary disease.[71] However, no corrections were made for multiple comparisons, and this observation requires confirmation in an independent series.

However, it is not only the extent of sickling that is important but also the interaction of the sickled cells with the endothelium and other blood cells (see "Blood Flow in the Microvasculature" below).

Concentration of Hemoglobin S in the Red Cell   A correlation exists between the concentration of sickle hemoglobin within a red cell and the susceptibility of the cell to sickling. The red cells of the sickle cell carrier, who is virtually symptom-free, always contain less than 50 percent Hb S; the remainder is largely normal adult hemoglobin. The exact proportions vary from one individual to another. It was proposed more than 50 years ago that the distribution of the concentration of sickle hemoglobin in the red cells of subjects with the sickle cell trait was bimodal.[72] Subsequent studies confirmed the existence of more than a single mode and indicated that the distribution might actually be trimodal.[73] The reason for such a discontinuous distribution has become apparent with the recognition of the very high frequency of α-thalassemia in persons of African ancestry. Individuals carrying α-thalassemic genes have a higher ratio of hemoglobin A to hemoglobin S than those who have four normal copies of the α locus.[74] Apparently the affinity of α-chains for β^A-chains is higher than the affinity for β^S-chains,[75] possibly because of differences in the charge of the two chains.[76] Thus, when the number of α-chains become limiting in the formation of hemoglobin tetramers, a higher proportion $\alpha_2\beta_2^A$ tetramers than $\alpha_2\beta_2^S$ tetramers is formed. Interaction of the α-thalassemic gene and the sickle gene also may influence the course of sickle cell disease: the lower corpuscular hemoglobin concentration in the red cells in α-thalassemia would be expected to protect against sickling.

It has been suggested that such an interaction may influence the severity of sickle cell disease in African-Americans[74,77,78] and that it may play an important role in producing the very mild clinical manifestation of sickle cell anemia in Saudi Arabia.[79]

Presence of Other Hemoglobins in the Cell   Other hemoglobins present in a red cell containing sickle hemoglobin are not inert bystanders in the sickling process.[80] Some hemoglobins, such as F, Korle-Bu, and A₂, interact less effectively with hemoglobin S than does hemoglobin A in the sickling process. Two common abnormal hemoglobins, Hb C and Hb D, and the relatively rare hemoglobin O$_{Arab}$ become involved in the formation of the sickling tubule. The interaction of these hemoglobins with sickle hemoglobin increases the propensity of red cells to sickle. Moreover, the red cells of patients with SC disease characteristically have an increased MCHC, presumably due to a transport defect, and this, too, greatly increases sickling.[81,82]

Other hemoglobins do not appear to play an active role in the sickling process, and their presence in the red cell can greatly reduce the clinical severity of sickle cell anemia. Fetal hemoglobin, for example, protects the red cell from sickling.[83] It is distributed heterogeneously in the red cells of an SS homozygote,[84,85] and those cells with the largest amount are least susceptible to sickling.[84,85] The relatively mild clinical manifestations of patients in the Middle East with sickle cell anemia has been ascribed, at least in part, to the high level of fetal hemoglobin present in their red cells.[86–88] In the United States, however, no significant correlation exists between fetal hemoglobin levels and the severity of the clinical manifestations of sickle cell anemia.[89] Even in the Arab population the relationship is not always clear,[90] although the effect may be obscured by a threshold phenomenon,[91] that is, a favorable effect of fetal hemoglobin concentration is observed only above a certain level. In adults heterozygous for hemoglobin S and hereditary persistence of hemoglobin F, hemoglobin S constitutes more than 70 percent of the hemoglobin, but the high concentration of hemoglobin F inhibits sickling because the distribution is such that each cell contains a considerable amount of hemoglobin F, and the patients experience a benign clinical course.[92] The presence of the abnormal hemoglobin Memphis ($\alpha^{23Glu \rightarrow Gln}\beta_2$) also decreases the clinical severity of sickle cell disease,[93] presumably by inhibiting the formation of the sickle tubule.

There is great variability among patients with sickle disease with respect to the number of cells containing high concentrations of hemoglobin F (F-cells). Numerous efforts have been made to find modifying genes, and it has been proposed that such genes might exist on the X chromosome[94] or on chromosome 6q,[95] but no such genes have yet been identified (see Chap. 46).

Interaction of Sickling and Thalassemia   The interaction of β-thalassemia with sickling is discussed in Chapter 46, and that with α-thalassemia is considered in "Concentration of Hemoglobin S in the Red Cell" above.

Glucose-6-Phosphate Dehydrogenase Deficiency   It has been suggested that glucose-6-phosphate dehydrogenase (G-6-PD) deficiency has a beneficial effect on the clinical course of sickle cell anemia,[96–99] but this correlation has not been confirmed in other studies.[19,100–107] It has also been proposed that hemolytic crises are more common in patients with sickle cell disease who are also G-6-PD deficient.[108] However, it seems unlikely that the G-6-PD–deficient cells of such a patient would be particularly sensitive in hemolytic stress; G-6-PD A- is very age labile (see Chap. 45) and, because the erythrocytes are young, they have relatively normal G-6-PD activity. In Jamaica,[105] the United States,[106] and Brazil,[107] G-6-PD deficiency did not influence parameters of disease severity, such as hemoglobin concentration, reticulocyte count, hemoglobin F concentration, irreversibly sickled cell counts, or plasma hemoglobin concentration, and there was no relationship between clinical severity and presence or absence of G-6-PD deficiency.

Deoxygenation   Deoxygenation for a sufficient period of time is the most important factor determining the occurrence of sickling in a red cell containing hemoglobin S. The degree of deoxygenation required to produce sickling varies with the percentage of hemoglobin S in the cells. Red cells from patients with sickle cell anemia begin to sickle at an oxygen tension of about 40 torr.[109] Changes that impair adequate oxygenation of the blood may be deleterious to any person whose red cells contain sickle hemoglobin.

An arterial oxygen tension of approximately 66 torr is found at approximately 10,000 ft (3048 m). Hypoxemia also may result from flying in unpressurized aircraft. However, most commercial aircraft maintain an atmospheric pressure in the cabin equivalent to that encountered at an altitude of 5000 to 7000 ft (1524 to 2134 m). Occasional patients with sickle cell anemia or hemoglobin SC disease have been reported to experience painful crises or splenic infarctions under such circumstances.[110] However, there is no evidence that persons with sickle cell trait are at risk in a pressurized airplane.[111] The oxygen content of the air may also be reduced during anesthesia or when using an artificial breathing apparatus, as in scuba diving. If pulmonary or cardiac function deteriorates (e.g., in pneumonia or cardiac failure), any resulting reduction in arterial oxygen tension may prove hazardous to a patient with sickle cell disease.

Vascular Stasis   The PO_2 level producing *in vitro* sickling of cells containing Hb S bears only an indirect relationship to clinical measurements of arterial and venous PO_2. This is because the PO_2 in the larger peripheral vessels does not accurately reflect the oxygen tension in areas of vascular stasis, such as the sinusoids of the spleen, in which hypoxemia is common and sickling is likely to occur. Although a period of 2 to 4 minutes is required for development of marked red cell distortion[35,112] and rigidity, the red cells normally remain within the venous circulation for only about 10 to 15 seconds. For this reason, red cells in areas of vascular stasis are more vulnerable to sickling. Once sickling has occurred, increased blood viscosity[113] results in further vascular stasis, further sickling, possible vascular occlusion, and infarction. This course of events leads to tissue death, manifested clinically as a painful crisis.

Although no organ of the body is immune to vasoocclusion resulting from *in vivo* sickling, certain sites notorious for circulatory stasis are characteristically affected. Splenic and marrow infarctions resulting from vascular stasis are particularly frequent, and priapism may occur in males. The role of vascular stasis in the development of leg ulcers and of retinal and renal lesions is discussed below (see "Clinical Features"). Studies from Jamaica indicated the incidence of peptic ulcer was greatly increased in patients with sickle cell disease.[114] Ulceration was identified in 30.5 percent of male patients over age 25 years, but this finding could not be confirmed in a West African population.[115] It is possible that *Helicobacter pylori* infections play a role in peptic ulceration in these patients.[116]

Temperature   Even though cold temperatures retard hemoglobin polymerization, on the basis of anecdotal observations low temperatures have been thought to precipitate sickle crises, presumably because of the accompanying vasoconstriction. However, this impression has not been confirmed in epidemiologic studies.[117]

Acidosis   Hydrogen ions produce a right shift in the oxygen dissociation curve (the Bohr effect), presumably by displacing the equilibrium between the high-affinity oxy conformation and the low-affinity deoxy conformation toward the deoxy conformation of hemoglobin. Since it is sickle hemoglobin in the deoxy conformation that aggregates, the lowered pH profoundly affects the sickling of red cells, even when the percent oxygenation is maintained at a constant level.[118,119] Alkalosis, on the other hand, by shifting the equilibrium toward the oxy conformation, tends to retard sickling but impairs oxygen release to tissue.

Corpuscular Hemoglobin Concentration   The tendency of hemoglobin S solutions to aggregate is proportional to the 30th power of the concentration.[37,120] Accordingly, sickling of red cells is markedly influenced by the concentration of sickle hemoglobin in the cells. Suspending sickle cells in a hyperosmolar medium increases the intracellular hemoglobin concentration as the cell is dehydrated. This phenomenon may account in part for sickling in renal papillae.[121,122] Conversely, any agent that causes increased red cell volume will retard the sickling process by decreasing MCHC. Marked dehydration results in both vascular stasis and hypertonicity and can precipitate a crisis.

Blood Flow in the Microvasculature   In the last analysis, vasoocclusion is the result of a variety of factors on blood flow in the microvasculature. The factors that influence the rheologic properties of blood that contains sickle cells are extremely complex. For example, shear stresses, such as those that occur in the circulation, break down gel structure.[123] However, this results in the creation of more nucleation centers and results in a decrease in the delay time. In the circulation, flow properties of blood are influenced not only by factors such as the rigidity of the erythrocytes but also by the adherence of sickle cells to the endothelium,[124,125] which may involve band 3,[126] and to each other.[127] Variations in such factors, modifying the rheologic consequences of the sickling process, undoubtedly play a role in determining when vasoocclusive episodes will occur. Granulocytes, too, manifest increased adherence to endothelium, and this has been attributed to increased expression of CD64.[128]

The sequence of events that lead to occlusion of blood vessels by sickle cells is thus complex.[129,130] One essential factor is the aggregation of sickle hemoglobin with the consequent changes in the rheologic properties of the erythrocytes (see "Biochemical Basis of Sickling" above). The overall viscosity of the blood is a function of the hematocrit, and occlusion is more likely when hematocrit levels are relatively high. Adhesion of sickle cells to the vascular endothelium is an important factor and may be related to exposure of vascular endothelial adhesion molecules, such as vascular cell adhesion molecule-1, and to the levels of plasma factors that enhance adhesion, including fibrinogen, factor VIII, fibronectin, von Willebrand factor, and thrombospondin. The adhesion receptors very late activation antigen-4 and CD36 are found in unusually high numbers on sickle cell reticulocytes, and they help mediate adhesion of sickle RBC to endothelium.[64,131] Abnormalities in NO-induced vascular relaxation have also been indirectly implicated. Leukocytes probably also participate in this complex process, perhaps by releasing cytokines that up-regulate adhesive endothelial glycoproteins, and it has been suggested that a part of the therapeutic effect of hydroxyurea may be related to reduction of the leukocyte count.[132]

Infections   Infections are common in patients with sickle cell disease,[133] and vasoocclusive crises may be precipitated by infections. In many cases, the mechanism by which infection increases sickling is easily discernible: fever, vomiting, and diarrhea may produce dehydration; lack of food intake may produce acidosis; and hypoxemia may result from pneumonia. Other, more subtle mechanisms also may be responsible for precipitation of crises in patients with sickle diseases with infections.

INHERITANCE

A patient with sickle cell anemia is homozygous for the gene for sickle hemoglobin and has therefore inherited one abnormal gene from each parent. If 7.8 percent of a population are sickle cell trait carriers,[19] as in the African-American population, there is a 1:164 chance that two carriers will marry, and the chances that an offspring of such a marriage will have sickle cell anemia is 1:4. In such a population, about 1 in 650 will have sickle cell anemia.

Similarly, persons with hemoglobin SC disease must have one parent with a sickle hemoglobin gene and another with a hemoglobin C gene. Because these genes are allelic β-chain mutations, persons with hemoglobin SC disease have no normal β polypeptide chain gene and therefore have no hemoglobin A. The carrier rate for hemoglobin C in African-Americans is about 2.3 percent.[19] If 7.8 percent of a population carries the hemoglobin S gene, then the probability of a sickle cell trait and hemoglobin C trait mating is approximately 1 in 280; therefore, 1 in approximately 1120 newborns will inherit hemoglobin SC disease. The same principles apply for inheritance of sickle cell β-thalassemia because the β-thalassemia gene also is allelic to the gene for sickle hemoglobin. In African-Americans, the frequency of β-thalassemia is approximately 0.8 percent,[134] so the expected birth frequency of sickle cell β-thalassemia is approximately 1 in 3200.

Although sickle cell anemia is regarded as the prototype of the sickle cell diseases, in the African-American population only approximately half of patients with sickle cell diseases have sickle cell anemia (homozygous SS disease). This fact is important from the point of view of genetic counseling: about half of all children with sickle cell disease arise from matings in which only one parent carries the sickle cell gene. Moreover, because early mortality rates probably are higher in sickle cell anemia than in the other sickle cell diseases, an even smaller proportion of adults with these sickle cell diseases actually are homozygous for hemoglobin S.

ANIMAL MODELS

No naturally occurring animal models of sickle cell disease have been described. Some deer have red cells that undergo sickling when the cells are oxygenated,[135] but not under physiologic conditions of pH and P_{O_2}. Cells from patients with sickle cell anemia have been infused into rats,[136] and this model system has been used to study the effect of various therapeutic agents. However, this approach is limited by the short time that the cells survive in the circulation of the heterologous species. The development of transgenic technologies (see Chap. 9) has made it possible to produce mice with red cells that carry a high percentage of sickle hemoglobin. Some of these models consist of mice with a combination of murine and human globin chains. In one model, the hemoglobin β^S Antilles transgene is used. Other models have been devised in which only human globin chains are produced. The various models differ in the severity of the genotype that is produced and some are more suitable for gene transfer studies, others for study of pathogenesis.[137]

CLINICAL FEATURES

The infant is protected during the first 8 to 10 weeks of life by the high level of fetal hemoglobin in the red cells. As the level declines, the clinical manifestations of sickle cell disease appear, and the hematologic manifestations of sickle disease are apparent by 10–12 weeks of age.[138]

CRISES

Many patients with sickle cell anemia are in reasonably good health much of the time, achieving a steady-state level of fitness. This state of relative well-being is periodically interrupted by a crisis that may have a sudden onset and, occasionally, a fatal outcome. The early recognition and subsequent clinical assessment of sickle crises are greatly facilitated by familiarity with the patient's steady state.

Various types of crises occur, and these may be classified as follows: vasoocclusive (painful) crisis, aplastic crises, sequestration crisis, and hemolytic crisis.

Vasoocclusive Crisis The vasoocclusive crisis is the most common and is the hallmark of the patient with sickle cell disease.[139] The frequency with which such crises occur varies from almost daily to less than once per year. The vasoocclusive crises result from complex interactions between endothelium, plasma factors, leukocytes, and rigid, sickled red cells leading to the obstruction of blood vessels (see "Blood Flow in the Microvasculature" above). Tissue hypoxia occurs and ultimately leads to tissue death and localized pain. It is important to distinguish the pain of a vasoocclusive crisis from the pain caused by other, sometimes more treatable disorders. Appendicitis must be considered in some cases, but it is notable that the incidence of appendicitis has been suggested to be lower in patients with sickle cell diseases than in the general population.[140] Fever is often present, even in the absence of demonstrable infection. Sickle cell crisis is, to a large extent, a diagnosis by exclusion.[141] Vasoocclusive crises may affect any tissue, but the pain occurs especially in bones, chest, and abdomen. Infarctions in the spleen, which may be a cause of abdominal pain, are so common in sickle cell anemia that after age 6 to 8 the spleen usually becomes very small because of scarring (autosplenectomy).[138] Myonecrosis is unusual but has been documented.[142]

Infarction of cerebral vessels, leading to stroke, is the most serious type of vasoocclusive complication (see "Central Nervous System" below).

Aplastic Crises Aplastic crises in sickle cell disease are of the type familiar in patients with other hemolytic disorders, in which the reticulocyte count falls to low levels, indicating that red cell production has decreased dramatically. Depression of erythropoiesis is generally associated with infections. Infections with Parvovirus B19 appear to be the most important cause of such crises[143] and may be accompanied by extensive marrow necrosis.[144] Because of the short red cell life span in sickle cell disease, even in the steady state, a temporary depression of marrow activity can cause a catastrophic fall in hemoglobin level manifesting as an aplastic crisis. Marrow output failure also may result from a deficiency of folic acid, especially during late pregnancy, and has sometimes been designated a *megaloblastic crisis.*

Sequestration Crisis The sequestration crisis occurs particularly in infants and young children,[145] but it can occur in adults with splenomegaly, particularly in those with hemoglobin SC disease or sickle β-thalassemia.[146–148] It is characterized by sudden massive pooling of red cells, especially in the spleen. Hypovolemic shock and cardiovascular failure may develop rapidly.[145] A major acute sequestration crisis is considered to be one in which the hemoglobin level is less than 6 g/dl and the hemoglobin level has fallen more than 3 g/dl compared with the baseline value. A minor acute sequestration crisis is an episode in which the hemoglobin level is higher than 6 g/dl.[149] In a study of children with sickle disease born in Los Angeles, California, in the 1960s and 1970s, such crises were responsible for 10 to 15 percent of deaths in the first 10 years of life.[138]

Hemolytic Crisis The red cell life span is shortened in all the varieties of sickle cell disease. The life span may suddenly be further reduced, probably for a variety of reasons. The increased rate of hemolysis is designated a *hemolytic crisis.* The resulting increase in jaundice is associated with a falling hemoglobin level and an elevated reticulocyte count. Such crises are very rare. In most instances, changes regarded to be caused by increased hemolysis represent some other complication of sickle cell disease.[150] It has been suggested that concurrent G-6-PD deficiency may be a factor leading to hemolytic crises[108] but likely is not[100]; the young red cell population of patients with sickle cell disease has normal or near-normal G-6-PD activity even when G-6-PD deficiency is present.

An increased level of jaundice is not necessarily an indication of increased hemolysis (see "Liver" below). Other causes of jaundice, such as hepatitis, cirrhosis, and gallstones, should be sought. Patients with chronic hemolytic anemia are especially likely to form bilirubin stones, which may cause extrahepatic biliary obstruction.

OTHER CLINICAL MANIFESTATIONS

Growth　Young children with sickle cell anemia reportedly are shorter than normal[151,152] and taller than normal.[153] Puberty is delayed, but considerable growth occurs in late adolescence so that adults with sickle cell anemia are at least as tall as normal.[152]

Bony Abnormalities　Chronic hemolytic anemia with erythroblastic hyperplasia results in widening of the medullary spaces, thinning of the cortices, and sparseness of the trabecular pattern.[154] Although these changes are recognizable in the skull, they usually are not as marked as the typical "hair-on-end" appearance characteristic of patients with thalassemia major (see Chap. 46). The vertebral bodies may show biconcavities of the upper and lower surfaces (codfish spine). Pressure from the nucleus pulposus into an area of bone infarction may result in step-like depressions, as if a coin had been pushed into the vertebral body. This x-ray picture is highly suggestive of sickle cell disease. A slight decrease in mineral bone density has been documented in adult patients.[155]

Crisis with bone pain may be followed by the appearance of periosteal reaction, and irregular areas of osteosclerosis may be seen, representing areas of bone infarction. Bone scans with technetium-99m (^{99m}Tc) are not helpful in delineating areas involved in painful crisis.[156] However, magnetic resonance imaging seems more promising.[157–159]

Sickle cell dactylitis probably results from limited avascular necrosis of marrow. Nearly half of children with sickle cell anemia suffer from this painful disorder, manifesting swelling of the dorsal surfaces of the hands and/or feet (Fig. 47-7). Dactylitis occurs almost entirely in the first 4 years of life, with a peak incidence at approximately 1 year.[160] Environmental cold is considered an important precipitating factor.

In later life, necrosis of the head of the femur resulting from infarction of the nutrient artery is common and may be responsible for severe pain and serious disturbances of gait. Osteonecrosis of the head of the humerus occurs in approximately 5 percent of patients with

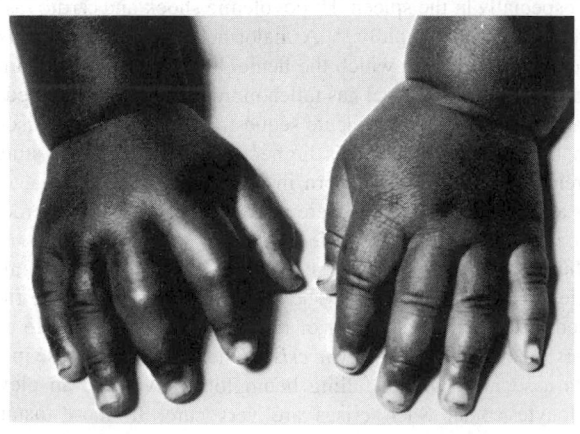

FIGURE 47-7　Sickle cell dactylitis (hand-foot syndrome). Note the swelling of the right hand involving the thumb and first and second fingers. (From LW Diggs,[545] with permission).

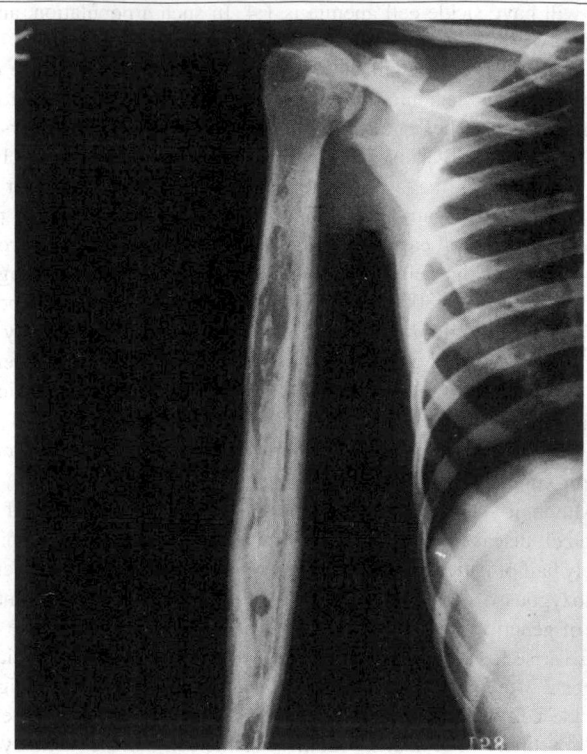

FIGURE 47-8　*Salmonella typhimurium* osteomyelitis in a patient with hemoglobin SC disease. (From GL River, AB Robbins, SO Schwartz,[546] with permission.)

sickle disease. Although the incidence in various genotypes is the same, onset tends to be earliest in those with the SS genotype, latest in those with sickle cell β-thalassemia, and intermediate in those with SC disease.[161,162] Chondrolytic arthritis has also been observed.[163] The bone manifestations of sickle cell disease may closely mimic osteomyelitis or arthritis.

The presence of necrotic marrow may favor the development of infection, especially with *Staphylococcus aureus*[164] and *Salmonella* (Fig 47-8).[165] Necrotic marrow may embolize the lung, producing the "chest syndrome" or, in some cases, sudden death.[166]

Genitourinary System　The renal medulla is an area that is particularly susceptible to damage in sickle cell disease. Its unique environment, characterized by anoxia, hyperosmolarity, and low pH, predisposes to sickling. The kidney is highly susceptible to the effects of the sickling phenomena and is the only organ commonly affected in the generally benign sickle cell trait. The ability to concentrate urine is lost in patients with sickle cell trait and in those with sickle cell disease.[167] Infarctions also may occur, with renal papillary necrosis (Fig. 47-9) in patients with SS disease and in those with sickle cell trait.[168] Approximately 50 percent of patients with sickle cell anemia have enlarged kidneys as judged by radiologic examination, and calyceal abnormalities of various types are common.[169] Renal failure is a late complication of sickle cell disease.[170] In one study, an increased incidence of renal carcinoma was observed in patients with sickle cell disease.[171]

Priapism is a serious complication of sickle cell disease[172–174] and is relatively common, occurring in approximately 35 percent of patients. The first episode usually occurs before age 20 years.[175] It is more common in patients with the SS genotype than in patients with other sickle disease genotypes. It often results in permanent impotence in adults. Prepubertal males have shorter episodes and a good prognosis for future erectile function.

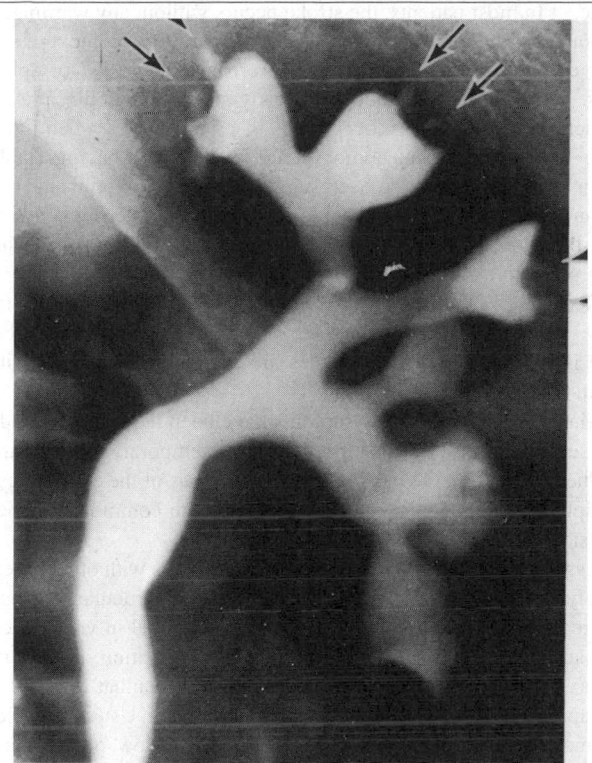

FIGURE 47-9 Renal papillary necrosis in a patient with sickle cell trait. Note the small medullary cavities in the upper three calyces of the left kidney *(arrows)*. (From BR Harrow, JA Sloane, NC Lichman,[547] with permission.)

Underdeveloped genitalia and hypogonadism may occur, and it has been suggested, but not proven, the underdevelopment could result from zinc deficiency.[176,177]

Spleen Splenomegaly is prominent in early childhood, but splenic function is impaired,[178] presumably as a result of the high incidence of bacteremic infections.[179] Infections of the splenic remnant itself, sometimes with abscess formation, have been documented.[180,181] In adults in the United States, splenomegaly is uncommon because of splenic fibrosis. Repeated infarctions of the spleen lead to fibrosis, calcifications, and autosplenectomy. In Africa, splenomegaly is observed in almost one fourth of patients with SS disease, probably because of infection with organisms such as *Plasmodia*.[182] In the United States, splenomegaly commonly persists into adult life in patients with sickle cell diseases other than SS disease (sickle cell thalassemia or hemoglobin SC disease).

Liver Jaundice and hepatomegaly are common in sickle cell anemia.[183] The liver may be enlarged, sometimes extending to the iliac crest, particularly in young children and again in middle age, at which time there may be evidence of hepatic dysfunction. The small number of sickled cells found in the hepatic vein after passage through the liver suggests the cells most susceptible to sickling are trapped by their rigidity and engulfed by phagocytes during their passage through the hepatic sinusoids, where the oxygen content of the blood is extremely low. The liver may transiently increase in size during a painful crisis.[184] Sickle cell intrahepatic cholestasis is a rare, catastrophic complication characterized by sudden onset of right upper quadrant pain, progressive hepatomegaly, and a serum bilirubin level that may rise to well over 100 mg/dl. The outcome usually is fatal, although recovery has been reported after exchange transfusion.[185] In sickle cell disease, excretion of urobilinogen usually is greater than normal. Approximately 50 to 70 percent of adult patients may have bilirubin gallstones,[186] and gallstones have also been found in children as young as 6 years.[187] Patients who have received transfusions may develop hepatitis that sometimes is mistaken for a hemolytic crisis. Although approximately one third of patients with sickle cell disease manifest liver dysfunction,[188] the cause is multifactorial.[186,188–190] Excess iron deposition is common, but frank hemochromatosis is encountered only occasionally.[189–193] The degree of iron overload seems unrelated to *HFE* mutations.[194] The degree of jaundice is related to inheritance of the common uridine diphosphate-glucuronosyltransferase promoter mutation responsible for Gilbert disease.[195,196]

Cardiopulmonary System The heart is frequently the site of some of the most prominent physical findings in sickle cell disease.[197] During crisis, striking tachycardia may occur because of the combination of fever and anemia. The precordium demonstrates the overactivity similar to that seen with marked hyperthyroidism. The point of maximal impulse usually is forceful and pounding in nature, and the heart frequently is enlarged to both the left and the right. Systolic and diastolic flow murmurs are often heard.

The blood pressure of patients with sickle cell anemia and, to a lesser degree, those with SC disease is significantly lower than published norms for age, race, and sex, and the difference increases with age.[198] Stroke was associated with higher systolic but not diastolic pressure.

Pulmonary infarctions are common in patients with sickle cell disease and may lead to repeated episodes of chest pain, unexplained dyspnea, or "atypical pneumonia." A combination of fever, chest pain, increased white blood cell count, and appearance of a pulmonary infiltrate in patients with sickle diseases is referred to as the *acute chest syndrome*.[199] Age exerts a marked effect on the clinical picture of acute chest syndrome. In children, acute chest syndrome is milder and more likely results from infection, whereas in adults it more likely is severe, is associated with pain, and has a higher mortality rate. The clinical and roentgenologic features observed in patients do not aid in differentiating pulmonary infarction from pulmonary infection, but thin-section computed tomography may be more helpful.[200] Rib infarctions are commonly observed on bone scan, and it has been suggested that they may play a role in the pathogenesis of the acute chest syndrome.[201] This disorder is regarded as multifactorial, with infection, infarction, and pulmonary fat embolism all factors that may play a role.[202] As pointed out in "Factors that Influence the Severity of Sickle Cell Disease" above, the claim that an eNOS polymorphism is a risk factor[71] requires independent confirmation.

The combination of increased flow rate and pulmonary vascular occlusions may result in increased pulmonary pressure and eventually cor pulmonale.[203–205] Systemic marrow fat embolism has been associated with pulmonary hypertension.[206] However, it has been suggested that patients with recurrent episodes of the acute chest syndrome are not particularly prone to develop pulmonary hypertension.[207]

Eye Retinal vessel obstruction is followed by neovascularization with arteriovenous aneurysms. These may eventually result in hemorrhage, scarring, retinal detachment, and blindness.[208] These changes occur at the periphery and may initially be difficult to visualize through an ophthalmoscope, even with a fully dilated pupil. At the early stage of retinal disease, vision is therefore not impaired. The retinal changes, collectively termed *sickle retinopathy*, have been divided into nonproliferative and proliferative groups. Nonproliferative changes include so-called "salmon patch" hemorrhages, iridescent spots, and black sunbursts. The latter term is used to describe lesions that occur in the peripheral retina. As the retina becomes ischemic, neovascular growth starts at abnormal arterial venous anastomoses resulting from vascular occlusions. These vascular growths extend toward the periphery. Because these abnormal vascular fronds resemble the marine invertebrate *Gorgonia flabellum*, the lesions are called "sea fans."

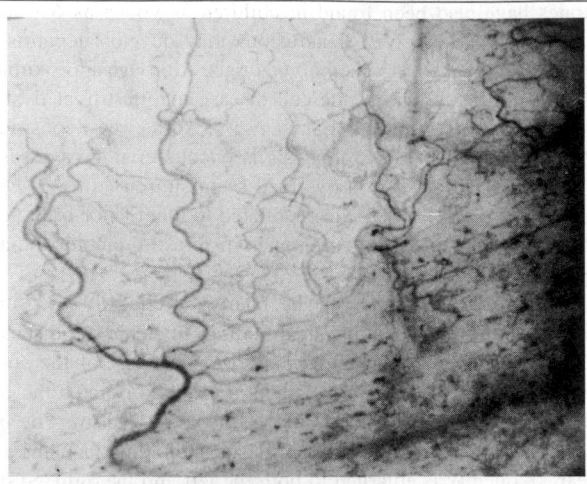

FIGURE 47-10 Lower bulbar conjunctiva in a patient with sickle cell anemia, showing many segmentations. (From D Paton,[548] with permission.)

Examination of the conjunctiva may reveal multiple, short comma-shaped capillary segments that often appear isolated from the vascular network because the afferent and efferent lumens are empty. These transient sites of tightly clumped intravascular erythrocytes are found on the bulbar conjunctiva underneath the eyelids (Fig. 47-10). They occasionally disappear during the course of a lengthy examination because of the warmth of the light. Visual loss is most common in SC disease and is due principally to vitreous hemorrhage, secondary to bleeding from the neovascularized areas.

The orbital compression syndrome, consisting of fever, headache, orbital swelling, and optic nerve dysfunction, has been documented in a number of patients with sickle cell disease.[209] The most common cause appears to be orbital marrow infarctions.

A single case of retinal vein occlusion has been documented, but the patient had concurrent protein S deficiency.[210]

Central Nervous System Cerebrovascular accidents are one of the most devastating complications of sickle cell disease. Once thought to be caused by obstruction of small blood vessels, cerebrovascular accidents now appear to be caused by lesions of major vessels, particularly the internal carotid and anterior and middle cerebral arteries.[211,212] Studies of the brain by magnetic resonance imaging (MRI) and of vasculopathy by magnetic resonance angiography in children with hemoglobin SS show that brain damage is very common.[213,214] At an average age of 10 years, the estimated prevalence of infarction, ischemic damage, or atrophy in SS patients was 46 percent and of vasculopathy was 64 percent. Only 28 percent of patients were normal by both modalities. However, the prevalence of frank cerebrovascular accidents has been found to be 4.01 percent and the incidence 0.61 per 100 patient-years in sickle cell anemia (SS) patients, and cardiovascular accidents occur at somewhat lower frequencies in other common genotypes.[215–218] Stroke has even been reported in more than a dozen children and adults with sickle trait, but the cause and effect relationship must be considered unproven.[219,220] The incidence of infarctive cerebrovascular accidents is lowest in sickle cell anemia patients 20 to 29 years of age and higher in children and older patients. On the other hand, the incidence of hemorrhagic stroke in SS patients is highest among patients 20 to 29 years old. The mortality rate was 26 percent in the 2 weeks after hemorrhagic stroke. The incidence of stroke among patients with hemoglobin SC disease is significantly lower, approximately 2 percent.[215–218] Measurement of the velocity of cerebral blood flow by transcranial Doppler ultrasonography has some predictive value with respect to the probability of developing a

stroke.[221] In most patients, the stroke occurs without any warning, but in about one quarter of cases, the stroke occurs in the context of some other complication, such as a painful crisis, priapism,[217] or aplastic crisis.[222] Risk factors include low steady-state hemoglobin, previous transient ischemic attacks, occurrence of priapism,[215,223] silent infarctions,[224] increased plasma homocysteine levels,[225] and having a sibling with a stroke.[218] It has also been suggested that polymorphisms at the human leukocyte antigen (HLA) loci,[226] of the angiotensin gene,[224,226] or of the IL4R 503, TNF (-308), and ADRB2 27 genes[227] may have some predictive value.

Recurrence of strokes is a prominent feature of this complication; 46–90 percent of patients who have one stroke will suffer at least one more if untreated.[228] Such episodes are particularly common within the first 36 months after a stroke.[216]

Many other neurologic symptoms have been described, including drowsiness, coma, convulsions, headache, temporary or permanent blindness, cranial nerve palsies, and paresthesias of the extremities.[229] Multiple cerebral aneurysms appear to be more common in patients with sickle cell disease.[230]

Leg Ulcers Although encountered in patients with other types of hemolytic disease, ulcers around the ankles are a particularly common feature of sickle cell disease.[231,232] They are unusual in younger children, and stasis clearly plays some part in their formation. They usually start as a small break in the skin or blister-like area that breaks down and rapidly extends to form a painful, indolent ulcer. Usually the ulcers become infected, and the base is covered with a yellow, purulent layer. They may extend deeply enough to expose muscle. Once formed, leg ulcers do not heal spontaneously, and they become a major source of morbidity for affected patients.

Infections Patients with sickle cell disease are particularly prone to develop infections, and this may be the single most common reason for hospitalization.[233] Because of functional asplenia, impaired phagocytic function,[234] and a defect in activation of the alternate complement pathway, infections may be quite hazardous, particularly in children. The risk varies significantly from patient to patient with some patients having very few infections. Pneumonia seems to be the most common infection encountered and often is of pneumococcal origin, particularly in children. Mycoplasma infections are not uncommon[235] and may play a role in the acute chest syndrome. As noted in "Bony Abnormalities" above, osteomyelitis due to *Staphylococcus* and to *Salmonella* also is relatively common.[164] Babesiosis has been reported to occur in one patient, possibly as a result of the impaired splenic function.[236]

Pregnancy Pregnancy in women with sickle cell anemia is accompanied by an increased incidence of pyelonephritis, pulmonary infarction, pneumonia, acute chest syndrome, antepartum hemorrhage, prematurity, and fetal death.[237] Megaloblastic anemia responsive to folic acid, especially in late pregnancy, also occurs with increased frequency. The birth weight of infants born of mothers with sickle cell anemia is below average,[238,239] and the fetal wastage is high.[240,241] The cause of neonatal death is obscure but may sometimes result from vasoocclusion of the placenta.[238] Postmortem findings are those of intrapartum anoxia.[242] Maternal mortality in sickle cell disease was formerly prohibitively high, with rates averaging 33 percent, but now is much lower, averaging about 1.5 percent in various series.[243–246] Higher mortality rates are still observed in some parts of the world, however, with maternal mortality rates up to 9.2 percent and perinatal mortality up to 19.5 percent.[247–250]

LABORATORY FEATURES

The steady-state hemoglobin level of patients with sickle cell anemia is usually between 5 and 11 g/dl. The anemia is normochromic and normocytic despite the elevated reticulocyte count.[251] In comparison with patients with similarly increased reticulocyte counts, patients with SS disease may be considered to have a "microcytic" anemia, presumably because the sickle mutation impairs the efficiency of production of hemoglobin. The range of red cell densities is increased in sickle cell anemia,[252] but the average cellular MCHC is normal. In SC disease, however, the average MCHC is increased.[252] Erythropoietin levels may be reduced relative to the degree of anemia[253] but have also been reported to be appropriate.[254] The anemia is accompanied by laboratory signs of hemolysis, with increased indirect-reacting serum bilirubin, reticulocytosis, and often circulating nucleated red cells. As in any hemolytic anemia, endogenous CO production is increased[255] and haptoglobin is absent. Sickled erythrocytes are often evident on inspection of the blood film. Target cells may be present, particularly in sickle cell hemoglobin C disease and sickle cell β-thalassemia. In sickle cell hemoglobin C disease, folded cells are sometimes seen (Figs. 47-11 and 47-12). Examination of the red cells by inference phase-contrast microscopy reveals surface indentations, presumably resulting from splenic hypofunction, in approximately 20 percent of

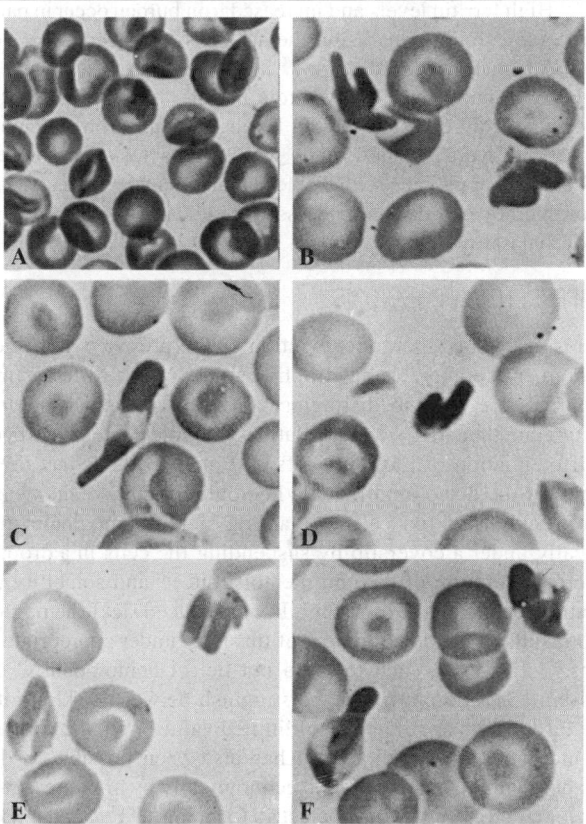

FIGURE 47-12   Bizarre-shaped erythrocytes in the blood film of patient with hemoglobin SC disease. (A) "Fat sickle cells." (B) Crescent-shaped erythrocyte with three deep-hued crystals (center left). Two bizarre condensed hemoglobin masses in a red blood cell (lower right). (C) Elongated red corpuscle with concentration of hemoglobin at each end and hemoglobin-free central area (center). (D) Red cell with two parallel, dark, crystal-like structures of different lengths, terminating in a pyramid tip (center). (E) Erythrocyte with two parallel formations separated by a clear area (upper right). Red cell with one elongated mass (lower left). (F) Erythrocyte with densely stained hemoglobin masses (upper right). Red cell with one dark, elongated, rounded bulge and one small triangular hemoglobin mass, leaving two areas relatively free of hemoglobin (lower left). (From LW Diggs, A Bell,[549] with permission.)

cells.[178] A modest polymorphonuclear leukocytosis with a left shift is common even in the steady state[256,257] and may result in part from redistribution of leukocytes from the marginal to the circulating granulocyte pool.[256] The finding does not necessarily signify an infection. Thrombocytosis is also common, but evidence of intravascular coagulation with thrombocytopenia has been noted rarely during crisis.[258]

The marrow shows erythroid hyperplasia. Immunoglobulin levels are frequently increased. IgA levels are particularly elevated in all forms of sickle cell disease. Elevations of IgG levels are also sometimes seen, while IgM levels appear to be elevated, particularly in patients with sickle cell thalassemia and in individuals with other combinations such as hemoglobin SC disease.[259] A decreased number of T lymphocytes and increased B lymphocytes in the blood have been reported.[260] Activation in the alternative complement pathway has been detected in some patients,[261] apparently as a result of phosphatidylserine exposure by erythrocytes.[66] This may be responsible, in part, for increased susceptibility to infection.

Plasma tocopherol[262] and zinc[263,264] levels often are low, the latter possibly because of zincuria.[176,264] Serum ferritin levels are normal in the first two decades of life but tend to rise in older patients, and modest elevations in plasma iron concentration are frequently encoun-

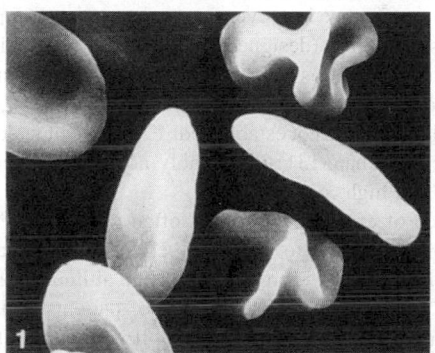
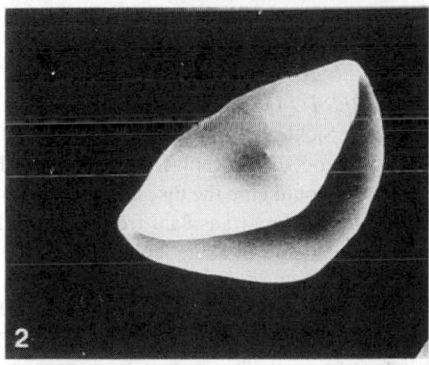
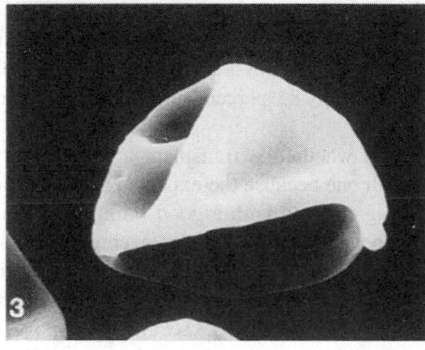

FIGURE 47-11   Scanning electron microscopy of individual SC cells: (1) multifolded cells; (2) unifolded cell resembling pita bread and most likely the same as the "fat cell" shown in Fig. 47-12, (3) tridimpled cell, also called a triangular cell. (From C Lawrence, ME Fabry, RL Nagel,[81] with permission.)

tered.[265] High ferritin levels and increased iron burden occur in patients who receive chronic transfusion therapy. Iron overload is not nearly so frequent in sickle cell disease as in thalassemia. Mutations of the *HFE* gene do not seem to play a role in determining which patients develop markedly elevated ferritin levels.[194] Frank iron deficiency is not rare, and overt iron deficiency with microcytosis has sometimes been observed in patients with sickle cell anemia.[266,267] Thus, the presence of microcytosis does not necessarily indicate the concurrent presence of thalassemia.

DIFFERENTIAL DIAGNOSIS

Diagnosis depends upon documentation of the presence of sickle hemoglobin, preferably by electrophoresis.[268] Many different media and buffers are used to distinguish different mutant hemoglobins from one another, but several relatively simple systems suffice for the differentiation of most variants.[269] Rapid methods that are less reliable for the detection of sickle hemoglobin include the observation of sickling of red cells containing sickle hemoglobin microscopically under a coverslip by suspending the cells in a droplet of a 2 percent solution of sodium metabisulfite[270] and solubility tests. The latter depend on the low solubility of reduced sickle hemoglobin, which results in the development of turbidity under appropriate conditions.[271] However, such tests do not detect hemoglobin C or β-thalassemia and do not reliably distinguish between sickle trait and sickle disease and are therefore of limited value. With the refinement and automation of techniques, it has also been possible to detect sickle hemoglobin accurately and economically by high-pressure liquid chromatography and by isoelectric focusing.[272] Use of the polymerase chain reaction to detect sickle hemoglobin is the method of choice for prenatal diagnosis.[273]

Because there are no normal β polypeptide chain genes, patients with sickle cell anemia or hemoglobin SC disease have no normal adult hemoglobin. In the heterozygote for the sickle cell gene and β-thalassemia, no hemoglobin A is found, but small amounts of normal hemoglobin are present in the compound heterozygote for the sickle cell and β^+-thalassemia genes. The concentration of fetal hemoglobin usually is increased in sickle cell β-thalassemia and is heterogeneously distributed among the red cells. The quantitation of hemoglobin A_2 is valuable in differentiating sickle cell anemia from sickle cell β^0-thalassemia; hemoglobin A_2 levels tend to be increased in the latter condition. Family studies are particularly helpful to clearly differentiate sickle cell β^0-thalassemia from sickle cell anemia.

Sickle cell anemia can be diagnosed at birth by subjecting cord blood samples to electrophoresis.[274] Ideally, all babies of ethnic groups with a high frequency of the sickle cell gene should be screened at birth because of a demonstrated decrease in mortality of very young children when the diagnosis is made.[275] The cost effectiveness of screening depends on the composition of the target population; it has been estimated to be $206,000 per death averted in Alaska. Screening is particularly desirable if the mother has sickle cell trait.

Chorionic villus biopsy has been used extensively to obtain fetal DNA for diagnosis in the first trimester.[276] The availability of techniques for amplification of genomic DNA makes feasible DNA-based prenatal diagnosis of sickle cell disease (see Chap. 9). The mutant or normal sequence can be differentiated with an appropriate restriction endonuclease or by the use of synthetic oligonucleotide probes.[273,277]

THERAPY

An authoritative guide for the management of patients with sickle cell diseases has been published under the auspices of the Heart, Lung, and Blood institute of the National Institutes of Health.[268]

GENERAL MEASURES

Because no fully satisfactory, specific treatments for the sickle cell disorders have yet become available, physicians must concentrate their therapeutic efforts in the direction of continuous and effective general medical care and appropriate management of complications as they arise.[278,279] Folic acid supplementation has been suggested, but there is little evidence that it is beneficial[280] except in pregnancy and in patients with other disorders that increase the requirement for folate. Transfusions are usually not required in special circumstances such as stroke, abnormal transcranial Doppler findings, leg ulcers, or intractable or frequently recurring painful crises.[281] Prophylactic transfusion does, as expected, decrease the frequency of crises,[191] but subjects patients to the risk of complications of transfusion such as alloimmunization[282] and transmission of infection. However, although the development of hemochromatosis has been reported,[190] it seems to be a relatively uncommon complication, even in extensively transfused patients. Such patients who are iron overloaded may be treated with desferrioxamine[268,283,284] or, where available, with deferiprone (see Chap. 40). A randomized, double-blind study showed that conservative transfusion therapy (designed to keep the hemoglobin level over 10 g/dl) was as effective in preventing perioperative complications as more aggressive therapy (designed to maintain the hemoglobin S level under 30 percent) and was safer.[285] Acute neurologic symptoms have been reported to occur after partial exchange transfusion, but a cause and effect relationship is not established.[286] The use of neocytes (young erythrocytes; see Chap. 131) is probably not justified because of inconvenience and high cost.

Avoidance of exposure to cold is often counseled,[268] but a controlled study was unable to show any effect of temperature on the prevalence of emergency room visits.[117] High altitudes can precipitate sickle crises. Special vocational training of patients with sickle cell anemia for suitable occupations is useful. It is important that patients live as normal a life as possible. Occupations that do not require heavy manual labor and in which occasional absences from work are practical may be excellent and can make them productive members of society.

SPECIFIC MEASURES TO DECREASE SICKLING

Transplantation Sickle cell disease is fundamentally a disease of the hemopoietic stem cell, and replacing the genetically defective cell with a normal one should cure the disease. One patient with sickle cell disease received a marrow transplant from a sib with sickle cell trait in the course of treatment of acute leukemia.[287] As expected, the sickle cell disease was cured—converted into sickle cell trait.

Subsequently, a considerable number of patients with sickle cell disease have undergone marrow transplantation. By 2003, more than 200 patients with sickle cell disease had been transplanted worldwide.[288] As might be expected, the best results are obtained in young children with HLA-matched sibs, with a disease-free survival of 93 percent. Even including less favorable patients, disease-free survival rates ranging from 80 to 85 percent have been obtained in various centers.

The decision of whether to transplant a patient with sickle cell disease is a difficult one because the expected mortality rate for transplantation in young children with a good family donor match is still appreciable, and potential morbidity from chronic graft-versus-host disease needs also to be taken into account. Thus, the initial focus has been upon those children with a poor prognosis, and apart from those who have already suffered a stroke, accurate prognostication is impossible.[289–291]

Agents with Antisickling Activities Many attempts have been made to modify red cells containing hemoglobin S in a manner that will suppress the sickling process. Examples of this approach included conversion of hemoglobin to carboxyhemoglobin[292–294] or methemoglobin,[295] acetylation of the hemoglobin molecules with aspirin,[296,297] methyl acetyl phosphate,[298] or succinyldisalicylate,[299] cross-linking hemoglobin molecules with dimethylapidimidate,[300,301] and use of carbonic anhydrase inhibitors to reduce the formation of H_2CO_3.[302] Distilled water has been given intravenously to lower MCHC[303] and glutamine to change the oxidative state of the cell.[304] Other antisickling agents that have been studied for a possible therapeutic effect include urea,[305] cyanate,[306] O-carbamoylsalicylates,[307] methyl acetyl phosphate,[308] lysyl-phenylalanine,[309] procaine,[310] zinc,[311] pyridoxine[312,313] and its derivatives,[314,315] phenothiazines,[316] steroids,[300] nitrogen mustard,[317] glyceraldehyde,[318] hexamethylenetetramine,[319] vitamin E,[320] lawsone,[321] substituted benzaldehydes,[322] bepridil,[323] cetiedil,[324] L-arginine,[325] and Nix-0699 (a Nigerian herbal extract).[326] The usefulness of none of these has been confirmed.

Only a relatively small proportion of antisickling agents have been examined in clinical trials. The induction of methemoglobinemia[295] by administration of sodium nitrite or p-aminopropiophenone lengthened the life span of sickle cells, and the inhalation of CO was found to have a similar effect.[294] A patient with sickle cell anemia who was accidentally exposed to CO levels presented with a hematocrit level that rose to 46 percent. A fatal outcome was attributed to extreme hyperviscosity that occurred as the carboxyhemoglobin was converted to oxyhemoglobin and the cells again began to sickle.[327] Pyridoxine, in contrast, did not influence red cell life span.[312] The use of alkali to counteract the Bohr effect (reduction of oxygen affinity of hemoglobin at acid pH[328]) has been thought to have some therapeutic value, but no beneficial effect could be demonstrated in controlled trials.[329] The rationale for use of urea was the ability of this chemical to dissociate hydrophobic molecular bonds and thus interfere with the sickling process. The concentration required to achieve such an effect cannot be reached in vivo, and clinical trials have proved disappointing.[255] Carbamylation of the hemoglobin molecule by cyanate increases the affinity of the hemoglobin for oxygen.[330] Because the sickling process requires the hemoglobin to be in the deoxy conformation, any agent capable of affecting the equilibrium between the oxy and deoxy conformations and thereby increasing the avidity of hemoglobin for oxygen must have an antisickling effect.[118] Unfortunately, in clinical trials, cyanate provoked polyneuropathy,[331] retinal changes,[331] and cataracts[332] and therefore appears to be too toxic for systemic use. A number of substituted benzaldehyde compounds have been given experimentally to patients, producing a left shift in the oxygen dissociation curve and suggestive evidence of a decrease in hemolysis.[322,333] It has been suggested that their effect may result not only from stabilization of the oxy conformation of hemoglobin but also from decreasing potassium loss.[322]

Because sickling is highly concentration dependent, efforts to treat the disorder by swelling the red cells have been made. These have included the administration of distilled water intravenously[303] and the lowering of serum sodium by the administration of a long-acting vasopressin derivative and vigorous hydration.[334,335] The effectiveness and safety of the latter treatment has been questioned.[336,337] Another approach to limiting cellular dehydration has been to attempt to block the Gardos channel with agents such as clotrimazole[338,339] or more recently developed more specific inhibitors such as ICA-17043, now in phase II/III clinical trials.[339]

Increasing the Level of Fetal Hemoglobin   Efforts have also been made to ameliorate the sickling process by stimulating the formation of fetal hemoglobin. Attempted originally by the administration of chorionic gonadotropin and estrogens,[295] more modern efforts have focused on 5-azacytidine, a drug that inhibits the methylation of DNA and was shown to increase fetal hemoglobin concentrations of the red cells of baboons.[340] The administration of 5-azacytidine to patients with sickle cell anemia resulted in an increased concentration of

fetal hemoglobin[341,342] and in a rise in the hemoglobin concentration of the blood.[341,342] More recently, encouraging results have been obtained with 5-aza 2′-deoxycytidine.[343] Other antineoplastic agents, including cytosine arabinoside[344,345] and hydroxyurea[344,346-348] or hydroxyurea in combination with erythropoietin,[349] and erythropoietin alone[350] also increase the fetal hemoglobin level. Butyric acid and related compounds[351-353] increase fetal hemoglobin production in progenitor cells, experimental animals, and humans. However, isobutyramide given orally was not found to be useful.[354] In vitro, interferon gamma has also been shown to increase fetal hemoglobin production.[355] Poloxamer 188, a nonionic surfactant with hemorrheologic properties, has been tested in a double-blind randomized trial and found to decrease the severity of painful sickle crises.[356]

Of these agents, hydroxyurea is the one that has been tested most extensively and that has been introduced selectively into clinical practice. A large number of studies using this agent have been carried out, and beneficial effects ranging from reduction in the frequency of painful crises, episodes of acute chest syndromes, and decrease in blood transfusions have been observed.[357,358] The usual approach has been to begin therapy with 10–15 mg/kg once daily, with blood counts monitored every 2 weeks. Dosage is then increased by 5 mg/kg/day every 12 weeks if the neutrophil count remains above 2×10^9/liter, the hemoglobin above 4.5 g/dl, and reticulocyte count above 80×10^9/liter. As marrow suppression occurs, the dose is restarted at 2.5 mg/kg/day less than the dose causing suppression.

Careful supervision is obviously required in the administration of a myelosuppressive agent. Compliance among children appears to be quite satisfactory.[358,359] Myelosuppression is the most common side effect of hydroxyurea therapy. Other toxic side effects have also been observed. These include nail and skin hyperpigmentation and possibly nausea, gastrointestinal upsets, and rash, although in randomized trials the latter are no more common than with placebo.[360] Because hydroxyurea is potentially a teratogen, contraceptive precautions are recommended for both men and women. However, more than 14 cases of pregnancy have been described in women taking hydroxyurea without observing any congenital abnormalities.[361]

Hydroxyurea was first used in the treatment of sickle cell disease because of its effect in increasing the level of fetal hemoglobin. However, the correlation between fetal hemoglobin levels and the clinical effect is relatively poor[360] and therefore other mechanisms have been sought to explain the effect. For example, it is possible that the reduced leukocyte counts improve blood rheology and lead to reduced levels of proinflammatory cytokines. It has also been proposed that reduced red cell–endothelial interactions, improved red cell rheology, or nitric oxide release might play a role in the beneficial effect.[357]

Management of Specific Clinical Manifestations   *Acute chest syndrome.*   Rapid and correct diagnosis is of paramount importance. It has been recommended that if normal flora is seen on Gram-stained sputum in a patient who is not seriously affected with the acute chest syndrome, no antibiotics should be used. However, more symptomatic patients with sputum production should receive antibiotics based on the organisms found in the Gram-stained sputum. In adults, in contrast to children, such pulmonary events rarely appear to result from infection with pneumococci.[362] Because of the life-threatening nature of the acute chest syndrome, some clinicians prefer a more aggressive approach, immediately instituting empiric antibiotic therapy including erythromycin because of the frequent involvement of bacterial such as chlamydia or mycoplasma.[202] Adequate hydration is important, but fluid overload resulting in pulmonary edema occurs not infrequently; thus, careful monitoring of fluid balance is required.[202] Exchange transfusion has been advocated,[363,364] and intratracheal DNAse has been used in one child.[365]

Infections. Administration of pneumococcal vaccine is recommended,[133] but a number of failures of the vaccine to protect children with sickle cell disease against infection with pneumococcus have been reported, and children with sickle disease should receive pneumococcal vaccine and penicillin prophylaxis at least until age 5.[133,268,366] Other infectious diseases against which patients with sickle diseases should be immunized include hepatitis B, diphtheria, tetanus, pertussis, poliomyelitis, and *Haemophilus influenzae*.[133,268] Infections should be treated vigorously with antibiotics. Because patients with sickle cell anemia are unable to concentrate urine adequately, dehydration during the course of infection represents a special risk to be avoided by adequate fluid administration.

Crises. Once a small blood vessel is totally obstructed by sickled cells in the development of a painful crisis, the obstruction probably is irreversible. Yet the function of neighboring blood vessels in the areas obstructed by rigid sickled cells may be preserved by a number of therapeutic measures. The patient should be kept warm, and adequate hydration should be maintained by the oral or intravenous route. The role of oxygen therapy in the treatment of vasoocclusive crises is poorly defined. Although administration of oxygen was once considered contraindicated because of a putative negative effect on erythropoiesis, it seems doubtful that it does any harm aside from the minor discomfort incident to its administration and may be useful in patients with decreased arterial oxygen saturation. Hyperbaric oxygen usually fails to benefit the patient,[367] although occasional success using this treatment has been claimed.[368]

The anticoagulants dicumarol[369] and the debrinating enzyme Arvin[370] have been tried without success. Intravenous administration of magnesium sulfate has been reported to be beneficial,[371] although a therapeutic effect has not been confirmed.[372] Promising results of the treatment of sickle crisis with pentoxifylline, a drug reported to increase erythrocyte deformability, were reported in a double-blind study[373] but could not be confirmed.[374] Oral sodium bicarbonate or sodium citrate therapy has been tried in the treatment of an established vasoocclusive crisis as well as in its prevention,[372] but its efficacy could not be confirmed in a controlled study.[375]

Management with analgesics of the pain of infarctive crises represents a particularly difficult problem for the physician[268,376,377] and is discussed in Chapter 27. In most instances, the manifestations of vasoocclusive crisis may gradually disappear over a period of hours or days on symptomatic management.

Splenic sequestration crises are a life-threatening complication that must be treated vigorously. Transfusion with red cells (exchange transfusions if there is respiratory distress) and splenectomy have been recommended.[145,149]

Strokes. Because of the high recurrence rates of strokes, special attention has been paid to this group of high-risk patients. Regular transfusion programs to maintain the sickle hemoglobin concentration at 30 percent of the total hemoglobin reduce recurrence rates.[192] Allowing no more than 50 percent of the hemoglobin to be sickle hemoglobin may provide similar protection.[378] Although children at high risk for stroke can be identified by transcranial Doppler ultrasound studies, it is not yet clear that red cell transfusions prevent a first stroke.[379,380]

Hypersplenism and splenectomy. Because of "autosplenectomy," hypersplenism is seldom a problem in sickle cell anemia. Hypersplenism may be suspected in other forms of sickle disease if a long-term transfusion program becomes necessary to maintain life or if leukopenia and thrombocytopenia are associated with a palpable spleen. Under these circumstances, splenectomy may very occasionally be warranted. It has been recommended that splenectomy be performed in all children older than 2 years in whom one major or two minor splenic sequestration crises have occurred, because of the danger of recurrent crises.[149,268]

Cholelithiasis. It is useful to examine adolescent and adult sickle cell anemia patients for the presence of gallstones. It has been suggested that elective cholecystectomy be performed when stones are present,[381] but since 50–70 percent of adult patients with sickle disease have been found to have gallstones,[186] gallstones that do not cause symptoms should probably not be removed. Laparoscopic cholecystectomy has been found to be safe and effective in children[382] and adults.[383]

Contraception and pregnancy. Oral contraception may offer some additional hazard of thromboembolism in patients with sickle hemoglobin,[384] but the risk is probably small compared to the risk of pregnancy itself. The contraceptives medroxyprogesterone acetate (Depo-Provera) given parenterally monthly for 3 months and then every month or levonorgestrel plus ethinylestradiol (Microgynon 30) given daily were associated with a decrease in the number of attacks of pain in one study.[385]

Although very high maternal mortality rates have been greatly reduced with good prenatal care, pregnancy and the postpartum period are still potentially hazardous for a mother with sickle cell disease.[386] The patient should be closely supervised during pregnancy.[387] Although prophylactic blood transfusions have been given to some patients with what appear to be satisfactory results,[388–391] the effectiveness of this type of therapy is not proven.[386,392] Studies demonstrating that exchange transfusions are not required have been presented[393] and contested.[390,394]

Leg ulcers. Leg ulcers may respond to conservative treatment, such as bed rest, elevation of the affected limb, zinc sulfate pressure dressings, or maintenance transfusion, or they may require surgical grafting.[232] No difference in the rate of healing has been demonstrated with any of the different treatment modalities.[231,395]

Bone and joint disease. Joint replacement may be helpful to patients who have suffered osteonecrosis, but the number of complications and the number of revisions needed are extraordinary, so the risk to benefit ratio has been high.[396] However, some more encouraging results have been reported.[397] Core decompression has been found to be useful in the management of early avascular necrosis of the hip.[398]

Retinal changes. Vitreous hemorrhages and subsequent blindness may be the end result of the neovascularization that follows retinal infarction. Laser photocoagulation of new vessels may help to prevent this complication.[208] When hemorrhages have occurred, vitrectomy may be indicated. The administration of nifedipine seemed to improve conjunctival and retinal perfusion and color vision performance in patients with sickle cell disease.[399] Retinal detachment can be treated by fluorescein angiography and laser photocoagulation.[400] Occlusion of the central retinal artery, presenting as acute loss of vision, is an emergency. Immediate red cell transfusion and referral to an ophthalmologist have been recommended.[400]

Priapism. Surgical intervention is commonly practiced, particularly in postpubertal patients with priapism. However, there is no clear evidence of benefit from shunting procedures.[172] Hydration and exchange transfusions have been associated with detumescence,[174] and it has been suggested that oral administration of the α-adrenergic agent etilefrine prevents recurrence of priapism.[401] Sildenafil has been used to treat episodes of priapism in three patients.[402] Penile prostheses have been found to be useful when impotence resulted from priapism.[403,404]

Anesthesia and surgery. The patient with sickle cell disease is at increased risk during anesthesia. If surgery is indicated, scrupulous care is needed to avoid factors known to precipitate crisis, including hypoxemia, dehydration, circulatory stasis, acidosis, cold, and infections.[405–408]

Preoperative transfusion with packed red cells may help prevent complications in patients with sickle cell disease undergoing major surgery. Partial exchange transfusion has been advocated,[191,409] and this has the advantage of immediate removal from the circulation of sickle cells that may obstruct the microcirculation. However, this more complex procedure probably has little, if any, advantage over simple transfusion if surgery is elective as might be the case with patients requiring cholecystectomy or hip replacement.[406] Exchange transfusion requires more blood to achieve an equivalent increment in the blood hemoglobin level and therefore entails more risk than simple transfusion. Elevation of the hemoglobin level of the blood will markedly reduce the production of sickle cells by the marrow and, in view of the short life span of the patient's own circulating erythrocytes, few sickle cells will remain in the circulation after a week or two. The complication rate of patients receiving exchange transfusions is, in point of fact, no lower than that observed in patients receiving simple transfusions.[410] Exchange transfusion provides an advantage if iron overload is a concern or if removal of sickle cells is desired within a period of less than 5 to 7 days. In a controlled multicenter study, conservative transfusional therapy (i.e., transfusing to a hemoglobin concentration of 10 g/dl) was as effective as aggressive therapy (i.e., reducing the sickle hemoglobin concentration to 30 percent).[285]

COURSE AND PROGNOSIS

For a number of years, it was unclear why sickle cell anemia was relatively common in the North-American black and yet appeared to be a rare disease in Central Africa. Subsequently it was recognized that the early mortality associated with sickle cell anemia in Central Africa[411,412] was responsible for its apparent rarity: the surveys of the distribution of sickle hemoglobin in Africa did not include the afflicted who had died. With good medical care, patients with sickle cell anemia usually survive to middle age.[413–415] Assessment of the overall mortality of sickle cell anemia must take into account the fact that cases first diagnosed in late childhood, adolescence, or adult life likely will result in a preponderance of the clinically more benign patients. In the two and one-half decades after 1968, mortality rates of African-American children with sickle cell disease decreased considerably.[416] In the 1- to 4-year age group, the mortality had fallen from 37 in 1000 persons in those born between 1967 and 1969 to 22 in 1000 among those born between 1986 and 1988. Corresponding figures for the 5- to 9-year age group were 19 in 1000 and 10 in 1000 and for the 10- to 14-year age group were 17 in 1000 and 8 in 1000.[416] These improvements in survival probably can best be ascribed to newborn screening programs, penicillin prophylaxis of disease caused by *Streptococcus pneumoniae*, and perhaps use of pneumococcal vaccines.[417] There were considerable regional differences. The mortality was considerably higher in Florida than in Maryland and Pennsylvania, probably related to the health care facilities available in different regions.[418] Astonishingly, in California and Illinois, mortality from all causes among African-American children born from 1990 to 1994 with sickle cell disease was slightly less than overall mortality for all African-American children born in the same time period.[419]

The morphologic evidence of the cause of death was studied in 306 autopsies of sickle cell disease accrued between 1929 and 1996. Infection was the most common cause of death for all sickle variants, accounting for 33 to 48 percent of deaths. Infection as a cause of death did not become less common with the passage of time, but the age at which the autopsy had been performed increased from an average of 11 years in the 1950s to 24 years in the 1980s. Other causes of death included stroke (9.8%), therapy complications (7.0%), splenic sequestration (6.6%), pulmonary emboli/thrombi (4.9%), renal failure (4.1%), pulmonary hypertension (2.9%), hepatic failure (0.8%), mas-

sive hemolysis/red cell aplasia (0.4%), and left ventricular failure (0.4%). Sudden, unexpected death occurred in 40.8 percent of patients.[420]

PREVENTION

Prevention of some of the sequelae of sickle cell diseases can be achieved by newborn screening (see "Differential Diagnosis" above). Another form of prevention is based on prenatal diagnosis. Parents can be screened and, if they are carriers, they can be provided with genetic counseling and educated about the options of not having children or of having pregnancies monitored for the occurrence of a sickle cell disease in the fetus. Because approximately half of the children with sickle cell diseases have only one parent with sickle hemoglobin, effective screening programs must do more than merely detect the presence of this abnormal hemoglobin. They also must use means that permit detection of hemoglobin C and of β-thalassemia trait. Because of the benign clinical nature of β-thalassemia, hemoglobin C, and sickle cell traits, no useful purpose other than genetic counseling seems to be served by screening populations for these carrier states. Indeed, misunderstanding concerning the significance of the carrier states has harmed individuals who are detected as carriers in screening programs.[421]

Many screening programs have been implemented, and the number and background of participants have been described.[422] However, only scant data permitting assessment of the actual effect of screening programs on birth frequency of infants with sickle cell disorders are available. In Guadalupe, 62 percent of the group of mothers at risk for bearing children with sickle disease underwent prenatal diagnosis, which allowed identification of 27 SS fetuses, with an induced abortion rate of 70 percent.[565] Such data are, of course, highly culture dependent, and very different results might be obtained elsewhere.

SICKLE CELL TRAIT

DEFINITION AND HISTORY

Sickle cell trait is the heterozygous state for the sickle cell diseases and is the most benign form of the sickling disorders.

ETIOLOGY AND PATHOGENESIS

The properties of sickle hemoglobin have been described above in "Biochemical Basis of Sickling." In sickle cell trait, less than half of the hemoglobin in each red cell is hemoglobin S. The abundance of normal hemoglobin A in the cell prevents sickling under most physiologic circumstances; sickle cell trait cells sickle at an oxygen tension of approximately 15 torr.[109]

Sickle cell trait is inherited as an autosomal dominant disorder. It affects approximately 8 percent of African-Americans and an even higher percentage of the population in Africa. Interaction between α-thalassemia and sickle cell trait in modifying the amount of sickle hemoglobin has been described in "Concentration of Hemoglobin S in the Red Cell" above.

CLINICAL FEATURES

Sickle cell trait does not produce any abnormalities of the blood counts and is an exceedingly rare cause of morbidity. Red cell life span is normal in normoxic persons with sickle cell trait.[423] Not only patients but even physicians[424] often appear to believe that sickle cell trait represents a mild type of sickle cell disease. Cerebral thrombosis, mishaps during anesthesia, and sudden death attract little notice when occurring in a person who does not have a known genetic variant, but the same occurrence in the 1 of 12 African-Americans who have this trait immediately raises the question of a cause and effect relationship. Thus, there is a legion of anecdotal reports suggesting that sickle cell trait contributed to a patient's illness.[219,220,425–431] There may, however, be certain situations in which a risk is plausible. Thus, in severe cyanotic congenital heart diseases, such as tetralogy of Fallot, patients with sickle cell trait may show signs of hemolysis.[432] In reality, the morbidity and possible mortality associated with sickle cell trait are very low and therefore difficult to document accurately. It seems to be limited largely to renal lesions (see Fig. 47-9) leading to hematuria that is otherwise unexplained and possibly to thromboembolic episodes involving the lung. In a massive study encompassing more than 65,000 consecutively admitted African-American male patients in 13 U.S. Veterans Administration hospitals,[19] slightly higher incidences were found for only hematuria of unspecified cause (2.5% vs. 1.3%) and pulmonary embolism (2.2% vs. 1.5%). No age stratification was found, indicating that the life span of patients with sickle cell trait is normal. Surgical patients with sickle cell trait had no greater perioperative mortality, no longer postoperative stay, and no greater mortality than those with normal hemoglobin. Similar conclusions have been drawn in other studies.[433] It has not been possible to document any differences from normal in cardiovascular function of sickle cell trait subjects, even when subjected to maximum exercise[434–438]; indeed, persons with sickle trait were overrepresented among champion athletes in the Ivory Coast.[439]

In a blinded study, data have been obtained that suggest that brain magnetic resonance angiography disclosed more arterial tortuosity in children with sickle trait than in controls. Tortuosity tended to be greater in children with a higher concentration of hemoglobin S.[440] A larger survey in Oman[441] suggested that there was an increased incidence of anemia, abortion, and neonatal death among women with sickle trait.

Sudden death resulting from rhabdomyolysis has been reported anecdotally in numerous subjects with sickle cell trait following severe exercise.[428,442–446] An extensive investigation of episodes of sudden death showed a statistically significant excess in the number of patients with sickle cell trait.[447] It is believed that the hyposthenuria (see "Genitourinary System" above) in combination with heat and extreme stress may trigger this catastrophic and usually fatal event.

Because of reports of splenic infarction in individuals thought to have sickle cell trait who were flying in unpressurized aircraft[448,449] or who ascended to very high altitudes,[450,451] there has been concern about the safety of permitting persons with sickle cell trait to fly. Because commercial aircraft maintain a cabin pressure equivalent to that encountered at 5000 to 7000 feet (1524–2134 m), this concern is unwarranted.[111] It appears that when splenic infarction does occur at high altitudes, non-African persons with sickle trait are much more likely to be affected than are Africans.[110,451] It has been suggested that coinheritance of sickle cell trait and hereditary spherocytosis leads to splenic infarction. Approximately 20 cases with both disorders have been documented, and several suffered from splenic infarctions.[452,453]

LABORATORY FEATURES

The diagnosis of sickle cell trait depends upon demonstration of the presence of hemoglobin S and hemoglobin A in the affected individual. The amount of hemoglobin S always is less than the concentration of hemoglobin A. In contrast, in sickle cell β^+-thalassemia the amount of hemoglobin S exceeds the concentration of hemoglobin A.

THERAPY

Because of its benign features, sickle cell trait does not require treatment and does not appear to affect life span.[19]

COURSE AND PROGNOSIS

Sickle cell trait does not appear to affect life span.[19]

HEMOGLOBIN C DISEASE

DEFINITION AND HISTORY

Hemoglobin C was the second abnormal hemoglobin to be described, not long after the description of hemoglobin S.[454] The homozygous state (CC disease) was described independently by Spaet and colleagues[455] and Ranney and colleagues[456] in 1953. Hemoglobin C trait is the heterozygous state in which hemoglobin C is inherited with normal hemoglobin. The combination with sickle cell hemoglobin, SC disease, has been described above in "The Sickle Cell Diseases."

ETIOLOGY AND PATHOGENESIS

In hemoglobin C, glutamic acid in the sixth position from the N terminal of the β-chain has been replaced by lysine.[457] Red cells containing principally hemoglobin C are more rigid than normal,[458] and their fragmentation in the circulation may result in the formation of microspherocytes. Intraerythrocytic crystals of oxygenated hemoglobin C are found in the red cells, especially in splenectomized patients,[458,459] and the formation of crystals is inhibited by hemoglobin F.[460] Red cell life span is shortened to a mean of 30 to 35 days.[461] The rate of hemoglobin production in hemoglobin C disease has been reported to be 2.5 to 3 times normal.[462] Erythrocytes from patients with hemoglobin C disease have a low oxygen affinity, possibly because of reduction, for unknown reasons, of the intracellular pH.[463] This may contribute to the mild anemia that usually is present.

CLINICAL FEATURES

Splenomegaly is a fairly constant feature of hemoglobin C disease and may be associated with fleeting abdominal pain. However, there is little evidence for clinically significant hemodynamic disturbances.[464] Women with hemoglobin C disease appear to tolerate pregnancy well.[465] Children have mild anemia with few symptoms and normal growth.[466]

LABORATORY FEATURES

In hemoglobin C disease, the hemoglobin level ranges from 8 to 12 g/dl. There is a marked increase in the number of target cells in the blood film (see Fig. 47-12). Some target cells also are present in the trait. Occasionally, intraerythrocytic hemoglobin crystals are seen on the blood film. The crystals may appear in larger numbers if the red cells have been dehydrated either by drying or by suspension in a hypertonic solution (see Chap. 28). The osmotic fragility of the red cells may be decreased.

DIFFERENTIAL DIAGNOSIS

The diagnosis of homozygous hemoglobin C disease is achieved by electrophoresis, hemoglobin C moving in the same position as hemoglobin A_2, hemoglobin E, and hemoglobin O_{Arab} at an alkaline pH. Hemoglobin C is readily distinguished from other hemoglobins by acid agar gel electrophoresis.

THERAPY

No specific therapy is available or required for patients with hemoglobin C disease. Uncommonly, severe splenic pain has led to splenectomy.[467]

COURSE AND PROGNOSIS

Anemia may be more severe following infections, but the overall prognosis is considered excellent.

HEMOGLOBIN D DISEASE

DEFINITION AND HISTORY

In his early studies of the hemoglobinopathies, Itano[468] encountered a white family with an abnormal hemoglobin that migrated at the same rate as hemoglobin S but did not sickle. Its solubility in the reduced state resembled that of hemoglobin A, and this new abnormal hemoglobin was designated hemoglobin D. Subsequently, this name was given to any hemoglobin variant that manifested the same electrophoretic properties as hemoglobin S at an alkaline pH but had normal solubility properties.

ETIOLOGY AND PATHOGENESIS

With the exact chemical analysis of hemoglobin variants, it became apparent that hemoglobin $D_{Los Angeles}$ was identical to hemoglobin D_{Punjab}, both manifesting a substitution of glutamate for lysine at the 121st position in the β-chain. Another "D" hemoglobin, $G_{Philadelphia}$, is, on the other hand, an α-chain variant with a substitution of asparagine for lysine at the 68th position.

Like the other structural mutations of hemoglobin, hemoglobin D trait is the heterozygous state for hemoglobin D and hemoglobin A, whereas the homozygous state for hemoglobin D is designated hemoglobin D disease.

CLINICAL FEATURES

The heterozygous state for hemoglobin D is entirely asymptomatic.[469] The abnormal hemoglobin constitutes between 35 and 50 percent of the total hemoglobin. Homozygous hemoglobin D disease is very rare, and some patients originally believed to be homozygous for hemoglobin D[470] subsequently were found to be heterozygous for hemoglobin

D and β-thalassemia. A small number of true homozygotes have been described, however, and the clinical consequences are very mild.[471] Hemoglobin S/$D_{Punjab/Los Angeles}$ disease is a relatively severe sickle cell disease.[472]

DIFFERENTIAL DIAGNOSIS

The diagnosis depends upon demonstrating the existence of hemoglobin D in the red cells.

THERAPY, COURSE, AND PROGNOSIS

The prognosis is excellent, and no therapy is required.

HEMOGLOBIN E DISEASE

DEFINITION AND HISTORY

Hemoglobin E was first described in 1954, independently by Itano and colleagues[473] and by Chernoff and colleagues.[474]

ETIOLOGY AND PATHOGENESIS

Hemoglobin E is the result of the β-chain mutation $\alpha_2\beta_2$ 26Glu→Lys.[475] The amino acid substitution not only produces a hemoglobin that is somewhat unstable when subjected to oxidative stress,[476] perhaps because of weakening of the bonds between the monomers constituting the hemoglobin tetramer, but the nucleotide substitution also creates a new potential splicing sequence so that some of the messenger may be spliced improperly.[477] The formation of unstable messenger accounts for the thalassemia-like nature of hemoglobin E trait and disease.

The inheritance of hemoglobin E is the same as that of the other β-chain mutants. Heterozygotes for hemoglobin E and hemoglobin A have hemoglobin E trait, whereas homozygotes for hemoglobin E are designated as having hemoglobin E disease. Hemoglobin E, like hemoglobin S and hemoglobin C, occurs with sufficient frequency to be considered a polymorphism. Figure 47-13 illustrates the distribution

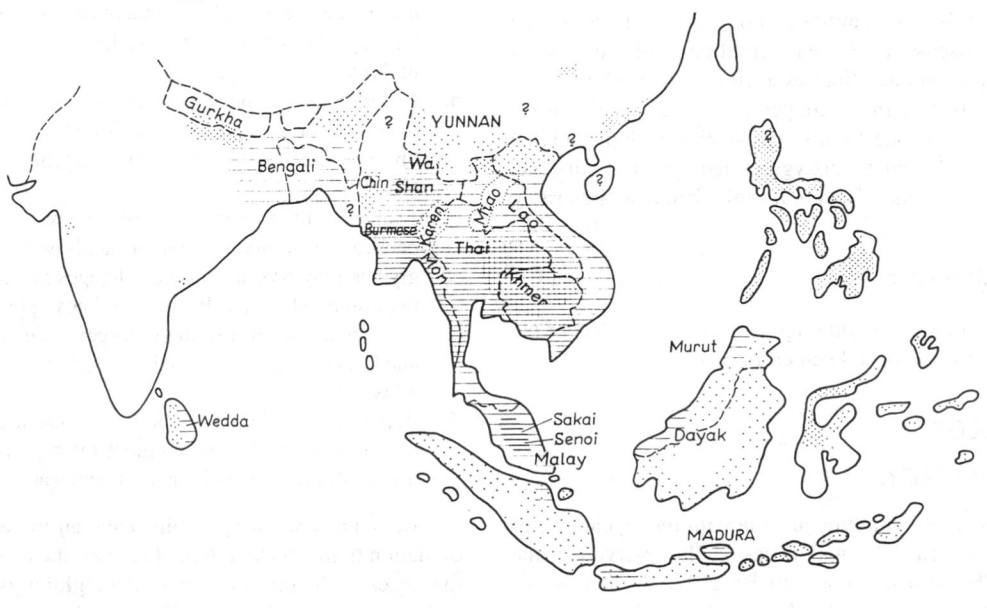

FIGURE 47-13   Distribution of hemoglobin E in Southeast Asia. Gene frequencies: *cross-hatching* indicates >0.2 percent; *narrow hatching* indicates 0.1 to 0.2 percent; *wide hatching* indicates 0.02 to 0.1 percent; *dotted area* indicates <0.02 percent and sporadic occurrence. (From G Flatz,[25] with permission.)

of the gene for this β-chain mutation. Decreased *Falciparum malaria* parasitemia has been documented in patients with hemoglobin E trait,[478] and resistance to malaria may be the advantage that has led to high gene frequencies.

CLINICAL FEATURES

Although the prevalence of the gene for hemoglobin E is quite high in Southeast Asia (see Fig. 47-13), relatively few patients with homozygous E disease, as distinguished from hemoglobin E β-thalassemia, have been described.[479–481] When homozygous E disease is encountered, it is associated with marked microcytosis and hypochromia, but the anemia usually is mild. Splenomegaly is unusual, and the red cell life span is normal. Clinically, the state closely resembles β-thalassemia minor.[482] In the hemoglobin E carrier state, 30 to 45 percent of the hemoglobin is hemoglobin E,[474] and such carriers are asymptomatic but do manifest microcytosis.

The clinical manifestations of the heterozygous state between hemoglobin E and β-thalassemia are remarkably variable in severity.[481,483] The disease phenotype is essentially that of β-thalassemia. Onset usually is in the first decade of life, but approximately 8 percent of patients are not diagnosed until after age 20 years. Characteristic findings include growth retardation, mongoloid faces, moderate splenomegaly, and often a transfusion requirement. Iron overload is almost universal, and cardiovascular complications are common. There is an increased susceptibility to infection, particularly in patients who have undergone splenectomy. Pulmonary arterial occlusions are commonly found at autopsy.

LABORATORY FEATURES

Hemoglobin E is electrophoretically slow in an alkaline medium, comigrating with hemoglobins C and A_2. The characteristic blood change is microcytosis—mild in the trait and more severe in the homozygous state and in hemoglobin E β-thalassemia. There is a modest decrease in the α-/non–α-globin chain synthetic ratio[480] and a minimal decrease in whole blood oxygen affinity.[474,479]

THERAPY

The prognosis seems to be good, although no thorough studies of the natural history of the disease have been carried out. Splenectomy increases red cell life span and ameliorates anemia in hemoglobin E β-thalassemia,[484,485] but its role in homozygous hemoglobin E disease has not been delineated. In one family manifesting both pyrimidine 5′-nucleotidase deficiency and homozygous hemoglobin E disease, those with both defects had more severe anemia than those inheriting only one.[486]

COURSE AND PROGNOSIS

The prognosis seems to be good, although no thorough studies of the natural history of the disease have been carried out.

UNSTABLE HEMOGLOBINS

DEFINITION AND HISTORY

The sporadic occurrence of hemolytic anemia with the appearance of inclusion bodies in the red cells was occasionally observed in the 1940s and 1950s,[487–489] but it was not until 1962[490,491] that it was recognized that such patients had abnormal hemoglobins that spontaneously denatured within the circulating red cell. The unstable hemoglobins discussed in this chapter are those resulting from a mutation that changes the amino acid sequence of one of the globin chains. Homotetramers of normal β-chains (hemoglobin H) or normal γ-chains (hemoglobin Bart's) also are unstable hemoglobins. These unstable hemoglobins occur in patients with α-thalassemia and are discussed in Chapter 46. *Hyperunstable hemoglobins*[492] have defects that are so severe that the globin chain is not found in the red cells, but their formation can be deduced from the DNA sequence.

ETIOLOGY AND PATHOGENESIS

The tetrameric hemoglobin molecule has evolved so that a variety of noncovalent forces maintain the structure of each subunit and bind the subunits to each other. A delicate balance allows the molecule to change from one state to another, facilitating its oxygen-binding function while maintaining its structural integrity, has been discussed in "Structure and Function of the Hemoglobin Molecule." It is not surprising that a variety of amino acid substitutions or deletions weaken the forces that maintain the structure of hemoglobin. When this occurs, the hemoglobin molecule denatures and precipitates as insoluble globins. These precipitates often attach to the cell membrane and are recognized as Heinz bodies (see Chap. 28).

Instability of hemoglobin can arise from any one of the following processes:

1. Replacement of an amino acid that contacts the heme group or produces a change in the property of the heme pocket often results in an unstable molecule with a tendency to lose heme from the abnormal globin chains. $Hb_{Hammersmith}$,[493,494] $Hb_{Sendagi}$,[495] Hb_{Alesha},[496] and $Hb_{La Roche-sur-Yon}$[497] are examples of this type of unstable hemoglobin.

2. Replacement of nonpolar by polar residues at the interior of the molecule results in gross distortion of the protein, particularly if the new polar residue remains in the interior portion of the molecule, as in $Hb_{Bristol}$[498] and Hb_{Volga}.[499]

3. Deletions or insertions of additional amino acids, particularly when critical helical regions of the sequence are involved, creates instability, as in $Hb_{Niteroi}$[500] and $Hb_{Montreal}$.[501]

4. Replacements at intersubunit contacts, particularly those between the α_1- and β_1-chains, create instability so that dissociation into monomers may occur. Hb_{Philly}[502] and Hb_{Tacoma}[503] are mildly unstable for this reason. Replacements at the contact between the α_1- and β_2-globin monomers usually result in hemoglobins with a high oxygen affinity.

5. If proline is introduced into an α helix beyond the third residue, distortion of the helix results in instability.[504] Variants in which proline substitution results in instability include Hb_{Duarte}[505] and $Hb_{Santa Ana}$.[506]

6. In areas of the hemoglobin molecule where atoms are very tightly packed, substitution of amino acids with larger side chains for glycine may produce marked changes in stability. In particular, at the points where the B and E helices approach each other, there is no room for substitution of larger amino acids for glycine at B6 and E8. $Hb_{Riverdale-Bronx}$,[507] $Hb_{Savannah}$,[508] and Hb_{Moscva}[509] arise in such a fashion.

7. Replacement of a hydrophobic residue that normally fits into a hydrophobic pocket with a more hydrophilic amino acid, such as the substitution of histidine for leucine at β81 in $Hb_{La Roche-sur-Yon}$.[497]

Many unstable hemoglobins have an increased susceptibility to oxidation to methemoglobin. However, the exact sequence of events that leads to the precipitation of hemoglobin is not fully understood and very likely varies with different unstable hemoglobins. The formation of hemichromes may be involved. These are compounds in which heme has been removed from its normal binding site and has become bonded to another part of the globin molecule.[510] These pigments can be shown to form during *in vitro* denaturation of some abnormal hemoglobins,[511] and they are present in hemoglobin H inclusion bodies.[512] The release of activated oxygen in the form of superoxide radicals with the subsequent formation of peroxide and the hydroxyl radicals[513,514] may also play a role. The attachment of Heinz bodies to the cell membrane impairs the deformability of the erythrocyte and impedes its ability to negotiate the narrow spaces between the endothelial cells lining the splenic sinuses. The "pitting" of Heinz bodies from the erythrocyte results in loss of membrane and ultimately in destruction of the red cells. Although Heinz bodies are formed, their presence in the blood does not become a prominent feature, except in patients who have been splenectomized (see "Laboratory Features" below). Table 47-2 lists selected unstable hemoglobins that have been characterized. Detailed tabulations are available.[515]

Hyperunstable hemoglobins are characterized by β-globin formation that is so defective that no β-chains are found. However, they differ from the β-thalassemias in that inheritance is dominant, that is,

a single copy of the mutant gene is all that is required to give the clinical phenotype. They may result from single base substitution, deletion of codons, frameshifts leading to elongated β-chains, or premature terminations.[516]

MODE OF INHERITANCE

Unstable hemoglobins are generally inherited as autosomal dominant disorders. Affected individuals are usually heterozygotes who have inherited the defect from one of their parents and who on the average will transmit it to one half of their offspring. Because unstable hemoglobins produce a disease state, genes for these disorders are subjected to negative selection, and the continued existence of the unstable hemoglobinopathies in the population is the result of such new mutations. Thus, occasionally patients with an unstable hemoglobin, neither of whose parents had the abnormality, are encountered. The homozygous state for the unstable hemoglobins Hb$_{Sun\ Prairie}$[517] and Hb$_{Bushwick}$[518] has been observed, and a homozygous-like state can occur when an unstable β-chain mutation is inherited together with a β°-thalassemic gene.[505,519]

More than 80 percent of unstable hemoglobins that have been characterized affect the β-chain. This probably reflects the fact that the normal genome contains four copies of the α-chain. The clinical effects of such mutants, affecting only one fourth of the total hemoglobin formed, are apt to be less pronounced than those of β-chain mutants, in which half of the hemoglobin produced is abnormal. Thus, many α-globin mutations are likely to be overlooked.

Although most patients with unstable hemoglobins have been found to have a combination of hemoglobin A and the unstable hemoglobin in their red cells, there are a number of reports of the inheritance of unstable hemoglobins with other hemoglobinopathies.[505,520–524]

CLINICAL FEATURES

A broad spectrum of clinical manifestations can be induced by unstable hemoglobins. In most cases, hemolysis is well compensated, and some hemoglobins that are unstable *in vitro* (e.g., Hb$_{Muscat}$[525]) are not associated with hemolysis at all. When an unstable hemoglobin also has a left-shifted oxygen dissociation curve, that is, an increased O_2 affinity, the hemoglobin level may be in the upper portion of the normal range. Episodes of infection and treatment with "oxidant" drugs are likely to precipitate hemolytic episodes in persons whose anemia is well compensated under ordinary circumstances. It is at this juncture that the diagnosis is often first made. In the case of patients who have particularly unstable variants, such as Hb$_{Hammersmith}$,[493] Hb$_{Bristol}$,[498] Hb$_{Santa\ Ana}$,[506] or Hb$_{Madrid}$,[526] a chronic hemolytic anemia may become evident during the first year of life as γ-chain production is replaced by production of the mutant β-chain. In contrast, in the rare instances where the γ-chain bears the abnormality,[527] the hemolytic anemia is evident at birth and disappears as normal β-chains are formed.

Physical findings include jaundice, splenomegaly, and, when the anemia is severe, pallor. In some patients, dark urine has been observed, probably as a result of the excretion of dipyrrole pigments derived from the catabolism of free heme groups or of Heinz bodies.[528] In some instances, methemoglobinemia may develop and cyanosis may then be evident. Priapism has been observed in one patient who had co-inherited Hb$_{Perth}$ and factor V Leiden.[529]

LABORATORY FEATURES

The hemoglobin concentration of the blood may be normal or decreased. The mean corpuscular hemoglobin is usually diminished

TABLE 47-2 UNSTABLE HEMOGLOBINS

HEMOGLOBIN	SUBSTITUTION
Torino	α3 Phe→Val
Hasharon* (Sinai, Sealy)	α47 Asp→His
Iwata	α87 His→Arg
Petah Tikva	α100 Ala→Asp
Freiburg	β23 Val deleted
Riverdale-Bronx	β24 Gly→Arg
Yokohama	β31 Leu→Pro
Castilla	β32 Leu→Arg
Perth* (Abraham Lincoln)	β32 Leu→Pro
Philly	β35 Tyr→Phe
Hammersmith	β42 Phe→Ser
Bucuresti* (Louisville)	β42 Phe→Leu
Niteroi	β42-44, or β43-45 Phe, Glu, Ser deleted
Duarte	β62 Ala→Pro
Zürich	β63 His→Arg
Bristol	β67 Val→Asp
Sydney	β67 Val→Ala
Mizuho	β68 Leu→Pro
Seattle	β70 Ala→Asp
Christchurch	β71 Phe→Ser
Shepherd's Bush	β74 Gly→Asp
Bushwick	β74 Gly→Val
Buenos Aires* (Bryn Mawr)	β85 Phe→Ser
Santa Ana	β88 Leu→Pro
Redondo	β92 His→Asn→Asp
St. Etienne* (Istanbul)	β92 His→Gln
Gun Hill	β91-95 or 92-96 or 93-97 Leu, Cys, Asp, His deleted
Köln* (Ube I)	β98 Val→Met
Djelfa	β98 Val→Ala
Presbyterian	β108 Asn→Lys
Shelby (Deaconess)	β131 Gln→Lys
North Shore	β134 Val→Glu
Coventry	β141 Leu deleted
Tak	Elongation of β-chain C-terminus
Cranston	Elongation of β-chain C-terminus
La Grange	β101 Glu→Lys
Poole	β130 Trp→Gly

* Parentheses indicate alternative names for these variants but are not intended to suggest that one or the other name is preferred.

because of the loss of hemoglobin from the red cells as a result of its denaturation and subsequent pitting from the erythrocytes. The blood film may show slight hypochromia, and in addition, poikilocytosis, polychromasia, anisocytosis, and some basophilic stippling may be evident. Hyperunstable hemoglobins, in particular, are associated with severe hypochromia of the erythrocytes and present clinically as dominant β-thalassemia. Reticulocytosis often is out of proportion to the severity of the anemia, particularly when the abnormal hemoglobin has a high oxygen affinity. After splenectomy, many Heinz bodies may be found in the circulation. Hemoglobin F levels may be increased.[530]

Diagnosis of this disorder usually depends upon the demonstration of the presence of an unstable hemoglobin. Three tests are used for this purpose. The most convenient is the isopropanol stability test.[531] The heat stability test also is useful[532] but is somewhat more difficult to interpret. It has been found, however, that at least one unstable hemoglobin, Hb_Olmsted, can be detected by heat stability but not isopropanol stability.[533] Finally, incubation of blood with brilliant cresyl blue generates Heinz bodies in hemoglobin H disease.[534,535] Further identification of unstable hemoglobins is aided by procedures such as hemoglobin electrophoresis; however, the electrophoretic pattern often is normal, and the diagnosis of the hemoglobinopathy cannot be ruled out in this way. The oxygen affinity of unstable hemoglobins is often altered, and the determination of P_{50} may help in detecting and characterizing the unstable hemoglobin. In the final analysis, unstable hemoglobins can be identified only by DNA analysis[496,530,536,537] or by physical separation of the abnormal hemoglobin from the normal hemoglobin, followed by globin chain separation and peptide analysis.

DIFFERENTIAL DIAGNOSIS

The possibility that an unstable hemoglobin is present should be considered in all patients who present with the clinical picture of hereditary nonspherocytic hemolytic anemia (see Chap. 45), particularly when hypochromia of the red cells is present and when the extent of the reticulocytosis is out of keeping with the degree of anemia. Not all patients with a positive test for unstable hemoglobins should be classified as having this disorder. The stability of methemoglobin, hemoglobin F, and sickle hemoglobin is appreciably less than that of hemoglobin A, and false-positive isopropanol stability tests may be obtained in patients with increased quantities of these hemoglobins. Hemoglobin H (β_4) and hemoglobin Bart's (γ_4) are unstable. These fast-moving hemoglobins can be detected on electrophoresis. Patients whose red cells contain these hemoglobins are diagnosed as having α-thalassemia (see Chap. 46).

Sometimes the hemoglobins are so unstable that none of the protein can be detected.

TREATMENT

As with other hemolytic states, gallstones are common, and cholecystectomy may be required. Hemolytic episodes may be precipitated by infection or by the ingestion of "oxidative" drugs. Treatment is not usually required. As in the case of other hemolytic disorders, folic acid in a dose of 1 mg/day often is given, but its usefulness has not been established. "Oxidant" drugs, such as those listed in Table 45-6, should be avoided. In addition, the use of all sulfonamides should be eschewed, particularly in the case of those variants that have been associated with drug-induced hemolysis. Splenectomy has proven to be useful in some patients with splenomegaly and severe hemolysis,[538,539] whereas others have enjoyed little benefit.[533] In view of the fact that patients with high-oxygen-affinity unstable hemoglobin have died after a splenectomy[505] and that thromboembolic complications have been

reported in a number of other patients,[540] it is probably best to avoid splenectomy. Preliminary results suggested that hydroxyurea therapy might be useful,[539] presumably by increasing the level of fetal hemoglobin. Hydroxyurea has also been administered to lower the platelet count after splenectomy.[529]

COURSE AND PROGNOSIS

Most patients with unstable hemoglobins follow a relatively benign course. As noted above under "Treatment," splenectomy has been associated with mortality in several patients. Priapism was observed in one patient who also had the factor V Leiden mutation.[529]

OTHER HEMOGLOBINOPATHIES

In comparison with hemoglobins S, C, D, and E, other abnormal hemoglobins are rare. Some, such as hemoglobins producing erythrocytosis (see Chap. 56) and those producing cyanosis (see Chap. 48), are of clinical importance. Many of the other hemoglobins do not produce significant clinical alterations but nonetheless have been important in clarifying the role of individual amino acids in the structure and function of the hemoglobin molecule. Some of the more common hemoglobin variants are summarized in Table 47-3. Complete compendia of mutations affecting hemoglobin have been published,[515] and further sources are available at *http://globin.cse.psu.edu/globin/hbvar/menu.html*.

TABLE 47-3 SOME REPRESENTATIVE HEMOGLOBIN VARIANTS

AMINO ACID (SEQUENTIAL NUMBER)	AMINO ACID SUBSTITUTION	NAME	MAJOR ABNORMAL PROPERTY	REFERENCE
α-Chain Variants				
5	Ala→Asp	J_Toronto		550
16	Lys→Glu	I		551
23	Glu→Gln	Memphis		93
30	Glu→Gln	G_Honolulu		552
87	His→Arg	Iwata	(3)	553
β-Chain Variants				
6	Glu→Val	S	(5)	554
6	Glu→Lys	C		555
24	Gly→Asp	Moscva	(3)(2)	509
62	Ala→Pro	Duarte	(3)(1)	505
63	His→Arg	Zürich	(3)(1)	556
6	Glu→Val	C_Harlem		557
73	Asp→Asn			
102	Asn→Thr	Kansas	(2)(4)	558
121	Glu→Gln	D_Los Angeles	(1)	559
*γ-Chain Variants				
6	Glu→Lys	F_TexasII		560
Fusion Hemoglobins				
		Lepore_Hollandia		561
		Lincoln Park		562
Stop Codon Mutations				
		Constant Spring		563
δ-Chain Variants				
22	Ala→Glu	A_2-Flatbush		564

(1) ↑ O_2 affinity; (2) ↓ O_2 affinity; (3) unstable; (4) ↑ dissociation; (5) sickling.

REFERENCES

1. Herrick JB: Peculiar elongated and sickle-shaped red corpuscles in a case of severe anemia. *Arch Intern Med* 6:517, 1910.

2. Emmel VE: A study of the erythrocytes in a case of severe anemia with elongated and sickle-shaped red blood corpuscles. *Arch Intern Med* 20: 586, 1917.

3. Hahn EV, Gillespie EB: Report of a case greatly improved by splenectomy; experimental study of sickle cell formation. *Arch Intern Med* 39: 233, 1927.

4. Taliaferro WH, Huck JG: The inheritance of sickle-cell anemia in man. *Genetics* 8:594, 1923.

5. Neel JV: The inheritance of sickle cell anemia. *Science* 110:64, 1949.

6. Beet EA: The genetics of the sickle-cell trait in a Bantu tribe. *Ann Eugen (Lond)* 14:279, 1949.

7. Pauling L, Itano HA, Singer SJ, Wells IC: Sickle cell anemia, a molecular disease. *Science* 110:543, 1949.

8. Ingram VM: Gene mutations in human haemoglobin. The chemical difference between normal and sickle cell haemoglobin. *Nature* 180:326, 1957.

9. Conley CL: Sickle-cell anemia. The first molecular disease, in *Blood, Pure and Eloquent*, edited by MM Wintrobe, p 319. McGraw-Hill, New York, 1980.

10. Ad Hoc Committee on Mutation Nomenclature: Update on nomenclature for human gene mutations. *Hum Mutat* 8:197, 1996.

11. Beaudet AL, Tsui LC: A suggested nomenclature for designating mutations. *Hum Mutat* 4:245, 1993.

12. Dunston T, Rowland R, Huntsman RG, Yawson GI: Sickle-cell haemoglobin C disease and sickle-cell beta thalassaemia in white South Africans. *S Afr Med J* 46:1423, 1972.

13. Luzzatto L: Genetics of red cells and susceptibility to malaria. *Blood* 54:961, 1979.

14. Lapouméroulie C, Dunda O, Ducrocq R, et al: A novel sickle cell mutation of yet another origin in Africa: The Cameroon type. *Hum Genet* 89:333, 1992.

15. Labie D, Srinivas R, Dunda O, et al: Haplotypes in tribal Indians bearing the sickle gene: Evidence for the unicentric origin of the beta S mutation and the unicentric origin of the tribal populations of India. *Hum Biol* 61:479, 1989.

16. Nagel RL: Beta-globin-gene haplotypes, mitochondrial DNA, the Y-chromosome: Their impact on the genetic epidemiology of the major structural hemoglobinopathies. *Cell Mol Biol* 50:5, 2004.

17. Edington GN, Lehmann H: A case of sickle cell hemoglobin C disease in a survey of hemoglobin C incidence in West Africa. *Trans R Soc Trop Med Hyg* 48:332, 1954.

18. Labie D, Richin C, Pagnier J, et al: Hemoglobins S and C in Upper Volta. *Hum Genet* 65:300, 1984.

19. Heller P, Best WR, Nelson RB, Becktel J: Clinical implications of sickle-cell trait and glucose-6-phosphate dehydrogenase deficiency in hospitalized Black male patients. *N Engl J Med* 300:1001, 1979.

20. Schneider RG: Incidence of hemoglobin C trait in 505 normal Negroes: A family with homozygous hemoglobin C and sickle-cell trait union. *J Lab Clin Med* 44:133, 1954.

21. Diggs LW, Kraus AP, Morrison DB, Rudnicki RPT: Intraerythrocytic crystals in a white patient with hemoglobin C in the absence of other types of hemoglobin. *Blood* 9:1172, 1954.

22. Fairhurst RM, Fujioka H, Hayton K, et al: Aberrant development of Plasmodium falciparum in hemoglobin CC red cells: Implications for the malaria protective effect of the homozygous state. *Blood* 101:3309, 2003.

23. Almeida AM, Henthorn JS, Davies SC: Neonatal screening for haemoglobinopathies: The results of a 10-year programme in an English Health Region. *Br J Haematol* 112:32, 2001.

24. Lachant NA: Hemoglobin E: An emerging hemoglobinopathy in the United States. *Am J Hematol* 25:449, 1987.

25. Flatz G: Hemoglobin E: Distribution and population dynamics. *Humangenetik* 3:189, 1967.

26. Kazazian HH Jr, Waber PG, Boehm CD, et al: Hemoglobin E in Europeans: Further evidence for multiple origins of the beta^E-globin gene. *Am J Hum Genet* 36:212, 1984.

27. Chotivanich K, Udomsangpetch R, Pattanapanyasat K, et al: Hemoglobin E: A balanced polymorphism protective against high parasitemias and thus severe P falciparum malaria. *Blood* 100:1172, 2002.

28. Manning JM, Dumoulin A, Li X, Manning LR: Normal and abnormal protein subunit interactions in hemoglobins. *J Biol Chem* 273:19359, 1998.

29. Wajcman H, Kister J, Galacteros F, et al: Hb Montefiore (126(H9)Asp→Tyr). High oxygen affinity and loss of cooperativity secondary to C-terminal disruption. *J Biol Chem* 271:22990, 1996.

30. Zuck TF, Riess JG: Current status of injectable oxygen carriers. *Crit Rev Clin Lab Sci* 31:295, 1994.

31. Cao Z, Liao D, Mirchev R, et al: Nucleation and polymerization of sickle hemoglobin with Leu beta 88 substituted by Ala. *J Mol Biol* 265:580, 1997.

32. Mirchev R, Ferrone FA: The structural link between polymerization and sickle cell disease. *J Mol Biol* 265:475, 1997.

33. Rodgers DW, Crepeau RH, Edelstein SJ: Pairings and polarities of the 14 strands in sickle cell hemoglobin fibers. *Proc Natl Acad Sci U S A* 84:6157, 1987.

34. Watowich SJ, Gross LJ, Josephs R: Intermolecular contacts within sickle hemoglobin fibers. *J Mol Biol* 209:821, 1989.

35. Mozzarelli A, Hofrichter J, Eaton WA: Delay time of hemoglobin S polymerization prevents most cells from sickling in vivo. *Science* 237: 500, 1987.

36. Samuel RE, Salmon ED, Briehl RW: Nucleation and growth of fibres and gel formation in sickle cell haemoglobin. *Nature* 345:833, 1990.

37. Eaton WA, Hofrichter J, Ross PD: Delay time of gelation: A possible determinant of clinical severity in sickle cell disease. *Blood* 47:621, 1976.

38. Goodman SR: The irreversibly sickled cell: A perspective. *Cell Mol Biol* 50:53, 2004.

39. Jensen M, Shohet SB, Nathan DG: The role of red cell energy metabolism in the generation of irreversible sickled cells in vitro. *Blood* 42: 835, 1973.

40. Bookchin RM, Ortiz OE, Lew VL: Evidence for a direct reticulocyte origin of dense red cells in sickle cell anemia. *J Clin Invest* 87:113, 1991.

41. Serjeant GR, Serjeant BE, Milner PF: The irreversibly sickled cell: A determinant of haemolysis in sickle-cell anaemia. *Br J Haematol* 17: 527, 1969.

42. Lande WM, Andrews DL, Clark MR, et al: The incidence of painful crisis in homozygous sickle cell disease: Correlation with red cell deformability. *Blood* 72:2056, 1988.

43. Ballas SK, Larner J, Smith ED, et al: Rheologic predictors of the severity of the painful sickle cell crisis. *Blood* 72:1216, 1988.

44. Tosteson DC, Carlsen E, Dunham ET: The effects of sickling on ion transport: I. Effect of sickling on potassium transport. *J Gen Physiol* 39: 31, 1955.

45. Dzandu JK, Johnson RM: Membrane protein phosphorylation in intact normal and sickle cell erythrocytes. *J Biol Chem* 255:6382, 1980.

46. Beutler E, Guinto E, Johnson C: Human red cell protein kinase in normal subjects and patients with hereditary spherocytosis, sickle cell disease, and autoimmune hemolytic anemia. *Blood* 48:887, 1976.

47. Hosey MM, Tao M: Altered erythrocyte membrane phosphorylation in sickle cell disease. *Nature* 263:424, 1976.

48. Bookchin RM, Lew VL: Progressive inhibition of the Ca pump and Ca: Ca exchange in sickle red cells. *Nature* 284:561, 1980.

49. Eaton JW, Jacob HS, White JG: Membrane abnormalities of irreversibly sickled cells. *Semin Hematol* 16:52, 1979.

50. Steinberg MH, Eaton JW, Berger E, et al: Erythrocyte calcium abnormalities and the clinical severity of sickling disorders. *Br J Haematol* 40:533, 1978.

51. Lew VL, Hockaday A, Sepulveda MI, et al: Compartmentalization of sickle-cell calcium in endocytic inside-out vesicles. *Nature* 315:586, 1985.

52. Williamson P, Puchulu E, Penniston JT, et al: Ca2+ accumulation and loss by aberrant endocytic vesicles in sickle erythrocytes. *J Cell Physiol* 152:1, 1992.

53. Hebbel RP: Auto-oxidation and a membrane-associated "Fenton reagent": A possible explanation for development of membrane lesions in sickle erythrocytes. *Clin Haematol* 14:129, 1985.

54. Hebbel RP, Eaton JW, Balasingam M, Steinberg MH: Spontaneous oxygen radical generation by sickle erythrocytes. *J Clin Invest* 70:1253, 1982.

55. Repka T, Hebbel RP: Hydroxyl radical formation by sickle erythrocyte membranes: Role of pathologic iron deposits and cytoplasmic reducing agents. *Blood* 78:2753, 1991.

56. Rank BH, Carlsson J, Hebbel RP: Abnormal redox status of membrane-protein thiols in sickle erythrocytes. *J Clin Invest* 75:1531, 1985.

57. Schacter L, Warth JA, Gordon EM, et al: Altered amount and activity of superoxide dismutase in sickle cell anemia. *FASEB J* 2:237, 1988.

58. Zerez CR, Lachant NA, Lee SJ, Tanaka KR: Decreased erythrocyte nicotinamide adenine dinucleotide redox potential and abnormal pyridine nucleotide content in sickle cell disease. *Blood* 71:512, 1988.

59. Vasseur C, Leclerc L, Hilly M, Bursaux E: Decreased G3PDH binding to erythrocyte membranes in sickle cell disease. *Nouv Rev Fr Hematol* 34:155, 1992.

60. Liu SC, Derick LH, Zhai S, Palek J: Uncoupling of the spectrin-based skeleton from the lipid bilayer in sickled red cells. *Science* 252:574, 1991.

61. Hebbel RP, Miller WJ: Phagocytosis of sickle erythrocytes: Immunologic and oxidative determinants of hemolytic anemia. *Blood* 64:733, 1984.

62. Kuypers FA, Lewis RA, Hua M, et al: Detection of altered membrane phospholipid asymmetry in subpopulations of human red blood cells using fluorescently labeled annexin V. *Blood* 87:1179, 1996.

63. Tait JF, Gibson D: Measurement of membrane phospholipid asymmetry in normal and sickle-cell erythrocytes by means of annexin V binding. *J Lab Clin Med* 123:741, 1994.

64. Ataga KI, Orringer EP: Hypercoagulability in sickle cell disease: A curious paradox. *Am J Med* 115:721, 2003.

65. Chiu D, Lubin B, Roelofsen B, Van Deenen LL: Sickled erythrocytes accelerate clotting in vitro: An effect of abnormal membrane lipid asymmetry. *Blood* 58:398, 1981.

66. Wang RH, Phillips G Jr, Medof ME, Mold C: Activation of the alternative complement pathway by exposure of phosphatidylethanolamine and phosphatidylserine on erythrocytes from sickle cell disease patients. *J Clin Invest* 92:1326, 1993.

67. Andrade FL, Annichino-Bizzacchi JM, Saad ST, et al: Prothrombin mutant, factor V Leiden, and thermolabile variant of methylenetetrahydrofolate reductase among patients with sickle cell disease in Brazil. *Am J Hematol* 59:46, 1998.

68. Kordes U, Janka-Schaub G, Schneppenheim R: Homozygous Factor V Leiden mutation in sickle cell anaemia. *Br J Haematol* 116:236, 2002.

69. Ballas SK, Smith ED: Red blood cell changes during the evolution of the sickle cell painful crisis. *Blood* 79:2154, 1992.

70. Poillon WN, Kim BC, Castro O: Intracellular hemoglobin S polymerization and the clinical severity of sickle cell anemia. *Blood* 91:1777, 1998.

71. Sharan K, Surrey S, Ballas S, et al: Association of T-786C eNOS gene polymorphism with increased susceptibility to acute chest syndrome in females with sickle cell disease. *Br J Haematol* 124:240, 2004.

72. Itano HA: Qualitative and quantitative control of adult hemoglobin synthesis: A multiple allele hypothesis. *Am J Hum Genet* 5:34, 1953.

73. Huisman THJ: Sickle cell anemia as a syndrome: A review of diagnostic features. *Am J Hematol* 6:173, 1979.

74. Steinberg MH, Embury SH: Alpha-thalassemia in Blacks: Genetic and clinical aspects and interactions with the sickle hemoglobin gene. *Blood* 68:985, 1986.

75. Shaeffer JR, Kingston RE, McDonald MJ, Bunn HF: Competition of normal beta chains and sickle hemoglobin beta chains for alpha chains as a post-translational control mechanism. *Nature* 276:631, 1978.

76. Bunn HF, McDonald MJ: Electrostatic interactions in the assembly of human hemoglobin. *Nature* 306:498, 1983.

77. Embury SH, Dozy AM, Miller J, et al: Concurrent sickle-cell anemia and alpha-thalassemia. Effect on severity of anemia. *N Engl J Med* 306:270, 1982.

78. Stevens MCG, Maude GH, Beckford M, et al: Alpha thalassemia and the hematology of homozygous sickle cell disease in childhood. *Blood* 67:411, 1986.

79. El-Hazmi MAF: On the nature of sickle-cell disease in the Arabian peninsula. *Hum Genet* 52:323, 1979.

80. Bookchin RM, Nagel RL: Interactions between human hemoglobins: Sickling and related phenomena. *Semin Hematol* 11:577, 1974.

81. Lawrence C, Fabry ME, Nagel RL: The unique red cell heterogeneity of SC disease: Crystal formation, dense reticulocytes, and unusual morphology. *Blood* 78:2104, 1991.

82. Fabry ME, Kaul DK, Raventos-Suarez C, et al: SC erythrocytes have an abnormally high intracellular hemoglobin concentration. Pathophysiological consequences. *J Clin Invest* 70:1315, 1982.

83. Noguchi CT, Rodgers GP, Serjeant G, Schechter AN: Levels of fetal hemoglobin necessary for treatment of sickle cell disease. *N Engl J Med* 318:96, 1988.

84. Bradley TB, Brawner JN III, Conley CL: Further observations on an inherited anomaly characterized by persistence of fetal hemoglobin. *Johns Hopkins Med J* 110:242, 1962.

85. Shepard MK, Weatherall DJ, Conley CL: Semiquantitative estimation of fetal hemoglobin in red cell populations. *Johns Hopkins Med J* 110:293, 1962.

86. Ali SA: Milder variant of sickle-cell disease in Arabs in Kuwait associated with unusually high levels of foetal haemoglobin. *Br J Haematol* 19:613, 1970.

87. Perrine RP, Pembrey ME, John P, et al: Natural history of sickle cell anemia in Saudi Arabs. *Ann Intern Med* 88:1, 1978.

88. El-Hazmi MAF, Al-Swailem AR, Bahakim HM, et al: Effect of alpha thalassaemia, G6PD deficiency and Hb F on the nature of sickle cell anaemia in south-western Saudi Arabia. *Trop Geogr Med* 42:241, 1990.

89. Powars DR, Schroeder WA, Weiss JN, et al: Lack of influence of fetal hemoglobin levels or erythrocyte indices on the severity of sickle cell anemia. *J Clin Invest* 65:732, 1980.

90. Padmos MA, Roberts GT, Sackey K, et al: Two different forms of homozygous sickle cell disease occur in Saudi Arabia. *Br J Haematol* 79:93, 1991.

91. Powars DR, Weiss JN, Chan LS, Schroeder WA: Is there a threshold level of fetal hemoglobin that ameliorates morbidity in sickle cell anemia? *Blood* 63:921, 1984.

92. Conley CL, Weatherall DJ, Richardson SN, et al: Hereditary persistence of fetal hemoglobin: A study of 79 affected persons in 15 Negro families in Baltimore. *Blood* 21:261, 1963.

93. Kraus LM, Miyaji T, Iuchi I, Kraus AP: Characterization of alpha23GluNH2 in hemoglobin Memphis. Hemoglobin Memphis/S, a new variant of molecular disease. *Biochemistry* 5:3701, 1966.

94. Chang YC, Smith KD, Moore RD, et al: An analysis of fetal hemoglobin variation in sickle cell disease: The relative contributions of the X-linked factor, β-globin haplotypes, α-globin gene number, gender, and age. *Blood* 85:1111, 1995.

95. Wyszynski DF, Baldwin CT, Cleves MA, et al: Polymorphisms near a chromosome 6Q QTL area are associated with modulation of fetal hemoglobin levels in sickle cell anemia. *Cell Mol Biol* 50:23, 2004.

96. Lewis RA, Hathorn M: Correlation of S hemoglobin with glucose-6-phosphate dehydrogenase deficiency and its significance. *Blood* 26:176, 1965.

97. Piomelli S, Reindorf CA, Arzanian MT, Corash LM: Clinical and biochemical interactions of glucose-6-phosphate dehydrogenase deficiency and sickle-cell anemia. *N Engl J Med* 287:213, 1972.

98. El-Hazmi MAF, Warsy AS: Aspects of sickle cell gene in Saudi Arabia: Interaction with glucose-6-phosphate dehydrogenase deficiency. *Hum Genet* 68:320, 1984.

99. El-Hazmi MAF, Warsy AS: The effects of glucose-6-phosphate dehydrogenase deficiency on the haematological parameters and clinical manifestations in patients with sickle cell anaemia. *Trop Geogr Med* 41:52, 1989.

100. Nagel RL, Steinberg MH: Role of epistatic (modifier) genes in the modulation of the phenotypic diversity of sickle cell anemia. *Pediatr Pathol Mol Med* 20:123, 2001.

101. Naylor J, Rosenthal I, Grossman A, et al: Activity of glucose-6-phosphate dehydrogenase in erythrocytes of patients with various abnormal hemoglobins. *Pediatrics* 26:285, 1960.

102. Milner PF, Sergeant GR: Laboratory studies in sickle cell anaemia. *Blood* 34:729, 1969.

103. Lewis RA: Glucose-6-phosphate dehydrogenase electrophoresis in Ghanaians with AA and SS haemoglobin. *Acta Haematol (Basel)* 50:105, 1973.

104. Beutler E, Johnson C, Powars D, West C: Prevalence of glucose-6-phosphate dehydrogenase deficiency in sickle cell disease. *N Engl J Med* 290:826, 1974.

105. Gibbs WN, Wardle J, Serjeant GR: Glucose-6-phosphate dehydrogenase deficiency and homozygous sickle cell disease in Jamaica. *Br J Haematol* 45:73, 1980.

106. Steinberg MH, West MS, Gallagher D, et al: Effects of glucose-6-phosphate dehydrogenase deficiency upon sickle cell anemia. *Blood* 71:748, 1988.

107. Saad STO, Costa FF: Glucose-6-phosphate dehydrogenase deficiency and sickle cell disease in Brazil. *Hum Hered* 42:125, 1992.

108. Smits HL, Oski FA, Brody JI: The hemolytic crisis of sickle cell disease: The role of glucose-6-phosphate dehydrogenase deficiency. *J Pediatr* 74:544, 1969.

109. Harris JW, Brewster HH, Ham TH, Castle WB: Studies on the destruction of red blood cells: X. The biophysics and biology of sickle-cell disease. *Arch Intern Med* 97:145, 1956.

110. Lane PA, Githens JH: Splenic syndrome at mountain altitudes in sickle cell trait. *JAMA* 253:2251, 1985.

111. Green RL, Huntsman RG, Serjeant GR: The sickle-cell and altitude. *BMJ* 2:593, 1971.

112. Charache S, Conley CL: Rate of sickling of red cells during deoxygenation of blood from persons with various sickling disorders. *Blood* 24:25, 1964.

113. Charache S, Conley CL: Factors leading to vascular occlusion in sickle cell anemia. *Prog Clin Biol Res* 1:343, 1975.

114. Serjeant GR, May H, Patrick A, Slifer ED: Duodenal ulceration in sickle cell anaemia. *Trans R Soc Trop Med Hyg* 67:59, 1973.

115. Bates I, De Caestecker J: Sickle cell disease and risk of peptic ulceration. *Trans R Soc Trop Med Hyg* 90:292, 1996.

116. Woods KF, Onuoha A, Schade RR, Kutlar A: Helicobacter pylori infection in sickle cell disease. *J Natl Med Assoc* 92:361, 2000.

117. Smith WR, Coyne P, Smith VS, Mercier B: Temperature changes, temperature extremes, and their relationship to emergency department visits and hospitalizations for sickle cell crisis. *Pain Manag Nurs* 4:106, 2003.

118. Beutler E: Hypothesis: Changes in the O_2 dissociation curve and sickling: A general formulation and therapeutic strategy. *Blood* 43:297, 1974.

119. Poillon WN, Kim BC: 2,3-Diphosphoglycerate and intracellular pH as interdependent determinants of the physiologic solubility of deoxyhemoglobin S. *Blood* 76:1028, 1990.

120. Noguchi CT, Schechter AN: The intracellular polymerization of sickle hemoglobin and its relevance to sickle cell disease. *Blood* 58:1057, 1981.

121. Akinla O: Pregnancy and the skeletal complications of sickle cell disease. *Postgrad Med J* 49:255, 1973.

122. Perillie PE, Epstein FH: Sickling phenomenon produced by hypertonic solutions: A possible explanation for the hyposthenuria in sicklemia. *J Clin Invest* 42:570, 1963.

123. Briehl RW, Nikolopoulou P: Kinetics of hemoglobin S polymerization and gelation under shear: I. Shape of the viscosity progress curve and dependence of delay time and reaction rate on shear rate and temperature. *Blood* 81:2420, 1993.

124. Hebbel RP: Endothelial adhesivity of sickle red blood cells. *J Lab Clin Med* 120:503, 1992.

125. Parise LV, Telen MJ: Erythrocyte adhesion in sickle cell disease. *Curr Hematol Rep* 2:102, 2003.

126. Thevenin BM, Crandall I, Ballas SK, et al: Band 3 peptides block the adherence of sickle cells to endothelial cells in vitro. *Blood* 90:4172, 1997.

127. Morris CL, Rucknagel DL, Joiner CH: Deoxygenation-induced changes in sickle cell-sickle cell adhesion. *Blood* 81:3138, 1993.

128. Fadlon E, Vordermeier S, Pearson TC, et al: Blood polymorphonuclear leukocytes from the majority of sickle cell patients in the crisis phase of the disease show enhanced adhesion to vascular endothelium and increased expression of CD64. *Blood* 91:266, 1998.

129. Ballas SK, Mohandas N: Pathophysiology of vaso-occlusion. *Hematol Oncol Clin North Am* 10:1221, 1996.

130. Kaul DK, Fabry ME, Nagel RL: The pathophysiology of vascular obstruction in the sickle syndromes. *Blood Rev* 10:29, 1996.

131. Styles LA, Lubin B, Vichinsky E, et al: Decrease of very late activation antigen-4 and CD36 on reticulocytes in sickle cell patients treated with hydroxyurea. *Blood* 89:2554, 1997.

132. Charache S, Barton FB, Moore RD, et al: Hydroxyurea and sickle cell anemia: Clinical utility of a myelosuppressive "switching" agent. *Medicine* 75:300, 1996.

133. Wong WY: Prevention and management of infection in children with sickle cell anaemia. *Paediatr Drugs* 3:793, 2001.

134. Goldstein MA, Patpongpanij N, Minnich V: The incidence of elevated hemoglobin A_2 levels in the American negro. *Ann Intern Med* 60:95, 1964.

135. Taylor WJ: Sickled red cells in the Cervidae. *Adv Vet Sci Comp Med* 27:77, 1983.

136. Castro O, Roth R, Orlin J, Finch SC: Human sickle cells in a heterologous species: A model for the screening of anti-sickling agents. *Prog Clin Biol Res* 1:455, 1975.

137. Nagel RL, Fabry ME: The panoply of animal models for sickle cell anaemia. *Br J Haematol* 112:19, 2001.

138. Powars DR: Natural history of sickle cell disease: The first ten years. *Semin Hematol* 12:267, 1975.

139. Serjeant GR, Ceulaer CDE, Lethbridge R, et al: The painful crisis of homozygous sickle cell disease: Clinical features. *Br J Haematol* 87:586, 1994.

140. Antal P, Gauderer M, Koshy M, Berman B: Is the incidence of appendicitis reduced in patients with sickle cell disease? *Pediatrics* 101:e7, 1998.

141. Charache S: The treatment of sickle cell anemia. *Arch Intern Med* 133: 698, 1974.

142. Mani S, Duffy TP: Sickle myonecrosis revisited. *Am J Med* 95:525, 1993.

143. Smith-Whitley K, Zhao H, Hodinka RL, et al: Epidemiology of human parvovirus B19 in children with sickle cell disease. *Blood* 103:422, 2004.

144. Godeau B, Galactéros F, Schaeffer A, et al: Aplastic crisis due to extensive bone marrow necrosis and human parvovirus infection in sickle cell disease. *Am J Med* 91:557, 1991.

145. Kinney TR, Ware RE, Schultz WH, Filston HC: Long-term management of splenic sequestration in children with sickle cell disease. *J Pediatr* 117:194, 1990.

146. Solanki DL, Kletter GG, Castro O: Acute splenic sequestration crises in adults with sickle cell disease. *Am J Med* 80:985, 1986.

147. Bowcock SJ, Nwabueze ED, Cook AE, et al: Fatal splenic sequestration in adult sickle cell disease. *Clin Lab Haematol* 10:95, 1988.

148. Koduri PR, Agbemadzo B, Nathan S: Hemoglobin S-C disease revisited: Clinical study of 106 adults. *Am J Hematol* 68:298, 2001.

149. Vichinsky E, Lubin BH: Suggested guidelines for the treatment of children with sickle cell anemia. *Hematol Oncol Clin North Am* 1:483, 1987.

150. Diggs LW: Crises in sickle cell anemia. *Am J Clin Pathol* 26:1109, 1956.

151. Whitten CF: Growth status of children with sickle-cell anemia. *Am J Dis Child* 102:355, 1961.

152. Ashcroft MT, Serjeant GR, Desai P: Heights, weights, and skeletal age of Jamaican adolescents with sickle cell anaemia. *Arch Dis Child* 47: 519, 1972.

153. Patey RA, Sylvester KP, Rafferty GF, et al: The importance of using ethnically appropriate reference ranges for growth assessment in sickle cell disease. *Arch Dis Child* 87:352, 2002.

154. Moseley JE: The Anemias, in *Bone Changes in Hematologic Disorders (Roentgen Aspects)*, p 12. Grune & Stratton, New York, 1963.

155. Nelson DA, Rizvi S, Bhattacharyya T, et al: Trabecular and integral bone density in adults with sickle cell disease. *J Clin Densitom* 6:125, 2003.

156. Sain A, Sham R, Silver L: Bone scan in sickle cell crisis. *Clin Nucl Med* 3:85, 1978.

157. Rao VM, Fishman M, Mitchell DG, et al: Painful sickle cell crisis: Bone marrow patterns observed with MR imaging. *Radiology* 161:211, 1986.

158. Mankad VN, Williams JP, Harpen MD, et al: Magnetic resonance imaging of bone marrow in sickle cell disease: Clinical, hematologic, and pathologic correlations. *Blood* 75:274, 1990.

159. Howlett DC, Hatrick AG, Jarosz JM, et al: The role of CT and MR in imaging the complications of sickle cell disease. *Clin Radiol* 52:821, 1997.

160. Stevens MCG, Padwick M, Serjeant GR: Observations on the natural history of dactylitis in homozygous sickle cell disease. *Clin Pediatr* 20: 311, 1981.

161. Milner PF, Kraus AP, Sebes JI, et al: Osteonecrosis of the humeral head in sickle cell disease. *Clin Orthop* 289:136, 1993.

162. David HG, Bridgman SA, Davies SC, et al: The shoulder in sickle-cell disease. *J Bone Joint Surg Br* 75B:538, 1993.

163. Schumacher HR Jr, Van Linthoudt D, Manno CS, et al: Diffuse chondrolytic arthritis in sickle cell disease. *J Rheumatol* 20:385, 1993.

164. Epps CH Jr, Bryant DD III, Coles MJM, Castro O: Osteomyelitis in patients who have sickle-cell disease. Diagnosis and management. *J Bone Joint Surg Am* 73A:1281, 1991.

165. Hook EW, Campbell CG, Weens HS, Cooper GR: Salmonella osteomyelitis in patients with sickle-cell anemia. *N Engl J Med* 257:403, 1957.

166. Shelley WM, Curtis EM: Bone marrow and fat embolism in sickle-cell anemia and sickle-cell hemoglobin C disease. *Johns Hopkins Med J* 103: 8, 1958.

167. Kontessis P, Mayopoulou-Symvoulidis D, Symvoulidis A, Kontopoulou-Griva I: Renal involvement in sickle cell-beta thalassemia. *Nephron* 61:10, 1992.

168. Zadeii G, Lohr JW: Renal papillary necrosis in a patient with sickle cell trait. *J Am Soc Nephrol* 8:1034, 1997.

169. Minkin SD, Oh KS, Sanders RC, Siegelman SS: Urologic manifestations of sickle hemoglobinopathies. *South Med J* 72:23, 1979.

170. Wong WY, Elliott-Mills D, Powars D: Renal failure in sickle cell anemia. *Hematol Oncol Clin North Am* 10:1321, 1996.

171. Baron BW, Mick R, Baron JM: Hematuria in sickle cell anemia—Not always benign: Evidence for excess frequency of sickle cell anemia in African-Americans with renal cell carcinoma. *Acta Haematol (Basel)* 92:119, 1994.

172. Sharpsteen JR Jr, Powars D, Johnson C, et al: Multisystem damage associated with tricorporal priapism in sickle cell disease. *Am J Med* 94: 289, 1993.

173. Chakrabarty A, Upadhyay J, Dhabuwala CB, et al: Priapism associated with sickle cell hemoglobinopathy in children: Long-term effects on potency. *J Urol* 155:1419, 1996.

174. Miller ST, Rao SP, Dunn EK, Glassberg KI: Priapism in children with sickle cell disease. *J Urol* 154:844, 1995.

175. Adeyoju AB, Olujohungbe AB, Morris J, et al: Priapism in sickle-cell disease: Incidence, risk factors and complications—An international multicentre study. *BJU Int* 90:898, 2002.

176. Prasad AS, Ortega J, Brewer GJ, et al: Trace elements in sickle cell disease. *JAMA* 22:2396, 1976.

177. Abbasi AA, Prasad AS, Ortega J, et al: Gonadal function abnormalities in sickle cell anemia. Studies in adult male patients. *Ann Intern Med* 85: 601, 1976.

178. Pearson HA, McIntosh S, Ritchey AK, et al: Developmental aspects of splenic function in sickle cell diseases. *Blood* 53:358, 1979.

179. Gill FM, Sleeper LA, Weiner SJ, et al: Clinical events in the first decade in a cohort of infants with sickle cell disease. *Blood* 86:776, 1995.

180. Cavenagh JD, Joseph AE, Dilly S, Bevan DH: Splenic sepsis in sickle cell disease. *Br J Haematol* 86:187, 1994.

181. Al-Salem AH, Qaisaruddin S, Al Jam'a A, et al: Splenic abscess and sickle cell disease. *Am J Hematol* 58:100, 1998.

182. Adekile AD, McKie KM, Adeodu OO, et al: Spleen in sickle cell anemia: Comparative studies of Nigerian and U.S. patients. *Am J Hematol* 42:316, 1993.

183. Krauss JS, Freant LJ, Lee JR: Gastrointestinal pathology in sickle cell disease. *Ann Clin Lab Sci* 28:19, 1998.

184. Green TW, Conley CL, Berthrong M: The liver in sickle cell anemia. *Johns Hopkins Med J* 92:99, 1953.

185. Sheehy TW, Law DE, Wade BH: Exchange transfusion for sickle cell intrahepatic cholestasis. *Arch Intern Med* 140:1364, 1980.

186. Schubert TT: Hepatobiliary system in sickle cell disease. *Gastroenterology* 90:2013, 1986.

187. Mintz AA, Pugh DP: Choledocholithiasis in sickle cell anemia. *South Med J* 63:1498, 1970.

188. Johnson CS, Omata M, Tong MJ, et al: Liver involvement in sickle cell disease. *Medicine* 64:349, 1985.

189. Omata M, Johnson CS, Tong M, Tatter D: Pathological spectrum of liver diseases in sickle cell disease. *Dig Dis Sci* 31:247, 1986.

190. Bauer TW, Moore GW, Hutchins GM: The liver in sickle cell disease. A clinicopathologic study of 70 patients. *Am J Med* 69:833, 1980.

191. Laulan S, Bernard JF, Boivin P: Systematic blood transfusions in adult homozygous sickle-cell anaemia. *Presse Med* 19:785, 1990.

192. Miller ST, Jensen D, Rao SP: Less intensive long-term transfusion therapy for sickle cell anemia and cerebrovascular accident. *J Pediatr* 120: 54, 1992.

193. Conrad ME: Sickle cell disease and hemochromatosis. *Am J Hematol* 38:150, 1991.

194. Jeng MR, Adams-Graves P, Howard TA, et al: Identification of hemochromatosis gene polymorphisms in chronically transfused patients with sickle cell disease. *Am J Hematol* 74:243, 2003.

195. Heeney MM, Howard TA, Zimmerman SA, Ware RE: UGT1A promoter polymorphisms influence bilirubin response to hydroxyurea therapy in sickle cell anemia. *J Lab Clin Med* 141:279, 2003.

196. Passon RG, Howard TA, Zimmerman SA, et al: Influence of bilirubin uridine diphosphate-glucuronosyltransferase 1A promoter polymorphisms on serum bilirubin levels and cholelithiasis in children with sickle cell anemia. *J Pediatr Hematol Oncol* 23:448, 2001.

197. Miller GJ, Sergeant GR, Sivapragasam S, Petch M: Cardiopulmonary responses and gas exchange during exercise in adults with homozygous sickle cell disease. *Clin Sci* 44:113, 1973.

198. Pegelow CH, Colangelo L, Steinberg M, et al: Natural history of blood pressure in sickle cell disease: Risks for stroke and death associated with relative hypertension in sickle cell anemia. *Am J Med* 102:171, 1997.

199. Vichinsky EP, Styles LA, Colangelo LH, et al: Acute chest syndrome in sickle cell disease: Clinical presentation and course. *Blood* 89:1787, 1997.

200. Bhalla M, Abboud MR, McLoud TC, et al: Acute chest syndrome in sickle cell disease: CT evidence of microvascular occlusion. *Radiology* 187:45, 1993.

201. Gelfand MJ, Daya SA, Rucknagel DL, et al: Simultaneous occurrence of rib infarction and pulmonary infiltrates in sickle cell disease patients with acute chest syndrome. *J Nucl Med* 34:614, 1993.

202. Golden C, Styles L, Vichinsky E: Acute chest syndrome and sickle cell disease. *Curr Opin Hematol* 5:89, 1998.

203. Powars D, Weidman JA, Odom-Maryon T, et al: Sickle cell chronic lung disease: Prior morbidity and the risk of pulmonary failure. *Medicine* 67:66, 1988.

204. Gladwin MT, Sachdev V, Jison ML, et al: Pulmonary hypertension as a risk factor for death in patients with sickle cell disease. *N Engl J Med* 350:886, 2004.

205. Vichinsky EP: Pulmonary hypertension in sickle cell disease. *N Engl J Med* 350:857, 2004.

206. Castro O: Systemic fat embolism and pulmonary hypertension in sickle cell disease. *Hematol Oncol Clin North Am* 10:1289, 1996.

207. Denbow CE, Chung EE, Serjeant GR: Pulmonary artery pressure and the acute chest syndrome in homozygous sickle cell disease. *Br Heart J* 69:536, 1993.

208. To KW, Nadel AJ: Ophthalmologic complications in hemoglobinopathies. *Hematol Oncol Clin North Am* 5:535, 1991.

209. Curran EL, Fleming JC, Rice K, Wang WC: Orbital compression syndrome in sickle cell disease. *Ophthalmology* 104:1610, 1997.

210. Hasan S, Elbedawi M, Castro O, et al: Central retinal vein occlusion in sickle cell disease. *South Med J* 97:202, 2004.

211. Stockman JA, Nigro MA, Mishkin MM, Oski FA: Occlusion of large cerebral vessels in sickle-cell anemia. *N Engl J Med* 287:846, 1972.

212. Russell MO, Goldberg HI, Hodson A, et al: Effect of transfusion therapy on arteriographic abnormalities and on recurrence of stroke in sickle cell disease. *Blood* 63:162, 1984.

213. Steen RG, Xiong XP, Langston JW, Helton KJ: Brain injury in children with sickle cell disease: Prevalence and etiology. *Ann Neurol* 54:564, 2003.

214. Steen RG, Emudiabughe T, Hankins GM, et al: Brain imaging findings in pediatric patients with sickle cell disease. *Radiology* 228:216, 2003.

215. Ohene-Frempong K, Weiner SJ, Sleeper LA, et al: Cerebrovascular accidents in sickle cell disease: Rates and risk factors. *Blood* 91:288, 1998.

216. Powars D, Wilson B, Imbus C, et al: The natural history of stroke in sickle cell disease. *Am J Med* 65:461, 1978.

217. Ohene-Frempong K: Stroke in sickle cell disease: Demographic, clinical, and therapeutic considerations. *Semin Hematol* 28:213, 1991.

218. Driscoll MC, Hurlet A, Styles L, et al: Stroke risk in siblings with sickle cell anemia. *Blood* 101:2401, 2003.

219. Riggs JE, Ketonen LM, Wang DD, Valanne LK: Cerebral infarction in a child with sickle cell trait. *J Child Neurol* 10:253, 1995.

220. Partington MD, Aronyk KE, Byrd SE: Sickle cell trait and stroke in children. *Pediatr Neurosurg* 20:148, 1994.

221. Adams RJ, McKie VC, Carl EM, et al: Long-term stroke risk in children with sickle cell disease screened with transcranial Doppler. *Ann Neurol* 42:699, 1997.

222. Balkaran B, Char G, Morris JS, et al: Stroke in a cohort of patients with homozygous sickle cell disease. *J Pediatr* 120:360, 1992.

223. Siegel JF, Rich MA, Brock WA: Association of sickle cell disease, priapism, exchange transfusion and neurological events: Aspen syndrome. *J Urol* 150:1480, 1993.

224. Miller ST, Macklin EA, Pegelow CH, et al: Silent infarction as a risk factor for overt stroke in children with sickle cell anemia: A report from the Cooperative Study of Sickle Cell Disease. *J Pediatr* 139:385, 2001.

225. Houston PE, Rana S, Sekhsaria S, et al: Homocysteine in sickle cell disease: Relationship to stroke. *Am J Med* 103:192, 1997.

226. Styles LA, Hoppe C, Klitz W, et al: Evidence for HLA-related susceptibility for stroke in children with sickle cell disease. *Blood* 95:3562, 2000.

227. Hoppe C, Klitz W, Cheng S, et al: Gene interactions and stroke risk in children with sickle cell anemia. *Blood* 103:2391, 2004.

228. Adams RJ, McKie VC, Brambilla D, et al: Stroke prevention trial in sickle cell anemia. *Controlled Clin Trials* 19:110, 1998.

229. Baird RL: Studies in sickle cell anemia: XXI. Clinicopathological aspects of neurological manifestations. *Pediatrics* 34:92, 1964.

230. Diggs LW, Brookoff D: Multiple cerebral aneurysms in patients with sickle cell disease. *South Med J* 86:377, 1993.

231. Koshy M, Entsuah R, Koranda A, et al: Leg ulcers in patients with sickle cell disease. *Blood* 74:1403, 1989.

232. Morgan AG: Sickle cell leg ulcers. *Int J Dermatol* 24:643, 1985.

233. Barrett-Conner E: Bacterial infection and sickle cell anemia. *Medicine* 50:97, 1971.

234. Boghossian SH, Wright G, Webster AD, Segal AW: Investigations of host defense in patients with sickle cell disease. *Br J Haematol* 59:523, 1985.

235. Neumayr L, Lennette E, Kelly D, et al: Mycoplasma disease and acute chest syndrome in sickle cell disease. *Pediatrics* 112:87, 2003.

236. Klein P, McMeeking AA, Goldenberg A: Babesiosis in a patient with sickle cell anemia. *Am J Med* 102:416, 1997.

237. McCurdy PR: Abnormal hemoglobins and pregnancy. *Am J Obstet Gynecol* 90:891, 1964.

238. Serjeant GR: Sickle haemoglobin and pregnancy. *BMJ* 287:628, 1983.

239. Anderson M, Went LN, MacIver JE, Dixon HG: Sickle cell disease in pregnancy. *Lancet* 2:516, 1960.

240. Poddar D, Maude GH, Plant MJ, et al: Pregnancy in Jamaican women with homozygous sickle cell disease. Fetal and maternal outcome. *Br J Obstet Gynaecol* 93:727, 1986.

241. Powars DR, Sandhu M, Niland-Weiss J, et al: Pregnancy in sickle cell disease. *Obstet Gynecol* 67:217, 1986.

242. Anderson MF: The foetal risks in sickle cell anaemia. *West Indian Med J* 2:288, 1971.

243. Howard RJ, Tuck SM, Pearson TC: Pregnancy in sickle cell disease in the U.K.: Results of a multicentre survey of the effect of prophylactic blood transfusion on maternal and fetal outcome. *Br J Obstet Gynaecol* 102:947, 1995.

244. Koshy M: Sickle cell disease and pregnancy. *Blood Rev* 9:157, 1995.

245. Smith JA, Espeland M, Bellevue R, et al: Pregnancy in sickle cell disease: Experience of the cooperative study of sickle cell disease. *Obstet Gynecol* 87:199, 1996.

246. Sun PM, Wilburn W, Raynor BD, Jamieson D: Sickle cell disease in pregnancy: Twenty years of experience at Grady Memorial Hospital, Atlanta, Georgia. *Am J Obstet Gynecol* 184:1127, 2001.

247. Dare FO, Makinde OO, Faasuba OB: The obstetric performance of sickle cell disease patients and homozygous hemoglobin C disease patients in Ile-Ife, Nigeria. *Int J Gynaecol Obstet* 37:163, 1992.

248. Idrisa A, Omigbodun AO, Adeleye JA: Pregnancy in hemoglobin sickle cell patients at the University College Hospital, Ibadan. *Int J Gynaecol Obstet* 38:83, 1992.

249. El-Shafei AM, Dhaliwal JK, Sandhu AK: Pregnancy in sickle cell disease in Bahrain. *Br J Obstet Gynaecol* 99:101, 1992.

250. Odum CU, Anorlu RI, Dim SI, Oyekan TO: Pregnancy outcome in HbSS-sickle cell disease in Lagos, Nigeria. *West Afr J Med* 21:19, 2002.

251. Glader BE, Propper RD, Buchanan GR: Microcytosis associated with sickle cell anemia. *Am J Clin Pathol* 72:63, 1979.

252. Mohandas N, Johnson A, Wyatt J, et al: Automated quantitation of cell density distribution and hyperdense cell fraction in RBC disorders. *Blood* 74:442, 1989.

253. Sherwood JB, Goldwasser E, Chilcote R, et al: Sickle cell anemia patients have low erythropoietin levels for their degree of anemia. *Blood* 67:46, 1986.

254. Erslev AJ, Wilson J, Caro J: Erythropoietin titers in anemic, nonuremic patients. *J Lab Clin Med* 109:429, 1987.

255. Bensinger TA, Mahmood L, Conrad ME, McCurdy PR: The effect of oral urea administration on red cell survival in sickle cell disease. *Am J Med Sci* 264:283, 1972.

256. Boggs DR, Hyde F, Srodes C: An unusual pattern of neutrophil kinetics in sickle cell anemia. *Blood* 41:59, 1973.

257. Buchanan GR, Glader BE: Leukocyte counts in children with sickle cell disease. Comparative values in the steady state, vaso-occlusive crisis, and bacterial infection. *Am J Dis Child* 132:396, 1978.

258. Corvelli AI, Binder RA, Kales A: Disseminated intravascular coagulation in sickle cell crisis. *South Med J* 72:23, 1979.

259. Ballas SK, Burka ER, Lewis CN, Krasnow SH: Serum immunoglobulin levels in patients having sickle cell syndromes. *Am J Clin Pathol* 73:394, 1980.

260. Glassman AB, Deas DV, Berlinsky FS, Bennett CE: Lymphocyte blast transformation and peripheral lymphocyte percentages in patients with sickle cell disease. *Ann Clin Lab Sci* 10:9, 1980.

261. Corry JM, Polhill RB Jr, Edmonds SR, Johnston RB Jr: Activity of the alternative complement pathway after splenectomy: Comparison to activity in sickle cell disease and hypogammaglobulinemia. *J Pediatr* 95:964, 1979.

262. Natta C, Machlin L: Plasma levels of tocopherol in sickle cell anemia subjects. *Am J Clin Nutr* 32:1359, 1979.

263. Karayalcin G, Lanzkowsky P, Kazi AB: Zinc deficiency in children with sickle cell disease. *Am J Pediatr Hematol Oncol* 1:283, 1979.

264. Niell HB, Leach BE, Kraus AP: Zinc metabolism in sickle cell anemia. *JAMA* 242:2686, 1979.

265. O'Brien RT: Iron burden in sickle cell anemia. *J Pediatr* 92:579, 1978.

266. Haddy TB, Castro O: Overt iron deficiency in sickle cell disease. *Arch Intern Med* 142:1621, 1982.

267. Davies S, Henthorn J, Brozovic M: Iron deficiency in sickle cell anaemia. *J Clin Pathol* 36:1012, 1983.

268. Reid CD, Charache S, Lubin B, Johnson C, Ohene-Frempong K: *Management and Therapy of Sickle Cell Disease*, p 96. National Institutes of Health, Heart Lung and Blood Institute, Bethesda, 1995.

269. International Committee for Standardization in Haematology: Simple electrophoretic system for presumptive identification of abnormal hemoglobins. *Blood* 52:1058, 1978.

270. Daland GA, Castle WB: A simple and rapid method for demonstrating sickling of the red blood cells: The use of reducing agents. *J Lab Clin Med* 33:1082, 1948.

271. Henry RL, Nalbandian RM, Nichols BM, et al: Modified Sickledex tube test: A specific test for S hemoglobin. *Clin Biochem* 4:196, 1971.

272. Mario N, Baudin B, Aussel C, Giboudeau J: Capillary isoelectric focusing and high-performance cation-exchange chromatography compared for qualitative and quantitative analysis of hemoglobin variants. *Clin Chem* 43:2137, 1997.

273. Steinberg MH: DNA diagnosis for the detection of sickle hemoglobinopathies. *Am J Hematol* 43:110, 1993.

274. Van Baelen H, Vandepitte J, Eeckels R: Observations on sickle cell anaemia and haemoglobin Bart's in Congolese neonates. *Ann Soc Belg Med Trop* 49:157, 1969.

275. Consensus conference. Newborn screening for sickle cell disease and other hemoglobinopathies. *JAMA* 258:1205, 1987.

276. Old JM, Fitches A, Heath C, et al: First-trimester fetal diagnosis for haemoglobinopathies: Report on 200 cases. *Lancet* 2:763, 1986.

277. Conner BJ, Reyes AA, Morin C, et al: Detection of sickle cell β^S-globin allele by hybridization with synthetic oligonucleotides. *Proc Natl Acad Sci U S A* 80:278, 1983.

278. Davies SC, Oni L: Fortnightly review: Management of patients with sickle cell disease. *BMJ* 315:656, 1997.

279. Steinberg MH: Review: Sickle cell disease: Present and future treatment. *Am J Med Sci* 312:166, 1996.

280. Carmel R: Folate supplementation in sickle cell anemia: Reply. *N Engl J Med* 349:813, 2003.

281. Wayne AS, Kevy SV, Nathan DG: Transfusion management of sickle cell disease. *Blood* 81:1109, 1993.

282. Rosse WF, Gallagher D, Kinney TR, et al: Transfusion and alloimmunization in sickle cell disease. *Blood* 76:1431, 1990.

283. Silliman CC, Peterson VM, Mellman DL, et al: Iron chelation by deferoxamine in sickle cell patients with severe transfusion-induced hemosiderosis: A randomized, double-blind study of the dose-response relationship. *J Lab Clin Med* 122:48, 1993.

284. Reed W, Vichinsky EP: New considerations in the treatment of sickle cell disease. *Annu Rev Med* 49:461, 1998.

285. Vichinsky EP, Haberkern CM, Neumayr L, et al: A comparison of conservative and aggressive transfusion regimens in the perioperative management of sickle cell disease. The Preoperative Transfusion in Sickle Cell Disease Study Group. *N Engl J Med* 333:206, 1995.

286. Rackoff WR, Ohene-Frempong K, Month S, et al: Neurologic events after partial exchange transfusion for priapism in sickle cell disease. *J Pediatr* 120:882, 1992.

287. Johnson FL, Look AT, Gockerman J, et al: Bone-marrow transplantation in a patient with sickle-cell anemia. *N Engl J Med* 311:780, 1984.

288. Vermylen C: Hematopoietic stem cell transplantation in sickle cell disease. *Blood Rev* 17:163, 2003.

289. Beutler E: Bone marrow transplantation for sickle cell anemia: Summarizing comments. *Semin Hematol* 28:263, 1991.

290. Davies SC: Bone marrow transplant for sickle cell disease—The dilemma. *Blood Rev* 7:4, 1993.

291. Platt OS, Guinan EC: Bone marrow transplantation in sickle cell anemia—The dilemma of choice. *N Engl J Med* 335:426, 1996.

292. Sirs JA: The use of carbon monoxide to prevent sickle-cell formation. *Lancet* 1:971, 1963.

293. Puruggganan HB, McElfresh AE: Failure of carbonmonoxy sickle-cell haemoglobin to alter the sickle state. *Lancet* 1:79, 1964.

294. Beutler E: The effect of carbon monoxide on red cell life span in sickle cell disease. *Blood* 46:253, 1975.

295. Beutler E: The effect of methemoglobin formation in sickle cell disease. *J Clin Invest* 40:1856, 1961.

296. Paniker NV, Ben-Bassat I, Beutler E: Evaluation of sickle hemoglobin and desickling agents by falling ball viscometry. *J Lab Clin Med* 80:282, 1972.

297. Shamsuddin M, Mason RG, Ritchey JM, et al: Sites of acetylation of sickle cell hemoglobin by aspirin. *Proc Natl Acad Sci U S A* 71:4693, 1974.

298. Ueno H, Yatco E, Benjamin LJ, Manning JM: Effects of methyl acetyl phosphate, a covalent antisickling agent, on the density profiles of sickle erythrocytes. *J Lab Clin Med* 120:152, 1992.

299. Zaugg RH, King LC, Klotz IM: Acylation of hemoglobin by succinyldisalicylate, a potential crosslinking reagent. *Biochem Biophys Res Commun* 64:1192, 1975.

300. Isaacs WA, Hayhoe FGJ: Steroid hormones in sickle cell disease. *Nature* 215:1139, 1967.

301. Waterman MR, Yamaoka K, Chuang AH, Cottam GL: Anti-sickling nature of dimethyl adipimidate. *Biochem Biophys Res Commun* 63:580, 1975.

302. Hilkowitz G: Sickle cell disease: New method for treatment: Preliminary report. *BMJ* 2:266, 1957.

303. Knochel JP: Hematuria in sickle cell trait. *Arch Intern Med* 123:160, 1969.

304. Niihara Y, Zerez CR, Akiyama DS, Tanaka KR: Oral L-glutamine therapy for sickle cell anemia: I. Subjective clinical improvement and favorable change in red cell NAD redox potential. *Am J Hematol* 58:117, 1998.

305. Nalbandian RM, Shultz G, Lusher JM, et al: Sickle cell crisis terminated by intravenous urea in sugar solutions—a preliminary report. *Am J Med Sci* 261:309, 1971.

306. Gillette PN, Manning JM, Cerami A: Increased survival of sickle cell erythrocytes after treatment in vitro with sodium cyanate. *Proc Natl Acad Sci U S A* 68:2791, 1971.

307. Parameswaran KN, Shi GY, Klotz IM: O-carbamoylsalicylates: Agents for modification of hemoglobins. *J Med Chem* 30:936, 1987.

308. Ueno H, Benjamin LJ, Manning JM: Effects of methyl acetyl phosphate on hemoglobin S: A novel acetylating agent directed towards the DPG binding site. *Prog Clin Biol Res* 240:105, 1987.

309. Franklin IM, Cotter RI, Cheetham RC, et al: A potent new dipeptide inhibitor of cell sickling and haemoglobin S gelation. *Eur J Biochem* 136:209, 1983.

310. Baker R, Powars D, Haywood J: Restoration of the deformability of "irreversibly" sickled cells by procaine hydrochloride. *Biochem Biophys Res Commun* 59:548, 1974.

311. Brewer GJ, Brewer LF, Prasad AS: Suppression of irreversibly sickled erythrocytes by zinc therapy in sickle cell anemia. *J Lab Clin Med* 90:549, 1977.

312. Beutler E, Paniker NV, West CJ: Pyridoxine administration in sickle cell disease: An unsuccessful attempt to influence the properties of sickle hemoglobin. *Biochem Med* 6:139, 1972.

313. Kark JA, Tarassoff PG, Bongiovanni R: Pyridoxal phosphate as an antisickling agent in vitro. *J Clin Invest* 71:1224, 1983.

314. Kark JA, Kale MP, Tarassoff PG, et al: Inhibition of erythrocyte sickling in vitro by pyridoxal. *J Clin Invest* 62:888, 1978.

315. Benesch R, Benesch RE, Edalji R, Suzuki T: 5'-Deoxypyridoxal as a potential anti-sickling agent. *Proc Natl Acad Sci U S A* 74:1721, 1977.

316. Bounameaux Y: Action inhibitrice de la nivaquine et de divers antihistaminiques sur la formation d'hematies en faucilles dans l'anemie drepanocytaire. *C R Soc Biol (Paris)* 155:425, 1961.

317. Fung LWM, Ho C, Roth EF Jr, Nagel RL: The alkylation of hemoglobin S by nitrogen mustard: High resolution proton nuclear magnetic resonance studies. *J Biol Chem* 250:4786, 1975.

318. Nigen AM, Manning JM: Inhibition of erythrocyte sickling in vitro by DL-glyceraldehyde. *Proc Natl Acad Sci U S A* 74:367, 1977.

319. Ross PD, Subramanian S: Hexamethylenetetramine: A powerful and novel inhibitor of gelation of deoxyhemoglobin S. *Arch Biochem Biophys* 190:736, 1978.

320. Natta CL, Machlin LJ, Brin M: A decrease in irreversibly sickled erythrocytes in sickle cell anemia patients given vitamin E. *Am J Clin Nutr* 33:968, 1980.

321. Clarke DT, Jones GR, Martin MM: The anti-sickling drug lawsone (2-OH-1,4-naphthoquinone) protects sickled cells against membrane damage. *Biochem Biophys Res Commun* 139:780, 1986.

322. Stone PCW, Nash GB, Stuart J: Substituted benzaldehydes (12C79 and 589C80) that stabilize oxyhaemoglobin also protect sickle cells against calcium-mediated dehydration. *Br J Haematol* 81:419, 1992.

323. Reilly MP, Asakura T: Antisickling effect of bepridil. *Lancet* 1:848, 1986.

324. Asakura T, Ohnishi ST, Adachi K, et al: Effect of cetiedil on erythrocyte sickling: New type of antisickling agent that may affect erythrocyte membranes. *Proc Natl Acad Sci U S A* 77:2955, 1980.

325. Romero JR, Suzuka SM, Nagel RL, Fabry ME: Arginine supplementation of sickle transgenic mice reduces red cell density and Gardos channel activity. *Blood* 99:1103, 2002.

326. Iyamu EW, Turner EA, Asakura T: In vitro effects of NIPRISAN (Nix-0699): A naturally occurring, potent antisickling agent. *Br J Haematol* 118:337, 2002.

327. Charache S, De La Monte S, MacDonald V: Increased blood viscosity in a patient with sickle cell anemia. *Blood Cells* 8:103, 1982.

328. Greenberg MS, Kass EH: Studies on the destruction of red blood cells: XIII. Observations on the role of pH in the pathogenesis and treatment of painful crisis in sickle-cell disease. *Arch Intern Med* 101:355, 1958.

329. Rhodes RS, Revo L, Hara S, et al: Therapy for sickle cell vaso-occlusive crises. Controlled clinical trials and cooperative study of intravenously administered alkali. *JAMA* 228:1129, 1974.

330. Kilmartin JV, Rossi-Bernardi L: The binding of carbon dioxide by horse haemoglobin. *Biochem J* 124:31, 1971.

331. Peterson CM, Tsairis P, Ohnishi A, et al: Sodium cyanate induced polyneuropathy in patients with sickle-cell disease. *Ann Intern Med* 81:152, 1974.

332. Nicholson DH, Harkness DR, Benson WE, Peterson CM: Cyanate-induced cataracts in patients with sickle-cell hemoglobinopathies. *Arch Ophthalmol* 94:927, 1976.

333. Keidan AJ, White RD, Huehns ER, et al: Effect of BW12C on oxygen affinity of haemoglobin in sickle-cell disease. *Lancet* 1:831, 1986.

334. Rosa RM, Bierer BE, Thomas R, et al: A study of induced hyponatremia in the prevention and treatment of sickle-cell crisis. *N Engl J Med* 303:1138, 1980.

335. Baldree LA, Ault BH, Chesney CM, Stapleton FB: Intravenous desmopressin acetate in children with sickle trait and persistent macroscopic hematuria. *Pediatrics* 86:238, 1990.

336. Leary M, Abramson N: Induced hyponatremia for sickle-cell crisis. *N Engl J Med* 304:844, 1981.

337. Charache S, Walker WG: Failure of desmopressin to lower serum sodium or prevent crisis in patients with sickle cell anemia. *Blood* 58:892, 1981.

338. Brugnara C, De Franceschi L, Alper SL: Inhibition of Ca^{2+}-dependent K^+ transport and cell dehydration in sickle erythrocytes by clotrimazole and other imidazole derivatives. *J Clin Invest* 92:520, 1993.

339. De Franceschi L, Corrocher R: Established and experimental treatments for sickle cell disease. *Haematologica* 89:348, 2004.

340. DeSimone J, Heller P, Hall L, Zwiers D: 5-Azacytidine stimulates fetal hemoglobin synthesis in anemic baboons. *Proc Natl Acad Sci U S A* 79:4428, 1982.

341. Charache S, Dover G, Smith K, et al: Treatment of sickle cell anemia with 5-azacytidine results in increased fetal hemoglobin production and is associated with nonrandom hypomethylation of DNA around the gamma-delta-beta globin gene complex. *Proc Natl Acad Sci U S A* 80:4842, 1983.

342. Ley TJ, DeSimone J, Noguchi C, et al: 5-Azacytidine increases gamma-globin synthesis and reduces the proportion of dense cells in patients with sickle cell anemia. *Blood* 62:370, 1983.

343. Saunthararajah Y, Hillery CA, Lavelle D, et al: Effects of 5-aza-2'-deoxycytidine on fetal hemoglobin levels, red cell adhesion, and hematopoietic differentiation in patients with sickle cell disease. *Blood* 102:3865, 2003.

344. Veith R, Galanello R, Papayannopoulou T, Stamatoyannopoulos G: Stimulation of F-cell production in Hb S patients treated with Ara-C or hydroxyurea. *N Engl J Med* 313:1571, 1985.

345. Platt OS, Orkin SH, Dover G, et al: Hydroxyurea enhances fetal hemoglobin production in sickle cell anemia. *J Clin Invest* 74:652, 1984.

346. Dover GJ, Humphries RK, Moore JG, et al: Hydroxyurea induction of hemoglobin F production in sickle cell disease: Relationship between cytotoxicity and F-cell production. *Blood* 67:735, 1986.

347. Kaufman RE: Hydroxyurea: Specific therapy for sickle cell anemia. *Blood* 79:2503, 1992.

348. Charache S, Dover GJ, Moore RD, et al: Hydroxyurea: Effects on hemoglobin F production in patients with sickle cell anemia. *Blood* 79:2555, 1992.

349. Rodgers GP, Dover GJ, Uyesaka N, et al: Augmentation by erythropoietin of the fetal-hemoglobin response to hydroxyurea in sickle cell disease. *N Engl J Med* 328:73, 1993.

350. Nagel RL, Vichinsky E, Shah M, et al: F reticulocyte response in sickle cell anemia treated with recombinant human erythropoietin. A double-blind study. *Blood* 81:9, 1993.

351. Perrine SP, Faller DV, Swerdlow P, et al: Stopping the biologic clock for globin gene switching. *Ann N Y Acad Sci* 612:134, 1990.

352. Dover GJ, Brusilow S, Samid D: Increased fetal hemoglobin in patients receiving sodium 4-phenylbutyrate. *N Engl J Med* 327:569, 1992.

353. Perrine SP, Ginder GD, Faller DV, et al: A short-term trial of butyrate to stimulate fetal-globin-gene expression in the β-globin disorders. *N Engl J Med* 328:81, 1993.

354. Saleh AW Jr, Van Goethem A, Jansen R, et al: Isobutyramide therapy in patients with sickle cell anemia. *Am J Hematol* 49:244, 1995.

355. Miller BA, Olivieri N, Hope SM, et al: Interferon-gamma modulates fetal hemoglobin synthesis in sickle cell anemia and thalassemia. *J Interferon Res* 10:357, 1990.

356. Adams-Graves P, Kedar A, Koshy M, et al: RheothRx (poloxamer 188) injection for the acute painful episode of sickle cell disease: A pilot study. *Blood* 90:2041, 1997.

357. Davies SC, Gilmore A: The role of hydroxyurea in the management of sickle cell disease. *Blood Rev* 17:99, 2003.

358. Zimmerman SA, Schultz WH, Davis JS, et al: Sustained long-term hematologic efficacy of hydroxyurea at maximum tolerated dose in children with sickle cell disease. *Blood* 103:2039, 2004.

359. Olivieri NF, Vichinsky EP: Hydroxyurea in children with sickle cell disease: Impact on splenic function and compliance with therapy. *J Pediatr Hematol Oncol* 20:26, 1998.

360. Charache S, Terrin ML, Moore RD, et al: Effect of hydroxyurea on the frequency of painful crises in sickle cell anemia. Investigators of the Multicenter Study of Hydroxyurea in Sickle Cell Anemia. *N Engl J Med* 332:1317, 1995.

361. Byrd DC, Pitts SR, Alexander CK: Hydroxyurea in two pregnant women with sickle cell anemia. *Pharmacotherapy* 19:1459, 1999.

362. Charache S, Scott JC, Charache P: "Acute chest syndrome" in adults with sickle cell anemia. Microbiology, treatment, and prevention. *Arch Intern Med* 139:67, 1979.

363. Davies SC, Brozovic M: The presentation, management and prophylaxis of sickle cell disease. *Blood Rev* 3:29, 1989.

364. Lombardo T, Rosso R, La Ferla A, et al: Acute chest syndrome: The role of erythro-exchange in patients with sickle cell disease in Sicily. *Transfus Apheresis Sci* 29:39, 2003.

365. Manna SS, Shaw J, Tibby SM, Durward A: Treatment of plastic bronchitis in acute chest syndrome of sickle cell disease with intratracheal rhDNase. *Arch Dis Child* 88:626, 2003.

366. Ahonkhai VI, Landesman SH, Fikrig SM, et al: Failure of pneumococcal vaccine in children with sickle-cell disease. *N Engl J Med* 301:26, 1979.

367. Laszlo J, Obenour W, Saltzman HA: Effects of hyperbaric oxygenation on sickle syndromes. *South Med J* 62:453, 1969.

368. Reynolds JDH: Painful sickle cell crisis: Successful treatment with hyperbaric oxygen therapy. *JAMA* 216:1977, 1971.

369. Henderson AB: Sickle cell disease: Studies on "in vivo" sickling and the effect of certain pharmacological agents. *Am J Med Sci* 221:628, 1951.

370. Mann JR, Deeble TJ, Breeze GR, Stuart J: Ancrod in sickle cell crisis. *Lancet* 1:934, 1972.

371. Hugh-Jones K, Lehmann H, McAlister JM: Some experiences in managing sickle cell anaemia in children and young adults, using alkalis and magnesium. *BMJ* 2:226, 1964.

372. Barreras L, Diggs LW: Sodium citrate orally for painful sickle cell crises. *JAMA* 215:762, 1971.

373. Teuscher T, Weil von der Ahe C, Baillod P, Holzer B: Double-blind randomized clinical trial of pentoxiphyllin in vaso-occlusive sickle cell crisis. *Trop Geogr Med* 41:320, 1989.

374. Billett HH, Kaul DK, Connel MM, et al: Pentoxifylline (Trental) has no significant effect on laboratory parameters in sickle cell disease. *Nouv Rev Fr Hematol* 31:403, 1989.

375. Cooperative Urea Trials Group: Clinical trials of therapy for sickle cell vaso-occlusive crises. *JAMA* 228:1120, 1974.

376. Okpala I: The management of crisis in sickle cell disease. *Eur J Haematol* 60:1, 1998.

377. Rees DC, Olujohungbe AD, Parker NE, et al: Guidelines for the management of the acute painful crisis in sickle cell disease. *Br J Haematol* 120:744, 2003.

378. Cohen AR, Martin MB, Silber JH, et al: A modified transfusion program for prevention of stroke in sickle cell disease. *Blood* 79:1657, 1992.

379. Abboud MR, Cure J, Granger S, et al: Magnetic resonance angiography in children with sickle cell disease and abnormal transcranial Doppler ultrasonography enrolled in the "STOP" study. *Blood* 103:2822, 2004.

380. Adams RJ, Brambilla DJ, Granger S, et al: Stroke and conversion to high risk in children screened with transcranial Doppler ultrasound during the STOP Study. *Blood* 2004.

381. Solanki DL, McCurdy PR: Cholelithiasis in sickle cell anemia: A case for elective cholecystectomy. *Am J Med Sci* 277:319, 1979.

382. Seguier-Lipszyc E, De Lagausie P, Benkerrou M, et al: Elective laparoscopic cholecystectomy. *Surg Endosc* 15:301, 2001.

383. Bonatsos G, Birbas K, Toutouzas K, Durakis N: Laparoscopic cholecystectomy in adults with sickle cell disease. *Surg Endosc* 15:816, 2001.

384. Greenwald JG: Stroke, sickle cell trait and oral contraceptives. *Ann Intern Med* 72:960, 1970.

385. De Abood M, De Castillo Z, Guerrero F, et al: Effect of Depo-Provera(R) or Microgynon(R) on the painful crises of sickle cell anemia patients. *Contraception* 56:313, 1997.

386. Charache S, Scott J, Niebyl J, Bonds D: Management of sickle cell disease in pregnant patients. *Obstet Gynecol* 55:407, 1980.

387. Koshy M, Burd L: Management of pregnancy in sickle cell syndromes. *Hematol Oncol Clin North* Am 5:585, 1991.

388. Morrison JC, Schneider JM, Whybrew WD, et al: Prophylactic transfusions in pregnant patients with sickle hemoglobinopathies: Benefit versus risk. *Obstet Gynecol* 56:274, 1980.

389. Cunningham FG, Pritchard JA: Prophylactic transfusions of normal red blood cells during pregnancies complicated by sickle cell hemoglobinopathies. *Am J Obstet Gynecol* 135:994, 1979.

390. Cunningham FG, Pritchard JA, Mason R: Pregnancy and sickle cell hemoglobinopathies: Results with and without prophylactic transfusions. *Obstet Gynecol* 62:419, 1983.

391. Morrison JC, Morrison FS: Prophylactic transfusions in pregnant patients with sickle cell disease. N Engl J Med 320:1286, 1989.

392. Morrison JC, Foster H: Transfusion therapy in pregnant patients with sickle-cell disease: A National Institutes of Health consensus development conference. Ann Intern Med 91:122, 1979.

393. Koshy M, Burd L, Wallace D, et al: Prophylactic red-cell transfusions in pregnant patients with sickle cell disease: A randomized cooperative study. N Engl J Med 319:1447, 1988.

394. Moussaoui DR, Chouhou L, Guelzim K, et al: Severe sickle cell disease and pregnancy. Systematic prophylactic transfusions in 16 cases. Med Trop (Mars) 62:603, 2002.

395. Cackovic M, Chung C, Bolton LL, Kerstein MD: Leg ulceration in the sickle cell patient. J Am Coll Surg 187:307, 1998.

396. Acurio MT, Friedman RJ: Hip arthroplasty in patients with sickle-cell haemoglobinopathy. J Bone Joint Surg Br 74B:367, 1992.

397. Ilyas I, Moreau P: Simultaneous bilateral total hip arthroplasty in sickle cell disease. J Arthroplasty 17:441, 2002.

398. Styles LA, Vichinsky EP: Core decompression in avascular necrosis of the hip in sickle-cell disease. Am J Hematol 52:103, 1996.

399. Rodgers GP, Roy MS, Noguchi CT, Schechter AN: Is there a role for selective vasodilation in the management of sickle cell disease? Blood 71:597, 1988.

400. Claster S, Vichinsky EP: Managing sickle cell disease. BMJ 327:1151, 2003.

401. Virag R, Bachir D, Lee K, Galacteros F: Preventive treatment of priapism in sickle cell disease with oral and self-administered intracavernous injection of etilefrine. Urology 47:777, 1996.

402. Bialecki ES, Bridges KR: Sildenafil relieves priapism in patients with sickle cell disease. Am J Med 113:252, 2002.

403. Upadhyay J, Shekarriz B, Dhabuwala CB: Penile implant for intractable priapism associated with sickle cell disease. Urology 51:638, 1998.

404. Monga M, Broderick GA, Hellstrom WJG: Priapism in sickle cell disease: The case for early implantation of the penile prosthesis. Eur Urol 30:54, 1996.

405. Ware R, Filston HC, Schultz WH, Kinney TR: Elective cholecystectomy in children with sickle hemoglobinopathies: Successful outcome using a preoperative transfusion regimen. Ann Surg 208:17, 1988.

406. Banerjee AK, Layton DM, Rennie JA, Bellingham AJ: Safe surgery in sickle cell disease. Br J Surg 78:516, 1991.

407. Derkay CS, Bray G, Milmoe GJ, Grundfast KM: Adenotonsillectomy in children with sickle cell disease. South Med J 84:205, 1991.

408. Esseltine DW, Baxter MR, Bevan JC: Sickle cell states and the anaesthetist. Can J Anaesth 35:385, 1988.

409. Neumayr L, Koshy M, Haberkern C, et al: Surgery in patients with hemoglobin SC disease. Am J Hematol 57:101, 1998.

410. Bischoff RJ, Williamson A III, Dalali MJ, et al: Assessment of the use of transfusion therapy perioperatively in patients with sickle cell hemoglobinopathies. Ann Surg 207:434, 1988.

411. Lambotte-Legrand J, Lambotte-Legrand C: Le prognostic de l'anemie drepanocytaire au Congo Belge (a propos de 300 cas et de 150 deces). Ann Soc Belg Med Trop 35:53, 1955.

412. Trowell HC, Raper AB, Welbourn HF: The natural history of homozygous sickle cell anaemia in Central Africa. Q J Med 25:401, 1957.

413. Sydenstricker VP, Kemp JA, Metts JC: Prolonged survival in sickle cell disease. Am Pract 13:584, 1962.

414. Serjeant GR, Richards RR, Barbor PHH, Milner PF: Relatively benign sickle anaemia in 60 patients over 30 in the West Indies. BMJ 2:86, 1968.

415. Platt OS, Brambilla DJ, Rosse WF, et al: Mortality in sickle cell disease—Life expectancy and risk factors for early death. N Engl J Med 330:1639, 1994.

416. Davis H, Schoendorf KC, Gergen PJ, Moore RM: National trends in the mortality of children with sickle cell disease 1968 through 1992. Am J Public Health 87:1317, 1997.

417. Powars D: Diagnosis at birth improves survival of children with sickle cell anemia. Pediatrics 83:830, 1989.

418. Davis H, Gergen PJ, Moore RJ: Geographic differences in mortality of young children with sickle cell disease in the United States. Public Health Rep 112:52, 1997.

419. Israel JB, Arias IM: Inheritable disorders of bilirubin metabolism. Adv Intern Med 21:77, 1976.

420. Manci EA, Culberson DE, Yang YM, et al: Causes of death in sickle cell disease: An autopsy study. Br J Haematol 123:359, 2003.

421. Beutler E, Boggs DR, Heller P, et al: Hazards of indiscriminate screening for sickling. N Engl J Med 285:1485, 1971.

422. Davies SC, Cronin E, Gill M, et al: Screening for sickle cell disease and thalassaemia: A systematic review with supplementary research. Health Technol Assess 4:i99, 2000.

423. Barbedo MMR, McCurdy PR: Red cell life span in sickle cell trait. Acta Haematol (Basel) 51:339, 1974.

424. Kellon DB, Beutler E: Physician attitudes about sickle cell. JAMA 227:71, 1974.

425. Sears DA: The morbidity of sickle cell trait. Am J Med 64:1021, 1978.

426. Humphries JE, Wheby MS: Case report: Sickle cell trait and recurrent deep venous thrombosis. Am J Med Sci 303:112, 1992.

427. Genet P, Pulik M, Lionnet F, et al: Multiple spontaneous vascular infarcts in sickle-cell trait: A case report. Am J Hematol 51:173, 1996.

428. Gozal D, Lorey FW, Chandler D, et al: Incidence of sudden infant death syndrome in infants with sickle cell trait. J Pediatr 124:211, 1994.

429. Von Känel R, Pirovino M: Non-hypoxemic splenic infarction in sickle cell trait. Schweiz Med Wochenschr 128:1614, 1998.

430. Bock H, Seidl S, Hausmann R, Betz P: Sudden death due to a haemoglobin variant. Int J Legal Med 2003.

431. Spear SL, Carter ME, Low M, et al: Sickle cell trait: A risk factor for flap necrosis. Plast Reconstr Surg 112:697, 2003.

432. Smith EW, Conley CL: Clinical manifestations of sickle-cell disease, in Conference on Hemoglobin 2–3 May 1957, p 276, National Academy of Sciences–National Research Council, Washington, DC, 1958.

433. Atlas SA: The sickle cell trait and surgical complications. JAMA 229:1078, 1974.

434. Francis CK, Bleakley DW: The risk of sudden death in sickle cell trait: Noninvasive assessment of cardiac response to exercise. Cathet Cardiovasc Diagn 6:73, 1980.

435. Weisman IM, Zeballos RJ, Johnson BD: Cardiopulmonary and gas exchange responses to acute strenuous exercise at 1,270 meters in sickle cell trait. Am J Med 84:377, 1988.

436. Gozal D, Thiriet P, Mbala E, et al: Effect of different modalities of exercise and recovery on exercise performance in subjects with sickle cell trait. Med Sci Sports Exerc 24:1325, 1992.

437. Nuss R, Loehr JP, Daberkow E, et al: Cardiopulmonary function in men with sickle cell trait who reside at moderately high altitude. J Lab Clin Med 122:382, 1993.

438. Le Gallais D, Prefaut C, Mercier J, et al: Sickle cell trait as a limiting factor for high-level performance in a semi-marathon. Int J Sports Med 15:399, 1994.

439. Bilé A, Le Gallais D, Mercier J, et al: Sickle cell trait in Ivory Coast athletic throw and jump champions 1956-1995. Int J Sports Med 19:215, 1998.

440. Steen RG, Hankins GM, Xiong X, et al: Prospective brain imaging evaluation of children with sickle cell trait: Initial observations. Radiology 228:208, 2003.

441. Hamdi IM, Kamakshi KS, Ghani EA: Pregnancy outcome in women with sickle cell trait. Saudi Med J 23:1455, 2002.

442. Jones SR, Binder RA, Donowho EM Jr: Sudden death in sickle-cell trait. *N Engl J Med* 282:323, 1970.

443. Koppes GM, Daly JJ, Coltman CA Jr, Butkus DE: Exertion-induced rhabdomyolysis with acute renal failure and disseminated intravascular coagulation in sickle cell trait. *Am J Med* 63:313, 1977.

444. Kerle KK, Nishimura KD: Exertional collapse and sudden death associated with sickle cell trait. *Mil Med* 161:766, 1996.

445. Le Gallais D, Bile A, Mercier J, et al: Exercise-induced death in sickle cell trait: Role of aging, training, and deconditioning. *Med Sci Sports Exerc* 28:541, 1996.

446. Murray MJ, Evans P: Sudden exertional death in a soldier with sickle cell trait. *Mil Med* 161:303, 1996.

447. Kark JA, Posey DM, Schumacher HR, Ruehle CJ: Sickle-cell trait as a risk factor for sudden death in physical trainees. *N Engl J Med* 317:781, 1987.

448. O'Brien RT, Pearson HA, Godley JA, Spencer RP: Splenic infarct and sickle (cell) trait. *N Engl J Med* 287:720, 1972.

449. Nichols SD: Splenic and pulmonary infarction in a Negro athlete. *Rocky Mt Med J* 65:49, 1968.

450. Rywlin AM, Benson J: Massive necrosis of the spleen with formation of a pseudocyst: Report of a case in a white man with sickle cell trait. *Am J Clin Pathol* 36:142, 1961.

451. Franklin QJ, Compeggie M: Splenic syndrome in sickle cell trait: Four case presentations and a review of the literature. *Mil Med* 164:230, 1999.

452. Ustun C, Kutlar F, Holley L, et al: Interaction of sickle cell trait with hereditary spherocytosis: Splenic infarcts and sequestration. *Acta Haematol (Basel)* 109:46, 2003.

453. Vicari P, Arantes AM, Figueiredo MS: Sickle cell trait associated with hereditary spherocytosis: A potentially life-threatening coexistence. *Acta Haematol (Basel)* 110:223, 2003.

454. Itano HA, Neel JV: A new inherited abnormality of human hemoglobin. *Proc Natl Acad Sci U S A* 36:613, 1950.

455. Spaet TH, Alway RH, Ward G: Homozygous type "C" hemoglobin. *Pediatrics* 12:483, 1953.

456. Ranney HM, Larson DL, McCormack GH Jr: Some clinical, biochemical and genetic observations on hemoglobin C. *J Clin Invest* 32:1277, 1953.

457. Hunt JA, Ingram VM: Allelomorphism and the chemical differences of the human hemoglobins A S, and C. *Nature* 181:1062, 1958.

458. Fabry ME, Kaul DK, Raventos C, et al: Some aspects of the pathophysiology of homozygous Hb CC erythrocytes. *J Clin Invest* 67:1284, 1981.

459. Hirsch RE, Raventos-Suarez C, Olson JA, Nagel RL: Ligand state of intraerythrocyte circulating Hb C crystals in homozygote CC patients. *Blood* 66:775, 1985.

460. Hirsch RE, Lin MJ, Nagel RL: The inhibition of hemoglobin C crystallization by hemoglobin F. *J Biol Chem* 263:5936, 1988.

461. Thomas ED, Motulsky AG, Walters DH: Homozygous hemoglobin C disease. *Am J Med* 18:832, 1955.

462. Movitt ER, Pollycove M, Mangum JF, Porter WR: Hemoglobin C disease: Quantitative determination of iron kinetics and hemoglobin synthesis. *Am J Med Sci* 247:558, 1964.

463. Murphy JR: Hemoglobin CC erythrocytes: Decreased intracellular pH and decreased O_2 affinity—anemia. *Semin Hematol* 13:177, 1976.

464. Fort JA, Graham-Pole JR, Chopik J: Vasoocclusion with homozygous hemoglobin-C disease. *Am J Pediatr Hematol Oncol* 10:323, 1988.

465. Maberry MC, Mason RA, Cunningham FG, Pritchard JA: Pregnancy complicated by hemoglobin CC and C-beta-thalassemia disease. *Obstet Gynecol* 76:324, 1990.

466. Olson JF, Ware RE, Schultz WH, Kinney TR: Hemoglobin C disease in infancy and childhood. *J Pediatr* 125:745, 1994.

467. Bruyneel M, De Caluwe JP, Des Grottes JM, Collart F: Hemoglobinopathy C and splenomegaly in an Ivory Coast patient. Value of splenectomy. *Rev Med Brux* 24:105, 2003.

468. Itano HA: A third abnormal hemoglobin associated with hereditary hemolytic anemia. *Proc Natl Acad Sci U S A* 37:775, 1951.

469. Chernoff AI: HgB D syndromes. *Blood* 13:116, 1958.

470. Bird GWG, Lehmann H: Haemoglobin D in India. *BMJ* 1:514, 1956.

471. Adekile AD, Kazanetz EG, Leonova JY, et al: Co-inheritance of Hb D-Punjab (codon 121; GAA→CAA) and beta (0) -thalassemia (IVS-II-1; G→A). *J Pediatr Hematol Oncol* 18:151, 1996.

472. Kelleher JFJ, Park JO, Kim HC, Schroeder WA: Life-threatening complications in a child with hemoglobin SD-Los Angeles disease. *Hemoglobin* 8:203, 1984.

473. Itano HA, Bergren WR, Sturgeon P: Identification of fourth abnormal human hemoglobin. *J Am Chem Soc* 76:2278, 1954.

474. Chernoff AI, Minnich V, Na Nakorn S, et al: Studies on hemoglobin E: I. The clinical, hematologic and genetic characteristics of the hemoglobin E syndromes. *J Lab Clin Med* 47:455, 1956.

475. Hunt JA, Ingram VM: Abnormal human haemoglobins: VI. The chemical difference between haemoglobins A and E. *Biochim Biophys Acta* 49:520, 1961.

476. Frischer H, Bowman J: Hemoglobin E, an oxidatively unstable mutation. *J Lab Clin Med* 85:531, 1975.

477. Orkin SH, Kazazian HH Jr, Antonarakis SE, et al: Abnormal RNA processing due to the exon mutation of beta^E-globin gene. *Nature* 300:768, 1982.

478. Oo M, Tin-Shwe, Marlar-Than, O'Sullivan WJ: Genetic red cell disorders and severity of falciparum malaria in Myanmar. *Bull World Health Organ* 73:659, 1995.

479. Fairbanks VF, Oliveros R, Brandabur JH, et al: Homozygous hemoglobin E mimics beta-thalassemia minor without anemia or hemolysis: Hematologic, functional, and biosynthetic studies of first North American cases. *Am J Hematol* 8:109, 1980.

480. Wong SC, Ali MAM: Hemoglobin E diseases: Hematological, analytical, and biosynthetic studies in homozygotes and double heterozygotes for alpha-thalassemia. *Am J Hematol* 13:15, 1982.

481. Tyagi S, Pati HP, Choudhry VP, Saxena R: Clinico-haematological profile of HbE syndrome in adults and children. *Hematology* 9:57, 2004.

482. Fairbanks VF, Gilchrist GS, Brimhall B, et al: Hemoglobin E trait reexamined: A cause of microcytosis and erythrocytosis. *Blood* 52:109, 1979.

483. Fucharoen S, Winichagoon P: Clinical and hematologic aspects of hemoglobin E beta-thalassemia. *Curr Opin Hematol* 7:106, 2000.

484. Ruymann FB, Popejoy LA, Brouillard RB: Splenic sequestration and ineffective erythropoiesis in hemoglobin E-beta-thalassemia disease. *Pediatr Res* 12:1020, 1978.

485. Hathirat P, Isarangkura P, Numhom S, et al: Results of the splenectomy in children with thalassemia. *J Med Assoc Thai* 72(suppl 1):133, 1989.

486. Rees DC, Duley J, Simmonds HA, et al: Interaction of hemoglobin E and pyrimidine 5' nucleotidase deficiency. *Blood* 88:2761, 1996.

487. Cathie IAB: Apparent idiopathic Heinz body anaemia. *Great Ormond St J* 3:343, 1952.

488. Lange RD, Akeroyd JH: Congenital hemolytic anemia with abnormal pigment metabolism and red cell inclusion bodies: A new clinical syndrome. *Blood* 13:950, 1958.

489. Schmid R, Brecher G, Clemens T: Familial hemolytic anemia with erythrocyte inclusion bodies and a defect in pigment metabolism. *Blood* 14:991, 1959.

490. Grimes AJ, Meisler A: Possible cause of Heinz bodies in congenital Heinz-body anaemia. *Nature* 194:190, 1962.

491. Frick PG, Hitzig WH, Betke K: Hemoglobin Zurich: I. A new hemoglobin anomaly associated with acute hemolytic episodes with inclusion bodies after sulfonamide therapy. *Blood* 20:261, 1962.

492. Thein SL: Dominant beta thalassaemia: Molecular basis and pathophysiology. *Br J Haematol* 80:273, 1992.

493. Dacie JV, Shinton NK, Gaffney PJ, et al: Haemoglobin Hammersmith (42(CD1) Phe 6 Ser). *Nature* 216:663, 1967.

494. Rahbar S, Feagler RJ, Beutler E: Hemoglobin Hammersmith associated with severe hemolytic anemia. *Hemoglobin* 5:97, 1981.

495. Ogata K, Ito T, Okazaki T, et al: Hemoglobin Sendagi (beta 42 Phe→Val): A new unstable hemoglobin variant having an amino acid substitution at CD1 of the beta-chain. *Hemoglobin* 10:469, 1986.

496. Molchanova TP, Postnikov YV, Pobedimskaya DD, et al: Hb Alesha or Alpha$_2$Beta$_2$67(E11)Val→Met: A new unstable hemoglobin variant identified through sequencing of amplified DNA. *Hemoglobin* 17:217, 1993.

497. Wajcman H, Kister J, Vasseur C, et al: Structure of the EF corner favors deamidation of asparaginyl residues in hemoglobin: The example of Hb La Roche-sur-Yon [81 (EF5) Leu→His]. *Biochim Biophys Acta* 1138: 127, 1992.

498. Sakuragawa M, Ohba Y, Miyaji T, et al: A Japanese boy with hemolytic anemia due to an unstable hemoglobin (Hb Bristol). *Nippon Ketsueki Gakkai Zasshi* 47:896, 1984.

499. Idelson LI, Didkovsky NA, Filippova AV, et al: Haemoglobin Volga, beta 27 (B9) Ala→Asp: A new highly unstable haemoglobin with a suppressed charge. *FEBS Lett* 58:122, 1975.

500. Praxedes H, Wiltshire BG, Lehmann H: Proceedings of the International Symposium on Standardization in Haematology and Clinical Pathology, Medical Edition Archivio, "Casa Sollievo della Sofferenza," edited by SG Rotondo, p 11. CI.SMEL, Foggia, 1972.

501. Plaseska D, Dimovski AJ, Wilson JB, et al: Hemoglobin Montreal: A new variant with an extended beta chain due to a deletion of Asp, Gly, Leu at positions 73, 74, and 75, and an insertion of Ala, Arg, Cys, Glu at the same location. *Blood* 77:178, 1991.

502. Rieder RF, Oski FA, Clegg JB: Hemoglobin Philly (beta 35 tyrosine→phenylalanine): Studies in the molecular pathology of hemoglobins. *J Clin Invest* 48:1627, 1969.

503. Idelson LI, Didkowsky NA, Casey R, et al: Structure and function of haemoglobin Tacoma (beta 30 Arg→Ser) found in a second family. *Acta Haematol (Basel)* 52:303, 1974.

504. Perutz MF, Kendrew JC, Watson HC: Structure and function of haemoglobin: II. Some relations between polypeptide chain configuration and amino acid sequence. *J Mol Biol* 13:669, 1965.

505. Beutler E, Lang A, Lehmann H: Hemoglobin Duarte: ($_2$ β_2 $6^{[E6]Ala\ Pro}$): A new unstable hemoglobin with increased oxygen affinity. *Blood* 43: 527, 1974.

506. Fairbanks VF, Opfell RW, Burgert EO: Three families with unstable hemoglobinopathies (Köln, Olmsted and Santa Ana) causing hemolytic anemia with inclusion bodies and pigmenturia. *Am J Med* 46:344, 1969.

507. Ranney HM, Jacobs AS, Udem L, Zalusky R: Hemoglobin Riverdale-Bronx, an unstable hemoglobin resulting from the substitution of arginine for glycine at helical residue B6 of the beta polypeptide chain. *Biochem Biophys Res Commun* 33:1004, 1968.

508. Huisman THJ, Brown AK, Efremov GD, et al: Hemoglobin Savannah (B6(24) beta glycine→valine): An unstable variant causing anemia with inclusion bodies. *J Clin Invest* 50:650, 1971.

509. Idelson LI, Didkowsky NA, Casey R, et al: New unstable haemoglobin Hb Moscva, beta 24(B6) Gly→Asp found in the USSR. *Nature* 249: 768, 1974.

510. Winterbourn CC: Oxidative denaturation in congenital hemolytic anemias: The unstable hemoglobins. *Semin Hematol* 27:41, 1990.

511. Rachmilewitz EA, White JM: Haemichrome formation during the in vitro oxidation of haemoglobin Köln. *Nat New Biol* 241:115, 1973.

512. Rachmilewitz EA, Peisach J, Bradley TB, Blumberg WE: Role of haemichromes in the formation of inclusion bodies in haemoglobin H disease. *Nature* 222:248, 1969.

513. Carrell RW, Winterbourn CC, Rachmilewitz EA: Activated oxygen and haemolysis. *Br J Haematol* 30:259, 1975.

514. Winterbourn CC, McGrath BM, Carrell RW: Reactions involving superoxide and normal and unstable haemoglobins. *Biochem J* 155:493, 1976.

515. Huisman THJ, Carver MFH, Efremov GD: *A Syllabus of Human Hemoglobin Variants*. The Sickle Cell Anemia Foundation, Augusta, 1996.

516. Cao A, Galanello R, Rosatelli MC: Genotype-phenotype correlations in beta-thalassemias. *Blood Rev* 8:1, 1994.

517. Ho PJ, Rochette J, Rees DC, et al: Hb Sun Prairie: Diagnostic pitfalls in thalassemic hemoglobinopathies. *Hemoglobin* 20:103, 1996.

518. Srivastava P, Kaeda JS, Roper D, et al: Severe hemolytic anemia associated with the homozygous state for an unstable hemoglobin variant (Hb Bushwick). *Blood* 86:1977, 1995.

519. Loukopoulos D, Fessas P, Kister J, et al: Hemoglobin Köln occurring in association with a beta zero thalassemia: Hematologic and functional consequences. *Blood* 74:496, 1989.

520. King MAR, Wiltshire BG, Lehmann H, Morimoto H: An unstable haemoglobin with reduced oxygen affinity: Haemoglobin Peterborough beta-111 (G13) valine→phenylalanine, its interaction with normal haemoglobin and haemoglobin Lepore. *Br J Haematol* 22:125, 1972.

521. Casey R, Lang A, Lehmann H, Shinton NK: Double heterozygosity for two unstable haemoglobins: Hb Sydney beta-67(E11)Val→Ala and Hb Coventry beta-141(H19) Leu deleted. *Br J Haematol* 33:143, 1976.

522. Lutcher CL, Huisman THJ: Hemoglobin Leslie, an unstable variant due to deletion of Gln beta-131 occurring in combination with beta-thalassemia, Hb S and Hb C. *Clin Res* 23:278A, 1975.

523. Beuzard Y, Basset P, Braconnier F, et al: Haemoglobin Saki alpha$_2$beta$_2^{Leu→Pro(A11)}$ structure and function. *Biochim Biophys Acta* 393: 182, 1975.

524. Tentori L: Three examples of double heterozygosis: Beta-thalassemia and rare hemoglobinopathies, in *Hematologic Contributions to Fetal Health*, p 68. Istanbul, 1974.

525. Ramachandran M, Gu LH, Wilson JB, et al: A new variant, HB Muscat [alpha 2 beta (2)32(B14)Leu→Val] observed in association with HB S in an Arabian family. *Hemoglobin* 16:259, 1992.

526. Outeirino J, Casey R, White JM, Lehmann H: Haemoglobin Madrid beta 115 (G17) alanine→proline: An unstable variant associated with haemolytic anaemia. *Acta Haematol (Basel)* 52:53, 1974.

527. Lee-Potter JP, Deacon-Smith RA, Simpkiss MJ, et al: A new cause of haemolytic anaemia in the newborn. A description of an unstable fetal haemoglobin F Poole, $\alpha_2{}^G\gamma_2$ 130 tryptophan→glycine. *J Clin Pathol* 28: 317, 1975.

528. Kreimer-Birnbaum M, Pinkerton PH, Bannerman RM, Hutchison HE: Dipyrolic urinary pigments in congenital Heinz-body anaemia due to Hb Köln and thalassaemia. *BMJ* 2:396, 1966.

529. Gyan E, Darre S, Jude B, et al: Acute priapism in a patient with unstable hemoglobin Perth and Factor V Leiden under effective oral anticoagulant therapy. *Hematol J* 2:210, 2001.

530. Keeling MM, Bertolone SJ, Baysal E, et al: Hb Mizuho or alpha 2 beta (2)68(E12)Leu→Pro in a Caucasian boy with high levels of Hb F; identification by sequencing of amplified DNA. *Hemoglobin* 15:477, 1991.

531. Carrell RW, Kay R: A simple method for the detection of unstable haemoglobins. *Br J Haematol* 23:615, 1972.

532. Dacie JV, Grimes AJ, Meisler A, et al: Hereditary Heinz-body anaemia. A report of studies on five patients with mild anaemia. *Br J Haematol* 10:388, 1964.

533. Phyliky RL, Fairbanks VF: Thromboembolic complication of splenectomy in unstable hemoglobin disorders: Hb Olmsted, Hb Koln. *Am J Hematol* 55:53, 1997.

534. Skogerboe KJ, West SF, Smith C, et al: Screening for alpha-thalassemia. Correlation of hemoglobin H inclusion bodies with DNA-determined genotype. *Arch Pathol Lab Med* 116:1012, 1992.

535. Winterbourn CC, Carrell RW: Studies of hemoglobin denaturation and Heinz body formation in the unstable hemoglobins. *J Clin Invest* 54: 678, 1974.

536. Girodon E, Ghanem N, Vidaud M, et al: Rapid molecular characterization of mutations leading to unstable hemoglobin β-chain variants. *Ann Hematol* 65:188, 1992.

537. Landin B, Astrom M: Unstable haemoglobin causing haemolytic anaemia: De novo mutation in Sweden identified by PCR. *J Intern Med* 233: 299, 1993.

538. Vichinsky EP, Lubin BH: Unstable hemoglobins, hemoglobins with altered oxygen affinity, and M-hemoglobins. *Pediatr Clin North Am* 27: 421, 1980.

539. Rose C, Bauters F, Galacteros F: Hydroxyurea therapy in highly unstable hemoglobin carriers. *Blood* 88:2807, 1996.

540. Thuret I, Bardakdjian J, Badens C, et al: Priapism following splenectomy in an unstable hemoglobin: Hemoglobin Olmsted beta141 (H19) Leu→Arg. *Am J Hematol* 51:133, 1996.

541. Allison AC: Abnormal haemoglobin and erythrocyte enzyme-deficiency traits, in *Genetical Variations in Human Populations*, edited by GA Harrison, p 16. Pergamon, New York, 1961.

542. Gelin BR, Lee AW, Karplus M: Hemoglobin tertiary structural change on ligand binding. Its role in the co-operative mechanism. *J Mol Biol* 171:489, 1983.

543. Perutz MF, Wilkinson AJ, Paoli M, Dodson GG: The stereochemical mechanism of the cooperative effects in hemoglobin revisited. *Annu Rev Biophys Biomol Struct* 27:1, 1998.

544. Edelstein SJ: Structure of the fibers of hemoglobin S. *Tex Rep Biol Med* 81:221, 1980.

545. Diggs LW: Sickle-cell crises. *Am J Clin Pathol* 44:1, 1965.

546. River GL, Robbins AB, Schwartz SO: SC hemoglobin: A clinical study. *Blood* 18:385, 1961.

547. Harrow BR, Sloane JA, Liebman NC: Roentgenologic demonstration of renal papillary necrosis in sickle-cell trait. *N Engl J Med* 268:969, 1963.

548. Paton D: Conjunctival sign of sickle cell disease. *Arch Ophthalmol* 68: 627, 1962.

549. Diggs LW, Bell A: Intraerythrocytic hemoglobin crystals in sickle cell hemoglobin C disease. *Blood* 25:218, 1958.

550. Crookston JH, Irvine D, Beale D, Lehmann H: A new haemoglobin JToronto (5 alanine 6 aspartic acid). *Nature* 208:1059, 1965.

551. Schneider RG, Alperin JB, Beale D, Lehmann H: Hemoglobin I in an American Negro family: Structural and hematologic studies. *J Lab Clin Med* 68:940, 1966.

552. Schneider RG, Jim RTS: A new haemoglobin variant (the "Honolulu type") in a Chinese. *Nature* 190:454, 1961.

553. Ohba Y, Miyaji T, Hattori Y, et al: Unstable hemoglobins in Japan. *Hemoglobin* 4:307, 1980.

554. Ingram VM: Abnormal human haemoglobins: III. The chemical difference between normal and sickle cell haemoglobins. *Biochim Biophys Acta* 36:402, 1959.

555. Hunt JA, Ingram VM: Abnormal human haemoglobins: IV. The chemical difference between normal human haemoglobin and haemoglobin C. *Biochim Biophys Acta* 42:409, 1960.

556. Muller CJ, Kingma S: Haemoglobin Zurich: Alpha$_2$beta$_2$^{63Arg}. *Biochim Biophys Acta* 50:595, 1961.

557. Bookchin RM, Nagel RL, Ranney HM, Jacobs AS: Hemoglobin C Harlem: A sickling variant containing amino acid substitutions in two residues of the beta-polypeptide chain. *Biochem Biophys Res Commun* 23: 122, 1966.

558. Bonaventura J, Riggs A: Hemoglobin Kansas, a human hemoglobin with a neutral amino acid substitution and an abnormal oxygen equilibrium. *J Biol Chem* 243:980, 1968.

559. Wasi P, Pootrakul S, Na-Nakorn S, et al: Haemoglobin D-beta Los Angeles (D Punjab, alpha-2-beta-2 121 Glu NH2) in a Thai family. *Acta Haematol (Basel)* 39:151, 1968.

560. Larkin IL, Baker T, Lorkin PA, et al: Haemoglobin F Texas II (alpha-2 gamma-2, 6 Glu-Lys), the second of the haemoglobin F Texas variants. *Br J Haematol* 14:233, 1968.

561. Barnabas J, Muller CJ: Haemoglobin-Lepore$_{HOLLANDIA}$. *Nature* 194:931, 1962.

562. Honig GR, Shamsuddin M, Mason RG, Vida LN: Hemoglobin Lincoln Park: A betadelta fusion (anti-Lepore) variant with an amino acid deletion in the delta chain-derived segment. *Proc Natl Acad Sci U S A* 75: 1475, 1978.

563. Clegg JB, Weatherall DJ, Milner PF: Haemoglobin Constant Spring—a chain termination mutant? *Nature* 234:337, 1971.

564. Jones RT, Brimhall B, Huisman TH: Structural characterization of two delta chain variants. Hemoglobin A′-2 (B2) and hemoglobin Flatbush. *J Biol Chem* 242:5141, 1967.

565. Alexandre L, Keclard L, Romana M, et al: Efficiency of prenatal counselling for sickle cell disease in Guadeloupe. *Genet Couns* 8:25, 1997.

METHEMOGLOBINEMIA AND OTHER CAUSES OF CYANOSIS

ERNEST BEUTLER

Cyanosis, blue discoloration of the skin and mucous membranes, is usually due to a change in the color of hemoglobin. Commonly this is due to a high concentration of deoxyhemoglobin because of cardiorespiratory failure or right-to-left shunting. Cyanosis also may indicate that an abnormal hemoglobin is present or that there is an increased concentration of a normally present hemoglobin derivative. Methemoglobin is a reversible oxidation product of hemoglobin and can be present in excess amounts either because of rapid oxidation of hemoglobin by drugs or toxic chemicals or because of a hereditary defect in the methemoglobin-reducing system. Hemoglobins M are mutant hemoglobins that cannot be adequately reduced by the enzymatic systems of the red cell. Sulfhemoglobins are irreversible denaturation products of hemoglobin that can produce cyanosis, even when present in relatively low and harmless quantities. Toxic methemoglobinemia is effectively treated by intravenous infusion of methylene blue, which links the highly efficient reduced nicotinamide adenine dinucleotide phosphate (NADPH)-reducing system to methemoglobin. In hereditary methemoglobinemia the level of methemoglobin can be diminished by the administration of ascorbic acid and, in some cases, by riboflavin.

DEFINITION AND HISTORY

A bluish discoloration of the skin and mucous membrane, designated *cyanosis*, has been recognized since antiquity as a manifestation of lung or heart disease. Cyanosis resulting from drug administration has also been recognized since before 1890.[1] Toxic methemoglobinemia occurs when various drugs or toxic substances either oxidize hemoglobin directly in the circulation or facilitate its oxidation by molecular oxygen.

In 1912 Sloss and Wybauw[2] reported a case of a patient with idiopathic methemoglobinemia. Later Hitzenberger[3] suggested that a hereditary form of methemoglobinemia might exist, and subsequently numerous such cases were reported.[4] In 1948 Hörlein and Weber[5] described a family in which eight members over four generations manifested cyanosis. The absorption spectrum of methemoglobin was abnormal. They demonstrated that the defect must reside in the globin portion of the molecule. Subsequently Singer[6] suggested that such abnormal hemoglobins be given the designation hemoglobin M. The cause of another form of methemoglobinemia that occurs independently of drug administration and without the existence of any abnormality of the globin portion of hemoglobin was first explained by Gibson,[7] who clearly pointed to the site of the enzyme defect, nicotin-

amide adenine dinucleotide (reduced form) (NADH) diaphorase, also designated as methemoglobin reductase, and currently cytochrome b_5 reductase. More than 50 years after Gibson's insightful studies, the mutation that he had predicted was verified at the DNA level.[8]

The existence of abnormal hemoglobins that cause cyanosis through quite another mechanism was first recognized in 1968 with the description of hemoglobin Kansas.[9] Here the cyanosis resulted not from methemoglobin, as occurs in hemoglobin M, but rather from an abnormally low oxygen affinity of the mutant hemoglobin. Thus, at normal oxygen tensions, a large amount of deoxygenated hemoglobin is present in the blood.

Sulfhemoglobinemia refers to the presence in the blood of hemoglobin derivatives that are defined by their characteristic absorption of light at 620 nm, even in the presence of cyanide.

EPIDEMIOLOGY

Methemoglobinemia occurring as a result of NADH-diaphorase deficiency is more common among Native Americans, both in Alaska and in the continental United States, and among the Yakuts of Russian Siberia than in other ethnic groups.[10-12] Methemoglobinemia resulting from hemoglobins M is sporadic in nature, as is the occurrence of toxic methemoglobinemia, although the latter is clearly related to industrial exposure, and is therefore most common among workers in the chemical industry.

ETIOLOGY AND PATHOGENESIS

Methemoglobinemia decreases the oxygen-carrying capacity of blood, because the oxidized iron cannot reversibly bind oxygen. Moreover, when one or more iron atoms have been oxidized, the conformation of hemoglobin is changed so as to increase the oxygen affinity of the remaining ferrous heme groups. In this way methemoglobinemia exerts a dual effect in impairing the supply of oxygen to tissues.[13]

TOXIC METHEMOGLOBINEMIA

Hemoglobin is continuously oxidized *in vivo* from the ferrous to the ferric state. The rate of such oxidation is accelerated by many drugs and toxic chemicals, including sulfonamides, lidocaine and other aniline derivatives, and nitrites. A vast number of chemical substances may cause methemoglobinemia.[14-16] Table 48-1 lists some of the agents that are responsible for clinically significant methemoglobinemia in current clinical practice. The most common offenders include benzocaine and lidocaine.[36-38,45-51] In some cases, the patients have been unaware that they have been ingesting one of the drugs known to produce methemoglobinemia; dapsone is apparently used in some "street drugs."[21,22] Nitrates and the nitrites contaminating water supplies or used as preservatives in foods are also common offending agents.[29-31,52-57]

NADH-DIAPHORASE DEFICIENCY

NADH diaphorase catalyzes a step in the major pathway for methemoglobin reduction. This enzyme reduces cytochrome b_5, using NADH as a hydrogen donor. The reduced cytochrome b_5 reduces, in turn, methemoglobin to hemoglobin (see Chap. 45). A steady-state methemoglobin level is achieved when the rate of methemoglobin formation equals the rate of methemoglobin reduction either through the NADH-diaphorase system or through the relatively minor auxiliary mechanisms such as direct chemical reduction by ascorbate and reduced glutathione. A reduced nicotinamide adenine dinucleotide phosphate (NADPH)-linked enzyme, NADPH diaphorase does not play a role in methemoglobin reduction except when a linking dye such as methylene blue is supplied (see "Therapy, Course, and

TABLE 48-1   SOME DRUGS THAT CAUSE METHEMOGLOBINEMIA

Phenazopyridine (Pyridium)[17–19]
Sulfamethoxazole[20]
Dapsone[21–23]
Aniline[24,25]
Paraquat/monolinuron[26,27,44]
Nitrate[28–31]
Nitroglycerin[17,32]
Amyl nitrite[33]
Isobutyl nitrite[34]
Sodium nitrite[30,35]
Benzocaine[36–38]
Prilocaine[39–41]
Methylene blue[42]
Chloramine[43,44]

Prognosis" below). A marked diminution in the activity of NADH diaphorase will result in the accumulation of the brown pigment in circulating erythrocytes.

Accordingly, hereditary deficiency of the enzyme that reduces cytochrome b_5, NADH diaphorase (also designated cytochrome b_5 reductase), is one of the causes of methemoglobinemia. A great many mutations of NADH diaphorase have been identified at the nucleotide level,[8,58,59–66] and the functional effect of some of these have been deduced from the structure of the enzyme.[58,65,67] In addition, a common polymorphism (allele frequency = 0.023) has been identified in African-Americans; it does not appear to impair the activity of the enzyme.[68] Most of the patients with NADH-diaphorase deficiency merely have methemoglobinemia, and these have been classified as having type I disease. Type II disease deficiency also exists in nonerythroid cells, such as fibroblasts and lymphocytes.[69] Patients with this form of disease are afflicted, in addition to methemoglobinemia, with a progressive encephalopathy and mental retardation. The finding that fatty acid elongation is defective in the platelets and leukocytes of such patients[70] may provide a clue to the type of defect that could occur in the central nervous system, where fatty acid elongation plays an important role in myelination. Occasionally, patients with deficiency of NADH diaphorase in nonerythroid cells do not suffer any neurologic disorder, and it has been suggested that they be designated as having type III disease.[71,72]

A combination of both increased hemoglobin oxidation and decreased methemoglobin reduction also may occur. Since the activity of NADH diaphorase is normally low in newborn infants,[73] they are particularly susceptible to the development of methemoglobinemia. Thus, serious degrees of methemoglobinemia have been observed in infants as a result of toxic materials, such as aniline dyes used on diapers,[74] and the ingestion of nitrate-contaminated water[31,57] and even of beets.[75] Bacterial action in the intestinal tract may reduce nitrates to nitrites, which, in turn, cause methemoglobinemia. In rural areas, fatal methemoglobinuria in infants caused by drinking water from wells contaminated with nitrates still occurs.[76]

Methemoglobinemia occurring in acidotic infants with diarrhea is a syndrome that may have a fatal outcome.[77–81] Such infants have normal red cell NADH-diaphorase activity, and the mechanism by which methemoglobinemia occurs is unknown. However, the syndrome seems most common when soy formula is being fed[82] and breast-feeding appears to protect.[76]

Heterozygotes for NADH-diaphorase deficiency are not usually clinically methemoglobinemic. However, under the stress of administration of drugs that normally induce only slight, clinically unimportant, methemoglobinemia, such persons may become severely cy-

anotic because of methemoglobinemia.[83] This occurrence seems to be quite uncommon.

An animal model of NADH-diaphorase deficiency has been described in the cat[84–86] and dog.[87,88]

CYTOCHROME B_5 DEFICIENCY

Rarely the defect may not be in the diaphorase that transfers hydrogen to the cytochrome b_5, but rather to a deficiency in the cytochrome itself.[84–86]

HEMOGLOBINS M

The molecular mechanisms by which hemoglobin binds oxygen and releases it are discussed in Chapter 47. Heme is held in a hydrophobic "heme pocket" between the E and F α-helices of each of the four globin chains. The iron atom in the heme forms four bonds with the pyrrole nitrogen atoms of the porphyrin ring and a fifth covalent bond with the imidazole nitrogen of a histidine residue in the nearby F α-helix (Fig. 48-1).[89] This histidine, residue 87 in the α chain and 92 in the β chain, is designated as the proximal histidine. On the opposite side of the porphyrin ring the iron atom lies adjacent to another histidine residue to which, however, it is not covalently bonded. This distal histidine occupies position 58 in the α chain and position 63 in the β chain. Under normal circumstances oxygen is occasionally discharged from the heme pocket as a superoxide anion, removing an electron from the iron and leaving it in the ferric state. The enzymatic machinery of the red cell efficiently reduces the iron to the divalent form, converting the methemoglobin to hemoglobin (see Chap. 45).

In most of the hemoglobins M, tyrosine has been substituted for either the proximal or the distal histidine. Tyrosine can form an iron-phenolate complex that resists reduction to the divalent state by the normal metabolic systems of the erythrocyte. Four hemoglobins M are a consequence of substitution of tyrosine for histidine in the proximal

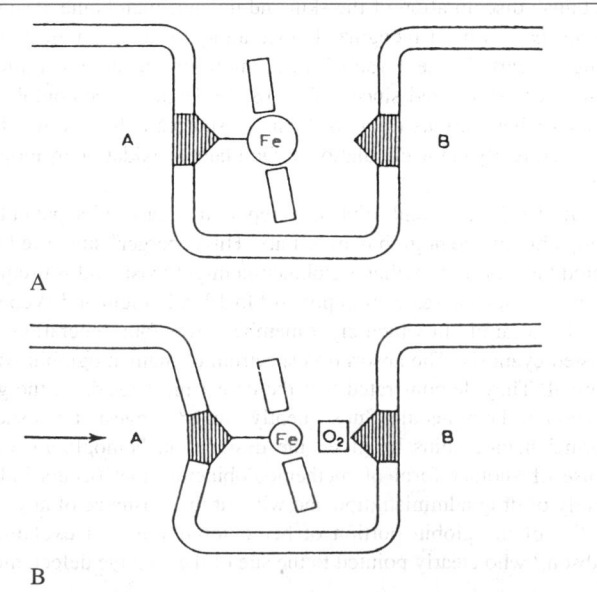

FIGURE 48-1   Diagrammatic representation of the heme group inserted into the heme pocket. A, proximal histidine; B, distal histidine. (A) In the deoxygenated form the larger ferrous atom lies out of the place of the porphyrin ring. (B) In the oxygenated form the now smaller "ferric-like" atom can slip into the plane of the porphyrin ring. As a result, the proximal histidine, and helix F into which it is incorporated, are displaced. (From Lehmann and Huntsman,[89] with permission.)

and distal sites of the α and β chains. As Table 48-2 shows, these four hemoglobins M have been designated by the geographic names Boston, Saskatoon, Iwate, and Hyde Park. Analogous His→Tyr substitutions in the γ chain of fetal hemoglobin have also been documented and have been designated hemoglobin FM-Osaka[95] and FM-Fort Ripley.[97]

Another hemoglobin M, Hb M_Milwaukee, is formed by substitution of glutamic acid for valine in the sixty-seventh residue of the β chain, rather than substitution of tyrosine for histidine. The glutamic acid side chain points toward the heme group and its γ-carboxyl group interacts with the iron atom, stabilizing it in the ferric state.

It is rare for methemoglobinemia to occur as a result of hemoglobinopathies other than hemoglobin M, but Hemoglobin_Chile (β28 Leu→Met) is such a hemoglobin. Producing hemolysis only with drug administration, this unstable hemoglobin is characterized clinically by chronic methemoglobinemia.[98]

LOW-OXYGEN AFFINITY HEMOGLOBINS: A CAUSE OF CYANOSIS

In some hemoglobin variants the deoxy conformation of the hemoglobin molecule is favored because the angle of the heme is altered from that found normally in deoxyhemoglobin. Such changes occur in Hb_Hammersmith, Hb_Bucuresti, Hb_Torino, and Hb_Peterborough. In other instances the quaternary conformation is changed by mutations involving the $\alpha_1\beta_2$ contact (Hb_Kansas, Hb_Titusville, and Hb_Yoshizuka). Properties of abnormal hemoglobins associated with low oxygen affinity are summarized in Table 48-3. In response to the improved tissue oxygen supply brought about by a right-shifted oxygen dissociation curve, the "oxygen sensor" of the body decreases the output of erythropoietin.[99] As a result, the steady-state level of hemoglobin is diminished; mild anemia is characteristic of patients with hemoglobins with a decreased oxygen affinity.

SULFHEMOGLOBIN

Sulfhemoglobin derives its name from the fact that it can be produced *in vitro* from the action of hydrogen sulfide on hemoglobin[101] and that the feeding of dogs with elemental sulfur has been associated with sulfhemoglobinemia.[102] Sulfhemoglobin may contain one excess sulfur atom.[103–105] The sulfur atom appears to be bound to a β-pyrrole carbon atom at the periphery of the porphyrin ring.[103–105] Sulfhemoglobinemia has been associated with the ingestion of various drugs, particularly sulfonamides, phenacetin, acetanilid, and phenazopyridine.[106,107] It also occurs independently of drug use, and has been thought to be related to chronic constipation or to purging.[108] Some patients with sulfhemoglobinemia or a past history of this disorder appear to have increased levels of red blood cell reduced glutathione

TABLE 48-2 PROPERTIES OF HEMOGLOBINS M

HEMOGLOBIN	AMINO ACID SUBSTITUTION	OXYGEN DISSOCIATION AND OTHER PROPERTIES	CLINICAL EFFECT	REFERENCE
Hb M_Boston	α58 (E7)His→Tyr	Very low O_2 affinity, almost nonexistent heme-heme interaction, no Bohr effect	Cyanosis resulting from formation of methemoglobin	90
Hb M_Saskatoon	β63 (E7)His→Tyr	Increased O_2 affinity, reduced heme-heme interaction, normal Bohr effect, slightly unstable	Cyanosis resulting from methemoglobin formation, mild hemolytic anemia exacerbated by ingestion of sulfonamides	90, 91
Hb M_Iwate	α87 (F8)His→Tyr	Low O_2 affinity, negligible heme-heme interaction, no Bohr effect	Cyanosis resulting from formation of methemoglobin	90, 92
Hb M_Kankakee				
Hb M_Oldenburg				
Hb M_Sendai				
Hb M_Hyde Park	β92 (F8)His→Tyr	Increased O_2 affinity, reduced heme interaction, normal Bohr effect, slightly unstable	Cyanosis resulting from formation of methemoglobin, mild hemolytic anemia	93
Hb Milwaukee 2				
Hb M_Akita				
Hb M_Milwaukee	β67 (E11)Val→Glu	Low O_2 affinity, reduced heme-heme interaction, normal Bohr effect, slightly unstable	Cyanosis resulting from methemoglobin formation	94
Hb FM_Osaka	$^G\gamma$63His→Tyr	Low O_2 affinity, increased Bohr effect. Methemoglobinemia	Cyanosis at birth	95
Hb FM_Fort Ripley	$^G\gamma$92His→Tyr	Slightly increased O_2 affinity	Cyanosis at birth	96

TABLE 48-3 SOME ABNORMAL HEMOGLOBINS ASSOCIATED WITH LOW OXYGEN AFFINITY

HEMOGLOBIN	AMINO ACID SUBSTITUTION	OXYGEN DISSOCIATION AND OTHER PROPERTIES	CLINICAL EFFECT	REFERENCE
Hb Seattle	β70 (E14)Ala→Asp	Decreased O_2 affinity, normal heme-heme interaction	Mild chronic anemia associated with reduced urinary erythropoietin; physiologic adaptation to more efficient oxygen release to tissues	99
Hb Kansas	β102 (G4)Asn→Thr	Very low O_2 affinity, low heme-heme interaction, dissociates into dimers in ligand form	Cyanosis resulting from deoxyhemoglobin, mild anemia	100

(GSH).[109] The reason for this and its relationship to sulfhemoglobinemia is not clearly understood, but it may be of significance that some of the types of drugs that have been associated with sulfhemoglobinemia cause an elevation of red cell GSH levels,[110] probably by activating the enzyme glutathione synthetase[110] or by increasing intracellular glutamate levels.[111]

MODE OF INHERITANCE

Cyanosis resulting from abnormal hemoglobins is inherited as an autosomal dominant disorder. In contrast, hereditary methemoglobinemia resulting from NADH-diaphorase deficiency is inherited in an autosomal recessive fashion. Evidence for the occurrence of hereditary sulfhemoglobinemia is not convincing,[112] and it is likely that the single family reported represents a hemoglobin M hemoglobinopathy.

CLINICAL FEATURES

Methemoglobinemia may be chronic or acute. Severe acute methemoglobinemia, usually the consequence of drug ingestion or toxic exposure, can produce symptoms of anemia, since methemoglobin lacks the capacity to transport oxygen. Symptoms may include shortness of breath, palpitations, and vascular collapse. Chemicals that induce methemoglobinemia are often also capable of causing hemolysis, and a combination of hemolytic anemia and methemoglobinemia may occur.

Chronic methemoglobinemia, whether a result of exposure to drugs or toxins or to hereditary causes, is usually asymptomatic. In instances when the methemoglobin levels are very high (>20% of the total pigment) mild erythrocytosis is occasionally noted. Patients with hemoglobins M or with low oxygen affinity hemoglobin also manifest cyanosis. In the case of α-chain variants, the dusky color of the infants will be noted at birth, but the clinical manifestations of β-chain variants become apparent only after β chains have largely replaced the fetal γ chains at 6 to 9 months of age. In spite of the impaired hemoglobin function, no cardiopulmonary symptoms are observed and there is no clubbing. In the case of Hb M$_{Saskatoon}$ and Hb M$_{Hyde Park}$, hemolytic anemia with jaundice may be present. The hemolytic state may be exacerbated by administration of sulfonamides.[113] Hereditary methemoglobinemia resulting from NADH-diaphorase deficiency may, as noted above, be associated with mental retardation. In one case skeletal anomalies were documented as well.[114]

Sulfhemoglobinemia is characterized by cyanosis. Drugs that cause sulfhemoglobinemia often have the capacity to produce accelerated red cell destruction as well. Thus, mild hemolysis is sometimes observed in patients with sulfhemoglobinemia.

LABORATORY FEATURES

TOXIC METHEMOGLOBINEMIA

In toxic methemoglobinemia an elevated level of methemoglobin is found, but the activity of NADH diaphorase is normal. Methemoglobin levels are best measured using the change of absorbance of methemoglobin at 630 nm that occurs when cyanide is added, converting the methemoglobin to cyanmethemoglobin.[115,116] Errors in diagnosis are frequently made when automated instruments designed to estimate levels of reduced hemoglobin, oxygenated hemoglobin, methemoglobin, and carboxyhemoglobin are used. Most automated instruments do not properly make this distinction,[107,117] and direct spectrophotometric analysis should be used when methemoglobinemia or sulfhemoglobinemia is suspected. This is achieved by lysing the blood in a slightly acid buffer and measuring the optical density at 630 nm before and after adding a small amount of neutralized cyanide. The absorption of methemoglobin at this wavelength disappears when it is converted to cyanmethemoglobin. If sulfhemoglobin is to be measured a reading is also made at 620 nm. Although this method was described in 1938,[115] it remains the most accurate technique for the estimation of methemoglobin and sulfhemoglobin levels in the blood. Details of its performance can be found in an earlier edition of this text[118] and elsewhere.[113]

NADH-DIAPHORASE DEFICIENCY

In hereditary methemoglobinemia resulting from NADH-diaphorase deficiency, between 8 and 40 percent of the hemoglobin is in the oxidized (methemoglobin) form. The blood may have a chocolate-brown color. NADH-diaphorase activity is best measured using ferricyanide as a receptor, measuring the rate of oxidation of NADH.[119,120] The residual level of enzyme activity is usually less than 20 percent of normal in patients with methemoglobinemia resulting from deficiency of this enzyme. An immunoassay has been described,[121] but such an assay would not detect mutants in which enzyme molecules with impaired catalytic activity are present. For unknown reasons, glutathione reductase activity is usually also diminished.[122] Cytochrome b_5 assays may be useful if diaphorase activity is normal.[123]

ABNORMAL HEMOGLOBINS

OPTICAL SPECTRUM

The spectrum of normal methemoglobin A at pH 7.0 is illustrated in Figure 48-2.[124] Hemoglobins M may be differentiated from methemoglobin formed from hemoglobin A by its absorption spectrum in the range of 450 to 750 nm. Since only some 20 to 35 percent of the total hemoglobin will ordinarily be the hemoglobin M, the mixed spectra of methemoglobin A and the hemoglobin M may be difficult to interpret. Therefore, it is preferable to perform these spectral studies on purified hemoglobin M isolated by electrophoretic or chromatographic means.[89]

ELECTROPHORESIS

All hemoglobin M samples should be converted to methemoglobin so that any difference found in electrophoresis will be the result of the

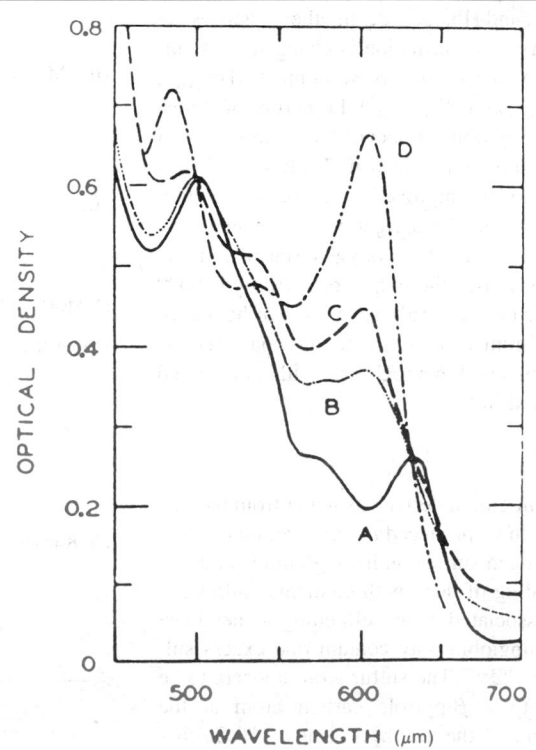

FIGURE 48-2   Absorption spectra at pH 7.0. A, methemoglobin A; B, methemoglobin M$_{Boston}$; C, methemoglobin M$_{Saskatoon}$; D, methemoglobin A fluoride complex. For purposes of comparison, all the optical densities have been made equal to 0.61 at 500 nm. (From Gerald and George,[124] with permission of the American Association for the Advancement of Science.)

amino acid substitution and not the different charge of the iron atom. Electrophoresis at pH 7.1 is most useful for separation of hemoglobins M since the imidazole groups of histidine have a net positive charge at this pH while at higher pH levels the histidines and the substituting tyrosines are both neutral.

OTHER STUDIES

The hemoglobins M differ in their reactivity to cyanide and to azide ions.[125] This property may help to identify the subunit affected, since the iron-phenolate bonds are stronger in the α-chain variants than in the β-chain variants. However, definitive identification of the variant requires peptide or DNA analysis. Hemoglobins that cause cyanosis because of a diminished oxygen affinity may be detected by determining the oxygen dissociation curve of blood, being certain that the 2,3-bisphosphoglycerate (2,3-BPG) level is normal, or by estimating the oxygen dissociation curve of hemoglobin, which has been stripped of 2,3-BPG by extensive dialysis against an appropriate buffer. Many of the hemoglobins with decreased oxygen affinity are unstable and will precipitate in the isopropanol stability test.[125] In many laboratories it may be easier to analyze the coding sequence of the globin chains at the DNA level than to attempt to determine the properties of the hemoglobin.[93]

SULFHEMOGLOBINEMIA

Sulfhemoglobin is detected in the lysate of blood treated with ferricyanide, cyanide, and ammonia by comparing the optical density at 620 nm with that at 540 nm.[115,116]

DIFFERENTIAL DIAGNOSIS

Cyanosis resulting from methemoglobinemia or sulfhemoglobinemia should be differentiated from cyanosis resulting from cardiac or pulmonary disease particularly when right-to-left shunting is present. In the latter instances the arterial oxygen tension will be low, while in methemoglobinemia and sulfhemoglobinemia it should be normal. One should be certain, however, that the oxygen tension was measured directly and not deduced from the percent saturation of hemoglobin. Blood from a patient with cyanosis because of arterial oxygen desaturation promptly becomes bright red upon being shaken with air. In addition, these causes of cyanosis are readily differentiated by carrying out quantitative blood methemoglobin and sulfhemoglobin levels. Because of the potential lethal nature of high levels of methemoglobin and because prompt treatment may be life saving, a high index of suspicion is important. A patient with cyanosis whose arterial blood is brown with a PO_2 that is found to be normal on blood gas examination is likely to have methemoglobinemia. One should not rely on the readings of a pulse oximeter, since false readings may be obtained in the presence of methemoglobin. Rapid examination of a blood sample using an automatic analyzer such as a CoOximeter™ is the first step in confirming the diagnosis. Treatment should not be delayed, but, as pointed out above in "Laboratory Features," direct spectrophotometric analysis should be carried out on the pretreatment sample as soon as possible to distinguish between methemoglobinemia and sulfhemoglobinemia.

A family history is usually helpful in differentiating hereditary methemoglobinemia as a result of NADH-diaphorase deficiency from hemoglobin M disease. The former has a recessive mode of inheritance, the latter a dominant mode. Thus, cyanosis in successive generations suggests the presence of hemoglobin M; normal parents but possibly affected sibs implies the presence of NADH-diaphorase deficiency. Cosanguinity is more common in NADH-diaphorase deficiency. In NADH-diaphorase deficiency, incubation of the blood with small amounts of methylene blue will result in rapid reduction of the methemoglobin; in hemoglobin M disease, such reduction does not take place. The absorption spectra of methemoglobin and its derivatives are normal in NADH-diaphorase deficiency; they are abnormal in hemoglobin M disease. In the case of toxic methemoglobinemia, cyanosis is generally of relatively recent origin, and a history of exposure to drug or toxin may usually be obtained; in hereditary methemoglobinemia a history of lifelong cyanosis may usually be elicited.

THERAPY, COURSE, AND PROGNOSIS

TOXIC METHEMOGLOBINEMIA

Acute toxic methemoglobinemia may represent a serious medical emergency. Because of the loss of oxygen-carrying capacity of the blood and because of the left shift in the oxygen dissociation curve that occurs when methemoglobin is present in high concentration,[126] acute methemoglobinemia may be life-threatening when the level of the pigment exceeds half of the total circulating hemoglobin. Levels of methemoglobin exceeding 60 to 70 percent of the total pigment may be associated with vascular collapse, coma, and death,[28,35] but recovery was documented in one patient with a level as high as 81.5 percent of the total pigment.[127]

Methylene blue[128] is an effective treatment for patients with methemoglobinemia because NADPH formed in the hexose monophosphate pathway can rapidly reduce this dye to leukomethylene blue in a reaction catalyzed by NADPH diaphorase. Leukomethylene blue, in turn, nonenzymatically reduces methemoglobin to hemoglobin.[129] An exception to the efficacy of this treatment exists in those patients who are glucose-6-phosphate dehydrogenase deficient (see Chap. 45). In these subjects methylene blue would not only fail to give the desired effect on methemoglobin levels but might compound the patient's difficulty by inducing an acute hemolytic episode[130] or by increasing the level of methemoglobin.[42] In patients with acute toxic methemoglobinemia who are symptomatic or whose methemoglobin level is rising rapidly, the intravenous administration of 1 or 2 mg methylene blue per kilogram body weight over a period of 5 minutes is the preferred treatment because of its very rapid action.[24] Use of excessive amounts of methylene blue should be avoided: the administration of repeated doses of 2 mg methylene blue per kilogram body weight has produced acute hemolysis even in patients with normal glucose-6-phosphate dehydrogenase levels.[25] The response to treatment is so rapid, with marked lowering or normalization of methemoglobin levels within an hour or two that no other treatment is usually needed, but the patient should be observed carefully, because continued absorption of a toxic substance from the gastrointestinal tract may cause recurrence of the methemoglobinemia. In patients who are in shock, blood transfusion may be helpful. Cimetidine, used as a selective inhibitor of N-hydroxylation, may decrease the methemoglobinemia produced by dapsone in patients with dermatitis herpetiformis.[131]

The course of hereditary methemoglobinemia is benign, but patients with this disorder should be shielded from exposure to aniline derivatives, nitrites, and other agents that may, even in normal persons, induce methemoglobinemia. Hereditary methemoglobinemia resulting from NADH-diaphorase deficiency is readily treated by the administration of ascorbic acid, 300 to 600 mg orally daily divided into three or four doses. While intravenously administered methylene blue is very effective in correcting this type of methemoglobinemia, it is not suitable for the long-term therapy that needs to be given if the state is to be treated at all. Riboflavin administration seems to benefit some patients[132] but not others.[133]

The iron phenolate complex that exists in the hemoglobins M prevents the reduction of ferric to ferrous iron. For this reason the methemoglobinemia does not respond to administration of ascorbic acid or of methylene blue. No effective treatment exists for the cyanosis that is present in patients with abnormal hemoglobins with reduced oxygen affinity.

Sulfhemoglobinemia is almost always a benign disorder. Unlike methemoglobin, sulfhemoglobin does not produce a left shift in the oxygen dissociation curve but rather decreases the affinity of hemoglobin for oxygen.[106] The disorder tends to recur in the same persons after exposure to drugs but does not generally appear to affect their overall health. Unlike methemoglobin, sulfhemoglobin cannot be converted to hemoglobin. Thus, once sulfhemoglobinemia occurs, it will persist until the erythrocytes carrying the abnormal pigment reach the end of their life span.

REFERENCES

1. Hsieh HS, Jaffe ER: The metabolism of methemoglobin in human erythrocytes, in *The Red Blood Cell*, edited by DM Surgenor, p 799. Academic Press, New York, 1975.
2. Sloss A, Wybauw R: Un Cas de methemoglobinemie idiopathique. *Ann Soc R Sci Med Nat Bruxettes* 70:206, 1912.
3. Hitzenberger K: Autotoxische Zyanose: Intraglobulare Methämoglobinamie. *Wien Arch Inn Med* 23:85, 1932.
4. Jaffe ER: Hereditary methemoglobinemias associated with abnormalities in the metabolism of erythrocytes. *Am J Med* 41:786, 1966.
5. Hörlein H, Weber G: Über Chronische familiare Methämoglobinamie und eine neue Modification des Methämoglobins. *Dtsch Med Wochenschr* 73:476, 1948.
6. Singer K: Hereditary hemolytic disorders associated with abnormal hemoglobins. *Am J Med* 18:633, 1955.
7. Gibson QH: The reduction of methemoglobin in red blood cells and studies on the cause of idiopathic methemoglobinemia. *Biochem J* 42:13, 1948.
8. Percy MJ, Gillespie MJ, Savage G, et al: Familial idiopathic methemoglobinemia revisited: Original cases reveal 2 novel mutations in NADH-cytochrome b5 reductase. *Blood* 100:3447, 2002.
9. Bonaventura J, Riggs A: Hemoglobin Kansas, a human hemoglobin with a neutral amino acid substitution and an abnormal oxygen equilibrium. *J Biol Chem* 243:980, 1968.
10. Scott EM, Hoskins DD: Hereditary methemoglobinemia in Alaskan Eskimos and Indians. *Blood* 13:795, 1958.
11. Balsamo P, Hardy WR, Scott EM: Hereditary methemoglobinemia to diaphorase deficiency in Navajo Indians. *J Pediatr* 65:928, 1964.
12. Nazarenko LP, Sazhenova EA, Nazarenko SA, Banshchikova ES: A search for mutations in the DIA1 gene in case of hereditary methemoglobinemia type I in the Iakut population. *Genetika* 39:858, 2003.
13. Sorensen PR: The influence of pH, pCO2 and concentrations of dyshemoglobins on the oxygen dissociation curve (ODC) of human blood determined by non-linear least squares regression analysis. *Scand J Clin Lab Invest Suppl* 203:163, 1990.
14. Bodansky O: Methemoglobinemia and methemoglobin-producing compounds. *Pharmacol Rev* 3:144, 1951.
15. Kiese M: The biochemical production of ferrihemoglobin-forming derivatives from aromatic amines, and mechanisms of ferrihemoglobin formation. *Pharmacol Rev* 18:1091, 1966.
16. Dean BS, Lopez G, Krenzelok EP: Environmentally-induced methemoglobinemia in an infant. *J Toxicol Clin Toxicol* 30:127, 1992.
17. Paris PM, Kaplan RM, Stewart RD, Weiss LD: Methemoglobin levels following sublingual nitroglycerin in human volunteers. *Ann Emerg Med* 15:171, 1986.
18. Gavish D, Knobler H, Gottehrer N, et al: Methemoglobinemia, muscle damage and renal failure complicating phenazopyridine overdose. *Isr J Med Sci* 22:45, 1986.

19. Christensen CM, Farrar HC, Kearns GL: Protracted methemoglobinemia after phenazopyridine overdose in an infant. *J Clin Pharmacol* 36:112, 1996.
20. Damergis JA, Stoker JM, Abadie JL: Methemoglobinemia after sulfamethoxazole and trimethoprim. *JAMA* 249:590, 1983.
21. Falkenhahn M, Kannan S, O'Kane M: Unexplained acute severe methaemoglobinaemia in a young adult. *Br J Anaesth* 86:278, 2001.
22. Lee SW, Lee JY, Lee KJ, et al: A case of methemoglobinemia after ingestion of an aphrodisiac, later proven as dapsone. *Yonsei Med J* 40:388, 1999.
23. Wagner A, Marosi C, Binder M, et al: Fatal poisoning due to dapsone in a patient with grossly elevated methaemoglobin levels. *Br J Dermatol* 133:816, 1995.
24. Kearney TE, Manoguerra AS, Dunford JV Jr: Chemically induced methemoglobinemia from aniline poisoning. *West J Med* 140:282, 1983.
25. Harvey JW, Keitt AS: Studies of the efficacy and potential hazards of methylene blue therapy in aniline-induced methaemoglobinaemia. *Br J Haematol* 54:29, 1983.
26. Ng LL, Naik RB, Polak A: Paraquat ingestion with methaemoglobinaemia treated with methylene blue. *BMJ* 284:1445, 1982.
27. Proudfoot AT: Methaemoglobinaemia due to monolinuron—not paraquat. *BMJ* 285:812, 1983.
28. Johnson CJ, Bonrud PA, Dosch TL, et al: Fatal outcome of methemoglobinemia in an infant. *JAMA* 257:2796, 1987.
29. Johnson CJ, Kross BC: Continuing importance of nitrate contamination of groundwater and wells in rural areas. *Am J Ind Med* 18:449, 1990.
30. Chan TY: Food-borne nitrates and nitrites as a cause of methemoglobinemia. *Southeast Asian J Trop Med Public Health* 27:189, 1996.
31. Knobeloch L, Proctor M: Eight blue babies. *WMJ* 100:43, 2001.
32. Gibson GR, Hunter JB, Rabbe DS, et al: Methemoglobinemia produced by high-dose intravenous nitroglycerin. *Ann Intern Med* 96:615, 1982.
33. Forsyth RJ, Moulden A: Methaemoglobinaemia after ingestion of amyl nitrite. *Arch Dis Child* 66:152, 1991.
34. Guss DA, Normann SA, Manoguerra AS: Clinically significant methemoglobinemia from inhalation of isobutyl nitrite. *Am J Emerg Med* 1:46, 1985.
35. Ellis M, Hiss Y, Shenkman L: Fatal methemoglobinemia caused by inadvertent contamination of a laxative solution with sodium nitrite. *Isr J Med Sci* 28:289, 1992.
36. Kuschner WG, Chitkara RK, Canfield J Jr, et al: Benzocaine-associated methemoglobinemia following bronchoscopy in a healthy research participant. *Respir Care* 45:953, 2000.
37. Abdallah HY, Shah SA: Methemoglobinemia induced by topical benzocaine: A warning for the endoscopist. *Endoscopy* 34:730, 2002.
38. Novaro GM, Aronow HD, Militello MA, et al: Benzocaine-induced methemoglobinemia: Experience from a high-volume transesophageal echocardiography laboratory. *J Am Soc Echocardiogr* 16:170, 2003.
39. Nilsson A, Engberg G, Henneberg S, et al: Inverse relationship between age-dependent erythrocyte activity of methaemoglobin reductase and prilocaine-induced methaemoglobinaemia during infancy. *Br J Anaesth* 64:72, 1990.
40. Duncan PG, Kobrinsky N: Prilocaine-induced methemoglobinemia in a newborn infant. *Anesthesiology* 59:75, 1983.
41. Lloyd CJ: Chemically induced methaemoglobinaemia in a neonate. *Br J Oral Maxillofac Surg* 30:63, 1992.
42. Bilgin H, Özcan B, Bilgin T: Methemoglobinemia induced by methylene blue perturbation during laparoscopy. *Acta Anaesthesiol Scand* 42:594, 1998.
43. Davidovits M, Barak A, Cleper R, et al: Methaemoglobinaemia and haemolysis associated with hydrogen peroxide in a paediatric haemodialysis centre: A warning note. *Nephrol Dial Transplant* 18:2354, 2003.

44. DeTorres JP, Strom JA, Jaber BL, Hendra KP: Hemodialysis-associated methemoglobinemia in acute renal failure. *Am J Kidney Dis* 39:1307, 2002.

45. Collins JF: Methemoglobinemia as a complication of 20% benzocaine spray for endoscopy. *Gastroenterology* 98:211, 1990.

46. Cooper HA: Methemoglobinemia caused by benzocaine topical spray. *South Med J* 90:946, 1997.

47. Guerriero SE: Methemoglobinemia caused by topical benzocaine. *Pharmacotherapy* 17:1038, 1997.

48. Klein SL, Nustad RA, Feinberg SE, Fonseca RJ: Acute toxic methemoglobinemia caused by a topical anesthetic. *Pediatr Dent* 5:107, 1983.

49. McGuigan MA: Benzocaine-induced methemoglobinemia. *Calif Med Assoc J* 125:816, 1983.

50. O'Donohue WJ, Moss LM, Angelillo VA: Acute methemoglobinemia induced by topical Benzocaine and Lidocaine. *Arch Intern Med* 140:1508, 1980.

51. Postiglione KF, Herold DA: Benzocaine-adulterd street cocaine in association with methemoglobinemia *Clin Chem* 38:596, 1992.

52. Askew GL, Finelli L, Genese CA, et al: Boilerbaisse: An outbreak of methemoglobinemia in New Jersey in 1992. *Pediatrics* 94:381, 1994.

53. Bakshi SP, Fahey JL, Pierce LE: Sausage cyanosis. Acquired methemoglobinemia nitrite poisoning. *N Engl J Med* 277:1072, 1967.

54. Bradberry SM, Whittington RM, Parry DA, Vale JA: Fatal methemoglobinemia due to inhalation of isobutyl nitrite. *J Toxicol Clin Toxicol* 32:179, 1994.

55. Bradberry SM, Gazzard B, Vale JA: Methemoglobinemia caused by the accidental contamination of drinking water with sodium nitrite. *J Toxicol Clin Toxicol* 32:173, 1994.

56. Harris JC, Rumack BH, Peterson RG, McGuire BM: Methemoglobinemia resulting from absorption of nitrates. *JAMA* 242:2869, 1979.

57. Lukens JN: The legacy of well-water methemoglobinemia. *JAMA* 257:2793, 1987.

58. Dekker J, Eppink MH, van Zwieten R, et al: Seven new mutations in the nicotinamide adenine dinucleotide reduced-cytochrome b(5) reductase gene leading to methemoglobinemia type I. *Blood* 97:1106, 2001.

59. Grabowska D, Plochocka D, Jablonska-Skwiecinska E, et al: Compound heterozygosity of two missense mutations in the NADH-cytochrome b5 reductase gene of a Polish patient with type I recessive congenital methaemoglobinaemia. *Eur J Haematol* 70:404, 2003.

60. Higasa K, Manabe J, Yubisui T, et al: Molecular basis of hereditary methaemoglobinaemia, types I and II: Two novel mutations in the NADH-cytochrome b_5 reductase gene. *Br J Haematol* 103:922, 1998.

61. Wu YS, Huang CH, Wan Y, et al: Identification of a novel point mutation (Leu72Pro) in the NADH-cytochrome b5 reductase gene of a patient with hereditary methaemoglobinaemia type I. *Br J Haematol* 102:575, 1998.

62. Manabe J, Arya R, Sumimoto H, et al: Two novel mutations in the reduced nicotinamide adenine dinucleotide (NADH) cytochrome b5 reductase gene of a patient with generalized type, hereditary methemoglobinemia. *Blood* 88:3208, 1996.

63. Vieira LM, Kaplan J-C, Kahn A, Leroux A: Four new mutations in the NADH-cytochrome b5 reductase gene from patients with recessive congenital methemoglobinemia type II. *Blood* 85:2254, 1995.

64. Shirabe K, Fujimoto Y, Yubisui T, Takeshita M: An in-frame deletion of codon 298 of the NADH-cytochrome b_5 reductase gene results in hereditary methemoglobinemia type II (generalized type). A functional implication for the role of the COOH-terminal region of the enzyme. *J Biol Chem* 269:5952, 1994.

65. Kugler W, Pekrun A, Laspe P, et al: Molecular basis of recessive congenital methemoglobinemia, types I and II: Exon skipping and three novel missense mutations in the NADH-cytochrome b5 reductase (diaphorase 1) gene. *Hum Mutat* 17:348, 2001.

66. Kedar PS, Colah RB, Ghosh K, Mohanty D: Congenital methemoglobinemia due to NADH-methemoglobin reductase deficiency in three Indian families. *Haematologia (Budap)* 32:543, 2002.

67. Bewley MC, Marohnic CC, Barber MJ: The structure and biochemistry of NADH-dependent cytochrome b5 reductase are now consistent. *Biochemistry* 40:13574, 2001.

68. Jenkins MM, Prchal JT: A high-frequency polymorphism of NADH-cytochrome b5 reductase in African-Americans. *Hum Genet* 99:248, 1997.

69. Tanishima K, Tomoda A, Yoneyama Y, Ohkuwa H: Three types of hereditary methemoglobinemia due to NADH-cytochrome b_5 reductase deficiency. *Adv Clin Enzymol* 5:81, 1987.

70. Takeshita M, Tamura M, Kugi M, et al: Decrease of palmitoyl-CoA elongation in platelets and leukocytes in the patient of hereditary methemoglobinemia associated with mental retardation. *Biochem Biophys Res Commun* 148:384, 1987.

71. Tanishima K, Tanimoto K, Tomoda A, et al: Hereditary methemoglobinemia due to cytochrome b5 reductase deficiency in blood cells without associated neurologic and mental disorders. *Blood* 66:1288, 1985.

72. Katsube T, Sakamoto N, Kobayashi Y, et al: Exonic point mutations in NADH-cytochrome B5 reductase genes of homozygotes for hereditary methemoglobinemia, types I and III: Putative mechanisms of tissue-dependent enzyme deficiency. *Am J Hum Genet* 48:799, 1991.

73. Lo SC-L, Agar NS: NADH-methemoglobin reductase activity in the erythrocytes of newborn and adult mammals. *Experientia* 42:1264, 1986.

74. Graubarth J, Bloom CJ, Coleman FC, Solomon HN: Dye poisoning in the nursery: A review of seventeen cases. *JAMA* 128.1155, 1945.

75. Sanchez-Echaniz J, Benito-Fernandez J, Mintegui-Raso S: Methemoglobinemia and consumption of vegetables in infants. *Pediatrics* 107:1024, 2001.

76. Hanukoglu A, Danon PN: Endogenous methemoglobinemia associated with diarrheal disease in infancy. *J Pediatr Gastroenterol Nutr* 23:1, 1996.

77. Yano S, Danish E, Hsia YE: Transient methemoglobinemia with acidosis in infants. *J Pediatr* 100:415, 1982.'

78. Bricker T, Jefferson LS, Mintz AA: Methemoglobinemia in infants with enteritis. *J Pediatr* 102:161, 1983.

79. Hanukoglu A, Fried D, Bodner D: Methemoglobinemia in infants with enteritis. *J Pediatr* 102:161, 1983.

80. Seeler RA: Methemoglobinemia in infants with enteritis. *J Pediatr* 102:162, 1983.

81. Danish EH: Methemoglobinemia in infants with enteritis. *J Pediatr* 102:162, 1983.

82. Murray KF, Christie DL: Dietary protein intolerance in infants with transient methemoglobinemia and diarrhea. *J Pediatr* 122:90, 1993.

83. Cohen RJ, Sachs JR, Wicker DJ, Conrad ME: Methemoglobinemia provoked by malarial chemoprophylaxis in Vietnam. *N Engl J Med* 279:1127, 1968.

84. Hegesh E, Hegesh J, Kaftory A: Congenital methemoglobinemia with a deficiency of cytochrome b5. *N Engl J Med* 314:757, 1986.

85. Mansouri A, McClellan JL: Congenital methemoglobinemia with cytochrome b_5 deficiency. *N Engl J Med* 315:893, 1986.

86. Tauber AI, Blanchard RA: Congenital methemoglobinemia with cytochrome b_5 deficiency. *N Engl J Med* 315:894, 1986.

87. Fine DM, Eyster GE, Anderson LK, Smitley A: Cyanosis and congenital methemoglobinemia in a puppy. *J Am Anim Hosp Assoc* 35:33, 1999.

88. Harvey JW, Ling GV, Kaneko JJ: Methemoglobin reductase deficiency in a dog. *J Am Vet Med Assoc* 164:1030, 1974.

89. Lehmann H, Huntsman RG: *Man's Haemoglobins*, p 213. Lippincott, Philadelphia, 1974.

90. Gerald PS, Efron ML: Chemical studies of several varieties of Hb M. *Proc Natl Acad Sci U S A* 47:1758, 1961.

91. Staven P, Strome J, Lorkin PA, Lehmann H: Haemoglobin M Saskatoon with slight constant haemolysis, markedly increased by sulphonamides. *Scand J Haematol* 9:566, 1972.

92. Hayashi N, Motokawa Y, Kikuchi G: Studies on relationships between structure and function of hemoglobin M Iwate. *J Biol Chem* 241:79, 1966.

93. Hutt PJ, Pisciotta AV, Fairbanks VF, et al: DNA sequence analysis proves Hb M-Milwaukee-2 is due to beta-globin gene codon 92 (CAC→TAC), the presumed mutation of Hb M-Hyde Park and Hb M-Akita. *Hemoglobin* 22:1, 1998.

94. Horst J, Schafer R, Kleihauer E, Kohne E: Analysis of the Hb M Milwaukee mutation at the DNA level. *Br J Haematol* 54:643, 1983.

95. Hayashi A, Fujita T, Fujimura M, Titani K: A new abnormal fetal hemoglobin, Hb FM-Osaka (alpha$_2$gamma$_2$$^{63His\rightarrow Tyr}$). *Hemoglobin* 4:447, 1980.

96. Hain RD, Chitayat D, Cooper R, et al: Hb FM-Fort Ripley: Confirmation of autosomal dominant inheritance and diagnosis by PCR and direct nucleotide sequencing. *Hum Mutat* 3:239, 1994.

97. Priest JR, Watterson J, Jones RT, et al: Mutant fetal hemoglobin causing cyanosis in a newborn. *Pediatrics* 83:734, 1989.

98. Hojas-Bernal R, McNab-Martin P, Fairbanks VF, et al: Hb Chile [beta 28(B10)Leu→Met]: An unstable hemoglobin associated with chronic methemoglobinemia and sulfonamide or methylene blue-induced hemolytic anemia. *Hemoglobin* 23:125, 1999.

99. Stamatoyannopoulos G, Parer JT, Finch CA: Physiologic implication of a hemoglobin with decreased oxygen affinity (hemoglobin Seattle). *N Engl J Med* 281:915, 1969.

100. Reissmann KR, Ruth WE, Namura T: A human hemoglobin with lowered oxygen affinity and impaired heme-heme interactions. *J Clin Invest* 40:1826, 1971.

101. Lemberg R, Legge JW: *Hematin Compounds and Bile Pigments*. Interscience Publishers, New York, 1949.

102. Harrop GA Jr, Waterfield RL: Sulphemoglobinemia. *JAMA* 95:647, 1930.

103. Nichol AW, Hendry I, Morell DB: Mechanism of formation of sulphhaemoglobin. *Biochim Biophys Acta* 156:97, 1968.

104. Berzofsky JA, Peisach J, Horecker BL: Sulfheme proteins: IV. The stoichiometry of sulfur incorporation and the isolation of sulfhemin, the prosthetic group of sulfmyoglobin. *J Biol Chem* 247:3783, 1972.

105. Berzofsky JA, Peisach J, Blumberg WE: Sulfheme proteins: II. The reversible oxygenation of ferrous sulfmyoglobin. *J Biol Chem* 246:7366, 1971.

106. Park CM, Nagel RL: Sulfhemoglobinemia. Clinical and molecular aspects. *N Engl J Med* 310:1579, 1984.

107. Halvorsen SM, Dull WL: Phenazopyridine-induced sulfhemoglobinemia: Inadvertent rechallenge. *Am J Med* 91:315, 1991.

108. Discombe G: Sulphaemoglobinaemia and glutathione. *Lancet* 2:371, 1960.

109. McCutcheon AD, Melb MD, Flack EH: Sulphaemoglobinaemia and glutathione. *Lancet* 2:240, 1960.

110. Paniker NV, Beutler E: The effect of methylene blue and diaminodiphenylsulfone on red cell reduced glutathione synthesis. *J Lab Clin Med* 80:481, 1972.

111. Smith JE, Mahaffey E, Lee M: Effect of methylene blue on glutamate and reduced glutathione of rabbit erythrocytes. *Biochem J* 168:587, 1977.

112. Miller AA: Congenital sulfhemoglobinemia. *J Pediatr* 51:233, 1957.

113. Dacie JV, Lewis SM: Chemical and physico-chemical methods of Haematological importance, in *Practical Haematology*, p 476. Grune & Stratton, New York, 1998.

114. Yawata Y, Ding L, Tanishima K, Tomoda A: New variant of cytochrome b5 reductase deficiency (b5R$_{Kurashiki}$) in red cells, platelets, lymphocytes, and cultured fibroblasts with congenital methemoglobinemia, mental and neurological retardation, and skeletal anomalies. *Am J Hematol* 40:299, 1992.

115. Evelyn KA, Malloy HT: Microdetermination of oxyhemoglobin, methemoglobin, and sulfhemoglobin in a single sample of blood. *J Biol Chem* 126:655, 1938.

116. Beutler E: Carboxyhemoglobin, methemoglobin, and sulfhemoglobin determinations, in *Hematology*, edited by E Beutler, MA Lichtman, BS Coller, TJ Kipps, p L50. McGraw-Hill, New York, 1995.

117. Watcha MF, Connor MT, Hing AV: Pulse oximetry in methemoglobinemia. *Am J Dis Child* 143:845, 1989.

118. Beutler E, Gelbart T: Carboxyhemoglobin, methemoglobin, and sulfhemoglobin determinations, in *Hematology*, edited by WJ Williams, E Beutler, AJ Erslev, MA Lichtman, p 1732. McGraw-Hill, New York, 1990.

119. Beutler E: *Red Cell Metabolism: A Manual of Biochemical Methods*. Grune & Stratton, New York, 1984.

120. Board PG: NADH-ferricyanide reductase, a convenient approach to the evaluation of NADH-methaemoglobin reductase in human erythrocytes. *Clin Chim Acta* 109:233, 1981.

121. Lan FH, Tang YC, Huang CH, et al: Antibody-based spot test for NADH-cytochrome b5 reductase activity for the laboratory diagnosis of congenital methemoglobinemia. *Clin Chim Acta* 273:13, 1998.

122. Das Gupta A, Vaidya MS, Bapat JP, et al: Associated red cell enzyme deficiencies and their significance in a case of congenital enzymopenic methemoglobinemia. *Acta Haematol (Basel)* 64:285, 1980.

123. Kaftory A, Hegesh E: Improved determination of cytochrome b5 in human erythrocytes. *Clin Chem* 30:1344, 1984.

124. Gerald PS, George P: A second spectroscopically abnormal methemoglobin associated with hereditary cyanosis. *Science* 129:393, 1959.

125. Carrell RW, Kay R: A simple method for the detection of unstable haemoglobins. *Br J Haematol* 23:615, 1972.

126. Darling RC, Roughton FJW: The effect of methemoglobin on the equilibrium between oxygen and hemoglobin. *Am J Physiol* 137:56, 1942.

127. Caudill L, Walbridge J, Kuhn G: Methemoglobinemia as a cause of coma. *Ann Emerg Med* 19:677, 1990.

128. Clifton J, Leikin JB: Methylene blue. *Am J Ther* 10:289, 2003.

129. Beutler E, Baluda MC: Methemoglobin reduction. Studies of the interaction between cell populations and of the role of methylene blue. *Blood* 22:323, 1963.

130. Rosen PJ, Johnson C, McGehee WG, Beutler E: Failure of methylene blue treatment in toxic methemoglobinemia. Association with glucose-6-phosphate dehydrogenase deficiency. *Ann Intern Med* 75:83, 1971.

131. Coleman MD, Rhodes LE, Scott AK, et al: The use of cimetidine to reduce dapsone-dependent methaemoglobinaemia in dermatitis herpetiformis patients. *Br J Clin Pharmacol* 34:244, 1992.

132. Kaplan JC, Chirouze M: Therapy of recessive congenital methaemoglobinaemia by oral riboflavine. *Lancet* 2:1043, 1978.

133. Beutler E: Important recent advances in the field of red cell metabolism: Practical implications, in *Erythrocytes, Thrombocytes, Leukocytes*, edited by E Gerlach, K Moser, E Deutsch, W Wilmanns, p 123. George Thieme Verlag, Stuttgart, 1973.

HEMOLYTIC ANEMIA RESULTING FROM PHYSICAL INJURY TO RED CELLS

KELTY R. BAKER

JOEL MOAKE

Extensive erythrocyte fragmentation and hemolysis occur when red blood cells are forced at high shear stress through partial vascular occlusions or abnormal vascular surfaces. "Split" red cells, or schistocytes, are prominent on blood films under these conditions. Considerable quantities of lactate dehydrogenase are released from traumatized red cells into the bloodstream. In the high-flow microvascular or arterial circulation, vascular obstructions or impediments include platelet aggregates in the systemic microvascular during episodes of thrombotic thrombocytopenic purpura, platelet-fibrin thrombi in the renal microvasculature with hemolytic uremic syndrome, and malfunction of a cardiac prosthetic valve in valve-related hemolysis. Less extensive red cell fragmentation, hemolysis, and schistocytosis occur under conditions of more modest vascular occlusion or vascular surface abnormality or conditions of lower shear stress. These latter entities include excessive fibrin polymer formation and secondary fibrinolysis in the arterial or venous circulation (disseminated intravascular coagulation) or in the placental vasculature in hemolysis, elevated liver enzymes, and low platelets (HELLP) syndrome, preeclampsia or eclampsia, and with metastatic cancers and cavernous hemangiomas. Thrombotic thrombocytopenic purpura (see Chap. 124), hemolytic uremic syndrome (see Chap. 110), and disseminated intravascular coagulation (see Chap. 121) are discussed elsewhere in this book, but this chapter discusses the remaining entities.

HELLP SYNDROME, ECLAMPSIA, AND PREECLAMPSIA

DEFINITION AND HISTORY

In 1922, Stahnke[1] first noted in the German literature a life-threatening condition of pregnancy denoted by eclampsia, hemolysis, and thrombocytopenia. Subsequently, Pritchard et al.[2] described three cases in the English literature and suggested that an immunologic process accounted for both the preeclampsia or eclampsia and the hematologic abnormalities. Although the condition initially was known as edema-proteinuria-hypertension gestosis type B,[3] a catchier phrase—HELLP

(hemolysis, elevated liver function tests, and low platelets) syndrome—ultimately was coined by Louis Weinstein[4] in 1982.

EPIDEMIOLOGY

HELLP syndrome is seen in five of 1000 pregnancies overall,[5] in 4 to 12 percent of pregnancies complicated by preeclampsia and in 30 to 50 percent of pregnancies complicated by eclampsia. However, 15 percent of patients ultimately diagnosed with HELLP syndrome do not present with either hypertension or significant proteinuria.[6] Two thirds of patients are diagnosed antepartum, with 70 percent of diagnoses made between 27 and 37 weeks. The remaining third of patients are diagnosed postpartum, anywhere from a few hours to 6 days following delivery, although the majority of cases are seen within 48 hours.[7,8] Established risk factors for HELLP syndrome are white ethnicity, multiparity, and older maternal age (older than 34 years).[5] Although the homozygous presence of the 677 (C→T) polymorphism of the methylenetetrahydrofolate reductase gene may be a modest risk factor for development of preeclampsia, such an association does not exist for HELLP syndrome.[9] Whether or not an increased prevalence of mutations in the factor V Leiden and prothrombin 20210 genes is seen in women affected by HELLP syndrome is controversial.[10–12]

ETIOLOGY AND PATHOGENESIS

A developing embryo must acquire a supply of maternal blood to survive. During a normal pregnancy, the first wave of trophoblastic invasion into the decidua occurs at 10 to 12 days. This event is followed by a second wave at 16 to 22 weeks, when the specialized placental epithelial cells replace the endothelium of the uterine spiral arteries and intercalate within the muscular tunica, increasing the vessels' diameters while decreasing their resistance. As a result, the spiral arteries are remodeled into unique hybrid vessels composed of fetal and maternal cells. The vasculature is converted into a high-flow, low-resistance system resistant to vasoconstrictors circulating in the maternal bloodstream.[13] In a preeclamptic pregnancy, the second wave fails to completely penetrate the spiral arteries of the uterus, perhaps because of reduced placental expression of syncytin and subsequent altered cell fusion processes during placentogenesis.[14] The resultant poorly perfused placenta releases factors such as soluble fms-like tyrosine kinase-1 (sFlt-1), an antiangiogenic protein that binds to placental growth factor and vascular endothelial growth factor, preventing their interaction with endothelial receptors and inducing endothelial dysfunction.[15] Key sequelae include increased vascular tone, enhanced platelet aggregation, and an altered ratio of thromboxane to prostacyclin. Thrombin-induced activation of the coagulation cascade results in fibrin deposition in the capillaries, multiorgan microvascular injury, microangiopathic hemolytic anemia, elevated liver enzymes because of hepatic necrosis, and thrombocytopenia.[5]

CLINICAL FEATURES

Ninety percent of patients present with malaise and right upper quadrant or epigastric pain. Between 45 and 86 percent have nausea or vomiting, 55 to 67 percent have edema, 31 to 50 percent have headache, and a smaller percentage complain of visual changes. Fever typically is not seen. Although hypertension is found in 85 percent of patients, 15 percent of patients with HELLP syndrome do not present with either hypertension or proteinuria.[6]

LABORATORY FEATURES

The blood film reveals schistocytes, helmet cells, and burr cells consistent with microangiopathic hemolytic anemia in 54 to 86 percent of patients.[6] Reticulocytosis is rarely reported in the literature but can be present. Low haptoglobin levels are sensitive and specific for confirming the presence of hemolysis[16,17] and return to normal 24 to 48 hours postpartum.[17]

Lactate dehydrogenase (LDH) level usually is greater than 600 units. The ratio of LDH-5 (an isoenzyme found specifically in the liver) to total LDH is elevated in proportion to the severity of preeclampsia.[18] The high LDH level seen in patients with this condition most likely results from liver damage rather than red cell hemolysis.[17] Levels of aspartate transaminase (AST) and alanine transaminase (ALT) can be up to 100 times higher than normal, whereas levels of alkaline phosphatase typically are only twice normal, and total bilirubin levels range between 1.2 and 5 mg/dl. In most cases, elevated liver enzymes return to baseline values within 3 to 5 days postpartum.[6]

The degree of thrombocytopenia has been utilized in a classification scheme to predict maternal morbidity and mortality, rapidity of postpartum disease recovery, risk of disease recurrence, perinatal outcome, and need for plasmapheresis. The so-called "Mississippi triple class system" places patients with platelet counts less than 50,000/μl in class 1 (with an associated 13 percent incidence of bleeding), patients with platelet counts between 50,000 and 100,000/μl in class 2 (with an associated 8 percent incidence of bleeding), and patients with platelet counts greater than 100,000/μl in class 3 (with no increased incidence of bleeding).[7] Not surprisingly, patients with class 1 HELLP syndrome suffer the highest incidence of perinatal morbidity and mortality and endure the most protracted recovery periods postpartum.[19] A direct correlation between the degree of thrombocytopenia and measures of liver function has been reported,[20] but no such association was seen upon review of the underlying hepatic histopathologic abnormalities.[21] Abundant megakaryocytes are found if marrow aspiration and biopsy are performed, consistent with a consumptive thrombocytopenia with resultant reduction of the normal platelet life span to 3 to 5 days.[19] The platelet count nadir occurs 23 to 29 hours postpartum, with subsequent normalization within 6 to 11 days.[7]

Prothrombin time (PT) and partial thromboplastin time (PTT) usually are within normal limits, although some investigators reported an elevated PTT can be found in 50 percent of patients. Although low fibrinogen levels are inconsistently found, other measures of increased fibrinolysis may be present, including decreased protein C and antithrombin III (AT-III) levels and increased D-dimer and thrombin–AT-III levels.[22] Although von Willebrand factor (vWF) antigen levels increase in proportion to the severity of the disease, reflecting the extent of endothelial damage, no unusually large vWF multimers are present compared to thrombotic thrombocytopenic purpura (TTP). Consistent with this observation, the thrombi found in organs affected by HELLP syndrome contain increased fibrin levels and low vWF levels.[23]

In patients with significant liver involvement, hepatic ultrasonography reveals large, irregular, fairly well-demarcated (or "geographical") areas of increased echogenicity.[24] Upon biopsy, periportal or focal necrosis, fibrin deposits in the sinusoids, and vascular microthrombi are found. As the disease progresses, large areas of necrosis coalesce and dissect into the liver capsule, leading to subcapsular hematomas and even hepatic rupture.[5]

DIFFERENTIAL DIAGNOSIS

HELLP syndrome may be confused with other complications of pregnancy, such as TTP and hemolytic uremic syndrome (see Chap. 110), sepsis (see Chap. 20), disseminated intravascular coagulation (DIC) (see Chap. 121), connective tissue disease, antiphospholipid antibody syndrome (see Chap. 123), and acute fatty liver of pregnancy. This latter entity also is seen in the last trimester or postpartum. It presents with thrombocytopenia and right upper quadrant pain, but the levels of AST and ALT rise to only one to five times normal, and PT and PTT both are prolonged. Oil-red-O staining of liver biopsies demon-

strates fat in the cytoplasm of centrilobular hepatocytes, whereas routine stains show inflammation and patchy hepatocellular necrosis. Because HELLP can cause right upper quadrant pain and nausea, HELLP also has been misdiagnosed as viral hepatitis, biliary colic, esophageal reflux, cholecystitis, and gastric ulcer. Conversely, other conditions misdiagnosed as HELLP syndrome include cardiomyopathy, dissecting aortic aneurysm, acute cocaine intoxication, essential hypertension and renal disease, and alcoholic liver disease.[19]

THERAPY

Supportive care of HELLP includes intravenous administration of magnesium sulfate to prevent eclamptic seizures, control of hypertension, scrupulous management of fluids and electrolytes, judicious transfusion of blood products, stimulation of fetal lung maturity with beclomethasone, and delivery of the fetus as soon as possible.[19] Indications for delivery include severe disease presentation, maternal DIC, fetal distress, and gestational age greater than 32 weeks with evidence of lung maturity.[6] Cesarean section under general anesthesia is utilized in 60 to 97 percent of cases, but vaginal delivery after induction can be attempted if the fetus is older than 32 weeks and the mother's cervix is favorable. Whether or not postpartum curettage is helpful in lowering mean arterial pressure and increasing urine output and platelet count is controversial.[19,25]

Adjunctive therapy for HELLP consists of dexamethasone administration and plasma exchange. Dexamethasone 10 mg given intravenously every 12 hours results in increased urine output and platelet counts, decreased AST and LDH levels, decreased time to delivery, and a trend toward reduced neonatal morbidity and mortality.[26] Dexamethasone does not affect the rate of infection or change the rate of maternal recovery postpartum, although the drug should be continued for at least 2 days following delivery to prevent a "rebound" of elevated liver enzymes, LDH, thrombocytopenia, and oliguria.[19] Plasma exchange cannot arrest or reverse HELLP syndrome when it is utilized antepartum, but it minimizes hemorrhage and morbidity when it is used peripartum. Plasma exchange can be tried postpartum if the patient does not spontaneously improve within 72 to 96 hours of delivery, as seen in 5 percent of patients, usually those who are younger than 20 years or are nulliparous.[7] Liver transplantation may be necessary in those cases complicated by large hematomas or massive hepatic necrosis.[27]

COURSE AND PROGNOSIS

Most patients stabilize within 24 to 48 hours following delivery, but death may occur in 3 to 5 percent of patients, with mortality rates as high as 25 percent reported in the literature prior to 1980. Events leading to maternal death include cerebral hemorrhage, cardiopulmonary arrest, DIC, adult respiratory distress syndrome, and hypoxic ischemic encephalopathy.[5] Other complications include infection, placenta abruptio, postpartum hemorrhage, intraabdominal bleeding, and subcapsular liver hematomas with resultant rupture, a fatal event in 50 percent of patients in whom it occurs.[6] Patients complain of right-sided shoulder pain and are found to be in shock with ascites or pleural effusions. The hematoma usually is present in the anterosuperior aspect of the right lobe of the liver. If the hematoma is unruptured when it is discovered, abdominal palpation, seizures, and emesis should be avoided. Emergent surgical consultation is required because hepatic artery embolization or ligation, lobectomy, and even liver transplantation may be necessary in those cases complicated by massive hepatic necrosis.[5,19]

Renal complications of HELLP include transient elevation of serum creatinine, acute renal failure, hyponatremia, and nephrogenic diabetes insipidus as a result of impaired hepatic metabolism of vasopressinase and resultant "resistance to vasopressin."[28] The small subset of patients with continued deterioration of renal function after delivery may require either temporary or permanent hemodialysis.[19] Pulmonary complications consist of pleural effusions, pulmonary edema, and adult respiratory distress syndrome. Other sequelae include retinal detachment, postictal cortical blindness, and hypoglycemic coma.[28]

In the past, fetal morbidity and mortality ranged from 5 to 100 percent but now ranges between 9 and 24 percent.[6] Complications usually result from prematurity, placental abruption, and intrauterine asphyxia. Thirty-nine percent of infants have intrauterine growth retardation, and one third have concomitant thrombocytopenia. Fortunately, intraventricular hemorrhage is seen in only 4 percent of patients with thrombocytopenia and is typically grade I or II, never grade III or IV.[29]

HELLP syndrome reportedly recurs in as many as 27 percent of patients with subsequent pregnancies,[30] but the more commonly reported range is 2 to 5 percent of women.[5] Other hypertensive disorders of pregnancy (preeclampsia or pregnancy-induced hypertension) are relatively common in future pregnancies, seen in 27 percent of women.[31]

DISSEMINATED MALIGNANCY

DEFINITION AND HISTORY

The relationship between widespread malignancy and hemolytic anemia associated with pathologic changes in small blood vessels was first noted by Brain and associates[32] in 1962.

EPIDEMIOLOGY

Malignancy associated microangiopathic hemolytic anemia (MAHA) has been described in a wide variety of malignancies (Table 49-1). However, MAHA is found only in the setting of metastatic disease and not with localized cancers or benign tumors.[33] Approximately 80 percent of reported tumors are mucinous adenocarcinomas of the stomach (55 percent), breast (13 percent), or lung (10 percent). The median age at diagnosis is 50 years, with a slight male predominance (male to female ratio 1.3:1).[34]

TABLE 49-1   CANCERS ASSOCIATED WITH MICROANGIOPATHIC
                       HEMOLYTIC ANEMIA

Gastric (55%)[34,36]

Breast (13%)[102]

Lung (10%)[32]

Other adenocarcinomas

  Unknown primary[35]

  Prostate[32]

  Colon[35]

  Gallbladder

  Pancreas

  Ovary

Other malignancies

  Erythroleukemia[103]

  Hemangiopericytoma[33]

  Hepatoma

  Melanoma

  Small cell cancer of the lung[104]

  Testicular cancer

  Squamous cell cancer of the oropharynx

  Thymoma

ETIOLOGY AND PATHOGENESIS

MAHA as a result of malignancy arises from two distinct mechanisms: DIC or intravascular tumor emboli.[32,35] In the former situation, a protease found in the mucin secreted by adenocarcinomas directly activates factor X. Subsequent activation of the coagulation cascade results in deposition of fibrin, formation of intravascular hyaline thrombi, shearing of the red blood cells upon strands of fibrin, and consumption of platelets. In the latter situation, intravascular tumor emboli disrupt the endothelium, promoting deposition of fibrin, adherence of platelets, intimal hyperplasia, and vascular hypertrophy.[32,34,35]

LABORATORY FEATURES

Patients with cancer-associated MAHA present with a rapidly progressive, moderate-to-severe anemia wherein the blood film reveals schistocytes (accounting for 4.6–21 percent of the red cells), helmet cells, burr cells, microspherocytes (formed by contraction of the aforementioned schistocytes), polychromasia, and nucleated red cells.[35] The reticulocyte count may be high but is unreliable in proving the presence of hemolysis, as extensive replacement of the marrow by metastatic tumor may prevent the reticulocytosis expected with MAHA.[34,35] Instead, other indirect measures of hemolysis, such as increased levels of serum bilirubin and LDH, plasma hemoglobin, or urine urobilinogen and hemoglobin, can be sought.[34] Low levels of haptoglobin may be seen, but haptoglobin is an acute phase reactant that may be increased in malignancy.[35] The Coombs' test is negative.[34,36]

Additional findings in MAHA usually include thrombocytopenia, with a reported mean platelet count of 50,000/μl (range 3.2–225/μl),[34] resulting from a markedly shortened platelet life span without demonstrable sequestration of platelets in the liver or spleen.[35] However, because some patients with tumors may have thrombocytosis,[37] a superimposed MAHA may reduce the platelet count only to "normal" values, although evidence of increased platelet consumption is present.[35] A normal to high white cell count with a left-shifted differential count may be seen.[34-36] In the absence of uremia or malignant hypertension, the presence of leukoerythroblastosis and MAHA is highly suggestive of metastatic malignancy.[35] Marrow aspiration and biopsy reveal erythroid hyperplasia, normal to high numbers of megakaryocytes, and tumor invasion in 55 percent of patients.[36]

Laboratory evidence of DIC has been reported in approximately 50 percent of patients with MAHA resulting from malignancy. Findings have included low levels of fibrinogen (mean 177 gm/dl, range 8–490 mg/dl), increased numbers of fibrin split products, and elevated prothrombin and thrombin times.[34] Despite reports to the contrary,[38] cancer-associated MAHA is not associated with severe deficiency of the vWF-cleaving protease.[39]

DIFFERENTIAL DIAGNOSIS

The most common cause of anemia in the setting of malignancy is anemia of chronic disease. Other diagnostic considerations include blood loss, myelophthisis resulting from disease metastatic to the marrow, DIC, and autoimmune hemolytic anemia, especially in the setting of lymphoproliferative disease but also with carcinoma of the stomach, colon, breast, and cervix.[40] In addition, treatment of cancer can induce anemia, resulting from myelosuppression, oxidative hemolysis (doxorubicin, pentostatin), autoimmune hemolysis (cisplatin, chlorambucil, cyclophosphamide, melphalan, teniposide, methotrexate), or microangiopathic hemolytic anemia (mitomycin C, cisplatin).

THERAPY

Multiple therapeutic interventions have been attempted for malignancy-associated MAHA. However, heparin, glucocorticoids, dipyridamole, indomethacin, and ε-aminocaproic acid have all been tried without success. Plasmapheresis is of questionable benefit, but treatment of the underlying malignancy with either hormonal therapy or chemotherapy may be beneficial.

COURSE AND PROGNOSIS

MAHA as a result of cancer usually is a preterminal event. The median life expectancy following diagnosis is 21 days.[34]

CARDIAC VALVE HEMOLYSIS

DEFINITION AND HISTORY

Anemia arising after cardiac valve replacement was first described in 1954,[41] soon after corrective valvular surgery became possible. The anemia subsequently was shown to result from erythrocyte shearing and fragmentation as the red cells traversed the turbulent flow through or around the prosthetic valve.[42] Preventing irreversible red cell injury has been a goal of new prosthesis designs. As a result, the incidence of clinically significant valve-associated hemolysis has declined from 5 to 15 percent in the 1960s and 1970s[43,44] to less than 1 percent with newer-generation prostheses such as the Omnicarbon valve.[45] However, compensated hemolysis can occur with any type of valve prosthesis and can be detected in almost every patient depending on the type of prosthetic device.[43,46,47] In addition, intravascular hemolysis can be seen in unoperated patients with underlying valvular disease (reviewed in ref. 43).

EPIDEMIOLOGY

Factors that increase the chance of valvular hemolysis include the presence of central or paravalvular regurgitation,[44,48] placement of small valve prostheses with resultant high transvalvular pressure gradients,[44] and regurgitation as a result of bioprosthetic valve failure, seen especially when the valve is older than 10 to 15 years.[48] Patients with ball-and-cage valves,[46] bileaflet valves versus tilting disc valves,[49] mechanical valve prostheses versus xenograft tissue prostheses,[50] and double compared to single valve replacement[49] more likely experience clinically significant hemolysis. Some studies have reported no difference in the degree of hemolysis with aortic and mitral valve prostheses,[47,49] whereas other studies have found that the aortic position is associated with slightly greater hemolysis than the mitral position.[51–53]

ETIOLOGY AND PATHOGENESIS

Valve-related hemolysis occurs when red cells are exposed to the shearing stresses created by turbulent blood flow through and around a valve prosthesis, impaction against foreign surfaces or cardiac structures such as the wall of the atrial appendage,[48] and large pressure fluctuations between cardiac chambers. A transvalvular pressure gradient greater than 50 mmHg can generate shearing forces exceeding 4000 dynes/cm^2, which is more than the 3000 dynes/cm^2 usually needed to cause red cell fragmentation.[54] In a study of malfunctioning mitral valve prostheses, sophisticated computer modeling using transesophageal echocardiography demonstrated a maximal shear value of 6000 dynes/cm^2 when the regurgitant jet was divided by a solid structure such as a loose suture or dehisced annuloplasty ring ("fragmentation"). A maximal shear rate of 4500 dynes/cm^2 was found when the regurgitant jet was suddenly decelerated by a solid structure such as the left atrial appendage ("collision") or when the blood was regurgitated through a small orifice (<2 mm in diameter) such as a leaflet perforation or a paravalvular leak ("rapid acceleration").[48] Lack of endothelialization of the prosthetic ring may contribute to the severity

of hemolysis following valve repair or replacement, but whether this situation is primary or secondary to the high-velocity jet of blood preventing fibrous incorporation of the prosthetic materials is unclear.[48,55] Similarly, lack of endothelialization of the Teflon patch can result in clinically significant hemolysis necessitating reoperation following repair of a ventricular septal defect.[56] These sorts of surface interactions appear to be more important at lower shear stresses (<1500 dynes/cm^2) when the amount of hemolysis depends more directly on contact surface area and exposure time.[57] Finally, excessive wear of the cloth covering caged-ball prostheses, such as the Starr-Edwards valve, can cause ballooning of the material into the bloodstream jet, with resultant turbulence and hemolysis.[58]

CLINICAL FEATURES

Patients with valve-induced hemolysis present with symptoms resulting from anemia or congestive heart failure, pallor, icterus, and dark urine (described variously as red, brown, or black). Predictably, urine during periods of physical activity may be darker than urine produced at rest.[59] Valve dysfunction is suggested by a change in the intensity or quality of a previously audible sound, the appearance of a new murmur, or a change in the characteristics of a preexisting murmur.[60]

LABORATORY FEATURES

Helpful laboratory studies include review of the blood film, which reveals moderate poikilocytosis, schistocytosis, and polychromasia.[43] The red cells usually are normochromic and normocytic but occasionally are hypochromic and microcytic as a result of iron deficiency from long-standing urinary iron loss[43] and increased erythropoiesis from ongoing hemolysis.[44] The reticulocyte count, urine hemosiderin, plasma hemoglobin, and serum total and indirect bilirubin and LDH levels all are elevated, whereas the serum haptoglobin level is depressed. Both the number of schistocytes in the blood[43,46] and the elevated LDH level[46,47,61,62] correlate with hemolysis severity. Hemoglobinuria usually is seen only in patients with particularly severe hemolysis and high LDH levels.[46,47] No correlation is seen between hemolysis severity and bilirubin levels.[47] Whether the reticulocyte count is helpful in assessing hemolysis severity is controversial.[46,47] Criteria utilizing the aforementioned laboratory tests have been proposed as a means for determining the degree of hemolysis and guiding management (Table 49-2).[46]

Red cell labeling studies confirm that erythrocyte life span is markedly shortened to between 6 and 13 days,[56,59] with a normal erythrocyte life span between 25 and 35 days.[59] Marrow aspiration shows erythroid hyperplasia.[55,59] As a result of hemosiderin deposition, magnetic resonance imaging of the kidneys reveals reduced signal intensity of the renal cortex compared with the medulla on T1- and T2-weighted images both with and without gadolinium enhancement.[63]

TABLE 49-2 SEVERITY OF PROSTHETIC VALVE HEMOLYSIS

	MILD	MODERATE	SEVERE
Hemosiderinuria	Present	Present	Marked
Hemoglobinuria	Absent	Absent	Absent
Schistocytosis	<1%	>1%	>>1%
Reticulocytosis[a]	<5%	>5%	>>5%
Haptoglobins	Decreased	Absent	Absent
LDH	<500 units	>500 units	>>500 units

[a] If hemosiderinuria and hemoglobinuria lead to iron deficiency, the reticulocyte count will be lower than expected.
SOURCE: Adapted from Eyster et al.[46]

DIFFERENTIAL DIAGNOSIS

Factors that can promote valve-associated hemolysis or worsen the anemia include iron deficiency (because hypochromic red cells are more fragile than normal), folate deficiency arising from increased erythropoiesis, anemia of chronic disease resulting from endocarditis, anticoagulant-induced gastrointestinal hemorrhage, and increased cardiac output as a result of strenuous physical exertion.[60]

THERAPY

Appropriate therapy for hemolytic anemia arising from valvular dysfunction consists of iron and folate replacement if their levels are deficient, and surgical repair or replacement of the malfunctioning prosthesis if indicated.[64] Adjunctive measures to be attempted include β-blockade to slow the velocity of the circulation,[65] erythropoietin therapy to further stimulate erythropoiesis,[66] and pentoxifylline therapy to increase the deformability of red cells.[67]

Although some authors have not found pentoxifylline to be beneficial,[60] several case reports have described amelioration of valve-related hemolysis and a decreased need for red blood cell transfusion in patients receiving pentoxifylline.[69–71] A prospective study of 40 individuals with double (mitral and aortic) valve replacement randomized patients to receive either no treatment or pentoxifylline 400 mg orally three times daily for 120 days. The group of patients who received pentoxifylline had significantly higher hemoglobin and haptoglobin levels and significantly lower LDH, total and indirect bilirubin, and corrected reticulocyte levels after 4 months of treatment. Of the nine patients with severe hemolysis (LDH >1500 U), six individuals had improvement or complete resolution of their disease, whereas three patients had persistence of their hemolysis, suggesting that pentoxifylline therapy is beneficial in 60 percent of patients with valve-related hemolysis.[72]

Between 15 and 30 percent of patients develop pigment gallstones following valve surgery, the majority within 6 months of the procedure.[73] Whether this occurrence results from acute hemolysis associated with use of the heart-lung machine[73] or from chronic hemolysis resulting from the valve replacement itself[74,75] is uncertain. However, therapy with ursodeoxycholic acid (UCDA) 600 mg daily beginning 1 week before surgery significantly decreases the incidence of gallstone formation from 29.2 percent in patients who were left untreated to 8.4 percent in patients who received UCDA (P < 0.01).[76]

COURSE AND PROGNOSIS

Evidence of hemolysis can be seen within days[42] or weeks[46,56,59] following valve surgery. If reoperation is required, reported mortality rates range between 0 and 6 percent.[55,77] Hemolytic anemia can recur occasionally.[42,77]

OTHER CAUSES OF NONIMMUNE HEMOLYSIS

MARCH HEMOGLOBINURIA

In 1881, Fleischer[78] first described a German soldier in whom hemoglobinuria was brought on by marching. March hemoglobinuria usually is reported in young males, no doubt because of their more frequent participation in severe and prolonged exertion, but march hemoglobinuria also can be seen in women.[79,80] The presenting complaint is passage of dark urine immediately following physical exertion in the upright position, occasionally accompanied by nausea, abdominal cramps, aching in the back or legs, a "stitch in the side," or a burning feeling in the soles of the feet. Physical examination usually is unrevealing, although hepatosplenomegaly and transient jaundice have been rarely reported.[81]

Davidson[81] proved definitively in 1969 that march hemoglobinuria results from red cell trauma within the vessels of the soles of the feet, and its severity is influenced by the hardness of the running surface, the distance run, the heaviness of the athlete's stride, and the protective adequacy of the athletic footwear.[81] Davidson also showed that the condition could be prevented by using padded insoles, a finding later substantiated by other authors.[82,83] Interestingly, however, hemoglobinuria also has been seen following other types of trauma in activities as diverse as repetitive slapping of the forehead,[84] karate exercises,[85] playing basketball and then beating on congo drums,[86] and kendo (a Japanese martial art where heavily padded combatants strike each other repeatedly with bamboo swords).[79]

Because the estimated quantity of blood hemolyzed in an average paroxysm is only 6 to 40 ml, anemia is uncommon; if present, the anemia usually is mild.[81] Morphologic evidence of red cell damage typically is not seen, although one patient had poikilocytes and occasional "four-leaf clover" cells after exercise.[87] Renal damage is infrequent, but cases of acute tubular necrosis and resultant acute renal insufficiency have been described.[88–91]

KASABACH-MERRITT PHENOMENON

Kasabach-Merritt phenomenon was first described in 1940.[92] Kasabach-Merritt phenomenon is a syndrome that develops in infancy and is characterized by thrombocytopenia, microangiopathic hemolytic anemia, consumptive coagulopathy, and hypofibrinogenemia as a result of an enlarging kaposiform hemangioendothelioma or tufted angioma.[93] Endothelial cell abnormalities and vascular stasis are postulated to lead to activation of platelets and the coagulation cascade within the tumor's vessels, with subsequent depletion of platelets and clotting factors. Microangiopathic hemolytic anemia results from mechanical trauma sustained by the erythrocytes traversing the tumor's abnormal, partially thrombosed vascular channels.[94]

Although numerous therapies have been utilized, the mortality rate of Kasabach-Merritt phenomenon can be as high as 30 percent.[95] Surgical resection is always followed by normalization of hematologic parameters, but many lesions are too large to be resected without severe disfigurement. Other treatments include corticosteroids, interferon alpha, antifibrinolytic agents, antiplatelet agents, low molecular weight heparin, embolization, radiation, laser therapy, and chemotherapy utilizing drugs such as vincristine and cyclophosphamide (reviewed in refs. 93, 94, and 96).

MISCELLANEOUS

Microangiopathic hemolytic anemia has been seen in malignant systemic hypertension, pulmonary hypertension,[97] giant cavernous hemangiomas of the liver,[98] and various vasculitides including Wegener granulomatosis,[99,100] and giant cell arteritis.[101]

REFERENCES

1. Stahnke E: Über das Verhalten der Blutplättchen bei Eklampsie. *Zentralbl Gynäkol* 46:391, 1922.
2. Pritchard JA, Weisman R Jr, Ratnoff OD, Vosburgh GJ: Intravascular hemolysis, thrombocytopenia and other hematologic abnormalities associated with severe toxemia of pregnancy. *N Engl J Med* 250:89, 1954.
3. Goodlin RC, Cotton DB, Haesslein HC: Severe edema-proteinuria-hypertension gestosis. *Am J Obstet Gynecol* 132:595, 1978.
4. Weinstein L: Syndrome of hemolysis, elevated liver enzymes, and low platelet count: A severe consequence of hypertension in pregnancy. *Am J Obstet Gynecol* 142:159, 1982.
5. Rahman TM, Wendon J: Severe hepatic dysfunction in pregnancy. *Q J Med* 95:343, 2002.

6. Rath W, Faridi A, Dudenhausen JW: HELLP syndrome. *J Perinat Med* 28:249, 2000.

7. Martin JN Jr, Magann EF, Blake PG, et al: Analysis of 454 pregnancies with severe preeclampsia/eclampsia HELLP syndrome using the 3-class system of classification. *Am J Obstet Gynecol* 68:386, 1993.

8. Sibai BM, Ramadan MK, Usta I, et al: Maternal morbidity and mortality in 442 pregnancies with hemolysis, elevated liver enzymes, and low platelets (HELLP) syndrome. *Am J Obstet Gynecol* 169:1000, 1993.

9. Zusterzeel PLM, Visser W, Blom HJ, et al: Methylenetetrahydrofolate reductase polymorphisms in preeclampsia and the HELLP syndrome. *Hypertens Pregnancy* 19:299, 2000.

10. Krauss T, Augustin HG, Osmers R, et al: Activated protein C resistance and factor V Leiden in patients with haemolysis, elevated liver enzymes, low platelets syndrome. *Obstet Gynecol* 92:457, 1998.

11. Bozzo M, Carpani G, Leo L, et al: HELLP syndrome and factor V Leiden. *Eur J Obstet Gynecol Reprod Biol* 95:55, 2001.

12. Benedetto C, Marozio L, Salton L, et al: Factor V Leiden and factor II G20210A in preeclampsia and HELLP syndrome. *Acta Obstet Gynecol Scand* 81:1095, 2002.

13. Zhou Y, McMaster M, Woo K, et al: Vascular endothelial growth factor ligands and receptors that regulate human cytotrophoblast survival are dysregulated in severe preeclampsia and hemolysis, elevated liver enzymes, and low platelets syndrome. *Am J Pathol* 160:1405, 2002.

14. Knerr I, Beinder E, Rascher W: Syncytin, a novel human endogenous retroviral gene in human placenta: Evidence for its dysregulation in preeclampsia and HELLP syndrome. *Am J Obstet Gynecol* 186:210, 2002.

15. Levine RJ, Maynard SE, Qian C, et al: Circulating angiogenic factors and the risk of preeclampsia. *N Engl J Med* 350:672, 2004.

16. Marchand A, Galen RS, Lonte VF: The predictive value of serum haptoglobin in haemolytic disease. *JAMA* 243:1909, 1980.

17. Wilke G, Rath W, Schutz E, et al: Haptoglobin as a sensitive marker of hemolysis in HELLP syndrome. *Int J Gynaecol Obstet* 39:29, 1992.

18. Shukla PK, Sharma D, Mandal RK: Serum lactate dehydrogenase in detecting liver damage associated with preeclampsia. *Br J Obstet Gynaecol* 85:40, 1978.

19. Magann EF, Martin JN Jr: Twelve steps to optimal management of HELLP syndrome. *Clin Obstet Gynecol* 42:532, 1999.

20. Thiagarajah S, Bourgeois FJ, Harbert GM, Caudle MR: Thrombocytopenia in preeclampsia: Associated abnormalities and management principles. *Am J Obstet Gynecol* 150:1, 1984.

21. Barton JR, Riely CA, Adamed TA, et al: Hepatic histopathologic condition does not correlate with laboratory abnormalities in HELLP syndrome (hemolysis, elevated liver enzymes, and low platelet count). *Am J Obstet Gynecol* 167:1538, 1992.

22. De Boer K, Büller HR, Ten Cate JW, Treffers PE: Coagulation studies in the syndrome of haemolysis, elevated liver enzymes, and low platelets. *Br J Obstet Gynaecol* 98:42, 1991.

23. Thorp JM Jr, Gilbert GC II, Moake JL, Bowes WA Jr: Von Willebrand factor multimeric levels and patterns in patients with severe preeclampsia. *Obstet Gynecol* 75:163, 1990.

24. Thomas EA, Copplestone JA, Dubbins PA, Friend JR: The radiologist cries "HELLP"! *Br J Radiol* 64:964, 1991.

25. Schlenzig C, Maurer S, Goppelt M, et al: Postpartum curettage in patients with HELLP syndrome does not result in accelerated recovery. *Eur J Obstet Gynecol Reprod Biol* 91:25, 2000.

26. Magann EF, Bass D, Chauhan SP, et al: Antepartum corticosteroids: Disease stabilization in patients with the syndrome of hemolysis, elevated liver enzymes, and low platelets (HELLP). *Am J Obstet Gynecol* 171:1148, 1994.

27. Erhard J, Lange R, Niebel W, et al: Acute liver necrosis in the HELLP syndrome: Successful outcome after orthotopic liver transplantation. A case report. *Transpl Int* 6:179, 1993.

28. Reubinoff BE, Schenker JG: HELLP syndrome—a syndrome of hemolysis, elevated liver enzymes, and low platelet count—complicating preeclampsia-eclampsia. *Suppl Int J Gynaecol Obstet* 36:95, 1991.

29. Harms K, Rath W, Herting E, Kuhn W: Maternal hemolysis, elevated liver enzymes, low platelet count, and neonatal outcome. *Am J Perinatol* 12:1, 1995.

30. Sullivan CA, Magann EF, Perry KG Jr, et al: The recurrence risk of the syndrome of hemolysis, elevated liver enzymes, and low platelets: Subsequent pregnancy outcome and long-term prognosis. *Am J Obstet Gynecol* 172:125, 1995.

31. van Pampus MG, Wolf H, Mayruhu G, et al: Long-term follow-up in patients with a history of HELLP syndrome. *Hypertens Pregnancy* 20:15, 2001.

32. Brain MC, Dacie JV, Hourihane DO: Microangiopathic haemolytic anemia: The possible role of vascular lesions in pathogenesis. *Br J Haematol* 8:358, 1962.

33. Kupers EC, Friedman NB, Lee S, Wolfstein RS: Metastatic hemangiopericytoma associated with microangiopathic hemolytic anemia: Review and report of a case. *J Am Geriatr Soc* 23:411, 1975.

34. Antman KH, Skarin AT, Mayer RJ, et al: Microangiopathic hemolytic anemia and cancer: A review. *Medicine* 58:377, 1979.

35. Lohrmann HP, Adam W, Heymer B, Kubanek B: Microangiopathic hemolytic anemia in metastatic carcinoma. Report of eight cases. *Ann Intern Med* 79:368, 1973.

36. Lynch EC, Bakken CL, Casey TH, Alfrey CP Jr: Microangiopathic hemolytic anemia in carcinoma of the stomach. *Gastroenterology* 52:88, 1967.

37. Silvis SE, Turkbas N, Doscherholmen A: Thrombocytosis in patients with lung cancer. *JAMA* 87:416, 1970.

38. Oleksowicz L, Bhagwati N, DeLeon-Fernandez M: Deficient activity of von Willebrand's factor-cleaving protease in patients with disseminated malignancies. *Cancer Res* 59:2244, 1999.

39. Fontana S, Gerritsen HE, Hovinga JK, et al: Microangiopathic haemolytic anaemia in metastasizing malignant tumours is not associated with a severe deficiency of the von Willebrand factor-cleaving protease. *Br J Haematol* 113:100, 2001.

40. Ellis LD, Westerman MP: Autoimmune hemolytic anemia and cancer. *JAMA* 193:962, 1965.

41. Rose JC, Hufnagel CA, Fries ED, et al: The hemodynamic alterations produced by plastic valvular prosthesis for severe aortic insufficiency in man. *J Clin Invest* 33:891, 1954.

42. Rodgers BM, Sabiston DC Jr: Hemolytic anemia following prosthetic valve replacement. *Circulation* 39:155, 1969.

43. Marsh GW, Lewis SM: Cardiac haemolytic anaemia. *Semin Hematol* 6:133, 1969.

44. Kloster FE: Diagnosis and management of complications of prosthetic heart valves. *Am J Cardiol* 872, 1975.

45. Iguro Y, Moriyama Y, Yamaoka A, et al: Clinical experience of 473 patients with the Omnicarbon prosthetic heart valve. *J Heart Valve Dis* 8:674, 1999.

46. Eyster E, Rothchild J, Mychajliw O: Chronic intravascular hemolysis after aortic valve replacement. *Circulation* 44:657, 1971.

47. Crexells C, Aerichide N, Bonny Y, et al: Factors influencing hemolysis in valve prosthesis. *Am Heart J* 84:161, 1972.

48. Garcia MJ, Vandervoort P, Stewart WJ, et al: Mechanisms of hemolysis with mitral prosthetic regurgitation. *J Am Coll Cardiol* 27:399, 1996.

49. Skoularigis J, Essop MR, Skudicky D, et al: Frequency and severity of intravascular hemolysis after left-sided cardiac valve replacement with Medtronic Hall and St. Jude Medical prostheses, and influence of prosthetic type, position, size, and number. *Am J Cardiol* 71:587, 1993.

50. Chang H, Lin FY, Hung CR, Chu SH: Chronic intravascular hemolysis after valvular surgery. *J Formos Med Assoc* 89:880, 1990.

51. Yacoub MH, Keeling DH: Chronic haemolysis following insertion of ball valve prostheses. *Br Heart J* 30:676, 1968.

52. Falk RH, Mackinnon J, Wainscoat J, et al: Intravascular haemolysis after valve replacement: Comparative study between Starr-Edwards (ball valve) and Bjork-Shiley (disc valve) prosthesis. *Thorax* 34:746, 1979.

53. Febres-Roman PR, Bourg WC, Crone RA, et al: Chronic intravascular hemolysis after aortic valve replacement with Ionescu-Shiley xenograft: Comparative study with Bjork-Shiley prosthesis. *Am J Cardiol* 46:735, 1980.

54. Nevaril CG, Lynch EC, Alfrey CP, et al: Erythrocyte damage and destruction induced by shearing stress. *J Lab Clin Med* 71:784, 1968.

55. Cerfolio RJ, Orszulak TA, Daly RC, Schaff HV: Reoperation for hemolytic anaemia complicating mitral valve repair. *Eur J Cardiothorac Surg* 11:479, 1997.

56. Sayed HM, Dacie JV, Handley DA, et al: Haemolytic anaemia of mechanical origin after open heart surgery. *Thorax* 16:356, 1961.

57. Leverett LB, Hellums JD, Alfrey CP, Lynch EC: Red blood cell damage by shear stress. *Biophys J* 12:257, 1972.

58. Murakami M, Tanaka H, Watanabe M, et al: Severe hemolysis due to cloth wear 23 years after aortic valve replacement on a Starr-Edwards ball valve model 2320. *Cardiovasc Surg* 10:284, 2002.

59. Sears DA, Crosby WH: Intravascular hemolysis due to intracardiac prosthetic devices. *Am J Med* 39:341, 1965.

60. Maraj R, Jacobs LE, Ioli A, Kotler MN: Evaluation of hemolysis in patients with prosthetic heart valves. *Clin Cardiol* 21:387, 1998.

61. Myhre E, Rasmussen K, Andersen A: Serum lactic dehydrogenase activity in patients with prosthetic heart valves: A parameter of intravascular hemolysis. *Am Heart J* 80:463, 1970.

62. Thompson ME, Lewis JH, Prokolab FL, et al: Indexes of intravascular hemolysis quantification of coagulation factors, and platelet survival in patients with porcine heterograft valves. *Am J Cardiol* 51:489, 1983.

63. Lee JW, Kim SH, Yoon CJ: Hemosiderin deposition on the renal cortex by mechanical hemolysis due to malfunctioning prosthetic cardiac valve: Report of MR findings in two cases. *J Comput Assist Tomogr* 23:445, 1999.

64. Amidon TM, Chou TM, Rankin JS, Ports TA: Mitral and aortic paravalvular leaks with hemolytic anemia. *Am Heart J* 125:122, 1993.

65. Okita Y, Miki S, Kusuhara K, et al: Propranolol for intractable hemolysis after open heart operation. *Ann Thorac Surg* 52:1158, 1991.

66. Shapira Y, Bairey O, Vatury M, et al: Erythropoietin can obviate the need for repeated heart valve replacement in high-risk patients with severe mechanical hemolytic anemia: Case reports and literature review. *J Heart Valve Dis* 10:431, 2001.

67. Ward A, Clissold SP: Pentoxifylline: A review of its pharmacodynamic and pharmacokinetic properties, and its therapeutic efficacy. *Drugs* 34: 50, 1987.

68. Okita Y, Miki S: Reply to the editor. *Ann Thorac Surg* 54:7, 1992.

69. Jim RT: New therapy for cardiac valve prosthesis caused by microangiopathic hemolytic anemia: A case report. *Hawaii Med J* 47:285, 1988.

70. Golino A, Stassano P, Spampinato N: Hemolysis after open heart operations [letter]. *Ann Thorac Surg* 54:1246, 1992.

71. Geller S, Gelber R: Pentoxifylline treatment for microangiopathic hemolytic anemia caused by mechanical heart valves. *Md Med J* 48:173, 1999.

72. Golbasi I, Turkay C, Timuragaoglu A, et al: The effect of pentoxifylline on haemolysis in patients with double cardiac prosthetic valves. *Acta Cardiol* 58:379, 2003.

73. Azemoto R, Tsuchiya Y, Ai T, et al: Does gallstone formation after open cardiac surgery result only from latent hemolysis by replaced valves? *Am J Gastroenterol* 91:2185, 1996.

74. Merendino KA, Manhas DR: Man-made gallstones: A new entity following cardiac valve replacement. *Ann Surg* 177:694, 1973.

75. Harrison EC, Roschke EJ, Meyers HI, et al: Cholelithiasis: A frequent complication of artificial heart valve replacement. *Am Heart J* 95:483, 1978.

76. Ai T, Azemoto R, Saisho H: Prevention of gallstones by ursodeoxycholic acid after cardiac surgery. *J Gastroenterol* 38:1071, 2003.

77. Lam B-K, Cosgrove DM, Bhudia SK, Gillinov AM. Hemolysis after mitral valve repair: mechanisms and treatment. *Ann Thorac Surg* 77: 191, 2004.

78. Fleischer R: Ueber eine neue Form von Haemoglobinurie beim Menschen. *Berl Klin Wschr* 18:691, 1881.

79. Urabe M, Hara Y, Hokama A, et al: A female case of march hemoglobinuria induced by kendo (Japanese fencing) exercise. *Nippon Naika Gakkai Zasshi* 75:1657, 1986.

80. Gilligan A: March hemoglobinuria in a woman. *N Engl J Med* 243:944, 1950.

81. Davidson RJL. March or exertional haemoglobinuria. *Semin Hematol* 6:150, 1969.

82. Buckle RM: Exertional (march) haemoglobinuria: Reduction of haemolytic episodes by use of sorbo-rubber insoles in shoes. *Lancet* 68: 1136, 1965.

83. Sagov SE: March hemoglobinuria treated with rubber insoles: Two case reports. *J Am Coll Health Assoc* 19:146, 1970.

84. Ensor CW, Barrett JOW: Paroxysmal haemoglobinuria of traumatic origin. *Medico-Chirurgical Trans* 86:165, 1903.

85. Streeton JA: Traumatic haemoglobinuria caused by karate exercises. *Lancet* 2:191, 1967.

86. Schwartz KA, Flessa HC: March hemoglobinuria. Report of a case after basketball and congo drum playing. *Ohio State Med J* 69:448, 1973.

87. Watson EM, Fischer LC: Paroxysmal "march" haemoglobinuria with a report of a case. *Am J Clin Pathol* 5:151, 1935.

88. Pollard TD, Weiss IW: Acute tubular necrosis in a patient with march hemoglobinuria. *N Engl J Med* 283:803, 1970.

89. Susa S, Dumovic B, Pantovic R: March hemoglobinuria associated with acute renal failure. *Vojnosanit Pregl* 29:407, 1972.

90. Ciko Z, Radojicic B, Lazic D: Pathogenesis of acute renal insufficiency in march hemoglobinuria. *Vojnosanit Pregl* 30:198, 1973.

91. Yashpal M, Abdulkader TA, Chatterji JC: Acute tubular necrosis in march haemoglobinuria. *J Assoc Physicians India* 28:145, 1980.

92. Kasabach HH, Merritt KK: Capillary hemangioma with extensive purpura: Report of a case. *Am J Dis Child* 59:1063, 1940.

93. Haisley-Royster C, Enjolras O, Frieden IJ, et al: Kasabach-Merritt phenomenon: A retrospective study of treatment with vincristine. *J Pediatr Hematol Oncol* 24:459, 2002.

94. Ortel TL, Onorato JJ, Bedrosian CL, Kaufman RE: Antifibrinolytic therapy in the management of the Kasabach Merritt syndrome. *Am J Hematol* 29:44, 1988.

95. Esterly NB: Kasabach-Merritt syndrome in infants. *J Am Acad Dermatol* 8:504, 1983.

96. Hall GW: Kasabach-Merritt syndrome: Pathogenesis and management. *Br J Haematol* 112:851, 2001.

97. Stuard DI, Heusinkveld RS, Moss AJ: Microangiopathic hemolytic anemia and thrombocytopenia in primary pulmonary hypertension. *N Engl J Med* 287:869, 1972.

98. Shimizu M, Miura J, Itoh H, Saitoh Y: Hepatic giant cavernous hemangioma with microangiopathic hemolytic anemia and consumption coagulopathy. *Am J Gastroenterol* 85:1411, 1990.

99. Crummy CS, Perlin E, Moquin RB: Microangiopathic hemolytic anemia in Wegener's granulomatosis. *Am J Med* 51:544, 1971.

100. Jordan JM, Manning M, Allen NB: Multiple unusual manifestations of Wegener's granulomatosis: Breast mass, microangiopathic hemolytic

anemia, consumptive coagulopathy, and low erythrocyte sedimentation rate. *Arthritis Rheum* 29:1527, 1986.

101. Zauber NP, Echikson AB: Giant cell arteritis and microangiopathic hemolytic anemia. *Am J Med* 73:928, 1982.

102. Stratford EC, Tanaka KR: Microangiopathic hemolytic anemia in metastatic carcinoma. Report of a case and biochemical studies. *Arch Intern Med* 116:346, 1965.

103. Atkins JN, Muss HB: Case report: Schistocytes in erythroleukemia. *Am J Med Sci* 289:110, 1985.

104. Davis S, Rambotti P, Grignani F, Steinhouse K: Microangiopathic hemolytic anemia and pulmonary small-cell carcinoma [letter]. *Ann Intern Med* 103:638, 1985.

HEMOLYTIC ANEMIA RESULTING FROM CHEMICAL AND PHYSICAL AGENTS

ERNEST BEUTLER

Arsenic, lead, copper, chlorates, and a variety of other chemicals can cause severe red cell destruction, and hemolytic anemia is a part of the clinical syndrome associated with intoxication by these substances. Arsenic may cause hemolysis by interacting with sulfhydryl groups. Lead inhibits a variety of red cell enzymes, including several enzymes of porphyrin metabolism and pyrimidine 5′-nucleotidase. The anemia that it produces is usually not primarily hemolytic in nature. Copper inhibits a number of red cell enzymes and catalyzes the oxidation of intracellular reduced glutathione (GSH). Chlorates produce methemoglobin and Heinz bodies. There are many drugs that have appeared to cause hemolytic anemia, usually by unknown or poorly defined mechanisms. Animal toxins, such as those elaborated by insects, spiders, and snakes, may also cause hemolytic anemia. Hemolytic anemia is a common accompaniment of severe burns, probably as a result of direct damage to erythrocytes by heat.

Many drugs and a variety of toxins have been associated with red cell destruction. Chapters 45 and 47 discuss hemolysis that results when certain drugs are administered to patients deficient in glucose-6-phosphate dehydrogenase (G-6-PD) or with unstable hemoglobins. Immune mechanisms may also play a role in drug- or toxin-induced hemolytic anemias. Chapter 52 discusses such hemolytic anemias. Microangiopathic hemolytic anemias (see Chap. 49) may also be caused by drugs such as mitomycin.

The present chapter deals with drugs, toxins, and other physical agents that can cause red cell destruction by other mechanisms or by mechanisms that are not understood at present.

ARSENIC HYDRIDE

The inhalation of arsine gas (arsenic hydride [AsH_3]) is a well-recognized cause of hemolytic anemia.[1,2] Arsine is formed during many industrial processes. Most commonly it results from the reaction of nascent hydrogen, generated by the action of acid on metal, with arsenic compounds. The arsenic is usually present as a contaminant of either the acid or the metal, so that the contact with arsenic compounds may not be apparent from the history. Exposure to sufficient amounts of the gas will lead to severe anemia, jaundice, and hemoglobinuria. The mechanism of hemolysis is not clearly understood, although the well-known reactions of arsenic compounds with sulfhydryl groups in the cell membrane may play an important role.

Acronyms and abbreviations that appear in this chapter include: ALA, aminolevulinic acid; EDTA, ethylenediaminetetraacetic acid; G-6-PD, glucose-6-phosphate dehydrogenase; GSH, reduced glutathione; NADPH, reduced nicotinamide adenine dinucleotide phosphate.

LEAD

HISTORY

Lead poisoning (plumbism) has been recognized since antiquity. The ingestion of beverages containing lead leached from highly soluble lead glazes or earthenware containers has been blamed for the decline and fall of the Roman aristocracy and is even now an occasional cause of lead intoxication.[3] The distillation of alcohol in leaded flasks is another rare cause of plumbism in certain areas, although the practice was prohibited in 1723 by the Massachusetts Bay Colony after it was noticed that consumption of rum so distilled resulted in abdominal pain known as the "dry gripes."[3] Among the earliest published descriptions of lead poisoning is a letter written in 1786 by Benjamin Franklin,[4,5] who had learned as a printer that working over small furnaces of melted metal or drying racks of wet type in front of a fire might cause pain in the hands.

EPIDEMIOLOGY

Today, lead intoxication in children generally results from ingestion of flaking lead paint or from chewing lead-painted articles. It tends to be more severe in iron-deficient children, even when appropriate corrections are made for differing exposure.[6] Conversely a negative influence of *HFE* mutations on blood lead levels has been found.[7] In adults, it occurs primarily as the result of inhalation of lead compounds used or produced in industrial processes[8] as in battery manufacture,[9] but poisoning may occur as a result of leaching from pottery or dishes that come in contact with food.[10,11] Restoring tapestries and producing pottery and tiles[12,13] have also caused lead poisoning.

ETIOLOGY AND PATHOGENESIS

Modest shortening of red cell life span is a relatively constant feature of the disorder.[14,15] *In vitro* treatment of red cells with lead produces measurable membrane damage: lead interferes with the cation pump,[16,17] possibly in inhibiting membrane ATPase.[18,19] It is not at all clear, however, that the hemolysis observed in lead poisoning is caused by these changes. In some children with lead poisoning, an electrophoretically fast moving hemoglobin indistinguishable from hemoglobin A_3 comprises approximately 15 percent of the total pigment.[20]

The anemia of lead intoxication is not usually due primarily to hemolysis. Lead apparently interferes with the normal production of erythrocytes, probably through a combination of mechanisms. Heme synthesis is markedly abnormal in patients with lead poisoning. Several enzymes of heme synthesis are inhibited, including δ-aminolevulinic acid (ALA) synthetase, ALA dehydrase, heme synthetase, porphyrinogen deaminase, uroporphyrinogen decarboxylase, and coproporphyrinogen oxidase.[14,21] ALA dehydrase has been considered particularly sensitive to inhibition, showing decreased activity in erythrocytes at blood lead levels in the upper portions of the normal range,[18] but its sensitivity at low blood lead levels has been questioned.[22] Increased amounts of δ-aminolevulinic acid and coproporphyrin are found in the urine,[23] and the free protoporphyrin levels[24] of the erythrocytes are strikingly increased, presumably as a result of inhibition of the heme biosynthetic enzymes. It may be presumed that iron entering the developing erythroblast fails to be incorporated into heme at a normal rate, either because of lead-induced impairment of heme synthesis or because of the direct effect of lead on mitochondria.

Marked inhibition of the enzyme pyrimidine 5′-nucleotidase is also observed.[25,26] In the absence of this enzyme, pyrimidine nucleotides accumulate in the red cells and normal depolymerization of reticulocyte ribosomal RNA does not occur. In hereditary pyrimidine 5′-nucleotidase deficiency, basophilic stippling of erythrocytes is a characteristic finding (see Chap. 45), and it has been suggested that inhibition of pyrimidine 5′-nucleotidase by lead may be responsible for the basophilic stippling of erythrocytes that occurs in plumbism (see "Laboratory Findings" below). Correlation between pyrimidine 5′-nucleotidase levels in lead-exposed workers has been interpreted as a possible cause and effect relationship between the enzyme and the anemia.[27] Inhibition of activity of the hexose monophosphate shunt has been documented.[28] Synthesis of α- and β-globin chains seems to be defective in lead poisoning,[29] and this may play a contributory role in the anemia of lead poisoning.

CLINICAL FEATURES

Most patients with lead poisoning manifest some degree of anemia, although anemia is only rarely the predominant clinical manifestation.[21] However, examination of the blood often provides the key diagnostic clue, and thus the hematologic findings are of special interest. Remarkably complete observations of the acute hematologic changes occurring after the intravenous injection of lead in an attempt to treat malignant disease were published in 1928.[30] Distortion of red cells was observed both in blood films and in wet preparations made immediately after infusion of lead. This was characterized by "folding" so as to appear as semicircles, clumping, and the presence of "bite cells." The anemia of chronic lead poisoning is usually mild in the adult but is frequently more severe in children. A relatively close relationship exists between blood lead levels and the hematocrit.[31]

LABORATORY FINDINGS

The red cells are normocytic and slightly hypochromic. The hypochromia may result from coexisting iron deficiency.[32] Basophilic stippling of the erythrocytes may be fine or coarse, and the number of granules seen in each cell may be quite variable. When blood is collected in ethylenediaminetetraacetic acid (EDTA; "purple top" tube), as is commonly done, the stippling may disappear.[33] Young polychromatophilic cells are most likely to be stippled. Electron microscopic studies have demonstrated that the basophilic granules represent abnormally aggregated ribosomes.[34] Ringed sideroblasts are frequently found in the marrow (see Chap. 28). Iron-laden mitochondria are present[34] but do not appear to contribute to the basophilic stippling that is observed on light microscopy.

TREATMENT

Meso 2,3-dimercaptosuccinic acid, an orally administered chelating agent, has been used to treat lead poisoning.[35,36]

COPPER

Hemolysis has also resulted from ingestion of copper sulfate in suicide attempts and from accumulation of toxic amounts from hemodialysis fluid contaminated by copper pipes.[37,38] Hemolysis in Wilson disease has been attributed to the elevated plasma copper levels characteristic of that disorder,[39–41] and hemolytic anemia may be the presenting symptom.[42] The pathogenesis of this hemolytic anemia may be related to oxidation of intracellular reduced glutathione (GSH), hemoglobin, and reduced nicotinamide adenine dinucleotide phosphate (NADPH) and inhibition of G-6-PD by copper.[43] However, the amount of copper required to inhibit G-6-PD is large, and copper in much lower concentrations inhibits pyruvate kinase,[44] hexokinase, phosphogluconate dehydrogenase, phosphofructokinase, and phosphoglycerate kinase.[45] Plasma exchange has been used successfully to treat the hemolytic anemia of Wilson disease.[46]

CHLORATES

Sodium and potassium chlorate are oxidative drugs that have been known to produce methemoglobinemia, Heinz bodies, and hemolytic anemia.[47] While it might be presumed that the mechanism of hemolysis is similar to that resulting from other oxidative drugs, no cases have been observed in patients deficient in G-6-PD. The rare instances of chlorate poisoning that have been reported usually resulted from prescription errors in which sodium chlorate was dispensed instead of sodium chloride.[48] Hemolytic anemia with Heinz body formation has also occurred in patients undergoing dialysis when the tap water used contained a substantial amount of chloramines. Oxidative damage of the red cells of these patients was demonstrated by the presence of Heinz bodies, a positive ascorbate-cyanide test, and methemoglobinemia.[49,50] Leaching of formaldehyde from plastic used in a water filter employed for hemodialysis is also a cause of hemolytic anemia. It was suggested that the effect of the low levels of formaldehyde found in the water was not mediated through a fixative effect but rather by inducing metabolic changes in the red cells.[51]

MISCELLANEOUS DRUGS AND CHEMICALS

There are also isolated reports of hemolytic anemia occurring after the administration of a variety of other substances (Table 50-1).

Hemolytic anemia produced by phenazopyridine is often associated with "bite cells" and "blister cells."[72] When large amounts of distilled water gain access to the systemic circulation, either by intravenous injection or when used as an irrigating solution during surgery, hemolysis will occur.[73] Severe hemolysis may also result from water inhalation in near-drowning.[74]

OXYGEN

Hemolytic anemia has been observed in astronauts exposed to 100 percent oxygen; a reduction of red cell volume also occurs when the O_2 tension is maintained at normal atmospheric levels and this is believed to be due in some unknown way to weightlessness.[75] In at least one patient, hyperbaric oxygenation was associated with acute hemolysis.[76] It was suggested that hemolysis in this instance may have

TABLE 50-1   DRUGS AND CHEMICALS THAT HAVE BEEN REPORTED TO CAUSE CLINICALLY SIGNIFICANT HEMOLYTIC ANEMIA

Chemicals
   Aniline[52]
   Apiol[53]
   Dichlorprop (herbicide)[54]
   Formaldehyde[51]
   Hydroxylamines[55]
   Lysol[56]
   Mineral spirits[57]
   Nitrobenzene[58]
   Resorcin[59]
Drugs
   Amyl nitrite[60,61]
   Mephenesin[62]
   Methylene blue[63,64]
   Omeprazole[65]
   Pentachlorophenol[66]
   Phenazopyridine (Pyridium)[67,68]
   Salicylazosulfapyridine (Azulfidine)[69,70]
   Tacrolimus[71]

resulted from abnormal peroxidation of lipids in the erythrocytes, but evidence supporting this view was indirect and equivocal. Ozone, which has been widely used in some countries for a variety of therapeutic purposes, had no effect on red cell enzymes and intermediates at the 30 μg/ml concentration commonly infused, but did produce some *in vitro* hemolysis at that concentration.[77]

INSECT, SPIDER, AND SNAKE VENOMS

Bee[78,79] and wasp[80-82] stings have been associated with severe hemolysis, and spider or scorpion bites have occasionally been followed by hemolytic anemia and hemoglobinuria.[83-88] Occasionally this may occur without a discernible skin lesion.[89] The spiders usually thought to be responsible are *Loxosceles laeta* and *Loxosceles reclusa*. It is unknown why some patients suffer hemolysis after insect bites whereas others do not. The venom preferentially hydrolyzes band 3 red cell membrane protein.[90] Although snake venom may cause hemolysis *in vitro* by converting lecithin to lysolecithin (see Chap. 44), hemolysis does not often result from snake bites,[91] and when it does occur, it may represent microangiopathic hemolytic anemia associated with coagulation abnormalities induced by the venom.[92]

HEAT

It has been known for more than 100 years that heating blood to temperatures above 47°C rapidly produces visible damage to erythrocytes. The sequence of events has been defined in detail.[93] Cells damaged by heating not only show morphologic changes and increases in osmotic and mechanical fragility but are also removed rapidly after reinjection into the circulation.[94] These observations explain the severe hemolytic anemia that occurs in patients with extensive burns. Spherocytosis and increased osmotic fragility are found in many patients, and blood films may show fragmentation, budding, spherocytosis, and severe microspherocytosis. These changes are particularly evident if films are made promptly after the burn occurs. Alterations of red cell lipids have been documented,[95] but it is not clear whether these play any physiologic role in erythrocyte survival. Gross hemoglobinemia was observed in 11 of 40 patients with second- and third-degree burns involving 15 to 65 percent of the body surface.[96] It seems likely that the acute hemolytic anemia occurring within the 24 hours following a burn results from the direct effect of heat on circulating erythrocytes. Hemolysis occurring more than 24 hours after the burn may sometimes result from the infusion of isoagglutinins (particularly anti-A) in pooled plasma, when this has been administered to the patient as part of treatment,[97] or be the result of infection or coagulation disorders that are common complications of extensive burn injury.

RADIATION

Although reduced red cell survival is a part of the complex series of events occurring after administration of large doses of total body radiation,[98] erythrocytes appear to be very resistant to the direct effects of radiation.[99] Such shortened red cell survival as may occur after radiation is probably related largely to red cell loss through internal bleeding and to various secondary events such as infection.

REFERENCES

1. Phoon WH, Chan MO, Goh CH, et al: Five cases of arsine poisoning. *Ann Acad Med Singapore* 13(2 suppl):394, 1984.
2. Romeo L, Apostoli P, Kovacic M, et al: Acute arsine intoxication as a consequence of metal burnishing operations. *Am J Ind Med* 32:211, 1997.
3. Klein M, Namer R, Harpur E, Corbin R: Earthenware containers as a source of fatal lead poisoning. *N Engl J Med* 283:669, 1970.
4. *The Complete Works of Benjamin Franklin.* Putnam, New York, 1888.
5. Andreasen NJC: Benjamin Franklin: Physicus et medicus. *JAMA* 236:57, 1976.
6. Bradman A, Eskenazi B, Sutton P, et al: Iron deficiency associated with higher blood lead in children living in contaminated environments. *Environ Health Perspect* 109:1079, 2001.
7. Wright RO, Silverman EK, Schwartz J, et al: Association between hemochromatosis genotype and lead exposure among elderly men: The normative aging study. *Environ Health Perspect* 112:746, 2004.
8. Staudinger KC, Roth VS: Occupational lead poisoning. *Am Fam Physician* 57:719, 1998.
9. Froom P, Kristal-Boneh E, Benbassat J, et al: Predictive value of determinations of zinc protoporphyrin for increased blood lead concentrations. *Clin Chem* 44:1283, 1998.
10. Autenrieth T, Schmidt T, Habscheid W: Lead poisoning caused by a Greek ceramic cup. *Dtsch Med Wochenschr* 123:353, 1998.
11. Kakosy T, Hudak A, Naray M: Lead intoxication epidemic caused by ingestion of contaminated ground paprika. *J Toxicol Clin Toxicol* 34:507, 1996.
12. Fischbein A, Wallace J, Sassa S, et al: Lead poisoning from art restoration and pottery work: Unusual exposure source and household risk. *J Environ Pathol Toxicol Oncol* 11:7, 1992.
13. Vahter M, Counter SA, Laurell G, et al: Extensive lead exposure in children living in an area with production of lead-glazed tiles in the Ecuadorian Andes. *Int Arch Occup Environ Health* 70:282, 1997.
14. Waldron HA: The anaemia of lead poisoning: A review. *Br J Ind Med* 23:83, 1966.
15. Westerman MP, Pfitzer E, Ellis LD, Jensen WN: Concentrations of lead in bone in plumbism. *N Engl J Med* 273:1246, 1965.
16. Khalil-Manesh F, Tartaglia-Erler J, Gonick HC: Experimental model of lead nephropathy: IV. Correlation between renal functional changes and hematological indices of lead toxicity. *J Trace Elem Electrolytes Health Dis* 8:13, 1994.
17. Vincent PC, Blackburn CRB: The effects of heavy metal ions on the human erythrocyte: I. Comparisons of the action of several heavy metals. *Aust J Exp Biol Med Sci* 36:471, 1958.
18. Hernberg S, Nikkanen J: Enzyme inhibition by lead under normal urban conditions. *Lancet* 1:63, 1970.
19. Hasan J, Vihko V, Hernberg S: Deficient red cell membrane Na+ + K+-ATPase in lead poisoning. *Arch Environ Health* 14:313, 1967.
20. Charache S, Weatherall DJ: Fast hemoglobin in lead poisoning. *Blood* 28:377, 1966.
21. Harris JW, Kellermeyer RW: Acquired abnormality: Porphyrinuria, in *The Red Cell*, p 35. Harvard University Press, Cambridge, 1970.
22. Chalevelakis G, Bouronikou H, Yalouris AG, et al: Delta-Aminolaevulinic acid dehydratase as an index of lead toxicity. Time for a reappraisal? *Eur J Clin Invest* 25:53, 1995.
23. Goldberg A: Annotation. Lead poisoning and haem biosynthesis. *Br J Haematol* 23:521, 1972.
24. McElvaine MD, Orbach HG, Binder S, et al: Evaluation of the erythrocyte protoporphyrin test as a screen for elevated blood lead levels. *J Pediatr* 119:548, 1991.
25. Paglia DE, Valentine WN, Dahlgren JG: Effects of low-level lead exposure on pyrimidine 5′-nucleotidase and other erythrocyte enzymes. *J Clin Invest* 56:1164, 1975.
26. Aly MH, Kim HC, Renner SW, et al: Hemolytic anemia associated with lead poisoning from shotgun pellets and the response to Succimer treatment. *Am J Hematol* 44:280, 1993.

27. Kim Y, Yoo CI, Lee CR, et al: Evaluation of activity of erythrocyte pyrimidine 5'-nucleotidase (P5N) in lead exposed workers: With focus on the effect on hemoglobin. *Ind Health* 40:23, 2002.

28. Lachant N, Tomoda A, Tanaka KR: Inhibition of the pentose phosphate shunt by lead: A potential mechanism for hemolysis in lead poisoning. *Blood* 63:518, 1984.

29. White JM, Harvey DR: Defective synthesis of alpha and beta globin chains in lead poisoning. *Nature* 236:71, 1972.

30. Brookfield RW: Blood changes occurring during the course of treatment of malignant disease by lead, with special reference to punctate basophilia and the platelets. *J Pathol* 31:277, 1928.

31. Schwartz J, Landrigan PJ, Baker EL Jr, et al: Lead-induced anemia: Dose-response relationships and evidence for a threshold. *Am J Public Health* 80:165, 1990.

32. Clark M, Royal J, Seeler R: Interaction of iron deficiency and lead and the hematologic findings in children with severe lead poisoning. *Pediatrics* 81:247, 1988.

33. White JM, Selhi HS: Lead and the red cell. *Br J Haematol* 30:133, 1975.

34. Jensen WN, Moreno GD, Bessis MC: An electron microscopic description of basophilic stippling in red cells. *Johns Hopkins Med J* 25:933, 1965.

35. Berlin CMJ: Lead poisoning in children. *Curr Opin Pediatr* 9:173, 1997.

36. Miller AL: Dimercaptosuccinic acid (DMSA), a non-toxic, water-soluble treatment for heavy metal toxicity. *Altern Med Rev* 3:199, 1998.

37. Klein WJ Jr, Metz EN, Price AR: Acute copper intoxication. A hazard of hemodialysis. *Arch Intern Med* 129:578, 1972.

38. Manzler AD, Schreiner AW: Copper-induced acute hemolytic anemia. A new complication of hemodialysis. *Ann Intern Med* 73:409, 1970.

39. McIntyre N, Clink HM, Levi AJ, et al: Hemolytic anemia in Wilson's disease. *N Engl J Med* 276:439, 1967.

40. Deiss A, Lee GR, Cartwright GE: Hemolytic anemia in Wilson's disease. *Ann Intern Med* 73:413, 1970.

41. Hansen PB: Wilson's disease presenting with severe haemolytic anaemia. *Ugeskr Laeger* 150:1229, 1988.

42. Grudeva-Popova JG, Spasova MI, Chepileva KG, Zaprianov ZH: Acute hemolytic anemia as an initial clinical manifestation of Wilson's disease. *Folia Med (Plovdiv)* 42:42, 2000.

43. Fairbanks VF: Copper sulfate-induced hemolytic anemia. *Arch Intern Med* 120:428, 1967.

44. Blume KG, Hoffbauer RW, Löhr GW, Rüdiger HW: Genetische und biochemische Aspekte der Pyruvatkinase menschlicher Erythrozyten (E.C.2.7.1.40). *Verh Dtsch Ges Inn Med* 75:450, 1969.

45. Boulard M, Blume K, Beutler E: The effect of copper on red cell enzyme activities. *J Clin Invest* 51:459, 1972.

46. Kiss JE, Berman D, Van Thiel D: Effective removal of copper by plasma exchange in fulminant Wilson's disease. *Transfusion* 38:327, 1998.

47. Eysseric H, Vincent F, Peoc'h M, et al: A fatal case of chlorate poisoning: Confirmation by ion chromatography of body fluids. *J Forensic Sci* 45:474, 2000.

48. Jackson RC, Elder WJ, McDonnell H: Sodium-chlorate poisoning complicated by acute renal failure. *Lancet* 2:1381, 1961.

49. Eaton JW, Kolpin CF, Swofford HS, et al: Chlorinated urban water: A cause of dialysis-induced hemolytic anemia. *Science* 181:463, 1973.

50. Caterson RJ, Savdie E, Raik E, et al: Heinz-body haemolysis in haemodialysed patients caused by chloramines in Sydney tap water. *Med J Aust* 2:367, 1982.

51. Orringer EP, Mattern WD: Formaldehyde-induced hemolysis during chronic hemodialysis. *N Engl J Med* 294:1416, 1976.

52. Lubash GD, Phillips RE, Shields JD, Bonsnes RW: Acute aniline poisoning treated by hemodialysis. *Arch Intern Med* 114:530, 1964.

53. Lowenstein L, Ballew DH: Fatal acute haemolytic anaemia, thrombocytopenic purpura, nephrosis and hepatitis resulting from ingestion of a compound containing apiol. *Can Med Assoc J* 78:195, 1958.

54. Schroder C, Kruger E, Abel J: Acute poisoning caused by the herbicide dichlorprop (preparation SYS 67 PROP). *Kinderarztl Prax* 59:81, 1991.

55. Martin H, Woerner W, Rittmeister B: Hämolytische Anämie durch Inhalation von Hydroxylaminen. *Klin Wochenschr* 42:725, 1964.

56. Fisher B: The significance of Heinz bodies in anemias of obscure etiology. *Am J Med Sci* 143, 1955.

57. Nierenberg DW, Horowitz MB, Harris KM, James DH: Mineral spirits inhalation associated with hemolysis, pulmonary edema, and ventricular fibrillation. *Arch Intern Med* 151:1437, 1991.

58. Hunter D: Industrial toxicology. *Q J Med* 12:185, 1943.

59. Gasser VC: Perakute hamolytische Innenkorperanamie mit Methamoglobinamie nach behandlung eines Sauglingsekzems mit Resorcin. *Helvetica Paediatrica Acta* 9:285, 1954.

60. Brandes JC, Bufill JA, Pisciotta AV: Amyl nitrite-induced hemolytic anemia. *Am J Med* 86:252, 1989.

61. Graves TD, Mitchell S: Acute haemolytic anaemia after inhalation of amyl nitrite. *J R Soc Med* 96:594, 2003.

62. Pugh JI, Enderby GEH: Haemoglobinuria after intravenous myanesin. *Lancet* 2:387, 1947.

63. Poinsot J, Guillois B, Margis D, et al: Neonatal hemolytic anemia after intra-amniotic injection of methylene blue. *Arch Fr Pediatr* 45:657, 1988.

64. Sills MR, Zinkham WH: Methylene blue-induced Heinz body hemolytic anemia. *Am J Dis Child* 148:306, 1994.

65. Davidson S, Seldon M, Jones B: Omeprazole and Heinz-body haemolytic anaemia. *Aust N Z J Med* 27:441, 1997.

66. Hassan AB, Seligmann H, Bassan HM: Intravascular hemolysis induced by pentachlorophenol. *BMJ* 291:21, 1985.

67. Adams JG, Heller P, Abramson RK, Vaithianathan T: Sulfonamide-induced hemolytic anemia and hemoglobin Hasharon. *Arch Intern Med* 137:1449, 1977.

68. Greenberg MS: Heinz body hemolytic anemia. *Arch Intern Med* 136:153, 1976.

69. Kaplinsky N, Frankl O: Salicylazosulphapyridine-induced Heinz body anemia. *Acta Haematol (Basel)* 59:310, 1978.

70. Ward PCJ, Schwartz BS, White JG: Heinz-body anemia: "Bite cell" variant—A light and electron microscopic study. *Am J Hematol* 15:135, 1983.

71. Lin CC, King KL, Chao YW, et al: Tacrolimus-associated hemolytic uremic syndrome: A case analysis. *J Nephrol* 16:580, 2003.

72. Yoo D, Lessin LS: Drug-associated "bite cell" hemolytic anemia. *Am J Med* 92:243, 1992.

73. Landsteiner EK, Finch CA: Hemoglobinuria accompanying transurethral resection of the prostate. *N Engl J Med* 237:310, 1947.

74. Rath CE: Drowning hemoglobinuria. *Blood* 8:1099, 1953.

75. Tavassoli M: Anemia of spaceflight. *Blood* 60:1059, 1982.

76. Mengel CE, Kann HE Jr, Heyman A, Metz E: Effects of in vivo hyperoxia on erythrocytes: II. Hemolysis in a human after exposure to oxygen under high pressure. *Blood* 25:822, 1965.

77. Zimran A, Wasser G, Forman L, et al: Effect of ozone on red blood cell enzymes and intermediates. *Acta Haematol (Basel)* 102:148, 2000.

78. Dacie JV: *The Haemolytic Anaemias*. Grune & Stratton, New York, 1967.

79. Bresolin NL, Carvalho LC, Goes EC, et al: Acute renal failure following massive attack by Africanized bee stings. *Pediatr Nephrol* 17:625, 2002.

80. Monzon C, Miles J: Hemolytic anemia following a wasp sting. *J Pediatr* 96:1039, 1980.

81. Schulte KL, Kochen MM: Haemolytic anaemia in an adult after a wasp sting. *Lancet* 2:478, 1981.

82. Vachvanichsanong P, Dissaneewate P, Mitarnun W: Non-fatal acute renal failure due to wasp stings in children. *Pediatr Nephrol* 11:734, 1997.

83. Nance WE: Hemolytic anemia of necrotic arachnidism. *Am J Med* 31:801, 1961.

84. Madrigal GC, Ercolani RL, Wenzl JE: Toxicity from a bite of the brown spider (Loxosceles reclusus). Skin necrosis, hemolytic anemia, and hemoglobinuria in a nine-year-old child. *Clin Pediatr* 11:641, 1972.

85. Chadha JS, Leviav A: Hemolysis, renal failure, and local necrosis following scorpion sting. *JAMA* 241:1038, 1979.

86. Barretto OCO, Cardoso JL, De Cillo D: Viscerocutaneous form of loxoscelism and erythrocyte glucose-6-phosphate deficiency. *Rev Inst Med Trop Sao Paulo* 27:264, 1985.

87. Wasserman GS, Siegel C: Loxoscelism (brown recluse spider bites): A review of the literature. *Clin Toxicol* 14:353, 1979.

88. Wright SW, Wrenn KD, Murray L, Seger D: Clinical presentation and outcome of brown recluse spider bite. *Ann Emerg Med* 30:28, 1997.

89. Hostetler MA, Dribben W, Wilson DB, Grossman WJ: Sudden unexplained hemolysis occurring in an infant due to presumed Loxosceles envenomation. *J Emerg Med* 25:277, 2003.

90. Barretto OC, Satake M, Nonoyama K, Cardoso JL: The calcium-dependent protease of Loxosceles gaucho venom acts preferentially upon red cell band 3 transmembrane protein. *Braz J Med Biol Res* 36:309, 2003.

91. Reid HA: Cobra-bites. *BMJ* 2:540, 1964.

92. Gillissen A, Theakston RD, Barth J, et al: Neurotoxicity, haemostatic disturbances and haemolytic anaemia after a bite by a Tunisian saw-scaled or carpet viper (Echis "pyramidum"-complex): Failure of anti-venom treatment. *Toxicon* 32:937, 1994.

93. Ham TH, Shen SC, Fleming EM, Castle WB: Studies on the destruction of red blood cells: IV. *Blood* 3:373, 1948.

94. Wagner HN Jr, Razzak MA, Gaertner RA, et al: Removal of erythrocytes from the circulation. *Arch Intern Med* 110:90, 1962.

95. Pratt VC, Tredget EE, Clandinin MT, Field CJ: Fatty acid content of plasma lipids and erythrocyte phospholipids are altered following burn injury. *Lipids* 36:675, 2001.

96. Shen SC, Ham TH, Fleming EM: Studies on the destruction of red blood cells: III. Mechanism and complications of hemoglobinuria in patients with thermal burns: Spherocytosis and increased osmotic fragility of red blood cells. *N Engl J Med* 229:701, 1943.

97. Topley E, Bull JP, Maycock WDA, et al: The relation of the isoagglutinins in pooled plasma to the haemolytic anaemia of burns. *J Clin Pathol* 16:79, 1963.

98. Stohlman F Jr, Brecher G, Schneiderman M, Cronkite EP: The hemolytic effect of ionizing radiations and its relationship to the hemorrhagic phase of radiation injury. *Blood* 12:1061, 1957.

99. Jin YS, Anderson G, Mintz PD: Effects of gamma irradiation on red cells from donors with sickle cell trait. *Transfusion* 37:804, 1997.

HEMOLYTIC ANEMIA RESULTING FROM INFECTIONS WITH MICROORGANISMS

ERNEST BEUTLER

Hemolytic anemia is a prominent part of the clinical presentation of patients infected with organisms such as the malaria parasites, *Babesia*, and *Bartonella*, which directly invade the erythrocyte. Malaria is probably the most common cause of hemolytic anemia on a worldwide basis, and much has been learned about how the parasite enters the erythrocyte. Falciparum malaria, in particular, can cause severe and sometimes fatal hemolysis (blackwater fever). Other organisms cause hemolytic anemia by producing a hemolysin (e.g., *Clostridium Welchii*), by stimulating an immune response (e.g., *Mycoplasma pneumoniae*), by enhancing macrophage recognition and hemophagocytosis, or by as yet unknown mechanisms. The many different infections that have been associated with hemolytic anemia are tabulated and references to the original studies provided.

Shortening of erythrocyte life span occurs commonly in the course of inflammatory and infectious diseases. This may occur particularly in patients with glucose-6-phosphate dehydrogenase (G-6-PD) deficiency (see Chap. 45), splenomegaly (see Chap. 55), and in the microvascular fragmentation syndrome (see Chap. 121). In some infections, however, rapid destruction of erythrocytes represents a prominent part of the overall clinical picture (Table 51-1). This chapter deals only with the latter states.

Several distinct mechanisms may lead to hemolysis during infections.[49] These include direct invasion of erythrocytes by the infecting organism, as in malaria, babesiosis, and bartonellosis; elaboration of hemolytic toxins, as by *Clostridium perfringens*; and development of antibodies either autoantibodies against red cell antigens or deposition of microbial antigens or immune complexes on erythrocytes.[50]

MALARIA

Known since antiquity, malaria is the world's most common cause of hemolytic anemia.[36] After the host is bitten by an infected female *Anopheles* mosquito, the sporozoites invade the liver and possibly other internal organs in the asymptomatic tissue stage of malaria. Merozoites, emerging at first from the tissues and later from previously parasitized red cells, bind to glycophorins A and B by means of a 175-kDa protein that has been designated the erythrocyte binding antigen (EBA-175).[51-53] A complex series of events, not yet fully understood, eventuates in invasion of the interior of the red cell by the parasite.[35,51]

Acronyms and abbreviations that appear in this chapter include: CR, complement receptor; EBA, erythrocyte binding antigen; ICAM, intercellular adhesion molecule; PfEMP, *Plasmodium falciparum* erythrocyte membrane protein; VCAM, vascular cell adhesion molecule.

Having entered the erythrocyte, the parasite grows intracellularly, nourished by the cell's contents. Erythrocytes infected with *Plasmodium falciparum* develop surface knobs[54,55] that contain receptors, especially the *P. falciparum* erythrocyte membrane protein-1 (PfEMP1), for endothelial proteins. All parasites bind to CD36 antigen (platelet glycoprotein IV) and thrombospondin found on endothelial surfaces, whereas some bind to the intercellular adhesion molecule-1 (ICAM-1), and a few bind to the vascular cell adhesion molecule (VCAM)[56-60] and mediate the adherence of parasitized cells to endothelium. Rosetting of parasitized cells with unparasitized cells also occurs through another mechanism mediated by complement receptor-1 (CR1) on uninfected erythrocytes.[61] One of the membrane proteins of *P. falciparum* binds specifically to the spectrin on the inner surface of the red cell membrane.[62] A large number of genetic polymorphisms that interfere with invasion of erythrocytes by parasites and their proliferation have developed in areas where malaria has been a leading cause of death for many generations.[61,63-65] These include G-6-PD deficiency, Southeast Asian ovalocytosis, CR1, the thalassemias, and hemoglobinopathies.

Plasmodium vivax invades only young red cells, while *P. falciparum* attacks both young and old cells. Thus, anemia tends to be more severe in the latter form of malaria.[35] The degree to which anemia develops often seems to be out of proportion to the number of cells infected with the parasite; the reason for this apparent destruction of uninvaded cells is not clear. Osmotic fragility is increased in nonparasitized cells as well as cells containing plasmodia.[66] The erythrocyte cation permeability is altered in monkeys with malaria.[67] Positive Coombs' tests have been reported, but the role of antibodies in the etiology of the anemia is not clear.[68] It has been suggested that oxidative damage to red cell lipids occurs[69,70] and that there is an abnormality in the phosphorylation of membranes of parasitized red cells.[71] *Plasmodium falciparum*-infected red cells have a highly irregular surface defect. This may be produced by the intracellular growth of the plasmodium, or it could represent the site of parasite entry. Nonparasitized cells often have similar surface defects,[72] suggesting a phenomenon known to occur in simian malaria,[73] the "pitting" of parasites from an infected cell.

Destruction of parasitized red cells appears to occur largely in the spleen, and splenomegaly is typically present in chronic malarial infection. The "pitting" of parasites from infected erythrocytes may also occur in the spleen.[74] The fever associated with malaria is characteristically cyclic, varying in frequency according to the malaria type. Although classic periodicity is often absent, febrile paroxysms of *P. vivax* malaria tend to occur every 48 hours, those of *P. malariae* infection occur each 72 hours, and those of *P. falciparum* malaria, daily. Falciparum malaria is occasionally associated with particularly severe hemolysis and may result in the passage of dark, almost black, urine. This disorder, also called blackwater fever, is no longer common. At one time it was seen frequently among Europeans in Africa and in India, usually after quinine was given to treat malaria. The relative roles of the malarial infection and of the drug have never been clarified.[75]

Diagnosis of malaria depends upon demonstration of the parasites on the blood film[76] (see Color Plates I-11,12) or demonstration of the appropriate DNA sequences in the blood.[77,78] The morphologic differentiation of *P. falciparum* from other forms of malaria, principally *P. vivax*, is clinically important since *P. falciparum* infection may constitute a clinical emergency. If more than 5 percent of the red cells infected contain parasites, the infection is almost certainly with *P. falciparum*. In an infection with this organism, rings are practically the only form of parasite evident on the blood film. The finding of two or more rings within the same red cells is regarded as pathognomic of *P. falciparum*.[78]

Eradication of blood forms is achieved with quinine, chloroquine,

TABLE 51-1 ORGANISMS CAUSING HEMOLYTIC ANEMIA

Aspergillus[1]
Bacillus anthracis[2]
Babesia microti and *Babesia divergens*[3]
Bartonella bacilliformis[4,5]
Campylobacter jejuni[6,7]
Clostridium welchii[8,9]
Coxsackie virus[10]
Cytomegalovirus[11]
Diplococcus pneumoniae[12]
Epstein-Barr virus[13,14]
Escherichia coli[15,16]
Fusobacterium necrophorum[17]
Haemophilus influenzae[12,23]
Hepatitis A[18–20]
Hepatitis B[19,21]
Hepatitis C[22]
Herpes simplex virus[10]
Human immunodeficiency virus[24–26] (see Chap. 83)
Influenza A virus[27,28]
Leishmania donovani[30]
Leptospira ballum and/or *Leptospira butembo*[29]
Mumps virus[31]
Mycobacterium tuberculosis[12,32]
Mycoplasma pneumoniae[33]
Neisseria intracellularis (meningococci)[12]
Parvovirus B19[34]
Plasmodium falciparum[35]
Plasmodium malariae[35]
Plasmodium vivax[36]
Rubella virus[37,38]
Rubeola virus[10]
Salmonella[12,39]
Shigella[40,41]
Streptococcus[12,42–45]
Toxoplasma[12]
Trypanosoma brucei[46]
Varicella virus[10,47]
Vibrio cholerae[12]
Yersinia enterocolitica[48]

or various sulfones or sulfonamides given together with pyrimethamine. Tissue stages of vivax malaria are effectively treated with primaquine. This drug, as well as certain sulfones used in the treatment of malaria, produces severe hemolysis in patients with G-6-PD deficiency (see Chap. 45).

When acute, unusually severe hemolysis occurs in the course of falciparum malaria (blackwater fever), the physician should be certain that a hemolytic drug is not being administered to a G-6-PD–deficient individual. Transfusions may be needed with severe hemolysis, and if renal failure occurs, extracorporeal dialysis may be required. With early institution of therapy the prognosis in malaria is excellent. However, when treatment is delayed or the strain is resistant to the administered agent, falciparum malaria may follow a rapid fatal course.

BARTONELLOSIS (OROYA FEVER)

In 1885, Daniel A. Carrión, a medical student, inoculated himself with blood obtained from a verrucous node of the skin of a patient with verruca peruviana. He developed a fatal hemolytic anemia with the characteristics of Oroya fever, a disease that had first been observed

some years earlier among workers in a railroad construction project near the city of Oroya in the Peruvian Andes. This fatal self-experiment established the identity of the verrucosa form and the hemolytic phase of human bartonellosis, an infection that now bears the name Carrión's disease.[5] Human bartonellosis is transmitted by the sand fly. The red blood cells become infected with *Bartonella bacilliformis*. It is believed that the organism does not grow within the red cell but rather adheres to its exterior surface: when infected red cells are washed with citrated plasma, free organisms are found but the red cells are not hemolyzed. In hanging-drop cultures, masses of organisms are clearly seen outside the erythrocytes, while the cells themselves are intact.[79] The osmotic fragility of the red cells is normal.[5] They are rapidly removed from the circulation, apparently both by liver and spleen. Normal red cells transfused into patients with bartonellosis meet a similar fate.[4] A 130-kD *Bartonella* protein that causes erythrocytes to acquire trenches, indentations, and invaginations has been purified from culture broths and has been called *deformin*.[80] In addition, two *Bartonella bacilliformis* genes, designated *ialA* and *ialB*, predicted to encode polypeptides of 170 amino acids (20.1 kDa) and of 186 amino acids (19.9 kDa), respectively, have been shown to greatly enhance the ability of *Escherichia coli* to invade erythrocytes.[81]

As demonstrated by Carrión's experiment, bartonellosis has two clinical stages. The acute hemolytic anemia, *Oroya fever*, represents the early, invasive stage of a chronic granulomatous disorder, the late stage of which is designated *verruca peruviana*. Most patients manifest no clinical symptoms during the Oroya fever phase, but when anemia does occur, its onset is dramatic. Red counts as low as 750,000/ μL have been documented.[82] In addition to symptoms of anemia, patients manifest thirst, anorexia, sweating, and generalized lymphadenopathy. Spleen and liver enlargement is unusual. Large numbers of nucleated red cells appear in the blood film, and reticulocytosis is often striking. The white cell count is variable. Diagnosis is established by demonstrating the presence of the organism *B. bacilliformis* on the erythrocytes. Giemsa-stained blood films reveal red-violet rods varying in length from 1 to 3 μm and in width from 0.25 to 0.2 μm.

The mortality rate among untreated patients is very high, but those who do survive undergo a sudden transitional period in which the *Bartonellae* change from an elongated to a coccoid form, the number of parasitized cells decreases, and the red cell count increases. Lymphocytosis and a right shift in the granulocyte series are observed with disappearance of the fever and abatement of other symptoms. Oroya fever responds well to treatment with penicillin, streptomycin, chloramphenicol, and the tetracyclines. The second stage of *Bartonella* infection, verruca peruviana, is a nonhematologic disorder characterized by an eruption over the face and extremities developing into bleeding warty tumors.

Other species of *Bartonella* cause febrile infections such as "cat-scratch fever," but these disorders are not ordinarily associated with severe hemolytic anemia.[83]

BABESIOSIS

Babesia are intraerythrocytic protozoa known as piroplasms. They are transmitted by ticks that may infect many species of wild and domestic animals. Humans occasionally become infected with *Babesia microti* or *Babesia divergens*, species that normally parasitize rodents and cattle, respectively.[84] Other *Babesia*-like piroplasms, such as WA1, first isolated from a patient in the state of Washington, and MO-1, isolated in Missouri, may also produce human disease.[85] Once thought to be rare, babesiosis is being recognized with increasing frequency.[86,87] The disease is usually tick-borne in man but has also been transmitted by transfusion.[88–93] Presumably because of the distribution of the vector, in the United States the disease is most common in the Northeastern coastal region where it became known as "Nantucket fever," but has also been encountered in the Midwest.[94] Infections with *B. divergens* usually occur in splenectomized patients, but this is not the case with *B. microti* infections.[3]

The disease generally has a gradual onset with malaise, anorexia, and fatigue, followed by fever, sweats, and muscle and joint pains. A moderate degree of hemolytic anemia is usually present; on occasion it has been sufficiently severe to cause hypotension,[95] and transfusion has occasionally been required.[84] Parasites can be seen in the red cells in Giemsa-stained thin blood films (see Color Plate I-10). Serologic tests for antibodies to *Babesia* have been described,[96] and polymerase chain reaction-based diagnostic tests are also available.[3] It has responded to chemotherapy with clindamycin and quinine,[97] but failure to respond to antibiotics has also been encountered.[89] A combination of atovaquone-azithromycin has also been suggested as treatment.[85,98] Whole-blood exchange was used with a marked improvement.[88]

CLOSTRIDIUM WELCHII

Clostridium perfringens (welchii) sepsis is most likely to occur in patients who have undergone septic abortion. It has also been observed following acute cholecystitis[99] and as a result of an intrahepatic abscess.[9] The α toxin of *C. welchii* is a lecithinase that may react with lipoprotein complexes at cell surfaces, liberating potent hemolytic substances, lysolecithins. It has also been suggested that erythrocyte membrane proteolysis plays an important role in hemolysis.[100] Severe, often fatal hemolysis occurs in patients with *C. welchii* septicemia. Striking hemoglobinemia and hemoglobinuria occur. The serum may become a brilliant red, and the urine is a dark brown mahogany color. The high plasma hemoglobin may produce a marked dissociation between the blood hemoglobin and hematocrit level. Microspherocytosis is prominent, and leukocytosis with a left shift as well as thrombocytopenia are often present. Acute renal and hepatic failure usually develops, and the prognosis is grave; more than half of the patients die, even with extensive treatment (see Chap. 121).[8,101] Therapy consists of high-dose penicillin and surgical debridement.[102]

OTHER INFECTIONS

A variety of other infections have occasionally been associated with hemolytic anemia. The mechanisms involved vary. Some organisms, among them such common pathogens as *Haemophilus influenzae*, *E. coli*, and *Salmonella* species, can produce red cell agglutination *in vitro*, but it is not known whether this phenomenon is important in initiating *in vivo* hemolysis.[103] Bacteria may also produce destruction of red cells indirectly when bacterial polysaccharides are adsorbed onto erythrocytes. Action of an antibody directed against the antigen-coated cells results in their agglutination[104] or in complement-mediated lysis.[23] The unmasking of T-type antigens by bacteria renders the cell polyagglutinable. This may be a rare cause of hemolysis occurring in the course of bacterial infections.[105,106]

Many different types of microorganisms may play a role in precipitating autoimmune hemolytic disease (see Chap. 52). In one study of 234 patients,[10] 55 were found to have an antecedent bacterial infection, 18 of these exhibiting an "unequivocal etiologic relationship" of infection to anemia. However, the principal evidence for such a relationship was a temporal one. A number of viral agents, including measles, cytomegalovirus, varicella, herpes simplex, influenza A and B, Epstein-Barr, human immunodeficiency virus[24–26] (see Chap. 83), and coxsackie virus have also been associated with immune hemolytic disease.[10,107] Various mechanisms have been postulated, including absorption of immune complexes and complement, cross-reacting antigen, and a true autoimmune state with possible loss of tolerance secondary to the infectious organism.[10] Histopathologic and sometimes virologic evidence of infection with cytomegalovirus has been reported in a high percentage of children with lymphadenopathy and hemolytic anemia.[108] A positive antiglobulin reaction was demonstrated in some of these patients, and it has been suggested that some cases of "idiopathic autoimmune hemolytic anemia" are in reality due to cytomegalovirus infection.[108]

The high cold agglutinin titer that sometimes develops in the course of *Mycoplasma pneumoniae* pneumonia (see Chap. 52) may occasionally result in hemolytic anemia[1,33] or compensated hemolysis, although most patients with high cold agglutinin titers do not become anemic. The red cells of a number of patients with kala azar were found to be agglutinated with anticomplement and anti-non–γ-globulin serum.[30] Both splenic and hepatic sequestration of red cells appears to occur in this disease.[13]

Microangiopathic hemolytic anemia is discussed in detail in Chapter 49. This disorder may be triggered by a variety of infections, some of which are caused by well-characterized organisms such as species of *Shigella*,[109,110] *Campylobacter*,[111] and *Aspergillus*.[1]

REFERENCES

1. Robboy SJ, Salisbury K, Ragsdale B, et al: Mechanism of aspergillus-induced microangiopathic hemolytic anemia. *Arch Intern Med* 128:790, 1971.

2. Freedman A, Afonja O, Chang MW, et al: Cutaneous anthrax associated with microangiopathic hemolytic anemia and coagulopathy in a 7-month-old infant. *JAMA* 287:869, 2002.

3. Pruthi RK, Marshall WF, Wiltsie JC, Persing DH: Human babesiosis. *Mayo Clin Proc* 70:853, 1995.

4. Reynafarje C, Ramos J: The hemolytic anemia of human bartonellosis. *Blood* 17:562, 1961.

5. Ricketts WE: Bartonella bacilliformis anemia (Oroya fever). A study of thirty cases. *Blood* 3:1025, 1948.

6. Smith MA, Shah NR, Lobel JS, Hamilton W: Methemoglobinemia and hemolytic anemia associated with Campylobacter jejuni enteritis. *Am J Pediatr Hematol Oncol* 10:35, 1988.

7. Damani NN, Humphrey CA, Bell B: Haemolytic anaemia in Campylobacter enteritis. *J Infect* 26:109, 1993.

8. Rogstad B, Ritland S, Lunde S, Hagen AG: *Clostridium perfringens* septicemia with massive hemolysis. *Infection* 21:54, 1993.

9. Kreidl KO, Green GR, Wren SM: Intravascular hemolysis from a Clostridium perfringens liver abscess. *J Am Coll Surg* 194:387, 2002.

10. Pirofsky B: Infectious disease and autoimmune hemolytic anemia, in *Autoimmunization and the Autoimmune Hemolytic Anemias*, p 147. Waverly Press, Baltimore, 1969.

11. van Spronsen DJ, Breed WP: Cytomegalovirus-induced thrombocytopenia and haemolysis in an immunocompetent adult. *Br J Haematol* 92: 218, 1996.

12. Dacie JV: Secondary or symptomatic hemolytic anemias, in *The Haemolytic Anaemias, Part III*, edited by JV Dacie, p 908. Grune & Stratton, New York, 1967.

13. Tonkin AM, Mond HG, Alford FP, Hurley TH: Severe acute haemolytic anaemia complicating infectious mononucleosis. *Med J Aust* 2:1048, 1973.

14. Whitelaw F, Brook MG, Kennedy N, Weir WR: Haemolytic anaemia complicating Epstein-Barr virus infection. *Br J Clin Pract* 49:212, 1995.

15. Ludwig K, Ruder H, Bitzan M, et al: Outbreak of Escherichia coli O157: H7 infection in a large family. *Eur J Clin Microbiol Infect Dis* 16:238, 1997.

16. Pennings CM, Seitz RC, Karch H, Lenard HG: Haemolytic anaemia in association with Escherichia coli O157 infection in two sisters. *Eur J Pediatr* 153:656, 1994.

17. Chand DH, Brady RC, Bissler JJ: Hemolytic uremic syndrome in an adolescent with Fusobacterium necrophorum bacteremia. *Am J Kidney Dis* 37:E22, 2001.

18. Gundersen SG, Bjoerneklett A, Bruun JN: Severe erythroblastopenia and hemolytic anemia during a hepatitis A infection. *Scand J Infect Dis* 21:225, 1989.

19. Kanematsu T, Nomura T, Higashi K, Ito M: Hemolytic anemia in association with viral hepatitis. *Nippon Rinsho Jpn J Clin Med* 54:2539, 1996.

20. Urganci N, Akyildiz B, Yildirmak Y, Ozbay G: A case of autoimmune hepatitis and autoimmune hemolytic anemia following hepatitis A infection. *Turk J Gastroenterol* 14:204, 2003.

21. Gurgey A, Yuce A, Ozbek N, Kocak N: Acute hemolysis in association with hepatitis B infection in a child with beta-thalassemia trait. *Turk J Pediatr* 36:259, 1994.

22. Etienne A, Gayet S, Vidal F, et al: Severe hemolytic anemia due to cold agglutinin complicating untreated chronic hepatitis C: Efficacy and safety of anti-CD20 (rituximab) treatment. *Am J Hematol* 75:243, 2004.

23. Shurin SB, Anderson P, Zollinger J, Rathbun RK: Pathophysiology of hemolysis in infections with Hemophilus influenzae type B. *J Clin Invest* 77:1340, 1986.

24. Rheingold SR, Burnham JM, Rutstein R, Manno CS: HIV infection presenting as severe autoimmune hemolytic anemia with disseminated intravascular coagulation in an infant. *J Pediatr Hematol Oncol* 26:9, 2004.

25. Koduri PR, Singa P, Nikolinakos P: Autoimmune hemolytic anemia in patients infected with human immunodeficiency virus-1. *Am J Hematol* 70:174, 2002.

26. Saif MW: HIV-associated autoimmune hemolytic anemia: An update. *AIDS Patient Care STDS* 15:217, 2001.

27. Watanabe T: Hemolytic uremic syndrome associated with influenza A virus infection. *Nephron* 89:359, 2001.

28. Asaka M, Ishikawa I, Nakazawa T, et al: Hemolytic uremic syndrome associated with influenza A virus infection in an adult renal allograft recipient: Case report and review of the literature. *Nephron* 84:258, 2000.

29. Trowbridge AA, Green JB III, Bonnett JD, et al: Hemolytic anemia associated with leptospirosis. Morphologic and lipid studies. *Am J Clin Pathol* 76:493, 1981.

30. Woodruff AW, Topley E, Knight R, Downie CGB: The anaemia of kala azar. *Br J Haematol* 22:319, 1972.

31. Ozen S, Damarguc I, Besbas N, et al: A case of mumps associated with acute hemolytic crisis resulting in hemoglobinuria and acute renal failure. *J Med* 25:255, 1994.

32. Kuo PH, Yang PC, Kuo SS, Luh KT: Severe immune hemolytic anemia in disseminated tuberculosis with response to antituberculosis therapy. *Chest* 119:1961, 2001.

33. Fiala M, Myhre BA, Chinh LT, et al: Pathogenesis of anemia associated with Mycoplasma pneumoniae. *Acta Haematol (Basel)* 51:297, 1974.

34. Chambers LA, Rauck AM: Acute transient hemolytic anemia with a positive Donath-Landsteiner test following parvovirus B19 infection. *J Pediatr Hematol Oncol* 18:178, 1996.

35. Weatherall DJ, Miller LH, Baruch DI, et al: Malaria and the red cell. *Hematology (Am Soc Hematol Educ Program)* 35, 2002.

36. White NJ: The treatment of malaria. *N Engl J Med* 335:800, 1996.

37. Moriuchi H, Yamasaki S, Mori K, et al: A rubella epidemic in Sasebo, Japan in 1987, with various complications. *Acta Paediatr Jpn* 32:67, 1990.

38. Yoneda S, Yoshikawa M, Yamane Y, et al: A case of rubella complicated by hemolytic anemia. *Kansenshogaku Zasshi* 74:724, 2000.

39. Albaqali A, Ghuloom A, Al Arrayed A, et al: Hemolytic uremic syndrome in association with typhoid fever. *Am J Kidney Dis* 41:709, 2003.

40. Houdouin V, Doit C, Mariani P, et al: A pediatric cluster of Shigella dysenteriae serotype 1 diarrhea with hemolytic uremic syndrome in 2 families from France. *Clin Infect Dis* 38:e96, 2004.

41. Kavaliotis J, Karyda S, Konstantoula T, et al: Shigellosis of childhood in northern Greece: Epidemiological, clinical and laboratory data of hospitalized patients during the period 1971-1996. *Scand J Infect Dis* 32: 207, 2000.

42. Shepherd AB, Palmer AL, Bigler SA, Baliga R: Hemolytic uremic syndrome associated with group A beta-hemolytic streptococcus. *Pediatr Nephrol* 18:949, 2003.

43. Apilanez UM, Areses TR, Ruiz Benito MA, et al: Hemolytic uremic syndrome secondary to Streptococcus pneumoniae pulmonary infection. *An Esp Pediatr* 57:378, 2002.

44. Reynolds E, Espinoza M, Monckeberg G, Graf J: Hemolytic-uremic syndrome and Streptococcus pneumoniae. *Rev Med Chil* 130:677, 2002.

45. Brandt J, Wong C, Mihm S, et al: Invasive pneumococcal disease and hemolytic uremic syndrome. *Pediatrics* 110:371, 2002.

46. Wéry M, Mulumba PM, Lambert PH, Kazyumba L: Hematologic manifestations, diagnosis, and immunopathology of African trypanosomiasis. *Semin Hematol* 19:83, 1982.

47. Papalia MA, Schwarer AP: Paroxysmal cold haemoglobinuria in an adult with chicken pox. *Br J Haematol* 109:328, 2000.

48. Von Knorring J, Pettersson T: Haemolytic anaemia complicating Yersinia enterocolitica infection. Report of a case. *Scand J Haematol* 9:149, 1972.

49. Berkowitz FE: Hemolysis and infection: Categories and mechanisms of their interrelationship. *Rev Infect Dis* 13:1151, 1991.

50. Seitz RC, Buschermohle G, Dubberke G, et al: The acute infection-associated hemolytic anemia of childhood: Immunofluorescent detection of microbial antigens altering the erythrocyte membrane. *Ann Hematol* 67:191, 1993.

51. Pasvol G, Clough B, Carlsson J: Malaria and the red cell membrane. *Blood Rev* 6:183, 1992.

52. Orlandi PA, Klotz FW, Haynes JD: A malaria invasion receptor, the 175-kilodalton erythrocyte binding antigen of Plasmodium falciparum recognizes the terminal Neu5Ac(alpha 2-3)Gal-sequences of glycophorin A. *J Cell Biol* 116:901, 1992.

53. Sim BKL, Chitnis CE, Wasniowska K, et al: Receptor and ligand domains for invasion of erythrocytes by *Plasmodium falciparum. Science* 264:1941, 1994.

54. Nakamura K, Hasler T, Morehead K, et al: Plasmodium falciparum-infected erythrocyte receptor(s) for CD36 and thrombospondin are restricted to knobs on the erythrocyte surface. *J Histochem Cytochem* 40: 1419, 1992.

55. Aikawa M, Kamanura K, Shiraishi S, et al: Membrane knobs of unfixed Plasmodium falciparum infected erythrocytes: New findings as revealed by atomic force microscopy and surface potential spectroscopy. *Exp Parasitol* 84:339, 1996.

56. Newbold C, Warn P, Black G, et al: Receptor-specific adhesion and clinical disease in Plasmodium falciparum. *Am J Trop Med Hyg* 57:389, 1997.

57. Baruch DI, Ma XC, Singh HB, et al: Identification of a region of PfEMP1 that mediates adherence of Plasmodium falciparum infected erythrocytes to CD36: Conserved function with variant sequence. *Blood* 90:3766, 1997.

58. Pasloske BL, Howard RJ: Malaria, the red cell, and the endothelium. *Annu Rev Med* 45:283, 1994.

59. Udomsangpetch R, Taylor BJ, Looareesuwan S, et al: Receptor specificity of clinical Plasmodium falciparum isolates: Nonadherence to cell-bound E-selectin and vascular cell adhesion molecule-1. *Blood* 88:2754, 1996.

60. McCormick CJ, Craig A, Roberts D, et al: Intercellular adhesion molecule-1 and CD36 synergize to mediate adherence of Plasmodium falciparum-infected erythrocytes to cultured human microvascular endothelial cells. *J Clin Invest* 100:2521, 1997.

61. Cockburn IA, MacKinnon MJ, O'Donnell A, et al: A human comple-

ment receptor 1 polymorphism that reduces Plasmodium falciparum rosetting confers protection against severe malaria. *Proc Natl Acad Sci U S A* 101:272, 2004.

62. Herrera S, Rudin W, Herrera M, et al: A conserved region of the MSP-1 surface protein of *Plasmodium falciparum* contains a recognition sequence for erythrocyte spectrin. *EMBO J* 12:1607, 1993.

63. Mombo LE, Ntoumi F, Bisseye C, et al: Human genetic polymorphisms and asymptomatic Plasmodium falciparum malaria in Gabonese schoolchildren. *Am J Trop Med Hyg* 68:186, 2003.

64. Clegg JB, Weatherall DJ: Thalassemia and malaria: New insights into an old problem. *Proc Assoc Amer Phys* 111:278, 1999.

65. Zimmerman PA, Patel SS, Maier AG, et al: Erythrocyte polymorphisms and malaria parasite invasion in Papua New Guinea. *Trends Parasitol* 19:250, 2003.

66. George JN, Wicker DJ, Fogel BJ, et al: Erythrocytic abnormalities in experimental malaria. *Proc Soc Exp Biol Med* 124:1086, 1967.

67. Overman RR: Reversible cellular permeability alterations in disease. In vivo studies on sodium, potassium and chloride concentrations in erythrocytes of the malarious monkey. *Am J Physiol* 152:113, 1948.

68. Lefrancois G, Bras JL, Simonneau M, et al: Anti-erythrocyte autoimmunisation during chronic falciparum malaria. *Lancet* 1:661, 1981.

69. Clark IA, Hunt NH: Evidence for reactive oxygen intermediates causing hemolysis and parasite death in malaria. *Infect Immun* 39:1, 1983.

70. Stocker R, Cowden WB, Tellan RL, et al: Lipids from *Plasmodium vinckei*-infected erythrocytes and their susceptibility to oxidative damage. *Lipids* 22:51, 1987.

71. Yuthavong Y, Limpaiboon T: The relationship of phosphorylation of membrane proteins with the osmotic fragility and filterability of Plasmodium berghei-infected mouse erythrocytes. *Biochim Biophys Acta* 929:278, 1987.

72. Balcerzak SP, Arnold JD, Martin DC: Anatomy of red cell damage by Plasmodium falciparum in man. *Blood* 40:98, 1972.

73. Conrad ME: Pathophysiology of malaria. Hematologic observations in human and animal studies. *Ann Intern Med* 70:134, 1969.

74. Angus BJ, Chotivanich K, Udomsangpetch R, White NJ: In vivo removal of malaria parasites from red blood cells without their destruction in acute falciparum malaria. *Blood* 90:2037, 1997.

75. Zuckerman A: Autoimmunization and other types of indirect damage to host cells as factors in certain protozoan diseases. *Exp Parasitol* 15:138, 1964.

76. Anthony RL, Bangs MJ, Anthony JM, Purnomo: On-site diagnosis of Plasmodium falciparum, P. vivax, and P. malariae by using the quantitative buffy coat system. *J Parasitol* 78:994, 1992.

77. Weiss JB: DNA probes and PCR for diagnosis of parasitic infections. *Clin Microbiol Rev* 8:113, 1995.

78. Oliveira DA, Holloway BP, Durigon EL, et al: Polymerase chain reaction and a liquid-phase, nonisotopic hybridization for species-specific and sensitive detection of malaria infection. *Am J Trop Med Hyg* 52:139, 1995.

79. Aldana L: Bacteriologia de la enfermedad de carrion. *Cronica Med* 46:235, 1929.

80. Xu YH, Lu ZY, Ihler GM: Purification of deformin, an extracellular protein synthesized by Bartonella bacilliformis which causes deformation of erythrocyte membranes. *Biochim Biophys Acta* 1234:173, 1995.

81. Mitchell SJ, Minnick MF: Characterization of a two-gene locus from Bartonella bacilliformis associated with the ability to invade human erythrocytes. *Infect Immun* 63:1552, 1995.

82. Weinman D: Human Bartonella infection and African sleeping sickness. *Bull N Y Acad Med* 22:647, 1946.

83. Patel UD, Hollander H, Saint S: Clinical problem-solving. Index of suspicion. *N Engl J Med* 350:1990, 2004.

84. Reubush TK II, Cassaday PB, Marsh HJ, et al: Human babesiosis on Nantucket Island. *Ann Intern Med* 86:6, 1977.

85. Krause PJ: Babesiosis. *Med Clin North Am* 86:361, 2002.

86. Krause PJ, McKay K, Gadbaw J, et al: Increasing health burden of human babesiosis in endemic sites. *Am J Trop Med Hyg* 68:431, 2003.

87. Herwaldt BL, McGovern PC, Gerwel MP, et al: Endemic babesiosis in another eastern state: New Jersey. *Emerg Infect Dis* 9:184, 2003.

88. Jacoby GA, Hunt JV, Kosinski KS, et al: Treatment of transfusion-transmitted babesiosis by exchange transfusion. *N Engl J Med* 303:1098, 1980.

89. Smith RP, Evans AT, Popovsky M, et al: Transfusion-acquired babesiosis and failure of antibiotic treatment. *JAMA* 256:2726, 1986.

90. Herwaldt BL, Kjemtrup AM, Conrad PA, et al: Transfusion-transmitted babesiosis in Washington State: First reported case caused by a WA1-type parasite. *J Infect Dis* 175:1259, 1997.

91. Nelson R: Blood on demand. *Am Heritage Invention Technol* 19:24, 2004.

92. Dobroszycki J, Herwaldt BL, Boctor F, et al: A cluster of transfusion-associated babesiosis cases traced to a single asymptomatic donor. *JAMA* 281:927, 1999.

93. Kjemtrup AM, Lee B, Fritz CL, et al: Investigation of transfusion transmission of a WA1-type babesial parasite to a premature infant in California. *Transfusion* 42:1482, 2002.

94. Steketee RW, Eckman MR, Burgess EC, et al: Babesiosis in Wisconsin. A new focus of disease transmission. *JAMA* 253:2675, 1985.

95. Cheng D, Yakobi-Shvilli R, Fernandez J: Life-threatening hypotension from babesiosis hemolysis. *Am J Emerg Med* 20:367, 2002.

96. Chisholm ES, Sulzer AJ, Ruebush TK II: Indirect immunofluorescence test for human Babesia microti infection: Antigenic specificity. *Am J Trop Med Hyg* 35:921, 1986.

97. Wittner M, Rowin KS, Tanowitz HB, et al: Successful chemotherapy of transfusion babesiosis. *Ann Intern Med* 96:601, 1982.

98. Weiss LM: Babesiosis in humans: A treatment review. *Expert Opin Pharmacother* 3:1109, 2002.

99. Clancy MT, OBriain S: Fatal Clostridium welchii septicaemia following acute cholecystitis. *Br J Surg* 62:518, 1975.

100. Simpkins H, Kahlenberg A, Rosenberg A, et al: Structural and compositional changes in the red cell membrane during Clostridium welchii infection. *Br J Haematol* 21:173, 1971.

101. Mahn HE, Dantuono LM: Postabortal septicotoxemia due to Clostridium welchii. *Am J Obstet Gynecol* 70:604, 1955.

102. Moustoukas NM, Nichols RL, Voros D: Clostridial sepsis: Unusual clinical presentations. *South Med J* 78:440, 1985.

103. Neter E: Bacterial hemagglutination and hemolysis. *Bacteriol Rev* 20:166, 1956.

104. Ceppellini R, De Gregorio M: Crisi emolitica in animali batterio-immuni transfusi con sangue omologo sensibilizzato in vitro mediante l'antigene batterico specifico. *Boll Ist Sieroter Milan* 32:445, 1953.

105. Dausset J, Moullec J, Bernard J: Acquired hemolytic anemia with polyagglutinability of red blood cells due to a new factor. *Blood* 14:1079, 1959.

106. Klein PJ, Vierbuchen M, Roth B, et al: Hemolytic anemia in infections caused by neuraminidase-producing bacteria. *Verh Dtsch Ges Pathol* 67:415, 1983.

107. McGinniss MH, Macher AM, Rook AH, Alter HJ: Red cell autoantibodies in patients with acquired immune deficiency syndrome. *Transfusion* 26:405, 1986.

108. Zuelzer WW, Stulberg CS, Page RH, et al: The Emily Cooley lecture. Etiology and pathogenesis of acquired hemolytic anemia. *Transfusion* 6:438, 1966.

109. Ullis KC, Rosenblatt RM: Shiga bacillus dysentery complicated by bacteremia and disseminated intravascular coagulation. *J Pediatr* 83:90, 1973.

110. Chesney R, Kaplan BS: Hemolytic-uremic syndrome with shigellosis. *J Pediatr* 84:312, 1974.

111. Dickgiesser A: Campylobacter infection and the hemolytic-uremic syndrome. *Immun Infekt* 11:71, 1983.

HEMOLYTIC ANEMIA RESULTING FROM IMMUNE INJURY

CHARLES H. PACKMAN

Autoimmune hemolytic anemia (AHA) is characterized by shortened red blood cell (RBC) survival and the presence of autoantibodies directed against autologous RBCs. A positive direct antiglobulin test (DAT, also known as the Coombs test) is essential for diagnosis. Most patients with AHA (80%) exhibit warm-reactive antibodies of the IgG isotype. Most of the remainder of patients exhibit cold-reactive autoantibodies. Two types of cold-reactive autoantibodies to RBCs are recognized: cold agglutinins and cold hemolysins. Cold agglutinins are generally of IgM isotype, whereas cold hemolysins usually are of IgG isotype. The DAT may detect IgG, proteolytic fragments of complement (mainly C3), or both on the RBCs of patients with warm-antibody AHA. In cold-antibody AHA, only complement is detected because the antibody dissociates from the RBCs during washing of the cells. About half of patients with AHA have no underlying associated disease; these cases are termed primary or idiopathic. Secondary cases are associated with underlying autoimmune, malignant, or infectious diseases or with ingestion of certain drugs.

Although most patients do not require transfusion of RBCs, transfusion should not be withheld from those with symptomatic anemia. In warm-antibody AHA, glucocorticoids are effective in slowing the rate of hemolysis. Splenectomy is indicated for patients who require an unacceptably high maintenance dose or prolonged administration of glucocorticoids. Intravenous immunoglobulin may provide short-term control of hemolysis. Immunosuppressive drugs and danazol have been used successfully in refractory cases. In cold agglutinin- and cold hemolysin-mediated hemolysis, keeping the patient warm and treating underlying lymphoproliferative disorders usually are effective. Rituximab has been effective in reported cases of both warm and cold AHA. Drug-immune hemolytic anemia usually is ameliorated by discontinuation of the offending drug.

DEFINITION AND HISTORY

The two main features of immune red blood cell (RBC) injury are (1) shortened RBC survival *in vivo* and (2) evidence of host antibodies reactive with autologous RBCs, most frequently demonstrated by a positive direct antiglobulin test (DAT), also known as the Coombs test. Most cases in adults are mediated by warm-reactive autoantibodies. A smaller proportion of patients exhibit cold-reactive autoantibodies or drug-related antibodies.

Acronyms and abbreviations that appear in this chapter include: AHA, autoimmune hemolytic anemia; CLL, chronic lymphocytic leukemia; DAF, decay-accelerating factor; DAT, direct antiglobulin test; HIV, human immunodeficiency virus; HLA, human leukocyte antigen; HRF, homologous restriction factor; HS, hereditary spherocytosis; IAT, indirect antiglobulin test; Ig, immunoglobulin; PNH, paroxysmal nocturnal hemoglobinuria; RBC, red blood cell; SLE, systemic lupus erythematosus.

By the early 20th century, reticulocytes, spherocytes, and osmotic fragility of RBCs had been described. Clinicians could diagnose hemolytic anemia, but the distinction between congenital and acquired forms was imprecise. Some clinicians even doubted the existence of acquired hemolytic anemia.[1] The sera of some patients with hemolytic anemia directly agglutinated saline suspensions of normal or autologous human RBCs. These serum factors, later shown to be specific antibodies (largely of the immunoglobulin [Ig]M class), were termed *direct* or *saline agglutinins*. In a smaller proportion of cases, the patients' sera could mediate lysis of the test RBCs in the presence of fresh serum as a complement source. The heat-stable factors (antibodies) necessary for *in vitro* complement-mediated lysis were called *hemolysins*. However, in the majority of cases of hemolytic anemia, neither direct agglutinins nor hemolysins could be demonstrated. In 1945, Coombs and colleagues[2] reported that RBCs coated with nonagglutinating Rh antibodies (now known to be of the IgG isotype) could be agglutinated by rabbit antiserum to human γ-globulin. That is, the rabbit antiglobulin serum cross-linked IgG antibody-coated RBCs to produce visible agglutination. Addition of rabbit antiglobulin serum to a suspension of washed RBCs isolated from patients with suspected autoimmune hemolytic anemia (AHA) produced agglutination in many cases, including those patients lacking saline agglutinins or hemolysins. RBCs from patients with congenital hemolytic anemia did not agglutinate.[3,4] This procedure now is termed the *direct antiglobulin (Coombs) test*. Subsequent studies established that positive direct antiglobulin reactions in AHA are attributable to coating of the RBCs with immunoglobulins (mainly IgG) and/or complement proteins. When the RBCs are coated chiefly with complement proteins, a positive DAT depends upon the presence of anticomplement (principally anti-C3) in the antiglobulin reagent.

Cryopathic hemolytic syndromes are caused by autoantibodies that bind RBCs optimally at temperatures less than 37°C (98.6°F) and usually less than 31°C (87.8°F). Two major types of "cold antibody" may produce AHA. Cold agglutinins mediate cold agglutinin disease. The Donath-Landsteiner autoantibody, which is not an agglutinin but a potent hemolysin, mediates paroxysmal cold hemoglobinuria. In both cryopathic syndromes, the complement system plays a major role in RBC injury; however, much greater potential exists for direct intravascular hemolysis than in warm-antibody–mediated AHA.

Cold agglutinins were first described by Landsteiner[5] in 1903. However, recognition of the connection among cold agglutinins, hemolytic anemia, and Raynaud-like peripheral vascular phenomena evolved slowly. In 1918, Clough and Richter[6] detected cold agglutinins in a patient with pneumonia. In 1925 and 1926, Iwai and Mei-Sai[7,8] reported two patients with cold agglutinins and Raynaud phenomenon and showed that flow of blood through capillary tubes *in vitro* or in superficial capillaries *in vivo* was impeded at low temperatures. During the late 1940s and early 1950s, the observations of many workers gradually established the pathogenic importance of cold agglutinins in RBC injury. Schubothe[9] introduced the term *cold agglutinin disease* in 1953 and clearly distinguished the disorder from other acquired hemolytic syndromes.

In current usage, cold agglutinin disease pertains to patients with chronic AHA in which the autoantibody directly agglutinates human RBCs at temperatures below body temperature, maximally at 0 to 5°C (32–41°F). Fixation of complement to a patient's RBCs by cold agglutinins *in vivo* occurs at higher temperatures but generally less than 37°C (98.6°F). Cold agglutinins typically are IgM, although occasionally they may be immunoglobulins of other isotypes. The cold agglutinins in chronic cold agglutinin disease generally are monoclonal. Most cold agglutinins have specificity for oligosaccharide antigens (I or i) of the RBC (see "Origin of Cold Agglutinins" below).

Donath and Landsteiner first described the cold hemolysin that bears their name in 1904. The Donath-Landsteiner antibody is responsible for complement-mediated hemolysis in paroxysmal cold hemoglobinuria, a very rare form of AHA in adults. The disorder is characterized by recurrent episodes of massive hemolysis following cold exposure.[10,11] A related form of hemolytic anemia occurs much more commonly in children (or young adults) as an acute, self-limited hemolytic process following several types of viral syndromes.[10,12–16] The disease was recognized during the latter half of the 19th century, when the disease was more common because of its association with congenital or tertiary syphilis. With the advent of effective therapy for syphilis, this cause of paroxysmal cold hemoglobinuria has almost disappeared. Now, recurrent paroxysmal cold hemoglobinuria occurs very rarely in a chronic idiopathic form.[10,11] An increasing proportion of Donath-Landsteiner autoantibody-mediated hemolytic anemias occurs as a single postviral episode in children, without recurrent attacks (paroxysms). The prognosis for such cases is excellent. Thus, rather than paroxysmal cold hemoglobinuria, a proposed term for this latter entity is *Donath-Landsteiner hemolytic anemia*.[13,14]

The first example of drug-related immune blood cell destruction was Ackroyd's description of Sedormid purpura in 1949.[17] In 1953, Snapper and coworkers[18] described a case of immune hemolysis and pancytopenia in a patient treated with mephenytoin (Mesantoin). Hemolysis ceased upon withdrawal of the drug. In 1956, Harris[19] reported what are now classic studies of a patient who developed immune hemolytic anemia during a second course of stibophen administered for treatment of schistosomiasis. Since then, many drugs have been implicated in the production of positive DATs and accelerated RBC destruction.

CLASSIFICATION

AHA can be classified in two complementary ways (Table 52-1). The majority of cases (80–90% in adults) are mediated by warm-reactive autoantibodies[10,11,20] or antibodies displaying optimal reactivity with human RBCs at 37°C (98.6°F). A smaller proportion of cases is attributable to cold-reactive autoantibodies exhibiting greater affinity for RBCs at temperatures less than 37°C (98.6°F). The distinction is important, not only because of differences in the pathophysiology of RBC injury but also in the therapeutic approaches required. An even smaller proportion of patients with AHA exhibit both cold-reactive and warm-reactive autoantibodies,[21,22] which apparently recognize different antigens on the RBC membrane.[23] RBC destruction is generally more severe in mixed cases.

Classification of AHA based on the presence or absence of underlying diseases also is useful (see Table 52-1). When no recognizable underlying disease is present, the AHA is termed *primary* or *idiopathic*. When AHA appears to be a manifestation or complication of an underlying disorder, the term *secondary AHA* is applied. Lymphocytic malignancies, particularly chronic lymphocytic leukemia (CLL) and lymphomas, account for about half of all secondary AHA cases and for the majority of AHA cases mediated by cold agglutinins.[24] Systemic lupus erythematosus (SLE) and other autoimmune diseases account for a lesser but considerable proportion of secondary AHA cases. A large proportion of patients with mixed cold and warm autoantibodies have SLE.[21,22] Infectious mononucleosis and *Mycoplasma pneumoniae* occasionally are associated with cryopathic AHA. Despite the frequent occurrence of immune thrombocytopenia and positive DATs in patients infected with the human immunodeficiency virus (HIV), AHA is relatively rare in these patients.[25–27] Table 52-1 lists other associated diseases that are less commonly reported. The etiologic and pathogenic significance of these associations is poorly understood, but most of the associated diseases involve components of the immune system, either by neoplasia or by aberrant immunopathologic responses.

TABLE 52-1   CLASSIFICATION OF HEMOLYTIC ANEMIA AS A RESULT OF IMMUNE INJURY

I. Warm-autoantibody type: autoantibody maximally active at body temperature (37°C)
   A. Primary or idiopathic warm AHA
   B. Secondary warm AHA
      1. Associated with lymphoproliferative disorders (e.g., Hodgkin disease, lymphoma)
      2. Associated with the rheumatic disorders, particularly SLE
      3. Associated with certain nonlymphoid neoplasms (e.g., ovarian tumors)
      4. Associated with certain chronic inflammatory diseases (e.g., ulcerative colitis)
      5. Associated with ingestion of certain drugs (e.g., α-methyldopa)
II. Cold-autoantibody type: autoantibody optimally active at temperatures <37°C
   A. Mediated by cold agglutinins
      1. Idiopathic (primary) chronic cold agglutinin disease
      2. Secondary cold agglutinin hemolytic anemia
         a. Postinfectious (e.g., *Mycoplasma pneumoniae* or infectious mononucleosis)
         b. Associated with malignant B cell lymphoproliferative disorder
   B. Mediated by cold hemolysins
      1. Idiopathic (primary) paroxysmal cold hemoglobinuria (very rare)
      2. Secondary
         a. Donath-Landsteiner hemolytic anemia, usually associated with an acute viral syndrome in children (relatively common)
         b. Congenital or tertiary syphilis in adults (very rare)
III. Mixed cold and warm autoantibodies
   A. Primary or idiopathic mixed AHA
   B. Secondary mixed AHA
      1. Associated with the rheumatic disorders, particularly SLE
IV. Drug-immune hemolytic anemia
   A. Hapten or drug adsorption mechanism
   B. Ternary (immune) complex mechanism
   C. True autoantibody mechanism

Certain drugs also mediate immune injury to RBCs, and three general mechanisms are recognized (see Table 52-1 and Fig. 52-1). This classification is based on the effector mechanism of RBC injury, because the induction mechanism for formation of drug-related RBC antibodies is unknown. Two of the mechanisms, hapten/drug adsorption and ternary complex formation, involve drug-dependent antibodies. In the third mechanism, the drugs in question appear to induce formation of true autoantibodies capable of reacting with human RBCs in the absence of the inciting drug. These types of drug-mediated immune injury to RBCs often are referred to collectively as *drug-immune hemolytic anemia* to distinguish them from *de novo* AHA. Distinguishing among the mechanisms is not always possible, and some cases involve a combination of mechanisms. In addition, drug-related nonimmunologic protein adsorption by RBCs may result in a positive DAT without actual RBC injury. This phenomenon should be distinguished from the other three forms of drug-immune RBC injury. Table 52-2 lists drugs documented to cause either immune injury or a positive DAT.

EPIDEMIOLOGY

The annual incidence of warm-antibody AHA is one per 75,000 to 80,000 population.[11] Estimates of the frequency of primary (idiopathic) AHA vary from 20 to 80 percent of all types of AHA, depending on the referral patterns of the reporting center.[11,20,105,106] In general, AHA is considered secondary (1) when AHA and the underlying disease occur together with greater frequency than can be accounted for by chance alone; (2) when the AHA reverses simulta-

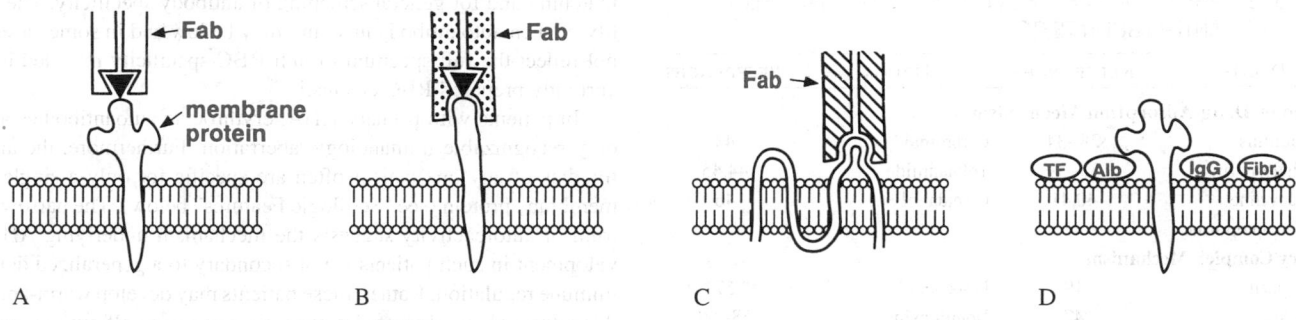

FIGURE 52-1   Effector mechanisms by which drugs mediate a positive direct antiglobulin test. Relationships of drug, antibody-combining site, and red blood cell membrane protein are shown. Panels *A*, *B*, and *C* show only a single immunoglobulin Fab region (bearing one combining site). *(A)* Drug adsorption/hapten mechanism. The drug (▼) binds avidly to an unknown red blood cell membrane protein *in vivo*. Antidrug antibody (usually IgG) binds to the protein-bound drug. The membrane protein is not known to be part of the epitope recognized by the antidrug antibody. The direct antiglobulin test (with anti-IgG) detects IgG antidrug antibody on the patient's circulating (drug-coated) red blood cells. The indirect antiglobulin test detects antibody in the patient's serum only when the test red blood cells have been previously coated with the drug by incubation *in vitro*. *(B)* Ternary complex mechanism. Drug binds loosely or in undetectable amounts to red blood cell membrane. However, in the presence of appropriate antidrug antibody, a stable trimolecular (ternary) complex is formed by drug, red blood cell membrane protein, and antibody. In general, the antibody-combining site (Fab) recognizes both drug and membrane protein components but binds only weakly to either drug or protein unless both are present in the reaction mixture. In this mechanism, the direct antiglobulin test typically detects only red blood cell–bound complement components (e.g., C3 fragments) that are bound covalently and in large number to the patient's red blood cells *in vivo*. The antibody itself escapes detection, possibly because of its low concentration but also because washing of the red cells (in the antiglobulin test procedure) apparently dissociates antibody and drug from the cells, leaving only the covalently bound C3 fragments. The indirect antiglobulin test also detects complement proteins on the test red blood cells when both antibody (patient serum) and a complement source (fresh patient serum or fresh normal serum) are present in the reaction mixture together with the drug. *(C)* Autoantibody induction. Some drug-induced antibodies can bind avidly to red blood cell membrane proteins (usually Rh proteins) in the absence of the inducing drug and are indistinguishable from the autoantibodies of patients with autoimmune hemolytic anemia. The direct antiglobulin test detects the IgG antibody on the patient's red blood cells. The indirect antiglobulin test usually detects antibody in the serum of patients with active hemolysis. *(D)* Drug-induced nonimmunologic protein adsorption. Certain drugs cause plasma proteins to attach nonspecifically to the red blood cell membrane. The direct antiglobulin test detects nonspecifically bound IgG and complement components. If special antiglobulin reagents are used, other plasma proteins, such as transferrin, albumin, and fibrinogen, also may be detected. In contrast to the other mechanisms of drug-induced red blood cell injury, this mechanism does not shorten red blood cell survival *in vivo*.

neously with correction of the associated disease; or (3) when AHA and the associated disease are related by evidence of immunologic aberration.[11] Using these criteria, the frequency of primary warm-antibody AHA probably is closer to 50 percent of all cases. Careful followup of patients with primary AHA is essential, because hemolytic anemia may be the presenting finding in a patient who subsequently develops overt evidence of an underlying disorder. For example, in one series, 18 of 107 patients with AHA developed a malignant lymphoproliferative disorder at a median of 26.5 months after diagnosis of the AHA.[107]

Warm-antibody AHA has been diagnosed in people of all ages, from infants to the elderly. The majority of patients are older than 40 years, with peak incidence around the seventh decade. This age distribution probably reflects, in part, the increased frequency of lymphoproliferative malignancies in the elderly, resulting in an age-related increase in the frequency of secondary AHA. Although multiple cases are occasionally observed in families,[108–110] most cases of primary AHA arise sporadically. Development of AHA does not have an apparent association with any particular HLA haplotype or other genetic factor.

Cold agglutinin disease is less common than warm-antibody AHA, with a prevalence of approximately 14 per million,[24] accounting for only 10 to 20 percent of all cases of AHA.[10,11,111] Women are affected more commonly than men..[10,11] No genetic or racial factors are known to contribute to the pathogenesis of this disease.

Secondary cold agglutinin disease is seen most commonly in adolescents or young adults as a self-limited process associated with *M. pneumoniae* infections or infectious mononucleosis and, rarely, in children with chickenpox. The term also has been used to describe a chronic disorder occurring in older patients with known malignant lymphoproliferative diseases. On the other hand, idiopathic (primary) chronic cold agglutinin disease has its peak incidence after age 50 years. This disorder, with its characteristic monoclonal IgM cold agglutinins, may be considered a special form of monoclonal gammopathy. Nearly all of these patients exhibit clonal B lymphocyte proliferation.[24] As with other "essential" or idiopathic monoclonal gammopathies, some patients in this group gradually develop features of a B cell lymphoproliferative disorder resembling Waldenström macroglobulinemia. Thus, the distinction between primary and secondary types of chronic cold agglutinin disease is not absolute.

Although the majority of patients with mycoplasma pneumonia have significant cold agglutinin titers, they only infrequently develop clinical hemolytic anemia.[112–114] However, subclinical RBC injury may occur. In one series of *M. pneumoniae* infections, weakly positive direct antiglobulin reactions and/or mild reticulocytosis were noted in the absence of anemia in a substantial number of cases.[112] Cold agglutinins occur in more than 60 percent of patients with infectious mononucleosis, but again hemolytic anemia is rare.[115–117]

Medical centers that receive many referrals report that paroxysmal cold hemoglobinuria constitutes 2 to 5 percent of all cases of AHA.[10,11] Among children, however, Donath-Landsteiner hemolytic anemia accounted for 32.4 percent of 68 immune hemolytic syndromes diagnosed over a 4-year period.[15] Commonly, the diagnosis is missed because of lack of physicians' awareness or failure to perform the proper serologic studies (see "Serologic Features" below).[12,15] Thus, the true incidence may be higher. Although familial occurrence has been reported, no racial or genetic risk factors are known.[10] As noted, most childhood cases follow either specific viral infections or upper respiratory infections of undefined etiology.[10–15]

Older series report that drug-immune hemolytic anemia accounts

TABLE 52-2   ASSOCIATION BETWEEN DRUGS AND POSITIVE DIRECT ANTIGLOBULIN TESTS

Drugs	References	Drugs	References
Hapten or Drug Adsorption Mechanism			
Penicillins	28–34	Carbromal	43
Cephalosporins	35–39	Tolbutamide	44,45
Tetracycline	40,41	Cianidanol	46
6-Mercaptopurine	42		
Ternary Complex Mechanism			
Stibophen	19	Probenecid	57
Quinine	47	Nomifensine	58–60
Quinidine	48,49	Cephalosporins	37–39,61
Chlorpropamide	50,51	Diethylstilbestrol	62
Rifampicin	52,53	Amphotericin B	63
Antazoline	54	Doxepin	64
Thiopental	55	Diclofenac	65,66
Tolmetin	56	Etodolac	67
Autoantibody Mechanism			
Cephalosporins	39	Cianidanol	46
Tolmetin	56	Latamoxef	79
Nomifensine	58	Glafenine	79
α-Methyldopa	68–71	Procainamide	80
L-Dopa	72–76	Diclofenac	65,81
Mefenamic acid	77,78	Pentostatin	82
Teniposide	79	Fludarabine	83
		Chlorodeoxyadenosine	84
Nonimmunologic Protein Adsorption			
Cephalosporins	85,86	Cisplatin	87
Uncertain Mechanism of Immune Injury			
Mesantoin	18	Streptomycin	95
Phenacetin	47	Ibuprofen	96
Insecticides	88	Triamterene	97
Chlorpromazine	89	Erythromycin	98
Melphalan	90	5-Fluorouracil	99
Isoniazid	91	Nalidixic acid	100
p-Aminosalicylic acid	92	Sulindac	101
Acetaminophen	93	Omeprazole	102
Thiazides	94	Temafloxacin	103
		Carboplatin	104

for 12 to 18 percent of immune hemolytic anemias.[11] The disorder is much less common now that α-methyldopa and mega-unit doses of penicillin are rarely used. The current incidence of drug-immune hemolytic anemia is estimated at one per million population, approximately 88 percent of which result from the second- and third-generation cephalosporins, cefotetan, and ceftriaxone.[118]

ETIOLOGY AND PATHOGENESIS

ETIOLOGY

WARM-ANTIBODY AUTOIMMUNE HEMOLYTIC ANEMIA
The etiology of AHA is unknown. In warm-antibody AHA, the autoantibodies that mediate RBC destruction are predominantly (but not exclusively) IgG globulins possessing relatively high binding affinity for human RBCs at 37°C. As a result, the major share of plasma autoantibody is bound to the patient's circulating RBCs. Eluates prepared from the patient's washed, autoantibody-coated RBCs constitute an important source of purified autoantibody for investigation of specificity, immunoglobulin structure, or other properties. In addition, sera from patients with warm AHA often are used in blood banks for cross-

matching and for general screening of antibody specificity. The quantity of such autoantibody in serum may be low and in some cases may not reflect the full spectrum of anti-RBC specificity revealed in concurrently prepared RBC eluates.[119]

In patients with primary AHA, erythrocyte autoantibodies are the only recognizable immunologic aberration. Furthermore, the autoantibodies of any one patient often are specific for only a single RBC membrane protein (see "Serologic Features" below). The narrow spectrum of autoreactivity suggests the mechanism underlying AHA development in such patients is not secondary to a generalized defect in immune regulation. Rather, these patients may develop warm-antibody AHA through an aberrant immune response to a self-antigen or to an immunogen that mimics a self-antigen.

In patients with secondary AHA, the disease may be associated with a fundamental disturbance in the immune system, for example, when in the setting of lymphoma, CLL, SLE, primary agammaglobulinemia (common variable immunodeficiency), or hyper-IgM immunodeficiency syndrome. In these settings, warm-antibody AHA most likely arises through an underlying defect in immune regulation, although the contribution of an aberrant immune response to self-antigen cannot be excluded. AHA seems especially frequent in patients with low-grade lymphoma or CLL treated with fludarabine[83] or 2-chlorodeoxyadenosine (cladribine).[84] The T lymphocytopenia induced by these drugs may exacerbate the preexisting tendency of patients to form autoantibodies.

A still unexplained observation is that certain drugs, such as α-methyldopa, can induce warm-reacting IgG anti-RBC autoantibodies in otherwise normal persons. The autoantibodies induced by α-methyldopa have Rh-related serologic[120] and immunochemical[121] specificity similar to that of autoantibodies arising in many patients with "spontaneous" AHA. A critical difference is that the drug-associated autoantibodies subside when the drug is discontinued, suggesting that (1) the latent potential to form this type of anti-RBC autoantibody is present in many immunologically normal individuals, and (2) the steps required to generate such autoantibodies do not necessarily create a sustained autoimmune state. On the other hand, maintenance of chronic idiopathic AHA may be either secondary to a continuing (but unknown) stimulus or induced by a short stimulus to which the patient continues to respond.

Normal subjects sometimes have a positive DAT when they volunteer to donate blood.[122,123] The positive DAT in these normal donors often results from warm-reacting IgG autoantibodies, similar in serologic specificity[119] and in IgG subclass[122] to the autoantibodies occurring in AHA. Although many of these donors remain Coombs positive without developing overt hemolytic anemia, a few have been documented to develop AHA.[122,123] The prevalence of positive DATs in normal blood donors is approximately one in 10,000.[122,124] Because blood donation *per se* likely does not contribute to an increased risk of developing autoantibodies, the one in 10,000 proportion likely is the approximate frequency of positive DATs in the entire population. A substantial proportion of patients who present with clinically overt primary AHA may come from a subset of asymptomatic individuals who are innately DAT positive, but this notion is not established.

Several concepts have been developed to explain immunologic tolerance to self-antigens.[125–127] Relevant to warm-antibody AHA, membrane-bound antigens expressed in a multivalent array at high concentration may induce tolerance by effecting clonal deletion of autoreactive B cells.[128] Both the Rh-related and the non-Rh types of RBC antigens targeted by AHA autoantibodies (see "Serologic Features" below) are expressed normally by human fetal erythrocytes, as early as 10 to 12 weeks of life.[129] However, because new B cells develop daily in the marrow throughout life and because B cells may somatically mutate their Ig receptors, self-tolerance in the B cell compartment is never assured. Analogy to observations in NZB mice[130,131] suggests the peritoneal cavity is a privileged compartment that shelters autoreactive B cells from host RBC, allowing them to escape deletion, later to produce anti-RBC autoantibodies with appropriate T cell help.[132] The strong predominance of IgG antibodies in AHA suggests B cell isotype switching, which is consistent with the idea of an antigen-driven process. Moreover, because T cell help is necessary for inducing B cell isotype switching, the pathway(s) to autoantibody induction in AHA also may involve an abnormal or unique mode of antigen presentation to T cells.[133]

ORIGIN OF COLD AGGLUTININS

A high proportion of monoclonal IgM cold agglutinins with either anti-I or anti-i specificity have heavy-chain variable regions encoded by V_H4-34, formerly designated $V_H4.21$.[134–136] This V_H gene encodes a distinct idiotype identified by the rat monoclonal antibody 9G4. This idiotype is expressed both by the cold agglutinins themselves and on the surface immunoglobulin of B cells synthesizing cold agglutinins or related immunoglobulins possessing V_H4-34 sequences.[137] Using the 9G4 monoclonal antibody as a probe, this idiotype was found not only in a very high proportion of circulating B cells and marrow lymphoplasmacytoid cells of patients with lymphoma-associated chronic cold agglutinin disease but also in a smaller proportion of B cells in the blood and lymphoid tissues of normal adult donors and in the spleens of 15-week human fetuses.[137] These data suggest B cells expressing the V_H4-34 gene (or a closely related sequence) are present throughout ontogeny. Therefore, chronic cold agglutinin disease may represent a marked, unregulated expansion of a subset (clone) of such B cells.

Light-chain V-region gene use in anti-I cold agglutinins is highly selective. A strong bias toward use of the κ III variable region subgroup (V_κ-III) is observed.[135,138] Light-chain selection among anti-i cold agglutinins, however, is much more variable and includes the lambda type.[135,139]

Observations that pathologic cold agglutinins are synthesized with distinct and highly selected V-region sequences must be viewed against the background of two other subsequent observations. First, V_H4-34 or related V_H genes also may encode the heavy-chain variable regions of other types of antibodies, such as rheumatoid factor autoantibodies and alloantibodies to a variety of blood group antigens, including polypeptide determinants such as Rh.[140] Second, normal human antibodies to an exogenous carbohydrate antigen, *Haemophilus influenzae* type b capsular polysaccharide, also are encoded by a restricted set of V_H genes[141] and Ig light-chain V genes.[142] Thus, regulation of Ig gene use for production of anti-I or anti-i cold agglutinins may not differ fundamentally from normal antibody formation to other carbohydrate antigens.

In the setting of B cell lymphoma or Waldenström macroglobulinemia, cold agglutinins may be produced by the malignant clone itself. Two patients with lymphoma and monoclonal cold agglutinin were identified as having a karyotypically abnormal B cell clone that produced a cold agglutinin identical to that found in their sera.[143,144] Trisomy 3 has been the most frequently observed karyotypic abnormality in patients with non-Hodgkin lymphoma and cold agglutinins.[143–145]

Normal human sera generally have naturally occurring cold agglutinins in low titer (usually 1/32 or less). Otherwise healthy persons may develop elevated titers of cold agglutinins specific for I/i antigens during certain infections (e.g., *M. pneumoniae*, Epstein-Barr virus, cytomegalovirus). In contrast to other forms of cold agglutinin disease, hyperproduction of these postinfectious cold agglutinins is transient. Some evidence indicates postinfectious cold agglutinins may be less clonally restricted than those occurring in chronic cold agglutinin dis-

ease,[146] but this finding is not universal.[147] Whether V_H4-34 also encodes most heavy-chain variable regions of all naturally occurring or postinfectious cold agglutinins remains to be determined.

The increased production of cold agglutinins in response to infection with *M. pneumoniae* may be secondary to the fact that the oligosaccharide antigens of the I/i type serve as specific *Mycoplasma* receptors.[148] This process may lead to altered antigen presentation involving a complex between a self-antigen (I/i) and a non–self-antigen (*Mycoplasma*). Alternatively, the anti-i cold agglutinins may arise as a consequence of polyclonal B cell activation, as occurs in infectious mononucleosis (see Chap. 84).

The mechanism(s) whereby dissimilar infectious agents (e.g., spirochetes and several types of virus) induce the immune system to produce Donath-Landsteiner antibodies with specificity for the human P blood group antigen (see "Serologic Features" below) is not known.

PATHOGENESIS

PATHOGENIC EFFECTS OF WARM ANTIBODIES

Warm autoantibodies to RBCs in AHA are pathogenic. In contrast to autologous RBCs, labeled RBCs lacking the antigen targeted by the autoantibodies may survive normally in patients with warm-antibody AHA.[10,149,150] Furthermore, transplacental passage of IgG anti-RBC autoantibodies from a mother with AHA to the fetus can induce intrauterine or neonatal hemolytic anemia.[151] Finally, despite notable exceptions and differences related to IgG subclass of the autoantibody, in general, an inverse relationship between the quantity of RBC-bound IgG antibody and RBC survival is noted in serial studies performed on a given patient.[152–157]

In warm-antibody AHA, the patient's RBCs typically are coated with IgG autoantibodies with or without complement proteins. Autoantibody-coated RBCs are trapped by macrophages in the Billroth cords of the spleen and, to a lesser extent, by Kupffer cells in the liver (see Chap. 67).[149,152,153,155–159] The process leads to generation of spherocytes and fragmentation and ingestion of antibody-coated RBCs.[160,161] The macrophage has surface receptors for the Fc region of IgG, with preference for the IgG1 and IgG3 subclasses[162,163] and surface receptors for opsonic fragments of C3 (C3b and C3bi) and C4b.[164–166] When present together on the RBC surface, IgG and C3b/C3bi appear to act cooperatively as opsonins to enhance trapping and phagocytosis.[155,156,165–169] Although RBC sequestration in warm-antibody AHA occurs primarily in the spleen,[149,156–158] very large quantities of RBC-bound IgG[152,153,159] or the concurrent presence of C3b on the RBCs[152,155,156] may favor trapping in the liver.

Interaction of a trapped RBC with splenic macrophages may result in phagocytosis of the entire cell. More commonly, a type of partial phagocytosis results in spherocyte formation. As RBCs adhere to macrophages via the Fc receptors, portions of RBC membrane are internalized by the macrophage. Because membrane is lost in excess of contents, the noningested portion of the RBC assumes a spherical shape, the shape with the lowest ratio of surface area to volume.[160,161,170] Spherical RBCs are more rigid and less deformable than normal RBCs. As such, spherical RBCs are fragmented further and eventually destroyed in future passages through the spleen. Spherocytosis is a consistent and diagnostically important hallmark of AHA,[171] and the degree of spherocytosis correlates well with the severity of hemolysis.[10]

Direct complement-mediated hemolysis with hemoglobinuria is unusual in warm-antibody AHA, even though many warm autoantibodies fix complement. The failure of C3b-coated RBCs to be hemolyzed by the terminal complement cascade (C5–C9) has been attributed, at least in part, to the ability of complement regulatory proteins (factors I and H) in plasma and C3b receptors on the RBC surface to alter the hemolytic function of cell-bound C3b and C4b.[172] Glycosyl-phosphatidylinositol-linked erythrocyte membrane proteins, such as decay-accelerating factor ([DAF] CD55) and homologous restriction factor ([HRF] CD59), may limit the action of autologous complement on autoantibody-coated RBCs.[173-175] DAF inhibits the formation and function of cell-bound C3-converting enzyme,[173] thus indirectly limiting formation of C5-converting enzyme. HRF, on the other hand, impedes C9 binding and formation of the C5b–9 membrane attack complex.[174]

Cytotoxic activities of macrophages and lymphocytes also may play a role in the destruction of RBCs in warm-antibody AHA. Monocytes can lyse IgG-coated RBCs *in vitro* independently of phagocytosis.[176,177] Cell-bound complement is neither necessary nor sufficient for such cytotoxicity, but bound C3b/C3d can potentiate the effects of IgG.[177] In one study, cytotoxicity, but not phagocytosis, was inhibited by hydrocortisone *in vitro*.[176] Lymphocytes also can lyse IgG antibody-coated RBCs *in vitro*.[178-180] The relative contribution of antibody-dependent monocyte- and lymphocyte-mediated cytotoxicity to RBC destruction in patients with warm-antibody AHA is not known.

PATHOGENIC EFFECTS OF COLD AGGLUTININS AND HEMOLYSINS

Most cold agglutinins are unable to agglutinate RBCs at temperatures higher than 30°C (86°F). The highest temperature at which these antibodies cause detectable agglutination is termed the *thermal amplitude*. The value varies considerably among patients. Generally, patients with cold agglutinins with higher thermal amplitudes have a greater risk for cold agglutinin disease.[9] For example, active hemolytic anemia has been observed in patients with cold agglutinins of modest titer (e.g., 1:256) and high thermal amplitudes.[181]

The pathogenicity of a cold agglutinin depends upon its ability to bind host RBCs and to activate complement.[10,167,182-186] This process is called *complement fixation*. Although *in vitro* agglutination of the RBCs may be maximal at 0 to 5°C (32–41°F), complement fixation by these antibodies may occur optimally at 20 to 25°C (68–77°F) and may be significant at even higher physiologic temperatures.[10,181,182] Agglutination is not required for the process. The great preponderance of cold agglutinin molecules are IgM pentamers, but small numbers of IgM hexamers with cold agglutinin activity are found in patients with cold agglutinin disease. Hexamers fix complement and lyse RBCs more efficiently than do pentamers, suggesting that hexameric IgM plays a role in the pathogenesis of hemolysis in these patients.[187]

Cold agglutinins may bind to RBCs in superficial vessels of the extremities, where the temperature generally ranges between 28 and 31°C (82.4–87.8°F), depending upon ambient temperature.[183] Cold agglutinins of high thermal amplitude may cause RBCs to aggregate at this temperature, thereby impeding RBC flow and producing acrocyanosis. In addition, the RBC-bound cold agglutinin may activate complement via the classic pathway. Once activated complement proteins are deposited onto the RBC surface, the cold agglutinin must remain bound to the RBCs for hemolysis to occur. Instead, the cold agglutinin may dissociate from the RBCs at the higher temperatures in the body core and again be capable of binding other RBCs at the lower temperatures in the superficial vessels. As a result, patients with cold agglutinins of high thermal amplitude tend toward a sustained hemolytic process and acrocyanosis.[188] In contrast, patients with antibodies of lower thermal amplitude require significant chilling to initiate complement-mediated injury of RBCs. This sequence may result in a burst of hemolysis with hemoglobinuria.[188] Combinations of these clinical patterns also occur. Cold agglutinins of the IgA isotype, an isotype that does not fix complement, may cause acrocyanosis but not hemolysis.[189] Thus, the relative degree of hemolysis or impeded RBC flow

is influenced significantly by the properties and quantity of the cold agglutinins in a given patient.

Complement fixation by cold agglutinins may effect RBC injury by two major mechanisms: (1) direct lysis and (2) opsonization for hepatic and splenic macrophages. Both mechanisms probably operate to varying degrees in any patient. Direct lysis requires propagation of the full C1-to-C9 sequence on the RBC membrane. If this process occurs to a significant degree, the patient may experience intravascular hemolysis leading to hemoglobinemia and hemoglobinuria. Intravascular hemolysis of this severity is relatively rare because phosphatidylinositol-linked RBC membrane proteins (DAF and HRF) protect against injury by autologous complement components. Thus, the complement sequence on many RBCs is completed only through the early steps, leaving opsonic fragments of C3 (C3b/C3bi) and C4 (C4b) on the cell surface. The fragments provide only a weak stimulus for phagocytosis by monocytes *in vitro*.[169,190] However, activated macrophages may ingest C3b-coated particles avidly.[191] Accordingly, RBCs heavily coated with C3b (and/or C3bi) may be removed from the circulation by macrophages either in the liver or, to a lesser extent, the spleen.[156,182,184,192] The trapped RBCs may be ingested entirely or released back into the circulation as spherocytes after losing plasma membrane.

In vivo studies of the fate of ^{51}Cr-labeled C3b-coated RBCs[155,182,184,185] indicate many of the erythrocytes trapped in the liver or spleen gradually may reenter the circulation. The released cells generally are coated with the opsonically inactive C3 fragment C3dg. Conversion of cell-bound C3b or C3bi to C3dg results from the action of the naturally occurring complement inhibitor factor I in concert with factor H or CR1 receptors.[166] The surviving C3dg-coated RBCs circulate with a near-normal life span[155,182,184,185] and are resistant to further uptake of cold agglutinins or complement.[182,184,193] However, C3dg-coated RBCs also may react *in vitro* with anticomplement (anti-C3) serum in the DAT. In fact, most of the antiglobulin-positive RBCs of patients with cold agglutinin disease are coated with C3dg.

In paroxysmal cold hemoglobinuria, the mechanism of hemolysis probably parallels *in vitro* events (see "Serologic Features" below). During severe chilling, blood flowing through skin capillaries is exposed to low temperatures. The Donath-Landsteiner antibody and early-acting complement components presumably bind to RBCs at the lowered temperatures. Upon return of the cells to 37°C (98.6°F) in the central circulation, the cells are lysed by propagation of the terminal complement sequence through C9. The Donath-Landsteiner antibody itself dissociates from the RBCs at 37°C (98.6°F). However, prior to dissociation, the antibody initiates the classic pathway of complement. Erythrocyte membrane proteins that restrict C5b–9 assembly (e.g., HRFs) may be less effective in controlling Donath-Landsteiner antibody-initiated complement activation than that initiated by cold agglutinins.

PATHOGENESIS OF DRUG-MEDIATED IMMUNE INJURY

Table 52-3 summarizes the three mechanisms of drug-mediated immune injury to RBCs. Drugs also may mediate protein adsorption to RBCs by nonimmune mechanisms, but RBC injury does not occur.

Hapten or Drug Adsorption Mechanism   This mechanism applies to drugs that can bind firmly to proteins, including RBC membrane proteins. The classic setting is very-high-dose penicillin therapy,[28-34] which is encountered less commonly today than in previous decades.

Most individuals who receive penicillin develop IgM antibodies directed against the benzylpenicilloyl determinant of penicillin, but this antibody plays no role in penicillin-related immune injury to RBCs. The antibody responsible for hemolytic anemia is of the IgG class, occurs less frequently than the IgM antibody, and may be di-

TABLE 52-3   MAJOR MECHANISMS OF DRUG-RELATED HEMOLYTIC ANEMIA AND POSITIVE DIRECT ANTIGLOBULIN TESTS

	HAPTEN/DRUG ADSORPTION	TERNARY COMPLEX FORMATION	AUTOANTIBODY BINDING	NONIMMUNOLOGIC PROTEIN ADSORPTION
Prototype drug	Penicillin	Quinidine	α-Methyldopa	Cephalothin
Role of drug	Binds to red cell membrane	Forms ternary complex with antibody and red cell membrane component	Induces formation of antibody to native red cell antigen	Possibly alters red cell membrane
Drug affinity to cell	Strong	Weak	None demonstrated to intact red cell but binding to membranes reported	Strong
Antibody to drug	Present	Present	Absent	Absent
Antibody class predominating	IgG	IgM or IgG	IgG	None
Proteins detected by direct antiglobulin test	IgG, rarely complement	Complement	IgG, rarely complement	Multiple plasma proteins
Dose of drug associated with positive antiglobulin test	High	Low	High	High
Presence of drug required for indirect antiglobulin test	Yes (coating test red cells)	Yes (added to test medium)	No	Yes (added to test medium)
Mechanism of red cell destruction	Splenic sequestration of IgG-coated red cells	Direct lysis by complement plus splenic–hepatic clearance of C3b-coated red cells	Splenic sequestration	None

rected against the benzylpenicilloyl[31] or, more commonly, nonbenzyl-penicilloyl determinants.[28–30,32] Other manifestations of penicillin sensitivity usually are not present.

All patients receiving high doses of penicillin develop substantial coating of RBCs with penicillin. The penicillin coating itself is not injurious. If the penicillin dose is very high (10–30 × 10⁶ units per day, or less in the setting of renal failure) and promotes cell coating and if the patient has an IgG antipenicillin antibody, the antibody binds to the RBC–bound penicillin molecules and the DAT with anti-IgG becomes positive[29,31,32,48,194] (see Fig. 52-1A). Antibodies eluted from patients' RBCs or present in their sera react in the indirect antiglobulin test (IAT) only against penicillin-coated RBCs. This step is critical in distinguishing these drug-dependent antibodies from true autoantibodies.

Significantly, not all patients receiving high-dose penicillin develop a positive DAT reaction or hemolytic anemia because only a small proportion of such individuals produce the requisite antibody. Destruction of RBCs coated with penicillin and IgG antipenicillin antibody occurs mainly through sequestration by splenic macrophages.[30,195] In some patients with penicillin-induced immune hemolytic anemia, blood monocytes and presumably splenic macrophages may lyse the IgG-coated RBCs without phagocytosis.[196] Hemolytic anemia resulting from penicillin typically occurs only after the patient has received the drug for 7 to 10 days and ceases a few days to 2 weeks after the patient discontinues taking the drug.

Low molecular weight substances, such as drugs, generally are not immunogenic in their own right. Induction of antidrug antibody is thought to require firm chemical coupling of the drug (as a hapten) to a protein carrier. In the case of penicillin, the carrier protein involved in antibody induction need not be the same as the erythrocyte membrane protein to which penicillin is coupled in the effector phase, that is, when the IgG antipenicillin antibodies bind to penicillin-coated RBCs. In contrast to growing evidence on the ternary complex mechanism, no present evidence indicates the drug-dependent antibodies responsible for RBC injury in this hapten/drug adsorption mechanism also recognize native erythrocyte membrane structures.

Cephalosporins have antigenic cross-reactivity with penicillin[197–199] and bind firmly to RBC membranes, as do semisynthetic penicillins.[33,34] Hemolytic anemia similar to that seen with penicillin has been ascribed to cephalosporins[35–39] and some semisynthetic penicillins.[33,34] Tetracycline[40,41] and tolbutamide[44,45] also may cause hemolysis by this mechanism. Carbromal causes positive IgG antiglobulin reactions by a similar mechanism,[43] but hemolytic anemia has not been described.

Ternary Complex Mechanism: Drug–Antibody–Target Cell Interaction   Many drugs can induce immune injury not only of RBCs but also of platelets or granulocytes by a process that differs in several ways from the mechanism of hapten/drug adsorption (see Table 52-3). First, drugs in this group (see Table 52-2) exhibit only weak direct binding to blood cell membranes. Second, a relatively small dose of drug is capable of triggering destruction of blood cells. Third, cellular injury appears to be mediated chiefly by complement activation at the cell surface. The cytopathic process induced by such drugs previously has been termed the *innocent bystander* or *immune complex mechanism*. The terminology reflected the prevailing notion that, *in vivo*, drug–antibody complexes formed first (immune complexes) and then became secondarily bound to target blood cells as "innocent bystanders," either nonspecifically or possibly via membrane receptors (e.g., Fcγ receptors on platelets or C3b receptors on red cells), with the potential for subsequent activation of complement by bound complexes.

The "immune complex" and "innocent bystander" terminology now seems less appropriate because of models developed from research on analogous drug-dependent platelet injury[200–202] (see Chap. 110) and a series of relevant serologic observations on drug-mediated immune hemolytic anemia. These studies suggest blood cell injury is mediated by a cooperative interaction among three reactants to generate a ternary complex (see Fig. 52-1B) involving (1) the drug (or drug metabolite in some cases), (2) a drug-binding membrane site on the target cell, and (3) antibody. For example, several patients possess drug-dependent antibodies that exhibited specificity for RBCs bearing defined alloantigens such as those of the Rh, Kell, or Kidd blood groups. That is, even in the presence of drug, the antibodies were selectively nonreactive with human RBCs lacking the alloantigen in question.[55,79,203–205] In each case, high-affinity drug binding to cell membrane could not be demonstrated. The drug-dependent antibody is thought to bind, through its Fab domain, to a compound neoantigen consisting of loosely bound drug and a blood group antigen intrinsic to the red cell membrane. Elegant studies on quinidine- or quinine-induced immune thrombocytopenia have demonstrated the IgG antibodies implicated in this disorder bind through their Fab domains, not by their Fc domains to platelet Fcγ receptors.[206,207]

The data elucidate how one patient with quinidine sensitivity may have selective destruction of platelets and another may have selective destruction of RBCs. This process occurs because the pathogenic antibody recognizes the drug only in combination with a particular membrane structure of the RBC (e.g., a known alloantigen) or of the platelet (e.g., α domain of the glycoprotein Ib complex). Therefore, at least in these cases, the target cell does not appear to be purely an innocent bystander. Binding of the drug itself to the target cell membrane is weak until the attachment of the antibody to *both* drug and cell membrane is stabilized. Yet the binding of the antibody is drug dependent. Such a three-reactant interdependent "troika" is unique to this mechanism of immune cytopenia.

The foregoing discussion depicting drugs as creating a "self + nonself" neoantigen on the target cell applies to the effector phase as opposed to the induction phase of the process. However, the same drug-binding membrane protein appears to be involved in forming the immunogen that induces the antibody, as evidenced by drug-dependent antibodies exhibiting selective reactivity with defined red cell alloantigens (carrier specificity).[55,79,203–205] How this process is accomplished in the absence of evidence for strong, covalent binding of the drugs in this group to a host membrane protein remains to be elucidated.

RBC destruction by this mechanism may occur intravascularly after completion of the whole complement sequence, resulting in hemoglobinemia and hemoglobinuria. Some destruction of intact C3b-coated RBCs may be mediated by splenic and liver sequestration via the C3b/C3bi receptors on macrophages. The DAT is positive usually only with anticomplement reagents, but exceptions occur. Sometimes, however, the drug-dependent antibody itself can be detected on the RBCs if the offending drug (or its metabolites) is included in all steps of the antiglobulin test, including washing.[208]

Autoantibody Mechanism　　A variety of drugs induce the formation of autoantibodies reactive with autologous (or homologous) RBCs in the absence of the instigating drug (see Tables 52-2 and 52-3). The most studied drug in this category has been α-methyldopa, an antihypertensive agent that no longer is commonly used.[68–71] Levodopa and several unrelated drugs also have been implicated.[39,46,56,58,65,72–81] Patients with CLL treated with pentostatin,[82] fludarabine,[83] or chlorodeoxyadenosine[84] are particularly predisposed to autoimmune hemolysis, which usually is severe and sometimes fatal.

Positive DAT reactions (with anti-IgG reagents) in patients taking α-methyldopa vary in frequency from 8 to 36 percent. Patients taking higher doses of the drug develop positive reactions with greater frequency.[68,70,71] A lag period of 3 to 6 months exists between the start of therapy and development of a positive antiglobulin test. The delay is not shortened when the drug is administered to patients who previously had positive antiglobulin tests while taking α-methyldopa.[70]

In contrast to the frequent observation of positive antiglobulin reactions, less than 1 percent of patients taking α-methyldopa exhibit hemolytic anemia.[69] Development of hemolytic anemia does not depend on drug dose. The hemolysis usually is mild to moderate and occurs chiefly by splenic sequestration of IgG-coated RBCs. α-Methyldopa has been proposed to suppress splenic macrophage function in some patients, and normal survival of antibody-coated RBCs in such patients may be related, in part, to this effect of the drug.[209]

The DAT reaction usually is positive only for IgG.[11,210] Occasionally, weak anticomplement reactions also are encountered.[11] Patients with immune hemolytic anemia resulting from α-methyldopa therapy typically exhibit strongly positive DAT reactions and serum antibody, evidenced by the IAT reaction.[11] Antibodies in the serum or eluted from RBC membranes react optimally at 37°C (98.6°F) with unaltered

autologous or homologous RBCs in the absence of drug[69,71,211] (Fig. 52-1C). Frequently the autoantibodies are reactive with determinants of the Rh complex,[69,71,211] and at least some appear to target the same 34-kDa Rh-related polypeptide targeted by the autoantibodies in many cases of "spontaneously arising" AHA.[121] Thus, distinguishing these drug-induced antibodies from similar warm-reacting autoantibodies in idiopathic AHA currently is not possible.

The mechanism by which a drug induces formation of an autoantibody is unknown. Radiolabeled α-methyldopa does not react directly with the membranes of intact human RBCs.[71,212] However, both α-methyldopa and levodopa reportedly bind to isolated RBC membranes. Binding of the drug to membranes of intact RBCs is inhibited by RBC superoxide dismutase and probably by hemoglobin.[212,213] Although not formally demonstrated, these drugs probably bind to membrane antigens of cells that are relatively hemoglobin free, for example, cells at the early proerythroblast stage or RBC stroma. In any case, the resulting altered membrane antigens then may induce autoantibodies. The concept that a drug–membrane compound neoantigen could lead to production of an autoantibody is supported by studies of patients receiving drugs unrelated to α-methyldopa. Patients simultaneously developed a drug-dependent antibody and an autoantibody, both of which showed specificity for the same RBC alloantigen.[79] Another hypothesis is that α-methyldopa interacts with human T lymphocytes, resulting in loss of suppressor cell function.[214] However, subsequent studies have failed to demonstrate any evidence for such a mechanism.[215]

Uncommonly, patients with CLL treated with the purine analogues fludarabine or chlorodeoxyadenosine develop autoimmune hemolysis.[83,84] Risk factors for autoimmune hemolysis include previous therapy with a purine analogue, a positive DAT prior to therapy, and hypogammaglobulinemia. Purine analogues are potent suppressors of T lymphocytes. These drugs may accelerate the preexisting T cell immune suppression that normally occurs during progression of CLL, exacerbating the underlying tendency to autoimmunity in CLL. However, the degree of depletion of T cell subsets is similar in patients who develop hemolysis and in patients who do not.

Nonimmunologic Protein Adsorption　　Fewer than 5 percent of patients receiving cephalosporin antibiotics develop positive antiglobulin reactions[11] as a result of nonspecific adsorption of plasma proteins to their RBC membranes.[85,86,216] This process may occur within 1 to 2 days after the drug is instituted. Multiple plasma proteins, including immunoglobulins, complement, albumin, fibrinogen, and others, may be detected on RBC membranes in such cases.[216,217] Hemolytic anemia resulting from this mechanism has not been reported. The clinical importance of this phenomenon is its potential to complicate cross-match procedures unless the drug history is considered. Cephalosporin antibiotics also may induce RBC injury by the hapten mechanism, by the ternary complex mechanism, and by the autoantibody mechanism. The latter reactions are more serious but apparently occur less frequently than the nonimmunologic reaction.

CLINICAL FEATURES

WARM-ANTIBODY AUTOIMMUNE HEMOLYTIC ANEMIA

Presenting complaints of warm-antibody AHA usually are referable to the anemia itself, although occasionally jaundice is the immediate cause for the patient to seek medical advice. Symptom onset usually is slow and insidious over several months, but occasionally a patient has sudden onset of symptoms of severe anemia and jaundice over a period of a few days. In secondary AHA, the symptoms and signs of the underlying disease may overshadow the hemolytic anemia and associated features.

In idiopathic AHA with only mild anemia, results of physical examination may be normal. Even patients with relatively severe hemolytic anemia may have only modest splenomegaly. However, in very severe cases, particularly those of acute onset, patients may present with fever, pallor, jaundice, hepatosplenomegaly, hyperpnea, tachycardia, angina, or heart failure.

Clinical warm-antibody AHA may be aggravated or first become apparent during pregnancy.[151,218,219] Most cases are mild, however, and the prognosis for the fetus is generally good, provided the mother is treated early.[218]

COLD-ANTIBODY AUTOIMMUNE HEMOLYTIC ANEMIA

Most patients with cold agglutinin hemolytic anemia have chronic hemolytic anemia with or without jaundice. In other patients, the principal feature is episodic, acute hemolysis with hemoglobinuria induced by chilling (see discussion of thermal amplitude in "Pathogenic Effects of Cold Agglutinins and Hemolysins," above). Combinations of these clinical features may occur. Acrocyanosis and other cold-mediated vasoocclusive phenomena affecting the fingers, toes, nose, and ears are associated with sludging of RBCs in the cutaneous microvasculature. Skin ulceration and necrosis are distinctly unusual. Hemolysis occurring in *M. pneumoniae* infections is acute in onset, typically appearing as the patient is recovering from pneumonia and coincident with peak titers of cold agglutinins. The hemolysis is self-limited, lasting 1 to 3 weeks.[11] Hemolytic anemia in infectious mononucleosis develops either at the onset of symptoms or within the first 3 weeks of illness.[116]

Other physical findings are variable, depending upon the presence of an underlying disease. Splenomegaly, a characteristic finding in lymphoproliferative diseases or infectious mononucleosis, may be observed in idiopathic cold agglutinin disease.

In paroxysmal cold hemoglobinuria, constitutional symptoms are prominent during a paroxysm. A few minutes to several hours after cold exposure, the patient develops aching pains in the back or legs, abdominal cramps, and perhaps headaches. Chills and fever usually follow. The first urine passed after onset of symptoms typically contains hemoglobin. The constitutional symptoms and hemoglobinuria generally last a few hours. Raynaud phenomenon and cold urticaria sometimes occur during an attack; jaundice may follow.

DRUG-IMMUNE HEMOLYTIC ANEMIA

A careful history of drug exposure should be obtained from all patients with hemolytic anemia and/or a positive DAT. As in idiopathic AHA, the clinical picture in drug-immune hemolytic anemia is quite variable. The severity of symptoms largely depends upon the rate of hemolysis. In general, patients with hapten/drug adsorption (e.g., penicillin) and autoimmune (e.g., α-methyldopa) types of drug-induced hemolytic anemia exhibit mild to moderate hemolysis, with insidious onset of symptoms developing over a period of days to weeks. In contrast, the ternary complex mechanism (e.g., cephalosporins or quinidine) often causes sudden, severe hemolysis with hemoglobinuria. In the latter setting, hemolysis can occur after only one dose of the drug in a patient previously exposed to the drug. Acute renal failure may accompany severe hemolysis by the ternary complex mechanism.[39,53,55,59,60,81,210] Several reports indicate second- and third-generation cephalosporins may cause severe, even fatal, hemolysis by the ternary complex mechanism.[37–39,61]

LABORATORY FEATURES

GENERAL FEATURES

By definition, patients with AHA present with anemia, the severity of which ranges from life threatening to very mild. Patients with warm-antibody AHA may present with hematocrit levels less than 10 percent or may have compensated hemolytic anemia and a near-normal hematocrit. For the latter patients, the predominant laboratory features are an increased reticulocyte count and a positive DAT. Occasionally, the patient has leukopenia and neutropenia.[10,220] Platelet counts typically are normal. Rarely, severe immune thrombocytopenia is associated with warm-antibody AHA. This constellation is termed *Evans syndrome.*[221] In this syndrome, the RBC and platelet antibodies are apparently distinct.[222]

Patients with classic chronic cold agglutinin disease exhibit mild to moderate, fairly stable anemia, with hematocrit levels only occasionally as low as 15 to 20 percent. In contrast, patients with paroxysmal cold hemoglobinuria have hematocrit levels that decrease rapidly during a paroxysm. During a paroxysm, leukopenia is noted early, followed by leukocytosis. Complement titers frequently are depressed because of consumption of complement proteins during hemolysis.

In drug-immune hemolytic anemia of the hapten/drug adsorption and true autoantibody types, the hematologic findings are similar to those described for spontaneously occurring warm-antibody AHA. Most patients exhibit anemia and reticulocytosis. Leukopenia and thrombocytopenia may be noted in cases of ternary complex-mediated hemolysis.

Evaluation of the blood film can reveal several features related to all types of AHA. Polychromasia indicates a reticulocytosis, reflecting an increased rate of reticulocyte egress from the marrow. Spherocytes are seen in patients with moderate to severe hemolytic anemia (see Color Plate I-6). Unless hereditary spherocytosis cannot be excluded, this finding suggests an immune hemolytic process. RBC fragments, nucleated RBCs, and occasionally erythrophagocytosis by monocytes may be seen in severe cases. Most patients have mild leukocytosis and neutrophilia. Patients with cold-antibody AHA may exhibit RBC autoagglutination in the blood film and in chilled anticoagulated blood.

The reticulocyte count usually is elevated. Nevertheless, early in the course of the disease, more than one third of all patients may have transient reticulocytopenia despite a normal or hyperplastic erythroid marrow.[223–226] The mechanism is unknown, but autoantibodies reactive against antigens on reticulocytes are speculated to lead to their selective destruction.[227] One unusual patient with warm-antibody AHA, reticulocytopenia, and marrow erythroid aplasia had a serum autoantibody that inhibited erythroid colony formation *in vitro.*[227] The aplastic crisis remitted after the serum IgG level was lowered by immunoadsorption. Reticulocytopenia also may be seen in patients with marrow function compromised by an underlying disease, parvovirus infection, toxic chemicals, or nutritional deficiency. Marrow examination usually reveals erythroid hyperplasia and may provide evidence of an underlying lymphoproliferative disorder.

Hyperbilirubinemia (chiefly unconjugated) is highly suggestive of hemolytic anemia, although its absence does not exclude the diagnosis. Total bilirubin is only modestly increased (up to 5 mg/dl) and, with rare exceptions, the conjugated (direct) fraction constitutes less than 15 percent of the total. Urinary urobilinogen is increased regularly, but bile is not detected in the urine unless serum conjugated bilirubin is increased. Usually, serum haptoglobin levels are low, and lactate dehydrogenase levels are elevated. Hemoglobinuria is encountered in rare patients with warm-antibody AHA and hyperacute hemolysis, more commonly in patients with cold agglutinin disease, and characteristically in patients with paroxysmal cold hemoglobinuria and with drug-immune hemolytic anemia mediated by the ternary complex mechanism.

DIRECT ANTIGLOBULIN TEST PATTERN

Diagnosis of AHA or drug-immune hemolytic anemia requires demonstration of immunoglobulin and/or complement bound to the pa-

TABLE 52-4   MAJOR REACTION PATTERNS OF THE DIRECT ANTIGLOBULIN
TEST AND ASSOCIATED TYPES OF IMMUNE INJURY

REACTION PATTERN	TYPE OF IMMUNE INJURY
IgG alone	Warm antibody autoimmune hemolytic anemia
	Drug-immune hemolytic anemia: hapten drug adsorption type or autoantibody type
Complement alone	Warm antibody autoimmune hemolytic anemia with subthreshold IgG deposition
	Cold-agglutinin disease
	Paroxysmal cold hemoglobinuria
	Drug-immune hemolytic anemia: ternary complex type
IgG plus complement	Warm antibody autoimmune hemolytic anemia
	Drug-immune hemolytic anemia: autoantibody type (rare)

tient's RBCs. As a screening procedure, use of a "broad-spectrum" antiglobulin (Coombs) reagent, that is, one that contains antibodies directed against human immunoglobulin and complement components (principally C3), is customary. If agglutination is noted with a broad-spectrum reagent, antisera reacting selectively with IgG (the "gamma" Coombs) or with C3 (the "nongamma" Coombs) are used to define the specific pattern of RBC sensitization. Monospecific antisera to IgM or IgA also have been used in selected cases.

Three possible *major* patterns of direct antiglobulin reaction in AHA and drug-immune hemolytic anemia exist: (1) RBCs coated with only IgG, (2) RBCs coated with IgG and complement components, and (3) RBCs coated with complement components without detectable immunoglobulin.[10,111,228,229] In patterns 2 and 3, the complement components most readily detected are C3 fragments (mainly C3dg). Each pattern is associated with accelerated RBC destruction. Positive antiglobulin reactions with anti-IgA or anti-IgM are encountered less commonly, often in association with bound IgG and/or complement.[230–236] Table 52-4 summarizes the diagnostic significance of each of these major patterns (see "Serologic Features" below).

SEROLOGIC FEATURES

WARM-ANTIBODY AUTOIMMUNE HEMOLYTIC ANEMIA

Free versus Bound Autoantibody   The autoantibody molecules in patients with warm-antibody AHA exist in a reversible, dynamic equilibrium between RBCs and plasma.[237,238] In addition to the major portion of autoantibody bound to the patient's RBCs (detected by the DAT), "free" autoantibody may be detected in the plasma or serum of these patients by the IAT. In the IAT, the patient's serum or plasma is incubated with normal donor erythrocytes at the appropriate temperature (in this case, 37°C). The cells are washed, suspended in saline solution, and then tested for agglutination by antiglobulin serum. The presence of unbound autoantibody in plasma depends upon the total amount of antibody being produced and the binding affinity of the antibody for RBC antigens. In general, patients whose RBCs are heavily coated with IgG more likely exhibit plasma autoantibody. Protease-modified RBCs are more sensitive than native RBCs in detecting plasma autoantibody, but such data must be interpreted with caution, because alloantibodies, naturally occurring antibodies to cryptic antigens, and other serum components may interact with enzyme-modified RBCs. Patients with a positive IAT as a result of a warm-reactive autoantibody should also have a positive DAT. A patient with a serum anti-RBC antibody (positive IAT) and a negative DAT probably does not have an autoimmune process but rather an alloantibody stimulated by prior transfusion or pregnancy.

Quantity of RBC-Bound Autoantibody   Figure 52-2 relates the intensity of the direct antiglobulin reaction, using specific anti-IgG

serum, to the number of IgG molecules bound per RBC. The latter was determined by a sensitive antibody-consumption method.[239] A trace-positive antiglobulin reaction (read macroscopically) detects 300 to 400 molecules of IgG per cell.[239,240] In another laboratory, a trace-positive antiglobulin reaction with anti-C3 was obtained with 60 to 115 molecules C3 per cell.[167]

More sensitive methods for quantifying RBC-bound IgG allow identification of AHA patients having all the usual hallmarks of warm-antibody AHA but a negative DAT with anti-immunoglobulin and anticomplement reagents.[239–241] In many patients, the RBCs are coated with quantities of IgG autoantibody that are too low to give a positive DAT (subthreshold IgG). However, the specialized methods (e.g., anti-IgG consumption assays, automated enhanced agglutination techniques, enzyme-linked immunoassays, radioimmunoassays) detect very small quantities of cell-bound IgG. In such cases, studies with highly concentrated RBC eluates confirm these IgG molecules are warm-reacting anti-RBC autoantibodies.[239] Patients generally have relatively mild hemolysis and often respond favorably to glucocorticoid therapy. By these specialized methods, subthreshold IgG also may be detected in a significant number of patients exhibiting the "complement alone" pattern of direct antiglobulin reaction in the absence of drug sensitivity or cold agglutinins. In such cases, studies with concentrated RBC eluates suggest subthreshold quantities of bound IgG antibodies are capable of fixing much larger quantities of C3 to the cell membrane.[239]

Nature of the Autoantibodies and RBC Target Antigens   In any series of warm-antibody AHA patients, the correlation between the strength of the antiglobulin reaction (IgG molecules per RBC) and the rate of RBC destruction is variable. The IgG subclass of warm autoantibodies apparently influences the degree to which these antibodies shorten RBC survival. IgG1 is the most commonly encountered subclass, either alone or in combination with other IgG subclasses.[230,242] IgG1 and IgG3 autoantibodies appear to be more effective in decreasing RBC life span than do those of the IgG2 or IgG4 subclass.[230,243]

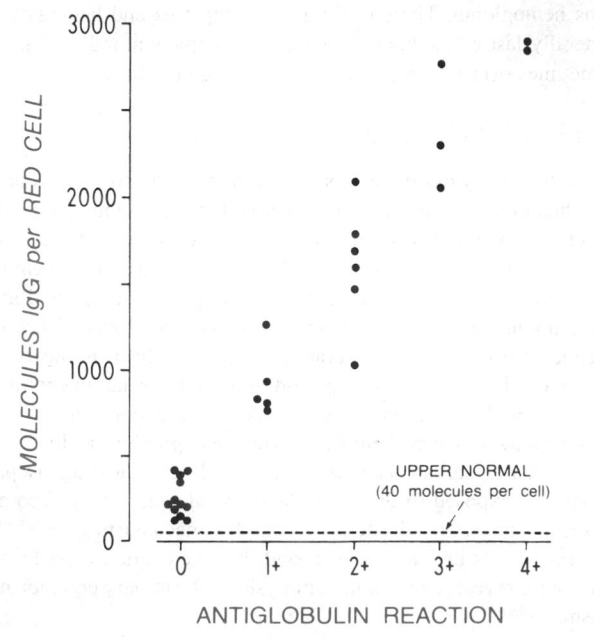

FIGURE 52-2   Comparison of direct antiglobulin reactions (with anti-IgG serum) with molecules of red blood cell–bound IgG determined by a quantitative antibody consumption assay (method described by Gilliland et al.[239]). The two assays were conducted concurrently on the same blood specimen. The antiglobulin reactions were performed manually and read macroscopically.

The difference may result from the greater affinity of macrophage Fc receptors for IgG1 and IgG3[162,163] and the higher complement-fixing activity of IgG1 or IgG3 antibodies relative to the activity of IgG2 or IgG4 antibodies.[172]

Autoantibodies eluted from patients' RBCs or present in their plasma typically bind to all the common types of human RBCs represented in test panels used by blood banks and thus might appear to be nonspecific. However, the antibodies of any one patient typically recognize one or more antigenic determinants (epitopes) that are common to almost all human RBCs, that is, "public" antigens. These antibodies have been useful for evaluating RBC membrane structures and for identifying rare RBC phenotypes, namely, RBCs that lack a common blood group antigen(s). Nearly half of all AHA patients have autoantibodies specific for epitopes on Rh proteins.[10,11,119,244-246] The autoantibodies of such patients commonly do not react with human Rh$_{null}$ RBCs, which lack expression of the Rh complex. Occasionally, the anti-Rh autoantibodies have anti-e, anti-E, or anti-c (or, more rarely, anti-D) specificity. Patients who have autoantibodies with selective specificity (e.g., anti-e) nearly always have other autoantibodies reactive with all human RBCs, except Rh$_{null}$. Autoantibodies with such specificity are designated collectively as Rh related.[121,246]

The remaining patients with warm-antibody AHA have IgG autoantibodies that are fully reactive with Rh$_{null}$ RBCs.[10,11,119,244-246] The exact specificity of the autoantibodies for many of these patients is undefined. However, in other instances, autoantibody specificity for serologically defined blood group antigens outside the Rh system has been identified (using RBCs of appropriate antigen-deficient phenotype) including anti-Wr^b,[119] anti-En^a,[247] anti LW,[248] anti-U,[249] anti-Ge,[235,250] anti-Sc1,[251] or antibodies to Kell blood group antigens.[252] For ease of reference, the entire group of autoantibodies is designated non–Rh related.[121,246]

Immunochemical studies indicate the autoantibodies from almost any AHA patient react with individual membrane proteins. The major target of Rh-related autoantibodies is a 32- to 34-kDa nonglycosylated polypeptide lacking on Rh$_{null}$ RBCs.[121,253] This polypeptide is similar, if not identical, to the polypeptide expressing the Rh(e) alloantigen. Many α-methyldopa–induced autoantibodies also react with this polypeptide.[121] Autoantibodies with non-Rh serologic specificity react with the band 3 anion transporter[121,254] or with both band 3 and glycophorin A.[121] The latter autoantibodies may react with an epitope formed through the interaction of these two proteins on the RBC membrane.[255] It is interesting to note that anti-RBC autoantibodies in NZB mice exhibit anti–band 3 specificity.[256] Furthermore, naturally occurring anti–band 3 IgG autoantibodies are found in almost all humans.[257,258] These autoantibodies may play a role in the clearance of senescent RBCs by reacting with neoantigens formed on these cells by proteolytic alteration[257] or aggregation[258] of band 3 proteins. Such neoantigens are not found on younger RBCs. An important but unanswered question concerns the possible relationship between naturally occurring and pathologic anti–band 3 autoantibodies.

COLD-ANTIBODY HEMOLYTIC ANEMIA

Cold agglutinins are distinguished by their ability to directly agglutinate saline-suspended human RBCs at low temperature, maximally at 0 to 5°C (32−41°F). The reaction is reversible by warming. In chronic cold agglutinin disease, serum titers are commonly 1:10,000 or higher and may reach 1:1,000,000 or more. Cold agglutinins are characteristically IgM. IgA or IgG cold agglutinins have been reported,[11,189,259] sometimes in combination with IgM.[260] In mixed warm- and cold-antibody AHA, warm-reactive IgG autoantibodies are found in association with IgM cold agglutinins.[21]

The DAT result is positive with anticomplement reagents. The antibody itself, however, is not detected by the DAT because the cold agglutinins readily dissociate from the RBCs both *in vivo* and during the washing steps of the standard antiglobulin procedure. In contrast, C4b and C3b are covalently bound to target RBCs via thioester linkages. In one unusual case, a low-titer IgG cold agglutinin could be detected by washing the patient's RBCs in ice-cold saline solution and performing the DAT at 4°C (39.2°F).[259]

The majority of cold agglutinins are reactive with oligosaccharide antigens of the I/i system, which are precursors of the ABH and Lewis blood group substances.[261-263] The I/i determinants are bound to erythrocyte membrane glycoprotein (band 3 anion transporter) or to glycolipids.[262,263] Anti-I and anti-i reportedly bind solubilized RBC glycoproteins at 37°C (98.6°F), suggesting the temperature dependence of cold agglutination of intact RBCs may be a function of temperature-induced conformational effects on the cell surface.[264,265]

I antigens are expressed strongly on adult RBCs but weakly on neonatal (cord) RBCs. The converse is true of i antigens, indicating I/i antigen expression is developmentally regulated.[262] The differences between adult and cord blood RBCs allow evaluation of the serologic specificity of cold agglutinins.[10,11,189] I/i antigens, or structurally related analogues, occur in human saliva, milk, amniotic fluid, and hydatid cyst fluid[189] and are expressed on human lymphocytes, neutrophils, and monocytes.[266]

Anti-I is the predominant specificity of cold agglutinins in idiopathic cold agglutinin disease, in patients with *M. pneumoniae*, and in some cases of lymphoma. Cold agglutinins with anti-i specificity are found in patients with infectious mononucleosis and in some patients with lymphoma. A small percentage of cold agglutinin-containing sera react equally well with adult and neonatal RBC. These antibodies recognize antigens outside the I/i system, including Pr antigens, consisting of carbohydrate epitopes of glycophorins that are inactivated by protease treatment[189] and, less commonly, the M or P blood group antigens.[267,268] Most cold agglutinins associated with chickenpox exhibit anti-Pr specificity. A single case with anti-I specificity has been observed.[269] Hemolysis resulting from a cold agglutinin with anti-Pr specificity occurred following an allogeneic marrow transplant.[270]

In hemolytic anemia associated with infectious mononucleosis, the patient's serum may contain IgM anti-i cold agglutinins or cold-reactive nonagglutinating IgG anti-i with IgM cold-reactive anti-IgG antibodies ("rheumatoid factors") that may cross-link the IgG-coated RBCs to produce agglutination.[271]

In paroxysmal cold hemoglobinuria, the direct antiglobulin reaction usually is positive during and briefly following an acute attack because of the coating of surviving RBCs with complement, primarily C3dg fragments. The Donath-Landsteiner antibody is responsible for complement deposition on the cells; it is a nonagglutinating IgG that binds RBCs only in the cold. It readily dissociates from the RBCs at room temperature. In adults subject to recurring episodes in association with cold exposure, the DAT result remains negative between attacks. The antibody is detected by the biphasic Donath-Landsteiner test, in which the patient's fresh serum is incubated with RBCs initially at 4°C (39.2°F) and the mixture is then warmed to 37°C (98.6°F).[11] Intense hemolysis occurs. Addition of fresh guinea pig serum or ABO-compatible human serum may be necessary to serve as a source of fresh complement if the patient's serum has been stored or is complement depleted. Antibody titers rarely exceed 1:16. The Donath-Landsteiner antibody typically has specificity for the P blood group antigen, a glycosphingolipid structure.[263] The P antigen also occurs on lymphocytes and skin fibroblasts.[16] The latter finding might be related in some way to the occurrence of cold urticaria in paroxysmal cold hemoglobinuria, a phenomenon that may be transferred passively by serum to normal skin.[10] Antibody specificities for RBC antigens other than the P blood group have been noted.[272]

DRUG-IMMUNE HEMOLYTIC ANEMIA

In the hapten/drug adsorption mechanism of immune injury associated with cephalosporins or penicillin, the patient's drug-coated RBCs bind drug-specific IgG antibody and exhibit positive DAT reactions with anti-IgG. Rarely, both anti-IgG and anti-C3d antisera produce positive DAT reactions. Such cases could have superficial resemblance to warm-antibody AHA. The key serologic difference is that, in this form of drug-immune hemolytic anemia, the antibodies in the patient's serum or eluted from the patient's RBCs react *only* with drug-coated RBCs. In contrast, the IgG antibodies in warm-type AHA react with unmodified human RBCs and may show preference for certain known blood groups (e.g., within the Rh complex). Such serologic distinction and the history of exposure to high blood levels of penicillin or a cephalosporin should be decisive.

In hemolysis mediated by the ternary complex mechanism, the DAT is positive with anticomplement serum. Immunoglobulins are only rarely detectable on the patient's RBCs. This pattern is similar to that encountered in AHA mediated by cold agglutinins. Moreover, the brisk type of hemolysis in the ternary complex mechanism also is seen in certain cases of cold-antibody AHA. In the drug-induced cases, however, the cold agglutinin titer and the Donath-Landsteiner test result are normal, and demonstration of serum antibody acting on human RBCs depends upon the presence of the drug in the test system. Thus, the IAT reaction with anticomplement serum may be positive only if the incubation mixture permits interaction of (1) normal RBCs; (2) antidrug antibody from the patient's serum; (3) the relevant drug, either still in the patient's serum or added *in vitro* in appropriate concentration; and (4) a source of complement, that is, fresh normal serum or the patient's own serum if freshly obtained. A negative result does not necessarily absolve the suspected drug because the critical determinant may be a metabolite of the drug in question. In some cases, use of urine or serum (of the patient or a volunteer taking the drug) as a source of drug metabolite has permitted successful demonstration of a drug-dependent mechanism.[58,204,208,273]

In patients with true autoantibodies as result of α-methyldopa, the DAT reaction is strongly positive for IgG, but complement only rarely is detected on the patient's RBCs. Autoantibody to RBCs is regularly present in the serum of patients and mediates a positive IAT reaction with unmodified human RBCs, often showing specificity related to the Rh complex. No presently available specific serologic test can separate idiopathic warm-reacting IgG autoantibodies with Rh-related specificities from those induced by α-methyldopa administration. The evidence must be circumstantial, with the helpful knowledge that discontinuation of α-methyldopa, without any form of immunosuppressive therapy, consistently permits a slow recovery from anemia and a gradual disappearance of anti-RBC antibodies.

Drugs now not known to cause immune RBC injury will be implicated in the future. In any patient with a clinical picture compatible with drug-related immune hemolysis, a reasonable approach is stopping any drug that is suspect while serologic studies are being performed. The patient should be monitored for improvement in hematocrit level, decrease in reticulocytosis, and gradual disappearance of the positive DAT. Repeat challenge with the suspected drug may confirm the diagnosis, but this measure is seldom necessary in patient management and may be unsafe. Therefore, rechallenge to exclude a drug-immune hemolytic anemia should be undertaken only for compelling reasons, such as the need to use the specific drug for the patient's illness.

DIFFERENTIAL DIAGNOSIS

Several nonautoimmune diseases may result in spherocytic anemia, such as hereditary spherocytosis (HS), Zieve syndrome, clostridial sep-

sis, and the hemolytic anemia preceding Wilson disease. Among the hereditary hemolytic anemias, HS can resemble acquired AHA most closely because the spherocytic anemia associated with HS may be detected first in adulthood (see Chap. 44). In addition, splenomegaly may be prominent in both HS and AHA. Family studies of patients with HS, however, usually can identify other affected individuals. Most important, in hereditary hemolytic anemia the DAT is negative.

In hemolytic anemia accompanied by a positive DAT, serologic characterization of the autoantibody may distinguish warm-antibody AHA from cold-reacting autoantibody syndromes. Diagnosis of a drug-immune hemolytic anemia depends upon a history of appropriate drug intake supported by compatible serologic findings. In patients who recently received a transfusion, a positive DAT reaction may reflect the binding of a newly formed alloantibody to donor RBCs in the patient's circulation (delayed transfusion reaction; see Chap. 131). This finding could lead to a false impression of an autoimmune process.

Recent recipients of allogeneic blood stem cell transplants or solid organ transplants may develop autoimmune hemolysis.[274] In the former, antibodies are produced by the stem cell graft against RBCs also produced by the stem cell graft, that is, both antibodies and RBCs are of donor origin. In the case of solid organ transplants, the recipient's own lymphocytes make antibody against recipient RBCs. In both situations, the autoimmunity is thought to arise from immunosuppressive therapy causing delayed reconstitution or dysfunction of T cell immunity, leading to development of antibodies autologous to the offended immune system.

Recipients of organ transplants may also develop an *allo*immune hemolytic anemia that mimics warm-antibody AHA. The problem is seen in kidney, liver, or marrow transplants and usually occurs when an organ from a blood group O donor is transplanted into a blood group A recipient. B lymphocytes present in the donated organ or marrow form alloantibodies against recipient RBCs.[275-279] Patients of blood group O who receive a marrow transplant from a donor of blood group A or B may develop a transiently positive DAT and hemolysis of RBCs made by the marrow graft because of temporary persistence of previously synthesized host anti-A or anti-B.[280] Furthermore, some group O marrow transplant recipients exhibit mixed hematopoietic chimerism with persistence of host B lymphocytes that can make alloantibodies directed against RBCs made by the marrow graft.[280] In these settings, the findings of hemolysis and a positive DAT as a result of anti-A and anti-B probably are diagnostic of an alloimmune process, because *auto*antibodies directed against the major blood group antigens A and B are extremely rare.

Other acquired types of hemolytic anemia are less easily confused with either warm- or cold-antibody AHA because spherocytes are not prominent on the blood film and the DAT is negative. Patients with paroxysmal nocturnal hemoglobinuria (PNH) may complain of dark urine (hemoglobinuria). This finding is unusual in patients with warm-antibody AHA but can occur in patients with the cold-antibody syndromes. Decreased levels of CD55 and CD59 on blood cells, detected by flow analysis, is characteristic of PNH but not AHA (see Chap. 38). Microangiopathic hemolytic disorders, such as thrombotic thrombocytopenic purpura and hemolytic uremic syndrome, can be distinguished from AHA by examining the blood film. In the former diseases, the blood film displays marked RBC fragmentation and minimal spherocytosis. In addition, microangiopathic hemolytic anemia more frequently is associated with thrombocytopenia than is either warm- or cold-antibody AHA.

The clinical and laboratory features of chronic cold agglutinin disease are sufficiently distinctive so that the diagnostic possibilities are limited. In general, a high-titer cold agglutinin ($>$1:10,000) and a positive DAT with anticomplement serum (but not with anti-IgG) are consistent with cold agglutinin disease. In many instances of drug-immune hemolytic anemia, the DAT result also is positive only for complement. The drug history and a low (or absent) cold agglutinin titer, however, help to distinguish drug-immune hemolytic anemia from cold agglutinin disease. If the patient has an elevated cold agglutinin level and a positive DAT result with both anti-IgG and anti-C3, then the patient may have a mixed-type AHA. Warm-antibody AHA, hereditary hemolytic disorders, and PNH should be excluded in cases exhibiting primarily a chronic hemolytic anemia. The pattern of antiglobulin reaction, family history, the result of acid or sucrose hemolysis test, and analysis of CD55/CD59 on blood cells provide additional help in difficult cases. When the hemolysis is episodic, paroxysmal cold hemoglobinuria, march hemoglobinuria, and PNH also should be considered. When cold-induced peripheral vasoocclusive symptoms are predominant, the differential diagnosis should include cryoglobulinemia and Raynaud phenomenon, with or without an associated rheumatic disease. Infectious mononucleosis, M. pneumoniae infection, or lymphoma may be considered in appropriate clinical settings.

Paroxysmal cold hemoglobinuria must be distinguished from the subset of cases of chronic cold agglutinin disease manifesting episodic hemolysis and hemoglobinuria. This distinction is made primarily in the laboratory. In general, patients with paroxysmal cold hemoglobinuria lack high titers of cold agglutinins. Furthermore, the Donath-Landsteiner antibody is a potent in vitro hemolysin, in contrast to most cold agglutinins, which are weak hemolysins. Warm-antibody AHA, march hemoglobinuria, myoglobinuria, and PNH can be distinguished through the history and appropriate laboratory studies.

Immune hemolysis caused by drugs should be distinguished from (1) the warm- or cold-antibody types of idiopathic AHA, (2) congenital hemolytic anemias such as hereditary spherocytosis, and (3) drug-mediated hemolysis resulting from disorders of red cell metabolism, such as glucose-6-phosphate dehydrogenase deficiency. Patients with drug-immune hemolytic anemia have a positive DAT that distinguishes this group from patients with inherited RBC defects.

THERAPY

GENERAL

TRANSFUSION

The clinical consequences of AHA or drug-immune hemolytic anemia are related to the severity of the anemia and acuity of its onset. Many patients develop anemia over a period sufficient to allow for cardiovascular compensation and hence do not require RBC transfusions. However, RBC transfusions may be necessary and should not be withheld from a patient with an underlying disease complicating the anemia, such as symptomatic coronary artery disease, or a patient who rapidly develops severe anemia with signs and/or symptoms of circulatory failure, as in paroxysmal cold hemoglobinuria or ternary complex drug-immune hemolysis.

Transfusion of RBCs in immune hemolytic anemia presents two difficulties: (1) cross-matching and (2) the short half-life of the transfused RBCs (see Chap. 131). Finding truly serocompatible donor blood is nearly always impossible except in rare cases when the autoantibody is specific for a defined blood group antigen (see "Serologic Features" above). Otherwise, donor RBCs that are least incompatible with the patient's serum in cross-match testing must be selected. Before transfusing an incompatible unit, the patient's serum must be tested carefully for an alloantibody that could cause a severe hemolytic transfusion reaction against donor RBCs, especially in patients with a history of pregnancy or prior transfusion.[246,281–283] Use of prophylactic antigen-matched donor RBCs for transfusion has been proposed as a means of preventing alloimmunization in patients with AHA.[284] This

process is feasible only in institutions with access to a good selection of phenotyped RBC units and a reference laboratory.[285] Consultation between the clinician and the blood bank physician is useful.

Once selected, the packed RBCs should be administered slowly. During the transfusion, the patient should be monitored for signs of a hemolytic transfusion reaction (see Chap. 131). The transfused cells may be destroyed as fast as or perhaps even faster than the patient's own cells. However, the increased oxygen-carrying capacity provided by the transfused cells may be sufficient to maintain the patient during the acute interval required for other modes of therapy to become effective.

THERAPY OF WARM-ANTIBODY AUTOIMMUNE HEMOLYTIC ANEMIA

GLUCOCORTICOIDS

Therapy with glucocorticoids has reduced the mortality associated with severe idiopathic warm-antibody AHA. Glucocorticoids were first used for this disorder more than 50 years ago.[286] Glucocorticoids can cause dramatic cessation or marked slowing of hemolysis in about two thirds of patients.[10,11,111,287,288] Approximately 20 percent of treated patients with warm-antibody AHA achieve complete remission. Approximately 10 percent show minimal or no response to glucocorticoids. The best responses are seen in idiopathic cases or in those related to SLE.

Most patients should be treated with oral prednisone at an initial daily dose of 60 to 100 mg. Critically ill patients with rapid hemolysis may receive intravenous methylprednisolone 100 to 200 mg in divided doses over the first 24 hours. High doses of prednisone may be required for 10 to 14 days. When the hematocrit stabilizes or begins to increase, the prednisone dose can be decreased in rapid-step dose reductions to approximately 30 mg/day. With continued improvement, the prednisone dose can be further decreased at a rate of 5 mg/day every week, to a dose of 15 to 20 mg/day. These doses should be administered for 2 to 3 months after the acute hemolytic episode has subsided, after which the patient can be weaned from the drug over 1 to 2 months or treatment switched to an alternate-day therapy schedule (e.g., 20–40 mg every other day). Alternate-day therapy reduces glucocorticoid side effects but should be attempted only after the patient has achieved stable remission on daily prednisone in the range from 15 to 20 mg/day. Therapy should not be stopped until the DAT becomes negative. Although many patients achieve full remission of their first hemolytic episode, relapses may occur after the glucocorticoids are discontinued. Therefore, patients should be followed for at least several years after treatment. A relapse may require repeat glucocorticoid therapy, splenectomy, or immunosuppression.

Occasionally, patients who present with only a positive DAT, minimal hemolysis, and stable hematocrit require no treatment. However, these patients should be observed for clinical deterioration because the rate of RBC destruction may increase spontaneously.

Glucocorticoids may influence hemolysis in warm-antibody AHA by several mechanisms. Earlier investigators noted that hematologic improvement was often, but not always, accompanied by reduction in the strength of the DAT.[10] The subsequent observation of a decrease in cell-bound and/or free serum autoantibody during stable glucocorticoid-induced remission suggested improved RBC survival following treatment with glucocorticoids resulted from a decrease in synthesis of anti-RBC autoantibodies.[154,237] However, this finding cannot explain why glucocorticoid-treated patients often improve within 24 to 72 hours, a time much shorter than the half-life of anti-RBC autoantibody. Rather, glucocorticoids may suppress RBC sequestration by splenic macrophages.[156,157,168,289] A quantitative decrease in one of the three known classes of Fcγ receptors[162,163] has been observed in the blood monocytes of AHA patients during glucocorticoid therapy.[290]

SPLENECTOMY

Nearly one third of patients with warm-antibody AHA require prednisone chronically in doses greater than 15 mg/day to maintain an acceptable hemoglobin concentration. These patients are candidates for splenectomy.

Splenectomy removes the primary site of RBC trapping. Investigations in human[154] and animal[156] subjects confirm that maintenance of a given rate of RBC destruction requires six to 10 times more RBC-bound IgG in splenectomized subjects than in nonsplenectomized subjects. Continuation of hemolysis after splenectomy is partly related to persisting high levels of autoantibody, favoring RBC destruction in the liver by hepatic Kupffer cells.[154,156,159]

Several investigators noted the amount of RBC-bound autoantibody decreased in AHA patients following splenectomy.[10,287,291] However, a significant proportion of patients show no change in cell-bound autoantibody following splenectomy. The processes determining the rate of autoantibody production are poorly understood. The beneficial effect of splenectomy may be related to several factors interacting in complex fashion.[292]

A patient's clinical data currently constitute the best selection criteria for splenectomy. Attempts to select potential responders by ^{51}Cr-RBC sequestration studies have been disappointing.[10,287,293] In most cases, a reasonable approach is to continue glucocorticoids for 1 to 2 months while waiting for a maximal response. However, if no response is noted within 3 weeks, the patient's condition deteriorates, or the anemia is very severe, splenectomy should be performed sooner.

Results of splenectomy are variable. Approximately two thirds of AHA patients have a partial or complete remission following splenectomy.[287,292,294] However, the relapse rate is disappointingly high. Many patients require further glucocorticoid therapy to maintain acceptable hemoglobin levels, although often at a lower dose than required prior to splenectomy.[10,111,287] Alternate-day therapy is preferable to daily therapy in these cases if adequate control of the anemia can be achieved.

The immediate mortality and morbidity from splenectomy depend upon the presence of underlying disease and the preoperative clinical status but generally are quite low.[295] Following splenectomy, children, more than adults, have an increased risk for developing sepsis as a result of encapsulated organisms.[296] Vaccination against *H. influenzae* type b and pneumococcal and meningococcal organisms is recommended 2 weeks prior to surgery.[297]

RITUXIMAB

Rituximab is a monoclonal antibody directed against the CD20 antigen expressed on B lymphocytes and used for treatment of B cell lymphoma. Its use for treatment of AHA is based on the antibody's ability to eliminate B lymphocytes, including presumably those making autoantibodies to RBCs. In the largest series to date,[298] 13 of 15 children with warm-antibody AHA responded to rituximab 375 mg/m[2] weekly for 2 to 4 weeks. More than 30 other case reports support the use of rituximab in adults, although the actual response rate is not known.

IMMUNOSUPPRESSIVE DRUGS

Cytotoxic drugs such as cyclophosphamide, 6-mercaptopurine, azathioprine, and 6-thioguanine have been given to patients with AHA to suppress synthesis of autoantibody. Direct evidence of such an effect is lacking. Although immunosuppressive therapy is not universally accepted, beneficial responses to immunosuppressive drugs have been observed in some patients who did not respond to glucocorticoids.[11,299] Importantly, the majority of patients with warm-antibody AHA respond to glucocorticoids and/or splenectomy and usually are not candidates for immunosuppressive therapy. At present, immunosuppressive therapy should be reserved primarily for patients who do not

respond to glucocorticoids and splenectomy or for patients who are poor surgical risks.[299]

The most successful approach used high-dose cyclophosphamide 50 mg/kg ideal body weight/day for 4 consecutive days, with granulocyte colony stimulating factor support.[300] Of nine patients, eight of whom had warm autoantibodies, all became transfusion independent. All patients had prolonged severe cytopenias and required hospitalization for a median of 21 days.

For patients who may not tolerate prolonged cytopenias, the drugs of choice are cyclophosphamide 60 mg/m[2] or azathioprine 80 mg/m[2], given daily. If the patient tolerates the drug, continue treatment for up to 6 months while waiting for a response. When response occurs, the patient can be weaned slowly from the drug. If no response is observed, the alternative drug can be tried. Because cyclophosphamide and azathioprine suppress hematopoiesis, blood counts including reticulocyte count must be monitored with extra care during therapy. Treatment with either agent increases the risk of subsequent neoplasia. Cyclophosphamide may cause severe hemorrhagic cystitis.

OTHER THERAPIES

For patients with chronic compensated hemolysis, treatment with folate at 1 mg/day is recommended to satisfy the increased demands for the vitamin because of increased red cell production. Plasma exchange or plasmapheresis has been used in patients with warm-antibody AHA. Improvement has been reported in a few cases, but use of the method is controversial.[301,302] Thymectomy has been reported useful in a few children who were refractory to glucocorticoids and splenectomy.[299] Selective injury to splenic macrophages by administration of vinblastine-loaded, IgG-sensitized platelets reportedly was successful in a few patients.[303] Several anecdotal reports and a case series indicate short-term successful treatment of patients with AHA using high-dose intravenous γ-globulin.[304-308] Uncontrolled studies indicate danazol, a nonvirilizing androgen, may be useful in patients with AHA.[309,310] Danazol may eliminate the need for splenectomy when danazol is combined with prednisone and may allow for a shorter duration of prednisone therapy.[310] Some patients with ulcerative colitis and AHA unresponsive to glucocorticoids and splenectomy may respond to colectomy.[311] In patients with AHA associated with an ovarian dermoid cyst, cyst removal produces remission of the hemolysis.[312] Patients with refractory AHA have been treated effectively with the purine analogue 2-chlorodeoxyadenosine (cladribine).[313]

THERAPY OF COLD-ANTIBODY HEMOLYTIC ANEMIA

Keeping the patient warm, particularly the patient's extremities, is moderately effective in providing symptomatic relief. This action may be the only measure required in patients with mild chronic hemolysis. In symptomatic patients, rituximab is effective and well tolerated. In a prospective trial, 14 of 27 patients responded to rituximab 375 mg/m[2] weekly for 4 weeks, with a median increase in hemoglobin levels of 4.0 gm/dl.[314] Patients who relapsed responded to a second course of rituximab at about the same rate. Chlorambucil or cyclophosphamide may be helpful for patients with symptomatic chronic cold agglutinin disease.[9-11,315,316] One patient treated with interferon-α experienced rapid resolution of acrocyanosis and hemolytic anemia, associated with a marked decrease in cold agglutinin titer,[317] but treatment failures also have been noted. Treatment with interferon-α also has proved beneficial in patients with type II cryoglobulinemia involving monoclonal IgM anti-IgG.[318] Results of splenectomy[10,11,319] or use of glucocorticoids[10,11] generally have been disappointing, although exceptions have been reported,[10,181,259,260] particularly in atypical cases. Experimental[156] and clinical[181] bases exist for considering very high doses of glucocorticoids in seriously ill patients. RBC transfusions generally are reserved for patients with severe anemia of rapid onset who are in danger of cardiorespiratory complications.[259] Washed RBCs often are used to avoid replenishing depleted complement components and reactivating the hemolytic process. In critically ill patients, plasma exchange (with replacement by albumin-containing saline solution) may provide transient amelioration of hemolysis.[320–322]

Most contemporary cases of paroxysmal cold hemoglobinuria are self-limited. Acute attacks in both chronic and transient forms of paroxysmal cold hemoglobinuria may be prevented by avoiding cold exposure. Glucocorticoid therapy and splenectomy have not been useful. When paroxysmal cold hemoglobinuria is associated with syphilis, effective treatment of the infection may result in complete remission. Antihistaminic and adrenergic agents may relieve symptoms of cold urticaria.

THERAPY OF DRUG-IMMUNE HEMOLYTIC ANEMIA

Discontinuation of the offending drug often is the only treatment needed. This measure is essential and may be life saving in patients with severe hemolysis mediated by the ternary complex mechanism.

If high-dose penicillin is the treatment of choice in a life-threatening infection and alternative antibiotic regimens are clearly inferior to penicillin, the drug need not be discontinued because of a positive direct antiglobulin reaction alone. A change in therapy is indicated only in the presence of overt hemolytic anemia. For example, lowering the penicillin dose by coadministering other antibiotics may allow continuation of the drug in some cases, particularly if hemolysis is not severe.

In patients taking α-methyldopa in the absence of hemolysis, a positive DAT has not necessarily been an indication for stopping the drug. However, given all the choices available, considering alternative antihypertensive therapy is prudent. Because less information on the natural history of autoantibodies induced by drugs other than α-methyldopa is available, discontinuation of the offending drug is advisable unless no suitable alternative exists.

Glucocorticoids are generally unnecessary, and their efficacy is questionable. However, prednisone is effective in patients with CLL and autoimmune hemolysis caused by purine analogues.[83,84] Transfusions should be given in the unusual circumstance of severe, life-threatening anemia. Problems with cross-matching, similar to those encountered in warm-antibody AHA, may occur in patients with a strongly positive IAT, for example, in α-methyldopa–related cases. Patients with hemolytic anemia resulting from the hapten/drug adsorption mechanism should have a compatible cross-match because the serum antibody reacts only with drug-coated cells. However, if therapy with the offending drug is still in progress, transfused cells may be destroyed at an increased rate as they become coated with drug *in vivo*.

Several cases of transfusion-associated graft-versus-host disease as a result of purine analogues have been reported in CLL patients transfused for hemolysis.[84,323,324] Such patients should receive irradiated blood products.

COURSE AND PROGNOSIS

Patients with idiopathic warm-antibody AHA have unpredictable clinical courses characterized by relapses and remissions. No particular feature of the illness has been a consistent predictor of outcome. Despite a rather high initial rate of response to glucocorticoids and splenectomy, the overall mortality rate was significant (up to 46%) in several older series but much lower in more recent studies.[10,11,287,325,326] The actuarial survival at 10 years reportedly is 73 percent.[325] Pulmonary emboli, infection, and cardiovascular collapse are causes of death.

Thromboembolic episodes in the form of deep vein thrombosis or splenic infarcts are relatively common during active phases of the disease.[287,326] In one series, eight of 30 patients with AHA developed venous thromboembolism; 19 of the patients had antiphospholipid antibodies, including six of the eight patients with thromboembolism.[327] In another retrospective analysis of 36 exacerbations of severe AHA in 28 patients, only six of whom were tested and found negative for antiphospholipid antibodies, venous thromboembolism occurred in five of 15 exacerbations without anticoagulation and one of 21 with anticoagulation.[328] The contribution of antiphospholipid antibodies to morbidity and mortality in AHA is not clear from these data. However, considering prophylactic anticoagulation for patients with AHA and antiphospholipid antibodies or other risk factors for venous thromboembolism seems prudent.

The prognosis in secondary warm-antibody AHA largely depends upon the course of the underlying disease.

In children, warm-antibody AHA frequently follows an acute infection or immunization.[291,329,330] Most of these patients exhibit a self-limited course and respond rapidly to glucocorticoids. Children with chronic AHA tend to be older.[330,331] Those who recover from the initial hemolytic episode have a good prognosis and are unlikely to relapse, although exceptions are known. The overall mortality rate is lower than in adults, ranging from 10 to 30 percent,[291,329–333] with higher mortality rates in those with chronic AHA[291,333] and associated autoimmune thrombocytopenia (Evans syndrome).[334]

Patients with idiopathic cold agglutinin disease often have a relatively benign course and survive for many years.[9,11,316] Occasionally, death results from infection or severe anemia or, not uncommonly, from an underlying lymphoproliferative process.

The postinfectious forms of cold agglutinin disease typically are self-limited. Recovery generally occurs in a few weeks. A few cases with massive hemoglobinuria have been complicated by acute renal failure, requiring temporary hemodialysis.

Postinfectious forms of paroxysmal cold hemoglobinuria terminate spontaneously within a few days to weeks after onset,[12–15] although the Donath-Landsteiner antibody may persist in low titer for several years.[10] Most patients with chronic idiopathic paroxysmal cold hemoglobinuria survive for many years despite occasional paroxysms of hemolysis.

Immune hemolysis in response to drugs usually is mild, and the prognosis is good. Occasional episodes of exceptionally severe hemolysis with renal failure or death have been reported, usually because of drugs operating through the ternary complex mechanism or purine analogues in patients with CLL.[39,53,55,59–62,64,81,100,101,210] In hemolysis resulting from ternary complex or hapten/drug adsorption mechanisms, the DAT becomes negative shortly after the drug is discontinued, that is, soon after the drug clears from the circulation. In addition, the hemolysis associated with α-methyldopa-induced autoantibodies ceases promptly after drug cessation. However, a positive DAT of gradually diminishing intensity may remain for weeks or months.

REFERENCES

1. Packman C: Historical review: The spherocytic haemolytic anaemias. *Br J Haematol* 112:888, 2001.
2. Coombs RRA, Mourant AE, Race EE: A new test for the detection of weak and incomplete Rh agglutinins. *Br J Exp Pathol* 26:255, 1945.
3. Boorman KE, Dodd BE, Loutit JF: Haemolytic icterus (acholuric jaundice), congenital and acquired. *Lancet* 1:812, 1946.
4. Loutit JF, Mollison PL: Haemolytic icterus (acholuric jaundice), congenital and acquired. *J Pathol Bacteriol* 58:711, 1946.
5. Landsteiner K: Uber Beziehungen zwischen dem Blutserum und den Körperzeller. *Munch Med Wochenschr* 50:1812, 1903.

6. Clough MC, Richter IM: A study of an autoagglutinin occurring in a human serum. *Johns Hopkins Hosp Bull* 29:86, 1918.

7. Iwai S, Mei-Sai N: Etiology of Raynaud's disease: A preliminary report. *Jpn Med World* 5:119, 1925.

8. Iwai S, Mei-Sai N: Etiology of Raynaud's disease. *Jpn Med World* 6: 345, 1926.

9. Schubothe H: The cold hemagglutinin disease. *Semin Hematol* 3:27, 1966.

10. Dacie JV: *The Haemolytic Anaemias*, vol 3, *The Autoimmune Haemolytic Anaemias*, 3d ed. Churchill Livingstone, New York, 1992.

11. Petz LD, Garratty G: *Acquired Immune Hemolytic Anemias*. Churchill Livingstone, London, 1980.

12. Nordhagen R, Stensvold K, Winsnes A, et al: Paroxysmal cold hemoglobinuria. The most frequent autoimmune hemolytic anemia in children? *Acta Paediatr Scand* 73:258, 1984.

13. Wolach B, Heddle N, Barr RD, et al: Transient Donath-Landsteiner hemolytic anemia. *Br J Haematol* 48:425, 1981.

14. Sokol RJ, Hewitt S, Stamps BK: Autoimmune hemolysis associated with Donath-Landsteiner antibodies. *Acta Haematol* 68:268, 1982.

15. Gottsche B, Salama A, Mueller-Eckhardt C: Donath-Landsteiner autoimmune hemolytic anemia in children: A study of 22 cases. *Vox Sang* 58:281, 1990.

16. Fellous M, Gerbal A, Tessier C, et al: Studies on the biosynthetic pathway of human P erythrocyte antigens using somatic cells in culture. *Vox Sang* 26:518, 1974.

17. Ackroyd JF: The pathogenesis of thrombocytopenic purpura due to hypersensitivity to Sedormid (allylisopropyl-acetylcarbamide). *Clin Sci* 7: 249, 1949.

18. Snapper I, Marks D, Schwartz L, Hollander L: Hemolytic anemia secondary to Mesantoin. *Ann Intern Med* 39:619, 1953.

19. Harris JW: Studies on the mechanism of drug-induced hemolytic anemia. *J Lab Clin Med* 47:760, 1956.

20. Sokol RJ, Hewitt S, Stamps BK: Autoimmune haemolysis: An 18 year study of 865 cases referred to a regional transfusion centre. *Br Med J* 282:2023, 1981.

21. Sokol RJ, Hewitt S, Stamps BK: Autoimmune haemolysis: Mixed warm and cold antibody type. *Acta Haematol* 69:266, 1983.

22. Shulman IA, Branch DR, Nelson JM, et al: Autoimmune hemolytic anemias with both cold and warm autoantibodies. *JAMA* 253:1746, 1985.

23. Kajii E, Miura Y, Ikemoto S: Characterization of autoantibodies in mixed-type autoimmune hemolytical anemia. *Vox Sang* 60:45, 1991.

24. Berentsen S, Bo K, Shammas F, et al: Chronic cold agglutinin disease of the "idiopathic" type is a premalignant or low-grade malignant lymphoproliferative disease. *APMIS* 105:354, 1997.

25. Telen MJ, Roberts KB, Bartlett JA: HIV-associated autoimmune hemolytic anemia: Report of a case and review of the literature. *J Acquir Immune Defic Syndr* 3:933, 1990.

26. Rapoport AP, Rowe JM, McMican A: Life-threatening autoimmune hemolytic anemia in patient with acquired immune deficiency syndrome. *Transfusion* 28:190, 1988.

27. Saif M: HIV Associated autoimmune hemolytic anemia: An update. *AIDS Patient Care* 15:217, 2001.

28. VanArsdel PP Jr, Gilliland BC: Anemia secondary to penicillin treatment: Studies on two patients with non-allergic serum hemagglutinins. *J Lab Clin Med* 65:277, 1965.

29. Petz LD, Fudenberg HH: Coombs-positive hemolytic anemia caused by penicillin administration. *N Engl J Med* 274:171, 1966.

30. Swanson MA, Chanmougan D, Schwartz RS: Immuno-hemolytic anemia due to antipenicillin antibodies. *N Engl J Med* 274:178, 1966.

31. Levine B, Redmond A: Immunochemical mechanisms of penicillin-induced Coombs positivity and hemolytic anemia in man. *Int Arch Allergy Appl Immunol* 1:594, 1967.

32. White JM, Brown DL, Hepner GW, Worlledge SM: Penicillin-induced hemolytic anaemia. *Br Med J* 3:26, 1968.

33. Seldon MR, Bain B, Johnson CA, Lennox CS: Ticarcillin-induced immune haemolytic anaemia. *Scand J Haematol* 28:459, 1982.

34. Tuffs L, Manoharan A: Flucloxacillin-induced haemolytic anaemia. *Med J Aust* 144:559, 1986.

35. Gralnick HR, McGinnis MH, Elton W, McCurdy P: Hemolytic anemia associated with cephalothin. *JAMA* 217:1193, 1971.

36. Branch DR, Berkowitz LR, Becker RL, et al: Extravascular hemolysis following the administration of cefamandole. *Am J Hematol* 18:213, 1985.

37. Chambers LA, Donovan BA, Kruskall MS: Ceftazidime-induced hemolysis patient with drug-dependent antibodies reactive by immune complex and drug adsorption mechanisms. *Am J Clin Pathol* 95:393, 1991.

38. Gallagher NI, Schergen AK, Sokol-Anderson ML, et al: Severe immune-mediated hemolytic anemia secondary to treatment with cefotetan. *Transfusion* 32:266, 1992.

39. Garratty G, Nance S, Lloyd M, Domen R: Fatal immune hemolytic anemia due to cefotetan. *Transfusion* 32:269, 1992.

40. Wenz B, Klein RL, Lalezari P: Tetracycline-induced immune hemolytic anemia. *Transfusion* 14:265, 1974.

41. Simpson MB, Pryzbylik J, Innis B, Denham MA: Hemolytic anemia after tetracycline therapy. *N Engl J Med* 312:840, 1985.

42. Pujol M, Fernandez F, Sancho JM, et al: Immune hemolytic anemia induced by 6-mercaptopurine. *Transfusion* 40:75, 2000.

43. Steanini M, Johnson NL: Positive antihuman globulin test in patients receiving carbromal. *Am J Med Sci* 259:49, 1970.

44. Bird GWG, Ecles GH, Litchfield JA, et al: Haemolytic anaemia associated with antibodies to tolbutamide and phenacetin. *Br Med J* 1:728, 1972.

45. Malacarne P, Castaldi G, Bertusi M, Zavagli G: Tolbutamide-induced hemolytic anemia. *Diabetes* 26:156, 1977.

46. Salama A, Mueller-Eckhardt C: Cianidanol and its metabolites bind tightly to red cells and are responsible for the production of auto- and/ or drug-dependent antibodies against these cells. *Br J Haematol* 66:263, 1987.

47. Muirhead EE, Halden ER, Granes M: Drug-dependent Coombs (antiglobulin) test and anemia: Observations on quinine and acetophenetidine (phenacetin). *Arch Intern Med* 101:827, 1958.

48. Croft JD Jr, Swisher SN, Gilliland BC, et al: Coombs test positivity induced by drugs: Mechanisms of immunologic reactions and red cell destruction. *Ann Intern Med* 68:176, 1968.

49. Freedman AL, Barr PS, Brody E: Hemolytic anemia due to quinidine: Observations on its mechanism. *Am J Med* 20:806, 1956.

50. Logue GL, Boyd AE, Rosse WF: Chlorpropamide-induced immune hemolytic anemia. *N Engl J Med* 283:900, 1970.

51. Kopicky JA, Packman CH: The mechanisms of sulfonylurea-induced immune hemolysis. Case report and review of the literature. *Am J Hematol* 23:283, 1986.

52. Lakshminarayan S, Sahn SA, Hudson LD: Massive hemolysis caused by rifampicin. *Br Med J* 2:282, 1973.

53. Pereira A, Sanz C, Cervantes F, Castillo R: Immune hemolytic anemia and renal failure associated with rifampicin-dependent antibodies with anti-I specificity. *Ann Hematol* 63:56, 1991.

54. Bengtsson U, Staffan A, Aurell M, Kaijser B: Antazoline-induced immune hemolytic anemia, hemoglobinuria and acute renal failure. *Acta Med Scand* 198:223, 1975.

55. Habibi B, Basty R, Chodez S, Prunat A: Thiopental-related immune hemolytic anemia and renal failure. *N Engl J Med* 312:353, 1985.

56. Squires JE, Mintz PD, Clark S: Tolmetin-induced hemolysis. *Transfusion* 25:410, 1985.

57. Sosler SD, Behzad V, Garratty G, et al: Immune hemolytic anemia associated with probenecid. *Am J Clin Pathol* 84:391, 1985.

58. Salama A, Mueller-Eckhardt C: Two types of nomifensine-induced immune haemolytic anaemias: Drug-dependent sensitization and/or auto-immunization. *Br J Haematol* 64:613, 1986.

59. Habibi B, Cartron JP, Bretagne M, et al: Anti-nomifensine antibody causing immune hemolytic anemia and renal failure. *Vox Sang* 40:79, 1981.

60. Fulton JD, Briggs JD, Dominiczak AF, et al: Intravascular haemolysis and acute renal failure induced by nomifensine. *Scott Med J* 31:242, 1986.

61. Garratty G, Postoway N, Schwellenbach J, McMahill PC: A fatal case of ceftriaxone (Rocephin)-induced hemolytic anemia associated with intravascular immune hemolysis. *Transfusion* 31:176, 1991.

62. Rosenfeld CS, Winters SJ, Tedrow HE: Diethylstilbestrol-associated hemolytic anemia with a positive direct antiglobulin test result. *Am J Med* 86:617, 1989.

63. Salama A, Burger M, Mueller-Eckhardt C: Acute immune hemolysis induced by a degradation product of amphotericin B. *Blut* 58:59, 1989.

64. Wolf B, Conradty M, Grohmann R, et al: A case of immune complex hemolytic anemia, thrombocytopenia, and acute renal failure associated with doxepin use. *J Clin Psychiatry* 50:99, 1989.

65. Salama A, Kroll H, Wittmann G, Mueller-Eckhardt C: Diclofenac-induced immune haemolytic anaemia: Simultaneous occurrence of red blood cell autoantibodies and drug-dependent antibodies. *Br J Haematol* 95:640, 1996.

66. Bougie D, Johnson ST, Weitekamp LA, Aster RH: Sensitivity to metabolite of diclofenac as a cause of acute immune hemolytic anemia. *Blood* 90:407, 1997.

67. Cunha PD, Lord RS, Johnson ST, et al: Immune hemolytic anemia caused by sensitivity to a metabolite of etodolac, a nonsteroidal anti-inflammatory drug. *Transfusion* 40:663, 2000.

68. Carstairs KC, Breckenridge A, Dollery CT, Worlledge SM: Incidence of a positive direct Coombs test in patients on alpha-methyldopa. *Lancet* 2:133, 1966.

69. Worlledge SM, Carstairs KC, Dacie JV: Autoimmune haemolytic anaemia associated with α-methyldopa therapy. *Lancet* 2:135, 1966.

70. Breckenridge A, Dollery CT, Worlledge SM, et al: Positive direct Coombs tests and antinuclear factors in patients treated with methyldopa. *Lancet* 2:1265, 1967.

71. Lo Buglio AF, Jandl JH: The nature of alpha-methyldopa red cell antibody. *N Engl J Med* 276:658, 1967.

72. Cotzias GC, Papavasiliou PS: Autoimmunity in patients treated with levodopa. *JAMA* 207:1353, 1969.

73. Henry RE, Goldberg LS, Sturgeon P, Ansel RD: Serologic abnormalities associated with *l*-dopa therapy. *Vox Sang* 20:306, 1971.

74. Joseph C: Occurrence of positive Coombs test in patients treated with levodopa. *N Engl J Med* 286:1400, 1972.

75. Gabor EP, Goldberg LS: Levodopa-induced Coombs positive haemolytic anaemia. *Scand J Haematol* 11:201, 1973.

76. Territo MC, Peters RW, Tanaka KR: Autoimmune hemolytic anemia due to levodopa therapy. *JAMA* 226:1347, 1973.

77. Scott GL, Myles AB, Bacon PA: Autoimmune haemolytic anaemia and mefenamic acid therapy. *Br Med J* 3:543, 1968.

78. Robertson JH, Kennedy CC, Hill CM: Haemolytic anaemia associated with mefenamic acid. *Irish J Med Sci* 140:226, 1971.

79. Habibi B: Drug-induced red blood cell autoantibodies co-developed with drug-specific antibodies causing a hemolytic anaemia. *Br J Haematol* 61:139, 1985.

80. Kleinman S, Nelson R, Smith L, Goldfinger D: Positive direct antiglobulin tests and immune hemolytic anemia in patients receiving procainamide. *N Engl J Med* 311:809, 1984.

81. Kramer MR, Levene C, Hershko C: Severe reversible autoimmune haemolytic anaemia and thrombocytopenia associated with diclofenac therapy. *Scand J Haematol* 36:118, 1986.

82. Byrd JC, Hertler AA, Weiss RB, et al: Fatal recurrence of autoimmune hemolytic anemia following pentostatin therapy in a patient with a history of fludarabine-associated hemolytic anemia. *Ann Oncol* 6:300, 1995.

83. Weiss R, Freiman J, Kweder S, et al: Hemolytic anemia after fludarabine therapy for chronic lymphocytic leukemia. *J Clin Oncol* 16:1885, 1998.

84. Chasty RC, Myint H, Oscier DG, et al: Autoimmune haemolysis in patients with B-CLL treated with chlorodeoxyadenosine (CDA). *Leuk Lymphoma* 29:391, 1998.

85. Gralnick HR, Wright LD, McGinnis MH: Coombs' positive reactions associated with sodium cephalothin therapy. *JAMA* 199:725, 1967.

86. Molthan L, Reidenberg MM, Eichman MF: Positive direct Coombs' tests due to cephalothin. *N Engl J Med* 277:123, 1967.

87. Zeger G, Smith L, McQuiston D, Goldfinger D: Cisplatin-induced non-immunologic adsorption of immunoglobulin by red cells. *Transfusion* 28:493, 1988.

88. Muirhead EE, Groves M, Guy R, et al: Acquired hemolytic anemia, exposures to insecticides and positive Coombs' test dependent on insecticide preparations. *Vox Sang* 4:277, 1959.

89. Lindberg LG, Norden A: Severe hemolytic reaction to chlorpromazine. *Acta Med Scand* 170:195, 1961.

90. Eyster ME: Melphalan (Alkeran) erythrocyte agglutinin and hemolytic anemia. *Ann Intern Med* 66:573, 1967.

91. Robinson MG, Foadi M: Hemolytic anemia with positive Coomb's test. Association with isoniazid therapy. *JAMA* 208:656, 1969.

92. Mueller-Eckhardt C, Kretschmer V, Coburg KH: Allergic, immuno-hemolytic anemia due to para-aminosalicylic acid (PAS). Immunohematologic studies of three cases. *Dtsch Med Wochenschr* 97:234, 1972.

93. Manor E, Marmor A, Kaufman S, Leiba H: Massive hemolysis caused by acetaminophen. *JAMA* 236:2777, 1976.

94. Vilal JM, Blum L, Dosik H: Thiazide-induced immune hemolytic anemia. *JAMA* 236:1723, 1976.

95. Letona JM-L, Barbolla L, Frieyro E, et al: Immune haemolytic anaemia and renal failure induced by streptomycin. *Br J Haematol* 35:561, 1977.

96. Korsager S, Sorensen H, Jensen OH, Falk JV: Antiglobulin tests for determination of autoimmunohaemolytic anaemia during long-term treatment with ibuprofen. *Scand J Rheumatol* 10:174, 1981.

97. Takahashi H, Tsukada T: Triamterene-induced immune hemolytic anemia with acute intravascular hemolysis and acute renal failure. *Scand J Haematol* 23:169, 1979.

98. Wong KY, Boose GM, Issitt CH: Erythromycin-induced hemolytic anemia. *J Pediatr* 98:647, 1981.

99. Sandvei P, Nordhagen R, Michaelsen TE, Wolthuis K: Fluorouracil (5-FU) induced acute immune haemolytic anaemia. *Br J Haematol* 65:357, 1987.

100. Tafani O, Mazzoli M, Landini G, Alterini B: Fatal acute immune haemolytic anaemia caused by nalidixic acid. *Br Med J* 285:936, 1982.

101. Angeles ML, Reid ME, Yacob UA, et al: Sulindac-induced immune hemolytic anemia. *Transfusion* 34:255, 1994.

102. Marks DR, Joy JV, Bonheim NA: Hemolytic anemia associated with the use of omeprazole. *Am J Gastroenterol* 86:217, 1991.

103. Blum MD, Graham DJ, McCloskey CA: Temafloxacin syndrome: Review of 95 cases. *Clin Infect Dis* 18:946, 1994.

104. Marani TM, Trich MB, Armstrong KS, et al: Carboplatin-induced immune hemolytic anemia. *Transfusion* 36:1016, 1996.

105. Dacie JV: *The Haemolytic Anemias, Congenital and Acquired*, vol 3, *Secondary or Symptomatic Haematolytic Anaemias*, 2d ed. Grune & Stratton, New York, 1967.

106. Chaplin H, Avioli LV: Autoimmune hemolytic anemia. *Arch Intern Med* 137:346, 1977.

107. Sallah S, Wan J, Hanrahan L: Future development of lymphoproliferative disorders in patients with autoimmune hemolytic anemia. *Clin Cancer Res* 7:791, 2001.

108. Pirofsky B: Hereditary aspects of autoimmune hemolytic anemia: A retrospective analysis. *Vox Sang* 14:334, 1968.

109. Dobbs CE: Familial auto-immune hemolytic anemia. *Arch Intern Med* 116:273, 1965.

110. Cordova MS, Baez-Villasenor J, Mendez JJ, Campos E: Acquired hemolytic anemia with positive antiglobulin (Coombs' test) in mother and daughter. *Arch Intern Med* 117:692, 1966.

111. Eyster ME, Jenkins DE Jr: Erythrocyte coating substances in patients with positive direct antiglobulin reactions: Correlation of γG globulin and complement coating with underlying diseases, overt hemolysis and response to therapy. *Am J Med* 46:360, 1969.

112. Feizi T: Cold agglutinins, the direct Coombs' test and serum immunoglobulins in *Mycoplasma pneumoniae* infection. *Ann N Y Acad Sci* 143:801, 1967.

113. Jacobson LB, Longstreth GF, Edington TS: Clinical and immunologic features of transient cold agglutinin hemolytic anemia. *Am J Med* 54:514, 1973.

114. Murray HW, Masur H, Senterfit LB, Roberts RB: The protean manifestations of *Mycoplasma pneumoniae* infection in adults. *Am J Med* 58:229, 1975.

115. Rosenfield RE, Schmidt PJ, Calvo RC, McGinniss MH: Anti-i, a frequent cold agglutinin in infectious mononucleosis. *Vox Sang* 10:631, 1965.

116. Worlledge SM, Dacie JV: Haemolytic and other anaemias in infectious mononucleosis, in *Infectious Mononucleosis*, edited by RL Carter, HG Penman, p 82. Blackwell Science, Oxford, 1969.

117. Hossaini AA: Anti-i in infectious mononucleosis. *Am J Clin Pathol* 53:198, 1970.

118. Arndt P, Garratty G: Cross-reactivity of cefotetan and ceftriaxone antibodies, associated with hemolytic anemia, with other cephalosporins and penicillin. *Coagul Transfusion Med* 118:256, 2002.

119. Issitt PD, Pavone BG, Goldfinger D, et al: Anti-Wr^b and other autoantibodies responsible for positive direct antiglobulin test in 150 individuals. *Br J Haematol* 34:5, 1976.

120. Worlledge SM: Immune drug-induced haemolytic anaemias. *Semin Hematol* 6:181, 1969.

121. Leddy JP, Falany JL, Kissel GE, et al: Erythrocyte membrane proteins reactive with human (warm-reacting) anti-red cell autoantibodies. *J Clin Invest* 91:1672, 1993.

122. Gorst DW, Rawlinson VI, Merry AH, Stratton F: Positive direct antiglobulin test in normal individuals. *Vox Sang* 38:99, 1980.

123. Bareford D, Langster G, Gilks L, Demick-Torey LA: Follow-up of normal individuals with a positive antiglobulin test. *Scand J Haematol* 35:348, 1985.

124. Worlledge SM: The interpretation of a positive direct antiglobulin test. *Br J Haematol* 39:157, 1978.

125. Nossal GJV: B-cell selection and tolerance. *Curr Opin Immunol* 3:193, 1991.

126. Basten A, Brink R, Peake P, et al: Self-tolerance in the B-cell repertoire. *Immunol Rev* 122:5, 1991.

127. Kroemer G, Martinez-A C: Mechanisms of self-tolerance. *Immunol Today* 13:401, 1992.

128. Hartley SB, Crosbie J, Brink R, et al: Elimination from peripheral lymphoid tissue of self-reactive B lymphocytes recognizing membrane bound antigens. *Nature* 353:765, 1991.

129. Leddy JP: Reactivity of human γG erythrocyte autoantibodies with fetal, autologous and maternal red cells. *Vox Sang* 17:525, 1969.

130. Okamoto M, Murakami M, Shimizu A, et al: A transgenic model of autoimmune hemolytic anemia. *J Exp Med* 175:71, 1992.

131. Murakami M, Tsubata T, Okamoto M, et al: Antigen-induced apoptotic death of Ly-1 B cells responsible for autoimmune disease in transgenic mice. *Nature* 357:77, 1992.

132. Leddy JP: Immune hemolytic anemia, in *Clinical Immunology: Principles and Practice*, edited by RR Rich, TA Fleisher, WT Shearer, et al, p 1273. Mosby, St. Louis, 1996.

133. Lin RH, Mamula MJ, Hardin JA, Janeway CA: Induction of autoreactive B cells allows priming of autoreactive T cells. *J Exp Med* 173:1433, 1991.

134. Silverman GJ, Carson DA: Structural characterization of human monoclonal cold agglutinins: Evidence for a distinct primary sequence-defined V$_H$4 idiotype. *Eur J Immunol* 20:351, 1990.

135. Silberstein LE, Jefferies LC, Goldman J, et al: Variable region gene analysis of pathologic human autoantibodies to the related i and I red blood cell antigens. *Blood* 78:2372, 1991.

136. Pascual V, Victor K, Spellerberg M, et al: V$_H$ restriction among human cold agglutinins: The V$_H$4−21 gene segment is required to encode anti-I and anti-i specificities. *J Immunol* 149:2337, 1992.

137. Stevenson FK, Smith GJ, North J, et al: Identification of normal B-cell counterparts of neoplastic cells which secrete cold agglutinins of anti-I and anti-i specificity. *Br J Haematol* 72:9, 1989.

138. Silverman GJ, Chen PP, Carson DA: Cold agglutinins: Specificity, idiotypy and structural analysis, in *Idiotypes in Biology and Medicine: Chemistry and Immunology*, vol 48, edited by DA Carson, PP Chen, TJ Kipps, p 109. Karger, Basel, 1990.

139. Feizi T: Lambda chains in cold agglutinins. *Science* 156:111, 1987.

140. Thompson KM, Sutherland J, Barden G, et al: Human monoclonal antibodies against blood group antigens preferentially express a V$_H$4−21 variable region gene-associated epitope. *Scand J Immunol* 34:509, 1991.

141. Adderson EE, Shackelford PG, Quinn A, et al: Restricted immunoglobulin VH usage and VDJ combinations in the human response to *Haemophilus influenzae* type b capsular polysaccharide: Nucleotide sequences of monospecific anti-*Haemophilus* antibodies and polyspecific antibodies cross-reacting with self-antigens. *J Clin Invest* 91:2734, 1993.

142. Adderson EE, Shackelford PG, Insel RA, et al: Immunoglobulin light chain variable region gene sequences for human antibodies to *Haemophilus influenzae* type b capsular polysaccharide are dominated by a limited number of V$_\kappa$ and V$_\lambda$ segments and VJ combinations. *J Clin Invest* 89:729, 1992.

143. Silberstein LE, Robertson GA, Hannam-Harris AC, et al: Etiologic aspects of cold agglutinin disease: Evidence of cytogenetically defined clones of lymphoid cells and the demonstration that an anti-Pr cold autoantibody is derived from an aberrant B cell clone. *Blood* 67:1705, 1986.

144. Gordon J, Silberstein LE, Moreau L, Nowell PC: Trisomy 3 in cold agglutinin disease. *Cancer Genet Cytogenet* 46:89, 1990.

145. Michaux L, Dierlamm J, Wlodarska I, et al: Trisomy 3q11-q29 is recurrently observed in B-cell non-Hodgkin's lymphomas associated with cold agglutinin syndrome. *Ann Hematol* 76:201, 1998.

146. Harboe M, Lind K: Light chain types of transiently occurring cold haemagglutinins. *Scand J Haematol* 3:269, 1966.

147. Feizi T: Monotypic cold agglutinins in infection by *Mycoplasma pneumoniae*. *Nature* 215:540, 1967.

148. Feizi T, Loveless W: Carbohydrate recognition by *Mycoplasma pneumoniae* and pathologic consequences. *Am J Respir Crit Care Med* 154:S133, 1996.

149. Mollison PL: Measurement of survival and destruction of red cells in haemolytic syndromes. *Br Med Bull* 15:59, 1959.

150. Holländer L: Erythrocyte survival time in a case of acquired haemolytic anaemia. *Vox Sang* 4:164, 1954.

151. Chaplin H, Cohen R, Bloomberg G, et al: Pregnancy and idiopathic autoimmune haemolytic anaemia: A prospective study during 6 months gestation and 3 months "post-partum." *Br J Haematol* 24:219, 1973.

152. Mollison PL, Crome P, Hughes-Jones NC, Rochna E: Rate of removal from the circulation of red cells sensitized with different amounts of antibody. *Br J Haematol* 11:461, 1965.

153. Mollison PL, Hughes-Jones NC: Clearance of Rh-positive red cells by low concentration of Rh antibody. *Immunology* 12:63, 1967.

154. Rosse WF: Quantitative immunology of immune hemolytic anemia: II. The relationship of cell-bound antibody to hemolysis and the effect of treatment. *J Clin Invest* 50:734, 1971.

155. Schreiber AD, Frank MM: Role of antibody and complement in the immune clearance and destruction of erythrocytes: I. In vivo effects of IgG and IgM complement-fixing sites. *J Clin Invest* 51:575, 1972.

156. Atkinson JP, Schreiber AD, Frank MM: Effects of corticosteroids and splenectomy on the immune clearance and destruction of erythrocytes. *J Clin Invest* 52:1509, 1973.

157. Atkinson JP, Frank MM: Complement independent clearance of IgG sensitized erythrocytes: Inhibition by cortisone. *Blood* 44:629, 1974.

158. Jandl JH, Richardson-Jones A, Castle WB: The destruction of red cells by antibodies in man: I. Observations on the sequestration and lysis of red cells altered by immune mechanisms. *J Clin Invest* 36:1428, 1957.

159. Jandl JH, Kaplan ME: The destruction of red cells by antibodies in man: III. Quantitative factors influencing the pattern of hemolysis in vivo. *J Clin Invest* 39:1145, 1960.

160. Abramson N, LoBuglio AF, Jandl JH, Cotran RS: The interaction between human monocytes and red cells: Binding characteristics. *J Exp Med* 132:1191, 1970.

161. LoBuglio AF, Cotran RS, Jandl JH: Red cells coated with immunoglobulin G: Binding and sphering by mononuclear cells in man. *Science* 158:1582, 1967.

162. Anderson CL, Looney RJ: Human leukocyte IgG Fc receptors. *Immunol Today* 7:264, 1986.

163. Ravetch JV, Kinet J-P: Fc receptors. *Annu Rev Immunol* 9:457, 1991.

164. Gigli I, Nelson RA: Complement-dependent immune phagocytosis: I. Requirements of C1, C4, C2, C3. *Exp Cell Res* 51:45, 1968.

165. Lay WF, Nussenzweig V: Receptors for complement on leukocytes. *J Exp Med* 128:991, 1968.

166. Ross GD: Opsonization and membrane complement receptors, in *Immunobiology of the Complement System*, edited by GD Ross, p 87. Academic Press, Orlando, 1986.

167. Fischer JT, Petz LD, Garratty G, Cooper NR: Correlations between quantitative assay of red cell bound C3, serologic reactions, and hemolytic anemia. *Blood* 44:359, 1974.

168. Schreiber AD, Parsons J, McDermott P, Cooper RA: Effect of corticosteroids on the human monocyte IgG and complement receptors. *J Clin Invest* 56:1189, 1975.

169. Ehlenberger AG, Nussenzweig V: The role of membrane receptors for C3b and C3d in phagocytosis. *J Exp Med* 145:357, 1977.

170. Rosse WF, De Boisfleury A, Bessis M: The interaction of phagocytic cells and red cells modified by immune reactions: Comparison of antibody and complement coated red cells. *Blood Cells* 1:345, 1975.

171. Dameshek W, Schwartz SO: Acute hemolytic anemia (acquired hemolytic icterus, acute type). *Medicine* 19:231, 1940.

172. Leddy JP, Rosenfeld SI: Role of complement in hemolytic anemia and thrombocytopenia, in *Immunobiology of the Complement System*, edited by GD Ross, p 213. Academic Press, Orlando, 1986.

173. Nicholson-Weller A, Burge J, Fearon DT, et al: Isolation of a human erythrocyte membrane glycoprotein with decay-accelerating activity for C3 convertases of the complement system. *J Immunol* 129:184, 1982.

174. Lachmann PJ: The control of homologous lysis. *Immunol Today* 12:312, 1991.

175. Packman CH: Pathogenesis and management of paroxysmal nocturnal hemoglobinuria. *Blood Rev* 12:1, 1998.

176. Fleer A, Van Schaik MLJ, Von dem Borne AEG Kr, Engelfriet CP: Destruction of sensitized erythrocytes by human monocytes in vitro:

177. Kurlander RJ, Rosse WF, Logue WL: Quantitative influence of antibody and complement coating of red cells on monocyte-mediated cell lysis. *J Clin Invest* 61:1309, 1978.

178. Urbaniak SJ: Lymphoid cell dependent (K-cell) lysis of human erythrocytes sensitized with rhesus alloantibodies. *Br J Haematol* 33:409, 1976.

179. Handwerger BS, Kay NW, Douglas SD: Lymphocyte-mediated antibody-dependent cytolysis: Role in immune hemolysis. *Vox Sang* 34:276, 1978.

180. Milgrom H, Shore SL: Lysis of antibody-coated human red cells by peripheral blood mononuclear cells: Altered effector cell profile after treatment of target cells with enzymes. *Cell Immunol* 39:178, 1978.

181. Schreiber AD, Herskovitz BS, Goldwein M: Low-titer cold-hemagglutinin disease. *N Engl J Med* 296:1490, 1977.

182. Evans RS, Turner F, Bingham M, Woods R: Chronic hemolytic anemia due to cold agglutinins: II. The role of C' in red cell destruction. *J Clin Invest* 47:691, 1968.

183. Logue GL, Rosse WF, Gockerman JP: Measurement of the third component of complement bound to red blood cells in patients with the cold agglutinin syndrome. *J Clin Invest* 52:493, 1973.

184. Jaffe CH, Atkinson JP, Frank MM: The role of complement in the clearance of cold agglutinin-sensitized erythrocytes in man. *J Clin Invest* 58:942, 1976.

185. Atkinson JP, Frank MM: Studies on in vivo effects of antibody: Interaction of IgM antibody and complement in the immune clearance and destruction of erythrocytes in man. *J Clin Invest* 54:339, 1974.

186. Kirschfink M, Fritze H, Roelcke D: Complement activation by cold agglutinins. *Vox Sang* 63:220, 1992.

187. Hughey CT, Brewer JW, Colosia AD, et al: Production of IgM hexamers by normal and autoimmune B cells: Implications for the physiologic role of hexameric IgM. *J Immunol* 161:4091, 1998.

188. Evans RS, Turner E, Bingham M: Studies with radioiodinated cold agglutinins of ten patients. *Am J Med* 38:378, 1965.

189. Roelcke D: Cold agglutination: Antibodies and antigens. *Clin Immunol Immunopathol* 2:266, 1974.

190. Mantovani B, Rabinovitch M, Nussenzweig V: Phagocytosis of immune complexes by macrophages: Different roles of the macrophage receptor sites for complement (C3) and for immunoglobulin (IgG). *J Exp Med* 135:780, 1972.

191. Silverstein SC, Steinman RM, Cohn ZA: Endocytosis. *Annu Rev Biochem* 46:669, 1977.

192. Brown DL, Nelson DA: Surface microfragmentation of red cells as a mechanism for complement-mediated immune spherocytosis. *Br J Haematol* 24:301, 1973.

193. Evans RS, Turner E, Bingham M: Chronic hemolytic anemia due to cold agglutinins: I. The mechanism of resistance of red cells to C' hemolysis by cold agglutinins. *J Clin Invest* 46:1461, 1967.

194. Kerr RO, Cardamone J, Dalmasso AP, Kaplan ME: Two mechanisms of erythrocyte destruction in penicillin-induced hemolytic anemia. *N Engl J Med* 287:1322, 1972.

195. Nesmith LW, Davis JW: Hemolytic anemia caused by penicillin. *JAMA* 203:27, 1968.

196. Yust I, Frisch B, Goldsher N: Simultaneous detection of two mechanisms of immune destruction of penicillin-treated human red blood cells. *Am J Hematol* 13:53, 1982.

197. Brandriss MW, Smith JW, Steinman HG: Common antigenic determinants of penicillin G, cephalothin and 6-aminopenicillanic acid in rabbits. *J Immunol* 94:696, 1965.

198. Abraham GN, Petz LD, Fudenberg HH: Immuno-hematological cross-allergenicity between penicillin and cephalothin in humans. *Clin Exp Immunol* 3:343, 1968.

Effects of cytochalasin B, hydrocortisone and colchicine. *Scand J Immunol* 8:515, 1978.

199. Petz LD: Immunologic cross reactivity between penicillins and cephalosporins: A review. *J Infect Dis* 137:S74, 1978.
200. Kunicki TJ, Russell N, Nurten AT, et al: Further studies of the human platelet receptor for quinine- and quinidine-dependent antibodies. *J Immunol* 126:398, 1981.
201. Christie DJ, Aster RH: Drug-antibody-platelet interaction in quinine- and quinidine-induced thrombocytopenia. *J Clin Invest* 70:989, 1982.
202. Berndt MC, Chong BH, Bull HA, et al: Molecular characterization of quinine/quinidine drug-dependent antibody platelet interaction using monoclonal antisera. *Blood* 66:1292, 1985.
203. Sosler SD, Behzad O, Garratty G, et al: Acute hemolytic anemia associated with a chlorpropamide-induced apparent auto-anti-Jk$_a$. *Transfusion* 24:206, 1984.
204. Salama A, Mueller-Eckhardt C: Rh blood group-specific antibodies in immune hemolytic anemia induced by nomifensine. *Blood* 68:1285, 1986.
205. Salama A, Mueller-Eckhardt C: On the mechanisms of sensitization and attachment of antibodies to RBC in drug-induced immune hemolytic anemia. *Blood* 69:1006, 1987.
206. Christie DJ, Mullen PC, Aster RH: Fab-mediated binding of drug-dependent antibodies to platelets in quinidine- and quinine-induced thrombocytopenia. *J Clin Invest* 75:310, 1985.
207. Smith ME, Reid DM, Jones CE, et al: Binding of quinine- and quinidine-dependent drug antibodies to platelets is mediated by the Fab domain of immunoglobulin G and is not Fc dependent. *J Clin Invest* 29:912, 1987.
208. Salama A, Mueller-Eckhardt C: The role of metabolite-specific antibodies in nomifensine-dependent immune hemolytic anemia. *N Engl J Med* 313:469, 1985.
209. Kelton JG: Impaired reticuloendothelial function in patients treated with methyldopa. *N Engl J Med* 313:596, 1985.
210. Worlledge SM: Immune drug-induced hemolytic anemias. *Semin Haematol* 10:327, 1973.
211. Bakemeier RF, Leddy JP: Erythrocyte autoantibody associated with alpha-methyldopa: Heterogeneity of structure and specificity. *Blood* 32:1, 1968.
212. Green FA, Jung CY, Rampal A, Lorusso DJ: Alpha-methyldopa and the erythrocyte membrane. *Clin Exp Immunol* 40:554, 1980.
213. Green Fa, Jung CY, Hui H: Modulation of alpha-methyldopa binding to the erythrocyte membrane by superoxide dismutase. *Biochem Biophys Res Commun* 95:1037, 1980.
214. Kirtland HH III, Mohler DN, Horwitz DA: Methyldopa inhibition of suppressor-lymphocyte function. A proposed cause of autoimmune hemolytic anemia. *N Engl J Med* 302:825, 1980.
215. Garratty G, Arndt P, Prince HE, Schulman IA: The effect of methyldopa and procainamide on suppressor cell activity in relation to red cell autoantibody production. *Br J Haematol* 84:310, 1993.
216. Spath P, Garratty G, Petz LD: Studies on the immune response to penicillin and cephalothin in humans: II. Immunohematologic reactions to cephalothin administration. *J Immunol* 107:860, 1971.
217. Garratty G, Petz L: Drug-induced hemolytic anemia. *Am J Med* 58:398, 1975.
218. Sokol RJ, Hewitt S, Stamps BK: Erythrocyte autoantibodies, autoimmune haemolysis and pregnancy. *Vox Sang* 43:169, 1982.
219. Issaragrisil S, Kruatrachue M: An association of pregnancy and autoimmune haemolytic anaemia. *Scand J Haematol* 31:63, 1983.
220. Evans RS, Duane RT: Acquired hemolytic anemia: I. The relation of erythrocyte antibody production to activity of the disease: II. The significance of thrombocytopenia and leukopenia. *Blood* 4:1196, 1949.
221. Evans RS, Takahashi K, Duane RT, et al: Primary thrombocytopenic purpura and acquired hemolytic anemia: Evidence for a common etiology. *Arch Intern Med* 87:48, 1951.
222. Pegels JG, Helmerhorst FM, vanLeeuwen EF, et al: The Evans syndrome: Characterization of the responsible autoantibodies. *Br J Haematol* 51:445, 1982.
223. Liesveld JL, Rowe JM, Lichtman MA: Variability of the erythropoietic response in autoimmune hemolytic anemia: Analysis of 109 cases. *Blood* 69:820, 1987.
224. Hegde UM, Gordon-Smith EC, Worlledge SM: Reticulocytopenia and absence of red cell autoantibodies in immune haemolytic anaemia. *Br Med J* 2:1444, 1977.
225. Conley CL, Lippman SM, Ness P: Autoimmune hemolytic anemia with reticulocytopenia: A medical emergency. *JAMA* 244:1688, 1980.
226. Greenberg J, Curtis-Cohen M, Gill FM, Cohen A: Prolonged reticulocytopenia in autoimmune hemolytic anemia of childhood. *J Pediatr* 97:784, 1980.
227. Mangan KF, Besa EC, Shadduck RK, et al: Demonstration of two distinct antibodies in autoimmune hemolytic anemia with reticulocytopenia and red cell aplasia. *Exp Hematol* 12:788, 1984.
228. Leddy JP: Immunological aspects of red cell injury in man. *Semin Hematol* 3:48, 1966.
229. Engelfriet CP, von dem Borne AEG Kr, Vander Giessen M, et al: Autoimmune haemolytic anaemias: I. Serological studies with pure anti-immunoglobulin reagents. *Clin Exp Immunol* 3:605, 1968.
230. Engelfriet CP, von dem Borne AEG Kr, Beckers D, van Loghem JJ: Autoimmune haemolytic anaemia: Serological and immunochemical characteristics of the autoantibodies: Mechanisms of cell destruction. *Ser Haematol* 7:328, 1974.
231. Suzuki S, Amano T, Mitsunaga M, et al: Autoimmune hemolytic anemia associated with IgA autoantibody. *Clin Immunol Immunopathol* 21:247, 1981.
232. Wolf CF, Wolf DJ, Peterson P: Autoimmune hemolytic anemia with predominance of IgA autoantibody. *Transfusion* 22:238, 1982.
233. Szymanski IO, Teno R, Rybak ME: Hemolytic anemia due to a mixture of low-titer IgG lambda and IgM lambda agglutinins reacting optimally at 22°C. *Vox Sang* 51:112, 1986.
234. Reusser P, Osterwalder B, Burri H, Speck B: Autoimmune hemolytic anemia associated with IgA: Diagnostic and therapeutic aspects in a case with long-term follow-up. *Acta Haematol* 77:53, 1987.
235. Göttsche B, Salama A, Mueller-Eckhardt C: Autoimmune hemolytic anemia associated with an IgA autoanti-Gerbich. *Vox Sang* 58:211, 1990.
236. Girelli G, Perrone MP, Adorno G, et al: A second example of hemolysis due to IgA autoantibody with anti-c specificity. *Haematologica* 75:182, 1990.
237. Evans RS, Bingham M, Boehni P: Autoimmune hemolytic disease: Antibody dissociation and activity. *Arch Intern Med* 108:338, 1961.
238. Evans RS, Bingham M, Turner E: Autoimmune hemolytic disease: Observations of serological reactions and disease activity. *Ann N Y Acad Sci* 124:422, 1965.
239. Gilliland BC, Leddy JP, Vaughan JH: The detection of cell-bound antibody on complement-coated human red cells. *J Clin Invest* 49:898, 1970.
240. Gilliland BC, Baxter E, Evans RS: Red cell antibodies in acquired hemolytic anemia with negative antiglobulin serum tests. *N Engl J Med* 285:252, 1971.
241. Gilliland BC: Coombs-negative immune hemolytic anemia. *Semin Hematol* 13:267, 1976.
242. Sokol RJ, Hewitt S, Booker DJ, Bailey A: Erythrocyte autoantibodies, subclasses of IgG and autoimmune haemolysis. *Autoimmunity Rev* 6:99, 1990.
243. von dem Borne AE Kr, Beckers D, van der Meulen W, Engelfriet CP: IgG$_4$ autoantibodies against erythrocytes, without increased hemolysis: A case report. *Br J Haematol* 37:137, 1977.
244. Weiner W, Vos GH: Serology of acquired hemolytic anemia. *Blood* 22:606, 1963.

245. Vos GH, Petz L, Funenberg HH: Specificity of acquired haemolytic anaemia autoantibodies and their serological characteristics. *Br J Haematol* 19:57, 1970.

246. Leddy JP, Peterson P, Yeaw MA, Bakemeier RF: Patterns of serologic specificity of human γG erythrocyte autoantibodies. *J Immunol* 105:677, 1970.

247. Bell CA, Zwicker H: Further studies on the relationship of anti-En^a and anti-Wr^b in warm autoimmune hemolytic anemia. *Transfusion* 18:572, 1978.

248. Celano MJ, Levine P: Anti-LW specificity in autoimmune acquired hemolytic anemia. *Transfusion* 7:265, 1967.

249. Marsh WL, Reid ME, Scott EP: Autoantibodies of U blood group specificity in autoimmune haemolytic anaemia. *Br J Haematol* 22:625, 1972.

250. Shulman IA, Vengelen-Tyler V, Thompson JC, et al: Autoanti-Ge associated with severe autoimmune hemolytic anemia. *Vox Sang* 59:232, 1990.

251. Owen I, Chowdhury V, Reid ME, et al: Autoimmune hemolytic anemia associated with anti-Sc1. *Transfusion* 32:173, 1992.

252. Marsh WL, Oyen R, Alicea E, et al: Autoimmune hemolytic anemia and the Kell blood groups. *Am J Hematol* 7:155, 1979.

253. Barker RN, Casswell KM, Reid ME, et al: Identification of autoantigens in autoimmune haemolytic anaemia by a non-radioisotope immunoprecipitation method. *Br J Haematol* 82:126, 1992.

254. Victoria EJ, Pierce SW, Branks MJ, Masouredis SP: IgG red blood cell autoantibodies in autoimmune hemolytic anemia bind to epitopes on red blood cell membrane band 3 glycoprotein. *J Lab Clin Med* 115:74, 1990.

255. Telen MJ, Chasis JA: Relationship of the human erythrocyte Wr^b antigen to an interaction between glycophorin A and band 3. *Blood* 76:842, 1990.

256. Barker RN, De la Sa Oliveira GG, Elson CJ, et al: Pathogenic autoantibodies in the NZB mouse are specific for erythrocyte band 3 protein. *Eur J Immunol* 23:1723, 1993.

257. Kay MMB, Marchalonis JJ, Hughes J, et al: Definition of a physiologic aging autoantigen by using synthetic peptides of membrane protein band 3: Localization of the active antigenic sites. *Proc Natl Acad Sci U S A* 87:5734, 1990.

258. Turrini F, Mannu F, Arese P, et al: Characterization of autologous antibodies that opsonize erythrocytes with clustered integral membrane proteins. *Blood* 181:3146, 1993.

259. Curtis BR, Lamon J, Roelcke D, Chaplin H: Life threatening, antiglobulin test-negative, acute autoimmune hemolytic anemia due to a non-complement-activating IgG 1k cold antibody with Pr$_a$ specificity. *Transfusion* 30:838, 1990.

260. Silberstein LE, Berkman EM, Schreiber AD: Cold hemagglutinin disease associated with IgG cold reactive antibody. *Ann Intern Med* 106:238, 1987.

261. Feizi T, Kabat EA, Vicari G, et al: Immunochemical studies on blood groups: XLVII. The I antigen complex precursors in the A, B, H, Le^a and Le^b blood group system: Hemagglutination inhibition studies. *J Exp Med* 133:39, 1971.

262. Hakomori S: Blood group ABH and Ii antigens of human erythrocytes: Chemistry, polymorphism, and their developmental change. *Semin Hematol* 18:39, 1981.

263. Marcus DM: A review of the immunogenic and immunomodulatory properties of glycosphingolipids. *Mol Immunol* 21:1083, 1984.

264. Rosse WF, Lauf PK: Reaction of cold agglutinins with I antigen solubilized from human red cells. *Blood* 36:777, 1970.

265. Lauf PK, Rosse WF: The reactivity of red blood cell membrane glycophorin with "cold-reacting" antibodies. *Clin Immunol Immunopathol* 4:1, 1975.

266. Pruzanski W, Shumak KH: Biologic activity of cold-reacting autoantibodies. *N Engl J Med* 297:583, 1977.

267. Chapman J, Murphy MF, Waters AH: Chronic cold hemagglutinin disease due to an anti-M-like autoantibody. *Vox Sang* 42:272, 1982.

268. von dem Borne AEG Kr, Mol JJ, Joustra-Maas N, et al: Autoimmune hemolytic anemia with monoclonal IgM (K) anti-P cold autohemolysins. *Br J Haematol* 50:345, 1982.

269. Terada K, Tanaka H, Mori R, et al: Hemolytic anemia associated with cold agglutinin during chickenpox and a review of the literature. *J Pediatr Hematol Oncol* 20:149, 1998.

270. Tamura T, Kanamori H, Yamazaki E, et al: Cold agglutinin disease following allogeneic bone marrow transplantation. *Bone Marrow Transplant* 13:321, 1994.

271. Capra JD, Dowling P, Cook S, Kunkel HG: An incomplete cold-reactive λ-G antibody with i specificity in infectious mononucleosis. *Vox Sang* 16:10, 1969.

272. Shirey RS, Park K, Ness PM, et al: An anti-i biphasic hemolysin in chronic paroxysmal cold hemoglobinuria. *Transfusion* 26:62, 1986.

273. Salama A, Santoso S, Mueller-Eckhardt C: Antigenic determinants responsible for the reactions of drug-dependent antibodies with blood cells. *Br J Haematol* 78:535, 1991.

274. Sokol R, Stamps R, Booker D, et al: Posttransplant immune-mediated hemolysis. *Transfusion* 42:198, 2002.

275. Lundgren G, Asaba H, Bergström J, et al: Fulminating anti-A autoimmune hemolysis with anuria in a renal transplant recipient: A therapeutic role of plasma exchange. *Clin Nephrol* 16:211, 1981.

276. Ramsey G, Nusbacher J, Starzl TE, Lindsay GD: Isohemagglutinins of graft origin after ABO-unmatched liver transplantation. *N Engl J Med* 311:1167, 1984.

277. Mangal AK, Growe GH, Sinclair M, et al: Acquired hemolytic anemia due to "auto"-anti-a or "auto"-anti-b induced by group O homograft in renal transplant recipients. *Transfusion* 24:201, 1984.

278. Hazlehurst GR, Brenner MK, Wimperis JZ, et al: Haemolysis after T-cell depleted bone marrow transplantation involving minor ABO incompatibility. *Scand J Haematol* 37:1, 1986.

279. Solheim BG, Albrechtsen D, Egeland T, et al: Auto-antibodies against erythrocytes in transplant patients produced by donor lymphocytes. *Transplant Proc* 6:4520, 1987.

280. Sniecinski IJ, Oien L, Petz LD, Blume KG: Immunohematologic consequences of major ABO-mismatched bone marrow transplantation. *Transplantation* 45:530, 1988.

281. Issitt PD: Autoimmune hemolytic anemia and cold hemagglutinin disease: Clinical disease and laboratory findings. *Prog Clin Pathol* 7:137, 1978.

282. Wallhermfechtel MA, Pohl BA, Chaplin H: Alloimmunization in patients with warm autoantibodies: A retrospective study employing three donor alloabsorptions to aid in antibody detection. *Transfusion* 24:482, 1984.

283. Branch DR, Petz LD: Detecting alloantibodies in patients with autoantibodies. *Transfusion* 39:6, 1999.

284. Shirey RS, Boyd JS, Parwani AV, et al: Prophylactic antigen matched donor blood for patients with warm autoantibodies: An algorithm for transfusion management. *Transfusion* 42:1435, 2002.

285. Garratty G, Petz LD: Approaches to selecting blood for transfusion to patients with autoimmune hemolytic anemia. *Transfusion* 42:1390, 2002.

286. Dameshek W, Rosenthal MC, Schwartz SO: The treatment of acquired hemolytic anemia with adrenocorticotrophic hormone (ACTH). *N Engl J Med* 244:117, 1951.

287. Allgood JW, Chaplin H Jr: Idiopathic acquired autoimmune hemolytic anemia: A review of forty-seven cases treated from 1955 to 1965. *Am J Med* 43:254, 1967.

288. Meyer O, Stahl D, Beckhove P, et al: Pulsed high-dose dexamethasone in chronic autoimmune haemolytic anaemia of warm type. *Br J Haematol* 98:860, 1997.

289. Greendyke RM, Bradley EB, Swisher SN: Studies of the effects of administration of ACTH and adrenal corticosteroids on erythrophagocytosis. *J Clin Invest* 44:746, 1965.

290. Fries LF, Brickman CM, Frank MM: Monocyte receptors for the Fc portion of IgG increase in number in autoimmune hemolytic anemia and other hemolytic states and are decreased by glucocorticoid therapy. *J Immunol* 131:1240, 1983.

291. Habibi B, Homberg JC, Schaison G, Salmon C: Autoimmune hemolytic anemia in children: A review of 80 cases. *Am J Med* 56:61, 1974.

292. Christensen BE: The pattern of erythrocyte sequestration in immunohaemolysis: Effects of prednisone treatment and splenectomy. *Scand J Haematol* 10:120, 1973.

293. Parker AC, MacPherson AIS, Richmond J: Value of radiochromium investigation in autoimmune haemolytic anemia. *Br Med J* 1:208, 1977.

294. Bowdler AJ: The role of the spleen and splenectomy in autoimmune hemolytic disease. *Semin Hematol* 13:335, 1976.

295. Schwartz SI, Bernard RP, Adams JT, Bauman AW: Splenectomy for hematologic disorders. *Arch Surg* 101:338, 1970.

296. Eichner ER: Splenic function: Normal, too much and too little. *Am J Med* 66:311, 1979.

297. Centers for Disease Control and Prevention: Recommended adult immunization schedule–United States 2003–2004. *MMWR Morb Mortal Wkly Rep* 52:965, 2003.

298. Zecca M, Nobili B, Ramenghi U, et al: Rituximab for the treatment of refractory autoimmune hemolytic anemia in children. *Blood* 101:3857, 2003.

299. Murphy S, LoBuglio AF: Drug therapy of autoimmune hemolytic anemia. *Semin Hematol* 13:323, 1976.

300. Moyo VM, Smith D, Brodsky I, et al: High-dose cyclophosphamide for refractory autoimmune hemolytic anemia. *Blood* 100:704, 2002.

301. Shumak KH, Rock GA: Therapeutic plasma exchange. *N Engl J Med* 310:762, 1984.

302. Council Report: Current status of therapeutic plasmapheresis and related techniques. *JAMA* 253:819, 1985.

303. Ahn YS, Harrington WJ, Byrnes JJ, et al: Treatment of autoimmune hemolytic anemia with vinca-loaded platelets. *JAMA* 249:2189, 1983.

304. Leickly FE, Buckley RH: Successful treatment of autoimmune hemolytic anemia in common variable immunodeficiency with high-dose intravenous gamma globulin. *Am J Med* 82:159, 1987.

305. Oda H, Honda A, Sugita K, et al: High-dose intravenous intact IgG infusion in refractory autoimmune hemolytic anemia (Evans syndrome). *J Pediatr* 107:744, 1985.

306. Bussel JB, Cunningham-Rundles C, Abraham C: Intravenous treatment of autoimmune hemolytic anemia with very high dose gammaglobulin. *Vox Sang* 41:264, 1986.

307. Besa EC: Rapid transient reversal of anemia and long-term effects of maintenance intravenous immunoglobulin for autoimmune hemolytic anemia in patients with lymphoproliferative disorders. *Am J Med* 84:691, 1988.

308. Flores G, Cunningham-Rundles C, Newland AC, Bussel JB: Efficacy of intravenous immunoglobulin in the treatment of autoimmune hemolytic anemia: Results in 73 patients. *Am J Hematol* 44:237 1993.

309. Ahn YS, Harrington WJ, Mylvaganam R, et al: Danazol therapy for autoimmune hemolytic anemia. *Ann Intern Med* 102:298, 1985.

310. Pignon J-M, Poirson E, Rochant H: Danazol in autoimmune haemolytic anaemia. *Br J Haematol* 83:343, 1993.

311. Giannadaki E, Potamianos S, Roussomoustakaki M, et al: Autoimmune hemolytic anemia and positive Coombs' test associated with ulcerative colitis. *Am J Gastroenterol* 92:1872, 1997.

312. Cobo F, Pereira A, Nomdedeu B, et al: Ovarian dermoid cyst-associated autoimmune hemolytic anemia. *Am J Clin Pathol* 105:567, 1996.

313. Beutler E: New chemotherapeutic agent: 2-Chlorodeoxyadenosine. *Semin Hematol* 31:40, 1994.

314. Berentsen S, Ulvestad E, Gjertsen BT, et al: Rituximab for primary cold agglutinin disease: A prospective study of 37 courses of therapy in 27 patients. *Blood* 103:2925, 2004.

315. Hippe E, Jensen KB, Olesen H, et al: Chlorambucil treatment of patients with cold agglutinin syndrome. *Blood* 35:68, 1970.

316. Evans RS, Baxter E, Gilliland BC: Chronic hemolytic anemia due to cold agglutinins: A 20-year history of benign gammopathy with response to chlorambucil. *Blood* 42:463, 1973.

317. O'Connor BM, Clifford JS, Lawrence WD, Logue GL: Alpha-interferon for severe cold agglutinin disease. *Ann Intern Med* 111:255, 1989.

318. Nydegger UE, Kazatchkine MD, Miescher PA: Immunopathologic and clinical features of hemolytic anemia due to cold agglutinins. *Semin Hematol* 28:66, 1991.

319. Bell CA, Zwicker H, Sacks HJ: Autoimmune hemolytic anemia. *Am J Clin Pathol* 60:903, 1973.

320. Taft EG, Propp RP, Sullivan SA: Plasma exchange for cold agglutinin hemolytic anemia. *Transfusion* 17:173, 1977.

321. Brooks BD, Steane EA, Sheehan RG, Frenkel EP: Therapeutic plasma exchange in the immune hemolytic anemias and immunologic thrombocytopenic purpura. *Prog Clin Biol Res* 106:317, 1982.

322. Silberstein LE, Berkman EM: Plasma exchange in antoimmune hemolytic anemia (AIHA). *J Clin Apheresis* 1:238, 1983.

323. Zulian GB, Roux E, Tiercy J-M, et al: Transfusion-associated graft-versus-host disease in a patient treated with cladribine (2-chlorodeoxy-adenosine): Demonstration of exogenous DNA in various tissue extracts by PCR analysis. *Br J Haematol* 89:83, 1995.

324. Briz M, Cabrera R, Sanjuan I: Diagnosis of transfusion-associated graft-versus-host disease by polymerase chain reaction fludarabine-treated B-chronic lymphocytic leukaemia. *Br J Haematol* 91:409, 1995.

325. Silverstein MN, Gomes MR, Elveback LR, et al: Idiopathic acquired hemolytic anemia: Survival in 117 cases. *Arch Intern Med* 129:85, 1972.

326. Dausset J, Colombani J: The serology and the prognosis of 128 cases of autoimmune hemolytic anemia. *Blood* 14:1280, 1959.

327. Pullarkat V, Ngo M, Iqbal S, et al: Detection of lupus anticoagulant identifies patients with autoimmune haemolytic anaemia at increased risk of venous thromboembolism. *Brt J Haematol* 118:1166, 2002.

328. Hendrick AM: Auto-immune haemolytic anaemia—A high-risk disorder for thromboembolism? *Hematology* 8:53, 2003.

329. Buchanan GR, Boxer LA, Nathan DG: The acute and transient nature of idiopathic immune hemolytic anemia in childhood. *J Pediatr* 88:780, 1976.

330. Zupanska B, Lawkowicz W, Gorska B, et al: Autoimmune haemolytic anemia in children. *Br J Haematol* 34:511, 1976.

331. Heisel MA, Ortega JA: Factors influencing prognosis in childhood autoimmune hemolytic anemia. *Am J Pediatr Hematol Oncol* 5:147, 1983.

332. Carapella de Luca E, Casadei AM, DiPero G, et al: Autoimmune haemolytic anemia in childhood: Follow-up in 29 cases. *Vox Sang* 36:13, 1979.

333. Sokol RJ, Hewitt S, Stamps BK, Hitchen PA: Autoimmune haemolysis in childhood and adolescence. *Acta Haematol* 72:245, 1984.

334. Wang WC: Evans syndrome in childhood: Pathophysiology, clinical course, and treatment. *Am J Pediatr Hematol Oncol* 10:330, 1988.

ALLOIMMUNE HEMOLYTIC DISEASE OF THE NEWBORN

JAYASHREE RAMASETHU

NAOMI L.C . LUBAN

Alloimmune hemolytic disease of the fetus and newborn is caused by the action of transplacentally transmitted maternal immunoglobulin (Ig) G antibodies on paternally inherited antigens present on fetal red cells but absent on the maternal red cells. Maternal IgG antibodies bind to fetal red cells, causing hemolysis. As a consequence of the hemolytic process, anemia, extramedullary hematopoiesis, and neonatal hyperbilirubinemia sometimes result in fetal loss or neonatal death or disability. Collaboration among maternal-fetal medicine specialists, hematologists, radiologists, and neonatologists has substantially reduced perinatal mortality and morbidity resulting from this condition. Antenatal diagnostic methods identify fetuses at risk for developing hemolysis and assess disease severity in affected fetuses. After birth, phototherapy and exchange transfusions prevent serum bilirubin from rising to levels that could produce bilirubin encephalopathy and resultant brain damage (kernicterus). Severely affected fetuses who in the past died before birth, secondary to severe anemia and hydrops, now are saved by vigilant antenatal monitoring and intrauterine transfusions. Anti-D prophylaxis protocols have successfully prevented alloimmune hemolytic disease resulting from RhD sensitization, but alloimmune hemolytic disease resulting from other red cell antibodies still occur. Advances in immunohematology and molecular biology may offer new avenues for prevention and treatment in the future.

DEFINITION AND HISTORY

Alloimmune hemolytic disease of the newborn is a disorder in which the life span of fetal and/or neonatal red cells is shortened as a result of binding of transplacentally transferred maternal immunoglobulin (Ig) G antibodies on fetal red cell antigens foreign to the mother, inherited by the fetus from the father.

The condition was described in newborn infants as early as the 1600s. In 1932, Diamond and colleagues[1] recognized that the clinical syndromes of stillbirth with unusual erythroblastic activity in the extramedullary sites and blood, fetal hydrops, anemia in the newborn, and "icterus gravis neonatorum" were closely related and probably were caused by the same underlying disturbance of the hematopoietic system. The discovery of the rhesus (Rh) factor by Landsteiner and Weiner[2] in 1940 led to further elucidation of the condition by Levine and colleagues,[3] who established that erythroblastosis fetalis was caused by immunization of an Rh-negative mother by the red blood cells from an Rh-positive fetus. Antibodies produced by the sensitized mother crossed the placenta in the next pregnancy and coated the fetal

Acronyms and abbreviations that appear in this chapter include: DAT, direct antiglobulin test; Ig, immunoglobulin; ΔOD_{450}, change in optical density at 450 nm; Rh, rhesus.

Rh-positive cells, leading to hemolysis and thus to anemia, hydrops, and severe neonatal jaundice secondary to hemolysis.

Neonatal mortality from Rh hemolytic disease of the newborn decreased considerably with the development of exchange transfusion techniques for correction of severe anemia and hyperbilirubinemia.[4] However, severely affected fetuses continued to die *in utero* before 34 weeks' gestation. In 1961, Liley[5] demonstrated the prognostic value of amniotic fluid spectrophotometry in identifying infants at risk and then showed that intrauterine transfusions could prevent fetal deaths. The most dramatic reduction in the incidence of Rh hemolytic disease of the newborn was achieved in the 1960s and 1970s with the development of postpartum and antepartum anti-D prophylaxis to prevent Rh sensitization.[6] Progress in the diagnosis and management of both the fetus and the affected newborn infant and prevention of Rh hemolytic disease of the newborn has resulted in a hundredfold decrease in deaths as a result of Rh hemolytic disease of the newborn in the past century.[7] However, the disease has not disappeared, and cases of hemolytic disease of the newborn resulting from red cell antibodies directed toward antigens other than the Rh blood group system are being increasingly recognized.[8–11]

ETIOLOGY AND PATHOGENESIS

CAUSATIVE ANTIBODIES

More than 40 different red cell antigens are associated with maternal alloimmunization.[8–11] Antenatal screening programs detect clinically significant antibodies in 0.24 to 1 percent of pregnant women.[8–10] These antibodies can be categorized into three main classes: (1) antibodies directed against the D antigen in the Rh blood group system, (2) antibodies directed against the A and B antigens, and (3) antibodies directed against the remaining red cell antigens. Despite the success of Rh prophylaxis, anti-D antibodies still constitute a large proportion of the antibodies detected. When D and ABO are excluded, non-D Rh antibodies (c, C, e, E, cc, and Ce) and antibodies belonging to the Kell, Duffy, Kidd, and MNS systems are most frequently involved.

Antigen-negative women may have naturally occurring antibodies to certain red cell antigens (anti-A or anti-B) or may develop antibodies as a result of exposure to foreign antigens through blood transfusion or, more often, by silent fetomaternal hemorrhage during delivery. Only IgG antibodies capable of crossing the placenta have the potential to affect the fetus. The clinical severity of hemolytic disease in the fetus and newborn infant may be affected by the class and subclass of IgG antibody, the concentration of antibody in the maternal circulation, and the rate of transplacental transfer. Fetal factors having a significant impact on the severity of hemolysis in the presence of maternal alloantibodies include the presence and concentration of antigens on the surface of fetal red cells, the competing effect of similar antigens present in fetal tissues other than fetal red cells, and the competency of the fetal mononuclear phagocyte system. In addition, the incidence of hemolytic disease of the newborn in response to antigens may vary among races, resulting in differences in clinical severity and outcome in different populations.

Rh hemolytic disease is discussed first because it is archetypal of this condition. The distinguishing features of the other classes of alloimmune hemolytic disease are highlighted.

RH HEMOLYTIC DISEASE

Genetics Inheritance of the three major Rh antigens (C/c, D, E/e) is determined by two genes on the short arm of chromosome 1: the RhD gene encoding the protein carrying the D antigen, and the *RHCE* gene encoding the proteins carrying the C/c antigens and E/e antigens (see Chap. 128). There is no "d" antigen; the letter "d" designates the absence of D. The presence or absence of D determines the Rh-positive or Rh-negative status of the individual. In Caucasian Rh-negative individuals, the RhD gene usually is deleted. The Rh-negative phenotype in people of African ancestry may result from an inactive RhD pseudogene, an important distinction to consider during genotyping.[12] Considerable racial variability exists in the prevalence of Rh negativity. Approximately 15 percent of Caucasians are Rh negative,[13] compared to 7 to 8 percent of American blacks, 5 percent of Asian Indians,[14] and 0.3 percent of Chinese people.[15]

Rh-positive individuals may be homozygous for D (DD), having inherited the D antigen from both parents, or they may be heterozygous for D (Dd), having inherited a D-containing set from one parent and a non–D-containing set of Rh antigens from the other parent. Therefore, all the offspring of a homozygous Rh-positive (DD) man and an Rh-negative (dd) woman are Rh or D positive (Dd). A fetus produced by a heterozygous Rh-positive (Dd) father and an Rh-negative mother (dd) can be either Rh positive (Dd) or Rh negative (dd).

Immunization   Isoimmunization of Rh-negative women by Rh-positive transfusions is rare since the mandatory institution of Rh-matched blood transfusions. The potential for immunization of the mother is determined by the existence of maternal-fetal blood group incompatibility and by the extent of fetomaternal hemorrhage. Asymptomatic transplacental passage of fetal red cells occurs in 75 percent of pregnant women at some time during pregnancy or during labor and delivery.[16] The incidence of fetomaternal transfusion increases with advancing gestation: from 3 percent in the first trimester, 12 percent in the second trimester, and 45 percent in the third trimester to 64 percent at delivery. The average volume of fetal blood in the maternal circulation after delivery is approximately 0.1 ml in most women and less than 1 ml in 96 percent of women.[17] Intrapartum fetomaternal hemorrhage of more than 30 ml may occur in up to 1 percent of deliveries.[18] Massive fetomaternal hemorrhage may present with decreased fetal movement and sinusoidal heart rhythm; however, it also may be clinically silent, with no clinical signs differentiating such deliveries from those with minimal fetomaternal hemorrhage.[18,19] Fetomaternal transfusion can result from invasive obstetric procedures such as chorionic villus sampling, amniocentesis, funipuncture, therapeutic abortion, cesarean section, and manual removal of the placenta, and from pathologic conditions such as abdominal trauma, spontaneous abortion, or ectopic pregnancy.[17,20–22]

The presence of D-positive red cells in a D-negative mother initially provokes a primary immune response that is weak and slow and consists of IgM antibodies that do not cross the placenta. Subsequently, anti-D IgG antibodies capable of crossing the placenta are produced. Repeated exposure to Rh-positive fetal red blood cells, as in a second Rh-positive pregnancy in a sensitized Rh-negative woman, produces a secondary immune response marked by rapid production of large amounts of anti-D IgG antibody by maternal memory B lymphocytes. The volume of blood required to cause sensitization usually is minuscule. Primary sensitization has been reported in 80 percent of individuals injected with 0.5 ml of Rh-positive cells. Secondary immune responses may occur with as little as 0.03 ml of Rh-positive cells. Repetitive exposure to D-positive cells in D-negative women who abuse intravenous drugs and share needles with Rh-positive partners leads to severe Rh sensitization.[23]

In the absence of Rh Ig prophylaxis, sensitization occurs in 7 to 16 percent of women at risk, within 6 months after delivery of the first Rh-positive ABO-compatible fetus, and in 2 percent after delivery of an ABO-incompatible fetus.[24] Fetomaternal ABO incompatibility offers some protection against primary Rh immunization because incompatible fetal red cells are destroyed rapidly by maternal anti-A and anti-B antibodies, reducing maternal exposure to RhD antigenic sites. ABO incompatibility confers no protection against the secondary immune response once sensitization has occurred.[24]

The reason why most women who are at risk for development of anti-D are not sensitized is unclear.

Hemolysis   Binding of transplacentally transferred maternal anti-D IgG antibodies to D-antigen sites on the fetal red cell membrane is followed by adherence of the coated red cells to the Fcγ R receptors of macrophages with rosette formation, leading to extravascular non-complement-mediated phagocytosis and lysis, predominantly in the spleen.[25,26] Although Rh antigens are found on fetal cells as early as week 7 of gestation, active transport of IgG across the placenta is slow until week 24 of gestation. The degree of hemolysis may be influenced by the functional immaturity of the fetal mononuclear phagocyte system prior to 20 weeks of gestation, maternal IgG levels, the IgG subclass, and the rate of transplacental transfer.[27,28] Although IgG anti-D consists mainly of IgG1 and IgG3 subclasses, the relative contribution of each of these subclasses to the severity of hemolytic disease in the newborn remains controversial.[25–28] Occasionally, women who are severely alloimmunized deliver babies with unexpectedly mild hemolysis. Protection from severe hemolytic disease in the fetuses of such women may result from inhibitory anti-HLA antibodies with specificity for allogeneic monocytes, which block Fcγ receptors on mononuclear phagocytic cells.[29,30]

Fetal anemia secondary to hemolysis results in compensatory extramedullary hematopoiesis in the liver, spleen, kidneys, and adrenal glands, associated with an outpouring of immature nucleated red blood cells in the fetal circulation. Increased fetal plasma erythropoietin levels have been reported with severe fetal anemia.[31] The marked increase in erythropoiesis may be accompanied by down-modulation of platelet and neutrophil production.[32] Extensive extramedullary hemopoiesis in the liver and spleen may cause portal and umbilical venous hypertension, leading to ascites, pleural effusions, and consequent pulmonary hypoplasia secondary to compression of the lungs.[33] Trophoblastic hypertrophy and placental edema cause impaired placental function. Hypoproteinemia as a result of liver dysfunction leads to generalized edema. "Hydrops fetalis," a state of anasarca, is the end result of a combination of anemia, hypoproteinemia, cardiac failure, elevated venous pressures, increased capillary permeability, and impaired lymphatic clearance.[34] Prior to the institution of intrauterine transfusions, most of these fetuses died *in utero* or soon after birth.

Although fetal bilirubin levels are elevated secondary to hemolysis,[35] the placenta effectively transports most of the lipid-soluble unconjugated fetal bilirubin, so the baby is not clinically jaundiced at birth. In severe cases, bilirubin secreted from the fetal trachea stains the amniotic fluid, umbilical cord, and vernix caseosa. At birth, the newborn infant's immature liver is incapable of handling the large bilirubin load that results from the ongoing destruction of antibody-coated neonatal red cells, and unconjugated bilirubin levels rise.

Some infants with hemolytic disease develop anemia beyond the immediate neonatal period lasting up to age 8 to 12 weeks. Delayed anemia is related to continuing hemolysis because of persistence of maternal antibodies and a hyporegenerative component with decreased red cell production, associated with low serum concentrations of erythropoietin.[36–38]

ABO HEMOLYTIC DISEASE

ABO hemolytic disease of the newborn is limited to mothers who are blood group type O and whose babies are group A or B. Table 53-1 lists the differences between Rh and ABO hemolytic disease of the newborn. Although ABO incompatibility exists in 15 percent of O group pregnancies, ABO hemolytic disease is estimated to occur in only approximately 3 percent of all births. Although far more common than Rh hemolytic disease of the newborn, ABO hemolytic disease of the newborn usually is mild and rarely responsible for fetal deaths. A higher incidence and greater severity are reported in southeast Asians,

TABLE 53-1   COMPARISON OF RH AND ABO INCOMPATIBILITY

CHARACTERISTIC	Rh	ABO
Blood groups		
Mother	Negative	O
Infant	Positive	A or B
Type of antibody	IgG1 and/or IgG3	IgG2
Clinical aspects		
Occurrence in firstborn	5%	40–50%
Predictable severity in subsequent pregnancies	Usually	Not always
Stillbirth and/or hydrops	Frequent	Rare
Severe anemia	Frequent	Rare
Degree of jaundice	+ + +	+
Hepatosplenomegaly	+ + +	+
Laboratory findings		
Maternal antibodies	Always present	Not clearcut
Direct antiglobulin test (infant)	+	+
Spherocytes	0	+
Treatment		
Antenatal measures	Yes	No
Exchange transfusions or red cell transfusions	Common	Rare
Donor blood type	Rh negative, group specific when possible	Group O only
Incidence of late anemia	Common	Rare

Hispanics, Arabs, and South African and American Blacks. However, even in these populations the clinical phenomenon usually is early neonatal jaundice requiring phototherapy or exchange transfusions.[39–43] The increased incidence and severity of hyperbilirubinemia in certain populations may result from the presence of a variant uridine diphosphate (UDP) glucuronyltransferase gene promoter.[44] Severe fetal anemia with hydrops has been rarely reported.[45,46]

Unlike Rh disease, ABO hemolytic disease of the newborn may affect the first-born ABO incompatible infant because IgG anti-A and anti-B antibodies may be present normally in group O adults. A recurrence rate of 88 percent has been reported in siblings having the same blood type as the affected index baby. Sixty-two percent of the affected siblings require therapy.[47] The low incidence of ABO hemolytic disease of the newborn despite considerable fetomaternal ABO incompatibility may be because most anti-A and anti-B antibodies are of the IgM type incapable of crossing the placenta. Only a small proportion of group O individuals produce anti-A and anti-B antibodies of the IgG type that can cross the placenta. The severity of the disease in the infant may be partly related to the level of IgG anti-A or anti-B in the mother and the IgG subclass. IgG2 constitutes a significant component of anti-A and anti-B antibody. This subclass of IgG is transported less readily across the placenta than is IgG1 or IgG3 and is a less efficient mediator of macrophage-induced red cell clearance.[13,48] However, antenatal testing of anti-A and anti-B levels in group O mothers has no value in predicting ABO hemolytic disease in the newborn infant.[49] The lack of predictive value may be a consequence of the small number of fully developed A or B antigen sites on fetal red blood cells and the fact that the effect of anti-A and anti-B antibodies on red cells is further diluted by other fetal tissues bearing these surface antigens.

Anti-A and anti-B IgG antibodies do not bind complement on the fetal red cell membrane. Hemolysis occurs by noncomplement-mediated phagocytosis of Ig-coated red cells, similar to Rh hemolytic disease of the newborn. The blood film in ABO hemolytic disease of the newborn is marked by the presence of microspherocytes, a feature not usually seen in Rh hemolytic disease of the newborn.[50] The spherocytosis is attributed to loss of membrane surface area when the spleen removes antigen–antibody complexes from the affected cell.

HEMOLYTIC DISEASE CAUSED BY OTHER RED CELL ANTIBODIES

Antenatal screening programs detect clinically significant antibodies in 0.24 to 1 percent of pregnant women.[8–10] Table 53-2 lists the seroprevalence of red blood cell antibodies in three large population studies. When the D antibodies are excluded, the non-D Rh antibodies (E, C, and c) and those belonging to the Kell, Duffy, Kidd, and MNS systems are most frequently involved. The mere presence of antibodies on screening tests may not be clinically significant, because only some antibodies are implicated in hemolytic disease of the newborn. For example, the antibodies may be IgM, the antibodies may be incapable of crossing the placenta, or the corresponding antigens may be poorly expressed on the fetal and neonatal red cells, as in the case of the Lewis or Chido antigens, and do not induce an antibody response. A review of the fetal and neonatal outcome of pregnancies associated with alloimmunization to non–anti-D antigens showed that although many antibodies reportedly cause hemolysis, case reports in the literature appear to be biased toward the more severe cases, whereas large published series of patients with non-D alloimmunization show that most fetuses are unaffected or minimally affected. However, anti-Kell, anti-c, and anti-E may cause hemolytic disease of the newborn as severe as that seen in anti-D disease.[11]

Kell hemolytic disease accounts for approximately 10 percent of antibody-mediated severe fetal anemia cases. The Kell blood group system consists of at least 24 discrete antigens, of which eight are associated with hemolytic disease of newborn. The most common of these antigens, the Kell antigen (K or K1), is expressed by erythroid progenitor cells and mature erythroid cells, but is expressed in only 9 percent of Caucasians and 2 percent of blacks. Almost all Kell-positive individuals are heterozygous.[51] Alloimmunization in Kell-negative women more often results from blood transfusion rather than sensitization by fetomaternal hemorrhage from a Kell-positive fetus.[52–55] Kell

TABLE 53-2   RED BLOOD CELL ANTIBODY SEROPREVALENCE IN WOMEN

ANTIBODY	SWEDEN[10] 1980–1991 (12 YEARS)	NEW YORK[8] 1993–1995 (2.5 YEARS)	MERSEY AND NORTH WALES[9] 1993–1995 (1 YEAR)
D	159 (19.0%)	101 (18.4%)	100 (40.9%)
E	51 (6.1%)	77 (14.0%)	29 (11.9%)
C	36 (4.3%)	26 (4.7%)	15 (6.1%)*
C^w	10 (1.2%)	1 (0.2%)	
c	38 (4.5%)	32 (5.8%)	28 (11.5%)†
e	1 (0.1%)		1 (0.4%)
Kell	48 (5.7%)	121 (22%)	42 (17.2%)
Duffy	26 (3.1%)	31 (5.6%)	9 (3.7%)
MNS	35 (4.2%)	26 (4.7%)	10 (4.1%)
Kidd	10 (1.2%)	8 (1.5%)	10 (4.1%)
Lutheran	13 (1.6%)	7 (1.3%)	
P$_1$	48 (5.7%)	1 (0.2%)	
Le^a, Le^b	241 (28.8%)	113 (20.5%)	
I		5 (0.9%)	
Others	120 (14.4%)	1 (0.2%)	
Total antibodies	836	550	244
Blood samples	110,765	37,506‡	22,264

* Includes C^w.
† Includes c plus e.
‡ Racial distribution of this population: Caucasian 70%, Black 20%, other 10%.

hemolytic disease is uncommon even in alloimmunized pregnancies because fetal anemia resulting from transplacentally transmitted antibodies can occur only in a Kell-positive fetus. The partners of Kell-negative women likely are Kell positive in less than 10 percent of pregnancies, and only half of these pregnancies likely are incompatible because of paternal heterozygosity. Published results on the outcome of maternal Kell alloimmunization indicate between 2.5 and 10 percent of Kell-immunized pregnancies end in the delivery of affected infants; approximately half the infants require intervention.[52,55] Unlike RhD hemolytic disease, fetal anemia in anti-Kell alloimmunization does not result solely from hemolysis but also is secondary to suppression of fetal erythropoiesis. This finding is evident from clinical observations of inappropriately low levels of circulating reticulocytes and normoblasts for the degree of anemia in affected fetuses and by *in vitro* studies showing that growth of Kell-positive erythroid progenitor cells is inhibited by monoclonal IgG and IgM anti-Kell antibodies.[56] Anti-Kell antibodies also are postulated to cause fetal anemia by promoting the immune destruction of K+ erythroid early progenitor cells by macrophages in the fetal liver.[57]

CLINICAL FEATURES

Anemia, jaundice, and hepatosplenomegaly are the hallmarks of hemolytic disease of the newborn. The clinical spectrum of affected infants is highly variable. In Rh hemolytic disease of the newborn, half of the infants have very mild disease and do not require intervention. One fourth of affected infants are born at term with moderate anemia and develop severe jaundice. In the days prior to intrauterine intervention, hydrops developed *in utero* in the remaining one fourth of infants; half became hydropic prior to 34 weeks' gestation. Hydrops recurs in 90 percent of affected pregnancies, often at an earlier gestation. In Kell hemolytic disease of the newborn, the clinical spectrum of hemolytic disease of the newborn is less predictable, ranging from mild anemia or hyperbilirubinemia to frank hydrops. Anemia, jaundice, and hepatosplenomegaly also are seen in ABO hemolytic disease of the newborn, but the disease usually is milder than is Rh hemolytic disease of the newborn.

ANEMIA

Infants with mild hemolytic disease of the newborn have cord blood hemoglobin concentrations slightly lower than the age-related normal range. Hemoglobin values usually continue to fall after birth in all affected infants. Hemolysis continues until all incompatible red cells and/or circulating maternal alloantibody are eliminated from the circulation. Physical examination in infants having moderate to severe anemia reveals pallor, tachypnea, and tachycardia. Signs of cardiovascular collapse and tissue hypoxia appear with severe anemia (hemoglobin <4 g/dl, hematocrit 15 percent).

JAUNDICE

Most infants with hemolytic disease are not jaundiced at birth, although the umbilical cord and vernix caseosa may be stained with bilirubin from the amniotic fluid in severely affected infants. Clinical icterus usually develops during the first day of life, often in the first few hours of life in severely affected infants. The icterus progresses in a cephalopedal direction with rising bilirubin levels. In patients with mild disease, the serum indirect bilirubin peaks by the fourth or fifth day and then declines slowly. Premature infants may have higher levels of serum bilirubin for a longer duration because of lower hepatic glucuronyl transferase activity. Conjugated hyperbilirubinemia at birth

is sometimes noted in infants who received multiple intrauterine transfusions.

An important complication of elevated serum levels of indirect bilirubin in the neonate is the development of bilirubin encephalopathy.[58] This disorder, also termed *kernicterus*, is caused by bilirubin pigment deposition, leading to neuronal necrosis, in the basal ganglia and brainstem nuclei. Acute bilirubin encephalopathy is initially marked by lethargy, poor feeding, and hypotonia. With increasing severity, the infant develops a high-pitched cry, fever, hypertonia progressing to frank opisthotonos, and irregular respiration. The hypertonia becomes less pronounced gradually. The infants then develop any or all of the classic sequelae of kernicterus: choreoathetoid cerebral palsy, gaze abnormalities, especially in upward gaze, sensorineural hearing loss, and cognitive deficits. The clinical presentation of bilirubin encephalopathy in preterm infants may be less distinctive. Abnormal or absent brainstem auditory evoked potentials and magnetic resonance imaging scans demonstrating the characteristic bilateral lesions of the globus pallidus help confirm the clinical diagnosis of kernicterus.

Infants with hemolytic disease of the newborn, particularly those with alloimmune hemolytic disease, are at higher risk for kernicterus than are other infants with the same bilirubin level. Heme pigments produced during active hemolysis are hypothesized to inhibit bilirubin–albumin binding. Alternatively, many conditions that potentially compromise the blood–brain barrier, such as prematurity, acidosis, hypoxemia, hypothermia, and hypoglycemia, are present in severely affected infants, making them more vulnerable to bilirubin encephalopathy.

OTHER CLINICAL FEATURES

Hepatosplenomegaly usually is present. Marked enlargement is seen in newborn infants with hydrops. Hydropic babies also have peripheral edema, and they may have ascites and pleural and pericardial effusions. Respiratory distress may be present as a result of pulmonary hypoplasia, pleural and/or pericardial effusions, or surfactant deficiency. Purpura associated with thrombocytopenia is sometimes seen in severely affected infants and may be a bad prognostic sign. The placenta is thickened, enlarged, and pale.

Babies who received intrauterine transfusions may still have hepatosplenomegaly and anemia at birth and may develop significant hyperbilirubinemia.[59]

OBSTETRIC HISTORY

The course and outcome of prior pregnancies are of paramount importance in the initial evaluation of an alloimmunized pregnancy. The history of early fetal deaths or hydrops is ominous. In Rh alloimmunization, the severity of hemolytic disease of the newborn either remains the same or worsens in subsequent affected pregnancies. Hydrops recurs in 90 percent of affected pregnancies, often at an earlier gestation. Jaundice as a result of hemolysis likely recurs to the same degree of severity in subsequent affected siblings. The history of prior blood transfusions may be obtained in women sensitized to antigens other than D, especially if Kell alloimmunization is detected. Establishment of paternity for each pregnancy is particularly relevant in both Rh and Kell alloimmunization, because the fetus is at risk only if the father is positive for the antigen in question. ABO hemolytic disease of the newborn may affect the first-born ABO-incompatible infant. Although rare, severe ABO hemolytic disease of the newborn may recur in subsequent ABO-incompatible pregnancies.[45]

LABORATORY FEATURES

MATERNAL IMMUNOHEMATOLOGIC TESTING

The aims of antenatal serologic testing are to identify Rh-negative women and to detect maternal alloimmunization. If alloimmunization is found, maternal serologic testing will help determine the risk to the fetus and aid in further diagnosis and management.

The practice guidelines for prenatal and perinatal immunohematologic testing have been revised by the Scientific Section Coordinating Committee of the American Association of Blood Banks.[60] Table 53-3 summarizes current recommendations for prenatal testing.

Every obstetric patient should undergo ABO and RhD typing and be tested for irregular serum antibodies, irrespective of Rh type, at the initial prenatal visit, preferably by 12 to 16 weeks' gestation. Testing is recommended for each pregnancy. No further D testing is necessary once concordant results are obtained on blood samples collected on two separate occasions, but D type should be confirmed by serologic testing at the beginning of each subsequent pregnancy. The American Association of Blood Banks Standards for Blood Banks and Transfusion testing recommends repeat Rh testing if red blood cell transfusion is requested.[61] Testing for the weak-D phenotype is optional because the benefit these women would receive from Rh Ig therapy is unclear. Severe hemolytic disease in patients with partial D has been reported but is rare.[62]

All women, irrespective of Rh type, should be tested at the first prenatal visit, during each pregnancy, for clinically significant unexpected antibodies. Tests with enzyme-treated red cells or polyspecific antihuman globulin sera are not recommended (see Chaps. 128 and 130). Antibody screening can be repeated at 26 to 28 weeks' gestation in Rh-negative women, prior to Rh Ig prophylaxis, but the cost effectiveness of this measure is uncertain, given the low incidence of D

TABLE 53-3 RECOMMENDATIONS FOR PRENATAL TESTING[60]

TESTING AND CONDITION	TIMING
ABO	
First pregnancy	Initial visit
Subsequent pregnancies	Initial visit
Other	Pretransfusion testing
Rh (test for weak D optional)	
First pregnancy	Initial visit and at 26–28 weeks' gestation
Subsequent pregnancies	Initial visit
Other	Pretransfusion testing
Unexpected antibodies	
All pregnancies	Initial visit
D-negative pregnancies	Before Rh immunoglobulin therapy (optional)
D-positive pregnancies	Third trimester if transfused or history of unexpected antibodies
Other	For pretransfusion testing
Antibody identification	
Unexpected antibodies present	Upon initial detection
Confirmatory testing	At time of titration
Antibody titration	
Rh antibodies	Upon initial detection
	Repeat at 18–20 weeks' gestation
	Repeat at 2- to 4-week intervals if below critical titer (16–32)
Other potentially significant antibodies	As above, with discussion with obstetrician

Reproduced from ref. 60 with permission.

alloimmunization between the first trimester visit and 28 weeks' gestation.[60,63] Routine testing for unexpected antibodies in the third trimester or at delivery appears to be superfluous, because large studies have shown that the incidence of potentially significant antibodies detected for the first time during delivery is less than 0.5 percent, with no consequent neonatal complications.[64,65] Third trimester testing is advocated in the case of a history of significant antibodies, blood transfusion, or traumatic deliveries.[60]

If a pregnant woman has unexpected antibodies at any time during pregnancy, the specificity of the antibody and its ability to cause hemolytic disease of the newborn must be determined. The indirect antiglobulin test is performed (see Chaps. 128 and 130) using a saline antiglobulin procedure utilizing specific donor red cells and anti-IgG. The result is reported as the reciprocal of the highest dilution step at which agglutination is observed.[51] Titration of potentially significant antibodies is recommended primarily as a screening test to determine the need for further evaluation of the fetus, by direct amniocentesis or cordocentesis. Testing is performed every 2 to 4 weeks from 18 weeks' gestation or as soon as antibody is detected.[26,60] Figure 53-1 shows an algorithm for the overall clinical management of the sensitized pregnancy. In the first pregnancy with Rh alloimmunization, rapidly rising levels or a critical titer of 16 dictates further investigation, although the critical titer may vary from 8 to 32 in different laboratories.[60] In the United Kingdom, anti-D levels are quantified by continuous flow analyzer, such as an Autoanalyzer, with critical titers of 15 IU/ml warranting additional investigation for fetal anemia.[66] Once the critical titer is reached and a decision is made to monitor the fetus by amniocentesis or cordocentesis, further antibody titration plays no role in assessment of fetal status. Antibody titration is not useful for monitoring pregnancies after the first affected pregnancy.

The significance of titer levels for antibodies other than D have not been defined. Maternal anti-Kell titers, in particular, correlate poorly with fetal outcome.[56] In a review of 156 anti-Kell positive pregnancies over 37 years, McKenna and colleagues[52] found that all severely affected fetuses had a titer of at least 1:32. Bowman and colleagues[55] also noted that a titer of 1:32 or greater was present in 16 of 17 severely affected pregnancies, but one patient with a titer of 1:8 had a grossly hydropic fetus at 23 weeks' gestation. Some authors recommend further testing of the fetus if a critical titer of 1:8 is attained and paternal red cell typing is K+.[11,55] In a case series of women with anti-c isoimmunization, a titer of 1:32 or greater was invariably associated with severe fetal or neonatal disease.[67]

However, in a review of 418 antenatal cases with primary isoimmunization, 50 percent of babies born to mothers with titers of 16 or greater needed only phototherapy or no therapy at all.[68] The use of "critical titers" as an indication for further assessment of fetal status by invasive tests such as amniocentesis or cordocentesis has been questioned, because these procedures carry significant risks to the fetus.[26,68]

The imperfect predictive value of serologic tests has led to the development of functional cellular assays that measure the ability of maternal antibodies to cause red cell destruction, thus providing better noninvasive differentiation of pregnancies at increased risk of fetal anemia. In these assays, red blood cells sensitized with maternal antibodies are incubated with effector cells carrying Fcγ receptors, such as lymphocytes or monocytes, to measure cellular interaction, such as binding, phagocytosis, or cytotoxic lysis.[25,26] Many authors have reported on the superiority of the monocyte monolayer assay,[69] the chemiluminescence test,[70] and the antibody-dependent cell-mediated cytotoxicity assay,[71] compared to serologic tests, in predicting severity of hemolytic disease in the fetus and newborn. However, these tests are complex, difficult to standardize, and have not gained wide acceptance in the United States.[60,72]

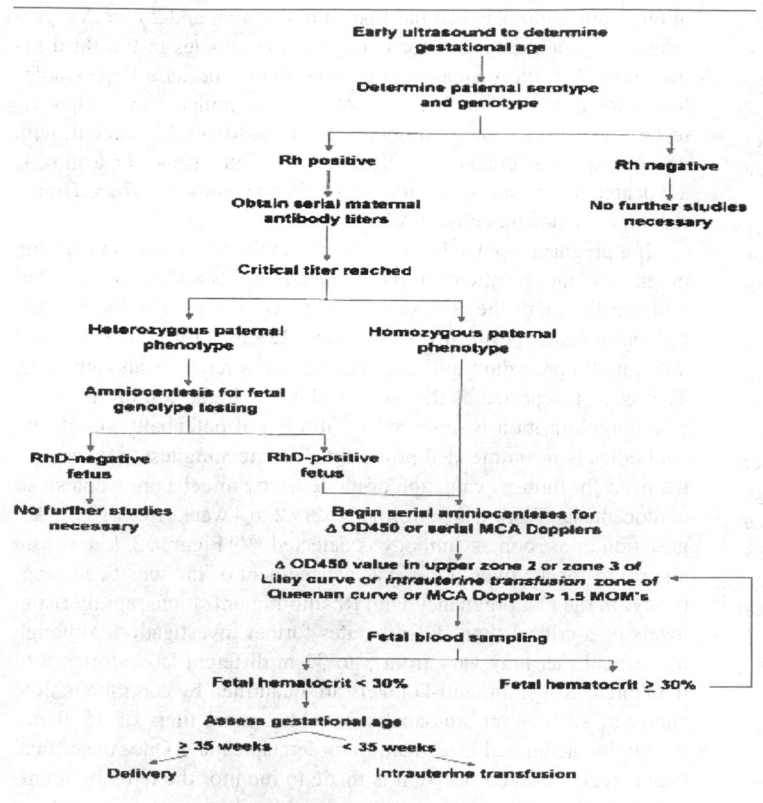

FIGURE 53-1   Algorithm for clinical management of alloimmunized pregnancy. MCA, middle cerebral artery; MOM, multiples of the median for gestational age; ΔOD, deviation in amniotic fluid optical density; Rh, rhesus. (Reproduced from ref. 97 with permission.)

DETERMINATION OF PATERNAL ZYGOSITY AND FETAL BLOOD TYPE

The child of an Rh-negative mother and a heterozygous Rh-positive father has a 50 percent chance of being Rh negative and thus being unaffected by prior maternal Rh alloimmunization. When the father is heterozygous or paternal zygosity is unknown, determination of fetal blood type early in pregnancy allows early institution of monitoring and therapy in RhD-positive fetuses who are at risk and avoidance of invasive procedures in Rh-negative fetuses.

The probable RhD zygosity in Rh-positive persons may be inferred from serologic phenotyping studies, based on gene frequencies in certain populations, and the fact that the C/c and E/e antigens are closely linked to the RhD locus.[13,73] Elucidation of the genetic structure of the prevalent RhD locus and the deletion responsible for RhD-negative phenotypes in Caucasians has led to the development of more direct and robust methods of determination of RhD zygosity by polymerase chain reaction tests performed on DNA extracted from white blood cells.[74] These tests likely will be used more frequently in the future but must be interpreted with caution in certain populations.[75]

If paternal heterozygosity is suspected or confirmed, determination of fetal blood type is helpful in planning further management. However, fetal blood sampling for serologic blood typing is associated with a 40 percent risk of fetomaternal hemorrhage and worsening maternal sensitization and up to 2 percent risk of fetal loss.[22] The fetal blood type can be ascertained by polymerase chain reaction amplification of fetal DNA obtained by amniocentesis.[76] Results of genotyping may not be concordant with serologic phenotyping because of rearrangements in the paternal RhD locus, which have been noted in approximately 2 percent of individuals.[77] Testing of a sample of the paternal

blood for gene rearrangements with the same primers used for fetal testing will prevent mislabeling an Rh-positive fetus as Rh negative. In 66 percent of black South Africans, 24 percent of African Americans, and 17 percent of South Africans of mixed race, the RhD-negative phenotype is associated with an inactive pseudogene or a partial RHD gene at the locus that could result in Rh-positive results on fetal genotyping, leading to unnecessary intervention.[12] Testing a maternal sample for an RhD pseudogene clarifies this error. Both amniocentesis and chorionic villus sampling for fetal genetic typing carry a significant risk of fetomaternal hemorrhage with increased risk of augmenting maternal sensitization; they also are associated with risk of fetal loss.[20,21] These risks have been eliminated by noninvasive methods of prenatal diagnosis of fetal RhD status, by using fetal cells isolated from the maternal blood,[78,79] and by using fetal DNA extracted from maternal plasma as early as the first trimester of pregnancy.[80,81]

Prenatal determination of the Kell genotype is necessary for assessing the possible risk to the fetus in Kell alloimmunization. Determination can be made by either flow cytometry or DNA amplification of fetal tissue obtained by chorionic villus sampling or from amniocytes.[82–84]

AMNIOTIC FLUID SPECTROPHOTOMETRY

In 1961, the spectrophotometric analysis of amniotic fluid for bilirubin was shown to be useful in predicting the severity of fetal anemia from 27 weeks to term.[85] Elevations of optical density at 450 nm (ΔOD_{450}) reflect the concentration of amniotic fluid bilirubin derived from fetal tracheal and pulmonary secretions. The change in optical density is quantified by measuring the elevation of the optical density at 450 nm above a line connecting the optical density values obtained at 375 and 550 nm and then plotting it against gestational age. Contamination of amniotic fluid samples with blood or meconium can alter ΔOD_{450} readings, but this problem can be solved by chloroform extraction of amniotic fluid. Liley defined three zones: readings in zone 3, the upper zone, indicate severe fetal disease with hydrops or impending fetal death; readings in zone 1, the lowest zone, indicate mild or no hemolytic disease with a 10 percent risk of needing a postnatal exchange transfusion; and readings in zone 2 indicate moderate disease. Serial determinations of ΔOD_{450} can achieve a sensitivity of 95 percent in detecting the severity of fetal anemia in the third trimester of pregnancy.[86] Linear extrapolations of the graph to the second trimester were unreliable.[87] Deviations in amniotic fluid optical density at 450 nm in Rh-isoimmunized pregnancies from 14 to 40 weeks' gestation led to the design of a reference chart with four zones, with the lowest zone representing unaffected fetuses and the highest zone associated with increased risk of intrauterine death (Fig. 53-2).[88] However, the Queenan graph also may overestimate the possible risk to the fetus, particularly before 28 weeks' gestation.[89]

ULTRASONOGRAPHY

Ultrasonography is noninvasive, can be performed serially, and can be combined with other diagnostic studies to assess the fetal condition, estimate the need for further aggressive management, and obtain a biophysical profile of the fetus to determine fetal well-being. As hydrops develops in the anemic fetus, a consistent pattern may be noted on ultrasonography. Polyhydramnios appears first, followed by placental enlargement, hepatomegaly, pericardial effusion, ascites, scalp edema, and pleural effusions in succession.[90] Nevertheless, in the absence of overt hydrops, ultrasonographic parameters, such as intrahepatic and extrahepatic vein diameters, abdominal and head circumference, head to abdominal circumference ratio, intraperitoneal volume, splenic size, and liver length have not been reliable in distinguishing mild from severe fetal anemia.[90,91] In the anemic fetus, decreased viscosity of the blood and increased cardiovascular output lead to a hyperdynamic circulation. Cerebral blood flow increases further in response to hypoxemia, resulting in increased blood flow velocity. Doppler flow velocity measurement in the middle cerebral artery is the most accurate predictor of fetal anemia, if the measurement is obtained strictly in accordance with the prescribed technique. Values greater than 1.5 multiples of the median for gestational age correlate highly with moderate or severe fetal anemia (Fig. 53-3).[91–93] This noninvasive technique likely will reduce, if not entirely eliminate, the need for serial amniocentesis and for diagnostic blood sampling in nonanemic fetuses.[90,93,94]

FETAL BLOOD SAMPLING

Fetal blood sampling (also called *percutaneous umbilical blood sampling* or *cordocentesis*) allows direct measurement of blood indices to specifically evaluate the degree of severity of fetal hemolytic disease as early as 17 to 18 weeks' gestation.[93] Indications for fetal blood sampling in alloimmunized pregnancies include fetal blood typing, confirmation of severe fetal anemia suspected based on amniocentesis with ΔOD_{450} measurements in Liley zone 3 or in the "intrauterine death zone" in the Queenan graph, elevated peak middle cerebral artery Doppler velocities, or ultrasonographic evidence of early or frank hydrops.[88,96] The procedure is performed under local anesthesia. A 20- to 22-gauge spinal needle is inserted into the umbilical vein at the level of cord insertion into the placenta, under ultrasonographic guidance. Specimens of fetal blood are obtained for direct measurement of complete blood count, reticulocyte count, red cell antigen phenotyping, direct antiglobulin test (DAT), bilirubin, blood gases, and lactate to assess acid–base status (Fig. 53-4). To exclude maternal blood contamination, fetal blood should be examined using a number of fetal-specific markers, such as red cell size, hemoglobin F, and/or expression of the i and I red cell antigens.[97] Blood should be available for immediate intrauterine transfusion when the procedure is being performed for suspected severe fetal anemia. Complications of fetal blood sampling include fetal loss, with procedure-related rates ranging from 0 to 4.9 percent, umbilical cord bleeding, chorioamnionitis, and significant risk of fetomaternal hemorrhage with anamnestic maternal sensitization.[98]

LABORATORY TESTS IN THE NEONATE

A sample of cord blood should be collected from all newborns at the time of delivery. However, specific testing of cord blood samples is performed only if the mother is Rh negative, if the maternal serum

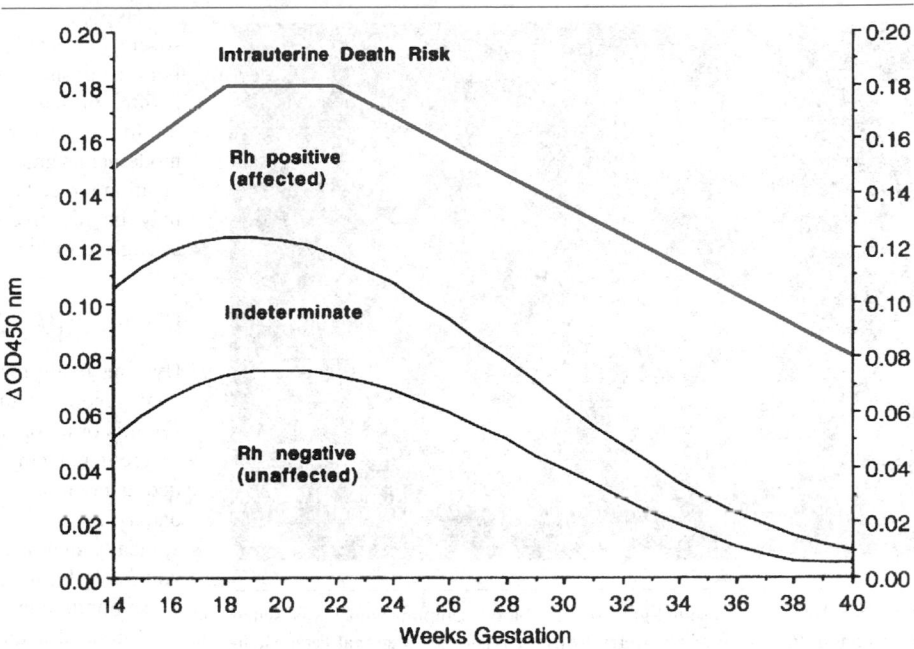

FIGURE 53-2   Queenan curve for ΔOD_{450} values from 14 to 40 weeks' gestation. (Reproduced from ref. 88 with permission.)

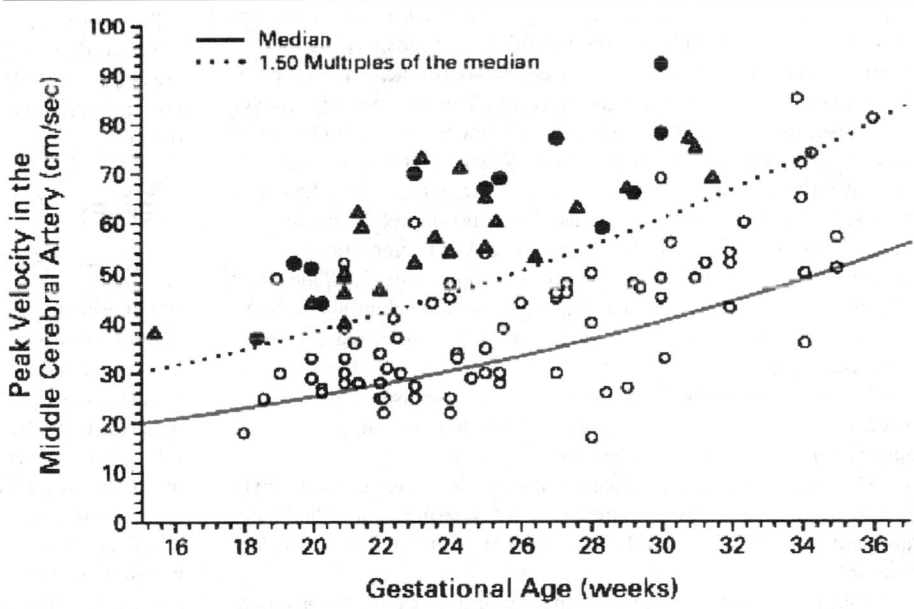

FIGURE 53-3   Peak velocity of systolic blood flow in the middle cerebral artery in 111 fetuses at risk for anemia as a result of maternal alloimmunization. *Open circles*, fetuses with either mild or no anemia; *solid circles*, fetuses with hydrops; *triangles*, fetuses with moderate or severe anemia. (Reproduced from ref. 92 with permission.)

contains red cell alloantibodies of potential clinical significance, or if the neonate develops signs of hemolytic disease.[60] Tests should include ABO and Rh typing and a DAT. Many birth hospitals routinely test cord blood for the infant's blood type and DAT if the mother is O Rh positive in order to detect ABO alloimmunization before the infant is discharged home.

In severe Rh alloimmunization, high titers of maternal antibody may block Rh-antigenic sites on the neonatal red cells, leading to false-negative Rh typing.

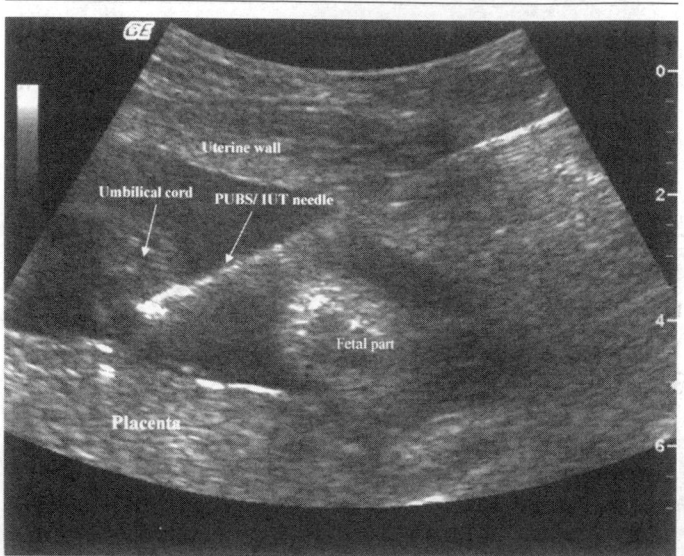

FIGURE 53-4   Ultrasound-guided fetal blood sampling and intravascular transfusion. (Courtesy of Dr. Kerry Lewis, Division of Maternal-Fetal Medicine, Georgetown University Hospital, Washington, D.C.)

Antepartum Rh Ig given to the mother may cause a weakly positive DAT result in the infant at birth. Contamination of the cord blood sample with Wharton's jelly during collection can result in a false-positive DAT result. Although the DAT usually is positive in all forms of alloimmune hemolytic disease of the newborn, the test cannot predict reliably the degree of clinical severity. This is especially true for cases resulting from ABO sensitization. The cord blood DAT may be only weakly positive in ABO disease. When fetomaternal ABO incompatibility is present, the presence of maternally derived IgG anti-A or anti-B in the infant's serum can be demonstrated by the indirect antiglobulin test to support the diagnosis of ABO hemolytic disease.[60] On the other hand, hemolysis in ABO-incompatible, DAT-negative infants may result from hematologic causes other than alloimmunization or from red cell membrane defects.[99] Elution of maternal antibody from the infant's red cells, followed by tests to determine the specificity of the antibody in the eluate, may be useful, particularly when several antibodies are present in the maternal serum or when the maternal antibody screen is negative.

Measurement of end-tidal carbon monoxide, corrected for ambient carbon monoxide levels, provides a direct measurement of heme catabolism to confirm a hemolytic process, but this test is not widely available.[100]

Cord blood hemoglobin and indirect bilirubin determinations more closely reflect disease severity. Most infants with cord hemoglobin levels within the age-adjusted normal range do not require exchange transfusion. Usually, a cord hemoglobin level less than 11 g/dl in a term newborn and/or a cord-indirect bilirubin level greater than 4.5 to 5 mg/dl indicates severe hemolysis and often warrants early exchange transfusion. Early exchange transfusion also may be indicated if the rate of rise of bilirubin, measured every 4 to 6 hours, exceeds 0.5 mg/dl/hour.

The reticulocyte count usually is greater than 6 percent and may approach 30 to 40 percent in severe Rh disease. The blood smear in Rh disease is characterized by increased nucleated red blood cell counts, polychromasia, and anisocytosis. Severely affected infants may develop thrombocytopenia with platelet counts less than 30,000/ml. Spherocytosis is seen primarily in ABO hemolytic disease. Low reticulocyte counts disproportionate to the low hematocrit may be noted in Kell hemolytic disease of the newborn.

Hypoglycemia, secondary to hyperinsulinemia, may be seen in severely affected infants. Arterial blood gas analysis may reveal metabolic acidosis and/or respiratory decompensation. Hypoalbuminemia is often present.

Infants who received intrauterine transfusions may have mild or moderate anemia with little reticulocytosis. Because most of their circulating red cells are transfused antigen-negative cells, the DAT result may be negative, but the indirect antiglobulin test result will be strongly positive.

DIFFERENTIAL DIAGNOSIS

Hydrops fetalis may be secondary to cardiac anomalies or arrhythmias, fetal genetic or metabolic disorders, intrauterine infections such as syphilis or toxoplasmosis, or any of a multitude of causes that lead to severe derangements in fetal homeostasis. These disorders are classified as nonimmune hydrops and are differentiated from anasarca secondary to hemolytic disease of the newborn by the absence of any clinically significant red cell alloantibodies in the mother's blood. Parvovirus B19 infection of the mother at any time during gestation can cause nonimmune hydrops, profound fetal anemia, and death.

Neonatal anemia caused by intrinsic red cell defects such as hereditary spherocytosis (see Chap. 44), red cell enzyme deficiencies (see Chap. 45), and specific hemoglobinopathies (see Chaps. 46 and 47) can give a similar clinical picture to hemolytic disease of the newborn.[101] The absence of maternal red cell alloantibodies, a negative DAT result, and detection of the specific defect determining the disorder clarify the diagnosis.

Disorders of bilirubin metabolism, either indirect or direct, usually are not associated with anemia. Hepatitis or obstructive biliary diseases present with direct hyperbilirubinemia, most often after the first week of life.

THERAPY

INTRAUTERINE FETAL TRANSFUSION

Intrauterine transfusions correct fetal anemia and may reduce the risk of congestive heart failure and hydrops fetalis. Fetal bilirubin is cleared very efficiently by the placenta and the mother, so bilirubin removal is not necessary. The first fetal blood sampling with transfusion ideally is performed when the fetus is anemic but before hydrops develops. Intraperitoneal fetal transfusion has been largely replaced by direct intravascular fetal transfusion, either through the umbilical cord, at its placental insertion (see Fig. 53-4), or in the intrahepatic portion of the umbilical vein.[96] Other techniques of fetal transfusion include combinations of intravascular with intraperitoneal transfusions and even intracardiac transfusion as a last resort. The intravascular technique offers precise diagnostic evaluation of the fetal status (see "Fetal Blood Sampling" above) and is effective, even in hydropic fetuses, by circumventing the problem of erratic and often poor absorption of red blood cells from the peritoneal cavity in such fetuses. Intraperitoneal transfusions may be necessary when intravascular access is difficult, as in early pregnancy when the umbilical vessels are narrow or later when increased fetal size prevents access to the umbilical cord. The relative merits of direct simple intravascular transfusion versus intravascular exchange transfusion have been debated,[102] but the shorter procedure time associated with direct simple intrauterine intravascular transfusion has made it the procedure of choice at most centers. The nonhydropic fetus can tolerate rapid blood infusions of 5 to 7 ml/minute because of the capacitance of the placenta. The hydropic fetus requires slower transfusion rates and can tolerate only smaller, more frequent transfusions.

Transfusions are given at fetal hematocrit levels of 25 to 30 percent or less, or if the hematocrit is less than two standard deviations below the mean for gestational age. Generally, the hematocrit drops by 1 to 2 percent per day in the transfused hydropic fetus. The fall in hematocrit is rapid in fetuses with severe hemolytic disease, often necessitating a second transfusion within 7 to 14 days. The interval between subsequent transfusions usually is 21 to 28 days. Very low pretransfusion fetal hematocrit levels, rapid large increases in posttransfusion hematocrit level, and increases in umbilical venous pressure during intrauterine transfusions are associated with fetal death after transfusion.[103,104]

Freshly packed, O-negative red blood cells that are antigen negative for any other identified antibody, cytomegalovirus seronegative, or leukodepleted, irradiated, and cross-matched against the mother's blood are used.[105,106] Fetuses are at risk for posttransfusion cytomegalovirus and graft-versus-host disease. Some centers use maternal blood, supporting serial maternal donations with iron and folate therapy.[107] Rigorous testing for infectious markers is indicated, and red cells should be free of maternal serum. Maternal blood has the potential advantage of decreasing the risk of sensitization to new red cell antigens associated with exposure to donor units. Maternal red cells are postulated to last longer than random donor red cells because of the reticulocytosis produced by repeated donations.[107,108]

Blood is transfused to increase the fetal hematocrit to between 40 and 45 percent. The blood should be as fresh as possible, washed free of additive solutions, warmed, and packed to a hematocrit of 70 to 85 percent in a volume calculation based on estimated fetal placental blood volume, fetal hematocrit, and hematocrit of donor blood. Various nomograms and formulas for the calculation of donor blood volume have been published.[109,110] If the hematocrit of the donor unit is approximately 75 percent, multiplying the estimated fetal weight in grams (estimated by ultrasound) by a factor of 0.02 provides a fairly accurate estimate of the volume of blood to be transfused to achieve a fetal hematocrit increment of 10 percent.[111]

DELIVERY

The decision regarding the appropriate time to deliver the baby is based on gestational age, fetal weight and lung maturity, fetal response to the intrauterine transfusions, ease of performing the transfusions, and antenatal ultrasound and Doppler studies for fetal anemia. Transfusions usually are provided up to 35 weeks in order to prolong gestation safely until the risks of preterm birth and its attendant complications are minimized.[112] Amniocentesis may be repeated late in gestation, at approximately 37 weeks, to study ΔOD_{450} values and assess fetal lung maturity prior to delivery.[96]

IMMUNOMODULATION

In women with severe alloimmunization and with fetal losses or hydrops very early in pregnancy, a variety of methods have been used to suppress the antibody response and prolong survival of the fetus until intrauterine transfusions become technically feasible.[113,114] The techniques include intravenous IgG, serial plasmapheresis, plasmapheresis combined with intravenous immunoglobulin, glucocorticoids, oral enteric-coated D-positive erythrocytes, and promethazine hydrochloride. The observation that alloimmunized women with offspring who exhibit mild hemolytic disease have significantly higher incidence of anti-HLA A, anti-B, anti-C, and anti-DR antibodies than mothers of children with severe hemolytic disease has given rise to the hypothesis that severe hemolytic disease can be prevented in women lacking anti-HLA antibodies by injecting them with the father's leukocytes before or at the beginning of a new pregnancy to provoke anti-

HLA antibody production, thus providing another avenue of immunomodulation.[29,30,115]

TREATMENT OF THE AFFECTED NEONATE

Results of antenatal monitoring and obstetric interventions during pregnancy and the history of the outcome of previous pregnancies allow the neonatal team to anticipate the needs of the infant born with hemolytic disease. In infants with severe hemolytic disease, severe anemia and hydrops are the immediate life-threatening concerns and often are accompanied by perinatal asphyxia, surfactant deficiency, hypoglycemia, acidosis, and thrombocytopenia. The next pressing problem is preventing bilirubin encephalopathy resulting from severe unconjugated hyperbilirubinemia. Exchange transfusions and phototherapy are the mainstays of treatment.

Resuscitation and stabilization of hydropic infants often is difficult and usually necessitates prompt intubation and positive-pressure ventilation with oxygen. Drainage of pleural effusions and ascites may be required to facilitate gas exchange. Metabolic acidosis and hypoglycemia should be corrected. A partial exchange transfusion can be performed using packed red cells to improve hemoglobin levels and oxygenation. A double-volume exchange transfusion is contemplated only after the initial stabilization.

Infants who received multiple intrauterine transfusions are delivered closer to term and often require less phototherapy and fewer exchange transfusions in the neonatal period.[59] However, some infants still have significant hemolytic anemia at birth, and a few require additional packed red cell transfusions for severe and prolonged hyporegenerative anemia secondary to suppression of fetal erythropoiesis.[38,116–118] In a study of 191 infants born alive after intrauterine transfusions between 1988 and 1999, the hematocrit at birth ranged from 13 to 51 percent. Endotracheal ventilation was required more often in babies who had been severely hydropic *in utero*, but the requirements for exchange transfusion (range 0–9) or simple transfusion (range 0–8) did not differ between babies who had been hydropic *in utero* and those without evidence of hydrops.[118]

EXCHANGE TRANSFUSION

Exchange transfusion corrects anemia, removes bilirubin and free maternal antibody in the plasma, and, when a double blood volume exchange is performed (calculated as 2×80 ml/kg in a term infant and 2×100 ml/kg in a preterm infant), replaces 90 percent of the infant's blood volume with antigen-negative red blood cells that should have normal *in vivo* survival.

The indications for early exchange transfusions performed within 9 to 12 hours of birth are debated but have remained essentially unchanged over the last 40 years, with minor modifications. Cord hemoglobin levels 110 g/liter or less, cord bilirubin levels 5.5 mg/dl or greater, and rapidly rising bilirubin levels 0.5 mg/dl/hour or greater despite phototherapy are commonly used criteria for early exchange transfusions. Early exchange transfusion has the advantage of replacing sensitized red cells with normal cells, thereby removing not only bilirubin but also the source of future bilirubin. Because bilirubin is distributed in the extracellular fluids, efficiency is enhanced by removing sensitized cells early in the process. "Late" exchange transfusions are performed when serum bilirubin levels threaten to exceed approximately 20 to 22 mg/dl in term infants. Considering that bilirubin levels rise steadily from birth and peak at approximately 72 to 96 hours of age, exchange transfusion may be considered within 24 hours of birth if serum bilirubin levels reach 15 mg/dl in an infant at least 35 weeks' gestation or 17 mg/dl in an infant at least 38 weeks' gestation despite intensive phototherapy. Immediate exchange transfusion is recommended in infants showing signs of acute bilirubin encephalopathy, even if bilirubin levels are falling.[119]

Conjugated or direct bilirubin values are not subtracted from total bilirubin levels when considering levels for exchange transfusions. A bilirubin albumin ratio (total serum bilirubin mg/dl to albumin g/dl) of 6.8 or higher may be considered an additional factor in determining the need for exchange transfusion.[119] Exchange transfusions are performed at lower bilirubin levels in premature infants, particularly those with hypoxemia, acidosis, and hypothermia, but little data are available to guide intervention in these infants. In infants with birth weights of at least 1500 g, exchange transfusions usually are performed at bilirubin levels of 13 to 16 mg/dl but may be considered even at levels as low as 8.8 mg/dl in sick babies of 24 weeks' gestation.[120]

A double-volume exchange should eliminate more than 50 percent of the intravascular bilirubin. However, the amount of bilirubin often is less, reflecting the equilibrating tissue-bound pool. Infusion of salt-poor albumin prior to the exchange transfusion may help bilirubin binding, thus increasing the amount of bilirubin removed. Equilibration of extravascular and intravascular bilirubin and continued breakdown of sensitized and newly formed red cells by persisting maternal antibodies result in a rebound of bilirubin following initial exchange transfusion, often necessitating repeated exchange transfusions in severe hemolytic disease.

Blood chosen for the exchange should be ABO compatible, Rh negative, negative for the antigen responsible for the hemolytic disease, and cross-matched against the mother's blood. Irradiated citrate-phosphate-dextrose blood is prepared as whole blood or reconstituted whole blood (red cells suspended in saline solution, albumin, or plasma) with a hematocrit of 40 to 50 percent. Additive solution anticoagulants should not be used, and the blood should be as fresh as possible (<7 days) to maximize the in vivo survival of the transfused red cells.[105]

Exchange transfusions can be performed by the traditional push–pull method with a single vascular access, usually the umbilical vein, or by isovolumetric techniques utilizing two access sites for simultaneous removal of the infant's blood and administration of new blood.[121] Aliquots of 5 to 20 ml, with a maximum of 5 ml/kg, are withdrawn or infused in the discontinuous method at a rate not exceeding 5 ml/kg every 3 minutes to prevent rapid fluctuations in arterial pressure, which are accompanied by changes in intracranial pressure. During an isovolumetric exchange, volumes to be removed or reinfused should not exceed 2 ml/kg/minute. The exchange usually lasts 1 to 2 hours.

Potential complications of exchange transfusion include hypocalcemia, hyperglycemia, hypoglycemia, thrombocytopenia, dilutional coagulopathy, neutropenia, disseminated intravascular coagulation, umbilical venous and/or arterial thrombosis, necrotizing enterocolitis, and infection. Despite advances in the management of critically ill newborn infants, morbidity and mortality associated with exchange transfusions remain high, particularly in infants who are premature, sick, or both. The risk of death or permanent serious sequelae reportedly is as high as 12 percent in sick infants compared with less than 1 percent in healthy infants in a retrospective review of exchange transfusions performed in two neonatal intensive care units between 1981 and 1995.[122] In another retrospective study of 55 neonates who underwent 66 exchange transfusions in two perinatal centers between 1992 and 2002, 74 percent of exchange transfusions were temporally associated with an adverse event, the majority of which were laboratory abnormalities. The most common events were thrombocytopenia (44 percent), hypocalcemia (29 percent), and metabolic acidosis (24 percent). Adverse events occurred more frequently in preterm infants and in infants who had preexisting neonatal morbidity prior to the exchange transfusion.[123] Careful clinical judgment is required to bal-

ance the potential risk of adverse events from exchange transfusion with the risk of bilirubin encephalopathy in sick neonates.

PHOTOTHERAPY

Exposure of bilirubin to light results in structural and configurational isomerization of bilirubin to less toxic and less lipophilic products that are excreted efficiently without hepatic conjugation. Phototherapy is the mainstay of treatment for unconjugated hyperbilirubinemia; the objective of treatment is preventing bilirubin neurotoxicity. The effectiveness of phototherapy is influenced by the wavelength and irradiance of light, the surface area of exposed skin, and the duration of exposure. Intensive phototherapy involves the use of high levels of irradiance ($\geq$30 μW/cm^2) in the 430- to 490-nm band, delivered to as much of the infant's surface area as possible. Intensive phototherapy effectively reduces bilirubin levels and decreases the need for exchange transfusions for hyperbilirubinemia in ABO and Rh hemolytic disease of the newborn.[124,125] Earlier protocols called for early institution of phototherapy in all infants with hemolytic disease, resulting in the unnecessary, albeit usually benign, treatment of large numbers of infants with mild hemolytic disease whose bilirubin levels would not have risen to nonphysiologic levels even without treatment. Nonetheless, early and intensive phototherapy should be initiated in infants with moderate or severe hemolysis or in infants with rapidly rising bilirubin levels (>0.5 mg/dl/hour). In infants of at least 38 weeks' gestation with alloimmune hemolytic disease, intensive phototherapy should be initiated if total bilirubin levels are 5 mg/dl or greater at birth, 10 mg/dl at 24 hours after birth, or approximately 13 to 15 mg/dl at 48 to 72 hours after birth.[119] Phototherapy is recommended at lower levels for preterm or sick infants. Therapy often is initiated at bilirubin levels less than 5 mg/dl in preterm infants with alloimmune hemolytic disease in order to avoid potentially risky exchange transfusions.[119,120]

OTHER TREATMENTS

Administration of high-dose intravenous immunoglobulin, as soon as possible after the diagnosis of neonatal immune hemolytic disease is made, decreases the need for phototherapy and exchange transfusions.[126,127] The decreased bilirubin levels in infants treated with intravenous immunoglobulin is attributed to reduction in hemolysis secondary to blockade of reticuloendothelial Fc receptors. Administration of 0.5 to 1 g/kg over 2 hours is recommended if total serum bilirubin levels continue to rise despite intensive phototherapy or the total serum bilirubin level is within 2 to 3 mg/dl of the exchange transfusion level. The dose can be repeated in 12 hours if necessary.[119]

Synthetic heme analogues suppress bilirubin production by competitively inhibiting the activity of heme oxygenase, the rate-limiting enzyme in the catabolism of heme to biliverdin. Sn-protoporphyrin, a potent heme oxygenase inhibitor, blunts the postnatal rise and peak bilirubin levels in term newborns with ABO hemolytic disease.[128] In a meta-analysis of randomized controlled trials of metalloporphyrins for treatment of unconjugated jaundice in term and preterm infants, metalloporphyrin-treated infants appeared to have short-term benefits compared to controls, including lower maximum bilirubin levels in one study, lower frequency of severe hyperbilirubinemia in one study, decreased need for phototherapy, and a shorter duration of hospitalization. However, there are insufficient data to support or refute the possibility that treatment with a metalloporphyrin decreases the risk of neonatal kernicterus or long-term neurodevelopmental impairment as a result of bilirubin encephalopathy.[129] In addition, metalloporphyrins are photochemically active, and a transient erythematous rash in some tin mesoporphyrin-treated infants who received phototherapy has been reported. Further documentation of safety and effectiveness of heme analogues is required, particularly because the option of phototherapy for treatment of jaundice is widely accepted and usually safe.

Recombinant human erythropoietin decreases the need for postnatal transfusions in infants with late hyporegenerative anemia of Rh hemolytic disease and in neonates with Kell hemolytic disease.[37,130,131] In 103 patients with Rh hemolytic disease, administration of 200 units/kg of recombinant erythropoietin subcutaneously, three times per week for 6 weeks, reportedly reduced the number of erythrocyte transfusions to a mean of 1.5, and 55 percent of patients did not require any transfusions.[132]

COURSE AND PROGNOSIS

In Manitoba, Canada, perinatal mortality from hemolytic disease dropped from 100 per year in the 1940s in a population of one million to one death every 3 years in the mid 1990s.[7] Similar reductions have been reported in the United States and United Kingdom. Prior to the development of treatment measures in the 1940s, almost half of all newborn infants with Rh hemolytic disease died or were severely handicapped. Perinatal survival rates greater than 90 percent have been achieved with intrauterine transfusions in nonhydropic fetuses with severe Rh hemolytic disease.[133] The overall survival rate for hydropic fetuses is lower (78 percent) despite intrauterine transfusions.[118] An 11-year study from 1988 to 1999 examined 80 fetuses with immune hydrops. The survival rate for fetuses with mild hydrops was 98 percent, with intrauterine reversal of hydrops in 88 percent of the fetuses. The outcome in severe fetal hydrops was poor, with reversal of hydrops in 39 percent of cases. The survival rate for fetuses with persistent hydrops was only 26 percent.[118] This study underscores the importance of early diagnosis and treatment of fetal anemia, before hydrops develops.

The neurodevelopmental outcome for infants saved by intrauterine transfusion has generally been excellent; more than 90 percent of survivors are free of disability.[59,134,135] Perinatal asphyxia and lower cord hemoglobin level at birth have been associated with an increased risk for neurologic abnormalities. Cerebral palsy and hearing disabilities have been noted in survivors.[59,134] No difference has been noted in the neurologic outcome of infants with hydrops fetalis compared with nonhydropic infants.[134,135]

The incidence of kernicterus in infants with Rh hemolytic disease, derived from the 1950s literature, reportedly is 8 percent in those with bilirubin concentrations of 19 to 24 mg/dl and rises to 33 percent in infants with bilirubin levels of 25 to 29 mg/dl and 73 percent in infants with bilirubin levels of 30 to 40 mg/dl.[136] Recent data indicate the mortality in term and near-term infants with kernicterus in the United States is approximately 4 percent.[137] Although preterm and low-birth-weight infants are generally believed to be more vulnerable to brain damage from increased bilirubin levels than are term neonates, data from follow-up studies have not provided clear proof of this assumption.

PREVENTION

Transfusion of blood compatible not only with the D antigen but also with Kell and other Rh antigens has been advocated for premenopausal women to prevent alloimmunization.[8,9]

Use of Rh Ig is the mainstay of prevention of maternal D immunization. Prophylaxis similar to Rh Ig does not exist for alloimmunization to antigens other than D. Postpartum administration of Rh Ig to all nonsensitized Rh-negative women who deliver an Rh-positive infant decreases the incidence of Rh isoimmunization from 12 percent to approximately 2 percent.[138] However approximately 1.8 percent of Rh-negative women apparently are sensitized from small asymptomatic transplacental hemorrhages during pregnancy. Further reduction in the incidence of Rh-isoimmunization to 0.1 percent has been achieved by antepartum Rh Ig prophylaxis at 28 weeks' gestation, and this is the current standard recommendation in the United States.[63]

The mechanism by which Rh Ig prevents sensitization to the D antigen is not understood. One theory proposes passively administered anti-D attaches to the D-antigen sites on Rh-positive red blood cells in the circulation and interferes with the host's primary immune response to the foreign antigen. Rh Ig also may inhibit antigen-induced B cell responsiveness by stimulating an increase in suppressor T cells.

The standard dose of 300 μg Rh Ig (1500 IU) in the United States affords protection against a fetomaternal transfusion of 15 ml of Rh-positive red blood cells or 30 ml of Rh-positive whole blood. However, fetomaternal hemorrhage in excess of 30 ml may occur in women without predisposing risk factors.[18,19] The blood of all Rh-negative nonimmunized women should be tested for fetomaternal hemorrhage approximately 1 hour after delivery of an Rh-positive baby.[60,63] During the antenatal period, testing is indicated after 20 weeks' gestation if clinical circumstances suggest the possibility of excessive transplacental hemorrhage (e.g., abdominal trauma or abruptio placentae). Screening for fetomaternal hemorrhage can be performed by the rosette test, which detects as little as 2.5 ml of whole blood.[139] If the rosette test result is positive, the number of fetal red cells should be determined. The Kleihauer-Betke test, the standard test used in most laboratories, permits quantification of fetal hemoglobin-containing red cells in a maternal blood sample.[140] The test is based on the resistance of fetal hemoglobin to acid elution, unlike adult hemoglobin. False-positive results can be obtained in maternal conditions associated with increased fetal hemoglobin, such as hereditary persistence of fetal hemoglobin, sickle cell disease, or sickle cell trait. Flow cytometric methods appear to offer increased accuracy and reliability and have been used for both screening and quantification of fetal red cells.[141]

The recommended dose of Rh Ig should be administered as soon as possible, within 72 hours of delivery of an Rh-positive baby. If Rh Ig is accidentally omitted, some protection still can be obtained with administration up to 13 days and possibly up to 28 days after delivery. Rh Ig is ineffective once alloimmunization to RhD antigen has occurred.

Rh Ig is indicated following pregnancy termination, miscarriage, amniocentesis, chorionic villus sampling, or other manipulation during pregnancy. A smaller 50-μg dose is adequate if pregnancy is terminated at less than 12 weeks' gestation.[63] No definite evidence-based recommendations are available regarding administration of Rh Ig to women with threatened abortion and a live fetus or embryo at or before 12 weeks' gestation. If therapeutic or spontaneous abortion occurs after the first trimester, the standard 300-μg dose is recommended.[63]

If a woman was exposed to more than 30 ml of D-positive blood, either secondary to fetomaternal hemorrhage or as a result of inadvertent transfusion of D-positive cells, the dose of Rh Ig should be calculated to cover the volume of D-positive cells to prevent immunization. Multiple doses of Rh Ig, calculated to cover the volume of exposure, can be given intramuscularly every 12 hours until the total dose is administered.[138] Alternatively, WinRho SDF (Calgene Corporation, Winnipeg, Canada), an intravenous preparation of Rh Ig, can be administered with much less discomfort to the patient.[142] WinRho SDF is a sterile, freeze-dried γ-globulin fraction containing antibodies to RhD antigen, prepared from human plasma by anion-exchange column chromatography. A 300-μg (1500-IU) vial contains sufficient anti-RhD to effectively suppress the immunizing potential of roughly 17 ml of D-positive red blood cells. The recommended dose, calculated as 9 μg/ml of whole blood or 18 μg/ml of red cells, can be administered as 600 μg intravenously every 8 hours until the total dose is given.

RhD alloimmunization occurs despite recommended prophylaxis in 0.1 percent of pregnancies. Many cases of preventable Rh alloimmunization continue to occur because of failure to implement immunoprophylaxis protocols.

MONOCLONAL ANTIBODY

Rh Ig currently is produced from the plasma of D-negative male volunteers injected with D-positive red blood cells. Although polyclonal Rh Ig is extremely safe, concerns exist regarding potential transmission of infectious agents and a possible shortage of supplies.[63] Monoclonal anti-D antibodies produced by Epstein-Barr virus immortalization of B lymphoblastoid cell lines or from heterohybridomas are being evaluated for their potential to replace polyclonal Rh Ig for RhD prophylaxis.[143] In a study of 95 D-negative male volunteers given a mixture of two human monoclonal anti-D antibodies (IgG1 and IgG3) 24 hours after injection of 5 ml of D-positive red cells, one definite and one possible failure of protection were observed. Further trials are necessary before monoclonal anti-D antibodies will be available for therapeutic use.

REFERENCES

1. Diamond LK, Blackfan KD, Baty JM: Erythroblastosis fetalis and its association with universal edema of the fetus, icterus gravis neonatorum and anemia of the newborn. *J Pediatr* 1:269, 1932.
2. Landsteiner K, Wiener AS: An agglutinable factor in human blood recognized by immune sera for Rhesus blood. *Proc Soc Exp Biol Med* 43:223, 1940.
3. Levine P, Katzin EM, Burnham L: Isoimmunization in pregnancy: Its possible bearing on the etiology of erythroblastosis fetalis. *JAMA* 116:825, 1941.
4. Diamond LK, Allen FH Jr, Thomas WO Jr: Erythroblastosis fetalis: VII. Treatment with exchange transfusion. *N Engl J Med* 244:39, 1951.
5. Liley AW: The use of amniocentesis and fetal transfusion in erythroblastosis fetalis. *Pediatrics* 35:836, 1965.
6. Wegmann A, Gluck R: The history of Rhesus prophylaxis with anti-D (classical article). *Eur J Pediatr* 155:835, 1996.
7. Bowman J: The management of hemolytic disease in the fetus and newborn. *Semin Perinatol* 21:39, 1997.
8. Geifman-Holtzman O, Wojtowycz M, Kosmas E, Artal R: Female alloimmunization with antibodies known to cause hemolytic disease. *Obstet Gynecol* 89:272, 1997.
9. Howard H, Martlew V, McFadyen I, et al: Consequences for fetus and neonate of maternal red cell alloimmunization. *Arch Dis Child Fetal Neonatal Ed* 78;F62, 1998.
10. Filbey D, Hanson U, Wesstrom G: The prevalence of red cell antibodies in pregnancy correlated to the outcome of the newborn. *Acta Obstet Gynecol Scand* 74:687, 1995.
11. Moise KJ Jr: Non anti-D antibodies in red cell alloimmunization. *Eur J Obstet Gynecol Reprod Biol* 92:75, 2000.
12. Singleton BK, Green CA, Avent ND, et al: The presence of RhD pseudogene containing a 37 base pair duplication and a nonsense mutation in Africans with the RhD negative blood group phenotype. *Blood* 174:818, 2000.
13. Issit PD, Anstee DJ: *Applied Blood Group Serology*, 4th ed. Montgomery Scientific Publications, Durham, 1998.
14. Joseph KS: Controlling Rh haemolytic disease of the newborn in India. *Br J Obstet Gynaecol* 98:369, 1991.
15. Mak KH, Yan KF, Cheng SS, Yuen MY: Rh phenotypes of Chinese blood donors in Hong Kong, with special reference to weak D antigens. *Transfusion* 33:348, 1993.
16. Bowman JM, Pollack JM, Penston LE: Fetomaternal transplacental hemorrhage during pregnancy and after delivery. *Vox Sang* 51:117, 1986.
17. Sebring ES, Polesky HF: Fetomaternal hemorrhage: Incidence, risk factors, time of occurrence, and clinical effects. *Transfusion* 30:344, 1990.
18. Ness PM, Baldwin ML, Niebyl JR: Clinical high-risk designation does not predict excess fetomaternal hemorrhage. *Am J Obstet Gynecol* 156:154, 1987.
19. Pourbak S, Rund CR, Crookston KP: Three cases of massive fetomaternal hemorrhage presenting without clinical suspicion. *Arch Pathol Lab Med* 128:463, 2004.
20. Jansen MWJC, Brandenburg H, Wildshut HIJ, et al: The effect of chorionic villus sampling on the number of fetal cells isolated from maternal blood and on maternal serum alpha-fetoprotein levels. *Prenat Diagn* 17:953, 1997.
21. Bowman JM, Pollack JM: Transplacental fetal hemorrhage after amniocentesis. *Obstet Gynecol* 66:749, 1985.
22. Bowman JM, Pollock JM, Peterson LE, et al: Fetomaternal hemorrhage following funipuncture: Increase in severity of maternal red-cell alloimmunization. *Obstet Gynecol* 84:839, 1994.
23. Bowman J, Harman C, Manning F, et al: Intravenous drug abuse causes Rh immunization. *Vox Sang* 61:96, 1991.
24. Bowman JM: Fetomaternal ABO incompatibility and erythroblastosis fetalis. *Vox Sang* 50:104, 1986.
25. Engelfriet CP, Overbeeke MAM, Dooren MC, et al: Bioassays to determine the clinical significance of red cell alloantibodies based on Fc receptor induced destruction of red cells sensitized by IgG. *Transfusion* 34;617, 1994.
26. Hadley AG: Laboratory assays for predicting the severity of haemolytic disease of the fetus and newborn. *Transpl Immunol* 10:191, 2002.
27. Palfi M, Hilden J, Gottval T, Selbing A: Placental transport of maternal immunoglobulin G in pregnancies at risk of Rh(D) hemolytic disease of the newborn. *Am J Reprod Immunol* 39;323, 1998.
28. Lambin P, Debbia M, Puillandre P, Brossard Y: IgG1 and IgG3 in maternal serum and on the RBCs of infants suffering from HDN: Relationship with the severity of the disease. *Transfusion* 42:1537, 2002.
29. Neppert J, v Witzleben-Schurholz E, Zupanski B, et al: High incidence of maternal HLA A B and C antibodies associated with a mild course of haemolytic disease of the newborn. Group for the Study of Protective Maternal HLA Antibodies in the Clinical Course of HDN. *Eur J Haematol* 63:120, 1999.
30. Shepard SL, Noble AL, Filbey D, Hadley AG: Inhibition of monocyte chemiluminescent response to anti-D sensitized red cells by Fc gamma RI-blocking antibodies which ameliorate the severity of haemolytic disease of the newborn. *Vox Sang* 70:157, 1996.
31. Thilaganathan B, Salvesan D, Abbas A, et al: Fetal plasma erythropoietin concentration in red blood cell–isoimmunized pregnancies. *Am J Obstet Gynecol* 167:1292, 1992.
32. Koenig JM, Christensen RD: Neutropenia and thrombocytopenia in infants with Rh hemolytic disease. *J Pediatr* 114:625, 1989.
33. Nicolaides KH: Studies in fetal physiology and pathophysiology in Rhesus disease. *Semin Perinatol* 13:328, 1989.
34. Phibbs RH: Hydrops fetalis and other causes of neonatal edema and ascites, in *Fetal and Neonatal Physiology*, 2nd ed, edited by RA Polin, WW Fox, p 1730. WB Saunders, Philadelphia, 1998.
35. Weiner CP: Human fetal bilirubin levels and fetal hemolytic disease. *Am J Obstet Gynecol* 166:1449, 1992.
36. Hayde M, Widness JA, Pollack A, et al: Rhesus isoimmunization: Increased hemolysis during early infancy. *Pediatr Res* 41:716, 1997.
37. Al-Alaiyan S, Al Omran A: Late hyporegenerative anemia in neonates with rhesus hemolytic disease. *J Perinat Med* 27:112, 1999.
38. Pessler F, Hart D: Hyporegenerative anemia associated with Rh hemolytic disease: Treatment failure of recombinant erythropoietin. *J Pediatr Hematol Oncol* 24:689, 2002.
39. Jadhav M, Devarajan LV: ABO hemolytic disease: An important cause of neonatal morbidity. *Indian Pediatr* 9:246, 1972.

40. Lin M, Broadberry RE: ABO Hemolytic disease of the newborn is more severe in Taiwan than in white populations. *Vox Sang* 68:136, 1995.

41. Cariani L, Romano EL, Martinez N, et al: ABO-haemolytic disease of the newborn (ABO-HDN): Factors influencing its severity and incidence in Venezuela. *J Trop Pediatr* 41:14, 1995.

42. Vos GH, Adhikari M, Coovadia HM: A study of ABO incompatibility and neonatal jaundice in Black South African newborn infants. *Transfusion* 21:744, 1981.

43. Dudin AA, Ramboud–Cousson A, Badawi S, et al: ABO and Rh(D) blood group distribution and their implications for feto-maternal incompatibility among the Palestinian population. *Ann Trop Pediatr* 13:249, 1993.

44. Kaplan M, Hammerman C, Renbaum P, et al: Gilbert's syndrome and hyperbilirubinemia in ABO incompatible neonates. *Lancet* 356:652, 2000.

45. Stiller RJ, Herzlinger R, Siegel S, Whetham JCG: Fetal ascites associated with ABO incompatibility: Case report and review of the literature. *Am J Obstet Gynecol* 175:1371, 1996.

46. McDonnell M, Hannam S, Devane SP: Hydrops fetalis due to ABO incompatibility. *Arch Dis Child Fetal Neonatal Ed* 78:F220, 1998.

47. Katz MA, Kanto WP, Korotkin JH: Recurrence rate of ABO hemolytic disease of the newborn. *Obstet Gynecol* 59:611, 1982.

48. Brouwers HAA, Overbeeke MAM, Gemke RJBJ, et al: Sensitive methods for determining subclasses of IgG anti-A and anti-B in sera of blood group O women with a blood group A or B child. *Br J Haematol* 66:267, 1987.

49. Brouwers HAA, Overbeeke MAM, van Ertbruggen I, et al: What is the best predictor of the severity of ABO haemolytic disease of the newborn? *Lancet* ii:641, 1988.

50. Oski FA, Naiman JL: Erythroblastosis fetalis, in *Hematologic Problems in the Newborn*, 4th ed, p 283. WB Saunders, Philadelphia, 1982.

51. Brecher ME: *AABB Technical Manual 50th Anniversary Edition 1953-2003*, p14. AABB Publications, Bethesda, 2002.

52. McKenna DS, Nagaraja HN, O'Shaughnessy R: Management of pregnancies complicated by anti-Kell isoimmunization. *Obstet Gynecol* 93:667, 1999.

53. Caine ME, Mueller-Heubach E: Kell sensitization in pregnancy. *Am J Obstet Gynecol* 154:85, 1986.

54. Leggat HM, Gibson JM, Barron SL, Reid MM: Anti-Kell in pregnancy. *Br J Obstet Gynaecol* 98:162, 1991.

55. Bowman JM, Pollack JM, Manning FA, et al: Maternal Kell blood group alloimmunization. *Obstet Gynecol* 79:239, 1992.

56. Vaughan JI, Manning M, Warwick RM, et al: Inhibition of erythroid progenitor cells by anti-Kell antibodies in fetal alloimmune anemia. *N Engl J Med* 338:798, 1998.

57. Daniels G, Hadley A, Green CA: Causes of fetal anemia in hemolytic disease due to anti-K. *Transfusion* 43:115, 2003.

58. Shapiro SM: Bilirubin toxicity in the developing nervous system. *Pediatr Neurol* 29:410, 2003.

59. Janssens HM, deHaan MJJ, van Kamp IL, et al: Outcome for children treated with fetal intravascular transfusions because of severe blood group antagonism. *J Pediatr* 131:373, 1997.

60. Judd WJ, Scientific Section Coordinating Committee of the AABB: Practice guidelines for prenatal and perinatal immunohematology, revisited. *Transfusion* 41:1445, 2001.

61. AABB: *Standards for Blood Banks and Transfusion Services*, 22nd ed. AABB, Bethesda, 2003.

62. Cannon M, Pierce R, Taber EB, Schucker J: Fatal hydrops fetalis caused by anti-D in a mother with partial D. *Obstet Gynecol* 102:1143, 2003.

63. American College of Obstetrics and Gynecology. *ACOG Practice Bulletin. Prevention of RhD alloimmunization, number 4 (replaces educational bulletin number 14, October 1990)*. Clinical Management Guidelines for Obstetricians and Gynecologists, 1999.

64. Anderson AS, Praetorius L, Jorgensen HL, et al: Prognostic value of screening for irregular antibodies late in pregnancy in rhesus positive women. *Acta Obstet Gynecol Scand* 81:407, 2002.

65. Heddle NM, Klama L, Frassetto R, et al: A retrospective study to determine the risk of red cell alloimmunization and transfusion during pregnancy. *Transfusion* 23:217, 1993.

66. Nicolaides KH, Rodeck CH: Maternal serum anti-D antibody concentration and assessment of Rhesus isoimmunization. *Br Med J* 304:1155, 1992.

67. Hackney DN, Knudtson EJ, Rossi KQ, et al: Management of pregnancies complicated by anti-c isoimmunization. *Obstet Gynecol* 103:24, 2004.

68. van Dijk BA, Dooren MC, Overbeeke AM: Red cell antibodies in pregnancy: There is no critical titre. *Transfus Med* 4:199, 1995.

69. Larson PJ, Thorp JM Jr, Miller RC, Hoffman M: The monocyte monolayer assay: A non-invasive technique for predicting the severity of in utero hemolysis. *Am J Perinatol* 12:157, 1995.

70. Hadley AG, Wilkes A, Goodrick J, et al: The ability of the chemiluminescence test to predict clinical outcome and the necessity for amniocentesis in pregnancies at risk of haemolytic disease of the newborn. *Br J Obstet Gynaecol* 105:231, 1998.

71. Oepkes D, van Kemp IL, Simon MJG, et al: Clinical value of an antibody dependent cell mediated cytotoxicity assay in the management of RhD alloimmunization. *Am J Obstet Gynecol* 184:1015, 2001.

72. Engelfriet CP, Reesink HW: International forum: Laboratory procedures for the prediction of the severity of hemolytic disease of the newborn. *Vox Sang* 69:61, 1995.

73. Kanter MH: Derivation of new mathematic formulas for determining whether a D-positive father is heterozygous or homozygous for the D antigen. *Am J Obstet Gynecol* 166:61, 1992.

74. Chiu RWK, Murphy MF, Fidler C, et al: Determination of RhD zygosity: Comparison of a double amplification refractory mutation system approach and a multiplex real-time quantitative PCR approach. *Clin Chem* 47:667, 2001.

75. Matheson KA, Denomme GA: Novel 3' Rhesus box sequences confound RhD zygosity assignment. *Transfusion* 42:645, 2002.

76. Van den Veyver IB, Subramanian SB, Hudson KM, et al: Prenatal diagnosis of the RhD fetal blood type on amniotic fluid polymerase chain reaction. *Obstet Gynecol* 87:419, 1996.

77. Simsek S, Faas BH, Bleeker PM, et al: Rapid Rh typing by polymerase chain reaction based amplification of DNA. *Blood* 85:2975, 1995.

78. Lo YMD, Bowell PJ, Selinger M, et al: Prenatal determination of fetal Rh-D status by analysis of peripheral blood of Rhesus negative mothers. *Lancet* 341:1147, 1993.

79. Geifman-Holtzman O, Bernstein IM, Berry SM, et al: Fetal Rh-D genotyping in fetal cells flow sorted from maternal circulation. *Am J Obstet Gynecol* 174:818, 1996.

80. Finning KM, Martin PG, Soothill PW, Avent ND: Prediction of fetal D status from maternal plasma: Introduction of a new non-invasive fetal RhD genotyping service. *Transfusion* 42:1079, 2002.

81. Turner MJ, Martin CM, O'Leary JJ: Detection of fetal Rhesus D gene in whole blood of women booking for routine antenatal care. *Eur J Obstet Gynecol Reprod Biol* 108:29, 2003.

82. Nelson M, Forsyth C, Popp H, Gibson J: Rapid detection of Rh-D- or K-positive fetal red cells in chorionic villus samples by a flow cytometric technique. *Transfus Med* 4:297, 1994.

83. Faas BH, Maaskant-Van Wijk PA, von dem Borne AE, et al: The applicability of different PCR based methods for fetal RH and K1 genotyping: A prospective study. *Prenat Diagn* 20:453, 2000.

84. Van der Schoot CE, Tax GH, Rijnders RJ, et al: Prenatal typing of Rh and Kell blood group system antigens: The edge of a watershed. *Transfus Med Rev* 17:31, 2003.

85. Liley AW: Liquor amnii analysis in the management of the pregnancy

complicated by Rhesus sensitization. *Am J Obstet Gynecol* 82:1359, 1961.

86. Bowman JM: The management of Rh-isoimmunization. *Obstet Gynecol* 52:1, 1978.

87. Nicolaides KH, Rodeck CH, Mibashan RS, Kemp JR: Have Liley charts outlived their usefulness? *Am J Obstet Gynecol* 155:90, 1986.

88. Queenan JT, Tomai TP, Ural SH, King JC: Deviation in amniotic fluid optical density at a wavelength of 450 nm in Rh-immunized pregnancies from 14 to 40 weeks' gestation: A proposal for clinical management. *Am J Obstet Gynecol* 168:1370, 1993.

89. Spinnato JA, Clark AL, Ralston KK, et al: Hemolytic disease of the fetus: A comparison of the Queenan and extended Liley methods. *Obstet Gynecol* 92:441, 1998.

90. Whitecar PW, Moise KJ Jr: Sonographic methods to detect fetal anemia in red blood cell alloimmunization. *Obstet Gynecol Surv* 55:240, 2000.

91. Dukler D, Oepkes D, Seaward G, et al: Noninvasive tests to predict fetal anemia: A study comparing Doppler and ultrasound parameters. *Am J Obstet Gynecol* 188:1310, 2003.

92. Mari G, Deter RL, Carpenter RL, et al: For the Collaborative Group for Doppler Assessment of the Blood Velocity in Anemic Fetuses. Noninvasive diagnosis by Doppler ultrasonography of fetal anemia due to maternal red cell alloimmunization. *N Engl J Med* 342:9, 2000.

93. Pereira L, Jenkins TM, Berghella V: Conventional management of maternal red cell alloimmunization compared with management by Doppler assessment of middle cerebral artery peak systolic velocity. *Am J Obstet Gynecol* 189:1002, 2003.

94. Oepkes D: Invasive versus noninvasive testing in red cell alloimmunized pregnancies. *Eur J Obstet Gynecol Reprod Biol* 92:83, 2000.

95. Daffos F, Capella-Pavlovsky M, Forestier F: Fetal blood sampling during pregnancy with use of a needle guided by ultrasound: A study of 606 consecutive cases. *Am J Obstet Gynecol* 153:655, 1985.

96. Steiner EA, Judd WJ, Oberman HA, et al: Percutaneous umbilical blood sampling and umbilical vein transfusions. Rapid serological differentiation of fetal blood from maternal blood. *Transfusion* 30:104, 1990.

97. Moise KJ Jr: Management of rhesus alloimmunization in pregnancy. *Obstet Gynecol* 100:600, 2002.

98. Ghidini A, Sepulveda W, Lockwood CJ, Romero R: Complications of fetal blood sampling. *Am J Obstet Gynecol* 168:1339, 1993.

99. Herschel M, Karrison T, Wen M, et al: Isoimmunization is unlikely to be the cause of hemolysis in ABO incompatible but direct antiglobulin test negative neonates. *Pediatrics* 110:127, 2002.

100. Herschel M, Karrison T, Wen M, et al: Evaluation of the direct antiglobulin (Coombs') test for identifying newborns at risk for hemolysis as determined by end tidal carbon monoxide concentration (ETCO$_c$); and comparison of the Coombs' test with ETCO$_c$ for detecting significant jaundice. *J Perinatol* 22:341, 2002.

101. Ramasethu J: Hemolytic disease of the newborn, in *Handbook of Pediatric Transfusion Medicine*, edited by CD Hillyer, RG Strauss, NLC Luban, pp 191–208. Elsevier Academic, 2004.

102. Poissonnier MH, Picone O, Brossard Y, Lepercq J: Intravenous fetal exchange transfusion before 22 weeks gestation in early and severe red cell fetomaternal alloimmunization. *Fetal Diang Ther* 18:467, 2003.

103. Radunovic N, Lockwood CJ, Alvarez M, et al: The severely anemic and hydropic isoimmune fetus: Changes in fetal hematocrit associated with intrauterine death. *Obstet Gynecol* 79:390, 1992.

104. Hallak M, Moise KJ, Hesketh DE, et al: Intravascular transfusion of fetuses with Rhesus incompatibility: Prediction of fetal outcome by changes in umbilical venous pressure. *Obstet Gynecol* 80:286, 1992.

105. Wong ECC, Luban NLC: Intrauterine, neonatal and pediatric transfusion, in *Transfusion Therapy: Clinical Principles and Practice*, 2nd ed, edited by PD Mintz. pp 159–201, AABB Press, Bethesda, 2005.

106. Gibson BE, Todd A, Roberts I, et al: British Committee for Standards in Haematology Transfusion Task Force: Writing Group. Transfusion guidelines for neonates and older children. *Br J Haematol* 124:433, 2004.

107. Gonsoulin WJ, Moise KJ Jr, Milam JD, et al: Serial maternal blood donations for intrauterine transfusions. *Obstet Gynecol* 75:158, 1990.

108. el-Azeem SA, Samuels P, Rose RL, et al: The effect of the source of transfused blood on the rate of consumption of transfused red blood cells in pregnancies affected by red blood cell alloimmunization. *Am J Obstet Gynecol* 177:753, 1997.

109. Nicolaides KH, Clewell WH, Rodeck CH: Measurement of human fetoplacental blood volume in erythroblastosis fetalis. *Am J Obstet Gynecol* 157:50, 1987.

110. Hoogeven M, Meerman RH, Pasman S, Egberts J: A new method to determine the fetoplacental volume based on dilution of fetal hemoglobin and an estimation of plasma fluid loss after intrauterine intravascular transfusion. *BJOG* 109:1132, 2002.

111. Giannina G, Moise KJ Jr, Dorman K: A simple method to estimate the volume for fetal intrauterine transfusion. *Fetal Diagn Ther* 13:94, 1998.

112. Klumper FJ, van Kamp IL, Vandenbussche FPHA, et al: Benefits and risks of fetal red cell transfusion after 32 weeks. *Eur J Obstet Gynecol Reprod Biol* 92:91, 2000.

113. Noia G, De Santis M, Romano D, et al: Complementary therapy for severe Rh-alloimmunization. *Clin Exp Obstet Gynecol* 29:297, 2002.

114. Collinet P, Subtil D, Puech F, Vaast P: Successful treatment of extremely severe fetal anemia due to Kell isoimmunization. *Obstet Gynecol* 100: 1102, 2002.

115. Whitecar PW, Farb R, Subramanyam L, et al: Paternal leukocyte alloimmunization as a treatment for hemolytic disease of the newborn in a rabbit model. *Am J Obstet Gynecol* 187:977, 2002

116. Weiner CP, Williamson RA, Wenstrom KD, et al: Management of fetal hemolytic disease by cordocentesis: II. Outcome of treatment. *Am J Obstet Gynecol* 165:1302, 1991.

117. Millard DD, Gidding SS, Socol ML, et al: Effects of intravascular intrauterine transfusion on prenatal and postnatal hemolysis and erythropoiesis in severe fetal isoimmunization. *J Pediatr* 117:447, 1990.

118. Van Kamp IL, Klumper FJCM, Bakkum RSLA, et al: The severity of immune fetal hydrops is predictive of fetal outcome after intrauterine treatment. *Am J Obstet Gynecol* 185:668, 2001.

119. American Academy of Pediatrics: Clinical Practice Guideline. Subcommittee on Hyperbilirubinemia. Management of hyperbilirubinemia in the newborn infant 35 or more weeks gestation. *Pediatrics* 114:297, 2004.

120. Maisels MJ, Watchko JF: Treatment of jaundice in low birth weight infants. *Arch Dis Child Fetal Neonatal Ed* 88:F459, 2003.

121. Ramasethu J: Exchange transfusions. In *Atlas of Procedures in Neonatology*, 3rd ed, edited by MG MacDonald, J Ramasethu, pp 348–356. Lippincott, Williams & Wilkins, Philadelphia, 2002.

122. Jackson JC: Adverse events associated with exchange transfusion in healthy and healthy and ill newborns. *Pediatrics* 99:e7, 1997.

123. Patra K, Storfer-Isser A, Siner B, et al: Adverse events associated with neonatal exchange transfusion in the 1990s. *J Pediatr* 144:626, 2004.

124. Tan KL, Lim GC, Boey KW: Phototherapy for ABO haemolytic hyperbilirubinemia. *Biol Neonate* 61:358, 1992.

125. Ebbesen F: Evaluation of the indications for early exchange transfusion in Rhesus haemolytic disease during phototherapy. *Eur J Pediatr* 133: 37, 1980.

126. Gottstein R, Cooke RWI: Systematic review of intravenous immunoglobulin in haemolytic disease of the Newborn. *Arch Dis Child Fetal Neonatal Ed* 88:F6, 2003.

127. Alcock GS, Liley H: Immunoglobulin infusion for isoimmune haemolytic disease in neonates. *Cochrane Database Syst Rev* 3:CD003313, 2002.

128. Kappas A, Drummond GS, Manola T, et al: Sn-protoporphyrin use in the management of hyperbilirubinemia in term newborns with direct Coombs-positive ABO incompatibility. *Pediatrics* 81:485, 1988.

129. Suresh GK, Martin CL, Soll RF: Metalloporphyrins for treatment of unconjugated hyperbilirubinemia in neonates. *Cochrane Database Syst Rev* 2:CD004207, 2003.

130. Ovaly F, Samancy N, Dagoglu T: Management of late anemia in rhesus hemolytic disease: Use of recombinant human erythropoietin (a pilot study). *Pediatr Res* 39:831, 1996.

131. Dhodapkar KM, Blei F: Treatment of hemolytic disease of the newborn caused by anti-Kell antibody with recombinant erythropoietin. *J Pediatr Hematol Oncol* 23:69, 2003.

132. Ovaly F: Late anemia in Rh haemolytic disease. *Arch Dis Child Fetal Neonatal Ed* 88:F 444, 2003.

133. Schumacher B, Moise KJ Jr: Fetal transfusion for red blood cell alloimmunization in pregnancy. *Obstet Gynecol* 88:137, 1996.

134. Hudon L, Moise KJ Jr, Hegemier SE, et al: Long-term neurodevelopmental outcome after intrauterine transfusion for the treatment of fetal hemolytic disease. *Am J Obstet Gynecol* 179:858, 1998.

135. Grab D, Paulus WE, Bommer A, et al: Treatment of fetal erythroblastosis by intravascular transfusions: Outcome at 6 years. *Obstet Gynecol* 93:165, 1999.

136. Volpe JJ: Bilirubin and brain injury, in *Neurology of the Newborn*, 4th ed, edited by J Volpe, p 521. WB Saunders, Philadelphia, 2001.

137. Johnson L, Brown AK: A pilot registry for acute and chronic kernicterus in term and near term infants. *Pediatrics* 104:736, 1999.

138. Bowman J: Thirty-five years of Rh prophylaxis. *Transfusion* 43:1661, 2003.

139. Sebring ES, Polesky HG: Detection of fetal maternal hemorrhage in Rh immune globulin candidates: A rosetting technique using enzyme-treated Rh_2Rh_2 indicator erythrocytes. *Transfusion* 22:468, 1982.

140. Kleihauer E, Braun H, Betki K: Demonstration von fetalem Hämoglobin in den Erythrocyten eines Blutausstrichs. *Klin Wochenschr* 35:637, 1957.

141. Nelson M, Zarkos K, Popp H, Gibson J: A flow-cytometric equivalent of the Kleihauer test. *Vox Sang* 75:234, 1998.

142. Anderson B, Shad AT, Gootenberg JE, Sandler SG: Successful prevention of posttransfusion Rh alloimmunization by intravenous Rho (D) immuneglobulin (WinRhoSD). *Am J Hematol* 69:245, 1999.

143. Kumpel BM: Monoclonal anti-D development programme. *Transpl Immunol* 10:199, 2002.

ACUTE BLOOD LOSS ANEMIA

ROBERT S. HILLMAN

CHAIM HERSHKO

The clinical manifestations of acute blood volume loss reflect adjustments in cardiac output and vascular tone that help prevent circulatory collapse and maintain oxygen supply to vital organs. The first requirement in the management of a patient with acute hemorrhage is maintaining adequate blood volume and preventing shock. This goal can be accomplished by intravenous infusion of crystalloid solutions, colloid expanders, or, when available, whole blood. When blood loss is relatively slow and the total blood volume is maintained by natural or artificial means, anemia becomes a problem. The importance of this problem depends on a number of variables, including the patient's general condition, the nature of the complicating illness, the ability of the cardiovascular system to compensate, and the flow characteristics of vital vascular pathways. A decision on blood transfusion is not based on any specific hemoglobin level but rather on a thoughtful evaluation of the anemic individual. Preexisting cardiac or pulmonary disease, advanced age, hypertension, a history of heavy smoking, or use of β-adrenergic antagonists all may indicate increased morbidity risk and justify a more liberal approach to blood transfusion. Massive hemorrhage, in association with trauma or surgery, is a special case, requiring well-coordinated volume support, red blood cell transfusion, and replacement of plasma, platelets, and coagulation factors. Once hemorrhage ceases, recovery of the red cell mass to normal usually is accomplished gradually by increased red cell production.

A hemorrhage of major proportions represents a double threat to the homeostasis of the organism. First, acute severe blood loss can decrease the blood volume to a point of cardiovascular collapse, irreversible shock, and death. In this situation, the loss of circulating red cells is of far less importance than the sudden depletion of the blood volume. Second, when blood loss is more gradual, the circulating red cell mass may be so depleted as to impair oxygen delivery to vital organs. The response to these threats involves a number of physiologic mechanisms, including adjustments in cardiovascular dynamics, blood volume, red cell production, and oxygen transport by erythrocytes.[1]

VOLUME LOSS AND REPLACEMENT

CLINICAL MANIFESTATIONS

The clinical manifestations of acute blood volume loss reflect adjustments in cardiac output and vascular tone that help prevent circulatory collapse and maintain oxygen supply to vital organs. Table 54-1 outlines how a normal person can rapidly lose up to 20 percent of the blood volume without signs or symptoms of anemia or cardiovascular collapse. If the hemorrhage exceeds 20 percent, signs of cardiovascular distress appear. At first, distress is limited to tachycardia with exercise and postural hypotension. When the blood loss exceeds 30 to 40 percent of the blood volume, a fall in cardiac output and gradual onset of shock ensue. The patient becomes immobile and exhibits air hunger; a rapid, thready pulse; and cold, clammy skin. Unless further hemor-

rhage is prevented and effective therapy is initiated, organ damage and death ensue. A very rapid blood loss that exceeds 50 percent of the patient's blood volume carries a high mortality rate unless immediate volume replacement therapy is initiated. With acute hemorrhage, the hemoglobin or hematocrit does not reflect the quantity of blood lost.

With more gradual blood loss, sufficient restoration of plasma volume can occur, permitting losses of even larger volumes of blood without the onset of shock. However, unless the physician intercedes with volume replacement therapy, plasma volume expansion is a relatively slow process. Following a sudden loss of 20 percent of the total volume, 20 to 60 hours are necessary to restore a normal blood volume by endogenous plasma replacement.[2,6,7] In humans, restoration is accomplished acutely by mobilizing albumin-containing fluid from extracellular sites.[7] For this reason, the hematocrit falls gradually over a period of 2 to 3 days after a sudden, single hemorrhage (Fig. 54-1). At the same time, normal individuals can produce enough albumin to tolerate chronic blood losses of 1000 ml or more each week.

REPLACEMENT THERAPY

The first requirement in the management of a patient with acute hemorrhage is maintaining an adequate blood volume and preventing shock. This goal can be accomplished by intravenous infusion of crystalloid (electrolyte) solutions; colloid solutions of plasma proteins, albumin, or hydroxyethyl starch; or, when available, whole blood. The choice of solution depends on the clinical setting, including factors such as the severity and rate of hemorrhage, the patient's age and cardiovascular status, and the duration of hypotension. With hemorrhagic shock of short duration, losses are primarily from the intravascular space, with little change in extracellular and intracellular fluid compartments. In this situation, infusion of a crystalloid solution can rapidly restore blood volume and circulation. With more prolonged hypotension, extracellular fluid shifts into both the intravascular and the intracellular fluid spaces. The latter reflects a failure of the active adenosine triphosphatase-dependent membrane sodium pump, with resultant increases in intracellular sodium, chloride, and water levels and an increase in extracellular potassium level.[8,9] To adequately resuscitate a patient suffering from severe hemorrhagic shock, large volumes of crystalloid and colloid solutions must be given quickly to replete both intravascular and extracellular fluid compartments and restore circulation to the point where cellular membrane transport can recover.

Based on this scenario, a crystalloid solution—isotonic saline or Ringer lactate—is the first choice in the emergency treatment of an

TABLE 54-1 REACTION TO ACUTE BLOOD LOSS OF INCREASING SEVERITY

VOLUME LOST UP TO		
TOTAL BLOOD VOLUME (%)	**ML***	**CLINICAL SIGNS**
10	500	None. Rarely seen, vasovagal syncope in blood bank donors.[1]
20	1000	Impossible to detect volume loss with patient at rest. Tachycardia is usual with exercise, and a slight postural drop in blood pressure may be evident.[2,3]
30	1500	Neck veins are flat when patient is supine. Postural hypotension and exercise tachycardia are generally present, but the resting, supine blood pressure and pulse still can be normal.
40	2000	Central venous pressure, cardiac output, and arterial blood pressure are below normal even when the patient is supine and at rest.[4,5] The patient usually demonstrates air hunger; a rapid, thready pulse; and cold, clammy skin.
50	2500	Severe shock, death.

* For a normal 70-kg person with a 5000-ml total blood volume.

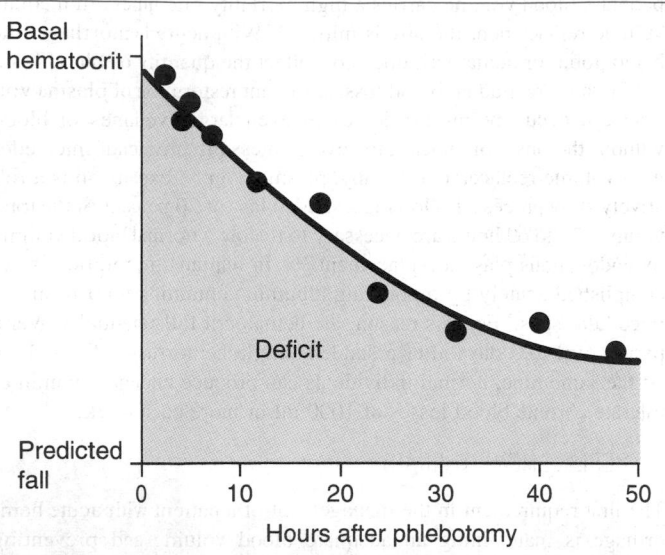

FIGURE 54-1   After a sudden loss of whole blood, the fall in hematocrit level is a gradual process that depends on the rate of mobilization of albumin from extravascular sites.[7] Full expansion of the blood volume and the lowest hematocrit value may not be appreciated for up to 72 hours.

acutely hemorrhaging patient.[10] Because crystalloid solutions are rapidly distributed between the intravascular and extravascular compartments, they must be infused at a volume two to four times the estimated blood loss. In patients with relatively normal cardiovascular status, this infusion quickly returns hemodynamic parameters toward normal, including the mean arterial pressure, cardiac output, systemic vascular resistance, and tissue oxygen consumption. Infusion of large volumes of crystalloid to elderly patients or to patients with heart disease is associated with a risk of fluid overload and pulmonary edema. However, whether colloid solutions are any better than crystalloid solutions in supporting the blood volume is debatable.[11] In pathologic states such as respiratory distress syndrome, capillary membrane integrity is altered, resulting in increased permeability of fluids with leakage of albumin into the pulmonary interstitial space. Consequently, administration of colloidal fluids in such patients may result in development of pulmonary edema.[12]

When the volume of blood lost is very large, treatment with a colloid solution such as 5 percent albumin or hydroxyethyl starch may be necessary.[13] Both 5 percent albumin in isotonic saline and a comparable product, "purified protein fraction," provide volume-for-volume expansion in hypovolemic patients. Neither product transmits hepatitis B, hepatitis C, or human immunodeficiency virus. Infusion of a 6 percent solution of hydroxyethyl starch produces a volume expansion slightly larger than the volume infused and maintains its effect as long as 24 to 36 hours. The starch polymer solution contains a spectrum of molecules with different molecular weights, the smaller of which are rapidly excreted in the urine, whereas larger molecules require molecular degradation. The half-life of hydroxyethyl starch is 17 days, and traces of the material can be detected in the circulation for many months.[14] Hydroxyethyl starch solutions are used frequently in surgery when patients undergo elective cardiac procedures and as a volume replacement fluid in pheresis therapy. Acute reactions to the starch polymer are unusual, and volumes of 2 to 3 liters of 6 percent hydroxyethyl starch can be administered with only minor impact on platelet function and coagulation. For emergency situations, hydroxyethyl starch is a reliable, readily available colloid expander and is relatively inexpensive.

Reliance on whole blood or packed red cells plus fresh-frozen plasma for emergency treatment of acute blood loss should be discouraged. Its use requires constant availability of large amounts of type O Rh-negative whole blood or type-specific blood. The requirement for typing and cross-match procedures prior to transfusion introduces an unnecessary and possibly dangerous delay in therapy. In addition, whole blood cannot always be relied upon to produce adequate volume expansion. A reaction to allergenic substances within the plasma or to the cells in whole blood can interfere with volume expansion and even produce plasma volume contraction.[15] Therefore, transfusion of whole blood or red blood cells should be reserved for specific treatment of a low red cell mass where tissue hypoxia is a potential threat.

RED CELL LOSS AND REPLACEMENT

CLINICAL MANIFESTATIONS

With precipitous hemorrhage, the immediate effects of volume depletion are more important than the loss of circulating red blood cells. Anemia becomes a problem only when blood loss is relatively slow and the total blood volume is maintained by natural or artificial means. How much of a problem depends on a number of variables, including the rate and volume of blood loss, the patient's general physical condition, the nature of the complicating illness, the ability of the cardiovascular system to compensate, and the flow characteristics of vital vascular pathways.[1] In trauma patients, mortality roughly correlates with volume of blood transfused during the first 24 hours. In a case study of patients receiving more than 20 units of blood, survival varied from 40 to 70 percent for those transfused with 20 to 40 units to 0 percent for those receiving more than 50 units, even in the absence of prolonged hypotension and preexisting disease.[16]

Although the change in hematocrit after hemorrhage occurs relatively slowly, a rapid increase in the numbers of circulating leukocytes and platelets occurs during the bleeding episode. The leukocyte count can rise to levels between 10,000 and 30,000/μl (10 and 30 $\times$ 10^9/liter) within a few hours as a result of a shift of marginated leukocytes into the circulation and a release of white cells from the marrow. The platelet count can rise to levels approaching 1,000,000/μl (1000 $\times$ 10^9/liter). In severe hemorrhage accompanied by shock and tissue hypoxia, immature elements—metamyelocytes, myelocytes, and nucleated red blood cells—may enter the circulation.

If no ready reserve of mature red cells to replace the lost red cell mass is available, oxygen supply to tissues is initially maintained by a shift in the hemoglobin oxygen dissociation curve and adjustments in cardiovascular dynamics. With sudden blood volume loss, reflex arteriolar constriction occurs in oxygen-insensitive areas such as skin and kidneys, and vascular resistance decreases in sensitive organs where oxygen delivery is essential. At the tissue level, changes in pH shift the oxygen dissociation curve to the right—the Bohr effect—and result in a greater release of oxygen. Over the next several hours and days, red cell levels of 2,3-bisphosphoglycerate increase to sustain the shift in the curve. Although this mechanism can be of importance in chronic anemias,[17] its effectiveness as a compensatory mechanism immediately after a hemorrhage remains to be defined. Plasma levels of erythropoietin also increase according to the severity of the anemia. A linear fall in the hemoglobin level is accompanied by a logarithmic rise in plasma erythropoietin.[18] This hormone is responsible for the subsequent increase in red cell production by the erythroid marrow (see Chap. 30).

Massive blood loss, especially when associated with severe tissue injury, can be complicated by a consumptive coagulopathy. This condition usually is accompanied by a diffuse bleeding tendency that cannot be controlled with local measures. Depletion of platelets and co-agulation factors can be worsened by transfusion of packed red cells and colloid or factor-poor plasma, resulting in dilutional coagulopathy. This complication must be anticipated by monitoring coagulation function and, in the case of massive transfusion, automatically replacing platelets and consumable coagulation factors such as factors V, VIII, and fibrinogen.

ERYTHROPOIETIC RESPONSE

Replacement of the red cell mass by increased red cell production is a gradual process. In response to erythropoietin stimulation, marrow progenitor cells must first proliferate and then mature over a period of 2 to 5 days prior to their delivery to the circulation as adult red cells. Therefore, a considerable time lag exists before red cell production appreciably increases the red cell mass.

Erythropoietin has a specific effect on the progenitor cells, and a rising tide of erythropoietin initiates proliferation and maturation of early erythroblasts. The response of the erythroid marrow can be recognized as early as the second day by examination of a marrow aspirate. A surge in erythropoietin also appears to cause premature delivery of marrow reticulocytes to the circulation.[19-21] The latter event can be detected within 6 to 12 hours of the onset of a hemorrhagic anemia as an increase in reticulocyte counts.[21] A full level of marrow production as estimated from the absolute reticulocyte count occurs only after 8 to 10 days, at which time the erythroid hyperplasia of the marrow and the absolute reticulocyte count are increased to the same extent.[22]

The severity of the anemia is important in determining the degree of marrow response. As long as the marrow structure is intact and iron supply to the red cell precursors is not rate limiting, the observed increase in red cell production usually reflects the severity of the anemia. However, damage to the kidneys, inflammation, or a hypometabolic state can markedly interfere with the response.[23,24] A normal individual with an intact erythropoietin mechanism increases marrow production by a factor of two to three times normal when the hematocrit falls below 30 percent. With progressively more severe anemia, plasma erythropoietin levels rise even higher, and marrow production can increase to levels three to five times normal if iron supply is sufficient.[22]

In the majority of individuals in whom marrow structure and erythropoietin response mechanisms are normal, the amount of iron available to the erythroid marrow is the prime determinant of the level of marrow production (Fig. 54-2).[22-24] With increasing anemia, the level of marrow response directly reflects the number of available iron supply pools and the rate of iron delivery from those pools.[22] For example, following a gastrointestinal hemorrhage, a normal individual can deliver sufficient iron to support a marrow production level of no greater than three times normal despite increasingly severe anemia. This response reflects the maximum rate of mobilization and delivery of storage iron from the monocyte-macrophage system. Furthermore, if these iron stores are exhausted, as is often seen with chronic blood loss, the patient cannot increase red cell production even to this level, and the proliferative response of the marrow is severely restricted. This effect on marrow production is the earliest sign of absolute iron deficiency. It antedates by weeks or months the typical microcytosis and hypochromia of long-standing iron deficiency. In contrast, when additional iron supply pools are available, as in a subject who bleeds internally and can mobilize iron from the degraded red cells, marrow production may attain levels four to five times normal. When large numbers of red cells are destroyed in the monocyte-macrophage system, as with a hemolytic anemia, the iron recovered from the degraded hemoglobin is even more rapidly returned to the erythroid marrow so as to permit

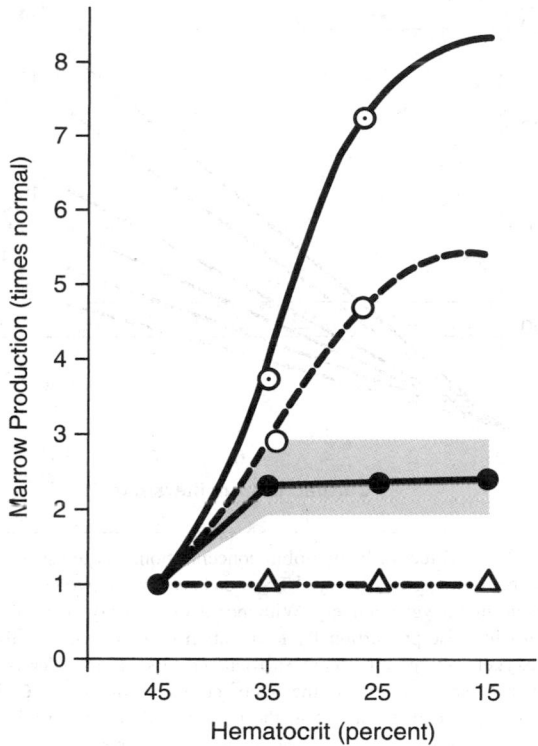

FIGURE 54-2   Rate of red blood cell production after hemorrhage reflects the severity of the anemia and the rate of iron delivery from various sources. With red cell mass depletions of 20 percent or less, marrow production increases to two to three times normal regardless of the source of iron. However, at lower hematocrit levels, production reflects the type of iron supply. A normal individual who must rely on hemosiderin stores in the monocyte-macrophage system cannot increase production further (*solid circles, shaded area*). In contrast, in patients with a hemolytic process (*circled dots*) or with more than one source of iron supply (*open circles*), production can increase to levels four to seven times normal when the hematocrit falls to 25 percent. Iron-deficient patients fail to show a marrow production increase at either hematocrit level (*triangles*).

marrow production levels exceeding five times normal. These characteristics of marrow production must be recognized in order to predict the rate of recovery of the patient's hematocrit and plan proper therapy.

THERAPY

The primary objective of red blood cell transfusions is the restoration of normal oxygen delivery to tissues.[25] However, the hemoglobin level is only one of several variables determining oxygen delivery (Fig. 54-3). The addition of oxygen to inhaled respiratory gases and an increase in cardiac output achieved by optimizing cardiopulmonary hemodynamics with fluid therapy or pharmacologic intervention can compensate for acute blood loss. These interventions and the subsequent evaluation of therapeutic response should precede the decision to transfuse blood.

HOMOLOGOUS BLOOD TRANSFUSION

The hemoglobin level at which a blood transfusion is justified is flexible. The traditional practice of transfusing blood preoperatively when hemoglobin concentration is less than 10 g/dl or hematocrit less than 30 percent can no longer be supported. An expert National Institutes of Health panel has proposed a "transfusion trigger" of less than 7.0

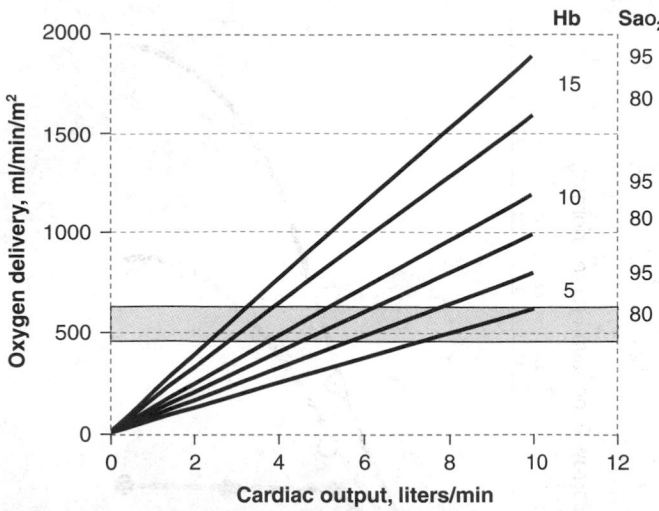

FIGURE 54-3   Effect of hemoglobin concentration, oxygen saturation, and cardiac output on oxygen delivery.[25] The area between the two *horizontal lines* represents normal oxygen delivery. With increasing severity of anemia, cardiac output must increase proportionally to maintain normal oxygen delivery. Increasing oxygen saturation (percent SaO$_2$) also offers a limited degree of compensation, but cardiac output is the major compensatory force. Conversely, failure to increase cardiac output in the presence of severe anemia leads to inadequate oxygen delivery. Hb, hemoglobin in grams per deciliter.

g/dl, with recommendations for more liberal transfusion criteria in patients at increased risk for suffering damage as a result of decreased oxygen-carrying capacity.[26] In resting healthy subjects, isovolemic reductions of blood hemoglobin concentration to 5.0 g/dl produce no evidence of inadequate oxygen delivery because of effective compensation by a shift in the hemoglobin oxygen dissociation curve, a decrease in systemic vascular resistance, and increases in heart rate and stroke volume.[27]

However, patients presenting with acute blood loss are not healthy resting subjects. Hence, a decision on blood transfusion cannot be based on any specific hemoglobin level but rather on a thoughtful evaluation of the anemic individual. Preexisting cardiac or pulmonary disease, advanced age, hypertension, a history of heavy smoking, or use of β-adrenergic antagonists all may indicate increased morbidity risk and justify a more liberal approach to blood transfusion.[28] Similarly, increased temperature, heart rate, sympathetic activity, or metabolic state may alter the balance between oxygen delivery and oxygen consumption, resulting in an increased transfusion requirement.[29]

Packed red blood cells are the preferred component for restoring oxygen-carrying capacity in patients with a normal coagulation status and a stable blood volume. Each unit contains about 200 ml of red blood cells with a hematocrit of about 70 to 80 percent. The infusion of one unit should raise the hematocrit of the average-size adult by 2 to 3 percent. Packed red cells do not provide significant amounts of coagulation factors or platelets. For massive transfusion therapy, whole blood or packed red cells with fresh-frozen plasma and platelets are preferable to packed red blood cells alone. As a rule, for every four to six units of packed red blood cells transfused, two units of fresh-frozen plasma and one unit of pheresed platelets or a pool of six units of random donor platelets should be given. When coagulation testing suggests a complicating consumptive coagulopathy, additional platelet transfusions and infusions of cryoprecipitate may be needed to support the platelet count and raise the fibrinogen level. Administration of activated recombinant factor VII has shown promise in massive trans-

fusion patients, reducing the blood requirement and improving overall survival.[30]

In emergency situations, large volumes of blood may be administered rapidly using large-bore intravenous catheters, multiple infusion sites, and infusion under pressure. The rate of infusion can be further increased by mixing red blood cells with normal saline. When transfusing large volumes of blood, careful hemodynamic monitoring and frequent hematocrit measurements are mandatory.[31] Hypothermia during massive blood transfusion can be prevented by warming the blood to 37°C using high-flow blood-warming devices. Citrate intoxication can occur when massive amounts of blood are given; it can be prevented by infusing calcium gluconate (see Chap. 131). The impact of homologous blood transfusion on survival in general and in surgical patients in particular was eloquently demonstrated by a major study of survival in 1958 surgical patients who declined blood transfusion for religious reasons.[32] The 30-day postoperative mortality was 1.3 percent in patients with a hemoglobin of 12 g/dl or greater and 33.3 percent in patients with a hemoglobin of less than 6 g/dl. The adjusted odds ratio for mortality by cardiovascular disease according to preoperative hemoglobin showed only a modest increase in patients without cardiovascular disease as hemoglobin levels decreased from 12 to 6 g/dl but increased 16-fold in patients with cardiovascular disease, defined by a history of angina, myocardial infarction, congestive heart failure, or peripheral vascular disease. This study illustrates the importance of identifying patients at risk in whom the ability to compensate for anemia by increased cardiac output is limited and in whom correction of anemia by blood transfusion may be life saving.

A patient's refusal to receive blood transfusion based on religious grounds may result in an apparent conflict between the right of a person not to accept a service and the professional values of the physician involved in the patient's management. Remember, however, that if surgical blood loss is limited to less than 500 ml, low hemoglobin levels may be well tolerated.[33] Likewise, minimizing perioperative diagnostic phlebotomies, effective use of combined iron and erythropoietin treatment to correct anemia preoperatively, and use of intraoperative blood salvage methods may limit significantly the risks of "bloodless surgery."[34] Finally, if a patient insists on avoiding transfusion after being informed of the possible consequences of such refusal, as in the case of severe anemia in a patient with cardiovascular disease, a physician is not obligated to violate his or her own professional and moral values. Arrangements can be made to transfer responsibility to another physician who is more comfortable with the patient's decision.[35,36]

MAXIMIZING RED CELL OUTPUT

Every effort should be made to evaluate the adequacy of the patient's marrow production response and institute appropriate therapy to maximize red cell output. Primarily, therapy involves an evaluation of iron supply and the use of oral or parenteral iron preparations when indicated. For example, in selected patients, such as individuals with an impaired erythropoietin response because of renal disease or chronic inflammation (the anemia of chronic disease), treatment with recombinant erythropoietin can speed recovery.[37]

Studies of the rate of hemoglobin regeneration in iron-deficient patients given either oral or parenteral iron have shown no significant advantage for either form of iron.[38,39] Marrow production studies[22,40] show a greater increase in red cell production immediately after intravenous infusions of large amounts of iron dextran than is seen with oral iron. However, this response is sustained for only 10 to 14 days. The major portion of the injected iron dextran is made available by the action of macrophages at a rate no greater than the level of iron absorbed from four oral iron tablets containing 60 mg of elemental iron each per day. Therefore, in the final analysis, a single source of iron, whether normal macrophage storage iron, oral iron, or parenteral iron injections, provides approximately the same iron supply, enough for a maximum red cell production level of three times normal. To exceed this limit, several sources of iron must be provided simultaneously. Thus, a combination of an oral iron supplement and macrophage or parenchymal iron deposits may improve iron delivery and permit marrow production to increase to levels four to five times normal.

Once hemorrhage ceases, recovery of the red cell mass to normal usually is accomplished gradually without inconvenience to the patient. Serious attempts at increasing iron supply by combination therapy should be reserved for situations where a rapid maximum response is essential, as in preparation of a patient for surgery or in the treatment of prolonged, continuous hemorrhage. Blood transfusion should be reserved for instances where normal response mechanisms and iron supplementation are insufficient to sustain an adequate red cell mass or the acuteness of the situation demands an immediate response.

REFERENCES

1. Finch CA, Lenfant G: Oxygen transport in man. *N Engl J Med* 286:407, 1972.
2. Ebert RV, Stead EA Jr, Gibson JG: Response of normal subjects to acute blood loss. *Arch Intern Med* 68:578, 1941.
3. Theyl RA, Tuohy GF: Hemodynamics and blood volume during operation with ether anesthesia and unreplaced blood loss. *Anesthesiology* 25:6, 1964.
4. Howarth S, Sharpey-Schafer EP: Low blood pressure phases following hemorrhage. *Lancet* 1:19, 1947.
5. Tovey GH, Lennon GG: Blood volume studies in accidental hemorrhage. *J Obstet Gynecol Br Commonw* 5:749, 1962.
6. Lister J, McNeill IF, Marshall VC, et al: Transcapillary refilling after hemorrhage in normal man: Basal rates and volumes; effect of norepinephrine. *Ann Surg* 158:698, 1963.
7. Adamson J, Hillman RS: Blood volume and plasma protein replacement following acute blood loss in normal man. *JAMA* 205:609, 1968.
8. Gann DS, Carlson DE, Brynes GJ: Impaired restitution of blood volume after large hemorrhage. *J Trauma* 21:598,1981.
9. Shires GT, Cunningham JN, Barker CRF: Alterations in cellular membrane function during hemorrhagic shock in primates. *Ann Surg* 176:288, 1972.
10. Maier RV, Carrico CJ: Developments in the resuscitation of critically ill surgical patients. *Adv Surg* 19:271, 1986.
11. Shine KI, Kuhn M, Young LS, Tillisch JH: Aspects of the management of shock. *Ann Intern Med* 93:723, 1980.
12. Velanovich VIC: Crystalloid vs colloid fluid resuscitation: a metaanalysis of mortality. *Surgery* 105:65, 1989.
13. Lamke LO, Liljedal SO: Plasma volume changes after infusion of various plasma expanders. *Resuscitation* 5:93,1977.
14. Thompson WL, Fukishima T, Rutherford RB, Walton RP: Intravascular persistence, tissue storage, and excretion of hydroxyethyl starch. *Surg Gynecol Obstet* 131:965, 1970.
15. Hutchison JK, Freedman JO, Richards BA, Burgen ASV: Plasma volume expansion and reactions after infusion of autologous and nonautologous plasma in man. *J Lab Clin Med* 56:734, 1960.
16. Wilson RF, Dulchavsky SA, Soullier G, Beckman B: Problems with 20 or more blood transfusions in 24 hours. *Am Surg* 53:410, 1987.

17. Torrance J, Jacobs P, Restrepo A, et al: Intraerythrocytic adaptation to anemia. *N Engl J Med* 283:165, 1970.
18. Erslev AJ: Erythropoietin. *N Engl J Med* 324:1339, 1991.
19. Hillman RS: Characteristics of marrow production and reticulocyte maturation in normal man in response to anemia. *J Clin Invest* 48:443, 1969.
20. Hillman RS, Finch CA: Erythropoiesis: Normal and abnormal. *Semin Hematol* 4:327, 1967.
21. Hillman RS, Finch CA: *Red Cell Manual*, 7th ed. FA Davis, Philadelphia, 1997.
22. Hillman RS, Henderson PA: Control of marrow production by the level of iron supply. *J Clin Invest* 48:454, 1969.
23. Hillman RS: The importance of iron supply in thalassemic erythropoiesis. *Ann N Y Acad Sci* 165:100, 1969.
24. Erslev AJ, McKenna PJ: Effect of splenectomy on red cell production. *Ann Intern Med* 67:990, 1967.
25. Greenburg AG: A physiologic basis for red blood cell transfusion decision. *Am J Surg* 170(suppl 44S):6A, 1995.
26. NIH Consensus Conference: Perioperative red blood cell transfusion. *JAMA* 260:2700, 1988.
27. Weiskopf RB, Viele MK, Feiner J, et al: Human cardiovascular and metabolic response to acute, severe isovolemic anemia. *JAMA* 279:217, 1998.
28. Carson JL: Morbidity risk assessment in the surgically anemic patient. *Am J Surg* 170:32S, 1995.
29. Strauss RG, Weiskopf RB, AuBuchon JP: Physiology and practice of red blood cell transfusions for surgical patients, in *Hematology 1998*, edited by JR McArthur, GP Schechter, SL Schrier, p 454. American Society of Hematology Education Program Book, Miami Beach, 1998.
30. Martinowitz U, Kenet G, Lubetski A et al. Possible role of recombinant activated factor VII (rFVIIa) in the control of hemorrhage associated with massive trauma. *Can J Anaesth* 49:S15, 2002.
31. Reiner AP: Massive transfusion, in *Perioperative Transfusion Medicine*, edited by BD Spiess, RB Counts, SA Gould, p 351. Williams & Wilkins, Baltimore, 1995.
32. Carson JL, Duff A, Poses RM, et al: Effect of anaemia and cardiovascular disease on surgical mortality and morbidity. *Lancet* 348:1055, 1996.
33. Spence RK, Carson JA, Poses R, et al: Elective surgery without transfusion: Influence of preoperative hemoglobin level and blood loss on mortality. *Am J Surg* 159:320, 1990.
34. Rosengart TK, Helm RE, DeBois WJ, et al: Open heart operations without transfusion using a multimodality blood conservation strategy in Jehovah's witness patients: Implications for a "bloodless" surgical technique. *J Am Coll Surg* 184:618, 1997.
35. Goldman EB: Legal considerations for allogeneic blood transfusion. *Am J Surg* 170:27S, 1995.
36. Alving BM, Spivak JL, DeLoughery TG: Consultative hematology: Hemostasis and transfusion issues in surgery and critical care medicine, in *Hematology 1998*, edited by JR McArthur, GP Schechter, SL Schrier, p 320. American Society of Hematology Education Program Book, Miami Beach, 1998.
37. Watanabe Y, Fuse K, Naruse Y, et al: Subcutaneous use of erythropoietin in heart surgery. *Ann Thorac Surg* 54:479, 1992.
38. Cope W, Gillhespy RO, Richardson RW: Treatment of iron-deficiency anemia: Comparisons of methods. *Br Med J* 2:638, 1956.
39. Bothwell TH, Charlton RW, Cook JD, Finch CA: *Iron Metabolism in Man*. Blackwell Scientific, Oxford, 1979.
40. Henderson PA, Hillman RS: Characteristics of iron dextran utilization in man. *Blood* 24:357, 1969.

C H A P T E R   5 5

HYPERSPLENISM AND HYPOSPLENISM

JAIME CARO

The spleen culls aged and abnormal cells from the blood; removes intraerythrocytic inclusions through a process called *pitting*; sequesters approximately one third of the normal intravascular platelet pool; removes bacteria, foreign particles, and tumor cells from the blood; and by virtue of the T and B lymphocytes and macrophages in the white pulp plays a role in immune surveillance and antibody formation. Exaggeration or impairment of some or all of these splenic functions results in hypersplenism or hyposplenism, respectively. Hypersplenism can be caused by splenic enlargement as a result of vascular engorgement or cellular infiltration. Infiltrative splenomegaly as seen in chronic myeloproliferative disease may cause segmental vascular insufficiency, splenic infarction, and abdominal pain. Splenomegaly resulting from vascular engorgement, such as portosplenal vein hypertension, or from infiltrative disease commonly leads to a combination of neutropenia, thrombocytopenia, and anemia. Hypersplenism also can be caused by moderate or minimal splenic enlargement as a result of exaggerated removal of physically abnormal (e.g., hereditary spherocytosis) or antibody-coated blood cells (e.g., immune thrombocytopenia). Splenectomy may be indicated if cytopenias are severe and require chronic cell replacement or lead to infection or bleeding. Splenectomy may be justified in the case of massive splenomegaly, infarction or disabling symptoms of pain, and compression of neighboring structures. In some circumstances, benefit can be achieved by partial destruction of splenic tissue by embolization using intraarterial infusion of gel microparticles. Hyposplenism can result from agenesis, atrophy, surgical removal of the spleen, or reduction of splenic function by disease. In the latter case, disturbance in splenic circulation disrupts the specific architecture required for the spleen's culling, phagocytic, and pitting functions. Hyposplenism may be suspected by alterations in red cell morphology, such as target cells or acanthocytes; red cell inclusions, such as Howell-Jolly bodies and Pappenheimer bodies (siderotic granules highlighted with polychrome stains); pitted red cells; or an elevated platelet count. The presence of pitted red cells identified by interference-contrast microscopy is perhaps the most specific blood finding of hyposplenism, followed by Howell-Jolly bodies. The most devastating consequence of hyposplenism—sudden overwhelming sepsis by encapsulated bacteria— is unexpected. Immunizations and prophylactic antibiotics can decrease the risk of sepsis. A high awareness and prompt antibiotic treatment of febrile episodes are warranted.

Acronyms and abbreviations that appear in this chapter include: Ig, immunoglobulin.

HYPERSPLENISM

HISTORY

The spleen has intrigued physicians and philosophers since ancient times.[1] The spleen has been assigned mysterious powers, but its association with destruction of blood cells was not elucidated until the turn of the twentieth century. The exaggerated and unfounded worry about somatic complaints often reflected by the sense of pain in the spleen (left hypochondrium) led to the term *hypochondriac*. In 1899, Chauffard[2] proposed that increased splenic activity causes hemolysis. This proposal provided the impetus for therapeutic splenectomy, which was performed first in 1910 by Sutherland and Burghard[3] in a patient with splenic anemia (hereditary spherocytosis) and subsequently by Kaznelson[4] in a patient with essentieller thrombopenia (immune thrombocytopenic purpura) in 1916.

DEFINITION

The designation *hypersplenism* refers to exaggeration of the spleen's normal filtration and phagocytic functions. The disorder can occur primarily by enlargement of the spleen from vascular congestion, histiophagocytic hyperplasia, cellular infiltration, or secondarily by the inability of physically abnormal red cells, such as sickle cells, or antibody-coated cells, such as in immune thrombocytopenia purpura, to navigate the circulation or avoid engulfment by the mononuclear phagocyte population of the normal spleen.[5] Hypersplenism usually is associated with the triad of splenomegaly, blood cytopenias, and compensatory marrow hyperplasia; it is characteristically corrected by splenectomy.[6]

ONTOGENY

The embryonic spleen appears in the first trimester of gestation as a multiply lobulated condensation of highly vascular mesenchyme interposed in the arterial circulation in the dorsal mesogastrium. The full scope of the molecular basis of splenic organogenesis is not known. The *Hox11 and WT1* genes are essential for its formation and defects in their expression result in hyposplenia or asplenia.[7–9]

The lymphoid compartment, the white pulp, begins its development early in the second trimester of gestation, when mature T cells, principally CD4+, form a continuous layer along the length of the vessels (periarteriolar sheaths). CD8+ cells reside in splenic cords (see Chap. 5). A specialized subset of $\gamma\delta$T cells homes to the pulp. IgD+ and IgG+ B lymphocytes form localized deposits, the primary lymph follicles. Secondary follicles arise later in life, after exposure to immunologic stimuli, and have a distinctive structure that includes a germinal center, a mantle zone, and a marginal zone containing IgM+ and IgG+.[10,11]

STRUCTURE AND FUNCTIONAL ORGANIZATION

The normal adult spleen weighs 135 ± 30 g and has a blood flow that is approximately 4 to 5 percent of the cardiac output. The spleen's principal structure is organized around an arborizing array of arterioles that branch and narrow until they terminate in either (1) the stroma of cords, forming the open circulation, or (2) the sinusoids, forming the closed circulation of the spleen (see Chap. 5). The cordal elements include histiocytes, antigen-presenting cells, pericytes, fibroblasts, and other cells necessary to maintain the discontinuous basal lamina that separates cords from lumen.[12] Lymphatic tissue is inconspicuous and found in T cell rich zones in the periarteriolar lymphoid sheaths.

The arterial vascular tree, which is lined by conventional CD31+ and CD34+ endothelial cells, branches into arterioles that terminate abruptly in caps of cordal macrophages. Blood cells must pass clusters of macrophages to enter the sinusoids.[12] The sinusoids, the origin of the venous circulation, are lined by specialized cells having combined phagocytic and endothelial activities and a distinctive CD31+, CD34−, CD68+, CD8+ phenotype. A principal function of the spleen is serving as a filter, retaining defective blood cells and foreign particles in the bed of phagocytic cells. This function is accomplished by diverting part of the splenic blood supply into the red pulp, where the blood slowly percolates through the nonendothelialized mesh studded with macrophages. The blood then reenters the circulation through narrow slits, measuring 1 to 3 μm, in the endothelium of the venous sinuses. The bulk of the blood is rapidly channeled through nonspecialized vessels that link the arterioles with the venous sinuses. This blood is not filtered or modified.[13] In many animals, such as dogs and horses, the red pulp is a reservoir for red cells, and splenic contraction provides the red cell volume with a functionally important boost.[14] In humans, however, the splenic capsule is poorly contractile, and the spleen does not store red cells to any significant degree.[15] On the other hand, a large fraction of the circulating neutrophil pool is marginated in the spleen,[16] and about one third of platelets normally are sequestered at any time.[17]

The slow transit of blood through the red pulp permits macrophages to recognize and destroy antibody- or complement-coated cells and microorganisms and to ingest poorly deformable cells or particles retained mechanically by the narrow exit slits in the venous sinuses.

PATHOPHYSIOLOGY

Filtration and elimination of defective cells occur notably in hereditary abnormalities of the red cell membranes, such as spherocytosis, elliptocytosis, or stomatocytosis, or with antibody-coated red cells, neutrophils, or platelets. In these circumstances, cytopenias of varying severity may ensue. In the case of removal of antibody-coated cells, the spleen itself produces anticell antibodies, especially antiplatelet antibodies.[18] Thus, the spleen contributes to immunizing the cells via its immune function and removing them through the Fc recognition function of the large macrophage population.

Splenomegaly increases the proportion of blood channeled through the red pulp, causing inappropriate hypersplenic sequestration of normal and abnormal blood cells.[12] Spleen enlargement may result from expansion of the red pulp compartment in any red cell sequestration process; extramedullary hematopoiesis, notably in idiopathic myelofibrosis; hyperplasia or neoplasia involving the white pulp, such as infectious mononucleosis or lymphoma, respectively; or histiophagocytic hyperplasia.

The increased size of the filtering bed is more pronounced when the splenomegaly is caused by congestion (as in portal hypertension) than when it is caused by cellular infiltration (as in leukemias, thalassemias, or amyloidosis). Nevertheless, even in space-occupying disorders such as Gaucher disease and myelofibrosis, splenomegaly may be associated with severe hypersplenic sequestration of normal cells.

Splenomegaly increases the vascular surface area and thereby the marginated neutrophil pool. Platelets are especially likely to be sequestered in an enlarged spleen, and up to 90 percent of the total number of platelets in blood may be found in massively enlarged spleens. However, sequestered white cells and platelets survive in the spleen and may be available when increased demand requires neutrophils or platelets, although their release may be slow.[19]

Red cells, on the other hand, often are destroyed prematurely in the red pulp.[20] Anemia in patients with splenomegaly has been considered the result of dilution of red cells in an expanded plasma volume.[21] However, expansion, as measured by radiolabeled albumin or fibrinogen, results more from an increase in the splenic pool of protein rather an increase in circulating plasma volume.[22]

Varying amounts of erythrophagocytosis are present, reflecting the normal culling of senescent red cells. Erythrophagocytosis increases as a result of hemolytic anemia and viral infections, and in alloimmunized transfusion recipients. Macrophages within the sinusoids contain red cell fragments. When the process is pronounced, the littoral cells become cuboidal and stand out on the basement membrane ("hobnails"). Sickle cell disease and red cell membrane disorders such as hereditary spherocytosis lead to sequestration of the poorly deformable red cells in the cords but little extrasinusoidal erythrophagocytosis, in contrast to immune hemolytic anemia where macrophage erythrophagocytosis is prominent.[12]

The increased blood flow from an enlarged spleen expands the splenic and portal veins. A significant increase in portal venous pressure may occur when hepatic vessel compliance is decreased, as in cirrhosis or myelofibrosis. This process initiates a vicious cycle in which portal hypertension contributes to splenomegaly, which in turn increases portal pressure as a result of increased arterial flow in response to organ enlargement.

Table 55-1 lists the many and varied causes of splenomegaly. Table 55-2 lists the causes of massive splenic enlargement.

CLINICAL FEATURES

Slight to moderate enlargement of the spleen usually does not produce local symptoms. Even massive splenomegaly can be well tolerated. However, not infrequently, the patient complains of a sagging feeling or other types of abdominal discomfort, early satiety from gastric encroachment, and trouble sleeping on one or the other side. Pleuriticlike pain in the left upper quadrant or referred to the left shoulder may accompany splenic infarcts, which may be recurrent.

In children with sickle cell anemia or patients with malaria, the spleen may become acutely enlarged and painful as a result of a sudden increase in red cell pooling and sequestration. These sequestration crises can follow infections and are characterized by sudden aggravation

TABLE 55-1   CLASSIFICATION AND MOST COMMON CAUSES OF SPLENOMEGALY WITH HYPERSPLENISM

SPLENOMEGALY WITH APPROPRIATE HYPERSPLENISM	SPLENOMEGALY WITH INAPPROPRIATE HYPERSPLENISM
Hereditary hemolytic anemias	Congestion (Banti syndrome)
Hereditary spherocytosis	Cirrhosis of the liver
Hereditary elliptocytosis	Portal vein thrombosis
Thalassemia	Splenic vein obstruction
Sickle cell anemia (infants)	Budd-Chiari syndrome
	Congestive heart failure
Autoimmune cytopenias	
Idiopathic thrombocytopenia	Infiltrative disease
Essential neutropenia	Leukemias, chronic and acute
Acquired hemolytic anemia	Lymphomas
	Polycythemia vera
Infections and inflammations	Agnogenic myeloid metaplasia
Infectious mononucleosis	Gaucher disease
Subacute bacterial endocarditis	Niemann-Pick disease
Miliary tuberculosis	Glycogen storage disease
Rheumatoid arthritis (Felty syndrome)	Amyloidosis
Lupus erythematosus	
Sarcoidosis	
Brucellosis	
Leishmaniasis	
Schistosomiasis	
Malaria	

TABLE 55-2 CAUSES OF MASSIVE SPLENOMEGALY*

Chronic myeloid leukemia
Gaucher disease
Hairy cell leukemia
Idiopathic and secondary myelofibrosis
Leishmaniasis (kala azar)
Lymphoma
Malaria
Thalassemia major

* The spleen may extend into one or both lower quadrants of the abdomen.

of the anemia. Splenic rupture is uncommon but can occur spontaneously with most causes of splenic enlargement or after blunt trauma. Splenic rupture in infectious mononucleosis is a classic example of such an occurrence.

The volume of an enlarged spleen is difficult to assess by palpation and percussion. Children and thin patients with low diaphragms may have a palpable spleen tip without splenomegaly.[23] Generally, a palpable spleen signifies splenomegaly and is measured by the number of centimeters the spleen extends below the left costal margin. Splenic size is most accurately measured with abdominal ultrasound or computed tomographic scans. Magnetic resonance imaging is used primarily to identify cysts, abscesses, and infarcts.[24]

A wandering spleen (splenoptosis) is an uncommon phenomenon in which the spleen hangs by a long pedicle of mesentery. The condition may present in three ways: (1) an asymptomatic mass in the pelvis, (2) intermittent abdominal pain with or without gastrointestinal symptoms, or (3) less often, an acute abdomen resulting from torsion. In the former case, the diagnosis may be made coincidentally on an imaging study.[25] The condition may be accompanied by signs of hypersplenism, hyposplenism, or neither and often is initially mistaken for a pelvic or lower abdominal tumor.

LABORATORY FEATURES

The characteristic triad of hypersplenism is (1) splenomegaly, (2) blood cytopenias, and (3) hyperplasia of the corresponding lineage in the marrow. The blood cell morphology usually is normal, although a few spherocytes may result from metabolic conditioning of red cells during repeated slow transits through the expanded red pulp. A compensatory increase in red cell production usually is evident by an increased reticulocyte count. This finding may be quantitatively less evident because the spleen preferentially sequesters reticulocytes. The presence of a compensatory increase in neutrophil or platelet production is more difficult to identify morphologically. Tests such as epinephrine mobilization have been used to distinguish sequestration from ineffective cellular production. Epinephrine releases neutrophils and platelets from the spleen, but the test may be difficult to interpret since epinephrine also releases the cells from marginal pools.[26] The pathophysiology usually can be inferred from the associated clinical findings and other tests including the marrow examination.

Pancytopenia is a common finding in patients with hepatic cirrhosis and portal hypertension.[27] However, why some patients with cirrhosis develop marked cytopenias and others do not is not clear. About one third of patients with cirrhosis develop severe hypersplenism, defined as a platelet count less than $70,000/\mu l$ (70×10^9/liter) and/or a neutrophil count less than $2000/\mu l$ (2×10^9/liter).[27,28] Decompensated liver disease and history of alcohol consumption are independent risk factors for hypersplenism. The presence of hypersplenism in patients with chronic liver disease increases the probability of variceal bleeding.

THERAPY, COURSE, AND PROGNOSIS

TOTAL SPLENECTOMY

Splenectomy is indicated as an emergency procedure after abdominal trauma and partial rupture of the spleen. It also may be indicated when splenic size or infarcts causes sustained left upper abdominal pain or discomfort. Splenectomy can be useful for treatment of functionally significant cytopenias (see Table 55-1).[29] In such circumstances, splenectomy may result in dramatic restoration of blood counts to normal levels within days to weeks after surgery. Splenectomy is not indicated when the spleen is enlarged unless significant consequences of hypersplenism are present. Ultrasound-guided fine needle biopsy of the spleen can be useful in circumstances in which the spleen holds the tissue required for diagnosis, such as splenic lymphoma. Aspiration cytology and core biopsy can be obtained with relative safety in experienced hands using image-guided fine needles.[30]

Splenectomy for hypersplenism in patients with a massive spleen size (>1500 g), especially in idiopathic myelofibrosis, is accompanied by higher morbidity and mortality than is removal of spleens for immune cytopenias.[82] Possible postoperative complications include extensive adhesions with collateral blood vessels, concomitant hemostatic disturbances, a tendency to hepatic or portal vein thrombosis, injury to the tail of the pancreas, operative site infections, and subdiaphragmatic abscesses.

Hereditary spherocytosis, immune thrombocytopenic purpura, and immune hemolytic anemia are the most common indications for splenectomy. In autoimmune neutropenias, thrombocytopenias, and hemolytic anemias, splenectomy may not only remove an inappropriate sequestration site but also may decrease autoantibody production. Hypersplenic cytopenias may aggravate and complicate the hemolytic anemia of thalassemia major. In such cases, splenectomy may improve the response to transfusion. Some children with sickle cell anemia may benefit from splenectomy if repeated sequestration crises and abdominal pains occur before autosplenectomy renders the spleen inactive.[31] Splenectomy can reduce the volume of blood flowing into the portal circulation and thus decrease the degree of portal hypertension.[32] However, intrahepatic or extrahepatic portosystemic shunts can reduce both excessive blood flow and congestive hypersplenic sequestration and thus are the preferable therapeutic options.[33,34]

In some diseases, such as Gaucher disease, the spleen serves a useful function as a sink for indigestible glycocerebrosides. In other conditions, such as idiopathic myelofibrosis or chronic lymphocytic leukemia, the spleen contributes to the cytopenias that develop because of the additive effect of sequestration in the face of inadequate hematopoiesis. Partial splenectomy has been explored because it may minimize the risks of immediate postsplenectomy thrombocytosis and overwhelming sepsis that may result from a complete absence of protective splenic filtering.[34–38]

The thrombocytopenia of liver failure largely results from a failure of thrombopoietin synthesis and secretion. Splenectomy may be of little benefit in this setting, but the cytopenia improves as a result of liver transplantation.

The response to transfusions of blood products, especially platelets, may be significantly impaired in patients with massive splenomegaly.[29]

Laparoscopic splenectomy performed by experienced surgeons for suitable hematologic conditions can result in less abdominal trauma and pain, shorter hospital stays, and smaller abdominal scars.[39,83] An advantage of open splenectomy in hematologic conditions such as the treatment of immune thrombocytopenic purpura is the increased ease of searching assiduously for accessory spleens.

PARTIAL SPLENECTOMY

Partial surgical removal of the spleen has been performed with ligation of some of the splenic arteries or the intraarterial infusion of Gelfoam particles (partial arterial embolization,).[36–38] These procedures induce large splenic infarcts and reduce the active splenic mass. Arterial embolization can be performed percutaneously or intravascularly, but the patients must be observed closely for a number of days to weeks to detect signs of intraabdominal rupture of the splenic infarcts. The long-term results have been encouraging.[40–42] Treatment with partial arterial embolization for recurrent thrombocytopenia in adults and children was safe and effective in temporarily improving the platelet count in approximately 70 percent of patients.[43]

SPLENIC RADIATION

Splenic radiation for treatment of an enlarged spleen is used sparingly. The procedure is associated with severe thrombocytopenia initially (abscopal effect). It can be used in patients with an absolute contra-indication to splenectomy who might benefit from massive splenic enlargement with its accompanying symptoms. Radiation dose must be carefully selected to suit the condition and purpose, which almost always is palliative.[44]

HYPOSPLENISM

DEFINITION

Hyposplenism is the designation for decreased splenic function resulting from diseases that impair function or from the absence of splenic tissue because of agenesis, atrophy (e.g., autoinfarction of sickle cell disease), or splenectomy. In the former case, the hypofunction may or may not be associated with a reduction in splenic size. A classic example is the infant or child with sickle cell disease in whom the vasculature of the spleen is affected by sequestered sickle cells such that blood is shunted through the organ, impairing the filtering function. In some cases, engorgement of ingested materials impairs the macrophagic-dependent functions of the spleen. Impaired filtering function may cause a mild thrombocytosis. Functional or anatomical asplenia, especially after surgical removal in infants and children, increases the risk of an overwhelming bacterial infection. The filtering and immunogenic functions of the spleen are reduced to a varying degree in a number of illnesses and are absent after splenectomy (Table 55-3).

CLINICAL FEATURES

The normal neonate and the geriatric adult may demonstrate findings suggestive of impaired splenic function.[45] These findings include the presence of Howell-Jolly bodies and erythrocyte pits (see "Laboratory Features" below). However, the clinical significance of functional hyposplenism is uncertain.[46–48]

Congenital asplenia may be found in infants with situs inversus and other developmental abnormalities.[29] Autoimmune disorders, such as glomerulonephritis,[49] systemic lupus erythematosus,[50,51] and rheumatoid arthritis,[52] are associated with laboratory evidence (Howell-Jolly bodies and erythrocyte pits, increased white cell and platelet counts) and clinical manifestations (impaired clearance of sensitized cells, overwhelming sepsis with encapsulated bacteria) of functional hyposplenism. The same is true for chronic graft-versus-host disease,[53,54] sarcoidosis,[55] alcoholic liver cirrhosis,[56,57] and hepatic amyloidosis.[58,59] Hyposplenism occurs in 30 to 50 percent of patients with celiac disease[60,61] and commonly occurs in inflammatory bowel disease.[62,63] The mechanisms for these associations are unknown.

Large anatomical lesions such as cysts or tumors may cause hyposplenism, but compensatory hypertrophy of the remaining normal tissue prevents the effect in many cases. Splenic replacement by neo-

TABLE 55-3 CONDITIONS ASSOCIATED WITH HYPOSPLENISM

Normal infants	Gastrointestinal disorders
Congenital asplenia	Celiac disease
Old age	Regional enteritis
Repeated sequestration crises	Ulcerative colitis
Sickle hemoglobinopathies	Dermatitis herpetiformis
Essential thrombocytosis	Tumors and cysts
Malaria	Amyloidosis
Thrombosis of splenic artery	Splenic irradiation
or vein	Postsplenectomy
Autoimmune disorders	
Glomerulonephritis	
Systemic lupus erythematosus	
Rheumatoid arthritis	
Graft-versus-host disease	
Sarcoidosis	

plastic cells, as in lymphomas and leukemias, usually does not cause hyposplenism, although splenic sequestration may be less than anticipated in view of the enlarged spleen. Splenic irradiation[64] and vascular obstruction[65] also may lead to functional hyposplenism; however, sickle cell anemia and surgical splenectomy are the most common causes. The hyposplenism of sickle cell anemia may be functional in infants and children with enlarged spleens and disordered circulation and may be the result of atrophy after repeated infarcts have destroyed splenic tissue in older children and adults.

Although the presence of an enlarged spleen usually suggests hypersplenism, spleen size is not a reliable index of splenic function. Complete splenic replacement by cysts, neoplastic tissues, or amyloid is an example of hyposplenic splenomegaly.[66] In addition, acute sequestration crises, which occur occasionally in patients with malaria[67] and often in infants and children with sickle hemoglobinopathies,[68] may clog the red cell pulp with cellular debris. The result is hypersplenic sequestration that may be followed by transient or permanent hyposplenism (see Chap. 47).

CLINICAL FEATURES

OVERWHELMING SEPSIS

If the spleen is totally destroyed or removed, serious infections may ensue. Because the spleen is a major component of the mononuclear phagocyte system and has substantial lymphatic tissue in the white pulp, hyposplenism or splenectomy can reduce antibody synthesis at least temporarily. This condition rarely causes a problem and actually may be beneficial in autoimmune disorders in which the spleen in part synthesizes pathologic autoantibodies. However, removal of an efficient filtering bed in which opsonized organisms are exposed to macrophages may lead to overwhelming sepsis. The responsible organism usually is an encapsulated bacterium, such as pneumococcus, meningococcus, or *Haemophilus influenzae*. Unrestrained *in vivo* proliferation of such microorganisms may cause fatal septicemia.[69–71] The risk is greatest among infants whose general immunologic tolerance has not matured enough to counteract bacterial infections, although the risk is present, albeit at reduced rates, regardless of the patient's age at removal. For this reason, splenectomy in children should be deferred until after age 5 years if possible. The risk is different depending on the reason for the splenectomy. In a child with an underlying immune disorder, such as Wiskott-Aldrich syndrome, the risk is very high. The risk is higher in children with thalassemia than in those with hereditary spherocytosis and lowest in those with splenectomy for splenic trauma. The risk is reduced by the use of pneumococcal and *H. influenzae* vaccines prior to splenectomy and prophylactic penicillin therapy.[72]

LABORATORY FEATURES

The reduction or absence of normal splenic function is accompanied by a slight to moderate increase in white cell and platelet counts. Howell-Jolly bodies, target cells, stippled red cells (Pappenheimer bodies), and occasional acanthocytes often are present in the blood film. The finding of pitted erythrocytes in wet preparations is of the greatest diagnostic specificity of all the blood findings.[73] Target cell formation reflects an increased red cell surface area causing buckling.[74] Target cells almost always are present in the asplenic state, but only one of 100 to 1000 red cells is affected. A sensitive indication of hyposplenism is the appearance of pits or pocks on the cell surface.[75] These pits consist of submembranous vacuoles and can be seen only in wet preparations of red cells using direct interference-contrast microscopy. Intracellular vesiculation containing hemoglobin is a normal occurrence during aging of the red cell in the circulation. This process is intensified in the last half of the erythrocyte life span and leads to a decreased mean cell hemoglobin level as the vesicles are removed (pitted) by the spleen. In asplenic individuals the vesicles are more numerous and enlarge, forming vacuoles that are evident by interference-phase microscopy.[76] This finding is the most specific evidence of hyposplenism, followed by the presence of DNA inclusions in circulating red cells (Howell-Jolly bodies).

Oxidative drugs may produce Heinz bodies even in normal individuals, but the spleen effectively removes these red cell inclusions. Heinz bodies may be observed in supravitally stained blood films after splenectomy. Nucleated red cells rarely are seen on blood films after splenectomy, except in patients with hemolytic disorders in whom the number of nucleated red cells may increase dramatically. The reticulocyte count remains within normal values, and the life span of red cells is unchanged as other organs take up the function of removing senescent erythrocytes.

Technetium-99m sulfur colloid particles are used for spleen scanning, a reliable measure of the capacity of the spleen to clear particulate matter from the bloodstream.[77]

THERAPY, COURSE, AND PROGNOSIS

Prophylactic immunization with polyvalent pneumococcal, *H. influenzae*, and meningococcal vaccines have significantly reduced, but not eliminated, the risk of overwhelming infection.[72,78-80] Vaccinations should be given to all patients with hyposplenism and to all patients before surgical splenectomy.[81] No current recommendation exists for revaccination with *H. influenzae* or meningococcal vaccine. Pneumococcal vaccine probably should be readministered every 5 years in children. Older patients may have exaggerated local reactions to revaccination, and the recommendations are indefinite. The vaccine against *H. influenzae* is not a requirement in adults. Pediatricians recommend oral penicillin as prophylaxis for every asplenic child or adult. Physicians should advise all asplenic patients that no febrile episode (>100°C) should be considered trivial. A physician or medical facility should be contacted immediately and blood cultures drawn, followed by daily antibiotics, until the culture results are known. Some physicians instruct hyposplenic patients to take amoxicillin or a comparable agent upon the onset of symptoms prior to a medical evaluation, which should be done as soon as possible. The decision should consider duration of symptoms, travel distance, and similar factors. Dental work, especially tooth extraction, should be preceded by broad-spectrum antibiotics, such as amoxicillin, if the patient is not taking prophylactic penicillin.

REFERENCES

1. Crosby WH: The spleen, in *Blood, Pure and Eloquent*, edited by MM Wintrobe, p 96. McGraw-Hill, New York, 1980.

2. Chauffard AME: Des hepatites d'origine splenique. *Semin Med* 19:177, 1899.

3. Sutherland GA, Burghard FF: The treatment of splenic anaemia by splenectomy. *Lancet* 2:1819, 1910.

4. Kaznelson P: Verschwinden der hamorrhagischen Diathesis bei einen falle von "Essentieller Thrombopenia." *Wien Klin Wochesnchr* 29:1451, 1916.

5. Crosby WH: Hypersplenism. *Annu Rev Med* 13:127, 1962.

6. Dameshek W: Hypersplenism. *Bull N Y Acad Sci* 31:113;1955.

7. Roberts CW, Shutter JR, Korsmeyer SJ: Hox11 controls the genesis of the spleen. *Nature* 368:747, 1994.

8. Dear TN, Colledge WH, Carlton MB, et al: The Hox11 gene is essential for cell survival during spleen development. *Development* 121:2909, 1995.

9. Roberts CW, Sonder AM, Lumsden A, et al: Developmental expression of HOV11 and specification of splenic cell fate. *Am J Pathol* 146:1089, 1995.

10. Steininger B, Barth P, Herbst B, et al: The species-specific structure of microanatomical compartments in the human spleen. *Immunology* 92:307, 1997.

11. Bourdessoule D, Gaulard P, Mason DY: Preferential localization of human lymphocytes bearing γ/δ T cell receptors to the red pulp of the spleen. *J Clin Pathol* 43:461, 1990.

12. Kraus MD: Splenic histology and histopathology: An update. *Semin Diagn Pathol* 20:84, 2003.

13. Rosse WF: The spleen as a filter [editorial]. *N Engl J Med* 317:704, 1987.

14. Areas Elenas N, Ewald R, Crosby WH: The reservoir function of the spleen and its relation to postsplenectomy anemia of the dog. *Blood* 24:299, 1964.

15. Wadenvik H, Kutti J: The spleen and pooling of blood cells. *Eur J Haematol* 41:1, 1988.

16. Aster RH: Pooling of platelets in the spleen: Role in the pathogenesis of "hypersplenic thrombocytopenia." *J Clin Invest* 45:645, 1966.

17. Bowdler AJ: Splenomegaly and hypersplenism. *Clin Haematol* 12:467, 1983.

18. Karpatkin S: The spleen and thrombocytopenia. *Clin Haematol* 12:591, 1983.

19. Brubaker LH, Johnson CA: Correlation of splenomegaly and abnormal neutrophil pooling (margination). *J Lab Clin Med* 92:508, 1978.

20. Christensen BE: Quantitative determination of splenic red cell blood destruction in patients with splenomegaly. *Scand J Haematol* 14:295, 1975.

21. Hess CE, Ayers CR, Sandusky WR, et al: Mechanism of dilutional anemia in massive splenomegaly. *Blood* 47:629, 1976.

22. Zhang B, Lewis SM: Splenic hematocrit and the splenic plasma pool. *Br J Haematol* 66:97, 1987.

23. McIntyre OR, Ebaugh FA: Palpable spleens in college freshmen. *Ann Intern Med* 66:301, 1967.

24. Sty JR, Wells RG: Imaging the spleen, in *Disorders of the Spleen: Pathophysiology and Management*, edited by C Pochedly, RH Sills, AD Schwartz, p 355. Marcel Dekker, New York, 1989.

25. Buehner M, Baker MS: The wandering spleen. *Surg Gynecol Obstet* 175:373, 1992.

26. Joyce RA, Boggs DR, Hasiba U, Srodes CH: Marginal neutrophil in the pool size in normal subjects as measured by epinephrine infusion. *J Lab Clin Med* 88:614, 1976.

27. Peck-Radosavljevic M: Hypersplenism. *Eur J Gastroenterol Hepatol* 13:317, 2001.

28. Liangpunsakul S, Ulmer BJ, Chalasani N: Predictors and implications of severe hypersplenism in patients with cirrhosis. *Am J Med Sci* 326:111, 2003.

29. Pochedly C, Sills RH, Schwartz A: *Disorders of the Spleen: Pathophysiology and Management*. Marcel Dekker, New York, 1989.

30. Civardi G, Vallisa D, Bertè R, et al: Ultrasound guided fine needle biopsy of the spleen: High clinical efficacy and low risk in a multicenter Italian study. *Am J Hematol* 67:93, 2001.

31. Al-Salem AH, Qaisaruddin S, Nasserallah Z, et al: Splenectomy in patients with sickle-cell disease. *Am J Surg* 172:254, 1996.

32. Shah SH, Hayes PC, Allan PL, et al: Measurement of spleen size and its relation to hypersplenism and portal hemodynamics in portal hypertension due to hepatic cirrhosis. *Am J Gastroenterol* 91:2580, 1996.

33. Liu QD, Ma KS, He ZP, et al: Experimental study on the feasibility and safety of radiofrequency ablation for secondary splenomegaly and hypersplenism. *World J Gastroenterol* 9:813, 2003.

34. Alvarez OA, Lopera GA, Patel V, et al: Improvement of thrombocytopenia due to hypersplenism after transjugular intrahepatic portosystemic shunt placement in cirrhotic patients. *Am J Gastroenterol* 91:134, 1996.

35. Sanyal AJ, Freedman AM, Purdum PP, et al: The hematologic consequences of transjugular intrahepatic portosystemic shunts. *Hepatology* 23:32, 1996.

36. Jalan R, Redhead DN, Simpson KJ, et al: Transjugular intrahepatic portosystemic stent-shunt (TIPSS): Long term follow-up. *Q J Med* 87:565, 1994.

37. Banani SA: Partial dearterialization of the spleen in thalassemia major. *J Pediatr Surg* 33:449, 1998.

38. Bar-Moor JA: Partial splenectomy in Gaucher's disease. *J Pediatr Surg* 28:686, 1993.

39. Caprotti R, Porta G, Franciosi C, et al: Laparoscopic splenectomy for hematological disorders. *Int Surg* 83:303, 1998.

40. Stanley P, Shen TC: Partial embolization of the spleen in patients with thalassemia. *J Vasc Interv Radiol* 6:137, 1995.

41. Palsson B, Hallen M, Forsberg AM, Alwmark A: Partial splenic embolization: Long-term outcome. *Langenbecks Arch Surg* 387:421, 2003.

42. Petersons A, Volrats O, Bernsteins A: The first experience with nonoperative treatment of hypersplenism in children with portal hypertension. *Eur J Pediatr Surg* 12:299, 2002.

43. Watanabe Y, Todani T, Noda T: Changes in splenic volume after partial splenic embolization in children. *J Pediatr Surg* 31:241, 1996.

44. Paulino AC, Reddy AC: Splenic irradiation in the palliation of patients with lymphoproliferative and myeloproliferative disorders. *Am J Hosp Palliat Care* 13:32, 1996.

45. Freedman RM, Johnston D, Mahoney MJ, et al: Development of splenic reticuloendothelial function in neonates. *J Pediatr* 96:466, 1980.

46. Padmanabhan J, Risemberg HM, Rome RD: Howell-Jolly bodies in the peripheral blood of full-term and premature neonates. *Johns Hopkins Med J* 132:146, 1973.

47. Markus HS, Toghill PJ: Impaired splenic function in elderly people. *Age Ageing* 20:287, 1991.

48. Ravaglia G, Forti P, Biagi F, et al: Splenic function in old age. *Gerontology* 44:91, 1998.

49. Lawrence SE, Pussell BA, Charlesworth JA: Splenic function in primary glomerulonephritis. *Adv Exp Med Biol* 641:1, 1982.

50. Webster J, Williams BD, Smith AP, et al: Systemic lupus erythematosus presenting as pneumococcal septicemia and septic arthritis. *Ann Rheum Dis* 49:181, 1990.

51. Liote F, Angle J, Gilmore N, Osterland CK: Asplenism and systemic lupus erythematosus. *Clin Rheumatol* 14:220, 1995.

52. Jarolim DR: Asplenia and rheumatoid arthritis [letter]. *Ann Intern Med* 97:61, 1982.

53. Kalhs P, Panzer S, Kletter K, et al: Functional asplenia after bone marrow transplantation. *Ann Intern Med* 109:461, 1988.

54. Cuthbert RJ, Iqbal A, Gates A, et al: Functional hyposplenism following allogeneic bone marrow transplantation. *J Clin Pathol* 48:257, 1995.

55. Stone RW, McDaniel WR, Armstrong EM, et al: Acquired functional asplenia in sarcoidosis. *J Natl Med Assoc* 77:930, 1985.

56. Muller AF, Toghill PJ: Splenic function in alcoholic liver disease. *Gut* 33:1386, 1992.

57. Muller AF, Toghill PJ: Functional hyposplenism in alcoholic liver disease: A toxic effect of alcohol? *Gut* 35:679, 1994.

58. Gertz MA, Kyle RA: Hepatic amyloidosis (primary [AL], immunoglobulin light chain): The natural history in 80 patients. *Am J Med* 85:73, 1988.

59. Powsner RA, Simms RW, Chudnovsky A, et al: Scintigraphic functional hyposplenism in amyloidosis. *J Nucl Med* 39:221, 1998.

60. Robinson PJ, Bullen AW, Hall R, et al: Splenic size and functions in adult coeliac disease. *Br J Radiol* 53:532, 1980.

61. O'Grady JG, Stevens FM, Harding B, et al: Hyposplenism and gluten-sensitive enteropathy. *Gastroenterology* 87:1316, 1984.

62. Palmer KR, Sherriff SB, Holdsworth CD, et al: Further experience of hyposplenism in inflammatory bowel disease. *Q J Med* 50:461, 1981.

63. Muller AF, Toghill PJ: Hyposplenism in gastrointestinal disease. *Gut* 36:165, 1995.

64. Dailey MO, Coleman CN, Kaplan HS: Radiation-induced splenic atrophy in patients with Hodgkin disease and non-Hodgkin lymphoma. *N Engl J Med* 302:215, 1990.

65. Spencer RP, Sziklas JJ, Turner JW: Functional obstruction of splenic blood vessel in adults: A radiocolloid study. *Int J Nucl Med Biol* 9:208, 1982.

66. Steinberg MH, Gatling RR, Tavassoli M: Evidence of hyposplenism in the presence of splenomegaly. *Scand J Haematol* 31:437, 1983.

67. Looareesuwan S, Ho M, Wallanagoon Y, et al: Dynamic alteration in splenic function during acute falciparum malaria. *N Engl J Med* 317:675, 1987.

68. Emond AM, Callis R, Darvill D, et al: Acute splenic sequestration in homozygous sickle cell disease: Natural history and management. *J Pediatr* 107:201, 1985.

69. Torres J, Bisno AL: Hyposplenism and pneumococcemia. *Am J Med* 55:851, 1973.

70. Cavenagh JD, Joseph AE, Dilly S, Bevan DH: Splenic sepsis in sickle cell disease. *Br J Haematol* 86:187, 1994.

71. Gopal V, Bisno AL: Fulminant pneumococcal infections in "normal" asplenic hosts. *Arch Intern Med* 137:1526, 1977.

72. Konradsen HB, Henrichsen J: Pneumococcal infections in splenectomized children are preventable. *Acta Paediatr Scand* 80:423, 1991.

73. Corazza GR, Ginaldi L, Zoli G, et al: Howell-Jolly body counting as a measure of splenic function: A reassessment. *Clin Lab Haematol* 12:269, 1990.

74. Holroyde CP, Oski FA, Gardner FH: The "pocked" erythrocytes. *N Engl J Med* 281:516, 1969.

75. Reinhart WH, Chien S: Red cell vacuoles: Their size and distribution under normal conditions and after splenectomy. *Am J Hematol* 27:265, 1988.

76. Willekens FLA, Roerdinkholder-Stoelwinder B, Groen-Döpp YAM: Hemoglobin loss from erythrocytes in vivo result from spleen-facilitated vesiculation. *Blood* 101:747, 2003.

77. Rutland MD: Correlation of splenic function with the splenic uptake rate of Tc-colloids. *Nucl Med Commun* 13:843, 1992.

78. Ward KM, Celebi JT, Gmyrek R, Grossman ME: Acute infectious purpura fulminans associated with asplenism or hyposplenism. *J Am Acad Dermatol* 47:493, 2002.

79. Sumaraju V, Smith LG, Smith SM: Infectious complications in asplenic hosts. *Infect Dis Clin North Am* 15:551, 2001.

80. Castagnola E, Fioredda F: Prevention of life-threatening infections due to encapsulated bacteria in children with hyposplenia or asplenia: A brief review of current recommendations for practical purposes. *Eur J Haematol* 71:319, 2003.

81. Kobel DE, Friedl A, Cerny T, et al: Pneumococcal vaccine in patients with absent or dysfunctional spleen. *Mayo Clin Proc* 75:749, 2000.

82. Mohren M, Markman I, Dworschak U, et al: Thromboembolic complications after splenectomy for hematologic diseases. *Am J Hematol* 76:143, 2004.

83. Delaitre B, Champault G, Barrat C, et al: Laparoscopic splenectomy for hematologic diseases. Study of 275 cases. *Ann Chir* 125:522, 2000.

PRIMARY AND SECONDARY POLYCYTHEMIAS (ERYTHROCYTOSIS)

JOSEF T. PRCHAL

ERNEST BEUTLER

Polycythemia is characterized by an increased red cell volume. Primary polycythemias are caused by acquired or inherited mutations causing changes within hematopoietic stem cells or erythroid progenitors leading to an accumulation of red cells. The most common primary polycythemia is polycythemia rubra vera, a clonal neoplastic disorder. In contrast, secondary polycythemias result from either appropriate or inappropriate increases in the red cell mass because of augmented levels of erythropoiesis-promoting substances such as erythropoietin, insulin growth factor 1, and cobalt. These polycythemias can also be either acquired (right to left cardiac shunt) or hereditary (e.g., high O_2 affinity hemoglobin). Although primary and secondary polycythemias are different disorders, they are discussed together because their clinical presentations may be quite similar, but distinguishing among them is important for proper management. Determining the molecular basis of polycythemic states aids accurate diagnoses and therapy.

Polycythemia vera is characterized by increases not only of the numbers of red cells but also of granulocytes and platelets and by splenomegaly. These findings are not usually present in secondary polycythemia. Control of hematocrit, but not other features of both types of polycythemia, can be achieved by phlebotomy. Myelosuppressive therapy is usually prescribed only in polycythemia vera, where drugs such as hydroxyurea, busulfan, chlorambucil, and interferon may be useful not only in controlling the hemoglobin levels of blood but also markedly elevated platelet count. Anagrelide may also be used for the latter problem.

Enalapril will control postrenal transplant erythrocytosis.

DEFINITION AND HISTORY

The term *polycythemia*, denoting an increased amount of blood, has traditionally been applied to those conditions in which the mass of erythrocytes is increased. *Erythrocytosis* is an alternative term that has been applied to an increase in red cell mass not accompanied by an increase in neutrophils and platelets, the latter characteristic of polycythemia vera. Although this usage has much to recommend it, no

consensus about terminology has been reached and the term polycythemia is used interchangeably with erythrocytosis by many physicians as an alternative term. In some instances, however, time-honored terms such as *postrenal transplant erythrocytosis* will be used. Table 32-2 presents a classification of the polycythemias.

Polycythemia vera, the sole clonal form of primary polycythemia, a prototype of the primary polycythemias, was first described in 1892 by Vaquez.[1] In 1903 Osler[2] reviewed four cases of his own and an additional five from the literature. He wrote, "The condition is characterized by chronic cyanosis, polycythemia, and moderate enlargement of the spleen. The chief symptoms have been weakness, prostration, constipation, headache, and vertigo."[2] The increased proliferation of granulocyte precursors and megakaryocytes was first described by Türk[3] in 1904. *Primary familial and congenital polycythemia (PFCP)*, also known as *autosomal dominant erythrocytosis* or *benign familial erythrocytosis*, is also a primary polycythemic disorder in that the defect is intrinsic to erythropoiesis.[4–6]

Secondary polycythemia, more appropriately *secondary erythrocytosis*, refers to those conditions in which only the erythrocyte mass is increased as a result of increased erythropoietin production. Although the term *secondary erythrocytosis* is more descriptive of this group of disorders, secondary polycythemia is a time-honored name and will be used interchangeably with secondary erythrocytosis.

Secondary polycythemia is a term that describes a group of disorders characterized by an increased red cell mass brought about by enhanced stimulation of red cell production by a physiologic mediator such as erythropoietin. Secondary polycythemia can be subdivided into *appropriate polycythemia*, in which erythropoiesis is responding normally to hypoxia, and *inappropriate polycythemia*, in which erythropoiesis is being stimulated by the aberrant production of or response to erythropoietin.

In his important monograph on barometric pressure published in 1878, Paul Bert[7] showed that the physiologic impairment observed at high altitude resulted from a reduction in the oxygen content of air. A few years earlier his friend and mentor Dennis Jourdanet[8] had observed an increase in the number of red corpuscles in the blood of the highlanders of Mexico, and Bert recognized that such an increase would tend to ameliorate the effect of atmospheric hypoxia. However, neither Bert nor Jourdanet suspected a cause–effect relationship. It was not until 1890, when Viault[9] observed a prompt increase in the number of his own red corpuscles after having traveled from Lima, Peru at sea level, to Morococha at 4570 m (15,000 ft) above sea level, that altitude erythrocytosis was accepted as a compensatory adaptation to hypoxia.[10] At approximately the same time, it was observed that many patients with cyanosis were also polycythemic. Both the *cardiacos negros*[11] with severe pulmonary failure and arterial oxygen desaturation and the children with *morbus caeruleus*, or right-to-left shunt through a congenital cardiac malformation, were found to have increased red cell counts.[12] Mechanical or neurogenic hypoventilation as a cause of cyanosis and polycythemia was first popularized in 1956 with the classic description of the Pickwickian syndrome by Burwell and colleagues.[13,14] Polycythemia associated with carboxyhemoglobinuria resulting from hypoxemia caused by smoking and with tissue hypoxia because of inherited abnormal hemoglobins with high oxygen affinity was recognized more recently. The erythrocytosis associated with abnormal hemoglobins with an increased affinity to oxygen also represents an appropriate response to hypoxia first noted by Charache and colleagues[15] in 1966 when they described hemoglobin Chesapeake.

Inappropriate polycythemia may be acquired as a result of aberrant erythropoietin production by the kidney, by certain tumors, and by ingestion of cobalt. Alternatively, it may be hereditary. *Familial secondary polycythemias* constitute a heterogeneous group of autosomal dominant or recessive diseases. *Chuvash polycythemia* is a special type of familial polycythemia having features of both primary and secondary polycythemia.

In addition to appropriate and inappropriate secondary polycythemia, there are some patients with mild erythrocytosis in whom neither the cause nor the clinical significance is clear. These patients do not have an increased red cell mass, and their erythrocytosis is the result of decreased plasma volume. Therefore, the disorder is not a true polycythemia and is designated *apparent, spurious,* or *relative polycythemia.* In 1905, Gaisbock reported that a number of hypertensive patients had plethora and an elevated red cell count but no splenomegaly, a condition he termed *polycythemia hypertonica* and that was sometimes called *Gaisbock syndrome.*[16] In 1952 direct measurement of the blood volume in patients with polycythemia led Lawrence and Berlin[17] to identify a subgroup of patients with a normal red cell volume but a reduced plasma volume. Although some members of this group were hypertensive, the authors were more impressed by their tense and anxious behavior and coined the term *stress polycythemia.*

EPIDEMIOLOGY

PRIMARY POLYCYTHEMIAS

POLYCYTHEMIA VERA
Mayo clinic data indicate that 2.8 per 100,000 men and 1.3 per 100,000 women have polycythemia vera,[18] estimates that are similar to those from epidemiologic data in Sweden.[19] Although most patients with polycythemia vera do not have a family history, familial incidence of the disorder occurs.[20] This inherited predisposition must interact with acquired somatic mutation(s) for disease onset.[21,22]

PRIMARY FAMILIAL AND CONGENITAL POLYCYTHEMIA
The disorder that has been designated PFCP is uncommon and is inherited as autosomal dominant disorder.

SECONDARY POLYCYTHEMIAS

INAPPROPRIATE TISSUE ELABORATION OF ERYTHROPOIETIN
The prevalence of the various types of secondary polycythemia is a function of the underlying cause, such as the geographical location of the patient or the presence of a causative neoplasm. Approximately 1 to 3 percent of all patients with hypernephromas have erythrocytosis.[24] Although uterine leiomyomas in premenopausal women are common, having been estimated at 20 to 40 percent, the occurrence of erythrocytosis ranges from 0.02 to 0.5 percent.[25] Isolated instances of polycythemia have been attributed to a myxoma of the atrium,[26] hamartoma of the liver,[27] and focal hyperplasia of the liver.[28] Erythrocytosis and inappropriate secretions of erythropoietin may be found in approximately 15 percent of patients with cerebellar hemangiomas.[29,30]

POSTRENAL TRANSPLANT ERYTHROCYTOSIS
This syndrome, defined as a persistent elevation of the hematocrit over 51 percent, is a relatively common condition found in approximately 5 to 10 percent of renal allograft recipients.[31,32] Postrenal transplant erythrocytosis usually develops within 8 to 24 months after successful transplantation and resolves spontaneously within 2 years in approximately 25 percent of patients, despite good function of the allograft.[33] Factors that increase the likelihood of its development are lack of erythropoietin therapy prior to transplantation, a history of smoking, diabetes mellitus, renal artery stenosis, low serum ferritin levels, and normal or higher pretransplant erythropoietin levels. Postrenal trans-

plant erythrocytosis is also more frequent in patients who are not undergoing graft rejection. Postrenal transplant erythrocytosis is more common in males and may recur in the same patient after a successful second transplantation.[34]

CHUVASH POLYCYTHEMIA
A Russian hematologist, Lydia A. Polyakova, described polycythemia in the Chuvash population (an ethnic isolate of Asian descent in the mid-Volga River region of Russia) in the early 1960s,[35] and by 1974, 103 cases from 81 families had been described.[35] Since then, more cases have come to light. Hundreds of children and adults suffer from this condition, indicating that Chuvash polycythemia is the most common congenital polycythemia in the world.

ETIOLOGY AND PATHOGENESIS

PRIMARY POLYCYTHEMIAS

POLYCYTHEMIA VERA
Polycythemia vera arises from the transformation of a single hematopoietic stem cell into a cell with a selective growth advantage that gradually becomes the predominant myeloid progenitor. The clonal origin of polycythemia vera has been demonstrated in women heterozygous for the polymorphic X chromosome marker glucose-6-phosphate dehydrogenase (see Chap. 9).[36] In each case, all hematopoietic cell lineages express either the enzyme encoded by the maternal or paternal X chromosome, whereas nonhematopoietic cells are a mosaic of both enzyme types.

Marrow-derived colonies contain burst forming unit–erythroid (BFU-E) with normal erythropoietin sensitivity along with colonies that grow in the absence of erythropoietin.[37,38] However, most of the progenitors with normal erythropoietin sensitivity are also part of the polycythemia vera clone.[37,38] Other abnormalities that have been described include (1) decreased levels of the platelet thrombopoietin receptor,[39] (2) deregulation of Bcl-x, an inhibitor of apoptosis,[40] (3) increased expression of protein tyrosine phosphatase activity by red cell precursors,[41] (4) increased mRNA levels of the polycythemia rubra vera *(PRV)-1* gene in granulocytes,[42] and (5) acquired loss of heterozygosity of chromosome 9p because of uniparenteral disomy.[22] The fibroblasts that accumulate in the marrow of patients with polycythemia vera as the disease progresses are not a part of the abnormal clone. Rather, they seem to be a response to the proliferating marrow cells, perhaps to the platelet-derived fibroblast growth factor (and other mediators) elaborated by megakaryocytes (see Chap. 89).[43]

In late 2004, William Vainchenker's group in France made an important discovery of a somatic mutation in a gene on chromosome 9p in the majority of polycythemia vera patients.[303,304] This gene encodes for tyrosine kinase—*JAK*, which is normally activated by erythropoietin activation of the erythropoietin receptor (see Chap. 32). This single nucleotide change of the *JAK2 gene* transforms this kinase into a constitutively active form that in reporter transfected cells has been shown to emulate the *in vitro* behavior of native polycythemia vera progenitors. About 30% of polycythemia vera patients have both *JAK2 alleles* mutated by previously described loss of heterozygosity created by uniparenteral disomy.[22] This important milestone in understanding the molecular basis of polycythemia vera was subsequently confirmed by several other groups in 2005.[305-307] The same mutation has also been found in a smaller fraction of patients with essential thrombocythemia and agnogenic myeloid metaplasia (see Chaps. 89 and 111); it is not clear whether these patients have variants of polycythemia vera, or early or late stages of polycythemia vera, respectively.

Fewer than 25 percent of patients have karyotypic abnormalities at diagnosis,[44-48] but the incidence rises with increasing duration of the disease.[45,49] Most patients have a normal karyotype at the time of diagnosis; gross genetic rearrangements do not seem to be the cause of the disease but are secondary changes.[50] Genetic factors may influence susceptibility to polycythemia vera.[22]

PRIMARY FAMILIAL AND CONGENITAL POLYCYTHEMIA

In contrast to polycythemia vera, PFCP results from germline rather than somatic mutations. It is congenital and manifests autosomal dominant inheritance.[5] Like polycythemia vera it is primary in that the defect is in the erythroid progenitor, and erythropoietin levels are low.

To date, 12 mutations of the erythropoietin receptor *(EPOR)* associated with PFCP have been described (Table 56-1). Nine of the 12 result in truncation of the EPOR cytoplasmic carboxyl terminal and are the only mutations convincingly linked with PFCP. Such truncations lead to a loss in the negative regulatory domain of the *EPOR* (see Chaps. 30 and 32). Three missense *EPOR* mutations have also been described, but these have not been linked to PFCP or any other disease phenotype (Table 56-1). In most PFCP families, mutations of gene(s) other than *EPOR* are responsible for the disease phenotype; the identities of these genes are not known.[51,52]

Erythropoietin-mediated activation of erythropoiesis involves several steps (see Chap. 30). First, erythropoietin activates its receptor by inducing conformational changes of its dimers. These changes lead to initiation of an erythroid-specific cascade of events. The first signal is initiated by binding of a tyrosine kinase to the EpoR and its phosphorylation and activation of the transcription factor STAT5, which regulates erythroid-specific genes. This "on" signal is negated by dephosphorylation of EpoR by the hematopoietic phosphatase HCP, that is, the "off" signal. EpoR truncations lead to loss of the negative regulatory domain of the EpoR, a binding site for hematopoietic cell phosphatase HCP, leading to a gain-of-function mutation of *EPOR* (Fig. 56-1).

SECONDARY POLYCYTHEMIAS

The morbidity that attends marked erythrocytosis presumably is related to the increase in blood viscosity.[53] However, the effect of blood viscosity on oxygen delivery often is oversimplified, and the emphasis on the hematocrit alone may lead to inappropriate therapeutic interventions. In the normovolemic state, the blood viscosity increases very rapidly as hematocrit levels rise above 50 percent. Absolute polycythemia is not a normovolemic state, however; it is accompanied by an increase in blood volume, which, in turn, enlarges the vascular bed and decreases the peripheral resistance (see Chap. 32). Thus hypervolemia can increase oxygen transport, and the optimum for oxygen transport occurs at higher hematocrit values than in normovolemic states. Consequently, despite the attendant increase in viscosity, an increase in hematocrit may be of benefit in some polycythemias. However, at some point the high viscosity causes an increase in the work of the heart and a reduction in blood flow to most tissues and may be responsible for cerebral and cardiovascular impairment.

APPROPRIATE POLYCYTHEMIAS

High-Altitude Polycythemia   The adaptive adjustments of humans living at high altitude involve a series of steps that reduce the steepness of the oxygen gradient between the atmosphere and the mitochondria (Fig. 56-2).[54] The initial oxygen gradient between atmospheric and alveolar air can be reduced by an increase in respiratory rate and volume. Because dead space and water vapor pressure are constant and acclimatized individuals do not ventilate excessively, the normal sea level gradient of approximately 60 mmHg is only reduced to approximately 40 mmHg at Morococha at 4540 m (14,900 ft) above sea level.[54] Further reduction can be achieved, and at the top of Mount Everest extreme hyperventilation reduces the gradient to less than 10 mmHg. A shift in the oxygen dissociation curve to the right, which represents decreased affinity of hemoglobin for oxygen, may be of benefit for short-term high-altitude acclimatization,[55] but its usefulness for chronic acclimatization probably has been

TABLE 56-1   SUMMARY OF ERYTHROPOIETIN RECEPTOR GENE MUTATIONS

TYPE OF MUTATION	MUTATION	STRUCTURAL DEFECT	ASSOCIATION WITH PFCP	REFERENCE
Deletion (7 bp)	Del5985-5991	Frameshift→ter truncation	Yes	288, 289
Duplication (8 bp)	5968-5975	Frameshift→ter truncation	Yes	290
Nonsense	G6002	Trp439→ter truncation	Yes	291
Nonsense	5986C→T	Gln435→ter truncation	Yes	292
Nonsense	5964C→G	Tyr426→ter truncation	Yes	293
Nonsense	5881C→T	Glu399→ter truncation	Yes	294
Nonsense	5959G→T	Glu425→ter truncation	Yes	295
Insertion (G)	5974insG	Frameshift→ter truncation	Yes	296
Insertion (T)	5967insT	Frameshift→ter truncation	Yes	297
Substitution	6148C→T	Pro488→Ser	No	289, 298
Substitution	6146A→G	Asn487→Ser	No	299
Substitution	2706A→T	Unknown	No	295

Adapted from Kralovics et al.[289]
Ter = termination codon.

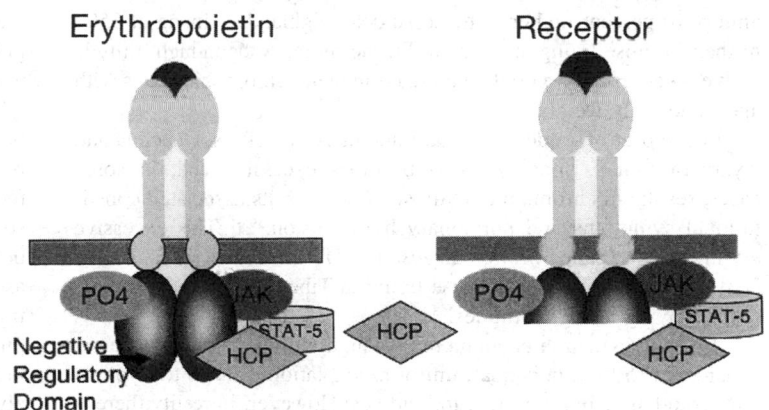

FIGURE 56-1   *(Left)* Erythropoietin binding to a normal erythropoietin receptor results in interaction of a protein kinase (JAK) with the receptor. The interaction leads to phosphorylation of the receptor and initiates a cascade of signaling that ultimately results in erythroid progenitor proliferation and differentiation. This process is self-regulatory. Activated signal transduction molecules, hematopoietic cell phosphatase (HCP), bind to the C-terminal of the erythropoietin receptor (EPOR), which is a negative regulatory domain. This interaction dephosphorylates the receptor and turns off the signaling, resulting in cessation of erythroid progenitor proliferation. *(Right)* Patients with mutated gain-of-function *EPOR* gene lack the C-terminal portion of the receptor that contains the negative regulatory domain. Erythropoietin binds, and the signal transduction pathway is activated by change of configuration of erythropoietin receptor dimer, but because there is no structure for HCP to bind on the activated erythropoietin receptor dimer, the receptor is left in the activated position, resulting in unbridled erythroid proliferation and an elevated red cell mass.

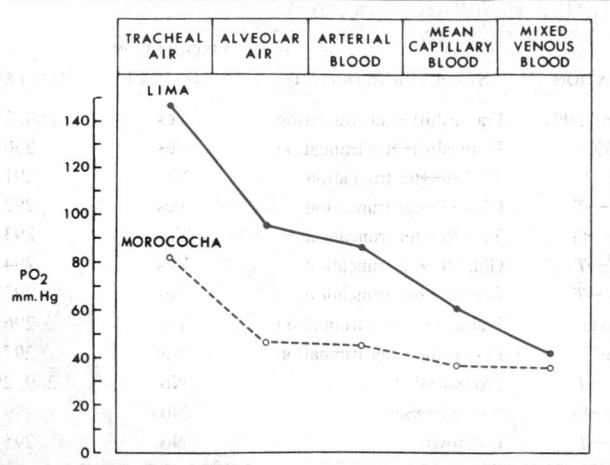

FIGURE 56-2 Oxygen gradient from atmospheric air to the tissues in individuals living at sea level and in Morococha, Peru, at 4540 m (14,900 ft) above sea level.

exaggerated.[56] In the unacclimatized subject exposed acutely to high altitude, hyperventilation alkalosis leads initially to a shift of the oxygen dissociation curve to the left, representing an increased affinity of hemoglobin for oxygen, and to additional tissue hypoxia. The alkalosis and the hypoxia in turn promote red cell synthesis of 2,3-BPG and cause the oxygen dissociation curve to shift back to a normal or even a right-shifted position (see Chap. 47). In chronic acclimatization, the blood pH is slightly increased, and when this is taken into account the dissociation curve is shifted approximately to normal.[57] It seems questionable if a shift to the right would be to the advantage of high-altitude dwellers.[58] There is a relationship between higher altitude and hemoglobin concentration response best studied among Andean highlanders and in Europeans in the United States. Hemoglobin concentration is almost 10 percent higher in those Andean highlanders living at 5500 m than in those living at 4355 m. Furthermore, Andean high-altitude native dwellers have a gradual increase in their hemoglobin levels with age[59] and body weight.[60]

In a subset of Andean high-altitude native dwellers, Quechua and Ayamara Indians, polycythemia becomes excessive and, in some cases, results in chronic mountain sickness with its associated constitutional symptoms and pulmonary hypertension.[59,61] This excessive erythrocytosis, called *Monge disease* or *chronic mountain sickness*,[61] is also described in Han Chinese living in Tibet[62] and occurs in Caucasians living in high altitudes.[63]

The polycythemia encountered by high-altitude dwellers often is considered to be a universal, uniform adaptation process to hypoxia that would arise in all normal individuals. However, in reality there is marked variability in erythropoietin levels and the subsequent polycythemic response to chronic hypoxia,[59] suggesting that some of these factors may be genetically determined. The same degree of hypoxia induces substantial differences in erythropoietin production in response to high altitude.[64–66] Three distinct adaptations to high altitude appear to have evolved. Andean highlanders have higher oxygen saturation than Tibetans at the same altitude.[67] Tibetan mean resting ventilation and hypoxic ventilatory response are higher than Andean Aymaras, whereas the mean Tibetan hemoglobin concentration is below the Andean means. It has been suggested that high levels of nitric oxide in the exhaled breath of Tibetans may improve oxygen delivery by inducing vasodilatation and increasing blood flow to tissues, thus making the compensatory increased red cell volume unnecessary.[68] As reported and paraphrased from Beall and colleagues[68]: "the Tibetan and

Andean patterns of oxygen transport appear equally effective functionally as evaluated by birth weight and maximal aerobic capacity across a range of altitudes. Another distinct successful pattern of human adaptation to high-altitude hypoxia that contrasts with both the Andean 'classic' (arterial hypoxemia with polycythemia) and the Tibetan (arterial hypoxemia with normal venous hemoglobin concentration) patterns evolved in Ethiopia. Although Ethiopian high dwellers have normal average hemoglobin concentration (15.9 and 15.0 g/dl for males and females, respectively), they have surprisingly high oxygen saturation of hemoglobin of 95.3 percent despite their hypoxic environment. Thus, Ethiopian highlanders maintain venous hemoglobin concentrations and arterial oxygen saturation within the ranges of sea level populations, despite the decrease in the ambient oxygen tension at high altitude."[69–72] This individual variability likely is a function of genetic differences in hypoxia sensing and hypoxia response pathways (see Chaps. 30 and 32); the exact mechanism remains to be identified.[60,73] Tibetans and Ethiopians have lived as mountain dwellers much longer than the Quechua or Ayamara Indians (and Han Chinese moving to Tibet and Caucasians moving to high altitudes), suggesting that extreme elevation of the red cell mass is a maladaptation that Tibetans avoided by evolving a more efficient, or less detrimental, compensatory mechanism than that causing Monge disease.

Understanding the etiology of polycythemia of high altitude is made more complex by a study of inhabitants of the Peruvian mining community of Cerro de Pasco (altitude 4280 m) with excessive erythrocytosis (mean hematocrit 76%, range 66%–91%). About half of those with a hematocrit greater than 75 percent had toxic serum cobalt levels,[74] suggesting that other erythropoiesis-promoting factors, such as cobalt,[75] can augment hypoxia induction of erythropoietin causing the extreme polycythemias. Most high-altitude dwellers, however, do not have measurable levels or a history of exposure to cobalt or other heavy metals.[76]

Pulmonary and Cardiac Disease Degrees of arterial hypoxia comparable to those observed in individuals at high altitudes are observed in patients with right-to-left shunting because of cardiac or intrapulmonary shunts or ventilation defects, as in chronic obstructive pulmonary disease (COPD). Patients with right-to-left shunting develop a degree of erythrocytosis that is comparable to that observed with similar degrees of desaturation at high altitudes,[77] but many patients with COPD with severe cyanosis are not polycythemic. This has been attributed to the infection that is often present in the lungs of these patients and to an increase in plasma volume; however, why some patients with lung disease and congenital heart disease develop polycythemia, whereas others do not, is not clear. COPD is frequently associated with cyanosis, clubbing, and arterial oxygen desaturation.[78,79] Central alveolar hypoventilation because of an impaired respiratory center has been reported following cerebral thrombosis, Parkinsonism, encephalitis, and barbiturate intoxication.[80] Peripheral alveolar hypoventilation because of mechanical impairment of the chest may be seen in patients with myotonic dystrophy, poliomyelitis, or severe spondylitis.[81,82] Eisenmenger syndrome, characterized by elevated pulmonary vascular resistance and right-to-left shunting of blood, usually is accompanied by polycythemia.[83]

Sleep Apnea-Induced Polycythemia In the colorful Pickwickian syndrome,[14] now more widely known as *sleep apnea syndrome*, the polycythemia is characterized by association with extreme obesity and somnolence. The sleep apnea syndrome[84] can, if severe, cause arterial hypoxemia and hypercapnia, somnolence, and secondary polycythemia.[85] Although the evidence is largely anecdotal,[86] secondary polycythemia is a widely recognized complication of long-standing sleep apnea, found in 5 to 10 percent of those with nocturnal apnea and hypopnea.[87] The mechanism by which sleep apnea causes polycythemia is unclear. No difference in erythropoietin levels was found between normoxic and hypoxemic patients referred for suspected sleep apnea.[88] In a later study, no statistically significant differences in erythropoietin levels were found between sleep apnea patients with and without polycythemia and age- and sex-matched healthy controls.[87]

Smoker's Polycythemia Heavy smoking will result in the formation of carboxyhemoglobin, which does not transport oxygen and causes an increase in oxygen affinity of the remaining normal hemoglobin. This leads to tissue hypoxia, erythropoietin production, and stimulation of red cell production.[89] Smoking also may cause a reduction in plasma volume,[90] and either augmentation of the red cell mass or shrinkage of plasma volume could easily explain the rise in the hematocrit. Chronic carbon monoxide poisoning is an important but generally unappreciated cause of mild polycythemia.[91]

Polycythemia Secondary to Mutant (High-Affinity) Hemoglobins Hemoglobins with certain amino acid substitutions manifest an increased affinity for oxygen, producing tissue hypoxia and a compensatory erythrocytosis (see Chap. 47). Mutations affecting the amino acids of the $\alpha_1\beta_2$ globin chain contact affect normal rotation within the molecule and impair the rate of deoxygenation. Changes in the carboxy-terminal and penultimate amino acids will also impair intramolecular motions and tend to keep the molecules in a high-affinity state. Alterations in the amino acids lining the central cavity of hemoglobin will destabilize the binding of 2,3-BPG in this cavity and lead to increased oxygen affinity. Finally, some heme pocket mutations interfere with deoxygenation; however, most hemoglobins with mutations involving amino acids in the heme pocket are unstable and associated with hemolytic anemia and cyanosis. The inheritance of these disorders is autosomal dominant. An up-to-date listing that includes such hemoglobin variants can be found at *http://www.ncbi.nlm.nih.gov/entrez/dispomim.cgi?id=141900* and *http://www.ncbi.nlm.nih.gov/entrez/dispomim.cgi?id=141850*.

Polycythemia Secondary to Red Cell Enzyme Deficiencies Deficiencies of red cell enzymes in early steps of glycolysis sometimes cause marked decreases in the levels of 2,3-BPG (see Chap. 45). This results in an increased oxygen affinity of hemoglobin and, in some cases, polycythemia. Polycythemia is particularly likely to occur in bisphosphoglyceromutase deficiency[92] and in phosphofructokinase deficiency.[93] Polycythemia has also been observed in the "high ATP syndrome" associated with an abnormality of pyruvate kinase[94]; however, in this particular family, decreased 2,3-BPG was found and was a likely culprit. Occasionally mild polycythemia occurs in patients with methemoglobinemia resulting from cytochrome b_5 reductase (methemoglobin reductase) deficiency (see Chap. 48).[77]

Chemically Induced Tissue Hypoxia A number of chemicals have been suspected of causing histotoxic anoxia and secondary polycythemia, but the only chemical with a predictable capacity to cause erythrocytosis is cobalt.[75] Cobalt administration increases the oxygen tension in subcutaneous air pockets in rats[77] and erythropoietin production.[77] It seems likely that it acts by inhibiting oxidative metabolism. This erythropoietic effect has led to the therapeutic administration of 60 to 150 mg cobalt chloride to patients with refractory anemias such as the anemias of chronic infection, cancer, or uremia.[95]

INAPPROPRIATE POLYCYTHEMIAS

Chuvash Polycythemia Chuvash polycythemia is the only known endemic congenital polycythemia. Chuvash polycythemia results from an abnormality in the oxygen-sensing pathway. The condition causes thrombotic and hemorrhagic vascular complications, which lead to early mortality; survival beyond the age of 60 years is uncommon.[35,96] The inheritance is autosomal recessive, and affected patients tend to have normal blood gases, normal calculated P_{50}, normal to increased erythropoietin levels, absence of genetic linkage to erythropoietin and *EPOR* loci, and no evidence of abnormal hemoglo-

bin.[96] Molecular studies in patients with Chuvash polycythemia indicate that von Hippel-Landau *(VHL)* 598C→T leads to impairment of the interaction of pVHL with hypoxia-inducible factor (HIF)-1α, reducing the rate of ubiquitin-mediated degradation of HIF-1α (see Chap. 30) and resulting in increased expression of downstream target genes including erythropoietin, *SLC2A1* (also known as *GLUT*-1, encoding facilitated glucose transporter member 1 of solute carrier family 2), transferrin *(TF)*, transferrin receptor *(TFRC*, encoding p90, CD71), and vascular endothelial growth factor *(VEGF)*.[97,98] Figure 56-3 depicts the effect of this mutation on hypoxic sensing. The role of circulating erythropoietin in the Chuvash polycythemia phenotype is indisputable; however, there must be other factors associated with the Chuvash polycythemia *VHL* mutation that contribute to the polycythemic phenotype because the erythroid progenitors of Chuvash polycythemia are hypersensitive *in vitro* to extrinsic erythropoietin; the mechanism of this observation remains unexplained. Thus, Chuvash polycythemia has features of both primary and secondary polycythemias.[97,98]

Other Congenital Polycythemias Characterized by VHL Mutations Other congenital polycythemias around the world are also caused by defects in the oxygen-sensing pathway and many of them by mutations in *VHL* (Table 56-2). These have been described in Caucasians in the United States and Europe and in people of Punjabi/Bangladeshi Asian ancestry. Some patients with congenital polycythemia have proved to be compound heterozygotes for the Chuvash mutation and other *VHL* mutations, including *VHL* 598C→T and 562C→G, *VHL* 598C→T and 574C→T, and *VHL* 598C→T and 388C→G. Additionally, a Croatian boy was homozygous for *VHL* 571C→G, the first example of a homozygous *VHL* germline mutation other than *VHL* 598C→T causing polycythemia.[99,105]

A small number of cases of congenital polycythemia that appear to have mutation of only one *VHL* allele confound an obvious pathophysiologic explanation. In a Ukrainian family, two children with polycythemia were heterozygotes for *VHL* 376G→T (D126Y), but the father with the same mutation was not polycythemic.[100] An English patient was a heterozygote for *VHL* 598C→T[106]; however, the inheritance of deletion of a *VHL* allele, or null *VHL* allele, in a trans position was not excluded. Subsequently, two polycythemic *VHL* heterozygous patients were described in whom a null *VHL* allele was more rigor-

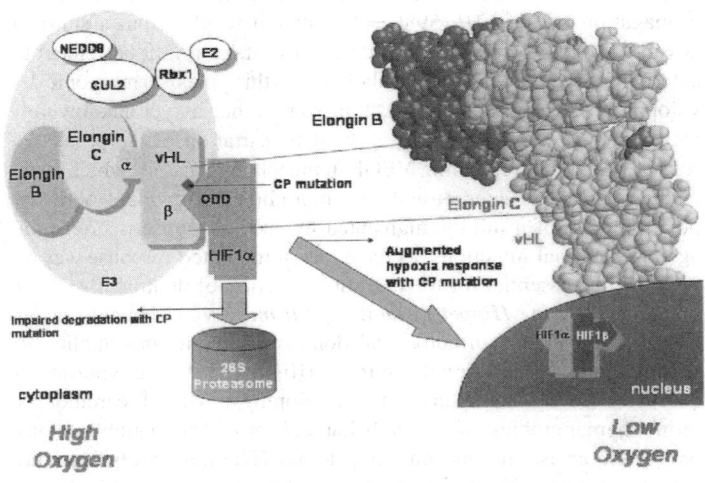

FIGURE 56-3 Elongins B and C and proteins Rbx1, Cul2, E2, and NEDD8 are interacting proteins that facilitate von Hippel-Landau (vHL) function. Interaction of mutated vHL protein with HIF-1α. The Chuvash *VHL* mutation leads to impaired interaction with HIF-1α, which results in impaired degradation in 26S proteasome and augmented hypoxia sensing.

TABLE 56-2 *VHL* MUTATIONS ASSOCIATED WITH CONGENITAL
POLYCYTHEMIA

VHL GENOTYPE	ETHNICITIES	REFERENCE	CLINICAL FEATURES
235 C→T/586 C→G	Caucasian	102	
598 C→T/598 C→T	Chuvash, Danish, US (white), Bangladeshi, Pakistani, Russian, Turkish	101, 102, 300–302	Frequent thrombotic complications
598 C→T/574 C→T	Caucasian	102	
598 C→T/562 C→G	US (white)	302	
598 C→T/388 G→C	US (white)	300	
571 C→G/571 C→G	Croatian	302	
311 G→T/wild-type	German (?)	101	
376 G→T/wild-type	Ukrainian	300	?vHL syndrome
598 C→T/wild-type	English, German	101	
523 A→G/wild-type	Portuguese	102	AT patient

AT=ataxia-telangiectasia; vHL = von Hippel-Lindau.

ously excluded[101,102]; the molecular mechanism of their polycythemic phenotype remains to be elucidated.

To address the question of whether the *VHL* 598C→T substitution occurred in a single founder or resulted from recurrent mutational events, haplotype analysis of eight highly informative single nucleotide polymorphic markers covering 340 kb spanning the *VHL* gene was performed on 101 subjects bearing the *VHL* 598C→T mutation and 447 normal unrelated individuals from Chuvash, Southeast Asian, Caucasian, Hispanic, and African American ethnic groups.[107] Polymorphism of the *VHL* locus in normal controls (having a wild *VHL* 598C* allele) and subjects bearing Chuvash polycythemia *VHL 598T* were in strong linkage disequilibrium. These studies indicated that in most individuals, the *VHL* 598C→T mutation arose in a single ancestor between 51,000 and 12,000 years ago. However, this is not the case for a Turkish polycythemic family with a *VHL* 598C→T mutation wherein the *VHL* 598C→T mutation occurred independently.[101]

Chuvash polycythemia homozygotes have decreased survival because of thrombotic complications[108] and thus are under negative selection pressure. The high frequency of the mutation in some areas may result from random factors ("drift"), but it is also possible that propagation of the *VHL* 598C→T mutation results from a survival advantage for heterozygotes. Such an advantage might be related to subtle improvement of iron metabolism, erythropoiesis, embryonic development, energy metabolism,[109] or some other as yet unknown effect. An intriguing possibility is the demonstration of the protective role of HIF-1α in regulating VEGF in preeclampsia,[110,111] which is the leading cause of maternal and fetal mortality worldwide.[112] Another potential role of a mildly augmented hypoxic response is protection against bacterial infections, as the hypoxia-mediated response was reported to be essential for the bactericidal action of neutrophils.[113]

Classic von Hippel-Lindau Syndrome   von Hippel-Landau (vHL) syndrome is an autosomal dominant genetic abnormality affecting the posttranslational control of HIF-1α.[114–116] The syndrome is characterized by a propensity for developing renal cell carcinomas, retinal hemangioblastomas, cerebellar and spinal hemangioblastomas, pancreatic cysts, and pheochromocytomas. The tumors result from a somatic mutation in addition to the germline mutation, that is, loss of heterozygosity. Polycythemia is not part of the vHL syndrome; however, hemangioblastomas of the central nervous system, and less commonly pheochromocytoma and renal cancer, have long been associated with polycythemia.[114] The *VHL* gene codes for 213 amino acids, and more than 130 germline mutations associated with classic vHL syn-

drome have been identified, virtually all of them 5′ to the codon 200 position that is mutated in Chuvash polycythemia.[117] Figure 56-4 depicts the schematic effect of the Chuvash polycythemia mutation in the context of other previously found *VHL* mutations.

Congenital Polycythemia Resulting from Altered Oxygen Sensing but without Mutation of VHL   More than half of patients with congenital polycythemia with inappropriately normal, or elevated, erythropoietin levels do not have *VHL* mutations; typically such cases are sporadic or recessively inherited. However, some such families show dominant inheritance.[118] The molecular basis of these cases remains to be elucidated. Lesions in genes linked to oxygen-dependent gene regulation and their interacting proteins are leading candidates for mutation; however, many of the candidate genes have been excluded by sequencing and/or genetic means.[118]

Renal Polycythemia and Postrenal Transplant Erythrocytosis   Absolute erythrocytosis has been observed in a considerable number of patients with solitary renal cysts, polycystic renal disease, or hydronephrosis.[119] In most of these cases, erythropoietin assays on cyst fluid, serum, or urine have disclosed the presence of erythropoietin.[120] Patients with polycystic disease have a hematocrit value slightly higher than normal and definitely higher than expected of patients with uremia. In some patients on prolonged dialysis treatment, cystic transformation occurs in the native kidneys. This acquired cystic disease is occasionally associated with marked erythrocytosis.[121] In patients with hypernephromas and erythrocytosis, erythropoietin assays of serum and urine have disclosed higher than normal levels, and the erythrocytosis most likely is caused by excessive erythropoietin secretion by the tumor. This assumption has been supported by the presence of erythropoietin mRNA in tumor cells.[122] Wilms tumors[123] and metanephric adenomas[124] are also occasionally associated with an erythrocytosis. However, many of these cases may have a somatic *VHL* gene mutation that, in combination with a germline mutation of another allele, may constitute an unrecognized vHL syndrome.

Partial obstruction of the renal artery would be expected to cause renal tissue hypoxia and a physiologic stimulation of erythropoietin production. Nevertheless, it has proved quite difficult to induce erythrocytosis in laboratory animals by placing a Goldblatt clamp on the renal arteries.[125] Only a few of the many patients who have arteriosclerotic narrowing of the renal arteries have been reported to have been polycythemic.[126]

Postrenal Transplantation Erythrocytosis   Although the full molecular basis of postrenal transplant erythrocytosis remains unknown, angiotensin II (see Chap. 30) plays an important role in its pathogenesis.[127] There is growing evidence that increased activity of angiotensin II–angiotensin receptor 1 pathway makes the erythroid progenitors hypersensitive to angiotensin II.[128,129] Further, angiotensin II can modulate release of erythropoiesis stimulatory factors (see Chap. 30), including erythropoietin and insulin-like growth factor-1.[130,131] Studies of venous effluents have determined that the native rather than the transplanted kidneys are the source of the inappropriate production of erythropoietin,[132] and in some patients removal of the native kidneys has led to rapid restoration of normal hematocrit values.[133]

Polycythemia with Connective Tissue Tumors   Occasionally there is an association of erythrocytosis with large uterine myomas.[25] Usually the tumor has been huge, and extirpation has routinely been followed by a hematologic "cure." The suggestion that the tumor interferes with pulmonary ventilation has not been supported by the normal arterial gas findings in the few patients so studied. Another possible mechanism is that the large abdominal mass causes mechanical interference with the blood supply to the kidneys, resulting in renal hypoxia and erythropoietin production. Inappropriate erythropoietin secretion by smooth muscle cells has been demonstrated both in uterine myomas and in one case of cutaneous leiomyoma.[25,134] Rare cases

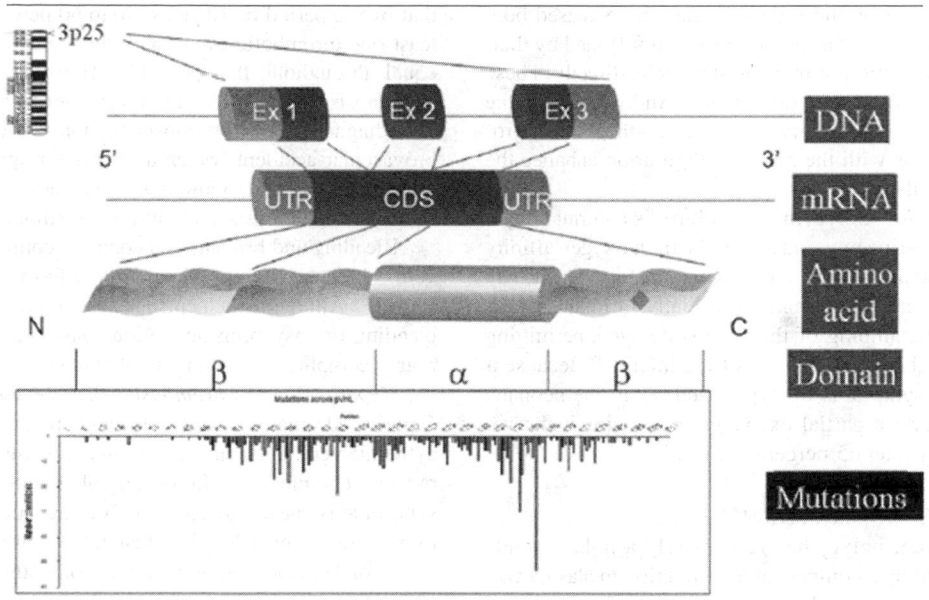

FIGURE 56-4   von Hippel-Lindau *(VHL)* gene structure and mutation. Three exons of *VHL* genes are depicted encoding for UTR (untranslated portion of mRNA) and coding sequences (CDS). vHL domains β, α, and β are shown. The relative numbers of reported *VHL* gene mutations are depicted as *vertical lines*. The location of the CP mutation is depicted by the *diamond*.

of polycythemia attributed to a myxoma of the atrium,[26] hamartoma of the liver,[27] and focal hyperplasia of the liver[28] have been documented.

Brain Tumors In adequately studied patients with erythrocytosis and cerebellar hemangiomas, the arterial gas tensions have been normal. That the tumors are directly responsible for the polycythemia can be surmised from the identification of erythropoietin in cyst fluid and stromal cells and from a case in which erythropoietin mRNA was present in the tumor.[135] Although in these cases a mutation of the *VHL* gene was not sought, these tumors likely were a manifestation of an underlying vHL syndrome because cerebellar hemangiomas are an integral feature of vHL syndrome.

Hepatoma In 1958, McFadzean and coworkers[136] reported that almost 10 percent of patients in Hong Kong with hepatocarcinoma developed erythrocytosis. Since then, this association has been recognized as an important clinical clue in the diagnostic consideration of patients with liver disease.[137] The cause of erythrocytosis probably is inappropriate production of erythropoietin by the neoplastic cells.[138] Normal hepatocytes and to a lesser degree nonparenchymal liver cells produce small amounts of erythropoietin both constitutively and in response to hypoxia.

Endocrine Disorders Pheochromocytomas,[139] aldosterone-producing adenomas,[140] Bartter syndrome,[141] and dermoid cyst of the ovary[142] have been described in association with erythrocytosis. Erythropoietin levels were elevated in the serum and returned to normal after extirpation of the tumors. A number of pathogenetic mechanisms have been suggested (see Chap. 36), including decreased plasma volume; mechanical interference with renal blood supply; hypertensive damage to renal parenchyma; functional interaction between aldosterone, renin, and erythropoietin; and inappropriate secretion of erythropoietin by the tumors. Mild polycythemia may be present in patients with Cushing syndrome; however, its pathophysiologic basis is not entirely clear.

The erythropoietic effect of androgens is of considerable practical importance. For many years, it was assumed that the higher red cell count in males was caused by androgens because the hemoglobin lev-

els of boys and girls were identical up until the time of puberty. It was not until pharmacologic doses of testosterone were administered to women with carcinoma of the breast that the full erythropoietic potency of androgens was appreciated.[143] Since then, various androgen preparations have been used in the treatment of refractory anemias,[144,145] occasionally causing dramatic overshoots into the polycythemic range (Fig. 56-5).

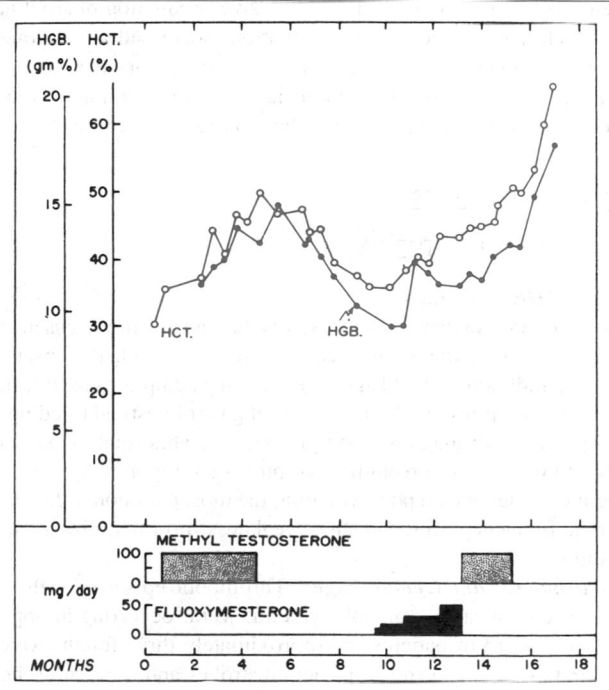

FIGURE 56-5   Erythropoietic response to testosterone derivatives in a patient with myelofibrosis.

The erythropoietic effect of androgens appears to be caused both by their capacity to stimulate erythropoietin production[146] and by their capacity to induce differentiation of marrow stem cells directly. These two effects have specific structural requirements. Androgens with the 5α-H configuration stimulate renal and extrarenal erythropoietin production, whereas androgens with the 5β-H configuration enhance the differentiation of stem cells.[146]

Neonatal Polycythemia Polycythemia at birth is a normal physiologic response to intrauterine hypoxia and to the high oxygen affinity of red cells containing hemoglobin F (see Chap. 6). However, it may become excessive and even symptomatic, especially in infants of diabetic mothers, or if the clamping of the cord is delayed, permitting placental blood to boost the blood volume of the infant.[147] Because it is difficult to recognize symptoms of hyperviscosity in the neonate, many pediatricians perform a partial exchange transfusion if the venous hematocrit is higher than 65 percent at birth.[148]

APPARENT (RELATIVE) POLYCYTHEMIA

Some believe that apparent polycythemia is merely a mild absolute polycythemia accentuated by a compensatory reduction in plasma volume. Others suggest that it is caused by a primary reduction in plasma volume and have associated it with hypertension, obesity, and stress. When the red cell volume is documented to be normal, spurious polycythemia is also an appropriate term. Its clinical significance has also been disputed. The high hematocrit with its associated high viscosity is believed by some to be a risk factor heralding cerebral and cardiac complications, whereas others believe it is merely a well-tolerated blemish. Because the designation *apparent polycythemia*[149] is noncommittal, it is used here.

The main clinical associations with apparent polycythemia are obesity, hypertension, and smoking. In obese patients the finding of a normal red cell volume may be spurious because if the volume is expressed in terms of lean body weight, some of these patients would have a significant increase in red cell mass. In hypertensive patients there is no adequate explanation for the apparent increase in red cell production or decrease in plasma volume. Sleep apnea (common in patients with congestive failure), excessive production of atrial natriuretic factor, increased adrenal activation, decreased aldosterone secretion, and hypoxic vasoconstriction are all factors that have been invoked,[150–152] but with little enthusiasm. Chronic administration of diuretics to treat hypertension may be a more likely cause.[152]

CLINICAL FEATURES

PRIMARY POLYCYTHEMIAS

POLYCYTHEMIA VERA

Onset Polycythemia vera usually has an insidious onset, most commonly during the sixth decade of life, although the onset may occur in childhood or in old age.[153] Presenting symptoms include headache, plethora, pruritus, thrombosis, and gastrointestinal bleeding, but some patients are diagnosed simply because abnormal blood counts are found on routine screening. Symptoms are reported by at least 30 percent of patients with polycythemia; the most common in decreasing order of frequency are headache, weakness, pruritus, dizziness, and sweating.[153]

Thrombosis and Hemorrhage Thrombotic episodes are the most common complications of polycythemia vera, occurring in approximately one third of patients.[154] Approximately three fourths were arterial and one fourth venous. Ischemic strokes and transient ischemic attacks accounted for the majority of arterial complications. Of the 164 patients who died in one series, thrombosis accounted for 41 percent of deaths and bleeding for 7 percent. In some studies it has been stated

that over a period of 10 years, 40 to 60 percent of patients develop at least one thrombotic event, with the annual incidence approximately equal throughout this period.[155] However, in prospective studies thrombosis was most common just prior to and in the first few years after diagnosis.[156,157] The most common serious complication is a cerebrovascular accident, which accounts for approximately one third of thrombotic events, followed in frequency by myocardial infarction, deep vein thrombosis, and pulmonary embolism.[155]

Bleeding and bruising is a common complication of polycythemia vera, observed in approximately one fourth of the patients in some series.[154] Although such episodes usually are minor, such as gingival bleeding or easy bruising, serious gastrointestinal and other hemorrhagic complications with a fatal outcome also occur.[50,158,159]

Hepatic Vein Thrombosis (Budd-Chiari Syndrome) Budd-Chiari syndrome is a catastrophic and often fatal complication of polycythemia vera, occurring in 10 percent of 140 patients in one series[160] but less common in a European collaborative study.[159] Budd-Chiari syndrome is caused by thrombosis of hepatic venous outflow leading to ischemia from reduced perfusion through hepatic arterioles and necrosis of hepatocytes, ascites, with or without right upper quadrant abdominal pain, hepatosplenomegaly, and jaundice. The Budd-Chiari syndrome may be the first clinical manifestation of polycythemia vera preceding the elevated blood counts; however, erythropoietin-independent erythroid colony formation has been described in many of these yet nonpolycythemic patients. Polycythemia vera is the most frequent underlying disease associated with Budd-Chiari syndrome. In some series it accounts for the majority of this serious and frequently liver transplant-requiring condition.[161–163]

Cutaneous Pruritus occurs in approximately 40 percent of patients.[164] It usually is aggravated by bathing or showering and may be so severe as to markedly compromise the patient's quality of life. Its cause in unclear, and it has been attributed to increased numbers of mast cells in the skin[165] and to elevated histamine levels,[166] although these associations were refuted by others.[167]

Several patients have developed the dermatologic disorder acute febrile neutrophilic dermatosis (Sweet syndrome).[168,169]

Erythromelalgia Erythromelalgia is a syndrome of warmth of the extremities, painful, reddened digits, and burning sensation and erythema of the hands and feet that is associated with thrombocytosis and, characteristically, responds rapidly (within hours) to low-dose aspirin therapy. In severe cases, it results in ischemic necrosis of digits and may lead to their amputation. This syndrome occurs in less than 5 percent of polycythemia vera patients.[158,159] It is not specific to polycythemia vera or other myeloproliferative disorders; in one series of 168 patients with erythromelalgia, less than 10 percent had polycythemia vera.[170] It is frequently associated with essential thrombocythemia, and a role for transient microvascular occlusion by platelet aggregates has been proposed (see Chap. 111).[171,172]

Gastrointestinal The occurrence of Budd-Chiari syndrome was discussed in "Hepatic Vein Thrombosis (Budd-Chiari Syndrome)" above. Portal hypertension and varices are not uncommon[173] and are often caused by unrecognized splenic or hepatic vein thromboses. The incidence of peptic ulcer is four to five times as great as in the general population.[174]

Cardiovascular Cardiovascular symptoms include angina, myocardial infarction, and congestive heart failure.[50,156,159]

Pulmonary Hypertension Pulmonary hypertension occurs in a higher than expected frequency in patients with polycythemia vera. The suggested etiologies include smooth muscle hyperplasia induced by release of platelet-derived growth factor from activated platelets, obstruction of pulmonary circulation by megakaryocytes, extramedullary hematopoiesis, and unrecognized recurrent thrombotic events[175,176]; however, none of these etiologies is clearly established.

Neurologic Neurologic symptoms, such as dizziness, are very common.[50,156,158,159,177] Spinal cord compression secondary to extramedullary hematopoiesis has been documented.[178]

Other Organ Systems The increased nucleic acid turnover that results from excessive proliferation of marrow cells often leads to an increase in blood uric acid concentration, and gout is a frequent complication.[50]

Surgery More than 75 percent of patients with uncontrolled polycythemia vera develop complications during or after major surgery because both bleeding and thrombosis are common.[179]

Pregnancy Polycythemia vera complications in pregnancy are discussed in Chapter 7.

Spent Phase of Polycythemia Vera The spent phase of polycythemia vera, also known as *postpolycythemia myeloid metaplasia*, is a frequent and often terminal complication of polycythemia vera.[157,159,180] It is characterized by a combination of anemia, recent and often progressive increase of splenic size, and marrow fibrosis (see Chap. 89). The other frequently associated features are thrombocytosis, leukocytosis often with immature cells, and leukopenia. The affected individuals are frequently symptomatic from anemia, infection, bleeding, and splenic enlargement, and most become transfusion dependent.[50,156,158,159,180] The anemia that characterizes the spent phase of polycythemia vera usually is multifactorial in origin. Splenomegaly results in pooling of red cells, expansion of the plasma volume, and shortening of red cell survival (see Chaps. 5 and 55). Development of the "spent phase" is associated with an increased risk of leukemic transformation. In the PVSG-01 study, the incidence of acute leukemia was 24 percent versus 7 percent in patients without myelofibrosis.[157]

Leukemic and Myelodysplastic Transformation of Polycythemia Vera Patients with polycythemia vera have an increased risk for developing leukemia. This contrasts with other polycythemic disorders wherein progression to leukemia is not part of the disease process. Acute leukemia, usually myeloid, is a fatal complication of polycythemia vera. The European multicenter observational study of 1638 patients reported a 6.3 relative risk of developing leukemia 10 years after the diagnosis of polycythemia vera.[159] In the PVSG-01 randomized trial, the incidence of acute leukemia at 18 years of followup was 1.5 percent on the phlebotomy only arm, 10 percent on the ^{32}P arm, and 13 percent on the chlorambucil arm.[158]

PRIMARY FAMILIAL AND CONGENITAL POLYCYTHEMIA

Although PFCP is uncommon, it is more prevalent than congenital polycythemia because of high oxygen affinity hemoglobin mutants or 2,3-BPG.[23] Unlike those with polycythemia vera, patients with PFCP lack splenomegaly, neutrophilia, and thrombocytosis and do not progress to acute leukemia. Generally thought to be benign, it is possible that this condition predisposes patients to severe cardiovascular problems.[181] An increased incidence of cardiovascular disease was observed in affected members of PFCP families.[182] Erythrocytosis may be very severe with hemoglobin levels that typically are greater than 20 g/dl. Headaches are commonly present. Hypertension, coronary artery disease, and strokes have been reported to occur but do not appear to be clearly related to an elevated hematocrit as they also occur in aggressively phlebotomized patients with normal hematocrit[183]; these are not a constant feature of the disorder.[184]

CHUVASH POLYCYTHEMIA

The recessive polycythemia that is endemic in Chuvashia is characterized by elevations of the hemoglobin level to a mean of 22.6 with a standard deviation of 1.4 g/liter.[96] Some patients are symptomatic with headache and fatigue and with signs including clubbing, thrombosis, and peptic ulcer. There is an approximately threefold increase

in incidence of thrombotic events that do not appear to be ameliorated by phlebotomies.[108]

Because Chuvash polycythemia is characterized by a germline mutation in the *VHL* gene, it was expected that homozygotes for this mutation may develop certain vascular tumors similar to those associated with classic vHL syndrome. In a matched cohort study, *VHL 598C→T* homozygosity was associated with varicose veins, lower blood pressures, elevated serum VEGF, and premature mortality related to cerebral vascular events and peripheral thrombosis.

Tumors typical of classic vHL syndrome, such as spinocerebellar hemangioblastomas, renal carcinomas, and pheochromocytomas, were not found, indicating that increased expression of HIF-1α and VEGF is not sufficient for tumorigenesis.[108] Chuvash polycythemia is associated with a history of thrombosis, relatively low blood pressure (also seen in heterozygotes), and varicose veins.[96,97,108] As yet, no significant association of thrombosis and hematocrit has been found. Imaging studies in 33 *VHL 598C→T* homozygotes revealed unsuspected cerebral ischemic lesions in 45 percent but no spinocerebellar hemangioblastomas, renal carcinomas, or pheochromocytomas. Benign vertebral body hemangiomas (a distinct entity from hemangioblastoma) were found in 55 percent of patients with Chuvash polycythemia versus 21 percent of control Chuvash individuals without polycythemia ($p = 0.006$).[108]

SECONDARY ACQUIRED POLYCYTHEMIA

Tolerance to high altitudes varies greatly, but most normal individuals have no discomfort at altitudes of up to 2130 m (7000 ft). Above this level, and especially if the ascent is rapid, some manifestations of cerebral hypoxia are common. Headaches, sleeplessness, and palpitations are frequently encountered, and weakness, nausea, vomiting, and mental dullness may be present. More severe manifestations include pulmonary and cerebral edema, which may lead to death. Cheyne-Stokes respiration commonly occurs, especially during sleep. These symptoms constitute the syndrome of *acute mountain sickness*.[185]

Ruddy cyanosis and physiologic emphysema are the two characteristic features of some humans living at high altitudes. Venous and capillary engorgement can be observed readily in the conjunctiva, mucous membranes, and skin and may contribute to the remarkable capacity of Tibetan Sherpas to walk barefoot and sleep on ice and snow.[186] Asymptomatic retinal hemorrhages are seen frequently at high altitudes but rarely at altitudes of 3000 m (9000 ft) or less.[187] Splenomegaly and jaundice are unusual, although the sustained erythrocytosis is associated with an increased rate of red cell destruction and bilirubin generation. It has been stated that Monge disease includes low fertility[61,63]; however, this finding may not be universal. High-altitude native resident Tibetans exhibit two distinct genotypes for increased oxygen affinity of hemoglobin. Women with genotypes for high oxygen saturation have more surviving children.[72] This finding suggests that high-altitude hypoxia is acting as an agent of natural selection on the locus for oxygen saturation of hemoglobin by the mechanism of higher infant survival of Tibetan women with high oxygen saturation genotypes.[69–72,188]

The polycythemia associated with smoking is generally asymptomatic, but there may be an increase in thrombotic events, which may be caused by the smoking rather than polycythemia.

Large studies of patients with Eisenmenger syndrome[83] and other patients with cyanotic heart disease[189] caution against routine phlebotomy for asymptomatic elevation of the hematocrit; in fact, thrombotic complications were not observed in these studies. Animal studies support these recommendations; transgenic mice with extreme polycythemia (hematocrit 85%) because of constitutive overexpression of erythropoietin did not develop the expected thrombotic complications.[190]

RENAL POLYCYTHEMIA AND POSTRENAL TRANSPLANT ERYTHROCYTOSIS

The erythrocytosis of renal disease and of the postrenal transplant state can be very severe. Erythrocyte counts may be as high as $8 \times 10^{12}/$ liter and be associated with hypertension and congestive failure.[191] At higher hematocrit levels (usually >60%), thrombotic events may complicate the clinical course[32–34]; however, frequent comorbidities that are associated or causative of renal failure are frequently also factors predisposing to thrombosis.

Tumors The erythrocytosis that occurs with tumors is generally mild,[135] and the predominating clinical manifestations are those of the tumor itself. Even moderate elevations to a hematocrit of 64 percent have been encountered without symptoms referable to the polycythemia.[28]

Neonatal Polycythemia Of 55 infants with neonatal polycythemia, 85 percent had signs and symptoms attributed to this disorder. These included "feeding problems" (21.8%), plethora (20.0%), lethargy (14.5%), cyanosis (14.5%), respiratory distress (9.1%), jitteriness (7.3%), and hypotonia (7.3%). Other findings included hypoglycemia (40.0%) and hyperbilirubinemia (21.8%). In a larger group of nearly 1000 infants, six had an intracranial hemorrhage.[147]

LABORATORY FEATURES

POLYCYTHEMIA VERA

MARROW

The marrow is characteristically hypercellular, with involvement of all myeloid lineages. Although the marrow morphology is a part of World Health Organization diagnostic criteria of polycythemia vera,[192–194] the morphologic features that have been described to be specific for polycythemia vera[308] have not as yet been validated by blinded studies and may be subject to interobserver and intraobserver variations. An absence of marrow iron stores is virtually a constant finding in polycythemia vera. There are no characteristic cytogenetic findings, but occasional clonal chromosomal changes, none of which are specific for polycythemia vera, are observed in a minority of patients (see Chap. 10).

ERYTHROCYTES

The erythrocyte count and hematocrit usually are increased, and in patients who have undergone phlebotomy or who have had gastrointestinal bleeding episodes, the erythrocyte count may be increased out of proportion to the increase in the hemoglobin and hematocrit because they may have marked hypochromia and microcytosis. The plasma iron in such patients is decreased, the iron binding capacity is increased, and plasma ferritin levels are low. The red cell mass usually is increased in proportion to the hematocrit value (Fig. 56-6). The effect of the elevated hematocrit on blood viscosity is discussed in "Therapy" below.

In the spent phase, there is marked anisocytosis and poikilocytosis, and teardrop cells (dacryocytes) are abundant (see Chap. 28). Alterations in red cell glycolytic metabolism have been documented[195,196] but are not unique or of any diagnostic value.

The P_{O_2} of the arterial blood often is lower than normal. Levels as low as 63 mmHg were encountered in more than 10 percent of patients, and the percent saturation with oxygen was accordingly slightly reduced,[197] complicating differential diagnosis from secondary polycythemia resulting from hypoxia.

LEUKOCYTES

An absolute neutrophilia occurs in approximately two thirds of patients.[153] Occasional myelocytes and metamyelocytes are often present in the blood, and considerable degrees of immaturity are often present in patients with long-standing, advanced disease. Basophilia occurs in approximately two thirds of patients with uncontrolled disease.[50,158,198] In polycythemia vera, the proportion of activated neutrophils is increased,[199] and it is possible that neutrophils may be an important factor in polycythemia vera-associated thrombosis.

The leukocyte alkaline phosphate level is elevated in approximately 70 percent of patients with polycythemia vera.[153]

PLATELETS

The platelet count is increased in approximately half of patients at the time of diagnosis and in approximately 10 percent is greater than 1000 $\times 10^9/$liter.[153] In contrast to normal individuals, in whom phlebotomy results in an increase in the platelet count, platelet levels usually are not affected by phlebotomy in patients with polycythemia vera.[200] There are no consistent abnormalities of thrombopoietin levels.[201] A significant proportion of polycythemia vera patients first present with isolated thrombocytosis without elevated hematocrit and are considered to have essential thrombocythemia.[202]

Qualitative abnormalities of the platelets have been described. Patients with polycythemia vera, essential thrombocythemia, and other myeloproliferative disorders have a very unusual, nearly pathognomic defect in the primary wave of platelet aggregation induced by epinephrine.[203] In contrast there is increased platelet thromboxane A_2 generation[204] and increased excretion of thromboxane metabolites,[205] even though the response to thromboxane A_2 may be subnormal.[206] Platelet factor-4 levels are elevated,[207] and platelet survival is normal[208] or shortened.[200,207] Fibrinogen binding after stimulation with platelet activating factor is diminished,[209] and there is reduced expression of the thrombopoietin receptor.[39] However, none of these changes is specific for polycythemia vera.

In a prospective study, the Pl^{A2} polymorphism of the platelet glycoprotein (Gp) IIIa was associated with an increased risk for arterial thrombosis in polycythemia vera patients.[210] However, polymorphisms of GpIb and GpIa, or the presence of the prothrombin G20210A mutation or factor V Leiden mutation, did not correlate with thrombohemorrhagic events.[210]

PLASMA

Serum lysozyme levels are slightly increased in some patients[211] and, because of the increased leukocyte turnover, levels of vitamin B_{12} usually are increased.[212] Hyperuricemia, a consequence of hyperproliferative myelopoiesis, is frequently encountered.[50]

PRIMARY FAMILIAL AND CONGENITAL POLYCYTHEMIA

Characteristic laboratory findings of PFCP are (1) an increased red blood cell mass without increased leukocyte or platelet counts, (2) normal vitamin B_{12} levels, (3) a normal hemoglobin-oxygen dissociation curve, (4) low serum erythropoietin levels, and (5) in vitro hypersensitivity of erythroid progenitors to erythropoietin.[5] PFCP often is misdiagnosed as polycythemia vera. Many of these patients have been treated with radioactive phosphorus and/or chemotherapy. Occasionally, this use leads to a second clonal myeloid disease. Whereas the leukocytes typically are normal, platelet counts often are mildly decreased, presumably by dilution of the normal platelet mass by an often dramatic increase of red cell and whole blood volumes. Some patients come to attention because of concurrent medical problems that may cause leukocytosis and secondary thrombocytosis, falsely suggesting the phenotype of polycythemia vera.

CHUVASH POLYCYTHEMIA

This type of polycythemia is associated with high serum erythropoietin, total plasminogen-activator inhibitor-1 (an HIF-1 regulated gene),

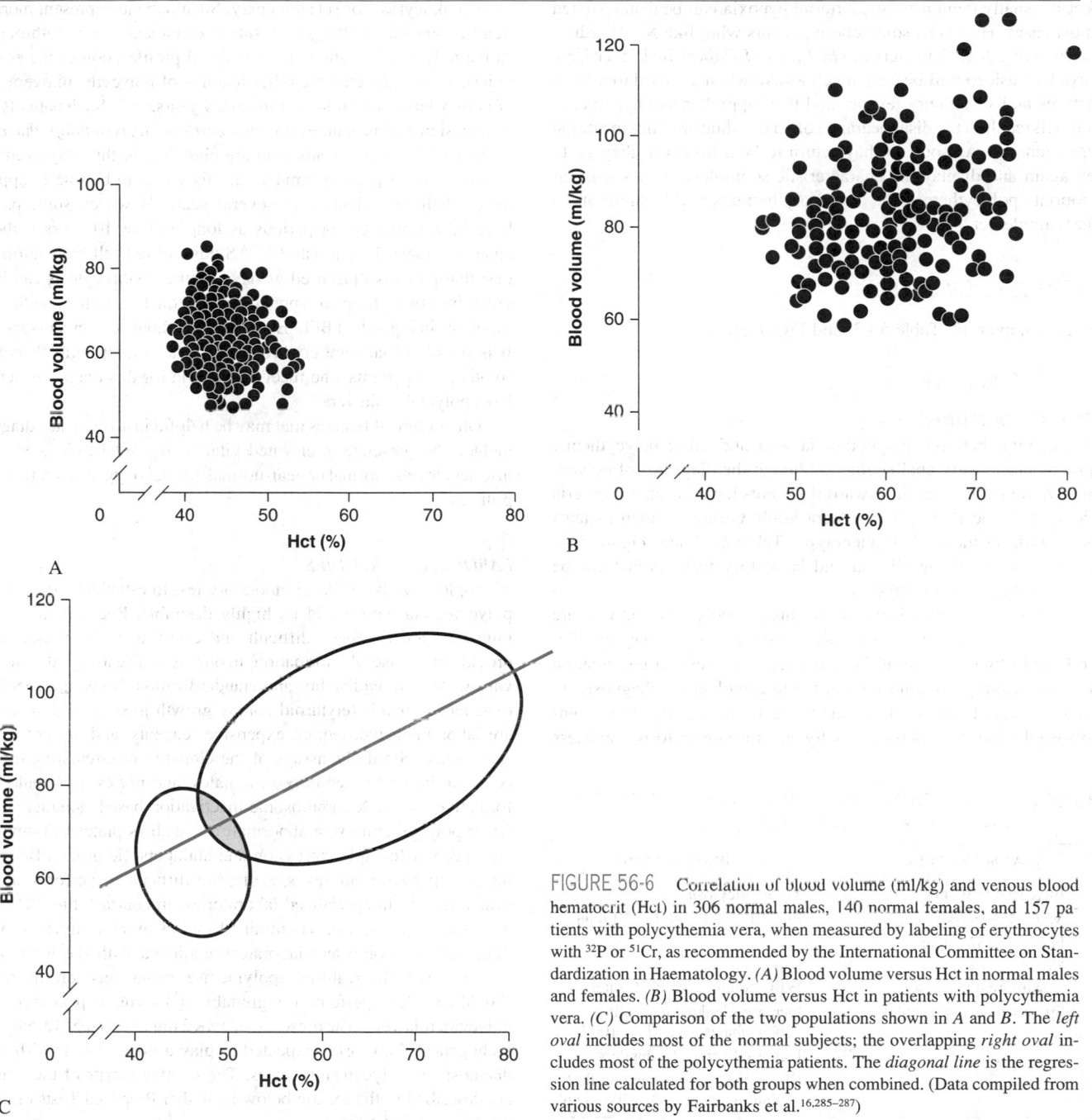

FIGURE 56-6   Correlation of blood volume (ml/kg) and venous blood hematocrit (Hct) in 306 normal males, 140 normal females, and 157 patients with polycythemia vera, when measured by labeling of erythrocytes with ^{32}P or ^{51}Cr, as recommended by the International Committee on Standardization in Haematology. *(A)* Blood volume versus Hct in normal males and females. *(B)* Blood volume versus Hct in patients with polycythemia vera. *(C)* Comparison of the two populations shown in *A* and *B*. The *left oval* includes most of the normal subjects; the overlapping *right oval* includes most of the polycythemia patients. The *diagonal line* is the regression line calculated for both groups when combined. (Data compiled from various sources by Fairbanks et al.[16,285–287])

and serum VEGF levels.[96,97,108] Hemoglobin-adjusted serum erythropoietin concentrations were approximately 10-fold higher in *VHL* 598C→T homozygotes than in controls.[97,98,108]

The serum ferritin and circulating transferrin receptor levels are higher in Chuvash polycythemia homozygotes compared to their unaffected relatives and spouses.[97,98,108] The ferritin-adjusted transferrin receptor concentration was approximately threefold higher in *VHL* 598C→T homozygotes than in unaffected participants ($p < 0.0005$), which is consistent with up-regulation by HIF-1. This finding indicates that storage iron is similar between *VHL* 598C→T homozygotes and unaffected controls despite the dramatically higher hemoglobin concentrations and phlebotomy therapy in Chuvash polycythemia patients.

Chuvash polycythemia is a recently described disorder, so additional laboratory findings resulting from augmentation of hypoxia sensing are expected to be described.

SECONDARY POLYCYTHEMIA

Characteristically only the numbers of erythrocytes in the blood are increased. Increase in the leukocyte count and splenomegaly may be present as other features of the underlying disease, such as pulmonary infection in chronic obstructive lung disease with *cor pulmonale*, or as seen in Monge disease among Andean high dwellers and patients inheriting high-affinity hemoglobin that is also unstable (see Chaps. 32 and 47). In patients with appropriate polycythemia the underlying defect is usually demonstrable. Arterial hypoxia can be demonstrated in most cases. However, some obese patients who, like Mr. Wardle's proverbial boy Joe, characters in *The Pickwick Papers* by Dickens, are always half asleep will be very much awake when exposed to arterial punctures and ventilatory testing, and their apprehensive hyperventilation will result in the disappearance of all the abnormalities in arterial oxygen tension. As soon as they return to bed, however, they go to sleep again and display the characteristic somnolent cyanosis. In inappropriate polycythemia, the laboratory findings will be those of the underlying defect.

DIFFERENTIAL DIAGNOSIS

See also Chapter 32, Table 56-3, and Figure 56-7.

POLYCYTHEMIA VERA

CLINICAL FEATURES
Distinguishing between polycythemia vera and other polycythemic disorders can be very challenging. Although the diagnosis of polycythemia vera may be straightforward if patients have the classic criteria as defined by the Polycythemia Vera Study Group,[157] often patients present with an incomplete phenotype. Table 56-3 and Figure 56-7 summarize some of the clinical and laboratory features that can be helpful for differential diagnosis.

The most important diagnostic features of polycythemia vera are *erythrocytosis, leukocytosis, thrombocytosis,* and *splenomegaly*. Frequently only two or three of these features are found at presentation and, if sufficiently pronounced, suffice to establish the diagnosis. In some patients only one of these features is found initially, most commonly erythrocytosis, but occasionally only thrombocytosis[202] and less

often leukocytosis or splenomegaly. Such patients represent more difficult diagnostic challenges. A subset of patients with erythrocytosis as the only manifestation of unregulated proliferation of the erythropoiesis do not develop the other features of polycythemia vera, even after they have been followed for many years.[213,214] Such patients have been designated as manifesting *pure erythrocytosis* or *idiopathic erythrocytosis*.[215] Some patients who are classified in this way eventually develop typical polycythemia vera; this seems to be true in approximately half of patients after several years. However, some patients have been observed for periods as long as 8 or 10 years without a change in their clinical state.[214–216] Studies of red cell progenitors suggest that patients diagnosed as having pure erythrocytosis can be divided into two groups of approximately equal size: those with erythropoietin-independent BFU-E and those without such precursors.[214,216] It is possible that pure erythrocytosis is a distinct entity[309] but that some of the patients who meet the criteria for this diagnosis actually have polycythemia vera.

Other clinical features that may be helpful in arriving at a diagnosis include the presence of elevated vitamin B_{12} levels, elevated serum uric acid levels, normal or near-normal arterial oxygen saturations, and pruritus.

LABORATORY STUDIES
A simple, readily available laboratory test to establish a diagnosis of polycythemia vera would be highly desirable. Red cell mass determinations are relatively difficult and costly to perform and do not provide much useful information, in our view. The assays that are used vary widely in availability and standardization. Some are specific in experienced hands (erythroid colony growth in semisolid media) but are labor intensive, require expensive reagents, and are not easy to standardize. Similarly, assays of the clonality of circulating myeloid cells can be performed only in females, and not every female is informative for the X chromosome inactivation-based clonality studies. Other polycythemia vera abnormalities, such as platelet thrombopoietin receptor (c-Mpl) expression and antiapoptotic protein Bcl-x erythroid expression, are not specific, are difficult to perform, and are available only in specialized laboratories. In contrast, the PRV-1 test is conceptually simple, has minimal interassay and intraassay variation, and any competent laboratory equipped with the increasingly widely available real-time polymerase chain reaction instrument should be able to perform it; regrettably it does not appear specific for polycythemia vera. The presence of JAK2 mutation (see "Etiology and Pathogenesis" above) is expected to play a major role in differential diagnosis of polycythemic states. The relative merits of these assays are described in the section below in "Other Proposed Tests of Potential Diagnostic Utility."

Red Cell Mass Determination The polycythemia vera study group has used direct determination of the red cell mass as the *sine qua non* of the diagnosis of polycythemia vera in patients entered into their studies.[155] It has been suggested that even in the routine clinical setting, this procedure should be performed on all patients to establish the diagnosis.[155,217] Unfortunately, the determination of the red cell mass is expensive and, when performed by the inexperienced, often inaccurate.[218] It is not useful for distinguishing polycythemia vera from secondary polycythemia, the differentiation that is usually needed, because it is increased in both disorders. The principal value of a red cell mass determination might then be to distinguish apparent or spurious polycythemia from polycythemia vera and secondary polycythemia. Ideally, the red cell volume and plasma volume should be measured separately. Unfortunately the ^{131}I-labeled albumin necessary to measure the plasma volume often is unavailable. Fortunately, in most cases the diagnosis of polycythemia

TABLE 56-3 *A.* POLYCYTHEMIA VERA STUDY GROUP CRITERIA FOR THE DIAGNOSIS OF POLYCYTHEMIA VERA

	MAJOR CRITERIA		MINOR CRITERIA
A1	Increased RBC mass Male: ≥36 ml/kg Female: ≥32 ml/kg	B1	Thrombocytosis Platelet count >400 × 10⁹/liter
A2	Normal arterial O_2 saturation (> 92%)	B2	Leukocytosis WBC count > 12 × 10⁹/liter
A3	Splenomegaly (palpable)	B3	Increased leukocyte alkaline phosphatase* (LAP > 100 U)
		B4	Increased serum B_{12}/binders* (B_{12} > 900 pg/ml; unbound B12 binding capacity > 2200 pg/ml)

Diagnosis virtually certain if all three major criteria *or* A1 + A2 + any two minor criteria.

B. WORLD HEALTH ORGANIZATION CRITERIA FOR THE DIAGNOSIS OF POLYCYTHEMIA VERA

Elevated RBC mass without obvious spontaneous erythroid colony growth in culture
AND

One of the following	*or*	*Two of the following*
Splenomegaly		Platelet count >400 × 10⁹/liter
Karyotypic abnormality other than t9:22		WBC >12 × 10⁹/liter
Endogenous erythroid colony formation		Bone marrow showing panmyelosis
		Low serum erythropoietin level

* Not specific for polycythemia vera; see text.
  RBC=red blood cell; WBC=white blood cell.

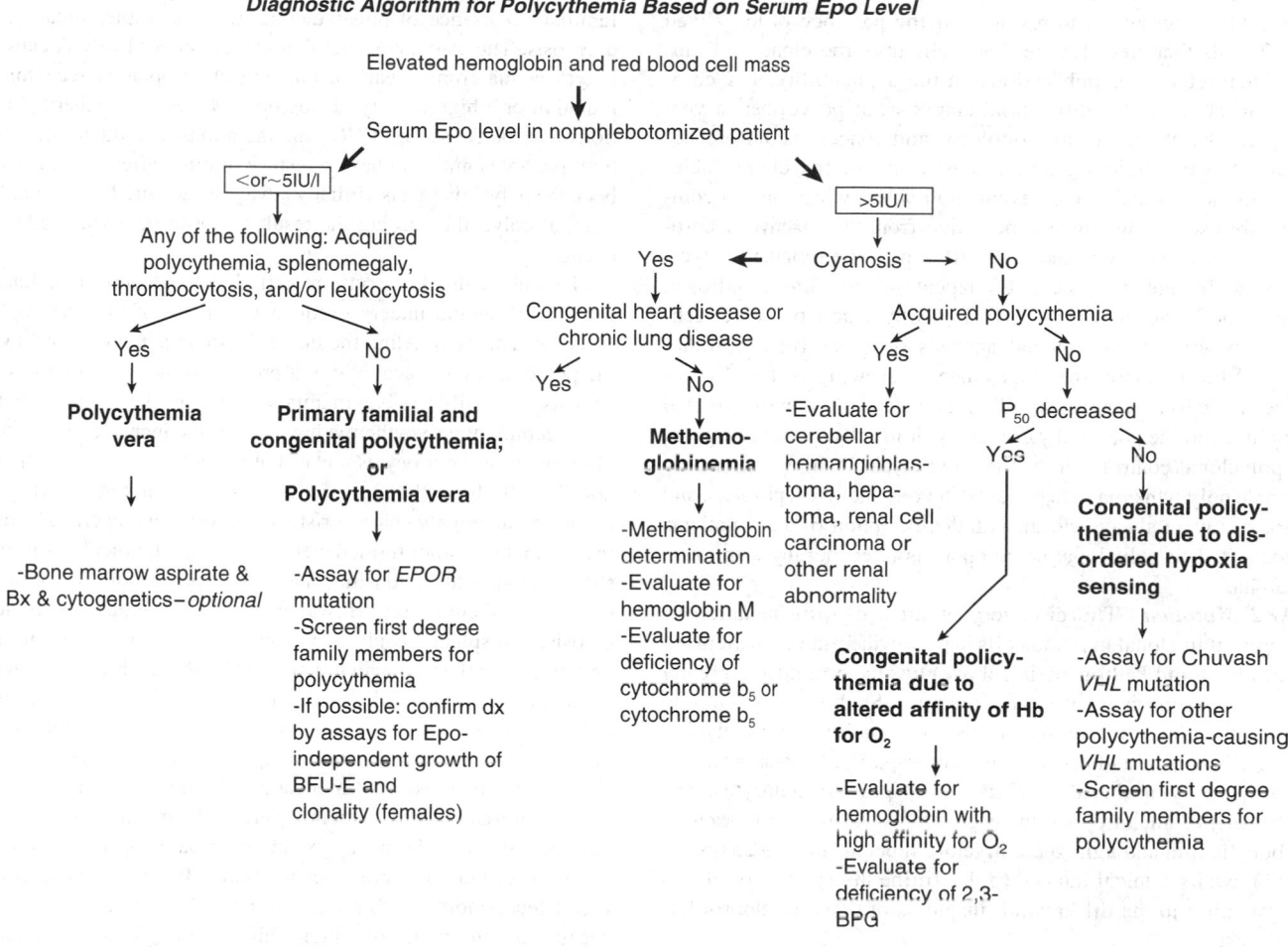

FIGURE 56-7   Diagnostic algorithm for polycythemia based on erythropoietin (Epo) level. BFU-E, burst forming unit–erythroid; 2,3-BPG, 2,3-bisphosphoglycerate; *EPOR*, erythropoietin receptor gene; *VHL*, von Hippel-Landau gene.

vera can be established with confidence without measuring the red cell volume.

Erythroid Colony Cultures   *In vitro* assays of erythroid progenitor cells permit the study of their responsiveness to erythropoietin. This can be applied to polycythemia vera and erythroid progenitor growth without added erythropoietin,[219] referred to as "endogenous erythroid colonies." Detection of endogenous erythroid colonies in cultures of marrow or blood may be the most specific test for polycythemia vera.[22,220,221] In one study, all patients with polycythemia vera but none with secondary or other causes of polycythemia had endogenous erythroid colonies.[216] Rare endogenous erythroid colonies may at times be observed in PFCP and in Chuvash polycythemia, but unlike the endogenous erythroid colonies of polycythemia vera, these are abrogated by pretreatment with erythropoietin and erythropoietin receptor blocking antibodies.[183,222]

In experienced hands, endogenous erythroid colonies is a specific and sensitive means for detecting polycythemia vera and may be useful in diagnosing patients with unusual presentations of polycythemia vera, such as Budd-Chiari syndrome[161,162,223,224] or isolated thrombocytosis.[202] However, this test has not been standardized, is expensive and laborious, and technical variations make interlaboratory results difficult to compare.

Erythropoietin Levels   Because polycythemia vera is distinguished by the fact that erythroid cells proliferate even in the absence of substantial levels of erythropoietin, one would expect that at high

hematocrit levels the production of erythropoietin would be inhibited and the serum levels consequently reduced. Older erythropoietin assays were too insensitive to detect subnormal levels of erythropoietin; however, using improved technology, several studies have documented serum erythropoietin levels below the normal reference range in patients with polycythemia vera.[225–227] Erythropoietin levels remain low even after phlebotomy,[225] which increases erythropoietin levels in normal individuals. Patients with secondary polycythemia usually have normal to elevated erythropoietin levels, although considerable overlap exists in the range of erythropoietin levels between patients with polycythemia vera and those with secondary polycythemia.[227,228] Although an elevated erythropoietin level, or inappropriately normal erythropoietin level for an elevated hematocrit, generally excludes the diagnosis of polycythemia vera, a low erythropoietin level is not pathognomonic of polycythemia vera because patients with PFCP have as low or lower erythropoietin levels; however, erythropoietin level is a valuable laboratory tool in the differential diagnosis of polycythemic disorders.[23,310]

Clonality in Female Subjects Using Assays Based on X Chromosome-Based Polymorphism   Polycythemia vera results from an acquired mutation in a pluripotential hematopoietic progenitor cell. Clonality studies based on the phenomenon of X chromosome inactivation[229] have shown that red cells, granulocytes, platelets, monocytes, and B lymphocytes all are part of the clone.[36,230] The majority of T lymphocytes and natural killer cells are polyclonal, but a small proportion of these cells are also derived from the polycythemia vera clone.[21] This is presumed to result from the presence of long-lived normal T cells that preceded the development of the clone. Unfortunately, interpretation of publications on the applicability of X chromosome inactivation for differential diagnosis of polycythemia vera is hampered by the many methodologic and conceptual differences that have drawn conflicting conclusions. Some of the discrepancies result from the fact that two different approaches, which are not comparable, are used to distinguish the active from the inactive X chromosome: one using X chromosome differential methylation,[231] typically using the polymorphic CAG repeat in the human androgen receptor gene,[232] versus the more biologically sound but more technically demanding transcriptional analysis of the active X chromosome.[233,234] Furthermore, the wide range of skewing of the X chromosome allelic usage that is normally present[235] is often misinterpreted as clonality, and the potentially clonal myeloid cells are not compared to the polyclonal control cells of the same origin.[221] In approximately 100 female polycythemia vera patients, the reticulocytes, platelets, and granulocytes were always clonal with the exception of a few patients who converted to polyclonal hematopoiesis after therapy with interferon alpha.[221]

JAK2 Mutation   The discovery of an activating mutation of JAK2 present in clonal myeloid cells in polycythemia vera patients[303] (see "Etiology and Pathogenesis" above) has the potential to greatly improve the diagnosis of polycythemia vera. Studies are ongoing to determine the diagnostic utility of this mutation by either analyzing genomic DNA of blood leukocytes versus purified clonal granulocytes or quantifying the level of its transcript in granulocytes. The presence of this mutation in those patients with apparent essential thrombocythemia and agnogenic myeloid metaplasia (see Chaps. 89 and 111) awaits clinical studies to determine the specificity of this JAK2 mutation in the differential diagnosis of these myeloproliferative diseases.

Other Proposed Tests of Potential Diagnostic Utility   *c-Mpl.* Thrombopoietin, a potent stimulator of platelet production, is produced at a constant rate, and its levels are regulated by binding to its receptor c-Mpl. Levels of c-Mpl on platelets and megakaryocytes have been reported to be decreased in patients with polycythemia vera.[39] The major limitations of an assay of c-Mpl levels in the diagnosis of polycythemia vera are its difficulty and nonspecificity.[22]

bcl-x.   Increased expression of *bcl-x,* an antiapoptotic gene, occurs in polycythemia vera erythroid progenitors,[40] but this finding is not specific for polycythemia vera.

Polycythemia Rubra V-1.   Increased mRNA levels of a receptor named polycythemia rubra vera-1 (PRV-1) has been reported in polycythemia vera granulocytes but not their progenitors.[42] The exact function of PRV-1 in normal hematopoiesis is unclear, and it likely plays no significant role in polycythemia vera pathophysiology because no differences in the amount of this protein between normal and polycythemia vera progenitors are noted; however, it may be a useful diagnostic marker of the disease. Depending on the report, 80 to 100 percent of polycythemia vera patients have increased granulocyte PRV-1 mRNA. However, elevations are also seen after granulocyte colony stimulating factor therapy, and because it is also observed in patients with other polycythemias, PRV-1 mRNA levels cannot reliably discriminate polycythemia vera from congenital polycythemias and various disorders with thrombocytoses.[22,221,236]

OTHER POLYCYTHEMIAS

The clinical history is of the utmost importance for the differential diagnosis of polycythemic states. The differentiation of an acquired from a congenital disorder and a distinction between sporadic versus familial occurrence of polycythemia, when possible, streamline the diagnosis. Thus, an autosomal dominant disorder likely is caused by polycythemia from a gain-of-function erythropoietin receptor gene mutation or a high-affinity hemoglobin. Recessively inherited conditions may be caused by *VHL* gene mutations. Although rare patients with polycythemia vera have a history of other affected family members, the polycythemia is virtually always an acquired condition. Many familial polycythemias are the result of yet-to-be-discovered genetic events.

Patients with a low erythropoietin level and autosomal dominant inheritance should undergo sequence analysis of the erythropoietin receptor. This will define the defect in some patients with PFCP. If the polycythemia is acquired and present in multiple relatives, a diagnosis of familial polycythemia vera should be pursued. Patients with secondary polycythemia have a genuine increase in the number of circulating erythrocytes and of the red cell mass. Such patients do not typically have the increase in the platelet and leukocyte counts or the splenomegaly characteristic of polycythemia vera. The lack of involvement of other formed elements in hematopoietic proliferation should arouse suspicion that the patient has a polycythemia other than polycythemia vera. However, reactive thrombocytosis, leukocytosis, and splenomegaly may occasionally also be present in secondary polycythemia, which then renders the distinction from polycythemia vera more difficult. In patients in whom secondary polycythemia is caused by lung or cardiac disease, clubbing is often present. In some cases, determining the arterial oxygen saturation clarifies the diagnosis, but modest arterial oxygen desaturation may also be present in polycythemia vera.[77,197] Imaging of the kidneys may reveal a neoplasm or cyst in some patients. Determining the oxygen dissociation curve, or estimation of P_{50} from venous blood,[237] will detect abnormalities related to increased oxygen affinity, either because of inheritance of a high-affinity hemoglobin (see Chap. 47) or because of very rare 2,3-BPG depletion, as in phosphoglyceromutase deficiency (see Chap. 45). The mild polycythemia associated with hereditary methemoglobinemia (see Chap. 48) is readily diagnosed because of coexistent cyanosis.

In patients with elevated erythropoietin or erythropoietin levels inappropriately normal for the degree of hemoglobin elevation, analysis of *VHL* gene may be in order. Some of these patients may have a history of autosomal recessive inheritance, and they have a typical history of congenital polycythemia. It may also be useful to determine the carboxyhemoglobin level of the blood if smoker's polycythemia is suspected.

SPURIOUS POLYCYTHEMIA

The erythrocytosis observed in patients with spurious polycythemia (apparent polycythemia, stress polycythemia) is a consequence of a decrease in the plasma volume.[149] The erythrocytosis that is observed does not represent a true increase in the red cell mass. Usually the increase in the hematocrit is very modest. Such patients do not have an increased white blood count, thrombocytosis, or splenomegaly. The arterial oxygen saturation is normal. Estimation of the red cell mass and plasma volume is required to establish a diagnosis of spurious polycythemia, but it should be recognized that during the natural history of patients who develop primary or secondary polycythemia their red cell mass is, at some point, within the normal range while it is rising to abnormal values. However, because of the significant error rate of red cell volume measurement, it is recommended that both red cell volume and plasma volume be measured simultaneously.

THERAPY

POLYCYTHEMIA VERA

PLETHORIC PHASE

The treatment of patients in the plethoric phase of the disease is aimed at ameliorating symptoms and decreasing the risk of thrombosis or bleeding by reducing the blood counts. The red count and hematocrit can be controlled in some patients by periodic phlebotomy, but administration of drugs that suppress marrow activity also is required to control the platelet and white counts. Both treatment modalities are used in most patients. Table 56-4 summarizes the advantages and disadvantages of various forms of therapy.

Phlebotomy The usual initial treatment for most patients is phlebotomy.[50,238] The rationale for phlebotomy therapy of polycythemia vera is based on a widely quoted paper that suggested that the risk of thrombosis in polycythemia vera was proportional to the elevation in hematocrit.[239] The underlying mechanisms causing thrombosis in polycythemia vera are not fully known, but the hematocrit likely is not the only, and may not even be the principal, risk factor. Large studies of patients with polycythemia of high altitude or resulting from Eisenmenger syndrome[83] and other cyanotic heart diseases[189] argue against hematocrit as the only factor causing thrombosis. When 100 cyanotic patients with congenital heart disease were observed for a total of 748 patient-years, no patient with polycythemia developed cerebral arterial thrombosis.[240] Shibata and colleagues[190] studied a transgenic mouse with extreme polycythemia resulting from constitutive overexpression of erythropoietin. They expected this to be a useful model for thrombotic complications that are a major cause of mortality and morbidity of individuals with polycythemia vera, but this was not observed. Additionally, the increased risk of strokes in Chuvash polycythemia does not appear to be statistically different in those affected patients whose hematocrit is controlled by phlebotomies. Further, the European Collaboration on Low-Dose Aspirin in Polycythemia Vera study, which included 1638 patients from 12 participating countries and 94 centers, did not find differences in thrombotic complications when hematocrit ranged between 40 and 50.

When phlebotomy is instituted, the hematocrit may be reduced to normal or near-normal values by removal of 450 to 500 ml of blood at intervals of 2 to 4 days for average-size patients, with smaller amounts removed from patients weighing less than 50 kg. The shorter interval is appropriate for patients with hematocrit values over 64 percent, whereas less energetic bleeding suffices for those who have only a modest increase in hematocrit. Patients with impaired cardiovascular functions are better treated with smaller phlebotomies at more frequent intervals.

The immediate effect of phlebotomies is to reduce the hematocrit, which results in improvement of symptoms such as headaches. It neither reduces the leukocyte or platelet count nor affects symptoms such as pruritus or gout. Iron deficiency is the usual consequence of repeated phlebotomy. The deficient state helps to control the hematocrit; when iron is administered to polycythemia vera patients who have been rendered iron deficient by phlebotomy, rapid increase of the hemoglobin level and hematocrit usually occurs. The iron deficiency that results from repeated phlebotomies causes striking microcytosis, but the viscosity of the blood is a function of the hematocrit and appears to be independent of the number of red cells,[241] and the deformability of iron-deficient erythrocytes appears to be normal.[242] Phlebotomy clearly

is an effective way to normalize the viscosity of the blood of patients with polycythemia vera.

A randomized study comparing phlebotomy alone with treatment with ^{32}P and with chlorambucil indicated that the life span of patients treated only with phlebotomy is better than that of patients treated with chlorambucil and no worse than that of patients given ^{32}P.[155,243] However, patients undergoing phlebotomy suffered more thrombotic episodes than patients treated with myelosuppressive therapy, although the risk seemed to be limited to the first 3 years of therapy.[157] This documented increased risk of phlebotomy is balanced by a lower incidence of leukemia late in the disease course. Surprisingly, there was no correlation between the level of the platelet count and the development of thrombotic complications. Apparently many patients can be well controlled by phlebotomy alone during much or all of their course, and the role of myelosuppressive therapy in the treatment of polycythemia vera has sometimes been questioned.[244] It has been suggested that patients younger than 50 years who have no prior history of thrombosis might be treated with phlebotomy alone,[245] but no rigorous data are available to support this recommendation.

Myelosuppression Although treatment with some myelosuppressive agents appears to increase the incidence of leukemic transformation of patients with polycythemia vera, patients usually are treated with such drugs when the platelet count rises to levels higher than 800 to 1000 × 10^9/liter. Platelet counts at these levels usually cause concern for the risk of bleeding and thrombosis. Myelosuppressive therapy is also considered when thrombotic or bleeding complications occur, when the patient requires phlebotomy at intervals exceeding one every 1 or 2 months, and in patients with severe pruritus.

Hydroxyurea. Hydroxyurea (Hydrea) is the most commonly used myelosuppressive agent for treatment of polycythemia vera. Hydroxyurea is effective therapy for controlling erythrocyte, leukocyte, and platelet counts and decreasing the risk of thrombosis during the first few years of therapy compared to a historical cohort treated with phlebotomy alone.[157] Its suppressive effect is of short duration. Thus, continuous rather than intermittent therapy is required. Because hydroxyurea is short acting, it is relatively safe to use. When excessive marrow suppression occurs, the blood counts rise within a few days or weeks of discontinuing the drug. Moreover, because it is not an alkylating agent, it is believed to have much less potential for causing leukemic transformation than other myelosuppressive agents. When used in conjunction with phlebotomy, the incidence of thrombotic complications appeared to be decreased. After approximately 7-year maximum followup, the incidence of leukemia was slightly higher

TABLE 56-4 TREATMENT OF POLYCYTHEMIA VERA

TREATMENT	ADVANTAGES	DISADVANTAGES
Phlebotomy	Low Risk. Simple to perform.	Does not control thrombocytosis or leukocytosis.
Hydroxyurea	Controls leukocytosis and thrombocytosis. Low leukemogenic risk.	Continuous therapy required.
Busulfan	Easy to administer. Prolonged remissions. Risk of leukemogenesis probably not high.	Overdose produces prolonged marrow suppression. Risks of leukemogenesis, long-term pulmonary and cutaneous toxicity.
^{32}P	Patient compliance not required. Prolonged control of thrombocytosis and leukocytosis.	Expensive and relatively inconvenient. Moderate leukemogenic risk.
Chlorambucil	Easy to administer. Good control of thrombocytosis and leukocytosis.	High risk of leukemogenesis.
Interferon	Low leukemogenic potential. Effect on pruritus.	Inconvenient, costly, frequent side effects.
Anagrelide	Selective effect on platelets.	Selective effect on platelets.

than that in patients treated with phlebotomy alone, but not significantly so.[246] Experience with the use of hydroxyurea for treatment of essential thrombocythemia has indicated a marked reduction of thrombosis to approximately 30 percent of background.[247] Although in most studies hydroxyurea had a higher risk for leukemia transformation, it never reached statistical significance, and its use in sickle cell disease has not shown increase of leukemia or other malignancies.[248]

Busulfan. Administration of busulfan (Myleran) is a convenient and effective means for treatment of polycythemia vera. Marrow suppression produced by this drug is long lasting, so it can be given intermittently. Administration of 2 or 4 mg daily over a period of several weeks is usually sufficient to normalize the blood counts; the counts continue to fall for several weeks after drug administration is discontinued. The counts may then remain normal for many months or even years. In one large study, the median first remission duration of busulfan-treated patients was 4 years.[249]

The prolonged depression of marrow activity that is brought about by busulfan is its major advantage in the treatment of polycythemia vera, but it also poses a hazard. If therapy is continued too long or given at too high a dose, the marrow suppression that results may persist for many months or even 1 year. For this reason it is safer not to exceed a daily dose of 4 mg but to extend the period of treatment rather than to increase the daily dose. The incidence of transformation to acute leukemia in patients treated intermittently with busulfan is relatively low. Of 145 patients followed from 2 to 11 years, only three developed acute leukemia.[249]

Radioactive phosphorus. ^{32}P therapy was one of the first effective modes of treatment used. Extensive investigations of the long-term outcome of treatment with ^{32}P have been documented.[155,250] Good control of the disease usually can be achieved with initial doses of 2 to 4 mC ^{32}P given intravenously, followed in 6 to 8 weeks by doses that are based upon the response to the first dose. ^{32}P treatment is associated with a moderate increase in the incidence of leukemic transformation, similar in magnitude to that observed with busulfan.[249] Because the treatment is administered directly by a physician, it is more suitable than busulfan for patients who cannot be relied upon to take their medication as prescribed. However, the logistics of ^{32}P administration have made it an inconvenient and expensive mode of therapy. Consultation with a radiotherapist is usually required, and each dose must be ordered especially for the patient. It is largely for this reason and because it is generally supposed that the leukemogenic potential of hydroxyurea is lower than that of radioactive phosphorus that the latter has been used less frequently. Some investigators, however, consider it the treatment of choice, especially in older patients.[251,252]

Interferon. Administration of interferon alpha at a starting dose of 3,000,000 U given three times weekly produces a therapeutic response in 50 percent[253] or more[180,254,255] of patients with polycythemia vera. A decrease in the red cell mass, the leukocyte count, and the platelet count has been documented, and it seems effective in ameliorating the pruritus that is common in polycythemia vera. The amelioration of the pruritus does not seem directly related to the hematologic response.[255] It is not clear whether this treatment, which requires frequent injections of a drug that causes toxicity that is troublesome to patients, has any advantage over less costly, more convenient therapies. However, the possibility exists that the incidence of both leukemia and myelofibrosis may be lower in interferon-treated patients,[255] and in the small number of patients studied thus far the clonal hematopoiesis converted to a polyclonal state.[221] It appears to be a drug of choice in pregnant patients (see Chap. 7).

Pipobroman. Although it was described in the early 1960s and appears to be effective in controlling polycythemia vera, pipobroman (Vercyte) has not been used as frequently as ^{32}P, busulfan, or hydroxyurea. However, it remains in active use in some countries.[256–258] Hem-

atologic remission is achieved in more than 90 percent of previously untreated patients[259,260] and is maintained for long periods of time. Gastrointestinal intolerance can be a problem.[204,257] The risk of leukemia is relatively high, observed in 6 and 9 percent of patients at 5 and 7 years of treatment and in 27 percent at 14 years in one study[257] and in the European Collaboration on Low-Dose Aspirin in Polycythemia Vera study.[159]

Anagrelide. Among 113 patients with polycythemia vera who had thrombocytosis, administration of anagrelide (Agrylin) produced a platelet response in 85 (75%).[261] It was suggested that the higher rates of response might be expected when the drug was administered by those more skilled in its use. The starting dose was 0.5 or 1.0 mg given four times daily, and a response was noted in most patients within 1 week. The average dose required to control the platelet count was 2.4 mg/day. Adverse events included headache, palpitations, diarrhea, and fluid retention and were occasionally sufficiently severe to require discontinuation of the treatment.[262] The United Kingdom randomized trial claims superior results for hydroxyurea compared to anagrelide for control of elevated platelet count, myelofibrosis, and hemorrhagic complications in essential thrombocythemia.[48]

Imatinib mesylate. Imatinib mesylate (Gleevec) is a tyrosine kinase inhibitor that can inactivate kinases resulting from cancer-causing somatic mutations. It has been very effective in the therapy of chronic myelogenous leukemia in which the tyrosine kinase mutation is the result of a chromosomal translocation. Diseases including chronic myelomonocytic leukemia (see Chap. 88), chronic eosinophilic leukemia, formerly hypereosinophilic syndrome (see Chap. 88), mastocytosis (see Chap. 63), Langerhans cell histiocytosis (see Chap. 72), and gastrointestinal stromal tumors have responded to the drug.[263,264] An imatinib mesylate-sensitive tyrosine phosphokinase has been identified in the leukocytes of some patients with polycythemia vera.[265] Early trials of imatinib have indicated that its use may decrease phlebotomy requirements in patients with polycythemia, but there is no evidence as yet that it can be used as primary therapy.

Symptomatic Therapy for Pruritus Many of the symptoms of polycythemia are controlled either by phlebotomy or by controlling the number of red cells and platelet mass with myelosuppressive therapy. Pruritus is a frequent exception. It tends to be more severe when the disease is active and becomes milder or disappears when control is achieved by myelosuppression. Nonetheless, in some patients it becomes a nearly intolerable annoyance. Because the itching usually is intensified by bathing or showering, often the best advice that can be offered is to bathe less frequently. Photochemotherapy with psoralens and ultraviolet light has been found to be helpful.[266] Antihistamines usually are not very effective. Aspirin[267] and cyproheptadine[198] each has been recommended. Interferon alpha has been helpful in some patients.[253,254,268]

Aspirin Because thromboembolic episodes represent a major source of morbidity and mortality in patients with polycythemia, attempts using aspirin and dipyridamole to prevent such episodes have been made. The results of early trials using 300 mg of aspirin daily have indicated an increase in the incidence of bleeding without a favorable impact on the incidence of thrombotic episodes.[269] Administration of low-dose aspirin has been suggested in patients with a vascular occlusion.[270] A pilot controlled trial showed that low-dose aspirin was well tolerated by polycythemia vera patients and is sufficient to fully inhibit synthesis of the platelet-aggregating compound thromboxane but not the endothelial cell protectant prostacyclin.[271] The European Collaboration on Low-Dose Aspirin in Polycythemia Vera study showed that daily low-dose aspirin decreases arterial and venous thromboses, albeit to a small extent.[159] Because most of the thrombotic complications were not prevented, this study suggests that only a minor fraction of thromboses are attributable to platelets and raises a question regarding the mechanism of thrombosis in polycythemia vera. Is the elevated leukocyte count a contributing factor to thrombotic complications? Multivariate analysis of a study of hydroxyurea in sickle cell disease revealed a benefit to decreasing neutrophils in preventing sickle cell vascular events.[272] The possibility that cytoreductive agents affect platelets and/or endothelial cells is an inadequately explored area.

Hydration Because dehydration may be a precipitating factor for thrombosis, patients should be kept well hydrated when they develop intercurrent gastrointestinal disorders.

SPENT PHASE

Ultimately, sometimes after only a few years and sometimes after 20 or more years, the erythrocytosis of patients with polycythemia vera who have not succumbed to other complications gradually abates, phlebotomy requirements decrease and then end, and anemia develops. During this "spent" phase of the disease, marrow fibrosis becomes more marked, and the spleen often becomes greatly enlarged. Instead of phlebotomies, transfusions now may be required. The platelet count may remain high or may decline, even to thrombocytopenic levels. Marked leukocytosis may occur with the appearance of immature granulocytes in the blood. At this point the disease mimics closely idiopathic myelofibrosis (see Chap. 89). Treatment of this phase of the disease is almost entirely symptomatic. Irradiation of the spleen usually is not helpful, and use of chemotherapy with busulfan or hydroxyurea is precluded by the advancing thrombocytopenia.

Splenectomy Occasionally splenectomy may be warranted, particularly if there is severe thrombocytopenia, the transfusion requirement becomes very high, or a greatly enlarged spleen produces severe physical discomfort.[273] However, a large Mayo clinic series reported a significant mortality and morbidity associated with splenectomy.[274]

Thalidomide Thalidomide and antiangiogenic agents that may ameliorate anemia, thrombocytopenia, and splenomegaly are under investigation. However, this response occurs only in a small proportion of patients, and side effects are common.[158]

Marrow Transplantation A few younger patients have undergone successful allogeneic marrow transplantation.[275] Nonmyeloablative stem cell transplantation, a procedure that may be performed in otherwise fit people in the sixth and seventh decades of life (see Chap. 22), has shown promise.[276]

JAK2 Targeted Inhibitors Taking lessons from the successful therapy of chronic myelocytic leukemia with imatinib mesylate, it is possible that similar compounds will be developed to inhibit constitutively active JAK2 tyrosine kinase activity associated with the JAK2 mutation present in polycythemia vera.

OTHER POLYCYTHEMIAS

Treatment of patients with postrenal transplant erythrocytosis using drugs that suppress the renal-angiotensin system has virtually eliminated the need for therapeutic phlebotomy. The maximal reduction of hemoglobin and hematocrit levels usually manifests by 6 months after starting therapy with either the angiotensin-converting enzyme inhibitor enalapril or the angiotensin II receptor type 1 blocker losartan.[127] Some patients are exquisitely sensitive and may become severely anemic.

High-altitude polycythemia is also associated with proteinuria and elevated blood pressure. The prospective randomized trial of enalapril reported decreased hemoglobin concentration, proteinuria, and beneficial effect on elevated blood pressure.[277]

When erythrocytosis is secondary to a renal tumor or cyst, pheochromocytoma, myoma, or brain tumor, removal of the neoplasm usually has resulted in disappearance of the erythrocytosis.

Lowering the hematocrit to a normal or near-normal level by phlebotomy is the usual treatment of secondary polycythemia[278,279] but should always be viewed in the context of a particular polycythemic subject.[83,189] The appropriate level is that at which the patient becomes asymptomatic. Although cytotoxic agents are sometimes used for this purpose, phlebotomy is preferred because of the leukemogenic risk of the agents used in polycythemia vera.

One should phlebotomize only those patients who are symptomatic from the elevated red cell mass and continue to do so cautiously only if symptoms respond promptly to phlebotomy.

COURSE AND PROGNOSIS

POLYCYTHEMIA VERA

Thrombotic complications discussed in preceding sections are the dominant cause of morbidity and mortality of polycythemia vera. However, in contrast to other polycythemic disorders, polycythemia vera has a increased risk of evolution to leukemia. Although several clinical stages of polycythemia vera are recognized (plethoric or proliferative phase, stable phase, spent phase, postpolycythemic myeloid metaplasia phase, acute leukemia), it is not clear that these stages represent a sequential progression of the disease.

The Polycythemia Vera Study Group[155] found that the median survival from the beginning of treatment was 13.9 years for patients treated by phlebotomy alone, 11.8 years for ^{32}P-treated patients, and 8.9 years for chlorambucil-treated patients. Thrombosis was the most common cause of death, accounting for 31 percent of fatalities. Nineteen percent of the patients died of acute leukemia, 15 percent of other neoplasms, and approximately 5 percent each from hemorrhage or development of the spent phase. Similarly, a large French study revealed a median survival of 13.5 years of polycythemia vera patients initially treated with ^{32}P, only slightly less that the 15.2 years of age-matched controls.[255] Others suggested that polycythemia vera is a disease that is compatible with normal or near-normal life for many years.[280,281] However, most studies agree that there is excess mortality of polycythemia vera and that is attributable to thrombotic complications and leukemia transformation as a direct consequence of polycythemia vera.[159] Leukemia occurs even in patients who have been treated only by phlebotomy, although its incidence is increased by the various forms of cytotoxic therapy used (Table 56-4). Although acute myeloid leukemia is most common, acute lymphoid leukemia[282] and chronic neutrophilic leukemia[283] also have been documented.

CHUVASH POLYCYTHEMIA

In a study of 96 patients with Chuvash polycythemia diagnosed before 1977, 65 spouses and 79 community members of the same age, sex, and village of birth, the estimated survival to 65 years was no greater than 31 percent for Chuvash polycythemia patients versus 67 percent and greater for spouses and community members ($p \leq 0.002$).[108]

OTHER POLYCYTHEMIAS

The clinical course of secondary polycythemia is largely a function of the underlying disorder. In patients with PFCP secondary to mutations of the erythropoietin receptor gene, coronary artery disease and strokes have been reported,[183] although not in all series.[184] However, the rarity of PFCP secondary to mutations of the erythropoietin receptor gene and polycythemias from globin mutations and/or red cell enzyme deficiencies precludes any meaningful prognostic evaluation; however, the effect of gain of function of erythropoietin receptor mutation is currently being evaluated in animal models of this disorder.[284]

REFERENCES

1. Vaquez MH: Sur une forme spéciale de cyanose s'accompagnant d'hyperglobulie excessive et persistante. *CR Soc Biol* 44:384, 1892.

2. Osler W: Chronic cyanosis, with polycythemia and enlarged spleen: A new clinical entity. *Am J Med Sci* 126:187, 1903.

3. Türk W: Beitrage zur Kenntnis des Symptomenbildes Polycythamie mit Milztumor und Zyanose. *Wien Klin Wochenschr* 17:153, 1904.

4. Perrine GM, Prchal JT, Prchal JF: Study of a polycythemic family. *Blood* 50:134, 1977.

5. Prchal JT, Crist WM, Goldwasser E, et al: Autosomal dominant polycythemia. *Blood* 66:1208, 1985.

6. Juvonen E, Ikkala E, Fyhrquist F, Ruutu T: Autosomal dominant erythrocytosis caused by increased sensitivity to erythropoietin. *Blood* 78:3066, 1991.

7. Bert P: *La Pression Barometrique.* Masson, Paris, 1878.

8. Jourdanet D: *De l'anemie des altitudes et de l'anemie en general dans ses rapports avec la pression l'atmosphere.* Bailliere, Paris, 1863.

9. Viault F: Sur l'augmentation considerable du nombre des globules rouges dans le sang chez les habitants des hauts plateaux de l'Amerique du Sud. *CR Acad Sci* 111:917, 1890.

10. Erslev AJ: Blood and mountains, in: *Blood, Pure and Eloquent*, edited by MM Wintrobe, p 257. McGraw-Hill, New York, 1980.

11. Leopold SS: The etiology of pulmonary arteriosclerosis (Ayerza's syndrome). *Am J Med* 219:152, 1950.

12. Abbott ME: *Atlas of Congenital Heart Disease.* American Heart Association, New York, 1936.

13. Burwell CS, Robin ED, Whaley RD, Bickelman AG: Extreme obesity associated with alveolar hypoventilation: A Pickwickian syndrome. *Am J Med* 21:811, 1956.

14. Kuhl W: History of clinical research on the sleep apnea syndrome. The early days of polysomnography. *Respiration* 64(suppl 1):5-10:5, 1997.

15. Charache S, Weatherall DJ, Clegg JB: Polycythemia associated with a hemoglobinopathy. *J Clin Invest* 45:813, 1966.

16. Fairbanks VF, Klee GG, Wiseman GA, et al: Measurement of blood volume and red cell mass: Re-examination of ^{51}Cr and ^{125}I methods. *Blood Cells Mol Dis* 22:169, 1996.

17. Lawrence JH, Berlin NI: Relative polycythemia—The polycythemia of stress. *Yale J Biol Med* 24:498, 1952.

18. Ania BJ, Suman VJ, Sobell JL, et al: Trends in the incidence of polycythemia vera among Olmsted County, Minnesota residents, 1935-1989. *Am J Hematol* 47:89, 1994.

19. Kutti J, Ridell B: Epidemiology of the myeloproliferative disorders: Essential thrombocythaemia, polycythaemia vera, and idiopathic myelofibrosis. *Pathol Biol (Paris)* 49:164, 2001.

20. Miller RL, Purvis JD, Weick JK: Familial polycythemia vera. *Cleve Clin J Med* 56:813, 1989.

21. Kralovics R, David W, Stockton DW, Prchal JT: Clonal hematopoiesis in familial polycythemia vera suggests the involvement of multiple mutational events in the early pathogenesis of the disease. *Blood*. 15; 102(10):3793, 2003.

22. Kralovics R, Guan Y, Prchal JT: Acquired uniparental disomy of chromosome 9p is a frequent stem cell defect in polycythemia vera. *Exp Hematol* 30:229, 2002.

23. Prchal JT: Classification and molecular biology of polycythemias (erythrocytoses) and thrombocytosis. *Hematol Oncol Clin North Am* 17:1151, 2003.

24. Thorling EB: Paraneoplastic erythrocytosis and inappropriate erythropoietin production. A review. *Scand J Haematol* 17(suppl):1, 1972.

25. LevGur M, Levie MD: The myomatous erythrocytosis syndrome: A review. *Obstet Gynecol* 86:1026, 1995.

26. Levinson JP, Kinkaid OW: Myxoma of the right atrium associated with polycythemia. Report of successful excision. *N Engl J Med* 264:1187, 1961.

27. Josephs BN, Robbins G, Levine A: Polycythemia secondary to hamartoma of the liver. *JAMA* 179:867, 1961.

28. Sandler A, Rivlin L, Filler R, et al: Polycythemia secondary to focal nodular hyperplasia. *J Pediatr Surg* 32:1386, 1997.

29. Sharma RR, Cast IP, O'Brien C: Supratentorial haemangioblastoma not associated with Von Hippel Lindau complex or polycythaemia: Case report and literature review. *Br J Neurosurg* 9:81, 1995.

30. Constans JP, Meder F, Maiuri F, et al: Posterior fossa hemangioblastomas. *Surg Neurol* 25:269, 1986.

31. Dagher FJ, Ramos E, Erslev AJ, et al: Are the native kidneys responsible for erythrocytosis in renal allorecipients? *Transplantation* 28:496, 1979.

32. Kessler M, Hestin D, Mayeux D, et al: Factors predisposing to postrenal transplant erythrocytosis. A prospective matched-pair control study. *Clin Nephrol* 45:83, 1996.

33. Gaston RS, Julian BA, Curtis JJ: Posttransplant erythrocytosis: An enigma revisited. *Am J Kidney Dis* 24:1, 1994.

34. Lezaic V, Biljanovic-Paunovic L, Pavlovic-Kentera V, Djukanovic L: Erythropoiesis after kidney transplantation: The role of erythropoietin, burst promoting activity and early erythroid progenitor cells. *Eur J Med Res* 6:27, 2001.

35. Polyakova LA: Familial erythrocytosis among inhabitants of the Chuvash ASSR. *Probl Gematol* 10:30, 1974.

36. Adamson JW, Fialkow PJ, Murphy S, et al: Polycythemia vera: Stem-cell and probable clonal origin of the disease. *N Engl J Med* 295:913, 1976.

37. Prchal JF, Adamson JW, Murphy S, et al: Polycythemia vera. The in vitro response of normal and abnormal stem cell lines to erythropoietin. *J Clin Invest* 61:1044, 1978.

38. Eaves CJ, Eaves AC: Erythropoietin (Ep) dose-response curves for three classes of erythroid progenitors in normal human marrow and in patients with polycythemia vera. *Blood* 52:1196, 1978.

39. Moliterno AR, Hankins WD, Spivak JL: Impaired expression of the thrombopoietin receptor by platelets from patients with polycythemia vera. *N Engl J Med* 338:572, 1998.

40. Silva M, Richard C, Benito A, et al: Expression of Bcl-x in erythroid precursors from patients with polycythemia vera. *N Engl J Med* 338:564, 1998.

41. Sui X, Krantz SB, Zhao Z: Identification of increased protein tyrosine phosphatase activity in polycythemia vera erythroid progenitor cells. *Blood* 90:651, 1997.

42. Klippel S, Strunck E, Busse CE, et al: Biochemical characterization of PRV-1, a novel hematopoietic cell surface receptor, which is overexpressed in polycythemia rubra vera. *Blood* 100:2441, 2002.

43. Groopman JE: The pathogenesis of myelofibrosis in myeloproliferative disorders. *Ann Intern Med* 92:857, 1980.

44. Wurster-Hill D, Whang-Peng J, McIntyre OR, et al: Cytogenetic studies in polycythemia vera. *Semin Hematol* 13:13, 1976.

45. Diez-Martin JL, Graham DL, Petitt RM, Dewald GW: Chromosome studies in 104 patients with polycythemia vera. *Mayo Clin Proc* 66:287, 1991.

46. Bench AJ, Nacheva EP, Champion KM, Green AR: Molecular genetics and cytogenetics of myeloproliferative disorders. *Baillieres Clin Haematol* 11:819, 1998.

47. Najfeld V, Montella L, Scalise A, Fruchtman S: Exploring polycythaemia vera with fluorescence in situ hybridization: Additional cryptic 9p is the most frequent abnormality detected. *Br J Haematol* 119:558, 2002.

48. Green A, Campbell P, Buck G, et al: The Medical Research Council PT1 Trial in Essential Thrombocythemia. *Blood* 104(suppl 1):5a, 2004.

49. Swolin B, Weinfeld A, Westin J: A prospective long-term cytogenetic study in polycythemia vera in relation to treatment and clinical course. *Blood* 72:386, 1988.

50. Spivak JL: Polycythemia vera: Myths, mechanisms, and management. *Blood* 100:4272, 2002.

51. Kralovics R, Indrak K, Stopka T, et al: Two new EPO receptor mutations: Truncated EPO receptors are most frequently associated with primary familial and congenital polycythemias. *Blood* 90:2057, 1997.

52. Kralovics R, Prchal JT: Genetic heterogeneity of primary familial and congenital polycythemia. *Am J Hematol* 68:115, 2001.

53. Chetty KG, Light RW, Stansbury DW, Milne N: Exercise performance of polycythemic chronic obstructive pulmonary disease patients. Effect of phlebotomies. *Chest* 98:1073, 1990.

54. Hurtado A: Acclimatization of high altitudes, in: *Physiological Effects of High Altitude*, edited by WH Weihe, p. 1. Macmillan, New York, 1964.

55. Moore LG, Brewer GJ: Beneficial effect of rightward hemoglobin-oxygen dissociation curve shift for short-term high-altitude adaptation. *J Lab Clin Med* 98:145, 1981.

56. Finch CA, Lenfant C: Oxygen transport in man. *N Engl J Med* 286:407, 1972.

57. Winslow RM, Monge CC, Statham NJ, et al: Variability of oxygen affinity of blood: Human subjects native to high altitude. *J Appl Physiol* 51:1411, 1981.

58. Eaton JW, Skelton TD, Berger E: Survival at extreme altitude: Protective effect of increased hemoglobin-oxygen affinity. *Science* 183:743, 1974.

59. Leon-Velarde F, Gamboa A, Chuquiza JA, et al: Hematological parameters in high altitude residents living at 4,355, 4,660, and 5,500 meters above sea level. *High Alt Med Biol* 1:97, 2000.

60. Mejia OM, Prchal JT, Leon-Velarde F, et al: Genetic association analysis of chronic mountain sickness subjects in an Andean high-altitude population. *Haematologica* 90:13, 2005.

61. Monge CC: Life in the Andes and chronic mountain sickness. *Science* 95:79, 1942.

62. Pei SX, Chen XJ, Si Ren BZ, et al: Chronic mountain sickness in Tibet. *Q J Med* 71:555, 1989.

63. Winslow RM, Monge CC: *Hypoxia, Polycythemia and Chronic Mountain Sickness*. Johns Hopkins University Press, Baltimore, 1987.

64. Beall CM, Brittenham GM, Strohl KP, et al: Hemoglobin concentration of high-altitude Tibetans and Bolivian Aymara. *Am J Phys Anthropol* 106:385, 1998.

65. Winslow RM, Butler WM, Kark JA, et al: The effect of bloodletting on exercise performance in a subject with a high-affinity hemoglobin variant. *Blood* 62:1159, 1983.

66. Winslow RM, Chapman KW, Gibson CC, et al: Different hematologic responses to hypoxia in Sherpas and Quechua Indians. *J Appl Physiol* 66:1561, 1989.

67. Beall CM, Almasy LA, Blangero J, et al: Percent of oxygen saturation of arterial hemoglobin among Bolivian Aymara at 3,900-4,000 m. *Am J Phys Anthropol* 108:41, 1999.

68. Beall CM, Laskowski D, Strohl KP, et al: Pulmonary nitric oxide in mountain dwellers. *Nature* 414:411, 2001.

69. Beall CM: Oxygen saturation increases during childhood and decreases during adulthood among high altitude native Tibetians residing at 3,800-4,200 m. *High Alt Med Biol* 1:25, 2000.

70. Beall CM, Decker MJ, Brittenham GM, et al: An Ethiopian pattern of human adaptation to high-altitude hypoxia. *Proc Natl Acad Sci U S A* 99:17215, 2002.

71. Beall CM: High-altitude adaptations. *Lancet* 362(suppl):s14, 2003.

72. Beall CM, Song K, Elston RC, Goldstein MC: Higher offspring survival among Tibetan women with high oxygen saturation genotypes residing at 4,000 m. *Proc Natl Acad Sci U S A* 101:14300, 2004.

73. Jedlickova K, Stockton DW, Chen H, et al: Search for genetic determinants of individual variability of the erythropoietin response to high altitude. *Blood Cells Mol Dis* 31:175, 2003.

74. Jefferson JA, Escudero E, Hurtado ME, et al: Excessive erythrocytosis, chronic mountain sickness, and serum cobalt levels. *Lancet* 359:407, 2002.

75. Goldwasser E, Jacobson LO, Fried W, Plzak L: Mechanism of the erythropoietic effect of cobalt. *Science* 125:1085, 1957.

76. Bernardi L, Roach RC, Keyl C, et al: Ventilation, autonomic function, sleep and erythropoietin. Chronic mountain sickness of Andean natives. *Adv Exp Med Biol* 543:161, 2003.

77. Murray JF: Classification of polycythemic disorders. With comments on the diagnostic value of arterial blood oxygen analysis. *Ann Intern Med* 64:892, 1966.

78. Flenley DC: Chronic obstructive pulmonary disease. *Dis Mon* 34:537, 1988.

79. Limthongkul S, Wongthim S, Udompanich V, et al: Chronic obstructive pulmonary disease at Chulalongkorn Hospital: An analysis of 400 episodes. *J Med Assoc Thai* 74:639, 1991.

80. Rodman T, Close HP. The primary hypoventilation syndrome. *Am J Med* 26:808, 1959.

81. Fishman AP, Turino GO, Bevgofsky EF: The syndrome of alveolar hypoventilation. *Am J Med* 23:233, 1957.

82. Alexander JK, Amad KH, Cole VW: Observations on some clinical features of extreme obesity with particular reference to cardio-respiratory effects. *Am J Med* 32:512, 1962.

83. Vongpatanasin W, Brickner ME, Hillis LD, Lange RA: The Eisenmenger syndrome in adults. *Ann Intern Med* 128:745, 1998.

84. Block AJ, Boysen PG, Wynne JW, Hunt LA: Sleep apnea, hypopnea and oxygen desaturation in normal subjects. A strong male predominance. *N Engl J Med* 300:513, 1979.

85. Moore-Gillon JC, Treacher DF, Gaminara EJ, et al: Intermittent hypoxia in patients with unexplained polycythaemia. *BMJ* 293:588, 1986.

86. Hoffstein V, Mateika S: Differences in abdominal and neck circumferences in patients with and without obstructive sleep apnoea. *Eur Respir J* 5:377, 1992.

87. Carlson JT, Hedner J, Fagerberg B, et al: Secondary polycythaemia associated with nocturnal apnoea—A relationship not mediated by erythropoietin? *J Intern Med* 231:381, 1992.

88. McKeon JL, Saunders NA, Murree-Allen K, et al: Urinary uric acid: Creatinine ratio, serum erythropoietin, and blood 2,3-diphosphoglycerate in patients with obstructive sleep apnea. *Am Rev Respir Dis* 142:8, 1990.

89. Smith JR, Landaw A: Smokers' polycythemia. *N Engl J Med* 298:6, 1978.

90. Stonesifer LD: How carbon monoxide reduces plasma volume [letter]. *N Engl J Med* 299:311, 1978.

91. Aitchison R, Russell N: Smoking—A major cause of polycythemia. *J R Soc Med* 81:89, 1998.

92. Galactéros F, Rosa R, Prehu M-O, et al: Deficit en diphosphoglycerate mutase: Nouveaux cas associes a une polyglobulie. *Nouv Rev Fr Hematol* 26:69, 1984.

93. Vora S, Corash L, Engel WK, et al: The molecular mechanism of the inherited phosphofructokinase deficiency associated with hemolysis and myopathy. *Blood* 55:629, 1980.

94. Beutler E, Westwood B, van Zwieten R, Roos D: G→T transition at cDNA nt 110 (K37Q) in the PKLR (pyruvate kinase) gene is the molecular basis of a case of hereditary increase of red blood cell ATP. *Hum Mutat* 9:282, 1997.

95. Gardner FH: The use of cobaltous chloride in the anemia associated with chronic renal disease. *N Engl J Med* 41:56, 1998.

96. Sergeyeva A, Gordeuk VR, Tokarev YN, et al: Congenital polycythemia in Chuvashia. *Blood* 89:2148, 1997.

97. Ang SO, Chen H, Gordeuk VR, et al: Endemic polycythemia in Russia: Mutation in the VHL gene. *Blood Cells Mol Dis* 28:57, 2002.

98. Ang SO, Chen H, Hirota K, et al: Disruption of oxygen homeostasis underlies congenital Chuvash polycythemia. *Nat Genet* 32:614, 2002.

99. Collins TS, Arcasoy MO: Iron overload due to X-linked sideroblastic anemia in an African American man. *Am J Med* 116:501, 2004.

100. Pastore YD, Jelinek J, Ang S, et al: Mutations in the VHL gene in sporadic apparently congenital polycythemia. *Blood* 101:1591, 2003.

101. Cario H, Schwarz K, Jorch N, et al: Mutations in the von-Hippel-Lindau (vHL) tumor suppressor gene and vHL-haplotype analysis in patients with presumable congenital erythrocytosis. *Haematologica* 90:19, 2005.

102. Bento MC, Chang KT, Guan YL, et al: Five new Caucasian patients with congenital polycythemia due to heterogenous VHL gene mutations. *Haematologica* 90:130, 2005.

103. Gordeuk VR, Stockton DW, Prchal JT: Congenital polycythemias/erythrocytoses. *Haematologica* 90:102, 2005.

104. Percy MJ, Beard ME, Carter C, Thein SL: Erythrocytosis and the Chuvash von Hippel-Lindau mutation. *Br J Haematol* 123:371, 2003.

105. Pastore Y, Jedlickova K, Guan YL, et al: Mutations of von Hippel-Lindau tumor-suppressor gene and congenital polycythemia. *Am J Hum Genet* 73:412, 2003.

106. Percy MJ, McMullin MF, Jowitt SN, et al: Chuvash-type congenital polycythemia in 4 families of Asian and Western European ancestry. *Blood* 102:1097, 2003.

107. Liu E, Percy MJ, Amos CI, et al: The worldwide distribution of the VHL 598C→T mutation indicates a single founding event. *Blood* 103:1937, 2004.

108. Gordeuk VR, Sergueeva AI, Miasnikova GY, et al: Congenital disorder of oxygen sensing: Association of the homozygous Chuvash polycythemia VHL mutation with thrombosis and vascular abnormalities but not tumors. *Blood* 103:3924, 2004.

109. Semenza GL: HIF-1 and mechanisms of hypoxia sensing. *Curr Opin Cell Biol* 13:167, 2001.

110. Laughner E, Taghavi P, Chiles K, et al: HER2 (neu) signaling increases the rate of hypoxia-inducible factor 1alpha (HIF-1alpha) synthesis: Novel mechanism for HIF-1-mediated vascular endothelial growth factor expression. *Mol Cell Biol* 21:3995, 2001.

111. Luttun A, Carmeliet P: Soluble VEGF receptor Flt1: The elusive preeclampsia factor discovered? *J Clin Invest* 111:600, 2003.

112. VanWijk MJ, Kublickiene K, Boer K, VanBavel E: Vascular function in preeclampsia. *Cardiovasc Res* 47:38, 2000.

113. Cramer T, Yamanishi Y, Clausen BE, et al: HIF-1alpha is essential for myeloid cell-mediated inflammation. *Cell* 112:645, 2003.

114. Krieg M, Marti HH, Plate KH: Coexpression of erythropoietin and vascular endothelial growth factor in nervous system tumors associated with von Hippel-Lindau tumor suppressor gene loss of function. *Blood* 92:3388, 1998.

115. Friedrich CA: Von Hippel-Lindau syndrome. A pleomorphic condition. *Cancer* 86:2478, 1999.

116. Haase VH, Glickman JN, Socolovsky M, Jaenisch R: Vascular tumors in livers with targeted inactivation of the von Hippel-Lindau tumor suppressor. *Proc Natl Acad Sci U S A* 98:1583, 2001.

117. Richards FM: Molecular pathology of von Hippel-Lindau disease and the vHL tumour suppressor gene. *Expert Rev Mol Med* 2001:1, 2001.

118. Maran J, Jedlickova K, Stockton D, Prchal JT: Finding the novel molecular defect in a family with high erythropoietin autosomal dominant polycythemia. *Blood* 102:162b, 2003.

119. Bailey RR, Shand BI, Walker RJ: Reversible erythrocytosis in a patient with a hydronephrotic horseshoe kidney. *Nephron* 70:104, 1995.

120. Hammond D, Winnick S: Paraneoplastic erythrocytosis and ectopic erythropoietins. *Ann N Y Acad Sci* 230:219, 1974.

121. Navarro J, Aguilera A, Liano F, et al: Phlebotomy for polycythemia associated with acquired cystic renal disease in a patient on hemodialysis. *Nephron* 62:110, 1992.

122. Da Silva JL, Lacombe C, Bruneval P, et al: Tumor cells are the site of erythropoietin synthesis in human renal cancers associated with polycythemia. *Blood* 75:577, 1990.

123. Lal A, Rice A, al Mahr M, et al: Wilms tumor associated with polycythemia: Case report and review of the literature. *J Pediatr Hematol Oncol* 19:263, 1997.

124. Grignon DJ, Eble JN: Papillary and metanephric adenomas of the kidney. *Semin Diagn Pathol* 15:41, 1998.

125. Fisher JW, Samuels AI: Relationship between renal blood flow and erythropoietin production in dogs. *Proc Soc Exp Biol Med* 125:482, 1967.

126. Beebe HG, Chesebro K, Merchant F, Bush W: Results of renal artery balloon angioplasty limit its indications. *J Vasc Surg* 8:300, 1988.

127. Mrug M, Julian BA, Prchal JT: Angiotensin II receptor type 1 expression in erythroid progenitors: Implications for the pathogenesis of postrenal transplant erythrocytosis. *Semin Nephrol* 24:120, 2004.

128. Mrug M, Stopka T, Julian BA, et al: Angiotensin II stimulates proliferation of normal early erythroid progenitors. *J Clin Invest* 100:2310, 1997.

129. Danovitch GM, Jamgotchian NJ, Eggena PH, et al: Angiotensin-converting enzyme inhibition in the treatment of renal transplant erythrocytosis. Clinical experience and observation of mechanism. *Transplantation* 60:132, 1995.

130. Gossmann J, Burkhardt R, Harder S, et al: Angiotensin II infusion increases plasma erythropoietin levels via an angiotensin II type 1 receptor-dependent pathway. *Kidney Int* 60:83, 2001.

131. Glicklich D, Burris L, Urban A, et al: Angiotensin-converting enzyme inhibition induces apoptosis in erythroid precursors and affects insulin-like growth factor-1 in posttransplantation erythrocytosis. *J Am Soc Nephrol* 12:1958, 2001.

132. Thevenod F, Radtke HW, Grutzmacher P, et al: Deficient feedback regulation of erythropoiesis in kidney transplant patients with polycythemia. *Kidney Int* 24:227, 1983.

133. Friman S, Nyberg G, Blohme I: Erythrocytosis after renal transplantation; treatment by removal of the native kidneys. *Nephrol Dial Transplant* 5:969, 1990.

134. Venencie PY, Puissant A, Boffa GA, et al: Multiple cutaneous leiomyomata and erythrocytosis with demonstration of erythropoietic activity in the cutaneous leiomyomata. *Br J Dermatol* 107:483, 1982.

135. Trimble M, Caro J, Talalla A, Brain M: Secondary erythrocytosis due to a cerebellar hemangioblastoma: Demonstration of erythropoietin mRNA in the tumor. *Blood* 78:599, 1991.

136. McFadzean AJS, Todd D, Tsang KC: Polycythemia in primary carcinoma of the liver. *Blood* 13:427, 1958.

137. Davidson CS: Hepatocellular carcinoma and erythrocytosis. *Semin Hematol* 13:115, 1976.

138. Muta H, Funakoshi A, Baba T, et al: Gene expression of erythropoietin in hepatocellular carcinoma. *Intern Med* 33:427, 1994.

139. Shulkin BL, Shapiro B, Sisson JC: Pheochromocytoma, polycythemia, and venous thrombosis. *Am J Med* 83:773, 1987.

140. Mann DL, Gallagher NI, Donati RM: Erythrocytosis and primary aldosteronism. *Ann Intern Med* 66:335, 1967.

141. Erkelens DW, Statius vEL: Bartter's syndrome and erythrocytosis. *Am J Med* 55:711, 1973.

142. Ghio R, Haupt E, Ratti M, Boccaccio P: Erythrocytosis associated with a dermoid cyst of the ovary and erythropoietic activity of the tumour fluid. *Scand J Haematol* 27:70, 1981.

143. Gardner FH, Nathan DG, Piomelli S, Cummins JF: The erythrocythaemic effects of androgen. *Br J Haematol* 14:611, 1968.

144. Piedras J, Hernandez G, Lopez-Karpovitch X: Effect of androgen therapy and anemia on serum erythropoietin levels in patients with aplastic anemia and myelodysplastic syndromes. *Am J Hematol* 57:113, 1998.

145. Gardner FH, Pringle JC Jr: Androgens and erythropoiesis: II. Treatment of myeloid metaplasia. *N Engl J Med* 264:103, 1961.

146. Besa EC: Hematologic effects of androgens revisited: An alternative therapy in various hematologic conditions. *Semin Hematol* 31:134, 1994.

147. Wiswell TE, Cornish JD, Northam RS: Neonatal polycythemia: Frequency of clinical manifestations and other associated findings. *Pediatrics* 78:26, 1986.

148. Black VD, Lubchenco LO, Koops BL, et al: Neonatal hyperviscosity: Randomized study of effect of partial plasma exchange transfusion on long-term outcome. *Pediatrics* 75:1048, 1985.

149. Pearson TC: Apparent polycythaemia. *Blood Rev* 5:205, 1991.

150. Chrysant SG, Frolich SG, Adamopoulos PN, et al: Pathologic significance of "stress" or relative polycythemia in essential hypertension. *Am J Cardiol* 37:1069, 1976.

151. Isbister JP: The contracted plasma volume syndromes (relative polycythemias) and their haemoheological significance. *Baillieres Clin Haematol* 1:66S, 1987.

152. Leth A: Changes in plasma and extracellular fluid volumes in patients with essential hypertension during long-term treatment with hydrochlorothiazide. *Circulation* 42:479, 1970.

153. Berlin NI: Diagnosis and classification of the polycythemias. *Semin Hematol* 12:339, 1975.

154. Wehmeier A, Daum I, Jamin H, Schneider W: Incidence and clinical risk factors for bleeding and thrombotic complications in myeloproliferative disorders. A retrospective analysis of 260 patients. *Ann Hematol* 63:101, 1991.

155. Berk PD, Goldberg JD, Donovan PB, et al: Therapeutic recommendations in polycythemia vera based on Polycythemia Vera Study Group protocols. *Semin Hematol* 23:132, 1986.

156. Gruppo Italian Studio Policitemia Polycythemia vera: The natural history of 1213 patients followed for 20 years. *Ann Intern Med* 123:664, 1995.

157. Berk P, Wasserman L, Fruchtman S: Treatment of polycythemia vera. A summary of clinical trials conducted by the Polycythemia Study Group, in *Polycythemia Vera and the Myeloproliferative Disorders*, edited by L Wasserman, P Berk, N Berlin, p 166. WB Saunders, Philadelphia, 1995.

158. Spivak JL, Barosi G, Tognoni G, et al: Chronic myeloproliferative disorders. *Hematology (Am Soc Hematol Educ Program)*, p. 200, 2003.

159. Landolfi R, Marchioli R, Kutti J, et al: Efficacy and safety of low-dose aspirin in polycythemia vera. *N Engl J Med* 350:114, 2004.

160. Anger BR, Seifried E, Scheppach J, Heimpel H: Budd-Chiari syndrome and thrombosis of other abdominal vessels in the chronic myeloproliferative diseases. *Wien Klin Wochenschr* 67:818, 1989.

161. Valla D, Casadevall N, Lacombe C, et al: Primary myeloproliferative disorder and hepatic vein thrombosis. A prospective study of erythroid colony formation in vitro in 20 patients with Budd-Chiari syndrome. *Ann Intern Med* 103:329, 1985.

162. De SV, Teofili L, Leone G, Michiels JJ: Spontaneous erythroid colony formation as the clue to an underlying myeloproliferative disorder in patients with Budd-Chiari syndrome or portal vein thrombosis. *Semin Thromb Hemost* 23:411, 1997.

163. Srinivasan P, Rela M, Prachalias A, et al: Liver transplantation for Budd-Chiari syndrome. *Transplantation* 73:973, 2002.

164. Murphy S: Polycythemia vera. *Dis Mon* 38:158, 1992.

165. Jackson N, Burt D, Crocker J, Boughton B: Skin mast cells in polycythaemia vera: Relationship to the pathogenesis and treatment of pruritus. *Br J Dermatol* 116:21, 1987.

166. Steinman HK, Kobza-Black A, Lotti TM, et al: Polycythaemia rubra vera and water-induced pruritus: Blood histamine levels and cutaneous fibrinolytic activity before and after water challenge. *Br J Dermatol* 116:329, 1987.

167. Buchanan JG, Ameratunga RV, Hawkins RC: Polycythemia vera and water-induced pruritus: Evidence against mast cell involvement. *Pathology* 26:43, 1994.

168. Furukawa T, Takahashi M, Shimada H, et al: Polycythaemia vera with Sweet's syndrome. *Clin Lab Haematol* 11:67, 1989.

169. Cox NH, Leggat H: Sweet's syndrome associated with polycythemia rubra vera. *J Am Acad Dermatol* 23:1171, 1990.

170. Davis MD, O'Fallon WM, Rogers RS III, Rooke TW: Natural history of erythromelalgia: Presentation and outcome in 168 patients. *Arch Dermatol* 136:330, 2000.

171. van Genderen PJ, Lucas IS, Van Strik R, et al: Erythromelalgia in essential thrombocythemia is characterized by platelet activation and endothelial cell damage but not by thrombin generation. *Thromb Haemost* 76:333, 1996.

172. van Genderen PJ, Michiels JJ: Erythromelalgia: A pathognomonic microvascular thrombotic complication in essential thrombocythemia and polycythemia vera. *Semin Thromb Hemost* 23:357, 1997.

173. Wanless IR, Peterson P, Das A, et al: Hepatic vascular disease and portal hypertension in polycythemia vera and agnogenic myeloid metaplasia: A clinicopathological study of 145 patients examined at autopsy. *Hepatology* 12:1166, 1990.

174. Tinney WS, Hall BE, Giffin HZ: Polycythemia vera and peptic ulcer. *Mayo Clin Proc* 18:24, 1943.

175. Garcia-Manero G, Schuster SJ, Patrick H, Martinez J: Pulmonary hypertension in patients with myelofibrosis secondary to myeloproliferative diseases. *Am J Hematol* 60:130, 1999.

176. Dingli D, Utz JP, Krowka MJ, et al: Unexplained pulmonary hypertension in chronic myeloproliferative disorders. *Chest* 120:801, 2001.

177. Newton LK: Neurologic complications of polycythemia and their impact on therapy. *Oncology* 4:59, 1990.

178. Jackson A, Burton IE: Retroperitoneal mass and spinal cord compression due to extramedullary haemopoiesis in polycythaemia rubra vera. *Br J Radiol* 62:944, 1989.

179. Wasserman LR, Gilbert HS: Surgical bleeding in polycythemia vera. *Ann N Y Acad Sci* 115:122, 1964.

180. Gilbert HS: Modern treatment strategies in polycythemia vera. *Semin Hematol* 40:26, 2003.

181. Queisser W, Heim ME, Schmitz JM, Worst P: Idiopathic familial erythrocytosis. Report on a family with autosomal dominant inheritance. *Dtsch Med Wochenschr* 113:851, 1988.

182. Prchal JT, Semenza GL, Prchal J, Sokol L: Familial polycythemia. *Science* 268:1831, 1995.

183. Kralovics R, Sokol L, Prchal JT: Absence of polycythemia in a child with a unique erythropoietin receptor mutation in a family with autosomal dominant primary polycythemia. *J Clin Invest* 102:124, 1998.

184. Arcasoy MO, Degar BA, Harris KW, Forget BG: Familial erythrocytosis associated with a short deletion in the erythropoietin receptor gene. *Blood* 89:4628, 1997.

185. Zafren K, Honigman B: High-altitude medicine. *Emerg Med Clin North Am* 15:191, 1997.

186. Bishop BC: Wintering in the high Himalayas. *National Geographic* 122:503, 1962.

187. Botella de Maglia J, Martinez-Costa R: High altitude retinal hemorrhages in the expeditions to 8,000 meter peaks. A study of 10 cases. *Med Clin (Barc)* 110:457, 1998.

188. Beall CM: Tibetan and Andean contrasts in adaptation to high-altitude hypoxia. *Adv Exp Med Biol* 475:63, 2000.

189. Thorne SA: Management of polycythaemia in adults with cyanotic congenital heart disease. *Heart* 79:315, 1998.

190. Shibata J, Hasegawa J, Siemens HJ, et al: Hemostasis and coagulation at a hematocrit level of 0.85: Functional consequences of erythrocytosis. *Blood* 101:4416, 2003.

191. Stefenelli T, Silberbauer K, Ulrich W, et al: Cardial decompensation caused by hypertension and polyglobulia associated with multiple renal oncocytomas. *Clin Nephrol* 23:307, 1985.

192. Michiels JJ, Juvonen E: Proposal for revised diagnostic criteria of es-

sential thrombocythemia and polycythemia vera by the Thrombocythemia Vera Study Group. *Semin Thromb Hemost* 23:339, 1997.

193. Thiele J, Kvasnicka HM, Zankovich R, Diehl V: The value of bone marrow histology in differentiating between early stage polycythemia vera and secondary (reactive) polycythemias. *Haematologica* 86:368, 2001.

194. Michiels JJ, Thiele J: Clinical and pathological criteria for the diagnosis of essential thrombocythemia, polycythemia vera, and idiopathic myelofibrosis (agnogenic myeloid metaplasia). *Int J Hematol* 76:133, 2002.

195. Arnaud J, Pris J, Brun H, Constans J: Consequences of moderate hypoxia on red cell glycolytic metabolism in polycythemia rubra vera. *Ann Biol Clin (Paris)* 49:9, 1991.

196. Avissar N, Farkash Y, Shaklai M: Erythrocyte enzymes in polycythemia vera: A comparison to erythrocyte enzyme activities of patients with iron deficiency anemia. *Acta Haematol (Basel)* 76:37, 1986.

197. Lertzman M, Frome BM, Israels LG, Cherniack RM: Hypoxia in polycythemia vera. *Ann Intern Med* 60:409, 1964.

198. Gilbert HS, Warner RRP, Wasserman LR: A study of histamine in myeloproliferative disease. *Blood* 28:795, 1966.

199. Falanga A, Marchetti M, Evangelista V, et al: Polymorphonuclear leukocyte activation and hemostasis in patients with essential thrombocythemia and polycythemia vera. *Blood* 96:4261, 2000.

200. Kutti M, Weinfield A: Platelet survival in active polycythaemia vera with reference to the haematocrit level. An experimental study before and after phlebotomy. *Scand J Haematol* 8:405, 1971.

201. Cerutti A, Custodi P, Duranti M, et al: Thrombopoietin levels in patients with primary and reactive thrombocytosis. *Br J Haematol* 99:281, 1997.

202. Shih LY, Lee CT: Identification of masked polycythemia vera from patients with idiopathic marked thrombocytosis by endogenous erythroid colony assay. *Blood* 83:744, 1994.

203. Yamamoto K, Sekiguchi E, Takatani O: Abnormalities of epinephrine-induced platelet aggregation and adenine nucleotides in myeloproliferative disorders. *Thromb Haemost* 52:292, 1984.

204. Mehta P, Mehta J, Ross M, et al: Decreased platelet aggregation but increased thromboxane A2 generation in polycythemia vera. *Arch Intern Med* 145:1225, 1985.

205. Landolfi R, Ciabattoni G, Patrignani P, et al: Increased thromboxane biosynthesis in patients with polycythemia vera: Evidence for aspirin-suppressible platelet activation in vivo. *Blood* 80:1965, 1992.

206. Ushikubi F, Ishibashi T, Narumiya S, Okuma M: Analysis of the defective signal transduction mechanism through the platelet thromboxane A2 receptor in a patient with polycythemia vera. *Thromb Haemost* 67:144, 1992.

207. Berild D, Hasselbalch H, Knudsen JB: Platelet survival, platelet factor-4 and bleeding time in myeloproliferative disorders. *Scand J Clin Lab Invest* 47:497, 1987.

208. Harker LA, Finch CA: Thrombokinetics in man. *J Clin Invest* 48:963, 1969.

209. Le Blanc K, Lindahl T, Rosendahl K, Samuelsson J: Impaired platelet binding of fibrinogen due to a lower number of GPIIB/IIIA receptors in polycythemia vera. *Thromb Res* 91:287, 1998.

210. Afshar-Kharghan V, Lopez JA, Gray LA, et al: Hemostatic gene polymorphisms and the prevalence of thrombotic complications in polycythemia vera and essential thrombocythemia. *Blood Coagul Fibrinolysis* 15:21, 2004.

211. Binder RA, Gilbert HS: Muramidase in polycythemia vera. *Blood* 36:228, 1970.

212. Gilbert HS, Krauss S, Pasternack B, et al: Serum vitamin B_{12} content and unsaturated vitamin B_{12}-binding capacity in myeloproliferative disease. Value in differential diagnosis and as indicators of disease activity. *Ann Intern Med* 71:719, 1969.

213. Najean Y, Triebel F, Dresch C: Pure erythrocytosis: Reappraisal of a study of 51 cases. *Am J Hematol* 10:129, 1981.

214. Clement S, Eberlin A, Najean Y, Chedeville A: Two different in vitro growth patterns for erythroid precursors in 18 patients with pure erythrocytosis. *Scand J Haematol* 29:319, 1982.

215. Pearson TC, Wetherley-Mein G: The course and complications of idiopathic erythrocytosis. *Clin Lab Haematol* 1:189, 1979.

216. Shih LY, Lee CT, See LC, et al: In vitro culture growth of erythroid progenitors and serum erythropoietin assay in the differential diagnosis of polycythaemia. *Eur J Clin Invest* 28:569, 1998.

217. Spivak JL: Diagnosis of the myeloproliferative disorders: Resolving phenotypic mimicry. *Semin Hematol* 40:1, 2003.

218. Beutler E: Polycythemia. *Med Grand Rounds* 3:142, 1984.

219. Prchal JF, Axelrad AA: Letter: Bone-marrow responses in polycythemia vera. *N Engl J Med* 290:1382, 1974.

220. Weinberg RS: In vitro erythropoiesis in polycythemia vera and other myeloproliferative disorders. *Semin Hematol* 34:64, 1997.

221. Liu E, Jelinek J, Pastore YD, et al: Discrimination of polycythemias and thrombocytoses by novel, simple, accurate clonality assays and comparison with PRV-1 expression and BFU-E response to erythropoietin. *Blood* 101:3294, 2003.

222. Fisher MJ, Prchal JF, Prchal JT, D'Andrea AD: Anti-erythropoietin (EPO) receptor monoclonal antibodies distinguish EPO-dependent and EPO-independent erythroid progenitors in polycythemia vera. *Blood* 84:1982, 1994.

223. Pagliuca A, Mufti GJ, Janossa-Tahernia M, et al: In vitro colony culture and chromosomal studies in hepatic and portal vein thrombosis—Possible evidence of an occult myeloproliferative state. *Q J Med* 76:981, 1990.

224. Acharya J, Westwood NB, Sawyer BM, et al: Identification of latent myeloproliferative disease in patients with Budd-Chiari syndrome using X-chromosome inactivation patterns and in vitro erythroid colony formation. *Eur J Haematol* 55:315, 1995.

225. Birgegard G, Wide L: Serum erythropoietin in the diagnosis of polycythaemia and after phlebotomy treatment. *Br J Haematol* 81:603, 1992.

226. Mossuz P, Girodon F, Donnard M, et al: Diagnostic value of serum erythropoietin level in patients with absolute erythrocytosis. *Haematologica* 89:1194, 2004.

227. Messinezy M, Westwood NB, El Hemaidi I, et al: Serum erythropoietin values in erythrocytoses and in primary thrombocythaemia. *Br J Haematol* 117:47, 2002.

228. Remacha AF, Montserrat I, Santamaria A, et al: Serum erythropoietin in the diagnosis of polycythemia vera. A follow-up study. *Haematologica* 82:406, 1997.

229. Beutler E, Yeh M, Fairbanks VF: The normal human female as a mosaic of X-chromosome activity: Studies using the gene for G-6-PD deficiency as a marker. *Proc Natl Acad Sci U S A* 48:9, 1962.

230. Prchal JT: Pathogenetic mechanisms of polycythemia vera and congenital polycythemic disorders. *Semin Hematol* 38:10, 2001.

231. Vogelstein B, Fearon ER, Hamilton SR, Feinberg AP: Use of restriction fragment length polymorphisms to determine the clonal origin of human tumors. *Science* 227:642, 1985.

232. Allen RC, Zoghbi HY, Moseley AB, et al: Methylation of HpaII and HhaI sites near the polymorphic CAG repeat in the human androgen-receptor gene correlates with X chromosome inactivation. *Am J Hum Genet* 51:1229, 1992.

233. Curnutte JT, Hopkins PJ, Kuhl W, Beutler E: Studying X-inactivation. *Lancet* 339:749, 1992.

234. Prchal JT, Guan YL, Prchal JF, Barany F: Transcriptional analysis of the active X-chromosome in normal and clonal hematopoiesis. *Blood* 81:269, 1993.

235. Prchal JT, Prchal JF, Belickova M, et al: Clonal stability of blood cell lineages indicated by X-chromosomal transcriptional polymorphism. *J Exp Med* 183:561, 1996.

236. Tefferi A, Lasho TL, Wolanskyj AP, Mesa RA: Neutrophil PRV-1 expression across the chronic myeloproliferative disorders and in secondary or spurious polycythemia. *Blood* 103:3547, 2004.

237. Lichtman MA, Murphy MS, Adamson JW: Detection of mutant hemoglobins with altered affinity for oxygen. A simplified technique. *Ann Intern Med* 84:517, 1976.

238. Tefferi A: Polycythemia vera: A comprehensive review and clinical recommendations. *Mayo Clin Proc* 78:174, 2003.

239. Pearson TC, Wetherley-Mein G: Vascular occlusive episodes and venous haematocrit in primary proliferative polycythaemia. *Lancet* 2:1219, 1978.

240. Perloff JK, Marelli AJ, Miner PD: Risk of stroke in adults with cyanotic congenital heart disease. *Circulation* 87:1954, 1993.

241. Van de Pette JEW, Guthrie DL, Pearson TC: Whole blood viscosity in polycythaemia: The effect of iron deficiency at a range of haemoglobin and packed cell volumes. *Br J Haematol* 63:369, 1986.

242. Reinhart WH: The influence of iron deficiency on erythrocyte deformability. *Br J Haematol* 80:550, 1992.

243. Berlin NI, Wasserman LR: Polycythemia vera: A retrospective and reprise. *J Lab Clin Med* 130:365, 1997.

244. Nand S, Messmore H, Fisher SG, et al: Leukemic transformation in polycythemia vera: Analysis of risk factors. *Am J Hematol* 34:32, 1990.

245. Hocking WG, Golde DW: Polycythemia: Evaluation and management. *Blood Rev* 3:59, 1989.

246. Kaplan ME, Mack K, Goldberg JD, et al: Long-term management of polycythemia vera with hydroxyurea: A progress report. *Semin Hematol* 23:167, 1986.

247. Cortelazzo S, Finazzi G, Ruggeri M, et al: Hydroxyurea for patients with essential thrombocythemia and a high risk of thrombosis. *N Engl J Med* 332:1132, 1995.

248. Steinberg MH, Barton F, Castro S, et al: Effect of hydroxyurea on mortality and morbidity in adult sickle cell anemia—Risks and benefits up to 9 years of treatment. *JAMA* 289:1645, 2003.

249. "Leukemia and Hematosarcoma" Cooperative Group, European Organization for Research on Treatment of Cancer (E.OR.TC): Treatment of polycythaemia vera by radiophosphorus or busulphan: A randomized trial. *Br J Cancer* 44:75, 1981.

250. Randi ML, Fabris F, Varotto L, et al: Haematological complications in polycythaemia vera and thrombocythaemia patients treated with radiophosphorus (32P). *Folia Haematol (Leipzig)* 117:461, 1990.

251. Balan KK, Critchley M: Outcome of 259 patients with primary proliferative polycythaemia (PPP) and idiopathic thrombocythaemia (IT) treated in a regional nuclear medicine department with phosphorus-32—A 15 year review. *Br J Radiol* 70:1169, 1997.

252. Roberts BE, Smith AH: Use of radioactive phosphorus in haematology. *Blood Rev* 11:146, 1997.

253. Foa P, Massaro P, Caldiera S, et al: Long-term therapeutic efficacy and toxicity of recombinant interferon-alpha 2a in polycythaemia vera. *Eur J Haematol* 60:273, 1998.

254. Ozturk A, Gunay A, Uskent N: Therapeutic efficacy of recombinant interferon-alpha in polycythaemia vera. *Acta Haematol (Basel)* 99:89, 1998.

255. Silver RT: Interferon alfa: Effects of long-term treatment for polycythemia vera. *Semin Hematol* 34:40, 1997.

256. Petti MC, Spadea A, Avvisati G, et al: Polycythemia vera treated with pipobroman as single agent: Low incidence of secondary leukemia in a cohort of patients observed during 20 years (1971-1991). *Leukemia* 12:869, 1998.

257. Najean Y, Rain JD: Treatment of polycythemia vera: The use of hydroxyurea and pipobroman in 292 patients under the age of 65 years. *Blood* 90:3370, 1997.

258. Passamonti F, Brusamolino E, Lazzarino M, et al: Efficacy of pipob-

259. Brusamolino E, Salvaneschi L, Canevari A, Bernasconi C. Efficacy trial of pipobroman in polycythemia vera and incidence of acute leukemia. *J Clin Oncol* 2:558, 1984.

260. Najman A, Stachowiak J, Parlier Y, et al: Pipobroman therapy of polycythemia vera. *Blood* 59:890, 1982.

261. Petitt RM, Silverstein MN, Petrone ME: Anagrelide for control of thrombocythemia in polycythemia and other myeloproliferative disorders. *Semin Hematol* 34:51, 1997.

262. Storen EC, Tefferi A: Long-term use of anagrelide in young patients with essential thrombocythemia. *Blood* 97:863, 2001.

263. Pardanani A, Tefferi A: Imatinib targets other than bcr/abl and their clinical relevance in myeloid disorders. *Blood* 104:1931, 2004.

264. Demetri GD, von Mehren M, Blanke CD, et al: Efficacy and safety of imatinib mesylate in advanced gastrointestinal stromal tumors. *N Engl J Med* 347:472, 2002.

265. Banerji L, Churchill W, Griffin J: Identification of an imatinib mesylate sensitive phosphoprotein in primary polycythemia vera. *Blood* 102:644a, 2003.

266. Swerlick RA: Photochemotherapy treatment of pruritus associated with polycythemia vera. *J Am Acad Dermatol* 13:675, 1985.

267. Bircher AJ: Water-induced itching. *Dermatologica* 181:83, 1990.

268. de Wolf JT, Hendriks DW, Egger RC, et al: Alpha-interferon for intractable pruritus in polycythaemia vera. *Lancet* 337:241, 1991.

269. Tartaglia A, Goldberg J, Berk P, Wasserman L: Adverse effects of antiaggregating platelet therapy in the treatment of polycythemia vera. *Semin Hematol* 23:172, 1986.

270. Willoughby S, Pearson TC: The use of aspirin in polycythaemia vera and primary thrombocythaemia. *Blood Rev* 12:12, 1998.

271. Landolfi R, Marchioli R: European Collaboration on Low-dose Aspirin in Polycythemia Vera (ECLAP): A randomized trial. *Semin Thromb Hemost* 23:473, 1997.

272. Buchanan GR, Debaun MR, Quinn CT, Steinberg MH: Sickle cell disease. *Hematology (Am Soc Hematol Educ Program)* 35, 2004.

273. Rosenthal DS: Clinical aspects of chronic myeloproliferative diseases. *Am J Med Sci* 304:109, 1992.

274. Tefferi A, Mesa RA, Nagorney DM, et al: Splenectomy in myelofibrosis with myeloid metaplasia: A single-institution experience with 223 patients. *Blood* 95:2226, 2000.

275. Anderson JE, Sale G, Appelbaum FR, et al: Allogeneic marrow transplantation for primary myelofibrosis and myelofibrosis secondary to polycythaemia vera or essential thrombocytosis. *Br J Haematol* 98:1010, 1997.

276. Devine SM, Hoffman R, Verma A, et al: Allogeneic blood cell transplantation following reduced-intensity conditioning is effective therapy for older patients with myelofibrosis with myeloid metaplasia. *Blood* 99:2255, 2002.

277. Plata R, Cornejo A, Arratia C, et al: Angiotensin-converting-enzyme inhibition therapy in altitude polycythaemia: A prospective randomised trial. *Lancet* 359:663, 2002.

278. Piccirillo G, Fimognari FL, Valdivia JL, Marigliano V: Effects of phlebotomy on a patient with secondary polycythemia and angina pectoris. *Int J Cardiol* 44:175, 1994.

279. Manglani MV, DeGroff CG, Dukes PP, Ettinger LJ: Congenital erythrocytosis with elevated erythropoietin level: An incorrectly set "erythrostat"? *J Pediatr Hematol Oncol* 20:560, 1998.

280. Rozman C, Giralt M, Feliu E, et al: Life expectancy of patients with chronic nonleukemic myeloproliferative disorders. *Cancer* 67:2658, 1991.

281. Passamonti F, Malabarba L, Orlandi E, et al: Polycythemia vera in young patients: A study on the long-term risk of thrombosis, myelofibrosis and leukemia. *Haematologica* 88:13, 2003.

282. Camos M, Cervantes F, Montoto S, et al: Acute lymphoid leukemia following polycythemia vera. *Leuk Lymphoma* 32:395, 1999.

283. Higuchi T, Oba R, Endo M, et al: Transition of polycythemia vera to chronic neutrophilic leukemia. *Leuk Lymphoma* 33:203, 1999.

284. Divoky V, Prchal JT: Mouse surviving solely on human erythropoietin receptor (EpoR): Model of human EpoR-linked disease. *Blood* 99:3873, 2002.

285. Berlin NI, Lawrence JH, Gartland J: Blood volume in polycythemia as determined by P^{32} labeled red blood cells. *Am J Med* 9:747, 1950.

286. Huber H, Lewis SM, Szur L: Die Indikation zur Bestimmung von blutvolumen und zirkulierender Erythrozytenmenge bei Polycythaemia vera und Polyglobulien. *Acta Haematol (Basel)* 34:116, 1965.

287. Najean Y, Dresch C, Rain J, et al: Radioisotope investigations for the diagnosis and follow-up of polycythemic patients, in *Polycythemia Vera and the Myeloproliferative Disorders*, edited by LR Wasserman, PD Berk, NI Berlin, p 361. WB Saunders, Philadelphia, 1995.

288. Arcasoy MO, Degar BA, Harris KW, Forget BG: Familial erythrocytosis associated with a short deletion in the erythropoietin receptor gene. *Blood* 89:4628, 1997.

289. Kralovics R, Indrak K, Stopka T, et al: Two new EPO receptor mutations: Truncated EPO receptors are most frequently associated with primary familial and congenital polycythemias. *Blood* 90:2057, 1997.

290. Watowich SS, Xie X, Klingmuller U, et al: Erythropoietin receptor mutations associated with familial erythrocytosis cause hypersensitivity to erythropoietin in the heterozygous state. *Blood* 94:2530, 1999.

291. de la Chapelle A, Traskelin AL, Juvonen E: Truncated erythropoietin receptor causes dominantly inherited benign human erythrocytosis. *Proc Natl Acad Sci U S A* 90:4495, 1993.

292. Furukawa T, Narita M, Sakaue M, et al: Primary familial polycythaemia associated with a novel point mutation in the erythropoietin receptor. *Br J Haematol* 99:222, 1997.

293. Kralovics R, Sokol L, Prchal JT: Absence of polycythemia in a child with a unique erythropoietin receptor mutation in a family with autosomal dominant primary polycythemia. *J Clin Invest* 102:124, 1998.

294. Arcasoy MO, Harris KW, Forget BG: A human erythropoietin receptor gene mutant causing familial erythrocytosis is associated with deregulation of the rates of Jak2 and Stat5 inactivation. *Exp Hematol* 27:63, 1999.

295. Kralovics R, Prchal JT: Genetic heterogeneity of primary familial and congenital polycythemia. *Am J Hematol* 68:115, 2001.

296. Sokol L, Luhovy M, Guan Y, et al: Primary familial polycythemia: A frameshift mutation in the erythropoietin receptor gene and increased sensitivity of erythroid progenitors to erythropoietin. *Blood* 86:15, 1995.

297. Kralovics R, Sokol L, Broxson EH Jr, Prchal JT: The erythropoietin receptor gene is not linked with the polycythemia phenotype in a family with autosomal dominant primary polycythemia. *Proc Assoc Am Physicians* 109:580, 1997.

298. Sokol L, Prchal JF, D'Andrea A, et al: Mutation in the negative regulatory element of the erythropoietin receptor gene in a case of sporadic primary polycythemia. *Exp Hematol* 22:447, 1994.

299. Le Couedic JP, Mitjavila MT, Villeval JL, et al: Missense mutation of the erythropoietin receptor is a rare event in human erythroid malignancies. *Blood* 87:1502, 1996.

300. Pastore YD, Jelinek J, Ang S, et al: Mutations in the VHL gene in sporadic apparently congenital polycythemia. *Blood* 101:1591, 2003.

301. Hultberg B, Sjoblad S, Öckerman PA: Properties of five acid hydrolases in human skin fibroblast cultures. *Acta Paediatr Scand* 62:474, 1973.

302. Pastore Y, Jedlickova K, Guan Y, et al: Mutations of von Hippel-Lindau tumor-suppressor gene and congenital polycythemia. *Am J Hum Genet* 73:412, 2003.

303. James C, Ugo V, Le Couedic JP, et al. A unique clonal JAK2 mutation leading to constitutive signalling causes polycythaemia vera. *Nature* 434:1145, 2005.

304. Ugo V, Marzac C, Teyssandier I, et al. Multiple signaling pathways are involved in erythropoietin-independent differentiation of erythroid progenitors in polycythemia vera. *Exp Hematol* 32:179, 2004.

305. Levine RL, Wadleigh M, Cools J, et al: Activating mutation in the tyrosine kinase JAK2 in polycythemia vera, essential thrombocythemia, and myeloid metaplasia with myelofibrosis. *Cancer Cell* 4:387, 2005.

306. Kralovics R, Passamonti F, Buser AS, et al: A gain-of-function mutation of JAK2 in myeloproliferative disorders. *N Engl J Med* 352:1779, 2005.

307. Baxter EJ, Scott LM, Campbell PJ, et al. Acquired mutation of the tyrosine kinase JAK2 in human myeloproliferative disorders. *Lancet* 365:1054, 2005.

308. Thiele J, Kvasnicka H, Orazi A. Bone marrow in myeloproliferative disorders. *Seminars in Hematology,* 2005, in press.

309. Finazi G, Gregg XT, Barbui T, Prchal JT: Idiopathic Erythrocytosis and other non-clonal polycythemias. *Bailliere's Clinical Haematology. International Practice and Research,* Vol. 18, 2005, in press.

310. Gordeuk V, Prchal JT. Erythropoietin in Polycythemias. *Haemotologica,* 2005, in press.

THE HEMATOLOGIC ASPECTS OF PORPHYRIA

SHIGERU SASSA

The porphyrias are both inherited and acquired disorders in which the activities of the enzymes of the heme biosynthetic pathway are partially or almost totally deficient. Eight enzymes are involved in the synthesis of heme. With the exception of the first enzyme, an enzymatic defect at every step leads to tissue accumulation and excessive excretion of porphyrins and/or their precursors, such as δ-aminolevulinic acid (ALA) and porphobilinogen (PBG). Heme, the final product of the biosynthetic pathway, is biologically important. Porphyrins and their precursors not only are useless but they also are toxic.

Porphyrias can be classified as either photosensitive or neurologic, depending on their manifestations, although some types have both features. Alternatively, they can be classified as either hepatic or erythropoietic, depending on the principal site of expression of the specific enzymatic defect, but some also show overlapping expression. Tissue-specific expression of porphyrias largely is a result of tissue-specific control of heme pathway gene expression. Congenital erythropoietic porphyria (CEP), although rare, is a major erythropoietic porphyria in its expression and severity. It is inherited in an autosomal recessive fashion and is characterized by marked skin photosensitivity and hemolytic anemia. The genetic defect is a marked deficiency of uroporphyrinogen III cosynthase activity. The hemolytic anemia is photosensitive in nature, usually manifests at birth, and results from massive accumulation of isomer I uroporphyrinogen and coproporphyrin in erythrocytes. Increased erythropoietic activity further stimulates porphyrin production in the marrow. Hemolysis may improve after splenectomy. The clinical symptoms of CEP are indistinguishable from those of hepatoerythropoietic porphyria (HEP); hence, some HEPs may be confused with CEP.

Erythropoietic protoporphyria (EPP), another erythropoietic porphyria, is inherited in an autosomal dominant fashion. In contrast to CEP, EPP is relatively common. EPP results from a deficiency of ferrochelatase activity to less than 50 percent of normal activity. The deficiency results in excessive accumulation of protoporphyrin in erythrocytes and massive excretion of protoporphyrin into the stool. The disease is characterized by mild to moderate photosensitivity. Usually no

hematologic manifestations are seen. Clinical expression is highly variable, such that some carriers have only mildly elevated red cell protoporphyrin levels but no skin photosensitivity. EPP is generally a mild disease, but some patients develop porphyrin-rich gallstones and hepatic failure, resulting in death.

In contrast to CEP and EPP, δ-aminolevulinate dehydratase deficiency porphyria (ADP) is an acute hepatic porphyria characterized by severe neurologic disturbances. It may involve the gastrointestinal and respiratory systems but does not produce skin photosensitivity. ADP results from a marked deficiency of δ-aminolevulinate dehydratase activity. Patients with ADP excrete a large amount of ALA, but not PBG, into urine. ADP is the least frequent form of porphyria; only four well-documented cases have been reported.

Acute intermittent porphyria (AIP) is the most common and important acute hepatic porphyria. It is inherited in an autosomal dominant fashion, but disease expression is highly variable. Both clinically affected and asymptomatic carriers of AIP have an approximately 50 percent deficiency of PBG deaminase activity, but only clinically affected individuals excrete a large amount of ALA and PBG into the urine. Many heterozygotes (approximately 90 percent) are asymptomatic throughout their lives. Patients present with severe neurologic symptoms but never develop cutaneous photosensitivity. AIP almost always is latent before puberty. Symptoms occur more frequently in females than in males. Hormonal, drug, and nutritional factors may aggravate the disease, probably by inducing hepatic ALA synthase, the rate-limiting enzyme in the heme biosynthetic pathway.

Hereditary coproporphyria (HCP) is also an acute hepatic porphyria. Its symptoms are similar to but generally milder than the symptoms of ADP and AIP. In contrast, HCP patients may display skin photosensitivity. The underlying genetic defect in HCP is an approximately 50 percent deficiency of coproporphyrinogen oxidase activity, which is inherited in an autosomal dominant fashion. Patients excrete an excessive amount of ALA, PBG, and coproporphyrin into their urine and coproporphyrin into their stool. Harderoporphyria is a variant form of HCP, which produces harderoporphyrin III rather than coproporphyrin III. Neonatal hemolytic anemia has been reported with harderoporphyria. Clinical expression of HCP is dependent upon the same metabolic and chemical factors that influence expression of the gene defect in AIP.

Variegate porphyria (VP) has been recognized in many populations but is most common in South African whites; thus, it is also called the South African porphyria. The underlying defect is an approximately 50 percent deficiency of protoporphyrinogen oxidase, which is inherited in an autosomal dominant fashion. Clinical expression and symptoms are similar to those of HCP but often more severe. Patients with VP excrete a large amount of ALA and PBG into their urine and protoporphyrin into their stool. The same spectrum of factors that activate other acute hepatic porphyrias also induce VP. In South Africa, many patients with VP have the same R59W mutation of the protoporphyrinogen oxidase gene, and apparently all are descendants of a single Dutch settler in 1680. Clinical management of VP is the same as that for other acute hepatic porphyrias.

Porphyria cutanea tarda (PCT) is the most common form of porphyria and usually begins in middle or late adult life. It is neither an erythropoietic nor an acute hepatic porphyria. Instead, PCT is a chronic hepatic porphyria. Most PCT occurs as an acquired disease, whereas some occur as an inherited

Acronyms and abbreviations that appear in this chapter include: ADP, δ-aminolevulinate dehydratase deficiency porphyria; AIP, acute intermittent porphyria; ALA, δ-aminolevulinic acid; ALAS-E, erythroid-specific δ-aminolevulinic acid synthase; ALAS-N, nonspecific δ-aminolevulinic acid synthase; CEP, congenital erythropoietic porphyria; CPO, coproporphyrinogen oxidase; CPRE, coproporphyrinogen oxidase gene promoter regulatory element; CRIM, cross-reactive immunologic material; EPP, erythropoietic protoporphyria; HCP, hereditary coproporphyria; HEP, hepatoerythropoietic porphyria; PBG, porphobilinogen; PCB, polychlorinated biphenyl; PCT, porphyria cutanea tarda; SCS-βA, β-subunit of ATP-specific succinyl coenzyme A synthetase; TCDD, 2,3,7,8-tetrachlorodibenzo-p-dioxin; UROD, uroporphyrinogen decarboxylase; VP, variegate porphyria; XLSA, X-linked sideroblastic anemia.

disease. All patients with PCT A have a deficiency of hepatic uroporphyrinogen decarboxylase activity. PCT patients have mild to severe photosensitivity and often have overt liver disease but no neurologic symptoms. PCT patients excrete a large amount of 8- and 7-carboxylated porphyrins into their urine and isocoproporphyrin into their stool, but not ALA or PBG. Alcohol, estrogens, and hepatic siderosis are common factors aggravating PCT. Some PCT patients coinherit the hemochromatosis gene. PCT can be successfully treated by phlebotomy, which reduces hepatic iron stores. Polyhalogenated aromatic hydrocarbons have been associated with development of acquired PCT in both man and animals. Homozygous deficiency of uroporphyrinogen decarboxylase is known as HEP. Patients with this condition are characterized by severe photosensitivity, which is indistinguishable from that of CEP. Both PCT and HEP result from the same uroporphyrinogen decarboxylase deficiency. The heterozygous defect in PCT leads to a chronic hepatic porphyria, whereas the homozygous defect in HEP results in a hepatic and erythropoietic porphyria, including photosensitive hemolytic anemia.

Molecular analysis of the gene defects in the porphyrias demonstrated numerous types of mutations for each porphyria. Many clinically "homozygous" porphyrias actually result from heteroallelic mutations, that is, compound heterozygosity for two distinct mutations, but very rare homoallelic mutations exist. The existence of rare homozygous (or compound heterozygous) deficiencies has been recognized in all dominantly inherited forms of porphyrias. Porphyrias occur not only as inherited diseases but also as acquired diseases resulting from exposure to environmental chemicals or in association with other defects. Clinically unaffected gene carriers of porphyrias may be at greater risk for infertility and intoxication by environmental chemicals, such as lead or dioxin, than are normal subjects.

DEFINITION AND HISTORY

The porphyrias are metabolic diseases resulting from deficiencies, usually of a genetic nature, in the activity of specific enzymes in the heme biosynthetic pathway. The intermediates of this pathway—porphyrinogens, porphyrins, and their precursors such as δ-aminolevulinic acid (ALA) or porphobilinogen (PBG)—are produced in excess and accumulate in tissues, resulting in neurologic, photocutaneous, or both types of symptoms. These disorders are classified as either *erythropoietic* or *hepatic*, depending on the principal site of expression of the specific enzymatic defect. Erythropoietic porphyrias include congenital erythropoietic porphyria (CEP) and erythropoietic protoporphyria (EPP). Hepatic porphyrias are further classified into *acute* and *chronic* forms. *Acute hepatic porphyrias* refer to a condition that exhibits acute attacks, mostly neurologic, related to deranged porphyrin biosynthesis in the liver. They are represented by ALA dehydratase deficiency porphyria, acute intermittent porphyria (AIP), hereditary coproporphyria (HCP), or variegate porphyria (VP). In contrast, chronic hepatic porphyrias are characterized by chronic skin photosensitivity as a result of overproduction of porphyrins, but without acute attacks, as represented by porphyria cutanea tarda (PCT). Hepatoerythropoietic porphyria (HEP) is an intermediate form expressing the defect in the liver and erythroid cells. Eight enzymes are involved in the synthesis of heme. With the exception of the first enzyme, ALA synthase, each enzymatic defect is associated with a specific form of porphyria (Table 57-1 and Fig. 57-1). This chapter describes the genetic defect or disturbances of heme biosynthesis for *erythropoietic porphyrias, acute*

TABLE 57-1   THE PORPHYRIAS AND THEIR ENZYMATIC DEFECTS

ENZYME DEFICIENCY	PORPHYRIA	PRINCIPAL SITE OF EXPRESSION	MODE OF TRANSMISSION
ALA dehydratase	ADP	Liver	Recessive
PBG deaminase	AIP		Dominant
	Type I	Liver and bone marrow	
	Type II	Marrow	
	Type III	Liver and marrow	
Uro'gen cosynthase	CEP	Marrow	Recessive
Uro'gen decarboxylase	PCT	Liver	
	Type I		Acquired
	Type II		Dominant
	Type III		Dominant
	HEP	Liver and marrow	Recessive
Copro'gen oxidase	HCP	Liver	Dominant
Proto'gen oxidase	VP	Liver	Dominant
Ferrochelatase	EPP	Marrow	Dominant

hepatic porphyrias, and *chronic hepatic porphyrias*. Table 57-2 summarizes the major clinical and laboratory features of the porphyrias. Table 57-3 summarizes the hematologic features of the porphyrias.

Perhaps the first published case of the acute hepatic porphyria was an elderly woman described by Stokvis[1] in 1889. The patient excreted dark red urine and later died after taking sulphonal.[1] Subsequently, two brothers (ages 23 and 26 years) who most likely had CEP were described by T. McCall Anderson[2] in 1898. Since early childhood, these patients suffered from attacks of *hydroa aestivale*, a cutaneous vesicular eruption associated with pruritus and burning that occurs on skin surfaces exposed to the sun. The attacks recurred each summer. The urine of the younger brother was persistently red, while that of the elder brother was said to be normal in color during the intervals between attacks of hydroa. Their skin was extensively scarred in regions exposed to light, and loss of substance of their ears and noses was observed. F. Harris[3] demonstrated that the urine of both patients contained a substance related to the hematoporphyrin group. Although characterization of the nature of porphyrins was understandably primitive, other descriptions match perfectly with those of CEP or HEP. In a monograph published in 1911, Hans Günther[4] classified porphyrias into four different groups: (1) those that have an acute onset without association with drug ingestion, (2) those that are caused by sulphonal or trional, (3) hematoporphyria congenita, and (4) chronic hematoporphyria. These groups probably correspond to (1) drug-unrelated relapse of acute hepatic porphyrias (ALA dehydratase deficiency porphyria, AIP, HCP, or VP), (2) drug-induced relapse (ALA dehydratase deficiency porphyria, AIP, HCP, or VP), (3) CEP (or HEP), and (4) PCT (or HEP), respectively. In 1923, Archibald Garrod[5] proposed the term *inborn errors of metabolism* for a group of inherited metabolic disorders that included porphyrias.

ETIOLOGY AND PATHOGENESIS

HEME

Heme is essential for the function of all aerobic cells. In addition to hemoglobin, heme serves as the prosthetic group of heme proteins such as myoglobin, mitochondrial and microsomal cytochromes, catalase, peroxidase, tryptophan pyrrolase, and nitric oxide synthase. Heme proteins are involved in the transport of oxygen and electrons, in the oxidative metabolism of various endogenous and exogenous chemicals, in the decomposition of hydrogen peroxide and organic peroxides, and in the oxidation of tryptophan. Most organisms have the ability to synthe-

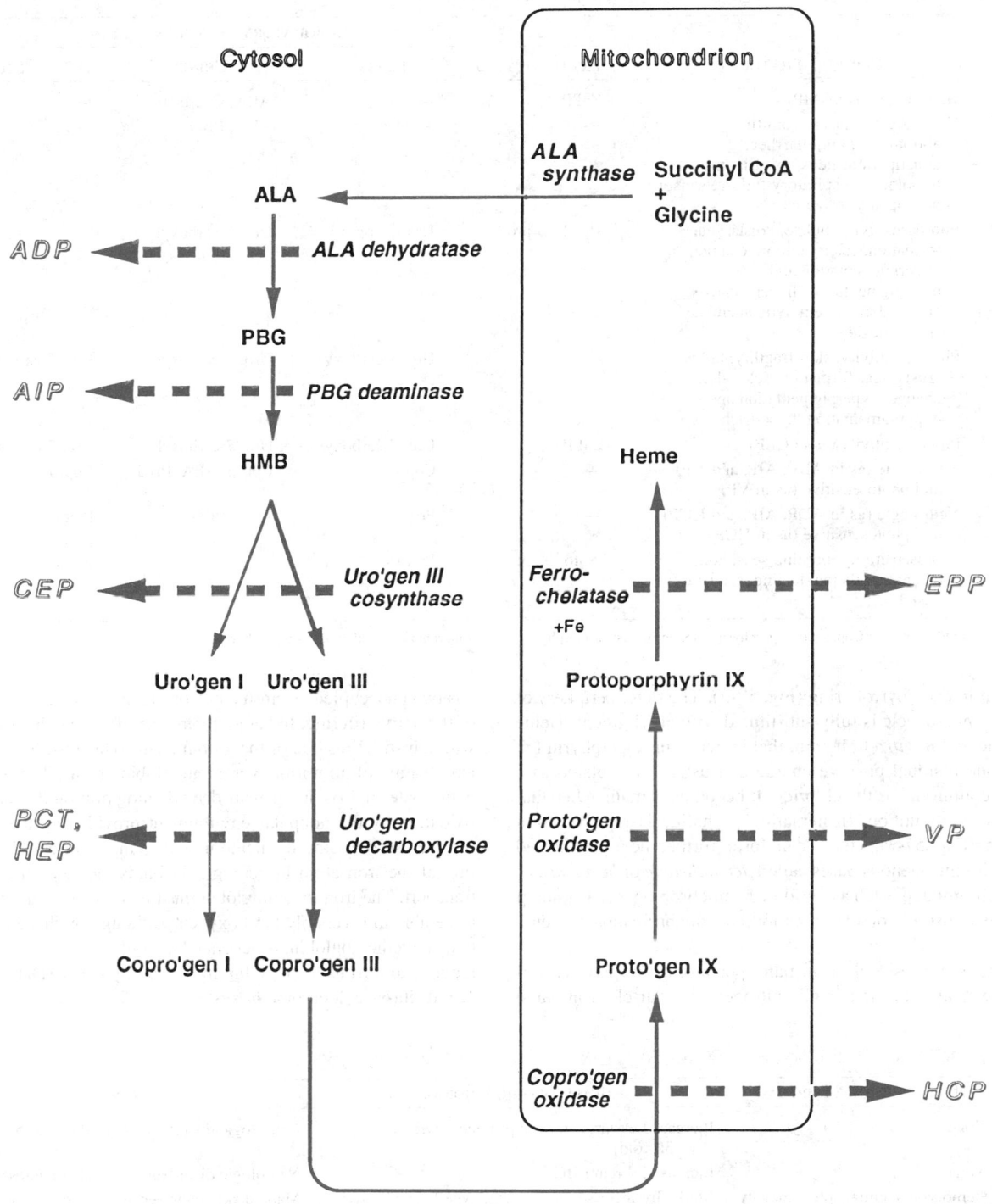

FIGURE 57-1   Enzymatic defects in the porphyrias. The enzymatic defect in each porphyria is shown by a *broken line*. In patients, the substrate for the defective enzymatic step accumulates in the tissue (e.g., erythrocytes) and in the plasma and is excreted in large excess into urine and/or stool. In addition, excretion of porphyrin precursors (ALA and PBG) may be increased in patients with acute hepatic porphyrias as a result of derepression of ALA synthase activity in the liver.

size heme and apohemeproteins. Exogenously administered heme can be incorporated, although rarely, into certain heme proteins such as hemoglobin[6] and cytochrome P450.[7] Approximately 500 to 700 g of hemoglobin (of which 3.8 percent is heme) is present in a normal man with 70-kg body weight.[8] Approximately 85 percent of heme is synthesized in the erythropoietic marrow; the remainder is synthesized largely by the liver.[9] In the liver, the majority of heme synthesized is incorpo-

rated into microsomal cytochrome P450s, which perform important biotransformations of a variety of chemicals, including carcinogens, steroids, vitamins, fatty acids, and prostaglandins.[10]

STRUCTURE OF HEME

Heme, that is, ferrous protoporphyrin IX, is composed of an iron atom coordinated to the four pyrrole rings of protoporphyrin through the

TABLE 57-2 CLINICAL AND LABORATORY FEATURES OF THE PORPHYRIAS

		LABORATORY FEATURES			
PORPHYRIA	CLINICAL FEATURES	ERYTHROCYTES	PLASMA	URINE	STOOL
ADP	Neurologic (as in AIP)	ZnPP	—	ALA, Copro III	—
AIP	Neurologic: nausea, vomiting, abdominal pain, diarrhea, constipation, ileus, dysuria, muscle hypotonia, respiratory failure, sensory neuropathy, seizures	—	—	ALA, PBG	—
CEP	Photosensitivity: bullae, crusts, scar formation, sclerodermoid change, hyperpigmentation and hypopigmentation, hypertrichosis, erythrodontia, hemolytic anemia, splenomegaly	Uro I, Copro I	Uro I, Copro I	Uro, 7-carboxyl	—
PCT	Photosensitivity: skin fragility, bullae, crusts, scar formation, sclerodermoid change, hyperpigmentation and hypopigmentation, hypertrichosis	—	Uro, 7-carboxyl	Uro, 7-carboxyl	Uro, 7-carboxyl, isocopro
HEP	Photosensitivity (as in CEP)	ZnPP	Uro, 7-carboxyl	Uro, 7-carboxyl	Uro, 7-carboxyl, isocopro
HCP	Neurologic (as in ADP, AIP, and VP) and photosensitive (as in VP)	—	Copro	Copro, ALA, PBG	Copro
VP	Neurologic (as in ADP, AIP, and HCP) and photosensitive (as in HCP)	—	Proto	ALA, PBG	Proto
EPP	Photosensitivity: burning sensation, edema, erythema, itching, scarring vesicles	Proto	Proto	—	Proto

7-Carboxyl, 7-carboxylporphyrin; Copro, coproporphyrin; Isocopro, isocoproporphyrin; Uro, uroporphyrin; ZnPP, zinc protoporphyrin.

nitrogen atom in each pyrrole ring (Fig. 57-2). The outer periphery of the porphyrin macrocycle is fully substituted with alkyl groups. Heme is readily oxidized *in vitro* to hemin, that is, ferric protoporphyrin IX. Hemin has one residual positive charge and usually is isolated as a halide, most commonly as the chloride. It becomes hematin when dissolved in alkaline solution. In hematin, the halide is replaced by a hydroxyl ion (Fig. 57-3). Heme can form further hexacoordinated complexes with nitrogenous bases called *hemochrome* or *hemochromogen*. Hemochromogen, such as pyridine hemochromogen, has a sharp spectrum and is useful for identification and quantification of heme proteins.

Ferrous ions have six electron pairs per atom. The ferrous iron atom in heme, bound to the pyrrolic nitrogen via four electron pairs,

has two unoccupied electron pairs, one above and one below the plane of the porphyrin ring. In hemoglobin, one of these pairs is coordinated with a histidyl residue of the globin chain. This histidine is an invariable feature of all normal vertebrate globin chains. The other coordination site of iron is open in deoxyhemoglobin and protected from oxidation by the nonpolar environment provided by the amino acid residues surrounding the heme moiety. This sixth coordination position of the iron atom in hemoglobin binds the oxygen molecule for transport. The iron in hemoglobin must be in the ferrous state in order to be able to reversibly bind oxygen. Although oxidized hemoglobin, that is, methemoglobin, is generated in erythrocytes, it is continuously reduced to ferrous hemoglobin in the cell by the NADH–cytochrome b_5 reductase–cytochrome b_5 system (see Chap. 47).

TABLE 57-3 HEMATOLOGIC SYMPTOMS AND LABORATORY FINDINGS IN THE PORPHYRIAS

PORPHYRIA	HEMATOLOGIC SYMPTOMS	HEMATOLOGIC FINDINGS	REMARKS
ADP	None	Increased erythrocyte zinc protoporphyrin (~30-fold)	Neurologic disturbances, no skin photosensitivity
AIP	None	Increased serum PBG	Neurologic disturbances, no skin photosensitivity
CEP	Hemolytic anemia, splenomegaly, marrow erythroid hyperplasia	Markedly increased erythrocyte type I uroporphyrin and coproporphyrin	Marked skin photosensitivity, no neurologic disturbances
PCT	None	Increased serum ferritin and porphyrin	Skin photosensitivity, no neurologic disturbances, most occur sporadically but some occur in families, often coinherited with mutations of the *HFE* gene, phlebotomy improves the condition
HEP	Hemolytic anemia, splenomegaly, marrow erythroid hyperplasia	Increased serum and erythrocyte porphyrins, normal serum ferritin concentration	Marked skin photosensitivity, no neurologic disturbances, phlebotomy has little effect
HCP	None	Increased serum coproporphyrin	Skin photosensitivity and neurologic disturbances, neonatal hemolytic anemia was associated with harderoporphyria, a variant form of HCP
VP	None	Increased serum protoporphyrin	Skin photosensitivity and neurologic disturbances, rare homozygous variants are associated with malformation and/or growth retardation but without anemia
EPP	None	Increased erythrocyte free protoporphyrin	Skin photosensitivity, no neurologic disturbances

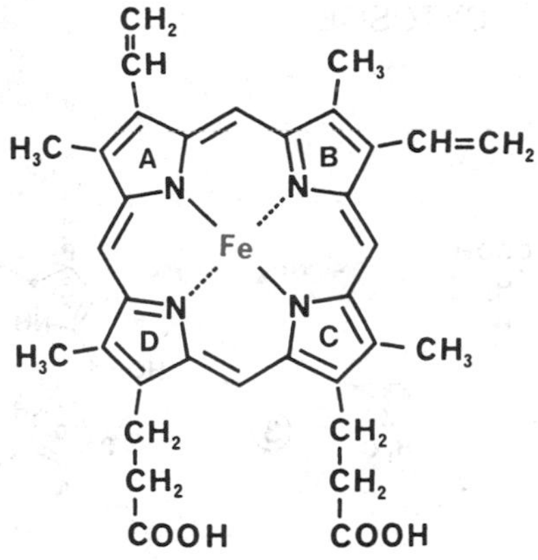

FIGURE 57-2 Structure of heme. The pyrole rings are labeled A through D.

BIOSYNTHESIS OF HEME

Figure 57-4 illustrates the steps involved in heme biosynthesis. In eukaryote cells, the first step and the last three steps occur in mitochondria. The four intermediate steps occur in the cytosol. The two major organs involved in heme synthesis are the bone marrow and the liver. In the bone marrow, heme is made in erythroblasts and reticulocytes, which contain mitochondria. Circulating erythrocytes lack the ability to form heme. The first intermediate of the heme biosynthetic pathway is ALA, a 5-carbon aminoketone, which is formed by the condensation of glycine and succinyl CoA. Two molecules of ALA combine to form the monopyrrole PBG. Four molecules of PBG then are combined to form uroporphyrinogen, a cyclic tetrapyrrole. Uroporphyrinogen is converted to coproporphyrinogen and subsequently to protoporphyrin IX. Finally, ferrous ion is inserted into protoporphyrin IX to form heme. Protoporphyrin IX is the immediate precursor of the various hemes and of the chlorophylls.

Step 1. Formation of ALA [δ-Aminolevulinate Synthase (Succinyl CoA: Glycine C-Succinyl Transferase) (Decarboxylating) (EC 2.3.1.37)] The first enzyme in the heme biosynthetic pathway is ALA synthase. ALA synthase catalyzes the condensation of glycine and succinyl CoA to form ALA (see Fig. 57-4, step 1). In mammalian cells, the enzyme is localized in the inner membrane of the mitochondria.[11] The enzyme reaction requires pyridoxal 5′-phosphate as a co-

factor. The enzyme is synthesized as a precursor protein in the cytosol and transported into mitochondria. Two separate ALA synthase genes—ALAS1 and ALAS2—encode nonspecific (ALAS-N) and erythroid-specific (ALAS-E) isoforms, respectively.[12,13] The human ALAS2 gene encodes a precursor of 587 amino acids, with an M_r of 64,600. Nucleotide sequences for the ALAS2 and the ALAS1 isoforms are approximately 60 percent similar. No homology is observed in the amino-terminal region, whereas high homology (approximately 73 percent) is seen after the hepatic residue 197.[14] The two human ALA synthase genes appear to have evolved by duplication of a common ancestral gene that encoded a primitive catalytic site, with subsequent addition of DNA sequences encoding variable functions, mostly at the amino termini.[15] The gene locus for human ALAS1 is at 3p.21. The gene locus for the erythroid ALA synthase is at Xp11.2.[13]

The promoter in the human ALAS2 gene contains several putative erythroid-specific cis-acting elements including both a GATA-1 and an NF-E2 binding site.[15] Both GATA-1 and NF-E2 are erythroid transcription factors that also bind to multiple DNA sites, such as the promoter of the human β-globin gene and the erythroid PBG deaminase gene.[16] These findings suggest ALAS2 gene expression likely is under the regulatory influence of erythroid transcription factors such as GATA-1. Additionally, ALAS2 mRNA contains an iron-responsive element in its 5′-untranslated region,[15] similar to mRNAs encoding ferritin[16] and transferrin receptor[17] (see Chap. 40). Gel retardation analysis showed that the iron-responsive element in ALAS2 mRNA is functional and suggests that translation of the erythroid-specific mRNA can be up-regulated by the availability of iron, or heme, in erythroid cells.[18]

The ALAS-N level in the liver is under positive and negative control by porphyrogenic chemicals and hemin, respectively.[19] Its level increases dramatically when the liver must make more heme in response to various chemical treatments. Enzyme synthesis also is derepressed in heme deficiency during relapse of acute hepatic porphyrias. Stimuli that increase hepatic heme demands, such as induction of cytochrome P450 by various drugs and/or hormones or induction of heme oxygenase by stress or fever, usually are associated with clinical aggravation of these disorders. In contrast, administration of hemin[20] or inhibitors of heme oxygenase activity[21] induces clinical remission. At heme concentrations much higher than the concentrations that repress enzyme synthesis, heme induces microsomal heme oxygenase, resulting in its enhanced catabolism.[22] Thus, maintenance of hepatic heme concentration by a balance between the synthesis of ALAS-N

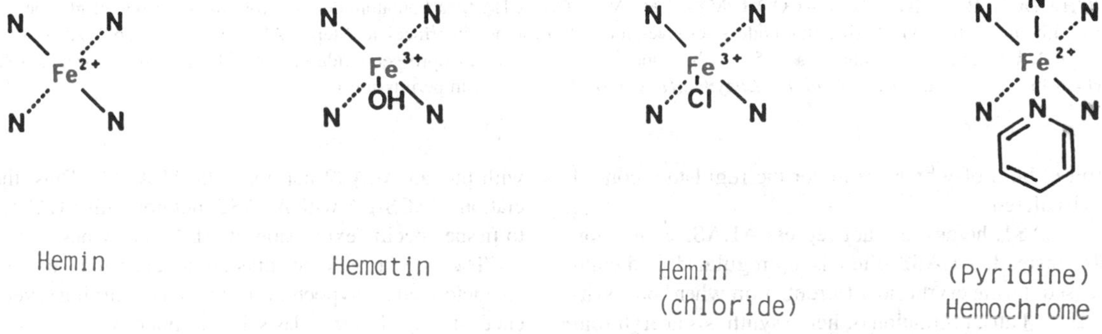

FIGURE 57-3 Forms of iron protoporphyrin IX. The nitrogen atom indicates the pyrrolic nitrogen.

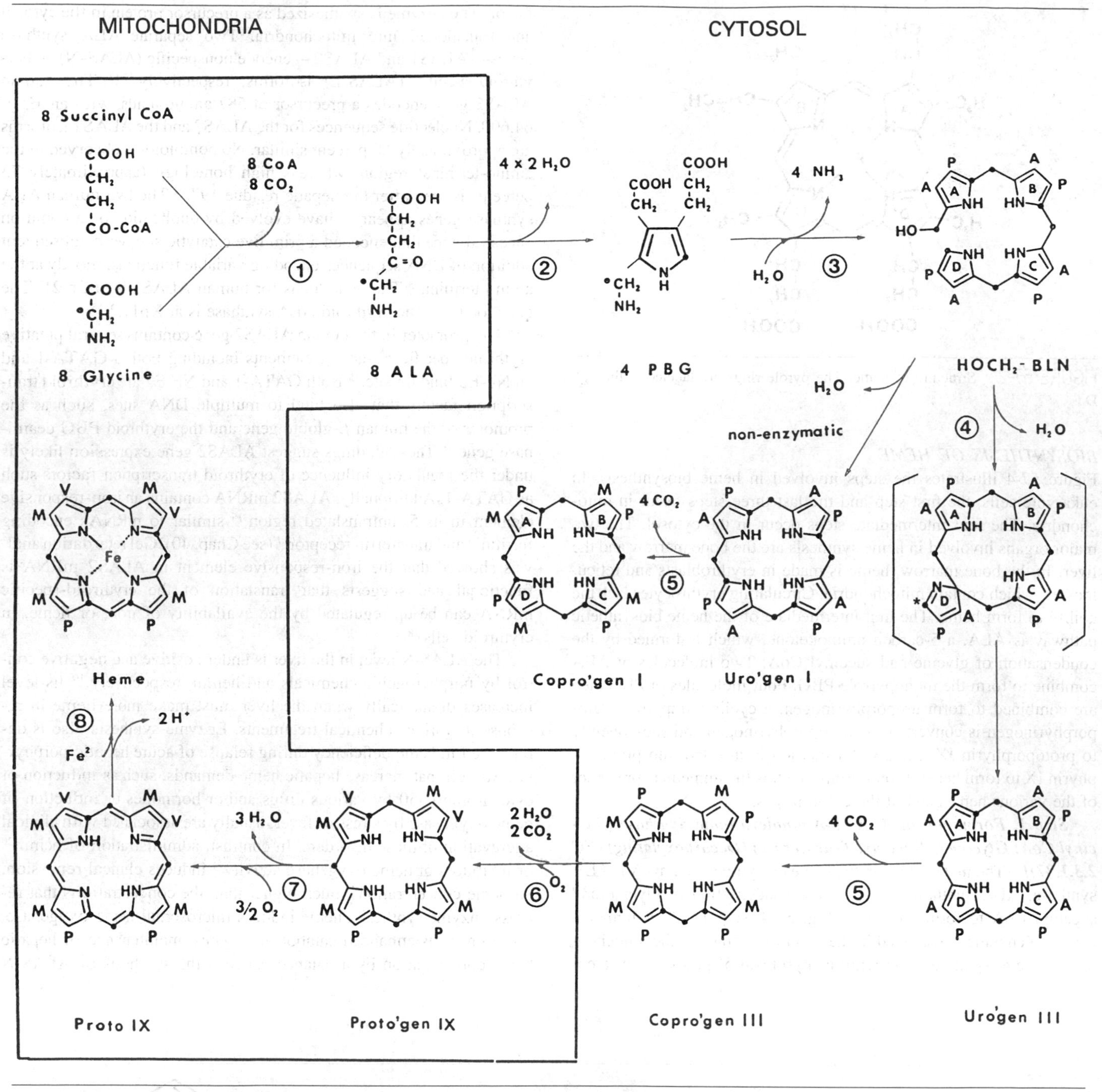

FIGURE 57-4   Heme biosynthesis pathway. Subcellular distribution of enzymes and intermediates are shown. ALA, δ-aminolevulinic acid; PBG, porpho-bilinogen; HOCH₂—BLN, hydroxymethylbilane; Uro'gen, uroporphyrinogen; Copro'gen, coproporphyrinogen; Proto'gen, protoporphyrinogen; Proto, proto-porphyrin. A, —CH₂COOH; P, —CH₂—CH₂—COOH; M, —CH₃; V, —CH=CH₂; •, carbon atom derived from the α-carbon of glycine; *, location of the α-carbon atom from glycine in the pyrrole ring that undergoes reversion; [ ], presumed intermediate. Step 1, ALA synthase; step 2, ALA dehydratase; step 3, PBG deaminase; step 4, Uro'gen III cosynthase; step 5, Uro'gen decarboxylase; step 6, Copro'gen oxidase; step 7, Proto'gen oxidase; step 8, ferrochelatase. (Modified from Hayashi N, *Protein, Nucleic Acid and Enzyme (Tokyo)* 32:797, 1987, with permission.)

and heme oxygenase, both of which are under the regulatory control of heme, can be visualized.

In contrast to ALAS1, heme does not repress ALAS2 expression in erythroid cells. Instead, ALAS2 often is up-regulated by hemin treatment or increased during erythroid differentiation when heme synthesis is increased.[23,24] Thus, regulation of heme synthesis in erythroid cells is distinct from regulation in the liver.[25] The β-subunit of human ATP-specific succinyl coenzyme A synthetase (SCS-βA) associates

with human ALAS2 but not with ALAS1.[26] Thus, the distinct association of SCS-βA with ALAS2, but not with ALAS1, may contribute to tissue-specific expression of ALAS isozymes.

The sideroblastic anemias are a heterogeneous group of disorders characterized by hypochromic anemia of varying severity and the presence of ringed sideroblasts in the bone marrow (see Chap. 58). X-linked sideroblastic anemia (XLSA) is the most common form of the inherited forms of sideroblastic anemia. Approximately 20 different point mutations of the ALAS2 gene have been reported in this disorder. Mutations frequently, but not necessarily, are in exon 9 of the ALAS2 gene, which contains the binding site for pyridoxal 5'-phosphate (K391), the essential cofactor for ALA synthase. The ALAS mutant D190V, identified in a patient with pyridoxine-refractory XLSA,[27] failed in association with SCS-βA, whereas other ALAS2 mutants were able to associate with SCS-βA. When ALAS2 was transcribed, translated, and transported into mitochondria, the mature D190V mutant protein, but not its precursor protein, underwent abnormal processing, resulting in an array of smeared bands. This process suggests appropriate association of SCS-βA and ALAS2 is necessary for proper functioning of ALAS2 in mitochondria, and a mutation in the SCS-βA may represent a novel mechanism for XLSA.[26]

Step 2. Formation of PBG [δ-Aminolevulinate Dehydratase; δ-Aminolevulinate Hydrolase (EC 4.2.1.24)] ALA dehydratase is a cytosolic enzyme that catalyzes the condensation of two molecules of ALA to form the monopyrrole PBG, with removal of two molecules of water (see Fig. 57-4, step 2). ALA dehydratase activity requires an intact sulfhydryl group and a zinc atom in the enzyme. Enzyme activity is inhibited by sulfhydryl reagents[28] or by lead, which displaces zinc.[29] Patients with lead poisoning show marked inhibition of ALA dehydratase activity in erythrocytes, excrete excessive amounts of ALA into urine, and exhibit various neurologic symptoms that often mimic those of acute hepatic porphyria.[30] The most potent inhibitor of the enzyme activity is 4,6-dioxoheptanoic acid (succinylacetone). This compound, which is found in urine and blood of patients with hereditary tyrosinemia,[31] is a substrate analogue and a potent inhibitor of the enzyme.[32,33] Patients with tyrosinemia show little ALA dehydratase activity in blood and liver and present symptoms similar to those of acute hepatic porphyria.[31,34]

Human ALA dehydratase is encoded by mRNA with an openreading frame of 990 bp, corresponding to a protein with an M_r of 36,274, and has a high degree of homology to the rat enzyme.[34,35] Sequences are essential for enzymatic activity, such as those for the active lysine residue and for the cysteine- and histidine-rich zinc binding sites.[36] The gene for human ALA dehydratase (ALAD) is localized at chromosome 9p34.[37]

Studies using [5-^{14}C]-ALA have shown that, of the two ALA molecules used as substrate, the ALA molecule contributing the propionic acid side is initially bound to the enzyme.[38] The tertiary structure of the yeast ALAD has been solved to 2.3-Å resolution, revealing that each subunit adopts a TIM barrel fold with a 39-residue N-terminal arm. Pairs of monomers then wrap their arms around each other to form compact dimers, and these dimers associate to form a 422 symmetric octamer.[39] All eight active sites are on the surface of the octamer and possess two lysine residues (210 and 263). The Lys263 residue forms a Schiff base link to the substrate. The two lysine side chains are close to two zinc binding sites. One binding site is formed by three cysteine residues; the other involves Cys234 and His142.

Unlike ALA synthase, no tissue-specific isozyme for ALA dehydratase is known. However, ALA dehydratase mRNA occurs in housekeeping (1A) and erythroid-specific (1B) forms, and significant tissue-specific control of these transcripts exists, namely, both GATA-1 and ALA dehydratase 1B mRNA are significantly up-regulated during erythroid differentiation in mice.[40] The fact that the promoter region upstream of exon 1B contains GATA-1 sites in both man and mouse may account for this finding.[40]

Human ALA dehydratase is a polymorphic enzyme.[41] It has two common alleles (allele 1 and allele 2) that result in three distinct charge isozyme phenotypes: 1-1, 1-2, and 2-2. The allele 2 sequence is different from the allele 1 sequence only by a G → C transversion of nucleotide 177 in the coding region.[42] This base substitution results in

replacement of lysine by asparagine, an amino acid change consistent with the more electronegative charge of the allele 2 subunit.

Step 3. Formation of Uroporphyrinogen I [PBG Deaminase; PBG Ammonia-Lyase (Polymerizing) (EC 4.3.1.8)] PBG deaminase catalyzes the condensation of four molecules of PBG to yield the linear tetrapyrrole hydroxymethylbilane[43] (see Fig. 57-4, step 3). In the absence of uroporphyrinogen III cosynthase, the subsequent enzyme in the pathway, the bilane spontaneously forms the ring structure uroporphyrinogen I. The type I porphyrinogen isomers do not produce any useful metabolites, whereas the type III isomers are the precursor for heme synthesis. Although PBG deaminase used to be referred to as *uroporphyrinogen I synthase*, the term is incorrect because PBG deaminase does not form uroporphyrinogen I. PBG deaminase should be called either *PBG deaminase* or *hydroxymethylbilane synthase*, because the enzyme furnishes hydroxymethylbilane by deaminating four PBG molecules.

The gene locus encoding human PBG deaminase is at chromosome 11q23→11qter.[44] The human PBG deaminase gene is split into 15 exons spread over 10 kb of DNA.[45] Two distinct molecular forms of PBG deaminase exist: the erythroid-specific and the nonspecific isoforms.[46] The two distinct mRNAs are produced through alternative splicing of two primary transcripts arising from two promoters. The upstream promoter is active in all tissues; thus, the enzyme encoded by the larger transcript is termed the *nonspecific*, or *housekeeping*, PBG deaminase. The size of the human housekeeping isoform predicted from its cDNA is 344 amino acids, with an M_r of 37,627.[47] The other promoter, located approximately 3 kb downstream, is active only in erythroid cells. Erythroid-specific *trans*-acting factors, such as GATA-1 and NF-E2, recognize sequences in the PBG deaminase erythroid promoter.[48] A 1320-bp stretch of perfect identity is present between the erythroid and the nonerythroid PBG deaminase, but with a mismatch in the first exon at their 5' extremities. An additional inframe AUG codon present 51 bp upstream from the initiating codon of the erythropoietic cDNA accounts for the additional 17 amino acid residues at the N-terminus of the nonerythropoietic isoform. Accordingly, a splice site mutation at the last position of exon 1, or a base transition in intron 1, in certain patients with AIP results in decreased PBG deaminase expression in nonerythroid tissues including the liver, but not in erythroid cells, because transcription of the gene in erythroid cells starts downstream of the site of mutation.

Step 4. Formation of Uroporphyrinogen III (Uroporphyrinogen III Cosynthase) Uroporphyrinogen III cosynthase, a cytosolic enzyme, catalyzes the formation of uroporphyrinogen III from hydroxymethylbilane. The process involves an intramolecular rearrangement that affects only ring D of the porphyrin macrocycle[43] (see Fig. 57-4, step 4). The protein predicted from a human uroporphyrinogen III cosynthase cDNA, which has an open-reading frame of 798 bp, consists of 263 amino acid residues, with an M_r of 28,607.[49] The amino acid compositions of the hepatic uroporphyrinogen III cosynthase and the purified erythrocyte enzyme are essentially identical, suggesting that the enzyme in the liver and in erythroid cells is identical.

Step 5. Formation of Coproporphyrinogen [Uroporphyrinogen Decarboxylase (EC 4.1.1.37)] A cytosolic enzyme, uroporphyrinogen decarboxylase (UROD), catalyzes the sequential removal of the four carboxylic groups of the carboxymethyl side chains in uroporphyrinogen to yield coproporphyrinogen (see Fig. 57-4, step 5). The single enzyme catalyzes four successive decarboxylation reactions yielding 7-, 6-, 5-, and 4-carboxylated porphyrinogens. The occurrence of all these intermediates has been identified in urine and stool. The enzyme activity in the liver can be inhibited by environmental chemicals such as polyhalogenated aromatic hydrocarbons. Human UROD is a 42-kDa polypeptide encoded by a single gene containing 10 exons spread over 3 kb.[50] The gene has been mapped to chromosome 1p34.

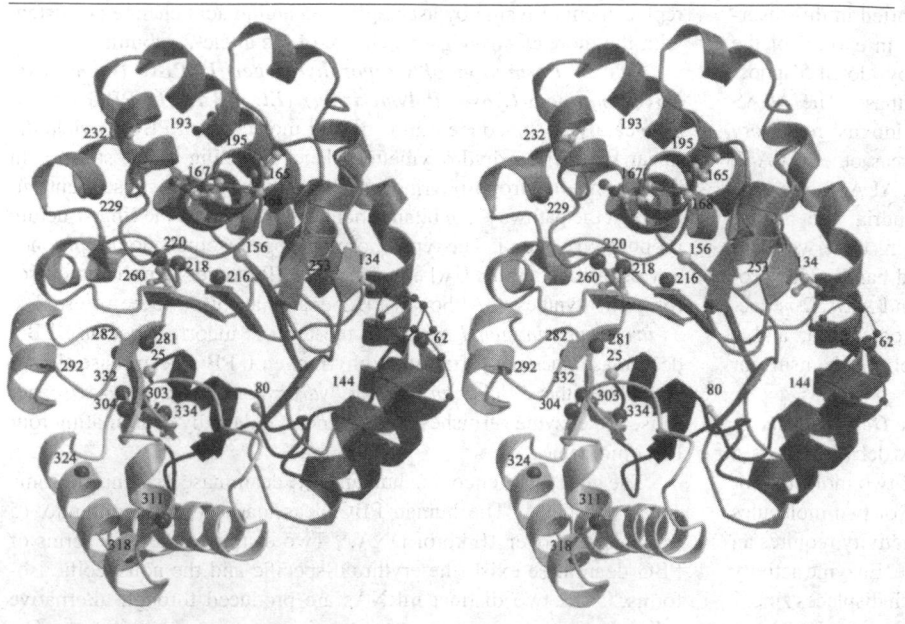

FIGURE 57-5   Crystal structure of human uroporphyrinogen decarboxylase (UROD) and the location of mutations in the UROD structure. View of a UROD monomer approximately along the axis of the β-barrel, looking at the active site cleft. Two adjacent monomers form an active dimer, creating an extended cleft. The large cleft can accommodate one or two substrate molecules and might enable intermediates to shuttle between monomers during the four-step decarboxylation of uroporphyrinogen. The disordered loop is shown as a *thin dark line with spheres* on the Cα positions. *Numbers* indicate the positions of mutant residues. Mutated amino acids that have been identified in PCT or HEP are depicted as *spheres*. More details are shown in color in reference 197. (Reproduced from JD Phillips, TL Parker, HL Schubert, et al.,[197] with permission.)

Although it contains two initiation sites, both sites are used with the same frequencies in all tissues, and the gene is transcribed into a unique mRNA.[51] Recombinant human UROD purified to homogeneity has been crystallized, and its crystal structure was determined at 1.60-Å resolution.[52] The purified protein is a dimer with a dissociation constant of 0.1 μM.[53] Figure 57-5 shows the 40.8-kDa polypeptide forms a single domain with a distorted $(\beta/\alpha)_8$-barrel fold, and a distinctive deep cleft for the enzyme's active site is formed by loops at the C-terminal ends of the barrel strands. One active-site cleft per monomer is located adjacent to its neighbor in the dimer. The structure creates a single extended cleft that is large enough to accommodate two substrate molecules in close proximity or to allow reaction intermediates to shuttle between monomers during the four-step decarboxylation of uroporphyrinogen.

Step 6. Formation of Protoporphyrinogen IX (Coproporphyrinogen Oxidase)   Coproporphyrinogen oxidase (CPO) in mammalian cells is a mitochondrial enzyme that catalyzes the removal of the carboxyl group and two hydrogens from the propionic groups of pyrrole rings A and B of coproporphyrinogen III to form vinyl groups at these positions, yielding protoporphyrinogen IX (see Fig. 57-4, step 6). The gene for human CPO has been assigned to chromosome 3q12, spans approximately 14 kb, and consists of seven exons and six introns.[54] cDNA cloning for this enzyme has been reported in mouse erythroleukemia cells.[55] The predicted protein comprises 354 amino acid residues ($M_r = 40,647$), with a putative leader sequence of 31 amino acid residues. The result is a mature protein consisting of 323 amino acid residues ($M_r = 37,225$).[55] Potential regulatory elements exist in the GC-rich promoter region on the gene, such as six Sp1, four GATA, one CACCC site, and the *CPO* gene promoter regulatory element (CPRE).[56] CPRE binds specifically to a CPRE-binding protein, which has a leucine-zipper-like structure and serves as a DNA sequence-

specific transcription factor that regulates gene expression.[56] Tissue-specific expression of CPO is significant. For example, binding proteins to the Sp1-like element, CPRE and GATA-1, cooperatively function in *CPO* gene expression in erythroid cells. The CPRE-binding protein by itself plays a principal role in basal expression of CPO in nonerythroid cells.[57] *CPO* mRNA increases during erythroid cell differentiation.[58,59] Newly synthesized human CPO contains a 110-amino-acid N-terminal signal peptide,[60] which is removed during transport into the intermembrane space of mitochondria, yielding a mature protein of 354 amino acid residues ($M_r = 36,842$). A five-base insertional mutation in the middle of this presequence has been described in one patient with HCP.[61]

Step 7. Formation of Protoporphyrin IX [Protoporphyrinogen Oxidase (EC 1.3.3.4)]   The penultimate step in heme biosynthesis, that is, the oxidation of protoporphyrinogen IX to protoporphyrin IX, is mediated by the mitochondrial enzyme *protoporphyrinogen oxidase*, which catalyzes the removal of six hydrogen atoms from the porphyrinogen nucleus (see Fig. 57-4, step 7). Human protoporphyrinogen oxidase cDNA has been cloned.[62] The gene is present as a single copy per haploid genome, at chromosome 1q22.[63] Protoporphyrinogen oxidase consists of 477 amino acids with an M_r of 50,800. The deduced protein exhibits a high degree of homology over its entire length to the amino acid sequence of protoporphyrinogen oxidase encoded by the *HEMY* gene of *Bacillus subtilis*. Protoporphyrinogen oxidase is a monomer with no apparent transport-specific leader sequence but is ultimately localized in mitochondria.[62]

Step 8. Formation of Heme [Ferrochelatase; Protoheme-Ferrolyase (EC 4.99.1.1)]   The final step of heme biosynthesis is the insertion of iron into protoporphyrin IX. This reaction is catalyzed by the mitochondrial enzyme *ferrochelatase* (see Fig. 57-4, step 8). Unlike other enzymatic steps in the heme biosynthetic pathway, ferrochelatase utilizes protoporphyrin IX, rather than its reduced form, as substrate. However, ferrous, not ferric, ion is utilized for insertion into protoporphyrin IX.[64] The gene encoding human ferrochelatase has been assigned to chromosome 18q.[65,66] Two ferrochelatase mRNA species, approximately 2.5 kb and approximately 1.6 kb in size, are derived from the utilization of two alternative polyadenylation sites in the mRNA. The human ferrochelatase gene contains a total of 11 exons and has a minimum size of approximately 45 kb.[65] A major site of transcription initiation is at an adenine, 89 bp upstream from the translation-initiating ATG. The promoter region contains a potential binding site for several transcription factors, Sp1, NF-E2, and GATA-1, but not a typical TATA or CAAT sequence. The transcripts are identical in all tissues examined.

The crystal structure of *B. subtilis* ferrochelatase has been determined at 1.9-Å resolution.[67] Ferrochelatase seems to have a structurally conserved core region that is common to the enzyme from bacteria, plants, and mammals. The porphyrin and the metal appear to bind in the identical cleft.

CONTROL OF HEME SYNTHESIS IN THE LIVER AND ERYTHROID CELLS

The rate of heme synthesis in the liver is largely regulated by the level of ALAS-N activity. The synthesis of ALAS-N in turn is under feedback control by heme. Compounds that increase hepatic cytochrome P450 synthesis, accelerate destruction of heme, or inhibit heme formation induce ALAS-N. Regulation of ALAS-N by heme occurs at least at four different levels: (1) transcription, (2) translation, (3) transfer into mitochondria, and (4) enzyme inhibition. The last mechanism appears least important, whereas the other three mechanisms may play an important role in regulating ALAS-N levels.

ALAS-E is not inducible by drugs that induce ALAS-N.[68] Unlike ALAS-N, the synthesis of ALAS-E is uninfluenced, or often up-regulated, by hemin treatment, both at the transcriptional and the translational levels.[18,23,69] Hemin treatment of rats strongly inhibits the synthesis of hepatic cytochrome P450,[70] but the same treatment of marrow cultures increases erythroid colony forming units.[71] A distinct difference exists in the association of SCS-βA with ALAS isoforms, namely, SCS-βA associates with ALAS-E[26] but not with ALAS-N, suggesting tissue-specific control in the mitochondrial transport between these isoforms. Thus, regulation of ALA synthase expression in these two major heme-synthesizing organs may be distinct at several levels. Table 57-4 summarizes other aspects of tissue-specific regulation of heme biosynthesis.

ERYTHROPOIETIC PORPHYRIAS

CONGENITAL ERYTHROPOIETIC PORPHYRIA

DEFINITION AND HISTORY

CEP is an erythropoietic porphyria that is inherited in an autosomal recessive fashion. The primary abnormality is almost total deficiency of uroporphyrinogen III cosynthase activity, which results in accumulation and massive excretion of type I porphyrins (see Table 57-1 and Fig. 57-1). After the first two cases of CEP described by Anderson[2] in 1898, approximately 130 cases have been reported,[75] but some of these individuals may have had HEP. Patients with CEP suffer from symptoms resulting from phototoxic reactions, including cutaneous lesions and hemolytic anemia.

PATHOPHYSIOLOGY

Remarkable molecular heterogeneity of the uroporphyrinogen III cosynthase defects in CEP exists. To date, 18 different mutations of the uroporphyrinogen cosynthase gene have been reported in CEP. The mutations include deletions, insertions, rearrangements, splicing ab-

normalities, and both missense and nonsense mutations. Six of the mutations are found in exon 4, four in exon 10, and three in both exons 2 and 9.[76] Of the 12 single base substitutions, four (T228M, G225S, A66V, A104V) were hot spot mutations, occurring at CpG dinucleotides. With the exception of V82F, all CEP missense mutations occurred in amino acid residues that are conserved in both the mouse and the human uroporphyrinogen cosynthase.

Genotype–phenotype comparison of the uroporphyrinogen cosynthase was studied using the prokaryotic expression of mutant cDNAs. Mean activities of the mutant enzymes ranged from 0 to 36 percent of the activity expressed in *Escherichia coli* by the normal cDNA. The majority of the mutant cDNAs expressed polypeptides with null enzyme activity. Only V82F, A66V, A104V, and V99A showed 36, 15, 8, and 6 percent enzyme activity, respectively, compared with the normal control. A66V and V82F were thermodynamically unstable mutants.[76] Homoallelism for C73R, the most common mutation, was found in five patients and is associated clinically with the most severe phenotype, hydrops fetalis, and/or transfusion dependency from birth.

PATHOGENESIS OF THE CLINICAL FINDINGS

Most marrow normoblasts display fluorescence, principally in the nuclei.[77] Marrow-derived porphyrins become distributed throughout the body and account for the multiple pathologies of the integument. Splenomegaly is frequently observed in CEP and is presumed to be secondary to the hemolytic process. Hemolysis of erythrocytes may result from photolysis as porphyrin-laden cells are exposed to light in the dermal capillaries.

CLINICAL FEATURES

Early onset of cutaneous photosensitivity exacerbated by exposure to sunlight is characteristic. Subepidermal bullous lesions progress to crusted erosions that heal with scarring and either hyperpigmentation or hypopigmentation. Hypertrichosis and alopecia are common, and erythrodontia (with red porphyrin fluorescence under ultraviolet light) is virtually pathognomonic of CEP. Hemolytic anemia may be accompanied by splenomegaly and porphyrin-rich gallstones. Compensatory expansion of the marrow may result in pathologic fractures, vertebral compression or collapse, shortness of stature, and, rarely, osteolytic and sclerotic lesions in the skeleton.

TABLE 57-4 TISSUE-SPECIFIC REGULATION OF ENZYMES IN THE HEME BIOSYNTHETIC PATHWAY

ENZYME	ERYTHROID CELLS	LIVER	REMARKS	REFERENCE
ALA synthase	ALAS2 mRNA, ALAS2 protein	ALAS1 mRNA, ALAS1 protein	ALAS1 and ALAS2 are two separate gene products. ALAS1 expression is suppressed, whereas ALAS2 expression is up-regulated by heme.	72
ALA dehydratase	ALAD1B mRNA	ALAD1A mRNA	Although their protein product is identical, ALAD1A and ALAD1B mRNA are subject to tissue-specific regulation.	40
PBG deaminase	PBGD-E mRNA, PBGD-E protein	PBGD-N mRNA, PBGD-N protein	Two mRNAs are the result of alternate splicing arising from two promoters. PBGD-E expression is controlled by GATA-1 and NF-E2.	48
Uroporphyrinogen cosynthase	The same enzyme is expressed in these two tissues.		No tissue-specific regulation.	
Uroporphyrinogen decarboxylase	The same enzyme is expressed in these two tissues.		Uroporphyrinogen decarboxylase mRNA increases during erythroid cell differentiation, although its mechanism is unknown.	73
Coproporphyrinogen oxidase	The same enzyme is expressed in these two tissues.		Potential distinct regulation between the two tissues by tissue-specific *trans*-acting factors.	
Protoporphyrinogen oxidase	The same enzyme is expressed in these two tissues.		No tissue-specific regulation.	
Ferrochelatase	The same enzyme is expressed in these two tissues.		Ferrochelatase mRNA increases during erythroid cell differentiation, although its mechanism is unknown.	74

DIAGNOSIS

CEP can be recognized *in utero* by dark brownish amniotic fluid enriched in porphyrins. The diagnosis of CEP in infants can be made by pink to dark brown staining of the diapers because of large amounts of urinary porphyrins. Severe cutaneous photosensitivity in infancy (or rarely in adults) suggests the diagnosis of CEP. Urinary porphyrin levels are always elevated 20- to 60-fold above normal. Uroporphyrin levels are increased more than coproporphyrin levels. Type I isomers of uroporphyrin and coproporphyrin series predominate, but type III isomer levels also are elevated. Fecal porphyrin excretion usually is increased and is predominantly coproporphyrin I. Anemia may be present, and erythrocytes may exhibit polychromasia, poikilocytosis, anisocytosis, and basophilic stippling. Demonstration of elevated urinary and fecal porphyrins of type I isomers and of free erythrocyte uroporphyrin and coproporphyrins are diagnostic of CEP. HEP may present as photosensitivity in childhood. Porphyrin excretion is elevated, but elevated fecal levels of isocoproporphyrin and 5-carboxylic porphyrins distinguish HEP from CEP.

THERAPY

Patients should be advised to avoid sunlight, trauma to the skin, and infections. Topical sunscreens and oral treatment with β-carotene may helpful.[78] Transfusions with packed erythrocytes transiently decrease hemolysis and its attendant drive to increased erythropoiesis.[79] Splenectomy has been performed on many patients but has resulted in only short-term reductions in hemolysis, porphyrin excretion, and skin manifestations. Treatment with charcoal for 9 months in a man with CEP reportedly lowered porphyrin levels in plasma and skin and resulted in complete clinical remission during therapy.[80] Oral administration of the free radical scavenger ascorbic acid and α-tocopherol reportedly was effective in improving anemia.[75]

ERYTHROPOIETIC PROTOPORPHYRIA

DEFINITION AND HISTORY

EPP is characterized by a partial deficiency of ferrochelatase activity. The disease generally is inherited in an autosomal dominant fashion with a variable degree of clinical expression (see Table 57-1 and Fig. 57-1). The defect results in massive accumulations of protoporphyrin in erythrocytes, plasma, and feces. Clinically, the disease is characterized by childhood onset of cutaneous photosensitivity in light-exposed areas, but skin lesions are milder and less disfiguring than those seen in CEP, PCT, HEP, and VP. EPP is the most common form of erythropoietic porphyria. By 1976, approximately 300 case reports had been published.[81] No racial or sexual predilection has been noted, and onset typically occurs in childhood.

PATHOPHYSIOLOGY

Molecular analysis of the ferrochelatase gene in patients with EPP has revealed missense mutations, splicing mutations, intragenic deletions, and possible nonsense mutations associated with functional deficiency of ferrochelatase.[82] Splicing mutations are most common. In a proband's family, typically one parent is classified as a carrier of the disease because of elevated erythrocyte and stool protoporphyrin levels. In many cases, the mode of inheritance is autosomal dominant, but it often is vague or has a variable degree of penetrance. Parent-to-offspring transmission of the clinical disease occurs in less than 10 percent of cases.[83] In addition to the typical dominant inheritance, a few cases of EPP with recessive inheritance have been confirmed.[84] Disease expression is influenced by other factors, including pregnancy.[85] These findings suggest EPP is a heterogeneous disorder.

A C→T transition at position -23 in intron 1 was first reported in a patient with EPP.[86] A later study showed that the -23C→T transition

was found invariably in all EPP patients and in some normal controls. A second mutation in patients with EPP likely is responsible for the disease.[87] Based on these findings, both a mutant allele and the C→T transition in *trans* are proposed to be necessary for EPP expression. However, the enzymatic activity encoded by the 23C→T transition has not been examined by heterologous expression; thus, whether the transition represents a mutation or a polymorphism remains uncertain.

Recombinant human ferrochelatase, which had been engineered to have individual exon skipping corresponding to exons 3 through 11, lacks significant enzyme activity when it is expressed in *E. coli*. All these mutants, with the exception of F417S, did not contain the [2Fe-2S] cluster or have enzyme activity.[88]

Despite the molecular findings on the defect of the *ferrochelatase* gene, incomplete penetrance and variable clinical expression remain puzzling features of EPP. No strict correlation between the genetic defects and the erythrocyte protoporphyrin levels, or between the abnormal ferrochelatase activity and EPP disease severity, has been demonstrated. For example, the same mutation found among four unrelated Swiss patients (Q59X) was associated with symptoms ranging from mild photosensitivity to terminal liver disease.[89] The genetic background of individuals contributes to the variable expression of the disease. An EPP family has been described in which a ferrochelatase allele with a normal coding sequence was expressed at a lower than normal level.[90] Other studies showed five more families with EPP had a low-expression normal ferrochelatase allele and a mutant allele.[91] The low-expression allele, which has a particular 5' haplotype (*-251A/G, IVS1-23C/T, IVS2μsatAn$_{1-10}$, 798G/C,* and *1520C/T*), is present in approximately 10 percent of the Caucasian population. Thus, inheritance of a ferrochelatase mutation in *cis* and the low-expression allele in *trans* could provide an explanation for the low ferrochelatase activity and clinical expression of the disease.

PATHOGENESIS OF THE CLINICAL FINDINGS

Histologic examinations of skin biopsies from EPP patients show thickened capillary walls in the papillary dermis surrounded by amorphous hyaline-like deposits, immunoglobulin, complement, and periodic acid Schiff (PAS)-positive mucopolysaccharides.[92] Basement membrane abnormalities are observed in EPP but are quantitatively less marked than in other forms of porphyria.[93] Thus, EPP may be suggested by, but not positively identified from, skin biopsies. Light-excited porphyrins generate free radicals and singlet oxygen,[94] which then lead to peroxidation of lipids[95] and cross-linking of membrane proteins.[96] Marrow reticulocytes may display fluorescence, but protoporphyrin content and fluorescence of circulating reticulocytes are nonuniform and decrease with age.[97] Erythrocyte protoporphyrin in EPP is free and not complexed with zinc, unlike other conditions associated with increased erythrocyte protoporphyrin content. The content of free protoporphyrin in these cells declines much more rapidly with red cell age than it does in conditions of increased erythrocyte zinc protoporphyrin.[98] In lead poisoning and iron deficiency, the excess erythrocyte zinc protoporphyrin is bound to hemoglobin and persists in the red cell as long as it circulates, whereas free protoporphyrin in EPP binds less readily to hemoglobin and diffuses more rapidly into the plasma. Interestingly, free protoporphyrin, but not zinc protoporphyrin, is released from erythrocytes following irradiation, which may explain why lead intoxication and iron deficiency, which are associated with elevated erythrocyte zinc protoporphyrin levels, are not associated with photosensitivity.[99] Skin irradiation in EPP patients leads to complement activation and polymorphonuclear chemotaxis. This event also may contribute to the pathogenesis of skin lesions in EPP.[100]

Light and electron microscopic examination of liver biopsies from EPP patients have revealed widely variable findings, ranging from complete normality to periportal fibrosis and severe cirrhosis. Abnormally elevated, sometimes massive, accumulations of protoporphyrin have been detected as brown pigment in hepatocytes, Kupffer cells, and biliary canaliculi and are doubly refractive under polarizing lenses.[101] As many as 20 patients with EPP have developed hepatic failure resulting in death, presumably secondary to protoporphyrin damage. A high ratio of protoporphyrin to bile acids in bile may be indicative of patients with EPP who have advanced liver disease.[102]

CLINICAL FEATURES

Table 57-5 lists the most common symptoms in a series of 32 patients with EPP. Symptoms usually are worse during spring and summer and occur in light-exposed areas, especially of the face and hands. Within 1 hour of sun exposure, stinging or painful burning sensations occur in the skin, followed several hours later by erythema and edema. Petechiae or, more rarely, purpura, vesicles, and crusting may develop and persist for several days after sun exposure. Some patients experience burning sensations in the absence of objective signs of cutaneous phototoxicity. Artificial lights may cause photosensitivity.[103] Severe sun exposure may result in onycholysis, leathery hyperkeratotic skin over the dorsae of the hands, and mild scarring. Bullae, skin fragility, hypertrichosis, hyperpigmentation, severe scarring, and mutilation are unusual in EPP. Gallstones, sometimes presenting at an unusually early age, are fairly common. Hepatic disease, although unusual, may be severe and associated with significant morbidity. Anemia is uncommon but has been reported in some cases. No precipitating factors or neurovisceral manifestations are known. Conversely, pregnancy is known to lower erythrocyte protoporphyrin levels and increase tolerance to sunlight.[85]

DIAGNOSIS

Photosensitivity suggests the diagnosis, which can be confirmed by demonstrating elevated concentrations of free protoporphyrin in erythrocytes, plasma, and stool, in association with normal urinary porphyrins. The presence of protoporphyrin in both plasma and erythrocytes is specific for EPP. Fluorescent reticulocytes on examination of peripheral blood smear suggest the diagnosis. Evidence favors the marrow and the newly released reticulocytes or erythrocytes as the major source of elevated protoporphyrin concentrations.[97] Mild anemia with hyperchromia and microcytosis may occur. Mild hypertriglyceridemia occurs with increased frequency in patients with EPP.

THERAPY

Avoidance of the sun and use of topical sunscreen agents may be helpful. Oral administration of β-carotene may afford photoprotection, resulting in improved, but highly variable, tolerance to the sun. The recommended serum β-carotene level of 600 to 800 μg/dl[104] usually is achieved with daily oral doses of 120 to 180 mg. Beneficial effects

TABLE 57-5 COMMON CLINICAL FEATURES OF ERYTHROPOIETIC PROTOPORPHYRIA FROM A SERIES OF 32 CASES[81]

SYMPTOMS AND SIGNS	INCIDENCE (% OF TOTAL)
Burning	97
Edema	94
Itching	88
Erythema	69
Scarring	19
Vesicles	3
Anemia	27
Cholelithiasis	12
Abnormal liver function results	4

typically are seen 1 to 3 months after the onset of therapy. β-Carotene probably quenches activated oxygen radicals.[105] Hypertransfusion therapy has been advocated to suppress erythropoiesis,[106] but the potential hazards of transfusion are a drawback. Cholestyramine reportedly improves photosensitivity and reduces hepatic protoporphyrin content.[107] Several patients who developed hepatic failure have been treated by liver transplantation, with only temporary relief of deranged liver function and accumulation of protoporphyrin in the liver.[108]

HEPATIC PORPHYRIA

ACUTE HEPATIC PORPHYRIAS

ALA DEHYDRATASE DEFICIENCY PORPHYRIA

Definition and History δ-Aminolevulinate dehydratase deficiency porphyria (ADP) is an autosomal recessive disorder resulting from an almost complete deficiency of ALA dehydratase activity (see Table 57-1 and Fig. 57-1). This is the rarest form of the porphyrias; only four well-documented cases have been reported.[109] Two cases were German males with onset in their teens,[110] the third case was a Swedish infant with severe acute hepatic porphyria,[111] and the fourth was a Belgian male with a late onset.[112]

Pathophysiology The molecular defect of ALA dehydratase in the first German patient was compound heterozygosity for two distinct point mutations of the ALA dehydratase gene, one at each allele.[113] One, termed G2, was a base substitution of A→G at nucleotide 820, which resulted in an amino acid change, Ala274→Thr. The other, termed G1, was a C→T transition at nucleotide 718, resulting in an amino acid change, Arg240→Trp.[114] The G1 mutation was located within the substrate binding site. The G2 mutation was present downstream of this site. Expression of G1 cDNA in Chinese hamster ovary cells produced ALA dehydratase protein with little activity. G2 cDNA produced the enzyme with approximately 50 percent normal enzyme activity. Pulse-labeling studies demonstrated that the G1 enzyme had a normal half-life, whereas the G2 enzyme had a markedly decreased half-life. These findings demonstrated that the proband was a compound heterozygote for two separate point mutations in each ALA dehydratase allele and accounted for the almost complete lack of enzymatic activity in the proband's cells and the half-normal activity in cells from the family members.

The molecular defect in the Swedish infant with ADP was reported.[115] A maternal G→A transition at nucleotide 397 predicted a Gly133→Arg change, which occurred at the carboxyl end of the zinc binding site in the enzyme. The paternal mutation was a G→A transition at nucleotide 823, resulting in the amino acid change Val275→Met.

The fourth patient was a Belgian male who was unique because he developed ADP at age 63 years.[112] He also developed polycythemia at that time. His erythrocyte ALAD activity was less than 1 percent of normal, whereas his lymphocytes had ALAD activity greater than 20 percent. Sequence analysis of ALAD cDNA in this subject revealed two base transitions in one allele, G177 to C, resulting in K59N, and G397 to A, resulting in G133R. The other allele was entirely normal. This finding indicates the proband was heterozygous for ALAD deficiency. All family members of the proband who had decreased ALAD activity (approximately 50 percent of normal) had the same set of two base transitions. Expression of ALAD cDNAs in CHO cells revealed that K59N cDNA produced a protein with normal ALAD activity, whereas G133R and K59N/G133R cDNA produced proteins with 8 percent and 16 percent ALAD activity, respectively, compared with that expressed by the wild-type cDNA. Heterozygous ALAD deficiency, which should be clinically silent, nevertheless produced clinical ADP in this patient, presumably because of clonal expansion of the polycythemia clone in his erythroid cells, which carried the mutant ALAD allele.[116]

The healthy asymptomatic Swedish girl had markedly decreased ALAD activity (12 percent of normal) determined by neonatal ALAD screening for hereditary tyrosinemia.[117] The molecular analysis of cloned *ALAD* cDNA revealed that this subject had C36 to G base transition and T168 to C base transition in one allele; the other allele was normal. The former transition resulted in F12L amino acid substitution, whereas the latter transition was silent, representing polymorphism. *F12L* mutant cDNA produced a protein that undergoes premature processing resulting in no enzymatic activity.[117] These findings suggest ALAD mutations in ADP are highly heterogeneous and that heterozygous ALAD deficiency usually does not result in clinical consequences but may be precipitated, although rarely, if clonal expansion of the mutant ALAD allele is present.

Clinical Features The symptomatology is similar to that seen in AIP. The two German male patients with onset in their teens were characterized by vomiting, pain in the legs, and neuropathy. One patient also had abdominal pain.[110] The second patient later developed paralysis of the arms, legs, and respiratory muscles. Both patients displayed clinical exacerbation following stress, decreased food intake, or alcohol ingestion. Despite these problems, the two patients fared well even 20 years after disease onset.[118] The Swedish infant was diagnosed at age 2 years and had a stormy course characterized by general muscle hypotonia, respiratory insufficiency, and bilateral paralysis of the legs.[111] The Belgian patient developed porphyria-related symptoms for the first time at age 63 years. This patient also had a myeloproliferative disorder.[112]

Diagnosis Definitive diagnosis of ADP is dependent on the demonstration of markedly deficient erythrocyte ALA dehydratase activity and the enzyme protein in the proband and intermediate decreases in the proband's relatives. Supportive evidence for the diagnosis includes massive elevations in urinary ALA and substantial elevation of porphyrins in urine and erythrocytes. In contrast, urinary PBG excretion is within the normal range. Urinary and erythrocyte porphyrins, predominantly coproporphyrin III and zinc protoporphyrin IX, respectively, are markedly elevated (approximately 100-fold). No explanation has satisfactorily accounted for this observation. Erythrocyte ALA dehydratase activity is markedly decreased (less than 2 percent of normal) in the proband and intermediately decreased (approximately 50 percent of normal) in the parents' erythrocytes.

Lead poisoning can be differentiated by increased blood lead and zinc protoporphyrin, excessive urinary excretion of ALA and coproporphyrin, and markedly inhibited ALA dehydratase activity in erythrocytes, which, however, can be restored to normal by the addition of reduced glutathione or by dithiothreitol *in vitro*. No reduction in the amount of ALA dehydratase protein is observed in lead poisoning,[119] which differentiates it from ADP.[109]

Hereditary tyrosinemia I is caused by an inherited deficiency of fumaryl acetoacetate hydrolase.[31] Patients with this condition excrete large amounts of ALA into urine, but not PBG. Diagnosis of tyrosinemia can be made by demonstrating succinylacetone in urine, for example, by showing inhibition of ALA dehydratase activity of normal blood by the addition of a patient's urine. No reduction in the amount of ALA dehydratase protein is observed in this disease.[120]

Therapy The clinical similarities of ADP to AIP suggest the clinical guidelines for treatment of ADP probably should follow that of AIP. However, the reported responses to treatment of the four cases varied greatly. One German patient responded to intravenous glucose, whereas the Swedish child failed to respond to glucose or intravenous hematin. This child finally required liver transplantation at age 7 years. The transplantation did not suppress urinary ALA excretion but im-

proved the patient's condition so that the child could withstand several porphyrogenic challenges.[121]

ACUTE INTERMITTENT PORPHYRIA

Definition and History An autosomal dominant disorder resulting from a partial deficiency of PBG deaminase activity (see Table 57-1 and Fig. 57-1), AIP is the major porphyria both in its incidence and severity. In the majority of patients (more than 90 percent), the deficient enzyme activity (approximately 50 percent of normal) is found in all tissues, including erythrocytes. This finding is consistent with a heterozygous enzyme deficiency in affected individuals. The first case of porphyria described in 1889 by Stokvis[1] probably was a sulphonal-induced AIP. Since then, many cases of AIP, with or without drug ingestion, have been described. The prevalence of AIP was estimated to be one to two per 100,000 in Europe,[122] or 2.4 per 100,000 in Finland.[123] A cluster of AIP exists in northern Sweden (one per 1500[124]). The frequency of low PBG deaminase activity, which additionally includes latent gene carriers of AIP, is as high as one per 500 in the general population of Finland.[125] Based on molecular defect analysis, the minimal prevalence of the AIP gene has been calculated to be one per 1675 in France.[126]

Pathophysiology More than 90 different abnormalities of the PBG deaminase gene in AIP have been reported since 1989.[127] The prevalence of specific defective alleles among AIP families appears to vary depending on the population studied. Founder effects likely account for a high frequency of a single mutation in Finland and, to a lesser extent, in Holland, whereas many other mutations have only been found once, each of them in a single family. Both negative and positive types of cross-reactive immunologic material (CRIM) were reported among AIP patients. Table 57-6 summarizes the three subtypes of AIP classification, which is based upon these findings.

Type I. Patients with this subtype are characterized by a *CRIM-negative* mutation of PBG deaminase. Patients exhibit intermediately reduced enzyme activity and protein content (approximately 50 percent of normal). The mutations include single base substitutions, deletions that result in a single amino acid change or truncated proteins produced by splicing defects or frameshift mutations.

Type II. Patients with type II AIP (less than 5 percent of all AIP) are characterized by partially decreased PBG deaminase activity in nonerythroid cells but *normal erythrocyte PBG deaminase activity*. A G→A transition was reported at the first position of the first intron of the PBG deaminase gene in a Dutch family. This transition modified the normal splice consensus sequence CGGTGAGT to CGATGAGT. A single base substitution (CG→CT) that resulted in a splicing defect at the last position of exon 1 was found in a Finnish family. Both mutations had no consequence on the expression of PBG deaminase in erythroid cells because transcription of the gene in this cell type starts downstream of the mutation site.

Type III. Patients with type III AIP are characterized by a *CRIM-positive mutation*, that is, decreased activity with the presence of a structurally abnormal enzyme protein.[128] Type III consists of patients with moderately increased CRIM (type IIIa)[129] and those with markedly increased CRIM (type IIIb)[130] (see Table 57-6).

TABLE 57-6   CLASSIFICATION OF AIP

	ACTIVITY	MASS	MASS/ACTIVITY	CRIM
Type I	50	50	1	Negative
Type II	100	100	1	Negative
Type IIIa	50	85	1.7	Positive
Type IIIb	50	280	5.7	Superpositive

Pathogenesis of the Clinical Findings The symptomatology of AIP principally results from neurologic dysfunction. However, post-mortem findings are unremarkable, suggesting the symptoms have a metabolic nature. Various theories accounting for the pathogenesis of neuropathy in AIP have been proposed: (1) PBG deaminase deficiency in the nervous system tissues could limit the synthesis of heme for brain heme proteins; (2) deficiency in heme synthesis in the liver may adversely influence heme protein formation in the brain; (3) heme pathway intermediates, such as ALA, PBG, or their metabolites, may be toxic to nerve cells; and (4) in acute attacks, hepatic heme deficiency may lead to decreased activity of hepatic tryptophan pyrrolase, resulting in enhanced plasma levels and brain uptake of tryptophan and ultimately to increased synthesis of 5-hydroxytryptamine, a neurotransmitter.

Precipitating Factors Up to 90 percent of individuals with documented deficiencies of PBG deaminase activity remain asymptomatic throughout their lifetimes. However, some individuals with PBG deaminase deficiency may have acute attacks precipitated by various endogenous or exogenous factors. At least five different classes of precipitating factors exist.

Inducers of hepatic ALA synthase. Most precipitating factors are inducers of ALAS-N. An increased metabolic demand for hepatic heme synthesis leads to induction of ALAS-N and overproduction of ALA. The partial deficiency of PBG deaminase activity (approximately 50 percent of normal) then becomes rate limiting.

Endocrine factors. Hormonal factors play a major role in induction of ALAS-N activity. Clinical expression of AIP is virtually absent before puberty. The clinical disease is more common in women, especially at the time of menses. A subset of female patients experience regular perimenstrual exacerbation of their disease. Synthetic estrogens and progesterone induce porphyria.

Caloric intake. Reduced caloric intake leads to exacerbation of AIP; conversely, carbohydrate-rich diets decrease PBG excretion and suppress clinical attacks.[131]

Drugs and foreign chemicals. Many chemicals, particularly barbiturates, exacerbate AIP. They are inducers of hepatic cytochrome P450, resulting in enhanced demand for *de novo* heme synthesis and derepression of hepatic ALA synthase activity.

Stress. Various forms of stress, including intermittent illnesses, infections, alcoholic excess, and surgery, may contribute to the genesis of an acute attack via induction of hepatic heme oxygenase, which then results in heme depletion.

Clinical Features Table 57-7 summarizes the clinical findings from three large series of AIP patients (total number of patients = 417[132–134]). The course of an acute AIP attack is highly variable; attacks last from a few days to several months. Abdominal pain almost always is present and often is the initial symptom of an acute attack. The pain may be generalized or localized. In severe cases, the pain mimics an acute surgical abdomen and may lead to inappropriate laparotomy. Chest, back, and limb pain may occur. Pains usually are intermittent but they also may be chronic; the severity may fluctuate. Gastrointestinal features are common and include nausea, vomiting, constipation or diarrhea, abdominal distention, and ileus. The incidence of hepatocellular carcinoma is increased.[135] Urinary incontinence, dysuria, frequency, and urinary retention may occur. The urine may appear "port-wine red" because of the high content of porphobilin, an autooxidation product of PBG and some porphyrins that are formed by nonenzymatic cyclization of PBG.

Neuropathy, particularly of the motor type, is a common feature of AIP, but any type of neuropathy may occur. Motor neuropathy may involve the cranial nerves (most commonly the seventh and tenth) or lead to bulbar paralysis, respiratory impairment, and death. Rarely, AIP presents as respiratory failure.[136] Acute attacks of AIP often are

TABLE 57-7   SIGNS AND SYMPTOMS OF AIP

SYMPTOMS & SIGNS	WALDENSTRÖM[132] 321 CASES (% OF TOTAL)	GOLDBERG[133] 50 CASES (% OF TOTAL)	STEIN & TSCHUDY[134] 46 CASES (% OF TOTAL)
Abdominal pain	85	94	95
Vomiting	59	88	43
Constipation	48	84	48
Diarrhea	9	12	5
Limb, head, neck, or chest pain	—	52	50
Muscle weakness	42	68	60
Sensory loss	9	38	26
Convulsions	10	16	20
Respiratory paralysis	14	10	9
Mental symptoms	55	58	40
Hypertension	40	54	36
Tachycardia	28	64	80
Fever	37	14	9

accompanied by seizures, especially in patients with hyponatremia as a result of vomiting, inappropriate fluid therapy, or the syndrome of inappropriate antidiuretic hormone release.

Diagnosis Diagnosis can be established by demonstrating reduced PBG deaminase activity (approximately 50 percent of normal) in erythrocytes. The exception is type II AIP patients, who show normal erythrocyte PBG deaminase activity. However, PBG deaminase activity in type II patients is reduced in nonerythroid cells such as fibroblasts or lymphocytes.[137,138] The distinction among (1) silent gene carriers, (2) clinically latent but biochemically manifest carriers, and (3) clinically and biochemically fully expressed patients depends on the demonstration of elevated urinary excretion of PBG and ALA and on the history of the individual subject. Patients with the clinically expressed disease and some latent gene carriers excrete increased amounts of ALA and PBG in the urine, often even during clinical remission. The onset of an acute attack is accompanied by further massive increases in excretion of these precursors (ALA 25 to 100 mg/day; PBG 50 to 200 mg/day).[139] The Watson-Schwartz test is widely used as a screening test for urinary PBG. The column method of Mauzerall and Granick[140] should be used to quantify the amount of ALA and PBG in urine. Elevated levels of ALA and PBG may be seen in HCP and VP. Urinary and stool porphyrin assays differentiate these conditions from AIP. Patients with ADP show elevated ALA in urine, but not PBG.[109]

Therapy Treatments of AIP, ADP, HCP, and VP are essentially identical. Treatment between attacks comprises adequate nutritional intake, avoidance of drugs known to exacerbate porphyria, and prompt treatment of other conditions, such as starvation, intermittent diseases, or infections. Unresponsive patients should be admitted to the hospital and intravenous administration of carbohydrate initiated with dextrose to provide a minimum of 300 g of carbohydrate per day. Use of intravenous hematin now is considered the treatment of choice. Intravenous hematin curtails urinary excretion of ALA and PBG, acute attacks, and perhaps the severity of neuropathy. Nasal or subcutaneous administration of long-acting agonists of luteinizing hormone-releasing hormone (LHRH) inhibits ovulation and greatly reduces the incidence of perimenstrual attacks of AIP in such women.[141] Pain, which is invariably present and severe, can be treated with frequent regular doses of narcotic analgesics.

HEREDITARY COPROPORPHYRIA

Definition   HCP is a disease caused by a partial deficiency of CPO activity (approximately 50 percent of normal) inherited in an autosomal dominant manner (see Table 57-1 and Fig. 57-1). Clinically expressed HCP is much less common than is clinically expressed AIP. In Denmark, the incidence of HCP has been estimated to be two per 1,000,000.[142] However, more gene carriers for this condition have been recognized with the improvement of laboratory techniques such as quantitative high-performance liquid chromatography (HPLC) of porphyrins and a radioactive assay of CPO activity.

Pathophysiology   Clinically, the disease is similar to ADP or AIP, although HCP often is milder. Additionally, HCP may be associated with photosensitivity as a result of coproporphyrin accumulation in the tissue. Expression of the disease is variable and influenced by the same precipitating factors responsible for exacerbation of AIP. Very rarely, homozygous deficiency of this enzyme occurs and is associated with a more severe form of the disease.[143]

Clinical Features   The principal symptoms of HCP are neurologic dysfunctions that are indistinguishable from those of ADP, AIP, and VP. Abdominal pain, vomiting, constipation, neuropathy, and psychiatric manifestations are common. Approximately 30 percent of patients with HCP have photocutaneous symptoms. Clinical attacks can be precipitated by pregnancy, the menstrual cycle, and contraceptive steroids, but the most common precipitating factor is administration of drugs, such as phenobarbital.

Diagnosis   HCP should be suspected in patients with the signs, symptoms, and clinical course characteristic of the acute hepatic porphyria but in whom erythrocyte PBG deaminase activity is normal. Urinary excretion of porphyrin precursors is similar in HCP and VP, but the predominance of coproporphyrin III is highly suggestive of HCP. Fecal coproporphyrin concentrations are markedly elevated. Excessive excretion of ALA, PBG, and uroporphyrin into the urine is common during acute attacks. However, in contrast to AIP, these findings generally normalize between attacks. Two rare variant forms of HCP have been described. One is harderoporphyria, which results from a homozygous defect of a structurally altered CPO. The other is homozygous HCP, which results from a homozygous deficiency of the normal enzyme. Fecal or urinary predominance of harderoporphyrin, with greatly reduced CPO activity, indicates harderoporphyria. Interestingly, harderoporphyria with K404E substitution in the *CPO* gene, either in the homozygous or compound heterozygous state and associated with a mutation leading to the absence of functional mRNA or protein, was responsible for neonatal hemolytic anemia.[144]

Therapy   The identification and avoidance of precipitating factors is essential. Treatment of acute attacks is similar to the treatment of AIP.

VARIEGATE PORPHYRIA

Definition and History   VP is caused by a partial deficiency in protoporphyrinogen oxidase activity and is inherited in an autosomal dominant manner (see Table 57-1 and Fig. 57-1). The incidence of VP is particularly high in South Africa at three per 1000. In 1980, an estimated 10,000 individuals in South Africa were affected,[145] and evidence suggests they all are descendants of a single Dutch settler in 1680.[146] However, the disease is recognized worldwide and probably has no racial or geographical predilection, with the exception of South Africa. Incidence in Finland is reported at 1.3 per 100,000.[147]

Pathophysiology   Patients with VP may show neurovisceral symptoms, photosensitivity, or both, as a result of a partial deficiency in protoporphyrinogen oxidase activity.[148] Disease expression is highly influenced by factors similar to those precipitating the acute attack of AIP.

Clinical Features   The neurovisceral symptomatology is indistinguishable from that of ADP, AIP, and HCP. Photosensitivity is more common, and cutaneous symptoms tend to be more chronic in VP than in HCP. Lesions are clinically and histologically indistinguishable from PCT. In the absence of neurovisceral symptoms, the diagnosis of VP is easily overlooked. Skin manifestations are less frequently observed in cold climates (e.g., 45 percent in a series from Finland[147]) than in hot climates (e.g., 85 percent in a series from South Africa[145]). The same spectrum of factors that activate ADP, AIP, and HCP also induce VP.

Diagnosis   VP should be considered in the differential diagnosis of acute hepatic porphyria (ADP, AIP, and HCP). If PBG deaminase activity is normal in a patient with an acute hepatic porphyria syndrome, VP and type II AIP must be evaluated. Characteristic plasma porphyrin fluorescence usually is seen in VP.[149] The differentiation of VP from HCP usually is possible by fecal porphyrin analysis. In patients with only cutaneous manifestations, the demonstration of urinary 8- and 7-carboxylic porphyrins and isocoproporphyrin usually is sufficient for differentiation of PCT from VP. If protoporphyrinogen oxidase assay is not available, screening of family members is best achieved by measuring fecal porphyrin concentrations and profiles.

Four homozygous cases of VP have been described. Parents of the patients had approximately 50 percent protoporphyrinogen oxidase activity but did not have clinical symptoms. Clinical features of these patients were severe photosensitivity, growth and mental retardation, and marked neurologic abnormalities in two cases; onset was in childhood in all cases. None of the patients were anemic, which suggests the principal site of protoporphyrinogen oxidase deficiency occurs in the liver, not erythroid cells.

Therapy   Identification and avoidance of precipitating factors is essential. Photosensitivity can be minimized by protective clothing. Canthaxanthin (a β-carotene analogue) may be helpful.[150] Treatment of neurovisceral symptoms is identical to that described for AIP.

CHRONIC HEPATIC PORPHYRIAS

PORPHYRIA CUTANEA TARDA

Definition   PCT results from a partial deficiency of UROD activity (see Table 57-1 and Fig. 57-1). PCT is the most common of all the porphyrias—genetic and acquired combined—but its exact incidence is not clear. The disease is recognized worldwide, with no racial predilection except among the Bantus in South Africa, secondary to their high incidence of hemosiderosis. Previously, PCT was more common in men than in women, partly because of higher alcohol intake in men, but the incidence in women has approached that of men, perhaps because of increased use of contraceptive steroids, postmenopausal estrogens, and alcohol. PCT can be classified into three subtypes (Table 57-8). The hallmark of all types of PCT is cutaneous photosensitivity resulting from increased accumulation of uroporphyrin and 7-carboxylic porphyrin.

Pathophysiology   **Type I.** Patients with type I PCT are characterized by the lack of family history and normal erythrocyte UROD activity and concentrations but decreased enzyme activity in the liver. Type I PCT typically presents in adults, either spontaneously or, more commonly, in conjunction with precipitating environmental factors

TABLE 57-8   CLASSIFICATION OF PCT

TYPE	FAMILIAL OCCURRENCE	URO'GEN DECARBOXYLASE ACTIVITY	
		ERYTHROCYTES	LIVER
I	–	Normal	Decreased
II	+	50% of normal	50% of normal
III	+	Normal	50% of normal

such as alcohol, estrogen, drug use, iron overload, or in association with other disorders.

Type II. In type II PCT patients, the catalytic activity and the concentration of UROD both are approximately 50 percent of normal in all tissues. The enzyme deficiency segregates as an autosomal dominant trait in the patient's pedigree.

Type III. Patients with type III PCT are characterized by normal erythrocyte UROD activity and concentrations but decreased hepatic UROD activity. This abnormality is found in more than one member in the same family.

Familial (types II and III) PCT is associated with heterozygous UROD deficiency. In contrast, HEP results from a homozygous or compound heterozygous state for mutations of the gene encoding this enzyme. Most UROD mutations in HEP have not been found in familial PCT and are associated with residual UROD activity. The heterozygous UROD mutations in most cases of familial PCT appear to be more critical to the enzyme activity than those found in HEP. However, a few families with cases of both HEP and PCT have been described. Heterozygosity for mutant UROD alleles in mice is a risk factor for development of PCT because heterozygous mice are much more sensitive to porphyrinogenic stimuli than wild-type animals.[151] In both heterozygous mice and humans that display porphyric phenotypes, hepatic UROD protein is half normal, but the catalytic activity of the enzyme is reduced to approximately 20 percent, suggesting the existence of an inhibitor of hepatic UROD.[151,152]

Pathogenesis of the Clinical Findings The initial event in bullous formation is the appearance of membrane-limited vacuoles in the superficial dermis. Porphyrin biosynthesis in the skin of PCT patients is increased compared to normal controls. Thus, phototoxic porphyrins in the skin may be derived from the liver and locally from the skin. Activation of the complement system after irradiation has been demonstrated in PCT patients both *in vivo* and *in vitro* in sera[153] and is thought to result from generation of reactive oxygen species. Bullous fluid contains prostaglandin E$_2$, and photoactivation of uroporphyrin damages lysosomes. These factors may result in inflammation and autolysis.

Liver biopsy specimens from patients with PCT, particularly those with type I, almost invariably display siderosis. Red autofluorescence and needle-like cytoplasmic inclusion bodies, representing crystallized porphyrins, have frequently been recognized. Most cases of type I PCT have evidence of cirrhosis at autopsy. The incidence of hepatocellular carcinoma in PCT is greater than normal.[154] Rarely, primary hepatomas secrete porphyrins and simulate PCT.[155]

Precipitating Factors Sporadic PCT often is triggered by exposure to environmental factors, such as alcohol, estrogens, iron, and polychlorinated aromatic hydrocarbons. Ethanol has long been known to exacerbate PCT, and the incidence of heavy alcohol intake reportedly ranges from 25 to 100 percent. The mechanisms by which alcohol exacerbates PCT are unclear, but alcohol reportedly increases iron uptake,[156] which may aggravate the disease.

Estrogen administration has been associated with clinical relapse of PCT.[157] Pregnancy may aggravate PCT.[158] PCT has been associated with the hyperestrogenic condition Klinefelter syndrome.[159]

Iron plays an important role in the pathogenesis of PCT. Serum iron and ferritin concentrations frequently are elevated in PCT patients.[160] Iron absorption and its turnover reportedly are either normal or elevated. Hemosiderosis is seen in approximately 80 percent of liver biopsy specimens from patients with PCT.[160] Phlebotomy induces clinical remission, whereas iron supplementation may lead to PCT relapse.[161] Addition of iron to *in vitro* systems reportedly either inhibits[162] or stimulates UROD activity.[163]

The cause of the hepatic siderosis and mild iron overload in PCT remains elusive. An association between human leukocyte antigen (HLA)-linked hereditary hemochromatosis and PCT has been suggested but also has been contested. The major histocompatibility complex class I-like gene *HFE* has been identified. Two missense variants, 845 G6A (C282Y) and 187 C6G (H63D), were found in the majority of unselected patients with hereditary hemochromatosis (see Chap. 40). A high prevalence of the C282Y mutation is observed in patients with PCT,[164,165] suggesting the *HFE* gene is involved in the pathogenesis of PCT.[166]

Polyhalogenated aromatic hydrocarbons have been associated with development of PCT in man and in laboratory animals. 2,3,7,8-Tetrachlorodibenzo-*p*-dioxin (TCDD) reportedly caused PCT in 11 chemical factory workers in Czechoslovakia.[167] Three cases of PCT were reported from a factory manufacturing the herbicides 2,4-dichloro- and trichlorophenoxyacetic acid,[168] and one janitor developed PCT after accidental exposure to polychlorinated biphenyls (PCBs) in a disinfectant.[169] A massive outbreak of approximately 4000 cases of PCT occurred following ingestion of hexachlorobenzene-contaminated wheat in Turkey from 1956 to 1961.[170,171] A number of studies on the porphyrinogenic effects of TCDD, hexachlorobenzene, and PCB suggest that metabolic activation of the compounds (probably by cytochrome P450) is required to decrease UROD activity.

PCT has been observed in association with hemodialysis,[172] systemic lupus erythematosus, Sjögren syndrome,[173] rheumatoid arthritis,[174] diabetes mellitus,[175] viral hepatitis,[176] Wilson disease,[177] striopallidodentate calcinosis (Fahr disease),[178] tumors and reticulosis,[179] thalassemia minor, and hemophilia.[180,181] PCT reportedly developed after treatment with cyclophosphamide[182] and bone marrow transplantation for chronic myelogenous leukemia.[183] An increasing number of patients with PCT in association with HIV infection has been reported, and positive links between PCT and AIDS have been suggested.[184]

Clinical Features Sporadic PCT (type I) almost exclusively presents in adults, whereas types II and III PCT may also occur in childhood. Patients have increased skin fragility such that minor trauma results in erosions from shearing of the skin. Sun exposure may lead to formation of vesicles and bullae, which crust over, take weeks to heal, and leave a scar. Milia may develop in the skin where bullae have healed. Hyperpigmentation, melanosis, and violaceous-brownish discolorations may develop on light-exposed areas. Facial hypertrichosis slowly develops and is most noticeable in women. Alopecia may develop at sites of repeated trauma or bullous formation. Hypopigmented indurated plaques of skin may develop and may appear as scleroderma-like changes.

Diagnosis The clinical picture of PCT is fairly specific, and its diagnosis usually is not difficult. However, PCT must be differentiated from other cutaneous photosensitivity syndromes. Clinical suspicion of PCT should lead to examination of the urine for fluorescence under an ultraviolet light and to quantitation of porphyrins. Uroporphyrin greater than coproporphyrin favors PCT; the reverse favors VP or HCP and may be associated with elevated urinary ALA and PBG concentrations. Plasma porphyrins invariably are elevated in PCT and in other photosensitizing porphyrias. Isocoproporphyrin in feces represents the most important diagnostic criterion for PCT (see Table 57-2).[185] In the presence of UROD deficiency, 5-carboxylate porphyrinogen III accumulates and undergoes metabolism by CPO to yield dehydroisocoproporphyrinogen. This product also accumulates because its conversion to harderoporphyrinogen is impaired by decarboxylase deficiency. Isocoproporphyrins then are generated by the autooxidation of the dehydro compound. Measurement of erythrocytic and hepatic UROD activity is usually a research procedure, and decreased erythrocyte enzyme activity identifies only those patients with type II PCT.

Therapy First-line treatment consists of the identification and avoidance of precipitating factors. Phlebotomy reduces urinary porphyrin concentrations and induces clinical remissions. Strong evidence indicates the beneficial effects of phlebotomy result from a diminution in the stores of body iron. Typically, 450 ml of blood is withdrawn at each phlebotomy, and this process initially is repeated 1 to 2 times per week. Remission usually is achieved after a total of approximately 4 to 10 liters of blood has been withdrawn. The best objective indices of progress is the serum iron or preferably the ferritin level, which should be reduced to the lower limit of normal.

If phlebotomy is contraindicated by the presence of other diseases such as anemia or cardiopulmonary disorders, chloroquine therapy may be considered. Low-dose chloroquine (125 mg twice weekly) and high-dose therapy (500 mg daily) in refractory cases have been beneficial. Both treatment regimens transiently induce increases in plasma and urinary porphyrin concentrations and in liver transaminases. Continued therapy eventually leads to reduced porphyrin excretion. Clinical improvement, or remission, may occur typically in 6 to 9 months.

HEPATOERYTHROPOIETIC PORPHYRIA

Definition and History HEP is a rare form of porphyria resulting from a homozygous defect in UROD activity (see Table 57-1 and Fig. 57-1). Clinically, HEP is indistinguishable from CEP and is characterized by childhood onset of severe photosensitivity and skin fragility. HEP is extremely rare. After the first report of HEP by Gunther in 1967,[186] only about 20 cases have been reported worldwide to date.[187]

Pathophysiology The UROD mutation in the first patient studied consisted of an 860 G→A change in the cDNA sequence that led to a Gly281→Glu change in the amino acid sequence. *In vitro* experiments showed that the cDNA with this mutation encoded a polypeptide that was very rapidly degraded in the presence of cell lysates. Two other point mutations were recognized. One was the replacement of Glu167→Lys, which produced a protein having an unstable phenotype.[188] The other mutation was a Arg292→Gly change.[189] The majority of the mutations found in familial PCT and HEP are distinct.

The molecular defect in familial PCT is heterogeneous. A Gly281→Val substitution with unstable phenotype,[190] a splice-site mutation,[191] and exon 6 deletion (unstable phenotype) have been described.[191] The exon 6 deletion was found in five of 22 pedigrees examined and is the only mutation having more than one pedigree with PCT. HEP patients represent individuals with homozygous or compound heterozygous deficiency of UROD, which is, however, stable enough to meet the requirements for heme synthesis.[190] In contrast, patients with familial PCT who are heterozygous for UROD deficiency may carry mutations with little enzyme activity or with a very unstable protein. One patient with HEP was heteroallelic for Val134→Gln substitution as a result of three sequential point mutations (T417G418T419→CCA) and His220→Pro substitution as a result of A677→C.[192] Interestingly, the same Val134→Gln substitution also was found in another pedigree as familial PCT,[193] suggesting that a cellular factor influences expression of a UROD defect.

Clinical Features The clinical findings are similar to those seen in CEP: pink urine, severe photosensitivity leading to scarring and mutilation of sun-exposed areas of skin, sclerodermoid changes, hypertrichosis, erythrodontia, anemia (often hemolytic), and hepatosplenomegaly. Unlike PCT, onset of HEP usually is in early infancy or childhood,[187] but occasional adult onset has been described.[194] Curiously, some of the cases with onset in childhood showed spontaneous resolution of their photosensitivity,[195] and others experienced relatively mild symptoms from onset despite markedly elevated urinary porphyrin concentrations.[187] In contrast to PCT, serum iron concentrations usually are normal in HEP patients, and phlebotomy does little to improve symptoms. Elevated erythrocyte protoporphyrin level and occasional fluorescent normoblasts suggest the bone marrow is a source of porphyrins.[196]

Diagnosis The diagnosis must be considered in patients with severe photosensitivity, such as CEP. Diagnostic criteria include elevated levels of fecal or urinary isocoproporphyrin and erythrocyte zinc protoporphyrin. Patients with EPP, who also have elevated erythrocyte protoporphyrin levels, can be distinguished from HEP because they excrete normal amounts of urinary porphyrins. EPP is clinically milder than HEP. Measurement of erythrocyte or fibroblast UROD activities typically shows reductions to 2 to 10 percent of normal control values, with intermediate reductions of UROD activities in family members. As in the case of PCT, isocoproporphyrin concentrations equal to or greater than coproporphyrin levels are the characteristic of HEP. Elevated erythrocyte protoporphyrin (usually zinc protoporphyrin) has also been a feature of several cases of HEP. In contrast to PCT, serum iron is usually normal.

Therapy Avoidance of the sun and the use of topical sunscreens are the only measures that can be offered to these patients at present. Patients with HEP do not respond to phlebotomy.[187]

REFERENCES

1. Stokvis BJ: Over Twee Zeldsame Kleuerstoffen in Urine van Zicken. *Ned Tijdschr Geneeskd* 13:409, 1889.
2. Anderson TM: Hydroa aestivale in two brothers, complicated with the presence of haematoporphyrin in the urine. *Br J Dermatol* 10:1, 1898.
3. Harris DF: Haematoporphyrinuria and its relations to the source of urobilin. *J Anat Physiol* 31:383, 1897.
4. Günther H: Die Hämatoporphyrie. *Dtsch Arch Klin Med* 105:89, 1911.
5. Garrod AE: *Inborn Errors of Metabolism.* Hodder & Stoughton, London, 1923.
6. Granick JL, Sassa S: Hemin control of heme biosynthesis in mouse Friend virus-transformed erythroleukemia cells in culture. *J Biol Chem* 253:5402, 1978.
7. Correia MA, Farrell GC, Schmid R, et al: Incorporation of exogenous heme into hepatic cytochrome P-450 in vivo. *J Biol Chem* 254:15, 1979.
8. Berk PD, Howe RB, Berlin NI: Disorders of bilirubin metabolism, in *Duncan's Diseases of Metabolism,* edited by PK Bondy, LE Rosenberg, p 825. WB Saunders, Philadelphia,1974.
9. Granick S, Sassa S: δ-Aminolevulinic acid synthetase and the control of heme and chlorophyll synthesis, in *Metabolic Regulation,* edited by HJ Vogel, p 77. Academic Press, New York, 1971.
10. Sassa S, Kappas A: Genetic, metabolic, and biochemical aspects of the porphyrias, in *Advances in Human Genetics,* edited by H Harris, K Hirschhorn, p 121. Plenum Publications, New York, 1981.
11. McKay R, Druyan R, Getz GS, Rabinowitz M: Intramitochondrial localization of δ-aminolevulinate synthase and ferrochelatase in rat liver. *Biochem J* 114:455, 1969.
12. Riddle RD, Yamamoto M, Engel JD: Expression of δ-aminolevulinate synthase in avian cells: Separate genes encode erythroid-specific and nonspecific isozymes. *Proc Natl Acad Sci U S A* 86:792, 1989.
13. Bishop DF, Astrin KH, Ioannou YA: Human δ-aminolevulinate synthase: Isolation, characterization, and mapping of house-keeping and erythroid-specific genes. *Am J Hum Genet* 45:A176, 1989.
14. Bishop DF: Two different genes encode δ-aminolevulinate synthase in humans: Nucleotide sequences of cDNAs for the housekeeping and erythroid genes. *Nucleic Acids Res* 18:7187, 1990.
15. Cox TC, Bawden MJ, Martin A, May BK: Human erythroid 5-aminolevulinate synthase: Promoter analysis and identification of an iron-responsive element in the mRNA. *EMBO J* 10:1891, 1991.
16. Aziz N, Munro HN: Iron regulates ferritin mRNA translation through a segment of its 5' untranslated region. *Proc Natl Acad Sci U S A* 84:8478, 1987.
17. Casey JL, Di Jeso B, Rao K, et al: The promoter region of the human transferrin receptor gene. *Ann N Y Acad Sci* 526:54, 1988.

18. Melefors O, Goossen B, Johansson HE, et al: Translational control of 5-aminolevulinate synthase mRNA by iron-responsive elements in erythroid cells. *J Biol Chem* 268:5974, 1993.

19. Elferink CJ, Srivastava G, Maguire DJ, et al: A unique gene for 5-aminolevulinate synthase in chickens. Evidence for expression of an identical messenger RNA in hepatic and erythroid tissues. *J Biol Chem* 262:3988, 1987.

20. Bonkowsky HL, Tschudy DP, Collins A, et al: Repression of the overproduction of porphyria precursors in acute intermittent porphyria by intravenous infusions of hematin. *Proc Natl Acad Sci U S A* 68:2725, 1971.

21. Galbraith RA, Kappas A: Pharmacokinetics of tin-mesoporphyrin in man and the effects of tin-chelated porphyrins on hyperexcretion of heme pathway precursors in patients with acute inducible porphyria. *Hepatology* 9:882, 1989.

22. Kitchin KT: Regulation of rat hepatic δ-aminolevulinic acid synthetase and heme oxygenase activities: Evidence for control by heme and against mediation by prosthetic iron. *Int J Biochem* 15:479, 1983.

23. Fujita H, Yamamoto M, Yamagami T, et al: Erythroleukemia differentiation. Distinctive responses of the erythroid-specific and the nonspecific δ-aminolevulinate synthase mRNA. *J Biol Chem* 266:17494, 1991.

24. Dandekar T, Stripecke R, Gray NK, et al: Identification of a novel iron-responsive element in murine and human erythroid δ-aminolevulinic acid synthase mRNA. *EMBO J* 10:1903, 1991.

25. Sassa S: Heme stimulation of cellular growth and differentiation. *Semin Hematol* 25:312, 1988.

26. Furuyama K, Sassa S: Interaction between succinyl CoA synthetase and the heme-biosynthetic enzyme ALAS-E is disrupted in sideroblastic anemia. *J Clin Invest* 105:757, 2000.

27. Furuyama K, Fujita H, Nagai T, et al: Pyridoxine refractory X-linked sideroblastic anemia caused by a point mutation in the erythroid 5-aminolevulinate synthase gene. *Blood* 90:822, 1997.

28. Sassa S: δ-Aminolevulinic acid dehydratase assay. *Enzyme* 28:133, 1982.

29. Tsukamoto I, Yoshinaga T, Sano S: The role of zinc with special reference to the essential thiol groups in δ-aminolevulinic acid dehydratase of bovine liver. *Biochim Biophys Acta* 570:167, 1979.

30. Granick JL, Sassa S, Kappas A: Some biochemical and clinical aspects of lead intoxication, in *Advances in Clinical Chemistry*, edited by O Bodansky, AL Latner, p 287. Academic Press, New York, 1978.

31. Lindblad B, Lindstedt S, Steen G: On the genetic defects in hereditary tyrosinemia. *Proc Natl Acad Sci U S A* 74:4641, 1977.

32. Tschudy DP, Hess RA, Frykholm BD: Inhibition of δ-aminolevulinic acid dehydratase by 4,6-dioxoheptanoic acid. *J Biol Chem* 256:9915, 1981.

33. Sassa S, Kappas A: Hereditary tyrosinemia and the heme biosynthetic pathway. Profound inhibition of δ-aminolevulinic acid dehydratase activity by succinylacetone. *J Clin Invest* 71:625, 1983.

34. Wetmur JG, Bishop DF, Ostasiewicz L, Desnick RJ: Molecular cloning of a cDNA for human δ-aminolevulinate dehydratase. *Gene* 43:123, 1986.

35. Bishop TR, Cohen PJ, Boyer SH, et al: Isolation of a rat liver delta-aminolevulinate dehydrase (ALAD) cDNA clone: Evidence for unequal ALAD gene dosage among inbred mouse strains. *Proc Natl Acad Sci U S A* 83:5568, 1986.

36. Gibbs PN, Jordan PM: Identification of lysine at the active site of human 5-aminolaevulinate dehydratase. *Biochem J* 236:447, 1986.

37. Potluri VR, Astrin KH, Wetmur JG, et al: Human 5-aminolevulinate dehydratase: Chromosomal localization to 9q34 by in situ hybridization. *Hum Genet* 76:236, 1987.

38. Jordan PM, Seehra JS: Mechanism of action of δ-aminolevulinic acid dehydratase. Stepwise order of addition of the two molecules of delta-aminolevulinic acid in the enzyme synthesis of porphobilinogen. *J Chem Soc Chem Commun* 5:240, 1980.

39. Erskine PT, Senior N, Awan S, et al: X-ray structure of 5-aminolaevulinate dehydratase, a hybrid aldolase. *Nat Struct Biol* 4:1025, 1997.

40. Bishop TR, Miller MW, Beall J, et al: Genetic regulation of delta-aminolevulinate dehydratase during erythropoiesis. *Nucleic Acids Res* 24:2511, 1996.

41. Wetmur JG, Bishop DF, Cantelmo C, Desnick RJ: Human delta-aminolevulinate dehydratase: Nucleotide sequence of a full-length cDNA clone. *Proc Natl Acad Sci U S A* 83:7703, 1986.

42. Wetmur JG, Kaya AH, Plewinska M: Molecular characterization of the human delta-aminolevulinate dehydratase 2 (ALAD2) allele: Implications for molecular screening of individuals for genetic susceptibility to lead poisoning. *Am J Hum Genet* 49:757, 1991.

43. Battersby AR, Fookes CJR, Matcham GWJ, McDonald E: Biosynthesis of the pigments of life-formation of the macrocyle. *Nature* 285:17, 1980.

44. Wang AL, Arredondo-Vega FX, Giampietro PF, et al: Regional gene assignment of human porphobilinogen deaminase and esterase A4 to chromosome 11q23 leads to 11qter. *Proc Natl Acad Sci U S A* 78:5734, 1981.

45. Chretien S, Dubart A, Beaupain D, et al: Alternative transcription and splicing of the human porphobilinogen deaminase gene result either in tissue-specific or in housekeeping expression. *Proc Natl Acad Sci U S A* 85:6, 1988.

46. Grandchamp B, Beaumont C, de Verneuil H, et al: Genetic expression of porphobilinogen deaminase and UROD during the erythroid differentiation of mouse erythroleukemic cells, in *Porphyrins and Porphyrias*, edited by Y Nordmann, p 35. John Libbey & Company, London, 1986.

47. Raich N, Romeo PH, Dubart A, et al: Molecular cloning and complete primary sequence of human erythrocyte porphobilinogen deaminase. *Nucleic Acids Res* 14:5955, 1986.

48. Mignotte V, Eleouet JF, Raich N, Romeo P-H: Cis- and trans-acting elements involved in the regulation of the erythroid promotor of the human porphobilinogen deaminase gene. *Proc Natl Acad Sci U S A* 86:6548, 1989.

49. Tsai SF, Bishop DF, Desnick RJ: Human uroporphyrinogen III synthase: Molecular cloning, nucleotide sequence, and expression of a full-length cDNA. *Proc Natl Acad Sci U S A* 85:7049, 1988.

50. Romana M, Dubart A, Beaupain D, et al: Structure of the gene for human uroporphyrinogen decarboxylase. *Nucleic Acids Res* 15:7343, 1987.

51. Romeo P-H, Raich N, Dubart A, et al: Molecular cloning and nucleotide sequence of a complete human uroporphyrinogen decarboxylase cDNA. *J Biol Chem* 261:9825, 1986.

52. Whitby FG, Phillips JD, Kushner JP, Hill CP: Crystal structure of human uroporphyrinogen decarboxylase. *EMBO J* 17:2463, 1998.

53. Phillips JD, Whitby FG, Kushner JP, Hill CP: Characterization and crystallization of human uroporphyrinogen decarboxylase. *Protein Sci* 6:1343, 1997.

54. Cacheux V, Martasek P, Fougerousse F, et al: Localization of the human coproporphyrinogen oxidase gene to chromosome band 3q12. *Hum Genet* 94:557, 1994.

55. Kohno H, Furukawa T, Yoshinaga T, et al: Coproporphyrinogen oxidase: Purification, molecular cloning, and induction of mRNA during erythroid differentiation. *J Biol Chem* 268:21359, 1993.

56. Takahashi S, Furuyama K, Kobayashi A, et al: Cloning of a coproporphyrinogen oxidase promoter regulatory element binding protein: Differential regulation of coproporphyrinogen oxidase gene between erythroid and nonerythroid cells. *Biochem Biophys Res Commun* 273:596, 2000.

57. Takahashi S, Taketani S, Akasaka J, et al: Differential regulation of mouse coproporphyrinogen oxidase gene expression in erythroid and non-erythroid cells. *Blood* 92:3436, 1998.

58. Conder LH, Woodard SI, Dailey HA: Multiple mechanisms for the regulation of haem synthesis during erythroid cell differentiation. Possible role for coproporphyrinogen oxidase. *Biochem J* 275:321, 1991.

59. Taketani S, Yoshinaga T, Furukawa T, et al: Induction of terminal enzymes for heme biosynthesis during differentiation of mouse erythroleukemia cells. *Eur J Biochem* 230:760, 1995.

60. Martasek P, Camadro JM, Delfau-Larue MH, et al: Molecular cloning, sequencing, and functional expression of a cDNA encoding human coproporphyrinogen oxidase. *Proc Natl Acad Sci U S A* 91:3024, 1994.

61. Lamoril J, Deybach JC, Puy H, et al: Three novel mutations in the coproporphyrinogen oxidase gene. *Hum Mutat* 9:78, 1997.

62. Nishimura K, Taketani S, Inokuchi H: Cloning of a human cDNA for protoporphyrinogen oxidase by complementation in vivo of a hemG mutant of Escherichia coli. *J Biol Chem* 270:8076, 1995.

63. Taketani S, Inazawa J, Abe T, et al: The human protoporphyrinogen oxidase gene (PPOX): Organization and location to chromosome 1. *Genomics* 29:698, 1995.

64. Porra RJ, Jones OTG: Studies on ferrochelatase 1. Assay and properties of ferrochelatase from a pig liver mitochondrial extract. *Biochem J* 87:181, 1963.

65. Taketani S, Inazawa J, Nakahashi Y, et al: Structure of the human ferrochelatase gene: Exon/intron gene organization and location of the gene to chromosome 18. *Eur J Biochem* 205:217, 1992.

66. Whitcombe DM, Carter NP, Albertson DG, et al: Assignment of the human ferrochelatase gene (FECH) and a locus for protoporphyria to chromosome 18q22. *Genomics* 11:1152, 1991.

67. Al-Karadaghi S, Hansson M, Nikonov S, et al: Crystal structure of ferrochelatase: The terminal enzyme in heme biosynthesis. *Structure* 5:1501, 1997.

68. Wada O, Sassa S, Takaku F, et al: Different responses of the hepatic and erythropoietic delta-aminolevulinic acid synthetase of mice. *Biochim Biophys Acta* 148:585, 1967.

69. Ross J, Sautner D: Induction of globin mRNA accumulation by hemin in cultured erythroleukemic cells. *Cell* 8:513, 1976.

70. Marver HS: The role of heme in the synthesis and repression of microsomal protein, in *Microsomes and Drug Oxidations*, edited by JR Gillette, AH Conney, GJ Cosmides, RW Estabrook, JR Fouts, GJ Manning, p 495. Academic Press, New York, 1969.

71. Porter PN, Meints RH, Mesner K: Enhancement of erythroid colony growth in culture by hemin. *Exp Hematol* 7:11, 1979.

72. Sassa S, Nagai T: The role of heme in gene expression. *Int J Hematol* 63:167, 1996.

73. Romana M, Le Boulch P, Romeo PH: Rat uroporphyrinogen decarboxylase cDNA: Nucleotide sequence and comparison to human uroporphyrinogen decarboxylase. *Nucleic Acids Res* 15:5487, 1987.

74. Fukuda Y, Fujita H, Taketani S, Sassa S: Haem is necessary for a continued increase in ferrochelatase mRNA in murine erythroleukaemia cells during erythroid differentiation. *Br J Haematol* 85:670, 1993.

75. Fritsch C, Bolsen K, Ruzicka T, Goerz G: Congenital erythropoietic porphyria [review]. *J Am Acad Dermatol* 36:594, 1997.

76. Desnick RJ, Glass IA, Xu W, et al: Molecular genetics of congenital erythropoietic porphyria [review]. *Semin Liver Dis* 18:77, 1998.

77. Watson CJ, Perman V, Spurrel FA, et al: Some studies of the comparative biology of human and bovine porphyria erythropoietia. *Trans Assoc Am Physicians* 71:196, 1958.

78. Seip M, Thune PO, Eriksen L: Treatment of photosensitivity in congenital erythropoietic porphyria (CEP) with beta-carotene. *Acta Derm Venereol Suppl (Stockh)* 54:239, 1974.

79. Haining RG, Cowger ML, Labbe RF, Finch CA: Congenital erythrpoietic porphyria: II. The effects of induced polycythemia. *Blood* 36:297, 1970.

80. Pimstone NR, Gandhi SN, Mukerji SK: Therapeutic efficacy of oral charcoal in congenital erythropoietic porphyria. *N Engl J Med* 316:390, 1987.

81. DeLeo VA, Poh-Fitzpatrick MB, Mathews-Roth MM, Harber LC: Erythropoietic protoporphyria 10 years experience. *Am J Med* 60:8, 1976.

82. Cox TM, Alexander GJ, Sarkany RP: Protoporphyria. *Semin Liver Dis* 18:85, 1998.

83. Went LN, Klasen EC: Genetic aspects of erythropoietic protoporphyria. *Ann Hum Genet* 48:105, 1984.

84. Lamoril J, Boulechfar S, de Verneuil H, et al: Human erythropoietic protoporphyria: Two point mutations in the ferrochelatase gene. *Biochem Biophys Res Commun* 181:594, 1991.

85. Poh-Fitzpatrick MB: Human protoporphyria: Reduced cutaneous photosensitivity and lower erythrocyte porphyrin levels during pregnancy. *J Am Acad Dermatol* 36:40, 1997.

86. Nakahashi Y, Fujita H, Taketani S, et al: The molecular defect of ferrochelatase in a patient with erythropoietic protoporphyria [abstract]. Fourth Congress of the European Society for Photobiology 197, 1991.

87. Wang X, Poh-Fitzpatrick M, Taketani S, et al: Screening for ferrochelatase mutations: Molecular heterogeneity of erythropoietic protoporphyria. *Biochim Biophys Acta* 1225:187, 1994.

88. Sellers VM, Dailey TA, Dailey HA: Examination of ferrochelatase mutations that cause erythropoietic protoporphyria. *Blood* 91:3980, 1998.

89. Rufenacht UB, Gouya L, Schneider-Yin X, et al: Systematic analysis of molecular defects in the ferrochelatase gene from patients with erythropoietic protoporphyria. *Am J Hum Genet* 62:1341, 1998.

90. Gouya L, Deybach JC, Lamoril J, et al: Modulation of the phenotype in dominant erythropoietic protoporphyria by a low expression of the normal ferrochelatase allele. *Am J Hum Genet* 58:292, 1996.

91. Gouya L, Puy H, Lamoril J, et al: Inheritance in erythropoietic protoporphyria: A common wild-type ferrochelatase allelic variant with low expression accounts for clinical manifestation. *Blood* 93:2105, 1999.

92. Ryan EA: Histochemistry of the skin in erythropoietic protoporphyria. *Br J Dermatol* 78:43, 1966.

93. Poh-Fitzpatrick MB: The erythropoietic porphyrias. *Dermatol Clin* 4:291, 1986.

94. Spikes JD: Porphyrins and related compounds as photodynamic sensitizers. *Ann N Y Acad Sci* 244:496, 1975.

95. Goldstein BD, Harber LC: Erythropoietic protoporphyria: Lipid peroxidation and red cell membrane damage associated with photohemolysis. *J Clin Invest* 51:892, 1972.

96. Schothorst AA, Van Steveninck J, Went IN, Suurmond D: Photodynamic damage of the erythrocyte membrane caused by protoporphyrin in protoporphyria and in normal red blood cells. *Clin Chim Acta* 39:161, 1972.

97. Bottomley SS, Tanaka M, Everett MA: Diminished erythroid ferrochelatase activity in protoporphyria. *J Lab Clin Med* 86:126, 1975.

98. Piomelli S, Lamola AA, Poh-Fitzpatrick MF, et al: Erythropoietic protoporphyria and lead intoxication: The molecular basis for difference in cutaneous photosensitivity: I. Different rates of disappearance of protoporphyrin from the erythrocytes, both in vivo and in vitro. *J Clin Invest* 56:1519, 1975.

99. Sandberg S, Brun A, Hovding G, et al: Effect of zinc on protoporphyrin induced photohaemolysis. *Scand J Clin Lab Invest* 40:185, 1980.

100. Lim HW, Poh-Fitzpatrick MB, Gigli I: Activation of the complement system in patients with porphyrias after irradiation in vivo. *J Clin Invest* 74:1961, 1984.

101. Bloomer JR, Enrichez R: Evidence that hepatic crystalline deposits in a patient with protoporphyria are composed of protoporphyrin. *Gastroenterology* 82:569, 1982.

102. Morton KO, Schneider F, Weimer MK, et al: Hepatic and bile porphyrins in patients with protoporphyria and liver failure. *Gastroenterology* 94:1488, 1988.

103. Mooney B, Tennant F: Operating theatre lights as hazard in photosensitive patients. *Br Med J* 287:1028, 1983.

104. Mathews-Roth MM: Systemic photoprotection. *Dermatol Clin* 4:335, 1986.

105. Mathews-Roth MM, Pathak MA, Fitzpatrick TB, et al: Beta carotene therapy for erythropoietic protoporphyria and other photosensitivity diseases. Arch Dermatol 113:1229, 1977.

106. Bechtel MA, Bertolone SJ, Hodge SJ: Transfusion therapy in a patient with erythropoietic protoporphyria. Arch Dermatol 117:99, 1981.

107. Bloomer JR: Pathogenesis and therapy of liver disease in protoporphyria. Yale J Biol Med 52:39, 1979.

108. Samuel D, Boboc B, Bernuau J, et al: Liver transplantation for protoporphyria. Evidence for the predominant role of the erythropoietic tissue in protoporphyrin overproduction. Gastroenterology 95:816, 1988.

109. Sassa S: ALAD porphyria, in Seminars in Liver Disease, edited by PD Berk, p 95. Thieme, New York, 1998.

110. Doss M, Von Tiepermann R, Schneider J, Schmid H: New type of hepatic porphyria with porphobilinogen synthase defect and intermittent acute clinical manifestation. Klin Wochenschr 57:1123, 1979.

111. Thunell S, Holmberg L, Lundgren J: Aminolevulinate dehydratase porphyria in infancy. A clinical and biochemical study. J Clin Chem Clin Biochem 25:5, 1987.

112. Hassoun A, Verstraeten L, Mercelis R, Martin J-J: Biochemical diagnosis of an hereditary aminolaevulinate dehydratase deficiency in a 63-year-old man. J Clin Chem Clin Biochem 27:781, 1989.

113. Ishida N, Fujita H, Noguchi T, et al: Message amplification phenotyping of an inherited delta-aminolevulinate dehydratase deficiency in a family with acute hepatic porphyria. Biochem Biophys Res Commun 172:237, 1990.

114. Ishida N, Fujita H, Fukuda Y, et al: Cloning and expression of the defective genes from a patient with delta-aminolevulinate dehydratase porphyria. J Clin Invest 89:1431, 1992.

115. Plewinska M, Thunell S, Holmberg L, et al: δ-Aminolevulinate dehydratase deficient porphyria: Identification of the molecular lesions in a severely affected homozygote. Am J Hum Genet 49:167, 1991.

116. Akagi R, Nishitani C, Harigae H, et al: Molecular analysis of delta-aminolevulinate dehydratase deficiency in a patient with an unusual late-onset porphyria. Blood 96:3618, 2000.

117. Akagi R, Yasui Y, Harper P, Sassa S: A novel mutation of delta-aminolaevulinate dehydratase in a healthy child with 12% erythrocyte enzyme activity. Br J Haematol 106:931, 1999.

118. Gross U, Sassa S, Jacob K, et al: 5-Aminolevulinic acid dehydratase deficiency porphyria: A twenty-year clinical and biochemical follow-up. Clin Chem 44:1892, 1998.

119. Fujita H, Sato K, Sano S: Increase in the amount of erythrocyte δ-aminolevulinic acid dehydratase in workers with moderate lead exposure. Int Arch Occup Environ Health 50:287, 1982.

120. Sassa S, Fujita H, Kappas A: Succinylacetone and δ-aminolevulinic acid dehydratase in hereditary tyrosinemia: Immunochemical study of the enzyme. Pediatrics 86:84, 1990.

121. Thunell S, Henrichson A, Floderus Y, et al: Liver transplantation in a boy with acute porphyria due to aminolaevulinate dehydratase deficiency. Eur J Clin Chem Clin Biochem 30:599, 1992.

122. Goldberg A, Moore MR, McColl KEL, Brodie MJ: Porphyrin metabolism and the porphyrias, in Oxford Textbook of Medicine, edited by JGG Ledingham, DA Warrell, DJ Weatherall, p 9136. Oxford University Press, Oxford, 1987.

123. Mustajoki P, Koskelo P: Hereditary hepatic porphyrias in Finland. Acta Med Scand 200:171, 1976.

124. Wetterberg L: A neuropsychiatric and genetical investigation of acute intermittent porphyria [PhD thesis]. Scandinavian University Books, Stockholm, 1967.

125. Mustajoki P, Kauppinen R, Lannfelt L, et al: Frequency of low erythrocyte porphobilinogen deaminase activity in Finland. J Intern Med 231:389, 1992.

126. Nordmann Y, Puy H, Da SV, et al: Acute intermittent porphyria: Prevalence of mutations in the porphobilinogen deaminase gene in blood donors in France. J Intern Med 242:213, 1997.

127. Grandchamp B: Acute intermittent porphyria. Semin Liver Dis 18:17, 1998.

128. Grandchamp B, Picat C, de Rooij F, et al: A point mutation G A in exon 12 of the porphobilinogen deaminase gene results in exon skipping and is responsible for acute intermittent porphyria. Nucleic Acids Res 17:6637, 1989.

129. Desnick RJ, Ostasiewicz LT, Tishler PA, Mustajoki P: Acute intermittent porphyria: Characterization of a novel mutation in the structural gene for porphobilingen deaminase. Demonstration of noncatalytic enzyme intermediates stabilized by bound substrate. J Clin Invest 76:865, 1985.

130. Wilson JHP, de Rooij FWM, Te Velde K: Acute intermittent porphyria in the Netherlands: Heterogeneity of the enzyme porphobilingen deaminase. Neth J Med 29:393, 1986.

131. Welland FH, Hellman ES, Gaddis EM, et al: Factors affecting the excretion of porphyrin precursors by patients with acute intermittent porphyria: I. The effects of diet. Metabolism 13:232, 1964.

132. Waldenstrom J: The porphyrias as inborn errors of metabolism. Am J Med 22:758, 1957.

133. Goldberg A: Acute intermittent porphyria: A study of 50 cases. Q J Med 28:183, 1959.

134. Stein JA, Tschudy DP: Acute intermittent porphyria: A clinical and biochemical study of 46 patients. Medicine 49:1, 1970.

135. Kauppinen R, Mustajoki P: Acute hepatic porphyria and hepatocellular carcinoma. Br J Cancer 57:117, 1988.

136. Greenspan GH, Block AJ: Respiratory insufficiency associated with acute intermittent porphyria. South Med J 74:954, 1981.

137. Sassa S, Solish G, Levere RD, Kappas A: Studies in porphyria: IV. Expression of the gene defect of acute intermittent porphyria in cultured human skin fibroblasts and amniotic cells: Prenatal diagnosis of the porphyric trait. J Exp Med 142:722, 1975.

138. Sassa S, Zalar GL, Kappas A: Studies in porphyria: VII. Induction of uroporphyrinogen-I synthase and expression of the gene defect of acute intermittent porphyria in mitogen-stimulated human lymphocytes. J Clin Invest 61:499, 1978.

139. Granick S, van den Schreieck HG: Porphobilinogen and delta-aminolevulinic acid in acute porphyria. Proc Soc Exp Biol Med 88:270, 1955.

140. Gorschein A: Determination of delta-aminolaevulinic acid in biological fluids by gas-liquid chromatography with electron-capture detection. Biochem J 219:883, 1984.

141. Anderson KE, Spitz IM, Sassa S, et al: Prevention of cyclical attacks of acute intermittent porphyria with a long-acting agonist of luteinizing hormone-releasing hormone. N Engl J Med 311:643, 1984.

142. With TK: Hereditary coproporphyria and variegate porphyria in Denmark. Dan Med Bull 30:106, 1983.

143. Grandchamp B, Phung N, Nordmann Y: Homozygous case of hereditary coproporphyria [letter]. Lancet 2:1348, 1977.

144. Lamoril J, Puy H, Gouya L, et al: Neonatal hemolytic anemia due to inherited harderoporphyria: Clinical characteristics and molecular basis. Blood 91:1453, 1998.

145. Eales L, Day RS, Blekkenhorst GH: The clinical and biochemical features of variegate porphyria: An analysis of 300 cases studied at Groote Schuur Hospital, Cape Town. Int J Biochem 12:837, 1980.

146. Dean G: The Porphyrias. A Study of Inheritance and Environment. Pitman Medical, London, 1971.

147. Mustajoki P: Variegate porphyria. Twelve years' experience in Finland. Q J Med 194:191, 1980.

148. Anderson KE, Sassa S, Bishop DF, Desnick RJ: Disorders of heme biosynthesis: X-linked sideroblastic anemia and the porphyrias, in The Metabolic & Molecular Bases of Inherited Disease, edited by CR Scriver, AL Beaudet, WS Sly, D Valle, p 2991. McGraw-Hill, New York, 2001.

149. Longas MO, Poh-Fitzpatrick MB: A tightly bound protein-porphyrin complex isolated from the plasma of a patient with variegate porphyria. *Clin Chim Acta* 118:219, 1982.

150. Eales L: The effects of canthaxanthin on the photocutaneous manifestations of porphyrias. *S Afr Med J* 54:1050, 1978.

151. Phillips JD, Jackson LK, Bunting M, et al: A mouse model of familial porphyria cutanea tarda. *Proc Natl Acad Sci U S A* 98:259, 2001.

152. Elder GH, Lee GB, Tovey JA: Decreased activity of hepatic uroporphyrinogen decarboxylase in sporadic porphyria cutanea tarda. *N Engl J Med* 299:274, 1978.

153. Pigatto PD, Polenghi MM, Altomare GF, et al: Complement cleavage products in the phototoxic reaction of porphyria cutanea tarda. *Br J Dermatol* 114:567, 1986.

154. Pierach CA: Porphyria and hepatocellular carcinoma. *Br J Cancer* 55:111, 1987.

155. Tio TH, Leijnse B, Jarrett A, Rimington C: Acquired porphyria from a liver tumor. *Clin Sci Mol Med* 16:517, 1959.

156. Felsher BF, Kushner JP: Hepatic siderosis and porphyria cutanea tarda: Relation of iron excess to the metabolic defect. *Semin Hematol* 14:243, 1977.

157. Domonkos AN: Porphyria cutanea tarda induced by estrogen therapy. *Arch Dermatol* 102:229, 1970.

158. Lamon JM, Frykholm BC: Pregnancy and porphyria cutanea tarda. *Johns Hopkins Med J* 145:235, 1979.

159. Saced-Uz-Zafar M, Gronewald WR, Bluhm GB: Co-existent Klinefelter's syndrome, acquired cutaneous hepatic porphyria and systemic lupus erythematosus. *Henry Ford Hosp Med J* 18:227, 1970.

160. Grossman ME, Bickers DR, Poh-Fitzpatrick MB, et al: Porphyria cutanea tarda: Clinical features and laboratory findings in forty patients. *Am J Med* 67:277, 1979.

161. Lundvall O: The effect of replenishment of iron stores after phlebotomy therapy in porphyria cutanea tarda. *Acta Med Scand* 189:51, 1971.

162. Kushner JP, Steinmuller DP, Lee GR: The role of iron in the pathogenesis of porphyria cutanea tarda. II. Inhibition of uroporphyrinogen decarboxylase. *J Clin Invest* 56:661, 1975.

163. Blekkenhorst GH, Eales L, Pimstone NR: Activation of uroporphyrinogen decarboxylase by ferrous iron in porphyria cutanea tarda. *S Afr Med J* 56:918, 1979.

164. Chiaverini C, Halimi G, Ouzan D, et al: Porphyria cutanea tarda, C282Y, H63D, and S65C HFE gene mutations and hepatitis C infection: A study from Southern France. *Dermatology* 206:212, 2003.

165. Tannapfel A, Stolzel U, Kostler E, et al: C282Y and H63D mutations of the hemochromatosis gene in German porphyria cutanea tarda patients. *Virchows Arch* 439:1, 2001.

166. Bulaj ZJ, Phillips JD, Ajioka RS, et al: Hemochromatosis genes and other factors contributing to the pathogenesis of porphyria cutanea tarda. *Blood* 95:1565, 2000.

167. Buckberg AM, Kinniburgh AJ: Induction of liver apoliprotein A-IV mRNA in porphyric mice. *Nucleic Acids Res* 13:1953, 1985.

168. Poland AP, Smith D, Metter G, Possick P: A health survey of workers in a 2,4,-D and 2,4,5-T plant. *Arch Environ Health* 22:316, 1971.

169. Lynch RE, Lee GR, Kushner JP: Porphyria cutanea tarda associated with disinfectant misuse. *Arch Intern Med* 135:549, 1975.

170. Cam C, Nigogoysan G: Acquired toxic porphyria cutanea tarda due to hexachlorobenzene. *JAMA* 183:88, 1963.

171. Schmid R: Cutaneous porphyria in Turkey. *N Engl J Med* 263:397, 1960.

172. Goldsman CI, Taylor JS: Porphyria cutanea tarda and bullous dermatoses associated with chronic renal failure: A review. *Cleve Clin Q* 50:151, 1983.

173. Ramasamy R, Kubik MM: Porphyria cutanea tarda in association with Sjogren's syndrome. *Practitioner* 226:1297, 1982.

174. Nyman CR: Porphyria cutanea tarda, carcinoma of the lung, rheumatoid arthritis, right hydronephrosis. *Proc R Soc Med* 65:688, 1972.

175. Franks AGJ, Pulini M, Bickers DR, et al: Carbohydrate metabolism in porphyria cutanea tarda. *Am J Med Sci* 277:163, 1979.

176. Coburn PR, Coleman JC, Cream JJ, et al: Porphyria cutanea tarda and porphyria variegata unmasked by viral hepatitis. *Clin Exp Dermatol* 10:169, 1985.

177. Chesney TM, Wardlaw LL, Kapalna RJ, Chow JF: Porphyria cutanea tarda complicating Wilson's disease. *J Am Acad Dermatol* 4:64, 1981.

178. Beall SS, Patten BM, Mallette L, Jankovic J: Abnormal systemic metabolism of iron, porphyrin, and calcium in Fahr's syndrome. *Ann Neurol* 26:569, 1989.

179. Grossman ME, Bickers DR: Porphyria cutanea tarda. A rare cutaneous manifestation of hepatic tumors. *Cutis* 21:782, 1978.

180. Burnett JW, Lamon JM, Levin J: Haemophilia, hepatitis and porphyria. *Br J Dermatol* 97:453, 1977.

181. Chapman RWG: Porphyria cutanea tarda and beta-thalassaemia minor with iron overload in mother and daughter. *Br Med J* 280:1255, 1980.

182. Manzione NC, Wolkoff AW, Sassa S: Development of porphyria cutanea tarda after treatment with cyclophosphamide. *Gastroenterology* 95:1119, 1988.

183. Guyotat D, Nicolas JF, Augey F, et al: Porphyria cutanea tarda after allogeneic bone marrow transplantation for chronic myelogenous leukemia. *Am J Hematol* 34:69, 1990.

184. Wissel PS, Sordillo P, Anderson KE, et al: Porphyria cutanea tarda associated with the acquired immune deficiency syndrome. *Am J Hematol* 25:107, 1987.

185. Elder GH: The metabolism of porphyrins of the isocoproporphyrin series. *Enzyme* 17:61, 1974.

186. Gunther WW: The porphyrias and erythropoietic protoporphyria: An unusual case. *Australas J Dermatol* 9:23, 1967.

187. Toback AC, Sassa S, Poh-Fitzpatrick MB, et al: Hepatoerythropoietic porphyria: Clinical, biochemical, and enzymatic studies in a three-generation family lineage. *N Engl J Med* 316:645, 1987.

188. Romana M, Grandchamp B, Dubart A, et al: Identification of a new mutation responsible for hepatoerythropoietic porphyria. *Eur J Clin Invest* 21:225, 1991.

189. de Verneuil H, Bourgeois F, de Rooij F, et al: Characterization of a new mutation (R292G) and a detection at the human uroporphyrinogen decarboxylase locus in two patients with hepatoerythropoietic porphyria. *Hum Genet* 89:548, 1992.

190. Garey JR, Hansen JL, Harrison LM, et al: A point mutation in the coding region of uroporphyrinogen decarboxylase associated with familial porphyria cutanea tarda. *Blood* 73:892, 1989.

191. Garey JR, Harrison LM, Franklin KF, et al: Uroporphyrinogen decarboxylase: A splice site mutation causes the deletion of exon 6 in multiple families with porphyria cutanea tarda. *J Clin Invest* 86:1416, 1990.

192. Meguro K, Fujita H, Ishida N, et al: Molecular defects of uroporphyrinogen decarboxylase in a patient with mild hepatoerythropoietic porphyria. *J Invest Dermatol* 102:681, 1994.

193. McManus JF, Begley CG, Sassa S, Ratnaike S: Three new mutations in the uroporphyrinogen decarboxylase gene in familial porphyria cutanea tarda. Mutation in brief no 237. Online. *Hum Mutat* 13:412, 1999.

194. Simon N, Berko GY, Schneider I: Hepatoerythropoietic porphyria presenting as scleroderma and acrosclerosis in a sibling pair. *Br J Dermatol* 96:663, 1977.

195. Czarnecki DB: Hepatoerythropoietic porphyria. *Arch Dermatol* 116:307, 1980.

196. Pinol-Aguade J, Herrero C, Almeida J, et al: Porphyrie hepatoerythrocytaire. Une nouvelle forme de porphyrie. *Ann Dermatol Syphiligr (Paris)* 102:129, 1975.

197. Phillips JD, Parker TL, Schubert HL, et al: Functional consequences of naturally occurring mutations in human uroporphyrinogen decarboxylase. *Blood* 98:3179, 2001.

HEREDITARY AND ACQUIRED SIDEROBLASTIC ANEMIAS

ERNEST BEUTLER

Sideroblastic anemias are characterized by the presence of ring sideroblasts in the marrow. These cells are erythroid precursors that have accumulated abnormal amounts of mitochondrial iron. A variety of abnormalities of porphyrin metabolism in affected erythroid cells have been documented. Hereditary sideroblastic anemias are usually X linked, the result of mutations in the erythroid form of δ-aminolevulinic acid (ALA) synthase. Inherited autosomal and mitochondrial forms are also occasionally seen. Acquired sideroblastic anemias can occur as a result of the ingestion of drugs, alcohol, or toxins such as lead or zinc. Ring sideroblasts are also a feature of myelodysplastic states, discussed in Chap. 86. Patients with sideroblastic anemia may respond to pharmacologic doses of pyridoxine that are often given together with folic acid. Iron loading is common in the sideroblastic anemias and can be treated by phlebotomy when the anemia is mild or with Desferal when it is more severe.

DEFINITION AND HISTORY

Sideroblastic anemias are a heterogeneous group of disorders that have as common features the presence of large numbers of ringed sideroblasts in the marrow, ineffective erythropoiesis, increased levels of tissue iron, and varying proportions of hypochromic erythrocytes in the blood. They may be acquired or hereditary (Table 58-1).

Acquired sideroblastic anemia may be a neoplastic disease, that is, a clonal disorder that can progress to acute leukemia. This subject is considered in Chapter 86, in which clonal, preleukemic disorders are discussed. Sideroblastic anemia may also develop as a result of the administration of certain drugs, exposure to toxins, or coincident to neoplastic or inflammatory disease. Hereditary sideroblastic anemias include X-linked, autosomal, and mitochondrial entities. Occasionally a patient with apparently familial disease has developed a myelodysplastic syndrome later,[41,42] but with these rare exceptions disorders are distinct and do not coexist or evolve one from the other.

Although the perinuclear distribution of siderotic granules in the nucleated red cells of patients with various types of anemia was described in 1947,[43,44] the concept of sideroblastic anemia as a generic designation was not generally accepted until the publications of Björkman,[45] Dacie and colleagues,[46] Heilmeyer and associates,[47,48] Bernard and colleagues,[49] and Mollin.[19] After description of the primary adult form of refractory sideroblastic anemia,[45,46] similarity to the morphologic and erythrokinetic changes in hereditary (sex-linked) hypochromic anemia was recognized. Cooley[50] described a patient with an anemia with ovalocytosis who was shortly thereafter shown to have inherited a hereditary sex-linked disorder,[51] that we now know resulted from an aminolevulinic acid (ALA) synthase mutation.[52] Autosomally

inherited cases were also described,[53] and prominent sideroblastic changes of the marrow were found in Pearson marrow-pancreas syndrome, a disorder that is associated with mutations of the mitochondrial DNA.[54–58] Subsequently, it became evident that similar abnormalities were associated with a wide variety of diseases,[20] therapy with antituberculosis drugs,[2,59] and lead intoxication.[13,15–17] In some patients the anemia responded to large doses of pyridoxine and was designated "pyridoxine-responsive anemia."[19,60–62] These "secondary" acquired disorders were then incorporated into the classification.

EPIDEMIOLOGY

All of the hereditary forms are rare, and no particular ethnic predilection is known. Drug-induced forms occur sporadically among subjects taking the drugs listed in Table 58-1.

ETIOLOGY AND PATHOGENESIS

MORPHOLOGIC ASPECTS: THE SIDEROBLASTS

Sideroblasts are erythroblasts containing aggregates of nonheme iron appearing as one or more Prussian blue-positive granules on light microscopy.[63] The morphology of these cells in normal and abnormal states is discussed in detail in Chapter 28. In normal subjects, 30 to 50 percent of marrow erythroblasts contain such granules, which, when viewed by electron microscopy, are seen to be neither within mitochondria nor associated with other cytoplasmic organelles.[64] In contrast to the normal cytoplasmic location of siderotic granules, the pathologic sideroblasts in the sideroblastic anemias exhibit large amounts of iron deposited as dust or plaque-like ferruginous micelles between the cristae of mitochondria (see Fig. 28-11).[65] The iron-loaded mitochondria are distorted and swollen, their cristae are indistinct, and the identification of mitochondria may itself be difficult. In humans, the mitochondria of the erythroblast are distributed perinuclearly,[13] and this accounts for the distinctive "ringed" sideroblast identified by Prussian blue staining when mitochondrial iron overload is present (see Fig. 28-11 and Color Plate XVIII-7). The morphologic features that characterize pathologic sideroblasts in various disorders have been summarized.[66]

TABLE 58-1 CLASSIFICATION OF SIDEROBLASTIC ANEMIAS

I. Acquired
   A. Primary sideroblastic anemia (myelodysplastic syndromes) (see Chap. 86)
   B. Sideroblastic anemia secondary to
      1. Isoniazid[1]
      2. Pyrazinamide[2,3]
      3. Cycloserine[2,3]
      4. Chloramphenicol[2,4–6]
      5. Ethanol[2,7–12]
      6. Lead[13–18]
      7. Chronic neoplastic and inflammatory disease[2,19–23]
      8. Triethylene tetramine dihydrochloride[24,25]
      9. Zinc[26–30]
      10. D-Penicillamine[31]
      11. Progesterone[32]
      12. Fusidic acid[33]
II. Hereditary
   A. X chromosome-linked
      1. ALAS2 deficiency[34]
      2. Hereditary sideroblastic anemia with ataxia: Mitochondrial ATP binding cassette (*ABC7*) mutations
   B. Autosomal
      1. Mitochondrial myopathy and sideroblastic anemia (*PSU1* mutations)[35]
   C. Mitochondrial
      1. Pearson marrow-pancreas syndrome[36–38]
      2. Subunit 1 of the mitochondrial cytochrome oxidase[39,40]

Acronyms and abbreviations that appear in this chapter include: ALA, aminolevulinic acid; ATP, adenosine triphosphate.

PATHOGENESIS

The pathogenesis of most of the sideroblastic anemias is not well understood.[34,67] It is not clear whether the basic mechanism by which abnormal accumulations of intramitochondrial iron occur is the same in inherited and acquired forms of the disease. However, it seems appropriate, given the present state of knowledge, to discuss both forms together. The pathogenesis of the disorder may be viewed from two standpoints: the underlying biochemical lesions and the mechanism(s) of the anemia itself.

BIOCHEMICAL LESIONS AND GENETICS

In the search for the biochemical lesions responsible for the development of sideroblastic anemia, attention has been focused upon an intramitochondrial defect in heme synthesis and on possible disturbances in pyridoxine metabolism.

Heme Synthesis The possible role of defects in heme biosynthesis have occupied central stage since the early studies of Garby and colleagues,[68] who postulated that such a defect might exist and demonstrated that the level of free erythrocyte protoporphyrin was decreased and that of coproporphyrin was increased. Subsequently, a variety of abnormalities of the levels of precursors and of their rate of incorporation into heme was documented.[69–74] However, the findings have not all been consistent, since levels of free erythrocyte protoporphyrin have often been increased,[75,76] not diminished. The role of mitochondria in the etiology of sideroblastic anemia gained further credence when mutations of the mitochondrial genome were found in patients with Pearson syndrome.[54–58]

Sideroblastic anemia with deficiency of ALA synthase of marrow erythroid cells has been documented in subjects both with the congenital disorder and the acquired disease.[77–79] Identification of the defect at the DNA level in the X-linked gene for erythroid-specific ALA synthase (ALAS2) establishes that hereditary X-linked cases result from structural mutations in this enzyme.[34] Hereditary sideroblastic anemia with spinocerebellar degeneration with ataxia is an X-linked syndrome that appears to be distinct from the other forms of sideroblastic anemia.[80–83] An X-linked adenosine triphosphate (ATP)-binding cassette has been identified as a likely cause for this rare disorder.[82,84,85]

Heteroplasmic point mutations in subunit 1 of the mitochondrial cytochrome oxidase have been documented in two patients with sideroblastic anemia.[39,40]

Rare autosomal forms of inherited sideroblastic anemia have been reported.[86,87] In one or more additional patients with sideroblastic anemia, a deficiency of uroporphyrinogen decarboxylase[4,88] and heme synthetase,[70,71,89–91] enzymes also necessary for the synthesis of heme (see Chap. 57), has been identified, but the defect in heme synthetase could simply result from the inhibitory effect of mitochondrial iron overload on enzyme activity.[71] The suggestion[68] that a defect in coproporphyrinogen oxidase might be responsible for sideroblast formation could not be confirmed by direct measurement.[92] Increased levels of uroporphyrinogen 1 synthase are commonly encountered.[74] Alcohol, a common cause of secondary sideroblastic anemia, inhibits heme synthesis at several steps.[73] In many instances, no abnormalities in the protoporphyrin synthetic pathway have been demonstrable.[93]

No single defect in heme synthesis accounts for sideroblast formation in this heterogeneous group of disorders. Moreover, a simple defect in heme synthesis fails to explain certain commonly encountered features, such as megaloblastoid and other dyserythropoietic features, the frequently low serum folate levels, and, at times, partial responses to folate administration.

Pyridoxine Metabolism The possibility of a role for pyridoxine has been fostered by the clear demonstration that pyridoxine deficiency in animals is a prototype of sideroblastic anemia.[65] Sideroblastic anemia can be induced by drugs that reduce the level of pyridoxal phosphate in blood and decrease the δ-ALA synthetase activity in normoblasts.[59,70,72] Moreover, certain sideroblastic disorders, though clearly not due to pyridoxine deficiency in a conventional sense, are nonetheless responsive to pharmacologic doses of pyridoxine.[79,94–96] Pyridoxal phosphate is a necessary coenzyme for the initial reaction of protoporphyrin synthesis, the condensation of glycine and succinyl CoA to form ALA, a reaction mediated by ALA synthetase (see Chap. 57). Furthermore, pyridoxal phosphate is a factor in the enzymatic conversion of serine to glycine (see Chap. 39). This reaction generates a form of folate coenzyme necessary for the formation of thymidylate, an important step in DNA synthesis. Pyridoxal 5'-phosphate, the active form of the coenzyme, must itself be enzymatically synthesized from pyridoxine. Deficiencies in its biosynthesis have also been invoked as the possible cause of certain sideroblastic anemias,[62,97] but direct measurements of pyridoxal kinase failed to confirm that the postulated lesion was present.[98] There are additional abnormalities that are difficult to rationalize in terms of defects in heme synthesis or abnormalities of pyridoxine metabolism. Sideroblastic anemia has been found in a patient with apparent antibody-mediated red cell aplasia.[99] Dramatically altered activity ratios of a wide diversity of enzymes have been described.[23,100] There are alterations in red cell antigen patterns frequently with an increase of i and a loss of A_1,[22] and, in some instances, a variety of metabolic abnormalities. Similar findings occur in certain hereditary and acquired refractory anemias with cellular marrows but without ringed sideroblasts.[23] Such dyscrasias are also characterized by ineffective erythropoiesis and, except for the lack of ringed sideroblasts, may in some instances be virtually indistinguishable from their sideroblastic counterparts.[101]

MECHANISM OF ANEMIA[102]

The dominant factor producing anemia is ineffective erythropoiesis; the rate of red cell destruction is usually near-normal or only moderately accelerated to levels for which a normally functioning marrow could easily compensate. The half-time of disappearance of intravenously injected tracer doses of radioactive iron may be normal, but it usually is rapid (25–50 minutes; normal mean, 90–100 minutes). The plasma iron turnover tends to be increased (1.5–5.9 mg per deciliter of whole blood per day; normal, approximately 0.30–0.70 mg), but incorporation of radioactive iron into heme and its delivery to the blood as newly synthesized hemoglobin are depressed (15–30% of tracer dose; normal, 70–90%). Red cell survival, as determined by the ^{51}Cr technique, varies from a half-time of 15 days to normal, corresponding to a mean erythrocyte life span of approximately 40 to 120 days. As in other kinds of anemia characterized by ineffective erythropoiesis, the total fecal stercobilin excreted per day may be greater than can be accounted for by the daily catabolism of circulating hemoglobin.

CLINICAL AND LABORATORY FEATURES

PRIMARY ACQUIRED SIDEROBLASTIC ANEMIA

Chapter 86 describes the features of primary acquired sideroblastic anemia.

SECONDARY ACQUIRED SIDEROBLASTIC ANEMIA

The administration of certain drugs and the ingestion of alcohol may cause sideroblastic anemia (Table 58-1). The drugs that are most commonly associated with this type of anemia are isonicotinic acid hydrazide,[1] pyrazinamide,[2,3,59] and cycloserine,[2,3,59] all pyridoxine antagonists. Although plasma pyridoxal phosphate levels are often low in alcoholic patients, there is no correlation between these levels and the appearance of ringed sideroblasts in the marrow.[103]

Anemia secondary to drugs may be quite severe, even necessitating transfusion,[59] but characteristically the anemia improves rapidly when the patient is given pyridoxine and/or when administration of the offending drug is discontinued. The red cells are hypochromic, and commonly a dimorphic appearance of the erythrocytes in the blood film, that is, two populations of red cells, can be distinguished. The reticulocyte count is low or normal.[104] In rare instances, a sideroblastic anemia first observed during the course of drug administration has progressed in the face of discontinuing the putative offending drug. In such cases, the patient presumably was suffering from an underlying myelodysplastic disorder.

HEREDITARY SIDEROBLASTIC ANEMIA

Hereditary sideroblastic anemia is very uncommon. More instances of the X-chromosome linked varieties than of apparently autosomally inherited cases have been documented.[105] The disorder is heterogeneous. In some of the cases of hereditary iron loading anemia that are cited below, either the presence of the sideroblasts in the marrow or the hereditary nature of the disorder is presumed; it has not been clearly documented in each case.

Anemia is usually apparent during the first few months[106] or years[68,69] of life; it may even occur prenatally.[107] However, remarkable patients in whom microcytic anemia first became evident in the eighth and ninth decade of life and were found to have a microcytic, pyridoxine response anemia apparently related to inherited mutations of the *ALAS2* gene have been documented.[108,109]

Pallor is the most prominent physical finding; splenomegaly may be present[78] but not universally so.[68,106] The anemia is characteristically microcytic and hypochromic, and prominent dimorphism of the red cell population has been noted in carrier females of the sex-linked form of the anemia.[51,106,110] This has been regarded as evidence of X-inactivation affecting the locus responsible for this disorder,[69,106,110,111] but it is notable that marked dimorphism sometimes is seen in the red cells of affected males as well[51,68] and in autosomal forms of the disease.[112] The degree of anisocytosis and poikilocytosis is usually striking. Sometimes the anemia can be macrocytic,[41,113] especially in mitochondrial forms of the disease. The red cells show marked heterogeneity with respect to resistance to osmotic lysis: a flattened curve indicates that cells with both increased and decreased resistance to lysis are present.[68,114] The white cell count is usually normal or slightly decreased, unless splenectomy has been performed. Then it may be greatly elevated.[115] Splenomegaly is present in most cases.[115] In one family, a platelet function abnormality resembling a storage pool defect was noted,[116] but this could have been an independently inherited disorder.

Pearson marrow-pancreas syndrome is a refractory sideroblastic anemia with vacuolization of marrow precursors and exocrine pancreatic dysfunction occurring during infancy.[36,117] Most patients die in infancy, although there is considerable phenotypic variation, presumably depending upon the number of mitochondria affected and their tissue distribution.

TREATMENT

Most patients with hereditary sideroblastic anemia appear to have some response to treatment with pyridoxine in doses of 50 to 200 mg/day,[51,106,110,115,118–120] but failures have also been observed.[47,68,76] Some patients have responded to doses as low as 2.5 mg/day.[115] An additional effect may be achieved by the administration of folic acid.[106] Very rarely patients have been reported to respond to a crude liver

extract, and it has been suggested that tryptophane may be an active principle, enhancing the effect of pyridoxine.[121,122] Responses to pyridoxine may result in an increase in the steady-state hemoglobin level of the blood or a decrease in the transfusion requirement, but normalization of the hemoglobin level does not usually occur and the anemia relapses when pyridoxine administration is discontinued.

Iron overloading regularly accompanies this disorder and may be the cause of death[71] (see Chap. 40). Iron storage may be enhanced when the mutations of hereditary hemochromatosis are co-inherited.[123] If the anemia is not too severe or if it can be partially corrected by the administration of pyridoxine, phlebotomy may be used to diminish the iron burden.[124,125] Otherwise it may be advisable to attempt to decrease the amount of body iron by the use of desferrioxamine (see Chap. 40).

Marrow transplantation, both ablative[126] and nonmyeloblative,[127] has been used on rare occasions to treat hereditary sideroblastic anemia.

REFERENCES

1. Lowe JG, Johnston RN: Anti-tuberculous drugs and sideroblastic anaemia. *Br J Clin Pract* 44:706, 1990.
2. Hines JD, Grasso JA: The sideroblastic anemias. *Semin Hematol* 7:86, 1970.
3. Harris EB, MacGibbon BH, Mollin DL: Experimental sideroblastic anemia. *Br J Haematol* 11:99, 1965.
4. Goodman JR, Hall SG: Accumulation of iron in mitochondria of erythroblasts. *Br J Haematol* 13:335, 1967.
5. Beck EA, Ziegler G, Schmid R, Lüdin H: Reversible sideroblastic anemia caused by chloramphenicol. *Acta Haematol (Basel)* 38:1, 1967.
6. Firkin FC: Mitochondrial lesions in reversible erythropoietic depression due to chloramphenicol. *J Clin Invest* 51:2085, 1972.
7. Hines JD: Reversible megaloblastic and sideroblastic marrow abnormalities in alcoholic patients. *Br J Haematol* 16:87, 1969.
8. Hines JD, Cowan DH: Studies on the pathogenesis of alcohol-induced sideroblastic bone-marrow abnormalities. *N Engl J Med* 283:441, 1970.
9. Eichner ER, Hillman RS: The evolution of anemia in alcoholic patients. *Am J Med* 50:218, 1971.
10. Anderson BB, Fulford-Jones CE, Child JA, et al: Conversion of vitamin B₆ compounds to active forms in the red blood cell. *J Clin Invest* 50: 1901, 1971.
11. Hines JD: Altered phosphorylation of vitamin B₆ in alcoholic patients induced by oral administration of alcohol. *J Lab Clin Med* 74:882, 1969.
12. Lumeng L, Li TK: Vitamin B₆ metabolism in chronic alcohol abuse. Pyridoxal phosphate levels in plasma and the effects of acetaldehyde on pyridoxal phosphate synthesis and degradation in human erythrocytes. *J Clin Invest* 53:693, 1974.
13. Bessis MC, Jensen WN: Sideroblastic anaemia, mitochondria and erythroblastic iron. *Br J Haematol* 11:49, 1965.
14. Dacie JV, Mollin DL: Siderocytes, sideroblasts, and sideroblastic anaemia. *Acta Med Scand* 179(suppl)445:237, 1966.
15. Jensen WN, Moreno G: Les Ribosomes et les ponctuations basophiles des érythrocytes dans l'intoxication par le plomb. *C R Acad Sci (Paris)* 258:3596, 1964.
16. Jensen WN, Moreno GD, Bessis MC: An electron microscopic description of basophilic stippling in red cells. *Johns Hopkins Med J* 25:933, 1965.
17. Griggs RC: Lead poisoning: Hematologic aspects, in *Progress in Hematology*, vol 4, edited by CV Moore, EB Brown, p 117. Grune & Stratton, New York, 1964.
18. Goldberg A: Lead poisoning as a disorder of heme synthesis. *Semin Hematol* 5:424, 1968.
19. Mollin DL: Sideroblasts and sideroblastic anaemia. *Br J Haematol* 11: 41, 1965.

20. MacGibbon BH, Mollin DL: Sideroblastic anaemia in man: Observations on seventy cases. *Br J Haematol* 11:59, 1965.

21. Hayhoe FGJ, Quaglino D: Refractory sideroblastic anaemia and erythremic myelosis: Possible relationship and cytochemical observations. *Br J Haematol* 6:381, 1960.

22. Rochant H, Dreyfus B, Bouguerra M, Hoi T-H: Hypothesis: Refractory anemias, preleukemic conditions, and fetal erythropoiesis. *Blood* 39: 721, 1972.

23. Valentine WN, Konrad PN, Paglia DE: Dyserythropoiesis, refractory anemia, and "preleukemia": Metabolic features of the erythrocytes. *Blood* 41:857, 1973.

24. Condamine L, Hermine O, Alvin P, et al: Acquired sideroblastic anaemia during treatment of Wilson's disease with triethylene tetramine dihydrochloride. *Br J Haematol* 83:166, 1993.

25. Perry AR, Pagliuca A, Fitzsimons EJ, et al: Acquired sideroblastic anaemia induced by a copper-chelating agent. *Int J Hematol* 64:69, 1996.

26. Greist A, Tricot G, Hoffman R: Excessive zinc ingestion. A reversible cause of sideroblastic anemia and bone marrow depression. *JAMA* 264: 1441, 1990.

27. Irving JA, Mattman A, Lockitch G, et al: Element of caution: A case of reversible cytopenias associated with excessive zinc supplementation. *CMAJ* 169:129, 2003.

28. Schwartz J, Landrigan PJ, Baker EL Jr, et al: Lead-induced anemia: Dose-response relationships and evidence for a threshold. *Am J Public Health* 80:165, 1990.

29. Ramadurai J, Shapiro C, Kozloff M, Telfer M: Zinc abuse and sideroblastic anemia. *Am J Hematol* 42:227, 1993.

30. Fiske DN, McCoy HE III, Kitchens CS: Zinc-induced sideroblastic anemia: Report of a case, review of the literature, and description of the hematologic syndrome. *Am J Hematol* 46:147, 1994.

31. Ramselaar AC, Dekker AW, Huber-Bruning O, Bijlsma JW: Acquired sideroblastic anaemia after aplastic anaemia caused by D-penicillamine therapy for rheumatoid arthritis. *Ann Rheum Dis* 46:156, 1987.

32. Brodsky RA, Hasegawa S, Fibach E, et al: Acquired sideroblastic anaemia following progesterone therapy. *Br J Haematol* 87:859, 1994.

33. Vial T, Grignon M, Daumont M, et al: Sideroblastic anaemia during fusidic acid treatment. *Eur J Haematol* 72:358, 2004.

34. Fleming MD: The genetics of inherited sideroblastic anemias. *Semin Hematol* 39:2002.

35. Bykhovskaya Y, Casas K, Mengesha E, et al: Missense mutation in pseudouridine synthase 1 (PUS1) causes mitochondrial myopathy and sideroblastic anemia (MLASA). *Am J Hum Genet* 74:1303, 2004.

36. Seneca S, De Meirleir L, De Schepper J, et al: Pearson marrow pancreas syndrome: A molecular study and clinical management. *Clin Genet* 51: 338, 1997.

37. Muraki K, Goto Y, Nishino I, et al: Severe lactic acidosis and neonatal death in Pearson syndrome. *J Inherit Metab Dis* 20:43, 1997.

38. Santorelli FM, Barmada MA, Pons R, et al: Leigh-type neuropathology in Pearson syndrome associated with impaired ATP production and a novel mtDNA deletion. *Neurology* 47:1320, 1996.

39. Bröker S, Meunier B, Rich P, et al: MtDNA mutations associated with sideroblastic anaemia cause a defect of mitochondrial cytochrome *c* oxidase. *Eur J Biochem* 258:132, 1998.

40. Gattermann N, Retzlaff S, Wang YL, et al: Heteroplasmic point mutations of mitochondrial DNA affecting subunit I of cytochrome c oxidase in two patients with acquired idiopathic sideroblastic anemia. *Blood* 90: 4961, 1997.

41. Tuckfield A, Ratnaike S, Hussein S, Metz J: A novel form of hereditary sideroblastic anaemia with macrocytosis. *Br J Haematol* 97:279, 1997.

42. Kardos G, Veerman AJ, de Waal FC, et al: Familial sideroblastic anemia with emergence of monosomy 5 and myelodysplastic syndrome. *Med Pediatr Oncol* 26:54, 1996.

43. Dacie JV, Doniach I: The basophilic property of the iron-containing granules in siderocytes. *J Pathol Bacteriol* 59:684, 1947.

44. McFadzean AJS, Davis LJ: Iron-staining erythrocyte inclusions with special reference to acquired haemolytic anaemia. *Glasg Med J* 28:237, 1947.

45. Björkman SE: Chronic refractory anemia with sideroblastic bone marrow: A study of four cases. *Blood* 11:250, 1956.

46. Dacie JV, Smith MD, White JC, Mollin DL: Refractory normoblastic anaemia: A clinical and haematologic study of seven cases. *Br J Haematol* 5:56, 1959.

47. Heilmeyer L, Keiderling W, Bilger R, Bernauer H: Über chronische refractare Anämien mit sideroblastischen Knochenmark (anaemia refractoria sideroblastica). *Folia Haematol (Frankfurt)* 2:49, 1958.

48. Heilmeyer L, Emmrich J, Hennemann HH, et al: Über eine chronische hypochrome Anämie bei zwei Gerschwistern auf der Grundlage einer Eisenverwertungs-störung (anaemia hypochromica sideroachrestica hereditaria). *Folia Haematol (Frankfurt) (N F)* 2:61, 1958.

49. Bernard J, Lortholary P, Levy JP, et al: Les Anémies normochromes sidéroblastiques primitives. *Nouv Rev Fr Hematol* 3:723, 1963.

50. Cooley TB: A severe type of hereditary anemia with elliptocytosis. Interesting sequence of splenectomy. *Am J Med Sci* 209:561, 1945.

51. Rundles RW, Falls HF: Hereditary (sex-linked) anemia. *Am J Med Sci* 211:641, 1946.

52. Cotter PD, Rucknagel DL, Bishop DF: X-linked sideroblastic anemia: Identification of the mutation in the erythroid-specific delta-aminolevulinate synthase gene (ALAS2) in the original family described by Cooley. *Blood* 84:3915, 1994.

53. Kasturi J, Basha HM, Smeda SH, Swehli M: Hereditary sideroblastic anaemia in 4 siblings of a Libyan family—Autosomal inheritance. *Acta Haematol (Basel)* 68:321, 1982.

54. Gürgey A, Rötig A, Gümrük F, et al: Pearson's marrow-pancreas syndrome in 2 Turkish children. *Acta Haematol (Basel)* 87:206, 1992.

55. McShane MA, Hammans SR, Sweeney M, et al: Pearson syndrome and mitochondrial encephalomyopathy in a patient with a deletion of MtDNA. *Am J Hum Genet* 48:39, 1991.

56. Rötig A, Cormier V, Blanche S, et al: Pearson's marrow-pancreas syndrome. A multisystem mitochondrial disorder in infancy. *J Clin Invest* 86:1601, 1990.

57. Cormier V, Rötig A, Quartino AR, et al: Widespread multi-tissue deletions of the mitochondrial genome in the Pearson marrow-pancreas syndrome. *J Pediatr* 117:599, 1990.

58. Jakobs C, Rotig A, Munnich A, Veerman AJ: Pearson's syndrome: A multi-system disorder based on a MtDNA deletion. *Tijdschr Kindergeneeskd* 59:196, 1991.

59. Verwilghen R, Reybrouck G, Callens L, Cosemans J: Antituberculous drugs and sideroblastic anaemia. *Br J Haematol* II:92, 1965.

60. Harris JW, Whittington RM, Weisman RJ, Horrigan DL: Pyridoxine responsive anemia in the human adult. *Proc Soc Exp Biol Med* 91:427, 1956.

61. Horrigan DL, Harris JW: Pyridoxine-responsive anemia in man. Vitam Horm 26:549, 1968

62. Gehrmann G: Pyridoxine responsive anaemias. *Br J Haematol* 11:86, 1965.

63. Cartwright GE, Deiss A: Sideroblasts, siderocytes, and sideroblastic anemia. *N Engl J Med* 292:185, 1975.

64. Bessis MC: *Living Blood Cells and Their Ultrastructure*, translated by RI Weed. Springer-Verlag, New York, 1973.

65. Hammond E, Deiss A, Carnes WH, Cartwright GE: Ultrastructural characteristics of siderocytes in swine. *Lab Invest* 21:292, 1969.

66. Koc S, Harris JW: Sideroblastic anemias: Variations on imprecision in diagnostic criteria, proposal for an extended classification of sideroblastic anemias. *Am J Hematol* 57:1, 1998.

67. Furuyama K, Sassa S: Multiple mechanisms for hereditary sideroblastic anemia. *Cell Mol Biol* 48:5, 2002.

68. Garby L, Sjölin S, Vahlquist B: Chronic refractory hypochromic anaemia with disturbed haem-metabolism. *Br J Haematol* 3:55, 1957.
69. Lee GR, MacDiarmid WD, Cartwright GE, Wintrobe MM: Hereditary, X-linked, sideroachrestic anemia. The isolation of two erythrocyte populations differing in Xga blood type and porphyrin content. *Blood* 32:59, 1968.
70. Konopka L, Hoffbrand AV: Haem synthesis in sideroblastic anaemia. *Br J Haematol* 42:73, 1979.
71. Vogler WR, Mingioli ES: Porphyrin synthesis and heme synthetase activity in pyridoxine-responsive anemia. *Blood* 32:979, 1968.
72. Tanaka M, Bottomley SS: Bone marrow delta-aminolevulinic acid synthetase activity in experimental sideroblastic anemia. *J Lab Clin Med* 84:92, 1974.
73. McColl KEL, Thompson GG, Moore MR, Goldberg A: Acute ethanol ingestion and haem biosynthesis in healthy subjects. *Eur J Clin Invest* 10:107, 1980.
74. Pasanen AVO, Vuopio P, Borgström GH, Tenhunen R: Haem biosynthesis in refractory sideroblastic anaemia associated with the preleukaemic syndrome. *Scand J Haematol* 27:35, 1981.
75. Kushner JP, Lee GR, Wintrobe MM, Cartwright GE: Idiopathic refractory sideroblastic anemia: Clinical and laboratory investigation of 17 patients and review of the literature. *Medicine* 50:139, 1971.
76. Heilmeyer L: *Disturbances in Heme Synthesis.* Charles C. Thomas, Springfield, 1966.
77. Aoki Y, Urata G, Wada O, Takaku F: Measurement of delta-aminolevulinic acid synthetase activity in human erythroblasts. *J Clin Invest* 53:1326, 1974.
78. Buchanan GR, Bottomley SS, Nitschke R: Bone marrow delta-aminolaevulinate synthase deficiency in a female with congenital sideroblastic anemia. *Blood* 55:109, 1980.
79. Cotter PD, Baumann M, Bishop DF: Enzymatic defect in "X-linked" sideroblastic anemia: Molecular evidence for erythroid delta-aminolevulinate synthase deficiency. *Proc Natl Acad Sci U S A* 89:4028, 1992.
80. Pagon RA, Bird TD, Detter JC, Pierce I: Hereditary sideroblastic anaemia and ataxia: An X linked recessive disorder. *J Med Genet* 22:267, 1985.
81. Raskind WH, Wijsman E, Pagon RA, et al: X-linked sideroblastic anemia and ataxia: Linkage to phosphoglycerate kinase at Xq13. *Am J Hum Genet* 48:335, 1991.
82. Allikmets R, Raskind WH, Hutchinson A, et al: Mutation of a putative mitochondrial iron transporter gene (ABC7) in X-linked sideroblastic anemia and ataxia (XLSA/A). *Hum Mol Genet* 8:743, 1999.
83. Hellier KD, Hatchwell E, Duncombe AS, et al: X-linked sideroblastic anaemia with ataxia: Another mitochondrial disease? *J Neurol Neurosurg Psychiatry* 70:65, 2001.
84. Shimada Y, Okuno S, Kawai A, et al: Cloning and chromosomal mapping of a novel ABC transporter gene (hABC7), a candidate for X-linked sideroblastic anemia with spinocerebellar ataxia. *J Hum Genet* 43:115, 1998.
85. Maguire A, Hellier K, Hammans S, May A: X-linked cerebellar ataxia and sideroblastic anaemia associated with a missense mutation in the ABC7 gene predicting V411L. *Br J Haematol* 115:910, 2001.
86. Jardine PE, Cotter PD, Johnson SA, et al: Pyridoxine-refractory congenital sideroblastic anaemia with evidence for autosomal inheritance: Exclusion of linkage to ALAS2 at Xp11.21 by polymorphism analysis. *J Med Genet* 31:213, 1994.
87. Casas K, Bykhovskaya Y, Mengesha E, et al: Gene responsible for mitochondrial myopathy and sideroblastic anemia (MSA) maps to chromosome 12q24.33. *Am J Med Genet* 127A:44, 2004.
88. Kushner JP, Barbuto AJ: Decreased activity of hepatic uroporphyrinogen decarboxylase (Urodecarb) in porphyria cutanea tarda (PCT). *Clin Res* 22:178, 1974.
89. Lee GR, Cartwright GE, Wintrobe MM: The response of free erythrocyte protoporphyrin to pyridoxine therapy in a patient with sideroachrestic (sideroblastic) anemia. *Blood* 27:557, 1966.
90. Chauhan MS, Dakshinamurti K: Fluorometric assay of B6 vitamers in biological material. *Clin Chim Acta* 109:159, 1981.
91. Pasanen AVO, Salmi M, Vuopio P, Tenhunen R: Heme biosynthesis in sideroblastic anemia. *Int J Biochem* 12:969, 1980.
92. Pasanen AVO, Eklöf M, Tenhunen R: Coproporphyrinogen oxidase activity and porphyrin concentrations in peripheral red blood cells in hereditary sideroblastic anaemia. *Scand J Haematol* 34:235, 1985.
93. Vavra JD, Poff SA: Heme and porphyrin synthesis in sideroblastic anemia. *J Lab Clin Med* 69:904, 1967.
94. Murakami R, Takumi T, Gouji J, et al: Sideroblastic anemia showing unique response to pyridoxine. *Am J Pediatr Hematol Oncol* 13:345, 1991.
95. Barton JR, Shaver DC, Sibai BM: Successive pregnancies complicated by idiopathic sideroblastic anemia. *Am J Obstet Gynecol* 166:576, 1992.
96. Breton-Gorius J, Bachir D, Rochant H: Congenital sideroblastic anemia without clinical iron overload. A case report. *Am J Hematol* 32:298, 1989.
97. Mason DY, Emerson PM: Primary acquired sideroblastic anaemia: Response to treatment with pyridoxal-5-phosphate. *BMJ* 1:389, 1973.
98. Chillar RK, Johnson CS, Beutler E: Erythrocyte pyridoxine kinase levels in patients with sideroblastic anemia. *N Engl J Med* 295:881, 1976.
99. Ritchey AK, Hoffman R, Dainiak N, et al: Antibody-mediated acquired sideroblastic anemia: Response to cytotoxic therapy. *Blood* 54:734, 1979.
100. Nishibe H, Yamagata K, Gotoh H: A case of sideroblastic anaemia associated with marked elevation of erythrocytic arginase activity. *Scand J Haematol* 15:17, 1975.
101. Geschke W, Beutler E: Refractory sideroblastic and nonsideroblastic anemia. A review of 27 cases. *West J Med* 127:85, 1977.
102. Singh AK, Shinton NK, Williams JDF: Ferrokinetic abnormalities and their significance in patients with sideroblastic anaemia. *Br J Haematol* 18:67, 1970.
103. Pierce HI, McGuffin RG, Hillman RS: Clinical studies in alcoholic sideroblastosis. *Arch Intern Med* 136:283, 1976.
104. McCurdy PR, Donohoe RF: Pyridoxine-responsive anemia conditioned by isonicotinic acid hydrazide. *Blood* 27:352, 1966.
105. Nusbaum NJ: Concise review: Genetic bases for sideroblastic anemia. *Am J Hematol* 37:41, 1991.
106. Weatherall DJ, Pembrey ME, Hall EG, et al: Familial sideroblastic anaemia: Problem of Xg and X chromosome inactivation. *Lancet* 2:744, 1970.
107. Andersen K, Kaad PH: Congenital sideroblastic anaemia with intrauterine symptoms and early lethal outcome. *Acta Paediatr Scand* 81:652, 1992.
108. Cotter PD, May A, Fitzsimons EJ, et al: Late-onset X-linked sideroblastic anemia. *J Clin Invest* 96:2090, 1995.
109. Furuyama K, Harigae H, Kinoshita C, et al: Late-onset X-linked sideroblastic anemia following hemodialysis. *Blood* 101:4623, 2003.
110. Prasad AS, Tranchida L, Konno ET, et al: Hereditary sideroblastic anemia and glucose-6-phosphate dehydrogenase deficiency in a Negro family. *J Clin Invest* 47:1415, 1968.
111. Beutler E: The distribution of gene products among populations of cells in heterozygous humans. *Cold Spring Harb Symp Quant Biol* 29:261, 1964.
112. van Waveren Hogervorst GD, van Roermund HP, Snijders PJ: Hereditary sideroblastic anaemia and autosomal inheritance of erythrocyte dimorphism in a Dutch family. *Eur J Haematol* 38:405, 1987.
113. Fitzsimons EJ, May A: The molecular basis of the sideroblastic anemias. *Curr Opin Hematol* 3:167, 1996.

114. Seip M, Gjessing LR, Lie SO: Congenital sideroblastic anaemia in a girl. *Scand J Haematol* 8:505, 1971.

115. Horrigan DL, Harris JW: Pyridoxine-responsive anemia: Analysis of 62 cases. *Adv Intern Med* 12:103, 1964.

116. Soslau G, Brodsky I: Hereditary sideroblastic anemia with associated platelet abnormalities. *Am J Hematol* 32:298, 1989.

117. Smith OP, Hann IM, Woodward CE, Brockington M: Pearson's marrow/pancreas syndrome: Haematological features associated with deletion and duplication of mitochondrial DNA. *Br J Haematol* 90:469, 1995.

118. Bishop RC, Bethell FH: Hereditary hypochromic anemia with transfusion siderosis treated with pyridoxine. *N Engl J Med* 261:486, 1959.

119. Harris JW, Horrigan DL: Pyridoxine responsive anemia: The prototype and variations on the theme. *Vitam Horm* 22:721, 1964.

120. Vogler WR, Mingioli ES: Heme synthesis in pyridoxine responsive anemia. *N Engl J Med* 273:347, 1965.

121. Horrigan DL: Pyridoxine-responsive anemia: Influence of tryptophane on pyridoxine responsiveness. *Blood* 42:187, 1973.

122. Albahary C, Boiron M: Anémie primitive réfractaire avec hypersidérose sanguine médullaire et hépatique—(cas féminin). *Acta Med Scand* 163:429, 1959.

123. Yaouanq J, Grosbois B, Jouanolle AM, et al: Haemochromatosis Cys282Tyr mutation in pyridoxine-responsive sideroblastic anaemia. *Lancet* 349:1475, 1997.

124. Weintraub LR, Conrad ME, Crosby WH: Iron-loading anemia. Treatment with repeated phlebotomies and pyridoxine. *N Engl J Med* 275:169, 1966.

125. French TJ, Jacobs P: Sideroblastic anaemia associated with iron overload treated by repeated phlebotomy. *S Afr Med J* 50:594, 1976.

126. Urban C, Binder B, Hauer C, Lanzer G: Congenital sideroblastic anemia successfully treated by allogeneic bone marrow transplantation. *Bone Marrow Transplant* 10:373, 1992.

127. Medeiros BC, Kolhouse JF, Cagnoni PJ, et al: Nonmyeloablative allogeneic hematopoietic stem cell transplantation for congenital sideroblastic anemia. *Bone Marrow Transplant* 31:1053, 2003.

NEUTROPHILS, EOSINOPHILS, BASOPHILS, AND MAST CELLS

MORPHOLOGY OF NEUTROPHILS, EOSINOPHILS, AND BASOPHILS

DOROTHY FORD BAINTON

Early in precursor development in the marrow, cells destined to be leukocytes of the granulocytic series—neutrophils, eosinophils, and basophils—synthesize proteins and store them as cytoplasmic granules. The synthesis of primary or azurophilic granules defines the conversion of the myeloblast, a virtually agranular, primitive cell that is the earliest granulocyte precursor identifiable by light microscopy, into the promyelocyte, which is rich in azurophilic granules. Synthesis and accumulation of secondary or specific granules follow. The appearance of specific granules marks the progression of the promyelocyte to a neutrophilic, eosinophilic, or basophilic myelocyte. Thereafter, the cell continues maturation into an amitotic cell with a segmented nucleus, capable of ameboid motility, phagocytosis, and microbial killing. Mature granulocytes develop cytoplasmic and surface structures that permit them to attach to and penetrate the wall of venules. The mature granulocytes enter the blood from the marrow, circulate briefly, and move to the tissues to perform out their major function of host defense. The neutrophil is highly phagocytic and can kill a variety of microorganisms. The eosinophil and basophil are specialized to participate in allergic inflammatory responses. The stages of maturation from promyelocyte to mature cell can be recognized on a stained film of marrow using a light microscope. This chapter discusses details of granulocyte structure and inherited and acquired abnormalities of neutrophil granules. Granulocytes must be normal in quantity and quality to function effectively in host defense.

NEUTROPHILS

In the normal adult human, the life of neutrophils is spent in three environments: marrow, blood, and tissues. Marrow is the site of differentiation of hematopoietic stem cells into neutrophil progenitors and of proliferation and terminal maturation of neutrophilic granulocytes (myeloblast to segmented neutrophils) (Fig. 59-1).[1-4] Precursor cell proliferation, which consists of approximately five divisions, occurs only during the first three stages of neutrophil maturation (blast, promyelocyte, and myelocyte). After the myelocyte stage, the cells are no longer capable of mitosis and enter a large marrow storage pool. After 5 days, they are released into the blood, where they circulate for a few hours before entering tissues (see Chap. 61).[5,6]

Acronyms and abbreviations that appear in this chapter include: AGE, advanced glycation end product; AML, acute myelogenous leukemia; CML, chronic myelogenous leukemia; HLA, human leukocyte antigen; IgE, immunoglobulin E; LAMP, lysosomal-associated membrane protein.

LIGHT MICROSCOPY AND PEROXIDASE HISTOCHEMISTRY

Figure 59-1 is a diagrammatic representation of the stages of neutrophil maturation.[1-3] The myeloblast is an immature cell with a large, oval nucleus, sizable nucleoli, and few or no granules. The cell, derived from hematopoietic stem cells (see Chap. 15), matures into the promyelocyte. In the promyelocyte stage, the azurophilic or primary granules, large peroxidase-positive granules that stain metachromatically (reddish-purple) with a polychromatic stain such as Wright stain, are formed. During the next, or myelocyte, stage of maturation, the specific or secondary granules, which are peroxidase negative, are formed. The metamyelocyte and band neutrophils are nonproliferating cells that precede the development of the mature neutrophil. The mature, segmented neutrophilic cells contain primary, peroxidase-positive granules and specific peroxidase-negative granules in a 1:2 ratio. The nucleus of the circulating neutrophil is segmented, usually into two to four interconnected lobes.

During the myelocyte stage, the larger, metachromatic, azurophilic granules lose their intense staining properties and are no longer evident by light microscopy of stained blood films. Diminution of the metachromatic staining results from an increase in acid mucin-containing molecules that form complexes with basic proteins of the azurophilic granules.[7] However, the presence of large (approximately 500 nm), peroxidase-positive, azurophilic granules in mature neutrophils is evident by electron microscopy.[2] Thus, the violet-colored granules seen with light microscopy in mature neutrophils on Wright-stained blood films are azurophilic granules whose staining characteristics altered during maturation. Therefore, with light microscopy, the most reliable method for identifying azurophilic granules on blood films is staining the cells for peroxidase. The size of most of the peroxidase-negative granules (approximately 200 nm) is at the limit of resolution of the light microscope. The granules cannot be distinguished individually but are responsible for the pink background color of neutrophil cytoplasm during and after the myelocyte stage.

The purpose of nuclear segmentation is not known. Fluorescence *in situ* hybridization with chromosome-specific probes has shown that chromosomes are randomly distributed among the nuclear lobes.[8] Some mature neutrophils in women have drumstick- or club-shaped nuclear appendages. These appendages contain the inactivated X chromosome. An X chromosome-specific nucleic acid probe has confirmed the position of the X chromosomes in the drumstick structure of leukocyte nuclei by *in situ* hybridization.[9]

ELECTRON MICROSCOPY AND PEROXIDASE CYTOCHEMISTRY

The peroxidase reaction has become a key tool for studying the formation of the azurophilic granule. The dense product of the peroxidase reaction serves as a marker of azurophilic granules in human marrow and blood cells for electron and for light microscopy.[2]

THE MYELOBLAST
The earliest precursor in the evolution of the neutrophil from the colony forming unit is an immature cell with a large nucleus and multiple nucleoli. The nucleolus is the site of assembly of ribosomal proteins and rRNA and is a prominent feature of early maturing cells. The scant cytoplasm contains reaction product for peroxidase within the rough-surfaced endoplasmic reticulum and Golgi cisternae and, sometimes, in early developing azurophilic granules.

THE PROMYELOCYTE
Figure 59-2 shows that the promyelocyte produces and accumulates a large population of peroxidase-positive granules. Most of the granules are spherical and have a diameter of 500 nm, but ellipsoid, crystalline forms and small granules connected by filaments also are present.[10]

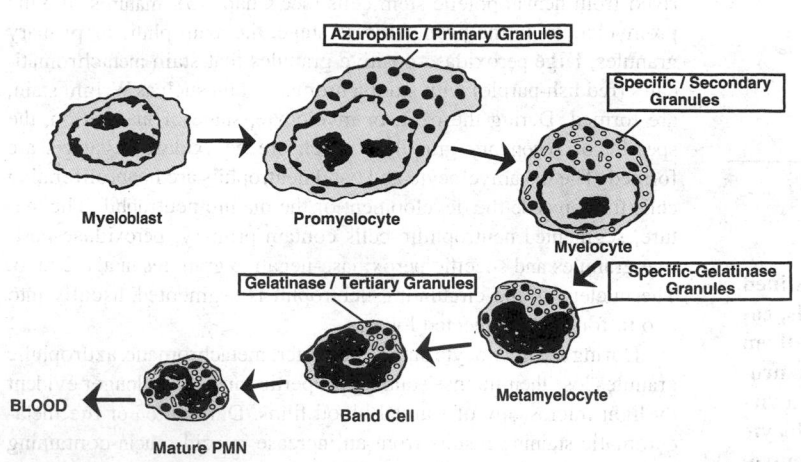

FIGURE 59-1　　Diagrammatic representation of neutrophil [polymorphonuclear neutrophil (PMN)] life span and stages of maturation (see text for discussion). Of every 100 nucleated cells in marrow, 0.5 percent are myeloblasts, 5 percent are promyelocytes, 12 percent are myelocytes, 22 percent are metamyelocytes and bands, and 20 percent are maturing and mature neutrophilic cells, yielding a total of approximately 60 percent of cells representing developing neutrophils in normal human marrow. The azurophilic (primary) granules, which are peroxidase positive, are shown as *solid black dots*. The other granules are shown as *open dots* and are discussed in greater detail in the text. Basically, the peroxidase-negative granules can be divided into specific/secondary granules and gelatinase/tertiary granules based on their relative content of lactoferrin and gelatinase. (Reproduced with permission from Bainton.[3])

As with other secretory cells, peroxidase is present throughout the secretory apparatus of the promyelocyte, for example, in cisternae of the rough endoplasmic reticulum, in all Golgi cisternae, in some vesicles, and in all developing granules.[2]

THE NEUTROPHILIC MYELOCYTE

At the end of the promyelocyte stage, peroxidase abruptly disappears from rough endoplasmic reticulum and Golgi cisternae, and the production of azurophilic granules ceases. The myelocyte stage begins with production of peroxidase-negative specific granules.

Figure 59-3 shows that the only peroxidase-positive elements at this stage are the azurophilic granules. The specific granules are formed by the Golgi complex. The granules vary in size and shape but typically are spherical (approximately 200 nm) or rod shaped (130 × 1000 nm). Figure 59-4 shows the cell also labeled with immunogold particles to illustrate the presence of lactoferrin, a specific granule marker. Approximately three cell divisions occur at this stage of maturation. Mitoses can be observed (Fig. 59-5), and the two types of granules appear to be distributed to the daughter cells in fairly equal numbers.

METAMYELOCYTE, BAND, AND MATURE NEUTROPHIL

The late stages of maturation consist of nondividing cells that can be distinguished by their nuclear morphology, mixed granule populations, small Golgi regions, and accumulations of glycogen particles. On average, an electron micrograph of a neutrophil displays 200 to 300 granules, and approximately one third are peroxidase positive (Fig. 59-6).

Peroxidase-negative granules are more numerous than peroxidase-positive granules during the myelocyte stage because peroxidase granule formation ceases after the promyelocyte stage, the number of per-

oxidase-positive granules per cell is reduced by mitoses, and peroxidase-negative granules continue to be produced by each myelocyte generation.[1]

OTHER CYTOPLASMIC CHANGES DURING MATURATION

MICROPEROXISOMES

Microperoxisomes are present from the promyelocyte stage through the development of mature neutrophils.[11] These organelles are small membrane-bound vesicles that contain catalase. Although this enzyme destroys hydrogen peroxide (H_2O_2), it also can act as a peroxidase. Its exact function in neutrophils has not been determined.

SURFACE MARKERS AND CYTOSKELETON

Changes in cell surface carbohydrates, glycoproteins, glycolipids, and human leukocyte antigens (HLAs) occur during maturation (reviewed in ref. 12). For example, the densities of membrane HLA-A, HLA-B, and HLA-C antigens decrease with granulocyte maturation. Some surface antigens appear during neutrophil maturation. Development of chemotactic and recognition capabilities parallels the acquisition of certain membrane receptors.[13,14] Fc receptors either are not present or are poorly expressed on progenitors younger than myelocytes, whereas greater than 90 percent of mature neutrophils have Fc receptors. Mature neutrophils possess at least two classes of receptors for fragments of the complement component C3—CRI and CR3. Other maturational changes occur in cytoskeletal elements, such as microtubules,[15] and in biophysical features, such as deformability and surface charge.[12,16] During early myeloid development, direct interactions must occur between hematopoietic cells and the components of the marrow microenvironment, both cellular and extracellular matrix.[17–25] Most of the known matrix protein receptors belong to the β_1-integrin family. On CD34+ marrow cells, $\alpha 4b_1$ and $\alpha 5b_1$ are expressed. During myeloid differentiation $\alpha 5b_1$ is lost at the myelocytic–metamyelocyte stage, before the loss of $\alpha 4b_1$ at the band stage.[21] Intercellular adhesion molecule -1, a member of the immunoglobulin superfamily, is detected on blasts and promyelocytes but is lost at later stages of myeloid maturation.[21] One of the members of the new adhesion molecule family of selectins, L-selectin, can be detected as early as the colony forming unit for granulocytes and monocytes,[24] through the mature neutrophil stage, until it is shed within minutes after activation (see Chap. 61). Neutrophils also express Toll-like receptors[25] that permit detection of the presence of a pathogen through receptors that recognize microbe-associated molecular patterns.

EXPRESSION OF mRNA TRANSCRIPTS

During granulocytic maturation, numerous genes that encode proteins important for the specific functions of mature cells are expressed (see Chap. 60).[26,27] Myeloperoxidase and elastase mRNA transcripts are found almost exclusively at the promyelocyte stage, but myeloperoxidase mRNA disappears earlier than does elastase mRNA.[28] Lactoferrin mRNA transcripts are detected later in neutrophil maturation, marking the beginning of the myelocyte stage (Fig. 59-7).[28] Mature neutrophils are capable of synthesizing and secreting interleukin-1 and tumor necrosis factor alpha.[29] In addition, bacterial infection induces nitric oxide synthase in human neutrophils.[30]

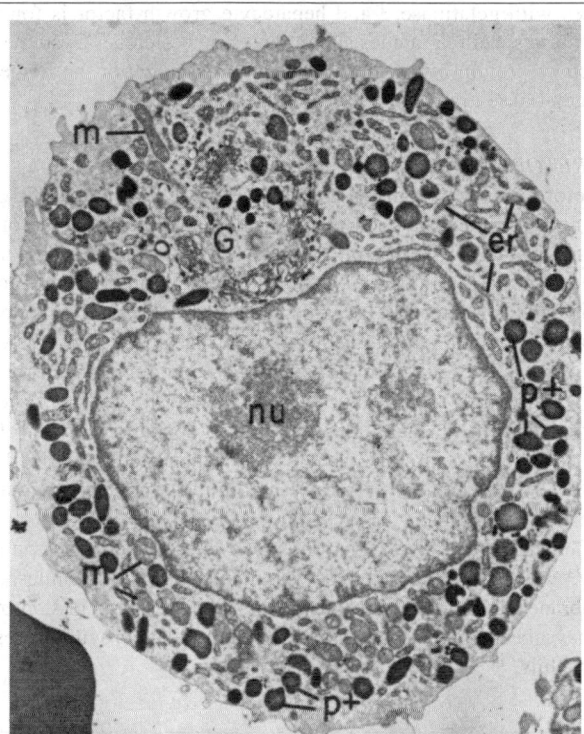

FIGURE 59-2 Electron micrograph of a neutrophilic promyelocyte from normal human marrow reacted for peroxidase. This cell is the largest of the neutrophilic series. It has a sizable, slightly indented nucleus with a nucleolus (nu), a prominent Golgi region (G), and cytoplasm packed with dense peroxidase-positive (p+) azurophilic granules of varying shapes and sizes. Peroxidase reaction product is visible in less concentrated form within all compartments of the secretory apparatus—endoplasmic reticulum (er), perinuclear cisterna, and Golgi cisternae (G). No reaction product is apparent in the cytoplasmic matrix or mitochondria (m) (×8000).

APOPTOSIS

Programmed cell death, or apoptosis, is a physiologic phenomenon associated with elimination of mature cells (see Chap. 11). Apoptosis is characterized biochemically by internucleosomal DNA fragmentation and morphologically by nuclear and cytoplasmic condensation. It plays an important role in cell removal.[31,32] Evidence indicates senescent neutrophils and eosinophils undergo apoptosis. One of the key features of programmed cell death in many tissues is the phagocytosis of apoptotic cells by macrophages. Ingestion of intact apoptotic granulocytes by macrophages may prevent the release of their toxic intracellular contents extracellularly, thereby promoting resolution of inflammation.

CONTENTS OF NEUTROPHIL GRANULES

Initially, the granules were classified into two major types, based on their content of peroxidase. Now granules can be further subdivided based on other granular and membrane proteins (Fig. 59-8).

The components of human neutrophilic granules have been analyzed by cytochemical and fractionation procedures[2,28,33–98] and are discussed extensively in Chaps. 60 and 66.

PRIMARY OR AZUROPHILIC GRANULES

In addition to myeloperoxidase, the azurophilic granule contains numerous lysosomal enzymes. Elastase,[64–66] proteinase-3,[66,67] and α_1-

antitrypsin[78] colocalize with some peroxidase-positive granules. Bactericidal factors such as defensins,[46,56,59,98] azurophil-derived bactericidal factors,[47] and bactericidal permeability-increasing protein,[40] which previously were called cationic proteins, have been found in some azurophilic granules.[52] Lysozyme has been found in both azurophilic and specific granules.[68–70] Presenilin-1, required for proteolytic processing of β-amyloid precursor protein, has been found in azurophilic granules.[71]

Of the 10 antimicrobial proteins of known sequence in the human azurophil granules,[55] two have unique primary structures (lysozyme and bactericidal permeability-increasing protein). The remaining eight fall into two families of four members each: (1) the defensins (which comprise 30–50 percent of granule proteins) and (2) cathepsin G, elastase, proteinase-3, and azurocidin (or heparin-binding protein).[98] The

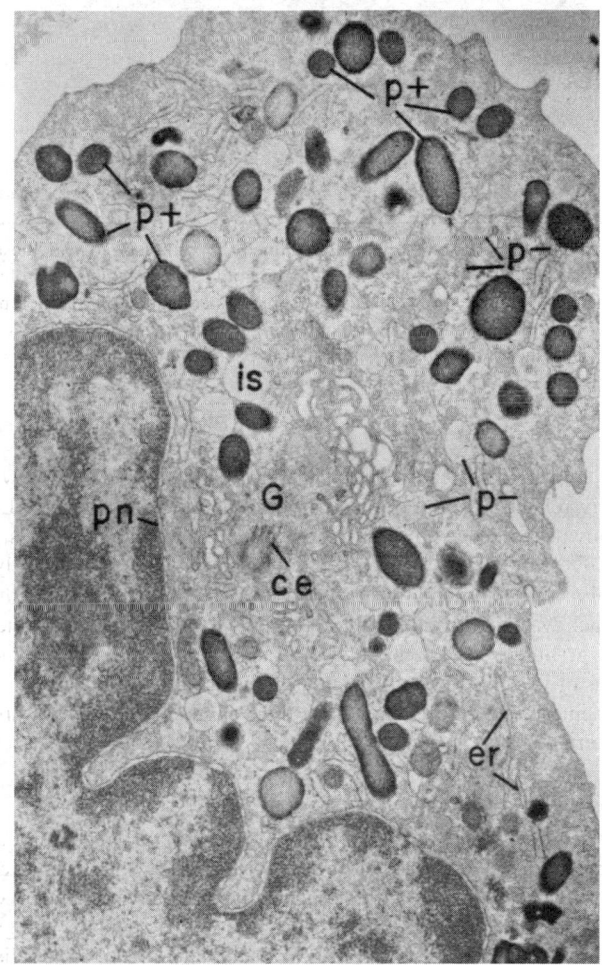

FIGURE 59-3 Neutrophilic myelocyte reacted for peroxidase. At this stage, the cell is smaller than the promyelocyte, the nucleus is more indented, and the cytoplasm contains two different types of granules: (1) large, peroxidase-positive azurophilic granules (p+) and (2) generally smaller specific granules (p−), which do not stain for peroxidase. A number of immature specific granules that are larger, less compact, and more irregular in contour than mature granules appear in the Golgi region (G). Note that peroxidase reaction product is present only in azurophilic granules and not in the rough-surfaced endoplasmic reticulum (er), perinuclear cisterna (pn), or Golgi cisternae (G). This finding is in keeping with the fact that azurophilic granule production has ceased and only peroxidase-negative specific granules are produced during the myelocyte stage (×20,000). ce, centriole.

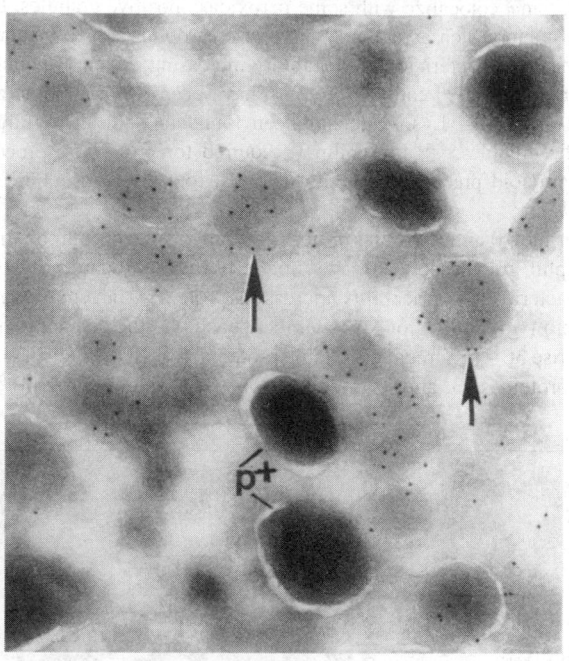

FIGURE 59-4   Portion of cytoplasm stained for peroxidase to mark the azurophil granules and then immunolabeled with gold particles to detect lactoferrin. The peroxidase-positive (p+) azurophil granules contain dense reaction product, whereas the lighter specific granules are peroxidase negative. Many of the peroxidase-negative granules (*arrows*) have gold label within their matrix (×70,000).

latter four proteins can be termed "serprocidins," to denote they are closely related to serine proteases with microbicidal activity.[55] Little is known about the limiting membrane of azurophilic granules, but CD63[80,92] and CD68[79] are present. We had anticipated that the lysosomal-associated membrane proteins (LAMPs) would be found there, but such was not the case.[77,93] Rather, LAMPs were absent in all identified granule populations but were consistently found in the membranes of vesicles, in multivesicular bodies, and in multilaminar compartments, which are identified by their content of concentric arrays of internal membranes.[93]

SECONDARY OR SPECIFIC GRANULES

The specific or secondary granule, which by definition does not contain peroxidase, contains lactoferrin, lysozyme, B_{12}-binding proteins, and other proteins.[28,89] These peroxidase-negative granules vary greatly in size, shape, electron lucency, isopycnic density, and granule content. However, they can be loosely categorized by the distribution of the two proteins lactoferrin and gelatinase. Approximately 16 percent of the peroxidase-negative granules contain only lactoferrin, 24 percent only gelatinase, and 60 percent contain both marker enzymes. Thus, based on ultrastructure alone, three types of peroxidase-negative granules can be identified: peroxidase-negative granules, which contain gelatinase but no lactoferrin; peroxidase-negative granules, which contain lactoferrin but no gelatinase; and peroxidase-negative granules, which contain both lactoferrin and gelatinase.[88] This heterogeneity may result from overlapping synthesis and packaging of different granule proteins during granulopoiesis. The heterogeneity is functionally significant as the gelatinase-containing granules are released from the cells by certain inflammatory mediators more readily than those containing lactoferrin.[28] NRAMP1 lo-

calizes with gelatinase,[82] and hepatocyte growth factor is found in gelatinase/specific granules and in secretory vesicles.[83] Cysteine-rich secretory protein-3 also has overlapping localization with specific and gelatinase granules.[84]

SECRETORY VESICLES

Secretory vesicles are distinct from the azurophilic or specific granules and have been defined as intracellular organelles that contain CD35 and latent alkaline phosphatase.[28,88,89] The latter enzyme is located on the luminal side of the vesicle membrane; therefore, in the presence of detergent it can be identified as latent alkaline phosphatase. This localization also was demonstrated by enzyme cytochemistry.[73] These secretory vesicles also contain plasma proteins, such as albumin, that are not synthesized by the cells but are endocytosed from plasma. They represent a specialized form of endocytic vesicle. Secretory vesicles are transported to the cell surface after the stimulus of formyl methionyl-leucyl phenylalanine or certain cytokines.[89]

Chapters 60 and 66, various reviews,[28,89] and other publications[33–98] discuss other proteins found in neutrophil granules. Two membrane adhesion proteins—L-selectin and P-selectin glycoprotein-1—have been found on the tips of neutrophil microvilli in resting neutrophils.[94–96]

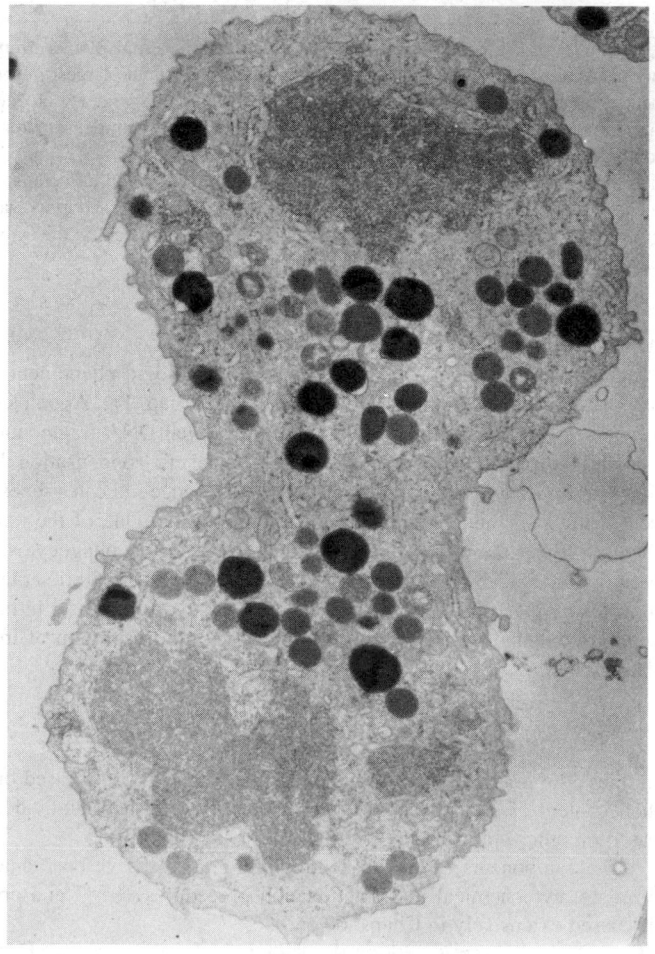

FIGURE 59-5   Myelocyte from rabbit marrow in the late stage of mitosis. This myelocyte is in telophase. Note that the granules are relatively equally distributed to the daughter cells (×15,000).

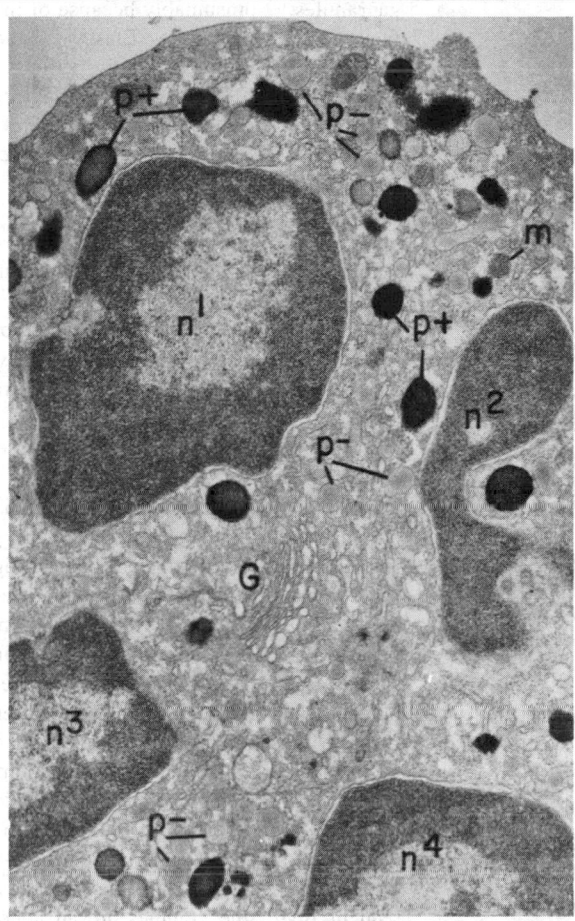

FIGURE 59-6 Mature neutrophil from normal human marrow reacted for peroxidase. The cytoplasm is filled with granules of the two basic types: (1) the smaller, pale, peroxidase-negative granules (p−) and (2) the large, dense, peroxidase-positive granules (p+). The nucleus is condensed and lobulated (n¹−n⁴), the Golgi region (G) is small and without any forming granules, the endoplasmic reticulum is scant, and mitochondria (m) are few (×21,000).

PATHOLOGIC ALTERATIONS OF GRANULES

Leukemic cells can be shown to contain chemical properties unique for a given normal cell line and thus are considered to be of that particular cell lineage. This finding has been particularly helpful in subdividing the acute leukemias. For example, peroxidase is recognized as one of the earliest synthetic products of granulocytic precursor cells. Production of this enzyme by leukemic cells has been the hallmark for distinguishing acute lymphocytic from myelogenous leukemia.[99] Chloroacetate esterases appear early in maturation and are used to detect the origin of the immature cells in granulocyte sarcomas. Naphthyl AS-D chloroacetate, the substrate used for this incubation, is a general substrate of neutrophil proteinases. Lactoferrin is recognized as a marker of specific granules.

Pathologic neutrophil granulations can be classified as a selective abnormality of a granule type.[100,101] Pathologic granules in hereditary or acquired disease states can be classified as abnormalities of either azurophilic granules or specific granules (Table 59-1).

ABNORMALITIES OF AZUROPHILIC GRANULES

Quantitative Neutrophils sometimes contain either fewer or more than normal numbers of azurophilic granules, or the azurophilic granule population may be missing. Some mature neutrophils lack azurophilic granules in acute myelogenous leukemia (AML)[102,103] or in the blast crisis of chronic myelogenous leukemia (CML).[104] Children with severe congenital neutropenia and repeated life-threatening infections have neutrophilic abnormalities that include (1) defective synthesis or degeneration of azurophilic (primary) granules, (2) an absence or marked deficiency of specific (secondary) granules, and (3) autophagia. This rare disease has been called congenital dysgranulopoietic neutropenia.[105]

Absence of Granule Contents In some instances, azurophilic granules lacking one or more enzymes or other substances form. For example, in hereditary myeloperoxidase deficiency, the azurophilic granules of neutrophils and monocytes,[106,107] but not eosinophils or basophils, lack peroxidase (Fig. 59-9). The deficiency occurs in one in 2000 to 5000 persons[108,109] and usually is not associated with clinical abnormalities. Although not detectable with enzyme assays, peroxidase can be revealed by immunologic methods in the neutrophils of persons with the deficiency.[110] Molecular analysis of cells from family members with this deficiency has revealed mutations of the gene(s) that resides on chromosome 17 and encodes a protein that is incapable of posttranslational processing and thus is enzymatically inactive.[111,112] Peroxidase deficiency also has been observed in refractory anemia,[113] preleukemia,[114,115] and the blast crisis of CML.[104] In these examples of peroxidase deficiency, both types of granules are present and apparently normal; only the enzyme is missing. In the hereditary deficiency, all the neutrophils are peroxidase negative, whereas in the refractory anemias and leukemias,[116,117] the percentage of peroxidase negative neutrophils varies. Neutrophils lacking peroxidase are observed in AML and in blast cell transformation of CML.[104] When present, this abnormality affects 8 to 70 percent of the circulating neutrophils. The deficient neutrophils may originate from the leukemic precursors. High neutrophil peroxidase activity is present in the neutrophils of patients with megaloblastic anemia.[118] Finally, immunologic techniques for peroxidase are useful in the diagnosis of minimally differentiated acute myeloid leukemia (AML-M0).[119]

Abnormal Variants Auer bodies are found in the immature cells of some patients with AML. They are abnormally large, elongated, azurophilic granules that contain peroxidase, lysosomal enzymes, and large crystalline inclusions.[99,103,120–122] Although they are similar to normal azurophilic granules in content and staining properties, Auer bodies are "abnormal" because they are so large (Fig. 59-10). Auer body formation in leukemic blasts and promyelocytes differs markedly from the normal secretory process of azurophilic granule formation in that Golgi cisternae contain very little peroxidase.[103,120] More Auer bodies can be detected on marrow and blood films from patients with AML when special stains, such as peroxidase, chloroacetate esterase, acid phosphatase, or Sudan black, are applied than when the Romanowsky stain is used. Not all Auer bodies exhibit all of these staining characteristics at the same time. Auer rod formation may be an occasional but normal phenomenon in fetal hematopoiesis.[123] Auer rod-like inclusions also can be seen at the light microscopic level in certain B cell neoplasms, but the inclusions are peroxidase negative.[124]

The Chédiak-Higashi anomaly or syndrome is a rare autosomal recessive disease. It is characterized clinically by oculocutaneous albinism and increased susceptibility to infection and microscopically by the presence of abnormally large lysosome-like organelles in most granule-containing cells (see Chap. 66). The large inclusions in the neutrophils of persons with Chédiak-Higashi syndrome are enormous abnormal azurophilic granules.[125,126] Early in neutrophil maturation, normal azurophilic granules form but then fuse together

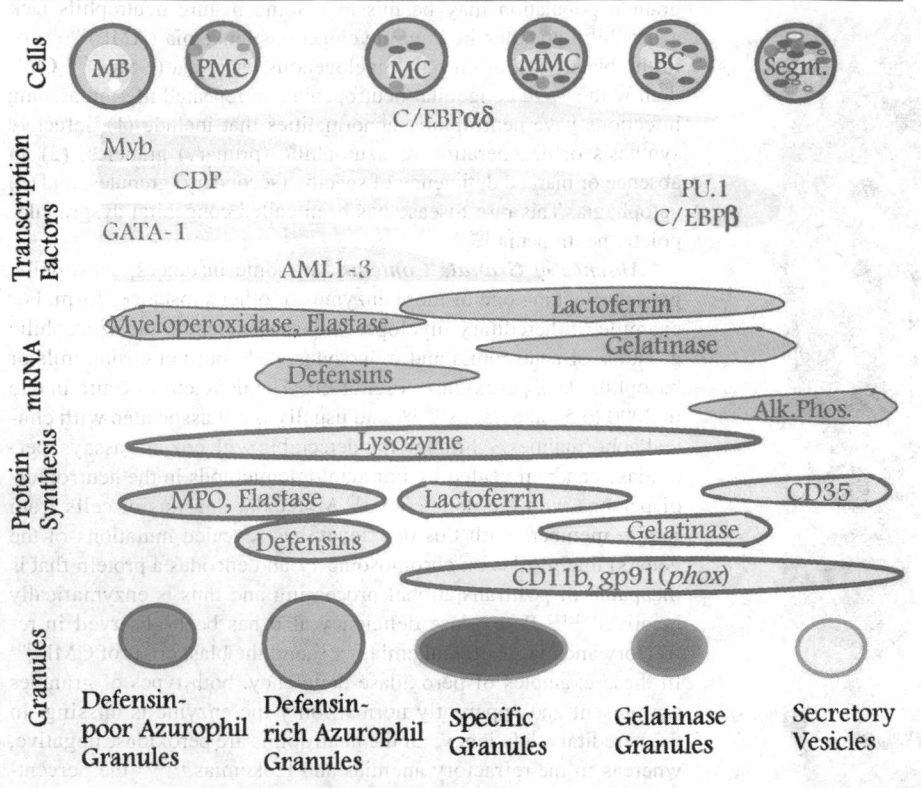

FIGURE 59-7   Granules defined by timing of biosynthesis of their characteristic proteins. The granules formed at any given stage of maturation of neutrophil precursors will be composed of the granule proteins synthesized at that time. BC, band cell; MB, myeloblast; MC, myelocyte; MMC, metamyelocyte; PMC, promyelocyte; Segm., segmented cell. (From Borregaard and Cowland,[28] with permission.)

to form megagranules. Later, during the myelocyte stage, normal specific granules form. The mature neutrophils contain both the abnormal azurophilic granules and the normal specific granules (Fig. 59-11). The contents of specific granules can be present in the me-

Characteristic Proteins					
		Cytochrome b558			
		Lysozyme			
	Myeloperoxidase	Lactoferrin		CD35	
		Defensins	Gelatinase		

Granule Subsets	Peroxidase Pos.		Peroxidase Neg.		Secretory Vesicles
	Azurophil		Specific	Gela.	
	Primary		Secondary	Tert.	
	Def.-Neg.	Def.-Pos.			

FIGURE 59-8   Classification of granules in neutrophils. Peroxidase-positive (azurophilic or primary) granules are characterized by their content of myeloperoxidase and can be further divided based on their content of defensins into large, defensin-rich granules and the smaller defensin-poor granules. The peroxidase-negative granules can be divided into specific (secondary) granules and gelatinase (tertiary) granules based on their relative content of lactoferrin and gelatinase. All granules contain lysozyme. Secretory vesicles share some of their membrane proteins with peroxidase-negative granules, whereas others are unique to secretory vesicles. Def., defensins; Gela., gelatinase; Tert., tertiary. (From Borregaard and Cowland,[28] with permission.)

gagranules,[127] presumably because of limited fusion with megagranules. Elastase, cathepsin G, and defensin are absent in patients with Chédiak-Higashi syndrome.[128] Positional cloning and YAC complementation have resulted in the identification of the Beige and CHS1/LYS genes.[129]

Giant peroxidase-positive granules have been observed in the neutrophils of a patient with neutrophil dysfunction.[130,131] The granules were structurally similar to those seen in Chédiak-Higashi syndrome, but the neutrophils were biochemically different in that there was defective activation of the respiratory burst.

Giant round granules have been observed in Wright-stained cells from patients with acute myelomonocytic leukemia.[132] This acquired abnormality closely mimicked the giant round granules seen in the Chédiak-Higashi syndrome and is termed the *pseudo–Chédiak-Higashi anomaly.*[133,134] In marrow from patients with AML, enormous round pink inclusions resembling ingested erythrocytes in blasts and promyelocytes may be observed. Electron microscopy and peroxidase cytochemistry show the inclusions are homogeneous large, membrane-bound, peroxidase-positive granules that correspond to the abnormal granules seen in the pseudo–Chédiak-Higashi anomaly. Like the Auer rods also seen in AML, the granules are an abnormal variant of peroxidase-positive azurophils. Their lack of azurophilic staining results from the absence of sulfated glycosaminoglycan.[135]

Morphologic changes in blood neutrophils occur in certain inflammatory disorders. The best-known alteration is the "shift to the left," which denotes the presence of bands, metamyelocytes, and sometimes myelocytes in the blood. The mature neutrophil also can display cytoplasmic modifications, including (1) "toxic" granules, which stain more prominently than those of normal neutrophils; (2) light-blue, amorphous inclusions called Döhle bodies; and (3) vacuoles. Toxic granules are azurophilic granules that have an abnormal staining pat-

TABLE 59-1   PROPOSED CLASSIFICATION OF NEUTROPHIL GRANULE ABNORMALITIES

I.   Abnormalities of azurophil granules
   A.   Quantitative
      1.   None
      2.   Fewer than normal
      3.   More than normal
   B.   Qualitative
      1.   Contents of granule incomplete
         Example: hereditary peroxidase deficiency
      2.   Abnormal variants
         Examples: Auer bodies, Chédiak-Higashi syndrome
II.   Abnormalities of specific granules
   A.   Quantitative
      1.   None
      2.   Fewer than normal
      3.   More than normal
   B.   Qualitative
      1.   Contents of granule are incomplete
      2.   Abnormal variants

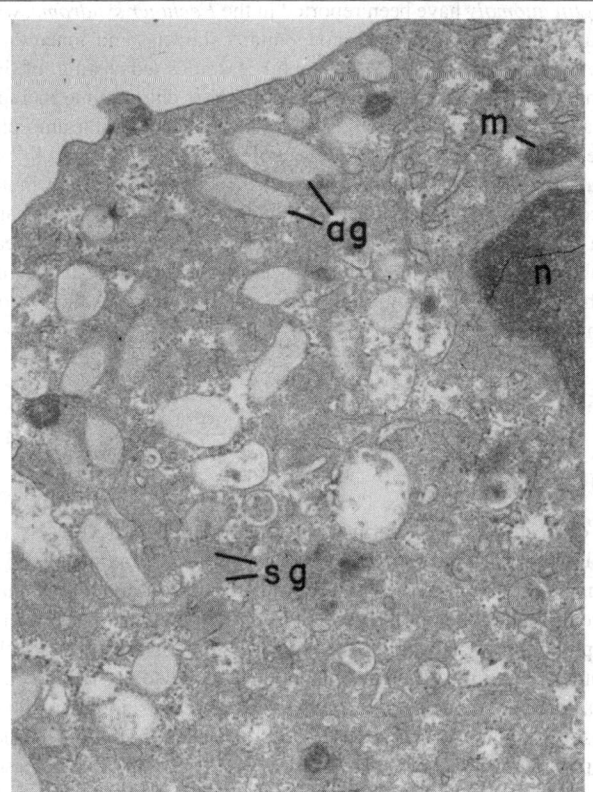

FIGURE 59-9 Neutrophil from the blood of a patient with hereditary peroxidase deficiency reacted for peroxidase. Note that the two types of granules are present: the large azurophilic granules (ag), pale because of the absence of peroxidase, and the small specific granules (sg) (×19,000). m, mitochondria; n, nucleus.

tern when viewed with the light microscope[136] but are indistinguishable from normal azurophilic granules when viewed by electron microscopy. Döhle bodies are not granules; rather, they are defined as several rows of rough endoplasmic reticulum. They stain as blue bodies in the cytoplasm because of the ribosomes bound to the membrane of the reticulum (Fig. 59-12). Toxic neutrophils have decreased chemotaxis and phagocytic and intracellular bactericidal activities.[137,138] Increased numbers of lipid bodies have been observed in inflammatory reactions,[139] and other inclusion bodies can be seen in certain hereditary conditions.[140-142]

An acquired azurophil granule abnormality occurs in neutrophils of patients with amiodarone pulmonary toxicity.[143] Some of the peroxidase-positive azurophil granules contain lamellar inclusions. The target antigen of anticytoplasmic antibodies in patients with Wegener granulomatosis is proteinase-3, located in azurophilic granules.[66,67,144-146]

ABNORMALITIES OF SPECIFIC GRANULES

Quantitative The three quantitative abnormalities of azurophilic granules described previously also apply to specific granules. Circulating neutrophils can have fewer or smaller than normal quantities of these granules, or they may lack them entirely.

The absence of specific granules was first observed in 1974 in a 14-year-old boy with recurrent infection whose neutrophils lacked leukocyte alkaline phosphatase.[147] More cases have been reported (see Chap. 64).[148-155] Patients have an abnormality that affects production of specific granules, their protein contents, and at least two additional proteins (gelatinase and defensins).[148-155] Abnormalities in the peroxidase-positive granules of these patients are seen.[152] In congenital dys-

granulocytic neutropenia, specific granules may be absent or markedly decreased in number.[105]

The absence of certain normal organelles from mature neutrophils in patients with acute leukemia has been documented by electron microscopic and cytochemical studies. Specific granules in neutrophils from patients with AML may be absent.[103] The absence or paucity of specific granules in the more mature segmented neutrophils in certain leukemic patients results from a cessation of cytoplasmic development after the promyelocytic stage, whereas nuclear maturation progresses in a fairly normal fashion. The abnormal neutrophils are frequent in AML with maturation (i.e., the M2 variety) and in myelodysplastic syndromes. After treatment of acute promyelocyte leukemia with all-*trans*-retinoic acid, aberrant peroxidase-positive granules, including Auer rods, have normalized, although the neutrophils lacked the specific (secondary) peroxidase-negative population.[156] Furthermore, neutrophils in patients with AML can be deficient in all granules.[157]

Absence of Granule Contents No examples in this category are well documented. The specific granules are present in normal numbers in all neutrophils of patients with CML.[158] The low leukocyte alkaline phosphatase score seen in most CML is associated with undetectable mRNA levels, so the protein is not being synthesized.[159] Two major antibacterial proteins, lysozyme and lactoferrin, can specifically bind glucose-modified proteins bearing advanced glycation end products (AGEs).[160] Exposure to AGE-modified proteins inhibits the enzymatic and bacterial activity of lysozyme and blocks the bacterial agglutination and bacterial killing activities of lactoferrin.

Abnormal Variants Morphologically abnormal variants of specific granules have not been reported. Other granule abnormalities[161] that cannot be subclassified include the Alder-Reilly anomaly, in which the cytoplasm of neutrophils contains prominent granules that stain a deep lilac color (see color plate in ref. 161). The inheritance pattern of this disorder is not clear but may be part of a general

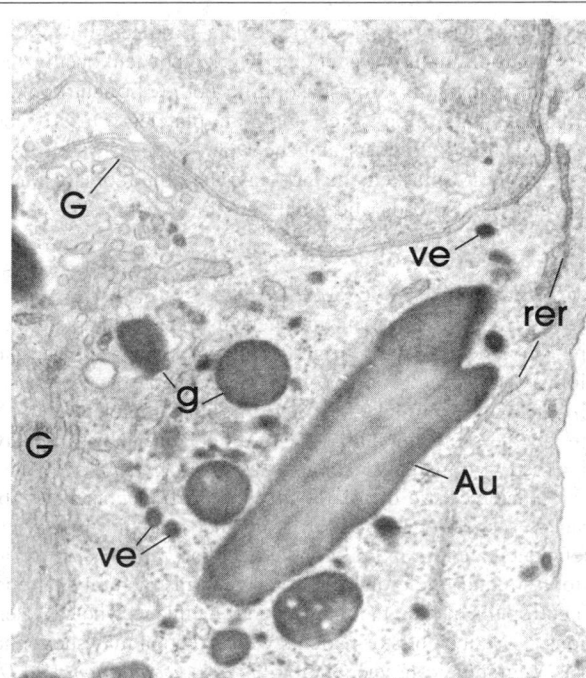

FIGURE 59-10 Peroxidase localization in an abnormal immature cell from a patient with acute myelogenous leukemia. Note the Auer body (Au) with its crystalline inclusion and a matrix containing peroxidase (×40,000). g, granule; G, Golgi cisternae; rer, rough endoplasmic reticulum; ve, vesicles.

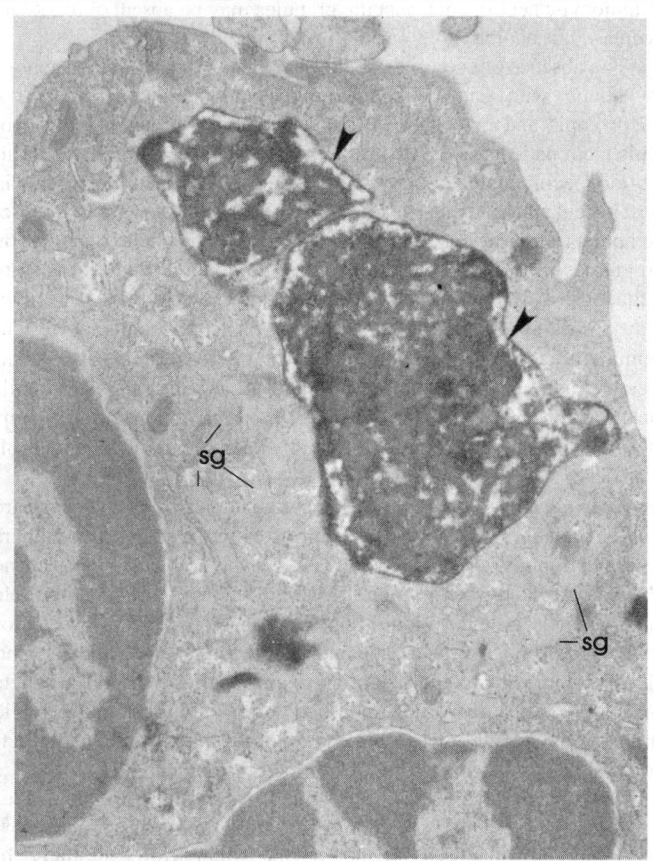

FIGURE 59-11   Peroxidase localization in a neutrophil from a patient with Chédiak-Higashi syndrome. Note the large megagranules are peroxidase positive (*arrows*), whereas the specific granules (sg) appear normal (×26,000).

metabolic disorder of polysaccharides. The May-Hegglin anomaly is an autosomal dominant disorder characterized by leukopenia and the presence of abnormally large basophilic bodies in neutrophils, eosinophils, basophils, monocytes, and giant platelets. Differences between these large inclusions and the Döhle bodies, which develop with infection, are marked. In the May-Hegglin anomaly, the blue area is occupied by rods and small granules, which may be ribosomes.[162]

OTHER CELLULAR ABNORMALITIES

The *Pelger-Huët anomaly*, an inherited disorder, is characterized by abnormal lobe development in granulocytes. Neutrophils can have a monolobed (homozygote) or bilobed (heterozygote) appearance. The abnormality can be mimicked in the neutrophils of patients with AML (acquired Pelger-Huët anomaly).[161] Acquired Pelger-Huët anomaly has been induced in transplant patients.[163] *Hypersegmentation* of neutrophils is a characteristic of folate and vitamin B$_{12}$ deficiencies, but it also can be seen after hydroxyurea or glucocorticoid therapy[164] and iron deficiency anemia in children.[165] Peculiar *fibrillary inclusions* of the cytoplasm and nuclei may be seen by ultrastructural examination in the neutrophils of human renal allograft recipients who have serious infections.[166] Neutrophils of patients with infection may show nuclear pyknosis, degranulation, vacuolation,[167] *toxic granulation*, and *Döhle bodies*. Döhle bodies may be found in the neutrophils of pregnant women for unexplained reasons.[168] Multiple persistent vacuoles can be seen in neutrophils, eosinophils, monocytes, and their precursors in *familial Jordan's anomaly*.[169] Döhle bodies and inclusions of May-

Hegglin anomaly have been reported in the *Fechtner syndrome*, which includes nephritis, deafness, congenital cataracts, and macrothrombocytopenia.[140] Abnormal neutrophil granules consisting of large membranous whirls have been observed after chloroquine therapy[170] and amiodarone toxicity.[143] In cryoglobulinemia, pale-blue amorphous material may be seen within the vacuoles of neutrophils and in extracellular deposits.[171] Toxic granulation in neutrophils can be induced by colony stimulating factor.[172] Unique neutrophil inclusions can be seen in a variant of the Sebastian platelet syndrome.[173] An increased number of apoptotic nuclei have been observed in systemic lupus erythematosus,[174] clozapine-induced agranulocytosis,[175] and glycogen storage disease.[176]

EOSINOPHILS

LIGHT MICROSCOPY OF EOSINOPHILS IN MARROW AND BLOOD FILMS

The earliest identifiable form of an eosinophilic leukocyte is as a late myeloblast or early promyelocyte. This cell is approximately 15 μm in diameter and has a large nucleus with nucleoli and a few blue or azurophilic granules in intensely basophilic cytoplasm. The later eosinophilic promyelocyte and myelocyte contain mostly acidophilic granules. The fully mature eosinophilic leukocyte has a bilobed nucleus, and its cytoplasm is filled with large eosinophilic granules whose rims stain for peroxidase and Sudan black. Multilobed nuclei, comparable to those of neutrophils, are rare. Eosinophils are susceptible to mechanical damage during preparation of blood films. Eosinophilic precursors may degranulate during maturation.[177] Lipid bodies can be found in eosinophils[178,179] and neutrophils.

ELECTRON MICROSCOPY AND CYTOCHEMISTRY

Eosinophils of the promyelocyte and myelocyte stages stain positively for peroxidase in all cisternae of the rough-surfaced endoplasmic reticulum, including transitional elements and the perinuclear cisterna; clusters of smooth vesicles at the periphery of the Golgi complex; all cisternae of the Golgi complex; and all immature and mature specific

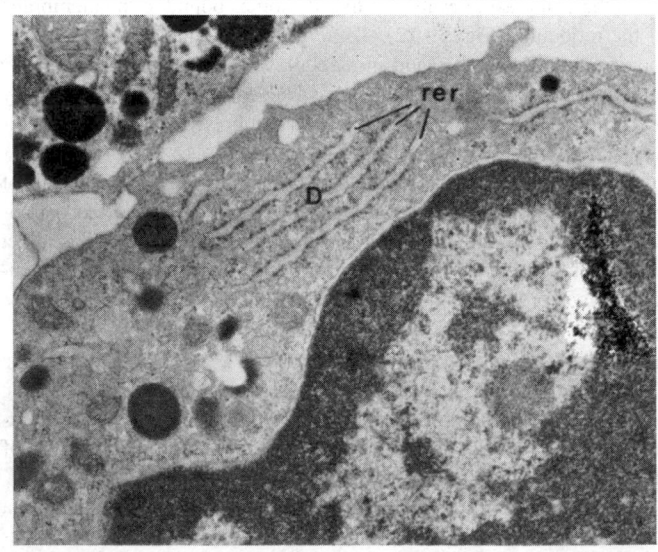

FIGURE 59-12   A portion of a neutrophil depicts a Döhle body (D), which consists of three stacks of rough endoplasmic reticulum (rer). The Döhle body stains blue by light microscopy because of the concentration of ribosomes.

granules.[4,180] Mature granules are completely filled with peroxidase except in areas occupied by centrally located crystals.

In the later stages of development, after granule formation has ceased, the eosinophils contain few of the organelles associated with the synthesis and packaging of secretory proteins. The endoplasmic reticulum is sparse or virtually nonexistent. The Golgi complex is small and inconspicuous. The cytoplasm of the mature eosinophil (Fig. 59-13) primarily contains granules and glycogen. Most of the granules are specific granules with crystals, which usually are centrally located. After the myelocyte stage, peroxidase can no longer be detected in the endoplasmic reticulum or Golgi elements of the eosinophil by any of the enzyme procedures; however, peroxidase can be found in the matrix of granules.[4,180]

GRANULES

CONTENTS

Eosinophil granules contain abundant peroxidase and lysosomal enzymes.[4] Eosinophil peroxidase is genetically and biochemically distinct from neutrophil peroxidase. It appears to play no role in the eosinophil's bactericidal activity.[181] Eosinophils have much less bactericidal activity than do neutrophils.[182,183] The specific granules of eosinophils are true peroxisomes in that they also contain catalase,[184] two enzymes of peroxisomal lipid β-oxidation (enoyl-CoA hydratase and ketoacyl-CoA thiolase[185]), and a flavoprotein (acyl-CoA oxidase[186]). All of these substances have been found in the matrix, but not the crystalloid, of the granule. Lectins have been identified in eosinophil granules, most heavily in the crystalloids.[187] The eosinophil granule contains several basic proteins: a major basic protein, eosinophil cationic protein, and eosinophil-derived neurotoxin.[188-191] More than half of the granule protein is the major basic protein, which con-

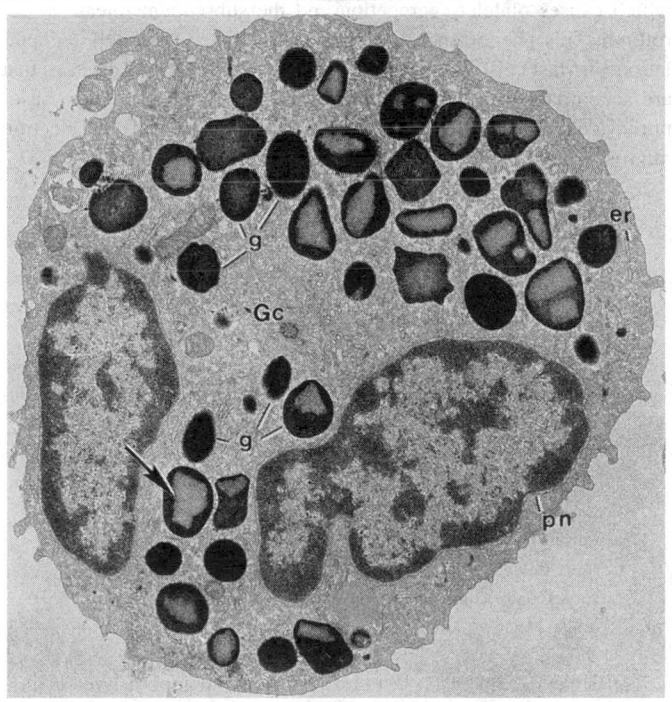

FIGURE 59-13 Human mature eosinophil incubated for peroxidase. Reaction product is present only in granules (g). The rough endoplasmic reticulum (er), including the perinuclear cisterna (pn) and the Golgi cisternae (Gc), does not contain reaction product. Most of the granules (*arrow*) contain the distinctive crystalline bar ($\times 8000$).

stitutes the crystalline core of the granule. It is cytotoxic to parasites and to normal mammalian cells and induces histamine release from basophils and mast cells.[192] The other two cationic proteins are found in the matrix of the granule.[188-190] Eosinophil cationic protein can cause the formation of transmembrane pores and thereby cause membrane damage.[192] The amino acid sequence of eosinophil cationic protein is homologous with that of eosinophil-derived neurotoxin. Both sequences show striking homology to that of ribonuclease.[193,194] Eosinophils also contain proteoglycans,[195] interleukin-6,[196] tumor necrosis factor alpha,[197] transforming growth factor alpha,[198] and granulocyte-macrophage colony stimulating factor.[199]

Charcot-Leyden crystals are bipyramidal crystals observed in fluids in association with eosinophilic inflammatory reactions. They possess lysophospholipase activity and compose 7 to 10 percent of total eosinophil protein.[200-205] The ultrastructural localization of this protein is in a large, crystal-free granule and supports the presence of a distinct primary granule population (approximately 5 percent) in mature eosinophils.[4,202,203]

ABNORMALITIES

Inherited Abnormalities of Eosinophils Four inherited abnormalities of eosinophils exist. (1) The absence of peroxidase and phospholipids in eosinophils is an autosomal recessive defect that produces no signs of disease.[206,207] (2) In Chédiak-Higashi syndrome,[125] almost all granulated cells, including eosinophils, contain large abnormal granules. (3) A family was found to have gray inclusions in eosinophils and basophils. This abnormality was autosomal dominant and had no clinical effects. Electron microscopy revealed cytoplasmic crystals and curved lamellar bodies in the cells.[208] (4) Neutrophil-specific granule deficiency, previously described, also involves eosinophils.[130]

Several acquired gross morphologic or cytochemical abnormalities of eosinophils have been observed in leukemias or in association with benign eosinophilias (see next section).

Cytochemistry of Abnormalities in Leukemias In a cytochemical study of eosinophils in acute leukemia,[209] the cells were considered normal when they did not show toluidine blue metachromasia or positivity for alkaline phosphatase, chloroacetate esterase, Astra blue, or periodic acid–Schiff but did show positivity for peroxidase and Sudan black and moderate reactivity with naphthol-AS or α-naphthyl esterase. Observation of chloroacetate esterase activity in some abnormal eosinophils is particularly interesting in view of the subsequent finding that abnormal marrow eosinophils in acute myelomonocytic leukemia are associated with inversion of chromosome 16.[210] Most of the patients studied had a higher than normal percentage of immature eosinophils containing a mixture of eosinophilic and basophilic granules. The eosinophilic granules showed abnormal reactivity for chloroacetate esterase and periodic acid–Schiff. None of the granules had well-formed central crystalloids.

An abnormality seen in patients with CML is the presence of basophilic and eosinophilic granules in eosinophilic myelocytes and occasionally in mature eosinophils.[211] Eosinophilic and basophilic granules are mutually exclusive markers of the respective granulocytic lineages. The presence of the two markers in CML cells is a sign of lineage infidelity.

Degranulated and light density eosinophils are associated with eosinophilia.[189,212,213] An expanding clinical spectrum of multisystem diseases is associated with eosinophilia[214] (see Chap. 62).

Intranuclear Crystals Associated with Abnormal Granules Eosinophils with abnormal granules and intranuclear crystalloids were observed in a 2-year-old girl with chronic benign neutropenia.[215] The father had the same morphologic abnormality but was asymptomatic and had normal leukocyte counts.

ACQUIRED EOSINOPHIL PSEUDO-PELGER-HUËT ANOMALY
Incomplete segmentation of the nucleus of mature eosinophils is seen
in AML[216] and myelodysplasia.[217] Eosinophil accumulation, activation, fate, and apoptosis have been reviewed[218-220] (see Chap. 62).

BASOPHILS AND MAST CELLS

Basophils and mast cells are distinct cell lines but have many functional similarities[221-225] (see Chap. 63). The granules of the two cell
types stain metachromatically but are distinct when examined by electron microscopy (Figs. 59-14 and 59-15). The cells can phagocytose
sensitized red cells but are less active phagocytes than the other granulocytes. They lack significant amounts of antibacterial or lysosomal
enzymes. Basophils are found in small numbers in blood (0.5%) and
can be seen in tissues in which inflammation resulting from hypersensitivity to proteins, contact allergy, or skin allograft rejection is
present.

Mast cells are normal residents of connective tissue throughout the
body. Mast cell granules contain various substances, including several
preformed biologically active substances such as histamine, which
causes increased vascular permeability; eosinophil chemotactic factor
of anaphylaxis; and heparin, which has antithrombin activity.[222-224]
This accounts for the metachromatic staining quality of the granules.
The generation of anaphylatoxin (C3a, C5a) or the interaction of allergen with immunoglobulin E (IgE) receptors of plasma membrane
can stimulate extracellular release of these granule contents and of
several newly formed substances, such as slow-reacting substance of
anaphylaxis, a leukotriene that causes contraction of human bronchi-

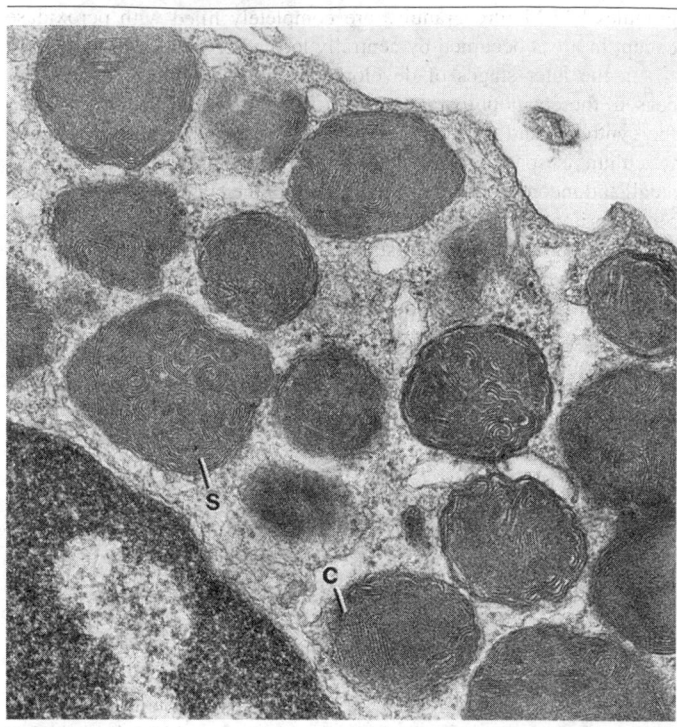

FIGURE 59-15   Portion of a mast cell from human bone marrow. Note the
granules are filled with scroll-like (s) and crystal (c) images and are distinct
from human basophil granules (see Fig. 59-14) in fine structural morphology
(×50,000).

oles and increased vascular permeability, and platelet-activating factor,
which causes platelet aggregation and the subsequent release of serotonin. This phenomenon is called IgE-mediated mast cell degranulation.[222] Mast cells also have been implicated in various diseases that
are accompanied by neovascularization (see Chap. 63). Acute basophilic leukemia is rare and diagnosed most definitively by electron
microscopy (see Chap. 87).[226]

REFERENCES

1. Bainton DF, Farquhar MG: Origin of granules in polymorphonuclear
   leukocytes: Two types derived from opposite faces of the Golgi complex
   in developing granulocytes. *J Cell Biol* 28:277, 1966.
2. Bainton DF, Ullyot JL, Farquhar MG: The development of neutrophilic
   polymorphonuclear leukocytes in human bone marrow: Origin and content of azurophil and specific granules. *J Exp Med* 134:907, 1971.
3. Bainton DF: Distinct granule populations in human neutrophils and lysosomal organelles identified by immuno-electron microscopy. *J Immunol Methods* 232:153,1999.
4. Bainton DF, Farquhar MG: Segregation and packaging of granule enzymes in eosinophilic leukocytes. *J Cell Biol* 45:54, 1970.
5. Cronkite EP, Vincent PC: Granulocytopoiesis. *Ser Haematol* 2:3, 1969.
6. Jamuar MP, Cronkite EP: The fate of granulocytes. *Exp Hematol* 8:884,
   1980.
7. Hardin JH, Spicer SS: Ultrastructural localization of dialyzed iron-re-
   active mucosubstance in rabbit heterophils, basophils, and eosinophils.
   J Cell Biol 48:368, 1971.
8. Sanchez AJ, Karni RJ, Wangh LJ: Fluorescent in situ hybridization
   (FISH) analysis of the relationship between chromosome location and
   nuclear morphology in human neutrophils. *Chromosoma* 106:168, 1997.
9. Hochstenbach PF, Scheres JM, Hustinx TW, Wieringa B: Demonstration of X chromatin in drumstick-like nuclear appendages of

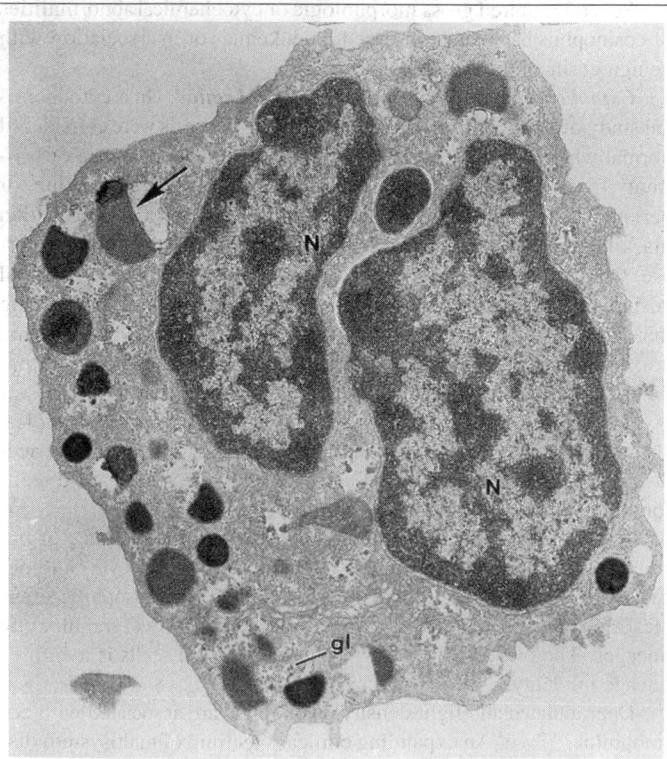

FIGURE 59-14   Mature basophil from human blood reacted for peroxidase.
Note unusually large nucleus (N) and scattered glycogen particles (gl). Human
basophil granules contain peroxidase, as illustrated by their density (as a result
of the presence of reaction product) in this type of preparation. They usually
are spherical, difficult to fix, and may be speckled in appearance (*arrow*)
(×17,000).

leukocytes by in situ hybridization on blood smears. *Histochemistry* 84: 383, 1986.

10. Pryzwansky KB, Breton-Gorius J: Identification of a subpopulation of primary granules in human neutrophils based upon maturation and distribution: Study by transmission electron microscopy cytochemistry and high voltage electron microscopy of whole cell preparations. *Lab Invest* 53:664, 1985.

11. Breton-Gorius J, Coquin Y, Guichard J: Cytochemical distinction between azurophils and catalase-containing granules in leukocytes. *Lab Invest* 38:21, 1978.

12. Wallace PJ, Packman CH, Lichtman MA: Maturation-associated changes in the peripheral cytoplasm of human neutrophils: A review. *Exp Hematol* 15:34, 1987.

13. Sullivan R, Griffin JD, Malech HL: Acquisition of formyl peptide receptors during normal human myeloid differentiation. *Blood* 70:1222, 1987.

14. Berger M, Wetzler EM, Welter E, et al: Intracellular sites for storage and recycling of C3b receptors in human neutrophils. *Proc Natl Acad Sci U S A* 88:3019, 1991.

15. Rothwell SW, Nath J, Wright DG: Interactions of cytoplasmic granules with microtubules in human neutrophils. *J Cell Biol* 108:2313, 1989.

16. Cramer EB: Cell biology of phagocyte migration from the bone marrow, out of the bloodstream, and across organ epithelia, in *Inflammation: Basic Principles and Clinical Correlates*, edited by JI Gallin, IM Goldstein, R Snyderman, p 341. Raven Press, New York, 1992.

17. Voura EB, Billia F, Iscove NN, Hawley RG: Expression mapping of adhesion receptor genes during differentiation of individual hematopoietic precursors. *Exp Hematol* 25:1172, 1997.

18. Soligo D, Schirò R, Luksch R, et al: Expression of integrins in human bone marrow. *Br J Haematol* 76:323, 1990.

19. Liesveld JL, Winslow JM, Frediani KE, et al: Expression of integrins and examinations of their adhesive function in normal and leukemic hematopoietic cells. *Blood* 81:112, 1993.

20. Prosper F, Verfaillie CM: Regulation of hematopoiesis through adhesion receptors. *J Leukoc Biol* 3:307, 2001.

21. Kerst JM, Sanders JB, Slaper-Cortenbach ICM, et al: Alpha 4 beta 1 and alpha 5 beta 1 are differentially expressed during myelopoiesis and mediate the adherence of human CD34+ cells to fibronectin in an activation-dependent way. *Blood* 81:344, 1993.

22. Arkin S, Naprstek B, Guarini L, et al: Expression of intercellular adhesion molecule-1 (CD-54) on hematopoietic progenitors. *Blood* 77:948, 1991.

23. Williams DA, Rios M, Stephens C, Patel VP: Fibronectin and VLA-4 in haematopoietic stem cell-microenvironment interactions. *Nature* 352: 438, 1991.

24. Griffin JD, Spertini O, Ernst TJ, et al: Granulocyte-macrophage colony-stimulating factor and other cytokines regulate surface expression of the leukocyte adhesion molecule-1 on human neutrophils, monocytes, and their precursors. *J Immunol* 145:576, 1990.

25. Hayashi F, Means TK, Luster AD: Toll-like receptors stimulate human neutrophil function. *Blood* 102:2660, 2003.

26. Lian Z, Wang L, Yamaga S, et al: Genomic and proteomic analysis of the myeloid differentiation program. *Blood* 98:513, 2001.

27. Bjerregaard MD, Jurlander J, Klausen P, et al: The in vivo profile of transcription factors during neutrophil differentiation in human bone marrow. *Blood* 101:4322, 2003.

28. Borregaard N, Cowland BJ: Granules of the human neutrophilic polymorphonuclear leukocyte. *Blood* 89:3503, 1997.

29. Dubravec DB, Spriggs DR, Mannick JA, Rodrick ML: Circulating human peripheral blood granulocytes synthesize and secrete tumor necrosis factor alpha. *Proc Natl Acad Sci U S A* 87:6758, 1990.

30. Wheeler MA, Smith SD, Garcia-Cardena G, et al: Bacterial infection induces nitric oxide synthase in human neutrophils. *J Clin Invest* 99: 110, 1997.

31. Hu S: Regulation of eosinophil and neutrophil apoptosis—similarities and differences. *Immunol Rev* 179:156, 2001.

32. Kobayashi SD, Braughton KR, Whitney AR, et al: Bacterial pathogens modulate an apoptosis differentiation program in human neutrophils. *Proc Natl Acad Sci U S A* 100:10948, 2003.

33. Klebanoff S: Myeloperoxidase. *Proc Assoc Am Physicians* 111:383, 1999.

34. Bendix-Hansen K: Annotation: Enzyme cytochemistry of neutrophil granulocytes. *Br J Haematol* 65:127, 1987.

35. Bretz U, Baggiolini M: Biochemical and morphological characterization of azurophil and specific granules of human neutrophilic polymorphonuclear leukocytes. *J Cell Biol* 63:251, 1974.

36. Spitznagel JK, Dalldorf FG, Leffell MS, et al: Character of azurophil and specific granule purified from human polymorphonuclear leukocytes. *Lab Invest* 30:774, 1974.

37. West BC, Rosenthal AS, Gelb NA, Kimball HR: Separation and characterization of human neutrophil granules. *Am J Pathol* 77:41, 1974.

38. Kane SP, Peters TJ: Analytical subcellular fractionation of human granulocytes with reference to the localization of vitamin B_{12}-binding proteins. *Clin Sci Mol Med* 49:171, 1975.

39. Borregaard N, Heiple JM, Simons ER, Clark RA: Subcellular localization of the b-cytochrome component of the human neutrophil microbicidal oxidase: Translocation during activation. *J Cell Biol* 97:52, 1983.

40. Ringel EW, Soter NA, Austen KF: Localization of histaminase to the specific granule of the human neutrophil. *Immunology* 52:649, 1984.

41. O'Shea JJ, Brown EJ, Seligmann E, et al: Evidence for distinct intracellular pools of receptors for C3b and C3bi in human neutrophils. *J Immunol* 134:2580, 1985.

42. Gabay JE, Heiple JM, Cohn ZA, Nathan CF: Subcellular location and properties of bactericidal factors from human neutrophils. *J Exp Med* 164:1407, 1986.

43. Heiple JM, Ossowski L: Human neutrophil plasminogen activator is localized in specific granules and is translocated to the cell surface by exocytosis. *J Exp Med* 164:826, 1986.

44. Rice WG, Kinkade JM, Parmley RT: High resolution of heterogeneity among human neutrophil granules: Physical, biochemical, and ultrastructural properties of isolated fractions. *Blood* 68:541, 1986.

45. Bjerrum OW, Bjerrum OJ, Borregaard N: Beta 2-microglobulin in neutrophils: An intragranular protein. *J Immunol* 138:3913, 1987.

46. Rice WG, Ganz T, Kinkade JM Jr, et al: Defensin-rich dense granules of human neutrophils. *Blood* 70:757, 1987.

47. Stevenson KB, Nauseef WM, Clark RA: The neutrophil glycoprotein Mo1 is an integral membrane protein of plasma membranes and specific granules. *J Immunol* 139:3759, 1987.

48. Weiss J, Olsson I: Cellular and subcellular localization of the bactericidal/permeability-increasing protein of neutrophils. *Blood* 69:652, 1987.

49. Yoon PS, Boxer LA, Mayo LA, et al: Human neutrophil laminin receptors: Activation-dependent receptor expression. *J Immunol* 138:259, 1987.

50. Lacal P, Pulido R, Sanchez-Madrid F, Mollinedo F: Intracellular location of T200 and Mo1 glycoproteins in human neutrophils. *J Biol Chem* 263:9946, 1988.

51. Bjerrum OW, Borregaard N: Dual granule localization of the dormant NADPH oxidase and cytochrome b559 in human neutrophils [published erratum appears in *Eur J Haematol* 8:270, 1989]. *Eur J Haematol* 43: 67, 1989.

52. Gabnay JE, Scott RW, Campanelli D: Antibiotic proteins of human polymorphonuclear leukocytes. *Proc Natl Acad Sci U S A* 86:5610, 1989.

53. Singer II, Scott S, Kawka DW, Kazazis DM: Adhesomes: Specific granule containing receptors for laminin, C3bi/fibrinogen, fibronectin, and vitronectin in human polymorphonuclear leukocytes and monocytes. *J Cell Biol* 109:3169, 1989.

54. Borregaard N, Christensen L, Bejerrum OW, et al: Identification of a highly mobilizable subset of human neutrophil intracellular vesicles that contains tetranectin and latent alkaline phosphatase. *J Clin Invest* 85: 408, 1990.

55. Campanelli D, Detmers PA, Nathan CF, Gabay JE: Azurocidin and a homologous serine protease from neutrophils. *J Clin Invest* 85:904, 1990.

56. Lehrer RI, Ganz T: Defensins of vertebrate animals. *Curr Opin Immunol* 14:96, 2002.

57. Pereira HA, Spitznagel JK, Winton EF, et al: The ontogeny of a 57-Kd cationic antimicrobial protein of human polymorphonuclear leukocytes: Localization to a novel granule population. *Blood* 76:825, 1990.

58. Spitznagel JK: Antibiotic proteins of human neutrophils. *J Clin Invest* 86:1381, 1990.

59. Ganz T: Defensins: Antimicrobial peptides of innate immunity. *Nat Rev Immunol* 3:710, 2003.

60. Cramer E, Pryzwansky KB, Villeval J-L, et al: Ultrastructural localization of lactoferrin and myeloperoxidase in human neutrophils by immunogold. *Blood* 65:423, 1985.

61. Bainton DF, Miller LJ, Kishimoto TK, Springer TA: Leukocyte adhesion receptors are stored in peroxidase-negative granules of human neutrophils. *J Exp Med* 166:1641, 1987.

62. Hibbs MS, Bainton DF: Human neutrophil gelatinase is a component of specific granules. *J Clin Invest* 84:1395, 1989.

63. Esaguy N, Aguas AP, Silva MT: High-resolution localization of lactoferrin in human neutrophils: Labeling of secondary granules and cell heterogeneity. *J Leukoc Biol* 46:51, 1989.

64. Damiano VV, Kucich U, Murer E, et al: Ultrastructural quantitation of peroxidase- and elastase-containing granules in human neutrophils. *Am J Pathol* 131:235, 1988.

65. Cramer EM, Beesley JE, Pulford KA, et al: Colocalization of elastase and myeloperoxidase in human blood and bone marrow neutrophils using a monoclonal antibody and immunogold. *Am J Pathol* 134:1275, 1989.

66. Calafat J, Goldschmeding R, Ringeling PL, et al: In situ localization by double-labeling immunoelectron microscopy of anti-neutrophil cytoplasmic autoantibodies in neutrophils and monocytes. *Blood* 75:242, 1990.

67. Csernok E, Lüdemann J, Gross WL, Bainton DF: Ultrastructural localization of proteinase 3, the target antigen of anti-cytoplasmic antibodies circulating in Wegener's granulomatosis. *Am J Pathol* 137:1113, 1990.

68. Cramer EM, Breton-Gorius J: Ultrastructural localization of lysozyme in human neutrophils by immunogold. *J Leukoc Biol* 41:242, 1987.

69. Livesey SA, Beuscher ES, Krannig GL: Human neutrophil granule heterogeneity: Immunolocalization studies using cryofixed, dried and embedded specimens. *Scanning Microsc* 3:231, 1989.

70. Mutasa HC: Combination of diaminobenzidine staining and immunogold labeling: A novel technical approach to identify lysozyme in human neutrophil cells. *Eur J Cell Biol* 49:319, 1989.

71. Mirinics ZK, Calafat J, Udby L, et al: Identification of the presenilins in hematopoietic cells with localization of presenilin 1 to neutrophil and platelet granules. *Blood Cells Mol Dis* 28:28, 2000.

72. Dewald B, Bretz U, Baggiolini M: Release of gelatinase from a novel secretory compartment of human neutrophils. *J Clin Invest* 70:518, 1982.

73. Robinson JM, Kobayashi TA: Novel intracellular compartment with unusual secretory properties in human neutrophils. *J Cell Biol* 113:743, 1991.

74. Rotrosen D, Gallin JI, Spiegel AM, Malech HL: Subcellular localization of Gi alpha in human neutrophils. *J Biol Chem* 263:10958, 1988.

75. Ginsel LA, Onderwater JJM, Fransen JAM, et al: Localization of the low-Mr subunit of cytochrome b558 in human blood phagocytes by immunoelectron microscopy. *Blood* 76:2105, 1990.

76. Jesaitis AJ, Buescher ES, Harrison D, et al: Ultrastructural localization of cytochrome b in the membranes of resting and phagocytosing human granulocytes. *J Clin Invest* 85:821, 1990.

77. Bainton DF, August JT: Multivesicular bodies of human neutrophils (PMN) not granules, immunolable with the two major lysosomal membrane glycoproteins hLAMP-1 and hLAMP-2. *J Histochem Cytochem* 36:953, 1988.

78. Mason DY, Cramer EM, Massé J-M, et al: Alpha1-antitrypsin is present within the primary granules of human polymorphonuclear leukocytes. *Am J Pathol* 139:623, 1991.

79. Saito N, Pulford KA, Breton-Gorius J, et al: Ultrastructural localization of the CD68 macrophage-associated antigen in human blood neutrophils and monocytes. *Am J Pathol* 139:1053, 1991.

80. Kuijpers TW, Tool ATJ, van der Schoot DE, et al: Membrane surface antigen expression on neutrophils: A reappraisal of the use of surface markers for neutrophil activation. *Blood* 78:1105, 1991.

81. VanWinkle BW: Lectinocytochemical specificity in human eosinophils and neutrophils: A reexamination. *J Histochem Cytochem* 39:1157, 1991.

82. Canonne-Hergauz F, Calafat J, Richer E, et al: Expression and subcellular localization of NRAMP1 in human neutrophil granules. *Blood* 100: 268, 2002.

83. Grenier A, Chollet-Martin S, Crestani B, et al. Presence of a mobilizable intracellular pool of hepatocyte growth actor in human polymorphonuclear neutrophils. *Blood* 99:2997, 2002.

84. Udby L, Calafat J, Sorensen OE, et al: Identification of human cysteine-rich secretory protein 3 (CRISP-3) as a matrix protein in a subset of peroxidase-negative granules of neutrophils and in the granules of eosinophils. *Leukoc Biol* 72:462, 2002.

85. Figueroa CD, Henderson LM, Kaufmann J, et al: Immunovisualization of high (HK) and low (LK) molecular weight kininogens on isolated human neutrophils. *Blood* 79:754, 1992.

86. Suchard SJ, Burton MJ, Stoehr SJ: Thrombospondin receptor expression in human neutrophils coincides with the release of a subpopulation of specific granules. *Biochem J* 284:513, 1992.

87. Ducker TP, Skubitz KM: Subcellular localization of CD66, CD67, and NCA in human neutrophils. *J Leukoc Biol* 52:11, 1992.

88. Kjeldsen L, Bainton DF, Sengelov H, Borregaard N: Structural and functional heterogeneity among peroxidase negative granules in human neutrophils: Identification of a distinct gelatinase containing granule subset by combined immunocytochemistry and subcellular fractionation. *Blood* 82:3183, 1993.

89. Borregaard N, Lollike K, Kjeldsen L, et al: Human neutrophil granules and secretory vesicles. *Eur J Haematol* 51:187, 1993.

90. Egesten A, Breton-Gorius J, Guichard J, et al: The heterogeneity of azurophil granules in neutrophil promyelocytes: Immunogold localization of myeloperoxidase, cathepsin G, elastase, proteinase 3, and bactericidal/permeability increasing protein. *Blood* 83:2985, 1994.

91. Peretz R, Shaft D, Yaari A, Nir E: Distinct intracellular lysozyme content in normal granulocytes and monocytes: A quantitative immunoperoxidase and ultrastructural immunogold study. *J Histochem Cytochem* 42:1471, 1994.

92. Cham BP, Gerrard JM, Bainton DF: Granulophysin is located in the membranes of azurophilic granules in human neutrophil and mobilizes to the plasma membrane following cell stimulation. *Am J Pathol* 144: 1369, 1994.

93. Cieutat A-M, Lobel P, August JT, et al: Azurophilic granules of human neutrophilic leukocytes are deficient in lysosome-associated membrane proteins but retain the mannose 6-phosphate recognition. *Blood* 91:1044, 1998.

94. Borregaard N, Kjeldsen L, Sengelov H, et al: Changes in subcellular localization and surface expression of L-selectin, alkaline phosphatase, and Mac-1 in human neutrophils during stimulation with inflammatory mediators. *J Leukoc Biol* 56:80, 1994.

95. Moore KL, Patel KD, Bruehl RE, et al: P-selectin glycoprotein ligand-1 mediates rolling of human neutrophils on P-selectin. *J Cell Biol* 128: 661, 1995.

96. Bruehl RE, Moore KL, Lorant DE, et al: Leukocyte activation induces surface redistribution of P-selectin glycoprotein ligand-1. *J Leukoc Biol* 61:489, 1997.

97. Le Cabec V, Cowland JB, Calafat J, Borregaard N: Targeting of proteins to granule subsets is determined by timing and not by sorting: The specific granule protein NGAL is localized to azurophil granules when expressed in HL-60 cells. *Proc Natl Acad Sci U S A* 93:6454, 1996.

98. Tapper H, Karlsson A, Morgelin M, et al: Secretion of heparin-binding protein from human neutrophils determined by its localization in azurophilic granules and secretory vesicles. *Blood* 99:1785, 2002.

99. Beckstead JH, Halverson PS, Ries CA, Bainton DF: Enzyme histochemistry and immunohistochemistry on biopsy specimens of pathologic human bone marrow. *Blood* 57:1088, 1981.

100. Bainton DF: Selective abnormalities of azurophil and specific granules of human neutrophilic leukocytes. *Fed Proc* 40:1443, 1981.

101. Zucker-Franklin D, Greaves MF, Grossi CE, Marmont AM: *Atlas of Blood Cells: Function and Pathology*, p 191. Lea and Febiger, Philadelphia, 1988.

102. Bainton DF: Abnormal neutrophils in acute myelogenous leukemia: Identification of subpopulations based on analysis of azurophil and specific granules. *Blood Cells* 1:191, 1975.

103. Bainton DF, Friedlander LM, Shohet SB: Abnormalities in granule formation in acute myelogenous leukemia. *Blood* 49:693, 1977.

104. Ullyot JL, Bainton DF: Azurophil and specific granules of blood neutrophils in chronic myelogenous leukemia: An ultrastructural and cytochemical analysis. *Blood* 44:469, 1974.

105. Parmley RT, Crist WM, Ragab AH, et al: Congenital dysgranulopoietic neutropenia. Clinical, serologic, ultra-structural, and in vivo proliferative characteristics. *Blood* 56:465, 1980.

106. Lehrer RI, Cline MJ: Leukocyte myeloperoxidase deficiency and disseminated candidiasis: The role of myeloperoxidase in resistance to *Candida* infection. *J Clin Invest* 48:1478, 1969.

107. Breton-Gorius J, Coquin MY, Guichard J: Activités péroxydasiques de certaines granulations des neutrophils dans deux cas de déficit congénital en myélopéroxidase. *C R Acad Sci Paris (D)* 280:1753, 1975.

108. Kitahara M, Eyre HJ, Simonian Y: Hereditary myeloperoxidase deficiency. *Blood* 57:888, 1981.

109. Parry MF, Root RK, Metcalf JA, et al: Myeloperoxidase deficiency. *Ann Intern Med* 95:293, 1981.

110. Ross DW, Kaplow LS: Myeloperoxidase deficiency: Increased sensitivity for immunocytochemical compared to cytochemical detection of enzyme. *Arch Pathol Lab Med* 109:1005, 1985.

111. Winterbourn CC, Vissers MC, Kettle AJ: Myeloperoxidase. *Curr Opin Hematol* 7:53, 2000.

112. Nauseef WM, Cogley M, McCormick S: Effect of R569W missense mutation on the biosynthesis of myeloperoxidase. *J Biol Chem* 271: 9546, 1996.

113. Lehrer RI, Goldberg LS, Apple MA, Rosenthal NP: Refractory megaloblastic anemia with myeloperoxidase and deficient neutrophils. *Ann Intern Med* 76:447, 1972.

114. Breton-Gorius J, Houssay D, Dryfux B: Partial myeloperoxidase deficiency in a case of preleukemia. *Br J Haematol* 30:273, 1975.

115. Davey FR, Erber WN, Gatter KC, Mason DY: Abnormal neutrophils in acute myeloid leukemia and myelodysplastic syndrome. *Hum Pathol* 19: 454, 1988.

116. Catovsky D, Galton DAG, Robinson J: Myeloperoxidase-deficient neutrophils in acute myeloid leukaemia. *Scand J Haematol* 9:142, 1972.

117. Elghetany MT, Peterson B, MacCallum J, et al: Deficiency of neutrophilic granule membrane glycoproteins in the myelodysplastic syndromes: A common deficiency in 216 patients studied by the Cancer and Leukemia Group B. *Leuk Res* 21:801, 1997.

118. Gulley ML, Bentley SA, Ross DW: Neutrophil myeloperoxidase measurement uncovers masked megaloblastic anemia. *Blood* 76:1004, 1990.

119. Venditti A, Del Poeta G, Buccisano F, et al: Minimally differentiated acute myeloid leukemia (AML-M0): Comparison of 25 cases with other French-American-British subtypes. *Blood* 89:621, 1997.

120. Breton-Gorius J, Houssay D: Auer bodies in acute promyelocytic leukemia: Demonstration of their fine structure and peroxidase localization. *Lab Invest* 28:135, 1973.

121. Tulliez M, Breton-Gorius J: Three types of Auer bodies in acute leukemia. *Lab Invest* 41:419, 1979.

122. Hassan HT, Rees JKH: Auer bodies in acute myeloid leukemia patients. *Pathol Res Pract* 186:293, 1990.

123. Newburger PE, Novak TJ, McCaffrey RP: Eosinophilic cytoplasmic inclusions in fetal leukocytes: Are Auer bodies a recapitulation of fetal morphology? *Blood* 61:593, 1983.

124. Juneja HS, Rajaraman S, Alperin JB, Bainton DF: Auer rod-like inclusions in prolymphocytic leukemia. *Acta Haematol* 77:115, 1987.

125. Davis WC, Douglas SD: Defective granule formation and function in the Chediak-Higashi syndrome in man and animals. *Semin Hematol* 9: 431, 1972.

126. Oliver C, Essner E: Formation of anomalous lysosomes in monocytes, neutrophils, and eosinophils from bone marrow of mice with Chediak-Higashi syndrome. *J Lab Invest* 32:17, 1975.

127. Rausch PG, Pryzwansky KB, Spitznagel JK: Immunocytochemical identification of azurophilic and specific granule markers in the giant granules of Chediak-Higashi neutrophils. *N Engl J Med* 298:694, 1978.

128. Ganz T, Metcalf JA, Gallin JI, et al: Microbicidal/cytotoxic proteins of neutrophils are deficient in two disorders: Chediak-Higashi syndrome and "specific" granule deficiency. *J Clin Invest* 82:552, 1988.

129. Ward DM, Shiflett SL, Kaplan J: Chediak-Higashi syndrome: A clinical and molecular view of a rare lysosomal storage disorder. *Curr Mol Med* 2:469, 2002.

130. Gale PF, Parkin JL, Quie PG, et al: Leukocyte granulation abnormality associated with normal neutrophil function and neurologic impairment. *Am J Clin Pathol* 86:33, 1986.

131. Newburger PE, Robinson JM, Pryzwansky KB, et al: Human neutrophil dysfunction with giant granules and defective activation of the respiratory burst. *Blood* 61:1247, 1983.

132. VanSlyck EJ, Rebuck JW: Pseudo-Chediak-Higashi anomaly in acute leukemia: A significant morphologic corollary? *Am J Clin Pathol* 62: 673, 1974.

133. Gorman AM, O'Connell LG: Pseudo-Chediak-Higashi anomaly in acute leukemia. *Am J Clin Pathol* 65:1030, 1976.

134. Efrati P, Nir E, Kaplan H, Dvilanski A: Pseudo-Chediak-Higashi anomaly in acute myeloid leukaemia: An electron microscopical study. *Acta Haematol (Basel)* 61:264, 1979.

135. Dittman WA, Kramer RJ, Bainton DF: Electron microscopic and peroxidase cytochemical analysis of pink pseudo-Chediak-Higashi granules in acute myelogenous leukemia. *Cancer Res* 40:4473, 1980.

136. McCall CE, Katayama I, Cotran RS, Finland M: Lysosomal ultrastructural changes in human "toxic" neutrophils during bacterial infection. *J Exp Med* 129:267, 1969.

137. McCall CE, Caves J, Cooper R, DeChatelet L: Functional characteristics of human toxic neutrophils. *J Infect Dis* 124:68, 1971.

138. McCall CE, DeChatelet LR, Cooper MR, Shannon C: Human toxic neutrophils: III. Metabolic characteristics. *J Infect Dis* 127:26, 1973.

139. Weller PF, Ackerman SJ, Nicholson-Weller A, Dvorak A: Cytoplasmic lipid bodies of human neutrophilic leukocytes. *Am J Pathol* 135:947, 1989.

140. Peterson LC, Rao KV, Crosson JT, White JG: Fechtner syndrome—a variant of Alport's syndrome with leukocyte inclusions and macrothrombocytopenia. *Blood* 65:397, 1985.

141. Heynen MJ, Blockmans D, Verwilghen RL, Vermylen J: Congenital macrothrombocytopenia, leukocyte inclusions, deafness and proteinuria: Functional and electron microscopic observations on platelets and megakaryocytes. *Br J Haematol* 70:441, 1988.

142. Seri M, Pecci A, Di Bari F, et al: MYH9-related disease: May-Hegglin anomaly, Sebastian syndrome, Fechtner syndrome, and Epstein syndrome are not distinct entities but represent a variable expression of a single illness. *Medicine* 82:203, 2003.

143. Dake MD, Madison JM, Montgomery CK, et al: Electron microscopic demonstration of lysosomal inclusion bodies in lung, liver, lymph nodes, and blood leukocytes of patients with amiodarone pulmonary toxicity. *Am J Med* 78:506, 1985.

144. Burkholder L, Bainton DF: Auto-antigens in Wegener's granulomatosis. *Blood* 75:1588, 1990.

145. Stummann WA, Kjeldsen L, Borregaard N, et al: The diversity of perinuclear antineutrophil cytoplasmic antibodies (pANCA) antigens. *Clin Exp Immunol* 101(suppl 1):15, 1995.

146. Kallenberg CG, Rarok A, Stegeman CA, Limburg PC: New insights into the pathogenesis of antineutrophil cytoplasm autoantibody-associated vasculitis. *Autoimmun Rev* 1:61, 2002.

147. Strauss RG, Bove KE, Jones JF, et al: An anomaly of neutrophil morphology with impaired function. *N Engl J Med* 290:478, 1974.

148. Komiyama A, Morosawa H, Nakahata T, et al: Abnormal neutrophil maturation in a neutrophil defect with morphologic abnormality and impaired function. *J Pediatr* 94:19, 1979.

149. Breton-Gorius J, Mason DY, Buriot D, et al: Lactoferrin deficiency as a consequence of a lack of specific granules in neutrophils from a patient with recurrent infections: Detection by immunoperoxidase staining for lactoferrin and cytochemical electron microscopy. *Am J Pathol* 99:413, 1980.

150. Rosenberg HF, Gallin JI: Neutrophil-specific granule deficiency includes eosinophils. *Blood* 82:268, 1993.

151. Malech HL, Gallin JI: Current concepts: Immunology. Neutrophils in human diseases. *N Engl J Med* 317:687, 1987.

152. Parmley RT, Gilbert CS, Boxer LA: Abnormal peroxidase-positive granules in "specific granule" deficiency. *Blood* 73:838, 1989.

153. Lomax KJ, Gallin JI, Rotrosen D, et al: Selective defect in myeloid cell lactoferrin gene expression in neutrophil specific granule deficiency. *J Clin Invest* 83:514, 1989.

154. Johnson JJ, Boxer LA, Berliner N: Correlation of messenger RNA levels with protein defects in specific granule deficiency. *Blood* 80:2088, 1992.

155. Holland SM, Gallin JI: Evaluation of the patient with recurrent bacterial infections. *Annu Rev Med* 49:185, 1998.

156. Miyauchi J, Ohyashiki K, Inatomi Y, Toyama K: Neutrophil secondary-granule deficiency as a hallmark of all-trans retinoic acid-induced differentiation of acute promyelocytic leukemia cells. *Blood* 90:2:803, 1997.

157. Repine JE, Clawson CC, Brunning RD: Abnormal pattern of bactericidal activity of neutrophils deficient in granules, myeloperoxidase, and alkaline phosphatase. *J Lab Clin Med* 88:788, 1976.

158. Thiele J, Timmer J, Jansen B, et al: Ultrastructure of neutrophilic granulopoiesis in the bone marrow of patients with chronic myeloid leukemia (CML). A morphometric study with special emphasis on azurophil (primary) and specific (secondary) granules. *Virchows Arch B Cell Pathol* 59:125, 1990.

159. Rambaldi A, Terao M, Bettoni S: Differences in the expression of alkaline phosphatase mRNA in chronic myelogenous leukemia and paroxysmal nocturnal hemoglobinuria polymorphonuclear leukocytes. *Blood* 73:1113, 1989.

160. Li YM, Tan AX, Vlassara H: Antibacterial activity of lysozyme and lactoferrin is inhibited by binding of advanced glycation-modified proteins to a conserved motif. *Nat Med* 1:1057, 1995.

161. Brunning RD: Morphologic alternations in nucleated blood and marrow cells in genetic disorders. *Hum Pathol* 1:99, 1970.

162. Cawley JJ, Hayhoe FGJ: The inclusions of the May-Hegglin anomaly and Döhle bodies of infection: An ultrastructural comparison. *Br J Haematol* 22:491, 1972.

163. Asmis LM, Hadaya K, Majno P, et al: Acquired and reversible Pelger-Huet anomaly of polymorphonuclear neutrophils in three transplant patients receiving mycophenolate mofetil therapy. *Am J Hematol* 73:244, 2003.

164. Eichacker P, Lawrence C: Steroid-induced hypersegmentation in neutrophils. *Am J Hematol* 18:41, 1985.

165. Sipahi T, Tavil B, Unver Y: Neutrophil hypersegmentation in children with iron deficiency anemia. *Pediatr Hematol Oncol* 19:235, 2002.

166. Valenzuela R, McMahon JT, Deodhar SD, Braun WE: Ultrastructural study of tissue and peripheral blood neutrophils in human renal allograft recipients. A clinicopathological description of an unusual abnormality discovered in three cases. *Hum Pathol* 12:355, 1981.

167. Malcolm ID, Flegel KM, Katz M: Vacuolization of the neutrophil in bacteremia. *Arch Intern Med* 139:675, 1979.

168. Abernathy MR: Döhle bodies associated with uncomplicated pregnancy. *Blood* 27:380, 1966.

169. Ulukutlu L, Koc ON, Tasyurekli M, et al: Persistent vacuoles in leukocytes: Familial Jordans anomaly. *Acta Paediatr Jpn* 37:177, 1995.

170. Fedorko M: Effect of chloroquine on morphology of cytoplasmic granules in maturing human leukocytes: An ultrastructural study. *J Clin Invest* 46:1932, 1967.

171. Laidlaw ST, Wagner B, Reilly JT: Neutrophil inclusions in cryoglobulinaemia. *Br J Haematol* 122:344, 2003.

172. Kabutomori O, Kanakura Y, Watani YI: Induction of toxic granulation in neutrophils by granulocyte colony-stimulating factor. *Eur J Haematol* 69:187, 2002.

173. White JG, Mattson JC, Nichols WL, et al: A variant of the Sebastian platelet syndrome with unique neutrophil inclusions. *Platelets* 13:121, 2002.

174. Ren Y, Tang J, Mok MY, et al: Increased apoptotic neutrophils and macrophages and impaired macrophage phagocytic clearance of apoptotic neutrophils in systemic lupus erythematosus. *Arthritis Rheum* 48:2888, 2003.

175. Loeffler S, Fehsel K, Henning U, et al: Increased apoptosis of neutrophils in a case of clozapine-induced agranulocytosis: A case report. *Pharmacopsychiatry* 36:37, 2003.

176. Kuijpers TW, Maianski NA, Tool ATJ, et al: Apoptotic neutrophils in the circulation of patients with glycogen storage disease type 1b (GSD1b). *Blood* 101:5021, 2003.

177. Butterfield JH, Ackerman SJ, Scott RE, et al: Evidence for secretion of human eosinophil granule major basic protein and Charcot-Leyden crystal protein during eosinophil maturation. *Exp Hematol* 12:163, 1984.

178. Weller PF, Monahan-Earley RA, Dvorak HF, Dvorak AM: Cytoplasmic lipid bodies of human eosinophils. *Am J Pathol* 138:141, 1991.

179. Bandeira-Melo C, Phoofolo M, Weller PF: Extranuclear lipid bodies, elicited by CCR3-ediated signaling pathways, are the sites of chemokine-enhanced leukotriene C4 production in eosinophils and basophils. *J Biol Chem* 276:22779, 2001.

180. Bainton DF: Developmental biology of neutrophils and eosinophils, in *Inflammation: Basic Principles and Clinical Correlates*, 2nd ed, edited by JI Gallin, IM Goldstein, R Snyderman, p 13. Raven Press, New York, 1992.

181. Bujak JS, Root RK: The role of peroxidase in the bactericidal activity of human blood eosinophils. *Blood* 43:727, 1974.

182. Yazdanbakhsh M, Eckmann CM, Bot AA, Roos D: Bactericidal action of eosinophils from normal human blood. *Infect Immun* 53:192, 1986.

183. Calafat J, Janssen H, Tool A, et al: The bactericidal/permeability-

increasing protein (BPI) is present in specific granules of human eosinophils. *Blood* 91:4770, 1998.

184. Iozzo RV, MacDonald GH, Wight TN: Immunoelectron microscopic localization of catalase in human eosinophilic leukocytes. *J Histochem Cytochem* 30:697, 1982.

185. Yokota S, Deimann W, Hashimoto T, Fahimi HD: Immunocytochemical localization of two peroxisomal enzyme of lipid beta-oxidation in specific granules of rat eosinophils. *Histochemistry* 78:425, 1983.

186. Yokota S, Deimann W, Hashimoto T, Fahimi HD: Specific granules of rat eosinophils contain peroxisomal acyl-CoA oxidase: Possible involvement in production of H$_2$O$_2$. *Histochem J* 16:573, 1984.

187. Eguchi M, Ozawa T, Suda J, et al: Lectins for electron microscopic distinction of eosinophils from other blood cells. *J Histochem Cytochem* 37:743, 1989.

188. Peters MS, Rodriguez M, Gleich GJ: Localization of human eosinophil granule major basic protein, eosinophil cationic protein, and eosinophil-derived neurotoxin by immunoelectron microscopy. *Lab Invest* 54:656, 1986.

189. Popken-Harris P, Checkel J, Loegering D, et al: Regulation and processing of a precursor form of eosinophil granule major basic protein (ProMBP) in differentiating eosinophils. *Blood* 92:623, 1998.

190. Walsh GM: Eosinophil granule proteins and their role in disease. *Curr Opin Hematol* 8:28, 2001.

191. McGrogan M, Simonsen C, Scott R, et al: Isolation of a complementary DNA clone encoding a precursor to human eosinophil major basic protein. *J Exp Med* 168:2295, 1988.

192. Young JD-E, Peterson CGB, Venge P, Cohn ZA: Mechanism of membrane damage mediated by human eosinophil cationic protein. *Nature* 321:613, 1986.

193. Plager DA, Stuart S, Gleich GJ: Human eosinophil granule major basic protein and its novel homolog. *Allergy* 53(suppl 45):33, 1998.

194. Rosenberg HF, Ackerman SJ, Tenen DG: Human eosinophilationic protein: Molecular cloning of a cytotoxin and helminthotoxin with ribonuclease activity. *J Exp Med* 170:163, 1989.

195. Rothenberg ME, Pomerantz JL, Owen WF Jr, et al: Characterization of a human eosinophil proteoglycan and augmentation of its biosynthesis and size by interleukin 3, interleukin 5, and granulocyte/macrophage colony stimulating factor. *J Biol Chem* 263:13901, 1988.

196. Hamid Q, Barkans J, Meng Q, et al: Human eosinophils synthesize and secrete interleukin-6, in vitro. *Blood* 80:1496, 1992.

197. Waltraud JB, Weller PF, Tzizik DM, et al: Ultrastructural immunogold localization of tumor necrosis factor-α to the matrix compartment of eosinophil secondary granules in patients with idiopathic hypereosinophilic syndrome. *J Histochem Cytochem* 41:1611, 1993.

198. Egesten A, Calafat J, Knol EF, et al: Subcellular localization of transforming growth factor-α in human eosinophil granulocytes. *Blood* 87:3910, 1996.

199. Levi-Schaffer F, Lacy P, Severs NJ, et al: Association of granulocyte-macrophage colony-stimulating factor with the crystalloid granules of human eosinophils. *Blood* 85:2579, 1995.

200. Weller PF, Bach DS, Austen KF: Biochemical characterization of human eosinophil Charcot-Leyden crystal protein (lysophospholipase). *J Biol Chem* 259:15100, 1984.

201. Zhou Z, Tenen DG, Dvorak AM, Ackerman SJ: The gene for human eosinophil Charcot-Leyden crystal protein directs expression of lysophospholipase activity and spontaneous crystallization in transiently transfected COS cells. *J Leukoc Biol* 52:587, 1992.

202. Dvorak AM, Letourneau L, Login GR, et al: Ultrastructural localization of the Charcot-Leyden crystal protein (lysophospholipase) to a distinct crystalloid-free granule population in mature human eosinophils. *Blood* 72:150, 1988.

203. Dvorak AM, Ackerman SJ, Weller PF: Subcellular morphological and biochemistry of eosinophils, in *Blood Cell Biochemistry, Megakaryocytes, Platelets, Macrophages, and Eosinophils*, vol 2, edited by JR Harris. Plenum Press, New York, 1990.

204. Calafat J, Janssen H, Knol EF, et al: Ultrastructural localization of Charcot-Leyden crystal protein in human eosinophils and basophils. *Eur J Haematol* 58:56, 1997.

205. Egesten A, Calafat J, Weller PF, et al: Localization of granule proteins in human eosinophil bone marrow progenitors. *Int Arch Allergy Immunol* 114:130, 1997.

206. Presentey B: Ultrastructure of human eosinophils genetically lacking peroxidase. *Acta Haematol* 71:334, 1984.

207. Zabucchi G, Soranzo MR, Menegazzi R, et al: Eosinophil peroxidase deficiency: Morphological and immunocytochemical studies of the eosinophil-specific granules. *Blood* 80:2903, 1992.

208. Tracey R, Smith H: An inherited anomaly of human eosinophils and basophils. *Blood Cells* 4:291, 1978.

209. Liso V, Troccoli G, Specchia G, Magno M: Cytochemical "normal" and "abnormal" eosinophils in acute leukemias. *Am J Hematol* 2:123, 1977.

210. LeBeau MM, Larson RA, Bitter MA, et al: Association of an inversion of chromosome 16 with abnormal marrow eosinophils in acute myelomonocytic leukemia. A unique cytogenetic-clinicopathology association. *N Engl J Med* 309:630, 1983.

211. Mlynek M-L, Leder L-D: Lineage infidelity in chronic myeloid leukemia: Demonstration and significance of hybridoid leukocytes. *Virchows Arch B Cell Pathol* 51:107, 1986.

212. Fauci AS: In the idiopathic hypereosinophilic syndrome: Clinical pathophysiologic, and therapeutic considerations. *Ann Intern Med* 97:78, 1982.

213. Caulfield JP, Hein A, Rothenberg ME, et al: A morphometric study of nomodense and hypodense human eosinophils that are derived in vivo and in vitro. *Am J Pathol* 137:27, 1990.

214. Prussin C, Metcalfe DD: IgE, mast cells, basophils, and eosinophils. *J Allergy Clin Immunol* 111(suppl 2):S486, 2003.

215. Parmley RT, Crist WM, Roper M, et al: Intranuclear crystalloids associated with abnormal granules in eosinophilic leukocytes. *Blood* 58:1134, 1981.

216. Chilosi M, Fossaluzza V, Tosato F: Eosinophilic acquired Pelger-Huét anomaly in acute myeloblastic leukemia. *Acta Haematol (Basel)* 61:198, 1979.

217. Fossaluzza V, Tosato F: Acquired Pelger-Huét anomaly limited to eosinophils. *Acta Haematol (Basel)* 63:295, 1980.

218. Walsh GM: Mechanisms of human eosinophil survival and apoptosis. *Clin Exp Allergy* 27:482, 1997.

219. Walsh GM: Human eosinophils: Their accumulation, activation and fate. *Br J Haematol* 97:701, 1997.

220. Rollins BJ: Chemokines. *Blood* 90:909, 1997.

221. Dvorak AM: Cell biology of the basophil. *Int Rev Cytol* 180:87, 1998.

222. Wedemeyer J, Tsai M, Galli SJ: Roles of mast cells and basophils in innate and acquired immunity. *Curr Opin Immunol* 12:624, 2000.

223. Marone G, Galli SJ, Kitamura Y: Probing the roles of mast cells and basophils in natural and acquired immunity, physiology and disease. *Trends Immunol* 23:425, 2002.

224. Dvorak AM: Histamine content and secretion in basophils and mast cells. *Prog Histochem Cytochem* 33:169, 1998.

225. Arock M, Schneider E, Boissan M, et al: Differentiation of human basophils: An overview of recent advances and pending questions. *J Leukoc Biol* 71:557, 2002.

226. Shvidel L, Shaft D, Stark B, et al: Acute basophilic leukaemia: Eight unsuspected new cases diagnosed by electron microscopy. *Br J Haematol* 120:774, 2003.

C H A P T E R 6 0

COMPOSITION OF NEUTROPHILS

C. WAYNE SMITH

Neutrophils are differentiated, relatively short-lived cells with an extensive array of surface receptors for response to inflammatory and phagocytic stimuli. A prominent feature of these cells is the presence of four distinguishable classes of cytoplasmic granules that contain a remarkable number of factors active in inflammation, tissue repair, and resistance to microbial infection. This chapter summarizes the major features of these receptors and factors. In addition, consideration is given to the fact that blood neutrophils are not end-stage cells but exhibit the capacity for changes in phenotypic characteristics and life span depending on the stimulating milieu of cytokines and chemokines. Gene expression profiling studies indicate the neutrophil is a transcriptionally active cell, responsive to environmental stimuli, and capable of a complex series of early and late changes in gene expression.

COMPOSITION OF NEUTROPHILS

Neutrophils are much more versatile cells than the terminally differentiated short-lived cells without transcriptional activities of earlier conceptualizations. Thus, consideration of the "composition" of the neutrophil should include (1) the prepackaged components of the cell that are released on acute stimulation (i.e., the classic attributes of the neutrophil) and (2) the phenotypic changes in various physiologic and pathologic environments that have functional significance. In addition, considerations of cell composition are most effectively expressed in

Acronyms and abbreviations that appear in this chapter include: ADP, adenosine diphosphate; AML1-3, transcription factor for various hematologic lineages; AMP, adenosine monophosphate; ATP, adenosine triphosphate; BPI, bactericidal/permeability-increasing protein; C5a, chemotactic fragment of complement component C5; CAP37, cationic protein of molecular weight 37; CCR, C-C chemokine receptor; C/EBPε, regulating factor of gene expression; CR3, complement receptor 3, also called CD11b/CD18, Mac-1 or integrin $\alpha_m\beta_2$; CR4, complement receptor 4, also called CD11c/CD18 or integrin $\alpha_X\beta_2$; CXC, chemokine IL-8; FcαR, receptor I for the Fc region of IgA; FcεRI, receptor I for the Fc region of IgE; FcγRI, receptor I for the Fc region of IgG; FcγRIIA, receptor IIA for the Fc region of IgG; FcγRIIIB, receptor IIIB for the Fc region of IgG; GATA-1, lineage-specific transcription factor; G-CSF, granulocyte colony stimulating factor; GM-CSF, granulocyte-monocyte colony stimulating factor; hCAP, human cationic peptide; HNP, human neutrophil peptide; ICAM, intercellular adhesion molecule; IgG, immunoglobulin G; IL, interleukin; IL-1RA, interleukin-1 receptor antagonist; JAK2, Janus-associated kinase 2; LFA-1, lymphocyte function antigen-1, also called CD11a/CD18 or integrin $\alpha_L\beta_2$; LPS, lipopolysaccharide; LTB$_4$, leukotriene B4; MMP-8, metalloproteinase-8, also called collagenase; MMP-9, metalloproteinase-9, also called gelatinase B; NAD, nicotinamide adenine dinucleotide; NADH, reduced form of nicotinamide adenine dinucleotide; NADP, nicotinamide adenine dinucleotide phosphate; NADPH, reduced form of nicotinamide adenine dinucleotide phosphate; NFκB1/p50, transcription factor; PAF, platelet-activating factor; PSGL, P-selectin glycoprotein ligand; PU.1, lineage-specific transcription factor; SNAP, soluble NSF (N-ethylmaleimide-sensitive factor)-attachment protein; TNF, tumor necrosis factor; TGF, transforming growth factor; u-PAR, urokinase-plasminogen activator receptor; VAMP, vesicle-associated membrane protein; VEGF, vascular endothelial growth factor.

This chapter is based in part on Chapter 65 by Dr. Ernest Beutler in the sixth edition of this text.

the context of pathways leading to significant physiologic and pathologic functions.

NEUTROPHIL GRANULES

A prominent characteristic of neutrophils is the abundance of cytoplasmic granules, the features of which are only partially defined. Cell fractionation and ultrastructural studies have revealed many of the contents of the four subsets of granules in mature neutrophils. Table 60-1 lists some of the components and illustrates the compartmentalization of diverse functionally significant receptors, enzymes, membrane constituents, and antimicrobial proteins. The granules function as intracellular stores of both membrane proteins and soluble proteins that may be incorporated into the plasma membrane or released, thereby assisting the neutrophil in diverse functionally important activities such as adhesion, migration, phagocytosis, and killing of microorganisms. Segregation of the proteins into different subpopulations of granules allows neutrophils to contain prestored proteins that could not exist in the same compartment, and the contents of the different granules are important at different times and places in the life of the cell.

The diversity of neutrophil granules appears to be linked to the timing of biosynthesis during myelopoiesis. The hypothesis is that the different subsets of granules are the result of differences in the biosynthetic windows of the various granule proteins during maturation[1] and not the result of specific sorting between individual granule subsets (see Chap. 66). The control of biosynthesis is exerted by transcription factors that control the expression of the genes for the various granule proteins. Several transcription factors have been identified as relevant in the timing of granule protein synthesis, including the lineage-specific transcription factor GATA-1, the lineage-specific transcription factor PU.1, transcription factor for various hematologic lineages AML1-3, and regulating factor of gene expression C/EBPε.[1-3] The importance of C/EBPε has been emphasized by the recognition of mutations in this protein in patients with the rare syndrome called "specific granule deficiency,"[4-6] a condition that leads to increased susceptibility to bacterial infections. In neutrophils from these patients, total cellular content and release of the secondary and tertiary granule markers (e.g., lactoferrin, B$_{12}$ binding protein, and lysozyme) are diminished, although levels of primary granule constituents (e.g., myeloperoxidase, β-glucuronidase) generally are normal.

The granular constituents are released from the membrane-enclosed granules into phagosomes or transported to the cell surface by a process of exocytosis following stimulation of the neutrophil.[7] The signal cascade following stimulation of specific receptors on the cytoplasmic membrane results in elevated intracellular Ca^{2+}, lipid remodeling, and protein kinase activation, which culminate in fusion of granules with phagosomes or the cell surface membrane. The process is rapid, highly efficient, and involves families of docking proteins related to those found in neurons (e.g., vesicle-associated membrane protein [VAMP]-2, syntaxin-4, soluble NSF (N-ethylmaleimide-sensitive factor)-attachment protein [SNAP]-23).[8]

The granule subsets appear to have a significant differential sensitivity to undergo exocytosis, ranging from secretory vesicles to tertiary, secondary, and primary granules, with primary granules being most resistant. The significance of this differential release is incompletely understood, but some aspects are apparent in the functions of the constituents within the granules and granular membranes. For example, secretory vesicles and tertiary granules contain receptors, such as CD11b/CD18 (adhesion molecule, Mac-1), formyl peptide receptor (chemotactic receptor), FcγRIIIB (Fc receptor), and gelatinase (metalloproteinase [MMP]-9), which potentially enhance extracellular interactions of the neutrophil. Primary granules contain

TABLE 60-1 NEUTROPHIL GRANULES

GRANULES/ENZYME MARKERS	MEMBRANE MARKERS	NADPH OXIDASE	RECEPTORS	ANTIMICROBIAL	ENZYMES	OTHER FACTORS
Primary (azurophilic) Myeloperoxidase	CD63 CD68 V-type H⁺-ATPase			BPI-protein Defensins (HNP 1-4) CAP37 Myeloperoxidase Lysozyme	Elastase Cathepsin G Proteinase 3 α-Mannosidase β-Glucuronidase β-Glycerophosphatase Sialidase N-Acetyl-β-glucosaminidase	Acid mucopolysaccharide α_1-antitrypsin
Secondary (specific) Lactoferrin	CD15 CD66 CD67 CD11b/CD18	gp91phox p22phox Rap1A Rap2	Formyl peptide R CR3 (CD11b/CD18) Fibronectin R G-protein α-subunit Laminin R Thrombospondin R TNF R u-PAR VAMP-2 Vitronectin R	Lactoferrin Lysozyme hCAP-18	Gelatinase B (MMP-9) Histaminase Sialidase Collagenase (MMP-8) Heparinase	β_2 microglobulin Vitamin B$_{12}$ binding protein Plasminogen activator NGAL (lipocalin)
Tertiary Gelatinase	CD11b/CD18 V-type H⁺-ATPase	gp91phox p22phox Rap1A	Formyl peptide R CR3 (CD11b/CD18) u-PAR VAMP-2	Lysozyme	Gelatinase B (MMP-9) Acetyltransferase Diacylglycerol-deacylating enzyme	β_2 microglobulin Oncostatin M
Secretory vesicles Alkaline phosphatase	CD11b/CD18 CD10 CD13 CD45 CD35 CD14	gp91phox p22phox Rap1A	Formyl peptide R CR1 (CD35) CR3 (CD11b/CD18) CR4 (CD11c/CD18) C1qR FcγRIIIB (CD16) u-PAR	CAP37	Proteinase 3	Plasma proteins (e.g., albumin) Decay accelerating factor

SOURCE: Data regarding antimicrobial factors from references 1,9–35. Data regarding enzymes from references 1,36–50.

microbicidal proteins and acid hydrolases, and the acidic environment of the phagolysosome creates an optimal pH for these enzymes.

BIOACTIVE FACTORS IN GRANULES

7980rophil granules are particularly rich in factors with antimicrobial activity. Some (e.g., myeloperoxidase) function in conjunction with the reduced form of nicotinamide adenine dinucleotide phosphate (NADPH) oxidase, whereas others (e.g., defensins) exhibit activity independent of the oxidative burst. Others are proteolytic enzymes,

surface opsonin receptors, and adhesion molecules. Chapters 59 and 66 provide detailed discussions of these factors. Tables 60-1 through 60-4 list and categorize the factors found within the neutrophils and on their surfaces and are provided as summaries of the prominent components of mature neutrophils.

WATER AND ELECTROLYTES

Approximately 82 percent of the leukocyte weight is water.[86] A remarkable paucity of data are available regarding the electrolyte content of neutrophils. The often quoted 1929 study of Endres and Hegert[86] was performed on mixed leukocytes from the blood of horses obtained at a slaughterhouse. They found an average of 2610 mg (113 mmol) sodium, 889 mg (22.7 mmol) potassium, 72 mg (1.8 mmol) calcium, 10.3 mg (0.18 mmol) iron, 2487 mg (70.2 mmol) chloride, and 299 mg (9.65 mmol) inorganic phosphate per liter of leukocytes. The copper content of neutrophils has been reported to average 4.69 nmol/10^9 cells,[87] zinc 109.2 nmol/10^9 cells[87] and 50.16 nmol/10^9 cells,[88] and magnesium 3.11 fmol/cell.[89] Little selenium is present in neutrophils; the median concentration reported is less than 0.0075 μmol/10^9 cells.[90] Otherwise, electrolyte determinations on human leukocytes appear to have been limited to leukemic cells and to pus.[91]

TABLE 60-2 OPSONIC RECEPTORS ON NEUTROPHILS

RECEPTOR	CHARACTERISTICS	LIGAND
FcγRI (CD64)	72 kDa, transmembrane, induced by IFN-γ	IgG1, high affinity
FcγRIIA (CD32)	40 kDa, transmembrane, constitutive, A isoform associates with CR3	IgG3 > IgG1, low affinity, binds polymeric IgG
FcγRIIIB (CD16)	50 kDa, GPI-linked, constitutive, associates with CR3	IgG1, low affinity, binds polymeric IgG
FcαR (CD89)	60 kDa, transmembrane, constitutive	IgA, polymeric (e.g., sIgA)
CR1 (CD35)	160–250 kDa, transmembrane, constitutive	C3b, C4b
CR3 (CD11b/CD18)	165/90 kDa, transmembrane, heterodimer, storage pool in granules	iC3b
CR4 (CD11c/CD18)	145/90 kDa transmembrane, heterodimer	iC3b

SOURCE: References 51–62.

TABLE 60-3 NEUTROPHIL ADHESION MOLECULES

NEUTROPHIL RECEPTOR	CLASSIFICATION	LIGANDS
L-selectin (CD62L)	Selectin family	PSGL-1, E-selectin
PSGL-1 (CD162)	Mucin family	E-selectin, P-selectin
sLe^X glycoproteins	Various glycoproteins	E-selectin
LFA-1 (CD11a/CD18)	$\alpha_L\beta_2$-Integrin	ICAM-1, ICAM-3
Mac-1 (CD11b/CD18)	$\alpha_M\beta_2$-Integrin	ICAM-1, GPIbα, factor X, fibrinogen, iC3b
CR4 (CD11c/CD18)	$\alpha_X\beta_2$-Integrin	Fibrinogen, iC3b
VLA-2 (CD49b/CD29)	$\alpha_2\beta_1$-Integrin	Collagen, laminin
VLA-3 (CD49c/CD29)	$\alpha_3\beta_1$-Integrin	Collagen, laminin, fibronectin, tenascin
VLA-4 (CD49d/CD29)	$\alpha_4\beta_1$-Integrin	VCAM-1, fibronectin
VLA-5 (CD49e/CD29)	$\alpha_5\beta_1$-Integrin	Fibronectin
VLA-6 (CD49f/CD29)	$\alpha_6\beta_1$-Integrin	Laminin
VLA-9	$\alpha_9\beta_1$-Integrin	VCAM-1, tenascin
$\alpha_V\beta_3$ (CD51/CD61)	β_3-Integrin	Vitronectin

SOURCE: References 56, 63–76.

CARBOHYDRATES

The rate of glucose metabolism by neutrophils is affected by insulin in diabetics but not in normal subjects.[92,93] The neutrophil is particularly rich in glycogen. The concentration of this complex polysaccharide has been reported to average 7.36 mg/10^9 cells.[94–96]

AMINO ACIDS, PEPTIDES, AND PROTEINS

The concentrations of most amino acids are higher in neutrophils than in the surrounding plasma.[97] Table 60-5 summarizes the amino acid concentration in neutrophils. The reduced glutathione content of neutrophils is 9.8 nmol/10^7 cells.[98]

The protein content of the neutrophil is 74.2 ± 3.1 (mean ± 1 SE) mg/10^9 cells.[99] These proteins include those of the structural matrix of the neutrophil; proteins required for its locomotion, chemotactic properties, and adhesiveness; and the many granule proteins with bactericidal, hydrolytic, and inflammatory functions.

LIPIDS

As in other cells, the plasma membrane and the membranes of the intracellular organelles are rich in lipids. Five percent of the wet weight

TABLE 60-4 CHEMOTACTIC RECEPTORS ON HUMAN NEUTROPHILS

RECEPTOR	LIGANDS
Formyl peptide receptor (FPR) (high affinity)	f-met-leu-phe (fMLP), other f-met peptides of bacterial origin
Formyl peptide receptor-like 1 (FPRL-1) (low affinity)	f-met peptides, LXA$_4$, SAA, HIV envelope domains
C5aR (high affinity)	C5a complement fragment
CXCR1 (high affinity)	IL-8 (CXCL8)
CXCR2 (high affinity)	GRO-α (CXCL1), GRO-β (CXCL2), ENA-78 (CXCL5)
CXCR4 in bone marrow (high affinity)	SDF-1α (CXCL12)
CCR2 (induced; high affinity)	MCP-1 (CCL2)
CCR6 (induced; high affinity)	LARC (CCL20), β-defensin
Platelet-activating factor R (low and high affinity)	Platelet-activating factor
BLT1 (high affinity)	LTB$_4$
BLT2 (low affinity)	LTB$_4$, other eicosanoids

SOURCE: References 77–85.

TABLE 60-5 BOUND AMINO ACID CONCENTRATIONS IN LEUKOCYTES (LYMPHOCYTES INCLUDED)

AMINO ACID	μMOL/KG WATER*
Alanine	2881 ± 256
Arginine	<290
Ergothioneine	<300
Ethanolamine	<250
Glutamic acid	2745 ± 251
Glutamine	2650 ± 251
Histidine	762 ± 70
Leucine plus isoleucine	1999 ± 195
Lysine	2111 ± 216
Methionine	391 ± 54
O-phosphoethanolamine	2651 ± 389
Ornithine	1767 ± 113
Phenylalanine	647 ± 105
Proline	862 ± 79
Serine plus glycine	13,021 ± 1480
Taurine	28,683 ± 2726
Threonine	2345 ± 174
Tryptophan	222 ± 31
Tyrosine	480 ± 97
Valine	1335 ± 132

* Mean ± 1 SD.
SOURCE: McMenamy et al.[97]

of neutrophils is lipid, which is distributed among various classes, as shown in Table 60-6.[100–104] The rare polyphosphoinositides are of special interest as sources of inositol 1,4,5-trisphosphate (a calcium-releasing mediator) and diacylglycerol (which activates protein kinase C).[105,106] The main glycolipid of neutrophils is lactosyl-ceramide.[107]

NUCLEOTIDES AND NUCLEIC ACIDS

Table 60-7 summarizes the levels of nucleotides in the neutrophils.[108,109]

Neutrophils contain all the forms of RNA needed for protein synthesis: transfer RNA, ribosomal RNA, and messenger RNA.[110,111] The DNA content of neutrophils is identical to that of all other haploid cells, at 0.7 pg DNA phosphorus per cell.[112]

VITAMINS AND COFACTORS

The average folic acid content of packed leukocytes of normal subjects was 0.1 μg/ml of packed leukocytes. Approximately 20 percent of the folic acid was free and the remainder conjugated.[115] The co-carbox-

TABLE 60-6 LIPID COMPOSITION OF NEUTROPHILS

LIPID	CONTENT (%)
Phospholipid	
Phosphatidylcholine	12
Phosphatidylethanolamine	12
Sphingomyelin	6.5
Phosphatidylserine	1.5
Phosphatidylinositol	1.5
Phosphatidic acid	1.5
Total	35
Triglyceride	20
Glycolipid	16
Cholesterol	10

SOURCE: Gottfried.[100]

TABLE 60-7   NUCLEOTIDES IN LEUKOCYTES (LYMPHOCYTES INCLUDED)

NUCLEOTIDE	NMOL/10^9 CELLS (MEAN ± SE)
NAD	32 ± 2.0*
NADH	25 ± 2.3*
NADP	8 ± 1.5*
NADPH	24 ± 39†
ATP	8800‡
ADP	1600‡
AMP	6100‡

SOURCE: *Silber et al.,[100] †Noyes et al.,[113] ‡Löhr et al.[114]

ylate content is 340 μg/10^{11} cells,[116] pyridoxal phosphate 0.24 to 0.38 ng/10^6 cells,[117] thiamine 67.5 ± 4.1 μg/100 ml,[115] ascorbic acid 16.5 ± 5.1 mg/100 ml,[118] and folate 92 ng/ml.[119]

METABOLISM OF NEUTROPHILS

CARBOHYDRATE METABOLISM

GLYCOLYSIS

Glycolytic (Embden-Meyerhof) Pathway   The main energy-producing pathway in the neutrophil is glycolysis, resulting in the conversion of glucose to lactate.[120–122] When intact or homogenized leukocytes are incubated with glucose uniformly labeled with ^{14}C, approximately 80 percent of the radioactivity is recovered in lactic acid.

Glycolysis is inhibited by cortisol. Table 60-8 summarizes the activities of the glycolytic enzymes of neutrophils.[123,124] In some cases, the conditions under which the neutrophils are disrupted have a significant effect on the activities measured.[124] Hexokinase is the rate-limiting enzyme of glycolysis in normal neutrophils.[121] The rate of glycolysis is not altered during phagocytosis,[122] but adenosine triphosphate (ATP) levels, normally 1.9 nmol/10^6 cells, fall to 0.8 nmol/10^6 cells. Both the glycogen stores of neutrophils and the glucose of the plasma can serve as the source of glucose. Galactose, mannose, and fructose can also be metabolized by leukocytes.[125]

Hexose Monophosphate Shunt Pathway   Neutrophils also metabolize glucose by way of the hexose monophosphate shunt,[126–128] thus accounting for some of the oxygen consumption of the cells. In resting cells, the amount of glucose metabolized via this route amounts to only 2 to 3 percent of the total glucose consumed by the cell.[127–129] The operation of the hexose monophosphate shunt, however, is of special importance to the neutrophil, because this pathway provides the NADPH needed for generation of microbicidal oxidants.

Glycogen Metabolism   Neutrophils contain a large quantity of glycogen arising mostly from glucose. Little net synthesis from substrates occurs at the triose phosphate level. Glycogen turnover increases when these cells are deprived of glucose, especially if they are engaged in phagocytosis, but resynthesis occurs when adequate glucose is added.[94,122,130] During phagocytosis by glucose-starved cells, glycogen phosphorylase activity rises, but phosphorylase kinase and glycogen synthase levels remain unchanged.[130] Glycogen first appears in myelocytes and increases with cell maturation.[131]

PROTEIN SYNTHESIS BY MATURE NEUTROPHILS

Mature neutrophils have been classically viewed as terminally differentiated cells without the ability to synthesize proteins. This view has changed as a result of numerous investigations *in vitro* and *in vivo* showing that neutrophils can synthesize numerous proteins (e.g., cytokines, chemokines, growth factors, interferons) potentially important to the inflammatory process and the regulation of immune reactions. Table 60-9 lists some of the factors expressed by mature neutrophils. The database for these observations has been extensively reviewed,[133,134] and some potentially important concepts are discussed here. As is evident from this list, the diversity is impressive, but the extent of production of each protein by individual neutrophils is limited when compared to mononuclear cells. However, because neutrophils make up the majority of infiltrating cells early in an acute inflammatory process, often emigrating in massive numbers, their aggregate synthetic ability may be significant to the course of the inflammatory or healing response. *In vitro*, an array of stimuli have been used to induce protein expression, including lipopolysaccharide (LPS), cytokines, chemotactic factors, adhesive ligands, opsonized particles, and modulatory cytokines such as interleukin (IL)-10 and IL-4.

TABLE 60-8   GLYCOLYTIC AND RELATED ENZYME ACTIVITIES IN NEUTROPHILS

ENZYME	ACTIVITY AT 37°C IN NEUTROPHILS*	ACTIVITY AT 30°C IN NEUTROPHILS†	ACTIVITY AT 25°C IN MIXED LEUKOCYTES‡
Hexokinase	78 ± 14	39.6 ± 27.3	—
Phosphofructokinase	36 ± 2	—	—
Aldolase	76 ± 7	118.7 ± 27.4	123
Glucosephosphate isomerase	4930 ± 716	—	—
Triosephosphate isomerase	7853 ± 323	—	2189
Glyceraldehyde dehydrogenase	3683 ± 124	—	242
Monophosphoglycerate mutase	508 ± 35	—	—
Phosphoglycerate kinase	3744 ± 197	—	890
Enolase	136 ± 17	—	734
Pyruvate kinase	173 ± 11	4125 ± 549	976
Lactate dehydrogenase	1128 ± 51	2981 ± 893	1165
Glucose-6-phosphate dehydrogenase	517 ± 11	596 ± 116.6	176
6-Phosphogluconate dehydrogenase	287 ± 5	—	—
Glutathione reductase	63 ± 7	—	—
Glutathione peroxidase	17 ± 3	—	—
Glutamic oxaloacetic transaminase	25 ± 2	—	43
Adenylate kinase	32 ± 2	163 ± 9.9	149
α-Glycerophosphate dehydrogenase	—	—	23
Isocitric dehydrogenase	—	—	47
Fructose 1,6-diphosphatase	—	0.76 ± 0.18	—
Isocitrate dehydrogenase	—	44.1 ± 6.4	—
Citrate synthase	—	32.0 ± 5.4	—
Malate dehydrogenase	—	482 ± 62.6	—
Transketolase	—	0.99 ± 0.27	—
Phosphorylase A	—	9.60 ± 2.66	—
Lipoamide dehydrogenase	—	29.7 ± 13.8	—
Ca^{2+} ATPase	—	—	28
Mg^{2+} ATPase	—	—	30

* IU/mg protein, [132]. † IU/liter, [124]. ‡ IU/mg protein, recalculated from Bücher units/10^{11} leukocytes, [114] assuming a protein content of 7.4 mg/10 leukocytes.

The signaling pathways leading to new protein synthesis are subjects of extensive studies and are briefly described here. Granulocyte colony stimulating factor (G-CSF), granulocyte-monocyte colony stimulating factor (GM-CSF), and IL-10 have the ability to activate signal transducer and activator of transcription (STAT) proteins in neutrophils. Both STAT-1 and STAT-3 and the upstream kinase Janus-associated kinase 2 (JAK2) are rapidly tyrosine phosphorylated.[135,136] Neutrophils express NFκB1/p50, p65/RelA, and c-Rel. Tumor necrosis factor alpha (TNF-α), IL-1β, and IL-15 lead to the rapid loss of IκBα and the concomitant nuclear accumulation of NFκB/Rel proteins. This pathway is not activated by G-CSF, GM-CSF, IL-8, or IL-10. PU.1 is expressed in mature neutrophils and constitutively binds DNA, and the AP-1 transcription factor is evident. Several of the inflammatory mediators produced by mature neutrophils are AP-1 driven (e.g., TNF, IL-1, IL-8, intercellular adhesion molecule [ICAM]).[136]

Production of the CXC chemokine IL-8 by neutrophils has been extensively studied, and a wide range of stimuli can induce its expression.[82] Cytokines such as TNF-α, IL-15, IL-1β, and GM-CSF; chemotactic factors such as C5a, platelet-activating factor (PAF), and leukotriene B4 (LTB$_4$); particles such as monosodium urate crystals; microbial products such as LPS and zymosan; interaction with antibody and complement opsonized bacteria and yeasts; and interactions with extracellular matrix molecules such as laminin and fibronectin all have been shown to induce synthesis of IL-8 by neutrophils. In most studies, release of significant amounts of protein from the neutrophils and synthesis of mRNA have been demonstrated. Immunocytochemistry and in situ hybridization studies have provided evidence of IL-8 production in neutrophils infiltrating inflammatory sites.

Some of the stimuli that induce expression of IL-8 also stimulate production by mature neutrophils of other proinflammatory agents, such as GRO-α, TNF-α, IL-1β, oncostatin M, and C-C chemokines. In addition, neutrophils may produce antiinflammatory agents such as IL-1 receptor antagonist (IL-1RA) and transforming growth factor (TGF)-β, and of interest is the observation that cytokines such as IL-10 may have some selectivity with regard to induction of antiinflammatory factors in neutrophils. Thus, considerable evidence exists for protein synthesis capability in neutrophils, but because this field of study is relatively new, much work remains to define the importance of the various proteins to inflammation, immune reactions and healing, the selectivity of the conditions, and disease states linked to the synthetic activities of neutrophils.

PHENOTYPIC CHANGES

Phenotypic changes occur in neutrophils under specific conditions.[137,138] Degranulation results in marked changes in surface expression of an array of proteins arriving at the surface from the storage pools of granules (e.g., CD11b/CD18, CD66, some β$_1$-integrins). These phenomena can be seen in degrees in circulating neutrophils. Exposure of neutrophils to activating factors results in surface and functional changes as a result of new synthesis (e.g., FcγRI following elevations in IFN-γ) or shedding (e.g., loss of L-selectin), also seen in circulating neutrophils. Cytokines (e.g., IL-15, IL-1, TNF) induce de novo synthesis of proteins (as noted in Table 60-9) to various degrees in blood neutrophils. Substantial changes occur once the neutrophil leaves the vasculature, increasing its expression of β$_1$-integrins, C-C chemokine receptors (CCRs), and protein synthesis.

TABLE 60-9 PROTEINS SYNTHESIZED BY NEUTROPHILS.

CYTOKINES	RECEPTORS	CHEMOKINES	GROWTH FACTORS	MISCELLANEOUS
TNF-α	IL-1 receptor antagonist (IL-1RA)	IL-8	G-CSF	Fas ligand
IL-1-β		GRO-α	M-CSF	CD40
IL-12	TGF-β	GRO-β	GM-CSF	CD83
IFN-α		IP-10	IL-3	CCR6
IL-6		MIP-1α	VEGF	CCR2
Oncostatin M		MIP-1β	TGF-β	HLA-DR
		MCP-1		

Evidence indicates that in response to specific combinations of cytokines (e.g., GM-CSF, TNF-α, IFN-γ), neutrophils can acquire phenotypic and functional characteristics of immature dendritic antigen-presenting cells.[137] Thus, any consideration of the "composition" of neutrophils requires a detailed understanding of the stage of development and the environment to which the neutrophil is exposed in vivo. The neutrophil is a remarkably versatile cell.

Gene expression profiling has provided rich insights into the capacity of the mature neutrophil to change in response to environmental stimuli. Following exposure to 10 ng/ml Escherichia coli LPS, 307 genes are activated or repressed.[139] These changes include transcription factors, cytokines, chemokines, interleukins, surface antigens, toll-like receptors, and members of immune mediator gene families. Neutrophils also show priming responses to LPS in which 97 genes change expression following exposure to LPS. Major changes in gene expression occur following LPS,[140] migration in wounds,[141] activation by phagocytosis,[142] or during the processes of apoptosis.[143] These findings indicate that the neutrophil is a transcriptionally active cell responsive to environmental stimuli and capable of a complex series of both early and late changes in gene expression.

REFERENCES

1. Borregaard N, Cowland JB: Granules of the human neutrophilic polymorphonuclear leukocyte. Blood 89:3503, 1997.
2. Gombart AF, Kwok SH, Anderson KL, et al: Regulation of neutrophil and eosinophil secondary granule gene expression by transcription factors C/EBP epsilon and PU.1. Blood 101:3265, 2003.
3. Lekstrom-Himes JA: The role of C/EBP(epsilon) in the terminal stages of granulocyte differentiation. Stem Cells 19:125, 2001.
4. Shiohara M, Gombart AF, Sekiguchi Y, et al: Phenotypic and functional alterations of peripheral blood monocytes in neutrophil-specific granule deficiency. J Leukoc Biol 75:190, 2004.
5. Lekstrom-Himes JA, Dorman SE, Kopar P, et al: Neutrophil-specific granule deficiency results from a novel mutation with loss of function of the transcription factor CCAAT/enhancer binding protein epsilon. J Exp Med 189:1847, 1999.
6. Gallin JI: Neutrophil specific granule deficiency. Annu Rev Med 36:263, 1985.
7. Brumell JH, Volchuk A, Sengelov H, et al: Subcellular distribution of docking/fusion proteins in neutrophils, secretory cells with multiple exocytic compartments. J Immunol 155:5750, 1995.
8. Mollinedo F, Martin-Martin B, Calafat J, et al: Role of vesicle-associated membrane protein-2, through Q-soluble N-ethylmaleimide-sensitive factor attachment protein receptor/R-soluble N-ethylmaleimide-sensitive factor attachment protein receptor interaction, in the exocytosis of specific and tertiary granules of human neutrophils. J Immunol 170:1034, 2003.
9. Brock JH: The physiology of lactoferrin. Biochem Cell Biol 80:1, 2002.

10. Farnaud S, Evans RW: Lactoferrin—A multifunctional protein with antimicrobial properties. *Mol Immunol* 40:395, 2003.

11. Chapple DS, Hussain R, Joannou CL, et al: Structure and association of human lactoferrin peptides with Escherichia coli lipopolysaccharide. *Antimicrob Agents Chemother* 48:2190, 2004.

12. Rocha-Pereira P, Santos-Silva A, Rebelo I, et al: The inflammatory response in mild and in severe psoriasis. *Br J Dermatol* 150:917, 2004.

13. Levy O: Impaired innate immunity at birth: Deficiency of bactericidal/permeability-increasing protein (BPI) in the neutrophils of newborns. *Pediatr Res* 51:667, 2002.

14. Nupponen I, Turunen R, Nevalainen T, et al: Extracellular release of bactericidal/permeability-increasing protein in newborn infants. *Pediatr Res* 51:670, 2002.

15. Schultz H, Weiss J, Carroll SF, et al: The endotoxin-binding bactericidal/permeability-increasing protein (BPI): A target antigen of auto-antibodies. *J Leukoc Biol* 69:505, 2001.

16. Watorek W: Azurocidin—Inactive serine proteinase homolog acting as a multifunctional inflammatory mediator. *Acta Biochim Pol* 50:743, 2003.

17. Gonzalez ML, Ruan X, Kumar P, et al: Functional modulation of smooth muscle cells by the inflammatory mediator CAP37. *Microvasc Res* 67:168, 2004.

18. Lee TD, Gonzalez ML, Kumar P, et al: CAP37, a neutrophil-derived inflammatory mediator, augments leukocyte adhesion to endothelial monolayers. *Microvasc Res* 66:38, 2003.

19. Tapper H, Karlsson A, Morgelin M, et al: Secretion of heparin-binding protein from human neutrophils is determined by its localization in azurophilic granules and secretory vesicles. *Blood* 99:1785, 2002.

20. Gray PW, Flaggs G, Leong SR, et al: Cloning of the cDNA of a human neutrophil bactericidal protein. Structural and functional correlations. *J Biol Chem* 264:9505, 1989.

21. Boman HG: Antibacterial peptides: Basic facts and emerging concepts. *J Intern Med* 254:197, 2003.

22. Niyonsaba F, Ogawa H, Nagaoka I: Human beta-defensin-2 functions as a chemotactic agent for tumour necrosis factor-alpha-treated human neutrophils. *Immunology* 111:273, 2004.

23. Oppenheim JJ, Biragyn A, Kwak LW, et al: Roles of antimicrobial peptides such as defensins in innate and adaptive immunity. *Ann Rheum Dis* 62(suppl 2):ii17, 2003.

24. Nizet V, Gallo RL: Cathelicidins and innate defense against invasive bacterial infection. *Scand J Infect Dis* 35:670, 2003.

25. Zanetti M: Cathelicidins, multifunctional peptides of the innate immunity. *J Leukoc Biol* 75:39, 2004.

26. Murakami M, Lopez-Garcia B, Braff M, et al: Postsecretory processing generates multiple cathelicidins for enhanced topical antimicrobial defense. *J Immunol* 172:3070, 2004.

27. Elssner A, Duncan M, Gavrilin M, et al: A novel P2X7 receptor activator, the human cathelicidin-derived peptide LL37, induces IL-1 beta processing and release. *J Immunol* 172:4987, 2004.

28. Davidson DJ, Currie AJ, Reid GS, et al: The cationic antimicrobial peptide LL-37 modulates dendritic cell differentiation and dendritic cell-induced T cell polarization. *J Immunol* 172:1146, 2004.

29. Ibrahim HR, Aoki T, Pellegrini A: Strategies for new antimicrobial proteins and peptides: lysozyme and aprotinin as model molecules. *Curr Pharm Des* 8:671, 2002.

30. Ganz T, Gabayan V, Liao HI, et al: Increased inflammation in lysozyme M-deficient mice in response to Micrococcus luteus and its peptidoglycan. *Blood* 101:2388, 2003.

31. Ganz T: Antimicrobial polypeptides. *J Leukoc Biol* 75:34, 2004.

32. Quinn MT, Gauss KA: Structure and regulation of the neutrophil respiratory burst oxidase: comparison with nonphagocyte oxidases. *J Leukoc Biol* 2004.

33. Klebanoff SJ: Myeloperoxidase. *Proc Assoc Am Physicians* 111:383, 1999.

34. Hampton MB, Kettle AJ, Winterbourn CC: Inside the neutrophil phagosome: oxidants, myeloperoxidase, and bacterial killing. *Blood* 92:3007, 1998.

35. Wheeler MA, Smith SD, Garcia-Cardena G, et al: Bacterial infection induces nitric oxide synthase in human neutrophils. *J Clin Invest* 99:110, 1997.

36. Shapiro SD: Neutrophil elastase: Path clearer, pathogen killer, or just pathologic? *Am J Respir Cell Mol Biol* 26:266, 2002.

37. Kawabata K, Hagio T, Matsuoka S: The role of neutrophil elastase in acute lung injury. *Eur J Pharmacol* 451:1, 2002.

38. Aprikyan AA, Liles WC, Boxer LA, et al: Mutant elastase in pathogenesis of cyclic and severe congenital neutropenia. *J Pediatr Hematol Oncol* 24:784, 2002.

39. Horwitz M, Benson KF, Duan Z, et al: Role of neutrophil elastase in bone marrow failure syndromes: Molecular genetic revival of the chalone hypothesis. *Curr Opin Hematol* 10:49, 2003.

40. Belaaouaj A: Neutrophil elastase-mediated killing of bacteria: Lessons from targeted mutagenesis. *Microbes Infect* 4:1259, 2002.

41. Hirche TO, Atkinson JJ, Bahr S, et al: Deficiency in neutrophil elastase does not impair neutrophil recruitment to inflamed sites. *Am J Respir Cell Mol Biol* 30:576, 2004.

42. Sennstrom MB, Brauner A, Bystrom B, et al: Matrix metalloproteinase-8 correlates with the cervical ripening process in humans. *Acta Obstet Gynecol Scand* 82:904, 2003.

43. Balbin M, Fueyo A, Tester AM, et al: Loss of collagenase-2 confers increased skin tumor susceptibility to male mice. *Nat Genet* 35:252, 2003.

44. Opdenakker G, Van den Steen PE, Dubois B, et al: Gelatinase B functions as regulator and effector in leukocyte biology. *J Leukoc Biol* 69:851, 2001.

45. Schonbeck U, Mach F, Libby P: Generation of biologically active IL-1 beta by matrix metalloproteinases: A novel caspase-1-independent pathway of IL-1 beta processing. *J Immunol* 161:3340, 1998.

46. Peppin GJ, Weiss SJ: Activation of the endogenous metalloproteinase, gelatinase, by triggered human neutrophils. *Proc Natl Acad Sci U S A* 83:4322, 1986.

47. Ogata Y, Enghild JJ, Nagase H: Matrix metalloproteinase 3 (stromelysin) activates the precursor for the human matrix metalloproteinase 9. *J Biol Chem* 267:3581, 1992.

48. Van den Steen PE, Husson SJ, Proost P, et al: Carboxyterminal cleavage of the chemokines MIG and IP-10 by gelatinase B and neutrophil collagenase. *Biochem Biophys Res Commun* 310:889, 2003.

49. Van den Steen PE, Wuyts A, Husson SJ, et al: Gelatinase B/MMP-9 and neutrophil collagenase/MMP-8 process the chemokines human GCP-2/CXCL6, ENA-78/CXCL5 and mouse GCP-2/LIX and modulate their physiological activities. *Eur J Biochem* 270:3739, 2003.

50. Pelus LM, Bian H, King AG, et al: Neutrophil-derived MMP-9 mediates synergistic mobilization of hematopoietic stem and progenitor cells by the combination of G-CSF and the chemokines GRObeta/CXCL2 and GRObetaT/CXCL2delta4. *Blood* 103:110, 2004.

51. Kwiatkowska K, Sobota A: Signaling pathways in phagocytosis. *Bioessays* 21:422, 1999.

52. Lee WL, Harrison RE, Grinstein S: Phagocytosis by neutrophils. *Microbes Infect* 5:1299, 2003.

53. Hogarth PM: Fc receptors are major mediators of antibody based inflammation in autoimmunity. *Curr Opin Immunol* 14:798, 2002.

54. Amigorena S, Bonnerot C: Fc receptor signaling and trafficking: a connection for antigen processing. *Immunol Rev* 172:279, 1999.

55. Chuang FY, Sassaroli M, Unkeless JC: Convergence of Fc gamma receptor IIA and Fc gamma receptor IIIB signaling pathways in human neutrophils. *J Immunol* 164:350, 2000.

56. Petty HR, Worth RG, Todd RF III: Interactions of integrins with their partner proteins in leukocyte membranes. *Immunol Res* 25:75, 2002.

57. Hamre R, Farstad IN, Brandtzaeg P, et al: Expression and modulation of the human immunoglobulin A Fc receptor (CD89) and the FcR gamma chain on myeloid cells in blood and tissue. *Scand J Immunol* 57:506, 2003.

58. Hoffmeyer F, Witte K, Schmidt RE: The high-affinity Fc gamma RI on PMN: Regulation of expression and signal transduction. *Immunology* 92:544, 1997.

59. Kakinoki Y, Kubota H, Yamamoto Y: CD64 surface expression on neutrophils and monocytes is significantly up-regulated after stimulation with granulocyte colony-stimulating factor during CHOP chemotherapy for patients with non-Hodgkin's lymphoma. *Int J Hematol* 79:55, 2004.

60. Pangburn MK, Rawal N: Structure and function of complement C5 convertase enzymes. *Biochem Soc Trans* 30:1006, 2002.

61. Sambandam T, Chatham WW: Ligation of CR1 attenuates Fc receptor-mediated myeloperoxidase release and HOCl production by neutrophils. *J Leukoc Biol* 63:477, 1998.

62. Ross GD: Role of the lectin domain of Mac-1/CR3 (CD11b/CD18) in regulating intercellular adhesion. *Immunol Res* 25:219, 2002.

63. Lindbom L, Werr J: Integrin-dependent neutrophil migration in extravascular tissue. *Semin Immunol* 14:115, 2002.

64. Takagi J, Springer TA: Integrin activation and structural rearrangement. *Immunol Rev* 186:141, 2002.

65. Hogg N, Henderson R, Leitinger B, et al: Mechanisms contributing to the activity of integrins on leukocytes. *Immunol Rev* 186:164, 2002.

66. McDowall A, Leitinger B, Stanley P, et al: The I domain of integrin leukocyte function-associated antigen-1 is involved in a conformational change leading to high affinity binding to ligand intercellular adhesion molecule 1 (ICAM-1) *J Biol Chem* 273:27396, 1998.

67. Grayson MH, Van der Vieren M, Sterbinsky SA, et al: $\alpha d\beta 2$ Integrin is expressed on human eosinophils and functions as an alternative ligand for vascular cell adhesion molecule 1 (VCAM-1). *J Exp Med* 188:2187, 1998.

68. Ortiz-Stern A, Rosales C: Cross-talk between Fc receptors and integrins. *Immunol Lett* 90:137, 2003.

69. Gonzalez-Amaro R, Sanchez-Madrid F: Cell adhesion molecules: Selectins and integrins. *Crit Rev Immunol* 19:389, 1999.

70. McEver RP, Cummings RD: Perspectives series: Cell adhesion in vascular biology. Role of PSGL-1 binding to selectins in leukocyte recruitment. *J Clin Invest* 100:485, 1997.

71. Urzainqui A, Serrador JM, Viedma F, et al: ITAM-based interaction of ERM proteins with Syk mediates signaling by the leukocyte adhesion receptor PSGL-1. *Immunity* 17:401, 2002.

72. van Buul JD, Mul FP, van der Schoot CE, et al: ICAM-3 activation modulates cell-cell contacts of human bone marrow endothelial cells. *J Vasc Res* 41:28, 2004.

73. Neelamegham S, Taylor AD, Shankaran H, et al: Shear and time-dependent changes in Mac-1, LFA-1, and ICAM-3 binding regulate neutrophil homotypic adhesion. *J Immunol* 164:3798, 2000.

74. Hart SP, Ross JA, Ross K, et al: Molecular characterization of the surface of apoptotic neutrophils: Implications for functional downregulation and recognition by phagocytes. *Cell Death Differ* 7:493, 2000.

75. Pluskota E, Soloviev DA, Bdeir K, et al: Integrin alphaMbeta2 orchestrates and accelerates plasminogen activation and fibrinolysis by neutrophils. *J Biol Chem* 279:18063, 2004.

76. Sitrin RG, Johnson DR, Pan PM, et al: Lipid raft compartmentalization of urokinase receptor signaling in human neutrophils. *Am J Respir Cell Mol Biol* 30:233, 2004.

77. Cicchetti G, Allen PG, Glogauer M: Chemotactic signaling pathways in neutrophils: from receptor to actin assembly. *Crit Rev Oral Biol Med* 13:220, 2002.

78. Paclet MH, Davis C, Kotsonis P, et al: N-Formyl peptide receptor subtypes in human neutrophils activate L-plastin phosphorylation through different signal transduction intermediates. *Biochem J* 377:469, 2004.

79. Bae YS, Yi HJ, Lee HY, et al: Differential activation of formyl peptide receptor-like 1 by peptide ligands. *J Immunol* 171:6807, 2003.

80. Bae YS, Park JC, He R, et al: Differential signaling of formyl peptide receptor-like 1 by Trp-Lys-Tyr-Met-Val-Met-CONH2 or lipoxin A4 in human neutrophils. *Mol Pharmacol* 64:721, 2003.

81. Wetsel RA: Structure, function and cellular expression of complement anaphylatoxin receptors. *Curr Opin Immunol* 7:48, 1995.

82. Cheng SS, Kunkel SL: The evolving role of the neutrophil in chemokine networks. *Chem Immunol Allergy* 83:81, 2003.

83. Ishii I, Izumi T, Tsukamoto H, et al: Alanine exchanges of polar amino acids in the transmembrane domains of a platelet-activating factor receptor generate both constitutively active and inactive mutants. *J Biol Chem* 272:7846, 1997.

84. Tager AM, Luster AD: BLT1 and BLT2: The leukotriene B(4) receptors. *Prostaglandins Leukot Essent Fatty Acids* 69:123, 2003.

85. Foxman EF, Kunkel EJ, Butcher EC: Integrating conflicting chemotactic signals. The role of memory in leukocyte navigation. *J Cell Biol* 147:577, 1999.

86. Endres G, Hegert L: Mineralzusammensetzung der bluplättchen und weissen blukörperchen. *Z Biol* 88:451, 1929.

87. Williams NR, Rajput-Williams J, West JA, et al: Plasma, granulocyte and mononuclear cell copper and zinc in patients with diabetes mellitus. *Analyst* 120:887, 1995.

88. Prasad AS, Mantzoros CS, Beck FW, et al: Zinc status and serum testosterone levels of healthy adults. *Nutrition* 12:344, 1996.

89. Loun B, Astles R, Copeland KR, et al: Intracellular magnesium content of mononuclear blood cells and granulocytes isolated from leukemic, infected, and granulocyte colony-stimulating factor-treated patients. *Clin Chem* 41.1768, 1995.

90. Rukgauer M, Zeyfang A, Uhland K, et al: Isolation of corpuscular components of whole blood for the determination of selenium in blood cells. *J Trace Elem Med Biol* 9:130, 1995.

91. Rigas DA: Electrolyte, nitrogen, and water content of human leukemic leukocytes: Relation to cell maturity. *J Lab Clin Med* 58:234, 1961.

92. Rauch HC, Loomis ME, Johnson ME, et al: In vitro suppression of polymorphonuclear leukocyte and lymphocyte glycolysis by cortisol. *Endocrinology* 68:375, 1961.

93. Martin SP, McKinney GR, Green R, et al: The influence of glucose, fructose, and insulin on the metabolism of leukocytes of healthy and diabetic subjects. *J Clin Invest* 32:1171, 1953.

94. Scott RB: Glycogen in human peripheral blood leukocytes. I. Characteristics of the synthesis and turnover of glycogen in vitro. *J Clin Invest* 47:344, 1968.

95. Scott RB, Still WJ: Glycogen in human peripheral blood leukocytes. II. The macromolecular state of leukocyte glycogen. *J Clin Invest* 47:353, 1968.

96. Esman V: The glycogen content of WBC from diabetic and nondiabetic subjects. *Scand J Lab Invest* 13:134, 1961.

97. McMenamy RH, Lund CC, Neville GJ, et al: Studies of unbound amino acid distributions in plasma, erythrocytes, leukocytes and urine of normal human subjects. *J Clin Invest* 39:1675, 1960.

98. Thornalley PJ, Bellavite P: Modification of the glyoxalase system during the functional activation of human neutrophils. *Biochim Biophys Acta* 931:120, 1987.

99. Beutler E, Kuhl W: 1991. Unpublished.

100. Gottfried EL: Lipids of human leukocytes: relation to cell type. *J Lipid Res* 8:321, 1967.

101. Gottfried EL: Lipid patterns of leukocytes in health and disease. *Semin Hematol* 9:241, 1972.

102. Boyd EM: The lipid content of the white blood cells in normal young women. *J Biol Chem* 101:623, 1933.

103. Boyd EM, Stephens DJ: A comparison of lipid composition with differential count of the white blood cells. *Proc Soc Exp Biol Med* 33:558, 1936.

104. Kidson C: Relation of leucocyte lipid metabolism to cell age: Studies in infective leucocytosis. *Br J Exp Pathol* 42:597, 1961.

105. Nishizuka Y: Studies and perspectives of protein kinase C. *Science* 233: 305, 1986.

106. Berridge MJ, Irvine RF: Inositol trisphosphate, a novel second messenger in cellular signal transduction. *Nature* 312:315, 1984.

107. Symington FW, Murray WA, Bearman SI, et al: Intracellular localization of lactosylceramide, the major human neutrophil glycosphingolipid. *J Biol Chem* 262:11356, 1987.

108. Willoughby HW, Waisman HA: Nucleic acid precursors and nucleotides in normal and leukemic blood. I. comparison of formic acid chromatograms. *Cancer Res* 17:942, 1957.

109. Silber R, Gabrio BW, Huennekens FM: Studies on normal and leukemic leukocytes. III. Pyridine nucleotides. *J Clin Invest* 41:230, 1962.

110. Silber R, Unger KW, Ellman L: RNA metabolism in normal and leukaemic leucocytes: further studies on RNA synthesis. *Br J Haematol* 14:261, 1968.

111. Tryfiates GP, Laszlo J: Human leukemic polyribosomes. *Proc Soc Exp Biol Med* 124:1125, 1967.

112. Garcia AM, Iorio R: Studies on DNA in leukocytes and related cells of mammals. V. The fast green-histone and the Feulgen-DNA content of rat leukocytes. *Acta Cytol* 12:46, 1968.

113. Noyes BE, Mevarech M, Stein R, et al: Detection and partial sequence analysis of gastrin mRNA by using an oligodeoxynucleotide probe. *Proc Natl Acad Sci U S A* 76:1770, 1979.

114. Löhr GW, Waller HD: Zellstoffwechsel und zellalterung. *Klin Wochenschr* 37:833, 1959.

115. Swendseid ME, Bethell FH, Bird OD: The concentration of folic acid in leukocytes; observations on normal subjects and persons with leukemia. *Cancer Res* 11:864, 1951.

116. Smits G, Florijn E: The aneurin pyrophosphate content of red and white blood corpuscles in the rat and in man, in various states of aneurin provision and in disease. *Biochim Biophys Acta* 3:44, 1949.

117. Boxer GE, Pruss MP, Goodhart RS: Pyridoxal-5-phosphoric acid in whole blood and isolated leukocytes of man and animals. *J Nutr* 63:623, 1957.

118. Barkhan P, Howard AN: Distribution of ascorbic acid in normal and leukaemic human blood. *Biochem J* 70:163, 1958.

119. Hoffbrand AV, Newcombe BF: Leucocyte folate in vitamin B12 and folate deficiency and in leukaemia. *Br J Haematol* 13:954, 1967.

120. Beck WS, Valentine WN: The aerobic carbohydrate metabolism of leukocytes in health and leukemia. I. Glycolysis and respiration. *Cancer Res* 12:818, 1952.

121. Beck WS: A kinetic analysis of the glycolytic rate and certain glycolytic enzymes in normal and leucemic leucocytes. *J Biol Chem* 216:333, 1955.

122. Borregaard N, Herlin T: Energy metabolism of human neutrophils during phagocytosis. *J Clin Invest* 70:550, 1982.

123. Lane TA, Beutler E, West C, et al: Glycolytic enzymes of stored granulocytes. *Transfusion* 24:153, 1984.

124. Fauth U, Schlechtriemen T, Heinrichs W, et al: The measurement of enzyme activities in the resting human polymorphonuclear leukocyte— Critical estimate of a method. *Eur J Clin Chem Clin Biochem* 31:5, 1993.

125. Stjernholm RL, Burns CP, Hohnadel JH: Carbohydrate metabolism by leukocytes. *Enzyme* 13:7, 1972.

126. Sbarra AJ, Karnovsky ML: The biochemical basis of phagocytosis. I. Metabolic changes during the ingestion of particles by polymorphonuclear leukocytes. *J Biol Chem* 234:1355, 1959.

127. Beck WS: Occurrence and control of the phosphogluconate oxidation pathway in normal and leukemic leukocytes. *J Biol Chem* 232:271, 1958.

128. Stjernholm RL, Manak RC: Carbohydrate metabolism in leukocytes. XIV. Regulation of pentose cycle activity and glycogen metabolism during phagocytosis. *J Reticuloendothel Soc* 8:550, 1970.

129. Wood HG, Katz J, Landau BR: Estimation of pathways of carbohydrate metabolism. *Biochem Z* 338:809, 1963.

130. Borregaard N, Juhl H: Activation of the glycogenolytic cascade in human polymorphonuclear leucocytes by different phagocytic stimuli. *Eur J Clin Invest* 11:257, 1981.

131. Wachstein M: The distribution of histochemically demonstrable glycogen in human blood and bone marrow cells. *Blood* 4:54, 1949.

132. Beutler E, West C: 1993. Unpublished.

133. Cassatella MA: Neutrophil-derived proteins: Selling cytokines by the pound. *Adv Immunol* 73:369, 1999.

134. Scapini P, Lapinet-Vera JA, Gasperini S, et al: The neutrophil as a cellular source of chemokines. *Immunol Rev* 177:195, 2000.

135. Boneberg EM, Hartung T: Molecular aspects of anti-inflammatory action of G-CSF. *Inflamm Res* 51:119, 2002.

136. Cloutier A, McDonald PP: Transcription factor activation in human neutrophils. *Chem Immunol Allergy* 83:1, 2003.

137. Galligan C, Yoshimura T: Phenotypic and functional changes of cytokine-activated neutrophils. *Chem Immunol Allergy* 83:24, 2003.

138. Girard D: Phenotypic and functional change of neutrophils activated by cytokines utilizing the common cytokine receptor gamma chain. *Chem Immunol Allergy* 83:64, 2003.

139. Tsukahara Y, Lian Z, Zhang X, et al: Gene expression in human neutrophils during activation and priming by bacterial lipopolysaccharide. *J Cell Biochem* 89:848, 2003.

140. Malcolm KC, Arndt PG, Manos EJ, et al: Microarray analysis of lipopolysaccharide-treated human neutrophils. *Am J Physiol Lung Cell Mol Physiol* 284:L663, 2003.

141. Theilgaard-Monch K, Knudsen S, Follin P, et al: The transcriptional activation program of human neutrophils in skin lesions supports their important role in wound healing. *J Immunol* 172:7684, 2004.

142. Kobayashi SD, Voyich JM, Braughton KR, et al: Gene expression profiling provides insight into the pathophysiology of chronic granulomatous disease. *J Immunol* 172:636, 2004.

143. Kobayashi SD, Voyich JM, Braughton KR, et al: Down-regulation of proinflammatory capacity during apoptosis in human polymorphonuclear leukocytes. *J Immunol* 170:3357, 2003.

PRODUCTION, DISTRIBUTION, AND FATE OF NEUTROPHILS

C. WAYNE SMITH

The neutrophil count in the blood is maintained in a normal steady state by the balance among neutropoiesis in the marrow, the distribution of neutrophils between the marginated pool in the microvasculature and the freely circulating pool in the blood, and the rate of egress from blood to tissues. Marrow production is regulated by three principal glycoprotein hormones, or cytokines: interleukin-3, granulocyte-monocyte colony stimulating factor, and granulocyte colony stimulating factors. The latter two cytokines are available as recombinant pharmaceutical products that can be administered therapeutically to ameliorate certain causes of neutropenia. Neutrophil interaction with endothelium is mediated by selectins, polypeptides that contain sugar-binding sites and enter tissues in response to inflammatory mediators by the up-regulation and exposure of integrins on the neutrophil and endothelial cell, permitting firm attachment to endothelium and emigration into tissues through intercellular junctions under the influence of chemoattractant chemicals. Neutrophils have a short life span in blood, with a half-disappearance time of approximately 7 hours. The process can be accelerated when inflammation is present and highlights the need for a sustained rate of production to maintain a normal blood neutrophil count. The pathogenesis of neutropenia is more complex to analyze kinetically than anemia or thrombocytopenia because at least four compartments are involved: marrow storage pool, circulating pool, marginated pool, and tissue pool. The latter is particularly difficult to assay. Measurements can be further complicated in the nonsteady state, when dramatic increases in turnover rates and distribution among the four principal pools are in disequilibrium, as occurs during acute inflammatory states.

INTRODUCTION

Neutrophils are produced in the marrow, where they arise from progenitor and precursor cells by a process of cellular proliferation and maturation. They differentiate from the pluripotential stem cell[1,2] through a series of progressively more committed progenitor or colony forming units, including the granulocyte-monocyte colony forming unit and the granulocyte colony forming unit, which give rise to neutrophils.[3,4] The early progenitor cells cannot be recognized under the microscope but can be identified by marrow culture (see Chap. 15). The earliest microscopically recognizable neutrophil precursor is the myeloblast. From there, the formal sequence of precursor development is myeloblast → promyelocyte → myelocyte → metamyelocyte → band neutrophil → segmented neutrophil (see Chap. 59). The term *granulocyte* often is loosely used to refer to neutrophils but strictly speaking includes eosinophils and basophils. Eosinophilic (see Chap. 62) and basophilic granulocytes (see Chap. 63) develop from progenitors in a manner analogous to the neutrophils, although commitment to neutrophilic, eosinophilic, or basophilic development probably is established at an early progenitor stage.

The normal human neutrophil production rate is 0.85 to 1.6×10^9 cells/kg/day. Mature neutrophils are stored in the marrow before they are released into the blood. They leave the circulation randomly, with a half-disappearance time of approximately 7 hours. The cells then enter the tissues and probably function for 1 or 2 days before their death or loss into the gastrointestinal tract through mucosal surfaces.

The neutropoietic system has a high production volume, yet it is finely modulated in the steady state and has a great capacity to increase production in response to inflammatory stimuli. This chapter outlines current concepts of neutrophil production, distribution, and survival. For detailed data and methods, the reader is referred to original articles and reviews on neutropoiesis and neutrophil kinetics.[5–17]

REGULATION OF NEUTROPHILIC GRANULOPOIESIS

Although the primary cellular manifestation of commitment is the expression of receptors for lineage-specific hematopoietins, the "decision" for a stem cell to self-renew or differentiate may be partly a random or stochastic event.[1,18] On the other hand, stromal elements, collectively referred to as the *hematopoietic microenvironment*, release short-range signals that regulate the process of commitment from multipotential stem cell pools. Although many details of hematopoietic stem cell regulation (see Chap. 4) remain to be elucidated, much is known regarding the interaction of hematopoietic cytokines with their receptors and actions on the committed granulocyte progenitor cells and their mature progeny.[19–24]

HUMORAL REGULATORS

The humoral regulators involved in granulopoiesis have been defined by *in vitro* culture systems.[20,21] Originally identified by their ability to stimulate colony formation from marrow progenitor cells, the hemopoietins (cytokines) came to be called *colony stimulating factors* (CSF).[25] With regard to neutrophil production, at least four human CSFs have been defined. Granulocyte-monocyte colony stimulating factor (GM-CSF) is a 22,000 relative molecular mass (M_r) glycoprotein that stimulates the production of neutrophils, monocytes, and eosinophils. Granulocyte colony stimulating factor (G-CSF) has an M_r of 20,000 and stimulates only the production of neutrophils. Interleukin-3 (IL-3), or multi-CSF, also has an M_r of 20,000 and acts relatively early in hematopoiesis, affecting pluripotential stem cells. Finally, stem cell factor (also known as c-*kit* ligand or steel factor), with an M_r of 28,000, acts in combination with IL-3 and/or GM-CSF to stimulate the proliferation of the early hematopoietic progenitor cells. In addition to their effects on neutrophil precursors, G-CSF and GM-CSF act directly on the neutrophil, enhancing its function. These cytokines regulate the production, survival, and functional activity of neutrophils.[21,22,26–28] The mature neutrophil lacks IL-3 receptors and thus is not affected by IL-3. However, IL-3 receptors are present on mature eosinophils and monocytes. IL-3 is produced by activated T lymphocytes and thus is expected to have a physiologic role in circumstances of cell-mediated immunity. GM-CSF also is produced by activated lymphocytes. However, like G-CSF, it also is elaborated by mononuclear phagocytes and endothelial and mesenchymal cells when these cell types are stimulated by certain cytokines, including IL-1 and tumor necrosis factor, or bacterial products, such as endotoxin.[29–31] Stem

---

cell factor is secreted by a variety of cells, including marrow stromal cells,[32,33] and affects the development of several kinds of tissues.[32,34]

The activities of exogenously administered biosynthetic (recombinant) human G-CSF and GM-CSF in humans are well documented.[22,27,35–37] G-CSF administration rapidly induces neutrophilia, whereas GM-CSF causes an increase in neutrophils, eosinophils, and monocytes. GM-CSF cannot be detected easily in normal plasma; thus, its role as a day-to-day, long-range modulator of neutrophil production is uncertain. Mice in which the GM-CSF gene is "knocked out" have generally normal hematopoiesis but show macrophage abnormalities, pulmonary alveolar proteinosis, and decreased resistance to microbial challenge.[38–41] However, G-CSF appears to be a critical regulator of neutrophil development, as giving an animal an antibody to G-CSF leads to profound neutropenia.[42] The G-CSF knockout mouse shows severe neutropenia.[43] Neutropenia that results from a production disturbance, such as exposure to cytotoxic drugs, is associated with high circulating serum concentrations of G-CSF.[44]

NEUTROPHIL KINETICS

Methods used to study granulocyte kinetics can be categorized as follows: (1) neutrophil depletion or destruction to determine the size and rate of mobilization of reserves and the level of compensatory neutropoiesis; (2) use of radioactive tracers to study neutrophil distribution, production rates, and survival times; (3) mitotic indices of marrow granulocytic cells to assess proliferative activity and cell cycle times; and (4) induced inflammatory lesions to study cell movement into the tissues. Of these categories, the most popular has been the use of radioactive tracers.

Neutrophil production and neutrophil kinetics usually are analyzed by describing neutrophil movement through a number of interconnected compartments. These compartments can be arranged into three major groups: the marrow, the blood, and the tissue (Fig. 61-1).

THE MARROW

Marrow neutrophils can be divided into the mitotic, or proliferative, compartment (see Color Plates X-1–8) and the maturation storage compartment. Myeloblasts, promyelocytes, and myelocytes are capa-

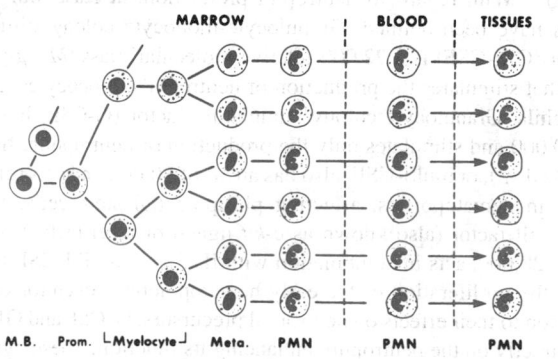

FIGURE 61-1   Scheme of maturation of neutrophil precursor cells. The myeloblast (MB) is the first recognizable precursor of neutrophils. Myeloblasts undergo division and maturation into promyelocytes (Prom) and thereafter into neutrophilic myelocytes (Myelocyte), after which stage mitotic capability is lost. The major compartments of precursor proliferation and distribution are indicated across the top of the figure: marrow, blood, and tissues. The marrow precursor compartment is made up of the proliferating compartment (myeloblasts through myelocytes) and the maturation and storage compartment [metamyelocytes (Meta) to mature polymorphonuclear neutrophils (PMN)]. Under normal conditions, cells do not return from the tissue compartment to the blood or marrow.

TABLE 61-1   MARROW NEUTROPHIL KINETICS

	FRACTION IN MITOSIS (MITOTIC INDEX)	FRACTION IN DNA SYNTHESIS (S PHASE)	TRANSIT TIME RANGE (H)	TOTAL CELLS ($\times 10^9$/kg)
Mitotic compartment				
Myeloblast	0.025	0.85	23	0.14
Promyelocyte	0.015	0.65	26–78	0.51
Myelocyte	0.011	0.33	17–126	1.95
Maturation storage compartment				
Metamyelocyte			8–108	2.7
Band			12–96	3.6
Polymorphonuclear neutrophil			0–120	2.5

SOURCE: Cronkite and Fliedner[11] and Donohue et al.[13]

ble of replication and constitute the mitotic compartment. Earlier progenitor cells are few in number, not morphologically identifiable, and usually neglected in kinetic studies. Metamyelocytes, bands, and mature neutrophils, none of which replicate, constitute the maturation storage compartment.

The number of cell divisions from the myeloblast to the myelocyte stage in the proliferative compartment has been estimated at between four and five.[45] Data obtained using radioactive diisopropyl fluorophosphate (DF^{32}P) suggest the existence of three divisions at the myelocyte stage, but the number of cell divisions at each step may not be constant. The major increase in neutrophil number probably occurs at the myelocyte level, because the myelocyte pool is at least four times the size of the promyelocyte pool. Because of the difficulties in measuring human intramarrow neutrophil kinetics, a precise model of the dynamics of the mitotic compartment is not available.

Table 61-1 lists the estimated sizes of the marrow neutrophil compartments and the transit times and cell cycle stages of the cells in the various compartments. Precise studies have measured a postmitotic pool of $(5.59 \pm 0.9) \times 10^9$ cells/kg and a mitotic pool (promyelocytes and myelocytes) of $(2.11 \pm 0.36) \times 10^9$ cells/kg. These studies led to a calculated normal marrow neutrophil production of 0.85×10^9 cells/kg/day. Radioautographic studies with [^{3}H]thymidine support the concept of an orderly progression from metamyelocytes to mature neutrophils within the maturation storage compartment. These studies also suggest a "first in, first out" pattern for cells leaving this compartment and entering the blood. Several labeling techniques indicate the myelocyte-to-blood transit time is 5 to 7 days.[12,46] Previous studies with DF^{32}P reported a range from 8 to 14 days.[9,45] During infections, however, the myelocyte-to-blood transit time may be as short as 48 hours.[47]

Whether the production of neutrophils in the mitotic compartment exactly equals the neutrophil turnover rate (NTR) is not known with certainty. Studies in dogs have suggested some immature neutrophils die in the marrow ("ineffective granulopoiesis").[48] Ineffective granulopoiesis has not been shown in normal humans,[14,49] although ineffective granulopoiesis occurs in some pathologic states. In the myelodysplastic syndromes,[50] substantial intramedullary cell death (see Chap. 86) probably occurs, as may occur in myelofibrosis and some of the idiopathic neutropenic disorders. At present, however, no convenient means of quantitating ineffective granulopoiesis is available.

On completion of maturation, the neutrophils are stored in the marrow and are referred to as the *mature neutrophil reserve*. The reserve contains many more cells than are normally circulating in the blood. Table 61-2 lists comparative data on the characteristics of the maturation storage compartment. Under stress, maturation time may

TABLE 61-2 COMPARATIVE DATA ON MARROW MATURATION STORAGE
COMPARTMENT

SIZE (CELLS × 10⁹ kg)	TRANSIT TIME (DAYS)	MEASUREMENT TECHNIQUE	REFERENCE
6.5–13	4–8	[³H]thymidine, in vitro DF³²P	5
3–23	8–14	In vivo and in vitro DF³²P	45
5.6	6.6	⁵⁹Fe and neutrophil/erythroid ratio	14

be shortened, divisions may be skipped, and release into the blood
may occur prematurely.

THE BLOOD

Neutrophils leave the marrow storage compartment and enter the blood
without significant reentry into the marrow. The total blood neutrophil
pool (TBNP) consists of all the neutrophils in the vascular spaces.
Some of these neutrophils are free in the circulation (the circulating
pool), while others roll along the endothelium of small vessels or are
temporarily sequestered in the alveolar capillaries of the lung[51,52] (the
marginated pool). Cells in the two pools are freely exchangeable.
When neutrophils labeled with DF³²P are injected into normal subjects,
approximately half can be accounted for in the circulating pool; the
remainder enters the marginated pool.[5–7] Neutrophils shift from the
marginated to the circulating pool with exercise, epinephrine injection,
or stress, but eventually the neutrophils leave the blood and enter the
tissues. Once the neutrophils enter the tissues, they do not normally
return to the blood. The flow of cells is unidirectional.

Rate of Neutrophil Disappearance DF³²P labeled neutrophils
disappear from the circulation with a half-time ($T_{1/2}$) of 6.7 hours.[7,53,54]
These data are supported by the finding that more than half of Pelger-
Huët cells infused into a normal individual disappeared after 6 to 8
hours.[55] Data obtained with ⁵¹Cr-labeled neutrophils give substantially
longer half-times.[56] The exponential disappearance of cells from the
blood suggests the cells leave in a random manner. Thus, neutrophils
newly released from the marrow are as likely to leave the blood as are
neutrophils that have been circulating for several hours. Neutrophils
also are eliminated by programmed cell death and disposed of by the
macrophage system.[47,57–59]

Direct observations of blood vessels have revealed some degree
of leukocyte rolling along the endothelium (first observed many years
ago by Atherton and Born[60]). Although the observation has been
clearly confirmed by numerous laboratories in different species of animals, the extent to which this phenomenon contributes to the marginated pool of neutrophils is uncertain.

The Marginated Pool A more compelling concept of the marginated pool is derived from investigations of the vascular bed of the
lung. A distinctive characteristic of this tissue is the complex inter-
connecting network of short capillary segments where the path from
arteriole to venule crosses several alveolar walls (often >8) and often
contains more than 50 capillary segments.[61–65] Compared to blood in
the large vessels of most vascular beds, the blood in this complex
network contains approximately 50-fold more neutrophils and even
more lymphocytes and monocytes.[66] Videomicroscopic study of these
vessels in animal models has revealed the transit of neutrophils
through this network required a median time of 26 seconds and mean
time of 6.1 seconds.[67,68] In contrast, the transit times of red blood cells
ranges from 1.4 to 4.2 seconds. The increased transit time results primarily from the time neutrophils are stopped within this vascular network. The longer time required for the neutrophils to pass through this
bed apparently accounts for their increased concentration.

Recruitment of neutrophils into the lungs through the alveolar capillary network contrasts with the recruitment of neutrophils through
postcapillary venules at sites of inflammation in a number of important
ways. The tethering mechanisms required to capture neutrophils from
flowing blood in larger vessels apparently are not necessary in the
alveolar capillary bed. The diameters of spherical neutrophils (6–8
μm) are larger than the diameters of many capillary segments (2–15
μm). Approximately 50 percent of the capillary segments would require neutrophils to change their shape in order to pass through.[68–71]
Given the large number of capillary segments through which a neutrophil must pass (often >50), most neutrophils must change shape
during transit from arteriole to venule. Morphometric analysis of neutrophils in the alveolar capillary beds has revealed significant deviation
from spherical shape.[68,69] Computational models of the capillary bed
describing flow, hematocrit, pressure gradients, and the effects of deformation on the capillary transit times of neutrophils support the concept that the structure of the capillary bed and the deformation of
neutrophils are critical under normal conditions. Thus, the enormous
lung vascular bed contains a substantial number of neutrophils that
can be mobilized into the systemic circulation with stimuli such as
epinephrine or exercise.

During inflammation, much of the sequestration and infiltration
occur through vessels so narrow that physical tapping is sufficient to
stop the flowing neutrophil.[64,68,72,73] Binding of mediators such as chemotactic factors (e.g., C5a, the chemotactic fragment of complement
component C5) to neutrophil receptors induces a transient resistance
of the cells to deformation.[74–79] Because neutrophils must deform to
pass through the capillary bed, leukocyte activation by inflammatory
mediators could affect further concentration of neutrophils at the alveolar walls.[61,72] The role of mechanical factors in the initial sequestration of neutrophils in the alveolar capillaries is supported by evidence that neither L-selectin nor β_2-integrins are required.[72,80,81] In
contrast, both selectins and β_2-integrins are required for localization
of neutrophils in postcapillary venules at sites of inflammation.

The events following the initial sequestration of neutrophils within
alveolar capillary beds apparently are influenced by adhesion molecules. For example, simple systemic activation of neutrophils by intravenous injection of chemotactic factors (e.g., IL-8 or C5a) results
in rapid (<1 minute) neutropenia with massive sequestration of neutrophils within alveolar capillaries. This event is not dependent on L-
selectin or β_2-integrins, but the retention times within this capillary
bed are influenced by these adhesion molecules.[72,81] Adhesion likely
is an interaction of leukocyte adhesion molecules and endothelial adhesion molecules. Blockade of the adhesive mechanism (e.g., using
blocking monoclonal antibodies) results in release of neutrophils from
the lungs.[72,80,82–84] Mediator-induced decreases in deformability are temporally correlated with up-regulation of β_2-integrins (e.g., both occurring within approximately 1 minute of exposure to IL-8). This allows
both physical trapping and sticking to the vascular wall within the
alveolar capillary bed. A similar phenomenon occurs in the liver where
sequestration is the result of physical trapping and liver injury is heavily dependent on adhesion of leukocytes through the β_2-integrins.[85]

Neutrophil Turnover Rate Assuming a random loss of neutrophils from the blood, NTR can be calculated from $T_{1/2}$ and TBNP:
NTR = 0.693 × TBNP/$T_{1/2}$. In the steady state, NTR measures the
rate of effective neutrophil production. Table 61-3 lists the definitions
and calculations related to blood neutrophil kinetics. Table 61-4 lists
data for normal human blood neutrophil kinetics. The high production
rate of neutrophils under normal conditions is remarkable, especially
given that the rate may increase several fold in response to inflammatory stimuli.

Effect of Glucocorticoids and Epinephrine Glucocorticoids increase TBNP by increasing influx from the marrow and decreasing

TABLE 61-3 DEFINITIONS AND CALCULATIONS RELATING TO BLOOD NEUTROPHIL KINETICS

Circulating neutrophil pool (CNP)	=	Blood neutrophil concentration × blood volume
Total blood neutrophil pool (TBNP)	=	All neutrophils in the circulation
Marginal neutrophil pool (MNP)	=	Total blood neutrophil pool less circulating pool (MNP = TBNP − CNP)
Blood clearance half-time ($T_{1/2}$)	=	Disappearance time of half the labeled neutrophils from circulation
Neutrophil turnover rate (NTR)	=	$\dfrac{0.693 \times \text{TBNP}}{T_{1/2}}$

efflux from the circulation. Five hours after a pharmacologic dose of glucocorticoid, the neutrophil count increases by approximately 4000/μl because of release from the marrow, demargination, and prolongation of $T_{1/2}$ to approximately 10 hours.[86-88] Consistent with the increase in $T_{1/2}$, prednisone reduces the accumulation of neutrophils at induced sites of skin inflammation.[71] With alternate-day, single-dose prednisone, neutrophil counts and kinetics are normal 24 hours after administration and during the day off.[89] Endotoxin causes a prompt neutropenia as a result of cell margination and sequestration, followed in 2 to 4 hours by a rebound neutrophilia as a result of cell release from the marrow. The size of the neutrophilic response correlates with the functional marrow reserves.[90-93] After epinephrine administration, a peak leukocytosis occurs in 5 to 10 minutes and rarely lasts more than 20 minutes. This finding reflects a shift of cells from the marginated to the circulating pool.

MIGRATION OF NEUTROPHILS INTO TISSUES

The migration of neutrophils from blood into tissue at sites of inflammation involves a series of sequential adhesive steps proceeding from tethering (rolling adhesion) on endothelium under shear conditions in postcapillary venules.[94] This model has been investigated in a variety of vascular beds[95] and *in vitro* with monolayers of endothelial cells in parallel plate flow chambers.[94] The tethering event in this model depends on adhesion molecules in the selectin family, E-selectin and P-selectin on the endothelium, L-selectin on the neutrophil, and ligands for the selectins expressed on both cell types. These adhesion molecules are necessary to efficiently initiate the cascade of adhesive steps ultimately leading to firm attachment of the neutrophils to endothelium. The cascade appears to be necessary for neutrophils to move from blood to tissues because the unstimulated neutrophil is not adhesive to endothelium.[94,96] The integrins necessary for firm adhesion and cell locomotion require stimulation to promote sufficient increases in avidity or affinity to support these functions.

LIFE SPAN OF NEUTROPHILS

After emigrating into tissue, the life span of neutrophils can be significantly prolonged (24–48 hours).[97] Programmed cell death (apoptosis) accounts for significant removal of tissue neutrophils through phagocytosis by macrophages. The constitutive rate of apoptosis of neutrophils is altered by inflammatory cytokines and chemokines. For example, tumor necrosis factor-α accelerates the rate, but endotoxin, G-CSF, GM-CSF, IL-15, and IL-3 inhibit the rate of apoptosis. The balance of these effects at specific inflammatory sites is poorly understood, but the functional life of neutrophils in tissue appears to be controlled by the rate of apoptosis. Apoptotic neutrophils lose the ability to release granular enzymes in response to external stimuli (see below), and marked changes in cell surface proteins occur (e.g., CD16, CD43, CD62L are greatly reduced). Although the loss of responsive-

ness may contribute to resolution of the inflammatory process, evidence indicates macrophages also are altered by the phagocytosis of apoptotic neutrophils. In contrast to the macrophage response to phagocytosis of microbes, where secretion of proinflammatory cytokines (e.g., IL-1β) and chemokines (e.g., IL-8) is stimulated, phagocytosis of apoptotic neutrophils fails to provoke secretion of proinflammatory factors; instead, phagocytosis stimulates release of factors that may suppress inflammatory responses (e.g., transforming growth factor-β and prostaglandin E_2). Macrophage recognition of apoptotic neutrophils is partially understood to involve the vitronectin receptor $\alpha_V\beta_3$ and the thrombospondin receptor CD36 on the macrophage surface. In addition, phosphatidylserine residues on the neutrophil are involved.[98]

As Chapter 60 noted, neutrophils are capable of phenotypic changes depending on the tissue and cytokine/chemokine milieu at the time of their migration into tissue. Because our understanding of neutrophil physiology is relatively new, knowing the extent of this phenomenon on neutrophil life span in tissues is not possible at present.

EVALUATION OF ADEQUACY OF NEUTROPHIL RESERVES

WHITE CELL COUNT AND MARROW CELLULARITY

White cell and absolute neutrophil counts are the most widely used guides to the status of neutrophil production. They are useful in evaluating the effects of cytotoxic chemotherapy, although they do not provide quantitative information on the rate of neutrophil production or destruction, the status of marrow reserves, or the presence of abnormalities in cell distribution.

Gauging neutrophil production by the appearance of marrow films, clot sections, or biopsies suffers from the limitations of sampling error and relatively poor correlation with kinetics, as measured by other techniques.[64] For example, the morphologic findings in the marrow of a "maturation arrest," with little neutrophil development beyond the promyelocyte or myelocyte stage, does not distinguish between a defect in precursor cell maturation and rapid mobilization of postmitotic cells from the marrow. Similarly, distinguishing by purely morphologic means neutropenic conditions resulting from ineffective neutropoiesis from conditions caused by peripheral destruction of neutrophils often is difficult. However, despite these limitations, when the absolute neutrophil count and marrow cellularity are used together, they provide a useful guide in most clinical settings. If the absolute neutrophil count is less than 1000/μl (1.0×10^9/liter) and multiple marrow aspirations and/or biopsies are hypocellular, the patient almost invariably has impaired production of marrow neutrophils. Very low neutrophil counts predispose to infections by bacteria and certain fungi (e.g., *Candida* and *Aspergillus*). Such infections become especially troublesome as the neutrophil count falls below 500/μl (0.5×10^9/liter). Unfortunately, the converse is not true. The finding of cellular marrow and

TABLE 61-4 DATA FOR HUMAN BLOOD NEUTROPHIL KINETICS

POOL	MEAN POOL SIZE × 10^7 kg	95% LIMITS
TBNP	70	14–160
CNP	31	11–46
MNP	39	0–85

	MEAN VALUE	95% LIMITS
Blood clearance $T_{1/2}$	6.7 h	4–10 h
NTR	63×10^7 kg/day	$50–340 \times 10^7$ kg/day

SOURCE: Athens et al.[5-7]
NOTE: For abbreviations, see Table 61-3.

neutrophil count greater than 1000/μl (>1.0 × 10⁹/liter) does not mean production is normal. Nevertheless, when marrow cellularity and absolute neutrophil count are considered together, they provide the most clinically useful assessment of neutrophil production.

FUNCTIONAL EVALUATION

Several agents that increase neutrophil numbers in circulation, including glucocorticoids, endotoxin, and etiocholanolone, have been used to evaluate neutrophil reserves in a clinical setting. These agents have been supplanted by recombinant human G-CSF, a remarkably nontoxic cytokine that, when given in therapeutic doses (5–8 μg/kg), increases the blood neutrophil count by stimulating neutropoiesis and accelerating neutrophil release from the marrow storage compartment (see Chap. 15). The increase in neutropoiesis results from a threefold increase in the number of cell divisions in the mitotic compartment and shortening of the maturation time from myelocyte to neutrophil from 4 to 5 days to less than 1 day.[99–101] Thus, as a byproduct of its therapeutic action, G-CSF administration directly tests an individual's capacity to produce neutrophils. This effect of G-CSF makes obsolete most of the older methods for evaluating neutrophil compartments.

G-CSF does not test the distribution of neutrophils between the marginated and circulating pools. On the rare occasions when such information is desirable, epinephrine stimulation can be used to assess the distribution. For this purpose, epinephrine 0.1 mg is infused intravenously over 5 minutes, and blood for white counts is obtained before and 1, 3, and 5 minutes after completion of the epinephrine infusion. Normally the neutrophils increase by approximately 50 percent after epinephrine infusion.[102]

REFERENCES

1. Kondo M, Wagers AJ, Manz MG, et al: Biology of hematopoietic stem cells and progenitors: Implications for clinical application. *Annu Rev Immunol* 21:759, 2003.
2. Spangrude GJ: When is a stem cell really a stem cell? *Bone Marrow Transplant* 32 (suppl 1):S7, 2003.
3. Smaaland R, Sothern RB, Laerum OD, et al: Rhythms in human bone marrow and blood cells. *Chronobiol Int* 19:101, 2002.
4. Metcalf D: Hematopoietic stem cells: Old and new. *Biomed Pharmacother* 55:75, 2001.
5. Athens JW: Neutrophilic granulocyte kinetics and granulopoiesis, in *Regulation of Hematopoiesis*, edited by AS Gordon, p 1143. Appleton-Century-Crofts, New York, 1970.
6. Athens JW, Raab SO, Haab OP, et al: Leukokinetic studies: III. The distribution of granulocytes in the blood of normal subjects. *J Clin Invest* 40:159, 1961.
7. Athens JW, Haab OP, Raab SO, et al: Leukokinetic studies: IV. The total blood, circulating and marginal granulocyte pools and the granulocyte turnover rate in normal subjects. *J Clin Invest* 40:989, 1961.
8. Boggs DR: The kinetics of neutrophilic leukocytes in health and in disease. *Semin Hematol* 4:359, 1967.
9. Cartwright GE, Athens JW, Boggs DR, et al: The kinetics of granulopoiesis in normal man. *Ser Haematol* 1:1, 1965.
10. Cronkite EP: Kinetics of granulocytopoiesis. *Clin Haematol* 8:351, 1979.
11. Cronkite EP, Fliedner TM: Granulocytopoiesis. *N Engl J Med* 270:1347, 1964.
12. Vincent PC: The measurement of granulocyte kinetics. *Br J Haematol* 36:1, 1977.
13. Donohue DM, Gabrio BW, Finch CA: Quantitative measurement of hematopoietic cells of the marrow. *J Clin Invest* 37:1564, 1958.
14. Dancey JT, Deubelbeiss KA, Harker LA, et al: Neutrophil kinetics in man. *J Clin Invest* 58:705, 1976.
15. Dresch C, Faille A, Rain JD, et al: Granulopoiesis: Comparison of several methods for studying production and bone marrow cellularity [author's translation]. *Nouv Rev Fr Hematol* 15:31, 1975.
16. Simon HU: Neutrophil apoptosis pathways and their modifications in inflammation. *Immunol Rev* 193:101, 2003.
17. Kuijpers TW: Clinical symptoms and neutropenia: The balance of neutrophil development, functional activity, and cell death. *Eur J Pediatr* 161(suppl 1):S75, 2002.
18. Ogawa M: Changing phenotypes of hematopoietic stem cells. *Exp Hematol* 30:3, 2002.
19. Friedman AD: Transcriptional regulation of myelopoiesis. *Int J Hematol* 75:466, 2002.
20. Metcalf D: Hematopoietic regulators: Redundancy or subtlety? *Blood* 82:3515, 1993.
21. Metcalf D: Neutrophilic granulocytes and macrophages: Molecular, cellular, and clinical aspects, in *Regulation of Hematopoiesis*, edited by AS Gordon, p 1143. Appleton-Century-Crofts, New York, 1970.
22. Lieschke GJ, Burgess AW: Granulocyte colony-stimulating factor and granulocyte-macrophage colony-stimulating factor (1). *N Engl J Med* 327:28, 1992.
23. Kaushansky K, Karplus PA: Hematopoietic growth factors: Understanding functional diversity in structural terms. *Blood* 82:3229, 1993.
24. Groopman JE, Molina JM, Scadden DT: Hematopoietic growth factors. Biology and clinical applications. *N Engl J Med* 321:1449, 1989.
25. Barreda DR, Hanington PC, Belosevic M: Regulation of myeloid development and function by colony stimulating factors. *Dev Comp Immunol* 28:509, 2004.
26. Welte K, Gabrilove J, Bronchud MH, et al: Filgrastim (r-metHuG-CSF): The first 10 years. *Blood* 88:1907, 1996.
27. Anderlini P, Przepiorka D, Champlin R, et al: Biologic and clinical effects of granulocyte colony-stimulating factor in normal individuals. *Blood* 88:2819, 1996.
28. Lopez AF, Williamson DJ, Gamble JR, et al: Recombinant human granulocyte-macrophage colony-stimulating factor stimulates in vitro mature human neutrophil and eosinophil function, surface receptor expression, and survival. *J Clin Invest* 78:1220, 1986.
29. Munker R, Gasson J, Ogawa M, et al: Recombinant human TNF induces production of granulocyte-monocyte colony-stimulating factor. *Nature* 323:79, 1986.
30. Zucali JR, Dinarello CA, Oblon DJ, et al: Interleukin 1 stimulates fibroblasts to produce granulocyte-macrophage colony-stimulating activity and prostaglandin E2. *J Clin Invest* 77:1857, 1986.
31. Metcalf D, Nicola NA, Mifsud S, et al: Receptor clearance obscures the magnitude of granulocyte-macrophage colony-stimulating factor responses in mice to endotoxin or local infections. *Blood* 93:1579, 1999.
32. Akin C, Metcalfe DD: The biology of Kit in disease and the application of pharmacogenetics. *J Allergy Clin Immunol* 114:13, 2004.
33. Heissig B, Werb Z, Rafii S, et al: Role of c-kit/Kit ligand signaling in regulating vasculogenesis. *Thromb Haemost* 90:570, 2003.
34. Wehrle-Haller B: The role of Kit-ligand in melanocyte development and epidermal homeostasis. *Pigment Cell Res* 16:287, 2003.
35. Lalami Y, Paesmans M, Aoun M, et al: A prospective randomized evaluation of G-CSF or G-CSF plus oral antibiotics in chemotherapy-treated patients at high risk of developing febrile neutropenia. *Support Care Cancer* 12:725, 2004.
36. De Waele M, Renmans W, Asosingh K, et al: Growth factor receptor profile of CD34 cells in normal bone marrow, cord blood and mobilized peripheral blood. *Eur J Haematol* 72:193, 2004.
37. Crawford J: Neutrophil growth factors. *Curr Hematol Rep* 1:95, 2002.
38. LeVine AM, Reed JA, Kurak KE, et al: GM-CSF-deficient mice are susceptible to pulmonary group B streptococcal infection. *J Clin Invest* 103:563, 1999.

39. Dranoff G, Crawford AD, Sadelain M, et al: Involvement of granulo-cyte-macrophage colony-stimulating factor in pulmonary homeostasis. *Science* 264:713, 1994.

40. Stanley E, Lieschke GJ, Grail D, et al: Granulocyte/macrophage colony-stimulating factor-deficient mice show no major perturbation of hematopoiesis but develop a characteristic pulmonary pathology. *Proc Natl Acad Sci U S A* 91:5592, 1994.

41. Huffman JA, Hull WM, Dranoff G, et al: Pulmonary epithelial cell expression of GM-CSF corrects the alveolar proteinosis in GM-CSF-deficient mice. *J Clin Invest* 97:649, 1996.

42. Hammond WP, Csiba E, Canin A, et al: Chronic neutropenia. A new canine model induced by human granulocyte colony-stimulating factor. *J Clin Invest* 87:704, 1991.

43. Lieschke GJ, Grail D, Hodgson G, et al: Mice lacking granulocyte colony-stimulating factor have chronic neutropenia, granulocyte and macrophage progenitor cell deficiency, and impaired neutrophil mobilization. *Blood* 84:1737, 1994.

44. Mempel K, Pietsch T, Menzel T, et al: Increased serum levels of granulocyte colony-stimulating factor in patients with severe congenital neutropenia. *Blood* 77:1919, 1991.

45. Warner HR, Athens JW: An analysis of granulocyte kinetics in blood and bone marrow. *Ann N Y Acad Sci* 113:523, 1964.

46. Dresch C, Faille A, Bauchet J, et al: Granulopoiesis: Comparison of different methods for studying maturation time and bone marrow storage. *Nouv Rev Fr Hematol* 13:5, 1973.

47. Fliedner TM, Cronkite EP, Robertson JS: Granulocytopoiesis: I. Senescence and random loss of neutrophilic granulocytes in human beings. *Blood* 24:402, 1964.

48. Patt HM, Maloney MA: Kinetics of neutrophil balance, in *The Kinetics of Cellular Proliferation*, edited by F Stohlman Jr, p 201. Grune & Stratton, New York, 1959.

49. Cronkite EP: Enigmas underlying the study of hemopoietic cell proliferation. *Fed Proc* 23:649, 1964.

50. Koeffler HP, Golde DW: Human preleukemia. *Ann Intern Med* 93:347, 1980.

51. Doerschuk CM: Mechanisms of leukocyte sequestration in inflamed lungs. *Microcirculation* 8:71, 2001.

52. Schwab AJ, Salamand A, Merhi Y, et al: Kinetic analysis of pulmonary neutrophil retention in vivo using the multiple-indicator-dilution technique. *J Appl Physiol* 95:279, 2003.

53. Mauer AM, Athens JW, Ashenbrucker H, et al: Leukokinetic studies: II. A method for labeling granulocytes in vitro with radioactive diisopropylfluorophosphate (DFP32). *J Clin Invest* 39:1481, 1960.

54. Bishop CR, Rothstein G, Ashenbrucker HE, et al: Leukokinetic studies: XIV. Blood neutrophil kinetics in chronic, steady-state neutropenia. *J Clin Invest* 50:1678, 1971.

55. Rosse WF, Gurney CW: The Pelger-Huet anomaly in three families and its use in determining the disappearance of transfused neutrophils from the peripheral blood. *Blood* 14:170, 1959.

56. Dresch C, Najean Y, Bauchet J: Kinetic studies of 51Cr and DF32P labeled granulocytes. *Br J Haematol* 29:67, 1975.

57. Maianski NA, Maianski AN, Kuijpers TW, et al: Apoptosis of neutrophils. *Acta Haematol* 111:56, 2004.

58. Edwards SW, Moulding DA, Derouet M, et al: Regulation of neutrophil apoptosis. *Chem Immunol Allergy* 83:204, 2003.

59. Fadeel B, Kagan VE: Apoptosis and macrophage clearance of neutrophils: Regulation by reactive oxygen species. *Redox Rep* 8:143, 2003.

60. Atherton A, Born GV: Effect of blood flow velocity on the rolling of granulocytes in venules. *J Physiol* 231:35P, 1973.

61. Hogg JC: Neutrophil kinetics and lung injury. *Physiol Rev* 67:1249, 1987.

62. Staub NC, Schultz EL: Pulmonary capillary length in dogs, cat, and rabbit. *Respir Physiol* 5:371, 1968.

63. Ambrus CM, Ambrus JL, Johnson GC, et al: Role of the lungs in regulation of the white blood cell level. *Am J Physiol* 178:33, 1954.

64. Doerschuk CM, Allard MF, Martin BA, et al: Marginated pool of neutrophils in rabbit lungs. *J Appl Physiol* 63:1806, 1987.

65. Lien DC, Wagner WW Jr, Capen RL, et al: Physiological neutrophil sequestration in the lung: Visual evidence for localization in capillaries. *J Appl Physiol* 62:1236, 1987.

66. Doerschuk CM, Downey GP, Doherty DE, et al: Leukocyte and platelet margination within microvasculature of rabbit lungs. *J Appl Physiol* 68:1956, 1990.

67. Presson RG Jr, Graham JA, Hanger CC, et al: Distribution of pulmonary capillary red blood cell transit times. *J Appl Physiol* 79:382, 1995.

68. Gebb SA, Graham JA, Hanger CC, et al: Sites of leukocyte sequestration in the pulmonary microcirculation. *J Appl Physiol* 79:493, 1995.

69. Doerschuk CM, Beyers N, Coxson HO, et al: Comparison of neutrophil and capillary diameters and their relation to neutrophil sequestration in the lung. *J Appl Physiol* 74:3040, 1993.

70. Martin BA, Wright JL, Thommasen H, et al: Effect of pulmonary blood flow on the exchange between the circulating and marginating pool of polymorphonuclear leukocytes in dog lungs. *J Clin Invest* 69:1277, 1982.

71. Hogg JC, McLean T, Martin BA, et al: Erythrocyte transit and neutrophil concentration in the dog lung. *J Appl Physiol* 65:1217, 1988.

72. Doerschuk CM: The role of CD18-mediated adhesion in neutrophil sequestration induced by infusion of activated plasma in rabbits. *Am J Resp Cell Mol Biol* 7:140, 1992.

73. Downey GP, Worthen GS, Henson PM, et al: Neutrophil sequestration and migration in localized pulmonary inflammation. Capillary localization and migration across the interalveolar septum. *Am Rev Respir Dis* 147:168, 1993.

74. Brown GM, Brown DM, Donaldson K, et al: Neutrophil sequestration in rat lungs. *Thorax* 50:661, 1995.

75. Buttrum SM, Drost EM, MacNee W, et al: Rheological response of neutrophils to different types of stimulation. *J Appl Physiol* 77:1801, 1994.

76. Downey GP, Doherty DE, Schwab B III, et al: Retention of leukocytes in capillaries: Role of cell size and deformability. *J Appl Physiol* 69:1767, 1990.

77. Downey GP, Worthen GS: Neutrophil retention in model capillaries: Deformability, geometry, and hydrodynamic forces. *J Appl Physiol* 65:1861, 1988.

78. Erzurum SC, Downey GP, Doherty DE, et al: Mechanisms of lipopolysaccharide-induced neutrophil retention. Relative contributions of adhesive and cellular mechanical properties. *J Immunol* 149:154, 1992.

79. Worthen GS, Schwab B III, Elson EL, et al: Mechanics of stimulated neutrophils: Cell stiffening induces retention of capillaries. *Science* 245:183, 1989.

80. Doyle NA, Bhagwan SD, Meek BB, et al: Neutrophil margination, sequestration, and emigration in the lungs of L-selectin-deficient mice. *J Clin Invest* 99:526, 1997.

81. Kubo H, Doyle NA, Graham L, et al: L- and P-selectin and CD11/CD18 in intracapillary neutrophil sequestration in rabbit lungs. *Am J Respir Crit Care Med* 159:267, 1999.

82. Doerschuk CM, Mizgerd JP, Kubo H, et al: Adhesion molecules and cellular biomechanical changes in acute lung injury: Giles F. Filley Lecture. *Chest* 116:37S, 1999.

83. Doerschuk CM, Quinlan WM, Doyle NA, et al: The role of P-selectin and ICAM-1 in acute lung injury as determined using blocking antibodies and mutant mice. *J Immunol* 157:4609, 1996.

84. Lundberg C, Wright SD: Relation of the CD11/CD18 family of leukocyte antigens to the transient neutropenia caused by chemoattractants. *Blood* 76:1240, 1990.

85. Jaeschke H, Farhood A, Fisher MA, et al: Sequestration of neutrophils in the hepatic vasculature during endotoxemia is independent of β_2 integrins and intercellular adhesion molecule-1. *Shock* 6:351, 1996.

86. Bishop CR, Athens JW, Boggs DR, et al: Leukokinetic studies 13. A non-steady-state kinetic evaluation of the mechanism of cortisone-induced granulocytosis. *J Clin Invest* 47:249, 1968.

87. Dale DC, Fauci AS, Guerry D, IV, et al: Comparison of agents producing a neutrophilic leukocytosis in man. Hydrocortisone, prednisone, endotoxin, and etiocholanolone. *J Clin Invest* 56:808, 1975.

88. Stausz I, Barcsak J, Kekes E, et al: Prednisone-induced acute changes in circulating neutrophil granulocytes: I. In cases of normal granulocyte reserves. *Haematologia* 1:319, 1993.

89. Dale DC, Fauci AS, Wolff SM: Alternate-day prednisone. Leukocyte kinetics and susceptibility to infections. *N Engl J Med* 291:1154, 1974.

90. Craddock CG Jr, Perry S, Ventzke LE, et al: Evaluation of marrow granulocytic reserves in normal and disease states. *Blood* 15:840, 1960.

91. Marsh JC, Perry S: The granulocyte response to endotoxin in patients with hematologic disorders. *Blood* 23:581, 1964.

92. DeConti RC, Kaplan SR, Calabresi P: Endotoxin stimulation in patients with lymphoma: Correlation with the myelosuppressive effects of alkylating agents. *Blood* 39:602, 1972.

93. Korbitz BC, Toren FA, Davis HL Jr, et al: The Piromen test: A useful assay of bone marrow granulocyte reserves. *Curr Ther Res Clin Exp* 11: 491, 1969.

94. Smith CW: Possible steps involved in the transition to stationary adhesion of rolling neutrophils: A brief review [in process citation]. *Microcirculation* 7(6 Pt 1):385, 2000.

95. Kubes P, Kerfoot SM: Leukocyte recruitment in the microcirculation: The rolling paradigm revisited. *News Physiol Sci* 16:76, 2001.

96. Ley K: Pathways and bottlenecks in the web of inflammatory adhesion molecules and chemoattractants. *Immunol Res* 24:87, 2001.

97. Haslett C: Granulocyte apoptosis and its role in the resolution and control of lung inflammation. *Am J Respir Crit Care Med* 160:S5, 1999.

98. Fadok VA, Henson PM: Apoptosis: Giving phosphatidylserine recognition an assist—With a twist. *Curr Biol* 13:R655, 2003.

99. Buescher ES, Gallin JI: Leukocyte transfusions in chronic granulomatous disease: Persistence of transfused leukocytes in sputum. *N Engl J Med* 307:800, 1982.

100. Lord BI, Bronchud MH, Owens S, et al: The kinetics of human granulopoiesis following treatment with granulocyte colony-stimulating factor in vivo. *Proc Natl Acad Sci U S A* 86:9499, 1989.

101. Lord BI, Gurney H, Chang J, et al: Haemopoietic cell kinetics in humans treated with rGM-CSF. *Int J Cancer* 50:26, 1992.

102. Buchanan MR, Crowley CA, Rosin RE, et al: Studies on the interaction between GP-180 deficient neutrophils and vascular endothelium. *Blood* 60:160, 1982.

EOSINOPHILS AND THEIR DISORDERS

ANDREW WARDLAW

The potential role of the eosinophil in asthma has resulted in intense research on this cell. The concept of the eosinophil as a cell that has protective effects against helminthic parasite infection but can cause tissue damage when inappropriately activated remains intact, although the evidence for the two roles remains circumstantial. Eosinophil production and function are profoundly influenced by interleukin-5 (IL-5). Thus, eosinophilia is associated with diseases characterized by T helper 2 (Th2)-mediated immune responses, including helminthic parasite infections and extrinsic asthma. However, eosinophilia also occurs in diseases not associated with Th2 dominance, such as intrinsic asthma, hypereosinophilic syndrome, and inflammatory bowel disease. IL-5 and other eosinophil mediators can be generated in various types of inflammatory response.

The eosinophil, like other leukocytes, can generate proinflammatory mediators. Eosinophil-specific granule proteins are toxic for a range of mammalian cells and parasitic larvae. Eosinophils, like mast cells, produce sulfidopeptide leukotrienes and other lipid mediators such as platelet-activating factor. Cytokine production by eosinophils broadens their potential functions, for example, in wound healing through the generation of transforming growth factor alpha. Synthesis of transforming growth factor beta may explain the propensity of eosinophils to be associated with fibrotic reactions such as endomyocardial fibrosis, characteristic of hypereosinophilic syndrome, and fibrosing alveolitis.

The selective accumulation of eosinophils in tissues results from a concerted and integrated series of events involving marrow egress, adhesion to endothelium, selective chemotaxis, and prolonged survival in tissues. The events are controlled, either directly or indirectly, by production of IL-4, IL-5, and IL-13.

The hypereosinophilic syndrome is a heterogenous group of disorders, principally neoplastic rather than inflammatory. A proportion of patients with hypereosinophilic syndrome have either a clonal abnormality in myeloid cells expressing largely the eosinophilic lineage resulting from a constitutively active tyrosine kinase (FLT1L1-PDGFR-α) (in effect chronic eosinophilic leukemia) or a subclinical clonal expansion of T cells (in effect a T cell lymphoma) liberating eosinophilic cytokines and inducing a reactive eosinophilia. Recognition of these disorders has provided new and more effective treatments for the condition and has given new insights into the control of eosinophil production.

Acronyms and abbreviations that appear in this chapter include: ECP, eosinophil cationic protein; EDN, eosinophil-derived neurotoxin; EPO, eosinophil peroxidase; GM-CSF, granulocyte-monocyte colony stimulating factor; HES, hypereosinophilic syndrome; HLA, human leukocyte antigen; ICAM, intercellular cell adhesion molecule; Ig, immunoglobulin; IL, interleukin; LAMP, lysosome-associated membrane protein; LIMP, lysosome integral membrane protein; LT, leukotriene; MAb, monoclonal antibody; MAdCAM-1, mucosal addressin cell adhesion molecule; MBP, major basic protein; PAF, platelet-activating factor; PECAM: platelet endothelial cell adhesion molecule; PSGL-1, P-selectin glycoprotein ligand-1; Siglec, sialic acid-recognizing lectin; TGF, transforming growth factor; T$_{reg}$, T regulatory; TRAIL, tumor necrosis factor-related apoptosis-inducing ligand; VCAM, vascular cell adhesion molecule; VLA, very late antigen.

BIOLOGY OF EOSINOPHILS

EOSINOPHIL MORPHOLOGY AND RECEPTOR PHENOTYPE

Eosinophils are 8-μm spherical diameter, end-stage, nondividing leukocytes derived from the marrow under the influence of granulocyte-monocyte colony stimulating factor (GM-CSF), interleukin (IL)-3, and IL-5. The electron microscopic morphology of the mature eosinophil has been well described (Figure 62-1).[1,2] Color Plate VII-3 depicts the light microscopic features of eosinophils. Chapter 59 provides a more detailed description of eosinophil ultrastructure. The relatively specific features that distinguish the eosinophil from other leukocytes are the bilobed nucleus, the approximately 20 specific granules with their electron-dense core, the paucity of mitochondria (approximately 20 per cell) and endoplasmic reticulum, and the dense network of cytoplasmic tubulovesicular structures or secretory vesicles that contain albumin and cytochrome b558 and are thought to be involved in superoxide production. Eosinophils also contain approximately five lipid bodies that are the major site of eicosanoid synthesis, primary granules, and small granules. Small granules are particularly prominent in tissue eosinophils and contain arylsulfatase B, acid phosphatase, and catalase. They can be derived from specific granules and act as a lysosomal compartment, especially as specific granules have been shown to express lysosome-associated membrane protein (LAMP)-1 and LAMP-2 and lysosome integral membrane protein-1 (LIMP-1: CD63).[3] Eosinophils also contain multilaminar bodies that contain transforming growth factor alpha (TGF-α). Eosinophil precursors derived from cord blood can be first identified morphologically when specific core-containing granules appear, although expression of Charcot-Leyden crystal protein and the basic granule proteins can be detected by immunohistochemistry or mRNA expression at the promyelocyte stage where they are found in the endoplasmic reticulum, Golgi apparatus, and large round coreless granules, most of which develop into specific granules. Electron microscopy can distinguish activated from resting blood eosinophils by the increased number of lipid bodies, primary and small granules, secretory vesicles, and endoplasmic reticulum. Cytoplasmic Charcot-Leyden crystal protein may be present. Activated eosinophils often are less dense than resting cells. However, with the advent of immunomagnetic selection rather than a density gradient to purify eosinophils, density is used less often as a marker of activation.[4] Eosinophils are weakly phagocytic, although they can ingest opsonized zymosan, which is taken up into phagolysosomes formed in part by fusion with specific granules. The eosinophil also degranulates onto large opsonized surfaces such as a Sephadex bead or parasitic larvae in a process called "frustrated phagocytosis."

The ultrastructure of in vitro-activated and tissue-infiltrating eosinophils has suggested three potential mechanisms of degranulation: necrosis or cytolytic degranulation, exocytosis or "classic degranulation," and piecemeal degranulation.[5] Cytolytic degranulation is associated with loss of eosinophil plasma membrane integrity and results in the release of clusters of free membrane-bound eosinophil granules. This is commonly observed in eosinophilic inflammation and is particularly marked in severe disease such as fatal cases of asthma where large quantities of basic proteins can be detected in the tissue by immunohistochemistry, often with relatively few intact eosinophils.[6] This type of degranulation is also a feature of milder disease such as allergic rhinitis[7,8] and Fc-mediated degranulation in vitro.[9] Exocytosis or classic degranulation occurs in mast cells and basophils after cross-linking of IgE receptors. It describes a process in which granules migrate to the plasma membrane and fuse with it, leading to extrusion of membrane-free granule contents. The process has been described for eosinophils in the gut but not the airway mucosa. Piecemeal degranulation was described in cord blood derived eosinophils.[10] The term describes the appearance of empty or partially empty granules that retain their structure and small granule protein-containing vesicles in the cyto-

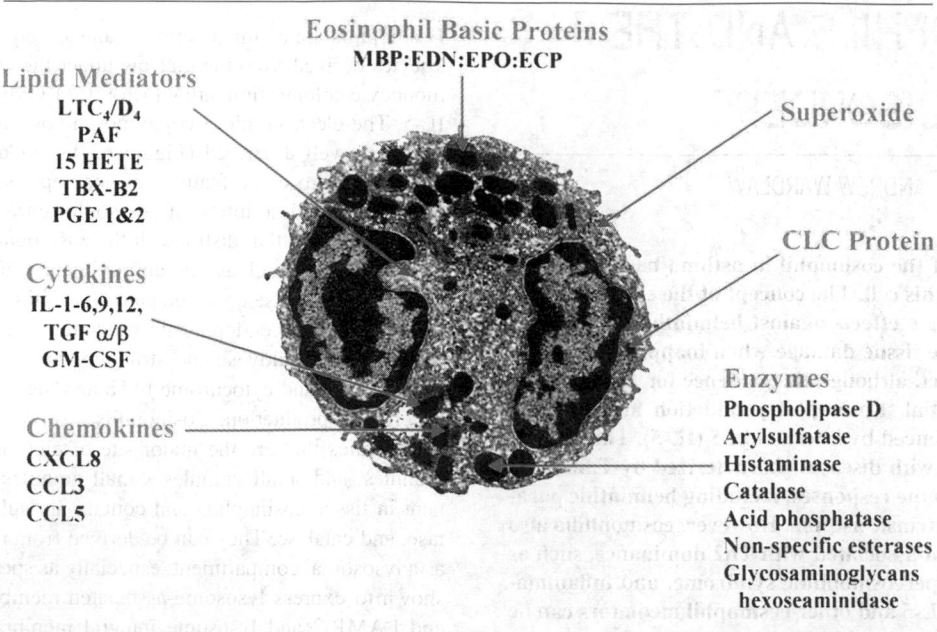

Eosinophil Basic Proteins
MBP:EDN:EPO:ECP

Lipid Mediators
LTC₄/D₄
PAF
15 HETE
TBX-B2
PGE 1&2

Superoxide

CLC Protein

Cytokines
IL-1-6,9,12,
TGF α/β
GM-CSF

Enzymes
Phospholipase D
Arylsulfatase
Histaminase
Catalase
Acid phosphatase
Non-specific esterases
Glycosaminoglycans
hexoseaminidase

Chemokines
CXCL8
CCL3
CCL5

FIGURE 62-1   Transmission electron micrograph of an eosinophil showing the characteristic specific granules with their electron-dense core (×10,000). (Courtesy of Dr. A Dewar, National Heart and Lung Institute).

plasm that transport the granule proteins to the cell surface, where they are released.[11] These appearances are common in tissue eosinophils in asthma and other allergic diseases.

A mouse model involves ovalbumin challenge to generate a lung eosinophilia and increased airway hyperresponsiveness. In this model, the lung eosinophils do not appear to have undergone degranulation either by cytolysis or piecemeal degranulation.[12] Immunostaining of the mouse lung in this model locates all the basic proteins within intact eosinophils, and bronchoalveolar lavage contains no free major basic protein (MBP).[13,14] This finding is quite unlike human disease, where cell free basic proteins can be readily detected in tissue and bronchoalveolar lavage. Consistent with this observation, mice in which the gene

for eosinophil peroxidase (EPO) or MBP has been deleted had the same phenotype as wild-type mice in this model.[15] The observation may explain in part the paucity of epithelial damage seen in the mouse asthma model. It also further calls into question the physiologic relevance of this type of experiment and emphasizes the complex and poorly understood relationship between eosinophil recruitment and degranulation.

Apoptotic eosinophils are small cells with a shrunken nucleus and condensed chromatin but an intact plasma membrane.[16] They are readily identifiable in aged cell populations *in vitro* and in cells from the airway lumen such as sputum but are more difficult to identify in tissue. This finding has led some investigators to argue that the majority of airway eosinophils, at least in asthma and rhinitis, are removed through luminal entry rather than by undergoing apoptosis in tissue.[5]

Like all leukocytes, eosinophils express a large number of membrane receptors that allow them to interact with the extracellular environment (Tables 62-1 and 62-2), including receptors required for locomotion, activation, growth, and mediator release. Most of the receptors are shared to some extent with other leukocytes, but some have a degree of specificity in terms of level of expression and function. An important feature of tissue eosinophils is that they express a different pattern of receptors to peripheral blood eosinophils consistent with a more activated phenotype, which includes induction of expression of

TABLE 62-1   EOSINOPHIL ADHESION RECEPTORS

| | LIGAND | |
RECEPTOR	ENDOTHELIAL	MATRIX PROTEIN
Integrins		
$\alpha_4\beta_1$(VLA-4)	VCAM-1	Fibronectin
$\alpha_4\beta_6$		Laminin
$\alpha_4\beta_7$	MAdCAM-1	Fibronectin
LFA-1($\alpha_L\beta_2$)	ICAM-1 through ICAM-3	
Mac-1($\alpha_M\beta_2$)	ICAM-1	
P150,95($\alpha_x\beta_2$)		
$\alpha_d\beta_2$	VCAM-1 (ICAM-3?)	
Selectins and Ligands		
PSGL-1	P-selectin (E-selectin)	
L-selectin	Gly-CAM-1, CD34, podocalyxin	
Other		
CD44		Hyaluronate
ICAM-3		
PECAM	PECAM	
Siglec-8		Sialic acid

ICAM, intercellular cell adhesion molecule; LFA, lymphocyte function-associated antigen; MAdCAM-1, mucosal addressin cell adhesion molecule-1; PECAM: platelet endothelial cell adhesion molecule; PSGL-1: P-selectin glycoprotein ligand-1; VCAM-1, vascular cell adhesion molecule.

TABLE 62-2   OTHER EOSINOPHIL RECEPTORS

Immunoglobulin receptors	Fcγ R11 (CD32); FcαR
Receptors for mediators	CCR3,* CCR1, PAF-R, LTC4/D4/E4-R, LTB4-R, C5a, C3a, IL-5,* IL-3, IL-4, IL-13
Receptors induced by cytokine stimulation	Fcγ RIII (CD16), Fcγ R1, CD69, HLA-DR, ICAM-1, CD25, CD4
Well-expressed miscellaneous receptors	CD9, CD45, CR1, CD154 (CD40 ligand), CD95 (Fas)

* Relatively selectively expressed by eosinophils.

C, complement; CCR, chemokine receptor; ICAM, intercellular cell adhesion molecule; LT, leukotriene; PAF, platelet activating factor; R, receptor.

CD69, intercellular cell adhesion molecule (ICAM)-1 and FcγR1 and increased expression of HLA-DR and Mac-1. Changes in expression can be induced *in vitro* by culture with cytokines such as IL-5 but also occur to some extent as the result of transmigration through endothelium.[17] A major difference between eosinophils and neutrophils that has been exploited to purify eosinophils by immunomagnetic selection is the expression of CD16 by neutrophils but not eosinophils. Another important difference is the expression of very late antigen (VLA)-4 by eosinophils but not to any great extent by neutrophils. Sialic acid-recognizing lectin (Siglec) 8 is a receptor expressed only by eosinophils, mast cells, and basophils.[18–20] Siglecs are sialic acid-recognizing animal lectins of the immunoglobulin superfamily. Eosinophils, monocytes, and a subset of dendritic cells also express Siglec 10.[21] In contrast, neutrophils express Siglec 9.[22] The function of Siglec 8 on eosinophils remains uncertain but may be involved in triggering apoptosis.[23]

EOSINOPHIL PRODUCTION

Eosinophils are nondividing, end-stage cells that, like other leukocytes, differentiate from the hematopoietic stem cell in the marrow. Eosinophils migrate into the blood, where they circulate with a half-life of approximately 18 hours before entering the tissues. Eosinophils are primarily tissue-dwelling cells. It has been estimated that there are approximately 100 tissue eosinophils for each eosinophil in the blood, although relatively few studies have been performed on eosinophil kinetics and even fewer studies have compared eosinophil turnover in health and disease.[24] Normal human adult marrow contains approximately 3 percent eosinophils, of which one third are mature and two thirds are precursors.

The development of eosinophilia is T cell dependent. In the 1970s, Basten and Beeson[25] established that T cell depletion abrogated the eosinophilic response to parasite infection. T cell–derived supernatants contained growth factors for eosinophils. This finding led to the characterization of IL-5 and awareness of the pivotal role this cytokine plays in eosinophil development.[26] IL-5 seems to be a rate limiting step for eosinophil production in that administration of IL-5 either exogenously or through transgenic manipulation in mice results in a marked eosinophilia[27] and anti–IL-5 in humans dramatically diminishes the blood eosinophil count in asthma.[28] Increased eosinophilopoiesis as a result of increased IL-5 synthesis appears to be a feature of a number of conditions, including parasitic and allergic diseases. For example, pulmonary eosinophilia as a result of *Necator americanus* infection in mice was IL-5 dependent,[29] and both eosinophilia and host defense to filariasis and *Trichinella spiralis* was markedly impaired in IL-5–deficient mice.[30] In asthma, IL-5 mRNA can be detected in increased amounts in the airways and in the serum of glucocorticoid-dependent asthmatics.[31,32] However, mice in which the IL-5 gene is deleted can sustain a baseline eosinophilia and can develop pulmonary eosinophilia after infection with paramyxovirus, demonstrating that cytokines other than IL-5 can cause late differentiation.[33] Therefore, an accepted paradigm is that a blood and tissue eosinophilia in IgE-mediated diseases, such as atopic asthma and helminthic parasite infections, result from antigen-dependent activation of Th2 cells, leading to IL-5 production and increased eosinophilopoiesis and tissue recruitment of eosinophils.

The control of Th2 and Th1 cell development may be related to (1) the cytokine milieu at the time of sensitization, (2) genetically regulated transcriptional control of IL-4, (3) route of sensitization, (4) the manner in which the antigen is presented,[34,35] and (5) the nature of the antigen. Many allergens have been purified and sequenced. No common structural features have been established that can explain their allergenicity, although many are proteases, which could influence their

immunogenicity.[36] The human leukocyte antigen (HLA) haplotype of individuals responsive to certain allergens has been investigated. A degree of restriction has been observed, particularly to more simple allergens, with, for example, the phenotype DR2.2 being overrepresented in individuals atopic to the ragweed allergen Amb aV. However, no clear pattern has emerged for the majority of allergens. Although HLA haplotypes may influence responses to individual allergens, they are unlikely to provide a universal explanation for Th2 type responsiveness.

Many eosinophilic diseases, including many cases of pulmonary eosinophilia, are not associated with atopy and IgE production and therefore do not entirely fit with the Th2-driven eosinophilic paradigm. Intrinsic asthma is generally assumed to associated with IL-5–producing T cells, but the supporting evidence is limited. A non-IgE associated eosinophilic disease is eosinophilic esophagitis caused by a defined food allergen in which there is no specific IgE.[37] In some of these cases, the patients are patch test positive to the food allergen, which raises the possibility of a Th2 type of type IV cell-mediated immunity.

T regulatory (T_{reg}) cells may control inappropriate immune responses, including those associated with Th2 cell activation. T_{reg} cells were first identified as mediating some aspects of immune tolerance and then were found to play an important role in suppressing immune-mediated inflammatory bowel disease in mice. The exact identity of T_{reg} cells is unclear; however, three T_{reg} cell types have been identified: CD4+CD25+ cells that require direct contact to mediate their immune suppressive effects, T_{reg} cells that produce TGF-β, and T_{reg} cells that produce IL-10.[38–40] Increasing understanding of the pivotal role that T_{reg} cells play in controlling immune responses has led to the interesting refinement of the "hygiene hypothesis." This hypothesis suggests the increase in allergic disease, which is paralleled by an increase in autoimmune disease, is not a consequence of a Th1 to Th2 switch as a result of lack of immune stimulation in infancy but rather a failure to develop T_{reg} responses, which leads to enhancement of both Th1 and Th2 immunity.[41–43] IL-10–producing T_{reg} cells are of particular interest in the context of pulmonary eosinophilia because of evidence that immunotherapy works by inducing expansion of antigen-specific IL-10–producing T_{reg} cells.[44] In addition, T_{reg} cells were able to suppress ovalbumin-induced pulmonary eosinophilia in mice.[45,46]

EOSINOPHIL HETEROGENEITY

Blood eosinophils from normal individuals are relatively dense cells that can be separated from other leukocytes by density gradient centrifuge. For many years, these differences were the basis for the standard method of purifying eosinophils. This method has been largely superseded by negative immunomagnetic selection based on the expression of the low-affinity (FcγRIII, CD16) IgG receptor by neutrophils but not eosinophils. This latter technique has the advantage of improved purity and cell yields. It also enables purification of eosinophils from individuals with low eosinophil counts.[47] A proportion of eosinophils from individuals with elevated eosinophil counts are less dense than eosinophils from normal subjects. So-called hypodense eosinophils[48] appear to be vacuolated and contain smaller granules although in an equal number to normal-density eosinophils. A correlation of eosinophil activation with hypodensity is a favored explanation, although the evidence supporting this relationship is contradictory.[4]

EOSINOPHIL TRAFFICKING AND TISSUE ACCUMULATION

TISSUE LOCALIZATION

Eosinophils are not normally found in tissues other than the gut but are a notable feature of the tissue pathology of a number of diseases.

The normal pattern of gut homing of eosinophils is mediated by eotaxin, which is constitutively expressed in the gut, and the integrin $\alpha_4\beta_7$ binding to mucosal addressin cell adhesion molecule (MAdCAM)-1, which is selectively expressed in the intestine.[49] Eosinophilia can accompany a general inflammatory response, as in idiopathic pulmonary fibrosis, in which increased numbers of eosinophils and neutrophils can be seen in bronchoalveolar lavage fluid. Eosinophilia often occurs without a marked increase in other leukocytes, raising the question of the mechanism behind the specific tissue accumulation of these leukocytes. Selective eosinophil accumulation occurs as a result of the coordinated effect of a number of adhesion, chemotactic, and growth/survival orientated signals at each stage in the cell's life cycle. In general, these events are controlled by mediators released by Th2 cells, particularly the cytokines IL-4, IL-5, IL-13, possibly IL-9, and most recently IL-25. This latter cytokine appears to act through an intermediate cell type to produce IL-5– and IL-13–dependent effects.[50]

EGRESS FROM THE MARROW

Eosinophil trafficking has been extensively investigated.[51–53] In addition to being crucial for differentiation, IL-5 is important in promoting emigration from the marrow. In particular, IL-5 acts as a priming factor for specific chemoattractants such as eotaxin.[54] Eosinophil emigration from the marrow in guinea pigs was inhibited by blocking anti-CD18 antibodies, but IL-5–dependent emigration was promoted by blocking anti–VLA-4 antibodies.[55] One explanation for this finding is that VLA-4/vascular cell adhesion molecule (VCAM)-1 is responsible for eosinophil precursors binding to marrow stromal cells, as has been shown for a range of cell types, although it has not been formally demonstrated in eosinophils. The observation that eotaxin decreased adhesion to VCAM-1 while increasing adhesion to the CD18 ligand BSA may be a mechanism for promoting egress from the marrow.[56] A localized inflammatory responses causing systemic effects has been demonstrated after allergen challenge in mice in which IL-5–producing cells (both T cells and non T cells) increased in the marrow.[57,58]

EGRESS FROM THE CIRCULATION

Accumulation of leukocytes in tissue is a highly regulated process so that the leukocytes respond effectively to noxious insults without causing an inappropriate inflammatory response. An obligate step in the migration of all leukocytes from the systemic circulation into tissue is their capture by endothelium as they flow at high shear rates through the postcapillary endothelium. A key receptor mediating eosinophil capture is P-selectin, whose low-level surface expression is selectively induced on endothelium by IL-4 and IL-13. Eosinophils express higher levels of P-selectin glycoprotein ligand-1 (PSGL-1, the primary receptor for P-selectin) than other leukocytes, which results in increased avidity for P-selectin compared to neutrophils, especially at the low levels of expression induced by Th2 cytokines.[59] Increased expression of PSGL-1 leading to enhanced recruitment has been reported in allergic disease.[60] IL-4 and IL-13 can induce low levels of VCAM-1 expression, which can bind eosinophils through VLA-4 and capture flowing cells albeit at lower shear stresses. VLA-4/VCAM-1 and PSGL-1/P-selectin cooperate as a major endothelial control point for selective eosinophil migration.[61] Once captured, eosinophils roll along the surface of the blood vessel until they are activated, which allows the CD18 integrins binding to ICAM-1 and ICAM-2 to nonselectively promote transmigration, although VLA-4/VCAM-1 can influence transmigration at this stage. The activation step mediated by chemoattractants expressed on the endothelial surface is another potential point of eosinophil selection, as shown by the effect of exogenously added chemoattractants such as eotaxin. The identity of the endoge-

nous chemoattractant involved and the extent to which it is selectively expressed in eosinophilic inflammation remain to be resolved.[62]

The blood supply to the bronchi via the bronchial arteries is part of the high-flow systemic circulation. In contrast, cell migration into the alveoli and interstitium of the lung occurs through the low-pressure pulmonary circulation, including the pulmonary capillaries. In this low-shear circulation, selectins are not necessary to mediate the capture step. Consistent with this finding, neither E- nor P-selectin is expressed on pulmonary capillaries, whereas P-selectin is well expressed in the bronchial circulation.[63,64] In some inflammatory insults in mice, such as *Streptococcus pneumoniae* infection, CD18 and VLA-4 integrins are not required for neutrophils to migrate into the alveolar bed.[65]

Once the eosinophil transmigrates through the endothelium, it migrates through the basement membrane and into the tissue. Chemokines and other eosinophil chemoattractants likely are central to this process (Table 62-3). In a mouse model in which CCR3, the major chemokine receptor on eosinophils, had been deleted, the cells migrated through the endothelium, suggesting that CCR3-binding chemokines, such as eotaxin, were not essential for the activation step. However, the cells did not migrate through the basement membrane, either because they lacked a chemotactic signal or they were unable to digest the extracellular matrix.[66]

PHYSIOLOGIC APOPTOSIS

Apoptosis is the universal mechanism by which cells undergo cell senescence in a manner that allows them to be efficiently removed by macrophages without inducing an inflammatory response. Morphologic observations have argued persuasively that eosinophil apoptosis is an unusual event in tissue and that most eosinophils either die by cytolysis or migrate into the gastrointestinal lumen, where they become apoptotic.[5,67] A slow rate of apoptosis in tissues is consistent with the survival signals delivered to eosinophils by the extracellular matrix as part of normal homeostasis and increased production of eosinophil growth factors during Th2-mediated inflammation.[68,69] The importance of prolonged survival of eosinophils in tissue as a mechanism for selective accumulation has been emphasized by studies using anti–IL-5, which effectively inhibits blood and sputum eosinophil numbers but has a much less marked effect on tissue eosinophils.[70] Glucocorticoids directly enhance the rate of eosinophil apoptosis through an unknown mechanism, unlike neutrophils where they prolong survival.[71] The effect of glucocorticoids in resolving eosinophilic inflammation, for example, in simple pulmonary eosinophilia, is a consequence of this direct effect. However, glucocorticoids only induce eosinophil apoptosis at high concentrations, and the effect is modest over and above the spontaneous rate of apoptosis. Glucocorticoids likely inhibit the production of eosinophil growth factors such as IL-5, IL-3, and GM-CSF generated both in an autocrine fashion by eosinophils in response to matrix signal and as part of the inflammatory process.[72] Tumor necrosis factor-related apoptosis-inducing ligand

TABLE 62-3   EOSINOPHIL CHEMOKINE RECEPTORS AND THEIR LIGANDS

RECEPTOR	CHEMOKINE
CCR1*	CCL3 (MIP-1a), CCL5 (RANTES)
CCR3	CCL11 (eotaxin1), CCL24 (eotaxin 2), CCL26 (eotaxin 3), CCL7,8,13 (MCP2–4), CCL5
CXCR1 and CYCR2	CXCL8 (IL-8†)

* Only expressed on eosinophils from some donors.
† Only active on *in vivo* activated or cytokine-primed eosinophils (may be indirect effect via neutrophils).
MIP, macrophage inflammatory protein; RANTES, regulated on activation, normal T cell expressed and secreted; MCP, monocyte chemotactic protein.

(TRAIL), another family of survival modulating mediators related to TNF, prolongs eosinophil survival both *in vitro* and *ex vivo* after allergen challenge.[73]

The biochemical mechanism by which growth factors mediate eosinophil survival is poorly understood. The effect is dependent on both new protein synthesis and phosphorylation events. The survival effects of IL-5 are dependent on activation of the Ras-Raf-MEC pathway and the Jak-2 Stat 1 and 5 pathway and involve lyn kinase, which binds to the IL-5R α-chain.[74] The roles of p38 and phosphoinositol 3 kinase are less clear. Wortmannin, which blocks phosphoinositol 3 kinase, had no effect on eosinophil apoptosis, although it did inhibit IL-5 enhancement of adhesion to fibrinogen. Eosinophils express significant amounts of the pro-apoptotic Bax and the anti-apoptotic Bcl-x$_L$ but very little Bad or Bcl-2.[75] As in other cell types, both spontaneous and Fas-induced eosinophil apoptosis are associated with the migration of Bax into the mitochondria, which leads to loss of mitochondrial membrane potential, cytochrome *c* release, and activation of downstream caspases. These events were inhibited by IL-5, demonstrating that IL-5 works by blocking Bax translocation.[76,77] Treatment of eosinophils with dexamethasone also leads to loss of mitochondrial permeability.[78] Pim-1 is one of the genes up-regulated by IL-5 in human blood eosinophils and in an IL-5–dependent cell line.[79] Pim-1 also was found to be relatively highly expressed in human eosinophils. Pim-1 is a serine/threonine kinase that was first identified as a putative lymphoma associated oncogene. Expression of Pim-1 in a myeloid leukemia cell line was found to be closely linked to IL-3 and GM-CSF stimulation.[80] Pim-1 subsequently was shown to be involved in IL-3–mediated survival, but not proliferation, of bone marrow-derived mouse mast cells downstream of Jak-2 and Stat 5 signaling.[81] In an IL-3–dependent murine cell line, ectopic Pim-1 expression was able to replace the survival-prolonging effects of IL-3 and to counteract the effects of overexpression of Bax on apoptosis.[82] Therefore, Pim-1 is a good candidate signaling molecule mediating the downstream effects of IL-5 and related growth factors on eosinophil survival.

LOCAL PROLIFERATION

Another potential mechanism involved in eosinophil tissue accumulation is *in situ* differentiation from eosinophil precursors. Eosinophil precursors can be identified in an IL-5Rα+CD34+ population in blood, which is increased after allergen challenge and in atopic disease. These cells have been found in asthmatic airways.[83]

TISSUE LIFE SPAN

Of equal importance as endothelial interactions to the kinetics of eosinophil migration are the factors controlling the fate of the eosinophil once it enters the tissue. Three outcomes are possible. (1) The eosinophil can remain in the tissue interacting with matrix proteins, other leukocytes, or structural cells such as the bronchial mucosa, epithelium, airway smooth muscle, mucus glands, and nerves. (2) The cell can migrate into the lumen of the gut or airway, where it likely undergoes apoptosis and is removed. (3) The cell can return to the circulation via the lymphatics. Limited evidence indicates eosinophils can recirculate, although they reportedly are present in lymph nodes where they are speculated to be involved in antigen presentation.[84] The length of time that eosinophils remain in tissue before migrating into the gut lumen is unclear because virtually no studies of the kinetics of eosinophil migration *in vivo* in humans are available. However, studies using anti–IL-5 in which significant tissue eosinophilia remains even after blood eosinophilia was almost completely inhibited suggest eosinophils can remain in the tissue for at least 12 weeks.[70] Anti–IL-5 also completely inhibited migration into the lumen, which suggests transepithelial migration is IL-5 dependent. In a mouse model of asthma, eosinophil migration into the lumen did not occur in the *MMP-2* gene-deleted mouse, which caused the animals to asphyxiate.[85] Therefore, IL-5 may be important in activating the eosinophils to digest the epithelial basement membrane in an MMP-2–dependent manner.[86] As shown with senescent neutrophils, when tissue eosinophils become senescent they start to alter their receptor phenotype in a way that inhibits tissue retention and promotes migration into the gastrointestinal lumen.[87] The factors controlling the retention and survival of eosinophils in tissue likely involve the integration of chemoattractant, adhesive and survival signals delivered by interactions with matrix proteins, and structural cells.

Few kinetic studies provide a basis for calculating which of the various mechanisms described above in "Tissue Life Span" make the largest contribution to eosinophil accumulation in tissues. In the mouse after allergen challenge, 80 percent of the eosinophils appeared to be newly arrived from the marrow.[57] In contrast, a study of anti–IL-5 suggested prolonged survival in tissues is of central importance.[88] Each pathway likely contributes, with the emphasis varying among individuals and over time within one individual.

ANIMAL MODELS OF EOSINOPHILIC DISEASE

Animal models, particularly the mouse model of ovalbumin challenge that results in selective and marked pulmonary eosinophilia, have been used extensively to analyze the molecular basis of eosinophil trafficking to the lung and its pathologic consequences. The combination of transgenic-, gene deletion-, and antibody-based manipulations in the mouse is a powerful tool for analyzing the biology of eosinophil migration, although the relevance of the findings to human disease must always be treated with caution. These studies have supported the concept of eosinophil migration resulting from a series of interlinked and obligate steps. IL-5 is necessary for providing a pool of circulating eosinophils, priming eosinophils for chemotactic responsiveness, and prolonging eosinophil survival. IL-4 and IL-13 control adhesion-related events in the endothelium and enhance the release of eosinophil chemoattractants, particularly CCR3-binding chemokines from mesenchymal cells within the airway.[89] However, a number of other studies are investigating other aspects of the immune response and challenging the concept by showing potential roles for innate immunity and other inflammatory mediators, such as platelet-activating factor (PAF), tryptase, and prostaglandin D$_2$.

EOSINOPHIL FUNCTIONS

PHAGOCYTOSIS

Although the eosinophil can phagocytose particles, its interactions with larval forms of helminthic parasites have formed the model by which eosinophil function has been described. In this situation, the eosinophil adheres tightly to the organism and releases its granule contents in high local concentrations onto the surface in a process described as frustrated phagocytosis. The paradigm of eosinophil effector function in host defense was developed from the observation that the basic granule proteins in particular were highly toxic for larval parasites. The paradigm was extended to include a proinflammatory role when the granules were also shown to be toxic for bronchial epithelium and therefore associated with epithelial desquamation, which is a well-established feature of severe asthma.

ANTIGEN PRESENTATION

The eosinophil has the capacity to present antigen to T cells, but how efficient they are compared to professional antigen-presenting cells is uncertain.[84]

CYTOKINE AND MEDIATOR RELEASE

Eosinophils can release a plethora of cytokines and chemokines, although many are generated in low amounts compared to other cells, and the extent to which they are important in eosinophil function is not clear.[90]

The eosinophil exerts its effects largely through its mediators (Fig. 62-2). The mediators are either newly generated, as with leukotrienes and other lipid mediators, or stored preformed in various compartments within the cytoplasm and released when the eosinophil receives a degranulating stimulus. The eosinophil is relatively biosynthetically inactive. Although new protein synthesis occurs, the majority of its protein mediators are stored.

Eosinophils can release a number of lipid mediators and are one of the relatively few sources of sulfidopeptide leukotrienes, although per cell they release about 10-fold less than mast cells and basophils.[91] This is in contrast to neutrophils, which produce large amounts of leukotriene (LT) B_4 but little, if any, LTC_4. LTC_4 generation by human eosinophils occurs after stimulation with opsonized zymosan and beads coated with IgG. Eosinophils can generate substantial quantities of 15-hydroperoxy-5,8,11,13-eicosatetraenoic acid via 15-lipoxygenase. Eosinophils also generate PAF after stimulation with either calcium ionophore or IgG-coated beads.[92] Eosinophils can generate mediators of the cyclooxygenase pathway, including prostaglandins E_1 and E_2 and thromboxane B_2. The principal sites of eicosanoid formation in eosinophils are the lipid bodies, which contain large amounts of arachidonic acid and enzymes required for eicosanoid synthesis, including 5-lipoxygenase, LTC_4 synthase, and cyclooxygenase.[93] Eo-

sinophils release significant amounts of TGF-β and TGF-α. This finding has stimulated interest in the potential role of eosinophils in causing structural changes in the lung that come under the heading of airway remodeling. Evidence indicates TGF-β released by eosinophils can promote generation of fibromyocytes, and anti–IL-5 reduced the amount of tenascin in the reticular subepithelial membrane.[88,94] Thickening of this membrane is closely associated with eosinophilic airway inflammation but not with airway hyperresponsiveness or airflow obstruction.[95]

EFFECTS OF GRANULE PROTEINS

A specific and important feature of eosinophils is the large amount of basic proteins— MBP, eosinophil cationic protein (ECP), EPO, and eosinophil-derived neurotoxin (EDN)—they contain within their specific granules. MBP has a molecular mass of 13.8 kDa and a pI of 10.9. Its 17 arginine residues account for its alkalinity in solution. MBP initially is synthesized as an acidic proprotein that is stored in the eosinophil granule.[96] MBP becomes toxic only after it is released and processed into its final form. Purified MBP is cytotoxic for the schistosomula of *Schistosoma mansoni*, and adherence of eosinophils to IgG-coated schistosomula results in secretion of MBP onto the tegument of the larvae, resulting in loss of viability.[97] MBP at concentrations as low as 10 μg/ml is toxic to both guinea pig and human respiratory epithelial cells and for rat and human pneumocytes.[98] The mechanism of action of MBP on epithelial cells appears to be mediated through inhibition of ATPase activity. MBP and EPO are strong agonists for platelet activation and for activation of mast cells, basophils,

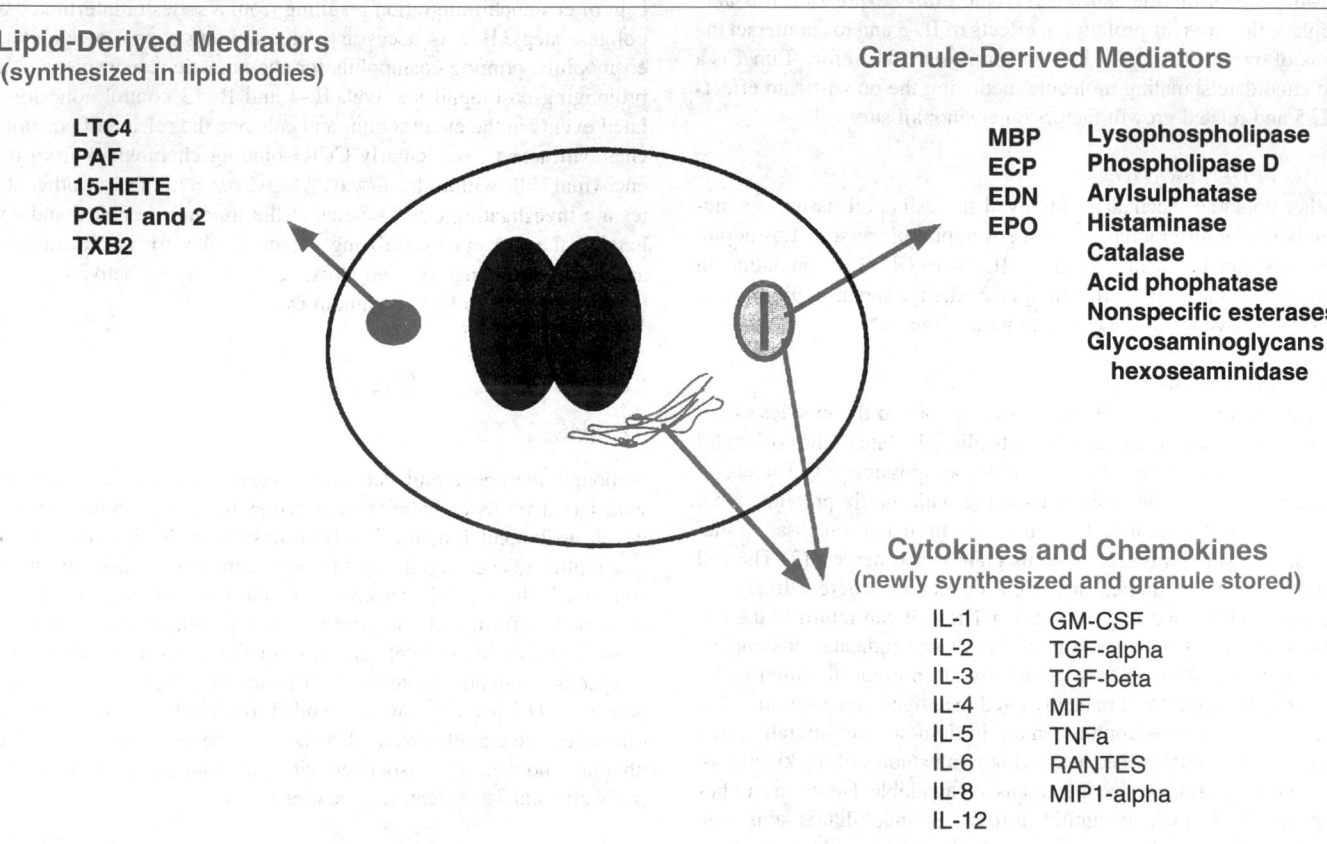

Lipid-Derived Mediators
(synthesized in lipid bodies)

LTC4
PAF
15-HETE
PGE1 and 2
TXB2

Granule-Derived Mediators

MBP Lysophospholipase
ECP Phospholipase D
EDN Arylsulphatase
EPO Histaminase
     Catalase
     Acid phophatase
     Nonspecific esterases
     Glycosaminoglycans
        hexoseaminidase

Cytokines and Chemokines
(newly synthesized and granule stored)

IL-1	GM-CSF
IL-2	TGF-alpha
IL-3	TGF-beta
IL-4	MIF
IL-5	TNFa
IL-6	RANTES
IL-8	MIP1-alpha
IL-12	

FIGURE 62-2   Schematic representation of eosinophil-derived mediators. MBP, major basic protein; ECP, eosinophil cationic protein; EDN, eosinophil-derived neurotoxin; EPO, eosinophil peroxidase; GM-CSF, granulocyte-monocyte colony stimulating factor; TGF, transforming growth factor; MIF, macrophage inhibition factor; TNF, tumor necrosis factor; MIP, macrophage inhibitory protein; PAF, platelet-activating factor. LTC, leukotriene C; HETE, hydroxyeicosatetraenoic acid; PGE, prostaglandin E; TXB, thromboxane B.

and neutrophils.[99] The mechanisms of action of MBP likely are related to its hydrophobicity and strong negative charge. Basophils also contain MBP but only about 2 percent the amount of eosinophils.

EPO is a heme-containing protein that is synthesized as a single protein and then cleaved into 14- and 58-kDa subunits.[100] The molecule shares a 68 percent identity in amino acid sequence with human neutrophil myeloperoxidase and other peroxidase enzymes. The substance is toxic for parasites, respiratory epithelium, and pneumocytes, either alone or (more potently) when combined with H_2O_2 and halide. The preferred ion in vivo is bromide. ECP is an arginine-rich protein. The cDNA encodes for a 27-amino-acid leader sequence and a 133-amino-acid mature polypeptide with a molecular mass of 15.6 kDa. ECP has 66 percent amino acid sequence homology with EDN and 31 percent homology with human pancreatic ribonuclease, but it has low ribonuclease activity compared to EDN.[101] ECP is toxic for helminthic parasites, isolated myocardial cells, and guinea pig tracheal epithelium. ECP also inhibits lymphocyte proliferation in vitro. ECP and EDN produce neurotoxicity (the Gordon phenomenon) when injected into the cerebrospinal fluid of experimental animals. ECP may damage cells by a colloid osmotic process, as it can induce non–ion-selective pores in both cellular and synthetic membranes.[102]

EDN, also called EPX, is a 16-kDa, glycosylated protein that possesses marked ribonuclease activity. The cDNA predicts a 134-amino-acid, mature polypeptide that is identical to human urinary ribonuclease. Like ECP, it is a member of a ribonuclease multigene family.[103] EDN expression is not restricted to eosinophils; it is found in mononuclear cells and possibly neutrophils. It probably also is secreted by the liver. It does not appear to be toxic to parasites or mammalian cells. Its only known effect, other than its ribonuclease activity, is neurotoxicity.

A major constituent of eosinophils is Charcot-Leyden crystal protein, which is a lysophospholipase. It constitutes up to 10 percent of eosinophil protein and is found in large quantities in basophils. It was thought to possess lysophospholipase activity, but this is not the case. It is a member of the galactin family (galectin 10).[104] Its precise function is unknown.

Vasoactive intestinal peptide has been detected in eosinophils in granulomas from mice infected with schistosomes. The eosinophil contains a number of granule-stored enzymes whose roles in eosinophil function are not clear. The enzymes include acid phosphatase, collagenase, arylsulfatase B, histaminase, phospholipase D, catalase, nonspecific esterases, vitamin B_{12}-binding proteins, and glycosaminoglycans. Eosinophils can undergo a respiratory burst with release of superoxide ion and H_2O_2 in response to stimulation with particulate stimuli, such as opsonized zymosan, and soluble mediators, such as leukotriene and phorbol myristate acetate. Eosinophils are twice as chemoluminescent as neutrophils.

EOSINOPHIL SECRETION AND ACTIVATION

A striking feature of eosinophil-rich inflammatory reactions is the high concentration of granule proteins, often in the presence of relatively small numbers of intact eosinophils. Mediator secretion can be triggered physiologically by engagement of immunoglobulin Fc receptors, especially after eosinophil activation has been primed with soluble mediators such as PAF and IL-5.[105] The eosinophil expresses receptors for IgG, IgA, and IgD. The eosinophil also binds IgE. Eosinophils can undertake a number of IgE-dependent functions, including killing of schistosomes opsonized with specific IgE. The receptor involved is unclear, but the accumulated evidence suggests eosinophils do not express either the low-affinity (FcγRII) or high-affinity (FcγRI) IgE receptor to any degree, although eosinophils do express high intracellular levels of the α-chain of FcγRI.[106]

Three receptors for IgG have been described: the high-affinity receptor FcγRI (CD64) and the two low-affinity receptors FcγRII (CDw32) and FcγRIII (CD16). CD16 is expressed as both a transmembrane form and a form with a phosphatidyl inositol anchor, transcribed from two distinct genes. Only FcγRII is constitutively expressed by eosinophils to any significant degree. A number of eosinophil functions are mediated via this receptor, including schistosomula killing, phagocytosis, secretion of granule proteins, and generation of newly formed, membrane-derived lipid mediators such as PAF and LTC$_4$. After stimulation for 2 days in vitro with interferon gamma, eosinophils express CD16, CD64, and CD32.[107] Perhaps the most potent stimulus for eosinophil degranulation is cross-linking of IgA receptors, especially when the cells have been primed with growth factors.[108] Consistent with the preference of eosinophils to secrete their mediators onto a large surface, Fc-mediated degranulation is enhanced if the eosinophils are adherent to a protein-coated surface via $\alpha_M\beta_2$.[109]

The killing of schistosomula opsonized with nonimmune serum presumably is mediated via the complement receptors CR1 and CR3. Incubation of eosinophils with serum-coated beads results in the release of 15 percent ECP. Similarly, opsonized zymosan interacts with eosinophils, causing generation of hydrogen peroxide and phagocytosis of zymosan. Soluble mediators such as PAF, LTB$_4$, and 5-oxo-eicosatetraenoate can elicit the direct secretion of granule proteins and lipid mediators, although only with highly activated eosinophils or when used in conjunction with cytochalasin B, which inhibits microtubule assembly. Eosinophils release their granule components by exocytosis, with individual granules fusing with the plasma membrane. The process involves a guanosine triphosphate-binding protein and is modulated by the intracellular calcium concentration.[110]

EOSINOPHILS IN DISEASE

MEASUREMENT OF EOSINOPHILS IN THE BLOOD

Eosinophils can be enumerated in the blood by "wet counts" in modified Neubauer chambers, differential counts on dried films, or automated cell counting by flow cytometry.[111] Automated counting that uses detection of EPO is the most accurate method, followed by counting in a cell chamber. Counting on films is least accurate because of the tendency for eosinophils to congregate at the margins of the slide. Common wet stains for eosinophils include eosin in acetone, phloxine, and Kimura stain, which originally was developed to stain basophils.[112] Many stains, including May-Grünwald-Giemsa, Romanowsky stain, Chromotrope 2R, and Biebrich scarlet, identify eosinophils in blood films, cytospin preparations, or tissues.

The eosinophil count should be evaluated in absolute numbers rather than as a percentage of white cells, as the latter depends on the total cell count. The normal eosinophil count is generally taken as less than 4000/μl (0.4 × 10^9/liter), although healthy medical students in the United States had a range from 15 to 650/μl (0.015–0.65 × 10^9/liter).[113] Eosinophil counts are higher in neonates. Eosinophil count varies with age, time of day, exercise status, and environmental stimuli, particularly allergen exposure. Blood eosinophil counts undergo diurnal variation, being lowest in the morning and highest at night. This effect results in a greater than 40 percent variation and may be related to the reciprocal diurnal variation in cortisol levels, which are highest in the morning. The factors that control blood eosinophil counts in health are imperfectly understood. Concentrations of eosinophil growth factors likely are important, but other factors may be involved. Normal counts vary by up to 40-fold. In populations where eosinophilia is common, such as endemically parasitized areas, blood eosinophil levels vary markedly, independent of the degree of infection. The variation is comparable to variations in IgE levels. No differences in eosinophil counts between ethnic groups have been observed.

The eosinophil count in hospitalized patients is less than 10 cells/μl (0.01 × 10^9/liter) in only 0.1 percent of patients. Eosinopenia can be ascribed to glucocorticoids or to disease in virtually all patients. Acute infection, or treatment with glucocorticoids or adrenaline, decreases eosinophil counts. In contrast, β-blockers inhibit adrenaline-induced eosinopenia and can cause a rise in the eosinophil count.

Several isolated cases of patients with absent eosinophils in the blood and marrow have been reported.[114] Several patients without eosinophils reportedly had allergic symptoms.[115] In one case, the symptoms occurred after drug-induced agranulocytosis.[116] In another case, a serum inhibitor of eosinophil colony formation was present.[117] A rare disorder, EPO deficiency, may be discovered by automatic counting that uses detection of EPO to count eosinophils. EPO deficiency does not have any adverse clinical consequences.[118]

CAUSES OF EOSINOPHILIA

The causes of eosinophilia can be classified according to the degree and frequency of occurrence (see Table 62-4). Division of eosinophil counts is arbitrary, but a mild eosinophilia can be regarded as less than 1500/μl (1.5 × 10^9/liter), a moderate elevation as 1500 to 5000/μl (1.5–5.0 × 10^9/liter), and a high count as greater than 5000/μl (5.0 × 10^9/liter). The most common cause of an eosinophilia worldwide is infection with helminthic parasites, which often can result in a very high eosinophil count. The most common causes of an eosinophilia in industrialized countries are the atopic allergic diseases, seasonal and perennial rhinitis, atopic dermatitis, and asthma. Allergic disease generally results in only a mild increase in eosinophil counts. A moderate or high eosinophil count in asthma raises the possibility of a complication such as Churg-Strauss syndrome or allergic bronchopulmonary aspergillosis.

EFFECTS OF EOSINOPHILS IN DISEASE

For years eosinophils were thought to ameliorate inflammatory response. Through the 1980s and 1990s, eosinophils were believed to cause tissue damage in some situations. Use of anti–IL-5 and tyrosine kinase inhibitors to inhibit eosinophil production has suggested a complex interaction between eosinophilic inflammation and target organ damage.[119] Eosinophils, partly through release of cytokines such as TGF-α, may have a homeostatic role in certain circumstances, such as wound healing and mammary gland development.[120,121] Evidence indicates eosinophils slow the rate of progression of solid tumors, presumably by their cytotoxicity to tumor cells,[122] although other studies have raised the possibility of a tumor-promoting role.[123] Eosinophils can cause severe tissue damage under certain circumstances. Chronically high eosinophil counts from many causes, including drug reactions, parasitic infections, eosinophilic leukemia, and hypereosinophilic syndrome (HES), are associated with endomyocardial fibrosis.[124] The observation in the mid-1970s that eosinophils could kill parasite targets led to the hypothesis that the principal role of eosinophils was to counter parasitic infection.[125] Therefore, eosinophils are associated with a number of different types of pathologic and reparative processes ranging from the permanent tissue damage seen in HES, the partly reversible tissue damage seen in asthma and pulmonary eosinophilia, and tissue repair characteristic of wound healing. The factors determining the role eosinophil adopts are unclear.

EOSINOPHILS AND ASTHMA

The relationship between airway inflammation and asthma is complex. In particular, no close relationship exists between the severity of eo-

sinophilic airway inflammation and the severity of symptoms, airway hyperresponsiveness, or abnormalities in forced expiratory volume-1.[126,127] A large number of studies have examined this relationship in endobronchial biopsies, sputum and bronchoalveolar lavage, and bronchial wash. The literature is generally consistent in showing a weak correlation at best. For example, we measured sputum eosinophilia in more than 200 patients attending our outpatient clinics with a diagnosis of asthma (ranging from mild to severe) and found only a weak correlation between sputum eosinophil in atopic subjects and no correlation at all in patients with nonatopic disease.[128] A caveat is that virtually all studies that investigated this relationship are cross-sectional. Longitudinal studies in clinical disease, relating changes in inflammation to changes in lung function and symptoms, are lacking. Another caveat is that the level of activation of leukocytes such as T cells and eosinophil may be more important than cell numbers, although eosinophils cell counts usually correlate well with concentrations of eosinophil-specific mediators in bronchoalveolar lavage. A reasonable correlation exists between changes in sputum eosinophils and airway hyperresponsiveness after allergen challenge and in a study of treatment with inhaled glucocorticoids.[129,130] However, even a better correlation between eosinophilic inflammation and severity of asthma within an individual still indicates considerable variability in the sensitivity to airway inflammation between individuals. Further support for the apparent dissociation between asthma and eosinophilic inflammation is provided by using an anti–IL-5 monoclonal antibody (MAb) that markedly reduced eosinophils in the blood and sputum but had no effect either on airway hyperresponsiveness or lung function in patients with mild asthma or on the late response to allergen challenge.[28] The interpretation of this and other studies using the anti–IL-5 antibody is complicated by the observation that anti–IL-5 only partially depletes the tissue eosinophilia.[70] Dissociation between airway hyperreactivity and eosinophilia has been seen in animal models of allergen challenge. For example anti–VLA-4 MAb was able to block ovalbumin-induced airway hyperreactivity but not airway eosinophilia when given by aerosol to mice.[131] Strikingly, in eosinophilic bronchitis, a condition in which patients have an eosinophilic airway inflammation but no evidence of asthma (no airway hyperresponsiveness or variable airflow obstruction), the asthma phenotype correlated with the number of mast cells in the airway smooth muscle. Tissue eosinophilia did not differ between the asthmatic and eosinophilic bronchitis groups.[95] Large numbers of eosinophils and mononuclear cells are found in and around the bronchi of patients who died of asthma, and their bronchial tissue contains large amounts of MBP.[6] The pathology of asthma deaths is at the extreme end of the pathology of asthma exacerbations. Increasing evidence indicates airway eosinophilia is closely associated with the risk of having exacerbations. In one study, treatment targeted at reducing chronic airway eosinophilia resulted in a considerable drop in the number of exacerbations compared to standard management.[132]

EOSINOPHILS AND THE SKIN

A large number of skin conditions are associated with infiltration by eosinophils.[133] Normal skin contains few eosinophils, so their presence usually is associated with pathology. The most common causes of eosinophilic infiltration of the skin is atopic dermatitis where, as with asthma, the relationship to pathogenesis remains contentious.[134] The skin is one of the most commonly affected organs in HES. Pruritus is the most common symptom. Ulceration can occur.

EOSINOPHILS AND THE GASTROINTESTINAL TRACT

Eosinophils are present in the normal gastrointestinal tract as a result of constitutive expression of eotaxin and MadCAM-1, the receptor for

TABLE 62-4 CAUSES OF EOSINOPHILIA

DISEASE	FREQUENCY OF CAUSE OF EOSINOPHILIA	USUAL DEGREE OF EOSINOPHILIA	COMMENT
Infections			
Parasitic disease	Common worldwide	Moderate to high	
Bacterial	Rare		Usually cause eosinopenia, although serum ECP levels may be raised, suggesting eosinophil involvement in tissue.
Mycobacterial	Rare		More often secondary to drug therapy.
Fungal	Rare		Apart from allergic reactions and coccidioidomycosis, in which as many as 88% of patients have an eosinophilia.
Rickettsial infections	Rare		
Yeast	Rare		*Cryptococcus* reported as causing CSF eosinophilia.
Viral infections	Rare		Occasional case reports of an eosinophilia in a variety of viral infections, including herpes and HIV infection.
Allergic Diseases			
Allergic rhinitis	Common worldwide	Mild	
Atopic dermatitis	Common especially in children	Mild	
Urticaria/angioedema	Common	Variable	Eosinophils seen in skin, even with normal count.
Asthma	Common	Mild	Syndrome of intrinsic asthma, nasal polyps, and aspirin intolerance associated with higher than usual eosinophil counts.
Drug Reactions			
Many drugs	Uncommon	Mild to high	Count usually returns to normal upon stopping drug.
Neoplasms			
Acute eosinophil leukemia	Rare	High	
Chronic myelogenous leukemia	Uncommon	Moderate to high	Increased eosinophil counts seen occasionally.
Chronic eosinophilic leukemia	Rare	High	Previously a subset of HES; now can be identified by chromosome abnormality.
Lymphomas (usually T cell lymphoma or Hodgkin lymphoma)	Uncommon	Moderate	Often intense tissue eosinophilia with moderate blood eosinophil count; Hodgkin lymphoma common most type.
Langerhans cell histiocytosis	Rare	Mild	Intense tissue eosinophilia in eosinophilic granuloma, but blood eosinophilia unusual.
Solid tumors	Uncommon	Mild to high	Many different tumors reported.
Musculoskeletal			
Rheumatoid arthritis	Rare	Mild to high	Occasional case reports; more usually secondary to therapy.
Fasciitis	Rare	High	
Gastrointestinal			
Eosinophilic gastroenteritis	Rare	Mild to moderate	As with many GI diseases, often a marked tissue eosinophilia with only a mild or absent blood eosinophilia.
Celiac disease	Uncommon	Normal	Tissue eosinophilia.
Inflammatory bowel disease			Eosinophils seen in biopsies in both Crohn and ulcerative colitis, but blood eosinophilia unusual.
Allergic gastroenteritis	Rare	Mild to high	Young children
Respiratory Tract (for *asthma* see *Allergic Diseases*)			
Churg-Strauss syndrome	Rare	Moderate to high	Syndrome of eosinophilic vasculitis and asthma.
Pulmonary eosinophilia	Uncommon	Mild to high	Syndrome of eosinophilia and lung imaging showing shadowing; apart from allergic bronchopulmonary aspergillosis, usually of unknown cause.
Bronchiectasis, cystic fibrosis	Uncommon	Mild	Often associated with asthma or allergic bronchopulmonary aspergillosis.
Skin Diseases (for *atopic dermatitis* see *Allergic Diseases*)			
Bullous pemphigoid	Uncommon	Moderate	
Miscellaneous Causes			
IL-2 therapy	Rare	Moderate to high	For renal cell carcinoma.
HES	Rare	High	
Endomyocardial fibrosis	Rare	High	Secondary to any cause of a high eosinophil count.
Hyper-IgE syndrome	Rare	Moderate to high	
Eosinophilia-myalgia and toxic oil syndromes	Rare	High	Two related conditions, one caused by poisoning with contaminated cooking oil in Spain and the other by a batch of tryptophan.

$\alpha_4\beta_7$, which is expressed by eosinophils.[49] A number of diseases are associated with gastrointestinal eosinophilia, including eosinophilic esophagitis, eosinophilic gastroenteritis, and inflammatory bowel disease.[135] Eosinophilic esophagitis is an increasingly recognized condition in children and adults. It is associated with food allergy often in the absence of specific IgE.[136] Case reports of successful treatment of this condition with anti–IL-5 suggest a proinflammatory role for eosinophils in the disease.[137]

EOSINOPHILS AND PARASITIC DISEASE

The role of eosinophils in parasitic disease has been reviewed.[125] Table 62-5 summarizes the most common helminthic causes of eosinophilia. Eosinophils can kill a number of opsonized parasites, including newborn larvae of *Trichinella spiralis*, larvae of *Nippostrongylus brasiliensis*, a gut parasite in the rat, larvae of *Fasciola hepatica*, and schistosomula of *S. mansoni*. *In vivo*, parasite larvae become opsonized with specific IgG and IgE antibodies and components of the complement cascade such as C3bi, which can promote adhesion and activation of eosinophils. Dead larvae of *Schistosoma haematobium* and other parasites have been detected in the skin surrounded by eosinophils and eosinophil granule products. Adult worms both *in vitro* and *in vivo* appear resistant to eosinophil-mediated damage. Despite the circumstantial evidence of eosinophil involvement in host defense against parasites, some doubt remains about their role. Except for schistosomiasis, no correlation between the degree of eosinophilia and protection against infection or reinfection is obvious.[138] A number of experiments have been performed in animal models of helminthic infection using IL-5 gene deletion, IL-5 transgenics, and anti–IL-5 antibodies to ablate the tissue eosinophilia. The studies suggested that eosinophils may have a protective role in *Strongyloides* and *Filariasis* but not in *Schistosoma*, *Nippostrongylus*, and *Trichuris* infections. For example, treatment of mice infected with *N. brasiliensis* or *S. mansoni* with neutralizing anti–IL-5 MAbs abolished the eosinophilia without modulating the disease process.[139] In contrast, using diffusion chambers, eosinophils were conclusively shown to be involved in killing the larvae of *Strongyloides stercoralis*.[140] The mechanism of eosinophilia in parasitic disease is thought to be similar to allergic disease, with a Th2-type response to helminthic antigens resulting in increased production of eosinophil growth factors, particularly IL-5.[141]

HYPEREOSINOPHILIC SYNDROMES

HYPEREOSINOPHILIC SYNDROME

Definition and History Idiopathic HES is an uncommon and potentially fatal disorder first described as a distinct entity by Hardy and Anderson[142] in 1968. It is defined as a persistent eosinophilia of greater than 1500/μl (1.5 x 10^9/liter) for more than 6 months with evidence of end-organ damage but no explanation after comprehensive investigation.[143] The major target organs for tissue damage are the skin, heart, and nervous system.[144,145]

Epidemiology HES has an incidence of approximately one in one million persons per year and prevalence of approximately one in 100,000 persons at any point in time. It occurs sporadically, and no geographic or environmental factors are correlated with its incidence. Males are affected more often than females.[145]

Etiology and Pathogenesis New insights into the classification, pathophysiology, and management of HES have been reported.[146] Three categories of HES have been discovered: (1) the most prevalent category is one in which a clonal expansion of myeloid cells with eosinophilic lineage predominance, akin to other lineage-dominant myelogenous leukemias (e.g., monocytic, erythroid, megakaryocytic), accounts for the eosinophilia; (2) a less prevalent category is one in which a clonal expansion of T lymphocytes is accompanied by over-

TABLE 62-5   HELMINTHIC CAUSES OF AN EOSINOPHILIA

PARASITE	COMMENT
Nematodes	
Ascariasis	Higher eosinophil counts in children. Larvae migrate from intestine to lungs where they cause Loeffler syndrome, a form of pulmonary eosinophilia.
Toxocara canis	Infective eggs are present in feces of puppies and pregnant bitches. Larvae in hosts such as chicken. Eosinophilia seen mainly in children <9 years. Can migrate to eye and cause blindness. Serologic evidence suggests infection not uncommon in industrialized countries.
Filariasis	Common. Invariably results in marked eosinophilia, especially Loa Loa infection. Filariasis is the cause of tropical pulmonary eosinophilia resulting from migration of adult worms to lung, elephantiasis resulting from involvement of lymphatics (*Wuchereria bancrofti* and *Brugia malayi*), and river blindness (*Onchocerca volvulus*). Treatment can result in systemic reaction called *Mazzotti reaction*, possibly resulting from massive eosinophil degranulation.
Ancylostomiasis	Hookworm infection. *Ancylostoma duodenale* and *Necator americanus*. One of the main causes of eosinophilia in patients returning from tropical countries. Counts in region of 2×10^9/liter.
Strongyloidiasis	Subclinical infection can persist for >20 years. Stool examinations often negative. Cause of eosinophilia in ex-servicemen who spent time in tropics. If strongyloides infection is not considered and these patients are given steroids for suspected HES or as trial of therapy, they can develop disseminated disease.
Trichinosis	Caused by ingestion of encysted muscle larvae of *Trichinella spiralis*. Most prominent eosinophilia seen during early stages of infection when larvae migrate into striated muscle via the blood. Fatal cases reported, of which only 20% were noted to have an eosinophilia.
Others	Other nematodes that can cause eosinophilia include *Trichuris trichiura*, *Capillaria*, and *Gnathostomiasis*. The thread worm *Enterobius vermicularis* occasionally causes an eosinophilia when it invades tissues.
Trematodes	
Schistosomiasis (Bilharzia)	Infection with a *Schistosoma* (blood flukes)—*S. mansoni*, *S. haematobium*, and *S. japonicum*—is perhaps the most common cause of a moderate to high eosinophilia worldwide, with 200 million people infected. Infection nearly always is associated with an eosinophilia.
Fascioliasis	Adult worms of *F. hepatica* reside in the bile ducts, where they are associated with abnormal liver function tests and an eosinophilia.
Cestodes	
Echinococcus	Eosinophilia occurs in 25–50% of patients with hydatid disease.

production of IL-5, engendering a reactive eosinophilia; and (3) a small residual third category includes cases not fitting into the first two categories (e.g., polyclonal T cell reaction accompanied by overelaboration of IL-5, and others awaiting definition). In effect, most cases of HES appear to be either chronic eosinophilic leukemia or a clonal T cell disorder.[146] Although several mutations have been described in the former disease, the prevalence of a chromosomal translocation involving the *PDGFR-*α gene, resulting in a mutant tyrosine kinase sensitive to imatinib mesylate, has provided a new and molecule-specific approach to therapy.[147] Precise studies of clonality are required to identify patients in the myeloid and lymphoid category of hypereosinophilia.

CHRONIC EOSINOPHILIC LEUKEMIA (MYELOID HES)

This is a clonal myeloid disorder resulting from a chromosomal abnormality in myeloid cells. Eosinophilia is a constant finding, often accompanied by anemia and mild splenomegaly, intense marrow hyperplasia of myelocytic and eosinophilic cells, and few if any blast cells in marrow and blood, unless progression to a more acute state is underway. Cardiac and neurologic involvement are poor prognostic factors in HES and are found mainly in this group of patients. A proportion of patients develop acute myeloid leukemia, sometimes with a predominantly eosinophilic phenotype. In one study, An interstitial deletion on 4q12 resulting in a fusion gene IP1L1P-PDGFR-α, which encodes a tyrosine kinase that is constitutively active, was present in eight of 15 patients with HES, all of whom responded to treatment with the tyrosine kinase inhibitor imatinib mesylate.[147] This mutation causes the Ba/F3 cell line to become IL-3 independent and is found in the EOL-1 cell line derived from a patient with eosinophilic leukemia.[148] The presence of this mutation and the good response to treatment with imatinib mesylate has been confirmed.[149] Imatinib mesylate also has been effective in other patients with chronic eosinophilic leukemia without this particular mutation, suggesting that other mutated tyrosine kinases sensitive to imatinib mesylate can cause the disease.[147,150] Standard karyotyping does not normally identify the cryptic 4q12 interstitial deletion and the PDGFR-α mutation. Serum tryptase appears to be a good marker of this disorder[151] (see Chap. 88 for further detailed description).

CLONAL T CELL LYMPHOMA (LYMPHOID HES)

This lymphoid disorder, previously part of the category HES, usually follows a more benign course than chronic eosinophilic leukemia.[152–154] Although the course may be indolent, the clone may progress to a more aggressive lymphoma. Patients tend to respond well to glucocorticoids or cladribine and are less likely to develop cardiac fibrosis and other severe complications of the disease. The clonally expanded T cells overproduce eosinophil growth factors, resulting in a reactive eosinophilia. Several different patterns of clonal T cell abnormalities have been found in association with this form of HES; a CD3+CD4−CD8− or a CD3−CD4+ population of clonally expanded T cells is most common.[146,152–154] These clones secrete increased amounts of eosinophil related cytokines, such as IL-5, IL-4, and IL-3. Clonality of the phenotypically aberrant T cells has been demonstrated in these cases, and some patients progress to frank malignancy. In the World Health Organization classification, eosinophil clonality or demonstration of a chromosomal or genic clonal marker identifies the eosinophilia as chronic eosinophilic leukemia. An alternative classification has been proposed.[149] This classification divides patients with hypereosinophilia into those with chronic eosinophilic leukemia who have the FIP1L1-PDGFR-α mutation[155] or other mutations associated with chronic eosinophilic leukemia and those with clonal T cell disorders (e.g., clonal immunophenotypic patterns by flow cytometry or rearrangement of a T cell receptor β- or γ-chain gene) and eosinophilia.[152–154] Some of these T cell clones have been associated with skin lesions and have evolved into cutaneous T cell lymphoma (e.g., Sézary syndrome). Eosinophilia with overt clonal lymphoid disorders, such as Hodgkin lymphoma, T cell lymphoblastic leukemia, and peripheral T cell lymphoma, have been described for decades, and eosinophilia has been thought to be reactive (prior to discovery of the role of IL-5 and other cytokines). In the latter cases, clonal lymphoid disease dominates the clinical picture, and eosinophilia is a secondary phenomenon.

By default, the third group of HES includes those that do not fall into the first two groups and await a molecular and cell pathophysiologic explanation for the persistent eosinophilia. For example, polyclonal T cell expansion may lead to hypereosinophilia. The relative prevalence of myeloid and lymphoid clonal diseases in a population of patients with HES is disputed, but the clonal lymphoid form probably is less frequent than the clonal myeloid form.

Clinical Features Patients with hypereosinophilia have a heterogeneous presentation, with persistent blood eosinophilia as the hallmark.[146,156] Patients usually present in the third or fourth decade of life, but they can present at any age, including, rarely, in childhood. Patients may be relatively asymptomatic, or they may have an aggressive course leading to death within months to years if the disease is not successfully treated. The more severe complications are generally found in the clonal myeloid disorder, especially those with elevated serum tryptase. Patients may present with nonspecific symptoms such as general malaise, weight loss, joint aches and pains, fever, and sweating attacks, or with one of the organ-specific features, such as cardiac failure or restrictive pulmonary disease. Cough is a common symptom, usually without bronchospasm and sometimes associated with pulmonary infiltrates. Skin symptoms are particularly common and include pruritus, sometimes associated with erythematous papules and urticaria.

Cardiac complications are common in the clonal myeloid disorder, particularly endomyocardial fibrosis, which leads to restrictive cardiomyopathy and left ventricular failure. Mitral incompetence can occur. Thromboembolic complications of large and small vessels are common in more severe disease, some originating from an endomyocardial clot. Many of the central neurologic features are embolic in origin. A variant of hypereosinophilia is Gleich syndrome, in which patients experience recurrent episodes of angioedema. The disorder can be associated with confusion, loss of memory, and ataxia. Peripheral nervous system signs, including mononeuritis multiplex, sensorimotor neuropathy, multifocal neuropathy, and radiculopathy, occur. The differential diagnosis with Churg-Strauss syndrome can be difficult. Patients can develop mucosal ulcerations but, as with the renal system, severe complications usually are not prominent.

Laboratory Features Investigations to exclude a reactive cause for the eosinophilia should be undertaken (see "Differential Diagnosis" below). Roufosse and colleagues[146] have suggested a scheme for investigation of patients with HES. The approach is aimed at locating evidence of myeloid clonality or an abnormal T cell clone. The approach includes full blood cell count with examination of a blood film, determination of serum immunoglobulins, serum vitamin B_{12} and tryptase, marrow examination, lymphocyte immunophenotyping, and, if available, analysis of relevant cytokine production, TCR gene rearrangement, karyotyping, and analysis of the presence of the FIP1L1-PDGFR-α fusion gene by reverse transcriptase polymerase chain reaction, or fluorescence in situ hybridization analysis. Chest imaging, spirometry, biochemical profile, echocardiogram, and cardiac and abdominal ultrasound also should be undertaken, with neurologic investigations where appropriate to assess the degree of organ-specific damage.

Differential Diagnosis Table 62-4 lists reactive causes of marked eosinophilia that must be excluded with appropriate investigations. Once these causes have been excluded, the differential diagnosis includes familial eosinophilia, which is rare condition that has been mapped to a region of chromosome 5q31-q33,[157] acute eosinophilic leukemia, eosinophilia secondary to a malignancy, Churg-Strauss syndrome, and chronic eosinophilic pneumonia.

Treatment The mainstay of treatment of HES had been glucocorticoids, which in many cases, particularly those with a clonal lymphoid disorder, may be effective at controlling the eosinophil count and target organ damage, albeit at the risk of long-term glucocorticoid side effects. Hydroxyurea is a useful second-line agent. Other cytotoxic drugs, such as vincristine, cyclophosphamide, cladribine, and cytarabine, have been used to lower the eosinophil count and decrease the risk of eosinophil-mediated tissue damage. Interferon alpha has been used with some success.[158] These approaches may be useful in the absence of a specific diagnosis, but identification of a clonal myeloid or clonal lymphoid disease, if present, is imperative so that a specific therapy can be used for each, as appropriate. Imatinib mesylate has changed the management of patients with chronic eosinophilic leukemia resulting from constitutive activation of a drug-sensitive tyrosine kinase.[147,149,155] This agent has been dramatically successful in a number of cases, with little toxicity and lower doses than required for treatment of CML (see Chap. 88). In one patient who developed resistance to imatinib mesylate, an alternative PDGFR-α tyrosine kinase inhibitor was effective.[159] Treatment with imatinib mesylate has been associated with acute left ventricular failure in some cases, and cardiac troponin may be useful in monitoring this adverse event.[160] Patients with hypereosinophilia but no apparent PDGFR-α mutation have responded to imatinib. The molecular basis for the response has not been described.[146]

In the case of eosinophilia secondary to a clonal lymphoid disease, suppression of the clone would be expected from drugs that are used in lymphoma (see Chap. 96). Cladribine, interferon, glucocorticoids, vincristine, and cyclophosphamide are among the drugs that have been used. No systematic approach to therapy has yet been presented because of the difficulty in performing therapeutic trials of rare diseases.

Another treatment approach to decrease the eosinophil count and the risk of tissue injury has been the use of anti–IL-5 MAb. This agent also causes a dramatic response in some patients, even in the absence of elevated serum IL-5 concentrations. To date this drug has been made available only on a compassionate use basis, so experience is limited.[137,161]

As in other clonal diseases that affect younger patients, hematopoietic stem cell transplantation can be considered in eligible patients if the course of the disease is progressive and potentially lethal.

Course and Prognosis   In a series reported in 1973, the outlook for patients with HES was poor. The 3-year survival rate was 12 percent, with cardiac failure accounting for much of the morbidity and mortality.[143] In a later report the outlook had improved, with a survival of 80 percent at 5 years.[149] However, the new approaches to diagnosis and treatment outlined above in the "Treatment" section suggests the prognosis for these patients is further improved. In addition, future assessments will stratify the underlying disease (e.g., lymphoid vs. myeloid) in determining prognosis.

TOXIC OIL SYNDROME

In 1981, more than 20,000 cases of a syndrome manifested by fever, cough, dyspnea, leukocytosis, neutrophilia, and an eosinophil count greater than 750 cells/μl (0.75 × 10⁹/liter) were reported in Spain.[162] Occasionally, the eosinophil count rose above normal only after the onset of pulmonary symptoms. Eosinophil degranulation was seen in the affected tissues.[163] Pulmonary infiltrates were evident on chest radiographs. Pleural effusion was common, and hypoxemia was frequent. In the cohort, 1500 deaths occurred. About half the patients went on to a chronic course that mimicked the eosinophilia-myalgia syndrome, with myalgias, eosinophilia, peripheral neuritis, scleroderma-like skin lesions, hair loss, and a sicca syndrome. Most patients improved from the acute or chronic symptoms and signs, but some residual nerve, muscle, or skin damage persisted. Endothelial cell proliferation, mononuclear cell infiltrates around blood vessels (vasculitis), and perineural inflammatory infiltrates were identified histopathologically. Glucocorticoid therapy may have decreased the pulmonary

symptomatology. The disease was thought to be a response to an unlabeled food oil, aniline-denatured rapeseed oil, marketed as pure olive oil.

REACTIVE HYPEREOSINOPHILIA AND NEOPLASMS

Exaggerated eosinophilia has been reported in association with a variety of lymphoid and solid tumors, particularly Hodgkin disease.[164] In these cases, the eosinophilia is thought to result from an increase in plasma IL-5 and other cytokines or chemokines elaborated by the tumor cells, although the expression of receptors of the TNF-α family by eosinophils suggest they also can regulate tumor growth. The eosinophilia may precede the clinical diagnosis of the tumor but usually is manifested concomitantly. In most cases of solid tumors with hypereosinophilia, the tumor is metastatic.[173] In some cases, successful treatment of the tumor is associated with amelioration of the eosinophilia. Angiolymphoid hyperplasia has been associated with eosinophilia.[165]

ACUTE EOSINOPHILIC LEUKEMIA

Chapter 87 describes this rare disorder.

EOSINOPHILIA, ANGIITIS, AND ASTHMA

A group of related diseases, including polyarthritis nodosa and allergic granulomatosis (Churg-Strauss angiitis), is associated with prominent eosinophilia.[166] In a review of subjects with asthma and necrotizing angitis, all patients had anemia and hypereosinophilia, with a mean blood eosinophil count greater than 8000 cells/μl (8 × 10⁹/liter).[167] Remission can be achieved in approximately 90 percent of patients. Approximately 10 percent of patients die of the vasculitis.[168] A number of case reports have suggested a link to leukotriene antagonists.[169] In subjects with asthma and exaggerated eosinophilia, development of multiorgan signs (skin, nervous system, kidney, joints, lung, heart, gastrointestinal tract) should lead to consideration of this disorder.

EOSINOPHILIC FASCIITIS

This syndrome can occur at any age in both sexes. It is characterized by stiffness, pain, and swelling of the arms, forearms, thighs, legs, hands, and feet in descending order of frequency. Malaise, fever, weakness, and weight loss occur.[170] Eosinophilia greater than 1000 cells/μl (1 × 10⁹/liter) is present in most patients but may be intermittent. A biopsy, usually required for the diagnosis, shows inflammation, edema, thickening, and fibrosis of the fascia. Synovial tissue may show similar changes. Aplastic anemia, isolated cytopenias, pernicious anemia, and leukemia have been associated with eosinophilic fasciitis.

EOSINOPHILURIA AND EOSINOPHILORRHACHIA

The urinary excretion of eosinophils is seen in several inflammatory disorders of the kidney but most often in urinary tract infection or acute interstitial nephritis.[171] Hansel stain is superior to Wright stain for identifying eosinophils in a stained urinary sediment. Cerebrospinal fluid eosinophilia may occur with infection, shunts, and allergic reactions involving the meninges.[172]

REFERENCES

1. Egesten A, Calafat J, Janssen H, et al: Granules of human eosinophilic leucocytes and their mobilization. *Clin Exp Allergy* 31:1173, 2001.
2. Dvorak AM, Weller PF: Ultrastructural analysis of human eosinophils. *Chem Immunol* 76:1, 2000.
3. Persson T, Calafat J, Janssen H, et al: Specific granules of human eosinophils have lysosomal characteristics: Presence of lysosome-associ-

ated membrane proteins and acidification upon cellular activation. *Biochem Biophys Res Commun* 291:844, 2002.

4. Wardlaw A: Eosinophil density: What does it mean? *Clin Exp Allergy* 25:1145, 1995.

5. Erjefalt JS, Persson CG: New aspects of degranulation and fates of airway mucosal eosinophils. *Am J Respir Crit Care Med* 161:2074, 2000.

6. Filley WV, Holley KE, Kephart GM, Gleich GJ: Identification by immunofluorescence of eosinophil granule major basic protein in lung tissues of patients with bronchial asthma. *Lancet* 2:11, 1982.

7. Erjefalt JS, Greiff L, Andersson M, et al: Allergen-induced eosinophil cytolysis is a primary mechanism for granule protein release in human upper airways. *Am J Respir Crit Care Med* 160:304, 1999.

8. Erjefalt JS, Greiff L, Andersson M, et al: Degranulation patterns of eosinophil granulocytes as determinants of eosinophil driven disease. *Thorax* 56:341, 2001.

9. Weiler CR, Kita H, Hukee M, Gleich GJ: Eosinophil viability during immunoglobulin-induced degranulation. *J Leukoc Biol* 60:493, 1996.

10. Dvorak AM, Furitsu T, Letourneau L, et al: Mature eosinophils stimulated to develop in human cord blood mononuclear cell cultures supplemented with recombinant human interleukin-5. Part I. Piecemeal degranulation of specific granules and distribution of Charcot-Leyden crystal protein. *Am J Pathol* 138:69, 1991.

11. Dvorak AM, Ackerman SJ, Furitsu T, et al: Mature eosinophils stimulated to develop in human-cord blood mononuclear cell cultures supplemented with recombinant human interleukin-5: II. Vesicular transport of specific granule matrix peroxidase, a mechanism for effecting piecemeal degranulation. *Am J Pathol* 140:795, 1992.

12. Malm Erjefalt M, Persson CG, Erjefalt JS: Degranulation status of airway tissue eosinophils in mouse models of allergic airway inflammation. *Am J Respir Cell Mol Biol* 24:352, 2001.

13. Denzler KL, Borchers MT, Crosby JR, et al: Extensive eosinophil degranulation and peroxidase-mediated oxidation of airway proteins do not occur in a mouse ovalbumin-challenge model of pulmonary inflammation. *J Immunol* 167:1672, 2001.

14. Stelts D, Egan RW, Falcone A, et al: Eosinophils retain their granule major basic protein in a murine model of allergic pulmonary inflammation. *Am J Respir Cell Mol Biol* 18:463, 1998.

15. Denzler KL, Farmer SC, Crosby JR, et al: Eosinophil major basic protein-1 does not contribute to allergen-induced airway pathologies in mouse models of asthma. *J Immunol* 165:5509, 2000.

16. Dvorak AM: Images in clinical medicine. An apoptotic eosinophil. *N Engl J Med* 340:437, 1999.

17. Yamamoto H, Sedgwick JB, Vrtis RF, Busse WW: The effect of transendothelial migration on eosinophil function. *Am J Respir Cell Mol Biol* 23:379, 2000.

18. Aizawa H, Plitt J, Bochner BS: Human eosinophils express two Siglec-8 splice variants. *J Allergy Clin Immunol* 109:176, 2002.

19. Kikly KK, Bochner BS, Freeman SD, et al: Identification of SAF-2, a novel siglec expressed on eosinophils, mast cells, and basophils. *J Allergy Clin Immunol* 105:1093, 2000.

20. Floyd H, Ni J, Cornish AL, et al: Siglec-8. A novel eosinophil-specific member of the immunoglobulin superfamily. *J Biol Chem* 275:861, 2000.

21. Munday J, Kerr S, Ni J, et al: Identification, characterization and leucocyte expression of Siglec-10, a novel human sialic acid-binding receptor. *Biochem J* 355:489, 2001.

22. Swystun VA, Gordon JR, Davis EB, et al: Mast cell tryptase release and asthmatic responses to allergen increase with regular use of salbutamol. *J Allergy Clin Immunol* 106:57, 2000.

23. Nutku E, Aizawa H, Hudson SA, Bochner BS: Ligation of Siglec-8: A selective mechanism for induction of human eosinophil apoptosis. *Blood* 101:5014, 2003.

24. Spry CJF: The natural history of eosinophils, in *The Immunopharma-*

cology of Eosinophils, edited by H Smith, RM Cook, p 1. Academic Press, London, 1993.

25. Basten A, Beeson PB: Mechanism of eosinophilia: II. Role of the lymphocyte. *J Exp Med* 131:1288, 1970.

26. Sanderson CJ: Interleukin-5, eosinophils, and disease. *Blood* 79:3101, 1992.

27. van Rensen EL, Stirling RG, Scheerens J, et al: Evidence for systemic rather than pulmonary effects of interleukin-5 administration in asthma. *Thorax* 56:935, 2001.

28. Leckie MJ, ten Brinke A, Khan J, et al: Effects of an interleukin-5 blocking monoclonal antibody on eosinophils, airway hyper-responsiveness, and the late asthmatic response. *Lancet* 356:2144, 2000.

29. Culley FJ, Brown A, Girod N, et al: Innate and cognate mechanisms of pulmonary eosinophilia in helminth infection. *Eur J Immunol* 32:1376, 2002.

30. Martin C, Al-Qaoud KM, Ungeheuer MN, et al: IL-5 is essential for vaccine-induced protection and for resolution of primary infection in murine filariasis. *Med Microbiol Immunol (Berl)* 189:67, 2000.

31. Humbert M, Corrigan CJ, Kimmitt P, et al: Relationship between IL-4 and IL-5 mRNA expression and disease severity in atopic asthma. *Am J Respir Crit Care Med* 156:704, 1997.

32. Alexander AG, Barkans J, Moqbel R, et al: Serum interleukin 5 concentrations in atopic and non-atopic patients with glucocorticoid-dependent chronic severe asthma. *Thorax* 49:1231, 1994.

33. Domachowske JB, Bonville CA, Easton AJ, Rosenberg HF: Pulmonary eosinophilia in mice devoid of interleukin-5. *J Leukoc Biol* 71:966, 2002.

34. Finotto S, Neurath MF, Glickman JN, et al: Development of spontaneous airway changes consistent with human asthma in mice lacking T-bet. *Science* 295:336, 2002.

35. Neurath MF, Finotto S, Glimcher LH: The role of Th1/Th2 polarization in mucosal immunity. *Nat Med* 8:567, 2002.

36. Hewitt CR, Horton H, Jones RM, Pritchard DI: Heterogeneous proteolytic specificity and activity of the house dust mite proteinase allergen Der p I. *Clin Exp Allergy* 27:201, 1997.

37. Rothenberg ME, Mishra A, Collins MH, Putnam PE: Pathogenesis and clinical features of eosinophilic esophagitis. *J Allergy Clin Immunol* 108:891, 2001.

38. McHugh RS, Shevach EM: The role of suppressor T cells in regulation of immune responses. *J Allergy Clin Immunol* 110:693, 2002.

39. Levings MK, Sangregorio R, Sartirana C, et al: Human CD25(+)CD4(+) T suppressor cell clones produce transforming growth factor beta, but not interleukin 10, and are distinct from type 1 T regulatory cells. *J Exp Med* 196:1335, 2002.

40. Curotto de Lafaille MA, Lafaille JJ: CD4(+) regulatory T cells in autoimmunity and allergy. *Curr Opin Immunol* 14:771, 2002.

41. Yazdanbakhsh M, Kremsner PG, van Ree R: Allergy, parasites, and the hygiene hypothesis. *Science* 296:490, 2002.

42. Wills-Karp M, Santeliz J, Karp CL: The germless theory of allergic disease: Revisiting the hygiene hypothesis. *Nat Rev Immunol* 1:69, 2001.

43. Umetsu DT, Akbari O, Dekruyff RH: Regulatory T cells control the development of allergic disease and asthma. *J Allergy Clin Immunol* 112:480, 2003.

44. Akdis CA, Blaser K: Mechanisms of interleukin-10-mediated immune suppression. *Immunology* 103:131, 2001.

45. Zuany-Amorim C, Sawicka E, Manlius C, et al: Suppression of airway eosinophilia by killed Mycobacterium vaccae-induced allergen-specific regulatory T-cells. *Nat Med* 8:625, 2002.

46. Suto A, Nakajima H, Kagami SI, et al: Role of CD4(+) CD25(+) regulatory T cells in T helper 2 cell-mediated allergic inflammation in the airways. *Am J Respir Crit Care Med* 164:680, 2001.

47. Hansel TT, De Vries IJ, Iff T, et al: An improved immunomagnetic procedure for the isolation of highly purified human blood eosinophils. *J Immunol Methods* 145:105, 1991.

48. Caulfield JP, Hein A, Rothenberg ME, et al: A morphometric study of normodense and hypodense human eosinophils that are derived in vivo and in vitro. *Am J Pathol* 137:27, 1990.

49. Mishra A, Hogan SP, Brandt EB, et al: Enterocyte expression of the eotaxin and interleukin-5 transgenes induces compartmentalized dysregulation of eosinophil trafficking. *J Biol Chem* 277:4406, 2002.

50. Hurst SD, Muchamuel T, Gorman DM, et al: New IL-17 family members promote Th1 or Th2 responses in the lung: In vivo function of the novel cytokine IL-25. *J Immunol* 169:443, 2002.

51. Bochner BS: Road signs guiding leukocytes along the inflammation superhighway. *J Allergy Clin Immunol* 106:817, 2000.

52. Wardlaw AJ: Molecular basis for selective eosinophil trafficking in asthma: A multistep paradigm. *J Allergy Clin Immunol* 104:917, 1999.

53. Rothenberg ME: Eosinophilia. *N Engl J Med* 338:1592, 1998.

54. Palframan RT, Collins PD, Williams TJ, Rankin SM: Eotaxin induces a rapid release of eosinophils and their progenitors from the bone marrow. *Blood* 91:2240, 1998.

55. Palframan RT, Collins PD, Severs NJ, et al: Mechanisms of acute eosinophil mobilization from the bone marrow stimulated by interleukin 5: The role of specific adhesion molecules and phosphatidylinositol 3-kinase. *J Exp Med* 188:1621, 1998.

56. Tachimoto H, Burdick MM, Hudson SA, et al: CCR3-active chemokines promote rapid detachment of eosinophils from VCAM-1 in vitro. *J Immunol* 165:2748, 2000.

57. Tomaki M, Zhao LL, Lundahl J, et al: Eosinophilopoiesis in a murine model of allergic airway eosinophilia: Involvement of bone marrow IL-5 and IL-5 receptor alpha. *J Immunol* 165:4040, 2000.

58. Inman MD: Bone marrow events in animal models of allergic inflammation and hyperresponsiveness. *J Allergy Clin Immunol* 106:S235, 2000.

59. Edwards BS, Curry MS, Tsuji H, et al: Expression of P-selectin at low site density promotes selective attachment of eosinophils over neutrophils. *J Immunol* 165:404, 2000.

60. Dang B, Wiehler S, Patel KD: Increased PSGL-1 expression on granulocytes from allergic-asthmatic subjects results in enhanced leukocyte recruitment under flow conditions. *J Leukoc Biol* 72:702, 2002.

61. Woltmann G, McNulty CA, Dewson G, et al: Interleukin-13 induces PSGL-1/P-selectin-dependent adhesion of eosinophils, but not neutrophils, to human umbilical vein endothelial cells under flow. *Blood* 95:3146, 2000.

62. Kitayama J, Mackay CR, Ponath PD, Springer TA: The C-C chemokine receptor CCR3 participates in stimulation of eosinophil arrest on inflammatory endothelium in shear flow. *J Clin Invest* 101:2017, 1998.

63. Ainslie MP, McNulty CA, Huynh T, et al: Characterization of adhesion receptors mediating lymphocyte adhesion to bronchial endothelium provides evidence for a distinct lung homing pathway. *Thorax* 57:1054, 2002.

64. Doerschuk CM: Leukocyte trafficking in alveoli and airway passages. *Respir Res* 1:136, 2000.

65. Doerschuk CM: Mechanisms of leukocyte sequestration in inflamed lungs. *Microcirculation* 8:71, 2001.

66. Humbles AA, Lu B, Friend DS, et al: The murine CCR3 receptor regulates both the role of eosinophils and mast cells in allergen-induced airway inflammation and hyperresponsiveness. *Proc Natl Acad Sci U S A* 99:1479, 2002.

67. Woolley KL, Gibson PG, Carty K, et al: Eosinophil apoptosis and the resolution of airway inflammation in asthma. *Am J Respir Crit Care Med* 154:237, 1996.

68. Simon HU, Yousefi S, Schranz C, et al: Direct demonstration of delayed eosinophil apoptosis as a mechanism causing tissue eosinophilia. *J Immunol* 158:3902, 1997.

69. Anwar AR, Moqbel R, Walsh GM, et al: Adhesion to fibronectin prolongs eosinophil survival. *J Exp Med* 177:839, 1993.

70. Flood-Page PT, Menzies-Gow AN, Kay AB, Robinson DS: Eosinophil's role remains uncertain as anti-interleukin-5 only partially depletes numbers in asthmatic airway. *Am J Respir Crit Care Med* 167:199, 2003.

71. Meagher LC, Cousin JM, Seckl JR, Haslett C: Opposing effects of glucocorticoids on the rate of apoptosis in neutrophilic and eosinophilic granulocytes. *J Immunol* 156:4422, 1996.

72. Walsh GM, Wardlaw AJ: Dexamethasone inhibits prolonged survival and autocrine granulocyte-macrophage colony-stimulating factor production by human eosinophils cultured on laminin or tissue fibronectin. *J Allergy Clin Immunol* 100:208, 1997.

73. Robertson NM, Zangrilli JG, Steplewski A, et al: Differential expression of TRAIL and TRAIL receptors in allergic asthmatics following segmental antigen challenge: Evidence for a role of TRAIL in eosinophil survival. *J Immunol* 169:5986, 2002.

74. Adachi T, Alam R: The mechanism of IL-5 signal transduction. *Am J Physiol* 275:C623, 1998.

75. Dewson G, Walsh GM, Wardlaw AJ: Expression of Bcl-2 and its homologues in human eosinophils. Modulation by interleukin-5. *Am J Respir Cell Mol Biol* 20:720, 1999.

76. Dewson G, Cohen GM, Wardlaw AJ: Interleukin-5 inhibits translocation of Bax to the mitochondria, cytochrome c release, and activation of caspases in human eosinophils. *Blood* 98:2239, 2001.

77. Letuve S, Druilhe A, Grandsaigne M, et al: Involvement of caspases and of mitochondria in Fas ligation-induced eosinophil apoptosis: Modulation by interleukin-5 and interferon-gamma. *J Leukoc Biol* 70:767, 2001.

78. Letuve S, Druilhe A, Grandsaigne M, et al: Critical role of mitochondria, but not caspases, during glucocorticosteroid-induced human eosinophil apoptosis. *Am J Respir Cell Mol Biol* 26:565, 2002.

79. Temple R, Allen E, Fordham J, et al: Microarray analysis of eosinophils reveals a number of candidate survival and apoptosis genes. *Am J Respir Cell Mol Biol* 25:425, 2001.

80. Lilly M, Le T, Holland P, Hendrickson SL: Sustained expression of the pim-1 kinase is specifically induced in myeloid cells by cytokines whose receptors are structurally related. *Oncogene* 7:727, 1992.

81. O'Farrell AM, Ichihara M, Mui AL, Miyajima A: Signaling pathways activated in a unique mast cell line where interleukin-3 supports survival and stem cell factor is required for a proliferative response. *Blood* 87:3655, 1996.

82. Lilly M, Sandholm J, Cooper JJ, et al: The PIM-1 serine kinase prolongs survival and inhibits apoptosis-related mitochondrial dysfunction in part through a bcl-2-dependent pathway. *Oncogene* 18:4022, 1999.

83. Robinson DS, Damia R, Zeibecoglou K, et al: CD34(+)/interleukin-5Ralpha messenger RNA+ cells in the bronchial mucosa in asthma: Potential airway eosinophil progenitors. *Am J Respir Cell Mol Biol* 20:9, 1999.

84. Shi HZ, Humbles A, Gerard C, et al: Lymph node trafficking and antigen presentation by endobronchial eosinophils. *J Clin Invest* 105:945, 2000.

85. Corry DB, Rishi K, Kanellis J, et al: Decreased allergic lung inflammatory cell egression and increased susceptibility to asphyxiation in MMP2-deficiency. *Nat Immunol* 3:347, 2003.

86. Okada S, Kita H, George TJ, et al: Transmigration of eosinophils through basement membrane components in vitro: Synergistic effects of platelet-activating factor and eosinophil-active cytokines. *Am J Respir Cell Mol Biol* 16:455, 1997.

87. Martin C, Burdon PC, Bridger G, et al: Chemokines acting via CXCR2 and CXCR4 control the release of neutrophils from the bone marrow and their return following senescence. *Immunity* 19:583, 2003.

88. Flood-Page P, Menzies-Gow A, Phipps S, et al: Anti-IL-5 treatment reduces deposition of ECM proteins in the bronchial subepithelial basement membrane of mild atopic asthmatics. *J Clin Invest* 112:1029, 2003.

89. Foster PS, Mould AW, Yang M, et al: Elemental signals regulating eosinophil accumulation in the lung. *Immunol Rev* 179:173, 2001.

90. Lacy P, Moqbel R: Eosinophil cytokines. *Chem Immunol* 76:134, 2000.

91. Bandeira-Melo C, Weller PF: Eosinophils and cysteinyl leukotrienes. *Prostaglandins Leukot Essent Fatty Acids* 69:135, 2003.

92. Cromwell O, Wardlaw AJ, Champion A, et al: IgG-dependent generation of platelet-activating factor by normal and low density human eosinophils. *J Immunol* 145:3862, 1990.

93. Bozza PT, Yu W, Penrose JF, Morgan ES, et al: Eosinophil lipid bodies: Specific, inducible intracellular sites for enhanced eicosanoid formation. *J Exp Med* 186:909, 1997.

94. Phipps S, Ying S, Wangoo A, Ong YE, et al: The relationship between allergen-induced tissue eosinophilia and markers of repair and remodeling in human atopic skin. *J Immunol* 169:4604, 2002.

95. Brightling CE, Bradding P, Symon FA, et al: Mast-cell infiltration of airway smooth muscle in asthma. *N Engl J Med* 346:1699, 2002.

96. Barker RL, Gleich GJ, Pease LR: Acidic precursor revealed in human eosinophil granule major basic protein cDNA. *J Exp Med* 168:1493, 1988.

97. Butterworth AE, Sturrock RF, Houba V, et al: Eosinophils as mediators of antibody-dependent damage to schistosomula. *Nature* 256:727, 1975.

98. Gleich GJ: Mechanisms of eosinophil-associated inflammation. *J Allergy Clin Immunol* 105:651, 2000.

99. Rohrbach MS, Wheatley CL, Slifman NR, Gleich GJ: Activation of platelets by eosinophil granule proteins. *J Exp Med* 172:1271, 1990.

100. Ten RM, Pease LR, McKean DJ, et al: Molecular cloning of the human eosinophil peroxidase. Evidence for the existence of a peroxidase multigene family. *J Exp Med* 169:1757, 1989.

101. Rosenberg HF, Ackerman SJ, Tenen DG: Human eosinophil cationic protein. Molecular cloning of a cytotoxin and helminthotoxin with ribonuclease activity. *J Exp Med* 170:163, 1989.

102. Young JD, Peterson CG, Venge P, Cohn ZA: Mechanism of membrane damage mediated by human eosinophil cationic protein. *Nature* 321:613, 1986.

103. Rosenberg HF, Tenen DG, Ackerman SJ: Molecular cloning of the human eosinophil-derived neurotoxin: A member of the ribonuclease gene family. *Proc Natl Acad Sci U S A* 86:4460, 1989.

104. Ackerman SJ, Liu L, Kwatia MA, et al: Charcot-Leyden crystal protein (galectin-10) is not a dual function galectin with lysophospholipase activity but binds a lysophospholipase inhibitor in a novel structural fashion. *J Biol Chem* 277:14859, 2002.

105. Kita H, Weiler DA, Abu-Ghazaleh R, et al: Release of granule proteins from eosinophils cultured with IL-5. *J Immunol* 149:629, 1992.

106. Seminario MC, Saini SS, MacGlashan DW Jr, Bochner BS: Intracellular expression and release of Fc epsilon RI alpha by human eosinophils. *J Immunol* 162:6893, 1999.

107. Hartnell A, Kay AB, Wardlaw AJ: IFN-gamma induces expression of Fc gamma RIII (CD16) on human eosinophils. *J Immunol* 148:1471, 1992.

108. Abu-Ghazaleh RI, Fujisawa T, Mestecky J, et al: IgA-induced eosinophil degranulation. *J Immunol* 142:2393, 1989.

109. Kaneko M, Horie S, Kato M, et al: A crucial role for beta 2 integrin in the activation of eosinophils stimulated by IgG. *J Immunol* 155:2631, 1995.

110. Nusse O, Lindau M, Cromwell O, et al: Intracellular application of guanosine-5'-O-(3-thiotriphosphate) induces exocytotic granule fusion in guinea pig eosinophils. *J Exp Med* 171:775, 1990.

111. Lavigne S, Bosse M, Boulet LP, Laviolette M: Identification and analysis of eosinophils by flow cytometry using the depolarized side scatter-saponin method. *Cytometry* 29:197, 1997.

112. Kimura I, Moritani Y, Tanizaki Y: Basophils in bronchial asthma with reference to reagin-type allergy. *Clin Allergy* 3:195, 1973.

113. Krause JR, Boggs DR: Search for eosinopenia in hospitalized patients with normal blood leukocyte concentration. *Am J Hematol* 24:55, 1987.

114. Juhlin L, Michaelsson G: A new syndrome characterized by absence of eosinophils and basophils. *Lancet* 1:1233, 1977.

115. Juhlin L, Venge P: Total absence of eosinophils in a patient with chronic urticaria and vitiligo. *Eur J Haematol* 40:368, 1988.

116. Telerman A, Amson RB, Delforge A, et al: A case of chronic aneosinocytosis. *Am J Hematol* 12:187, 1982.

117. Nakahata T, Spicer SS, Leary AG, et al: Circulating eosinophil colony-forming cells in pure eosinophil aplasia. *Ann Intern Med* 101:321, 1984.

118. Joshua H, Zucker A, Presentey B: Peroxidase and phospholipid deficiency in eosinophilic granulocytes among Arabs of the Nazareth district. *Isr J Med Sci* 12:71, 1976.

119. Bochner BS: Verdict in the case of therapies versus eosinophils: The jury is still out. *J Allergy Clin Immunol* 113:3, quiz 10, 2004.

120. Todd R, Donoff BR, Chiang T, et al: The eosinophil as a cellular source of transforming growth factor alpha in healing cutaneous wounds. *Am J Pathol* 138:1307, 1991.

121. Gouon-Evans V, Rothenberg ME, Pollard JW: Postnatal mammary gland development requires macrophages and eosinophils. *Development* 127:2269, 2000.

122. Munitz A, Levi-Schaffer F: Eosinophils: "New" roles for "old" cells. *Allergy* 59:268, 2004.

123. Wong DT, Bowen SM, Elovic A, et al: Eosinophil ablation and tumor development. *Oral Oncol* 35:496, 1999.

124. Weller PF: The idiopathic hypereosinophilic syndrome. *Arch Dermatol* 132:583, 1996.

125. Klion AD, Nutman TB: The role of eosinophils in host defense against helminth parasites. *J Allergy Clin Immunol* 113:30, 2004.

126. Chapman ID, Foster A, Morley J: The relationship between inflammation and hyperreactivity of the airways in asthma. *Clin Exp Allergy* 23:168, 1993.

127. Wardlaw AJ, Brightling C, Green R, et al: Eosinophils in asthma and other allergic diseases. *Br Med Bull* 56:985, 2000.

128. Green RH, Brightling CE, Woltmann G, et al: Analysis of induced sputum in adults with asthma: Identification of subgroup with isolated sputum neutrophilia and poor response to inhaled corticosteroids. *Thorax* 57:875, 2002.

129. Pin I, Freitag AP, O'Byrne PM, et al: Changes in the cellular profile of induced sputum after allergen-induced asthmatic responses. *Am Rev Respir Dis* 145:1265, 1992.

130. Pavord ID, Brightling CE, Woltmann G, Wardlaw AJ: Non-eosinophilic corticosteroid unresponsive asthma [letter]. *Lancet* 353:2213, 1999.

131. Henderson WR, Jr, Chi EY, Albert RK, et al: Blockade of CD49d (alpha4 integrin) on intrapulmonary but not circulating leukocytes inhibits airway inflammation and hyperresponsiveness in a mouse model of asthma. *J Clin Invest* 100:3083, 1997.

132. Green RH, Brightling CE, McKenna S, et al: Asthma exacerbations and sputum eosinophil counts: A randomized controlled trial. *Lancet* 360:1715, 2002.

133. Leiferman KM, Gleich GJ: Hypereosinophilic syndrome: Case presentation and update. *J Allergy Clin Immunol* 113:50, 2004.

134. Simon D, Braathen LR, Simon HU: Eosinophils and atopic dermatitis. *Allergy* 59:561, 2004.

135. Rothenberg ME: Eosinophilic gastrointestinal disorders (EGID). *J Allergy Clin Immunol* 113:11, quiz 29, 2004.

136. Straumann A, Spichtin HP, Grize L, et al: Natural history of primary eosinophilic esophagitis: A follow-up of 30 adult patients for up to 11.5 years. *Gastroenterology* 125:1660, 2003.

137. Garrett JK, Jameson SC, Thomson B, et al: Anti-interleukin-5 (mepolizumab) therapy for hypereosinophilic syndromes. *J Allergy Clin Immunol* 113:115, 2004.

138. Hagan P, Wilkins HA, Blumenthal UJ, et al: Eosinophilia and resistance to Schistosoma haematobium in man. *Parasite Immunol* 7:625, 1985.

139. Sher A, Coffman RL, Hieny S, Cheever AW: Ablation of eosinophil

and IgE responses with anti-IL-5 or anti-IL-4 antibodies fails to affect immunity against Schistosoma mansoni in the mouse. *J Immunol* 145: 3911, 1990.

140. Herbert DR, Lee JJ, Lee NA, et al: Role of IL-5 in innate and adaptive immunity to larval Strongyloides stercoralis in mice. *J Immunol* 165: 4544, 2000.

141. Limaye AP, Abrams JS, Silver JE, et al: Regulation of parasite-induced eosinophilia: Selectively increased interleukin 5 production in helminth-infected patients. *J Exp Med* 172:399, 1990.

142. Hardy WR, Anderson RE: The hypereosinophilic syndromes. *Ann Intern Med* 68:1220, 1968.

143. Chusid MJ, Dale DC, West BC, Wolff SM: The hypereosinophilic syndrome: Analysis of fourteen cases with review of the literature. *Medicine (Baltimore)* 54:1, 1975.

144. Weller PF, Bubley GJ: The idiopathic hypereosinophilic syndrome. *Blood* 83:2759, 1994.

145. Fauci AS, Harley JB, Roberts WC, et al: The idiopathic hypereosinophilic syndrome. Clinical, pathophysiologic, and therapeutic considerations. *Ann Intern Med* 97:78, 1982.

146. Roufosse F, Cogan E, Goldman M: Recent advances in pathogenesis and management of hypereosinophilic syndromes. *Allergy* 59:673, 2004.

147. Cools J, DeAngelo DJ, Gotlib J, et al: A tyrosine kinase created by fusion of the PDGFRA and FIP1L1 genes as a therapeutic target of imatinib in idiopathic hypereosinophilic syndrome. *N Engl J Med* 348: 1201, 2003.

148. Griffin JH, Leung J, Bruner RJ, et al: Discovery of a fusion kinase in EOL-1 cells and idiopathic hypereosinophilic syndrome. *Proc Natl Acad Sci U S A* 100:7830, 2003.

149. Gotlib J, Cools J, Malone JM 3rd, et al: The FIP1L1-PDGFRalpha fusion tyrosine kinase in hypereosinophilic syndrome and chronic eosinophilic leukemia: Implications for diagnosis, classification, and management. *Blood* 103:2879, 2004.

150. Musto P, Perla G, Minervini MM, et al: Imatinib-mesylate for all patients with hypereosinophilic syndrome? *Leuk Res* 28:773, 2004.

151. Klion AD, Noel P, Akin C, et al: Elevated serum tryptase levels identify a subset of patients with a myeloproliferative variant of idiopathic hypereosinophilic syndrome associated with tissue fibrosis, poor prognosis, and imatinib responsiveness. *Blood* 101:4660, 2003.

152. Cogan E, Schandene L, Crusiaux A, et al: Brief report: Clonal proliferation of type 2 helper T cells in a man with the hypereosinophilic syndrome. *N Engl J Med* 330:535, 1994.

153. Simon HU, Plotz SG, Dummer R, Blaser K: Abnormal clones of T cells producing interleukin-5 in idiopathic eosinophilia. *N Engl J Med* 341: 1112, 1999.

154. Roufosse F, Schandene L, Sibille C, et al: Clonal Th2 lymphocytes in patients with the idiopathic hypereosinophilic syndrome. *Br J Haematol* 109:540, 2000.

155. Pardanani A, Ketterling RP, Brockman SR, et al: CHIC2 deletion, a surrogate for FIP1L1-PDGFRA fusion, occurs in systemic mastocytosis

associated with eosinophilia and predicts response to imatinib mesylate therapy. *Blood* 102:3093, 2003.

156. Spry CJF: The idiopathic hypereosinophilic syndrome, in *Eosinophils, Biological and Clinical Aspects*, edited by S Makino, T Fukuda, chap 22, pp 403–421. CRC Press, Boca Raton, 1991.

157. Klion AD, Law MA, Riemenschneider W, et al: Familial eosinophilia: A benign disorder? *Blood* 103:4050, 2004.

158. Butterfield JH, Gleich GJ: Response of six patients with idiopathic hypereosinophilic syndrome to interferon alfa. *J Allergy Clin Immunol* 94: 1318, 1994.

159. Cools J, Stover EH, Boulton CL, et al: PKC412 overcomes resistance to imatinib in a murine model of FIP1L1-PDGFRalpha-induced myeloproliferative disease. *Cancer Cell* 3:459, 2003.

160. Pitini V, Arrigo C, Azzarello D, et al: Serum concentration of cardiac troponin T in patients with hypereosinophilic syndrome treated with imatinib is predictive of adverse outcomes. *Blood* 102:3456, 2003.

161. Klion AD, Law MA, Noel P, et al: Safety and efficacy of the monoclonal anti-interleukin-5 antibody SCH55700 in the treatment of patients with hypereosinophilic syndrome. *Blood* 103:2939, 2004.

162. Posada de la Paz M, Philen RM, Borda AI: Toxic oil syndrome: The perspective after 20 years. *Epidemiol Rev* 23:231, 2001.

163. Ten RM, Kephart GM, Posada M, et al: Participation of eosinophils in the toxic oil syndrome. *Clin Exp Immunol* 82:313, 1990.

164. Di Biagio E, Sanchez-Borges M, Desenne JJ, et al: Eosinophilia in Hodgkin disease: A role for interleukin 5. *Int Arch Allergy Immunol* 110:244, 1996.

165. Hallam LA, Mackinlay GA, Wright AM: Angiolymphoid hyperplasia with eosinophilia: Possible aetiological role for immunization. *J Clin Pathol* 42:944, 1989.

166. Hellmich B, Ehlers S, Csernok E, Gross WL: Update on the pathogenesis of Churg-Strauss syndrome. *Clin Exp Rheumatol* 21:S69, 2003.

167. Guillevin L, Guittard T, Bletry O, et al: Systemic necrotizing angiitis with asthma: Causes and precipitating factors in 43 cases. *Lung* 165: 165, 1987.

168. Guillevin L, Cohen P, Gayraud M, et al: Churg-Strauss syndrome. Clinical study and long-term follow-up of 96 patients. *Medicine (Baltimore)* 78:26, 1999.

169. Guilpain P, Viallard JF, Lagarde P, et al: Churg-Strauss syndrome in two patients receiving montelukast. *Rheumatology (Oxford)* 41:535, 2002.

170. Lakhanpal S, Ginsburg WW, Michet CJ, Doyle JA, Moore SB: Eosinophilic fasciitis: Clinical spectrum and therapeutic response in 52 cases. *Semin Arthritis Rheum* 17:221, 1988.

171. Corwin HL, Bray RA, Haber MH: The detection and interpretation of urinary eosinophils. *Arch Pathol Lab Med* 113:1256, 1989.

172. Hughes PA, Magnet AD, Fishbain JT: Eosinophilic meningitis: A case series report and review of the literature. *Mil Med* 168:817, 2003.

173. Stephanini M, Cvlaustro JC, Motos RA, Bendigo LL: Blood and marrow eosinophilia in malignant tumors. *Cancer* 68:543, 1991.

BASOPHILS AND MAST CELLS AND THEIR DISORDERS

STEPHEN J. GALLI

DEAN D. METCALFE

DANIEL A. ARBER

ANN M. DVORAK

Although basophils and mast cells share biochemical and functional characteristics, they are not identical. In humans, basophils are the least frequent of the three granulocytes, typically accounting for less than 0.5 percent of blood leukocytes. Basophils circulate as mature cells and can be recruited into tissues, particularly at sites of immunologic or inflammatory responses, but they ordinarily do not reside in tissues. By contrast, mast cells typically are derived from blood precursors that lack many of the characteristic features of the mature cells and complete their maturation in the tissues. The mature mast cells can reside in tissues for long periods of time. Mast cells are particularly abundant near blood vessels and nerves and in connective tissues beneath surfaces that are exposed to the external environment, such as the skin, gastrointestinal and urogenital tracts, and respiratory system. Tissue mast cell numbers can increase at sites of parasite infection or in association with certain chronic allergic diseases or other forms of pathology, by recruitment and local maturation of blood precursors and by proliferation of resident mast cells.

Mast cells and basophils express the high-affinity receptor for immunoglobulin (Ig) E (FcεRI) on their surface. Both cell types can be triggered to release potent mediators in response to activation via FcεRI, for example, when their cell-bound IgE recognizes bivalent or multivalent allergens. Accordingly, mast cells and basophils have long been regarded as important effector cells in asthma, hay fever, and other allergic disorders. It is thought that the cells' cytoplasmic granule-associated preformed mediators, including histamine and certain proteases, their lipid mediators (such as prostaglandin D_2 and leukotriene C_4), which are generated upon activation of the cells, and their cytokines, growth factors, and chemokines contribute to many of the characteristic signs and symptoms of these diseases. However, several lines of evidence indicate mast cells and basophils also contribute to protective host responses associated with IgE production, especially those directed against parasites. Mast cells also contribute to host defense in innate immune responses to certain bacterial infections and to pathology in certain T cell–associated immunologic disorders not thought to involve IgE, including some autoimmune diseases. Mast cells and basophils may express immunoregulatory functions through cytokine production and other mechanisms.

Although a variety of systemic disorders have been associated with changes in the numbers of blood basophils and many pathologic processes can be associated with changes in the numbers of tissue mast cells, patients with primary deficiencies in basophils appear to be exceedingly rare (if they exist at all). Patients with a primary deficiency of tissue mast cells have not been reported. By contrast, neoplastic processes can affect both of the lineages. Increased numbers of basophils may be present in association with myeloproliferative disorders and several forms of myelogenous leukemias. Increased numbers of basophils, sometimes to levels of 20 to 90 percent of blood leukocytes, occur in virtually all patients with chronic myelogenous leukemia. It is thought the basophils associated with cases of leukemia are themselves neoplastic. The management of patients with "basophilic leukemia" can be complicated by shock as a result of massive release of histamine and other mediators in association with acute cytolysis.

Disorders of mast cell hyperplasia/neoplasia include solitary mastocytomas, the pathogenesis of which is uncertain, the spectrum of disorders encompassed in the term *mastocytosis*, in which significantly increased numbers of mast cells occur in the skin and/or other organs, and mast cell leukemia. The most common form of mastocytosis, indolent systemic mastocytosis (ISM), typically presents with urticaria pigmentosa (UP) involving the skin, although other organs may be involved. Patients with ISM have the best prognosis and can expect a normal life span. The prognosis of systemic mastocytosis with associated clonal, hematologic non-mast cell lineage disease depends on the course of the associated disease. Patients with aggressive systemic mastocytosis have a guarded prognosis because of complications arising from rapid increases in tissue mast cell numbers. Patients with mast cell leukemia, who often present with large numbers of immature mast cells in the peripheral blood at the time of diagnosis, have a fulminant and rapidly fatal course. Most adult patients with mastocytosis have gain-of-function mutations affecting c-*kit*, which encodes the receptor for the major mast cell growth factor stem cell factor (also known as *kit ligand* and *mast cell growth factor*). Some pediatric patients with mastocytosis reportedly have the same Asp816Val gain-of-function c-*kit* mutation observed in most adult patients. Some pediatric patients have a dominant inactivating c-*kit* mutation, whereas others lack c-*kit* mutations entirely.

DISTINGUISHING FEATURES OF BASOPHILS AND MAST CELLS

BASOPHILS

Despite certain striking similarities in biochemistry and function, mammalian basophils and mast cells are not identical.[1–5] The distinction was appreciated by Paul Ehrlich, who described the histochemical staining characteristics of both of these cells in the late nineteenth century. Many lines of evidence indicate basophils share a common precursor with other granulocytes and monocytes.[1–5] Basophils have a short life span[6] and retain granulocytic features even after emigrating into tissues (Fig. 63-1).[7]

The human basophil is the least common blood granulocyte, with a prevalence of approximately 0.5 percent of total leukocytes and approximately 0.3 percent of nucleated marrow cells.[8] Although the basophil's prominent metachromatic cytoplasmic granules allow unmis-

Acronyms and abbreviations that appear in this chapter include: AML, acute myelogenous leukemia; ASM, aggressive systemic mastocytosis; CHS, contact hypersensitivity; CML, chronic myelogenous leukemia; gp120, glycoprotein 120; H&E, hematoxylin and eosin; IL, interleukin; MCL, mast cell leukemia; PUVA, psoralen ultraviolet A; SCF, stem cell factor; SCT, stem cell transplantation; SM-AHNMD, systemic mastocytosis with associated clonal hematologic non-mast cell disease; TLR, Toll-like receptor; TNF, tumor necrosis factor; UP, urticaria pigmentosa.

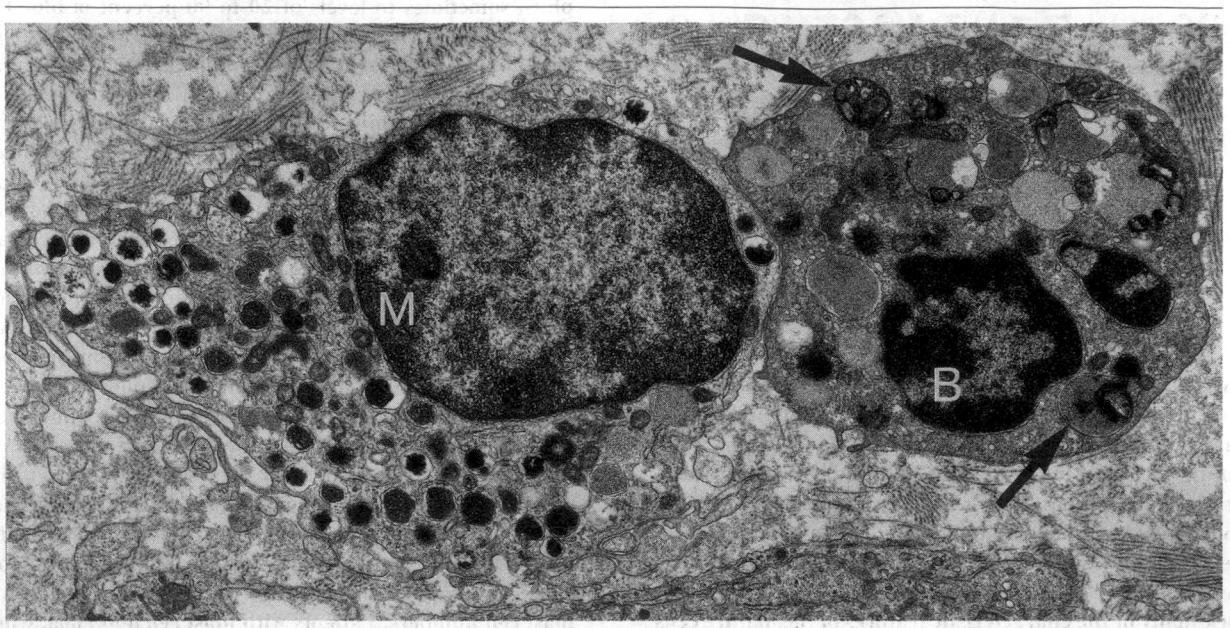

FIGURE 63-1   Mast cell (M) and basophil (B) in the ileal submucosa of a patient with Crohn disease. The mast cell is a larger, mononuclear cell with a more complex plasma membrane surface and cytoplasmic granules that are smaller and more numerous than those of the basophil. In this section plane, the basophil exhibits two nuclear lobes. Several basophil cytoplasmic granules contain whorls of membranes (arrows). Osmium collidine uranyl *en bloc* processing. (From Dvorak et al.,[7] with permission.)

takable identification in Wright-Giemsa–stained films of blood or marrow, accurate basophil determinations require absolute counting methods.[9] Differential counts of blood films yield valid results only if the percentage of basophils is substantially elevated or if many thousands of leukocytes are counted.

Interleukin (IL)-3 promotes the production and survival of human basophils *in vitro*[3,10] and can induce basophilia *in vivo*.[11] Findings in IL-3–/– mice indicate IL-3 is not necessary for the development of normal numbers of bone marrow or blood basophils but is important for the bone marrow and blood basophilia associated with certain T helper (Th)2 cell–associated immunologic responses.[12,13] Basophils also express receptors for several other cytokines (Table 63-1). IL-3 and some of the other cytokines can modulate basophil function, for example, by inducing mediator release directly and/or by augmenting the cells' ability to release mediators in response to challenge with IgE and specific antigen.[3,11,14,15]

MAST CELLS

Mast cells normally reside in the connective tissue, particularly beneath epithelial surfaces and around blood vessels and, in some species, in serous cavities.[1,2,4,5,17–19] Mast cells are derived from hematopoietic precursors.[17,20] Except for a numerically minor population of mast cells that resides in the marrow,[8] this lineage completes its program of maturation in the tissues.[1,2,4,17–20] Unlike basophils, mast cells are long-lived cells. At least some mast cells can locally proliferate in the tissues during a variety of inflammatory or reparative processes.[1,2,4,17–19]

Studies in murine rodents, nonhuman primates, and humans indicate many aspects of mast cell development are critically regulated by stem cell factor (SCF), the ligand for the c-*kit* tyrosine growth factor receptor.[12,18–22] SCF is produced in membrane-associated and in soluble forms, both of which are biologically active.[19,23] In addition to promoting the migration, survival, proliferation, and maturation of

cells in the mast cell lineage, SCF can directly promote mast cell mediator release[22,24–28] and, at even lower concentrations, can augment mast cell mediator release in response to stimulation by immunoglobulin (Ig) E and antigen.[25–27] Abnormalities affecting c-*kit* are involved in the pathogenesis of certain examples of mastocytosis (see below in "Disorders Affecting Mast Cells"). Moreover, alterations in the production of SCF by fibroblasts and other cells likely contribute to the changes in mast cell numbers that occur during many chronic inflammatory conditions and other pathologic responses.[18,19,21,29]

MAST CELL AND BASOPHIL HETEROGENEITY

Variation in the morphologic, biochemical, and/or functional characteristics of mast cells from different anatomic locations or from the same organ or site has been reported in several mammalian species, including humans.[1,2,5,17,19,30–32] This phenomenon, often referred to as *mast cell heterogeneity*, raises the possibility that mast cells of different phenotype express different functions in health or disease and may exhibit different sensitivities to pharmacologic manipulation. At least four mechanisms may account for phenotypic variation in mast cell populations: (1) factors promoting branching within the mast cell lineage; (2) factors influencing differentiation and maturation (within single pathways or, if they occur, within multiple pathways); (3) factors modulating mast cell function; and (4) factors influencing local concentrations of exogenous substances not derived from mast cells but taken up and stored in mast cell granules. Of these four mechanisms, experimental evidence has been obtained for all but the first.[31] Basophils can exhibit some variation in phenotypic characteristics, such as immunoreactivity for tryptase, chymase, and carboxypeptidase A,[16] or levels of expression of surface structures, including HLA-DR, CD32 (FcγRII), and receptors for cytokines.[33] Such variation in basophil mediator content and/or cell surface phenotype may reflect individual differences among different subjects and/or the effects of disease processes[16] or the consequences of immunotherapy.[33]

TABLE 63-1 NATURAL HISTORY, MAJOR MEDIATORS, AND SURFACE MEMBRANE STRUCTURES OF HUMAN MAST CELLS AND BASOPHILS

CHARACTERISTICS	BASOPHILS	MAST CELLS
Natural History		
Origin of precursor cells	Marrow	Marrow
Site of maturation	Marrow	Connective tissue (a few in marrow)
Mature cells in circulation	Yes (usually <1% of blood leukocytes)	No
Mature cells recruited into tissues from circulation	Yes (during immunologic, inflammatory responses)	No
Mature cells normally residing in connective tissues	No (not detectable by microscopy)	Yes
Proliferative ability of morphologically mature cells	None reported	Yes (limited; under certain circumstances)
Life span	Days (like other granulocytes)	Weeks to months (according to studies in rodents)
Major growth factor	IL-3	Stem cell factor (SCF)
Mediators		
Major mediators stored performed in cytoplasmic granules	Histamine, chondroitin sulfates, tryptase,* chymase,* carboxypeptidase A,* neutral protease with bradykinin-generating activity, β-glucuronidase, elastase, cathepsin G-like enzyme, major basic protein, Charcot-Leyden crystal protein	Histamine, heparin, and/or chondroitin sulfates; neutral proteases (chymase and/or tryptase), many acid hydrolases, cathepsin, carboxypeptidases
Major lipid mediators produced on appropriate activation	Leukotriene C_4	Prostaglandin D_2, leukotriene C_4, platelet-activating factor
Cytokines released on appropriate activation	IL-4, IL-13	TNF, macrophage inflammatory protein-1α, VPF/VEGF, IL-13, IL-16 (mouse and human mast cells can secrete many more; see text)
Surface Structures		
Ig receptors	FcϵRI, FcγRII (CDw32)	FcϵRI
Cytokine or growth factor receptors for:	IL-1, IL-2 (CD25), IL-3, IL-4, IL-5, and IL-8; chemokine and interferon receptors; SCF (basophils can express variable numbers of c-*kit* receptors)	SCF (c-*kit* receptor)
Cell adhesion structures (structures in italics are apparently expressed on just one of the two cell types)	P24 (CD9), *LFA-1α chain (CD11a), C3bi receptor/Mac-1α (CD11b)*, LFA-1β chain, β2 & β1 (CD18 & 29), *PECAM (CD31)*, leukosialin (CD43), Pgp-1 (CD44), VLA-4α, β1 (CD49d), VLA-5α, β1 (CD49e), ICAM-3 (CD50), ICAM-1 (CD54), CD58 (LFA-3), ICAM-2 (CD102)	CD09, CD29, CD43, CD44, CD49d, CD49e, CD50, *VNRα, β3 (CD51)*, CD54, CD58, *LFA 1β chain, β3 (CD61)*, CD102

* Basophil content of these (and perhaps other) mediators apparently can vary, e.g., in different subjects and/or in association with certain allergic diseases.[16]
ABBREVIATIONS: ICAM, intercellular adhesion molecule; IL, interleukin; LFA, lymphocyte function–associated antigen; SCF, stem cell factor; VLA, very late antigen; VNR, vitronectin receptor.
SOURCE: Modified from Galli[2] with permission; data regarding CD antigens are from analyses of blood basophils and lung or uterine mast cells.[3] NOTE: Expression of these and other surface structures, including chemokine receptors, can vary in different *in vitro*– or *in vivo*–derived basophil or mast cell populations.

RELATIONSHIP BETWEEN BASOPHILS AND MAST CELLS

Mature basophils and mast cells differ in morphology, natural history, tissue distribution, mediator production, cell surface phenotype, growth factor requirements, and responses to drugs (see Fig. 63-1 and Table 63-1).[1-5] Nevertheless, the two cells exhibit a number of striking similarities. These similarities, taken together with evidence from murine rodents indicating that tissue mast cells are derived from circulating marrow-derived precursors,[17,20] have suggested to some investigators that basophils represent the circulating precursor of mast cells. Although this hypothesis has not formally been excluded, current evidence greatly favors the view that mature basophils represent terminally differentiated granulocytes and not circulating mast cell precursors. In addition to the morphologic evidence discussed below, the latter position is supported by the following observations: (1) no actual evidence has been presented, in any species, indicating that mature circulating basophils are capable of either mitosis or differentiation into mast cells; (2) rare reports of patients with hereditary or acquired abnormalities affecting basophil numbers or morphology indicate that eosinophils also may be affected in these disorders but not mast cells[34-36]; and (3) morphologically identifiable human tissue mast cells can exhibit mitotic activity,[37] indicating this cell lineage is capable of replication independent of a stage resembling that of circulating basophils.

MORPHOLOGY OF BASOPHILS AND MAST CELLS

Routine methods of tissue fixation and processing are poorly suited for demonstration of basophils and mast cells (see Plate VII). Optimal visualization is achieved in appropriately prepared 1-μm sections or with an ultrastructural approach.[1,4] Ultrastructurally, human basophils are 5 to 7 μm in spherical diameter, exhibit a segmented or, in some cases, unsegmented nucleus with marked condensation of nuclear chromatin, and contain round or oval cytoplasmic granules. The granules are surrounded by a membrane and contain a substructure of dense particles, less dense matrix, and, in some granules, membrane whorls and Charcot-Leyden crystals (see Fig. 63-1).[1,4] A second, minor population of small, uniform granules is characteristically located close to the nucleus.[38] The cytoplasm of mature human basophils also contains glycogen particles, mitochondria, free ribosomes, and small membrane-bound vesicles. Lipid bodies are rarely present. Other organelles are inconspicuous.

In tissue sections, mast cells typically appear as either round or elongated cells, usually with a nonsegmented nucleus with moderate condensation of nuclear chromatin, and contain prominent cytoplasmic granules. Mast cell granules are smaller, more numerous, and generally more variable in appearance than in basophils and contain scroll-like structures, particles, and crystals, alone or in combination.[1,4] In contrast to the irregularly spaced blunt surface projections of basophils, mast cells are covered by uniformly distributed thin surface processes. Mast cells also differ from basophils in that they have many more cytoplasmic filaments and lack cytoplasmic glycogen deposits. Human mast cells can contain numerous cytoplasmic lipid bodies. Figure 63-1 shows an electron micrograph of a human basophil adjacent to a human mast cell in the same tissue, the ileal submucosa.

BIOCHEMISTRY AND ROLE IN IgE-ASSOCIATED IMMUNE RESPONSES

MEDIATORS

The cytoplasmic granules of basophils and mast cells contain proteoglycans, consisting of sulfated glycosaminoglycans covalently linked to a protein core.[39,40] Under appropriate conditions, these substances stain metachromatically with basic dyes. In humans and murine species, individual mast cell populations can contain variable mixtures of heparin and chondroitin sulfate proteoglycans.[17,31,39,40] Although the sulfated glycosaminoglycans of normal human blood basophils have not yet been characterized, two studies of the proteoglycans synthesized by blood leukocytes (containing 10–75 percent basophils) of five patients with myelogenous leukemia indicate that such cells may produce solely chondroitin sulfates[41] or a mixture of chondroitin sulfates (50–84 percent) and heparin (8–43 percent).[42] Normal guinea pig basophils synthesize predominantly (85 percent) chondroitin sulfates; the remainder is characterized as heparan sulfate rather than heparin.[43] Although the biologic functions of basophil and mast cell proteoglycans are not fully understood, in mice, heparin is required for normal packaging of certain neutral proteases in mast cell cytoplasmic granules.[44,45] Both human mast cells and basophils synthesize and store histamine.[1,16,39] Basophils represent the source of most (if not all) the histamine present in normal human blood.[46] Studies in mice indicate that mast cells represent the source of virtually all the histamine stored in normal tissues, with the notable exceptions of the glandular stomach and parts of the central nervous system.[47]

In addition to proteoglycans and histamine, basophils and mast cells generate many other mediators that can influence the course of inflammatory processes[1–3,5,39,48] (see Table 63-1). These substances are either preformed and granule associated (e.g., histamine, neutral proteases, proteoglycans) or produced during activation of the cell (e.g., prostaglandin D_2, leukotrienes and other metabolites of arachidonic acid, and platelet-activating factor). Appropriately stimulated mouse or human mast cells can release the cytokine tumor necrosis factor (TNF).[2,5,49–51] Mouse and perhaps human mast cells[2,5,51,52] and human basophils[5,53] can produce IL-4 and IL-13. Work with mouse and human mast cells indicates mast cells also may represent a potential source of many additional cytokines with effects on inflammation, immunity, hematopoiesis, tissue remodeling, and many other biologic processes.[5,51,54–60] By contrast, the spectrum of basophil-derived cytokines appears to be more limited but includes IL-4 and IL-13, and, at least in mice, several chemokines.[5,53,61,62]

ROLE IN ACUTE REACTIONS

Basophils and mast cells have specific, high-affinity plasma membrane receptors for the Fc region of homocytotropic immunoglobulins, which in humans is largely IgE.[63–65] When IgE antibodies bound to the basophil or mast cell surface are bridged by specific divalent or multivalent antigens, anaphylactic degranulation is triggered.[1,2,5,39,40,59,60,63–69] The critical signal in this event is the bridging of IgE receptors (FcεRI) on the plasma membrane. Antibodies to the receptors may substitute for IgE and antigen to initiate degranulation in vitro.[63–65] Antigen binding is independent of divalent cations. However, later steps in degranulation require both calcium and physiologic temperatures.[16,63–65] Morphologically, anaphylactic degranulation involves the fusion of plasma membranes with the membranes delimiting individual cytoplasmic granules or with groups of granules whose membranes have undergone fusion, leading to rapid noncytolytic release of granule contents, such as histamine and other preformed mediators.[1,4] The complex sequence of biochemical events associated with anaphylactic degranulation and the rationale of their pharmacologic manipulation have been reviewed.[66–70]

The sudden, massive release of mediators from basophils and mast cells is thought to provoke many of the clinical manifestations of acute immediate hypersensitivity reactions in disorders such as certain forms of bronchial asthma; urticaria; allergic rhinitis; and anaphylaxis to foods, drugs, insect stings, and other antigens.[1,2,16,39,70,71] Other diverse stimuli, including certain complement fragments (anaphylatoxins), neutrophil lysosomal proteins, a variety of basic peptides and peptide hormones, components of insect venoms, radiocontrast solutions, cold, calcium ionophores, and certain drugs such as narcotics and muscle relaxants, also may initiate rapid release of mediators from basophils and mast cells, independently of IgE.[5,16,39,71] The clinical reactions provoked by these agents can closely mimic those of immediate hypersensitivity. Certain agents, including protein Fv, a sialoprotein found in normal liver and released into the intestinal tract in patients with viral hepatitis, or the HIV glycoprotein 120 (gp120), can interact with the V_H3 domain of IgE and thereby induce release of histamine, IL-4, and IL-3 from human basophils and mast cells.[72,73] The extent to which such proposed "endogenous superallergen" functions of protein Fv or gp120 are important in host defense or in the pathogenesis of viral infections remains to be determined.[72–75]

ROLE IN LATE-PHASE REACTIONS AND THE MAST CELL–LEUKOCYTE CYTOKINE CASCADE

In addition to their roles in classic acute immediate hypersensitivity responses, such as anaphylaxis, mast cells and basophils can contribute to late-phase reactions. Late-phase reactions occur when antigen challenge is followed, hours after initial IgE-dependent mast cell activation, by recurrence of signs (e.g., cutaneous edema) and symptoms (e.g., bronchoconstriction).[71,76] Much of the morbidity associated with chronic allergic conditions, such as allergic asthma, is widely believed to reflect the actions of leukocytes that are recruited to sites of late-phase reactions.[71,76] Studies in mast cell knockin mice (genetically mast cell-deficient mice that have been selectively repaired of their mast cell deficiency) indicate mast cells are responsible for virtually all of the vascular permeability changes and leukocyte infiltration associated with cutaneous late-phase reactions and that TNF importantly contributes to these responses.[77] Mast cell TNF production also likely helps initiate late-phase reactions in humans,[2,5,50,51] and basophils, eosinophils, and other leukocytes that are recruited to these reactions likely produce cytokines and other mediators that regulate further development and, ultimately, resolution of these reactions.[2,5,51] This sequence of events in the pathogenesis of late-phase reactions is termed the *mast cell–leukocyte cytokine cascade*.[2,5,51]

ROLE IN CHRONIC CHANGES ASSOCIATED WITH ALLERGIC DISORDERS

Studies in mast cell knockin mice (see below in "Other Functions and Mast Cell Knockin Mice") indicate that mast cells can contribute importantly to many of the features of chronic asthma, as observed in mouse models of allergic inflammation involving the lungs. The features include the development of airway hyperreactivity to immunologically nonspecific agonists of bronchoconstriction such as methacholine[78,79]; infiltration of the airways and lung interstitium with inflammatory cells, including eosinophils and T cells[78,80]; development of increased deposition of collagen in the lungs and hyperplasia and/or hypertrophy of airway smooth muscle; and induction of increased numbers of mucus-producing goblet cells in the large airways.[80] Thus, such mouse models indicate mast cells and their products can promote the development of much of the pathology and pathophysiologic changes observed in long-standing asthma in humans. Analyses of biopsies of patients with asthma suggest the development of increased numbers of mast cells within the airway smooth muscle layer may be especially important in placing mast cells and their products in proximity to a major target cell in asthma, the bronchial smooth muscle cell.[81]

IGE-DEPENDENT UPREGULATION OF FCεRI EXPRESSION AND FCεRI-DEPENDENT FUNCTION

Notably, as plasma levels of IgE increase (as typically occurs in subjects with allergic diseases or parasite infections), levels of FcεRI expression on the surface of basophils and mast cells also increase.[82,83] Compared with cells with low "baseline" levels of $Fc_\varepsilon RI$ expression, such cells can bind more IgE, release mediators in response to lower concentrations of allergens, and produce significantly larger amounts of preformed and lipid mediators and cytokines.[55,82–85] Thus, basophils and mast cells in subjects with high levels of IgE may have significantly enhanced ability to express IgE-dependent and/or immunoregulatory functions.[70]

Exposure of mouse mast cells to certain monoclonal IgE antibodies, in the absence of exposure to the antigen for which the IgE is known to have specificity, can enhance the survival of the cells and, in some cases, induce the cells to release all three classes of mediators (preformed, lipid, cytokines).[86–88] Exposure to IgE in the absence of known antigen also can induce enhanced survival and cytokine and chemokine release in in vitro-derived human mast cells.[89] Although the mechanisms responsible for these intriguing findings are not fully understood, some types of IgE antibodies appear to induce aggregation of FcεRI in the absence of known antigen.[88] In some cases, this action may reflect the ability of the antigen-binding portion of the IgE to exist in at least two distinct isomeric forms, one binds the "known" antigen and the other binds an "unknown" antigen that may differ from the known antigen structurally and chemically.[90,91] The clinical implications of these findings, if any, remain to be defined. However, the observations raise the possibility that high levels of IgE per se may have biologic consequences, such as enhanced mast cell survival or mast cell mediator release, which can occur even in the absence of exposure to the antigens to which the patient is known to be allergic.

ROLES IN T CELL–DEPENDENT RESPONSES NOT INVOLVING IgE

Mast cell activation and/or infiltration of affected tissues with circulating basophils can occur during a variety of T cell–dependent immunologic responses in both humans and experimental animals.[1,92] Moreover, studies in mast cell knockin mice (see below in "Other Functions and Mast Cell Knockin Mice") show that mast cells can contribute to the expression of mouse models of certain T cell–associated disorders that are not thought to involve IgE, including experimental autoimmune encephalomyelitis (a mouse model of multiple sclerosis)[93] and an antibody-dependent form of destructive arthritis (a model of rheumatoid arthritis).[94] In such settings, mast cell function

may partly reflect the activation of these cells via IgG1 antibodies that recognize the experimental autoantigen, as mouse mast cells can be activated via aggregation of FcγRIII receptors (which bind IgG1 antibodies) and via IgE bound to FcγRI.[95–97]

Several groups have shown that mast cell-deficient mice can exhibit reduced expression of some models of T cell immunity, as in certain examples of contact hypersensitivity (CHS) or delayed hypersensitivity.[98,99] However, in other, apparently quite similar, models of CHS, genetically mast cell-deficient mice can express apparently unimpaired responses.[18,100] Whether or not mast cells are required for optimal expression of CHS, and presumably other T cell–associated responses, now appears to depend on factors such as the type, dose, and vehicle used to administer the hapten in the particular model of CHS tested.[101] One of the functions of mast cells in such settings is to promote the migration of dendritic cells from the skin to the draining lymph nodes during the sensitization phase of the response, when the subject is acquiring sensitivity to that hapten.[101,102] Accordingly, in certain settings, mast cells appear to be able to enhance the development of acquired immune responses. They perform this function by expressing roles (such as enhancing DC migration) that are distinct from the effector functions they may exhibit upon later reexposure to the antigen, when antigen-specific reactions are elicited in subjects who already are sensitized to the antigen of interest.[102]

BIOLOGIC FUNCTIONS OF BASOPHILS AND MAST CELLS

ROLES IN HOST DEFENSE

Basophils and mast cells have critical roles in the expression of host resistance to certain parasites. Whether the basophil or the mast cell represents the major effector cell type in these responses appears to vary according to factors such as species of parasite, species of host, and site of infection. Thus, in the guinea pig, basophils appear to be required for expression of immune resistance to infestation of the skin by larval ixodid Amblyomma americanum ticks,[92,103] whereas expression of IgE-dependent immune resistance to the cutaneous infestation of larval Haemaphysalis longicornis ticks in mice is dependent on mast cells.[104] Such findings support the notion that basophils and mast cells express similar or complementary functions in host defense against parasites and other agents.

Studies in "mast cell knockin mice" (see below in "Other Functions and Mast Cell Knockin Mice") have shown that mast cells can contribute to "innate immunity" to host defense against some bacterial infections.[105–108] The protective role of the mast cell in "natural immunity" in mice partly results from complement-dependent[109] or Toll-like receptor (TLR) 4-dependent[110,111] activation of mast cells and partly from TNF production by mast cells,[105–108,112] resulting in enhanced local recruitment of neutrophils and enhanced clearance of bacteria. Studies in mice indicate mast cells can phagocytose bacteria,[113] and mouse and human mast cells can produce antimicrobial peptides (cathelicidin LL-37 in humans).[114] However, mast cells also may contribute to survival during bacterial infection in mice by additional mechanisms, such as protease-dependent degradation of endothelin-1 and perhaps other endogenous peptides that are produced during infections and contribute to the pathology associated with the disorders.[115] On the other hand, some mast cell functions that may be expressed during bacterial infection in mice, such as the ability of cells to degrade IL-6, may have detrimental consequences.[116] Thus, mast cells may have complex roles in innate immune responses, with some actions promoting host defense and survival and others enhancing the pathology associated with the response.

Mast cells and basophils have been implicated in certain viral infections. Mast cell progenitors[117–119] and circulating basophils[117] can become infected with "M tropic" strains of HIV. Stimulation of cells with ligands for TLR2, TLR4, or TLR9 enhanced viral replication in both HIV-1–infected progenitor and latently infected more mature mast cells.[119] At least one HIV-derived protein, gp120, can induce mast cell or basophil mediator release (histamine and, in basophils, IL-4 and IL-13) by binding to and cross-linking cell-surface bound IgE.[73] Many patients infected with HIV develop high levels of IgE and can exhibit exacerbation of the symptoms and signs of their allergic disorders.[74] However, whether the infection of basophils or mast cells or their precursors with HIV or the activation of these cells in response to gp120 play important roles in the progression of disease in HIV-infected patients remain to be determined. Many potential secreted products of mast cells or basophils may have effects that enhance (or suppress) host responses to a variety of viruses or contribute to the pathology associated with the infections. Moreover, exposure of *in vitro*-derived human mast cells to live dengue virus together with virus-specific antibody induces the cells to release chemokines.[120] However, the extent to which mast cells contribute to host defense or pathology during viral infections is not clear.

OTHER FUNCTIONS AND MAST CELL KNOCKIN MICE

Factors capable of inducing basophil infiltration, mast cell proliferation, and/or basophil or mast cell degranulation are generated during a wide variety of immunologic or pathologic processes and immune responses to parasites.[1,12,16,31,70,71,92] As a result, speculation is considerable that basophils and mast cells express critical roles in diverse biologic responses. On the other hand, the precise functions of basophils and mast cells in most of the biologic responses in which the cells have been implicated are obscure.[18,47,70,108] In the mouse, mutant animals virtually devoid of mast cells and congenic normal mice can be used to define and quantify the contributions of mast cells to many different biologic responses.[2,17,18,47,70,107,108,121] A particularly useful approach is transferring cultured mast cells derived from the bone marrow of normal (WBB6F1-+/+) mice (or mast cells derived from hematopoietic precursors or embryonic stem cells with spontaneous or targeted mutations that affect mast cell development or function) into the skin or other tissues of WBB6F1-*W/W*ᵛ mice, which lack mast cells because of mutations at the *W/c-kit* locus.[17–19,70,107,108,115,121] After sufficient time has been allowed to permit the transferred mast cells to acquire phenotypic characteristics appropriate for their anatomical location, biologic responses can be elicited at sites where mast cell deficiency has been locally and selectively repaired and at paired ("control") mast cell-deficient sites.

Studies using such mast cell knockin mice have shown that mast cells are essential for certain IgE-dependent acute- or late-phase reactions in the skin,[2,77] gastrointestinal tract,[122] or respiratory system[123]; they can enhance the expression of certain IgE-independent immunologic responses to exogenous[95] or auto-antigens[93,94]; they can significantly augment innate immunity to certain bacterial infections[107,108]; and they contribute to certain other immunologically nonspecific acute inflammatory reactions.[2,18,70] However, no human patients devoid of mast cells have yet been identified. In addition, the clinical findings in the rare patients who express a deficiency of basophils are not easy to interpret. One human patient with a profound basopenia experienced persistent and severe infestation with scabies,[34] a finding that might be viewed as consistent with the role of basophils in resisting ectoparasites in humans. However, that patient also had eosinopenia, IgA deficiency, and multiple other clinical problems.[34] A second basophil-deficient patient had a history of recurrent bacterial and viral infections.[36] However, this patient also had a deficiency of eosinophils, hypogammaglobulinemia, abnormal suppressor T cell function *in vitro*, and a thymoma.[36]

BLOOD BASOPHIL COUNT

The normal blood basophil count is difficult to define precisely, but two studies place the normal range between 20 and 80/μl (0.020 and 0.080 × 10⁹/liter).[8,9,48,124] The blood basophil count reportedly varies by age,[125] gender,[125] and season.[126]

BASOPHILOPENIA

Because numbers of blood basophils can be very low even in apparently normal individuals,[8,9,48,124] determining whether examples of *basophilopenia* reflect pathologic processes as opposed to normal variation can be difficult. Nevertheless, reduced numbers of circulating basophils have been reported in several disorders (Table 63-2). Basophilopenia has been recorded in association with urticaria and anaphylaxis,[127,128] but the extent to which this finding represents a loss of metachromatic staining of circulating degranulated cells rather than a true decrease in the number of cells is undetermined. Basophilopenia occurs in conditions that also are associated with eosinophilopenia. These conditions often are associated with increased secretion of adrenal glucocorticoids.[48,124,129,130] Basophil counts may diminish, sometimes markedly, during leukocytosis accompanying infection, inflammatory states, immunologic reactions, neoplasia, or hemorrhage.[129] Basophil counts also are diminished in thyrotoxicosis or after pharmacologic administration of thyroid hormones. Conversely, basophil counts may be increased in myxedema or after ablation of thyroid

TABLE 63-2 CONDITIONS ASSOCIATED WITH ALTERATIONS IN NUMBERS OF BLOOD BASOPHILS[48,124,129]

Decreased Numbers (Basopenia)
Hereditary absence of basophils (very rare)
Elevated levels of glucocorticoids
Hyperthyroidism or treatment with thyroid hormones
Ovulation
Hypersensitivity reactions
   Urticaria
   Anaphylaxis
   Drug-induced reactions
Leukocytosis (in association with diverse disorders)
Increased Numbers (Basophilia)
Allergy or inflammation
   Ulcerative colitis
   Drug, food, inhalant hypersensitivity
   Erythroderma, urticaria
   Juvenile rheumatoid arthritis
Endocrinopathy
   Diabetes mellitus
   Estrogen administration
   Hypothyroidism (myxedema)
Infection
   Chickenpox
   Influenza
   Smallpox
   Tuberculosis
Iron deficiency
Exposure to ionizing radiation
Neoplasia
   "Basophilic leukemia" (see text)
Myeloproliferative diseases (especially chronic myelogenous leukemia; also polycythemia vera, idiopathic myelofibrosis, primary thrombocythemia)
Carcinoma

function.[48,129] A rapid and significant drop in blood basophil levels of up to 50 percent has been documented at ovulation.[131] A few patients with an apparent total lack of basophils have been reported.[34,36]

A morphologic abnormality expressed in the majority of eosinophils and basophils but not in other leukocytes or mast cells has been described as an autosomal dominant condition affecting four members of a family.[35] Cytoplasmic inclusions and crystals in basophils resembling the May-Hegglin anomaly have occurred in healthy individuals.

BASOPHILIA

Table 63-2 lists conditions associated with increased numbers of blood basophils (basophilia).

INFLAMMATORY AND IMMUNOLOGIC RESPONSES

An increased number of basophils is commonly associated with hypersensitivity disorders of the IgE-associated "immediate" type. This disorder often is accompanied by increased levels of IgE. Although serum IgE levels and basophil numbers are not directly related,[132] increased IgE levels are associated with increased expression of FcεRI on the surfaces of both basophils and mast cells.[82,83,133] Moreover, basophils can be recruited into tissues at sites of IgE-associated and other immunologic responses.[1,5,16,71,92] Basophil levels may be elevated in ulcerative colitis[134] and juvenile rheumatoid arthritis,[135] whereas many inflammatory conditions that cause a leukocytosis are associated with basophilopenia. Basophilia can occur in subjects exposed to ionizing radiation.[136]

CLONAL MYELOID DISEASES

Chronic Myeloproliferative Diseases The concentration of blood basophils is slightly increased in many patients with polycythemia vera (see Chap. 56), idiopathic myelofibrosis (see Chap. 89), and thrombocythemia (see Chap. 111). A slight increase in the absolute basophil count may be a useful early sign of a myeloproliferative disease. An increased absolute basophil count occurs in virtually all patients with chronic myelogenous leukemia (CML).[137–139] In some patients, basophils can represent 20 to 90 percent of blood leukocytes (see Chap. 88). Exaggerated basophilia of this type is a poor prognostic sign and may herald transformation to the accelerated phase of CML.[140] The basophil in myeloproliferative diseases is generally thought to be derived from the malignant clone and in CML can contain the Ph chromosome[141] and presumably also the breakpoint cluster gene rearrangement on chromosome 22. The basophils in CML exhibit a variety of ultrastructural and biochemical abnormalities.[142,143] In some cases, the abnormalities obscure the typical distinctions between basophils and mast cells.[144–147] Release of basophil-associated histamine can lead to episodes of flushing, pruritus, and hypotension in occasional patients with basophilic CML.[148,149] Severe peptic ulcer of the stomach and duodenum can occur in association with hypersecretion of gastric acid and pepsin.[150,151] Ph chromosome–positive acute basophilic leukemia may be a presenting manifestation of CML.[152]

Basophilic Leukemias The basis for designating some cases as basophilic leukemias as opposed to examples of myelogenous leukemia with an associated pronounced basophilia is not always clear. Accordingly, we refer to these conditions herein as *leukemias associated with basophilia*. Table 63-3 lists the leukemias associated with basophilia. In addition to extreme basophilia in chronic phase CML or as a manifestation of the accelerated phase of CML, acute basophilic leukemia can rarely occur *de novo*.[153–159] Thus, acute basophilic leukemia is included in the recent World Health Organization classification of acute myelogenous leukemias (AMLs), but the entity is poorly defined, with no recurring cytogenetic or molecular genetic abnormality described.[158,159] Some cases are recognized only by elec-

TABLE 63-3 LEUKEMIAS ASSOCIATED WITH BASOPHILIA

Chronic myelogenous leukemia with exaggerated basophilia[141,148–151]

Blast transformation, including acute basophilic transformation, of chronic myelogenous leukemia[148,158]

Acute myelogenous leukemia with t(9;22), t(6;9), t(3;6) or 12p abnormalities and marrow basophilia[158,160–164]

Acute promyelocytic leukemia with basophilic maturation[165–167]

"Acute basophilic leukemia"[152–159]

tron microscopy, a procedure not used routinely in the diagnosis or classification of leukemias.

Other types of acute myeloid leukemia that have an associated increase in basophils are more prevalent than acute basophilic leukemia. Such acute leukemias most commonly have t(9;22), t(6;9), t(3;6), or 12p abnormalities.[160–163] The t(9;22) AMLs have features similar to blast crisis of CML and may be more related to that disease. The t(6;9) AML often is associated with erythroid hyperplasia and dysplasia and has a poor prognosis.[164]

Rare cases of acute promyelocytic leukemia have been described with associated basophils,[165–167] but the so-called "hyperbasophilic microgranular variant" of this disease refers to cytoplasmic basophilia rather than the presence of basophilic granules,[168] which are unusual in this disease. Similarly, AML with inv(16) or t(16;16) are characteristically associated with cells having large basophilic granules, but these granules are generally thought to represent abnormal eosinophils rather than basophils.[169]

Although the clinical and pathologic features of acute basophilic leukemia are largely similar to the features of myelogenous leukemia, affected patients occasionally exhibit symptoms that result from release of mediators (especially histamine) derived from degranulating or dying basophils.[48,148,149,155,170] Remission induction therapy is similar to the therapy used for other types of AML, but management can be complicated by shock resulting from massive release of histamine and other mediators associated with acute cytolysis.

Chapter 87 provides further details on the acute leukemias associated with basophilia.

DISORDERS AFFECTING MAST CELLS

NORMAL MAST CELL LEVELS

Mast cells cannot be identified in the blood of healthy individuals using standard techniques. However, mast cells can be observed in the blood of monkeys that have been treated chronically with large amounts of the c-*kit* ligand SCF[21] and in the blood of some patients with systemic mastocytosis.[171] Increases in tissue mast cells can occur by a combination of enhanced progenitor influx and proliferation of resident mast cells in tissues.[5,17,172] Human mast cells have been classified according to their content of neutral proteases as MC_T, because the granules contain tryptase but not detectable chymase, and MC_{TC}, whose secretory granules contain both enzymes.[32] The former mast cell type ordinarily predominates in lung and gastrointestinal mucosal tissues and the latter type in dermis and submucosal tissues.[173–175] Mast cells that express chymase but little or no tryptase (MC_C) also have been described.[176]

SECONDARY CHANGES IN MAST CELL NUMBERS

Although long-term treatment with glucocorticoids (particularly topical treatment of the skin) can result in diminished mast cell numbers,[177] no clinical disorder whose primary feature is a reduction in levels of

TABLE 63-4   CONDITIONS ASSOCIATED WITH SECONDARY CHANGES IN MAST CELL NUMBERS

Decreased Numbers
  Long-term treatment with glucocorticoids
  Primary or acquired immunodeficiency disorders (certain mast cell populations, see text and ref. 135)
Increased Numbers
  IgE-associated "immediate hypersensitivity" reactions
    Rhinitis
    Asthma
    Urticaria
  Connective tissue disorders
    Rheumatoid arthritis
    Psoriatic arthritis
    Scleroderma
    Systemic lupus erythematosus
  Infectious diseases
    Tuberculosis
    Syphilis
    Parasitic diseases
  Neoplastic disorders
    Lymphoproliferative diseases *(Waldenström macroglobulinemia, lymphoma, chronic lymphocytic leukemia)
    Hematopoietic stem cell diseases* (acute or chronic myelogenous leukemias, preleukemia, idiopathic refractory sideroblastic anemia)
  Lymph nodes draining areas of tumor growth
  Osteoporosis*
  Chronic liver disease*
  Chronic renal disease*

* Can include increases in numbers of mast cells in the bone marrow.

tissue mast cells has been reported. Studies of small numbers of patients indicate that certain mast cell populations, namely, the MC_T mast cells in the gastrointestinal mucosa, can be strikingly reduced in numbers in subjects with genetically determined or acquired (HIV-induced) immunodeficiency.[178] Human mast cell precursors can be infected in vitro with so-called "M tropic" strains of HIV.[117–119] However, whether the susceptibility of mast cells or their precursors to infection with HIV contributes to the reduction in gastrointestinal mast cells observed in some subjects with HIV infection remains to be determined.

A number of disorders are associated with small to up to several-fold increases in mast cell numbers in or near the tissues affected by the disorder (Table 63-4). Tissues at sites of recurrent allergic reactions often exhibit increases in mast cell numbers, to levels as high as approximately fourfold normal.[174,179] Small increases in mast cell numbers have been observed at sites of pathology in rheumatoid arthritis, psoriatic arthritis, scleroderma, and systemic lupus erythematosus.[180,181] Mast cells have been reported to be increased in osteoporosis,[182] but the extent to which this increase reflects decreases in other cell types and/or a decrease in bone matrix is unclear. Numbers of marrow mast cells can be increased in patients with chronic liver or renal diseases.[183] Increases in mast cells also have been documented in infectious diseases, particularly at sites of infection with parasites such as Strongyloides, in which a greater than fourfold increase in mast cell numbers can occur.[184] In such settings, mast cell numbers can return toward normal upon resolution of the infection. Finally, mast cell numbers can be increased several-fold in lymph nodes draining areas of tumor growth[183,185] and in subjects with stem cell diseases and lymphoproliferative diseases, including lymphoma in the bone marrow and in association with CML.[183,186–188]

DISORDERS OF MAST CELLS: HYPERPLASIA AND NEOPLASIA

DEFINITION AND HISTORY

A group of systemic disorders associated with significant increases in mast cell numbers in the skin and internal organs have been brought together under the term mastocytosis. The first report of a primary mast cell disorder probably was that of Unna[189] in 1887. Unna found that the skin lesions of UP[190,191] contained numerous mast cells. However, it was not until 1949 that Ellis[192] recognized the systemic nature of the disorder. In addition to the systemic disorders classified as mastocytosis, localized cutaneous aggregates of mast cells, ranging from mast cells nevuses and mastocytomas in infants and children to multiple nodules in older children, may occur.[193,194] Solitary mastocytomas generally present before age 6 months and usually involute spontaneously, although in rare cases they are followed by UP.[194] The pathogenesis of such lesions has not been elucidated. Accordingly, the remainder of this section focuses on mastocytosis.

The clinical pattern of disease in mastocytosis and its prognosis can vary substantially among patients (see "Course and Prognosis" below). A consensus classification for mastocytosis has been developed to address the issue and to provide guidelines regarding prognosis and treatment (Table 63-5).[195] Patients with indolent disease, who compose the great majority of subjects with mastocytosis, can expect a normal life span. Patients with systemic mastocytosis with associated clonal, hematologic non-mast cell lineage disease (SM-AHNMD) have a prognosis determined by the associated hematologic disorder. Patients with aggressive systemic mastocytosis (ASM) generally have a 3- to 5-year survival. Mast cell leukemia (MCL) usually is rapidly fatal.

ETIOLOGY AND PATHOGENESIS

Activating mutations in KIT, which encodes the SCF receptor, have been documented in patients with mastocytosis. Several lines of evidence indicate such mutations can be involved in the pathogenesis of the disease. The most common of these mutations (Asp816Val), which results in ligand-independent activation of the KIT receptor, was first identified in a long-term cell line derived from a patient with mast cell leukemia.[196] It then was detected in mononuclear cells in the blood of patients with mastocytosis who had an associated hematologic disorder,[197] as a somatic mutation in lesional tissue obtained from one patient with an aggressive form of mastocytosis and from a second patient with an indolent form of UP,[198] and in the skin, but not the bone marrow and peripheral blood, of an 11-month-old child with mastocytosis.[199]

TABLE 63-5   WORLD HEALTH ORGANIZATION CLASSIFICATION OF SYSTEMIC MASTOCYTOSIS

Cutaneous mastocytosis
  Urticaria pigmentosa (UP)
  Maculopapular cutaneous mastocytosis (MPCM)
  Diffuse cutaneous mastocytosis
  Telangiectasia macularis eruptiva perstans (TMEP)
Indolent systemic mastocytosis (ISM)
Systemic mastocytosis with associated clonal, hematologic non-mast cell lineage disease (SM-AHNMD)
Aggressive systemic mastocytosis (ASM)
Mast cell leukemia (MCL)
Mast cell sarcoma (MCS)
Extracutaneous mastocytoma

* Modified from Valent et al. 2001.[195]

Taken together, these findings suggest the mutation occurs initially in a mast cell progenitor and that, as the clone expands, it first becomes detectable in mastocytosis skin lesions. In patients with more severe disease and thus with a larger clonal expansion, it also can be identified in circulating cells. The Asp816Val mutation, or similar 816 activating mutations that result in the substitution of valine or tyrosine for aspartate, now are believed to occur in almost all adult patients with mastocytosis, in whom the mutation can be readily identified in the skin lesions of UP.[200] Mutations at codon 816 (valine, tyrosine, or phenylalanine for aspartate) have been identified in a subset of pediatric patients, whereas other pediatric patients exhibit a dominant inactivating *KIT* mutation, in which lysine is substituted for glutamic acid in position 839, the site of a potential salt bridge.[200]

The extent to which the presence of various *KIT* mutations, and the anatomical distribution of the affected cells, can be used to predict prognosis or disease severity in patients with mastocytosis largely remains to be determined. Notably, some pediatric patients with mastocytosis appear to lack any *KIT* mutations.[200] Moreover, additional "gain-of-function" mutations of *KIT* in human subjects with mastocytosis may yet remain to be characterized. For example, a novel form of mastocytosis with a transmembrane *KIT* mutation (Phe522Cys) has been described.[201] In dogs, a species in which up to 20 percent of all neoplasms are mast cell tumors, many mast cell tumors exhibit tandem duplications involving exons 11 and 12 of *KIT*.[202,203] Analysis of a dog mastocytoma cell line indicates that such mutations, which affect the juxtamembrane portion of the cytoplasmic domain of the KIT receptor, result in ligand-independent activation of the receptor.[202] Gain-of-function mutations of c-*kit* also have been reported in gastrointestinal stromal tumors[204] and in one pedigree as a germ-line mutation.[205] Whether mast cell numbers are increased in these subjects is not clear.

CLINICAL FEATURES

The organs most frequently involved in systemic mastocytosis are the skin, lymph nodes, liver, spleen, marrow, and gastrointestinal tract.

THE SKIN

The usual presenting lesion of cutaneous mast cell disease is UP. UP lesions appear as small yellowish-tan to reddish-brown macules or slightly raised papules (Fig. 63-2), which can exhibit the Darier sign, that is, urticaria after mild friction of the skin.[193,206] The palms, soles, face, and scalp generally remain free of lesions. In many cases, UP develops before age 2 and subsides by puberty. In adults with UP, extracutaneous involvement by mastocytosis is common.[171,206–208] However, some patients, particularly those with SM-AHNMD, ASM, or MCL, entirely lack cutaneous lesions. In such cases, other organs must be biopsied to make the diagnosis. Diffuse cutaneous mastocytosis is an unusual manifestation of mastocytosis.[194,208] The skin appears yellowish-brown and is thickened. Young children with cutaneous disease may have bullous eruptions with hemorrhage.[194] Some adult patients develop prominent vascularity in association with the skin lesions, a condition termed *telangiectasia macularis eruptiva perstans*.[194]

LYMPH NODES

In one series, peripheral lymphadenopathy occurred in 26 percent and central lymphadenopathy in 19 percent of patients at diagnosis.[209] Lymphadenopathy tends to be most prominent in patients with SM-AHNMD or ASM. Mast cell infiltrates are observed in the node's paracortex, follicles, medullary cords, and sinuses. Additional findings include infiltrates of eosinophils, blood vessel proliferation in association with mast cells in the paracortical areas, and extramedullary hematopoiesis. In hematoxylin and eosin (H&E) stained sections, mast cell infiltrates in the lymph nodes may resemble T cell lymphomas in

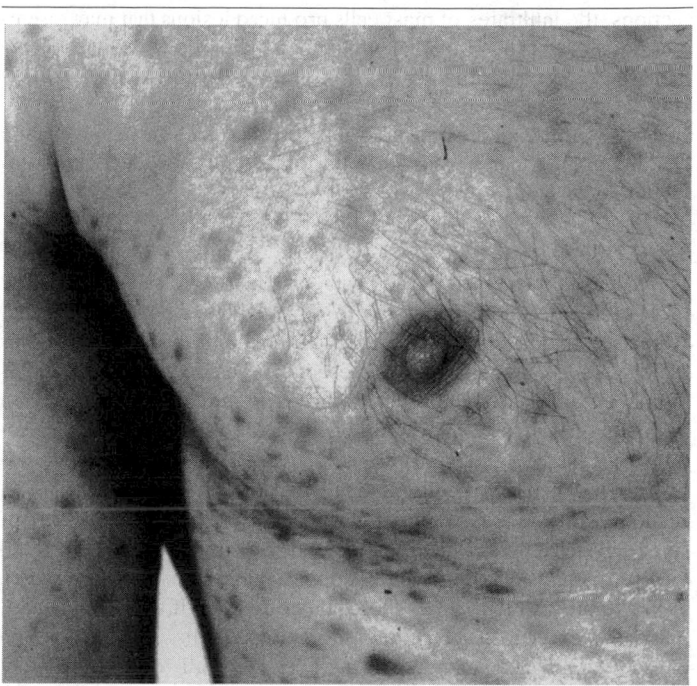

FIGURE 63-2 Urticaria pigmentosa in an adult man with indolent systemic mastocytosis. Multiple pigmented macules are present. If local pressure is applied to the skin, individual lesions show urtication and become raised, pruritic, and erythematous.

their pericortical distribution, the clear cytoplasm that is sometimes exhibited by the mast cells, and the associated vascular proliferation and eosinophilia.[209] Alternatively, when mast cells replace lymphoid follicles, the pattern may resemble follicular hyperplasia or follicular lymphoma.[209] Fibrosis may be observed in lymph nodes involved by mast cell infiltrates.

LIVER

Patients frequently exhibit infiltration of the liver with mast cells. Many of these individuals have some associated liver pathology, but severe liver disease is uncommon. When severe liver disease does occur, it typically affects patients with mastocytosis and an associated hematologic disorder or aggressive mastocytosis (SM-AHNMD or ASM). In one series of 41 patients, 61 percent had some liver disease.[210] Elevated alkaline phosphatase aminotransamidases, 5′ nucleotidase, or γ-glutamyl transpeptidase was detected in the serum of approximately half of the patients. Hepatomegaly, prominent infiltration of the liver with mast cells, and hepatic fibrosis are positively correlated with elevated levels of alkaline phosphatase and were observed more frequently in patients with aggressive disease; ascites or portal hypertension occurred in some of these individuals. Portal fibrosis was observed in 68 percent and was positively correlated with hepatic inflammation and mast cells infiltrates. Venopathy and associated venoocclusive disease was observed in four patients, all of whom had an associated hematologic disorder.

SPLEEN

Splenic involvement at diagnosis has been reported in approximately half of patients with systemic disease.[209,211] Mast cells most commonly occurred in a paratrabecular distribution, followed by perifollicular, follicular, and diffuse infiltrates. Trabecular and capsular fibrosis and eosinophilic infiltration also were observed, and extramedullary hematopoiesis was present in the majority of cases. On H&E stained sections, the infiltrates of mast cells produced lesions that may resemble those of T cell lymphoma, follicular hyperplasia, follicular lymphoma, Kaposi sarcoma, myeloproliferative disorder, hairy cell leukemia, or a granulomatous process. Splenomegaly also occurred in the absence of infiltration of the spleen by mast cells.[212] Increased splenic weights greater than 700 g generally occurred in patients within unfavorable categories of mastocytosis.

MARROW

More than 90 percent of adults with systemic mast cell disease have focal mast cell lesions in the marrow,[211,213–216] which typically appear as foci of spindle-shaped mast cells in a fibrotic background (Color Plate XIV-13), sometimes with associated eosinophils and T and B lymphocytes. The focal mast cell lesions constitute the major criterion in the diagnosis of systemic mastocytosis (Table 63-6). These collections of cells can occur in perivascular, paratrabecular, and intertrabecular locations. Reticulin staining may be increased, and Masson trichome staining may reveal collagen deposition. In specimens extensively involved by mast cell lesions, the bony trabeculae may be moderately to markedly thickened. Aggressive variants of mastocytosis, such as mast cell leukemia, should be considered if the percentage of mast cells exceeds 20 percent of all nucleated cells.

In H&E stained sections, the mast cells typically exhibit a spindle-shaped or oval nucleus (see Color Plate XIV-13A), and fine eosinophilic granules are apparent in the cytoplasm at high-power magnification (see Color Plate XIV-13B). Mast cells with bilobed nuclei may be seen in these lesions and is a finding associated with a poor prognosis.[211] Wright-Giemsa and toluidine blue stains can be used, especially with nondecalcified, plastic-embedded specimens, for more definitive visualization of mast cells. Unfortunately, these stains are less effective on ethylenediaminetetraacetic acid (EDTA)-decalcified, paraffin-embedded material. Mast cells also stain positively for chloracetate esterase and aminocaproate esterase and, in suitably processed specimens, for mast cell tryptase by immunohistochemistry (see Color Plate XIV-13D). This is the procedure of choice for visualizing mast cells. Mast cells exhibit immunoreactivity for a variety of paraffin section markers.[217,218] Although they do not express specific B or T lineage antigens, mast cells are positive for CD43 and CD68, which may cause confusion with histiocytes, T lymphocytes, or even blast cells. However, the lack of other T cell antigens, more specific histiocyte markers, or myeloperoxidase help to exclude those cell types. The more specific mast cell markers in paraffin tissues are CD117 (see Color Plate XIV-13C) and mast cell tryptase (see Color Plate XIV-13D). Although tryptase is the most specific paraffin marker, it is not used in many laboratories. Strong CD117 membrane staining is equally sensitive as tryptase for mast cells but is less specific. A subset of marrow myeloblasts gives strong membrane staining for CD117, but this cell type usually can be identified based on positive staining for myeloperoxidase.

Films of marrow aspirates or clot sections alone cannot be used to diagnose mast cell disease in the marrow. Although increased numbers of mast cells may be present in bone marrow aspirate films of patients with systemic mast cell diseases, similar findings have been reported in patients without mast cell disorders or in patients with a reactive increase in marrow mast cells. However, mast cells in reactive lesions usually are not spindle shaped, nor do they typically exhibit evidence of degranulation. On marrow films, a normal mast cell has a round or oval shape, a round and centrally located, nonlobated nucleus, and a fully granulated cytoplasm. Mast cells from patients with mastocytosis may exhibit phenotypic aberrations, such as a spindle shape, cytoplasmic projections, and hypogranulation. A multilobular and/or eccentrically located nucleus may be observed.[219] If at least 25 percent of all mast cells on aspirate smears have aberrant morphology, the findings are considered to support the diagnosis of systemic mastocytosis (minor criterion).[219] An aberrant mast cell phenotype also may be detected on flow cytometric analysis of the bone marrow aspirate. In patients with mastocytosis, mast cells may express CD2, CD25, and CD33 (minor criterion).[219]

Marrow involvement appears to be much less common in children. In a study of 17 children with cutaneous or disseminated mast cell disease, small focal mast cell lesions were observed in marrow biopsies in 10 individuals, and increased mast cells in marrow aspirate films were noted in five.[215] The focal lesions found in children were uniformly small and perivascular.

Progression of marrow involvement in systemic mast cell disease is variable. Many adults with indolent disease appear to have stable, or even decreasing, marrow involvement over time.[211] In contrast, a progressive increase in focal mast cell lesions is more commonly observed in patients with more aggressive patterns of disease.

CLINICAL PRESENTATION

Even though individuals differ in the specific pathogenesis of their disease, all patients within a given category of mastocytosis (see Table 63-5) generally exhibit similar clinical features. Manifestations of the disease largely reflect the local and systemic consequences of mediator release from tissue mast cells. Effects caused by disruption of normal structures by local collections of mast cells also may be seen.

At presentation, patients with mastocytosis may complain of vague and nonspecific constitutional symptoms, such as fatigue, weakness, flushing, and musculoskeletal pain. Some patients experience fever and/or weight loss.[171,208] A subset of patients may present with recurrent episodes of unexplained hypotension.[220] However, most patients with indolent mastocytosis and a hematologic disorder usually are diagnosed based on marrow biopsy findings, during the investigation of their hematologic disease.[208,211] Patients with aggressive disease often present with unexplained lymphadenopathy and splenomegaly and/or hepatomegaly.

Gastrointestinal disease and associated symptoms are commonly associated with systemic mastocytosis, either at presentation or as the disease progresses.[208,221] Findings include nausea, vomiting, abdominal pain, and diarrhea. Peptic ulcer disease, which is thought to reflect, at least in part, the promotion of gastric acid secretion by elevated histamine levels, occurs in up to 50 percent of patients with systemic

---

TABLE 63-6　DIAGNOSTIC CRITERIA FOR SYSTEMIC MASTOCYTOSIS

Major Criteria

Multifocal, dense infiltrates of mast cells (≥15 mast cells in an aggregate) detected in sections of bone marrow and/or other extracutaneous organ(s) and confirmed by tryptase immunohistochemistry (or other special stains)

Minor Criteria

a. In biopsy sections of bone marrow or other extracutaneous organs, >25% of the mast cells in the infiltrate are spindle shaped or have atypical morphology, or, of all mast cells in bone marrow aspirate smears, >25% are immature or atypical mast cells

b. Detection of c-*kit* mutation at codon 816 in bone marrow, blood, or other extracutaneous organs

c. Mast cells in bone marrow, blood, or other extracutaneous organs that coexpress CD117 with CD2 and/or CD25

d. Serum total tryptase persistently >20 ng/ml (if there is an associated myeloid disorder, this parameter is not valid)

The diagnosis of systemic mastocytosis can be made if one major and one minor criterion are present or if three minor criteria are met.

disease.[221] With progressive disease, patients may develop mild malabsorption.[221]

If systemic involvement is advanced at the time of diagnosis, patients may exhibit lymphadenopathy, hepatomegaly, and splenomegaly during the initial evaluation.[171,208] Because osteoporosis may accompany systemic disease, rare patients present with pathologic fractures.[222]

LABORATORY FEATURES

When mastocytosis is suspected following the history and results of physical examination, an evaluation in adults should consist of a gross and microscopic examination of the skin, bone marrow biopsy, and aspirate[171,195,208] and serum for total tryptase.[223] Total serum tryptase persistently greater than 20 ng/ml is a minor criterion in the diagnosis of systemic mastocytosis (see Table 63-6). Additional studies, as suggested by the need to assess the extent of disease or to evaluate pain, may include a bone scan and a skeletal survey. Gastrointestinal evaluation, involving radiographic studies of the upper gastrointestinal tract and small intestines, computed tomographic scan of the abdomen, and endoscopy also may be justified. In skin biopsies of sites that lack other causes of increased numbers of mast cells, such as chronic inflammatory processes, a 10-fold increase in mast cells numbers is generally considered diagnostic of cutaneous mastocytosis.[179,194,208] In patients with advanced SM-AHNMD or ASM disease, mast cells may be detectable in the peripheral blood. Patients with mast cell leukemia have significant numbers of mast cells in the blood.[208,211,224–227]

Plasma or urinary histamine levels frequently are increased in systemic mastocytosis.[228] However, the isolated findings of increased levels of histamine or histamine metabolites may reflect a number of other situations, including anaphylaxis. Further, the accuracy of laboratory measurement of histamine depends on the assay used. Urine histamine levels may be falsely elevated as a result of bacterial contamination, pharmacologic agents and their metabolites excreted in the urine, or diets rich in histamine or histamine precursors. Similarly, serum tryptase may be elevated after anaphylaxis. Thus, no single laboratory test is diagnostic of mastocytosis. Rather, the demonstration of mast cell mediators in blood or urine should prompt the clinician to investigate further for the presence of mastocytosis.

DIFFERENTIAL DIAGNOSIS

The differential diagnosis of systemic mastocytosis includes allergic diseases, the hyper-IgE syndrome, hereditary or acquired angioneurotic edema, idiopathic flushing or anaphylaxis, carcinoid tumor, and idiopathic capillary leak syndrome. When episodic hypertension is a major finding, pheochromocytoma should be considered. Significant unexplained gastroduodenal ulcer disease requires that Zollinger-Ellison gastrinoma syndrome be ruled out. *Helicobacter pylori* infection should be considered in all patients with ulcer disease, even in patients diagnosed with mastocytosis.

Some diseases have hematologic findings that overlap with those of systemic mastocytosis. The findings include tryptase-positive acute myeloid leukemia, chronic myeloid leukemia with accumulation of tryptase-positive cells, idiopathic myelofibrosis with mast cell accumulation, and acute or chronic basophilic leukemia.

A somatic mutation in *KIT* at codon 816 (most commonly Asp816Val) is associated especially with adult-onset systemic mastocytosis. Demonstration of a codon 816 gain-of-function mutation, where the most sensitive approach is to look for its presence in sorted bone marrow-derived mast cells, is a minor criterion in the diagnosis of mastocytosis (see Table 63-6).

THERAPY

Mastocytosis currently has no cure.[229] In addition, no evidence indicates symptomatic therapy significantly alters the course of the underlying disease.[229]

AVOIDING TRIGGERS

Management of mastocytosis includes instructing the patient on the avoidance of factors that may trigger symptoms (presumably by direct or indirect activation of mast cell mediator production). The factors can include temperature extremes, physical exertion, or, in some unusual cases, ingestion of ethanol, nonsteroidal antiinflammatory drugs, or opiate analgesics.[208,229]

EPINEPHRINE AND H_1 OR H_2 ANTIHISTAMINES

Anaphylaxis may follow insect stings, even in the absence of evidence of allergic sensitivity. Epinephrine-filled syringes and instructions on their use can be given to patients considered at risk for such a reaction. Patients with mast cell disease and a history of anaphylaxis should be advised to carry epinephrine-filled syringes, instructed on their use, and taught to self-medicate, if necessary. These patients also may benefit from the concurrent use of H_1 and H_2 antihistamines prophylactically. Patients may experience severe reactions to iodinated contrast materials. Thus, consideration should be given to premedicating mastocytosis patients with H_1 and H_2 antihistamines and prednisone. Nonsedative H_1 antihistamines decrease skin irritability and pruritus.[208,229–231] More potent H_1 blockers, such as hydroxyzine and doxepin,[232] may be useful in more severe cases. Pruritus may be relieved by approaches that maintain skin hydration. H_2 antihistamines, including ranitidine and famotidine, are used to treat the gastritis and peptic ulcer disease associated with mastocytosis.[208,229,231] H_2 antihistamines may be titrated based on symptom control or to a particular level of gastric secretion. Proton pump inhibitors (omeprazole) are useful for management of gastric hypersecretion.[208,229]

OTHER DRUG THERAPY

DISODIUM CROMOGLYCATE

Oral administration of disodium cromoglycate may be useful for treatment of gastrointestinal cramping and diarrhea.[195,230,233] The agent has been beneficial in cutaneous mast cell disease in children and infants.[234] Other symptoms, including headache, have improved with administration of cromolyn sodium.

KETOTIFEN

Ketotifen reportedly has been effective in relieving pruritus and wheal formation in cutaneous mastocytosis[235] and improving osteoporosis.[236] By contrast, one pediatric study found ketotifen was no more effective than hydroxyzine.[237] Similarly, in another study, azelastine offered only minimal benefit over chlorpheniramine.[238] Diphosphonates reportedly have been useful for treatment of osteopenia associated with mastocytosis.[239]

NONSTEROIDAL ANTIINFLAMMATORY AGENTS

Nonsteroidal antiinflammatory agents have been useful in some patients whose primary manifestations are recurrent episodes of flushing, syncope, or both.[229] However, these agents may exacerbate ulcer disease. Patients with a history of aspirin sensitivity should not be placed on this therapy unless they first undergo desensitization.

GLUCOCORTICOIDS OR METHOXYPSORALEN

Cutaneous lesions have been treated with either glucocorticoids[240] or 8-methoxypsoralen plus ultraviolet A (PUVA),[241,242] largely to reduce pruritus or for cosmetic improvement. No evidence indicates such approaches alter the progression of systemic disease. Relapses 3 to 6 months after cessation of PUVA therapy are common. Patients may experience a decrease in the intensity of lesions after exposure to natural sunlight. Repeated or extensive application of glucocorticoids may result in cutaneous atrophy or adrenocortical suppression.[240]

Systemic glucocorticoids are used to decrease significant malabsorption and ascites[243] in patients with advanced disease. In adults, oral prednisone (40–60 mg/day) usually results in decreased symptoms over a 2- to 3-week period. After initial improvement, steroids usually can be tapered to an alternate-day regimen. However, with time, the ascites frequently recurs. Such patients reportedly can benefit from a portacaval shunt.[243]

Patients with more advanced categories of systemic mastocytosis may be candidates for approaches directed at reducing the mast cell burden. None of these approaches has consistently resulted in cure of the disease. The most experience has been reported for interferon alpha.[244] Its mechanism of action on mastocytosis is not known, but it is presumed to act by restricting the proliferation of hematopoietic progenitor cells. Using proposed response criteria, one study determined that patients who appeared to have derived the most benefit from interferon alpha were those with aggressive systemic mastocytosis.[219] The overall response rate in 14 patients with aggressive systemic mastocytosis in this retrospective meta-analysis was 57 percent. Only 21 percent of the patients had a major response. However, interferon alpha failed to produce a beneficial effect in other studies.[245] Its use is not routinely recommended for patients with indolent systemic disease, who generally have a favorable prognosis.

CLADRIBINE
Cladribine (2-chlorodeoxyadenosine), a nucleoside analogue, reportedly induced major clinical and histopathologic response in one patient with systemic mastocytosis.[246] This drug does not require cells in active cell cycle to exert its cytotoxic activity and may be beneficial in slowly progressing neoplastic processes. The drug has myelosuppressive and immunosuppressive properties and thus cannot be recommended for patients with indolent disease.

HEMATOPOIETIC STEM CELL TRANSPLANTATION
Allogeneic stem cell transplantation (SCT) is under study as a treatment option for patients with advanced categories of mastocytosis associated with poor survival. SCT has been used to treat a hematologic disorder associated with mastocytosis in only a few cases.[247–249] Although these studies reported favorable responses of the associated hematologic disorders, complete remission of the mast cell disease was reported in only one study, which used non-T cell–depleted blood SCT in a patient with an associated myeloproliferative disorder.[249] The value of allogeneic SCT in mastocytosis may result from the immunotherapeutic effects of the donor marrow rather than the myeloablative conditioning regimen. A protocol utilizing nonmyeloablative blood SCT for treatment of advanced systemic mastocytosis is under investigation at the National Institutes of Health Clinical Center. Of three patients transplanted under this protocol to date, two have achieved a complete response of their clonal myeloid diseases and a partial response of their mast cell disease, with reduced tryptase levels but persistent mast cell collections in the bone marrow.[250]

TYROSINE KINASE INHIBITORS
The availability of small molecular weight inhibitors of tyrosine kinase suggested the mutated KIT tyrosine kinase in mastocytosis as a therapeutic target. Imatinib mesylate (Gleevec; Novartis, Basel, Switzerland) currently is the only such drug available. It has a specific inhibition profile that includes ABL, KIT, and PDGFR tyrosine

kinases.[251–253] Although the drug inhibits wild-type KIT and KIT-bearing juxtamembrane activating mutations similar to those found in gastrointestinal stromal tumors, it does not inhibit KIT bearing codon 816 mutations associated with most common forms of systemic mastocytosis.[254,255] This finding has been attributed to a conformational change in KIT bearing the codon 816 mutation, which interferes with the association of the drug with the ATP-binding domains of the receptor. Consistent with these observations, imatinib mesylate showed a strong in vitro cytotoxic effect on mast cells bearing wild-type KIT. Mast cells bearing a codon 816 mutation isolated from marrow of patients with mastocytosis were fairly resistant to the drug.[256] These studies suggest imatinib mesylate is unlikely to be an effective therapy for patients who carry codon 816 mutations. However, the drug might be of value in the unusual presentations of mastocytosis that are not associated with codon 816 mutations.

A patient with an unusual form of systemic mastocytosis associated with a c-kit mutation (Phe522Cys) affecting the transmembrane region of the receptor responded to treatment with imatinib.[201] Accordingly, a careful mutational analysis of a sample enriched for lesional mast cells appears to be essential in patients with mastocytosis before contemplating imatinib therapy. Other tyrosine kinase inhibitors that decrease the activity of KIT with codon 816 mutations are under development.[257]

Some patients with a variant of the chronic eosinophilic leukemia (clonal hypereosinophilic syndrome) exhibit elevated serum tryptase levels, increased numbers of mast cells in the marrow, some of which can appear atypical and spindle shaped, tissue fibrosis and, like other patients who have the FIP1L1-PDGFR-α fusion gene, are responsive to imatinib mesylate.[258,259] Although such patients have laboratory findings that may fulfill the diagnostic criteria for systemic mastocytosis, they exhibit clinical features that differ from the findings in patients with systemic mastocytosis related to gain-of-function mutations of KIT. For example, patients with systemic mastocytosis typically present with signs and symptoms related to mast cell infiltration of tissues and histamine release, and marrow mast cells from most patients coexpress CD2 and CD25.[258] By contrast, patients with hypereosinophilia and elevated serum tryptase typically develop end-organ damage associated with eosinophil infiltration of tissues including endomyocardial fibrosis and mucosal ulcerations (see Chap. 62). Such tissues typically do not show evidence of increased numbers of mast cells histologically but do exhibit eosinophil granule deposition in some instances. CD2 was not detected on their marrow mast cells.[258] The extent to which the findings involving mast cells in this subset of hypereosinophilic patients, including the elevations of serum tryptase, reflect consequences of eosinophilia as opposed to intrinsic effects of the FIP1L1-PDGFR-α fusion gene on the mast cell lineage remains to be determined.

SPLENECTOMY
Splenectomy has been performed on patients with severe aggressive mastocytosis in an attempt to improve their limiting cytopenias.[260] Based on comparisons to historical controls, splenectomy increased survival by an average of 12 months. Patients who had undergone splenectomy appeared to be better able to tolerate chemotherapy. Splenectomy is of no value in the management of indolent mast cell disease.[260]

COURSE AND PROGNOSIS

The prognosis of adult patients with mast cell disorders is related to the disease category. The vast majority of patients who present with UP and ISM have a chronic protracted course that responds to symptomatic medical management. A normal life span is expected. Few of these patients progress to more severe forms of the disease; some patients may even experience a diminution in the severity of skin lesions in later years.[261] However, elevated serum lactate dehydrogenase levels, a late age of onset, and, in patients with SM-AHNMD, presence of a significant hematologic abnormality (such as a myeloproliferative or myelodysplastic disorder or, more rarely, overt leukemia) are indicators of a poor prognosis and shortened survival.[211] The prognosis for patients with SM-AHNMD depends on the course of the associated hematologic disorder.[211] Patients with ASM have a guarded prognosis because of complications arising from rapid and profound increases in mast cell numbers. These patients usually have a 3- to 5-year survival.[211] Patients with mast cell leukemia also have a short survival.[225]

MAST CELL LEUKEMIA

This disorder develops in a small minority of patients with ISM or SM-AHNMD[224–227] but also can be the initial clinical presentation of the mast cell disorder.[195,262,263] Patients with mast cell leukemia may have fever, anorexia, weight loss, fatigue, severe abdominal cramping, nausea, vomiting, diarrhea, flushing, hypotension, pruritus, or bone pain. Peptic ulcer and gastrointestinal bleeding, hepatomegaly, splenomegaly, and lymph node enlargement are frequent findings. Anemia is a constant feature, and thrombocytopenia is nearly always present. The total leukocyte count varies from 10,000 to 150,000 μl (10 to 150 $\times$ 10^9/liter), and mast cells compose 10 to 90 percent of leukocytes. Marrow biopsy invariably shows a striking increase in mast cells, sometimes up to 90 percent of marrow cells, although the leukemic mast cells often are hypogranular or agranular. Leukemic mast cells are stained with Sudan black and Alcian blue. They are positive for chloracetate esterase and acid phosphatase and are negative in the peroxidase and α-naphthyl esterase reactions.[225,262]

MAST CELL SARCOMA

This is an exceedingly rare tumor, characterized by nodules at various cutaneous and mucosal sites.[183,219]

REFERENCES

1. Galli SJ, Dvorak AM, Dvorak, HF: Basophils and mast cells: Morphologic insights into their biology, secretory patterns, and function. *Prog Allergy* 34:1, 1984.
2. Galli, SJ: New concepts about the mast cell. *N Engl J Med* 328:257, 1993.
3. Valent P: Immunophenotypic characterization of human basophils and mast cells. *Chem Immunol* 61:34, 1995.
4. Dvorak AM: Blood cell biochemistry, in *Basophil and Mast Cell Degranulation and Recovery*, edited by JR Harris. Plenum, New York, 1991.
5. Costa J, Galli SJ: Mast cells and basophils, in *Clinical Immunology: Principles and Practice*, edited by TA Fleisher, WT Shearer, W Strober, p 408. Mosby, St. Louis, 1996.
6. Murakami I, Ogawa M, Amo H, et al: Studies on kinetics of human leucocytes in vivo with 3H-thymidine autoradiography: II. Eosinophils and basophils. *Nippon Ketsueki Gakkai Zasshi* 32:384, 1969.
7. Dvorak AM, Monahan RA, Osage JE, et al: Crohn's disease: Transmission electron microscopic studies: II. Immunologic inflammatory response. Alterations of mast cells, basophils, eosinophils, and the microvasculature. *Hum Pathol* 11:606, 1980.
8. Juhlin L: Basophil leukocyte differential in blood and bone marrow. *Acta Haematol* 29: 89, 1963.
9. Gilbert HS, Ornstein L: Basophil counting with a new staining method using Alcian blue. *Blood* 46:279, 1975.
10. Ishizaka T, Dvorak, AM, Conrad, DH, et al: Morphologic and immunologic characterization of human basophils developed in cultures of cord blood mononuclear cells. *J Immunol* 134:532, 1985.
11. Ganser A, Lindemann A, Seipelt G, et al: Effects of recombinant human interleukin-3 in patients with normal hematopoiesis and in patients with bone marrow failure. *Blood* 76:666, 1990.
12. Lantz CS, Boesiger J, Song CH, et al: Role for interleukin-3 in mast-cell and basophil development and in immunity to parasites. *Nature* 392: 90, 1998.
13. Lantz CS, Song CH, Dranoff G, et al: Interleukin-3 (IL-3) is required for blood basophilia, but not for increased IL-4 production, in response to parasite infection in mice [abstract]. *FASEB J* 13:A325, 1999.
14. Kurimoto Y, De Weck AL, Dahinden, CA: The effect of interleukin 3 upon IgE-dependent and IgE-independent basophil degranulation and leukotriene generation. *Eur J Immunol* 21:361, 1991.
15. Alam R, Welter JB, Forsythe PA, et al: Comparative effect of recombinant IL-1, -2, -3, -4, and -6, IFN-gamma, granulocyte-macrophage-colony-stimulating factor, tumor necrosis factor-alpha, and histamine-releasing factors on the secretion of histamine from basophils. *J Immunol* 142:3431, 1989.
16. Li L, Li Y, Reddel SW, et al: Identification of basophilic cells that express mast cell granule proteases in the peripheral blood of asthma, allergy, and drug-reactive patients. *J Immunol* 161:5079, 1998.
17. Kitamura Y: Heterogeneity of mast cells and phenotypic change between subpopulations. *Annu Rev Immunol* 7:59, 1989.
18. Galli SJ, Geissler EN, Wershil BK, et al: Insights into mast cell development and function derived from analyses of mice carrying mutations at beige, *W/c-kit* or *Sl/SCF* (c-kit ligand) loci, in *The Role of the Mast Cell in Health and Disease*, edited by MA Kaliner, p 129. Marcel Dekker, New York, 1992.
19. Galli SJ, Zsebo KM, Geissler EN: The kit ligand, stem cell factor. *Adv Immunol* 55:1, 1994.
20. Rodewald HR, Dessing M, Dvorak AM, et al: Identification of a committed precursor for the mast cell lineage. *Science* 271:818, 1996.
21. Galli SJ, Iemura A, Garlick DS, et al: Reversible expansion of primate mast cell populations in vivo by stem cell factor. *J Clin Invest* 91:148, 1993.
22. Costa JJ, Demetri GD, Harrist TJ, et al: Recombinant human stem cell factor (kit ligand) promotes human mast cell and melanocyte hyperplasia and functional activation in vivo. *J Exp Med* 183:2681, 1996.
23. Broudy VC: Stem cell factor and hematopoiesis. *Blood* 90:1345, 1997.
24. Wershil BK, Tsai M, Geissler EN, et al: The rat c-kit ligand, stem cell factor, induces c-kit receptor-dependent mouse mast cell activation in vivo. Evidence that signaling through the c-kit receptor can induce expression of cellular function. *J Exp Med* 175:245, 1992.
25. Columbo M, Horowitz EM, Botana LM, et al: The human recombinant c-kit receptor ligand, rhSCF, induces mediator release from human cutaneous mast cells and enhances IgE-dependent mediator release from both skin mast cells and peripheral blood basophils. *J Immunol* 149:599, 1992.
26. Coleman JW, Holliday MR, Kimber I, et al: Regulation of mouse peritoneal mast cell secretory function by stem cell factor, IL-3 or IL-4. *J Immunol* 150:556, 1993.
27. Bischoff SC, Dahinden CA: c-kit ligand: A unique potentiator of mediator release by human lung mast cells. *J Exp Med* 175:237, 1992.
28. Gagari E, Tsai M, Lantz CS, et al: Differential release of mast cell interleukin-6 via c-kit. *Blood* 89:2654, 1997.
29. Finotto S, Mekori YA, Metcalfe DD: Glucocorticoids decrease tissue mast cell number by reducing the production of the c-kit ligand, stem cell factor, by resident cells: In vitro and in vivo evidence in murine systems. *J Clin Invest* 99:1721, 1997.
30. Enerbäck L: Mast cell heterogeneity: The evolution of the concept of a specific mucosal mast cell, in *Mast Cell Differentiation and Heterogeneity*, edited by AD Befus, J Bienenstock, JA Denburg, p 1. Raven, New York, 1986.

31. Galli SJ: New insights into "the riddle of the mast cells": Microenvironmental regulation of mast cell development and phenotypic heterogeneity. *Lab Invest* 62:5, 1990.

32. Irani AA, Schechter NM, Craig SS, et al: Two types of human mast cells that have distinct neutral protease compositions. *Proc Natl Acad Sci U S A* 83:4464, 1986.

33. Siegmund R, Vogelsang H, Machnik A, et al: Surface membrane antigen alteration on blood basophils in patients with Hymenoptera venom allergy under immunotherapy. *J Allergy Clin Immunol* 106:1190, 2000.

34. Juhlin L, Michaelsson G: A new syndrome characterized by absence of eosinophils and basophils. *Lancet* 1:1233, 1977.

35. Tracey R, Smith H: An inherited anomaly of human eosinophils and basophils. *Blood Cells* 4:291, 1978.

36. Mitchell EB, Platts-Mills TA, Pereira RS, et al: Basophil and eosinophil deficiency in a patient with hypogammaglobulinemia associated with thymoma. *Birth Defects Orig Artic Ser* 19:331, 1983.

37. Dvorak AM, Mihm MC Jr, Dvorak, HF: Morphology of delayed-type hypersensitivity reactions in man: II. Ultrastructural alterations affecting the microvasculature and the tissue mast cells. *Lab Invest* 34:179, 1976.

38. Hastie R: A study of the ultrastructure of human basophil leukocytes. *Lab Invest* 31:223, 1974.

39. Schwartz LB, Austen KF: Structure and function of the chemical mediators of mast cells. *Prog Allergy* 34:271, 1984.

40. Stevens RL, Austen KF: Recent advances in the cellular and molecular biology of mast cells. *Immunol Today* 10:381, 1989.

41. Metcalfe DD, Bland CE, Wasserman SI: Biochemical and functional characterization of proteoglycans isolated from basophils of patients with chronic myelogenous leukemia. *J Immunol* 132:1943, 1984.

42. Rothenberg ME, Caulfield JP, Austen KF, et al: Biochemical and morphological characterization of basophilic leukocytes from two patients with myelogenous leukemia. *J Immunol* 138:2616, 1987.

43. Orenstein NS, Galli SJ, Dvorak AM, et al: Sulfated glycosaminoglycans of guinea pig basophilic leukocytes. *J Immunol* 121:586, 1978.

44. Humphries DE, Wong GW, Friend DS, et al: Heparin is essential for the storage of specific granule proteases in mast cells. *Nature* 400:769, 1999.

45. Forsberg E, Pejler G, Ringvall M, et al: Abnormal mast cells in mice deficient in a heparin-synthesizing enzyme. *Nature* 400:773, 1999.

46. Porter JF, Mitchell RG; Distribution of histamine in human blood. *Physiol Rev* 52:361, 1972.

47. Galli SJ, Kitamura Y: Genetically mast-cell-deficient *W/Wᵥ* and *Sl/Slᵈ* mice. Their value for the analysis of the roles of mast cells in biologic responses in vivo. *Am J Pathol* 127:191, 1987.

48. Parwaresch M: *The Human Blood Basophil*. Springer-Verlag, New York, 1976.

49. Gordon JR, Galli SJ: Mast cells as a source of both preformed and immunologically inducible TNF-alpha/cachectin. *Nature* 346:274, 1990.

50. Walsh LJ, Trinchieri G, Waldorf HA, et al: Human dermal mast cells contain and release tumor necrosis factor alpha, which induces endothelial leukocyte adhesion molecule 1. *Proc Natl Acad Sci U S A* 88:4220, 1991.

51. Galli SJ, Gordon JR, Wershil BK: Cytokine production by mast cells and basophils. *Curr Opin Immunol* 3:865, 1991.

52. Bradding P, Feather IH, Howarth PH, et al: Interleukin 4 is localized to and released by human mast cells. *J Exp Med* 176:1381, 1992.

53. Brunner T, Heusser CH, Dahinden CA: Human peripheral blood basophils primed by interleukin 3 (IL-3) produce IL-4 in response to immunoglobulin E receptor stimulation. *J Exp Med* 177:605, 1993.

54. Burd PR, Rogers HW, Gordon JR, et al: Interleukin 3-dependent and -independent mast cells stimulated with IgE and antigen express multiple cytokines. *J Exp Med* 170:245, 1989.

55. Yano K, Yamaguchi M, de Mora F, et al: Production of macrophage inflammatory protein-1alpha by human mast cells: Increased anti-IgE-dependent secretion after IgE-dependent enhancement of mast cell IgE-binding ability. *Lab Invest* 77:185, 1997.

56. Pawankar R, Okuda M, Yssel H, et al: Nasal mast cells in perennial allergic rhinitics exhibit increased expression of the Fc epsilonRI, CD40L, IL-4, and IL-13, and can induce IgE synthesis in B cells. *J Clin Invest* 99:1492, 1997.

57. Rumsaeng V, Cruikshank, WW, Foster B, et al: Human mast cells produce the CD4+ T lymphocyte chemoattractant factor, IL-16. *J Immunol* 159:2904, 1997.

58. Sayama K, Diehn M, Matsuda K, et al: Transcriptional response of human mast cells stimulated via the Fc(epsilon)RI and identification of mast cells as a source of IL-11. *BMC Immunol* 3, 2002. Available at http://www.biomedcentral.com/1471-2172/3/5

59. Nakajima T, Inagaki N, Tanaka H, et al: Marked increase in CC chemokine gene expression in both human and mouse mast cell transcriptomes following Fcepsilon receptor I cross-linking: An interspecies comparison. *Blood* 100:3861, 2002.

60. Okumura S, Kashiwakura J, Tomita H, et al: Identification of specific gene expression profiles in human mast cells mediated by Toll-like receptor 4 and FcepsilonRI. *Blood* 102:2547, 2003.

61. Li H, Sim TC, Alam R: IL-13 released by and localized in human basophils. *J Immunol* 156:4833, 1996.

62. Voehringer D, Shinkai K, Locksley RM: Type 2 immunity reflects orchestrated recruitment of cells committed to IL-4 production. *Immunity* 20:267, 2004.

63. Ishizaka T, Ishizaka K: Activation of mast cells for mediator release through IgE receptors. *Prog Allergy* 34:188, 1984.

64. Kinet JP: The high-affinity IgE receptor (Fc epsilon RI): From physiology to pathology. *Annu Rev Immunol* 17:931, 1999.

65. Beaven MA, Metzger H: Signal transduction by Fc receptors: The Fc epsilon RI case. *Immunol Today* 14:222, 1993.

66. Kawakami T, Galli SJ: Regulation of mast-cell and basophil function and survival by IgE. *Nat Rev Immunol* 2:773, 2002.

67. Rivera J: Molecular adapters in Fc(epsilon)RI signaling and the allergic response. *Curr Opin Immunol* 14:688, 2002.

68. Nadler MJ, Kinet, JP: Uncovering new complexities in mast cell signaling. *Nat Immunol* 3:707, 2002.

69. Siraganian RP: Mast cell signal transduction from the high-affinity IgE receptor. *Curr Opin Immunol* 15:639, 2003.

70. Galli SJ, Kalesnikoff J, Grimbaldeston MA, et al: Mast cells as "tunable" effector and immunoregulatory cells: Recent advances. *Annu Rev Immunol* 23:749, 2005.

71. Galli SJ, Lantz C: Allergy, in *Fundamental Immunology*, edited by W Paul, p 1137. Lippincott-Raven, Philadelphia, 1999.

72. Patella V, Giuliano A, Bouvet JP, et al: Endogenous superallergen protein Fv induces IL-4 secretion from human Fc epsilon RI+ cells through interaction with the VH3 region of IgE. *J Immunol* 161:5647, 1998.

73. Patella V, Florio G, Petraroli A, et al: HIV-1 gp120 induces IL-4 and IL-13 release from human Fc epsilon RI+ cells through interaction with the VH3 region of IgE. *J Immunol* 164:589, 2000.

74. Marone G, Florio G, Petraroli A, et al: Role of human FcepsilonRI+ cells in HIV-1 infection. *Immunol Rev* 179:128, 2001.

75. Marone G, Galli SJ, Kitamura Y: Probing the roles of mast cells and basophils in natural and acquired immunity, physiology and disease. *Trends Immunol* 23:425, 2002.

76. Lemanske RFJ, Kaliner MA: Late phase allergic reactions, in *Allergy: Principles and Practice*, edited by E Middleton Jr, CE Reed, EF Ellis, et al. Mosby, St. Louis, 1993.

77. Wershil BK, Wang ZS, Gordon JR, et al: Recruitment of neutrophils during IgE-dependent cutaneous late phase reactions in the mouse is mast cell-dependent. Partial inhibition of the reaction with antiserum against tumor necrosis factor-alpha. *J Clin Invest* 87:446, 1991.

78. Williams CM, Galli SJ: Mast cells can amplify airway reactivity and features of chronic inflammation in an asthma model in mice. *J Exp Med* 192:455, 2000.

79. Kobayashi T, Miura T, Haba T, et al: An essential role of mast cells in the development of airway hyperresponsiveness in a murine asthma model. *J Immunol* 164:3855, 2000.

80. Yu M, Tsai M, Tam S-Y, et al: Mast cells contribute to multiple features of a model of chronic asthma in mice. *JACI*, 2005, in press (abstr.).

81. Brightling CE, Bradding P, Symon FA, et al: Mast-cell infiltration of airway smooth muscle in asthma. *N Engl J Med* 346:1699, 2002.

82. Yamaguchi M, Lantz CS, Oettgen HC, et al: IgE enhances mouse mast cell Fc(epsilon)RI expression in vitro and in vivo: Evidence for a novel amplification mechanism in IgE-dependent reactions. *J Exp Med* 185:663, 1997.

83. MacGlashan DW Jr, Bochner BS, Adelman DC, et al: Down-regulation of Fc(epsilon)RI expression on human basophils during in vivo treatment of atopic patients with anti-IgE antibody. *J Immunol* 158:1438, 1997.

84. Boesiger J, Tsai M, Maurer M, et al: Mast cells can secrete vascular permeability factor/vascular endothelial cell growth factor and exhibit enhanced release after immunoglobulin E-dependent upregulation of Fc epsilon receptor I expression. *J Exp Med* 188:1135, 1998.

85. Yamaguchi M, Sayama K, Yano K, et al: IgE enhances Fc epsilon receptor I expression and IgE-dependent release of histamine and lipid mediators from human umbilical cord blood-derived mast cells: Synergistic effect of IL-4 and IgE on human mast cell Fc epsilon receptor I expression and mediator release. *J Immunol* 162:5455, 1999.

86. Kalesnikoff J, Huber M, Lam V, et al: Monomeric IgE stimulates signaling pathways in mast cells that lead to cytokine production and cell survival. *Immunity* 14:801, 2001.

87. Asai K, Kitaura J, Kawakami Y, et al: Regulation of mast cell survival by IgE. *Immunity* 14:791, 2001.

88. Kitaura J, Song J, Tsai M, et al: Evidence that IgE molecules mediate a spectrum of effects on mast cell survival and activation via aggregation of the FcepsilonRI. *Proc Natl Acad Sci U S A* 100:12911, 2003.

89. Matsuda K, Piliponsky, AM, Nakae S, et al: IgE enhances human mast cell survival and chemokine production: IL-4 augments the secretory response. 2005 [submitted].

90. James LC, Roversi P, Tawfik DS: Antibody multispecificity mediated by conformational diversity. *Science* 299:1362, 2003.

91. Foote J: Immunology. Isomeric antibodies. *Science* 299:1327, 2003.

92. Galli SJ, Askenase PW: Cutaneous basophil hypersensitivity, in *The Reticuloendothelial System: A Comprehensive Treatise SP*, edited by P Abramoff, NR Escobar. Plenum, New York, 1986.

93. Secor VH, Secor WE, Gutekunst CA, et al: Mast cells are essential for early onset and severe disease in a murine model of multiple sclerosis. *J Exp Med* 191:813, 2000.

94. Lee DM, Friend DS, Gurish MF, et al: Mast cells: A cellular link between autoantibodies and inflammatory arthritis. *Science* 297:1689, 2002.

95. Miyajima I, Dombrowicz D, Martin TR, et al: Systemic anaphylaxis in the mouse can be mediated largely through IgG1 and Fc gammaRIII. Assessment of the cardiopulmonary changes, mast cell degranulation, and death associated with active or IgE- or IgG1-dependent passive anaphylaxis. *J Clin Invest* 99:901, 1997.

96. Strait RT, Morris SC, Yang M, et al: Pathways of anaphylaxis in the mouse. *J Allergy Clin Immunol* 109:658, 2002.

97. Pedotti R, De Voss JJ, Steinman L, et al: Involvement of both "allergic" and "autoimmune" mechanisms in EAE, MS and other autoimmune diseases. *Trends Immunol* 24:479, 2003.

98. Askenase PW, Van Loveren H, Kraeuter-Kops S, et al: Defective elicitation of delayed-type hypersensitivity in *W/W^v* and *Sl/Sl^d* mast cell-deficient mice. *J Immunol* 131:2687, 1983.

99. Biedermann T, Kneilling M, Mailhammer R, et al: Mast cells control neutrophil recruitment during T cell-mediated delayed-type hypersensitivity reactions through tumor necrosis factor and macrophage inflammatory protein 2. *J Exp Med* 192:1441, 2000.

100. Galli SJ, Hammel I: Unequivocal delayed hypersensitivity in mast cell-deficient and beige mice. *Science* 226:710, 1984.

101. Bryce PJ, Miller ML, Miyajima I, et al: Immune sensitization in the skin is enhanced by antigen-independent effects of IgE. *Immunity* 20:381, 2004.

102. Tam S-Y, Tsai M, Snouwaert JN, Kalesnikoff J, et al: RabGEF1 is a negative regulator of mast cell activation and skin inflammation. *Nature Immunology* 5:844, 2004.

103. Brown SJ, Galli SJ, Gleich GJ, et al: Ablation of immunity to *Amblyomma americanum* by anti-basophil serum: Cooperation between basophils and eosinophils in expression of immunity to ectoparasites (ticks) in guinea pigs. *J Immunol* 129:790, 1982.

104. Matsuda H, Watanabe N, Kiso Y, et al: Necessity of IgE antibodies and mast cells for manifestation of resistance against larval *Haemaphysalis longicornis* ticks in mice. *J Immunol* 144:259, 1990.

105. Echtenacher B, Mannel DN, Hultner L: Critical protective role of mast cells in a model of acute septic peritonitis. *Nature* 381:75, 1996.

106. Malaviya R, Ikeda T, Ross E, et al: Mast cell modulation of neutrophil influx and bacterial clearance at sites of infection through TNF-alpha. *Nature* 381:77, 1996.

107. Galli SJ, Maurer M, Lantz CS: Mast cells as sentinels of innate immunity. *Curr Opin Immunol* 11:53, 1999.

108. Chatterjea D, Tsai M, Galli SJ: Roles of mast cells and basophils in innate immunity, in *The Innate Immune Response to Infection*, edited by SHE Kaufman, R Medzhitov, S Gordon, p 111. ASM Press, Berlin, 2004.

109. Prodeus AP, Zhou X, Maurer M, et al: Impaired mast cell-dependent natural immunity in complement C3-deficient mice. *Nature* 390:172, 1997.

110. Supajatura V, Ushio H, Nakao A, et al: Protective roles of mast cells against enterobacterial infection are mediated by Toll-like receptor 4. *J Immunol* 167:2250, 2001.

111. Supajatura V, Ushio H, Nakao A, et al: Differential responses of mast cell Toll-like receptors 2 and 4 in allergy and innate immunity. *J Clin Invest* 109:1351, 2002.

112. Maurer M, Echtenacher B, Hultner L, et al: The c-kit ligand, stem cell factor, can enhance innate immunity through effects on mast cells. *J Exp Med* 188:2343, 1998.

113. Malaviya R, Twesten NJ, Ross EA, et al: Mast cells process bacterial Ags through a phagocytic route for class I MHC presentation to T cells. *J Immunol* 156:1490, 1996.

114. Di Nardo A, Vitiello A, Gallo RL: Cutting edge: Mast cell antimicrobial activity is mediated by expression of cathelicidin antimicrobial peptide. *J Immunol* 170:2274, 2003.

115. Maurer M, Wedemeyer J, Metz M, et al: Mast cells promote homeostasis by limiting endothelin-1 induced toxicity *Nature* 432:512, 2004.

116. Mallen-St. Clair J, Pham CT, Villalta SA, et al: Mast cell dipeptidyl peptidase I mediates survival from sepsis. *J Clin Invest* 113:628, 2004.

117. Li Y, Li L, Wadley R, et al: Mast cells/basophils in the peripheral blood of allergic individuals who are HIV-1 susceptible due to their surface expression of CD4 and the chemokine receptors CCR3, CCR5, and CXCR4. *Blood* 97:3484, 2001.

118. Bannert N, Farzan M, Friend DS, et al: Human mast cell progenitors can be infected by macrophagetropic human immunodeficiency virus type 1 and retain virus with maturation in vitro. *J Virol* 75:10808, 2001.

119. Sundstrom JB, Little DM, Villinger F, et al: Signaling through toll-like receptors triggers HIV-1 replication in latently infected mast cells. *J Immunol* 172:4391, 2004.

120. King CA, Anderson R, Marshall JS: Dengue virus selectively induces human mast cell chemokine production. *J Virol* 76:8408, 2002.

121. Nakano T, Sonoda T, Hayashi C, et al: Fate of bone marrow-derived cultured mast cells after intracutaneous, intraperitoneal, and intravenous transfer into genetically mast cell-deficient *W/W^v* mice. Evidence that cultured mast cells can give rise to both connective tissue type and mucosal mast cells. *J Exp Med* 162:1025, 1985.

122. Wershil BK, Furuta GT, Wang ZS, et al: Mast cell-dependent neutrophil and mononuclear cell recruitment in immunoglobulin E-induced gastric reactions in mice. *Gastroenterology* 110:1482, 1996.

123. Martin TR, Takeishi T, Katz HR, et al: Mast cell activation enhances airway responsiveness to methacholine in the mouse. *J Clin Invest* 91:1176, 1993.

124. Shelley WB, Parnes HM: The absolute basophil count. *JAMA* 192:368, 1965.

125. Thonnard-Neumann E: Studies of basophils, variations with age and sex. *Acta Haematol* 30:221, 1963.

126. Chavance M, Herbeth B, Kauffmann F: Seasonal patterns of circulating basophils. *Int Arch Allergy Appl Immunol* 86:462, 1988.

127. Shelley WB, Juhlin L: New test for detecting anaphylactic sensitivity: Basophil reaction. *Nature* 191:1056, 1961.

128. Shelley WB: The circulating basophil as an indicator of hypersensitivity in man. Experimental novobiocin sensitization. *Arch Dermatol* 88:759, 1963.

129. Juhlin L: Basophil and eosinophil leukocytes in various internal disorders. *Acta Med Scand* 174:249, 1963.

130. Juhlin L: The effect of corticotrophin and corticosteroids on the basophil and eosinophil granulocytes. *Acta Haematol* 29:157, 1963.

131. Mettler L, Shirwani D: Direct basophil count for timing ovulation. *Fertil Steril* 25:718, 1974.

132. Malveaux FJ, Conroy MC, Adkinson NFJr, et al: IgE receptors on human basophils. Relationship to serum IgE concentration. *J Clin Invest* 62:176, 1978.

133. Lantz CS, Yamaguchi M, Oettgen HC, et al: IgE regulates mouse basophil Fc epsilon RI expression in vivo. *J Immunol* 158:2517, 1997.

134. Juhlin L: Basophil leukocytes in ulcerative colitis. *Acta Med Scand* 173:351, 1963.

135. Athreya BH, Moser G, Raghavan TE: Increased circulating basophils in juvenile rheumatoid arthritis. A preliminary report. *Am J Dis Child* 129:935, 1975.

136. Fredericks RE, Moloney WC: The basophilic granulocyte. *Blood* 14:571, 1959.

137. Spiers AS, Bain BJ, Turner JE: The peripheral blood in chronic granulocytic leukaemia. Study of 50 untreated Philadelphia-positive cases. *Scand J Haematol* 18:25, 1977.

138. Kamada N, Uchino H: Chronologic sequence in appearance of clinical and laboratory findings characteristic of chronic myelocytic leukemia. *Blood* 51:843, 1978.

139. Drewinko B, Bollinger P, Brailas C, et al: Flow cytochemical patterns of white blood cells in human haematopoietic malignancies: II. Chronic leukaemias. *Br J Haematol* 67:157, 1987.

140. Denburg JA, Browman G: The chronic myeloid leukemia study group: Prognostic implications of basophilic differentiation in chronic myeloid leukemia. *Am J Hematol* 27: 110, 1988.

141. Goh KO, Anderson FW: Cytogenetic studies in basophilic chronic myelocytic leukemia. *Arch Pathol Lab Med* 103:288, 1979.

142. Denburg JA, Wilson WE, Goodacre R, et al: Chronic myeloid leukaemia: Evidence for basophil differentiation and histamine synthesis from cultured peripheral blood cells. *Br J Haematol* 45:13, 1980.

143. Parkin JL, McKenna RW, Brunning RD: Philadelphia chromosome-positive blastic leukaemia: Ultrastructural and ultracytochemical evidence of basophil and mast cell differentiation. *Br J Haematol* 52:663, 1982.

144. Zucker-Franklin D: Ultrastructural evidence for the common origin of human mast cells and basophils. *Blood* 56:534, 1980.

145. Soler J, O'Brien M, de Castro JT, et al: Blast crisis of chronic granulocytic leukemia with mast cell and basophilic precursors. *Am J Clin Pathol* 83:254, 1985.

146. Weil SC, Hrisinko MA: A hybrid eosinophilic-basophilic granulocyte in chronic granulocytic leukemia. *Am J Clin Pathol* 87:66, 1987.

147. Gabriel LC, Escribano LM, Marie JP, et al: Peroxidase activity in circulating mast cells in blast crisis of chronic granulocytic leukemia. Comparative studies with basophils and cutaneous mast cells. *Am J Clin Pathol* 86:212, 1986.

148. Youman JD, Taddeini L, Cooper T: Histamine excess symptoms in basophilic chronic granulocytic leukemia. *Arch Intern Med* 131:560, 1973.

149. Rosenthal S, Schwartz JH, Canellos GP: Basophilic chronic granulocytic leukaemia with hyperhistaminaemia. *Br J Haematol* 36:367, 1977.

150. Valimaki M, Vuopio P, Salaspuro M: Plasma histamine and serum pepsinogen I concentrations in chronic myelogenous leukaemia. *Acta Med Scand* 217:89, 1985.

151. Anderson W, Helman CA, Hirschowitz BI: Basophilic leukemia and the hypersecretion of gastric acid and pepsin. *Gastroenterology* 95:195, 1988.

152. Xue YQ, Guo Y, Lu DR, et al: A case of basophilic leukemia bearing simultaneous translocations t(8;21) and t(9;22). *Cancer Genet Cytogenet* 51:215, 1991.

153. Cecio A, Dini E, Quattrin N: Initial electron microscopy studies in 2 cases of acute basophilic leukemia. *Boll Soc Ital Biol Sper* 46:459, 1970.

154. Dvorak AM, Dickersin GR, Connell A, et al: Degranulation mechanisms in human leukemic basophils. *Clin Immunol Immunopathol* 5:235, 1976.

155. Quattrin N: Follow-up of sixty two cases of acute basophilic leukemia. *Biomedicine* 28:72, 1978.

156. Wick MR, Li CY, Pierre RV: Acute nonlymphocytic leukemia with basophilic differentiation. *Blood* 60:38, 1982.

157. Lertprasertsuke N, Tsutsumi Y: An unusual form of chronic myeloproliferative disorder. Aleukemic basophilic leukemia. *Acta Pathol Jpn* 41:73, 1991.

158. Peterson LC, Parkin JL, Arthur DC, et al: Acute basophilic leukemia. A clinical, morphologic, and cytogenetic study of eight cases. *Am J Clin Pathol* 96:160, 1991.

159. Shvidel L, Shaft D, Stark B, et al: Acute basophilic leukaemia: Eight unsuspected new cases diagnosed by electron microscopy. *Br J Haematol* 120:774, 2003.

160. Pearson MG, Vardiman JW, Le Beau MM, et al: Increased numbers of marrow basophils may be associated with a t(6;9) in ANLL. *Am J Hematol* 18:393, 1985.

161. Horsman DE, Kalousek DK: Acute myelomonocytic leukemia (AML-M4) and translocation t(6;9)(p23;q34): Two additional patients with prominent myelodysplasia. *Am J Hematol* 26:77, 1987.

162. Matsuura Y, Sato N, Kimura F, et al: An increase in basophils in a case of acute myelomonocytic leukaemia associated with marrow eosinophilia and inversion of chromosome 16. *Eur J Haematol* 39:457, 1987.

163. Hoyle CF, Sherrington P, Hayhoe FG: Translocation (3;6)(q21;p21) in acute myeloid leukemia with abnormal thrombopoiesis and basophilia. *Cancer Genet Cytogenet* 30:261, 1988.

164. Alsabeh R, Brynes RK, Slovak ML, et al: Acute myeloid leukemia with t(6;9) (p23;q34): Association with myelodysplasia, basophilia, and initial CD34 negative immunophenotype. *Am J Clin Pathol* 107:430, 1997.

165. Moir DJ, Pearson J, Buckle VJ: Acute promyelocytic transformation in a case of acute myelomonocytic leukemia. *Cancer Genet Cytogenet* 12:359, 1984.

166. Umeda M, Nojima Z, Yamaguchi R, et al: Two cases of acute promyelocytic leukemia with marked basophilia— A variant type of APL with the capability of differentiating into basophils. *Rinsho Ketsueki* 28:2004, 1987.

167. Gotoh H, Murakami S, Oku N, et al: Translocations t(15;17) and t(9; 14)(q34;q22) in a case of acute promyelocytic leukemia with increased number of basophils. *Cancer Genet Cytogenet* 36:103, 1988.

168. McKenna RW, Parkin J, Bloomfield CD, et al: Acute promyelocytic leukaemia: A study of 39 cases with identification of a hyperbasophilic microgranular variant. *Br J Haematol* 50:201, 1982.

169. Le Beau MM, Larson RA, Bitter MA, et al: Association of an inversion of chromosome 16 with abnormal marrow eosinophils in acute myelomonocytic leukemia. A unique cytogenetic-clinicopathological association. *N Engl J Med* 309:630, 1983.

170. Lewis RA, Goetzl EJ, Wasserman SI, et al: The release of four mediators of immediate hypersensitivity from human leukemic basophils. *J Immunol* 114(1 Pt 1):87, 1975.

171. Travis WD, Li CY, Bergstralh EJ, et al: Systemic mast cell disease. Analysis of 58 cases and literature review. *Medicine (Baltimore)* 67: 345, 1988.

172. Tsai M, Shih LS, Newlands GF, et al: The rat c-kit ligand, stem cell factor, induces the development of connective tissue-type and mucosal mast cells in vivo. Analysis by anatomical distribution, histochemistry, and protease phenotype. *J Exp Med* 174:125, 1991.

173. Schwartz LB, Metcalfe DD, Miller JS, et al: Tryptase levels as an indicator of mast-cell activation in systemic anaphylaxis and mastocytosis. *N Engl J Med* 316:1622, 1987.

174. Irani AA, Garriga MM, Metcalfe DD, et al: Mast cells in cutaneous mastocytosis: Accumulation of the MC$_{TC}$ type. *Clin Exp Allergy* 20:53, 1990.

175. Weidner N, Horan RF, Austen KF: Mast-cell phenotype in indolent forms of mastocytosis. Ultrastructural features, fluorescence detection of avidin binding, and immunofluorescent determination of chymase, tryptase, and carboxypeptidase. *Am J Pathol* 140:847, 1992.

176. Weidner N, Austen KF: Heterogeneity of mast cells at multiple body sites. Fluorescent determination of avidin binding and immunofluorescent determination of chymase, tryptase, and carboxypeptidase content. *Pathol Res Pract* 189:156, 1993.

177. Lavker RM, Schechter NM: Cutaneous mast cell depletion results from topical corticosteroid usage. *J Immunol* 135:2368, 1985.

178. Irani AM, Craig SS, DeBlois G, et al: Deficiency of the tryptase-positive, chymase-negative mast cell type in gastrointestinal mucosa of patients with defective T lymphocyte function. *J Immunol* 138:4381, 1987.

179. Garriga MM, Friedman MM, Metcalfe DD: A survey of the number and distribution of mast cells in the skin of patients with mast cell disorders. *J Allergy Clin Immunol* 82(3 Pt 1):425, 1988.

180. Malone DG, Irani AM, Schwartz LB, et al: Mast cell numbers and histamine levels in synovial fluids from patients with diverse arthritides. *Arthritis Rheum* 29:956, 1986.

181. Malone DG, Wilder RL, Saavedra-Delgado AM, et al: Mast cell numbers in rheumatoid synovial tissues. Correlations with quantitative measures of lymphocytic infiltration and modulation by antiinflammatory therapy. *Arthritis Rheum* 30:130, 1987.

182. Frame B, Nixon RK: Bone-marrow mast cells in osteoporosis of aging. *N Engl J Med* 279:626, 1968.

183. Lennert K, Parwaresch MR: Mast cells and mast cell neoplasia: A review. *Histopathology* 3:349, 1979.

184. Barrett KE, Neva FA, Gam AA, et al: The immune response to nematode parasites: Modulation of mast cell numbers and function during *Strongyloides stercoralis* infections in nonhuman primates. *Am J Trop Med Hyg* 38:574, 1988.

185. Bowers HM Jr, Mahapatro RC, Kennedy JW: Numbers of mast cells in the axillary lymph nodes of breast cancer patients. *Cancer* 43:568, 1979.

186. Yoo D, Lessin LS, Jensen WN: Bone-marrow mast cells in lymphoproliferative disorders. *Ann Intern Med* 88:753, 1978.

187. Yoo D, Lessin LS: Bone marrow mast cell content in preleukemic syndrome. *Am J Med* 73:539, 1982.

188. Fohlmeister I, Reber T, Fischer R: Bone marrow mast cell reaction in preleukaemic myelodysplasia and in aplastic anaemia. *Virchows Arch A Pathol Anat Histopathol* 405:503, 1985.

189. Unna P: Beitrage zur anatomic und pathogenese der urticaria simplex und pigmentosa. *Mscch Prakt Dermatol Suppl Dermatol Stud* 3:9, 1887.

190. Nettleship E, Tay W: Rare forms of urticaria. *Br Med J* 2:323, 1869.

191. Sangster A: An anomalous mottled rash, accompanied by pruritus, factious urticaria and pigmentation, "urticaria pigmentosa (?)". *Trans Clin Soc Lond* 11:161, 1878.

192. Ellis JM: Urticaria pigmentosa: A report of a case with autopsy. *Arch Pathol Lab Med* 48:426, 1949.

193. Fine J: Mastocytosis. *Int J Dermatol* 19:117, 1980.

194. Soter NA: Mastocytosis and the skin. *Hematol Oncol Clin North Am* 14: 537, 2000.

195. Valent P, Horny HP, Li CY, et al: Mastocytosis, in *World Health Organization Classification of Tumours, Pathology and Genetics of Tumours of the Haematopoietic and Lymphoid tissues IIN*, edited by ES Jaffe, H Stein, JW Vardiman, p 291. IARC Press, Lyon, 2001.

196. Furitsu T, Tsujimura T, Tono T, et al: Identification of mutations in the coding sequence of the proto-oncogene c-kit in a human mast cell leukemia cell line causing ligand-independent activation of c-kit product. *J Clin Invest* 92:1736, 1993.

197. Nagata H, Worobec AS, Oh CK, et al: Identification of a point mutation in the catalytic domain of the protooncogene c-kit in peripheral blood mononuclear cells of patients who have mastocytosis with an associated hematologic disorder. *Proc Natl Acad Sci U S A* 92:10560, 1995.

198. Longley BJ, Tyrrell L, Lu SZ, et al: Somatic c-KIT activating mutation in urticaria pigmentosa and aggressive mastocytosis: Establishment of clonality in a human mast cell neoplasm. *Nat Genet* 12:312, 1996.

199. Nagata H, Okada T, Worobec, AS, et al: c-kit mutation in a population of patients with mastocytosis. *Int Arch Allergy Immunol* 113:184, 1997.

200. Longley BJ Jr, Metcalfe DD, Tharp M, et al: Activating and dominant inactivating c-KIT catalytic domain mutations in distinct clinical forms of human mastocytosis. *Proc Natl Acad Sci U S A* 96:1609, 1999.

201. Akin C, Fumo G, Yavuz AS, et al: A novel form of mastocytosis associated with a transmembrane c-kit mutation and response to imatinib. *Blood* 103:3222, 2004.

202. London CA, Galli SJ, Yuuki T, et al: Spontaneous canine mast cell tumors express tandem duplications in the proto-oncogene c-kit. *Exp Hematol* 27:689, 1999.

203. Downing S, Chien MB, Kass PH, et al: Prevalence and importance of internal tandem duplications in exons 11 and 12 of c-kit in mast cell tumors of dogs. *Am J Vet Res* 63: 1718, 2002.

204. Hirota S, Isozaki K, Moriyama Y, et al: Gain-of-function mutations of c-kit in human gastrointestinal stromal tumors. *Science* 279:577, 1998.

205. Nishida T, Hirota S, Taniguchi M, et al: Familial gastrointestinal stromal tumours with germline mutation of the KIT gene. *Nat Genet* 19:323, 1998.

206. Czarnetzki BM, Behrendt H: Urticaria pigmentosa: Clinical picture and response to oral disodium cromoglycate. *Br J Dermatol* 105:563, 1981.

207. Tharp MD: The spectrum of mastocytosis. *Am J Med Sci* 289:119, 1985.

208. Hartmann K, Metcalfe DD: Pediatric mastocytosis. *Hematol Oncol Clin North Am* 14: 625, 2000.

209. Travis WD, Li CY: Pathology of the lymph node and spleen in systemic mast cell disease. *Mod Pathol* 1:4, 1988.

210. Mican JM, Di Bisceglie AM, Fong TL, et al: Hepatic involvement in mastocytosis: Clinicopathologic correlations in 41 cases. *Hepatology* 22(4 Pt 1):1163, 1995.

211. Lawrence JB, Friedman BS, Travis WD, et al: Hematologic manifestations of systemic mast cell disease: A prospective study of laboratory and morphologic features and their relation to prognosis. *Am J Med* 91: 612, 1991.

212. Horny HP, Ruck MT, Kaiserling E: Spleen findings in generalized mastocytosis. A clinicopathologic study. *Cancer* 70:459, 1992.

213. Horny HP, Parwaresch MR, Lennert K: Bone marrow findings in systemic mastocytosis. *Hum Pathol* 16:808, 1985.

214. Ridell B, Olafsson JH, Roupe G, et al: The bone marrow in urticaria pigmentosa and systemic mastocytosis. Cell composition and mast cell density in relation to urinary excretion of tele-methylimidazoleacetic acid. *Arch Dermatol* 122:422, 1986.

215. Kettelhut BV, Parker RI, Travis WD, et al: Hematopathology of the bone marrow in pediatric cutaneous mastocytosis. A study of 17 patients. *Am J Clin Pathol* 91:558, 1989.

216. Parker RI: Hematologic aspects of systemic mastocytosis. *Hematol Oncol Clin North Am* 14:557, 2000.

217. Yang F, Tran TA, Carlson JA, et al: Paraffin section immunophenotype of cutaneous and extracutaneous mast cell disease: Comparison to other hematopoietic neoplasms. *Am J Surg Pathol* 24:703, 2000.

218. Natkunam Y, Rouse RV: Utility of paraffin section immunohistochemistry for C-KIT (CD117) in the differential diagnosis of systemic mast cell disease involving the bone marrow. *Am J Surg Pathol* 24:81, 2000.

219. Valent P, Horny HP, Escribano L, et al: Diagnostic criteria and classification of mastocytosis: A consensus proposal. *Leuk Res* 25:603, 2001.

220. Roberts LJ 2nd, Fields JP, Oates, JA: Mastocytosis without urticaria pigmentosa: A frequently unrecognized cause of recurrent syncope. *Trans Assoc Am Physicians* 95:36, 1982.

221. Cherner JA, Jensen RT, Dubois A, et al: Gastrointestinal dysfunction in systemic mastocytosis. A prospective study. *Gastroenterology* 95:657, 1988.

222. Rafii M, Firooznia H, Golimbu C, et al: Pathologic fracture in systemic mastocytosis. Radiographic spectrum and review of the literature. *Clin Orthop* 180:260, 1983.

223. Schwartz LB, Sakai K, Bradford TR, et al: The alpha form of human tryptase is the predominant type present in blood at baseline in normal subjects and is elevated in those with systemic mastocytosis. *J Clin Invest* 96:2702, 1995.

224. Joachim G: Über mastzellenleukämie. *Dtsch Arch Klin Med* 87:437, 1906.

225. Travis WD, Li CY, Hoagland HC, et al: Mast cell leukemia: Report of a case and review of the literature. *Mayo Clin Proc* 61:957, 1986.

226. Torrey E, Simpson K, Wilbur S, et al: Malignant mastocytosis with circulating mast cells. *Am J Hematol* 34:283, 1990.

227. Lennert K, Koster E, Martin H: Über die mastzellen-leukaemie. *Acta Haematol* 16: 255, 1956.

228. Friedman BS, Steinberg SC, Meggs WJ, et al: Analysis of plasma histamine levels in patients with mast cell disorders. *Am J Med* 87:649, 1989.

229. Valent P, Akin C, Sperr WR, et al: Diagnosis and treatment of systemic mastocytosis: State of the art. *Br J Haematol* 122:695, 2003.

230. Frieri M, Alling DW, Metcalfe DD: Comparison of the therapeutic efficacy of cromolyn sodium with that of combined chlorpheniramine and cimetidine in systemic mastocytosis. Results of a double-blind clinical trial. *Am J Med* 78:9, 1985.

231. Worobec AS: Treatment of systemic mast cell disorders. *Hematol Oncol Clin North Am* 14:659, 2000.

232. Sullivan TJ: Pharmacologic modulation of the whealing response to histamine in human skin: Identification of doxepin as a potent in vivo inhibitor. *J Allergy Clin Immunol* 69:260, 1982.

233. Soter NA, Austen KF, Wasserman SI: Oral disodium cromoglycate in the treatment of systemic mastocytosis. *N Engl J Med* 301:465, 1979.

234. Welch EA, Alper JC, Bogaars H, et al: Treatment of bullous mastocytosis with disodium cromoglycate. *J Am Acad Dermatol* 9:349, 1983.

235. Czarnetzki BM: A double-blind cross-over study of the effect of ketotifen in urticaria pigmentosa. *Dermatologica* 166:44, 1983.

236. Graves L 3rd, Stechschulte DJ, Morris DC, et al: Inhibition of mediator release in systemic mastocytosis is associated with reversal of bone changes. *J Bone Miner Res* 5:1113, 1990.

237. Kettelhut BV, Berkebile C, Bradley D, et al: A double-blind, placebo-controlled, crossover trial of ketotifen versus hydroxyzine in the treatment of pediatric mastocytosis. *J Allergy Clin Immunol* 83:866, 1989.

238. Friedman BS, Santiago ML, Berkebile C, et al: Comparison of azelastine and chlorpheniramine in the treatment of mastocytosis. *J Allergy Clin Immunol* 92:520, 1993.

239. Cundy T, Beneton MN, Darby AJ, et al: Osteopenia in systemic mastocytosis: Natural history and responses to treatment with inhibitors of bone resorption. *Bone* 8:149, 1987.

240. Barton J, Lavker RM, Schechter NM, et al: Treatment of urticaria pigmentosa with corticosteroids. *Arch Dermatol* 121:1516, 1985.

241. Kolde G, Frosch PJ, Czarnetzki BM: Response of cutaneous mast cells to PUVA in patients with urticaria pigmentosa: Histomorphometric, ultrastructural, and biochemical investigations. *J Invest Dermatol* 83:175, 1984.

242. Czarnetzki BM, Rosenbach T, Kolde G, et al: Phototherapy of urticaria pigmentosa: Clinical response and changes of cutaneous reactivity, histamine and chemotactic leukotrienes. *Arch Dermatol Res* 277:105, 1985.

243. Reisberg IR, Oyakawa S: Mastocytosis with malabsorption, myelofibrosis, and massive ascites. *Am J Gastroenterol* 82:54, 1987.

244. Kluin-Nelemans HC, Jansen JH, Breukelman H, et al: Response to interferon alfa-2b in a patient with systemic mastocytosis. *N Engl J Med* 326:19, 1992.

245. Worobec AS, Kirshenbaum AS, Schwartz LB, et al: Treatment of three patients with systemic mastocytosis with interferon alpha-2b. *Leuk Lymphoma* 22:501, 1996.

246. Tefferi A, Li CY, Butterfield JH, et al: Treatment of systemic mast-cell disease with cladribine. *N Engl J Med* 344:307, 2001.

247. Ronnov-Jessen AD, Nielsen, PL: Mastocytosis. *Ugeskr Laeger* 153:3131, 1991.

248. Fodinger M, Fritsch G, Winkler K, et al: Origin of human mast cells: Development from transplanted hematopoietic stem cells after allogeneic bone marrow transplantation. *Blood* 84:2954, 1994.

249. Przepiorka D, Giralt S, Khouri I, et al: Allogeneic marrow transplantation for myeloproliferative disorders other than chronic myelogenous leukemia: Review of forty cases. *Am J Hematol* 57:24, 1998.

250. Nakamura R, Akin C, Bahceci E, et al: Allogeneic non-myeloablative stem cell transplantation for advanced systemic mastocytosis: Possible induction of a graft versus mastocytosis effect [abstract]. *Biol Blood Marrow Transplant* 8:81, 2002.

251. Buchdunger E, Zimmermann J, Mett H, et al: Inhibition of the Abl protein-tyrosine kinase in vitro and in vivo by a 2-phenylaminopyrimidine derivative. *Cancer Res* 56:100, 1996.

252. Druker BJ, Tamura S, Buchdunger E, et al: Effects of a selective inhibitor of the Abl tyrosine kinase on the growth of Bcr-Abl positive cells. *Nat Med* 2:561, 1996.

253. Buchdunger E, Cioffi CL, Law N, et al: Abl protein-tyrosine kinase inhibitor STI571 inhibits in vitro signal transduction mediated by c-kit and platelet-derived growth factor receptors. *J Pharmacol Exp Ther* 295:139, 2000.

254. Ma Y, Zeng S, Metcalfe DD, et al: The c-KIT mutation causing human mastocytosis is resistant to STI571 and other KIT kinase inhibitors; kinases with enzymatic site mutations show different inhibitor sensitivity profiles than wild-type kinases and those with regulatory-type mutations. *Blood* 99:1741, 2002.

255. Zermati Y, De Sepulveda P, Feger F, et al: Effect of tyrosine kinase inhibitor STI571 on the kinase activity of wild-type and various mutated c-kit receptors found in mast cell neoplasms. *Oncogene* 22:660, 2003.

256. Akin C, Brockow K, D'Ambrosio C, et al: Effects of tyrosine kinase inhibitor STI571 on human mast cells bearing wild-type or mutated c-kit. *Exp Hematol* 31:686, 2003.

257. Liao AT, Chien MB, Shenoy N, et al: Inhibition of constitutively active forms of mutant kit by multitargeted indolinone tyrosine kinase inhibitors. *Blood* 100:585, 2002.

258. Klion AD, Noel P, Akin C, et al: Elevated serum tryptase levels identify a subset of patients with a myeloproliferative variant of idiopathic hypereosinophilic syndrome associated with tissue fibrosis, poor prognosis, and imatinib responsiveness. *Blood* 101:4660, 2003.

259. Pardanani A, Ketterling RP, Brockman SR, et al: CHIC2 deletion, a surrogate for FIP1L1-PDGFRA fusion, occurs in systemic mastocytosis associated with eosinophilia and predicts response to imatinib mesylate therapy. *Blood* 102:3093, 2003.

260. Friedman B, Darling G, Norton J, et al: Splenectomy in the management of systemic mast cell disease. *Surgery* 107:94, 1990.

261. Horan, RF, Austen, KF: Systemic mastocytosis: Retrospective review of a decade's clinical experience at the Brigham and Women's Hospital. *J Invest Dermatol* 96:5S, 1991.

262. Coser P, Quaglino D, De Pasquale A, et al: Cytobiological and clinical aspects of tissue mast cell leukaemia. *Br J Haematol* 45:5, 1980.

263. Dalton R, Chan L, Batten E, et al: Mast cell leukaemia: Evidence for bone marrow origin of the pathological clone. *Br J Haematol* 64:397, 1986.

CLASSIFICATION AND CLINICAL MANIFESTATIONS OF NEUTROPHIL DISORDERS

MARSHALL A . LICHTMAN

Neutrophil disorders can be grouped into deficiencies, or *neutropenia*, and excesses, or *neutrophilia*. Neutropenia can have the severe consequence of predisposing to infection, whereas neutrophilia usually is a manifestation of an underlying inflammatory or neoplastic disease: the neutrophilia, per se, having no specific consequences. Qualitative disorders of neutrophils may lead to infection as a result of defective chemotaxis to an inflammatory site or defective microbial killing. Neutropenia may reflect an inherited disease that usually is evident in childhood (such as congenital neutropenia), but more often it is acquired. The most common cause of neutropenia is the adverse effect of a drug. Some cases of neutropenia have no evident cause. The health consequence of neutropenia is a function of the severity of the decrease in the blood neutrophil count and the abruptness and duration of the decrease. Table 64-1 provides a comprehensive categorization of quantitative and qualitative neutrophil disorders.

CLASSIFICATION

Table 64-1 lists disorders that result from a primary deficiency in neutrophil numbers or function. Neutropenia or neutrophilia also occurs as part of a disorder that affects multiple blood cell lineages, as occurs in infiltrative diseases of the marrow or after cytotoxic drug therapy, but these diseases are not included in this classification and are discussed in other parts of this text. In this classification and in this chapter, we consider diseases resulting from neutrophil deficiencies in which the neutrophil is either the only cell type affected or is the dominant cell type affected.

A pathophysiologic classification of neutrophil disorders has proved elusive. Techniques for measuring mechanisms of impaired production or accelerated destruction of neutrophils are more difficult and complex than the techniques used for red cells or platelets. The low concentration of blood neutrophils, accentuated in neutropenic states, makes radioactive labeling techniques for studying the kinetics of autologous cells in neutropenic subjects technically difficult or not possible. The two compartments of neutrophils in the blood, the random disappearance of neutrophils from the circulation, the extremely short circulation time of neutrophils, the absence of practical techniques for measuring the size of the tissue neutrophil compartment, and the disappearance of neutrophils by apoptosis or excretion from the tissue compartment also make multicompartment kinetic analysis difficult. Also, neutropenic disorders are uncommon, and few laboratories are able, or prepared, to undertake the studies necessary to define the mechanisms of their development in sporadic cases. Therefore, efforts to understand the pathophysiology of neutropenia have been of limited success. Hence, the classification of neutrophil disorders is partly pathophysiologic and partly descriptive (see Table 64-1). Classification, although imperfect, does provide a language for commu-

nication and a basis for rectification as knowledge of the cause and mechanism of disease advances.

The classification is self-explanatory except in two areas. First, certain childhood syndromes listed under decreased neutrophilic granulopoiesis could have been listed under chronic hypoplastic neutropenia or chronic idiopathic neutropenia; however, they seem to hold a special interest. The pathogenesis becomes clarified as the mutant genes for the inherited syndromes are identified. Three childhood syndromes are associated with neutropenia but are omitted because the neutropenia is part of a more global suppression of hemopoiesis: Pearson syndrome,[1,2] Fanconi syndrome,[3,4] and dyskeratosis congenita.[4,5]

A second area requiring explanation is the chronic idiopathic neutropenias. This group includes (1) cases with normocellular marrows but an inadequate compensatory increase in granulopoiesis for the degree of neutropenia and (2) cases with hyperplastic granulopoiesis that apparently is ineffective. Unlike hypoplastic neutropenias in which the granulocyte precursors are markedly reduced or absent, precursors are present in the marrow in the idiopathic neutropenias, but the extent of effective granulopoiesis probably is low (see Chap. 65).

Qualitative disorders of neutrophils affect their ability to enter inflammatory exudates or to kill ingested microorganisms (see Chap. 66).

CLINICAL MANIFESTATIONS

The clinical manifestations of decreased concentrations or abnormal function of neutrophils principally result from infection.

The combined deficit of neutrophils and monocytes characteristic of aplastic anemia, hairy cell leukemia, and cytotoxic therapy leads to susceptibility to a broader spectrum of infectious agents. Increased concentrations of normal neutrophils per se have not been associated with clinical manifestations, although increased concentrations of leukemic neutrophil precursors can produce clinical manifestations of microcirculatory leukostasis (see Chap. 85).

NEUTROPENIA

The lower limit of the normal neutrophil count is approximately 1800/μl (1.8 $\times$ 10^9/liter) in subjects of European descent and 1400/μl (1.4 $\times$ 10^9/liter) in subjects of African descent.[148-154] This finding is especially striking in Yemenite Jews, another ethnic group with very low "normal" neutrophil counts.[155] A decrement in neutrophil concentration to 1000/μl (1.0 $\times$ 10^9/liter) usually poses little threat in the otherwise healthy individual. If the neutrophil count drops further, the risk of infection increases. Subjects who are chronically neutropenic as a result of a production abnormality with counts less than 500 neutrophils/μl (0.5 $\times$ 10^9/liter) are at risk for developing recurrent infections.[156]

The relationship of frequency or type of infection to neutrophil concentration is imperfect. The cause of the neutropenia, the coincidence of monocytopenia or lymphopenia, concurrent use of alcohol or glucocorticoids, and other factors can influence the likelihood of infection.

Infections in neutropenic subjects who are not otherwise compromised most likely result from gram-positive cocci and usually are superficial, involving skin, oropharynx, bronchi, anal canal, or vagina. However, any site can become infected, with gram-negative organisms, viruses, or opportunistic organisms possibly involved.

A decrease in neutrophil count can occur abruptly or gradually (see Chap. 65). One type of drug-induced neutropenia is distinguished by the rapidity of onset. Abrupt-onset neutropenia more likely is severe and leads to symptoms. If the neutrophil count approaches zero (agranulocytosis), high fever; chills; necrotizing, painful oral ulcers (agranulocytic angina); and prostration may occur, presumably as a result of sepsis.[157-159] As the disease progresses, headache, stupor, and rash may

TABLE 64-1   CLASSIFICATION OF NEUTROPHIL DISORDERS

I. Quantitative disorders of neutrophils
  A. Neutropenia
    1. Decreased neutrophilic granulopoiesis
      a. Congenital neutropenias (Kostmann syndrome and related disorders)[6-8]
      b. Reticular dysgenesis (congenital aleukocytosis)[9]
      c. Neutropenia and exocrine pancreas dysfunction (Shwachman-Diamond syndrome)[9,10,15-17]
      d. Neutropenia and immunoglobulin abnormality[8,18]
      e. Neutropenia and disordered cellular immunity (cartilage hair hypoplasia)[9,21,22]
      f. Mental retardation, anomalies, and neutropenia (Cohen syndrome)[10,11,23,24]
      g. X-linked cardioskeletal myopathy and neutropenia (Barth syndrome)[12,20,25,26]
      h. Myelokathexis[13,14,19,27,28]
      i. Neonatal neutropenia and maternal hypertension[30,31,188]
      j. Griscelli syndrome[29]
      k. Chronic hypoplastic neutropenia
        (1) Drug-induced[32-35]
        (2) Cyclic
          (a) Sporadic[36-40]
          (b) Familial[41-43]
        (3) Idiopathic
          (a) Sporadic[44]
          (b) Familial[44]
        (4) Branched-chain aminoacidemia[45]
      l. Acute hypoplastic neutropenia
        (1) Drug-induced[32-35]
        (2) Infectious[46,47]
      m. Chronic idiopathic neutropenia
        (1) Benign
          (a) Familial[48]
          (b) Sporadic[49-54]
        (2) Symptomatic[55,56]
    2. Accelerated neutrophil destruction
      a. Alloimmune neonatal neutropenia[57,58,189]
      b. Autoimmune neutropenia[59,60,189]
        (1) Idiopathic[61-63]
        (2) Drug-induced[32,33]
        (3) Felty syndrome[64-66]
        (4) Systemic lupus erythematosus[66]
        (5) Other autoimmune diseases[67,68]
        (6) Complement activation–induced neutropenia[69,70]
        (7) Pure white cell aplasia[71,72]
    3. Maldistribution of neutrophils
      a. Pseudoneutropenia[73]
  B. Neutrophilia
    1. Increased neutrophilic granulopoiesis
      a. Hereditary neutrophilia[74]
      b. Chronic idiopathic neutrophilia[75]
        (1) Asplenia[76]
      c. Neutrophilic leukemoid reactions[77]
        (1) Inflammation[77,176]
        (2) Infection[78,176]
        (3) Cancer[79,176,177,187]
        (4) Drugs (e.g., glucocorticoids, lithium, granulocyte- or granulocyte monocyte colony stimulating factor)[80,81,178,179]
        (5) Exercise[180,183]
      d. Sweets syndrome[82]
      e. Cigarette smoking[83,184]
    2. Decreased neutrophil circulatory egress
      a. Drugs (e.g., glucocorticoids)[40,179]
    3. Maldistribution of neutrophils
      a. Pseudoneutrophilia[84]
      b. Membrane CD11/18 deficiency[85]

TABLE 64-1   CLASSIFICATION OF NEUTROPHIL DISORDERS (CONTINUED)

II. Qualitative disorders of neutrophils[86-88]
  A. Defective adhesion of neutrophils
    1. Leukocyte adhesion deficiency types I and II[89-92,99]
    2. Drug-induced[93]
  B. Defective locomotion and chemotaxis[94,95]
    1. Lazy leukocyte syndrome[96]
    2. Actin polymerization abnormalities[97,98]
    3. Neonatal neutrophils[100]
    4. Interleukin-2 administration[101]
  C. Defective microbial killing[102,103]
    1. Chronic granulomatous disease[102-104]
    2. RAC-2 deficiency[181]
    3. Myeloperoxidase deficiency[104-106]
    4. Hyperimmunoglobulin E (Job) syndrome[107]
    5. Glucose-6-phosphate dehydrogenase deficiency[108]
    6. Extensive burns[109]
    7. Glycogen storage disease Ib[110,111]
    8. Ethanol toxicity[112]
    9. End-stage renal disease[113]
  D. Multiple or mixed disorders[86]
  E. Abnormal structure of the nucleus or of an organelle
    1. Hereditary macropolycytes[114]
    2. Hereditary hypersegmentation[115]
    3. Specific granule deficiency[116,117]
    4. Pelger-Huët anomaly[118]
    5. Alder-Reilly anomaly[119]
    6. May-Hegglin anomaly[120,182]
    7. Chédiak-Higashi disease[121,122]
III. Neutrophil-induced vascular or tissue damage[123-147,185,186]

Pus formation decreases in patients with severe neutropenia.[160,161] The failure to suppurate can mislead the clinician and delay identification of the infection site because minimal physical or radiographic findings develop. For example, lack of pneumonic consolidation is characteristic of pneumonia in granulocytopenic subjects. Exudate, swelling, heat, and regional adenopathy are much less prevalent in granulocytopenic patients. Fever is common, and local pain, tenderness, and erythema nearly always are present despite a marked reduction in neutrophils.[162-164]

The mechanism of neutropenia and the severity of the deficiency of cells play roles in clinical manifestations. *Chronic idiopathic (benign) neutropenia* is associated with normal granulopoiesis in the marrow and is asymptomatic even when the neutropenia has been present for prolonged periods, sometimes in the face of neutrophil counts approaching zero.[49] Presumably the delivery of neutrophils from marrow to tissues is sufficient to prevent infection despite the low blood pool size.[50,51] Monocyte counts are normal, which may aid in host defenses because monocytes are effective phagocytes.

Chronic idiopathic (symptomatic) neutropenia often is associated with pyoderma and otitis media in children.[55] The former usually is caused by *Staphylococcus aureus, Escherichia coli,* and *Pseudomonas* species, and the latter usually results from infection by pneumococci or *Pseudomonas aeruginosa.* Unexplained chronic gingivitis may be a manifestation of chronic neutropenia.[165] Pneumonia, lung abscesses, stomatitis, hepatic abscesses, or infections in other sites can occur.[56]

Chronic cyclic neutropenia is characterized by periodic oscillations in the number of neutrophils, with the nadir occurring at approximately 3-week intervals.[36,166] During neutropenia, patients develop malaise; fever; buccal, labial, or lingual ulcers; and cervical adenopathy. Furuncles, carbuncles, cellulitis, infected cuts with lymphangitis, chronic gingivitis, and abscesses of the axilla or groin may occur. Although severe infections may be fatal, life-threatening complications are uncommon (see Chap. 65).

develop. In the preantibiotic era, persistent agranulocytosis had a fatality rate approaching 100 percent. Even with bactericidal, broad-spectrum antibiotics, severe, sustained neutropenia or agranulocytosis is a serious illness with a high fatality rate.

Some individuals have neutropenia because a larger proportion of their blood neutrophils is in the marginal rather than the circulating pool. The total blood neutrophil pool is normal, and infections do not result from this atypical distribution of neutrophils.[167] This type of alteration has been called *pseudoneutropenia*.

QUALITATIVE NEUTROPHIL ABNORMALITIES

Neutrophil function depends on the ability of neutrophils to adhere to endothelium, move, respond to chemotactic gradients, ingest microorganisms, and kill ingested pathogens. Loss of any of these functions can predispose to infection (see Chap. 66). Defects in each step of the neutrophil's participation in the inflammatory response have been identified.[168,169] Defects in cytoplasmic contractile proteins, granule synthesis or contents, or intracellular enzymes may underlie a movement, ingestion, or killing defect. These defects may be congenital or acquired. Chronic granulomatous disease[102,103] and Chédiak-Higashi disease[121] are two examples of the congenital defects. Among the acquired disorders are those extrinsic to the cell, as in the movement, chemotactic, or phagocytic defects of diabetes mellitus,[168–171] alcohol abuse,[172,173] or glucocorticoid excess.[174] Acquired intrinsic disorders usually are manifestations of clonal hematopoietic disorders such as myelogenous leukemia[175] (see Chap. 85).

Severe defects in bacterial killing, as occur in chronic granulomatous disease, result in *S. aureus, Klebsiella-Aerobacter, E. coli,* and other catalase-positive bacterial infections. Suppurative lymphadenitis, pneumonia, dermatitis, hepatic abscesses, osteomyelitis, and stomatitis occur, and chronic granulomatous reactions in these sites give the disease its name. Fatality rates have been high. Functional disorders may be severe, as in chronic granulomatous disease. Mild functional disorders predispose to infections that occur infrequently and respond readily to antibiotics. Severe functional disorders result in suppurative lesions because neutrophil influx into inflammatory foci is not impaired, whereas agranulocytosis is associated with nonsuppurative lesions.

NEUTROPHILIA

An overabundance of neutrophils does not result in specific clinical manifestations. Neutrophils can transiently occlude capillaries, as determined by supravital microscopy, and such occlusions may reduce local blood flow transiently and contribute to the development of ischemia.[124] Impairment of reperfusion of the coronary microcirculation has been thought to be dependent, in part, on neutrophil plugging of myocardial capillaries.[123]

NEUTROPHIL-INDUCED VASCULAR OR TISSUE DAMAGE

Neutrophil products may contribute to the pathogenesis of inflammatory skin, bowel, synovial, glomerular, and bronchial and interstitial pulmonary diseases.[124–138] These products may act as mediators of tissue injury in myocardial infarction.[139–142] Highly reactive oxygen products of neutrophils may be mutagens that increase the risk of neoplasia.[144,145] This action may explain, for example, the development of carcinoma of the bowel in patients with chronic ulcerative colitis and the relationship between elevated leukocyte count and the occurrence of lung cancer, independent of the effect of cigarette usage.[146] The oxidants, especially hypochlorous acid and chloramines, released by the neutrophil are extremely short lived and may play a role in tissue injury by inactivating several protease inhibitors in tissue fluids, permitting proteases, especially elastase, collagenase, and gelatinase, to cause tissue injury.[129] Thrombogenesis also has been ascribed to leukocyte products.[143]

REFERENCES

1. Pearson HA, Lobel JS, Kocoshis SA, et al: A new syndrome of refractory sideroblastic anemia with vacuolization of marrow precursors and exocrine pancreatic dysfunction. *J Pediatr* 95:976, 1979.
2. van de Corput MP, van den Ouweland JM, Dirks RW, et al: Detection of mitochondrial DNA deletions in human skin fibroblasts of patients with Pearson's syndrome by two-color fluorescence in situ hybridization. *J Histochem Cytochem* 45:55, 1997.
3. Gordon-Smith EC, Rutherford TR: Fanconi anemia. *Ballères Clin Haematol* 2:139, 1989.
4. Bagby GC Jr: Genetic basis of Fanconi anemia. *Curr Opin Hematol* 10:68, 2003.
5. Srinavin C, Trowbridge A: Dyskeratosis congenita: Clinical features and genetic aspects. *J Med Genet* 12:339, 1975.
6. Dokal I: Severe aplastic anemia including Fanconi's anemia and dyskeratosis congenita. *Curr Opin Hematol* 3:453, 1996.
7. Kostmann R: Infantile genetic agranulocytosis. *Acta Pediatr Scand* 64:362, 1975.
8. Tidow N, Pilz C, Teichmann B, et al: Clinical relevance of point mutations in the cytoplasmic domain of granulocyte colony-stimulating factor receptor gene in patients with severe congenital neutropenia. *Blood* 89:2369, 1997.
9. Zetterstrom R: Kostman disease. *Acta Paediatr* 91:1397, 2002.
10. Ancliff PJ: Congenital neutropenia. *Blood Rev* 17:209, 2003.
11. Kolehmainen J, Black GC, Saarinen A, et al: Cohen syndrome is caused by mutations in a novel gene, COH1, encoding a transmembrane protein with a presumed role in vesicle-mediated sorting and intracellular protein transport. *Am J Hum Genet* 72:1359, 2003.
12. Weston B, Todd RF III, Axtell R, et al: Severe congenital neutropenia: Clinical effects and neutrophil function during treatment with granulocyte colony-stimulating factor. *J Lab Clin Med* 117:282, 1991.
13. Haas RJ, Niethammer D, Goldmann SF, et al: Congenital immunodeficiency and agranulocytosis (reticular dysgenesis). *Acta Paediatr Scand* 66:279, 1977.
14. Levinsky RJ, Tiedman K: Successful bone-marrow transplantation for reticular dysgenesis. *Lancet* 1:671, 1983.
15. Boocock GR, Morrison JA, Popovic M, et al: Mutations in SBDS are associated with Shwachman-Diamond syndrome. *Nat Genet* 33:97, 2003.
16. Woods WG, Roloff JS, Lukens JN: The occurrence of leukemia in patients with Shwachman syndrome. *J Pediatr* 99:425, 1981.
17. Azzarà A, Carulli G, Ceccarelli M, et al: In vivo effectiveness of lithium on impaired neutrophil chemotaxis in Shwachman-Diamond syndrome. *Acta Haematol* 85:100, 1991.
18. Lonsdale D, Doedhar SD, Mercer RD: Familial granulocytopenia associated with immunoglobulin abnormality. *J Pediatr* 71:760, 1967.
19. Wetzler M, Talpaz M, Kleinerman ES, et al: A new familial immunodeficiency disorder characterized by severe neutropenia, a defective marrow release mechanism, and hypogammaglobulinemia. *Am J Med* 89:663, 1990.
20. Kozlowski C, Evans DIK: Neutropenia associated with X-linked agammaglobulinemia. *J Clin Pathol* 44:388, 1991.
21. Lux SE, Johnston RB Jr, August CS, et al: Chronic neutropenia and abnormal cellular immunity in cartilage-hair hypoplasia. *N Engl J Med* 282:231, 1970.
22. Trojak JE, Polmar SH, Winkelstein JA: Immunologic studies of cartilage-hair hypoplasia in the Amish. *Johns Hopkins Med J* 148:157, 1981.
23. Olivieri O, Lombardi S, Russo C, Corrocher R: Increased neutrophil adhesive capability in Cohen syndrome, an autosomal recessive disorder associated with granulocytopenia. *Haematologia* 83:778, 1998.
24. Warburg M, Pedersen SA, Hønlyk H: The Cohen syndrome. *Ophthalmic Pediatr Genet* II:7, 1990.

25. Barth PG, Scholte HR, Berden JA, et al: An X-linked mitochondrial disease affecting cardiac muscle, skeletal muscle and neutrophil leukocytes. *J Neurol Sci* 62:327, 1983.

26. Bohurs PA, Hensels GW, Hulsebos TJM, et al: Mapping of the locus for the X-linked cardioskeletal myopathy with neutropenia and abnormal mitochondria (Barth syndrome) to Xq28. *Am J Hum Genet* 48:481, 1991.

27. Bassan R, Viero P, Minetti B, et al: Myelokathexis: A rare form of chronic benign neutropenia. *Br J Haematol* 58:115, 1984.

28. Wetzler M, Talpaz M, Kellagher MJ, et al: Myelokathexis. *JAMA* 267:2179, 1992.

29. Menasche G, Fischer A, de Saint Basile G: Griscelli syndrome types 1 and 2. *Am J Hum Genet* 71:1237, 2002.

30. Koenig JM, Christensen RD: Incidence, neutrophil kinetics and natural history of neonatal neutropenia associated with maternal hypertension. *N Engl J Med* 321:557, 1989.

31. Koenig JM, Christensen RD: The mechanism responsible for diminished neutrophil production in neonates delivered of women with pregnancy-induced hypertension. *Am J Obstet Gynecol* 165:467, 1991.

32. Hartl PW: Drug-induced agranulocytosis, in *Blood Disorders Due to Drugs and Other Agents*, edited by RH Girdwood, p 147. Excerpta Medica, Amsterdam, 1974.

33. Hine LK, Gerstman BB, Wise RP, Tsang Y: Mortality resulting from blood dyscrasias in the United States 1984. *Am J Med* 88:151, 1990.

34. Pisciotta AV: Drug-induced agranulocytosis peripheral destruction of polymorphonuclear leukocytes and their marrow precursors. *Blood Rev* 4:226, 1990.

35. Julia A, Olona M, Bueno J, et al: Drug-induced agranulocytosis. *Br J Haematol* 79:366, 1991.

36. Wright DG, Dale DC, Fauci AS, Wolff SM: Human cyclic neutropenia. *Medicine* 60:13, 1981.

37. Tefferi A, Solberg LA, Petett RM, Willis LG: Adult-onset cyclic bicy-topenia. *Am J Hematol* 30:181, 1989.

38. Loughran TP Jr, Clark EA, Hammond WP: Adult-onset cyclic neutropenia is associated with increased large granular lymphocytes. *Blood* 68:1082, 1986.

39. Hammond WP, Price TH, Souza LM, Dale DC: Treatment of cyclic neutropenia with granulocyte colony-stimulating factor. *N Engl J Med* 320:1306, 1989.

40. Marinone G, Roncoli B, Marinone MG: Pure white cell aplasia. *Semin Hematol* 28:298, 1991.

41. Morley AA, Carew JP, Baikie AG: Familial cyclic neutropenia. *Br J Haematol* 13:719, 1967.

42. Hammond WP, Chatta GS, Andrews RG, Dale DC: Abnormal responsiveness of granulocyte-committed progenitor cells in cyclic neutropenia. *Blood* 79:2536, 1992.

43. Dale DC, Hammond WP: Cyclic neutropenia: A clinical review. *Blood Rev* 2:178, 1988.

44. Spaet TH, Dameshek W: Chronic hypoplastic neutropenia. *Am J Med* 13:35, 1952.

45. Hutchinson R, Bunnell K, Thorne J: Suppression of granulopoietic progenitor cell proliferation by metabolites of the branched-chain amino acids. *J Pediatr* 106:62, 1985.

46. Murdock JMC, Smith CC: Haematologic aspects of systemic disease—infection. *Clin Haematol* 1:619, 1972.

47. Olson JP, Lichtman MA: Neutropenia, in *Hematology for Practitioners*, edited by MA Lichtman, p 105. Little, Brown, Boston, 1978.

48. Cutting HO, Lange JE: Familial-benign chronic neutropenia. *Ann Intern Med* 61:876, 1964.

49. Kyle RA: Natural history of chronic idiopathic neutropenia. *N Engl J Med* 302:908, 1970.

50. Wright DG, Meierovics AI, Foxley JM: Assessing the delivery of neutrophils to tissues in neutropenia. *Blood* 67:1023, 1986.

51. Mant MJ, Gordon PA, Akabotu JJ: Bone marrow granulocyte reserve in chronic benign idiopathic neutropenia. *Clin Lab Haematol* 9:281, 1987.

52. Logue GL, Shastri KA, Laughlin M, et al: Idiopathic neutropenia: Antineutrophil antibodies and clinical correlations. *Am J Med* 90:211, 1991.

53. Jonsson OG, Buchanan GR: Chronic neutropenia during childhood. *Am J Dis Child* 145:232, 1991.

54. Jakubowski AA, Souza L, Kelly F, et al: Effects of human granulocyte colony-stimulating factor in a patient with idiopathic neutropenia. *N Engl J Med* 320:38, 1989.

55. Pincus SH, Boxer LA, Stossel TP: Chronic neutropenia in childhood. *Am J Med* 61:849, 1976.

56. Dale DC, Guerry D IV, Wewerka JR, et al: Chronic neutropenia. *Medicine* 58:128, 1979.

57. Lalezari P: Alloimmune neonatal neutropenia, in *Clinical Immunology and Allergy*, edited by CP Engelfriet, AEG VondemBorne, p 423. Balliére Tindall, London, 1987.

58. Fromont P, Bettaieb A, Skouri H, et al: Frequency of the polymorphonuclear neutrophil Fc receptor III deficiency in the French population and its involvement in the development of neonatal alloimmune neutropenia. *Blood* 79:2131, 1992.

59. Shastri KA, Logue GL: Autoimmune neutropenia. *Blood* 81:1984, 1993.

60. Bux J, Behrens G, Jaeger G, Welte K: Diagnosis and clinical course of autoimmune neutropenia in infancy: Analysis of 240 cases. *Blood* 91:181, 1998.

61. Boxer LA, Greenberg MS, Boxer GJ, Stossel TP: Autoimmune neutropenia. *N Engl J Med* 293:748, 1975.

62. Hadley AG, Holdurn AM, Bunch C, Chapel H: Antigranulocyte opsonic activity and autoimmune neutropenia. *Br J Haematol* 63:581, 1986.

63. Hartman KR, Wright DG: Identification of autoantibodies specific for the neutrophil adhesion glycoproteins CD116/CD18 in parents with autoimmune neutropenia. *Blood* 78:1096, 1991.

64. Starkebaum G, Loughran TP Jr, Gaur LK, et al: Immunogenetic similarities between patients with Felty's syndrome and those with clonal expansion of large granular lymphocytes in rheumatoid arthritis. *Arthritis Rheum* 40:624, 1997.

65. Mason C, Perroux-Goummy L, Audran M: Felty's syndrome, pseudo-Felty's syndrome, monoclonal or polyclonal CD3 lymphocytosis of undetermined significance. *Rev Rhum Ed Fr* 63:5, 1996.

66. Hellmich B, Schnabel A, Gross WL: Treatment of severe neutropenia due to Felty's syndrome or systemic lupus erythematosus with granulocyte colony-stimulating factor. *Semin Arthritis Rheum* 29:82, 1999.

67. Yamato E, Fujioka Y, Masugi F, et al: Autoimmune neutropenia with anti-neutrophil autoantibody associated with Sjögren's syndrome. *Am J Med Sci* 300:102, 1990.

68. Stevens C, Peppercorn MA, Grand RJ: Crohn's disease associated with autoimmune neutropenia. *J Clin Gastroenterol* 13:328, 1991.

69. Zachee P, Daeleans R, Pollaris P, et al: Neutrophil adhesion molecules in chronic hemodialysis patients. *Nephron* 68:192, 1994.

70. Knudsen F, Nielsen AH, Pedersen JO, et al: Adult respiratory distress-like syndrome during hemodialysis: Relationship between activation of complement, leukopenia, and release of granulocyte elastase. *Int J Artif Organs* 8:187, 1985.

71. Firkin FC, Prewett EJ, Nicholls K, Moran J: Antithymocyte globulin therapy for pure white cell aplasia. *Am J Hematol* 25:101, 1987.

72. Mathieson PW, O'Neill JH, Durrant STS, et al: Antibody-mediated pure neutrophil aplasia, recurrent myasthenia gravis and previous thymoma. *Q J Med* 74:57, 1990.

73. Joyce RA, Boggs DR, Hasiba U, Srodes CH: Marginal neutrophil pool size in normal subjects and neutropenic patients as measured by epinephrine infusion. *J Lab Clin Med* 88:614, 1976.

74. Herring WB, Smith LG, Walker RI, Herion JC: Hereditary neutrophilia. *Am J Med* 56:729, 1974.

75. Ward HN, Reinhard EH: Chronic idiopathic leukocytosis. *Ann Intern Med* 75:193, 1971.

76. Joyce RA, O'Donnell J, Sanghvi J, Westerman MP: Asplenia and abnormal neutrophil kinetics in chronic idiopathic neutrophilia. *Am J Med* 69:633, 1980.

77. Hilts SV, Shaw CC: Leukemoid blood reactions. *N Engl J Med* 149:343, 1953.

78. Marsh JC, Boggs DR, Cartwright GE, Wintrobe MM: Neutrophil kinetics in acute infection. *J Clin Invest* 46:1943, 1967.

79. McKee LC: Excess leukocytosis (leukemoid reactions) associated with malignant diseases. *South Med J* 78:1475, 1985.

80. Bishop CR: Leukokinetic studies: XIII. A non-steady state kinetic evaluation of the mechanism of cortisone-induced granulocytosis. *J Clin Invest* 47:249, 1968.

81. Murphy DL, Goodwin FK, Bunney WE: Leukocytosis during lithium treatment. *Am J Psychiatry* 127:135, 1971.

82. Huang W, McNeely MC: Neutrophilic tissue reactions. *Adv Dermatol* 13:33, 1998.

83. Petitti DB, Kipp H: The leukocyte count: Association with intensity of smoking and persistence of effect after quitting. *Am J Epidemiol* 123:89, 1986.

84. Athens JW, Haab OP, Raab SO, et al: Leukokinetic studies: IV. The total blood, circulating and marginal granulocyte pools and the granulocyte turnover rate in normal subjects. *J Clin Invest* 40:989, 1961.

85. Arnaout MA, Pitt J, Cohen HJ, et al: Deficiency of membrane glycoprotein (gp 150) in a boy with recurrent bacterial infections. *N Engl J Med* 306:693, 1982.

86. Rotrosen D, Gallin JI: Disorders of phagocyte function. *Annu Rev Immunol* 5:127, 1987.

87. Klebanoff SJ, Clark RA: *The Neutrophil: Function and Clinical Disorders.* North-Holland, Amsterdam, 1978.

88. Yang KD, Hill HR: Neutrophil function disorders: Pathophysiology, prevention and therapy. *J Pediatr* 119:343, 1991.

89. Gallin J: Leukocyte adherence related glycoproteins LFA-1, Mo-1, and p 150,95: A new group of monoclonal antibodies, a new disease and a possible opportunity to understand the molecular basis of leukocyte adherence. *J Infect Dis* 152:661, 1985.

90. Anderson DC, Springer TA: Leukocyte adhesion deficiency: An inherited defect in Mac-1, LFA-1, and p150,95 glycoproteins. *Annu Rev Med* 38:175, 1987.

91. Etzioni A, Frydman M, Pollock S, et al: Recurrent severe infections caused by a novel leukocyte adhesion deficiency. *N Engl J Med* 327:1789, 1992.

92. Etzioni A, Tonetti M: Leukocyte adhesion deficiency II—from A to almost Z. *Immunol Rev* 178:138, 2000.

93. MacGregor RR, Spagnulo PJ, Lentnek AL: Inhibition of granulocyte adherence by ethanol, prednisone, and aspirin, measured with an assay system. *N Engl J Med* 291:642, 1974.

94. Clark RA: Disorders of granulocyte chemotaxis: An analytical review. *Clin Immunol Immunopathol* 15:52, 1980.

95. Rotrosen D, Gallen JI: Disorders of phagocyte function. *Annu Rev Immunol* 5:127, 1987.

96. Miller ME, Oski FA, Harris MB: Lazy-leucocyte syndrome. A new disorder of neutrophil function. *Lancet* 1:665, 1971.

97. Boxer LA, Hedley-White ET, Stossel TP: Neutrophil actin dysfunction and abnormal neutrophil behavior. *N Engl J Med* 291:1043, 1974.

98. Coates TD, Torkildson JC, Torres M, et al: An inherited defect of neutrophil motility and microfilamentous cytoskeleton associated with abnormalities in 47-Kd and 89-Kd proteins. *Blood* 78:1338, 1991.

99. Meyle J: Leukocyte adhesion deficiency and prepubertal periodontitis. *Periodontol 2000* 6:26, 1994.

100. Hill HR, Augustine NH, Jaffe HS: Human recombinant interferon gamma enhances neonatal PMN activation and movement increases free intracellular calcium. *J Exp Med* 173:767, 1991.

101. Klempner MS, Noring R, Meir JW, Atkins MB: An acquired chemotactic defect in neutrophils from patients receiving interleukin-2 immunotherapy. *N Engl J Med* 322:959, 1990.

102. Meischi C, Roos D: The molecular basis of chronic granulomatous disease. *Springer Semin Immunopathol* 19:417, 1998.

103. Segal AW: Biochemistry and molecular biology of chronic granulomatous disease. *J Inherit Metab Dis* 15:683, 1992.

104. Bogomolski-Yahalom V, Matzner Y: Disorders of neutrophil function. *Blood Rev* 9:183, 1995.

105. Lehrer RI, Cline MJ: Leukocyte myeloperoxidase deficiency and disseminated candidiasis: The role of myeloperoxidase in resistance to *Candida* infection. *J Clin Invest* 48:1478, 1989.

106. Gerber CE, Kuci S, Zipfel M, et al: Phagocytic activity and oxidative burst of granulocytes in persons with myeloperoxidase deficiency. *Eur J Clin Chem Clin Biochem* 34:901, 1996.

107. Jeppson JD, Jaffe HW, Hill HR: Use of recombinant human interferon gamma enhances neutrophil chemotactic responses in Job syndrome of hypergammaglobulin E and recurrent infections. *J Pediatr* 118:383, 1991.

108. Cooper MR, DeChatelet LR, McCall CE, et al: Complete deficiency of leukocyte glucose-6-phosphate dehydrogenase with defective bactericidal activity. *J Clin Invest* 51:769, 1972.

109. Ahmed S el-D, el-Shahat AS, Saad SO: Assessment of certain neutrophil receptors, opsonophagocytosis and soluble intercellular adhesion molecule-1 (ICAM-1) following thermal injury. *Burns* 25:395, 1999.

110. Couper R, Kapellushnik J, Griffiths AM: Neutrophil dysfunction in glycogen storage disease Ib: Association with Crohn's-like colitis. *Gastroenterology* 100:549, 1991.

111. Schroten H, Wendel U, Burdach S, et al: Colony-stimulating factors for neutropenia in glycogen storage disease Ib. *Lancet* 337:736, 1991.

112. Tamura DY, Moore EE, Patrick DA, et al: Clinically relevant concentrations of ethanol attenuate primed neutrophil bacteriocidal activity. *J Trauma* 44:320, 1998.

113. Porter CJ, Burden RP, Morgan AG, et al: Impaired bacterial killing and hydrogen peroxide production by polymorphonuclear neutrophils in end-stage renal failure. *Nephron* 77:479, 1997.

114. Davidson WM, Milner RDG, Lawlor SD: Giant neutrophil leukocytes: An inherited anomaly. *Br J Haematol* 6:339, 1960.

115. Undritz VE: Eine neue Sippe mit Erblich Konstitutioneller Hochsegmentierung der Neutrophilenkerne. *Schweiz Med Wochenschr* 94:1365, 1964.

116. Uzel G, Holland SM: White blood cell defects: Molecular discoveries and clinical management. *Curr Allergy Asthma Rep* 2:385, 2002.

117. Gombart AF, Koeffler HP: Neutrophil specific granule deficiency and mutations in the gene encoding transcription factor C/EBP (epsilon). *Curr Opin Humantology* 9:36, 2002.

118. Hoffmann K, Dreger CK, Olins AL, et al: Mutations in the gene encoding the laminin B receptor produce an altered nuclear morphology in granulocytes (Pelger-Hüet anomaly). *Nat Genet* 31:410, 2002.

119. Reilly WA, Lindsay S: Gargoylism (lipochondrodystrophy): A review of clinical observations in eighteen cases. *Am J Dis Child* 75:595, 1948.

120. Oski FA, Naiman JL, Allen DM, Diamond LK: Leukocytic inclusions—Döhle bodies-associated with platelet abnormality (the May-Hegglin anomaly): Report of a family and review of the literature. *Blood* 20:657, 1962.

121. Bara KY: Chédiak-Higashi syndrome. *Scand J Haematol* 37:1627, 1987.

122. Ganz T, Metcalf JA, Gallin JI, et al: Microbicidal/cytotoxic proteins of neutrophils are deficient in two disorders: Chédiak-Higashi syndrome and specific granule deficiency. *J Clin Invest* 82:552, 1988.

123. Dahlgren MD, Petersen MA, Engler RL, Schmid-Schönbein GW: Leukocyte rheology in cardiac ischemia, in *White Cell Mechanics: Basic Science and Clinical Aspects*, edited by H Meiselman, MA Lichtman, La Celle PL, p 271. Alan R. Liss, New York, 1984.

124. Schmid-Schönbein GN: Leukocyte kinetics in the microcirculation. *Biorheology* 24:139, 1987.

125. Gallin JI: Neutrophil specific granules: A fuse that ignites the inflammatory response. *Clin Res* 32:320, 1984.

126. Janoff A: Elastase in tissue injury. *Annu Rev Med* 36:207, 1985.

127. Smedly LA, Tonnesen MG, Sandhaus RA, et al: Neutrophil-mediated injury to endothelial cells: Enhancement by endotoxin and essential role of neutrophil elastase. *J Clin Invest* 77:1233, 1986.

128. Malech HL, Gallin JI: Neutrophils in human diseases. *N Engl J Med* 317:687, 1987.

129. Weiss SJ: Tissue destruction by neutrophils. *N Engl J Med* 320:365, 1989.

130. Meiselman H, Lichtman MA, La Celle PL: *White Cell Mechanics: Basic Science and Clinical Aspects.* Alan R. Liss, New York, 1984.

131. Swank DW, Moore SB: Roles of the neutrophil and other mediators in adult respiratory distress syndrome. *Mayo Clin Proc* 64:1118, 1989.

132. MacNee W, Wiggs B, Balzberg AS, Hogg JC: The effect of cigarette smoking on neutrophil kinetics in human lungs. *N Engl J Med* 321:924, 1989.

133. Parker CW: Neutrophil mechanisms. *Am Rev Respir Dis* 143:559, 1991.

134. Martin TR, Pistorese BP, Hudson LD, Maunder RJ: The function of lung and blood neutrophils in patients with the adult respiratory distress syndrome. Implication for the pathogenesis of lung infections. *Am Rev Respir Dis* 144:254, 1991.

135. Godek JE: Adverse effects of neutrophils on the lung. *Am J Med* 92(suppl 6A):27S, 1992.

136. Palmgren MS, deShazo RO, Cater RM, et al: Mechanisms of neutrophil damage to human alveolar extracellular matrix: The role of serine and metalloproteases. *J Allergy Clin Immunol* 89:905, 1992.

137. Boventre JV, Colvin RB: Adhesion molecules in renal disease. *Curr Opin Nephrol Hypertension* 5:254, 1996.

138. Weiss ST, Segal MR, Sparrow D, Wager C: Relation of FEV1 and peripheral blood leukocyte count to total mortality. *Am J Epidemiol* 142:493, 1995.

139. Bednar M, Smith B, Pinto A, Mullane KM: Nafazatrom-induced salvage of ischemic myocardium in anesthetized dogs is mediated through inhibition of neutrophil function. *Circ Res* 57:131, 1985.

140. Allan G, Bhattacherjee P, Brook CD, et al: Myeloperoxidase activity as a quantitative marker of polymorphonuclear leukocyte accumulation into an experimental myocardial infarct—The effect of ibuprofen on infarct size and polymorphonuclear leukocyte accumulation. *J Cardiovasc Pharmacol* 7:1154, 1985.

141. Ranjadayalan K, Umachandran V, Daviews SW, et al: Thrombolytic treatment in acute myocardial infarction: Neutrophil activation, peripheral leucocyte responses, and myocardial injury. *Br Heart J* 66:10, 1991.

142. Welbourn CRB, Goldman G, Paterson IS, et al: Pathophysiology of ischaemia reperfusion injury: Central role of the neutrophil. *Br J Surg* 78:651, 1991.

143. Schaub RG, Yamashita A, Simmons CA, et al: Leukocyte-mediated large vein injury and thrombosis: Pharmacologic intervention with lipoxygenase inhibitors, in *Leukocyte Emigration and Its Sequelae*, edited by HZ Morat, p 62. Karger, Basel, 1987.

144. Weitzman SA, Weitburg AB, Clark EP, Stossel TP: Phagocytes as carcinogens: Malignant transformation produced by human neutrophil. *Science* 227:1231, 1985.

145. Trush MA, Seed JL, Kensler TW: Oxidant-dependent metabolic activation of polycyclic aromatic hydrocarbons by phorbol ester–stimulated human polymorphonuclear leukocytes: Possible link between inflammation and cancer. *Proc Natl Acad Sci U S A* 82:5194, 1985.

146. Phillips AN, Neaton JD, Cook DG, et al: The leukocyte count and risk of lung cancer. *Cancer* 69:680, 1992.

147. Fadlon E, Vordermeier S, Pearson TC, et al: Blood polymorphonuclear leukocytes from the majority of sickle cell patients in the crisis phase

148. Orfanakis NG, Ostlund RE, Bishop CR, Athens JW: Normal blood leukocyte concentration values. *Am J Clin Pathol* 53:649, 1970.

149. Rumke CL, Brezemer PD, Kuik DJ: Normal values and least significant differences for differential leukocyte counts. *J Chronic Dis* 28:661, 1975.

150. England JM, Bain BJ: Total and differential leukocyte count. *Br J Haematol* 33:1, 1976.

151. Broun GO, Herbeg FK, Hamilton JR: Leukopenia in Negroes. *N Engl J Med* 275:1410, 1966.

152. Rippey JJ: Leukopenia in West Indians and Africans. *Lancet* 2:44, 1967.

153. Karakyalcin G, Rosner F, Saurtsky A: Pseudoneutropenia in Negroes. *N Y State J Med* 72:1815, 1972.

154. Reed WW, Diehl LF: Leukopenia, neutropenia, and reduced hemoglobin levels in healthy American Blacks. *Arch Intern Med* 151:501, 1991.

155. Shoenfeld Y, Weinberger A, Avishar R, et al: Familial leukopenia among Yemenite Jews. *Isr J Med Sci* 14:1271, 1978.

156. Bodey GP, Buckley M, Sathe YS: Quantitative relationships between circulating leukocytes and infection in patients with acute leukemia. *Ann Intern Med* 64:328, 1966.

157. Kracke RR: Recurrent agranulocytosis. *Am J Clin Pathol* 1:385, 1931.

158. Gorlin RJ, Chaudhry AP: The oral manifestations of cyclic (periodic) neutropenia. *Arch Dermatol* 82:344, 1960.

159. Levine S: Neutropenia with marked periodontal lesions. *Oral Surg* 12:310, 1959.

160. Boggs DR: The cellular composition of inflammatory exudates in human leukemia. *Blood* 15:466, 1960.

161. Dale DC, Wolff SM: Skin window studies of the acute inflammatory responses of neutropenic patients. *Blood* 38:138, 1971.

162. Sickles EA, Green WH, Wiernick PH: Clinical presentation of infection in granulocytopenic patients. *Arch Intern Med* 135:715, 1975.

163. Russin SJ, Fillipo BH, Adler AG: Neutropenia in adults. *Postgrad Med* 88:209, 1990.

164. Welte K, Boxer LA: Severe chronic neutropenia; pathophysiology and therapy. *Semin Hematol* 34:267, 1997.

165. Kyle RA, Linman JW: Gingivitis and chronic idiopathic neutropenia. *Mayo Clin Proc* 45:494, 1970.

166. Wright DG, Dale DC, Fauci AS, Wolff SM: Human cyclic neutropenia: Clinical review and long-term follow-up of patients. *Medicine* 60:1, 1981.

167. Joyce RA, Boggs DR, Hasiba U, Srodes CH: Marginal neutrophil pool size in normal subjects and neutropenic patients as measured by epinephrine infusion. *J Lab Clin Med* 88:614, 1976.

168. Baehner RL: Neutrophil dysfunction associated with states of chronic and recurrent infection. *Pediatr Clin North Am* 27:377, 1980.

169. Gallin JI, Wright DG, Malech HL, et al: Disorders of phagocyte chemotaxis. *Ann Intern Med* 92:520, 1980.

170. Mowat AG, Baum J: Chemotaxis of polymorphonuclear leukocytes from patients with diabetes mellitus. *N Engl J Med* 284:621, 1971.

171. Tan JS, Anderson JL, Watanakunakorn C, et al: Neutrophil dysfunction in diabetes mellitus. *J Lab Clin Med* 85:26, 1975.

172. Brayton RG, Stokes PE, Schwartz MS, Louria DB: Effect of alcohol and various diseases on leukocyte mobilization, phagocytosis, and intracellular killing. *N Engl J Med* 282:123, 1970.

173. Liu YK: The effect of alcohol on granulocytes and lymphocytes. *Semin Hematol* 17:130, 1980.

174. Dale DC, Fauci AS, Dupont G IV, Wolff SM: Comparison of agents producing a neutrophilic leukocytosis in man: Hydrocortisone, prednisone, endotoxin and etiocholanolone. *J Clin Invest* 56:808, 1975.

175. Breton-Gorius J: Abnormalities of granulocytes and megakaryocytes in preleukemic syndromes, in *Preleukemia*, edited by F Schmalzl, K-P Helbriegel, p 24. Springer-Verlag, Berlin, 1979.

of the disease show adhesion to vascular endothelium and increased expression of CD64. *Blood* 91:266, 1998.

176. Reding MT, Hibbs JR, Morrison VA, et al: Diagnosis and outcome of 100 consecutive patients with extreme granulocytic leukocytosis. *Am J Med* 104:12, 1998.

177. Watanabe M, Ono K, Ozeki Y, et al: Production of granulocyte-macrophage colony-stimulating factor in a patient with metastatic chest wall large cell carcinoma. *Jpn J Clin Oncol* 28:559, 1998.

178. Salloum E, Stoessel KM, Cooper DL: Hyperleukocytosis and retinal hemorrhages after chemotherapy and filgrastim administration for peripheral blood progenitor cell mobilization. *Bone Marrow Transplant* 21:835, 1998.

179. Crockard AD, Boylan MT, Droogan AG, et al: Methylprednisolone-induced neutrophil leukocytosis-down-modulation of neutrophil L-selectin and Mac-1 expression and induction of colony-stimulating factor. *Int J Clin Lab Invest* 28:110, 1998.

180. Ceddia MA, Price EA, Kohlmeier CK, et al: Differential leukocytosis and lymphocyte mitogenic response to acute maximal exercise in the young and old. *Med Sci Sport Exerc* 31:829, 1999.

181. Nunoi H, Yamazaki T, Kanegasaki S: Neutrophil cytoskeletal disease. *Int J Hematol* 74:119, 2001.

182. Seri M, Pecci A, Di Bari F, et al: MYH9-related disease: May-Hegglen anomaly, Sebastian syndrome, Fechtner syndrome, and Epstein syndrome are not distinct entities but represent a variable expression of a single illness. *Medicine* 82:203, 2003.

183. Kratz A, Lewandrowski KB, Siegel AJ: Effect of marathon running on hematologic and biochemical laboratory parameters, including cardiac markers. *Am J Clin Pathol* 118:856, 2002.

184. Iho S, Tanaka Y, Takauji R, et al: Nicotine induces human neutrophils to produce IL-8 through the generation of peroxynitrate and subsequent activation of NF-kappaB. *J Leukoc Biol* 74:942, 2003.

185. Kassirer M, Zeltser D, Gluzman B, et al: The appearance of L-selectin (low) polymorphonuclear leukocytes in the circulating pool of peripheral blood during myocardial infarction correlates with neutrophilia and the size of the infarct. *Clin Cardiol* 22:721, 1999.

186. Kyne L, Hausdorff JM, Knight E, et al: Neutrophilia and congestive heart failure after acute myocardial infarction. *Am Heart J* 139:32, 2000.

187. Sato T, Omura M, Saito J, et al: Neutrophilia associated with anaplastic carcinoma of the thyroid. *Thyroid* 10:1113, 2000.

188. Funke A, Berner K, Traichel B, et al: Frequency, natural course, and outcome of neonatal neutropenia. *Pediatrics* 106(Pt1)45, 2000.

189. Maheshwari A, Christensen RD, Calhoun DA: Immune neutropenia in the neonate. *Adv Pediatr* 49:317, 2002.

NEUTROPENIA AND NEUTROPHILIA

DAVID C. DALE

Neutropenia designates a blood absolute neutrophil count that is less than two standard deviations below the normal population mean. Neutropenia can be inherited or acquired. It usually results from decreased production of neutrophil precursor cells in the marrow. Neutropenia also can result from a shift of neutrophils from the circulating into the marginated cell pools in the circulation. Less commonly, neutropenia results from accelerated destruction of neutrophils or increased egress of neutrophils from the circulation into the tissues. Neutropenia can occur with anemia, thrombocytopenia, or both, in which case the condition is a bicytopenia or pancytopenia. When neutropenia is the sole or dominant abnormality, the condition is called "selective" or "isolated" neutropenia, such as chronic idiopathic neutropenia or drug-induced neutropenia. In some diseases, several cell lineages are mildly affected but the reduction in neutrophils is the most severe, such as Felty syndrome. Neutropenia may be an indicator of an underlying systemic disease, such as early vitamin B_{12} deficiency. Neutropenia, particularly severe neutropenia [counts less than 500 neutrophils/ μl (0.5×10^9/liter)], increases susceptibility to bacterial or fungal infections and impairs the resolution of these infections. Therapy with granulocyte colony-stimulating factor is helpful in increasing blood neutrophil counts for many types of neutropenia.

Neutrophilia is an increase in the absolute neutrophil count to a concentration greater than two standard deviations above the normal population mean value. Neutrophilia contributes to the inflammatory response and to resolution of infections. Inflammatory and infectious diseases are the most frequent causes of neutrophilia. Bacterial infections usually produce neutrophilia, whereas viral infections may not produce neutrophilia or may raise the neutrophil count only slightly. Solid tumors occasionally engender striking neutrophilia. When the neutrophil count is very high, it may be referred to as a leukemoid reaction. The rare neutrophilic variants of chronic myeloid leukemia and chronic neutrophilic leukemia may result in striking neutrophilia. Demargination of neutrophils or rapid release of neutrophils from a large marrow pool may transiently increase the blood neutrophil count. Sustained increases require increased production of these cells.

NEUTROPENIA

Neutropenia refers to an absolute blood neutrophil count (total leukocyte count per microliter × percent of neutrophils) that is less than

two standard deviations below the normal mean of the population. The terms *leukopenia*, a reduced total white blood cell count, and *granulocytopenia*, reduced numbers of blood granulocytes (neutrophils, eosinophils, and basophils), sometimes are imprecisely used as synonyms for neutropenia. *Agranulocytosis* literally means a complete absence of blood granulocytes, but this term often is used to indicate severe neutropenia, that is, counts less than $0.5 \times 10^3/\mu$l (0.5×10^9/ liter).

The concentration of neutrophils in blood is influenced by age, activity, and genetic and environmental factors (see Chap. 2). For children from 1 month to 10 years old, neutropenia is defined as a blood neutrophil count less than $1.5 \times 10^3/\mu$l (1.5×10^9/liter). For individuals older than 10 years, neutropenia is defined as a count less than approximately $1.8 \times 10^3/\mu$l (1.8×10^9/liter) (see Chap. 6 regarding levels in newborns). Healthy older persons have the same blood neutrophil counts as younger individuals (see Chap. 8). Some racial and ethnic groups, such as Africans, African-Americans, and Yemenite Jews, have lower mean neutrophil counts than persons of Asian or European ancestry (see Chap. 2, Table 2-2). The mean differences in neutrophils are modest and have no recognized health consequences.[1,2]

Severe neutropenia is a predisposing factor for infections. The organisms normally are found on the skin, in the nasopharynx, and as part of the intestinal flora. The risk of infections is inversely related to the severity of the neutropenia (see Chap. 20). Individuals with neutrophil counts of 1.0 to $1.8 \times 10^3/\mu$l ($1.0-1.8 \times 10^9$/liter) are at little risk. In general, neutrophil counts between 0.5×10^3 and $1.0 \times 10^3/\mu$l ($0.5-1.0 \times 10^9$/liter) are associated with only slight risk unless other contributing factors are present. Individuals with neutrophil counts less than $0.5 \times 10^3/\mu$l (0.5×10^9/liter) are at substantially greater risk, but the frequency of infections varies considerably, depending on the cause and duration of neutropenia. Severe acute neutropenia (i.e., developing over a few hours or days) usually is associated with greater risk of infection than severe chronic neutropenia (usually present for months or years). Neutropenia resulting from disorders of production that affect early hematopoietic precursor cells (e.g., aplastic anemia, severe congenital neutropenia) leads to greater susceptibility to infections than do conditions with adequate neutrophil precursors in the marrow and neutropenia attributed to accelerated turnover in the blood (e.g., rheumatoid arthritis, Felty syndrome, autoimmune neutropenia). For patients made severely neutropenic by cancer chemotherapy, the risk is greater when the neutrophils are decreasing than with similar counts when neutrophils are increasing. Neutropenia accompanied by monocytopenia, lymphocytopenia, or hypogammaglobulinemia is more serious than isolated neutropenia. Other factors, such as the integrity of the skin and mucous membranes, the vascular supply to tissues, and the nutritional status of the patient, also influence the risk of infections.

PATHOPHYSIOLOGIC MECHANISMS

GENERAL MECHANISMS

Neutropenia occurs because of (1) hypoplastic neutropoiesis, (2) ineffective neutropoiesis (resulting from exaggerated apoptosis of late precursors), (3) accelerated removal or utilization of circulating neutrophils, (4) shifts of cells from the circulating to the marginal blood pools, or (5) a combination of these mechanisms (Fig. 65-1). Some production disorders are caused by intrinsic abnormalities of hematopoietic progenitor cells (see Chap. 85). Other disorders in cell production are caused by extrinsic factors, including changes in the marrow environment, such as tumor infiltration, fibrosis, or irradiation. Myelotoxic chemotherapeutic drugs commonly cause neutropenia because of the high proliferative activity of neutrophil precursors in the marrow and short half-life of neutrophils in the blood. Production of neutrophils is defined as ineffective when, under a steady state of hematopoiesis, a relative abundance of early neutrophil precursors, a

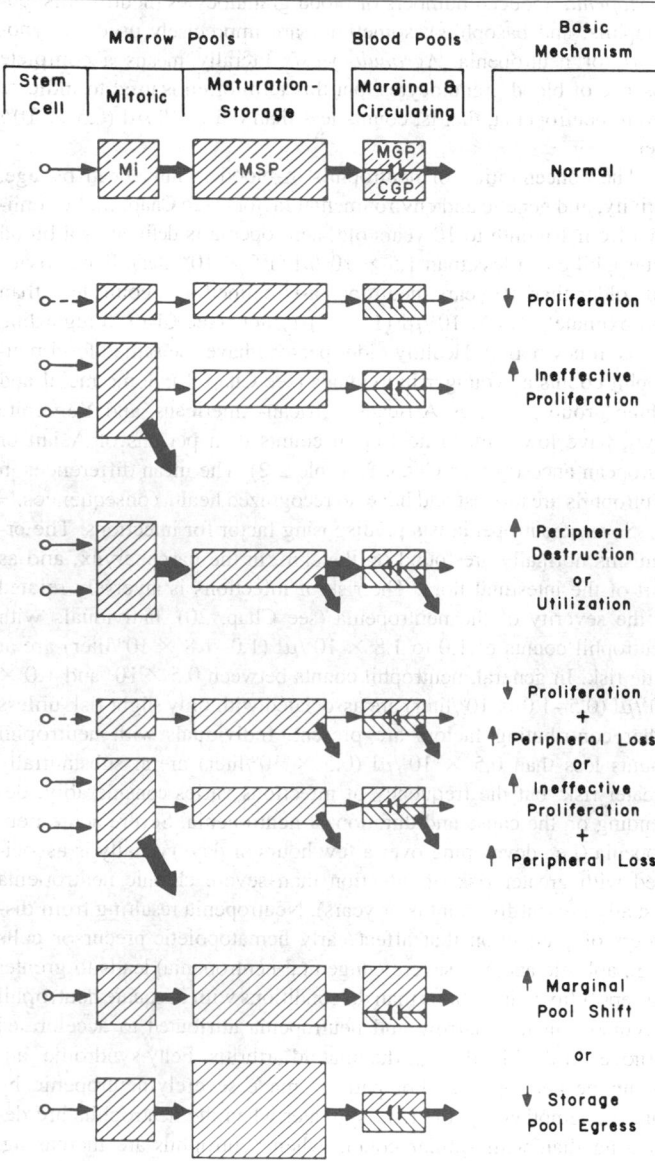

FIGURE 65-1 Mechanisms of neutropenia are shown schematically. The size of each pool is represented by the size of the *cross-hatched areas*. The rate of flow of cells through each compartment is represented by the size of the *arrows*. CGP, circulating granulocyte (neutrophil) pool; MGP, marginated granulocyte (neutrophil) pool; Mi, mitotic; MSP, maturation (marrow storage) pool.

paucity of late-maturing cells, and neutropenia occur. This condition has often been referred to as "maturation arrest," but it is almost always explained by either rapid release of segmented neutrophils because of exaggerated peripheral demands or the apoptotic loss of late precursors in the marrow as an intrinsic defect in cell maturation.

Accelerated neutrophil utilization occurs with autoimmune neutropenia and acute bacterial infections. When rapid neutrophil utilization and impaired production occur, acute severe neutropenia often develops. The condition is illustrated by the abrupt and sustained fall in neutrophils when an alcoholic patient develops pneumococcal pneumonia. Alcohol suppresses the marrow, and the infection consumes the available neutrophil supply. After myelotoxic cancer chemotherapy, the abrupt fall in blood neutrophils at the onset of infections reflects a similar mechanism: high demand and limited supply. With

idiosyncratic drug-induced neutropenia, the counts may fall abruptly because both blood and marrow cells are simultaneously damaged. Acute neutropenia that develops because of a shift of blood neutrophils from the circulating to the marginal blood pools, that is, increased margination (e.g., after injection of endotoxin, with exposure of blood to dialysis membranes, or after intravenous granulocyte colony stimulating factor [G-CSF] or granulocyte-macrophage–colony stimulating factor [GM-CSF]) usually is a transient event. The marginated cells reenter the circulating pool, and the blood supply of neutrophils is rapidly restored from the large reserves of marrow neutrophils entering the blood.

CELLULAR AND MOLECULAR MECHANISMS OF NEUTROPENIA

Our understanding of the mechanisms of neutropenia at the cellular and molecular levels is increasing rapidly because of advances in molecular genetics and cell biology. For many inherited forms of neutropenia, the chromosomal loci for the mutations causing these diseases are known, and the mutant protein products have been identified. Some mutations and acquired defects shorten the survival of the precursor cells, that is, they accelerate apoptosis. This form of cell loss now is thought to be the mechanism for "maturation arrest" in several diseases. Examples of increased apoptosis causing neutropenia include vitamin B_{12} deficiency,[3] clonal cytopenias (myelodysplasia),[4] myelokathexis,[5] congenital and cyclic neutropenia,[6,7] and the Shwachman-Diamond syndrome.[8] Neutrophils also can be depleted from the blood and the marrow as a result of extrinsic factors such antineutrophil antibodies and toxic cytokines generated by other cells.[9,10] Some disorders that cause neutropenia also perturb neutrophil function, such as glycogen storage disease type 1b,[11] Chédiak-Higashi syndrome,[12] and human immunodeficiency virus (HIV) infection.[13] Susceptibility to infection in these conditions relates to the combination of defects.

CAUSES OF NEUTROPENIA

Causes of neutropenia are classified physiologically as disorders of production, distribution, or turnover. Not every condition fits neatly into this scheme, but it provides a framework for understanding these diverse disorders.

DISORDERS OF PRODUCTION

Cytotoxic drugs given for cancer chemotherapy and as immunosuppressive agents regularly cause neutropenia by decreasing cell production (see Chap. 19). These drugs now are probably the most frequent cause of neutropenia in the United States. Neutropenia as a result of impaired production is a common feature of several diseases affecting hematopoietic stem cells, such as acute leukemia (see Chaps. 87 and 91), the myelodysplastic syndromes (see Chap. 86), and aplastic anemia (see Chap. 33). The selective causes of impaired production, progressing from disorders of early precursors to disorders presumed to involve defective maturation (ineffective production), are described briefly as follows.

Congenital Disorders *Kostmann Syndrome and Related Disorders.* In 1956, Kostmann described congenital neutropenia (agranulocytosis) as an autosomal recessive disease occurring in an extended family in northern Sweden.[14,15] Phenotypically similar sporadic cases and families with autosomal dominant congenital neutropenia have been reported.[16] In severe congenital neutropenia, symptoms and signs of otitis, gingivitis, pneumonia, enteritis, peritonitis, and bacteremia usually begin in the first months of life. At diagnosis, the neutrophil count usually is less than $0.2 \times 10^3/\mu l$ ($0.2 \times 10^9/$ liter).[17] Monocytosis, mild anemia, thrombocytosis, and splenomegaly frequently are present. Characteristically, the marrow shows early neutrophil precursors (myeloblasts, promyelocytes) but few or no myelocytes or mature neutrophils. Marrow eosinophilia is common. *In vitro* marrow culture studies show poor growth in response to various growth factors and with reduced numbers of marrow neutrophil and monocyte progenitor cell colonies.[18] Usually blood lymphocyte numbers are normal, immunoglobulin levels are normal or increased, and lymphocyte functions are intact. Up to 80 percent of patients with these clinical characteristics have heterozygous mutations of the gene for neutrophil elastase (also called *ELA-2*). A diversity of mutations have been identified from exons 2 through 5.[19] Clinical and laboratory studies have demonstrated that these mutations are the primary cause of most sporadic and autosomal dominant cases of severe congenital neutropenia.[20] A mutation of the *GFI-1* gene is a potential cause of severe congenital neutropenia.[21] Mutations in the gene for the receptor for G-CSF also occur in patients with severe congenital neutropenia[22]; however, most of these receptor mutations have caused truncations of the distal portion of the cytoplasmic domain of the receptor, an abnormality associated with altered sensitivity to G-CSF.[23] G-CSF receptor mutations and *RAS* mutations are part of the evolution to myelodysplasia or acute myelogenous leukemia and are not the primary cause of this neutropenia.[24] An exception may be a patient identified with a mutation in the external domain of the G-CSF receptor who responded to treatment with G-CSF and glucocorticoids and has not developed leukemia over several years of observation.[25]

G-CSF is a very effective therapy for severe congenital neutropenia, increasing the neutrophil counts and reducing recurrent fevers and infections.[26] Approximately 5 percent of patients do not respond to G-CSF. Hematopoietic transplantation is the only other therapy known to improve the clinical course for these patients.[27] Untreated patients and patients treated with G-CSF are at risk for developing acute myelogenous leukemia. Observational studies indicate the risk is approximately 2 percent per year.[28] Requirement for high daily doses of G-CSF appears to be a marker of disease severity and of the risk for leukemic transformation.

Congenital Immunodeficiency Diseases. Neutropenia is a feature of the congenital immunodeficiency diseases and a contributing factor to their susceptibility to infections (see Chap. 82). In X-linked agammaglobulinemia, which is attributed to defective B cell development and a mutation in a cytoplasmic (Bruton) tyrosine kinase *(BTK)*, severe neutropenia is present in approximately 25 percent of patients.[29] Children with common variable immunodeficiency often have neutropenia associated with thrombocytopenia and hemolytic anemia.[29] Neutropenia occurs in almost half of patients with the X-linked hyperimmunoglobulin M syndrome, a disorder caused by a mutation in the gene encoding the CD-40 ligand.[30] In severe combined immunodeficiency, neutropenia is not always present. The neutropenia varies over time in individual patients. Neutropenia is particularly prominent in the rarest of the immunodeficiencies, reticular dysgenesis.[29,31] Neutropenia is a less common feature of adenosine deaminase deficiency, the T−B+, T−B−, and Omenn syndromes.[29,32] Neutropenia occurs on an autoimmune basis in some cases of the Wiskott-Aldrich syndrome and can be a primary feature of the disease.[33,34] G-CSF therapy is effective in most patients with neutropenia associated with immunodeficiencies.[35,36]

Cartilage Hair Hypoplasia Syndrome. This rare autosomal recessive disorder is characterized by short-limbed dwarfism, hyperextensible digits, very fine hair, neutropenia, lymphopenia, and recurrent infections.[37] The genetic locus is at 9p13 and affects a gene coding for an endoribonuclease.[38] The degree of neutropenia is variable, with blood counts ranging from 0.1 to $2.0 \times 10^3/\mu l$ ($0.1–2.0 \times 10^9$/liter). An accompanying defect in T cell proliferation results from an abnormality in the transition from the G_0 to the G_1 phase of the mitotic cycle.[39] Patients have frequent bacterial and viral respiratory infec-

tions. Hematopoietic stem cell transplantation can correct the neutropenia and immune deficiency.[40]

Shwachman-Diamond Syndrome. This autosomal recessive disorder combines short stature, pancreatic exocrine deficiency, and neutropenia beginning early in the neonatal period.[41] Thrombocytopenia and anemia may be severe. The chromosomal locus of the mutation is at 7qll, and the mutation affects the *SBDS* gene.[42] The mutation causes a proliferative defect and increased apoptosis of early myeloid progenitor cells.[43] A chemotactic defect also occurs in mature neutrophils. The patients are malnourished, but the neutropenia is not corrected by improving the patients' nutritional status. Treatment with G-CSF raises blood neutrophil levels, and hematopoietic stem cell transplantation corrects the hematologic abnormalities.[44] Without transplantation, the risk of evolution to myelodysplastic syndrome and acute myelogenous leukemia is 20 percent or greater.

Diamond-Blackfan Syndrome. Neutropenia is a rare complication of hereditary hypoplastic anemia.[45] Other features include congenital anomalies of the head and upper limbs. Two genetic loci have been identified: 19q13.2 and 8p23.[46,47] The varying severity of neutropenia may reflect genetic heterogeneity among patients with this diagnosis (see Chap. 34).

Griscelli Syndrome. This rare autosomal recessive disorder is characterized by pigmentary dilution and variable degrees of cellular immunodeficiency.[48] The syndrome consists of three types. Neutropenia is a feature of type 2 but not types 1 or 3. In type 2, the neutropenia is relatively mild and associated with pancytopenia. These hematologic abnormalities are attributable to a mutation located at 15q21 affecting the *RAB27a* gene.[49] The gene product is a GTPase. The mutation also causes abnormal release of granule proteins and hematophagocytosis.[50] As in the Chédiak-Higashi syndrome, type 2 patients may develop an acute phase of uncontrolled lymphocyte and macrophage activation leading rapidly to death.[51] Hematopoietic stem cell transplantation can correct the hematologic features. Evolution to myelodysplasia has been reported.[52]

Chédiak-Higashi Syndrome. This rare autosomal recessive disorder is characterized by partial oculocutaneous albinism, giant granules in many cells (including granulocytes, monocytes, and lymphocytes), neutropenia, and recurrent infections[53,54] (see Chap. 66). This syndrome now is attributable to a chromosomal mutation at 1q43 affecting the *LYST* gene.[55] The product of this gene regulates lysosomal trafficking. In Chédiak-Higashi syndrome, the neutropenia usually is mild, and susceptibility to infection is attributed to neutropenia and defective microbicidal activity of the phagocytes[54] (see Chap. 66).

Myelokathexis, WHIM, and Related syndromes. Myelokathexis is a rare autosomal dominant or sporadically occurring disorder in which patients have severe neutropenia and lymphocytopenia, with total white blood cell counts often less than $1.0 \times 10^3/\mu l$ (1.0×10^9/liter).[56] WHIM syndrome, characterized by *w*arts, *h*ypogammaglobulinemia, *i*nfections, and *m*yelokathexis, now is attributable to a mutation in the gene encoding the receptor for stromal cell-derived factor-1 (SDF-1), called *CXCR-4*.[57,58] The ligand–receptor pair SDF-1/CXCR-4 is very important for regulating the trafficking of all type of leukocytes, including hematopoietic stem cells, from the marrow to the blood and tissues. In these syndromes, the marrow usually shows abundant precursors and developing neutrophils. Neutrophils in the marrow and the blood show hypersegmentation with pyknotic nuclei and cytoplasmic vacuoles. These morphologic changes and some molecular studies suggest cell loss in the marrow and blood caused by accelerated apoptosis.[5] Favorable responses to G-CSF and GM-CSF occur, as does evolution to the myelodysplastic syndrome.[59,60] A myelokathexis-like variant of myelodysplastic syndrome has been reported.[61]

Lazy Leukocyte Syndrome. In the 1970s, a condition called the "lazy leukocyte syndrome" was described in which the neutrophils also appeared to accumulate in the marrow. The neutrophils were morphologically normal. The neutropenia was attributed to defective chemotaxis of cells in the marrow to the blood.[62] No genetic or molecular mechanisms have been identified.

Glycogen Storage Diseases. These autosomal recessive disorders are characterized by hypoglycemia, hepatosplenomegaly, seizures, and failure to thrive in infants. Only type 1b is associated with neutropenia.[63] The genetic defect in type 1b maps to chromosome 11q23 and is attributed to an intracellular transport protein defect for glucose.[64] The marrow appears normal despite severely reduced blood neutrophils. The neutrophils have a reduced oxidative burst and defective chemotaxis.[65] Treatment with G-CSF is effective for correcting the neutropenia and improving the associated inflammatory bowel disease.[66,67]

Cyclic Neutropenia. Cyclic neutropenia is an autosomal dominant or sporadically occurring disease characterized by regularly recurring episodes of severe neutropenia, usually every 21 days.[68,69] Regular oscillations of other white blood cells, reticulocytes, and platelets are observed. Cyclic neutropenia now is attributable to mutations in the gene for neutrophil elastase (*NE* or *ELA-2*) at locus 19q3. Most mutations in the *NE* gene are in the regions of exons 4 and 5.[70] The diagnosis usually is made in the first year of life, especially in the presence of a family history of the condition.[71] The neutropenic periods last for 3 to 6 days and often are accompanied by fever, malaise, anorexia, mouth ulcers, and cervical lymphadenopathy. Cases of acquired cyclic neutropenia in adults, some of whom have an associated clonal proliferation of large granular lymphocytes, have been reported.[72]

The diagnosis of cyclic neutropenia can be made only by serial differential white cell counts, at least two or three times per week for a minimum of 6 weeks. Sequencing of the *NE* gene may be helpful in confirming the diagnosis.[73] Most affected children survive to adulthood, with symptoms often milder after puberty.[71] Fatal clostridial bacteremia has been reported in several cases, and careful observation is warranted with each neutropenic period in untreated patients. Treatment with G-CSF is very effective.[74] G-CSF does not abolish cycling, but it shortens the neutropenic periods sufficiently to prevent symptoms and infections.

Neutropenia Due to Genetic Defects of Folate, Cobalamin, and Transcobalamin II. A variety of congenital disorders lead to disturbed function of methylmalonyl CoA mutase and methionine synthetase, the two cobalamin-requiring enzymes. Each of these disorders causes neutropenia, anemia and thrombocytopenia as a result of ineffective hematopoiesis[75,76] (see Chap. 39).

Other Inherited Neutropenias. Several disorders, currently with only descriptive names, may be genetically determined forms of neutropenia. These cases often are called familial (benign) neutropenia and probably are autosomal dominant disorders.[77–79] Some cases of chronic benign neutropenia of childhood (usually a negative family history) may represent new mutations, and patients with chronic idiopathic neutropenia of adulthood may be childhood cases escaping early detection. Until better information is available, these conditions probably are best referred to as "idiopathic neutropenias."

Acquired Disorders *Neutropenia in Neonates of Hypertensive Mothers.* Hypertensive women often have low-birth-weight infants with low neutrophil counts, attributed to decreased production.[80] The neutropenia often is severe with a high risk of infection, particularly during the first few weeks of life. The neutropenia usually resolves within a few weeks. G-CSF elevates the neutrophil count in this form of neonatal neutropenia, but the clinical benefit of treatment remains to be determined.[81]

Neutropenia Due to Nutritional Deficiencies. Neutropenia is an early and consistent feature of megaloblastic anemias resulting from vitamin B_{12} or folate deficiency. When present it usually is accompanied by macrocytic anemia and mild thrombocytopenia (see Chap. 39). Copper deficiency can cause neutropenia in patients on total parenteral nutrition and in malnourished children[82–84] and can masquerade as myelodysplastic syndrome.

Neutropenia Due to Immune Suppression of Production. Pure white cell aplasia is a rare acquired disorder causing severe selective neutropenia. The marrow is devoid or nearly devoid of neutrophils and their precursors.[85] Ibuprofen, chlorpropamide, excessive zinc, and various infectious and inflammatory diseases are considered possible causes of this syndrome. Differential diagnosis includes aplastic anemia, myelodysplasia, hairy cell leukemia, neutropenia associated with the large granular lymphocyte syndrome, and Parvovirus B19 infection. Immunosuppressive therapy with antithymocyte globulin, glucocorticoids, and cyclosporine has been used in individual cases.

Chronic Idiopathic Neutropenia in Adults This is a distinct syndrome predominantly affecting young adult women aged 18 to 35 years; the female-to-male ratio is approximately 8:1.[77,78] The medical history (lack of episodes of fever, gingivitis, mouth sores, or other infections) and previous blood counts suggest the condition is acquired in most cases. Erythrocyte, reticulocyte, and platelet counts usually are normal. Mild leukopenia and lymphocytopenia may be present, and the spleen is normal or only minimally enlarged. The patients have no chromosomal abnormalities or other evidence of myelodysplasia.[86,87] Marrow examinations show a spectrum of abnormalities, ranging from normal cellularity to selective hypoplasia of the neutrophilic series. In most cases, quantitative marrow studies show the ratio of immature to mature cells is increased, suggesting loss of cells during the maturation process, that is, ineffective granulocytopoiesis.[88] Antineutrophil antibodies are not detected, and results of tests for other autoantibodies, including antinuclear or antimitochondrial antibodies, are negative.[89] Chronic idiopathic neutropenia in adults is the result of accelerated apoptosis of neutrophils and their precursors mediated via the Fas ligand or interferon gamma.[90] The disease mechanism, that is, activation of the extracellular apoptotic pathway, is similar to the mechanism described for patients with systemic lupus erythematosus.[91]

For most individual patients, the clinical course can be predicted from the level of blood neutrophils, marrow examination, and prior history of fevers and infections. In general, patients with the lowest levels of blood and marrow neutrophils have the most frequent problems. Long-term observations have shown, however, that some patients have very low blood neutrophil levels for long periods with few or no infections. Evolution to acute leukemia or aplastic anemia generally does not occur. G-CSF increases neutrophils in most patients and is a useful therapy for patients with recurrent fever and infections.[26,92]

DISORDERS AFFECTING NEUTROPHIL UTILIZATION AND TURNOVER

MECHANISMS OF IMMUNE NEUTROPENIA

Immune disorders primarily alter the distribution of neutrophils in the blood and accelerate neutrophil turnover. Antineutrophil antibodies cause transfusion reactions, alloimmune neonatal neutropenia, and autoimmune neutropenia. Antigen–antibody complexes, autoantibodies, and cytokine-mediated cellular injury are possible contributors to neutropenia of systemic lupus erythematosus and Felty syndrome. The association of neutropenia with increased numbers of circulating large granular lymphocytes demonstrates that cellular and humoral immune mechanisms can cause neutropenia (see Chap. 94).

Neutrophils share surface antigens with other tissues including the i-I antigens and HLA antigens. They also have some specific antigens, including NA-1, NA-2 (now recognized as isotypes of FcγRIII or CD-16), NB-1, NC-1, and 9a.[93–95]A number of other antigens can be identified on neutrophils and neutrophil precursors with monoclonal antibodies. The clearest associations of autoantibodies and neutropenia are with NA-1 and NA-2.[94,95]

Several tests are available for detecting antineutrophil antibodies, including agglutination and microagglutination, cytotoxicity, direct and indirect immunofluorescence, direct and indirect antiglobulin assays, and tests involving the binding of staphylococcal protein A to immunoglobulins on the surface of cells.[96] The agglutination tests are the oldest methods and depend on the propensity of immunoglobulin-coated cells to aggregate. Immunofluorescence tests utilize antihuman γ-globulin tagged with a fluorescein label. These tests can be adapted for quantitative studies with fluorescence-activated cell sorting. Immunofluorescence and staphylococcal protein A–binding tests also can be adapted for examining immunoglobulins bound to single cells, including marrow cells. Direct methods are used to detect the antibodies on the patient's neutrophils. Indirect methods are used to test the patient's plasma or serum against panels of normal cells. Use of paraformaldehyde to expose antigens and to preserve the neutrophils for multiple tests has been especially helpful. Appropriate controls are essential for proper interpretation of these studies. Measurements of apoptosis and cytokine-mediated cellular injury are done through research laboratories.

CAUSES OF IMMUNE-MEDIATED NEUTROPENIA

Alloimmune Neonatal Neutropenia   Newborn infants may have neutropenia for a variety of reasons.[97] In some cases, the disorder results from transplacental passage of maternal immunoglobulin (Ig) G antibodies that bind to the infant's neutrophil-specific antigens, usually the FcγRIII b (NA1, NA2, or 016) isotype inherited from the infant's father.[98,99] Other antigens, such as NB1, 5b, HLA, and unknown antigens, also may be involved.[100–103] Overall, this disorder occurs in approximately one in 2000 neonates. The disorder usually lasts 2 to 4 months and disappears as the passively acquired antibody wanes.

Immune neonatal neutropenia may be severe or relatively mild. It often is not recognized until bacterial infections occur in an otherwise healthy infant. The hematologic picture usually consists of severe neutropenia with normal to increased lymphocytes and normal monocytes, erythrocytes, and platelets. Marrow cellularity is normal or increased, with reduced numbers of mature neutrophils. Alloimmune neonatal neutropenia may be confused with neonatal sepsis because the latter condition also causes severe neutropenia. The diagnosis of alloimmune neutropenia usually is made using neutrophil agglutination or immunofluorescence tests. Treatment should be conservative; antibiotics are used only when necessary. Exchange transfusions to decrease antibody titers or neutrophil transfusions from the patient's mother are rarely needed.

Autoimmune Neutropenia   Neutrophil autoantibodies can decrease neutrophil survival and impair neutrophil production. From a clinical perspective, however, distinguishing autoimmune neutropenia from chronic idiopathic neutropenia often is difficult.[104] Patients diagnosed with autoimmune neutropenia have one or more positive tests for antineutrophil antibodies. Their cytopenia is selective; other blood cell counts are normal or near normal. Marrow morphology, colony forming cells, and other tests, including antinuclear antibody tests, are normal. In general, therapy should be conservative and expectant. Intravenous γ-globulin may transiently increase neutrophils, but the therapy is expensive and relatively ineffective. The response to glucocorticoid therapy is unpredictable. Daily or alternate-day G-CSF is

effective but should be reserved for patients with recurrent infections. Spontaneous remissions appear to occur much more commonly in children than adults.[105,106]

Systemic Lupus Erythematosus   Total leukocyte counts usually are between 2 and $5 \times 10^3/\mu l$ (2 to 5×10^9/liter) and neutrophils are less than 1.8×10^9/liter in approximately 50 percent of patients with systemic lupus erythematosus.[107,108] Mild neutropenia often is accompanied by monocytopenia and lymphocytopenia, anemia, thrombocytopenia, and mild degrees of splenomegaly. Marrow cellularity and maturation of cells usually are normal. An increased amount of IgG is present on the surface of neutrophils, and immune complexes are increased within the neutrophils.[109] Fas and tumor necrosis factor-related apoptosis-inducing ligand (TRAIL)–mediated apoptosis of neutrophils are important mechanisms.[110,111] Glucocorticosteriods, G-CSF, and GM-CSF elevate neutrophils in most patients with lupus, including patients on immunosuppressive therapies, but the mild neutropenia of these patients usually does not require treatment.[109]

Rheumatoid Arthritis, Sjögren Syndrome, and Felty Syndrome   Leukopenia in association with rheumatoid arthritis is unusual, occurring in less than 3 percent of large series of patients.[111] Approximately 1 percent of patients with rheumatoid arthritis develop additional features of Felty syndrome (splenomegaly, deforming rheumatoid arthritis, and leukopenia).[91] Usually, these patients have had active, deforming arthritis and very high rheumatoid factor titers. The neutropenia may be moderate to severe; occasionally patients are seen with no circulating neutrophils. The marrow usually is normal or hypercellular but occasionally is hypocellular. Granulopoiesis usually is marked by sufficient precursors but few band or segmented neutrophils. No clear relationship between spleen size and the neutrophil count is evident.

The incidence of bacterial infections in patients with Felty syndrome is low until the neutrophil count is less than $0.2 \times 10^3/\mu l$ (0.2 $\times 10^9$/liter), which has long suggested that neutrophils are made but that their blood kinetics are altered. The altered kinetics may result from high levels of circulating and intracellular immune complexes and IgG on the surface of neutrophils. Cellular injury via Fas-mediated apoptosis is an additional mechanism for cell loss from the marrow and blood.[110]

In Sjögren syndrome, approximately 30 percent of patients have moderate leukopenia. The total leukocyte count usually is 2 to $5 \times 10^3/\mu l$ (2 to 5×10^9/liter) with a normal differential count.[112,113] Rarely, severe neutropenia occurs in association with recurrent bacterial infections.

Therapeutic options for management of neutropenia in these autoimmune disorders include methotrexate, glucocorticoids, G-CSF, GM-CSF, and splenectomy. Results with these therapies are unpredictable.[109,114] Many specialists prefer weekly methotrexate because of its ease of administration, efficacy, and low toxicity. G-CSF or GM-CSF can increase neutrophils but may exacerbate arthralgias.[115] Combinations of these agents is another good alternative. Splenectomy is followed by a rapid increase in counts in approximately two thirds of cases, but approximately two thirds of patients who respond to splenectomy have recurrence of neutropenia.[116] A subset of patients with Felty syndrome has a high blood concentration of large granular lymphocytes with a phenotype characteristic of immature natural killer cells.[117] These patients tend to respond poorly to therapies directed toward increasing neutrophil levels but may respond to combinations of methotrexate and G-CSF. Several factors in addition to neutropenia predispose these patients to infections, including monocytopenia, hypocomplementemia, circulating immune complexes, and treatment with glucocorticoids or cytotoxic drugs. In general, treatments to correct neutropenia should be reserved for patients with documented infections.

Other Causes of Neutropenia Associated with Splenomegaly

In 1942 Wiseman and Doan[118] described a disorder they called primary splenic neutropenia. Since then, a variety of diseases are recognized as also possibly causing this type of neutropenia, or pseudoneutropenia. Diseases associated with splenomegaly and neutropenia include sarcoidosis, lymphoma, tuberculosis, malaria, kala azar, and Gaucher disease. Usually thrombocytopenia and anemia are present as well. Immune mechanisms in patients with inflammatory diseases are similar to the mechanisms observed in patients with lupus erythematosus, and Felty syndrome may be operative. In others patients, sluggish blood flow through the spleen with passive trapping of neutrophils in the congested red pulp probably is the primary cause. For the most part, the neutropenia in these patients is not sufficiently severe to be of clinical consequence. Removal of the spleen to raise the neutrophil count is rarely indicated.

DRUG-INDUCED NEUTROPENIA

Idiosyncratic drug reactions cause neutropenia with an estimated annual frequency of 3 to 12 cases per million population.[119,120] In 1922, Schultz[121] reported six cases of severe sore throat and prostration with absent blood neutrophils, which led rapidly to sepsis and death. A few years later, this syndrome was associated with the coal tar-derived drug aminopyrine.[122] Over the past 50 years, scores of other drugs have been recognized to cause this syndrome.

Two main types of idiosyncratic drug-induced neutropenia are recognized.[123,124] One type is a dose-related toxicity resulting from interference of the drug with protein synthesis or cell replication. This effect often is nonselective. It can involve the pluripotential hematopoietic stem cells and highly proliferative cells in other organs, such as the epithelial cells of the gastrointestinal tract. Prototype drugs for this type of reaction include phenothiazines, antithyroid drugs, chloramphenicol, and clozapine.[125] Similar effects on marrow cells may be mediated through free radicals and drug metabolites. Patients receiving multiple drugs and patients having high plasma concentration of drugs as a result of the dose administered, slow metabolism, or renal excretory impairment are more prone to these reactions.[126]

A second type of drug-induced neutropenia may not be dose related. The neutropenia is thought to be allergic or immunologic in origin, similar to drug-induced skin reactions and drug-initiated, antibody-mediated erythrocyte destruction. Many drugs can trigger this form of neutropenia.[119,120] Large studies suggest women are affected more often than men. Older patients are affected more frequently than younger patients. Patients with a history of allergies, including allergies to other drugs, are affected more often than individuals without allergies. Neutropenia may occur at any time but tends to occur relatively early in the course of treatment with drugs to which the patient has been previously exposed.

Our basic understanding of drug-induced neutropenia is limited, partly because of the unpredictable occurrence of cases, the myriad agents involved, and the lack of good animal models for research. Clinical studies suggest the rate of recovery can be roughly predicted from the degree of marrow hypoplasia present when neutropenia is discovered. In patients with sparse marrow neutrophils but normal-appearing precursor cells (promyelocytes and myelocytes), neutrophils reappear in the blood approximately 4 to 7 days after the offending drug is stopped. Often an increase in the blood monocyte count heralds marrow recovery, and an "overshoot" with marked neutrophilia follows. When early precursor cells are severely depleted, recovery may require considerably more time.

Symptomatic patients with drug-induced neutropenia usually present with fever, myalgia, and sore throat but usually no rash or evidence of allergy elsewhere. Blood examination shows few or absent neutrophils. Mild lymphopenia may be observed, but other cell counts usually are normal. A high level of suspicion and careful clinical history are critical to identifying the offending drug. Differential diagnosis includes acute viral infections, particularly infectious mononucleosis and infectious hepatitis, and acute bacterial sepsis. If other hematologic abnormalities also are present, acute leukemia and aplastic anemia should be considered. Treatment usually consists of supportive care, including broad-spectrum antibiotics for febrile patients. Hematopoietic growth factors may be beneficial, but their use in this setting has not been established in randomized trials.[125]

Table 65-1 lists some of the drugs frequently implicated in neutropenia. Given the rapidity of introduction of new agents, consult the manufacturer, a drug information center, or a poison control center when questions arise to learn if a drug can cause neutropenia.

TABLE 65-1   CLASSIFICATION OF WIDELY USED DRUGS ASSOCIATED WITH IDIOSYNCRATIC NEUTROPENIA

Analgesics and Antiinflammatory Agents	*Antimalarials*
Indomethacin*	Amodiaquine
Gold salts	Chloroquine
Pentazocine	Dapsone
Para-aminophenol derivatives*	Pyrimethamine
Acetaminophen	Quinine
Phenacetin	*Antithyroid Drugs**
Pyrazolone derivatives*	Carbimazole
Aminopyrine	Methimazole
Dipyrone	Propylthiouracil
Oxyphenbutazone	*Cardiovascular Drugs*
Phenylbutazone	Captopril
Antibiotics	Disopyramide
Cephalosporins	Hydralazine
Chloramphenicol*	Methyldopa
Clindamycin	Procainamide
Gentamicin	Propranolol
Isoniazid	Quinidine
Para-aminosalicylic acid	Tocainide
Penicillins and semisynthetic penicillins*	*Diuretics*
Rifampin	Acetazolamide
Streptomycin	Chlorthalidone
Sulfonamides*	Chlorothiazide
Tetracyclines	Ethacrynic acid
Trimethoprim-sulfamethoxazole	Hydrochlorothiazide
Vancomycin	*Hypoglycemic Agents*
Anticonvulsants	Chlorpropamide
Carbamazepine	Tolbutamide
Mephenytoin	*Hypnotics and Sedatives*
Phenytoin	Chlordiazepoxide and other
Antidepressants	benzodiazepines
Amitriptyline	Meprobamate
Amoxapine	*Phenothiazines**
Desipramine	Chlorpromazine
Doxepin	Phenothiazines
Imipramine	*Other Drugs*
Antihistamines—H₂ Blockers	Allopurinol
Cimetidine	Clozapine
Ranitidine	Levamisole
	Penicillamine
	Ticlopidine

* More frequently reported to cause neutropenia in epidemiologic studies.
NOTE: Documentation of the role of specific drugs in the causation of neutropenia is dependent on (1) the frequency of the occurrence among patients, (2) the timing of the event in relationship to drug use, (3) the absence of alternative explanations, or (4) the inadvertent or intentional reuse of the drug (rechallenges) with a similar response. Readers who require supplementary lists of putative drugs involved in the development of neutropenia or wish to read original references for these interactions are referred to: The International Agranulocytosis and Aplastic Anemia Study. Risks of agranulocytosis and aplastic anemia. *JAMA* 256:1749, 1986; Roeser HP: Drug-bone marrow interactions. *Med J Aust* 146:145, 1987; Hemopoietic system, in *Meyler's Side Effects of Drugs*, 10th ed, edited by MNG Dukes, pp 951–953, Elsevier, New York, 1984; Kaufman DW. Drugs in the aetiology of agranulocytosis and aplastic anaemia. *Eur J Haematol Suppl* 60:23, 1996.

NEUTROPENIA WITH INFECTIOUS DISEASES

Neutropenia can result from acute or chronic bacterial, viral, parasitic, or rickettsial diseases. Several mechanisms are involved. Certain viral infections, such as infectious mononucleosis, infectious hepatitis, Parvovirus B19, Kawasaki disease, and HIV infection, may cause severe or protracted neutropenia and pancytopenia resulting from infection of hematopoietic precursor cells. Other agents, such as *Rickettsia* and *Bartonella*, can infect endothelial cells. These agents may cause leukopenia, neutropenia, thrombocytopenia, and anemia as part of a generalized vasculitic process. Increased neutrophil adherence to altered endothelial cells may occur in dengue, measles, and other viral infections. With severe gram-negative bacterial infections, neutropenia probably results from increased adherence to the endothelium and increased utilization at the site of infection. Some chronic infections causing splenomegaly, such as tuberculosis, brucellosis, typhoid fever, malaria, and kala azar, probably cause neutropenia because of splenic sequestration and marrow suppression.

CLINICAL APPROACH TO THE PATIENT PRESENTING WITH NEUTROPENIA

Ordinarily, patients with acute onset of severe neutropenia present with fever, sore throat, and evidence of inflammation beneath the skin or mucous membranes. New respiratory or abdominal symptoms should heighten concern of an urgent clinical situation. Immediate investigation should include a careful history with particular attention to drugs. The physical examination should give careful attention to the oropharynx, sinuses, chest, abdomen, bones for evidence of tenderness, and size of the lymph nodes and spleen. Prompt blood counts and microbial cultures, institution of intravenous fluids, antibiotics, and other supportive measures may be lifesaving. In this situation, fever and infections usually result from surface bacteria sensitive to numerous broad-spectrum agents, unless the patient has been treated recently with antibiotics. A complete blood count should be obtained and a marrow examination considered, particularly if the cause of acute neutropenia is not known. The marrow may reveal fibrosis, selective or nonselective hypoplasia, excessive blasts, or atypical cells. With this information in hand and supportive care started, further diagnostic tests can be considered.

Chronic neutropenia often is discovered as a chance finding at a routine examination or during the course of investigation of a patient with recurrent fevers and infections. Determining if the neutropenia is chronic or cyclic and the mean level of blood cell counts when the patient is afebrile and relatively well is useful. Other important hematologic and immunologic data include the absolute monocyte, lymphocyte, eosinophil, and platelet counts; hematocrit or hemoglobin determination; and immunoglobulin levels. Patients with hypergammaglobulinemia usually have chronic and recurrent inflammation; patients with hypogammaglobulinemia and neutropenia usually are very susceptible to recurrent infections. Morphologic examination of the blood and marrow can identify some causes of benign neutropenia in children, the Chédiak-Higashi syndrome, and myelokathexis. The marrow examination is most useful for ruling out leukemia and myelodysplastic disorders and assessing the severity of the marrow defect.

In patients with chronic neutropenia, measurement of antinuclear antibodies (ANA) and rheumatoid factor titers and other serologic tests for autoimmune diseases may be useful. Usually, neutropenia associated with these disorders occurs in patients with obvious and severe disease, but occasionally patients are seen with occult splenomegaly, high ANA and rheumatoid factor titers, and a few other symptoms. Examination of the blood and marrow for large granular lymphocytes may be helpful. Infectious and nutritional causes of chronic neutropenia are rare and usually are evident at the time of patient evaluation. In adults, differentiation between chronic idiopathic neutropenia and the myelodysplastic syndromes may be the most difficult. Abnormalities in other cell lines (e.g., anemia with poikilocytosis and thrombocytopenia, pseudo-Pelger-Huët cells), atypical cells in the marrow, and clonal chromosomal abnormalities indicate myelodysplasia, particularly in older patients. Investigations of the mechanism of neutropenia with marrow and blood kinetic studies, *in vitro* marrow cultures, measurements of marrow granulocyte reserves, and indirect measurements of marrow proliferative activity may be useful in defining mechanisms of neutropenia but are not widely available.

NEUTROPHILIA

Neutrophilia is defined as an increase in the absolute blood neutrophil count to a level greater than two standard deviations above the mean value for normal individuals. For children 1 month or older and adults of all ages, this level is approximately $7.5 \times 10^3/\mu l$ ($7.5 \times 10^9/\text{liter}$) bands and mature neutrophils (see Chap. 2). At birth the mean neutrophil count is $12 \times 10^3/\mu l$ ($12 \times 10^9/\text{liter}$), and counts as high as $26 \times 10^3 \ \mu l/\text{liter}$ ($26 \times 10^9/\text{liter}$) are regarded as normal (see Chap. 6).

Several terms are used almost synonymously with neutrophilia, including *neutrophilic leukocytosis, polymorphonuclear leukocytosis,* and *granulocytosis. Leukocytosis* is used because an elevated number of neutrophils is the most frequent cause of an increased total white cell count. *Granulocytosis* is less specific than neutrophilia, because granulocytes include eosinophils and basophils as well as neutrophils. Extreme neutrophilia often is referred to as a *leukemoid reaction* because the height of the white cell count may suggest leukemia. This exaggerated reaction may be the result of segmented neutrophils or may be associated with band neutrophils, metamyelocytes, and myelocytes in smaller proportions.

In normal individuals, neutrophil counts follow a diurnal pattern of variation, with peak counts in the late afternoon. Neutrophil counts also rise slightly after meals, with erect posture, and with emotional stimuli. Ordinarily these changes are not sufficient to cause neutrophilia.[127]

MECHANISMS OF NEUTROPHILIA

Under normal circumstances, neutrophils follow an orderly progression from the marrow through the blood to tissue sites of utilization.[128] Neutrophilia may occur by several mechanisms: increased cell production, accelerated release of cells from the marrow into the blood, shift within the circulation from the marginal to the circulating pool, reduced egress of neutrophils from the blood to tissues, or a combination of these mechanisms. The time required for these events varies substantially. Shifts between the marginal and circulating pools take only a few minutes. Shifts of neutrophils from the marrow to the blood occur within a few hours. Increases in the production of neutrophils, even with intense stimulation, may take at least a few days (Fig. 65-2).

ACUTE NEUTROPHILIA

Pseudoneutrophilia (Demargination) Vigorous exercise and acute physical and emotional stress can substantially increase the number of blood neutrophils within a few minutes.[129,130] The response is mimicked by infusion of epinephrine and other catecholamines that increase heart rate and cardiac output.[131] The response is caused by a shift of cells from the marginal to the circulating pool; hence, it frequently is referred to as *demargination.* This response in humans is dependent partially on release of neutrophils from the spleen,[132] but redistribution from other vascular beds, particularly the pulmonary

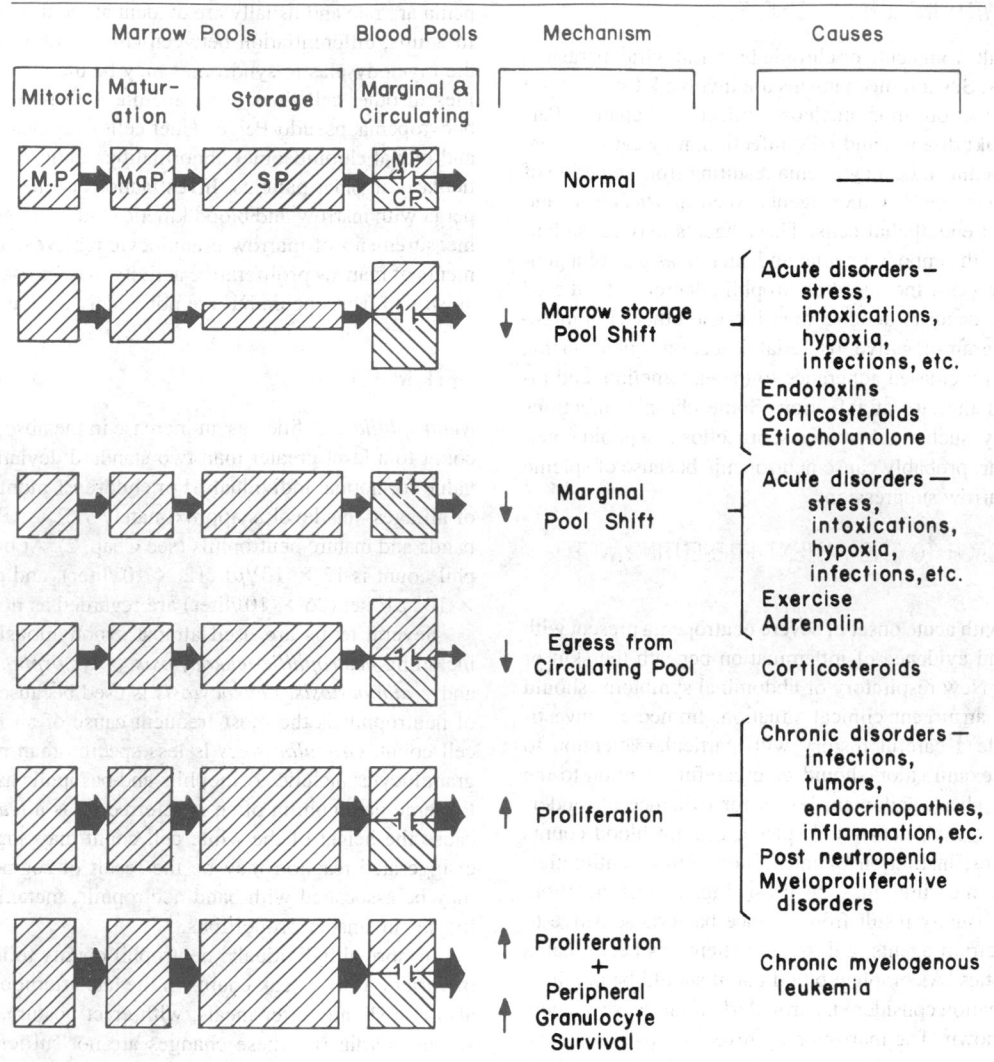

FIGURE 65-2   Mechanisms of neutrophilia are shown schematically. The rate of flow of cells through each compartment is represented by the size of the *arrows*. CP, circulating neutrophil pool; MaP, maturation (postmitotic) pool; M.P., mitotic pool; MP, marginated neutrophil pool; SP, storage pool (marrow reserves).

capillaries,[133] is quantitatively more important. The increase in lymphocytes, monocytes, and neutrophils that occurs with demargination may be helpful in distinguishing this type of neutrophilia from the response to infections, protracted stress, or glucocorticoid administration. With these conditions, neutrophil counts are elevated, but lymphocyte and monocyte counts generally are depressed.

Marrow Storage Pool Shift   Acute neutrophilia occurs as a consequence of release of neutrophils from the marrow storage pool, the *marrow neutrophil reserves*.[134] This mechanism produces acute neutrophilia in response to inflammation and infections. The marrow reserve pool consists principally of segmented neutrophils and bands. Metamyelocytes are not released to the blood except under extreme circumstances. The postmitotic marrow neutrophil pool is approximately 10 times the size of the blood neutrophil pool, and approximately half of these cells are band and segmented neutrophils.[128] In neutrophil production disorders, chronic inflammatory diseases, and malignancies, and with cancer chemotherapy, the size of this pool is reduced and the capacity to develop neutrophilia is impaired. Exposure of blood to foreign surfaces, such as hemodialysis membranes, activates the complement system and causes transient neutropenia, followed by neutrophilia resulting from release of marrow neutrophils.

Colony stimulating factors (G-CSF and GM-CSF) cause acute and chronic neutrophilia by mobilizing cells from the marrow reserves and stimulate neutrophil production.[135,136]

CHRONIC NEUTROPHILIA

Chronic neutrophilia follows a prolonged stimulus to proliferation of neutrophil precursors. It can be studied experimentally with repeated doses of endotoxin, glucocorticoids, or colony stimulating factors. Although the details of the mediators and mechanisms for the development of chronic neutrophilia are not understood fully, a general scheme for this response is now widely accepted (see Fig. 65-2). Expansion of cell production follows stimulation of cell divisions within the mitotic precursor pool, that is, divisions of promyelocytes and myelocytes. Subsequently, the size of the postmitotic pool increases. The changes cause an increase in the marrow granulocytic to erythroid ratio. In humans the neutrophil production rate increases several-fold with chronic infections. Even greater increases may occur in polycythemia vera, chronic myelogenous leukemia, and leukemoid reactions in response to nonhematologic malignancies[137] and to exogenously administered hematopoietic growth factors such as G-CSF,[135,136] with a maximum response taking at least 1 week to develop.

Neutrophilia resulting from decreased egress from the vascular compartment occurs infrequently. A prototype disorder illustrating this mechanism occurs in patients with the neutrophil cell membrane defect CD11a/CD18 deficiency.[138] The neutrophils do not adhere to the capillary endothelium normally, but cell production and marrow release apparently are normal. Because these patients cannot mobilize neutrophils to sites of inflammation when they develop infections, extreme neutrophilia is observed (see Chap. 66). Glucocorticoids may produce a functionally similar state, with neutrophils accumulating in the blood, at least transiently, after each dose is administered.[139,140] In patients recovering from infections, as the "tissue demand" for neutrophils diminishes, the persistence of neutrophilia may be attributed to this same mechanism. In chronic myelogenous leukemia, accumulation of neutrophils with a longer than normal half-life in the blood partially explains the extreme neutrophilia.[141]

DISORDERS ASSOCIATED WITH NEUTROPHILIA

NEUTROPHILIA IN RESPONSE TO INFLAMMATION AND STRESS

Table 65-2 lists the categories and causes of acute and chronic neutrophilia. Probably the most frequent causes of acute neutrophilia are

TABLE 65-2 MAJOR CAUSES OF NEUTROPHILIA

ACUTE NEUTROPHILIA	CHRONIC NEUTROPHILIA
Physical Stimuli	*Infections*
Cold, heat, exercise, convulsions, pain, labor, anesthesia, surgery	Persistence of infections that cause acute neutrophilia
Emotional Stimuli	*Inflammation*
Panic, rage, severe stress, depression	Most acute inflammatory reactions, such as colitis, dermatitis, drug-sensitivity reactions, gout, hepatitis, myositis, nephritis, pancreatitis, periodontitis, rheumatic fever, rheumatoid arthritis, vasculitis, thyroiditis, Sweet syndrome
Infections	*Tumors*
Many localized and systemic acute bacterial, mycotic, rickettsial, spirochetal, and certain viral infections	Gastric, bronchogenic, breast, renal, hepatic, pancreatic, uterine, and squamous cell cancers; rarely Hodgkin disease, lymphoma, brain tumors, melanoma, and multiple myeloma
Inflammation or Tissue Necrosis	*Drugs, Hormones, and Toxins*
Burns, electric shock, trauma, infarction, gout, vasculitis, antigen–antibody complexes, complement activation	Continued exposure to many substances that produce acute neutrophilia, lithium; rarely as a reaction to other drugs
Drugs, Hormones, and Toxins	*Metabolic and Endocrinologic Disorders*
Colony stimulating factors, epinephrine, etiocholanolone, endotoxin, glucocorticoids, smoking tobacco, vaccines, venoms	Eclampsia, thyroid storm, overproduction of adrenocorticotropic hormone
	Hematologic Disorders
	Rebound from agranulocytosis or therapy of megaloblastic anemia, chronic hemolysis or hemorrhage, asplenia, myeloproliferative disorders, chronic idiopathic leukocytosis
	Hereditary and Congenital Disorders
	Down syndrome, congenital

exercise, emotional stress, or any other circumstance that raises endogenous epinephrine, norepinephrine, or cortisol levels. Acute neutrophilia occurs in pregnant patients and may be especially notable at the time of entering labor. Acute neutrophilia occurs with induction of general or epidural anesthesia, with all types of surgery, and with other acute events such as seizures, gastrointestinal hemorrhage, subarachnoid hemorrhage, or other internal bleeding.

Neutrophilia occurs with many acute bacterial infections. It occurs less predictably with infections caused by viruses, fungi, and parasites. Many aspects of the complex interactions of microbes with the infected host are not fully understood. Most patients with gram-positive infections, such as pneumococcal pneumonia, staphylococcal abscesses, and streptococcal pharyngitis, have neutrophilia. Infections caused by gram-negative bacteria, particularly those resulting in bacteremia or septic shock, may cause neutropenia or extreme neutrophilia.[142] Increased circulating levels of activated complement components, G-CSF, tumor necrosis factor, and the interleukins (IL) IL-1, IL-6, and IL-8 may cause this response. Bacterial infections that have an insidious onset and cause splenomegaly, such as typhoid fever and brucellosis, characteristically do not show neutrophilia except in the initial or disseminated phase. Miliary tuberculosis is an important cause of leukemoid reactions. Neutrophilia is far less common with viral infections. In general, neutrophilia is seen in infections producing substantial tissue injury, evoked by toxins produced by the infecting organisms. Damage to host tissues also is the presumed mechanism of neutrophilia in thermal burns, electric shock, myocardial infarction, pulmonary embolism, sickle cell crisis, and systemic vasculitis.

Many chronic noninfectious conditions cause neutrophilia. Probably the most frequent cause is cigarette smoking.[143,144] Neutrophil counts of smokers are increased in proportion to the amount of exposure. Neutrophil counts of smokers inhaling two packs per day average twice the normal levels. Chronic inflammatory diseases, including dermatitis, bronchitis, rheumatoid arthritis, ulcerative colitis, and gout, may cause a persistent neutrophilia. Sweet syndrome is an unusual dermatologic condition manifested as intense neutrophil accumulation in the skin and persistent neutrophilia.[145]

NEUTROPHILIA IN ASSOCIATION WITH CANCER OR HEART DISEASE

Neutrophilia is associated with many nonhematologic malignancies, such as lung and gastrointestinal malignancies, particularly when they metastasize to the liver and lung.[137,146] In some cases, tumor cells produce colony stimulating factors that presumably cause the neutrophilia by direct marrow stimulation. Tumor necrosis and superinfections are other possible mechanisms. Neutrophilia is unusual in brain tumors, melanoma, prostate cancer, and lymphocytic malignancies.

Neutrophilia is a marker for the occurrence and severity of a variety of illnesses. Neutrophilia is associated with an increased incidence and severity of coronary heart disease independent of smoking status.[147,148] Similarly, elevated white cell counts have been associated with increased cancer mortality independent of smoking history.[149] In patients with cancer, subarachnoid hemorrhage, and other serious inflammatory conditions, neutrophilia portends a less favorable prognosis.

NEUTROPHILIA AS A MANIFESTATION OF AN HEMATOLOGIC DISORDER

In addition to the myeloproliferative syndromes including chronic neutrophilic leukemia and neutrophilic chronic myelogenous leukemia (see Chap. 88), several unusual hematologic conditions may be associated with neutrophilia. The mechanisms for most of these disorders remain obscure. In Down syndrome, transient neonatal leukemoid reactions resembling chronic myelogenous leukemia may occur.[150] This type of neutrophilia may be related to a defect in regulation of neutrophil production caused by chromosome 21 trisomy, but the precise mechanism is unknown. Idiopathic neutrophilic leukocytosis with a negative family history and a similar condition of hereditary neutrophilia with an autosomal dominant pattern of inheritance have been reported[151,152] but are very rare. Careful clinical examination and follow-up almost always reveal the cause of the neutrophilia.

NEUTROPHILIA ASSOCIATED WITH DRUGS

Many drugs cause neutropenia, but neutrophilia in response to drugs is uncommon except for the well-known effects of epinephrine, other catecholamines, and glucocorticoids. Lithium salts cause sustained neutrophilia.[153] The counts return to normal when the drug is discontinued. The drug increases levels of colony stimulating factor. Cases of neutrophilia have been reported with ranitidine and quinidine therapy, but such reactions are very uncommon.

CLINICAL APPROACH TO PATIENTS WITH NEUTROPHILIA

In most instances, the finding of neutrophilia, band neutrophils, and toxic granules in the mature cells can be related to an obvious ongoing inflammatory condition. Often the finding of neutrophilia helps confirm the diagnosis of appendicitis, cholecystitis, or bacterial pharyngitis. When the cause of neutrophilia is not readily apparent, especially if the neutrophilia is associated with fever or other signs of inflammation, more subtle infections such as tuberculosis or osteomyelitis should be considered. In addition, a history of smoking and evidence for a chronic anxiety state or an occult malignancy should be sought. If neutrophilia is accompanied by myelocytes and promyelocytes, increased basophils, and unexplained splenomegaly, the diagnosis of a myeloproliferative disease (e.g., chronic myelogenous leukemia, idiopathic myelofibrosis, or polycythemia vera) should be considered. Measurement of leukocyte alkaline phosphatase activity can be a useful screening test in cases of moderate neutrophilia ($15-25 \times 10^3$ neutrophils/μl [$15-25 \times 10^9$ neutrophils/liter]). Ordinarily the values are elevated with inflammation of any cause and in subjects receiving glucocorticoid therapy. The values are low in chronic myelogenous leukemia and variable with other myeloproliferative disorders. Serum vitamin B_{12} levels and B_{12}-binding proteins are elevated in both benign neutrophilia and chronic myelogenous leukemia. In unexplained neutrophilia, testing for the cytogenetic alterations and the BCR gene rearrangement is important in the diagnostic evaluation. Chapter 88 discusses the diagnosis of chronic myelogenous leukemia and other myeloproliferative disorders with prominent neutrophilia.

Except for the epidemiologic associations of neutrophilia with adverse effects of smoking, coronary artery disease, and malignancies, no direct adverse effect of an elevated circulating neutrophil count is known. In some inflammatory diseases, glucocorticoids and immunosuppressive therapies are used to reduce inflammation; a part of their mechanism is reducing the production and deployment of neutrophils and other leukocytes. For instance, glucocorticoids usually suppress the inflammation of the skin in Sweet syndrome. Otherwise, specific therapy to reduce the neutrophil counts generally is not indicated.

REFERENCES

1. Bain BJ: Ethnic and sex differences in the total and differential white cell count and platelet count. *J Clin Pathol* 49:664, 1996.
2. Weingarten MA, Pottick-Schwartz EA, Brauner A: The epidemiology of benign leucopenia in Yemenite Jews. *Isr J Med Sci* 29:297, 1993.
3. Koury MJ, Price JO, Hicks GG: Apoptosis in megaloblastic anemia occurs during DNA synthesis by a p53-independent, nucleoside-reversible mechanism. *Blood* 96:3249, 2000.
4. Parker JE, Mufti GJ: The myelodysplastic syndromes: A matter of life or death. *Acta Haematol* 111:78, 2004.
5. Aprikyan AA, Liles WC, Park JR, et al: Myelokathexis, a congenital disorder of severe neutropenia characterized by accelerated apoptosis and defective expression of bcl-x in neutrophil precursors. *Blood* 95:320, 2000.
6. Aprikyan AA, Liles WC, Rodger E, et al: Impaired survival of bone marrow hematopoietic progenitor cells in cyclic neutropenia. *Blood* 97:147, 2001.
7. Aprikyan AA, Kutyavin T, Stein S, et al: Cellular and molecular abnormalities in severe congenital neutropenia predisposing to leukemia. *Exp Hematol* 31:372, 2003.
8. Dror Y, Freedman MH: Shwachman-Diamond syndrome marrow cells show abnormally increased apoptosis mediated through the Fas pathway. *Blood* 97:3011, 2001.
9. Bux J: Molecular nature of antigens implicated in immune neutropenias. *Int J Hematol* 76:399, 2002.
10. Papadaki HA, Eliopoulos AG, Kosteas T, et al: Impaired granulocytopoiesis in patients with chronic idiopathic neutropenia is associated with increased apoptosis of bone marrow myeloid progenitor cells. *Blood* 101:2591, 2003.
11. Kannourakis G: Glycogen storage disease. *Semin Hematol* 39:103, 2002.
12. Introne W, Boissy RE, Gahl WA: Clinical, molecular, and cell biological aspects of Chediak-Higashi syndrome. *Mol Genet Metab* 68:283, 1999.
13. Kaul D, Coffey MJ, Phare SM, Kazanjian PH: Capacity of neutrophils and monocytes from human immunodeficiency virus-infected patients and healthy controls to inhibit growth of Mycobacterium bovis. *J Lab Clin Med* 141:330, 2003.
14. Pitrak DL, Bak PM, DeMarais P, et al: Depressed neutrophil superoxide production in human immunodeficiency virus infection. *J Infect Dis* 167:1406, 1993.
15. Kostmann R: Infantile genetic agranulocytosis; agranulocytosis infantilis hereditaria. *Acta Paediatr* 45:1, 1956.
16. Bellanne-Chantelot C, Clauin S, Leblanc T, et al: Mutations in the ELA2 gene correlate with more severe expression of neutropenia: A study of 81 patients from the French Neutropenia Register. *Blood* 103:4119, 2004.
17. Zeidler C, Schwinzer B, Welte K: Congenital neutropenias. *Rev Clin Exp Hematol* 7:72, 2003.
18. Hestdal K, Welte K, Lie SO, et al: Severe congenital neutropenia: Abnormal growth and differentiation of myeloid progenitors to granulocyte colony-stimulating factor (G-CSF) but normal response to G-CSF plus stem cell factor. *Blood* 82:2991, 1993.
19. Dale DC, Person RE, Bolyard AA, et al: Mutations in the gene encoding neutrophil elastase in congenital and cyclic neutropenia. *Blood* 96:2317, 2000.
20. Ancliff PJ: Congenital neutropenia. *Blood Rev* 17:209, 2003.
21. Person RE, Li FQ, Duan Z, Benson KF, et al: Mutations in proto-oncogene GFI1 cause human neutropenia and target ELA2. *Nat Genet* 34:308, 2003.
22. Dong F, Hoefsloot LH, Schelen AM, et al: Identification of a nonsense mutation in the granulocyte-colony stimulating factor receptor in severe congenital neutropenia. *Proc Natl Acad Sci U S A* 91:4480, 1994.
23. Hermans MH, Antonissen C, Ward AC, et al: Sustained receptor activation and hyperproliferation in response to granulocyte colony-stimulating factor (G-CSF) in mice with a severe congenital neutropenia/acute myeloid leukemia-derived mutation in the G-CSF receptor gene. *J Exp Med* 189:683, 1999.
24. Germeshausen M, Ballmaier M, Welte K: Implications of mutations in hematopoietic growth factor receptor genes in congenital cytopenias. *Ann N Y Acad Sci* 938:305, 2001.

25. Dror Y, Ward AC, Touw IP, Freedman MH: Combined corticosteroid/granulocyte colony-stimulating factor (G-CSF) therapy in the treatment of severe congenital neutropenia unresponsive to G-CSF: Activated glucocorticoid receptors synergize with G-CSF signals. *Exp Hematol* 28: 1381, 2000.

26. Dale DC, Cottle TE, Fier CJ, et al: Severe chronic neutropenia: Treatment and follow-up of patients in the Severe Chronic Neutropenia International Registry. *Am J Hematol* 72:82, 2003.

27. Zeidler C, Welte K, Barak Y, et al: Stem cell transplantation in patients with severe congenital neutropenia without evidence of leukemic transformation. *Blood* 95:1195, 2000.

28. Freedman MH, Alter BP: Malignant myeloid transformation in congenital forms of neutropenia. *Isr Med Assoc J* 4:1011, 2002.

29. Cham B, Bonilla MA, Winkelstein J: Neutropenia associated with primary immunodeficiency syndromes. *Semin Hematol* 39:107, 2002.

30. Winkelstein JA, Marino MC, Ochs H, et al: The X-linked hyper-IgM syndrome: Clinical and immunologic features of 79 patients. *Medicine* 82:373, 2003.

31. Stephan JL, Vlekova V, Le Deist F, et al: Severe combined immunodeficiency: A retrospective single-center study of clinical presentation and outcome in 117 patients. *J Pediatr* 123:564, 1993.

32. Buckley RH, Schiff RI, Schiff SE, et al: Human severe combined immunodeficiency: Genetic, phenotypic, and functional diversity in one hundred eight infants. *J Pediatr* 130:378, 1997.

33. Dupuis-Girod S, Medioni J, Haddad E, et al: Autoimmunity in Wiskott-Aldrich syndrome: Risk factors, clinical features, and outcome in a single-center cohort of 55 patients. *Pediatric* 111:e622, 2003.

34. Devriendt K, Kim AS, Mathijs G, et al: Constitutively activating mutation in WASP causes X-linked severe congenital neutropenia. *Nat Genet* 27:313, 2001.

35. Calhoun DA, Christensen RD: Recent advances in the pathogenesis and treatment of nonimmune neutropenias in the neonate. *Curr Opin Hematol* 5:37, 1998.

36. Stein SM, Dale DC: Molecular basis and therapy of disorders associated with chronic neutropenia. *Curr Allergy Asthma Rep* 3:385, 2003.

37. McKusick VA, Eldridge R, Hostetler JA, et al: Dwarfism in the Amish: II. Cartilage hair hypoplasia. *Bull Johns Hopkins Hosp* 116:285, 1965.

38. Sulisalo T, Klockars J, Makitie O, et al: High-resolution linkage-disequilibrium mapping of the cartilage-hair hypoplasia gene. *Am J Hum Genet* 55:937, 1994.

39. Yel L, Aggarwal S, Gupta S: Cartilage-hair hypoplasia syndrome: Increased apoptosis of T lymphocytes is associated with altered expression of Fas (CD95), FasL (CD95L), IAP, Bax, and Bcl2. *J Clin Immunol* 19: 428, 1999.

40. Berthet F, Siegrist CA, Ozsahin H, et al: Bone marrow transplantation in cartilage-hair hypoplasia: Correction of the immunodeficiency but not of the chondrodysplasia. *Eur J Pediatr* 155:286, 1996.

41. Shwachman H, Diamond LK, Oski FA, Khaw KT: The syndrome of pancreatic insufficiency and bone marrow dysfunction. *J Pediatr* 65: 645, 1964.

42. Boocock GR, Morrison JA, Popovic M, et al: Mutations in SBDS are associated with Shwachman-Diamond syndrome. *Nat Genet* 33:97, 2003.

43. Dror Y, Freedman MH: Shwachman-Diamond syndrome marrow cells show abnormally increased apoptosis mediated through the Fas pathway. *Blood* 97:3011, 2001.

44. Dror Y, Freedman MH: Shwachman-diamond syndrome. *Br J Haematol* 118:701, 2002.

45. Schofield KP, Evans DI: Diamond-Blackfan syndrome and neutropenia. *J Clin Pathol* 44:742, 1991.

46. Orfali KA, Ohene-Abuakwa Y, Ball SE: Diamond Blackfan anaemia in the U.K.: Clinical and genetic heterogeneity. *Br J Haematol* 125:243, 2004.

47. Campagnoli MF, Garelli E, Quarello P, et al: Molecular basis of Diamond-Blackfan anemia: New findings from the Italian registry and a review of the literature. *Haematologica* 89:480, 2004.

48. Griscelli C, Durandy A, Guy-Grand D, et al: A syndrome associating partial albinism and immunodeficiency. *Am J Med* 65:691, 1978.

49. Menasche G, Pastural E, Feldmann J, et al: Mutations in RAB27A cause Griscelli syndrome associated with haemophagocytic syndrome. *Nat Genet* 25:173, 2000.

50. Sanal O, Ersoy F, Tezcan I, et al: Griscelli disease: Genotype-phenotype correlation in an array of clinical heterogeneity. *J Clin Immunol* 22:237, 2002.

51. Baumeister FA, Stachel D, Schuster F, et al: Accelerated phase in partial albinism with immunodeficiency (Griscelli syndrome): Genetics and stem cell transplantation in a 2-month-old girl. *Eur J Pediatr* 159:74, 2000.

52. Arico M, Zecca M, Santoro N, et al: Successful treatment of Griscelli syndrome with unrelated donor allogeneic hematopoietic stem cell transplantation. *Bone Marrow Transplant* 29:995, 2000.

53. Beguez Cesar A, Castellanos Fonseca E, Teixido Vaillant S: Taeniasis and hymenolepiasis in children. *Rev Cubana Pediatr* 24:735, 1952.

54. Blume RS, Wolff SM: The Chediak-Higashi syndrome: Studies in four patients and a review of the literature. *Medicine* 51:247, 1972.

55. Barbosa MD, Nguyen QA, Tchernev VT, et al: Identification of the homologous beige and Chediak-Higashi syndrome genes. *Nature* 382: 262, 1996.

56. Zuelzer WW: "Myelokathexis"—A new form of chronic granulocytopenia. Report of a case. *N Engl J Med* 270:699, 1964.

57. Gorlin RJ, Gelb B, Diaz GA, et al: WHIM syndrome, an autosomal dominant disorder: Clinical, hematological, and molecular studies. *Am J Med Genet* 91:368, 2000.

58. Hernandez PA, Gorlin RJ, Lukens JN, et al: Mutations in the chemokine receptor gene CXCR4 are associated with WHIM syndrome, a combined immunodeficiency disease. *Nat Genet* 34:70, 2003.

59. Weston B, Axtell RA, Todd RFIII, et al: Clinical and biologic effects of granulocyte colony stimulating factor in the treatment of myelokathexis. *J Pediatr* 118:229, 1991.

60. Wetzler M, Talpaz M, Kellagher MJ, et al: Myelokathexis: Normalization of neutrophil counts and morphology by GM-CSF. *JAMA* 267: 2179, 1992.

61. Sheridan BL, Pinkerton PH, Curtis JE, et al: The myelokathexis-like variant of the myelodysplastic syndrome—a second example. *Clin Lab Haematol* 13:81, 1991.

62. Patrone F, Dallegri F, Rebora A, Sacchetti C: Lazy leukocyte syndrome. *Blut* 39:265, 1979.

63. Narisawa K, Igarashi Y, Otomo H, Tada K: A new variant of glycogen storage disease type I probably due to a defect in the glucose-6-phosphate transport system. *Biochem Biophys Res Commun* 83:1360, 1978.

64. Annabi B, Hiraiwa H, Mansfield BC, et al: The gene for glycogen-storage disease type 1b maps to chromosome 11q23. *Am J Hum Genet* 62:400, 1998.

65. Visser G, Rake JP, Fernandes J, et al: Neutropenia, neutrophil dysfunction, and inflammatory bowel disease in glycogen storage disease type Ib: Results of the European Study on Glycogen Storage Disease type I. *J Pediatr* 13:187, 2000.

66. McCawley LJ, Korchak HM, Douglas SD, et al: In vitro and in vivo effects of granulocyte colony-stimulating factor on neutrophils in glycogen storage disease type 1B: Granulocyte colony stimulating factor therapy corrects the neutropenia and the defects in respiratory burst activity and Ca2+ mobilization. *Pediatr Res* 35:84, 1994.

67. Zuccotti GV, Longhi R, Flumine P, et al: Effect of granulocyte-colony stimulating factor in glycogen storage disease type Ib. *J Int Med Res* 21:276, 1993.

68. Leale M: Recurrent furunculosis in an infant showing an unusual blood picture. *JAMA* 1910:54, 1844.

69. Dale DC, Bolyard AA, Aprikyan A: Cyclic neutropenia. *Semin Hematol* 39:89, 2002.

70. Horwitz M, Benson KF, Person RE, et al: Mutations in ELA2, encoding neutrophil elastase, define a 21-day biological clock in cyclic haematopoiesis. *Nat Genet* 23:433, 1999.

71. Palmer SE, Stephens K, Dale DC: Genetics, phenotype, and natural history of autosomal dominant cyclic hematopoiesis. *Am J Med Genet* 66: 413, 1996.

72. Dale DC, Hammond WP IV: Cyclic neutropenia: A clinical review. *Blood Rev* 2:178, 1998.

73. Dale DC: ELA2-related neutropenia, in *GeneReviews: Genetic Disease Online Reviews at GeneTests-GeneClinics* [database online]. Copyright, University of Washington, Seattle. Available at *http:// www.geneclinics.org*.

74. Hammond WP IV, Price TH, Souza LM, Dale DC: Treatment of cyclic neutropenia with granulocyte colony-stimulating factor. *N Engl J Med* 320:1306, 1989.

75. Fowler B: Genetic defects of folate and cobalamin metabolism. *Eur J Pediatr* 157:S60, 1998.

76. Monagle PT, Tauro GP: Long-term follow up of patients with transcobalamin II deficiency. *Arch Dis Child* 72:237, 1995.

77. Dale DC, Guerry D 4th, Wewerka JR, et al: Chronic neutropenia. *Medicine* 58:128, 1979.

78. Kyle RA: Natural history of chronic idiopathic neutropenia. *N Engl J Med* 302:908, 1980.

79. Jonsson OG, Buchanan GR: Chronic neutropenia during childhood. A 13-year experience in a single institution. *Am J Dis Child* 145:232, 1991.

80. Juul SE, Haynes JW, McPherson RJ: Evaluation of neutropenia and neutrophilia in hospitalized preterm infants. *J Perinatol* 24:150, 2004.

81. Juul SE, Christensen RD: Effect of recombinant granulocyte colony-stimulating factor on blood neutrophil concentrations among patients with "idiopathic neonatal neutropenia": A randomized, placebo-controlled trial. *J Perinatol* 23:493, 2003.

82. Percival SS: Neutropenia caused by copper deficiency: Possible mechanisms of action. *Nutr Rev* 53:59, 1999.

83. Olivares M, Uauy R: Copper as an essential nutrient. *Am J Clin Nutr* 63:791S 1996.

84. Gregg XT, Reddy V, Prchal JT: Copper deficiency masquerading as myelodysplastic syndrome. *Blood* 100:1493, 2002.

85. Levitt LJ: Chlorpropamide-induced pure white cell aplasia. *Blood* 69: 394, 1987.

86. Palmblad JE, von dem Borne AE: Idiopathic, immune, infectious, and idiosyncratic neutropenias. *Semin Hematol* 39:113, 2002.

87. Papadaki HA, Palmblad J, Eliopoulos GD: Non-immune chronic idiopathic neutropenia of adult: An overview. *Eur J Haematol* 67:35, 2001.

88. Price TH, Lee MY, Dale DC, Finch CA: Neutrophil kinetics in chronic neutropenia. *Blood* 54:581, 1979.

89. Logue GL, Shastri KA, Laughlin M, et al: Idiopathic neutropenia: Antineutrophil antibodies and clinical correlations. *Am J Med* 90:211, 1991.

90. Papadaki HA, Eliopoulos AG, Kosteas T, et al: Impaired granulocytopoiesis in patients with chronic idiopathic neutropenia is associated with increased apoptosis of bone marrow myeloid progenitor cells. *Blood* 101:2591, 2003.

91. Matsuyama W, Yamamoto M, Higashimoto I, et al: TNF-related apoptosis-inducing ligand is involved in neutropenia of systemic lupus erythematosus. *Blood* 104:184, 2004.

92. Dale DC, Bonilla MA, Davis MW, et al: A randomized controlled phase III trial of recombinant human granulocyte colony-stimulating factor (filgrastim) for treatment of severe chronic neutropenia. *Blood* 81:2496, 1993.

93. Lalezari P, Radel E: Neutrophil-specific antigens: Immunology and clinical significance. *Semin Hematol* 11:281, 1974.

94. Bux J: Molecular nature of antigens implicated in immune neutropenias. *Int J Hematol* 76 (suppl 1):399, 2002.

95. Stroncek D: Neutrophil alloantigens. *Transfus Med Rev* 16:67, 2002.

96. Bux J, Chapman J: Report on the second international granulocyte serology workshop. *Transfusion* 37:977, 1997.

97. Maheshwari A, Christensen RD, Calhoun DA: Immune neutropenia in the neonate. *Adv Pediatr* 49:317, 2002.

98. Puig N, de Haas M, Kleijer M, et al: Isoimmune neonatal neutropenia caused by Fc gamma RIIIb antibodies in a Spanish child. *Transfusion* 35:683, 1995.

99. Maslanka K, Guz K, Uhrynowska M, Zupanska B: Isoimmune neonatal neutropenia due to anti-Fc(gamma) RIIIb antibody in a mother with an Fc(gamma) RIIIb deficiency. *Transfus Med* 11:111, 2001.

100. Bux J, Stein EL, Bierling P, et al: Characterization of a new alloantigen (SH) on the human neutrophil Fc gamma receptor IIIb. *Blood* 89:1027, 1997.

101. de Haas M, Muniz-Diaz E, Alonso LG, et al: Neutrophil antigen 5b is carried by a protein, migrating from 70 to 95 kDa, and may be involved in neonatal alloimmune neutropenia. *Transfusion* 40:222, 2000.

102. Hagimoto R, Koike K, Sakashita K, et al: A possible role for maternal HLA antibody in a case of alloimmune neonatal neutropenia. *Transfusion* 4:615, 2001.

103. Maheshwari A, Christensen RD, Calhoun DA: Resistance to recombinant human granulocyte colony-stimulating factor in neonatal alloimmune neutropenia associated with anti-human neutrophil antigen-2a (NB1) antibodies. *Pediatrics* 109:e64, 2002.

104. Palmblad JE, von dem Borne AE: Idiopathic, immune, infectious, and idiosyncratic neutropenias. *Semin Hematol* 39:113, 2002.

105. Taniuchi S, Masuda M, Hasui M, et al: Differential diagnosis and clinical course of autoimmune neutropenia in infancy: Comparison with congenital neutropenia. *Acta Paediatr* 91:1179, 2002.

106. Smith MA, Smith JG: Clinical experience with the use of rhG-CSF in secondary autoimmune neutropenia. *Clin Lab Haematol* 24:93, 2002.

107. Nossent JC, Swaak AJ: Prevalence and significance of haematological abnormalities in patients with systemic lupus erythematosus. *Q J Med* 80:605, 1991.

108. Bowman SJ: Hematological manifestations of rheumatoid arthritis. *Scand J Rheumatol* 31:251, 2002.

109. Starkebaum G: Chronic neutropenia associated with autoimmune disease. *Semin Hematol* 39:121, 2002.

110. Baier A, Meineckel I, Gay S, Pap T: Apoptosis in rheumatoid arthritis. *Curr Opin Rheumatol* 15:274, 2003.

111. Campion G, Maddison PJ, Goulding N, et al: The Felty syndrome: A case-matched study of clinical manifestations and outcome, serologic features, and immunogenetic associations. *Medicine (Baltimore)* 69:69, 1990.

112. Starkebaum G, Dancey JT, Arend WP: Chronic neutropenia: Possible association with Sjogren's syndrome. *J Rheumatol* 8:679, 1981.

113. Coppo P, Sibilia J, Maloisel F, et al: Primary Sjogren's syndrome associated agranulocytosis: A benign disorder? *Ann Rheum Dis* 62:476, 2003.

114. Wassenberg S, Herborn G, Rau R: Methotrexate treatment in Felty's syndrome. *Br J Rheumatol* 37:908, 1998.

115. Hellmich B, Schnabel A, Gross WL: Treatment of severe neutropenia due to Felty's syndrome or systemic lupus erythematosus with granulocyte colony-stimulating factor. *Semin Arthritis Rheum* 29:82, 1999.

116. Rashba EJ, Rowe JM, Packman CH: Treatment of the neutropenia of Felty syndrome. *Blood Rev* 10:177, 1996.

117. Bowman SJ, Geddes GC, Corrigall V, et al: Large granular lymphocyte expansions in Felty's syndrome have an unusual phenotype of activated CD45RA+ cells. *Br J Rheumatol* 35:1252, 1996.

118. Wiseman BK, Doan CA: A newly recognized granulopenic syndrome caused by excessive splenic leukolysis and successfully treated by splenectomy. *Ann Intern Med* 16:1097, 1942.

119. van Staa TP, Boulton F, Cooper C, et al: Neutropenia and agranulocytosis in England and Wales: Incidence and risk factors. *Am J Hematol* 72:248, 2003.

120. Andres E, Noel E, Kurtz JE, et al: Life-threatening idiosyncratic drug-induced agranulocytosis in elderly patients. *Drugs Aging* 21:427, 2004.

121. Schulz W: Ueber digenartige Halserkrankungen. *Dtch Med Wockenschr* 48:1495, 1922.

122. Kracke RR: Relation of drug therapy to neutropenic states. *JAMA* 111:1255, 1938.

123. Uetreicht JP: Reactive metabolites and agranulocytosis. *Eur J Haematol Suppl* 60:33, 1996.

124. Claas FH: Immune mechanisms leading to drug-induced blood dyscrasias. *Eur J Haematol Suppl* 60:64, 1996.

125. Carey PJ: Drug-induced myelosuppression: Diagnosis and management. *Drug Saf* 26:691, 2003.

126. Mauri MC, Rudelli R, Bravin S, et al: Clozapine metabolism rate as a possible index of drug induced granulocytopenia. *Psychopharmacology (Berl)* 35:459, 1998

127. Garrey WE, Bryan WR: Variations in white blood cell counts. *Physiol Rev* 15:597, 1935.

128. Dancey JT, Deubelbeiss KA, Harker LA, Finch CA: Neutrophil kinetics in man. *J Clin Invest* 58:705, 1976.

129. Moyna NM, Acker GR, Weber KM, et al: The effects of incremental submaximal exercise on circulating leukocytes in physically active and sedentary males and females. *Eur J Appl Physiol* 74:211, 1996.

130. Quindry JC, Stone WL, King J, Broeder CE: The effects of acute exercise on neutrophils and plasma oxidative stress. *Med Sci Sports Exerc* 35:1139, 2003.

131. Benschop RJ, Rodriquez-Feuerhahn M, Schedlowski M: Catecholamine-induced leukocytosis: Early observations, current research, and future directions. *Brain Behav Immun* 10:77, 1996.

132. Toft P, Helbo-Hansen HS, Tonnesen E, et al: Redistribution of granulocytes during adrenaline infusion and following administration of cortisol in healthy volunteers. *Acta Anaesthesiol Scand* 38:254, 1994.

133. Hogg JC, Doerschuk CM: Leukocyte traffic in the lung. *Ann Rev Physiol* 57:97, 1995.

134. Dale DC, Fauci, AS, Gerry D IV, Wolff SM: Comparison of agents producing neutrophilic leukocytosis in man. *J Clin Invest* 56:808, 1975.

135. Price TH, Chatta GS, Dale DC: The effect of recombinant granulocyte-colony stimulating factor on neutrophil kinetics in normal young and elderly humans. *Blood* 88:335, 1996.

136. Dale DC, Liles WC, Llewellyn C, Price TH: The effects of granulocyte macrophage colony stimulating factor (GM-CSF) on neutrophil kinetics and function in normal human volunteers. *Am J Hematol* 57:7, 1998.

137. Reding MT, Hibbs JR, Morrison VA, et al. Diagnosis and outcome of 100 consecutive patients with extreme granulocytic leukocytosis. *Am J Med* 104:12, 1998.

138. Etzioni A, Tonetti M: Leukocyte adhesion deficiency II-from A to almost Z. *Immunol Rev* 178:138, 2000.

139. Bishop CR, Athens JW, Boggs DR, et al: Leukokinetic studies: XIII. A non-steady state kinetic evaluation of the mechanism of cortisone-induced granulocytosis. *J Clin Invest* 47:249, 1968.

140. Crockard AD, Boylan MT, Droogan AG, et al: Methylprednisolone-induced neutrophil leukocytosis—down-modulation of neutrophil L-selectin and Mac-1 expression and induction of granulocyte colony-stimulating factor. *Int J Clin Lab Res* 28:110, 1998.

141. Cartwright GE, Athens JW, Haab OP, et al: Blood granulocyte kinetics in conditions associated with granulocytosis. *Ann N Y Acad Sci* 11:963, 1964.

142. Deulofeu F, Cervell'o B, Capell S, et al: Predictors of mortality in patients with bacteremia: The importance of functional status. *J Am Geriatr Soc* 46:14, 1998.

143. Parry H, Cohen S, Schlarb JE, et al: Smoking, alcohol consumption, and leukocyte counts. *Am J Clin Pathol* 107:64, 1997.

144. Miki K, Miki M, Nakamura Y, et al: Early-phase neutrophilia in cigarette smoke-induced acute eosinophilic pneumonia. *Intern Med* 42:839, 2003.

145. Weenig RH, Bruce AJ, McEvoy MT, et al: Neutrophilic dermatosis of the hands: Four new cases and review of the literature. *Int J Dermatol* 43:95, 2004.

146. Shoenfeld Y, Tal A, Berliner S, Pinkhas J: Leukocytosis in nonhematological malignancies—a possible tumor-associated marker. *J Cancer Res Clin Oncol* 111:54, 1986.

147. Zalokar JB, Richard JL, Claude JR: Leukocyte count, smoking, and myocardial infarction. *N Engl J Med* 304:465, 1981.

148. Kirtane AJ, Bui A, Murphy SA, et al: Association of peripheral neutrophilia with adverse angiographic outcomes in ST-elevation myocardial infarction. *Am J Cardiol* 93:532, 2004.

149. Grimm RH, Neaton JD, Ludwig W: Prognostic importance of the white blood cell count for coronary, cancer, and all-cause mortality. *JAMA* 254:1932, 1985.

150. Kwong YL, Cheng G, Tang TS, et al: Transient myeloproliferative disorder in a Down's neonate with rearranged T-cell receptor beta gene and evidence of in vivo maturation demonstrated by dual-colour flow cytometric DNA ploidy analysis. *Leukemia* 7:1667, 1993.

151. Ward HN, Reinhard EH: Chronic idiopathic leukocytosis. *Ann Intern Med* 75:193, 1971.

152. Herring WB, Smith LB, Walker R, Herion JC: Hereditary neutrophilia. *Am J Med* 56:729, 1974.

153. Ozdemir MA, Sofuoglu S, Tanrikulu G, et al: Lithium-induced hematologic changes in patients with bipolar affective disorder. *Biol Psychiatry* 35:210, 1994.

DISORDERS OF NEUTROPHIL FUNCTION

NIELS BORREGAARD

LAURENCE A . BOXER

The neutrophil circulates in blood as a quiescent cell. Its main function as a phagocytic and bactericidal cell is performed outside the circulation in tissues where microbial invasion occurs. Neutrophil function traditionally is viewed as chemotaxis, phagocytosis, and bacterial killing. Although these actions conceptionally represent distinct entities, they are functionally related and rely to a large extent on the same intracellular signal transduction mechanisms that result in localized rises in intracellular Ca^{2+}, changes in organization of the cytoskeleton, assembly of reduced nicotinamide adenine dinucleotide phosphate oxidase from its cytosolic and membrane integrated subunits, and fusion of granules with the phagosome or neutrophil plasma membrane. Clinical disorders of the neutrophil may arise from impaired function of these normal processes. The clinical presentation of a patient with a qualitative neutrophil abnormality may be similar to the presentation of a patient with an antibody or complement disorder. In general, evaluation for phagocyte cell disorders (Table 66-2) should be initiated among patients who have at least one of the four following clinical features: (1) two or more systematic bacterial infections; (2) frequent, serious respiratory infections, such as pneumonia or sinusitis, otitis media, or lymphadenitis; (3) infections

present at unusual sites (liver or brain abscess); and (4) infections associated with unusual pathogens (e.g., *Aspergillus* pneumonia, disseminated candidiasis, or infections with *Serratia marcescens*, *Nocardia* species, and *Burkholderia cepacia*).

NEUTROPHIL STRUCTURE AND FUNCTION

CHEMOTAXIS AND MOTILITY

The similarity between neutrophil locomotion and that of amebas was noted 70 years ago.[1] Neutrophils can respond to spatial gradients of chemotaxins with concentration differences as little as 1 percent,[2] although whether chemotaxis also requires temporal and spatial sensing is debated.[3] A broad range of responsiveness is found even with populations of cells as "morphologically homogenous" as neutrophils.[4] During locomotion toward a chemotactic source, neutrophils acquire a characteristic asymmetric shape (Fig. 66-1). In the front of the cell is a pseudopodium, referred to as the *lamellipodium*, which advances before the body of the cell and contains the nucleus and the cytoplasmic granules. At the rear of the moving cell is a knob-like tail. The lamellipodium undulates or "ruffles" as the neutrophil moves at rates up to 50 μm/min. The membrane lipids also flow during locomotion,[5] and enhanced cytosolic Ca^{2+} is observed along the membrane margin.[6] The lamellipodium, which is very thin, forms immediately when the cell encounters a gradient of chemotactic factor. As the cell moves, the cytoplasm behind the lamellipodium streams forward, almost obliterating it. At this point, some granules appear to contact the cell periphery and release granule contents in response to chemotactic agents. The lamellipodium extends again, and the process repeats itself. A flow of cortical materials, composed particularly of actin filaments, has been proposed to account for chemotaxis and other cellular movements.[7] This flow also may account for changes in cell viscosity.

INGESTION

When a neutrophil comes in contact with a particle, the pseudopodium flows around the particle and its extensions fuse, thereby encompassing the particle within the phagosome.[1] The ingestion phase extends from recognition to the end of pseudopodium fusion. The particle becomes enclosed within a phagosome into which granules are rapidly discharged (Fig. 66-1). As with locomotion, phagocytosis results in release of Ca^{2+} in the vicinity of the active membranes.[6] The number of ingested particles eventually may be limited by the availability of plasma membrane.[7] Locomotion is not a prerequisite for ingestion. If neutrophils collide with a particle not secreting a chemotactic substance, pseudopodia form abruptly at the contact point and envelop the particle. Ingested particles gradually move toward the cell interior, where they tumble about with the nucleus and cytoplasmic granules as the cell moves off. A small number of the phagocytosed particles are expelled.[8]

The formation of a lamellipodium is essential for neutrophil locomotion. The interior cytoplasm is squeezed in the direction of the lamellipodium, possibly by the peripheral cytoplasm in the rear of the cell. The lamellipodium also is required for ingestion. When dissolution of the lamellipodium occurs, the interior contents of the cell are allowed to contact the cell membrane. Granule discharge may occur. Fusion of membranes is a common feature of (1) ingestion, where pseudopodia fuse; (2) degranulation, where granules fuse with the phagosome; and possibly (3) locomotion, where some granules may fuse with the plasma membrane. Pseudopodia form whether neutrophils are suspended in liquid medium or are attached to a surface, but the cell can only move translationally when it is fixed to a surface; thus, the cell crawls but does not swim. Such "stickiness" is also a phase of ingestion.[7] The neutrophil membrane adheres firmly to in-

Acronyms and abbreviations that appear in this chapter include: ADP, adenosine diphosphate; ARF, ADP-ribosylation factor; ASC, apoptosis-associated speck-like protein with a caspase recruitment domain; ATP, adenosine triphosphate; ATPase, adenosine triphosphatase; BPI, bactericidal/permeability-increasing protein; cAMP, cyclic adenosine monophosphate; cANCA, cytoplasmic anti-neutrophil cytoplasmic antibody; CARD, caspase recruitment domain; c/EBP, CCAAT/enhancer binding protein; CGD, chronic granulomatous disease; CHS, Chédiak-Higashi syndrome; DAG, diacylglycerol; FAD, flavin prosthetic group; FMF, familial Mediterranean fever; fMLP, formyl-methionyl-leucyl-phenylalanine; G-6-PD, glucose-6-phosphate dehydrogenase; GDP, glucose diphosphate; GPI, glycosylphosphatidylinositol; GTP, guanosine triphosphate; GTPase, guanosine triphosphatase; H_2O_2, hydrogen peroxide; HBP, heparin-binding protein; HETE, hydroxyeicosatetraenoic acid; HLA, human leukocyte antigen; HNP, human neutrophil peptide; Ig, immunoglobulin; ICAM, intercellular adhesion molecule; IFN, interferon; IL, interleukin; IP_3, inositol triphosphate; ITAM, immunoreceptor tyrosine-based activation motif; LAD, leukocyte adhesion deficiency; LFA-1, leukocyte function-associated antigen-1; LPS, lipopolysaccharide; LSP-1, lymphocyte-specific protein-1; LTB_4, leukotriene B_4; MAPK, microtubule-associated protein kinases; MBL, mannose-binding lectin; MMP, matrix metalloproteinase; MPO, myeloperoxidase; NADPH, reduced nicotinamide adenine dinucleotide phosphate; NBT, nitroblue tetrazolium; NEM, N-ethyl maleimide; NF-κB, nuclear factor-κB; NGAL, neutrophil gelatinase-associated lipocalin; NK, natural killer; NSF, N-ethyl maleimide-sensitive fusion protein; PA, phosphatidic acid; PAF, platelet-activating factor; PCR, polymerase chain reaction; PECAM, platelet endothelial adhesion molecule; PI3K, phosphatidylinositide-3-kinase; PIP_1, phosphatidylinositol-4-monophosphate; PIP_2, phosphatidylinositol-4,5-bisphosphate; PKC, protein kinase C; PLC, phospholipase C; PLD, phospholipase D; phox, phagocyte oxidase; PSGL, P-selectin ligand; SGD, specific granule deficiency; SH3, Src homology 3; sLe^x, sialyl Lewis X; SNAP, soluble NSF attachment protein; SNARE, SNAP receptor; TLR, toll-like receptors; TNF, tumor necrosis factor; TRAPS, tumor necrosis factor receptor-associated periodic syndrome; VAMP-2, vesicle-associated membrane protein-2.

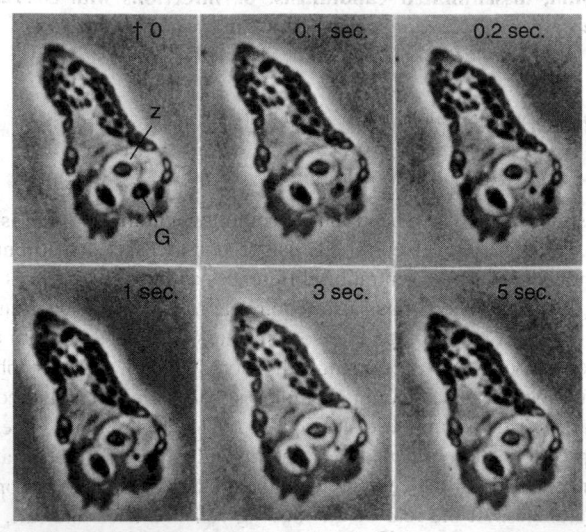

FIGURE 66-1 Cine microphotographic observation of granule lysis of a chicken neutrophil after phagocytosis of zymosan particles. Note lysis of the cytoplasmic granule (G) against one of two ingested zymosan particles (Z). The dense body of the granule disappears from view in an interval of 5 seconds (×1200). (From JG Hirsch, *J Exp Med* 116:827, 1962, with permission.)

gested particles, presumably to provide the frictional force needed to move pseudopodia around the particles. Thus, the formation of pseudopodia, membrane fusion, and membrane adhesiveness all are characteristics associated with the functional responses of neutrophils.

ADHESION

The dual neutrophil functions of immune surveillance and *in situ* elimination of microorganisms or cellular debris require rapid transition between a circulating nonadherent state to an adherent state allowing the cells to migrate into tissues when necessary. Initially neutrophils appear at sites on the endothelium adjacent to the site of inflammation. New adhesion molecules on endothelium are induced by inflammatory mediators released by damaged tissues, which result in local extravasation of the neutrophil. In postcapillary venules or pulmonary capillaries, the slow rate, which is further reduced by vessel dilation at sites of inflammation, permits a loose and somewhat transient adhesion referred to as *tethering* and results in the rolling of the neutrophil along the endothelium.[9] During the tethering step, neutrophils respond to ligands, primarily chemokines dispatched on the endothelial surface by a signaling event that acts to reorganize neutrophil microvilli exposing adhesion molecules, which in turn leads to sustained adhesion and spreading.

NEUTROPHIL MICROVILLI AND THEIR DYNAMICS

Circulating neutrophils contain surface microvilli of 0.3-μm diameter.[10] Moesin, ezrin, and p205 radixin are actin-binding proteins associated with neutrophil plasma membranes and likely are responsible for organization of microvilli on the surface of the cell.[11] These actin-binding proteins tether the primary adhesion proteins exposed on the microvilli, such as L-selectin and P-selectin ligand-1 (PSGL-1) to the tips of the microvilli.[12] L-selectin is a filamentous glycosylated protein protruding from the tips of the microvilli. L-selectin has a short transmembrane segment and cytosolic component, which can activate the microtubule-associated protein (MAP) kinase pathway.[13] L-selection, like the other selectins, including P-selectin, which is expressed on platelets and endothelial Weibel-Palade bodies, and E-selectin, which

is expressed in endothelial cells, binds with variable affinity to sialyl fucosylated oligosaccharides including sialyl Lewis X (sLe^x), which is present on multiple specific glycolipids and glycoproteins on leukocytes and inflamed endothelial cells.[14] P-selectin is localized to the membrane of Weibel-Palade bodies and is mobilized during inflammation to the endothelial cell luminal surface. Following expression on the endothelial cells surface, P-selectin makes contact with its major ligand, PSGL-1 on circulating neutrophils. PSGL-1, like L-selectin, is located on the tips of microvilli on neutrophils. It is a transmembrane, heavily O-glycosylated protein with a short transmembrane segment and an intracellular domain that likely transmits signals via the actin-binding proteins that tether it to the tip of the microvillus and to Syk protein kinase to initiate cell activation.[15]

ROLLING AND TETHERING

P-selectin is mobilized rapidly to the endothelial cell surface following stimulation by thrombin, histamine, or oxygen radicals. P-selectin interacts with neutrophil PSGL-1 to initiate neutrophil rolling.[14] Rolling subsequently involves newly expressed E-selectin, which appears on endothelial cells 1 to 2 hours after cell stimulation by interleukin (IL)-1, tumor necrosis factor alpha (TNF-α), or lipopolysaccharide (LPS). E-selectin counterreceptors include PSGL-1 and E-selectin ligand-1, which also is located on neutrophil microvilli.[16] Both P-selectin and L-selectin contribute sequentially to leukocyte rolling, but L-selectin is involved in prolonged neutrophil sequestration on inflamed microvasculature. L-selectin is constitutively present on neutrophils. Its binding capacity is rapid and transiently increased after neutrophil activation, possibly via receptor oligomerization. To date, only one inducible L-selectin counter receptor has been identified on inflamed endothelium. In addition to its binding to endothelial ligands, neutrophil PSGL-1 is a counterreceptor for L-selectin, which permits previously adherent neutrophils to recruit other neutrophils to inflamed endothelium.[9,14]

NEUTROPHIL ADHESION AND SPREADING

Figure 66-2 shows a sequence of molecular and biophysical events leading to neutrophil activation and increased adherence during acute inflammatory response *in vivo*. The inflamed endothelium produces chemoattractants such as platelet-activating factor (PAF), leukotriene B4 (LTB$_4$), and various chemokines, immobilized by proteoglycans on the luminal surface of endothelial cells.[17] Among these chemokines, IL-8 specifically attacks neutrophils. IL-8 is synthesized by endothelial cells in response to IL-1 or LPS and is stored in Weibel-Palade bodies. IL-8 then can be released by histamine or thrombin.[8] Additionally, IL-8 can be internalized by endothelial cells, transcytosed to the abluminal surface via vesicular caveolae, and presented to the tips of microvilli of the endothelial cell luminal surface.[19] Binding of signaling molecules such as PAF and IL-8 to surface receptors on the leukocytes activates them in a juxtacrine fashion and triggers changes in affinity or avidity of β_2-integrins (CD11/CD18) that become incorporated in the neutrophil plasma membrane from secretory vesicles.[9,14,20] β_2-integrins are recognized by counterligands on endothelial cells, including members of the intercellular adhesion molecule (ICAM) family ICAM-1 and ICAM-2. The ICAM glycoproteins are induced by cytokines including TNF and IL-1. The relative affinity of the β_2-integrins for ICAM is increased by exposure of neutrophils to numerous stimuli, including C5a, N-formylated bacterial peptides, IL-8, and LTB$_4$. Regulation of β_2-integrin avidity involves interactions of both α- and β-chains by their cytoplasmic tails with the cytoskeleton membrane and the subsequent "outside-in signaling."[14] Neutrophils integrate the signals of integrin engagement and those delivered simulta-

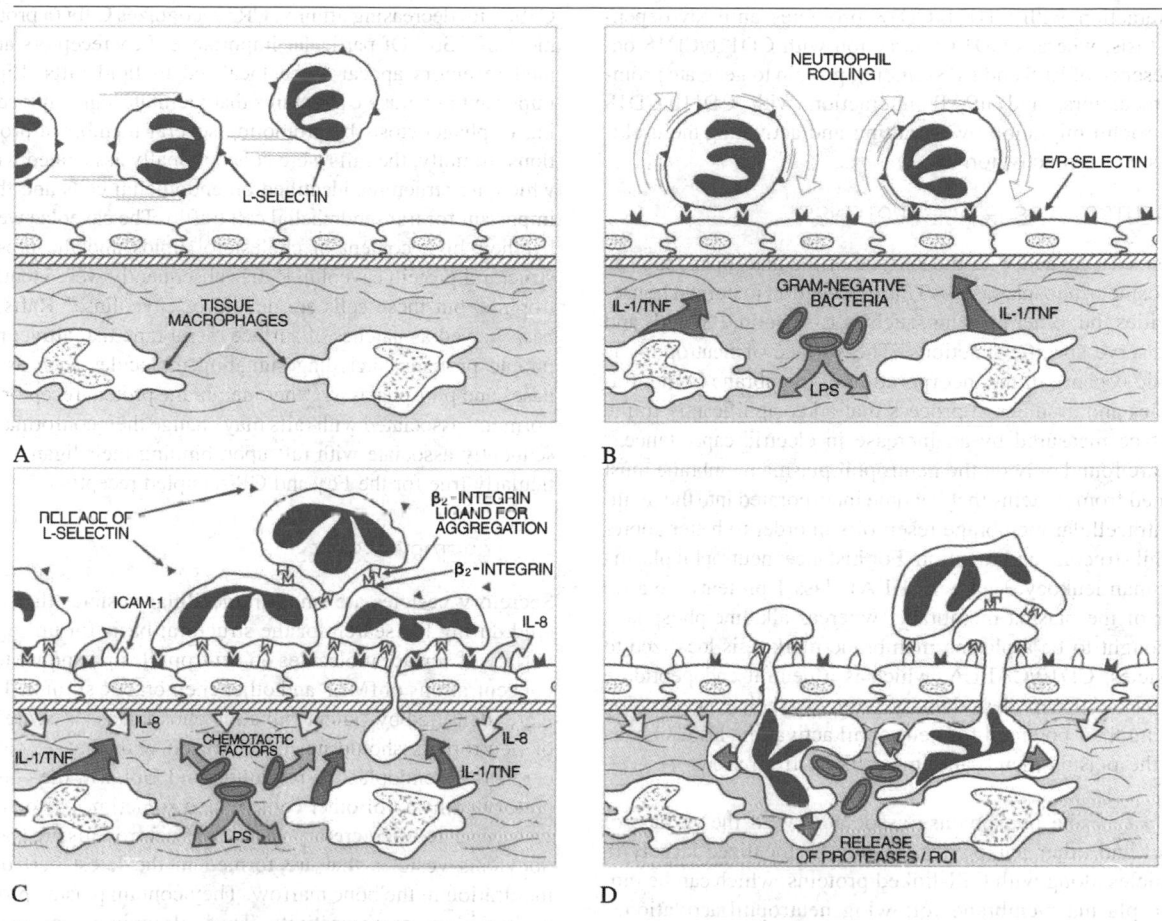

FIGURE 66-2   Neutrophil-mediated inflammatory response. *(A)* Initial tethering and rolling are dominantly mediated by selectin present on neutrophils and endothelial cells and their ligands. They also are present on leukocytes such as P-selectin glycoprotein ligand-1. *(B)* Invasion of gram-negative bacteria with release of polysaccharide stimulates tissue macrophages to secrete inflammatory monokines IL-1 and TNF, which in turn activate endothelial cells to express E- and P-selectin. E- and P-selectin serve as counter-receptors for the neutrophil P-selectin glycoprotein ligand-1. *(C)* Activated endothelial cells express ICAM-1 and ICAM-2, which serve as ligands for the neutrophil β_2-integrins. β_2-integrins mediate tight adhesion and arrest of leukocytes in cooperation with the selectins. Localized activation of neutrophils by juxtacrine signaling molecules or chemoattractants that bind to surface receptors is critical for inside-out signaling of β_2-integrins, making them adhesive for the ICAM ligands on the endothelium. *(D)* Neutrophil invasion through the vascular base membrane with release of proteases and reactive oxidative intermediates that cause local destruction of the extracellular matrix, thus allowing migration of neutrophils into tissues.

neously by inflammatory cytokines or chemoattractants to activate a cascade of intracellular events resulting in cell spreading (Fig. 66-2).

TRANSENDOTHELIAL MIGRATION

Neutrophil transmigration occurs predominately at the borders of endothelial cells. P-selectin concentrates along endothelial borders and may facilitate neutrophil adhesion. Extravasation requires discontinuation of endothelial cell-to-cell adherent junctions. Cellular activation by IL-8 reduces neutrophil tethering rates to P-selection under flow conditions. The precise molecular mechanisms remain undefined.[14] Tight adhesion mediated by β_2-integrins also is modified for a successful emigration that may involve RhoA kinase modulation of the cytoskeletal-dependent spreading.[21] At endothelial-type junctions, sequential molecular interactions occur after leukocyte transmigration from the apical surface has been initiated. Platelet endothelial adhesion molecule-1 (PECAM-1) is localized at junctions of tightly apposed endothelial cells and is involved in the transmigration of neutrophils. PECAM-1 also is expressed at the neutrophil surface, and PECAM-1/PECAM-1 homophilic interaction in a "zipper" model is suggested to

mediate in part the transmigration of leukocytes into the tissues.[9,14] Subsequently, the direction of neutrophil movement in the tissues is guided by the steepest local chemoattractant gradient and then regulated by successive receptor desensitization and attraction by secondary distant agonists. Finally, targeted attractants such as formyl-methionyl-leucyl-phenylalanine (fMLP) and C5a are dominant and override regulatory cell-derived attractants such as LTB_4 or IL-8.[22] This process permits the leukocytes recruited by endothelial chemoattractants to migrate away from the endothelial agonist source toward the final microbial target within tissue. Neutrophil migration through the extracellular matrix is mediated by β_2-integrins in concert with β_1-integrins.[17] Neutrophil migration requires continuous formation of new adhesive contacts at the cell front while the cell rear detaches from the adhesive substrate.

The CD11b/CD18 integrin (MAC-1) is known to interact in *cis* fashion with glycosylphosphatidylinositol (GPI)-anchored membrane proteins such as $Fc\gamma RIIIB$ (CD16), the LPS receptor (CD14), and the urokinase receptor uPAR (CD87). Integrins behave as transducers mediating signals transferred by the GPI-linked receptors.[23] For instance,

FcγRIIIB interaction with CD11b/CD18 promotes antibody-dependent phagocytosis, whereas CD14 interaction with CD11b/CD18 occurs in the presence of LPS and LPS-binding protein to generate proinflammatory mediators, and uPAR interaction with CD11b/CD18 mediates neutrophil migration by recruiting and activating the urokinase-type plasminogen activator.[17]

OTHER NEUTROPHIL SURFACE PROTEINS

Several proteins associated with the surface of the neutrophil, such as Na+/K+ adenosine triphosphatase (ATPase), function in normal housekeeping activities, but other proteins, such as L-selectin, PSGL-1, and the integrins, serve specific functions. The surface of neutrophils is highly dynamic because of the incorporation of membrane from intracellular vesicles and granules, a process that adds significantly to the total cell surface measured by an increase in electric capacitance.[24] Proteins that are found only on the neutrophil plasma membrane must be distinguished from proteins that become incorporated into the membrane from intracellular membrane reservoirs in order to better appreciate neutrophil structure and function. For instance, neutrophil plasma membrane human leukocyte antigen (HLA) class 1 proteins are a reliable marker of the plasma membrane, whereas alkaline phosphate, previously thought to be a plasma membrane marker, is localized to secretory vesicles. CD10/CALLA, which is a neutral endopeptidase that cleaves bacterial peptides, thereby reducing their concentration and diminishing their potential for neutrophil activation, also is incorporated into the plasma membrane, most likely from secretory vesicles.[25]

CD45 is a tyrosine phosphatase associated with the surface of the neutrophil and other leukocytes. It may be localized largely to secretory vesicles along with GPI-linked proteins, which can be mobilized to the plasma membrane following neutrophil activation.[25] CD45 may be involved in facilitating signals that promote L-selectin shedding.[26]

Toll-like receptors (TLRs) are type 1 transmembrane signaling receptors that interact with specific structures characteristic for microorganisms and generate signals that result in chemokine release. All 10 TLRs except TLR3 are expressed in human leukocytes. They recognize different pathogen-associated molecular patterns and share a conserved leucine-rich extracellular domain and a cytoplasmic domain with homology to the IL-1 receptor. TLRs in general transmit signals through the adaptor protein MyD88, which participates in activating MAP kinase and gene transcription via the nuclear factor-κB (NF-κB) pathway.[27] The known TLRs except for TLR3 are expressed on human neutrophils and likely contribute to neutrophil activation when they are engaged.

A variety of chemokine receptors, generally G-protein coupled receptors, are associated with the neutrophil. Other G-protein coupled receptors on neutrophils are the purine receptors for adenosine diphosphate (ADP) and adenosine triphosphate (ATP), the PAF receptor C5a, and fLMP receptors. Receptors not belonging to the G-protein coupled receptor family include receptors for IL-1, IL-10 and TNF-α, and the growth factors receptors for granulocyte colony stimulating factor and granulocyte-macrophage colony stimulating factor. Of course, both growth factor receptors are important for myeloid development, but they also may play an important role in enhancing neutrophil function and gene transcription.

SURFACE COMPONENTS FOR PHAGOCYTOSIS

Neutrophils express the Fcα receptor (CD89) for IgA and IgG receptors, FcγRIIA (CD32), and FcγRIII (CD16). Neutrophils also express receptors for the complement components, including CD1qR, CR1 (CD35), CR3 (CD11/CD18), and CR4. CR1 binds CD3b, C4b, and C3bi with decreasing affinity. CR3 recognizes C3bi (a proteolytic fragment of C3b). Of particular importance, Fcγ receptors and GPI-coupled receptors appear to be localized to lipid rafts. Lipid rafts are important but elusive structures that facilitate signal transduction leading to phagocytosis by promoting several membrane protein interactions. Initially, the rafts were conceptionally associated with caveolae, which are structures identified on endothelial cells and thought to be important for transendothelial cell traffic. The caveolae were identified by their high content of cholesterol lipids and the presence of the structural protein caveolin. Rafts subsequently were identified on neutrophils, but these cells are devoid of caveolins.[28] Rafts are perhaps best viewed as patches of surface membrane that attract many hydrophobic proteins, including signaling molecules such as tyrosine kinases and phosphatases. Other membrane protein receptors that are not normally associated with rafts may change their conformation and subsequently associate with raft upon binding their ligands. This is particularly true for the Fcγ and GPI-coupled receptors.

SECRETORY VESICLES

Secretory vesicles are small intracellular vesicles that were discovered during the search for the structural basis for up-regulation of a variety of surface molecules on neutrophils in response to nanomolar concentrations of fMLP and other chemotactic stimuli. They initially were identified by "latent" alkaline phosphatase.[29] Secretory vesicles of neutrophils should not be confused with the vesicles that carry cargo from endoplasmic reticulum and Golgi in the constitutive secretory pathway of other cells, which sometimes also are named secretory vesicles. Secretory vesicles of neutrophils are specialized endocytosis vesicles that are formed in the latest part of neutrophil maturation in the bone marrow. They contain plasma proteins, seemingly without any selectivity. Thus, albumin serves as a marker for secretory vesicles and has allowed their identification as small intracellular vesicles that are scattered throughout the cytoplasm of neutrophils just like granules. The plasma proteins inside secretory vesicles show no sign of degradation; thus, no fusion takes place with lysosomal structures.[30] The secretory vesicles behave like the traditional neutrophil granules. They require a specific signal for mobilization.[31] Secretory vesicles are not important for their cargo (plasma proteins) but for their membrane, which becomes fully incorporated into the plasma membrane of the neutrophil upon stimulation.[30,32–35] Secretory vesicles host most of the neutrophil chemotactic and GPI-coupled receptors and phospholipase D, one of the early-acting downstream effectors.[36] They enrich the plasma membrane with receptors for adhesion and signaling. They can be considered the structural basis for transition of neutrophils from circulating quiescent cells that do not respond well to stimuli such as phagocytosis to highly responsive cells capable of establishing firm contact with endothelium. The signals generated by tethering of selectins or PSGL-1 to the endothelium are sufficient to mobilize secretory vesicles. Secretory vesicles are completely mobilized *in vivo* during neutrophil diapedesis.[14,35]

Latent alkaline phosphatase, the first identified marker of secretory vesicles, is elevated in chronic myeloproliferative disorders except for chronic myelogenous leukemia, but the content of secretory vesicles in neutrophils from patients with chronic myeloproliferative disorders is not different from normal neutrophils.[37–39] The best marker for secretory vesicles is CD35 because CD35, in contrast to alkaline phosphatase, is absent from the plasma membrane of unstimulated neutrophils and because CD35 is absent from granules (in contrast to $\alpha_M\beta_2$).[20,34,40] Whether secretory vesicles contain lipid rafts is not known, but most GPI-linked proteins are raft associated[41] and are localized to secretory vesicles in neutrophils.

GRANULES

NOMENCLATURE OF NEUTROPHIL GRANULES

The neutrophil is known for its granules. When Paul Ehrlich introduced anilic dyes in histochemistry and discovered the different subsets of leukocytes, the neutrophil granules were divided into those that took up the azure dye—the azurophilic granules—and the others—the specific granules.[42,43] When the peroxidase reaction was introduced, the azurophil granules were found to be peroxidase positive as a result of the presence of the major myeloid cell protein myeloperoxidase (MPO); thus, the specific granules were named *peroxidase-negative granules*.[44,45] Because the azurophil granules are formed first, in the promyelocyte, and the specific granules later, in the myelocytes, they are also termed *primary* and *secondary granules*, respectively. From a study of rabbit neutrophils, a third granule subset termed *tertiary granules* was identified in subcellular fractions.[46] Using the same technology, a tertiary granule subset was identified in human neutrophils and shown to contain gelatinase,[47] but the ultrastructure was not determined until the issue of the neutrophil gelatinase (matrix metalloproteinase [MMP]-9) as a possible complex with neutrophil gelatinase-associated lipocalin (NGAL) was identified.[48,49]

Granules initially were viewed as small bags that emptied their content of bactericidal substances onto the ingested microorganisms when granules fused with the phagocytic vacuole during phagocytosis. However, later came knowledge that granules are important not only for their cargo, which may be emptied into the phagocytic vacuole or extracellularly, but also for their membranes because they contain proteins that become incorporated into the membrane of the phagocytic vacuole and into the surface membrane when the granules are mobilized.[50,51] If granules were classified by their content of matrix proteins and membrane proteins, the number of different granule subsets that exists in neutrophils would be meaninglessly high. Yet nature has provided a beautiful setting that allows the neutrophil to fine tune its response to a specific task. A priori, different subsets of granules exist for two reasons. One is to ensure that proteins, which cannot coexist, are segregated, that is, protease-sensitive proteins separate from proteases. The other reason is to separate proteins whose service is needed at one time from proteins whose service is needed at a different time.

HETEROGENEITY OF GRANULES

Among the peroxidase-positive granules, subsets can be identified that are rich in defensins and some that are not.[52,53] Functionally, no difference in terms of the regulation of exocytosis of these peroxidase-positive granule subsets has been identified.[54] Other constituents include the serine proteases elastase, cathepsin G, and proteinase-3 and the inactive serine protease azurocidin (or CAP37), the antimicrobial proteins, bactericidal/permeability-increasing protein (BPI), lysozyme, and the α-defensins (HNPs), which are by far the dominating species.[50] The membrane of the azurophil granules contains CD63 (granulophysin) and CD67, but their role in neutrophil function remains unclear.[55,56] Characteristically, many of the proteins present in peroxidase granules are proteolytically processed from inactive proforms to the active mature forms, which are stored in the granule matrix. The processing seems to take place in the trans Golgi, but the proteases responsible have not been identified.[57–59]

Peroxidase-negative granules can be divided into three subsets based on the distribution of the two marker proteins lactoferrin and gelatinase: (1) granules that contain lactoferrin but no gelatinase (15 percent of peroxidase-negative granules), (2) granules that contain both lactoferrin and gelatinase (60 percent), and granules that are rich in gelatinase but low (or absent) in lactoferrin (25 percent).[60] The latter

are named *gelatinase* or *tertiary granules*. Granules that contain lactoferrin are called *specific* or *secondary granules*. The specific granules can be further subdivided into those that contain CRISP3 and those that do not.[61] Characteristic of peroxidase-negative granules, the proteins present in their matrix are not proteolytically processed. The MMPs of peroxidase-negative granules are stored as a proform,[62] as is the major bactericidal protein hCAP18.[63,64] No major differences have been identified in the content of membrane proteins of the peroxidase-negative granule subsets. All contain the flavocytochrome p47^{phox}/gp91^{phox} complex, which is part of the reduced nicotinamide adenine dinucleotide phosphate (NADPH) oxidase. All contain the major β_2-integrin $\alpha_M\beta_2$, which are shared with the membrane of secretory vesicles.[20,65,66] The divalent cation transporter Nramp1 is localized only to gelatinase granules.[67] MMP-25, the membrane MMP leukolysin,[68] is shared between gelatinase granules and secretory vesicles. However, the subsets differ markedly in their propensity for exocytosis. Following neutrophil stimulation, gelatinase granules are exocytosed to a larger extent than granules containing both lactoferrin and gelatinase, and these again are more readily mobilized than granules containing lactoferrin but lacking gelatinase. These in turn are mobilized more readily than peroxidase-positive granules.[31,35,48,60,69] This organization of granule subsets with different content and set points for triggering exocytosis allows the neutrophil to mobilize MMPs and integrins necessary for movement through the basement membrane and tissue before the bactericidal and serine protease are called to play. However, an enormous burden is placed on the organization of the biosynthetic apparatus to ensure the right granule proteins are targeted to the granules with a given trigger for exocytosis.

TARGETING BY BIOSYNTHETIC TIMING

The extreme heterogeneity of neutrophil granules and their individual control of exocytosis can be explained simply by the timing of their biosynthesis. Granule proteins are synthesized during myelopoiesis from myeloblasts to band and segmented neutrophils in the bone marrow.[44,45,70] The window of biosynthesis of each granule protein is highly individually controlled by combinations of transcription factors that change as the cells differentiate and mature.[71,72] If all granule proteins are targeted to granules during synthesis, the content of newly formed granules changes as the cell matures because the profile of biosynthesis changes. This simple mechanism largely explains the heterogeneity of granules[73] and their contents, but it does not account for the differences in exocytotic rates among individualized subsets. By timing the biosynthesis of the proteins essential for fusion[74,75] to granules membranes during maturation, exocytosis rates can be regulated. The fusion protein vesicle-associated membrane protein-2 (VAMP-2) is present at a higher density on gelatinase granules than on specific granules and is expressed most highly on secretory vesicles.[76,77] This finding correlates with the ease of releasing granule subsets from the neutrophil following activation.

SORTING BETWEEN THE CONSTITUTIVE AND REGULATED EXOCYTOTIC PATHWAY

Although sorting by timing can explain the granule heterogeneity of neutrophil granules, it does not provide any clues to the mechanisms responsible for diverting newly synthesized proteins to granules as opposed to immediate (constitutive) secretion. Not all granule proteins are equally efficiently directed to granules. Lysozyme is poorly retained during biosynthesis.[78] This explains the high concentration of lysozyme in plasma.[79] MPO is efficiently retained, and the plasma level of MPO is consequently very low. A particular interesting observation pertains to α-defensins. α-Defensins are localized exclusively to azurophil granules, but their window of biosynthesis is very similar to that of lactoferrin.[72,78] Defensins and lactoferrin are con-

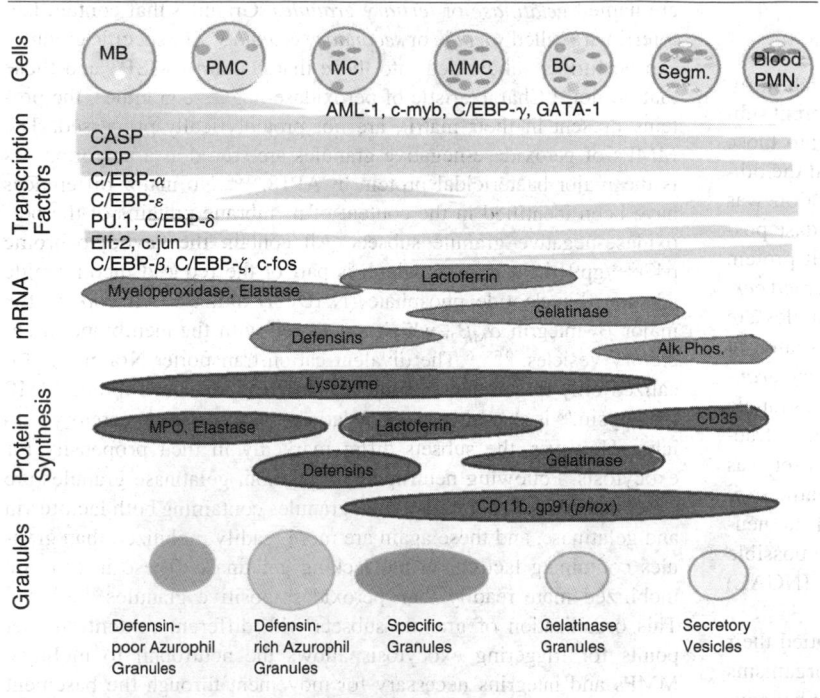

FIGURE 66-3   Formation of granule subsets during myelopoiesis and regulation of granule protein transcription. Difference in the appearance and disappearance of transcription factors regulates the individual window of granule protein gene transcription and translation into protein that is targeted to form granules, thus explaining the heterogeneity of neutrophil granules.

However, this does not preclude PU.1 from regulating transcription of individual granule proteins at a later stage of development.[86–89] The role of individual transcription factors in controlling granule protein expression can be difficult to establish. Consensus binding sites for the transcription factor must be modified in the promoters of target genes. This can be achieved only in myeloid cell lines; however, they do not display with high fidelity the normal sequence of granule protein synthesis during maturation.

Figure 66-3 shows the profile of important myeloid transcription factors during maturation of normal myeloid cells in the marrow *in vivo*. AML-1, c-myb, CASP, C/EBP-α, C/EBP-γ, GATA-1, and Elf-1 all are strongly expressed in the myeloblast and promyelocyte, and some of these factors are required for azurophil granule protein expression. c-myb, AML-1, GATA-1, and Elf-1 are down-regulated as the cells enter the myelocyte stages, heralded by a brisk and transient up-regulation of C/EBP-ε to initiate expression of peroxidase negative granule proteins.[71] This process is in agreement with the lack of specific granules in C/EBP–ε-/- mice and the observation of a C/EBP-ε mutation in patients with the rare specific granule deficiency (SGD).[80,81,90,91] PU.1, C/EBP-β, and C/EBP-δ also appear at the promyelocyte myelocyte transition, but in contrast to C/EBP-ε they continue to increase as the cells mature to neutrophils. Elf-1 reappears at the metamyelocyte stage followed by C/EBP-ξ, c-jun, and c-fos, which are expressed at the band cell stage and increase in content as the cells mature.[71]

trolled by the transcription factor CCAAT/enhancer binding protein (C/EBP-ε), which is absolutely required for biosynthesis of specific granule proteins.[80,81] The absence of defensins from specific granules despite active biosynthesis when other specific granule proteins are formed is explained by a complete lack of sorting of defensins to granules in myelocytes.[71,72,78] Only defensins synthesized at the late promyelocytic stage are routed to granules. Defensins synthesized at the myelocyte stage are secreted from cells after biosynthesis.[78] The defensins that are targeted to granules are processed to mature defensins, whereas the defensins that are secreted remain unprocessed. Because the processing of defensins removes a charge neutralizing propiece, sorting of defensins and other granule proteins to granules may depend on their ability to interact with negatively charged proteoglycans that are present in the matrix of granules.[82,83] No common denominator that fully explains why neutrophil proteins are sorted to granules has been identified. Perhaps the lack of efficient sorting to granules may not solely be taken as inefficiency but may secure a desirable level of antibiotic protein, such as lysozyme in plasma,[79] which renders the myeloid cells of the bone marrow as a major secretory organ.

CONTROL OF GRANULE PROTEIN EXPRESSION
Biosynthesis of neutrophil granule proteins is controlled at the transcriptional level and not the translational level because of complete congruence between protein biosynthesis and mRNA levels during myelopoiesis (Fig. 66-3).[70–72] Not all transcription factors involved have been identified, and the role of an individual transcription factor may be difficult to identify from gene knockout studies because transcription factors may work at multiple stages during myelopoiesis. The transcription factor PU.1 is essential for myelopoiesis because knockout mice do not form myeloid progenitors beyond myeloblasts.[84,85]

GRANULES AND LYSOSOMES
All cells contain granules, which are defined as membrane-bound organelles that contain proteinases. The distinction between lysosomes and granules in neutrophils may be a matter of semantics. Lysosomes are conceptually defined as organelles that contain acid hydrolases whose function is related to degradation of endocytosed material. This is in contrast to the secretory granules of endocrine and exocrine cells in which the granules do not receive endocytosed cargo and do not act as scavengers. Granules of platelets receive endocytosed material and discharge the material upon exocytosis. Similarly, neutrophil azurophil granules can incorporate endocytosed material into the granule matrix.[92] Thus, the distinction may not be as obvious. Disorders that interfere with trafficking of material to lysosomes and result in defects of lysosomal function affect neutrophil granules; thus, lysosomes and neutrophil granules are related and share some fundamental features. CD63 is a protein that is found on most lysosomes.[93] In neutrophils, this protein is associated with azurophil granules.[55] In contrast, Lamp1, another protein associated with lysosomes, is not found on azurophil granules. Instead, Lamp1 is associated with multivesicular bodies,[94] which are dynamic structures that are part of the endocytotic pathway and result from vesicle fusion. Multivesicular bodies are found even in resting neutrophils.[95] What role, if any, they play during phagocytosis is not clear. The mannose-6-phosphate receptor is important for sorting proteins irrespective of whether they are newly synthesized or endocytosed to lysosomes.[96] Defects in the mannose-6-phosphate receptor lead to dysfunctional lysosomes in liver cells.[97] Although this receptor clearly recognizes azurophil granule proteins,[94] defects do not affect neutrophils and targeting of mannose-6-phosphate containing proteins to azurophil granules is unaffected, again making a distinction between these and classic lysosomes.

FUNCTION OF INDIVIDUAL GRANULE PROTEINS AND THEIR ROLE IN OXIDATIVE AND NONOXIDATIVE MICROBIAL KILLING

PROTEINS OF AZUROPHIL GRANULES

MPO is the marker protein of azurophil granules. It is formed as a 90-kDa precursor with an internal disulfide bridge that forms a link between the 57- and the 13.5-kDa subunits, which are generated by the proteolytic processing that occurs during routing to granules (Table 66-1). The heme group, which is necessary for the redox functions of MPO, associates with the 90-kDa subunit.[98] This seems to be a necessary prerequisite for subsequent processing.[99] MPO reacts with hydrogen peroxide (H_2O_2), formed by the NADPH oxidase, and increases the toxic potential of this oxidant. Through oxidation of chloride, tyrosine, and nitrite, the H_2O_2-MPO system induces formation of hypochlorous acid, other chlorination products, tyrosine radicals, and reactive nitrogen intermediates, all off which can attack the surface membrane of microorganisms.[100,101]

MPO may be found on endothelial cells during inflammation and can inactivate nitric oxide (NO).[102] Plasma levels of MPO are predictive of an adverse outcome in patients with angina pectoris.[103] In addition to the activities of MPO itself, MPO is known for the anti-MPO autoantibodies that are characteristic of the perinuclear antineutrophil cytoplasmic antibodies found in vasculitides, particularly those that primarily affect kidneys.[104,105]

BPI is a 55-kDa protein with high homology to the LPS-binding protein of plasma. It is organized into two largely symmetric subdomains, one of which is responsible for binding of LPS and antimicrobial activity against gram-negative microorganisms. In contrast to LPS-binding protein, which presents endotoxin to CD14 and elicits a proinflammatory response, BPI delivers LPS independent of CD14 and neutralizes the effects of LPS.[106] A transgene expressing high levels of BPI has enhanced resistance against endotoxin.[107]

Defensins are small antibacterial cationic peptides with a broad spectrum of antibacterial activity.[108] They share a characteristic three-disulfide bond motif.[52,109,110] Based on this structure, mammalian defensins are divided into α-defensins, β-defensins, and the cyclical θ-defensins.[111] Only α-defensins are found in human neutrophils, and they reside exclusively in azurophil granules. Defensins also are named human neutrophil peptides (HNPs). They are by far the dominating proteins of azurophil granules, yet they are expressed in only a subset of granules that are formed late in the promyelocyte stage.[53,72,78] Three defensins— HNP-1 to HNP-3—have been isolated from azurophil granules.[52]

The serine proteases of azurophil granules include three major serine proteases: elastase, cathepsin G, and proteinase-3. Azurocidin, also called CAP37 or heparin-binding protein (HBP), is a fourth but enzymatically inactive serine protease.[112–116] Both elastase and cathepsin G have direct antibacterial activities that are not dependent on their enzymatic activity. Proteinase-3 expression leads to autoantibodies against itself in Wegener granulomatosis, which is known as cANCA (cytoplasmic antineutrophil cytoplasmic antibodies).[117] A secreted precursor of proteinase-3 has been suggested to inhibit normal myelopoiesis[118] and to play a role in myelopoiesis regulation. The only specific substrate of proteinase-3 identified to date is hCAP18, the cathelicidin of specific granules. Proteinase-3 activates hCAP18 by removing the cathelicidin part and unleashing the antibacterial activity of the C-terminal LL37 peptide.[64] HBP also is localized to secretory vesicles and may play a role in opening endothelial cells for neutrophil transmigration.[119]

The membrane of azurophil granules contains CD63 (granulophysin), which is implicated in transmembrane signaling with the β_2-integrins in the activated neutrophil.[55,56,120] The CD68 antigen[72,121] and presinilin appear localized exclusively to the membrane of azurophil granules,[122] whereas stomatin is found in the membrane of all granules,[123] and the vacuolar-type H^+-ATPase is shared among azurophil, gelatinase granules, and secretory vesicles.[124] These membrane proteins translocate to the phagocytic vacuole or the plasma membrane when neutrophils are activated and engaged in phagocytosis.

PROTEINS OF PEROXIDASE NEGATIVE GRANULES

Lactoferrin is the dominating protein of specific granules.[125] It is a 78-kDa iron-chelator, member of the transferrin protein family with a high affinity for iron and binding characteristics similar to ferritin (Table 66-1).[126,127] The antibacterial activity of lactoferrin does not depend exclusively on its ability to sequester iron because proteolytic fragments of lactoferrin, some of which are known as lactoferricin, are directly bactericidal.[128,129]

NGAL, or siderochalin, is a 25-kDa N-glycosylated member of the lipocalin protein family.[49] Lipocalins are transport proteins that bind small and often lipophilic substances in their canonical lipocalin pocket.[130] Some NGAL is associated with gelatinase (MMP-9) in a subset of specific granules,[131] but the majority is present either as a monomer or as a homodimer in specific granules. NGAL interferes with the activation and stability of MMPs,[132] but a major activity of NGAL is its behavior as a siderophore-binding protein. NGAL binds enterochalin/enterobactin with high affinity and blocks growth of *Escherichia coli* by sequestering siderophore–iron complexes.[133] This may not only be a neutrophil-specific antibacterial defense because NGAL can be induced in a variety of epithelial cells during inflammation by IL-1.[134]

Nramp1, the cation transporter, initially was identified in macrophages as an essential resistance factor against mycobacterial infection. It is present in neutrophil membranes of both specific and gelatinase granules.[67,135]

Lysozyme is a cationic antimicrobial peptide of 14 kDa.[136]. In agreement with its biosynthetic profile, lysozyme is present in all granule subsets, with peak concentrations in specific granules.[72,79] Lysozyme cleaves peptidoglycan polymers of bacterial cell walls and displays bactericidal activity towards the nonpathogenic gram-positive bacteria *Bacillus subtilis*.[137] Lysozyme also binds LPS[138] and reduces cytokine production and mortality caused by LPS in a murine model system of septic shock.[139] In contrast to many neutrophil granule proteins, lysozyme is inefficiently targeted to granules and circulates free in plasma in a substantial quantity that reflects normal myelopoietic activity.[78,79] Lysozyme also is secreted from activated macrophages,[140] and a aparticular elevated serum level is characteristic of the myelomonocytic leukemias.[141]

hCAP-18,[63] also known as LL-37,[142] is the only human member of a family of antimicrobial peptides known as *cathelicidins*. Cathelicidins typically are found in peroxidase-negative granules of mammalian neutrophils.[143] hCAP-18 is a prominent protein of neutrophil-specific granules present in equimolar concentrations with lactoferrin.[144] It also is present in plasma at a substantial concentration bound to lipoproteins.[145] In general, cathelicidins are proantibiotic peptides that share a common and highly conserved 14-kDa N-terminal region known as the *cathelin region*, whereas the C-terminal regions vary extensively among the different cathelicidins. To become antibacterial, the C-terminal peptides must be liberated from the cathelin part by proteolysis. In most species this action is performed by elastase, but in human neutrophils this action is performed by proteinase-3 from azurophil granules. The liberated C-terminal peptide is known as LL-37.[64,142] Like several other neutrophil proteins, hCAP-18 is formed by cells in other tissues, particularly epithelial cells.[64,146–148] It is constitutively expressed in the testis and is present in semen. The

TABLE 66-1   PHYSICAL-CHEMICAL AND FUNCTIONAL PROPERTIES OF NEUTROPHIL GRANULES

GRANULE PROTEIN	LOCALIZATION	PHYSICO-CHEMICAL PROPERTIES	FUNCTION
Myeloperoxidase	AG	Heme protein, 90-kDa proform with an internal disulfide bond between the 57- and 13.5-kDa subunits, generated by proteolytic processing that occurs during routing to granules	The MPO–halide–H_2O_2 system generates hypochlorous acid, other chlorination products, tyrosine radicals, and reactive nitrogen intermediates, all off which can attack the surface membrane of microorganisms
Bacterial/permeability-increasing protein	AG	55-kDa proteins with high homology to the LPS-binding protein of plasma	BPI is organized into two largely symmetric subdomains, one responsible for binding of LPS and antimicrobial activity against gram-negative microorganisms
Defensins: α-defensins HNP-1– HNP-3	AG	7-kDa proforms processed by proteolytic cleavage to mature 3-kDa defensins; proforms share a characteristic three-disulfide bond motif:1-6,2-4,3-5	Defensins are small amphipathic pore-forming antibacterial cationic peptides with a broad spectrum of antibacterial activity
Serine proteases of azurophil granules: elastase, cathepsin G, and proteinase-3 Azurocidin (CAP37 or HBP) is enzymatically inactive	AG	28-kDa proforms, processed to active proteases en route to azurophil granules	Serine proteases, but both elastase and cathepsin G have direct antibacterial activities that are not dependent on their enzymatic activity. Proteinase-3 liberates the antibacterial peptide LL-37 from hCAP-18. HBP is chemotactic for monocytes and may open endothelial cell tight junctions
Lysozyme	AG ~30% SG ~50% GG ~20%	Cationic antimicrobial 14-kDa peptide; in contrast to many neutrophil granule proteins, lysozyme is inefficiently targeted to granules and circulates free in plasma in a substantial quantity that reflects the normal myelopoietic activity	Lysozyme cleaves peptidoglycan-polymers of bacterial cell walls and displays bactericidal activity towards the nonpathogenic gram-positive bacteria *B. subtilis*; A very high serum level is characteristic for the myelomonocytic leukemias
Lactoferrin	SG	78-kDa iron-chelator, member of the transferrin protein family with a high affinity for iron and similar iron-binding characteristics as ferritin	Antibacterial activity of lactoferrin does not depend exclusively on its ability to sequester iron; proteolytic fragments, some of which are known as lactoferricin, are directly bactericidal
Neutrophil gelatinase-associated lipocalin (NGAL) or siderochalin	SG	25-kDa N-glycosylated member of the lipocalin protein family	NGAL is the first known siderophore-binding eukaryotic protein; binds enterochalin/enterobactin with high affinity; blocks growth of *E. coli* by sequestering siderophore–iron complexes
hCAP-18	SG	18 kDa; only human member of the cathelicidin protein family	Stored and released intact; binds endotoxin; C-terminal antibactericidal peptide LL-37 released by proteinase 3; active mainly against gram-positive bacteria; is chemotactic for T-cells, monocytes, and neutrophils; has angiogenetic properties
Neutrophil collagenase	SG	75-kDa MMP-8; like other MMPs, MMP-8 is stored inactive and must be N-terminally trimmed to remove the inhibitory peptide	Active against type I, II, and III collagen
Gelatinase	GG	92-kDa MMP-9; stored inactive	Active against type IV collagen
Leukolysin, which is distributed among resting neutrophils	SG ~10% GG ~40% SV ~30% PM ~20%	Leukolysin is a 56-kDa GPI anchored membrane-bound MMP (MT6-MMP/MMP-25)	Active against fibronectin, chondroitin sulfate proteoglycan, dermatin sulfate proteoglycan
Cytochrome b_{558}, (gp91^{phox}, p22^{phox})	SG ~60% GG ~25% SV ~15%	Heterodimeric flavo-heme protein: 91-kDa glycoprotein subunit (heme-flavin binding) and 22-kDa protein subunit, possibly heme binding	Together with p47^{phox}, p67^{phox}, and p40^{phos}, cytochrome b_{558} constitutes the superoxide generating NADPH oxidase of phagocytes
CD11b/CD18 (Mac-1, Mo1, CR3, $\alpha_M\beta_2$)	SG ~60% GG ~25% SV ~15%	Most prominent β_2-integrin in neutrophils; CD11B = α_M is a 170-kDa glycoprotein; CD18 = β_2 is 95-kDa glycoprotein	Multifunctional integrin that functions as an adhesion receptor binding to members of the immunoglobulin family ICAM-1, fibronectin, collagen; is important in mediating firm adhesion to vascular endothelial cells; functions as a phagocytosis receptor for C3bi-coated particles

AG = azurophil granule; GG = gelatinase granule; GPI = glycosylphosphatidylinositol; MMP = matrix metalloproteinase; PM = plasma membrane; SG = specific granule; SV = secretory vesicle.

activating protease is gastricin, a prostate protease that is active at low pH. Gastricin cleaves hCAP-18 to ALL-38, which has the same antibacterial spectrum as LL-37.[149] The cathelin part, which is released, has some protease inhibitory activity by itself.[150] LL-37 stimulates neutrophil, monocyte, and T cell chemotaxis via formyl peptide receptor-like–1.[151] In addition, hCAP-18/LL-37 has angiogenic[152] and endotoxin neutralizing properties.[153]

Three MMPs have been identified in neutrophils: neutrophil collagenase (MMP-8, 75 kDa), which is located in specific granules[154]; gelatinase (MMP-9, 92 kDa), which resides predominantly in gelatinase granules;[48,155] and leukolysin (MT6-MMP/MMP-25, 56kDa), which is distributed among specific granules (~10 percent), gelatinase granules (~40 percent), secretory vesicles (~30 percent), and the plasma membrane (~20 percent) of resting neutrophils.[68,156] The MMPs are stored as inactive proforms that are proteolytically activated following exocytosis. Together, the MMPs are capable of degrading major structural components of the extracellular matrix, including collagens, fibronectin, proteoglycans, and laminin. They are believed to be of central importance for the degradation of vascular basement membranes and interstitial structures during neutrophil extravasation and migration.

CRISP-3 is a novel cysteine-rich protein identified in peroxidase-negative granules. It is located in a subset of granules that contain both lactoferrin and gelatinase. No function has yet been ascribed to CRISP-3.[61]

Membrane proteins of peroxidase-negative granules are shared among the subsets of peroxidase-negative granules, which can be distinguished based on their matrix proteins, that is, into specific and azurophil granules. Two exceptions are Nramp1 and MMP-25, which both are present predominantly in the membrane of gelatinase granules and secretory vesicles.[67,68] Cytochrome b_{558}, which is composed of gp91phox and p22phox, forms the membrane component of the NADPH oxidase and is a prominent membrane protein of peroxidase-negative granules.[51,157] It codistributes with the major β_2-integrin of neutrophils, CD11b/CD18, with the major part in specific granules, some in gelatinase granules, and some in secretory vesicles. Bearing in mind that secretory vesicles are rapidly mobilized, and even though only 15 percent of the total cytochrome b_{588} and CD11b localizes to secretory vesicles, this fraction is primarily translocated to the plasma membrane during neutrophil diapesis.[20,35] The CD66 antigens found in the membrane of specific granules may play a role as bacterial receptors (galectin receptors) and generate signals to activate the NADPH oxidase.[158,159]

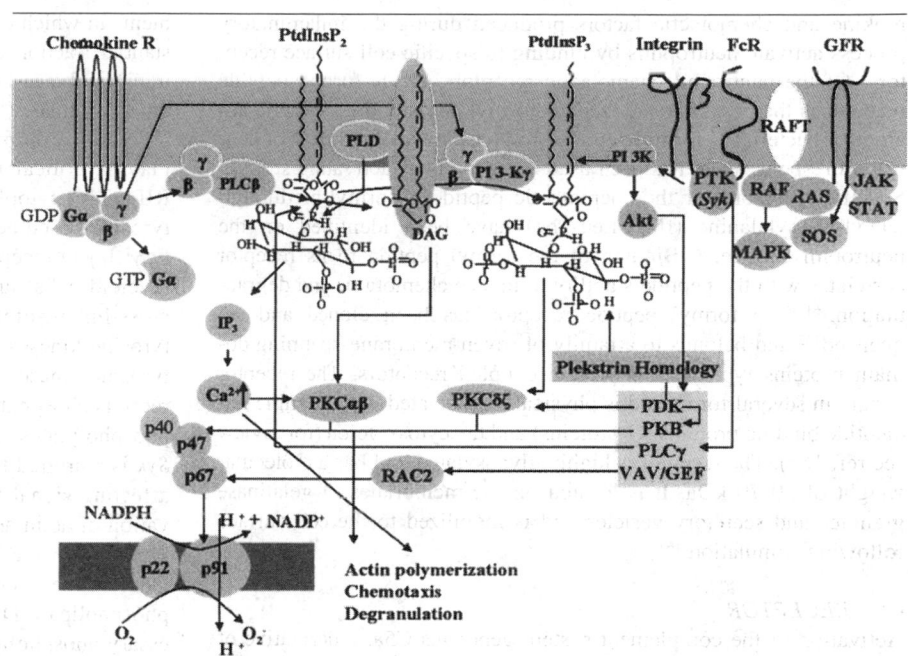

FIGURE 66-4 Signal transduction in neutrophils. G-protein coupled receptors are seven transmembrane receptors that couple to heterotrimeric GTP-binding (G) proteins. Agonist binding to the receptor triggers exchange of guanine diphosphate (GDP) for guanine triphosphate (GTP) on the G α-subunit of the G-protein and, consequently, the disassociation of the α-subunit for the $\beta\gamma$-dimer. Both subunits can regulate the activity of multiple effectors such as phospholipase Cβ (PLCβ). PLCβ cleaves an endogenous lipid, namely, phosphatidylinositol bisphosphate (PtdInsP$_2$), yielding DAG and IP$_3$, which liberate calcium from bound intracellular stores leading to a rise in intracellular free calcium (Ca^{2+})i. The increase in intracellular Ca^{2+} is augmented by an influx of Ca^{2+} from the extracellular space. Increased DAG, in concert with elevated Ca^{2+}, can activate protein kinase isozymes-α and -β (PKC-$\alpha\beta$), leading to their translocation to membranous sites. PLD can be activated by PKC converting phosphatidylcholine to PA. Elevations in PA can mobilize the cytosolic proteins p47, p67phox, and p40phox to bind to the membrane-bound proteins gp91phox and p22phox, which then reduces O$_2$ to O$_2^-$ in the presence of NADPH. The G-protein $\beta\gamma$ subunits also may activate phosphatidylinositol kinase-γ (PI3K-γ), which can phosphorylate PtdInsP$_2$ to phosphatidylinositol triphosphate (PtdInsP$_3$). PtdInsP$_3$ also can trigger the activation of protein kinases, for example, recruit and activate protein kinase B/Akt and PKC-δ and PKC-ζ. Downstream signaling by PI3K is generally considered to be mediated by molecules with a plecksum homology (PH) domain, which serves as a binding domain for polyphosphorylated phosphoinositides. Ligation of integrins or Fc receptors with their ligand leads to activation of proteins tyrosine kinases (PTK), of which Syk is prominent. In turn, Syk may further activate PI3K and the immunoreceptor tyrosine-base motifs (ITAMs) located on the cytoplasmic domain of Fc receptors. PtdInsP$_3$ can activate VAV, a guanine-nucleotide-exchange factor (GEF). VAV then can activate the GTPases such as Rac or CDC42. Rac2 is involved in NADPH activation, whereas Rac1 is involved in chemotaxis and degranulation. Growth factor receptors (GFRs) signal through janus kinases (JAKs), which bind to and phosphorylate tyrosine kinases, which in turn activate the transcription factors STAT leading to further activation of pathways mediated by the son of sevenless (SOS). Activation of receptors often results in their detergent insoluble phospholipid domains (RAFT) and further enhances movement into signal transduction. The process appears to be especially important for FcR, which upon activation uses the RAF, RAS, and microtubule-associated protein kinase (MAPK) pathways to initiate phagosome formation.

minating some of the underlying causes of defects in cell activation. Studies of neutrophil degranulation and oxidative metabolism have revealed transduction mechanisms common to a wide variety of other important secretory cell types, thereby greatly expanding the relevance of this work. The following sections discuss in greater depth the activation process, which is shown schematically in Fig. 66-4.

RECEPTOR–LIGAND INTERACTIONS

FORMYL PEPTIDE RECEPTOR

Neutrophil responses can be evoked by a variety of particulate and soluble stimuli. Opsonized particles, immune complexes, and che-

STIMULUS–RESPONSE COUPLING BY NEUTROPHILS

Stimulus–response coupling by neutrophils has been the subject of intense research for many years. The work has been fruitful in illumokine and chemotactic factors produced during the inflammatory process activate neutrophils by binding to specific cell surface receptors. Of the neutrophil chemotactic receptors, the N-formyl peptide receptor is the best characterized. N-formyl peptide, the synthetic analogs of bacterial N-formyl peptide products, induces a variety of neutrophil responses and has been used extensively as activating stimuli. Specific receptors for the chemotactic peptide N-formyl-methionyl-leucyl-phenylalanine (fMet-Leu-Phe) have been identified on the neutrophil surface.[160] Binding of the formyl peptide to its receptor correlates with the peptide's ability to induce chemotaxis and degranulation.[161] The formyl peptide receptor has been cloned and sequenced[162] and belongs to a family of seven membrane-spanning domain proteins typical of G-protein coupled receptors. The receptor occurs in several forms and is physically associated with guanine nucleotide binding proteins (G-proteins) and the cytoskeleton (for review see ref. 163). The receptor is highly glycosylated and has a molecular weight of 50–70 kDa. It is located on the membranes of gelatinase granules and secretory vesicles and is mobilized to the cell surface following stimulation.[164]

C5a RECEPTOR

Activation of the complement system generates C5a, a derivative of C5 and the most potent of the chemotactic proteins. C5a induces neutrophil chemotaxis, degranulation, and superoxide generation.[165] Responses to C5a result from interactions with specific receptors on the cell surface.[166] The receptor was identified as a single polypeptide in the plasma membrane with an apparent mass of 40 to 48 kDa.[167] Binding studies have demonstrated 50,000 to 113,000 receptor sites per cell with a dissociation constant (K_d) of 2×10^{-9} M. The C5a receptor has been isolated and cloned. It is a member of the seven membrane-spanning class of G-protein coupled receptors.[168]

C3 RECEPTORS

Neutrophils express receptors for the complement-derived chemotactic factors C3b and C3bi. Receptors for C3b and C3bi (also known as CR1 and CR3, respectively) are sparse on resting neutrophils but increase significantly in numbers following activation with several stimuli as a result of incorporation from secretory vesicles (CR1 and CR3) and gelatinase and specific granules (CR3).[20,40] The C3b receptor (CR1) is a glycoprotein with a molecular weight of 205 kDa and is located in secretory vesicles.[34,40]

INTEGRINS

CD11/CD18 integrins play an important role in cell signaling. Adhesion of cells to surfaces or to other cells can either activate neutrophils directly or "prime" them for an enhanced response to other stimuli. For example, the oxidative burst of neutrophils is very different in cells that are suspended versus those that are adherent to surfaces.[169] H_2O_2 production in response to chemotaxins is influenced by monoclonal antibodies to CD11b but not CD11a.[170]

Fc RECEPTORS

Neutrophils possess three different receptors for immunoglobulins. Unstimulated cells express FcγRIIA and FcγRIII, also known as CD32 and CD16, respectively. Functionally, the most important of the two receptors is FcγRIII for clearing immune complexes.[171] It is attached to the membrane by a GPI linkage.[171] The linkage is relatively labile, so the amount of FcγRIII on the membrane reflects a balance between shedding and mobilization from intracellular stores. FcγRIIA is a conventional protein that spans the plasma membrane.[172] The signal transduction pathways initiated by FcγRIII can cross-talk with the formyl peptide receptor, with CR3, and even with each other. A direct physical linkage between CD11b and FcγRIIIB was demonstrated by experi-

ments in which capping of one receptor resulted in co-capping a substantial fraction of the other receptor. CD11b can interact with the transmembrane FcγRII, and both of these molecules can modify each other's signals.[173]

The Src homology 2 domain containing tyrosine kinase (Syk) plays a critical role in the phagocytic pathway mediated by FcγRIIA.[174] A cytoplasmic amino acid motif, known as immunoreceptor tyrosine-based activation motif (ITAM), is present on FcγRIIA and FcγRI/γ (a receptor found on interferon gamma [IFN-γ]-stimulated myeloid cells) and is essential for the phagocytic response during cross-linking of these two Fc receptors. Binding of Src family protein tyrosine kinases to ITAM leads to activation of Src family protein tyrosine kinases and ITAM tyrosine phosphorylation. This process recruits phosphatidylinositol-3 kinase and Syk, which when activated phosphorylates multiple substrates including neighboring ITAMs. Syk is recruited from the cytosolic pool. The essential role of Syk in affecting signal transduction is reflected by ITAM-dependent activation of actin assembly. Other tyrosine kinases, which include Src kinases, especially Lyn, facilitate the formation of the phagosome.[175] Once active microfilaments are formed, they enhance the activity of phospholipase D (PLD) in generating phosphatidic acid (PA), a necessary phospholipid for phagocytosis.[176,177]

OTHER RECEPTORS

Three other important G-protein coupled receptors are PAF, IL-8, and LTB$_4$. PAF and IL-8 receptors have been cloned.[178,179] Their intracellular stores and signal transduction mechanisms are largely similar to those used by other G-protein coupled receptors (e.g., FMLP).[178] IL-8 has two related receptors for which slightly different signal transduction pathways have been detected.[180]

G-PROTEINS

The receptors for the chemotactic stimuli—fMet-Leu-Phe, C5a, LTB$_4$, and PAF—all are coupled to cellular responses through a guanine nucleotide binding protein similar to the inhibitory protein Gi of the adenylate cyclase system. Studies demonstrating that guanine nucleotides can regulate receptor affinity provide evidence linking a G-protein to these receptors.[181] A high-affinity guanosine triphosphatase (GTPase) located in neutrophil plasma membranes is stimulated by the same receptor-mediated stimuli.[182] The enzymatic activity likely is involved in terminating activation of the guanine nucleotide binding protein. Direct linkages between receptors and G-proteins have been observed.[162]

Studies using pertussis toxin have proved instrumental in demonstrating G-protein involvement in the proposed stimulus–response coupling pathway. Pertussis toxin ADP-ribosylates the α-subunit of Gi of the adenylate cyclase system and a 40- to 41-kDa protein in neutrophil plasma membranes.[183] Initial studies demonstrated a strong correlation between the ability of the toxin to catalyze the ADP-ribosylation of the membrane protein and its ability to affect cellular responses initiated by surface receptors. Further characterization of a guanine nucleotide binding protein in neutrophils indicate this protein differs structurally and immunochemically from previously reported guanine nucleotide binding proteins.[184] Not only can neutrophil responses be abolished by pertussis toxin, but stable guanine nucleotides can directly stimulate permeabilized neutrophils.[185] In other cells, heterotrimeric G-proteins may play a tonic inhibitory role in degranulation.[186] Although pertussis toxin inhibits fMet-Leu-Phe–induced secretion from intact cells, it does not inhibit degranulation in response to phorbol 12-myristate 13-acetate, Ca^{2+}, and guanine nucleotides in the permeabilized cell system, suggesting a second G-protein is involved at distal sites in secretion.[185] Potential candidates for this role are the family of small G-proteins (with molecular weight of 20–30 kDa) that has been reported in neutrophils. Some of these proteins include RhoA and ADP-ribosylation factor (ARF)-1, which probably are involved in vesicular traffic and reportedly translocate from cytosol to granules following neutrophil stimulation.[187]

PHOSPOLIPID METABOLISM AND TYROSINE KINASE ACTIVATION

The next step in signal transduction can be attributed to interactions of receptor-activated G-proteins or through FcγRIIA and tyrosine kinases with phospholipases.[188,189] For instance, a membrane-associated phosphoinositide-specific phospholipase is activated upon stimulation with chemotactic stimuli. In particular, phospholipase C hydrolyzes phosphatidylinositol-4,5-bisphosphate (PIP_2) and phosphatidylinositol-4-monophosphate (PIP_1) to the putative second messenger products inositol 1,4,5-trisphosphate (IP_3) and 1,2-diacylglycerol (DAG).[190] In permeabilized neutrophils, IP_3 interacts with a specific intracellular receptor, stimulates the release of Ca^{2+}, and opens Ca^{2+} channels on the plasma membrane, increasing intracellular Ca^{2+}.[191] Activation of the small guanosine triphosphate (GTP)-binding proteins of the Rac, Rho, and Cdc42 families regulate actin-dependent processes, such as membrane ruffling, formation of pseudopodia, and stress fibers leading to cell adhesion and motility. They appear critical in neutrophil function[192,193] and work in concert with the phospholipases.

Even in the absence of phospholipase C metabolism, significant increases in intracellular DAG and Ca^{2+} accompany phagocytosis.[194] Ca^{2+} is necessary for granule phagosome fusion, and DAG has been linked to particle ingestion and degranulation.[195] Both entities can be formed by activation of PLD, which hydrolyzes phosphatidylcholine to produce PA and choline. Activation of PLD is mediated by Rho and/or ARF.[187] DAG then is generated by PA phosphohydrolase, which catalyzes dephosphorylation of PA. The hallmark of phosphatidylcholine-derived DAG is the presence of 1-0-alkyl linkages. During PA formation by the action of PLD on phosphatidylcholine, PA can act as a Ca^{2+} ionophore and thereby initiates fusiogenic activity.[196] Thus, PA generated during phagocytosis may promote fusion of neutrophil granules with newly formed phagosomes.

Another downstream target of DAG in phagocytosis is the activation of protein kinase C (PKC), particularly PKCδ, a Ca^{2+}-independent isozyme of PKC found in neutrophils.[176] PKCδ is one of four PKCs isozymes that translocate to the plasma membrane during phagocytosis. During phagocytosis, PKCδ is translocated from the cytosol to the plasma membrane. Translocation of PKCδ to the membrane is accompanied by promotion of RAF-1 translocation. Following translocation of these two key components, MEK activation occurs, followed by activation of MAP kinase/extracellular signal-related protein kinase-2 and then myosin light chain kinase.[189] Following phosphorylation of myosin, reorganization of the actin cytoskeleton occurs, leading to phagocytosis. Concomitant with PLD activation, ceramide is generated by neutral sphingomyelinase activity found in the plasma membrane of neutrophils and most likely is important in attenuating the activity of the cells through inhibition of PLD.[194] Following engagement of the Fc receptors and *Syk* activation in the neutrophil, phosphatidylinositide-3-kinase (PI3K) is activated. Inhibition of PI3K activity impedes phagocytosis.[176]

Arachidonate Metabolism In addition to their participation as putative second messenger products in the stimulus–response coupling pathway, many lipid metabolites may be released from stimulated neutrophils and in turn modulate cell function by interacting with receptors on other neutrophils. Phospholipase A_2, which is present on the granules and plasma membranes of neutrophils[197] and the cytosol,[198] is activated during neutrophil stimulation, yielding arachidonic acid as one of the major end products. Arachidonic acid not only is released from stimulated neutrophils, but it also serves as a regulator of phospholipase A_2 activity and as a stimulus for these cells.[199] Sensitivity of the cells to other stimuli can be enhanced with arachidonic acid and other long-chain fatty acids.[200]

Arachidonic acid can be metabolized by the lipoxygenase pathway to produce hydroxyeicosatetraenoic acids (HETEs), including 5-HETE, 12-HETE, and 5,12-diHETE.[201] These compounds induce several neutrophil responses.[202] Stimulated neutrophils also produce the diHETE LTB_4 through the lipoxygenase pathway. LTB_4 and other leukotrienes can be released in response to a variety of stimuli.[203] Receptors for LTB_4 have been partially purified, and their activation serves as a potent stimulus for chemotaxis and adherence.[204]

Another potent mediator of inflammation produced by stimulated neutrophils is 1-O-alkyl-2-acetyl-sn-glyceryl-3-phosphoryl choline, also as known PAF.[14] Not only is PAF synthesized by neutrophils and activated endothelial cells, but it has been shown to induce degranulation, aggregation, and superoxide generation.[17] Inflamed endothelium generates PAF, which immobilizes neutrophils on the luminal surface of the endothelials and thereby facilitates the interaction of the neutrophil integrin receptors with the ICAM ligands on endothelial cells.

DEGRANULATION AND MEMBRANE FUSION

In stimulated cells, the signal transduction cascade activates G-proteins, followed by increased intracellular Ca^{2+}, lipid remodeling, and protein kinase activation. These events culminate in secretion. This ultimate event of fusion of granule membranes with phagosomes or the plasma membrane occurs rapidly and is highly efficient.

Fusion Proteins Over the past 15 years, the SNARE hypothesis has become the reigning paradigm for fusion of biomembranes.[75,205] The hypothesis centers around the N-ethyl maleimide (NEM)-sensitive fusion protein (NSF) and several soluble NSF-attachment protein receptors (SNAREs) on the participating membranes. The SNAREs are termed *v-SNAREs* and *t-SNAREs*. The v-SNAREs are found on vesicles or granules. The t-SNAREs are found on the *target* plasma membranes. The SNARE hypothesis has great predictive value because the constellation of fusion proteins and their interactions appears in almost all species and tissues. Increasing evidence indicates VAMP-2 is localized to the membranes of specific and gelatinase granule and secretory vesicles in resting human neutrophils.[76,77] Activation of neutrophils leads to degranulation of the secondary and gelatinase-containing granules, which is associated with interaction of VAMP-2 with the plasma membrane SNARE syntaxin 4 as shown by immunoelectron microscopy. The mechanisms underlying this secretion of primary granules is unknown. Fusion of the neutrophil granules with the plasma membrane represents a heterotypic fusion event. This event involves protein-to-protein interactions that dock a vesicle to its final destination, requiring proteins that favor the interaction between the phospholipid bilayer, the vesicle, and its target membrane.

CLINICAL DISORDERS OF NEUTROPHIL FUNCTION

CLASSIFICATION

Neutrophil dysfunction may arise from (1) absence of antibodies or complement components required to oxidase microorganisms, an interaction that provides a chemotactic signal; (2) abnormalities of cytoplasmic and granule movement that alter the chemotactic response or result in abnormalities of the plasma membrane affecting the cells in terms of capability to modulate movement; and (3) defective mi-

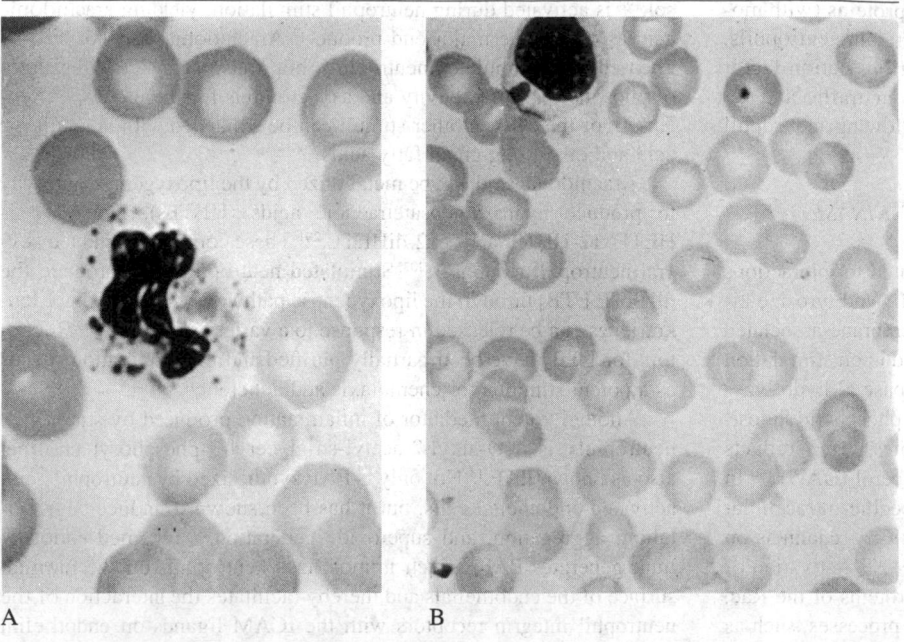

FIGURE 66-5   Blood films of patients with the Chédiak-Higashi syndrome. *(A)* The granulocyte contains large amorphic cytoplasmic granulations. *(B)* A large inclusion is easily seen in a lymphocyte.

crobicidal capability. Other comprehensive reviews of these syndromes are available to the interested reader.[206–208]

ABNORMALITIES OF THE SIGNAL MECHANISM AS A RESULT OF ANTIBODY OR COMPLEMENT DEFECTS

Because the synergistic action of immunoglobulins and complement proteins creates the opsonins that coat microorganisms and stimulate the development of chemotactic factors, a deficiency of either protein may result in impaired neutrophil function. The most profound disturbances arise from abnormalities in C3, because this protein is the focal point for generation of opsonins and chemotactic factors (see Chap. 16).[209,210] Opsonins such as C3b generated from cleavage of C3 coat bacteria. Opsonization in general refers to the coating of pathogens by serum proteins such that the pathogens more likely will be ingested. Activation of C3 can occur in the absence of either an antibody or the classic complement components C1, C4, and C2. Thus, disorders of these latter molecules result in less severe clinical conditions. C3 deficiency is inherited as an autosomal recessive disorder. Homozygotes have undetectable serum levels of C3 and suffer from recurrent severe pyrogenic infections. Asymptomatic heterozygotes have half the normal values.

A functional deficiency of C3 protease resulting in severe pyrogenic infections is seen in patients with a deficiency in C3b inactivator, a protein inhibitor of the alternative complement pathway. Unchecked activation of this pathway leads to hypercatabolism of C3 and factor B.[211] Properidin deficiency also results in a functional deficiency in C3.[212] Properidin is a serum protein that belongs to the alternative complement pathway. It is involved in the stabilization of the enzyme complex C3bBb. The protein is a multimeric glycoprotein with a subunit M_r of 56,000, the gene of which has been cloned.[213] Absence of properidin is associated with severe, often fatal pyrogenic infections, usually with meningococci.

Approximately 5 percent of the populations have low serum levels of mannose-binding lectin (MBL).[214] MBL is a serum lectin secreted by the liver. It binds mannose sugars present on the surface of bacteria, fungi, and some viruses. MBL is one of the collectin-soluble effector proteins that contribute to the basic armamentarium of nonclonal immunity. MBL can function as an opsonin when bound to the surfaces by activating the complement cascade. A deficiency of MBL has been reported in infants with frequent unexplained infection, chronic diarrhea, and otitis media.[214] Other studies have identified an increased susceptibility to infection by specific pathogens in MBL-deficient individuals, including human immunodeficiency virus, *Plasmodium falciparum, Cryptosporidium parvum,* and *Meningococcus meningitides.*[215] The deficiency in MBL largely results from three relatively common single point mutations in the exon of one of the genes, which leads to failure of MBL to activate complement.[216] In addition, the protein modulates disease severity, partly through complex, dose-dependent influence on cytokine production.

Because a large number of chemoattractants are generated during inflammation, establishing the relative significance of a given individual component is difficult. Furthermore, chemotactic factors and opsonins are involved in the activity of neutrophils and mononuclear phagocytes. Therefore, whether the clinical consequences of disorders involving these substances are unique to one or the other of these phagocytic cells is unclear. Patients with antibody- or complement-deficiency syndromes suffer mainly from infections with encapsulated pathogens such as *Haemophilus influenzae,* pneumococci, streptococci, and meningococci.[217] Splenectomized individuals deprived of an organ rich in mononuclear phagocytes have a small but finite risk of sepsis as the result of the same microorganisms. Encapsulated pathogens characteristically are not associated with neutropenic states. Antibody coating of encapsulated organisms facilitates their ingestion by mononuclear phagocytes but may be less important for their ingestion by neutrophils.

ABNORMALITIES OF CELLULAR RESPONSES AS THE RESULT OF DEFECTS IN CYTOPLASMIC MOVEMENT

DEGRANULATION ABNORMALITIES

Chédiak-Higashi Syndrome *Definition and History.* This rare autosomal recessive disease initially was recognized as a disorder in which neutrophils, monocytes, and lymphocytes contained giant cytoplasmic granules (Fig. 66-5).[218] Chédiak-Higashi syndrome (CHS) now is recognized as a disorder of generalized cellular dysfunction characterized by increased fusion of cytoplasmic granules.[219] Pigmentary dilution affecting the hair, skin, and ocular fundi results from pathologic aggregation of melanosomes and is associated with a decreased failure of decussation of the optic and auditory nerves (Table 66-2).[220] Patients with this syndrome exhibit an increased susceptibility to infection that begins in infancy. Infections most commonly involve the skin and respiratory systems. The susceptibility to infection can be explained in part by defects in neutrophil chemotaxis, degranulation, and bactericidal activity.[218] The presence of giant granules in the neutrophils interferes with their ability to traverse narrow passages between endothelial cells. Other features of the disease include neutropenia,[220] thrombocytopathy,[221] natural killer (NK) cell abnormalities,[218,222] and peripheral neuropathies.[223] Similar genetic syndromes have been described in mice, mink, cats, rats, cattle, and killer whales.[223]

TABLE 66-2   CLINICAL DISORDERS OF NEUTROPHIL FUNCTION

DISORDER	ETIOLOGY	IMPAIRED FUNCTION	CLINICAL CONSEQUENCE
Degranulation abnormalities			
Chédiak-Higashi syndrome	Autosomal recessive; disordered coalescence of lysosomal granules; autosomal recessive; disordered coalescence of liposomal granules, responsible gene is CHS1 or LYST, which encodes a protein hypothesized to regulate granule fusion	Decreased neutrophil chemotaxis, degranulation and bactericidal activity; platelet storage pool defect; impaired NK function; failure to disperse melanosomes	Neutropenia; recurrent pyogenic infections, propensity to develop marked hepatosplenomegaly in the accelerated phase; pigment dilution in skin and fundus and neuropathies
Specific granule deficiency	Autosomal recessive; functional loss of myeloid transcription factor arising from a mutation of C/EBP_ε, which regulates specific granule formation	Impaired chemotaxis and bactericidal activity; bilobed nuclei in neutrophils; reduced content of neutrophil defensins, gelatinase, collagenase, vitamin B_{12}-binding protein, lactoferrin	Recurrent deep-seated abscesses
Adhesion abnormalities			
Leukocyte adhesion deficiency-1	Autosomal recessive; absences of CD11/CD18 surface adhesive glycoprotein (β_2-integrins) on leukocyte membranes most commonly arising from failure to express CD18 mRNA	Decreased binding of C3bi to neutrophils and impaired adhesion to ICAM-1 and ICAM-2	Neutrophilia, recurrent bacterial infection associated with a lack of pus formation
Leukocyte adhesion deficiency-2	Autosomal recessive; loss of fucosylation of ligands for selectins and other glycol-conjugates arising from mutations of the GDP-fucose transporter	Decreased adhesion to activated endothelium expressing endothelial-leukocyte adhesion molecule	Neutrophilia; recurrent bacterial infection without pus
Neutrophil actin dysfunction	Altered polymerization of neutrophil cytoplasmic actin, perhaps arising from the presence of an inhibitor to F-actin formation	Impaired neutrophil adhesion, chemotaxis, and bacterial killing	Neutrophilia, recurrent bacterial infections without pus
Disorders of cell motility			
Enhanced motile responses			
Familial Mediterranean Fever	Autosomal recessive gene responsible for FMF on chromosome 16, which encodes for the protein "pyrin"; pyrin may modify macrophage activation and release of cytokines known to recruit neutrophils to sites of inflammation	Excessive accumulation of neutrophils at inflamed sites, which may result from neutrophil inhibiting C5a activity	Recurrent fever, peritonitis, pleuritis, arthritis, and amyloidosis
Depressed motile responses			
Defects in the generation of chemotactic signals	IgG deficiencies; C3 and properdin deficiency can arise from genetic or acquired abnormalities; mannose-binding protein deficiency predominantly in neonates	Deficiency of serum chemotaxis and opsonic activities	Recurrent pyogenic infections
Intrinsic defects of the neutrophil, e.g. leukocyte adhesion deficiency, Chédiak-Higashi syndrome, specific granule deficiency, neutrophil actin dysfunction, neonatal neutrophils	Neonatal neutrophil has diminished ability to express β_2-integrins and qualitative impairment in β_2-integrin function	Diminished chemotaxis	Propensity to develop pyogenic infections
Direct inhibition of neutrophil mobility, e.g. drugs	Ethanol, glucocorticoids, cAMP	Impaired locomotion, ingestion, and adherence	Possible cause for frequent infections; neutrophilia seen with epinephrine is the result of cAMP release from endothelium
Immune complexes	Bind to Fc receptors on neutrophils in patients with rheumatoid arthritis, systemic lupus erythematosus, other inflammatory states	Impaired chemotaxis	Recurrent pyogenic infections
Hyperimmunoglobulin E syndrome	Autosomal dominant; variable expression of a soluble inhibitor from mononuclear cells affecting neutrophil chemotaxis; high levels of antistaphylococcal IgE	Impaired chemotaxis at times; impaired IgG opsonization of *S. aureus*	Recurrent skin and sinopulmonary infections
Defects of microbicidal activity			
Chronic granulomatous disease	X-linked and autosomal recessive; failure to express functional gp91^{phox} in the phagocyte membrane in p22^{phox} (autosomal recessive); other autosomal recessive forms of CGD arise from failure to express protein p47^{phox} or p67^{phox}	Failure to activate neutrophil respiratory burst leading to failure to kill catalase-positive microbes	Recurrent pyogenic infections with catalase-positive microorganisms
G-6-PD deficiency	Less than 5% of normal activity of G-6-PD	Failure to activate NADPH-dependent oxidase	Infections with catalase-positive microorganisms
Myeloperoxidase deficiency	Autosomal recessive; failure to process modified precursor protein arising from missense mutation	H_2O_2-dependent antimicrobial activity not potentiated by myeloperoxidase	None
Rac2 deficiency	Autosomal recessive; dominant negative inhibitor by mutant protein of Rac2 mediated functions	Absent receptor mediated O_2^- generation and chemotaxis	Neutrophilia, recurrent bacterial infections
Deficiencies of glutathione reductase and glutathione synthetase	Failure to detoxify H_2O_2	Excessive formation of H_2O_2	Minimal problems with recurrent pyogenic infections

C = complement; CD = cluster designation; CGD = chronic granulomatous disease; FMF = familial Mediterranean fever; G-6-PD = glucose 6-phosphate dehydrogenase; ICAM = intracellular adhesion molecule; NK = natural killer.
Modified from Curnutte JT, Boxer LA: Clinically significant phagocytic cell defects, in *Current Clinical Topics in Infectious Diseases*, 6th ed, edited by JS Remington, MN Swartz, p. 144. McGraw-Hill, New York, 1985.

Although CHS carries the names of Moises Chédiak and Ototaka Higashi, the disorder was first described in 1943 by Béguez-César, a Cuban pediatrician.[224] Initially characterized by neutropenia and abnormal granules in leukocytes, the syndrome was further delineated in 1948 by Steinbrinck's description of a second case.[225] In 1952, Chédiak reported the hematologic characteristics of the disorder,[226] and in 1953 Higashi emphasized the giant peroxidase-containing granules within patients' neutrophils.[227] Besides the susceptibility of infections, patients often suffer a fatal lymphohistiocytic infiltration known as the accelerated phase, which occurs months after birth to several years later.[223]

Epidemiology.   In 1972, 59 cases of CHS were reported.[228] By 1989, 200 cases worldwide were described, with concentrations in the United States, Japan, Northern Europe, and Latin America.[223] Patients of African descent also have been described.

Etiology and Pathogenesis.   Although the basic mechanism underlying CHS is unknown, alterations in membrane fusion likely play an important role.[218,229–231] CHS appears to be caused by a fundamental defect in granule morphogenesis that results in abnormally large granules in multiple tissues. Giant granules are seen in Schwann cells, leukocytes, and macrophages of the liver and spleen and in certain cells of the pancreas, gastric mucosa, kidney, adrenal gland, and pituitary gland. Giant melanosomes form and prevent even distribution of melanin, which results in pigmentary dilution of the hair, skin, iris, and optic fundus. Although the giant lysosomes are the primary morphologic feature of the disorder, only cells relying on the secretion of these lysosomes manifest pathologic defects. In the early stages of myelopoiesis, some of the normal-sized azurophil granules coalesce to form giant granules that result in large secondary lysosomes containing reduced content of hydrolytic enzymes, including proteinases, elastase, and cathepsin G. Many of the myeloid precursors die in the marrow, resulting in a moderate neutropenia, with white cell counts of approximately 2.5×10^9/liter.[232] The marrow itself appears normal to hypercellular. Despite normal ingestion of particles and active oxygen metabolism, these neutrophils kill microorganisms relatively slowly. The delay reflects a slow and inconsistent delivery of diluted amounts of hydrolytic enzymes from the giant granules into the phagosomes, which may predispose the host to bacterial infection.[207,231] In this syndrome, monocytes have the same functional derangements as neutrophils.[218] In an analogous fashion, perforin-deficient NK cells show profoundly impaired cytotoxic activity and are unable to kill many targets.[233]

CHS blood cell membranes are more fluid than cells of normal individuals.[218,229] The altered membrane structure could lead to defective regulation of membrane activation. Conceivably, changes in membrane fluidity may affect cell function by altering expression of membrane receptors. This, in turn, could result in elevated levels of intracellular cyclic adenosine monophosphate, disordered assembly of microtubules, and defective interaction of microtubules with lysosome membranes, which appear in this disorder and are reflected in the reduced chemotactic responses.[218]

The gene that is mutated in CHS predicts protein of more than 400 kDa, known as CHS1 or *LYST*.[234] During early development, granule biogenesis is normal. Perforin in NK cells and granule enzymes in myeloid cells are synthesized and routed correctly to the granules. However, once formed the granules fuse to form giant organelles.[235] Several studies led to the suggestion that the enlarged lysosomes found in CHS cells result from abnormalities in membrane fusion, which could occur during the biogenesis of the lysosomes. This CHS1 protein has been hypothesized to interact with attachment proteins on lysosomes (v-SNAREs), with the mutated protein leading to indiscriminate interactions with v-SNARE and yielding uncontrolled fusion of lysosomes with each other.[236]

Clinical Features.   Patients with CHS characteristically have light skin and silvery hair. They frequently complain of solar sensitivity and photophobia. Other eye findings can include horizontal or rotatory nystagmus. Infections are common and involve the mucous membranes, skin, and respiratory tract. Patients are susceptible to gram-positive and gram-negative bacteria and to fungi, with *Staphylococcus aureus* the most common infecting organism. Attenuated NK function probably contributes to the increased susceptibility to infection. Neurologic signs and symptoms are variable in CHS and may include a peripheral and cranial neuropathy, autonomic dysfunction, weakness, and sensory deficit. Ataxia may be a prominent feature.

Patients with CHS have prolonged bleeding times with normal platelet counts resulting from impaired platelet aggregation associated with a deficiency of the storage pools of adenosine diphosphate and serotonin.[221] Electron micrographs reveal normal numbers of α-granules in platelets but decreased numbers of platelet dense bodies.[223]

The accelerated phase of CHS is characterized by lymphocytic proliferation in the liver, spleen, and bone marrow. The accelerated phase may occur at any age. Typically the patient develops hepatosplenomegaly and high fever in the absence of bacterial sepsis. Pancytopenia becomes worse at this stage, producing hemorrhage and an increased susceptibility to infection. Onset of the accelerated phase may be related to the inability of patients to contain and control the Epstein-Barr virus, leading to features simulating viral-mediated hemophagocytic syndrome (see Chap. 72).[237,238] Lymphocyte expansion into the tissue is associated with excessive cytokine production and massive tissue necrosis and organ failure leading to the propensity for recurrent bacterial viral infections, fever, and prostration usually resulting in death.[239] At autopsy, the lymphohistiocytic infiltrates in the liver, spleen, and lymph nodes are extensive but not neoplastic by histopathologic criteria.[218,239]

Laboratory Features.   Currently the only laboratory test diagnostic for CHS is examination of granular cell morphology. The pathognomonic feature is giant peroxidase-positive granules that can be seen in neutrophils.[227] Microscopic examination of hair shafts reveal large, speckled pigment clumps rather than the normal pattern of finally divided pigment of melanin spread along the length of the shaft.[223] Similar giant granules can be present in chronic myelogenous leukemia and acute myelocytic leukemia.[223] Molecular diagnosis of CHS remains difficult and is not commercially available. Heterozygotes for CHS are considered completely normal and cannot be detected clinically or biochemically.

Differential Diagnosis.   Diagnosis of CHS should be considered in individuals with partial albinism, normal bleeding, and recurrent infections. Patients with CHS must be distinguished from patients with Griscelli syndrome and Hermansky-Pudlak syndrome.

Griscelli syndrome is a rare disorder defined by partial ocular and cutaneous albinism, variable cellular and humeral immunodeficiency, variable neurologic involvement, and development of the accelerated phase. Individuals with Griscelli syndrome lack the giant granules present in CHS cells.[223] Hermansky-Pudlak syndrome is a disorder of ocular and cutaneous albinism, bleeding diathesis, and deposition of ceroid lipofuscin in various organs. In contrast to CHS, Hermansky-Pudlak syndrome cells lack giant granules, and patients are not predisposed to recurrent infections.[223]

Therapy, Course, and Prognosis.   High-dose ascorbic acid (200 mg/day for infants, 2 g/day for adults) improves the clinical status of some patients in the stable phase.[218] Although controversy exists regarding the efficacy of ascorbic acid, its administration to all patients seems reasonable given the safety of the vitamin.[223] CHS presents a therapeutic dilemma, particularly when the accelerated phase begins. Prophylactic antibiotics do not prevent infections. The only curative therapy for the accelerated phase is marrow transplantation from an

HLA-compatible donor or an unrelated donor compatible at the D locus.[240,241] Marrow transplantation constitutes normal hematopoietic and immunologic function and corrects the NK deficiency in patients entering the accelerated phase.[240] Ocular and cutaneous albinisms are not corrected after transplantation. Whether transplantation will prevent development of neuropathies remains to be determined.

Specific Granule Deficiency SGD has been described in five patients of both sexes and likely is inherited as an autosomal recessive disorder (see Table 66-2).[218] Besides the absence of specific granules, the nuclei of the neutrophils are bilobed. Patients are afflicted with recurrent infections primarily involving the skin and lungs. *Staphylococcus aureus* and *Pseudomonas aeruginosa* have been the most commonly observed pathogens, although *Candida albicans* also has been isolated. Specific granule-deficient neutrophils lack gelatinolytic activity in the tertiary granules; vitamin B_{12}-binding protein, lactoferrin, and collagenase in the specific granules; and defensins in the primary granules.[242–244] The disorder also extends to eosinophils that lack the characteristic eosinophil granule proteins: major basic protein, eosinophilic cationic protein, and eosinophil-derived neurotoxin (see Chap. 62).[245] Thus, the disorder is a global defect of phagocytic granules rather than limited to specific granules, as suggested by the name of the disorder. Neutrophils from these patients are defective in chemotaxis, possibly related to the absence of the intracellular pool of leukocyte adhesion molecules that normally reside in the tertiary and specific granules and a mild defect in bactericidal activity, possibly related to the deficiency of the granule constituents lactoferrin and defensins.[242,246] Impairment of granule protein synthesis affecting the granulocytic cells appears secondary to functional loss of the myeloid transcription factor C/EBP-ε, which has been identified in two patients.[80,247] In another case of SGD, detectable mutations in the C/EBP-ε genomic locus was not identified, indicating the disorder is a heterogenous disease arising from different underlying mechanisms.[248,249] The defect is restricted to blood cells, as normal lactoferrin secretion has been demonstrated in the nasal secretions of a SGD patient despite the abnormality present in his neutrophils.[243]

The diagnosis of SGD is suggested by the presence of neutrophils devoid of specific granules but containing azurophilic granules on the blood film.[218] Electron microscopy reveals small peroxidase-negative vesicles presumably representing empty specific granules.[250] The diagnosis can be confirmed by demonstrating a severe deficiency in either lactoferrin or vitamin B_{12}-binding protein. An acquired form of SGD can be observed in thermally injured patients or in individuals with myelodysplasia.[218,251] Treatment of SGD is symptomatic, with administration of parenteral antibiotics for acute infections and surgical drainage of refractory infections. Patients may survive into their adult years with aggressive medical management.

ADHESION ABNORMALITIES

LEUKOCYTE ADHESION DEFICIENCY

Definition and History Leukocyte adhesion deficiency (LAD) type 1 (LAD-1) is a rare autosomal recessive disorder of leukocyte function (see Table 66-2). Approximately 80 cases have been reported worldwide. The disease is characterized clinically by recurrent soft-tissue infections, delayed wound healing, and severely impaired pus formation despite striking blood neutrophilia.[252] Individuals with the disorder have decreased or absent expression of a family of structurally and functionally related leukocyte surface glycoproteins designated CD11/CD18 complex (also referred to as the β_2-integrin family of leukocyte adhesive proteins; Table 66-3). The proteins include lymphocyte function-associated antigen-1 (LFA-1; CD11a/CD18), Mo-1 or Mac-1 (CD11b/CD18), and p150,95 (CD11c/CD18).[252] The CD11 subunits are integral membrane glycoproteins, each spanning the

plasma membrane only once. They are approximately 40 percent homologous, suggesting they arise from a common primordial gene.[252] The three distinct genes encoding the γ-subunits occur in a cluster on chromosome 16, whereas the gene for the β-subunit is located on chromosome 21.[253]

The initial clinical report in 1979 described six children and two families with findings of delayed separation of the umbilical cord and delayed healing at the site of detachment of the cord, recurrent infections despite neutrophilia, neutrophilia persisting during infection-free periods, and impaired neutrophil chemotaxis.[254] The molecular basis for LAD-1 was first suggested by Crowley and colleagues,[255] who found that neutrophils from a patient with the disorder lacked a high molecular weight membrane glycoprotein. They suggested that the lack of the membrane protein impaired the neutrophil's functional responses. In 1982, Arnaout and co-workers[256] evaluated another patient and confirmed that the membrane glycoprotein with a molecular weight of 150 kDa was missing. They determined that clinically normal parents and siblings of the proband exhibited intermediate quantities of the glycoprotein, suggesting the existence of a heterozygous carrier state. The innate disorder then became known as LAD. Subsequently in 1984, Dana and colleagues[257] identified glycoprotein 150 as one subunit of a glycoprotein having two parts that served as a receptor for a plasma complement component. Subsequently other investigators found that two other related leukocyte membrane glycoproteins also were deficient. Each of the three glycoproteins then was determined to be heterodimers with one identical subunit and one subunit unique to each glycoprotein.[258] Springer and colleagues[259] established that synthesis of a defective subunit common to the three glycoproteins of CD11/CD18 complex resulted in loss of expression of all three heterodimers. The mutant gene led to expression of a defective subunit common to each of the three glycoproteins in the complex, yielding a deficiency of the entire complex. This observation provided the molecular explanation for the cellular defect. In 1985, Anderson and co-workers[258] correlated the extent of clinical severity and magnitude of the cellular abnormalities with the degree of CD11/CD18 deficiency, laying the groundwork for the direct relationship between glycoprotein deficiency and the clinical presentation.

Etiology and Pathogenesis Each of these molecules contains an α- and a β-subunit noncovalently associated in an αβ structure. They all have the same β-subunit and are distinguished by their α-subunits, which have different isoelectric points, molecular weights, and cell distribution (see Table 66-3).[252] The structure of CD11/CD18 has been deduced from molecular cloning of the various subunits.[258] These studies established that CD11/CD18 are members of a large gene family involved in cell-to-cell and cell-to-matrix adhesion (integrins).[260] Several subfamilies of integrins have been described and classified according to the type of their highly homologous β subunits.[261] The α-subunits also are homologous to each other but to a lesser degree than are the associated β-subunits. Within each subfamily, a single β-subunit usually is shared by several α-subunits. Certain α-subunits often share more than one β-subunit, which alters their specificity for various ligands.[258] The molecular defect involves all three members of the CD11 integrin subfamily. In patients with LAD-1 who have been evaluated at the molecular level, absent, diminished, or structurally abnormal β-subunits (CD18) have been identified.[258] A heterogeneous group of mutations confined to the gene on chromosome 21q22.3 has been identified.[258] Many patients have point mutations that result in single amino acid substitutions in CD18, which predominantly resides between amino acids 111 and 361.[258] This peptide domain is highly conserved among all β-subunits and appears to be important for interaction with the α-subunit. Several affected individuals are compound heterozygotes for two different mutant alleles, whereas others are homozygotes for a single mutant allele. Messenger RNA splicing

TABLE 66-3   BIOLOGICAL AND CLINICAL FEATURES OF LEUKOCYTE ADHERENCE DEFICIENCY

THE CD11/CD18 FAMILY	LEUKOCYTE FUNCTIONAL ABNORMALITIES*	CLINICAL FEATURES*
Mac-1 (CD11b/CD18): molecular mass of α-chain 170 kDa; found on monocytes; neutrophils, NK cells; receptor for C3bi (CR3) function, i.e., adherence, and antibody-dependent cellular cytotoxicity	Neutrophils: adherence, spreading, aggregation, chemotaxis receptor CR3 activities (C3bi-binding phagocytosis, respiratory burst, and degranulation in response to C3bi-coated particles), antibody-dependent cellular cytotoxicity	Autosomal recessive; delayed umbilical cord separation; neutrophilia; defective neutrophil mobilization; recurrent bacterial infection without pus; impaired wound recurrent bacterial (sometimes life-threatening) bacterial infections
LFA-1 (CD11a/CD18): molecular mass of α-chain 170 kDa; found on all human leukocytes; adhesion-promoting molecule for leukocytes; facilitates NK binding, cytolytic T-lymphocyte-mediated killing, and helper T-cell response p150,95 (CD11c/CD18): molecular mass of α-chain 150 kDa; found on monocytes and neutrophils; promotes neutrophil and monocyte adhesion	Monocytes: adherence, CR3 activities Lymphocytes: cytotoxic T-lymphocytes activities, NK activities, blastogenesis	

* These functional abnormalities and clinical features are a consequence of lack of the CD11/CD18 complex, which includes CD11a, CD11b, CD11c markers of three different α-chains and the common β-chain CD18 of molecular mass 95 kDa.

abnormalities described in two kindreds can result in either deletion or insertion of amino acids in the conserved extracellular domain of CD18. Small deletions within the coding sequences of the CD18 gene disrupting the reading frame or a nucleotide substitution resulting in a premature termination signal has been described. Mutations in CD18 disrupt the association in the $\alpha\beta$ subunits so that maturation, intracellular transport, and all cell surface assembly of functionally active $\alpha\beta$ molecules fail to occur.[258] Approximately half of patients exhibit a low level of CD11/CD18 cell surface molecules and moderate disease. The remainder of patients have totally absent surface expression of these proteins, which accounts for a profound impairment of neutrophil and monocyte adherence and adhesion-dependent functions in vitro, including cell migration, phagocytosis, and complement- or antibody-dependent cytotoxicity.[259,262]

Besides the requirement for surface expression of the CD11/CD18, the molecules must undergo posttranslational modification during leukocyte activation.[263] Two compound heterozygotes have a mutation that results in impaired expression and dysfunction of the β_2 gene and reportedly causes variant LAD-1.[264,265] The levels of β_2-integrins were approximately 60 percent of control in each case, which was sufficient for normal adhesive function.[258] Transfection studies indicated that each subject had one mutation that did not support surface expression in β_2 heterodimers, accounting for the reduced levels on the membrane of leukocytes, and a second allele that resulted in surface expression of heterodimers that did not bind ligands. Changes in confirmation in the function of the I-like domain of β_2, which is critical for ligand recognition, probably accounts for the adhesion defect.[9]

A second type of variant LAD-1 is consistent with impaired inside-out signaling. Sequence analysis of the β-chain from a patient who had an LAD-1–like phenotype and myelodysplasia[266] and another similar patient[267] revealed no mutations. However, primary leukocytes and transformed lymphoblasts from these patients were deficient in their ability to activate constitutively expressed surface β_2 heterodimers in response to extracellular stimuli, indicating intracellular inside-out signaling pathways were deficient. In one patient, platelets also were involved.[267] In the other patient, markedly impaired β_1-integrin adhesion[266] was observed, indicating the occurrence of defective inside-out signaling mediated by integrin $\alpha_2\beta_3$ on the platelets. The mechanism accounting for inside-out signaling of the β_1-, β_2-, and β_3-integrins remains elusive.

The bulk of the neutrophil Mac-1 glycoprotein is stored inside the cell in the membrane of neutrophil-specific gelatinase granules and in secretory vesicles.[20,268] Exposure of neutrophils to degranulating stimuli results in a 5- to 10-fold increase in the number of Mac-1 molecules on the cell surface, which parallels the fusion of granules to the plasma membrane.[268] Neutrophils from these patients fail to augment their surface adhesive glycoproteins, as the defect in β-subunit synthesis affects both membrane and granule pools of Mac-1.[269] In contrast to Mac-1 and p150,95, LFA-1 is predominantly confined to the neutrophil plasma membrane. Consequently, the cell surface levels of LFA-1 are not enhanced by neutrophil degranulation.

Lymphocytes deficient in CD11/CD18 can adhere to endothelial surfaces via expression on lymphocytes of very late activation-4 (VLA-4) integrin receptors, which bind to the vascular wall adhesion molecule-1 (VCAM-1) found on endothelial cells.[270] This residual adhesion may account for the paucity of clinical symptoms related to lymphocyte function.

The failure of LAD-1 neutrophils to migrate to the sites of inflammation outside of the lung and peritoneum arises from their inability to adhere firmly to surfaces and undergo transendothelial migration from venules.[271–273] Failure of LAD-1–deficient neutrophils to undergo transendothelial migration occurs because β_2-integrins bind to intercellular adhesion molecule-1 (CD54) and intercellular adhesion molecule-2 (ICAM-2) expressed on inflamed endothelial cells.[252,274] LAD-1 neutrophils can accumulate in the lung, perhaps through a process movement mediated by chimneying that does not require functional integrins.[275] The neutrophils that do arrive at inflammatory sites in the inflamed lung by CD11/CD18-independent processes fail to recognize microorganisms coated with the opsonic complement fragment C3bi (an important stable opsonin formed by cleavage of C3b by C3b inactivator).[252,260] Other neutrophil functions, such as degranulation and oxidative metabolism, normally triggered by C3bi binding, also are diminished or markedly compromised in patients from LAD-1.[252] Similarly, urokinase-plasminogen activator receptors and Fcγ RIII receptors, both phosphatidylinositol-linked proteins, are defective in their functions because these receptors transduce their signals through CD11/CD18.[173,276] Monocyte function also is impaired. Monocytes of affected individuals have poor fibrinogen-binding function, an activity promoted by the CD11/CD18 complex.[252,277] Consequently, such cells are not able to participate effectively in wound healing. Thus, impairment in neutrophil function underlies the propensity to recurrent infections, which is the clinical expression of this disease. Similar genetic syndromes have been discovered in Irish Setter dogs and Holstein cattle.[258] A CD11/CD18-deficient mouse with 2 to 6 percent normal β_2-integrin expression has been produced by gene targeting.[271,278]

Clinical Features   Activated leukocytes of patients with the most severe clinical form express less than 0.3 percent of the normal amount of the β_2-integrins. Activated leukocytes of patients with the moderate phenotype may express 2 to 7 percent of the normal number of β_2-integrin molecules.[252] Severely affected patients suffer from recurrent and chronic or even gangrenous soft-tissue infections (subcutaneous tissues or mucous membranes), generally by bacterial or fungal microorganisms such as *S. aureus, Pseudomonas* species and other gram-negative enteric rods, or *Candida* species. Patients with the moderate phenotype have fewer and less severe infections. Infectious susceptibility and impaired wound healing are related to diminished or delayed infiltration of neutrophils and monocytes into extravascular inflammatory sites. Severe progressive generalized periodontitis is present in all patients surviving infancy. Individuals who are clinically well but are heterozygous carriers of LAD have been identified. Their stimulated neutrophils express approximately 50 percent of the normal amount of the Mac-1 α-subunit and the common β-subunit.[252]

Laboratory Features The diagnosis is made most readily by flow cytometric measurement of surface CD11b in stimulated and unstimulated neutrophils using monoclonal antibodies directed against CD11b (Fig. 66-6). Assessment of neutrophil and monocyte adherence, aggregation, chemotaxis, C3bi-mediated phagocytosis, and cytotoxicity generally demonstrate striking abnormalities directly related to the molecular deficiency. Delayed-type hypersensitivity reactions are normal, and most individuals have normal specific antibody synthesis. The ability of lymphocytes to generate specific antibodies ex-

plains the self-limited course of varicella or viral respiratory infections. However, some patients have impaired T lymphocyte-dependent antibody responses, for example, to repeat vaccination with tetanus toxoid, diphtheria toxoid, and polio virus.

Patients with LAD-1 usually have blood neutrophil counts of 15 to 60 × 10⁹/liter. However, during infectious episodes, they commonly have neutrophil counts greater than 100 × 10⁹/liter and sometimes as high as 160 × 10⁹/liter. Granulocytic hyperplasia is a feature of the marrow examination and may be related to excessive production of IL-17 and granulocyte colony stimulating factor.[279] Despite elevated blood counts, neutrophils in inflammatory skin windows and biopsies of infected tissues are scarce.

Differential Diagnosis Five patients with neutrophilia, recurrent bacterial infections, and an inability to form pus have been described.[9] The patients also had the Bombay blood phenotype (deficiency in H blood group integrins) and mental retardation. Functionally, the neutrophils were unable to adhere to E-selectin or cytokine-activated endothelial cells and exhibited impaired chemotaxis and an inability to roll on postcapillary venules *in vivo*. The patients now are classified as having LAD type 2 (LAD-2). In contrast to LAD-1, in LAD-2 the patient's NK cell activity is normal. LAD-2 neutrophils express normal levels of CD18 integrins but are deficient in the carbohydrate structure sLeˣ, which renders the cells unable to roll on activated endothelial

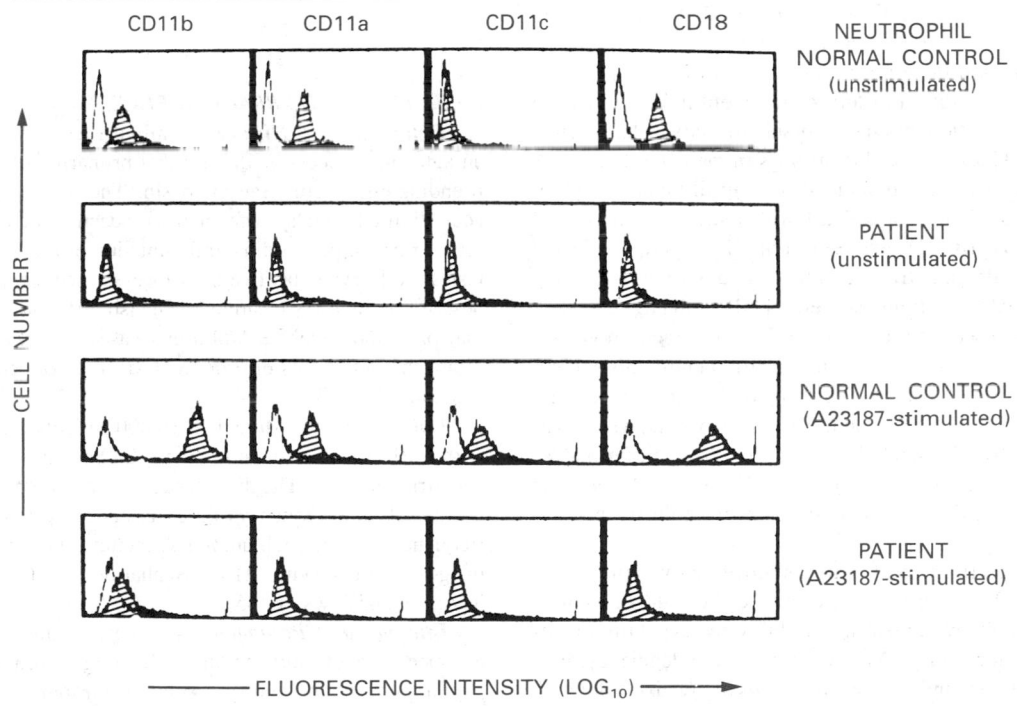

FIGURE 66-6 Specific diagnosis of CD11/CD18 glycoprotein deficiency by indirect immunofluorescence flow cytometric analysis. Blood neutrophils of a pediatric patient suspected of having CD11/CD18 glycoprotein deficiency and those of an abnormal individual were subjected to immunofluorescence staining for expression of the CD11b, CD11a, CD11c, and CD18 epitope *(cross-hatched histograms)* and compared with background immunofluorescence staining by isotype-identical negative-control antibodies *(open histograms)*. Neutrophils were stained either immediately after purification by Ficoll-Hypaque density centrifugation (unstimulated) or after exposure to calcium ionophore A23187 (1 mM) for 15 minutes at 37°C (A23187-stimulated). A23187 stimulation causes significant increase in CD11b and CD18 epitope staining (surface MO1 expression) by normal neutrophils compared with unstimulated normal cells. A23187 stimulation also causes a small increase in CD11b epitope expression of patient cells (CD11b cross-hatched histogram becomes distinguishable from background staining after A23187 stimulation), suggesting this patient has a "moderate" form of the disorder (capable of expressing small but detectable quantities of CD11/CD18 glycoproteins). Flow cytometric analysis was performed using a Coulter Electronics EPICS F C Flow Cytometer with a logarithmic amplifier. (From Todd R, Freyer DR, *Hematol Oncol Clin North Am* 2:13, 1988, with permission).

cells expressing E-selectin. Thus, neutrophils from the patients categorized as having LAD-2 are unable to tether to inflamed venules, which is necessary for subsequent activation (see Chap. 16). LAD-2 appears to be explained by a congenital disorder of fucosylation of ligands for selectins and other glycoconjugates. Each of the three selectins binds with variable affinity to sialylated and fucosylated oligosaccharides including sLe^X, which is present on multiple specific glycolipids and glycoproteins on leukocytes and activated endothelial cells.[9] Neutrophils from LAD-2 subjects lack sLe^X, which leads to impaired neutrophil rolling on endothelial cells. Other fucosylated determinants, including the H, Lewis, and secretor blood group antigens, also are lacking, suggesting a global defect in fucosylation. Diminished fucosylation arises from impaired transport of glucose diphosphate (GDP)-fucose from the cytoplasm to the Golgi lumen.[279] A human GDP-fucose transporter that localizes to the Golgi apparatus is defective secondary to distinct mutations in the gene encoding the transporter.[9] When fibroblasts and lymphoblastoid cells derived from an LAD-2 patient were grown in the presence of millimolar concentrations of fucose, cell surface fucosylation could be restored. Following this observation, oral administration of L-fucose to two Turkish patients led to normalization of neutrophil counts and functional E- and P-selectin ligands on myeloid cells.[9] In contrast to the Turkish patients, two Arab patients with different mutations of the gene encoding the putative GDP-fucose transporter did not respond to oral fucose.[9] Like the Turkish patients, a Brazilian LAD-2 patient initially benefited from oral fucose but, after expression of sLe^x on the myeloid cells, the patient developed autoimmune neutropenia.[280]

Therapy, Course, and Prognosis   Treatment of LAD-1 is largely supportive.[252,258] Patients with a history of recurrent infections can be maintained on prophylactic trimethoprim-sulfamethoxazole. Marrow transplantation with HLA-compatible siblings or parental donors has resulted in engraftment and restoration of neutrophil function and remains the treatment of choice for patients with a severe phenotype.[281]

Restoration of CD11/CD18 expression in CD34 peripheral stem cells from LAD-1 following transduction with a retrovirus bearing CD18 and induced to differentiate into neutrophils with growth factors indicates LAD-1 is caused by a defective CD18 gene and provides a basis for somatic gene therapy.[282] Not only did the neutrophils express the integrins, but the cells demonstrated improvement in their functional responses, such as adhesion and the respiratory burst when challenged with ligands for CD11/CD18. These results indicate that *ex vivo* transfer of the gene for CD18 into LAD-1 CD34+ cells followed by reinfusion of the transfused cells may represent a therapeutic approach for LAD.

The severity of infectious complications correlates with the degree of β_2 deficiency.[269] Patients with severe deficiency may die in infancy, and those surviving infancy have a susceptibility to severe life-threatening systemic infections. In patients with moderate deficiency, life-threatening infections are infrequent and survival relatively long.[269] Fetal blood sampling and flow cytometric analysis for expression of CD11/CD18 integrins can be used for prenatal diagnosis of LAD-1.[283] However, contamination of the sample by maternal blood can complicate interpretation of the analysis.

NEUTROPHIL ACTIN DYSFUNCTION

Like patients with LAD, patients with neutrophil actin dysfunction have recurrent pyogenic infections from birth as a result of defective chemotactic and phagocytic response (see Table 66-2). In one patient, actin isolated from blood and neutrophils could not polymerize under conditions that fully polymerized the actin of neutrophils from normal individuals.[284] Subsequent studies on the index patient's family confirmed that partial actin dysfunction was present in the parents and one sister.[285] One of the parents was a heterozygote for LAD but the

other was not.[286] Further studies established that LAD is not generally associated with defective actin filament assembly.[287] The basis of the defective polymerization of actin in the index patient remains unknown, but this disorder of phagocytes is distinct from LAD.

Defective actin polymerization has been described in a 2-month-old infant with severe recurrent bacterial infections associated with impaired chemotaxis and phagocytic response.[288] The patient's neutrophils showed increased expression of CD11b, which distinguished the patient's clinical problem from LAD-1. Morphologically the neutrophils displayed thin, filamentous projections of membrane with an underlying abnormal cytoskeletal structure. A 47-kDa protein that inhibited actin polymerization *in vitro* subsequently was purified.[289] Further biochemical studies revealed a markedly defective actin polymerization in the patient's neutrophils, a severe deficiency of an 89-kDa protein, and an elevated level of the 47-kDa protein. The 47-kDa protein has been identified as lymphocyte-specific protein-1 (LSP-1), which is an actin-binding protein present in normal neutrophils. Overexpression of LSP-1 has resulted in bundling of actin in cells, leading to an abnormal cytoskeletal structure and motility defects.[290] Because actin dysfunction is lethal, treatment requires restoration of normal neutrophil function by marrow replacement from a normal donor. Bone marrow transplantation was attempted in both infants. The bone marrow transplantation was not successful in the first infant but was successful in the second infant with neutrophil actin dysfunction associated with overexpression of the 47-kDa protein.[288,291]

DISORDERS OF NEUTROPHIL MOTILITY

FAMILIAL MEDITERRANEAN FEVER

Definition and History   Familial Mediterranean fever (FMF) is an autosomal recessive disease that primarily affects populations surrounding the Mediterranean basin. The disease is characterized by acute limited attacks of fever often accompanied by pleuritis, peritonitis, arthritis, pericarditis, inflammation of the tunica vaginalis of the testes, and erysipelas-like skin disease (see Table 66-2). The initial description in 1908 identified a Jewish girl who had episodic abdominal pain and fever.[292] Additional cases later were identified,[293] but establishment of this disorder as FMF did not occur for nearly a half a century.[294]

Epidemiology   More than 10,000 patients worldwide are affected with FMF. It occurs predominantly in Sephardic Jews, Arabs, Turks, and Armenians.[292] The disorder can occur in other populations, but it is unusual. The frequency of the susceptibility gene varies widely. The frequency is very high among Armenians (1:7 ratio of persons with the gene to those without) and Sephardic Jews (1:5–1:16) but is lower in Ashkenazi Jews (1:135).

Etiology and Pathogenesis   The pathologic finding in FMF is nonspecific acute inflammation affecting serosal tissues such as the pleura, peritoneum, and synovium. Neutrophilic infiltration predominates in the affected tissues. Physical and emotional stress, menstruation, and a high-fat diet may trigger the attacks.[295]

The gene responsible for FMF is located on chromosome 16. It encodes for a 781-amino-acid protein called pyrin or marenostrin.[296,297] The MEFV gene is predominantly expressed in myeloid cells, and its expression is up-regulated by IFN-γ and TNF and by the process of myeloid differentiation itself.[298] At least 29 mutations in the MEFV gene have been described, most of which are clustered on exons 2 and 10. Founder effects in FMF have been established. The two most common mutations, V726A and M694V, are suggested to originate from common ancestors who lived in the Middle East about 2500 years ago.[296]

The precise function of pyrin is not well defined. One of the four domains of pyrin (known as PYRIN) is suggested to bear homology to a number of proteins involved in apoptosis and inflammation and to be similar to a member of the six-helix-bundle, death domain superfamily, which includes death domains and death effector domains known as caspase recruitment domains (CARDs).[299] The pyrin domain appears to allow for interaction of macromolecular complexes by PYRIN–PYRIN interactions. The interaction has led to identification of pyrin's ability to interact specifically with another PYRIN domain protein termed apoptosis-associated speck-like protein with a CARD (ASC).[300] Besides the amino-terminal pyrin domain, ASC has a C-terminal CARD domain that allows binding to the CARD of procaspase-1 (IL-1β–converting enzyme), which results in procaspase-1 autoactivation.[299] Activated caspase-1 then metabolizes pro–IL-1β to IL-1β, which in turn is secreted and interacts with the IL-1 receptor to mediate inflammation. Pyrin may act as an antiinflammatory molecule by inhibiting ASC-induced IL-1 processing, which in turn could be defective in FMF. This hypothesis is supported by the observation of increased IL-1 processing and impaired lipopolysaccharide and IL-4–induced apoptosis in peritoneal macrophages from pyrin knockout mice. The puzzle remains as to why serosal tissues are the main targets of inflammation in FMF, but aberrant functioning macrophages may be responsible for recruiting neutrophils to the serosal tissue.

Clinical Features The duration and frequency of attacks may vary considerably even in the same patient.[295] Acute attacks frequently last 24 to 48 hours and recur once or twice per month. In some patients, attacks may recur as frequently as several times per week or as infrequently as once per year. Symptoms may persist as long as 1 week during individual episodes. Some patients experience spontaneous remission that persists for years, followed by recurrence of frequent attacks. Peritonitis as a result of FMF may resemble an acute abdomen, thereby leading to potential uncertainties about the clinical management of the acute abdominal episode. Attacks of pleuritic pain occur in approximately 25 to 80 percent of patients. Symptoms of pleuritis may precede abdominal pain, but some patients experience pleuritic attacks without abdominal symptoms. Recurrent pericarditis has been rarely reported. The course of peritonitis in FMF is similar to attacks at other serosal sites but tends to appear at a late stage of the disease. Mild arthralgia is a common feature of febrile attacks, and monoarticular or oligoarticular arthritis may occur. Arthritis usually affects large joints, particularly the knees, and effusions are common. As many as one third of patients experience transient erysipelas-like skin lesions that typically appear on the lower leg, ankle, or dorsum of the foot. The lesions are circumscribed, painful, erythematous areas of swelling that usually subside within 24 to 48 hours.

In approximately 25 percent of affected patients, a form of renal amyloidosis develops in which the amyloid derives from a normal serum protein called serum amyloid A (amyloidosis of the AA type; see Chap. 101). The amyloidosis progresses over a period of years to renal failure in almost all cases, and death in patients with FMF usually is attributed to this complication. Polymorphisms in the gene for serum amyloid A appear to increase the susceptibility to renal amyloidosis, and polymorphisms in a gene for the major histocompatibility complex class 1α chain appear to influence the severity of the disease.[294]

Laboratory Features Laboratory findings in FMF are nonspecific. Nonspecific findings include increases in renal inflammatory mediators such as amyloid A, fibrinogen, and C-reactive protein during febrile attacks.[294] Proteinuria greater than 0.5 g of protein per 24 hours in patients with FMF suggests amyloidosis.

Cloning of the FMF gene now allows a reliable diagnostic test. Using a set of polymerase chain reaction (PCR) primers enables identification of the mutations responsible for the disease. Five founder mutations account for 74 percent of FMF carrier chromosomes from typical populations known to harbor the disease.[301] Carrier rates for FMF mutations may be as high as 1:3 in some populations, suggesting

the disease often is underdiagnosed. Some amino acids that cause human disease often are present in wild-type primates.[302] The mutant is suggested to represent the reappearance of an ancestral amino acid state in response to positive selection not yet defined.

Differential Diagnosis The TNF receptor-associated periodic syndrome (TRAPS) was first described in 1982 in a large Irish family.[303] The affected family members had recurrent fever with localized myalgia and painful erythema. The response of TRAPS to corticosteroids and the autosomal dominant inheritance of TRAPS differentiate the disorder from FMF. Affected patients can have attacks that last for at least 1 or 2 days, but prolonged attacks lasting more than 1 week are common. Localized pain and tightness in one muscle group and a migratory pattern of the symptoms are prominent features. The disorder may be associated with colicky abdominal pain, diarrhea or constipation, nausea, and/or vomiting. Painful conjunctivitis, periorbital edema, or both are common; chest pain secondary to sterile pleuritis also is common.[294] During febrile attacks, painless skin lesions may develop on the trunk or extremities and may migrate distally. Missense mutations in the gene for the type 1 TNF 55-kDa cell membrane receptor have been identified. Patients with TRAPS respond dramatically to high doses of oral prednisone (>20 mg). However, the responses wane with time and require higher doses of corticosteroids. Standard doses of the p75:Fc fusion protein etanercept administered subcutaneously twice weekly decrease the frequency, duration, and severity of attacks. Thus, etanercept may provide a safer, more effective alternative than corticosteroids in controlling the disease.

Therapy, Course, and Prognosis Colchicine treatment is effective in FMF and may prevent the development of amyloidosis.[302] Prophylactic colchicine 0.6 mg orally given two to three times per day prevents or substantially reduces the acute attacks of FMF in most patients. Some patients can abort attacks with intermittent doses of colchicine beginning at the onset of attacks (0.6 mg orally every hour for 4 hours, then every 2 hours for four doses, and then every 12 hours for 2 days). In general, patients who benefit from intermittent colchicine therapy are those who experience a recognizable prodrome before developing fever and clear-cut acute symptoms.

The prognosis for normal longevity of patients has been excellent since the recognition of colchicine efficacy in this disease. Most patients can be maintained almost entirely symptom-free. Amyloidosis, if it develops, may be followed by the nephrotic syndrome or uremia. Unless the patient receives a renal transplant, the likelihood of eventual death from renal failure is high.

OTHER DISORDERS OF NEUTROPHIL MOTILITY

The directed migration of neutrophils from the circulation to an inflammatory site is a consequence of chemotaxis and leads to accumulation of an exudate. A complex series of events must be coordinated for normal chemotaxis to occur. Chemotactic factors must be generated in sufficient quantities to establish a chemotactic gradient. The neutrophils must have receptors for the chemotactic agents and mechanisms for discerning the direction of the chemotactic gradient. Depressed neutrophil chemotaxis has been observed in a wide variety of clinical conditions (see Table 66-2).[208] The conditions can be stratified as follows: (1) defects in the generation of chemotactic signals; (2) intrinsic defects of the neutrophil; and (3) direct inhibitors of neutrophil motility in response to chemotactic factors.

Older patients with chemotactic disorders may be infected by a variety of microorganisms, including fungi and gram-positive or gram-negative bacteria. *Staphylococcus aureus* is the most frequent bacterial offender. Typically, the skin, gingival mucosa, and regional lymph nodes are involved. Respiratory tract infections are frequent, but sepsis is rare. Delayed or inappropriate signs and symptoms of inflammation are common. Although the cells move slowly in Boyden chambers or other chemotactic assays, they accumulate in sufficient numbers in inflammatory sites and produce pus. However, detection of patients with neutrophils that have profound defects in chemotaxis usually is accomplished by other phagocytic assays.

Patients with the hereditary deficiency of complement factors C3, C5, or properidin exhibit an increased incidence of bacterial infections because they are unable to form the chemotactic peptide C5a.[304] The degree to which defective chemotaxis plays a role in C3 deficiency is unclear because opsonization and ingestion rates are abnormal in these disorders. Frequently, chemotactic disorders are associated with other impaired neutrophil functions. For instance, both glycogen storage disease type 1b[305] and Shwachman-Diamond syndrome[306] are chemotactic disorders frequently associated with an absolute neutrophil count less than 0.5×10^9/liter. Following restoration of a normal neutrophil count with granulocyte colony stimulating factor, patients no longer are predisposed to recurrent bacterial infections despite a persistent chemotactic defect. Thus, a chemotactic defect observed in vitro does not correlate invariably with decreased resistance to bacterial infections in vivo.

Among the impaired defense mechanisms of the neonate is neutrophil chemotaxis, as demonstrated by the in vitro response of neonatal neutrophils to a variety of chemotactic factors.[272] The impaired motility of the neonatal neutrophils partly arises from the diminished ability to mobilize neutrophil β_2-integrins following neutrophil activation.[307] In addition, the neonatal neutrophil may have a qualitative defect in β_2-integrin function, resulting in impaired neutrophil transendothelial migration for up to 1 month after birth.

DRUGS AND EXTRINSIC AGENTS THAT IMPAIR NEUTROPHIL MOTILITY

Although many pharmacologic agents can influence neutrophil function, few drugs used in clinical medicine affect neutrophil behavior in vivo. Ethanol is an inhibitor of phospholipase D that, in concentrations occurring in human blood, can inhibit neutrophil locomotion and ingestion.[308] Glucocorticoids, especially at high and sustained doses, inhibit neutrophil locomotion, ingestion, and degranulation.[309] Administration of glucocorticoids on alternate days does not interfere with neutrophil movement.[310] Epinephrine does not have a direct effect on neutrophil adhesion.[311] Cyclic adenosine monophosphate (cAMP), which is released from endothelial cells following exposure to epinephrine, can depress neutrophil adherence. Similarly, elevated cAMP levels following epinephrine administration may impair neutrophil adherence, leading to diminished neutrophil margination and apparent neutrophilia. Immune complexes, as seen in patients with rheumatoid arthritis or other autoimmune diseases, can inhibit neutrophil movement by binding to neutrophil Fc receptors.

HYPERIMMUNOGLOBULIN E SYNDROME

Definition and History   Hyperimmunoglobulin E syndrome is a disorder characterized by markedly elevated serum IgE levels, chronic dermatitis, and serious recurrent bacterial infections.[312] The skin infections seen in patients are remarkable for their absence of surrounding erythema, leading to the formation of "cold abscesses." Neutrophils and monocytes from patients with this syndrome exhibit a variable but at times profound chemotactic defect that appears extrinsic to the neutrophil (see Table 66-2).

The syndrome originally was described in 1966 in two red-haired, fair-skinned females who had "cold abscesses" and hyperextensible joints, which led to the appellation "Job syndrome."[313] Buckley and co-workers[314] subsequently documented the association of levels of immunoglobulin E with undue susceptibility to infection.

Epidemiology   More than 200 cases have been documented.[314,315] Hyperimmunoglobulin E syndrome occurs in persons from diverse ethnic backgrounds and does not seem to be more common in any specific population.

Etiology and Pathogenesis   Both males and females are affected, as are members of succeeding generations, suggesting the disorder is autosomal dominant with an incomplete penetrance form of inheritance.[315] The syndrome may be caused by mutation of a single gene, common mutations, and different genes in different families, or deletion of contiguous genes in a short chromosomal region. The molecular basis for the syndrome is unknown. Some believe the immunologic basis of hyperimmunoglobulin E syndrome arises from insufficient suppressor T cells, which is manifested partly by reduced production of IFN-γ and TNF.[314] The proposed T cell defect could explain the hyperproduction of IgE and the abnormal antibody responses documented in some patients in response to various vaccines. On the other hand, other investigators have not found deficient IFN-γ production by T cells from patients with hyperimmunoglobulin E syndrome; therefore, the results leave in doubt the existence of T cell defects. The predisposition to bacterial infections may arise from impaired anamnestic IgG antibody responses and poor responses to neoantigens. Other immune abnormalities have been described, including defective neutrophil chemotaxis and abnormalities in T lymphocyte subgroups; however, no specific defect in the immune system has been found in all patients.

Clinical Features   Hyperimmunoglobulin E syndrome may begin as early as day 1 of life.[314] The syndrome is characterized by chronic eczematoid rashes, which typically are papular and pruritic. The rash generally involves the face and extensor surfaces of the arms and legs. Skin lesions frequently are sharply demarcated and usually lack surrounding erythema. By age 5 years, all patients have experienced recurrent skin abscess formation with recurrent pneumonias, chronic otitis media, and sinusitis. Patients may develop septic arthritis, cellulitis, or osteomyelitis. The major offending pathogen generally is S. aureus. Other pathogens commonly infecting patients are C. albicans, H. influenzae, and pneumococci. Other associated features include coarse facial features, including a prominent forehead, deep-set eyes, a broad nasal bridge, a wide fleshly nasal tip, mild prognathism facial asymmetry, and hemihypertrophy.[315] High incidences of scoliosis and hyperextensible joints and delayed shedding of the primary teeth are observed.[315] Occasionally unexplained osteopenia is present and often is complicated by recurrent bone fractures.

Laboratory Features   Eosinophilia in the blood and sputum has been a consistent finding in all patients. Serum IgE levels range from 3 to 80 times the upper limit of normal.[314] Usually patients have normal concentrations of IgG, IgA, and IgM but may have elevated levels of IgD. Patients often have abnormally low anamnestic antibody response and poor antibody and cell-mediated responses to neoantigens. At times the neutrophils and monocytes of patients have a profound chemotactic defect.

Therapy, Course, and Prognosis   No known therapy is curative, and management decisions are based on the clinical findings. Prophylactic trimethoprim-sulfamethoxazole is effective in reducing infections with S. aureus.[314] Type and route of antibiotic therapy are dictated by the results of the gram stain and culture in patients with acute bacterial infections. Incision and drainage are essential for management of abscesses, including superinfected pneumatoceles. Eczematoid dermatitis can be controlled with topical glucocorticoids to reduce inflammation and antihistamines to control pruritus. Plasmapheresis reportedly is effective in patients who do not respond to more conservative approaches.[312] Based on observations that IFN-γ inhibits murine IL-4–induced IgE synthesis and on confirmation in humans, a trial of IFN-γ was initiated in patients with hyperimmunoglobulin IgE syndrome. A decline in the serum IgE levels was observed in two of five patients given high doses of IFN-γ, but no clinical benefit was noted.[316]

If hyperimmunoglobulin IgE syndrome is recognized and the patient is maintained on chronic antistaphylococcal antibiotic therapy, the prognosis remains good. Many patients who reached maturity indicate the syndrome is compatible with prolonged survival. On the other hand, if the diagnosis is delayed and the patient develops infected giant pneumatoceles, secondary fungal infections may occur and lead to a morbid state.[314]

DEFECTS IN MICROBICIDAL ACTIVITY

CHRONIC GRANULOMATOUS DISEASE

Definition and History Chronic granulomatous disease (CGD) is a genetic disorder that affects neutrophil and monocyte function. These phagocytic cells can ingest but cannot kill catalase-positive microorganisms because of an inability to generate antimicrobial oxygen metabolites (see Table 66-2). CGD is caused by mutations involving one of several genes encoding a component of NADPH oxidase.[317]

In 1957, two pediatric groups caring for six male infants reported a clinical disorder of chronic suppurative lymphadenitis and recurrent fevers leading to premature death of the children.[318,319] In the same time period, three observations assisted in providing the framework for understanding the defect in the phagocytes of patients with CGD. Scientists reported that particle ingestion by phagocytes resulted in a striking increase in oxygen consumption that was not related to mitochondrial oxygen metabolism.[320] In addition, the process of phagocytosis was accompanied by the formation of large quantities of H_2O_2 in the cell.[321] Subsequently, Iyer and Quastel[322] reported that homogenates of phagocytes consume oxygen when they are incubated with pyridine nucleotides. These observations indicated an oxidase enzyme or enzymes in the phagocytes activated during phagocytosis converted molecular oxygen into H_2O_2. Phagocytes from patients with CGD then were determined to be able to ingest but not to kill the catalase-positive organisms.[322] Building on previous studies reporting a neutrophil oxidase mediates the increase in oxygen consumption, a pyridine-dependent oxidase was found to be deficient in neutrophils of patients with CGD and led to their inability to reduce the dye nitroblue tetrazolium (NBT) during phagocytosis of particles.[323] Collectively these studies laid the groundwork for subsequent studies unraveling the biochemical and genetic defects in CGD.

Epidemiology The incidence of CGD in the United States is one per 200,000 births, based on data from the National Institutes of Allergy and Infectious Disease Registry.[324] Data from the Registry indicate 86 percent of patients are male and 14 percent female; 80 percent are classified as white, 11 percent black, and 3 percent Asian or mixed race. Of the 340 patients in the Registry with information adequate for determining genetic transmission, 70 percent had the X-linked recessive form of the disease.

Etiology and Pathogenesis Several laboratory tests are used to classify forms of CGD and to aid in understanding its pathogenesis (Table 66-4). The diagnosis of CGD is based on a compatible clinical history and demonstration of a defective respiratory burst. Several methods detect the production of reactive oxidants. The NBT method relies on intracellular reduction of NBT by superoxide anion to a blue formazan precipitate that can be seen microscopically.[317] More sensitive methods rely on the reaction of oxidants with specific chemiluminescent and fluorescent probes. Patients with CGD may have a

TABLE 66-4 DIAGNOSTIC CLASSIFICATION OF CHRONIC GRANULOMATOUS DISEASE

AFFECTED COMPONENT	INHERITANCE	SUBTYPE	CYTOCHROME B_{558}*	P47phox*	P67phox*
gp91phox	X	X91^0	Not detectable	Normal	Normal
		X91$^+$	Normal quantity	Normal	Normal
		X91$^-$	Defective gp91phox Low quality	Normal	Normal
p22phox	A	A22$^-$	Not detectable Normal quality	Normal	Normal
p47phox	A	A22$^+$	Normal quantity	Normal	Normal
p67phox	A	A47^0	Defective p22phox Normal	Not detectable	Normal
		A67^0	Normal	Normal	Not detectable

* Detected by spectral analysis or immunoblotting. In this nomenclature, the first letter represents the node of inheritance (X-linked [X] or autosomal recessive [A]). The number indicates the *phox* component, which is genetically affected. The superscript symbols indicate whether the level of protein of the affected component is undetectable (0), diminished (−), or normal as measured by immunoblot or spectral analysis.

heterogeneous array of regular symptoms and severities, depending on which subunit is defective and the nature of the genetic mutation.

NADPH Oxidase Function. Engulfment of microbes by phagocytic cells is associated with a burst of oxygen consumption that is important for microbicidal killing and digestion. The respiratory burst is accompanied not by mitochondrial respiration but by a unique electron transport chain called NADPH oxidase. Prior to stimulation, the components of the oxidase are physically separated into two major subcellular locations (Fig. 66-7). The membrane-bound portion of the NADPH oxidase contains a heterodimeric cytochrome b_{558} composed of a large, heavily glycosylated subunit with an M_r of 91 kDa, known as gp91phox (91-kDa glycoprotein of the phagocyte oxidase [phox]), and a 22-kDa protein known as p22phox.[317,325] The heavy chain of cytochrome b contains sites for heme binding, flavin prosthetic (FAD) groups, and NADPH binding.[326–329] The three-dimensional structure of cytochrome b_{558} indicates the carboxyl terminal half of the peptide contains sequences for flavin and NADPH binding.[330] Heme groups, amino-linked glycosylation sites, and a proton conduction channel within the amino-terminus of gp91phox are present.[331] The amino-half of the molecule is hydrophobic and contains the histidines that coordinate heme binding.[332] p22phox also contains a site for heme binding.[326] Synthesis of the p22phox peptide is absolutely required for stability of gp91phox and for oxidase activity in the membrane.[317] p22phox contains proline-rich regions that have consensus structure for binding SH3 ([Src homology 3]-type domains) found in p47phox.[132] Three other proteins vital to the function of this oxidase system reside in the cytosol of the resting phagocyte. Upon stimulation, translocation of p47phox occurs. Phosphorylated p47phox and two other cytoplasmic components of the oxidase, p67phox and a low molecular weight guanosine triphosphate Rac2, translocate to the membrane, where they interact with cytoplasmic domains of the transmembrane cytochrome b_{558} to form the active oxidase.[333,334] Both p47phox and p67phox contain two SH3 domains that may participate in intramolecular and intermolecular binding with consensus proline-rich regions in p47phox.[135] Phosphorylation, which occurs on serines in the cationic C-terminal region of p47phox, might serve to disrupt this intermolecular interaction, making the SH3 regions available for binding to p22phox. Another cytoplasmic component with homology to p47phox has been identified as p40phox, which appears to interact with p67phox before and during oxidase assembly.[335] An inhibitory role for p40phox in regulating oxidase activation has been suggested.[336]

The cell-free system for activating the oxidase has permitted dissection of the enzyme system into its components and evaluation of each unit's function.[337–343] Cytosolic and membrane proteins are re-

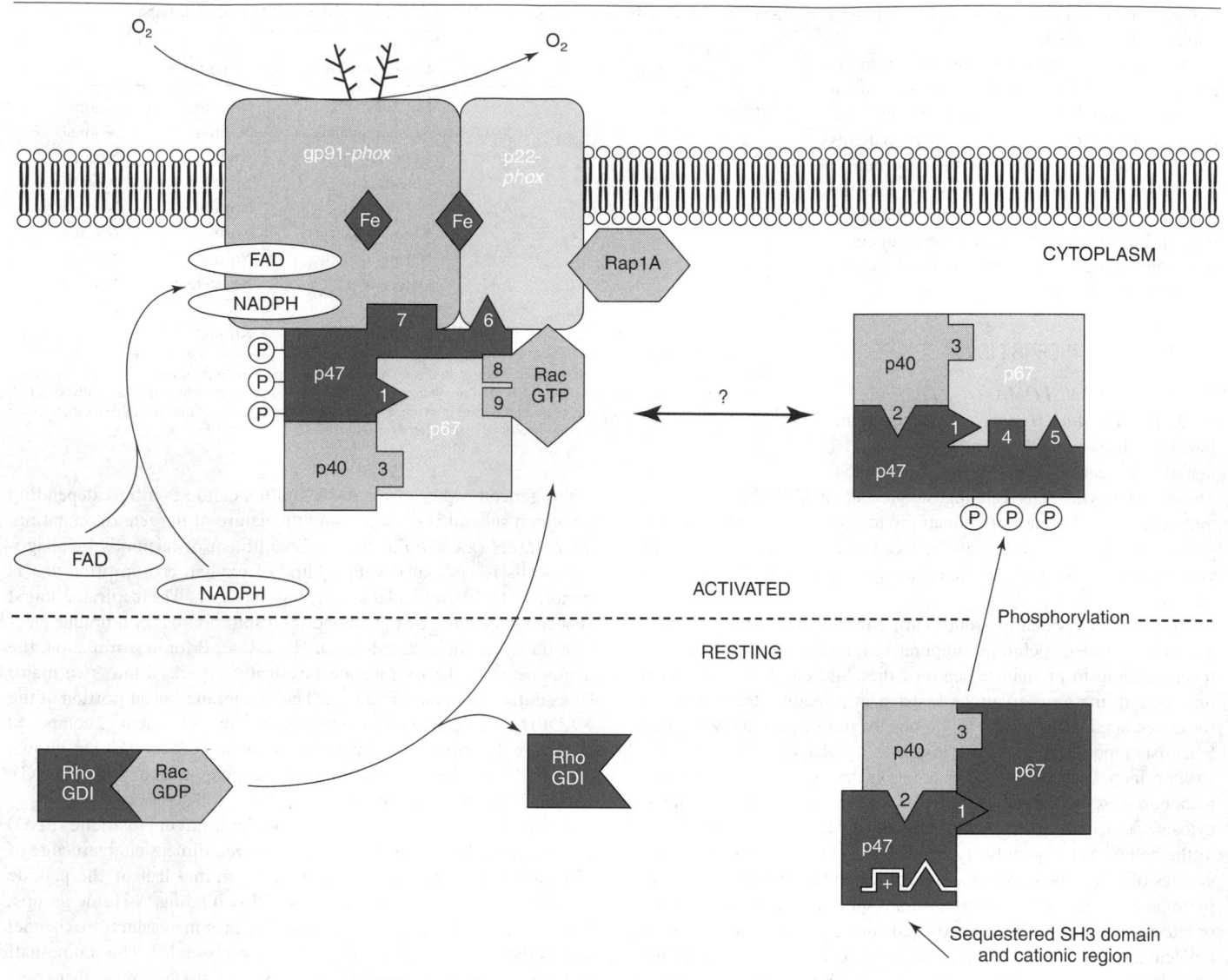

FIGURE 66-7   Possible mechanisms for production of superoxide anion in polymorphonuclear leukocytes. Oxygen is reduced to superoxide (O_2^-) by an NADPH oxidase. The oxidase appears to be a composite of (1) a 47-kDa cytosolic protein (p47); (2) a 67-kDa cytosolic protein (p67); (3) a 40-kDa cytosolic protein (p40); (4) one or more low molecular weight cytosolic G-proteins, such as Rac2 and Rap1A; and (5) a membrane-bound cytochrome b_{558}. Cytochrome b consists of a 22-kDa protein subunit and a 91-kDa glycoprotein subunit, both of which contain heme. The gp91 subunit is an FAD-dependent flavoprotein that contains the NADPH binding site and ultimately shuttles electrons to molecular oxygen, forming O_2^-. The cytosol components also reportedly translocate to the membrane and may serve to alter the tertiary structure of cytochrome b, permitting the flow of electrons from NADPH to O_2. The p47 subunit can be phosphorylated to various extents, but the significance of this phosphorylation is unclear. The low molecular weight G-protein is important in stabilizing the oxidase complex. (From DeLeo FR, Quinn MT, *J Leukoc Biol* 60:677, 1996, with permission.)

quired for oxidase activation, and all patients with CGD have defects involving cytochrome b or the cytosolic components p47[phox] or p67[phox].[317] The membrane and cytosol interaction for oxidase activation in the cell-free system defines the genetic heterogeneity of CGD.[317] Table 66-4 illustrates this point. The neutrophil membrane fractions from patients with XO (X-linked, cytochrome b-negative) and AO (autosomal recessive, cytochrome b-negative) CGD do not support oxidase activation even upon addition of normal cytosol, whereas the corresponding patient's cytosol functions normally.[344] The membrane defect in the two types of CGD results from the absence of cytochrome b. In the case of A+ CGD (autosomal recessive, cytochrome b-positive), the membrane fraction is normal, whereas the cytosol is severely defective.

Genetic Alterations Affecting Cytochrome b.   The most frequent form of CGD occurs in 70 percent of patients and is caused by mu-

tations in the gp91[phox] gene located on chromosome Xp21.1.[317,345] These mutations lead to the X-linked form. Large interstitial deletions causing other X-linked disorders, such as retinitis pigmentosa, Duchenne muscular dystrophy, McLeod hemolytic anemia, and ornithine transcarbamylase deficiency, have been reported in a few patients with X-linked CGD.[324,346–348] Mutation analysis of the gene encoding gp91 and a large group of X-linked CGD kindreds has documented many distinct defects, including point mutations, inversions, deletions, or insertions that disrupt the reading frame and nonsense mutations that create a premature stop codon.[345] Some splice site defects have been identified. In this situation, short deletions in gp91[phox] mRNA are caused by point mutations that produce partial or complete exon skipping during mRNA splicing.[349] This abnormality is a common cause of X-linked CGD. In the remaining patients, point mutations that generate either premature stop codons or amino acid substitutions that apparently disrupt protein stability or function and lead to a complete lack of detectable cytochrome b_{558} protein in phagocytic cells in most patients with X-linked CGD have been identified.[350] In some situations, low levels of functional cytochrome b are present, whereas in others, normal levels of dysfunctional cytochrome b_{558} occur.[350] In the latter situation, some clustering of defects occurs in regions of known function, such as the NADPH- or flavin-binding consensus regions.[351,352]

A similar array of mutations has been identified in the 5 percent of CGD patients who have abnormalities in the p22phox gene located on chromosome 16q24.[317,352,353] In this autosomal disorder, mutations in the p22phox gene result in deletions, frameshifts, and/or missense mutations. Two patients have been identified as homozygous for missense mutations as a result of consanguineous heritage. Patients with a defective p22phox gene do not express the other cytoplasmic unit polypeptide. In one patient, p22phox peptide was associated with normal amounts of cytochrome b with normal heme spectrum, but p47phox translocation membrane did not occur and no oxidase activation was observed. The mutation affected a proline-rich region thought to mediate binding to one of the SH3 domains of p47phox. In gp91phox-deficient patients, p22phox mRNA is present but is not translated, which is consistent with the notion that either cytochrome subunit polypeptide is dependent upon stable expression of the other subunit.[317]

Genetic Alterations Affecting Cytosolic Proteins. Two other proteins have been identified as vital to the function of the NADPH-oxidase system. Their absence results in the syndrome of CGD.[354] These proteins have molecular masses of 47 and 67 kDa, respectively, and are located in the cytosol of resting cells. Defects in the genes for p47phox found on chromosome 7q11 are responsible for the majority of cases of autosomal recessive CGD, whereas inherited defects for the gene for neutrophil p67phox account for a small subgroup of autosomal recessive CGD.[317] The function of *p47phox* and p67phox in regulating the respiratory burst oxidase is thought to involve activation of the electron transport function of cytochrome b_{558}. Mutation analysis of patients with p47phox-deficient forms of CGD reveals an unusual pattern, in that more than 90 percent of mutant alleles have guanine-thymine dinucleotide deletion at the start of exon 2, resulting in frameshift and premature stop.[352,355] The truncated protein is unstable in that it cannot be detected immunologically. The majority of patients appear to be homozygous for this mutation without any history of consanguinity. The p47phox gene occurs in an area of chromosome 7 that has a high degree of evolutionary duplication in normal individuals because a pseudogene highly homologous to the normal p47phox gene exists in the normal genome in this region of duplication. The pseudogene contains the same GT deletion associated with most cases of p47phox CGD. This finding implied that recombination of the normal gene and pseudogene with conversion of the normal gene to partial pseudotype sequence in that region was responsible for the high relative rate of this specific mutation in diverse racial groups, which proved to be the case.[351]

A second rare form of CGD is caused by mutations in the gene for the p67phox cytosolic component.[350] The p67phox gene, which has

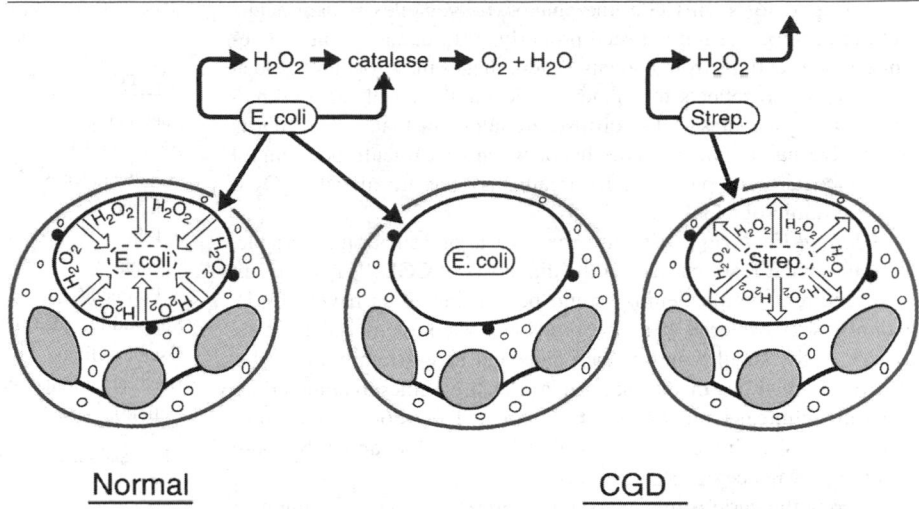

FIGURE 66-8 Pathogenesis of chronic granulomatous disease. Schematic diagram of the manner in which the metabolic deficiency of the CGD neutrophil predisposes the host to infection. Normal neutrophils accumulate hydrogen peroxide in the phagosome containing ingested *Escherichia coli*. Myeloperoxidase is delivered to the phagosome by degranulation, as indicated by the *closed circles*. In this setting, hydrogen peroxide acts as a substrate for myeloperoxidase to oxidize halide to hypochlorous acid and chloramines, which kill the microbes. The quantity of hydrogen peroxide produced by normal neutrophils is sufficient to exceed the capacity of catalase, a hydrogen peroxide-catabolizing enzyme of many aerobic microorganisms, including most gram-negative enteric bacteria, *S. aureus*, *C. albicans*, and *Aspergillus* species. When organisms such as *E. coli* gain entry into the CGD neutrophils, they are not exposed to hydrogen peroxide because the neutrophils do not produce it, and the hydrogen peroxide generated by microbes themselves is destroyed by their own catalase. When CGD neutrophils ingest streptococci or pneumococci, the organisms generate enough hydrogen peroxide to result in a microbicidal effect. On the other hand, as indicated in the *middle figure*, catalase-positive microbes, such as *E. coli*, can survive within the phagosome of the CGD neutrophil.

been mapped to the long arm of chromosome 1, spans 37 kb and contains 16 exons. The mutations identified in p67phox-deficiency CGD have included missense mutations and spliced junction mutations affecting mRNA processing, which led to nondetectable p67phox protein by immunologic means.[352]

Predisposition to Infection. Mutations in the gene for cytochrome b_{558} or the cytosolic factors involved in activating the cytochrome have been associated with the CGD phenotype. Figure 66-8 shows the manner in which the metabolic deficiency of CGD neutrophil predisposes the host to infection. Normal neutrophils accumulate H_2O_2 and other oxygen metabolites in the phagosomes containing ingested microorganisms. MPO is delivered to the phagosome by degranulation. In this setting, H_2O_2 acts as a substrate for MPO to oxidize halide to hypochlorous acid and chloramines, which kill the microbes. The quantity of H_2O_2 produced by the normal neutrophils is sufficient to exceed the capacity of catalase, an H_2O_2-catabolizing enzyme produced by many aerobic microorganisms, including *S. aureus*, most gram-negative enteric bacteria, *C. albicans*, and *Aspergillus* species. In contrast, H_2O_2 is not produced by CGD neutrophils, and any H_2O_2 generated by the microbes themselves may be destroyed by their own catalase. Thus, catalase-positive microbes can multiply inside CGD neutrophils, where they are protected from most circulating antibiotics, and can be transported to distant sites and released to establish new foci of infection.[354] Activation of the oxidase also has a pronounced effect on the pH within the phagocytic vacuole. Whether activation of the respiratory burst is associated with an alkaline phase is controversial, but the pH of the phagocytic vacuole becomes much more acidic in CGD patients than in normals.[356] The alkaline phase may be important for the antimicrobial and digestive functions of the neutral hydrolases released from the cytoplasmic granules into the vacuole upon phagocytosis. In CGD, the phagocytic vacuoles remain acidic and the bacteria are not digested properly.[357] In hematoxylin and eosin–stained sections from patients, macrophages may contain a golden pigment, which reflects this abnormal accumulation of ingested material and contributes to the diffuse granulomata that give CGD its descriptive name. On the other hand, when CGD neutrophils ingest pneumococci or streptococci, the organisms generate enough H_2O_2 to result in a microbicidal effect.

Clinical Features   Although the clinical presentation is variable, several clinical features suggest the diagnosis of CGD.[317] Any patient with recurrent lymphadenitis should be considered as having CGD. Patients with bacterial hepatic abscesses, osteomyelitis at multiple sites or in the small bones of the hands and feet, a family history of recurrent infections, or unusual catalase-positive microbial infections all require clinical evaluation for the disorder. Table 66-5 lists the most common clinical infections that afflict CGD patients and Table 66-6 lists the prevalence of the infections.

Among the various infections, only perirectal abscess, suppurative adenitis, and bacteremia/fungemia differ significantly in prevalence in X-linked recessive and autosomal recessive CGD patients.[324] Each of these conditions was twice as common with the X-linked form.

The onset of clinical signs and symptoms may occur from early infancy to young adulthood. Although the majority of patients with CGD (76 percent) are diagnosed before age 5 years, approximately 10 percent are not diagnosed until the second decade of life or, on rare occasions, in the third decade or later.[324] The organisms infecting CGD patients have changed considerably from those initially reported from 1957 to 1976. *Staphylococcus* caused most of the infections in the initial cases; *Klebsiella* and *E. coli* were the next most common pathogens. Now *Aspergillus* is the prominent organism causing pneumonia and is the leading cause of death in patients.[317]

TABLE 66-5   COMMON INFECTING ORGANISMS ISOLATED FROM CHRONIC GRANULOMATOUS DISEASE PATIENTS

INFECTION TYPE	ORGANISM	XLR (%)	AR (%)
Pneumonia	*Aspergillus* species	41	29
	Staphylococcus species	11	13
	Burkholderia cepacia	7	11
	Nocardia species	6	13
	Serratia species	4	5
Abscess			
Subcutaneous	*Staphylococcus* species	28	21
	Serratia species	19	9
	Aspergillus species	7	0
Liver	*Staphylococcus* species	52	52
	Serratia species	6	4
	Candida species	12	0
Lung	*Aspergillus* species	27	18
Perirectal	*Staphylococcus* species	9	15
Brain	*Aspergillus* species	75	25
Suppurative adenitis	*Staphylococcus* species	29	12
	Serratia species	9	15
	Candida species	7	4
Osteomyelitis	*Serratia* species	32	12
	Aspergillus species	25	18
Bacteremia/fungemia	*Salmonella* species	20	13
	Burkholderia cepacia	13	0
	Candida species	9	25
	Staphylococcus species	11	0

AR = autosomal recessive; XLR = X-linked recessive; Data adapted from reference 124.

TABLE 66-6   PREVALENCE OF INFECTION COMPLICATION OF CHRONIC GRANULOMATOUS DISEASE PATIENTS

INFECTION TYPE	XLR (%)	AR (%)
Pneumonia	80	77
Abscess (all)	68	70
Subcutaneous	43	42
Liver	26	33
Lung	16	14
Brain	3	5
Perirectal	17	7
Suppurative adenitis	59	32
Osteomyelitis	27	21
Bacteremia/fungemia	21	10
Cellulitis	7	5

AR = autosomal recessive; XLR = X-linked recessive; Data adapted from reference 124.

Invasive *Aspergillosis* can occur in the first few months of life in healthy infants and inpatients of any age with CGD. Although *Aspergillosis* is the most common infecting fungus in CGD, *Candida* and several other fungal strains are invasive in this disorder. *Burkholderia cepacia* is another leading cause of death in patients with CGD. *Serratia marcescens* is the third leading organism that commonly infects patients with CGD. Infections are characterized by microabscesses and granuloma formation. The presence of pigmented histiocytes is helpful in establishing the diagnosis. Patients may suffer from the consequences of chronic infections, including the anemia of chronic disease, lymphadenopathy, hepatosplenomegaly, chronic purulent dermatitis, restrictive lung disease, gingivitis, hydronephrosis, and gastroenteral narrowing.[324] Patients with CGD also are at risk for developing colitis, chorioretinitis, and discoid lupus erythematosus.[324]

Several mothers of patients with established X-linked inheritance had an illness resembling systemic lupus erythematosus.[324] Both X-linked and autosomal recessive patients with CGD have a similar disorder.[358] Possibly the cells of these mothers and patients are unable to clear immune complexes sufficiently, which is a characteristic feature of CGD cells *in vitro*.[359] Variant alleles of MBL and FcγRIIA, especially in combination, are associated with rheumatologic disorders in patients with CGD.[360]

Laboratory Features   The defect in respiratory burst is best determined by measuring superoxide or H_2O_2 production in response to both soluble and particulate stimuli. An applicable test is flow cytometry using dihydrorhodamine 123 fluorescence.[361] Dihydrorhodamine fluorescence detects oxidant production because it increases fluorescence upon oxidation. In most cases, no superoxide or H_2O_2 generation is detectable with either type of stimulus. In the variant form of CGD, on the other hand, superoxide may be produced at rates between 0.5 and 10 percent of control.[362]

An alternative method for measuring respiratory burst activity is the NBT test. This assay is performed by microscopically assessing the ability of individual cells to reduce NBT to purple formazan crystals following stimulation. Commonly no NBT reduction occurs in most forms of CGD. In some of the variant forms, however, a high percentage of cells may contain some formazan, a finding indicative of a greatly diminished respiratory burst in most of the neutrophils. This test also permits detection of the carrier state in X-linked CGD when as few as 5 to 10 percent of the cells are NBT negative.[363]

Most sophisticated procedures can identify the molecular defect. Cytochrome *b* content can be measured in extracts of detergent-disrupted neutrophils by a spectrophotometric assay.[363] The activity of a patient's membrane and cytosol in the cell-free oxidase system can be measured. Immunoblotting for a cytochrome b subunit and cytosol oxidase component can be used to characterize X-linked from autosomal recessive forms of CGD. The genotype can be determined once the diagnosis of CGD is made. A mosaic population of oxidation that has positive and negative neutrophils in the mother and sister of male patients strongly suggests X-linked CGD. Lack of a mosaic pattern among female relatives does not rule out the X-linked mode of inheritance because the defect can arise spontaneously. Prenatal diagnosis of CGD is established by performing analysis of DNA neutrophil oxidant production from umbilical blood samples obtained by fetoscopy.[364] Alternatively, DNA can be analyzed from amniocytes or chorionic villus samples. Restriction fragment length polymorphisms have been successful for diagnosing gp91[phox] and p67[phox] deficiency in informative families.[365] In other families, PCR technology can be used to analyze fetal DNA if a family's specific mutation is known.

Differential Diagnosis Leukocytes from patients with CGD have normal glucose-6-phosphate dehydrogenase (G-6-PD) activity. However, a few individuals with apparent CGD have neutrophils that lack or almost lack G-6-PD activity.[366,367] The erythrocytes of these patients also lack the enzyme, and the patients have chronic hemolysis. In cases of severe neutrophil G-6-PD deficiency, an attenuated respiratory burst progressively decreases because of depletion of intracellular NADPH, which is the primary substrate for the respiratory burst oxidase. CGD and G-6-PD deficiency can be distinguished from one another by the hemolytic anemia seen in the latter disorder and by the finding of normal erythrocyte G-6-PD activity in CGD versus markedly reduced activity in G-6-PD deficiency.[350]

A variety of studies have indicated the small GTPase Rac2 plays an essential role in activity of NADPH and the actin cytoskeleton in human neutrophils.[324] A toddler who presented with a perirectal abscess at age 5 weeks has been described. The patient subsequently had necrosis of the periumbilical skin and fascia, and his surgical wounds did not heal properly. Functionally his neutrophils had defective chemotaxis that failed to release primary azurophil granules upon stimulation with a chemotactic peptide and undergo the respiratory burst using the same stimulus.[368,369] These cells also failed to adhere properly to ligands for sLe^x. Molecular analysis identified the asparagine for aspartic acid mutation at amino acid 57 of one allele of the Rac2 gene.[368,369] Mutant Rac2 did not bind GTP. It inhibited and behaved as a dominant negative, impairing Rac2-mediated activation of respiratory burst.[369] Fortunately, the toddler was successfully transplanted with marrow from a HLA-identical older brother.[369]

Therapy, Course, and Prognosis Because marrow transplantation is the only known cure for CGD, vigorous supportive care and use of rIFN-γ continues to be the foundation of treatment.[317] Cultures must be obtained as soon as infection is suspected, as unusual organisms are commonly the source of infection and may grow promptly *in vitro*. Most abscesses require surgical drainage for therapeutic and diagnostic purposes, and prolonged use of antibiotics often is required. If fever occurs, obtaining certain studies that aid in the management of septic episodes is advisable. The studies include roentgenograms of the chest and skeleton and computed tomographic scan of the liver because of the frequency of pneumonia, osteomyelitis, and liver abscesses.[324] Arrangements should be made for prompt medical attention at the first signs of infection. With early intervention, many lesions can be managed by conservative medical means. For example, enlarging lymph nodes often regress when they are treated with local heat and orally administered antistaphylococcal

antibiotics. Obtaining a microbiologic diagnosis is important, and fine needle aspiration may be helpful in this regard. In general, antibiotic therapy for the offending organisms is indicated, and purulent masses should be drained. The cause of fever and prostration cannot always be established, and empiric treatment with broad-spectrum parenteral antibiotics is required. Often prolonged treatment with antibiotics is necessary until the initial sedimentation rate approaches normal values. Infection with *Aspergillus* species requires treatment with amphotericin B or, in refractory cases, granulocyte transfusions.[317] Glucocorticoids may be useful for treatment of patients with antral and urethral obstruction. The risk of *Aspergillus* infection can be reduced by avoiding marijuana smoke and decaying plant material, such as mulch and hay, both of which contain numerous fungal spores.[370]

Long-term oral prophylaxis with trimethoprim-sulfamethoxazole (trimethoprim 5 mg/kg/day) is an accepted practice in the management of patients with CGD.[317] Patients have prolonged infection-free periods that result from prevention of infections by *S. aureus*, without increasing the incidence of fungal infections. Prophylactic use of itraconazole has reduced the development of fungal infections.[371]

IFN-γ (50 μg/m^2, three times per week) can reduce the number of serious bacterial and fungal infections.[372] IFN-γ–enhanced neutrophil function *in vitro* has not been correlated with improved activity of the neutrophil respiratory burst in patients totally lacking the ability to generate superoxide. On the other hand, use of IFN-γ increases neutrophil expression of the high-affinity Fcγ receptor-1 and monocyte expression of Fcγ RI, Fcγ RII, Fcγ RIII, CD11/CD18, and HLA-DR.[373] The IFN-γ protective effect in patients with CGD may involve improved microbial clearance, as suggested by the enhanced phagocytic activity by neutrophils of opsonized *S. aureus*. In rare X-linked CGD patients able to generate some superoxide, IFN-γ programs granulocyte cells to increase their expression of cytochrome b, which results in normal superoxide generation.[374] With current prophylactic treatments, the mortality of CGD has been reduced to two patient deaths per year per hundred patients followed.[317]

Patients with CGD mutations that result in 5 to 10 percent of normal functioning amounts of NADPH have a mild phenotype and better clinical prognosis than patients with complete absence of NADPH oxidase activity.[375,376] Similarly, female carriers of X-linked CGD who have only 3 to 5 percent oxidase-normal neutrophils rarely get serious infections suggestive of the CGD clinical phenotype.[377] Thus, even low levels or partial correction of CGD by gene therapy likely provides clinical benefits. In support of that hypothesis, mouse models of X-linked and p47[phox]-deficient CGD have been developed by gene targeting.[378,379] Studies in gp91[phox]- and p47[phox]-deficient mouse models of CGD have shown that retrovirus-mediated gene therapy targeting of marrow progenitor cells *ex vivo* can correct defects in oxidant production *in vivo* in peripheral blood neutrophils after radiation conditioning and transplantation of marrow stem cells.[380,381] Protection from infection challenge occurred even when oxidase-corrected cells composed less than 10 percent of circulating neutrophils. These promising results suggest somatic gene therapy can be used to correct defective phagocyte oxidase function in selected patients with CGD. In a phase I clinical trial of gene therapy for p47[phox]-deficiency CGD, five adult patients received intravenous infusions of autologous blood stem cells that were *ex vivo* transduced using a retrovirus encoding normal p47[phox].[382] Although conditioning therapy was not given prior to stem cell infusion, functionally corrected neutrophils were detectable in peripheral blood 3 to 6 weeks after the single infusion and ranged from 0.004 to 0.05 percent of total blood neutrophils. The corrected cells were detectable as long as 6 months after infusion in some patients. These results indicate a promise for gene therapy in the future to correct phagocytic oxidase function in selected patients with CGD.

MYELOPEROXIDASE DEFICIENCY

The functional and immunochemical absence of the enzyme MPO from granules of neutrophils and monocytes, but not eosinophils, is inherited as an autosomal recessive trait, with a prevalence of 1:2000.[383] MPO, an enzyme that catalyzes the production of hypochlorous acid in the phagosome, causes microbicidal deficiency of the neutrophils early after ingestion of microorganisms (see Table 66-2). However, normal microbicidal activity is observed approximately 1 hour after a variety of organisms are ingested.[382] Thus, the MPO-deficient neutrophil uses an MPO-independent system for killing bacteria that is slower than the MPO– H_2O_2–halide system that eventually is effective in eliminating bacteria. MPO-deficient neutrophils accumulate more H_2O_2 than do normal neutrophils. The higher peroxide concentration improves the bactericidal activity of the affected neutrophils. In contrast to retardation of bactericidal activity, candidacidal activity in MPO-deficient neutrophils is absent.[383,384] The most significant clinical manifestation in a few patients with diabetes mellitus and MPO deficiency has been severe infection with C. albicans. Because the disorder is so common in phagocytes, the vast majority of patients with this genetic disorder have not been unusually susceptible to pyogenic infections and do not require therapy.

The cDNA encoding human MPO has been cloned and the gene structure, including promoter and regulatory elements, delineated.[385,386] The gene consists of 12 exons and 11 introns and is located on the long arm of chromosome 17. Its expression is finely coordinated with expression of genes encoding other lysosomal proteins. Expression of genes for human neutrophil elastase and MPO is very similar. Expression is low in myeloblasts, peaks during the promyelocyte stage, and eventually drops to low levels in myelocytes. MPO is a symmetric molecule composed of four peptides; each half consists of a heavy-chain and a light-chain heterodimer.[387] Each heavy- and light-chain heterodimer starts as a single peptide that is cleaved during the posttranslational process, yielding the heavy and light chains that form half of the mature molecules. The two halves of the molecule are associated by a disulfide linkage between heavy-subunit residues at position C319.

The primary translation product of the gene is a single-chain 80-kDa peptide that undergoes cotranslational glycosylation at several asparagine residues, followed by a series of modifications of the oligosaccharides. The apopromyeloperoxidase exists for a prolonged time in the endoplasmic reticulum, where it associates reversibly with several endoplasmic reticulum-resident proteins known as molecular chaperones.[388,389] Subsequent to heme insertion, the enzymatically active promyeloperoxidase undergoes proteolytic cleavage of the pro region. Then, in a prelysosomal compartment, the single peptide is cleaved into the heavy and light subunits, which remain linked. During final sorting within the azurophil lysosome compartment, dimerization of half-molecules occurs, forming the mature MPO.[389]

Most patients with MPO deficiency have a missense mutation in the gene that results in replacement of arginine 569 with tryptophan.[390] The mutation results in a precursor that associates with molecular chaperones but does not incorporate heme, leading to maturational arrest during processing at the stage of an inactive enzymatic apopromyeloperoxidase. Other patients are compound heterozygotes in whom one allele bears the common mutation and the other is normal, resulting in partial deficiency.[389] To date, four genotypes have been reported as causing inherited MPO deficiency, each of which results in missense mutations. In the genotype Y173C, a missense mutation results in replacement of a tyrosine at codon 173 with a cysteine residue, leading to retention of the mutant precursor in the endoplasmic reticulum by virtue of its prolonged interaction with the chaperone calnexin and eventual degradation of the mutant precursor in a proteosome.[390] In the process, the quality control system operating in the endoplasmic reticulum retrieves malfolded MPO precursors from the biosynthetic pathway and creates the biochemical phenotype of MPO deficiency. In another patient, a missense mutation resulted in an intact MPO molecule that acquired heme but failed to undergo proteolytic processing to a mature molecule.[391]

Acquired disorders are with associated MPO deficiency. Reported states include lead intoxication, ceroid lipofuscinosis, myelodysplastic syndromes, and acute myelogenous leukemia.[383] Half of untreated patients with acute myelogenous leukemia and 20 percent of patients with chronic myelogenous leukemia may have MPO deficiency.[383,384]

DEFICIENCIES OF GLUTATHIONE REDUCTASE AND GLUTATHIONE SYNTHETASE

Neutrophils contain enzymes capable of inactivating potentially damaging reduced oxygen byproducts. Disposal of superoxide anion is accomplished through superoxide dismutase, a soluble enzyme that converts superoxide to H_2O_2. H_2O_2 is detoxified by catalase and by the glutathione peroxidase–glutathione reductase system, which converts H_2O_2 to water and oxygen.[392] In addition to the soluble enzymes, cellular vitamin E serves as an antioxidant to prevent damage to the surface of activated neutrophils upon H_2O_2 release.[392] Single cases of profound deficiencies in glutathione reductase[392] and glutathione synthetase[393] have been associated with impaired neutrophil bactericidal activity (see Table 66-2). Both deficiencies are associated with hemolysis under conditions of oxidative stress (see Chap. 45). Glutathione synthetase deficiency also has been associated with intermittent neutropenia during times of mild infection. Vitamin E has been used to ameliorate hemolysis and improve neutrophil function in a patient with glutathione synthetase deficiency.[394] Like patients with MPO-deficient neutrophils, patients with glutathione reductase deficiency and glutathione synthetase deficiency are not unusually susceptible to bacterial infections.

DIAGNOSTIC APPROACH TO PATIENTS WITH SUSPECTED NEUTROPHIL DYSFUNCTION

An increased susceptibility to pyogenic infections must be viewed in light of a number of factors: (1) adequacy of host defense, (2) microbes to which the host is exposed, and (3) conditions of the exposure. Establishing a diagnosis of a specific neutrophil dysfunction based on clinical grounds alone may be difficult. Patients with recurrent pyogenic infections often yield no clues as to why they are afflicted, and patients with established deficiency of a defense mechanism may have an unimpressive clinical history. On the other hand, patients may be suspected of having a neutrophil dysfunction if they have a history of frequent bacterial or severe infections. Recurrent pulmonary infections, hepatic abscesses, and perirectal abscesses should alert the clinician to consider further diagnostic evaluation of neutrophil function. For example, identification of unusual catalase-positive bacteria and fungi, such as B. cepacia, S. marcescens, Nocardia, and Aspergillus, could be indicative of CGD.

Because many of the tests of neutrophil function are bioassays with great variability, the test results must be interpreted in light of the patient's clinical condition. For instance, isolated chemotactic defects usually do not explain the patient's propensity for recurrent severe infections. Furthermore, bioassay variations often are intensified by inflammation or infection. Figure 66-9 provides an algorithm for evaluating the patient with recurrent infection.

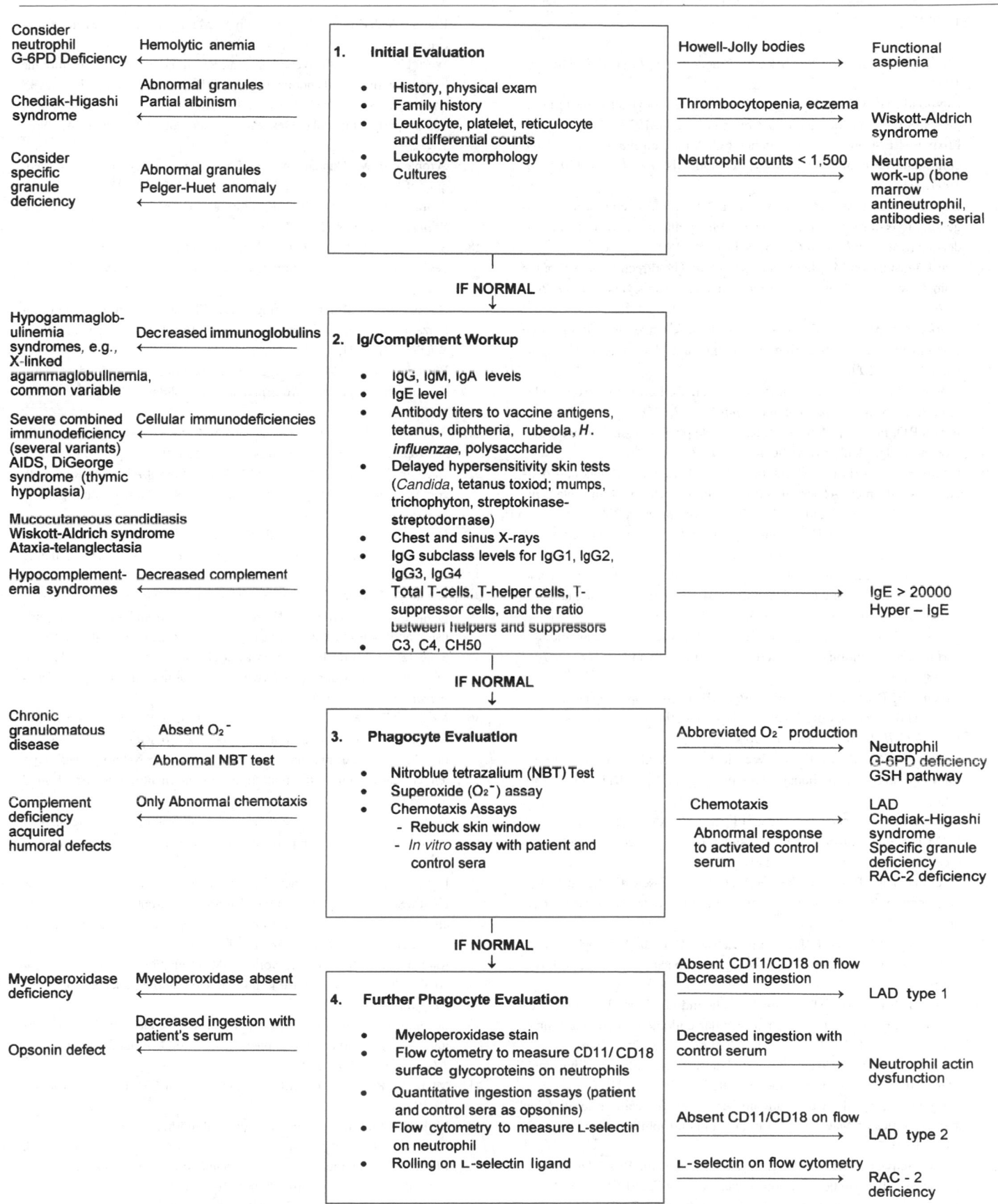

FIGURE 66-9   Algorithm for clinical evaluation of patients with recurrent infections. CBC, complete blood count; G-6-PD, glucose-6-phosphate dehydrogenase; Ig, immunoglobulin; LAD, leukocyte adhesion deficiency.

REFERENCES

1. Mudd S, McCutcheon S, Lucke B: Phagocytosis. *Physiol Rev* 14:210, 1934.

2. Zigmond SH: Ability of polymorphonuclear leukocytes to orient in gradients of chemotactic factors. *J Cell Biol* 75:606, 1977.

3. Foxman EF, Campbell JJ, Butcher EC: Multistep navigation and the combinatorial control of leukocyte chemotaxis. *J Cell Biol* 139:1349, 1997.

4. Quitt M, Torres M, McGuire W, et al: Neutrophil chemotactic heterogeneity to N-formyl-methionyl-leucyl-phenylalanine detected by the under-agarose assay. *J Lab Clin Med* 115:159, 1990.

5. Lee J, Gustafsson M, Magnusson KE, et al: The direction of membrane lipid flow in locomoting polymorphonuclear leukocytes. *Science* 247:1229, 1990.

6. Marks PW, Maxfield FR: Local and global changes in cytosolic free calcium in neutrophils during chemotaxis and phagocytosis. *Cell Calcium* 11:181, 1990.

7. Stossel TP, Hartwig JH, Janmey PA, et al: Cell crawling two decades after Abercrombie. *Biochem Soc Symp* 65:267, 1999.

8. Berlin RD, Fera JP, Pfeiffer JR: Reversible phagocytosis in rabbit polymorphonuclear leukocytes. *J Clin Invest* 63:1137, 1979.

9. Bunting M, Harris ES, McIntyre TM, et al: Leukocyte adhesion deficiency syndromes: Adhesion and tethering defects involving beta 2 integrins and selectin ligands. *Curr Opin Hematol* 9:30, 2002.

10. Shao JY, TingBeall HP, Hochmuth RM: Static and dynamic lengths of neutrophil microvilli. *Proc Natl Acad Sci U S A* 95:6797, 1998.

11. Pestonjamasp K, Amieva MR, Strassel CP, et al: Moesin, ezrin, and p205 are actin-binding proteins associated with neutrophil plasma membranes. *Mol Biol Cell* 6:247, 1995.

12. Bruehl RE, Moore KL, Lorant DE, et al: Leukocyte activation induces surface redistribution of P-selectin glycoprotein ligand-1. *J Leukoc Biol* 61:489, 1997.

13. Green CE, Pearson DN, Christensen NB, et al: Topographic requirements and dynamics of signaling via L-selectin on neutrophils. *Am J Physiol Cell Physiol* 284:C705, 2003.

14. McIntyre TM, Prescott SM, Weyrich AS, et al: Cell-cell interactions: Leukocyte-endothelial interactions. *Curr Opin Hematol* 10:150, 2003.

15. Urzainqui A, Serrador JM, Viedma F, et al: ITAM-based interaction of ERM proteins with Syk mediates signaling by the leukocyte adhesion receptor PSGL-1. *Immunity* 17:401, 2002.

16. Steegmaier M, Borges E, Berger J, et al: The E-selectin-ligand ESL-1 is located in the Golgi as well as on microvilli on the cell surface. *J Cell Sci* 110:687, 1997.

17. Witko-Sarsat V, Rieu P, Descamps-Latscha B, et al: Neutrophils: Molecules, functions and pathophysiological aspects. *Lab Invest* 80:617, 2000.

18. Wolff B, Burns AR, Middleton J, et al: Endothelial cell "memory" of inflammatory stimulation: Human venular endothelial cells store interleukin 8 in Weibel-Palade bodies. *J Exp Med* 188:1757, 1998.

19. Middleton J, Neil S, Wintle J, et al: Transcytosis and surface presentation of IL-8 by venular endothelial cells. *Cell* 91:385, 1997.

20. Sengeløv H, Kjeldsen L, Diamond MS, et al: Subcellular localization and dynamics of Mac-1 ($\alpha_m\beta_2$) in human neutrophils. *J Clin Invest* 92:1467, 1993.

21. Liu L, Schwartz BR, Lin N, et al: Requirement for RhoA kinase activation in leukocyte de-adhesion. *J Immunol* 169:2330, 2002.

22. Foxman EF, Kunkel EJ, Butcher EC: Integrating conflicting chemotactic signals. The role of memory in leukocyte navigation. *J Cell Biol* 147:577, 1999.

23. Petty HR, Todd RF: Integrins as promiscuous signal transduction devices. *Immunol Today* 17:209, 1996.

24. Booth JW, Trimble WS, Grinstein S: Membrane dynamics in phagocytosis. *Semin Immunol* 13:357, 2001.

25. Werfel T, Sonntag G, Weber M, et al: Rapid increases in the membrane expression of neutral endopeptidase (CD10), aminopeptidase N (CD13), tyrosine phosphatase (CD45), and Fcτ-RIII (CD16) upon stimulation of human peripheral leukocytes with human C5a. *J Immunol* 147:3909, 1991.

26. Wroblewski M, Hamann A: CD45-mediated signals can trigger shedding of lymphocyte L-selectin. *Int Immunol* 9:555, 1997.

27. Akira S, Sato S: Toll-like receptors and their signaling mechanisms. *Scand J Infect Dis* 35:555, 2003.

28. Sengeløv H, Voldstedlund M, Vinthen J, et al: Human neutrophils are devoid of the integral membrane protein caveolin. *J Leukoc Biol* 63:563, 1998.

29. Borregaard N, Miller L, Springer TA: Chemoattractant-regulated mobilization of a novel intracellular compartment in human neutrophils. *Science* 237:1204, 1987.

30. Borregaard N, Kjeldsen L, Rygaard K, et al: Stimulus-dependent secretion of plasma proteins from human neutrophils. *J Clin Invest* 90:86, 1992.

31. Sengeløv H, Kjeldsen L, Borregaard N: Control of exocytosis in early neutrophil activation. *J Immunol* 150:1535, 1993.

32. Chaudhuri S, Kumar A, Berger M: Association of ARF and Rabs with complement receptor type-1 storage vesicles in human neutrophils. *J Leukoc Biol* 70:669, 2001.

33. Dahlgren C, Karlsson A, Sendo F: Neutrophil secretory vesicles are the intracellular reservoir for GPI-80, a protein with adhesion-regulating potential. *J Leukoc Biol* 69:57, 2001.

34. Kumar A, Wetzler E, Berger M: Isolation and characterization of complement receptor type 1 (CR1) storage vesicles from human neutrophils using antibodies to the cytoplasmic tail of CR1. *Blood* 89:4555, 1997.

35. Sengeløv H, Follin P, Kjeldsen L, et al: Mobilization of granules and secretory vesicles during in vivo exudation of human neutrophils. *J Immunol* 154:4157, 1995.

36. Morgan CP, Sengelov H, Whatmore J, et al: ADP-ribosylation-factor-regulated phospholipase D activity localizes to secretory vesicles and mobilizes to the plasma membrane following N-formylmethionyl-leucyl-phenylalanine stimulation of human neutrophils. *Biochem J* 325:581, 1997.

37. Borregaard N, Kjeldsen L, Sengeløv H: Mobilization of granules in neutrophils from patients with myeloproliferative disorders. *Eur J Haematol* 50:189, 1993.

38. Dotti G, Garattini E, Borleri G, et al: Leucocyte alkaline phosphatase identifies terminally differentiated normal neutrophils and its lack in chronic myelogenous leukaemia is not dependent on p210 tyrosine kinase activity. *Br J Haematol* 105:163, 1999.

39. Rambaldi A, Masuhara K, Borleri GM, et al: Flow cytometry of leucocyte alkaline phosphatase in normal and pathologic leucocytes. *Br J Haematol* 96:815, 1997.

40. Sengeløv H, Kjeldsen L, Kroeze W, et al: Secretory vesicles are the intracellular reservoir of complement receptor 1 in human neutrophils. *J Immunol* 153:804, 1994.

41. Muniz M, Riezman H: Intracellular transport of GPI-anchored proteins. *EMBO J* 19:10, 2000.

42. Ehrlich P: Beiträge zur kenntniss der anilinfärbunden und ihrer verwendung in der mikroskopizchen technik. *Arch Mikrosk Anat* 13:263, 1878.

43. Ehrlich P: Über die specifischen granulationen des blutes. *Arch Anat Physiol Physiologische Abteilung* 571(suppl):1879.

44. Bainton DF, Farquhar MG: Origin of granules in polymorphonuclear leukocytes. *J Cell Biol* 28:277, 1966.

45. Bainton DF, Ullyot JL, Farquhar M: The development of neutrophilic polymorphonuclear leukocytes in human bone marrow. *J Exp Med* 143:907, 1971.

46. Baggiolini M, Hirsch JG, de Duve C: Resolution of granules from rabbit heterophil leukocytes into distinct populations by zonal sedimentation. *J Cell Biol* 40:529, 1969.

47. Dewald B, Bretz U, Baggiolini M: Release of gelatinase from a novel secretory compartment of human neutrophils. *J Clin Invest* 70:518, 1982.

48. Kjeldsen L, Sengeløv H, Lollike K, et al: Isolation and characterization of gelatinase granules from human neutrophils. *Blood* 83:1640, 1994.

49. Kjeldsen L, Johnsen AH, Sengeløv H, et al: Isolation and primary structure of NGAL, a novel protein associated with human neutrophil gelatinase. *J Biol Chem* 268:10425, 1993.

50. Borregaard N, Cowland JB: Granules of the human neutrophilic polymorphonuclear leukocyte. *Blood* 89:3503, 1997.

51. Borregaard N, Heiple JM, Simons ER, et al: Subcellular localization of the b-cytochrome component of the human neutrophil microbicidal oxidase: Translocation during activation. *J Cell Biol* 97:52, 1983.

52. Ganz T, Selsted M, Szklarek D, et al: Defensins. Natural peptide antibiotics of human neutrophils. *J Clin Invest* 76.1427, 1985.

53. Rice WG, Ganz T, Kinkade JM, et al: Defensin-rich dense granules of human neutrophils. *Blood* 70:757, 1987.

54. Faurschou M, Sorensen OE, Johnsen AH, et al: Defensin-rich granules of human neutrophils: Characterization of secretory properties. *Biochim Biophys Acta* 1591:29, 2002.

55. Cham BP, Gerrard JM, Bainton DF: Granulophysin is located in the membrane of azurophilic granules in human neutrophils and mobilizes to the plasma membrane following cell stimulation. *Am J Pathol* 144:1369, 1994.

56. Skubitz KM, Campbell KD, Iida J, et al: CD63 associates with tyrosine kinase activity and CD11/CD18, and transmits an activation signal in neutrophils. *J Immunol* 157:3617, 1996.

57. Andersson E, Hellman L, Gullberg U, et al: The role of the propeptide for processing and sorting of human myeloperoxidase. *J Biol Chem* 273:4747, 1998.

58. Bulow E, Gullberg U, Olsson I: Structural requirements for intracellular processing and sorting of bactericidal/permeability-increasing protein (BPI): Comparison with lipopolysaccharide-binding protein. *J Leukoc Biol* 68:669, 2000.

59. Gullberg U, Bengtsson N, Bulow E, et al: Processing and targeting of granule proteins in human neutrophils. *J Immunol Methods* 232:201, 1999.

60. Kjeldsen L, Bainton DF, Sengeløv H, et al: Structural and functional heterogeneity among peroxidase-negative granules in human neutrophils: Identification of a distinct gelatinase containing granule subset by combined immunocytochemistry and subcellular fractionation. *Blood* 82:3183, 1993.

61. Udby L, Calafat J, Sorensen OE, et al: Identification of human cysteine-rich secretory protein 3 (CRISP-3) as a matrix protein in a subset of peroxidase-negative granules of neutrophils and in the granules of eosinophils. *J Leukoc Biol* 72:462, 2002.

62. Kjeldsen L, Bjerrum OW, Hovgaard D, et al: Human neutrophil gelatinase: A marker for circulating blood neutrophils. Purification and quantitation by enzyme linked immunosorbent assay. *Eur J Haematol* 49:180, 1992.

63. Cowland JB, Johnsen AH, Borregaard N: HCAP-18, a cathelin/bactenecin like protein of human neutrophil specific granules. *FEBS Lett* 368:173, 1995.

64. Sorensen OE, Follin P, Johnsen AH, et al: Human cathelicidin, hCAP-18, is processed to the antimicrobial peptide LL-37 by extracellular cleavage with proteinase 3. *Blood* 97:3951, 2001.

65. Borregaard N, Kjeldsen L, Sengeløv H, et al: Changes in the subcellular localization and surface expression of L-selectin, alkaline phosphatase, and Mac-1 in human neutrophils during stimulation with inflammatory mediators. *J Leukoc Biol* 56:80, 1994.

66. Borregaard N, Lollike K, Kjeldsen L, et al: Human neutrophil granules and secretory vesicles. *Eur J Haematol* 51:187, 1993.

67. Canonne Hergaux F, Calafat J, Richer E, et al: Expression and subcellular localization of NRAMP1 in human neutrophil granules. *Blood* 100:268, 2002.

68. Kang T, Yi J, Guo A, et al: Subcellular Distribution and cytokine- and chemokine-regulated secretion of leukolysin/MT6-MMP/MMP-25 in neutrophils. *J Biol Chem* 276:21960, 2001.

69. Kjeldsen L, Bjerrum OW, Askaa J, et al: Subcellular localization and release of human neutrophil gelatinase, confirming the existence of separate gelatinase-containing granules. *Biochem J* 287:603, 1992.

70. Borregaard N, Sehested M, Nielsen BS, et al: Biosynthesis of granule proteins in normal human bone marrow cells. Gelatinase is a marker of terminal neutrophil differentiation. *Blood* 85:812, 1995.

71. Bjerregaard MD, Jurlander J, Klausen P, et al: The in vivo profile of transcription factors during neutrophil differentiation in human bone marrow. *Blood* 101:4322, 2003.

72. Cowland JB, Borregaard N: The individual regulation of granule protein mRNA levels during neutrophil maturation explains the heterogeneity of neutrophil granules. *J Leukoc Biol* 66:989, 1999.

73. Le Cabec V, Cowland JB, Calafat J, et al: Targeting of proteins to granule subsets determined by timing not by sorting: The specific granule protein NGAL is localized to azurophil granules when expressed in HL-60 cells. *Proc Natl Acad Sci U S A* 93:6454, 1996.

74. Goda Y: SNAREs and regulated vesicle exocytosis. *Proc Natl Acad Sci U S A* 94:769, 1997.

75. Rothman JE: *Molecular and Cellular Mechanisms of Neurotransmitter Release*, edited by L Stjärne, P Greengard, S Grillner, T Hökfelt, D Ottoson, p 81. Raven Press, New York, 1994.

76. Brumell JH, Volchuk A, Sengelov H, et al: Subcellular distribution of docking/fusion proteins in neutrophils, secretory cells with multiple exocytic compartments. *J Immunol* 155:5750, 1995.

77. Mollinedo F, Martin-Martin B, Calafat J, et al: Role of vesicle-associated membrane protein-2, through q-soluble N-ethylmaleimide-sensitive factor attachment protein receptor/r-soluble N-ethylmaleimide-sensitive factor attachment protein receptor interaction, in the exocytosis of specific and tertiary granules of human neutrophils. *J Immunol* 170:1034, 2003.

78. Arnljots K, Sorensen O, Lollike K, et al: Timing targeting and sorting of azurophil granule proteins in human myeloid cells. *Leukemia* 12:1789, 1998.

79. Lollike K, Kjeldsen L, Sengeløv H, et al: Lysozyme in human neutrophils and plasma. A parameter of myelopoietic activity. *Leukemia* 9:159, 1995.

80. Gombart AF, Shiohara M, Kwok SH, et al: Neutrophil-specific granule deficiency: Homozygous recessive inheritance of a frameshift mutation in the gene encoding transcription factor CCAAT/enhancer binding protein-epsilon. *Blood* 97:2561, 2001.

81. Verbeek W, Wachter M, Lekstrom-Himes J, et al: C/EBP epsilon -/- mice: Increased rate of myeloid proliferation and apoptosis. *Leukemia* 15:103, 2001.

82. Liu L, Ganz T: The pro region of human neutrophil defensin contains a motif that is essential for normal subcellular sorting. *Blood* 85:1095, 1995.

83. Lemansky P, Gerecitano-Schmidek M, Das RC, et al: Targeting myeloperoxidase to azurophilic granules in HL-60 cells. *J Leukoc Biol* 74:542, 2003.

84. Anderson KL, Smith KA, Conners K, et al: Myeloid development is selectively disrupted in PU.1 null mice. *Blood* 91:3702, 1998.

85. Fisher RC, Lovelock JD, Scott EW: A critical role for PU.1 in homing and long-term engraftment by hematopoietic stem cells in the bone marrow. *Blood* 94:1283, 1999.

86. Eklund EA, Jalava A, Kakar R: PU.1, interferon regulatory factor 1, and interferon consensus sequence-binding protein cooperate to increase gp91(phox) expression. *J Biol Chem* 273:13957, 1998.

87. Gombart AF, Kwok SH, Anderson KL, et al: Regulation of neutrophil and eosinophil secondary granule gene expression by transcription factors C/EBP epsilon and PU.1. *Blood* 101:3265, 2003.

88. Oelgeschlager M, Nuchprayoon I, Luscher B, et al: C/EBP, c-Myb, and PU.1 cooperate to regulate the neutrophil elastase promoter. *Mol Cell Biol* 16:4717, 1996.

89. Simon MC, Olson M, Scott E, et al: Terminal myeloid gene expression and differentiation requires the transcription factor PU.1. *Curr Top Microbiol Immunol* 211:113, 1996.

90. Yamanaka R, Barlow C, Lekstrom-Himes J, et al: Impaired granulopoiesis, myelodysplasia, and early lethality in CCAAT/enhancer binding protein epsilon-deficient mice. *Proc Natl Acad Sci U S A* 94:13187, 1997.

91. Morosetti R, Park DJ, Chumakov AM, et al: A novel, myeloid transcription factor, C/EBP epsilon, is upregulated during granulocytic, but not monocytic, differentiation. *Blood* 90:2591, 1997.

92. Zabucchi G, Menegazzi R, Soranzo MR, et al: Uptake of human eosinophil peroxidase by human neutrophils. *Am J Pathol* 124:510, 1986.

93. Guarnieri FG, Arterburn LM, Penno MB, et al: The motif Tyr-X-X-hydrophobic residue mediates lysosomal membrane targeting of lysosome-associated membrane protein 1. *J Biol Chem* 268:1941, 1993.

94. Cieutat AM, Lobel P, August JT, et al: Azurophilic granules of human neutrophilic leukocytes are deficient in lysosome-associated membrane proteins but retain the mannose 6-phosphate recognition marker. *Blood* 91:1044, 1998.

95. Bainton DF: Distinct granule populations in human neutrophils and lysosomal organelles identified by immuno-electron microscopy. *J Immunol Method* 232:153, 1999.

96. Ghosh P, Dahms NM, Kornfeld S: Mannose 6-phosphate receptors: New twists in the tale. *Nat Rev Mol Cell Biol* 4:202, 2003.

97. Dittmer F, Hafner A, Ulbrich EJ, et al: I-cell disease-like phenotype in mice deficient in mannose 6-phosphate receptors. *Transgenic Res* 7:473, 1998.

98. Arnljots K, Olsson I: Myeloperoxidase precursors incorporate heme. *J Biol Chem* 262:10430, 1987.

99. Nauseef WM, McCormick S, Yi H: Roles of heme insertion and the mannose-6-phosphate receptor in processing of the human myeloid lysosomal enzyme, myeloperoxidase. *Blood* 80:2622, 1992.

100. Klebanoff SJ: Myeloperoxidase. *Proc Assoc Am Physicians* 111:383, 1999.

101. Klebanoff SJ, Nathan CF: Nitrite production by stimulated human polymorphonuclear leukocytes supplemented with azide and catalase. *Biochem Biophys Res Commun* 197:192, 1993.

102. Eiserich JP, Baldus S, Brennan ML, et al: Myeloperoxidase, a leukocyte-derived vascular NO oxidase. *Science* 296:2391, 2002.

103. Brennan ML, Penn MS, Van Lente F, et al: Prognostic value of myeloperoxidase in patients with chest pain. *N Engl J Med* 349:1595, 2003.

104. Savige J, Davies D, Falk RJ, et al: Antineutrophil cytoplasmic antibodies and associated diseases: A review of the clinical and laboratory features. *Kidney Int* 57:846, 2000.

105. Tervaert JW, Goldschmeding R, Elema JD, et al: Association of autoantibodies to myeloperoxidase with different forms of vasculitis. *Arthritis Rheum* 33:1264, 1990.

106. Levy O, Elsbach P: Bactericidal/permeability-increasing protein in host defense and its efficacy in the treatment of bacterial sepsis. *Curr Infect Dis Rep* 3:407, 2001.

107. Alexander S, Bramson J, Foley R, et al: Protection from endotoxemia by adenoviral-mediated gene transfer of human bactericidal/permeability-increasing protein. *Blood* 2003.

108. Ganz T: Defensins: Antimicrobial peptides of innate immunity. *Nat Rev Immunol* 3:710, 2003.

109. Selsted ME, Harwig SSL, Ganz T, et al: Primary structures of three human neutrophil defensins. *J Clin Invest* 76:1436, 1985.

110. Selsted ME, Tang Y-Q, Morris WL, et al: Purification, primary structures, and antibacterial activities of β-defensins, a new family of antimicrobial peptides from bovine neutrophils. *J Biol Chem* 268:6641, 1993.

111. Tang YU, Yuan J, Ösapay G, et al: A cyclic antibicrobial peptide produced in primate leukocytes by the ligation of two truncated α-defensins. *Science* 286:498, 1999.

112. Almeida RP, Vanet A, Witkosarsat V, et al: Azurocidin, a natural antibiotic from human neutrophils: Expression, antimicrobial activity, and secretion. *Protein Express Purif* 7:355, 1996.

113. Campanelli D, Detmers PA, Nathan CF, et al: Azurocidin and a homologous serine protease from neutrophils. Differential antimicrobial and proteolytic properties. *J Clin Invest* 85:904, 1990.

114. Flodgaard H, Østergaard E, Bayne S, et al: Covalent structure of two novel neutrophile leucocyte derived proteins of porcine and human origin. Neutrophile elastase homologues with strong monocyte and fibroblast chemotactic activities. *Eur J Biochem* 197:535, 1991.

115. Gautam N, Olofsson AM, Herwald H, et al: Heparin-binding protein (HBP/CAP37): A missing link in neutrophil-evoked alteration of vascular permeability. *Nat Med* 7:1123, 2001.

116. Tapper H, Karlsson A, Morgelin M, et al: Secretion of heparin-binding protein from human neutrophils is determined by its localization in azurophilic granules and secretory vesicles. *Blood* 99:1785, 2002.

117. Goldschmeding R, Tervaert JW, Dolman KM, et al: ANCA: A class of vasculitis-associated autoantibodies against myeloid granule proteins: Clinical and laboratory aspects and possible pathogenetic implications. *Adv Exp Med Biol* 297:129, 1991.

118. Skold S, Rosberg B, Gullberg U, et al: A secreted proform of neutrophil proteinase 3 regulates the proliferation of granulopoietic progenitor cells. *Blood* 93:849, 1999.

119. Edens HA, Parkos CA: Neutrophil transendothelial migration and alteration in vascular permeability: Focus on neutrophil-derived azurocidin. *Curr Opin Hematol* 10:25, 2003.

120. Skubitz KM, Campbell KD, Skubitz APN: CD63 associates with CD11/CD18 in large detergent-resistant complexes after translocation to the cell surface in human neutrophils. *FEBS Lett* 469:52, 2000.

121. Saito N, Pulford KAF, Breton-Gorius J, et al: Ultrastructural localization of the CD68 macrophage-associated antigen in human blood neutrophils and monocytes. *Am J Pathol* 139:1053, 1991.

122. Mirinics ZK, Calafat J, Udby L, et al: Identification of the presenilins in hematopoietic cells with localization of presenilin 1 to neutrophil and platelet granules. *Blood Cells Mol Dis* 28:28, 2002.

123. Feuk-Lagerstedt E, Samuelsson M, Mosgoeller W, et al: The presence of stomatin in detergent-insoluble domains of neutrophil granule membranes. *J Leukoc Biol* 72:970, 2002.

124. Nanda A, Brumell JH, Nordstrom T, et al: Activation of proton pumping in human neutrophils occurs by exocytosis of vesicles bearing vacuolar-type H+-ATPases. *J Biol Chem* 271:15963, 1996.

125. Masson PL, Heremans JF, Schonne E: Lactoferrin, an iron-binding protein in neutrophilic leukocytes. *J Exp Med* 130:643, 1969.

126. Baveye S, Elass E, Mazurier J, et al: Lactoferrin: A multifunctional glycoprotein involved in the modulation of the inflammatory process. *Clin Chem Lab Med* 37:281, 1999.

127. Farnaud S, Evans RW: Lactoferrin: A multifunctional protein with antimicrobial properties. *Mol Immunol* 40:395, 2003.

128. Aguilera O, Ostolaza H, Quiros LM, et al: Permeabilizing action of an antimicrobial lactoferricin-derived peptide on bacterial and artificial membranes. *FEBS Lett* 462:273, 1999.

129. Nibbering PH, Ravensbergen E, Welling MM, et al: Human lactoferrin and peptides derived from its N terminus are highly effective against infections with antibiotic-resistant bacteria. *Infect Immun* 69:1469, 2001.

130. Flower DR: The lipocalin protein family: Structure and function. *Biochem J* 318:1, 1996.

131. Kjeldsen L, Bainton DF, Sengeløv H, et al: Identification of neutrophil gelatinase-associated lipocalin as a novel matrix protein of specific granules in human neutrophils. *Blood* 83:799, 1994.

132. Yan L, Borregaard N, Kjeldsen L, et al: The high molecular weight urinary matrix metalloproteinase (MMP) activity is a complex of gelatinase B/MMP-9 and neutrophil gelatinase-associated lipocalin (NGAL). Modulation of MMP-9 activity by NGAL. *J Biol Chem* 276:37258, 2001.

133. Goetz DH, Holmes MA, Borregaard N, et al: The neutrophil lipocalin NGAL is a bacteriostatic agent that interferes with siderophore-mediated iron acquisition. *Mol Cell* 10:1033, 2002.

134. Cowland JB, Sorensen OE, Sehested M, et al: Neutrophil gelatinase-associated lipocalin is up-regulated in human epithelial cells by IL-1beta, but not by TNF-alpha. *J Immunol* 171:6630, 2003.

135. Cellier M, Govoni G, Vidal S, et al: Human natural resistance-associated macrophage protein: CDNA cloning, chromosomal mapping, genomic organization, and tissue-specific expression. *J Exp Med* 180:1741, 1994.

136. Fleming A: On a remarkable bacteriolytic element found in tissues and excretions. *Proc R Soc Med* 93:306, 1922.

137. Selsted ME, Martinez RJ: Lysozyme: Primary bactericidin in human plasma serum active against Bacillus subtilis. *Infect Immun* 20:782, 1978.

138. Tanida N, Onho N, Adachi Y, et al: Binding of lysozyme to synthetic monosaccharide lipid A analogue, GLA60. *Biol Pharm Bull* 16:288, 1993.

139. Takada K, Ohno N, Yadomae T: Binding of lysozyme to lipopolysaccharide suppresses tumor necrosis factor production in vivo. *Infect Immun* 62:1171, 1994.

140. Keshav S, Chung P, Milon G, et al: Lysozyme is an inducible marker of macrophage activation in murine tissues as demonstrated by in situ hybridization. *J Exp Med* 174:1049, 1991.

141. Sexton C, Buss D, Powell B, et al: Usefulness and limitations of serum and urine lysozyme levels in the classification of acute myeloid leukemia: An analysis of 208 cases. *Leuk Res* 20:467, 1996.

142. Gudmundsson GH, Agerberth B, Odeberg J, et al: The human gene FALL39 and processing of the cathelin precursor to the antibacterial peptide LL-37 in granulocytes. *Eur J Biochem* 238:325, 1996.

143. Zanetti M: Cathelicidins, multifunctional peptides of the innate immunity. *J Leukoc Biol* 2003.

144. Sorensen O, Arnljots K, Cowland JB, et al: The human antibacterial cathelicidin, hCAP-18, is synthesized in myelocytes and metamyelocytes and localized to specific granules in neutrophils. *Blood* 90:2796, 1997.

145. Sorensen O, Bratt T, Johnsen AH, et al: The human antibacterial cathelicidin, hCAP-18, is bound to lipoproteins in plasma. *J Biol Chem* 274:22445, 1999.

146. Frohm-Nilsson M, Sandstedt B, Sorensen O, et al: The human cationic antimicrobial protein (hCAP18), a peptide antibiotic, is widely expressed in human squamous epithelia and colocalizes with interleukin-6. *Infect Immun* 67:2561, 1999.

147. Heilborn JD, Nilsson MF, Kratz G, et al: The cathelicidin anti-microbial peptide LL-37 is involved in re-epithelialization of human skin wounds and is lacking in chronic ulcer epithelium. *J Invest Dermatol* 120:379, 2003.

148. Sorensen OE, Cowland JB, Theilgaard-Monch K, et al: Wound healing and expression of antimicrobial peptides/polypeptides in human keratinocytes, a consequence of common growth factors. *J Immunol* 170:5583, 2003.

149. Sorensen OE, Gram L, Johnsen AH, et al: Processing of seminal plasma hCAP-18 to ALL-38 by gastricsin: A novel mechanism of generating antimicrobial peptides in vagina. *J Biol Chem* 278:28540, 2003.

150. Zaiou M, Nizet V, Gallo RL: Antimicrobial and protease inhibitory functions of the human cathelicidin (hCAP18/LL-37) prosequence. *J Invest Dermatol* 120:810, 2003.

151. Yang D, Chen Q, Schmidt AP, et al: LL-37, the neutrophil granule- and epithelial cell-derived cathelicidin, utilizes formyl peptide receptor-like-1 (FPRL1) as a receptor to chemoattract human peripheral blood neutrophils, monocytes, and T cells. *J Exp Med* 192:1069, 2000.

152. Koczulla R, von Degenfeld G, Kupatt C, et al: An angiogenic role for the human peptide antibiotic LL-37/hCAP-18. *J Clin Invest* 111:1665, 2003.

153. Scott MG, Davidson DJ, Gold MR, et al: The human antimicrobial peptide LL-37 is a multifunctional modulator of innate immune responses. *J Immunol* 169:3883, 2002.

154. Murphy G, Reynolds JJ, Bretz U, et al: Collagenase is a component of the specific granules of human neutrophil leucocytes. *Biochem J* 162:195, 1977.

155. Murphy G, Bretz U, Baggiolini M, et al: The latent collagenase and gelatinase of human polymorphonuclear neutrophil leucocytes. *Biochem J* 192:517, 1980.

156. Pei D: Leukolysin/MMP25/MT6-MMP: A novel matrix metalloproteinase specifically expressed in the leukocyte lineage. *Cell Research* 9:291, 1999.

157. Ginsel LA, Onderwater JJM, Fransen JAM, et al: Localization of the low-M_r subunit of cytochrome b_{558} in human blood phagocytes by immunoelectron microscopy. *Blood* 76:2105, 1990.

158. Feuk-Lagerstedt E, Jordan ET, Leffler H, et al: Identification of CD66a and CD66b as the major galectin-3 receptor candidates in human neutrophils. *J Immunol* 163:5592, 1999.

159. Karlsson A, Follin P, Leffler H, et al: Galectin-3 activates the NADPH-oxidase in exudated but not peripheral blood neutrophils. *Blood* 91:3430, 1998.

160. Williams LT, Snyderman R, Pike MC, et al: Specific receptor sites for chemotactic peptides on human polymorphonuclear leukocytes. *Proc Natl Acad Sci U S A* 74:1204, 1977.

161. Schiffmann E, Aswanikumar S, Venkatasubramanian K, et al: Some characteristics of the neutrophil receptor for chemotactic peptides. *FEBS Lett* 117:1, 1980.

162. Boulay F, Tardif M, Brouchon L, et al: The human N-formylpeptide receptor. Characterization of two cDNA isolates and evidence for a new subfamily of G-protein-coupled receptors. *Biochemistry* 29:11123, 1990.

163. Prossnitz ER, Ye RD: The N-formyl peptide receptor: A model for the study of chemoattractant receptor structure and function. *Pharmacol Ther* 74:73, 1997.

164. Sengeløv H, Boulay F, Kjeldsen L, et al: Subcellular localization and translocation of the receptor for N-formyl-methionyl-leucyl-phenylalanine in human neutrophils. *Biochem J* 299:473, 1994.

165. Hugli TE: Structure and function of the anaphylatoxins. *Springer Semin Immunopathol* 7:193, 1984.

166. Chenoweth DE, Hugli TE: Demonstration of specific C5a receptor on intact human polymorphonuclear leukocytes. *Proc Natl Acad Sci U S A* 75:3943, 1978.

167. Rollins TE, Springer MS: Identification of the polymorphonuclear leukocyte C5a receptor. *J Biol Chem* 260:7157, 1985.

168. Boulay F, Mery L, Tardif M, et al: Expression cloning of a receptor for C5a anaphylatoxin on differentiated HL-60 cells. *Biochemistry* 30:2993, 1991.

169. Nathan CF: Neutrophil activation on biological surfaces. Massive secretion of hydrogen peroxide in response to products of macrophages and lymphocytes. *J Clin Invest* 80:1550, 1987.

170. Shappell SB, Toman C, Anderson DC, et al: Mac-1 (CD11b/CD18) mediates adherence-dependent hydrogen peroxide production by human and canine neutrophils. *J Immunol* 144:2702, 1990.

171. Kew RR, Grimaldi CM, Furie MB, et al: Human neutrophil Fc gamma RIIIB and formyl peptide receptors are functionally linked during formyl-methionyl-leucyl-phenylalanine-induced chemotaxis. *J Immunol* 149:989, 1992.

172. Leeuwenberg JF, Van De Winkel JG, Jeunhomme TM, et al: Functional polymorphism of IgG FcRII (CD32) on human neutrophils. *Immunology* 71:301, 1990.

173. Sehgal G, Zhang K, Todd RFIII, et al: Lectin-like inhibition of immune complex receptor-mediated stimulation of neutrophils. Effects on cytosolic calcium release and superoxide production. *J Immunol* 150:4571, 1993.

174. Indik ZK, Park JG, Hunter S, et al: The molecular dissection of Fc gamma receptor mediated phagocytosis. *Blood* 86:4389, 1995.

175. Strzelecka-Kiliszek A, Kwiatkowska K, Sobota A: Lyn and Syk kinases are sequentially engaged in phagocytosis mediated by Fc gamma R. *J Immunol* 169:6787, 2002.

176. Raeder EM, Mansfield PJ, Hinkovska-Galcheva V, et al: Syk activation initiates downstream signaling events during human polymorphonuclear leukocyte phagocytosis. *J Immunol* 163:6785, 1999.

177. Kusner DJ, Barton JA, Wen KK, et al: Regulation of phospholipase D activity by actin. Actin exerts bidirectional modulation of mammalian phospholipase D activity in a polymerization-dependent, isoform-specific manner. *J Biol Chem* 277:50683, 2002.

178. Didsbury JR, Uhing RJ, Tomhave E, et al: Receptor class desensitization of leukocyte chemoattractant receptors. *Proc Natl Acad Sci U S A* 88:11564, 1991.

179. Nakamura M, Honda Z, Izumi T, et al: Molecular cloning and expression of platelet-activating factor receptor from human leukocytes. *J Biol Chem* 266:20400, 1991.

180. Jones SA, Wolf M, Qin SX, et al: Different functions for the interleukin 8 receptors (IL-8R) of human neutrophil leukocytes: NADPH oxidase and phospholipase D are activated through IL-8R1 but not IL-8R2. *Proc Natl Acad Sci U S A* 93:6682, 1996.

181. Sklar LA, Bokoch GM, Button D, et al: Regulation of ligand-receptor dynamics by guanine nucleotides. Real-time analysis of interconverting states for the neutrophil formyl peptide receptor. *J Biol Chem* 262:135, 1987.

182. Pelz C, Matsumoto T, Molski TF, et al: Characterization of the membrane-associated GTPase activity: Effects of chemotactic factors and toxins. *J Cell Biochem* 39:197, 1989.

183. Bokoch GM, Bickford K, Bohl BP: Subcellular localization and quantitation of the major neutrophil pertussis toxin substrate, G_n. *J Cell Biol* 106:1927, 1988.

184. Kanaho Y, Kanoh H, Nozawa Y: Activation of phospholipase D in rabbit neutrophils by fMet-Leu-Phe is mediated by a pertussis toxin-sensitive GTP-binding protein that may be distinct from a phospholipase C-regulating protein. *FEBS Lett* 279:249, 1991.

185. Barrowman MM, Cockcroft S, Gomperts BD: Two roles for guanine nucleotides in the stimulus-secretion sequence of neutrophils. *Nature* 319:504, 1986.

186. Ohnishi H, Ernst SA, Yule DI, et al: Heterotrimeric G-protein Gq/11 localized on pancreatic zymogen granules is involved in calcium-regulated amylase secretion. *J Biol Chem* 272:16056, 1997.

187. Mansfield PJ, Carey SS, Hinkovska-Galcheva V, et al: Ceramide inhibition of phospholipase D and its relationship to RhoA and ARF1 translocation in GTP gamma S-stimulated polymorphonuclear leukocytes. *Blood* 103:2363, 2004.

188. Dusi S, Donini M, Dellabianca V, et al: Tyrosine phosphorylation of phospholipase c-gamma 2 is involved In the activation of phosphoinositide hydrolysis by Fc receptors in human neutrophils. *Biochem Biophys Res Commun* 201:1100, 1994.

189. Mansfield PJ, Shayman JA, Boxer LA: Regulation of polymorphonu-clear leukocyte phagocytosis by myosin light chain kinase after activation of mitogen-activated protein kinase. *Blood* 95:2407, 2000.

190. Cockcroft S, Baldwin JM, Allan D: The Ca2+-activated polyphosphoinositide phosphodiesterase of human and rabbit neutrophil membranes. *Biochem J* 221:477, 1984.

191. Favre CJ, Lew DP, Krause KH: Rapid heparin-sensitive Ca2+ release following Ca(2+)-ATPase inhibition in intact HL-60 granulocytes. Evidence for Ins(1,4,5)P3-dependent Ca2+ cycling across the membrane of Ca2+ stores. *Biochem J* 302 (Pt 1):155, 1994.

192. Cox D, Chang P, Zhang Q, et al: Requirements for both Rac1 and Cdc42 in membrane ruffling and phagocytosis in leukocytes. *J Exp Med* 186:1487, 1997.

193. Roberts AW, Kim C, Zhen L, et al: Deficiency of the hematopoietic cell-specific Rho family GTPase Rac2 is characterized by abnormalities in neutrophil function and host defense. *Immunity* 10:183, 1999.

194. Mansfield PJ, Hinkovska-Galcheva V, Carey SS, et al: Regulation of polymorphonuclear leukocyte degranulation and oxidant production by ceramide through inhibition of phospholipase D. *Blood* 99:1434, 2002.

195. Blackwood RA, Smolen JE, Transue A, et al: Phospholipase D activity facilitates Ca2+-induced aggregation and fusion of complex liposomes. *Am J Physiol* 272:C1279, 1997.

196. English D, Cui Y, Siddiqui RA: Messenger functions of phosphatidic acid. *Chem Phys Lipids* 80:117, 1996.

197. Diez E, Balsinde J, Mollinedo F: Subcellular distribution of fatty acids, phospholipids and phospholipase A2 in human neutrophils. *Biochim Biophys Acta* 1047:83, 1990.

198. Pessach I, Leto TL, Malech HL, et al: Essential requirement of cytosolic phospholipase A(2) for stimulation of NADPH oxidase-associated diaphorase activity in granulocyte-like cells. *J Biol Chem* 276:33495, 2001.

199. Naccache PH, Showell HJ, Becker EL, et al: Arachidonic acid induced degranulation of rabbit peritoneal neutrophils. *Biochem Biophys Res Commun* 87:292, 1979.

200. Hardy SJ, Robinson BS, Ferrante A, et al: Polyenoic very-long-chain fatty acids mobilize intracellular calcium from a thapsigargin-insensitive pool in human neutrophils. The relationship between Ca2+ mobilization and superoxide production induced by long- and very-long-chain fatty acids. *Biochem J* 311(Pt 2):689, 1995.

201. Borgeat P, Hamberg M, Samuelsson B: Transformation of arachidonic acid and homo-gamma-linolenic acid by rabbit polymorphonuclear leukocytes. Monohydroxy acids from novel lipoxygenases. *J Biol Chem* 251:7816, 1976.

202. Naccache PH, Sha'afi RI, Borgeat P, et al: Mono- and dihydroxyeicosatetraenoic acids alter calcium homeostasis in rabbit neutrophils. *J Clin Invest* 67:1584, 1981.

203. Palmer RM, Salmon JA: Release of leukotriene B4 from human neutrophils and its relationship to degranulation induced by N-formyl-methionyl-leucyl-phenylalanine, serum-treated zymosan and the ionophore A23187. *Immunology* 50:65, 1983.

204. Palmblad J, Malmsten CL, Uden AM, et al: Leukotriene B4 is a potent and stereospecific stimulator of neutrophil chemotaxis and adherence. *Blood* 58:658, 1981.

205. Rothman JE: Mechanisms of intracellular protein transport. *Nature* 372:55, 1994.

206. Lekstrom-Himes JA, Gallin JI: Immunodeficiency diseases caused by defects in phagocytes. *N Engl J Med* 343:1703, 2000.

207. Andrews T, Sullivan KE: Infections in patients with inherited defects in phagocytic function. *Clin Microbiol Rev* 16:597, 2003.

208. Lakshman R, Finn A: Neutrophil disorders and their management. *J Clin Pathol* 54:7, 2001.

209. Botto M, Fong KY, So AK, et al: Molecular basis of hereditary C3 deficiency. *J Clin Invest* 86:1158, 1990.

210. Frank MM: Complement deficiencies. *Pediatr Clin North Am* 47:1339, 2000.

211. Alper CA, Abramson N, Johnston RB Jr, et al: Studies in vivo and in vitro on an abnormality in the metabolism of C3 in a patient with increased susceptibility to infection. *J Clin Invest* 49:1975, 1970.

212. Densen P, Weiler JM, Griffiss JM, et al: Familial properdin deficiency and fatal meningococcemia. Correction of the bactericidal defect by vaccination. *N Engl J Med* 316:922, 1987.

213. Nolan KF, Schwaeble W, Kaluz S, et al: Molecular cloning of the cDNA coding for properdin, a positive regulator of the alternative pathway of human complement. *Eur J Immunol* 21:771, 1991.

214. Super M, Thiel S, Lu J, et al: Association of low levels of mannan-binding protein with a common defect of opsonisation. *Lancet* 2:1236, 1989.

215. Jack DL, Klein NJ, Turner MW: Mannose-binding lectin: Targeting the microbial world for complement attack and opsonophagocytosis. *Immunol Rev* 180:86, 2001.

216. Turner MW: The role of mannose-binding lectin in health and disease. *Mol Immunol* 40:423, 2003.

217. Buckley RH: Immunodeficiency diseases. *JAMA* 268:2797, 1992.

218. Boxer LA, Smolen JE: Neutrophil granule constituents and their release in health and disease. *Hematol Oncol Clin North Am* 2:101, 1988.

219. Ward DM, Shiflett SL, Kaplan J: Chediak-Higashi syndrome: A clinical and molecular view of a rare lysosomal storage disorder. *Curr Mol Med* 2:469, 2002.

220. Creel D, Boxer LA, Fauci AS: Visual and auditory anomalies in Chediak-Higashi syndrome. *Electroencephalogr Clin Neurophysiol* 55:252, 1983.

221. Boxer GJ, Holmsen H, Robkin L, et al: Abnormal platelet function in Chediak-Higashi syndrome. *Br J Haematol* 35:521, 1977.

222. Abo T, Roder JC, Abo W, et al: Natural killer (HNK-1+) cells in Chediak-Higashi patients are present in normal numbers but are abnormal in function and morphology. *J Clin Invest* 70:193, 1982.

223. Introne W, Boissy RE, Gahl WA: Clinical, molecular, and cell biological aspects of Chediak-Higashi syndrome. *Mol Genet Metab* 68:283, 1999.

224. Beguez-Cesar A: Neutropenia cronica maligna familiar con granulaciounes atipicas de los leucocitos. *Bol Soc Cubana Pediatr* 15:900, 1943.

225. Steinbrinck W: Über ene neue granulations anomalie der leukocyten. *Dtsch Arch Klin Med* 193:577, 1948.

226. Chediak MM: New leukocyte anomaly of constitutional and familial character. *Rev Hematol* 7:362, 1952.

227. Higashi O: Congenital gigantism of peroxidase granules; the first case ever reported of qualitative abnormity of peroxidase. *Tohoku J Exp Med* 59:315, 1954.

228. Blume RS, Wolff SM: The Chediak-Higashi syndrome: Studies in four patients and a review of the literature. *Medicine (Baltimore)* 51:247, 1972.

229. Ingraham LM, Burns CP, Boxer LA, et al: Fluidity properties and liquid composition of erythrocyte membranes in Chediak-Higashi syndrome. *J Cell Biol* 89:510, 1981.

230. Ostlund RE Jr, Tucker RW, Leung JT, et al: The cytoskeleton in Chediak-Higashi syndrome fibroblasts. *Blood* 56:806, 1980.

231. White JG, Clawson CC: The Chediak-Higashi syndrome: The nature of the giant neutrophil granules and their interactions with cytoplasm and foreign particulates. *Am J Pathol* 98:151, 1980.

232. Blume RS, Bennett JM, Yankee RA, et al: Defective granulocyte regulation in the Chediak-Higashi syndrome. *N Engl J Med* 279:1009, 1968.

233. Trambas CM, Griffiths GM: Delivering the kiss of death. *Nat Immunol* 4:399, 2003.

234. Barbosa MD, Barrat FJ, Tchernev VT, et al: Identification of mutations in two major mRNA isoforms of the Chediak-Higashi syndrome gene in human and mouse. *Hum Mol Genet* 6:1091, 1997.

235. Stinchcombe JC, Page LJ, Griffiths GM: Secretory lysosome biogenesis in cytotoxic T lymphocytes from normal and Chediak-Higashi syndrome patients. *Traffic* 1:435, 2000.

236. Tchernev VT, Mansfield TA, Giot L, et al: The Chediak-Higashi protein interacts with SNARE complex and signal transduction proteins. *Mol Med* 8:56, 2002.

237. Nair MP, Gray RII, Boxer LA, et al: Deficiency of inducible suppressor cell activity in the Chediak-Higashi syndrome. *Am J Hematol* 26:55, 1987.

238. Rubin CM, Burke BA, McKenna RW, et al: The accelerated phase of Chediak-Higashi syndrome. An expression of the virus-associated hemophagocytic syndrome? *Cancer* 56:524, 1985.

239. de Saint BG, Fischer A: The role of cytotoxicity in lymphocyte homeostasis. *Curr Opin Immunol* 13:549, 2001.

240. Haddad E, Le Deist F, Blanche S, et al: Treatment of Chediak-Higashi syndrome by allogenic bone marrow transplantation: Report of 10 cases. *Blood* 85:3328, 1995.

241. Virelizier JL, Lagrue A, Durandy A, et al: Reversal of natural killer defect in a patient with Chediak-Higashi syndrome after bone-marrow transplantation. *N Engl J Med* 306:1055, 1982.

242. Ganz T, Metcalf JA, Gallin JI, et al: Microbicidal/cytotoxic proteins of neutrophils are deficient in two disorders: Chediak-Higashi syndrome and "specific" granule deficiency. *J Clin Invest* 82:552, 1988.

243. Lomax KJ, Gallin JI, Rotrosen D, et al: Selective defect in myeloid cell lactoferrin gene expression in neutrophil specific granule deficiency. *J Clin Invest* 83:514, 1989.

244. Johnston JJ, Boxer LA, Berliner N: Correlation of messenger RNA levels with protein defects in specific granule deficiency. *Blood* 80:2088, 1992.

245. Rosenberg HF, Gallin JI: Neutrophil-specific granule deficiency includes eosinophils. *Blood* 82:268, 1993.

246. Gallin JI, Fletcher MP, Seligmann BE, et al: Human neutrophil-specific granule deficiency: A model to assess the role of neutrophil-specific granules in the evolution of the inflammatory response. *Blood* 59:1317, 1982.

247. Lekstrom-Himes JA, Dorman SE, Kopar P, et al: Neutrophil-specific granule deficiency results from a novel mutation with loss of function of the transcription factor CCAAT enhancer binding protein epsilon. *J Exp Med* 189:1847, 1999.

248. Gombart AF, Koeffler HP: Neutrophil specific granule deficiency and mutations in the gene encoding transcription factor C/EBP(epsilon). *Curr Opin Hematol* 9:36, 2002.

249. Lekstrom-Himes JA: The role of C/EBP(epsilon) in the terminal stages of granulocyte differentiation. *Stem Cells* 19:125, 2001.

250. Parmley RT, Tzeng DY, Baehner RL, et al: Abnormal distribution of complex carbohydrates in neutrophils of a patient with lactoferrin deficiency. *Blood* 62:538, 1983.

251. Kuriyama K, Tomonaga M, Matsuo T, et al: Diagnostic significance of detecting pseudo-Pelger-Huet anomalies and micro-megakaryocytes in myelodysplastic syndrome. *Br J Haematol* 63:665, 1986.

252. Arnaout MA: Leukocyte adhesion molecules deficiency: Its structural basis, pathophysiology and implications for modulating the inflammatory response. *Immunol Rev* 114:145, 1990.

253. Corbi AL, Larson RS, Kishimoto TK, et al: Chromosomal location of the genes encoding the leukocyte adhesion receptors LFA-1, Mac-1 and p150,95. Identification of a gene cluster involved in cell adhesion. *J Exp Med* 167:1597, 1988.

254. Hayward AR, Harvey BA, Leonard J, et al: Delayed separation of the umbilical cord, widespread infections, and defective neutrophil mobility. *Lancet* 1:1099, 1979.

255. Crowley CA, Curnutte JT, Rosin RE, et al: An inherited abnormality of neutrophil adhesion. Its genetic transmission and its association with a missing protein. *N Engl J Med* 302:1163, 1980.

256. Arnaout MA, Pitt J, Cohen HJ, et al: Deficiency of a granulocyte-membrane glycoprotein (gp150) in a boy with recurrent bacterial infections. *N Engl J Med* 306:693, 1982.

257. Dana N, Todd RF III, Pitt P, et al: Deficiency of a surface membrane glycoprotein (Mo1) in man. *J Clin Invest* 73:153, 1984.

258. Anderson DC, Smith CW: Leukocyte adhesion deficiencies, in *The Metabolic and Molecular Basis of Inherited Disease*, 8th ed, edited by C Scriver, A Beaudet, W Sly, D Valle, B Childs, K Kinzler, B Vogelstein, p 4829. McGraw-Hill, New York, 2001.

259. Springer TA, Thompson WS, Miller LJ, et al: Inherited deficiency of the Mac-1, LFA-1, p150,95 glycoprotein family and its molecular basis. *J Exp Med* 160:1901, 1984.

260. Arnaout MA: Structure and function of the leukocyte adhesion molecules CD11/CD18. *Blood* 75:1037, 1990.

261. Cheresh DA, Smith JW, Cooper HM, et al: A novel vitronectin receptor integrin (alpha v beta x) is responsible for distinct adhesive properties of carcinoma cells. *Cell* 57:59, 1989.

262. Anderson DC, Schmalstieg FC, Finegold MJ, et al: The severe and moderate phenotypes of heritable Mac-1, LFA-1 deficiency: Their quantitative definition and relation to leukocyte dysfunction and clinical features. *J Infect Dis* 152:668, 1985.

263. Larson RS, Springer TA: Structure and function of leukocyte integrins. *Immunol Rev* 114:181, 1990.

264. Hogg N, Stewart MP, Scarth SL, et al: A novel leukocyte adhesion deficiency caused by expressed but nonfunctional beta2 integrins Mac-1 and LFA-1. *J Clin Invest* 103:97, 1999.

265. Mathew EC, Shaw JM, Bonilla FA, et al: A novel point mutation in CD18 causing the expression of dysfunctional CD11/CD18 leucocyte integrins in a patient with leucocyte adhesion deficiency (LAD). *Clin Exp Immunol* 121:133, 2000.

266. Harris ES, Shigeoka AO, Li WH, et al: A novel syndrome of variant leukocyte adhesion deficiency involving defects in adhesion mediated by beta(1) and beta(2) integrins. *Blood* 97:767, 2001.

267. Kuijpers TW, vanLier RAW, Hamann D, et al: Leukocyte adhesion deficiency type 1 (LAD-1)/variant: A novel immunodeficiency syndrome characterized by dysfunctional beta(2) integrins. *J Clin Invest* 100:1725, 1997.

268. Petrequin PR, Todd RF III, Devall LJ, et al: Association between gelatinase release and increased plasma membrane expression of the Mo1 glycoprotein. *Blood* 69:605, 1987.

269. Anderson DC, Springer TA: Leukocyte adhesion deficiency: An inherited defect in the Mac-1, LFA-1, and p150,95 glycoproteins. *Annu Rev Med* 38:175, 1987.

270. Schwartz BR, Wayner EA, Carlos TM, et al: Identification of surface proteins mediating adherence of CD11/CD18-deficient lymphoblastoid cells to cultured human endothelium. *J Clin Invest* 85:2019, 1990.

271. Mizgerd JP, Kubo H, Kutkoski GJ, et al: Neutrophil emigration in the skin, lungs, and peritoneum: Different requirements for CD11/CD18 revealed by CD18-deficient mice. *J Exp Med* 186:1357, 1997.

272. Anderson DC, Rothlein R, Marlin SD, et al: Impaired transendothelial migration by neonatal neutrophils: Abnormalities of Mac-1 (CD11b/CD18)-dependent adherence reactions. *Blood* 76:2613, 1990.

273. Mulligan MS, Varani J, Dame MK, et al: Role of endothelial-leukocyte adhesion molecule 1 (ELAM-1) in neutrophil-mediated lung injury in rats. *J Clin Invest* 88:1396, 1991.

274. Wertheimer SJ, Myers CL, Wallace RW, et al: Intercellular adhesion molecule-1 gene expression in human endothelial cells. Differential regulation by tumor necrosis factor-alpha and phorbol myristate acetate. *J Biol Chem* 267:12030, 1992.

275. Malawista SE, de Boisfleury CA, Boxer LA: Random locomotion and chemotaxis of human blood polymorphonuclear leukocytes from a patient with leukocyte adhesion deficiency-1: Normal displacement in close quarters via chimneying. *Cell Motil Cytoskeleton* 46:183, 2000.

276. Cao D, Mizukami IF, Garni-Wagner BA, et al: Human urokinase-type plasminogen activator primes neutrophils for superoxide anion release. Possible roles of complement receptor type 3 and calcium. *J Immunol* 154:1817, 1995.

277. Altieri DC, Bader R, Mannucci PM, et al: Oligospecificity of the cellular adhesion receptor Mac-1 encompasses an inducible recognition specificity for fibrinogen. *J Cell Biol* 107:1893, 1988.

278. Wilson RW, Ballantyne CM, Smith CW, et al: Gene targeting yields a CD18-mutant mouse for study of inflammation. *J Immunol* 151:1571, 1993.

279. Forlow SB, Schurr JR, Kolls JK, et al: Increased granulopoiesis through interleukin-17 and granulocyte colony-stimulating factor in leukocyte adhesion molecule-deficient mice. *Blood* 98:3309, 2001.

280. Hidalgo A, Ma S, Peired AJ, et al: Insights into leukocyte adhesion deficiency type 2 from a novel mutation in the GDP-fucose transporter gene. *Blood* 101:1705, 2003.

281. Fischer A, Lisowska-Grospierre B, Anderson DC, et al: Leukocyte adhesion deficiency: Molecular basis and functional consequences. *Immunodefic Rev* 1:39, 1988.

282. Bauer TR Jr, Hickstein DD: Gene therapy for leukocyte adhesion deficiency. *Curr Opin Mol Ther* 2:383, 2000.

283. Kral V, Bartunkova J, Svorc K, et al: The first case of leukocyte integrin deficiency syndrome in the Czech Republic and successful prenatal diagnosis in the affected family. *Cas Lek Cesk* 135:154, 1996.

284. Boxer LA, Hedley-Whyte ET, Stossel TP: Neutrophil actin dysfunction and abnormal neutrophil behavior. *N Engl J Med* 291:1093, 1974.

285. Southwick FS, Dabiri GA, Stosse TP: Neutrophil actin dysfunction is a genetic disorder associated with partial impairment of neutrophil actin assembly in three family members. *J Clin Invest* 82:1525, 1988.

286. Malech HL, Gallin JI: Current concepts: Immunology neutrophils in human diseases. *N Engl J Med* 317:687, 1987.

287. Southwick FS, Howard TH, Holbrook T, et al: The relationship between CR3 deficiency and neutrophil actin assembly. *Blood* 73:1973, 1989.

288. Coates TD, Torkildson JC, Torres M, et al: An inherited defect of neutrophil motility and microfilamentous cytoskeleton associated with abnormalities in 47-Kd and 89-Kd proteins. *Blood* 78:1338, 1991.

289. Howard T, Li Y, Torres M, et al: The 47-kD protein increased in neutrophil actin dysfunction with 47-and 89-kD protein abnormalities is lymphocyte-specific protein. *Blood* 83:231, 1994.

290. Howard TH, Hartwig J, Cunningham C: Lymphocyte-specific protein 1 expression in eukaryotic cells reproduces the morphologic and motile abnormality of NAD 47/89 neutrophils. *Blood* 91:4786, 1998.

291. Camitta BM, Quesenberry PJ, Parkman R, et al: Bone marrow transplantation for an infant with neutrophil dysfunction. *Exp Hematol* 5:109, 1977.

292. Samuels J, Aksentijevich I, Torosyan Y, et al: Familial Mediterranean fever at the millennium. Clinical spectrum, ancient mutations, and a survey of 100 American referrals to the National Institutes of Health. *Medicine* 77:268, 1998.

293. Siegal S: Benign paroxysural peritonitis. *Ann Intern Med* 23:1, 1945.

294. Drenth JP, van der Meer JW: Hereditary periodic fever. *N Engl J Med* 345:1748, 2001.

295. Ben Chetrit E, Levy M: Familial Mediterranean fever. *Lancet* 351:659, 1998.

296. Ancient missense mutations in a new member of the RoRet gene family are likely to cause familial Mediterranean fever. The International FMF Consortium. *Cell* 90:797, 1997.

297. A candidate gene for familial Mediterranean fever. The French FMF Consortium. *Nat Genet* 17:25, 1997.

298. Centola M, Wood G, Frucht DM, et al: The gene for familial Mediterranean fever, MEFV, is expressed in early leukocyte development and is regulated in response to inflammatory mediators. *Blood* 95:3223, 2000.

299. Hull KM, Shoham N, Chae JJ, et al: The expanding spectrum of systemic autoinflammatory disorders and their rheumatic manifestations. *Curr Opin Rheumatol* 15:61, 2003.

300. Richards N, Schaner P, Diaz A, et al: Interaction between pyrin and the apoptotic speck protein (ASC) modulates ASC-induced apoptosis. *J Biol Chem* 276:39320, 2001.

301. Touitou I: The spectrum of Familial Mediterranean Fever (FMF) mutations. *Eur J Hum Genet* 9:473, 2001.

302. Schaner P, Richards N, Wadhwa A, et al: Episodic evolution of pyrin in primates: Human mutations recapitulate ancestral amino acid states. *Nat Genet* 27:318, 2001.

303. Williamson LM, Hull D, Mehta R, et al: Familial Hibernian fever. *Q J Med* 51:469, 1982.

304. Perlmutter DH, Colten HR: Molecular basis of complement deficiencies. *Immunodefic Rev* 1:105, 1989.

305. Kannourakis G: Glycogen storage disease. *Semin Hematol* 39:103, 2002.

306. Smith OP: Shwachman-Diamond syndrome. *Semin Hematol* 39:95, 2002.

307. Jones DH, Schmalstieg FC, Dempsey K, et al: Subcellular distribution and mobilization of MAC-1 (CD11b/CD18) in neonatal neutrophils. *Blood* 75:488, 1990.

308. Brayton RG, Stokes PE, Schwartz MS, et al: Effect of alcohol and various diseases on leukocyte mobilization, phagocytosis and intracellular bacterial killing. *N Engl J Med* 282:123, 1970.

309. Oseas RS, Allen J, Yang HH, et al: Mechanism of dexamethasone inhibition of chemotactic factor induced granulocyte aggregation. *Blood* 59:265, 1982.

310. Dale DC, Fauci AS, Wolff SM: Alternate-day prednisone. Leukocyte kinetics and susceptibility to infections. *N Engl J Med* 291:1154, 1974.

311. Boxer LA, Allen JM, Baehner RL: Diminished polymorphonuclear leukocyte adherence. Function dependent on release of cyclic AMP by endothelial cells after stimulation of beta-receptors by epinephrine. *J Clin Invest* 66:268, 1980.

312. Leung DY, Geha RS: Clinical and immunologic aspects of the hyperimmunoglobulin E syndrome. *Hematol Oncol Clin North Am* 2:81, 1988.

313. Davis SD, Schaller J, Wedgwood RJ: Job's syndrome. Recurrent, "cold", staphylococcal abscesses. *Lancet* 1:1013, 1966.

314. Buckley RH: The hyper-IgE syndrome. *Clin Rev Allergy Immunol* 20:139, 2001.

315. Grimbacher B, Holland SM, Gallin JI, et al: Hyper-IgE syndrome with recurrent infections—an autosomal dominant multisystem disorder. *N Engl J Med* 340:692, 1999.

316. King CL, Gallin JI, Malech HL, et al: Regulation of immunoglobulin production in hyperimmunoglobulin E recurrent-infection syndrome by interferon gamma. *Proc Natl Acad Sci U S A* 86:10085, 1989.

317. Segal BH, Leto TL, Gallin JI, et al: Genetic, biochemical, and clinical features of chronic granulomatous disease. *Medicine* 79:170, 2000.

318. Berendes H, Bridges RA, Good RA: A fatal granulomatosus of childhood: The clinical study of a new syndrome. *Minn Med* 40:309, 1957.

319. Landing BH, Shirkey HS: A syndrome of recurrent infection and infiltration of viscera by pigmented lipid histiocytes. *Pediatrics* 20:431, 1957.

320. Sbarra AJ, Karnovsky ML: The biochemical basis of phagocytosis: I. Metabolic changes during the ingestion of particles by polymorphonuclear leukocytes. *J Biol Chem* 234:1355, 1959.

321. Iyer GY, Quastel JH: Biochemical aspects of phagocytosis. *Nature* 192:535, 1961.

322. Iyer GY, Quastel JH: NADPH and NADH oxidation by guinea pig polymorphonuclear leucocytes. *Can J Biochem Physiol* 41:427, 1963.

323. Baehner RL, Nathan DG: Quantitative nitroblue tetrazolium test in chronic granulomatous disease. *N Engl J Med* 278:971, 1968.

324. Winkelstein JA, Marino MC, Johnston RB Jr, et al: Chronic granulomatous disease. Report on a national registry of 368 patients. *Medicine* 79:155, 2000.

325. Parkos CA, Allen RA, Cochrane CG, et al: Purified cytochrome b from human granulocyte plasma membrane is comprised of two polypeptides with relative molecular weights of 91,000 and 22,000. *J Clin Invest* 80:732, 1987.

326. Quinn MT, Mullen ML, Jesaitis AJ: Human neutrophil cytochrome b contains multiple hemes. Evidence for heme associated with both subunits. *J Biol Chem* 267:7303, 1992.

327. Rotrosen D, Yeung CL, Leto TL, et al: Cytochrome b_{558}: The flavin-binding component of the phagocyte NADPH oxidase. *Science* 256:1459, 1992.

328. Segal AW, West I, Wientjes F, et al: Cytochrome b_{-245} is a flavocytochrome containing FAD and the NADPH-binding site of the microbicidal oxidase of phagocytes. *Biochem J* 284:781, 1992.

329. Sumimoto H, Sakamoto N, Nozaki M, et al: Cytochrome b558, a component of the phagocyte NADPH oxidase, is a flavoprotein. *Biochem Biophys Res Commun* 186:1368, 1992.

330. Zhen L, Yu L, Dinauer MC: Probing the role of the carboxyl terminus of the gp91phox subunit of neutrophil flavocytochrome b558 using site-directed mutagenesis. *J Biol Chem* 273:6575, 1998.

331. Henderson LM, Thomas S, Banting G, et al: The arachidonate-activatable, NADPH oxidase-associated H+ channel is contained within the multi-membrane-spanning N-terminal region of gp91-phox. *Biochem J* 325:701, 1997.

332. Shatwell KP, Dancis A, Cross AR, et al: The FRE1 ferric reductase of Saccharomyces cerevisiae is a cytochrome b similar to that of NADPH oxidase. *J Biol Chem* 271:14240, 1996.

333. Deleo FR, Quinn MT: Assembly of the phagocyte NADPH oxidase: Molecular interaction of oxidase proteins. *J Leukoc Biol* 60:677, 1996.

334. Segal AW: The NADPH oxidase and chronic granulomatous disease. *Mol Med Today* 2:129, 1996.

335. Wientjes FB, Hsuan JJ, Totty NF, et al: P40phox, a third cytosolic component of the activation complex of the NADPH oxidase to contain Src homology 3 domains. *Biochem J* 296:557, 1993.

336. Sathyamoorthy M, de M I, Adams AG, et al: P40(phox) down-regulates NADPH oxidase activity through interactions with its SH3 domain. *J Biol Chem* 272:9141, 1997.

337. Abo A, Boyhan A, West I, et al: Reconstitution of neutrophil NADPH oxidase activity in the cell-free system by four components: P67-phox, p47-phox, p21rac1, and cytochrome b-245. *J Biol Chem* 267:16767, 1992.

338. Clark RA, Volpp BD, Leidal KG, et al: Two cytosolic components of the human neutrophil respiratory burst oxidase translocate to the plasma membrane during cell activation. *J Clin Invest* 85:714, 1990.

339. Heyworth PG, Curnutte JT, Nauseef WM, et al: Neutrophil nicotinamide adenine dinucleotide phosphate oxidase assembly. Translocation of p47-phox and p67-phox requires interaction between p47-phox and cytochrome b_{558}. *J Clin Invest* 87:352, 1991.

340. Knaus UG, Morris S, Dong HJ, et al: Regulation of human leukocyte p21-activated kinases through g protein-coupled receptors. *Science* 269:221, 1995.

341. Bromberg Y, Pick E: Unsaturated fatty acids stimulate NADPH-dependent superoxide production by cell-free system derived from macrophages. *Cell Immunol* 88:213, 1984.

342. Curnutte JT: Activation of human neutrophil nicotinamide adenine dinucleotide phosphate, reduced (triphosphopyridine nucleotide, reduced)

oxidase by arachidonic acid in a cell-free system. *J Clin Invest* 75:1740, 1985.

343. McPhail LC, Shirley PS, Clayton CC, et al: Activation of the respiratory burst enzyme from human neutrophils in a cell-free system. Evidence for a soluble cofactor. *J Clin Invest* 75:1735, 1985.

344. Curnutte JT: Molecular basis of the autosomal recessive forms of chronic granulomatous disease. *Immunodefic Rev* 3:149, 1992.

345. Heyworth PG, Curnutte JT, Rae J, et al: Hematologically important mutations: X-linked chronic granulomatous disease [second update]. *Blood Cells Mol Dis* 27:16, 2001.

346. Francke U, Ochs HD, de Martinville B, et al: Minor Xp21 chromosome deletion in a male associated with expression of Duchenne muscular dystrophy, chronic granulomatous disease, retinitis pigmentosa, and McLeod syndrome. *Am J Hum Genet* 37:250, 1985.

347. Royer-Pokora B, Kunkel LM, Monaco AP, et al: Cloning the gene for an inherited human disorder-chronic granulomatous disease-on the basis of its chromosomal location. *Nature* 322:32, 1986.

348. Frey D, Mächler M, Seger R, et al: Gene deletion in a patient with chronic granulomatous disease and McLeod syndrome: Fine mapping of the Xk gene locus. *Blood* 71:252, 1988.

349. de Boer M, Bolscher BG, Dinauer MC, et al: Splice site mutations are a common cause of X-linked chronic granulomatous disease. *Blood* 80:1553, 1992.

350. Curnutte JT, Orkin S, Dinauer MC: Genetic disorders of phagocyte function, in *The Molecular Basis of Blood Diseases*, 2nd ed, edited by G Stammatoyannopoulos, p 493. WB Saunders, Philadelphia, 1994.

351. Roos D: X-CGDbase: A database of X-CGD-causing mutations. *Immunol Today* 17:517, 1996.

352. Roos D, Deboer M, Kuribayashi F, et al: Mutations in the x-linked and autosomal recessive forms of chronic granulomatous disease. *Blood* 87:1663, 1996.

353. Dinauer MC, Pierce EA, Bruns GAP, et al: Human neutrophil cytochrome b light chain (p22-phox). Gene structure, chromosomal location, and mutations in cytochrome-negative autosomal recessive chronic granulomatous disease. *J Clin Invest* 86:1729, 1990.

354. Segal AW: Biochemistry and molecular biology of chronic granulomatous disease. *J Inherit Metab Dis* 15:683, 1992.

355. Casimir CM, Bu-Ghanim HN, Rodaway AR, et al: Autosomal recessive chronic granulomatous disease caused by deletion at a dinucleotide repeat. *Proc Natl Acad Sci U S A* 88:2753, 1991.

356. Jankowski A, Scott CC, Grinstein S: Determinants of the phagosomal pH in neutrophils. *J Biol Chem* 277:6059, 2002.

357. Reeves EP, Lu H, Jacobs HL, et al: Killing activity of neutrophils is mediated through activation of proteases by K+ flux. *Nature* 416:291, 2002.

358. Johnston RB Jr: Clinical aspects of chronic granulomatous disease. *Curr Opin Hematol* 8:17, 2001.

359. Petty HR, Francis JW, Boxer LA: Deficiency in immune complex uptake by chronic granulomatous disease neutrophils. *J Cell Sci* 90:425, 1988.

360. Foster CB, Lehrnbecher T, Mol F, et al: Host defense molecule polymorphisms influence the risk for immune-mediated complications in chronic granulomatous disease. *J Clin Invest* 102:2146, 1998.

361. Crockard AD, Thompson JM, Boyd NA, et al: Diagnosis and carrier detection of chronic granulomatous disease in five families by flow cytometry. *Int Arch Allergy Immunol* 114:144, 1997.

362. Newburger PE, Luscinskas FW, Ryan T, et al: Variant chronic granulomatous disease: Modulation of the neutrophil defect by severe infection. *Blood* 68:914, 1986.

363. Curnutte JT: Chronic granulomatous disease: The solving of clinical riddle at the molecular level. *Clin Immunol Immunopathol* 67:S2, 1993.

364. Newburger PE, Cohen HJ, Rothchild SB, et al: Prenatal diagnosis of chronic granulomatous disease. *N Engl J Med* 300:178, 1979.

365. Pelham A, O'Reilly MA, Malcolm S, et al: RFLP and deletion analysis for X-linked chronic granulomatous disease using the cDNA probe: Potential for improved prenatal diagnosis and carrier determination. *Blood* 76:820, 1990.

366. Cooper MR, DeChatelet LR, McCall CE, et al: Complete deficiency of leukocyte glucose-6-phosphate dehydrogenase with defective bactericidal activity. *J Clin Invest* 51:769, 1972.

367. Vives Corrons JL, Feliu E, Pujades MA, et al: Severe-glucose-6-phosphate dehydrogenase (G6PD) deficiency associated with chronic hemolytic anemia, granulocyte dysfunction, and increased susceptibility to infections: Description of a new molecular variant (G6PD Barcelona). *Blood* 59:428, 1982.

368. Ambruso DR, Knall C, Abell AN, et al: Human neutrophil immunodeficiency syndrome is associated with an inhibitory Rac2 mutation. *Proc Natl Acad Sci U S A* 97:4654, 2000.

369. Williams DA, Tao W, Yang FC, et al: Dominant negative mutation of the hematopoietic-specific Rho GTPase, Rac2, is associated with a human phagocyte immunodeficiency. *Blood* 96:1646, 2000.

370. Chusid MJ, Gelfand JA, Nutter C, et al: Letter: Pulmonary aspergillosis, inhalation of contaminated marijuana smoke, chronic granulomatous disease. *Ann Intern Med* 82:682, 1975.

371. Gallin JI, Alling DW, Malech HL, et al: Itraconazole to prevent fungal infections in chronic granulomatous disease. *N Engl J Med* 348:2416, 2003.

372. A controlled trial of interferon gamma to prevent infection in chronic granulomatous disease. The International Chronic Granulomatous Disease Cooperative Study Group. *N Engl J Med* 324:509, 1991.

373. Schiff DE, Rae J, Martin TR, et al: Increased phagocyte Fc gammaRI expression and improved Fc gamma-receptor-mediated phagocytosis after in vivo recombinant human interferon-gamma treatment of normal human subjects. *Blood* 90:3187, 1997.

374. Woodman RC, Erickson RW, Rae J, et al: Prolonged recombinant interferon-gamma therapy in chronic granulomatous disease: Evidence against enhanced neutrophil oxidase activity. *Blood* 79:1558, 1992.

375. Seger RA, Tiefenauer L, Matsunaga T, et al: Chronic granulomatous disease due to granulocytes with abnormal NADPH oxidase activity and deficient cytochrome-b. *Blood* 61:423, 1983.

376. Styrt B, Klempner MS: Late-presenting variant of chronic granulomatous disease. *Pediatr Infect Dis* 3:556, 1984.

377. Malech HL, Bauer TR, Hickstein DD: Prospects for gene therapy of neutrophil defects. *Semin Hematol* 34:355, 1997.

378. Pollock JD, Williams DA, Gifford MAC, et al: Mouse model of x-linked chronic granulomatous disease, an inherited defect in phagocyte superoxide production. *Nat Genet* 9:202, 1995.

379. Jackson SH, Gallin JI, Holland SM: The p47(phox) mouse knock-out model of chronic granulomatous disease. *J Exp Med* 182:751, 1995.

380. Mardiney M III, Jackson SH, Spratt SK, et al: Enhanced host defense after gene transfer in the murine p47phox-deficient model of chronic granulomatous disease. *Blood* 89:2268, 1997.

381. Bjorgvinsdottir H, Ding CJ, Pech N, et al: Retroviral-mediated gene transfer of gp91(phox) into bone marrow cells rescues defect in host defense against Aspergillus fumigatus in murine X-linked chronic granulomatous disease. *Blood* 89:41, 1997.

382. Malech HL, Maples PB, Whitingtheobald N, et al: Prolonged production of NADPH oxidase-corrected granulocytes after gene therapy of chronic granulomatous disease. *Proc Natl Acad Sci U S A* 94:12133, 1997.

383. Nauseef WM: Myeloperoxidase deficiency. *Hematol Pathol* 4:165, 1990.

384. Nauseef WM: Myeloperoxidase deficiency. *Hematol Oncol Clin North Am* 2:135, 1988.

385. Austin GE, Zhao WG, Zhang W, et al: Identification and characterization of the human myeloperoxidase promoter. *Leukemia* 9:848, 1995.

386. Morishita K, Tsuchiya M, Asano S, et al: Chromosomal gene structure of human myeloperoxidase and regulation of its expression by granulocyte colony-stimulating factor. *J Biol Chem* 262:15208, 1987.

387. Zeng J, Fenna RE: X-ray crystal structure of canine myeloperoxidase at 3 A resolution. *J Mol Biol* 226:185, 1992.

388. Nauseef WM, Mccormick SJ, Clark RA: Calreticulin functions as a molecular chaperone in the biosynthesis of myeloperoxidase. *J Biol Chem* 270:4741, 1995.

389. Nauseef WM: Insights into myeloperoxidase biosynthesis from its inherited deficiency. *J Mol Med* 76:661, 1998.

390. Nauseef WM: Quality control in the endoplasmic reticulum: Lessons from hereditary myeloperoxidase deficiency. *J Lab Clin Med* 134:215, 1999.

391. Deleo FR, Goedken M, Mccormick SJ, et al: A novel form of hereditary myeloperoxidase deficiency linked to endoplasmic reticulum proteasome degradation. *J Clin Invest* 101:2900, 1998.

392. Boxer LA: The role of antioxidants in modulating neutrophiln functional responses, in *Advances in Experimental Medicine* edited by A Bendich, M Philip, P Tengedy, p 19. Plenum Press, New York, 1990.

393. Roos D, Weening RS, Voetman AA, et al: Protection of phagocytic leukocytes by endogenous glutathione: Studies in a family with glutathione reductase deficiency. *Blood* 53:851, 1979.

394. Boxer LA, Oliver JM, Spielberg SP, et al: Protection of granulocytes by vitamin E in glutathione synthetase deficiency. *N Engl J Med* 301:901, 1979.

PART VII

MONOCYTES
AND
MACROPHAGES

CHAPTER 67

MORPHOLOGY OF MONOCYTES AND MACROPHAGES

STEVEN D. DOUGLAS
WEN-ZHE HO

The monocyte is a spherical cell with prominent surface ruffles and blebs when examined by scanning electron microscopy. When reconstructed from sections examined under transmission electron microscopy, the monocyte has a reniform nucleus containing a small nucleolus. The cytoplasm has many mitochondria, microtubules, and microfilaments. The Golgi apparatus is well developed and has neighboring centrioles. Numerous microvilli and microcytotic vesicles are evident at or near the cell surface. The cytoplasm contains scattered granules, akin to lysosomes. The granule contents share features with the primary granules of neutrophils, although, in contrast to the neutrophil, the monocyte granule is characterized by fluoride-inhibitable esterases. As the monocyte enters the tissue and differentiates into a macrophage, the cell volume and number of cytoplasmic granules increase. Cell shape varies depending on the tissue type in which the macrophage resides (e.g., lung, liver, spleen, brain, etc.). A characteristic feature of macrophages is their prominent electron-dense membrane-bound lysosomes, which can be seen fusing with phagosomes to form secondary lysosomes. The latter contain ingested cellular and noncellular material in stages of degradation. A broad range of surface receptors for many ligands, including the Fc portion of immunoglobulin, complement proteins, cytokines, chemokines, lipoproteins, and others are on the cell surface. Macrophages differ in appearance, biochemistry, and function based on the environment in which they mature from monocytes. These differences are exemplified by the diversity among dendritic cells of lymph nodes, histiocytes of connective tissue, osteoclasts of bone, Kupffer cells of liver, microglia of the central nervous system, and macrophages of the serosal surfaces, each fashioned to meet the local needs of the mononuclear phagocyte system, which plays a role in inflammation and host defense against microbes.

MONONUCLEAR PHAGOCYTE SYSTEM

Modern study of mammalian phagocytes began with Metchnikoff in the 19th century. An understanding of the ontogeny, kinetics, and function of phagocytic cells in animals led to the concept of the mononuclear phagocyte system.[1,2] The system consists of marrow mononuclear blasts and promonocytes, blood monocytes, and both free and fixed-tissue macrophages. Vascular endothelium, reticular cells, and dendritic cells of lymphoid germinal centers usually are not included in the mononuclear phagocyte system, although the now-obsolete term *reticuloendothelial system*[3] denoted these cells as playing some complementary part with mononuclear phagocytes. Studies indicate monocytes can differentiate into dendritic cells *in vitro*.[4] Monocytes and macrophages comprise the functional system formerly thought to be the reticuloendothelial system. Tissue macrophages share many functional characteristics, such as phagocytic and microbial killing capabilities and adherence to glass or plastic surfaces *in vitro*. Kinetic studies indicate macrophages are transformed monocytes and that the monocyte is derived from differentiation of the hematopoietic stem cell (see Chap. 15).

The blood monocyte is a medium to large motile cell that can marginate along vessel walls and has a propensity for adherence to surfaces. Monocytes respond to inflammation and chemotactic stimuli by active diapedesis across vessel walls into inflammatory foci, where they can mature into macrophages, with greater phagocytic capacity and increased content of hydrolytic enzymes. Free macrophages also are present in mammary glands, alveolar spaces, pleura, peritoneum, and synovia. The somewhat less motile fixed-tissue macrophages are found in different tissues and serous cavities (Table 67-1). The functions of mononuclear phagocytes include the following: phagocytosis and digestion of microorganisms, particulate material, or tissue debris; secretion of chemical mediators and regulators of the inflammatory response; interaction with antigen and lymphocytes in the generation of the immune response; cytotoxicity, such as killing of some tumor cells; and other functions specific for macrophages of particular tissues.

The development of techniques to isolate monocytes from blood of adult subjects led to the discovery that monocytes are heterogeneous with regard to cell volumes. Isolation of purified monocytes by adherence to glass substrates or to gelatin-coated flasks or by centrifugal elutriation reveals distinct populations of monocytes.[1,2] In addition to the usual 12- to 15-μm diameter (when measured on a dried blood film) monocyte, so-called "regular monocytes," a somewhat smaller cell that is less active than its larger, more mature counterpart has been identified. This cell is referred to as a *small immature monocyte*, but its functional significance is not clear.

Monocytes continuously emigrate from the blood into peripheral tissue, with a half-life in the blood of approximately 1 day in mice.[5] Nondividing monocytes can be induced to differentiate into dendritic-

TABLE 67-1 DISTRIBUTION OF MONONUCLEAR PHAGOCYTES

Marrow	Tissues
Monoblasts	Liver (Kupffer cells)
Promonocytes	Lung (alveolar macrophages)
Monocytes	Connective tissue (histiocytes)
Macrophages	Spleen (red pulp macrophages)
Blood	Lymph nodes
Monocytes	Thymus
Body cavities	Bone (osteoclasts)
Pleural macrophages	Synovium (type A cells)
Peritoneal macrophages	Mucosa-associated lymphoid tissue
Inflammatory tissues	Gastrointestinal tract
Epithelioid cells	Genitourinary tract
Exudate macrophages	Endocrine organs
Multinucleate giant cells	Central nervous system (microglia)
	Skin (histiocyte/dendritic cells)

SOURCE: Adapted from Angen and Ross, in Lewis and McGee,[2] with permission. Refer to references 7, 67, 68.

like cells *in vitro*. However, this process requires culture of the cells for 7 to 10 days with exogenous cytokines, typically interleukin-4 (IL-4) and granulocyte-monocyte colony stimulating factor (GM-CSF).[6] In the presence of endothelial cells grown on an extracellular matrix, monocytes differentiate along two distinct pathways: toward dendritic cells or macrophages. Monocytes that migrate across endothelium in an abluminal to luminal direction differentiate into dendritic cells. In contrast, monocytes that remain in the subendothelial matrix differentiate into macrophages.

MORPHOLOGY OF MONOCYTE PRECURSORS

Monoblasts and promonocytes are the precursors of monocytes, bearing finely dispersed nuclear chromatin and nucleoli when observed in the stained film of the blood or marrow. The monoblast is a very-low-prevalence marrow cell, indistinguishable by light microscopy from the myeloblast. Promonocytes are 12 to 18 μm in diameter (as measured on dried blood films) and have characteristic deeply indented, irregularly shaped nuclei with condensed chromatin and numerous cytoplasmic microfilaments.

In animal studies, a small percentage of marrow cells are phagocytic, synthesize DNA, adhere to glass surfaces, and contain nonspecific esterases.[7] These cells have been referred to as *promonocytes* and considered as intermediate between monoblasts and the monocytes of the blood.[7] Cytochemical studies identify the promonocyte in normal human marrow. These cells have deeply indented and irregularly shaped nuclei and bundled and scattered single filaments in the cytoplasm. These morphologic features distinguish the promonocyte from the progranulocyte.[8,9] Peroxidase is present throughout the cell secretory apparatus in all cisternae of the rough-surfaced endoplasmic reticulum, the Golgi complex, associated vesicles, and all immature and mature granules. Cytochemical reaction products for acid phosphatase and arylsulfatase also are deposited throughout the secretory apparatus of the promonocyte.

MORPHOLOGY OF MONOCYTES

LIGHT MICROSCOPY

The morphology of monocytes has been investigated by light and phase-contrast optics,[10] scanning and transmission electron microscopy, and freeze-fracture and freeze-etch procedures.[11]

On the stained blood film, the monocyte has a diameter of 12 to 15 μm. The monocyte nucleus occupies approximately half the area of the cell and usually is eccentrically placed. The nucleus most often is reniform but may be round or irregular. It contains a characteristic chromatin net with fine strands bridging small chromatin clumps. Chromatin aggregates are arranged along the internal aspect of the nuclear membrane. The nuclear chromatin pattern has been called "raked" because of its fine-stranded appearance. The cytoplasm is spread out, stains grayish-blue with Wright stain, and contains a variable number of fine, pink-purple granules, which at times are sufficiently numerous to give the entire cytoplasm a pink hue. Clear cytoplasmic vacuoles and a variable number of larger azurophilic granulations often are encountered in these cells.

PHASE MICROSCOPY

The monocyte nucleus has a distinct chromatin pattern on a cloudy background when examined by phase-contrast microscopy. The cytoplasm is clear gray. Mitochondria are extremely fine and occasionally form a small, juxtanuclear rosette surrounding the centrosome. The phase-dense cytoplasmic granules, varying in number, are generally at the limit of resolution of light microscopy and appear as fine

intracytoplasmic dust. Monocytes contain several types of cytoplasmic vacuoles. The reniform nucleus with a juxtanuclear depression filled by a centrosome and its active undulating movement similar to that of other leukocytes are characteristic of the monocyte. The locomotion of the monocyte has the same pattern of undulating cytoplasmic veils seen in macrophages. The monocyte generally assumes a triangular shape as it moves, with one point trailing behind and the other two points advancing before the cell. Blood monocytes undergo adherence and cytoplasmic spreading following attachment to glass surfaces.[12] The extent of spreading increases in the presence of antigen–antibody complexes, certain divalent metals, and proteolytic enzymes.[12,13] The spread form of the monocyte reveals the nucleus and granules are located centrally and the abundant hyaloplasm is in the periphery of the cell, terminating in a fringed border that displays undulating movement. The small monocyte may be difficult to distinguish from the large lymphocyte when examined by phase-contrast microscopy.

A striking feature on phase-contrast microscopy is the ruffled plasma membrane that forms prominent phase-dense folds at the cell surface and edges. Some cells have a dense thickening at the edge of the cytoplasm, with microextensions on the thickened edge.

SCANNING ELECTRON MICROSCOPY

The monocyte surface has very prominent ruffles and small surface blebs.[14,15] Extensive ruffling on the monocyte plasma membrane is of functional significance. The monocyte is both motile and phagocytic, and these functions require physical contact with particles or cell surfaces. Reduction in the radius of curvature of the cell surface by formation of ruffles or microvilli may reduce repulsive forces when surface negative-charge groups on the cell approach and contact a negatively charged substratum or cell. In addition, redundancy of the cell membrane may provide reserve membrane required for locomotion and phagocytosis.

TRANSMISSION ELECTRON MICROSCOPY

The nucleus of the monocyte contains one or two small nucleoli surrounded by nucleolar-associated chromatin (Fig. 67-1).[16] The cytoplasm contains a relatively small quantity of endoplasmic reticulum and a variable quantity of ribosomes and polysomes. The mitochondria are numerous, small, and elongated. The Golgi complex is well developed and is situated about the centrosome within the nuclear indentation. Centrioles and filamentous centriolar satellites are often visualized in this region. Microtubules are numerous, and microfibrils are found in bundles surrounding the nucleus. In cultured macrophages, collections of microfilaments are present underneath the plasma membrane near sites of cell attachment either to a substratum or to phagocytizable particles.[17] The cell surface is characterized by numerous microvilli and vesicles of micropinocytosis. The cytoplasmic granules resemble the small granules found in the granulocytic series, measuring approximately 0.05 to 0.2 μm in diameter. They are dense and homogeneous and are surrounded by a limiting membrane. These granules, as with the lysosomal granules of other leukocytes, are packaged by the Golgi apparatus after their enzymatic content has been produced by the ribosomal complex of the cell.[7,8,18] These cytoplasmic granules contain acid phosphatase and arylsulfatase and therefore are primary lysosomes. After endocytosis, lysosomes fuse with the phagosome, forming secondary lysosomes. Some monocyte granules stain positive for peroxidase, whereas others are peroxidase negative.[7,8]

FREEZE-FRACTURE MICROSCOPY

In this technique, a cell suspension is frozen, placed in a high-vacuum chamber, and struck with a blunt edge, thus producing a fracture

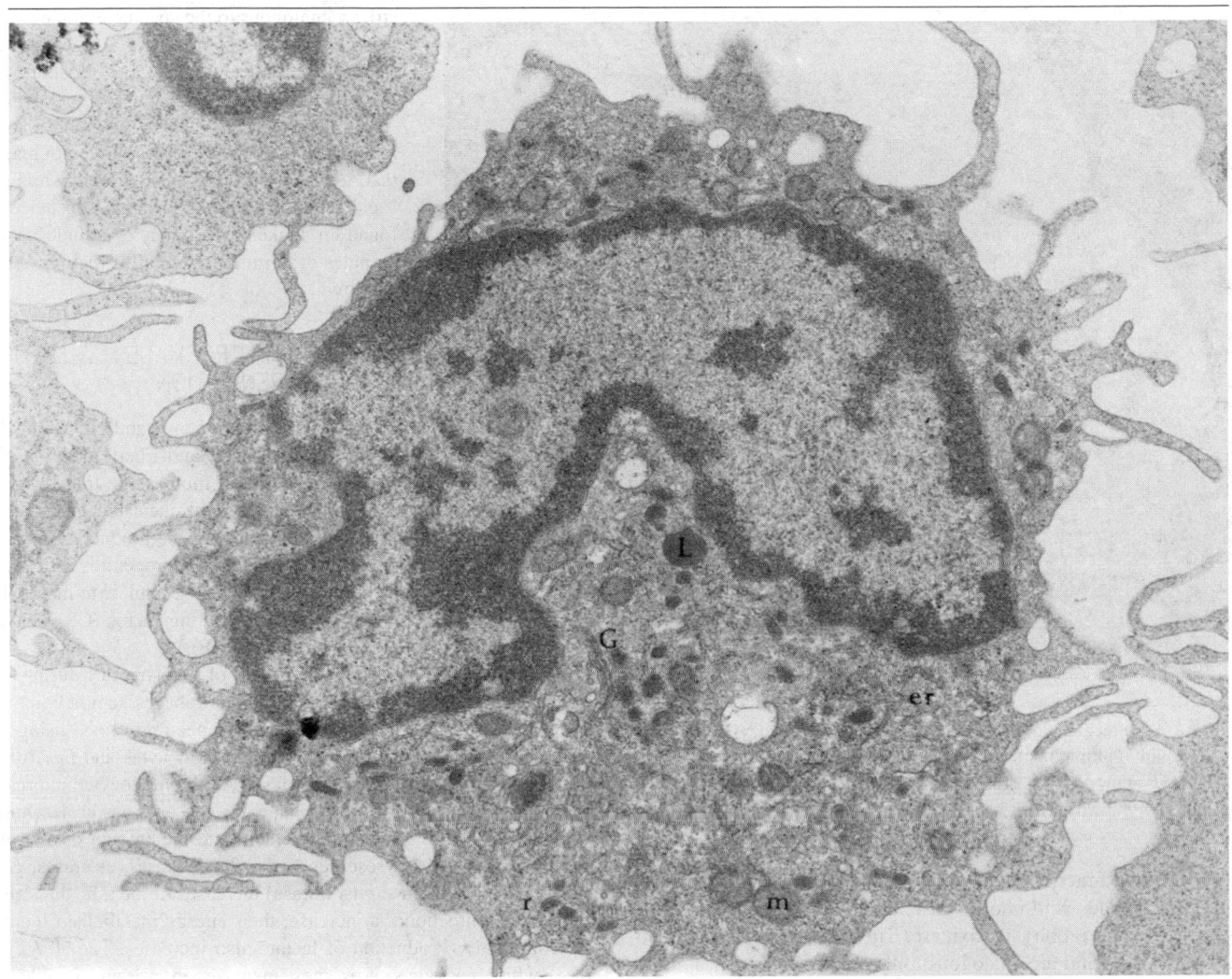

FIGURE 67-1   Transmission electron micrograph of a monocyte. The eccentric reniform nucleus has a thinly dispersed chromatin pattern. The Golgi complex (G) is in a juxtanuclear position. Small electron-dense granules can be seen evolving in the Golgi complex. Small amounts of rough endoplasmic reticulum (er) and polyribosomes (r) are present, particularly about the cell periphery. Mitochondria (m) are concentrated in the region of the Golgi apparatus; they also are scattered in the cell periphery. Lysosomes (L) are small, electron-dense granules surrounded by a limiting membrane. The irregular ruffled cell margin is apparent with numerous microprojections. (×24,000)

that propagates through the frozen specimen. The utility of the procedure comes from the remarkable finding that when the fracture encounters a cell, the fracture tends to propagate along the interior of the plasma membrane and thus split the lipid bilayer into its two constituent layers. After fracture, the specimen is coated with platinum, which is electron dense when viewed with transmission electron microscopy. All cell types examined thus far by the freeze-fracture technique reveal intramembrane particles (IMP) as the predominant topographic feature of the interior of the bilayer. Studies of the erythrocyte have shown that at least some particles contain intercalated membrane proteins, and this has been assumed to be the case for nucleated cells as well. The distribution of IMP is dramatically altered in a number of cell systems by physiologic stimuli, for example, hormonal stimulation.

Profound changes in the distribution of IMP on mononuclear phagocytes occur following binding of antibody-coated erythrocytes.[11] Because redistribution of IMP also occurs in some nonphagocyte Fc receptor (FcR)-bearing cells[11] and after exposure to aggregated IgG, this alteration in IMP presumably reflects interaction with FcR. Freeze-etch electron micrographs of the monocyte show nuclear pores tra-

versing both lamellae of the nuclear membrane and contours of cytoplasmic lysosomes and mitochondria (Fig. 67-2).

HISTOCHEMISTRY OF MONOCYTES

Table 67-2 compares the hydrolytic enzyme contents of monocytes, neutrophils, and lymphocytes. Monocytes also give a weak but positive periodic acid–Schiff reaction (for polysaccharides) and Sudan black B reaction (for lipids).

Nonspecific esterase[19–21] is frequently used as a marker for monocytes. Monocyte esterases are inhibited by sodium fluoride, whereas the esterases of the granulocytic series are not. The nonspecific esterase reaction is positive in promyelocytes and myelocytes; therefore, analysis of fluoride inhibition is necessary to distinguish marrow monocytes from early myelocytes. Monocyte granules, although heterogeneous in size (0.3–0.6 μm), are not separable into populations by routine electron microscopic criteria (except in the rat).[22] Identification of monocyte granule populations has depended on subcellular localization of monocyte enzymes by electron microscopic cytochemistry.[8] Human marrow promonocytes and blood monocytes contain granules

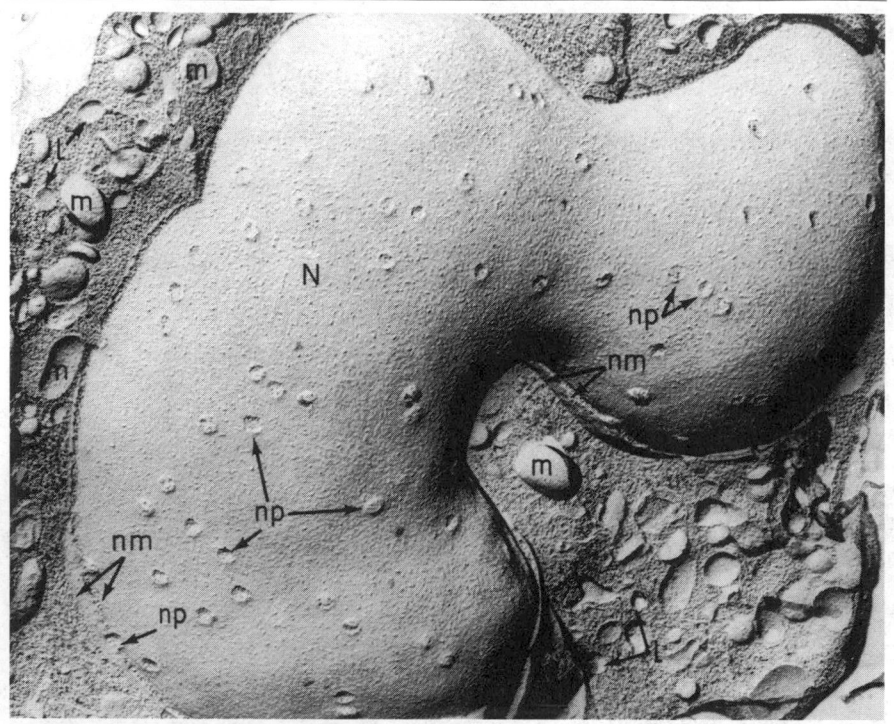

FIGURE 67-2   Freeze-etch electron micrograph of a monocyte. Fracture plane displays the large nucleus (N), with multiple nuclear pores (np) and the two lamellae of the fractured nuclear membrane (nm) evident in some regions. Membrane and cleaved surfaces of mitochondria (m) and lysosomal granules (L) can be identified in the cytoplasm.

that comprise two functionally distinct populations.[8,9] One population contains the enzymes acid phosphatase, arylsulfatase, and, in the human (but not in the rabbit), peroxidase. These granules are modified primary lysosomes and are analogous to the azurophil granules of the neutrophil. The monocyte azurophil granule population is heterogeneous in cytochemical reactivity for peroxidase, acid phosphatase, and arylsulfatase.[23,24] Moreover, primary granules that are morphologically identical with other vesicles can be identified as lysosomes cytochemically. The content of the other population of monocyte granules is unknown; however, they lack alkaline phosphatase[23] and hence are not

strictly analogous to the specific granules of neutrophils. The lysosomes have a digestive function, whereas the function of the second population is unknown.

Approximately 10 percent of granules in normal human blood monocytes stain with reagents that identify complex acid carbohydrates, or "acid mucosubstances."[25] These substances are found in leukemic monocyte granules and in granules of normal neutrophils. Their function is unknown.

MONOCYTE/MACROPHAGE MATURATION AND DIFFERENTIATION

The classic studies of Lewis and Lewis[26] in 1926, Maximow[27] in 1932, and Ebert and Florey[28] in 1939 showed that monocytes transform into macrophages and multinucleated giant cells *in vitro*. Macrophages can be produced from monocytes or hematopoietic progenitor cells culture in cytokines, such as granulocyte-macrophage (GM) colony stimulating factor (CSF) or macrophage-CSF (M-CSF).[29]

The alterations of ultrastructure during transformation into macrophages, epithelioid cells, and giant cells have been described using purified populations of monocytes and *in vitro* culture techniques.[16] As the monocyte matures into the macrophage, the cell enlarges in size, and the lysosomal content and the amount of hydrolytic enzymes within the lysosomes (e.g., phosphatases, esterases, β-glucuronidase, lysozyme, arylsulfatase) increase. At the time the size and number of mitochondria increase, their energy metabolism increases concomitantly. Production of lactate also increases. The Golgi complex, which packages lysosomes, increases in size and vesicle complexity (Figs. 67-3 and 67-4). Several stimuli (e.g., phorbol myristate acetate) induce formation of multinucleated giant cells from monocytes.[30]

MORPHOLOGY OF MACROPHAGES

Macrophage characteristics are heralded by a significant increase in cell size, increase in the number of cytoplasmic granules, increase in the heterogeneity of cell size and shape, and increase in the number of cytoplasmic clear vacuoles.

MOTILITY

An effective monocyte response to infection is predicated upon the ability to migrate and accumulate at sites of inflammation and infection. Monocytes are capable of both random and directed movement. Random migration is nondirected movement that occurs in the absence of attracting substances. Directed movement, as a result of chemotaxis, refers to monocyte migration that occurs in response to soluble factors or stimuli and that is mediated by different types of receptors on phagocyte cell surfaces.[31] A number of different methods have been used to study macrophage movement both *in vivo*[32] and *in vitro*.[33]

LIGHT AND PHASE-CONTRAST MICROSCOPY

In vitro culture of monocytes purified from adult human blood has provided an opportunity to observe the maturation of these cells into mature macrophages.

TABLE 67-2   CYTOCHEMICAL REACTIONS OF LEUKOCYTE ENZYMES

CHEMICAL	MONOCYTES	NEUTROPHILS	LYMPHOCYTES
Acid phosphatase	+ +	+	+
β-Glucuronidase	+ +	+	0 to +
Sulfatase	+	+	0
N-Acetylglucosaminidase	+ +	+ +	0
Lysozyme*	+ +	+ +	0
Naphthylamidase	+ +	+	0 to +
α-Naphthyl butyrate esterase†	+ +	0 to +	0
Naphthol AS-D chloroacetate esterase	0 to +	+ +	0
Peroxidase	+	+ +	0
Alkaline phosphatase	0	0 to +	0

* Most lysozyme produced by mononuclear phagocytes is secreted rather than stored intracellularly.
† α-Naphthyl acetate and α-naphthyl butyrate esterase activities may appear in human T lymphocytes under certain conditions.
SOURCE: Modified from Braunsteiner and Schmalzl[20] and Li et al.[21]

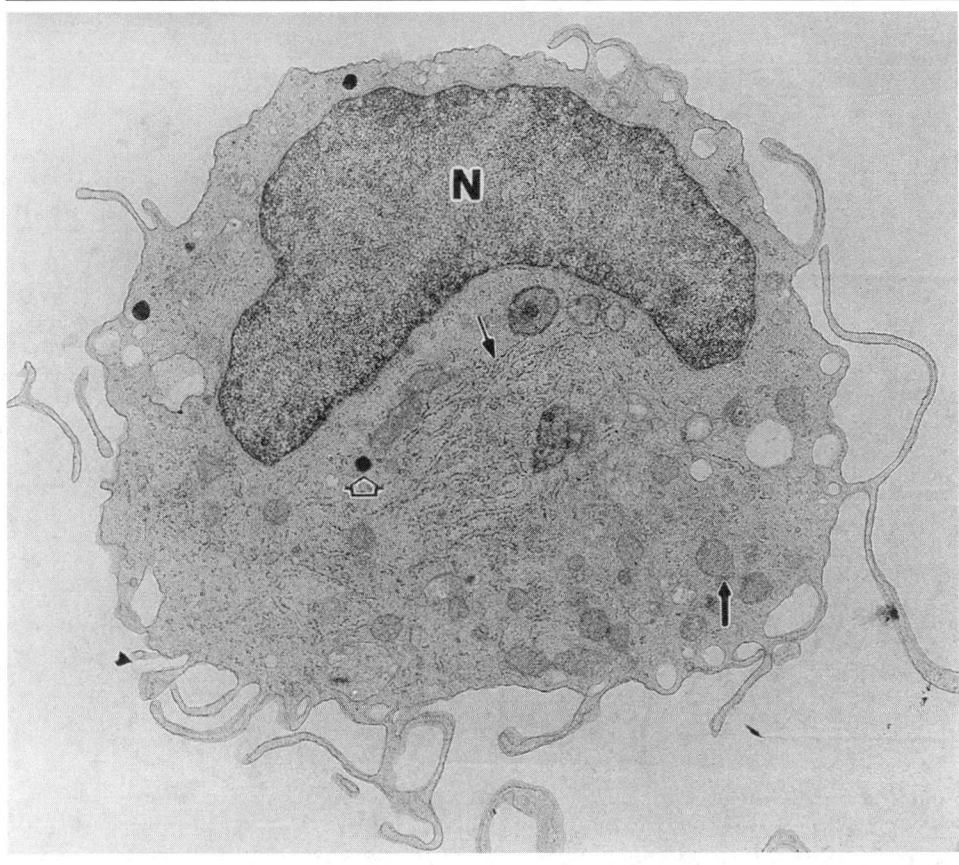

FIGURE 67-3   Electron micrograph of monocytes cultured *in vitro* for 2 days. *Thin arrow* indicates endoplasmic reticulum; *thick arrow* indicates mitochondria; *open arrow* indicates lysosomes. N, Nucleus.

The macrophages of the pulmonary alveoli, peritoneal and pleural cavities, and inflammatory exudates are hypermature cells that have undergone *in vivo* stimulation and maturation. This process results in enhanced bactericidal activity[1,2] because of augmentation of lysosome number and acid hydrolase content.

Macrophages display attributes of morphologic specialization specific to their location and function. The fixed macrophages of the spleen (littoral cells) are involved in the sequestration and destruction of effete or abnormal red cells and exhibit stages of erythrophagocytosis and intracytoplasmic aggregates of ferritin (see Chap. 5). The macrophages of the marrow, the "nurse cells" of the erythroblastic island, play a similar role in erythrophagocytosis and iron storage and transfer (see Chaps. 4 and 28). Hepatic macrophages (Kupffer cells), found in liver sinusoids, also phagocytize red cells and other cellular elements and are important sites of iron storage. Macrophages of the pulmonary alveoli, the lamina propria of the gastrointestinal tract, and the peritoneal and pleural fluids reflect in their morphology a specific function of phagocytosis of microorganisms, cells, and cellular and noncellular debris, characteristic of the specific organ location.

Most macrophages are 25 to 50 μm in diameter on Wright-stained films. They have an eccentrically placed reniform or fusiform nucleus with one or two distinct nucleoli and finely dispersed, loosely stranded nuclear chromatin that tends to clump in the nuclear interior and along the internal aspect of the nuclear membrane. A juxtanuclear clear zone (Golgi complex) is well defined. The cytoplasm shows fine granules and multiple pink-purple, large azurophil granules. The cytoplasmic borders are irregularly serrated. Cytoplasmic vacuoles are present near the cell periphery, reflecting the active pinocytosis in these cells.

On phase-contrast microscopy, living macrophages are large cells with a propensity to adhere to and spread on glass surfaces. Thus, the cell organelles are concentrated within the central portion of the cell and clear veils of hyaloplasm spread about the cell, with intense ruffling of the membrane borders. Vesicles and contractile vacuoles are seen about the cell periphery and in the cell interior. The juxtanuclear clear zone bearing the centrosome and the Golgi complex is particularly dynamic and displays an undulating motion.

ELECTRON MICROSCOPY

Macrophages show a variable degree of differentiation, nuclear "maturity," ribosomes, mitochondria, and lysosome content. In thin sections, the nucleus varies from horseshoe shaped to fusiform. The heterochromatin is disposed in fine clumps in the interior of the nucleus and along the internal aspect of the nuclear membrane. Clear spaces between membrane-fixed chromatin aggregates mark the sites of nuclear pores that are relatively abundant on freeze-etch electron micrographs of macrophages and monocytes (see Fig. 67-2). Polyribosomes and scant smooth and rough endoplasmic reticulum are seen about the cell periphery. A well-developed Golgi complex is in a juxtanuclear location. It often is multicentric and contains a concentration of vesicles, some with dense inclusions that mark them as early lysosomes. A relatively constant feature of cells engaged in endocytosis is the large number of microvilli at the cell surface, forming the equivalent of a "brush border." The degree of development of this surface adaptation is related to the phagocytic activity of the cell and its rate of pinocytosis.

The number and size of mitochondria vary with the phagocytic and hence metabolic activity of the cell. Mitochondria tend to be

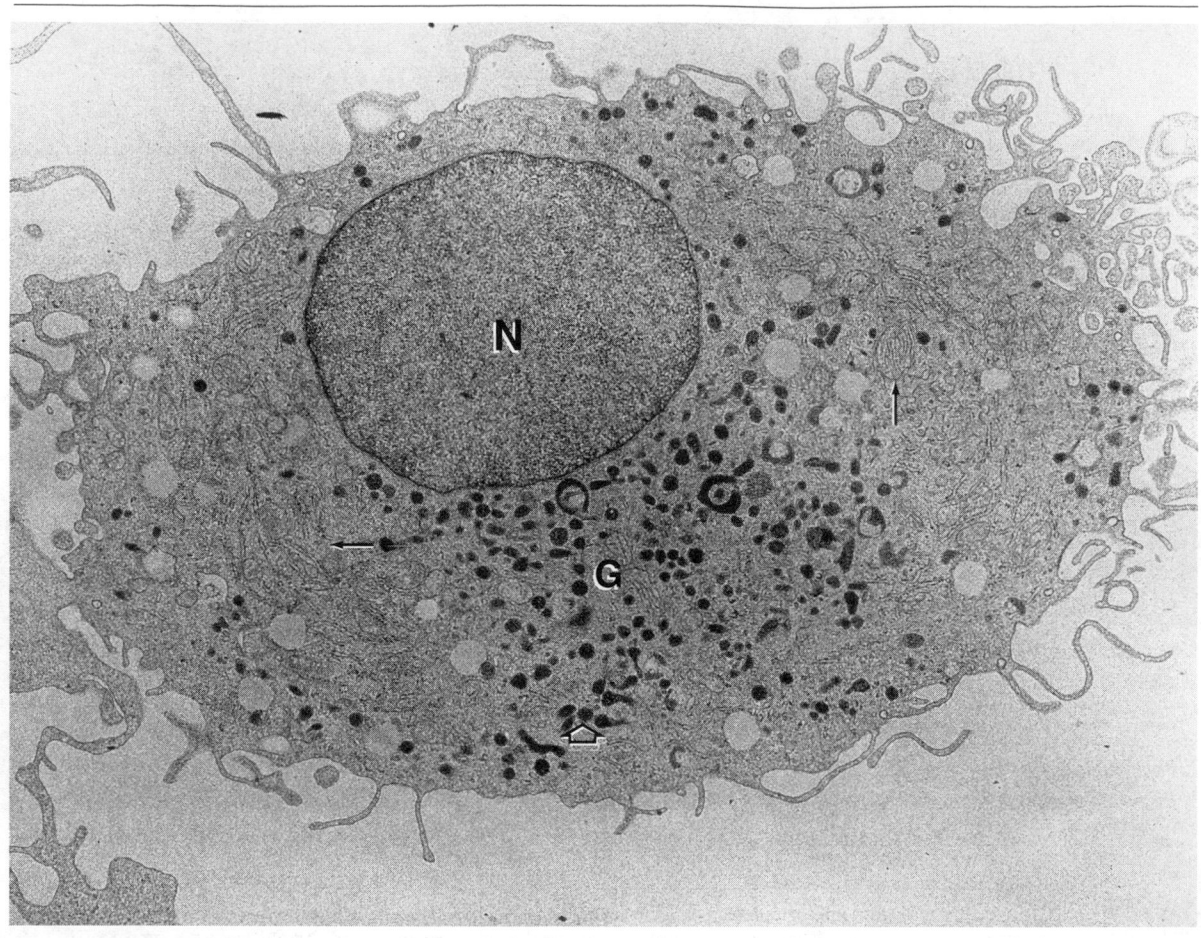

FIGURE 67-4   Electron micrograph of monocyte-derived macrophage cultured *in vitro* for 9 days. G, Golgi zone; N, nucleus. *Arrow on right* indicates endoplasmic reticulum; *arrow on left* indicates mitochondria; *open arrow* indicates lysosomes. (×7,600).

grouped about the region of the Golgi complex, although several usually are seen dispersed about the cell periphery, presumably supplying energy for the active endocytic processes occurring there.

The most constant and characteristic ultrastructural features of macrophages are the electron-dense membrane-bound lysosomes that often can be seen fusing with phagosomes to form secondary lysosomes. Within the secondary lysosomes, ingested cellular, bacterial, and noncellular material can be seen in various stages of degradation, often recognizable as degenerating mitochondria or nuclear material. These secondary lysosomes also contain partially degraded material from the late stages of the endocytic process, often appearing as multilamellar lipid bodies.

Microtubules and microfilaments are prominent in macrophages. Actin- and myosin-like proteins have been isolated from monocytes and partially characterized.

Resting macrophages have irregular cell borders and pseudopodia pushed out in all directions. Their cytoplasm has rough endoplasmic reticulum and Golgi complex in the perinuclear area. Lipid globules, primary lysosomes, and mitochondria are characteristically prominent. Activated monocytes/macrophages are motile cells that extend a leading pseudopod as they move forward.[34]

MONOCYTE/MACROPHAGE SURFACE RECEPTORS

Monocyte/macrophage cells have surface receptors that have been characterized by their binding to specific monoclonal antibodies.

These receptors (Table 67-3) are markers for origin, growth, differentiation,[35] activation, recognition, migration, and function of the monocyte/macrophage.

RECEPTORS FOR PEPTIDES AND SMALL MOLECULES

FC RECEPTORS

FcRs for IgG are expressed on the surface of mononuclear cells, macrophages, granulocytes, and platelets.[36,37] FcRs are divided into three distinct classes: FcRI, FcRII, and FcRIII. These receptors have broad ranges of expression on different cells. The first IgG receptor, FcRI (CD64), is a receptor found on monocytes, macrophages, and activated neutrophils. This receptor binds monomeric IgG through the Fc portion of the molecule. This immunoglobulin receptor has increased expression on activated monocytes and macrophages. CD64 allows for receptor-mediated endocytosis of IgG–antigen complexes for presentation to T cells, can trigger the release of cytokines and reactive oxygen intermediates, and can play a role in granulocyte-mediated antibody-dependent cytotoxicity. The second IgG receptor, FcRII (CD32), is a widely distributed receptor present on many cell types, including monocytes, platelets, neutrophils, B cells, some T cells, and some capillary endothelium. This receptor can bind complexed IgG rather than monomeric IgG. This FcR regulates B cell function when coengaged with the B cell receptor for antigen, namely, surface Ig. It also can induce mediator release from myeloid cells and phagocytosis of Ig-coated particles *in vitro*. Finally, this FcR also can target antigen into presenting pathways. The third IgG receptor, FcRIII (CD16), is ex-

TABLE 67-3 SURFACE RECEPTORS OF MONOCYTES AND MACROPHAGES

Fc receptors
  IgG2a, IgG2b/IgG1, IgG3, IgA, IgE
Complement receptors
  C3b, C3bi, C5a, C1q
LPS receptors
  CD14
Cytokine receptors
  MIF, MAF, LIF, CF, MFF, TNF-α, IL-1, IL-2, IL-3, IL-4,
  IL-10, IL-18, INF-α, INF-β, INF-γ, GM-CSF, M-CSF/CSF-1
Chemokine receptors
  CCR1, CCR2A, CCR2B, CCR3, CXCR4, CCR5
Macrophage growth factor receptors
  M-CSF, GM-CSF
Receptors for peptides and small molecules
  Neurokinin-1
  II$_1$, II$_2$, 5-IIT
  1,2,5-Dihydroxy vitamin D$_3$
  N-Formylated peptides
  Enkephalins/endorphins
  Substance P
  Hemokinin-1
  Arg-vasopressin
Hormone receptors
  Insulin
  Glucocorticoids
  Angiotensin
Transferrin and lactoferrin receptors
Lipoprotein lipid receptors
  Anionic low-density lipoproteins
  PGE$_2$, LTB$_4$, LTC$_4$, PAG
  Apolipoproteins B and E (chylomicron remnants, VLDL)
Receptors for coagulants and anticoagulants
  Fibrinogen/fibrin
  Coagulation factor VII
  α_1-Antithrombin
  Heparin
  Integrins (CD11b, CD18)
Fibronectin receptors
Laminin receptors
Mannosyl, fucosyl, galactosyl residue
α_2-Macroglobulin-proteinase complex receptors
Toll-like receptors
  TLR2, TLR4, TLR5, TLR9
Others
Cholinergic agonists
α_1-Adrenergic agonists
β_2-Adrenergic agonists

Ig, immunoglobulin; C, complement; MIF, macrophage inhibitory factor; MAF, macrophage-activating factor; LIF, leukocyte migration inhibition factor; MFF, macrophage fusion factor; IL, interleukin; INF, interferon; GM, granulocyte macrophage; H$_1$, histamine; 5-HT, 5-hydroxytryptamine; PG, prostaglandin; LT, leukotriene; PAG, platelet-activating factor; VLDL, very low density lipoprotein
SOURCE: Adapted from Angen and Ross, in Lewis and McGee,[2] with permission. Refer to references 69 to 75.

pressed by neutrophils, natural killer cells, and tissue macrophages.[38] This receptor can bind Ig in immune complexes and Ig bound to cell surface membranes. It is the main FcR responsible for antibody-dependent cellular cytotoxicity. All three FcRs specifically bind the human IgG subclasses IgG1 and IgG3 (see Chap. 77). The interaction of FcR on macrophages with immune complexes results in cell "activa-

tion," with an increase in phagocytosis, superoxide production, and prostaglandin and leukotriene release.

COMPLEMENT RECEPTORS
Activation of the complement system results in liberation of numerous ligands that bind to specific receptors on mononuclear phagocytes. Four receptors that bind fragments of the complement component C3 have been identified.[39] Complement receptor 1 (CR1, or CD35) binds dimeric C3bi and is found on both monocytes and macrophages. Complement receptor 3 (CR3, or CD11b) binds the complement fragment C3b. CR3 is a heterodimeric glycoprotein that is composed of two noncovalently linked polypeptides. The α-chain of the polypeptide has an M_r of 185,000, and the β-subunit has an M_r of 95,000. This receptor and the leukocyte antigens lymphocyte function-associated antigen (CD11a) and alpha-X integrin chain (CD11c) compose a family of heterodimers that share a common β-subunit (CD18).[40] This family is designated the *leukocyte integrin (β_2) subfamily*.[41] These heterodimers are involved in cell–cell interactions, including leukocyte trafficking into the tissues, binding of opsonized particles and plasma proteins, and attachment to various substrates. They also may modulate intercellular adhesion. Elimination of the integrin β_2 subunit causes leukocyte adhesion deficiency.[76]

TOLL-LIKE RECEPTORS
Toll-like receptors (TLRs), identified on macrophages in mammals, recognize a specific pattern of pathogen components, including endotoxins (lipopolysaccharide [LPS]) and viral nucleic acids. For example, TLR4 is part of a recognition couple for LPS. Pathogen recognition by TLRs activates the innate immune system through the signaling pathway and provokes inflammatory responses, such as cytokine production.[77]

MONOCYTE/MACROPHAGE SURFACE ANTIGEN RECEPTORS

HUMAN LEUKOCYTE ANTIGEN CLASS II RECEPTORS
Monocytes and macrophages serve an important function as antigen-presenting cells. They bear the class II glycoproteins of the major histocompatibility gene complex, human leukocyte antigen (HLA)-DR, HLA-DP, and HLA-DQ. Expression of major histocompatibility complex (MHC) class II antigens on macrophages from different tissues varies widely. Splenic macrophages contain a high percentage of HLA-DR-positive cells (50 percent), whereas peritoneal macrophages have relatively few (10–20 percent).[42] The proportion of Ia-positive alveolar macrophages is only approximately 5 percent.[43] Lymphokines, primarily interferon gamma, can induce macrophages to express higher levels of MHC class II antigens,[44] whereas prostaglandin E, α-fetoprotein, and glucocorticoids[45] down-regulate HLA-DR antigen expression on macrophages.

CD11 RECEPTORS
CD11 defines a family of three accessory adhesion surface glycoproteins: CD11a, CD11b, and CD11c. These proteins are distinct α-subunits for three heterodimeric surface glycoproteins, each sharing a common β-subunit, designated CD18. The α-subunits have different isoelectric points, molecular weights, and cell distribution[46] (see Chap. 14). Whereas CD11a is expressed on all leukocytes, CD11b and CD11c are expressed predominantly on monocytes and macrophages, a minor subset of B lymphocytes, and most polymorphonuclear leukocytes. CD11b is expressed on greater than 95 percent of fresh human monocytes and macrophages but declines rapidly on cells maintained *in vitro*. Antibodies specific for CD11b, such as OKM1 or Mo1, may block this complement receptor's ability to bind to CD3bi.[47] Accord-

ingly, these antibodies strongly inhibit complement receptor-mediated rosetting of erythrocyte-IgM antibody–complement complexes.

CD14, CD16, AND CD68 RECEPTORS

The CD14 molecule is one of the most characteristic surface antigens of the monocyte lineage. It is a polypeptide of 356 amino acids that is anchored to the plasma membrane by a phosphoinositol linkage.[48] It is expressed strongly on the surface of monocytes and weakly on the surface of granulocytes and most tissue macrophages. It can be detected on some nonmyeloid cells (e.g., hepatocytes and some epithelial cells). CD14 functions as a receptor for endotoxin (LPS). LPS binds to a serum protein, LPS-binding protein, which facilitates the binding of LPS to CD14. The coreceptor MD2 and TLR4 also are vital in this process. When LPS binds to CD14/MD-2/TLR4 expressed by monocytes or neutrophils, the cells become activated and release cytokines such as tumor necrosis factor and up-regulate cell surface molecules, including adhesion molecules. *In vitro*, soluble CD14 binds to LPS, and the complex stimulates cells that do not express CD14 to secrete cytokines and coregulate adhesion molecules.[49]

A subset of human blood monocytes that express low levels of CD14 molecules and high levels of the Fcγ receptor III (FcγR III) CD16 has been identified.[50–52] These CD14+CD16+ monocytes resemble alveolar but not peripheral macrophages. CD14+CD16+ monocytes represent 5 to 10 percent of peripheral blood monocytes in normal individuals and can be dramatically expanded in pathologic conditions, such as sepsis, HIV infection, and cancer. CD16+ monocytes produce high levels of proinflammatory cytokines and may represent dendritic cell precursors *in vivo*, because CD16+ monocytes preferentially differentiate into dendritic cells.[53,54] The mechanisms of CD16+ monocyte recruitment into tissues remains unknown.[55]

The CD68 antigen is a specific marker of monocytes and macrophages. Antibodies against the antigen label macrophages and other members of the mononuclear phagocyte lineage in routinely processed tissue sections and have been used to stain a range of lymphoid, histiocytic, and myelomonocytic proliferation.[56]

CD4 RECEPTORS

T lymphocytes express several surface receptors. The surface antigen CD4 is expressed exclusively in T helper lymphocytes (see Chap. 78). CD4 and its corresponding mRNA have been demonstrated on monocytes, macrophages, and the monocyte-like cell line U-937.[57] Although CD4 is present at low concentrations in blood monocytes, the proportion of cells that display this plasma membrane determinant ranges from less than 5 percent to 90 percent. Several monoclonal antibodies that react with different epitopes of the CD4 antigen have been described.[58] The CD4 molecule is involved in induction of T lymphocyte helper functions (T4) and T proliferative responses to antigen stimulation; however, its role in the function of monocyte/macrophages has not been determined. An important aspect of the monocyte/macrophage phenotype is the presence of CD4 molecules on the surface of monocytes that can act as receptors for HIV type 1 (HIV-1). HIV-1 utilizes the CD4 receptors as an entry pathway for infection of monocyte/macrophages.[59]

CHEMOKINE RECEPTORS

Chemokines mediate their activities by binding to target cell surface chemokine receptors that belong to a large family of G-protein coupled, seven transmembrane domain receptors. Human monocytes/macrophages express several chemokine receptors (see Table 67-3). The chemokine receptor CCR5 has been implicated in HIV infection of monocytes/macrophages.[60–64] CCR5 is a major coreceptor on monocytes/macrophages for M-tropic HIV infection. A 32-nucleotide deletion within the CCR5 gene has a highly protective role against acquisition of HIV.[65,66]

REFERENCES

1. van Furth R: *Mononuclear Phagocytes: Characteristics, Physiology and Function.* Martinus Nijhoff, Dordrecht, 1985.
2. Lewis CE, McGee JO'D: *The Macrophage.* Oxford University Press, New York, 1992.
3. Aschoff L: Das reticulo-endotheliale System. *Ergeb Inn Med Kinderheilkd* 26:1, 1924.
4. Randolph GJ, Beaulieu S, Lebecque S, et al: Differentiation of monocytes into dendritic cells in a model of transendothelial trafficking. *Science* 282:480, 1998.
5. van Furth R, Cohn ZA: The origin and kinetics of mononuclear phagocytes. *J Exp Med* 128:415, 1968.
6. Sallusto F, Lanzavecchia A: Efficient presentation of soluble antigen by cultured human dendritic cells is maintained by granulocyte/macrophage colony-stimulating factor plus interleukin 4 and downregulated by tumor necrosis factor-α. *J Exp Med* 179:1109, 1994.
7. van Furth R: Phagocytic cells: Development and distribution of mononuclear phagocytes in normal steady state and inflammation, in *Inflammation: Basic Principles and Clinical Correlates,* 2nd ed, edited by JI Gallin, R Snyderman, pp 325–341. Raven, New York, 1992.
8. Nichols BA, Bainton DF, Farquahr MG: Differentiation of monocytes: Origin, nature and fate of their azurophil granules. *J Cell Biol* 50:498, 1971.
9. Nichols BA, Bainton DF: Differentiation of human monocytes in bone marrow and blood: Sequential formation of two granule populations. *Lab Invest* 29:27, 1973.
10. Ploem JS: Reflection contrast microscopy as a tool in investigations of the attachment of living cells to a glass surface, in *Mononuclear Phagocytes in Immunity, Infection, and Pathology,* edited by R van Furth, p 405. Blackwell, Oxford, 1975.
11. Douglas SD: Alterations in intramembrane particle distribution during interaction of erythrocyte-bound ligands with immunoprotein receptors. *J Immunol* 120:151, 1978.
12. Rabinovitch M, DeStefano MJ: Macrophage spreading in vitro: I. Inducers of spreading. *Exp Cell Res* 77:323, 1973.
13. Douglas SD: Human monocyte spreading in vitro: Inducers and effects on Fc and C3 receptors. *Cell Immunol* 21:344, 1976.
14. Ackerman SK, Douglas SD: Purification of human monocytes on microexudate-coated surfaces. *J Immunol* 120:1372, 1978.
15. Zuckerman SH, Ackerman SK, Douglas SD: Long-term peripheral blood monocyte cultures: Establishment and morphology of primary human monocyte-macrophage cell culture. *Immunology* 38:401, 1979.
16. Sutton JS, Weiss L: Transformation of monocytes in tissue culture into macrophages, epithelioid cells and multinucleated giant cells. *J Cell Biol* 29:303, 1966.
17. Reaven EP, Axline SG: Subplasmalemmal microfilaments and microtubules in resting and phagocytizing cultivated macrophages. *J Cell Biol* 29:303, 1966.
18. Cohn ZA, Benson B: The differentiation of mononuclear phagocytes: Morphology, cytochemistry, and biochemistry. *J Exp Med* 121:153, 1965.
19. Wachstein M, Wolf G: The histochemical demonstration of esterase activity in human blood and bone marrow smears. *J Histochem Cytochem* 6:457, 1958.
20. Braunsteiner H, Schmalzl F: Cytochemistry of monocytes and macrophages, in *Mononuclear Phagocytes,* edited by R van Furth, p 62. Blackwell, Oxford, 1970.
21. Li CY, Lam KW, Yam LT: Esterases in human leukocytes. *J Histochem Cytochem* 21:1, 1973.

22. van der Rhee HJ, de Winter CPM, Daems WT: Fine structure and peroxidative activity of rat blood monocytes. *Cell Tissue Res* 185:1, 1977.

23. Dodel PT, Nichols BA, Bainton DF: Appearance of peroxidase reactivity within the rough ER of blood monocytes after surface adherence. *J Exp Med* 145:264, 1977.

24. Nichols BA, Bainton DF: Ultrastructure and cytochemistry of mononuclear phagocytes, in *Mononuclear Phagocytes in Immunity, Infection and Pathology*, edited by R van Furth, p 17. Blackwell, Oxford, 1975.

25. Parmley RT, Spicer SS, O'Dell RF: Ultrastructural identification of acid complex carbohydrate in cytoplasmic granules of normal and leukemic human monocytes. *Br J Haematol* 39:33, 1978.

26. Lewis MR, Lewis WH: Transformation of mononuclear blood-cells into macrophages, epithelioid cells, and giant cells in hanging-drop blood-cultures from lower vertebrates. Carnegie Institute of Washington, Pub 96. *Contrib Embryol* 18:95, 1926.

27. Maximow AA: The macrophages or histiocytes, in *Special Cytology: The Form and Functions of the Cell in Health and Disease*, vol II, 2nd ed, edited by EV Cowdry, p 711. Hoeber-Harper, New York, 1932.

28. Ebert RH, Florey HW: The extravascular development of the monocyte observed in vitro. *Br J Exp Pathol* 20:341, 1939.

29. Unanue ER: Macrophages, antigen-presenting cells, and the phenomena of antigen handling and presentation, in *Fundamental Immunology* 3rd ed, edited by WE Paul, p 111. Raven Press, New York, 1993.

30. Hassan NF, Kamani N, Messaros M, Douglas SD: Induction of multinucleated giant cell formation from human blood-derived monocytes by phorbol myristate acetate in in vitro culture. *J Immunol* 143:2179, 1989.

31. Snyderman R, Pike MC: Structure and function of monocytes and macrophages, in *Arthritis and Allied Conditions*, edited by DJ McCarty, p 306. Lea & Febiger, Philadelphia, 1989.

32. Rebuck JW, Crowley JH: A method of studying leukocytic functions in vivo. *Ann N Y Acad Sci* 59:757, 1955.

33. Boyden S: The chemotactic effect of mixtures of antibody and antigen on polymorphonuclear leukocytes. *J Exp Med* 115:453, 1962.

34. Fawcett DW, Raviola E: *Bloom and Fawcett: A Textbook of Histology*. Chapman and Hall, New York, 1994.

35. Russell SW, Gordon S: *Macrophage Biology and Activation*. Springer-Verlag, New York, 1992.

36. Metzger H: *Fc Receptors and the Action of Antibodies*. American Society for Microbiology, Washington, DC, 1990.

37. Anderson CL, Guyre PM, Whitin JC, et al: Monoclonal antibodies to Fc receptors for IgG on human mononuclear phagocytes. *J Biol Chem* 261:12856, 1986.

38. Looney RJ, Abraham GN, Anderson CL: Human monocytes and U-937 cells bear two distinct Fc receptors for IgG. *J Immunol* 136:1641, 1986.

39. Wright SD, Griffin FM Jr: Activation of phagocytic cells' C3 receptors for phagocytosis. *J Leukoc Biol* 38:327, 1985.

40. Kishimoto TK, Hollander N, Roberts TM, et al: Heterogenous mutations in the β subunit common to the LFA-1, Mac-1, and p150,95 glycoproteins cause leukocyte adhesion deficiency. *Cell* 50:193, 1987.

41. Hynes RO: Integrins: A family of cell surface receptors. *Cell* 48:549, 1987.

42. Cowing C, Schwartz BD, Dickler HB: Macrophage Ia antigens: I. Macrophage populations differ in their expression on Ia antigens. *J Immunol* 120:378, 1978.

43. Unanue ER, Allen PM: The basis for the immunoregulatory role of macrophages and other accessory cells. *Science* 236:551, 1987.

44. Belle ID: Functional significance of the regulation of macrophage Ia expression. *Eur J Immunol* 14:138, 1984.

45. Snider DD, Ulnae ER: Corticosteroids inhibit murine macrophages, Ia expression and interleukin-1 production. *J Immunol* 129:1803, 1982.

46. Sanchez-Madrid F, Nagy JA, Robbins E, et al: A human leukocyte differentiation antigen family with distinct alpha subunits and a common beta subunit: The lymphocyte-function associated antigen (LFA-1). The C3bi complement receptor (OKM1/Mac) and the p150,95 molecule. *J Exp Med* 158:1785, 1983.

47. Beller DI, Springer TA, Schreiber RD: Anti-Mac-1 selectively inhibits the mouse and human type three complement receptor. *J Exp Med* 156:1000, 1982.

48. Kazazi F, Mathijs J-M, Foley P, Cunningham AL: Variations in CD4 expression by human monocytes and macrophages and their relationship to infection with the human immunodeficiency virus. *Gen Virol* 70:2661, 1989.

49. Yu B, Hailman E, Wright SD: Lipopolysaccharide binding protein and soluble CD14 catalyze exchange of phospholipid. *J Clin Invest* 99:315, 1997.

50. Passlick B, Flieger D, Ziegler-Heitbrock HW: Identification and characterization of a novel monocyte subpopulation in human peripheral blood. *Blood* 74:2527, 1989.

51. Ziegler-Heitbrock HW, Fingerle G, Strobel M, et al: The novel subset of CD14+/CD16+ monocytes exhibits features of tissue macrophages. *Eur J Immunol* 23.2053, 1993.

52. Ziegler-Heitbrock HW: Heterogeneity of human blood monocytes: The CD14+CD16+ subpopulation. *Immunol Today* 17:424, 1996.

53. Grage-Griebenow E, Flad HD, Ernst M: Heterogeneity of human peripheral blood monocyte subsets. *J Leukoc Biol* 69:11, 2001.

54. Randolph GJ, Sanchez-Schmitz G, Liebman RM, Schakel K: The CD16+ (Fc RIII+) subset of human monocytes preferentially becomes migratory dendritic cells in a model tissue setting. *J Exp Med* 196:517, 2002.

55. Ancuta P, Rao R, Moses A, et al: Fractalkine preferentially mediates arrest and migration of CD16+ monocytes. *J Exp Med* 197:1701, 2003.

56. Collman R, Godfrey B, Cutilli J, et al: Macrophage-tropic strains of human immunodeficiency virus type 1 utilize the CD4 receptor. *J Virol* 64:4468, 1990.

57. Haziot A, Chen S, Ferrero E, et al: The monocyte differentiation antigen, CD14, is anchored to the cell membrane by a phosphatidylinositol linkage. *J Immunol* 141:547, 1988.

58. Schneider EM, Lorenz I, Kogler G, Wernet P: Modulation of monocyte function by CD14-specific antibodies in vitro, in *Leukocyte Typing*, vol IV, edited by W Knapp, B Dörken, WR Gilks, et al, p 794. Oxford University Press, New York, 1989.

59. Warnke RA, Pulford KAF, Pallesen G, et al: Diagnosis of myelomonocytic and macrophage neoplasms in routinely processed tissue biopsies with monoclonal antibody KP1. *Am J Pathol* 135:1089, 1989.

60. Alkhatib G, Combadiere C, Broder CC, et al: Ckr5: A rantes, mip-1a, receptor as a fusion cofactor for macrophage-tropic HIV. *Science* 272:1955, 1996.

61. Hill CM, Littman DR: Natural resistance to HIV. *Nature* 382:668, 1996.

62. Deng HK, Liu F, Ellmeier W, et al: Identification of a major co-receptor for primary isolates of HIV. *Nature* 381:661, 1996.

63. Huang Y: The role of a mutant CCR5 allele in HIV transmission and disease progression. *Nat Med* 2:1240, 1996.

64. Dragic T, Litwin V, Allaway GP, et al: HIV entry into CD4 cells is mediated by the chemokine receptor CC-CKR-5. *Nature* 381:667, 1996.

65. Samson M, Libert F, Doranz BJ, et al: Resistance to HIV infection in Caucasian individuals bearing mutant alleles of the CCR-5 chemokine receptor gene. *Nature* 382:722, 1996.

66. Liu R, Paxton WA, Choe S, et al: Homozygous defect in HIV-1 co-receptor accounts for resistance of some multiply-exposed individuals to HIV-1 infection. *Cell* 86:367, 1996.

67. Gordon S, Fraser I, Nath D, et al: Macrophages in tissues and in vitro. *Curr Opin Immunol* 4:25, 1992.

68. Lasser AP: The mononuclear phagocyte system: A review. *Hum Pathol* 14:1080, 1983.

69. Fogelman AM, van Lenten BJ, Warden C, et al: Macrophage lipoprotein receptors. *J Cell Sci* 9(suppl):135, 1988.

70. Adams DO, Hamilton TA: Phagocytic cells. Cytotoxic activities of macrophages, in *Inflammation. Basic Principles and Clinical Correlates*, 2nd ed, edited by JI Galin, IM Goldstein, R Snyderman, p 471. Raven Press, New York, 1992.

71. Werb Z, Goldstein IM: Phagocytic cells: Chemotactic and effector functions of macrophages and granulocytes, in *Basic and Clinical Immunology*, 7th ed, edited by DP Stites, AI Terr, p 96. Appleton and Lange, Norwalk, 1991.

72. Papadimitriou JM, Ashman RB: Macrophages: Current views on their differentiation, structure and function. *Ultrastruct Pathol* 13:343, 1989.

73. Gordon S, Perry H, Rabinowitz S, et al: Plasma membrane receptors of the mononuclear phagocyte system. *J Cell Sci* 9(suppl):1, 1988.

74. Law SKA: C3 receptors on macrophages. *J Cell Sci* 9(suppl):67, 1988.

75. Hume DA, Ross IL, Himes SR, et al: The mononuclear phagocyte system revisited. *J Leukoc Biol* 72:621, 2002.

76. Etzioni A, Doerschuk CM, Harlan JM: Of man and mouse: Leukocyte and endothelial adhesion molecule deficiencies. *Blood* 94:3281, 1999.

77. Athman R, Philpott D: Innate immunity via Toll-like receptors and Nod proteins. *Curr Opin Microbiol* 7:25, 2004.

BIOCHEMISTRY AND FUNCTION OF MONOCYTES AND MACROPHAGES

ROBERT I. LEHRER

TOMAS GANZ

Mononuclear phagocytes play central roles in resistance to many infectious diseases, including tuberculosis, leishmaniasis, typhoid fever, and systemic mycoses. Unlike short-lived and biosynthetically quiescent neutrophils, macrophages exhibit a prodigious capacity for macromolecular synthesis, can survive within tissues for weeks and even months, and provide a preferred intracellular niche for specialized parasitic microbes. Macrophages secrete numerous bioactive molecules and are highly responsive to signals from surrounding tissues. The function of macrophages is modulated through their receptors responding to cytokines, such as interferon gamma and tumor necrosis factor alpha, secreted by other host defense cells. Additional surface receptors enhance their phagocytic properties by recognizing various host-derived factors, including immunoglobulins, complement, and integrins. Other macrophage receptors recognize molecular motifs characteristic of microbes, including lipopolysaccharide (LPS), lipopeptides, bacterial DNA, mannans, and (lipo)teichoic acids. These pattern recognition receptors allow macrophages to distinguish potential pathogens from more inert particles and initiate target-appropriate host defense and inflammatory responses. The antimicrobial mechanisms of macrophages are mediated largely, but not exclusively, by various oxidants produced by their NADPH-oxidase and/or inducible nitric oxide synthase systems.

Mononuclear phagocytes (monocytes and macrophages) are relatively large phagocytic cells with abundant cytoplasm and a round to reniform nucleus (see Chap. 67). The morphology can vary under the influence of tissue-specific differentiating signals or the effects of pathologic processes. Altered macrophages bear eponyms, such as *Gaucher* or *Kupffer cells*, or have pseudonyms, such as *foam* (lipid-laden) or epithelioid cells. Mononuclear phagocytes combine prodigious biosynthetic and secretory abilities with an ability to vary their output in response to local conditions and chemical mediators. Dendritic cells are transiently phagocytic cells closely related to macrophages but specialized in antigen presentation to T lymphocytes.[1] Because of their fundamental role in adaptive immunity, dendritic cells merit separate consideration (see Chap. 18). Although cells of the monocyte/macrophage lineage may undergo malignant transformation or exuberant proliferation (see Chap. 72), most often their routine duties—host defense, antigen presentation, and removal of detritus—are performed away from the spotlight of disease.

To analyze macrophage biochemistry and function in humans,[2,3] investigators can readily obtain blood monocytes, macrophages generated from these monocytes in cell culture, and bronchoalveolar macrophages, but most other human macrophage populations are less accessible. Consequently, much of our information about macrophages derives from *in vivo* experiments on mice and from *in vitro* experiments with cultured murine blood monocytes or murine macrophages recovered from marrow, peritoneum, lungs, or minced solid organs.[2,3] Several human and murine cell lines have been used as models of macrophage function.[4] This chapter reviews selected aspects of the biology of mononuclear phagocytes, including their endocytic and phagocytic behavior, receptors, secretory properties, and microbicidal and cytotoxic mechanisms. Chapter 69 discusses the production, distribution, and fate of monocytes and macrophages.

MOTILITY AND CHEMOTAXIS

Many mononuclear phagocytes are present in or near the surfaces of organs regularly exposed to microbes, including the intestinal and genitourinary tracts, skin, and lungs. Local tissue populations of macrophages are rapidly augmented by entry of blood monocytes responding to various signals that arise during infection and inflammation. Macrophage motility depends on the contractile properties of actin and myosin, regulated by many additional proteins, including profilin, gelsolin, acumentin, tropomyosin, actin-binding protein, and calmodulin.[5]

Chemotaxis refers to the ability of cells to orient in and move along a chemical gradient. Many molecules generated during infection or injury are recognized by the surface receptors of monocytes and macrophages and trigger chemotactic responses.[6] Such substances include N-formylated peptides produced by bacteria,[7] complement component C5a,[8] leukotriene B4 and other eicosanoids, collagen and elastin fragments,[9] thrombin, platelet factor 4, platelet-derived growth factor (PDGF), and several neutrophil proteins and peptides, including cathepsin G, azurocidin, and defensins.[10,11]

Chemokines (i.e., chemotactic cytokines) are important mediators of chemotactic and migratory behavior.[12] These 8- to 10-kDa molecules contain four conserved cysteines that are linked by disulfide bonds. They are divided into two groups, based on their homology and the spacing of their first two cysteine residues. In CXC chemokines, also called *α-chemokines*, an amino acid is interposed between these cysteines. In CC chemokines, also called *β-chemokines*, these cysteines are adjacent. The genes for CXC and CC chemokines are clustered on human chromosomes 4 and 17, respectively. Whereas CXC chemokines such as interleukin (IL)-8 act primarily on neutrophils, CC chemokines, such as monocyte chemotactic protein (MCP)-1 to MCP-4, macrophage inhibitory protein (MIP)-1α, MIP-β, and regulated upon activation, normal T cell expressed and secreted (RANTES), are potent activators of monocytes and T lymphocytes.[12,13]

Multiple, structurally related receptors for chemokines have been identified. Typically, these receptors have seven transmembrane domains and signal through heterotrimeric guanosine triphosphate (GTP)-binding proteins. Chemokines and their receptors vary with respect to binding specificity. Many chemokines bind to more than one receptor, and most chemokine receptors bind more than one chemokine. Expression of chemokine receptors is regulated by the ambient cytokine environment, thereby allowing complex and graded responses.

Certain chemokine receptors have been subverted by pathogens in ways detrimental to the host. For example, CCR5, the macrophage receptor for RANTES, MIP-1α, and MIP-1β, is used by monocyte/ macrophage-tropic strains of HIV-1 as a coreceptor for intracellular entry.[14] Additionally, many members of the poxvirus, herpesvirus, and retrovirus families have captured genes encoding cytokine or chemokine receptors and modified them in ways that enhance viral pathogenicity.[15] For example, molluscum contagiosum virus secretes a modified CC chemokine that interferes with the chemotactic response of human leukocytes to multiple CC and CXC chemokines, thereby blunting the *in vivo* inflammatory response to the virus. Human herpesvirus 8, a Kaposi sarcoma–associated herpesvirus, appears to use similar strategies to deliver signals that initiate inappropriate growth or transformation.

ENERGETICS AND ENDOCYTOSIS

Mononuclear phagocytes derive most of their metabolic energy from glycolytic metabolism. In alveolar macrophages, this process is augmented substantially by oxidative phosphorylation. Macrophages imbibe extracellular fluid continually by a process known as *pinocytosis* (literally, "cell drinking"). Their fluid uptake occurs in several types of vesicles, including macropinosomes that are larger than 0.2 μm in diameter, clathrin-coated vesicles, and small uncoated vesicles. Receptor-mediated endocytosis takes place principally via clathrin-coated vesicles.[16] The content of degradative enzymes in macrophages increases after they take up digestible substances by endocytosis or phagocytosis. Although proteins retained within the lysosomal apparatus emerge only after extensive degradation, regulated endocytic mechanisms specialized for antigen presentation allow partially degraded antigens to be displayed on the macrophage cell membrane, bound to major histocompatibility complex (MHC) molecules.[17]

SECRETION

Certain secretory products of macrophages, such as lysozyme, are produced regularly and in large amounts. Most other products are produced and released in a highly controlled fashion, determined by the functional state of the cell and its exposure to regulatory stimuli. In addition to many cytokines (e.g., IL-1α, IL-1β, IL-6, tumor necrosis factor alpha [TNF-α], and interferons alpha, beta, and gamma [α, β, and γ]) and chemokines, macrophages produce numerous growth factors, including granulocyte colony stimulating factor, granulocyte-monocyte colony stimulating factor, transforming growth factor β, PDGF, and fibroblast growth factor.[18] By secreting classic and alternative pathway complement factors, macrophages can augment local tissue concentrations of these host defense molecules. Macrophages release various enzymes (e.g., plasminogen activator, elastase, collagenases, and acid hydrolases) that participate in tissue remodeling and wound healing. They also produce matrix proteins such as fibronectin, thrombospondin, proteoglycans, and diverse lipid mediators, including prostaglandins (PGE$_2$, PGF$_{2\alpha}$), prostacyclin, and various lipoxygenase products.[19]

RECEPTORS

Receptors allow mononuclear phagocytes to recognize and respond to other cells. They also permit macrophages to adhere to extracellular matrix, bind and ingest microorganisms, and respond to various cytokines and growth factors. Expression of membrane receptors varies according to the macrophage's functional state and reflects its prior exposure to cytokines. When receptor ligand binding occurs, the event is communicated to the intracellular machinery by transduction pathways that ultimately impinge on molecules that regulate transcription. Transcription factors that prominently regulate macrophage synthetic repertoire during inflammation include NF-κB, NF-IL6, PU.1, interferon regulatory factor-1, Egr-1, and Stat-1. Like other cells, macrophages respond to a large number of regulatory molecules, such as macrophage colony-stimulating factor (M-CSF), hormones, leukotrienes, other eicosanoids, coagulation factors, transport proteins, antiproteases, and many other bioactive molecules[20] that regulate macrophage growth, nutrient uptake, differentiation. and survival.

ADHESIVE MOLECULES

Monocytes and macrophages can adhere reversibly to various surfaces, including endothelial cells and extracellular matrix proteins. This property allows monocytes and macrophages to migrate on such surfaces and is imparted by adhesive plasma membrane glycoprotein receptors called *adhesins*. At least three families of adhesins participate in these processes—selectins, integrins, and intercellular adhesion molecules (ICAMs).[21] Mononuclear phagocytes and other leukocytes contain "homing receptors" called L-selectins or leukocyte endothelial cell adhesion molecules, which bind to corresponding glycans on endothelial surfaces. The endothelial surfaces display E- and P-selectins that bind to glycans on leukocytes. These lectin–glycan interactions mediate an initial, low-affinity rolling type of adhesion between leukocytes and vascular endothelium, before stronger connections are made via integrins. The integrin superfamily is composed of heterodimeric molecules with noncovalently associated α- and β-chains. Several β_2-integrins are prominent in macrophages, including lymphocyte function-associated antigen (LFA)-1 (CD11a/CD18), MAC-1 (CD11b/CD18), and p150/95 (CD 11c/CD18). The ligands (often called *counterreceptors*) of these adhesins include ICAM-1, ICAM-2, and ICAM-3 (LFA-1); fibrinogen and fibronectin (MAC-1); and iC3b (p150,95). Several β_1-integrins (very late activation antigen [VLA]-4, VLA-5, and VLA-6) expressed by monocytes are fibronectin receptors that may promote recruitment of monocytes to inflammatory foci. Leukocyte adhesion deficiency—a complex inherited disorder that results from a marked deficiency of β_2-integrins, is associated with frequent and severe infections, poor wound healing, and diminished accrual of leukocytes at sites of infection. Diapedesis of monocytes through the endothelium depends on homotypic interactions between platelet endothelial cell adhesion molecules-1 (PECAM, CD31) located on both monocytes and endothelia.[22]

RECEPTORS INVOLVED IN DETECTION AND PHAGOCYTOSIS OF MICROBES

Macrophages detect and phagocytize microbes based on "tags" attached to microbial surfaces consequent to their recognition by humoral innate and adaptive immune systems. These "tags," collectively called *opsonins*, include various immunoglobulins and components of complement. The surface membranes of mononuclear phagocytes contain specific receptors for immunoglobulins, including immunoglobulin G1 (IgG1) and other IgG subtypes, IgA, and IgE. IgG binds organisms via its Fab sites and binds the macrophage's Ig receptors via its Fc portion. IgG receptors promote both attachment and ingestion of immunoglobulin-coated particles. Macrophages also display receptors for several complement components, including C3b, C3bi, C3a, and C5a. The C3b receptor (also called *CR1* and *CD35*) also is found on neutrophils. It recognizes opsonized particles and accelerates C3b breakdown by factor I. CR1 mediates attachment without ingestion unless small amounts of IgG are present or the macrophages are otherwise stimulated.[23] The C3bi receptor (also called *CR3, Mac1,* and *CD 11b/CD18*) recognizes an Arg-Gly-Asp (RGD) triplet in its ligand C3bi,[24] and in fibrinogen and fibrin. CR3 binds many other ligands (including molecules found on bacteria, fungi, and protozoans), ICAM-1, and other ligands of endothelial cells. The contact sites of the C3bi receptor for several such ligands partially overlap. Fc and complement receptors allow macrophages to recognize, ingest, and usually destroy microorganisms opsonized by deposition of immunoglobulin and/or complement on their surface. *In vivo* administration of interferon-γ to normal subjects significantly increases the expression of Ig receptors (FcγRI, FcγRII, FcγRIII), integrins (CD11a/CD18, CD11b/CD18), and human leukocyte antigen-DR by monocytes.[25]

Certain macrophage receptors recognize molecules or molecular arrays that typically are found on microbes and can be classified as "pattern recognition receptors."[26] Toll-like receptors (TLRs) are a family of receptors found on the cell and phagosomal membranes of macrophages, dendritic cells, and other cell types involved in host defense. The 10 known human TLRs exist as homodimers and heterodimers that associate with other membrane and signaling molecules to detect microbe-specific components such as LPS, lipopeptides, bacterial DNA, flagellin, and double-stranded viral RNA.[27,28] Another well-studied example is the macrophage mannose receptor—a 180-kDa transmembrane protein with eight tandem carbohydrate recognition domains.[29] Two of these domains interact with linear or branched-chain mannosyl and fucosyl residues, allowing the mannose receptor to recognize a wide variety of bacteria, mycobacteria, yeasts, and parasites and to initiate phagocytic, endocytic, or antigen capture responses. Members of the Nod family of cytosolic microbial sensors, exemplified by the Nod2 protein of macrophages and intestinal Paneth cells, participate in detection of intracellular microbes, probably by sensing peptidoglycan fragments.[30] Collectively, pattern recognition receptors allow macrophages to distinguish potentially pathogenic microbes from relatively inert targets (e.g., inorganic particles, apoptotic cells). In response to microbe-specific molecules but much less so to inert targets, macrophages produce and release many inflammatory mediators, including reactive oxygen and nitrogen intermediates, prostaglandins, and various proinflammatory cytokines, including TNF-α, IL-1β, IL-6, and IL-8.

SCAVENGER RECEPTORS

Macrophages contain several types of receptors that recognize various negatively charged macromolecules. They originally were described as macrophage receptors that mediated the uptake of cholesterol from modified low-density lipoprotein, but their specificity turned out to be much broader, hence the name "scavenger receptors." Based on structural features, they were subdivided into several classes (A, B, C) and types (e.g., class A, type 1). Although they have been studied mostly because of their involvement in the pathophysiology of atherosclerosis, their primary role probably is in innate immunity (pathogen recognition) or in removal of apoptotic cells.[31]

ANTIMICROBIAL MECHANISMS

Experimental studies of murine listeriosis were instrumental in developing the concept of "activated macrophages."[32] In this model, bacterial numbers increased logarithmically in the liver and spleen for 3 days after intravenous inoculation of *Listeria monocytogenes*. Thereafter, net bacterial growth ceased, and viable bacteria declined sharply in numbers, disappearing by the next week. These beneficial changes were accompanied by the appearance of delayed hypersensitivity. An altered phenotype was evident in the peritoneal macrophages, which enlarged, became more phagocytic, and more effectively resisted *in vitro* challenge by *L. monocytogenes*. Similar changes were noted after mice were infected with *Brucella abortus, Salmonella typhimurium,* or *Mycobacterium bovis*. The antimicrobial efficacy of these macrophages was nonspecific. Infection by any one of these intracellular pathogens engendered macrophages with an enhanced ability to inhibit intracellular replication by all of them. Although such activated macrophages reverted to their basal state after 1 to 2 weeks, the phenotypic changes recurred within 24 hours after a challenge by the same organism that had initiated the original infection. *In vivo* resistance was not transferred from immune to naive mice by serum, but the transfer of splenic T lymphocytes conferred protection.

During the ensuing decades, much has been learned about the events responsible for these phenomena. Mononuclear phagocytes possess multiple mechanisms that allow them to kill ingested microorganisms or restrict their replication. Ingested microbes are sequestered within membrane-bounded compartments, called *phagocytic vacuoles* or *phagosomes*, which can be acidified to a pH of approximately 4.5. Within such phagosomes, the microbes are exposed to a mixture of lysolipids, macrophage-derived enzymes and proteins, and various oxidants. Moreover, macrophages activate mechanisms that starve the phagocytized microbes for micronutrients that are essential for their growth, especially iron[33,34] and tryptophan.[35,36] Although entrapment within phagolysosomes is a lethal event for most microbes, successful pathogens have developed stratagems that allow them to survive and even thrive in this environment. Some pathogens, such as *L. monocytogenes*, escape from phagosomes and enter the cytoplasmic compartment, where they co-opt the host cell's actin and use it to propel themselves into adjacent cells.[37] Other microbes actively enter other vacuolar compartments that are more hospitable than the phagosomes.[38] Yet other pathogens moderate their phagosomal microenvironments[39] by inhibiting vacuolar acidification or phagolysosomal fusion or undergo phenotypic changes that enhance their resistance to this environment.[40,41]

DEPLETION OF IRON AND OTHER DIVALENT METALS

Natural resistance-associated macrophage protein-1 (Nramp1), a macrophage protein that contributes substantially to innate resistance to intracellular infections, was identified by detailed genetic analysis of inbred mice with different resistances to infection by different microbes. Nramp1 (also called SLC11A1) is a hydrophobic, integral membrane protein that is encoded by the *Lsh/Ity/Bcg* gene, which regulates resistance to *Leishmania, Salmonella,* and *Mycobacteria*. Expression of Nramp1 in mice is restricted to macrophages and is enhanced by treatment with interferon-γ and LPS. Nramp1 also is found in late endosomal and lysosomal vesicular compartments of the macrophage. By pumping protons in and divalent metals out of the phagosomes, the protein may enhance vacuolar acidification and act to deplete the phagosomal environment of iron or other trace metals needed for microbial growth and pathogenicity.[42] Intracellular pathogens, such as mycobacteria, can interfere with phagosome-lysosome fusion, thereby preventing vacuolar acidification and reducing the delivery of Nramp1 to phagosomes.[34] Nramp1 affects other aspects of macrophage function, including MHC expression, their production of proinflammatory cytokines and chemokines, and their production of antimicrobial oxidants.[43]

REACTIVE OXYGEN INTERMEDIATES

Macrophages with enhanced antimicrobial or cytotoxic activity generally show increased production of reactive oxygen intermediates.[44] To generate these oxidants, phagocytes, including monocytes and macrophages, contain multiple protein components that, when assembled and activated, form an nicotinamide adenine dinucleotide phosphate [(reduced form) NADPH] oxidase complex that transfers electrons to molecular oxygen from intracellular NADPH. Activation of NADPH oxidase is triggered by protein kinases and involves translocation to the plasma membrane of several cytosolic components, including p67^{phox}, p47^{phox}, and p40^{phox}.[45] The fully active NADPH oxidase complex also includes several small GTP-binding proteins. In the plasma membrane, the several cytosolic components interact via proline-rich and SH3 domains with the flavo-hemoprotein cytochrome b$_{558}$, which is composed of large and small subunits called gp91^{phox} and p22^{phox}, respectively. Superoxide (O$_2^-$) anions generated by NADPH oxidase are unstable and undergo various reactions, including dismutation to form hydrogen peroxide (H$_2$O$_2$) and oxygen.

Chronic granulomatous disease (CGD) refers to a group of uncommon disorders associated with defective activation and assembly of NADPH oxidase by neutrophils and mononuclear phagocytes.[46,47,48] The neutrophils and monocytes of children with CGD fail to produce superoxide and H$_2$O$_2$ and show markedly impaired antimicrobial activity against many bacteria and fungi in vitro. The most common variant of CGD is transmitted with X-linked inheritance and affects male children only. It results from the absence or abnormality of gp91^{phox}, whose gene is located on the X chromosome at Xp21.1. Defects in p47^{phox} (chromosome 7q11.23) are transmitted autosomally and account for approximately 30 percent of total CGD cases. It affects males and females equally. Primary genetic defects involving p22^{phox}, p67^{phox}, and gp91 have been described and account for the remaining cases of CGD. Children affected by CGD sustain repeated infections, most often caused by Staphylococcus aureus but also by bacteria and fungi of limited pathogenic potential (e.g., Serratia marcescens, Burkholderia cepacia, and Aspergillus fumigatus). Prophylactic administration of antibiotics, such as trimethoprim-sulfamethoxazole, and of interferon-γ decreases the frequency and severity of infections in patients with all forms of CGD (see Chap. 66).

MYELOPEROXIDASE

Like neutrophils, blood monocytes contain myeloperoxidase (MPO) and use it to convert H$_2$O$_2$ into microbicidal oxidants.[49] Their MPO is lost when monocytes differentiate into macrophages. Hereditary deficiency of MPO is relatively common, perhaps affecting as many as one in 2000 individuals.[50] Neutrophils and monocytes of affected individuals lack MPO and are unable to convert the H$_2$O$_2$ produced by dismutation of superoxide into more potent oxidants such as hypochlorite or chloramines. Neutrophils and monocytes from subjects with hereditary MPO deficiency show selectively impaired microbicidal activity in vitro. Several such patients (typically with additional predisposing factors, such as diabetes mellitus) have developed disseminated Candida albicans infections.

NITRIC OXIDE

Nitric oxide (NO) and other reactive nitrogen intermediates play important roles in restricting the growth of many pathogenic organisms

in mice and in murine macrophages.[51,52] NO is both diffusible and unstable. It reacts with oxygen and water to yield equimolar amounts of nitrite and nitrate. It reacts with other molecules to form S-nitrosothiols. NO and superoxide (O$_2^-$) can interact to form peroxynitrite (ONOO$^-$), a potent oxidant that also may mediate antimicrobial activity.

Distinct NO synthase enzymes are responsible for the constitutive and inducible production of NO. In murine macrophages, stimulation by LPS or cytokines such as interferon-γ leads to the expression of an inducible NO synthase, called iNOS or NOS2. This heme-containing enzyme converts L-arginine to citrulline plus NO, using NADPH and oxygen as additional substrates and flavin adenine dinucleotide (FAD), flavin mononucleotide (FMN), calmodulin, and tetrahydrobiopterin as cofactors.

In rodent macrophages, pathogens killed or inhibited by NO include Cryptococcus neoformans, Francisella tularensis, Leishmania major, and Schistosoma manson.[53] iNOS knockout mice show increased susceptibility to acute infection by many, but not all, organisms.[51] Human lung macrophages from patients with tuberculosis express iNOS, and inflammatory human macrophages have been induced to express iNOS in vitro.[54] However, inducing human macrophages to produce microbicidal amounts of NO in vitro is difficult.[55] In humans, NO contributes to innate immunity,[53,55] but whether it functions as a regulator of host defense responses, a microbicidal effector, or both is uncertain.

INTERACTIONS OF MACROPHAGES WITH TUMORS

Many human tumors are infiltrated by macrophages, and most investigators assumed these cells were mediating host resistance to the tumor. The relationship between macrophages and tumors is much more complex. Macrophages are capable of either supporting tumor growth through the production of growth and angiogenic factors or inhibiting tumor growth by releasing cytostatic or cytocidal substances.[56,57] The role of chronic inflammation and macrophages in promoting carcinogenesis, first proposed by Virchow in the 19th century, is receiving increased attention given the effectiveness of antiinflammatory agents in preventing some cancers.[58]

Macrophage infiltration into tumors correlates with the expression of CC chemokine ligand-2 (also called MCP-1), vascular endothelial growth factor (VEGF), and M-CSF.[56,59] MCP-1 and VEGF act as chemotactic factors for monocytes, whereas M-CSF also induces maturation of monocytes into macrophages and promotes macrophage survival.[59]

Whether macrophages support or oppose tumor growth depends on the specific signals they receive. At one extreme, macrophages exposed to LPS and interferon-γ show increased production of TNF-α and reactive oxygen and nitrogen products. They also show increased ability to kill microbes and tumor cells. Such macrophages have been described as "activated" or M1 macrophages.[59] At the opposite extreme, macrophages exposed to IL-4, IL-13, and IL-10, termed "alternatively activated" or M2, scavenge dead cells and debris and promote angiogenesis and tissue repair.[60,61] Some tumor environments polarize macrophages predominantly to M2. These tumor-associated macrophages generate little cytotoxic activity[62] and can provide important growth factor and angiogenic support for the tumor.[63]

MACROPHAGES AS SCAVENGERS

Apoptotic clearance is the programmed and regulated process by which damaged, senescent, or developmentally redundant cells are broken up and eventually removed by macrophages.[64,65] A key event in apoptosis is the redistribution of phospholipids that normally are found only on the inner leaflet of the cell membrane. The appearance of these lipids on the outer leaflet and their access to extracellular fluid generates important signals for both chemotaxis of macrophages to apoptotic cells and their subsequent phagocytosis.[66] Lysophosphatidylcholine, generated by the action of phospholipase A_2, is a lipid released by apoptotic cells that serves as a chemotactic signal attracting macrophages.[67] However, other substances released from apoptotic cells also can contribute to the signal.[66] In many situations, subsequent cell clearance by macrophages depends on the appearance of oxidized phosphatidylserine in the external leaflet of the target cell membrane[64,68] and its recognition by a macrophage phosphatidylserine receptor.[65,69] However, other target cell surface alterations and macrophage receptors[70] also can contribute to phagocytosis of apoptotic cells. In general, clearance of apoptotic cells, unlike clearance of microbes, does not trigger inflammation or release proinflammatory cytokines.

A related important function of macrophages is removal of senescent erythrocytes and recycling of their iron content.[71] As is the case with apoptotic cells, phosphatidylserine exposure is a prominent feature of red cell senescence[72] and leads to phagocytic clearance by splenic and other macrophages.[73] Other molecules expressed on senescent erythrocytes and implicated in their phagocytic clearance include clustered band 3 protein, targeted by natural antibodies, and modified carbohydrate moieties that expose binding sites for natural antibodies or alter erythrocyte surface charge. Chapters 31 and 52 address the mechanisms of erythrocyte destruction and clearance in hemolytic anemias.

Alveolar macrophages clear inhaled particles that reach the alveoli. Although some of these particles contain microbial material that can engage microbial clearance mechanisms, other particles are inert. Inert particles also are avidly phagocytized by alveolar macrophages, by scavenger receptors including prominently *macrophage receptor with collagenous structure* (MARCO).[74,75]

The scavenger function of macrophages is intimately involved in the pathogenesis of atherosclerosis.[76,77] In subjects with high concentrations of low-density lipoproteins (LDL), LDL molecules penetrate the artery wall, are trapped in proteoglycan matrix, and subsequently are oxidized by one of several candidate enzymes, including MPO, lipoxygenases, iNOS, or NADPH oxidase. Oxidized LDLs act as monocyte chemotactic factors that attract monocytes into nascent atherosclerotic lesions. Once in the lesions, monocytes transform into macrophages, and they and other cells within the lesions generate CC chemokines that attract additional monocytes into the lesions. Uptake of oxidized LDLs by macrophage scavenger receptors causes engorgement of macrophages with cholesterol, the formation of "foam cells" within the plaques, and progression and expansion of the lesions. Thus, atherosclerosis can be considered a side effect of the homeostatic function of macrophages in host defense and in the clearance of particles and apoptotic cells.

MACROPHAGES AND NEUTROPHILS

One of the striking features of phagocyte biology is the apparent duplication of some functions between macrophages and neutrophils. Both cell types are highly mobile, use similar chemotactic mechanisms to home in on their targets, are actively phagocytic, use similar or identical receptors for phagocytosis, and generate reactive oxygen products as microbicidal effectors. However, closer examination of the differences provides some clues to the distinct roles of the short-lived neutrophils (tissue half-life of approximately 1 day) and the longer-lived macrophages (life span of weeks to months). Neutrophils emerge from the marrow with an arsenal of hydrolytic and (per)oxidative en-

zymes, augmented by multiple antimicrobial peptides and proteins stored in various types of cytoplasmic granules (see Chap. 60). However, mature neutrophils have only a limited capacity to synthesize nucleic acids and proteins, which limits their life span and their ability to adapt to differing functional requirements and tissue environments. Their short life span and lack of biosynthetic capacity also make neutrophils unattractive to parasitization by most microbes and viruses that depend on the host cell for their metabolic and reproductive functions. The short life span and lack of replicative potential of neutrophils also requires that a large part of the hematopoietic capacity of the bone marrow be dedicated to neutrophil production. In contrast, macrophages possess an active protein and nucleic acid synthetic machinery, lack a large cytoplasmic granule storage compartment, and make their microbicidal effectors and lytic enzymes on demand. They are self-replicating, are able to remodel and adapt to differing tissue environments, and can fulfill multiple distinct functions. Their broad synthetic repertoire allows them to function as coordinators of host defense, inflammation, and tissue repair. However, their longer life span, large variety of receptors and transport processes, and high synthetic capacity make them vulnerable to parasitization by microbes and viruses.

REFERENCES

1. Banchereau J, Steinman RM: Dendritic cells and the control of immunity. *Nature* 392:245, 1998.
2. Herscowitz HB, Holden HTBJA, Ghaffar A: *Manual of Macrophage Methodology.* Marcel Dekker, New York, 1981.
3. Adams DO, Edelson PJ, Koren H: *Methods for Studying Mononuclear Phagocytes.* Academic Press, New York, 1981.
4. Walker WS: Establishment of mononuclear phagocyte cell lines. *J Immunol Methods* 174:25, 1994.
5. Stossel TP, Hartwig JH, Janmey PA, et al: Cell crawling two decades after Abercrombie. *Biochem Soc Symp* 65:267, 1999.
6. Snyderman R, Pike MC: Chemoattractant receptors on phagocytic cells. *Annu Rev Immunol* 2:257, 1984.
7. Le Y, Oppenheim JJ, Wang JM: Pleiotropic roles of formyl peptide receptors. *Cytokine Growth Factor Rev* 12:91, 2001.
8. Riedemann NC, Guo RF, Ward PA: A key role of C5a/C5aR activation for the development of sepsis. *J Leukoc Biol* 74:966, 2003.
9. Hunninghake GW, Davidson JM, Rennard S, et al: Elastin fragments attract macrophage precursors to diseased sites in pulmonary emphysema. *Science* 212:925, 1981.
10. Yang D, Chen Q, Chertov O, et al: Human neutrophil defensins selectively chemoattract naive T and immature dendritic cells. *J Leukoc Biol* 68:9, 2000.
11. Wu Z, Hoover DM, Yang D, et al: Engineering disulfide bridges to dissect antimicrobial and chemotactic activities of human beta-defensin 3. *Proc Natl Acad Sci U S A* 100:8880, 2003.
12. Baggiolini M: Chemokines and leukocyte traffic. *Nature* 392:565, 1998.
13. Boulay F, Naik N, Giannini E, et al: Phagocyte chemoattractant receptors. *Ann N Y Acad Sci* 832:69, 1997.
14. Berger EA, Murphy PM, Farber JM: Chemokine receptors as HIV-1 coreceptors: Roles in viral entry, tropism, and disease. *Annu Rev Immunol* 17:657, 1999.
15. Alcami A: Viral mimicry of cytokines, chemokines and their receptors. *Nat Rev Immunol* 3:36, 2003.
16. Mukherjee S, Ghosh RN, Maxfield FR: Endocytosis. *Physiol Rev* 77:759, 1997.
17. Lennon-Dumenil AM, Bakker AH, Wolf-Bryant P, et al: A closer look at proteolysis and MHC-class-II-restricted antigen presentation. *Curr Opin Immunol* 14:15, 2002.

18. Nathan CF: Secretory products of macrophages. *J Clin Invest* 79:319, 1987.

19. Funk CD: Prostaglandins and leukotrienes: Advances in eicosanoid biology. *Science* 294:1871, 2001.

20. Gordon S, Perry VH, Rabinowitz S, et al: Plasma membrane receptors of the mononuclear phagocyte system. *J Cell Sci Suppl* 9:1, 1988.

21. Beekhuizen H, van Furth R: Monocyte adherence to human vascular endothelium. *J Leukoc Biol* 54:363, 1993.

22. Muller WA, Randolph GJ: Migration of leukocytes across endothelium and beyond: Molecules involved in the transmigration and fate of monocytes. *J Leukoc Biol* 66:698, 1999.

23. Krych-Goldberg M, Atkinson JP: Structure-function relationships of complement receptor type 1. *Immunol Rev* 180:112, 2001.

24. Todd RF III: The continuing saga of complement receptor type 3 (CR3). *J Clin Invest* 98:1, 1996.

25. Schiff DE, Rae J, Martin TR, et al: Increased phagocyte Fc gammaRI expression and improved Fc gamma-receptor-mediated phagocytosis after in vivo recombinant human interferon-gamma treatment of normal human subjects. *Blood* 90:3187, 1997.

26. Gordon S: Pattern recognition receptors: Doubling up for the innate immune response. *Cell* 111:927, 2002.

27. Takeda K, Kaisho T, Akira S: Toll-like receptors. *Annu Rev Immunol* 21:335, 2003.

28. Aderem A: Phagocytosis and the inflammatory response. *J Infect Dis* 187(suppl 2):S340, 2003.

29. Ezekowitz RA: Role of the mannose-binding lectin in innate immunity. *J Infect Dis* 187(suppl 2):S335, 2003.

30. Girardin SE, Hugot JP, Sansonetti PJ: Lessons from Nod2 studies: Towards a link between Crohn's disease and bacterial sensing. *Trends Immunol* 24:652, 2003.

31. Peiser L, Mukhopadhyay S, Gordon S: Scavenger receptors in innate immunity. *Curr Opin Immunol* 14:123, 2002.

32. Mackaness GB: Reflections on the history of the macrophage, in *Mononuclear Phagocytes in Cell Biology*, edited by G Lopez-Bernstein, J Klostergaard, p 1. CRC Press, Boca Raton, 1993.

33. Byrd TF, Horwitz MA: Interferon gamma-activated human monocytes downregulate transferrin receptors and inhibit the intracellular multiplication of Legionella pneumophila by limiting the availability of iron. *J Clin Invest* 83:1457, 1989.

34. Forbes JR, Gros P: Divalent-metal transport by NRAMP proteins at the interface of host-pathogen interactions. *Trends Microbiol* 9:397, 2001.

35. Daubener W, MacKenzie CR: IFN-gamma activated indoleamine 2,3-dioxygenase activity in human cells is an antiparasitic and an antibacterial effector mechanism. *Adv Exp Med Biol* 467:517, 1999.

36. Murray HW, Szuro-Sudol A, Wellner D, et al: Role of tryptophan degradation in respiratory burst-independent antimicrobial activity of gamma interferon-stimulated human macrophages. *Infect Immun* 57:845, 1989.

37. Portnoy DA, Auerbuch V, Glomski IJ: The cell biology of Listeria monocytogenes infection: The intersection of bacterial pathogenesis and cell-mediated immunity. *J Cell Biol* 158:409, 2002.

38. Rosenberger CM, Finlay BB: Phagocyte sabotage: Disruption of macrophage signaling by bacterial pathogens. *Nat Rev Mol Cell Biol* 4:385, 2003.

39. Amer AO, Swanson MS: A phagosome of one's own: A microbial guide to life in the macrophage. *Curr Opin Microbiol* 5:56, 2002.

40. Ernst RK, Guina T, Miller SI: How intracellular bacteria survive: Surface modifications that promote resistance to host innate immune responses. *J Infect Dis* 179(suppl 2):S326, 1999.

41. Groisman EA, Saier MH Jr: Salmonella virulence: New clues to intramacrophage survival. *Trends Biochem Sci* 15:30, 1990.

42. Forbes JR, Gros P: Iron, manganese, and cobalt transport by Nramp1 (Slc11a1) and Nramp2 (Slc11a2) expressed at the plasma membrane. *Blood* 102:1884, 2003.

43. Blackwell JM, Goswami T, Evans CA, et al: SLC11A1 (formerly NRAMP1) and disease resistance. *Cell Microbiol* 3:773, 2001.

44. Nathan CF: Secretion of oxygen intermediates: Role in effector functions of activated macrophages. *Fed Proc* 41:2206, 1982.

45. Babior BM: NADPH oxidase: An update. *Blood* 93:1464, 1999.

46. Roos D: The genetic basis of chronic granulomatous disease. *Immunol Rev* 138:121, 1994.

47. Segal AW: The molecular and cellular pathology of chronic granulomatous disease. *Eur J Clin Invest* 18:433, 1988.

48. Segal BH, Leto TL, Gallin JI, et al: Genetic, biochemical, and clinical features of chronic granulomatous disease. *Medicine (Baltimore)* 79:170, 2000.

49. Klebanoff SJ, Rosen H: The role of myeloperoxidase in the microbicidal activity of polymorphonuclear leukocytes. *Ciba Found Symp* 263, 1978.

50. Nauseef WM, Root RK, Malech HL: Biochemical and immunologic analysis of hereditary myeloperoxidase deficiency. *J Clin Invest* 71:1297, 1983.

51. MacMicking J, Xie QW, Nathan C: Nitric oxide and macrophage function. *Annu Rev Immunol* 15:323, 1997.

52. Nathan C, Shiloh MU: Reactive oxygen and nitrogen intermediates in the relationship between mammalian hosts and microbial pathogens. *Proc Natl Acad Sci U S A* 97:8841, 2000.

53. Fang FC: Perspectives series: Host/pathogen interactions. Mechanisms of nitric oxide-related antimicrobial activity. *J Clin Invest* 99:2818, 1997.

54. Nathan C: Inducible nitric oxide synthase: What difference does it make? *J Clin Invest* 100:2417, 1997.

55. Fang FC, Vazquez-Torres A: Nitric oxide production by human macrophages: There's NO doubt about it. *Am J Physiol Lung Cell Mol Physiol* 282:L941, 2002.

56. Bingle L, Brown NJ, Lewis CE: The role of tumour-associated macrophages in tumour progression: Implications for new anticancer therapies. *J Pathol* 196:254, 2002.

57. Klimp AH, de Vries EGE, Scherphof GL, et al: A potential role of macrophage activation in the treatment of cancer. *Crit Rev Oncol Hematol* 44:143, 2002.

58. Balkwill F, Mantovani A: Inflammation and cancer: Back to Virchow? *Lancet* 357:539, 2001.

59. Mantovani A, Sozzani S, Locati M, et al: Macrophage polarization: Tumor-associated macrophages as a paradigm for polarized M2 mononuclear phagocytes. *Trends Immunol* 23:549, 2002.

60. Goerdt S, Politz O, Schledzewski K, et al: Alternative versus classical activation of macrophages. *Pathobiology* 67:222, 1999.

61. Stein M, Keshav S, Harris N, et al: Interleukin 4 potently enhances murine macrophage mannose receptor activity: A marker of alternative immunologic macrophage activation. *J Exp Med* 176:287, 1992.

62. DiNapoli MR, Calderon CL, Lopez DM: The altered tumoricidal capacity of macrophages isolated from tumor-bearing mice is related to reduced expression of the inducible nitric oxide synthase gene. *J Exp Med* 183:1323, 1996.

63. Crowther M, Brown NJ, Bishop ET, et al: Microenvironmental influence on macrophage regulation of angiogenesis in wounds and malignant tumors. *J Leukoc Biol* 70:478, 2001.

64. Fadok VA, Bratton DL, Henson PM: Phagocyte receptors for apoptotic cells: Recognition, uptake, and consequences. *J Clin Invest* 108:957, 2001.

65. Grimsley C, Ravichandran KS: Cues for apoptotic cell engulfment: Eat-me, don't eat-me and come-get-me signals. *Trends Cell Biol* 13:648, 2003.

66. Fadok VA: The sirens' call. *Nat Cell Biol* 5:697, 2003.

67. Lauber K, Bohn E, Krober SM, et al: Apoptotic cells induce migration of phagocytes via caspase-3-mediated release of a lipid attraction signal. *Cell* 113:717, 2003.

68. Fadeel B: Programmed cell clearance. *Cell Mol Life Sci* 60:2575, 2003.

69. Fadok VA, Bratton DL, Rose DM, et al: A receptor for phosphatidyl-serine-specific clearance of apoptotic cells. *Nature* 405:85, 2000.

70. Giles KM, Hart SP, Haslett C, et al: An appetite for apoptotic cells? Controversies and challenges. *Br J Haematol* 109:1, 2000.

71. Knutson M, Wessling-Resnick M: Iron metabolism in the reticuloen-dothelial system. *Crit Rev Biochem Mol Biol* 38:61, 2003.

72. Boas FE, Forman L, Beutler E: Phosphatidylserine exposure and red cell viability in red cell aging and in hemolytic anemia. *Proc Natl Acad Sci U S A* 95:3077, 1998.

73. Schroit AJ, Madsen JW, Tanaka Y: In vivo recognition and clearance of red blood cells containing phosphatidylserine in their plasma membranes. *J Biol Chem* 260:5131, 1985.

74. Palecanda A, Paulauskis J, Al Mutairi E, et al: Role of the scavenger receptor MARCO in alveolar macrophage binding of unopsonized environmental particles. *J Exp Med* 189:1497, 1999.

75. Palecanda A, Kobzik L: Receptors for unopsonized particles: The role of alveolar macrophage scavenger receptors. *Curr Mol Med* 1:589, 2001.

76. Greaves DR, Gough PJ, Gordon S: Recent progress in defining the role of scavenger receptors in lipid transport, atherosclerosis and host defence. *Curr Opin Lipidol* 9:425, 1998.

77. Li AC, Glass CK: The macrophage foam cell as a target for therapeutic intervention. *Nat Med* 8:1235, 2002.

PRODUCTION, DISTRIBUTION, AND FATE OF MONOCYTES AND MACROPHAGES

TOMAS GANZ
ROBERT I. LEHRER

Macrophages are ancient, mesoderm-derived host defense cells. During embryogenesis, they appear first in the yolk sac, then in the liver, and finally in the marrow—a sequence that recapitulates the phylogeny of blood-forming tissues in vertebrates. Large populations of tissue macrophages exist in the small intestine, liver (Kupffer cells), and lungs. Tissue macrophages can replicate sufficiently to sustain steady-state macrophage populations. Blood monocytes arise in the marrow from precursor cells (monoblasts) that are derived from the differentiation of multipotential progenitors. Blood monocytes rapidly enter inflamed or infected tissues, where they can mature into macrophages and substantially augment resident macrophage populations. Monocytes also can mature into dendritic cells that efficiently present antigen to T cells.

IDENTIFICATION AND KINETIC STUDIES OF MONOCYTES AND MACROPHAGES

Monocytes and macrophages are recognized outside the marrow as smaller (spread diameter of 10–18 μm) and larger (20–80 μm) cells that are mononuclear and phagocytic (see Chap. 71). Among the histochemical markers characteristic of mammalian monocytes and macrophages, "lipase" (a nonspecific esterase usually detected by its hydrolysis of α-naphthyl butyrate) and myeloperoxidase (detected by peroxidation of diaminobenzidine) have been the most useful. Human monocytes and macrophages both express lipase activity, but only monocytes and immature macrophages contain granules that react with peroxidase substrates. Marrow macrophages and monocytes are morphologically and histochemically similar to their extramyeloid counterparts. Myeloid lineage-specific genes that encode transcription factors regulate macrophage development. The transcription factor PU.1, encoded by a member of the *ETS* family, appears to be central in macrophage development. Transcription factor gene expression probably is induced by exogenous cytokine stimulation, especially by monocyte colony stimulating factor (M-CSF), interacting with granulocyte-monocyte colony stimulating factor (GM-CSF), and interleukin (IL)-3.[43] Promonocytes, monocyte precursors in the marrow, are weakly phagocytic mononuclear cells 10 to 20 μm in diameter that contain cytoplasmic filaments visible under electron microscopy and a small number of peroxidase-positive cytoplasmic granules.[1,2] Mono-

Acronyms and abbreviations that appear in this chapter include: FIM, factor increasing monocytopoiesis; GM-CSF, granulocyte-monocyte colony stimulating factor; IL, interleukin; M-CSF, monocyte colony stimulating factor; PECAM, platelet endothelial cell adhesion molecule; TNF, tumor necrosis factor.

clonal antibodies and lectins variably specific for monocytes and macrophages have been developed.[3]

Monocytes or macrophages can be isolated from body fluids, labeled with lipophilic dyes or radioactive compounds, then reinfused and their fate followed by repeated sampling of blood or tissues. Alternatively, genetic markers can be used to follow the fate of infused monocytes, macrophages, or marrow cells. Concerns have been raised about the effects of *in vitro* handling on the fate of reinfused cells. The kinetics of monocytes and macrophages after marrow transplantation also may be altered from normal by the effects of radiation and conditioning drugs on the recipient.[4]

Experimental animals treated with a brief infusion of ^{3}H-thymidine incorporate the radioactive nucleotide into cells undergoing DNA replication. The labeled cells and their descendants can be detected by overlaying tissue sections, imprints, or thin films with photographic emulsions where the beta particles emitted by tritium cause black "grains" to develop. Cells that have divided more than once after incorporating tritiated (^{3}H)-thymidine are less radioactive, because each division splits the labeled DNA equally between the daughter cells. The films or tissue sections can be conventionally stained to allow classification of the labeled cells according to their morphologic and staining characteristics. When a nondividing population arises only by maturation of a dividing precursor cell population, most of the precursors incorporate tritiated thymidine abundantly, but the mature descendants incorporate comparatively little. As the precursors mature, the number of labeled precursors decreases while their labeled descendants increase. Quantitative analysis can yield kinetic models of traffic between various cell populations and their rates of proliferation. Because macrophages are labeled both directly (dividing macrophages) and indirectly (macrophages arising from dividing earlier marrow precursors), interpretation of the experimental data can be complex and has led to controversy.[4,5]

Dual *in vivo* labeling of macrophage populations is largely avoided by using parabiotic animals[4] whose blood circulations are joined by a permanent cutaneous connection. The skin tunnel between the two animals can be clamped to temporarily separate their circulations while only one animal is infused with tritiated thymidine. When labeling is complete, cross-circulation is allowed to resume. In this case, the macrophages of the recipient animal that was not injected with tritiated thymidine are labeled only if they develop from labeled donor-derived circulating cells.

PHYLOGENY AND ONTOGENY OF MACROPHAGES

Large mononuclear phagocytic cells of mesodermal origin (macrophages) are the principal host defense cells in invertebrates[6] (e.g., mollusks, crustaceans, or insects), where they usually are referred to as *amebocytes* or *hemocytes*. The premyeloid phylogenetic origin of macrophages may be mirrored during embryonic development. Primitive (weakly phagocytic) macrophages with an ameboid shape that react with the monocyte-macrophage lineage-specific monoclonal antibody F4/80 are found in the developing yolk sac when blood vessels and blood cells first appear.[7–9] Promonocytes and monocyte-like cells appear subsequently. Before hematopoiesis shifts from the yolk sac to the liver, macrophages become more phagocytic, develop lysosomal structures, display lipase activity, and divide rapidly as indicated by incorporation of tritiated thymidine into DNA. At the same time, macrophages identified morphologically and by staining with *Griffonia simplicifolia* isolectin B4 already are present in the developing liver, brain, and lungs and persist there throughout embryonic development.[8,9] Whether these tissue macrophages are of yolk sac origin or arise independently is not clear. Normal tissue macrophage populations can undergo prominent expansion in response to postnatal influences. For example, rabbit alveolar macrophages exposed to ambient microbes, their products, and various particulates proliferate rapidly during the first 2 weeks of life.[10]

TISSUE DISTRIBUTION OF MONOCYTES AND MACROPHAGES

In the adult, the major macrophage populations are found in the lamina propria of the small intestine, in the liver (Kupffer cells), the lungs (alveolar and interstitial macrophages), the spleen, the lymph nodes, the bone marrow, the serosal cavities (peritoneal and pleural), the kidney and endocrine glands, and in the brain (microglia).[11,46] The heart and the muscles are relatively macrophage poor. Additional cells thought to be closely related to macrophages functionally, antigenically, and developmentally are found in the skin (Langerhans or dendritic cells) and in the bone (osteoclasts). The precise lineage relationship of the latter two cells to monocytes is complex.[47,48,51] Dendritic cells arise from both myeloid and lymphoid progenitors,[51,53] and osteoclasts may develop from myeloid progenitors at an early stage.[48] In the absence of inflammation, monocytes are found principally in the marrow and blood. Monocytes migrate from blood into inflammatory lesions, where they differentiate into typical macrophages.[12–15] Macrophages, whether resident or inflammatory, assume different morphologic and functional features depending on their location in organs and tissues. The determinants of this tissue-specific differentiation are not known.

DEVELOPMENT OF MONOCYTES IN THE MARROW

Blood monocytes arise from progenitor cells in the marrow,[15,16] since they do not incorporate tritiated thymidine into their DNA, do not undergo mitosis while in blood, and carry the genotype of the donor after marrow transplantation. Labeled monocytes do not appear in blood for 13 to 24 hours after intravenous injection of tritiated thymidine,[17] indicating that blood monocytes arise from precursors that divided at least 13 hours previously. Because blood monocytes have myeloperoxidase-containing granules, monocyte precursors in the marrow were sought among dividing cells that synthesized myeloperoxidase and resembled monocytes morphologically. The immediate monocyte precursors, promonocytes, were identified by intense thymidine labeling, peroxidase staining of rough endoplasmic reticulum and Golgi, and the presence of cytoplasmic filaments and cleft nuclei.[1,2,18] Although similar to myelocytes under light microscopy, they could be distinguished from the latter under electron microscopy: promonocyte cell membranes displayed many finger-like projections and cytoplasmic filaments, and they contained many fewer and smaller granules than did the myelocytes. The putative precursors of promonocytes, termed *monoblasts*, were recognized in macrophage-forming colonies as smaller dividing cells that contained large nuclei, scant cytoplasm, and few peroxidase-positive granules.[19] Monoblasts probably develop from multipotential granulocyte-monocyte progenitors.[20] A model of monocyte development has been proposed in which each monoblast gives rise to two promonocytes, each of which then divides into two monocytes.[21]

KINETICS OF MONOCYTES IN CIRCULATION AND IN INFLAMMATORY LESIONS

Human monocytes appear in the circulation 13 to 26 hours after the last round of promonocyte DNA synthesis, followed by mitotic division. They leave the circulation at random times with a half-life that has been estimated at 8 to 70 hours.[17,22,23] The shorter half-lives were obtained in experiments in which monocytes were removed from blood, labeled, and reinfused, manipulations that may have shortened the half-life of labeled cells. The longer half-life was seen after labeling monocytes *in vivo*.[17] The calculated basal monocyte output is approximately 9.4×10^8 cells per day for the average adult. In rabbits, a large pool of monocytes is transiently trapped in the lung vasculature, but whether human monocytes are similarly marginated is not known. Within a few hours of the onset of infection or inflammation, monocytes migrating from the bloodstream are found in the lesions, although initially they are much less numerous than neutrophils. In model lesions, monocytes begin to predominate over neutrophils after 12 hours.[24] Endothelial transmigration is mediated by platelet endothelial cell adhesion molecule (PECAM)-1 and other surface molecules.[49] In rats, hematogenous infection with *Salmonella enteritidis* elicits transient monocytopenia followed by prolonged monocytosis.[25] The monocytosis is a combined effect of the release of immature monocytes into the circulation, shortened monocyte generation time, and an expanded monocyte precursor pool. In this model of infection, the half-life of monocytes in blood is shortened to 50 percent of normal, probably as a result of more rapid efflux into tissues.

The interleukins IL-3 and IL-6, the colony-stimulating factors GM-CSF and M-CSF, many cytokines, and a less extensively characterized protein named *factor increasing monocytopoiesis* (FIM) induce monocytosis in experimental animals,[5,26–29] but the role of these factors in the physiologic regulation of monocyte and macrophage production and kinetics is not yet fully understood. Release of cytokines and hematopoietic growth factors by macrophages engaged in host defense contributes to the increase in monocyte/macrophage production during infections. Pharmacologic doses of glucocorticoids induce monocytopenia and diminish monocyte recruitment into test skin lesions.[30]

DIFFERENTIATION OF MONOCYTES INTO MACROPHAGES

Monocytes in cell culture[12] and in tissues[31] spontaneously transform into macrophages, and it is well established that monocytes migrating into inflamed tissues give rise to most of the reactive macrophage population[13,16,32] Nevertheless, macrophages are capable of cell division, and resident (noninflammatory) macrophage populations may be largely self-sustaining.[4] Serial analysis of gene expression during cytokine-induced maturation of human blood monocytes to macrophages has found a high frequency of expressed genes involved in lipid metabolism.[50] In human marrow transplant recipients, alveolar and liver macrophages (Kupffer cells) eventually are replaced by donor-derived cells,[33,34] occurring in the case of alveolar macrophages over a period of approximately 100 days. Whether the influx of donor-derived cells results from tissue inflammation or from damage to resident macrophages caused by radiation or cytotoxic therapy or reflects the natural dynamics of macrophage populations is not certain. The former possibilities are supported by studies on parabiotic mice and rats, wherein macrophage replacement from the cross-circulating monocytes is not seen unless inflammation is induced.[4,35,36] In human liver transplant recipients, liver macrophages (Kupffer cells) were replaced by recipient-derived cells over a period of several months.[37] The migration of macrophage precursors into donor tissue likely was stimulated by the inflammation associated with low-grade transplant rejection.

MULTINUCLEATED GIANT CELLS

Multinucleated giant cells are phagocytic, microbicidal cells found in areas of chronic tissue inflammation. They arise from macrophages either by cell fusion or perhaps by a process in which nuclear division occurs without cell division. *In vitro*, transformation of macrophages to giant cells occurs by fusion after approximately 1 to 2 weeks of culture[12] and is stimulated by interferon γ or IL-3 or macrophage adherence to surfaces.[38]

DENDRITIC CELLS AND THEIR RELATIONSHIP TO MONOCYTES AND MACROPHAGES

Dendritic cells are found in peripheral tissues where they take up proteins and particulates, process them, then migrate into lymph nodes where they present antigenic fragments to T lymphocytes.[39,40] Their ability to present antigen very efficiently and their characteristic morphology have been used as the defining characteristics of this cell type. *In vivo*, dendritic cells are especially important during primary immunization. "Veiled cells" are dendritic cells that migrate in lymph vessels to lymph nodes. Studies in animals pulsed with ^{3}H-thymidine show that these cells arose from precursors that last divided a few days before. This time course can be reproduced in an *in vitro* model, where maturation of monocytes into dendritic cells takes place within 48 hours after exposure to particles or microorganisms followed by a signal from endothelial cells during transmigration of monocytes from the luminal surface to the subendothelial matrix.[41] In the absence of the second signal, monocytes develop into macrophages. Slower differentiation of marrow precursors or blood monocytes to dendritic cells occurs under the influence of mixtures of cytokines, typically including GM-CSF with IL-4 or tumor necrosis factor (TNF)-α.[42–45,52,53] Using different mixtures of cytokines not including GM-CSF, dendritic cells can also be generated *in vitro* from lymphoid cells.[47,51] Dendritic cells of lymphoid origin are abundant in the thymus and may participate in presenting self-antigens during lymphocyte selection.[51,53] Dendritic cell development and differentiation are an active and rapidly evolving area of research.[54]

FATE OF MONOCYTES AND MACROPHAGES

The fate of monocytes under noninflammatory conditions is not known with certainty. Some may develop into macrophages, whereas others may be destroyed in as yet unknown disposal sites. Alveolar macrophages leave the body in swallowed mucus from the airways, and other macrophages may migrate to local lymph nodes.[42] However, the ultimate destination of the majority of senescent macrophages is not known. The lymph nodes appear to be the principal final destination of dendritic cells.[39–41]

REFERENCES

1. Van Furth R, Hirsch JG, Fedorko ME: Morphology and peroxidase cytochemistry of mouse promonocytes, monocytes, and macrophages. *J Exp Med* 132:794, 1970.
2. Nichols BA, Bainton DF: Differentiation of human monocytes in bone marrow and blood. *Lab Invest* 29:27, 1973.
3. Lawson GL, Rabinowitz PR, Morris L, Perry VH: Antigen markers of macrophage differentiation in murine tissues. *Curr Top Microbiol Immunol* 181:1, 1992.
4. Volkman A: Disparity in origin of mononuclear phagocyte populations. *J Reticuloend Soc* 19:249, 1976.
5. Van Furth R: Production and migration of monocytes and kinetics of macrophages, in *Mononuclear Phagocytes*, edited by R van Furth, p 3. Kluwer, Netherlands, 1992.
6. Metchnikoff E: *Immunity in Infective Diseases*. University Press, Cambridge, 1905.
7. Sorokin SP, Hoyt RF, Blunt DG, McNelly NA: Macrophage development: II. Early ontogeny of macrophage populations in brain, liver, and lungs of rat embryos as revealed by a lectin marker. *Anat Rec* 232:527, 1992.
8. Sorokin SP, McNelly NA, Hoyt RF: CFU-rAM, the origin of lung macrophages, and the macrophage lineage. *Am Physiol Soc* 263:L299, 1992.
9. Takahashi K, Yamamura F, Naito M: Differentiation, maturation, and proliferation of macrophages in the mouse yolk sac: A light-microscopic, enzyme-cytochemical, immunohistochemical, and ultrastructural study. *J Leukoc Biol* 45:87, 1989.
10. Evans MJ, Sherman MP, Campbell LA, Shami SG: Proliferation of pulmonary alveolar macrophages during postnatal development of rabbit lung. *Am Rev Respir Dis* 136:384, 1987.
11. Hume DA, Robinson AP, Macpherson GC, Gordon S: The mononuclear phagocyte system of the mouse defined by immunohistochemical localization of antigen F4/80. *J Exp Med* 158:1522, 1983.
12. Sutton JS, Weiss L: Transformation of monocytes in tissue culture into macrophages, epithelioid cells, and multinucleated giant cells. *J Cell Biol* 28:303, 1966.
13. Van Furth R, Diesselhoff-den Dulk MMC, Mattie H: Quantitative study on the production and kinetics of mononuclear phagocytes during an acute inflammatory reaction. *J Exp Med* 138:1314, 1973.
14. Volkman A: The origin and turnover of mononuclear cells in peritoneal exudates in rats. *J Exp Med* 124:241 1966.
15. Van Furth R, Cohn ZA: The origin and kinetics of mononuclear phagocytes. *J Exp Med* 128:415 1968.
16. Volkman A, Gowans JL: The production of macrophages in the rat. *Br J Exp Pathol* 46:50 1965.
17. Whitelaw DM: Observations on human monocyte kinetics after pulse labeling. *Cell Tissue Kinet* 5:311, 1972.
18. Van der Meer JWM, Beelen RHJ, Fluitsma DM, van Furth R: Ultrastructure of mononuclear phagocytes developing in liquid bone marrow cultures. *J Exp Med* 149:17, 1979.
19. van der Meer JWM, van de Gevel JS, Beelen RHJ, et al: Culture of human bone marrow in the Teflon culture bag: Identification of the human monoblast. *J Reticuloend Soc* 32:355, 1982.
20. Metcalf D, Burgess AW: Clonal analysis of progenitor cell commitment to granulocyte or macrophage production. *J Cell Physiol* 111:275, 1982.
21. Van Furth R, Diesselhoff-den Dulk MMC: The kinetics of promonocytes and monocytes in the bone marrow. *J Exp Med* 132:813, 1970.
22. Meuret G, Batara E, Fürste HO: Monocytopoiesis in normal man: Pool size, proliferation activity, and DNA synthesis time of promonocytes. *Acta Haematol* 54:261, 1975.
23. Meuret G, Hoffmann G: Monocyte kinetic studies in normal and disease states. *Br J Haematol* 24:275, 1973.
24. Issekutz TB, Issekutz AC, Movat HZ: The in vivo quantitation and kinetics of monocyte migration into acute inflammatory tissue. *Am J Pathol* 103:47, 1981.
25. Volkman A, Collins FM: The cytokinetics of monocytosis in acute salmonella infection in the rat. *J Exp Med* 139:264, 1974.
26. Ulich TR, del Castillo J, Watson LR, et al: In vivo hematologic effects of recombinant human macrophage colony-stimulating factor. *Blood* 75:846, 1990.
27. Andrews RG, Knitter GH, Bartelmez SH, et al: Recombinant human stem cell factor, a *c-kit* ligand, stimulates hematopoiesis in primates. *Blood* 78:1975, 1991.
28. Ulich TR, del Castillo J, Busser K, et al: Acute in vivo effects of IL-3 alone and in combination with IL-6 on the blood cells in circulation and bone marrow. *Am J Pathol* 135:663, 1989.
29. Ulich TR, del Castillo J, McNiece I, et al: Hematologic effects of recombinant murine granulocyte-macrophage colony-stimulating factor on the peripheral blood and bone marrow. *Am J Pathol* 137:369, 1990.
30. Dale DC, Fauci AS, Wolff SM: Alternate-day prednisone. Leukocyte kinetics and susceptibility to infection. *N Engl J Med* 291:1154, 1993.
31. Ryan GB, Spector WG: Macrophage turnover in inflamed connective tissue. *Proc R Soc Lond* 175:269, 1970.

32. van Furth R, Nibbering PH, van Dissel JT, Diesselhoff-den Dulk MMC: The characterization, origin, and kinetics of skin macrophages during inflammation. *J Invest Dermatol* 85:398, 1985.

33. Thomas ED, Ramberg RE, Sale GE, et al: Direct evidence for a bone marrow origin of the alveolar macrophage in man. *Science* 192:1016, 1976.

34. Gale RP, Sparkes RS, Golde DW: Bone marrow origin of hepatic macrophages (Kupffer cells) in humans. *Science* 201:937, 1978.

35. Sawyer RT: The ontogeny of pulmonary alveolar macrophages in parabiotic mice. *J Leukoc Biol* 40:347, 1986.

36. Collins FM, Auclair LK: Mononuclear phagocytes within the lungs of unstimulated parabiotic rats. *J Reticuloend Soc* 27:429, 1980.

37. Porter KA: Origin of Kupffer cells and endothelial cells in long-surviving human hepatic homografts, in *Experience in Hepatic Transplantation*, edited by TE Starzl, p 464. WB Saunders, Philadelphia, 1969.

38. Enelow RI, Sullivan GW, Carper HT, Mandell GL: Induction of multinucleated giant cell formation from in vitro culture of human monocytes with interleukin-3 and interferon-gamma: Comparison with other stimulating factors. *Am J Respir Cell Mol Biol* 6:57, 1992.

39. Hart DN: Dendritic cells: Unique leukocyte populations which control the primary immune response. *Blood* 90:3245, 1997.

40. Shortman K, Maraskovsky E: Developmental options. *Science* 282:424, 1998.

41. Randolph GJ, Beaulieu S, Lebecque S, et al: Differentiation of monocytes into dendritic cells in a model of transendothelial trafficking. *Science* 282:480, 1998.

42. Lauweryns JW, Baert JH: Alveolar clearance and the role of the pulmonary lymphatics. *Am Rev Respir Dis* 115:625, 1977.

43. Valledor AF, Borràs FE, Cullell-Young M, Celada A: Transcription factors that regulate monocyte/macrophage differentiation. *J Leukoc Biol* 63:405, 1998.

44. Lane PJ, Brocker T: Developmental regulation of dendritic cell function. *Curr Opin Immunol* 11:308, 1999.

45. Banyer JL, Hapel AJ: Myb-transformed hematopoietic cells as a model for monocyte differentiation into dendritic cells and macrophages. *J Leukoc Biol* 66:217, 1999.

46. Kennedy DW, Abkowitz JL: Kinetics of central nervous system microglial and macrophage engraftment: Analysis using a transgenic bone marrow transplantation model. *Blood* 90:986, 1997.

47. Anjùere F, Martinez del Hoyo G, Martin P, Ardavín: Langerhans cells develop from a lymphoid-committed precursor. *Blood* 96:1633, 2000.

48. Muguruma Y, Lee MY: Isolation and characterization of murine clonogenic osteoclast progenitors by cell surface phenotype analysis. *Blood* 91:1272, 1998.

49. Muller WA, Randolph GJ: Migration of leukocytes across endothelium and beyond: Molecules involved in the transmigration and fate of monocytes. *J Leukoc Biol* 66:698, 1999.

50. Hashimoto S-I, Suzuki T, Dong H-Y, et al: Serial analysis of gene expression in human monocytes and macrophages. *Blood* 94:837, 1999.

51. Young JW: Dendritic cells: Expansion and differentiation in the hematopoietic growth factors. *Curr Opin Hematol* 6:135, 1999.

52. Steinman R, Inaba K: Myeloid dendritic cells. *J Leukoc Biol* 66:205, 1999.

53. Santiago-Schwarz F: Positive and negative regulation of the myeloid dendritic cell lineage. *J Leukoc Biol* 66:209, 1999.

54. Shortman K, Liu Y: Mouse and human dendritic cell subtypes. *Nat Rev Immunol* 2:151, 2002.

CLASSIFICATION AND CLINICAL MANIFESTATIONS OF DISORDERS OF MONOCYTES AND MACROPHAGES

MARSHALL A . LICHTMAN

Disorders that result in abnormalities of monocytes, macrophages, or dendritic histiocytes exclusively are uncommon and usually are referred to pathologically as *histiocytosis*. These disorders may be inherited, such as familial hemophagocytic lymphohistiocytosis; inflammatory, such as infectious hemophagocytic syndrome; or neoplastic, such as Langerhans cell histiocytosis; or they may result from an inherited enzyme insufficiency in macrophages that leads to exaggerated storage of macromolecules, as in Gaucher disease. A variety of hematopoietic neoplasms may have a phenotype that expresses a large proportion of monocytes. Idiopathic (clonal) monocytosis is an uncommon myelodysplastic syndrome. Some cases of myelogenous leukemia have progenitor cells that mature preferentially into leukemic monocytes, including acute monoblastic or monocytic leukemia, chronic myelomonocytic leukemia, and juvenile myelomonocytic leukemia. Two acquired diseases, hairy cell leukemia and aplastic anemia, result in severe depression of blood monocytes and other blood cell types. Inherited disorders affecting white cells, such as chronic granulomatous disease and Chédiak-Higashi syndrome, result in impaired monocyte function. Monocyte dysfunction may accompany a variety of severe illnesses, such as sepsis, trauma, and cancer. Monocytes may play a pathogenetic role in other complex, acquired disorders, such as thrombosis and atherogenesis. Table 70-1 categorizes the qualitative and quantitative abnormalities of monocytes, macrophages, and dendritic histiocytes.

CLASSIFICATION

Classification of monocytic disorders is difficult because few abnormalities result solely in a disturbance of monocytes or macrophages. However, the presence of monocytopenia or monocytosis may be an important diagnostic feature or contribute to the functional abnormality in the patient.

The terms *histiocyte* and *macrophage* have been synonymous. The latter term is customary when discussing the biology of the cells of the mononuclear phagocyte system, which is the total pool of marrow, blood, and tissue monocytes and macrophages (formerly referred to as the *reticuloendothelial system*). In disease nosology, the terms *histiocytosis* and *histiocyte* still are used for diseases that principally involve

Acronyms and abbreviations that appear in this chapter include: IL, interleukin; Th, T helper.

cells derived from blood monocytes, that is, macrophages and dendritic cells.

The physician must consider the absolute monocyte count and not the percent of cells that are monocytes when evaluating the differential blood cell count before concluding the content of blood monocytes is inappropriate (see Chap. 71).

Table 70-1 lists a classification of monocyte, macrophage, and dendritic disorders of relevance to hematologists. Isolated cutaneous or organ involvement not affecting hematolymphopoiesis is not included.

MONOCYTOPENIA

Table 70-1 contains a comprehensive list of causes of monocytopenia. Two notable examples of disorders accompanied by severe monocytopenia are aplastic anemia and hairy cell leukemia. Pancytopenia is usual in both conditions, but the predisposition to serious infection is heightened by the deficiency in monocyte production. In hairy cell leukemia, the severe monocytopenia represents an important diagnostic clue because of its constancy.

MONOCYTOSIS AND HISTIOCYTOSIS

Table 70-1 contains a comprehensive list of causes of monocytosis. Monocytosis often is the manifestation of an inflammatory or neoplastic disease. Certain hematopoietic tumors, especially acute monocytic and chronic myelomonocytic leukemia, have as their principal manifestation a predominance of monocytic cells in blood and marrow. Occasionally, chronic idiopathic monocytosis precedes the onset of acute myelogenous leukemia, representing an uncommon manifestation of the myelodysplastic syndromes. Dendritic cell variants of acute myelogenous leukemia have been discovered with the more frequent use of immunophenotyping and genotyping of acute leukemias. In some cases of monocytic leukemia, the malignant clone does not appear to include precursors of red cells and platelets and thus likely does not result from a mutation in the multipotential hematopoietic cell. Thus, so-called progenitor cell monocytic leukemia and other histiocytic or dendritic cell tumors support the concept that primitive cells, committed to the monocyte/macrophage lineage, undergo malignant transformation.

Several uncommon types of histiocytosis are serious systemic diseases and may mimic malignant disease; however, the cytopathologic changes in monocytes or macrophages are not indicative of a malignant transformation and presumably are not clonal in origin. Familial and sporadic hemophagocytic lymphohistiocytosis, infection-induced hemophagocytic syndromes, and sinus histiocytosis with massive lymphadenopathy are among such disorders (see Chap. 72). Infectious hemophagocytic histiocytosis caused by Epstein-Barr virus may be a hybrid disease because, in addition to striking hemophagocytic histiocytes, an underlying monoclonal or oligoclonal proliferation of virus-infected lymphocytes may be present. Tumors of histiocytes or dendritic cells are rare but can be classified into several groups using a combination of morphologic and immunophenotypic markers (see Chap. 72).

QUALITATIVE DISORDERS OF MONOCYTES

Inherited abnormalities of macrophages can result in ineffective macrophage function. In these situations, the abnormality usually is shared by other cells, as in chronic granulomatous disease, which results from a defect in oxygen-dependent microbial killing, and in Chédiak-Higashi disease, which results from an abnormality of the membranes of cell granules (see Chap. 66). An indomethacin-sensitive monocyte killing defect in children has been associated with a predisposition to atypical mycobacterial disease (see Table 70-1). Enzyme deficiencies

TABLE 70-1　DISORDERS OF MONOCYTES AND MACROPHAGES

I. Monocytopenia (see Chap. 71)
   A. Aplastic anemia[1]
   B. Hairy cell leukemia[2,3]
   C. Glucocorticoid therapy[4]
II. Monocytosis (see Chap. 71)
   A. Benign
     1. Reactive monocytosis[5]
   B. Clonal monocytosis
     1. Indolent
       a. Chronic idiopathic monocytosis[6]
       b. Oligoblastic myelogenous leukemia (myelodysplasia)[7]
     2. Progressive
       a. Acute monocytic leukemia[8–10]
       b. Terminal deoxynucleotide transferase-positive acute monocytic leukemia[11]
       c. Dendritic cell leukemia[12,13]
       d. Progenitor cell monocytic leukemia[14]
       e. Chronic myelomonocytic leukemia[15,16]
       f. Juvenile myelomonocytic leukemia[17]
III. Macrophage Deficiency
   A. Osteopetrosis (isolated osteoclast deficiency)[18,19]
IV. Inflammatory Histiocytosis (see Chap. 72)
   A. Primary hemophagocytic lymphohistiocytosis[20–22]
     1. Familial
     2. Sporadic
   B. Infectious hemophagocytic histiocytosis[22,23]
   C. Tumor-associated hemophagocytic histiocytosis[24]
   D. Drug-associated hemophagocytic histiocytosis[24]
   E. Disease-associated hemophagocytic histiocytosis[25–27]
   F. Sinus histiocytosis with massive lymphadenopathy[28,29]
V. Storage Histiocytosis (see Chap. 73)
   A. Gaucher disease[30]
   B. Niemann-Pick disease[31]
   C. Gangliosidosis[32]
   D. Sea-blue histiocytosis syndrome[33]
VI. Clonal (Neoplastic) Histiocytosis (see Chap. 72)
   A. Langerhans cell histiocytosis[34,35]
     1. Localized
     2. Systemic
   B. Tumors or sarcomas of histiocytes and dendritic cells[36]
     1. Histiocytic sarcoma
     2. Langerhans cell sarcoma
     3. Interdigitating dendritic cell sarcoma
     4. Follicular dendritic cell sarcoma
VII. Monocyte and Macrophage Dysfunction[37–39]
   A. α_1-Proteinase inhibitor deficiency[40]
   B. Chédiak-Higashi syndrome[41]
   C. Chronic granulomatous disease[42]
   D. Chronic lymphocytic leukemia[43]
   E. Disseminated mucocutaneous candidiasis[44,45]
   F. Glucocorticoid therapy[46]
   G. Kawasaki disease[47]
   H. Malakoplakia[48]
   I. Mycobacteriosis syndrome[49–52]
   J. Posttraumatic[53–55]
   K. Septic shock induced[56,57]
   L. Solid tumors[58,59]
   M. Tobacco smoking[60]
   N. Marijuana smoking or cocaine inhalation[61]
   O. Whipple disease[62,63]
   P. Human IL-10 effects; Epstein-Barr virus IL-10–like gene product (vIL-10)[64,65]
VIII. Atherogenesis[66,67]
IX. Thrombogenesis[68,69]
X. Obesity[70]

in macrophages can result in accumulation of undegraded macromolecules, leading to various types of storage diseases. A classic example is Gaucher disease, a disorder that results from an inherited deficiency of the enzyme glucocerebrosidase (see Chap. 73).

Acquired functional abnormalities of monocytes have been reported in a variety of diseases and circumstances (see Monocyte and Macrophage Dysfunction in Table 70-1). Several alterations in monocyte function occur after severe trauma, after sepsis, in other critically ill patients, and in cancer patients. The abnormalities in monocyte responses correlate with the severity of the trauma or sepsis. For example, in trauma patients, monocyte IL-12 production is decreased, which leads to a decrease in the T helper (Th) 1/Th2 lymphocyte ratio and concomitant altered immune responses. Maturation to dendritic cells also is impaired in trauma patients. In patients with breast cancer, IL-12 production and dendritic cell maturation are impaired; this abnormality is reversed after excision of the tumor. IL-10 secretion by Th2 lymphocytes can block cytokine elaboration by T cells and natural killer cells. This effect is mediated by inhibition of macrophage accessory cell function. A viral IL-10–like molecule encoded by the Epstein-Barr virus *BCRF1* gene may play a role in the pathogenesis of the viral infection and act in part by inhibiting monocyte function. Tobacco smoking and marijuana smoking result in impaired alveolar macrophage function. In several diseases, including chronic lymphocytic leukemia, Kawasaki disease, Whipple disease, and malakoplakia, specific abnormalities of monocyte function play a significant role in the immune impairment of each disorder.

CLINICAL MANIFESTATIONS OF MONOCYTE DISORDERS
MONOCYTOPENIA OR MONOCYTE DYSFUNCTION

Isolated monocytopenia does not occur. Thus, the manifestations of such a clinical state must be inferred. Neutrophils, endothelial cells, and other cell types can substitute in part for some monocyte functions. Monocytes have antibacterial, antiviral, antifungal, and antiparasitic capabilities. They are effective phagocytes involved in the ingestion of organisms such as mycobacteria, *Listeria, Brucella,* trypanosomes, and other granuloma-producing organisms. Thus, their deficiency or functional abnormality predisposes to such infections. Macrophages can serve as a reservoir for the human immunodeficiency virus and is the principal locus for the virus in brain and neural tissue.

Deficiency in a specific subset of macrophages, the osteoclasts, results in *osteopetrosis*, an imbalance in bone metabolism that favors accretion. Osteoclasts normally play a key role in the closely regulated process of bone resorption.

Macrophages and their derivatives, dendritic cells, process and present antigens and play a role in immune regulation. In complex systems, such as that of antibody production, abnormal macrophages might lead to faulty modulation of antibody synthetic rates. Activated monocytes secrete more than 50 chemical mediators or monokines, which, among other things, play a vital role in cellular immunity. The absence of monocytes from the inflammatory response and the failure to elaborate or the inappropriate elaboration of monokines such as IL-1, α_1-proteinase inhibitor, prostaglandins, leukotrienes, plasminogen activator, elastase, tumor necrosis factor, IL-6, IL-12, and others may cause or contribute to disease manifestations. A deficiency or impairment of monocytes has the potential to influence several functions and systems because monocytes are important sources of inflammatory cytokines.

Monocytopenia and decreased monocyte entry into inflammatory sites occur after glucocorticoid administration. This process may explain why patients treated with glucocorticoids are predisposed to infections in which monocytes play a protective role, such as infections resulting from fungal, mycobacterial, and other opportunistic organisms. Dysfunctional monocytes, which are incapable of killing ingested microorganisms, are present in chronic granulomatous disease (see Chap. 66) and in hematopoietic stem cell diseases such as acute myelogenous leukemia.

TISSUE EFFECTS OF MONOCYTOSIS

Benign monocytosis is not associated with specific clinical manifestations. All forms of myelogenous leukemia with a predominance of monocytes are associated with a predisposition to troublesome tissue infiltrates, especially in the skin, gingiva, lymph nodes, meninges, and anal canal. The higher the monocyte count and the proportion of leukemic monocytes, the more prevalent is tissue infiltration. In some cases, tissue infiltration of leukemic monocytes can produce symptoms, such as lung dysfunction, laryngeal obstruction, and intracranial vessel rupture. Release of procoagulants leading to intravascular coagulation also occurs in myelogenous leukemia with a high proportion of monocytes (see Chap. 87).

EFFECTS OF HISTIOCYTOSIS

Histiocytosis usually refers to the accumulation of activated macrophages (histiocytes) in tissue sites. The cells may become cytophagocytic. Ingestion of red cells and occasionally of leukocytes, platelets, erythroblasts in marrow, or cells in other tissue sites is an important feature of certain inflammatory histiocytosis (see Chap. 72). Because morphology has been misleading, the diagnosis of histiocytosis requires identification of specific cell markers. A histiocytosis may be inflammatory (polyclonal) or neoplastic (clonal). Because tissue macrophages can take on highly specialized phenotypes and localize in different tissues, histiocytosis is further defined by whether they carry markers of these cell types (e.g., Langerhans cells, interdigitating dendritic cells) (see Chap. 72).

REFERENCES

1. Twomey JJ, Douglas CC, Sharkey O Jr: The monocytopenia of aplastic anemia. *Blood* 41:187, 1973.
2. Golomb HM, Catovsky D, Golde DW: Hairy cell leukemia: A clinical review based on 71 cases. *Ann Intern Med* 89:667, 1978.
3. Paoletti M, Bitter MA, Vardiman JW: Hairy cell leukemia: Morphologic, cytochemical, and immunologic features. *Clin Lab Med* 8:179, 1988.
4. Fauci AS, Dale DC: The effect of in vivo hydrocortisone on subpopulations of human lymphocytes. *J Clin Invest* 53:240, 1974.
5. Maldonado GE, Hanlon DG: Monocytosis. *Mayo Clin Proc* 40:248, 1965.
6. Jaworkowsky LI, Solovey DY, Rhausova LY, Udris OY: Monocytosis as a sign of subsequent leukemia in patients with cytopenias (preleukemia). *Folia Hematol* 110:395, 1983.
7. Rigolin GM, Cuneo A, Roberti MG, et al: Myelodysplastic syndrome with monocytic component: Hematologic and cytologic characterization. *Haematologica* 82:25, 1997.
8. Fung H, Shepherd JD, Naiman SC, et al: Acute monocytic leukemia. *Leuk Lymphoma* 19:259, 1995.
9. Haferlach T, Schoch C, Schnittger S, et al: Distinct genetic patterns can be identified in acute monoblastic leukaemia (FAB AML M5a and M5b): A study of 124 patients. *Br J Haematol* 118:426, 2002.
10. de Fonseca LM, Brunetti IL, Campa A, et al: Assessment of monocytic component in acute myelomonocytic and monocytic/monoblastic leukemias by a chemoluminescence assay. *Hematol J* 4:26, 2003.
11. Cuttner J, Seremetis S, Najfeld V, et al: TDT-positive acute leukemia with monocytoid characteristics. *Blood* 64:237, 1984.
12. Santiago-Schwartz F, Coppock DL, Hindenberg AA, Kern J: Identification of a malignant counterpart of the monocytic-dendritic cell progenitor in an acute myeloid leukemia. *Blood* 84:3054, 1994.
13. Srivastava HI, Srivistava A, Srivastava MD: Phenotype, genotype and cytokine production in acute leukemia involving progenitors of dendritic Langerhans' cell. *Leuk Res* 18:499, 1994.
14. Ferraris AM, Broccia G, Meloni T, et al: Clonal origin of cells restricted to monocytic differentiation in acute nonlymphocytic leukemia. *Blood* 64:817, 1984.
15. Cambier N, Baruchel A, Schlageter MH, et al: Chronic myelomonocytic leukemia: From biology to therapy. *Hematol Cell Ther* 39:41, 1997.
16. Onida F, Kantarjian HM, Smith TL, et al: Prognostic scoring factors and scoring systems in chronic myelomonocytic leukemia: A retrospective analysis of 213 patients. *Blood* 99:840, 2002.
17. Aricò M, Biondi A, Pui C-H: Juvenile myelomonocytic leukemia. *Blood* 90:479, 1997.
18. Teitelbaum SI: The osteoclast and osteopetrosis. *Mt Sinai J Med* 63:399, 1996.
19. Helfrich MH: Osteoclast diseases. *Microsc Res Tech* 61:514, 2003.
20. Filipovich AH: Hemophagocytic lymphohistiocytosis. *J Pediatr* 130:337, 1997.
21. Aricò M, Janka G, Fischer A, et al, for the FHL Study Group of the Histiocyte Society: Hemophagocytic lymphohistiocytosis. Report of 122 children from the international registry. *Leukemia* 10:197, 1996.
22. Tsuda H: Hemophagocytic syndrome (HPS) in children and adults. *Int J Hematol* 65:215, 1997.
23. Imashuku S: Differential diagnosis of hemophagocytic syndrome: Underlying disorders and selection of the most effective treatment. *Int J Hematol* 66:135, 1997.
24. Reiner AP, Spivak JL: Hematophagic histiocytosis. *Medicine* 67:369, 1988.
25. Stephan JL, Zeller J, Hubert P, et al: Macrophage activation syndrome and rheumatic diseases in childhood. *Clin Exp Rheumatol* 11:451, 1993.
26. Favara BE, Feller AC, Pauli M, et al: Contemporary classification of histiocytic disorders. *Med Pediatr Oncol* 29:157, 1997.
27. Imashuku S: Clinical features and treatment strategies of Epstein-Barr virus-associated hemophagocytic lymphohistiocytosis. *Crit Rev Oncol Hematol* 44:259, 2002.
28. Foucar E, Rosai J, Dorfman RF: Sinus histiocytosis with massive lymphadenopathy. *Cancer* 54:1834, 1984.
29. Pauli M, Bergamashi G, Tonon L, et al: Evidence of a polyclonal nature of the cell infiltrate in sinus histiocytosis with massive lymphadenopathy (Rosai-Dorfman disease). *Br J Haematol* 91:415, 1995.
30. Balicki D, Beutler E: Gaucher disease. *Medicine* 74:305, 1995.
31. Weisz B, Spirer Z, Reif S: Niemann-Pick disease: Newer classification based on genetic mutation of the disease. *Adv Pediatr* 41:415, 1994.
32. Sandhoff K, Harzer K, Fürst W: Lysosomal enzymes (part 12), in *The Metabolic and Molecular Bases of Inherited Disease*, 6th ed, edited by CR Scriver, AL Beaudet, WS Sly, D Valle, p 2427. McGraw-Hill, New York, 1995.
33. Hirayama Y, Kohada K, Andoh M, et al: Syndrome of the sea-blue histiocyte. *Intern Med* 35:419, 1996.
34. Egler RM, Favera BE, Van Meurs M, et al: Differential in situ cytokine profiles of Langerhans-like cells and T-cells in Langerhans cell histiocytosis. Abundant expression of cytokines relevant to disease and treatment. *Blood* 94:4195, 1999.
35. Egeler RM, Nesbit ME: Langerhans cell histiocytosis and other disorders of monocyte-histiocyte lineage. *Crit Rev Oncol Hematol* 18:9, 1995.
36. Jaffe ES, Harris NL, Stein H, Vardiman JW: Tumors of haematopoietic and lymphoid tissues, Chapter 10. Histiocytic and dendritic cell neoplasms, in *World Health Organization Classification of Tumors*, edited by ES Jaffe, NL Harris, JW Vardiman, p 273. IARC Press, Lyon, 2001.
37. Lopez-Berestein G, Klostergaard J: *Mononuclear Phagocytes in Cell Biology*. CRC Press, Boca Raton, 1993.
38. Cline MJ: Histiocytes and histiocytosis. *Blood* 84:2840, 1994.
39. Asherson GL, Zembala M: Monocyte abnormalities in disease, in *Human Monocytes*, edited by M Zembala, GL Asherson, p 395. Academic Press, London, 1989.

40. Perlmutter DH, Travis J, Punsal PI: Elastase regulates the synthesis of its inhibitor, alpha 1-proteinase inhibitor, and exaggerates the defect in homozygous pizz alpha 1 PI deficiency. *J Clin Invest* 81:1774, 1998.

41. Dinauer MC: The phagocyte system and disorders of granulopoiesis and granulocyte function, in *Nathan and Oski's Hematology of Infancy and Childhood*, 5th ed, edited by DG Nathan, SH Orkin, p 826. WB Saunders, Philadelphia, 1998.

42. Davis WC, Huber H, Douglas SD, Fudenberg HH: A defect in circulating mononuclear phagocytes in chronic granulomatous disease of childhood. *J Immunol* 101:1093, 1968.

43. Orsini E, Guarini A, Chiaretti S, et al: The circulating dendritic cell compartment in patients with chronic lymphocytic leukemia is severely defective and unable to stimulate an effective T cell response. *Cancer Res* 63:4497, 2003.

44. Snyderman R, Altman LC, Frankel A, Blaese RM: Defective mononuclear leukocyte chemotaxis. *Ann Intern Med* 78:509, 1973.

45. Komiyama A, Ichikawa M, Kanda H, et al: Defective interleukin 1 production in a familial monocyte disorder with a combined abnormality of mobility and phagocytosis-killing. *Clin Exp Immunol* 73:500, 1988.

46. Rinehart JJ, Sagone AL, Balcerzak SP, et al: Effects of corticosteroid therapy on human monocyte function. *N Engl J Med* 292:236, 1975.

47. Ichiyama T, Yoshitoma T, Nishikawa M, et al: NF-kappaB activation in peripheral blood monocytes/macrophages and T cells during acute Kawasaki Disease. *Clin Immunol* 99:373, 2001.

48. Van Crevel R, Curfs J, van der Ven AJ, et al: Functional and morphological monocyte abnormalities in a patient with malakoplakia. *Am J Med* 105:74, 1998.

49. Uchiyama N, Green GR, Warren BJ, Morzumi PA, et al: Possible monocyte killing defect in familial mycobacteriosis. *J Pediatr* 98:785, 1981.

50. Mason UG III, Greenberg LE, Yen SS, Kirkpatrick CH: Indomethacin-responsive mononuclear cell dysfunction in "atypical" mycobacteriosis. *Cell Immunol* 71:54, 1982.

51. Ridgeway D, Wolff LJ, Wall M, Bouzy MS, et al: Indomethacin-sensitive monocyte killing defect in a child with disseminated atypical mycobacterial disease. *J Clin Immunol* 11:357, 1991.

52. Onwubalili JK: Defective monocyte chemotactic responsiveness in patients with active tuberculosis. *Immunol Lett* 16:39, 1987.

53. Kampalath B, Cleveland RP, Chang CC, Kass L: Monocytes with altered phenotypes in posttrauma patients. *Arch Pathol Lab Med* 127:1580, 2003.

54. Spolarics Z, Siddiqi M, Siegel JH, et al: Depressed interleukin-12-producing activity by monocytes correlates with adverse clinical course and a shift toward Th2-type lymphocyte pattern in severely injured male trauma patients. *Crit Care Med* 31:1722, 2003.

55. De AK, Laudanski K, Miller-Graziano CL: Failure of monocytes of trauma patients to convert to immature dendritic cells is related to preferential macrophage-colony-stimulating factor-driven macrophage differentiation. *J Immunol* 170:6355, 2003.

56. Calandra T, Baumgartner J-D, Grau GE, et al: Prognostic value of tumor necrosis factor/cachectin, interleukin-1, interferon and interferon-8 in the serum of patients with septic shock. *J Infect Dis* 161:982, 1990.

57. Fumeaux T, Pugin J: Role of interleukin-10 in the intracellular sequestration of human leukocyte antigen-DR in monocytes during septic shock. *Am J Respir Crit Care Med* 166:1475, 2002.

58. Anastosopoulos E, Reclos GJ, Boxevanis CN, et al: Monocyte disorders associated with T cell defects in patients with solid tumors. *Anticancer Res* 12:489, 1992.

59. Elgert KD, Alleva DG, Mullins DW: Tumor-induced immune dysfunction: The macrophage connection. *J Leukoc Biol* 64:275, 1998.

60. Ryder MI, Saghizadeh M, Ding Y, et al: Effects of tobacco smoke on secretion of interleukin 1-beta, tumor necrosis factor-alpha, and transforming growth-beta from peripheral blood mononuclear cells. *Oral Microbiol Immunol* 17:331, 2002.

61. Shay AH, Choi R, Whittaker K, et al: Impairment of antimicrobial activity and nitric acid production by alveolar macrophages from smokers of marijuana and cocaine. *J Infect Dis* 187:700, 2003.

62. Bjerknes R, Laerum OP, Degaards S: Impaired bacterial degradation of monocytes and macrophages from a patient with treated Whipple's disease. *Gastroenterology* 89:1139, 1985.

63. Marth T, Neurath M, Cuccherini BA, Strober W: Defects of monocyte interleukin 12 production an humoral immunity in Whipple's disease. *Gastroenterology* 113:442, 1997.

64. Moore KW, de Waal Maleyt R, Coffman RL, O'Garra A: Interleukin-10 and the interleukin 10 receptor. *Annu Rev Immunol* 19:683, 2001.

65. Dobrovolskaia MA, Vogel SN: Toll receptors, CD14, and macrophage activation and deactivation by LPS. *Microbes Infect* 4:903, 2002.

66. Gidron Y, Gilutz H, Berger R, Huleihel M: Molecular and cellular interface between behavior and acute coronary syndromes. *Cardiovasc Res* 56:15, 2002.

67. Tousoulis D, Davies G, Stefanadis C, et al: Inflammatory and thrombotic mechanisms in coronary atherosclerosis. *Heart* 89:993, 2003.

68. Spillent CR, Lazaro EJ: Contribution of the monocyte to thrombotic potential. *Agents Actions* 34:28, 1991.

69. Osterud B: The role of platelets in decrypting monocyte tissue factor. *Semin Hematol* 38(suppl 12):2, 2001.

70. Weisberg SP, McCann D, Desai M, et al: Obesity is associated with macrophage accumulation in adipose tissue. *J Clin Invest* 112:1796, 2003.

MONOCYTOSIS AND MONOCYTOPENIA

MARSHALL A. LICHTMAN

The blood monocyte is in transit between the marrow and tissues, where it transforms (matures) into a macrophage. In tissues, the monocyte develops a phenotype characteristic of the specific tissue of residence (e.g., Kupffer cells of liver, microglia of brain, osteoclasts of marrow). The monocyte participates in virtually all inflammatory and immune reactions. Its concentration can increase in many such conditions, including autoimmune diseases, gastrointestinal disorders, sarcoidosis, and several viral and bacterial infections. Monocytosis, an increase in the blood absolute monocyte count to greater than 800 × 10⁶/liter, may occur in some patients with cancer and several unrelated conditions, such as postsplenectomy states, inflammatory bowel disease, and chronic infections such as bacterial endocarditis, tuberculosis, and brucellosis. The inconsistency and unpredictability in blood monocyte concentration among patients with the same disease is a function of the monocyte's relatively small blood pool size, the dampening effect of a large tissue pool, the monocyte's relatively long life span, the number and complexity of effectors in the relevant cytokine network that can influence the response, and, perhaps, the ability to expand macrophage numbers by local mitosis in tissues. The most striking increase in blood monocyte concentration occurs with hematopoietic malignancies, especially clonal monocytosis (myelodysplastic syndrome), and monocytic or myelomonocytic leukemia. Depression, myocardial infarction, parturition, thermal injuries, and marathon competition are closely associated with monocytosis. Table 71-1 gives a comprehensive list of diseases associated with monocytosis. Monocytopenia as an isolated finding is rare. However, monocytopenia is notable in patients with aplastic anemia or hairy cell leukemia as a feature of pancytopenia. Although other cytopenias accompany the monocytopenia, the latter contributes significantly to the predisposition to infection and aids in the diagnosis of hairy cell leukemia because of its constancy.

The blood monocyte is a cell in transit from marrow to tissues.[1] The two major populations of blood monocytes are (1) a smaller population that represents a less mature stage, has a higher buoyant density, a smaller volume, lacks Fc receptors, and has greater tumoricidal activity; and (2) a larger population that represents a more mature stage, has a lower buoyant density, is larger in volume, displays Fc receptors, expresses more peroxidase activity, secretes larger amounts of interleukin-1, presents antigen, and mediates antibody-dependent cell-mediated cytotoxicity more efficiently. The larger population, which comprises approximately 90 percent of blood monocytes, strongly expresses cluster of differentiation (CD)14 (lipo-

polysaccharide receptor) but does not express CD16 (FcγRIII), the CD14++CD16-subset. The other 10 percent of blood monocytes has weak expression of CD14 and strong expression of CD16, the CD14+CD16++ subset.[2] The latter subset contains dendritic cell precursors.[3] The two major subsets each can be further stratified based on the expression of CD64 (FcγR1).[4]

In tissues, the monocyte is capable of transformation, under the influence of local environmental factors, into a macrophage. The monocyte plays an important role in acute and chronic inflammatory reactions, including granulomatous inflammation; immunologic reactions, including those involved in delayed hypersensitivity; tissue repair and reorganization; atheroma formation; and the reaction to neoplasia and allografts. Because of the monocyte's key role in a variety of pathophysiologic reactions, blood monocyte count can increase modestly in many disparate conditions. In addition, in circumstances where tissue sites require large increases in the number of macrophages, the demand may be met by local proliferation of macrophages and may not be reflected either in increased transit of monocytes through the blood compartment from marrow to tissue or in an increased concentration of blood monocytes.[5] The evidence for local proliferation of macrophages is suggestive but inconclusive. Occasionally, T cell clones release only monocyte/macrophage colony stimulating factor (M-CSF). Their conditioned medium stimulates growth of only macrophage colonies, providing a hypothetical model for local control of macrophage proliferation.[6]

NORMAL BLOOD MONOCYTE CONCENTRATION

In the first 2 weeks of life, the average absolute blood monocyte count is approximately 1000/μl (1 × 10⁹/liter) (see Chap. 6). The normal monocyte count gradual decreases to a mean of 400/μl (0.4 × 10⁹/liter) in adulthood, at which time monocytes constitute 1 to 9 percent (mean 4 percent) of blood leukocytes (see Chap. 2). Monocytosis is present when the absolute count is greater than 800/μl (0.8 × 10⁹/liter) in adults. Men tend to have slightly higher monocyte counts than women.[7] Increments in the number of blood monocytes correlate directly with increases in the total blood monocyte pool and the monocyte turnover rate.[8] The blood monocyte count cycles with a periodicity of 5 days.[9] Older persons have a striking decrease in the proportion of CD14++CD16- to CD14+CD16+ monocytes compared with younger persons.[10]

DISORDERS ASSOCIATED WITH MONOCYTOSIS

Table 71-1 outlines the diseases reported to be associated with monocytosis. In one review, hematologic disorders represented more than 50 percent, collagen vascular diseases approximately 10 percent, and malignant disease approximately 8 percent of cases of monocytosis.[11]

HEMATOLOGIC DISORDERS

About one fourth of patients with myelodysplastic states exhibit an increase in absolute monocyte count.[12–14] Occasional patients with a myelodysplastic state develop an absolute monocyte count as high as 30,000/μl (30 × 10⁹/liter).[15] Chronic monocytosis may be the principal feature of a clonal myeloid disease and precede by years the development of acute myelogenous leukemia.[16,17] Patients with myelodysplasia and monocytosis have a high propensity to evolve into acute or chronic myelomonocytic leukemia.[14] The number of promonocytes and monocytes may increase in patients with acute myelogenous leukemia of the monocytic[18–20] or myelomonocytic type.[21,22] Patients with chronic myelomonocytic leukemia by definition have an increased proportion of monocytes in the blood. The monocytosis may be striking in some cases.[21,22] Juvenile myelomonocytic leukemia also is defined in part by the increased proportion of monocytes in the

TABLE 71-1 DISORDERS ASSOCIATED WITH MONOCYTOSIS

Hematologic disorders	Inflammatory and immune disorders
Hematopoietic stem cell disorders	Connective tissue diseases
Myelodysplastic states[13–17]	Rheumatoid arthritis[50]
Acute myelogenous leukemia	Systemic lupus erythematosus[51]
Monocytic type[18–20]	Temporal arteritis[11]
Myelomonocytic type[21]	Myositis[11]
Histiocytic type[42]	Polyarteritis nodosa[11]
Chronic myelogenous leukemia	Gastrointestinal disorders
Myelomonocytic type[22]	Alcoholic liver disease[79]
m-BCR–positive type[25,26]	Inflammatory bowel disease[66]
Polycythemia vera[11]	Sprue[11]
Lymphocytic tumors	Sarcoidosis[67,68]
Lymphoma[39]	Infections
Hodgkin lymphoma[40]	Cytomegalovirus infection[64]
Macroglobulinemia[45]	Varicella-zoster virus[65]
Multiple myeloma[43,44]	Mycobacterial infections[52–55]
Immune hemolytic anemia[11]	Subacute bacterial
Idiopathic thrombocytopenic	endocarditis[56–57]
purpura[11]	Syphilis[62,63]
Chronic neutropenias[27,29,–32]	Nonhematopoietic malignancies[69–72]
Postsplenectomy state[48,49]	Miscellaneous conditions
	Tetrachloroethane poisoning[80]
	Glucocorticoid administration[86–88]
	Parturition[81,82]
	Drug related[33–36,47]
	Depression[89–91]
	Myocardial infarction[83,84]
	Cardiac bypass surgery[85]
	Thermal injury[97,98]
	Marathon running[92,93]
	Exogenous cytokine
	administration[73–78]

blood.[23] In some cases of monocytic leukemia, the monocytes are immature and have features of monoblasts or promonocytes; however, in many cases the monocytes are indistinguishable from normal blood monocytes by light microscopy. Some automated instruments are dependent on the α-naphthol acetate esterase reaction to detect the proportion of monocytes in white cell differential counts. These instruments may underestimate leukemic monocytes counts, especially in cases of chronic myelomonocytic leukemia, because leukemic monocytes have a decreased activity of the enzyme.[24] A rare variant of Ph-positive chronic myelogenous leukemia (CML), expressing a p190 BCR-ABL transcript, is associated with a striking monocytosis in approximately 50 percent of cases.[25,26]

Monocytosis occurs in a number of neutropenic states: cyclic neutropenia,[27] chronic granulocytopenia of childhood,[28] familial benign chronic neutropenia,[29] infantile genetic agranulocytosis,[30,31] and chronic hypoplastic neutropenia.[32] In human cyclic neutropenia, monocytes oscillate reciprocal to the neutrophil cycle. Peak monocytosis, which often is greater than 2000×10^9/liter, occurs at the end of the neutropenic period. Monocyte levels often remain greater than 500×10^9/liter throughout the cycle. In the variety of other neutropenias, monocytopoiesis often is preserved despite the neutropenia. Transient elevations of monocyte count have been reported in the acute phases of drug-induced agranulocytosis.[33,34] Monocytosis characteristically appears later in the recovery phase of agranulocytosis.[35,36] Several reports[33,35,36] have indicated that normal or increased numbers of monocytes are a harbinger of recovery from agranulocytosis, but another

study found monocyte counts were of no prognostic value.[37] Monocytosis reportedly precedes agranulocytosis resulting from chlorpromazine use.[38]

Monocytosis can occur with lymphomas and can increase with exacerbation of disease activity.[39] Monocytosis has been observed in approximately 25 percent of cases of Hodgkin disease, although monocytosis occurrence does not correlate with prognosis.[40] In contrast, one treatise on the disease reports the hematologic values of patients with Hodgkin disease at the time of diagnosis and indicates only four of 100 have nominal increases in absolute blood monocyte counts.[41] Blood monocytosis may occur in cases of true malignant histiocytosis with a leukemic pattern.[42] A statistically significant increase in blood monocyte concentration has been reported in multiple myeloma[43,44] and has been correlated with the presence of γ light chains containing monoclonal immunoglobulin.[44] Rare cases of M-CSF–secreting lymphoid tumors have been associated with monocytosis.[45,46] Pseudolymphoma syndrome induced by drugs such as carbamazepine, phenytoin, phenobarbital, or valproic acid is associated with monocytosis.[47]

SPLENECTOMY

Monocytosis is a common feature in individuals who have undergone splenectomy.[48,49]

INFLAMMATORY AND IMMUNE DISORDERS

Collagen vascular disease, including rheumatoid arthritis,[50] systemic lupus erythematosus, temporal arteritis, myositis, and periarteritis nodosa, may be associated with monocytosis, although monocytosis is not common in these diseases. The usual alterations of white cell count in systemic lupus erythematosus, for example, are neutropenia and lymphopenia, but 10 percent of patients have a mild monocytosis.[51]

Infectious diseases are an uncommon cause of monocytosis. Only a few instances of infection were noted in a comprehensive review of causes of monocytosis, including tonsillitis, dental infection, recurrent liver abscesses, candidiasis, and one instance of tuberculous peritonitis.[11] Tuberculosis once was a leading cause of monocytosis because of the role of monocytes in granuloma (tubercle) formation. Neither the monocyte count nor the ratio of monocytes to lymphocytes correlates with the stage or activity of tuberculosis.[52–54] Mycobacterium fortuitum infection, usually in the setting of acquired immunodeficiency disease (AIDS), also is associated with monocytosis.[55]

Monocytosis is found in 15 to 20 percent of patients with subacute bacterial endocarditis[58] but is not correlated with the presence of blood macrophages, which may be present in this disease.[59]

A number of infections formerly thought to be associated with monocytosis are not when examined systematically. These infections include rickettsial diseases, leishmaniasis, typhoid fever, malaria, and disseminated candidiasis. Brucellosis can be accompanied by monocytosis.[60]

Monocytosis in the resolution phase of acute infections has been noted.[61] Monocytosis appears in neonatal, primary, and secondary syphilis.[62,63] Certain viruses, especially cytomegalovirus and varicella-zoster virus, induce an increase in blood monocyte level.[64,65]

Sprue, ulcerative colitis, and regional enteritis are associated with monocytosis.[1,66] Elevated blood monocyte count occurs in sarcoidosis[67] and is inversely related to a reduction in circulating T lymphocytes.[68] A similar correlation has been noted in patients with malignant disease.[69]

NONHEMATOPOIETIC MALIGNANCIES

Sixty percent of patients with nonhematologic malignancy exhibit a monocytosis that is independent of the presence or absence of metastatic disease.[70] Reports of hematologic values in metastatic colon cancer and soft tissue sarcoma have reemphasized the frequency of monocytosis in cancer.[71,72] If *unexplained* monocytosis persists, malignancy should be considered.

EXOGENOUS CYTOKINE ADMINISTRATION

Administration of granulocyte-monocyte colony stimulating factor,[73] interleukin-10,[74] or granulocyte colony stimulating factor[75] may result in mildly increased blood monocyte counts. Administration of macrophage colony stimulating factor (M-CSF)[76,77] results in an invariable increase in blood monocytes. At doses of 40 to 120 μg/kg/day, the peak increase, which may reach threefold to fourfold baseline, is reached in approximately 8 days. Administration of human macrophage inflammatory protein-1α to patients or normal volunteers is associated with a brief monocytopenia followed by a monocytosis that is proportional to the dose administered.[78]

MISCELLANEOUS CONDITIONS

Other disorders associated with monocytosis include alcoholic liver disease[79] and tetrachloroethane poisoning.[80] Monocytosis is a frequent finding at the time of parturition.[81,82] Monocytosis occurs after myocardial infarction and peaks on day 3. A correlation exists between creatine kinase and monocyte count, indicating a relationship between extent of infarction and monocytosis.[83] After myocardial infarction, persistent monocytosis correlates with pump failure.[84] Monocytosis is a frequent finding after cardiopulmonary bypass surgery.[85] In the latter circumstance, CD14 (endotoxin receptor) is markedly decreased on the monocyte surface and plasma soluble CD14 is increased, indicating monocyte activation. An increase in blood monocytes occurs in healthy volunteers[86,87] or rarely in patients with myelodysplasia[88] given moderately high, therapeutic-level doses of glucocorticoids. Psychiatric depression is associated with a conjoint increase in neutrophils and monocytes.[89,90] The monocytosis in depressive and anxiety disorders is associated with high plasma levels of β-endorphins and dysfunctional (hypophagocytic) monocytes.[91] Competitive marathon runners have a monocytosis associated with elevated plasma levels of several cytokines, including M-CSF.[92,93]

BLOOD MONOCYTE SUBSET COUNTS IN DISEASE

Differential monocyte subset responses (Cd14++CD16- vs. CD14+CD16+) without deviation of total monocyte counts outside the normal range have been observed in older subjects and in patients with sepsis, AIDS, allergic disorders, dermatitides, hemodialysis, and atherosclerosis.[4,10,71,85,101] These refinements usually are not measured in clinical laboratories.

DISORDERS ASSOCIATED WITH MONOCYTOPENIA

Although monocytopenia can occur in any hematopoietic stem cell disease associated with pancytopenia (e.g., myelogenous leukemia), a decrease in monocytes is notable and constant in aplastic anemia.[94] It is a constant and important feature of hairy cell leukemia, in which monocytopenia can be a helpful diagnostic clue and is a contributor to the predisposition to infection, which is an important, morbid feature of the disease.[95] Monocytopenia occurs in a small proportion of patients with chronic lymphocytic leukemia. These patients may have a higher frequency of infections, especially by viruses.[96] Cyclic neutropenia is notable for intermittent periods of monocytopenia. Severe thermal injuries can result in monocytopenia.[97,98] Rare cases of conjoint severe neutropenia and monocytopenia occur.[99,100] Transient

monocytopenia is a feature of hemodialysis, but monocyte counts return to normal within hours after the procedure ends.[101]

Automated blood cell counts in large numbers of subjects have demonstrated that decreased absolute monocyte counts occur frequently in patients with rheumatoid arthritis,[102] systemic lupus erythematosus,[103] and human immunodeficiency virus infection.[104]

Glucocorticoid hormones produce a transient monocytopenia approximately 6 hours after administration to human volunteers[105] or to patients.[86,106] Administration of interferon alpha and tumor necrosis factor alpha also may also cause monocytopenia.[107] Monocytopenia may occur after radiotherapy.[108]

BLOOD DENDRITIC CELL COUNTS

Blood dendritic cells are composed of two phenotypic subtypes: myeloid derived (CD11c+CD123+) and lymphoid derived (CD11c-CD123+). The total blood dendritic cell count can be measured by flow cytometry measuring CMRF 44 positive cells.[109,110] Dendritic cells compose approximately 0.6 percent of blood cells (range 0.15–1.30 percent) and represent 14×10^6 cells/liter (range 3.0–30×10^6 cells/liter). One third of these cells are lymphoid-derived type and two thirds are myeloid-derived type.[111] Blood dendritic cell counts increase with surgical stress (and presumably other stressful reactions) in relation to cortisol levels. Fluctuations in blood dendritic cells are independent of changes in total blood monocyte count.

REFERENCES

1. Turpin JA, Lopez-Bernstein G: Differentiation, maturation, and activation of monocytes and macrophages: Functional activity is controlled by a continuum of activation, in *Mononuclear Phagocytes in Cell Biology*, edited by G Lopez-Berestein, J Klostergaard, p 71. CRC Press, Boca Raton, 1993.
2. Zeigler-Heitbrock HW: Heterogeneity of human blood monocytes: The CD14+ CD16+ subpopulation. *Immunol Today* 17:424, 1996.
3. Thomas R, Lipsky PE: Human peripheral blood dendritic cell subsets. Isolation and characterization of precursor and mature antigen-presenting cells. *J Immunol* 153:4016, 1994.
4. Grage-Griebenow E, Flad H-D, Ernst M: Heterogeneity of peripheral blood monocyte subsets. *J Leukoc Biol* 69:11, 2001.
5. Hume DA, Ross IL, Himes SR, et al: The mononuclear phagocyte system revisited. *J Leukoc Biol* 72:621, 2001.
6. Griffin JD, Meuer SC, Schlossman SF, Reinherz EL: T-cell regulation of myelopoiesis: Analysis at a clonal level. *J Immunol* 133:1863, 1984.
7. Munan L, Kelly A: Age-dependent changes in blood monocyte populations in man. *Clin Exp Immunol* 35:161, 1979.
8. Meuret G, Hoffman G: Monocyte kinetic studies in normal and disease states. *Br J Haematol* 24:275, 1973.
9. Meuret G, Bremer C, Bammert J, Ewen J: Oscillation of blood monocyte counts in healthy individuals. *Cell Tissue Kinet* 7:223, 1974.
10. Sadeghi HM, Schnelle JF, Thoma JK, et al: Phenotypic and functional characteristics of circulating monocytes of elderly persons. *Exp Gerontol* 34:959, 1999.
11. Maldonado JE, Hanlon DG: Monocytosis: A current appraisal. *Mayo Clin Proc* 40:248, 1965.
12. Rigolin GM, Cuneo A, Roberti MG, et al: Myelodysplastic syndromes with monocytic component: Hematologic and cytogenetic characterization. *Haematologia* 82:25, 1997.
13. Cunningham I, MacCallum SJ, Nicholls MD, et al: The myelodysplastic syndromes: An analysis of prognostic factors in 226 cases from a single institution. *Br J Haematol* 90:602, 1995
14. Castaldi G, Rigolin GM: The monocytic component in myelodysplastic syndromes. *Cancer Treat Res* 108:81, 2001.

15. Weitberg AB: A monocytic leukemoid reaction in a patient with my-elodysplasia. *CA Cancer J Clin* 35:308, 1985.

16. Pretlow TG II: Chronic monocytic dyscrasia culminating in acute leukemia. *Am J Med* 46:130, 1969.

17. Jaworkowsky LI, Solovey DY, Rhausova LY, Udris OY: Monocytosis as a sign of subsequent leukemia in patients with cytopenias (preleukemia). *Folia Hematol (Frankf)* 110:395, 1983.

18. Janvier M, Tobelem G, Daniel MT, et al: Acute monoblastic leukaemia. Clinical, biological data, and survival in 45 cases. *Scand J Haematol* 32:385, 1984.

19. Scott CS, Stark AN, Limbert HJ, et al: Diagnostic and prognostic factors in acute monocytic leukaemia. *Br J Haematol* 69:247, 1988.

20. Odom LF, Lampkin BC, Tannous R, et al: Acute monoblastic leukemia. *Leuk Res* 14:1, 1990.

21. Larson RA, Williams SF, LeBeau MM, et al: Acute myelomonocytic leukemia with abnormal eosinophils and inv (16) or t (16;16) has favorable prognosis. *Blood* 68:1242, 1986.

22. Onida F, Kantajarian HM, Smith TL, et al: Prognostic factors and scoring systems in chronic myelomonocytic leukemia: A retrospective analysis of 213 patients. *Blood* 99:840, 2002.

23. Arico M, Biondi A, Pui C-H: Juvenile myelomonocytic leukemia. *Blood* 90:479, 1997.

24. Frew ME, Donaldson K: Monocyte analysis in chronic myelomonocytic leukaemia. *Br J Biomed Sci* 54:244, 1997.

25. Ohsaka A, Shiina S, Kobayashi M, et al: Philadelphia chromosome-positive chronic myeloid leukemia expressing p190(BCR-ABL). *Intern Med* 41:1092, 2002.

26. Hur M, Song HM, Kang SH, et al: Lymphoid predominance and the absence of basophilia and splenomegaly are frequent in m-bcr-positive chronic myelogenous leukemia. *Ann Hematol* 81:219, 2002.

27. Wright D, Dale DC, Fauci AS, Wolff SM: Human cyclic neutropenia: Clinical review and long-term follow-up of patients. *Medicine* 60:1, 1981.

28. Zuelzer WW, Bajoghli M: Chronic granulocytopenia in childhood. *Blood* 23:359, 1964.

29. Cutting HO, Lang JE: Familial benign chronic neutropenia. *Ann Intern Med* 61:876, 1964.

30. Krill CE, Mauer AM: Congenital agranulocytosis. *J Pediatr* 68:361, 1966.

31. Lang JE, Cutting HO: Infantile genetic agranulocytosis. *Pediatrics* 35:596, 1965.

32. Spaet TH, Dameshek W: Chronic hypoplastic neutropenia. *Am J Med* 13:35, 1952.

33. Cassileth PA: Monocytosis in chlorpromazine-associated agranulocytosis: Termination in acute leukemia. *Am J Med* 43:471, 1967.

34. Graf M, Tarlov A: Agranulocytosis with monohistiocytosis associated with ampicillin therapy. *Ann Intern Med* 69:91, 1968.

35. Reznikoff P: The etiologic importance of fatigue and the prognostic significance of monocytosis in neutropenia (agranulocytosis). *Am J Clin Pathol* 6:205, 1936.

36. Rosenthal N, Abel HA: The significance of the monocytes in agranulocytosis (leukopenic infectious agranulocytosis). *Am J Clin Pathol* 6:205, 1936.

37. Pretty HM, Gosselin G, Colprian G, Long LA: Agranulocytosis: A report of 30 cases. *Can Med Assoc J* 93:1058, 1965.

38. Lutz EG: Monocytosis, blood dyscrasia and chlorpromazine toxicity. *Int J Neuropsych* 1:76, 1965.

39. Rosenberg SA, Diamond HD, Jaslowitz B, Craver LF: Lymphosarcoma: A review of 1269 cases. *Medicine* 40:31, 1961.

40. Ultmann JE: Clinical features and diagnosis of Hodgkin's disease. *Cancer* 9:297, 1966.

41. Kaplan HS: *Hodgkin's Disease*, 2nd ed, p 127. Harvard University Press, Cambridge, 1980.

42. Laurencet FM, Chapius B, Roux-Lombard P, et al: Malignant histiocytosis in the leukaemic stage: A new entity (M5c-AML) in the FAB classification? *Leukemia* 8:502, 1994.

43. Sewell RL: Lymphocyte abnormalities in myeloma. *Br J Haematol* 36:545, 1977.

44. Blom J, Nielsen H, Larsen SO, et al: A study of certain functional parameters of monocytes from patients with multiple myeloma: Comparison with monocytes from healthy individuals. *Scand J Haematol* 33:425, 1984.

45. Nakajima H, Mori S, Takeuchi T, et al: Monocytosis and high serum macrophage colony-stimulating factor in Waldenstrom's macroglobulinemia. *Blood* 86:2863, 1995.

46. Tokioka T, Shimamoto Y, Motoyoshi K, Yamaguchi M: Clinical significance of monocytosis and human monocytic colony stimulating factor in patients with adult T-cell leukaemia/lymphoma. *Haematologia* 26:1, 1994.

47. Choi TS, Doh KS, Kim SH, et al: Clinicopathological and genotypic aspects of anticonvulsant-induced pseudolymphoma syndrome. *Br J Dermatol* 148:730, 2003.

48. Durig M, Landmann RMA, Harder F: Lymphocyte subsets in human peripheral blood after splenectomy and autotransplantation of splenic tissue. *J Lab Clin Med* 104:110, 1984.

49. Lanng Nielson J, Romer FK, Ellegaard J: Serum angiotensin-converting enzyme and blood monocytes in splenectomized individuals. *Acta Haematol* 67:132, 1982.

50. Buchan GS, Palmer DG, Gibbins BL: The response of human peripheral blood mononuclear phagocytes to rheumatoid arthritis. *J Leukoc Biol* 37:221, 1985.

51. Budman DR, Steinberg AD: Hematologic aspects of systemic lupus erythematosus. Current concepts. *Am Intern Med* 86:220, 1977.

52. Stobie W, England NJ, McMenemy WH: The interpretation of haemograms in pulmonary tuberculosis. *Am Rev Tuberc* 46:1, 1942.

53. Flinn JW: A study of the differential blood count in 1000 cases of active pulmonary tuberculosis. *Ann Intern Med* 2:622, 1929.

54. Singh KJ, Ahluwalia G, Sharma SK, et al: Significance of haematological reactions in patients with tuberculosis. *J Assoc Physicians India* 49:788, 2001.

55. Smith MB, Schnadig VJ, Boyars MC, Woods GL: Clinical and pathological features of Mycobacterium fortuitum infections: An emerging pathogen in patients with AIDS. *Am J Clin Pathol* 116:225, 2001.

56. Daland GA, Gottlieb L, Wallerstein RO, et al: Hematologic observations in bacterial endocarditis. *J Lab Clin Med* 48:827, 1956.

57. Hill RW, Bayrd ED: Phagocytic reticuloendothelial cells in subacute bacterial endocarditis with negative cultures. *Ann Intern Med* 52:310, 1960.

58. Myhre EB, Braconier JH, Sjögren U: Automated cytochemical differential leukocyte count in patients hospitalized with acute bacterial infections. *Scand J Infect Dis* 17:201, 1985.

59. Horsfall FL Jr, Tamm I: *Viral and Rickettsial Diseases of Man*, 4th ed. Lippincott, Philadelphia, 1965.

60. Tsolia M, Drakonaki S, Messaritaki A, et al: Clinical features, complications and treatment outcome of childhood brucellosis in central Greece. *J Infect* 44:257, 2002.

61. Hickling RA: The monocytes in pneumonia: A clinical and hematologic study. *Arch Intern Med* 40:594, 1927.

62. Rosahn PD, Pearce L: The blood cytology in untreated and treated syphilis. *Am J Med Sci* 187:88, 1934.

63. Karyalcin G, Khanijou A, Kim KY, et al: Monocytosis in congenital syphilis. *Am J Dis Child* 131:782, 1977.

64. Klemola E: Cytomegalovirus infection in previously healthy adults. *Ann Intern Med* 79:267, 1973.

65. Tsukahara T, Yogushi A, Horiuchi Y: Significance of monocytosis in varicella herpes zoster. *J Dermatol* 19:94, 1992.

66. Mees AS, Berney J, Jewell DP: Monocytes in inflammatory bowel disease: Absolute monocyte counts. *J Clin Pathol* 33:917, 1980.

67. Goodwin JS, DeHaratius R, Israel H, et al: Suppressor cell function in sarcoidosis. *Ann Intern Med* 90:169, 1979.

68. Daniele RP, Dauber JH, Rossman MD: Immunologic abnormalities in sarcoidosis. *Ann Intern Med* 92:406, 1980.

69. Wood GW, Neff JE, Stephens R: Relationship between monocytosis and T-lymphocyte function in human cancer. *J Natl Cancer Inst* 63:587, 1979.

70. Barrett O'N Jr: Monocytosis in malignant disease. *Ann Intern Med* 73:991, 1970.

71. Melichar B, Touskova M, Vesely P: Effect of irinotecan on the phenotype of peripheral blood leukocyte populations in patients with metastatic colorectal cancer. *Hepatogastroenterology* 49:967, 2002.

72. Ruka W, Rutkowski P, Kaminska J, et al: Alterations of routine blood tests in adult patients with soft tissue sarcomas: Relationships to cytokine serum levels and prognostic significance. *Ann Oncol* 12:1423, 2001.

73. Schmitz LL, McClure JS, Litz CE, et al: Morphologic and quantitative changes in blood and marrow cells following growth factor therapy. *Am J Clin Pathol* 101:67, 1994.

74. Chernoff AE, Granowitz EV, Shapiro L, et al: A randomized controlled trial of IL-10 in humans. *J Immunol* 154:5492, 1995.

75. Ranaghan L, Drake M, Humphreys MW, Morris TC: Leukaemoid monocytosis in M4 AML following chemotherapy: G-CSF. *Clin Lab Haematol* 20:49, 1998.

76. Weiner LM, Li W, Holmes M, et al: Phase I trial of recombinant macrophage colony-stimulating factor and recombinant gamma-interferon: Toxicity, monocytosis, and clinical effects. *Cancer Res* 54:4084, 1994.

77. Minasian LM, Yao TJ, Steffens TA, et al: A phase I study of anti-GD3 ganglioside monoclonal antibody R24 and recombinant human macrophage-colony stimulating factor in patients with metastatic melanoma. *Cancer* 75:2251, 1995.

78. Marshall E, Howell AH, Powles R, et al: Clinical effects of human macrophage inflammatory protein-1 alpha MIP-1 alpha (LD78) administration in humans. *Eur J Cancer* 34:1023, 1998.

79. McKeever UM, O'Mahoney C, Lawlor E, et al: Monocytosis: A feature of alcoholic liver disease. *Lancet* 2:1492, 1983.

80. Minot GR, Smith LW: The blood in tetrachloroethane poisoning. *Arch Intern Med* 28:687, 1921.

81. Siegal I, Gleichner N: Peripheral white blood cells alterations in early labor. *Diagn Gynecol Obstet* 3:123, 1981.

82. Buchan GS, Gibbins BL, Griffin JFT: The influence of parturition on peripheral blood mononuclear phagocyte subpopulation in pregnant women. *J Leukoc Biol* 37:231, 1985.

83. Meisel SR, Panzner H, Schecter M, et al: Peripheral monocytosis following myocardial infarction. *Cardiology* 90:52, 1998.

84. Maekawa Y, Anzai T, Yoshikawa T, et al: Prognostic significance of peripheral monocytosis after reperfusion acute myocardial infarction: Possible role for left ventricular remodeling. *J Am Coll Cardiol* 16:241, 2002.

85. Fingerle-Rowson G, Auers J, Kreuzer E, et al: Down-regulation of surface monocyte lipopolysaccharide-receptor CD14 in patients on cardiopulmonary bypass undergoing aorta-coronary bypass operation. *J Thorac Cardiovasc Surg* 115:1172, 1998.

86. Rinehard JJ, Sagone AL, Balcerzak SP, et al: Effects of corticosteroid therapy on human monocyte function. *N Engl J Med* 292:236, 1975.

87. Shoenfeld Y, Gurewich Y, Gallant LA, et al: Prednisone-induced leukocytosis. *Am J Med* 71:773, 1981.

88. Morales M, Wilkes J, Lowder JN: Monocytic leukemoid reaction, glucocorticoid therapy, and myelodysplastic syndrome. *Cleve Clin J Med* 6:571, 1990.

89. Maes M, VanDerPlanken M, Stevens WJ, et al: Leukocytosis, monocytosis and neutrophilia: Hallmarks of severe depression. *J Psychiat Res* 26:125, 1992.

90. Maes M, Lambrechts J, Suy E, et al: Absolute number and percentage of circulating natural killer, non-MHC-restricted T cytotoxic, and phagocytic cells in unipolar depression. *Neuropsychobiology* 29:157, 1994.

91. Castilla-Cortazar I, Castilla A, Gurpegui M: Opioid peptides and immunodysfunction in a patient with major depression and anxiety disorders. *J Physiol Biochem* 54:203, 1998.

92. Kratz A, Lewandrowski KB, Siegel AJ, et al: Effect of marathon running on hematologic and biochemical laboratory parameters, including cardiac markers. *Am J Clin Pathol* 118:856, 2002.

93. Suzuki K, Nakaji S, Yamadi M, et al: Impact of a competitive marathon race on systemic cytokine and neutrophil responses. *Med Sci Sports Exerc* 35:348, 2003.

94. Twormey JJ, Douglas CC, Sharkey O Jr: The monocytopenia of aplastic anemia. *Blood* 41:187, 1973.

95. den Ottolander GJ, van der Burgh FJ, Lopes Cardozo P, et al: The Hemalog D automated differential counter in the diagnosis of hairy cell leukemia. *Leuk Res* 7:309, 1983.

96. DeRossi G, Mauro FR, Ialongo P, et al: Monocytopenia and infections in chronic lymphocytic leukemia (CLL). *Eur J Haematol* 46:119, 1991.

97. Peterson V, Hensbrough J, Buerk C, et al: Regulation of granulopoiesis following severe thermal injury. *J Trauma* 23:19, 1983.

98. Santangelo S, Gamelli RL, Shankar R: Myeloid commitment shifts toward monocytopoiesis after thermal injury and sepsis. *Ann Surg* 233:97, 2001.

99. Adams WH, Liu YK: Periodic neutropenia and monocytopenia. *Am J Hematol* 13:73, 1982.

100. Marinone G, Roncoli B, Marinone MG Jr: Pure white cell aplasia. *Semin Hematol* 28:298, 1991.

101. Nockher WA, Wiemer J, Scherberich JE: Hemodialysis monocytopenia: Differential sequestration kinetics of CD14+CD16+ and CD14++ blood monocyte subsets. *Clin Exp Immunol* 123:49, 2001.

102. Isenberg DA, Martin P, Hajirousou V, et al: Haematological reassessment of rheumatoid arthritis using an automated method. *Br J Rheumatol* 25:152, 1986.

103. Isenberg DA, Patterson KG, Todd-Pokropek A, et al: Haematological aspects of systemic lupus erythematosus: A reappraisal using automated methods. *Acta Haematol* 67:242, 1982.

104. Treacy M, Lai L, Costello C, et al: Peripheral blood and bone marrow abnormalities in patients with HIV related disease. *Br J Haematol* 65:289, 1987.

105. Steer JH, Vuong Q, Joyce DA: Suppression of human monocyte tumor necrosis factor-alpha release by glucocorticoid therapy: Relationship to systemic monocytopenia and cortisol suppression. *Br J Clin Pharmacol* 43:383, 1997.

106. Fauci AS, Dale DC: Monocytopenia after prednisone. *N Engl J Med* 292:928, 1975.

107. Aulitzky WE, Tilg H, Vogel W, et al: Acute hematologic effects of interferon alpha, interferon gamma, tumor necrosis factor alpha and interleukin 2. *Ann Hematol* 62:25, 1991.

108. Rotman M, Ansley H, Rogow L, et al: Monocytosis: A new observation during radiotherapy. *Int J Radiat Oncol Biol Phys* 2:117, 1977.

109. Fearnley DB, Whyte LF, Carnoutosis SA, et al: The monitoring of human blood dendritic cell numbers. *Blood* 93:728, 1999.

110. Ho CSK, López JA, Vuckovic S, et al: Surgical and physical stress increases circulatory blood dendritic cell counts independently of monocyte counts. *Blood* 98:140, 2001.

111. Szabolcs P, Park K-D, Reese M, et al: Absolute values of dendritic cell subsets in bone marrow, cord blood, and peripheral blood enumerated by a novel method. *Stem Cells* 21:269, 2003.

INFLAMMATORY AND MALIGNANT HISTIOCYTOSIS

MARSHALL A. LICHTMAN

Clinical disorders that are the consequence of a primary proliferation of histiocytes (macrophages) may result from a metabolic, inflammatory, or neoplastic pathogenetic mechanism. This chapter discusses the latter two mechanisms. Chapter 73 discusses the former mechanism.

Three principal inflammatory disorders of macrophages affect the marrow or lymph nodes and are relevant to hematologists. The first disorder is familial hemophagocytic lymphohistiocytosis, an autosomal recessive disease that develops during infancy in most cases. Consanguineous parentage is common, and approximately two thirds of cases occur in siblings. Thirty percent of cases have mutations in the perforin gene. Fever and hepatosplenomegaly are common. Neurologic manifestations, jaundice, and ascites may develop. Anemia and thrombocytopenia are constant features. Marrow, hepatic, or splenic biopsy specimens contain macrophages with ingested blood cells or their precursors. Left untreated, the disorder is rapidly fatal. Glucocorticoids and etoposide combined with cyclosporine may induce remission. Hematopoietic stem cell transplantation is the most successful form of treatment and can be curative. The second disorder is infectious hemophagocytic histiocytosis, an infrequent but severe and dramatic reaction to viral (especially Epstein-Barr virus), bacterial, fungal, or protozoal infection. It may accompany drug reactions, inflammatory, or neoplastic diseases, especially lymphoma. Fever, myalgias, lethargy, and hepatosplenomegaly often are present. Bicytopenia or pancytopenia is common. Activated macrophages ingesting blood cells or their precursors are abundant in the marrow specimen. In its most severe form, the disorder produces a severe systemic illness that includes cytokine storm, multiorgan failure, and disseminated intravascular clotting. The clinical syndrome may resolve in weeks if the underlying infection is treated successfully or resolves. When caused by Epstein-Barr virus, oligoclonal T cell expansion may require chemotherapy. The third disorder is sinus histiocytosis with massive lymphadenopathy (Rosai-Dorfman syndrome), which is a polyclonal disorder that usually manifests as massive, painless cervical lymph node enlargement. Other nodes or extranodal sites are involved in many patients. Localized disease may occur in virtually any organ or tissue and mimic cancer at that site; however, biopsy of an involved area shows engorgement of sinuses or tissue by activated, phagocytic macrophages. The disease usually is self-limited and regresses spontaneously at various times within approximately 18 months. Progressive disease can be treated with glucocorticoids or chemotherapy. Surgical excision of lymphatic masses compressing vital organs may be required.

Clonal histiocytic disorders include Langerhans cell histiocytosis and malignant histiocytosis. Langerhans cell histiocytosis can be localized to skin, bone, or other sites, or the disorder can be widespread, involving almost any organ. Diabetes insipidus is common in the latter form. The diagnosis requires localization of S-100 protein, CD1a, or langerin on the histiocytic cells in the infiltrate and identification of Langerhans cell (Birbeck) granules by electron microscopy. In the localized form, observation, excisional biopsy, or local treatment may suffice. In the progressive or disseminated form, multidrug chemotherapy or stem cell transplantation may be required. Malignant histiocytosis had been overdiagnosed before stringent criteria, including absence of evidence for immunoglobulin or T lymphocyte receptor–chain gene rearrangement, were used to eliminate lymphoma masquerading as histiocytoma. The neoplastic cell type may have phenotypic features of a macrophage, Langerhans cell, or interdigitating or follicular dendritic cell. The disease may present with lymph node enlargement or other single organ involvement, or the disease may be disseminated, involving marrow, lymph nodes, liver, and spleen. Therapy usually involves multidrug chemotherapy and, in younger patients, stem cell transplantation if a donor is available.

INTRODUCTION

Diseases associated with the proliferation of histiocytes can be grouped into three categories: inflammatory disorders, neoplastic (clonal) disorders, and storage diseases (Table 72-1). Chapter 73 describes the storage diseases. This chapter describes histiocytic disorders that can be evaluated by hematologists. The large number of histiocytoses that principally affect the skin are not discussed.[1]

The terms *macrophage* and *histiocyte* are synonyms. The former designation is favored for discussions of the cell biology and pathophysiology of the mature cell found in tissues in the monocyte-macrophage system. In the medical literature, the terms histiocyte and histiocytosis are used to describe histopathologic lesions of macrophage or dendritic cell disorders. Cells derived from the monocyte-macrophage lineage can include varied and highly distinctive phenotypes. These specialized cells may be free, or they may localize to specific tissues (e.g., Kupffer cells of the liver, Langerhans cells of the skin, dendritic cells of the lymph node). Macrophages are phagocytic and rich in lysosomes. Five types of dendritic cells derived from the monocyte lineage have been characterized: Langerhans, follicular dendritic, interstitial dendritic, veiled, and interdigitating dendritic cells. These cells are nonphagocytic, lysosome poor, and specialized to engage, process, and present antigen to lymphocytes (see Chaps. 18 and

TABLE 72-1   HISTIOCYTIC DISORDERS

Hemophagocytic histiocytosis (macrophage activation syndrome*)
- Familial (inherited) hemophagocytic lymphohistiocytosis
- Infectious hemophagocytic histiocytosis (e.g., viral, bacterial, fungal, protozoal)
- Tumor-associated hemophagocytic histiocytosis (e.g., lymphoma, carcinoma)
- Drug-associated hemophagocytic histiocytosis (e.g., phenytoin)

Sinus histiocytosis with massive lymphadenopathy (Rosai-Dorfman disease)

Clonal histiocytosis
- Langerhans cell histiocytosis
- Malignant histiocytosis (histiocytic and dendritic cell tumors)

Storage diseases (see Chap. 73)

NOTE: The disorders listed are those most likely to be encountered by a hematologist. Histiocytic disorders that do not usually involve lymph nodes, blood, or marrow are not considered.

* Synonym of hemophagocytic histioocytosis.[254]

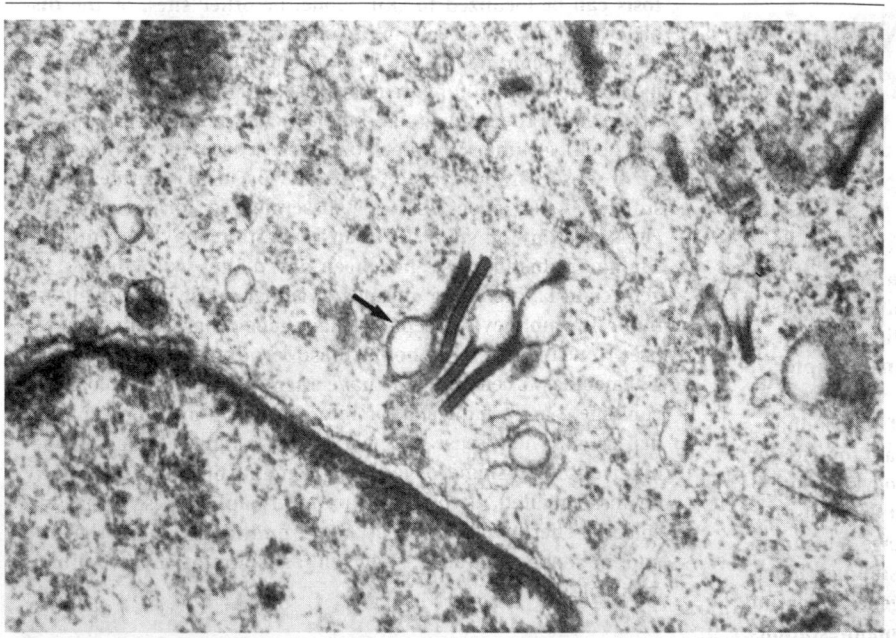

FIGURE 72-1   Transmission electron micrograph of a pathologic Langerhans cell from a bone lesion. The cell contains typical cytoplasmic Langerhans granules (Birbeck bodies; *arrow*). The latter have a characteristic racquet shape. (From BE Favara, ER Jaffe, *Hematol Oncol Clin North Am* 1:75, 1987, with permission.)

67). Histiocytic diseases may reflect these distinctions; specific diagnosis requires careful assessment of cell phenotype and genotype. Some investigators use the term histiocyte, in contradistinction to macrophage, specifically to describe cells that process antigen and dendritic cells that present antigen, focusing solely on the role of these cells in the immune system.[2]

Considerable confusion existed in the classification of disorders of histiocytes when morphologic characterization of pathologic specimens using light microscopy was the principal basis for diagnosis. Use of electron microscopy to identify the specific granules in Langerhans cells (Birbeck bodies) (Fig. 72-1) and development of a series of antibodies and immunocytochemical techniques that recognize cluster of differentiation (CD) sites present on macrophages and dendritic cells or other novel intracellular features have clarified the classification of these diseases.[2] These tools, coupled with studies of T and B lymphocyte gene rearrangements to exclude diseases of lymphocytes that are phenocopies of histiocytic disorders, have led to improved diagnostic accuracy. In addition, refined phenotyping has permitted discrimination between disorders of dendritic histiocytes, for example, Langerhans cell histiocytosis, and nondendritic histiocytes involved in the secondary hemophagocytic syndromes.

INFLAMMATORY DISORDERS OF HISTIOCYTES

FAMILIAL (INHERITED) HEMOPHAGOCYTIC LYMPHOHISTIOCYTOSIS

DEFINITION AND HISTORY
Familial hemophagocytic lymphohistiocytosis was first described in 1952. It also has been referred to as familial reticulosis and familial erythrophagocytic lymphohistiocytosis. The disease is an inherited immune regulatory disorder resulting in ineffective activation of cytotoxic lymphocytes and natural killer (NK) cells, accompanied by poorly regulated secretion of inflammatory cytokines. Inadequate apoptotic activity in the immune system results in expansion of lym-

phocytes and histiocytes in liver, spleen, lymph nodes, and other sites and multiorgan dysfunction. Left untreated, the disease usually is lethal.

EPIDEMIOLOGY
The annual incidence in Sweden is approximately one per million children, or one per 50,000 live births.[3] Males and females are equally affected. The disease affects neonates and infants; 90 percent of patients are symptomatic by age 2 years. More than two thirds of cases occur in siblings.[4] Occasionally a second affected sibling does not become symptomatic until the child becomes a teenager.[5] Parents of patients admit consanguinity in approximately one fourth of cases. The frequency of affected siblings and consanguineous parents is consistent with autosomal recessive inheritance.

PATHOGENESIS
Approximately 30 percent of cases have a mutation in the perforin gene (FHL2 locus on chromosome 10q21-22) and 10 percent in the FHL1 locus on chromosome 9q21.3-22.[6–8] The mutations in the remaining cases are assumed to involve other genes that affect immune function in a similar manner.[9,10] Normally, perforin is secreted by cytotoxic lymphocytes and NK cells, inserts itself into target cell membranes creating channels through which granzymes enter, triggering the caspase cascade and apoptosis of the target cell.[11] Patients have defective cytotoxic cell activation, defective apoptotic regulation of mononuclear cells, and expansion of lymphocytes and histiocytes in tissues with resulting organomegaly and tissue damage.[11–13] Aberrant secretion of proinflammatory cytokines by Th1 lymphocytes contributes to the symptom complex.[14–19]

CLINICAL FINDINGS
The most frequent signs in infants are fever, failure to thrive, irritability, and vomiting. Hepatic or splenic enlargement is present in almost all cases. The spleen can become greatly enlarged. As the condition progresses, lymphadenopathy, jaundice, ascites, and edema can occur. Neurologic abnormalities such as meningitis, seizures, hemiplegia, and coma may become prominent. In infants, bulging fontanelles, hypotonia, or hypertonia may be evident. Atypical presentations such as encephalitis or hepatitis may occur.[3,20,21]

LABORATORY FINDINGS
Blood and Marrow Findings   Anemia, reticulocytopenia, and thrombocytopenia are present in most patients. Leukopenia and neutropenia are less common. With progression of the disease, pancytopenia is the rule.[4] Cytotoxic T cell and NK cell concentrations are normal, but cytotoxic assays show a moderate to marked decrease in activity.[12]

Results of marrow examination may be normal and erythrophagocytic histiocytes inconspicuous early after onset. However, later in the course of the disease the marrow contains decreased numbers of normal precursors and increased numbers of macrophages ingesting blood cells (hemophagocytic histiocytes).[20,21] Prominent hemophagocytosis develops in nearly all patients.

Plasma Abnormalities   Serum alanine aminotransferase and bilirubin levels may be elevated. Serum ferritin and triglyceride concentrations frequently are elevated. Serum albumin, sodium, and fibrinogen levels often are low, and overt disseminated intravascular coagulation occurs frequently.[4,20,21]

Increased serum concentrations of interleukin (IL)-12, interferon gamma (IFN-γ), tumor necrosis factor alpha (TNF-α), soluble IL-2 receptor (IL-2R), soluble FAS ligand, and soluble CD8 are evident in most affected children. Increased IL-6 occurs in approximately one third of children.[14–19]

Spinal Fluid Abnormalities The cerebrospinal fluid frequently has an increased concentration of mononuclear cells, primarily lymphocytes. Some macrophages may be present. The spinal fluid protein is elevated in most children.[22]

Histopathologic Findings The diagnosis of the clinical syndrome in infants is supported by biopsies showing an infiltrate of T lymphocytes and macrophages in the liver, spleen, lymph nodes, or marrow. The macrophages do not have the morphologic features of malignant cells but are engorged with phagocytosed erythrocytes and occasionally neutrophils, lymphocytes, platelets, or erythroblasts. Early in the disease, histiocytes are prominent in the T cell zones and sinuses of lymph nodes. Later, lymphoid depletion in the paracortex of lymph nodes and the white pulp of the spleen is characteristic.[4,20,23]

DNA Abnormalities Identification of a mutation in the perforin gene (approximately 30 percent) or the FHL1 locus on chromosome 9q21.3-22 (approximately 10 percent) confirms the diagnosis in the approximately 40 percent of patients who carry these mutations.[6,7,24]

DIFFERENTIAL DIAGNOSIS

An early diagnosis enhances the effect of treatment because irreversible organ damage, especially neurologic injury, may be prevented. The disease is uncommon and unexpected; therefore, the disease often is unrecognized. Atypical presentations, such as encephalitis or hepatitis, may be confusing. Other hemophagocytic syndromes associated with viral infections, particularly Epstein-Barr virus, cytomegalovirus, and parvovirus, those associated with leishmaniasis, and those associated with the accelerated phase of Chédiak-Higashi disease or the X-linked lymphoproliferative disease, each of which has increased susceptibility to Epstein-Barr virus infection, may mislead the diagnostician. The cytopenias and hepatosplenomegaly may be confused with neonatal leukemia or lymphoma. The distinction from a hemophagocytosis syndrome secondary to infection is made more difficult by the presence of infection in approximately one fifth of patients at the time of diagnosis.[25] Low cytotoxicity assays of cytotoxic T lymphocytes and NK cells favor familial hemophagocytic lymphohistiocytosis compared to infection-induced hemophagocytic syndrome.[24] Identification of a perforin gene mutation is diagnostic.[24] The neurologic findings may mimic the findings seen with physical child abuse and have led to misdiagnosis and wasted time and emotional trauma charging parents of severely ill children with abuse.[26] Table 72-2 lists the most prevalent findings in familial hemophagocytic lymphohistiocytosis.

THERAPY

Etoposide, teniposide, vinca alkaloids, glucocorticoids, and methotrexate have been used as single or multiple agents with or without intrathecal methotrexate, followed by cranial irradiation to treat central nervous system disease. Splenectomy, plasmapheresis, plasma exchange transfusion, cyclosporine A, and antithymocyte globulin have been used in individual patients. Remissions as a result of such therapies have occurred in a very small proportion of patients.[4]

The preferred treatment is high-dose dexamethasone, etoposide, cyclosporine A, and intrathecal methotrexate, if the latter is indicated (spinal fluid or central nervous system abnormalities), followed by hematopoietic stem cell transplantation.[27] Hematopoietic stem cell transplantation should be used if an appropriate matched-related, matched-unrelated, or haploidentical donor can be identified.[28–30] It is

TABLE 72-2 KEY DIAGNOSTIC FINDINGS OF FAMILIAL HEMOPHAGOCYTIC LYMPHOHISTIOCYTOSIS

SIGN	APPROXIMATE FREQUENCY (%)
Hemophagocytosis (marrow, liver, spleen)	95
Fever	90
Anemia	90
Thrombocytopenia	90
Splenomegaly	90
Hypertriglyceridemia	80
Perforin gene or FHL1 locus mutation	40
History of prior sibling affected	25
Parental consanguinity	20

the only potentially curative therapy. Combined liver and stem cell transplantation has been successful for patients with severe, irreversible liver injury.[31] Intrauterine etoposide and dexamethasone have been administered, followed by cesarian section at 32 weeks, and successful hematopoietic stem cell transplantation.[19] Prenatal diagnosis should become available for families carrying a mutated perforin gene or another identifiable mutation.

COURSE

Left untreated, the disease is rapidly fatal. Remission or substantial improvement can occur with the combination immunochemotherapy. Cure can result from hematopoietic stem cell transplantation. The estimated 5-year survival rate for patients treated with stem cell transplantation (approximately 65 percent) in uncontrolled studies compared to that for chemotherapy alone (approximately 10 percent), highlights the value of early transplantation. The theoretical possibility of future gene therapy also exists.

INFECTION-, DISEASE-, OR DRUG-INDUCED HEMOPHAGOCYTIC HISTIOCYTOSIS

ETIOLOGY

Since the mid-1970s, an acquired syndrome of exaggerated histiocytic proliferation and activation has been defined that usually is associated with systemic viral infection,[32,33] especially with Epstein-Barr virus[34–39] and occasionally with bacterial, fungal, or protozoal infections.[40–46] The disease affects children and adults. Epstein-Barr virus, human herpesvirus-6, cytomegalovirus, varicella-zoster virus, adenovirus, influenza virus, human immunodeficiency virus, dengue virus, parvovirus, measles vaccine, enteric bacteria, streptococcus, staphylococcus, rickettsia, mycobacteria, *Candida, Histoplasma, Cryptococcus*, leishmania, and Babesia have been implicated.

Hemophagocytic histiocytosis can occur as a result of Epstein-Barr virus infection during the X-linked lymphoproliferative syndrome or the accelerated phase of Chédiak-Higashi syndrome. A similar syndrome can occur in patients with a variety of malignancies, perhaps as a result of the enhanced susceptibility to infection or the immunosuppressed state associated with cancer, chemotherapy, radiotherapy, and inanition.[42,44–48] This syndrome also has developed with lymphomas as a result of cytokines released by lymphoma cells that stimulate histiocyte proliferation and phagocytosis.[49–53] The syndrome has developed in patients with lupus erythematosus[54] or other autoimmune diseases,[55] including juvenile arthritis,[56,57] after phenytoin administration,[58] and in association with other miscellaneous disorders.

PATHOGENESIS

Unlike familial hemophagocytic lymphohistiocytic syndrome, which is initiated by a gene mutation that results in immune dysregulation, these syndromes are provoked by another primary disease: infection, cancer, or autoimmunity. In some cases, an underlying disorder such as X-linked lymphoproliferative disease may enhance susceptibility. Because these immune deficiency states may be related to gene mutations, for example, as in the IL-2 receptor γ-chain gene mutated in combined immunodeficiency disorder, the mutation in X-linked lymphoproliferative disease, *SH2D1A*, or the gene for purine nucleoside phosphorylase, resulting in diminished T lymphocyte function, any or all of these mutations may predispose to the acquired hemophagocytic syndrome resulting from viral infection.[252] The manifestations are a mixture of the primary disease, such as infection, and the manifestations that result from the release of proinflammatory cytokines.[15–17,37] These processes account for much of the resultant effects on blood cell counts, organ dysfunction, and intravascular coagulation.

In this syndrome, Epstein-Barr virus can enter T lymphocytes.[18,37] The virus DNA can be found in monoclonal or oligoclonal proliferating T and NK cells.[35–37] Proliferation of these cells leads to disruption of immune regulation and cytokine storm. Elevated levels of TNF-α, soluble IL-2R, IL-1, IL-10, IL-18, and FAS ligand are associated with the severity of the manifestations.[10–12,15–17,37,59] Soluble IL-2R is thought to contribute to immune impairment by negating the effect of IL-2.[37] Endothelial cell activation and capillary leakage coupled with hepatic injury from histiocyte infiltration, bile acids, and the FAS/FAS ligand pathway may combine to account for hypoalbuminemia and hypofibrinogenemia. Endothelial cell injury may induce microvascular thrombosis and consumption of labile coagulation factors, which contributes to hypofibrinogenemia and coagulopathy. Cytopenias may result from the effects of elevated concentrations of IFN-γ, TNF-α, or transforming growth factor beta–mediated suppression of the marrow, and monocyte colony stimulating factor–mediated accelerated clearance of platelets by histiocytes.[60,61]

Major organ failure of liver, kidneys, or lung may ensue as a consequence of hypercytokinemia.[37]

The severity of the syndrome varies from mild to severe and lethal.[41,42,44,62]

CLINICAL FINDINGS

The signs and symptoms of this syndrome include fever, severe malaise, myalgias, lethargy, and often hepatic and splenic enlargement.[32,33,44] The last two findings are less prevalent in adults. Children

also may have prominent lymphadenopathy. Pulmonary infiltrates develop occasionally.

LABORATORY FINDINGS

Blood, Marrow, Lymph Node, and Tissue Findings Severe anemia (<90 g/liter), leukopenia [<2.5 × 10⁹/liter], and thrombocytopenia [<50 × 10⁹/liter], or a combination of two cytopenias is seen in nearly all cases.[32,33,37,44] A careful search may uncover macrophages in the blood film. CD3+, HLA-DR+ cells in the blood are elevated in Epstein-Barr virus–induced hemophagocytic syndrome. The marrow often is hypocellular, and granulopoiesis and erythropoiesis, in particular, may be markedly decreased. The number of megakaryocytes in the marrow are normal or reduced slightly.

An increase in marrow macrophages is a constant finding. The presence of macrophages ranges from a slightly greater prominence to replacement of hematopoietic tissue.[32,33,37,44] The macrophages often are vacuolated, with ingested cellular material in varying stages of digestion. Ingestion of erythrocytes and erythroblasts is usual, but phagocytosis of platelets and, rarely, neutrophils can occur (Fig. 72-2). A lymph node biopsy contains increased hemophagocytic histiocytes, but lymph node architecture is not effaced. Occasionally, histiocytic proliferation involves the meninges, gastrointestinal tract, lung, and other sites.

Plasma Findings During the acute phase of the illness, the plasma concentrations of proinflammatory cytokines and acute-phase reactants are elevated. IFN-γ, TNF-α, and IL-6 levels often are markedly elevated, as is soluble IL-2R. Hypertriglyceridemia, hyperferritinemia, and elevated lactic dehydrogenase are frequent. Plasma fibrinogen and plasminogen activator inhibitor-1 levels often are very low, and these changes may reflect disseminated intravascular clotting.

The disease can be distinguished from malignant histiocytosis by clinical and serologic evidence of an antecedent viral infection, the clinical setting in which the disease occurs, the absence of cytologic evidence of malignant histiocytes (see "Malignant Tumors of Histiocytes and Dendritic Cells"), and the absence of effacement of lymph node architecture.

TREATMENT AND COURSE

The severity of the clinical disorder depends on the presence of some or all of the following conditions: (1) cytokine storm, (2) multiorgan failure, (3) disseminated intravascular coagulation, (4) reversibility of

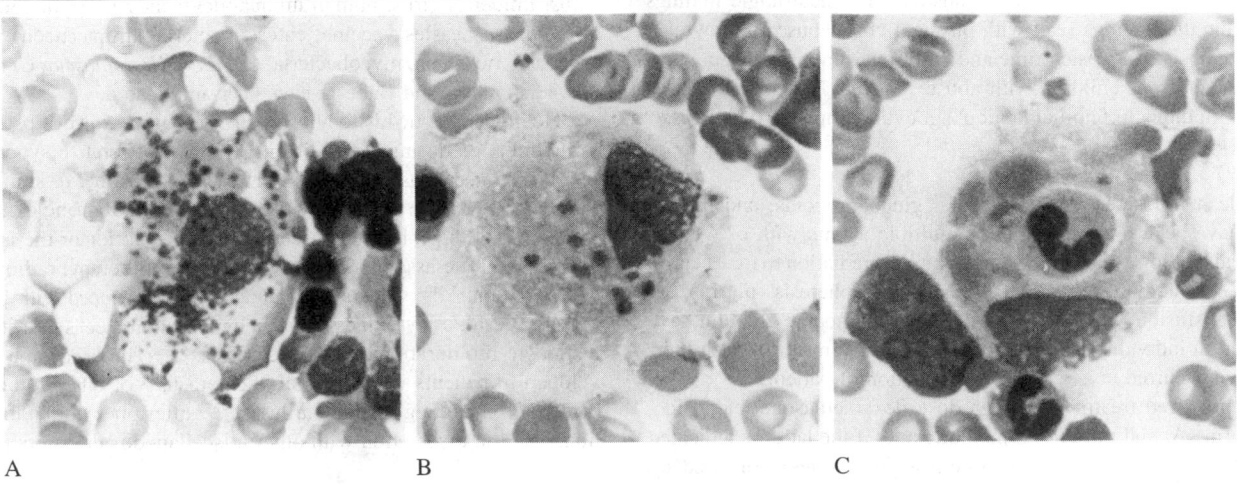

A   B   C

FIGURE 72-2   Composite showing macrophages from a patient with histiocytosis. These macrophages show (A) erythrophagocytosis, (B) platelet phagocytosis, and (C) band neutrophil (and erythro) phagocytosis.

the underlying disease, (5) control of opportunistic infection, and (6) in the case of Epstein-Barr virus infection, the presence of an expanded population of oligoclonal or monoclonal cytotoxic lymphocytes and NK cells. Patients who have mild to moderate disease may recover in weeks if the infectious agent is treatable with antimicrobial therapy, or the disease may resolve naturally if the patient has a normal immune system. Complete disappearance of the histopathologic evidence of histiocytosis follows in months.[32,41,42,46] In patients in whom disease- or drug-induced immunodeficiency is present, as in renal transplant patients, immunosuppressive therapy may need to be decreased or stopped until the viral infection subsides.[33] In the severe Epstein-Barr virus–induced syndrome, treatment for up to 8 weeks with dexamethasone, etoposide, and cyclosporine A can be used to suppress cytokine release and reverse oligoclonal proliferation of T and NK cells.[37] Therapy to curtail disseminated intravascular coagulation also may be required (see Chap. 121). This aggregate therapy has resulted in striking improvement of severe Epstein-Barr virus–associated hemophagocytic syndrome.[37,62,63] Etoposide alone,[64] antithymocyte globulin,[65] and γ-globulin[65–68] also have been used for less severe syndromes.

Disease severity is positively correlated with underlying immune deficiency, chronic active Epstein-Barr virus infection, older age, severe anemia or neutropenia, intravascular coagulation, high cytokine levels, and elevated plasma ferritin, β_2-microglobulin, or serum bilirubin concentration.[37,62]

SINUS HISTIOCYTOSIS WITH MASSIVE LYMPHADENOPATHY (ROSAI-DORFMAN SYNDROME)

DEFINITION AND HISTORY
Sinus histiocytosis with massive lymphadenopathy usually is a self-limited disorder of unknown etiology that first was described in 1969 by Rosai and Dorfman.[69] The disorder principally occurs in the first two decades of life but can occur at any age. The disease is self-limited in the majority of patients. However, it can be recurrent or progressive and can lead to death in some patients.[70,71]

CLINICAL FINDINGS
Signs and Symptoms The typical presentation is characterized by massive bilateral, painless cervical lymphadenopathy, which may be isolated or associated with generalized adenopathy. Early, the nodes may be discrete, but they often progress to adherent, multinodular masses. Axillary and inguinal adenopathy may develop in approximately half of patients. Fever is frequent, and weight loss may occur. Extranodal involvement is present in nearly half of patients, especially in the head and neck region, involving the skin, soft tissue, orbit, eye lids, uvea, lacrimal glands, paranasal sinuses, salivary glands, thyroid, or oral cavity. The respiratory tract, breast, mediastinum, thymus, heart, liver, kidneys, testes, synovia, bone, meninges, and spinal cord also may be involved.[70]

LABORATORY FINDINGS
Blood, Marrow, and Plasma Findings Patients frequently have signs of chronic inflammation, such as anemia, neutrophilia, elevated erythrocyte sedimentation rate, hypoalbuminemia, and polyclonal hypergammaglobulinemia. Marrow examination usually is uninformative, and histiocytic proliferation usually is not present.[70]

Histopathology Excisional biopsy or needle aspiration of a lymph node or an extranodal site can provide specimens for diagnostic study.[70–72] The histopathologic features in the lymph node biopsy, such as marked fibrosis in the capsular and pericapsular areas and distention and engorgement of medullary and subcapsular sinusoids by phagocytic histiocytes, usually are diagnostic. Lymphophagocytosis and

erythrophagocytosis by histiocytes in the lymph node sinus are characteristic.[70] The active phagocyte is a histiocyte that is positive for S-100 protein, CD11c, CD14, CD33, CD68, acid phosphatase, and non-specific esterase.[70,71,73,74] Lymphocytes and plasma cells are prominent in the intersinusoidal spaces. Eosinophils are absent or rare. Later in the disease, continued proliferation can lead to effacement of the node. The histiocytic proliferation is polyclonal.[75] The histopathologic appearance of extranodal biopsies is strikingly similar to that of lymph nodes.

COURSE AND PROGNOSIS
The course of the disease is influenced by the degree of coexistent immune impairment or dysfunction. A significant number of occurrences are seen in children with underlying immunologic disorders, including Wiskott-Aldrich syndrome, autoimmune hemolytic disease, polyarthritis, glomerulonephritis, or severe pneumonia.[70,76,77] In other cases, no specific immune abnormality characterizes the disease.

Lymph node enlargement usually progresses for weeks to months, reaches a maximum, and then gradually recedes so that most patients have little or no residual evidence of disease 9 to 18 months after onset.[70] Some patients have persistent lymphadenopathy but stable disease; other patients have progressive disease and may have a fatal outcome. The latter patients usually have an accompanying immunologic disease and/or widespread nodal involvement that may encroach on vital organs.[70,78]

THERAPY
Most patients require no therapy other than excisional biopsy for diagnosis because the disease runs its course and abates. Glucocorticoids, cytotoxic agents, radiotherapy, and antibiotics have no consistent effect on disease duration.[70,79,80] Surgical excision of masses compromising critical organ function often is successful.[80] Patients with severe or progressive disease have been successfully treated with acyclovir,[81] glucocorticoids,[82,83] IFN-α,[84,85] thalidomide,[86] or combination chemotherapy,[79,87,88] but these approaches do not always result in benefit. No clinical trials have described a treatment algorithm in patients who do not have spontaneous resolution.

CLONAL DISORDERS OF HISTIOCYTOSIS

LANGERHANS CELL HISTIOCYTOSIS

DEFINITION AND HISTORY
Langerhans cells are dendritic cells with irregularly shaped nuclei. They normally are present in the epidermis, oral and vaginal mucosa, and lungs.[89,90] They derive from the hematopoietic stem cells in marrow, as do all other types of macrophages.[91] Langerhans cells differ from other tissue cells in their racquet-shaped ultrastructural inclusions (Birbeck bodies),[92] their content of the β-chain of the neuroprotein S-100,[93] fascin,[94] neuronal-specific enolase,[95] and langerin,[96] and cell surface CD 1a immunoreactivity (Table 72-3).[97,98]

The Langerhans cell is an immature dendritic cell that is a specialized component of the immune accessory cell system. It processes antigens, migrates from the skin to the lymph nodes, transforms to a mature dendritic phenotype, and presents antigen to paracortical T cells. The antigen-presenting cells partially degrade antigen and express peptides on the cell surface in association with human leukocyte antigen (HLA) molecules, making them recognizable to T lymphocytes.[77,89,90,98] The veiled cell of afferent lymphatics may represent a Langerhans cell in transit. After antigen presentation, the Langerhans cell may alter its phenotype to an interdigitating dendritic cell.[77,89,90]

In 1868, Paul Langerhans[99] described the cell in the epidermis. In 1973, the histiocytes (dendritic cells) of "histiocytosis X" were rec-

TABLE 72-3   FEATURES OF LANGERHANS CELLS

Ultrastructural marker
    Birbeck bodies*
Histochemical markers
    α-Naphthyl acetate esterase
    α-Naphthyl butyrate esterase
    Acid phosphate
    Adenosine triphosphatase*
    Adenosine diphosphatase*
    α-D-Mannosidase*
Immunologic markers
    HLA-DR
    Fc receptors
    C3b receptors
    CD1a*
    MT1, KP1, Mac
    Peanut lectin receptor*
    Langerin (CD207)*
Protein markers
    S-100 β-subunit*
    Neuronal-specific enolase*
    Fascin*

* Specific markers for Langerhans cells. Monocytes and macrophages are positive for 5'-nucleotidase, peroxidase, and lysozyme, but Langerhans cells are not.

ognized as having the characteristics of epidermal Langerhans cells.[100] The preferred term *Langerhans cell histiocytosis* should be used for all the eponymic diseases Lichtenstein embraced with the term *histiocytosis X*,[101] including eosinophilic granuloma, Abt-Letterer-Siwe disease, and Hand-Schüller-Christian disease, and several diseases added since the time of his writing, including self-healing histiocytosis, eosinophilic xanthomatous granuloma, pure cutaneous histiocytosis, Langerhans cell granulomatosis, type II histiocytosis, Hashimoto-Pritzker syndrome, eosinophilic xanthomatosis of the normocholesterolemic type, and nonlipid reticuloendotheliosis.

ETIOLOGY AND PATHOGENESIS

The etiology and nature of Langerhans cell histiocytosis have been enigmatic. The syndrome was thought to be inflammatory, with granulomatous, xanthomatous, or fibrotic elements observed during the evolution of the histopathologic lesions. These cellular changes were thought to be the manifestation of an autoimmune process. The cells do not appear malignant, although a high mitotic index is not uncommon. An infectious etiology has not been identified.

A neoplastic etiology was suggested in 1940 based on the x-ray appearance of bone lesions[102] and in 1986 when aneuploidy was demonstrated by flow cytometric study of the DNA content of cutaneous Langerhans cells from a patient.[103] These speculations were proved when molecular studies indicated the proliferating histiocytes represent a monoclonal population. Monoclonality was evident whether the lesions examined were localized or widespread.[104] Thus, the disorder is a neoplasm, which can be localized and nonprogressive or disseminated and progressive but which often behaves like a chronic inflammatory disease, because the cells involved can secrete a variety of inflammatory cytokines inappropriately.[104,105] The loss of E-cadherin expression on Langerhans cells has been associated with dissemination from the skin.[106] The down-regulation of the chemokine CCR6 and up-regulation of CCR7 may favor migration of Langerhans cells from skin to lymph nodes.[107]

Initially the lesions contain many pathologic Langerhans cells. Macrophages, eosinophils, and lymphocytes frequently participate in the formation of granulomatous lesions. Pathologic Langerhans cells express an immature dendritic cell marker CCR6 and overexpress CCL20/MIP-3a, the ligand for CCR6. The lesional Langerhans cells also produce CCL5/Rantes and CXCL11/1TAC. These secretory products set up an autocrine loop that fosters retention of Langerhans cells in the lesion and a paracrine loop that attracts eosinophils and T lymphocytes.[108] The masses proliferate and can be destructive. Later in the course of the disease, the lesions may become less cellular, xanthomatous, and fibrotic.[77,109,110]

The lesions usually involve bone, especially the flat bones of the skull, face, ribs, and pelvis, and the skin, lungs, liver, marrow, lymph nodes, spleen, thymus, central nervous system, and pituitary gland. Occasionally, the gastrointestinal tract is involved.[77,109–111]

EPIDEMIOLOGY

The disease has been reported in siblings and identical twins, but most cases are sporadic. A strong genetic influence is not apparent, consistent with the presumptive neoplastic pathogenesis.[112]

The incidence of Langerhans cell histiocytosis is estimated to be one per 200,000 children. Seventy-five percent of patients are diagnosed before age 10 years and 90 percent before age 30 years. Males are affected more frequently (3:1) by limited or nonprogressive disease. Females and males are affected equally by chronic progressive or fatal disease. Approximately 90 percent of cases with multisystem involvement occur before age 20 years.[113,114]

Patients in Scandinavia with single organ involvement have a significantly higher frequency of HLA-A*03 and a higher occurrence of haplotype HLA-A3*01, B*08, and DRB1*03. The latter haplotype has been associated with immune disorders, such as lupus erythematosus and Graves disease.[115] This haplotype was thought to reduce the risk of multisystem disease.

CLINICAL FINDINGS

Symptoms and Signs Lesions fulfill common histopathologic criteria, but the extent of disease and the clinical features vary.[109–111] The disease may be localized to a bone or to a soft tissue site, multifocal involving only bone, or multifocal involving bone and other sites.[116–118]

The expression of the disease is correlated frequently with the age of the patient at onset. Infants may present with fever, otitis media, or mastoiditis.[119] Enlargement of the liver, spleen, and lymph nodes is frequent. Dermatitis also occurs frequently. The self-limited syndrome benign cephalic histiocytosis can occur during the first year of life. Papules and macules, which reveal a histiocytic infiltrate when biopsied, occur on forehead, ears, and cheeks. They occur elsewhere later and then resolve spontaneously in weeks to months.[120]

Skin lesions can resemble seborrheic, eczematoid, pustular, or nodular dermatitis and often involve the scalp in infants. Tumors limited to the skin can be the sole manifestation of the disease.[121,122] Lesions of the bones or soft tissues of the head and neck are present in greater than 75 percent of children.[123,124] In children and adolescents, pain, tenderness, and swelling in the head, face, leg, back, chest, or groin may be the only evidence of an osteolytic lesion involving the skull, orbit, jaw, femur, vertebra, rib, or pelvis.[116–118] Protrusion of the eye may occur. Gastrointestinal tract involvement in children can result in vomiting, diarrhea, ulceration, and bleeding.[125,126] Hepatic involvement is uncommon.[127,128] Polyuria and polydipsia can signal hypothalamic involvement and the onset of diabetes insipidus (Fig. 72-3).[129–132] Diabetes insipidus occurs in approximately one fourth of cases, usually in patients with multisystem disease and involvement of skull, temporal, or orbital bones, and usually during the course of the disease, not as an initial manifestation.[109,110]

Primary pulmonary involvement, which is rare in children, is seen predominately in male adults.[133,134] Chronic nonproductive cough, chest pain, shortness of breath, and wheezing are the most common symptoms. The presence of greater than 5 percent CD1a-positive cells in bronchoalveolar lavage fluid is evidence favoring pulmonary involvement by Langerhans cell histiocytosis.[135] A lung biopsy can provide definitive histologic evidence of the disease. The radiographic picture initially shows a reticular pattern but can progress to cystic changes.[136–140] Pneumothoraces tend to occur and recur, especially when honeycomb changes are present on the chest x-ray film. Although adult pulmonary Langerhans cell histiocytosis affects middle-aged persons who are almost invariably heavy smokers, the role of smoking is unclear but it may contribute to the initiation of a Langerhans cell tumor. Smoking is not associated with extrapulmonary lesions, and smoking cessation has not affected the course of the disease.[134] Pulmonary disease is associated with an unusually high frequency of pulmonary hypertension. A high prevalence of other pulmonary cancers has been associated with pulmonary histiocytosis.[141] Isolated generalized lymphadenopathy is more common in adults than children.[143] Langerhans cells may occur incidentally in lymphomatous lesions, thus creating a diagnostic problem.[144]

Magnetic resonance imaging has increased the identification of central nervous system involvement. Langerhans cell histiocytosis has a predilection for the hypothalamic-pituitary area. The cerebellum is the second most frequent site of involvement. A late neurologic syndrome that includes cerebellar ataxia occurs in patients years after they appeared to be disease-free.[145] Autopsy studies indicate active disease of neurologic tissue rather than damage from therapy is the usual mechanism. Involvement of the dentate nucleus often is prominent. Space-occupying lesions in gray or white matter may occur. Rare cases of diffuse cerebral involvement occur, although intracranial involvement is limited primarily to the hypothalamus and secondarily to the cerebellum.[146,147]

The female genital tract usually is involved in young women but may become involved in childhood. The ovary, endometrium, cervix, vagina, or vulva may be involved.[148,149] The disease may be localized or represent one site of multicentric involvement. Pregnancy presents special problems in women with Langerhans cell histiocytosis.[150] The most common complication is the onset or exacerbation of diabetes insipidus. Involvement of the vagina, vulva, or pelvic bones may interfere with a normal vaginal delivery. Reactivation of the disease after years of remission has been reported during pregnancy. Reduced fecundity can occur, possibly from hypothalamic-pituitary axis involvement, resulting in decreased gonadotropins and elevated prolactin levels.

In affected adults, the disease involves principally the skin, lungs, bone, pituitary, and lymph nodes. Diabetes insipidus is common.[151,152]

LABORATORY FINDINGS

Neutrophilia, increased sedimentation rate, and increased serum alkaline phosphatase levels may occur. Serum levels of IL-1R antagonist and TNF-α are elevated in patients with multisystem disease.[153] The diagnosis is based on a biopsy of involved organs, especially skin, bone, liver, or lymph node, whichever is most involved and most accessible.[109–111] Imaging studies of bone lesions can be strongly sug-

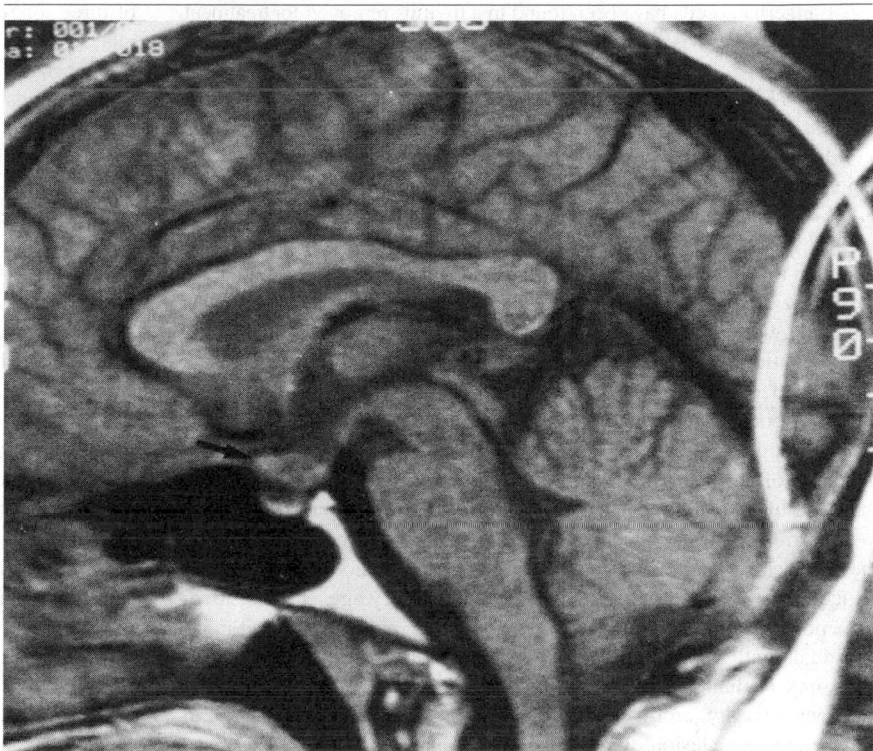

FIGURE 72-3 Magnetic resonance imaging study demonstrating hypothalamic involvement by Langerhans cell histiocytosis. *Arrow* indicates the anterior pole of the greatly enlarged hypothalamic region, expanded by the tumor mass.

gestive of the disease. The key diagnostic feature is the presence of pathologic Langerhans cells, which may be abundant in proliferative lesions or scarce in fibrotic, hypocellular lesions. Giant cells with multiple nuclei resembling osteoclasts are features of the lesion, but they are not derived from Langerhans cells. Marker studies for the presence of S-100, CD1a, langerin, fascin, peanut lectin binding, and adenosinetriphosphatase and ultrastructural studies for Birbeck bodies are used to conclusively identify the Langerhans cells.[77,90,94–107,110,154]

DIFFERENTIAL DIAGNOSIS

The differential diagnosis in adult patients depends on the site of involvement. The differential diagnosis includes a chronic infectious (granulomatous) disease, lymphoma, collagen-vascular disease, pneumoconiosis, and amyloidosis.[109,110] Several diseases associated with proliferative histiocytes not involving Langerhans cells may need to be differentiated from Langerhans cell histiocytosis, including xanthogranuloma,[155] histiocytic necrotizing lymphadenitis (Kikuchi disease),[156] and Erdheim-Chester disease.[157,158] Biopsy specimens from these entities usually can be distinguished by an experienced pathologist using immunophenotyping.

Langerhans cell tumors or sarcomas are discussed in "Tumors of Malignant Histiocytes and Dendritic Cells." They are derived from the same cell and are neoplasms, but in most cases they have different clinical manifestations. However, a gradient exists between Langerhans cell histiocytosis and Langerhans cell tumors, with some overlapping features.

Langerhans cells may be present in the biopsies of patients with solid tumors, Hodgkin or non-Hodgkin lymphoma, or chronic lymphocytic leukemia.[159–166] The focal nature of Langerhans cell lesions and their absence from most other cancers suggest they are a reaction to the lymphoma.[160,167]

Langerhans cells have been found in a thymus removed for treatment of myasthenia gravis[167] and in a variety of dermatologic disorders.[168]

TREATMENT

If possible, physicians treating patients diagnosed with Langerhans cell histiocytosis should access clinical trials through the Histiocytosis Society (www.histio.org/society/).

Spontaneous fluctuations and remissions are features of the disease.[77,109,110,169] Treatment should be considered in patients with symptomatic localized or progressive multifocal disease. However, these generalizations should be amplified by contact with the Histiocytosis Society, which can provide the most effective protocols for an individual patient depending on age and distribution of disease.

Localized disease can be managed by local means in many cases. Isolated bone lesions in the skull, especially the temporal or orbital bones, should be treated systemically (e.g., vinblastine and prednisone) because of the risk of associated neurologic involvement, especially because of the risk of diabetes insipidus. Isolated lymph node disease can be treated by excisional biopsy. Patients with bone lesions should be assessed for pathologic fractures. Curettage, excision,[170] intralesional glucocorticoids,[171] or nonsteroidal antiinflammatory agents can be used, depending on circumstances. Physical exertion may be restricted in individuals with vertebral or other lesions who are at risk for pathologic fractures. Radiation therapy must be individualized according to the size, number, severity, and location of bone lesions.[172–174] Radiotherapy can be used for bone lesions that are painful, are inaccessible, or compromise vital organs or for large lesions in weight-bearing bones.[116,117,169] The usual dose is between 400 and 800 cGy. Grafts may also be required for large lesions in weight-bearing bones. Extension from a vertebra to the spinal cord requires the urgent use of radiation therapy. Bisphosphonates may be useful to decrease bone pain from osteolysis, but these reports have been largely anecdotal.[175]

Localized skin disease can be treated by excisional biopsy, which often is required for diagnosis. Mild skin lesions may respond to topical or interlesional therapy. Use of an aqueous solution of mustine hydrochloride (nitrogen mustard) can be effective and is especially useful in outpatients.[176,177] Psoralen coupled with ultraviolet A light treatment may be the most consistently effective therapy.[178] Intradermal IFN-β has been associated with resolution of skin lesions.[179,180] Glucocorticoids have been used frequently in the past, but they usually are of modest, short-term benefit. High-potency preparations are required for the best results. Radiation therapy should be restricted to local, obstinate lesions, especially if they result in a sinus tract from an underlying visceral lesion. Etoposide, isotretinoin, trimethoprim-sulfamethoxazole, and thalidomide may be useful for skin lesions but require further study. The former may be particularly useful for progressive, multiple sites of skin involvement.[181]

Chemotherapy may be useful for patients with progressive, multisystem disease.[169,182–184] Many agents have been used alone, but few systematic studies of single agents are available. Vinca alkaloids, alkylating agents, purine or pyrimidine antagonists, anthracycline antibiotics, epidophyllotoxins, adenosine deaminase inhibitors, cyclosporine, bisphosphonates (bone pain), and others may be useful single agents. Vinblastine and etoposide are of equivalent effectiveness as single agents.[185] The latter drug has been associated with an increased frequency of secondary acute myelogenous leukemia. Entanercept has been efficacious in a patient with multisystem disease.[186] This utility follows from the high plasma levels of TNF-α in most cases.[153] The distribution of the disease, threat to organ function, rate of progression, and patient age should be considered in deciding on the best approach to therapy. Etoposide can suppress multisystem disease and may have a special role in the treatment of disease in the skin or central nervous system.[173] For progressive multisystem disease, various combinations

of three- or four-drug therapy, given at regular intervals for approximately 6 to 9 months, have been used in a manner akin to treatment of higher-risk lymphomas.[169,183,184] Table 72-4 lists drugs and drug combinations that have been used to ameliorate this disorder.[187–205]

A case of cerebral Langerhans cell histiocytosis in an adult in which the cells were found to express high levels of platelet-derived growth factor-beta (PDGF-β) responded to imatinib mesylate. Given the overexpression of PDGF-β by Langerhans cells. This drug may have frequent applicability in treatment.[253]

In older children and adults, multisystem Langerhans cell histiocytosis often has a relapsing and remitting course and may regress. The decision to use systemic multidrug cytotoxic therapy requires integration of the extent and progression of disease with the potential adverse effects.

Controversy exists as to whether fully established diabetes insipidus requiring desmopressin therapy can be reversed by radiotherapy.[206] Radiotherapy treatment may prevent early partial diabetes insipidus associated with a mass lesion seen by computed tomography or magnetic resonance imaging, but reversal of fully developed diabetes insipidus, although reported, is improbable. Symptomatic therapy with desmopressin is required in virtually all cases.[207]

Blood-component therapy may be required in patients with marrow involvement and cytopenia. If the spleen is grossly enlarged, splenectomy may be useful in patients who require frequent red cell transfusions. Because this complication usually occurs in younger patients, the risk of postsplenectomy infection should be weighed against the risks of long-term, frequent red cell transfusions.

Marrow transplantation has benefited some patients with severe multisystem disease.[197,208,209] Progressive hepatic failure has been treated by liver transplantation.[210] Pulmonary failure has been treated with lung transplantation.

COURSE AND PROGNOSIS

The following factors are associated with a poor prognosis: disease onset during the first 2 years of life, fever not explained by infection, failure to thrive in infants, blood cytopenias, abnormalities of liver function tests, and splenic enlargement. Patients with a serum soluble IL-2R level greater than 17,500 pg/ml had a much shorter median survival than patients with lower levels.[211] A salutary response of multisystem disease to combination chemotherapy within 6 weeks identifies patients who likely will have a good long-term response to therapy. Isolated skin or bone lesions point to a good prognosis. The mortality rate in patients with multisystem disease, especially in those younger than 2 years, remains in the 25 percent range despite therapy.

TABLE 72-4   DRUGS USED FOR PROGRESSIVE LANGERHANS CELL HISTIOCYTOSIS

Bisphosphonates[175,205]

Cladrabine[187–190]

Cyclosporine[191,192]

Deoxycoformycin[193,197]

Etanercept[186]

Etoposide[185,194–196,202]

Imatinib mesylate[253]

Interferon-γ[198,202]

Thalidomide[199–201]

Vinblastine[185]

Vinblastine, etoposide, prednisone, and mercaptopurine or methotrexate[184]

Vincristine, cytarabine, prednisone[203]

Prednisone, etoposide, cyclosporine[204]

* Other drugs added in some cases.

Some patients achieve resolution of disease, and some show marked regression (approximately 50 percent). Others have an intermediate response, with some improvement of existing sites but with development of new sites. Long-term results await the follow-up of ongoing clinical trials.[169]

An association between Langerhans cell histiocytosis and acute lymphocytic leukemia and retinoblastoma is possible.[166] The high frequency of other cancers in patients may be the consequence of chemotherapy.

MALIGNANT TUMORS OF HISTIOCYTES AND DENDRITIC CELLS

DEFINITION AND HISTORY

In 1939, Scott and Robb-Smith[212,213] reported cases of a rapidly fatal disease associated with jaundice, lymphadenopathy, refractory anemia, leukopenia, and often hepatic and splenic enlargement that they called *histiocytic medullary reticulosis*. However, the suspected histiocytic cell proliferation could not be established beyond visual impression. Israels[214] expanded on the clinical description and histopathology and referred to the disease as *giant cell reticulosis*, based on the use of the term *reticulum cells* for large malignant cells that are determined to be either lymphocytes or histiocytes when assessed by more specific immunocytochemical techniques. In 1966, Rappaport[215] introduced the term *malignant histiocytosis* and focused on the nature of the malignant process, which he believed to be an invasive, progressive proliferation of neoplastic histiocytes, again based principally on the resemblance of the proliferating cells to histiocytes by light microscopy.

The introduction of techniques to characterize specific markers of macrophages and the requirement for the absence of immunoglobulin gene and T lymphocyte receptor–chain gene rearrangements before a diagnosis of histiocytic sarcoma can be made have resulted in the reclassification of most cases of malignant histiocytosis as anaplastic large T cell (CD30+) lymphoma or, less frequently, B cell lymphoma, or a tumor without definitive markers.[216–223] An estimated one of 250 cases of lymphoma is a histiocytic or dendritic cell malignancy, based on appropriate criteria.[219,220]

A comprehensive study by the International Lymphoma Study Group used a panel of 15 antibodies to study 61 cases of suspected histiocytic or dendritic cell tumors.[224] These cases could be subclassified into four groups. (1) histiocytic sarcoma (31 percent), (2) Langerhans cell tumor or sarcoma (46 percent), (3) follicular dendritic cell tumor or sarcoma (22 percent), and (4) interdigitating cell sarcoma (1 percent).

EPIDEMIOLOGY

The disease affects all age groups; the age of validated cases ranges from 2 to 74 years. The disease occurs more frequently from the third to the fifth decade of life and occurs more frequently in men than in women.[217,219,222,224,225]

CLINICAL FINDINGS

Signs and Symptoms Fever, headache, weakness, weight loss, dyspnea, and sweating occur commonly in most patients with generalized disease.[222,224–227] Splenomegaly, hepatomegaly, and lymphadenopathy are seen frequently.[222,224–227] Skin, central nervous system, and lung involvement may accompany the aforementioned findings. Localized presentation in the skin, a lymph node group, or the intestines may occur.[222–224,227–234] The appearance of malignant histiocytosis on a background of prior lymphoma may represent a biologic predisposition to progress to other hematolymphoid tumors or reflect a therapy-induced event.[231,232]

LABORATORY FINDINGS

Anemia and thrombocytopenia are common. Neutropenia occurs in the majority of cases, although the white cell count can be elevated. Marrow examination may show infiltration with histiocytic cells, and cytophagocytosis by histiocytes may be evident. The serum lactic dehydrogenase and serum bilirubin levels often are elevated, but liver-derived serum enzyme levels usually are not. Renal function usually is not disturbed.[225] Elevated serum levels of TNF, IL-6, IL-1α receptor, lysozyme, α_1-antitrypsin, and angiotensin-converting enzyme may be found.[225]

DIFFERENTIAL DIAGNOSIS

The diagnosis of malignant histiocytosis requires biopsy of a tumor mass in lymph node, skin, liver, intestine, marrow, or other involved site and verification of the cell phenotype using the markers listed in Table 72-5. The cells should not express T or B lymphocyte markers and should not show rearrangement of lymphoid lineage genes (immunoglobulin or T receptor chains).[224,227,235,236]

The principal diseases that can mimic malignant histiocytosis include anaplastic and other large-cell lymphomas,[219–221,223,227,234,237,238] Hodgkin lymphoma,[227] malignant fibrous histiocytoma (a myofibroblastic tumor),[227] hemangiopericytoma,[227] and inflammatory pseudotumor of lymph nodes.[227]

The malignant histiocytoses are related to other clonal myeloid progenitor cell disorders that express a monocytic or macrophagic phenotype. Variants such as Langerhans cell sarcoma, follicular dendritic cell tumors,[224,230,232] tumors derived from fixed compared to free histiocytes,[238] and leukemic presentation[239–242] or progression[243] of malignant histiocytosis occur, as do localized malignant histiocytomas.[224,244]

TREATMENT, COURSE, AND PROGNOSIS

No systematic multicenter clinical trials using stringent diagnostic criteria have been reported. The infrequency of this tumor makes single-

TABLE 72-5   MORPHOLOGIC AND IMMUNOPHENOTYPIC DISTINCTIONS AMONG MALIGNANT HISTIOCYTIC AND DENDRITIC TUMORS

PHENOTYPIC FEATURE	HISTIOCYTIC SARCOMA (18)	LANGERHANS CELL TUMOR/SARCOMA (26)	FOLLICULAR DENDRITIC CELL TUMOR/SARCOMA (13)	INTERDIGITATING CELL SARCOMA (4)
Birbeck granules	Absent	Present	Absent	Absent
Desmosomes	Absent	Absent	Present	Present
Complex cellular junctions	Absent	Absent	Absent	Present
CD1a	0%	100%	0%	0%
S-100 protein	33%	100%	54%	100%
CD21	0%	0%	100%	0%
CD35	0%	0%	100%	0%
CD68	100%	96%	61%	50%

Parentheses indicate number of cases studied. Desmosomes (syn. macula adherens) are anchoring cell-to-cell junctions that form particularly strong intercellular bonds. Data were taken from Pileri et al., *Histopathology* 41:1, 2002.[224]

center studies of limited value. Four-drug combinations, such as cyclophosphamide, doxorubicin, vincristine, and prednisone; lomustine, vincristine, bleomycin, and prednisone; or mechlorethamine hydrochloride, procarbazine, prednisone, and either vincristine or teniposide given at monthly intervals have been used for patients with generalized disease.[225] The disease has a broad spectrum of expression. Some cases are rapidly progressive, such as Langerhans cell sarcoma. Remissions are not infrequent, and some patients have sustained remission of long duration.[224] A remission duration of greater than 7 years has been reported in two patients.[225] Stem cell transplantation in younger patients with appropriate donors may be useful.[245]

Localized dendritic cell tumors can be excised with or without the use of local irradiation or chemotherapy.[233,234,246] Whether such additional therapy is beneficial is unclear.

MALIGNANT FIBROUS HISTIOCYTOMA AND GIANT CELL TUMOR OF THE BONE

The precise cell of origin of malignant fibrous histiocytoma and giant cell tumor of the bone has been the subject of dispute. A monocyte-macrophage and a fibroblast are the two principal cell types thought to undergo malignant transformation in both tumors. Gene expression profiling and immunophenotyping indicate that both types of malignancy are poorly differentiated fibrosarcomas, myosarcomas, fibromyosarcomas, or liposarcomas, not a type of malignant histiocytosis.[247–250] The histiocytes sometimes present in the tumor are reactive and may result from release of cytokines by the tumor cells that recruit macrophages.[251]

REFERENCES

1. Zelger B, Burgdorf WH: The cutaneous "histiocytoses." *Adv Dermatol* 17:77, 2001.
2. Favara BE, Feller AC, Pauli M, et al: Contemporary classification of histiocytic disorders. *Med Pediatr Oncol* 29:157, 1997.
3. Henter JI, Söder O, Öst Ä, Elinder G: Incidence and clinical features of familial hemophagocytic lymphohistiocytosis in Sweden. *Acta Paediatr Scand* 80:428, 1991.
4. Aricò M, Janka G, Fischer A, et al: Hemophagocytic lymphohistiocytosis: Report of 122 children from the international registry. *Leukemia* 10:197, 1996.
5. Allen M, De Fusco C, Legrand F, et al: Familial hemophagocytic lymphocytosis; how late can the onset be? *Haematologica* 86:499, 2002.
6. Stepp SE, Dufourcq-Lagelouse R, Le Diest F, et al: Perforin gene defects in familial hemophagocytic lymphohistiocytosis. *Science* 286:1957, 1999.
7. Grandsdotter Ericson KG, Fadell B, Nilsson-Ardnor S, et al: Spectrum of perforin mutations in familial hemophagocytic lymphohistiocytosis. *Am J Hum Genet* 68:590, 2001.
8. McCormick J, Flower DR, Strobel S, et al: Novel perforin gene mutations in a patient with hemophagocytic lymphohistiocytosis and CD45 abnormal splicing. *Am J Med Genet* 117A:255, 2003.
9. Grunebaum E, Roifman CM: Gene abnormalities in patients with hemophagocytic lymphohistiocytosis. *Isr Med Assoc J* 4:366, 2002.
10. Cesaro S, Messina C, Sainati L, et al: Del 22Q11.2 and hemophagocytic lymphohistiocytosis; a non-random association. *Am J Med Genet* 116A: 208, 2003.
11. Henter JI: Biology and treatment of familial hemophagocytic lymphohistiocytosis: Importance of perforin in lymphocyte-mediated cytotoxicity and triggering of apoptosis. *Med Pediatr Oncol* 38:305, 2002.
12. Imashuku S, Hyakuna N, Funabiki T, et al: Low natural killer cell activity and central nervous system disease: A high-risk prognostic indicator in young people with hemophagocytic lymphohistiocytosis. *Cancer* 94:3023, 2002.
13. Fadeel B, Orrenius S, Henter J-I: Induction of apoptosis and caspase activation in cells obtained from familial hemophagocytic lymphohistiocytosis patients. *Br J Haematol* 106:406, 1999.
14. Henter J-I, Elinder G, Söder O, et al: Hypercytokinemia in familial hemophagocytic lymphohistiocytosis. *Blood* 78:2918, 1991.
15. Hagasagawa D, Kojima S, Tatusumi E, et al: Elevation of the serum Fas ligand in patients with the hemophagocytic syndrome and Diamond-Blackfan anemia. *Blood* 91:2793, 1998.
16. Imashuka S, Hibi S, Sako M, et al: Soluble interleukin-2 receptor: A useful prognostic factor for patients with hemophagocytic histiocytosis. *Blood* 86:4706, 1995.
17. Fujimara F, Hibi S, Imashuku S: Hypercytokinemia in hemophagocytic syndrome. *Am J Pediatr Hematol Oncol* 15:92, 1993.
18. Osugi Y, Hara J, Tagawa S, et al: Cytokine production regulating Th1 and Th2 cytokines in hemophagocytic lymphohistiocytosis. *Blood* 89: 4100, 1997.
19. Henter J-I: Biology and treatment of familial hemophagocytic lymphohistiocytosis: Importance of perforin in lymphocyte-mediated cytotoxicity and triggering of apoptosis. *Med Pediatr Oncol* 38:305, 2002.
20. Henter J-L, Elinder G, the FHL Study Group of the Histiocyte Society, et al: Diagnostic guidelines for hemophagocytic syndrome. *Semin Oncol* 18:29, 1991.
21. Henter J-L, Nennesmo I: Neuropathological findings and neurological symptoms in 23 children with hemophagocytic lymphohistiocytosis. *J Pediatr* 130:358, 1997.
22. Haddad E, Sulis M-L, Jabado N, et al: Frequency and severity of central nervous system lesions in hemophagocytic lymphohistiocytosis. *Blood* 89:794, 1997.
23. Soffer D, Okon E, Rosen N, Stark B: Familial hemophagocytic lymphohistiocytosis in Israel: II. Pathologic findings. *Cancer* 54:2423, 1984.
24. Aricò M, Allen M, Brusa S, et al: Haemophagocytic lymphohistiocytosis: Proposal of a diagnostic algorithm based on perforin expression. *Br J Haematol* 119:180, 2002.
25. Sung L, Weitzman SS, Petric M, King SM: The role of infections in primary hemophagocytic lymphohistiocytosis: A case series and review of the literature. *Clin Infect Dis* 15:1644, 2001.
26. Rooms L, Fitzgerald N, McClain KL: Hemophagocytic lymphohistiocytosis masquerading as child abuse. *Pediatrics* 111:e636, 2003.
27. Henter J-I, Horne-Samuleson A, Arico M, et al: Treatment of hemophagocytic lymphohistiocytosis with HLH-94 immunotherapy and bone marrow transplantation. *Blood* 100:2367, 2002.
28. Jabado N, de Graeff-Meeder ER, Cavazzana-Calvo M, et al: Treatment of familial hemophagocytic lymphohistiocytosis with bone marrow transplantation from HLA genetically non-identical donors. *Blood* 90: 4743, 1997.
29. Baher KS, De Laat CA, Steinbush M, et al: Successful correction of hemophagocytic lymphohistiocytosis with related or unrelated bone marrow. *Blood* 89:3857, 1997.
30. Dürken M, Finckenstein FG, Janka GE: Bone marrow transplantation in hemophagocytic lymphohistiocytosis. *Leuk Lymphoma* 41:89, 2001.
31. Matthes-Martin S, Peters C, Konigsrainer A, et al: Successful stem cell transplantation following orthotopic liver transplantation from the same haploidentical family donor in a patient with hemophagocytic lymphohistiocytosis. *Blood* 96:3997, 2000.
32. Risdall RJ, McKenna RW, Nesbit ME, et al: Virus associated hemophagocytic syndrome: A benign histiocytic proliferation distinct from malignant histiocytosis. *Cancer* 44:993, 1979.
33. Grateau G, Bachmeyer C, Blanche P, et al: Haemophagocytic syndrome in patients infected with the human immunodeficiency virus: Nine cases and a review. *J Infect* 34:219, 1997.
34. Su I-J, Wang C-H, Cheng A-L, Chen R-L: Hemophagocytic syndrome in Epstein-Barr virus-associated T-lymphoproliferative disorders: Disease spectrum, pathogenesis, and management. *Leuk Lymphoma* 19:401, 1995.

35. Bird G, Peel D, McCarthy K, Williams H: Epstein-Barr virus–induced virus-associated hemophagocytic syndrome and monoclonal TCR-beta rearrangement: A case report. *Hematol Oncol* 15:47, 1997.

36. Chen JS, Tzeng CC, Tsao CJ, et al: Clonal karyotype abnormalities in EBV-associated hemophagocytic syndrome. *Haematologica* 82:572, 1997.

37. Imashuku S: Clinical features and treatment strategies of Epstein-Barr virus-associated hemophagocytic lymphohistiocytosis. *Crit Rev Oncol Hematol* 44:259, 2002.

38. Kawaguchi H, Miyashita T, Herbst H, et al: Epstein-Barr virus–infected T lymphocytes in Epstein-Barr-virus–associated hemophagocytic syndrome. *J Clin Invest* 92:1444, 1993.

39. Lay JD, Tsao CJ, Chen JY, et al: Upregulation of tumor necrosis factor-alpha gene by Epstein-Barr virus and activation of macrophages in Epstein-Barr virus–infected T cells in the pathogenesis of hemophagocytic syndrome. *J Clin Invest* 100:1069, 1997.

40. Risdall RJ, Brunning RD, Hernandez JL, et al: Bacteria-associated hemophagocytic syndrome. *Cancer* 54:2968, 1984.

41. Ningsanond V: Infection associated hemophagocytic syndrome: A report of 50 children. *J Med Assoc Thai* 83:1141, 2000.

42. Tsuda H: Hemophagocytic syndrome (HPS) in children and adults. *Int J Hematol* 65:215, 1997.

43. Palazzi DL, McClainn KL, Kaplan SL: Hemophagocytic syndrome in children: An important diagnostic consideration in fever of unknown origin. *Clin Infect Dis* 36:306, 2003.

44. Takahashi N, Chubachi A, Kume M, et al: A clinical analysis of 52 adult patients with hemophagocytic syndrome: The prognostic significance of the underlying disease. *Int J Hematol* 74:209, 2001.

45. Fisman DN: Hemophagocytic syndrome and infection. *Emerg Infect Dis* 6:601, 2000.

46. Imashuku S: Differential diagnosis of hemophagocytic syndrome: Underlying disorders and selection of most effective treatment. *Int J Hematol* 66:135, 1997.

47. Sakai T, Shiraki K, Deguchi M, et al: Hepatocellular carcinoma associated with hemophagocytic syndrome. *Hepatogastroenterology* 48:1464, 2001.

48. Urban C, Lackner H, Schwinger W, Beham-Schmid C: Fatal hemophagocytic syndrome as initial manifestation of a mediastinal germ cell tumor. *Med Pediatr Oncol* 40:247, 2003.

49. Stark R, Manoharan A: Haemophagocytic syndrome as the primary clinical symptom of acute lymphoblastic leukaemia. *Postgrad Med J* 65:249, 1989.

50. Takahishi N, Miura I, Chubachi A, et al: A clinicopathological study of 20 patients with T/natural killer (NK)-cell lymphoma-associated hemophagocytic syndrome with special reference to nasal and nasal-type NK/T-cell lymphoma. *Int J Hematol* 74:303, 2001.

51. Miyahara M, Sano M, Shibata K, et al: B-cell lymphoma-associated hemophagocytic syndrome. *Ann Hematol* 79:378, 2000.

52. Noguchi M, Kawano Y, Sato N, Oshimi K: T-cell lymphoma of CD3+ CD4+ CD56+ granular lymphocytes with hemophagocytic syndrome. *Leuk Lymphoma* 26:349, 1997.

53. Kojima H, Takei N, Mukai Y, et al: Hemophagocytic syndrome as the primary clinical symptom of Hodgkin's disease. *Ann Hematol* 82:53, 2003.

54. Papo T, Andre MH, Amoura Z, et al: The spectrum of hemophagocytic syndrome in systemic lupus erythematosus. *J Rheumatol* 99:927, 1999.

55. Kumakura S, Ishikura H, Umegae N, et al: Autoimmune-associated hemophagocytic syndrome. *Am J Med* 102:113, 1997.

56. Quesnel B, Catteau B, Aznar V, et al: Successful treatment of juvenile rheumatoid arthritis associated haemophagocytic syndrome by cyclosporin A with transient exacerbation by conventional-dose G-CSF. *Br J Haematol* 97:508, 1997.

57. Ravelli A: Macrophage activation syndrome. *Curr Opin Rheumatol* 14:548, 2002.

58. Pecero VMGR, Marquez RL, Lerchundi MAA, Jurado AF: Phenytoin-induced hemocytophagic histiocytosis indistinguishable from malignant histiocytosis. *South Med J* 84:649, 1991.

59. Takada H, Ohga S, Mizuno Y, et al: Oversecretion of IL-18 in hemophagocytic lymphohistiocytosis syndrome. A novel marker of disease activity. *Br J Haematol* 106:182, 1999.

60. Baker GR, Levin J: Transient thrombocytopenia produced by administration of macrophage colony-stimulating factor: Investigations of the mechanism. *Blood* 91:89, 1998.

61. Chapoval AI, Kamdar SJ, Kremlev SG, Evans R: CSF-1 (M-CSF) differentially sensitizes mononuclear phagocyte subpopulations to endotoxin in vivo: A potential pathway that regulates the severity of gram-negative infections. *J Leuk Biol* 63:245, 1998.

62. Kaito K, Kobayashi M, Ktayama T, et al: Prognostic factors of hemophagocytic syndrome in adults: Analysis of 34 cases. *Eur J Hematol* 59:247, 1997.

63. Imashuku S, Tabata Y, Teramura T, Hibi S: Treatment strategies for Epstein-Barr virus-associated hemophagocytic lymphohistiocytosis (EBV-HLH). *Leuk Lymphoma* 39:37, 2000.

64. Hanai M, Takei M, Yamazaki T, et al: Successful treatment with intermittent administration of etoposide for an adult case with recurrent hemophagocytic syndrome, developed in association with chronic EB virus related lymphoid hyperplasia in the small intestine. *Rinsho Ketsueki* 38:682, 1997.

65. Perel Y, Alos N, Ansoborlo S, et al: Dramatic efficacy of antithymocyte globulins in childhood EBV-associated haemophagocytic syndrome. *Acta Paediatr* 86:911, 1997.

66. Baldwin CL, Noris P, Loni C, Aiosa C: Hemophagocytic syndrome responding to high-dose gammaglobulin as presenting feature of sarcoidosis. *Am J Hematol* 54:88, 1997.

67. Freeman B, Rathore MH, Salman E, et al: Intravenously administered immune globulin for treatment of infection-associated hemophagocytic syndrome. *J Pediatr* 124:332, 1994.

68. Gill DS, Spencer A, Cobcroft RG: High-dose gamma-globulin therapy in the reactive haemophagocytic syndrome. *Br J Haematol* 88:204, 1994.

69. Rosai J, Dorfman RF: Sinus histiocytosis with massive lymphadenopathy: A newly recognized benign clinicopathologic entity. *Arch Pathol* 87:63, 1969.

70. Foucar E, Rosai J, Dorfman R: Sinus histiocytosis with massive lymphadenopathy (Rosai-Dorfman disease): Review of the entity. *Semin Diagn Pathol* 7:19, 1990.

71. Stastny JF, Wilkerson ML, Hamati HF, Kornstein MJ: Cytologic features of sinus histiocytosis with massive lymphadenopathy. *Acta Cytol* 41:871, 1997.

72. Ng WK, Cheung FM: Fine needle aspiration biopsy for definitive diagnosis of sinus histiocytosis with massive lymphadenopathy. *Acta Cytol* 46:1025, 2002.

73. Eisen RN, Buckley PJ, Rosai J: Immunophenotypic characterization of sinus histiocytosis with massive lymphadenopathy. *Semin Diagn Pathol* 7:74, 1990.

74. Paulli M, Rosso R, Kindl S, et al: Immunophenotypic characterization of the cell infiltrate in five cases of sinus histiocytosis with massive lymphadenopathy (Rosai-Dorfman disease). *Hum Pathol* 23:647, 1992.

75. Paulli M, Bergamaschi G, Tonon L, et al: Evidence for a polyclonal nature of the cells infiltrate in sinus histiocytosis with massive lymphadenopathy. *Br J Haematol* 91:415, 1995.

76. Maennle DL, Grierson HL, Gnarra DG, Weissenburger DD: Sinus histiocytosis with massive lymphadenopathy: A spectrum of disease associated with immune dysfunction. *Pediatr Pathol* 11:399, 1991.

77. Favara BE: Langerhans cell histiocytosis: Pathobiology and pathogenesis. *Semin Oncol* 18:3, 1991.

78. Foucar E, Rosai J, Dorfman RF: Sinus histiocytosis with massive lymphadenopathy: An analysis of 14 deaths occurring in a patient registry. *Cancer* 54:1834, 1984.

79. Komp DM: The treatment of sinus histiocytosis with massive lymphadenopathy. *Semin Diagn Pathol* 7:83, 1990.

80. Pulsoni A, Anghel G, Falucci P, et al: Treatment of sinus histiocytosis with massive lymphadenopathy (Rosai-Dorfman) disease): Report of a case and literature review. *Am J Hematol* 69:67, 2002.

81. Baildam EM, D'Souza SW, Stevens RF: Sinus histiocytosis with massive lymphadenopathy (Rosai-Dorfman disease): Response to acyclovir. *J R Soc Med* 85:179, 1992.

82. Sita G, Guffanti A, Colombi M, et al: Rosai-Dorfman syndrome with extranodal localizations and response to glucocorticoids: A case report. *Haematologica* 81:165, 1996.

83. Antonius JI, Farid SM, Baez-Giangreco A: Steroid responsive Rosai-Dorfman disease. *Pediatr Hematol Oncol* 13:563, 1996.

84. Lohr HF, Godderz W, Wolfe T, et al: Long-term survival in a patient with Rosai-Dorfman disease treated with interferon-alpha. *Eur J Cancer* 31A:2427, 1995.

85. Palomera L, Domingo JM, Olave T, et al: Sinus histiocytosis with massive lymphadenopathy: Complete response to low-dose interferon-alpha. *J Clin Oncol* 15:2176, 1997.

86. Viraben R, Dupre A, Gourget B: Pure cutaneous histiocytosis resembling sinus histiocytosis. *Clin Exp Dermatol* 13:197, 1988.

87. Colleoni M, Gaion F, Perasole A, et al: Evidence of responsiveness to chemotherapy in aggressive Rosai-Dorfman disease. *Eur J Cancer* 31A:424, 1995.

88. Horneff G, Jurgens H, Hort W, et al: Sinus histiocytosis with massive lymphadenopathy (Rosai-Dorfman disease): Response to methotrexate and mercaptopurine. *Med Pediatr Oncol* 27:187, 1996.

89. Foucar K, Foucar E: The mononuclear phagocyte and immunoregulatory effector (M-PIRE) system: Evolving concepts. *Semin Diagn Pathol* 7:4, 1994.

90. Chu T, Jaffe R: The normal Langerhans cell and the LCH. *Br J Cancer* 70:S4, 1994.

91. Reid CDL, Fryer PR, Clifford C, et al: Identification of hematopoietic progenitors of macrophages and dendritic Langerhans cells (DL-CFU) in human bone marrow and peripheral blood. *Blood* 76:1139, 1990.

92. Birbeck MS, Breathnach AS, Eversall JD: An electron microscope study of basal melanocytes and high-level clear cells (Langerhans cells) in vitiligo. *J Invest Dermatol* 37:51, 1961.

93. Nakajima T, Watanabe S, Sato Y, et al: S-100 protein in Langerhans cells, interdigitating reticulum cells and histiocytosis X cells. *Gann* 73:429, 1982.

94. Pinkus GS, Lones MA, Matsumura F, et al: Langerhans cell histiocytosis immunochemical expression of fascin, a dendritic cell marker. *Am J Clin Pathol Immunol* 118:335, 2002.

95. Kanitakis J, Fantini F, Pincelli C, et al: Neuron-specific enolase as a marker of cutaneous Langerhans cell histiocytosis. *Anticancer Res* 11:635, 1991.

96. Vallideau J, Ravel O, Dezutter-Dambauyant C, et al: Langerin, a novel C-type lectin specific to Langerhans cells as an endocytotic receptor that induces the formation of Birbeck granules. *Immunity* 12:71, 2000.

97. Emile JF, Wechsler J, Brousse N, et al: Langerhans cell histiocytosis: Definitive diagnosis with the use of the monoclonal antibody 010 on routine paraffin-embedded samples. *Am J Surg Pathol* 19:626, 1995.

98. Hance AJ: Accessory cell-lymphocyte interactions, in *The Lung: Scientific Foundations*, edited by RG Crystal, JB West, p 483. Raven Press, New York, 1991.

99. Langerhans P: Ueber die nerven der menschlichen Haut. *Virchows Arch [A]* 44:325, 1868.

100. Nezelof C, Basset F, Rousseau MF, et al: Histiocytosis X: Histogenetic arguments for a Langerhans' cell origin. *Biomedicine* 18:365, 1973.

101. Lichtenstein L: Histiocytosis X: Integration of eosinophilic granuloma of bone, "Letterer-Siwe disease" and "Schuller-Christian disease" as related manifestations of a single nosologic entity. *Arch Pathol Lab Med* 56:84, 1953.

102. Otani S, Ehrlich J: Solitary granuloma of bone simulating primary neoplasm. *Am J Pathol* 16:479, 1940.

103. Goldberg NS, Bauer K, Rosen ST, et al: Histiocytosis X: Flow analysis. *Arch Dermatol* 122:446, 1986.

104. Willman CL, McClain KL: An update on clonality, cytokines, and viral etiology in Langerhans cell histiocytosis. *Hematol Oncol Clin North Am* 12:407, 1998.

105. deGraaf JH, Egeler RM: New insights into the pathogenesis of Langerhans cell histiocytosis. *Curr Opin Pediatr* 9:46, 1997.

106. Geissman F, Emile JF, Andig P, et al: Lack of expression of E-cadherin is associated with dissemination of Langerhans cell histiocytosis and poor outcome. *J Pathol* 181:301, 1997.

107. Fleming MD, Pinkus JL, Alexander SW, et al: Coincident expression of chemokine receptors CCR6 and CCR7 by pathologic Langerhans cells in Langerhans cell histiocytosis. *Blood* 101:2473, 2003.

108. Annels NE, de Costa CET, Prins FA, et al: Aberrant chemokine receptor expression and chemokine production by Langerhans cell underlies the pathogenesis of Langerhans cell histiocytosis. *J Exp Med* 197:1358, 2003.

109. Komp DM: Langerhans cell histiocytosis. *N Engl J Med* 316:747, 1987.

110. Aricò M, Egeler RM: Clinical aspects of Langerhans cell histiocytosis. *Hematol Oncol Clin North Am* 12:247, 1998.

111. Broadbent V, Egeler RM, Nesbit ME: Langerhans cell histiocytosis: Clinical and epidemiological aspects. *Br J Cancer* 70(suppl):S11, 1994.

112. Aricò M, Nichols K, Whitlock JA, et al: Familial clustering of Langerhans cell histiocytosis. *Br J Haematol* 883, 1999.

113. Carstensen H, Ornvold K: The epidemiology of LCH in Denmark: 1975–1989. *Med Pediatr Oncol* 21:387, 1993.

114. Bhatia S, Nesbit ME, Egeler RM, et al: Epidemiologic study of Langerhans cell histiocytosis in children. *J Pediatr* 130:774, 1997.

115. Fadell B, Henter J-I: Langerhans-cell histiocytosis. Neoplasia or unbridled inflammation? *Trends Immunol* 24:409, 2003.

116. Berry DH, Gresik M, Maybee D, Marcus R: Histiocytosis X in bone only. *Med Pediatr Oncol* 18:292, 1990.

117. Bollini G, Jouve JL, Gentet JC, et al: Bone lesions in histiocytosis X. *J Pediatr Orthop* 11:469, 1991.

118. David R, Orio RA, Kumar R, et al: Radiology features of eosinophilic granuloma of bone. *AJR Am J Roentgenol* 153:1021, 1989.

119. Cunningham MJ, Curtin HD, Jaffe R, Stool SE: Otologic manifestations of Langerhans cell histiocytosis. *Arch Otolaryngol Head Neck Surg* 115:807, 1989.

120. deLuna ML, Flikin I, Golberg J, et al: Benign cephalic histiocytosis. *Pediatr Dermatol* 6:198, 1989.

121. Santhosh-Kumar CR, Almomen A, Ajarim DSS, et al: Unusual skin tumors in Langerhans cell histiocytosis. *Arch Dermatol* 126:1617, 1990.

122. Camacho-Martinez F: Unusual skin tumors in Langerhans cell histiocytes. *Arch Dermatol* 127:1237, 1991.

123. Cochrane LA, Prince M, Clarke K: Langerhans cell histiocytosis in the paediatric population: Presentation and treatment of head and neck manifestations. *J Otolaryngol* 32:33, 2003.

124. DeVaney RO, Putzi MJ, Forlito A, Rinaldo A: Head and neck Langerhans cell histiocytosis. *Ann Otorhinolaryngol* 106:526, 1997.

125. Egeler RM, Schipper MEI, Heymans HSA: Gastrointestinal involvement in Langerhans cell histiocytosis (histiocytosis X). *Eur J Pediatr* 149:325, 1990.

126. Lee RG, Brozial RM, Stenzel P: Gastrointestinal involvement in Langerhans cell histiocytosis. *Mod Pathol* 3:154, 1990.

127. Radin DR: Langerhans cell histiocytosis of the liver: Imaging findings. *AJR Am J Roentgenol* 159:63, 1992.

128. Heyn RM, Hamoudi A, Newton WA Jr: Pretreatment liver biopsy in 20 children with histiocytosis X. *Med Pediatr Oncol* 18:110, 1990.

129. Dünger DB, Broadbent V, Yeoman E, et al: The frequency and natural history of diabetes insipidus in children with Langerhans cell histiocytosis. *N Engl J Med* 321:1157, 1989.

130. O'Sullivan RM, Sheehan M, Poskett KJ, et al: Langerhans cell histiocytosis of hypothalamus and optic chiasm: CT and MR studies. *J Comput Assist Tomogr* 15:52, 1991.

131. Tabarin A, Corcuff J-B, Dautheribes M, et al: Histiocytosis X of the hypothalamus. *J Endocrinol Invest* 14:139, 1991.

132. MacCumber MW, Hoffman PN, Wand GS, et al: Ophthalmic involvement in aggressive histiocytosis X. *Ophthalmology* 97:22, 1990.

133. Nondahl SR, Finlay JL, Farrell PM, et al: A case report and literature review of "primary" pulmonary histiocytosis X of childhood. *Med Pediatr Oncol* 14:57, 1986.

134. Sundar KM, Gosselin MV, Chung HL, Cahill BC: Pulmonary Langerhans cell histiocytosis. *Chest* 123:1673, 2003.

135. Auerswald U, Barth J, Magnussen H: Value of CD-1 positive bronchoalveolar lavage fluid for the diagnosis of pulmonary histiocytosis. *Lung* 169:305, 1991.

136. Brauner MW, Granier P, Mouelki MM, et al: Pulmonary histiocytosis X: Evaluation of high-resolution CT. *Radiology* 172:255, 1989.

137. Brambilla E, Fontaine E, Pison CM, et al: Pulmonary histiocytosis X with mediastinal lymph node involvement. *Am Rev Respir Res* 142:1216, 1990.

138. Moore ADA, Godwin JD, Muller NC, et al: Pulmonary histiocytosis X: Comparison of radiographic and CT findings. *Radiology* 172:249, 1989.

139. Soler P, Kambouchner M, Valeyre D, Hance AJ: Pulmonary Langerhans cell granulomatosis. *Ann Rev Med* 43:105, 1992.

140. Ha SY, Helms P, Fletcher M, et al: Lung involvement in Langerhans' cell histiocytosis: Prevalence, clinical features, and outcome. *Pediatrics* 89:466, 1992.

141. Tomashefski JF, Khiyami A, Kleinerman J: Neoplasms associated with eosinophilic granuloma. *Arch Pathol Lab Med* 115:499, 1991.

142. Motoi M, Helbron D, Kaiserling E, Lennert K: Eosinophilic granuloma of lymph nodes: A variant of histiocytosis X. *Histopathology* 4:585, 1980.

143. Williams JW, Dorfman RF: Lymphadenopathy as the initial manifestation of histiocytosis X. *Am J Surg Pathol* 3:405, 1979.

144. Neumann MP, Fizzera G: The coexistence of Langerhans's cell granulomatosis and malignant lymphoma may take different forms. *Hum Pathol* 17:1060, 1986.

145. Adornato BT, Eil C, Head GL, Lorioux DL: Cerebellar involvement in multifocal eosinophilic granuloma: Demonstration by computerized tomographic scanning. *Ann Neurol* 7:125, 1980.

146. Grois NG, Favera BE, Mostbeck GH, Prayer D: Central nervous system disease in Langerhans cell histiocytosis. *Hematol Oncol Clin North Am* 12:287, 1998.

147. Burn DJ, Watson JDG, Roddie M, et al: Langerhans' cell histiocytosis and the nervous system. *J Neurol* 239:345, 1992.

148. Axiotis CA, Merino MJ, Duray PH: Langerhans cell histiocytosis of the female genital tract. *Cancer* 67:1650, 1991.

149. Otis CN, Fischer RA, Johnson N, et al: Histiocytosis X of the vulva: A case report and review of the literature. *Obstet Gynecol* 75:555, 1990.

150. Ogburn PL, Cefalo RC, Nagel T, Okagahi T: Histiocytosis X and pregnancy. *Obstet Gynecol* 58:513, 1981.

151. Malpas JS: Langerhans cell histiocytosis in adults. *Hematol Oncol Clin North Am* 12:259, 1998.

152. McLelland J, Chu AC: Multisystem Langerhans-cell histiocytosis in adults. *Clin Exp Dermatol* 15:79, 1990.

153. Rosso DA, Ripoli MF, Ray A, et al: Serum levels of interleukin-1 receptor antagonist and tumor necrosis factor-alpha are elevated in children with Langerhans cell histiocytosis. *J Pediatr Hematol Oncol* 25:480, 2003.

154. Hashimoto K, Nagetsu N, Tamguchi Y, et al: Immunohistochemistry and electron microscopy in Langerhans cell histiocytosis confined to skin. *J Am Acad Dermatol* 25:1044, 1991.

155. Nascimento AG: A clinicopathologic and immunohistochemical comparative study of cutaneous and intramuscular forms of juvenile xanthogranuloma. *Am J Surg Pathol* 2:645, 1997.

156. Kumar BN, Walsh RM, Walter NN, Little JT: Histiocytic necrotizing lymphadenitis (Kikuchi's disease) of the cervical lymph nodes. *ORL J Otorhinolaryngol Relat Spec* 59:176, 1997.

157. Shamburek RD, Brewer HB Jr, Gochuico BR: Erdheim-Chester disease: A rare multisystem histiocytic disorder associated with interstitial lung disease. *Am J Med Sci* 321:66, 2001.

158. Kenn W, Eck M, Allolio B, et al: Erdheim-Chester disease: Evidence for a disease entity different from Langerhans cell histocytosis? *Hum Pathol* 31:734, 2000.

159. Burns BF, Colby TV, Dorfman RF: Langerhans' cells granulomatosis (histiocytosis X) associated with malignant lymphomas. *Am J Surg Pathol* 7:529, 1983.

160. Almanaseer IY, Kosova L, Pellettiere EV: Composite lymphoma with immunoblastic features and Langerhans's cell granulomatosis (histiocytosis X). *Am J Clin Pathol* 85:111, 1986.

161. Colby TV, Hoppe RT, Warnke RA: Hodgkin disease: A clinicopathologic study of 659 cases. *Cancer* 49:1848, 1981.

162. Bonetti F, Knowles DM, Chilosi M, et al: A distinctive cutaneous malignant neoplasm expressing the Langerhans's cell phenotype: Synchronous occurrence of B-chronic lymphocytic leukemia. *Cancer* 55:2417, 1985.

163. Favara BE, Jaffe R: The histopathology of Langerhans cell histiocytosis. *Br J Cancer* 70(suppl XXIII):S17, 1994.

164. Shin MS, Buchalter SE, Kang-Jey H: Langerhans histiocytosis associated with Hodgkins disease. *J Natl Med Assoc* 86:65, 1994.

165. Egeler RM, Neglia JP, Pucetti DM, et al: Association of Langerhans histiocytosis with malignant neoplasms. *Cancer* 71:865, 1993.

166. Egeler RM, Neglia JP, Aricò M, et al: The relationship of Langerhans cell histiocytosis to acute leukemia, lymphomas, and other solid tumors. *Hematol Oncol Clin North Am* 12:369, 1998.

167. Bramwell NH, Burns BF: Histiocytosis X of the thymus in association with myasthenia gravis. *Am J Clin Pathol* 86:224, 1986.

168. Goldberg NS: Histiocytosis X. *Arch Dermatol* 122:446, 1986.

169. Broadbent V, Gadner H: Current therapy for Langerhans cell histiocytosis. *Hematol Oncol Clin North Am* 12:327, 1998.

170. Greis PE, Hanken FM: Eosinophilic granuloma: The management of solitary lesions of bone. *Clin Orthop* 257:204, 1990.

171. Wirtschafter JD, Nesbit M, Anderson P, et al: Intralesion methylprednisolone for Langerhans cell histiocytosis of the orbit and cranium. *J Pediatr Ophthalmol Strabismus* 24:194, 1987.

172. El-Sayed S, Brewin TB: Histiocytosis X: Does radiotherapy still have a role? *Clin Oncol* 4:27, 1992.

173. Minehan KJ, Chen MG, Zimmerman D, et al: Radiation therapy for diabetes insipidus caused by Langerhans cell histiocytosis. *Int J Radiat Oncol Biol Phys* 23:519, 1992.

174. Gramatovici R, D'Angio GJ: Radiation therapy in soft-tissue lesions in histiocytosis X (Langerhans cell histiocytosis). *J Med Pediatr Oncol* 16:259, 1988.

175. Farran AP, Zaretski E, Egeler RM: Treatment of Langerhans cell histiocytosis with pamidronate. *J Pediatr Hematol Oncol* 23:54, 2001.

176. Hadfield PJ, Birchall MA, Albert DM: Otitis externa in Langerhans cell histiocytosis: The successful use of topical nitrogen mustard. *Int J Pediatr Otorhinolaryngol* 30:143, 1994.

177. Sheehan MP, Atherton DJ, Broadbeat V, et al: Topical nitrogen mustard: An effective treatment for cutaneous Langerhans cell histiocytosis. *J Pediatr* 119:317, 1991.

178. Sahai H, Ibe M, Takahashi H, et al: Satisfactory remission achieved by PUVA therapy in Langerhans cell histiocytosis in an elderly patient. *J Dermatol* 23:42, 1996.

179. Matsushima Y, Baba T: Resolution of cutaneous lesions of histiocytosis X by intralesional injections of interferon beta. *Int J Dermatol* 30:373, 1991.

180. Jakobson AM, Kreuger A, Harberg H, Sundstrome C: Treatment of Langerhans cell histiocytosis with alpha-interferon. *Lancet* 26:1520, 1987.

181. Munn S, Chu AC: Langerhans histiocytosis of the skin. *Hematol Oncol Clin North Am* 12:269, 1998.

182. Arceci RJ, Brenner MK, Pritchard J: Controversies and new approaches to Langerhans cell histiocytosis. *Hematol Oncol Clin North Am* 12:339, 1998.

183. Ceci A, de Terlizzi M, Collela R, et al: Langerhans cell histiocytosis in childhood: Results from the Italian cooperative AIEOP-CNR-HX83 study. *Med Pediatr Oncol* 21:265, 1993.

184. Gadner H, Heitger A, Grois N, et al: Treatment strategy for disseminated Langerhans cell histiocytosis. *Med Pediatr Oncol* 23:72, 1994.

185. Gadner H, Grois N, Aricò M, et al: A randomized trial of treatment for multisystem Langerhans' cell histiocytosis. *J Pediatr* 138:728, 2001.

186. Henter J-I, Karlen J, Calming U, et al: Successful treatment of Langerhans-cell histiocytosis with etanercept. *N Engl J Med* 345:1577, 2001.

187. Saven A, Burian C: Cladribine activity in adult Langerhans-cell histiocytosis. *Blood* 93:4125, 1999.

188. Stine KC, Saylors RL, Williams LL, Becton DL: 2-Chlorodeoxyadenosine (2-CA) for the treatment of refractory Langerhans cell histiocytosis (LCH) in pediatric patients. *Med Pediatr Oncol* 29:288, 1997.

189. Goh NS, McDonald CE, MacGregor DP, et al: Successful treatment of Langerhans cell histiocytosis with 2-chlorodeoxyadenosine. *Respirology* 8:91, 2003.

190. Rodriguez-Galindo C, Kelly P, Jeng M, et al: Treatment of children with Langerhans-cell histiocytosis with 2-chlorodeoxyadenosine. *Am J Hematol* 69:179, 2002.

191. Minkov M, Grois N, Broadbent V, et al: Immunosuppressive treatment for chemotherapy-resistant multisystem Langerhans cell histiocytosis. *Med Pediatr Oncol* 40:253, 2003.

192. Arico M, Colella R, Conter V, et al: Cyclosporine therapy for refractory Langerhans cell histiocytosis. *Med Pediatr Oncol* 25:12, 1995.

193. McCowage GB, Frush DP, Kurtzberg J: Successful treatment of two children in the Langerhans cell histiocytosis with 2-deoxycoformycin. *J Pediatr Hematol Oncol* 18:154, 1996.

194. Viana MB, Oliveria BM, Silva CM, Leite VHR: Etoposide in the treatment of six children with Langerhans cell histiocytosis (histiocytosis X). *Med Pediatr Oncol* 19:289, 1991.

195. Broadbent V, Pritchard J, Yeomans E: Etoposide (VP16) in the treatment of multisystem Langerhans cell histiocytosis (histiocytosis X). *Med Pediatr Oncol* 17:97, 1989.

196. Mayou SC, Chu AC, Munro DD, et al: Langerhans cell histiocytosis: Excellent response to etoposide. *Clin Exp Dermatol* 16:292, 1991.

197. Arceci RJ: New approaches for patients with Langerhans cell histiocytosis. Available at www.histio.org/society/.

198. Bellmunt J, Albanell J, Salud A, et al: Interferon and disseminated Langerhans cell histiocytosis. *Med Pediatr Oncol* 20:336, 1992.

199. Thomas L, Ducros B, Secchi T, et al: Successful treatment of adult's Langerhans cell histiocytosis with thalidomide. *Arch Dermatol* 129:1261, 1993.

200. Misery L, Larbe B, Lyonnet S, et al: Remission of Langerhans cell histiocytosis with thalidomide treatment [letter]. *Clin Exp Dermatol* 18:48, 1993.

201. Meunier L, March Y, Ribeyre L, et al: Adult cutaneous Langerhans cell histiocytosis: Remission with thalidomide treatment [letter]. *Br J Dermatol* 132:168, 1995.

202. Čulić S, Jakobson Ä, Čulić V, et al: Etoposide as the basic and interferon-a as the maintenance therapy for Langerhans cell histiocytosis: A RTC. *Pediatr Hematol Oncol* 18:291, 2001.

203. Egeler RM, Kraher J, Voûte PA: Cytosine-arabinoside, vincristine, and prednisone in the treatment of children with disseminated Langerhans cell histiocytosis in the organ dysfunction: Experience at a single institution. *Med Pediatr Oncol* 21:265, 1993.

204. Körholz D, Jansen G, Göbel U: Treatment of relapse Langerhans cell histiocytosis by cyclosporine combined with etoposide and prednisone. *Pediatr Hematol Oncol* 14:443, 1997.

205. Kanuzono J, Okada Y, Shirahata A, Tanaka Y: Bisphosphonate induces remission of refractory osteolysis in Langerhans cell histiocytosis. *J Bone Miner Res* 17:1926, 2002.

206. Broadbent V, Pritchard J: Diabetes insipidus associated with Langerhans cell histiocytosis. *Med Pediatr Oncol* 28:289, 1997.

207. Katsas GA, Fowles TB, Evanson J, et al: Hypothalamic-pituitary abnormalities in adult patients with Langerhans cell histiocytosis. *J Clin Endocrinol Metab* 85:1370, 2000.

208. Storb R, Sanders JE, Petersen FB: Marrow transplantation for treatment of multisystem progressive Langerhans cell histiocytosis. *Bone Marrow Transplant* 10:39, 1992.

209. Morgan G: Myeloablative therapy and bone marrow transplantation for Langerhans cell histiocytosis. *Br J Cancer* 70(suppl XXIII):S52, 1994.

210. Concepcion W, Esquirel CO, Terry A, et al: Liver transplantation in Langerhans cell histiocytosis. *Semin Oncol* 18:24, 1991.

211. Rosso DA, Roy A, Zelasko M, Braier JL: Prognostic value of soluble interleukin 2 receptor levels in Langerhans cell histiocytosis. *Br J Haematol* 117:54, 2002.

212. Scott RB, Robb-Smith AHT: Histiocytic medullary reticulosis. *Lancet* ii:194, 1939.

213. Robb-Smith AHT: Before our time: Half a century of histiocytic medullary reticulosis: A T-cell teaser? *Histopathology* 17:279, 1990.

214. Israels MCG: The reticuloses: A clinicopathologic study. *Lancet* ii:526, 1953.

215. Rappaport H: Tumors of the hemopoietic system, in *Atlas of Tumor Pathology*, p 49. Armed Forces Institute of Pathology, Washington, DC, 1966.

216. Weiss LM, Trela MJ, Cleary ML, et al: Frequent immunoglobulin and T cell receptor rearrangements in "histiocytic" neoplasms. *Am J Pathol* 121:369, 1985.

217. Wright DH: Histiocytic malignancies, in *Malignant Lymphomas*, edited by JA Habeshaw, I Lauder, p 217. Churchill-Livingstone, Edinburgh, 1988.

218. Cattoretti G, Villa A, Vezzoni P, et al: Malignant histiocytosis: A phenotypic and genotypic investigation. *Am J Pathol* 136:1009, 1990.

219. Wilson MS, Weiss LM, Gatter KC, et al: Malignant histiocytosis: A reassessment of cases reported in 1975 based on paraffin section immunophenotyping studies. *Cancer* 66:530, 1990.

220. Aozasa K, Ohsawa M, Saeki K, et al: Histiocytic neoplasms: Immunohistochemical evaluation of their frequencies among malignant lymphoma and related conditions in Japan. *J Surg Oncol* 47:215, 1991.

221. Ornvold K, Carstensen H, Junge J, et al: Tumors classified as "malignant histiocytosis" in children are T-cell neoplasms. *APMIS* 100:558, 1992.

222. Lauritzen AF, Delsol G, Hansen NE, et al: Histiocytic sarcomas and monoblastic leukemias. *Am J Clin Pathol* 102:45, 1994.

223. Egeler RM, Schmitz L, Sonneveld P, et al: Malignant histiocytosis: A reassessment of cases formerly classified as histiocytic neoplasms and review of the literature. *Med Pediatr Oncol* 25:1, 1995.

224. Pileri SA, Grogan TM, Harris NL, et al: Tumours of histiocytes and accessory dendritic cells: An immunochemical approach to classification

from the International Lymphoma Study Group based on 61 cases. *Histopathology* 41:1, 2002.

225. Sonneveld P, VanLom K, Kappers-Klunne M, et al: Clinicopathological diagnosis and treatment of malignant histiocytosis. *Br J Haematol* 75:511, 1990.

226. Kemelow OW, Gocke CD, Kell DL, et al: True histiocytic lymphoma: A study of 12 cases based on current definition. *Leuk Lymphoma* 18:81, 1995.

227. Sun W, Nordberg ML, Fowler MR: Histiocytic sarcoma involving the central nervous system. *Am J Surg Pathol* 27:258, 2003.

228. Milchgrub S, Kamel OW, Wiley E, et al: Malignant histiocytic neoplasms of the small intestines. *Am J Surg Pathol* 16:11, 1992.

229. Patrizi A, Pileri S, Rivano MT, Di Lernia V: Malignant histiocytosis presenting as erythroderma. *Int J Dermatol* 29:214, 1990.

230. Hollowood K, Stamp G, Zouvani I, Fletcher CD: Extranodal follicular dendritic cell sarcoma of the gastrointestinal tract. *Am J Clin Pathol* 103:90, 1995.

231. Chan JK, Tsang WY, Ng CS, et al: Follicular dendritic cell tumors of the oral cavity. *Am J Surg Pathol* 18:148, 1994.

232. Miettinen M, Fletcher CDM, Lasota J: True histiocytic lymphoma of the small intestines. *Am J Clin Pathol* 100:285, 1993.

233. Osborne BM, Mackay B: True histiocytic lymphoma with multiple skin nodules. *Ultrastround Pathol* 18:241, 1994.

234. Fonesca R, Tefferi A, Strickler JG: Follicular dendritic cell sarcoma mimicking diffuse large cell lymphoma: A case report. *Am J Hematol* 55:148, 1997.

235. Soslow RA, Davis RE, Warnke RA, et al: True histiocytic lymphoma following therapy for lymphoblastic neoplasms. *Blood* 87:5207, 1996.

236. Rodilla CM, Acenero JF, Mayor LP, Carmona AA: True histiocytic lymphoma as a second neoplasm in a follicular centroblastic-centrocytic lymphoma. *Pathol Res Pract* 193:319, 1997.

237. Bucksky P, Favera B, Feller AC, et al: Malignant histiocytosis and large cell anaplastic (Ki-1) lymphoma in childhood: Guidelines for differential diagnosis. Report of the Histiocyte Society. *Med Pediatr Oncol* 22:200, 1994.

238. Hsu S M, Ho Y S, Hsu P-L: Lymphomas of true histiocytic origin. *Am J Pathol* 138:1389, 1991.

239. Laurencet FM, Chapuis B, Roux-Lombard P, et al: Malignant histiocytosis in the leukaemic stage: A new entity (M5c-AML) in the FAB classification? *Leukemia* 8:502, 1994.

240. Santiago-Schwartz F, Coppock DL, Hindenberg AA, Kern J: Identification of a malignant counterpart of the monocytic-dendritic cell progenitor in an acute myeloid leukemia. *Blood* 84:3054, 1994.

241. Srivastava HI, Srivastava A, Srivastava MD: Phenotype, genotype and cytokine production in acute leukemia involving progenitors of dendritic Langerhans' cells. *Leuk Res* 18:499, 1994.

242. Ohno T, Sugiyama T, Furukawa H, et al: Malignant histiocytosis associate with autoimmune thrombocytopenia. *Am J Hematol* 45:244, 1994.

243. Esteve J, Rozman M, Campo E, et al: Leukemia after true histiocytic lymphoma: Another type of acute monocytic leukemia with histiocytic differentiation (AML-M5c)? *Leukemia* 9:1389, 1995.

244. Lauritzen AF, Ralfkiaer E: Histiocytic sarcoma. *Leuk Lymphoma* 18:73, 1995.

245. Kao W-Y, Hwang W-S: Bone marrow transplantation for malignant histiocytosis. *Transplant Proc* 24:1524, 1992.

246. Misery L, Godard W, Hamzeh H, et al: Malignant Langerhans cell tumor: A case with a favorable outcome associated with absence of blood dendritic cell proliferation. *J Am Acad Dermatol* 49:527, 2003.

247. Chibon F, Mariani O, Mairal A, et al: The use of clustering software for the classification of comparative genomic hybridization data, an analysis of 109 malignant fibrous histiocytomas. *Cancer Genet Cytogenet* 141:75, 2003.

248. Lee YF, John M, Edwards S, et al: Molecular classification of synovial sarcomas, leiomyosarcomas and malignant fibrous histiocytomas by gene expression profiling. *Br J Cancer* 24:510, 2003.

249. Gazziola C, Cordani N, Wasserman B, et al: Malignant fibrous histiocytoma: A proposed cellular origin and identification of its characterizing gene transcripts *Int J Oncol* 23:343, 2003.

250. Hasegawa T, Hasegawa F, Hirose T, et al: Expression of smooth muscle markers in so called malignant fibrous histiocytomas. *J Clin Pathol* 56:666, 2003.

251. Mantovani A. The interplay between primary and secondary cytokines: Cytokines involved in the regulation of monocyte recruitment. *Drugs* 54(suppl 1):15, 1997.

252. Grunebaum E, Rifman CM: Gene abnormalities in patients with hemophagocytic lymphohistiocytosis. *Isr Med Assc J* 4:366, 2002.

253. Montella L, Insabato L, Palmieri G: Imatinib mesylate for cerebral Langerhan's-cell histiocytosis. *N Eng J Med* 351:1034, 2004.

254. Billiau AD, Roskams T, van Damme-Lombaerts R, et al: Macrophage activation syndrome. *Blood* 105:1648, 2005.

LIPID STORAGE DISEASES

ERNEST BEUTLER

Gaucher disease and Niemann-Pick disease are the two lipid storage disorders that are most likely to be encountered by the hematologist, because both may cause splenomegaly and cytopenias. Gaucher disease is the most common of the lipid storage diseases. It is most prevalent among Ashkenazi Jews, in whom the disease genotype occurs at a rate of approximately one per 1000 births. Deficiency of the enzyme glucocerebrosidase results in accumulation of the glycolipid glucocerebroside in the cells of the macrophage-monocyte system. Patients with the common type 1 disease have no primary neurologic symptoms, but the central nervous system is involved in type 2 and type 3 disease. Diagnosis of Gaucher disease depends upon demonstration of a deficiency of glucocerebrosidase, an acid β-glucosidase, or of mutations of the glucocerebrosidase gene. Disease manifestations include hepatosplenomegaly, thrombocytopenia, anemia, osteoporosis and infarctive bone lesions, and, uncommonly, pulmonary lesions. Many patients with type 1 disease do not require treatment, particularly those who are homozygous for the common Jewish mutation 1226C→G (N370S). For those who have sufficiently severe disease manifestations, the replacement of the missing enzyme by infusions is an effective and safe, but very costly, therapy. The administration of Miglustat, an inhibitor of glucocerebroside synthesis, is also effective in reducing disease manifestations. Splenectomy corrects the thrombocytopenia that commonly occurs in Gaucher disease. Diphosphonates have been used to treat bone involvement. The prognosis for patients with type 1 disease is usually excellent, but a small proportion of the patients are severely affected; there is generally little or no progression in adults.

Niemann-Pick disease is a heterogeneous group of disorders. Type A and B disease result from deficiency of the enzyme sphingomyelinase, while types C, D, and E result from a mutation in the *NPC1* or *NPC2* gene, genes that appear to be involved with cholesterol trafficking; not only sphingomyelin but also cholesterol accumulates in these disorders. Type A disease is associated with severe neurologic disease, and patients general die during the first few years of life. Type B disease has a later onset, and neurologic disease is usually absent. Type C disease is associated with neurologic symptoms and often hepatosplenomegaly. There is currently no treatment for Niemann-Pick disease, but some patients have benefited from liver transplantation. The sea-blue histiocyte syndrome is a heterogeneous group of disorders, characterized by the presence in the marrow of macrophages that contain granules that stain a bright blue color. These cells are found in some patients with Niemann-Pick disease and are occasionally seen in a variety of hematologic disorders.

Acronyms and abbreviations that appear in this chapter include: cDNA, complementary DNA.

DEFINITIONS AND HISTORY

The lipid storage diseases are hereditary disorders in which one or more tissues become engorged with a lipid. The type of lipid and its distribution have a characteristic pattern in each disorder; this chapter deals only with those disorders in which lipid storage in the macrophages causes major clinical manifestations. These disorders are Gaucher disease, in which glucocerebroside is stored, and Niemann-Pick disease, in which the storage material is sphingomyelin and/or cholesterol.

GAUCHER DISEASE

HISTORY

Gaucher disease was first described by Philippe Gaucher, who thought that the peculiar large cells in the spleen were evidence of a primary neoplasm.[1] Although it was believed at one time that the glycolipid that accumulated in Gaucher disease was a galactocerebroside, it was shown in 1934 that glucocerebroside accumulated.[2] In 1965, the primary defect was recognized as the inability to degrade glucocerebroside.[3,4]

EPIDEMIOLOGY

Gaucher disease is inherited as an autosomal recessive disorder. It is most common in the Ashkenazi Jewish population, in which the gene frequency is 0.034.[5] Thus, approximately 6.8 percent of the Jewish population is heterozygous for Gaucher disease, and the expected birth frequency is 1:1000. Gaucher disease is also relatively common in a population isolate in Norrbottnia in Northern Sweden.[6]

Gaucher disease, Niemann-Pick disease, and Tay-Sachs disease all occur with elevated frequencies among Ashkenazi Jews. The high frequency of these genes is almost certainly the result of some advantage enjoyed by heterozygotes, analogous to that found in sickle cell anemia and glucose-6-phosphate dehydrogenase deficiency among African and Mediterranean peoples (see Chaps. 45 and 47). The basis for such a possible heterozygote advantage in Gaucher disease is unknown.

ETIOLOGY AND PATHOGENESIS

ENZYMATIC BASIS OF LYSOSOMAL STORAGE DISEASES

In the course of normal growth, development, and senescence, parts of cells or whole cells are continually replaced in all tissues. Breakdown of the complex constituents of cells requires sequential, enzymatic degradation. Such degradation takes place largely in secondary lysosomes, organelles formed by the fusion of primary lysosomes with the phagocytic vacuole containing the ingested material.

Gaucher disease is the result of a hereditary deficiency in the activity of one of the lysosomal enzymes required for glycolipid degradation, *viz.*, glucocerebrosidase. The parent substance is either a globoside or a ganglioside (Fig. 73-1). In the degradation of globosides and gangliosides, it is necessary for the carbohydrate portion to be removed before hydrolysis of the sphingosine–fatty acid complex ceramide. Removal of carbohydrate always proceeds from the free end of the polysaccharide chain: the distal glycosidic linkage must be cleaved with removal of the terminal sugar before the other glycosidic linkages can be enzymatically hydrolyzed. In the glycolipid storage diseases, the hereditary lack of a lysosomal enzyme required for hydrolysis of one of the glycosidic bonds results in the accumulation of the glycolipid that serves as a substrate for the missing enzyme. As shown in Fig. 73-1, the absence of the β-glucosidase that cleaves glucocerebroside (glucocerebrosidase) will result in accumulation of glucocerebroside. Storage of this glycolipid results in Gaucher disease.

While Gaucher disease is almost always characterized by a deficiency of β-glucocerebrosidase, a lysosomal β-glucosidase,[7] in very

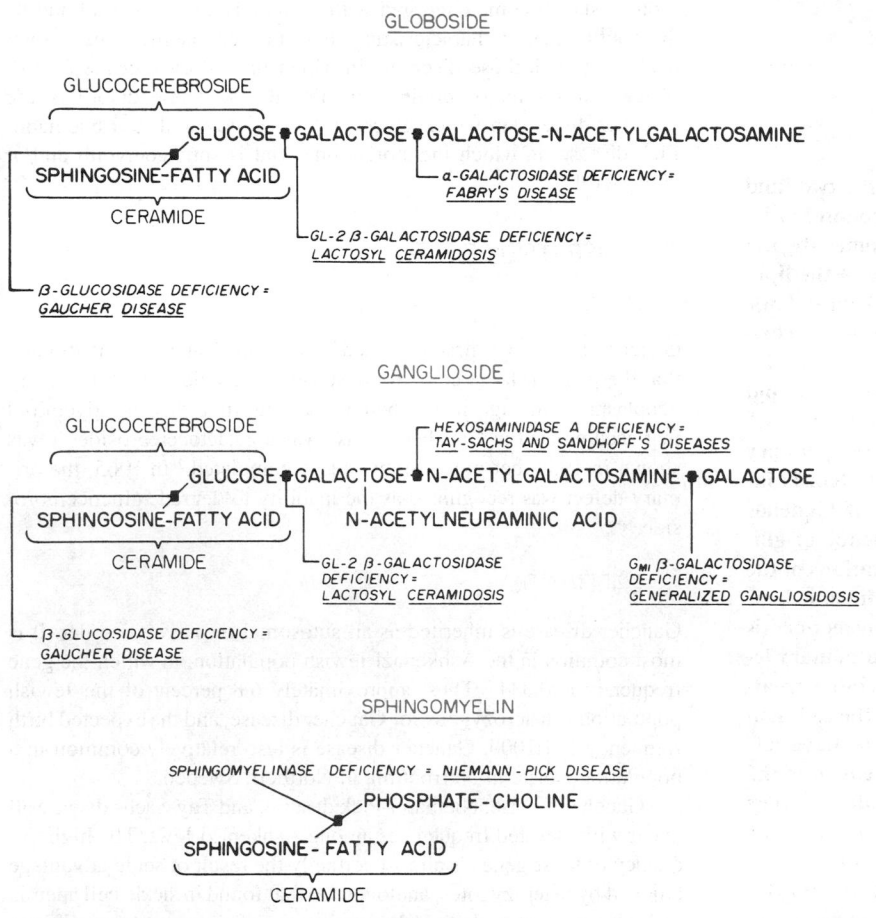

GLOBOSIDE

GLUCOCEREBROSIDE

GLUCOSE ● GALACTOSE ● GALACTOSE-N-ACETYLGALACTOSAMINE

SPHINGOSINE-FATTY ACID

CERAMIDE

└── α-GALACTOSIDASE DEFICIENCY = *FABRY'S DISEASE*

└── GL-2 β-GALACTOSIDASE DEFICIENCY = *LACTOSYL CERAMIDOSIS*

└── β-GLUCOSIDASE DEFICIENCY = *GAUCHER DISEASE*

GANGLIOSIDE

GLUCOCEREBROSIDE

HEXOSAMINIDASE A DEFICIENCY = *TAY-SACHS AND SANDHOFF'S DISEASES*

GLUCOSE ● GALACTOSE ● N-ACETYLGALACTOSAMINE ● GALACTOSE

SPHINGOSINE-FATTY ACID   N-ACETYLNEURAMINIC ACID

CERAMIDE

└── GL-2 β-GALACTOSIDASE DEFICIENCY = *LACTOSYL CERAMIDOSIS*

G_{MI} β-GALACTOSIDASE DEFICIENCY = *GENERALIZED GANGLIOSIDOSIS*

└── β-GLUCOSIDASE DEFICIENCY = *GAUCHER DISEASE*

SPHINGOMYELIN

SPHINGOMYELINASE DEFICIENCY = *NIEMANN-PICK DISEASE*

PHOSPHATE-CHOLINE

SPHINGOSINE-FATTY ACID

CERAMIDE

FIGURE 73-1   Structure of some of the lipids involved in lipid storage diseases. *Solid squares* indicate the bonds that fail to be cleaved in the diseases specified. The globosides are sometimes designated GL-1, GL-2, etc., the number designating the number of sugar residues attached to ceramide. There are many systems of nomenclature for the gangliosides; the designation G_{M2} is commonly applied to the ganglioside that accumulates in Tay-Sachs disease.

rare instances a severe neuronopathic form of the disease occurs as a result of a deficiency of saposin, a heat-stable glucocerebrosidase cofactor.[8]

GENETIC BASIS OF GAUCHER DISEASE

The glucocerebrosidase gene is located on chromosome 1. A pseudogene has been identified approximately 16 kB downstream from the functional gene. Well over 100 mutations causing Gaucher disease have been described[9] (see *http://www.tau.ac.il/~racheli/genedis/gaucher/gaucher.html#point__89*). Most of these are point mutations, but one very common mutation represents the insertion of a single guanine at nucleotide (nt) 84 of the cDNA. Deletions, gene fusion events, and gene conversions involving the pseudogene also have been documented. In the Ashkenazi Jewish population, the predominant mutation is at cDNA nucleotide 1226, where it causes a Asp→Ser substitution at amino acid 370 (N370S). This mutation accounts for approximately 75 percent of the mutant alleles in Jewish patients and approximately 30 percent of the alleles in non-Jewish patients. It is relatively mild, both with respect to the amount of residual enzyme that can be detected in cells of affected individuals and in its phenotypic effect. A frameshift mutation resulting in the insertion of a guanine nucleotide at nt84 is also common in the Jewish population and is phenotypically much more severe. The five most common mutations account for approximately 97 percent of the alleles in the Jewish pop-

ulation but only for approximately 75 percent of the alleles in the non-Jewish population.[5,10,11] The common mutation in the Norrbottnian population (see "Epidemiology" above) is at nt1448, and this mutation, which represents the normal pseudogene sequence, is also common in other ethnic groups.

CLINICAL FEATURES

Three major types of Gaucher disease have been differentiated clinically.[7] All are characterized by mutations of the gene encoding glucocerebrosidase, deficiency of glucocerebrosidase, and accumulation of glucocerebroside, but they are clinically quite distinct; patients with at least one "mild" mutation have type 1 disease, while those who have only "severe" or "null" mutations will generally inherit type 2 or type 3 disease.[12] Type 1 ("adult") Gaucher disease occurs in children as well as in adults but is clearly differentiated from type 2 (acute infantile neuronopathic) and type 3 disease by the absence of primary neurologic symptoms. Type 2 disease is exceedingly rare, does not occur predominantly in Jewish families, and is characterized by rapid neurologic deterioration and early death. Type 3 (juvenile) Gaucher disease is a less well-defined subacute neuronopathic disorder with later onset of neurologic symptoms and a better prognosis than the acute infantile neuronopathic type. The prototype of this type of the disease is the Norrbottnian form of the disorder.[6] Type 3 disease has been subdivided into three further subtypes: a, b, and c.

The clinical manifestations of Gaucher disease are produced by the accumulation of Gaucher cells (Fig. 73-2), glucocerebroside-laden macrophages, in spleen, liver, and marrow and the reaction of the body to these cells. In type 2 and type 3 disease, storage of glycolipid also occurs in the brain.

There is enormous variability in the severity of all types of Gaucher disease. Type 1 disease may be entirely asymptomatic, discovered in the course of a population survey[5] or accidentally in the course of investigation of an unrelated hematologic disorder. In those patients who do have clinical manifestations, the spleen may be barely palpable, or it may be massively enlarged and produce symptoms, both as a result of its great bulk and by sequestering formed elements of the blood. Chronic fatigue is a common complaint. Hepatic enlargement, like splenic enlargement, may cause mechanical symptoms, and liver fibrosis accompanied by functional abnormalities and varices may develop. In children, growth retardation is common. Severe pulmonary disease with cyanosis and clubbing occurs in some patients with advanced liver involvement, probably because of shunting through the lung secondary to the liver disease. Direct involvement of the lungs with Gaucher cells also has been observed.[13,14] Pulmonary hypertension occurs in some patients and has been noted particularly after enzyme replacement therapy has been initiated.[15–19] Contrariwise, it has been suggested that pulmonary hypertension is more common in untreated patients.[20] Mild pulmonary hypertension as documented by Doppler echocardiography is present in many Gaucher disease patients, and splenectomy seems to be a risk factor for developing severe pulmonary hypertension.[20]

Skeletal lesions are often widespread. Patchy areas of bone demineralization and areas of infarction are found, and widening of the distal femur gives rise to a typical "Erlenmeyer flask" deformity opacities, and cardiac valve calcification, but generally have little visceral disease.

Neoplastic disorders are somewhat more common in patients with Gaucher disease than in the general population.[38] Especially notable are lymphoproliferative diseases, including chronic lymphocytic leukemia,[27,39–41] multiple myeloma,[42–46] lymphoma,[47] and Hodgkin lymphoma.[48,49] The existence of monoclonal immunoglobulin spikes in the serum also has been documented in a high proportion of patients

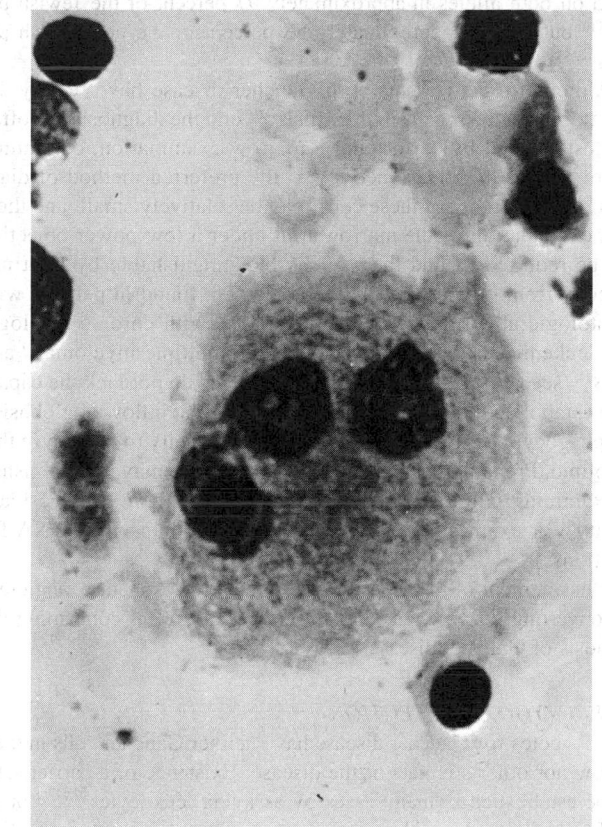

FIGURE 73-2   Gaucher disease cell from the marrow (×915).

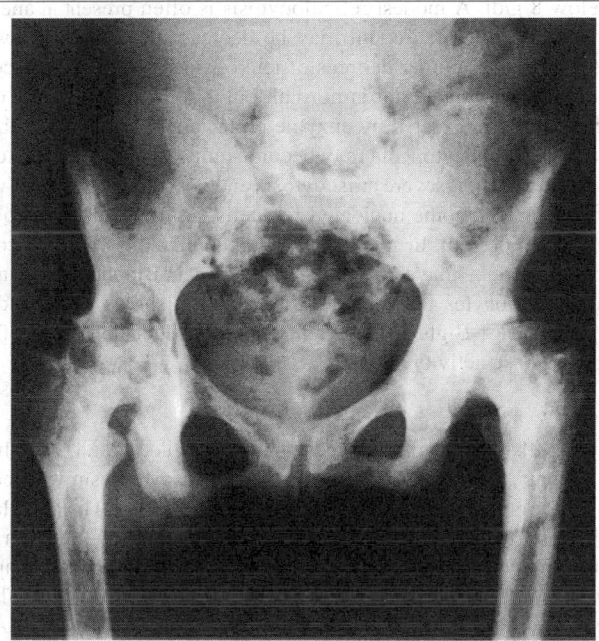

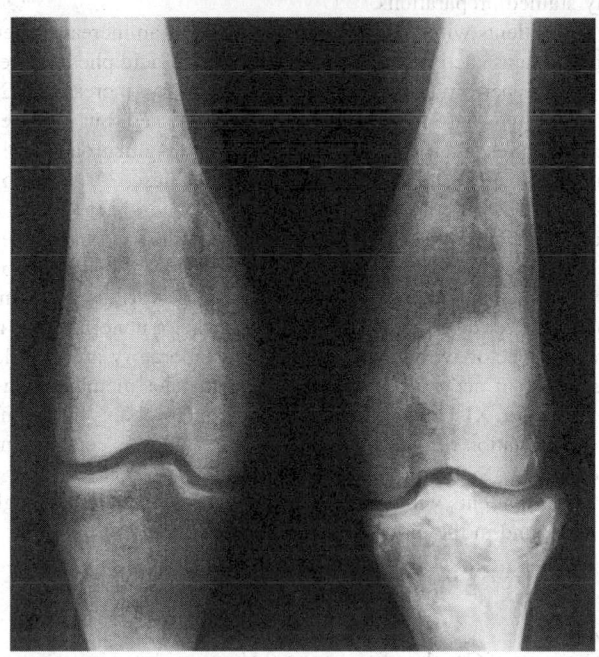

FIGURE 73-3   X-ray films of distal femora and pelvis of a 27-year-old woman with Gaucher disease. The distal femur shafts are flared with thinning bone trabeculae, scattered sclerotic zones, and bone infarcts. The most extensive changes are seen in the left tibia proximally. The pelvis and upper femurs demonstrate extensive cystic and sclerotic changes with collapse of both femoral heads and of the right acetabulum. (X-ray films courtesy of Dr. Hyman Gildenhorn, City of Hope Medical Center.)

(Fig. 73-3). Various markers of bone metabolism have suggested that bone resorption predominates,[21] but the mechanism underlying the development of bone lesions is poorly understood. Bone pain is probably the most troublesome clinical manifestation of Gaucher disease. Pain may occur anywhere. It generally has a deep, somewhat dull character and may be very severe. Bone pain may occur in areas with no involvement detectable by x-ray examination. It may last for weeks or months but usually subsides spontaneously, only to reappear later in the same or in another location. Aseptic necrosis of the femoral heads and vertebral collapse are particularly common, crippling complications.[22,23]

Many organs other than the liver, spleen, and bones may be affected. Brownish masses of Gaucher cells have been reported to occur at the corneoscleral limbus of the eye.[24] Gaucher cells have been found in a colonic polyp[25] and the maxillary sinus.[26] Fever may occur in patients in whom a meticulous search fails to reveal evidence of infection, often[27,28] but not always[29] in connection with bone crises,[27,28] and hypermetabolism has been documented.[30] Severe neonatal ichthyosis ("collodion babies") has been described in infants with acute neuronopathic Gaucher disease.[31]

Neurologic symptoms are the hallmark of type 2 and type 3 disease. Particularly notable are oculomotor abnormalities, hypertonia of the neck muscles with extreme arching of the neck (opisthotonus), bulbar signs, limb rigidity, seizures, and sometimes choreoathetoid movements. Patients with type 3a disease[32] have progressive neurologic disease dominated by myoclonus and dementia; those with type 3b disease[32] have aggressive visceral and skeletal disease, but with neurologic manifestations largely limited to horizontal supranuclear gaze palsy; those with type 3c disease[33–37] have neurologic manifestations largely limited to horizontal supranuclear gaze palsy, corneal with Gaucher disease older than 50 years.[50–53] Cohort control studies showed that the risk of hematologic neoplasms in Gaucher disease patients was 14.7 (confidence limits 5.2–41.7) times that of controls.[54]

LABORATORY FEATURES

BLOOD

The blood of patients with Gaucher disease may be normal or may manifest effects of hypersplenism. A normocytic, normochromic anemia is frequently present, but hemoglobin levels only uncommonly fall below 8 g/dl. A modest reticulocytosis is often present in anemic patients. The white cell count may be decreased to levels as low as $1000/\mu l$, although milder degrees of leukopenia are much more common. The differential count is normal, but a defect of leukocyte chemotaxis[55] that is corrected by enzyme replacement therapy[56] has been reported. Thrombocytopenia may become quite severe. If splenectomy has been carried out, severe anisocytosis and poikilocytosis occur, with many target cells, some nucleated red cells, and Howell-Jolly bodies usually being present. In splenectomized patients, the white cell count and platelet count may be higher than normal. Biochemical examination of leukocytes for β-glucosidase activity shows a severe deficiency of a pH 4 β-glucosidase and a much milder deficiency of pH 5 β-glucosidase activity.[57,58]

GAUCHER CELLS

Gaucher cells, found mainly in the marrow, spleen, and liver, have small, usually eccentrically placed nuclei and cytoplasm with characteristic crinkles or striations (see Color Plate IX-5). The cytoplasm is stained by the periodic acid–Schiff technique (PAS). Electron microscopy reveals that the cytoplasm contains spindle- or rod-shaped, membrane-bound inclusion bodies 0.6 to 4 μm in diameter. These bodies appear to consist of numerous small tubules 130 to 750 Å in diameter that are seen to be composed of twisted multilayers in negatively stained preparations.[59,60]

Most patients with Gaucher disease manifest an increase in serum acid phosphatase activity. Since measurement of acid phosphatase activity can be performed in any clinical laboratory, increased activity of this acid hydrolase is the one most often detected, but activities of other hydrolases, such as β-hexosaminidase,[61] β-glucuronidase,[61] angiotensin-converting enzyme,[61] and chitotriosidase,[59,60] are also increased in the serum of most patients with Gaucher disease. The latter may be a particularly sensitive indicator of disease activity, since the percentage increase of chitotriosidase is greater than that of the other analytes. When liver involvement is extensive, various biochemical stigmata of liver disease, including clotting factor abnormalities, may be present. Factor IX deficiency may be a laboratory artifact related to the effect of accumulated lipid on the platelet membrane on the assay.[62] Factor XI deficiency is common but probably represents a chance association of two disorders, each of which is common in the Ashkenazi Jewish population.[63]

In older patients with Gaucher disease, monoclonal immunoglobulins are found in the plasma more frequently than expected.[50,51]

DIFFERENTIAL DIAGNOSIS

DIAGNOSIS

The diagnosis of Gaucher disease should be considered in patients with splenomegaly, particularly if the splenomegaly has been present for an extended period of time. The definitive diagnosis is established by determining leukocyte[57] or cultured fibroblast[64] β-glucosidase activity or by demonstrating the presence of known Gaucher mutations in the patient's DNA. The latter method of diagnosis can usually establish the diagnosis in Jewish patients but cannot exclude it: if the DNA is examined for the most common five mutations, mutations will be detected on both alleles in approximately 97 percent of the Jewish patients[10] but in only approximately 55 percent of the non-Jewish patients.[65,66]

Although most patients with Gaucher disease have readily demonstrable Gaucher cells in their marrow and the diagnosis has often been established by performing a marrow examination, determination of the β-glucosidase activity is the preferred method of diagnosis.[65] The number of these cells may be relatively small, and thorough examination of the marrow film under a low-power objective may be required to find them. Cells indistinguishable by light microscopy from typical Gaucher cells also are found in patients with hematologic abnormalities, including those with chronic myelogenous leukemia,[67,68] Hodgkin lymphoma,[69] multiple myeloma,[70] and AIDS[71] (see Color Plate IX-6). These patients do not lack the capacity to catabolize glucocerebroside,[72] but the great inflow of globoside into phagocytic cells exceeds their normal capacity to hydrolyze this glycolipid. Prenatal diagnosis of Gaucher disease may be established by examining cultured amniocentesis cells for their β-glucosidase activity[64] or examining amniocentesis or chorionic villus DNA for mutations.

Measurement of the activity of serum acid phosphatase, angiotensin-converting enzyme, or chitotriosidase is useful in confirming the diagnosis of Gaucher disease.

HETEROZYGOTE DETECTION

Heterozygotes for Gaucher disease have neither Gaucher cells in their marrow nor other stigmata of the disease. Existence of a carrier state can be established in many cases by assaying leukocytes[57,73,74] or fibroblasts[64] for β-glucosidase activity and demonstrating the reduction in the activity of the enzyme to approximately half of normal. However, regardless of the method used, there is an overlap between the measured enzyme activity in heterozygous individuals and the normal range. Definitive diagnosis of the heterozygous state can only be established by DNA analysis.

THERAPY

SYMPTOMATIC TREATMENT

Thrombocytopenia and leukopenia in Gaucher disease are more frequently the consequence of hypersplenism than of marrow replacement by Gaucher cells. These cytopenias respond very satisfactorily to splenectomy. However, with the availability of enzyme replacement therapy, splenectomy is considered as a therapeutic option much less frequently. The pathophysiology of Gaucher disease suggests that splenectomy be avoided as long as possible. The body must continue to metabolize all of the globoside that is formed; after the spleen has been removed, the glucocerebroside that accumulates as the result of incomplete globoside metabolism is deposited in the liver and marrow. Bone lesions may progress more rapidly following surgical removal of the spleen,[75–77] but this impression is difficult to quantitate and cannot be verified experimentally, and no worsening of bone lesions after splenectomy could be documented in one study.[38] Conservatism is advised, however, in recommending splenectomy. Partial splenectomy has been introduced in an attempt to preserve a glycolipid-sequestering site.[78] The results of such surgery have been reported in a number of patients,[79–88] without conclusive data being obtained regarding the merits of the procedure.[89]

When bone lesions result in fractures, orthopedic procedures may be required. Hip replacement surgery is often successful, allowing some severely incapacitated patients to return to normal activity. Radiation therapy has been credited with relief of bone pain.[90,91] However, radiotherapy more often fails to produce a satisfactory response[92,93] and therefore is not recommended.

Liver transplantation has been carried out in a few patients with severe hepatic failure.[94–97]

ENZYME REPLACEMENT

Enzyme replacement therapy for Gaucher disease has been attempted intermittently since the middle 1970s[98–101] but did not become successful until the commercial production of enzyme was undertaken. Alglucerase (Ceredase) is a mannose terminated form of the enzyme extracted from placenta. It has been replaced by imiglucerase (Cerezyme), the recombinant product. The removal of sugars to expose inner mannose residues was designed to take advantage of the mannose receptor of macrophages to target the enzyme. However, alglucerase and presumably imiglucerase are inefficiently taken up by macrophages, both in vivo and in vitro. A calcium-independent mannose receptor, distinct from the classic mannose receptor found on macrophages, is ubiquitously present in large numbers in many tissues and probably binds most of the enzyme in vivo.[102]

Nonetheless, the response to enzyme replacement therapy is gratifying.[103–110] Decrease in the size of the liver and spleen and increase in the hemoglobin levels of anemic patients and the platelet levels of patients with thrombocytopenia occur within 6 months in most of the patients. The platelet count of patients with massively enlarged spleens often requires a longer period of therapy to respond, and in some patients there is sufficient splenic scarring that no appreciable response occurs.[111] Response of bony lesions is much slower than that of visceral lesions, but improvement may be evident after treatment for approximately 2 years, regardless of the dose that is used.[106,112–115] The expense of enzyme replacement therapy is daunting, particularly when administered on the high dose/low frequency schedule (60 U/kg every 2 weeks) recommended by the manufacturer and by some investigators.[116] Enzyme alone, given on this schedule to an average adult, costs one-half million dollars per year. Giving enzyme infusions one to three times weekly requires much less enzyme and therefore is much more economical. One unit per kilogram every day or 2.3 U/kg three times weekly has been shown to be fully as effective as a dose more than four times as large given every 2 weeks.[107] This greater effectiveness of small doses is expected for a preparation for which a few high-affinity and many lower-affinity receptors compete. Moreover, the intracellular life span of the administered enzyme is very short, so that infrequent administration provides therapeutic levels for only a very small proportion of the time. Even half of this dose was found to be fully effective in most or all patients.[117,118] The practicality and effectiveness of frequent administration of enzyme replacement have been questioned,[119,120] but the results obtained have been amply confirmed,[106–108,121,122] and home therapy with enzyme has been shown to be feasible and safe.[123]

In view of the very high cost and inconvenience of enzyme replacement therapy and that, as with any treatment, there are unknown risks, the treatment should be reserved for patients with at least moderately severe disease. These would include patients with marked organomegaly, severe or moderately severe cytopenias, or extensive skeletal involvement. The criteria should be broadened somewhat for children younger than 15 years, since, unlike adults, they may have progressive disease. At present, imiglucerase therapy of the many patients who have clinically mild disease cannot be endorsed. The recommended starting dose for patients who do need treatment is 3.75 to 7.5 U/kg body weight given weekly.

MARROW TRANSPLANTATION

Because the macrophage is a descendant of the hematopoietic stem cell, allogeneic marrow transplantation might be expected to cure Gaucher disease. This has, indeed, been accomplished several times.[6,124–131] Although some enthusiasm has been expressed for this approach,[126] the very considerable short-term risk of marrow transplantation markedly limits the number of patients who might be suitable candidates for this therapeutic approach. The availability of effective enzyme replacement therapy further limits the appropriateness of marrow transplantation. However, because of its lower cost and the potential for cure, transplantation may occasionally be considered for the management of severe Gaucher disease and for patients with type 3 disease. The visceral disease in the latter patients responds quite well to enzyme replacement, but the response of neurologic disease is less clear.[132,133]

INHIBITORS OF GLUCOCEREBROSIDE SYNTHESIS

The amount of glucocerebroside accumulating in macrophages represents the balance that is achieved between the rate of synthesis and the rate of degradation. The possibility that decreasing the formation of glucocerebroside from ceramide and glucose might favorably affect the disease was proposed in the 1970s.[134] Among a number of potential inhibitors, only Miglustat (N-butyldeoxynojirimycin, Zavesca, Vevesca) has undergone clinical evaluation and has been licensed for the treatment of Gaucher disease in patients unwilling or unable to receive enzyme replacement therapy. Inhibiting glucocerebroside synthesis has been somewhat euphemistically designated as "substrate balance therapy"[135] or perhaps more accurately as substrate reduction therapy.[136–140] Miglustat is effective in reducing the size of the liver and spleen of patients with Gaucher disease when given at an initial dose of 100 mg three times daily with as much as 300 mg three times a day given to some patients.[141] The response is dose sensitive, and some improvement, although suboptimal, has been documented with a dose as low as 50 mg given three times daily.[135] The convenience of oral treatment is undeniable, but a number of toxic side effects have been ascribed to Miglustat. These include diarrhea, which usually subsides with continued treatment, weight loss, peripheral neuropathies, and tremor. The neurologic symptoms appear to be reversible with discontinuation of therapy, and since some patients with type 1 Gaucher disease have neurologic symptoms not primarily related to Gaucher disease,[142] the cause and effect relationship is not always clear.

OTHER THERAPIES

Autologous transplantation after gene transfer into hematopoietic cells has received considerable attention as a possible alternative form of therapy.[143–147] Despite some exaggerated claims, there is no credible evidence of benefit to any patient; in vivo studies showed that a minimal number of cells carried the transgene.[148]

Decreasing globoside inflow by repeated phlebotomy has not yielded clinically significant results,[149] probably because most of the glucocerebroside is formed from sequestered white cells. Splenic transplantation was attempted in one patient, without success.[150]

Bone disease appears to respond to the administration of biphosphonates such as aminohydroxypropylidene bisphosphonate (pamidronate).[151–153] In fact, the response to this form of treatment seems to be more rapid than that achieved by enzyme replacement. Orally administered treatment with alendronate disodium has been found in a double-blind study to be effective in decreasing osteopenia in Gaucher disease patients.[154]

A new approach to the treatment of lysosomal storage diseases is the use of "chaperone therapy." This type of treatment depends upon the assumption that some of the mutant enzymes misfold and are destroyed in their passage through the endoplasmic reticulum to the lysosomes. Under these circumstances, a loosely binding inhibitor may stabilize the enzyme so that it can reach the lysosomes, the inhibitor then diffusing away from the enzyme.[155] A subinhibitory concentration of N-(n-nonyl)deoxynojirimycin leads to a twofold increase in the activity of the N370S mutant enzyme in the cultured fibroblasts from a homozygote. Interestingly, the N-butyl derivative, the compound that is effective as an inhibitor of glucocerebroside synthesis, does not appear to have any chaperoning effect on the N370S mutant.

COURSE AND PROGNOSIS

The age of onset, severity of clinical manifestations, and degree of progression are related to the genotype of the patient. Patients with the 1226G/1226G (N370S/N370S) genotype tend to have late-onset disease (Fig. 73-4), relatively mild manifestations, and virtually no progression of disease during adult life. In contrast, patients who have the 1226G (N370S)/84GG, 1226G (N370S)/1448C (N 444P), and 1226G (N370S)//IVS2(+1) genotypes tend to have much earlier onset of disease, usually in the first decade of life, and show gradual progression even during adult life.[113,156] Patients who are homozygous for the 1448C mutation generally develop neurologic symptoms, but some possible exceptions have been noted.[157,158]

Although the genotype of the patient does provide a guide to the prognosis, there is, unfortunately, much variability among patients with the same genotype—even between sibs. Other, as yet unknown genetic or environmental factors are important in determining the actual course of the disease in an individual patient. However, whatever the genotype, the severity of the disease does not change after early childhood.[113,156,159] Progression, when it does occur, is gradual, except, of course insofar that complications such as aseptic necrosis and collapse of vertebrae may represent acute events.

In severely affected patients with type 1 disease or those with type 3 disease, death may occur as a result of liver disease, bleeding, or sepsis. In type 2 disease, death usually results from the neurologic manifestations and occurs in the first or second year of life. This type of disease can be fatal in the perinatal period.[160] The fact that no patient homozygous for the 84GG mutation has ever been encountered in spite of the relative high frequency with which this mutation occurs in the Jewish population suggests that a total lack of glucocerebrosidase may not be compatible with extrauterine life. This deduction is supported by the fact that a "knockout" mouse that has been deprived of a gene for glucocerebrosidase is not capable of extrauterine life.[161]

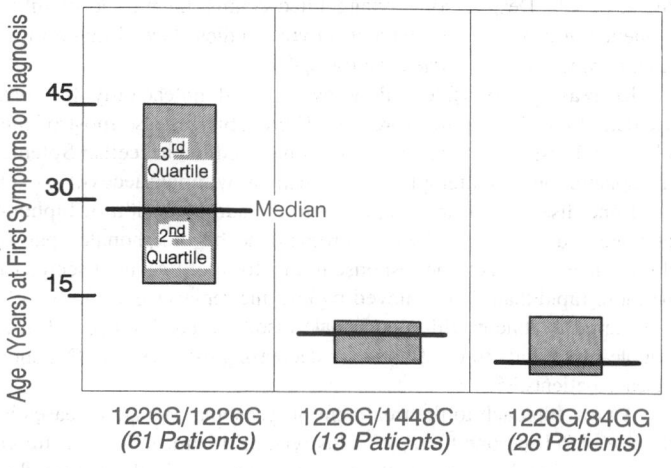

FIGURE 73-4 Median and second and third quartiles of the distribution of the age at first symptoms or diagnosis of Gaucher disease in patients with three different genotypes. (Permission from *Science.* Beutler, E. Gaucher disease: New molecular approaches to diagnosis and treatment. *Science* 256:794–799, 1992).

NIEMANN-PICK DISEASE

HISTORY AND CLASSIFICATION

Niemann, a Berlin pediatrician, reported the case of an infant who died at age 18 months with a disorder that seemed to be unique because of its early onset and rapid course, which seemed atypical for Gaucher disease.[162] The predominant phospholipid accumulating in this disorder is sphingomyelin. In 1966, a deficiency of sphingomyelinase activity was demonstrated in a patient with Niemann-Pick disease.[163] However, there is not a single Niemann-Pick disease but rather a group of disorders that are related in that sphingomyelin storage occurs. Type A and type B disease, the classic forms of the disorder, are the results of mutations in the sphingomyelinase gene and represent an infantile neuropathic and a later-onset non-neuronopathic form, respectively.[164] Type C, the most common form of Niemann-Pick disease, is a neuronopathic disorder, usually with onset in early childhood, that results from an abnormality in cholesterol transport.[165] The sphingomyelinase gene is normal in type C disease, but mutations occur in one of two genes that have been designated *NPC1* and *NPC2*. The designation *type D disease* was once applied to a population isolate in Nova Scotia,[165] but with the demonstration that these individuals also had a *NPC1* mutation, this term is no longer used.

EPIDEMIOLOGY

Type A and type B Niemann-Pick disease occur more frequently among people with Ashkenazi Jewish ancestry than in the general population.[166] There are no reliable data regarding either the prevalence or ethnic predilection of patients with type C disease, except for the fact that there is an isolate in Nova Scotia with a high prevalence.[165,167]

ETIOLOGY AND PATHOGENESIS

Type A and type B disease are autosomal recessive diseases caused by mutations of the gene for sphingomyelinase,[168–170] required to cleave the bond between ceramide and phosphorylcholine (see Fig. 73-1). Nonsense mutations seem to cause the more severe type A disease, while missense mutations are found in the milder type B disorder.[168] Although sphingomyelinase is believed to be a part of an apoptosis-signaling pathway by generating ceramide from sphingomyelin,[171] no relationship between the disease manifestations and this pathway has been established.

Type C disease also shows autosomal recessive inheritance and is caused by mutations in either the *NPC1*[172,173] or *NPC2*[173] gene, the function of which is not fully understood but that presumably plays a role in intracellular cholesterol transport and homeostasis.[173,174] The *NPC1* mutations account for more than 95 percent of the cases.[175] A naturally occurring murine model of the disease exists.[176]

PATHOLOGY AND CLINICAL MANIFESTATIONS

The most characteristic histopathologic feature of the various forms of Niemann-Pick disease is the presence of foam histiocytes (Fig. 73-5) (see Color Plate IX-4). These cells are found mainly in lymphoid tissues, but they may be present throughout the body. The foam cells contain largely sphingomyelin and cholesterol, the storage of cholesterol being more prominent in type C disease.

Type A Niemann-Pick disease is an affliction of infancy. During the first months of life, affected infants gain weight poorly, the abdomen enlarges, and development is delayed. They usually do not learn to sit and lose those capabilities already achieved. They may become blind and deaf. Some infants have a protracted course of jaundice of unknown cause. During the second year of life, the child lies

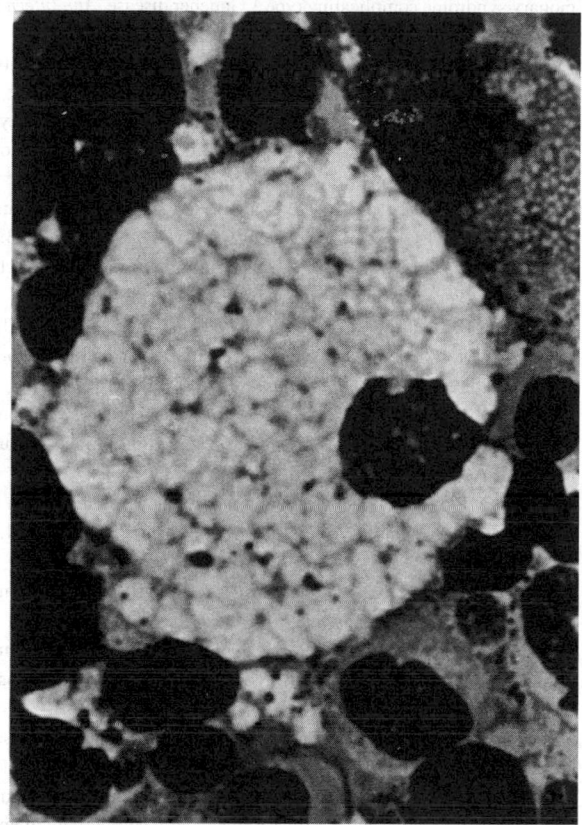

FIGURE 73-5 Foam cell from the marrow of a patient with Niemann-Pick disease (×875).

still with nearly flaccid hyporeflexic extremities, an abdomen enlarged with enormous spleen and liver, mild lymphadenopathy, and often a fine xanthomatous rash. Bone lesions may be present but are less prominent than in Gaucher disease.

Patients with type B disease generally present in the first decade of life with hepatosplenomegaly, but in mild cases abnormalities may not be noted until adult life. Neurologic manifestations are usually absent; pulmonary infiltrates are common. Sea-blue histiocytes are sometimes found in the marrow, and a number of patients have been diagnosed as having sea-blue histiocytosis before a deficiency in sphingomyelinase was demonstrated to be present.[177]

Patients with type C disease often have neonatal jaundice, develop normally in early childhood, and then develop dementia, ataxia, dysarthria, dystonia, and seizures. Hepatosplenomegaly is often, but not always, present.[165] This form of the disease can present at any age, even the seventh decade.[178]

LABORATORY FEATURES AND DIFFERENTIAL DIAGNOSIS

The hemoglobin concentration of the blood may be normal, or mild anemia may be present. Typically, approximately 75 percent of the blood lymphocytes contain one to nine vacuoles. These measure approximately 2 μm in diameter. Electron microscopy reveals that these vacuoles are lipid-filled lysosomes.[179]

The marrow contains typical foam cells ranging from 20 to 100 μm in diameter and containing small droplets throughout the cytoplasm (see Fig. 73-5). The cytoplasm of these cells stains only very faintly with the periodic acid-Schiff reagent. Phase microscopy of unstained preparations clearly reveals droplets in the cytoplasm of Niemann-Pick foam cells that distinguish them from Gaucher cells. In

polarized light the droplets may be birefringent, and in ultraviolet light they manifest a greenish-yellow fluorescence.[180] Foam cells resembling those seen in Niemann-Pick disease also are observed in generalized gangliosidosis, and foamy histiocytes, primarily involving the bone, are seen in the rare Erdheim-Chester disease, a non-Langerhans form of histiocytosis.[181] Occasionally the storage cells in Gaucher disease may present a somewhat vacuolated appearance and thereby may be misinterpreted. The occurrence of sea-blue histiocytes in the spleen and marrow has been documented.[177,182–184]

Type A and type B Niemann-Pick disease can be distinguished from other disorders by identification of the lipid as sphingomyelin and by demonstration of sphingomyelinase deficiency in leukocytes or cultured fibroblasts. Heterozygotes may be detected by measurement of sphingomyelinase activity of cultured fibroblasts.[185] Prenatal diagnosis by amniocentesis has been achieved.[185,186] An artificial substrate that is very useful for measurement of sphingomyelinase activity has been introduced,[187,188] but its reliability has been questioned.[189] In type C disease, studies of cholesterol uptake by cultured fibroblasts are diagnostic[190] but cumbersome and not readily available. The identification of the *NPC1* and *NPC2* genes has facilitated the diagnosis of type C disease.

TREATMENT

There is no effective treatment for Niemann-Pick disease. Splenectomy is only rarely required, because death usually occurs from other manifestations of the disease before hypersplenism becomes clinically important. Liver transplantation was carried out with encouraging results.[96] Repeated implantations of amniotic epithelial cells as a source of exogenous sphingomyelinase has been claimed to be associated with clinical improvement.[191] In mice, infusion of enzyme had a corrective effect on visceral but not neurologic manifestations of the disease.[192]

COURSE AND PROGNOSIS

The prognosis in type A Niemann-Pick disease is very poor; death nearly always occurs before the third year of life.[164] Patients with type B disease may survive into childhood or adult life.[164] Patients with type C disease usually die in the second decade of life,[165] but some patients with mild disease live out a normal life span.[178]

SEA-BLUE HISTIOCYTE SYNDROME

HISTORY

According to Sawitsky and colleagues,[193] Moeschlin, in his 1947 book on splenic puncture, described a 29-year-old man with unexplained splenomegaly whose spleen contained macrophages with closely packed granules colored deep azure blue with May-Grünwald stain. He named these *blauen pigmentmakrophagen* (blue pigment macrophages) (see Color Plate IX-9). These cells have subsequently been found in marrow as well as spleen, and in 1954 Sawitsky and colleagues[194] suggested that two cases they observed and Moeschlin's might represent a syndrome.

ETIOLOGY AND PATHOGENESIS

Although sea-blue histiocytes are found in Niemann-Pick disease, presumably particularly in the type B disorder, sea-blue histiocytes are also found in patients who do not have any well-defined disorder. They have been reported in the marrow of patients with immune thrombocytopenic purpura,[195] in patients receiving parenteral nutrition,[196] and in patients with chronic myelogenous leukemia,[197] as well as patients with Niemann-Pick disease.[182–184,198,199]

CLINICAL FEATURES

In patients without other underlying disorders, the sea-blue histiocyte syndrome is often characterized by hepatosplenomegaly and thrombocytopenia and usually by a mild chronic course. Most patients are below the age of 40 when diagnosed, and there is usually not a clear family history.[193]

THERAPY, COURSE, AND PROGNOSIS

There is no treatment except that which can be offered for the underlying disease. In cases associated with parenteral nutrition, there has been improvement when the dose was decreased. In those cases in which there is no known cause, the course is generally a chronic, stable one.[193]

REFERENCES

1. Gaucher PCE: De l'epithelioma primitif de la rate, hypertrophie idiopathique del la rate san leucemie. University of Paris, 1882.
2. Aghion H: *La maladie de Gaucher dans l'enfance [PhD Thesis]*. Paris, 1934.
3. Brady RO, Kanfer JN, Shapiro D: Metabolism of glucocerebrosides: II. Evidence of an enzymatic deficiency in Gaucher's disease. *Biochem Biophys Res Commun* 18:221, 1965.
4. Patrick AD: Short communications: A deficiency of glucocerebrosidase in Gaucher's disease. *Biochem J* 97:17C, 1965.
5. Beutler E, Nguyen NJ, Henneberger MW, et al: Gaucher disease: Gene frequencies in the Ashkenazi Jewish population. *Am J Hum Genet* 52:85, 1993.
6. Svennerholm L, Erikson A, Groth CG, et al: Norrbottnian type of Gaucher disease—Clinical, biochemical and molecular biology aspects: Successful treatment with bone marrow transplantation. *Dev Neurosci* 13:345, 1991.
7. Beutler E, Grabowski G: Gaucher disease, in: *The Metabolic and Molecular Bases of Inherited Disease*, edited by CR Scriver, AL Beaudet, WS Sly, D Valle, p 3635. McGraw-Hill, New York, 2001.
8. Schnabel D, Schröder M, Sandhoff K: Mutation in the sphingolipid activator protein 2 in a patient with a variant of Gaucher disease. *FEBS Lett* 284:57, 1991.
9. Beutler E, Gelbart T: Hematologically important mutations: Gaucher disease. *Blood Cells Mol Dis* 24:2, 1998.
10. Beutler E, Gelbart T, Kuhl W, et al: Mutations in Jewish patients with Gaucher disease. *Blood* 79:1662, 1992.
11. Beutler E, Gelbart T: Gaucher disease mutations in non-Jewish patients. *Br J Haematol* 85:401, 1993.
12. Beutler E, Gelbart T, Demina A, et al: Five new Gaucher disease mutations. *Blood Cells Mol Dis* 21:20, 1995.
13. Smith RL, Hutchins GM, Sack GH Jr, et al: Unusual cardiac, renal and pulmonary involvement in Gaucher's disease. Interstitial glucocerebroside accumulation, pulmonary hypertension and fatal bone marrow embolization. *Am J Med* 65:352, 1978.
14. Schneider EL, Epstein CJ, Kaback MJ, et al: Severe pulmonary involvement in adult Gaucher's disease. *Am J Med* 63:475, 1977.
15. Belmatoug N, Launay O, Carbon C, et al: Pulmonary hypertension in type 1 Gaucher's disease. *Lancet* 352:240, 1998.
16. Elstein D, Klutstein MW, Lahad A, et al: Echocardiographic assessment of pulmonary hypertension in Gaucher's disease. *Lancet* 351:1544, 1998.
17. Harats D, Pauzner R, Elstein D, et al: Pulmonary hypertension in two patients with type I Gaucher disease while on alglucerase therapy. *Acta Haematol (Basel)* 98:47, 1997.
18. Dawson A, Elias DJ, Rubenson D, et al: Development of pulmonary hypertension after alglucerase therapy in two patients with hepatopul-

monary syndrome complicating type 1 Gaucher disease. *Ann Intern Med* 125:901, 1996.
19. Kerem E, Elstein D, Abrahamov A, et al: Pulmonary function abnormalities in type I Gaucher disease. *Eur Respir J* 9:340, 1996.
20. Mistry PK, Sirrs S, Chan A, et al: Pulmonary hypertension in type I Gaucher's disease: Genetic and epigenetic determinants of phenotype and response to therapy. *Mol Genet Metab* 77:91, 2002.
21. Ciana G, Martini C, Leopaldi A, et al: Bone marker alterations in patients with type 1 Gaucher disease. *Calcif Tissue Int* 72:185, 2003.
22. Elstein D, Itzchaki M, Mankin HJ: Skeletal involvement in Gaucher's disease. *Baillieres Clin Haematol* 10:793, 1997.
23. Lachiewicz PF: Gaucher's disease. *Orthop Clin North Am* 15:765, 1984.
24. Petrohelos M, Tricoulis D, Kotsiras I, et al: Ocular manifestations of Gaucher's disease. *Am J Ophthalmol* 80:1006, 1975.
25. Henderson JM, Gilinsky NH, Lee EY, et al: Gaucher's disease complicated by bleeding esophageal varices and colonic infiltration by Gaucher cells. *Am J Gastroenterol* 86:346, 1991.
26. Schwartz MR, Weycer JS, McGavran MH: Gaucher's disease involving the maxillary sinuses. *Arch Otolaryngol Head Neck Surg* 114:203, 1988.
27. Amstutz HC, Carey EJ: Skeletal manifestations and treatment of Gaucher's disease. *J Bone Joint Surg Am* 48:670, 1966.
28. Draznin SZ, Singer K: Legg-Perthes' disease: A syndrome of many etiologies? With clinical and roentgenographic findings in a case of Gaucher's disease. *AJR Am J Roentgenol* 60:490, 1948.
29. Billings AA, Post M, Shapiro CM: Febrile reaction of Gaucher's disease. *Ill Med J* 145:222, 1973.
30. Barton DJ, Ludman MD, Benkov K, et al: Resting energy expenditure in Gaucher's disease type 1: Effect of Gaucher's cell burden on energy requirements. *Metabolism* 38:1238, 1989.
31. Fujimoto A, Tayebi N, Sidransky E: Congenital ichthyosis preceding neurologic symptoms in two sibs with type 2 Gaucher disease. *Am J Med Genet* 59:356, 1995.
32. Patterson MC, Horowitz M, Abel RB, et al: Isolated horizontal supranuclear gaze palsy as a marker of severe systemic involvement in Gaucher's disease. *Neurology* 43:1993, 1993.
33. Uyama E, Takahashi K, Owada M, et al: Hydrocephalus, corneal opacities, deafness, valvular heart disease, deformed toes and leptomeningeal fibrous thickening in adult siblings: A new syndrome associated with beta-glucocerebrosidase deficiency and a mosaic population of storage cells. *Acta Neurol Scand* 86:407, 1992.
34. Abrahamov A, Elstein D, Gross-Tsur V, et al: Gaucher's disease variant characterized by progressive calcification of heart valves and unique genotype. *Lancet* 346:1000, 1995.
35. Chabas A, Cormand B, Grinberg D, et al: Unusual expression of Gaucher's disease: Cardiovascular calcifications in three sibs homozygous for the D409H mutation. *J Med Genet* 32:740, 1995.
36. Beutler E, Kattamis C, Sipe J, et al: The 1342C mutation in Gaucher's disease. *Lancet* 346:1637, 1995.
37. Mistry PK: Genotype/phenotype correlations in Gaucher's disease. *Lancet* 346:982, 1995.
38. Lee RE: The pathology of Gaucher disease, in *Gaucher Disease: A Century of Delineation and Research*, edited by RJ Desnick, S Gatt, GA Grabowski, p 177. Alan R. Liss, New York, 1982.
39. Chang-Lo M, Yam LT, Rubenstone AI, et al: Gaucher's disease associated with chronic lymphocytic leukaemia, gout and carcinoma. *J Pathol* 116:203, 1975.
40. Mark T, Dominguez C, Rywlin AM: Gaucher's disease associated with chronic lymphocytic leukemia. *South Med J* 75:361, 1982.
41. Kaufman S, Rozenfeld V, Yona R, et al: Gaucher's disease associated with chronic lymphocytic leukaemia. *Clin Lab Haematol* 8:321, 1986.
42. Garfinkel D, Sidi Y, Ben-Bassat M, et al: Coexistence of Gaucher's disease and multiple myeloma. *Arch Intern Med* 142:2229, 1982.

43. Lamon J, Miller W, Tavassoli M, et al: Specialty conference: Multiple myeloma complicating Gaucher's disease. *West J Med* 136:122, 1982.

44. Ruestow PC, Levinson DJ, Catchatourian R, et al: Coexistence of IgA myeloma and Gaucher's disease. *Arch Intern Med* 140:1115, 1980.

45. Benjamin D, Joshua H, Djaldetti M, et al: Nonsecretory IgD-kappa multiple myeloma in a patient with Gaucher's disease. *Scand J Haematol* 22:179, 1979.

46. Gal R, Gukovsky-Oren S, Floru S, et al: Sequential appearance of breast carcinoma, multiple myeloma and Gaucher's disease. *Haematologica* 73:63, 1988.

47. Paulson JA, Marti GE, Fink JK, et al: Richter's transformation of lymphoma complicating Gaucher's disease. *Hematol Pathol* 3:91, 1989.

48. Bruckstein AH, Karanas A, Dire JJ: Gaucher's disease associated with Hodgkin's disease. *Am J Med* 68:610, 1980.

49. Cho SY, Sastre M: Coexistence of Hodgkin's disease and Gaucher's disease. *Am J Clin Pathol* 65:103, 1976.

50. Shoenfeld Y, Berliner S, Pinkhas J, et al: The association of Gaucher's disease and dysproteinemias. *Acta Haematol (Basel)* 64:241, 1980.

51. Pratt PW, Estren F, Kochwa S: Immunoglobulin abnormalities in Gaucher's disease. Report of 16 cases. *Blood* 31:633, 1968.

52. Turesson I, Rausing A: Gaucher's disease and benign monoclonal gammapathy. A case report with immunofluorescence study of bone marrow and spleen. *Acta Med Scand* 197:507, 1975.

53. Liel Y, Hausmann MJ, Mozes M: Case report: Serendipitous Gaucher's disease presenting as elevated erythrocyte sedimentation rate due to monoclonal gammopathy. *Am J Med Sci* 301:393, 1991.

54. Shiran A, Brenner B, Laor A, et al: Increased risk of cancer in patients with Gaucher disease. *Cancer* 72:219, 1993.

55. Aker M, Zimran A, Abrahamov A, et al: Abnormal neutrophil chemotaxis in Gaucher disease. *Br J Haematol* 83:187, 1993.

56. Zimran A, Abrahamov A, Aker M, et al: Correction of neutrophil chemotaxis defect in patients with Gaucher disease by low-dose enzyme replacement therapy. *Am J Hematol* 43:69, 1993.

57. Beutler E, Kuhl W: The diagnosis of the adult type of Gaucher's disease and its carrier state by demonstration of deficiency of beta-glucosidase activity in peripheral blood leukocytes. *J Lab Clin Med* 76:747, 1970.

58. Beutler E: Gaucher disease: New developments, in *Current Hematology and Oncology*, edited by VF Fairbanks, p 6. Year Book Medical Publishers, Chicago, 1988.

59. Brady RO, King FM: Gaucher's disease, in *Lysosomes and Storage Diseases*, edited by HG Hers, F Van Hoof, p 381. Academic Press, New York, 1973.

60. Naito M, Takahashi K, Hojo H: An ultrastructural and experimental study on the development of tubular structures in the lysosomes of Gaucher cells. *Lab Invest* 58:590, 1988.

61. Öckerman PA, Köhlin P: Acid hydrolases in plasma in Gaucher's disease. *Clin Chem* 15:61, 1969.

62. Boklan BF, Sawitsky A: Factor IX deficiency in Gaucher disease. An in vitro phenomenon. *Arch Intern Med* 136:489, 1976.

63. Berrebi A, Malnick SDH, Vorst EJ, et al: High incidence of Factor XI deficiency in Gaucher's disease. *Am J Hematol* 40:153, 1992.

64. Beutler E, Kuhl W, Trinidad F, et al: Beta-glucosidase activity in fibroblasts from homozygotes and heterozygotes for Gaucher's disease. *Am J Hum Genet* 23:62, 1971.

65. Beutler E, Saven A: Misuse of marrow examination in the diagnosis of Gaucher disease. *Blood* 76:646, 1990.

66. Beutler E: Modern diagnosis and treatment of Gaucher's disease. *Am J Dis Child* 147:1175, 1993.

67. Rosner F, Dosik H, Kaiser SS, et al: Gaucher cell in leukemia. *JAMA* 209:935, 1969.

68. Hopfner C, Potron G, Adnet JJ, et al: Histiocytes bleus et "cellules de Gaucher" avec surcharges splenique et ganglionnaire au cours d'une leucemie myeloide chronique. *Nouv Rev Fr Hematol* 14:607, 1974.

69. Zidar BL, Hartsock RJ, Lee RE, et al: Pseudo-Gaucher cells in the bone marrow of a patient with Hodgkin's disease. *Am J Clin Pathol* 87:533, 1987.

70. Scullin DC Jr, Shelburne JD, Cohen HJ: Pseudo-Gaucher cells in multiple myeloma. *Am J Med* 67:347, 1979.

71. Solis OG, Belmonte AH, Ramaswamy G, et al: Pseudogaucher cells in Mycobacterium avium intracellulare infections in acquired immune deficiency syndrome (AIDS). *Am J Clin Pathol* 85:233, 1986.

72. Kattlove HE, Williams JC, Gaynor E, et al: Gaucher cells in chronic myelocytic leukemia: An acquired abnormality. *Blood* 33:379, 1969.

73. Beutler E, Kuhl W, Matsumoto F, et al: Acid hydrolases in leukocytes and platelets of normal subjects and in patients with Gaucher's and Fabry's disease. *J Exp Med* 143:975, 1976.

74. Raghavan SS, Topol J, Kolodny EH: Leukocyte beta-glucosidase in homozygotes and heterozygotes for Gaucher disease. *Am J Hum Genet* 32:158, 1980.

75. Silverstein MN, Kelly PJ: Osteoarticular manifestations of Gaucher's disease. *Am J Med Sci* 253:569, 1967.

76. Ashkenazi A, Zaizov R, Matoth Y: Effect of splenectomy on destructive bone changes in children with chronic (type I) Gaucher disease. *Eur J Pediatr* 145:138, 1986.

77. Shiloni E, Bitran D, Rachmilewitz E, et al: The role of splenectomy in Gaucher's disease. *Arch Surg* 118:929, 1983.

78. Beutler E: Newer aspects of some interesting lipid storage diseases: Tay-Sachs and Gaucher's diseases. *West J Med* 126:46, 1977.

79. Stellin GP, Lilly JR, Githens JH: On partial splenectomy in Gaucher's disease. *Pediatrics* 77:618, 1986.

80. Rubin M, Yampolski I, Lambrozo R, et al: Partial splenectomy in Gaucher's disease. *J Pediatr Surg* 21:125, 1986.

81. Rodgers BM, Tribble C, Joob A: Partial splenectomy for Gaucher's disease. *Ann Surg* 205:693, 1987.

82. Guzzetta PC, Connors RH, Fink J, et al: Operative technique and results of subtotal splenectomy for Gaucher disease. *Surg Gynecol Obstet* 164:359, 1987.

83. Morgenstern L, Phillips EH, Fermelia D, et al: Near-total splenectomy for massive splenomegaly due to Gaucher disease: A new surgical approach. *Mt Sinai J Med* 53:501, 1986.

84. Kyllerman M, Conradi N, Månsson J E, et al: Rapidly progressive type III Gaucher disease: Deterioration following partial splenectomy. *Acta Paediatr Scand* 79:448, 1990.

85. Guzzetta PC, Ruley EJ, Merrick HFW, et al: Elective subtotal splenectomy. Indications and results in 33 patients. *Ann Surg* 211:34, 1990.

86. Thomas WEG, Winfield DA: Partial splenectomy for massive splenomegaly secondary to Gaucher's disease. *Postgrad Med J* 67:1072, 1991.

87. Zer M, Freud E: Subtotal splenectomy in Gaucher's disease: Towards a definition of critical splenic mass. *Br J Surg* 79:742, 1992.

88. Cohen IJ, Katz K, Freud E, et al: Long-term follow-up of partial splenectomy in Gaucher's disease. *Am J Surg* 164:345, 1992.

89. Zimran A, Elstein D, Schiffmann R, et al: Outcome of partial splenectomy for type I Gaucher disease. *J Pediatr* 126:596, 1995.

90. Amstutz HC: The hip in Gaucher's disease. *Clin Orthop* 90:83, 1973.

91. Davies FWT: Gaucher's disease in bone. *J Bone Joint Surg Br* 34B:454, 1952.

92. Schein AJ, Arkin AM: The classic: Hip-joint involvement in Gaucher's disease. *Clin Orthop* 90:4, 1973.

93. Moore M Jr, Coley BL: Bone lesions in Gaucher's disease. *J Tenn Med Assoc* 40:101, 1947.

94. Carlson DE, Busuttil RW, Giudici TA, et al: Orthotopic liver transplantation in the treatment of complications of type I Gaucher disease. *Transplantation* 49:1192, 1990.

95. DuCerf C, Bancel B, Caillon P, et al: Orthotopic liver transplantation for type 1 Gaucher's disease. *Transplantation* 53:1141, 1992.

96. Smanik EJ, Tavill AS, Jacobs GH, et al: Orthotopic liver transplantation in two adults with Niemann-Pick and Gaucher's diseases: Implications for the treatment of inherited metabolic disease. *Hepatology* 17:42, 1993.

97. Starzl TE, Demetris AJ, Trucco M, et al: Chimerism after liver transplantation for type IV glycogen storage disease and type 1 Gaucher's disease. *N Engl J Med* 328:745, 1993.

98. Brady RO, Pentchev PG, Gal AE, et al: Replacement therapy for inherited enzyme deficiency. Use of purified glucocerebrosidase in Gaucher's disease. *N Engl J Med* 291:989, 1974.

99. Beutler E, Dale GL: Enzyme replacement therapy, in *Covalent and Noncovalent Modulation of Protein Function*, edited by D Atkinson, CF Fox, p 449. Academic Press, New York, 1979.

100. Beutler E, Dale GL, Guinto E, et al: Enzyme replacement therapy in Gaucher's disease: Preliminary clinical trial of a new enzyme preparation. *Proc Natl Acad Sci U S A* 74:4620, 1977.

101. Belchetz PE, Crawley JCW, Braidman IP, et al: Treatment of Gaucher's disease with liposome-entrapped glucocerebroside: Beta-glucosidase. *Lancet* 2:116, 1977.

102. Sato Y, Kuhl W, Beutler E: Binding, internalization and degradation of mannose-terminated glucocerebrosidase by macrophages. *Blood* 80(suppl 1):100a, 1992.

103. Barton NW, Brady RO, Dambrosia JM, et al: Replacement therapy for inherited enzyme deficiency—Macrophage-targeted glucocerebrosidase for Gaucher's disease. *N Engl J Med* 324:1464, 1991.

104. Beutler E, Kay A, Saven A, et al: Enzyme replacement therapy for Gaucher disease. *Blood* 78:1183, 1991.

105. Zimran A, Elstein D, Kannai R, et al: Low-dose enzyme replacement therapy for Gaucher's disease: Effects of age, sex, genotype, and clinical features on response to treatment. *Am J Med* 97:3, 1994.

106. Elstein D, Hadas-Halpern I, Itzchaki M, et al: Effect of low-dose enzyme replacement therapy on bones in Gaucher disease patients with severe skeletal involvement. *Blood Cells Mol Dis* 22:104, 1996.

107. Beutler E: Enzyme replacement therapy for Gaucher disease. *Baillieres Clin Haematol* 10:711, 1997.

108. Elstein D, Abrahamov A, Hadas-Halpern I, et al: Low-dose low-frequency imiglucerase as a starting regimen of enzyme replacement therapy for patients with type I Gaucher disease. *Q J Med* 91:483, 1998.

109. Petrides PE: Mobus Gaucher. Aktueller Stand der Therapie. *Arzneimitteltherapie* 2:49, 1998.

110. McCabe ERB, Fine BA, Golbus MS, et al: Gaucher disease—Current issues in diagnosis and treatment. *JAMA* 275:548, 1996.

111. Krasnewich D, Dietrich K, Bauer L, et al: Splenectomy in Gaucher disease: New management dilemmas. *Blood* 91:3085, 1998.

112. Beutler E: Effect of low-dose enzyme replacement therapy on bones in Gaucher disease patients with severe skeletal involvement—Commentary. *Blood Cells Mol Dis* 22:113, 1996.

113. Beutler E, Demina A, Laubscher K, et al: The clinical course of treated and untreated Gaucher disease. A study of 45 patients. *Blood Cells Mol Dis* 21:86, 1995.

114. Rosenthal DI, Doppelt SH, Mankin HJ, et al: Enzyme replacement therapy for Gaucher disease: Skeletal responses to macrophage-targeted glucocerebrosidase. *Pediatrics* 96(Pt 1):629, 1995.

115. Cohen IJ, Katz K, Kornreich L, et al: Low-dose high-frequency enzyme replacement therapy prevents fractures without complete suppression of painful bone crises in patients with severe juvenile onset type I Gaucher disease. *Blood Cells Mol Dis* 24:296, 1998.

116. Barton NW, Brady RO, Murray GJ, et al: Enzyme-replacement therapy for Gaucher's disease: Reply. *N Engl J Med* 325:1811, 1991.

117. Hollak CEM, Aerts JMFG, Goudsmit R, et al: Individualized low-dose alglucerase therapy for type 1 Gaucher's disease. *Lancet* 345:1474, 1995.

118. Beutler E: Treatment regimens in Gaucher's disease. *Lancet* 346:581, 1995.

119. Barton NW, Brady RO, Dambrosia JM: Treatment of Gaucher's disease. *N Engl J Med* 328:1564, 1993.

120. Moscicki RA, Taunton-Rigby A: Treatment of Gaucher's disease. *N Engl J Med* 328:1564, 1993.

121. Zimran A, Hadas-Halpern I, Zevin S, et al: Low dose high frequency enzyme replacement therapy for very young children with Gaucher disease. *Br J Haematol* 85:783, 1993.

122. Hollak CEM, Aerts JMFG, van Oers MHJ: Treatment of Gaucher's disease. *N Engl J Med* 328:1565, 1993.

123. Zimran A, Hollak CEM, Abrahamov A, et al: Home treatment with intravenous enzyme replacement therapy for Gaucher disease: An international collaborative study of 33 patients. *Blood* 82:1107, 1993.

124. Rappeport JM, Ginns EI: Bone-marrow transplantation in severe Gaucher disease. *N Engl J Med* 311:84, 1984.

125. Groth CG, Ringden O: Transplantation in relation to the treatment of inherited disease. *Transplantation* 38:319, 1984.

126. Hobbs JR, Shaw PJ, Jones KH, et al: Beneficial effect of pre-transplant splenectomy on displacement bone marrow transplantation for Gaucher's syndrome. *Lancet* 1:1111, 1987.

127. Tsai P, Lipton JM, Sahdev I, et al: Allogenic bone marrow transplantation in severe Gaucher disease. *Pediatr Res* 31:503, 1992.

128. Gluckman E, Esperou H, Devergie A, et al: Pediatric bone marrow transplantation for leukemia and aplastic anemia. Report of 222 cases transplanted in a single center. *Nouv Rev Fr Hematol* 31:111, 1989.

129. Young E, Chatterton C, Vellodi A, et al: Plasma chitotriosidase activity in Gaucher disease patients who have been treated either by bone marrow transplantation or by enzyme replacement therapy with alglucerase. *J Inherit Metab Dis* 20:595, 1997.

130. Ringdén O, Groth CG, Erikson A, et al: Ten years' experience of bone marrow transplantation for Gaucher disease. *Transplantation* 59:864, 1995.

131. Chan KW, Wong LTK, Applegarth D, et al: Bone marrow transplantation in Gaucher's disease: Effect of mixed chimeric state. *Bone Marrow Transplant* 14:327, 1994.

132. Altarescu G, Hill S, Wiggs E, et al: The efficacy of enzyme replacement therapy in patients with chronic neuronopathic Gaucher's disease. *J Pediatr* 138:539, 2001.

133. Aoki M, Takahashi Y, Miwa Y, et al: Improvement of neurological symptoms by enzyme replacement therapy for Gaucher disease type IIIb. *Eur J Pediatr* 160:63, 2001.

134. Radin NS: Chemical models and chemotherapy in the sphingolipidoses, in *Current Trends in Sphingolipidoses and Allied Disorders*, edited by BW Volk, L Schneck, p 453. Plenum Press, New York, 1976.

135. Heitner R, Elstein D, Aerts J, et al: Low-dose N-butyldeoxynojirimycin (OGT 918) for type I Gaucher disease. *Blood Cells Mol Dis* 28:127, 2002.

136. Lachmann RH: Miglustat. Oxford GlycoSciences/Actelion. *Curr Opin Investig Drugs* 4:472, 2003.

137. Butters TD, Mellor HR, Narita K, et al: Small-molecule therapeutics for the treatment of glycolipid lysosomal storage disorders. *Philos Trans R Soc Lond B Biol Sci* 358:927, 2003.

138. Moyses C: Substrate reduction therapy: Clinical evaluation in type 1 Gaucher disease. *Philos Trans R Soc Lond B Biol Sci* 358:955, 2003.

139. Zimran A, Elstein D: Gaucher disease and the clinical experience with substrate reduction therapy. *Philos Trans R Soc Lond B Biol Sci* 358:961, 2003.

140. McCormack PL, Goa KL: Miglustat. *Drugs* 63:2427, 2003.

141. Cox T, Lachmann R, Hollak C, et al: Novel oral treatment of Gaucher's disease with N-butyldeoxynojirimycin (OGT 918) to decrease substrate biosynthesis. *Lancet* 355:1481, 2000.

142. Pastores GM, Barnett NL, Bathan P, et al: A neurological symptom survey of patients with type I Gaucher disease. *J Inherit Metab Dis* 26:641, 2003.

143. Takiyama N, Mohney T, Swaney W, et al: Comparison of methods for retroviral mediated transfer of glucocerebrosidase gene to CD34⁺ hematopoietic progenitor cells. *Eur J Haematol* 61:1, 1998.

144. Schuening F, Longo WL, Atkinson ME, et al: Retrovirus-mediated transfer of the cDNA for human glucocerebrosidase into peripheral blood repopulating cells of patients with Gaucher's disease. *Hum Gene Ther* 8:2143, 1997.

145. Dunbar C, Kohn D, Karlsson S, et al: Retroviral mediated transfer of the cDNA for human glucocerebrosidase into hematopoietic stem cells of patients with Gaucher disease. A phase I study. *Hum Gene Ther* 7: 231, 1996.

146. Nolta JA, Sender LS, Barranger JA, et al: Expression of human glucocerebrosidase in murine long-term bone marrow cultures after retroviral vector-mediated transfer. *Blood* 75:787, 1990.

147. Sorge J, Kuhl W, West C, et al: Gaucher disease: Retrovirus-mediated correction of the enzymatic defect in cultured cells. *Cold Spring Harb Symp Quant Biol* 60:1041, 1986.

148. Kohn DB: Gene therapy for genetic haematological disorders and immunodeficiencies. *J Intern Med* 249:379, 2001.

149. Beutler E, Southgate MT: Clinical pathological conference: Hepatosplenomegaly, abdominal pain, anemia, and bone lesions. *JAMA* 224: 502, 1973.

150. Groth CG, Dreborg S, Öckerman PA, et al: Splenic transplantation in a case of Gaucher's disease. *Lancet* 1:1260, 1971.

151. Ciana G, Cuttini M, Bembi B: Short-term effects of pamidronate in patients with Gaucher's disease and severe skeletal involvement. *N Engl J Med* 337:712, 1997.

152. Ostlere L, Warner T, Meunier PJ, et al: Treatment of type 1 Gaucher's disease affecting bone with aminohydroxypropylidene bisphosphonate (pamidronate). *Q J Med* 79:503, 1991.

153. Harinck HIJ, Bijvoet OLM, van der Meer JWH, et al: Regression of bone lesions in Gaucher's disease during treatment with aminohydroxypropylidene bisphosphonate. *Lancet* 2:513, 1984.

154. Wenstrup RJ, Bailey L, Grabowski GA, et al: Gaucher disease: Alendronate disodium improves bone mineral density in adults receiving enzyme therapy. *Blood* 104:1253, 2004.

155. Fan JQ: A contradictory treatment for lysosomal storage disorders: Inhibitors enhance mutant enzyme activity. *Trends Pharmacol Sci* 24:355, 2003.

156. Balicki D, Beutler E: Gaucher disease. *Medicine* 74:305, 1995.

157. Sidransky E, Tsuji S, Martin BM, et al: DNA mutation analysis of Gaucher patients. *Am J Med Genet* 42:331, 1992.

158. Masuno M, Tomatsu S, Sukegawa K, et al: Non-existence of a tight association between a ⁴⁴⁴leucine to proline mutation and phenotypes of Gaucher disease: High frequency of a NciI polymorphism in the non-neuronopathic form. *Hum Genet* 84:203, 1990.

159. Zimran A, Kay AC, Gelbart T, et al: Gaucher disease: Clinical, laboratory, radiologic and genetic features of 53 patients. *Medicine* 71:337, 1992.

160. Ginsburg SJ, Groll M: Hydrops fetalis due to infantile Gaucher's disease. *J Pediatr* 82:1046, 1973.

161. Tybulewicz VLJ, Tremblay ML, LaMarca ME, et al: Animal model of Gaucher's disease from targeted disruption of the mouse glucocerebrosidase gene. *Nature* 357:407, 1992.

162. Niemann A: Ein unbekanntes Krankheitsbild. *Jahrbuch Kinderheilkunde* 79:1, 1914.

163. Brady RO, Kanfer JN, Mock MB, et al: The metabolism of sphingomyelin II. Evidence of an enzymatic deficiency in Niemann-Pick disease. *Proc Natl Acad Sci U S A* 55:366, 1966.

164. Schuchman EH, Desnick RJ: Niemann-Pick disease types A and B: Acid sphingomyelinase deficiencies, in *The Metabolic and Molecular Bases of Inherited Disease*, edited by CR Scriver, AL Beaudet, WS Sly, D Valle, p 2601. McGraw-Hill, New York, 1995.

165. Pentchev PG, Vanier MT, Suzuki K, et al: Niemann-Pick disease type C: A cellular cholesterol lipidosis, in *The Metabolic and Molecular Bases of Inherited Disease*, edited by CR Scriver, AL Beaudet, WS Sly, D Valle, p 2625. McGraw-Hill, New York, 1995.

166. Crocker A, Farber S: Niemann-Pick disease: A review of eighteen patients. *Medicine* 37:1, 1958.

167. Greer WL, Riddell DC, Murty S, et al: Linkage disequilibrium mapping of the Nova Scotia variant of Niemann-Pick disease. *Clin Genet* 55:248, 1999.

168. Takahashi T, Suchi M, Desnick RJ, et al: Identification and expression of five mutations in the human acid sphingomyelinase gene causing types A and B Niemann-Pick disease. Molecular evidence for genetic heterogeneity in the neuronopathic and non-neuronopathic forms. *J Biol Chem* 267:12552, 1992.

169. Ida H, Rennert OM, Maekawa K, et al: Identification of three novel mutations in the acid sphingomyelinase gene of Japanese patients with Niemann-Pick disease type A and B. *Hum Mutat* 7:65, 1996.

170. Sikora J, Pavlu-Pereira H, Elleder M, et al: Seven novel acid sphingomyelinase gene mutations in Niemann-Pick type A and B patients. *Ann Hum Genet* 67:63, 2003.

171. De Maria R, Rippo MR, Schuchman EH, et al: Acidic sphingomyelinase (ASM) is necessary for fas-induced GD3 ganglioside accumulation and efficient apoptosis of lymphoid cells. *J Exp Med* 187:897, 1998.

172. Carstea ED, Morris JA, Coleman KG, et al: Niemann-Pick C1 disease gene: Homology to mediators of cholesterol homeostasis. *Science* 277: 228, 1997.

173. Park WD, O'Brien JF, Lundquist PA, et al: Identification of 58 novel mutations in Niemann-Pick disease type C: Correlation with biochemical phenotype and importance of PTC1-like domains in NPC1. *Hum Mutat* 22:313, 2003.

174. Liscum L, Klansek JJ: Niemann-Pick disease type C. *Curr Opin Lipidol* 9:131, 1998.

175. Millat G, Chikh K, Naureckiene S, et al: Niemann-Pick disease type C: Spectrum of HE1 mutations and genotype/phenotype correlations in the NPC2 group. *Am J Hum Genet* 69:1013, 2001.

176. Loftus SK, Morris JA, Carstea ED, et al: Murine model of Niemann-Pick C disease: Mutation in a cholesterol homeostasis gene. *Science* 277: 232, 1997.

177. Golde DW, Schneider EL, Bainton EL, et al: Pathogenesis of one variant of sea-blue histiocytosis. *Lab Invest* 33:371, 1975.

178. Patterson MC: A riddle wrapped in a mystery: Understanding Niemann-Pick disease, type C. *Neurologist* 9:301, 2003.

179. Lazarus SS, Vethamany VG, Schneck L, et al: Fine structure and histochemistry of peripheral blood cells in Niemann-Pick disease. *Lab Invest* 17:155, 1967.

180. Brady RO: Sphingomyelin lipidoses: Niemann-Pick disease, in *The Metabolic Basis of Inherited Disease*, edited by JB Stanbury, JB Wyngaarden, DS Fredrickson, JL Goldstein, MS Brown, p 831. McGraw-Hill, New York, 1983.

181. Veyssier-Belot C, Cacoub P, Caparros-Lefebvre D, et al: Erdheim-Chester disease. Clinical and radiologic characteristics of 59 cases. *Medicine* 75:157, 1996.

182. Landas S, Foucar K, Sando GN, et al: Adult Niemann-Pick disease masquerading as sea blue histiocyte syndrome: Report of a case confirmed by lipid analysis and enzyme assays. *Am J Hematol* 20:391, 1985.

183. Briere J, Calman F, Lageron A, et al: Maladie de Niemann-Pick de l'adulte suivie de la naissance a l'age de 26 ans. Forme viscerale pure avec surcharge en sphingomyeline et deficit en sphingomyelinase. *Nouv Rev Fr Hematol* 16:185, 1976.

184. Dewhurst N, Besley GTN, Finlayson NDC, et al: Sea blue histiocytosis in a patient with chronic non-neuropathic Niemann-Pick disease. *J Clin Pathol* 32:1121, 1979.

185. Brady RO, King FM: Niemann Pick disease, in *Lysosomes and Storage Diseases*, edited by HG Hers, F Van Hoof, p 439. Academic Press, New York, 1973.

186. Epstein CJ, Brady RO, Schneider EL, et al: In utero diagnosis of Niemann-Pick disease. *Am J Hum Genet* 23:533, 1971.

187. Gal AE, Brady RO, Hibberg SR, et al: A practical chromogenic procedure for the detection of homozygotes and heterozygous carriers of Niemann-Pick disease. *N Engl J Med* 293:632, 1975.

188. Levade T, Salvayre R, Douste-Blazy L: Sphingomyelinases and Niemann-Pick disease. *J Clin Chem Clin Biochem* 24:205, 1986.

189. Harzer K, Rolfs A, Bauer P, et al: Niemann-Pick disease type A and B are clinically but also enzymatically heterogeneous: Pitfall in the laboratory diagnosis of sphingomyelinase deficiency associated with the mutation Q292 K. *Neuropediatrics* 34:301, 2003.

190. Roff CF, Goldin E, Comly ME, et al: Niemann-Pick type-C disease: Deficient intracellular transport of exogenously derived cholesterol. *Am J Med Genet* 42:593, 1992.

191. Bembi B, Comelli M, Scaggiante B, et al: Treatment of sphingomyelinase deficiency by repeated implantations of amniotic epithelial cells. *Am J Med Genet* 44:527, 1992.

192. Miranda SRP, He X, Simonaro CM, et al: Infusion of recombinant human acid sphingomyelinase into Niemann-Pick disease mice leads to visceral, but not neurological, correction of the pathophysiology. *FASEB J* 14:1988, 2000.

193. Sawitsky A, Rosner F, Chodsky S: The sea-blue histiocyte syndrome, a review: Genetic and biochemical studies. *Semin Hematol* 9:285, 1972.

194. Sawitsky A, Hyman GA, Hyman JB: An unidentified reticuloendothelial cell in bone marrow and spleen. Report of two cases with histochemical studies. *Blood* 9:977, 1954.

195. Baumgartner C, Bucher U: Blaue Pigmentmakrophagen (sea blue histiocytes) and Gaucher-aehnliche Zellen. Vorkommen und Bedeutung. *Blut* 30:309, 1975.

196. Bigorgne C, Le Tourneau A, Vahedi K, et al: Sea-blue histiocyte syndrome in bone marrow secondary to total parenteral nutrition. *Leuk Lymphoma* 28:523, 1998.

197. Kelsey PR, Geary CG: Sea-blue histiocytes and Gaucher cells in bone marrow of patients with chronic myeloid leukaemia. *J Clin Pathol* 41:960, 1988.

198. Zelingher J, Shouval D: Liver failure and the sea-blue histiocyte/adult Niemann-Pick disease. Case report and review of the literature. *J Clin Gastroenterol* 2:146, 1992.

199. Candoni A, Grimaz S, Doretto P et al: Sea-blue histiocytosis secondary to Niemann-Pick disease type B: A case report. *Ann Hematol* 80:620, 2001.

LYMPHOCYTES AND PLASMA CELLS

MORPHOLOGY OF LYMPHOCYTES AND PLASMA CELLS

STEPHEN M. BAIRD

Lymphocytes are a heterogeneous collection of cells that can be distinguished easily from other leukocytes by their characteristic morphology. However, this morphology is shared by all three major blood lymphocyte subsets, namely, T cells, B cells, and natural killer cells. Although B cells can differentiate into plasma cells that have a distinctive morphology, most morphologic changes that occur during differentiation or activation are not unique to any one of the three major subgroups. Instead, other means such as flow cytometry are required to distinguish the major subsets and sub-subsets of lymphocytes. This distinction has been achieved through the advent of monoclonal antibodies and the characterization of surface membrane antigens that are distinctive for each lymphocyte subset. This chapter describes the morphologic features that distinguish lymphocytes from other leukocytes and the membrane antigens that most commonly are used to distinguish the major lymphocyte subsets.

DEFINITION AND HISTORY

Lymphocytes and plasma cells first were described morphologically in 1774 and 1875, respectively.[1] Later investigations of these cells until the 1960s primarily further defined their morphology. Subsequently, lymphocytes were found to make immunoglobulins (Igs) and to be necessary for cell-mediated immunity.[2–6] With the advent of monoclonal antibodies and flow cytometry, the refinement of *in vitro* functional assays, and the application of molecular techniques, major advances in the understanding of lymphocytes have been made. Membrane antigens that assist in the designation of lymphocyte subsets and function have been identified. Three major blood lymphocyte subsets have been identified: T lymphocytes, B lymphocytes, and natural killer (NK) cells. Further, there are small numbers of circulating hematopoietic stem cells that resemble lymphocytes and that are capable of differentiating into any one of the various lymphocyte subsets.

MICROSCOPY AND HISTOCHEMISTRY OF NORMAL BLOOD LYMPHOCYTES

LIGHT MICROSCOPY

Classic studies of blood and tissues have demonstrated populations of spherical and/or ovoid cells that have diameters from 6 to 15 μm when flattened on glass slides.[3] Some of these studies described small lym-

Acronyms and abbreviations that appear in this chapter include: CD, clusters of differentiation; Ig, immunoglobulin; IL-2R, interleukin-2 receptor; LFA-3, lymphocyte function-associated antigen-3; MHC, major histocompatibility complex; NK, natural killer; PAS, periodic acid–Schiff; TCR, T cell antigen receptor.

phocytes with diameters of 6 to 9 μm, and large lymphocytes, with diameters of 9 to 15 μm. Patients with acute viral illnesses or certain genetic immunologic deficiencies, particularly the Wiskott-Aldrich syndrome, have increased numbers of circulating large lymphocytes. The mean absolute number of circulating small lymphocytes in normal adults is 2.5×10^9/liter (range 1.5–4.0), or 35 percent of the total leukocytes (range 20–50 percent).

The typical small lymphocyte as observed with Romanowsky polychromatic stains (e.g., Giemsa or Wright) has an ovoid or kidney-shaped nucleus that stains purple, has densely packed nuclear chromatin, and occupies approximately 90 percent of the cell area (see Color Plates I-1,2,3,7,8,9). A small rim of cytoplasm stains blue. Although nucleoli rarely are observed in Giemsa-stained films, they can be demonstrated with methyl green-pyronine stains. Cytoplasmic basophilia is related to RNA content. The cytoplasm of some lymphocytes, particularly large lymphocytes, contains a number of coarse pink granules, usually 5 to 15 per cell, and occasional clear vacuoles. Cytoplasmic glycogen is detected with periodic acid–Schiff (PAS) and methenamine-silver techniques. A number of enzymes, including phosphorylase, acid hydrolases, nucleases, and mitochondrial enzymes, are in the lymphocyte cytoplasm.[7] Peroxidase reactions are negative in lymphocytes.[8]

In a normal adult, approximately 3 percent of blood lymphocytes are large granular lymphocytes[9] (see Color Plate XX-3). These cells are a mixed population consisting of NK cells and some of the CD8 subset of mature T cells. However, the majority of mature T lymphocytes show a localized "dot" staining pattern for acid phosphatase, acid and neutral nonspecific esterases, β-glucuronidase, and N-acetyl-β-glucosaminidase.[10–12] B lymphocytes either lack esterase and acid phosphatase or show scattered granular staining.

Enzymes in the purine salvage pathways are expressed differently in lymphocyte subsets. The enzyme 5'-nucleotidase is detectable on plasma membranes of both B and T cells. In contrast, more adenosine deaminase and purine nucleoside phosphorylase are present in the cytoplasm of T cells than in the cytoplasm of B cells.[13,14] Terminal deoxynucleotidyl transferase is present in cortical thymocytes, stem cells starting to differentiate, and the malignant cells of acute lymphoid leukemias.[15,16]

PHASE-CONTRAST MICROSCOPY

Active movement of lymphocytes is studied by phase-contrast, or interference-contrast, microscopy. Lymphocytes move slowly with a "hand mirror" appearance. Cytoplasmic spreading does not occur. However, during cell movement a thickening occurs in the cytoplasmic rim (the Hof region), a region that houses most of the cell's organelles, including the Golgi. Lymphocytes from patients with chronic lymphocytic leukemia have decreased movement.[17]

TRANSMISSION ELECTRON MICROSCOPY AND CYTOCHEMISTRY

The circulating lymphocyte measures approximately 5 μm in diameter as visualized by transmission electron microscopy.[18–20] The nucleus has an abundance of electron-dense, condensed heterochromatin, a feature characteristic of nonproliferating cells. The nucleoli are round in section, approximately 1.0 to 1.5 μm in diameter. They are composed of three distinct and concentrically arranged structural units: the central region or agranular zone; the middle, fibrillar region; and the granular zone, which contains intranucleolar chromatin. The lymphocyte's nuclear membrane contains nuclear pores and a perinuclear space.

The cytoplasmic organelles of the lymphocytes are characteristic of eukaryotic cells.[18–20] Some organelles, such as the Golgi zone, are poorly developed. The cytoplasm contains free ribosomes, occasional ribosome clusters, and strands of rough-surfaced endoplasmic reticu-

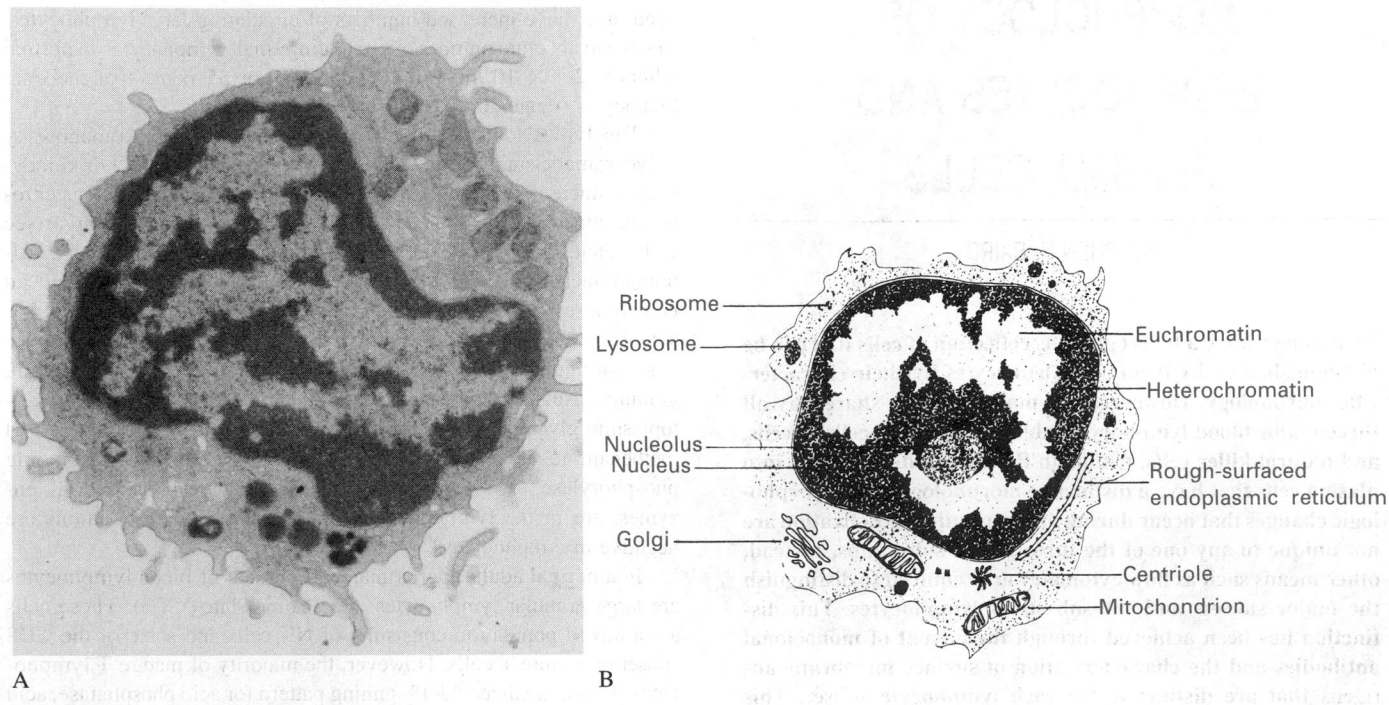

FIGURE 74-1   (A) Electron micrograph of normal human blood lymphocyte (×12,000). (B) Diagrammatic representation of normal blood lymphocyte, with organelles labeled.

lum (Fig. 74-1). Centrioles, mitochondria, microtubules (diameter approximately 0.25 μm), and microfilaments (diameter approximately 0.07 μm) are present in the cytoplasm adjacent to the cell membrane. The cytoplasm also contains lysosomes, which are approximately 0.4 μm in diameter, are electron opaque, and contain classic lysosomal enzymes (e.g., acid phosphatase, β-glucuronidase, and acid ribonuclease).[7] The lymphocyte plasma membrane stains with colloidal iron, a marker for membrane sialic acid. Lymphocyte cell membranes and cell coat glycoproteins are shown with other electron-dense markers, including phosphotungstic acid, lanthanum colloid, and ruthenium red.

SCANNING ELECTRON MICROSCOPY

Scanning electron microscopy provides three-dimensional information.[21] However, the resolution achieved with scanning electron microscopy, approximately 0.1 μm, is considerably less than that possible with transmission electron microscopy, generally 0.002 to 0.0039 μm. Normal blood lymphocytes, washed and collected onto silver membranes and fixed in glutaraldehyde, have a spherical topography with varying numbers of stubby or finger-like microvilli (Fig. 74-2).[22] In contrast, monocytes are much larger, have few microvilli, and display ruffled membranes and ridge-like profiles. T lymphocytes have smaller numbers of microvilli than B lymphocytes.[22] However, the surface morphology of B lymphocytes is heterogeneous. Many B cells have moderate to markedly villous surfaces, but approximately 10 to 20 percent of B cells are smooth with few microvilli and thus are indistinguishable from most T lymphocytes.[23] Furthermore, human blood lymphocytes fixed in suspension appear uniformly covered with short microvilli, and no differences between T and B cells are demonstrable.

MORPHOLOGIC CHANGES ASSOCIATED WITH ACTIVATION

Lymphocyte stimulation is associated with a complex sequence of morphologic and biochemical events, culminating in the transformation of small lymphocytes into blast or plasmacytoid cells (Figs. 74-3 and 74-4). Plant lectins, bacterial products, polymeric substances, and enzymes stimulate lymphocyte mitosis. Such agents are called *mitogens*. Some mitogens are specific for either B cells or T lymphocytes, whereas other mitogens stimulate both. The responses of specific lymphocyte subpopulations to various mitogens are complex.[24] Nucleolar changes become evident as early as 4 hours after exposure to phytomitogens (e.g., phytohemagglutinin, which stimulates T cells). These morphologic changes consist of increases in nucleolar size and in the number and concentration of granules in the granular zone. These changes are followed by an increase in fibrillar zones and increased intranucleolar chromatin. Nucleolar

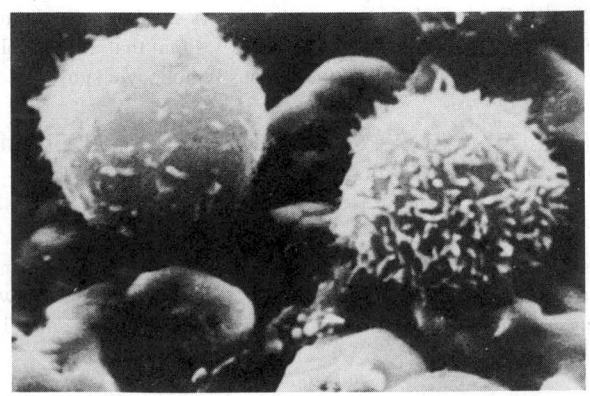

FIGURE 74-2   Scanning electron micrograph of normal blood lymphocytes separated by the Ficoll-Hypaque method. Cells show varying numbers of microvilli (×5000). (Figs. 74-2, 74-4, and 74-5 provided by Dr. Aaron Polliack of the Department of Hematology, Hebrew University Hadassah Medical School, Jerusalem, Israel.)

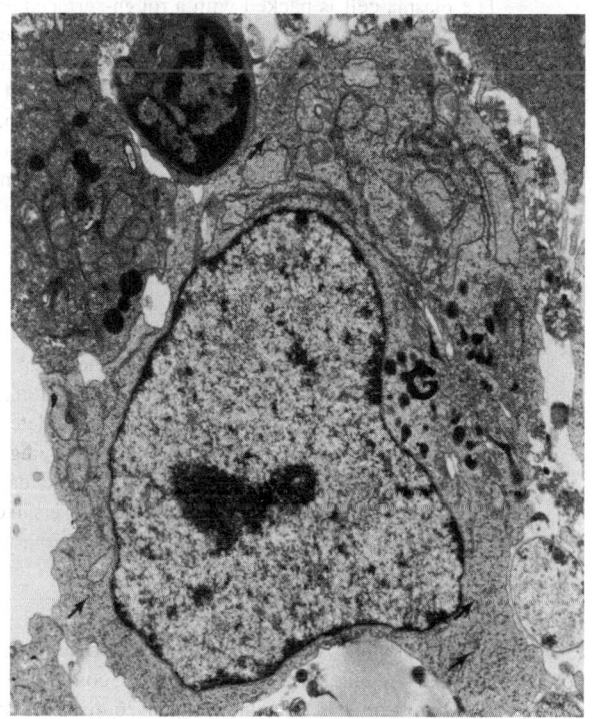

FIGURE 74-3   Transmission electron micrograph of lymphocyte from normal individual incubated with phytohemagglutinin (PHA) for 3 days. The transformed cell has a large Golgi zone (G) and many ribosomal aggregates (arrows). The nucleus is euchromatic (×7500).

chromatin becomes more electron lucent or dispersed. Electron microscopic autoradiography demonstrates that tritiated thymidine, incorporated into newly synthesized DNA, is spread throughout the nucleoplasm but is most concentrated at the nuclear membrane. From 48 to 72 hours following the addition of phytohemagglutinin, the size of the cytoplasm increases. In addition, the cytoplasm contains an increased number of ribosomal clusters and more rough-surfaced endoplasmic reticulum. The transformed cell (lymphoblast) has increased numbers of lysosomes and a larger Golgi complex with more components.[18–20] Under some circumstances (e.g., cultures of human lymphocytes stimulated for 7–10 days with pokeweed mitogen), some cells form well-developed Golgi and plasmacytoid features.[25] Similar plasmacytoid cells are observed in antigen-stimulated lymph nodes, during graft rejection *in vivo*, and in some *in vitro* systems, including the mixed lymphocyte culture. In lymph nodes, the stimulated lymphoid cells may be referred to by various authors as lymphoblasts, immunoblasts, centroblasts, or large lymphoid cells. Morphologic criteria for these cells overlap.

Following stimulation with antigen or mitogens, the lymphocyte enters the cell cycle. Figure 74-5 summarizes the cell-cycle phases and accompanying genetic or morphologic changes. These parallel genetic and morphologic alterations are necessary correlates of the cell-cycle phases. The fate and function of lymphocytes that traverse the cell cycle can be divided into two pathways. Some lymphocytes undergo several mitotic cycles and then return to the G_0 phase, indistinguishable in morphology from the original nonactivated cells. Some of them then become memory cells, programmed to remember the stimulating antigen and thus respond more rapidly to reexposure to the original antigen. Alternatively, they become terminally differentiated lymphocytes, such as plasma cells or cytotoxic T cells.

MICROSCOPY AND HISTOCHEMISTRY OF PLASMA CELLS

MORPHOLOGIC STUDIES

Plasma cells derive from small B lymphocytes after antigenic stimulation and T cell help. Several sequential mitotic divisions occur during cellular differentiation from the resting lymphocyte to the plasmablast to the immature plasma cell. Immature plasma cells also can undergo successive waves of mitosis in the medullary cords of lymph nodes in response to antigen.[26] Cell transfer experiments demonstrated that these transformed cells later mature into antibody-producing plasma cells.[27]

Pokeweed mitogen induces B lymphocytes to transform into plasma cells after 7 to 10 days of culture.[28] These plasma cells infrequently contain large electron-dense inclusions (Russell bodies), which may measure 2 to 3 μm in diameter (Fig. 74-6).[29] Russell bodies, cytoplasmic Ig in the endoplasmic reticulum, sometimes are dissolved during the Giemsa staining procedure. They usually occur in pathologic states but may be found in normal lymph nodes or marrow. When cytoplasmic Ig becomes detectable, the same Ig isotype is present in the cytoplasm as on the cell membrane.

LIGHT MICROSCOPY, HISTOCHEMISTRY, AND ELECTRON MICROSCOPY

When treated with a polychrome stain, the mature plasma cell has a characteristic basophilic cytoplasm and an eccentric nucleus. The nuclear polarity is attributable to a large paranuclear zone, which corresponds to the Golgi apparatus. The typical mature plasma cell spread on a slide usually is round or oval and has a diameter of 9 to 20 μm, with a mean cell diameter of 14.4 μm and a mean nuclear diameter of

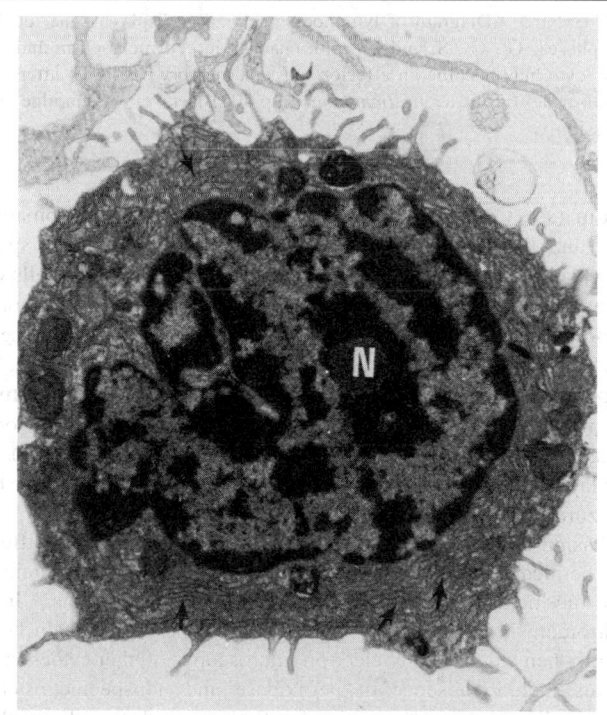

FIGURE 74-4   Transmission electron micrograph of plasmacytoid cell present in culture of lymphocytes from a patient with chronic lymphocytic leukemia incubated with pokeweed mitogen for 7 days. The nucleolus (N) and rough-surfaced endoplasmic reticulum (arrows) are evident (×9000). (From Cohnen, Douglas, Konig, et al: Pokeweed mitogen response of lymphocytes in chronic lymphocytic leukemia. *Blood* 42:591, 1973, with permission.)

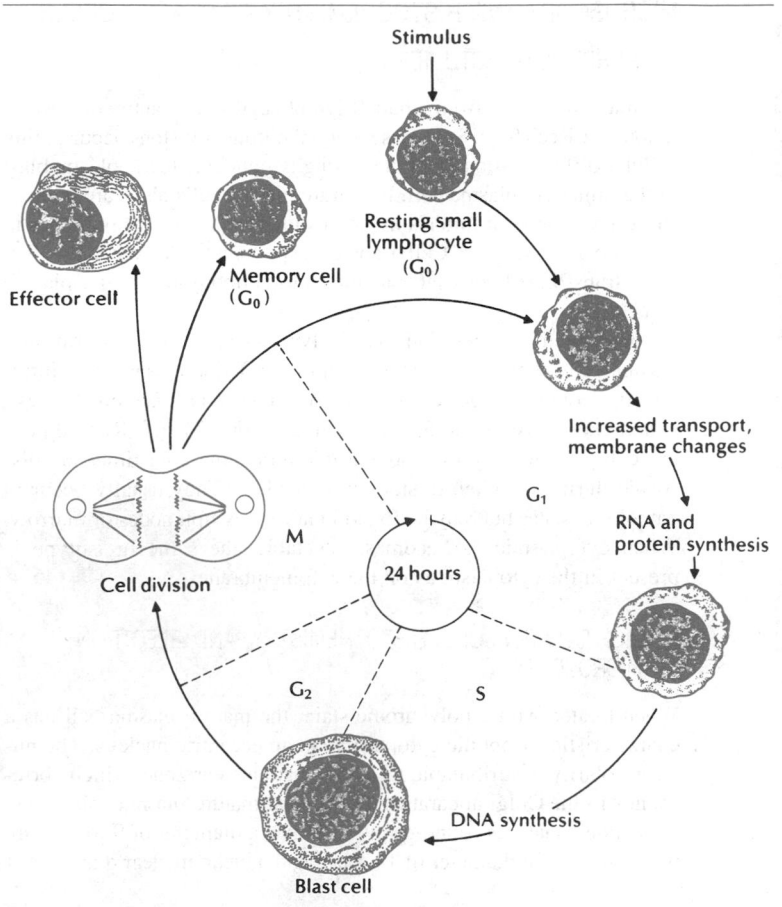

FIGURE 74-5 Diagram of lymphocyte activation displaying the relationship of cell-cycle phases (G_0, G_1, S, and M) with changes in cell metabolism and cell function. A lymphocyte may become an effector cell or a memory cell in G_0 after having traversed the cell cycle. (From Klein, *Immunology*, p 40. Blackwell, Cambridge, MA, 1990, with permission.)

The plasma cell is packed with a rough-surfaced endoplasmic reticulum having numerous attached ribosomes as seen by electron microscopy. A large circumscribed Golgi zone forms a paranuclear halo when observed by light microscopy. The nucleus has dense areas of heterochromatin. The Golgi zone contains lamellae, vesicles, vacuoles, and a number of granules. Mitochondria are located between the strands of endoplasmic reticulum (Fig. 74-7).[35]

ANTIGENS OF HUMAN LYMPHOCYTES

Human blood lymphocytes possess an array of different membrane antigens. Standardization of monoclonal antibody reagents by identifying clusters of differentiation (CD) and the advent of flow cytometry have facilitated detection of lymphocyte subsets (see Chap. 14). The following sections discuss the surface antigens and morphologic features that help define the major human lymphocyte subsets in clinical practice.

B-LYMPHOCYTE ANTIGENS

Table 74-1 summarizes the expression of CD antigens on cells of the B lymphocyte lineage, including committed progenitor B cells and pre-B cells. Chapter 76 discusses these cells and the maturation stages they represent. Table 74-1 also lists antigens that are expressed or increased upon B cell activation. Chapter 14 (see Table 14-1) discusses the physiology, structure, and distribution of each of the CD antigens listed in Table 74-1.

Of the B cell-associated antigens that are commonly used, only a few are restricted to cells of the B lineage (see Chap. 14). Of these antigens, only CD20, CD79a, and CD79b are not found on other cell types. The latter two antigens associate with Ig to facilitate surface Ig expression and surface Ig-mediated signal transduction and are ex-

8.5 μm (see Color Plate XXI-1).[30] The nuclear heterochromatin is coarse and distributed in a pattern that sometimes resembles the spokes of a wheel (cartwheel nucleus) on paraffin sections. Plasma cells with two or more nuclei occasionally are seen in the marrow of normal individuals. The nucleus stains blue-green with methyl green. The cytoplasm is characterized by an intense affinity for cationic dyes. The cytoplasm, basophilic because of ribonucleoprotein, stains selectively with methyl green-pyronine. The cytoplasm stains red with pyronine because of the high content of ribonucleoprotein (pyroninophilia). The cytoplasm also stains with several basic dyes, including toluidine blue and azures.

Plasma cells in patients with certain diseases may have different histochemical properties. These cells may be larger and contain cytoplasmic inclusions that may be observed with PAS stains.[31] In hemochromatosis and hemosiderosis, plasma cells may contain hemosiderin when examined by electron microscopy.[32] Other cytochemical features include absence of peroxidase and nonspecific esterase. Plasma cells are strongly positive for β-glucuronidase and mitochondrial enzyme markers.[33] Plasma cell size and morphology may be altered substantially in myeloma and macroglobulinemia (see Color Plates XXI-4–XXI-9). Cells with two or three nuclei may be seen more frequently than in adults without plasma cell dyscrasias. Under some circumstances, amyloid inclusions in plasma cells have been detected by electron microscopy.[34]

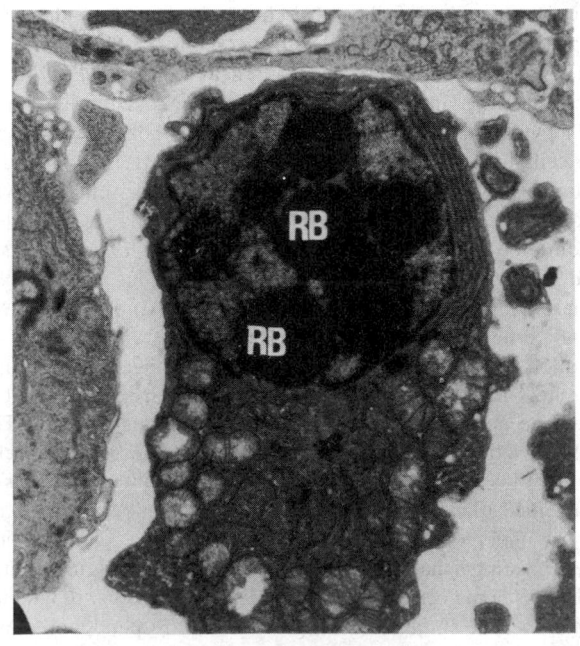

FIGURE 74-6 Intranuclear electron-dense bodies (Russell bodies [RB]) in plasma cell from the marrow of a patient with multiple myeloma (×7000).

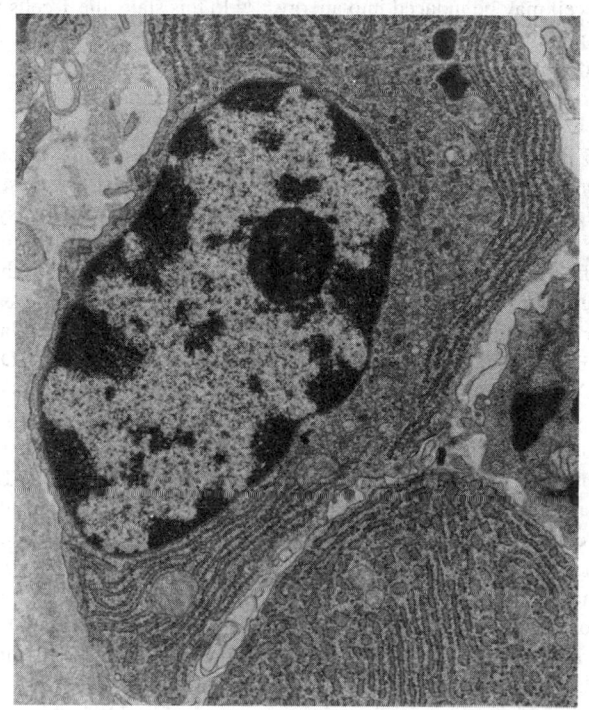

A

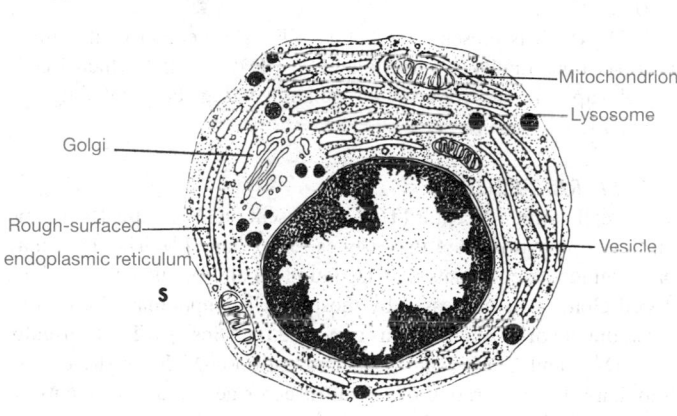

Golgi

Rough-surfaced
endoplasmic reticulum

S

Mitochondrion

Lysosome

Vesicle

B

FIGURE 74-7   *(A)* Electron micrograph of mature plasma cells in normal human lymph node (×9000). *(B)* Diagrammatic representation of normal plasma cell with organelles labeled.

pressed only by cells that produce Ig, an exclusive function of B lymphocytes and plasma cells (see Chap. 77). Demonstration of monoclonal surface Ig allows diagnosis of clonal, neoplastic B cells. CD20 is the target of monoclonal antibody commonly used for treatment of B cell neoplasms. CD19 is restricted mostly to B cells but may be expressed weakly by follicular dendritic cells. However, CD19 is expressed by B cells at all stages of maturation, including the committed B cell progenitor. As such, it is the best-defined pan-B cell surface antigen. Cytoplasmic CD22 is perhaps the broadest mature B cell marker.

In addition to the CD antigens and Igs, B cells express the three major histocompatibility complex (MHC) class II antigens: DR, DP, DQ. These antigens are heterodimers of α heavy chains and β light chains that are encoded by genes within the D complex of the HLA complex (see Chap. 129). MHC class I antigens are expressed on all nucleated cells.

B-1 B CELLS

A subset of normal B cells express CD5, a 67-kDa transmembrane glycoprotein that is more brightly expressed by T cells (see Chap. 14). These cells are designated CD5 B cells or now B-1 B cells.[36,37] B-1 B cells do not express other T cell markers but do express all other pan-B cell surface antigens.[37] Various agents modulate B cell expression of CD5.[38] B-1 B cells are found in umbilical cord blood,[39] adult blood, the pleura and peritoneum, and all major secondary lymphoid organs; they are rare in the marrow.[40] These cells apparently are enriched for cells that spontaneously produce polyreactive autoantibodies.[41–43]

PLASMA CELLS

Most B cell differentiation antigens are not expressed by the mature plasma cell, including surface Ig and HLA class II antigens (see Table 74-1). Of the cells of the B lineage, plasma cells are distinctive in that they express CD38 and PCA-1. CD38 is found on marrow plasma cells and myeloma cell lines.[44] PCA-1 also is found on human plasma cells[44] and may function as a threonine-specific protein kinase.[45] This latter function may assist in phosphorylation of secretory proteins. PCA-1 is present at low density on granulocytes and monocytes. In contrast to mature B lymphocytes, plasma cells do not bear surface Ig but express CD38, CD138, and very high levels of CD43 and CD85 (see Table 74-1).

T LYMPHOCYTE ANTIGENS

CD1

CD1 is a family of three membrane glycoproteins, CD1a, CD1b, and CD1c, of 49, 45, and 43 kDa, respectively. CD1 is found on all cortical thymocytes (see Chap. 14). CD1 also can be expressed on monocytes following activation and on Langerhans cells.[46] CD1 has a structural relationship to HLA class I and class II proteins. This structural association suggests CD1 is involved in T cell interaction with accessory/antigen-presenting cells, perhaps presenting hydrophobic antigens such as lipids.

CD2

This T cell antigen is expressed early in T cell development. It is a 50-kDa surface glycoprotein that facilitates T lymphocyte target cell interactions and T lymphocyte activation.[47] Lymphocyte function-associated antigen-3 (LFA-3) (CD58) is a ligand for CD2 (see Chaps. 14 and 78). Cross-linking CD2 may activate T cells through a pathway that is distinct from that used by the T cell receptor for antigen. This

TABLE 74-1   B LYMPHOCYTE ANTIGENS USED IN CLINICAL MEDICINE

CELL TYPE	ANTIGEN
Committed progenitor	CD34, CD19, CD40, CD45, CD72, HLADR
Early pre-B cell	CD10, CD19, CD20, CD34 terminal deoxynucleotidyl transferase (TdT), cytoplasmic CD22,HLADR
Pre-B cell	Add cytoplasmic μ-chain to early pre-B antigens
Mature B cell	CD10 (weak and only on germinal center B cells), CD19, CD20, CD21, CD22 (α- and β-isoforms), CD5 (B-1 cell subset, weak), and CD11c (subset) Surface IgM, IgD, CD79a, 79b
Activated B cells	CD23 (usually germinal center B cells), CD38, CD39, weak CD5 Cytoplasmic Ig shifts to IgG, IgA, or IgE Surface IgM and IgD are lost
Mammary-type B cell	CD27, CD19
Plasma cell	CD38, CD138, PCA-1, BB4, cytoplasmic immunoglobulin (IgM, IgG, IgA, or IgE)

activation may result in augmentation of the immune response in the absence of additional antigenic stimulation. Because anti-CD2 monoclonal antibodies activate early T lymphocyte progenitors, CD2 antigen probably is a receptor used in the activation of thymocytes prior to appearance of a functional T cell receptor.[48]

CD3

CD3 is a three-subunit complex expressed by early thymocytes and mature T cells.[49] It is tightly linked to the T cell antigen receptor (see Chap. 78). The CD3 complex serves as a signal transduction unit after T cell receptor activation. This complex frequently is expressed in T cell acute lymphoblastic leukemia.

CD5

CD5 is found on all T cells and appears to be a signal transducer. It appears early in T lymphocyte ontogeny.[50,51] CD5 also may be detected on a subset of adult blood and umbilical cord B cells.

CD7

CD7 is a 40-kDa glycoprotein that is expressed very early in T cell ontogeny.[51] The antigen is lost during the terminal stage of T cell maturation. The function of CD7 is not known. CD7 also is expressed on monocytes and NK cells.[52]

CD4 AND CD8

CD8 is first expressed at low levels on thymocytes. CD4 then is expressed with CD8 on thymocytes (see Chaps. 76 and 78). Mature T cells express either CD4 or CD8. CD4, a member of the Ig supergene family, is a single-chain transmembrane glycoprotein.[53] CD8 is a 34-kDa dimeric transmembrane glycoprotein.[54] Most T cells express the α- and β-subunits of CD8. Some cells, often malignant T cells, express a homodimer of β-chains. Each molecule also is associated with the T cell-specific tyrosine kinase p56.[55] CD4 and CD8 act as coreceptors during T cell activation by antigen. CD4 recognizes MHC II and CD8 recognizes MHC I (see Chap. 78). CD4 also is a coreceptor for the human immunodeficiency virus[56] (see Chap. 83), as are CCR5 and CXCR4.

CD25

CD25 originally was defined as a component of the interleukin-2 receptor (IL-2R).[57] This antigen is expressed on activated T and B cells. CD25 also is found on thymocytes and monocytes. IL-2R is composed of three distinct proteins: α-chain (CD25), β-chain (CD122), and γ-chain, which also is a component of the receptors for IL-4, IL-7, IL-9, IL-13, and IL-15. When IL-2 is bound to the α-chain alone, IL-2 binds with higher affinity to the IL-2R β-chain. The result is formation of a high-affinity complex of IL-2 bound to both IL-2R α- and β-chains.[58] The γ-chain is involved in signaling to the cell after IL-2 binding. IL-2 binding to the high-affinity receptor signals T cells to proliferate and differentiate into specific effector T cells (e.g., helper T or cytotoxic T cells). Absence of the γ-chain causes one form of severe combined immune deficiency disease.

CD28

CD28 is a 44-kDa homodimer that is expressed on resting T cells. CD28 is a surface receptor for a cyclosporine-resistant T cell signal transduction pathway.[59] CD28 binds the CD80 (B7/BB1) antigen expressed by activated B cells and professional antigen-presenting cells (see Chap. 78).[60] The interaction provides a second costimulatory signal to T cells that are activated by the cross-linking of their T cell antigen receptors in response to specific interactions with antigenic peptide bound to the major histocompatibility antigens expressed by antigen-presenting cells.[61,62] Without this second costimulatory signal,

the T cell may be induced into anergy.[63,64] In this state, the T cells fail to respond to the antigen(s) presented by the antigen-presenting cell because of a block in IL-2 gene expression.

CD45

CD45 is tyrosine-specific phosphatase.[65] It is expressed by virtually all hematopoietic cells. However, different isoforms exist because of alternative splicing of the CD45 transcript and differential glycosylation.[66] These different isoforms of CD45 are expressed differentially by different cell subsets (see Chap. 78). CD4+ helper T cells can be divided into functionally disparate subsets based on their expression of the different CD45 isoforms and CD29 (the VLA β-chain). Naive CD4+ helper T cells are CD45RA+ and express low levels of CD29. The CD4+ T cells can induce CD8+ T cells to down-regulate B cell IgG synthesis. After activation, T cell expression of CD45RA is diminished, but expression of CD29 and CD45RO (a lower-molecular-weight isoform of CD45) is enhanced.[67,68] CD4+ CD45RO+ CD29 high-affinity T cells are called *memory-helper T cells*, in that they apparently facilitate induction of B cell IgG synthesis in response to secondary challenge with antigen. In addition, CD45 is necessary for activation of either CD4+ or CD8+ T cells. T cells that lack expression of CD45 do not respond well to various activation stimuli.[68] In acute lymphoblastic leukemia of the early pre-B cell type, CD45 often is absent or significantly weaker than on normal cells.

CD154

CD154, which is present on CD4 T cells, is a member of the tumor necrosis alpha family. It is the ligand for CD40, through which T cells signal help to B cells for growth regulation and Ig class switching (see Chap. 14).

T CELL RECEPTOR

The T cell antigen receptor (TCR) is present on all mature T cells and on developing immature thymocytes (see Chap. 78). The TCR may have unique determinants that are found on all T cells within a given T cell clone. It is expressed by most T cell lymphomas. Two forms exist: dimers of α- and β-chains or γ- and δ-chains. γ/δ T cells usually are CD4− and CD8− and associated with non-MHC−restricted cytotoxicity. Demonstration of clonal receptor gene rearrangements allows diagnosis of clonal T cell neoplasms.

NK CELLS

The NK cell is defined as an effector cell that is not MHC restricted and has the capacity for spontaneous cytotoxicity toward various target cells (see Chap. 79). The large granular lymphocyte was identified as the blood cell responsible for NK cell function because these cells, when enriched by sedimentation, accounted for almost all the blood NK cell activity.[69] However, not all NK cells have large granular lymphocyte morphology.

Large granular lymphocytes have a unique morphology (see Plate XX-3). These cells typically have round or indented nuclei and abundant pale cytoplasm containing a few coarse pink granules (diameter 1.0–2.0 μm).[70] Large granular lymphocytes have membrane-bound granules that stain for acid hydrolases, including acid phosphatase, α-naphthyl acetate esterase, and β-glucuronidase. These granules may be related to the cytolytic capacity of these cells. These cells do not express surface Ig and lack adherent or phagocytic properties. They may form rosettes with sheep erythrocytes and express Ig Fc receptors.[71] Despite their relative morphologic homogeneity, they comprise several subpopulations with distinct phenotypes. NK cells express class I but not class II antigens of the MHC. Human NK cells characteristically express CD16 (FcγRIII) and CD56 but not CD3.[72,73]

CD16 (FcγRIII) is a low-affinity receptor that binds to IgG, which is bound specifically to antigens present on cells targeted for destruction in antibody-dependent cell-mediated cytotoxicity. CD16 is expressed on all NK cells, neutrophils, and tissue macrophages. CD56 is the neural cell adhesion molecule (N-CAM) and is seen on most NK cells, albeit at low density.[74] This 200-kDa protein is expressed at higher levels following activation.

NK cells have some T cell antigens on their cell membranes, including CD8, found on approximately 30 to 50 percent of NK cells. The CD8 is weak on flow cytometry and is of the β-homodimer form. CD2 is present on about half of all NK cells, and CD38 is present at low density on most NK cells. However, NK cells do not express CD4.[75] Upon activation, NK cells express increased levels of CD25, CD56, and class II antigens of the MHC. Three cytokines that can activate NK cells are IL-2, interferon alpha, and IL-12. IL-2 also can induce NK cells and some T cells to differentiate into lymphokine-activated killer cells *in vitro* (see Chaps. 78 and 79).

REFERENCES

1. Hewson W, Johnson J: No. 72, Pauls Church Yard London, 1774, in *Lymphatics, Lymph and Lymphomyeloid Complex*, 3rd ed, edited by JM Yoffey, FC Courtice, p 3. Harvard University Press, Cambridge, 1970.

2. Everett NB, Caffey RW, Rieke WO: Recirculation of lymphocytes. *Ann N Y Acad Sci* 113:887, 1964.

3. Ford WL, Gowans JL: The traffic of lymphocytes. *Semin Hematol* 6:67, 1969.

4. Nossal GJV, Makela O: Elaboration of antibodies by single cells. *Annu Rev Microbiol* 16:53, 1962.

5. Miller RG: Physical separation of lymphocytes in the lymphocyte structure and function, in *Immunology Series*, vol 5, edited by JJ Marchalonis, p 205. Marcel Dekker, New York, 1977.

6. Ackerman GA: Structural studies of the lymphocyte and lymphocyte development, in *Regulation of Hematopoiesis*, vol 2, edited by AS Gordon, p 1297. Appleton Century Crofts, New York, 1970.

7. Brottinger G, Hirschhorn R, Douglas SD, Weissmann G: Studies on lysosomes: XI. Characterization of a hydrolase-rich fraction from human lymphocytes. *J Cell Biol* 37:394, 1968.

8. Yam LT, Li CY, Crosby WH: Cytochemical identification of monocytes and granulocytes. *Am J Clin Pathol* 55:283, 1971.

9. Timonen T, Ortaldo JR, Herberman RB: Characteristics of' human large granular lymphocytes and relationship to natural killer and K cells. *J Exp Med* 153:569, 1981.

10. Bevan A, Burns GF, Gray L, Cawley JC: Cytochemistry of human T-cell subpopulations. *Scand J Immunol* 11:223, 1980.

11. Basso G, Cocito MG, Semenzato G, et al: Cytochemical study of thymocytes and T lymphocytes. *Br J Haematol* 44:577, 1980.

12. Machin GA, Halper JP, Knowles DM: Cytochemically demonstrable β-glucuronidase activity in normal and neoplastic human lymphoid cells. *Blood* 56:1111, 1980.

13. Tung R, Silber R, Quagliata F, et al: ADA activity in chronic lymphocytic leukemia: Relationship to B- and T-cell subpopulations. *J Clin Invest* 57:756, 1976.

14. Rowe M, deGast GG, Platts-Mills TA, et al: 5'-nucleotidase of B and T lymphocytes isolated from human peripheral blood. *Clin Exp Immunol* 36:97, 1979.

15. Greenwood MF, Coleman MS, Hutton JJ, et al: Terminal deoxynucleotidyl transferase distribution in neoplastic and hematopoietic cells. *J Clin Invest* 59:889, 1977.

16. Bollum FJ: Terminal deoxynucleotidyl transferase as a hematopoietic cell marker. *Blood* 54:1203, 1979.

17. Cohen HJ: Human lymphocyte surface immunoglobulin capping: Normal characteristics and anomalous behavior of chronic lymphocytic leukemic lymphocytes. *J Clin Invest* 55:84, 1975.

18. Douglas SD: Human lymphocyte growth in vitro: Morphologic, biochemical and immunologic significance. *Int Rev Exp Pathol* 10:42, 1971.

19. Tanaka Y, Goodman JR: *Electron Microscopy of Human Blood Cells*. Harper & Row, New York, 1972.

20. Douglas SD, Cohnen G, Brittinger G: Ultrastructural comparison between phytomitogen transformed normal and chronic lymphocytic leukemic lymphocytes. *J Ultrastruct Res* 44:11, 1973.

21. Hayes TL: Scanning electron microscope techniques in biology, in *Advanced Techniques in Biological Electron Microscopy*, edited by JK Koehler, p 153. Springer, New York, 1973.

22. Polliack A, Lampen N, Clarkson BD, et al: Identification of human B and T lymphocytes by scanning electron microscopy. *J Exp Med* 138:607, 1973.

23. Polliack A, Hammerling V, Lampen N, DeHarven E: Surface morphology of murine B and T lymphocytes: A comparative study by scanning electron microscopy. *Eur J Immunol* 5:32, 1975.

24. Handwerger BS, Douglas SD: The cell biology of blastogenesis, in *Handbook of Inflammation*, vol 2, edited by G Weissman, p 609. Elsevier, North Holland, 1980.

25. Douglas SD, Fudenberg HH: In vitro development of plasma cells from lymphocytes following pokeweed mitogen stimulation: A fine structural study. *Exp Cell Res* 54:277, 1969.

26. Sainte-Marie G: Study on plasmocytopoiesis: Description of plasmocytes and of their mitoses in the mediastinal lymph nodes of ten-week-old rats. *Am J Anat* 114:207, 1964

27. Sainte-Marie G, Coons AH: Studies on antibody production: X. Mode of formation of plasmocytes in cell transfer experiments. *J Exp Med* 119:742, 1964.

28. Parkhouse RME, Janossy G, Greaves MF: Selective stimulation of IgM synthesis in mouse B lymphocytes by pokeweed mitogen. *Nat New Biol* 235:21, 1972.

29. Welsh RA: Electron microscopic localization of Russell bodies in the human plasma cell. *Blood* 16:1307, 1960.

30. Sachetti D: Le plasmacellule nel midollo osseo delluomo nella norma e nella pathologia: Richerche quantitative citometriche et auxologiche. *Haematologica* 35:13, 1951.

31. Quaglino D, Torelli V, Sauli S, Mauri C: Cytochemical and autoradiographic investigations on normal and myelomatous plasma cells. *Acta Haematol (Basel)* 38:79, 1967.

32. Lerner RG, Parker JW: Dysglobulinemia and iron in plasma cells: Ferrokinetics and electron microscopy. *Arch Intern Med* 121:284, 1968.

33. Suzuki A, Shibata A, Onodera S, et al: Histochemical study on plasma cells. *Tohoku J Exp Med* 97:1, 1969.

34. Franklin EC, Zucker-Franklin D: Current concepts on amyloid. *Adv Immunol* 15:249, 1972.

35. Bessis MC: Ultrastructure of lymphoid and plasma cells in relation to globulin and antibody formation. *Lab Invest* 10:1040, 1961.

36. Allison A, Alt F, Arnold L, et al: A new nomenclature for B cells. *Immunol Today* 12:383, 1991.

37. Kipps TJ: The CD5 B cell. *Adv Immunol* 47:117, 1989.

38. Defrance T, Vanbervliet B, Durand I, Banchereau J: Human interleukin 4 down-regulates the surface expression of CD5 on normal and leukemic B cells. *Eur J Immunol* 19:293, 1989.

39. Durandy A, Thuillier L, Forveille M, Fischer A: Phenotype and functional characteristics of human newborns' B lymphocytes. *J Immunol* 144:60, 1990.

40. Caligaris-Cappio F, Gobbi M, Bofill M, Janossy G: Infrequent normal B lymphocytes express features of B-chronic lymphocytic leukemia. *J Exp Med* 155:623, 1982.

41. Casali P, Prabhakar BS, Notkins AL: Characterization of multireactive autoantibodies and identification of LEU-1+ B lymphocytes as cells making antibodies binding multiple self and exogenous molecules. *Int Rev Immunol* 3:17, 1988.

42. Hayakawa K, Hardy RR, Honda M, et al: Ly-1 B cells: Functionally distinct lymphocytes that secrete IgM autoantibodies. *Proc Natl Acad Sci U S A* 81:2494, 1984.

43. Stoegher ZM, Wakai M, Tse DB, et al: Production of autoantibodies by CD5-expressing B lymphocytes from patients with chronic lymphocytic leukemia. *J Exp Med* 169:255, 1989.

44. Anderson KC, Park EK, Bates MP, et al: Antigens on human plasma cells identified by monoclonal antibodies. *J Immunol* 130:1132, 1983.

45. Rebbe NF, Tong BD, Finley EM, Hickman S: Identification of nucleotide pyrophosphatase/alkaline phosphodiesterase I activity associated with the mouse plasma cell differentiation antigen PC-1. *Proc Natl Acad Sci U S A* 88:5192, 1991.

46. Fithian E, Kuag P, Goldstein G, et al: Receptivity of Langerhans cells with hybridoma antibody. *Proc Natl Acad Sci U S A* 78:2541, 1988.

47. Siciliano R, Pratt JC, Schmidt RE, et al: Activation of cytolytic T lymphocyte and natural killer cell function through the T11 sheep erythrocyte binding protein. *Nature* 317:428, 1985.

48. Fox DA, Hussey RE, Fitzgerald KA, et al: Activation of human thymocytes via the 50-kD T11 sheep erythrocyte binding protein induces the expression of interleukin 2 receptors on both T3+ and T3− populations. *J Immunol* 134:330, 1985.

49. Keegan A, Paul W: Multichain immune recognition receptors: Similarities in structure and signaling pathways. *Immunol Today* 13:63, 1992.

50. Link M, Warnke R, Finlay J, et al: A single monoclonal antibody identifies T-cell lineage of childhood lymphoid malignancies. *Blood* 2:722, 1983.

51. Haynes BF, Martin ME, Kay HH, Kuntzborg J: Early events in human T cell ontogeny. *J Exp Med* 168:1061, 1988.

52. Chabannon C, Wood P, Torak-Storg B: Expression of CD7 normal human myeloid progenitors. *J Immunol* 149:2110, 1992.

53. Madden PJ, Littman DR, Godfrey M, et al: The isolation and nucleotide sequence of a cDNA encoding the T cell surface protein T4: A new member of the immunoglobulin gene family. *Cell* 42:93, 1985.

54. Snow PM, Terhorst C: The T8 antigen is a multimeric complex of two distinct subunits as human thymocytes but consists of homomultimeric forms on peripheral blood T lymphocytes. *J Biol Chem* 258:14675, 1983.

55. Luo K, Sefton BM: Cross linking of T cell surface molecules CD4 and CD8 stimulates phosphorylation of the lck tyrosine phosphorylation kinase at the autophosphorylation site. *Mol Cell Biol* 10:5305, 1990.

56. Dalgleish AG, Beverley PCL, Clapham PR, et al: The CD4(T4) antigen is an essential component of the receptor for the AIDS retrovirus. *Nature* 312:763, 1984.

57. Greene WC, Leonard WJ: The human interleukin-2 receptor, in *Annual Review of Immunology*, vol 4, edited by WE Paul, CG Fathman, H Metzger, p 69. Annual Reviews, Palo Alto, 1986.

58. Arima N, Kamio M, Okuma M, et al: The IL-2 receptor α-chain alters the binding of IL-2 to the β-chain. *J Immunol* 147:3396, 1991.

59. van Lier RA, Brouwer M, Aarden LA: Signals involved in T cell activation. T cell proliferation through the synergistic action of anti-CD28 and anti-CD2 monoclonal antibodies. *Eur J Immunol* 18:167, 1988.

60. Linsley PS, Brady W, Grosmaire L, et al: Binding of the B cell activation antigen B7 to CD28 costimulates T cell proliferation and interleukin 2 mRNA accumulation. *J Exp Med* 173:721, 1991.

61. Koulova L, Clark EA, Shu G, Dupont B: The CD28 ligand B7/BB1 provides costimulatory signal for alloactivation of CD4+ T cells. *J Exp Med* 173:759, 1991.

62. Gimmi CD, Freeman GJ, Gribben JG, et al: B-cell surface B7 provides a costimulatory signal that induces T cells to proliferate and secrete interleukin 2. *Proc Natl Acad Sci U S A* 88:6575, 1991.

63. Linsley PS, Wallace PM, Johnson J, et al: Immunosuppression in vivo by a soluble form of the CTLA-4 T cell activation molecule. *Science* 257:792, 1992.

64. Kang S-M, Beverly B, Tran A-C, et al: Transactivation by AP-1 is a molecular target of T cell clonal anergy. *Science* 257:1134, 1992.

65. Tonks NK, Charbonneau H, Diltz CD, et al: Demonstration that the leucocyte common antigen (CD45) is a protein tyrosine phosphatase. *Biochemistry* 27:8695, 1989.

66. LeFrancois L, Thomas ML, Beran MJ, Trowbridge IS: Different classes of T lymphocytes have different mRNAs for the leucocyte-common antigen T200. *J Exp Med* 163:1337, 1986.

67. Ievata S, Ohashi Y, Kamiguchi K, Morimoto C: Beta 1-integrin mediated cell signaling in T lymphocytes. *J Dermatol Sci* 23:75, 2000.

68. Janeway CA: The T cell receptor as a multicomponent signaling machine: CD4/CD8 coreceptors and CD45 in T cell activation. *Annu Rev Immunol* 10:645, 1992.

69. Timonen T, Jaksela E: Isolation of human natural killer cells by density gradient centrifugation. *J Immunol Methods* 36:285, 1980.

70. Grossi CE, Ferrarini M: Morphology and cytochemistry of human large granular lymphocytes, in *NK Cells and Other Natural Effector Cells*, edited by RB Herberman, p 1. Academic Press, New York, 1982.

71. West WH, Cannon GB, Kay HD, et al: Natural cytotoxic reactivity of human lymphocytes against a myeloid cell line: Characterization of effector cells. *J Immunol* 118:355, 1977.

72. Lanier LL, Phillips JH, Hackett J, et al: Opinion and natural killer cells: Definition of a cell type rather than a function. *J Immunol* 137:2735, 1986.

73. Hercend T, Griffin JD, Bensussan A, et al: Generation of monoclonal antibodies to a human natural killer clone: Characterization of two natural killer associated antigens, NKH1a and NKH2, expressed on subsets of large granular lymphocytes. *J Clin Invest* 75:932, 1985.

74. Lanier LL, Le AM, Phillips JH, et al: Subpopulations of human natural killer cells defined by expression of the Leu7 (HNK-1) and Leu11 (NK-15) antigens. *J Immunol* 131:1789, 1983.

75. Hercend T, Schmidt RE: Characteristics and uses of natural killer cells. *Immunol Today* 9:292, 1988.

COMPOSITION AND BIOCHEMISTRY OF LYMPHOCYTES AND PLASMA CELLS

THOMAS J. KIPPS

DENNIS A. CARSON

Mature lymphocytes can be divided into several functional types and subtypes. The major classes of lymphocytes are the T cells, B cells, and natural killer cells. T lymphocytes are derived from the thymus (see Chaps. 5 and 76) and are responsible for cell-mediated cytotoxic reactions and for delayed hypersensitivity responses (see Chap. 78). They also produce the cytokines that regulate immune responses and provide helper activity for B cells. B lymphocytes can concentrate and present antigens to T cells and are the precursors of immunoglobulin-secreting plasma cells (see Chap. 77). Natural killer cells account for innate immunity against infectious agents and transformed cells that have altered expression of transplantation antigens (see Chap. 79). This chapter describes methods for isolating lymphocytes and discusses their physical and biochemical properties.

ISOLATION OF LYMPHOCYTES

LYMPHOCYTE DENSITY

Lymphocytes can be isolated from the blood using density gradient centrifugation. Most commonly, density gradient centrifugation is performed using a step gradient composed of a mixture of the carbohydrate polymer Ficoll and the dense iodine-containing compound sodium metrizoate.[1] This technique takes advantage of the low density of lymphocytes (1.07 g/ml) relative to that of erythrocytes (1.09–1.10 g/ml), granulocytes (1.08–1.09 g/ml), and monocytes (1.08 g/ml).

A Ficoll solution adjusted to a density of 1.077 g/ml is ideal for isolating human lymphocytes. Whole blood is layered onto a cushion of Ficoll-sodium metrizoate prior to centrifugation at 400g for 30 minutes. The denser red blood cells and granulocytes sediment to the bottom of the tube, and the monocytes enter into the Ficoll cushion. The lymphocytes can be collected from the interface formed between the Ficoll-sodium metrizoate cushion and the plasma above, which con-

tains the lighter-density platelets (1.04–1.06 g/ml). This layer contains lymphocytes and some monocytes, which can be removed by plating the cells in culture flasks and harvesting the lymphocytes that are not adherent to plastic.

LYMPHOCYTE SURFACE ANTIGENS

Lymphocyte subsets generally cannot be distinguished from one another by morphology. Most resting lymphocytes appear as small round cells with a dense nucleus and little cytoplasm (see Chap. 74). However, this homogeneous appearance is deceptive, as these cells compose many functionally distinct subpopulations.

These subsets can be distinguished through the differential expression of cell surface proteins, each of which can be recognized by a specific monoclonal antibody. Coupled with the biochemical analyses of the surface molecules that are recognized by each of these antibodies, many lymphocyte surface antigens have been defined (see Chap. 14).

Typically, coexpression of two or more cell surface proteins must be monitored to define a functional subset of lymphocytes. The same cell surface protein often is expressed by more than one cell subset. For example, both helper and cytotoxic T cells express CD3, the proteins associated with the T cell receptor for antigen (see Chap. 78). Expression of both CD3 and CD4 helps to distinguish mature helper T cells from cytotoxic T cells that express CD3 and CD8 and from other cells, such as dendritic cells, that express CD4 but lack expression of CD3.[2] Another subset of T cells with immunoregulatory function (sometimes referred to *Treg cells*) is defined by the coexpression of CD3, CD4, and CD25, the low-affinity receptor for interleukin-2. For these and other types of lymphocytes, the expression of a characteristic constellation of surface molecules, rather than the expression of any one particular surface marker, generally helps to distinguish one subset of lymphocytes from another (see Chap. 14).

Fluorescent probes also can be used to identify antigen-specific lymphocytes.[3] Each clone of B lymphocytes expresses immunoglobulin capable of binding a particular antigen (see Chap. 77). The frequencies of B cells specific for one antigen have been estimated to range from one in 100,000 to 1,000,000 cells or less. Populations of lymphocytes enriched for B cells binding to a specific antigen can be stained using antigen coupled to probes allowing for the detection and isolation of antigen-specific B cells using flow cytometry.[4] T lymphocytes, on the other hand, generally recognize antigen in the form of peptides nestled into molecules of the major histocompatibility complex (MHC) (see Chap. 78). Identification and isolation of antigen-specific T cells therefore require more complex probes using multimeric complexes composed of specific peptide antigen complexed with the relevant MHC molecule.[3]

FLOW CYTOMETRY

The flow cytometer is a highly effective tool for defining these lymphocyte subsets.[5] This instrument is based on the principle of fluorescence, or the emission of light resulting from the release of energy gained through the absorption of light at a different wavelength. Monoclonal antibodies specific for desired cell surface proteins each can be coupled to a fluorescent dye, called a *fluorochrome*, that fluoresces with a defined spectrum of light when excited by light at a certain wavelength.[6] The flow cytometer can detect cells labeled with such fluorochrome-conjugated antibodies as they pass in a liquid stream through a beam of laser light of defined wavelength. As each cell passes through the laser beam, the laser light is scattered and excites any dye molecules bound to the cell, causing it to fluoresce. Sensitive photomultiplier tubes can detect the scattered light and the fluorescence emissions, providing information on each cell's granularity and the extent to which it bound a given fluorescence dye, respectively.

This technique is the most common means used for distinguishing the lymphocyte subsets from one another.

The flow cytometer also can be used to isolate lymphocytes that express selected surface antigens. This process requires a *fluorescent-activated cell sorter* (FACS). With this instrument, the fluorescence signals of cells passing through the laser light are passed back to a computer. This process in turn triggers an electric charge that passes from the nozzle through the liquid stream at the precise time the stream is breaking up into droplets containing the desired cell.[7] Therefore, the droplets have a positive or negative charge, allowing for their deflection from the main stream of droplets as they pass between plates of opposite charge. In this way, different subsets of cells can be isolated from each other and from the unsorted cells in nondeflected droplets.

In addition, the flow cytometer can be used to monitor for lymphocyte cell division[3,8] and/or to identify lymphocyte subsets that produce specific cytokines[3] or express specific intracellular proteins or enzymes.[9,10] Using monoclonal antibodies specific for particular phosphoproteins, flow cytometry can be used to monitor the biochemical events that occur within lymphocytes that are stimulated with antigen or by cross-linking one or more surface receptor molecules.[11] The advent of these new technologies should allow for better understanding of how different lymphocyte subpopulations respond to various microenvironmental signals that occur during the immune response to antigen (see Chap. 78).[12]

OTHER SEPARATION TECHNIQUES

An effective way of isolating lymphocyte subpopulations is to expose them to paramagnetic beads coated with a monoclonal antibody specific for a surface molecule that is differentially expressed by the desired versus the undesired cell subpopulation.[13] The tube of cells then is placed in a strong magnetic field, thereby attracting the cells that are attached to the beads. The cells attached to the beads are retained, allowing for decanting of the cells that lack the specific surface molecule. The decanted cells lacking the surface molecule are designated as being isolated via *negative selection*. Bead-bound cells can be harvested and released from the magnetic beads by adding an antibody that reacts with the antibody attached to the magnetic beads, thereby displacing the cells that are bound to the magnetic-bound antibody. The released cells are said to have been isolated via *positive selection*.

Lymphocyte subsets also can be isolated by binding the cells to plates that are coated with antibodies to a selected surface antigen or with selected surface proteins,[14] a technique known as *panning*. Alternatively, cells binding a specific complement-fixing antibody can be lysed with complement, leaving behind those cells that lack expression of the targeted surface antigen. All these techniques can be used to enrich for a selected cell subset or to deplete an undesired subset, prior to sorting using the FACS.

COMPOSITION OF LYMPHOCYTES

Unfortunately, few studies of the composition and biochemistry of lymphocytes have used purified lymphocyte subpopulations. Because mature helper T cells are the predominant blood lymphocyte of normal adults, many reported biochemical parameters are most relevant to this subpopulation.

ION AND WATER CONTENT

The resting blood lymphocyte has a mean cell volume of 200 μm^3 and contains 71 ± 1.2 percent by weight of water.[15] The total lymphocyte cation content is 35 fm per cell, of which 22 to 28 fm per cell is potassium and 7.9 ± 3.2 fm per cell is sodium.[16] Lymphocyte membranes have both voltage-gated and calcium-activated potassium channels that regulate cell volume. Pharmacologic inhibition of these channels blocks T cell activation. The calcium content of resting lymphocytes has been estimated at 580 to 800 $pmol/10^6$ cells.[17] Cytosolic free calcium concentrations are relatively low in resting lymphocytes (approximately 10^{-7} M) but increase several-fold after activation.[18]

LYMPHOCYTE MEMBRANE

The lymphocyte plasma membrane is composed of equal parts by weight of protein and glycosphingolipids and 6 percent by weight of carbohydrate.[19] The molar ratio of cholesterol to phospholipid is approximately 0.5.[20,21] Phosphatidylcholine is the predominant phospholipid in the lymphocyte plasma membrane, but phosphatidylethanolamine, phosphatidylinositol, phosphatidylserine, and sphingomyelin also are present. Approximately half the membrane fatty acids are saturated. The membrane proteins usually are glycosylated.

The glycosphingolipids and protein receptors of lymphocytes often are organized in glycolipoprotein microdomains termed *lipid rafts*.[22,23] Such lipid rafts sequester various protein receptors, coreceptors, and accessory molecules that together are involved in lymphocyte cell signaling, cytoskeletal reorganization, and/or membrane trafficking.[24] As such, the surface molecules on lymphocytes are not randomly distributed.

EXTRACELLULAR MEMBRANE-ASSOCIATED ENZYMES (ECTOENZYMES)

Exposed on the exterior surface of lymphocytes are several enzymes called *ectoenzymes* (Table 75-1). Generally, the number of surface enzyme molecules is low compared with the number of other surface molecules, such as those involved in lymphocyte adhesion (see Chap. 14). This finding probably reflects the fact that these molecules are catalytic and have a higher functional specific activity than do molecules involved in adhesion events, where multiple interactions over large surface areas are required. As such, it is possible that many more enzymes are present than the enzymes currently recognized because they are expressed at levels that are not detectable by conventional methods using monoclonal antibodies and flow cytometry.

Some of the surface enzymes are involved in nucleotide metabolism (see Table 75-1). For example, CD73 is an ecto-5'-nucleotidase that catalyzes the 5' dephosphorylation of purine and pyrimidine ribonucleoside and deoxyribonucleoside monophosphates to nucleosides that can be taken up by transport systems.[25] This ecto-5'-nucleotidase is attached to the plasma membrane by a glycerol phosphatidylinositol anchor (see Chap. 14). In addition, lymphocytes express a membrane-associated adenosine deaminase, the levels of which are increased after activation.[26] The shedding of adenosine deaminase by stimulated cells may explain why plasma levels of this enzyme are increased in early HIV infection and in other diseases associated with immune activation.[27]

The ectoenzymes of nucleotide metabolism may regulate lymphocyte and granulocyte function at sites of inflammation. Activated T lymphocytes can release adenosine 5'-triphosphate (ATP), which in turn can bind to specific plasma membrane ATP receptors.[27] In addition, CD38 can catalyze the transient formation of cyclic adenosine 5'-diphosphate (ADP)-ribose, a new second messenger molecule directly involved in the control of calcium homeostasis by means of receptor-mediated release of calcium from ryanodine-sensitive intracellular stores.[28] The consequent increase in calcium mobilization and phospholipid breakdown can provoke activation or death, depending on the target cell. Subsequently, dephosphorylation of ATP generates adenosine, which can interact with A2 receptors on the plasma membranes of neutrophils, monocytes, and lymphocytes. The engagement

TABLE 75-1   ECTOENZYMES EXPRESSED BY LYMPHOCYTES

SURFACE MOLECULE	ENZYMATIC ACTIVITY	FUNCTION	REFERENCE
CD10	Neutral endopeptidase, EC 3.4.24.11	Metalloproteinase that may also play a role in the metabolic stability of glucagon-like peptide-1	30
CD13	Aminopeptidase N, EC 3.4.11.2	Aminopeptidase involved in trimming peptides bound to MHC class II molecules and cleaving MIP-1 chemokine to alter target cell specificity; also served as receptor for coronavirus.	91
CD26	Dipeptidylpeptidase IV, EC 3.4.14.5	Serine peptidase that may be involved in T cell signaling and T cell activation	32
CD38	ADP-ribosyl cyclase, EC 3.4.14.5	Ectoenzyme with NAD glycohydrolase, ADP ribosyl cyclase, and cyclic ADP ribose hydrolase activities	92
CD39	Ecto (Ca^{2+}, Mg^{2+})-apyrase (ecto-ATPase)	Ectoenzyme with ADPase and ATPase activities that plays a role in regulating platelet aggregation	93
CD73	Ecto-5′-nucleotidase	Ecto-5′-nucleotidase that may play a role in T cell signaling	25
CD143	Peptidyl-dipeptide hydrolase (angiotensin-converting enzyme [ACE])	Peptidyl-dipeptide hydrolase that is involved in the metabolism of vasoactive peptides angiotensin II and bradykinin	94
CD156a	ADAM8 metalloprotease	Matrix metalloprotease that may play a role in leukocyte extravasation	34
CD156b	ADAM17 metalloprotease	Metalloprotease that cleaves membrane-bound tumor necrosis factor (TNF) and transforming growth factor α to release the soluble cytokine	35
CD157	ADP ribosyl cyclase and cyclic ADP ribose hydrolase	ADP ribosyl cyclase and cyclic ADP ribose hydrolase that may play a role in lymphocyte development; like CD38, this enzyme also is involved in NAD metabolism	95
CD224	γ-Glutamyl transpeptidase, EC 2.3.2.2	γ-Glutamyl transpeptidase role in γ-glutamyl cycle involving degradation and neosynthesis of glutathione	96

of A2 receptors elevates cyclic adenosine 3′,5′-monophosphate (cAMP) levels, counteracting the effects of ATP on cell activation.[29] The deamination of adenosine permits the cycle to begin anew.

The ectodomains of several other surface antigens can possess proteolytic activity. For example, CD10 (or CALLA) also has neutral endopeptidase activity,[30] and CD26 has dipeptidyl peptidase IV activity.[31,32] These enzymes may play a role in modulating the binding of lymphocytes to other cells and to the extracellular matrix. In addition, inhibition of the catalytic activity of CD26 can provoke many cellular effects, including induction of tyrosine phosphorylation and p38 MAP kinase activation, suppression of DNA synthesis, and reduced production of various cytokines. As such, these ectoenzymes may play an important role in lymphocyte activation.

Some membrane-bound proteases have a disintegrin and a metalloprotease (ADAM) domain.[33,34] One member of this family of proteins is the tumor necrosis factor-α converting enzyme (TACE), otherwise known as ADAM17 (CD156b).[35] These enzymes cleave other surface molecules, such as tumor necrosis factor, thereby releasing the soluble active cytokine.[36] In addition, they may play an important role in modifying the activity of cytokines or other cell surface molecules that are present in the vicinity of the plasma membrane.

INTRACELLULAR MEMBRANE-ASSOCIATED ENZYMES

Transmembrane proteins that have cytoplasmic regions with kinase or phosphatase activities are common in biology, although relatively few of these are restricted to lymphocytes. Nevertheless, many cytoplasmic domains of transmembrane proteins interact directly with enzymes that are restricted or preferentially expressed by lymphocytes or lymphocyte subsets (see Chaps. 76 and 77). For example, B lymphocytes selectively express Bruton tyrosine kinase (Btk), a tyrosine kinase that plays a critical role in signal transduction via surface immunoglobulin receptors.[37] Moreover, mutations that disrupt the function of such kinases can impair B cell development, leading to dysregulated B cell function or immune deficiency.[38,39] On the other hand, T cell development and function rely heavily on cytoplasmic receptor-associated tyrosine kinases, such as the zeta-associated protein of 70 kDa (ZAP-70) or leukocyte tyrosine kinase (lck).[40,41] ZAP-70 interacts with the T cell receptor for antigen, whereas lck is an Src-family tyrosine kinase

that interacts with cytoplasmic domains of CD2,[42] CD4,[43] CD8,[43] CD44,[44] CD50,[45] and CD137.[46] Through such interactions, these receptor protein tyrosine kinases play important roles in signal transduction following immune recognition and/or cognate intercellular immune interactions.

In addition, lymphocytes possess an important class of intracellular molecules known collectively as *adapter proteins*, which have no intrinsic enzymatic activity.[47–49] These adaptor proteins can serve as a scaffolding for the assembly of kinases and other signaling molecules following antigen-receptor ligation. One important adaptor protein expressed in B lymphocytes is B cell linker protein (BLNK) (see Chap. 77).[50] On the other hand, T cells use a distinct adaptor protein called *linker for activation of T cells* (LAT).[51] These molecules couple proximal biochemical events initiated by surface-receptor ligation with more distal signaling pathways by recruiting other cytosolic proteins (see Chaps. 77 and 78).

CYTOPLASMIC STRUCTURES

CYTOMATRIX

Beneath the lymphocyte's plasma membrane is a fully developed cytomatrix with several different structural and mechanical proteins, including tubulin, actin, myosin, tropomyosin, α-actinin, filamin, and a spectrin-like molecule. These proteins are arranged into typical microfilaments, microtubules, and intermediate filaments.[52] Lymphocyte activation by antigens or mitogens can lead to changes in the interaction of membrane components with the cytoskeleton, allowing for antigen processing, immunoglobulin secretion, or cell-mediated cytotoxic reactions.

ORGANELLES

In large part, the composition and metabolism of long-lived blood T lymphocytes reflects their resting state. The T cells have a high nuclear to cytoplasmic ratio, few ribosomes or mitochondria, and scant endoplasmic reticulum. Glycogen stores are meager. The DNA content of the resting small lymphocyte, 8 pg per cell, is the same amount as in other diploid cells. In contrast, the RNA content averages 2.5 pg per cell, yielding an RNA to DNA ratio of approximately 0.32.[53] This value is less than in most other human cells because of the small amount of ribosomal RNA in lymphocytes.

In contrast to most lymphocytes, however, plasma cells have a high RNA to DNA ratio. These cells are the end products of B cell differentiation and are committed to the synthesis, assembly, and secretion of immunoglobulin. Accordingly, these cells have a well-developed rough endoplasmic reticulum and Golgi apparatus but lack many of the surface receptors found on lymphocytes. Mature plasma cells probably are terminally differentiated and have a low rate of DNA synthesis and abundant RNA, reflecting the plasma cell's high-level synthesis of immunoglobulin protein.

LYSOSOMES

The few lysosomes in blood lymphocytes contain several different acid hydrolases, including acid phosphatase, β-glucuronidase, β-galactosidase, β-hexosaminidase, α-arabinosidase, α-galactosidase, α-mannosidase, α-glucosidase, and β-glucosidase.[54] Acid hydrolase activities are generally higher in T cells than in non-T lymphocytes. Lysosomal acid esterase, assayed histochemically with α-naphthyl acetate as substrate, has a characteristic punctate appearance in mature T lymphocytes.[55]

CYTOPLASMIC GRANULES

In contrast to other lymphocytes, cytotoxic T lymphocytes and natural killer cells possess abundant cytoplasmic granules. These granules contain the pore-forming proteolytic enzyme *perforin* and a series of serine proteinases with specific proapoptotic activity, called *granzymes*.[56] To protect against possible autolysis by granule contents, cytotoxic lymphocytes possess serine proteinase inhibitors, termed *serpins*.[57] As an additional safeguard, the granzymes of resting lymphocytes are stored as inactive proenzymes.

Cytotoxic lymphocytes rely primarily on the perforin/granzyme system to kill their targets.[58,59] Upon contact with its target cell, the cytotoxic lymphocyte converts the granzymes into active forms by a lysosomal cysteine protease called *dipeptidyl peptidase I* (DPPI).[60] Then perforin introduces a pore in the membrane, allowing the activated granzymes and other granule contents to pass into the cytoplasm and then the nucleus of the cell targeted for destruction.[61,62] *In vitro* studies indicate granzyme nuclear import is independent of ATP, cannot be inhibited by nonhydrolyzable guanosine triphosphate analogues, and involves binding within the nucleus, unlike conventional signal-dependent nuclear protein import. The perforin-dependent nuclear entry of granzymes precedes the nuclear events of apoptosis, such as DNA fragmentation and breakdown of the nuclear envelope (see Chap. 11).

LYMPHOCYTE METABOLISM

FATTY ACID AND LIPID SYNTHESIS

Normal lymphocytes synthesize phospholipids from acetate. The cells contain phospholipases A_1, A_2, C, and D and the enzymes of the inositol phosphate metabolic cycle.[63]

In contrast to monocytes, small lymphocytes probably do not synthesize prostaglandins or leukotrienes; however, small lymphocytes may contain prostaglandin receptors. Prostaglandins synthesized by macrophages inhibit lymphocyte function and may be partially responsible for the impaired immunity associated with chronic inflammatory states such as Hodgkin disease or systemic fungal infections.[64] Certain natural fatty acid precursors of prostaglandins, such as γ-linoleic acid, suppress immune function and may be useful for treatment of autoimmune disorders.[65] However, some prostaglandins may facil-

itate immunoglobulin class switching and synthesis of selected cytokines or cytokine receptors.[66]

CARBOHYDRATE METABOLISM

Quiescent blood lymphocytes have few or no insulin receptors, although these receptors appear following activation. The rate of glucose metabolism is limited by the rate of entry of glucose into the cells by facilitated diffusion. Lymphocytes contain all the enzymes of the glycolytic pathway and the tricarboxylic acid cycle. Although resting lymphocytes consume only small amounts of oxygen *in vitro*, their mitochondria typically have coupled electron transport chains.

The resting lymphocyte requires energy to maintain its ionic milieu, to replace degraded proteins and lipids, and for active locomotion.[67,68] The recirculation of long-lived lymphocytes through the vascular space to the interstitial tissues and back from the lymphatic drainage system requires directed cell movement and utilizes considerable amounts of ATP. Lymphocytes treated with nonlethal concentrations of drugs that specifically inhibit mitochondrial respiration, but not with agents that inhibit glycolysis, recirculate sluggishly. This finding suggests that the energy for lymphocyte locomotion is derived largely from oxidative phosphorylation.[68]

The enzymes of the pentose phosphate pathway account for only a small fraction of energy production in resting lymphocytes.[69] As in other cell types, the pathway provides lymphocytes with phosphorylated ribose derivatives necessary for purine and pyrimidine synthesis and with a source of reducing energy in the form of reduced nicotinamide adenine dinucleotide phosphate (NADPH).

PROTEIN SYNTHESIS AND AMINO ACID METABOLISM

Human blood lymphocytes actively incorporate radioactive amino acids into protein. The protein synthesis is necessary for survival, and inhibition with cycloheximide or puromycin leads to the rapid death of lymphocytes.

The metabolic pathways for the synthesis of two normally nonessential amino acids, L-cysteine and L-asparagine, are inadequate in thymic lymphocytes and probably in blood T cells.[70,71] A similar L-asparagine requirement among certain null and T cell leukemias is responsible for the L-asparaginase sensitivity of these neoplasms.

NUCLEIC ACID SYNTHESIS AND REPAIR

RNA SYNTHESIS

Blood lymphocytes incorporate radioactive uridine into RNA at a slow but measurable rate. The cells contain the heterogeneous ribonucleoprotein particles that are important for RNA transport and splicing. In B cells, different species of RNA direct the synthesis of immunoglobulin light and heavy chains that are either inserted into the plasma membrane or secreted.[72] The former predominate in nonstimulated B cells. These RNA species undergo extensive processing in the cytoplasm prior to translation, including generation of 5'-terminal cap structures, internal methylations, and selective removal of intervening sequences.[72]

NUCLEOTIDE METABOLISM

The enzymes for the early pathways of *de novo* purine and pyrimidine synthesis have very low activity in blood lymphocytes, consistent with the small nucleotide requirements of these nondividing cells. The lymphocytes also have minimal ribonucleotide reductase activity and a concomitantly low rate of deoxyribonucleotide synthesis. In contrast, enzymes for purine and pyrimidine intraconversion are easily detectable, with the exception of xanthine oxidase and guanase, which are absent in lymphocytes. The lymphocytes have the capacity to utilize preformed purines and pyrimidines in the plasma, when they are available. However, patients with genetic deficiencies of the purine salvage enzymes hypoxanthine-guanine phosphoribosyltransferase (Lesch-Nyhan syndrome) and adenine phosphoribosyltransferase have normal numbers of lymphocytes and adequate immune function. Hence, the purine salvage pathways are not absolutely necessary for lymphocyte survival.

Genetic deficiencies in two enzymes of purine metabolism, adenosine deaminase and purine nucleoside phosphorylase, are associated with a specific impairment of the development and function of the lymphoid system.[73] The primary function of these enzymes is the catabolism of the potentially toxic nucleosides deoxyadenosine and deoxyguanosine. In adenosine deaminase- and purine nucleoside phosphorylase-deficient patients, phosphorylated derivatives of deoxyadenosine and deoxyguanosine may accumulate in lymphocytes. Compared with other cell types, the lymphocytes have high levels of deoxycytidine kinase, for which the purine deoxyribonucleosides are alternative substrates, and low levels of cytoplasmic deoxynucleotidase.

HORMONES AND VITAMINS

Lymphocytes have receptors for several biologically active peptides, including adrenocorticotropic hormone, corticotrophin-releasing hormone, calcitonin, calcitonin gene-related peptide, melatonin, endorphins, enkephalins, vasopressin, oxytocin, thyrotropin, the tachykinins, bombesin, prolactin, growth hormone, somatostatin, vasoactive intestinal peptide, and chemokines.[74-77] The various neuropeptides can deliver both positive and negative activation signals to lymphocytes. For example, the tachykinin substance P, which is released by peripheral nerves at sites of injury or inflammation, enhances lymphocyte activation by monocytes.[78] Immune function is inhibited by the dopamine D2 receptor-agonist bromocriptine, which causes hypoprolactinemia. Antibodies against prolactin block lymphocyte mitogenesis.[75]

Lymphocyte activation and proliferation require enhanced cell metabolism, leading to an increased requirement for cofactors required for DNA and protein synthesis. For example, proliferating lymphocytes generally increase biotin uptake presumably to provide adequate coenzyme for biotin-dependent carboxylases.[79] Also, the receptor density for peptide hormones on lymphocytes generally increases markedly following activation of the cells.

Glucocorticoids in pharmacologic concentrations have a unique lympholytic effect that is not dependent upon cell division, and they are potent immunosuppressive agents.[80] Among normal lymphocyte subsets, immature T cells in the thymus are most sensitive. Lymphocytes contain high-affinity receptors for glucocorticoids that may direct and enhance immune functions when they interact with glucocorticoids at physiologic concentrations.[81] The glucocorticoid-receptor complexes bind to specific DNA sequences and induce mRNA for proteins that inhibit glucose transport and phospholipid hydrolysis.[82] Exposure of lymphocytes to high concentrations of glucocorticoids causes endonuclease activation and DNA fragmentation.[83-86] Glucocorticoids also profoundly inhibit the synthesis of interleukin-2 by activated T cells and of interleukin-1 by monocytes.[87] The latter two effects offer an attractive explanation for the immunosuppressive effects of the hormones.

Lymphocytes presumably have receptors for androgens and estrogens, given that the sex hormones can modulate immune function.[88] The incidence of many autoimmune diseases is higher in females than in males. Androgen therapy may benefit some women with systemic lupus erythematosus but frequently causes unacceptable masculinizing side effects. The androgens may inhibit formation of proinflammatory cytokines by lymphocytes and monocytes, either directly or through release of transforming growth factor β_1.

The natural adrenal steroid dehydroepiandrosterone (DHEA) stimulates lymphocyte function in old mice, perhaps by interaction with a DHEA receptor complex on T cells.[89] Plasma levels of DHEA in people decline with age.[90] Whether DHEA supplementation can enhance immune responses in aged humans is not known.

REFERENCES

1. Bøyum A: Isolation of mononuclear cells and granulocytes from human blood. Isolation of mononuclear cells by one centrifugation, and of granulocytes by combining centrifugation and sedimentation at 1 g. *Scand J Clin Lab Invest Suppl* 97:77, 1968.

2. O'Doherty U, Steinman RM, Peng M, et al: Dendritic cells freshly isolated from human blood express CD4 and mature into typical immunostimulatory dendritic cells after culture in monocyte-conditioned medium. *J Exp Med* 178:1067, 1993.

3. Thiel A, Scheffold A, Radbruch A: Antigen-specific cytometry—New tools arrived! *Clin Immunol* 111:155, 2004.

4. Kodituwakku AP, Jessup C, Zola H, Roberton DM: Isolation of antigen-specific B cells. *Immunol Cell Biol* 81:163, 2003.

5. Jennings CD, Foon KA: Recent advances in flow cytometry: Application to the diagnosis of hematologic malignancy. *Blood* 90:2863, 1997.

6. Cunningham RE: Overview of flow cytometry and fluorescent probes for cytometry. *Methods Mol Biol* 115:249, 1999.

7. Orfao A, Ruiz-Arguelles A: General concepts about cell sorting techniques. *Clin Biochem* 29:5, 1996.

8. Lyons AB: Analysing cell division in vivo and in vitro using flow cytometric measurement of CFSE dye dilution. *J Immunol Methods* 243:147, 2000.

9. Francis C, Connelly MC: Rapid single-step method for flow cytometric detection of surface and intracellular antigens using whole blood. *Cytometry* 25.58, 1996.

10. Crespo M, Bosch F, Villamor N, et al: ZAP-70 expression as a surrogate for immunoglobulin-variable-region mutations in chronic lymphocytic leukemia. *N Engl J Med* 348:1764, 2003.

11. Krutzik PO, Irish JM, Nolan GP, Perez OD: Analysis of protein phosphorylation and cellular signaling events by flow cytometry: Techniques and clinical applications. *Clin Immunol* 110:206, 2004.

12. Perez OD, Krutzik PO, Nolan GP: Flow cytometric analysis of kinase signaling cascades. *Methods Mol Biol* 263:67, 2004.

13. Thiel A, Scheffold A, Radbruch A: Immunomagnetic cell sorting—Pushing the limits. *Immunotechnology* 4:89, 1998.

14. Hoellman JR, Suttles J, Stout RD: Panning T cells on vascular endothelial cell monolayers: A rapid method for enriching naive T cells. *Immunobiology* 203:769, 2001.

15. Segel GB, Cokelet GR, Lichtman MA: The measurement of lymphocyte volume: Importance of reference particle deformability and counting solution tonicity. *Blood* 57:894, 1981.

16. Segel GB, Simon W, Lichtman MA: Regulation of sodium and potassium transport in phytohemagglutinin-stimulated human blood lymphocytes. *J Clin Invest* 64:834, 1979.

17. Lichtman AH, Segel GB, Lichtman MA: An ultrasensitive method for the measurement of human leukocyte calcium: Lymphocytes. *Clin Chim Acta* 97:107, 1979.

18. Komada H, Nakabayashi H, Nakano H, et al: Measurement of the cytosolic free calcium ion concentration of individual lymphocytes by microfluorometry using quin 2 or fura-2. *Cell Struct Funct* 14:141, 1989.

19. Crumpton MJ, Snary D: Preparation and properties of lymphocyte plasma membrane. *Contemp Top Mol Immunol* 3:27, 1974.

20. Goppelt M, Eichhorn R, Krebs G, Resch K: Lipid composition of functional domains of the lymphocyte plasma membrane. *Biochim Biophys Acta* 854:184, 1986.

21. Johnson SM, Robinson R: The composition and fluidity of normal and leukaemic or lymphomatous lymphocyte plasma membranes in mouse and man. *Biochim Biophys Acta* 558:282, 1979.

22. Pierce SK: Lipid rafts and B-cell activation. *Nat Rev Immunol* 2:96, 2002.

23. Thomas S, Preda-Pais A, Casares S, Brumeanu TD: Analysis of lipid rafts in T cells. *Mol Immunol* 41:399, 2004.

24. Dykstra M, Cherukuri A, Sohn HW, et al: Location is everything: Lipid rafts and immune cell signaling. *Annu Rev Immunol* 21:457, 2003.

25. Galmarini CM, Jordheim L, Dumontet C: Role of IMP-selective 5′-nucleotidase (cN-II) in hematological malignancies. *Leuk Lymphoma* 44:1105, 2003.

26. Kameoka J, Tanaka T, Nojima Y, et al: Direct association of adenosine deaminase with a T cell activation antigen, CD26. *Science* 261:466, 1993.

27. Apasov S, Redegeld F, Sitkovsky M: Cell-mediated cytotoxicity: Contact and secreted factors. *Curr Opin Immunol* 5:404, 1993.

28. De Flora A, Guida L, Franco L, Zocchi E: The CD38/cyclic ADP-ribose system: A topological paradox. *Int J Biochem Cell Biol* 29:1149, 1997.

29. Jacobson KA, van Galen PJ, Williams M: Adenosine receptors: Pharmacology, structure-activity relationships, and therapeutic potential. *J Med Chem* 35:407, 1992.

30. Plamboeck A, Holst JJ, Carr RD, Deacon CF: Neutral endopeptidase 24.11 and dipeptidyl peptidase IV are both involved in regulating the metabolic stability of glucagon-like peptide-1 in vivo. *Adv Exp Med Biol* 524:303, 2003.

31. Kahne T, Lendeckel U, Wrenger S, et al: Dipeptidyl peptidase IV: A cell surface peptidase involved in regulating T cell growth. *Int J Mol Med* 4:3, 1999.

32. Reinhold D, Hemmer B, Gran B, et al: Dipeptidyl peptidase IV (CD26): Role in T cell activation and autoimmune disease. *Adv Exp Med Biol* 477:155, 2000.

33. Arribas J, Coodly L, Vollmer P, et al: Diverse cell surface protein ectodomains are shed by a system sensitive to metalloprotease inhibitors. *J Biol Chem* 271:11376, 1996.

34. Yamamoto S, Higuchi Y, Yoshiyama K, et al: ADAM family proteins in the immune system. *Immunol Today* 20:278, 1999.

35. Black RA: Tumor necrosis factor-alpha converting enzyme. *Int J Biochem Cell Biol* 34:1, 2002.

36. Blobel CP: Metalloprotease-disintegrins: Links to cell adhesion and cleavage of TNF alpha and Notch. *Cell* 90:589, 1997.

37. Kurosaki T: Genetic analysis of B cell antigen receptor signaling. *Annu Rev Immunol* 17:555, 1999.

38. Rawlings DJ: Bruton's tyrosine kinase controls a sustained calcium signal essential for B lineage development and function. *Clin Immunol* 91:243, 1999.

39. Harnett M: Syk deficiency—A knockout for B-cell development. *Immunol Today* 17:4, 1996.

40. Chu DH, Morita CT, Weiss A: The Syk family of protein tyrosine kinases in T-cell activation and development. *Immunol Rev* 165:167, 1998.

41. Elder ME: ZAP-70 and defects of T-cell receptor signaling. *Semin Hematol* 35:310, 1998.

42. Bell GM, Fargnoli J, Bolen JB, et al: The SH3 domain of p56lck binds to proline-rich sequences in the cytoplasmic domain of CD2. *J Exp Med* 183:169, 1996.

43. Zamoyska R: The CD8 coreceptor revisited: One chain good, two chains better. *Immunity* 1:243, 1994.

44. Taher TE, Smit L, Griffioen AW, et al: Signaling through CD44 is mediated by tyrosine kinases. Association with p56lck in T lymphocytes. *J Biol Chem* 271:2863, 1996.

45. Juan M, Viñas O, Pino-Otín MR, et al: CD50 (intercellular adhesion molecule 3) stimulation induces calcium mobilization and tyrosine phosphorylation through p59fyn and p56lck in Jurkat T cell line. *J Exp Med* 179:1747, 1994.

46. Kim YJ, Pollok KE, Zhou Z, et al: Novel T cell antigen 4-1BB associates with the protein tyrosine kinase p56lck1. *J Immunol* 151:1255, 1993.

47. Clements JL, Boerth NJ, Lee JR, Koretzky GA: Integration of T cell receptor-dependent signaling pathways by adapter proteins. *Annu Rev Immunol* 17:89, 1999.

48. Wollscheid B, Wienands J, Reth M: The adaptor protein SLP-65/BLNK controls the calcium response in activated B cells. *Curr Top Microbiol Immunol* 246:283, 1999.

49. Rudd CE: Adaptors and molecular scaffolds in immune cell signaling. *Cell* 96:5, 1999.

50. Tsukada S, Baba Y, Watanabe D: Btk and BLNK in B cell development. *Adv Immunol* 77:123, 2001.

51. Sommers CL, Samelson LE, Love PE: LAT: A T lymphocyte adapter protein that couples the antigen receptor to downstream signaling pathways. *Bioessays* 26:61, 2004.

52. Braun J, Unanue ER: The lymphocyte cytoskeleton and its control of surface receptor functions. *Semin Hematol* 20:322, 1983.

53. Glen AC: Measurement of DNA and RNA in human peripheral blood lymphocytes. *Clin Chem* 13:299, 1967.

54. Pangalis GA, Kuhl W, Waldman SR, Beutler E: Acid hydrolases in normal B and T blood lymphocytes. *Acta Haematol* 59:285, 1978.

55. Kulenkampff J, Janossy G, Greaves MF: Acid esterase in human lymphoid cells and leukaemic blasts: A marker for T lymphocytes. *Br J Haematol* 36:231, 1977.

56. Smyth MJ, O'Connor MD, Trapani JA: Granzymes: A variety of serine protease specificities encoded by genetically distinct subfamilies. *J Leukoc Biol* 60:555, 1996.

57. Bird PI: Regulation of pro-apoptotic leucocyte granule serine proteinases by intracellular serpins. *Immunol Cell Biol* 77:47, 1999.

58. Shresta S, Pham CT, Thomas DA, et al: How do cytotoxic lymphocytes kill their targets? *Curr Opin Immunol* 10:581, 1998.

59. Kajino K, Kajino Y, Greene MI: Fas- and perforin-independent mechanism of cytotoxic T lymphocyte. *Immunol Res* 17:89, 1998.

60. Pham CT, Ley TJ: Dipeptidyl peptidase I is required for the processing and activation of granzymes A and B in vivo. *Proc Natl Acad Sci U S A* 96:8627, 1999.

61. Spaeny-Dekking EH, Hanna WL, Wolbink AM, et al: Extracellular granzymes A and B in humans: Detection of native species during CTL responses in vitro and in vivo. *J Immunol* 160:3610, 1998.

62. Blink EJ, Trapani JA, Jans DA: Perforin-dependent nuclear targeting of granzymes: A central role in the nuclear events of granule-exocytosis-mediated apoptosis? *Immunol Cell Biol* 77:206, 1999.

63. Morimoto K, Kanoh H: The role of the de novo synthetic pathway in forming molecular species of phospholipids in resting lymphocytes from human tonsils. *Biochim Biophys Acta* 617:51, 1980.

64. Olding LB, Papadogiannakis N, Barbieri B, Murgita RA: Suppressive cellular and molecular activities in maternofetal immune interactions: Suppressor cell activity, prostaglandins, and alpha-fetoproteins. *Curr Top Microbiol Immunol* 222:159, 1997.

65. Callegari PE, Zurier RB: Botanical lipids: Potential role in modulation of immunologic responses and inflammatory reactions. *Rheum Dis Clin North Am* 17:415, 1991.

66. Phipps RP, Stein SH, Roper RL: A new view of prostaglandin E regulation of the immune response. *Immunol Today* 12:349, 1991.

67. Segel GB, Androphy EJ, Lichtman MA: Increased ouabain-sensitive glycolysis of lymphocytes treated with phytohemagglutinin: Relationship to potassium transport. *J Cell Physiol* 97:407, 1978.

68. Freitas AA, Bognacki J: The role of locomotion in lymphocyte migration. *Immunology* 36:247, 1979.

69. Hedeskov CJ: Early effects of phytohaemagglutinin on glucose metabolism of normal human lymphocytes. *Biochem J* 110:373, 1968.

70. Miller HK, Krakoff IH, Salser JS, Balis ME: Sensitivity to L-asparaginase and amino acid metabolism. *J Natl Cancer Inst* 44:1129, 1970.

71. Kamatani N, Carson DA: Differential cyst(e)ine requirements in human T and B lymphoblastoid cell lines. *Int Arch Allergy Appl Immunol* 68:84, 1982.

72. Harriman W, Völk H, Defranoux N, Wabl M: Immunoglobulin class switch recombination. *Annu Rev Immunol* 11:361, 1993.

73. Carson DA, Carrera CJ: Immunodeficiency secondary to adenosine deaminase deficiency and purine nucleoside phosphorylation deficiency. *Semin Hematol* 27:260, 1990.

74. Goetzl EJ, Adelman DC, Sreedharan SP: Neuroimmunology. *Adv Immunol* 48:161, 1990.

75. Clevenger CV, Freier DO, Kline JB: Prolactin receptor signal transduction in cells of the immune system. *J Endocrinol* 157:187, 1998.

76. Baird AM, Gerstein RM, Berg LJ: The role of cytokine receptor signaling in lymphocyte development. *Curr Opin Immunol* 11:157, 1999.

77. Cyster JG, Ngo VN, Ekland EH, et al: Chemokines and B-cell homing to follicles. *Curr Top Microbiol Immunol* 246:87, 1999.

78. Lotz M, Vaughan JH, Carson DA: Effect of neuropeptides on production of inflammatory cytokines by human monocytes. *Science* 241:1218, 1988.

79. Zempleni J, Mock DM: Utilization of biotin in proliferating human lymphocytes. *J Nutr* 130:335S 2000.

80. Cupps TR, Gerrard TL, Falkoff RJ, et al: Effects of in vitro corticosteroids on B cell activation, proliferation, and differentiation. *J Clin Invest* 75:754, 1985.

81. Wilckens T, De Rijk R: Glucocorticoids and immune function: Unknown dimensions and new frontiers. *Immunol Today* 18:418, 1997.

82. Miller AH, Pariante CM, Pearce BD: Effects of cytokines on glucocorticoid receptor expression and function. Glucocorticoid resistance and relevance to depression. *Adv Exp Med Biol* 461:107, 1999.

83. Cohen JJ, Duke RC: Glucocorticoid activation of a calcium-dependent endonuclease in thymocyte nuclei leads to cell death. *J Immunol* 132:38, 1984.

84. Evans-Storms RB, Cidlowski JA: Regulation of apoptosis by steroid hormones. *J Steroid Biochem Mol Biol* 53:1, 1995.

85. Montague IW, Cidlowski JA: Glucocorticoid-induced death of immune cells: Mechanisms of action. *Curr Top Microbiol Immunol* 200:51, 1995.

86. Scudeletti M, Lanza L, Monaco E, et al: Immune regulatory properties of corticosteroids: Prednisone induces apoptosis of human T lymphocytes following the CD3 down-regulation. *Ann N Y Acad Sci* 876:164, 1999.

87. Northrop JP, Crabtree GR, Mattila PS: Negative regulation of interleukin 2 transcription by the glucocorticoid receptor. *J Exp Med* 175:1235, 1992.

88. Grossman CJ, Roselle GA, Mendenhall CL: Sex steroid regulation of autoimmunity. *J Steroid Biochem Mol Biol* 40:649, 1991.

89. Meikle AW, Dorchuck RW, Araneo BA, et al: The presence of a dehydroepiandrosterone-specific receptor binding complex in murine T cells. *J Steroid Biochem Mol Biol* 42:293, 1992.

90. Orentreich N, Brind JL, Rizer RL, Vogelman JH: Age changes and sex differences in serum dehydroepiandrosterone sulfate concentrations throughout adulthood. *J Clin Endocrinol Metab* 59:551, 1984.

91. Tani K, Ogushi F, Huang L, et al: CD13/aminopeptidase N, a novel chemoattractant for T lymphocytes in pulmonary sarcoidosis. *Am J Respir Crit Care Med* 161:1636, 2000.

92. Mehta K, Shahid U, Malavasi F: Human CD38, a cell-surface protein with multiple functions. *FASEB J* 10:1408, 1996.

93. Schulte am Esch J 2nd, Sevigny J, Kaczmarek E, et al: Structural elements and limited proteolysis of CD39 influence ATP diphosphohydrolase activity. *Biochemistry* 38:2248, 1999.

94. Bauvois B: Transmembrane proteases in cell growth and invasion: New contributors to angiogenesis? *Oncogene* 23:317, 2004.

95. Ortolan E, Vacca P, Capobianco A, et al: CD157, the Janus of CD38 but with a unique personality. *Cell Biochem Funct* 20:309, 2002.

96. Stark AA, Porat N, Volohonsky G, et al: The role of gamma-glutamyl transpeptidase in the biosynthesis of glutathione. *Biofactors* 17:139, 2003.

LYMPHOPOIESIS

TUCKER W. LEBIEN

The functional mammalian immune system consists of three major lymphocyte populations with different antigen recognition systems: thymus-derived (T) cells; bursal or marrow-derived (B) cells; and natural killer (NK) cells. The three populations mediate complex and distinct immune effector functions. The development and manifestation of immune effector functions reflect differences in patterns of gene expression in T, B, and NK cells. Of primary importance in T and B cells are receptor complexes that mediate antigen recognition: the T cell receptor on T cells and the B cell receptor on B cells. NK cells do not express antigen-specific receptors; rather, specificity of NK cell recognition is provided by inhibitory signals transduced by receptors recognizing class I major histocompatibility complex molecules. The differences in effector functions and organ distribution can be traced to differences in early ontogeny. This chapter reviews lymphocyte ontogeny. The genesis, gene expression, developmental options, and proliferation requirements of T, B, and NK cells are emphasized. Chapters 77, 78, and 79 provide A more extensive discussion of B cell, T cell, and NK cell function, respectively.

LYMPHOCYTE DEVELOPMENT FROM HEMATOPOIETIC STEM CELLS

The most primitive mammalian blood-forming cell is designated the *hematopoietic stem cell* (HSC). HSCs have the capacity to develop into all populations of blood cells. Chapter 15 discusses HSCs in greater detail. HSC have two fundamental developmental options: self-renewal and differentiation. *Self-renewal* refers to the capacity of a cell to divide and give rise to two daughter cells that exhibit an indistinguishable pattern of gene expression. Self-renewal requires that HSC in a quiescent state receive the appropriate stimulus to divide (i.e., proliferate). *Differentiation* refers to the sequence of events wherein cells undergo orderly changes in gene expression, culminating in the development of a more mature cell. Differentiation can occur coincident with, or independent of, proliferation. The closer two cells are in a developmental pathway, the more subtle their differences in gene expression. The developmental stage and cell cycle status of a cell can dictate the cell's vulnerability to undergoing apoptosis.

For many years, the extraembryonic yolk sac (i.e., tissue outside the embryo proper) was considered the reservoir of self-renewing HSCs that contribute to lifelong lymphohematopoiesis.[1] This concept was proven incorrect when murine intraembryonic tissue encompassing *paraaortic splanchnopleura* and derived aorta-gonad-mesoneph-

ros was shown to harbor HSC prior to their appearance in fetal liver.[2,3] Furthermore, murine lymphoid precursors were identified in the paraaortic splanchnopleura prior to the onset of circulation.[2,4]

In vitro colony-forming assays initially were used to demonstrate that human hematopoiesis can be detected in the yolk sac at week 3 of gestation and shifts to fetal liver at approximately week 5.[5] Two subsequent studies used the cell surface sialomucin CD34 as a marker to identify candidate HSC in human embryonic tissue. In one study, highly proliferating CD34+ stem cells were identified in 5-week-old human embryonic tissue devoid of yolk sac and liver anlage.[6] In a second study, clusters of CD34+ hematopoietic-like cells were detected in the ventral aortic endothelium at 27 days of gestation.[7] CD34+ hematopoietic cells clustered in the ventral aortic endothelium were analyzed by *in situ* hybridization and were shown to express transcription factors and growth factor receptors important in early hematopoiesis.[8] A subsequent study revealed that intraembryonic splanchnopleural mesoderm and derived aorta from days 19 to 24 of gestation gave rise to myeloid cells and CD19+ B lineage cells.[9] In contrast, 3-week-old yolk sac gave rise only to myeloid cells. Thus, human HSC with multilineage developmental potential exist in 3-week-old intraembryonic tissue but not 3-week-old extraembryonic tissue.

COMMON LYMPHOID PROGENITORS

T, B, and natural killer (NK) lymphoid cells ultimately develop from HSC. However, the existence of a common lymphoid progenitor (CLP) restricted to developing into T, B, or NK cells (but not myeloid and erythroid cells) has been a point of historical controversy. Data from the study of alterations in the hypoxanthine guanine phosphoribosyl transferase gene in blood mononuclear cells from an atomic bomb survivor were among the first evidence that T, B, and NK cells are derived from a common progenitor.[10] However, whether the progenitor was lymphoid restricted or it also harbored the capacity to differentiate into myeloid and erythroid cells was unclear.[10] Two subsequent reports provided stronger evidence supporting the existence of a CLP in humans and mice. Fluorescence-activated cell sorting (FACS) was used to isolate a rare population of CD34+/CD10+/CD19− lymphoid progenitors from human adult and fetal marrow.[11] These CD34+/CD10+/CD19− progenitors were capable of developing into B, NK, and lymphoid dendritic cells (and possibly T lineage cells) but not myeloid or erythroid cells.[11] A second study used FACS to isolate a rare population of murine marrow lymphoid cells expressing the interleukin-7 (IL-7) receptor and demonstrated that a single such cell could generate at least T and B cells but not myeloid cells.[12] Studies using FACS to purify candidate CLP from human cord blood isolated a rare CD34+/CD38−/CD7+ population shown to differentiate into B, NK, and dendritic cells but not myeloid or erythroid cells.[13] In contrast to studies using adult marrow,[11] CD10 expression was not useful for discriminating cord blood CLP from myeloid progenitors.[13] A similar study confirmed that cord blood CD34+/CD38−/CD7+ CLP have no phenotypic counterpart in adult marrow.[14] Figure 76-1 shows the existence of CLP in the adult marrow and cord blood and the developmental potential of each. Whether CLP with the respective phenotypes in marrow and cord blood are poised to migrate to the thymus and initiate T cell development is unknown.

The developmental scheme shown in Figure 76-1 may be an oversimplification. Studies in the mouse suggest a more complex hierarchy of CLP.[15] A population of cells designated early T lineage progenitors were shown to develop independently of CLP.[16] Thus, an alternative model[15] posits the existence of "pre-CLPs" with equal potential to develop into B or T lineage cells. Slightly more differentiated progenitors are identified as CLP-B (B lineage development favored over T lineage) and CLP-T (T lineage development favored over B lineage development).

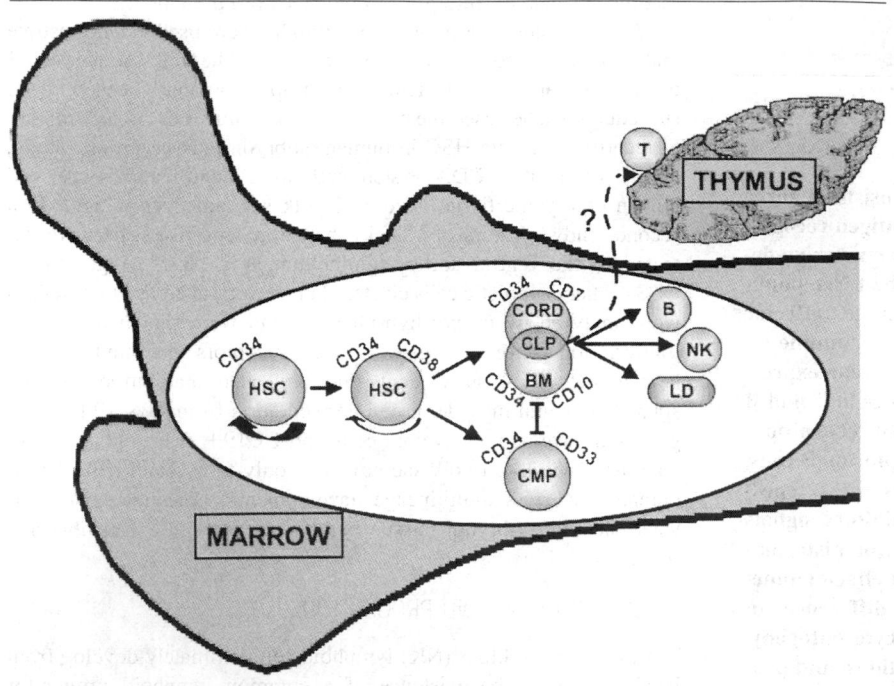

FIGURE 76-1   Origin and developmental potential of human CLP. Long-term self-renewing (CD34+) and short-term self-renewing (CD34+/CD38+) HSC differentiate into CLP or common myeloid progenitors (CMP). The CLP is shown as a CD34+/CD7+ progenitor in cord blood[13] and a CD34+/CD10+ progenitor in adult marrow.[11] CLP are shown as two overlapping cells because their developmental potentials are very similar. Single CLP can differentiate into B, NK, or lymphoid dendritic (LD) cells, and possibly T lineage cells, assuming migration to the thymus. The *thicker arrow* beneath the CD34+ HSC indicates a high degree of self-renewal compared to the CD34+/CD38+ HSC *(thinner arrow)*. The *blocking symbol* between CMP and CLP indicates a reciprocal inability to transdifferentiate. This scheme is intended to depict developmental options of normal lymphohematopoietic progenitors only. Completed pathways for B, T, and NK development are shown in Figs. 76-2, 76-3 and 76-4, respectively. Suppressed differentiation in leukemia and greater developmental plasticity observed in certain gene-targeted mice would not necessarily be consistent with the pathways shown in this scheme.

B CELL DEVELOPMENT

The hallmark characteristic of a mature B cell circulating in blood or residing in secondary lymphoid tissue is the expression of cell surface immunoglobulin (Ig). The cell surface Ig consists of μ, δ, γ, α, or ε heavy chains disulfide-linked to κ or λ light chains (see Chap. 77). The cell surface Ig and the associated signaling molecules Igα (dC79a) and Igβ (CD79b) are referred to as the *B cell receptor* (BCR). Precursor (pre-) B cells are defined by the presence of cytoplasmic μ heavy chains in the absence of cell surface BCR. Progenitor (pro-) B cells are defined by the absence of cytoplasmic μ heavy chains and cell surface BCR. This minimal definition of pro-B, pre-B, and B cells[17,18] forms the basis of the current detailed model of human B cell development. B cell development can be divided into two stages: an antigen-independent stage that occurs primarily in fetal liver and fetal and adult marrow, and an antigen-dependent stage that occurs primarily in secondary lymphoid tissue, such as spleen and lymph node.

ORGANS INVOLVED IN B CELL DEVELOPMENT

Human fetal liver and omentum are the main sites of B cell development from 8 to 14 weeks' gestation. Fetal omentum is a thin, vascularized, membranous fold of peritoneum. Fetal omentum is considered part of the lymphoid system because it contains aggregates of lymphoid cells called *milk spots*. Pre-B cells are present in fetal liver at 7 to 8 weeks' gestation[19] and in fetal omentum at 10 weeks' gestation.[20]

Second-trimester B cell development is multifocal; pro-B, pre-B, and immature B cells can be detected in the marrow and liver and, to a lesser extent, the lung and kidney.[21] From the end of the second trimester throughout adult life, marrow is the exclusive site of B cell development. The frequency of early B lineage cells as a percentage of the total nucleated lymphohematopoietic cell pool is higher in fetal than in adult marrow.[21,22] However, the ratio between pro-B, pre-B, and immature B cells and the mitotic activity within these fractions is relatively constant.[14]

IMMUNOGLOBULIN GENE REARRANGEMENT AND EXPRESSION

The hallmark of marrow B cell development is the ordered rearrangement of gene segments that encode the variable portion of the antibody molecule (see Chap. 77 for additional details). The process typically begins with germ-line transcription of the μ heavy-chain locus, followed by the joining of one of 30 D_H segments to one of six J_H segments.[23] Once DJ_H rearrangement is complete, one of approximately 130 upstream V_H gene segments[24] can join to form a completed VDJ_H rearrangement. If the VDJ_H rearrangement is functional or "in frame," meaning it is capable of encoding a full-length μ heavy-chain protein, VDJ rearrangement ceases. This process is termed *allelic exclusion*. Targeted disruption of the μ heavy-chain locus in mice leads to loss of allelic exclusion,[25] but the precise mechanism remains unknown. If the initial VDJ_H rearrangement is nonfunctional (i.e., the rearrangement does not encode a full-length μ heavy-chain protein), then rearrangement can occur on the other heavy-chain allele. If a nonfunctional VDJ_H rearrangement occurs on both alleles, the cell undergoes apoptosis and is phagocytized by marrow macrophages.

Recombination at the light-chain locus generally follows completion of a functional heavy-chain rearrangement.[23] This usually begins with germ-line transcription of the κ locus followed by the rearrangement of a V_κ to J_κ. If an initial VJ_κ rearrangement is functional, the light-chain locus also undergoes allelic exclusion. If not, rearrangement occurs on the other κ allele. If recombination at both κ alleles fails to yield a functional rearrangement, the λ light-chain locus rearranges.[23] An alternative model proposes that light-chain rearrangement begins at κ and λ loci simultaneously.[26] Because of a difference in recombination rate, the κ locus usually finishes recombining first, potentially explaining the high ratio of κ- to λ-expressing B cells in the mouse.[26]

Heavy- and light-chain Ig gene rearrangements occur at different stages of human B cell development (Fig. 76-2). DJ_H rearrangements initially occur in CD34+/CD10+/−/CD19− CLP in adult marrow and cord blood.[27-29] CD19+/CD34+ pro-B cells harbor VDJ_H rearrangements,[27] and a functional VDJ_H rearrangement results in differentiation to the large pre-B cell stage. The large pre-B compartment is enriched for cells in cycle that express the pre-BCR. Cessation of heavy-chain rearrangement and expression of the pre-BCR signal the differentiation of large pre-B cells to small pre-B cells. The small pre-B compartment undergoes V to J_κ light-chain rearrangement, and small pre-B cells with functional light-chain rearrangements differentiate

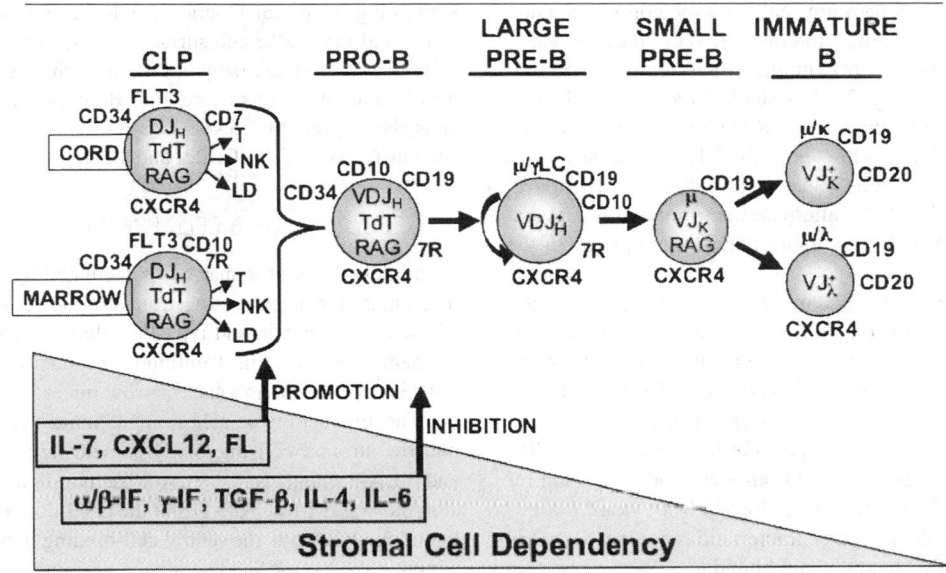

FIGURE 76-2   B cell development in human marrow. The CLP corresponds to the CLP in Figure 76-1 with multilymphoid lineage developmental potential. The TdT, RAG, and μ designations within the cells indicate nuclear (TdT and RAG) and cytoplasmic (μ) expression of these proteins. The *curved arrow* juxtaposed to the large pre-B cell indicates that this population undergoes a high degree of proliferation. A *plus superscript* in large pre-B and immature B cells indicates a successful rearrangement of the heavy- and light-chain loci, respectively, leading to expression of μ heavy chain proteins and κ or λ light-chain proteins. 7R refers to the IL-7 receptor. Cytokine production by stromal cells that promote or inhibit proliferation and differentiation are shown. Stromal cell dependency is shown as decreasing in importance *(slanted line)* as B cell development proceeds. A comprehensive review of human B cell development is given in references 17 and 18.

into immature B cells expressing μ/κ or μ/λ BCR. Ig gene rearrangement generally proceeds through an ordered progression, beginning with the μ heavy-chain gene and proceeding through κ and (if necessary) λ light-chain genes.[30] Alternative pathways have been described in which light-chain rearrangement precedes heavy-chain rearrangement[31] and λ light-chain rearrangement precedes κ light-chain rearrangement.[32]

SURROGATE LIGHT CHAIN

The surrogate light chain (ψLC) genes λ5 and Vpre-B originally were discovered in the mouse and are restricted in expression to the B lineage.[33] Homologous genes in humans[34,35] encode Vpre-B and λ5 proteins that form a heterodimer and associate with μ heavy chain. ψLC genes exhibit significant sequence homology with conventional λ light chains but do not undergo rearrangement.[33] The μ-ψLC complex associates with the Igα and Igβ signaling molecules to form the pre-BCR.[31] The Vpre-B protein initially is expressed in the cytoplasm of CD19− early B lineage cells prior to the expression of μ heavy chain,[36] but the relationship of these Vpre-B+/CD19− cells to CLP is unknown (see Fig. 76-2). However, surface expression of the pre-BCR is restricted to a subset of large pre-B cells in marrow.[37] Interestingly, a rare population of peripheral blood B cells coexpress ψLC and conventional light chains,[38] and approximately 70 percent of these dual light-chain–expressing B cells produce autoreactive antibodies.[39]

The importance of the ψLC in B cell development was first demonstrated in mice with a targeted disruption of the λ5 gene.[40] λ5-Deficient mice exhibit a block in B cell development at the pro-B to pre-B transition, presumably because the cells fail to receive a survival signal in the absence of a functional pre-BCR.[40] Patients with mutations in the λ5 gene exhibit a profound block in pro-B to pre-B cell

differentiation,[41] confirming the importance of the μ-ψLC in human B cell development.

Large pre-B cells undergo a process called *positive selection* by virtue of pre-BCR expression, that is, pre-BCR expression is a requisite for pre-B cell proliferation and differentiation. A major controversy has been whether the pre-BCR has a ligand, and whether a potential ligand transduces a signal to the pre-B cell via cross linking the pre-BCR. Support for and against a role for ligand exist. An elegant study reported that a human marrow stromal cell S-type lectin, designated *galectin-1*, binds to the ψLC component of the pre-BCR.[42] In cooperation with other unidentified glycosylated surface molecules on pre-B cells and stromal cells, the galectin-1/pre-BCR interaction induces tyrosine kinase activation and signal transduction in pre-B cells. A murine stromal cell molecule distinct from galectin-1 binds to the pre-BCR.[43] A ligand-independent pre-BCR signaling model is supported by evidence indicating that charged domains of the λ5 and Vpre-B subunits can undergo electrostatic interaction in the absence of any source of potential ligand, thereby transducing a survival signal in a pre-B cell autonomous manner.[44]

EXPRESSION OF RECOMBINATION-ASSOCIATED GENES

Two genes designated *recombination activating gene-1 (RAG-1)* and *recombination activating gene-2 (RAG-2)* are required for Ig and T cell receptor (TCR) gene rearrangements.[45] Mice deficient in either RAG-1 or RAG-2 have severe disruptions in early B cell development.[46,47] Furthermore, mutations in the RAG genes have been identified in some patients with severe combined immunodeficiency.[48] *In vitro* studies have shown that the RAG-1 and RAG-2 proteins bind to recombination signal sequences and introduce double-stranded DNA breaks during initiation of the recombination cleavage reaction.[45,49]

Double-stranded DNA breaks then are sealed by the concerted action of six nonhomologous end-joining proteins.[49] RAG expression vacillates during B cell development. Maximum expression occurs in pro-B and small pre-B cells (see Fig. 76-2), coincident with active heavy- and light-chain gene rearrangement.[18,30] RAG expression has been detected in rare murine splenic B lineage cells.[50] This observation was used to argue that mature B cells can reinduce RAG expression in order to edit autoreactive BCR. An alternate interpretation asserts that RAG activity occurs in B cell precursors that have migrated to the spleen.

The enzyme terminal deoxynucleotidyl transferase (TdT) is not required for the recombination reaction but is necessary for the generation of antigen-receptor diversity. TdT inserts non–template-encoded nucleotides (so-called *N-region insertions*) at the D_H to J_H and V_H to DJ_H junctions of heavy chains.[51] N-region insertions increase the diversity of the antigen-receptor repertoire to encode greater than 1×10^8 different specificities. A limited number of κ light-chain rearrangements contain TdT N-region insertions.[52] Mice bearing a targeted deletion of the TdT gene lack characteristic N-region insertions at the D_H to J_H and V_H to DJ_H heavy-chain boundaries.[53,54] TdT protein initially is expressed in CLPs.[55] Figure 76-2 shows the CD19+/CD34+ pro-B cell population is TdT+, but expression is turned off in pre-B cells.[30,56] Reduction in TdT expression at the pro-B to pre-B transition explains why light-chain gene rearrangements have relatively few N-region insertions.

B LINEAGE-ASSOCIATED SURFACE ANTIGENS

Although Ig gene rearrangement provides the most precise molecular definition of B cell development, monoclonal antibodies recognizing cell surface molecules have been essential for characterizing and isolating specific stages by flow cytometry and cell sorting. Figure 76-2 shows the expression of several cell surface molecules that have been useful in characterizing different stages of human B cell development.[17,18] Chapter 14 provides a more in-depth discussion of the CD antigens. Analysis of CD34+/CD10+/CD19− marrow lymphoid cells revealed expression of cytoplasmic Vpre-B[36] and DJ_H rearrangements.[27,28] Thus, some of these cells may comprise an early-B cell compartment. Furthermore, a CD34+/CD10−/CD19− cord blood progenitor expressing cytoplasmic CD79a and DJ_H rearrangements can develop into B lineage cells (and NK cells and macrophages).[29] These collective results indicate that cells having the greatest generative potential for commitment to the B lineage may exhibit a different phenotype in adult marrow as compared to cord blood.

Pro-B cells are characterized by expression of cell surface CD10, CD34, and the B lineage-restricted molecule CD19. A small percentage (approximately 10 percent) of CD34+/CD19+ cells express the Vpre-B component of the pre-BCR on their cell surface.[36,37] However, this population is cytoplasmic $\mu +$,[37] indicating they represent a small fraction of pre-B cells that have not fully down-regulated CD34. The next major compartment is the large pre-B cell, which is characterized by the expression of CD19, loss of CD34 and TdT, and acquisition of μ heavy chain in more than 90 percent of the cells.[17,18] The pre-B cell population can be subdivided into large cycling cells and small quiescent cells based on cell cycle analysis.[1,37] A subset of large pre-B cells express the μ-ψLC pre-BCR[30,37] in association with a heterodimer designated Igα/CD79a and Igβ/CD79b. The Igα/Igβ heterodimer initiates signal transduction following cross-linking of the pre-BCR and BCR.[57,58] Igα and Igβ are expressed in CD10+/CD19− lymphoid cells prior to the appearance of functional VDJ_H rearrangements.[59] The function of Igα and Igβ in these lymphoid cells and their level of commitment to the B lineage are unknown. Mice with a targeted disruption of the Igβ gene are blocked at the level of DJ_H rearrangement,[60]

suggesting a critical function for the Igβ protein separate from its functional role in the cell surface μ-ψLC pre-BCR. Once small pre-B cells successfully rearrange κ or λ light-chain genes, they differentiate into immature B cells expressing BCR (see Fig. 76-2). Immature B cells also express high levels of B cell-restricted cell surface molecules such as CD20, CD21, CD22, and CD40.

REGULATION OF B CELL PRECURSOR DEVELOPMENT

B cell development in marrow is regulated by a complex interplay of molecular signals emanating from stromal cells, the extracellular matrix (e.g., fibronectin and type IV collagen), and possibly other lymphohematopoietic cells. Continuous production of B cells throughout life[14,21] depends on an intact marrow microenvironment.

The interaction or adhesion of human B cell precursors to the marrow stromal cell microenvironment is mediated through VLA-4 and VLA-5 integrins.[61,62] VLA-4 has two ligands: vascular cell adhesion molecule-1 (VCAM-1) and the CS-1 domain of fibronectin.[63] The ligand for VLA-5 is the central cell-binding domain of fibronectin that contains the amino acid sequence arginine-glycine-aspartic acid, or RGD.[63] Marrow stromal cells constitutively express VCAM-1.[61,62] Functional expression of VCAM-1 can be positively regulated by IL-1β and IL-4 and negatively regulated by transforming growth factor β (TGF-β).[62] Similarly, adhesion of B cell precursors to VCAM-1 can be sustained by binding of the stromal cell-derived chemokine CXCL12 (also known as stromal cell-derived factor-1) to its CXCR4 receptor on B lineage cells.[64] Thus, VLA-4–mediated adhesion of B cell precursors to stromal cell VCAM-1 can be regulated by marrow-derived cytokines and chemokines.

Despite the wealth of progress in characterizing the cytokines and colony-stimulating factors that regulate survival and proliferation of hematopoietic cells, gaps remain in our understanding of how human B lymphopoiesis is regulated. IL-7 facilitates the stromal cell-dependent proliferation of CD19+/CD34+ pro-B cells *in vitro*[65] and triggers decreased expression of RAG-1, RAG-2, and TdT.[66,67] However, IL-7 alone has no effect. The combination of IL-7 and the flt-3 ligand (FL) imparts a modest proliferative stimulus to human marrow pro-B cells.[67] The requirement for IL-7 signaling differs in human and murine B cell development. Adult murine B cell development has an absolute requirement for IL-7 to IL-7 receptor interaction and subsequent downstream signaling involving the γ_c subunit of the IL-7 receptor and the JAK-3 tyrosine kinase.[68] In contrast, IL-7 does not appear to be essential for human B cell development. X-linked severe combined immunodeficiency patients with mutations in the γ_c cytokine–receptor subunit exhibit profound thymic hypoplasia and an absence of NK cells but normal or elevated numbers of B cells.[69] Immunodeficiency patients with mutations in JAK-3[70,71] or the IL-7 receptor[72] also have normal numbers of blood B cells. Furthermore, an *in vitro* model of human B cell development is IL-7 independent.[73] These collective results indicate IL-7 is not essential for at least the numerically normal development of human B cells. CXCR4 may play a role in B cell development beyond promoting adhesion of B cell precursors to marrow stromal cells. Some patients afflicted with an autosomal dominant disorder designated WHIM (warts, hypogammaglobulinemia immunodeficiency, and myelokathexis) exhibit deficiencies in B cell development, and these patients have mutations in CXCR4.[74] Thus, CXCR4 may play a role in proliferation and differentiation of B cell precursors. Nonetheless, the identity of the human marrow-derived molecule or molecules that provide the essential proliferative stimulus for human pro-B cells is unknown. Conversely, cytokines that suppress proliferation and/or differentiation of developing B lineage cells (and other hematopoietic cells) also are produced by marrow stromal cells (see Fig. 76-2). Serial analysis of gene expression of marrow pre-B cells revealed expression of genes such as platelet-derived growth factor receptor-α and Wnt16 that could provide fresh clues to the identity of potentially important surface receptors and signaling pathways.[75]

T CELL DEVELOPMENT

B cell development can be detected in 7- to 8-week human fetal liver. The marrow is the primary source of B cell development from the end of the second trimester throughout life.[14,21] A fundamental distinction between mammalian B and T cell development is that the latter requires the migration of a fetal liver or fetal or postnatal marrow lymphoid progenitor (the CLP?) to the thymus (see Fig. 76-1). Our understanding of the mechanisms underlying migration of marrow lymphoid precursors to the thymus are incomplete, but chemokines produced by thymic stromal cells likely play a role.[76]

ORGANS INVOLVED IN T CELL DEVELOPMENT

FETAL LIVER AND MARROW

A challenging problem in studies of mammalian T cell development has been identifying the phenotype of the fetal liver or marrow progenitor poised to migrate to the thymus and the commitment status of such a progenitor regarding the capacity to develop into T cells, vis-à-vis, other lymphoid cells. CD7 is a cell surface molecule expressed throughout T cell development. CD7+ lymphoid cells expressing cytoplasmic CD3ε are present in fetal liver at 7 to 8 weeks' gestation.[77,78] Furthermore, CD7+/cytoplasmic CD3ε+ progenitors are present in fetal liver and fetal thorax just prior to colonization of the epithelial thymic rudiment.[77] Rare CD34+/CD7+ lymphoid cells also are present in fetal marrow.[79] However, CD7 also is expressed on NK progenitors and some myeloid cells and therefore is not a T lineage-specific marker. CD34+/CD7- cord blood progenitors can differentiate into T lineage cells, but their absence of T cell receptor (TCR) rearrangements implies they are not T lineage committed.[80] The identification of rare adult marrow lymphoid cells expressing the pre-TCR and harboring TCRβ rearrangements suggests that commitment to the T lineage occurs prior to thymic migration,[81] although this likely is a rare event. Similarly, an alternative pathway of T cell development that occurs in marrow has been described in the mouse.[82] Extrathymic T cell maturation also occurs in human fetal liver[83] and fetal intestine.[84]

THYMUS

The human thymic microenvironment begins to develop at approximately 4 weeks' gestation[85] and then undergoes three developmental phases.[86] The first phase occurs between 4 and 8 weeks' gestation. Transient outpocketing of the pharyngeal endoderm (third pharyngeal pouch) and contributions from the ectoderm and neural crest-derived mesoderm lead to expansion of thymic epithelial cells (TEC).[87] The second phase occurs between 9 and 15 weeks' gestation and is characterized by the development of subcapsular, cortical, and medullary regions. Colonization by fetal liver-derived progenitors begins at approximately week 9. The third phase occurs from 16 weeks' gestation until age 1 to 2 years and is characterized by robust intrathymic T cell maturation.

A prevailing historical viewpoint has held that the thymus only functions in young humans and mice because of its well-known involution during puberty.[88] This viewpoint has been challenged following the development of a method that can measure thymic emigrants throughout life. A polymerase chain reaction assay was developed that detects extrachromosomal DNA circles called *TCR rearrangement excision circles* (TRECs).[89] TRECs are a product of TCR gene rearrangement and represent a molecular marker of thymic function. Using the TREC assay, thymic function was observed to decline by five-fold at age 35 years and 50-fold by age 65 years, but TRECs still are present in the blood T cells of individuals older than 70 years.[90] Therefore, the T cell pool is replenished by a functional thymus (albeit in an age-dependent manner) throughout life, similar to the lifelong development of marrow-derived B lineage cells.

Thymocyte maturation is a complex series of steps that culminates in the development of a functional T cell repertoire.[80] In addition to thymocytes at multiple stages of development, the thymic microenvironment is composed of numerous nonlymphoid cells.[91] The subcapsular, cortical, and medullary regions of the thymus contain heterogeneous populations of TEC, macrophages, and dendritic/interdigitating cells. Cortical and medullary TEC are derived from a TEC progenitor and perform distinct functions in regulating thymocyte development.[91] Current models suggest positive selection (the process by which T cells are selected following low-affinity interactions with self-peptides associated with MHC) and negative selection (the process by which T cells are deleted following high-affinity recognition of self-peptides) occur when developing thymocytes interact with TEC and dendritic/interdigitating cells, respectively.[91] Human medullary TEC express a highly diverse set of genes encoding many tissue- and disease-associated autoantigens, which may explain the development of some autoimmune spectra following failure of T cells to be negatively selected.[92]

T CELL RECEPTOR GENE REARRANGEMENT AND EXPRESSION

Similar to the BCR, the TCR is encoded by distinct gene segments (V, D, J, and C) that undergo rearrangement during T cell development.[80] TCR genes encode polypeptides designated α, β, γ, and δ. The α and β protein pair with one another to form the TCR$\alpha\beta$. The γ and δ proteins pair with one another to form the TCR$\gamma\delta$. The TCR$\alpha\beta$ and TCR$\gamma\delta$ are noncovalently associated with a family of proteins called the *CD3 complex*. CD3 performs a crucial role in signal transduction following TCR cross-linking, analogous to the role of Igα/Igβ in mediating signal transduction following BCR cross-linking. Chapter 78 provides a more detailed description of TCR genes and proteins.

Rearrangement of TCR genes generally occurs in a hierarchical manner during thymocyte development.[93–95] The CD34+/CD1a+ thymocytes (pre-T) compartment contains TCRγ and δ rearrangements with TCRβ genes in germ-line configuration (Fig. 76-3).[80,96] The next stage of human thymocyte development is the CD4 single-positive (SP) stage. These cells have complete TCRδ and γ rearrangements and begin to undergo TCRβ rearrangements.[93,94] If the TCRβ rearrangement is functional, the encoded TCRβ protein assembles into a complex called the *pre-TCR*.[96] Cells expressing the pre-TCR are designated *early double-positive (DP) thymocytes* because they express cell surface CD4 and CD8. If the TCRβ rearrangement is nonfunctional, the early SP thymocytes undergo apoptosis. The elimination of early SP thymocytes by this mechanism mirrors the elimination of pro-B cells that fail to make a functional VDJ$_H$ rearrangement. The pre-TCR consists of TCRβ protein, the CD3 signal transduction protein complex, and an invariant chain designated pTα.[96] The pTα gene originally was cloned in the mouse[97] and subsequently in humans.[98] The pre-TCR functions as a sensor and facilitates the survival and expansion of pre-TCR+ thymocytes in a process called β-selection.[80,96] The pre-TCR has no known ligand, and "constitutive signaling" occurs as a consequence of spontaneous clustering of the TCR with lipid raft-associated molecules leading to internalization.[96] Rearrangement of TCRα genes subsequently occurs in intermediate DP thymocytes, eventually culminating in expression of low levels of surface TCR$\alpha\beta$ in late DP thymocytes (Fig. 76-3).

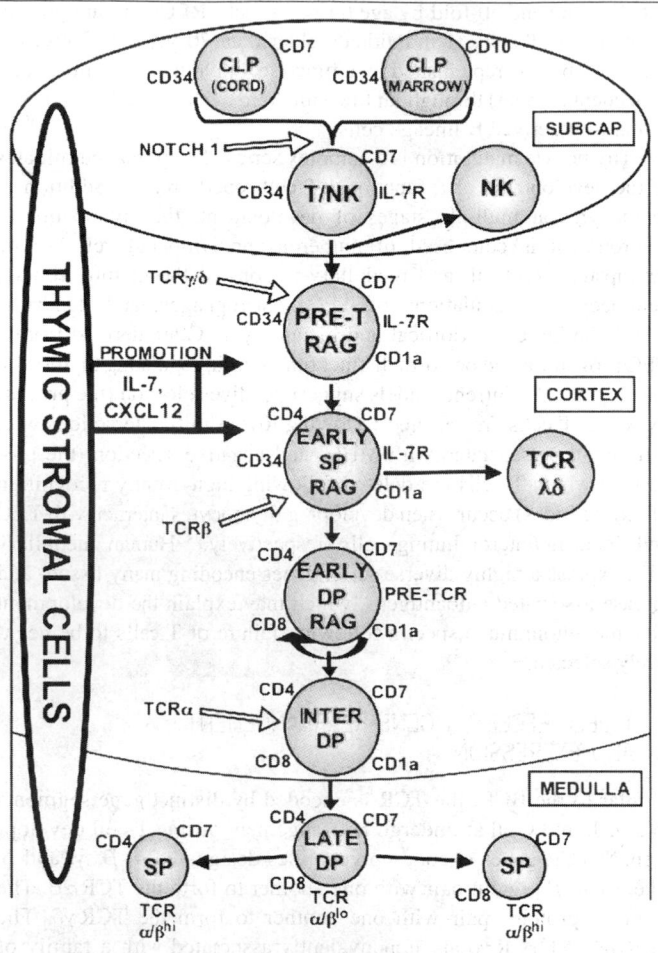

FIGURE 76-3   T cell development in human thymus. The CLP correspond to the CLP in Figure 76-1, with multilymphoid lineage developmental potential, assuming that both can migrate to the thymus. The subcapsule, cortex, and medulla are shown as approximate thymic microenvironmental boundaries. NOTCH 1 refers to a Notch1-mediated signal that promotes commitment of a CLP to the T lineage. *Open arrows* point to stages of thymocyte development where specific TCR rearrangements first occur. The *curved arrow* juxtaposed to the early DP thymocyte expressing the pre-TCR indicates this population undergoes a high degree of proliferation. Thymic stromal cells (representing multiple distinct cell types; see text) are shown as a constant requirement throughout thymocyte development, but this is an oversimplification. A comprehensive review of human T cell development is given in references 80, 91, and 96.

EXPRESSION OF RECOMBINATION-ASSOCIATED GENES

The roles of RAG-1, RAG-2, and TdT in the rearrangement and diversification of the TCR repertoire is similar to their roles in rearrangement and diversification of the BCR repertoire. Mice deficient in RAG-1 and RAG-2 exhibit profound disruptions in normal thymocyte development because of failure to initiate TCR rearrangement.[46,47] Likewise, TdT-deficient mice lack N-region insertions and exhibit restricted diversification of the TCR repertoire.[53,54] RAG gene expression oscillates during murine thymocyte development, corresponding to two waves of rearrangement involving TCRβ, γ, δ, and TCRα.[99] Northern blot and reverse transcriptase polymerase chain reaction analysis of human thymocyte subpopulations indicate RAG-1 and RAG-2 are expressed in multiple stages of thymocytes development but are down-regulated in CD4+ and CD8+ SP thymocytes following positive selection.[100]

T LINEAGE-ASSOCIATED SURFACE ANTIGENS

The earliest definable lymphoid progenitors in the thymus are multi-potential.[80] The cell surface phenotype of the fetal liver or postnatal lymphoid progenitor that migrates to the thymus is unknown. However, several studies demonstrated that CD34+/CD7+/CD1a− thymic progenitors can develop into T, NK, and lymphoid dendritic cells. This multilineage potential is lost following acquisition of CD1a.[101-104] Thus, assuming a marrow-derived CD34+/CD7+ or CD34+/CD10+ CLP (see Fig. 76-1) is the cell that migrates to the thymus (and this remains conjecture), upon arrival this cell must undergo additional differentiation prior to becoming committed to the T lineage.

Notch receptors are a highly conserved family of transmembrane molecules that regulate cell fate decisions in organisms ranging from *Drosophila* to man.[105] Notch receptors (e.g., Notch1) bind multiple membrane-associated ligands such as Delta/Serrate and Jagged.[105] The outcome of ligand binding is a unique sequence of proteolytic cleavage events within the Notch1 transmembrane domain and just cytosolic to the transmembrane domain, which culminate in an activated intracellular fragment of Notch. This intracellular fragment then translocates to the nucleus and functions as a transcriptional regulator. Studies in the mouse have demonstrated that Notch activation in early multilineage thymic emigrants concomitantly suppresses B cell development and promotes T cell development.[106] Studies of human T cell development have reported similar results.[107,108]

Figure 76-3 shows that acquisition of cell surface CD1 defines an important checkpoint in T cell development. The CD34+/CD1a+ pre-T cell population preferentially develops into the T lineage.[80] The next developmental stage is the early CD4+/CD8− SP thymocyte. Early SP thymocytes are fully committed to the T lineage and can give rise to TCR$\alpha\beta$- or TCR$\gamma\delta$- expressing T cells.[80] Early SP thymocytes differentiate into early CD4+/CD8+ DP thymocytes. Early DP thymocytes are easily distinguished from their early SP precursors by the expression of CD8 and the pre-TCR.[80,96] Figure 76-3 shows three DP stages (early, intermediate, and late) that likely reflect a linear developmental pathway. Early DP thymocytes expressing the pre-TCR expand substantially in cell numbers. The pre-TCR is lost at the intermediate DP thymocyte stage, coincident with the onset of TCRα rearrangement and subsequent expression of low levels of TCR$\alpha\beta$ (the late DP thymocyte). Distinct subcompartments in the DP thymocyte pool have been identified. Late DP thymocytes differentiate into CD4+/CD8− SP and CD4−/CD8+ SP thymocytes expressing high levels of cell surface TCR$\alpha\beta$. These two populations correspond to helper/inducer and cytotoxic T cells that make up the blood and secondary lymphoid organ T cell pool. Chapter 78 discusses T lymphocytes in more detail.

REGULATION OF T CELL PRECURSOR/THYMOCYTE DEVELOPMENT

The developmental fate of thymocytes is regulated through physical interaction with thymic stromal cells (i.e., TEC, fibroblasts, and dendritic/interdigitating cells) and cytokines produced by thymic stromal cells. TEC synthesize and secrete a complex array of cytokines, including IL-1, IL-3, IL-6, IL-7, stem cell factor, leukemia inhibitory factor, CXCL12, and TGF-β.[109-113] Cytokine stimulation likely occurs in the localized microenvironment between a thymocyte and a thymic epithelial cell. The stimulation may be accomplished through adhesive interactions mediated by thymocyte CD2 and through CD11a interaction with thymic epithelial cell CD58 and CD54.[114,115] Thymocytes also express VLA-4,[79] and thymic stromal cell VCAM-1 or fibronectin likely serves as the counterreceptor to facilitate adhesion.

Which cytokines support thymocyte proliferation? In contrast to human B cell precursors, IL-7 to IL-7 receptor interaction and downstream signaling events appear to be essential for normal human thymocyte development.[116] Immunodeficiency patients with mutations in the γ_c subunit of the IL-2, IL-4, IL-7, IL-9, and IL-15 receptors[69]; patients with mutations in JAK-3[70,71]; and patients with mutations in the IL-7 receptor[72] all exhibit a profound block in thymocyte development. The importance of IL-7 in these experiments of nature has been reproduced using a chimeric human–mouse fetal thymic organ culture.[117] IL-7 transduces a survival/proliferation stimulus to CD34+/CD1a− thymocytes, protects CD4+/CD8+ thymocytes from glucocorticoid-induced apoptosis, and stimulates proliferation in mature CD3+/CD4+ and CD3+/CD8+ thymocytes.[118] IL-7 at least partially exerts its effect on human thymocytes by activating phosphatidylinositol-3 kinase,[116] a lipid kinase essential to many mitogenic pathways. Interestingly, IL-7 also up-regulates expression of CXCR4 on CD34+ thymocytes. Subsequent stimulation with CXCL12 enhances the survival and proliferation of these cells.[113]

Studies in the mouse provide additional clues about the function of IL-7. Mice deficient in expression of the IL-7 receptor α-chain exhibit a severe block in thymocyte development, but this deficiency can be overcome by enforced expression of the antiapoptotic protein Bcl-2.[119,120] Furthermore, mice deficient in IL-7 exhibit a profound loss of Bcl-2 in immature thymocytes (i.e., CD3−/CD4−/CD8−), but short-term culture of these cells with IL-7 increases expression of Bcl-2 and promotes cell survival.[121] These collective results indicate IL-7 enhances Bcl-2 levels in early thymocytes, thereby transmitting a survival signal essential for continuing thymocyte development. Whether human thymocyte survival is mediated by a similar IL-7–dependent mechanism is unknown.

NK CELL DEVELOPMENT

NK cells are large granular lymphocytes that account for approximately 5 percent of blood and splenic lymphocytes. NK cells play an important role in the innate immune response to viral infection and some tumors (see Chap. 79). Considerable progress has been made in identifying and characterizing receptors on NK cells that transduce inhibitory and activation signals.[122] Precise characterization of NK cell development has been difficult because of the paucity of NK-specific cell surface markers. However, with the increased ability to isolate CLP by FACS and the development of human *in vitro* and murine *in vivo* models for analyzing differentiation of CLP into lymphoid lineages, our understanding of the regulation of NK cell development has increased.

ORGANS INVOLVED IN NK CELL DEVELOPMENT

NK cell development originates from CD34+ HSC present in yolk sac, aorta/gonad/mesonephros, fetal liver, fetal thymus, cord blood, and adult marrow.[123] Whether these tissues generate discrete subsets of NK cells or reflect a shift in the site of NK cell development as a function of ontogeny is unclear. NK cells can be detected at 6 weeks' gestation in fetal liver,[124] prior to the development of a functional thymus.[86] Consistent with this ontology, fetal liver CD34+ HSC can differentiate into NK cells *in vitro*.[125] A close ontogenic relationship exists between NK cells and thymocytes.[123] The development of NK cells from CD34+ thymic progenitors and the supportive capacity of the thymic microenvironment for NK cell development provide direct evidence for a thymic origin of at least some NK cells.[126–128] The immediate precursor of an NK-committed progenitor could be a T/NK or dendritic cell/NK bipotential progenitor. Evidence supporting both progenitors have been published.[126–129] CD34+ HSC isolated from adult marrow and cord blood can develop into functional cytolytic NK cells using a variety of *in vitro* culture systems containing cytokines

and stromal cells.[130–134] The CLP likely is the immediate precursor. Marrow is the primary if not exclusive source of NK cell development in adults.[122]

NK RECEPTORS AND RECOMBINATION-ASSOCIATED GENES

Unlike T and B cells, NK cell development does not require a process of receptor gene rearrangement mediated by RAG-1 and RAG-2. Thus, NK cell development is essentially normal in mice deficient in RAG-1 or RAG-2.[46,47] Target-cell recognition by human NK cells is mediated by cell surface molecules representing two receptor families.[135,136] The first family recognizes polymorphic class I major histocompatibility molecules and is designated the *killer cell Ig-like receptors* (KIR) or CD158. The second family recognizes molecules of pathogen or host origin that are homologous to class I MHC and is designated CD94/NKG2. The KIR (CD158) family is made up of at least 14 distinct genes that encode molecules with Ig-like superfamily domains. In contrast, the CD94 family encodes molecules with a C-type lectin structure. Following binding to ligand, these two receptor families can transduce activation or inhibitory signals that regulate NK cell-mediated cytotoxicity and cytokine production. Chapter 79 provides a more detailed discussion of these receptors and their functions.

NK LINEAGE-ASSOCIATED SURFACE ANTIGENS

Studies of NK cell development have been hampered by the absence of NK lineage-specific cell surface markers. Cell surface molecules on NK cells, such as CD16, CD56, CD94, and CD158, are also variably expressed on T lineage cells.[123] Likewise, cell surface molecules commonly found on T cells, such as CD5, CD7, and CD28, are variably expressed on NK cells. However, combinations of markers have provided the means to trace the NK lineage. Figure 76-4 shows a developmental scheme for human NK cells in marrow. The CLP is a likely precursor of cells committed to the NK lineage. CLP isolated from marrow[11] and cord blood[13] are restricted to lymphoid development, including NK cells. The most useful marker for identifying cells committed to the NK lineage is CD122, the β-subunit of the IL-2/IL-15 receptors.[133] The NK progenitor expressing CD122 does not express CD7 or several other cell surface molecules that are acquired during later stages of NK cell development. The next developmental compartment is defined by the acquisition of the CD161 NK cell receptor protein and CD2.[123,137] Acquisition of CD56 and CD94 and the appearance of cytoplasmic granules define the next stage of development, which is followed by the appearance of a fully mature NK cell expressing CD16 and various members of the KIR family.[125,138,139] Classification of these populations as distinct developmental stages may be an oversimplification; considering these stages as a developmental continuum may be more appropriate. The mature NK cell population (i.e., the population in blood) is composed of two subpopulations. The predominant subpopulation (approximately 95 percent of mature NK cells) expresses CD16, low amounts of CD56, and both inhibitory receptor families (CD94 and CD158). The minority subpopulation (approximately 5 percent of mature NK cells) expresses high levels of CD56 and CD94 but is CD158− and CD16−. Ample evidence supports a functional distinction between these two populations based on chemokine responsiveness, tissue distribution, and cytolytic capability.[122] However, no evidence indicates that a precursor/progeny relationship exists between them.

REGULATION OF NK CELL DEVELOPMENT

NK cells, like B and T cells, require the complex milieu of the marrow or thymic microenvironment for proliferation and differentiation. A large number of cytokines enhance the development of NK cells from

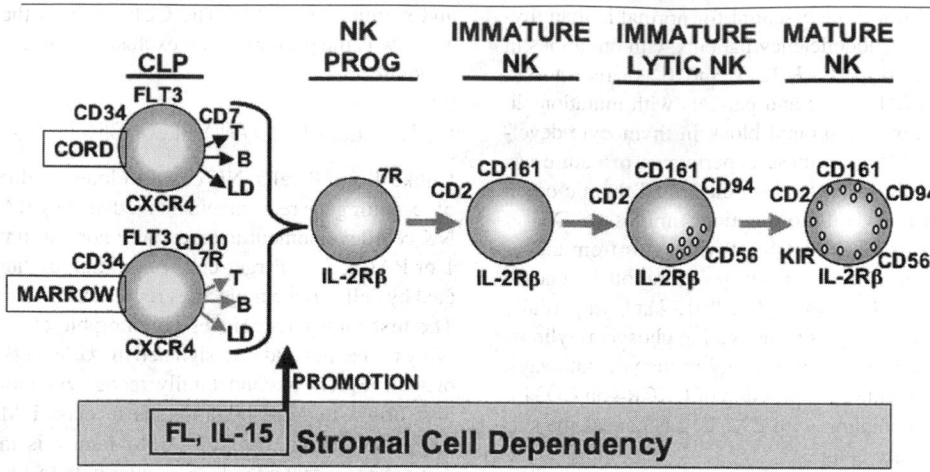

FIGURE 76-4   NK cell development in human marrow. The CLP correspond to the CLP in Figure 76-1 with multilineage developmental potential. The *small circles* in the immature lytic and mature NK cells represent cytolytic granules. Stromal cell support is shown as a constant requirement throughout NK cell development, but this is likely an oversimplification. A comprehensive review of human NK cell development is given in references 122 and 123.

CD34+ stem cells *in vitro*. The cytokines include IL-1α, IL-2, IL-6, IL-7, IL-15, FL, stem cell factor, and granulocyte-macrophage colony stimulating factor.[125,126,129–134,140,141] Determining the precise role of each cytokine in promoting CLP commitment to the NK lineage and promoting proliferation/differentiation of the various NK progenitors has been difficult because of expression of the cognate receptors on many lymphohematopoietic cells.

NK cell development from CD34+ marrow HSC has been a useful model for evaluating the contribution of marrow stromal cell products to NK cell development. Initial studies demonstrated that NK cell development from human HSC requires stromal cell contact.[130] A subsequent study showed that stem cell factor, FL, and IL-7[133] were sufficient to support NK cell development from HSC. Further development is mediated by IL-15. IL-15 binds to a receptor complex consisting of a unique α-chain, a β-chain (CD122) that is used by IL-15 and IL-2, and the common γ-chain (γ$_c$) that is used by IL-2, IL-4, IL-7, IL-9, and IL-15. Human marrow stromal cells produce IL-15, which promotes the development of CD56+ NK cells from CD34+ marrow stem cells.[130] FL also promotes the development of CD56+ NK cells from CD34+ marrow stem cells.[134,140] A potential hierarchical effect of FL and IL-15 may be sufficient for NK development from HSC and subsequent expansion and differentiation of cells committed to the NK lineage. FL reportedly induces the expression of CD122 and IL-15 receptor α-transcripts on CD34+ marrow stem cells.[134] The FL-stimulated CD34+ stem cells then can respond to IL-15 and differentiate into CD56+/CD158+ NK cells with cytolytic activity.[134] In another study, human thymic progenitors cultured in IL-15 gave rise to NK cells.[133] These *in vitro* studies are consistent with experiments of nature. Severe combined immunodeficiency patients with mutations in the γ$_c$ subunit or JAK-3 tyrosine kinase do not develop NK cells.[69] These mutations negate the function of IL-2, IL-4, IL-7, IL-9, and IL-15. IL-7 likely is not essential for NK cell development given that patients with mutations in the IL-7 receptor have normal NK cell development.[73] IL-2 likely is not essential, and IL-4 and IL-9 have no known roles in NK cell development. However, mice deficient in IL-15 and IL-15 receptor α-chain lack NK cells.[142] These collective data indicate that IL-15 plays a pivotal role in NK cell development. Definitive evidence for a role of IL-15 may require the identification of an immunodeficient patient having an IL-15 gene mu-

tation. Interestingly, two patients with an apparent autosomal recessive syndrome exhibited severe prenatal and postnatal growth failure and no detectable NK cells.[143] The genetic basis for this syndrome was not identified.

REFERENCES

1. Zon LI: Developmental biology of hematopoiesis. *Blood* 86:2876, 1995.
2. Godin IE, Garcia-Porrero JA, Coutinho A, et al: Para-aortic splanchnopleura from early mouse embryos contains B1a cell progenitors. *Nature* 364:67, 1993.
3. Medvinksy AL, Samoylina NL, Muller AM, Dzierzak EA: An early preliver intraembryonic source of CFU-S in the developing mouse embryo. *Nature* 364:64, 1993.
4. Cumano A, Dieterlen-Lièvre F, Godin I: Lymphoid potential, probed before circulation in mouse, is restricted to caudal intraembryonic splanchnopleura. *Cell* 86:907, 1996.
5. Migliaccio G, Migliaccio AR, Petti S, et al: Human embryonic hemopoiesis: Kinetics of progenitors and precursors underlying the yolk sac→liver transition. *J Clin Invest* 78:51, 1986.
6. Huyhn A, Dommergues M, Izac B, et al: Characterization of hematopoietic progenitors from human yolk sacs and embryos. *Blood* 86:4474, 1995.
7. Tavian M, Coulombel L, Luton D, et al: Aorta-associated CD34+ hematopoietic cells in the early human embryo. *Blood* 87:67, 1996.
8. Labastie M-C, Cortés F, Roméo P-H, et al: Molecular identity of hematopoietic precursor cells emerging in the human embryo. *Blood* 92:3624, 1998.
9. Tavian M, Robin C, Coulombel L, Peault B: The human embryo, but not its yolk sac, generates lympho-myeloid stem cells: Mapping multipotent hematopoietic cell fate in intraembryonic mesoderm. *Immunity* 15:487, 2001.
10. Hakoda M, Hirai Y, Shimba H, et al: Cloning of phenotypically different human lymphocytes originating from a single stem cell. *J Exp Med* 169:1265, 1989.
11. Galy A, Travis M, Cen Z, Chen B: Human T B, natural killer and dendritic cells arise from a common marrow progenitor cell subset. *Immunity* 3:459, 1995.

12. Kondo M, Weissman IL, Akashi K: Identification of clonogenic common lymphoid progenitors in mouse marrow. *Cell* 91:661, 1997.

13. Hao Q-L, Zhu J, Price MA, et al: Identification of a novel, human multilymphoid progenitor in cord blood. *Blood* 97:3683, 2001.

14. Rossi MID, Yokota T, Medina KL, et al: B lymphopoiesis is active throughout human life, but there are developmental age-related changes. *Blood* 101:576, 2003.

15. Montecino-Rodriguez E, Dorshkind K: To T or not to T: Reassessing the common lymphoid progenitor. *Nat Immunol* 4:100, 2003.

16. Allman D, Samgandam A, Kim S, et al: Thymopoiesis independent of common lymphoid progenitors. *Nat Immunol* 4:168, 2003.

17. LeBien TW: Fates of human B-cell precursors: *Blood* 96:9, 2000.

18. Burrows PD, LeBien TW, Zhang Z, et al: The development of human B lymphocytes, in *Molecular Biology of B Cells*, edited by FW Alt, T Honjo, M Neuberger, p 141. Elsevier Academic Press, London, 2004.

19. Gathings WE, Lawton AR, Cooper MD: Immunofluorescent studies of the development of pre-B-cells, B lymphocytes, and immunoglobulin isotype diversity in humans. *Eur J Immunol* 7:804, 1977.

20. Solvason N, Kearney JF: The human fetal omentum: A site of B cell generation. *J Exp Med* 175:397, 1992.

21. Nunez C, Nishimoto N, Gartland LG, et al: B cells are generated throughout life in humans. *J Immunol* 156:866, 1996.

22. Brashem CJ, Kersey JH, Bollum FJ, LeBien TW: Ontogenic studies of human lymphoid progenitor cells in human marrow. *Exp Hematol* 10:886, 1982.

23. Hesslein DGT, Schatz DG: Factors and forces controlling V(D)J recombination. *Adv Immunol* 78:169, 2001.

24. Matsuda F, Ishii K, Bourvagnet P, et al: The complete nucleotide sequence of the human immunoglobulin heavy chain variable region locus. *J Exp Med* 188:2151, 1999.

25. Kitamura D, Rajewsky K: Targeted disruption of μ chain membrane exon causes loss of heavy chain allelic exclusion. *Nature* 356:154, 1992.

26. Ramsden DA, Wu GE: Mouse κ light-chain recombination signal sequences mediate recombination more frequently than those of λ light chain. *Proc Natl Acad Sci U S A* 88:10721, 1991.

27. Bertrand FE III, Billips LG, Burrows PD, et al: IgH gene segment transcription and rearrangement prior to surface expression of the pan B-cell marker CD19 in normal human marrow. *Blood* 90:738, 1997.

28. Davi F, Faili A, Gritti C, et al: Early onset of immunoglobulin heavy chain gene rearrangements in normal human marrow CD34+ cells. *Blood* 90:4014, 1997.

29. Reynaud D, Lefort N, Manie E, et al: In vitro identification of human pro-B cells that give rise to macrophages, natural killer cells, and T cells. *Blood* 101:4313, 2003.

30. Ghia P, Ten Boekel E, Sanz E, et al: Ordering of human marrow B lymphocyte precursors by single-cell polymerase chain reaction analyses of the rearrangement status of the immunoglobulin H and L chain gene loci. *J Exp Med* 184:2217, 1996.

31. Kubagawa H, Cooper MD, Carroll AJ, Burrows PD: Light-chain gene expression before heavy-chain gene rearrangement in pre-B cells transformed by Epstein-Barr virus. *Proc Natl Acad Sci U S A* 86:2356, 1989.

32. Pauza ME, Rehmann JA, LeBien TW: Unusual patterns of immunoglobulin gene rearrangement and expression during human B-cell ontogeny: Human B cells can simultaneously express cell surface κ and λ light chains. *J Exp Med* 178:139, 1993.

33. Karasuyama H, Rolink A, Melchers F: Surrogate light chain in B-cell development. *Adv Immunol* 63:1, 1996.

34. Hollis GF, Evans RJ, Stafford-Hollis JM, et al: Immunoglobulin λ light-chain-related genes 14.1 and 16.1 are expressed in pre-B cells and may encode the human immunoglobulin ω light-chain protein. *Proc Natl Acad Sci U S A* 88:5552, 1989.

35. Bossy D, Milili M, Zucman J, et al: Organization of the λ-like genes that contribute to the μ-ψ light chain complex in human pre-B cells. *Int Immunol* 3:1081, 1991.

36. Wang YH, Nomura J, Faye-Peterson OM, Cooper MD: Surrogate light chain production during B-cell differentiation: Differential intracellular versus cell surface expression. *J Immunol* 161:1132, 1998.

37. Wang Y-H, Stephan RP, Scheffold A, et al: Differential surrogate light chain expression governs B-cell differentiation. *Blood* 99:2459, 2002.

38. Meffre E, Davis E, Schiff C, et al: Circulating human B cells that express surrogate light chains and edited receptors. *Nat Immunol* 1:207, 2000.

39. Meffre E, Schaefer A, Wardemann H, et al: Surrogate light chain expressing human peripheral B cells produce self-reactive antibodies. *J Exp Med* 199:145, 2004.

40. Kitamura D, Kudo A, Schaal S, et al: A critical role of λ5 protein in B-cell development. *Cell* 69:823, 1992.

41. Minegishi Y, Coustan-Smith E, Wang YH, et al: Mutations in the human lambda 5/14.1 gene result in B-cell deficiency and agammaglobulinemia. *J Exp Med* 187:71, 1998.

42. Gauthier L, Rossi B, Roux F, et al: Galectin-1 is a stromal cell ligand of the pre-B cell receptor (BCR) implicated in synapse formation between pre-B and stromal cells and in pre-BCR triggering. *Proc Nat Acad Sci U S A* 99:13014, 2002.

43. Bradl H, Hans-Martin J: Surrogate light chain-mediated interaction of a soluble pre-B cell receptor with adherent cell lines. *J Immunol* 167:6403, 2001.

44. Ohnishi K, Melchers F: The nonimmunoglobulin portion of λ5 mediates cell-autonomous pre-B cell receptor signaling. *Nat Immunol* 4:849, 2003.

45. Pavavasiliou FN, Schatz DG: Somatic hypermutation of immunoglobulin genes: Merging mechanisms for genetic diversity. *Cell* 109:535, 2002.

46. Mombaerts P, Iacomini J, Johnson RS, et al: RAG-1-deficient mice have no mature B and T lymphocytes. *Cell* 68:869, 1992.

47. Shinkai Y, Rathbun G, Lam K-P, et al: RAG-2-deficient mice lack mature lymphocytes owing to inability to initiate V(D)J rearrangement. *Cell* 68:855, 1992.

48. Schwarz KG, Gauss GH, Ludwig L, et al: RAG mutations in human B cell-negative SCID. *Science* 274:97, 1996.

49. Jung D, Alt F: Unraveling V(D)J recombination: Insights into gene regulation. *Cell* 116:299, 2004.

50. Nemazee D: Receptor selection in B and T lymphocytes. *Annu Rev Immunol* 18:19, 2000.

51. Desiderio SV, Yancopoulos G, Paskind M, et al: Insertion of N regions into heavy-chain genes is correlated with expression of terminal deoxynucleotidyl transferase in B cells. *Nature* 311:752, 1984.

52. Bridges SL, Lee SK, Johnson ML, et al: Somatic mutation and CDR3 lengths of immunoglobulin kappa light chains expressed in patients with rheumatoid arthritis and in normal individuals. *J Clin Invest* 96:831, 1995.

53. Komori T, Okada A, Stewart V, Alt F: Lack of N regions in antigen receptor variable region genes of TdT-deficient lymphocytes. *Science* 261:1171, 1993.

54. Gilfillan S, Dierich A, Lemeur M, et al: Mice lacking TdT: Mature animals with an immature lymphocyte repertoire. *Science* 261:1175, 1993.

55. Gore SD, Kastan MB, Civin CI: Normal human marrow precursors that express terminal deoxynucleotidyl transferase include T-cell precursors and possible lymphoid stem cells. *Blood* 77:1681, 1991.

56. LeBien TW, Wörmann B, Villablanca JG, et al: Multiparameter flow cytometric analysis of human fetal marrow B cells. *Leukemia* 4:354, 1990.

57. Reth M: Antigen receptors on B lymphocytes. *Annu Rev Immunol* 10:97, 1992.

58. DeFranco AL: The complexity of signaling pathways activated by the BCR. *Curr Opin Immunol* 9:296, 1997.

59. Dworzak MN, Fritsch G, Fröschl G, et al: Four-color flow cytometric investigation of terminal deoxynucleotidyl transferase-positive lymphoid precursors in pediatric marrow: CD79a expression precedes CD19 in early B-cell ontogeny. *Blood* 92:3203, 1998

60. Gong S, Nussenzweig MC: Regulation of an early developmental checkpoint in the B-cell pathway by Ig beta. *Science* 272:411, 1996.

61. Ryan DH, Nuccie BL, Abboud CN, Winslow JM: Vascular cell adhesion molecule-1 and the integrin VLA-4 mediate adhesion of human B-cell precursors to cultured marrow adherent cells. *J Clin Invest* 88:995, 1991.

62. Dittel BN, McCarthy JB, Wayner EA, LeBien TW: Regulation of human B-cell precursor adhesion to marrow stromal cells by cytokines that exert opposing effects on the expression of vascular cell adhesion molecule-1 (VCAM-1). *Blood* 81:2272, 1993.

63. Hynes RO: Integrins, versatility, modulation, and signaling in cell adhesion. *Cell* 69:11, 1992.

64. Glodek AM, Honczarenko M, Le Y, et al: Sustained activation of cell adhesion is a differentially regulated process in B lymphopoiesis. *J Exp Med* 197:461, 2003.

65. Dittel BN, LeBien TW: The growth response to IL-7 during normal human B-cell ontogeny is restricted to B-lineage cells expressing CD34. *J Immunol* 154:58, 1995.

66. Billips LG, Nunez CA, Bertrand FE III, et al: Immunoglobulin recombinase gene activity is modulated reciprocally by interleukin 7 and CD19 in B-cell progenitors. *J Exp Med* 182:973, 1995.

67. Namikawa R, Muench MO, deVries JE, Roncarolo MG: The FLK2/FLT3 ligand synergizes with interleukin-7 in promoting stromal-cell-independent expansion and differentiation of human fetal pro-B cells in vitro. *Blood* 87:1881, 1996.

68. Candeias S, Muegge K, Durum SK: IL-7 receptor and VDJ recombination: Trophic versus mechanistic actions. *Immunity* 6:501, 1997.

69. Leonard W: Cytokines and immunodeficiency diseases. *Nat Rev Immunol* 1:200, 2001.

70. Macchi P, Villa A, Giliani S, et al: Mutations of Jak-3 gene in patients with autosomal severe combined immune deficiency (SCID). *Nature* 377:65, 1995.

71. Russell SM, Tayebi N, Nakajima H, et al: Mutation of Jak3 in a patient with SCID: Essential role of Jak3 in lymphoid development. *Science* 270:797, 1995.

72. Puel A, Ziegler SF, Buckley RH, Leonard WJ: Defective IL7R expression in T(−)B(+)NK(+) severe combined immunodeficiency. *Nat Genet* 20:394, 1998.

73. Pribyl JAR, LeBien TW: IL-7 independent development of human B cells. *Proc Natl Acad Sci U S A* 93:10348, 1996.

74. Hernandez PA, Gorlin RJ, Lukens JN, et al: Mutations in the chemokine receptor gene CXCR4 are associated with WHIM syndrome, a combined immunodeficiency disease. *Nat Genet* 34:70, 2003.

75. Muschen M, Lee S, Zhou G, et al: Molecular portraits of B cell lineage commitment. *Proc Nat Acad Sci U S A* 99:10014, 2002.

76. Baggiolini M: Chemokines and leukocyte traffic. *Nature* 392:565, 1998.

77. Haynes BF, Martin ME, Kay HH, Kurtzberg J: Early events in human T cell ontogeny: Phenotypic characterization and immunohistologic localization of T-cell precursors in early human fetal tissues. *J Exp Med* 168:1061, 1988.

78. Campana D, Janossy G, Constan-Smith E, et al: The expression of T-cell receptor-associated proteins during T-cell ontogeny in man. *J Immunol* 142:57, 1989.

79. Terstappen LWMM, Huang S, Picker LJ: Flow cytometric assessment of human T cell differentiation in thymus and marrow. *Blood* 79:666, 1992.

80. Spits H: Development of alphabeta T cells in the human thymus. *Nat Rev Immunol* 2:760, 2002.

81. Klein F, Feldhahn N, Lee S, et al: T lymphoid differentiation in human bone marrow. *Proc Nat Acad Sci U S A* 100:6747, 2003.

82. Garcia-Ojeda ME, Dejbakhsh-Jones S, Weissman IL, Strober S: An alternate pathway for T cell development supported by the marrow microenvironment: Recapitulation of thymic maturation. *J Exp Med* 187:1813, 1998.

83. McVay LD, Carding SR: Extrathymic origin of human γδ T cells during fetal development. *J Immunol* 157:2873, 1996.

84. Howie D, Spencer J, DeLord D et al: Extrathymic T cell differentiation in the human intestine early in life. *J Immunol* 161:5862, 1998.

85. Weller GL: Development of the thyroid, parathyroid, and thymus gland in man. *Contrib Embryol Carnegie Inst* 24:95, 1933.

86. Haynes BF: The human thymic microenvironment. *Adv Immunol* 36:87, 1984.

87. Manley NR, Blackburn CC: A developmental look at thymus organogenesis: Where do the non-hematopoietic cells in the thymus come from? *Curr Opin Immunol* 15:225, 2003.

88. Rodewald H-R: The thymus in the age of retirement. *Nature* 396:630, 1998.

89. Kong F, Chen CH, Cooper MD: Thymic function can be accurately monitored by the level of recent T cell emigrants in the circulation. *Immunity* 8:97, 1998.

90. Douek DC, McFarland RD, Keiser PH, et al: Changes in thymic function with age and during treatment of HIV infection. *Nature* 396:690, 1998.

91. Gill J, Malin M, Sutherland J, et al: Thymic generation and regeneration. *Immunol Rev* 195:28, 2003.

92. Jörn Gotter J, Brors B, Hergenhahn M, et al: Medullary epithelial cells of the human thymus express a highly diverse selection of tissue-specific genes colocalized in chromosomal clusters. *J Exp Med* 199:155, 2004.

93. Blom B, Verschuren MCM, Heemskerk MHM, et al: TCR gene rearrangements and expression of the pre-T cell receptor complex during human T-cell differentiation. *Blood* 93:3033, 1999.

94. Ktorza S, Sarun S, Rieux-Laucat F, et al: CD34-positive early human thymocytes: T cell receptor and cytokine receptor gene expression. *Eur J Immunol* 25:2471, 1995.

95. Krangel MS, Yssel H, Brocklehurst C, Spits H: A distinct wave of human T-cell receptor λδ lymphocytes in the early fetal thymus: Evidence for controlled gene rearrangement and cytokine production. *J Exp Med* 172:847, 1990.

96. Carrasco YR, Navarro MN, de Yebenes VG, et al: Regulation of surface expression of the human pre-T cell receptor complex. *Semin Immunol* 14:325, 2002.

97. Saint-Ruf C, Ungewiss K, Groettrup M, et al: Analysis and expression of a cloned pre-T cell receptor gene. *Science* 266:1208, 1994.

98. Del Porto P, Bruno L, Mattei MG, et al: Cloning and comparative analysis of the human pre-T-cell receptor alpha-chain gene. *Proc Natl Acad Sci U S A* 92:12105, 1995.

99. Wilson A, Held W, MacDonald HR: Two waves of recombinase gene expression in developing thymocytes. *J Exp Med* / 179:1355, 1994.

100. Trigueros C, Ramiro AR, Carrasco YR, et al: Identification of a late stage of small noncycling pTα− pre-T cells as immediate precursors of T cell receptor α/β+ thymocytes. *J Exp Med* 188:1401, 1998.

101. Galy A, Barcena A, Verma S, Spits H: Precursors of CD3+CD4+CD8+ in the human thymus are defined by expression of CD34: Delineation of early events in human thymic development. *J Exp Med* 178:391, 1993.

102. Sánchez M-J, Muench MO, Roncarolo MG, et al: Identification of a common T/NK cell progenitor in human fetal thymus. *J Exp Med* 180:569, 1994.

103. Res P, Martínez Cáceres E, Jaleco AC, et al: CD34+CD38dim cells in the human thymus can differentiate into T, natural killer and dendritic cells but are distinct from stem cells. *Blood* 87:5196, 1996.

104. Márquez C, Trigueros C, Franco JM, et al: Identification of a common developmental pathway for thymic natural killer cells and dendritic cells. *Blood* 91:2760, 1998.

105. Artavanis-Tsakonas S, Rand MD, Lake RJ: Notch signaling: Cell fate control and signal integration in development. *Science* 284:770, 1999.

106. Maillard I, Adler SH, Pear WS: Notch and the immune system. *Immunity* 19:781, 2003.

107. De Smedt M, Reynvoet K, Kerre T, et al: Active form of Notch imposes T cell fate in human progenitor cells. *J Immunol* 169:3021, 2002.

108. García-Peydró M, De Yébenes VG, Toribio ML: Sustained Notch1 signaling instructs the earliest human intrathymic precursors to adopt a γδT-cell fate in fetal thymus organ culture. *Blood* 102:2444, 2003.

109. Galy AHM, Spits H: IL-1, IL-4 and IFN-γ differentially regulate cytokine production and cell surface molecule expression in cultured human thymic epithelial cells. *J Immunol* 147:3823, 1991.

110. Le PT, Lazorick S, Whichard LP, et al: Regulation of cytokine production in the human thymus: Epidermal growth factor and transforming growth factor α regulate mRNA levels of IL1α, IL1β and IL6 in human thymic epithelial cells at a post-transcriptional level. *J Exp Med* 174: 1147, 1991.

111. Le PT, Lazorick S, Whichard LP, et al: Human thymic epithelial cells produce IL-6, granulocyte-monocyte CSF and leukemia inhibitory factor. *J Immunol* 145:3310, 1990.

112. Dalloul AH, Arock M, Fourcade C, et al: Human thymic epithelial cells produce interleukin-3. *Blood* 77:69, 1991.

113. Hernández-López C, Varas A, Sacedón A, et al: Stromal cell-derived factor 1/CXCR4 signaling is critical for early human T-cell development. *Blood* 99:546;2002.

114. Vollger LW, Tuck DT, Springer TA, et al: Thymocyte binding to human thymic epithelial cells is inhibited by monoclonal antibodies to CD2 and LFA3 antigens. *J Immunol* 138:358, 1987.

115. Singer KH, Denning SM, Whichard LP, Haynes BF: Thymocyte LFA-1 and thymic epithelial cell ICAM-1 molecules mediate binding of activated human thymocytes to thymic epithelial cells. *J Immunol* 143: 3944, 1989.

116. Fry TJ, Mackall CL: Interleukin-7: From bench to clinic. *Blood* 99:3892, 2002.

117. Plum J, De Smedt M, Leclercq G, et al: Interleukin-7 is a critical growth factor in early human T-cell development. *Blood* 88:4239, 1996.

118. Napolitano LA, Stoddart CA, Hanley MB, et al: Effects of IL-7 on early human thymocyte progenitor cells in vitro and in SCID-hu thy/liv mice. *J Immunol* 171:645, 2003.

119. Akashi K, Kondo M, Von Freeden-Jeffry U, et al: Bcl-2 rescues T lymphopoiesis in interleukin-7 receptor-deficient mice. *Cell* 89:1033, 1997.

120. Maraskovsky E, O'Reilly LA, Teepe M, et al: Bcl-2 can rescue T lymphocyte development in interleukin-7 receptor-deficient mice but not in mutant rag-1-/-mice. *Cell* 89:1011, 1997.

121. von Freeden-Jeffry U, Solvason N, Howard M, Murray R: The earliest T lineage-committed cells depend on IL-7 for Bcl-2 expression and normal cell cycle progression. *Immunity* 7:147, 1997.

122. Colucci F, Di Santo JP, Leibson P: Natural killer cell activation in mice and men: Different triggers for similar weapons? *Nat Immunol* 3:807, 2002.

123. Colucci F, Caligiuri MA, Di Santo JP. What does it take to make a natural killer? *Nat Rev Immunol* 3:413, 2003.

124. Phillips JH, Hori T, Nagler A, et al: Ontogeny of human natural killer (NK) cells: Fetal NK cells mediate cytolytic function and express cytoplasmic CD3 epsilon, delta proteins. *J Exp Med* 175:1055, 1992.

125. Jaleco AC, Blom B, Res P, et al: Fetal liver contains committed NK progenitors, but is not a site for development of CD34+ cells into T cells. *J Immunol* 159:694, 1997.

126. Sanchez MJ, Muench MO, Roncarolo MG, et al: Identification of a common T/natural killer cell progenitor in human fetal thymus. *J Exp Med* 180:569, 1994.

127. Barcena A, Galy AH, Punnonen J, et al: Lymphoid and myeloid differentiation of fetal liver CD34+ lineage-cells in human thymic organ culture. *J Exp Med* 180:123, 1994.

128. Plum J, de Smedt M, Verhasselt B, et al: In vitro intrathymic differentiation kinetics of human fetal liver CD34+CD38− progenitors reveals a phenotypically defined dendritic/T-NK precursor split. *J Immunol* 162: 60, 1999.

129. Márquez C, Trigueros C, Franco JM, et al: Identification of a common developmental pathway for thymic natural killer cells and dendritic cells. *Blood* 91:2760, 1998.

130. Miller JS, Alley KA, McGlave P: Differentiation of NK cells from human primitive marrow progenitors. *Blood* 83:2594, 1994.

131. Silva MRG, Hoffman R, Srour EF, Ascensao JL: Generation of human natural killer cells from immature progenitors does not require marrow stromal cells. *Blood* 84:841, 1994.

132. Shibuya A, Nagayoshi K, Nakamura K, Nakauchi H: Lymphokine requirement for the generation of natural killer cells from CD34+ hematopoietic progenitor cells. *Blood* 85:3538, 1995.

133. Mrozek E, Anderson P, Caligiuri MA: Role of interleukin-15 in the development of human CD56+ natural killer cells from CD34+ hematopoietic progenitor cells. *Blood* 87:2632, 1996.

134. Yu H, Fehniger TA, Fuchshuber P, et al: Flt3 ligand promotes the generation of a distinct CD34(+) human natural killer cell progenitor that responds to interleukin-15. *Blood* 92:3647, 1998.

135. Lanier LL: On guard: Activating NK cell receptors. *Nat Immunol* 2:23, 2001.

136. McQueen KL, Parham P: Variable receptors controlling activation and inhibition of NK cells. *Curr Opin Immunol* 14:615, 2002.

137. Bennett IM, Zatsepina O, Zamai L, et al: Definition of a natural killer NKR-P1A+/CD56−/CD16− functionally immature human NK cell subset that differentiates in vitro in the presence of interleukin 12. *J Exp Med* 184:1845, 1996.

138. Yu H, Fehniger TA, Fuchshuber P, et al: Flt3 ligand promotes the generation of a distinct CD34+ human natural killer cell progenitor that responds to interleukin-15. *Blood* 92:3647, 1998.

139. Sivori S, Falco M, Marcenaro E, et al: Early expression of triggering receptors and regulatory role of 2B4 in human natural killer cell precursors undergoing in vitro differentiation. *Proc Nat Acad Sci U S A* 99: 4526, 2002.

140. Miller JS, McCullar V, Punzel M, et al: Single adult human CD34+/ Lin−/CD38− progenitors give rise to natural killer cells, B-lineage cells, dendritic cells, and myeloid cells. *Blood* 93:96, 1999.

141. Leclercq G, Debacker V, De Smedt M, Plum J: Differential effects of interleukin-15 and interleukin-2 on differentiation of bipotential T/natural killer progenitor cells. *J Exp Med* 184:325, 1996.

142. Sevilir Williams N, Klem J, Puzanov IJ, et al: Natural killer cell differentiation: Insights from knockout and transgenic mouse models and in vitro systems. *Immunol Rev* 165:47, 1998.

143. Bernard F, Picard C, Cormier-Daire V, et al: A novel developmental and immunodeficiency syndrome associated with intrauterine growth retardation and lack of natural killer cells. *Pediatrics* 113:136, 2004.

FUNCTIONS OF B LYMPHOCYTES AND PLASMA CELLS IN IMMUNOGLOBULIN PRODUCTION

THOMAS J. KIPPS

Much of our immune defense against invading organisms is predicated upon the tremendous diversity of immunoglobulin molecules. Immunoglobulins are glycoproteins produced by B lymphocytes and plasma cells. These molecules can be considered receptors because the primary function of the immunoglobulin molecule is to bind antigen. A single person can synthesize 10 to 100 million different immunoglobulin molecules, each having a distinct antigen-binding specificity. The great diversity in this so-called humoral immune system allows us to generate antibodies specific for a variety of substances, including synthetic molecules not naturally present in our environment. Despite the diversity in the specificities of antibody molecules, the binding of antibody to antigen initiates a limited series of biologically important effector functions, such as complement activation and/or adherence of the immune complex to receptors on leukocytes. The eventual outcome is the clearance and degradation of the foreign substance. This chapter describes the structure of immunoglobulins and outlines the mechanisms by which B cells produce molecules of such tremendous diversity with defined effector functions.

IMMUNOGLOBULIN STRUCTURE AND FUNCTION

BASIC STRUCTURE

All naturally occurring immunoglobulin molecules are composed of one or several basic units consisting of two identical heavy (H) chains and two identical light (L) chains (Fig. 77-1). The four polypeptides are held in a bilaterally symmetrical, Y-shaped structure by disulfide

Acronyms and abbreviations that appear in this chapter include: AID, activation-induced deaminase; BiP, immunoglobulin "binding protein"; BLNK, *B* cell *link*er protein; Btk, Bruton tyrosine kinase; C, constant; CDR, complementarity-determining region; CRI, cross-reactive idiotype; CSR, class switch recombination; D, diversity; DNA-PK, DNA protein kinase; FR, framework region; H, heavy; HMG, high-mobility group protein; Ig, immunoglobulin; IL, interleukin; ITAM, immunoreceptor tyrosine-based activation motif; ITIM, immunoreceptor tyrosine-based inhibitory motif; κ, immunoglobulin kappa light chain; Kde, kappa-deleting element; λ, immunoglobulin lambda light chain; L, light; mRNA, messenger RNA; NHEJ, nonhomologous DNA end-joining; N-nucleotide, non–template-encoded nucleotide; NK, natural killer; PLC, phospholipase C; P-nucleotide, palindromic nucleotide; *RAG*, recombination activating gene; RSS, recombination signal sequences; SCID, severe combined immunodeficiency; SHP-1, Src homology 2 domain-containing protein tyrosine phosphatase-1; UNG, uracil-DNA glycosylase; V, variable-region gene; VDJ, exon created by a rearranged immunoglobulin heavy-chain variable-region gene, diversity gene segment, and joining gene segment.

bonds and noncovalent interactions.[1,2] The internal disulfide bonds of the heavy and light chains cause the polypeptides to fold into compact globe-shaped regions called *domains*, each containing approximately 110 to 120 amino acid residues.[3] Each domain forms a common fold of a type of protein structure known as *beta-pleated sheets* and is stabilized by a conserved disulfide bond (Fig. 77-1). The light chains have two domains; the heavy chains have four or five domains. The amino-terminal domains of the heavy and light chains are designated the *variable (V) regions* because their primary structure varies markedly among different immunoglobulin molecules.[4] The carboxy-terminal domains are referred to as *constant (C) regions* because their primary structure is the same among immunoglobulins of the same class or subclass. The amino acids in the light- and heavy-chain variable regions interact to form an antigen-binding site.[1,5] Each four-chain immunoglobulin basic unit has two identical binding sites. The constant-region domains of the heavy and light chains provide stability for the immunoglobulin molecule. The heavy-chain constant regions also mediate the specific effector functions of the different immunoglobulin classes (Table 77-1).[6]

LIGHT CHAINS

Immunoglobulin light chains have an approximate M_r of 23,000. They are divided into two types, κ and λ, based upon multiple amino acid sequence differences in the single constant-region domain.[4] The λ-chains are divided further into subclasses. The proportion of κ- to λ-chains in adult human plasma is approximately 2:1. The immunoglobulin light-chain constant region has no known effector function. Its main purpose may be to allow for proper assembly and release of an intact immunoglobulin molecule. Soon after synthesis, the antibody light-chain constant region associates with the nascent immunoglobulin heavy chain (see Fig. 77-1), releasing the latter from the immunoglobulin "binding protein" (BiP). BiP is a heat shock protein that, in the absence of antibody light chain, binds the first constant-region domain of the newly synthesized heavy chain, thereby retaining the heavy-chain polypeptide in the cell's endoplasmic reticulum.[7]

HEAVY CHAINS

Immunoglobulin heavy chains have an M_r of 50,000 to 70,000, depending upon the number and length of the constant-region domains. The five major isotypes of heavy chains—γ, α, μ, δ, and ε—determine the five corresponding classes of immunoglobulin (Ig): IgG, IgA, IgM, IgD, and IgE. The individual immunoglobulin molecules of each isotype may contain either κ- or λ-light chains, but not both. Tables 77-1 and 77-2 summarize the distinct physical and functional properties of the human immunoglobulin classes.

IgG

Approximately 80 percent of the immunoglobulins in adult plasma are IgG. The IgG molecule is composed of the basic 150-kDa immunoglobulin four-chain structure plus approximately 3 percent carbohydrate. IgG is the predominant antibody produced during the secondary immune response. IgG molecules effectively penetrate extravascular spaces and readily cross the placental barrier to provide passive immunity to the newborn.

Near the junction of the two arms of the Y-shaped immunoglobulin molecule, the two heavy chains interact to form a flexible "hinge" region (see Fig. 77-1). Exposed between constant-region globular domains, the hinge region is attacked readily by the proteolytic enzyme papain or pepsin. Figure 77-1 shows the cleavage sites. Digestion of IgG with papain yields three fragments. The single Fc piece contains the carboxy-terminal region of both heavy chains. The two identical F(ab) pieces contain the entire light chain and the amino-terminal portion of the heavy chain.

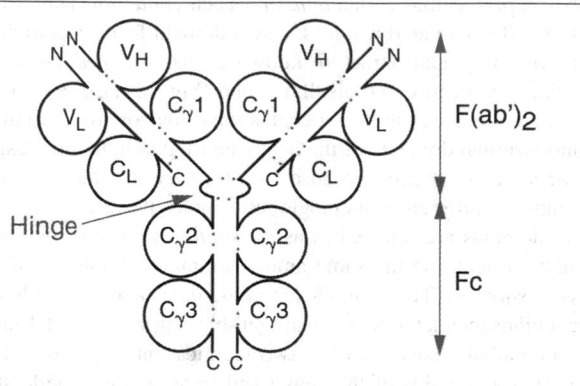

FIGURE 77-1 Schematic model of an IgG molecule. The light-chain domains V_L and C_L and the heavy-chain domains V_H, $C_\gamma 1$ (or $C_H 1$), $C_\gamma 2$ (or $C_H 2$), and $C_\gamma 3$ (or $C_H 3$) are labeled inside the respective immunoglobulin domain. *Dotted colored lines* indicate intrachain and interchain disulfide bonds. The amino-terminus (N) and carboxyl-terminus (C) of each polypeptide is indicated. The hinge region also is indicated. Digestion by pepsin cleaves the molecule at the carboxyl side of the hinge region, which generates Fc and $F(ab')_2$ fragments, as indicated on the *right*. The $F(ab')_2$ fragment is bivalent, as it is held together by the disulfide bridges in the hinge region. On the other hand, digestion of the molecule by papain degrades the Fc portion and generates monovalent Fab fragments, as the cleavage site for papain is on the amino-terminal side of the disulfide bridges of the hinge region.

Within the IgG class are four major subclasses, designated IgG1, IgG2, IgG3, and IgG4. Each subclass has a distinct heavy-chain constant region and mediates different effector functions (Table 77-3).[6] The average half-life of circulating IgG molecules is approximately 21 days, although the exact value varies among the IgG subclasses (Table 77-3). The most abundant subclass is IgG1, which constitutes 65 percent of the total IgG in plasma. Whereas IgG1 and IgG3 proteins activate complement via the classic pathway, IgG2 molecules fix complement poorly and IgG4 proteins not at all. IgG3 myeloma protein may aggregate spontaneously to produce a hyperviscosity syndrome.

Either aggregated IgG or antigen–antibody complexes may bind to specific receptors for the Fc fragment, designated FcRI (CD64), FcRII (CD32), and FcRIII (CD16). Of the IgG subclasses, IgG1 binds best to FcRI (CD64) and FcRII (CD32), with affinities (K_d) of 1×10^{-8} M and 5×10^{-7} M, respectively (see Table 77-3). IgG1 and IgG3 bind equally well to FcRIII (CD16), with a K_d of 2×10^{-6} M (see Table 77-3). This is the Fc receptor expressed by natural killer (NK)

cells (or K cells), which mediate antibody-dependent cell-mediated cytotoxicity. Proteins of the IgG4 or IgG2 subclass bind poorly to FcRI (CD64) or FcRII (CD32) and bind not at all to FcRIII (CD16) (see Table 77-3).

IgA

IgA composes approximately 13 percent of plasma immunoglobulins (see Table 77-1). Specific IgA antibodies are synthesized during secondary immune responses. IgA circulates as a monomer, dimer, or higher polymer containing approximately 8 percent carbohydrate. Within the IgA class are two major subclasses, designated IgA1 and IgA2. The most abundant subclass is IgA1, which constitutes approximately 85 percent of the total IgA in plasma. The half-life of circulating IgA of either subclass is approximately 6 days.

The primary role for IgA is in mucosal immunity.[8,9] A modified form of IgA is the principal antibody in saliva, tears, colostrum, and the fluids of the gastrointestinal, respiratory, and urinary tracts. These secreted immunoglobulins consist of an IgA dimer bound to the J-(joining) chain polypeptide and a secretory protein of 70 kDa. The J chain is required for proper hepatic transport of IgA.[10] The secretory component actually is part of an Fc receptor for dimeric IgA that is not synthesized by B cells but rather by epithelial cells of organs such as the intestine. This protein facilitates transport of the IgA protein across the epithelial cell and may protect the secreted IgA molecule from proteolytic digestion by enzymes in the intestinal lumen. IgA antibodies do not cross the placenta, fix complement via the classic pathway, or bind efficiently to cell surfaces. Their main function may be to prevent foreign substances from adhering to mucosal surfaces and entering the blood.

IgM

In a normal adult, approximately 6 percent of the total plasma immunoglobulins belong to the IgM class (see Tables 77-1 and 77-2). IgM molecules classically are termed *macroglobulins* because of their large molecular weight. Circulating IgM molecules contain 12 percent carbohydrate and are formed through the linkage of five identical immunoglobulin units by disulfide bonds and by a J chain (Fig. 77-2).[10] IgM represents the predominant immunoglobulin class formed during a primary immune response. IgM macroglobulins do not penetrate easily into extravascular spaces or readily cross the placenta. Compared to monomeric IgG antibodies, pentavalent IgM antibodies fix complement more efficiently. A single IgM molecule on the surface of a red blood cell can initiate complement-mediated hemolysis. IgM is catabolized rapidly, with a plasma half-life of only 6 days. The monomeric form of IgM, with only two heavy and two light

TABLE 77-1 PHYSICAL PROPERTIES OF HUMAN IMMUNOGLOBULINS

	IgG	IgA	IgM	IgD	IgE
Heavy-chain class	γ	α	μ	δ	ε
Heavy chain subclass	$\gamma 1, \gamma 2, \gamma 3, \gamma 4$	$\alpha 1, \alpha 2$	—	—	—
No. of H-chain domains	4	4	5	4	5
Secretory form	Monomer	Monomer, dimer	Pentamer	Monomer	Monomer
Molecular mass (Da)	150,000	160,000 (monomer) 400,000 (secretory)	900,000	184,000	188,000
Antigen-binding valency	2	2 (monomer) 4 (secretory)	10	2	2
Serum concentration (mg/ml)	8–16	1.4–4.0	0.5–2.0	0–0.4	17–450 ng/ml
Percent of total immunoglobulin	80	13	6	1	0.002
Electrophoretic mobility	γ	Fast γ to β	Slow γ	Fast γ	Fast γ
Percent carbohydrate	3	8	12	13	12

TABLE 77-2   BIOLOGIC PROPERTIES OF HUMAN IMMUNOGLOBULINS

	IgG	IgA	IgM	IgD	IgE
Percent of body pool in intravascular space	45	42	76	75	51
Percent of intravascular pool catabolized per day	6.7	25	18	37	89
Normal synthetic rate (mg/kg/day)	33	24	6.7	0.4	0.02
Serum half-life (days)	21	5.8	10	2.8	2.3
Placental transfer	Yes	No	No	No	No
Cytophilic for mast cells and basophils	No	No	No	No	Yes
Binding to macrophages and other phagocytes	Yes	No	No	No	Yes
Reactivity with staphylococcal protein A	Yes	No	No	No	No
Antibody-dependent cell-mediated cytoxicity	Yes	No	No	No	No
Complement fixation					
Classic pathway	Yes	No	Yes	No	No
Alternative pathway	No	Yes	No	No	No

chains, is the major immunoglobulin expressed on the B cell surface (Fig. 77-3).

IgD

IgD is a trace serum protein that composes less than 1 percent of plasma immunoglobulins. IgD is expressed on most peripheral B cells, as is IgM. The molecule has the basic four-chain constant region and contains 11 percent carbohydrate (see Tables 77-1 and 77-2). IgD antibodies are sensitive to proteolytic degradation. They do not penetrate extravascular spaces efficiently, cross the placental barrier, or fix complement via the classic pathway. Rather, IgD functions primarily as a B cell membrane receptor for antigen that facilitates recruitment of B cells into specific antigen-driven responses.[11]

IgE

Although four human IgE isoforms can be produced by alternative splicing of the epsilon primary transcript,[12] each isoform appears to have similar function. IgE has been called *reaginic* antibody to denote its association with immediate hypersensitivity. It normally constitutes only 0.004 percent of total plasma immunoglobulin (see Tables 77-1 and 77-2). In patients with parasitic infestation and in some children with atopic diseases, plasma IgE levels may rise to five to 20 times normal. The IgE molecule consists of a four-chain basic unit plus 12 percent carbohydrate. Monomeric IgE binds via the Fc region to high-affinity receptors on the surface membranes of basophils and mast

TABLE 77-3   CHARACTERISTICS OF MAJOR IgG SUBCLASSES

	IgG1	IgG2	IgG3	IgG4
Heavy-chain subclass	γ1	γ2	γ3	γ4
Serum concentration (mg/ml)	9	3	1	0.5
Percent of total IgG	67	22	7	4
Serum half-life (days)	21	20	7	21
Complement fixation				
Classic pathway	++	+/−	+++	−
Alternative pathway	−	−	−	−
FcRI (CD64) binding	++++	+/−	++	+
FcRII (CD32) binding	+++	+/−	+	+
FcRIII (CD16) binding	+	−	+	−
Antibody-dependent cell-mediated cytotoxicity	+	−	+	−
Heterologous skin sensitization	+	−	+	+

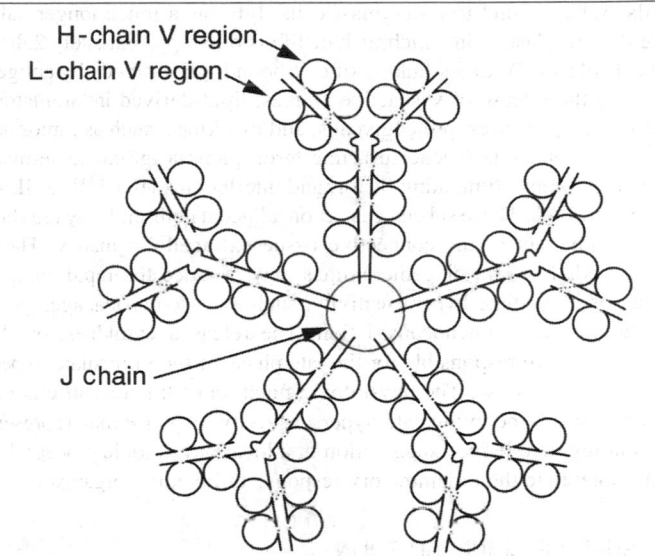

FIGURE 77-2   Schematic model of an IgM pentamer. IgM has 10 binding sites for antigen, each composed of a heavy-chain variable region (H-chain V region) and a light-chain variable region (L-chain V region). Five bivalent IgM molecules are held together by the single joining (J) chain. *Broken colored lines* indicate intrachain and interchain disulfide bonds.

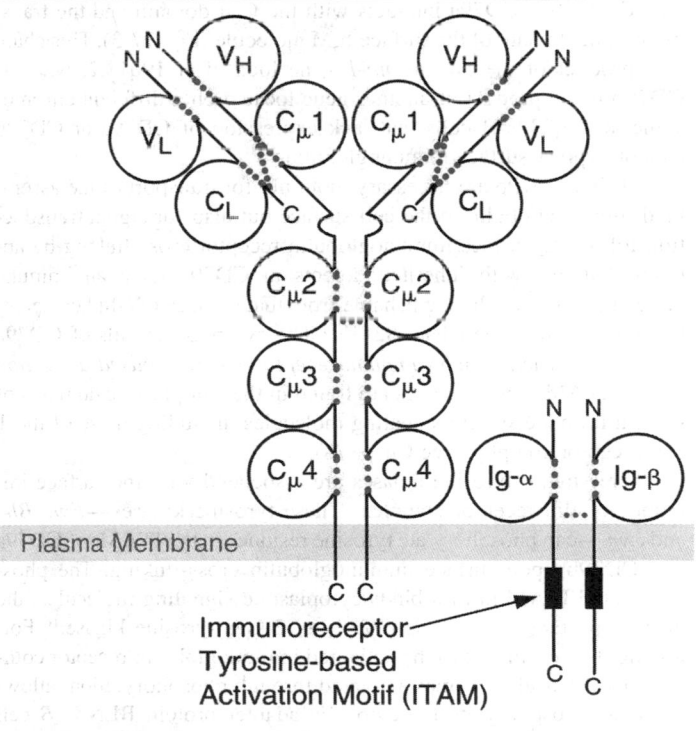

FIGURE 77-3   Schematic model of membrane IgM and its associated accessory proteins Ig-α (CD79a) and Ig-β (CD79b). The light-chain domains V_L and C_L and the heavy-chain domains V_H, $C_\mu 1$ (or $C_H 1$), $C_\mu 2$ (or $C_H 2$), $C_\mu 3$ (or $C_H 3$), and $C_\mu 4$ (or $C_H 4$) are labeled inside the respective immunoglobulin domain. The cytoplasmic domains of Ig-α (CD79a) and Ig-β (CD79b) each has an immunoreceptor tyrosine-based activation motif (ITAM) depicted by a *black rectangle*. These ITAMs play a critical role in the signaling events that are initiated by ligation of surface immunoglobulin by antigen. *Dotted colored lines* indicate intrachain and interchain disulfide bonds.

cells. When bound to tissue mast cells, IgE has a much longer half-life than in plasma, in which its half-life is only approximately 2 days (see Table 77-2). Cross-linking of cell-bound IgE antibody by antigen induces the release of vasoactive amines, lipid-derived inflammatory mediators, proteases, proteoglycans, and cytokines, such as tumor necrosis factor alpha (cachectin), interferon gamma, granulocyte-macrophage colony stimulating factor, and interleukins (IL)-1, IL-3, IL-4, IL-5, and IL-6. These substances act on adjacent cells and may regulate the metabolism of the connective tissue extracellular matrix. These lipid mediators and biogenic amines may produce the rapid components of immediate hypersensitivity, such as vascular leakage, vasodilatation, and bronchoconstriction. The released cytokines, on the other hand, are responsible for the late phase of the immediate hypersensitivity response. The physiologic function of this response is not clear. Instead, the immediate hypersensitivity response may represent a pathologic systemic exaggeration of a local physiologic process that may potentiate the inflammatory response to invading organisms.

SURFACE IMMUNOGLOBULIN

Any one of the immunoglobulin isotypes may serve as a B cell membrane receptor for antigen. However, most B cells express surface IgM with or without IgD. Each immunoglobulin is expressed on the surface membrane as a monomer complexed noncovalently with disulfide-linked heterodimeric glycoproteins that, together with surface immunoglobulin, form the B cell antigen–receptor complex (Fig. 77-3).[13] For surface IgM, each heterodimer is composed of CD79a, an IgM α-chain of 33 kDa, complexed with CD79b, an Ig β-chain of 37 kDa (see Chap. 14). CD79a interacts with the C_H4 domain and the transmembrane domain of the surface IgM molecule (Fig. 77-3). This chain is a product of the human *mb-1* gene located at 19q13.2, whereas CD79b is the product of another gene located on a different chromosome at 17q23.[13] B cells that lack expression of CD79a or CD79b cannot express surface immunoglobulin.

CD79a/CD79b are necessary, not only for transport of the assembled immunoglobulin to the cell surface but also for signal transduction following surface immunoglobulin-receptor cross-linking by antigen. Patients with inherited defects in CD79a have an immune deficiency that is indistinguishable from that of classic X-linked agammaglobulinemia (see Chap. 82).[14,15] The cytoplasmic tails of CD79a and CD79b each contain *immunoreceptor tyrosine-based activation motifs* (ITAMs). Such motifs are found in the cytoplasmic domains of several immune system signaling molecules, including those of the T cell receptor complex (see Chap. 78).

Three major tyrosine kinases are associated with the surface immunoglobulin receptor complex. These tyrosine kinases—*Fyn, Blk,* and *Lyn*—can phosphorylate tyrosine residues in the ITAMs of CD79a and CD79b upon surface immunoglobulin cross-linking. The phosphorylated ITAM in turn binds cytoplasmic signaling molecules, the most important of which is p72^{Syk}, a 72-kDa tyrosine kinase.[16] Following its recruitment to the activated immunoglobulin receptor complex, p72^{Syk} itself becomes activated through phosphorylation, allowing it to phosphorylate the cytosolic adapter protein BLNK (*B* cell *link*er protein, also known as SLP-65, BASH, or BCA).[17] BLNK serves as a docking site for a number of important signaling molecules, including Bruton tyrosine kinase (Btk), Vav-1, Vav-2, and phospholipase C gamma (PLCγ).[18,19] Dual phosphorylation and activation of PLCγ by Btk and p72^{Syk} allows PLCγ to effect hydrolysis of the polyphosphoinositides into inositol 1,4,5-trisphosphate and diacylglycerol, which in turn increase intracellular Ca^{2+} and activate protein kinase C and Ras, respectively.[20] This leads to activation of B cells that is seen following ligation of their surface immunoglobulin receptors by antigen.[21] The importance of these activation events in B cell signaling

and development is underscored by patients with inherited defects in Btk, who lack B cell development and have X-linked agammaglobulinemia (see Chap. 82).[22]

To mitigate the problem of accidental initiation of signal transduction, the signaling cascade is subject to negative controls.[23,24] The quantity and quality of immunoglobulin receptor signaling are modulated by several transmembrane proteins that are associated with the immunoglobulin-CD79a/CD79b receptor complex. These associated proteins can be either costimulatory[25] (e.g., CD19) or inhibitory[26,27] (e.g., CD22 and CD72, see Chap. 14). In contrast to CD79a and CD79b, CD22 and CD72 have cytoplasmic domains with *immunoreceptor tyrosine-based inhibitory motifs* (ITIMs). When ITIMs are phosphorylated by activated Lyn kinase,[28] the domains recruit *Src homology 2 (SH2) domain-containing protein tyrosine phosphatase 1* (SHP-1),[29] otherwise known as *protein tyrosine phosphatase 1c*. Bound SHP-1 can remove the phosphate group from the phosphorylated (and thereby activated) tyrosine kinases, returning these kinases to their inactive state so that they no longer trigger B cell activation.[30,31] The importance of SHP-1 in limiting B cell activation is demonstrated by mutant mice that lack this phosphatase.[32] The B lymphocytes of such animals are stimulated by much lower concentrations of antigen than the B lymphocytes of normal mice.[33] Because of this situation, these mice have excessive B cell proliferation, autoimmune disease, and early mortality.

GENETICS OF IMMUNOGLOBULINS

IMMUNOGLOBULIN GENE COMPLEXES

Immunoglobulin genes are inherited in three unlinked gene complexes: one for the heavy-chain classes, one for κ light chains, and one for λ light chains. The immunoglobulin heavy-chain gene complex is located at band q32 of the long arm of chromosome 14. This complex is composed of 39 functional heavy-chain variable-region (V_H) genes, more than 120 nonfunctional V_H pseudogenes, 25 functional diversity (D) segments, six functional J_H minigenes, and exons encoding the constant regions for each of the immunoglobulin heavy-chain isotypes (Fig. 77-4).[34] The κ light-chain gene complex is contained within band p12 on the short arm of chromosome 2. This gene complex consists of approximately 40 functional κ light-chain variable-region genes (V_κ genes), more than 30 nonfunctional V_κ pseudogenes, five J_κ segments, one constant-region exon, and one kappa-deleting element (Kde) (Fig. 77-5).[35,36] Many of the V_κ genes in the so-called "p region" most proximal to the J_κ segments are in the opposite orientation of the J_κ segments, thus requiring that the V_κ exons in the proximal region undergo inversion during immunoglobulin gene rearrangement (Fig. 77-5). The λ light-chain gene complex is located at band q11.2 on the long arm of chromosome 22, six megabases from the centromere.[37] This gene complex consists of approximately 41 functional λ light-chain variable-region genes (V_λ genes), more than 30 V_λ pseudogenes, four functional λ constant-region genes ($C_\lambda 1, C_\lambda 2, C_\lambda 3, C_\lambda 7$), and three λ constant-region pseudogenes ($C_\lambda 4, C_\lambda 5, C_\lambda 6$), each associated with one J_λ segment (Fig. 77-5).[38] The constant-region elements of the heavy-chain gene complex are proximal to variable-region segments on chromosome 14, whereas the constant-region segments of the two light chains are in the opposite orientation, telomeric to the variable-region genes.

Each germ-line V gene, D element, and J segment is flanked by recognition sequences that are necessary to direct site-specific recombination. Such sequences consist of a highly conserved palindromic heptamer (5'-CACAGTG-3'), a nonconserved spacer of 12 or 23 bp, and a conserved nonamer (5'-ACAAAAACC-3').[39] Joining usually occurs only between segments flanked by recognition sequences with

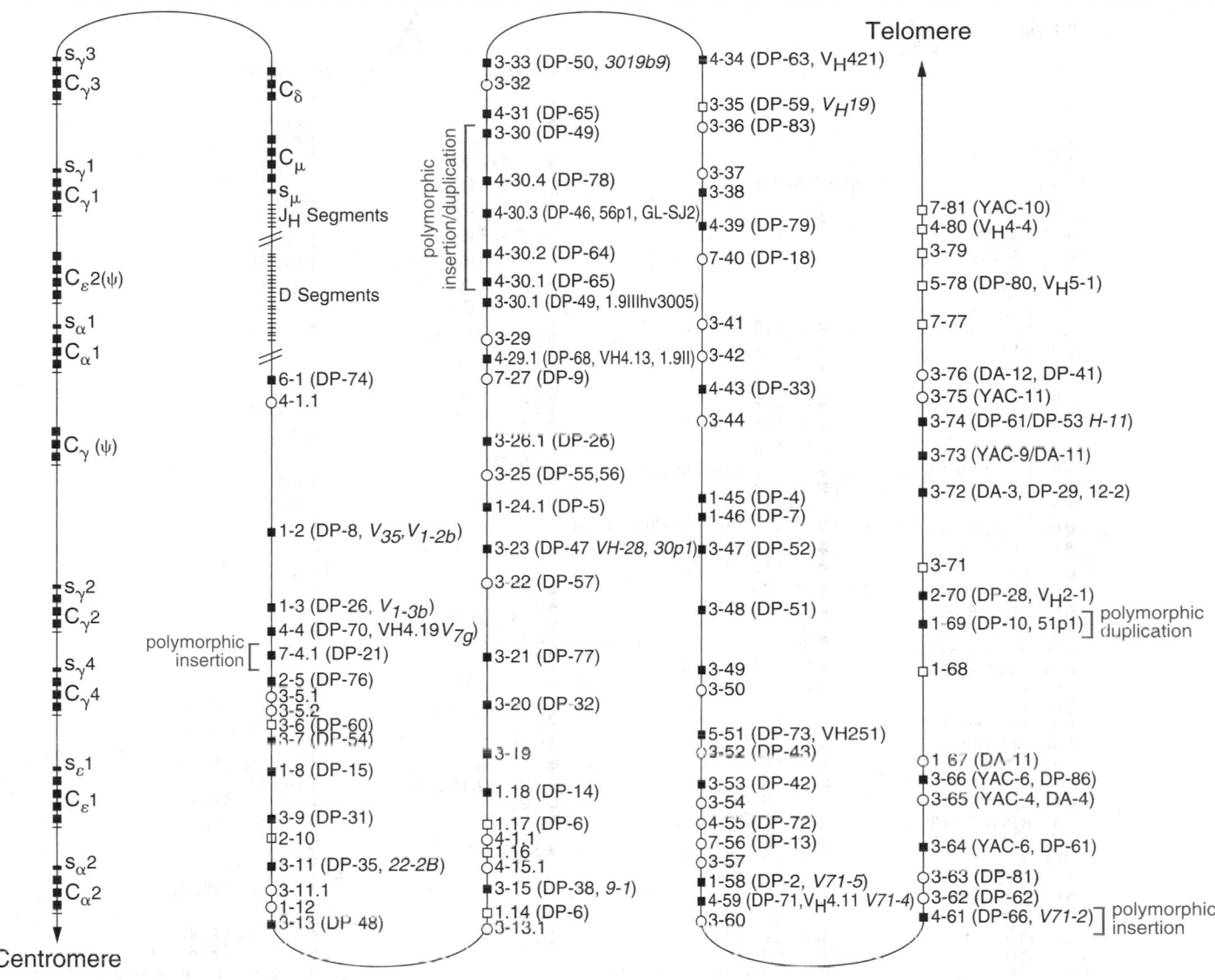

FIGURE 77-4 Human heavy-chain immunoglobulin gene complex on chromosome 14q32. The heavy-chain exons encoding the constant regions are represented by *black boxes*, and the associated intronic switch regions (S) each is depicted as a *line*. These exons are labeled to the *right* of these symbols. A ψ symbol next to the heavy-chain isotype designation indicates the gene is a pseudogene. J_H segments and D segments are indicated by *lines*. Each V_H gene is labeled on the *right* of each symbol. By convention, the loci encoding each of the various V_H genes are assigned a number corresponding to the V_H gene subgroup, followed by a hyphen and then the rank order distance from the heavy-chain D segments. The alternative names that have been used to designate each locus are listed in *parentheses*. Identified polymorphic insertions and/or duplications are indicated with *brackets. Black squares* represent V_H gene loci that are known to be functional. *Open circles* represent V_H pseudogenes. *Open boxes* depict V_H exons that appear to be functional but rarely are found to encode a functional heavy-chain gene rearrangement and, in fact, may be pseudogenes. *Arrows* at the end of the line containing the symbols indicate the direction to the centromere or the telomere.

unequal spacers.[40–42] Each recognition sequence consists of a dyad symmetric heptamer, an A/T–rich nonamer, and a spacer region of conserved length, either 12 bp or 23 bp $\pm$ 1 bp. This sequence is referred to as the *12/23 joining rule*. The consensus sequences for the heptamer (CACAGTG) and nonamers (ACAAAAACC) are optimal for rearrangement, but considerable deviation from the consensus sequence is observed and tolerated.[43] Each spacer varies in sequence, but its length is conserved and corresponds to one or two turns of the DNA double helix. Each spacer brings the heptamer and nonamer sequences to one side of the DNA helix, where they can be bound by the protein complex that catalyzes recombination. Similar recognition sequences flank the elements that rearrange to form the T cell antigen receptor (see Chap. 78). Because all segments of a particular type (e.g., Vκ gene segments) are flanked by one type of signal sequence and all

the segments to which they should be joined (e.g., Jκ segments) are flanked by the opposite type of signal sequence, the 12/23 rule ensures that the joining is restricted to events that could be biologically productive. Such heptamer-spacer-nonamer sequences, often called recombination signal sequences (RSS), are targets of lymphocyte-specific enzymes encoded by recombination activating gene (*RAG*)-*1* and *RAG-2*.[41,42]

IMMUNOGLOBULIN GENE REARRANGEMENT AND EXPRESSION DURING B CELL DEVELOPMENT

IMMUNOGLOBULIN GENE REARRANGEMENT

During B cell ontogeny, the first immunoglobulin gene rearrangements generally occur within the heavy-chain gene complex (Fig.

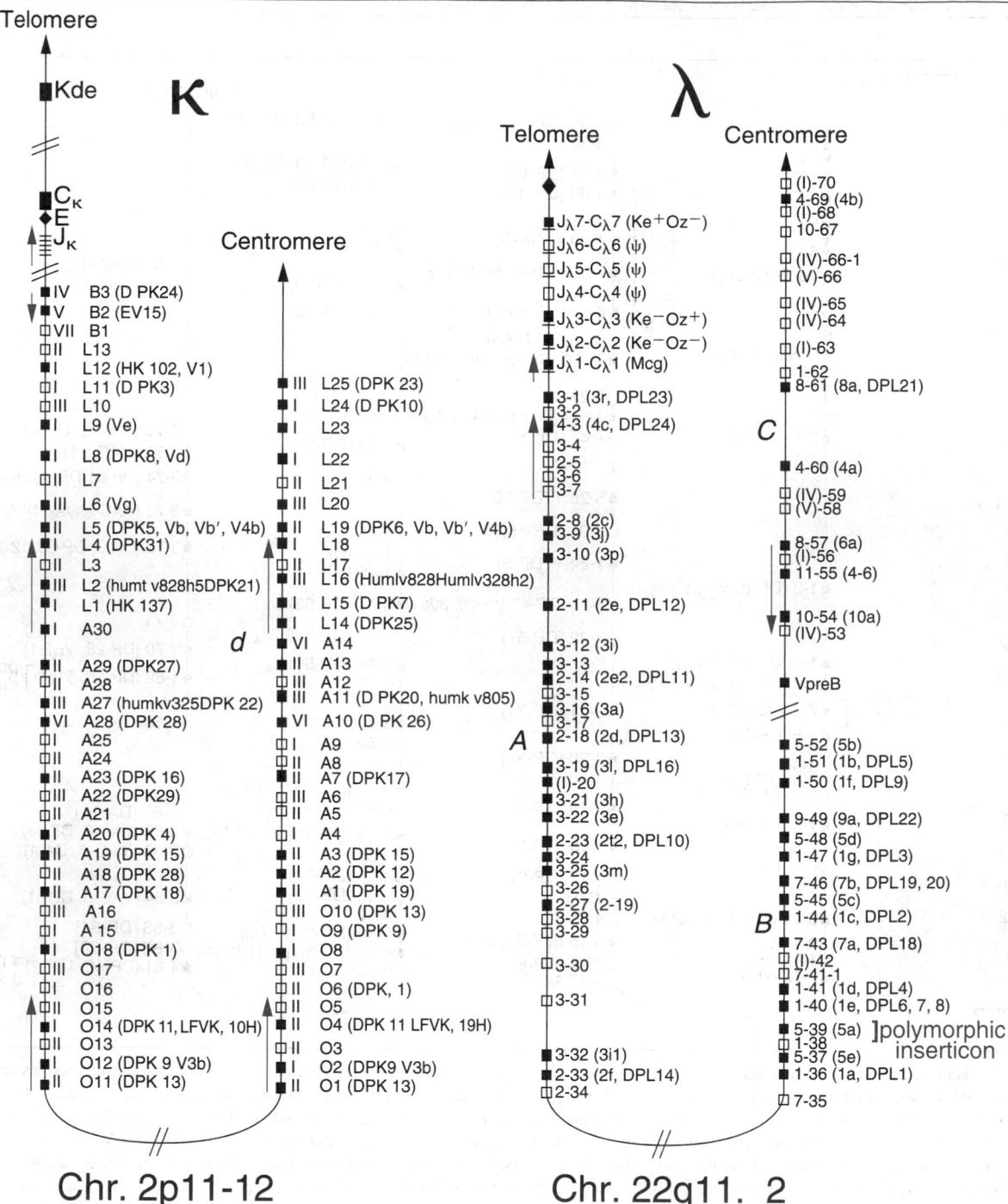

κ Telomere
■ Kde

■ Cκ
◆ E
≡ Jκ

■I IV B3 (D PK24)
■ V B2 (EV15)
□VII B1
□II L13
■I L12 (HK 102, V1)
□I L11 (D PK3)
□III L10
■I L9 (Ve)
■I L8 (DPK8, Vd)
□II L7
■III L6 (Vg)
■II L5 (DPK5, Vb', V4b)
■I L4 (DPK31)
□II L3
■III L2 (humt v828h5DPK21)
■I L1 (HK 137)
■I A30

■II A29 (DPK27)
■II A28
■III A27 (humkv325DPK 22)
■VI A28 (DPK 28)
□I A25
□II A24
■II A23 (DPK 16)
□III A22 (DPK29)
□II A21
■I A20 (DPK 4)
■I A19 (DPK 15)
□II A18 (DPK 28)
■II A17 (DPK 18)
□III A16
□I A 15
■I O18 (DPK 1)
□III O17
□I O16
□II O15
■I O14 (DPK 11, LFVK, 10H)
□II O13
■I O12 (DPK 9 V3b)
■II O11 (DPK 13)

Centromere
■III L25 (DPK 23)
■I L24 (D PK10)
■I L23
■I L22
□II L21
■III L20
■II L19 (DPK6, Vb, Vb', V4b)
■I L18
□II L17
■III L16 (Humlv828Humlv328h2)
■I L15 (D PK7)
■I L14 (DPK25)

d
■VI A14
■II A13
■III A12
■III A11 (D PK20, humk v805)
■VI A10 (D PK 26)
□I A9
■II A8
■II A7 (DPK17)
□III A6
□II A5
■I A4
■II A3 (DPK 15)
■II A2 (DPK 12)
■II A1 (DPK 19)
□III O10 (DPK 13)
□I O9 (DPK 9)
□I O8
□III O7
□II O6 (DPK, 1)
□II O5
■II O4 (DPK 11 LFVK, 19H)
□II O3
■I O2 (DPK9 V3b)
■II O1 (DPK 13)

Chr. 2p11-12

λ Telomere

Centromere

◆
■ Jλ7-Cλ7 (Ke+Oz−)
□ Jλ6-Cλ6 (ψ)
□ Jλ5-Cλ5 (ψ)
□ Jλ4-Cλ4 (ψ)
■ Jλ3-Cλ3 (Ke−Oz+)
■ Jλ2-Cλ2 (Ke−Oz−)
■ Jλ1-Cλ1 (Mcg)
■ 3-1 (3r, DPL23)
□ 3-2
■ 4-3 (4c, DPL24)
□ 3-4
□ 2-5
□ 3-6
□ 3-7
■ 2-8 (2c)
■ 3-9 (3j)
■ 3-10 (3p)
■ 2-11 (2e, DPL12)
A
■ 3-12 (3i)
■ 3-13
■ 2-14 (2e2, DPL11)
□ 3-15
■ 3-16 (3a)
□ 3-17
■ 2-18 (2d, DPL13)
■ 3-19 (3l, DPL16)
■ (I)-20
■ 3-21 (3h)
■ 3-22 (3e)
■ 2-23 (2t2, DPL10)
□ 3-24
■ 3-25 (3m)
□ 3-26
■ 2-27 (2-19)
□ 3-28
□ 3-29
□ 3-30
□ 3-31
■ 3-32 (3i1)
■ 2-33 (2f, DPL14)
□ 2-34

□ (I)-70
■ 4-69 (4b)
□ (I)-68
□ 10-67
□ (IV)-66-1
□ (V)-66
□ (IV)-65
□ (IV)-64
□ (I)-63
□ 1-62
■ 8-61 (8a, DPL21)
C
■ 4-60 (4a)
□ (IV)-59
□ (V)-58
■ 8-57 (6a)
□ (I)-56
■ 11-55 (4-6)
■ 10-54 (10a)
□ (IV)-53
■ VpreB
■ 5-52 (5b)
■ 1-51 (1b, DPL5)
■ 1-50 (1f, DPL9)
■ 9-49 (9a, DPL22)
■ 5-48 (5d)
■ 1-47 (1g, DPL3)
■ 7-46 (7b, DPL19, 20)
■ 5-45 (5c)
■ 1-44 (1c, DPL2)
B
■ 7-43 (7a, DPL18)
□ (I)-42
□ 7-41-1
■ 1-41 (1d, DPL4)
■ 1-40 (1e, DPL6, 7, 8)
■ 5-39 (5a)
□ 1-38
■ 5-37 (5e)
■ 1-36 (1a, DPL1)
□ 7-35

] polymorphic inserticon

Chr. 22q11. 2

FIGURE 77-5   Immunoglobulin light-chain gene complexes. *(Left)* κ Light-chain gene complex on chromosome 2p11-12. *Black boxes* represent the Kde element or the Cκ constant-region exon as indicated to the *right* of each box. The κ light-chain enhancer *(E)* is positioned between the Cκ constant-region exon and the Jκ segments. Jκ segments are indicated by *lines.* The Vκ genes are clustered in two regions centromeric to the Jκ and Cκ exons, each region spanning approximately 500 kb. Approximately 800 kb separate the two regions. The region proximal to Jκ and Cκ, designated *p*, contains 40 Vκ genes (B3→B1, L13→L1, A30→A15, O18→O11). The distal region, designated *d*, contains 36 gene segments (O1→O10, A1→A14, L14→L25). Vκ genes that can encode functional κ light chains are represented by *black boxes* and are labeled to the *right* of each symbol. Thirty-two of the 76 Vκ genes are pseudogenes *(open boxes).* The *d* region apparently arose through duplication of a large portion of the *p* region. Consequently, 33 pairs of Vκ genes share 95 to 100 percent nucleic acid sequence homology, accounting for 66 of the 76 Vκ genes in the κ light-chain complex. Vκ genes can be grouped further into four clusters: A, B, L, and O. Three of the clusters (A, L, O) are duplicated and found in both the Jκ-proximal *p* region and the Jκ-distal *d* region. The B cluster, containing Vκ genes B1, B2 (EV15), and B3 (DPK26), is found only in the Jκ-proximal *p* region. Each Vκ gene can be assigned to one of three main subgroups (I–III) and several smaller subgroups (IV–VII) based on nucleotide sequence homology. The largest subgroup is Vκ1, with 21 functional genes, depicted as *black boxes.* The next largest subgroups are Vκ2, with 11 functional genes, and Vκ3, with seven functional genes. The Vκ6 subgroup has three functional genes, and the Vκ4 and Vκ5 subgroups each has one functional gene. The Vκ7 subgroup consists of one of the nonfunctional pseudogenes, which are depicted as *open squares. Black arrows* indicate the transcriptional orientation of the V genes in the complex. *Arrows* at the end of the line

77-6a).[40] One or more D segments may rearrange and become juxtaposed with a single J_H element, generating a DJ_H complex that then may rearrange with one of the 39 functional V_H genes. Subsequently, gene rearrangements occur in the light-chain loci (Fig. 77-6b). One of the 40 functional V_κ genes can rearrange with any one of five J_κ segments. Should these gene rearrangements fail to generate a functional $V_\kappa J_\kappa$ exon, the Kde may rearrange to a site in or immediately downstream of the $V_\kappa J_\kappa$ exon, thus deleting the kappa light-chain constant-region exon. Subsequent to κ light-chain gene rearrangement, one of the 41 functional V_λ exons can rearrange with any one of the four functional $J_\lambda C_\lambda$ exons to generate a gene that can encode a λ light chain (Fig. 77-6).[38]

Somatic V region gene recombination involves introduction of double-strand DNA breaks at RSS, juxtaposition of the broken ends, and then religation through a process called *nonhomologous DNA end-joining (NHEJ)*. The most common mode of recombination involves the looping out and deletion of the DNA intervening between two gene segments on the same chromosome. The ends of the heptamer sequences are joined precisely in a head-to-head configuration to form a *signal joint* in a circular piece of DNA that then is lost from the genome when the cell divides. However, when the RSS are oriented in the same direction along the chromosome, the segments undergo recombination via inversion, in which case the intervening DNA is retained.

The first cleavage step requires a specialized heterodimeric endonuclease encoded by *RAG-1* and *RAG-2*.[44] *RAG-1* and *RAG-2* are adjacent genes located on the short arm of chromosome 11 (11p13-p12). They were isolated based on their ability to enable fibroblasts to catalyze V(D)J recombination of nonrearranged immunoglobulin genes that were cointroduced via gene transfer.[45] *RAG-1* has sequence similarities to bacterial *topoisomerases* that catalyze the breakage and rejoining of DNA. *RAG-1* and *RAG-2* normally are coexpressed only in developing lymphocytes that are undergoing receptor gene rearrangement. Mice with either *RAG* gene knocked out cannot undergo immunoglobulin or T cell receptor gene rearrangements and consequently fail to produce mature B or T lymphocytes.[46] Mutations that impair, but do not completely abolish, the function of *RAG-1* or *RAG-2* in humans result in a form of combined immune deficiency called *Omenn syndrome*.[47]

The RAG-1/RAG-2 endonuclease recognizes either the 12-mer–spaced or 23-mer–spaced RSS and then introduces double-stranded DNA breaks. After introducing these breaks, the RAG-1/RAG-2 complex remains bound to the DNA. Mutations that affect the ability of the RAG proteins to bind and maintain the broken ends in a stable postcleavage complex can lead to misrepair of the double-strand breaks, thereby enhancing the risk for oncogenic chromosomal aberrations.[48,49] Several proteins are involved in the processing and juxtaposition of these double-strand breaks, including high-mobility group protein-1 (HMG1) and high-mobility group protein 2 (HMG2). HMG1 and HMG2 are widely expressed, abundant nuclear proteins that bind and bend DNA without sequence specificity, thereby playing an important role in the assembly of nucleoprotein complexes involved in DNA repair and transcription.[50] HMG1 may facilitate the bending of the DNA to allow the components of one double-stranded-break-RAG complex to bind and cleave the DNA at a different RSS, thus bringing together two disparate RSS in accordance with the 12/23 joining rule.[41,42]

The double-stranded-break RAG complex also binds at least six other proteins, including Ku70, Ku80, DNA-dependent protein kinase (DNA-PK), XRCC4, DNA ligase IV (Lig4), and Artemis.[51,52] DNA-PK is a serine-threonine protein kinase that is activated by DNA double-stranded breaks and is essential for the normal repair of DNA breaks induced by ionizing radiation, chemical agents, and during VDJ (exon created by a rearranged immunoglobulin heavy-chain variable-region gene, diversity gene segment, and joining gene segment) recombination.[53] Mice deficient in DNA-PK can make only trivial amounts of immunoglobulin or T cell receptors and are called *severe combined immunodeficiency* (SCID) mice.[54] Mice deficient in Artemis have a "leaky" SCID phenotype and develop some T and B cells in later life.[53] Ku-deficient mice also are deficient in T and B cells but have a small stature and other nonimmunologic defects, suggesting that these proteins also play important roles in normal development.[55,56] Defects resulting from mutation in Ku, XRCC4, Lig4, Artemis, or DNA-PK predispose to lymphomagenesis in mice.[57,58]

The process of recombination allows for generation of "*junctional diversity*" in the sequence of the rearranged gene segments. DNA ends generated by the RAG-1/RAG-2 endonuclease cleavage reaction each is fused by the NHEJ pathway involving the proteins mentioned in the preceding paragraph. The hairpinned termini of gene segments that give rise to the *coding joint* each is subsequently cleaved at random sites by an endonuclease. Cleavage of a hairpin away from its apex generates an overhanging flap that, if incorporated into the joint, results in addition of palindromic (P) nucleotides that contribute to junctional diversity. The opened hairpin ends can be modified further by nucleases that can remove a self-complementary overhang or cut further into the original coding sequence. In addition, a lymphocyte-specific enzyme, terminal deoxynucleotidyl transferase, can add *non–template-encoded (N) nucleotides*.[59] Finally, additional junctional diversity comes from the nucleolytic activities that remove potential coding end nucleotides prior to the final ligation of the DNA breaks into one intact recombination joint.[60] Such processes contribute to immunoglobulin diversity and are the principal mechanism responsible for somatic diversification of the T cell repertoire (see Chap. 78).

Under normal conditions, a B lymphocyte or plasma cell synthesizes only one species of light chain and heavy chain, even though the cell has two different sets of immunoglobulin gene complexes that initially undergo seemingly independent immunoglobulin gene rearrangements. The specificity of the humoral immune response depends upon antigenic selection of unique clones of B cells, each clone expressing a homogeneous set of immunoglobulin receptors. Such restriction is achieved by limiting a given B cell to functional rearrangement and expression of only a single heavy-chain allele and a single

---

FIGURE 77-5 (CONTINUED) connecting the symbols indicate the direction to the centromere or the telomere. *(Right)* λ Light-chain gene complex on chromosome 22q11.2. *Black boxes* represent functional genes. *Open boxes* represent pseudogenes. The $J_\lambda C_\lambda$ exon pairs are labeled to the *right* of each symbol. *Black boxes* also indicate the 39 functional V_λ genes centromeric to the λ constant regions. These V_λ genes are arranged into 10 subgroups, each composed of V_λ genes sharing greater than 75 percent nucleotide sequence homology. The *first number* in the labels to the right of each V_λ gene is the number of the subgroup, followed by a hyphen and then the relative rank order of the V gene from the constant-region exons. Note that the V_λ genes have been mapped into three clusters within 860 kb of the J_λ and C_λ genes, which are separated from one another in the figure by *double lines*. The cluster most proximal to the $J_\lambda C_\lambda$ exons, designated A, is composed of 18 functional V_λ genes mostly belonging to the $V_\lambda 2$ and $V_\lambda 3$ gene subgroups. The next cluster, B, contains 15 functional V_λ genes of the $V_\lambda 1$, $V_\lambda 5$, $V_\lambda 7$, and $V_\lambda 9$ gene subgroups. The third cluster, C, contains six functional V_λ genes of the $V_\lambda 4$, $V_\lambda 6$, $V_\lambda 8$, $V_\lambda 10$, and $V_\lambda 11$ gene subgroups and the exon encoding VpreB. Some individuals have an insertion of a functional V_λ gene, 5-39 (5a), marked as *polymorphic insertion*. *Black arrows* indicate the transcriptional orientation of the V genes in the complex.

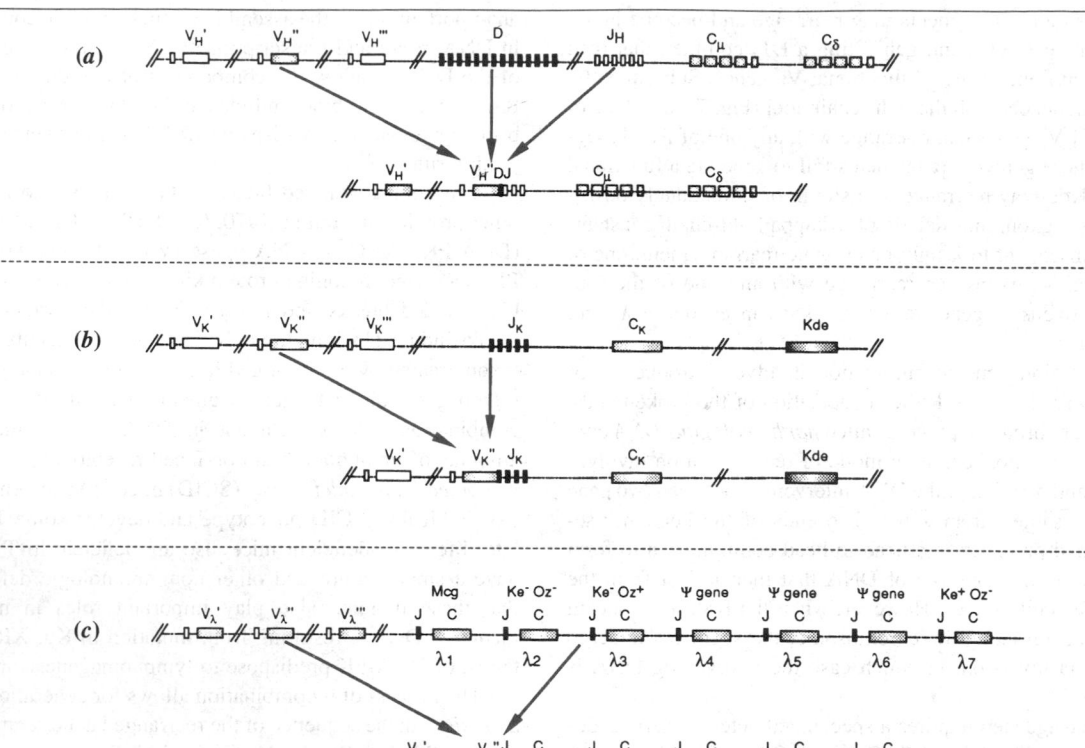

FIGURE 77-6   Immunoglobulin gene complexes and rearrangement. *Diagonal double lines* indicate a large DNA distance between the flanking genes depicted as *rectangular boxes* (not drawn to scale). The *upper diagrams* in *(a), (b),* and *(c)* show the germ-line DNA configuration of the immunoglobulin heavy-chain genes, κ light-chain genes, and λ light-chain genes, respectively. Exemplary immunoglobulin heavy-chain variable-region genes (V_H', V_H'', V_H'''), immunoglobulin κ light-chain genes (V_κ', V_κ'', V_κ'''), and immunoglobulin λ light-chain variable-region genes (V_λ', V_λ'', V_λ''') are depicted on the *left side* of each immunoglobulin gene complex. *D* denotes the diversity gene segments of the antibody heavy-chain locus. J_H, J_κ, and J_λ indicate the joining gene segments of the antibody heavy chain, κ light chain, and λ light chain, respectively. C_μ and C_δ denote the constant-region exons of the μ and δ heavy chains, respectively. Below each is a possible immunoglobulin gene rearrangement composed of a VDJ for the antibody heavy chain or a $V_\kappa J_\kappa$ or $V_\lambda J_\lambda$ for the κ or λ light-chain gene, respectively. Below the representative λ constant-region loci in row *C* are listed the names of the λ nonallelic genetic markers Mcg, Ke$-$Oz$-$, Ke$-$Oz$+$, and Ke$+$Oz$-$ on $C_\lambda 1$, $C_\lambda 2$, $C_\lambda 3$, and $C_\lambda 7$, respectively. As indicated, $C_\lambda 4$, $C_\lambda 5$, and $C_\lambda 6$ are pseudogenes (ψ gene) that do not encode protein.

light-chain allele. This phenomenon is called *allelic exclusion.* Although occasional neoplastic B cell populations lack allelic exclusion and express both immunoglobulin alleles, allelic exclusion generally is observed with most B cell tumors.[61]

SURROGATE λ LIGHT CHAINS

Precursor B cells that only have rearranged D and J_H elements are referred to as *progenitor B cells* or *"pro-B cells."* The term *pre-B cells* is reserved for precursor B cells that have completed immunoglobulin heavy-chain gene rearrangement and have a functional VDJ complex. Both pro-B cells and pre-B cells have immunoglobulin light-chain loci in germ-line configuration.

Despite this situation, pre-B cells express some immunoglobulin μ chains in association with "surrogate" λ light chains. One of these proteins, called λ_5, has similarity with known C_λ light-chain domains.[62] Another protein is called *VpreB* because it resembles a V domain but bears an extra N-terminal protein sequence. Both proteins are encoded by genes located on chromosome 22. The λ_5 gene is situated within a λ-like locus that is telomeric to the true λ light-chain locus. The *VpreB* gene is located within the cluster of immunoglobulin V_λ genes (see Fig. 77-5), defined by breakpoints of chromosomal translocations found in a few leukemias and lymphomas.[62] Together,

VpreB and λ_5 pair with the μ heavy chains. Subsequent covalent linkages via an S-S bond between the λ_5 and the first C_H1 domain of the μH chain allow VpreB and λ_5 μ heavy chains to form a primitive immunoglobulin receptor that, with CD79a and CD79b, may be expressed on the surface membrane of the developing pre-B cell.[63,64] Monoclonal antibodies that recognize λ_5 or VpreB specifically bind to pre-B cells and can react with B lineage acute lymphocytic leukemias.[65]

The pre-B cell receptor complex is expressed only transiently, as production of λ_5 ceases as soon as it is formed. Nevertheless, this protein plays an important role in normal B cell development. In normal mice, the appearance of the pre-B cell receptor coincides with inactivation of the *RAG-2* protein by phosphorylation and degradation of *RAG-1* and *RAG-2* messenger (m)RNA, suggesting that this receptor plays a role in suppressing further immunoglobulin gene rearrangement. However, expression of the pre-B cell receptor on the surface membrane is associated with cell activation and proliferation, leading to generation of small, resting pre-B daughter cells that again express *RAG-1* and *RAG-2*. This situation leads to subsequent light-chain gene rearrangement. As such, expression of the pre-B cell receptor appears to signal that a complete μ heavy-chain gene has been formed, that further rearrangements at this locus should be suppressed, and that development to the next stage can proceed. Therefore, the surrogate light chains play a critical role in normal B cell development. This observation is underscored by studies on transgenic mice that lack functional λ_5 genes.[66] In these mice, B cell development in the marrow is blocked at the pre-B cell stage, thereby markedly reducing the numbers of functional mature B lymphocytes in the blood and lymphoid tissues.[67] Similarly, humans that have inactivating mutations in the λ_5 genes on both alleles of chromosome 22 have agammaglobulinemia and markedly reduced numbers of B cells.[68]

HEAVY-CHAIN CLASS SWITCHING

During differentiation, a single B lymphocyte can synthesize heavy chains with different constant regions coupled to the same variable region.[69] As pre-B cells develop into mature B cells, intact IgM monomers are inserted into the plasma membrane, followed by IgD molecules with the same antigen-binding specificity. The IgM and IgD constant-region genes are closely linked in embryonic DNA (see Fig. 77-4) and may be transcribed together. The differential splicing of the transcript allows simultaneous synthesis of the two immunoglobulin heavy chains from a single species of mRNA. As such, the expression of IgD that occurs during B cell maturation only rarely involves deletion of $C\mu$.

The switch from IgM to IgG, IgA, or IgE requires active transcription of the downstream constant-region exons encoding the future immunoglobulin isotype. This process requires prior interaction of B lymphocytes with antigen or mitogen and ligation of CD40 via the ligand for CD40 (CD154) expressed by activated T cells. Patients with inherited defects in CD40 or CD154 have an immune deficiency (hyper-IgM syndrome type I) characterized by normal to high serum levels of IgM with extremely low serum levels of other immunoglobulin isotypes (see Chap. 82).[70] Interleukins provided by antigen-reactive T lymphocytes strongly influence (1) which B cells differentiate into IgM-secreting plasma cells and (2) which B cells switch to synthesizing the heavy chain of another immunoglobulin isotype, such as IgG and IgA.[69,71]

Immunoglobulin class switch recombination (CSR) occurs in or near the switch region located in the intron between the rearranged VDJ$_H$ sequence and the μ gene and any one of similar regions located upstream of the C genes encoding each of the other heavy-chain isotypes, with the exception of the δ gene (see Fig. 77-4). The μ switch region, designated S$_\mu$, consists of approximately 150 repeats of the sequence (GAGCT)$_n$(GGGGG), where n is generally three but can be as many as seven. The sequences of the other switch regions (S$_\lambda$, S$_\delta$, S$_\varepsilon$) are similar in that they also contain repeats of the GAGCT and GGGGGT sequences. The switch in heavy-chain classes results from DNA recombination between S$_\mu$ and S$_\lambda$, S$_\delta$, or S$_\varepsilon$, accompanied by the deletion of intervening DNA segments and the apposition of the previously rearranged variable-region gene next to the new constant-region gene.

In contrast to VDJ recombination, which mostly occurs in the G$_0$ and/or G$_1$ stage of the cell cycle, CSR seems to require DNA replication. Also, unlike VDJ recombination, CSR requires expression of activation-induced deaminase (AID), an enzyme expressed in activated B cells that also is required for somatic hypermutation.[72,73] Patients with inherited defects in AID have an immune deficiency (hyper-IgM syndrome type II) characterized by relatively high serum levels of IgM and negligible serum levels of other immunoglobulin isotypes.[74] AID is expressed in germinal centers of peripheral lymphoid organs, the site where CSR occurs in B cells activated in response to antigen. AID most likely deaminates the closely positioned cytosines (dC) in the S-region DNA, converting the dC to uracils (dU), which in turn are removed by uracil-DNA glycosylase (UNG). The importance of UNG is underscored by patients who have inherited defects in this enzyme,

resulting in an autosomal recessive form of the hyper-IgM immunodeficiency syndrome similar to that of patients with inherited defects in AID (see Chap. 82).[75] The abasic sites generated by UNG are cleaved by AP endonuclease, resulting in closely positioned staggered nicks in the DNA that may result in double-stranded DNA breaks.[76] The end processing, repair, and joining mechanisms for these DNA breaks apparently involve mechanisms and proteins similar to those involved in NHEJ used for VDJ recombination. Because the CSR occurs in the intron between the variable-region exon and the exon encoding the first constant-region domain, this process does not generate mutations in the regions encoding the variable or constant regions of the newly generated immunoglobulin heavy chain.

MECHANISMS FOR GENERATING ANTIBODY DIVERSITY

Several mechanisms contribute to the generation of diversity among immunoglobulin polypeptide variable regions.[40] The mechanisms are (1) the presence in the germ-line DNA of multiple different V, J, and D gene segments; (2) the random joining of these DNA segments to produce a complete variable-region exon; (3) junctional diversity; (4) the coming together of the heavy- and light-chain polypeptides to produce a complete immunoglobulin monomer capable of binding antigen; and (5) somatic mutations within the rearranged DNA segments themselves. The latter occurs through a process called somatic hypermutation.

Somatic hypermutation is not active in all B cells and cannot be triggered merely by mitogen-induced B cell activation. However, during discrete stages of B cell differentiation, expressed immunoglobulin V genes may incur new mutations at rates as high as 10^{-3} base substitutions per base pair per generation over several cell divisions, particularly during the secondary humoral immune response to antigen. Hypermutations begin on the 5' end of rearranged V genes downstream of the transcription initiation site and continue through the V gene and into the 3' flanking region before tapering off. As such, the mutations are clustered in the region spanning from 300 bp 5' of the rearranged variable-region exon to approximately 1 kb 3' of the rearranged minigene J segment. A high frequency of mutations are clustered around "hotspots" defined by the primary DNA sequence. The sequence RGYW (R = purine, A or G; Y = pyrimidine, C or T; W = A/T) and its complement, for example, is a hotspot for mutation that is conserved among species.[77]

The process of somatic hypermutation requires the activity of AID through a process that has some similarly with CSR. In addition to having the hyper-IgM immunodeficiency syndrome type II, patients who have inherited defects in AID have B cells that lack the capacity to undergo somatic hypermutation (see Chap. 82).[73,74] As with CSR, somatic hypermutation requires active transcription of the genes undergoing mutation. AID most likely deaminates the cytosines (dC) in the region encompassing the rearranged variable-region gene, converting the dC to uracils (dU), which are converted to T after DNA replication, giving rise to C/G to T/A transitions. Alternatively, the dU are removed by UNG, resulting in abasic sites that subsequently are cleaved by AP endonuclease. This process generates staggered nick cleavage of the DNA. Repair of these staggered nicks may involve low-fidelity DNA synthesis, giving rise to frequent mutations. DNA cleaving enzymes and DNA repair enzymes (e.g., mismatch repair enzymes, base-excision repair enzymes, proteins involved in NHEJ, etc.) form a complex called the "mutasome," which also apparently binds the target DNA to reduce its tendency to incur complete double-stranded DNA breaks. As a consequence of this process, mostly transitional mutations are introduced at high frequency in the expressed immunoglobulin V genes and in other transcriptionally active genes with "hotspots" that can serve as a substrate for AID, UNG, and the

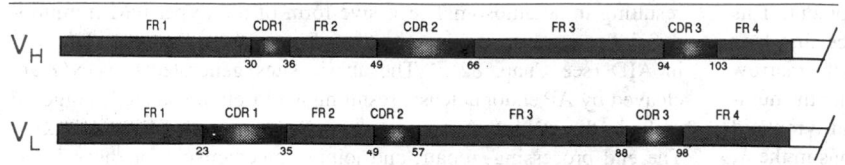

FIGURE 77-7 Schematic diagrams depicting each FR and CDR of the immunoglobulin heavy chain (V_H) or light chain (V_L). The first, second, third, and fourth framework regions are labeled FR1, FR2, FR3, and FR4, respectively. Similarly, the first, second, and third CDRs are labeled CDR1, CDR2, and CDR3, respectively. The *numbers* beneath each diagram indicate the numbers of the amino acid residues that define the borders between these regions according to Kabat and colleagues.[4]

mutasome.[78] Subsequent selection of the B cell and its daughter cells that express mutated V genes encoding an immunoglobulin variable region with improved fitness for binding antigen allows for "affinity maturation" of the antibodies expressed during the immune response to antigen. Such selection enhances the frequency of nonconservative base substitutions in the DNA sequences encoding the complementarity-determining region (CDRs) that serves as the contact site for antigen binding.[79]

IMMUNOGLOBULIN VARIABLE-REGION STRUCTURE

IMMUNOGLOBULIN VARIABLE-REGION SUBGROUPS

Despite the large number of different immunoglobulin variable regions that can be generated through the mechanisms, each antibody polypeptide can be assigned to one of a relatively small number of variable-region subgroups.[4] Comparisons of the amino acid sequences of a large number of different monoclonal immunoglobulin proteins reveal four segments of limited amino acid sequence diversity between different antibody heavy- or light-chain variable regions. These segments are designated the *immunoglobulin variable-region frameworks* (FRs) (Fig. 77-7). Each immunoglobulin polypeptide can be assigned to one of a relatively small number of variable-region subgroups based upon the primary structure of its first three frameworks. Moreover, each subgroup has characteristic framework sequences that distinguish it from other variable-region subgroups.

Satisfying expectations that immunoglobulin subgroups defined families of highly related antibody V genes, variable-region amino acid subgroup homologies extend to the nucleic acid sequence level.[80–82] Cloned immunoglobulin V genes whose deduced amino acid sequences belong to a given subgroup generally share greater than 80 percent nucleic acid sequence homology. The human heavy-chain variable regions can be grouped into seven subgroups, whereas κ or λ light chains can be divided into six or 11 subgroups, respectively.

Crystallographic data of immunoglobulin variable regions indicate that amino acids within the first and third FRs of either the light or heavy chain form beta bonds on the external surface of the molecule.[5,83] These regions form relatively compact structures on the external solvent-accessible face of the antibody molecule that are not adjacent to the classic antibody-combining site for antigen. Accordingly, amino acid differences noted between the different variable-region subgroups are amenable to recognition by antisubgroup antibodies.[84]

IMMUNOGLOBULIN IDIOTYPES

Antisubgroup antibodies must be distinguished from antiidiotypic antibodies. Positioned between the FRs are three segments of extreme hypervariability in both light- and heavy-chain sequences.[4] The third hypervariable region is generated through the recombinatorial process that joins the antibody light-chain V gene with the J segment of the light chain or the V_H gene with the somatically generated DJ_H segment of the antibody heavy chain. The diversity in first and second hypervariable regions in part reflects germ-line DNA-encoded differences between disparate antibody V genes, a diversity often noted even between V genes of the same subgroup.[4,34] During an immune response, somatic hypermutation subsequent to V gene rearrangement also may play an important role in increasing the amino acid sequence diversity noted within these regions. These hypervariable regions on both chains fold together to form the antigen combining site.[3,50] Hence, each of these regions of hypervariability is designated a CDR (see Fig. 77-7).

During secondary immune responses, extensive amino acid substitutions may occur in the CDRs. In contrast, amino acid replacement mutations occur much less frequently in the FRs than would be anticipated if the nucleic acid substitutions were occurring randomly. As aconsequence, the subgroup determinants that characterize an entire variable-region subgroup may be relatively resilient to somatic hypermutation. On the other hand, the CDRs may form determinants of unique specificity that contribute to the epitopes recognized by antiidiotypic antibodies.

Despite the tremendous potential for diversity in Ig V gene expression and genetic polymorphism, antibodies produced by B cell malignancies or normal B cells of unrelated persons may share common idiotypic determinants.[85] These common idiotypes, designated cross-reactive idiotypes (CRIs), were defined initially on IgM autoantibodies, such as rheumatoid factors. However, CRIs may be found on antibodies that do not have anti–self-reactivity. Molecular studies have demonstrated several of these CRIs represent serologic markers for expression of conserved immunoglobulin variable-region genes with little or no somatic mutation.[86]

IMMUNOGLOBULIN ALLOTYPES

HEAVY-CHAIN ALLOTYPES

Human immunoglobulins have inherited differences in structure, termed *allotypes*. These genetic markers usually are detected with agglutinating sera from individuals naturally immunized through transfusion or pregnancy. These antibodies recognize minor amino acid sequence variations in the constant regions of γ, α, and κ chains.[87,88] No definite allotypic differences have been detected on μ or δ chains. On ε chains, a monoclonal antibody to IgE defined an allotype that was common to persons of all races except for a few individuals of Asian or Melanesian background.

The κ light-chain allotypes are designated *Km allotypes* (formerly called *inv*). At least three major Km allotypes exist, designated Km(1), Km(1,2), and Km(3), which may be recognized serologically or, more recently, via the polymerase chain reaction.[89] The α-chain allotypes, designated *Am allotypes*, are on the heavy chains of the IgA2 subclass.[88] The γ-chain allotypes are on the heavy chains of the IgG1, IgG2, and IgG3 subclasses and are designated *G1m*, *G2m*, and *G3m*, respectively. More than 24 Gm allotypic markers have been identified serologically.[88] All the heavy-chain constant-region genes reside on chromosome 14. Therefore, different combinations of heavy-chain allotype markers are inherited as haplotypic units, in an autosomal codominant manner. The frequency of the various allelic markers differs among ethnic groups.

λ LIGHT-CHAIN ISOTYPES

The λ light chains have four isotypes, termed Mcg+, Ke−Oz−, Ke−Oz+, and Ke+Oz−, which were defined based on their reactivity with the Oz, Kern, and Mcg antisera raised against λ Bence Jones proteins.[90] These isotypes reflect minor nonallelic amino acid differences in the λ light-chain constant regions that each is encoded by one of the multiple constant-region genes in the λ light-chain complex.[91] Mcg+, Ke−Oz−, Ke−Oz+, and Ke+Oz− isotypes each is associated with the $C_\lambda1$, $C_\lambda2$, $C_\lambda3$, or $C_\lambda7$ λ light-chain constant region, respectively (see Fig. 77-6).

IMMUNOGLOBULIN SYNTHESIS AND SECRETION

IMMUNOGLOBULIN SYNTHESIS

The total IgG content of the adult human body is approximately 75 g, of which 2.2 g is synthesized each day. Most immunoglobulin is produced by mature plasma cells, which have abundant rough endoplasmic reticulum, a well-developed Golgi apparatus, and high-level transcription of the immunoglobulin genes because of the convergence of multiple regulatory pathways involving Blimp1, Bcl6, XBP-1, and other transcription factors.[92]

The final mRNAs for immunoglobulin light and heavy chains are derived by the processing of large nuclear RNA transcripts. In plasma cells, the rearranged and spliced mRNA molecules for the heavy- and light-chain polypeptides are translated on separate ribosomal complexes. An amino-terminal leader peptide approximately 18 to 30 residues long is cleaved prior to the release of the completed light and heavy chains in the cisternae of the endoplasmic reticulum. In that location, the heavy-chain immunoglobulin polypeptides interact via their C_H1 domains with BiP, a heat-shock chaperone protein that allows for proper folding of the heavy-chain polypeptide and prevents its transport into the Golgi.[93] The nascent immunoglobulin light chain can displace BiP and then spontaneously combine with the heavy chain to form immunoglobulin half molecules that are stabilized by disulfide bonds.[94] The joining of two identical half molecules by disulfide bonds yields a basic four-chain immunoglobulin unit, which then is allowed to transport to the Golgi for glycosylation.

Glycosyltransferase enzymes add a defined sequence of sugars to the assembled immunoglobulin unit to form branched-chain oligosaccharides composed of N-acetyl-glucosamine, mannose, galactose, fructose, and sialic acid. The oligosaccharides are attached covalently to the immunoglobulin heavy chain at several sites. The carbohydrate facilitates the transport of the antibody molecule across the plasma membrane and into the extracellular space and increases the solubility of the secreted protein.[95]

Five monomeric units of IgM combine to form a pentameric macroglobulin linked by disulfide bonds and a single J-chain polypeptide. Usually polymerization immediately precedes or occurs simultaneously with IgM secretion. Similarly, IgA molecules form dimers and polymers linked by the J chain just prior to secretion from the plasma cell.

REGULATION OF IMMUNOGLOBULIN SYNTHESIS

A normal adult has preexisting B lymphocytes that can interact with almost any foreign antigen. In the presence of accessory T lymphocytes and macrophages, an antigen-binding clone of B lymphocytes may transform into antibody-secreting plasma cells or memory B cells, which can be readily reactivated during an immune to antigen.[96,97] Most plasma cells are terminally differentiated and do not divide.[98] Therefore, the continued production of antibody depends upon the rate

of plasma cell generation, the functional life span of the plasma cell, and the half-life of the immunoglobulin in the body.[99]

B lymphocytes are produced throughout life by differentiation of hematopoietic cells in the marrow and proliferation of B lymphocytes in secondary lymphoid tissues.[100] Many B lymphocytes survive for only a few weeks without stimulation by antigen and activated accessory T lymphocytes.[101] Without antigen to cross-link their surface immunoglobulin receptors, B lymphocytes that home to the germinal centers of secondary lymphoid tissues undergo apoptosis, or programmed cell death, within a matter of hours in vitro.[102–104] Not only does this process select for B lymphocytes that have surface immunoglobulin with high affinity for antigen,[105] but the requirement for antigen-directed surface immunoglobulin cross-linking also allows for secreted specific antibody to regulate its own production. Under normal short-term exposure to antigen, newly formed B lymphocytes must compete with secreted antibody and other antigen-specific B lymphocytes for ever-decreasing amounts of circulating antigen.[106] By preventing the interaction of antigen with immunoglobulin receptors on B lymphocytes, secreted antibody may inhibit the production of more plasma cells.

REFERENCES

1. Edelman GM: Antibody structure and molecular immunology. *Scand J Immunol* 34:1, 1991.
2. Virella G, Wang AC: Immunoglobulin structure. *Immunol Ser* 58:75, 1993.
3. Perkins SJ, Ashton AW, Boehm MK, Chamberlain D: Molecular structures from low angle X-ray and neutron scattering studies. *Int J Biol Macromol* 22:1, 1998.
4. Kabat E, Wu TT, Perry HM, et al: *Sequences of Proteins of Immunological Interest*, 5th ed, U.S. Department of Health and Human Services, Bethesda, 1991.
5. Harris LJ, Larson SB, Hasel KW, et al: The three-dimensional structure of an intact monoclonal antibody for canine lymphoma. *Nature* 360: 369, 1992.
6. Jefferis R, Lund J, Goodall M: Recognition sites on human IgG for Fc gamma receptors: The role of glycosylation. *Immunol Lett* 44:111, 1995.
7. Lee YK, Brewer JW, Hellman R, Hendershot LM: BiP and immunoglobulin light chain cooperate to control the folding of heavy chain and ensure the fidelity of immunoglobulin assembly. *Mol Biol Cell* 10:2209, 1999.
8. Lamm ME, Nedrud JG, Kaetzel CS, Mazanec MB: IgA and mucosal defense. *APMIS* 103:241, 1995.
9. Corthesy B, Kraehenbuhl JP: Antibody-mediated protection of mucosal surfaces. *Curr Top Microbiol Immunol* 236:93, 1999.
10. Niles MJ, Matsuuchi L, Koshland ME: Polymer IgM assembly and secretion in lymphoid and nonlymphoid cell lines: Evidence that J chain is required for pentamer IgM synthesis. *Proc Natl Acad Sci U S A* 92: 2884, 1995.
11. Roes J, Rajewsky K: Immunoglobulin D (IgD)-deficient mice reveal an auxiliary receptor function for IgD in antigen-mediated recruitment of B cells. *J Exp Med* 177:45, 1993.
12. Lyczak JB, Zhang K, Saxon A, Morrison SL: Expression of novel secreted isoforms of human immunoglobulin E proteins. *J Biol Chem* 271: 3428, 1996.
13. Cambier JC, Campbell KS: Membrane immunoglobulin and its accomplices: New lessons from an old receptor. *FASEB J* 6:3207, 1992.
14. Minegishi Y, Coustan-Smith E, Rapalus L, et al: Mutations in Igalpha (CD79a) result in a complete block in B-cell development. *J Clin Invest* 104:1115, 1999.

15. Wang Y, Kanegane H, Sanal O, et al: Novel Igalpha (CD79a) gene mutation in a Turkish patient with B cell-deficient agammaglobulinemia. *Am J Med Genet* 108:333, 2002.

16. Law CL, Sidorenko SP, Chandran KA, et al: Molecular cloning of human Syk. A B cell protein-tyrosine kinase associated with the surface immunoglobulin M-B cell receptor complex. *J Biol Chem* 269:12310, 1994.

17. Kabak S, Skaggs BJ, Gold MR, et al: The direct recruitment of BLNK to immunoglobulin alpha couples the B-cell antigen receptor to distal signaling pathways. *Mol Cell Biol* 22:2524, 2002.

18. Chiu CW, Dalton M, Ishiai M, et al: BLNK: Molecular scaffolding through "cis"-mediated organization of signaling proteins. *EMBO J* 21:6461, 2002.

19. Doody GM, Bell SE, Vigorito E, et al: Signal transduction through Vav-2 participates in humoral immune responses and B cell maturation. *Nat Immunol* 2:542, 2001.

20. Fluckiger AC, Li Z, Kato RM, et al: Btk/Tec kinases regulate sustained increases in intracellular Ca2+ following B-cell receptor activation. *EMBO J* 17:1973, 1998.

21. Kurosaki T: Genetic analysis of B cell antigen receptor signaling. *Annu Rev Immunol* 17:555, 1999.

22. Fruman DA, Satterthwaite AB, Witte ON: Xid-like phenotypes: A B cell signalosome takes shape. *Immunity* 13:1, 2000.

23. Healy JI, Goodnow CC: Positive versus negative signaling by lymphocyte antigen receptors. *Annu Rev Immunol* 16:645, 1998.

24. Cornall RJ, Goodnow CC, Cyster JG: Regulation of B cell antigen receptor signaling by the Lyn/CD22/SHP1 pathway. *Curr Top Microbiol Immunol* 244:57, 1999.

25. Fearon DT, Carroll MC: Regulation of B lymphocyte responses to foreign and self-antigens by the CD19/CD21 complex. *Annu Rev Immunol* 18:393, 2000.

26. Poe JC, Fujimoto M, Jansen PJ, et al: CD22 forms a quaternary complex with SHIP, Grb2, and Shc. A pathway for regulation of B lymphocyte antigen receptor-induced calcium flux. *J Biol Chem* 275:17420, 2000.

27. Kumanogoh A, Kikutani H: The CD100-CD72 interaction: A novel mechanism of immune regulation. *Trends Immunol* 22:670, 2001.

28. Chan VW, Lowell CA, DeFranco AL: Defective negative regulation of antigen receptor signaling in Lyn-deficient B lymphocytes. *Curr Biol* 8:545, 1998.

29. Doody GM, Justement LB, Delibrias CC, et al: A role in B cell activation for CD22 and the protein tyrosine phosphatase SHP. *Science* 269:242, 1995.

30. Plas DR, Thomas ML: Negative regulation of antigen receptor signaling in lymphocytes. *J Mol Med* 76:589, 1998.

31. Siminovitch KA, Neel BG: Regulation of B cell signal transduction by SH2-containing protein-tyrosine phosphatases. *Semin Immunol* 10:329, 1998.

32. Shultz LD, Rajan TV, Greiner DL: Severe defects in immunity and hematopoiesis caused by SHP-1 protein-tyrosine-phosphatase deficiency. *Trends Biotechnol* 15:302, 1997.

33. Cyster JG, Goodnow CC: Protein tyrosine phosphatase 1C negatively regulates antigen receptor signaling in B lymphocytes and determines thresholds for negative selection. *Immunity* 2:13, 1995.

34. Matsuda F, Ishii K, Bourvagnet P, et al: The complete nucleotide sequence of the human immunoglobulin heavy chain variable region locus. *J Exp Med* 188:2151, 1998.

35. Tomlinson IM, Cox JP, Gherardi E, et al: The structural repertoire of the human V kappa domain. *EMBO J* 14:4628, 1995.

36. Kawasaki K, Minoshima S, Nakato E, et al: Evolutionary dynamics of the human immunoglobulin kappa locus and the germline repertoire of the Vkappa genes. *Eur J Immunol* 31:1017, 2001.

37. Dunham I, Shimizu N, Roe BA, et al: The DNA sequence of human chromosome 22. *Nature* 402:489, 1999.

38. Pallarès N, Frippiat JP, Giudicelli V, Lefranc MP: The human immunoglobulin lambda variable (IGLV) genes and joining (IGLJ) segments. *Exp Clin Immunogenet* 15:8, 1998.

39. Bassing CH, Alt FW, Hughes MM, et al: Recombination signal sequences restrict chromosomal V(D)J recombination beyond the 12/23 rule. *Nature* 405:583, 2000.

40. Tonegawa S: The Nobel Lectures in Immunology. The Nobel Prize for Physiology or Medicine 1987. Somatic generation of immune diversity [classical article]. *Scand J Immunol* 38:303, 1993.

41. Gellert M: Recent advances in understanding V(D)J recombination. *Adv Immunol* 64:39, 1997.

42. Steen SB, Gomelsky L, Speidel SL, Roth DB: Initiation of V(D)J recombination in vivo: Role of recombination signal sequences in formation of single and paired double-strand breaks. *EMBO J* 16:2656, 1997.

43. Lewis SM: The mechanism of V(D)J joining: Lessons from molecular, immunological, and comparative analyses. *Adv Immunol* 56:27, 1994.

44. Oettinger MA, Schatz DG, Gorka C, Baltimore D: RAG-1 and RAG-2, adjacent genes that synergistically activate V(D)J recombination. *Science* 248:1517, 1990.

45. Oettinger MA, Stanger B, Schatz DG, et al: The recombination activating genes, RAG 1 and RAG 2, are on chromosome 11p in humans and chromosome 2p in mice. *Immunogenetics* 35:97, 1992.

46. Shinkai Y, Rathbun G, Lam KP, et al: RAG-2-deficient mice lack mature lymphocytes owing to inability to initiate V(D)J rearrangement. *Cell* 68:855, 1992.

47. Villa A, Santagata S, Bozzi F, et al: Omenn syndrome: A disorder of Rag1 and Rag2 genes. *J Clin Immunol* 19:87, 1999.

48. Huye LE, Purugganan MM, Jiang MM, Roth DB: Mutational analysis of all conserved basic amino acids in RAG-1 reveals catalytic, step arrest, and joining-deficient mutants in the V(D)J recombinase. *Mol Cell Biol* 22:3460, 2002.

49. Tsai CL, Drejer AH, Schatz DG: Evidence of a critical architectural function for the RAG proteins in end processing, protection, and joining in V(D)J recombination. *Genes Dev* 16:1934, 2002.

50. Thomas JO, Travers AA: HMG1 and 2, and related "architectural" DNA-binding proteins. *Trends Biochem Sci* 26:167, 2001.

51. Ma Y, Pannicke U, Schwarz K, Lieber MR: Hairpin opening and overhang processing by an Artemis/DNA-dependent protein kinase complex in nonhomologous end joining and V(D)J recombination. *Cell* 108:781, 2002.

52. Lieber MR, Ma Y, Pannicke U, Schwarz K: Mechanism and regulation of human non-homologous DNA end-joining. *Nat Rev Mol Cell Biol* 4:712, 2003.

53. Taccioli GE, Amatucci AG, Beamish HJ, et al: Targeted disruption of the catalytic subunit of the DNA-PK gene in mice confers severe combined immunodeficiency and radiosensitivity. *Immunity* 9:355, 1998.

54. Khanna KK, Jackson SP: DNA double-strand breaks: Signaling, repair, and the cancer connection. *Nat Genet* 27:247, 2001.

55. Gu Y, Sekiguchi J, Gao Y, et al: Defective embryonic neurogenesis in Ku-deficient but not DNA-dependent protein kinase catalytic subunit-deficient mice. *Proc Natl Acad Sci U S A* 97:2668, 2000.

56. Ouyang H, Nussenzweig A, Kurimasa A, et al: Ku70 is required for DNA repair but not for T cell antigen receptor gene recombination in vivo. *J Exp Med* 186:921, 1997.

57. Bassing CH, Suh H, Ferguson DO, et al: Histone H2AX: A dosage-dependent suppressor of oncogenic translocations and tumors. *Cell* 114:359, 2003.

58. Celeste A, Difilippantonio S, Difilippantonio MJ, et al: H2AX haploinsufficiency modifies genomic stability and tumor susceptibility. *Cell* 114:371, 2003.

59. Komori T, Okada A, Stewart V, Alt FW: Lack of N regions in antigen receptor variable region genes of TdT-deficient lymphocytes. *Science* 261:1171, 1993.

60. Grawunder U, West RB, Lieber MR: Antigen receptor gene rearrangement. *Curr Opin Immunol* 10:172, 1998.

61. Rassenti LZ, Kipps TJ: Lack of allelic exclusion in B cell chronic lymphocytic leukemia. *J Exp Med* 185:1435, 1997.

62. Melchers F, Karasuyama H, Haasner D, et al: The surrogate light chain in B-cell development. *Immunol Today* 14:60, 1993.

63. ten Boekel E, Yamagami T, Andersson J, et al: The formation and selection of cells expressing pre-B cell receptors and B cell receptors. *Curr Top Microbiol Immunol* 246:3, 1999.

64. Melchers F, ten Boekel E, Seidl T, et al: Repertoire selection by pre-B-cell receptors and B-cell receptors, and genetic control of B-cell development from immature to mature B cells. *Immunol Rev* 175:33, 2000.

65. Tsuganezawa K, Kiyokawa N, Matsuo Y, et al: Flow cytometric diagnosis of the cell lineage and developmental stage of acute lymphoblastic leukemia by novel monoclonal antibodies specific to human pre-B-cell receptor. *Blood* 92:4317, 1998.

66. Kitamura D, Kudo A, Schaal S, et al: A critical role of lambda 5 protein in B cell development. *Cell* 69:823, 1992.

67. Corcos D, Dunda O, Butor C, et al: Pre-B-cell development in the absence of lambda 5 in transgenic mice expressing a heavy-chain disease protein. *Curr Biol* 5:1140, 1995.

68. Minegishi Y, Coustan-Smith E, Wang YH, et al: Mutations in the human lambda5/14.1 gene result in B cell deficiency and agammaglobulinemia. *J Exp Med* 187:71, 1998.

69. Stavnezer J: Immunoglobulin class switching. *Curr Opin Immunol* 8:199, 1996.

70. Ferrari S, Plebani A: Cross-talk between CD40 and CD40L: Lessons from primary immune deficiencies. *Curr Opin Allergy Clin Immunol* 2:489, 2002.

71. Lorenz MG, Radbruch A: Insights into the control of immunoglobulin class switch recombination from analysis of targeted mice. *Res Immunol* 148:460, 1997.

72. Honjo T, Kinoshita K, Muramatsu M. Molecular mechanism of class switch recombination: Linkage with somatic hypermutation. *Annu Rev Immunol* 20:165, 2002.

73. Muramatsu M, Kinoshita K, Fagarasan S, et al: Class switch recombination and hypermutation require activation-induced cytidine deaminase (AID), a potential RNA editing enzyme. *Cell* 102:553, 2000.

74. Revy P, Muto T, Levy Y, et al: Activation-induced cytidine deaminase (AID) deficiency causes the autosomal recessive form of the hyper-IgM syndrome (HIGM2). *Cell* 102:565, 2000.

75. Imai K, Slupphaug G, Lee WI, et al: Human uracil-DNA glycosylase deficiency associated with profoundly impaired immunoglobulin class-switch recombination. *Nat Immunol* 4:1023, 2003.

76. Chen X, Kinoshita K, Honjo T: Variable deletion and duplication at recombination junction ends: Implication for staggered double-strand cleavage in class-switch recombination. *Proc Natl Acad Sci U S A* 98:13860, 2001.

77. Rogozin IB, Sredneva NE, Kolchanov NA: Somatic hypermutagenesis in immunoglobulin genes: III. Somatic mutations in the chicken light chain locus. *Biochim Biophys Acta* 1306:171, 1996.

78. Storb U, Shen HM, Michael N, Kim N: Somatic hypermutation of immunoglobulin and non-immunoglobulin genes. *Philos Trans R Soc Lond B Biol Sci* 356:13, 2001.

79. Dorner T, Foster SJ, Brezinschek HP, Lipsky PE: Analysis of the targeting of the hypermutational machinery and the impact of subsequent selection on the distribution of nucleotide changes in human VHDJH rearrangements. *Immunol Rev* 162:161, 1998.

80. Cook GP, Tomlinson IM: The human immunoglobulin VH repertoire. *Immunol Today* 16:237, 1995.

81. Kipps TJ: Human B cell biology. *Int Rev Immunol* 15:243, 1997.

82. Frippiat JP, Williams SC, Tomlinson IM, et al: Organization of the human immunoglobulin lambda light-chain locus on chromosome 22q11.2. *Hum Mol Genet* 4:983, 1995.

83. Poljak RJ: Structure of antibodies and their complexes with antigens. *Mol Immunol* 28:1341, 1991.

84. Jefferis R: Nomenclature of V-region markers [comment]. *Immunol Today* 16:207, 1995.

85. Kipps TJ, Carson DA: Autoantibodies in chronic lymphocytic leukemia and related systemic autoimmune diseases. *Blood* 81:2475, 1993.

86. Kipps TJ: Immunologic and therapeutic implications of anti-idiotype antibodies, in *Chronic Lymphocytic Leukemia*, edited by BD Cheson, p 123. Marcel Dekker, New York, 1992.

87. Williams RC Jr, Malone CC, Solomon A: Conformational dependency of human IgG heavy chain-associated Gm allotypes. *Mol Immunol* 30:341, 1993.

88. Schanfield MS, van Loghem E: Human immunoglobulin allotypes, in *Handbook of Experimental Immunology—Genetics and Molecular Immunology*, 4th ed, edited by DM Weir, LA Herzenberg, C Blackwell, L Herzenberg, p 1. Blackwell Scientific Publications, Oxford, 1986.

89. Moxley G, Gibbs RS: Polymerase chain reaction-based genotyping for allotypic markers of immunoglobulin kappa shows allelic association of Km with kappa variable segment. *Genomics* 13:104, 1992.

90. Hess M, Hilschmann N, Rivat L, et al: Isotypes in human immunoglobulin lambda-chains. *Nat New Biol* 234:58, 1971.

91. Walker MR, Solomon A, Weiss DT, et al: Immunogenic and antigenic epitopes of Ig: XXV. Monoclonal antibodies that differentiate the Mcg+/Mcg− and Oz+/Oz− C region isotypes of human lambda L chains. *J Immunol* 140:1600, 1988.

92. Shaffer AL, Lin KI, Kuo TC, et al: Blimp-1 orchestrates plasma cell differentiation by extinguishing the mature B cell gene expression program. *Immunity* 17:51, 2002.

93. Hendershot LM, Kearney JF: A role for human heavy chain binding protein in the regulation of immunoglobin transport. *Mol Immunol* 25:585, 1988.

94. Reddy PS, Corley RB: The contribution of ER quality control to the biologic functions of secretory IgM. *Immunol Today* 20:582, 1999.

95. Rudd PM, Elliott T, Cresswell P, et al: Glycosylation and the immune system. *Science* 291:2370, 2001.

96. Gray D. Immunologic memory. *Annu Rev Immunol* 11:49, 1993.

97. Bernasconi NL, Traggiai E, Lanzavecchia A: Maintenance of serological memory by polyclonal activation of human memory B cells. *Science* 298:2199, 2002.

98. Manz RA, Thiel A, Radbruch A: Lifetime of plasma cells in the bone marrow. *Nature* 388:133, 1997.

99. Virella G, Wang AC: Biosynthesis, metabolism and biological properties of immunoglobulins. *Immunol Ser* 58:91, 1993.

100. Nunez C, Nishimoto N, Gartland GL, et al: B cells are generated throughout life in humans. *J Immunol* 156:866, 1996.

101. Benschop RJ, Cambier JC: B cell development: Signal transduction by antigen receptors and their surrogates. *Curr Opin Immunol* 11:143, 1999.

102. Choi YS: Differentiation and apoptosis of human germinal center B-lymphocytes. *Immunol Res* 16:161, 1997.

103. Liu YJ, de Bouteiller O, Fugier-Vivier I: Mechanisms of selection and differentiation in germinal centers. *Curr Opin Immunol* 9:256, 1997.

104. Hollowood K, Goodlad JR: Germinal centre cell kinetics. *J Pathol* 185:229, 1998.

105. Przylepa J, Himes C, Kelsoe G: Lymphocyte development and selection in germinal centers. *Curr Top Microbiol Immunol* 229:85, 1998.

106. Freitas AA, Rocha B: Population biology of lymphocytes: The flight for survival. *Annu Rev Immunol* 18:83, 2000.

CHAPTER 78

FUNCTIONS OF
T LYMPHOCYTES: T CELL
RECEPTORS FOR ANTIGEN

THOMAS J. KIPPS

All T cells express a receptor for antigen that is formed by two polymorphic polypeptides that invariably are associated with a collection of invariant proteins called CD3γ, CD3δ, CD3ε, and CD247. The invariant proteins are necessary for surface expression and signaling by the T cell receptor. The two polypeptides forming the T cell receptor on most T cells are termed α and β. A small subset of T cells have receptors formed by different polypeptides called γ and δ. The polypeptides of the T cell receptor have a diversity comparable to that estimated for immunoglobulin molecules. However, unlike immunoglobulins, T cell receptors recognize small fragments of antigen, usually peptides, which are nestled in defined peptide-binding groves of major histocompatibility complex molecules that are present on the plasma membrane of another cell. As such, T cell immune recognition generally requires cognate intercellular interactions between a T cell and another cell, sometimes called the *antigen-presenting cell* (APC). The response of the T cell to antigen depends upon the intensity of the signal generated by ligation of the T cell receptor. In addition, this signal is modified by the simultaneous ligation of other T cell receptors for accessory molecules on the plasma membrane of the APC. Because of this, the outcome of T cell antigen recognition can range from immune activation and T cell proliferation to specific T cell tolerance and/or programmed cell death.

T LYMPHOCYTE ANTIGEN RECEPTORS

T CELL RECEPTOR HETERODIMERS

The receptor proteins of the T cell antigen receptor are structurally related to immunoglobulin molecules.[1] The receptor for antigen on

Acronyms and abbreviations that appear in this chapter include: AP-1, activation protein-1; APC, antigen-presenting cell; CTLs, cytolytic T lymphocytes; DAG, diacylglycerol; ERK, extracellular receptor-activated kinase; FKBP, FK-506 binding protein; GM-CSF, granulocyte-macrophage colony stimulating factor; GDP, guanosine diphosphate; GTP, guanosine triphosphate; HIV, human immunodeficiency virus; ICAMs, intercellular adhesion molecules; IFN-γ, interferon gamma; Ig, immunoglobulin; IL, interleukin; IP$_3$, inositol 1,4,5-triphosphate; ITAMs, immunoreceptor tyrosine-based activation motifs; ITIMs, immunoreceptor tyrosine-based inhibitory motifs; JNK, c-Jun N-terminal kinase; LAG-3, lymphocyte activation gene-3; LAT, linker of activation of T cells; LFA, lymphocyte function-associated; MAP, mitogen-activated protein; MHC, major histocompatibility complex; NFAT, nuclear factor of activated T cells; NK, natural killer; PI3K, phosphatidylinositide 3 kinase; PIP$_2$, phosphatidylinositol 4,5-biphosphate; PKC, protein kinase C; PLC-γ1, phospholipase C-gamma 1; SAP, stress-activated kinase; SH2, Src homology 2; SH3, Src homology 3; SLP-76, SH2-binding leukocyte phosphoprotein of 76 kDa; Sos, homolog to son of sevenless; STAT, signal transducer of activated T cells; TNF, tumor necrosis factor; T$_{reg}$, CD4+CD25+ regulatory T cells; V-like, variable region-like; VLA, very late activation; ZAP-70, zeta-associated protein of 70 kDa.

most T cells is formed by two polypeptides, termed α and β, which are linked together via disulfide bonds and associated with a collection of invariant proteins called CD3 (see Chap. 14). Following the rule of allelic exclusion, the T cell receptor is clonally distributed, with each T cell expressing a single α-chain and a single β-chain. Each chain has a hydrophobic leader sequence of 18 to 29 amino acids and an amino-terminal domain of 102 to 119 amino acids termed the *variable region*. This designation reflects the variation in the primary structure of these domains among different T cell receptor polypeptides. Furthermore, each chain has a carboxyl-terminal region segment of 87 to 113 amino acids, termed the *constant region* because the region is invariant among chains of the same class. Because of their role as surface-membrane receptors, each chain also has a small connecting peptide, a transmembrane region of 20 to 24 amino acids, and a small cytoplasmic region of 5 to 12 residues at the carboxyl-terminus.

Like the immunoglobulin domains, the variable and constant regions each contains cysteine residues at positions consistent with the presence of a centrally located disulfide loop of 63 to 69 amino acids. Sequence comparisons indicate that several amino acids that are highly conserved in immunoglobulins, including those involved in domain–domain interactions, also are conserved in the T cell receptor chains. Furthermore, the T cell receptor chains fold into tertiary structures that are very similar to the structures of the light and heavy chains of the immunoglobulin molecule. The structural similarities of the T cell receptor justifiably place the genes encoding these receptor proteins in the so-called immunoglobulin supergene family.[2]

$\alpha\beta$-HETERODIMERS

Greater than 90 percent of mature T cells express an $\alpha\beta$-heterodimer, making this the major class of T cell receptor. Without glycan side chains, each α-or β-polypeptide has a size of only 27 or 32 kDa, respectively. However, within minutes after being translated into protein, both chains are glycosylated and assembled into a heterodimer composed of a single acidic α-glycoprotein of 39 to 46 kDa linked to a more basic 40- to 44-kDa β-glycoprotein via a disulfide bond between the constant regions of the two chains (Fig. 78-1).

$\gamma\delta$-HETERODIMERS

Less than 10 percent of blood T cells and thymocytes exclusively express a different T cell receptor heterodimer composed of two glycoproteins designated γ and δ.[3] The development of $\gamma\delta$-expressing T cells appears distinct from that of $\alpha\beta$-expressing T cells.[4,5] T cells bearing $\gamma\delta$-receptors apparently constitute a distinct cell lineage that can undergo relative expansion in response to infection with certain organisms, such as *Listeria monocytogenes*.[6] In secondary lymphoid tissues (see Chap. 5), only approximately 1 to 5 percent of CD3-positive T cells express $\gamma\delta$-receptors. However, in epithelial tissues most T cells express $\gamma\delta$-receptors, especially in the epidermis and small intestine of the mouse.

The amino acid sequence of the γ-chain is more like that of the T cell receptor β-chain, whereas the amino acid sequence of the δ-chain is more like that of the α-chain. Like the $\alpha\beta$-heterodimer and immunoglobulins, the $\gamma\delta$-heterodimer is clonally distributed. Like the homologous $\alpha\beta$-heterodimer, the $\gamma\delta$-heterodimer also is associated with the CD3 complex and appears capable of stimulating T cell activation when bound to a specific ligand. Together these two chains have structural and size characteristics similar to those of the $\alpha\beta$-heterodimer. However, the tertiary structure of variable regions of $\gamma\delta$-T cell receptors has a closer resemblance to immunoglobulin variable regions than to the variable regions of $\alpha\beta$-T cell receptors.[7]

GENETICS OF T CELL RECEPTOR HETERODIMERS

Similar to the immunoglobulin genes, each chain of the T cell receptors is encoded by discrete genetic elements that rearrange during de-

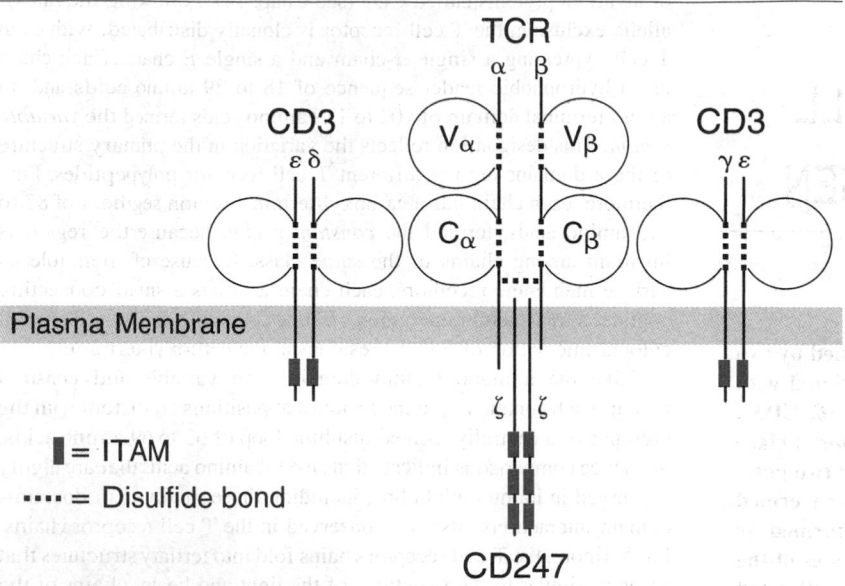

FIGURE 78-1   Schematic diagram of the $\alpha\beta$-T cell receptor (TCR) complex. The two chains of the $\alpha\beta$-T cell receptor are depicted under the heading TCR and labeled α and β. The variable (V) domain and constant (C) domains of each chain are depicted within the loop representing the immunoglobulin-like domain of each chain. The heterodimers composed of CD3ε and CD3δ or CD3γ and CD3ε are depicted to the **left** and **right** of the two chains of the $\alpha\beta$-T cell receptor, respectively, each under the heading CD3 and labeled ε and δ or γ and ε, respectively. The ζ chain (CD247) homodimer is depicted between the two chains of $\alpha\beta$-T cell receptor. *Dotted lines* represent intrachain or interchain disulfide bridges, as indicated in the legend in the **lower left-hand corner**. The plasma membrane spanned by each of these chains is indicated. *Boxes* indicate the immunoreceptor tyrosine-based activation motifs (ITAMs) in the cytoplasmic domains of the CD3 polypeptides and the ζ chain.

velopment (Fig. 78-2) (see Chap. 77). Evaluation for T cell receptor gene rearrangements can distinguish between patients having clonal T cell lymphoproliferative diseases from those having nonneoplastic polyclonal T cell expansion.[8] Furthermore, molecular analysis for clonal T cell receptor gene rearrangements can be used to detect minimal residual disease in patients treated for clonal T cell disorders.[9]

Located at band q35 on the long arm of chromosome 7, the β-chain complex has two closely linked genes, each capable of encoding the β-chain constant region. Each constant region gene is associated with a cluster of functional J_β gene segments and a single D_β segment.

The functional gene encoding the variable region of the β-chain is constructed from the rearrangement of any of approximately 50 variable region gene segments to either one of the two D_β regions and one of 13 J_β regions. The α-chain complex is located at band q11.2 on the long arm of chromosome 14 and thus is linked to the immunoglobulin heavy-chain complex. The α-chain gene complex consists of one constant region gene and at least 50 different variable region gene segments. The functional gene encoding the α-chain variable region is derived from the juxtaposition of any one of the variable region gene segments with one of the many J_α segments through rearrangement that generally involves deletion of the intervening DNA.

The organization of the γ- and δ-genes is similar to that of the α- and β-genes except for some significant differences. First, the gene complex encoding the δ-genes is located entirely within the α-chain gene complex between the V_α and J_α gene segments.[10] Consequently, any rearrangement of the α-chain genes inactivates the genes encoding the δ-chain. Second, many fewer V gene segments are present in the γ- and δ-gene complexes than at either the T cell receptor α or γ gene loci. For example, the γ-gene complex on band p15 on the short arm of chromosome 7 has only approximately 12 V_γ gene segments, two virtually identical J_γ segments, and two constant region gene segments.[11] Moreover, the δ-gene complex has only approximately four V_δ gene segments, three D_δ gene segments, three J_δ gene segments, and a single constant region gene. Consequently, most of the variability in the γ- and δ-chains is found in the junctional region formed during the process of $\gamma\delta$-T cell receptor gene rearrangement. The amino acids encoded by this region form the center of the T cell receptor-binding site.

ANTIGENS RECOGNIZED BY T CELL RECEPTOR HETERODIMERS

Although they are highly similar in structure, T cell receptors and immunoglobulins recognize antigen in important different ways.[1] Whereas immunoglobulins can bind antigens directly, T cell receptors generally recognize peptide antigens that are bound to a molecule of the major histocompatibility complex (MHC) on the surface of another cell.[12]

MHC molecules are divided into two basic classes. Class I MHC molecules bind peptides that generally are derived from proteins synthesized and degraded in the cytosol. The human histocompatibility antigens HLA-A, HLA-B, and HLA-C are class I molecules. Class II MHC molecules, such as the HLA-D antigens DP, DQ, and DR, generally bind peptides derived from exogenous proteins that are degraded in the intracellular vesicles. Peptides that bind to MHC class I molecules usually are 8 to 10 amino acids long. Binding of the peptides is stabilized by contacts between atoms in the free amino- and carboxyl-termini of the peptide and the peptide-binding groove of all MHC class I molecules. In contrast, peptides that bind to MHC class II molecules generally

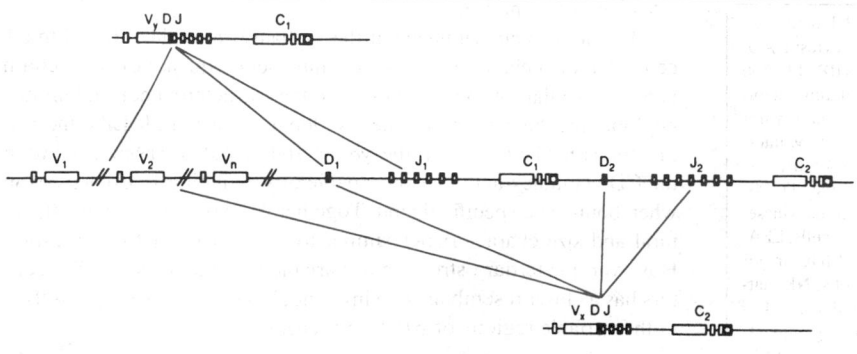

FIGURE 78-2   Schematic diagram of possible rearrangements of the T cell receptor (TCR) β-chain genes. The TCR β-chain genes in the germ-line DNA configuration are depicted in the **middle**. Possible recombination of either the first constant region (C_1, **top**) or the second constant region (C_2, **bottom**) with the variable region (V), diversity (D), or joining (J) segments are indicated by the *lines*.

are 13 or more amino acids long because MHC class II molecules do not bind the two ends of the peptide as do the MHC class I molecules.

Nevertheless, for either class I or class II molecules, a discrete binding site for the peptide lies in a cleft between two α-helices of the MHC molecule. Steric factors, hydrogen bonding, and hydrophobic interactions between the peptide and the particular MHC molecule tether the peptide within this cleft, generating a tertiary structure that is formed by amino acid residues of both the MHC and the peptide antigen. This tertiary structure is recognized by the T cell receptor for antigen.

There are several genes for each class of MHC molecule, and each gene is highly polymorphic with many different alleles (see Chap. 129). The particular combination of MHC alleles found on an individual chromosome is the *MHC haplotype*. Maternal and paternal MHC haplotypes are expressed concomitantly. Polymorphism in the MHC molecules primarily is found in the amino acids lining the clefts that cradle the peptide antigen, allowing the MHC molecules encoded by each allele to bind a distinctive array of different peptides. Structural studies show the T cell receptor can recognize the bound peptide and the amino acid residues that surround the peptide-binding pocket of self- or allogeneic MHC molecules.[13,14]

Each MHC allele encodes an MHC molecule that can bind a restricted set of peptides with a discrete *sequence motif*. Moreover, different alleles of the same MHC molecule bind peptides with different sequence motifs. This polymorphism combined with biallelic expression of MHC genes and the degeneracy of MHC molecules on any given MHC haplotype ensure that a wide variety of different peptides can be presented to the T cell for immune recognition. Because T cells actually interact with a tertiary structure that is largely dictated by a particular MHC molecule, T cells manifest MHC-restricted antigen recognition.

Some T cells do not recognize peptide bound to a given MHC molecule. Such T cells recognize nonpeptide antigens that are presented by MHC class I–like molecules encoded by genes that map outside the MHC region. One such family of molecules is *CD1*, the first defined cluster of differentiation antigen (see Chap. 14). CD1 molecules can present nonpeptide antigens to T cells.[15] For example, in cells infected with mycobacteria, CD1 molecules can bind and present mycobacterial membrane components such as lipoarabinomannan or mycolic acid. T cells that recognize these complexes play an important role in the immune response to *Mycobacterium tuberculosis*.

Structural studies show that $\gamma\delta$-T cell receptors assume a different tertiary structure than $\alpha\beta$-T cell receptors.[7] As such, T cells that express $\gamma\delta$-receptors (so-called $\gamma\delta$-T cells) apparently do not recognize peptides bound to classic MHC class I molecules.[16] Some $\gamma\delta$-T cells recognize products of certain *MHC class IB genes*, or variants of the standard MHC class I genes that have little polymorphism (see Chap. 129). Other $\gamma\delta$-receptors apparently recognize antigen directly, as immunoglobulin molecules do. Finally, $\gamma\delta$-T cells can recognize determinants presented by CD1 molecules.[15] Because increased numbers of $\gamma\delta$-T cells have been found in a variety of infectious and autoimmune diseases, $\gamma\delta$-T cells are speculated to play an immunoregulatory role that is complementary to the function of T cells bearing the more conventional $\alpha\beta$-T cell receptor.[16]

GENERATION OF T CELL RECEPTOR DIVERSITY

Diversity of the T cell receptor for antigen is achieved by several mechanisms, some of which are the same as those that generate diversity among immunoglobulin molecules[17] (see Chap. 77). The joining of different V, D, and J elements to produce a complete V gene, the presence of uncorrected errors made during recombination of these

genetic elements, and the combinatorial diversity afforded by the random pairing of two chains encoded by separated gene complexes all enhance the diversity of the T cell antigen receptor repertoire.[18,19] An important difference between T cells and B cells in how they may enhance receptor diversity is that B cells are capable of somatic hypermutation (see Chap. 77). This process requires expression of activation-induced deaminase and other enzymes that are expressed primarily by B cells within the germinal center of secondary lymphoid tissue during the immune response to antigen (see Chaps. 5 and 77).

The fact that T cell receptor genes do not undergo somatic mutation probably relates to the central role of T cells in directing host immune defenses. During differentiation, immature precursors to $\alpha\beta$-expressing T cells pass through the thymus, where they are "educated" to distinguish self from nonself *vis-à-vis* the cell-surface proteins of MHC[20] (see Chaps. 5 and 76). Because the ligand for the $\alpha\beta$-T cell receptor is "processed" antigen presented by the proteins of the MHC,[21] close interaction with the molecules of the MHC might be lost if the variable region genes of the T cell receptor were allowed to diverge significantly from the inherited germ-line repertoire. Furthermore, somatic mutation of expressed T cell receptor variable region genes may lead to constitutive T cell activation to processed self-antigen presented by self-MHC molecules. Such a scenario could lead to a breakdown in tolerance to self-antigens and autoimmunity.

THE T CELL RECEPTOR COMPLEX

COMPOSITION

Closely associated with and required for surface expression of the two polypeptides of the T cell receptor is the CD3 complex of polypeptides and CD247, known as the zeta-chain (ζ-chain) of the T cell receptor.[22] Unlike T cell receptor heterodimers, these polypeptides are invariant and are found on all T cells that express $\alpha\beta$- or $\gamma\delta$-heterodimers. The CD3 polypeptides are designated CD3γ, CD3δ, CD3ε. The CD3ε chain couples with either the CD3γ or CD3δ chain to generate heterodimers that each forms a tight association with the $\alpha\beta$-receptor (or $\gamma\delta$-receptor) heterodimer on the T cell surface (see Fig. 78-1). Each CD3 polypeptide has a negatively charged amino acid in the central portion of the hydrophobic transmembrane region that stabilizes the CD3 complex with the two chains of the T cell receptor. The ζ-chain (CD247), on the other hand, forms a disulfide-like homodimer that primarily associates with the two T cell receptor chains and only weakly associates with the CD3 complex. As such, it cannot be co-immunoprecipitated readily with antibodies to the CD3 polypeptides. Very little of the ζ-chain is present on the T cell surface (see Fig. 78-1).

MOLECULAR FEATURES OF THE T CELL RECEPTOR COMPLEX

The genes encoding CD3γ, CD3δ, or CD3ε chains are clustered in band q23 on the long arm of chromosome 11. CD3γ has a 16-kDa polypeptide backbone that is heavily glycosylated to assume a final molecular mass of 25 to 28 kDa. CD3δ and CD3ε are each 20 kDa in molecular mass. The CD3δ is a glycoprotein consisting of 30 percent carbohydrate. In contrast, CD3ε is not glycosylated. CD3δ and CD3γ are highly homologous at the protein and nucleic acid sequence levels. The nucleic acid sequence of each predicts CD3δ and CD3γ to have typical signal peptides, respective hydrophilic extracellular domains of 79 to 89 amino acids, hydrophobic transmembrane regions of 27 amino acids, and hydrophilic intracellular domains of 44 to 55 amino acids. CD3ε is similar, with a 22-residue signal peptide, an extracellular domain of 104 amino acids, a transmembrane domain, and a comparatively long intracellular domain of 81 amino acids. Each CD3 polypeptide has one immunoglobulin-like domain in its extracellular domain that is defined by an intrachain disulfide bond (see Fig. 78-1), indicating that these polypeptides are members of the immunoglobulin superfamily. However, unlike the $\alpha\beta$- or $\gamma\delta$-chains of the T cell receptor, no variability is present in the extracellular domains of the CD3 proteins, indicating these molecules do not contribute to the specificity of antigen recognition.

The ζ-chain has no sequence or structural homology to the other three CD3 chains. It is a nonglycosylated protein of 16-kDa molecular mass that is encoded by a gene found on chromosome 1. The ζ-chain has only a very short extracellular domain of six to nine amino acids, a transmembrane domain of 21 amino acids, and a long intracellular domain of 113 amino acids.

The cytoplasmic domains of all the CD3 polypeptides and the ζ-chain each contains sequences called *immunoreceptor tyrosine-based activation motifs* (ITAMs). Each ITAM contains two copies of the sequence tyrosine-X-X-leucine separated by six to eight amino acid residues, in which X represents an unspecified amino acid. The cytoplasmic domains of each CD3 polypeptide contain one ITAM, whereas each ζ-chain contains three ITAMs (see Fig. 78-1). These sequences allow CD3 proteins to associate with cytosolic protein tyrosine kinases following T cell receptor ligation, thus transducing a signal to the interior of the T cell. The cytoplasmic domains of CD3ε and CD3ζ are particularly important in this regard.

SIGNAL TRANSDUCTION VIA THE T CELL RECEPTOR COMPLEX

The CD3 polypeptides and the ζ-chain are responsible for signal transduction from the T cell receptor heterodimer to intracellular proteins.[23] Upon binding to specific ligand, the T cell receptor $\alpha\beta$- (or $\gamma\delta$-) heterodimer undergoes steric changes that result in phosphorylation of the ITAMs of the ζ-chain and each of the CD3 polypeptides (see Fig. 78-1). When the tyrosine residues in the ITAMs become phosphorylated, they can act as docking sites for adapter proteins or tyrosine kinases, such as the zeta-associated protein of 70 kDa (ZAP-70), which possesses a pair of Src homology 2 (SH2) domain and an Src homology 3 (SH3) domain. Following ligation of the T cell receptor, recruitment and activation of a Src family protein tyrosine kinase (e.g., Lck) in turn differentially phosphorylate the ITAMs of the accessory molecules in the T cell receptor complex.[24] ZAP-70 is recruited to the phosphorylated ITAMs of the ζ-chain via its SH2 and SH3 domains and subsequently is activated.[25] Activated ZAP-70 can recruit and phosphorylate a membrane-anchored adapter protein called *linker of activation of T cells* (LAT).[26] Activated LAT in turn can recruit several other adapter proteins, including the SH2-binding leukocyte phosphoprotein of 76 kDa (SLP-76) and Grb2 to the site of T cell receptor clustering.[27] Grb2 in turn can recruit a Ras guanosine triphosphate/guanosine diphosphate (GTP/GDP) exchange factor called *Sos* (because of its structural homology to the *Drosophila* protein called "*son of sevenless*"), which catalyzes GTP for GDP exchange on Ras. This process generates a GTP-bound form of Ras that functions as an allosteric activator of successive mitogen-activated protein (MAP) kinases, culminating in activation of extracellular receptor-activated kinase (ERK)-1 and ERK-2. Activated ERK phosphorylates the protein Elk, which in turn stimulates transcription of Fos, a component of the activation protein-1 (AP-1) factor that is a necessary component of the transcription factor complex required for expression of interleukin (IL)-2.

In parallel with activation of ERK, the adapter proteins that are phosphorylated and recruited to the T cell receptor complex also recruit and activate another GTP/GDP exchange protein called *Vav*, which in turn acts on a 21-kDa guanine nucleotide-binding protein

called Rac. The newly generated GTP-bound form of Rac activates another MAP kinase, called p38, and initiates a parallel enzymatic cascade, resulting in activation of yet another MAP kinase called c-Jun N-terminal kinase (JNK), otherwise known as stress-activated kinase (SAP). Activated JNK phosphorylates c-Jun, the second component of the AP-1 transcription factor required for IL-2 transcription. The GTP-bound form of Rac also induces cytoskeletal reorganization, thereby facilitating the clustering of the T cell receptor complex, accessory molecules, and other accessory proteins at the site(s) of contact between the T cell and the APC.

The activated adapter proteins recruited to the T cell receptor complex also can induce calcium signaling and activation of protein kinase C (PKC) and the phosphoinositide 3 kinase (PI3K).[28] Upon its phosphorylation by ZAP-70, the recruited LAT molecule can directly bind phospholipase C-gamma 1 (PLC-γ1), which in turn is activated through phosphorylation by activated ZAP-70. Activated PLC-γ1 mediates hydrolysis of a plasma membrane phospholipid called phosphatidylinositol 4,5-biphosphate (PIP$_2$), generating inositol 1,4,5-triphosphate (IP$_3$) and diacylglycerol (DAG), which induce a rapid increase in cytosolic free calcium and activation of the ϕ isoform of PKC, respectively. Cytosolic free calcium binds to a ubiquitous calcium-dependent regulatory protein called calmodulin. The calcium–calmodulin complex activates the cytoplasmic phosphatase called *calcineurin*, which in turn catalyzes removal of an inhibitory phosphate group on the *nuclear factor of activated T cells* (NFAT) that retains NFAT proteins in the cytoplasm. Removal of phosphates from NFAT-1 and NFAT-2 by activated calcineurin allows these transcription factors to translocate into the nucleus, where they can enhance transcription of several activation-induced genes, including those encoding IL-2, IL-4, and tumor necrosis factor (TNF). The importance of this pathway in T cell activation is underscored by the strong immunosuppressive activity of the drugs *cyclosporine* and *FK-506*, which can bind cyclophilin and FK-506 binding protein (FKBP), respectively, to form complexes that inhibit the phosphatase activity of calcineurin.

CD4 AND CD8

STRUCTURE OF CD4 AND CD8

CD4 and CD8 are glycoproteins that share structural features with other receptor molecules of the immunoglobulin superfamily. CD8 is expressed as a heterodimer of CD8α and CD8β or as a CD8α/CD8α homodimer. Each chain contains a single immunoglobulin-like domain linked to the membrane by a segment of polypeptide chain that could have an extended conformation. These chains are encoded by genes that are linked closely to the immunoglobulin κ light-chain locus at band p12, on the short arm of chromosome 2. The protein sequence of the amino-terminal domains of each CD8 chain shares greater than 28 percent homology with κ light-chain variable regions. As such, these domains are called the variable region-like (V-like) domains. Following this V-like domain, the CD8 molecule has a short region, rich in proline, threonine, and serine, that resembles the immunoglobulin hinge region. This region also contains sites for O-linked glycosylation. A hydrophobic transmembrane region anchors this hinge-like region. The CD8 molecule has a 25-amino-acid cytoplasmic tail consisting of highly basic residues. Two cysteines within the V-like domain form a disulfide bridge that stabilizes the immunoglobulin-like fold. An additional cysteine residue is located each within the V-like domain, the hinge region, the transmembrane segment, and cytoplasmic domain. These cysteines form intermolecular disulfide bridges between two CD8 molecules, thereby stabilizing the CD8α/CD8β heterodimers or CD8α/CD8α homodimers expressed on the T cell surface. The cell-surface CD8 heterodimer shares structural geometry with the heterodimers formed by the pairing of light-chain and heavy-chain immunoglobulin.

CD4, on the other hand, is expressed as a monomer on the surface of a subset of peripheral T cells, mononuclear phagocytes, and some blood-derived dendritic cells. CD4 is a 55-kDa monomeric glycoprotein encoded by a gene that maps to the short arm of chromosome 12. It consists of five external domains, a stretch of hydrophobic transmembrane residues, and a highly basic cytoplasmic tail of 38 residues. Similar to CD8, the amino-terminal domain of CD4 has extensive homology to immunoglobulin light-chain variable regions. However, following this immunoglobulin-like domain is a domain of 270 amino acids that bears little resemblance to other proteins of the immunoglobulin superfamily.

The cytoplasmic regions of CD4 and CD8 are conserved among vertebrates, which suggests these regions are essential for the function of these molecules. The cytoplasmic region of CD4 contains five serines and threonines, one or more of which is phosphorylated by PKC upon activation of T cells by phorbol esters or exposure to antigen. Subsequent to phosphorylation, the CD4 glycoprotein is internalized concomitant with T cell activation. Similarly, the CD8 protein possesses a highly charged and conserved cytoplasmic domain that may be involved in transmembrane signal transduction. In this light, CD4 and CD8 may be integral components of the functional T cell receptor complex required to trigger T cell activation and/or function upon exposure to specific antigen.

FUNCTION OF CD4 AND CD8

CD4 and CD8 facilitate T cell antigen recognition by interacting with the glycoproteins of MHC.[29] Moreover, during antigen recognition, CD4 and CD8 molecules associate on the plasma membrane with components of the T cell receptor for antigens. For these reasons, the molecules are considered coreceptors of the T cell receptor for antigen.

CD8 molecules bind to the nonpolymorphic $\alpha3$ domain of the HLA class I molecule (HLA-A, HLA-B, or HLA-C),[30] whereas the CD4 molecule binds to the nonpolymorphic $\beta2$ domain of HLA class II molecules (HLA-D region-encoded molecules: DP, DQ, and DR).[31] CD8 or CD4 enhance by more than 100-fold the adhesion between the T cell's CD3/T cell receptor complex and the MHC glycoproteins expressed by an APC or target cell. The molecules apparently focus MHC molecules of the APC or target cell onto the T cell surface, allowing for specific recognition of "processed" antigen that is cradled within the MHC glycoproteins. Because CD4 and CD8 differ in their MHC-binding specificities, T cells expressing CD4 or CD8 generally recognize antigens presented by class II or class I MHC glycoproteins, respectively.[32] The selectivity is underscored by studies on knockout mice lacking expression of either of the accessory molecules. Mice lacking CD4 or CD8 fail to develop class II-restricted or class I-restricted T cells, respectively, indicating the coreceptors play essential roles in the maturation of T cells in the thymus. A similar defect is observed in patients with the bear lymphocyte syndrome, who have a congenital immune deficiency caused by genetic defects in their capacity to make MHC class II molecules.[33] Although patients have normal numbers of B cells and T cells, they have markedly reduced numbers of CD4+ T cells, which partly accounts for their profound immune deficiency.

In addition to serving as coreceptors, CD4 or CD8 molecules enhance antigen responsiveness by transducing a signal either directly or in concert with the CD3/T cell receptor complex.[34] Such signal transducing functions are mediated through their interaction with the Src family tyrosine kinase called Lck. Lck is noncovalently associated with the cytoplasmic tails of CD4 and/or CD8. When a T cell recog-

nizes a peptide antigen presented by an appropriate MHC antigen, the interaction of CD4 or CD8 with the MHC molecule brings Lck close to the T cell receptor complex. Lck then phosphorylates the tyrosine residues in the ITAMs of CD3 polypeptides and the ζ chain, thereby initiating the receptor signaling required for T cell activation.

Finally, CD4 also is a coreceptor molecule for the human immunodeficiency virus (HIV).[35,36] Binding of CD4 along with a chemokine receptor facilitates virus entry into T cells that are stimulated specifically in an antigen-driven immune response. Monoclonal antibodies specific for the CD4 glycoprotein can block infection by HIV. Moreover, genetically engineered soluble CD4 can compete with cell-surface CD4 for HIV binding. Finally, disease progression in patients infected with HIV correlates with depletion of blood T cells that express CD4 (see Chap. 83).

T CELL SUBSETS

PRECURSOR THYMOCYTES

CD4 and CD8 are expressed by nearly all T cell precursors. Only a fraction of thymocytes express neither CD4 nor CD8. These cells are thought to be the marrow-derived precursors to the vast majority of thymocytes that express both CD4 and CD8. More mature thymocytes and all peripheral T cells express either CD4 or CD8, but not both (see Chap. 76).

HELPER AND SUPPRESSOR (CYTOLYTIC) T CELLS

The mutually exclusive expression of CD4 or CD8 defines two major blood T cell subsets. Blood T cells that express CD8 are designated suppressor T cells. These cells normally constitute 25 to 35 percent of the peripheral T cell population. Suppressor T cells more appropriately should be designated cytolytic T lymphocytes (CTLs) because one of their main functions is to lyse cells, termed target cells, which bear surface antigens for which they are specific. Blood T cells that solely express the CD4 surface antigen are designated helper T cells. These cells normally compose 65 percent of blood T cells. Generally, helper T cells produce lymphokines upon activation by foreign antigens presented by MHC molecules expressed on the surface of APCs.

CD4+ T CELL SUBSETS

Th1 AND Th2 CELLS
Mature CD4+ T cells can be divided into at least two subsets, each able to elaborate a distinctive profile of cytokines upon activation.[37,38] The primary differences between the subsets are that Th1 cells are the major helper T cell source of IL-2, interferon gamma (IFN-γ), and TNF-β,[39] whereas Th2 cells are the predominate producers of IL-4 and IL-5[40] (Table 78-1). In addition, Th1 cells may be the major helper T cell source of TNF-α and granulocyte-macrophage colony stimulating factor (GM-CSF), whereas Th2 cells apparently are the major T cell producers of IL-10 and IL-13. A third cell subset, designated Th0, is composed of CD4+ helper T cells that may elaborate all of these cytokines and may represent a precursor population to the other two subsets. Although these subsets initially were considered mutually exclusive, individual T cells now are recognized as possibly expressing various mixtures of cytokines. As such, more T cell subpopulations have more heterogeneous patterns of cytokine expression.

The CD4+ T cell subsets are distinguished most effectively by the cytokines they produce and not by the surface antigens or cytokine receptors they express. Nevertheless, human Th1 cells preferentially express CD26, membrane IFN-γ, and the chemokine receptors CCR5 and CXCR3.[41] Moreover, Th1 cells may express higher levels of *lymphocyte activation gene-3 (LAG-3)*, a ligand for MHC class II antigens

TABLE 78-1   MAJOR CD4+ T-CELL SUBSETS

	CD4+ T-CELL SUBSET	
	TH1	TH2
Cytokine Production		
IL-2	+	−
IFN-γ	++	−
TNF-β	++	−
IL-4	−	++
IL-5	−	++
TNF-α	++	+
GM-CSF	++	+
IL-10	+/−	++
IL-13	−	++
Functions		
B cell help		
Total Ig	+	+++
IgE	−	++
Mast cell production	−	++
Eosinophil production	−	++
Macrophage activation	++	−
Delayed-type hypersensitivity	++	−

that is structurally related to CD4.[42] Th2 cells, on the other hand, preferentially express CD62L, CD30, and the chemokine receptors CCR3, CCR4, CCR8, and, to some extent, CXCR4.[41,43,44] Distinctive expression levels of these chemokine receptors and distinctive binding activities for various endothelial selectins may account for the differences in the tissue-specific migration of the helper T cell subsets.[45]

Each of the two T cell subsets has a discrete function.[46] The principle functions of Th1 cells are to activate macrophages to kill microorganisms and to induce B cells to make subclasses of immunoglobulin (Ig) G antibodies that are very effective at opsonizing extracellular pathogens for uptake by phagocytic cells. In addition, Th1 cells are the major helper T cells involved in delayed-type hypersensitivity. The cytokines elaborated by Th1 cells stimulate macrophage Fc receptor expression, phagocytosis, and antigen presentation, enhancing the capacity of macrophages to kill intracellular pathogens. Th2 cells, on the other hand, initiate the antibody response to antigen by activating naive antigen-specific B cells to produce IgM antibodies and subsequently stimulate the production of switched immunoglobulin isotypes, including IgA, IgE, and neutralizing and/or weakly opsonizing subtypes of IgG (see Chap. 77). In addition to stimulating the production of IgE antibodies, the cytokines made by Th2 cells induce differentiation of mast cells and eosinophils. Although these effects may contribute to development of allergy,[47,48] these responses may be protective in helminth infections.[49,50] Studies demonstrate that eosinophilia and elevated IgE accompanying infection with Schistosoma mansoni, for example, result from induction of Th2-type cells in the immune response to parasite ova.[51,52] In addition, because Th2 cells express the B cell stimulatory/growth factor IL-4, Th2 cells appear better suited than Th1 cells to induce B cell responses to antigen.

The cytokines produced by each subset stimulate differentiation of additional T cells of the same subset. For example, the IFN-γ and IL-12 elaborated by Th1 cells promote further Th1 differentiation and inhibit proliferation of Th2 cells. The Th1 cytokines IFN-γ or IL-12 respectively induce or activate Tbet and signal transducer of activated T cells-4 (STAT4), transcription factors that play critical roles in Th1 cell differentiation.[39,53,54] On the other hand, IL-4, the archetypical Th2 cytokine, respectively activates or enhances expression of STAT6 and GATA-3, transcription factors that play important roles in Th2 cell

development.[55,56] Another Th2 cytokine, IL-10, inhibits Th1 cell activation, thereby limiting production of Th1-type cytokines. Because of these self-amplifying and mutually excluding feedback loops, an immune response becomes increasingly polarized once it develops along a Th1 or Th2 pathway, particularly upon protracted stimulation by chronic infection or prolonged exposure to environmental antigens.

Extracellular antigens tend to stimulate generation of Th2 cells, whereas pathogens that accumulate in large numbers inside macrophage vesicles tend to stimulate differentiation of Th1 cells.[57] CD4+ T cells secrete minute amounts of IL-4 during their initial activation. If the antigen is present at high concentrations and does not trigger inflammation and attendant production of IL-12, then the local concentration of IL-4 increases over time, inducing differentiation of Th2 cells. Because of this process, Th2 cells typically develop in response to helminth infections or noninflammatory environmental allergens.[40] On the other hand, pathogens that induce inflammation and/or engage Toll-like receptors on accessory cells and macrophages can promote production of IFN-γ and IL-12, thereby stimulating development of the immune response down the Th1 pathway.[39] Immune responses restricted to that of Th1 cells, for example, are observed in patients with leprosy who have developed cellular immunity to *Mycobacterium leprae*[58] or in patients with arthritis triggered by infection with either *Borrelia burgdorferi* (Lyme disease)[59] or *Yersinia enterocolitica*.[60]

CD4+CD25+ REGULATORY T CELLS
Another subset of CD4 T cells apparently functions to suppress immune responses rather than to provide the helper activity that typically is associated with CD4 T cells. In addition to CD3 and CD4, these cells have surface expression of CD25, the low-affinity receptor for IL-2 (see Chap. 14). These cells sometimes are referred to as "T_{reg}" cells, which is an abbreviation of the term *CD4+CD25+ regulatory T cells*.[61] T_{reg} cells can suppress immune responses to self-antigens and environmental antigens. They are thought to play a role in maintaining tolerance to self-antigens and in preventing runaway immune responses to environmental antigens that might evolve into cross-reactive autoimmunity.[62,63]

MEMORY T CELLS

Following a successful immune response to antigen, antigen-specific T lymphocytes may differentiate into memory T cells.[64–66] These cells may have less stringent requirements for activation and an enhanced capacity for lymphokine production upon rechallenge with the same antigen.[67] Alternatively, these cells may develop an impaired responsiveness to antigen when stimulated in the absence of certain costimulatory factors, thus rendering the cells "anergic."[68] In any case, naive and memory CD4+ or CD8+ T lymphocytes apparently differ in surface phenotypes, response to recall antigens, rate of cycling, and migration.[69,70] These subsets may be distinguished using antibodies specific for isoforms of CD45.[71,72]

CD45, also known as *leukocyte common antigen* or *T200*, consists of a family of membrane glycoproteins, ranging from 180 to 220 kDa, that are expressed on all leukocytes. Each member is the product of a single complex gene on chromosome 1 that contains 34 exons. Exons 3 through 7 can be spliced differently at the RNA transcript level to generate several distinct mRNA and protein products. The deduced amino acid sequences of these protein products have extracellular domains ranging from 391 to 552 amino acids, a transmembrane region, and a highly conserved cytoplasmic domain of 705 amino acids. This large cytoplasmic domain contains an intrinsic tyrosine phosphatase activity that is important in the regulation of various activation pathways involving tyrosine kinase activity, such as those involved in signal transduction via the T cell receptor for antigen.[73–75]

Differential glycosylation of the CD45 peptide backbone contributes further to the heterogeneity of the members of this protein family. Different isoforms of CD45 have distinct patterns of expression during lymphocyte ontogeny and activation.[76] Monoclonal antibodies have been developed that recognize individual members of this family that are expressed on physiologically distinct lymphocyte subsets (see Chap. 14). Isoforms of CD45 that are expressed on such distinct subsets of cells are designated *CD45R*.

Naive CD4+ T cells express a form of CD45R, called *CD45RA*, whereas memory CD4+ T cells and CD8+ T cells express another isoform of CD45R, designated *CD45RO*. These isoforms can be recognized by monoclonal antibodies 2H4 and UCHL1, respectively.[77] Evaluation for the expression level of another isoform of CD45, designated *CD45RB*, can be useful for distinguishing memory T cells. Within the CD4+ memory T cell population, for example, increased helper activity is associated with the shift from a CD45RB[bright] to a CD45RB[dim] phenotype.[78] In addition, relative to naive T cells, memory T cells express lower levels of L-selectin (CD62L) and higher levels of CD29 and CD44[65] (see Chap. 14). Whether the differentiation of CD4+ T cells with the "naive" phenotype (i.e., CD4+CD45RA+CD29[low]CD44[low]) to cells having the "memory" phenotype (i.e., CD4+CD45RO+CD29[high]CD44[high]) is irreversible[77] and whether these phenotypic changes are valid for all Th1- and Th2-type CD4+ T cells[79] are uncertain.

Memory T cells express higher levels of certain adhesion molecules, such as integrins and CD44, which facilitate the homing and migration of memory cells to sites of inflammation or secondary lymphoid tissues. Some memory T cells migrate preferentially to lymph nodes, where they can be activated rapidly in response to reexposure to antigen. Other memory T cells circulate in the blood or reside in mucosal or dermal tissue, from where they can be recruited to distant or to local sites of inflammation, respectively.

T CELL ACCESSORY MOLECULES

IMMUNE MODULATORY MOLECULES

CD28

CD28 is a 44-kDa disulfide-linked homodimer that is expressed on most resting T cells and plasma cells.[80,81] Mature thymocytes have higher levels of CD28 than immature cells. Among peripheral T cells, more than 90 percent of CD4+ T cells and approximately 50 percent of CD8 T cells express CD28. In general, activation of T cells induces enhanced expression of CD28, but ligation of CD28 leads to transient T cell down-regulation.[81]

CD28 is another member of the immunoglobulin superfamily that is an important receptor for CD80 and CD86. It binds to CD80 and CD86 using a highly conserved motif (MYPPPY) in a loop that resembles the third complementarity-determining region of immunoglobulin molecules.[82] CD28 binds to CD80 with relatively low affinity ($K_d = 4 \mu M$) and dissociates very rapidly ($K_{off} = 1.6 s^{-1}$).[83] Its binding to CD86 may be even weaker.[84]

CD28 is one of the major costimulatory molecules important in T cell activation.[85] CD28 may enhance signaling by the T cell receptor complex by stabilizing and prolonging the synapse between T cells and APCs. More importantly, ligation of CD28 by CD80, CD86, or anti-CD28 antibodies activates distinct signaling pathways that function with the signals induced by ligation of the T cell receptor to allow for T cell activation and proliferation.[80,86–89] Following coligation of CD28, the Src kinases Lck and Fyn may phosphorylate a tyrosine within an ITAM found in the cytoplasmic domain of CD28, allowing the latter to bind and activate PI3K via its SH2 domains.[28] CD28 signaling also facilitates GTP/GDP exchange in Ras, resulting in acti-

vation of the MAP kinase pathway, activation of Akt kinase, and activation of the adapter protein Vav and the associated Rac pathway.[28] These signals enhance the transcription of IL-2 and the stability of IL-2 transcripts, thereby stimulating T cell proliferation.[90] Although mice lacking CD28 can mount effective T cell responses, they are defective in T cell-dependent antibody responses, suggesting that CD28 is necessary for T cell to B cell interactions and the proficient generation of antibody responses to antigen.[91]

The requirement that the same cell present both the specific antigen and the costimulatory signal plays an important role in preventing destructive autoimmune responses to self-tissues.[92] Initiation of T cell responses requires simultaneous ligation of the T cell receptor and CD28. This requirement restricts the initiation of T cell responses to APCs that express both the peptide antigen in the context of self-MHC molecules and the ligands for CD28, namely, CD80 and CD86. This is important, as not all self-reactive T cells undergo deletion in the thymus because not all self-peptides are presented in the thymus (see Chap. 5). This is especially true for specialized tissues that express proteins that are never expressed in the thymus. If simultaneous ligation of the T cell receptor and CD28 was not required, then T cells that recognize the self-peptide expressed by the MHC of such specialized tissues could become activated, leading to autoimmune rejection of the specialized tissue. Instead, ligation of the T cell receptor in the absence of CD28 ligation leads to a state of anergy in which the T cell expressing that receptor becomes refractory to activation.[93] Anergic T cells are unable to produce IL-2 following ligation of their antigen receptors. This inability prevents the T cells from proliferating and differentiating into effector cells when they encounter antigen. This is an important basis for development of peripheral tolerance for self-antigens that are not expressed in the thymus (see Chaps. 5 and 76).

CTLA-4 (CD152)

CTLA-4 (CD152) is another receptor for CD80 and CD86. It is a 50-kDa disulfide-linked homodimer that shares 31 percent identity with CD28. The gene encoding this receptor is closely linked with the gene encoding CD28 on the long arm of chromosome 2 at 2q33-q34. However, in contrast to the constitutive expression of CD28, T cells express CD152 only upon activation. Expression of CD152 peaks approximately 24 hours after activation and then subsides by 72 hours but is always approximately 30- to 50-fold lower than that of CD28. Ligation of CD28 is particularly effective in inducing CD152.

CD152 binds to CD80 and CD86 using the same highly conserved motif (MYPPPY) used by CD28, which, like CD28, is in a loop that resembles the third complementarity-determining region of immunoglobulin molecules. However, CD152 binds to CD80 and CD86 approximately 20 times more avidly than does CD28, with K_d values of .4 and 2.2 μM, respectively.[83,84]

In contrast to CD28, ligation of CD152 transmits a negative signal to T cell activation.[27] Instead of an ITAM in its cytoplasmic domain, CD152 possesses an "*immunoreceptor tyrosine-based inhibitory motif*" (or ITIM) in its cytoplasmic domain. Ligation of CD152 induces tyrosine phosphorylation of the ITIM, which in turn recruits the tyrosine phosphatase SHP-2 that can deactivate the phosphorylated ITAMs of the ξ chains (CD247) of the T cell receptor complex.[88,94] Mice made genetically deficient in CD152 develop a fatal disorder characterized by massive lymphocyte proliferation,[95,96] indicating CD152 serves as an important brake on runaway T cell activation. On the other hand, anti-CD152 monoclonal antibodies that block the interaction of CD152 with CD80 and CD86 can enhance T cell responses *in vitro* and *in vivo*,[97,98] prompting their evaluation as immune-enhancing agents in vaccine studies or clinical trials in active immune therapy.

1072

PART VIII LYMPHOCYTES AND PLASMA CELLS

Antigen-Presenting Cell

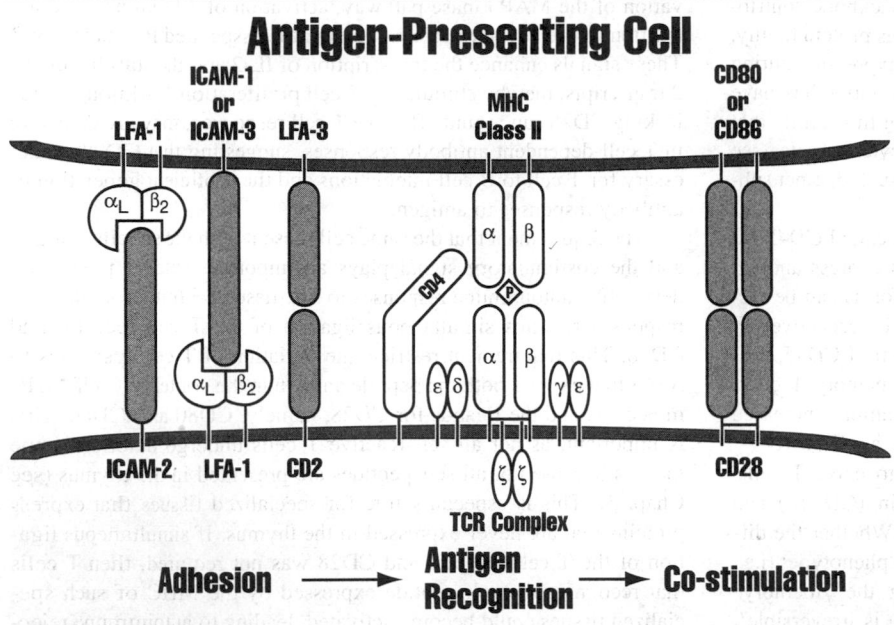

FIGURE 78-3 Schematic diagram of T cell interactions with an antigen-presenting cell (APC). *Thick gray lines* depict the plasma membranes of the interacting cells. The molecules of the APC (namely, LFA-1, ICAM-1, or ICAM-3, LFA-3; MHC class II; and CD80 or CD86) are displayed on **top**. T cell antigens (ICAM-2, LFA-1, CD2, CD4, T cell receptor [TCR] complex, and CD28) are shown on the **bottom**. *Thin lines* connecting the stick figures indicate disulfide bridges. The TCR complex consists of the αβ heterodimer, which is noncovalently coupled with the δ-, ε-, γ-, and ζ-chains of CD3, as indicated. This complex can recognize peptide antigen (designated by the *diamond* labeled P), which is cradled by the α- and β-chains of the MHC class II molecule of the APC. The avidity of this interaction is enhanced by CD4 on the T cell surface that interacts with nonpolymorphic determinants on the MHC class II molecule. The interaction steps between the T cell and the APC are listed at the **bottom** of the figure. T cell molecules ICAM-2 (CD102), LFA-1 (CD11a/CD18), and CD2 bind to LFA-1, ICAM-1 (CD54) or ICAM-3 (CD50), or LFA-3 (CD58), respectively, which are present on the surface of the APC. These molecules provide for better adhesion between the T cell and the APC (adhesion), allowing time for the TCR receptor complex to find the MHC molecule bearing a specific peptide antigen (antigen recognition). Should the APC express CD80 or CD86, then simultaneous ligation of CD28 occurs (costimulation), leading to activation of the reactive T cell.

OTHER MEMBERS OF THE CD28 RECEPTOR FAMILY
Homology-based cloning strategies have identified other proteins that are structurally related to CD28/CTLA-4 or its ligand CD80. These proteins are considered members of the CD28 or CD80 (B7) families, respectively. All of these proteins are members of the larger immunoglobulin superfamily. Two more recently identified members of the CD28 family are *ICOS* (for "*inducible costimulator*" because of its expression on activated T cells) and *PD-1* (for "*programmed death-1*" because this molecule initially was thought to regulate programmed cell death of T cells).[99] Whereas ICOS is found primarily on activated T cells, PD-1 can be found on activated T cells, B cells, and some myeloid cells. ICOS or PD-1 binds to the ICOS ligand (ICOS-L) or the PD ligands PD-L1 or PD-L2, respectively. ICOS-L, PD-L1, and PD-L2 belong to the CD80 (B7) family of surface molecules and are found or can be induced on B cells, APCs, and other tissues. Whereas ICOS primarily functions as a costimulatory molecule for cells bearing ICOS-L, PD-1 apparently plays a negative regulatory role on activated T cells. Like CD152, PD-1 possesses an ITIM motif in its cytoplasmic tail that, upon phosphorylation, can recruit the tyrosine phosphatase SHP-2. In this regard, PD-1 may play a role similar to that of CD152, helping to brake cellular activation when expressed in the context of cells expressing PD-L1 or PD-L2.

T CELL ADHESION MOLECULES

DEFINITION

Besides the CD3/T cell receptor molecules and CD4 or CD8, several other surface proteins are required for efficient T cell antigen recognition.[100] Some of these surface proteins can be termed *adhesion molecules*, in that they facilitate the adhesion of the T cell to its appropriate APC or target cell (Fig. 78-3).[101] By facilitating cell adhesion, these accessory molecules permit the T cell antigen receptor complex to interact better with the MHC glycoproteins of the other cell, allowing for efficient T cell antigen recognition and activation. Because each member of this group of accessory molecules has distinctive affinities for the surface molecules expressed by the APC or target cell, differential expression of the accessory molecules may pattern differences in the antigenic specificities and/or cell types with which a given T cell best may interact. As such, the differential expression of these accessory molecules by peripheral T cells may define physiologically distinct T cell subsets.

LYMPHOCYTE FUNCTION-ASSOCIATED GLYCOPROTEINS

The lymphocyte function-associated (LFA) molecules are an important family of glycoproteins that facilitate efficient cell–cell adhesion.[102,103] The molecules were first identified with monoclonal antibodies that could block T cell function, such as cytotoxic T cell-mediated killing of target cells. From these early experiments, three major surface molecules were identified and designated *LFA-1, LFA-2,* and *LFA-3*. Following international convention, LFA-2 is referred to as CD2.

LFA-1 belongs to a family of three related glycoproteins: LFA-1, MAC-1, and p150,95 (see Chap. 14). These proteins also are called *integrins* because they are hypothesized to coordinate the binding of cells to other cell types and to extracellular proteins.[104] Each protein consists of a distinct α-subunit noncovalently associated with the common β2-subunit glycoprotein of 95 kDa, designated *CD18*. Because they share a common β2-subunit, these molecules also are referred to as the β2-*integrins*. The α subunit of LFA-1, designated *CD11a*, is a 180-kDa glycoprotein (see Chap. 14). Coupled with the common β2-subunit, this 180-kDa molecule is expressed on more than one third of all marrow cells, all T cells, B cells, and natural killer (NK) cells. The α-subunit of MAC-1 is a glycoprotein of 170 kDa, designated *CD11b*. MAC-1 is expressed on NK cells, monocytes, macrophages, granulocytes, and small subpopulations of T and B cells. The α-subunit of p150,95, designated *CD11c*, is a 150-kDa glycoprotein that is not expressed by T lymphocytes.

The LFA-1 family of glycoproteins is composed of important adhesion molecules.[102,105] The shared β2-subunit (CD18) has extensive sequence homology to the β3-subunit (CD61) of the platelet adhesion receptor glycoprotein IIb/IIIa (CD41/CD61) and the β1-subunit (CD29) of a family of related adhesion proteins termed *very late activation* (VLA) antigens. Many of these receptors function in cell–cell interactions and recognize their ligands at sites that contain the amino acid sequence Arg-Gly-Asp. In addition, the α-subunit provides some selectivity. LFA-1, because of its α-subunit, binds best to cell surface ligands called *intercellular adhesion molecules* (ICAMs), namely, ICAM-1 (CD54), ICAM-2 (CD102), and ICAM-3 (CD50) (see Chap. 14). ICAM-1 and ICAM-2 are expressed on endothelial cells and APCs. Binding of LFA-1 on lymphocytes to these molecules allows lymphocytes to migrate through blood vessel walls. ICAM-3 is expressed only on leukocytes, including T cells, and is thought to play an important role in adhesion of T cells with LFA-1 expressed on APCs (see Fig. 78-3).

LFA glycoproteins are required for proper T cell function and host immunity. Monoclonal antibodies specific for LFA-1 may inhibit T cell-directed cytolysis of target cells. Furthermore, a few CD8+ or CD4+ cytolytic T cell clones express MAC-1. Antibodies to CD11b may inhibit conjugate formation between these T cell clones and their specific target cells and thus block cytotoxic T lymphocyte-mediated killing. Finally, patients with an inherited deficiency in the ability to produce the common β_2-subunit (CD18) suffer from recurrent life-threatening bacterial and fungal infections and rarely survive beyond childhood.

LFA molecules are important for initial T cell interactions with APCs. LFA-1, CD2, and ICAM-3 on the T cell interact with ICAM-1, ICAM-2, LFA-1, and LFA-3 on the APC (see Fig. 78-3). This process provides time for the T cell to sample large numbers of MHC molecules on the plasma membrane of the APC for the presence of specific peptide antigen. When a naive T cell recognizes its specific peptide in the context of the MHC, signaling through the T cell receptor induces a conformational change in LFA-1 that greatly increases its affinity for ICAM-1 and ICAM-2. This change stabilizes the association between the antigen-specific T cell and the APC. This association can last for several days during which time the naive T cell proliferates, forming daughter cells that also adhere to the APC and differentiate into armed effector T cells.

VERY LATE ACTIVATION ANTIGENS

The VLA molecules are β_1 integrins in that that each shares a common β_1 unit (CD29) that is paired with any one of six different α chains (α_1–α_6), designated CD49a to CD49f (see Chap. 14). CD49a, CD49b, CD49c, CD49d, CD49e, and CD49f form molecules called VLA-1, VLA-2, VLA-3, VLA-4, VLA-5, and VLA-6, respectively, when paired with CD29. These molecules are called *"very late antigens"* because the first identified VLA molecules, namely, VLA-1 and VLA-2, initially were found on T cells only weeks after repetitive stimulation *in vitro*. However, some of these VLA molecules, most notably VLA-4, also are expressed constitutively by some T cells and are rapidly induced on others. VLA-4 plays an important role in facilitating the attachment of cells that bear this molecule to the endothelium through its binding to vascular cell adhesion molecule-1 (VCAM-1), designated CD106 (see Chap. 14). CD106 can be up-regulated by various proinflammatory cytokines. Up-regulation of CD106 allows VLA-4 to play an important role in facilitating the homing of T cells to endothelium at sites of inflammation.

CD2

CD2 is a glycoprotein of approximately 50 kDa found on all T lymphocytes, large granular lymphocytes, and thymocytes.[106] CD2 facilitates cell–cell adhesion by binding to LFA-3, a 55- to 70-kDa surface glycoprotein expressed on erythrocytes, leukocytes, and endothelial, epithelial, and connective tissue cells in most organ studies (see Fig. 78-3 and see Chap. 14). Monoclonal antibodies that bind CD2 may inhibit a variety of T lymphocyte functions, including antigen-specific T lymphocyte-proliferative responses to lectins, alloantigens, and soluble antigens. Anti-CD2 inhibits cytotoxic T lymphocyte-mediated

cell killing by binding to the T cell rather than to the target, which generally does not express CD2. On the other hand, antibodies directed against LFA-3 inhibit cytotoxic T lymphocyte-mediated cell killing by binding to LFA-3 on the target cell, blocking interaction of CD2 with LFA-3. T cells can be activated by certain monoclonal antibodies to CD2, apparently independent of the CD3/T cell receptor complex.[107] Thus, in addition to being a receptor for LFA-3, CD2 plays a role in transmembrane signal transduction leading to T cell activation in response to antigen.

REFERENCES

1. Garcia KC, Teyton L, Wilson IA: Structural basis of T cell recognition. *Annu Rev Immunol* 17:369, 1999.
2. Barclay AN, Brown MH, Alex Law SK, et al: Protein superfamilies and cell surface molecules, in *The Leucocyte Antigen Facts Book*, 2nd ed, p 32. San Diego: Academic Press, San Diego, 1997.
3. Kabelitz D, Wesch D, Hinz T: Gamma delta T cells, their T cell receptor usage and role in human diseases. *Springer Semin Immunopathol* 21:55, 1999.
4. Kang J, Raulet DH: Events that regulate differentiation of alpha beta TCR+ and gamma delta TCR+ T cells from a common precursor. *Semin Immunol* 9:171, 1997.
5. Hayday AC, Barber DF, Douglas N, Hoffman ES: Signals involved in gamma/delta T cell versus alpha/beta T cell lineage commitment. *Semin Immunol* 11:239, 1999.
6. Jouen-Beades F, Paris E, Dieulois C, et al: In vivo and in vitro activation and expansion of gammadelta T cells during Listeria monocytogenes infection in humans. *Infect Immun* 65:4267, 1997.
7. Allison TJ, Winter CC, Fournie JJ, et al: Structure of a human gammadelta T-cell antigen receptor. *Nature* 411:820, 2001.
8. Rockman SP: Determination of clonality in patients who present with diagnostic dilemmas: A laboratory experience and review of the literature. *Leukemia* 11:852, 1997.
9. Dibenedetto SP, Lo Nigro L, Di Cataldo A, Schilirò G: Detection of minimal residual disease: Methods and relationship to outcome in T-lineage acute lymphoblastic leukemia. *Leuk Lymphoma* 32:65, 1998.
10. Lefranc MP: Organization of the human T-cell receptor genes. *Eur Cytokine Netw* 1:121, 1990.
11. Krangel MS, Hernandez-Munain C, Lauzurica P, et al: Developmental regulation of V(D)J recombination at the TCR alpha/delta locus. *Immunol Rev* 165:131, 1998.
12. Housset D, Malissen B: What do TCR-pMHC crystal structures teach us about MHC restriction and alloreactivity? *Trends Immunol* 24:429, 2003.
13. Marchalonis JJ, Jensen I, Schluter SF: Structural, antigenic and evolutionary analyses of immunoglobulins and T cell receptors. *J Mol Recognit* 15:260, 2002.
14. Whitelegg A, Barber LD: The structural basis of T-cell allorecognition. *Tissue Antigens* 63:101, 2004.
15. Brigl M, Brenner MB: CD1: Antigen presentation and T cell function. *Annu Rev Immunol* 22:817, 2004.
16. Carding SR, Egan PJ: Gammadelta T cells: Functional plasticity and heterogeneity. *Nat Rev Immunol* 2:336, 2002.
17. Krangel MS, Hernandez-Munain C, Lauzurica P, et al: Developmental regulation of V(D)J recombination at the TCR alpha/delta locus. *Immunol Rev* 165:131, 1998.
18. Posnett DN: Environmental and genetic factors shape the human T-cell receptor repertoire. *Ann N Y Acad Sci* 756:71, 1995.
19. Theofilopoulos AN, Baccalà R, González-Quintial R, et al: T-cell repertoires in health and disease. *Ann N Y Acad Sci* 756:53, 1995.
20. Nikolich-Zugich J, Slifka MK, Messaoudi I: The many important facets of T-cell repertoire diversity. *Nat Rev Immunol* 4:123, 2004.

21. Germain RN, Margulies DH: The biochemistry and cell biology of antigen processing and presentation. *Annu Rev Immunol* 11:403, 1993.

22. Call ME, Wucherpfennig KW: Molecular mechanisms for the assembly of the T cell receptor-CD3 complex. *Mol Immunol* 40:1295, 2004.

23. Peterson EJ, Koretzky GA: Signal transduction in T lymphocytes. *Clin Exp Rheumatol* 17:107, 1999.

24. Guirado M, de Aos I, Orta T, et al: Phosphorylation of the N-terminal and C-terminal CD3-epsilon-ITAM tyrosines is differentially regulated in T cells. *Biochem Biophys Res Commun* 291:574, 2002.

25. Qian D, Weiss A: T cell antigen receptor signal transduction. *Curr Opin Cell Biol* 9:205, 1997.

26. Sommers CL, Samelson LE, Love PE: LAT: A T lymphocyte adapter protein that couples the antigen receptor to downstream signaling pathways. *Bioessays* 26:61, 2004.

27. Saito T, Yamasaki S: Negative feedback of T cell activation through inhibitory adapters and costimulatory receptors. *Immunol Rev* 192:143, 2003.

28. Kane LP, Weiss A: The PI-3 kinase/Akt pathway and T cell activation: Pleiotropic pathways downstream of PIP3. *Immunol Rev* 192:7, 2003.

29. Zamoyska R: CD4 and CD8: Modulators of T-cell receptor recognition of antigen and of immune responses? *Curr Opin Immunol* 10:82, 1998.

30. Gao GF, Jakobsen BK: Molecular interactions of coreceptor CD8 and MHC class I: The molecular basis for functional coordination with the T-cell receptor. *Immunol Today* 21:630, 2000.

31. Reinherz EL, Tan K, Tang L, et al: The crystal structure of a T cell receptor in complex with peptide and MHC class II. *Science* 286:1913, 1999.

32. Janeway CAJ: The co-receptor function of CD4. *Semin Immunol* 3:153, 1991.

33. Reith W, Mach B: The bare lymphocyte syndrome and the regulation of MHC expression. *Annu Rev Immunol* 19:331, 2001.

34. Miceli MC, Parnes JR: Role of CD4 and CD8 in T cell activation and differentiation. *Adv Immunol* 53:59, 1993.

35. Virelizier JL: Blocking HIV co-receptors by chemokines. *Dev Biol Stand* 97:105, 1999.

36. Berger EA, Murphy PM, Farber JM: Chemokine receptors as HIV-1 coreceptors: Roles in viral entry, tropism, and disease. *Annu Rev Immunol* 17:657, 1999.

37. Romagnani S: Human TH1 and TH2 subsets: Doubt no more. *Immunol Today* 12:256, 1991.

38. Powrie F, Coffman RL: Cytokine regulation of T-cell function: Potential for therapeutic intervention. *Immunol Today* 14:270, 1993.

39. O'Garra A, Robinson D: Development and function of T helper 1 cells. *Adv Immunol* 83:133, 2004.

40. Stetson DB, Voehringer D, Grogan JL, et al: Th2 cells: Orchestrating barrier immunity. *Adv Immunol* 83:163, 2004.

41. Annunziato F, Galli G, Cosmi L, et al: Molecules associated with human Th1 or Th2 cells. *Eur Cytokine Netw* 9:12, 1998.

42. Huard B, Mastrangeli R, Prigent P, et al: Characterization of the major histocompatibility complex class II binding site on LAG-3 protein. *Proc Natl Acad Sci U S A* 94:5744, 1997.

43. Zingoni A, Soto H, Hedrick JA, et al: The chemokine receptor CCR8 is preferentially expressed in Th2 but not Th1 cells. *J Immunol* 161:547, 1998.

44. Kim CH, Broxmeyer HE: Chemokines: Signal lamps for trafficking of T and B cells for development and effector function. *J Leukoc Biol* 65:6, 1999.

45. O'Garra A, McEvoy LM, Zlotnik A: T-cell subsets: Chemokine receptors guide the way. *Curr Biol* 8:R646, 1998.

46. Lucey DR: Evolution of the type-1 (Th1)-type-2 (Th2) cytokine paradigm. *Infect Dis Clin North Am* 13:1, 1999.

47. Del Prete G: Human Th1 and Th2 lymphocytes: Their role in the pathophysiology of atopy. *Allergy* 47:450, 1992.

48. van Reijsen FC, Bruijnzeel-Koomen CA, Kalthoff FS, et al: Skin-derived aeroallergen-specific T-cell clones of Th2 phenotype in patients with atopic dermatitis. *J Allergy Clin Immunol* 90:184, 1992.

49. Sher A, Coffman RL: Regulation of immunity to parasites by T cells and T cell-derived cytokines. *Annu Rev Immunol* 10:385, 1992.

50. King CL, Nutman TB: Biological role of helper T-cell subsets in helminth infections. *Chem Immunol* 54:136, 1992.

51. Vella AT, Pearce EJ: CD4+ Th2 response induced by Schistosoma mansoni eggs develops rapidly, through an early, transient, Th0-like stage. *J Immunol* 148:2283, 1992.

52. Contigli C, Silva-Teixeira DN, Del Prete G, et al: Phenotype and cytokine profile of Schistosoma mansoni specific T cell lines and clones derived from schistosomiasis patients with distinct clinical forms. *Clin Immunol* 91:338, 1999.

53. Fields PE, Kim ST, Flavell RA: Cutting edge: Changes in histone acetylation at the IL-4 and IFN-gamma loci accompany Th1/Th2 differentiation. *J Immunol* 169:647, 2002.

54. Nishikomori R, Usui T, Wu CY, et al: Activated STAT4 has an essential role in Th1 differentiation and proliferation that is independent of its role in the maintenance of IL-12R beta 2 chain expression and signaling. *J Immunol* 169:4388, 2002.

55. Rao A, Avni O: Molecular aspects of T-cell differentiation. *Br Med Bull* 56:969, 2000.

56. Zhou M, Ouyang W: The function role of GATA-3 in Th1 and Th2 differentiation. *Immunol Res* 28:25, 2003.

57. Constant SL, Bottomly K: Induction of Th1 and Th2 CD4+ T cell responses: The alternative approaches. *Annu Rev Immunol* 15:297, 1997.

58. Haanen JB, de Waal Malefijt R, Res PC, et al: Selection of a human T helper type 1-like T cell subset by mycobacteria. *J Exp Med* 174:583, 1991.

59. Yssel H, Shanafelt MC, Soderberg C, et al: Borrelia burgdorferi activates a T helper type 1-like T cell subset in Lyme arthritis. *J Exp Med* 174:593, 1991.

60. Lahesmaa R, Yssel H, Batsford S, et al: Yersinia enterocolitica activates a T helper type 1-like T cell subset in reactive arthritis. *J Immunol* 148:3079, 1992.

61. Walker LS: CD4+ CD25+ Treg: Divide and rule? *Immunology* 111:129, 2004.

62. Curotto de Lafaille MA, Lafaille JJ: CD4(+) regulatory T cells in autoimmunity and allergy. *Curr Opin Immunol* 14:771, 2002.

63. Stassen M, Schmitt E, Jonuleit H: Human CD(4+)CD(25+) regulatory T cells and infectious tolerance. *Transplantation* 77:S23, 2004.

64. Ahmed R, Gray D: Immunological memory and protective immunity: Understanding their relation. *Science* 272:54, 1996.

65. Sprent J, Tough DF, Sun S: Factors controlling the turnover of T memory cells. *Immunol Rev* 156:79, 1997.

66. Tanchot C, Rocha B: The organization of mature T-cell pools. *Immunol Today* 19:575, 1998.

67. Carter LL, Zhang X, Dubey C, et al: Regulation of T cell subsets from naive to memory. *J Immunother* 21:181, 1998.

68. Jenkins MK, Miller RA: Memory and anergy: Challenges to traditional models of T lymphocyte differentiation. *FASEB J* 6:2428, 1992.

69. Beverley P: Immunological memory in T cells. *Curr Opin Immunol* 3:355, 1991.

70. McHeyzer-Williams MG, Altman JD, Davis MM: Enumeration and characterization of memory cells in the TH compartment. *Immunol Rev* 150:5, 1996.

71. Plebanski M, Saunders M, Burtles SS, et al: Primary and secondary human in vitro T-cell responses to soluble antigens are mediated by subsets bearing different CD45 isoforms. *Immunology* 75:86, 1992.

72. Mason D: Subsets of CD4+ T cells defined by their expression of different isoforms of the leucocyte-common antigen, CD45. *Biochem Soc Trans* 20:188, 1992.

73. Janeway CAJ: The T cell receptor as a multicomponent signaling machine: CD4/CD8 coreceptors and CD45 in T cell activation. *Annu Rev Immunol* 10:645, 1992.

74. Turka LA, Kanner SB, Schieven GL, et al: CD45 modulates T cell receptor/CD3-induced activation of human thymocytes via regulation of tyrosine phosphorylation. *Eur J Immunol* 22:551, 1992.

75. Koretzky GA: Role of the CD45 tyrosine phosphatase in signal transduction in the immune system. *FASEB J* 7:420, 1993.

76. Dianzani U, Redoglia V, Malavasi F, et al: Isoform-specific associations of CD45 with accessory molecules in human T lymphocytes. *Eur J Immunol* 22:365, 1992.

77. Beverley PC: CD45 isoform expression: Implications for recirculation of naive and memory cells. *Immunol Res* 10:196, 1991.

78. Tortorella C, Schulze-Koops H, Thomas R, et al: Expression of CD45RB and CD27 identifies subsets of CD4+ memory T cells with different capacities to induce B cell differentiation. *J Immunol* 155:149, 1995.

79. Lee WT, Vitetta ES: Changes in expression of CD45R during the development of Th1 and Th2 cell lines. *Eur J Immunol* 22:1455, 1992.

80. Linsley PS, Ledbetter JA: The role of the CD28 receptor during T cell responses to antigen. *Annu Rev Immunol* 11:191, 1993.

81. Lenschow DJ, Walunas TL, Bluestone JA: CD28/B7 system of T cell costimulation. *Annu Rev Immunol* 14:233, 1996.

82. Peach RJ, Bajorath J, Brady W, et al: Complementarity determining region 1 (CDR1)- and CDR3-analogous regions in CTLA-4 and CD28 determine the binding to B7-1. *J Exp Med* 180:2049, 1994.

83. van der Merwe PA, Bodian DL, Daenke S, et al: CD80 (B7-1) binds both CD28 and CTLA-4 with a low affinity and very fast kinetics. *J Exp Med* 185:393, 1997.

84. Greene JL, Leytze GM, Emswiler J, et al: Covalent dimerization of CD28/CTLA-4 and oligomerization of CD80/CD86 regulate T cell costimulatory interactions. *J Biol Chem* 271:26762, 1996.

85. Watts TH, DeBenedette MA: T cell co-stimulatory molecules other than CD28. *Curr Opin Immunol* 11:286, 1999.

86. Boussiotis VA, Freeman GJ, Gribben JG, Nadler LM: The role of B7-1/B7-2:CD28/CLTA-4 pathways in the prevention of anergy, induction of productive immunity and down-regulation of the immune response. *Immunol Rev* 153:5, 1996.

87. Blair PJ, Riley JL, Carroll RG, et al: CD28 co-receptor signal transduction in T-cell activation. *Biochem Soc Trans* 25:651, 1997.

88. Lane P: Regulation of T and B cell responses by modulating interactions between CD28/CTLA4 and their ligands, CD80 and CD86. *Ann N Y Acad Sci* 815:392, 1997.

89. Greenfield EA, Nguyen KA, Kuchroo VK: CD28/B7 costimulation: A review. *Crit Rev Immunol* 18:389, 1998.

90. Powell JD, Ragheb JA, Kitagawa-Sakakida S, Schwartz RH: Molecular regulation of interleukin-2 expression by CD28 co-stimulation and anergy. *Immunol Rev* 165:287, 1998.

91. Shahinian A, Pfeffer K, Lee KP, et al: Differential T cell costimulatory requirements in CD28-deficient mice. *Science* 261:609, 1993.

92. Malvey EN, Telander DG, Vanasek TL, Mueller DL: The role of clonal anergy in the avoidance of autoimmunity: Inactivation of autocrine growth without loss of effector function. *Immunol Rev* 165:301, 1998.

93. Appleman LJ, Boussiotis VA: T cell anergy and costimulation. *Immunol Rev* 192:161, 2003.

94. Chambers CA, Allison JP: Costimulatory regulation of T cell function. *Curr Opin Cell Biol* 11:203, 1999.

95. Tivol EA, Borriello F, Schweitzer AN, et al: Loss of CTLA-4 leads to massive lymphoproliferation and fatal multiorgan tissue destruction, revealing a critical negative regulatory role of CTLA-4. *Immunity* 3:541, 1995.

96. Waterhouse P, Penninger JM, Timms E, et al: Lymphoproliferative disorders with early lethality in mice deficient in Ctla-4. *Science* 270:985, 1995.

97. Kearney ER, Walunas TL, Karr RW, et al: Antigen-dependent clonal expansion of a trace population of antigen-specific CD4+ T cells in vivo is dependent on CD28 costimulation and inhibited by CTLA-4. *J Immunol* 155:1032, 1995.

98. Leach DR, Krummel MF, Allison JP: Enhancement of antitumor immunity by CTLA-4 blockade. *Science* 271:1734, 1996.

99. Dong C, Nurieva RI, Prasad DV: Immune regulation by novel costimulatory molecules. *Immunol Res* 28:39, 2003.

100. van Seventer GA, Semnani RT, Palmer EM, et al: Integrins and T helper cell activation. *Transplant Proc* 30:4270, 1998.

101. Wang J, Springer TA: Structural specializations of immunoglobulin super family members for adhesion to integrins and viruses. *Immunol Rev* 163:197, 1998.

102. Springer TA: Adhesion receptors of the immune system. *Nature* 346:425, 1990.

103. de Fougerolles A, Springer TA: Ideas crystallized on immunoglobulin superfamily-integrin interactions. *Chem Biol* 2:639, 1995.

104. Larson RS, Springer TA: Structure and function of leukocyte integrins. *Immunol Rev* 114:181, 1990.

105. Springer TA: Traffic signals for lymphocyte recirculation and leukocyte emigration: The multistep paradigm. *Cell* 76:301, 1994.

106. Davis SJ, Ikemizu S, Wild MK, Van der Merwe PA: CD2 and the nature of protein interactions mediating cell-cell recognition. *Immunol Rev* 163:217, 1998.

107. Holter W, Schwarz M, Cerwenka A, Knapp W: The role of CD2 as a regulator of human T-cell cytokine production. *Immunol Rev* 153:107, 1996.

FUNCTIONS OF NATURAL KILLER CELLS

GIORGIO TRINCHIERI

LEWIS L. LANIER

Natural killer (NK) cells, with a predominant morphology of large granular lymphocytes, represent a third lineage of lymphoid cells with constitutive ability to mediate cytotoxicity of pathologic target cells and secrete cytokines. NK cells participate in the innate resistance to intracellular pathogens and malignancies and have a modulatory effect on adaptive immunity and hematopoiesis. NK cell activity is regulated by the opposite effects of activating and inhibitory receptors. Malignant expansions of NK cells, either acute or chronic, are rare but represent well-identified clinical entities.

IDENTIFICATION AND DEFINITION OF NATURAL KILLER CELLS

DEFINITION

Natural killer (NK) cells originally were identified in the blood and other lymphoid organs of humans and experimental animals as cells capable of killing a variety of cell types, including tumor-derived cell lines, virus-infected cells, and, in some instances, normal cells in the absence of previous deliberate or known sensitization.[1,2] NK cells currently are defined as cytotoxic cells with the predominant morphology of large granular lymphocytes (LGL) that (1) neither rearrange any of the genes encoding the T cell receptor (TCR) chains nor express on their surface the CD3 antigen complex or any TCR chain; (2) express on the majority of cells the CD16 (FcγRIIIA) and CD56 (N-CAM) antigens in humans, the NK1.1 (NKR-P1C) and DX5 (VLA-2/CD49d) antigens in the mouse, and the NKR-P1 antigen in the rat; (3) mediate cytolytic reactions even in the absence of major histocompatibility complex (MHC) class I or class II antigen expression on the target cells. The cytotoxicity mediated by NK cells is clearly distinct from the cytotoxicity mediated by cytotoxic T lymphocytes (CTL), which recognize specific antigenic peptides in association with MHC class I molecules. Cytotoxicity mediated by NK cells often is defined as non–MHC requiring, to distinguish it from the MHC-restricted cytotoxicity mediated by CTL. Nonetheless, the presence of MHC class I on target cells can affect NK cell recognition, in some cases inhibiting an NK cell response against cells expressing MHC class I. Certain T lymphocytes that express either an αβ or a γδ TCR may exhibit, particularly upon activation, TCR-independent cytolytic activity that resembles that of NK cells. Among the T lymphocytes displaying NK-like cytotoxicity or non–MHC-requiring cytotoxicity, NK T cells are a subset of cytotoxic T cells expressing in the mouse NK1.1 and with a restricted αβ TCR diversity. The majority of NK T cells recognize glycolipids presented by CD1d, a non-classic MHC molecule, and upon stimulation rapidly produce large amounts of interleukin (IL)-4, interferon gamma (IFN-γ), granulocyte-macrophage colony stimulating factor (GM-CSF), and IL-13.[3]

MORPHOLOGY

Human LGL are medium- to large-size lymphocytes with round or indented nuclei, condensed chromatin, and usually prominent nucleoli. The cytoplasm is abundant and contains a variety of organelles. Circular membrane-bound granules (primary lysosomes), which are characteristic of these cells, range in diameter from 50 to 800 nm and contain an electron-dense core (internum) surrounded by a layer of lesser opacity (externum). In addition to lysosomal enzymes, the granules contain phospholipids, proteoglycans, and proteins important for cytotoxic lymphocyte function, such as serine esterases (granzymes) and pore-forming proteins (perforin).[4] Although many NK cells have the morphology typical of LGL, a significant proportion of NK cells are indistinguishable from other lymphocytes and may even be agranular.[5]

ORIGIN AND TISSUE DISTRIBUTION

NK cells originate in the marrow. Most are short lived, with calculated life spans ranging from a few days to a few weeks.[6,7] NK cells derive from the common lymphoid progenitor cell that gives rise to T, B, and NK cells and some dendritic cells. The cytokine IL-15 and its receptor play a particularly important role in the differentiation and expansion of NK cells.[8,9] NK cell differentiation does not require the presence of the thymus, although NK cell progenitors can be demonstrated in the thymus, particularly during fetal development.[10] The increased number of NK cells and altered anatomical distribution in response to infection or other stimuli are primarily the result of increased NK cell production in the marrow and possibly partly proliferation of mature peripheral NK cells.[11]

Mature NK cells are present in blood, where they represent approximately 15 percent of lymphocytes (but with large individual variations). They also are present in the red pulp of the spleen and are found at a very low frequency in other lymphoid organs.[2,12] NK cells have been detected in lymph nodes. These NK cells display an antigenic phenotype distinct from NK cells in peripheral blood and predominantly lack expression of CD16.[13] In the marrow, NK cells represent less than 1 percent of the cells, indicating that a pool of preformed NK cells is not sequestered in the marrow. Small numbers of NK cells can be identified in the liver (pit cells), lung, and intestinal mucosa.[14,15] Upon activation, for example, in response to interferon or viral or bacterial infections, NK cells may accumulate in organs in which they normally are rare, particularly the liver and marrow.[12] Cells with characteristics of activated NK cells (decidual granulocytes) represent the predominant cell type present in the human early pregnancy decidua.[16] The physiologic significance of these cells in the decidua is not clear, but they may have a role in facilitating embryonic implantation, allowing placenta and embryo growth, monitoring mucosal integrity throughout the menstrual cycle, controlling trophoblast invasion during pregnancy, and modulating the maternal immune response against embryo antigens.

MECHANISMS OF NK CELL FUNCTIONS

CELL-MEDIATED CYTOTOXICITY

Cytotoxicity mediated by NK cells depends on binding to the target cells, followed by activation of the lytic mechanism, which usually involves secretion of the granules, including molecules with lytic ability, such as the pore-forming protein perforin and granzymes.[4] In some cases, cytotoxicity also is mediated through the interaction of surface molecules, for example, the interaction of Fas ligand or TNF-related apoptosis-inducing ligand (TRAIL) on NK cells with their death-inducing receptors on target cells. Lysis of the target cells results from alteration of membrane permeability and induction of apoptosis.[4]

The initial interaction between an NK cell and a potential target requires cell-to-cell contact, which often involves LFA-1 (CD11a/CD18) on the NK cell interacting with an intercellular adhesion molecule on the target cell. Several surface molecules on NK cells have been identified that, when stimulated, activate the cytotoxic mechanism and induce cytokine secretion (Fig. 79-1).[17] One of these molecules is the low-affinity receptor for the Fc fragment of immunoglobulin (Ig) G (FcγIIIA or CD16), which is expressed on most human NK cells in association with the signal-transducing CD3ξ or FcεRIγ chains. When CD16 is cross-linked by IgG antibodies bound to a target cell surface, it triggers antibody-dependent cell-mediated cytotoxicity.[18] CD16 is not required, in the absence of antibodies, for NK cell cytotoxicity.[17] In the case of "natural killing," this process can be accomplished using several different receptors, depending upon the presence of a relevant ligand on the potential target cell. NKG2D, a receptor expressed on all NK cells, has been implicated in NK cell recognition of transformed and virus-infected cells.[19] This receptor recognizes a family of MHC class I-related glycoproteins (including MICA, MICB, ULBP1, ULBP2, ULBP3, and ULBP4) that are absent or expressed at only low levels on healthy cells but are induced or up-regulated upon cell transformation or viral infection.[20] Some tumors secrete soluble forms of these NKG2D ligands, which serve as a decoy to avoid NK cell attack.[21] Certain viruses, such as cytomegalovirus, also have devised strategies to prevent the expression of NKG2D ligands in the infected cells,[22] presumably to escape NK cell-mediated immunity. NK cells express many other activating receptors that have been implicated in their recognition of tumors, including the "natural cytotoxicity" receptors NKp30, NKp44, and NKp46.[23] Ligands for these receptors have not been identified.

Based on the observation that NK cells preferentially kill certain tumor cells lacking expression of MHC class I molecules, NK cells may detect and eliminate autologous cells lacking MHC class I.[24] NK cells may be regulated by positive signals initiated by activating receptors and negative signals transmitted by interactions between inhibitory receptors for MHC class I on the NK cells and autologous MHC class I molecules on potential target cells. A mechanism for immune surveillance against cells that lose expression of MHC class I would be advantageous because, in the absence of class I, these abnormal cells would escape elimination by CTL. Numerous viruses inhibit the synthesis or transport of MHC class I proteins, presumably to avoid detection by CTL.[25] In addition, frequent loss of MHC class I expression on tumor cells has been documented.[26] However, NK cells are capable of killing cells expressing MHC class I if they received sufficiently strong activation signals.

Two families of NK cell receptors for MHC class I have been identified in humans. The killer cell Ig-like receptors (KIR) are encoded by approximately 15 genes present on human chromosome 19q13.4.[27] KIR genes are polymorphic and appear to be evolving rapidly and diversifying by gene duplication and conversion events. Certain KIR bind human leukocyte antigen (HLA)-C ligands, whereas other KIR recognize certain alleles of HLA-B or HLA-A. Another class of NK cell receptors are heterodimeric glycoproteins composed of a CD94 subunit that is disulfide bonded to an NKG2A molecule.[27] The CD94 and NKG2A genes are on human chromosome 12p12-p13 and are members of the C-type lectin superfamily. The CD94/NKG2A receptor binds to a nonclassic MHC class I molecule, HLA-E, which is unusual because the peptides present in the HLA-E binding groove usually are leader segments derived from HLA-A, HLA-B, HLA-C, or HLA-G proteins.[28] When synthesis of HLA-A, HLA-B, HLA-C, or HLA-G is disrupted, possibly by viral infection or transformation of the host cell, HLA-E cannot be transported to the cell surface for presentation to the CD94/NKG2A receptor. The various KIR and CD94/NKG2A receptors are expressed on overlapping subsets within the NK cell population and on certain memory T cells, usually CD8+ T cells. The observation that F1 mice reject marrow grafts from their parents can be explained by the existence of NK cell subpopulations in the F1 recipient that lack appropriate inhibitory NK cell receptors for the grafted parental cells.[29] The KIR molecules and the CD94/NKG2A receptor have an immunoreceptor tyrosine-based inhibitory motif (ITIM) sequence in their cytoplasmic domains, which binds to the cytoplasmic tyrosine phosphatase SHP-1, resulting in inhibition of NK cell cytotoxicity and cytokine secretion.[27] Therefore, the functional behavior of NK and T cells expressing KIR or CD94/NKG2A is regulated by the balance of positive signals transmitted by a variety of activating receptors and negative signals (resulting in phosphatase recruitment) provided by the inhibitory MHC class I receptors.

Certain receptors of the KIR and CD94/NKG2 families do not possess ITIM sequences and activate, rather than suppress, NK and T cell responses.[27] These receptors noncovalently associate with the homodimeric adapter protein DAP12.[30] Like the CD3ξ and the FcεRI-γ subunits, DAP12 contains an immunoreceptor tyrosine-based activation motif in the cytoplasmic domain. Upon receptor ligation, DAP12 becomes tyrosine phosphorylated, recruits the ZAP70 and Syk cytoplasmic tyrosine kinases, and induces cellular activation.[30] The physiologic role of activating NK cell receptors for MHC class I has not been determined, but these receptors may have consequences in allogeneic marrow transplantation. In mice, one activating receptor in the Ly49 family (the functional counterpart of KIR in humans) has been shown to recognize the m157 viral glycoprotein encoded by cytomegalovirus and protects the mice from this pathogen.[31,32] This finding suggests certain activating KIR in humans also recognize pathogens.

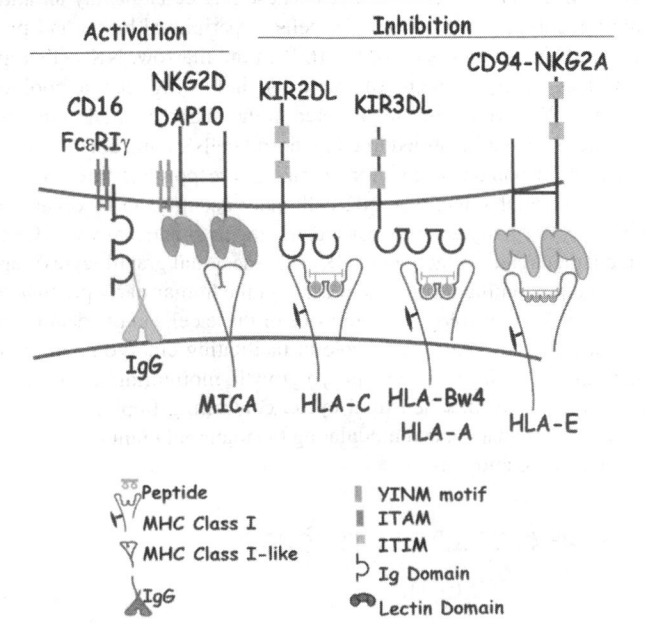

FIGURE 79-1   Schematic representation of selected inhibitory and activating NK cell receptors regulating NK cell responses.

Although resting blood NK cells are cytotoxic, their activity can be greatly enhanced by both *in vivo* or *in vitro* exposure to cytokines such as IFN-α/β, IL-2, IL-12, IL-15, and IL-18.[33–35] Resting NK cells express intermediate-affinity IL-2 receptors, and IL-2 induces the progression of most NK cells into the cell cycle.[36]

PRODUCTION OF CYTOKINES

Many of the physiologic functions of NK cells are mediated at least partly by their ability to secrete cytokines. NK cells are powerful producers of IFN-γ and GM-CSFs. They also can produce tumor necrosis factor alpha (TNF-α), macrophage colony stimulating factor (M-CSF), IL-3, IL-5, IL-8, IL-13, and other cytokines and chemokines. Stimulation by cytokines, such as IL-2, IL-12, IL-18, TNF-α, and IL-1,[2,34,37,38] and triggering by receptors, such as CD16 interacting with immune complexes, are among the stimuli that, acting individually or often in synergistic combination, induce NK cells to produce cytokines.[2,39,40]

PHYSIOLOGIC ROLES OF NK CELLS

NATURAL RESISTANCE

Because of their ability to respond to external stimuli without previous sensitization, NK cells can respond rapidly to the presence of infectious microorganisms or, in some cases, neoplastic cells (see Chap. 17). Together with phagocytic cells, NK cells are effectors of the innate or natural resistance, which represents the first line of defense against infection (Fig. 79-2).

The ability of NK cells to participate in the resistance against infection by certain viruses is well documented in experimental animals and is strongly suggested by the recurrent viral infections in the few patients described to have a selective deficiency of NK cells.[41] NK cells selectively kill virus-infected cells by a mechanism that is at least partly dependent on the production of IFN-α, a potent stimulator of NK cell activity.[42,43] *In vivo* virus infection and IFN production usually are accompanied by rapid activation of, and increase in the number of, NK cells, both systemically and localized in the infected area.[11] The NK response to virus infection usually peaks 2 to 3 days postinfection and is followed by an antigen-specific T helper and CTL response, which peaks 7 to 9 days postinfection.[11] The early NK response induces a significant reduction in the titer of certain viruses, including murine cytomegalovirus.[44,45] NK cells from certain resistant mouse strains specifically recognize the m157 protein of murine cytomegalovirus through the DAP12-linked activating receptor Ly49H and respond by killing the virus-infected cells and secreting IFN-γ.[32,45,46] Other viruses, such as lymphocytic choriomeningitis virus (LCMV), are resistant to the antiviral effects of NK cells. NK cell activation induced by these viruses has pathogenic effects.[44]

NK cells enhance the response of phagocytic cells to microorganisms, especially intracellular bacteria and parasites, by producing high levels of the phagocyte-activating cytokines IFN-γ and GM-CSF in response to the microorganisms themselves or to factors, such as IL-12 and TNF-α, produced by infected phagocytic cells.[47,48]

The observation that NK cells kill *in vitro*–transformed or tumor-derived cell lines has been used to support the theory that, in immune surveillance, NK cells, rather than T cells, can recognize and kill newly arising malignant tumor cells.[49] In experimental animals, the *in vivo* activity of NK cells against tumors was investigated by evaluating their effects on long-term growth of tumors, metastasis formation, and

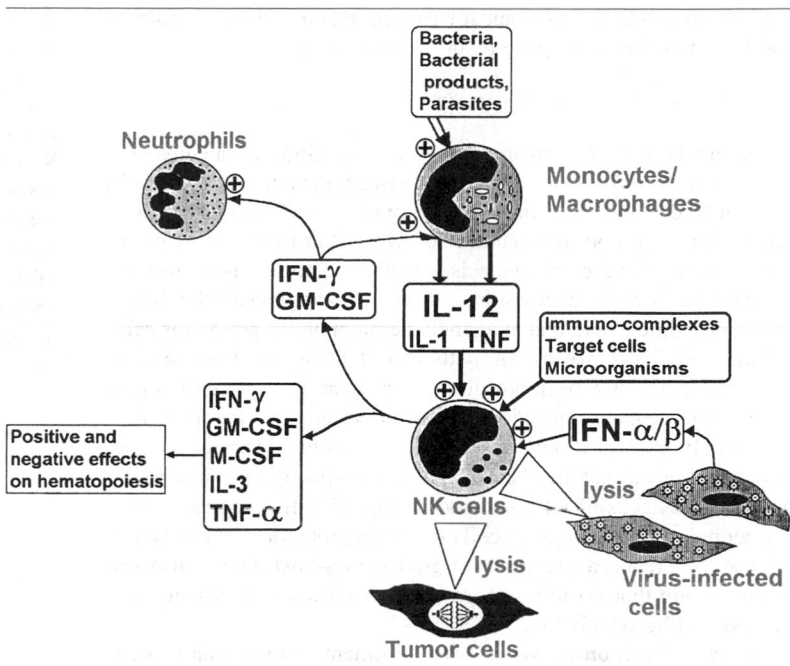

FIGURE 79-2   Schematic depiction of some of the functions and regulatory pathways of NK cells as effector cells of natural resistance. In addition to mediating cytotoxicity, NK cells exert their physiologic roles by releasing several cytokines that affect the functions of other cell types, including hematopoietic cells. Natural killer cell activity also is regulated by cytokines. Cytokines IFN-α/β, IL-2, and IL-12 enhance NK cell-mediated cytotoxicity. IL-2, IL-12, TNF, and IL-1 induce NK cell lymphokine production. IL-2 and IL-12 induce NK cell proliferation. *Arrows* with a plus (+) indicate stimulatory effects resulting in lymphokine secretion, enhancement of NK cell cytotoxic activity, or activation of phagocytic cells.

short-term elimination of radiolabeled tumor cells.[2] Experiments have clearly shown that NK cells can destroy tumor cells *in vivo*, and some evidence indicates an effective role of NK cells in resistance to spontaneously arising neoplastic cells.[50] An activating receptor expressed by NK cells (NKG2D) recognizes ligands that are up-regulated on tumor cells and virally infected cells but are not expressed well by normal cells.[51] NK-mediated rejection of tumor cells then may facilitate tumor antigen presentation to T cells and induce an antigen-specific antitumor immune response.[52,53] NK cell cytotoxic activity often is decreased in human cancer patients. Several studies have suggested that increased NK cell activity tends to correlate with increased survival times and longer intervals before metastasis.[54] However, the hypothesis of a role for NK cells in immune surveillance is not yet supported by statistical evidence indicating a correlation between low tumor incidence and high NK cell cytotoxic activity.[54,55]

REGULATION OF ADAPTIVE IMMUNITY

NK cells, by interacting with infectious agents and antigens early during the immune response, have either stimulatory or inhibitory effects on the function of B and T cells and antigen-presenting cells.[2] Evidence for an enhancing effect of NK cells on B cell responses has been shown both *in vitro* and *in vivo* by studies demonstrating that NK cells in the absence of T cells support antigen-specific B cell responses, partly by producing IFN-γ.[56,57] In certain infections, NK cells may be necessary for optimal induction of both a CD4 and CD8 T cell response.[58,59] NK cells stimulated by microorganisms or by cytokines, such as IL-12 and TNF, produce large amounts of IFN-γ and other cytokines that facilitate T helper cell type 1 development.[60] The reciprocal activating interaction between NK cells and the antigen-presenting dendritic cells is important for the regulation of innate resistance and the downstream adaptive response to pathogens.[61,62]

MODULATION OF HEMATOPOIESIS

Experimental observations in animals, clinical findings in human patients, and *in vitro* analyses provided strong evidence that NK cells are involved in the regulation of hematopoiesis.[63] The effector role of NK cells in rejection of parental marrow graft in irradiated F1 mice[64] and in suppressing erythropoiesis and phagocytopoiesis in mice infected with LCMV[65] demonstrated that *in vivo* activated NK cells can affect both allogeneic and syngeneic hematopoietic progenitor cells. Because of the ability of NK cells to kill malignant hematopoietic cells, NK cells have been postulated to play an important role in the graft-versus-leukemia reaction in allogeneic marrow transplantation but an only modest, if any, role in graft-versus-host disease.[66] In haploidentical or mismatched hematopoietic transplantation, the presence on donor NK cells of KIR not recognizing inhibiting ligands on host hematopoietic and malignant cells results in protection from leukemia relapse.[67] A reduced incidence of graft-versus-host disease also was observed and thought to result from the elimination of recipient antigen-presenting cells by donor NK cells.[67]

In vivo depletion of NK cells by treatment of mice with anti-NK cell antibodies produces differential effects on various lineages. NK cell depletion in normal mice increases phagocytopoiesis and decreases erythropoiesis and megakaryocytopoiesis.[68,69] Consistent with these results, depletion of NK cells in mice receiving myelosuppressive irradiation results in faster recovery of phagocytopoiesis and slower recovery of megakaryocytopoiesis and erythropoiesis.[70] Clinical evidence for a role of NK cells in the regulation of human hematopoiesis is provided by the demonstration that NK cells are the effector cells mediating suppression of hematopoiesis in some cases of acquired aplastic anemia in both acute and chronic monoclonal NK lymphocytosis and possibly in other clinical conditions.[63] *In vitro* studies have shown that NK cells have a prevalent inhibitory effect on colony formation from hematopoietic progenitor cells.[71,72] However, NK cells enhance formation of megakaryocytic colonies and, in some experimental conditions, of erythroid and granulocyte-macrophage colonies.[73,74] The effect of NK cells is mostly mediated by secretion of humoral factors and may require the participation of accessory cells.[72] NK cells, constitutively or upon activation, produce several lymphokines, some with mostly inhibitory effects on hematopoiesis, such as TNF and IFN-γ, and some with mostly positive effects, such as GM-CSF, M-CSF, and IL-3.[37,73]

PATHOLOGIC ALTERATIONS IN NK CELL NUMBER AND FUNCTIONS

NK cell function and NK cell numbers often are decreased in pathologic conditions, including cancer and AIDS.[55,75] The reduced activity or number of NK cells may contribute to disease pathology by decreasing the innate resistance against tumor growth and metastasis in cancer patients or against opportunistic infections in AIDS patients. An NK hyporesponsiveness is observed in patients with Chédiak-Higashi syndrome,[76] a rare autosomal recessive disease associated with cellular dysfunction, including fusion of cytoplasmic granules and defective degranulation of neutrophil lysosomes. NK cell numbers are normal in these patients, but the NK cells present a single, large granule in the cytoplasm and have a severely reduced ability to mediate cytotoxicity.[76]

Malignant acute expansion of NK cells is rare. It occurs in both the nasopharyngeal region and in non-nasal areas as an NK cell (CD2+, CD3−, CD56+, CD16−, CD57−) leukemia or lymphoma

that mostly affects extranodal tissues. It usually has an extremely aggressive clinical course. It may be associated with Epstein-Barr virus infection.[77–79] A chronic monoclonal proliferative disorder of LGL with a clinical course that is often relatively benign is more commonly observed.[80] Most patients have lymphocytic infiltration of the marrow. Severe neutropenia and anemia often are observed. Associated diseases, most commonly rheumatoid arthritis, hepatitis, or cancer, are present in up to half of patients.[80] Although cells from all these patients are characterized by an LGL morphology, in approximately two thirds of the cases they represent a monoclonal expansion of CD8+ T cells, and in only less than one third of cases they have the typical phenotype and genotype of CD3−, CD56+, CD57+, and, in some patients, CD16+ NK cells.[80]

REFERENCES

1. Takasugi M, Mickey MR, Terasaki PI: Reactivity of lymphocytes from normal persons on cultured tumor cells. *Cancer Res* 33:2898, 1973.
2. Trinchieri G: Biology of natural killer cells. *Adv Immunol* 47:187, 1989.
3. Kronenberg M, Gapin L: The unconventional lifestyle of NKT cells. *Nat Rev Immunol* 2:557, 2002.
4. Young JDE, Cohn ZA: Cellular and humoral mechanisms of cytotoxicity: Structural and functional analogies. *Adv Immunol* 41:269, 1987.
5. Ortaldo JR, Winkler-Pickett R, Kopp W, et al: Relationship of large and small CD3−CD56+ lymphocytes mediating NK-associated activities. *J Leukoc Biol* 52:287, 1992.
6. Miller SC: Production and renewal of murine killer cells in the spleen and bone marrow. *J Immunol* 129:2282, 1982.
7. Hochman PS, Cudkowicz G, Dausset J: Decline of natural killer cell activity in sublethally irradiated mice. *J Natl Cancer Inst* 61:265, 1978.
8. Williams NS, Klem J, Puzanov IJ, et al: Natural killer cell differentiation: Insights from knockout and transgenic mouse models and in vitro systems. *Immunol Rev* 165:47, 1998.
9. Liu CC, Perussia B, Young JD: The emerging role of IL-15 in NK-cell development. *Immunol Today* 21:113, 2000.
10. Lian RH, Kumar V: Murine natural killer cell progenitors and their requirements for development. *Semin Immunol* 14:453, 2002.
11. Biron CA, Turgiss LR, Welsh RM: Increase in NK cell number and turnover rate during acute viral infection. *J Immunol* 131:1539, 1983.
12. Perussia B, Acuto O, Terhorst C, et al: Human natural killer cells analyzed by B73.1, a monoclonal antibody blocking FcR functions: II. Studies of B73.1 antibody-antigen interaction on the lymphocyte membrane. *J Immunol* 130:2142, 1983.
13. Fehniger TA, Cooper MA, Nuovo GJ, et al: CD56 bright natural killer cells are present in human lymph nodes and are activated by T cell-derived IL-2: A potential new link between adaptive and innate immunity. *Blood* 101:3052, 2003.
14. Bouwens L, Wisse E: Pit cells in the liver. *Liver* 12:3, 1992.
15. Weissler JC, Nicod LP, Lipscomb MF, Toews GB: Natural killer cell function in human lung is compartmentalized. *Am Rev Respir Dis* 135:941, 1987.
16. Moffett-King A: Natural killer cells and pregnancy. *Nat Rev Immunol* 2:656, 2002.
17. Lanier LL: On guard−Activating NK cell receptors. *Nat Immunol* 2:23, 2001.
18. Sulica A, Morel P, Metes D, Herberman RB: Ig-binding receptors on human NK cells as effector and regulatory surface molecules. *Int Rev Immunol* 20:371, 2001.
19. Bauer S, Groh V, Wu J, et al: Activation of NK cells and T cells by NKG2D, a receptor for stress-inducible MICA. *Science* 285:727, 1999.
20. Cerwenka A, Lanier LL: NKG2D ligands: Unconventional MHC class I-like molecules exploited by viruses and cancer. *Tissue Antigens* 61:335, 2003.

21. Groh V, Wu J, Yee C, Spies T: Tumour-derived soluble MIC ligands impair expression of NKG2D and T-cell activation. *Nature* 419:734, 2002.

22. Cosman D, Mullberg J, Sutherland CL, et al: ULBPs, novel MHC class I-related molecules, bind to CMV glycoprotein UL16 and stimulate NK cytotoxicity through the NKG2D receptor. *Immunity* 14:123, 2001.

23. Moretta A, Bottino C, Vitale M, et al: Activating receptors and coreceptors involved in human natural killer cell-mediated cytolysis. *Annu Rev Immunol* 19:197, 2001.

24. Karre K, Ljunggren HG, Piontek G, Kiessling R: Selective rejection of H-2-deficient lymphoma variants suggests alternative immune defence strategy. *Nature* 319:675, 1986.

25. Ploegh HL: Viral strategies of immune evasion. *Science* 280:248, 1998.

26. Garcia-Lora A, Algarra I, Garrido F: MHC class I antigens, immune surveillance, and tumor immune escape. *J Cell Physiol* 195:346, 2003.

27. Long EO: Regulation of immune responses through inhibitory receptors. *Annu Rev Immunol* 17:875, 1999.

28. Braud VM, Allan DS, O'Callaghan CA, et al: HLA-E binds to natural killer cell receptors CD94/NKG2A Band C. *Nature* 391:795, 1998.

29. Yu YY, George T, Dorfman JRet al: The role of Ly49A and 5E6(Ly49C) molecules in hybrid resistance mediated by murine natural killer cells against normal T cell blasts. *Immunity* 4:67, 1996.

30. Lanier LL, Corliss BC, Wu J, et al: Immunoreceptor DAP12 bearing a tyrosine-based activation motif is involved in activating NK cells. *Nature* 391:703, 1998.

31. Brown MG, Dokun AO, Heusel JW, et al: Vital involvement of a natural killer cell activation receptor in resistance to viral infection. *Science* 292:934, 2001.

32. Arase H, Mocarski ES, Campbell AE, et al: Direct recognition of cytomegalovirus by activating and inhibitory NK cell receptors. *Science* 296:1323, 2002.

33. Trinchieri G, Santoli D: Antiviral activity induced by culturing lymphocytes with tumor-derived or virus-transformed cells. Enhancement of human natural killer cell activity by interferon and antagonistic inhibition of susceptibility of target cells to lysis. *J Exp Med* 147:1314, 1978.

34. Trinchieri G, Matsumoto-Kobayashi M, Clark SC, et al: Response of resting human peripheral blood natural killer cells to interleukin-2. *J Exp Med* 160:1147, 1984.

35. Kobayashi M, Fitz L, Ryan M, et al: Identification and purification of natural killer cell stimulatory factor (NKSF), a cytokine with multiple biologic effects on human lymphocytes. *J Exp Med* 170:827, 1989.

36. London L, Perussia B, Trinchieri G: Induction of proliferation in vitro of resting human natural killer cells: IL-2 induces into cell cycle most peripheral blood NK cells, but only a minor subset of low density T cells. *J Immunol* 137:3845, 1986.

37. Cuturi MC, Anegon I, Sherman F, et al: Production of hematopoietic colony-stimulating factors by human natural killer cells. *J Exp Med* 169:569, 1989.

38. Peritt D, Robertson S, Gri G, et al: Differentiation of human NK cells into NK1 and NK2 subsets. *J Immunol* 161:5821, 1998.

39. Anegon I, Cuturi MC, Trinchieri G, Perussia B: Interaction of Fcg receptor (CD16) with ligands induces transcription of IL-2 receptor (CD25) and lymphokine genes and expression of their products in human natural killer cells. *J Exp Med* 167:452, 1988.

40. Chan SH, Perussia B, Gupta JW, et al: Induction of IFN-g production by NK cell stimulatory factor (NKSF): Characterization of the responder cells and synergy with other inducers. *J Exp Med* 173:8691991.

41. Biron CA, Byron KS, Sullivan JL: Severe herpesvirus infections in an adolescent without natural killer cells. *N Engl J Med* 320:1731, 1989.

42. Santoli D, Trinchieri G, Koproswki H: Cell-mediated cytotoxicity in humans against virus-infected target cells: II. Interferon induction and activation of natural killer cells. *J Immunol* 121:532, 1978.

43. Bandyopadhyay S, Perussia B, Trinchieri G, et al: Requirement for HLA-DR positive accessory cells in natural killing of cytomegalovirus-infected fibroblasts. *J Exp Med* 164:180, 1986.

44. Welsh RM: Regulation of virus infections by natural killer cells. A review. *Nat Immun Cell Growth Regul* 5:169, 1986.

45. Arase H, Lanier LL: Virus-driven evolution of natural killer cell receptors. *Microbes Infect* 4:1505, 2002.

46. Smith HR, Heusel JW, Mehta IK, et al: Recognition of a virus-encoded ligand by a natural killer cell activation receptor. *Proc Natl Acad Sci U S A* 99:8826, 2002.

47. Bancroft GJ, Schreiber RD, Unanue ER: Natural immunity: A T-cell-independent pathway of macrophage activation, defined in the SCID mouse. *Immunol Rev* 124:5, 1991.

48. Gazzinelli RT, Hieny S, Wynn TA, et al: Interleukin 12 is required for the T-lymphocyte-independent induction of interferon gamma by an intracellular parasite and induces resistance in T-cell-deficient hosts. *Proc Natl Acad Sci U S A* 90:6115, 1993.

49. Bloom BR: Natural killers to rescue immune surveillance? *Nature* 300:214, 1982.

50. Smyth MJ, Hayakawa Y, Takeda K, Yagita H: New aspects of natural-killer-cell surveillance and therapy of cancer. *Nat Rev Cancer* 2:850, 2002.

51. Diefenbach A, Raulet DH: The innate immune response to tumors and its role in the induction of T-cell immunity. *Immunol Rev* 188:9, 2002.

52. Kelly JM, Darcy PK, Markby JL, et al: Induction of tumor-specific T cell memory by NK cell-mediated tumor rejection. *Nat Immunol* 3:83, 2002.

53. Mocikat R, Braumuller H, Gumy A, et al: Natural killer cells activated by MHC class I(low) targets prime dendritic cells to induce protective CD8 T cell responses. *Immunity* 19:561, 2003.

54. Brittenden J, Heys SD, Ross J, Eremin O: Natural killer cells and cancer. *Cancer* 77:1226, 1996.

55. Pross HF: Natural killer cell activity in human malignant disease, in *Natural Immunity Cancer and Biological Response Modification*, edited by E Lotzova, Oxford University Press, Oxford, UK, p 196. 1986.

56. Mond JJ, Brunswick M: A role for IFN-gamma and NK cells in immune response to T cell-regulated antigens types 1 and 2. *Immunol Rev* 99:105, 1987.

57. Yuan D, Koh CY, Wilder JA: Interactions between B lymphocytes and NK cells. *FASEB J* 8:1012, 1994.

58. Dowdell KC, Cua DJ, Kirkman E, Stohlman SA: NK cells regulate CD4 responses prior to antigen encounter. *J Immunol* 171:234, 2003.

59. Vankayalapati R, Klucar P, Wizel B, et al: NK cells regulate CD8+ T cell effector function in response to an intracellular pathogen. *J Immunol* 172:130, 2004.

60. Trinchieri G: Interleukin-12 and the regulation of innate resistance and adaptive immunity. *Nat Rev Immunol* 3:133, 2003.

61. Gerosa F, Baldani-Guerra B, Nisii C, et al: Reciprocal activating interaction between natural killer cells and dendritic cells. *J Exp Med* 195:327, 2002.

62. Moretta A: Natural killer cells and dendritic cells: Rendezvous in abused tissues. *Nat Rev Immunol* 2:957, 2002.

63. Trinchieri G: Natural killer cells in hematopoiesis, in *The Natural Immune System: Natural Killer Cells*, edited by CE Lewis, Oxford University Press, Oxford, UK, p 41. 1992.

64. Cudkowicz G, Hochman PS: Do natural killer cells engage in regulated reaction against self to ensure homeostasis? *Immunol Rev* 44:13, 1979.

65. Randrup-Thomsen A, Pisa P, Bro-Jorgensen K, Kiessling R: Mechanisms of lymphocytic choriomeningitis virus-induced hemopoietic dysfunction. *J Virol* 59:428, 1986.

66. Jiang YZ, Barrett AJ, Goldman JM, Mavroudis DA: Association of natural killer cell immune recovery with a graft-versus-leukemia effect in-

dependent of graft-versus-host disease following allogeneic bone marrow transplantation. *Ann Hematol* 74:1, 1997.

67. Velardi A, Ruggeri L, Moretta A, Moretta L: NK cells: A lesson from mismatched hematopoietic transplantation. *Trends Immunol* 23:438, 2002.

68. Hansson M, Petersson M, Koo GC, et al: In vivo function of natural killer cells as regulators of myeloid precursor cells in the spleen. *Eur J Immunol* 18:485, 1988.

69. Pantel K, Nakeff A: Differential effect of natural killer cells on modulating CFU-Meg and BFU-E proliferation in situ. *Exp Hematol* 17:1017, 1989.

70. Pantel K, Boertman J, Nakeff A: Inhibition of hematopoietic recovery from radiation-induced myelosuppression by natural killer cells. *Radiat Res* 122:168, 1990.

71. Hansson M, Beran M, Andersson B, Kiessling R: Inhibition of in vitro granulopoiesis by autologous and allogeneic human NK cells. *J Immunol* 129:126, 1982.

72. Degliantoni G, Murphy M, Kobayashi M, et al: Natural killer (NK) cell-derived hematopoietic colony-inhibiting activity and NK cytotoxic factor. Relationship with tumor necrosis factor and synergism with immune interferon. *J Exp Med* 162:1512, 1985.

73. Murphy WJ, Keller JR, Harrison CL, et al: Interleukin-2-activated natural killer cells can support hematopoiesis in vitro and promote marrow engraftment in vivo. *Blood* 80:670, 1992.

74. Gewirtz AM, Xu WY, Mangan KF: Role of natural killer cells, in comparison with T lymphocytes and monocytes, in the regulation of normal human megakaryocytopoiesis in vitro. *J Immunol* 139:2915, 1987.

75. Chehimi J, Starr SE, Frank I, et al: Natural killer (NK) cell stimulatory factor increases the cytotoxic activity of NK cells from both healthy donors and human immunodeficiency virus-infected patients. *J Exp Med* 175:789, 1992.

76. Haliotis T, Roder J, Klein M, et al: Chediak-Higashi gene in humans: I. Impairment of natural-killer function. *J Exp Med* 151:1039, 1980.

77. Kanavaros P, Lescs MC, Briere J, et al: Nasal T-cell lymphoma: A clinicopathologic entity associated with peculiar phenotype and with Epstein-Barr virus. *Blood* 81:2688, 1993.

78. Chan JK, Sin VC, Wong KF, et al: Nonnasal lymphoma expressing the natural killer cell marker CD56: A clinicopathologic study of 49 cases of an uncommon aggressive neoplasm. *Blood* 89:4501, 1997.

79. Jaffe ES: Classification of natural killer (NK) cell and NK-like T-cell malignancies. *Blood* 87:1207, 1996.

80. Reynolds CW, Foon KA: T gamma-lymphoproliferative disorders in man and experimental animals: A review of the clinical, cellular and functional characteristics. *Blood* 64:1146, 1984.

CLASSIFICATION AND CLINICAL MANIFESTATIONS OF LYMPHOCYTE AND PLASMA CELL DISORDERS

THOMAS J. KIPPS

This chapter outlines the major categories of lymphocyte and plasma cell disorders. The disorders can be sorted into three main groups. The first is composed of diseases caused by defects intrinsic to lymphoid cells. The second is caused by disorders that result from factors extrinsic to lymphoid cells. The third is composed of disorders caused by neoplastic or preoplastic lymphoid cells and is outlined in Chapter 95 using the World Health Organization classification of tumors of lymphoid tissues. The clinical manifestations of diseases in any one of the three groups may be difficult to distinguish, but this grouping can provide a framework with which to proceed in evaluating patients with known or suspected lymphocyte disorders. This chapter introduces the framework and presents a roadmap to other chapters in this book that discuss each of the disorders in greater detail.

CLASSIFICATION

Lymphocyte and plasma cell disorders can be classified into three major groups. The first group is composed of lymphocyte disorders caused by intrinsic defects in lymphoid cells that result in functional abnormalities of marrow-derived (B) lymphocytes, thymic-derived (T) lymphocytes, both (impaired humoral and cellular immunity), or natural killer (NK) cells (Table 80-1). These disorders primarily result from inborn errors in lymphocyte metabolism (see Chaps. 75 and 82) and/or receptor–ligand expression (see Chaps. 14 and 82). Table 80-1 groups these disorders together as "primary disorders." The second group consists of disorders caused by factors extrinsic to lymphocytes resulting in immune dysfunction. These conditions most commonly result from infection with viruses or other cellular pathogens (see Chaps. 81, 83, and 84), but they also may be caused by drugs or systemic disease of nonlymphoid cells. Table 80-1 lists these disorders as "acquired disorders." The third group of diseases is composed of preoplastic and neoplastic lymphocyte disorders (see Chap. 90).

Different categories of lymphocyte and plasma cell disorders may be difficult to distinguish clinically for several reasons. Lymphocyte disorders can have many clinical manifestations that are not restricted to cells of the immune system. Also, disparate disorders can have similar clinical manifestations, and any one disorder can be associated with a diverse array of clinical pathologies.

Acronyms and abbreviations that appear in this chapter include: Ig, immunoglobulin; NK, natural killer; Th, T helper.

In some cases, however, the classification of lymphocyte disorders is influenced by the manifestations of the disease. For example, autoimmune hemolytic disease (see Chap. 52) and autoimmune thrombocytopenia (see Chap. 110) are caused by inappropriate secretion of autoantibodies by B lymphocytes. The blood cell that is coated with autoantibody presumably is normal, yet we classify the disease that can result from hemolytic autoantibodies as an acquired hemolytic anemia because that aspect of the disease is more visible and better understood than is the inappropriate synthesis of antierythrocyte antibody by the disturbed lymphocyte population(s). These disorders are not considered here.

Many diseases, especially infection (e.g., tuberculous adenitis), inflammatory states (e.g., rheumatoid arthritis), autoimmune disease (e.g., systemic lupus erythematosus), and metastatic carcinoma can involve lymph nodes or the spleen as a secondary alteration. These disorders also may be associated with abnormal production of antibodies, such as those resulting in the lupus anticoagulant (see Chap. 123). These disorders also are not considered here because the primary disease is not generally considered a lymphocyte disorder per se.

CLINICAL MANIFESTATIONS

B LYMPHOCYTE DISORDERS

IMMUNOGLOBULIN DEFICIENCY

The clinical manifestations of B lymphocyte disorders include the consequences of B lymphocyte deficiency, dysfunction, or malignant transformation. The manifestations may consist of a specific deficiency of one of the Ig isotypes or of several or all normal Ig molecules (panhypogammaglobulinemia) (see Chap. 77). Inability to synthesize or secrete antibodies impairs the clearance of pathogens because of the inability to opsonize microorganisms for phagocytosis, resulting in immune deficiency (see Chap. 82).

ABNORMAL IMMUNOGLOBULIN PRODUCTION

Excess production of Ig by a clone of B cells can result in essential monoclonal gammopathy (see Chap. 99). This situation could result from a primary defect in the B cell clone or expansion of a clone in response to chronic antigen stimulation. Essential monoclonal gammopathy could be a harbinger for development of B cell neoplastic disease, such as plasma cell myeloma (see Chap. 100) or Waldenström macroglobulinemia (see Chap. 102). Production of abnormal Ig molecules or Ig fragments can be seen in association with chronic infection, leading to development of Ig heavy-chain disease (see Chap. 103). Deposition of Ig or Ig fragments can contribute to amyloid formation (see Chap. 101). Reactivity of the Ig with self-antigen(s), such as those found on the red cell membrane (see Chap. 52), can result in systemic autoimmune disease.

T LYMPHOCYTE DISORDERS

IMPAIRED IMMUNOREGULATION

The clinical manifestations of deficiencies or excesses of T lymphocytes depend on the subset of T lymphocytes involved. For example, delayed hypersensitivity normally is mediated by CD4-positive helper T cells (Th cells) and, more specifically, Th1-type cells (see Chap. 78). A deficit or functional disturbance in these T cells can impair the cellular immune response to mycobacteria, listeria, brucella, fungi, or other intracellular organisms associated with formation of immune granulomas. Th2-type CD4-positive helper T cells, on the other hand, appear better suited to induce B cell responses to antigen and direct the immune response against parasitic infestations (see Chap. 78). Depletion of CD4 T cells in patients infected with human immunodeficiency virus accounts in large part for the acquired immune deficiency that develops in patients infected with the virus (see Chap. 83).

TABLE 80-1 CLASSIFICATION OF DISORDERS OF LYMPHOCYTES AND PLASMA CELLS

I. Primary disorders
   A. B lymphocyte deficiency or dysfunction
      1. Agammaglobulinemia (see Chap. 82)
         a) Acquired agammaglobulinemia[8]
         b) Associated with plasma cell myeloma[9]
         c) Associated with celiac disease[10,11]
         d) X-linked agammaglobulinemia of Bruton [12–14]
      2. Selective agammaglobulinemia (see Chap. 82)
         a) IgM deficiency
            (1) Bloom syndrome[15]
            (2) Isolated[16]
            (3) Wiskott-Aldrich syndrome[17,18]
         b) IgA deficiency[19]
            (1) Isolated asymptomatic[20]
            (2) Steatorrheic[21]
         c) IgA and IgM deficiency[22]
      3. Hyper-IgA[23,24]
      4. Hyper-IgD[23,25,26]
      5. Hyper-IgE[27,28]
      6. Hyper-IgE associated with HIV infection[29]
      7. Hyper-IgM immunodeficiency[30]
      8. X-linked lymphoproliferative disease[31,32]
   B. T lymphocyte deficiency or dysfunction (see Chap. 82)[33]
      1. Cartilage-hair hypoplasia[34,35]
      2. Lymphocyte function antigen-1 deficiency[36]
      3. Thymic aplasia (DiGeorge syndrome)[37,38]
      4. Thymic dysplasia (Nezelof syndrome)[39]
      5. Thymic hypoplasia[40]
      6. Wiskott-Aldrich syndrome[17,41]
   C. Combined T and B cell deficiency or dysfunction (see Chap. 82)[42]
      1. Ataxia-telangiectasia[43]
      2. Combined immunodeficiency syndrome (see Chap. 82)
         a) Adenosine deaminase deficiency[44]
         b) Thymic alymphoplasia[45]
      3. Defective expression of major histocompatibility antigens—bare lymphocyte syndrome (see Chap. 82)[46–48]
      4. IgG and IgA deficiency and impaired cellular immunity (type I dysgammaglobulinemia)[49]
      5. Immunodeficiency with thymoma[50]
      6. Pyridoxine deficiency[51]
      7. Reticular agenesis (congenital aleukocytosis)[52]
      8. ZAP-70 deficiency[53]
   D. Natural killer cells (see Chaps. 79 and 94)
      1. Chronic natural killer cell lymphocytosis[1–7]
II. Acquired disorders
   A. Acquired immunodeficiency syndrome (see Chap. 83)
   B. Reactive lymphocytosis or plasmacytosis (see Chap. 81)[54]
      1. *Bordetella pertussis* lymphocytosis (see Chap. 81)[55]
      2. Cytomegalovirus mononucleosis (see Chap. 84)[54,56]
      3. Drug-induced lymphocytosis[57,58]
      4. Epstein-Barr virus mononucleosis (see Chap. 84)[59]
      5. Inflammatory (secondary) plasmacytosis of marrow
      6. Large granular lymphocytosis[60]
      7. Other viral mononucleosis (see Chap. 84)[54,61]
      8. Polyclonal lymphocytosis (see Chap. 81)[62]
      9. Serum sickness[63,64]
      10. T cell lymphocytosis associated with thymoma[65]
      11. *Toxoplasma gondii* mononucleosis (see Chap. 84)
      12. Viral infectious lymphocytosis[54,66]
   C. T lymphocyte dysfunction or depletion associated with systemic disease
      1. B cell chronic lymphocytic leukemia (see Chap. 92)
      2. Hodgkin lymphoma (see Chap. 97)
      3. Leprosy[67–69]
      4. Lupus erythematosus[70]
      5. Sjögren syndrome[71]
      6. Sarcoidosis[72,73]

T lymphocytes within a marrow allograft are responsible for initiation of the graft-versus-host reaction (see Chap. 22). The acute form of the reaction can lead to severe dermatitis, gastroenteritis, and hepatitis. The chronic syndrome simulates a collage of vascular diseases, such as scleroderma, xerophthalmia, xerostomia, and pulmonary insufficiency. Eosinophilia, hypergammaglobulinemia, development of autoantibodies, and plasmacytosis can occur. Infection with classic or opportunistic pathogens is a common complication of both acute and chronic graft-versus-host disease. A similar qualitative reaction, albeit more limited, is seen in mononucleosis resulting from Epstein-Barr virus infection (see Chap. 84).

NK CELL DISORDERS

CHRONIC NK CELL LYMPHOCYTOSIS

Chronic NK cell lymphocytosis is a rare proliferative disorder that can be distinguished from NK cell leukemia and lymphoma by its indolent nature.[1] Patients typically have neutropenia, anemia, vasculitic syndromes, fever of unknown origin, constitutional symptoms, and autoimmune disorders, including rheumatoid arthritis and/or polymyalgia rheumatica,[2] and often have cutaneous lesions.[3] Studies seeking to define this condition as a clonal disorder using X-linked gene analysis have not yielded consistent findings[4,5] (see Chap. 79).

The association of such conditions with chronic expansions in the numbers of NK cells implicates the NK cell as playing a role in autoimmunity. Consistent with this notion are animal studies implicating a deficiency of NK cells and/or NK-like T cells as a contributing factor in the pathogenesis of type 1 diabetes.[6] Moreover, NK cells play a role in regulating stem cell engraftment and in graft-versus-host disease following allogeneic hematopoietic stem cell transplantation.[7]

REFERENCES

1. Tefferi A: Chronic natural killer cell lymphocytosis. *Leuk Lymphoma* 20:245, 1996.
2. Sivakumaran M, Richards SJ, Scott CS: Clinical and laboratory characteristics of chronic natural killer cell lymphocytosis. *Blood* 87:1659, 1996.
3. Vanness ER, Davis MD, Tefferi A: Cutaneous findings associated with chronic natural killer cell lymphocytosis. *Int J Dermatol* 41:852, 2002.
4. Tefferi A, Greipp PR, Leibson PJ, Thibodeau SN: Demonstration of clonality, by X-linked DNA analysis, in chronic natural killer cell lymphocytosis and successful therapy with oral cyclophosphamide. *Leukemia* 6:477, 1992.
5. Nash R, McSweeney P, Zambello R, et al: Clonal studies of CD3- lymphoproliferative disease of granular lymphocytes. *Blood* 81:2363, 1993.
6. Kukreja A, Maclaren NK: NKT cells and type-1 diabetes and the "hygiene hypothesis" to explain the rising incidence rates. *Diabetes Technol Ther* 4:323, 2002.
7. Lowdell MW: Natural killer cells in haematopoietic stem cell transplantation. *Transfus Med* 13:399, 2003.
8. Ballow M: Primary immunodeficiency disorders: Antibody deficiency. *J Allergy Clin Immunol* 109:581, 2002.
9. Kyrtsonis MC, Mouzaki A, Maniatis A: Mechanisms of polyclonal hypogammaglobulinaemia in multiple myeloma (MM). *Med Oncol* 16:73, 1999.
10. Heneghan MA, Stevens FM, Cryan EM, et al: Celiac sprue and immunodeficiency states: A 25-year review. *J Clin Gastroenterol* 25:421, 1997.
11. Wong RC, Steele RH, Reeves GE, et al: Antibody and genetic testing in coeliac disease. *Pathology* 35:285, 2003.

12. Ochs HD, Smith CI: X-linked agammaglobulinemia. A clinical and molecular analysis. *Medicine (Baltimore)* 75:287, 1996.

13. Smith CI, Backesjo CM, Berglof A, et al: X-linked agammaglobulinemia: Lack of mature B lineage cells caused by mutations in the Btk kinase. *Springer Semin Immunopathol* 19:369, 1998.

14. Nonoyama S: Recent advances in the diagnosis of X-linked agammaglobulinemia. *Intern Med* 38:687, 1999.

15. Kaneko H, Kondo N: Clinical features of Bloom syndrome and function of the causative gene, BLM helicase. *Expert Rev Mol Diagn* 4:393, 2004.

16. Callard RE, Smith SH, Matthews DJ: Regulation of human B cell growth and differentiation: Lessons from the primary immunodeficiencies. *Chem Immunol* 67:114, 1997.

17. Sullivan KE: Recent advances in our understanding of Wiskott-Aldrich syndrome. *Curr Opin Hematol* 6:8, 1999.

18. Snapper SB, Rosen FS: The Wiskott-Aldrich syndrome protein (WASP): Roles in signaling and cytoskeletal organization. *Annu Rev Immunol* 17:905, 1999.

19. Etzioni A: Immune deficiency and autoimmunity. *Autoimmun Rev* 2:364, 2003.

20. Quartier P: IgA deficiency. *Arch Pediatr* 8:629, 2001.

21. Ojuawo A, St Louis D, Lindley KJ, Milla PJ: Non-infective colitis in infancy: Evidence in favour of minor immunodeficiency in its pathogenesis. *Arch Dis Child* 76:345, 1997.

22. Schroeder HW Jr, Schroeder HW 3rd, Sheikh SM: The complex genetics of common variable immunodeficiency. *J Investig Med* 52:90, 2004.

23. Klasen IS, Goertz JH, Van de Wiel GA, et al: Hyper-immunoglobulin A in the hyperimmunoglobulinemia D syndrome. *Clin Diagn Lab Immunol* 8:58, 2001.

24. Bermejo JF, Carbone J, Rodriguez JJ, et al: Macroamylasaemia, IgA hypergammaglobulinaemia and autoimmunity in a patient with Down syndrome and coeliac disease. *Scand J Gastroenterol* 38:445, 2003.

25. Yoshimura K, Wakiguchi H: Hyperimmunoglobulinemia D syndrome successfully treated with a corticosteroid. *Pediatr Int* 44:326, 2002.

26. Simon A, Mariman EC, Van der Meer JW, Drenth JP: A founder effect in the hyperimmunoglobulinemia D and periodic fever syndrome. *Am J Med* 114:148, 2003.

27. Salaria M, Poddar B, Parmar V: Hyperimmunoglobulin E syndrome. *Indian J Pediatr* 68:87, 2001.

28. Erlewyn-Lajeunesse MD: Hyperimmunoglobulin-E syndrome with recurrent infection: A review of current opinion and treatment. *Pediatr Allergy Immunol* 11:133, 2000.

29. Blanche P, Bachmeyer C, Buvry C, Sicard D: Hyperimmunoglobulinemia E syndrome in HIV infection. *J Am Acad Dermatol* 36:106, 1997.

30. Gilmour KC, Walshe D, Heath S, et al: Immunological and genetic analysis of 65 patients with a clinical suspicion of X linked hyper-IgM. *Mol Pathol* 56:256, 2003.

31. Engel P, Eck MJ, Terhorst C: The SAP and SLAM families in immune responses and X-linked lymphoproliferative disease. *Nat Rev Immunol* 3:813, 2003.

32. Gilmour KC, Gaspar HB: Pathogenesis and diagnosis of X-linked lymphoproliferative disease. *Expert Rev Mol Diagn* 3:549, 2003.

33. Elder ME: T-cell immunodeficiencies. *Pediatr Clin North Am* 47:1253, 2000.

34. Makitie O, Sulisalo T, de la Chapelle A, Kaitila I: Cartilage-hair hypoplasia. *J Med Genet* 32:39, 1995.

35. Cham B, Bonilla MA, Winkelstein J: Neutropenia associated with primary immunodeficiency syndromes. *Semin Hematol* 39:107, 2002.

36. Hogg N, Bates PA: Genetic analysis of integrin function in man: LAD-1 and other syndromes. *Matrix Biol* 19:211, 2000.

37. Perez E, Sullivan KE: Chromosome 22q11.2 deletion syndrome (DiGeorge and velocardiofacial syndromes). *Curr Opin Pediatr* 14:678, 2002.

38. Baldini A: DiGeorge syndrome: An update. *Curr Opin Cardiol* 19:201, 2004.

39. Nezelof C: Thymic pathology in primary and secondary immunodeficiencies. *Histopathology* 21:499, 1992.

40. Frick H, Munger DM, Fauchere JC, Stallmach T: Hypoplastic thymus and T-cell reduction in EECUT syndrome. *Am J Med Genet* 69:65, 1997.

41. Thrasher AJ: WASp in immune-system organization and function. *Nat Rev Immunol* 2:635, 2002.

42. Fischer A, Cavazzana-Calvo M, De Saint Basile G, et al: Naturally occurring primary deficiencies of the immune system. *Annu Rev Immunol* 15:93, 1997.

43. Perlman S, Becker-Catania S, Gatti RA: Ataxia-telangiectasia: Diagnosis and treatment. *Semin Pediatr Neurol* 10:173, 2003.

44. Hershfield MS: Genotype is an important determinant of phenotype in adenosine deaminase deficiency. *Curr Opin Immunol* 15:571, 2003.

45. Buckley RH: Immunodeficiency diseases. *JAMA* 268:2797, 1992.

46. Masternak K, Muhlethaler-Mottet A, Villard J, et al: Molecular genetics of the bare lymphocyte syndrome. *Rev Immunogenet* 2:267, 2000.

47. Reith W, Mach B: The bare lymphocyte syndrome and the regulation of MHC expression. *Annu Rev Immunol* 19:331, 2001.

48. Nekrep N, Fontes JD, Geyer M, Peterlin BM: When the lymphocyte loses its clothes. *Immunity* 18:453, 2003.

49. Sutor G, Fabel H: Sarcoidosis and common variable immunodeficiency. A case of a malignant course of sarcoidosis in conjunction with severe impairment of the cellular and humoral immune system. *Respiration* 67:204, 2000.

50. Granel B, Gayet S, Christides C, et al: Thymoma and hypogammaglobulinemia. Good's syndrome: Apropos of a case and review of the literature. *Rev Med Interne* 20:347, 1999.

51. Trakatellis A, Dimitriadou A, Trakatelli M: Pyridoxine deficiency: New approaches in immunosuppression and chemotherapy. *Postgrad Med J* 73:617, 1997.

52. Small TN, Wall DA, Kurtzberg J, et al: Association of reticular dysgenesis (thymic alymphoplasia and congenital aleukocytosis) with bilateral sensorineural deafness. *J Pediatr* 135:387, 1999.

53. Elder ME: SCID due to ZAP-70 deficiency. *J Pediatr Hematol Oncol* 19:546, 1997.

54. Brown KA: Nonmalignant disorders of lymphocytes. *Clin Lab Sci* 10:329, 1997.

55. Agarwal RK, Sun SH, Su SB, et al: Pertussis toxin alters the innate and the adaptive immune responses in a pertussis-dependent model of autoimmunity. *J Neuroimmunol* 129:133, 2002.

56. Drew WL, Lalezari JP: Cytomegalovirus: Disease syndromes and treatment. *Curr Clin Top Infect Dis* 19:16, 1999.

57. Holcombe RF: Drug-induced granulocytopenia with natural killer lymphocytosis after renal transplantation. *Acta Haematol* 83:96, 1990.

58. Toft P, Tonnesen E, Svendsen P, et al: The redistribution of lymphocytes during adrenaline infusion. An in vivo study with radiolabelled cells. *APMIS* 100:593, 1992.

59. Peter J, Ray CG: Infectious mononucleosis. *Pediatr Rev* 19:276, 1998.

60. Zambello R, Semenzato G: Large granular lymphocytosis. *Haematologica* 83:936, 1998.

61. Greenberg MS: Herpesvirus infections. *Dent Clin North Am* 40:359, 1996.

62. Troussard X, Flandrin G: Chronic B-cell lymphocytosis with binucleated lymphocytes (LWBL): A review of 38 cases. *Leuk Lymphoma* 20:275, 1996.

63. Erffmeyer JE: Serum sickness. *Ann Allergy* 56:105, 1986.

64. Virella G: Immune complex diseases. *Immunol Ser* 50:395, 1990.

65. Barton AD: T-cell lymphocytosis associated with lymphocyte-rich thymoma. *Cancer* 80:1409, 1997.

66. Saulsbury FT: B cell proliferation in acute infectious lymphocytosis. *Pediatr Infect Dis J* 6:1127, 1987.

67. Griffin G, Krishna S: Cytokines in infectious diseases. *J R Coll Physicians Lond* 32:195, 1998.

68. Gulle H, Schoel B, Chiplunkar S, et al: T-cell responses of leprosy patients and healthy contacts toward separated protein antigens of Mycobacterium leprae. *Int J Lepr Other Mycobact Dis* 60:44, 1992.

69. Walker KB, Butler R, Colston MJ: Role of Th-1 lymphocytes in the development of protective immunity against Mycobacterium leprae. Analysis of lymphocyte function by polymerase chain reaction detection of cytokine messenger RNA. *J Immunol* 148:1885, 1992.

70. Wenzel J, Gerdsen R, Uerlich M, et al: Lymphocytopenia in lupus erythematosus: Close in vivo association to autoantibodies targeting nuclear antigens. *Br J Dermatol* 150:994, 2004.

71. Mandl T, Bredberg A, Jacobsson LT, et al: CD4+ T-lymphocytopenia—A frequent finding in anti-SSA antibody seropositive patients with primary Sjogren's syndrome. *J Rheumatol* 31:726, 2004.

72. Morell F, Levy G, Orriols R, et al: Delayed cutaneous hypersensitivity tests and lymphopenia as activity markers in sarcoidosis. *Chest* 121:1239, 2002.

73. Gentil B, Cottin V, Girard P, Cordier JF: Ambivalence of CD4 lymphocytopenia in sarcoidosis. *Sarcoidosis Vasc Diffuse Lung Dis* 20:74, 2003.

LYMPHOCYTOSIS AND LYMPHOCYTOPENIA

THOMAS J. KIPPS

Lymphocytosis **is defined as an absolute lymphocyte count exceeding** 4×10^9**/liter (4000/**μ**l), whereas** *lymphocytopenia* **is defined as a total lymphocyte count less than** 1.0×10^9**/liter (1000/**μ**l). The causes of each are many and varied. Lymphocytosis can be categorized as either polyclonal or monoclonal.** *Monoclonal lymphocytosis* **generally reflects an underlying lymphoproliferative disease in which the numbers of lymphocytes are increased because of an intrinsic defect in the expanded lymphocyte population, whereas** *polyclonal lymphocytosis* **most commonly is secondary to stimulation or reaction to factors extrinsic to lymphocytes, generally infections and/or inflammation. Lymphocytopenia, on the other hand, typically reflects depletion of T cells, the most abundant lymphocyte in the blood. The most common cause of such T cell depletion is viral infection, such as infection with the human immunodeficiency virus, although other causes exist. This chapter outlines the conditions associated with abnormalities in the numbers of circulating lymphocytes in the blood. It also serves as a useful road map to other chapters in the book that describe in detail those conditions that commonly are associated with abnormalities in the absolute numbers of circulating lymphocytes.**

LYMPHOCYTOSIS

DEFINITION

Lymphocytosis is defined as an absolute lymphocyte count exceeding 4×10^9/liter (4000/μl), although somewhat higher threshold values (e.g., $>5.0 \times 10^9$/liter [$>5000/\mu$l]) are sometimes used. The normal absolute lymphocyte count is significantly higher in childhood. Chapter 2 describes the methods for determining the absolute lymphocyte count and the normal range for such counts.

The blood film of patients with lymphocytosis should be evaluated for a predominance of reactive lymphocytes associated with infectious mononucleosis (see Chap. 84), large granular lymphocytes associated with large granular lymphocytic leukemia (see Chap. 94), smudge cells associated with chronic lymphocytic leukemia (CLL; see Chap. 92), or blasts of acute lymphocytic leukemia (see Chap. 91). Chapter 74 provides a description of normal lymphocyte morphology.

Characterization of cell surface markers is valuable in distinguishing primary lymphocytosis (leukemic) from secondary lymphocytosis (reactive). New improvements in flow cytometric techniques and reagents have allowed clinical laboratories to perform flow cytometric immunophenotyping to distinguish benign from neoplastic lymphoproliferative disease (see Chap. 14). Analysis for immunoglobulin or

Acronyms and abbreviations that appear in this chapter include: CLL, chronic lymphocytic leukemia; EBV, Epstein-Barr virus; HIV, human immunodeficiency virus; Ig, immunoglobulin; NK, natural killer; PPBL, persistent polyclonal B cell lymphocytosis; PUVA, psoralen and ultraviolet A.

T cell receptor gene rearrangement also may provide evidence for monoclonal B cell or T cell proliferation, respectively.[1]

PRIMARY LYMPHOCYTOSIS

Primary lymphocytosis defines conditions associated with an increase in the absolute number of lymphocytes secondary to an intrinsic defect in the expanded lymphocyte population (Table 81-1). These conditions also are referred to as *lymphoproliferative disorders* and most commonly are secondary to the neoplastic accumulation of monoclonal B cells, T cells, natural killer (NK) cells,[2] or less fully differentiated cells of the lymphoid lineage. Table 81-1 lists the chapters describing each of these conditions.

Although patients with lymphocytosis secondary to lymphoproliferative disease generally maintain abnormal lymphocyte counts that may rise over time, this finding is not invariable. Patients with large granular lymphocytic leukemia (see Chap. 94) may have only transient lymphocytosis that is induced by stress or exercise.[3]

ESSENTIAL MONOCLONAL B CELL LYMPHOCYTOSIS

The advent of flow cytometric and molecular diagnostic techniques has identified a syndrome in patients who have expanded populations of monoclonal B cells without other associated clinical signs or symptoms.[4] High-sensitivity flow cytometric techniques, developed to monitor disease in patients with CLL undergoing treatment, have allowed for identification of monoclonal or oligoclonal B cell populations in a high proportion of healthy individuals from the general population and an even higher proportion of relatives of patients with familial CLL[5-7] (see Chap. 92). This syndrome may resemble that of patients with essential monoclonal gammopathy who otherwise do not have the clinical features of myeloma. Such patients also were identified after improved technology was introduced for evaluating serum immunoglobulins (see Chaps. 98 and 99). Similar to the latter, some patients who have expanded populations of monoclonal B cells may develop progressive neoplastic lymphoproliferative disease.[8]

PERSISTENT POLYCLONAL LYMPHOCYTOSIS OF B LYMPHOCYTES

Persistent polyclonal B cell lymphocytosis (PPBL) is defined as a chronic, moderate increase in absolute lymphocyte counts ($>4 \times 10^9$/liter) without evidence for infection or other conditions that can increase the lymphocyte count. In perhaps the most common manifestation of PPBL, the patients have an accumulation of polyclonal B cells that have an unusual binucleate appearance on the blood film.[9,10] These lymphocytes typically lack expression of CD5 or CD23[11,12] and are polyclonal with respect to light-chain expression and immunoglobulin heavy-chain gene rearrangements.[13] Patients may have mild splenomegaly and raised serum immunoglobulin (Ig)M levels. This disorder appears more common among cigarette smokers[14,15] and most typically is associated the HLA-DR7 haplotype.[9]

Patients with PPBL can have features resembling those of patients with various monoclonal B cell malignancies. In some cases, the marrow has modest infiltration of polyclonal B cells that can be mistaken for a neoplastic disease.[16] In possibly another manifestation of this syndrome, first identified in Japan as hairy B cell lymphoproliferative disorder,[17] the patients can present with anemia, thrombocytopenia, and splenomegaly and have an excess of polyclonal B lymphocytes that appear similar in morphology to the neoplastic B cells in hairy cell leukemia. In perhaps a related syndrome, some patients have an accumulation of polyclonal B cells that coexpress CD19, CD5, and CD23, thus displaying an immunophenotype similar to that of B cell CLL.[7,18] Other studies have identified expansions of B cells bearing the phenotype of memory-type B cells, namely, high-level expression of surface IgD and CD27, with increased proportions of B cells har-

TABLE 81-1 CAUSES OF LYMPHOCYTOSIS

I. Primary lymphocytosis
   A. Lymphocytic malignancies
      1. Acute lymphocytic leukemia (Chap. 91)
      2. Chronic lymphocytic leukemia and related disorders (Chap. 92)
      3. Prolymphocytic leukemia (Chap. 92)
      4. Hairy cell leukemia[133] (Chap. 93)
      5. Adult T cell leukemia (Chaps. 92 and 96)
      6. Lymphoma cell leukemia[134] (Chap. 96)
      7. Large granular lymphocytic leukemia[135] (Chap. 94)
         a. NK cell leukemia[136] (Chap. 94)
         b. CD8+ T cell large granular lymphocytic leukemia[137–139]
         c. CD4+ T cell large granular lymphocytic leukemia[53,140]
         d. γ/δ T cell large granular lymphocytic leukemia[141]
   B. Essential monoclonal B cell lymphocytosis[6] (Chap. 92)
   C. Persistent polyclonal B cell lymphocytosis[9,10]
II. Reactive lymphocytosis
   A. Mononucleosis syndromes (Chap. 84)
      1. Epstein-Barr virus[38,142–146]
      2. Cytomegalovirus[41,42,147–152]
      3. Human immunodeficiency virus[153–158]
      4. Herpes simplex virus type II
      5. Rubella virus
      6. Toxoplasma gondii[159]
      7. Adenovirus
      8. Infectious hepatitis virus
      9. Dengue fever virus[160–162]
      10. Human herpes virus type 6 (HHV-6)[77,163]
      11. Human herpes virus type 8 (HHV-8)[164]
      12. Varicella zoster virus[165]
   B. Bordetella pertussis[45]
   C. NK cell lymphocytosis[54–56,73,75,166–169]
   D. Stress lymphocytosis (acute)[69]
      1. Cardiovascular collapse[66]
         a. Acute cardiac failure
         b. Myocardial infarction
      2. Staphylococcal toxic shock syndrome[170]
      3. Drug-induced[68,77,171]
      4. Major surgery
      5. Sickle cell crisis[172]
      6. Status epilepticus
      7. Trauma[65,66]
   E. Hypersensitivity reactions
      1. Insect bites[73–75]
      2. Drugs[76,78,80,81,173]
   F. Persistent lymphocytosis (subacute or chronic)
      1. Cancer[84]
      2. Cigarette smoking[15,174]
      3. Hyposplenism[86]
      4. Chronic infection
         a. Leishmaniasis[175]
         b. Leprosy[176]
         c. Strongyloidiasis[58–60]
      5. Thymoma[83]

NK = natural killer.

boring the t(14;18) translocation of immunoglobulin genes and *BCL-2* that is associated with follicular lymphomas.[19]

The cause(s) of PPBL is unknown. The immunoglobulin variable-region genes used by the B cells in PPBL most commonly have evidence of somatic mutations, implying that the expanded B cells have undergone germinal center maturation in an immune response(s) to antigen(s).[20,21] Analyses of the immunoglobulin variable-region genes expressed by memory-type B cells of patients with PPBL failed to reveal evidence of positive antigenic selection, suggesting inappropriate clearance of B cells expressing low-affinity immunoglobulin receptors plays some role in this disorder.[20] Defective signaling via the Fas (CD95) death receptor has been implicated as causing insufficient clearance of B lymphocytes.[22]

Gender and genotype may be important in the pathogenesis, as the patients most commonly are young to middle-age women who often are HLA-DR7 positive.[9] In addition, shared cases of PPBL among identical twins[23] and in families[24] have been reported. Moreover, evaluation of first-degree relatives of individuals with PPBL may identify new patients who have all the criteria for diagnosis of PPBL or have slight increases in serum IgM,[25] suggesting a possible hereditary or genetic contribution to the pathogenesis.

Although the lymphocytosis of PPBL generally is not progressive, most patients have small numbers of blood B cells with chromosomal abnormalities. These abnormalities most commonly include an additional isochromosome +i(3q) and premature chromosome condensation,[10,26–28] although t(14;18) involving the *BCL-2* and immunoglobulin heavy-chain loci also have been detected.[13,24,25,29–31] In another study of 43 patients with PPBL, two thirds had lymphocytes with independent chromosomal abnormalities, such as del(6q), +der(8), +8, or other polyploidy karyotypic abnormalities.[32] In any one patient, these chromosomal abnormalities are restricted to B lymphocytes independent of their expression of immunoglobulin κ or λ light chain.[10] For PPBL associated with smoking, these cytogenetic abnormalities apparently persist after the discontinuation of tobacco use.[9] The finding of such chromosome abnormalities is consistent with the notion that PPBL represents a preneoplastic state. Occasional reports of clonal immunoglobulin rearrangements in this disorder suggest that polyclonal expansion in some cases may be followed by the emergence of one predominant clone.[9,16,33] Moreover, a small proportion of patients with PPBL ultimately develop monoclonal B cell lymphoma or B cell leukemia.[34–36]

SECONDARY (REACTIVE) LYMPHOCYTOSIS

Secondary lymphocytosis defines conditions associated with an increase in the absolute number of lymphocytes secondary to a physiologic or pathophysiologic response to infection, toxins, cytokines, or unknown factors.[37]

INFECTIOUS MONONUCLEOSIS

The most common reactive lymphocytosis is infectious mononucleosis (see Table 81-1). In cases of mononucleosis secondary to infection with Epstein-Barr virus (EBV), the atypical lymphocytes commonly consist of polyclonal populations of CD8+ T cells, γ/δ T cells, and CD16+CD56+ NK cells that are stimulated in response to EBV-infected B cells.[38] Typically, no changes in the absolute CD4+ T cell and CD19+ B cell counts are observed. Chapter 84 describes the syndrome.

ACUTE INFECTION LYMPHOCYTOSIS

A disorder possibly related to infectious mononucleosis is acute infection lymphocytosis, a contagious disease characterized by an increase in circulating lymphocytes, often to 20 to 30 × 10⁹/liter (20,000–30,000/µl)[39] and occasionally to 100 × 10⁹/liter (100,000/µl).[40] Patients usually are asymptomatic but may have fever, abdominal pain, or diarrhea. Lymph node enlargement and splenomegaly do not occur, and the patient's serum usually is negative for heterophil antibodies. In this regard, the disease resembles infectious mononucleosis caused by viruses other than EBV, such as cytomegalovirus (see Chap. 84).[41,42] Clinical symptoms last for a few days, but the lymphocytosis may persist for several weeks. Eosinophilia may be present.[43] Examination of marrow from a few patients has shown minimal increases in lymphocytes, but marked infiltration with lymphocytes also has been observed. In some cases, the lymphocytosis has been found in association with acute infection by coxsackievirus B2.[44]

BORDETELLA PERTUSSIS

A marked increase in the number of morphologically normal lymphocytes occurs in patients infected with the gram-negative bacterium

Bordetella pertussis. Absolute lymphocyte counts range from 8 to 70 × 10⁹/liter (8000–70,000/µl), with a mean of approximately 30 × 10⁹/liter (30,000/µl), involving all lymphocyte subsets.[45–47]

Lymphocytosis primarily results from failure of lymphocytes to leave the blood because of a toxin, termed *pertussis toxin*, released by the bacteria.[48] Pertussis toxin is an adenosine diphosphate ribosylase that modifies Gi proteins in mammalian lymphocytes and inhibits their capacity to traffic from blood into lymphoid tissues, primarily through inhibition of chemokine receptors.[49,50] Pertussis toxin also may stimulate egress of maturing T cells from the thymus[51] and may bind to neuraminic acid residues of T cell surface glycoproteins to induce T cell activation.[52]

LARGE GRANULAR LYMPHOCYTOSIS
Large granular lymphocytosis can result from expansions of NK cells, CD8⁺ T cells, or, more rarely, CD4+ T cells.[53] In the most common form, the lymphocytosis is secondary to CD3−CD16+CD56+ NK cells and is termed *NK lymphocytosis*, in which NK cell counts typically approximate 4 × 10⁹/liter (4000/µl) but can sometimes exceed 15 × 10⁹/liter (15,000/µl).[54] Patients with NK lymphocytosis frequently have recurrent cutaneous lesions, such as livedoid vasculopathy, urticarial vasculitis, or complex recurrent aphthous stomatitis.[55,56] Other reports noted an association between NK lymphocytosis and various cytopenias, including severe aplastic anemia.[54,57] Expansion of NK cells may represent an exaggerated response to systemic infection, with several reports describing an association between NK lymphocytosis and strongyloidiasis.[58–60]

A relatively high proportion of patients with rheumatoid arthritis and related disorders have large granular lymphocytosis. Occurring in less than 0.6 percent of patients with rheumatoid arthritis, large granular lymphocytic lymphocytosis almost invariably is associated with neutropenia in the absence of splenomegaly and thus may represent a subset disorder of patients with Felty syndrome.[61,62] Patients with autoimmune pure red cell aplasia or immune thrombocytopenia also may have large granular lymphocytosis secondary to expanded numbers of polyclonal T cells[63] or NK cells.[54,57,64]

STRESS LYMPHOCYTOSIS
Trauma, surgery, acute cardiac failure, septic shock, myocardial infarction, sickle cell crisis, or status epilepticus may be associated with an elevated lymphocyte count, often greater than 5 × 10⁹/liter (5000/µl),[65,66] which may revert to normal or below-normal levels within hours.[67] The increased lymphocyte count appears promptly after the event and appears secondary to lymphocyte redistribution affecting all major lymphocyte subsets.[68,69] A transient lymphocytosis can be induced by the adrenaline released and/or administered in response to the medical episode.[70–72] Characteristically, two phases are recognized after catecholamine administration: a quick (<30 minutes) mobilization of lymphocytes, followed by an increase in granulocyte numbers with decreasing lymphocyte numbers.[71]

HYPERSENSITIVITY REACTIONS
Delayed hypersensitivity reactions to insect bites, especially mosquitos, may be associated with a large granular lymphocytic lymphocytosis and adenopathy.[73–75] Idiosyncratic drug reactions also may be associated with subacute lymphocytosis.[76–80] An infectious mononucleosis-like syndrome can be induced in some patients by salazosulfapyridine[81] or sulfasalazine.[78]

PERSISTENT LYMPHOCYTOSIS
Patients may have subacute or chronic lymphocytosis, termed *persistent lymphocytosis*, in association with a variety of clinical conditions (see Table 81-1).

Cancer   Patients with lymphocytosis may have underlying neoplastic disease. Most notably, patients with malignant thymoma may have a polyclonal T cell lymphocytosis thought to be secondary to the aberrant release of thymic hormones by the neoplastic thymic epithelium.[82,83] A reactive lymphocytosis or plasmacytosis may be detected in a relatively high proportion of patients with acute myeloid leukemia[84] or systemic mastocytosis.[85]

Cigarette Smoking   Cigarette smokers may have a persistent lymphocytosis secondary to an increase in polyclonal CD4+ T cells and B cells, some of which have an unusual binuclear morphology.[15]

Postsplenectomy Lymphocytosis   Patients undergoing splenectomy for staging of Hodgkin disease may develop a chronic postoperative polyclonal lymphocytosis.[86] An absolute lymphocyte count ranging from 4.0 to 8.7 × 10⁹/liter often is noted 4 to 242 (median 70) months after splenectomy and can persist for prolonged periods (e.g., >50 months).[87]

Chronic Infections   A reactive lymphocytosis commonly is associated with many viral and certain bacterial infections, which, if protracted, can result in subacute or chronic lymphocytosis[37] (see Table 81-1).

LYMPHOCYTOPENIA

DEFINITION

Chapter 2 presents the methods for determining the absolute lymphocyte count and the normal range for such counts. *Lymphocytopenia* is defined as a total lymphocyte count less than 1.0 × 10⁹/liter (1000/µl), but some consider the lower limit of normal to be 1.5 × 10⁹/liter (1500/µl). Because approximately 80 percent of normal adult blood lymphocytes are T lymphocytes and nearly two thirds of blood T lymphocytes are CD4+ (helper) T lymphocytes, most patients with lymphocytopenia have reductions in the absolute numbers of T lymphocytes, particularly CD4+ T lymphocytes. The average absolute number of T lymphocytes in normal adult blood is 1.9 × 10⁹/liter (1900/µl), ranging from 1.0 to 2.3 × 10⁹/liter (1000–2300/µl).[88] The average absolute number of CD4+ T lymphocytes is 1.1 × 10⁹/liter (1100/µl), ranging from 7.2 to 14 × 10⁸/liter (720–1400/µl). The average absolute number of cells of the other major T cell subgroup, CD8+ T lymphocytes, is 6.5 × 10⁸/liter (650/µl), ranging from 3.8 to 9.7 × 10⁸/liter (380–970/µl). Some Asians and blacks may lack or be heterozygous for an epitope on the CD4 molecule that is recognized by the mouse monoclonal antibody OKT4A, thus making these patients appear to have a deficiency in the absolute number of CD4 T cells. Use of other anti-CD4 monoclonal antibodies (e.g., Leu-3a) that bind other epitopes of the CD4 molecule may help rule out factitious CD4+ T cell depletion.

Table 81-2 summarizes the conditions associated with lymphocytopenia. The mechanism of lymphocytopenia is not established for many of these disorders, and several possible mechanisms exist. Further discussion of lymphocytes and of the diseases associated with lymphocytopenia are presented in the cited reports (see Table 81-2).

The relative incidence of each of these conditions varies, depending upon the patient population. In one New Zealand survey of patients who had significant lymphocytopenia (<0.6 × 10⁹/liter), the patients fell into several categories with some overlap.[89] In order of decreasing frequency, the factors associated with lymphocytopenia were bacterial or fungal sepsis (250 patients), major surgery (228 patients), definite (153 patients) or suspected (53 patients) glucocorticoid therapy, malignancy (180 patients), cytotoxic therapy and/or radiotherapy (90 patients), recent trauma or hemorrhage (86 patients), renal allograft (38 patients), marrow allograft (35 patients), "viral infections" other than human immunodeficiency virus (HIV; 26 patients), or infection with

TABLE 81-2   CAUSES OF LYMPHOCYTOPENIA

I.   Inherited causes
    A.   Congenital immunodeficiency diseases[177] (Chap. 82)
        1.   Severe combined immunodeficiency disease[178]
            a.   Aplasia of lymphopoietic stem cells
            b.   Adenosine deaminase deficiency[179]
            c.   Absence of histocompatibility antigens[180]
            d.   Absence of CD4+ helper cells[181]
            e.   Thymic alymphoplasia with aleukocytosis (reticular dysgenesis)[182]
        2.   Common variable immune deficiency[183,184]
        3.   Ataxia-telangiectasia[185,186]
        4.   Wiskott-Aldrich syndrome[187]
        5.   Immunodeficiency with short-limbed dwarfism (cartilage-hair hypoplasia)[188]
        6.   Immunodeficiency with thymoma[189–191]
        7.   Purine nucleoside phosphorylase deficiency[192]
        8.   Immunodeficiency with venoocclusive disease of the liver[193]
    B.   Lymphopenia resulting from genetic polymorphism[91,92]
II.   Acquired causes
    A.   Aplastic anemia[194] (Chap. 33)
    B.   Infectious diseases
        1.   Viral diseases (Chap. 83)
            a.   Acquired immunodeficiency syndrome[195]
            b.   Severe acute respiratory syndrome (SARS)[98,99,196–199]
            c.   West Nile encephalitis[200–202]
            d.   Hepatitis[203]
            e.   Influenza[204,205]
            f.   Herpes simplex virus[206]
            g.   Herpes virus type 6 (HHV-6)[163,207]
            h.   Herpes virus type 8 (HHV-8)[208,209]
            i.   Measles virus[100,101]
            j.   Other[210]
        2.   Bacterial diseases
            a.   Tuberculosis[95–97,211]
            b.   Typhoid fever[212]
            c.   Pneumonia[213]
            d.   Rickettsiosis[214]
            e.   Ehrlichiosis[14]
            f.   Sepsis[215,216]
         3.   Parasitic diseases
            a.   Acute phase of malaria infection[217–219]
    C.   Iatrogenic
        1.   Immunosuppressive agents[220,221]
            a.   Antilymphocyte globulin therapy[222]
            b.   Alemtuzumab (CAMPATH 1-H)[223]
            c.   Glucocorticoids[224]
         2.   High-dose PUVA treatment[102]
        3.   Stevens-Johnson syndrome[225]
        4.   Chemotherapy[226,227]
        5.   Platelet or stem cell apheresis procedures[108,109]
        6.   Radiation[228,229]
        7.   Major surgery[230,231]
        8.   Extracorporeal bypass circulation[232]
        9.   Renal or marrow transplant[233]
        10.   Thoracic duct drainage[107]
        11.   Hemodialysis[234]
    D.   Systemic disease associated
        1.   Autoimmune diseases[110]
            a.   Arthritis[235]
            b.   Systemic lupus erythematosus[112,236]
            c.   Sjögren syndrome[111,237]
            d.   Myasthenia gravis[238]
            e.   Systemic vasculitis[239]
            f.   Behçet-like syndrome[240]
            g.   Dermatomyositis[241]
            h.   Wegener granulomatosis[242]
         2.   Hodgkin disease[243]
         3.   Carcinoma[244–247]
         4.   Idiopathic myelofibrosis[248]
         5.   Protein-losing enteropathy[249,250]
         6.   Renal failure[251]
         7.   Sarcoidosis[252–255]
         8.   Thermal injury[113]
         9.   Severe acute pancreatitis[256]
         10.   Strenuous exercise[257,258]
         11.   Silicosis[259]
         12.   Coeliac disease[260]
    E.   Nutritional and dietary
        1.   Ethanol abuse[116]
        2.   Zinc deficiency[114,115]
III.   Idiopathic
    A.   Idiopathic CD4+ T lymphocytopenia[117,120,127,131,132]

PUVA=psoralen plus ultraviolet A.

HIV (13 patients). Only one patient was suspected of having idiopathic CD4+ T lymphocytopenia.

INHERITED CAUSES

Patients with inherited immunodeficiency diseases may have associated lymphocytopenia (see Table 81-2 and see Chap. 82). Inherited immunodeficiency disorders may have a quantitative or qualitative stem cell abnormality, resulting in ineffective lymphopoiesis (see cited references in Table 81-2). Others, such as the Wiskott-Aldrich syndrome, have associated lymphopenia because of premature destruction of T cells secondary to a defect in the lymphocyte cytoskeleton.[90] Studies have reported that certain ethnic groups have lower CD4 T cell counts in the absence of other identified factors (e.g., Ethiopians[91] and Chukotka natives[92]).

ACQUIRED LYMPHOCYTOPENIA

Acquired lymphocytopenia defines syndromes associated with depletion of blood lymphocytes that are not secondary to inherited disease.

INFECTIOUS DISEASES

The most common infectious disease associated with lymphopenia is the acquired immunodeficiency syndrome. The lymphocytopenia results in part from destruction and/or clearance of CD4+ T cells infected with HIV-1 or HIV-2.[88,93,94] The lymphocytopenia also may reflect impaired lymphocyte production and proliferation secondary to loss of the normal thymic or lymphoid architecture and the high levels of transforming growth factor β that often are noted in patients with this disease (see Chap. 83).

Other viral and bacterial diseases may be associated with lymphocytopenia (see Table 81-2). Patients presenting with active tuberculosis often have lymphocytopenia that usually resolves 2 weeks after initiating appropriate antimicrobial therapy.[95–97] Patients with severe acute respiratory syndrome resulting from infection with coronavirus typically have lymphocytopenia that resolves following recovery.[47,98,99] Several other common viral diseases, such as measles,[100,101] typically are associated with transient lymphocytopenia during the acute phases of infection, which in turn is thought to contribute to a disease course-related immune deficiency that can predispose patients to infection with opportunistic infectious agents (see Table 81-2).

IATROGENIC

Radiotherapy, neoplastic chemotherapy, glucocorticoids, or administration of antilymphocyte globulin or alemtuzumab (CAMPATH-1 H) each can lead to lymphocytopenia by destroying circulating lymphocytes (see Table 81-2). Long-term treatment of psoriasis with psoralen and ultraviolet A (PUVA) irradiation may result in T lymphocyte lymphopenia, possibly through destruction of cells circulating through the cutaneous vasculature.[102] The mechanism by which glucocorticoids cause lymphocytopenia is not clear but may be secondary to a glucocorticoid-induced redistribution of lymphocytes[103,104] in addition to induced cell destruction.[104,105] Redistribution also may be responsible for the lymphocytopenia occurring after surgery.[106] In thoracic duct drainage, the lymphocytes are lost from the body.[107] Platelet or stem cell apheresis similarly lowers the lymphocyte count because of inadvertent removal of lymphocytes with the platelets.[108,109]

SYSTEMIC DISEASE ASSOCIATED WITH LYMPHOCYTOPENIA

Patients with systemic autoimmune disease can have lymphocytopenia, secondary to either the underlying disease or therapy.[110,111] The lymphocytopenia of patients with systemic lupus erythematosus may be autoantibody mediated.[112] Similarly, patients with primary Sjögren syndrome sometimes have lymphocytopenia.[111] In conditions such as protein-losing enteropathy, lymphocytes may be lost from the body. Severe thermal injury may result in profound T cell lymphopenia secondary to redistribution of blood T cells to the tissues.[113]

NUTRITIONAL OR DIETARY

Zinc is essential for normal T cell development and function.[114,115] Zinc therapy corrects the lymphocytopenia of zinc deficiency, and lymphocytic function is restored. Excessive intake of ethanol and/or chronic ethanol use may result in impaired lymphocyte proliferative responses and lymphopenia, which may resolve with abstinence from alcohol.[116]

IDIOPATHIC CD4+ T LYMPHOCYTOPENIA

The advent of immunophenotyping and HIV serologic testing has identified a syndrome of isolated CD4+ T cell depletion in the absence of evidence for retroviral infection. The syndrome, termed *idiopathic CD4+ T lymphocytopenia* by the Centers for Disease Control and Prevention in 1993, is defined by a CD4+ T lymphocyte count less than 3×10^8/liter (300/μl) on two separate occasions in patients without serologic or virologic evidence of HIV-1 or HIV-2 infection.[117] It is important to exclude congenital immunodeficiency diseases, such as common variable immunodeficiency, which may lead to altered CD4 T cell counts that are recognized in later life (see Chap. 82).[88,118] The pathogenesis of this disorder is not known, although one study found that the CD4+ T cells from patients with this abnormality were unusually sensitive to programmed cell death induced by T cell receptor cross-linking.[119]

Although some patients with idiopathic CD4+ T lymphocytopenia do not have any clinical manifestations,[120,121] more than half of all reported cases had prior opportunistic infections indicative of a cellular immunodeficiency (e.g., recurrent herpes zoster, pulmonary *Mycobacterium avium*, *Pneumocystis carinii* pneumonia, Toxoplasmosis, or cryptococcal infections).[122–127] Patients with a clinical history are classified by the World Health Organization as having idiopathic CD4+ T lymphocytopenia and severe unexplained HIV-seronegative immune suppression.[88]

The exact proportion of patients with this disorder is unknown because patients who are not affected clinically by the isolated CD4+ T cell depletion may not come to medical attention. There are several reports of this abnormality in aged individuals, suggesting that the incidence is increased in the aged population.[128–130] CD4+ T lymphocytopenic patients with this condition differ from those infected with HIV in that they generally have stable CD4+ counts over time and may manifest reductions in other lymphocyte subgroups.[131,132] Also, patients with this abnormality may have a complete or partial spontaneous reversal in the CD4+ T lymphocytopenia.[131]

REFERENCES

1. Rockman SP: Determination of clonality in patients who present with diagnostic dilemmas: A laboratory experience and review of the literature. *Leukemia* 11:852, 1997.
2. Zambello R, Semenzato G: Large granular lymphocytosis. *Haematologica* 83:936, 1998.
3. de Pasquale A, Ginaldi L, di Leonardo G, et al: Exercise-induced variations of lymphocytosis in the lymphoproliferative disease of large granular lymphocytes [letter]. *Br J Haematol* 82:178, 1992.
4. Kimby E, Mellstedt H, Bjorkholm M, Holm G: Clonal cell surface structures related to differentiation, activation and homing in B-cell chronic lymphocytic leukemia and monoclonal lymphocytosis of undetermined significance. *Eur J Haematol* 43:452, 1989.
5. Rawstron AC, Green MJ, Kuzmicki A, et al: Monoclonal B lymphocytes with the characteristics of "indolent" chronic lymphocytic leukemia are present in 3.5% of adults with normal blood counts. *Blood* 100:635, 2002.
6. Marti GE, Carter P, Abbasi F, et al: B-cell monoclonal lymphocytosis and B-cell abnormalities in the setting of familial B-cell chronic lymphocytic leukemia. *Cytometry* 52B:1, 2003.
7. Ghia P, Prato G, Scielzo C, et al: Monoclonal CD5+ and CD5– B-lymphocyte expansions are frequent in the peripheral blood of the elderly. *Blood* 103:2337, 2004.
8. Ritis K, Tsironidou V, Martinis G, et al: Development of CLL in individuals with mild lymphocytosis, without bone marrow infiltration, but with evidence of a monoclonally expanded population in peripheral blood. *Haematologica* 82:184, 1997.
9. Troussard X, Flandrin G: Chronic B-cell lymphocytosis with binucleated lymphocytes (LWBL): A review of 38 cases. *Leuk Lymphoma* 20:275, 1996.
10. Mossafa H, Malaure H, Maynadie M, et al: Persistent polyclonal B lymphocytosis with binucleated lymphocytes: A study of 25 cases. Groupe Français d'Hématologie Cellulaire. *Br J Haematol* 104:486, 1999.
11. Wang C, Amato D, Fernandes B: CD5-negative phenotype of monoclonal B-lymphocytosis of undetermined significance (MLUS). *Am J Hematol* 69:147, 2002.
12. Keung YK, Buss D, Pettenati M, Powell BL: CD5-negative chronic lymphocytic leukemia or monoclonal B-lymphocytosis of undetermined significance? *Am J Hematol* 70:334, 2002.
13. Delage R, Roy J, Jacques L, et al: Multiple bcl-2/Ig gene rearrangements in persistent polyclonal B-cell lymphocytosis. *Br J Haematol* 97:589, 1997.
14. Bakken JS, Aguero-Rosenfeld ME, Tilden RL, et al: Serial measurements of hematologic counts during the active phase of human granulocytic ehrlichiosis. *Clin Infect Dis* 32:862, 2001.
15. Delannoy A, Djian D, Wallef G, et al: Cigarette smoking and chronic polyclonal B-cell lymphocytosis. *Nouv Rev Fr Hematol* 35:141, 1993.
16. Feugier P, De March AK, Lesesve JF, et al: Intravascular bone marrow accumulation in persistent polyclonal lymphocytosis: A misleading feature for B-cell neoplasm. *Mod Pathol* 17:1087, 2004.
17. Machii T, Yamaguchi M, Inoue R, et al: Polyclonal B-cell lymphocytosis with features resembling hairy cell leukemia-Japanese variant. *Blood* 89:2008, 1997.
18. Lush CJ, Vora AJ, Campbell AC, Wood JK: Polyclonal CD5+ B-lymphocytosis resembling chronic lymphocytic leukaemia. *Br J Haematol* 79:119, 1991.
19. Himmelmann A, Gautschi O, Nawrath M, et al: Persistent polyclonal B-cell lymphocytosis is an expansion of functional IgD(+)CD27(+) memory B cells. *Br J Haematol* 114:400, 2001.
20. Loembe MM, Neron S, Delage R, Darveau A: Analysis of expressed V(H) genes in persistent polyclonal B cell lymphocytosis reveals absence of selection in CD27+IgM+IgD+ memory B cells. *Eur J Immunol* 32:3678, 2002.
21. Salcedo I, Campos-Caro A, Sampalo A, et al: Persistent polyclonal B lymphocytosis: An expansion of cells showing IgVH gene mutations and phenotypic features of normal lymphocytes from the CD27+ marginal zone B-cell compartment. *Br J Haematol* 116:662, 2002.
22. Roussel M, Roue G, Sola B, et al: Dysfunction of the Fas apoptotic signaling pathway in persistent polyclonal B-cell lymphocytosis. *Haematologica* 88:239, 2003.
23. Carr R, Fishlock K, Matutes E: Persistent polyclonal B-cell lymphocytosis in identical twins. *Br J Haematol* 96:272, 1997.
24. Himmelmann A, Ruegg R, Fehr J: Familial persistent polyclonal B-cell lymphocytosis. *Leuk Lymphoma* 41:157, 2001.
25. Delage R, Jacques L, Massinga-Loembe M, et al: Persistent polyclonal B-cell lymphocytosis: Further evidence for a genetic disorder associated with B-cell abnormalities. *Br J Haematol* 114:666, 2001.

26. Callet-Bauchu E, Renard N, Gazzo S, et al: Distribution of the cytogenetic abnormality +i(3)(q10) in persistent polyclonal B-cell lymphocytosis: A FICTION study in three cases. *Br J Haematol* 99:531, 1997.

27. Espinet B, Florensa L, Sole F, et al: Isochromosome +i(3)(q10) in a new case of persistent polyclonal B-cell lymphocytosis (PPBL). *Eur J Haematol* 64:344, 2000.

28. Samson T, Mossafa H, Lusina D, et al: Dicentric chromosome 3 associated with binucleated lymphocytes in atypical B-cell chronic lymphoproliferative disorder. *Leuk Lymphoma* 43:1749, 2002.

29. Granados E, Llamas P, Pinilla I, et al: Persistent polyclonal B lymphocytosis with multiple bcl-2/IgH rearrangements: A benign disorder. *Haematologica* 83:369, 1998.

30. Delage R, Roy J, Jacques L, Darveau A: All patients with persistent polyclonal B cell lymphocytosis present Bcl-2/Ig gene rearrangements. *Leuk Lymphoma* 31:567, 1998.

31. Lancry L, Roulland S, Roue G, et al: No BCL-2 protein over expression but BCL-2/IgH rearrangements in B cells of patients with persistent polyclonal B-cell lymphocytosis. *Hematol J* 2:228, 2001.

32. Mossafa H, Tapia S, Flandrin G, Troussard X: Chromosomal instability and ATR amplification gene in patients with persistent and polyclonal B-cell lymphocytosis (PPBL). *Leuk Lymphoma* 45:1401, 2004.

33. Chan MA, Benedict SH, Carstairs KC, et al: Expansion of B lymphocytes with an unusual immunoglobulin rearrangement associated with atypical lymphocytosis and cigarette smoking. *Am J Respir Cell Mol Biol* 2:549, 1990.

34. Roy J, Ryckman C, Bernier V, et al: Large cell lymphoma complicating persistent polyclonal B cell lymphocytosis. *Leukemia* 12:1026, 1998.

35. Radossi P, Dazzi F, De Franchis G, et al: Myasthenic syndrome and oligoclonal lymphocytosis: Evolution into chronic lymphocytic leukemia. *Ann Hematol* 76:45, 1998.

36. Bassan R, Spinelli O, Rambaldi A, Barbui T: The course of monoclonal "villous" lymphocytosis over 15 years of follow-up: Progression to SLVL or spontaneous clinical but not molecular remission. *Leukemia* 17:2243, 2003.

37. Brown KA: Nonmalignant disorders of lymphocytes. *Clin Lab Sci* 10:329, 1997.

38. Hudnall SD, Patel J, Schwab H, Martinez J: Comparative immunophenotypic features of EBV-positive and EBV-negative atypical lymphocytosis. *Cytometry* 55B:22, 2003.

39. Horwitz MS, Moore GT: Acute infectious lymphocytosis: An etiologic and epidemiologic study of an outbreak. *N Engl J Med* 279:399, 1968.

40. Scalletar HE, Maisel JE, Bramson M: Acute infectious lymphocytosis: Report of an outbreak. *Am J Dis Child* 88:15, 1954.

41. Labalette M, Salez F, Pruvot FR, et al: CD8 lymphocytosis in primary cytomegalovirus (CMV) infection of allograft recipients: Expansion of an uncommon CD8+ CD57− subset and its progressive replacement by CD8+ CD57+ T cells. *Clin Exp Immunol* 95:465, 1994.

42. Kunno A, Abe M, Yamada M, Murakami K: Clinical and histological features of cytomegalovirus hepatitis in previously healthy adults. *Liver* 17:129, 1997.

43. Roumier AS, Grardel N, Lai JL, et al: Hypereosinophilia with abnormal T cells, trisomy 7 and elevated TARC serum level. *Haematologica* 88:ECR24, 2003.

44. Arnez M, Cizman M, Jazbec J, Kotnik A: Acute infectious lymphocytosis caused by coxsackievirus B2. *Pediatr Infect Dis J* 15:1127, 1996.

45. Heininger U, Klich K, Stehr K, Cherry JD: Clinical findings in Bordetella pertussis infections: Results of a prospective multicenter surveillance study. *Pediatrics* 100:E10, 1997.

46. Hodge G, Hodge S, Markus C, et al: A marked decrease in L-selectin expression by leucocytes in infants with Bordetella pertussis infection: Leucocytosis explained? *Respirology* 8:157, 2003.

47. Lin PY, Chiu CH, Wang YH, et al: Bordetella pertussis infection in northern Taiwan 1997-2001. *J Microbiol Immunol Infect* 37:288, 2004.

48. Verschueren H, Dewit J, Van der Wegen A, et al: The lymphocytosis promoting action of pertussis toxin can be mimicked in vitro. Holotoxin but not the B subunit inhibits invasion of human T lymphoma cells through fibroblast monolayers. *J Immunol Methods* 144:231, 1991.

49. Passador L, Iglewski W: ADP-ribosylating toxins. *Methods Enzymol* 235:617, 1994.

50. Burnette WN: AB5 ADP-ribosylating toxins: Comparative anatomy and physiology. *Structure* 2:151, 1994.

51. Suzuki G, Sawa H, Kobayashi Y, et al: Pertussis toxin-sensitive signal controls the trafficking of thymocytes across the corticomedullary junction in the thymus. *J Immunol* 162:5981, 1999.

52. Witvliet MH, Vogel ML, Wiertz EJ, Poolman JT: Interaction of pertussis toxin with human T lymphocytes. *Infect Immunol* 60:5085, 1992.

53. Lima M, Almeida J, Dos Anjos Teixeira M, et al: TCRalphabeta+/CD4+ large granular lymphocytosis: A new clonal T-cell lymphoproliferative disorder. *Am J Pathol* 163:763, 2003.

54. Rabbani GR, Phyliky RL, Tefferi A: A long-term study of patients with chronic natural killer cell lymphocytosis. *Br J Haematol* 106:960, 1999.

55. Granjo E, Lima M, Fraga M, et al: Abnormal NK cell lymphocytosis detected after splenectomy: Association with repeated infections, relapsing neutropenia, and persistent polyclonal B-cell proliferation. *Int J Hematol* 75:484, 2002.

56. Vanness ER, Davis MD, Tefferi A: Cutaneous findings associated with chronic natural killer cell lymphocytosis. *Int J Dermatol* 41:852, 2002.

57. Kaito K, Otsubo H, Ogasawara Y, et al: Severe aplastic anemia associated with chronic natural killer cell lymphocytosis. *Int J Hematol* 72:463, 2000.

58. Speight EL, Myers B, Davies JM: Strongyloidiasis, angio-oedema and natural killer cell lymphocytosis. *Br J Dermatol* 140:1179, 1999.

59. del Giudice P: Strongyloidiasis and natural killer cell lymphocytosis. *Br J Dermatol* 142:1066, 2000.

60. Myers B, Speight EL, Huissoon AP, Davies JM: Natural killer-cell lymphocytosis and strongyloides infection. *Clin Lab Haematol* 22:237, 2000.

61. Stanworth SJ, Green L, Pumphrey RS, et al: An unusual association of Felty syndrome and TCR gamma delta lymphocytosis. *J Clin Pathol* 49:351, 1996.

62. Agarwal V, Sachdev A, Lehl S, Basu S: Unusual haematological alterations in rheumatoid arthritis. *J Postgrad Med* 50:60, 2004.

63. Grossi A, Nozzoli C, Gheri R, et al: Pure red cell aplasia in autoimmune polyglandular syndrome with T lymphocytosis [letter]. *Haematologica* 83:1043, 1998.

64. Garcia-Suarez J, Prieto A, Reyes E, et al: Persistent lymphocytosis of natural killer cells in autoimmune thrombocytopenic purpura (ATP) patients after splenectomy. *Br J Haematol* 89:653, 1995.

65. Pinkerton PH, McLellan BA, Quantz MC, Robinson JB: Acute lymphocytosis after trauma—Early recognition of the high-risk patient? *J Trauma* 29:749, 1989.

66. Teggatz JR, Parkin J, Peterson L: Transient atypical lymphocytosis in patients with emergency medical conditions. *Arch Pathol Lab Med* 111:712, 1987.

67. Thommasen HV, Boyko WJ, Montaner JS, et al: Absolute lymphocytosis associated with nonsurgical trauma. *Am J Clin Pathol* 86:480, 1986.

68. Toft P, Tonnesen E, Svendsen P, et al: The redistribution of lymphocytes during adrenaline infusion. An in vivo study with radiolabeled cells. *APMIS* 100:593, 1992.

69. Karandikar NJ, Hotchkiss EC, McKenna RW, Kroft SH: Transient stress lymphocytosis: An immunophenotypic characterization of the most common cause of newly identified adult lymphocytosis in a tertiary hospital. *Am J Clin Pathol* 117:819, 2002.

70. Tonnesen E, Hohndorf K, Lerbjerg G, et al: Immunological and hormonal responses to lung surgery during one-lung ventilation. *Eur J Anaesthesiol* 10:189, 1993.

71. Benschop RJ, Rodriguez-Feuerhahn M, Schedlowski M: Catecholamine-induced leukocytosis: Early observations, current research, and future directions. *Brain Behav Immun* 10:77, 1996.

72. Bergmann M, Sautner T: Immunomodulatory effects of vasoactive catecholamines. *Wien Klin Wochenschr* 114:752, 2002.

73. Chung JS, Shin HJ, Lee EY, Cho GJ: Hypersensitivity to mosquito bites associated with natural killer cell-derived large granular lymphocyte lymphocytosis: A case report in Korea. *Korean J Intern Med* 18:50, 2003.

74. Satoh M, Oyama N, Akiba H, et al: Hypersensitivity to mosquito bites with natural-killer cell lymphocytosis: The possible implication of Epstein-Barr virus reactivation. *Eur J Dermatol* 12:381, 2002.

75. Asada H, Miyagawa S, Sumikawa Y, et al: CD4+ T-lymphocyte-induced Epstein-Barr virus reactivation in a patient with severe hypersensitivity to mosquito bites and Epstein-Barr virus-infected NK cell lymphocytosis. *Arch Dermatol* 139:1601, 2003.

76. Sakai C, Takagi T, Oguro M, et al: Erythroderma and marked atypical lymphocytosis mimicking cutaneous T-cell lymphoma probably caused by phenobarbital. *Intern Med* 32:182, 1993.

77. Enomoto M, Ochi M, Teramae K, et al: Codeine phosphate-induced hypersensitivity syndrome. *Ann Pharmacother* 38:799, 2004.

78. Halmos B, Anastopoulos HT, Schnipper LE, Ballesteros E: Extreme lymphoplasmacytosis and hepatic failure associated with sulfasalazine hypersensitivity reaction and a concurrent EBV infection—Case report and review of the literature. *Ann Hematol* 83:242, 2004.

79. Choi TS, Doh KS, Kim SH, et al: Clinicopathological and genotypic aspects of anticonvulsant induced pseudolymphoma syndrome. *Br J Dermatol* 148:730, 2003.

80. Leslie KS, Gaffney K, Ross CN, et al: A near fatal case of the dapsone hypersensitivity syndrome in a patient with urticarial vasculitis. *Clin Exp Dermatol* 28:496, 2003.

81. Ohtani T, Hiroi A, Sakurane M, Furukawa F: Slow acetylator genotypes as a possible risk factor for infectious mononucleosis-like syndrome induced by salazosulfapyridine. *Br J Dermatol* 148:1035, 2003.

82. Medeiros LJ, Bhagat SK, Naylor P, et al: Malignant thymoma associated with T-cell lymphocytosis. A case report with immunophenotypic and gene rearrangement analysis. *Arch Pathol Lab Med* 117:279, 1993.

83. Cranney A, Markman S, Lach B, Karsh J: Polymyositis in a patient with thymoma and T cell lymphocytosis. *J Rheumatol* 24:1413, 1997.

84. Rosenthal NS, Farhi DC: Reactive plasmacytosis and lymphocytosis in acute myeloid leukemia. *Hematol Pathol* 8:43, 1994.

85. Horny HP, Lange K, Sotlar K, Valent P: Increase of bone marrow lymphocytes in systemic mastocytosis: Reactive lymphocytosis or malignant lymphoma? Immunohistochemical and molecular findings on routinely processed bone marrow biopsy specimens. *J Clin Pathol* 56:575, 2003.

86. Juneja S, Januszewicz E, Wolf M, Cooper I: Post-splenectomy lymphocytosis. *Clin Lab Haematol* 17:335, 1995.

87. Domingo P, Fuster M, Muñiz-Diaz E, et al: Spurious post-splenectomy CD4 and CD8 lymphocytosis in HIV-infected patients [letter]. *AIDS* 10:106, 1996.

88. Laurence J: T-cell subsets in health, infectious disease, and idiopathic CD4+ T lymphocytopenia. *Ann Intern Med* 119:55, 1993.

89. Castelino DJ, McNair P, Kay TW: Lymphocytopenia in a hospital population—What does it signify? *Australian N Z J Med* 27:170, 1997.

90. Molina IJ, Kenney DM, Rosen FS, Remold-O'Donnell E: T cell lines characterize events in the pathogenesis of the Wiskott-Aldrich syndrome. *J Exp Med* 176:867, 1992.

91. Wolday D, Tsegaye A, Messele T: Low absolute CD4 counts in Ethiopians. *Ethiop Med J* 40(suppl 1):11, 2002.

92. Gyrgolkay LA, Nikitin YP: Leukogram and white blood cells count in native people of Chukotka. *Int J Circumpolar Health* 60:534, 2001.

93. Phillips AN: CD4 lymphocyte depletion prior to the development of AIDS [editorial, comment]. *AIDS* 6:735, 1992.

94. Daniel V, Melk A, Süsal C, et al: CD4 depletion in HIV-infected haemophilia patients is associated with rapid clearance of immune complex-coated CD4+ lymphocytes. *Clin Exp Immunol* 115:477, 1999.

95. Pilheu JA, De Salvo MC, Gonzalez J, et al: CD4+ T-lymphocytopenia in severe pulmonary tuberculosis without evidence of human immunodeficiency virus infection. *Int J Tuberc Lung Dis* 1:422, 1997.

96. Singh KJ, Ahluwalia G, Sharma SK, et al: Significance of haematological manifestations in patients with tuberculosis. *J Assoc Physicians India* 49:788, 2001.

97. Olaniyi JA, Aken'Ova YA: Haematological profile of patients with pulmonary tuberculosis in Ibadan, Nigeria. *Afr J Med Med Sci* 32:239, 2003.

98. Peiris JS, Lai ST, Poon LL, et al: Coronavirus as a possible cause of severe acute respiratory syndrome. *Lancet* 361·1319, 2003.

99. Yang M, Li CK, Li K, et al: Hematological findings in SARS patients and possible mechanisms [review]. *Int J Mol Med* 14:311, 2004.

100. Okada H, Kobune F, Sato TA, et al: Extensive lymphopenia due to apoptosis of uninfected lymphocytes in acute measles patients. *Arch Virol* 145:905, 2000.

101. Am JS: Influenza A (H5N1) in Hong Kong: An overview. *Vaccine* 20(suppl 2):S77, 2002.

102. Borroni G, Zaccone C, Vignati G, et al: Lymphopenia and decrease in the total number of circulating CD3+ and CD4+ T cells during "long-term" PUVA treatment for psoriasis. *Dermatologica* 183:10, 1991.

103. Bloemena E, Weinreich S, Schellekens PT: The influence of prednisolone on the recirculation of peripheral blood lymphocytes in vivo. *Clin Exp Immunol* 80:460, 1990.

104. Bloemena E, Koopmans RP, Weinreich S, et al: Pharmacodynamic modeling of lymphocytopenia and whole blood lymphocyte cultures in prednisolone-treated individuals. *Clin Immunol Immunopathol* 57:374, 1990.

105. Braat MC, Oosterhuis B, Koopmans RP, et al: Kinetic-dynamic modeling of lymphocytopenia induced by the combined action of dexamethasone and hydrocortisone in humans, after inhalation and intravenous administration of dexamethasone. *J Pharmacol Exp Ther* 262:509, 1992.

106. Hauser GJ, Chan MM, Casey WF, et al: Immune dysfunction in children after corrective surgery for congenital heart disease. *Crit Care Med* 19:874, 1991.

107. Ueo T, Tanaka S, Tominaga Y, et al: The effect of thoracic duct drainage on lymphocyte dynamics and clinical symptoms in patients with rheumatoid arthritis. *Arthritis Rheum* 22:1405, 1979.

108. Prior CR, Coghlan PJ, Hall JM, Jacobs P: In vitro study of immunologic changes in long-term cytapheresis donors. *J Clin Apheresis* 6:69, 1991.

109. Novotny J, Kadar J, Hertenstein B, et al: Sustained decrease of peripheral lymphocytes after allogeneic blood stem cell aphereses. *Br J Haematol* 100:695, 1998.

110. Martin-Suarez I, D'Cruz D, Mansoor M, et al: Immunosuppressive treatment in severe connective tissue diseases: Effects of low dose intravenous cyclophosphamide. *Ann Rheum Dis* 56:481, 1997.

111. Mandl T, Bredberg A, Jacobsson LT, et al: CD4+ T-lymphocytopenia—A frequent finding in anti-SSA antibody seropositive patients with primary Sjogren's syndrome. *J Rheumatol* 31:726, 2004.

112. Wenzel J, Gerdsen R, Uerlich M, et al: Lymphocytopenia in lupus erythematosus: Close in vivo association to autoantibodies targeting nuclear antigens. *Br J Dermatol* 150:994, 2004.

113. Maldonado MD, Venturoli A, Franco A, Nunez-Roldan A: Specific changes in peripheral blood lymphocyte phenotype from burn patients. Probable origin of the thermal injury-related lymphocytopenia. *Burns* 17:188, 1991.

114. Taylor CG, Giesbrecht JA: Dietary zinc deficiency and expression of T lymphocyte signal transduction proteins. *Can J Physiol Pharmacol* 78: 823, 2000.

115. Fraker PJ, King LE: Reprogramming of the immune system during zinc deficiency. *Annu Rev Nutr* 24:277, 2004.

116. Kapasi AA, Patel G, Goenka A, et al: Ethanol promotes T cell apoptosis through the mitochondrial pathway. *Immunology* 108:313, 2003.

117. Smith DK, Neal JJ, Holmberg SD: Unexplained opportunistic infections and CD4+ T-lymphocytopenia without HIV infection. An investigation of cases in the United States. The Centers for Disease Control Idiopathic CD4+ T-lymphocytopenia Task Force. *N Engl J Med* 328:373, 1993.

118. al-Attas RA, Rahi AH, Ahmed el-FE: Common variable immunodeficiency with CD4+ T lymphocytopenia and overproduction of soluble IL-2 receptor associated with Turner's syndrome and dorsal kyphoscoliosis. *J Clin Pathol* 50:876, 1997.

119. Laurence J, Mitra D, Steiner M, et al: Apoptotic depletion of CD4+ T cells in idiopathic CD4+ T lymphocytopenia. *J Clin Invest* 97:672, 1996.

120. Spira TJ, Jones BM, Nicholson JK, et al: Idiopathic CD4+ T-lymphocytopenia—An analysis of five patients with unexplained opportunistic infections. *N Engl J Med* 328:386, 1993.

121. Cascio G, Massobrio AM, Cascio B, Anania A: Undefined CD4 lymphocytopenia without clinical complications. A report of two cases. *Panminerva Med* 40:69, 1998.

122. Sinicco A, Maiello A, Raiteri R, et al: Pneumocystis carinii in a patient with pulmonary sarcoidosis and idiopathic CD4+ T lymphocytopenia. *Thorax* 51:446, 1996.

123. Kumlin U, Elmqvist LG, Granlund M, et al: CD4 lymphopenia in a patient with cryptococcal osteomyelitis. *Scand J Infect Dis* 29:205, 1997.

124. Zanelli G, Sansoni A, Ricciardi B, et al: Muscular-skeletal cryptococcosis in a patient with idiopathic CD4+ lymphopenia. *Mycopathologia* 149:137, 2001.

125. Cheung MC, Rachlis AR, Shumak SL: A cryptic cause of cryptococcal meningitis. *CMAJ* 168:451, 2003.

126. Plonquet A, Bassez G, Authier FJ, et al: Toxoplasmic myositis as a presenting manifestation of idiopathic CD4 lymphocytopenia. *Muscle Nerve* 27:761, 2003.

127. Netea MG, Brouwer AE, Hoogendoorn EH, et al: Two patients with cryptococcal meningitis and idiopathic CD4 lymphopenia: Defective cytokine production and reversal by recombinant interferon-gamma therapy. *Clin Infect Dis* 39:e83, 2004.

128. Matsuyama W, Tsurukawa T, Iwami F, et al: Two cases of idiopathic CD4+ T-lymphocytopenia in elderly patients. *Intern Med* 37:891, 1998.

129. Belmin J, Ortega MN, Bruhat A, et al: CD4 lymphopenia in very elderly people [letter]. *Lancet* 347:328, 1996.

130. McBride M: CD4 lymphopenia in elderly patients [letter, comment]. *Lancet* 347:911, discussion 912, 1996.

131. Ho DD, Cao Y, Zhu T, et al: Idiopathic CD4+ T-lymphocytopenia—Immunodeficiency without evidence of HIV infection. *N Engl J Med* 328:380, 1993.

132. Duncan RA, von Reyn CF, Alliegro GM, et al: Idiopathic CD4+ T-lymphocytopenia—Four patients with opportunistic infections and no evidence of HIV infection. *N Engl J Med* 328:393, 1993.

133. Adley BP, Sun X, Shaw JM, Variakojis D: Hairy cell leukemia with marked lymphocytosis. *Arch Pathol Lab Med* 127:253, 2003.

134. Nelson BP, Variakojis D, Peterson LC: Leukemic phase of B-cell lymphomas mimicking chronic lymphocytic leukemia and variants at presentation. *Mod Pathol* 15:1111, 2002.

135. Lamy T, Loughran TP Jr: Clinical features of large granular lymphocyte leukemia. *Semin Hematol* 40:185, 2003.

136. Oshimi K: Leukemia and lymphoma of natural killer lineage cells. *Int J Hematol* 78:18, 2003.

137. Granjo E, Lima M, Correia T, et al: Cd8(+)/V beta 5.1(+) large granular lymphocyte leukemia associated with autoimmune cytopenias, rheumatoid arthritis and vascular mammary skin lesions: Successful response to 2-deoxycoformycin. *Hematol Oncol* 20:87, 2002.

138. Krishna MT, Hodges E, Lavender FL, et al: CD3+CD4−CD8+NK− large granular lymphocytosis with neutropenia and evidence for clonality and T-cell receptor gene rearrangement: Two pediatric cases. *J Pediatr Hematol Oncol* 24:495, 2002.

139. Narumi H, Kojima K, Matsuo Y, et al: T-cell large granular lymphocytic leukemia occurring after autologous peripheral blood stem cell transplantation. *Bone Marrow Transplant* 33:99, 2004.

140. Schleinitz N, Brunet C, Pascal V, et al: A CD4+ V(beta)13.6+ CD56+ large granular lymphocyte expansion with decreased expression of CD95 and an indolent clinical course. *Haematologica* 87:ECR35, 2002.

141. Vartholomatos G, Alymara V, Dova L, et al: T-cell receptor gamma-delta-large granular lymphocytic leukemia associated with an aberrant phenotype and TCR-Vbeta20 clonality. *Haematologica* 89:ECR16, 2004.

142. Chow KC, Nacilla JQ, Witzig TE, Li CY: Is persistent polyclonal B lymphocytosis caused by Epstein-Barr virus? A study with polymerase chain reaction and in situ hybridization. *Am J Hematol* 41: 270, 1992.

143. Ebell MH: Epstein-Barr virus infectious mononucleosis. *Am Fam Physician* 70:1279, 2004.

144. Ventura KC, Hudnall SD: Hematologic differences in heterophile-positive and heterophile-negative infectious mononucleosis. *Am J Hematol* 76:315, 2004.

145. Grotto I, Mimouni D, Huerta M, et al: Clinical and laboratory presentation of EBV positive infectious mononucleosis in young adults. *Epidemiol Infect* 131:683, 2003.

146. Rea TD, Russo JE, Katon W, et al: Prospective study of the natural history of infectious mononucleosis caused by Epstein-Barr virus. *J Am Board Fam Pract* 14:234, 2001.

147. Rodriguez-Bano J, Muniain MA, Borobio MV, et al: Cytomegalovirus mononucleosis as a cause of prolonged fever and prominent weight loss in immunocompetent adults. *Clin Microbiol Infect* 10:468, 2004.

148. Wong KF, Yip SF, So CC, et al: Cytomegalovirus infection associated with clonal proliferation of T-cell large granular lymphocytes: Causal or casual? *Cancer Genet Cytogenet* 142:77, 2003.

149. Nigro G, Anceschi MM, Cosmi EV: Clinical manifestations and abnormal laboratory findings in pregnant women with primary cytomegalovirus infection. *BJOG* 110:572, 2003.

150. Just-Nubling G, Korn S, Ludwig B, et al: Primary cytomegalovirus infection in an outpatient setting—Laboratory markers and clinical aspects. *Infection* 31:318, 2003.

151. Crowley B, Dempsey J, Olujohungbe A, et al: Unusual manifestations of primary cytomegalovirus infection in patients without HIV infection and without organ transplants. *J Med Virol* 68:237, 2002.

152. Mathew P, Hudnall SD, Elghetany MT, Payne DA: T-gamma gene rearrangement and CMV mononucleosis. *Am J Hematol* 66:64, 2001.

153. Itescu S: Diffuse infiltrative lymphocytosis syndrome in children and adults infected with HIV-1: A model of rheumatic illness caused by acquired viral infection. *Am J Reprod Immunol* 28:247, 1992.

154. Williams FM, Cohen PR, Jumshyd J, Reveille JD: Prevalence of the diffuse infiltrative lymphocytosis syndrome among human immunodeficiency virus type 1-positive outpatients. *Arthritis Rheum* 41:863, 1998.

155. Smith P, Helbert M, Raftery M, et al: Paraproteins and monoclonal expansion of CD3+CD8+ CD56-CD57+ T lymphocytes in a patient with HIV infection. *Br J Haematol* 105:85, 1999.

156. Johnson RW, Williams FM, Kazi S, et al: Human immunodeficiency virus-associated polymyositis: A longitudinal study of outcome. *Arthritis Rheum* 49:172, 2003.

157. Franco-Paredes C, Rebolledo P, Folch E, et al: Diagnosis of diffuse CD8+ lymphocytosis syndrome in HIV-infected patients. *AIDS Read* 12:408, 2002.

158. Smith PR, Cavenagh JD, Milne T, et al: Benign monoclonal expansion of CD8+ lymphocytes in HIV infection. *J Clin Pathol* 53:177, 2000.

159. Sijpkens YW, de Knegt RJ, van der Werf SD: Unusual presentation of acquired toxoplasmosis in an immunocompetent adult. *Nether J Med* 45:174, 1994.

160. Gawoski JM, Ooi WW: Dengue fever mimicking plasma cell leukemia. *Arch Pathol Lab Med* 127:1026, 2003.

161. Wiwanitkit V: Bleeding and other presentations in Thai patients with dengue infection. *Clin Appl Thromb Hemost* 10:397, 2004.

162. Liu CC, Huang KJ, Lin YS, et al: Transient CD4/CD8 ratio inversion and aberrant immune activation during dengue virus infection. *J Med Virol* 68:241, 2002.

163. Wang FZ, Linde A, Dahl H, Ljungman P: Human herpesvirus 6 infection inhibits specific lymphocyte proliferation responses and is related to lymphocytopenia after allogeneic stem cell transplantation. *Bone Marrow Transplant* 24:1201, 1999.

164. Bernit E, Veit V, Zandotti C, et al: Chronic lymphadenopathies and human herpes virus type 8. *Scand J Infect Dis* 34:625, 2002.

165. Buyukavci M, Tan H, Keskin Z: Profound lymphocytosis preceding chickenpox. *Pediatr Infect Dis J* 23:693, 2004.

166. Orange JS, Chehimi J, Ghavimi D, et al: Decreased natural killer (NK) cell function in chronic NK cell lymphocytosis associated with decreased surface expression of CD11b. *Clin Immunol* 99:53, 2001.

167. Morice WG, Leibson PJ, Tefferi A: Natural killer cells and the syndrome of chronic natural killer cell lymphocytosis. *Leuk Lymphoma* 41:277, 2001.

168. Choi YL, Makishima H, Ohashi J, et al: DNA microarray analysis of natural killer cell-type lymphoproliferative disease of granular lymphocytes with purified CD3−CD56+ fractions. *Leukemia* 18:556, 2004.

169. Warren HS, Christiansen FT, Witt CS: Functional inhibitory human leucocyte antigen class I receptors on natural killer (NK) cells in patients with chronic NK lymphocytosis. *Br J Haematol* 121:793, 2003.

170. Carulli G, Lagomarsini G, Azzara A, et al: Expansion of Tc-Ralphabeta+CD3+CD4−CD8− (CD4/CD8 double-negative) T lymphocytes in a case of staphylococcal toxic shock syndrome. *Acta Haematol* 111:163, 2004.

171. Tiberghien P, Racadot E, Deschaseaux ML, et al: Interleukin-2-induced increase of a monoclonal B-cell lymphocytosis. A novel in vivo interleukin-2 effect? *Cancer* 69:2583, 1992.

172. Groom DA, Kunkel LA, Brynes RK, et al: Transient stress lymphocytosis during crisis of sickle cell anemia and emergency trauma and medical conditions. An immunophenotyping study. *Arch Pathol Lab Med* 114:570, 1990.

173. Higa K, Hirata K, Dan K: Mexiletine-induced severe skin eruption, fever, eosinophilia, atypical lymphocytosis, and liver dysfunction. *Pain* 73:97, 1997.

174. Tollerud DJ, Brown LM, Blattner WA, et al: T cell subsets in healthy black smokers and nonsmokers. Evidence for ethnic group as an important response modifier. *Am Rev Respir Dis* 144:612, 1991.

175. Sever-Prebilic M, Prebilic I, Seili-Bekafigo I, et al: A case of visceral leishmaniasis in the Northern Adriatic region. *Coll Antropol* 26:545, 2002.

176. Halim NK, Ogbeide E: Haematological alterations in leprosy patients treated with dapsone. *East Afr Med J* 79:100, 2002.

177. Buckley RH: Primary cellular immunodeficiencies. *J Allergy Clin Immunol* 109:747, 2002.

178. Kalman L, Lindegren ML, Kobrynski L, et al: Mutations in genes required for T-cell development: IL7R, CD45, IL2RG, JAK3, RAG1, RAG2, ARTEMIS, and ADA and severe combined immunodeficiency: HuGE review. *Genet Med* 6:16, 2004.

179. Hartel C, Strunk T, Bucsky P, Schultz C: Failure to thrive in a 14-month-old boy with lymphopenia and eosinophilia. *Klin Padiatr* 216:24, 2004.

180. Touraine JL, Betuel H, Souillet G, Jeune M: Combined immunodeficiency disease associated with absence of cell-surface HLA-A and -B antigens. *J Pediatr* 93:47, 1978.

181. Freier S, Kerem E, Dranitzki Z, et al: Hereditary CD4+ T lymphocytopenia. *Arch Dis Child* 78:371, 1998.

182. Roper M, Parmley RT, Crist WM, et al: Severe congenital leukopenia (reticular dysgenesis). Immunologic and morphologic characterizations of leukocytes. *Am J Dis Child* 139:832, 1985.

183. Di Renzo M, Zhou Z, George I, et al: Enhanced apoptosis of T cells in common variable immunodeficiency (CVID): Role of defective CD28 co-stimulation. *Clin Exp Immunol* 120:503, 2000.

184. Sawabe T, Horiuchi T, Nakamura M, et al: Defect of lck in a patient with common variable immunodeficiency. *Int J Mol Med* 7:609, 2001.

185. Schubert R, Reichenbach J, Royer N, et al: Spontaneous and oxidative stress-induced programmed cell death in lymphocytes from patients with ataxia telangiectasia (AT). *Clin Exp Immunol* 119:140, 2000.

186. Nowak-Wegrzyn A, Crawford TO, Winkelstein JA, et al: Immunodeficiency and infections in ataxia-telangiectasia. *J Pediatr* 144:505, 2004.

187. Ochs HD: The Wiskott-Aldrich syndrome. *Semin Hematol* 35:332, 1998.

188. Yel L, Aggarwal S, Gupta S: Cartilage-hair hypoplasia syndrome: Increased apoptosis of T lymphocytes is associated with altered expression of Fas (CD95), FasL (CD95L), IAP, Bax, and Bcl2. *J Clin Immunol* 19:428, 1999.

189. Tarr PE, Sneller MC, Mechanic LJ, et al: Infections in patients with immunodeficiency with thymoma (Good syndrome). Report of 5 cases and review of the literature. *Medicine (Baltimore)* 80:123, 2001.

190. Montella L, Masci AM, Merkabaoui G, et al: B-cell lymphopenia and hypogammaglobulinemia in thymoma patients. *Ann Hematol* 82:343, 2003.

191. Yel L, Liao O, Lin F, Gupta S: Severe T- and B-cell immune deficiency associated with malignant thymoma. *Ann Allergy Asthma Immunol* 91:501, 2003.

192. Myers LA, Hershfield MS, Neale WT, et al: Purine nucleoside phosphorylase deficiency (PNP-def) presenting with lymphopenia and developmental delay: Successful correction with umbilical cord blood transplantation. *J Pediatr* 145:710, 2004.

193. Etzioni A, Benderly A, Rosenthal E, et al: Defective humoral and cellular immune functions associated with veno-occlusive disease of the liver. *J Pediatr* 110:549, 1987.

194. Zeng W, Maciejewski JP, Chen G, et al: Selective reduction of natural killer T cells in the bone marrow of aplastic anaemia. *Br J Haematol* 119:803, 2002.

195. Douek DC, Picker LJ, Koup RA: T cell dynamics in HIV-1 infection. *Annu Rev Immunol* 21:265, 2003.

196. Panesar NS: Lymphopenia in SARS. *Lancet* 361:1985, 2003.

197. Wang JT, Chang SC: Severe acute respiratory syndrome. *Curr Opin Infect Dis* 17:143, 2004.

198. Wang JT, Sheng WH, Fang CT, et al: Clinical manifestations, laboratory findings, and treatment outcomes of SARS patients. *Emerg Infect Dis* 10:818, 2004.

199. Hui DS, Chan MC, Wu AK, Ng PC: Severe acute respiratory syndrome (SARS): Epidemiology and clinical features. *Postgrad Med J* 80:373, 2004.

200. Cunha BA, Minnaganti V, Johnson DH, Klein NC: Profound and prolonged lymphocytopenia with West Nile encephalitis. *Clin Infect Dis* 31:1116, 2000.

201. Huhn GD, Sejvar JJ, Montgomery SP, Dworkin MS: West Nile virus in the United States: An update on an emerging infectious disease. *Am Fam Physician* 68:653, 2003.

202. Cunha BA, Sachdev B, Canario D: Serum ferritin levels in West Nile encephalitis. *Clin Microbiol Infect* 10:184, 2004.

203. Laurence J: CD4+ T-lymphocytopenia without HIV infection [letter]. *N Engl J Med* 328:1848, 1993.

204. Vuorinen T, Peri P, Vainionpaa R: Measles virus induces apoptosis in uninfected bystander T cells and leads to granzyme B and caspase activation in peripheral blood mononuclear cell cultures. *Eur J Clin Invest* 33:434, 2003.

205. Servet-Delprat C, Vidalain PO, Valentin H, Rabourdin-Combe C: Measles virus and dendritic cell functions: How specific response cohabits with immunosuppression. *Curr Top Microbiol Immunol* 276:103, 2003.

206. Wollenberg A, Zoch C, Wetzel S, et al: Predisposing factors and clinical features of eczema herpeticum: A retrospective analysis of 100 cases. *J Am Acad Dermatol* 49:198, 2003.

207. Yoshikawa T, Ihira M, Asano Y, et al: Fatal adult case of severe lymphocytopenia associated with reactivation of human herpesvirus 6. *J Med Virol* 66:82, 2002.

208. Mazzucchelli I, Vezzoli M, Ottini E, et al: A complex immunodeficiency. Idiopathic CD4+ T-lymphocytopenia and hypogammaglobulinemia associated with HHV8 infection, Kaposi's sarcoma and gastric cancer [letter]. *Haematologica* 84:378, 1999.

209. García-Silva J, Almagro M, Peña C, et al: CD4+ T-lymphocytopenia, Kaposi's sarcoma, HHV-8 infection, severe seborrheic dermatitis, and onychomycosis in a homosexual man without HIV infection [letter]. *Int J Dermatol* 38:231, 1999.

210. Kim SK, Welsh RM: Comprehensive early and lasting loss of memory CD8 T cells and functional memory during acute and persistent viral infections. *J Immunol* 172:3139, 2004.

211. Mert A, Bilir M, Tabak F, et al: Miliary tuberculosis: Clinical manifestations, diagnosis and outcome in 38 adults. *Respirology* 6:217, 2001.

212. Abdool Gaffar MS, Seedat YK, Coovadia YM, Khan Q: The white cell count in typhoid fever. *Trop Geogr Med* 44:23, 1992.

213. Kemp K, Bruunsgaard H, Skinhoj P, Klarlund Pedersen B: Pneumococcal infections in humans are associated with increased apoptosis and trafficking of type 1 cytokine-producing T cells. *Infect Immun* 70:5019, 2002.

214. Jensenius M, Fournier PE, Hellum KB, et al: Sequential changes in hematologic and biochemical parameters in African tick bite fever. *Clin Microbiol Infect* 9:678, 2003.

215. Hotchkiss RS, Tinsley KW, Swanson PE, et al: Sepsis-induced apoptosis causes progressive profound depletion of B and CD4+ T lymphocytes in humans. *J Immunol* 166:6952, 2001.

216. Le Tulzo Y, Pangault C, Gacouin A, et al: Early circulating lymphocyte apoptosis in human septic shock is associated with poor outcome. *Shock* 18:487, 2002.

217. Kern P, Dietrich M, Hemmer C, Wellinghausen N: Increased levels of soluble Fas ligand in serum in Plasmodium falciparum malaria. *Infect Immun* 68:3061, 2000.

218. Lee HK, Lim J, Kim M, et al: Immunological alterations associated with Plasmodium vivax malaria in South Korea. *Ann Trop Med Parasitol* 95:31, 2001.

219. Aubouy A, Deloron P, Migot-Nabias F: Plasma and in vitro levels of cytokines during and after a Plasmodium falciparum malaria attack in Gabon. *Acta Trop* 83:195, 2002.

220. Hutchinson P, Chadban SJ, Atkins RC, Holdsworth SR: Laboratory assessment of immune function in renal transplant patients. *Nephrol Dial Transplant* 18:983, 2003.

221. Bohler T, Waiser J, Schutz M, et al: FTY720 mediates apoptosis-independent lymphopenia in human renal allograft recipients: Different effects on CD62L+ and CCR5+ T lymphocytes. *Transplantation* 77:1424, 2004.

222. Schatz DA, Riley WJ, Silverstein JH, Barrett DJ: Long-term immunoregulatory effects of therapy with corticosteroids and anti-thymocyte globulin. *Immunopharmacol Immunotoxicol* 11:269, 1989.

223. Dearden C: Alemtuzumab in peripheral T-cell malignancies. *Cancer Biother Radiopharm* 19:391, 2004.

224. Buysmann S, van Diepen FN, Yong SL, et al: Mechanism of lymphocytopenia following administration of corticosteroids. *Transplant Proc* 27:871, 1995.

225. Wang L, Hong KC, Lin FC, Yang KD: Mycoplasma pneumoniae-associated Stevens-Johnson syndrome exhibits lymphopenia and redistribution of CD4+ T cells. *J Formos Med Assoc* 102:55, 2003.

226. Takada K, Danning CL, Kuroiwa T, et al: Lymphocyte depletion with fludarabine in patients with psoriatic arthritis: Clinical and immunological effects. *Ann Rheum Dis* 62:1112, 2003.

227. Borg C, Ray-Coquard I, Philip I, et al: CD4 lymphopenia as a risk factor for febrile neutropenia and early death after cytotoxic chemotherapy in adult patients with cancer. *Cancer* 101:2675, 2004.

228. Fujimori Y, Saheki K, Itoi H, et al: Increased expression of Fas (APO-1, CD95) on CD4+ and CD8+ T lymphocytes during total body irradiation. *Acta Haematol* 104:193, 2000.

229. Verastegui EL, Morales RB, Barrera-Franco JL, et al: Long-term immune dysfunction after radiotherapy to the head and neck area. *Int Immunopharmacol* 3:1093, 2003.

230. Bolla G, Tuzzato G: Immunologic postoperative competence after laparoscopy versus laparotomy. *Surg Endosc* 17:1247, 2003.

231. Leung KL, Tsang KS, Ng MH, et al: Lymphocyte subsets and natural killer cell cytotoxicity after laparoscopically assisted resection of rectosigmoid carcinoma. *Surg Endosc* 17:1305, 2003.

232. Tayama E, Hayashida N, Oda T, et al: Recovery from lymphocytopenia following extracorporeal circulation: Simple indicator to assess surgical stress. *Artif Organs* 23:736, 1999.

233. Ducloux D, Carron PL, Racadot E, et al: CD4 lymphocytopenia in long-term renal transplant recipients. *Transplant Proc* 30:2859, 1998.

234. Bhaskaran M, Ranjan R, Shah H, et al: Lymphopenia in dialysis patients: A preliminary study indicating a possible role of apoptosis. *Clin Nephrol* 57:221, 2002.

235. Wagner U, Kaltenhauser S, Pierer M, et al: B lymphocytopenia in rheumatoid arthritis is associated with the DRB1 shared epitope and increased acute phase response. *Arthritis Res* 4:R1, 2002.

236. Silva LM, Garcia AB, Donadi EA: Increased lymphocyte death by neglect-apoptosis is associated with lymphopenia and autoantibodies in lupus patients presenting with neuropsychiatric manifestations. *J Neurol* 249:1048, 2002.

237. Manganelli P, Fietta P: Apoptosis and Sjogren syndrome. *Semin Arthritis Rheum* 33:49, 2003.

238. Gerli R, Paganelli R, Cossarizza A, et al: Long-term immunologic effects of thymectomy in patients with myasthenia gravis. *J Allergy Clin Immunol* 103:865, 1999.

239. Sebnem Kilic S, Bostan O, Cil E: Takayasu arteritis. *Ann Rheum Dis* 61:92, 2002.

240. Venzor J, Hua Q, Bressler RB, et al: Behçet's-like syndrome associated with idiopathic CD4+ T-lymphocytopenia, opportunistic infections, and a large population of TCR alpha beta+ CD4− CD8− T cells. *Am J Med Sci* 313:236, 1997.

241. Viguier M, Fouere S, de la Salmoniere P, et al: Peripheral blood lymphocyte subset counts in patients with dermatomyositis: Clinical correlations and changes following therapy. *Medicine (Baltimore)* 82:82, 2003.

242. Izzedine H, Cacoub P, Launay-Vacher V, et al: Lymphopenia in Wegener's granulomatosis. A new clinical activity index? *Nephron* 92:466, 2002.

243. Ayoub JP, Palmer JL, Huh Y, et al: Therapeutic and prognostic implications of peripheral blood lymphopenia in patients with Hodgkin's disease. *Leuk Lymphoma* 34:519, 1999.

244. Melichar B, Touskova M, Solichova D, et al: CD4+ T-lymphocytopenia and systemic immune activation in patients with primary and secondary liver tumours. *Scand J Clin Lab Invest* 61:363, 2001.

245. Ruka W, Rutkowski P, Kaminska J, et al: Alterations of routine blood tests in adult patients with soft tissue sarcomas: Relationships to cytokine serum levels and prognostic significance. *Ann Oncol* 12:1423, 2001.

246. Ordemann J, Jacobi CA, Braumann C, et al: Immunomodulatory changes in patients with colorectal cancer. *Int J Colorectal Dis* 17:37, 2002.

247. Romano F, Caprotti R, Bravo AF, et al: Radical surgery does not recover immunodeficiency associated with gastric cancer. *J Exp Clin Cancer Res* 22:179, 2003.

248. Cervantes F, Hernandez-Boluda JC, Villamor N, et al: Assessment of peripheral blood lymphocyte subsets in idiopathic myelofibrosis. *Eur J Haematol* 65:104, 2000.

249. Garty BZ: Deficiency of CD4+ lymphocytes due to intestinal loss after Fontan procedure. *Eur J Pediatr* 160:58, 2001.

250. Chakrabarti S, Keeton BR, Salmon AP, Vettukattil JJ: Acquired combined immunodeficiency associated with protein losing enteropathy complicating Fontan operation. *Heart* 89:1130, 2003.

251. Meier P, Dayer E, Blanc E, Wauters JP: Early T cell activation correlates with expression of apoptosis markers in patients with end-stage renal disease. *J Am Soc Nephrol* 13:204, 2002.

252. Gupta D, Rao VM, Aggarwal AN, et al: Haematological abnormalities in patients of sarcoidosis. *Indian J Chest Dis Allied Sci* 44:233, 2002.

253. Morell F, Levy G, Orriols R, et al: Delayed cutaneous hypersensitivity tests and lymphopenia as activity markers in sarcoidosis. *Chest* 121:1239, 2002.

254. Yanardag H, Pamuk GE, Karayel T, Demirci S: Bone marrow involvement in sarcoidosis: An analysis of 50 bone marrow samples. *Haematologia (Budap)* 32:419, 2002.

255. Gentil B, Cottin V, Girard P, Cordier JF: Ambivalence of CD4 lymphocytopenia in sarcoidosis. *Sarcoidosis Vasc Diffuse Lung Dis* 20:74, 2003.

256. Takeyama Y, Takas K, Ueda T, et al: Peripheral lymphocyte reduction in severe acute pancreatitis is caused by apoptotic cell death. *J Gastrointest Surg* 4:379, 2000.

257. Mooren FC, Bloming D, Lechtermann A, et al: Lymphocyte apoptosis after exhaustive and moderate exercise. *J Appl Physiol* 93:147, 2002.

258. Steensberg A, Morrow J, Toft AD, et al: Prolonged exercise, lymphocyte apoptosis and F2-isoprostanes. *Eur J Appl Physiol* 87:38, 2002.

259. Subra JF, Renier G, Reboul P, et al: Lymphopenia in occupational pulmonary silicosis with or without autoimmune disease. *Clin Exp Immunol* 126:540, 2001.

260. Di Sabatino A, D'Alo S, Millimaggi D, et al: Apoptosis and peripheral blood lymphocyte depletion in coeliac disease. *Immunology* 103:435, 2001.

IMMUNODEFICIENCY DISEASES

HARRY W. SCHROEDER, JR.
MAX D. COOPER

Patients with immunodeficiency disorders typically come to medical attention because of a history of increased susceptibility to infections. More than 100 primary immunodeficiency syndromes have been identified since the first of these conditions were described in the early 1950s.[1-6] The majority of these syndromes reflect single gene defects that impair the function of one or more components of the immune system: T cells, B cells, natural killer cells, phagocytes, and complement or other elements of the innate immune response. Most of these disorders are relatively rare, with a prevalence of 1:50,000 or less. IgA deficiency, which occurs with a frequency of one in 600 individuals of European ancestry, is an exception. The latter immunodeficiency and the related disorder common variable immune deficiency appear to be multifactorial in origin, which adds complexity to the diagnosis.

This chapter focuses on defects that primarily affect the T and B lymphocyte arms of the adaptive immune response (Table 82-1). Abnormal B lymphocyte function leads to ineffective or absent immunoglobulin production, rendering patients susceptible to infection with pyogenic bacteria. In some B cell disorders, the immunoglobulin deficiency and infection become apparent in young infants after their maternally derived immunoglobulin is catabolized; immunodeficiency in others may not become apparent until adulthood. The more severe B cell disorders can be clinically controlled with intravenous infusions of γ-globulin with or without prophylactic antibiotics. Defects in T lymphocytes lead to deficiencies in cell-mediated immunity, rendering patients susceptible from birth to life-threatening opportunistic infections. Major T cell disorders often require intensive specialized therapy, extending to bone marrow transplantation or gene transfer. Disorders affecting both T cells and B cells, termed severe combined immunodeficiencies, are uniformly fatal without some form of cellular engineering.

PREDOMINANTLY ANTIBODY DEFICIENCY

Antibody deficiency disorders are best understood as being the product of specific defects in B cell differentiation. B cells are generated first

Acronyms and abbreviations that appear in this chapter include: ADA, adenosine deaminase; AID, activation-induced cytidine deaminase; AT, ataxia-telangiectasia; ATM, ataxia-telangiectasia mutated; BTK, Bruton tyrosine kinase; CVID, common variable immunodeficiency; dATP, deoxyadenosine triphosphate; dGTP, deoxyguanosine triphosphate; GVHD, graft-versus-host disease; IFN, interferon; Ig, immunoglobulin; IgAD, selective IgA deficiency; IVIG, intravenous immunoglobulin G or γ-globulin; JAK3, Janus-associated kinase 3; LRRC8, leucine-rich repeat-containing 8; MHC, major histocompatibility complex; *NEMO*, nuclear factor-κB essential modulator; NK, natural killer; PNP, purine nucleoside phosphorylase; SCID, severe combined immunodeficiency; TAP, ATP-binding cassette transporter; THI, transient hypogammaglobulinemia of infancy; UNG, uracil-DNA glycosylase; WAS, Wiskott-Aldrich syndrome; XLA, X-linked agammaglobulinemia; ZAP, zeta-associated protein.

in the fetal liver and then throughout life in the multipotential marrow (see Chap. 76). Multipotent hematopoietic stem cells are the source of all types of blood cells, including B lineage cells. Common lymphoid progenitor descendants of hematopoietic stem cells give rise to pro-B cells, which differentiate into pre-B cells that in turn give rise to the immature IgM$^+$ B cells. With maturation, B cells gain the expression of immunoglobulin D (IgD) as they enter the bloodstream and migrate into the spleen, lymph nodes, and other peripheral lymphoid tissues. In the germinal centers of these peripheral lymphoid organs, B cells respond to antigenic stimulation and T cell help with proliferation, a switch in their heavy (H) chain isotype, and somatic hypermutation of their variable domains (see Chap. 78). The latter leads to affinity maturation of the antibody response through positive selection of B cells that produce antibodies of higher affinity. The response to protein antigens, including toxins and viral proteins, typically requires T cell help. Contact with a polymeric cognate antigen, such as a polysaccharide, can induce activation of the mature B cell, with progression to either the memory or plasma cell stage. The antipolysaccharide antibodies typically are of IgM isotype and have relatively modest antigen binding affinity.

X-LINKED AGAMMAGLOBULINEMIA

X-linked agammaglobulinemia (XLA), also known as Bruton agammaglobulinemia, is the prototype for selective B lymphocyte deficiencies.[7] In 1952, Bruton[3] identified a young boy with recurrent bacterial infections and pan-hypogammaglobulinemia. Bruton went on to demonstrate that human γ-globulin replacement therapy could prevent recurrence of infection. This therapeutic approach is still the mainstay of treatment for humoral immune deficiency more than 50 years later.

ETIOLOGY AND PATHOGENESIS
Among patients with early onset of recurrent infections, profound hypogammaglobulinemia, and markedly reduced or absent B cells, greater than 90 percent have loss-of-function mutations in an Src family tyrosine kinase gene named Bruton tyrosine kinase (*BTK*).[8] Because *BTK* is located on the X chromosome at position Xq22, XLA is inherited as a mendelian X-linked recessive trait. Mutations in *BTK* prevent pre-B cells from progressing from the pre-B cell to the immature B cell stage. This severe blockage results in an almost complete absence of B cells in the periphery. With their consequent paucity of plasma cells, these patients usually produce very little immunoglobulin. T cell function appears to be normal in that delayed-type hypersensitivity, contact hypersensitivity, and homograft rejection are intact.

CLINICAL FEATURES
Neonates are protected by placental transfer of maternal IgG immunoglobulins.[9] In addition, breast-fed offspring receive IgA in breast milk. By age 6 months, most of the maternal antibodies are lost to catabolism; the half-life of IgG is approximately 25 days (see Chap. 77). Boys affected with XLA then begin to have infections with pyogenic organisms, including staphylococci, pneumococci, streptococci, and especially *Haemophilus influenzae*. Purulent otitis media, sinusitis, pneumonia, bacteremia, meningitis, and furunculosis may occur. These infections usually can be controlled with antibiotics, but they tend to recur repeatedly until immunoglobulin replacement is undertaken. The onset and frequency of infection can be influenced by the environment, including the presence or absence of older siblings and social contacts. A late diagnosis of agammaglobulinemia may result from an isolated upbringing, a negative family history, vigilant parental attention, and aggressive antimicrobial therapy.[10]

Because of their T cell integrity, agammaglobulinemic children usually overcome varicella in an ordinary fashion and have no diffi-

TABLE 82-1   COMMON PRIMARY IMMUNODEFICIENCIES - LABORATORY AND CLINICAL FEATURES*

| | Lymphocytes | | | Cellular Immunity | Humoral Immunity | | | | | |
| | | | | | Serum Immunoglobulins | | | | Antibody Responses | Common Infections |
	B	T	NK		M	G	A	E		
Predominantly Antibody Deficiency										
X-linked agammaglobulinemia	−	+	+	+	↓	↓	↓	↓	−	Bacteria, *Giardia lamblia*
Autosomal agammaglobulinemia										
Recessive (λ5, Igβ, or BLNK deficiency)	−	+	+	+	↓	↓	↓	↓	−	"
Dominant (ICOS, LRRC8)	−	+	+	+	↓	↓	↓	↓	−	"
Transient hypogammaglobulinemia of infancy	+	+	+	+	N/↓	N/↓	N/↓	N/↓	+/−	"
Selective IgA deficiency	+	+	+	+	N	N	↓	N	+/−	"
Common variable immune deficiency	+	+	+	+	N/↓	↓	↓	↓	−	"
IgG subclass deficiencies	+	+	+	+	N	N/↓	N/↓	N	+/−	Bacteria
Hyper-IgM syndrome										
Activation-induced cytidine deaminase deficiency	+	+	+	+	N/↑	↓	↓	↓	+/−	Bacteria
Uracil-DNA glycosylase deficiency	+	+	+	+	N/↑	↓	↓	↓	+/−	"
X-linked CD40 ligand deficiency	+	+	+	+	N/↑	↓	N/↓	↓	+/−	Bacteria, viruses, fungi
CD40 deficiency	+	+	+	+	N/↑	↓	N/↓	↓	+/−	"
X-linked IKK-gamma (NEMO) deficiency	+	+	+	+	N/↑	↓	↓	↓	+/−	"
Severe Combined Immunodeficiency (SCID)										
Interleukin receptor γ-chain deficiency (X-linked SCID)	+	−	−	−	N	↓	↓	↓	−	"
Janus-associated kinase 3 (JAK3) deficiency	+	−	−	−	N	↓	↓	↓	−	"
Interleukin-7 receptor α-chain deficiency	+	−	+	−	N	↓	↓	↓	−	"
Zap-70 tyrosine kinase deficiency	+	+/−	+	−	N	N/↓	N/↓	N/↓	+/−	"
Adenosine deaminase (ADA) deficiency	−	−	+	−	↓	↓	↓	↓	−	Bacteria, viruses, fungi
Purine nucleotide phosphorylase (PNP) deficiency	+	−	+	−	N	↓	↓	↓	+/−	"
Recombinase activating gene (RAG ½) deficiency	−	−	+	−	↓	↓	↓	↓	−	"
Artemis deficiency (SCIDA)	−	−	+	−	↓	↓	↓	↓	−	"
Reticular dysgenesis	−	−	−	−	↓	↓	↓	↓	−	"
Primary T Cell Deficiency										
Congenital thymic aplasia (DiGeorge syndrome)	+	−	+	−	N	N	N	N	+/−	Bacteria, viruses, fungi
MHC class II deficiency	+	+/−	+	+	N	↓	↓	↓	+/−	"
TAP-1 or TAP-2 deficiency (MHC class I deficiency)	+	+/−	+	−	N	N	N	N	+	"
TH1 deficiency										
Interferon-γ and interferon-γ receptor deficiency	+	+	+	+	N	N	N	N	+	Mycobacteria, *Salmonella*
Interleukin-12 and interleukin-12 receptor deficiency	+	+	+	+	N	N	N	N	+	"
Other Well-Defined Immunodeficiency Syndromes										
Ataxia-telangiectasia	+	+	+	+	N/↑	N/↓	N/↓	↓	+/−	Bacteria
Wiskott-Aldrich syndrome	+	+/−	+	+/−	↓	N	↑	↑	+/−	"

* Natural killer lymphocytes (NK), T cells (T), B cells (B).
Normal levels (+), reduced or absent levels (−); normal (N), elevated (↑), or reduced (↓) serum immunoglobulins.

culty with mycotic infections. In the absence of immunoglobulin replacement therapy, however, they remain susceptible to measles, mumps, and rubella after vaccination. Recurrent infection with latent viruses, such as herpes zoster, is common. Bronchiectasis may result from incomplete treatment of recurrent pulmonary infections. With chronic mucosal inflammation and scarring of the respiratory tract, the pattern of infection can expand to include enterococci and gram-negative bacilli. Susceptibility to these enteric bacteria may continue for patients with severe bronchiectasis even after high-dose γ-globulin replacement is initiated.

Untreated XLA patients are at risk for inflammatory arthritis of the large joints. This arthritis may reflect mycoplasma infection and typically resolves with appropriate antibiotics and γ-globulin replacement. A syndrome resembling dermatomyositis, with edema, ligneous induration of the muscles, weakness, and rash over extensor surfaces, has been observed. Central nervous system involvement may include a progressive and potentially fatal neurologic disease. Echovirus can be cultured from the cerebrospinal fluid of many of these patients.[11] High-dose intravenous γ-globulin and appropriate antiviral therapeutics can be effective in controlling this latter syndrome.

LABORATORY FEATURES

The hallmark of XLA is a profound deficit of both B cells and immunoglobulin, usually extending to all of the immunoglobulin isotypes, IgM, IgG, IgA, IgD, and IgE. *BTK* is expressed in neutrophils and in B lineage cells, although neutrophil function usually is normal in XLA patients. However, in the face of recurrent infections, XLA patients, like other hypogammaglobulinemic individuals, may suffer from severe neutropenia. Other constituents involved in resistance to infection, including serum complement, T cells, and natural killer (NK) cells, are normal. Early detection in neonates at risk for XLA typically is focused on the enumeration of CD19+ B cells and the measurement of the levels of non-IgG immunoglobulin isotypes, particularly IgM and IgA. Deficient expression of monocytes BTK protein can be evaluated by flow cytometry.[12] In cases where protein is present but the phenotype suggests XLA, sequence analysis of the *BTK* gene remains the definitive diagnostic procedure. Many different mutations have been found and collected in a disease-specific database known as BTKbase.[13] As with other X-linked lethal diseases, approximately one third of sporadic cases are caused by *de novo* mutations. Therefore, definitive diagnosis may require individual mutation analysis.

THERAPY, COURSE, AND PROGNOSIS

Intravenous administration of human IgG (IVIG) is effective in preventing severe recurrent pyogenic infections, arthritis, and latent viral infections. The optimal therapeutic dose must be determined in each case. IVIG typically is administered at monthly intervals, but clinical circumstances may require immunoglobulin infusions as frequently as weekly or biweekly. Dosage begins at 400 mg/kg/month, but up to 600 mg/kg/month may be required to achieve an optimal clinical remission of symptoms. Presently it is not possible to replace mucosal IgA. Hence, agammaglobulinemic patients often suffer with sinusitis, mild to moderate upper respiratory infections, especially with *Haemophilus influenza*, and inflammatory gastrointestinal disorders. Prophylactic therapy with antibiotics can diminish the frequency and severity of these infections, although complete resolution is rarely achieved. Patients can be acutely sensitive to the dose of γ-globulin and often benefit from an additional one-time infusion of 5 to 10 g of IVIG when they are recovering from a severe breakthrough infection. Excessive fatigue is a frequent symptom when serum immunoglobulin levels become very low.

With aggressive prophylactic IVIG and appropriate antibiotic therapy, the prognosis for agammaglobulinemic patients is excellent. However, insufficient or inadequate antimicrobial therapy can lead to chronic progressive bronchiectasis as a result of repeated pulmonary infections, ultimately leading to respiratory failure. Thus, annual assessment of pulmonary function is helpful in assessing efficacy of therapy. More severe complications, such as central nervous system infection with echovirus and the dermatomyositis-like syndrome, also may be controlled with high-dose intravenous γ-globulin and antiviral therapy.

AUTOSOMAL AGAMMAGLOBULINEMIA

Expression of the pre-B cell receptor is required for transition from the pro-B to the pre-B cell stage, and defects in components of the pre-B cell receptor account for 5 to 10 percent of patients with agammaglobulinemia and absent B cells.[8] These include loss-of-function mutations of the constant domain of the μ heavy chain,[14] λ14.1 (human λ5 equivalent), which is part of the surrogate light chain,[15] or Igα (CD792),[16] a transmembrane protein that partners with Igβ (CD796) and binds to μ heavy chains to form the membrane-bound B cell receptor. All three defects manifest as mendelian autosomal recessive traits and affect only the B cell lineage.

A young female patient with agammaglobulinemia, no B cells, and unusual facial features, including epicanthic folds, mild hypertelorism, high-arched palate, and lower ears, was reported to have a balanced translocation between chromosomes 9 and 20.[17] This situation resulted in the truncation of a novel gene, leucine-rich repeat-containing 8 (LRRC8), which is expressed in brain, heart, lung, liver, kidney, and T and B lineage cells. This mutation appears to have a mendelian dominant suppressor effect on B cell development.

TRANSIENT HYPOGAMMAGLOBULINEMIA OF INFANCY

As maternal immunoglobulin is catabolized,[9] infants must begin to rely on endogenous production of immunoglobulin. This transition leads to a physiologic nadir of serum immunoglobulin at age 4 to 6 months. This period is associated with susceptibility to mild upper respiratory infections and otitis media, even in infants with a normal immune system. The diagnosis of transient hypogammaglobulinemia of infancy (THI) is made when serum levels of the three major immunoglobulin classes fall below the fifth percentile for age on two or more occasions in infants who demonstrate normalization of serum immunoglobulin over time and who lack features consistent with other forms of primary immunodeficiency.[18] Thus, the diagnosis of THI can be made with certainty only in retrospect.

Most patients with the diagnosis of THI come to medical attention because of recurrent infections or as a result of routine screening studies of relatives of other immunodeficient patients.[18–20] Most patients with THI, especially those who present as a result of a positive family history or mild upper respiratory infections alone, exhibit fewer infections over time. Some children will not achieve normal levels of IgG for several years, and some will remain IgG subclass or IgA deficient. Treatment of transient hypogammaglobulinemia with IVIG is generally not warranted unless the child suffers from persistent, recurrent, invasive infections, including pneumonia.[20]

SELECTIVE IgA DEFICIENCY

Approximately one in 600 individuals of Caucasian ancestry is unable to produce detectable quantities of IgA, making selective IgA deficiency (IgAD) the most frequently recognized primary immunodeficiency in the Americas, Australia, Europe and the Middle East.[21] IgAD may be one twentieth as frequent in African-Americans[22] and even less common among Japanese and other Asian populations. Most IgA-deficient individuals have normal serum levels of IgM, normal or elevated levels of IgG, normal cell-mediated immunity, and no undue illness early in life. A minority of these patients have other evidence of immune dysfunction, including the inability to generate IgG_2 anticarbohydrate antibodies and frank IgG subclass deficiencies.

Among IgAD patients referred to immunology clinics, more than 85 percent present with recurrent pyogenic infections,[23] which are best treated with antibiotics. IgA-deficient individuals also have a high incidence of celiac disease, systemic lupus erythematosus, rheumatoid arthritis, and allergies.[21] Chronic intermittent diarrhea resulting from *Giardia lamblia* is a common problem. Some IgAD patients experience recurrent bronchitis, pneumonia, and even bronchiectasis. These patients also may have deficits in IgG2 and IgG4. Intravenous γ-globulin therapy should be reserved for those rare patients with significant IgG subclass deficiency and evidence of pulmonary dysfunction. Because IgA-deficient patients may also produce anti-IgA antibodies of IgG or IgE isotypes, these patients are at risk for adverse reactions following transfusion with blood products.

Susceptibility for IgAD appears to reside in the major histocompatibility complex (MHC) in most patients of European descent. Two susceptibility loci have been identified, one near the class II region[24] and one in the class III region near the class I region.[25,26] IgAD and common variable immune deficiency (CVID) have also been associated with congenital infection with rubella virus, cytomegalovirus, and *Toxoplasma gondii* and with treatment with certain drugs. Up to 20 percent of patients treated with phenytoin for idiopathic epilepsy experience a mild decrease in serum IgA levels, and a minority may become panhypogammaglobulinemic.[27,28] Gold salts, D-penicillamine, captopril, antimalarials, and other drugs also can inhibit antibody production. Recovery of normal immunoglobulin production may take months or years after cessation of the offending drug.

COMMON VARIABLE IMMUNE DEFICIENCY

EPIDEMIOLOGY

With an estimated prevalence of one in 50,000,[29] CVID is the most frequent type of primary immune deficiency requiring the care of clinical immunologists. Men and women are equally affected. As with IgAD, the prevalence among Americans of African descent is approximately one twentieth that of Americans of European descent. This immunodeficiency may become evident during childhood, but most patients are diagnosed in the third decade of life.[30] The typical patient begins to have recurrent sinusitis and bronchitis during adolescence. Repeated bouts of pneumonia as a young adult is the most common precipitating complaint that brings the patient to the attention of the clinical immunologist. Although CVID appears to be an acquired disorder, family studies have documented that susceptibility to the disease is inherited and that the degree of immunoglobulin deficiency may change over time.[30,31] Normal serum immunoglobulin concentrations may give way to IgA deficiency and progress to IgA deficiency with IgG subclass deficits and then to panhypogammafobulinemia as both sporadic occurrences and in familial cases.[22]

PATHOGENESIS

As with congenital agammaglobulinemia and absent B cells, CVID may represent a mixture of primary immunodeficiencies.[32] Homozygous loss-of-function mutations in *ICOS*, a gene associated with T cell reactivation, is an infrequent cause of adult-onset CVID.[31] Of those patients in whom no specific single gene defect has been identified, most have inherited all or a portion of two extended MHC haplotypes: HLA–DQ2, –DR7, –B44 or HLA–DQ2, –DR3(17), –B8. These patients, who are of European descent, exhibit a distinctive phenotype characterized by a broad deficiency of immunoglobulin isotypes despite the presence of normal numbers of surface immunoglobulin-bearing B cells. They are consistently IgA deficient and, by definition, have serum IgG levels of less than 500 mg/dl. Some IgG subclasses may be more affected than others, with the sequential order of involvement being IgG4 > IgG2 > IgG1 > IgG3. Most CVID patients are also deficient in IgM and IgE. Cell-mediated immunity usually is normal, although some patients may have evidence of T cell dysfunction[33] and dysfunction of other hematopoietic cell types.[34] The numbers of B cells are rarely reduced and never to the same extent as that seen in XLA or the agammaglobulinemia associated with thymoma.

CLINICAL MANIFESTATIONS

The clinical manifestations of CVID are similar but more severe than those seen in IgAD. In addition to the severe respiratory symptoms, gastrointestinal infections, and arthritis associated with agammaglobulinemia, some unfortunate patients develop a malabsorption syndrome that resembles celiac sprue but does not improve with gluten avoidance. Allergic disorders are rare in CVID, although affected individuals may produce sufficient IgE antibodies to cause anaphylactic reactions.[35] Although CVID patients often are anergic, as judged by

delayed-type hypersensitivity skin testing, only a minority suffer infections characteristic of cell-mediated immune dysfunction, such as mycobacteria, *Pneumocystis carinii*, and fungi. The latter often have reduced numbers of CD8+ cytotoxic/suppressor T cells.

Patients with CVID are at higher risk for developing a broad spectrum of autoimmune diseases, including pernicious anemia, autoimmune neutropenia, Graves disease, hypothyroidism, rheumatoid arthritis, systemic lupus erythematosus, Sjögren syndrome, and a Coombs-positive hemolytic anemia with idiopathic thrombocytopenic purpura (Evans syndrome). Patients may also develop a sarcoid-like syndrome characterized by noncaseating granulomas in the lung, lymph nodes, skin, marrow, and liver.[36] CVID patients in general have a higher incidence of gastrointestinal and lymphoid malignancies, especially B cell lymphomas.[37] Notably confounding the diagnosis of malignancy in these immunodeficient patients is their propensity to develop benign lymphoproliferative disorders. Atypical lymphoid hyperplasia can be difficult to differentiate from a malignant lymphoma. Because immunosuppressive chemotherapy may be particularly disastrous for immunodeficient individuals, assessment of clonality is very important to discriminate polyclonal immune responses from monoclonal lymphoid malignancies.

TREATMENT

Therapy for CVID requires the aggressive treatment of ongoing infections and the institution of prophylactic measures to prevent future infection, including intravenous γ-globulin and prophylactic antibiotics. The overwhelming majority of CVID patients require IVIG therapy for life.

Splenomegaly is common in untreated patients with CVID but responds to aggressive therapy with antibiotics and intravenous immunoglobulin in most patients. This finding suggests that the hypersplenism is secondary to reactive lymphoid hyperplasia in response to infection.[38] Rarely the development of the other hematologic manifestations of hypersplenism (refractory thrombocytopenia, anemia, neutropenia, lymphopenia) may require splenectomy as a last therapeutic resort.

IgA-deficient mothers fail to secrete IgA in their colostrum.[39] Although colostral IgM levels may be elevated in an attempt to compensate for the lack of maternal IgA, the newborn offspring of an IgA-deficient mother remains relatively unprotected against intestinal pathogens. Of even greater concern are the children of mothers with untreated CVID who are born in a state of humoral immunodeficiency and are at great risk for life-threatening sinopulmonary infection.[40] To compensate for the loss of IgG across the placenta and to provide the infant with the necessary passive immunity, the level of intravenous γ-globulin infusion should be increased to 600 mg/kg during the mother's third trimester of pregnancy.

IgG SUBCLASS DEFICIENCIES

Patients with recurrent bacterial infections may have selective deficiency of IgG1, IgG2, IgG3, IgG4, or a combination of these subclasses.[41] The basis of IgG subclass deficiency usually is not obvious, but in rare cases homozygous deletions of IgG and IgE constant region exons have been observed. Interestingly, most of the latter group of individuals do not have unusual difficulty with infections. When the IgG subclass deficiency is associated with recurrent infections, prophylactic antibiotics are the preferred form of therapy. Some patients may require treatment with intravenous γ-globulin.

HYPER-IgM SYNDROME

The secondary immune response is marked by class switching and affinity maturation. In class switching, nonhomologous recombination between constant domain genes allows the antibody to preserve the variable domain, and hence antigen binding characteristics, while altering effector function. In affinity maturation, somatic hypermutation of the variable region allows the antibody to enhance its affinity for its antigen while maintaining effector function. Both of these processes require the activity of activation-induced cytidine deaminase (AID),[42] the gene for which is located on chromosome 12 at 12p13, and uracil-DNA glycosylase (UNG),[43] the gene for which is located on chromosome 12 at 12q23-24.1. Homozygosity for loss-of-function mutations of either of these genes yields a deficiency of IgA and IgG that usually, but not always, is accompanied by increased IgM levels. The IgM levels in these patients can range up to 1000 mg/dl. For this reason, this disorder is commonly called the hyper-IgM syndrome or hyper-IgM immunodeficiency. The excessive IgM levels reflect exaggerated polyclonal responses to antigens in these patients. Individuals afflicted with the hyper-IgM syndrome resulting from either UNG or AID mutations nevertheless experience recurrent bacterial infections. The incidence of infection can be greatly reduced by IVIG replacement therapy.

Activation of class switching and somatic hypermutation requires that the B cell receive two signals from helper T cells. The first signal is a cytokine, such as interleukin-4 (for IgE synthesis), and the second signal involves the physical engagement of CD40 on the B cell with CD154 (CD40 ligand) on activated T cells. The *CD154* gene is located on the X chromosome at Xq26, and the inheritance of loss-of-function mutations is mendelian X-linked recessive.[44] *CD40* is located on chromosome 12 at 12p13 so that inheritance of loss-of-function mutations of this gene is mendelian autosomal recessive.[45] The signal transduction cascade triggered by CD40 ligation involves activity of the product of a gene termed nuclear factor-κB essential modulator (*NEMO*), which is located on the X chromosome at Xq28. Hence, inheritance of loss-of-function mutations in this gene is X-linked recessive. Loss of function of any one of these genes yields a hyper-IgM syndrome with susceptibility to opportunistic infections, including *P. carinii* pneumonia, and thrombocytopenia, neutropenia, aplastic anemia, or hemolytic anemia. Because these genes are active in cell types other than B and T cells, the consequences of their mutation may extend beyond deficient T and B cell function. As a result, prognosis is less favorable than with AID or UNG deficiency. Treatment begins with intravenous γ-globulin replacement and may include granulocyte-macrophage colony stimulating factor or plasma transfusions for neutropenia.[46] In patients with refractory disease, bone marrow transplantation may prove necessary.[47]

SEVERE COMBINED IMMUNODEFICIENCY

DEFINITION AND HISTORY

In 1950, Glanzmann and Riniker[2] described two unrelated infants who died of overwhelming infection during the second year of life after a succession of serious infections, including intractable diarrhea, thrush, and a persistent morbilliform rash. Infants with this clinical presentation have a profound lymphopenia and hypogammaglobulinemia or agammaglobulinemia. Untreated, this severe combined immunodeficiency (SCID) is uniformly fatal.

ETIOLOGY AND PATHOGENESIS

Family studies quickly demonstrated that SCID was a heterogeneous disorder with two common patterns of inheritance: X-linked and autosomal recessive. Increasingly sophisticated definition of the syndromes has disclosed that, in some cases, only the T cells are absent (termed $T^-B^+NK^+$ SCID), whereas in other cases both T and B cells are affected ($T^-B^-NK^+$ SCID). In those with the most severe lymphopenia, NK cells are also absent ($T^-B^-NK^-$ SCID). Because of the need for T cell help in generating an efficient antibody response against protein antigens, immunoglobulin production is impaired even when B cells are present.

Classic X-linked SCID composes approximately 45 percent of all SCID cases.[48] This $T^-B^+NK^+$ SCID is caused by a loss-of-function mutation in the gene for the γ-chain of the interleukin-2 receptor,[49] which is located at Xq13. This γ-chain is also an essential signal-transduction unit of the IL-4, IL-7, IL-9, and IL-15 cytokine receptors. This shared usage led to its designation as the common gamma (γc)-chain. Engagement of the IL-7 receptor is required for T cell development; hence, absence of the γc-chain leads to a profound T cell deficiency. When T cells are activated by IL-7, the γc-chain is phosphorylated by the tyrosine kinase Janus-associated kinase 3 (JAK3), the gene for which is located at 19p13.1. JAK3 deficiency, a $T^-B^+NK^+$ SCID,[50] composes approximately 6 percent of all SCID cases. The gene for the IL-7 receptor α-chain is located at 5p13. IL-7 receptor α-chain deficiency, another $T^-B^+NK^+$ SCID,[51] composes approximately 9 percent of all SCID cases. Zeta-associated protein kinase 70 (ZAP-70) associates with the CD3ζ chain of the TCR/CD3 complex and undergoes tyrosine phosphorylation following TCR stimulation. Loss-of-function mutations in the gene for ZAP-70, which is located at 2q12, also lead to a $T^-B^+NK^+$ SCID.[52]

Approximately 15 percent of infants with SCID have a deficiency of adenosine deaminase (ADA), the aminohydrolase that converts adenosine to inosine and thus plays a major role in DNA synthesis.[53] The gene for ADA is located at 20q13.11. Approximately 2 percent of SCID infants have a deficiency of purine nucleoside phosphorylase (PNP),[54] the gene for which is located at 14q13.1. In both ADA and PNP deficiency, the accumulation of toxic DNA metabolites, deoxyadenosine triphosphate (dATP) or deoxyguanosine triphosphate (dGTP), inhibits normal T and B lymphocyte development, resulting in a $T^-B^-NK^+$ SCID. $T^-B^-NK^+$ SCID also can result from mutations in enzymes that are involved in the nonhomologous end-joining reactions required for the VDJ joining that creates the variable domains of the T cell receptors and immunoglobulins. Loss-of-function mutations have been reported in the *RAG-1* and *RAG-2* genes (~3% of SCID cases), which catalyze VDJ recombination, and in *Artemis* (~1% of SCID cases), which encodes a DNA repair factor. Missense mutations in *RAG-1* and *RAG-2* can result in a variant of SCID called Omenn syndrome, which is characterized by marked erythrodermia, hyper-IgE, eosinophilia, and oligoclonal expansion of T cells.

Reticular dysgenesis is one of the rarest and most severe forms of SCID. It is a $T^-B^-NK^-$ SCID characterized by congenital agranulocytosis, lymphopenia, lymphoid hypoplasia, and thymic hypoplasia.[55] Cellular and humoral immune function is completely absent in affected newborns. Reticular dysgenesis is a rapidly fatal disorder unless treated by marrow transplantation. The etiology remains unclear.

CLINICAL FEATURES

The complete absence of T cell function impairs both cell-mediated immunity and humoral immunity. Infections begin early, between 3 and 6 months of age. Diarrhea, bronchitis, and pneumonia with failure to thrive are almost universal. Affected infants are highly susceptible to opportunistic organisms, including *Candida albicans, P. carinii,* adenovirus, respiratory syncytial virus, parainfluenza 3, Epstein-Barr virus, and cytomegalovirus.[56] Extensive moniliasis of the mouth or diaper area that persists beyond the neonatal period often is the first sign of the disease. Stool cultures frequently reveal strains of *Salmonella* or enteropathic *Escherichia coli*. Lung abscesses may contain *Pseudomonas aeruginosa*.

Affected infants are also at risk from several routine medical interventions. Vaccination can lead to death because the SCID patients are incapable of limiting or overcoming relatively benign viral or mycobacterial infections. Inoculation with vaccinia virus or bacille Calmette-Guérin (BCG) can result in a progressive, ultimately fatal infection. After whole-blood transfusion, donor lymphocytes can induce graft-versus-host disease (GVHD). GVHD also may result from the persistence of maternal lymphoid cells that have traversed the placental barrier. The onset of GVHD is marked by the appearance of a characteristic maculopapular rash, starting on the face in the second week after injection of immunocompetent histoincompatible cells. The rash spreads rapidly, ultimately involving all skin surfaces including the palms and soles. Thrombocytopenia, leukopenia, jaundice, anasarca, and death from hemorrhage may follow.

LABORATORY FEATURES

The number of lymphocytes in blood usually is less than $2000/\mu l$ (2×10^9/liter), and almost no CD3+ cells are present. When mature T cells are present, they usually are of maternal origin.[57] The variation of lymphocyte counts seen in SCID patients is largely the result of those who are able to generate B cells and NK cells. Thus, in affected neonates, lymphocyte counts may begin at normal neonatal levels (>$3000/\mu l$ [3×10^9/liter]), only to later develop into a profound lymphopenia. Accordingly, a single normal lymphocyte count in newborns cannot exclude the diagnosis of SCID. Platelet and neutrophil counts typically are in the normal range, but eosinophilia is common.

A deficiency of plasma cells, lymphocytes, and lymphoblasts is observed in the marrow. In the secondary lymphoid organs, germinal center elements, plasma cells, and lymphocytes are completely lacking. Tonsils may be rudimentary or absent, and the spleen, appendix, or intestinal tract is virtually devoid of lymphoid populations. Lymph node stroma may contain occasional mast cells and eosinophils. Rarely, small collections of lymphoid cells are seen without any apparent organization. Lymph node biopsies should not be performed to establish the diagnosis, however, as the biopsy site can serve as a portal of entry for infection.

Because the thymus fails to generate T cells, the thymus shadow is not visible on a chest x-ray film. The rudimentary thymus ordinarily weighs less than 1 g and is composed of primordial spindle-shaped cells that occasionally form swirls or rosettes. No Hassall corpuscles and few, if any, lymphocytes are present. Nevertheless, the thymus is capable of generating T cells when lymphoid progenitors are provided by marrow transplant or specific gene therapy.

Because of the absence of T cells, neither tuberculin nor chemical contact delayed-type hypersensitivity can be elicited. Blood mononuclear lymphocytes are unresponsive to phytohemagglutinin or allogenic stimulation, and skin allografts are not rejected. Patients with B cells are unable to generate a humoral response to protein antigens, including toxins and viral proteins.

THERAPY, COURSE, AND PROGNOSIS

If SCID is left untreated, infection and malnutrition lead inexorably to death of SCID patients within the first 2 years of life. Transplantation of marrow from MHC-matched siblings was the first successful therapy. Marrow transplant therapy for SCID has been revolutionized by the development of techniques for T cell depletion and the use of haploidentical donors, typically parents, in addition to MHC-matched sibling donors.[58,59] Because infants with SCID cannot reject allografts, marrow transplantation does not require pretransplant chemotherapeutic conditioning, except for cases where marrow "niche clearing" is necessary. Because of the high risk of hospital-acquired infection, patients may be transplanted as outpatients.

The accessibility of lymphoid progenitors has made SCID a model for gene therapy. Success has been achieved in X-linked SCID caused by deficiency of the common γ chain[60] and ADA deficiency,[61] although many pitfalls remain.[61]

PRIMARY T CELL DEFICIENCY

CONGENITAL THYMIC APLASIA (DIGEORGE SYNDROME)

During early embryonic development, neural crest cell migration into the third and fourth pharyngeal arches leads to the normal development of the thymus, parathyroid glands, outflow vessels of the heart, and facial features including the philtrum of the lip and the tubercles of the ear. Chromosomal deletions in 22q11.2 or 10p13 are associated with variable disruption of this process, giving rise to a spectrum of phenotypes that include thymic hypoplasia, parathyroid hypoplasia, cardiac defects (including tetralogy of Fallot, truncus arteriosus, and interrupted aortic arch), cleft palate, and facial anomalies.[62] Within this spectrum, the DiGeorge syndrome is characterized by hypocalcemia resulting from parathyroid dysfunction, T cell lymphopenia resulting from thymic hypoplasia, and cardiac outflow tract defects. DiGeorge syndrome patients often present with neonatal tetany, cardiac defects requiring surgical intervention, and a history of increased susceptibility to viral, fungal, and bacterial infections. Speech delay is a common finding. The variability of this syndrome is emphasized by the observation that up to one fourth of the patients with DiGeorge syndrome have an asymptomatic parent who also has a 22q11 deletion.[63]

A variable amount of parathyroid tissue and thymic tissue may be found in ectopic positions in the neck of DiGeorge syndrome patients. The extent of functioning thymic and parathyroid tissue exercises a strong influence on outcome. For patients with sufficient parathyroid tissue, the hypocalcemia tends to ameliorate with development during the first year of life. Patients have variable numbers of CD3+ T cells in the blood, and the severity of susceptibility to infection correlates with the T cell level. T cell numbers in the blood vary from normal in approximately one fifth of patients to total absence in less than one in 200 affected individuals. Delayed hypersensitivity to common antigens, such as *Candida* or *Trichophyton*, often is impaired. Skin allograft rejection is abnormally delayed or absent, and lymphocyte responses to stimulation with mitogens or allogenic cells are impaired.

Management of the immunodeficiency in DiGeorge syndrome is heavily influenced by the clinical spectrum of symptoms. No therapy is necessary in patients with only moderately impaired thymic function. In DiGeorge syndrome patients who have T cells, the bone marrow and secondary lymphoid organs may contain normal numbers of germinal centers and plasma cells. Antibody responses to many antigens may be preserved, and serum immunoglobulins levels usually are normal. At the other end of the spectrum, patients with severely impaired thymic function may require transplantation of thymic epithelial tissue that has been depleted of donor thymocytes.[64]

MHC CLASS II DEFICIENCY

Patients with MHC class II deficiency, or bare lymphocyte syndrome type II, may appear to have normal numbers of T cells and B cells. However, closer examination reveals a deficiency of CD4 T cells. The T cell deficiency in these patients typically is more obvious in lymphoid tissues than in the circulation. The three types of MHC class II molecules are HLA-DP, HLA-DQ, and HLA-DR. These molecules are constitutively expressed by B cells, monocytes, and dendritic cells, and they can be induced in T cells, fibroblasts, and other cells. The interaction of CD4 with MHC class II is required for the development and survival of CD4 T cells. The absence of these molecules does not result from structural deficits in the genes, which are located on 6p21.

Instead, their lack of expression can result from the absence of any one of four promoter binding proteins that are essential for MHC class II gene expression: RFXANK (19p12), RFX5 (1q21), RFXAP (13q14), and CIITA (16p13).[65] Thus, MHC class II deficiency is a disease of gene regulation. All four transcription factor disorders are inherited as mendelian autosomal recessive traits.

These patients have severe and repeated opportunistic infections that frequently are life-threatening. Without adequate numbers of helper CD4 T cells, their B cells cannot respond appropriately to protein antigens, including toxins and viral peptides. The *in vitro* response of their T cells to mitogens and allogeneic lymphocytes in mixed lymphocyte cultures is poor, although they may respond normally to stimulation with anti-CD3 and anti-CD2 monoclonal antibodies. Marrow transplantation can be successful in treating patients with this condition.

TAP-1 OR TAP-2 DEFICIENCY (MHC CLASS I DEFICIENCY)

TAP, the ATP-binding cassette transporter, is a heterodimeric protein composed of TAP-1 and TAP-2. The *TAP1* and *TAP2* genes are closely linked on chromosome 6p21.3 just upstream of the MHC class II locus. TAP translocates peptides derived from the cytosolic proteosomes into the endoplasmic reticulum to load the MHC class I molecules. This peptide loading of the MHC class I β-microglobulin complex is required for stabilization of the MHC class I complex and its transport to the cell surface. Therefore, loss-of-function mutations in *TAP1* or *TAP2* are associated with a severe deficit in cell surface expression of MHC class I molecules, which has been termed the *bare lymphocyte syndrome, type 1*. Because the presentation of peptides by MHC class I molecules is required for normal development and function of cytotoxic CD8 T cells, patients with *TAP1* or *TAP2* mutations are deficient in these cells. Affected patients often appear healthy in the first years of life,[66,67] but in late childhood they begin to have recurrent respiratory infections that may lead to bronchiectasis. Currently no satisfactory therapy exists for these patients beyond appropriate treatment of their infections and the attendant respiratory complications.

FUNCTIONAL DEFICIENCY OF THE TH1 SUBPOPULATION OF T CELLS

The production of interferon gamma (IFN-γ) by effector TH1 cells within the CD4 T cell subpopulation is required for effective elimination of intracellular pathogens. Interleukin-12, a heterodimeric cytokine, interacts with its receptor to play a dominant role in directing the development of Th1 cells. IFN-γ is also produced by NK cells and CD8 T cells. Patients who demonstrate abnormal induction of IFN-γ because of loss-of-function mutations of the *IFN-γ* gene (12q14) or the genes for the two IFN-γ receptor chains 6q23 and 21q22 exhibit an increased susceptibility to tuberculosis, atypical mycobacteria, and *Salmonella*.[68,69] Patients with loss-of-function mutations in either the genes for interleukin-12 (3p12 and 5q31) or the gene for the interleukin-12 receptor β1-chain (19p13) have similar types of infections. Patients suffering from these infections usually respond well to the appropriate antimicrobial therapy. For patients with affected defects that do not involve the IFN-γ receptor, treatment of their infections with IFN-γ in addition to antimicrobials may be beneficial.

OTHER WELL-DEFINED IMMUNODEFICIENCY SYNDROMES

ATAXIA-TELANGIECTASIA

Ataxia-telangiectasia (AT) is an autosomal recessive disease that results from mutations in the ataxia-telangiectasia mutated gene *(ATM)* (11q22-23).[70,71] ATM is involved in the repair of double-stranded DNA breaks. AT patients begin to have progressive cerebellar ataxia early in childhood. Affected individuals later develop conjunctival telangiectasias and sinopulmonary infections. In addition, they exhibit increased susceptibility to malignancy. Death from infection or lymphoreticular malignancy is common in the second or third decade of life. Heterozygous carriers, who compose an estimated 1.4 percent of the population, also appear to be at increased risk for malignancy.

AT patients may have both humoral and cell-mediated immunodeficiency. Serum IgG2 or IgA levels are reduced or absent in up to 80 percent of patients. The thymus is uniformly hypoplastic, and the numbers of α,β T cells are low, especially in the secondary lymphoid tissues. Delayed hypersensitivity reactions and skin allograft rejection are compromised as a reflection of their T cell deficiency. Immunoglobulin replacement and symptomatic measures may offer limited therapeutic benefit.

WISKOTT-ALDRICH SYNDROME

The Wiskott-Aldrich syndrome (WAS) is characterized by eczema, thrombocytopenia, and recurrent infections.[72] The gene for Wiskott-Aldrich syndrome protein *(WASP)* is located at Xp11.22, and the syndrome is inherited as a mendelian X-linked recessive. WAS patients have a specific inability to respond normally to polysaccharide antigens. Hence, serum IgM levels usually are low, whereas IgG and IgA levels can be normal or elevated. With increasing age, patients become lymphopenic and have severely impaired cell-mediated immunity. Because of their immunodeficiency, affected boys rarely survive beyond the first decade of life because of overwhelming infections with gram-positive and gram-negative bacteria, viruses, and fungi. WAS patients also may suffer from hemorrhage and lymphoreticular malignancies.

REFERENCES

1. Rosen FS: Immunodeficiency diseases, in: *Williams Textbook of Hematology*, edited by ME Replace, p 977, McGraw-Hill, New York, 1999.
2. Glanzmann E, Riniker P: Essentielle lymphocytophtose. Ein neues krankeitsbild aus der Sauglingspathologie. *Ann Paediatr* 175:1, 1950.
3. Bruton OC: Agammaglobulinemia. *Pediatrics* 9:722, 1952.
4. Ochs HD, Smith CIE, Puck JM: *Primary Immunodeficiency Diseases: A Molecular and Genetic Approach*. Oxford University Press, Oxford, 1999.
5. Buckley RH: Primary cellular immunodeficiencies. *J Allergy Clin Immunol* 109:747, 2002.
6. Conley ME: Diagnostic guidelines—An International Consensus document. *Clin Immunol* 93:189, 1999.
7. Smith CI, Backesjo CM, Berglof A, et al: X-linked agammaglobulinemia: Lack of mature B lineage cells caused by mutations in the Btk kinase. *Springer Semin Immunopathol* 19:369, 1998.
8. Conley ME: Genes required for B cell development. *J Clin Invest* 112: 1636, 2003.
9. Zinkernagel RM: Maternal antibodies, childhood infections, and autoimmune diseases. *N Engl J Med* 345:1331, 2001.
10. Conley ME, Howard V: Clinical findings leading to the diagnosis of X-linked agammaglobulinemia. *J Pediatr* 141:566, 2002.
11. Wilfert CM, Buckley RH, Mohanakumar T, et al: Persistent and fatal central-nervous-system echovirus infections in patients with agammaglobulinemia. *N Engl J Med* 296:1485, 1977.
12. Futatani T, Miyawaki T, Tsukada S, et al: Deficient expression of Bruton's tyrosine kinase in monocytes from X-linked agammaglobulinemia as evaluated by a flow cytometric analysis and its clinical application to carrier detection. *Blood* 91:595, 1998.
13. Vihinen M, Brandau O, Branden LJ, et al: BTKbase, mutation database for X-linked agammaglobulinemia (XLA). *Prog Nucleic Acid Res Mol Biol* 26:242, 1998.

14. Granados EL, Porpiglia AS, Hogan MB, et al: Clinical and molecular analysis of patients with defects in micro heavy chain gene. *J Clin Invest* 110:1029, 2002.

15. Minegishi Y, Coustan-Smith E, Wang YH, et al: Mutations in the human lambda5/14.1 gene result in B cell deficiency and agammaglobulinemia. *J Exp Med* 187:71, 1998.

16. Minegishi Y, Coustan-Smith E, Rapalus L, et al: Mutations in Igalpha (CD79a) result in a complete block in B-cell development. *J Clin Invest* 104:1115, 1999.

17. Sawada A, Takihara Y, Kim JY, et al: A congenital mutation of the novel gene LRRC8 causes agammaglobulinemia in humans. *J Clin Invest* 112:1707, 2003.

18. Tiller TL Jr, Buckley RH: Transient hypogammaglobulinemia of infancy: Review of the literature, clinical and immunologic features of 11 new cases, and long-term follow-up. *J Pediatr* 92:347, 1978.

19. Dressler F, Peter HH, Muller W, Rieger CH: Transient hypogamma-globulinemia of infancy: Five new cases, review of the literature and redefinition. *Acta Paediatr Scand* 78:767, 1989.

20. Dalal I, Reid B, Nisbet-Brown E, Roifman CM: The outcome of patients with hypogammaglobulinemia in infancy and early childhood. *J Pediatr* 133:144, 1998.

21. Burrows PD, Cooper MD: IgA Deficiency. *Adv Immunol* 65:245, 1997.

22. Johnson ML, Keeton LG, Zhu Z-B, et al: Age-related changes in serum immunoglobulins in patients with familial IgA deficiency and common variable immunodeficiency (CVID). *Clin Exp Immunol* 108:477, 1997.

23. Morell A, Muehlheim E, Schaad U, et al: Susceptibility to infections in children with selective IgA and IgA-IgG subclass deficiency. *Eur J Pediatr* 145:199, 1986.

24. Kralovicova J, Hammarstrom L, Plebani A, et al: Fine-scale mapping at IGAD1 and genome-wide genetic linkage analysis implicate HLA-DQ/DR as a major susceptibility locus in selective IgA deficiency and common variable immunodeficiency. *J Immunol* 170:2765, 2003.

25. de la Concha EG, Fernandez-Arquero M, Gual L, et al: MHC susceptibility genes to IgA deficiency are located in different regions on different HLA haplotypes. *J Immunol* 169:4637, 2002.

26. Schroeder HWJ, Zhu ZB, March RE, et al: Susceptibility locus for IgA deficiency and common variable immunodeficiency in the HLA-DR3, -B8, -A1 haplotypes. *Mol Med* 4:72, 1998.

27. Schroeder HW Jr: Genetics of IgA deficiency and common variable immunodeficiency. *Clin Rev Allergy Immunol* 19:127, 2000.

28. Bardana EJ, Gabourel JD, Davies GH, Craig S: Effects of phenytoin on man's immunity. Evaluation of changes in serum immunoglobulins, complement, and antinuclear antibody. *Am J Med* 74:289, 1983.

29. Fasth A: Primary immunodeficiency disorders in Sweden: Cases among children 1974-1979. *J Clin Immunol* 2:86, 1982.

30. Schroeder HW Jr, Schroeder HW III, Sheikh SM: The complex genetics of common variable immunodeficiency. *J Investig Med* 52:90, 2004.

31. Grimbacher B, Hutloff A, Schlesier M, et al: Homozygous loss of ICOS is associated with adult-onset common variable immunodeficiency. *Nat Immunol* 4:261, 2003.

32. Rosen FS, Wedgwood RJ, Eibl MM, et al: Primary immunodeficiency diseases: Report of a WHO Scientific Group. *Clin Exp Immunol* 109(suppl 1):S1, 1997.

33. Sneller MC, Strober W, Eisenstein E, et al: New insights into common variable immunodeficiency. *Ann Intern Med* 118:720, 1993.

34. Belickova M, Schroeder HW Jr, Guan YL, et al: Clonal hematopoiesis and acquired thalassemia in common variable immunodeficiency. *Mol Med* 1:56, 1994.

35. Loria RC, Jadidi S, Wedner HJ: Anaphylactic reaction to ampicillin in a patient with common variable immunodeficiency syndrome desensitized to penicillin. *Ann Allergy* 59:15,348, 1987.

36. Fasano MB, Sullivan KE, Sarpong SB, et al: Sarcoidosis and common variable immunodeficiency. Report of 8 cases and review of the literature. *Medicine* 75:251, 1996.

37. Cunningham Rundles C, Siegal FP, Cunningham Rundles S, Lieberman P: Incidence of cancer in 98 patients with common variable immunodeficiency. *J Clin Immunol* 7:294, 1987.

38. Prasad AS, Raeiner E, Watson DJ: Syndrome of hypogammaglobulinemia, splenomegaly, and hypersplenism. *Blood* 12:926, 1957.

39. Barros MD, Porto MH, Leser PG, et al: Study of colostrum of a patient with selective IgA deficiency. *Allergol Immunopathol (Madr)* 13:331, 1985.

40. Madsen DL, Catanzarite VA, Varela Gittings F: Common variable hypogammaglobulinemia in pregnancy: Treatment with high-dose immunoglobulin infusions. *Am J Hematol* 21:327, 1986.

41. Schur PH, Borel H, Gelfand EW, et al: Selective gamma-g globulin deficiencies in patients with recurrent pyogenic infections. *N Engl J Med* 283:631, 1970.

42. Revy P, Muto T, Levy Y, et al: Activation-induced cytidine deaminase (AICD) deficiency causes the autosomal recessive form of the hyper-IgM syndrome (HIGM2). *Cell* 102:565, 2000.

43. Imai K, Slupphaug G, Lee WI, et al: Human uracil-DNA glycosylase deficiency associated with profoundly impaired immunoglobulin class-switch recombination. *Nat Immunol* 4:1023, 2003.

44. Kroczek RA, Graf D, Brugnoni D, et al: Defective expression of CD40 ligand on T cells causes "X-linked immunodeficiency with hyper-IgM (HIGM1)." *Immunol Rev* 138:39, 1994.

45. Ferrari S, Giliani S, Insalaco A, et al: Mutations of CD40 gene cause an autosomal recessive form of immunodeficiency with hyper IgM. *Proc Natl Acad Sci U S A* 98:12614, 2001.

46. Dunn K, Lubens R, Stiehm ER: Reversal of neutropenia in X-linked immunodeficiency with hyper-IgM by large doses of plasma. *Clin Res* 30:125A, 1982.

47. Duplantier JE, Seyama K, Day NK, et al: Immunologic reconstitution following bone marrow transplantation for X-linked hyper IgM syndrome. *Clin Immunol* 98:313, 2001.

48. Buckley RH: A historical review of bone marrow transplantation for immunodeficiencies. *J Allergy Clin Immunol* 113:793, 2004.

49. Noguchi M, Yi H, Rosenblatt HM, et al: Interleukin-2 receptor gamma chain mutation results in X-linked severe combined immunodeficiency in humans. *Cell* 73:147, 1993.

50. Russell SM, Johnston JA, Noguchi M, et al: Interaction of IL-2R beta and gamma c chains with Jak1 and Jak3: Implications for XSCID and XCID. *Science* 266:1042, 1994.

51. Puel A, Ziegler SF, Buckley RH, Leonard WJ: Defective IL7R expression in T(-)B(+)NK(+) severe combined immunodeficiency. *Nat Genet* 20:394, 1998.

52. Colucci F, Schweighoffer E, Tomasello E, et al: Natural cytotoxicity uncoupled from the Syk and ZAP-70 intracellular kinases. *Nat Immunol* 3:288, 2002.

53. Giblett ER, Anderson JE, Cohen F, et al: Adenosine-deaminase deficiency in two patients with severely impaired cellular immunity. *Lancet* 2:1067, 1972.

54. Giblett ER, Ammann AJ, Wara DW, et al: Nucleoside-phosphorylase deficiency in a child with severely defective T-cell immunity and normal B-cell immunity. *Lancet* 1:1010, 1975.

55. Bertrand Y, Muller SM, Casanova JL, et al: Reticular dysgenesis: HLA non-identical bone marrow transplants in a series of 10 patients. *Bone Marrow Transplant* 29:759, 2002.

56. Buckley RH, Schiff RI, Schiff SE, et al: Human severe combined immunodeficiency: Genetic, phenotypic, and functional diversity in one hundred eight infants. *J Pediatr* 130:378, 1997.

57. Reinherz EL, Cooper MD, Schlossman SF, Rosen FS: Abnormalities of T cell maturation and regulation in human beings with immunodeficiency disorders. *J Clin Investig* 68:699, 1981.

58. Reisner Y, Kapoor N, Kirkpatrick D, et al: Transplantation for severe combined immunodeficiency with HLA-A,-B,-D,-DR incompatible parental marrow cells fractionated by soybean agglutinin and sheep red blood cells. *Blood* 61:341, 1983.

59. Buckley RH, Schiff SE, Schiff RI, et al: Hematopoietic stem-cell transplantation for the treatment of severe combined immunodeficiency. *N Engl J Med* 340:508, 1999.

60. Fischer A, Hacein-Bey S, Cavazzana-Calvo M: Gene therapy of severe combined immunodeficiencies. *Nat Rev Immunol* 2:615, 2002.

61. Muul LM, Tuschong LM, Soenen SL, et al: Persistence and expression of the adenosine deaminase gene for 12 years and immune reaction to gene transfer components: Long-term results of the first clinical gene therapy trial. *Blood* 101:2563, 2003.

62. Perez E, Sullivan KE: Chromosome 22q11.2 deletion syndrome (DiGeorge and velocardiofacial syndromes). *Curr Opin Pediatr* 14:678, 2002.

63. Levy A, Michel G, Lemerrer M, Philip N: Idiopathic thrombocytopenic purpura in two mothers of children with DiGeorge sequence: A new component manifestation of deletion 22q11? *Am J Med Genet* 69:356, 1997.

64. Markert ML, Boeck A, Hale LP, et al: Transplantation of thymus tissue in complete DiGeorge syndrome. *N Engl J Med* 341:1180, 1999.

65. Reith W, Mach B: The bare lymphocyte syndrome and the regulation of MHC expression. *Annu Rev Immunol* 19:331, 2001.

66. de la Salle H, Zimmer J, Fricker D, et al: HLA class I deficiencies due to mutations in subunit 1 of the peptide transporter TAP1. *J Clin Investig* 103:R9, 1999.

67. Moins-Teisserenc HT, Gadola SD, Cella M, et al: Association of a syndrome resembling Wegener's granulomatosis with low surface expression of HLA class-I molecules. *Lancet* 354:1598, 1999.

68. Jouanguy E, Doffinger R, Dupuis S, et al: IL-12 and IFN-gamma in host defense against mycobacteria and salmonella in mice and men. *Curr Opin Immunol* 11:346, 1999.

69. Rossouw M, Nel HJ, Cooke GS, et al: Association between tuberculosis and a polymorphic NFkappaB binding site in the interferon gamma gene. *Lancet* 361:1871, 2003.

70. Gatti RA, Boder E, Vinters HV, et al: Ataxia-telangiectasia: An interdisciplinary approach to pathogenesis. *Medicine* 70:99, 1991.

71. Xu Y: ATM in lymphoid development and tumorigenesis. *Adv Immunol* 72:179, 1999.

72. Kirchhausen T, Rosen FS; Disease mechanism: Unraveling Wiskott-Aldrich syndrome. *Curr Biol* 6:676, 1996.

HEMATOLOGIC ASPECTS OF HUMAN IMMUNODEFICIENCY SYNDROME

SOON THYE LIM
ALEXANDRA M. LEVINE

Significant advances have been made in the area of human immunodeficiency virus (HIV) and acquired immunodeficiency syndrome (AIDS) in terms of the molecular aspects of the virus and immunopathogenesis of the disease. Mechanisms of HIV transmission have been elucidated, with specific means to decrease the transmission to health care workers and children born to HIV-infected mothers. Detection of specific HIV RNA levels in the blood may provide prognostic information and help guide treatment decisions. Use of highly active antiretroviral therapy (HAART) has been associated with a marked decrease in new AIDS-defining illnesses and in mortality from AIDS. HIV may affect virtually all organ systems, with prominent abnormalities related to the marrow and blood. The hematologic abnormalities associated with HIV are numerous and profound, and many of these abnormalities may be prevented or corrected by the use of HAART. Malignancies associated with HIV include lymphoma, Kaposi sarcoma, and cervical cancer. The pathogenesis of these neoplastic disorders has been elucidated in large part, with new treatment strategies attempting to address the various steps involved in the development of these tumors.

Acronyms and abbreviations that appear in this chapter include: ABVD, adriamycin, bleomycin, vinblastine, dacarbazine; ACTG, AIDS Clinical Trials Group; AIDS, acquired immunodeficiency syndrome; AMC, AIDS Malignancy Consortium; ANC, absolute neutrophil count; AZT, zidovudine; BEACOPP, bleomycin, etoposide, doxorubicin, cyclophosphamide, vincristine, procarbazine, prednisone; CDC, Centers for Disease Control and Prevention; CI, confidence interval; CNS, central nervous system; EBER, Epstein-Barr early region; EBV, Epstein-Barr virus; ECOG, Eastern Cooperative Oncology Group; ELISA, enzyme-linked immunosorbent assay; G-6-PD, glucose-6-phosphate dehydrogenase; G-CSF, granulocyte colony stimulating factor; GI, gastrointestinal; GM-CSF, granulocyte-macrophage colony stimulating factor; Gp, glycoprotein; HAART, highly active antiretroviral therapy; HHV, human herpesvirus; HIV, human immunodeficiency virus; HL, Hodgkin lymphoma; IFN, interferon; Ig, immunoglobulin; IL, interleukin; ITP, immune thrombocytopenic purpura; IV, intravenous; IVIG, intravenous γ-globulin; KS, Kaposi sarcoma; LASA, linear analogue scale; MAC, Mycobacterium avium complex; m-BACOD, methotrexate, bleomycin, Adriamycin (doxorubicin), cyclophosphamide, Oncovin (vincristine) dexamethasone; MOS, Medical Outcomes Study; NK, natural killer; NCI, National Cancer Institute; OR, odds ratio; PCR, polymerase chain reaction; PET, positron emission tomography; PGL, persistent generalized lymphadenopathy; QOL, quality of life; RT-PCR, reverse transcriptase polymerase chain reaction; SIR, standardized incidence ratio; TNF, tumor necrosis factor; WHO, World Health Organization; WIHS, Women's Interagency HIV Study.

DEFINITION AND HISTORY

DEFINITION

The definition of acquired immunodeficiency syndrome (AIDS) initially was based exclusively upon clinical symptoms and signs.[1] As knowledge of the viral etiopathogenesis evolved, the case definition of AIDS underwent multiple revisions by the Centers for Disease Control and Prevention (CDC). Inclusion of specific clinical illnesses in a patient with serologic evidence of infection with the human immunodeficiency virus (HIV) was classified as "clinical AIDS," while an HIV-infected patient with a blood CD4 count of less than 200 cells/μl (0.2×10^9/liter) was considered to have "immunological AIDS."[2-4] The World Health Organization (WHO) adopted alternative case-definition systems for diagnosis of AIDS in resource-poor countries where serologic and immunologic testing is not readily available (Table 83-1).[5,6]

The WHO has estimated that more than 40 million people worldwide were infected by HIV through 2003.[5] The majority were infected by heterosexual contact, with homosexual contact and injection drug use the predominant modes of transmission in the United States and western Europe. Vertical transmission from infected mother to child is now decreasing in developed countries, although such transmission continues to increase in resource-poor regions of the world.

ETIOLOGY AND PATHOGENESIS

HUMAN IMMUNODEFICIENCY VIRUS 1

HIV-1 is a member of the primate Lentivirinae subfamily of retroviruses,[6,7] RNA viruses that induce a chronic cellular infection by converting their RNA genome into a DNA provirus that is integrated into the genome of the infected cell. Infection by these lentiviruses is characterized by long periods of clinical latency followed by a gradual onset of disease-related symptoms.[8-10]

TRANSMISSION OF HUMAN IMMUNODEFICIENCY VIRUS
HIV can be transmitted by sexual contact with an infected partner, parenteral drug use with a contaminated needle, exposure to infected blood or blood products, and perinatal exposure from an infected mother to her infant.

General Mechanisms of Sexual Transmission HIV-1 has been isolated from the semen of HIV-infected men[11] and from cell-free seminal fluid.[12] It can be detected during the first 2 to 4 weeks after primary infection.[13] Factors associated with increased viral burden in semen include more advanced symptomatic HIV disease, higher levels of HIV RNA in blood, CD4 cell counts less than 200/μl, and presence of seminal fluid leukocytosis. HIV infection has been reported after exposure to infected semen during artificial insemination.[14]

TABLE 83-1   DEFINITION OF AIDS IN THE UNITED STATES

Clinical AIDS-defining conditions in persons infected with human
   immunodeficiency syndrome
    Opportunistic infections
    Lymphomas
    Kaposi sarcoma
    Cervical cancer
    Wasting syndrome
    AIDS dementia syndrome
    Recurrent bacteria pneumonia ($\geq$2 episodes/yr)
    Mycobacterium tuberculosis
Immunologic AIDS
    CD4 cell counts <200/μl

AIDS = Acquired immunodeficiency syndrome

HIV has been recovered from cervical and vaginal secretions of HIV-infected women.[15,16] HIV-infected endothelial cells and macrophages have been detected in cervical biopsies.[17] Factors that influence the levels of HIV-1 in female genital tract secretions include the stage of HIV disease, menstruation status, hormonal parameters, concomitant vaginal infection, age, HIV-1 RNA level in plasma, and antiviral therapy.[18] Female-to-female transmission of HIV has been reported[19,20] but appears to be relatively unusual.

HIV transmission may be facilitated by the presence of other sexually transmitted diseases, both with and without ulceration,[21] and HIV has been isolated directly from genital ulcers.[22] Prevention or treatment of sexually transmitted disease has been associated with decreased HIV-1 transmission.[23]

Transmission Through Parenteral Drug Use   Sharing needles and syringes is an important mode of transmission among parenteral drug users.[24] Use of cocaine or other such nonparenteral drugs also has been associated with an increased risk for HIV infection,[25] through engagement in sexual risk-taking behaviors.

Transmission Through Infected Blood Products   The risk of infection with HIV after receiving 1 U of infected blood is approximately 90 percent.[26] Transfusion of blood products derived from multiple units of pooled blood can transmit HIV and accounts for the initially high prevalence of HIV infection among patients with hemophilia. Screening of all donated blood, beginning in March 1985, and the subsequent routine heat or solvent detergent treatment of clotting factor concentrates have resulted in a marked decrease in new transfusion-associated HIV infections. Guidelines for proper inactivation of HIV in clotting factor concentrates have been developed.[27,28] Currently, the risk of acquiring HIV through receipt of 1 U of blood that tests negative for antibodies to HIV-1 is approximately one in 493,000.[29]

Mother-to-Child Transmission   The risk of infection from mother to infant differs in various parts of the world, ranging from approximately 15 percent in Europe to 15 to 30 percent in the United States and 40 to 50 percent in Africa.[30–32] HIV-1 may be transmitted in utero,[33,34] intrapartum,[35,36] or postpartum through ingestion of HIV-1 infected mother's milk.[37,38] Several factors predict an increased risk of perinatal transmission. In terms of the mother, more advanced HIV disease,[39,40] higher HIV-1 viral load in the plasma,[41,42] cigarette smoking,[43] and active injected drug use[44] all have been associated with increased risk of transmission. In terms of the details of delivery, premature rupture of the amniotic membranes (>4 hours),[45,46] presence of chorioamnionitis,[44] and vaginal delivery, as opposed to elective cesarean section,[47,48] each has been associated with increased rates of transmission. In terms of the infant, breast-feeding, prematurity, and low gestational age are reported as risk factors.[45–49] The CDC has made formal recommendations regarding the optimal care for HIV-1 infected pregnant women.[50] These recommendations differ for resource-rich and resource-poor settings. In the United States, use of antiretroviral agents in pregnancy and delivery, with subsequent administration to the infant for the first 6 weeks of life, has resulted in a dramatically reduced rate of transmission, from approximately 25 to 8 percent with zidovudine alone and even lower with use of highly active antiretroviral therapy (HAART).[51] With the further use of elective cesarean section and avoidance of breast-feeding, transmission rates have dropped to approximately 2 percent.[47] The efficacy of shorter courses of zidovudine or nevirapine (a nonnucleoside reverse transcriptase inhibitor) have been demonstrated and may be more practically feasible in resource-poor regions of the world.[52,53] The long-term toxicities of in utero exposure to antiretroviral agents are unknown. Nonetheless, their use during pregnancy resulted in a 43 percent decrease in the number of children with perinatally acquired HIV infection in the United States when comparing data from 1992 and 1996.[54]

PATHOGENESIS OF HUMAN IMMUNODEFICIENCY VIRUS INFECTION

HIV infection results in aberrant immune regulation and immunodeficiency. The numerous in vitro and in vivo defects in cellular immune response observed with HIV infection include decreased lymphocyte proliferative response to soluble antigens in vitro,[55] decreased helper response in immunoglobulin (Ig) synthesis,[56] impaired delayed hypersensitivity,[1,2] decreased interferon (IFN)-γ production,[57] and decreased T cell-mediated cytotoxicity of virally infected cells.[58]

DEPLETION OF CD4+ T CELLS

Infection with HIV-1 results in a progressive loss of CD4-positive (CD4+) T lymphocytes, resulting from the direct cytopathic effect of HIV on these cells. Formation of syncytial multinucleated giant cells by a mechanism involving fusion of infected cells expressing viral gp120 with noninfected CD4+ T lymphocytes is another mechanism of CD4 depletion.[59] The propensity of certain viral stains to form syncytia appears to be associated with an aggressive clinical course.[58,59] Experimental data suggest that an HIV-1 phenotypic switch from a macrophage-tropic (nonsyncytial) to a T lymphocyte-tropic (syncytial) virus may be the central event in acceleration of HIV-induced immunodepletion.[60]

The host immunologic response against HIV-infected lymphocytes may contribute to the progressive loss of CD4+ lymphocytes by antibody-mediated and cytotoxic T cell-mediated mechanisms.[61,62] Noninfected lymphocytes may become "innocent bystander" targets for immunologic destruction by binding free gp120 to their surface CD4 protein.

Defective production of immunostimulatory cytokines, such as interleukin (IL)-2,[63–65] or exaggerated expression of inhibitors of T lymphocyte proliferation, such as transforming growth factor-β,[66] can contribute to the progressive decline in CD4 lymphocytes. High-level replication and budding of virus, resulting in membrane injury, has also been proposed as a mechanism for lymphocyte cytotoxicity.

Combination antiretroviral therapy has resulted in marked suppression of viral replication, with resulting reductions of blood and tissue viral reservoirs.[67,68] Efficient viral suppression has resulted in significant and prolonged immunologic reconstitution characterized by increased CD4+ lymphocyte numbers, reduced opportunistic infections, and prolonged survival.[69,70] However, significant deficits in the immunologic repertoire persist, and complete immunologic reconstitution has not yet been attained.[71,72]

DEFECTS IN B CELL IMMUNITY

A number of defects in humoral immunity have been associated with HIV infection. Pronounced polyclonal activation of B lymphocytes is common, resulting in polyclonal hypergammaglobulinemia.[73,74] Spontaneous proliferation of B cells is observed in patients with advanced HIV infection.[75] In contrast, antigen-specific B cell proliferation and antibody production are decreased in patients with AIDS.[76] This finding may result from the loss of helper T lymphocyte activity.

The aberrant B lymphocyte regulation in HIV infection is associated with a pronounced increase in autoimmune phenomena and an increased risk of B cell lymphomas.[77] In addition to an increased frequency of positive antiglobulin test results, antibodies against neutrophils,[78,79] lymphocytes,[80] and platelets[81–83] have been reported.

DEFECTS IN IMMUNE ACCESSORY CELLS AND NATURAL KILLER CELLS

Monocytes, macrophages, and follicular dendritic cells of the lymph nodes express CD4 antigen and can be infected by HIV.[84,85] Monocytes and macrophages are resistant to HIV-induced cytotoxicity and serve

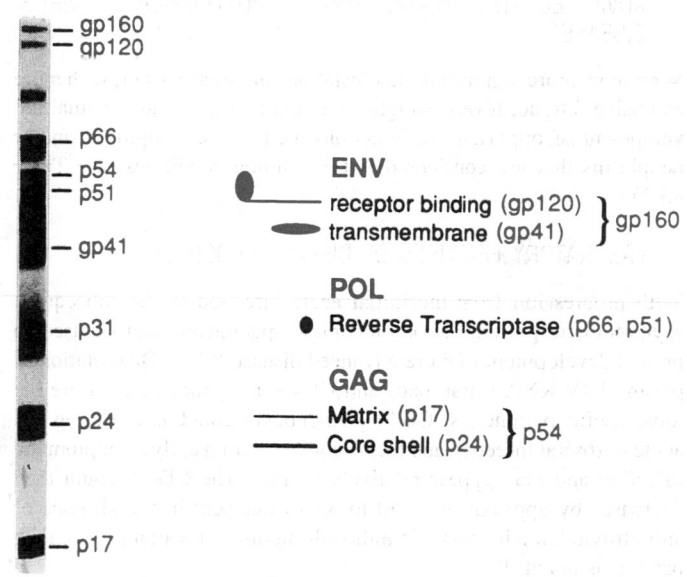

- gp160
- gp120

- p66
- p54
- p51

- gp41

- p31

- p24

- p17

ENV
— receptor binding (gp120)
— transmembrane (gp41) } gp160

POL
● Reverse Transcriptase (p66, p51)

GAG
— Matrix (p17)
— Core shell (p24) } p54

FIGURE 83-1 Western blot analysis of antibodies against human immuno-deficiency virus proteins from the serum of a patient with acquired immuno-deficiency syndrome.

as a chronic reservoir of HIV expression.[84] Although functional defects in the chemotaxis of HIV-infected monocytes have been reported,[86] most studies have failed to demonstrate consistent defects.[87,88] The follicular dendritic cells appear to play an important role in HIV clearance in early asymptomatic HIV disease. However, a progressive depletion of these cells is observed over time, resulting in increasing plasma viremia. The loss of follicular dendritic cells results in defective antigen processing in patients with advanced HIV disease.

Natural killer (NK) cell activity is decreased in the blood of HIV-infected individuals.[88,89] In combination with helper T lymphocyte depletion, decreased NK activity results in defective clearance of virally infected cells. Although the number of NK cells reportedly is nor-

mal,[88,89] the defect in NK activity appears to result from a deficiency in the signals for cell activation. The addition of exogenous IL-2 can improve NK lymphocyte function.[90]

DIAGNOSIS OF HUMAN IMMUNODEFICIENCY VIRUS INFECTION

The primary diagnostic screening tool for HIV infection is detection of antibody via the enzyme-linked immunosorbent assay (ELISA). However, because a positive ELISA result may not be specific for HIV-1 infection, all positive ELISA screening test results should be verified by immunoblotting HIV-1 antigens (Fig. 83-1).

By ELISA and immunoblot techniques, the median time from initial infection to first detection of HIV antibody has been estimated to be approximately 2 to 4 weeks. Ninety-five percent of patients are expected to seroconvert within 5.8 months (Fig. 83-2).[91] HIV infection for longer than 6 months without detectable antibody is extremely uncommon.[92-94]

The presence of the p24 antigen or HIV RNA in serum or plasma may precede seroconversion by several weeks.[95] This initial rise in p24 antigen correlates with the burst of viremia that occurs shortly after primary HIV infection.[96] Despite these observations, p24 antigen screening of donated units of blood appears to provide no benefit over conventional ELISA and immunoblot techniques.[97]

Testing by polymerase chain reaction (PCR) may detect presence of HIV within days or 1 week of initial infection. However, PCR is not used as a screening tool because false-positive results have been detected in as many as 9 percent of individuals.

COURSE AND PROGNOSIS

HIV infection results in a progressive process characterized by gradual depletion of immune function and eventual development of rather nonspecific symptoms, followed by specific infections and/or neoplastic disease. Patients who develop AIDS generally experience relentless deterioration in physical health and ultimately die of one or more complications secondary to acquired immunodeficiency, organ dysfunction, and/or malignancy associated with HIV infection.

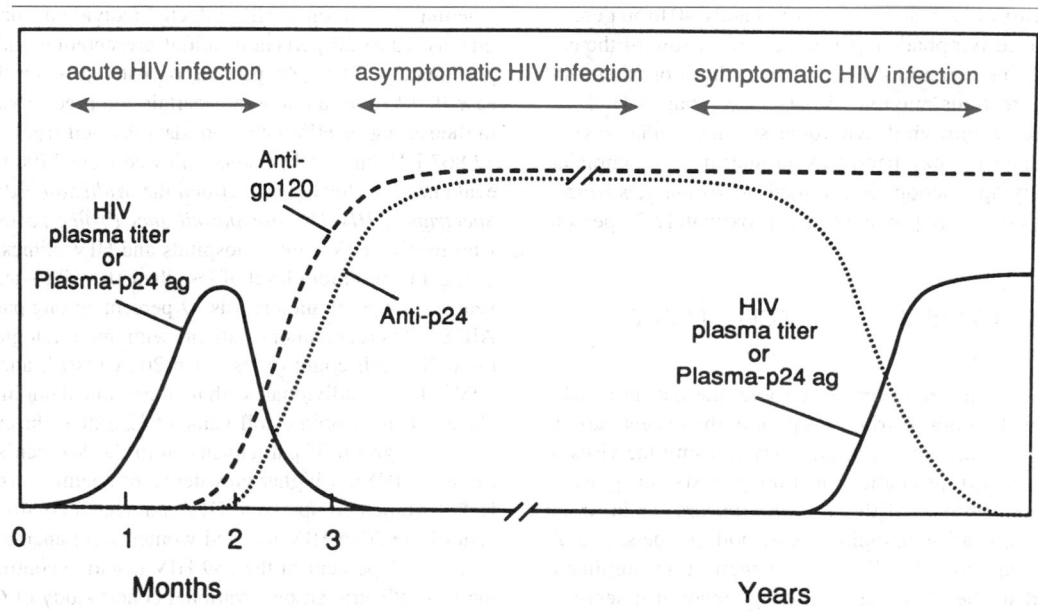

acute HIV infection · asymptomatic HIV infection · symptomatic HIV infection

Anti-gp120

HIV plasma titer or Plasma-p24 ag

Anti-p24

HIV plasma titer or Plasma-p24 ag

0 1 2 3

Months

Years

FIGURE 83-2 Virologic, serologic, and clinical course of human immunodeficiency virus (HIV) infection. Antibodies against HIV can first be detected between 2 and 5 months after infection.

Use of monitoring by assessment of the quantity of HIV-1 RNA in the plasma has allowed a more rational basis upon which to predict the course of disease in individual patients. In a study performed through the Multicenter AIDS Cohort, a longitudinal cohort study of HIV disease in homosexual and bisexual men, the earliest, baseline level of HIV RNA in plasma was found to correlate significantly with prognosis over time.[98] In a subsequent study, use of both viral load and CD4+ cells was found to more accurately predict the prognosis of HIV-infected men.[99] Current guidelines from the US Public Health Department suggest institution of HAART in all patients with symptomatic HIV or AIDS and in asymptomatic HIV-infected individuals when the CD4 count falls below 350 cells/μl (0.35×10^9/liter) or when the HIV viral load reaches 55,000 copies/cc or more.[100]

In addition to the use of viral load monitoring, the development of potent new antiretroviral agents, including the protease inhibitors,[101,102] has led to a remarkable improvement in the natural history of HIV infection.[70] The use of combinations of HAART was found to be associated with a 73 percent decrease in the incidence of new opportunistic infections and a 49 percent decrease in death resulting from AIDS when data from 1994 were compared to data from 1997 to 1998.[70] Remarkable decreases in the incidence of cytomegalovirus disease, atypical *Mycobacterium intracellulare* infection, and other serious opportunistic infections have occurred as a consequence of HAART therapy,[103] and improvement in immune function has been documented.[104] It may now be possible to discontinue the routine use of prophylaxis against *Pneumocystis carinii* or other opportunistic infections in patients who have been successfully treated with HAART.[105] These remarkable improvements in disease outcome have been maintained over time.[106]

ACUTE RETROVIRAL SYNDROME

An acute clinical illness often is associated with initial HIV infection, occurring in approximately 50 to 90 percent of individuals.[96,107,108] This syndrome begins approximately 1 to 3 weeks (range 5 days to 3 months) after primary infection and usually lasts for 1 to 2 weeks. Prominent symptoms include significant fatigue and malaise; fever, which may be as high as 40°C (104°F); headache; photophobia; myalgias; and a morbilliform rash, seen in approximately 40 to 50 percent of patients. Generalized lymphadenopathy may occur toward the end of the acute illness. The symptoms are similar to those of other viral illnesses, such as infectious mononucleosis (see Chap. 84). Most symptoms of this acute retroviral syndrome subside within several weeks. However, headache may persist as an intermittent complaint, as may generalized lymphadenopathy, termed *persistent generalized lymphadenopathy* (PGL), which occurs in approximately 75 percent of patients.[96,108]

EARLY ASYMPTOMATIC HUMAN IMMUNODEFICIENCY VIRUS DISEASE

After resolution of the acute retroviral syndrome, the patient usually returns to a state of well-being. During this period, the patient harbors HIV in blood and in genital secretions and may transmit the virus to others. This phase of asymptomatic infection persists for approximately 1 decade in the absence of therapy and appears similar in all racial and ethnic groups, all geographic areas, both genders, and all risk groups for HIV infection.[109–112] Certain genetic polymorphisms have been described in the chemokine receptor genes that serve as coreceptors for HIV (e.g., Δ32 deletion of CCR4), which predict for better prognosis and longer periods of AIDS-free survival.[113]

ADVANCED SYMPTOMATIC HUMAN IMMUNODEFICIENCY VIRUS DISEASE

With time, more significant manifestations of disease occur, with more extensive fatigue, fevers, weight loss, night sweats, and eventual development of opportunistic infections, neurologic symptoms, and/or neoplasms that are considered AIDS-defining conditions (see Table 83-1).

LABORATORY FEATURES OF DISEASE PROGRESSION

With progression from the initial acute infection to the subsequent asymptomatic period, various laboratory parameters can be used to predict development of more advanced disease.[98,99,114] Quantitation of plasma HIV RNA (viral load) and CD4+ lymphocyte count are the most useful parameters. CD4+ lymphocyte count falls during the acute retroviral infection and then stabilizes during early asymptomatic infection and may appear relatively normal. The CD4+ count then decreases by approximately 40 to 80 μl per year in the absence of antiretroviral medications,[115] although significant variability among patients is noted.[116]

An initial measurement of plasma viral load by reverse transcriptase (RT)-PCR or branched-DNA methods provides important prognostic information that can be useful in determining when to start antiretroviral medications.[98,99] Serial assessment of plasma HIV viral load also allows for rapid assessment of efficacy of antiretroviral medications. Changes in viral load usually precede significant alterations in CD4+ lymphocyte counts.[69,99]

Several nonspecific markers of disease progression have been defined, including β_2-microglobulin[117] and neopterin,[118] each of which has an independent predictive value in estimating the probability of progression to AIDS. However, each of these surrogate markers has been largely replaced by the more specific molecular assays to quantify plasma HIV viral load.

HEMATOLOGIC ABNORMALITIES

ANEMIA IN HUMAN IMMUNODEFICIENCY VIRUS INFECTION

INCIDENCE OF ANEMIA
Anemia is common in HIV-infected individuals, occurring in approximately 10 to 20 percent at initial presentation and diagnosed in approximately 70 to 80 percent of patients over the course of disease.[119–121] In an attempt to ascertain the precise incidence of anemia in the setting of HIV infection, data derived from the case records of 32,867 HIV-infected persons followed from 1990 through 1996 were evaluated.[121] This cohort, termed the *Multistate Adult and Adolescent Spectrum of HIV Disease Surveillance Project*, consists of individuals who receive HIV care in hospitals and HIV clinics in nine US cities. Using a hemoglobin level of less than 10 g/dl to define anemia, the 1-year incidence of anemia was 37 percent among patients with clinical AIDS; 12 percent among patients with immunologic AIDS, as defined by a CD4 cell count of less than 200 cells/μl; and 3 percent among HIV-infected individuals with neither clinical nor immunologic AIDS. Using a hemoglobin cutoff value of 12 g/dl as the criterion for anemia in a large group of participants from the Women's Interagency HIV Study (WIHS), a higher prevalence of anemia was found in HIV-infected women compared to HIV-uninfected controls.[122] Thus, 37 percent of the 2056 HIV infected women were anemic at baseline, compared to 17 percent of the 569 HIV negative controls ($p < 0.001$). In the HAART era, an observational cohort study of 6725 HIV-infected patients from across Europe also documented a high prevalence of anemia.[123] Thus, 58.2 percent had mild anemia, defined as hemoglobin

level of 8 to 14 g/dl in males or 8 to 12 g/dl in females; whereas 1.4 percent had severe anemia, defined as a hemoglobin level of less than 8 g/dl.[123] These data thus confirm the high incidence of anemia among HIV-infected patients in both the pre-HAART and HAART eras. Further, the frequency and severity of anemia in HIV-infected patients appear to correlate with HIV-related factors, such as CD4 cell counts less than 200 cells/μl (0.2 × 10^9/liter), higher plasma HIV-1 RNA levels, and a history of clinical AIDS-defining condition.[122,123]

CAUSES OF ANEMIA

Numerous causes for anemia exist in HIV-infected patients (Table 83-2).

Anemia Resulting from Decreased Production of Red Blood Cells   A decrease in red blood cell production may result from factors suppressing the CD34+ colony-forming unit–granulocyte-erythroid-monocyte-macrophage, such as inflammatory cytokines or the HIV virus itself.[119,120] In addition, blunted production of erythropoietin has been documented in anemic HIV-infected patients, similar to the suppression observed in other states of chronic infection or inflammation.[124] Infiltration of the marrow by tumor, such as lymphoma,[125] or infection, such as Mycobacterium avium complex (MAC), may lead to the decreased production of red cells. In addition, MAC may also be associated with cytokine-induced marrow suppression. Involvement of the gastrointestinal (GI) tract by various infections or tumors may lead to chronic blood loss, with eventual iron deficiency anemia. Another prominent cause of hypoproliferative anemia in patients with HIV infection is the common use of multiple medications, many of which may cause marrow and/or red cell suppression. Zidovudine (AZT), the first licensed antiretroviral agent, is uniformly associated with macrocytosis (mean cell volume >100 fm), which can be used

TABLE 83-2   MECHANISMS AND CAUSES OF ANEMIA IN HUMAN IMMUNODEFICIENCY VIRUS INFECTION

MECHANISM OF ANEMIA	CAUSE OF ANEMIA

Decreased red cell production	Neoplasm infiltrating the marrow
	   Lymphoma
	   Kaposi sarcoma
	   Other
	Infection
	   Atypical tuberculosis (*Mycobacterium avium intracellulare* or *Mycobacterium avium* complex)
	   Mycobacterium tuberculosis
	   Cytomegalovirus
	   B19 parvovirus
	   Fungal infection
	Medications
	HIV infection
	   • Abnormal growth of burst forming unit–erythroid
	   • Anemia of chronic disease
	   • Blunted erythropoietin production and response
	Iron deficiency anemia secondary to chronic blood loss

Ineffective production	Folic acid deficiency Vitamin B$_{12}$ deficiency

Increased red cell destruction	Coombs-positive hemolytic anemia
	Hemophagocytic syndrome
	Thrombotic thrombocytopenic purpura
	Disseminated intravascular coagulation
	Medications
	   Sulfonamides, dapsone
	   Oxidant drugs in glucose-6-phosphate dehydrogenase deficiency

as an objective indication that the patient has been compliant with this medication.[126] Of note, transfusion-dependent anemia (hemoglobin <8.5 g/dl) has been reported in approximately 30 percent of patients with full-blown AIDS who were receiving zidovudine at doses of 600 mg/day. However, the incidence of severe anemia is only 1 percent when the same dose of zidovudine is used in patients with asymptomatic HIV disease.[127]

Infection of the marrow by parvovirus B19 is another cause of hypoproliferative anemia in HIV-infected patients, resulting in specific infection of the pronormoblast.[128,129] Thus, although marrow failure affecting all three lines has been described in association with parvovirus B19 infection, a pure red cell aplasia is the usual consequence. Parvovirus infection usually is acquired during childhood, leading to "fifth disease," one of the common childhood exanthems. Exposure to the virus leads to an antibody response, with subsequent resistance to further infection. Approximately 85 percent of adults have serologic evidence of prior parvovirus infection. However, the seroprevalence of such antibodies among HIV-infected patients is only 64 percent. These individuals may have an ineffective immune response against newly acquired infection, or they may have lost prior seropositivity. The diagnosis of parvovirus B19 can be made on marrow examination, revealing giant pronormoblasts with clumped basophilic chromatin and clear cytoplasmic vacuoles. Diagnosis can be confirmed by *in situ* hybridization using sequence-specific DNA probes for parvovirus B19 (see Chap. 34). Therapy for parvovirus-induced red cell aplasia consists of infusions of intravenous (IV) γ-globulin (IVIG) that contain antibodies from plasma donors, most of whom have been exposed to parvovirus. Relapse of parvovirus B19-induced red cell aplasia may occur, necessitating retreatment in these individuals.[128,129]

Anemia Resulting from Increased Red Cell Destruction   Increased red cell destruction may be seen in HIV-infected patients with glucose-6-phosphate dehydrogenase (G-6-PD) deficiency who are exposed to oxidant drugs and in HIV-infected patients with disseminated intravascular coagulation or thrombotic thrombocytopenic purpura.[130] Presence of fragmented red cells and thrombocytopenia on blood film is seen in the latter two conditions, and Heinz bodies are seen in association with G-6-PD deficiency. Hemophagocytic syndrome has been described in association with HIV infection.[131,132] An additional cause of red cell destruction in HIV-infected patients is the development of autoantibodies, with resultant positive Coombs test and shortened red cell survival. Of interest, a positive direct Coombs test has been reported in 18 to 77 percent of HIV-infected patients, although the incidence of actual hemolysis is low.[133] When present, anti-i antibody and antibody against auto-U antigens have been described, occurring in 64 percent and 32 percent of HIV-infected patients, respectively.[133–135] A high incidence of positive direct Coombs test results has been detected in patients with other hypergammaglobulinemic states, indicating that positive Coombs test results in HIV may be secondary to the polyclonal hypergammaglobulinemia known to occur in the setting of HIV infection.[136]

Anemia Resulting from Ineffective Production of Red Cells (Vitamin B$_{12}$ and/or Folic Acid Deficiency)   Folic acid is absorbed in the jejunum and is responsible for one carbon transfer required in the synthesis of DNA. A deficiency of folic acid leads to a megaloblastic anemia, with large ovalocytes in the blood, hypersegmented neutrophils, and a decrease in all three lines, with resultant anemia, neutropenia, and thrombocytopenia (see Chap. 39). Because tissue stores of folate are relatively small, a deficiency of folate in the diet lasting as few as 3 to 6 months may lead to anemia. Thus, HIV-infected patients who are ill and not eating properly and those with underlying disease of the jejunum may be unable to absorb sufficient folic acid. The classic changes of megaloblastic anemia are detected upon examination of the bone marrow, whereas serum and red cell folate levels are low.

Ineffective production of red cells, with pancytopenia in the blood, elevated indirect bilirubin level, and low reticulocyte count may be seen in vitamin B_{12} deficiency (see Chap. 39). Absorption of vitamin B_{12} requires initial production of intrinsic factor by parietal cells in the stomach, with subsequent absorption of the complex of B_{12} and intrinsic factor within the ileum. Thus, malabsorption of vitamin B_{12} can occur in various disorders of the stomach, by production of antibodies to the H^+-K^+ ATP pump or to intrinsic factor (pernicious anemia), or by various disorders of the small bowel and ileum (infection or Crohn disease). Although vitamin B_{12} deficiency based on diet alone is highly unlikely, patients with HIV infection appear to be prone to vitamin B_{12} malabsorption, presumably because of the myriad of infections and other disorders that may occur in the small intestine. Negative vitamin B_{12} balance has been documented in approximately one third of patients with AIDS, the majority demonstrating defective absorption of the vitamin.[137] Diagnosis of vitamin B_{12} deficiency can be made by documenting low serum vitamin B_{12} levels. The earliest indication of negative vitamin B_{12} balance is the finding of low vitamin B_{12} levels in blood in patients taking transcobalamin II.[138] Monthly administration of parenteral vitamin B_{12} corrects the deficiency and the resultant anemia and pancytopenia in the peripheral blood. Because vitamin B_{12} deficiency may cause neurologic dysfunction (subacute combined degeneration of the cord), with motor, sensory, and higher cortical dysfunction, the possibility of vitamin B_{12} deficiency should be considered in HIV-infected patients with these neurologic symptoms and signs.

CONSEQUENCES OF ANEMIA IN HUMAN IMMUNODEFICIENCY VIRUS INFECTION

Decreased Survival Several large cohort studies have shown that anemia is an independent risk factor for shorter survival in HIV-infected patients.[139-142] In the Multistate Adult and Adolescent Spectrum of HIV Disease Surveillance Project, anemia, defined as a hemoglobin level less than 10 g/dl or a physician's diagnosis of anemia, was found to be associated with an increased risk of death for all CD4 ranges in this cohort.[139] However, the greatest risk of death was noted in patients with baseline CD4 cell counts greater than 200 cells/μl (0.2×10^9/ liter), with a relative risk of death 150 percent higher than for individuals in the same CD4 cell count strata without anemia (relative risk, RR, 2.3, $p < 0.001$). In comparison, the risk of death was increased by approximately 60 percent for anemic patients with baseline CD4 cell counts less than 200 cells/μl (0.2×10^9/liter). Recovery from anemia was shown to be independently associated with improved survival. Thus, among anemic patients with baseline CD4 counts less than 50 cells/μl (0.05×10^9/liter), those who remained anemic (hemoglobin level <10 g/dl) had a 160 percent higher risk of death than patients who recovered from anemia following treatment. In another series of 2348 HIV-infected patients from Baltimore, Maryland, development of any grade of anemia was found to be independently associated with decreased survival, with the risk of death approximately threefold increased in those with a hemoglobin level of 7 to 8 g/dl and fourfold increased in those with a hemoglobin level less than 6.5 g/dl.[140] Use of erythropoietin was associated with a decreased risk of death, as was use of antiretroviral therapy. Similarly, an additional study of 6725 European HIV-infected patients demonstrated that hemoglobin level at baseline, CD4 count, and viral load were independent prognostic factors for survival.[106] For each 1 g/dl decrease in hemoglobin level, the relative hazard of death was 1.39 (95% confidence interval [CI] 1.34-1.43; $p < 0.0001$). A large multicenter prospective study of 2056 HIV-infected women confirmed the independent association between anemia and decreased survival.[142] Further work is required to elucidate

the precise mechanisms underlying this strong prognostic association. It is conceivable that anemia may simply serve as a surrogate marker for more advanced systemic illness.

Disease Progression Anemia has been shown to be independently associated with more rapid clinical progression of HIV infection. In one large European study aimed at identifying predictive factors for disease progression among HIV-infected patients receiving HAART, the most recent measured hemoglobin level, CD4 cell count, and HIV-1 viral load, and a history of clinical AIDS before initiation of HAART all were independently related to the risk of disease progression.[143] Thus, with mild anemia (hemoglobin 8-14 g/dl for men and 8-12 g/dl for women) the relative hazard of disease progression or death was 2.2 (95% CI 1.6-2.9, $p < 0.0001$), whereas for severe anemia (hemoglobin <8 g/dl) the relative hazard was 7.1 (95% CI 2.5-20.1, $p = 0.0002$).

Quality-of-Life Parameters Anemia has been associated with decreases in quality of life (QOL), as measured by the linear analogue self-assessment (LASA) scale and other such instruments.[144,145]

PREVENTION OR CORRECTION OF ANEMIA WITH HIGHLY ACTIVE ANTIRETROVIRAL THERAPY

HAART can correct or improve the anemia of HIV infection. In a study of 6725 HIV-infected patients from across Europe,[141] use of HAART was statistically associated with improvement in hemoglobin levels. In addition, prolonged HAART use was associated with a greater likelihood of correcting anemia. Thus, 65.5 percent of the cohort were anemic before the use of HAART, 53 percent were anemic after 6 months of HAART, and 46 percent were anemic after 12 months of HAART. In a study of 905 HIV-infected patients from Baltimore, use of HAART was associated with an increase in hemoglobin levels after 1-year followup.[146] Among the patients with a baseline hemoglobin level less than 14 g/dl, 21 percent of patients receiving HAART recovered from anemia (hemoglobin >14 g/dl) compared to only 8 percent of patients not receiving HAART ($p = 0.0006$).[146] In multivariate analysis, use of HAART was strongly associated with freedom from anemia, after adjusting for CD4 cell count, HIV-1 RNA level, sex, race, history of injection drug use, and use of various therapies for anemia. Data from the WIHS demonstrated that use of HAART for as few as 6 months was independently associated with a higher likelihood of resolution of anemia, and longer use was associated with more profound improvements.[142] Additionally, use of HAART for at least 12 months was significantly associated with a reduced risk of developing anemia.[142]

The mechanisms whereby HAART may protect against development of anemia or correct preexisting anemia are not yet fully understood. Nonetheless, because HIV infection directly contributes to the development of anemia, it is conceivable that HAART may protect against or correct anemia simply by decreasing the level of HIV-1 viral burden and/or by overcoming the factors responsible for the anemia of chronic disease. Additionally, use of HAART has been associated with an increase in hematopoietic progenitor cell growth,[147] while ritonavir, a protease inhibitor, has been shown to directly stimulate progenitor cell growth and to inhibit apoptosis of hematopoietic progenitors *in vitro*.[148]

Use of Erythropoietin in Human Immunodeficiency Virus-Infected Patients with Anemia A blunted response to erythropoietin is extremely common in the setting of HIV infection.[141,149,150] The mechanism of this decreased production of erythropoietin likely is a post-transcriptional defect in production, as levels of messenger RNA for erythropoietin are normal although erythropoietin protein levels are decreased. In addition, development of autoantibodies to erythropoietin has been described in HIV-infected patients.[151] Multiple studies have confirmed the beneficial effect of erythropoietin in HIV-infected patients with anemia, in whom marrow function was suppressed as a result of HIV or other chronic infectious or inflammatory diseases.[140,152-154] Erythropoietin also is effective in treating anemia resulting from zidovudine or other medications, including cancer chemotherapy, which suppress the marrow.[154]

The baseline level of endogenous serum erythropoietin can predict which patients likely will respond to therapeutic use of erythropoietin. Thus, patients with a baseline endogenous erythropoietin level of 500 IU/liter or less are expected to respond to erythropoietin therapy, whereas those with endogenous levels greater than 500 IU/liter are not. Erythropoietin 100 to 200 U/kg body weight is administered subcutaneously three times per week until normalization of the red blood cell and then approximately once every week or every other week to maintain a hemoglobin concentration of approximately 12 g/dl. Clinical trials have demonstrated the equivalent efficacy of 40,000 U of erythropoietin given weekly compared with the original thrice-weekly schedule in anemic HIV-infected patients.[145]

Correction of anemia is associated with improvement in QOL measures after erythropoietin use,[144,145,155] with the mean LASA QOL score increasing by 41 percent and the Medical Outcomes Study-HIV (MOS-HIV) overall QOL score increasing by as much as 37 percent in one study.[144]

Toxicity of erythropoietin is uncommon, consisting primarily of local pain at the site of injection, mild fever, or rash. However, the prevalence of these side effects has been similar to the rates seen for placebo-treated patients. Development of pure red cell aplasia has been described in HIV-negative patients receiving the Eprex product (erythropoietin alfa) from Europe, although this complication is uncommon and has not been reported in the setting of HIV.[156]

Several prospective trials are evaluating the efficacy and toxicity of darbepoetin alfa, a novel erythropoiesis stimulating protein, in anemic HIV-infected patients. Compared to conventional erythropoietin, darbepoetin alfa has a longer terminal half-life because of the presence of an additional sialic acid residues; thus it offers the additional advantage of a less frequent dosing. Preliminary data from one study suggest that darbepoetin alfa 3.0 mg/kg given once every 2 weeks is effective in improving the hemoglobin level in the majority of HIV-infected patients and in maintaining hemoglobin levels and improving QOL measures.[157]

NEUTROPENIA

ETIOLOGY OF NEUTROPENIA AND DECREASED GRANULOCYTE FUNCTION IN HUMAN IMMUNODEFICIENCY VIRUS

Neutropenia is reported in approximately 10 percent of patients with early, asymptomatic HIV infection and in more than 50 percent of individuals with more advanced HIV-related immunodeficiency.[119,120,154] As with other blood cytopenias in the setting of HIV infection, multiple etiologies may be present, either singly or in combination.[158] Thus, decreased colony growth of the progenitor cell colony forming unit–granulocyte-macrophage[159] may lead to decreased production of both granulocytes and monocytes. Soluble inhibitory substances produced by HIV-infected cells have been noted to suppress neutrophil production in vitro, suggesting that autoimmunity plays a part in the development of neutropenia in HIV infection.[160] However, other studies have shown that the presence of neutrophil-bound Ig correlates best with stage of disease rather than with neutropenia per se.[161] Decreased serum levels of granulocyte colony stimulating factor (G-CSF) have been described in HIV-seropositive subjects with afebrile neutropenia (<1000 neutrophils/μl), indicating that a relative deficiency of this specific hematopoietic growth factor also may contribute to persistent neutropenia.[162] The other causes of

neutropenia in HIV infection include the presence of opportunistic infections, malignancies, and HIV-related myelodysplasia affecting marrow function.[163] Myelosuppression and neutropenia may result from any one of several medications that are commonly prescribed for HIV-infected patients.

Aside from absolute neutropenia, patients with HIV infection also may experience decreased function of granulocytes and monocytes. Thus, abnormal Fc processing by macrophages has been described. Decreased opsonization and intracellular killing of bacterial or fungal organisms by granulocytes also have been noted.[164]

RISK FACTORS FOR INFECTION IN NEUTROPENIC PATIENTS WITH HUMAN IMMUNODEFICIENCY VIRUS

In patients with cancer who receive chemotherapy, multiple studies have shown that the risk of bacterial infection rises when the absolute neutrophil count (ANC) falls below 1000 cells/μl and increases further when the ANC falls below 500 cells/μl.[165] Several studies have confirmed the same relationship in patients with HIV infection. Thus, Moore and colleagues[166] found that the risk of bacterial infection increased 2.3-fold for HIV-infected individuals with ANC less than 1000 cells/μl and rose by 7.9-fold in those with ANC levels less than 500 cells/μl. Lower ANCs have been associated with increased risk of hospitalization for serious infection, as shown in a review of 2047 HIV-positive patients.[167] On multivariate analysis, the severity and duration of neutropenia were found to be significant predictors of the incidence of hospitalization for serious bacterial infections.[167]

In a study of 62 HIV-infected patients with ANCs of 1000 cells/μl or less, 24 percent developed infectious complications, most commonly within 24 hours after onset of neutropenia.[168] On multivariate analysis, the three factors independently associated with infectious complications were presence of a central venous catheter, neutropenia in the previous 3 months, and a lower nadir of granulocyte count (250 cells/μl in those with infections vs. 622 cells/μl in those without infections). Among patients with medication-associated neutropenia, the most common cause was zidovudine, followed by trimethoprim-sulfamethoxazole and ganciclovir. Neutropenia was less likely to be associated with infection in these patients than in individuals who were neutropenic because of cancer chemotherapy.[168]

Another study, however, has suggested that the risk of serious infectious complications in neutropenic HIV-infected patients is low.[169] In this prospective study of neutropenia (defined as ANC ≤1000 cells/μl) in 87 consecutive HIV-infected patients, all except three episodes of neutropenia were associated with known myelosuppressive medications. The majority of patients had received cotrimoxazole (62%), lamivudine (56%), and/or zidovudine (40%).[169] The mean ANC of these individuals was 660 cells/μl (range 100–900 cells/μl), and the median duration of neutropenia was 13 days. However, severe neutropenia was uncommon; only three patients had ANC nadirs less than 200 cells/μl. Serious neutropenia-related sepsis in this setting was uncommon, with culture-proven infection occurring in only 8 percent of patients and presumed infection in another 8 percent. No patient died of infection. As expected, patients with infections had significantly lower ANC nadirs (mean 460 vs. 710 cells/μl) and significantly lower CD4 cell counts (mean 64 vs. 126/μl) but did not have a longer duration of neutropenia than patients who did not develop infection.

IMPACT OF EFFECTIVE ANTIRETROVIRAL THERAPY ON NEUTROPENIA

Evidence indicates that use of HAART may be associated with improvement of leukopenia and neutropenia in treated patients.[148] Thus, in a group of 66 HIV-infected patients treated with HAART, significant increases in total leukocyte counts and absolute granulocyte counts were seen after 6 months of treatment.[148] A direct stimulatory effect of protease inhibitors on human hematopoiesis has been demonstrated.[170] These data indicate that mild to moderate levels of neutropenia can be managed by use of HAART alone, although several months of therapy are required to achieve the desired effect.

USE OF GRANULOCYTE-MACROPHAGE COLONY STIMULATING FACTOR OR GRANULOCYTE COLONY STIMULATING FACTOR IN NEUTROPENIC PATIENTS WITH HUMAN IMMUNODEFICIENCY VIRUS INFECTION

When administered subcutaneously to HIV-infected patients with neutropenia, granulocyte-macrophage colony stimulating factor (GM-CSF) results in dose-dependent increases in granulocytes, monocytes, and eosinophils.[171,172] Therapy with GM-CSF may improve neutrophil function by enhancing phagocytosis, degranulation, leukotriene B$_4$ synthesis, release of arachidonic acid, superoxide anion generation, and antibody-dependent cellular cytotoxicity.[173–175] Although there were initial concerns that GM-CSF may increase HIV replication,[176] subsequent in vitro studies indicated that GM-CSF actually inhibits HIV-1 replication in monocytes and macrophages.[177]

Granulocyte-Macrophage Colony Stimulating Factor In one study comparing 123 HIV-positive leukopenic patients (defined as a white blood cell count $<3 \times 10^9/l$) treated with subcutaneous GM-CSF with 121 nontreated leukopenic HIV-positive controls, administration of GM-CSF for 12 weeks significantly increased the total leukocyte count of treated patients.[176] In patients receiving GM-CSF, the total leukocyte count increased by 22 percent at week 1 and by 65 percent at week 12 over baseline values ($p < 0.001$), whereas the circulating monocyte levels increased by twofold to threefold at week 12 ($p < 0.001$). In contrast, the total leukocyte count decreased by 24 percent below baseline values at week 12 ($p < 0.001$) in the control group. Of importance, no statistically significant change occurred in HIV p24 antigen levels in patients treated with GM-CSF, even among those who were not receiving antiretroviral therapy.[176–178]

The safety and efficacy of GM-CSF in HIV-infected patients receiving antiretroviral therapy has also been confirmed in another randomized placebo-controlled trial involving a group of 105 HIV-infected patients.[179] GM-CSF 125 μg/m^2 was given twice weekly for 6 months. Patients randomized to antiretroviral therapy plus GM-CSF achieved a greater reduction in plasma viral load, were more likely to achieve HIV-1 RNA levels below the limit of detection, and demonstrated a lower frequency of zidovudine resistance mutations than those who received antiretroviral agents plus placebo. Side effects of GM-CSF include primarily an influenza-like syndrome, with fever, bone pain, myalgia, fatigue, malaise, and headache.

Granulocyte Colony Stimulating Factor G-CSF has been shown to be effective at preventing severe neutropenia and reducing the incidence of bacterial infections and the number of days of hospitalization in neutropenic HIV-infected patients.[180] A study that randomized 258 such patients with CD4 counts less than 200 cells/mm^3 and moderate neutropenia (defined as ANC 750–1000/μl) to receive G-CSF (1 μg/kg/day or 300 μg three times per week) versus no treatment for 24 weeks.[180] Patients in the control group who developed severe neutropenia (ANC $<500/\mu$l) were re-randomized to receive G-CSF according to one of the two treatment groups. Treatment with G-CSF was effective at preventing the development of severe neutropenia and reducing the incidence of bacterial infections, independent of CD4 count, number of prior opportunistic infections and baseline use of zidovudine. Thus, in an intention-to-treat analysis, the incidence of severe neutropenia was 1.7 percent in the treated group versus 22 percent in the control group, whereas the incidence of bacterial infections was 31 percent lower in the treated group (2.93 vs. 4.25/1000 patient-days). Further, patients treated with G-CSF had 54 percent

fewer severe bacterial infections and 45 percent fewer hospital days for bacterial infections. Of importance, there was no difference between the groups in terms of toxicity or HIV RNA levels in plasma. The most frequently reported adverse events were fever, diarrhea, fatigue, nausea, headache, anemia, abdominal pain, vomiting, and myalgia. Thus, administration of G-CSF when patients are mildly neutropenic appears to be superior to waiting for patients to become severely neutropenic. However, effective use of HAART may be equally efficacious in resolving mild to moderate neutropenia.

The early recommendations for dosing of G-CSF included use of 5 μg/kg/day given subcutaneously. Evidence suggests, however, that much lower doses of G-CSF may be effective in HIV-infected persons. Thus, an initial dose of 1 μg/kg/day often is initiated and used until the neutrophil count rises to acceptable levels (>1000 cells/μl). This is followed by a titration of dosing, often requiring therapy only once or twice per week, as necessary to maintain the desired response.

Thus, use of G-CSF or GM-CSF to improve neutropenia in HIV-infected patients has been shown to be both safe and effective. Although patient survival has not increased as a consequence of G-CSF or GM-CSF,[181] these drugs allow safer administration of other necessary medications and potentially reduce both the incidence of bacterial infections and number of hospital days.[172,180,181]

THROMBOCYTOPENIA

Thrombocytopenia is relatively common during the course of HIV infection, occurring in approximately 40 percent of patients and serving as the first symptom or sign of infection in approximately 10 percent.[182,183] Evaluation of the 1-year incidence of thrombocytopenia ($<50,000/\mu$l) in a group of 30,214 HIV-infected patients as part of the retrospective Adult and Adolescent Spectrum of Disease Project[183] found the incidence of thrombocytopenia over 1 year was 8.7 percent in patients with clinical AIDS, 3.1 percent in patients with immunologic AIDS (CD4 <200 cells/μl), and 1.7 percent in patients with neither clinical nor immunologic AIDS. Development of thrombocytopenia was associated with (1) history of clinical or immunologic AIDS, (2) injection drug use, (3) history of anemia or lymphoma, and (4) being an American of African descent. After controlling for multiple factors (AIDS, CD4 count, anemia, neutropenia, antiviral therapy, receipt of prophylaxis against P. carinii), thrombocytopenia was significantly associated with shorter survival (risk ratio 1.7, 95% CI 1.6–1.8).[183]

The incidence of thrombocytopenia, defined as a platelet count less than 150,000/μl, was evaluated among 1990 HIV-infected and 553 HIV-negative women who were part of the WIHS. At baseline, 15 percent of HIV-positive women were thrombocytopenic compared to 1.6 percent of HIV-negative women ($p < 0.001$).[184] Factors associated with increased risk of thrombocytopenia included (1) HIV infection, (2) low CD4 levels, (3) increasing viral load, (4) smoking, and (5) being an American of European descent. The study also found thrombocytopenia was a significant predictor of both all-cause and AIDS-related mortality among women infected with HIV. Thus, HIV-infected women with a platelet count less than 50,000/μl had a fivefold increased risk of death from any cause compared to women with normal platelet counts (hazard ratio [HR] 5.10, 95% CI 2.71–9.58) and an approximate threefold increased risk of death from AIDS (HR 3.36, 95% CI 1.44–7.83).

MECHANISMS OF THROMBOCYTOPENIA IN HUMAN IMMUNODEFICIENCY VIRUS-RELATED IMMUNE THROMBOCYTOPENIC PURPURA

Increased Platelet Destruction As in de novo immune thrombocytopenic purpura (ITP), HIV-infected patients with ITP also demonstrate increased platelet destruction via phagocytosis by macrophages in the spleen.[185] In HIV-related ITP, however, several mechanisms for development of platelet-associated antibody have been described, often occurring simultaneously in a given patient. Thus, presence of platelet-specific antibodies, immunochemically characterized as anti-glycoprotein (Gp) IIb and/or GpIIIa, have been detected in HIV-infected patients with ITP, indicating a mechanism similar to that described in *de novo* disease.[186] However, cross-reactive antibody between HIV Gp160/120 and platelet GpIIb-IIIa has been demonstrated.[187] Thus, serum antibodies against HIV Gp160/120 could be eluted from platelets of patients with HIV-related ITP, and these HIV-specific antibodies shared a common epitope with antibodies against platelet GpIIb-IIIa on the platelet surface. Thus it is apparent that molecular mimicry between HIV Gp160/120 and platelet GpIIb-IIIa may be operative in the immune destruction of platelets in some cases of HIV-related ITP. A further mechanism of antibody-induced destruction of platelets arises from the absorption of immune complexes against HIV onto the platelet Fc receptor, thus providing a "free" Fc portion for subsequent macrophage binding and phagocytosis.[186]

Decreased Platelet Production Kinetic studies of platelet production and destruction have been performed in patients with HIV-related ITP, with results compared to a group of normal control subjects and to a group of patients with *de novo* ITP.[185] Mean platelet survival was significantly decreased in patients with HIV ITP, occurring to the same extent in patients receiving zidovudine and in those who were untreated. Mean platelet survival also was significantly decreased in HIV-infected patients with normal platelet counts. In addition to increased destruction of platelets, mean platelet production was significantly decreased in patients with untreated HIV ITP, although those patients receiving zidovudine demonstrated a subsequent increase in platelet production, occurring even in zidovudine-treated HIV-infected individuals without thrombocytopenia. Thus, patients with HIV ITP, while experiencing a moderate increase in platelet destruction, also face a significant decrease in platelet production, which occurs even in individuals with normal platelet counts.[185]

Infection of Megakaryocytes by Human Immunodeficiency Virus The cause of reduced production of platelets in the setting of HIV infection may be direct infection of the megakaryocyte by HIV. Human megakaryocytes bear a CD4+ receptor capable of binding HIV-1,[188] and HIV-1 can be internalized by human megakaryocytes.[189] The HIV-1 coreceptor CXCR4 is present on megakaryocytic progenitors, megakaryocytes, and platelets.[190] Using *in situ* hybridization techniques and a ^{35}S HIV riboprobe (antisense to an HIV *ENV* sequence), HIV transcripts have been detected in megakaryocytes of five of 10 patients with HIV ITP, indicating the megakaryocyte had been infected by HIV in these cases.[191] Expression of viral RNA was also detected in all 10 patients using *in situ* hybridization techniques. Specific ultrastructural damage in the HIV-infected megakaryocytes has been noted, consisting of blebbing and vacuolization of the surface membrane.[192] Documentation of significant increases in platelet production after receipt of zidovudine[193] would be consistent with the hypothesis that a major mechanism of this disorder is the direct infection of the megakaryocyte by HIV.

In three chimpanzees infected with HIV-1 who developed ITP associated with elevated levels of antibody against platelet GpIIIa, use of recombinant pegylated human megakaryocyte growth and development factor resulted in a decline in antiplatelet antibodies in serum, an increase in blood platelet counts, and an increase in the number of megakaryocytes and megakaryocyte progenitors in the marrow.[194] These changes imply that the mechanism of ITP in HIV-infected chimps includes insufficient compensatory increases in platelet production, similar to that decreased in humans.

THERAPY FOR HUMAN IMMUNODEFICIENCY VIRUS-RELATED IMMUNE THROMBOCYTOPENIC PURPURA

Zidovudine The Swiss Group for HIV Studies was the first to demonstrate the efficacy of zidovudine therapy in patients with HIV ITP.[193] Ten seropositive patients, with platelet counts ranging from 20,000 to 100,000/μl, received zidovudine 2 g/day for 2 weeks, followed by 1 g/day for 6 weeks. This treatment was followed by 8 weeks of placebo. All 10 patients experienced an increase in platelet counts while receiving zidovudine, with a mean increase of 54,600/μl (range 53,200–107,800/μl). In contrast, no patient experienced an increase in platelet count while receiving placebo. The time to onset of response was approximately 8 days, with full response achieved by day 30. These results were subsequently confirmed by other studies.[195,196]

The appropriate dose of zidovudine for treatment of HIV ITP was studied by comparing a dose of 500 mg/day in 35 patients with 1000 mg/day in another group of 36 individuals.[197] The majority of patients in both groups were injection drug users, with similar mean platelet counts (approximately 23,000/μl) and mean CD4+ counts (approximately 400 cells/μl). A response rate of 57 percent was achieved in the low-dose group, with 11 percent experiencing complete response. In contrast, a response rate of 72 percent was achieved in those receiving zidovudine 1000 mg/day, with complete response in 39 percent. At month 6, a significant difference remained between the groups, with a mean platelet count of 56,000/μl in the low-dose group versus 98,200/μl in those receiving high-dose zidovudine. It is apparent from this study that high-dose zidovudine is advantageous in patients with HIV ITP.[197]

Highly Active Antiretroviral Therapy in Immune Thrombocytopenic Purpura HAART has been shown to be effective for treatment of HIV-related ITP. In a report of 37 such patients, effective use of HAART was associated with a significantly increased platelet count after 3 months, independent of baseline platelet count or concomitant use of zidovudine.[198] Similarly, in a retrospective study involving 15 patients with HIV-related ITP treated with HAART, 11 (73%) had an increase in platelet count to values of 50,000/μl or greater, and 8 (53%) had an increase in platelet count to values of 100,000/μl or greater after 6 months of HAART therapy.[199] Consistent with these findings, data from the WIHS demonstrated a strong association between use of HAART and resolution of thrombocytopenia (defined as a platelet count >150,000/μl).[184] Thus, compared to thrombocytopenic women not receiving antiretroviral therapy, women taking a non–AZT-containing HAART regimen were nearly two times more likely to improve their thrombocytopenia (odds ratio [OR], 1.84, 95% CI 1.31–2.59, p < 0.001), whereas women taking an AZT-containing HAART regimen were even more likely to resolve their thrombocytopenia (OR 2.85, 95% CI 1.96–4.15, p < 0.0001).[184] Thus, HAART is an important treatment modality in patients with HIV-related ITP and should be the initial treatment of choice in these patients. Effective use of HAART probably significantly decreases HIV viral load and, in so doing, ameliorates many of the effects of HIV on megakaryocytes, platelet production, and destruction.

Interferon-α A prospective, randomized, double-blind, placebo-controlled trial of IFN-α 3,000,000 U given subcutaneously three times per week was conducted in 15 patients with HIV-related ITP.[200] A platelet response was documented in 66 percent, with a mean increase of 60,000/μl. The average time to response was 3 weeks. When IFN therapy was discontinued, platelet counts returned to baseline values within 3 months, indicating the necessity to maintain IFN-α therapy over time. IFN-α was found to prolong platelet survival, whereas no significant increase in platelet production was noted.[201]

High-Dose Intravenous γ-Globulin IVIG 1000 to 2000 mg/kg has been used effectively in pediatric and adult patients with *de novo*

ITP, resulting in a significant rise in platelet counts within 24 to 72 hours in the majority of individuals.[202] Twenty-two patients with HIV-related ITP were treated with IVIG 1 to 2 g/kg during a 2- to 5-day period, depending upon the platelet response.[203] The average platelet count prior to therapy was 22,000/μl and rose to a mean of 182,000/μl (range 10,000–404,000/μl) within 2 to 5 days. Only two patients did not respond, whereas 77 percent experienced an increase to greater than 100,000/μl, and 86 percent had an increase to greater than 50,000/μl. However, when IVIG was discontinued, only 25 percent of patients maintained the increased platelet count, whereas the remainder required repeat infusions approximately every 21 days. The major problem with IVIG appears to be its significant cost. For this reason, IVIG often is reserved for use in patients who are acutely bleeding or require an immediate increase in platelet count, for example, prior to an invasive procedure.

Anti-Rh Immunoglobulin Use of anti-Rh Ig in nonsplenectomized Rh-positive patients with HIV-related ITP is another potential mode of therapy.[204] Requirements for effective therapy with anti-Rh (D) include a baseline hemoglobin level adequate to permit a 1- to 2-g decrease, because of hemolysis, presence of Rh positivity in the patient, and presence of a spleen, the site at which red cells preferentially are phagocytized. Fourteen patients with HIV ITP were treated with 25 mg/kg IV over 30 minutes on 2 consecutive days.[205] Nine of 11 (83%) Rh-positive patients responded with a platelet count greater than 50,000/μl, with response first noted at a median of 4 days (range 3–12 days), and median response duration of 13 days (range 0–37 days). Maintenance therapy of 13 to 25 mg/kg IV was administered every 2 to 4 weeks, resulting in a long-term response (>6 months) in 70 percent of patients. Subclinical hemolysis occurred in all patients, with a decrease in hemoglobin of 0.4 to 2.2 g. These results were confirmed, and use of intramuscular anti-D IG was examined for maintenance treatment after successful induction therapy by the intravenous route.[204] Patients self-administered anti-Rh intramuscularly at a dosage of 6 to 13 mg/kg/week. After induction, 83 percent of patients had achieved a platelet count greater than 50,000/μl, a response that was maintained in 85 percent of patients over time. Thus it is apparent that anti-Rh Ig can be used safely and effectively in patients with HIV-related ITP, providing an alternative that in some institutions may be half the cost of high-dose IVIG.[204,205]

Splenectomy Splenectomy has been used effectively in patients with *de novo* ITP who are refractory to glucocorticoids. At the onset of the AIDS epidemic, several anecdotal case reports described a rapid progression of AIDS postsplenectomy, and the procedure was largely abandoned. Long-term experience with splenectomy in a cohort of 185 patients with HIV ITP has been reported.[206] Splenectomy eventually was performed in 68 such patients, at an average of 13 months from initial diagnosis of HIV ITP. The mean platelet count presplenectomy was 18,000/ml and rose to 223,000/ml postoperatively. A response was seen in 92 percent of patients, with complete response (platelet count >100,000/μl) in 85 percent. Maintenance of the elevated platelet count for longer than 6 months was documented in 82 percent. No difference was found when the survival or rate of progression to AIDS in the 68 splenectomized patients was compared with the rate in the 117 patients who did not undergo the procedure, indicating that splenectomy was not associated with more rapid progression of HIV disease. Another study reached similar conclusions.[207] However, 5.8 percent of patients who underwent splenectomy in one series experienced fulminant infection, consisting of *Streptococcus pneumoniae* meningitis in two and *Haemophilus influenzae* sepsis in one.[206] Thus it is apparent that patients should undergo prophylactic vaccination prior to splenectomy and that such surgery ultimately may be safer in HIV-infected patients who can still achieve an appropriate antibody response to vaccination against *S. pneumoniae* or *H. influenzae*.

Glucocorticoids Glucocorticoids remain the initial therapy of choice in patients with *de novo* ITP and at a dosage of 1 mg/kg/day are associated with an 80 to 90 percent response rate. Similar results were documented in patients with HIV-related disease. However, the immunosuppressive effects of high-dose glucocorticoids have made such therapy far from optimal in HIV-infected patients. Furthermore, the potential development of fulminant Kaposi sarcoma (KS) in dually HIV-infected and human herpes virus (HHV)-8–infected patients after use of corticosteroids has further dampened enthusiasm for this therapeutic modality.

THROMBOTIC DISEASE

Several cases of venous thrombosis occurring in HIV-infected patients have been reported, with an increased incidence of venous thromboembolic disease described in the setting of underlying HIV infection.[208–215] In the Multistate Adult and Adolescent Spectrum of HIV Disease Surveillance Project sponsored by the CDC, the incidence of thrombosis among 42,935 HIV-infected individuals was 2.6 per 1000 person-years.[212] The incidence was lower for individuals with immunologic AIDS (1.8 per 1000 person-years) or asymptomatic HIV infection (1.3 per 1000 person-years) than for persons with clinical AIDS (6.2 per 1000 person-years). Factors significantly associated with the risk of thrombosis included age 45 years or older, cytomegalovirus retinitis or other infection, other AIDS-defining opportunistic infections, hospitalization, use of megestrol acetate, and use of indinavir.[212] Use of other antiretroviral agents, sex, race, and a history of injection drug use were not associated with an increased risk for thrombosis.

However, in another study that directly compared the risk of venous thromboembolism in HIV-infected patients and HIV-negative controls, no statistically significant difference in the rate of thrombotic disease was reported between the groups (HIV-infected patients 2.8% vs. HIV-negative controls 1.8%).[214] Nonetheless, in patients younger than 50 years, the frequencies were significantly different (HIV-infected patients 3.31% vs. HIV-negative controls 0.53%, $p < 0.0001$).

In an attempt to determine the incidence of venous thrombosis in HIV-infected patients compared to individuals without HIV infection and to determine whether the introduction of combination antiretroviral therapy altered the rates of thrombotic disease, a retrospective review was conducted of the medical charts of 37,535 HIV-infected veterans and 37,535 age-, race-, and site-matched controls.[215] Compared to HIV-negative controls, HIV infection was associated with a 39 percent increased incidence of thromboembolism in the pre-HAART era (standardized incidence ratio [SIR] 1.39; 95% CI 1.26–1.52) and a 33 percent increased incidence in the post-1996 era (SIR 1.33; 95% CI 1.24–1.43). This increased risk of thrombosis was independent of a diagnosis of malignancy, HIV-related opportunistic infection, or use of central venous catheters. Furthermore, thrombosis was significantly associated with increased mortality in all groups. Thus, venous thrombotic disease is increased in the setting of HIV infection, independent of many of the more commonly known risk factors.

HIV infection is known to result in increased levels of proinflammatory cytokines, such as tumor necrosis factor (TNF)-α, IL-1, and IL-6, which can contribute to the development of a procoagulant state by increased levels of factor VIII and decreased levels of protein S.[216–218] These same cytokines have been shown to down-regulate the expression of numerous proteins necessary for fibrinolysis.[219] Several studies have suggested that progressive HIV infection may be associated with the development of such a hypercoagulable state. Thus, one study comparing 94 HIV infected women and 50 HIV-negative controls documented a clear relationship between progressive stages of HIV disease, progressive increases in factor VIII activity, and progressively decreasing levels of protein S; the latter two changes have been associated with increased risk of thromboembolism in HIV-infected individuals.[220] Other studies have reported abnormalities of coagulation proteins in HIV-infected patients, such as acquired deficiencies in protein S,[221–226] protein C,[226,227] and heparin cofactor II,[228] and higher titers of anticardiolipin antibodies.[229] Thus, although the mechanisms leading to thromboembolism in HIV are not completely elucidated, the progressive proinflammatory milieu of HIV infection may be operative.

Although the incidence of venous thrombotic events is clearly not as common as the other hematologic disorders, an increase in such events is expected in the setting of HIV infection, and clinicians should be alert to this possibility.

HUMAN IMMUNODEFICIENCY VIRUS-ASSOCIATED MALIGNANCIES

Greater than 40 percent of all HIV-infected patients eventually are diagnosed with cancer.[230] Furthermore, the spectrum of neoplastic disease appears to be wider than initially thought.[230–232] Three cancers currently are considered AIDS-defining in HIV-infected persons: (1) KS, associated with the epidemic from the onset in 1981; (2) intermediate- or high-grade B cell lymphoma, added to the case definition for AIDS in 1985; and (3) cervical carcinoma, which became an AIDS-defining condition on January 1, 1993. Although not considered an AIDS-defining condition, data from cohort studies have consistently shown an increased risk of Hodgkin lymphoma (HL) among patients infected with HIV.

ACQUIRED IMMUNODEFICIENCY SYNDROME RELATED LYMPHOMA

EPIDEMIOLOGY
Patients with AIDS have a risk of developing lymphoma that is nearly 100 times greater than that of the general population.[232–234] The incidence of lymphoma increases with prolonged survival in HIV and may approach 20 percent for patients with prolonged, far-advanced immunodeficiency.[235,236] In one study that linked AIDS and cancer registries in selected areas in the United States, the relative risk of developing lymphoma within 3 years of an AIDS diagnosis was increased by 165-fold compared to people without AIDS.[237] The same study also demonstrated that the increase in risk ranged from 652-fold for high-grade diffuse immunoblastic tumors to 261-fold for Burkitt lymphomas, 113-fold for intermediate-grade lymphomas, and 14-fold for low-grade lymphomas.

As a percentage of first AIDS-defining illness, lymphomas have increased since the widespread use of HAART.[238–241] In one prospective observational multicenter study of more than 7300 patients from Europe, the proportion of AIDS-defining illness attributable to AIDS-related lymphoma rose from less than 4 percent in 1994 to almost 16 percent in 1998.[239] A similar trend has been observed in the United States and Australia.[210,241]

Although use of HAART has led to a major and dramatic decline in the incidence of KS, results from studies evaluating the impact of HAART on the incidence of lymphoma have been inconsistent. The Swiss HIV Cohort study and the Multicenter AIDS Cohort Study (MACS) found no decline in the incidence rates of lymphoma between the pre-HAART and HAART eras,[242,243] but the International Collaboration on HIV and Cancer and the EuroSIDA studies documented a significant decline of lymphoma in the HAART era.[244,245] However, these studies have primarily examined the influence of HAART by dividing the study population into two different time intervals, without considering the actual effects of HAART on individual patients. Thus,

when HAART is effective in a population, data from a French study suggest that the incidence of lymphoma will decline. Using data from the French Hospital Database on HIV, the incidence of systemic AIDS-related lymphoma decreased from 86.0 per 10,000 person-years during the pre-HAART era (defined as 1993 to 1994) to 42.9 per 10,000 person-years during the HAART era (defined as 1997 to 1998).[246] In both the pre-HAART and HAART periods, patients with lower CD4 counts were more likely to develop lymphoma. Nonetheless, within strata of patients with similar CD4 cell counts, the French study showed no change in the incidence of AIDS-related lymphoma between the two periods.[246] Although the risk of lymphoma did not change between the periods among patients with similar CD4 counts, the proportion of patients with low CD4 cell counts (<200 cells/μl [0.2×10^9/liter]) decreased from 49.5 to 24.5 percent between the pre-HAART and HAART periods, thus decreasing the overall proportion of individuals at risk for AIDS-related lymphoma in the second period. The observed decrease in the incidence of lymphoma in the French study resulted from the overall decrease in the proportion of patients with low CD4 counts. Taken together, these data suggest that the incidence of AIDS-related lymphoma in a population depends on the effectiveness of HAART in improving the immune status of that population. If access to HAART is not uniformly available or if HAART is ineffective in increasing CD4 counts or decreasing HIV RNA levels, the incidence of lymphoma in that population will not decline.

ETIOLOGY AND PATHOGENESIS
The mechanisms underlying the development of lymphoma in the setting of HIV are not fully understood. One factor may be immune suppression itself, which is associated with an increased incidence of lymphoma in certain congenital immunodeficiency diseases,[247] autoimmune disorders,[248] or in patients chronically using immunosuppressive drugs, as in the setting of organ transplantation.[249,250] The lymphomas that develop in these settings are similar to the AIDS lymphomas in terms of the pathologic types, the high frequency of extranodal disease at presentation, and the relatively poor prognosis.

Infection by HIV is associated with a myriad of immunologic aberrations (Fig. 83-3). These abnormalities include functional and quantitative defects of CD4 T cells[66,73,251] and chronic antigenic stimulation of B lymphocytes by antigens, mitogens, or viruses, including Epstein Barr virus (EBV)[252] and HIV itself.[75,253] Ongoing B cell expansion and activation result in the development of reactive B cell hyperplasia in lymphoid tissues (PGL)[73,65,88,251] and polyclonal hypergammaglobulinemia in the serum.[74] Lymphomas may develop after acquisition of genetic errors occurring during the course of polyclonal B cell proliferation in the setting of underlying immunodeficiency. This finding has been observed in a primate model, in which high-grade B cell lymphoma develops between 5 and 15 months after infection with the simian immune deficiency virus, coincident with development of severe immunodeficiency.[254]

Cytokine Networks Dysregulated expression of cytokines may contribute to the chronic B cell proliferation that characterizes HIV disease. B cell proliferation and maturation may be induced by several cytokines, including IL-4, IL-6, IL-10, and TNF-α.[255] B cells from HIV-infected patients with hypergammaglobulinemia constitutively express TNF-α and IL-6.[256] High levels of IL-6 gene expression have been noted in myeloma, chronic lymphocytic leukemia, and both HIV-positive and HIV-negative cases of immunoblastic and large-cell lymphoma, independent of EBV status.[257–259] Although not unique to AIDS-related lymphoma, IL-6 may play a role in the pathogenesis of diverse types of B cell neoplasia. Moreover, elevated serum IL-6 levels can be detected in the sera of patients with symptomatic HIV infection who later develop large-cell lymphoma.[236]

IL-10 may play a role in the development of AIDS-related lym-

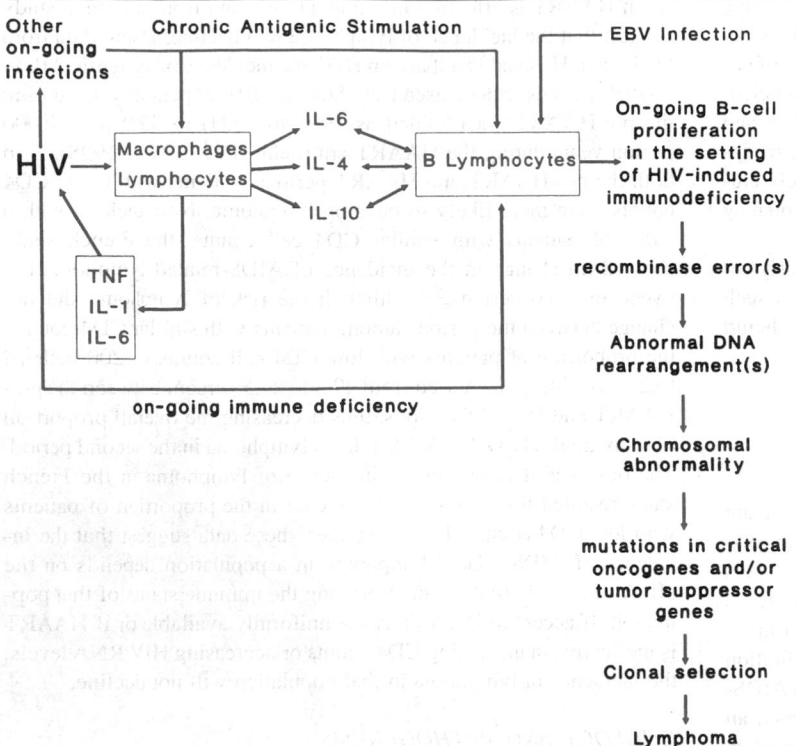

FIGURE 83-3   Schematic representation of the possible sequence of events resulting in the development of lymphoma in human immunodeficiency virus (HIV) disease. EBV, Epstein-Barr virus; IL, interleukin; TNF, tumor necrosis factor. (Modified from Martin et al.[379])

phoma. Constitutive expression of IL-10 has been shown in EBV-positive B cell lines derived from patients with AIDS-related Burkitt lymphoma,[260] and IL-10 has been shown to function as an autocrine growth factor in B cell lines.[261] HIV may induce aberrant expression of these cytokines,[262] thus stimulating pathologic B cell proliferation and differentiation and allowing for neoplastic transformation.

Epstein-Barr Virus   EBV is implicated in the pathogenesis of at least a subset of AIDS-related lymphoma, perhaps related to the impaired immunosurveillance against EBV-infected cells.[252] EBV DNA has been found in the affected lymph nodes of 35 percent of HIV-infected patients with reactive lymphadenopathy.[263] These individuals were shown to have an increased incidence of lymphoma over time.[263]

Patients with large-cell or immunoblastic lymphoma primary to the brain uniformly have latent EBV infections.[264] Epstein-Barr early region (EBER) protein can be detected in essentially all such patients and the latent membrane protein in 45 percent.[264] Latent membrane protein has transforming and oncogenic properties.[265]

Approximately 40 to 60 percent of systemic AIDS-related lymphoma cases have detectable EBV DNA within tumor nuclei.[266,267] Immunoblastic lymphomas and, to a lesser extent, diffuse large-cell lymphomas are most commonly EBV positive.[268] Evidence for clonal EBV infection has been demonstrated in all cases examined, indicating that EBV integration occurred before clonal B cell expansion.[269] This finding suggests, but does not prove, that EBV plays a role in the etiopathogenesis of these lymphomas.

Abnormal DNA Rearrangements   During AIDS-related B cell stimulation induced by HIV, EBV, and/or or other antigens, genetic "errors" in Ig gene rearrangement and/or expression may occur, leading to chromosomal translocations involving the Ig heavy- or light-chain genes. Thus, specific chromosomal translocations have been de-

scribed in AIDs-related Burkitt lymphoma, including t(8;14), t(8;22), and t(8;2).[270–272]

c-myc Dysregulation   Translocations involving chromosome 8 can result in dysregulation of the c-*myc* oncogene. Dependent upon the specific breakpoint position on chromosome 8 and the locus on chromosome 14, 2, or 22, different mechanisms for c-*myc* dysregulation might apply, as described in the distinct forms of Burkitt lymphoma and in distinct geographic regions of the world.[273,274] However, c-*myc* dysregulation is not seen in all cases of AIDS-related lymphoma. Activation of c-*myc* was detected in 100 percent of small noncleaved lymphomas in one series,[269] but such activation was found in only a minority of large-cell or immunoblastic lymphomas.[275] Moreover, the specific mechanisms leading to c-*myc* dysregulation appear to be diverse.[269,276,277] Thus, HIV-1 infection of immortalized B cell lines in itself can result in upregulation of c-*myc* transcripts,[278] whereas HIV may also affect cellular c-*myc* gene expression directly.[277] Whatever the mechanism, dysregulation of c-*myc* may contribute to transformation of human B cells *in vitro* and may cause B cell lymphoma in transgenic animals carrying Ig-*myc* chimeric constructs.[279,280]

bcl-6 Dysregulation and Other Genetic Abnormalities   In AIDS-related diffuse large-cell lymphoma, the primary molecular alteration involves mutations of *bcl*-6.[281,282] Although gross rearrangements or chromosomal translocations involving *bcl*-6 usually are absent, mutations in the 5' regions of the gene are detectable in as many as 60 percent of cases.[281–283] *bcl*-6 mutations are markers of germinal center derivation of B cells, indicating that diffuse large-cell lymphomas in AIDS are related to germinal center B cells.[284]

Aside from these genetic abnormalities, other molecular aberrations have been noted, including p53 mutations or deletions, which may occur in as many as 60 percent of AIDS-related small noncleaved lymphomas.[275,285] In addition, mutations of *ras* have been described in some cases of AIDS-related Burkitt lymphoma.[275]

Diverse molecular mechanisms are responsible for the various types of AIDS-related lymphoma.[284] Small noncleaved lymphomas are most often associated with c-*myc* aberrations, mutations in p53, and occasionally *ras*. Diffuse large-cell lymphomas are associated with mutations in the *bcl*-6 gene, whereas immunoblastic and large-cell lymphomas appear to be driven primarily by EBV.

PATHOLOGY

Eighty to ninety percent of lymphomas associated with AIDS are intermediate- or high-grade B cell tumors,[285–289] including immunoblastic or large-cell types and small noncleaved or Burkitt lymphoma, which is in sharp contrast to non–HIV-infected patients, in whom high-grade lymphomas are expected in only 10 to 15 percent.[290] In an effort to standardize the nomenclature, the WHO has classified AIDS-related lymphoma into three groups: (1) those occurring specifically in HIV-infected patients, (2) those also occurring in other immunodeficiency states, and (3) those that also arise in immunocompetent patients (Table 83-3).[291] The two most common histologic subtypes of lymphoma in HIV-infected patients are Burkitt lymphoma and diffuse large cell lymphoma.

Burkitt Lymphoma   In patients with HIV-related Burkitt lymphoma, histology may resemble classic Burkitt lymphoma as seen in the general population or, more commonly, may demonstrate atypical features.[292–295] Histologically, classic Burkitt lymphoma is characterized by sheets of intermediate-size lymphoid cells with regular round

TABLE 83-3 CATEGORIES OF HIV-ASSOCIATED LYMPHOMAS: WORLD HEALTH ORGANIZATION CLASSIFICATION

Lymphomas also occurring in immunocompetent patients
  Burkitt lymphoma
    Classic
  With plasmacytoid differentiation
    Atypical
  Diffuse large B cell lymphoma
    Centroblastic
    Immunoblastic
  Extranodal marginal zone B cell lymphoma of mucosa-associated
    lymphoid tissue (MALT) lymphoma (rare)
  Peripheral T cell lymphoma (rare)
  Classic Hodgkin lymphoma
Lymphomas occurring more specifically in patients who are HIV positive
  Primary effusion lymphoma
  Plasmablastic lymphoma of the oral cavity
Lymphomas occurring in other immunodeficiency states
  Polymorphic B cell lymphoma

HIV=human immunodeficiency virus.

or oval nuclear outlines or slight nuclear irregularities. A "starry-sky" appearance resulting from the presence of tangible body macrophages is characteristically described. The neoplastic cells have an extremely high mitotic rate, with a Ki67 score approaching 100 percent. In atypical Burkitt lymphoma, the cells are more varied in size and shape and show greater nuclear pleomorphism.[295] In some cases, the cells have a plasmacytoid appearance, characterized by medium-size cells with abundant cytoplasm and eccentric nuclei. This type of Burkitt lymphoma is termed *Burkitt lymphoma with plasmacytoid differentiation* in the WHO classification, an entity unique to patients with HIV.[296]

Diffuse Large B Cell Lymphoma In the WHO classification, AIDS-related diffuse large B cell lymphomas are divided into centroblastic and immunoblastic subtypes. The centroblastic subtype has features of large cell lymphomas similar to those seen in the general population without HIV. The immunoblastic subtype (approximately 20% of cases) is more typical of HIV infection. It is characterized by large cells, each containing a single prominent nucleolus and plasmacytoid features in the cytoplasm. Compared to the centroblastic subtype, the immunoblastic subtype more frequently involves extranodal sites, particularly the central nervous system (CNS), and is more commonly associated with EBV infection, with EBV-encoded LMP antigen found in 90 percent compared to 30 percent in the centroblastic variant.[268,297,298] Furthermore, amplification of *bcl-6* is associated with the centroblastic but usually not the immunoblastic subtype, whereas CD138/syndecan-1, normally expressed by B cells in late stages of B cell differentiation, is more commonly expressed in the immunoblastic subtype. These phenotypic differences suggest that the two variants of diffuse large B cell lymphoma have differing histogenesis, with the centroblastic subtype arising from germinal centers and the immunoblastic variant arising from postgerminal center lymphocytes.

Primary Effusion Lymphoma Primary effusion lymphoma and plasmablastic lymphoma of the oral cavity occur more specifically in patients with HIV infection. Primary effusion lymphoma is uncommon, representing only a small fraction of all AIDS lymphomas, and is caused by HHV-8.[299-301] Morphologically, primary effusion lymphoma is characterized by large neoplastic cells with cytologic features that range between immunoblastic, plasmablastic, and anaplastic large cells.[301] The malignant cell usually lacks B cell markers on its surface but is B lymphoid in origin, as Ig gene rearrangement is consistently present. In addition to HHV-8, the tumor cells often harbor EBV.[301]

Plasmablastic lymphoma of the oral cavity, another uncommon entity, is characterized by rapidly growing large lymphoid cells with marked plasma cell differentiation.[302,303] Phenotypically, these lymphomas usually do not express conventional B cell markers such as CD20 but stain strongly with plasma cell markers CD138/syndecan-1 and VS38c.[302,303] They are positive for EBV EBER by *in situ* hybridization, variably positive for EBV LMP-1, and negative for EBNA2; HHV-8 is negative.[304] However, plasmablastic lymphoma of the oral cavity remains a rare and poorly understood entity and the genetic mechanisms responsible for its pathogenesis remain to be elucidated.

T Cell Lymphoma Patients with AIDS are at an increased risk for developing T cell lymphomas. One study reported a 15-fold increased risk for developing T cell lymphoma 2 years after a diagnosis of AIDS.[235] The prevalence of T cell lymphomas among patients with AIDS-related lymphoma is approximately 3 percent.[235,305] A wide spectrum of T cell malignancies in the setting of HIV infection has been reported.[306-308] However, the majority of cases consist of peripheral T cell lymphomas, occurring in 45 percent, or anaplastic large cell lymphomas, occurring in 27 percent of a small series.[305] Morphologically, they resemble peripheral T cell lymphomas seen in the general population.

Low-Grade B Cell Lymphoma Occasional HIV-infected patients with low-grade B cell lymphomas have been reported,[285,289,309] as have relatively young individuals with multiple myeloma or solitary plasmacytoma.[310] The natural history of low-grade lymphoma appears similar in the presence or absence of underlying HIV infection.[309,311]

CLINICAL FEATURES

B symptoms, such as fever, night sweats, and weight loss, are present at diagnosis in 80 to 90 percent of patients with AIDS-related lymphoma,[312,313] and 61 to 90 percent have far-advanced disease presenting in extranodal sites.[285-289,310,313] This finding is in contrast to non–AIDS-related lymphoma, in which approximately 40 percent of individuals present with extranodal lymphomatous disease.[314]

Virtually any anatomic site may be involved.[312] The more common sites of initial extranodal disease include the CNS (17%–42%), GI tract (4%–28%), marrow (21%–33%), and liver (9%–26%).[285-289,312]

Staging evaluation should include computed tomographic scanning of the chest, abdomen, and pelvis; a gallium-67 scan[315] or positron emission tomography (PET) scan; marrow aspirate and biopsy; and other studies as clinically indicated. Lumbar puncture should routinely be performed, because approximately 20 percent of patients have leptomeningeal lymphoma, even in the absence of specific symptoms or signs.[316] Intrathecal methotrexate or cytosine arabinoside is often given to prevent isolated CNS relapse.[316]

Primary Central Nervous System Lymphoma Approximately 75 percent of patients with primary CNS lymphoma have far-advanced HIV disease, with median CD4 cell counts less than 50/μl, and a prior history of AIDS.[231,313,317-319] Initial symptoms and signs may be variable, with seizures, headache, and/or focal neurologic dysfunction noted in most patients. However, subtle changes in behavior may be the only presenting complaint.[317]

Radiographic scanning reveals relatively large mass lesions (2–4 cm), which tend to be few in number (one to three lesions). Ring enhancement may be seen.[318,319] There is no specific radiographic picture. PET scanning may be useful in differentiating cerebral lymphoma from toxoplasmosis.[320] In addition, thallium-201 single-photon emission computerized tomography scanning may be useful, with median T1 uptake index greater than 1.5 and lesion size greater than 2.5 cm serving as independent predictors of primary CNS lymphoma.[321]

Pathologically, almost all such lymphomas are of diffuse large-cell or immunoblastic subtypes and are uniformly associated with EBV infection within malignant cells.[322] Thus, detection of EBV DNA

(EBNA) in cerebrospinal fluid by polymerase chain reaction may be used as a diagnostic criterion for primary CNS lymphoma. One study reported a sensitivity of 80 percent and a specificity of 100 percent.[323]

Optimal therapy for primary CNS lymphoma remains to be defined. Use of cranial radiation is associated with a complete remission rate of only 50 percent and median survival of only 2 or 3 months. Although median survival times have not been prolonged with radiation, approximately 75 percent of patients experience an improvement in QOL.[306] No specific regimen of chemotherapy has yet proved efficacious, perhaps because of the severe level of immunocompromise in affected patients. Nonetheless, use of HAART has been associated with significantly prolonged survival of these patients.[324]

T Cell Lymphomas Systemic B symptoms, consisting of fever, drenching night sweats, and/or unexplained weight loss, are extremely common in patients with T cell lymphomas; one study reported such symptoms occurred in 82 percent of patients.[305] Like B cell lymphomas in the setting of HIV, T cell lymphomas also present with advanced lymphomatous disease, with stage IV disease confirmed in up to 90 percent.[305] Compared to HIV-infected patients with aggressive B cell lymphomas, patients with T cell lymphomas more likely present with cutaneous and bone marrow involvement.[305]

Primary Effusion Lymphoma Primary effusion lymphoma has been reported in both HIV-positive and HIV-negative patients but appears to be more common in the former. Of note, primary effusion lymphoma was diagnosed in an HIV-negative cardiac transplant recipient whose original explanted heart was retrospectively found to be infected by HHV-8.[325] Clinically, patients present with effusions in the pleura, pericardium, or peritoneal cavity. Most patients do not have mass lesions, although such masses have been reported, most commonly in the gastrointestinal tract. Optimal therapy is unknown. Outcome with polychemotherapy has generally been poor, with median survival of approximately 2 months.[326] Immune reconstitution with HAART likely plays an important role in the control of this condition. Several studies reported complete remissions in patients treated with HAART alone.[327–329]

PROGNOSTIC FACTORS IN ACQUIRED IMMUNODEFICIENCY SYNDROME-RELATED LYMPHOMA

Poor prognostic indicators for survival in AIDS-related lymphoma include a Karnofsky performance status less than 70 percent, history of AIDS prior to lymphoma, CD4 count less than 100 cells/μl (0.05 $\times$ 10^9/liter),[313,330] stage III or IV disease, elevated lactate dehydrogenase, history of injection drug use, and age over 35 years.[330] The age-adjusted International Prognostic Index was validated in a single institutional series of AIDS patients with lymphoma.[331] Thus, median survival for patients with low-risk, low- to intermediate-risk, high-intermediate risk, and high-risk lymphoma was 60 months, 17 months, 10.9 months, and 6.8 months respectively. Although not been previously shown to be an important prognostic factor, one retrospective study evaluating prognostic factors in 363 patients with systemic AIDS-related lymphoma treated with standard chemotherapy, such as CHOP (cyclophosphamide, doxorubicin, vincristine [Oncovin] prednisone) or m-BACOD (methotrexate bleomycin, doxorubicin [Adriamycin], cyclophosphamide, vincristine [Oncovin], dexamethasone), in the HAART era found that a histology of Burkitt lymphoma was an independent poor prognostic factor for survival.[332]

Patients with systemic lymphoma with leptomeningeal involvement have decreased survival.[333]

TREATMENT

Standard versus Low-Dose Chemotherapy At the outset of the AIDS epidemic, very dose-intensive regimens were used in patients with AIDS-related lymphoma but were associated with low complete remission rates (20%–33%) and high rates of serious infectious complications, leading to death in 28 to 78 percent of patients.[318,319,334,335] These observations led to the design and implementation of a low-dose modification of the m-BACOD regimen.[316] In an attempt to clarify the value of low-dose therapy, the AIDS Clinical Trials Group (ACTG) in the United States compared standard-dose m-BACOD and GM-CSF support with reduced-dose m-BACOD without GM-CSF in 198 HIV-infected patients with aggressive lymphomas.[336] No differences were found in either response rate (standard dose 52% vs. reduced dose 41%) or median survival (standard dose 6.8 months vs. reduced dose 7.7months). However, reduced dose m-BACOD was associated with a statistically superior toxicity profile. Thus in the pre-HAART era, this trial indicated that low-dose m-BACOD was preferable to standard-dose therapy in patients with AIDS lymphoma.[336]

Since these early efforts, a significant advance in the management of patients with AIDS-related lymphoma has been made, with survival of many of these patients now comparable to that of patients without HIV infection.[333,337] Apart from the contribution of HAART, this improvement in prognosis can be attributed to new initiatives in treatment, such as the use of effective infusional regimens and the feasibility of high-dose therapy with peripheral stem cell rescue for relapsed or refractory disease, and better supportive care. However, several controversial issues, such as the optimal timing of HAART with combination chemotherapy and the role of rituximab, remain.

Infusional Dose-Adjusted EPOCH Regimen and Optimal Timing of HAART Investigators at the National Cancer Institute (NCI) reported on the dose-adjusted EPOCH regimen (Table 83-4), used in 39 patients with newly diagnosed AIDS-related lymphoma. The regimen consists of a 96-hour continuous infusion of etoposide, vincristine, and doxorubicin, and a bolus of cyclophosphamide, which was dose adjusted based on the patient's CD4 cell count and neutrophil count at the nadir.[333] Oral prednisone also was given. HAART was omitted during the administration of chemotherapy to prevent potential drug interactions but was restarted immediately upon completion of chemotherapy. The overall complete remission rate was 74 percent. Among patients with CD4 cell counts greater than 100 cells/μl (0.1 $\times$ 10^9/liter), the complete remission rate was 87 percent, and the overall survival was 87 percent at 56 months. However, patients with CD4 cell counts less than 100 cells/μl (0.1 $\times$ 10^9/liter) continued to do poorly, with a complete remission rate of 56 percent and an overall survival of only 16 percent at 56 months. As expected, the median CD4 cell count fell significantly during chemotherapy while the median viral load increased by 0.87 log10 copies/ml by the time the last cycle of chemotherapy was given. Nonetheless, these values returned to baseline within 6 to 12 months following reinstitution of HAART at the completion of chemotherapy. These data suggest that good virologic control during chemotherapy may not be essential for optimal tumor response, and use of HAART may be safely omitted until com-

TABLE 83-4　DOSE-ADJUSTED EPOCH IN ACQUIRED IMMUNODEFICIENCY SYNDROME LYMPHOMA

AGENT	DOSE	DAY
Etoposide	50 mg/m^2/day	1–4
Oncovin	0.4 mg/m^2/day	1–4
Doxorubicin	10 mg/m^2/day	1–4
Prednisolone	60 mg/m^2/day	1–5
Cytoxan		
<100 CD4+cells	187 mg/m^2	5
>100 CD4+cells	375 mg/m^2	

SOURCE: Little et al.[333]

pletion of chemotherapy, at least in patients with baseline CD4 counts greater than 100 cells/μl (0.1 × 10^9/liter).

Optimal Timing of Highly Active Antiretroviral Therapy Consistent with the NCI data on dose-adjusted EPOCH, a prospective study evaluating the safety and efficacy of liposomal doxorubicin, cyclophosphamide, vincristine, and prednisone in 24 patients with AIDS-related lymphoma found no statistically significant relationship between virologic response to HAART and antitumor response to chemotherapy.[337] Nonetheless, in this study, concurrent use of HAART during administration of chemotherapy was generally well tolerated, and treatment-related toxicities were comparable to those previously reported with low-dose or standard-dose m-BACOD. In another study investigating the pharmokinetic interactions resulting from simultaneous combination chemotherapy (low-dose or standard-dose CHOP) and HAART for patients with AIDS-related lymphoma, no clinically significant interactions were documented, although the clearance of cyclophosphamide was 1.5-fold reduced compared to historical controls.[338] Thus, delaying HAART until completion of chemotherapy is reasonable but does not appear to be obligatory. Furthermore, including HAART therapy with chemotherapy in patients with CD4 cells less than 100/μl (0.1 × 10^9/liter) clearly seems important.

Although the optimal timing of HAART during chemotherapy remains controversial, use of HAART is clearly associated with improved survival in patients with AIDS-related lymphoma.[339,340] Thus, in a multicenter cohort study from Germany involving 203 patients, response to HAART therapy, defined as CD4 cell count increase to 100 cells/μl (0.1 × 10^9/liter) cells/mm^3 or greater and/or at least one viral load less than 500 copies/ml during the first 2 years following diagnosis of lymphoma, were independently associated with prolonged survival.[339] Among patients with both a response to HAART and complete tumor remission, 83 percent were still alive at 39 months. Complete remission to chemotherapy without a HAART response in terms of HIV resulted in significantly decreased survival compared to HAART responders. Similarly, a retrospective study from Italy also reported that a good virologic response to HAART therapy was associated with a prolongation in survival.[340] Interestingly, in contrast to the NCI data on dose-adjusted EPOCH, the Italian study showed that virologic response to HAART was the only factor correlated with response to chemotherapy; nonetheless, the study was retrospective with only a small number of patients.

Taken together, these data suggest that use of HAART, concurrently or sequentially with combination chemotherapy, clearly improves survival in patients with AIDS-related lymphoma, although attainment of virologic control does not appear to be mandatory for achievement of complete response to chemotherapy.

Role of Rituximab The role of rituximab in patients with AIDS-related lymphoma has been investigated. In a randomized phase III trial conducted by the AIDS Malignancy Consortium (AMC) of the NCI, standard-dose CHOP was compared to CHOP with rituximab (R-CHOP).[341] Although complete remission was higher in the 99 patients who received R-CHOP (58%) compared to the 50 patients who received CHOP alone (47%), this difference did not reach statistical significance. With a median followup of 137 weeks, the progression-free survival (R-CHOP 45 weeks vs. CHOP 38 weeks) and overall survival (R-CHOP 139 weeks vs. CHOP 110 weeks) were not statistically different. Of importance, this study documented a statistically increased risk of infectious deaths in the R-CHOP arm. Overall, 15 of the 16 infectious deaths occurred in the group receiving R-CHOP. However, nine of the 15 patients who died had a CD4 cell count less than 50 cells/μl (0.05 × 10^9/liter), suggesting that the higher infectious death rate observed was related to the severely immunodeficient state of these individuals. In this regard, CD4 cells less than 50 cells/μl (0.05 × 10^9/liter) have been associated with an increased risk of neu-

tropenia, neutropenic infections, and death in patients with HIV infection without lymphoma.[342]

Investigators in Europe have investigated the role of rituximab in patients with AIDS-related lymphoma.[343,344] The pooled results of three phase II trials evaluating rituximab in combination with 96-hour continuous infusion of cyclophosphamide (187.5–200 mg/m^2/day), doxorubicin (12.5 mg/m^2/day), and etoposide (60 mg/m^2/day) (R-CDE) in 74 patients with AIDS-related lymphoma has been reported.[343] All patients received G-CSF as prophylaxis, and most patients (76%) received concurrent HAART.[343] The overall response rate was 75 percent, with complete remission in 52 patients (70%) and partial remission in 4 (5%). With a median followup of 23 months, the estimated 2-year overall survival and disease-free survival rates were 64 percent (95% CI 52%–76%) and 89 percent (95% CI 81%–97%), respectively. These results were superior to the complete remission rate of 45 percent and 2-year overall survival rate of 38 percent reported in a multicenter trial of infusional CDE without rituximab in 55 patients with AIDS-related lymphoma conducted by the Eastern Cooperative Oncology Group (ECOG).[344]

With regard to the infectious complications of infusional R-CDE, 10 (14%) patients developed opportunistic infections during or within 3 months of completion of chemotherapy; 17 (23%) developed other infections. Although six deaths were related to infections (two bacterial sepsis and four opportunistic infections), three of the four opportunistic infections occurred more than 4 months after completion of chemotherapy. Compared to the infection rates in patients receiving infusional CDE in the ECOG study,[343,344] infusional R-CDE was associated with a higher incidence of grade 3 to 4 infection (31% vs. 20%) and lethal infection (2% vs. 0%), although no differences in the proportions of patients with grade 3 to 4 neutropenia (78% vs. 90%) were apparent. Thus, consistent with the AMC data on R-CHOP,[347] the study by Spina and colleagues[343] also suggested that rituximab increased the risk for severe and life-threatening infection when used in combination with chemotherapy in patients with AIDS, particularly in those who are severely immunocompromised. Importantly, the addition of rituximab to infusional CDE was associated with an improvement in complete remission rate and overall survival despite the higher rates of infectious complications.[343] Thus, although use of rituximab with chemotherapy may increase the risk of severe infectious complications, it is apparent from these trials that such a strategy also may result in superior tumor control and better overall survival.

The safety and efficacy of rituximab with chemotherapy currently is being addressed in an AMC ongoing randomized phase III trial, which compares concurrent administration of rituximab with EPOCH (R-EPOCH) to EPOCH followed sequentially by rituximab, given weekly for 6 weeks (EPOCH→R).

Role of Central Nervous System Prophylaxis The incidence of CNS involvement at presentation in patients with systemic AIDS-related lymphoma has ranged from 10 to 20 percent.[333] Although CNS chemoprophylaxis is generally recommended for patients with Burkitt lymphoma or in those with bone marrow, paraspinal, paranasal, epidural, testicular, or widespread systemic involvement,[345] our practice is to treat all patients with AIDS-related lymphoma using prophylactic intrathecal chemotherapy. Of importance, in the NCI trial of dose-adjusted EPOCH, CNS prophylaxis was not uniformly given.[333] However, CNS relapse occurred rather quickly in two patients, resulting in a change in the protocol to mandate such prophylaxis.[333]

Management of Relapsed or Refractory Acquired Immunodeficiency Syndrome-Related Lymphoma In the pre-HAART era, patients with relapsed or refractory lymphoma had little possibility of cure with standard-dose salvage regimens. Complete response rates with salvage chemotherapy ranged from 10 to 30 percent, with median survival ranging from 2 to 7 months. One study of 21 such patients treated with etoposide, mitoxantrone, and prednimustine (VMP) reported a complete response rate of 26 percent and an overall median survival of only 2 months.[346] Similarly, in another study involving 40 patients with resistant or recurrent AIDS-related lymphoma, infusional CDE was associated with a low complete remission rate of 10 percent and overall median survival of only 4 months.[347] Slightly more encouraging results were reported in another retrospective study evaluating the use of the ESHAP (etoposide, methylprednisolone, cytosine arabinoside, cisplatin) regimen as salvage therapy in patients with relapsed or refractory AIDS-related lymphoma.[348] Among the 13 treated patients, 4 patients (31%) achieved complete remission and 3 patients (23%) attained partial remission, with a median survival of 7.1 months. One of these patients remains well more than 5 years after completion of ESHAP after having failed three prior regimens.[348]

With the advent of HAART and improvement in supportive care, HIV-infected patients with relapsed or refractory lymphoma now can be effectively salvaged with high-dose chemotherapy and peripheral stem cell transplantation. In one reported series of 20 patients with relapsed or refractory patients with AIDS-related lymphoma, 17 (85%) remained alive and in complete remission a median of 31.8 months after transplantation.[349] Both the ability to collect adequate CD34+ cells and the time required for white cell engraftment were comparable to that in non–HIV-infected individuals. Encouraging results have been reported by other investigators.[350] These studies suggest that salvage chemotherapy followed by high-dose therapy with peripheral progenitor stem cell transplant is a viable option for selected patients with relapsed or refractory AIDS-related lymphoma.

HODGKIN LYMPHOMA IN THE SETTING OF HUMAN IMMUNODEFICIENCY VIRUS INFECTION

Epidemiology of Human Immunodeficiency Virus-Related Hodgkin lymphoma   HL is one of the most common non–AIDS-defining cancers in HIV-infected patients. Large epidemiologic studies have consistently indicated that HIV-infected individuals have an eightfold to 10-fold increased risk of developing HL than expected in the general population.[351–358] In a large linkage analysis performed in Italy, Franceschi and colleagues[353] observed an 8.9-fold increase in the standardized incidence ratio for HL (95% CI 4.4–16.0) among the 6067 persons with AIDS. Notably, of the 11 patients who developed HL, seven were of mixed cellularity type.

Immunosuppression and Human Immunodeficiency Virus-Related Hodgkin Lymphoma   Earlier studies reported a wide range of median CD4 cell counts in patients with HIV-related Hodgkin lymphoma (HIV-HL), ranging from a median of 113 cells/μl (0.11 × 10^9/liter) in a group of 21 patients treated prospectively as part of ACTG (study 149)[359] to 306 cells/μl (0.36 × 10^9/liter) in a comparable study from France.[360] The precise level of immune dysfunction in patients with HIV-HL from these earlier studies was uncertain. However, recent data have suggested that HIV-HL is associated with more profound immunodeficiency. A statistically increased risk of HIV-HL is present in the period after initial diagnosis of AIDS compared to the period immediately prior to diagnosis of AIDS.[361] Also, using linked population-based AIDS and cancer registry data from diverse areas in the United States, a fourfold increase in the relative risk of HL has been observed in the period immediately prior to development of AIDS (RR 9.8) compared to the period 60 to 25 months before development of AIDS (RR 2.6).[362] Similarly, in studies conducted in Australia, no case of HL was observed in the period 5 years prior to diagnosis of AIDS (SIR 0) compared to 10 cases in the period within 6 months following an AIDS diagnosis (SIR 59.1) and one case in the period 6 months to 2 years after diagnosis of AIDS (SIR 7.34).[363]

Pathology   In western series, nodular sclerosis disease is the most common subtype of *de novo* HL, described in 52 to 62 percent of patients.[364] Lymphocyte-predominant disease accounts for 8 to 21 percent, whereas mixed cellularity HL is seen in 24 percent and lymphocyte depletion subtype in 3 to 6 percent of patients.[364] In contrast, HIV-related HL is characterized by the preponderance of more aggressive histologic subtypes, with mixed cellularity HL and lymphocyte depletion HL diagnosed in 41 to 100 percent of patients.[360,364–369] Another distinguishing feature of HIV-HL is its close association with EBV, which can be detected within the nuclei of Reed-Sternberg cells in almost all cases.[297,370] In contrast, EBV is associated with only one third of *de novo* HL cases[371] and one half of *de novo* mixed cellularity cases.[372]

Clinical Features   Systemic B symptoms such as fever, drenching night sweats, and/or weight loss occur frequently in patients with HIV-HL, with 70 to 100 percent reporting these symptoms compared to 30 to 60 percent of patients with *de novo* HL.[355,360,364–367] Furthermore, compared to patients with *de novo* HL, those with HIV-related HL are more likely to present with advanced stages of disease.[357,360,368] Bone marrow involvement is particularly prominent in patients with underlying HIV infection, present in approximately 50 percent and often presenting with pancytopenia and systemic B symptoms.[373]

Staging evaluation should include a thorough history, physical examination, standard laboratory tests, CT scans of the chest, abdomen, and pelvis, gallium or PET scans, and bilateral bone marrow biopsies. Because determining the precise etiology of constitutional symptoms such as fever and night sweats often is difficult, microbiologic tests to exclude *Mycobacterium avium-intracellulare*, cytomegalovirus disease, and other opportunistic infections should be performed as clinically indicated.

Therapy   In the pre-HAART era, treatment of HIV-HL with chemotherapy was associated with poor treatment outcomes. Treatment-related toxicities, especially hematologic, were substantial, even when hematopoietic growth factors were used. The ACTG conducted a nonrandomized, prospective, multiinstitutional clinical trial in 21 HIV-infected patients with HL using the standard ABVD (adriamycin, bleomycin, vinblastine, dacarbazine) regimen with G-CSF.[359] No antiretroviral therapy was used. Between May 1992 and August 1996, 21 patients were accrued, with a median CD4 count of 113 cells/μl (0.11 × 10^9/liter)/mm^3. Stage IV HL was present in 67 percent, with bone marrow involvement in 12 (57%). Despite routine use of G-CSF, 10 patients (47.6%) experienced life-threatening neutropenia, with ANCs less than 500 cells/μl. In addition, nine opportunistic infections occurred in 6 patients (29%) during the study or shortly thereafter. Results were poor, with complete remission attained in only 43 percent of treated patients and a median survival of only 1.5 years.

Similarly, in another prospective study from Italy, a disappointing overall survival rate of 32 percent at 36 months in 35 HIV-infected patients with Hodgkin lymphoma (HL) treated with a regimen consisting of epirubicin, bleomycin, vinblastine, and prednisolone (EBVP) with concomitant antiretroviral therapy and G-CSF support was reported.[374]

With the availability of HAART, better treatment outcomes with combination chemotherapy have been reported. In a phase II study of the Stanford V regimen in 59 patients with HIV-HL, Spina and colleagues[375] reported an overall response rate of 89 percent and a complete response rate of 81 percent, with an estimated 3-year overall survival and disease-free survival of 51 percent and 68 percent, respectively. The regimen consisted of mechlorethamine (6 mg/m^2 on day 1), doxorubicin (25 mg/m^2 on days 1 and 15), vinblastine (6 mg/m^2 on 1 and 15), vincristine (2 mg/m^2 IV on days 8 and 22), bleomycin (5 U/m^2 on days 8 and 22), etoposide 60 mg/m^2 on days 15 and 16), and prednisone (40 mg/m^2 PO every other day), given every 28 days for a total of three cycles. Involved-field radiation was planned for all patients who achieved partial remission or who had initial bulky mediastinal disease. Of importance, 52 (88%) of the 59 patients received HAART concomitantly with the Stanford V regimen.

In another retrospective study evaluating the impact of HAART on patients with HIV-HL, an improvement in complete response rate from 64.5 percent in the pre-HAART to 74.5 percent in the HAART period was observed, with an improvement in the estimated 2-year survival probability from 45 percent to 62 percent, respectively.[376] Although the median survival of patients treated in the pre-HAART era was only 19 months, the median survival of patients treated in the post-HAART era had not been reached at a median followup of 20 months. Of interest, improvements in response rate and survival were achieved without significant change in the chemotherapy regimens used between the two periods. Further, Hoffman and colleagues[377] showed that response to HAART therapy, defined as CD4 cell count increase of at least 100 cells/μL (0.1×10^9/liter) and/or at least one viral load less than 500 copies/ml during the first 2 years following diagnosis of HIV-related HL, was associated with prolonged survival.

The German Hodgkin's Study Group (GHSG) reported results of a small phase II study evaluating the efficacy and safety of six cycles of a regimen consisting of bleomycin, etoposide, doxorubicin, cyclophosphamide, vincristine, procarbazine, and prednisone (BEACOPP) at standard doses in 12 patients with HIV-related HL.[378] The median age of the patients treated in this study was 33 years, and 92 percent had advanced stage disease. Eight of the 12 treated patients received the intended six cycles of BEACOPP. Overall, toxicity with BEA-COPP was moderate; grade 3 or 4 neutropenia occurred in 75 percent, and two patients died of opportunistic infections in the treatment period. Efficacy results from this study were impressive; all 12 patients attained complete remission of disease, although two died of infection. With a median followup of 49 months, nine patients remained alive and in continuous complete remission. Although the results of this trial are encouraging, further confirmation is required, especially considering the apparent toxicity encountered.

Although improved outcomes have been reported in the HAART era, results still are inferior compared to those in HIV-negative patients with HL, among whom even those with stage IV disease have a cure rate of approximately 70 percent. Nonetheless, at the current time, it is reasonable to treat patients with HIV-related HL using standard regimens such as ABVD or the Stanford V regimen.

REFERENCES

1. Centers for Disease Control: Case definition of acquired immunodeficiency syndrome. *MMWR Morb Mortal Wkly Rep* 30:250, 1981.
2. Centers for Disease Control: Revision of the case definition of acquired immunodeficiency syndrome for national reporting. *MMWR Morb Mortal Wkly Rep* 34:373, 1985.
3. Centers for Disease Control: Revision of the CDC surveillance case definition for acquired immunodeficiency syndrome. *MMWR Morb Mortal Wkly Rep* 36(1S):1, 1987.
4. Centers for Disease Control: New case definition of HIV/AIDS. *MMWR Morb Mortal Wkly Rep* 41:RR17, 1992.
5. Surendran A: AIDS infections, deaths hit record high in 2003. *Nat Med* 10:4, 2004.
6. Varmus H: Retroviruses. *Science* 240:1427, 1988.
7. Sharp PM, Robertson F, Gao F, Hahn B: Origins and diversity of human immunodeficiency viruses. *AIDS* 8(suppl 1):S27, 1994.
8. Gonda MA, Wong-Staal F, Gallo RC, et al: Sequence homology and morphologic similarity of HTLV-III and visna virus, a pathogenic lentivirus. *Science* 227:173, 1985.
9. Daniel MD, Letvin NL, King NW, et al: Isolation of T-cell tropic HTLV-III-like retrovirus from macaques. *Science* 228:1201, 1985.
10. Overbaugh J, Donahue PR, Quackenbush SL, et al: Molecular cloning of a feline leukemia virus that induces fatal immunodeficiency disease in cats. *Science* 239:906, 1988.
11. Ho DD, Schooley RT, Rota TR, et al: HTLV-III in the semen and blood of a healthy homosexual man. *Science* 226:451, 1984.
12. Levy JA: Human immunodeficiency viruses and the pathogenesis of AIDS. *JAMA* 261:2997, 1989.
13. Tindall B, Evans L, Cunningham P, et al: Identification of HIV-1 in semen following primary HIV-1 infection. *AIDS* 6:949, 1992.
14. Chiasson MA, Stoneburner RI, Joseph SC: Human immunodeficiency virus transmission through artificial insemination. *J Acquir Immune Defic Syndr* 3:69, 1990.
15. Vogt MW, Witt DJ, Craven DE, et al: Isolation of HTLV-III/LAV from cervical secretions of women at risk for AIDS. *Lancet* 1:525, 1986.
16. Wofsy C, Cohen J, Hauer I, et al: Isolation of AIDS associated retrovirus from genital secretions of women with antibodies to the virus. *Lancet* 1:527, 1986.
17. Pomerants RJ, de la Monte SM, Donegan SP, et al: Human immunodeficiency virus (HIV) infection of the uterine cervix. *Ann Intern Med* 108:321, 1988.
18. Anderson DA, Voeller B: AIDS and contraception, in *Clinical Perspective in Obstetrics and Gynecology*, edited by F Haseltine, D Shoupe, p 192. Springer-Verlag, New York, 1993.
19. Marmor M, Weiss LR, Lyden M, et al: Possible female to female transmission of human immunodeficiency virus. *Ann Intern Med* 105:969, 1986.
20. Monzon OT, Capellan JM: Female to female transmission of HIV. *Lancet* 2:40, 1987.
21. Stamm WE, Handsfield HH, Rompalo AM, et al: The association between genital ulcer disease and acquisition of HIV infection in homosexual men. *JAMA* 260:1429, 1988.
22. Kreiss JK, Coombs R, Plummer F, et al: Isolation of human immunodeficiency virus from genital ulcers in Nairobi prostitutes. *J Infect Dis* 160:380, 1989.
23. Grosskurth H, Mosha F, Todd J, et al: Impact of improved treatment of sexually transmitted diseases on HIV infection in rural Tanzania: Randomized controlled trial. *Lancet* 356:530, 1995.
24. Sasse H, Salmaso S, Conti S: First Drug User Multicenter Study Group: Risk behaviors for HIV-1 infection in Italian drug users: Report from a multicenter study. *J Acquir Immune Defic Syndr* 2:486, 1989.
25. Chaisson RE, Bacchetti P, Osmond D, et al: Cocaine use and HIV infection in intravenous drug users in San Francisco. *JAMA* 261:561, 1989.
26. Donegan E, Stuart M, Niland JC, et al: Infection with human immunodeficiency virus type 1 (HIV-1) among recipients of antibody-positive blood donations. *Ann Intern Med* 113:733, 1990.
27. Centers for Disease Control: Safety of therapeutic products used for hemophilia patients. *MMWR Morb Mortal Wkly Rep* 37:441, 1988.
28. Pierce GF, Lusher JM, Brownstein AP, et al: The use of purified clotting factor concentrates in hemophilia: Influence of viral safety, cost and supply on therapy. *JAMA* 261:3434, 1989.
29. Schreiber GB, Busch MP, Kleinman SH, Korelitz JJ: The risk of transfusion transmitted viral infections. *N Engl J Med* 334:1685, 1996.
30. Goedert JJ, Mendez H, Drummond JE, et al: Mother to infant transmission of human immunodeficiency virus type 1: Association with prematurity or low anti-gp 120. *Lancet* 2:1351, 1989.
31. Hira SK, Kamanga J, Bhat GJ, et al: Perinatal transmission of HIV-1 in Zambia. *BMJ* 299:1250, 1989.
32. European Collaborative Study: Risk factors for mother-to-child transmission of HIV-1. *Lancet* 339:1007, 1992.
33. Courgnaud V, Laure F, Brossard A, et al: Frequent and early in utero HIV-1 infection. *AIDS Res Hum Retroviruses* 7:337, 1991.
34. Rouzioux C, Costagliola D, Burgard M, et al: Timing of mother-to-child HIV-1 transmission depends on maternal status: The HIV infection in

newborns French Collaborative Study Group. *AIDS* 7(suppl 2):S49, 1993.

35. Burgard M, Mayaux MJ, Blanche S, et al: The use of viral culture and p24 antigen testing to HIV infection in neonates: The HIV infection in newborns French Collaborative Study Group. *N Engl J Med* 327:1192, 1992.

36. Ehrns A, Lindgren S, Dictor M, et al: HIV in pregnant women and their offspring: Evidence for late transmission. *Lancet* 337:203, 1991.

37. van de Perre P, Simonon A, Msellati P, et al: Postnatal transmission of human immunodeficiency virus type 1 from mother to infant: A prospective cohort study in Kigali, Rwanda. *N Engl J Med* 325:593, 1991.

38. Dunn DT, Newell ML, Ades AE, Peckham CS: Risk of human immunodeficiency virus type 1 transmission through breast-feeding. *Lancet* 340:585, 1992.

39. European Collaborative Study: Risk factors for mother-to-child transmission of HIV-1. *Lancet* 339:1007, 1992.

40. Mayzux M-J, Blanche S, Rouzioux C, et al: Maternal factors associated with perinatal HIV-1 transmission: The French cohort study, seven years of follow-up observation. *J Acquir Immune Defic Syndr* 8:188, 1995.

41. Fang G, Burger H, Grimson R, et al: Maternal plasma human immunodeficiency virus type 1 RNA level: A determinant and projected threshold for mother-to-child transmission. *Proc Natl Acad Sci U S A* 92:12100, 1995.

42. Weiser B, Nachman S, Tropper P, et al: Quantitation of human immunodeficiency virus type 1 during pregnancy: Relationship of viral titer to mother-to-child transmission and stability of viral load. *Proc Natl Acad Sci U S A* 91:8031, 1994.

43. Burns DN, Landesman S, Muenz LR, et al: Cigarette smoking, premature rupture of membranes, and vertical transmission of HIV-1 among women with low CD4 levels. *J Acquir Immune Defic Syndr* 7:718, 1994.

44. Nair P, Alger L, Hines S, et al: Maternal and neonatal characteristics associated with HIV infection in infants of seropositive women. *J Acquir Immune Defic Syndr* 6:298, 1993.

45. Landesman SH, Kalish LA, Burns DN, et al: Obstetrical factors and the transmission of human immunodeficiency virus type 1 from mother to child. *N Engl J Med* 334:1617, 1996.

46. Simonds RJ, Steketee R, Nesheim S, et al: Impact of zidovudine use on risk and risk factors for perinatal transmission of HIV. *AIDS* 12:301, 1998.

47. The International Perinatal HIV Group: The mode of delivery and the risk of vertical transmission of human immunodeficiency virus type 1: A meta-analysis of 15 prospective cohort studies. *N Engl J Med* 340:977, 1999.

48. European Collaborative Study: Caesarean section and the risk of vertical transmission of HIV-1 infection. *Lancet* 343:1464, 1994.

49. Stratton P, Tuomala RE, Abboud R, et al: Obstetric and newborn outcomes in a cohort of HIV-infected pregnant women: A report of the Women and Infants Transmission Study. *J Acquir Immune Defic Syndr Hum Retroviol* 20:179, 1999.

50. Centers for Disease Control and Prevention: Public Health Service Task Force recommendations for the use of antiretroviral drugs in pregnant women infected with HIV-1 for maternal health and for reducing perinatal HIV-1 transmission in the United States. *MMWR Morb Mortal Wkly Rep* 47:1, 1998.

51. Connor EM, Sperling RS, Gelver R, et al: Reduction of maternal-infant transmission of human immunodeficiency virus type 1 with zidovudine treatment. *N Engl J Med* 331:1173, 1994.

52. Shaffer N, Chauchoowong R, Mock PA, et al: Short-course zidovudine for perinatal HIV-1 transmission in Bangkok, Thailand: A randomized controlled trial. *Lancet* 353:773, 1999.

53. Jackson B, Fleming TR: Executive Summary, HIVNET 012. http://www.niaid.nih.gov/newsroom/simple/exec.htm. July 14, 1999.

54. Centers for Disease Control and Prevention: Update: Perinatally ac-

quired HIV/AIDS—United States 1997. *MMWR Morb Mortal Wkly Rep* 46:1086, 1997.

55. Pahwa SG, Quilop MTJ, Lane M, et al: Defective B-lymphocyte function in homosexual men in relation to the acquired immunodeficiency syndrome. *Ann Intern Med* 101:757, 1984.

56. Murry HW, Rubin BY, Masur H, Roberts RB: Impaired production of lymphokines and immune (gamma) interferon in the acquired immunodeficiency syndrome. *N Engl J Med* 310:883, 1984.

57. Rook AH, Masur H, Lane HC, et al: Interleukin-2 enhances the depressed natural killer and cytomegalovirus-specific cytotoxic activities of lymphocytes from patients with the acquired immunodeficiency syndrome. *J Clin Invest* 72:398, 1983.

58. Tersmette M, de Goede REY, Al BJM, et al: Differential syncytium-inducing capacity of human immunodeficiency virus isolates: Frequent detection of syncytium-inducing isolates in patients with acquired immunodeficiency syndrome (AIDS) and AIDS-related complex. *J Virol* 62:2026, 1988.

59. Pantaleo G, Graziosi C, Demarest JF, et al: HIV infection is active and progressive in lymphoid tissue during the clinically latent stage of disease. *Nature* 362:355, 1993.

60. Glushakova S, Grivel J-C, Fitzgerald W, et al: Evidence for the HIV-1 phenotype switch as a causal factor in acquired immunodeficiency. *Nat Med* 4:346, 1998.

61. Walker BD, Chakrabarti S, Moss B, et al: HIV-specific cytotoxic T lymphocytes in seropositive individuals. *Nature* 328:345, 1987.

62. Tsuchiya S, Imaizumi M, Minegishi M, et al: Lack of interleukin-2 production in a patient with OKT4+ T-cell deficiency. *N Engl J Med* 308:1294, 1983.

63. Ebert EC, Stoll DB, Cassens BJ, et al: Diminished interleukin production and receptor generation characterize the acquired immunodeficiency syndrome. *Clin Immunol Immunopathol* 37:283, 1985.

64. Prince HE, Kermani-Arab V, Fahey J: Depressed interleukin-2 receptor expression in acquired immune deficiency and lymphadenopathy syndromes. *J Immunol* 133:1313, 1984.

65. Kekow J, Wachsman W, Gross WL, et al: Transforming growth factor-beta and suppression of humoral immune responses in HIV infection. *J Clin Invest* 87:1010, 1991.

66. Ammann AJ, Abrams D, Conant M, et al: Acquired immune dysfunction in homosexual men: Immunologic profiles. *Clin Immunol Immunopathol* 27:315, 1983.

67. Wong JK, Gunthard HF, Havir DV, et al: Reduction of HIV-1 in blood and lymph nodes following potent antiretroviral therapy of HIV-1 infection. *Proc Natl Acad Sci U S A* 94:2574, 1997.

68. Cavert W, Notermans DW, Staskus K, et al: Kinetics of response in lymphoid tissues to antiretroviral therapy of HIV-1 infection. *Science* 276:960, 1997.

69. Hammer SM, Squires KE, Hughes MD, et al: A controlled trial of two nucleoside analogues plus indinavir in persons with human immunodeficiency virus infection and CD4 cell counts of 200 per cubic millimeter or less. *N Engl J Med* 337:725, 1997.

70. Palella FJ Jr, Delaney KM, Moorman AC, et al: Declining morbidity and mortality among patients with advanced human immunodeficiency virus infection. *N Engl J Med* 338:853, 1998.

71. Connors M, Kovacs JA, Krevat S, et al: HIV infection induces changes in CD4+ T-cell phenotype and depletions within the CD4+ T-cell repertoire that are not immediately restored by antiviral or immune-based therapies. *Nat Med* 3:533, 1997.

72. Gorochov G, Neumann AU, Kereveur A, et al: Perturbation of CD4+ and CD8+ T-cell repertoire during progression to AIDS and regulation of the CD4+ repertoire during antiviral therapy. *Nat Med* 4:215, 1998.

73. Chess Q, Daniels J, North E, et al: Serum immunoglobulin elevations in the acquired immunodeficiency syndrome (AIDS): IgG, IgA, IgM, and IgD. *Diagn Immunol* 2:148, 1984.

74. Lane HC, Masur H, Edgar LC, et al: Abnormalities of B-cell activation and immunoregulation in patients with the acquired immunodeficiency syndrome. *N Engl J Med* 309:453, 1983.

75. Pahwa S, Pahwa R, Saxinger C, et al: Influence of the human T-lymphotropic virus/lymphadenopathy–associated virus on functions of human lymphocytes: Evidence for immunosuppressive effects and polyclonal B-cell activation by banded viral preparations. *Proc Natl Acad Sci U S A* 82:8198, 1985.

76. Kopelman RG, Zolla-Pazner S: Association of human immunodeficiency virus infection and autoimmune phenomena. *Am J Med* 84:82, 1988.

77. Walsh CM, Nardi MA, Karpatkin S: On the mechanism of thrombocytopenic purpura in sexually active homosexual men. *N Engl J Med* 311:635, 1984.

78. van der Lelie J, Lange JMA, Vos JJE, et al: Autoimmunity against blood cells in human immunodeficiency virus infection. *Br J Haematol* 67:755, 1987.

79. Stricker RB, McHugh TM, Moody D, et al: An AIDS-related cytotoxic autoantibody reacts with a specific antigen on stimulated CD4+ cells. *Nature* 327:170, 1987.

80. Rossi G, Goria R, Stellini R, et al: Prevalence, clinical, and laboratory features of thrombocytopenia in HIV-infected individuals. *AIDS Res Hum Retroviruses* 6:261, 1990.

81. Murphy MF, Metcalfe P, Waters AH, et al: Incidence and mechanism of neutropenia and thrombocytopenia in patients with human immunodeficiency virus infection. *Br J Haematol* 66:337, 1987.

82. Ballem PJ, Belzberg A, Devine DV, et al: Kinetic studies of the mechanism of thrombocytopenia in patients with human immunodeficiency virus infection. *N Engl J Med* 327:1179, 1992.

83. Gartner S, Markovits P, Markovitz DM, et al: The role of mononuclear phagocytes in HTLV-III/LAV infection. *Science* 233:215, 1986.

84. Armstrong GA, Horne R: Follicular dendritic cells and virus-like particles in AIDS-related lymphadenopathy. *Lancet* 2:370, 1984.

85. Poli G, Bottazzi B, Acero R, et al: Monocyte function in intravenous drug abusers with lymphadenopathy syndrome and in patients with the acquired immunodeficiency syndrome: Selective impairment of chemotaxis. *Clin Exp Immunol* 62:136, 1985.

86. Murray HW, Gellene RA, Libby DM, et al: Activation of tissue macrophages from AIDS patients: In vitro response of alveolar macrophages to lymphokines and interferon gamma. *J Immunol* 135:1501, 1985.

87. Kleinerman ES, Ceccorulli LM, Zwelling LA, et al: Activation of monocyte-mediated tumoricidal activity in patients with acquired immunodeficiency syndrome. *J Clin Oncol* 3:1005, 1985.

88. Creemers PC, Stark DF, Boyko WJ: Evaluation of natural killer cell activity in patients with persistent generalized lymphadenopathy and acquired immunodeficiency syndrome. *J Clin Lab Immunol* 14:114, 1984.

89. Klatzman M, Lederman MM: Defective postbinding lysis underlies the impaired natural killer activity in factor VIII–treated human T lymphotropic virus type III seropositive hemophiliacs. *J Clin Invest* 45:406, 1986.

90. Reddy MM, Chinoy P, Grieco MH: Differential effects of interferon alpha and interleukin-2 on natural killer cell activity in patients with the acquired immune deficiency syndrome. *J Biol Response Mod* 3:379, 1984.

91. Horsburgh CR Jr, Ou CY, Jason J, et al: Duration of human immunodeficiency virus infection before detection of antibody. *Lancet* 2:637, 1989.

92. Imagawa DT, Lee MH, Wolinsky SM, et al: HIV-1 infection in homosexual men who remain seronegative for prolonged periods. *N Engl J Med* 320:1458, 1989.

93. Brettler DB, Somasundaran M, Forsberg AF, et al: Silent human immunodeficiency virus type 1 infection: A rare occurrence in a high-risk heterosexual population. *Blood* 80:2396, 1992.

94. Read S, Cassol S, Coates R, et al: Detection of incident HIV infection by PCR compared to serology. *J Acquir Immune Defic Syndr* 5:1075, 1992.

95. Goudsmit J, Lange JM, Krone WJ, et al: Pathogenesis of HIV and its implications for serodiagnosis and monitoring of antiviral therapy. *J Virol Methods* 17:19, 1987.

96. Tindall B, Cooper DA, Donovan B, et al: Primary human immunodeficiency virus infection: Clinical and serologic aspects. *Infect Dis Clin North Am* 2:329, 1988.

97. Alter HJ, Epstein JS, Swensen SG, et al: Prevalence of human immunodeficiency virus type 1 p24 antigen in U.S. blood donors: An assessment of the efficacy of testing in donor screening. *N Engl J Med* 323:1312, 1990.

98. Mellors JW, Rinaldo CR Jr, Gupta P, et al: Prognosis in HIV-1 infection predicted by the quantity of virus in plasma. *Science* 272:1167, 1996.

99. Mellors JW, Munoz A, Giorgi J, et al: Plasma viral load and CD4+ lymphocytes as prognostic markers of HIV-1 infection. *Ann Intern Med* 126:946, 1997.

100. Department of Health and Human Services: Guidelines for the use of antiretroviral agents of HIV-1-infected adults and adolescents. Available at http://www.aidsinfo.nih.gov, last accessed March 23, 2004.

101. Hammer SM, Squires KE, Hughes MD, et al: A controlled trial of two nucleoside analogues plus indinavir in persons with human immunodeficiency virus infection and CD4 cell counts of 200/mm³ or less. *N Engl J Med* 337:725, 1997.

102. Centers for Disease Control and Prevention: Guidelines for the use of antiretroviral agents in HIV-infected adults and adolescents. *MMWR Morb Mortal Wkly Rep* 48: 1999.

103. Tural C, Romeu J, Sirera G, et al: Long lasting remission of cytomegalovirus retinitis without maintenance therapy in human immunodeficiency virus infected patients. *J Infect Dis* 177.1080, 1998.

104. Li TS, Tubiana R, Katlama C, et al: Long-lasting recovery in CD4 T cell function and viral load reduction after highly active antiretroviral therapy in advanced HIV-1 disease. *Lancet* 351:1682, 1998.

105. Furrer H, Egger M, Opravil M, et al: Discontinuation of primary prophylaxis against *Pneumocystis carinii* pneumonia in HIV-1 infected adults treated with combination antiretroviral therapy. *N Engl J Med* 340:1301, 1999.

106. Mocroft A, Ledergerber B, Katlama C, et al: Decline in the AIDS and death rates in the EuroSIDA study: An observational study. *Lancet* 362: 22, 2003.

107. Cooper DA, Maclean P, Finlayson R, et al: Acute AIDS retrovirus infection. *Lancet* 1:537, 1985.

108. Fox R, Eldred LJ, Fuchs EJ, et al: Clinical manifestations of acute infection with human immunodeficiency virus in a cohort of gay men. *AIDS* 1:35, 1987.

109. Lemp GF, Payne SF, Rutherford GW, et al: Projections of AIDS morbidity and mortality in San Francisco. *JAMA* 263:1497, 1990.

110. Moss AR, Bacchetti P: Editorial review: Natural history of HIV infection. *AIDS* 3:55, 1989.

111. Schoenbaum EE, Hartel D, Friedland G: HIV infection and intravenous drug use. *Curr Opin Infect Dis* 3:80, 1990.

112. Volberding P: Clinical spectrum of HIV disease, in *AIDS: Etiology, Diagnosis, Treatment and Prevention*, 3rd ed, edited by VT DeVita Jr, S Hellman, SA Rosenberg, p 123. Lippincott, Philadelphia, 1992.

113. Samson M, Libert F, Doranz BJ: Resistance to HIV-1 infection in Caucasian individuals bearing mutant alleles of the CCR-5 chemokine receptor gene. *Nature* 382:722, 1996.

114. Phillips AN: Studies of prognostic markers in HIV infection: Implications for pathogenesis. *AIDS* 6:1391, 1992.

115. Munoz A, Carey V, Saah AJ, et al: Predictors of decline in CD4 lymphocytes in a cohort of homosexual men infected with human immunodeficiency virus. *J Acquir Immune Defic Syndr* 1:396, 1988.

116. Malone JL, Simms TE, Gray GC, et al: Sources of variability in repeated T-helper lymphocyte counts from human immunodeficiency virus type 1 infected patients: Total lymphocyte count fluctuations and diurnal cycle are important. *J Acquir Immune Defic Syndr* 3:144, 1990.

117. Anderson RE, Lang W, Shiboski S, et al: Use of beta 2 microglobulin level and CD4 lymphocyte count to predict development of acquired immunodeficiency syndrome in persons with human immunodeficiency virus infection. *Arch Intern Med* 150:73, 1990.

118. Melmed RN, Taylor JMG, Detels R, et al: Serum neopterin changes in HIV infected subjects: Indicator of significant pathology, CD4 T cell changes, and the development of AIDS. *J Acquir Immune Defic Syndr* 2:70, 1989.

119. Mitsuyasu R: *AIDS Clin Review 1993/4*, p 189. Marcel Dekker, New York, 1993.

120. Zon LI, Arkin C, Groopman JE: Hematologic manifestations of the human immunodeficiency virus (HIV). *Semin Hematol* 25:208, 1988.

121. Sullivan PS, Hanson DL, Chu SY, et al: Epidemiology of anemia in human immunodeficiency virus infected persons: Results from the Multistate Adult and Adolescent Spectrum of HIV Disease Surveillance Project. *Blood* 91:301, 1998.

122. Levine AM, Berhane K, Masri-Lavine L: Prevalence and correlates of anemia in a large cohort of HIV-infected women: Women's Interagency HIV Study. *J Acquir Immune Defic Syndr* 26:28, 2001.

123. Mocroft A, Kirk O, Barton SE, et al: Anaemia is an independent predictive marker for clinical prognosis in HIV infected patients from across Europe. *AIDS* 13:943, 1999.

124. Spivak JL, Barnes DC, Fuchs E, Quinn TC: Serum immunoreactive erythropoietin in HIV infected patients. *JAMA* 261:310, 1989.

125. Seneviratne LS, Tulpule A, Mummaneni M, et al: Clinical, immunological, and pathologic correlates of bone marrow involvement in 253 patients with AIDS-related lymphoma. *Blood* 92:244A, 1998.

126. Walker RE, Parker RI, Kovacs JA, et al: Anemia and erythropoiesis in patients with the acquired immunodeficiency syndrome (AIDS) and Kaposi sarcoma treated with zidovudine. *Ann Intern Med* 108:372, 1988.

127. Richman DD, Fischl MA, Grieco MH, et al: The toxicity of azidothymidine (AZT) in the treatment of patients with AIDS and AIDS-related complex: A double-blind, placebo-controlled trial. *N Engl J Med* 317:192, 1987.

128. Anderson LJ: Human parvoviruses. *J Infect Dis* 161:603, 1990.

129. Frickhofen N, Abkowitz JL, Safford M, et al: Persistent B19 parvovirus infection in patients infected with human immunodeficiency virus type 1 (HIV-1): A treatable cause of anemia in AIDS. *Ann Intern Med* 113:926, 1990.

130. Rarick MU, Espina B, Mocharnuk R, et al: Thrombotic thrombocytopenic purpura in patients with human immunodeficiency virus infection: A report of three cases and review of the literature. *Am J Hematol* 40:103, 1992.

131. Sasadeusz J, Buchanan M, Speed B: Reactive haemophagocytic syndrome in human immunodeficiency virus infection. *J Infect* 20:65, 1990.

132. Sproat LO, Pantanowitz L, Lu CM, et al: Human immunodeficiency virus-associated hemophagocytosis with iron-deficiency anemia and massive splenomegaly. *Clin Infect Dis* 37:170, 2003.

133. Telen MJ, Roberts KB, Bartlett JA: HIV associated autoimmune hemolytic anemia: Report of a case and review of the literature. *AIDS* 3:933, 1990.

134. McGinniss MH, Macher AM, Rook AH, Alter HJ: Red cell autoantibodies in patients with acquired immune deficiency syndrome. *Transfusion* 26:405, 1986.

135. Gupta S, Licorish K: The Coombs' test and the acquired immunodeficiency syndrome. *Ann Intern Med* 100:462, 1984.

136. Toy PTCY, Reid ME, Burns M: Positive direct antiglobulin test associated with hyperglobulinemia in AIDS. *Am J Hematol* 19:145, 1985.

137. Harriman GR, Smith PD, Horne MK, et al: Vitamin B_{12} malabsorption in patients with acquired immunodeficiency syndrome. *Arch Intern Med* 149:2039, 1989.

138. Herbert V, Fong W, Gulle V, Stopler T: Low holotranscobalamin II is the earliest serum marker for subnormal vitamin B_{12} (cobalamin) absorption in patients with AIDS. *Am J Hematol* 34:132, 1990.

139. Sullivan PS, Hanson DL, Chu SY, et al: Epidemiology of anemia in human immunodeficiency virus infected persons: Results from the Multistate Adult and Adolescent Spectrum of HIV Disease Surveillance Project. *Blood* 91:301, 1998.

140. Moore RD, Keruly JC, Chaisson RE: Anemia and survival in HIV infection. *J Acquir Immune Defic Syndr* 19:29, 1998.

141. Mocroft A, Kirk O, Barton SE, et al: Anaemia is an independent predictive marker for clinical prognosis in HIV infected patients from across Europe. *AIDS* 13:943, 1999.

142. Berhane K, Karim R, Cohen MH: Impact of highly active antiretroviral therapy on anemia and relationship between anemia and survival in a large cohort of HIV-infected women: Women's Interagency HIV Study. *J Acquir Immune Defic Syndr* 37:1245, 2004.

143. Lundgren JD, Mocroft A, Gatell JM, et al: A clinically prognostic scoring system for patients receiving highly active antiretroviral therapy: Results from the EuroSIDA Study. *J Infect Dis* 185:178, 2002.

144. Saag MS, Bowers P, Leitz GJ, et al: Once-weekly epoetin alfa improves quality of life and increases hemoglobin in anemic HIV+ patients. *AIDS Res Hum Retroviruses* 20:1037, 2004.

145. Grossman HA, Goon B, Bowers P, et al: Once-weekly epoetin alfa dosing is as effective as three times-weekly dosing in increasing hemoglobin levels and is associated with improved quality of life in anemic HIV-infected patients. *J Acquir Immune Defic Syndr* 34:368, 2003.

146. Moore RD, Forney D: Anemia in HIV-infected patients receiving highly active antiretroviral therapy. *J Acquir Immune Defic Syndr* 29:54, 2002.

147. Isgro A, Mezzaroma I, Aiuti A, et al: Recovery of hematopoietic activity in bone marrow from human immunodeficiency virus type 1 infected patients during highly active antiretroviral therapy. *AIDS Res Hum Retroviruses* 16:1471, 2000.

148. Huang SS, Barbour JD, Deeks SG, et al: Reversal of human immunodeficiency virus type 1 associated hematosuppression by effective antiretroviral therapy. *Clin Infect Dis* 30:504, 2000.

149. Spivak JL, Barnes DC, Fuchs E, et al: Serum immunoreactive erythropoietin in HIV-infected patients. *JAMA* 261:3104, 1989.

150. Moore RD: Human immunodeficiency virus infection, anemia, and survival. *Clin Infect Dis* 29:44, 1999.

151. Sipsas NV, Kokori SI, Ionnidis JPA, et al: Circulating autoantibodies to erythropoietin are associated with human immunodeficiency virus type 1 related anemia. *J Infect Dis* 180:2044, 1999.

152. Henry DH, Beall GN, Benson CA, et al: Recombinant human erythropoietin in the treatment of anemia associated with human immunodeficiency virus (HIV) infection and zidovudine therapy: Overview of four clinical trials. *Ann Intern Med* 117:739, 1992.

153. Demetri G, Wade J, Cella D, et al: Epoetin alfa improves quality of life in cancer patients receiving cytotoxic treatment independent of disease response: Prospective clinical trial results. *Blood* 90:175a, 1997.

154. Miles SA: The use of hematopoietic growth factors in HIV infection and AIDS-related malignancies. *Cancer Invest* 9:229, 1991.

155. Abrams DI, Steinhart C, Frascino R: Epoetin alfa therapy for anemia in HIV infected patients: Impact on quality of life. *Int J STD AIDS* 11:659, 2000.

156. Bennett CL, Luminari S, Nissenson AR, et al: Pure red-cell aplasia and epoetin therapy. *N Engl J Med* 351:1403, 2004.

157. Tulpule A, Dharmapala D, Burian P, et al: Treatment of Anemia with Aranesp® (Darbepoetin-alfa) given once every two weeks in HIV seropositive patients. *Blood* 104:2108a, 2004.

158. Murphy M, Metcalfe P, Waters A: Incidence and mechanism of neutropenia and thrombocytopenia in patients with human immunodeficiency virus infection. *Br J Haematol* 66:337, 1987.

159. Bagnara GP, Zauli G, Giovannini M, et al: Early loss of circulating hemopoietic progenitors in HIV-1 infected subjects. *Exp Hematol* 18:426, 1990.

160. Leiderman I, Greenberg M, Adelsberg B, et al: A glycoprotein inhibitor of in vitro granulopoiesis associated with AIDS. *Blood* 70:1267, 1987.

161. Klaassen RJ, Mulder JW, Vlekke AB, et al: Autoantibodies against peripheral blood cells appear early in HIV infection and their prevalence increases with disease progression. *Clin Exp Immunol* 81:11, 1990.

162. Mauss S, Steinmetz HT, Willers R, et al: Induction of granulocyte colony-stimulating factor by acute febrile infection but not by neutropenia in HIV seropositive individuals. *J Acquir Immune Defic Syndr* 14:430, 1997.

163. Karcher DS, Frost AR: The bone marrow in human immunodeficiency virus (HIV)-related disease. Morphology and clinical correlation. *Am J Clin Pathol* 95:63, 1991.

164. Elis M, Gupta S, Galant S, et al: Impaired neutrophil function in patients with AIDS or AIDS-related complex: A comprehensive evaluation. *J Infect Dis* 158:1268, 1988.

165. Bodey GP, Buckley M, Sathe US, et al: Qualitative relationships between circulating leukocytes and infection in patients with acute leukemia. *Ann Intern Med* 64:328, 1966.

166. Moore RD, Keruly J, Chaisson RE, et al: Neutropenia and bacterial infection in acquired immunodeficiency syndrome. *Arch Intern Med* 155:1965, 1995.

167. Jacobson MA, Cohen PT, Liu RC, et al: Risk of hospitalization for serious bacterial infection associated with neutropenia severity in patients with HIV [abstract 231]. 11th International Conference on AIDS, Vancouver, Canada, 1996.

168. Meynard J-L, Guiguet M, Arsac S, et al: Frequency and risk factors of infectious complications in neutropenic patients infected with HIV. *AIDS* 11:995, 1997.

169. Moore DAJ, Benepal T, Portsmouth S, et al: Etiology and natural history of neutropenia in human immunodeficiency virus disease: A prospective study. *Clin Infect Dis* 32:469, 2001.

170. Sloand EM, Maciejewski J, Kumar P, et al: Protease inhibitors stimulate hematopoiesis and decrease apoptosis and ICE expression in CD34+ cells. *Blood* 96:2735, 2000.

171. Groopman JE, Feder D: Hematopoietic growth factors in AIDS. *Semin Oncol* 19:408, 1992.

172. Groopman JE, Mitsuyasu RT, DeLeo MJ, et al: Effect of recombinant human granulocyte-macrophage colony stimulating factor on myelopoiesis in the acquired immunodeficiency syndrome. *N Engl J Med* 317:593, 1987.

173. Lieschke GJ, Burgess AW: Granulocyte colony-stimulating factor and granulocyte-macrophage colony-stimulating factor (1). *N Engl J Med* 327:28, 1992.

174. Lieschke GJ, Burgess AW: Granulocyte colony-stimulating factor and granulocyte-macrophage colony-stimulating factor (2). *N Engl J Med* 327:99, 1992.

175. Avalos BR, Parker JM, Ware DA, et al: Dissociation of the Jak kinase pathway from G-CSF receptor signaling in neutrophils. *Exp Hematol* 25:160, 1997.

176. Kaplan LD, Kahn JO, Crowe S, et al: Clinical and virologic effects of recombinant human granulocyte-macrophage colony-stimulating factor in patients receiving chemotherapy for human immunodeficiency virus-associated non-Hodgkin's lymphoma: Results of a randomized trial. *J Clin Oncol* 9:929, 1991.

177. Kedzierska K, Maerz A, Warby T, et al: Granulocyte-macrophage colony-stimulating factor inhibits HIV-1 replication in monocyte-derived macrophages. *AIDS* 14:1739, 2000.

178. Barbaro G, Di Lorenzo G, Grisorio B, et al: Effect of recombinant human granulocyte-macrophage colony-stimulating factor on HIV-related leukopenia: A randomized, controlled clinical study. *AIDS* 11:1453, 1997.

179. Brites C, Gilbert MJ, Pedral-Sampaio D, et al: A randomized, placebo-controlled trial of granulocyte-macrophage colony-stimulating factor and nucleoside analogue therapy in AIDS. *J Infect Dis* 182:1531, 2000.

180. Kuritzkes DR, Parenti D, Ward DJ, et al: Filgrastim prevents severe neutropenia and reduces infective morbidity in patients with advanced HIV infection: Results of a randomized, multicenter, controlled trial. G-CSF 930101 Study Group *AIDS* 12:65, 1998.

181. Keiser P, Higgs E, Scanton J: Neutropenia is associated with bacteremia in patients with HIV. *Am J Med Sci* 312:118, 1996.

182. Pechere M, Samii K, Hirschel B: HIV related thrombocytopenia. *N Engl J Med* 328:1785, 1993.

183. Sullivan PS, Hanson DL, Chu SY, et al: Surveillance for thrombocytopenia in persons infected with HIV: Results from the multistate Adult and Adolescent Spectrum of Disease Project. *J Acquir Immune Defic Syndr* 14:374, 1997.

184. Pearce CL, Wendy JM, Levine AM, et al: "Thrombocytopenia is a Strong Predictor of All-Cause and AIDS-Specific Mortality in Women with HIV: The Women's Interagency HIV Study." 46th Annual Meeting of the American Society of Hematology, San Diego, California, 2004.

185. Ballem PJ, Belzberg A, Devine DV, et al: Kinetic studies of the mechanism of thrombocytopenia in patients with human immunodeficiency virus infection. *N Engl J Med* 327:1779, 1992.

186. Walsh CM, Nardi MA, Karpatkin S: On the mechanism of thrombocytopenic purpura in sexually active homosexual men. *N Engl J Med* 311:635, 1984.

187. Bettaieb A, Fromont P, Louache F, et al: Presence of cross-reactive antibody between human immunodeficiency virus (HIV) and platelet glycoproteins in HIV related immune thrombocytopenic purpura. *Blood* 80:162, 1992.

188. Kouri Y, Borkowsky W, Nardi M, et al: Human megakaryocytes have a CD4+ molecule capable of binding human immunodeficiency virus-1. *Blood* 81:2664, 1993.

189. Zucker-Franklin D, Seremetis S, Heng ZY: Internalization of human immunodeficiency virus type I and other retroviruses by megakaryocytes and platelets. *Blood* 75:1920, 1990.

190. Wang J-F, Liu Z-Y, Groopman JE: The alpha-chemokine receptor CXCR4 is expressed on the megakaryocytic lineage from progenitor to platelets, and modulates migration and adhesion. *Blood* 92:756, 1998.

191. Zucker-Franklin D, Cao Y: Megakaryocytes of human immunodeficiency virus-infected individuals express viral RNA. *Proc Natl Acad Sci U S A* 86:5595, 1989.

192. Zucker-Franklin D, Termin CS, Cooper MC: Structural changes in the megakaryocytes of patients infected with the human immunodeficiency virus (HIV-1). *Am J Pathol* 134:1295, 1989.

193. Swiss Group for Clinical Studies on AIDS: Zidovudine for the treatment of thrombocytopenia associated with HIV: A prospective study. *Ann Intern Med* 109:718, 1988.

194. Harker LA, Marzec UM, Novembre F, et al: Treatment of thrombocytopenia in chimpanzees infected with HIV by pegylated recombinant human megakaryocyte growth and development factor. *Blood* 91:4427, 1998.

195. Oksenhendler E, Bierling P, Farcet JP, et al: Response to therapy in 37 patients with HIV related thrombocytopenic purpura. *Br J Haematol* 66:49, 1987.

196. Oksenhendler E, Bierling P, Ferchal F, et al: Zidovudine for thrombocytopenic purpura related to human immunodeficiency virus (HIV) infection. *Ann Intern Med* 110:365, 1989.

197. Landonio G, Cinque P, Nosari A, et al: Comparison of two dose regimens of zidovudine in an open, randomized, multicenter study for severe HIV related thrombocytopenia. *AIDS* 7:209, 1993.

198. Caso JAA, Mingo CS, Tena JG: Effect of highly active antiretroviral therapy on thrombocytopenia in patients with HIV infection. *N Engl J Med* 16:1239, 1999.

199. Carbonara S, Fiorentino G, Serio G, et al: Response of severe HIV-associated thrombocytopenia to highly active antiretroviral therapy including protease inhibitors. *J Infect* 42:251, 2001.

200. Marroni M, Gresele P, Landonio G, et al: Interferon-a is effective in the treatment of HIV-1 related, severe, zidovudine-resistant thrombocytopenia: A prospective, placebo-controlled, double-blind trial. *Ann Intern Med* 121:423, 1994.

201. Vianelli N, Catani L, Gugliotta L, et al: Recombinant alpha-interferon 2b in the treatment of HIV related thrombocytopenia. *AIDS* 7:823, 1993.

202. Imbach P, D'Apuzzo V, Hirt A, et al: High dose intravenous gammaglobulin for idiopathic thrombocytopenic purpura in childhood. *Lancet* 1:1228, 1981.

203. Bussel JB, Saimi JS: Isolated thrombocytopenia in patients infected with HIV: Treatment with intravenous gammaglobulin. *Am J Hematol* 28:79, 1998.

204. Gringeri A, Cattaneo M, Santagostino E, Mannucci PM: Intramuscular anti-D immunoglobulins for home treatment of chronic immune thrombocytopenic purpura. *Br J Hematol* 80:337, 1992.

205. Oksenhendler E, Bierling P, Brossard Y, et al: Anti-Rh immunoglobulin therapy for human immunodeficiency virus-related immune thrombocytopenic purpura. *Blood* 71:1499, 1988.

206. Oksenhendler E, Bierling P, Chevret S, et al: Splenectomy is safe and effective in human immunodeficiency virus related immune thrombocytopenia. *Blood* 82:29, 1993.

207. Kemeny MM, Cooke V, Melester TS, et al: Splenectomy in patients with AIDS and AIDS-related complex. *AIDS* 7:1063, 1993.

208. Becker DM, Saunders TJ, Wispelwey B, Schain DC: Case report: Venous thromboembolism in AIDS. *Am J Med Sci* 303;395, 1992.

209. Roberts SP, Haefs TMP: Central retinal vein occlusion in a middle aged adult with HIV infection. *Optom Vis Sci* 210:108, 1992.

210. Tanimowo M: Deep vein thrombosis as a manifestation of acquired immunodeficiency syndrome? A case report. *Cent Afr J Med* 42:327, 1996.

211. Narayanan TS, Narawane NM, Phadke AY, et al: Multiple abdominal venous thrombosis in HIV seropositive patient. *Indian J Gastroenterol* 17:105, 1998.

212. Sullivan PS, Dworkin MS, Jones JL, et al: Epidemiology of thrombosis in HIV-infected individuals. *AIDS* 14:321, 2000.

213. Jacobson MC, Dezube BJ, Aboulafia DM: Thrombotic complications in patients infected with HIV in the era of highly active antiretroviral therapy: A case series. *Clin Infect Dis* 39:1214, 2004.

214. Copur AS, Smith PR, Gomez V, et al: HIV infection is a risk factor for venous thromboembolism. *AIDS Patient Care STDS* 16:205, 2002.

215. Fultz SL, McGinnis KA, Skanderson M, et al: Association of venous thromboembolism with Human Immunodeficiency virus and mortality in Veterans. *Am J Med* 116:420, 2004.

216. Birx DL, Redfield RR, Tencer K, et al: Induction of interleukin 6 during human immunodeficiency virus infection. *Blood* 76:2303, 1990.

217. Emilie D, Peuchmaur M, Maillot MC, et al: Production of interleukins in HIV-1 replicating lymph nodes. *J Clin Invest* 86:148, 1990.

218. Hack EC: Tissue factor pathway of coagulation in sepsis. *Crit Care Med* 28 (suppl):25S, 2000.

219. Nawroth PP, Handley DA, Esmon CT, Stern DM: Interleukin 1 induces endothelial cell pro-coagulant while suppressing cell-surface anti coagulant activity. *Proc Natl Acad Sci U S A* 83:3460, 1986.

220. Levine AM, Vigen C, Gravink J, et al: Development of Prothrombotic Repertoire with Progressive HIV Disease: Data from the Women's Interagency HIV Study WIHS Program and abstracts of the 46th Annual Meeting of the American Society of Hematology [abstract 1057]. December 4, 2004; San Diego, California.

221. Iranzo A, Domingo P, Cadafalch J, Sambeat MA: Intracranial venous and dural sinus thrombosis due to protein S deficiency in a patient with AIDS. *J Neurol Neurosurg Psychiatry* 64:688, 1998.

222. Bissuel F, Berruyer M, Causse X, et al: Acquired Protein S deficiency: Correlation with advanced disease in HIV 1 infected patients. *J Acquir Immune Defic Syndr* 5:484, 1992.

223. Pulik M, Lebret-Lerolle D: Acquired protein S deficiency in HIV infections. *Ann Med Interne (Paris)* 143:57, 1992.

224. Stahl CP, Wideman CS, Spira TJ, et al: Protein S deficiency in men with long term human immunodeficiency virus infection. *Blood* 81:1801, 1993.

225. Sorice M, Griggi T, Acieri P, et al: Protein S and HIV infection. The role of anticardiolipin and anti-protein S antibodies. *Thromb Res* 73:165, 1992.

226. Erbe M, Rickerts V, Bauersachs RM, et al: Acquired protein C and protein S deficiency in HIV-infected patients. *Clin Appl Thromb Hemost* 9:325, 2003.

227. Feffer SE, Fox FL, Orsen MM, et al: Thrombotic tendencies and correlation with clinical status in patients infected with HIV. *South Med J* 88:1126, 1995.

228. Toulon P, Lamine M, Ledjev I, et al: Heparin cofactor II deficiency in patients infected with the human immunodeficiency virus. *Thromb Haemost* 70:730, 1993.

229. Bloom EJ, Abrams DI, Rodgers G, et al: Lupus anticoagulant in the Acquired Immunodeficiency Syndrome. *JAMA* 256:491, 1986.

230. Peters BS, Beck EJ, Coleman DG, et al: Changing disease patterns in patients with AIDS in a referral center in the United Kingdom: The changing face of AIDS. *BMJ* 302:203, 1991.

231. Pluda JM, Yarchoan R, Jaffe ES, et al: Development of non-Hodgkin's lymphoma in a cohort of patients with severe human immunodeficiency virus (HIV) infection on long-term antiretroviral therapy. *Ann Intern Med* 113:276, 1990.

232. Gail MH, Pluda JM, Rabkin CS, et al: Projections of the incidence of non-Hodgkin's lymphoma related to acquired immunodeficiency syndrome. *J Natl Cancer Inst* 83:695, 1991.

233. Rabkin CS, Biggar RJ, Horm JW: Increasing incidence of cancers associated with the human immunodeficiency virus epidemic. *Int J Cancer* 47:692, 1991.

234. Beral V, Peterman T, Berkelman R, Jaffe H: AIDS-associated non-Hodgkin lymphoma. *Lancet* 337:805, 1991.

235. Biggar RJ, Rabkin CS: The epidemiology of acquired immunodeficiency syndrome-related lymphomas. *Curr Opin Oncol* 4:883, 1992.

236. Pluda JM, Vanzon D, Tosato G, et al: Factors which predict for the development of non-Hodgkin's lymphoma in patients with HIV infection receiving antiretroviral therapy. *Blood* 78:285a, 1991.

237. Cote TR, Biggar RJ, Rosenberg PS, et al: Non-Hodgkin's lymphoma among people with AIDS: Incidence, presentation, and public health burden. AIDS/Cancer Study Group. *Int J Cancer* 73:645, 1997.

238. Franceschi S, Dal Maso L, La Vecchia C: Advances in the epidemiology of HIV-associated non-Hodgkin's lymphoma and other lymphoid neoplasms. *Int J Cancer* 83:481, 1999.

239. Mocroft A, Katlama C, Johnson AM, et al: AIDS across Europe 1994-98: The EuroSIDA study. *Lancet* 356:291, 2000.

240. Rabkin CS, Testa MA, Huang J, et al: Kaposi's sarcoma and non-Hodgkin's lymphoma incidence trends in AIDS Clinical Trial Group study participants. *J Acquir Immune Defic Syndr* 21(suppl 1):S31, 1999.

241. Dore GJ, Li Y, McDonald A, et al: Impact of highly active antiretroviral therapy on individual AIDS-defining illness incidence and survival in Australia. *J Acquir Immune Defic Syndr* 4:388, 2002.

242. Ledergerber B, Telenti A, Egger M, et al: Risk of HIV-related Kaposi's sarcoma and non-Hodgkin's lymphoma with potent antiretroviral therapy: Prospective cohort study. *BMJ* 319:23, 1999.

243. Jacobson LP: Impact of highly effective anti-retroviral therapy on the

incidence of malignancies among HIV infected individuals [abstract S5]. *J Acquir Immune Defic Syndr* 17:A39, 1998.

244. International Collaboration on HIV and Cancer: Highly active antiretroviral therapy and incidence of cancer in human immunodeficiency virus-infected adults. *J Natl Cancer Inst* 92:1823, 2000.

245. Kirk O, Pedersen C, Cozzi-Lepri A, et al: Non-Hodgkin lymphoma in HIV-infected patients in the era of highly active antiretroviral therapy. *Blood* 98:3406, 2001.

246. Besson C, Goubar A, Gabarre J, et al: Changes in AIDS-related lymphoma since the era of highly active antiretroviral therapy. *Blood* 98:2339, 2001.

247. Purtilo DT: Opportunistic non-Hodgkin's lymphoma in X-linked recessive immunodeficiency and lymphoproliferative syndromes. *Semin Oncol* 4:335, 1977.

248. Levine AM, Taylor CR, Schneider DR, et al: Immunoblastic sarcoma of T cell versus B cell origin: I. Clinical features. *Blood* 58:52, 1981.

249. Penn I: Tumors of the immunocompromised patient. *Annu Rev Med* 39:63, 1988.

250. Swinnen LJ, Costanzo-Nordin MR, Fisher SG, et al: Increased incidence of lymphoproliferative disorder after immunosuppression with the monoclonal antibody OKT3 in cardiac transplant recipients. *N Engl J Med* 323:1723, 1990.

251. Pantaleo G, Graziosi C, Fauci AS: Mechanisms of disease: The immunopathogenesis of human immunodeficiency virus infection. *N Engl J Med* 328:327, 1993.

252. Birx DI, Redfield RR, Tosato G: Defective regulation of Epstein-Barr virus infection in patients with acquired immunodeficiency syndrome (AIDS) or AIDS-related disorders. *N Engl J Med* 314:874, 1986.

253. Shear GM, Salahuddin SZ, Markham PD, et al: Prospective study of cytotoxic T lymphocyte responses to influenza virus and antibodies to human T lymphotropic virus-III in homosexual men: Selective loss of influenza-specific human leukocyte antigen-restricted cytotoxic lymphocyte response to human T lymphotropic virus-III positive individuals with symptoms of acquired immunodeficiency syndrome. *J Clin Invest* 76:1699, 1985.

254. Feichtinger H, Rutkonen P, Parravicini C, et al: Malignant lymphomas in *Cynomolgus* monkeys infected with simian immunodeficiency virus. *Am J Pathol* 137.1311, 1990.

255. Jelinek DF, Lipsky PE: Enhancement of human B cell proliferation and differentiation by tumor necrosis factor-alpha and interleukin 1. *J Immunol* 139:2970, 1987.

256. Fauci A, Schnittman SM, Poli G, et al: Immunopathogenetic mechanisms in human immunodeficiency virus (HIV) infection. *Ann Intern Med* 114:678, 1991.

257. Kawano M, Hirano T, Matsuda T, et al: Autocrine generation and requirement of BSF-2/IL-6 for human multiple myelomas. *Nature* 332:83, 1988.

258. Biondi A, Rossi V, Bassan R, et al: Constitutive expression of IL-6 gene in chronic lymphocytic leukemia. *Blood* 73:1279, 1989.

259. Emillie D, Coumbaras J, Raphael M, et al: IL-6 production in high grade B lymphomas: Correlation with presence of malignant immunoblasts in AIDS and in HIV-seronegative patients. *Blood* 80:498, 1992.

260. Benjamin D, Knobloch TJ, Abrams J, Dayton MA: Human B cell IL-10: B cell lines derived from patients with AIDS and Burkitt's lymphoma constitutively secrete large quantities of IL-10. *Blood* 78:384a, 1991.

261. Masood R, Bond M, Scadden D, et al: Interleukin-10: An autocrine B cell growth for human B-cell lymphomas and their progenitors. *Blood* 80:115a, 1992.

262. Poli G, Fauci AS: The effect of cytokines and pharmacologic agents on chronic HIV infection. *AIDS Res Hum Retroviruses* 8:191, 1992.

263. Shibata D, Weiss LM, Nathwani BN, et al: Epstein-Barr virus in benign lymph node biopsies from individuals infected with the human immunodeficiency virus is associated with concurrent or subsequent development of non-Hodgkin's lymphoma. *Blood* 77:1527, 1991.

264. MacMahon EME, Glass JD, Hayward SD, et al: Epstein-Barr virus in AIDS-related primary central nervous system lymphoma. *Lancet* 338:969, 1991.

265. Wang D, Liebowitz D, Kieff E: An EBV membrane protein expressed in immortalized lymphocytes transforms established rodent cells. *Cell* 43:831, 1985.

266. Subar M, Neri A, Inghirami G, et al: Frequent c-myc oncogene activation and infrequent presence of Epstein-Barr virus genome in AIDS-associated lymphoma. *Blood* 72:667, 1988.

267. Shibata D, Weiss LM, Hernandez AM, et al: Epstein-Barr virus–associated non-Hodgkin's lymphoma in patients infected with the human immunodeficiency virus. *Blood* 81:2102, 1993.

268. Hamilton-Dutoit SJ, Raphael M, Audouin M, et al: In situ demonstration of Epstein-Barr virus small RNAs (EBER 1) in AIDS related lymphomas: Correlation with tumor morphology and primary site. *Blood* 82:619, 1993.

269. Neri A, Barriga F, Inghirami G, et al: Epstein-Barr virus infection precedes clonal expansion in Burkitt's and acquired immunodeficiency associated lymphoma. *Blood* 77:1092, 1991.

270. Chaganti RSK, Jhanwar SC, Koziner B, et al: Specific translocations characterize Burkitt's-like lymphoma of homosexual men with the acquired immunodeficiency syndrome. *Blood* 61:1269, 1983.

271. Peterson JM, Tubbs RR, Savage RA, et al: Small noncleaved B cell Burkitt-like lymphoma with chromosome t(8;14) translocation and Epstein-Barr virus nuclear associated antigen in a homosexual man with acquired immunodeficiency syndrome. *Am J Med* 78:141, 1985.

272. Rechavi G, Ben-Bassat M, Berkowicz U, et al: Molecular analysis of Burkitt's leukemia in two hemophilic brothers with AIDS. *Blood* 70:1713, 1987.

273. Pelicci PG, Knowles DM, McGrath IT, Dalla-Favera R: Chromosomal breakpoints and structural alterations of the c-myc locus differ in endemic and sporadic forms of Burkitt lymphoma. *Proc Natl Acad Sci U S A* 83:2984, 1986.

274. Shiramizu B, Barriga F, Neequaye J, et al: Patterns of chromosomal breakpoint locations in Burkitt's lymphoma: Relevance to geography and Epstein-Barr virus association. *Blood* 77:1516, 1991.

275. Ballerini P, Gaidano G, Gong JZ, et al: Molecular pathogenesis of HIV-associated lymphomas. *AIDS Res Hum Retroviruses* 8:731, 1992.

276. Pelicci PG, Knowles DM II, Arlin ZA, et al: Multiple monoclonal B cell expansions and c-myc oncogene rearrangements in acquired immune deficiency syndrome-related lymphoproliferative disorders: Implications for lymphomagenesis. *J Exp Med* 164:2049, 1986.

277. Pauza CD, Galindo J, Richman DD: Human immunodeficiency virus infection of monoblastoid cells: Cellular differentiation determines the pattern of virus replication. *J Virol* 62:3558, 1988.

278. Laurence J, Astrin SM: Human immunodeficiency virus induction of malignant transformation in human B lymphocytes. *Proc Natl Acad Sci U S A* 88:7635, 1991.

279. Lombardi L, Newcomb EW, Dalla-Favera R: Pathogenesis of Burkitt lymphoma: Expression of an activated c-myc oncogene causes the tumorigenic conversion of EBV infected human B lymphoblasts. *Cell* 46:161, 1987.

280. Adams JM, Harris AW, Pinkert CA, et al: The c-myc oncogene driven by immunoglobulin enhancers induces lymphoid malignancy in transgenic mice. *Nature* 318:553, 1985.

281. Gaidano G, Lo Coco F, Ye BH, et al: Rearrangements of the BCL-6 gene in AIDS associated non-Hodgkin's lymphoma: Association with diffuse large cell subtype. *Blood* 84:397, 1994.

282. Gaidano G, Carbone A, Pastore C, et al: Frequent mutations of the 5′ noncoding region of the BCL-6 gene in acquired immunodeficiency syndrome-related non-Hodgkin's lymphomas. *Blood* 89:3755, 1997.

283. Gaidano G, Dalla-Favera R: Biologic aspects of human immunodeficiency virus-related lymphoma. *Curr Opin Oncol* 4:900, 1992.

284. Gaidano G, Carbone A, Dalla-Favera R: Pathogenesis of AIDS-related lymphomas: Molecular and histogenetic heterogeneity. *Am J Pathol* 152:623, 1998.

285. Ziegler JL, Beckstead JA, Volberding PA, et al: Non-Hodgkin's lymphoma in 90 homosexual men: Relation to generalized lymphadenopathy and the acquired immunodeficiency syndrome. *N Engl J Med* 311:565, 1984.

286. Kaplan LD, Abrams DI, Feigal E, et al: AIDS-associated non-Hodgkin's lymphoma in San Francisco. *JAMA* 261:719, 1989.

287. Knowles DM, Chamulak GA, Subar M, et al: Lymphoid neoplasia associated with the acquired immunodeficiency syndrome (AIDS): The New York University experience with 105 cases during 1981 through 1986. *Ann Intern Med* 108:744, 1988.

288. Lowenthal DA, Straus DJ, Campbell SW, et al: AIDS-related lymphoid neoplasia: The Memorial Hospital experience. *Cancer* 61:2325, 1988.

289. Ioachim HL, Dorsett B, Cronin W, et al: Acquired immunodeficiency syndrome associated lymphomas: Clinical, pathological, immunologic, and viral characteristics of 111 cases. *Hum Pathol* 22:659, 1991.

290. Lukes RJ, Parker JW, Taylor CR, et al: Immunologic approach to non-Hodgkin's lymphomas and related leukemias: Analysis of the results of multiparameter studies of 425 cases. *Semin Hematol* 15:322, 1978.

291. Jaffe ES, Harris NL, Stein H, Vardinan JW: *World Health Organization Classification of Tumors. Pathology & Genetics. Tumours of Haematopoietic and Lymphoma Tissues*, p 260. IARC Press, Lyon, 2001.

292. Bellas C, Santon A, Manzanal A, et al: Pathological, immunological, and molecular features of Hodgkin's disease associated with HIV infection. Comparison with ordinary Hodgkin's disease. *Am J Surg Pathol* 12:1520, 1996.

293. Raphael M, Gentilhomme O, Tulliez M, et al: Histopathologic features of high-grade non-Hodgkin's lymphomas in acquired immunodeficiency syndrome. The French Study Group of Pathology for Human Immunodeficiency Virus-Associated Tumors. *Arch Pathol Lab Med* 115:15, 1991.

294. Carbone A, Gloghini A, Gaidano G, et al: AIDS-related Burkitt's lymphoma. Morphologic and immunophenotypic study of biopsy specimens. *Am J Clin Pathol* 103:561, 1995.

295. Delecluse HJ, Raphael M, Magaud JP, et al: Variable morphology of human immunodeficiency virus-associated lymphomas with c-myc rearrangements. The French Study Group of Pathology for Human Immunodeficiency Virus-Associated Tumors I. *Blood* 82:552, 1993.

296. Davi F, Delecluse HJ, Guiet P, et al: Burkitt-like lymphomas in AIDS patients: Characterization within a series of 103 human immunodeficiency virus-associated non-Hodgkin's lymphomas. Burkitt's Lymphoma Study Group. *J Clin Oncol* 12:3788, 1998.

297. Ambinder RF: Epstein-Barr virus associated lymphoproliferations in the AIDS setting. *Eur J Cancer* 10:1209, 2001.

298. Carbone A, Gaidano G, Gloghini, et al: BCL-6 protein expression in AIDS-related non-Hodgkin's lymphomas: Inverse relationship with Epstein-Barr virus-encoded latent membrane protein-1 expression. *Am J Pathol* 1:155, 1997.

299. Nador RG, Cesarman E, Chadburn A, et al: Primary effusion lymphomas: A distinct clinicopathologic entity associated with the Kaposi's sarcoma-associated herpes virus. *Blood* 88:645, 1996.

300. Chang Y, Cesarman E, Pessin MS, et al: Identification of herpesvirus-like DNA sequences in AIDS associated Kaposi's sarcoma. *Science* 266:1865, 1994.

301. Cesarman E, Chang Y, Moore PS, et al: Kaposi's sarcoma associated herpesvirus like DNA sequences in AIDS-related body cavity based lymphomas. *N Engl J Med* 332:1186, 1995.

302. Flaitz CM, Nichols CM, Walling DM, et al: Plasmablastic lymphoma: An HIV-associated entity with primary oral manifestations. *Oral Oncol* 38:96, 2002.

303. Delecluse HJ, Anagnostopoulos I, Dallenbach F, et al: Plasmablastic lymphomas of the oral cavity: A new entity associated with the human immunodeficiency virus infection. *Blood* 89:1413, 1997.

304. Gaidano G, Cerri M, Capello D, et al: Molecular histogenesis of plasmablastic lymphoma of the oral cavity. *Br J Haematol* 119:622, 2002.

305. Arzoo KK, Bu X, Espina BM, et al: T-Cell lymphoma in HIV-infected patients. *J Acquir Immune Defic Syndr* 36:1020, 2004.

306. Jhala DN, Medeiros LJ, Lopez-Terrada D, et al: Neutrophil-rich anaplastic large cell lymphoma of T-cell lineage. A report of two cases arising in HIV-positive patients. *Am J Clin Pathol* 114:478, 2000.

307. Gonzalez-Clemente JM, Ribera JM, Campo E, et al: Ki-1+ anaplastic large-cell lymphoma of T-cell origin in an HIV-infected patient. *AIDS* 5:751 1991.

308. Arber DA, Chang KL, Weiss LM: Peripheral T-cell lymphoma with Touton like tumor giant cells associated with HIV infection: Report of two cases. *Am J Surg Pathol* 23:519, 1999.

309. Levine AM, Burkes RL, Walker M, et al: Development of B cell lymphoma in two monogamous homosexual men. *Arch Intern Med* 145:479, 1985.

310. Dezube BJ, Aboulafia DM, Pantanowitz L: Plasma cell disorders in HIV-infected patients: From benign gammopathy to multiple myeloma. *AIDS Read* 14:372,2004.

311. Horning SJ, Rosenberg SA: The natural history of initially untreated low grade non-Hodgkin's lymphomas. *N Engl J Med* 311:1471, 1984.

312. Levine AM: Acquired immunodeficiency syndrome-related lymphoma [review]. *Blood* 80:8, 1992.

313. Levine AM, Sullivan-Halley J, Pike MC, et al: HIV-related lymphoma: Prognostic factors predictive of survival. *Cancer* 68:2466, 1991.

314. Jones SE, Fuks Z, Bellm M, et al: Non-Hodgkin's lymphoma: IV. Clinicopathologic correlation of 405 cases. *Cancer* 31:806, 1973.

315. Podzamczer D, Ricat I, Bolao F, et al: Gallium-67 scan for distinguishing follicular hyperplasia from other AIDS associated diseases in lymph nodes. *AIDS* 4:683, 1990.

316. Levine AM, Wernz JC, Kaplan L, et al: Low dose chemotherapy with central nervous system prophylaxis and azidothymidine maintenance in AIDS-related lymphoma: A prospective multi-institutional trial. *JAMA* 266:84, 1991.

317. Gill PS, Levine AM, Meyer PR, et al: Primary central nervous system lymphoma in homosexual men: Clinical, immunologic, and pathologic features. *Am J Med* 78:742, 1985.

318. Gill PS, Graham RA, Boswell W, et al: A comparison of imaging, clinical, and pathologic aspects of space occupying lesions within the brain in patients with acquired immunodeficiency syndrome. *Am J Physiologic Imaging* 1:134, 1986.

319. Ciricillo SF, Rosenblum ML: Use of CT and MR imaging to distinguish intracranial lesions and to define the need for biopsy in AIDS patients. *J Neurosurg* 73:720, 1990.

320. Hoffman JM, Waskin HA, Schifter T, et al: PDG-PET in differentiating lymphoma from nonmalignant central nervous system lesions in patients with AIDS. *J Nucl Med* 34:567, 1993.

321. Alcaide FG, Lomena F, Cruceta A, et al: Predictive value of thallium-201 SPECT in the diagnosis of primary central nervous system lymphoma in AIDS patients [abstract 22291]. 12th World AIDS Conference, Geneva, Switzerland, 1998.

322. MacMahon EME, Glass JD, Hayward SDC, et al: Epstein-Barr virus in AIDS related primary central nervous system lymphoma. *Lancet* 338:969, 1991.

323. Cingolani A, De Luca A, Larocca LM, et al: Minimally invasive diagnosis of acquired immunodeficiency syndrome-related primary central nervous system lymphoma. *J Natl Cancer Inst* 5:364, 1998.

324. Ribera JM, Navarro JT, Oriol A, et al: Prognostic impact of highly active antiretroviral therapy in HIV-related Hodgkin's disease. *AIDS* 27:1973, 2002.

325. Jones D, Ballestas ME, Kaye KM, et al: Primary effusion lymphoma and Kaposi's sarcoma in a cardiac transplant recipient. *N Engl J Med* 339:444, 1998.

326. Simonelli C, Spina M, Cinelli R, et al: Clinical features and outcome of primary effusion lymphoma in HIV-infected patients: A single-institution study. *J Clin Oncol* 21:3948, 2003.

327. Oksenhendler E, Clauvel JP, Jouveshomme S, et al: Complete remission of a primary effusion lymphoma with antiretroviral therapy. *Am J Hematol* 57:266, 1998.

328. Hocqueloux L, Agbalika F, Oksenhendler E: Long-term remission of an AIDS-related primary effusion lymphoma with antiviral therapy. *AIDS* 15:280, 2001.

329. Spina M, Gaidano G, Carbone A: Highly active antiretroviral therapy in human herpesvirus-8-related body-cavity-based lymphoma. *AIDS* 12:955, 1998.

330. Straus DJ, Huang J, Testa MA, et al: Prognostic factors in the treatment of human immunodeficiency virus-associated non-Hodgkin's lymphoma: Analysis of AIDS Clinical Trials Group protocol 142: Low dose versus standard dose m-BACOD plus granulocyte-macrophage stimulating factor. *J Clin Oncol* 16:3601, 1998.

331. Rossi G, Donisi A, Casari S, et al: The International Prognostic Index can be used as a guide to treatment decisions regarding patients with human immunodeficiency virus-related systemic non-Hodgkin lymphoma. *Cancer* 86:239, 1999.

332. Lim ST, Espina B, Tulpulr A, et al: AIDS related small non-cleaved (Burkitt or atypical burkitt) lymphoma versus diffuse large cell lymphoma in the pre- and post-HAART eras: Significant differences in survival. 46th Annual Meeting of the American Society of Hematology, San Diego, California, December 6, 2004.

333. Little RF, Pittaluga S, Grant N, et al: Highly effective treatment of acquired immunodeficiency syndrome-related lymphoma with dose-adjusted EPOCH: Impact of antiretroviral therapy suspension and tumor biology. *Blood* 101:4653, 2003.

334. Dugan M, Subar M, Odajnyk C, et al: Intensive multiagent chemotherapy for AIDS related diffuse large cell lymphoma. *Blood* 68:124a, 1986.

335. Odajnyk C, Subar M, Dugan M, et al: Clinical features and correlates with immunopathology and molecular biology of a large group of patients with AIDS associated small non-cleaved lymphoma (SNCL). *Blood* 68:1331a, 1986.

336. Kaplan LD, Straus DH, Testa MA, et al: Low dose compared with standard dose m-BACOD chemotherapy for non-Hodgkin's lymphoma associated with human immunodeficiency virus infection. *N Engl J Med* 336:1641, 1997.

337. Levine AM, Tulpule A, Espina B, et al: Liposome-encapsulated doxorubicin in combination with standard agents (cyclophosphamide, vincristine, prednisone) in patients with newly diagnosed AIDS-related non-Hodgkin's lymphoma: Results of therapy and correlates of response. *J Clin Oncol* 22:2662, 2004.

338. Ratner L, Lee J, Tang S, et al: Chemotherapy for human immunodeficiency virus-associated non-Hodgkin's lymphoma in combination with highly active antiretroviral therapy. *J Clin Oncol* 19:2171, 2001.

339. Hoffmann C, Wolf E, Fatkenheuer G, et al: Response to highly active antiretroviral therapy strongly predicts outcome in patients with AIDS-related lymphoma *AIDS* 10:1521, 2003.

340. Antinori A, Cingolani A, Alba L, et al: Better response to chemotherapy and prolonged survival in AIDS-related lymphomas responding to highly active antiretroviral therapy. *AIDS* 15:1483, 2001.

341. Kaplan LD, Scadden DT: No benefit from rituximab in a randomized phase III trial of CHOP with or without rituximab for patients with HIV-associated non Hodgkin's lymphoma: AIDS Malignancies Consortium Study 010 [abstract 2268]. *Proc Am Soc Clin Oncol* 22:564, 2003.

342. Vlahov D, Graham N, Hoover D: Prognostic indicators for AIDS and infectious disease death in HIV-infected injection drug users: Plasma viral load and CD4+ cell count. *JAMA* 279:35,1998.

343. Spina M, Jaeger U, Sparano JA, et al: Rituximab plus infusional cyclophosphamide, doxorubicin, and etoposide in HIV-associated non-Hodgkin lymphoma: Pooled results from 3 phase 2 trials. *Blood* 105:1891, 2005.

344. Sparano JA, Bernardo P, Stephenson P, et al: Randomized phase III trial of marimastat versus placebo in patients with metastatic breast cancer who have responding or stable disease after first-line chemotherapy: Eastern Cooperative Oncology Group trial E2196. *J Clin Oncol* 22:4683, 2004.

345. Seneviratne L, Espina BM, Nathwani BN, et al: Clinical, immunologic, and pathologic correlates of bone marrow involvement in 291 patients with acquired immunodeficiency syndrome-related lymphoma. *Blood* 98:2358, 2001.

346. Tirelli U, Errante D, Spina M, et al: Second-line chemotherapy in human immunodeficiency virus-related non-Hodgkin's lymphoma: Evidence of activity of a combination of etoposide, mitoxantrone, and prednimustine in relapsed patients. *Cancer* 77:2127, 1996.

347. Spina M, Vaccher E, Juzbasic S, et al: Human immunodeficiency virus-related non-Hodgkin lymphoma: Activity of infusional cyclophosphamide, doxorubicin, and etoposide as second-line chemotherapy in 40 patients. *Cancer* 92:200, 2001.

348. Bi J, Espina BM, Tulpule A, et al: High-dose cytosine-arabinoside and cisplatin regimens as salvage therapy for refractory or relapsed AIDS-related non-Hodgkin's lymphoma. *J Acquir Immune Defic Syndr* 28:416,2001.

349. Krishnan A, Molina A, Zaia J, et al: Durable remissions with autologous stem cell transplantation for high risk HIV-associated lymphomas. *Blood* 105:874, 2004.

350. Re A, Cattaneo C, Michieli M, et al: High-dose therapy and autologous peripheral-blood stem-cell transplantation as salvage treatment for HIV-associated lymphoma in patients receiving highly active antiretroviral therapy. *J Clin Oncol* 23:4423, 2003.

351. Hessol NA, Katz MH, Liu JY, et al: Increased incidence of Hodgkin disease in homosexual men with HIV infection. *Ann Intern Med* 117:309, 1992.

352. Lyter DW, Bryant J, Thackeray R, et al: Incidence of human immunodeficiency virus-related and nonrelated malignancies in a large cohort of homosexual men. *J Clin Oncol* 13:2540, 1995.

353. Franceschi S, Dal Maso L, Arniabi S, et al: Risk of cancer other than Kaposi's sarcoma and non-Hodgkin's lymphoma in persons with AIDS in Italy. *Br J Cancer* 78:966, 1998.

354. Spina M, Vaccher E, Nasti G, Tirelli U: Human immunodeficiency virus-associated Hodgkin's disease. *Semin Oncol* 27:480, 2000.

355. Ames ED, Conjalka MS, Goldberg AF, et al: Hodgkin's disease and AIDS. Twenty-three new cases and a review of the literature. *Hematol Oncol Clin North Am* 5:343, 1991.

356. Re A, Casari S, Cattaneo C, et al: Hodgkin disease developing in patients infected by human immunodeficiency virus results in clinical features and a prognosis similar to those in patients with human immunodeficiency virus-related non-Hodgkin lymphoma. *Cancer* 92:2739, 2001.

357. Bellas C, Santon A, Manzanal A, et al: Pathological, immunological, and molecular features of Hodgkin's disease associated with HIV infection. Comparison with ordinary Hodgkin's disease. *Am J Surg Pathol* 20:1520, 1996.

358. Cooley TP: Non-AIDS-defining cancer in HIV-infected people. *Hematol Oncol Clin North Am* 17:889, 2003.

359. Levine AM, Li P, Cheung T, et al: Chemotherapy consisting of doxorubicin, bleomycin, vinblastine, and dacarbazine with granulocyte-colony-stimulating factor in HIV-infected patients with newly diagnosed Hodgkin's disease: A prospective, multi-institutional AIDS clinical trials group study (ACTG 149). *J Acquir Immune Defic Syndr* 24:444, 2000.

360. Andrieu JM, Roithmann S, Tourani JM, et al: Hodgkin's disease during HIV1 infection: The French registry experience. French Registry of HIV-associated tumors. *Ann Oncol* 4:635, 1993.

361. Goedert JJ, Cote TR, Virgo P, et al: Spectrum of AIDS-associated malignant disorders. *Lancet* 351:1833, 1998.

362. Frisch M, Biggar RJ, Engels EA, et al: Association of cancer with AIDS-related immunosuppression in adults. *JAMA* 285:1736, 2001.

363. Grulich AE, Li Y, McDonald A, et al: Rates of non-AIDS-defining cancers in people with HIV infection before and after AIDS diagnosis. *AIDS* 16:1155, 2002.

364. Rubio R. Hodgkin's disease associated with human immunodeficiency virus infection. A clinical study of 46 cases. Cooperative Study Group of Malignancies Associated with HIV Infection of Madrid. *Cancer* 73:2400, 1994.

365. Monfardini S, Tirelli U, Vaccher E, et al: Hodgkin's disease in 63 intravenous drug users infected with human immunodeficiency virus. Gruppo Italiano Cooperativo AIDS & Tumori (GICAT). *Ann Oncol* 2(suppl 2):201, 1991.

366. Gold JE, Altarac D, Ree HJ, et al: HIV-associated Hodgkin disease: A clinical study of 18 cases and review of the literature. *Am J Hematol* 36:93, 1991.

367. Ree HJ, Strauchen JA, Khan AA, et al: Human immunodeficiency virus-associated Hodgkin's disease. Clinicopathologic studies of 24 cases and preponderance of mixed cellularity type characterized by the occurrence of fibrohistiocytoid stromal cells. *Cancer* 67:1614, 1991.

368. Serrano M, Bellas C, Campo E, et al: Hodgkin's disease in patients with antibodies to human immunodeficiency virus. A study of 22 patients. *Cancer* 65:2248, 1990.

369. Tirelli U, Errante D, Vaccher E, et al: Hodgkin's disease in 92 patients with HIV infection: The Italian experience. GICAT (Italian Cooperative Group on AIDS & Tumors). *Ann Oncol* 3(suppl 4):69, 1992.

370. Dolcetti R, Boiocchi M, Gloghini A, et al: Pathogenetic and histogenetic features of HIV-associated Hodgkin's disease. *Eur J Cancer* 37:1276, 2001.

371. Glaser SL, Lin RJ, Stewart SL, et al: Epstein-Barr virus-associated Hodgkin's disease: Epidemiologic characteristics in international data. *Int J Cancer* 70:375, 1997.

372. Herbst H, Steinbrecher E, Niedobitek G, et al: Distribution and phenotype of Epstein-Barr virus-harboring cells in Hodgkin's disease. *Blood* 80:484, 1992.

373. Levine AM: Hodgkin's disease in the setting of human immunodeficiency virus infection. *J Natl Cancer Inst Monogr* 23:37,1998.

374. Errante D, Gabarre J, Ridolfo AL, et al: Hodgkin's disease in 35 patients with HIV infection: An experience with epirubicin, bleomycin, vinblastine and prednisone chemotherapy in combination with antiretroviral therapy and primary use of G-CSF. *Ann Oncol* 10:189, 1999.

375. Spina M, Gabarre J, Rossi G, et al: Stanford V regimen and concomitant HAART in 59 patients with Hodgkin disease and HIV infection. *Blood* 100:1984, 2002.

376. Gerard L, Galicier L, Boulanger E, et al: Improved survival in HIV-related Hodgkin's lymphoma since the introduction of highly active antiretroviral therapy. *AIDS* 17:81, 2003.

377. Hoffmann C, Chow KU, Wolf E, et al: Strong impact of highly active antiretroviral therapy on survival in patients with human immunodeficiency virus-associated Hodgkin's disease. *Br J Haematol* 125:455, 2004.

378. Hartmann P, Rehwald U, Salzberger B, et al: BEACOPP therapeutic regimen for patients with Hodgkin's disease and HIV infection. *Ann Oncol* 14:1562, 2003.

379. Martin JN, Ganem DE, Osmond DH, et al: Sexual transmission and the natural history of human herpesvirus 8 infection. *N Engl J Med* 338:948, 1998.

MONONUCLEOSIS SYNDROMES

ROBERT F. BETTS

The defining clinical features of a mononucleosis syndrome are fever and reactive lymphocytes in the blood. The two most common causes of mononucleosis are Epstein-Barr virus (EBV) and cytomegalovirus (CMV) infection. The clinical manifestations of EBV and CMV mononucleosis depend on a vigorous host response to the viral infection. Patients who become infected without a host response develop antibodies to the virus but no or minimal clinical manifestations. Several clinical similarities exist between EBV and CMV mononucleosis. Both infections have a febrile prodrome before the mononucleosis phase develops. Both infections can induce fever, an enlarged spleen, and an erythematous skin rash—the mononucleosis phase. The disease is self-limited in the vast majority of patients, although resolution may take several weeks, especially in older individuals. In both viral infections, lymphocytes represent greater than 50 percent of blood cells, and at least 10 percent are reactive lymphocytes. Differences in clinical and laboratory findings are observed. Severe pharyngitis and tender lymph node enlargement, often in several lymph node groups, occur in infection with EBV and perhaps with some unknown agents, but not to the same degree in infections with CMV. The majority of cases of EBV mononucleosis occur in teenagers and young adults, whereas CMV-induced disease occurs most commonly in adults in their 30s to 60s. A much larger percentage of adults have unrecognized primary infection with CMV than with EBV. EBV results in the development of heterophile antibodies, active against sheep and horse red cells among others, but this development does not occur in CMV. The pathway leading to lymphocytosis and reactive lymphocytes differs between the two agents. The B cell is infected in EBV infection, whereas the macrophage is infected in CMV. In both infections, the T lymphocyte is the reactive cell. Other agents, including _Toxoplasma gondii_, human immune deficiency virus type 1, and several other viruses, can cause a mononucleosis-like syndrome with reactive lymphocytes in the blood.

DEFINITION AND HISTORY

The first clinical description of a syndrome that probably was infectious mononucleosis was published in 1885 when Pfeiffer[1] described a disorder termed _Drüsenfieber_ (glandular fever). In 1920, Sprunt and Evans[2] introduced the term _infectious mononucleosis_ for an acute, self-limited syndrome of mononuclear leukocytosis in febrile patients. Paul had become interested in heterophil antibodies that were phylogenetically unrelated to the antigen with which they reacted, the so-called Forssman antigen. For this reason, he was studying human sera that reacted with sheep red cells. He inadvertently found that the highest

titer came from an individual recovering from infectious mononucleosis. In 1932, Paul and Bunnell[3] showed that the sera from patients with infectious mononucleosis agglutinated red cells from sheep and horses, a reaction that was termed the _heterophile antibody test_. Davidson showed that the heterophil antibody of infectious mononucleosis could be absorbed by guinea pig kidney cells. This demonstration of patient serum reactivity with sheep or horse cells but not after guinea pig kidney absorption of serum made this test very specific for EBV infection.[4] In 1964, Epstein, Ashong, and Barr reported the isolation of a virus from the cells of a patient with African Burkitt lymphoma. The virus later was named after two of the investigators. The etiologic role of EBV in infectious mononucleosis was discovered serendipitously in the laboratory of Gertrude and Werner Henle, who devised immunofluorescent assays for EBV-specific antibodies.[5] A technician in their laboratory whose serum had been negative for EBV antibodies was restudied (as a control) after she recovered from infectious mononucleosis. Her serum was found to contain antibodies to EBV. The association later was confirmed by large seroepidemiologic studies in college students.[6–9] Much of the clinical nature of mononucleosis was documented by Hoagland,[10] who reported studies of cadets at West Point. His studies led to mononucleosis being dubbed the "kissing disease," after he established that oral transmission was the principal route of viral transmission among teenagers and young adults. He also deduced the incubation period of the viral infection given the finding that cadets developed the disease approximately 6 weeks after they returned to West Point from their vacation.[11]

Although EBV-induced mononucleosis is the most prevalent type of this syndrome, other agents produced a febrile syndrome with a blood lymphocytosis, which could mimic some aspects of EBV mononucleosis. The first report of cytomegalovirus (CMV) infection in individuals other than newborns described chronic liver function abnormalities and hepatomegaly in young children.[12] Later, a mononucleosis syndrome attributed to CMV occurring in young adults was reported.[13]

GENERAL FEATURES OF THE INFECTIOUS MONONUCLEOSIS SYNDROME

The infectious mononucleosis syndrome most commonly is caused by one of two members of the herpes virus family: EBV or CMV. Occasionally, the human immune deficiency virus-1 (HIV) and, less commonly, the parasite _Toxoplasma gondii_ produce a febrile illness with lymphocytosis. Several other viral agents produce the blood picture of mononucleosis, but only infrequently (Table 84-1).

Distinct clinical, epidemiologic, and cytopathologic differences exist between EBV and CMV mononucleosis. CMV is more common in older individuals than in individuals in the age group from 15 to 25 years in which EBV occurs most commonly. Distinct differences in clinical manifestations of EBV are observed in the young versus the older population. In older individuals, EBV and CMV more closely

TABLE 84-1 ETIOLOGIC AGENTS ASSOCIATED WITH MONONUCLEOSIS SYNDROME

Epstein-Barr virus
Cytomegalovirus
Human immunodeficiency virus
Human herpes virus-6
Rubella
Hepatitis A
Adenovirus
Toxoplasma gondii
Bartonella henselae
Brucella abortus

Acronyms and abbreviations that appear in this chapter include: CMV, cytomegalovirus; EA, early antigen; EBNA, Epstein-Barr nuclear antigen; EBV, Epstein-Barr virus; HIV, human immunodeficiency virus; NK, natural killer; PCR, polymerase chain reaction; PTLD, posttransplantation lymphoproliferative disease; VCA, virus capsid antigen.

resemble one another in their clinical manifestations, whereas EBV in the younger population is different from either virus infections in older persons. Table 84-2 compares the clinical manifestations of EBV in the young population, EBV in the older population, and CMV.

After the early phase of fever, which lasts for 3 to 7 days, laboratory abnormalities include a blood lymphocyte proportion greater than 50 percent, often with greater than 10 percent reactive lymphocytes. Liver function test abnormalities indicating cholestasis predominate over hepatocellular changes. The abnormality is notable by elevations in alkaline phosphatase and proportionately lower elevations in transaminases. Bilirubin elevation is uncommon in EBV in the young but of similar frequency to that of CMV in the older age group. Severe jaundice is rare. Table 84-3 lists other complications of EBV and CMV mononucleosis.

EBV MONONUCLEOSIS

PATHOGENESIS

EBV is a DNA virus of the Gammaherpesvirinae subfamily. The virus is estimated to infect 90 percent of the world's population who carry the virus as a latent infection of B lymphocytes. EBV intercalates itself into the B cell and establishes lifelong residence in its host. It infects primarily the long-lived memory B cells and not naive B cells.[14,15] Early after infection, the virus is continuously shed into oral secretions. The virus then usually undergoes latency, but it may be reactivated periodically.[16] Within a few days to 1 week after onset of EBV infection, T lymphocytes recognize viral replicative antigens on the infected B cell as foreign, and an exuberant polyclonal cytotoxic T cell response ensues. The proliferative rate of CD8+T cells is estimated to be approximately 50 percent of this population of cells proliferating per day, which translates into a population doubling time of 1.5 days so that 5×10^9 CD8+ T cells per day appear in the blood. The later rate of appearance is two orders of magnitude greater than normal.[17] The surface activation marker SLAM-associated protein (SAP) on T lymphocytes engenders cell activation in response to a signal from CD244 and CD150 (SLAM) on the T cell surface.[18] In the healthy individual, the process subsides over days to weeks, the signs and symptoms of the infection subside, and the individual returns to normal.

EPIDEMIOLOGY

Close contact is required for transmission; epidemics rarely occur. Nonetheless, nearly all individuals in the society will become infected. This degree of infection is attributed to the frequent reactivation of EBV, which enhances its transmissibility. The age at which infection

TABLE 84-2 SIGNS AND SYMPTOMS OF EPSTEIN-BARR VIRUS AND CYTOMEGALOVIRUS MONONUCLEOSIS: EFFECT OF AGE (PERCENT OF PATIENTS)

SIGNS AND SYMPTOMS	EBV (AGE 14–35 YEARS*)	EBV (AGE 40–72 YEARS†)	CMV (AGE 30–70 YEARS‡)
Fever	95	94	85
Pharyngitis	95	46	15
Lymphadenopathy	98	49	24
Splenomegaly	65	33	3
Hepatomegaly	23	42	N/A
Jaundice	8	27	24

* Data from reference 30.
† Data from reference 29.
‡ Data from reference 89.

TABLE 84-3 COMPLICATIONS OF EPSTEIN-BARR VIRUS AND CYTOMEGALOVIRUS MONONUCLEOSIS

	EBV	CMV
Hemolytic anemia	++	+
Thrombocytopenia	+	+
Aplastic anemia	+	-
Splenic rupture	+	-
Jaundice (>age 25 years)	++	++
Guillain-Barré syndrome	+	++
Encephalitis*	++	+/-
Pneumonitis*	+/-	+
Myocarditis*	+	-
B cell lymphoma	+	-
Agammaglobulinemia	+	-

* Can occur without the mononucleosis syndrome.
++, Common; +, can occur; +/-, occasional; -, not observed.

first occurs varies widely based on socioeconomic conditions and geography. In the developing world and in the lowest socioeconomic strata of the developed world, nearly everyone is subclinically infected by age 5 years, and the disease is rarely apparent. In the upper socioeconomic strata of the developed world, persons avoid infection in infancy. As the individual reaches teenage years, infection is transmitted from a latently infected asymptomatic individual to a previously uninfected person. Characteristically, primary infection occurs in an individual a few months after he/she develops a relationship with an individual who has latent infection. The transmitter had been infected earlier in life, and the sporadically reactivated EBV is transmitted by intimate oral contact.[16] The most common age for occurrence of the mononucleosis syndrome is between 12 and 25 years. Individuals raised in more protected environments or in single-child families may reach their 30s before they are infected while they are dating or after they are married. If both individuals in a relationship are seronegative, years may pass before they become infected, usually from their children. Individuals who are seropositive usually do not develop clinical disease upon reexposure,[5] although a second infection with a different strain may occur.[19–21]

CLINICAL MANIFESTATIONS

Clinical manifestations vary according to the age at infection.[22–29] When young children acquire EBV, less than 10 percent develop the syndrome of infectious mononucleosis. Instead, they develop a typical childhood illness of respiratory tract infection (43 percent) otitis media (29 percent), pharyngitis (21 percent), and gastroenteritis (7 percent). Rashes and eyelid or periorbital swelling occur more frequently in younger children. A palpable spleen and liver occur more frequently in individuals younger than 40 years.

If serologic methods alone are used to identify the disease in teenagers and young adults, variability in the symptoms, signs, physical findings, and laboratory abnormalities are observed.[30] The earliest manifestations of disease—fever and lassitude—develop 30 to 45 days after patients become infected. Initial symptoms of pharyngitis, tonsillar enlargement, and fever result from infection and proliferation of the B lymphocytes that are found in the Waldeyer ring. Infection occurs via the virus cell surface CD21 glycoprotein, a 140-kDa complement receptor type 2, a process that induces polyclonal proliferation of infected B cells in the nodes of the pharynx. From the nodes of the pharynx, virus-infected cells make their way into the circulating lymphocyte pool.[31,32]

Subsequent massive T lymphocyte response to the neoantigens on infected B lymphocytes is evident by the lymphocytosis with reactive blood T lymphocytes and other disease manifestations, such as lymphadenopathy, hepatic inflammation, and splenomegaly.[33] The frequency of each clinical finding of the typical syndrome in newly infected patients is variable (see Table 84-2).[30]

The classic clinical syndrome includes fever, exudative pharyngitis, and enlarged tonsils, sometimes to the point where the tonsils touch in the midline and obstruct the airway. Diffuse lymphadenopathy, splenomegaly, and abnormal liver function test results, notably increased serum alkaline phosphatase, aspartate aminotransferase (serum glutamic oxalo-acetic transaminase), and alanine aminotransferase (serum glutamate pyruvate transaminase), but not usually hyperbilirubinemia, are typical of the classic picture.

Group A streptococcus infection occurs occasionally in concert with an EBV primary infection. Several studies have shown this co-occurrence is uncommon (3 and 4 percent of cases). Although treatment of the streptococcus eradicates the organism, the severe pharyngitis changes little, and the disease follows its usual course. Thus, treatment should be administered only if the test result for β streptococcus is positive. If ampicillin, amoxicillin, or other penicillin congeners are used to treat the pharyngitis, a rash almost always develops[34,35] and the patient may be labeled "penicillin allergic." The patient should be reevaluated after the mononucleosis resolves to determine if the patient has a true allergy.

The disease abates with the occurrence of a T cell-mediated counterresponse to the virus-induced initial polyclonal B cell proliferation. During this time, dramatic clinical improvement can occur. Subsequently, EBV remains in the patient's B cells throughout life but expresses only Epstein-Barr nuclear antigen-1 (EBNA-1), which does not elicit a T cell response because of a glycine alanine repeat that inhibits its processing.[36]

EBV is much less likely to be accompanied by lymphadenopathy and pharyngitis when the disease presents in elderly patients than in younger patients (see Table 84-2).[26–29] Fever is present in almost all older patients. Abdominal pain, hepatomegaly, and liver function abnormalities occur in substantial proportions, frequently leading to an initial clinical impression of hepatitis or an intraabdominal problem, such as cholecystitis. Older adults have less significant lymphocytosis and fewer reactive lymphocytes in the blood. Splenomegaly is less evident. The illness tends to be more prolonged in older adults.

LABORATORY ABNORMALITIES

ANTIBODY RESPONSES

A heterophile antibody response directed at sheep, horse, or another species red cell surface antigen occurs in approximately 85 percent of cases by week 3 of illness. Repeat testing may be necessary to detect late responders. The rapid slide test for heterophil antibody may be falsely negative in approximately 6 percent of patients,[37] especially in young children.[22] A variety of other antibodies also are produced nonspecifically because of polyclonal B cell activation. These antibodies include antiplatelet, anti-red cell (anti-i cold agglutinin), and antinuclear antibodies. Although the interaction of EBV with B lymphocytes elicits a polyclonal response, among the clones expanded are those preprogrammed to make specific antibody, including antibodies against other infectious agents, such as Brucellosis chlamydia, the yellow fever virus, and others. If the patient's disease is approached as a fever of unknown origin, the results can be misleading.

At the time clinical disease is evident, IgG and IgM antibodies to Epstein-Barr virus capsid antigen (VCA) usually are detectable. Later, antibody to early antigen (EA) develops. Even later, often during recovery, antibody to EBNA-1 evolves. For patients suspected of having infectious mononucleosis but who do not have a positive heterophile antibody test result, a positive reaction for IgG and IgM antibodies to

EBV and usually a negative antibody reaction to EBNA-1[38] are diagnostic of acute infection. In a study of 100 patients with EBV mononucleosis, IgM anti-VCA antibodies were positive in all patients, whereas only approximately 50 percent were positive for heterophile or IgG anti-VCA antibodies.[39] A real-time polymerase chain reaction (PCR) that measures serum or plasma EBV load is useful in seronegative patients, although this approach requires special adaptations to remove inhibitors of the assay in plasma.[40]

REACTIVE LYMPHOCYTOSIS

Expansion of cytotoxic T lymphocytes produces lymphocytosis. Reactive lymphocytes are larger than lymphocytes normally found in the blood. They have a vacuolated cytoplasm, lobulated and eccentrically placed nucleus, and a cell membrane that often is indented by neighboring erythrocytes (see Color Plates XX-1 and XX-2). A more darkly staining peripheral cytoplasm "skirting" occurs. Reactive lymphocytes are a hematologic hallmark of infectious mononucleosis, but they are not always found[30] and are not pathognomonic. They also are found in CMV infection, roseola (caused by human herpes virus-6), viral hepatitis, toxoplasmosis, rubella, mumps, and drug reactions.

Sheets of lymphocytes are noted on a stained slide preparation of tonsillar exudate. If β-streptococcal infection accompanies the EBV infection or is the etiology of the exudate, segmented neutrophils are seen. The immunophenotype of lymphocytes in mononucleosis syndromes assessed by multiparametric flow cytometry has confirmed that lymphocytosis results from CD8+ T cells. CD4+ cells and B cells are not increased. In EBV mononucleosis, the notable populations increased are CD8+CD57− and CD3+γδ+ T cells.[41]

SERUM ABNORMALITIES

Liver function abnormalities are common, predominantly elevated serum alkaline phosphatase and γ-aminotransferase activity with only no or only slight elevation of bilirubin in most patients. Studies in Israel have found a higher frequency of hyperbilirubinemia (15 percent), a lower incidence of leukocytosis (46 percent), and elevated liver enzymes (58 percent) than previously reported, but the differences may be geographical. Lymphadenopathy and reactive lymphocytes were each noted in approximately 90 percent of the 590 young adults studied.[30]

COMPLICATIONS OF EBV MONONUCLEOSIS

HEMATOLOGIC

Virtually all subjects with acute mononucleosis develop a mildly decreased platelet count (see Table 84-3). More severe hematologic complications occur infrequently, including severe immune thrombocytopenia with petechiae, immune hemolytic anemia, immune-mediated agranulocytosis, and aplastic anemia.[42–48] Hematologic complications stem from the array of antibody responses resulting from B lymphocyte activation. Uncommonly, the splenomegaly accentuates an underlying, previously undiagnosed hereditary spherocytosis.[49,50]

Splenic rupture is estimated to occur in one to five per 1000 cases. It is the leading cause of death from EBV mononucleosis.[51,52] Although most cases are spontaneous without an apparent traumatic cause, the risk of splenic rupture requires avoidance of athletic and other high-risk activities until the signs of the disease have disappeared and the spleen has returned to normal size.[52]

NEUROLOGIC

Neurologic complications include acute encephalitis, acute disseminated encephalomyelitis (Alice in Wonderland syndrome), acute cerebellar ataxia, viral meningitis, Guillain-Barré syndrome, transverse myelitis, and cranial nerve palsies.[47,48,53–55] Neurologic complications can occur in the absence of clinical mononucleosis. Diagnosis of EBV-induced disease requires studies of EBV-specific antibodies (see Laboratory Abnormalities above) and PCR for EBV on cerebrospinal fluid.[53] Neurologic disease can be associated with primary infection, reactivated infection, or chronic EBV infection.[53] Table 84-3 lists other complications.

SPECIAL COMPLICATIONS

Chronic Progressive EBV Infection, T or NK Lymphoproliferation and Lymphoma, and Hemophagocytic Syndrome Chronic EBV infection is a rare outcome of primary EBV infection.[56,57] It tends to occur in persons with an immune deficiency but occasionally develops in subjects without an apparent immune defect. In chronic EBV infection, fever, marrow hypoplasia, interstitial pneumonia, hepatosplenomegaly, persistent hepatitis often to the point of hepatic failure, lymphadenitis, and uveitis are frequent clinical manifestations. The syndrome may persist for months or years and has a relatively high fatality rate.[56] The EBV-related antibodies, including IgG to VCA, may be greater than 1:5120 and anti-EA greater than 1:640, accompanied by a low to undetectable EBNA-1 titer. In addition, persistently high EBV load in circulating lymphocytes is measured by PCR for EBV DNA. The more severe form of the syndrome may evolve into an NK or T cell lymphoproliferative disease[57–59] that ranges from chronic to fulminant.[60] EBV genomes are present in the T or NK cells and presumably result in clonal expansion of these cells and clinical lymphoma. EBV-induced hemophagocytic syndrome can be another concomitant feature of chronic active EBV infection. The latter disease is a severe multiorgan, inflammatory disease provoked by massive inflammatory cytokine elaboration and, in some cases, clonal lymphocyte expansion induced by EBV infection[61–63] (discussed in Chap. 72). The EBV-induced hemophagocytic syndrome can occur in apparently normal and in immunocompromised persons.

OTHER EBV-ASSOCIATED DISEASE PROCESSES

NEOPLASTIC POTENTIAL OF THE VIRUS
EBV was isolated from the cultured cells of a patient with African Burkitt lymphoma, subsequently was established as the etiologic agent in that disease, and was the first human tumor virus identified.[64] EBV can confer unlimited growth potential on infected B lymphocytes in culture. A single base pair mutation in the internal ribosome entry site element of the EBV nuclear antigen gene affects its expression and may be one factor contributing to the malignant potential of the virus.[65] EBV has since been associated with tumors other than Burkitt lymphoma: approximately one third of patients with Hodgkin lymphoma,[66–68] lymphoma in immunodeficient individuals, including the immunodeficiency state posttransplantation[69–71] and X chromosome-linked lymphoproliferative disease,[72,73] T cell and NK cell lymphomas that follow chronic EBV infection,[73–75] nasopharyngeal carcinoma in patients in the Far East,[76,77] leiomyomas and leiomyosarcomas in persons infected with HIV or immunodeficient posttransplantation,[78,79] and a small fraction of cases of gastric carcinoma[80] (Table 84-4). In the three principal lymphomas, Burkitt, Hodgkin, and posttransplant lymphomas, the cell mutated to produce the clonal disease is a germinal center B cell.[81] These tumors are characterized by the presence of circular viral genome in the tumor cells and the expression of EBV-encoded latent genes.[82]

EBV is detectable in the neoplastic B cells (Reed-Sternberg cells) of approximately 35 percent of patients with Hodgkin lymphoma.[66] The precise etiologic role of EBV in this subset of patients with Hodgkin lymphoma is uncertain.

In the case of posttransplantation lymphoproliferative disease (PTLD), the most characteristic clinical scenario involves an EBV se-

TABLE 84-4 SPECIAL PROBLEMS WITH EPSTEIN-BARR VIRUS OR CYTOMEGALOVIRUS INFECTION

EPSTEIN-BARR VIRUS	CYTOMEGALOVIRUS
Rare congenital infection[111,112]	Congenital infection[87]
Chronic progressive mononucleosis[56,57]	Posttransplant primary infection[92]
Hemophagocytic syndrome[61–63]	Graft-versus-host disease association[115]
X-linked B cell lymphoma[72,73]	Transfusion-related infection[113,114]
Post transplant lymphoproliferative disease[69–71]	*Aspergillus* and/or *Pneumocystis* infection[116]
T or NK lymphoproliferative disease[73–75]	
African Burkitt lymphoma[64]	
Approximately 20% of Burkitt lymphoma in the United States[73]	
Approximately 35% of Hodgkin lymphoma[66–68,73]	
Nasopharyngeal carcinoma[76,77]	
Approximately 5% of gastric carcinoma[80]	
Leiomyoma and leiomyosarcoma in HIV or immunosuppressed patients[78,79]	
Oral hairy leukoplakia[83]	

ronegative person receiving an organ from an EBV seropositive donor.[69] Disease becomes manifest usually within the first year after transplant and often sooner. Occasionally PTLD occurs in a subject known to be EBV seropositive pretransplant.[69,70] In its initial stages, the disease may respond to lowering the immunosuppressive medications. The abnormally proliferating cell almost always is a B cell. Although antiviral prophylaxis seems to reduce the incidence of PTLD,[71] antiviral therapy is ineffective once the disease develops. Primary therapy is a reduction in immunosuppressive medications and use of anti-CD20 therapy with rituximab.

In young males with an X-linked lymphoproliferative syndrome, primary EBV infection leads to unabated B cell proliferation and evolution into a frank B cell lymphoma, the so-called Duncan syndrome.[72,73] These young males do not develop a T cell response and hence do not develop mononucleosis. Although control of this effect of EBV infection by treatment with antiviral agents and/or chemotherapy has been attempted, the Duncan syndrome usually is fatal.

Oral hairy leukoplakia, a characteristic white lingual lesion with hairy projections seen in patients with HIV infection, results from EBV infection of the lingual epithelium.[83]

FUTURE THERAPEUTIC APPROACHES TO EBV INFECTION AND NEOPLASIA

Because of the severe consequences of EBV infection, several approaches to preventing or treating these disorders are underway, such as an EBV vaccine,[84] adoptive transfer of activated cytotoxic T cells,[117] and the development of peptides that inhibit viral replication.[85]

CYTOMEGALOVIRUS MONONUCLEOSIS

BACKGROUND

The early description of CMV-related disease was that of an uncommon congenital syndrome in which some individuals with the disease developed thrombocytopenia and petechiae and had abnormal liver function study results.[86] The recognition that young children had similar clinical findings led to the discovery that previously healthy young children with prolonged abnormal liver function, hepatosplenomegaly, lymphocytosis, and thrombocytopenia had a primary infection with CMV.[12] Subsequently, primary CMV infection was linked to a febrile mononucleosis syndrome.[13]

EPIDEMIOLOGY

In the developing world, CMV, like EBV, infects the majority of individuals at an early age as a result of transmission by teenage mothers carrying CMV in their cervix to their newborn children or after birth by transmission through their breast milk. In the United States, a small percent of individuals develop infection in association with birth or breast-feeding. Infection also occurs when children congregate in large urban families, in crowded conditions, or in day care centers. In virtually every society, 2 percent of newborns are infected with CMV *in utero*. Severe fetal abnormalities can occur if the mother acquires primary infection during pregnancy.[87] If the mother is seropositive prior to pregnancy and congenital infection occurs, the newborn child usually is asymptomatic. However, a significant percent of these children go on to develop unilateral or bilateral deafness.

The epidemiology of CMV in the older population is quite different from the epidemiology of EBV. For unexplained reasons, college-aged individuals and those in their early 30s are relatively resistant to primary CMV infection. In classic studies of students at Yale and at West Point,[8,88] seroconversion reflecting CMV infection was rare, whereas annual seroconversion to EBV was high. However, primary CMV infection, unlike EBV, continues into the eighth decade. CMV is much more likely than EBV to be transmitted by genital sexual contact, although it can be transmitted by oral contact. It is by the latter route that children in day care centers develop primary CMV infection from their playmates. They bring the virus home to their parents or grandparents, thus accounting for primary CMV infection in adults. If the mother is pregnant, primary infection can lead to congenital CMV. In grandparents, primary infection can lead to CMV mononucleosis. Although approximately 50 percent of the population in higher socioeconomic strata becomes infected between the ages of 20 and 70 years, symptomatic disease is uncommon.

Sexual transmission occurs because male semen has one of the highest concentrations of virus among the body fluids. Infected semen accounts for some of the cases of congenital CMV and perhaps explains why a previously seropositive mother delivers a child with congenital CMV infection. It also explains why nearly all homosexual males, but only 15 to 20 percent of heterosexual males, are infected by age 20 years. This genital infection has no symptoms.

CLINICAL MANIFESTATIONS

Like EBV, use of diagnostic serologic studies to identify the newly infected patient indicates primary infection with CMV has a broad spectrum of clinical manifestations.[89] Because no classic manifestation, such as severe exudative pharyngitis, is seen, the disease often is not considered in the differential diagnosis. Fever, weight loss, and associated malaise and myalgia are common. Because the disease occurs in the older population, including those older than 50 years, the causes of fever of unknown origin often are pursued in an expensive evaluation prior to the diagnosis.[90] The fever evaluation is compounded by the development of antinuclear factor and thrombocytopenia (Table 84-5) that often stimulates evaluation for a collagen vascular disease or, because of the splenomegaly, for lymphoma. The basic clinical disease is fever, often as high as 40°C, with a palpable spleen and laboratory abnormalities. Tables 84-2 and 84-3 list additional clinical findings and complications of CMV infection, respectively. As in EBV infection, administration of amoxicillin, ampicillin,

TABLE 84-5 LABORATORY FINDINGS IN MONONUCLEOSIS

	EBV	CMV
Heterophile antibody	+++	-
Lymphocytosis	+++	++
Atypical lymphocytes	+++	++
Abnormal liver function	++	++
Antinuclear factor	+	+
Cold agglutinins	+	+
Cryoglobulins	+	+
Decreased Platelets	++	+

+++, Characteristic; ++, common; +, occurs.

or other penicillins can result in development of a rash that is not a reflection of future sensitivity to the drugs.

LABORATORY ABNORMALITIES

Neutrophilia with band neutrophils in the blood is not uncommonly seen early in the infection. However, lymphocytosis that develops later is indistinguishable from that of EBV. Liver function changes mimic those of the older group of EBV primary infection (see Tables 84-2 and 84-3). Bilirubin elevation and jaundice may occur in up to 25 percent of patients.[87] Heterophile antibodies do not develop, but specific anti-CMV antibodies develop. Because the incubation period ranges between 30 and 40 days, IgM and IgG antibodies to CMV usually are positive at presentation. No recognized equivalent of the antibody to the EBV early antigen (anti-EA) or anti-EBNA antibody in patients infected with CMV is known. The PCR of a blood sample for CMV usually is positive, and CMV can be isolated from urine or saliva specimens.

COMPLICATIONS

Hemolytic anemia and thrombocytopenia occur in primary CMV infection and are other factors that may lead the clinician initially to consider a diagnosis of lymphoma. The most prominent neurologic complication is Guillain-Barré syndrome and less commonly transverse myelitis and aseptic meningitis (see Table 84-3).

The macrophage is the cell infected with CMV.[91] The T cell response to the macrophage neoantigen leads to reactive lymphocytosis. Because of the T cell response, evolution to unrestrained B cell replication, lymphoma, and PTLD do not occur.

Primary CMV infection is a major problem in organ transplantation. A special circumstance is possible for the development of CMV infection in organ transplantation. CMV infects all the major organs during primary infection. It then evolves to a latent state, presumably in the parenchymal cells. The majority of the potential recipient population is not infected. An uninfected individual requiring a transplantation may be transplanted with an organ that contains CMV, which becomes a source of primary infection.[92] The infection leads to organ-specific rejection and CMV-induced bowel disease in recipients. Superinfection for the seropositive recipient is less of a problem. In allogeneic stem cell transplantation, the situation is somewhat reversed. The recipient of the transplant may have previously been infected with CMV. They reactivate their CMV, which replicates in pulmonary macrophages. The previously uninfected donor T cells may recognize neoantigen on the infected macrophages and respond to that neoantigen. Thus, pneumonitis develops in concert with graft-versus-host disease. Both immune globulin and ganciclovir are required to control this process. IgG 400 mg/kg administered once per week for 4 weeks and ganciclovir 5 mg/kg every 12 hours for 2 weeks then once per day for 2 weeks is one of several approaches to therapy, depending on circumstances. For slightly different reasons, lung transplant recipients are at higher risk for CMV pneumonitis. The donor's CMV reactivates in the pulmonary macrophage and the recipient's immune cells in turn react against infected macrophages, releasing cytokines eventuating in pneumonitis.

PRIMARY HIV INFECTION

At the time of development of primary infection with HIV, an acute syndrome develops.[93,94] The frequency with which the HIV mononucleosis syndrome develops is uncertain, but for this discussion the difference in features is more important (Table 84-6). Fever is sudden in onset, followed by sore throat, lymphadenopathy, tonsillar hypertrophy, painful oral ulcerations, conjunctivitis, and rash. Nausea, vomiting, and diarrhea also occur. Leucopenia, thrombocytopenia, a relative increase in band neutrophils, and a small proportion of reactive lymphocytes usually can be identified on the blood film. Although absolute lymphocytosis is uncommon, the syndrome is referred to as *HIV mononucleosis*. Uncommonly, patients may also develop a heterophile antibody. Among a group of 563 heterophile antibody-positive patient samples retrospectively tested for HIV-1 RNA and p24 antigen, approximately 1 percent had evidence of primary HIV-1 infection.[95] In another study, none of 132 cases was positive.[96] The acute retroviral syndrome must be recognized for both the patient's health and the public health. In this situation, before an anti-HIV antibody response develops, HIV load in the blood should be measured by PCR to make a diagnosis of HIV infection. Usually, viral load is very high (greater than 50,000 viral particles per milliliter of blood). Early treatment may reduce the incidence of HIV-1 complications (see Chap. 83). Acute HIV-1 infection may be particularly contagious. Physician intervention may prevent further transmission.

OTHER AGENTS LINKED TO THE MONONUCLEOSIS SYNDROME

Human herpes virus-6 occasionally has been associated with a mononucleosis-type picture (see Table 84-1).[97] Hepatitis A and rubella virus infection have produced the typical lymphocytic changes. Pharyngitis is not a prominent feature in patients infected with *T. gondii*. Lymphocytosis is mild, and liver functions are normal even when the liver is enlarged. Usually toxoplasmosis presents as posterior cervical lymphadenopathy. In the United States, exposure to oocysts from cat feces is the primary route of infection. In overseas countries, ingestion of partially cooked meat, especially from sheep, is a route of infection. The IgM immunofluorescent antibody test for *T. gondii* is useful in diagnosing the disease.

Cat scratch disease, *Corynebacterium diphtheriae* pharyngitis, infection with brucellosis, or lymphoma can be mistaken for mononucleosis. Other as-yet unidentified agents probably produce the classic syndrome because laboratory studies do not implicate one of the several agents in a small percentage of mononucleosis cases.

TABLE 84-6   CLINICAL FINDINGS IN PRIMARY HIV INFECTION

FINDING	FREQUENCY (%)
Fever	79
Pharyngitis	48
Oral ulcers	29
Lymphadenopathy	44
Splenomegaly	5
Hepatomegaly	<1
Atypical lymphocytes	Uncommon

DIFFERENTIAL DIAGNOSIS

Age and the presence or absence of exudative pharyngitis play critical roles in the differential diagnosis. In the individual who is sexually active between the ages of 15 and 25 years and who has a febrile illness with lymphadenopathy, evidence for infection with EBV and HIV should be sought. Simultaneous infection with these two viruses, although not common, may occur. Mononucleosis-like changes in blood lymphocytes occur in HIV but are uncommon. Exudative pharyngitis suggests infection by EBV rather than by HIV, whereas intraoral ulcers suggest infection with HIV. Rarely, heterophile antibodies occur in conjunction with primary HIV.[95,96]

β-Hemolytic streptococcus, adenovirus, or *Arcanobacterium hemolyticum* also can produce exudative pharyngitis.

In adults in their 30s or 40s, mononucleosis more likely results from infection with CMV than EBV. Absence of exudative pharyngitis points to CMV. HIV must be considered in this age group. Patients infected with either CMV or HIV can present with blood neutrophilia with an increased proportion of band neutrophils. Rash or aseptic meningitis is more common in patients infected with HIV than CMV. In the middle-aged patient, primary CMV infection is by far the most important possibility, although the unusual individual who has escaped infection with EBV earlier in life can present with clinical manifestations similar to patients with primary CMV infection.[27–29]

THERAPY COURSE AND PROGNOSIS

For the majority of patients with primary CMV or EBV infection, treatment is supportive. Salicylates or other analgesics are appropriate for control of fever, headache, and sore throat. Splenic rupture can occur in the first few weeks after diagnosis. Thus, contact sports should be avoided until the spleen has returned to normal size. The vast majority of subjects improve and have resolution of most symptoms. Almost half of patients recovering from EBV mononucleosis still feel fatigued at 60 days and a small percent at six months. Severe fatigue can persist after CMV mononucleosis.

Antiviral or glucocorticoid therapy may be considered in special settings for treatment of EBV mononucleosis. The nucleoside analogue acyclovir blocks EBV replication through inhibition of viral DNA polymerase and can prevent viral shedding from the oropharynx.[98,99] However, acyclovir has little if any effect on the course of mononucleosis, presumably because the disease at that point results from the immunopathologic process and not virus proliferation. Antiviral therapy may be useful in chronic aggressive EBV infection and in EBV infection posttransplantation. Glucocorticoids have been used for management of specific complications. Their specific benefit is difficult to determine because glucocorticoids often are started only late in the clinical course, when immunologic reaction to infection is leading to improvement and the response is credited to the treatment. One carefully controlled trial showed little benefit from prednisone, and the treated group did less well at 30 days than the placebo group.[100] Nevertheless, treatment with glucocorticoid is indicated when the tonsils are touching in the midline and airway obstruction is imminent. For impending airway obstruction in patients with EBV, prednisone 40 to 60 mg/day can be given for 7 to 10 days, then rapidly tapered once a clinical response is achieved. Urgent tonsillectomy and adenoidectomy may be required.[101] The same regimen is used for severe immune hemolytic anemia, severe symptomatic immune thrombocytopenia,[102] neurologic complications, pancreatitis, and myocarditis.

The same dose of glucocorticoid has been used for the hematologic or neurologic complications of CMV mononucleosis. Results of ganciclovir 5 mg/kg/day given intravenously for 14 days for severe CMV mononucleosis occasionally have been dramatic. However, ganciclovir is seldom used because of the potential long-term risk to spermatogenesis (aspermia) or potentially on female fertility. Antiretroviral therapy has been suggested for severe HIV primary disease. However, when the disease appears to be self-limited, many therapists do not begin therapy. Therapy that already was started is stopped after a few weeks.

Acyclovir use for other manifestations of EBV infection not resulting from host response but from a high titer of EBV replication, such as oral hairy leukoplakia of AIDS, rapid resolves lingual lesions.[103] However, treatment with acyclovir does not appear to be effective for PTLD.[104]

MONONUCLEOSIS IN PREGNANCY

When EBV mononucleosis occurs during pregnancy, severe congenital abnormalities similar to those described in primary CMV infection during pregnancy can occur (see Table 84-4). Microcephaly, mental retardation, cataracts, hepatosplenomegaly, and fetal loss or postnatal death have been described. For CMV, immunity does not necessarily protect against congenital infection. Two percent of live births in all societies are infected at the time of birth, but most of the newborns are asymptomatic at birth. Some go on to develop unilateral or bilateral hearing loss. The fact that high titers of CMV are found in semen and that infection and conception may occur simultaneously may explain the failure of protection. If primary CMV infection occurs during gestation, severe abnormalities similar to those produced by EBV noted above may occur.[87] Antiviral therapy with famciclovir or valacyclovir has been used for EBV primary infection during pregnancy, but the number of patients treated is too small to draw conclusions. Ganciclovir for primary CMV infection is being studied.

Primary infection with HIV during pregnancy is seldom recognized because HIV antibody is absent early in infection, and the antibody screening process is performed at the first prenatal visit. If suspicion of primary infection is raised during pregnancy, then viral load should be measured. If positive, antiretroviral therapy for the mother to prevent HIV transmission to the fetus or newborn is indicated.[105]

Toxoplasma gondii producing primary infection during pregnancy can lead to congenital abnormalities. Although no controlled trials are available, treatment of the mother with pyrimethamine plus sulfonamides or spiramycin may eradicate parasites from the infant and the placenta.[106,107]

THE COMPROMISED HOST

CMV is a major problem in the immunocompromised host. CMV infection produces organ-specific disease (e.g., rejection in renal transplant, pneumonia in lung transplant). In all settings, it can produce a syndrome of fever, leukopenia, and inflammatory gastrointestinal disease. Clinically significant CMV infection often is followed by other opportunistic infections, such as *Pneumocystis carinii* or *Aspergillus* sp[108] (see Table 84-4). In solid organ transplants, the highest risk for symptomatic infection occurs when a CMV seronegative recipient receives an organ from a seropositive donor. The classic situation involves a parent donating a kidney to a seronegative child.[109,110] In marrow transplantation, CMV is closely linked to the development of graft-versus-host disease. In contrast to solid organ transplants, patients at highest risk are those who are seropositive and receive donor cells from a seronegative donor. Two approaches have been taken to mitigate this problem. One approach is treatment with ganciclovir for 90 days from the time of transplant. The other approach is monitoring either for evidence of CMV infection by measuring circulating CMV antigen or for CMV RNA/DNA using quantitative PCR. Therapy with ganciclovir is initiated when evidence for

infection is detected. No trial comparing these two approaches has been conducted, but use of the latter approach leads to treatment of far fewer subjects and a shorter course of therapy among the treated patients.

REFERENCES

1. Pfeiffer E: Drüsenfieber. *Jahrbuch für Kinderheilkunde* 23:257, 1885.
2. Sprunt TP, Evans FA: Mononucleosis in reaction to acute infections ("infectious mononucleosis"). *Johns Hopkins Bull* 31:410, 1920.
3. Paul JR, Bunnell WW: The presence of heterophile antibodies in infectious mononucleosis. *Am J Med Sci* 183:91, 1932.
4. Davidson I, Walker PH: The nature of the heterophile antibodies in infectious mononucleosis. *Am J Clin Pathol* 5:455, 1935.
5. Henle G, Henle W, Diehl V: Relation of Burkitt's tumor associated herpes type virus to infectious mononucleosis. *Proc Natl Acad Sci U S A* 59:94, 1968
6. Niederman JC, McCollum RW, Henle G, et al: Infectious mononucleosis: Clinical manifestations in relation to EB virus antibodies. *JAMA* 203:205, 1968.
7. Evans AS, Niederman JC, McCollum RW: Seroepidemiologic studies of infectious mononucleosis with EB virus. *N Engl J Med* 279:1121, 1968
8. Sawyer RN, Evans AS, Niederman JC, et al: Prospective studies of a group of Yale University freshman: I. Occurrence of infectious mononucleosis. *J Infect Dis* 123:263 1971.
9. University Health Physicians, PHLS Laboratories: A joint investigation of infectious mononucleosis and it relationship to EB virus antibody. *Br Med J* 4:643 1971.
10. Hoagland RJ: The clinical manifestations of infectious mononucleosis: A report of 200 cases. *Am J Med Sci* 240:55, 1960.
11. Hoagland RJ: The incubation period of infectious mononucleosis. *Am J Public Health* 54:1699, 1964.
12. Hanshaw JB, Betts RF, Simon G, Boynton RC: Acquired cytomegalovirus infection. *N Engl J Med* 272:602, 1965
13. Klemola E, Von Essen R, Henle G, et al: Infectious mononucleosis like disease with negative heterophile agglutination test. Clinical features in relation to Epstein-Barr virus and cytomegalovirus antibodies. *J Infect Dis* 121:608, 1970.
14. Macsween KF, Crawford DH: Epstein-Barr virus-recent advances. *Lancet Infect Dis* 3:131, 2003.
15. Hochberg D, Souza T, Catalina M, et al: Acute infection with Epstein-Barr virus targets and overwhelms peripheral memory B-cell compartment with resting, latently infected cells. *J Virol* 78:5194, 2004.
16. Yao QY, Rickinson AB, Epstein MA: A re-examination of the Epstein-Barr virus carrier state in healthy seropositive individuals. *Int J Cancer* 35:35, 1985.
17. Macallan DC, Wallace DL, Irvine AJ, et al: Rapid turnover of T cells in acute infectious mononucleosis. *Eur J Immunol* 33:2655, 2003.
18. Williams H, Macsween K, McAulay K, et al: Analysis of immune activation and clinical events in acute infectious mononucleosis. *J Infect Dis* 190:63, 2004.
19. Sixbey JW, Shirley P, Chesney PJ, et al: Detection of a second widespread strain of Epstein-Barr virus. *Lancet* 2:76, 1989.
20. Yao QY, Croom-Carter DSG, Tierney RJ, et al: Epidemiology of infection with Epstein-Barr virus types 1 and 2: Lessons from the study of a T cell immunocompromised hemophiliac cohort. *J Virol* 72:4352, 1998.
21. Pichler R, Berg J, Hengstschlager A, et al: Recurrent infectious mononucleosis caused by Epstein-Barr virus with persistent splenomegaly. *Mil Med* 166:733, 2001.
22. Sumaya CV, Ench Y: Epstein-Barr virus infectious mononucleosis in children: I. Clinical and general laboratory findings. *Pediatrics* 75:1003, 1985.

23. Sumaya CV, Ench Y: Epstein-Barr virus infectious mononucleosis in children: II. Heterophil antibody and viral specific responses. *Pediatrics* 75:1011, 1985.

24. Fleisher G, Henle W, Henle G, et al: Primary infection with Epstein-Barr virus in infants in the United States: Clinical and serologic observations. *J Infect Dis*139:553 1979.

25. Hickey SM, Strasburger VC: What every pediatrician should know about infectious mononucleosis in adolescents. *Pediatr Clin North Am* 44:1541 1997.

26. Auwaerter PG: Infectious mononucleosis in middle age. *JAMA* 281:454, 1999.

27. Axelrod P, Finestone AJ: Infectious mononucleosis in older adults. *Am Fam Physician* 42:1599, 1990.

28. Hurwitz CA, Henle W, Henle G, et al: Infectious mononucleosis in patients aged 40 to 72 years: Report of 27 cases, including 3 without heterophile-antibody responses. *Medicine* 62:256, 1983.

29. Schmader KE, van der Horst CM, Klotman ME: Epstein-Barr virus and the elderly host. *Rev Infect Dis* 11:64, 1989.

30. Grotto I, Mimouni D, Huerta M, et al: Clinical and laboratory presentation of EBV positive infectious mononucleosis in young adults. *Epidemiol Infect* 131:683, 2003.

31. Karajannis MA, Hummel M, Anagnostopoulos I, Stein H: Strict lymphotropism of Epstein-Barr virus during acute infectious mononucleosis in non-immunocompromised individuals. *Blood* 89:2856, 1997.

32. Yefenof E, Bakacs T, Einhorn L, et al: Epstein-Barr virus (EBV) receptors, complement receptors and EBV infectibility of different lymphocyte fractions of human peripheral blood: I. Complement receptor distribution and complement binding by separated lymphocyte subpopulations. *Cell Immunol* 35:34, 1978.

33. Thorley-Lawson DA: Immunological responses to Epstein-Barr virus infection and the pathogenesis of EBV-induced disease. *Biochim Biophys Acta* 948:263, 1988.

34. Renn CN, Straff W, Dorfmuller A, et al: Amoxicillin-induced exanthema in young adults with infectious mononucleosis: Demonstration of drug-specific lymphocyte reactivity. *Br J Dermatol* 147:1166, 2002.

35. Haverkos HW, Amsel Z, Drotman DP: Adverse virus-drug interactions. *Rev Infect Dis* 13:697, 1991.

36. Levitskaya J, Coram M, Levitsky V, et al: Inhibition of antigen processing by the internal repeat region of the Epstein-Barr virus nuclear antigen-1 *Nature* 375:685, 1995.

37. Linderholm M, Boman J, Juto P, Linde A: Comparative evaluation of nine kits for rapid diagnosis of infectious mononucleosis and Epstein-Barr virus-specific serology. *J Clin Microbiol* 32:259, 1994.

38. Rea TD, Ashley TL, Russo JE, Buchwald DS: A systematic study of Epstein-Barr virus serologic assays following acute infection. *Am J Clin Pathol* 117:156, 2002.

39. Brkic S, Jovanovic J, Preveden T, Vukobratov Z: Serologic profile of Epstein-Barr virus infection in acute infectious mononucleosis. *Med Pregl* 56:7, 2003.

40. Pitetti RD, Laus S, Wadowsky RM: Clinical evaluation of a quantitative realtime polymerase chain reaction assay for diagnosis of primary Epstein-Barr virus infection in children. *Pediatr Infect Dis J* 22:736, 2003.

41. Hudnall SD, Patel JU, Schwab H, Martinez J: Comparative immunophenotypic features of EBV-positive and EBV-negative atypical lymphocytosis. *Cytometry* 55B:22, 2003.

42. Matsukawa Y, Okano M, Ishikawa N, Imasi S: Severe thrombocytopenic purpura associated with primary Epstein-Barr virus infection. *J Infect* 29:107, 1994.

43. Whitelaw F, Brook MG, Kennedy N, Weir WR: Haemolytic anemia complicating Epstein-Barr virus infection. *Br J Clin Pract* 49:212, 1995.

44. Lazarus KH, Baehner RL: Aplastic anemia complicating infectious mononucleosis: A case report and review of the literature. *Pediatrics* 67:907, 1981.

45. Auvin S, Dalle JH, Ganga-Zandzou PS, Ythier H: Is agranulocytosis following infectious mononucleosis caused by autoimmunity? *Pediatr Hematol Oncol* 20:611, 2003.

46. Tanaka M, Kamijo T, Koike T, et al: Specific autoantibodies to platelet glycoprotein in Epstein-Barr virus-associated immune thrombocytopenia. *Int J Hematol* 78:168, 2003.

47. Evans AS: Infectious mononucleosis and related syndromes. *Am J Med Sci* 276:325, 1978.

48. Jones JF: A perspective on Epstein-Barr virus diseases. *Adv Pediatr* 36: 307, 1989.

49. Bhaskaran J, Harkness DR: Hereditary spherocytosis unmasked by infectious mononucleosis with autoimmune hemolytic anemia. *J Fla Med Assoc* 67:483, 1980.

50. Taylor JJ: Haemolysis in infectious mononucleosis: Inapparent congenital spherocytosis. *Br Med J* 4:525, 1973.

51. Asgari MM, Begos DG: Spontaneous splenic rupture in infectious mononucleosis: A review. *Yale J Biol Med* 70:175, 1997.

52. Kinderknecht JJ: Infectious mononucleosis and the spleen. *Curr Sports Med Rep* 1:116,2002

53. Fujimoto H, Asaoka K, Imaaizumi T, et al: Epstein-Barr virus infections of the central nervous system. *Intern Med* 42:33, 2003.

54. Connelly KP, DeWitt LD: Neurologic complications of infectious mononucleosis. *Pediatr Neurol* 10:181, 1994.

55. Jacobs BC, Rothbarth PH, van der Meche, et al: The spectrum of antecedent infections in Guillain-Barre syndrome. *Neurology* 51:1110, 1998.

56. Kimura H, Morishima T, Kanegane H, et al: Prognostic factors for chronic active Epstein-Barr virus infection. *J Infect Dis* 187:527, 2003.

57. Buchwald DS, Rea TD, Katon WJ, et al: Acute infectious mononucleosis: Characteristics of patients who report failure to recover. *Am J Med* 109:531,2000.

58. Okano M: Overview and problematic standpoints of severe chronic active Epstein-Barr virus infection syndrome. *Crit Rev Oncol Hematol* 44: 273, 2002.

59. Ohga S, Monura A, Takada H, Hara T: Immunological aspects of Epstein-Barr virus infection. *Crit Rev Oncol Hematol* 44:203, 2002.

60. Suzuki K, Ohshima K, Karube K, et al: Clinicopathological states of Epstein-Barr virus-associated T/NK cell proliferative disorders (severe chronic active EBV infection) of children and young adults. *Int J Oncol* 24:1165, 2004.

61. Chen CJ, Huang YC, Jaing TH, et al: Hemophagocytic syndrome: A review of 18 pediatric cases. *J Microbiol Immunol Infect* 37:157, 2004.

62. Imashuku S, Kuriyama K, Sakai R, et al: Treatment of Epstein-Barr virus-associated hemophagocytic lymphohistiocytosis (EBV-HLH) in young adults: A report from HLH study center. *Med Pediatr Oncol* 41:103, 2003.

63. Imashuku S, Teramura T, Tauchi H, et al: Longitudinal follow-up of patients with Epstein-Barr virus-associated hemophagocytic lymphohistiocytosis. *Haematologica* 89:183, 2004.

64. Pagano JS: Epstein-Barr virus: The first human tumor virus and its role in cancer. *Proc Assoc Am Physicians* 111:573, 1999.

65. Endo R, Kikuta H, Ebihara T, et al: Possible involvement in oncogenesis of a single base mutation in internal ribosome entry site of Epstein-Barr nuclear antigen 1 mRNA. *J Med Virol* 72:630, 2004.

66. Flavell KJ, Murray PG: Hodgkin disease and Epstein-Barr virus. *Mol Pathol* 53:262, 2000.

67. Hjalgrim H, Askling J, Rostgaard K, et al: Characteristics of Hodgkin's lymphoma after infectious mononucleosis. *N Engl J Med* 349:1324, 2003.

68. Jarrett RF: Risk factors for Hodgkin lymphoma by EBV status and significance of detection of EBV genomes in serum of patients with EBV-associated Hodgkin's lymphoma. *Leuk Lymphoma* 44(suppl 3):S27, 2003.

69. Zangwill SD, Hsu DT, Kichuk MR, et al: Incidence and outcome of Epstein-Barr virus infection and lymphoproliferative disease in pediatric heart transplant recipients. *J Heart Lung Transplant* 17:1161, 1998.

70. Gao SZ, Chapparro SV, Perlroth M, et al: Post-transplant lymphoprolifera-

tive disease in heart and heart-lung transplant recipients: 30 year experience at Stanford University. *J Heart Lung Transplant* 22:505, 2003.

71.   Malouf MA, Chajed PN, Hopkins P, et al: Anti-viral prophylaxis reduces the incidence of lymphoproliferative disease in lung transplant recipients. *J Heart Lung Transplant* 21:547, 2002.

72.   MacGinnitie AJ, Geha R: X-linked lymphoproliferative disease: Genetic lesions and clinical consequences. *Curr Allergy Asthma Rep* 2:361, 2002.

73.   Cohen JI: Benign and malignant Epstein-Barr virus-associated B-cell lymphoproliferative diseases. *Semin Hematol* 40:116, 2003.

74.   Yachie A, Kanegane H, Kasahara Y: Epstein-Barr virus associated T-/natural killer cell lymphoproliferative diseases. *Semin Hematol* 40:124, 2003.

75.   Kawa K, Okamura T, Yasui M, et al: Allogeneic hematopoietic stem cell transplantation for Epstein-Barr virus-associated T/NK-cell lymphoproliferative disease. *Crit Rev Oncol Hematol* 44:251, 2002.

76.   Cheng WM, Chan KH, Chen HL, et al: Assessing the risk of nasopharyngeal cancer on the basis of EBV antibody spectrum. *Int J Cancer* 97:489, 2002.

77.   Moss DJ, Khanna R, Bharadwaj M: Will a vaccine to nasopharyngeal carcinoma retain orphan status? *Dev Biol* 110:67, 2002.

78.   McClain K, Leach CT, Jenson HB, et al: Association of Epstein-Barr virus with leiomyosarcomas in young people with AIDS. *N Engl J Med* 332:12, 1995.

79.   Lee ES, Locker J, Nalesnik M, et al: The association of Epstein-Barr virus with smooth muscle tumors occurring after organ transplantation. *N Engl J Med* 332:19, 1995.

80.   Oda K, Koda K, Takiguchi N, et al: Detection of Epstein-Barr virus in gastric carcinoma cells and surrounding lymphocytes. *Gastric Cancer* 6:173, 2003.

81.   Kuppers R: B cells under influence: Transformation of B cells by Epstein-Barr virus. *Nat Rev Immunol* 3:801, 2003.

82.   Murry PG, Young LS: Epstein-Barr virus infection: Basis of malignancy and potential for therapy. *Expert Rev Mol Med* 15:2001, 2001.

83.   Greenspan JS, Greenspan D, Lennette ET: Replication of Epstein-Barr virus within epithelial cells of hairy oral leukoplakia an AIDS associated lesion. *N Engl J Med* 332:19, 1986.

84.   Bharadwaj M, Moss DJ: Epstein-Barr virus vaccine: A cytotoxic T-cell-based approach. *Expert Rev Vaccines* 1:467, 2002.

85.   Farrell CJ, Lee JM, Shin EC, et al: Inhibition of Epstein-Barr virus–induced growth proliferation by nuclear antigen EBNA-2 peptide. *Proc Natl Acad Sci U S A* 101:4625, 2004.

86.   Weller TH, Hanshaw JB: Virologic and clinical observations in cytomegalic inclusion disease. *N Engl J Med* 266:1233, 1962.

87.   Stagno S, Pass RF, Dworsky ME, et al: Congenital cytomegalovirus infection: The relative importance of primary or recurrent maternal infection. *N Engl J Med* 306:945, 1982.

88.   Hallee TJ, Evans AS, Niederman JC, et al: Infectious mononucleosis at the United States Military Academy. A prospective study of a single class over 4 years. *Yale J Biol Med* 47:182, 1974.

89.   Wreghitt TG, Teare O, Sule O, et al: Cytomegalovirus infection in immunocompetent patients. *Clin Infect Dis* 37:1603, 2003.

90.   Rodriguez-Bano J, Muniain MA, Borobio MV, et al: Cytomegalovirus mononucleosis as a cause of prolonged fever and prominent weight loss in immunocompetent adults. *Clin Microbiol Infect* 10:468, 2004.

91.   Smith MS, Bentz GL, Alexander JS, Yurochko AD: Human cytomegalovirus induces monocyte differentiation and migration as a strategy for dissemination and persistence. *J Virol* 78:4444, 2004.

92.   Betts RF, Freeman RB, Douglas RG Jr, et al: Transmission of cytomegalovirus with renal allograft. *Kidney Int* 8:385, 1975

93.   Tindall B, Cooper DA, Donovan B, Penny R: Primary human immunodeficiency infection. Clinical and serologic aspects. *Infect Dis Clin North Am* 2:329, 1988.

94.   Vanhems P, Allard R, Cooper DA, et al: Acute human immunodefi-

95.   Rosenberg ES, Caliendo AM, Walker BD: Acute HIV among patients tested for mononucleosis (letter). *N Engl J Med* 340:969, 1999.

96.   Walensky RP, Rosenberg ES, Ferraro MJ, et al: Investigation of primary human immunodeficiency virus infection in patients who test positive for heterophile antibody. *Clin Infect Dis* 33:570, 2001.

97.   Steeper TA, Horwitz CA, Ablashi DV, et al: The spectrum of clinical and laboratory findings resulting from human Herpesvirus-6 (HHV-6) in patients with mononucleosis-like illness not resulting from Epstein-Barr virus or cytomegalovirus. *Am J Clin Pathol* 93:776, 1990.

98.   Andersson J, Britton S, Ernberg I, et al: Effect of acyclovir on infectious mononucleosis: A double-blinded, placebo-controlled study. *J Infect Dis* 153:283, 1986.

99.   Torre D, Tambini R: Acyclovir for treatment of infectious mononucleosis: A meta-analysis. *Scand J Infect Dis* 31:543, 1999.

100.   Collins M, Fleisher G, Kreisberg J, Fager S: Role of steroids in the treatment of infectious mononucleosis in the ambulatory college student. *J Am Coll Health* 33:101, 1984.

101.   Chan SC, Dawes PJ: The management of severe infectious mononucleosis tonsillitis and upper airway obstruction. *J Laryngol Otol* 115:973;2001.

102.   Peter J, Ray GG: Infectious mononucleosis. *Pediatr Rev* 19:276, 1998.

103.   Walling DM, Flaitz CM, Nichols CM, et al: Persistent productive Epstein-Barr virus replication in normal epithelial cells in vivo. *J Infect Dis* 184:1499, 2001.

104.   Yao QY, Ogan P, Rowe M, et al: Epstein-Barr virus-infected B cells persist in the circulation of acyclovir-treated virus carriers. *Int J Cancer* 43:67, 1989.

105.   Connor EM, Sperling RS, Gelber R, et al: Reduction of maternal-infant transmission of human immunodeficiency virus type 1 with zidovudine treatment. Pediatrics AIDS Clinical Trials Group Protocol 076 Study Group *N Engl J Med* 331:1173, 1994.

106.   Cengir SD, Ortac F, Soylemez F: Treatment and results of chronic toxoplasmosis. Analysis of 33 cases. *Gynecol Obstet Invest* 33:105, 1992.

107.   Stray-Pedersen B: Treatment of toxoplasmosis in the pregnant mother and newborn child. *Scand J Infect Dis* 84:23, 1992.

108.   Schooley RT, Hirsch MS, Colvin RB, et al: Association of Herpesvirus infections with T lymphocyte subset alterations, glomerulopathy, and opportunistic infections after renal transplantation. *N Engl J Med* 308:307, 1983.

109.   Betts RF, Freeman RB, Douglas RG Jr, Talley TE: Clinical manifestations of renal allograft derived primary cytomegalovirus infection. *Am J Dis Child* 131:759, 1977.

110.   Ho M, Suwansirkul S, Dowling JN, et al. The transplanted kidney as a source of cytomegalovirus infection. *N Engl J Med* 293:1109, 1975.

111.   Goldberg GN, Fulginiti VA, Ray CG, et al: In utero Epstein-Barr virus (infectious mononucleosis) infection. *JAMA* 246:1579,1981.

112.   Fleisher G, Bologonese R: Epstein-Barr virus infections in pregnancy: A prospective study. *J Pediatr* 104:374, 1984.

113.   Ho M: Epidemiology of cytomegalovirus infections. *Rev Infect Dis* 12(suppl 7):S701, 1990.

114.   Yeager AS: Transfusion-acquired cytomegalovirus infection in newborn infants. *Am J Dis Child* 128:478, 1974.

115.   Meters JD, Spencer HC Jr, Watts JC, et al: Cytomegalovirus pneumonia after human marrow transplantation. *Ann Intern Med* 82:181, 1975.

116.   George MJ, Snydman DR, Werner BG, et al: The independent role of cytomegalovirus for invasive fungal disease in orthotopic liver transplant recipients: The Boston Center for Liver Transplantation CMV Ig-Study Group: Cytogam, MedImmune Inc., Gaithersburg, Md. *Am J Med* 103:106, 1997.

117.   Davis JE, Moss DJ: Treatment options for post-transplant lymphoproliferative disorders and other Epstein-Barr virus-associated malignancies. *Tissue Antigens* 63:285, 2004.

MALIGNANT DISEASES

CLASSIFICATION AND CLINICAL MANIFESTATIONS OF THE CLONAL MYELOID DISORDERS

MARSHALL A. LICHTMAN

The clonal myeloid disorders result from acquired mutations of DNA within a multipotential marrow cell or very early progenitor cell. The chromosomal alteration resulting from the primary mutation often is evident when cytogenetic analysis is performed. Translocations, inversions, and deletions of chromosomes can result in (1) the expression of fusion genes that encode fusion proteins that are oncogenic or (2) the overexpression or underexpression of genes that encode molecules critical to the control of cell growth or programmed cell death.

The different mutations may result in variable phenotypes that range from mild impairment of the steady-state levels of blood cells, insignificant functional impairment of cells, and little consequence on longevity to severe cytopenias and death in days, if the disorder is untreated. Although very mild disease expression can be considered a "benign" neoplasm compared to acute myelogenous leukemia, the term has not been used to classify disorders such as clonal sideroblastic anemia because they have measurable alterations in blood cells, may result in symptoms, and have a greatly increased risk to progress to acute myelogenous leukemia compared to age- and gender-matched unaffected persons.

The somatically mutated (neoplastic) multipotential cell from which the clonal expansion of hematopoietic cells derives retains the ability, with various degrees of imperfection, to differentiate and mature into each blood cell lineage. The particular syndrome may have altered blood cell numbers, structure, and function and may have a minimal to severe effect on a particular blood cell lineage. The effect on any one lineage occurs in an unpredictable way, even in subjects within the same category of disease. The resulting phenotypes are numerous and varied. In polycythemia vera or thrombocythemia, maturation of progenitors results in cells nearly normal in appearance and function but excessive in their level in the blood. Moreover, overlapping features are common, such as thrombocythemia as a feature of polycythemia or chronic myelogenous leukemia. The clonal anemias may be accompanied by insignificant or very severe neutropenia or thrombocytopenia or sometimes thrombocytosis. This finding reflects the unpredictable expression of the mutant multipotential cell's differentiation capabilities for which the genic explanations are largely unknown. Tight relationships between the cytogenetic alteration and the phenotype occur in only a few circumstances, and even these are imperfect, for example t(9;22)(q34;q11)(BCR-ABL) with chronic myeloge-

nous leukemia or t(15;17)(q22;q21)(PML-RARα) with acute promyelocytic leukemia. However, most patients can be grouped into the classic diagnostic designations listed in Table 85-1.

An important feature of the clonal myeloid diseases is the potentially reversible suppression of expression of normal stem cells by the clonally expanded cells. This coexistence and competition forms the basis for the remission-relapse pattern seen in acute myelogenous leukemia after intensive chemotherapy and for the reappearance of polyclonal, normal hematopoiesis in some patients with chronic myelogenous leukemia after imatinib mesylate therapy.

A wide array of clonal (neoplastic) syndromes or diseases can result from a somatic mutation in a multipotential or progenitor hematopoietic cell (Table 85-1). The diseases can be grouped, somewhat arbitrarily, by their degree of malignancy, using the classic terminology of experimental carcinogenesis, which logically considers the degree of loss of differentiation potential and the rate of progression of the disease. The term *deviation* relates to the relationship to normal cellular differentiation potential and the regulation of cell population homeostasis (birth and death rates). This terminology has been used to array the diagnostic categories of clonal hematopoietic diseases into a framework for the reader related to pathogenesis.

MINIMAL-DEVIATION MYELOID CLONAL DISORDERS

The neoplasms designated in Table 85-1 retain a higher degree of differentiating capability and usually permit life spans measured in decades without treatment or with minimally toxic treatment approaches.[1] Use of the term *minimal deviation* should not be construed as indicating these conditions do not have morbidity, shorten life, and have other consequences to the patient. The term is used relative to acute myelogenous leukemia (AML), which has an expected life span measured in days to weeks if left untreated.

INEFFECTIVE HEMATOPOIESIS (PRECURSOR APOPTOSIS) PROMINENT

Cytopenia resulting from ineffective hematopoiesis is the most characteristic feature of a subgroup of clonal hematopoietic multipotential cell diseases. A common secondary characteristic is striking dysmorphogenesis of blood cells. These cytologic abnormalities, characteristic of the clonal anemias, bicytopenias, or pancytopenias, include changes in the size (macrocytosis and microcytosis), shape (poikilocytosis), and nuclear or organelle structure (hypogranulation or hypergranulation, nuclear hypolobulation) of blood cells and their precursors (see Chap. 86). Abnormal maturation of blood cells leads to morphologic, biochemical, and functional alterations of the cells. Ineffective erythropoiesis, the intramedullary death of erythroblasts before they reach full maturation, is a common feature. Ineffective granulopoiesis and thrombopoiesis also occur. No distinction in the presenting manifestation or the course of clonal anemia with lesser (<15 percent) or greater (>15 percent) proportions of sideroblasts in the marrow exists. Therefore, this distinction has no functional utility, yet the World Health Organization has retained it.[2] Leukemic blast cells are not evident in these syndromes. If marrow blasts are elevated above the normal upper limit of 2 percent, the disorder should be considered oligoblastic leukemia (syn. *refractory anemia with excess blasts*). Because of the variability of marrow differential counts and marrow sampling, such distinctions may require several observations.

The term *hematopoietic dysplasia*, later simplified to *myelodysplasia*, has become ensconced as the category into which some of these

TABLE 85-1   NEOPLASTIC (CLONAL) MYELOID DISORDERS

Minimal-deviation neoplasms (no leukemic blast cells are evident in marrow)

Underproduction (apoptosis) of mature cells is prominent

Clonal sideroblastic anemia (Chap. 86)*

Clonal nonsideroblastic anemia (Chap. 86)*

Clonal multicytopenia (Chap. 86)*

Paroxysmal nocturnal hemoglobinuria (Chap. 38)

Overproduction of cells is prominent

Polycythemia vera (Chap. 56)

Primary thrombocythemia (Chap. 111)

Moderate-deviation neoplasms (small proportions of leukemic blast cells usually present in marrow)

Chronic myelogenous leukemia (Chap. 88)

Ph-positive *BCR* rearrangement positive CML

Ph-negative *BCR* rearrangement positive CML

Idiopathic myelofibrosis (Chap. 89)

Chronic eosinophilic leukemia (Chaps. 62 and 88)

Chronic neutrophilic leukemia (Chap. 88)

Moderately severe deviation neoplasms (moderate concentration of leukemic blast cells present in marrow)

Oligoblastic myelogenous leukemia (refractory anemia with excess myeloblasts)* (Chap. 86)

Subacute myelomonocytic leukemia (Chap. 88)

Juvenile myelomonocytic leukemia (Chap. 88)

Severe deviation neoplasms (leukemic blast cells frequent in the marrow)

Phenotypic variants of acute myelogenous leukemia (Chap. 87)

Myeloblastic (granuloblastic)

Myelomonocytic (granulomonoblastic)

Promyelocytic

Erythroid

Monocytic

Megakaryocytic

Eosinophilic[†]

Basophilic[‡]

Mastocytic[§]

Histiocytic or Dendritic[¶]

Recurring genotypic variants of acute myelogenous leukemia [t(8;21), Inv16 or t(16;16), t(15;17), or (11q23)][**]

Myeloid (granulocytic) sarcoma

Acute biphenotypic (myeloid and lymphoid markers) leukemia[††]

Acute leukemia with lymphoid markers evolving from a prior clonal myeloid disease

---

* The World Health Organization includes these disorders under the rubric of the "Myelodysplastic Syndrome," the classification of which is discussed in Chap. 86.

† Acute eosinophilic leukemia is rare. Most cases are subacute or chronic and formerly were included in the hypereosinophilic syndrome (see Chaps. 62, 87, and 88).

‡ Rare cases of basophilic leukemia are Ph-negative and are variants of AML. Most cases have the Ph chromosome and evolve from CML (see Chaps. 63, 87, and 88).

§ See Chap. 63.

¶ See Chap. 72.

** The World Health Organization has designated these subtypes as separate entities even though they also have phenotypes listed under phenotypic variants.[1]

†† Approximately 10 percent of cases of acute myeloblastic leukemia may be biphenotypic (myeloid and lymphoid markers on individual cells) when studied with antimyeloid and antilymphoid monoclonal antibodies (see Chap. 87).

---

syndromes, but not others, are grouped. In strict pathologic terms, a dysplasia is a polyclonal and thus nonmalignant change in the cells of a tissue. These myeloid syndromes are clonal, often have aneuploid or pseudodiploid cells in the clone, and can be associated with significant morbidity and premature death; thus, they are neoplasms rather than dysplasias. They demonstrate clonal instability, and each has a propensity to evolve into AML that far exceeds that of the general population. The term *dysplasia* was used at a time when the prominent dysmorphogenesis was thought to be the singular abnormality.

OVERPRODUCTION OF CELLS PROMINENT

Polycythemia vera (see Chap. 56) and primary thrombocythemia (see Chap. 111) are clonal myeloid disorders. They are so named because of the overaccumulation of red cells, neutrophils, and platelets in polycythemia and of platelets and to a lesser extent neutrophils in thrombocythemia. Each cell lineage is affected in each disorder, reflecting a multipotential cell origin, but the magnitude of the effects differs. The inhibiting effect on red cell production in thrombocythemia usually is slight. Polycythemia vera and primary thrombocythemia do not show morphologic evidence of leukemic hematopoiesis; differentiation and maturation are maintained. The proportion of blast cells in the marrow is not increased above normal, and blast cells are not present in the blood. The survival of cohorts of patients with these diseases is only slightly less than expected for age- and gender-matched unaffected persons.[1,3,4] An exception is the very uncommon onset of polycythemia vera in childhood in which shortened survival has been reported.[5]

MODERATE-DEVIATION CLONAL MYELOID DISORDERS

Chronic myelogenous leukemia (CML) (see Chap. 88) and idiopathic myelofibrosis (agnogenic myeloid metaplasia) (see Chap. 89) classically share the features of overproduction of granulocytes and platelets and impaired production of red cells. However, idiopathic myelofibrosis has a strong predisposition to marrow fibrosis and striking teardrop-shaped red cells. The cells in the disorder have no specific cytogenetic change. Whereas CML invariably has a rearrangement of *BCR* on chromosome 22, in approximately 90 percent of patients this mutation is reflected in t(9;22)(q34;q11)(*BCR-ABL*) by standard cytogenetic methods. Splenomegaly and a gradually progressive course are common to both. Blast cells are very slightly increased in marrow and blood in most patients with the two disorders. CML has a very high propensity to transform to acute leukemia. Idiopathic myelofibrosis terminates in acute leukemia in about one of six patients. Life span in these disorders usually is measured in years but is significantly decreased compared to age- and gender-matched unaffected cohorts. Therapy is required in virtually all cases of CML and in most cases of idiopathic myelofibrosis at the time of diagnosis. Both diseases can be cured only by stem cell transplantation, although life span has been increased significantly in CML with the use of imatinib mesylate and interferon alpha therapy.

MODERATELY SEVERE-DEVIATION CLONAL MYELOID DISORDERS

These disorders fall into a group that progresses less rapidly than acute leukemia and more rapidly than chronic leukemia. They have a predisposition to develop with a granulocytic and monocytic phenotype, either morphologically or cytochemically. These diseases also have been called *oligoblastic* or *smoldering myelogenous leukemia, refractory anemia with excess myeloblasts, subacute myelomonocytic leukemia,* and *atypical or unclassifiable myeloproliferative syndromes.* The latter designation is sometimes used for uncommon syndromes that do not fall into easily classifiable designations. They usually are seen in patients older than 65 years. The subacute syndromes produce more morbidity than do the chronic syndromes, and patients have a shorter life expectancy. These are leukemic states that have low or moderate concentrations of leukemic blast cells in marrow and often blood, anemia, thrombocytopenia, and sometimes prominent monocytic maturation of cells (see Chap. 86). The oligoblastic myelogenous leukemias compose approximately 60 to 80 percent of the cases that have been grouped under the title *myelodysplastic syndromes. Sub-*

acute myelomonocytic leukemia has been withdrawn from the category of myelodysplastic diseases, highlighting the confusion surrounding the term. In all other malignancies, the presence of tumor cells determines the diagnosis, such as carcinoma of the colon or the uterine cervix, whether *in situ*, invasive, or metastatic. Use of the percentage of leukemic cells as the basis of a diagnostic distinction is illogical, hence the preference for oligoblastic myelogenous leukemia rather than myelodysplasia for patients with increased blast cells (leukemia) and dysmorphic cell maturation.

SEVERE-DEVIATION CLONAL MYELOID DISORDERS

Morphologic, immunologic, histochemical, and cytogenetic characteristics of cells in the blood and marrow provide the major basis for recognition of AML and its subtypes (see Chaps. 10 and 87). Correlation among observers and between the morphologic method of classification and the monoclonal antibody reactivity-dependent classification of AML is imperfect.[6–8] The importance of these various approaches differs. The morphologic plus cytochemical approach is the most inclusive because virtually all cases can be placed into a morphologic subtype. Occasionally this requires supplementation by analysis of immunophenotype (the CD representation). Because immunophenotyping is a standard procedure in most laboratories, the results are readily available in any case. Classification by cytogenetics is more limited because many cases have infrequent abnormalities, making this approach complex. However, knowing the cytogenetic alterations is useful for estimating the prognosis (risk category), for example, t(8;21), t(16;16) or Inv16 AML, and in some cases determining treatment, for example, t(15;17). Thus, combined light microscopy of blood and marrow, cytochemistry, and immunophenotyping to designate the phenotypic subtype, supplemented by cytogenetics or molecular diagnostic methods, currently is the best approach. The polymerase chain reaction may be particularly useful for determining subclinical residual disease and monitoring therapy (see Chap. 87).

Gene chips containing thousands of genes can be used to further genotype and subclassify AML into prognostic groups. A study of patients with AML who had normal karyotypes by standard cytogenetic methods separated patients into two groups by hierarchical gene clustering with significantly different survival after current therapy.[9] In addition, patients with AML who have prevalent cytogenetic abnormalities, such as t(8;21), can be further stratified based on the hierarchical clusters of gene expression. Patients with AML also can be stratified into several prognostic groups using hierarchical gene cluster analysis.[10] These studies are important because they (1) identify genes that cooperate or interact to result in a fully malignant phenotype, (2) provide potential new targets for therapy, and (3) help identify patients who might benefit from early stem cell transplantation. At this time, these methods are complex and not available in most laboratories. Moreover, they require refinement based on the time during the course of the disease that genetic analyses are performed; gene abnormalities differ over time. Also, studies should focus on the most primitive multipotential cells in the clone to avoid secondary changes in the mass of leukemic cells.

TRANSITIONS AMONG CLONAL MYELOID DISEASES

Patients with minimal, moderate, and moderately severe clonal myeloid disorders have an increased likelihood of progressing to florid AML, with a frequency ranging from approximately less than 1 percent of patients with paroxysmal nocturnal hemoglobinuria, 10 percent of patients with clonal sideroblastic anemia, and approximately 35 percent of patients with clonal pancytopenia. Approximately 15 percent of patients with polycythemia vera evolve to a syndrome indis-

tinguishable from idiopathic myelofibrosis.[49] AML develops as a terminal event in approximately 1 percent of patients with polycythemia vera not treated with ^{32}P or an alkylating agent and in a larger proportion of patients who are treated.[50]

Approximately 5 percent of patients with primary thrombocythemia and approximately 15 percent of patients with idiopathic myelofibrosis progress to AML. The rate of conversion to AML in polycythemia and thrombocythemia is increased by prior radiotherapy or chemotherapy depending on the dose, duration, and type of drug. Virtually all patients with CML progress to AML, although in some cases the patient enters a phase that behaves like oligoblastic leukemia before it progresses to acute leukemia (see Chap. 88).

PATHOGENESIS OF CLONAL MYELOID DISEASES

In AML, a sequence of mutations in a single multipotential cell results in a clone that is severely defective and contains precursor cells that are unable to mature.[11] Proliferation of primitive progenitors is excessive when considered in absolute terms, that is, the total number of blast cells proliferating. AML is considered a clinical disease with many forms of morphologic expression. This variation of phenotype is consistent with the large number of genetic lesions identified and the behavior of the leukemic multipotential cell, which is capable of differentiation into all the blood cell lineages (Fig. 85-1). Hence, the asymmetrical and uncoordinated maturation of leukemic progenitor cells may allow one or another cell type to predominate. Little variation exists in the course of these different morphologic or cytogenetic variants of AML.

Important epiphenomena are related to special features of certain morphologic types of leukemia, such as tissue infiltration, including the central nervous system (monocyte leukemia), disseminated intravascular coagulation and hemorrhage (promyelocytic leukemia), heart and lung fibrosis (eosinophilic leukemia), intense marrow fibrosis (megakaryocytic leukemia), myeloid sarcomas [t(8;21) leukemia], and others (see Chap. 87). These morphologic subtypes and epiphenomena are determined by genic differences. The differences may be evident in gross cytogenic abnormalities that correlate with, and may determine, some phenotypes. The subtypes include t(15;17) promyelocytic leukemia, t(8;21) myelomonocytic leukemia, and Inv16 myelomonocytic leukemia with prominent eosinophilic maturation in the marrow (see Chap. 87).

In CML, injury to a single cell results in a clone in which there is an enormous expansion of progenitors for granulocytic and, often, megakaryocytic cells. Erythropoiesis is effective but decreased. Unlike AML, maturation of progenitor cells in CML is nearly normal; hence, the predominant leukemic cells in the blood are amitotic, mature, or partially matured cells, such as myelocytes and segmented neutrophils, erythrocytes, and platelets.

Because hematopoiesis is generated by a leukemic stem cell, erythropoiesis, thrombopoiesis, and granulopoiesis are leukemic in most patients with AML, CML, and other clonal myeloid diseases. The qualitative abnormalities of structure and function and clonal cytogenic abnormalities are present in erythroblasts, megakaryocytes, and granulocyte precursors in most cases of AML (see Chap. 87) and in all cases of CML (see Chap. 88).

PHENOTYPE OF MYELOID CLONAL DISEASES AS A RESULT OF THE MATRIX OF DIFFERENTIATION AND MATURATION

The phenotype of clonal myeloid diseases is a reflection of a neoplastic stem cell's abnormal capability to differentiate into committed progenitor cells and the ability of progenitor cells to mature into identifiable cells of the erythroid, granulocytic (neutrophilic, basophilic,

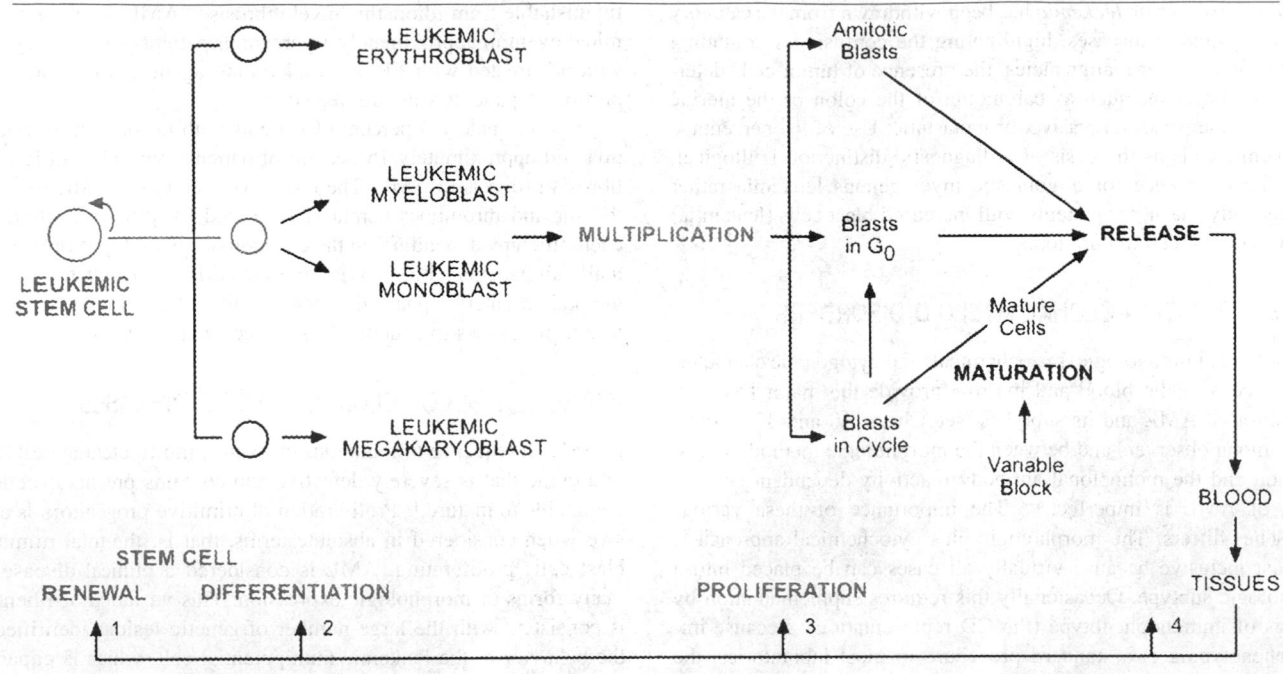

FIGURE 85-1   Hematopoiesis in acute myelogenous leukemia. The malignant process evolves from a single mutant multipotential cell.[12–14] This cell is represented at either level 1 or level 2 in Fig. 85-3. This cell is capable of multivariate commitment to leukemic erythroid, granulocytic, and megakaryocytic progenitors. In most cases, granulocytic commitment predominates, and myeloblasts and monoblasts or their immediate derivatives are the dominant cell types. Leukemic blast cells accumulate in the marrow. The leukemic blast cells may become amitotic (sterile) and undergo programmed cell death, may stop dividing for prolonged periods (blasts in G_0) but have the potential to reenter the mitotic cycle, or may divide and undergo varying degrees of maturation. Maturation may lead to mature cells, such as red cells, segmented neutrophils, monocytes, or platelets. A severe block in maturation is characteristic of AML, whereas a high proportion of leukemic blast cells mature in CML. The disturbance in commitment and maturation in myelogenous leukemia is quantitative, so many patterns are possible. At least four major steps in hematopoiesis are regulated: (1) stem cell self-renewal and (2) differentiation into hematopoietic cell lineages (red cells, granulocytes, platelets), (3) proliferation (multiplication) and maturation of progenitor and precursor cells, and (4) release of mature cells into the blood. These control points are defective in myelogenous leukemia. Premature or delayed apoptosis of cells may be another key abnormality contributing to cell accumulation or premature death.

mastocytic, eosinophilic), monocytic, or megakaryocytic lineage (Fig. 85-2).[12–14]

Under normal circumstances, differentiation represents the changes from a multipotential cell to multiple unipotential lineage progenitors. Maturation represents the physical and chemical changes from a unipotential progenitor through a sequence of precursors to the fully mature and functional blood cell, including progression from a burst forming unit–erythroid to proerythroblast to erythrocyte, a colony forming unit–granulocyte to myeloblast to segmented neutrophil, a colony forming unit–eosinophil to a segmented eosinophil, a colony forming unit–basophil to a mature basophil, a colony forming unit–mast cell to a mature mast cell, a colony forming unit–monocyte-macrophage to promonocyte to monocyte to macrophage or dendritic cell, a colony forming unit–megakaryocyte to a diploid megakaryoblast to the polyploid megakaryocyte. This matrix, which is composed of the options of commitment to different lineages and the progressive stages of maturation at which partial or complete arrest can occur, results in the potential for a wide array of morphologic syndromes by which a mutant (leukemic) stem cell can dominate hematopoiesis (see Fig. 85-2).

In the clonal myeloid diseases in which differentiation and maturation capability are retained, one of the cell lines, for example, erythrocytes, granulocytes, or platelets, tends to accumulate in the blood more prominently and results in a phenotypic expression of the disease that determines the nosology (e.g., primary thrombocythemia). In AML, the phenotypic expression may be predominantly myeloblastic (granuloblastic), erythroid, monocytic, megakaryocytic, or combina-

tions thereof. Certain patterns are favored. In AML, myeloblastic leukemia, monocytic leukemia, or mixtures of the two are more common than erythroid, megakaryocytic, or eosinophilic leukemia. However, AML usually has a disturbance in all cell lines. In myeloblastic or myelomonocytic leukemia, overt, qualitative abnormalities of erythroblasts and megakaryocytes may occur. The prevalence of the abnormalities in the latter two lineages may not be great enough or evident enough for the observer to designate a case as erythroid or megakaryocytic leukemia. In the latter two cases, identification of markers unique for erythroid or megakaryocytic cells, rather than reliance solely on light microscopy, has increased the frequency of identification of the variants.

The continuum of maturation can be completely or partially blocked at various levels, leading to morphologic variants such as acute myeloblastic, acute promyelocytic, subacute myelogenous, or CML.

PLURIPOTENTIAL STEM CELL POOL AS SITE OF THE LESION

Evidence points to a lesion in the pluripotential stem cell pool in most of the clonal myeloid diseases, especially in patients older than 50 years, who account for the great proportion of cases. In CML patients, the mutation is in the pluripotential stem cell. In other syndromes, evidence for involvement of B and T lymphocytes is variable. B lymphocytes are derived from the clone in many cases. The evidence for T lymphocyte involvement is less compelling. Evidence that affected

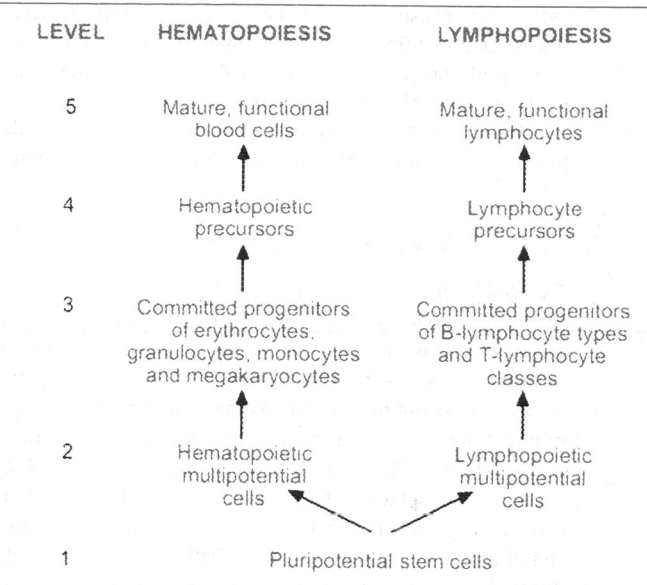

LEVEL	HEMATOPOIESIS	LYMPHOPOIESIS

FIGURE 85-2   Differentiation and maturation of hematopoietic stem cells. The functioning stem cell pool is thought to be at level 1, the pluripotential cells. In healthy humans, two multipotential progenitor cell pools may be operative (level 2). The multipotential progenitors differentiate further to unipotential progenitors, which are sensitive to cytokines (level 3). The committed progenitor cells are referred to as colony forming units or colony forming cells because they form colonies of cells in semisolid medium in the presence of the appropriate growth factors. These growth factors are capable of inducing proliferation and maturation of the committed progenitor cells so that they achieve level 4, at which the first morphologically identifiable precursors are present, such as myeloblasts and proerythroblasts, and ultimately level 5, the fully mature, functional blood cells.

T lymphocytes undergo apoptosis before entering the blood in patients with CML may explain their absence in blood lymphocytes in other clonal myeloid disorders.[15]

Thus, the mutation of the cell may be at level 1, between levels 1 and 2, or at level 2 in different patients (Fig. 85-3).

PROGENITOR CELL LEUKEMIA

Analysis of cases of AML in girls and women who were heterozygous for isotypes A and B of the enzyme glucose-6-phosphate dehydrogenase indicated that the AML clone in the girls was restricted to the granulocyte-monocyte pathway, whereas monoclonality was expressed in all cell lines in the women. These findings are in keeping with all prior CML and AML studies using enzymes or chromosome markers.[16,17] These findings support the possibility that a leukemic transformation in some (young) patients can occur in progenitor cells (e.g., colony forming unit granulocyte-monocyte) (level 3 in Fig. 85-3) and result in a true acute "granulocytic" leukemia. If progenitor cell leukemia is common in young people, this pattern could explain their better response to treatment. In a subset of patients with acute monocytic leukemia,[18] t(8;21) AML,[19] and t(15;17) AML, the leukemia derives from the neoplastic transformation of a progenitor cell.[20]

QUANTITATIVENESS OF CLONAL MYELOID DISEASES

The lesions of the primitive hematopoietic multipotential cell compartment are qualitative in the sense that distinct alteration from normal is seen in the function of the cell pool. The alteration reflects a change in the genome of one primitive hematopoietic cell.[11] This qual-

itative change, however, is such that the mutant multipotential cell can express all or some of the normal differentiation and maturation options. This expression can mimic the differentiation (commitment) and maturation expected of normal hematopoietic cells, as occurs in CML and polycythemia vera. Most cases tend to conform to readily recognized patterns, but the opportunity for a large number of variations on the most common themes is possible. Thus, some mixed and so-called in-between syndromes occur in which features of ineffective hematopoiesis and myeloproliferation of different cell lineages are present. For example, extreme thrombocytosis, usually confined to primary thrombocythemia, may accompany CML or idiopathic myelofibrosis. Erythrocytosis may rarely accompany CML. Atypical myeloproliferative syndromes or other clonal myeloid diseases may have mixtures of anemia, granulocytopenia, and thrombocytosis or of anemia, granulocytosis, and thrombocytopenia rather than pancytopenia. Qualitative abnormalities of red cell, granulocyte, or platelet structure or function may be more or less prominent in a given patient. For example, qualitative abnormalities of erythroblast development may result in acquired α-thalassemia (hemoglobin H disease) in patients with idiopathic myelofibrosis or other clonal myeloid diseases. In AML, unusual patterns of phenotypic expression occur frequently. For example, prominent leukemic erythroblasts and monocytes or eosinophils and monocytes may be seen in patients. So much opportunity for variation in disease expression exists among patients with AML that observation of patients in whom the phenotype of their leukemic cells is identical to the phenotype other patients is unusual. Choice of treatment is little affected by these variations. Decisions about whether to treat and which drugs to use are greatly influenced by whether a patient has a chronic, subacute, or acute clonal myeloid disease; by the rate of progression of the disease; by the extent of the leukemic blast cell infiltrate; and by the severity of the cytopenias. The diagnostician and therapist usually can identify variants as diseases of a clonal myeloid disorder and can manage the disorders as dictated by their manifestations regardless of precise subclassification.

INTERPLAY OF CLONAL AND POLYCLONAL HEMATOPOIESIS

Although potentially curative chemotherapy of myelogenous leukemia was introduced to kill "the last leukemic cell," two important factors were not explicitly discussed. The first was whether residual normal stem cells existed in marrow to restore polyclonal (normal) hematopoiesis if ablation of the leukemia was accomplished. The second was whether, given the early estimates of one trillion leukemic cells in a patient, the therapist had to eliminate all the leukemic cells in order to achieve cure. A corollary of the latter was whether the disease was the result of a mutant stem cell and, if so, was the mutant cell the only cell that mattered, ultimately, in the eradication process. We now recognize that remission results from sufficient suppression of the leukemic population by intensive chemotherapy to permit restitution of polyclonal hematopoiesis by normal stem cells.[21] Because relapse is the rule, two additional therapeutic approaches should include determining and interfering with the chemicals elaborated by leukemic cells that suppress normal hematopoiesis and assessing whether agents that foster normal stem cell recruitment can tip the balance in favor of those cells. Why monoclonal hematopoiesis is so difficult to subdue, even temporarily, with intensive chemotherapy (pre-imatinib therapy) in the chronic myeloid neoplasms (e.g., CML) compared to the acute myeloid neoplasms (AML) is unclear. Evidence has accumulated that sustained remission (clinical cure) may occur in some cases, with posttherapy minimal residual disease suggesting a new symbiotic relationship occurs after intensive therapy that suppresses the growth

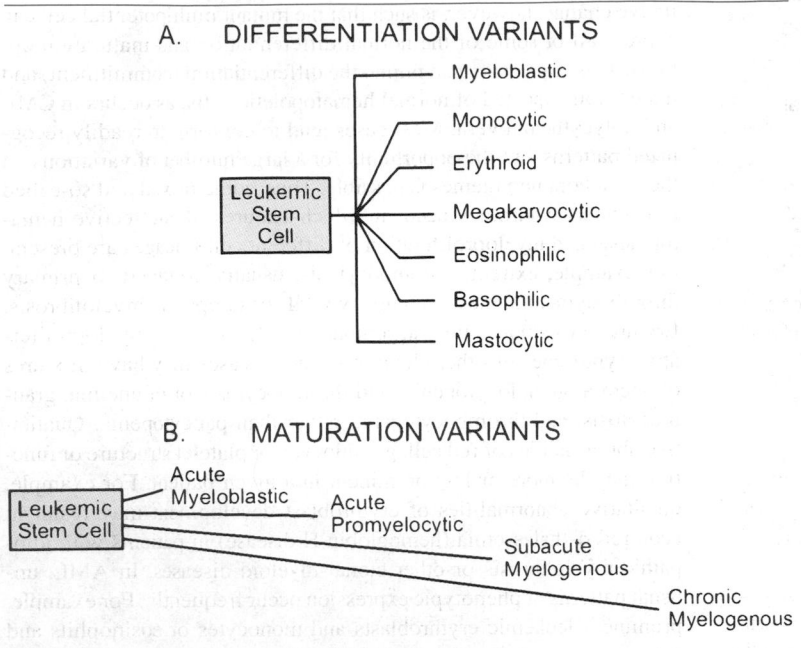

A. DIFFERENTIATION VARIANTS

Leukemic Stem Cell
- Myeloblastic
- Monocytic
- Erythroid
- Megakaryocytic
- Eosinophilic
- Basophilic
- Mastocytic

B. MATURATION VARIANTS

Leukemic Stem Cell
- Acute Myeloblastic
- Acute Promyelocytic
- Subacute Myelogenous
- Chronic Myelogenous

FIGURE 85-3 Phenotypic subtypes of acute myelogenous leukemia. Acute myelogenous leukemia has variable morphologic expression and a variable degree of maturation of leukemic cells into recognizable precursors of each blood cell type. This phenotypic variation results because the leukemic lesion resides in a cell normally capable of all the different commitment decisions. (A) Morphologic variants of AML can be considered differentiation variants in which the cells derived from one of the options of commitment accumulate prominently (e.g., leukemic erythroblasts, leukemic monocytes, leukemic megakaryocytes, etc.). In promyelocytic leukemia and some cases of acute leukemia in younger individuals, the somatic mutation may arise in a somewhat more differentiated progenitor. (B) Acute myeloblastic leukemia, promyelocytic leukemia, subacute leukemia, and chronic leukemia can be considered maturation variants in which blocks at different levels of maturation are present.

potential of leukemic cells. However, this phenomenon may be more evident in lymphoid than myeloid neoplasms.

CLINICAL MANIFESTATIONS

DEFICIENCY, EXCESS, OR DYSFUNCTION OF BLOOD CELLS

Alterations in blood cell concentration are the primary manifestations of clonal hematopoietic disorders. The clinical manifestations of deficiencies or excesses of individual blood cell types are described in the chapters on clinical manifestations of disorders of erythrocytes (see Chap. 32), granulocytes, and monocytes (see Chaps. 64 and 70), and platelets (see Chap. 109).

Several clonal hematopoietic diseases frequently manifest as qualitative abnormalities of blood cells. Abnormal red cell shapes, red cell or granulocyte enzyme deficiencies, abnormal neutrophil granules, bizarre nuclear configurations, disorders of neutrophil chemotaxis, phagocytosis or microbial killing, giant platelets, abnormal platelet granules, and disturbed platelet function can occur in some patients with oligoblastic myelogenous leukemia and idiopathic myelofibrosis. In oligoblastic myelogenous leukemia, the effects of severe cytopenia usually dominate. The disturbances of cell function are less important. In idiopathic myelofibrosis and primary thrombocythemia, functional platelet abnormalities may contribute to the hemorrhage diathesis, especially if surgery or injury occurs. Paroxysmal nocturnal hemoglobinuria is a hematopoietic stem cell disease in which a highly specific alteration in blood cell membranes renders the cells exquisitely sensitive to complement lysis (see Chap. 38). Patients with CML or poly-

cythemia vera usually do not have clinically significant functional abnormalities of cells, although in polycythemia vera neutrophils often are activated with heightened metabolic rates and enhanced phagocytosis.

Secondary clinical manifestations occur as a result of the proliferation and accumulation of the malignant (leukemic) cells.

EFFECTS OF LEUKEMIC BLAST CELLS

EXTRAMEDULLARY TUMORS

Myeloid (granulocytic) sarcomas (also called *chloromas* or *myeloblastomas*) are discrete tumors of leukemic cells that form in skin and soft tissues, periosteum and bone, lymph nodes, mediastinum, gastrointestinal tract, pleura, gonads, urinary tract, uterus, central nervous system, and other sites[22] (see Chap. 87). They can develop in patients with AML or the accelerated phase of CML and, occasionally, may be the first manifestation of AML, preceding the onset in marrow and blood by months or years.[23–25] Patients with AML with t(8;21) have a somewhat higher predisposition to developing myeloid sarcomas. Myeloid sarcomas can be mistaken for large-cell lymphomas because of the similarity of the histopathology in biopsy specimens from soft tissues. In the past, approximately 50 percent of cases that occur in the absence of blood and marrow involvement initially were misdiagnosed, usually as lymphoma.[23] The presence of eosinophils or other granulocytes may arouse suspicion of a myeloid sarcoma; however, immunohistochemistry should be used on such lesions to identify peroxidase, lysozyme, CD68, von Willebrand factor, CD31, CD61, and other relevant CD markers. One of four histopathologic patterns usually is evident by immunohistochemistry: myeloblastic, monoblastic, myelomonoblastic, or megakaryoblastic.[24]

More diffuse collections of leukemic promonocytes or monoblasts invade the skin, gingiva, anal canal, lymph nodes, or central nervous system of patients with AML of the monocytic subtype and may form tumors in those locations. Leukemic monocytes tend to mature to the point at which they develop many of the cytoplasmic and membrane features required for motility and tissue entry.[25–27] Moreover, monocytes proliferate and survive in tissues for long periods. Consequently, this AML phenotype has a higher frequency of overt infiltrative tissue lesions than do other forms of AML.

Extramedullary tumors may usher in the accelerated phase of CML. These tumors may be composed of myeloblasts or lymphoblasts, although in each case the Ph chromosome is present in the cells, indicating the *extramedullary Ph-positive lymphoblastomas* are the tissue variant of the predisposition of CML to transform into a terminal deoxynucleotidyl transferase-positive lymphoblastic leukemia in approximately 30 percent of patients who enter blast crisis (see Chap. 88).

RELEASE OF PROCOAGULANTS AND FIBRINOLYTIC ACTIVATORS

Microvascular thrombosis is a feature of AML of promyelocytic type, although the thrombosis can occur in other forms of acute leukemia, especially monocytic leukemia. The leukemic promyelocytes are thought to liberate tissue factor and a cancer procoagulant giving rise to disseminated intravascular coagulation and annexin II, which augments conversion of plasminogen to plasmin and results in fibrinolysis (see Chap. 121). Each may ultimately contribute to hypofibrinogenemia and hemorrhage. Thrombin generation may mediate the microvascular thrombotic aspect of this process, which can occur in acute promyelocytic, acute monocytic, or acute myelomonocytic leukemia, especially after cytotoxic treatment. Increased fibrinolytic activity further complicates coagulopathy in patients with promyelocytic leukemia[28] (see Chap. 87). Large-vessel arterial thrombosis is very rare as a presenting feature or complication of leukemia but has occurred in the setting of hyperleukocytosis or as a presenting feature of acute promyelocytic leukemia.[29]

HYPERLEUKOCYTIC SYNDROMES

A small proportion of patients with AML (5 percent) and CML (15 percent) manifest extraordinarily high blood leukocyte counts.[30,31] These patients present special problems because of the effects of blast cells in the microcirculation of the lung, brain, eye, ear, and penis and the metabolic effects that result when massive numbers of leukemic cells in blood, marrow, and tissues are simultaneously killed by cytotoxic drugs. Cell concentrations greater than 75,000/μl (75 × 10^9/liter) in AML and greater than 250,000/μl (250 × 10^9/liter) in CML usually are required to produce such problems. A respiratory distress syndrome attributed to pulmonary leukostasis occurs in some patients with acute promyelocytic leukemia after all-*trans*-retinoic acid therapy. The syndrome usually but not always is associated with neutrophilia.

The viscosity of blood is related to the total cytocrit and usually is not increased in hyperleukocytic leukemias because the reduced hematocrit compensates for increased leukocrit. Occasional patients with hyperleukocytic CML who are transfused with red cells may have an increased blood viscosity above normal.

Pathologic studies have identified leuko-occlusion and vascular invasion in small vessels of the lung, brain, or other sites. Because viscosity in the microcirculation is a function of the plasma viscosity and the deformability of individual cells in capillaries, leukocytes should transiently raise the viscosity in such small channels. Flow in microchannels decreases if poorly deformable blast cells enter capillary channels.[32] With high leukocyte counts, chronically reduced flow may reduce oxygen transport to tissues because the probability of leukocytes being in microchannels should increase as a function of white cell count. Moreover, trapped leukemic cells have an oxygen consumption rate that contributes to deleterious effects in the microcirculation. Leukocyte aggregation, leukocyte microthrombi, release of toxic products from leukocytes, endothelial cell damage, and microvascular invasion can contribute to vascular injury and flow impedance.

High leukemic blast cell counts in AML and CML may be associated with pulmonary, central nervous system, special sensory, or penile circulatory impairment (Table 85-2). Sudden death can occur in patients with hyperleukocytic acute leukemia as a result of intracranial hemorrhage.[33] Hyperleukocytosis should be treated promptly with leukapheresis and cytotoxic therapy, usually hydroxyurea (see Chaps. 87 and 88). In CML, leukapheresis reverses the hyperleukocytic syndrome, can be used immediately without waiting for the effect of allopurinol to reduce the risk of uric acid nephropathy, and can reduce the extent of cytolysis-induced hyperuricemia, hyperkalemia, and hyperphosphatemia by reducing tumor cell mass. The effect of leukapheresis in AML on the patient's ultimate duration of survival appears to be negligible, however.[34]

THROMBOCYTHEMIC SYNDROMES

Hemorrhagic or thrombotic episodes can develop during the course of primary thrombocythemia or thrombocythemia associated with other clonal myeloid diseases.[35,36] Arterial vascular insufficiency and venous thrombosis are the major vascular manifestations of thrombocythemia. Peripheral vascular insufficiency with gangrene and cerebral vascular thrombi can occur. Thrombosis of superficial or deep veins of the extremities occurs frequently. Mesenteric, hepatic, portal, splenic, or

TABLE 85-2   CLINICAL FEATURES OF THE HYPERLEUKOCYTIC SYNDROME

Pulmonary circulation
   Tachypnea, dyspnea, cyanosis
   Alveolar-capillary block
Pulmonary infiltrates
Postchemotherapy respiratory dysfunction
Central nervous system circulation
   Dizziness, slurred speech, delirium, stupor
   Intracranial (cerebral) hemorrhage
Special sensory organ circulation
Visual blurring
Papilledema
Diplopia
Tinnitus, impaired hearing
Retinal vein distention, retinal hemorrhages
Penile circulation
   Priapism
Spurious laboratory results
   Decreased blood PO$_2$; increased serum potassium
   Decreased plasma glucose; increased mean corpuscular volume, red cell count, hemoglobin, and hematocrit

penile venous thrombosis can develop. Hemorrhage is a frequent manifestation of thrombocythemia and often occurs concomitantly with thrombotic episodes. Gastrointestinal hemorrhage and cutaneous hemorrhage, the latter especially after trauma, occur most frequently, but bleeding from other sites also can occur (see Chap. 111).

Thrombotic complications occur in approximately one third of patients with polycythemia vera.[37] Erythrocytosis and thrombocytosis may interact and cause hypercoagulability, especially in the abdominal venous circulation. A syndrome of splanchnic venous thrombosis associated with endogenous erythroid colony growth, the latter characteristic of polycythemia vera, but without blood cell count changes indicative of a myeloproliferative disease has accounted for a very high proportion of patients with apparent idiopathic hepatic or portal vein thrombosis.[38,39] Thrombosis of the veins of the abdomen, liver, and other organs, characteristic complications of paroxysmal nocturnal hemoglobinuria, may result from complement-induced exposure of platelet sites, enhancing prothrombinase-related conversion of prothrombin to thrombin[40] (see Chap. 38).

SYSTEMIC SYMPTOMS

Fever, weight loss, and malaise occur as early manifestations of AML. At the time of diagnosis, low-grade fever is present in nearly 50 percent of patients.[41] Although minor infections may be present, systemic infection is relatively uncommon at the time of AML diagnosis.[42] However, fever during cytotoxic therapy, when neutrophil counts are extremely low, nearly always is a sign of infection. Fever also may be a manifestation of the acute leukemic transformation of CML and can occur in patients with oligoblastic leukemia.

Weight loss occurs in nearly one fifth of patients with AML.[42] Loss of well-being and intolerance to exertion may be out of proportion to the extent of anemia and may not be corrected by red cell transfusions. The pathogenesis of these effects is unknown.

METABOLIC SIGNS

Hyperuricemia and hyperuricosuria are common manifestations of AML and CML. Acute gouty arthritis and hyperuricosuric nephropathy are less common. If therapy is instituted without a reduction in plasma uric acid and without adequate hydration, saturation of the urine with uric acid can lead to precipitation of urate (gravel) and obstructive uropathy. If the uropathy is severe, urine flow can be obliterated, and renal failure ensues. Hyponatremia can occur in AML and in some cases results from inappropriate antidiuretic hormone secretion.[43] Hyponatremia also can result from an osmotic diuresis of urea, creatinine, urate, and other substances released from blast cells and wasting muscles. Hypokalemia is commonly seen in AML and has been thought to be caused by injury to the kidney by increased plasma and urine lysozyme and subsequent kaliuresis. Hypokalemia is related to excessive urinary potassium loss, but the correlation with lysozymuria is imperfect. Other mechanisms probably are responsible in most cases, including osmotic diuresis and tubular dysfunction. Kaliuretic antibiotics, often used by patients with AML, may accentuate the hypokalemia.

Hypercalcemia occurs in approximately 2 percent of patients with myelogenous leukemia. Several causes have been proposed, including bone resorption as a result of leukemic infiltration. This explanation is in keeping with the normal serum inorganic phosphate in most patients. Occasional patients had hypercalcemia and hypophosphatemia, and ectopic parathyroid hormone secretion by leukemic blast cells was strongly suggested in one carefully studied case. Lactic acidosis also has been observed in association with myelogenous leukemia, although the mechanism is obscure. Hypoxia can result from the hyperleukocytic syndrome as a consequence of pulmonary vascular leukostasis. Hypophosphatemia can occur because of rapid utilization of plasma inorganic phosphate in some cases of myelogenous leukemia with a high blood blast cell count and a high fraction of proliferative cells.

Increased serum concentrations of lipoprotein A and decreased concentrations of both low-density and high-density lipoproteins have been observed in a high proportion of patients with AML.[44] The increased level of lipoprotein A, which returns to normal after successful treatment, correlates with the presence of leukemic blast cells. Serum prolactin also is increased in patients with AML.[45] Leukemic blast cells may be an ectopic source of this hormone.[46]

Colony stimulating factor-1 is elevated in a variety of lymphoid and hemopoietic malignancies, including AML and CML.[47] The malignant cells have been proposed as the source of excess cytokine.

The plasma levels of protein C antigen, functional protein C, and free protein S are decreased in patients with AML. The changes are not related to liver disease or white cell count.[48]

FACTITIOUS LABORATORY RESULTS

Elevations of serum potassium levels have resulted from the release of potassium from platelets or, less often, leukocytes in patients with myeloproliferative diseases and extreme elevations in those blood cell concentrations. If blood is collected in a tube that contains an anticoagulant and the plasma is removed after high-speed centrifugation, the potassium concentration is normal. Glucose can be falsely decreased, especially because autoanalyzer techniques call for omission of glycolytic inhibitors such as sodium fluoride in collection tubes. Blood with high leukocyte counts that stands prior to separation of the plasma may have a significant amount of plasma glucose utilized by leukocytes. Factitious hypoglycemia also can occur as a result of red cell utilization of glucose, especially in polycythemic patients. True hypoglycemia has been observed rarely in patients with leukemia. Blood oxygen content also can be lowered spuriously as a result of *in vitro* utilization by large numbers of leukocytes.

SPECIFIC ORGAN INVOLVEMENT

Myeloproliferative diseases lead to disturbances principally in marrow, blood, and spleen. Although clusters of cells may be found in all organs, major infiltrates and organ dysfunction are unusual. In AML and the acute phase of CML, clinically significant infiltration of the larynx, central nervous system, heart, lungs, bone, joints, gastrointestinal tract, kidney, skin, or virtually any other organ can occur. Splenic enlargement is a feature of the acute and chronic myeloproliferative diseases. In AML, palpable splenomegaly is present in approximately one third of cases but usually is slight in extent. In the chronic myeloproliferative diseases, palpable splenomegaly is present in a high proportion of cases (polycythemia vera 80 percent, CML 90 percent, idiopathic myelofibrosis 100 percent). In primary thrombocythemia, splenic enlargement is present in approximately 60 percent of patients. A predisposition to silent splenic vascular thrombi and splenic atrophy analogous to that occurring in sickle cell anemia has been postulated as the cause of the lower frequency of splenic enlargement. Early satiety, left upper quadrant discomfort, splenic infarctions with painful perisplenitis, diaphragmatic pleuritis, and shoulder pain may occur in patients with splenomegaly, especially in the acute phase of CML and in myeloid metaplasia. In idiopathic myelofibrosis, the spleen can become enormous, occupying the left hemi-abdomen. Blood flow through the splenic vein can be so great as to lead to portal hypertension and gastroesophageal varices. Usually, reduced hepatic venous compliance also is present (see Chap. 89). Bleeding and occasional encephalopathy can result from portosystemic venous shunts.

REFERENCES

1. Rozman CGM, Feliu E, Rubio D, et al: Life expectancy of patients with chronic nonleukemic myeloproliferative disorders. *Cancer* 67:2658, 1991.

2. Jaffe ES, Harris NL, Stein H, Vardiman JW: *World Health Organization Classification of Tumours: Pathology and Genetics of Tumours of Haematopoietic and Lymphoid Tissues.* IARC Press, Lyon, 2001.

3. Kiladjian JJ, Gardin C, Renoux M, et al: Long-term outcomes of polycythemia vera patients treated with pipobroman as initial therapy. *Hematol J* 4:198, 2003.

4. Tefferi A, Fonesca R, Pereira DL, Hoagland HC: A long-term retrospective study of young women with essential thrombocythemia. *Mayo Clin Proc* 76:22, 2001.

5. Passamonti F, Malabarba L, Orlandi E, et al: Polycythemia in young patients: A study on the long-term risk of thrombosis, myelofibrosis and leukemia. *Haematologica* 88:13, 2003.

6. Barnard DR, Kalousek DK, Wiersma SR, et al: Morphologic, immunologic, and cytogenetic classification of acute myeloid leukemia and myelodysplastic syndrome in childhood. *Leukemia* 10:5,1996.

7. Bene MC, Castoldi G, Knapp W, et al: Proposals for the immunological classification of acute leukemias. *Leukemia* 9:1783, 1995.

8. Jennings CD, Foon KA: Recent advances in flow cytometry: Application to the diagnosis of hematologic malignancy. *Blood* 90:2863, 1997.

9. Bullinger L, Döhner K, Bair E, et al: Use of gene-expression profiling to identify prognostic subclasses in adult myeloid leukemia. *N Engl J Med* 350:1605, 2004.

10. Valk PJM, Verhaak RGW, Beijen A, et al: Prognostically useful gene-expression profiles in acute myeloid leukemia. *N Engl J Med* 350:1617, 2004.

11. Gilliland DG: Molecular genetics of human leukemias: New insights into therapy. *Semin Hematol* 39:6, 2002.

12. Ploemacher RE: Characterization and biology of normal human haematopoietic stem cells. *Haematologica* 84:4(EHA-4), 1999.

13. Bonnet D, Dick J: Human acute myeloid leukemia is organized as a hierarchy that originates from a primitive hematopoietic cell. *Nat Med* 3:730, 1997.

14. Lichtman MA: The stem cell in the pathogenesis and treatment of myelogenous leukemia: A perspective. *Leukemia* 15:1489, 2001.

15. Takahashi N, Maura I, Saitoh K, Miura AB: Lineage involvement of stem cells bearing the Philadelphia chromosome in chronic myeloid leukemia in the chronic phase as shown by combination of fluorescence activated cell sorting and fluorescence in situ hybridization. *Blood* 92: 4758, 1998.

16. Fialkow PJ, Singer JW, Adamson JW, et al: Acute nonlymphocytic leukemia: Expression in cells restricted to granulocytic and monocytic differentiation. *N Engl J Med* 301:1, 1979.

17. Fialkow PJ, Singer JW, Adamson JW, et al: Acute nonlymphocytic leukemia: Heterogeneity of stem cell origin. *Blood* 57:1068, 1981.

18. Ferraris AM, Broccia G, Meloni T, et al: Clonal origin of cells restricted to monocytic differentiation in acute nonlymphocytic leukemia. *Blood* 64:817, 1984.

19. Van Lom K, Hagenmaijer A, Vandekerckhove F, et al: Clonality analysis of hematopoietic cell lineages in acute myeloid leukemia and translocation (8;21): Only myeloid cells are part of the malignant clone. *Leukemia* 11:202, 1997.

20. Grimwade D, Enver T: Acute promyelocytic leukemia: Where does it stem from? *Leukemia* 18:375, 2004.

21. Lichtman MA: Interrupting the inhibition of normal hematopoiesis in myelogenous leukemia: An hypothetical approach to therapy. *Stem Cells* 18:304, 2000.

22. Yamauchi K, Yasuda M: Comparison of treatments on nonleukemic granulocytic sarcoma. *Cancer* 94:1739, 2002.

23. Menasce LP, Banerjee SS, Becket E, Harris M: Extramedullary myeloid tumor (granulocytic sarcoma) is often misdiagnosed. A study of 26 cases. *Histopathology* 34:391, 1999.

24. Audouin J, Comperat E, Le Tourneau A, et al: Myeloid sarcoma: Clinical and morphologic criteria useful for diagnosis. *Int J Surg Pathol* 11: 271, 2003.

25. Tsimberidou AM, Kantarjian HM, Estey E, et al: Outcome in patients with nonleukemic granulocytic sarcoma treated with chemotherapy with or without radiotherapy. *Leukemia* 17:1100, 2003.

26. Peterson L, Dekner LP, Brunning RD: Extramedullary masses as presenting features of acute monoblastic leukemia. *Am J Clin Pathol* 75: 140, 1981.

27. Tobelem G, Jacquillat C, Chastang C, et al: Acute monoblastic leukemia: A clinical and biologic study of 74 cases. *Blood* 55:71, 1980.

28. Lichtman MA, Weed RI: Peripheral cytoplasmic characteristics of leukemia cells in monocytic leukemia: Relationship to clinical manifestations. *Blood* 40:52, 1972.

29. Falanga A, Rickles FR: Pathogenesis and management of the bleeding diathesis in acute promyelocytic leukaemia. *Best Pract Res Clin Haematol* 16: 463, 2003.

30. Barbui T, Falanga A: Disseminated intravascular coagulation in acute leukemia. *Semin Thromb Hemost* 27:593, 2001.

31. Lichtman MA, Heal J, Rowe JM: Hyperleukocytic leukaemia: Rheological and clinical features and management. *Baillieres Clin Haematol* 1: 725, 1987.

32. Porcu P, Cripe LD, Ng EW, et al: Hyperleukocytic leukemias and leukostasis: A review of pathophysiology, clinical presentation and management. *Leuk Lymphoma* 39:1, 2000.

33. Östergren J, Fagrell B, Björkholm M: Hyperleukocytic effects on skin capillary circulation in patients with leukaemia. *J Intern Med* 231:19, 1992.

34. Dutcher JP, Schiffer CA, Wiernik PH: Hyperleukocytosis in adult acute nonlymphocytic leukemia: Impact on remission rate and duration, and survival. *J Clin Oncol* 5:1364, 1987.

35. Porcu P, Danielson CF, Orazi A, et al: Therapeutic leukapheresis in hyperleucocytic leukaemias: Lack of correlation between degree of cytoreduction and early mortality rate. *Br J Haematol* 98:433, 1997.

36. Cortelazzo S, Vicero P, Finazzi G, et al: Incidence and risk factors for thrombotic complications in a historical cohort of 100 patients with thrombocythemia. *J Clin Oncol* 8:556, 1990.

37. Landolfi R: Bleeding and thrombosis in myeloproliferative disorders. *Curr Opin Hematol* 5:327, 1998.

38. Anger B, Haugh U, Seidler R, Heimpel H: Polycythemia vera: A clinical study of 141 patients. *Blut* 59:493, 1989.

39. Teofili L, De Stefano V, Leone G, et al: Hematologic causes of venous thrombosis in young people: High incidence of myeloproliferative disorder as underlying disease in patients with splanchnic venous thrombosis. *Thromb Haemost* 67:297, 1992.

40. Vadher BD, Machin SJ, Paterson KG, et al: Life-threatening thrombotic and hemorrhagic problems associated with silent myeloproliferative disorders. *Br J Haematol* 85:213, 1993.

41. Wiedmer T, Hall SE, Ortel TL, et al: Complement-induced vesiculation and exposure of membrane prothrombinase sites in platelets of paroxysmal nocturnal hemoglobinuria. *Blood* 82:1192, 1993.

42. Burke PJ, Braine HG, Rathbun HK, Owens AH Jr: The clinical significance of fever in acute myelocytic leukemia. *Johns Hopkins Med J* 139: 1, 1976.

43. Burns CP, Armitage JO, Frey AL, et al: Analysis of the presenting features of adult acute leukemia. *Cancer* 47:2460, 1981.

44. Mir MA, Delamore JW: Metabolic disorders in acute myeloid leukaemia. *Br J Haematol* 40:79, 1978.

45. Niendorf A, Stang A, Beisiegel U, et al: Elevated lipoprotein (a) levels in patients with acute myeloblastic leukaemia decrease after successful chemotherapeutic treatment. *Clin Invest* 70:683, 1990.

46. Hatfill SJ, Kirby R, Hanley M, et al: Hyperprolactinemia in acute myeloid leukemia and indication of ectopic expression of human prolactin in blast cells of a patient of subtype M4. *Leuk Res* 14:57, 1990.

47. Janowska-Wieczarek A, Belch AR, Jacobs A, et al: Increased circulating colony-stimulating factor-1 in patients with preleukemia, leukemia and lymphoid malignancies. *Blood* 77:1796, 1991.

48. Troy K, Essex D, Rand J, et al: Protein C and S levels in acute leukemia. *Am J Hematol* 37:159, 1991.

49. Andrieux J, Demory JL, Caulier MT, et al: Karyotype abnormalities in myelofibrosis following polycythemia vera. *Cancer Genet Cytogenet* 140:118, 2003.

50. Finazzi G, Caruso V, Marchioli R, et al: Acute leukemia in polycythemia vera: An analysis of 1638 patients enrolled in a prospective observational study. *Blood* 105:2664, 2005.

MYELODYSPLASTIC SYNDROMES (CLONAL CYTOPENIAS AND OLIGOBLASTIC LEUKEMIA)

MARSHALL A. LICHTMAN

JANE L. LIESVELD

In contrast to florid acute myelogenous leukemia (AML) is a group of neoplastic (clonal) myeloid disorders that range from nonprogressive to more slowly progressive than AML. The disorders may appear in childhood, but the incidence increases exponentially after age 20 years. Most cases occur between the ages of 50 and 90 years. Most cases are sporadic, but a proportion result from stem cell injury during treatment of lymphomas or solid tumors with cytotoxic therapy. The disorder may develop in inherited syndromes that predispose to AML, such as Fanconi anemia. The disorders range from clonally derived (refractory) anemias to oligoblastic myelogenous leukemia (refractory anemia with excess blasts). The diseases share a propensity to (1) cytopenias, as a result of inappropriate apoptosis, usually of late-stage marrow precursors, and (2) multilineage dysmorphogenesis of blood cells. Red cells often have striking poikilocytosis, anisocytosis, anisochromia, and basophilic stippling. The marrow usually contains increased erythroid precursors with dysmorphic features, including nuclear distortions and scanty, poorly hemoglobinized cytoplasm. Ringed sideroblasts are almost a constant feature. Neutrophils have anomalies, including bilobed nuclei and hypogranulated cytoplasm, in association with increased marrow granulocyte precursors. Giant and microcytic platelets, often with abnormal granulation, in the blood are associated with megakaryocytic hyperplasia and atypical lobulation of the nucleus and decreased size of megakaryocytes in the marrow. In the nonprogressive syndromes, anemia may be accompanied by mild variations, usually decreases, in neutrophil and platelet levels, and blast cells are not increased to greater than 2 percent in the marrow. Clonal cytogenetic abnormalities occur in approximately three fourths of patients. Chromosomes 5, 7, and 8 are most frequently involved. The classic 5q- syndrome is categorized within the myelodysplastic disorders. The syndrome primarily affects older women, exhibiting anemia and hypercellular and dysmorphic erythropoiesis with lobulated erythroblast nuclei and hypolobulated micromegakaryocytes but usually normal or elevated platelet counts. It is the most indolent form of the myelodysplastic syndrome with the lowest propensity to evolve into AML. In the more progressive syndromes, leukemic blast cells are increased, cytopenias are more severe, and the disease has high morbidity and mortality from infection and bleeding. Each of the syndromes has a propensity to evolve into frank AML ranging from approximately 10 to 15 percent in the clonal (refractory) anemias to approximately 40 to 50 percent of patients with trilineage cytopenias and increased marrow blast cells. Mortality from infection is a high risk in patients with severe leukopenia. In the most indolent forms, therapy may not be required. Erythropoietin plus granulocyte–colony stimulating factor may improve the anemia or decrease transfusion requirements if clonal anemia is the principal feature. Cyclosporine or antithymocyte globulin may transiently improve the anemia in patients with clonal anemia and low blast counts. Therapy with cytotoxic drugs, red cell or platelet transfusions, and antibiotics may palliate the progressive syndrome (oligoblastic leukemia). Thalidomide congeners and inhibitors of DNA methylation, such as 5-azacytidine or decitabine, have been useful in some patients. Allogeneic stem cell transplantation may be curative in younger patients, and nonmyeloablative stem cell transplantation is being explored in older patients.

DEFINITION

Myelodysplasia is a term used to encompass a spectrum of clonal (neoplastic) myeloid disorders marked by ineffective hematopoiesis, cytopenias, qualitative disorders of blood cells and their precursors, clonal chromosomal abnormalities, and a variable predilection to undergo clonal evolution to florid acute myelogenous leukemia (AML).[1] The disorders range from relatively indolent clonally derived anemias, with a relatively lower frequency of progression to AML, to more troublesome clonal multilineage cytopenias or to oligoblastic myelogenous leukemias that often progress to overt AML. The somatic mutation leading to these disorders arises in a multipotential hematopoietic cell. *Dysplasia* is a term that classically implies a polyclonal and, therefore, nonneoplastic process. The choice of the term *myelodysplasia* to denote clonal (neoplastic) disorders was unfortunate because the term does not assist students and patients in understanding the relationship of myelodysplasia to other clonal stem cell disorders. In addition, diseases such as idiopathic myelofibrosis can have all the features of "myelodysplasia" but are ignored in its classification. Moreover, drawing diagnostic distinctions among 10, 20, and 30 percent leukemic blast cells is inconsistent with the biologic behavior of cancer and medicine's classification of cancer.[1] Separation of clonal anemias into two categories based on whether the anemia has greater than or less than 15 percent sideroblasts is arbitrary and is not based on the pathobiology of the two variants. The term *myelodysplasia* is, however, widely used.[2]

The term *clonal cytopenias* refers to (1) neoplasms arising in a multipotential hematopoietic marrow cell that result in diseases with no discernible leukemic blast cells in the marrow or blood (e.g., refractory anemias) and (2) *oligoblastic leukemia* (refractory anemia with excess blasts [RAEB]) in which an increased proportion of (leukemic) blast cells is present in the marrow but in which, untreated, the course is smoldering or subacute in contrast to AML.[3]

The boundary between clonal anemia and oligoblastic myelogenous leukemia may be indistinct because of the insensitivity of the marrow examination; however, continued observation clarifies the situation. If leukemic blast cells are evident in marrow, the diagnosis of oligoblastic leukemia can be made, maintaining the principle that the histopathologic diagnosis depends on the presence or absence of tumor cells and not the rate of progression or severity of the manifestations of the malignancy. The proportion of marrow myeloblasts is not increased in reactive states, for example, granulocytic hyperplasia as a result of infection, noninfectious inflammation, solid tumors, and drug-induced granulocytosis (e.g., glucocorticoids, lithium). The proportion of blasts usually falls to less than the normal value of 1.0 ± 0.4 SD percent. A finding of greater than 2.0 percent myeloblasts in a normal marrow is rare in older children and adults. Higher proportions, for example, greater than 2 percent, are mostly confined to cases of oligoblastic leukemia. The one exception to this rule is some patients treated with granulocytic growth factors who may have a slight transient increase in blast cells.

Clonal proliferation of multipotential hemopoietic cells in this group of disorders is accompanied by variable effects on all blood cell lineages and usually is associated with pathologically enhanced apoptosis of marrow precursor cells such that leukopenia and thrombocytopenia of varying severity often accompany the anemia. Qualitative abnormalities of cell shape, organelle structure, biochemical pathways, and function can occur in each lineage. The range of clinical expression is broad. Thus, clonal cytopenias can occur with isolated anemia and a nearly normal-appearing marrow or with severe pancytopenia, profoundly hypercellular marrow, and alterations in blood cell shape, size, and function. The more profound the disorder, the more likely the finding of oligoblastic leukemia on marrow examination.

HISTORY

At the beginning of the 20th century, reports of highly morbid cytopenic disorders that were refractory to treatment began to appear in the medical literature.[4] In 1942, Chevallier and colleagues[5] discussed formally the "odo-leukemias." They chose the Greek word *odo*, meaning threshold, to highlight disorders on the threshold of leukemia. Chevallier proposed *leucoses* as the generic term for the leukemias so that marked variations in white cell counts and other highly variable presenting features would not engender inappropriate terminology. His proposal was sage but neglected.

In 1949, Hamilton-Paterson[6] used the term *preleukemic anemia* to describe patients with refractory anemia antecedent to AML development. In 1953, Block and coworkers[7] expanded the concept to include cytopenias of all lineages and described cases that closely fit with our current concepts of a clonal myeloid hemopathy prior to evolution to overt AML. By mid-century, the relationship of acquired idiopathic cytopenias to the subsequent onset of AML had become broadly appreciated.[8-15] Terms such as *herald state of leukemia, refractory anemia, sideroachrestic anemia, idiopathic refractory sideroblastic anemia, pancytopenia with hyperplastic marrow,* and others were coined to describe the various manifestations of the hematopoietic derangement that preceded the onset of florid AML.

In 1975, at a conference on unclassifiable leukemias held in Paris, Marcel Bessis, Jean Bernard, and others suggested the term *hematopoietic dysplasia,* later shortened to *myelodysplasia,* for the group of disorders having a more indolent course than AML.[1,16] The concept that neoplasia is a tissue abnormality defined by its origin in the mutation(s) within a single cell (monoclonality) and that dysplasia is a polyclonal tissue change was ignored and took a back seat to the participants' primary interest in the dysmorphia of cells that characterized most of these syndromes, hence the application of the term "dysplasia," which has become entrenched.

CLASSIFICATION

The World Health Organization classification (WHO) designates five categories in the spectrum of the myelodysplastic syndromes (MDS): (1) refractory anemia, (2) refractory anemia with ringed sideroblasts, (3) refractory anemia with multilineage dysplasia, (4) RAEB, and (5) isolated 5q- abnormality. RAEB in transformation has been eliminated as a category and is included in the diagnosis of AML (Table 86-1). In addition, a category of disorders that cannot be pigeonholed, the *unclassifiable myelodysplastic syndromes,* is included.[2] MDSs include entities that have marrow blast percentages ranging from a mean of less than 2 percent in refractory anemia to a mean of approximately 10 percent and upper limit of 20 percent in RAEB.[17] The distinction between refractory anemia in which less than 15 percent of nucleated red cells in marrow are ringed sideroblasts and refractory anemia with ringed sideroblasts in which greater than 15 percent of nucleated red cells are ringed sideroblasts uses the same arbitrary boundary as does classifying a patient as having RAEB if less than 21 percent of nucleated marrow cells are blasts or as having AML if greater than 20 percent of nucleated marrow cells are myeloblasts. This approach to categorization is unfortunate because in no other neoplasm is the designation of the cancer, in this case myelogenous leukemia, which all such patients have, called by another name when a greater or fewer number of tumor cells are present. Thus, in actuality, *myelogenous leukemia,* not refractory anemia, is the name of the tumor whether the marrow has 5 percent or 50 percent blast cells. Chronic myelomonocytic leukemia and juvenile myelomonocytic leukemia are believed by some to be MDSs, especially in the parlance of pediatric hematologists, but appropriately are not included in the WHO classification. Chapter 88 discusses chronic myelogenous leukemias and related diseases.

Several laboratories that explored the use of flow cytometry in the classification of these heterogenous disorders have found it to be of limited value or largely confirmatory of the findings on blood film and marrow examination.[17,18]

EPIDEMIOLOGY

INCIDENCE BY AGE, SEX, AND OCCUPATION

Disease onset before age 50 years is uncommon except in cases preceded by irradiation or chemotherapy given for another malignancy.[21-24] MDS, as defined by the WHO classification, occurs in children aged 5 months to 15 years at a rate of approximately one per million children per year. In contrast to adults, most pediatric cases are oligoblastic myelogenous leukemia (RAEB); clonal sideroblastic anemia is rare.[25-28] A proportion of childhood cases evolve from inherited predisposing diseases, such as Down syndrome and Fanconi

TABLE 86-1   CLASSIFICATION OF THE MYELODYSPLASTIC SYNDROMES (CLONAL CYTOPENIAS AND OLIGOBLASTIC LEUKEMIA)

Classic 5q- syndrome

Clonal (refractory) nonsideroblastic anemia*

Clonal (refractory) sideroblastic anemia

Clonal bicytopenia or tricytopenia (overt multilineage dysmorphic cytopenias)

Oligoblastic leukemia (refractory anemia with excess myeloblasts)

Apparent clonal myeloid disease that does not fit in any category shown above (e.g., chronic clonal monocytosis)[19,20]

* No strong basis exists for the category "nonsideroblastic" anemia because almost all patients have ringed sideroblasts, and the manifestations and course of the disease are very similar in patients with a high or low prevalence of sideroblasts.
NOTE: Other acute and chronic clonal myeloid diseases are categorized in Table 85-1.

anemia. The annual incidence of MDS increases logarithmically after age 20 years from less than 1.0 per million persons to more than 20 per 100,000 persons in septuagenarians.[23] Males are affected approximately 1.5 times as often as females. Case control studies of possible occupational or environmental associations have provided many possible candidates as contributors to MDS, but none other than benzene has reached a level of scientific validity.[29,30]

ETIOLOGY AND PATHOGENESIS

ETIOLOGY

Not unexpectedly, the etiologic factors that increase the incidence of MDS are similar to the factors in AML. Exposure to benzene,[31,32] chemotherapeutic agents, particularly alkylating agents and topoisomerase inhibitors,[33–40] and radiation[41] increase the risk of these clonal hemopathies. These agents may cause DNA damage, impair DNA repair enzymes, and induce loss of chromosome integrity. Most cases of secondary or posttreatment MDS occur in patients treated for a lymphoma or solid tumor. Increasing reports of MDS as a complication of treatment of myeloid diseases, such as acute promyelocytic leukemia, reflect a second clonal myeloid disease from another stem cell injury following therapy.[40] The increased life span of patients with acute promyelocytic leukemia after effective therapy may make this event more common.

Inherited diseases, such as Fanconi anemia, known to predispose to AML development occasionally evolve instead into a clonal myeloid hemopathy.[42] In addition, as is the case in all hematologic malignancies,[43] familial myelodysplasia occurs rarely as a result of as-yet undefined germ-line susceptibility genes.[44–46]

PATHOGENESIS

These disorders arise from the clonal expansion of a multipotential hematopoietic cell. The clonal origin is supported by studies of women who were heterozygotes for glucose-6-phosphate dehydrogenase isoenzymes A and B and who had such a syndrome. The hematopoietic progenitors[47,48] and in some cases B lymphocytes[49] of such patients had only one isoenzyme present, supporting the concept of clonal expansion of a neoplastic marrow cell. Clonal studies using X-linked restriction length polymorphisms with probes for hypoxanthine phosphoribosyl transferase or phosphoglycerate kinase also supported the origin of these disorders from a single multipotential stem cell.[50–52]

Fluorescence *in situ* hybridization (FISH) of interphase blood cell populations with probes for chromosome 7 or 8 in patients with monosomy 7 or trisomy 8 indicates chromosome abnormalities may not be present in lymphoid populations.[52,53] Studies of immunoglobulin heavy-chain gene rearrangement and assay of the human androgen receptor and other genes on the X chromosome also have concluded that lymphocytes are not derived from the neoplastic clone.[51,54–56] However, pseudodiploidy has been observed in Epstein-Barr virus-stimulated cell populations of two patients with idiopathic refractory sideroblastic anemia,[57] suggesting that B lymphocytes may be derived from the affected stem cell in some patients.

The frequency of deletions of part or all of chromosomes 5, 7, 11, 12, 13, and 20 indicates a role for tumor suppressor genes in disease onset, but identification of these genes has been elusive (see "5q-Syndrome" below). Molecular genetic studies of patient's cells show identifiable gene mutations in approximately 60 percent of patients. Presumably, such mutations contribute to the apparent maintenance of proliferation of early progenitors, the abnormalities in maturation seen in each hematopoietic lineage, and the high proportional loss of mature cells in the marrow. Mutated RAS is most common,[58–62] and lower frequencies of FMS and p53 mutations are present. Codon 12 of RAS

and codon 969 of FMS are the predominant sites of alteration in the respective genes.[63,64] Hypermethylation of p15, an inhibitor of cyclin-dependent kinases 4 and 6, is present in more than one third of patients examined and may contribute to disease progression.[65] A variety of other mutations in protooncogenes, or genes encoding proteins involved in the cell cycle, or of transcription factors have been described sporadically.[63,64] Interpretation of these molecular studies is difficult because the mutations are present in patients with advanced disease and may be late changes, not seminal in the neoplastic transformation. Overexpression of DLK (delta-like) and GATA-1 and GATA-2 have been suggested as a marker for MDS in the former case and as contributing to the maturation abnormalities in the case of the latter two genes.[66,67] The role of mutations in mitochondrial DNA in the cells of older persons and in the hematopoietic cells of patients with MDS and AML has not been integrated into the pathogenesis of the disease.[68]

The major specific pathophysiologic mechanism in MDS is ineffective hemopoiesis, that is, defective maturation and death of marrow precursor cells.[69–71] The specific characteristics of ineffective erythropoiesis and granulopoiesis include a decreased proportion of cells in the DNA synthesis phase of the mitotic cycle and a marked increase in the fraction of late precursor cells undergoing apoptosis.[72] Increased levels of apoptotic mediators are present in cells, including tumor necrosis factor (TNF)-α, FAS antigen (CD95), and calcium-dependent nuclease activity.[73–75] Stepwise degradation of DNA, which is characteristic of apoptosis, is evident in late precursors.[73–75] The proliferation of progenitor and early precursor cells usually is normal or enhanced, resulting in a hypercellular marrow, but failure to accumulate adequate numbers of mature cells has been observed. Mild shortening of cell life span also contributes to the cytopenias.

Immune dysregulation involving B and T lymphocytes in MDS has been described. Heightened apoptosis of marrow B lymphocytes is a feature of the disease.[76] Depletion of autologous T lymphocytes in cultures of the marrow of patients with early MDS (clonal anemia) results in improved growth of marrow cells, apparently from residual normal stem cells.[77] The T cell inhibitory effect is highlighted by transient improvement in cell counts in a minority of patients with early disease after treatment with antithymocyte globulin (ATG) and cyclosporine.[78] However, evidence that lymphocytes are part of the leukemic clone has been contradictory.[54,78,79] Immune dysregulation may be secondary to the neoplasia and not a factor in its origin.[80]

CLINICAL FEATURES

SYMPTOMS AND SIGNS

Patients can be asymptomatic or, if anemia is more severe, can have pallor, weakness, loss of a sense of well-being, and exertional dyspnea.[14,81,82] A small proportion of patients have infections related to granulocytopenia or hemorrhage related to thrombocytopenia at the time of diagnosis. Patients with severe depressions of neutrophil and platelet counts at diagnosis usually have oligoblastic leukemia. Rarely, patients have fever unrelated to infection.[83] Arthralgias are the initial complaint in some patients.[75] Rarely, the presentation mimics a connective tissue disease.[84,85] Hepatomegaly or splenomegaly occurs in approximately 5 or 10 percent of patients, respectively.

SPECIAL CLINICAL FEATURES

Patients with an indolent phase (smoldering myelogenous leukemia) prior to overt AML may develop diabetes insipidus. Hypothalamic involvement can lead to polyuria, polydipsia, and decreased libido. Hypothalamic-posterior hypophysis insufficiency in clonal myeloid states has been associated with monosomy 7 in hematopoietic cells.[86,87] Hypodipsia can occur with extensive hypothalamic involvement. The syndrome lacks the signs of thirst, polyuria, and polydipsia because signals transmitted by the thirst center to the cerebral cortex are blocked.[87]

Acute neutrophilic dermatosis (Sweet disease) is an acute febrile illness characterized by erythematous patches on the arms, face, and legs that progress to painful brown plaques. The plaques may ulcerate and produce large necrotizing skin lesions. The histopathology of the skin is that of a dense dermal neutrophilic infiltrate.[88,89] The syndrome, which occurs principally in middle-aged women, lasts for 6 to 10 weeks, often is associated with blood neutrophilia, and may recur. At least 10 percent of patients with Sweet disease develop AML or another clonal myeloid disease. Occasional cases have been associated with monocytosis or cytogenic abnormalities in marrow cells prior to AML onset. Granulocyte–colony stimulating factor (G-CSF) and all-trans-retinoic acid (ATRA) administration has been followed by Sweet disease in some cases.[89] Other dermatopathic conditions also have been associated with clonal myeloid diseases.[90]

Immune or inflammatory syndromes may be seen in as many as 10 percent of patients. A symptom complex that mimics systemic lupus erythematosus ([LE]; fever, pleurisy, symmetric arthritis, plasma antinuclear antibody, and pancytopenia with a hyperplastic marrow) may precede AML.[84] Several patients with signs of LE and the LE cell phenomenon were reported in a review of the clonal myeloid syndromes.[84,91] Behçet disease, glomerulonephritis, seronegative arthritis, systemic vasculitis, polychondritis, polyneuropathy, panniculitis, and inflammatory bowel disease also have been associated with clonal myeloid disorders.[84,85,92–97]

The incidence of other cancers may be higher in subjects with myelodysplastic diseases.[98–100]

LABORATORY FEATURES

BLOOD (SEE COLOR PLATE XVIII 1–5)

RED CELLS

Anemia is present in greater than 85 percent of patients.[14,81,82] In approximately 4 percent of patients, the anemia results from erythroid aplasia.[101] Mean cell volume often is increased. Red cell shape abnormalities include oval, elliptical, teardrop, spherical, and fragmented cells. Red cell findings occur in a spectrum. Some patients have only slight anisocytosis. Elliptical red cells sometimes dominate. Basophilic stippling of red cells occurs. Nucleated red cells are seen in the blood film in approximately 10 percent of cases. Reticulocyte counts usually are low for the degree of anemia. Other abnormalities of red cells occur, such as an increased proportion of hemoglobin F[102] and decreased red cell enzyme activities, especially acquired pyruvate kinase deficiency.[103] Hemolysis has occurred in some patients with pyruvate kinase deficiency. Enhanced sensitivity of membranes to complement[104] and modification of red cell blood group antigens may be observed.[105] Acquired hemoglobin H disease results in red cell morphology similar to thalassemia (microcytosis, anisocytosis, basophilic stippling, poikilocytosis with target cells, fragmented cells, and teardrop cells). Intracellular precipitates of β-chain tetramers (identified by crystal violet stain) reflect an acquired decrease in the rate of α-chain synthesis in erythroblasts.[106–108] The decrease in α-globin chain synthesis is profound, involves each of the four α-chain loci, and results from a transcription abnormality. No gross alterations in genes (e.g., insertions, deletions) are seen in these cases.[106] Acquired hemoglobin H disease in this setting has been dubbed the α-thalassemia myelodysplastic syndrome and is the consequence of acquired mutations in ATRX.[108]

GRANULOCYTES AND MONOCYTES

Neutropenia is present in approximately 50 percent of patients at the time of diagnosis.[109] The proportion of monocytes often is increased, and monocytosis per se can be the dominant manifestation of the hematopoietic abnormality for months or years.[19,20,110] Morphologic abnormalities of neutrophils can occur, sometimes resulting in the acquired Pelger-Huët anomaly. In this condition, neutrophils have very condensed chromatin and unilobed or bilobed nuclei that often have a pince-nez shape. The neutrophils may be in the process of apoptosis.[111] Ring-shaped nuclei also occur in neutrophils.[112] Neutrophil alkaline phosphatase activity is decreased in some patients.[14] Expression of normal surface antigens on neutrophils and monocytes is decreased, and abnormal surface antigen expression occurs in some cases.[113] Defective primary granules of abnormal size and shape with decreased myeloperoxidase content can be present.[114] Specific neutrophil granules can be decreased in number, producing hypogranular cells.[115] Neutrophil granule membranes frequently are deficient in glycoprotein.[116] Chemotactic, phagocytic, and bactericidal capability may be impaired.[117–119] Formyl-leucyl-methionyl-phenylamine receptor signaling and actin polymerization can be abnormal.[120,121] Muramidase (lysozyme) activity in blood and urine may be increased, reflecting granulocytic hyperplasia, heightened monocytopoiesis, and monocyte turnover.

PLATELETS

Approximately 25 percent of patients have mild to moderate thrombocytopenia at the time of diagnosis.[14,109] Mild thrombocytosis also can occur.[14,109] Platelets may be abnormally large, have poor granulation, or have large, fused central granules.[122,123] Abnormal platelet function can contribute to a prolonged bleeding time, easy bruising, or exaggerated bleeding. Decreased platelet aggregation in response to collagen or epinephrine is a frequent functional abnormality.[124]

LYMPHOCYTES

Patients with clonal hemopathies may have immunologic deficiencies, such as a decreased in natural killer cells in the blood but no decrease in large granular lymphocytes,[125–128] a decrease in helper T lymphocytes,[126] and a decrease in Epstein-Barr virus receptors on B lymphocytes.[126–129] Antibody-dependent cellular cytotoxicity is normal.[126] Thymidine incorporation after mitogenic stimulation[130,131] and colony growth of T lymphocytes are decreased.[126] Lymphocytes may have an increased sensitivity to irradiation.[130] The defects in lymphoid cells could reflect the level of the somatic mutation in a primitive multipotential cell in different cases. Intrinsic, rather than secondary, alterations in lymphocytes are determined by whether no lymphocytes are generated from the clone, B cells are part of the clone, or B and T cells are part of the clone[57] (see "Pathogenesis" above).

PLASMA ABNORMALITIES

Serum iron, transferrin, and ferritin levels may be elevated. Lactic dehydrogenase and uric acid concentrations can be increased as a result of ineffective hemopoiesis and a high death fraction of maturing marrow precursors. Monoclonal gammopathy, polyclonal hypergammaglobulinemia, and hypogammaglobulinemia each occurs with increased frequency.[132,133] The frequency of autoantibodies was increased in one report[133] but not in another report.[132] β_2-microglobulin serum levels are increased in proportion to the prognostic category of the disease.[134]

MARROW (SEE COLOR PLATE XVIII 6–8)

MAGNETIC RESONANCE IMAGING

Magnetic resonance imaging scans of human femoral marrow correlate with disease severity. Approximately 85 percent of patients with refractory anemia have images consistent with fatty marrow, whereas approximately 85 percent of patients with oligoblastic leukemia have images showing marrow fat replaced by abnormal hematopoietic tissue.[135]

CELLULARITY

Marrow cellularity usually is normal or increased.[14,136–138] Occasionally, cellularity is decreased, simulating hypoplastic or aplastic anemia.[136,139] However, islands of dysmorphic cells, especially atypical megakaryocytes, usually are present. An increased proportion of blast cells in this setting suggests hypoplastic myelogenous leukemia (see Chap. 87).

ERYTHROPOIESIS

Erythroid hyperplasia is frequent. Very large or small erythroblasts, nuclear fragmentation, stippled erythroblasts, and poor hemoglobinization may be seen.[14,136–138] Proerythroblasts may be present in excess, and the marrow may lack normal clusters or islets of erythroblasts. Erythroblasts may resemble megaloblasts that have nuclear cytoplasmic maturation asynchrony, nuclear fragmentation, or cytoplasmic nuclear remnants. This pattern is referred to as *megaloblastoid erythropoiesis*. Erythroid aplasia seen in occasional cases results in a hypocellular marrow.[101]

Pathologic sideroblasts may be identified when the marrow is treated with Prussian blue stain. The sideroblasts include erythroblasts with an increased number and size of siderosomes (cytoplasmic ferritin-containing vacuoles), referred to as *intermediate sideroblasts*, or erythroblasts with mitochondrial iron aggregates that take the form of a partial or complete circumnuclear ring of iron globules, referred to as *ringed sideroblasts*. Macrophage iron often is increased. Ringed sideroblasts are uncommon or present only in very low proportions in clonal myeloid disorders other than refractory anemia.

GRANULOPOIESIS

Granulocytic hyperplasia is frequent.[14,109,136–138] Marrow monocytes may be increased in number. Abnormalities of granulocytes include hypogranulation, a monocytoid appearance of neutrophilic granulocytes, and the acquired Pelger-Huët nuclear abnormality of neutrophils.[111,140] Progranulocytes and myelocytes may be increased. The proportion of blast cells is not increased in clonal hemopathies that are categorized as refractory anemia (i.e., <2%); a blast percentage of greater than 2 percent is considered oligoblastic leukemia. Marrow biopsy may show abnormal localized immature precursors (ALIP),[141,142] which are clusters of immature myeloid (? blast) cells located centrally rather than subjacent to the endosteum. These clusters of atypical cells are present in almost all cases of oligoblastic leukemia where blast cells compose 3 or more percent of nucleated marrow cells (RAEB) and in approximately one third of patients with refractory anemia, suggesting these patients have a disorder closely approaching oligoblastic leukemia. Patients with this abnormality are more prone to develop overt AML. Vascular endothelial growth factor (VEGF) is expressed on cells forming ALIP clusters and has been proposed as providing an autocrine loop to promote leukemia progenitor cell formation.[143] The number of plasma cells may be slightly increased. Marrow basophilia or eosinophilia occurs in approximately one in seven patients and is associated with a higher probability of evolution to AML.[144]

THROMBOPOIESIS

Megakaryocytes are present in normal or increased numbers.[14,136–138] Micromegakaryocytes (dwarf megakaryocytes) may occur.[136–138,145,146] Megakaryocytes with unilobed or bilobed nuclei may be increased, and hypersegmented and hyposegmented megakaryocytes may be present. Clusters of megakaryocytes may be seen. Megakaryocytes may be distributed laterally from their usual parasinusoidal location.[147]

FIBROSIS AND ANGIOGENESIS

An increase in reticulin and collagen fibers of varying degree is common, especially in oligoblastic leukemias. When fibrosis is prominent, the disorder can resemble primary myelofibrosis, although, in contrast to the latter, splenomegaly usually is not marked. Because idiopathic myelofibrosis is an oligoblastic leukemia with striking dysmorphogenesis of cells, some confusion in classification with other fibrotic clonal myeloid disorders is expected.[148] Some physicians have proposed a category of myelofibrotic myelodysplasia, but all clonal myeloid diseases, including AML, chronic myelogenous leukemia (CML), and chronic myelomonocytic leukemia (CMML) may have within their spectrum of expression occasional cases with intense myelofibrosis. Like numerous other epiphenomena that occur in the expression of hematopoietic stem cell diseases, extending the general classifications is not warranted.

Increased angiogenesis is a feature of MDS. Microvessel density increases with more advanced stages of the disease.[149] Mast cell frequency and mast cell tryptase activity are highly correlated with microvessel density.[150]

CULTURE

Clonal growth of marrow progenitors in soft agar or other viscous culture systems usually is abnormal in patients with clonal hemopathies.[151] Most reports indicate growth of multipotential (colony forming unit–granulocyte-erythrocyte-monocyte megakaryocyte) and erythroid progenitors (burst forming unit–erythroid, colony forming unit–erythroid) in the blood or marrow is markedly decreased in subjects with clonal myeloid disorders.[151–154] Biochemical abnormalities of erythroid precursors also have been found. Colony forming units for granulocytes and monocytes (CFU-GM) are decreased.[151,152] Very small colonies or clusters with impaired maturation often dominate the cultures. Abnormally small and infrequent CFU-GM may be found when blood neutrophil and monocyte counts are nearly normal. Occasionally, overabundant growth is present. Usually, cell culture results become more abnormal as the blood cell abnormalities in the patient worsen.

In overt AML, CFU-GM growth usually is absent. Some studies indicate very abnormal growth of progenitors in culture (decreased colonies or predominance of small clusters) is a poor prognostic sign and may be a harbinger of overt leukemia.[155,156] Growth occurring in clonal myeloid hemopathies (and AML) usually remains dependent on growth factors such as erythropoietin and granulocyte-macrophage colony stimulating factor (GM-CSF).[157] Colony growth in children with the monosomy 7 syndrome may occur without added growth factors, supporting the view of autocrine and paracrine stimulation of progenitor cells.[158–161] Blast cell progenitors (CFU-BL) may be increased in patients with oligoblastic leukemia.[154] The long-term marrow initiating cell is decreased in some patients,[160,161] and the ability of marrow stromal layers to support *in vitro* hematopoiesis can be impaired.[162]

Circulating monocyte colony stimulating factor (CSF-1) is increased in some patients with MDS, AML, and other hematologic malignancies.[163] Interleukin (IL)-1α and GM-CSF levels have been undetectable in most patients. IL-6, G-CSF, and erythropoietin concentrations have been variable. TNF has been inversely related to hematocrit.[164] Stem cell factor (SCF), a multilineage hematopoietin, has been decreased in some patients.[165] The flt-3 ligand, another multilineage growth factor, is increased in patients with indolent clonal hemopathies but not oligoblastic leukemia.[166] The inverse relationship between platelet count and thrombopoietin levels is maintained in clonal anemia but not oligoblastic leukemia.[167]

CYTOGENETICS

An altered number or form of chromosomes may occur in up to 80 percent of patients with clonal hemopathies, depending on the severity of the syndrome.[168-171] The chromosome abnormalities are nonrandom and often involve chromosomes that are abnormal in patients with AML, although certain chromosomal rearrangements seen in AML, such as t(15;17), t(8;21), and inv16, are seen rarely[172-174] (see Chap. 10).

Chromosomal abnormalities involving virtually every chromosome have been noted in marrow cells. Common abnormalities include an extra chromosome 8; loss of the long arm of the chromosome 5, 7, 9, 20, or 21; and monosomy for chromosomes 7 and 9. Losses of part or all of chromosomes 5 and 7 and complex chromosome aberrations are particularly common in the oligoblastic myelogenous leukemias (and the overt leukemias) associated with prior treatment with cytotoxic drugs, radiation, or exposure to benzene.[29,39,175,176] In this circumstance, the deletion in 5q is at band 5q31.1, in distinction to the classic 5q- syndrome (see "5q- Syndrome" below) in which the deletions occur at band q32-33.3. The Ph chromosome t(9q+;22q) and a variety of other chromosome abnormalities rarely seen in MDS have been described on occasion.[177]

Categories of cytogenetic abnormalities correlated with median survival have been determined. The more favorable risk category includes a normal karyotype and isolated deletions of 5q32-33.3, 20q, or Y. The poor-risk category includes -5q31.1, -7, del (7q), and complex chromosomal abnormalities. The intermediate-risk group includes other abnormalities. In treatment-induced MDS, complex cytogenetic abnormalities are very common, whereas in *de novo* MDS abnormalities occur in approximately 15 percent of cases.[39,177]

The proportion of cases with chromosome abnormalities differs depending on the severity of clinical manifestations. Chromosome abnormalities are more frequent in patients with oligoblastic myelogenous leukemia (RAEB) than in patients with clonal (refractory) anemia. In general, prevalence of chromosome abnormalities and the likelihood of progression to overt AML each is a function of the number of cell lines involved, the severity of the cytopenias, and the proportion of blast cells present.

Allelotype analysis of chromosomes of patients with MDS using microsatellite markers mapped to most of the arms of autosomes have found loss of heterozygosity on chromosomes 5q, 7q, 17p, and 20q, in keeping with the most prevalent chromosome abnormalities in MDS patients. Loss of heterozygosity on three new segments, 1p, 1q, and 18q, also were identified. These segments are presumed to contain tumor suppressor genes that may play a role in the initiation of these neoplasms.[178]

Gene expression studies using primitive multipotential cells (CD34+) from patients with MDS and confirmed by real-time polymerase chain reaction studies have identified 11 selected genes by hierarchical clustering that differ from the CD34+ cells of normal persons.[179] In addition, distinctions in gene expression were identified that distinguished high-risk (more blast cells) from low-risk MDS patients. In low-risk patients three genes (retinoic acid-induced gene; radiation-inducible, immediate early response gene; stress-induced phosphoprotein 1 gene) were down-regulated. Apparently, MDS patients accumulate gene defects that interfere with hematopoietic regulation.

SPECIFIC MYELODYSPLASTIC SYNDROMES

These syndromes highlight the variability in expression of the MDS (see Table 86-1). Most patients have one of the syndromes described below.

5Q- SYNDROME

Patients with the 5q- syndrome have clonal anemia and dysmorphic cells in the marrow containing, as the sole cytogenetic abnormality, a deletion in the long arm of chromosome 5 (5q).[180-182] The deletion in chromosome 5 is at band 5q32-33.3, as distinguished from the 5q-syndrome associated with AML and oligoblastic leukemia (MDS), which is located at band 5q31.1. The anemia, observed most frequently in older women, is associated with marked dyserythropoiesis, erythroid multinuclearity, and hypolobulated and frequently small ("dwarf") megakaryocytes. Neutropenia and thrombocytopenia are highly uncommon. The syndrome occurs infrequently in children.

The somatic mutation in this syndrome resides in a very primitive multipotential cell, which has been defined as a myeloid progenitor in some studies[183,184] or as a lymphohematopoietic progenitor in other studies.[185,186] Patients with this disorder have a risk of developing AML (approximately 10%) that is similar to the risk of patients with clonal anemia and marrow cells without 5q-. Patients in whom 5q- is a single abnormality by FISH and patients who correspond to the WHO morphologic criteria for the 5q- syndrome have a median survival of approximately 7 years.[187] Patients who appear to have a solitary 5q- by standard cytogenetics but who have other abnormalities when studied by FISH have a median survival of less than 3 years. With the application of FISH, complex abnormalities involving 5q-unlikely represent the classic syndrome with its very favorable prognosis. The much less morbid course of the classic 5q- syndrome is associated with a lower degree of pathologic apoptosis.[188]

Deletion of 5q- may be a feature of other clonal cytopenias, oligoblastic myelogenous leukemia, or AML. In these situations, two of the classic features of the 5q- syndrome often are absent: macrocytic red cells and normal or elevated platelet count. Blast cells are evident in the oligoblastic leukemias, and basophilia and eosinophilia have been found in over half of patients.[189] The 5q- cytogenetic finding still confers a somewhat better prognosis in these atypical situations if the marrow blast percentage is less than 10. In some cases, the 5q deletion may be a translocation or insertion as judged by FISH.[190] Cells in cases of T cell or B cell acute lymphoblastic leukemia also have contained a 5q- abnormality.[182]

Extensive studies of the deleted region of chromosome long arm 5q have demonstrated a narrowing of the common deleted region and the spectrum of genes that may be involved in the initiation of this clonal syndrome. A 1.5-megabase segment, containing 24 known genes and 16 predicted genes and 3793 single nucleotide polymorphisms, has been the shortest common region described.[191] Of these genes, 33 are expressed in CD34+ hematopoietic cells as measured by reverse transcriptase polymerase chain reaction, giving them a high probability status as candidates for involvement in the 5q- syndrome. Several favored candidate genes in the initiation of a clonal myeloid disease containing the 5q- identified in this study include (1) a member of the E-cadherin family (e.g. α-catenin, β-catenin) and homologue of the *Drosophila fat* tumor suppressor gene and the gene encoding RAS guanosine triphosphatase-activating protein-binding protein. Mutations have not been found on the normal homologous region of chromosome 5, and an epigenetic change such as hypermethylation of the allelic gene likely accounts for the loss of tumor suppressor activity.

MONOSOMY 7 SYNDROME

Monosomy 7 is the second most frequent cytogenetic abnormality in the marrow cells of patients with myelodysplasia. It often occurs in marrow cells of subjects exposed to chemicals or radiation and is associated with a poor prognosis and rapid transformation to AML.[192-196] A critical region carrying the gene responsible for the neoplastic transformation may reside within bands 7q35-36.[197,198] Monosomy 7 syndromes are difficult to classify. The syndromes usually are not associated with special clinical features in adults, but in children they are characterized by an atypical myeloproliferative disorder or myelomonocytic leukemia with abnormal expression of the neurofibromatosis (NF1) and Wilms tumor (WT1) genes, unusual susceptibility to infection, and a rapid termination in acute leukemia.[192,195] Chapter 88 discusses juvenile chronic myelomonocytic leukemia. Monosomy 7 also occurs in a familial form and in the leukemic evolution of Down syndrome and Fanconi anemia.[198–201] A variant of the monosomy 7 syndrome, translocation 1;7, also is seen in adults and children and may be preceded by exposure to cytotoxic treatment.[192,202] The *ERB-B* gene, which encodes a shortened form of the epidermal growth factor receptor, is amplified in this syndrome.[203] Patients with aplastic anemia have a predisposition to evolving into a clonal myeloid disease with a monosomy 7 cytogenetic abnormality.[204,205]

CLONAL (REFRACTORY) SIDEROBLASTIC ANEMIA

HISTORY

The term *refractory anemia* has been used for nearly a century to define erythropoietic insufficiencies that cannot be assigned to a specific vitamin or mineral deficiency and thus are unresponsive to the known hematinics.[1] At the time, the knowledge base was insufficient to determine the disorder was a neoplasia behaving in a relatively benign fashion. One sage observer likened the disorder to an adenoma in relationship to a carcinoma.[1] In 1956, Bjorkman[206] defined a subset of refractory anemias by the presence of ringed sideroblasts in the marrow. The intramitochondrial location of the iron in the ringed sideroblasts was described 1 year later.[207] Because the finding of ringed sideroblasts was a constant feature of marrow stained with Prussian blue in this situation, the designation *refractory anemia with ringed sideroblasts* was coined.

PATHOGENESIS

The disorder is a clonal multipotential hemopoietic stem cell defect in which ineffective erythropoiesis with normal or slightly shortened red cell survival and only slight impairment of the maturation of other cell lineages occur. Plasma iron turnover is increased, but incorporation of radioactive iron into heme and its delivery to blood as newly synthesized hemoglobin are depressed. These early ferrokinetic studies presaged the evidence that erythroid precursors were subject to aberrant maturation and pathologic apoptosis.[69,70] The genes somatically mutated to initiate this disorder have not been identified, but the frequency of deleted chromosome arms suggests a tumor suppressor gene on the affected chromosome is involved.[170]

CLINICAL FEATURES

The disease is very uncommon in individuals younger than 50 years,[23,25,208] except in patients in whom the disease occurs as a result of radiotherapy or chemotherapy of a malignant tumor. The rare concurrence of familial sideroblastic anemia has been reported.[209] Males and females are affected almost equally. The signs and symptoms are those of anemia: pallor, easy fatigue, weakness, dyspnea, and palpitations on exertion.[207,208] In most patients the anemia is detected as a result of blood cell analysis for other medical reasons. The liver may be slightly enlarged. The spleen is slightly increased in size in approximately 5 percent of patients. Splenic and hepatic enlargement do not necessarily occur together, and more than slight enlargement is unusual.

LABORATORY FEATURES

Most patients have mild to severe macrocytic anemia.[207,208] The blood film often contains a population of hypochromic cells (dimorphic red cell changes).[207,210] Red cell anisocytosis, basophilic stippling, and slight poikilocytosis may be present. The total white cell count and platelet count usually are normal, but mild abnormalities may be seen, including a decreased white cell count and an increased or decreased platelet count. Occasionally, the white cell count or platelet count is increased markedly, or nucleated red cells are present in the blood film. The reticulocyte percentage usually is between 0.5 and 2.0. Hemoglobin F concentration may be increased slightly. The disease may express a subtle phenotype: either mild macrocytic anemia in older patients with few other features of clonal anemia [211,212] or patients with clonal cytogenetic abnormalities with cytopenia but no unequivocal morphologic evidence of clonal dysmorphic hematopoiesis.[213]

Marrow cellularity usually is increased as a result of erythroid hyperplasia. Evidence of dyserythropoiesis in the form of vacuolated, small, large, or binucleate erythroblasts may be present. Prussian blue stain of the marrow invariably shows pathologic sideroblasts. The latter may have Prussian blue-positive cytoplasmic granules in a partial or complete circumnuclear pattern (ringed sideroblasts) in 15 or more percent of cells or an increased number (more than five) of Prussian blue-positive granules in their cytoplasm. If the disease progresses to oligoblastic leukemia, sideroblasts may become less prominent.[214] Granulopoiesis and thrombopoiesis are not altered significantly in two thirds of patients.[210,215] In the other third of patients, dysgranulopoiesis (hypogranulation, acquired Pelger-Huët anomaly, hypersegmented nuclei, granule abnormalities) or dysmegakaryocytopoiesis (micromegakaryocytes, large lobulated cells) may be present. Marrow iron stores often are increased.

Cytogenetic abnormalities in marrow cells of patients with acquired refractory sideroblastic anemia provide evidence for the clonal character of the disease. Approximately half of the reported patients with sideroblastic anemia in whom cytogenetic studies have been performed have a chromosomal abnormality.[209] Involvement of chromosomes 8, 11, and 20 has been notable.[169,216,217] The Philadelphia chromosome has been reported.[218] Involvement of chromosome 3 has been associated with thrombocytosis.[219] The absence of the Y chromosome, only in the pathologic sideroblasts in one report (45;X/46;XY mosaic), substantiates the dimorphic nature of the erythroid lineage involvement and parallels the hypochromic and normochromic red cell populations.[220] Involvement of the X chromosome (a breakpoint at Xq13) of female patients with sideroblastic anemia[221] is noteworthy because a type of hereditary sideroblastic anemia is X chromosome linked (see Chap. 58).

Serum iron levels and saturation of transferrin are increased. Serum ferritin concentration is increased, reflecting an increase in body iron stores. Bilirubin-proteinase levels (indirect-reacting fraction) may be increased as a result of ineffective erythropoiesis and intramedullary hemolysis.

DIFFERENTIAL DIAGNOSIS

The principal considerations are the anemias with an inadequate reticulocyte response in which erythrocytes are hypochromic. Iron deficiency anemia in contradistinction to sideroblastic anemia is associated with low serum iron levels, saturation of transferrin of less than 16 percent, low serum ferritin concentration, elevated serum transferrin receptors, and absent marrow sideroblasts and macrophage iron. The anemia of chronic disease can simulate some features of clonal anemia, although the low serum iron in the former and the presence of an overt chronic inflammatory disease, such as rheumatoid arthritis, are important distinctions. β-Thalassemia minor is characterized by normal to elevated serum iron and ferritin, low mean red cell volume, elevated hemoglobin A$_2$ concentration, and evidence of the disease in a parent, siblings, or offspring. Detection of secondary forms of sideroblastic anemia requires evaluation for exposure to lead or other agents or diseases listed in Chapter 58, as do the hereditary sideroblastic anemias.

THERAPY

Some patients do not require treatment because the moderate decrease in hemoglobin concentration is tolerated without limitation of usual activities. Occasional patients who have low serum and red cell folate concentrations may have partial improvement in blood hemoglobin concentration after administration of folic acid (1 mg/day orally). Rare patients benefit temporarily from pharmacologic doses of pyridoxine (200 mg/day orally for at least 3 months) or danazol.[222] A therapeutic trial with folic acid and pyridoxine is worthwhile if the anemia is symptomatic, even though only a small percentage of patients are responsive. If anemia is severe or symptoms of heart failure or coronary insufficiency are present, periodic transfusion of red cells is required. Recombinant human erythropoietin generally is not useful unless the pretreatment serum erythropoietin level is low for the blood hemoglobin concentration, an infrequent finding in these patients.[223] The combination of G-CSF with erythropoietin may increase the response rate to greater than 40 percent.[224] Erythropoietin (20,000–40,000 units subcutaneously, once per week) and G-CSF (300 μg subcutaneously, two or three times per week) is one regimen that can be used if the cytopenias are not tolerated. Serum iron should be maintained at a normal level by oral supplementation, if needed to ensure an optimal response from erythropoietin administration. A controlled trial of erythropoietin (20,000 IU) and G-CSF (105 μg), each given subcutaneously three times per week, compared to supportive care resulted in a marked difference in the improvement in blood hemoglobin concentration in the treated group (10 of 24 patients) versus (0 of 26) in the group receiving supportive care. However, no difference in quality of life was evident.[462]

COURSE AND PROGNOSIS

In many patients, the disorder lasts for years without progression of the anemia or symptoms. A small proportion of patients may have progressive marrow failure, severe cytopenia, and morbidity from infections or hemorrhage. Iron overload is common, and some patients develop hemochromatosis.[225] The frequency of HLA-A$_3$ is significantly higher in patients who develop iron overload than in the general population. The frequency is comparable to that found in hereditary hemochromatosis,[226] suggesting the combination of a genetic predisposition plus sideroblastic anemia facilitates the expression of iron overload in these patients. Evidence supporting this linkage has not been found after search for mutations associated with hemochromatosis.[227] The appearance of hemochromatosis may be accelerated if frequent transfusions were required for a period of years.[225] Improvement of the anemia and the adverse effects of iron overload in parenchymal tissues can occur following cautious phlebotomy or chelation therapy.[228–230]

Over a 10- to 15-year period, approximately 10 percent of patients with clonal (sideroblastic) anemia develop AML.[224,231–234] Progression to leukemia is correlated with the degree of dyshematopoiesis and trilineage abnormalities.[187,214] Transformation to acute lymphocytic leukemia (ALL) also has occurred.[235] In one series of 37 patients, 25 had abnormalities confined to the erythroid series, transfusion dependence occurred in 26, and iron overload was common. Five patients progressed to marrow failure and five to AML. Median survival was 72 months.[236] Survival in other series has ranged from 21 to more than 85 months.[171,187] Survival is better in patients without significant abnormalities in lineages other than erythroid cells and with favorable cytogenetic findings.[236,237] This prognostic indicator also applies to clonal nonsideroblastic anemias and oligoblastic leukemia.[238]

CLONAL (REFRACTORY) NONSIDEROBLASTIC ANEMIA

This clonal disorder, another arbitrary misnomer, closely mimics clonal sideroblastic anemia. No significant difference is observed in any of comparative variables (age, gender, blood cell counts, marrow findings), except that the frequency of ringed sideroblasts is by definition less than 15 percent but usually present. The anemia is mild to moderate, with a tendency to macrocytosis. Leukopenia and thrombocytopenia, if present, usually are mild.[239] Hyposegmented and hypersegmented neutrophils, giant platelets, and red cell shape, size, and hemoglobinization abnormalities may be present. The marrow usually is cellular, and the precursors may show morphologic evidence of dyserythropoiesis. Because anemia predominates and other cytopenias are slight, the course and management are similar to those of clonal (refractory) sideroblastic anemia. Patients with low erythropoietin levels may have a significant increase in hemoglobin concentration with weekly injections of the hormone. The proportion of patients transforming into AML and the median survival of patients are similar to patients with clonal sideroblastic anemia.[237–239] Cytopenias and blood and marrow dysmorphic changes can become more severe, and the course and management in that instance are similar to clonal multilineal cytopenia.

In a study of 640 patients with MDS, 467 were categorized as clonal anemia (39%), clonal sideroblastic anemia (16%), or oligoblastic leukemia (45%). Ninety-four percent of clonal anemia patients were in the low or low–intermediate risk category of the International Prognostic Scoring System (IPSS), and 98 percent of patients with clonal sideroblastic anemia were so categorized. In each case, approximately 50 percent of patients were low risk, and approximately 50 percent were low–intermediate risk. The median survival of patients with clonal anemia who were categorized as low risk was 9 years and for patients categorized as low–intermediate risk was 5 years.[171] Because of equivalent numbers in each group, the overall median survival for patients with clonal anemia of either type was approximately 7 years.

CLONAL MULTILINEAL CYTOPENIAS

Approximately two thirds of patients with clonal cytopenia present with some degree of neutropenia and/or thrombocytopenia in addition to anemia. Patients with clonal multilineal cytopenias (refractory cytopenia with multilineal dysplasia) represent a subset of myelodysplastic disorders that are more morbid and have a significantly decreased life expectancy than the clonal anemias.

CLINICAL FINDINGS

Patients present with anemia, neutropenia, and thrombocytopenia; anemia and neutropenia; or anemia and thrombocytopenia. The blood and marrow features are as described in "Laboratory Features" above and lead to the diagnosis, especially in the patient older than 50 years.[14,15,240–242] The patient usually seeks medical attention for symptoms of anemia: fatigue, dyspnea, and palpitations on exertion, headache, or dizziness. Exaggerated bleeding associated with thrombocytopenia may be present. Mild hepatomegaly and/or splenomegaly may be present occasionally.

Dysmorphic blood and marrow cell changes are common. Myeloblasts are not increased in the marrow (<2%) and are absent from the blood. Cytogenetic abnormalities may be present as described in "Cytogenetics" above. If monocytosis is greater than 1000×10^6/liter, the disorder merges with chronic myelomonocytic leukemia (see Chap. 88).

DIFFERENTIAL DIAGNOSIS

Mild to moderate bicytopenia (anemia and neutropenia) and sometimes tricytopenia with dysmorphic blood and marrow findings and hypercellular marrow occur in patients with the acquired immune deficiency syndrome[243,244] but have not been associated with progression to acute leukemia. Pancytopenia with hyperplastic marrow has been associated with nonhemopoietic cancers (paraneoplastic syndrome).[245] Megaloblastic anemia can be simulated and distinguished by the normal concentration of serum or red cell folate and serum vitamin B_{12}. In the small proportion of patients with a hypocellular marrow, aplastic anemia or paroxysmal nocturnal hemoglobinuria should be considered (see "Relationship Among Aplastic Anemia, Paroxysmal Nocturnal Hemoglobinuria, and Clonal Myeloid Diseases" in Chap. 33).

TREATMENT

In patients with pancytopenia and hyperplastic marrow, cytopenias that are not troublesome should not be treated. Transfusion of blood components when necessary is the mainstay of treatment. Regular transfusion of red cells may be used for patients who do not adapt to moderate anemia or in whom medical conditions, such as angina pectoris, require a higher packed red cell volume. Erythropoietin with or without G-CSF administration may increase hemoglobin concentration and decrease transfusion frequency. Thrombocytopenia often is not so severe as to require treatment. If thrombocytopenic bleeding occurs, platelet transfusions should be used. Aminocaproic acid (Amicar) may be a useful adjunct to platelet transfusion for thrombocytopenic bleeding. IL-11 may increase platelet counts in some patients. SCF, IL-3, and thrombopoietin, each of which may improve blood cell counts, are not approved for clinical use. Amifostine, an aminothiol agent used for radioprotection, given in doses of 100 to 200 mg/m² three times per week may increase blood counts in some patients.[246] Asymptomatic neutropenia should not be treated, but fever should be evaluated promptly and suspected infection treated with broad-spectrum bactericidal antibiotics until the results of cultures are known. In appropriate situations, oral antibiotics can be used in patients treated at home.[247,248]

Androgens have not been generally useful. Rare cases may show minor improvement, but the likelihood of substantial or sustained improvement is low. Occasional cases have shown improvement in blood cell counts and, where present, resolution of myelofibrosis following administration of glucocorticoids (prednisone 40 mg/m² per day orally or 60 mg qd).[249,250] Protracted glucocorticoid use may increase the risk of infection, especially with opportunistic organisms, and has not been shown to increase survival.

For patients with symptomatic anemia and high transfusion requirements or severe, symptomatic neutropenia, therapeutic trials of erythropoietin[251–254] and/or GM-CSF,[255–257] G-CSF,[258,259] or IL-3[260] occasionally have been beneficial in increasing counts and improving neutrophil function. Cytokines have not been shown to increase survival and can produce troubling side effects, such as local skin reactions, fever, bone pain, and a capillary leak syndrome.[251,261] They also can lead to increased immature granulocytes, including blasts in the marrow and blood.[262]

In uncommon cases with hypoplastic marrows, cyclosporin A and ATG have been used,[263,264] analogous to the responsiveness of the hypoplasia of some cases of aplastic anemia to such approaches (see "Pathogenesis" above and "Immunotherapy" below). A variety of chemotherapeutic agents have been used, especially when the disease evolves to oligoblastic or frank AML (see "Oligoblastic Myelogenous Leukemia" and "Treatment" below).

COURSE AND PROGNOSIS

Morbidity is high in patients with multicytopenias. Lassitude, severe infections, exaggerated bleeding, and severe anemia may occur. Mortality from infection or hemorrhage occurs in approximately 25 percent of patients. AML develops in approximately 50 percent of patients. The likelihood of transformation to overt AML is greater if the patient has severe cytopenias, more overt qualitative disorders of cells, abnormal localized immature myeloid precursors in marrow, complex chromosome abnormalities, and abnormalities of marrow cell colony growth in culture (excessive growth or decreased growth).[238,265–268] Median survival of patients with clonal hemopathy and multicytopenias is approximately 20 to 40 months.[187,266,267]

OLIGOBLASTIC MYELOGENOUS LEUKEMIA (RAEB)

DEFINITION AND HISTORY

In 1963, the term *smoldering acute leukemia* was introduced to highlight a subset of patients, usually those older than 50 years, who had a low proportion of leukemic blast cells in marrow (3–20%) and blood (0–7%) and who survived for months or years without specific therapy for leukemia.[268–270] The terms "smoldering, pauciblastic, low-infiltrate, and oligoblastic" are synonyms. Oligoblastic leukemia is called *refractory anemia with excess myeloblasts*.[2,3,270,271] When the blast count increased to greater than 20 percent (formerly 30%), the phrase *in transformation* (to AML) had been used. The latter distinction has proved of little value in choosing treatment or predicting patient outcome and has been deleted from the WHO classification.[2] These patients have AML. Chronic myelomonocytic leukemia, previously included under the rubric myelodysplasia, is better linked to the subacute and chronic myelogenous leukemias discussed in Chap. 88. Elimination of RAEB-T and CMML in the WHO reclassification of MDS further minimizes the oxymoronic nomenclature that considers acute (RAEB-T) and subacute (CMML) myelogenous leukemias as dysplasias.

CLINICAL FINDINGS

Oligoblastic leukemia composes approximately 45 percent of all cases of myelodysplasia.[171] Most patients are older than 50 years. Males are affected more often than females by approximately 1.5:1. Reticulocytopenic anemia, granulocytopenia, and/or thrombocytopenia are present. Qualitative abnormalities of blood cells usually are overt (see "Laboratory Features" above). Myeloblasts constitute from 3 to 20 percent of nucleated marrow cells. Auer rods may be present in blast cells. Dysmorphic changes that occur in abnormal marrow precursor cells are described in "Laboratory Features" (above). This syndrome evolves into overt AML in more than 50 percent of cases.[171,272,273] Median survival of patients with oligoblastic leukemia is approximately 9 months, although occasional long-term survival has been reported.[171]

TREATMENT, COURSE, AND PROGNOSIS

Treatment of oligoblastic leukemia should be individualized. In some cases, no active treatment is required. Periodic evaluation is essential to detect deterioration in well-being or blood cell counts. Most patients require treatment in weeks to months (Table 86-2). The response to cytotoxic therapy is poor, and symptomatic therapy with component transfusion and antibiotics, as required, is the preferable management if that approach can sustain a reasonable functional status. If the disease progresses such that cytopenias lead to infection, hemorrhage, or anemia and require inordinate amounts of transfusions or if the disease progresses to polyblastic leukemia (AML) and the patient is fit, therapy for AML may be warranted (see Chap. 87). If the patient has a poor performance status or has comorbid medical conditions that would lower the tolerance for intensive cytotoxic therapy, attenuation of doses should be considered. Cytarabine combined with anthracycline antibiotics, etoposide, or topotecan has produced remissions in approximately half of a group of selected patients.[274–280] Recovery may

TABLE 86-2   AGENTS USED IN VARIOUS PHASES OF THE
MYELODYSPLASTIC SPECTRUM

Single Agents	**Immunotherapy**
Amifostine[246,355,365]	Antithymocyte globulin[78,264,320,323,324,322,328]
All-*trans*-retinoic acid[367]	Cyclosporine[263,321,327,329,331]
Arsenic troxide[377,378]	Glucocorticoids[249,250,331]
5-Azacytidine[281,282,334,336]	Combinations of three agents above
5-Aza-2′-deoxycytidine (decitabine)[337–339]	Etanercept (TNFR)[357–359]
CPT-11[344]	Mycophenolate mofetil[332]
Cytarabine, low or intermediate dose[317]	Inhibitors of TNF-α (Enbrel, Remicaid)[359,360]
Danazol[222,271,361]	VEGF receptor TK inhibitors[354]
Etoposide, low dose[341]	VEGF neutralizing antibody (bevacizumab)[354]
Farnesyl transferase inhibitors[387]	WT peptide vaccination[333]
Gemcitabine[343]	**Multiple Agents**[274,279,280,390]
Gemtuzumab ozogamicin[394,395]	Amifostine+pentoxifylline+ciprofloxacin[375]
Hexamethylene bisacetamide[364,374]	ATRA+IFN+G-CSF[302,368]
Idarubicin, oral[346]	ATRA+danazol+prednisone[362]
IFN[379–383]	Cytarabine+daunomycin
Imatinib mesylate[384,385]	Cytarabine+daunomycin+etoposide
Melphalan, low dose[342]	Cytarabine+daunomycin+thalidomide
Phenylbutyrate[340,365]	Cytarabine+idarubicin+amifostine[356]
SU5416 (TK inhibitor)[353]	Cytarabine, low dose+etoposide[276]
CC5013 (Revimid)[352]	Cytarabine, low dose+ATRA+VitD$_3$[373]
Thalidomide[347–351]	Cytarabine+idarubicin+topotecan or troxicitabine[345]
Topotecan[277]	Cytarabine+daunomycin (liposomal)+topotecan+/−thalidomide[391]
Vitamin D$_3$[369,370]	Cytarabine+idarubicin[275]
Cytokines[251,261,299]	Cytarabine+idarubicin+fludarabine+G-CSF[278]
EPO[223,252–254,296,304–307,309]	Daunomycin+topotecan+thalidomide
G-CSF,[258,259,296,311,314]	
GM-CSF[255,256]	**Stem Cell Transplantation**[407,408]
EPO+G-CSF, [224,257,310]	Matched related[283–285,396,398–400]
EPO+GM-CSF[298,308]	Matched unrelated[401,405,406,411]
IL-3[260]	Mismatched related[417]
rMGF, pegylated[316]	Nonmyeloablative[409,410,412]
	Autologous[286,399,413,414,416]

be slow, and remissions tend to be short, however. Patients with a poor performance status, of advanced age, or who choose not to be treated with combined-agent chemotherapy have been treated with low-dose cytarabine, 5-azacytidine or decitabine,[281,282] etoposide, hydroxyurea, retinoids, butyrates, or interferon (IFN) coupled with transfusion therapy for palliation of the disease. Although some patients have improved, these approaches have been of limited benefit. Patients younger than 50 years age with a histocompatible donor should be considered for allogeneic stem cell transplantation.[283–285] Other patients may be considered for nonmyeloablative allogeneic transplantation or, if in remission, intensive therapy and autologous stem cell rescue.[286]

TREATMENT OF MDS BASED ON PROGNOSTIC SCORE

The IPSS score assigned to patients at the time of diagnosis can be utilized to approximate the average time by which patients with those

characteristics will evolve to AML.[238,239,287] Multivariate analysis combines the impact of (1) three cytogenetic subgroups (favorable, unfavorable, intermediate), (2) percentage of marrow blasts, and (3) number of cytopenias. In large numbers of patients, the following frequency distribution of patients has been observed: low risk (i.e., longest time to evolve to AML) in 15 to 30 percent of patients, intermediate-1 risk in 30 to 40 percent of patients, intermediate-2 risk in 20 to 25 percent of patients, and high risk in 5 to 10 percent of patients.[238,239,287] The prognostic score should not be the sole guide to treatment because many patients deviate from the average expectation of disease behavior. Unexpected progression may necessitate changes in treatment approach and, in the case of patients who are candidates for stem cell transplantation, may prompt recommending the procedure.

Treatments for myelodysplasia can be considered (1) supportive care, (2) low-intensity therapy, or (3) high-intensity treatment.[288–290] Treatment response is judged based on the MDS subtype and IPSS score of the patient and the presence of treatment-induced (secondary) MDS.[291]

SUPPORTIVE CARE

Supportive care consists of improving quality of life with specific treatment of cytopenias or their complications and providing psychosocial support, while monitoring at intervals the patient's clinical status.[292,293] Red cell transfusions should be administered for symptomatic anemia. Chelation with deferoxamine may be necessary to prevent iron overload in patients receiving frequent transfusions. Platelet transfusions can be utilized for thrombocytopenic bleeding. Therapeutic rather than prophylactic transfusions lessen the risk of infectious disease transmission, blood cell immunization, and febrile transfusion reactions.[294] Antifibrinolytic agents such as aminocaproic acid can be used in patients who have bleeding despite platelet transfusion or to decrease the need of platelet transfusions.[295] Antibiotics are used to treat infections (see Chap. 20).

ERYTHROPOIETIN, GRANULOCYTE-MACROPHAGE COLONY STIMULATING FACTOR, GRANULOCYTE COLONY STIMULATING FACTOR, INTERLEUKIN-3, AND INTERLEUKIN-11

Randomized, double-blind studies have not shown that any cytokine prolongs survival or reduces morbidity in oligoblastic leukemia. Erythropoietin occasionally reduces transfusion requirement,[296] GM-CSF and G-CSF[297,298] increase neutrophil counts and functions in some patients, and IL-3[260] results in increased white cell count and, less frequently, increased red cell and platelet counts. Combined erythropoietin and G-CSF[257] or GM-CSF[298] can be useful. Responses have been seen in oligoblastic leukemias and clonal multicytopenia. Cytokines do not delay progression to acute leukemia; however, they increase the percentage of blasts in the blood in a proportion of patients, an event that is not always reversible with cessation of cytokine.[297,298] In one review, 22 of 83 reported cases of myelodysplasia treated with G-CSF or GM-CSF had an increase in marrow blast percentage, and AML evolved in 12 of 69 patients. An increased percentage of abnormal macrophages has been reported.[299] Use of these agents without chemotherapy in oligoblastic leukemias carries a risk of promoting expansion of leukemic blast cells.[300] Combinations of growth factors alone or coupled with maturing agents have not significantly improved response or survival rates.[301,302] IL-11 is being studied as a means of increasing the platelet count in patients with symptomatic thrombocytopenia.[303]

Recombinant erythropoietin can be utilized to treat anemia in patients who are transfusion dependent if the serum erythropoietin level is low for the hemoglobin level. Serum erythropoietin levels correlate with survival and predict response to erythropoietin. Responses are best with low erythropoietin levels, normal blast counts, and normal cytogenetics[304] and in patients who do not require transfusion.[305] Hemolysis or iron, B_{12}, or folate deficiency should be ruled out as a cause of anemia before erythropoietin therapy is started. Iron stores must be kept replete during erythropoietin therapy. Erythropoietin 150 to 300 units/kg/day and single weekly doses of 40,000 units are effective.[306] The probability of a response increases with duration of therapy, for example, best at 26 weeks compared to 12 weeks.[307] G-CSF combined with erythropoietin may produce a more frequent response.[308,309] Quality of life has been improved in patients who respond to treatment with the combination of erythropoietin and G-CSF.[310]

Low-dose G-CSF can improve neutropenia in MDS patients[311] and is generally well tolerated. Rare serious complications, such as splenic rupture, have been reported.[312] G-CSF receptor expression may be low in some patients with MDS and prevents a good response to endogenous or administered G-CSF.[313] Complete remissions have been reported in hypoplastic AML/MDS with G-CSF alone.[314] Granulocyte transfusions are rarely used in MDS.[315]

Pegylated recombinant human megakaryocyte growth and development factor improves blood counts in some patients with MDS. Platelet and red cell responses were noted.[316]

THERAPY FOR PATIENTS WITH LOW AND LOW–INTERMEDIATE PROGNOSTIC SCORES

LOWER-DOSE CYTARABINE

Low-dose cytarabine 5 to 20 mg/m²/ day by subcutaneous injection every 12 hours for up to 8 to 16 weeks or by continuous intravenous infusion has been used in lieu of intensive chemotherapy.[317,318] Although this approach led to remission in approximately 20 percent of patients with oligoblastic leukemia, the median duration of remission is approximately 10 months, and survival has not been prolonged compared with supportive care alone. Also, in contrast to AML, survival has not been influenced greatly by induction of remission. Moreover, low-dose cytosine arabinoside usually is cytotoxic, inducing marrow hypoplasia and worsening cytopenias. Often the patient requires hospitalization and blood cell component transfusion and antibiotic treatment analogous to that used for intensive treatment of AML. In some cases, outpatient therapy is possible with self-administration of subcutaneous cytarabine. Although occasional reports of remission following low-dose cytarabine have been consistent with an effect on leukemia cell maturation, most patients experience suppression of the malignant stem cell clone, leading to marrow repopulation with polyclonal hemopoiesis.[280,287,288] Combinations of low-dose cytarabine with growth factors have not shown a clear advantage over chemotherapy alone, and this treatment modality has fallen out of use.[288]

IMMUNOTHERAPY

Cyclosporine and Antithymocyte Globulin In some patients with MDS, T lymphocyte–mediated inhibition of hematopoiesis occurs and contributes to cytopenias. The cytopenias can be ameliorated by treatment with immunosuppressive agents.[319] In patients who recovered effective hematopoiesis after treatment, the Vβ (T cell receptor-β) spectra type representative of clonal or oligoclonal T cell populations reverted to normal patterns.[319] A nonclonal X-chromosome inactivation pattern in the marrow as assessed by the androgen receptor gene assay and the phosphoglycerated kinase-1 assay was associated with a response to ATG. This finding was attributed to incomplete

clonal expansion, with ATG improving normal hematopoiesis by relieving the immunologic pressure on the remaining normal progenitors.[320] Others have postulated that responses may result from suppression of IFN-γ secretion by CD4+ T cells.[321] Some series have reported response rates to ATG of 15 to 60 percent[322–324] and longer survival times in patients who respond. HLA-DR15 (DR2) is overrepresented in MDS and predicts a response to immunosuppressive therapy.[325] In one series of 60 patients treated with ATG and cyclosporine, 60 percent had hematologic improvement, and more responders had good karyotype or DRB1 1501.[326] Most of the patients in this series had refractory anemia and an IPSS score of intermediate-1. Most but not all responses have occurred in patients with hypocellular marrows.[327] Other groups have reported lack of response to ATG and prednisone. One study was stopped early because of lack of efficacy and development of adverse reactions.[328] Other studies also have reported lack of efficacy of single-agent cyclosporine.[329] Idiopathic thrombocytopenic purpura complicating MDS can respond to cyclosporine.[330]

High-Dose Glucocorticoids Responses to pulse methylprednisolone therapy have occurred in patients with normocellular and hypercellular marrows and in those with hypocellular marrows.[331]

Mycophenolate Mofetil In a case of autoimmune hemolytic anemia complicating MDS, the hemolysis and the underlying clonal disorder responded to treatment with mycophenolate mofetil.[332]

Vaccines The Wilms tumor protein WT1 is a tumor antigen for myelogenous leukemia. Peptide-based immunotherapy has been studied in clinical trials, and the peptide resulted in an increase in WT1-specific cytotoxic T lymphocytes, followed by rapid reduction in leukemic blast cells. Severe leukopenia and erythema at the injection site were noted.[333]

THERAPY FOR PATIENTS WITH HIGH–INTERMEDIATE PROGNOSTIC SCORES

5-AZACYTIDINE AND OTHER AGENTS AFFECTING METHYLATION STATUS

Oligoblastic and secondary myelogenous leukemias have a high prevalence of tumor suppressor gene hypermethylation.[334] 5-Azacytidine is a pyrimidine analogue that inhibits DNA methyltransferase, reduces cytosine methylation, and induces maturation of some leukemic cell lines. It also is an antiproliferative drug. It inhibits the release of oncostatin-M, IL-6, and IL-11 from mononuclear cells in patients with clonal anemia.[335] Administration of the drug and its congener decitabine has resulted in improvement of some patients with oligoblastic leukemia.[281,282] 5-Azacytidine at a dose of 75 mg/m² once per day given subcutaneously for 7 consecutive days each month provided significantly more frequent benefit to two thirds of patients than did supportive care. Quality of life was enhanced, and disease progression was delayed.[282] In another series,[336] subclasses of MDS did not predict for response to 5-azacytidine. A decrease in the white blood count during the initial cycle correlated with a higher response rate. The drug is available from the National Cancer Institute based on "compassionate use."

5-Aza-2′-deoxycytidine (decitabine) can be used for high-risk MDS. Seventeen percent of patients in one series had a major cytogenetic response on an intention-to-treat basis after a median of three courses. The median duration of cytogenetic response was 7.5 months in all IPSS groups.[337] Patients who responded had improved survival compared with patients in whom the cytogenetically abnormal clone persisted.[338,339] Decitabine probably works partly through demethylation, as it has resulted in demethylation of a hypermethylated p15/INK4B gene in patients.[338] Demethylation was associated with clinical responses.[339]

Inhibitors of histone deacetylation may have activity in MDS. So-dium phenylbutyrate has resulted in some partial responses in MDS, although hematopoiesis remained clonal.[340]

Other Single-Agent Cytotoxic Drugs Hydroxyurea and low-dose etoposide are useful in controlling leukemic cell proliferation but usually produce only partial responses and do not influence survival duration.[289] Occasional patients have achieved remissions with etoposide (50 mg as a 2-hour infusion, two to seven times weekly for 4 weeks; or 100 mg/day orally for 3 days and then 50 mg twice weekly).[341] Low-dose melphalan,[342] gemcitabine,[343] CPT-11, a DNA topoisomerase I inhibitor,[344] troxacitabine, an enantiomer of cytarabine,[345] and weekly doses of oral idarubicin[346] each has resulted in responses in some patients.

Antiangiogenesis Agents Thalidomide has shown effectiveness.[291] In one series in which patients received 100 to 400 mg/day for 12 or more weeks of therapy, no cytogenetic or complete responses were noted, but 16 patients had hematologic improvement.[347] In another series of 34 patients in whom 400 mg/day was the median dose tolerated, six patients had progressive disease, four patients had stable disease, and 11 patients had partial remissions (five major responses and six minor responses), accounting for a 56 percent response rate. Hematologic improvement was not noted until after a median of 2 months.[348] Cytogenetic responses have been seen in cases of monosomy 7, 5q- syndrome, and complex karyotypic abnormalities. Although thalidomide has antiangiogenesis activity, it also decreases VEGF and basic fibroblast growth factor levels.[349] The drug may have a particular role in patients with marrow fibrosis.[350] Thromboembolic events have occurred in patients receiving thalidomide in combination with darbepoietin-α.[351]

The thalidomide derivative CC-5013 (Revlimid) lowers levels of proangiogenic cytokines, inhibits attachment of stromal cells, promotes cell cycle arrest and apoptosis, and affects function of natural killer and cytotoxic T lymphocytes. In one early trial, CC-5013 reduced the need for red cell transfusions in 16 of 25 evaluable patients. This result occurred in 1 of 12 patients with early-stage clonal anemia and 15 of 21 with low-risk and intermediate-risk disease. In patients with 5q- syndrome, responses were noted in each of eight patients, and cells with the chromosome abnormality were undetectable in all who received CC-5013 25 mg/day. Unlike the case with thalidomide, dose reduction for myelosuppression often was required.[352]

The small molecule tyrosine kinase receptor inhibitor SU5416, which also inhibits VEGF, has only minimal activity in MDS.[353] The VEGF tyrosine kinase receptor inhibitor RTK474 and the anti-VEGF neutralizing antibody bevacizumab have entered clinical trials of patients with MDS.[354]

Anticytokine Therapies Anticytokine therapies have been utilized in MDS because excess local generation of inhibitory cytokines, such as TNF-α, may promote accelerated apoptotic loss of progenitor cells leading to ineffective maturation and ineffective hematopoiesis.

Amifostine Amifostine as a single agent given as 200 mg/m^2 intravenously three times per week for 3 weeks did not result in reduction of transfusions but did result in some blood count improvement.[355] Amifostine has been utilized with other chemotherapeutic agents in an attempt to minimize toxicities and to allow dose escalation of chemotherapeutic agents. When combined with high-dose cytarabine and idarubicin in patients with AML or high-risk MDS, amifostine did not allow dose escalation of idarubicin.[356]

Anti–Tumor Necrosis Factor Therapy The soluble TNF receptor fusion protein etanercept (p75 TNFR:Fc) has produced mixed results in MDS. In one pilot series, moderate improvement in cytopenias was noted,[357] whereas in another trial, no responses were noted in 10 patients.[358] In another pilot study with a 3-month duration, one patient

became temporarily transfusion independent, but overall efficacy was low.[359] The chimeric anti–TNF-α monoclonal antibody infliximab resulted in two sustained erythroid responses (one major and one minor), and a decreased percentage of apoptotic cells in marrow was noted.[360]

Danazol The attenuated androgen danazol reportedly has activity in MDS. An increased platelet count and a decreased frequency of platelet transfusions have been noted. Responses have been seen in all categories of MDS.[361] Danazol has been combined with retinoic acid and low-dose prednisone.[362]

RETINOIDS, VITAMIN D DERIVATIVES, AND OTHER POTENTIALLY MATURATION-ENHANCING AGENTS

Glucocorticoids, vitamin A analogues (retinoids), vitamin D analogues (dihydroxyvitamin D$_3$), pyrimidine analogues (cytarabine), hexamethylene bisacetamide, and IFNs among other agents can induce *in vitro* maturation of mouse and human leukemic cells.[363–365] Use of *cis*-retinoic acid 20 to 100 mg/m^2, isotretinoin 25 mg/m^2, or ATRA 45 mg/m^2 orally given daily for up to 3 months has produced only slight, transient (few weeks) improvement in a very small proportion of patients with oligoblastic leukemia.[366,367] Adverse effects of these vitamin A derivatives, which include dry skin, cheilitis, pruritus, lethargy, and arthralgia, usually disappear after discontinuation of the agent. ATRA combined with IFN-α and G-CSF resulted in responses in six of 17 patients with MDS.[368]

A regimen including dihydroxyvitamin D$_3$ 2.5 μg/day orally for at least 8 weeks has not been beneficial in patients with oligoblastic leukemia.[369,370] Hypercalcemia has been a dose-limiting factor. Analogues with less hypercalcemia-inducing capacity, such as α-calcidol, have shown some effect on reducing blasts and promoting monocytoid differentiation, whereas others have been inactive.[371,372]

A combination of low-dose cytarabine, retinoic acid, and 1,25-dihydroxyvitamin D$_3$ in 44 patients with oligoblastic leukemias produced 50 percent response rates, with longer survival in responders than in nonresponders.[373] Hexamethylene bisacetamide given at a dosage of 20 to 24 g/m^2/day intravenously for 10 days followed by an 18- to 75-day observation period produced increased neutrophil counts and reduced marrow blasts in only four of 16 patients with oligoblastic leukemia.[374] In another study, no responses were observed.[364] Sodium phenylbutyrate is an agent that has shown some activity against oligoblastic leukemia and is in clinical trials.[365]

Amifostine, pentoxifylline, and dexamethasone have shown effectiveness in prolonging patient survival. When ciprofloxacin was added to this regimen, 76 percent of patients had improvement in cytopenias, but some patients did not respond until after 12 months of therapy.[375] The combination is thought to reverse the exaggerated apoptosis of maturing precursor cells. Pentoxifylline is a xanthine derivative that interferes with the lipid-signaling pathway used by TNF, transforming growth factor, and IL-1. Ciprofloxacin reduces the hepatic degradation of pentoxifylline.

Trials of arsenic trioxide in MDS are in progress. Whether the drug affects cell maturation, apoptosis, or proliferation in this disease remains to be determined.[376–378]

INTERFERONS

IFNs have been used to treat oligoblastic leukemia.[379,380] Doses of IFN-α ranged from 3 × 10^6 units/day to 1 × 10^6 units/m^2 three times per week. Occasional reductions in blast percentages or transfusion requirements have occurred at the price of substantial toxicity. AML occurred in some patients. IFN-γ given at a dosage of 0.01 to 0.1 mg/m^2 three times per week improved counts and reduced blast percentages in approximately 40 percent of 30 patients with oligoblastic leukemia in one series. Median survivals were no longer than in untreated historical controls, although they were longer than in untreated concurrent patients. Other reports show little effect of IFN treatment.[381]

INTERLEUKIN-2

In one case of therapy-related oligoblastic leukemia that developed during a third complete remission of ALL, IL-2 given subcutaneously at 2.5 to 8 × 10[5] IU twice daily for 30 days enhanced natural killer cell activity and eliminated blasts in the marrow.[382] However, a phase II clinical trial failed to show improved blood counts or decreased transfusion requirement in treated patients.[383]

TYROSINE KINASE AND OTHER CELL-SIGNALING INHIBITORS

Imatinib mesylate, the tyrosine kinase inhibitor of c-abl, c-kit, and platelet-derived growth factor-receptor, has not resulted in clinical responses in patients with MDS.[384,385] Inhibitors of raf protein kinase and farnesyltransferase are under examination.[386] In 20 patients with MDS, two cycles of oral R115777, a farnesyl transferase inhibitor, produced an overall response rate of 30 percent.[387] Statins that inhibit geranylgeranylation are being studied for treatment of AML and MDS.[388] Progenitors involved in MDS rarely express flt-3,[389] so flt-3 inhibitors doubtfully have an important role in the treatment of MDS.

THERAPY FOR PATIENTS WITH HIGH-INTERMEDIATE OR HIGH-RISK PROGNOSTIC SCORES

ACUTE MYELOGENOUS LEUKEMIA CHEMOTHERAPY

Chemotherapeutic regimens containing standard doses of cytarabine, an anthracycline antibiotic, and/or etoposide (see Chap. 87) result in remission in fewer than 20 percent of patients with oligoblastic leukemia. Moreover, a proportion of patients become worse with intensive chemotherapy. The advanced age and the high frequency of cardiac, renal, immunologic, and other organ system impairment in most patients with oligoblastic leukemia are largely responsible for the poor outcome. Patients who are younger than 60 years have higher remission rates of up to 50 percent[390] and should be considered for intensive therapy. In addition to the standard combination of anthracycline and cytarabine, other regimens, such as liposomal daunorubicin and topotecan with or without thalidomide, did not result in clinical benefit in patients with AML or high-risk MDS.[391] Topotecan/ARA-C or idarubicin/ARA-C regimens also did not result in clinical benefit.[392] The so-called FLAG-Ida regimen (fludarabine, cytarabine, idarubicin, and GSF) resulted in 53 percent complete remissions and 11 percent improvement in 45 patients with high-risk myeloid malignancies, 13 of whom had MDS.[393] Gemtuzumab ozogamicin (Mylotarg), which is approved for treatment of relapsed AML in elderly patients, has not been useful for treatment of MDS.[394,395]

HEMATOPOIETIC STEM CELL TRANSPLANTATION

ALLOGENEIC STEM CELL TRANSPLANTATION

This approach has been used to treat various MDS in patients ranging in age from 1 month to 60 years.[396–403] It remains the only treatment with curative potential for MDS. Conditioning regimens have consisted of cyclophosphamide plus irradiation or busulfan plus cyclophosphamide. Most patients have received transplants from histocompatible sibling donors, although some experience with partially mismatched, related, and unrelated donors has been reported. A good representation of the results of this approach using marrow stem cells is a study of 93 patients (age range 1 month to older than 60 years, median 30 years). The patients were conditioned with cyclophosphamide and total body irradiation or busulfan and cyclophosphamide and transplanted with an identical twin donor (three patients), genotypically HLA-identical sibling (62 patients), HLA-matched family

member (two patients), one to three antigen HLA-mismatched family member (20 patients), or unrelated donor marrow (six patients). Twenty-nine patients were in the clonal anemia category, 47 recipients were in the oligoblastic leukemia category, and the remainder had miscellaneous disorders. Most patients received graft-versus-host disease prophylaxis with methotrexate and cyclosporine, with or without prednisone. The most favorable results were seen in patients younger than 40 years with shorter duration of disease and without blasts. These patients may have a disease-free survival of 60 percent at 4 years and an overall disease-free survival estimated at 40 percent. Older patients had higher peritransplant mortality and relapse rates. Actuarial relapse probability at 4 years was 30 percent for the entire group and 50 percent for patients with greater than 5 percent marrow blasts. Cytogenetic abnormalities did not predict outcome in this study, but adverse cytogenetics were an important prognostic factor in other studies.

An International Bone Marrow Transplant Registry report of 452 patients with MDS who received allogeneic transplantation found that young age and platelet counts greater then 100 × 10[9]/liter prior to transplantation were associated with lower transplant mortality, higher disease-free survival, and overall survival. Patients with higher percentage of blasts and high IPSS scores had higher relapse rates.[403] Blood or marrow stem cell sources can be utilized. One report showed superior results with mobilized blood versus marrow stem cells.[404]

The National Marrow Donor Program transplant experience in MDS included 510 patients. Median age was 38 years, and the probability of disease-free survival at 2 years was 29 percent (confidence interval [CI] 25–33%). The 2-year incidence of treatment-related mortality was 54 percent, which was the major barrier to success in this patient population.[405] Unrelated cord blood transplantation for adult and pediatric patients with MDS has been successfully performed,[406] but results with unrelated marrow donors are inferior to the results for other donor categories.

Stem cell transplantation for MDS should be performed before the disease progresses to AML.[407] The morbidity and mortality of various transplantation approaches remain high, and some patients are not candidates for ablative transplants because of age or comorbid conditions.[408]

Reduced intensity conditioning with allogeneic transplantation from HLA-identical family members in an attempt to minimize toxicity has been examined for MDS treatment.[409] In one series of 16 patients (median age 54 years) receiving a conditioning regimen of fludarabine and cyclophosphamide, no day 100 transplant-related mortality was observed, and the 2-year actuarial event-free survival was 56 percent (CI 30–68%). Other fludarabine-containing conditioning regimens have been reported.[410,411] One series compared reduced intensity to standard transplant in MDS patients and noted similar 2-year overall and disease-free survival with different patterns of toxicity.[412]

AUTOLOGOUS STEM CELL INFUSION

Patients with oligoblastic leukemia have been treated with their own stem cells after intensive chemotherapy.[413] The approach may be limited by contamination of the stem cell product with a repopulating leukemic cell and the absence of a graft-versus-leukemia effect. The absence of a graft-versus-host reaction makes the approach more applicable to the age group usually affected. In selected patients, peritransplant mortality with intensive therapy and stem cell rescue has been approximately 10 percent, and approximately 50 percent of selected patients had extended survivals.[414] The more advanced the disease at the time of treatment, the worse the outcome. Autologous transplantation can result in survival comparable to that of sibling donor allogeneic transplants.[415,416] However, in patients younger than 20 years, allogeneic transplantation may be the treatment of choice[417] to decrease the risk of relapse.

COURSE AND PROGNOSIS

The median survival in published series of patients with oligoblastic leukemia varied from 6 to 36 months, with survival of individual patients ranging from 1 to 160 months.[410-414] In a very large single series that included refractory anemia, median survival was 15 months.[270] Approximately half of the patients died of infection associated with severe neutropenia or dysfunctional neutrophils and monocytes, and approximately 25 percent died of bleeding complications resulting from thrombocytopenia. Approximately 30 percent of cases evolved into AML. Length of survival of patients with oligoblastic leukemia after diagnosis is inversely correlated with the severity of the cytogenetic abnormality, proportion of blast cells in the marrow, presence of N-ras mutations, presence of adverse cytogenetic patterns, severity of the neutropenia and thrombocytopenia, and serum level of β_2-microglobulin.[134,418-424]

A rare case of spontaneous disappearance of oligoblastic leukemia has been documented.[425]

UNCOMMON ACQUIRED SYNDROMES WITH INCREASED RISK OF ACUTE MYELOGENOUS LEUKEMIA

AMEGAKARYOCYTIC THROMBOCYTOPENIA

Amegakaryocytic thrombocytopenia is a very uncommon preleukemic syndrome (<1%), although bona fide cases have transformed into AML months or years after diagnosis.[426,427] Among 1220 cases of MDS, 11 cases of isolated thrombocytopenia associated with clonal chromosome abnormalities, usually involving chromosome 3, 5, 8, or 20, were identified. Antiplatelet antibodies were not present, and glucocorticoids were ineffective. Five of the 11 patients progressed to acute myelogenous leukemia[426] (Table 86-3). (See Chap. 110.)

ISOLATED NEUTROPENIA

Chronic neutropenic states are rare antecedents of AML.[428] Congenital neutropenia (Kostmann syndrome) has evolved into AML.[428,429] Evolution of Shwachman syndrome (neutropenia and exocrine pancreatic insufficiency) into oligoblastic or overt acute leukemia has been documented.[430] The related disorder Pearson syndrome (sideroblastic anemia, neutropenia, and exocrine pancreatic insufficiency) is a preleukemia disorder in children[431] (see Chap. 33).

CHRONIC MONOCYTOSIS

In a small proportion of patients, unexplained persistent monocytosis may be the most striking blood cell abnormality for months or years before development of acute leukemia.[19,20,110]

APLASTIC ANEMIA, PAROXYSMAL NOCTURNAL HEMOGLOBINURIA, AND EOSINOPHILIC FASCIITIS

AML or MDS occurs in a proportion of patients with acquired aplastic anemia.[432,433] Since the advent of immunotherapy, the propensity to

myelodysplasia and leukemia has increased, partly because of the greater longevity of patients and the often incomplete restitution of hematopoiesis. Patients who initially responded to immunosuppressive therapy have later developed MDS (see Chap. 33 for a discussion of the interrelationship among aplastic anemia, MDS, and paroxysmal nocturnal hemoglobinuria).[434]

Paroxysmal nocturnal hemoglobinuria is a clonal stem cell disease that often is associated with marrow hypoplasia (see Chap. 38). AML may ensue in approximately 0.5 percent of patients. It is a clonally derived syndrome with a low incidence of leukemic transformation relative to other clonal myeloid diseases. All chronic clonal hemopoietic stem cell disorders (e.g., polycythemia vera, essential thrombocythemia, idiopathic myelofibrosis, chronic myelogenous leukemia) have a propensity to undergo clonal evolution to AML (see Chap. 85). Patients with indolent myeloid clonal disorders may have a paroxysmal nocturnal hemoglobinuria-like defect of their blood cell membranes.

Eosinophilic fasciitis mimics the cutaneous manifestations of scleroderma. Symmetrical swelling and induration of arms and legs, sparing the hands and feet, are common.[435,436] Eosinophilia and hypergammaglobulinemia are frequent. Immune cytopenias, aplastic anemia, myelodysplasia, AML, and lymphoma have been associated with the disease.[437] An immune mechanism has been postulated for all the disease manifestations. The risk of developing AML is greatly increased compared with healthy individuals.[435-437] Marrow transplantation has been used to treat the aplastic anemia.[438]

PRODROMAL SYNDROMES ANTEDATING LYMPHOCYTIC LEUKEMIA

The indolent clonal disorder usually implies a condition that is an antecedent of myelogenous leukemia. AML often begins with a protracted period (weeks to months) of symptoms or signs preceding clinical diagnosis. A significant proportion of cases are preceded by an MDS. ALL usually begins explosively, and symptoms rarely present for more than a few weeks prior to diagnosis (see Chap. 91). Intermediate syndromes (e.g., smoldering or oligoblastic lymphocytic leukemia or prodromal clonal anemias) are rare, but the latter have been reported, especially in adults.[439-444]

Apparent aplastic anemia[445-449] or erythroid hypoplasia[450] has been described as an antecedent to ALL in a few children and a rare adult. The aplasia is promptly improved by glucocorticoids, and ALL ensues quickly, usually within 1 to 8 months. The brief interval between remission of aplastic anemia and onset of leukemia suggests the leukemia, although inapparent on marrow biopsy, in some way initiates the aplasia.[449] Remission of aplasia followed shortly by ALL has occurred in the absence of glucocorticoid or other specific therapy in several cases. The aplastic marrow prodrome of ALL may be distinguishable by its very high prevalence in females (approximately 90%), high prevalence of fibrosis on marrow biopsy (approximately 90%), frequent marrow lymphocytosis (approximately 60%), and spontaneous, temporary recovery (>90%).[451]

INDOLENT CLONAL MYELOID DISORDERS OR OLIGOBLASTIC (MYELOGENOUS) LEUKEMIA PRECEDING OR EMERGING IN LYMPHOID MALIGNANCIES OTHER THAN ACUTE LYMPHOCYTIC LEUKEMIA

Sideroblastic anemia sometimes associated with qualitative disorders of other blood cell lines (such as thrombopathy) has developed in patients who had, or later developed, a lymphoproliferative disease, such as hairy cell leukemia, lymphocytic lymphoma, myeloma, chronic lymphocytic leukemia, or Hodgkin disease.[452-460] The sidero-

TABLE 86-3   HYPOCELLULAR MARROW SYNDROMES THAT MAY PRECEDE ONSET OF ACUTE MYELOGENOUS LEUKEMIA

Amegakaryocytic thrombocytopenia (Chap. 110)

Chronic hypoplastic neutropenia (Chap. 65)

Apparent aplastic anemia with evidence of clonal hematopoiesis (Chap. 33)

Paroxysmal nocturnal hemoglobinuria–aplastic anemia syndrome (Chaps. 33 and 38) blastic anemia in these cases was not preceded by cytotoxic therapy. Similar associations have been reported in patients who received chemotherapy or radiotherapy for a lymphoproliferative disease or a solid tumor and who later developed a preleukemic syndrome presumed to result from the prior treatment. Other types of myelodysplasia can occur concurrent with B or T lymphocyte–derived tumors. [452–461]

REFERENCES

1. Lichtman MA: Myelodysplasia or myeloneoplasia: Thoughts on the nosology of the clonal myeloid disorders. *Blood Cells Mol Dis* 26:572, 2000.

2. Brunning RD, Head D, Bennett JM, et al: Myelodysplastic syndromes, in *World Health Organization Classification of Tumors; Tumors of Haematopoietic and Lymphoid Tissues, chap 2*, edited by E Jaffe, NL Harris, H Stein, JW Vardiman, p 63. IARC Press, Lyon, 2001.

3. Dreyfus B, Rochant H, Sultan C, et al: Les anémies refractaires avec excès de myeloblastes dans la moelle. Etude de onze observations. *La Presse Med* 78:359, 1970.

4. Layton DM, Mufti GJ: Myelodysplastic syndromes: Their history, evolution, and relation to acute myeloid leukemia. *Blut* 53:423, 1986.

5. Chevallier P: Sur la terminologie des leucoses et des affection frontieres. *Le Sang* 15:587, 1942.

6. Hamilton-Paterson JL: Preleukaemic anemia. *Acta Haematol* 2:309, 1949.

7. Block M, Jacobson LO, Bethard WJ: Preleukemic acute human leukemia. *JAMA* 152:1018, 1953.

8. Vilter RW, Jarrold T, Will JJ, et al: Refractory anemia with hyperplastic bone marrow. *Blood* 15:1, 1960.

9. Schiller M, Rachmilewitz EA, Izak G: Pancytopenia with hypercellular hemopoietic tissue. *Isr J Med Sci* 5:69, 1969.

10. Saarni MI, Linman JW: Preleukemia. *Am J Med* 55:38, 1973.

11. Linman JW, Saarni MI: The preleukemic syndrome. *Semin Hematol* 11:93, 1974.

12. Pierre RV: Preleukemic states. *Semin Hematol* 11:73, 1974.

13. Dreyfus B: Preleukemic states. *Blood Cells* 2:33, 1976.

14. Linman JW, Bagby GC Jr: The preleukemic syndrome: Clinical and laboratory features, natural course and management. *Blood Cells* 2:11, 1976.

15. Linman JW, Bagby GC Jr: The preleukemic syndrome (hemopoietic dysplasia). *Cancer* 42:854, 1978.

16. Bessis M, Bernard J: Hematopoietic dysplasias. *Blood Cells* 2:5, 1976.

17. Maynadie M, Picard F, Husson B, et al: Immunophenotypic clustering of myelodysplastic syndromes. *Blood* 100:2349, 2002.

18. Stetler-Stevenson M, Arthur DC, Jabbour N, et al: Diagnostic utility of flow cytometric immunophenotyping in myelodysplastic syndrome. *Blood* 98:979, 2001.

19. Jaworkowsky LI, Solovey DY, Rhausova LY, Udris OY: Monocytosis as a sign of subsequent leukemia in patients with cytopenias (preleukemia). *Folia Hematol (Frankf)* 110:395, 1983.

20. Friedland ML, Ward H, Wittels EG, Arlin ZA: A monocytic leukemoid reaction: A manifestation of preleukemia. *Rhode Island Med J* 68:173, 1985.

21. Groupe Francais de Morphologie Hématologique: French registry of acute leukemia and myelodysplastic syndromes. *Cancer* 60:1385, 1987.

22. Aul C, Gatterman N, Schneider W: Age-related incidence and other epidemiologic aspects of myelodysplastic syndrome. *Br J Haematol* 82:358, 1992.

23. McNally RJO, Rowland D, Roman E, Cartwright RA: Age and sex distributions of hematological malignancies in the U.K. *Hematol Oncol* 15:173, 1997.

24. Luna-Fineman S, Shannon KM, Atwater SK, et al: Myelodysplastic and myeloproliferative disorders of childhood: A study of 167 patients. *Blood* 93:459, 1999.

25. Novitzky N, Prindull G, for the European Society of Paediatric Haematology and Immunology: Myelodysplastic syndromes in children. *Am J Hematol* 63:212, 2000.

26. Hasle H, Niemeyer CM, Chessells JM, et al: A pediatric approach to the WHO classification of myelodysplastic and myeloproliferative diseases. *Leukemia* 17:277, 2003.

27. Sasaki H, Manabe A, Kojima S, et al: Myelodysplastic syndrome in childhood. *Leukemia* 15:713, 2001.

28. Kardos G, Baumann I, Passmore SJ, et al: Refractory anemia in childhood: A retrospective analysis of 67 patients with particular reference to monosomy 7. *Blood* 102:1997, 2003.

29. West RR, Stafford DA, White DT, et al: Cytogenetic abnormalities in the myelodysplastic syndromes and occupational or environmental exposure. *Blood* 95:2093, 2000.

30. Nisse C, Haguenoer JM, Grandbastien B, et al: Occupational and environmental risk factors of the myelodysplastic syndromes in the North of France. *Br J Haematol* 112:927, 2001.

31. Yin SN, Hayes RB, Linet MS, et al: A cohort study of cancer among benzene-exposed workers in China: Overall results. *Am J Ind Med* 29:227, 1996.

32. Snyder R: Benzene and leukemia. *Crit Rev Toxicol* 32:155, 2002.

33. Park DJ, Koeffler HP: Therapy related myelodysplastic syndromes. *Semin Hematol* 33:256, 1996.

34. Rigolin GM, Cuneo A, Roberti MG, et al: Exposure to myelotoxic agents and myelodysplasia: Case-control study and correlation with clinicobiological findings. *Br J Haematol* 103:189, 1998.

35. Sterkers Y, Preudhomme C, Lai JL, et al: Acute myeloid leukemia and myelodysplastic syndromes following essential thrombocythemia treated with hydroxyurea: High proportion of cases with 17p deletion. *Blood* 91:616, 1998.

36. Van Den Neste E, Louviaux I, Michaux JL, et al: Myelodysplastic syndrome with monosomy 5 and/or 7 following therapy with 2-chloro-2′-deoxyadenosine. *Br J Haematol* 105:268, 1999.

37. Krishnan A, Bhatia S, Slovak ML, et al: Predictors of therapy-related leukemia and myelodysplasia following autologous transplantation for lymphoma. *Blood* 95:1588, 2000.

38. Abruzzese E, Radford JE, Miller JS, et al: Detection of abnormal pretransplant clones in progenitor cells of patients who developed myelodysplasia after autologous transplantation. *Blood* 94:1814, 2000.

39. Smith SH, Le Beau MM, Huo D, et al: Clinical-cytogenetic associations in 306 patients with therapy-related myelodysplasia and myeloid leukemia: The University of Chicago series. *Blood* 102:43, 2003.

40. Lobe I, Rigal-Huguet F, Vekhoff A, et al: Myelodysplastic syndrome after acute promyelocytic leukemia: The European APL group experience. *Leukemia* 17:1600, 2003.

41. Nakanishi M, Tanaka K, Shintani T, et al: Chromosomal instability in acute myelocytic leukemia and myelodysplastic syndrome patients among atomic bomb survivors. *J Radiat Res (Toyko)* 40:159, 1999.

42. Alter BP: Cancer in Fanconi's anemia 1923-2001. *Cancer* 97:425, 2003.

43. Segel GB, Lichtman MA: Familial (inherited) leukemia, lymphoma, and myeloma. *Blood Cells Mol Dis* 32:2004.

44. Horwitz M, Sabath DE, Smithson WA, Radich J: A family inheriting different subtypes of acute myelogenous leukemia. *Am J Hematol* 52:295, 1996.

45. Pradhan A, Mijovic A, Mills K, et al: Differentially expressed genes in adult familial myelodysplastic syndromes. *Leukemia* 18:449, 2004.

46. Kumar T, Mandla SG, Greer WL: Familial myelodysplastic syndrome with early age onset. *Am J Hematol* 64:53, 2000.

47. Abkowitz JL, Fialkow PJ, Niebrugge DJ, et al: Pancytopenia as a clonal disorder of a multipotent hemopoietic stem cell. *J Clin Invest* 73:258, 1984.

48. Rasking WH, Tirumali N, Jacobson R, et al: Evidence for a multistep pathogenesis of a myelodysplastic syndrome. *Blood* 63:1318, 1984.

49. Mongkonsritragoon W, Letendre L, Li CY: Multiple lymphoid nodules in bone marrow have the same clonality as underlying myelodysplastic syndrome recognized with fluorescent in situ hybridization technique. *Am J Hematol* 59:252, 1998.

50. Janssen JWG, Buschle M, Layton M, et al: Clonal analysis of myelodysplastic syndromes: Evidence of multipotent stem cell origin. *Blood* 73:248, 1989.

51. Boultwood J, Weainscot JS: Clonality in the myelodysplastic syndromes. *Int J Hematol* 73:411, 2001.

52. Gerritsen WR, Donohue J, Bauman J, et al: Clonal analysis of myelodysplastic syndrome: Monosomy 7 is expressed in the myeloid lineage but not in the lymphoid lineage as detected by fluorescent in situ hybridization. *Blood* 80:217, 1992.

53. Anastasi J, Fang J, LeBeau MM, et al: Cytogenetic clonality in myelodysplastic syndromes studied with fluorescence in situ hybridization: Lineage, response to growth factor therapy, and clone expansion. *Blood* 81:1580, 1993.

54. Culligan DJ, Cachia P, Whittaker A, et al: Clonal lymphocytes are detectable in only some cases of MDS. *Br J Haematol* 81:346, 1992.

55. Abrahamson G, Boultwod J, Madden J, et al: Clonality of cell population in refractory anaemia using combined approach of gene loss and X-linked restricting fragment length polymorphism–methylation analysis. *Br J Haematol* 79:550, 1991.

56. Delforge M, Demuynck H, Verhoef G, et al: Patients with high-risk myelodysplastic syndrome can have polyclonal or clonal haemopoiesis in complete haematological remission. *Br J Haematol* 102:486, 1998.

57. Lawrence HJ, Broudy VC, Magenis RE, et al: Cytogenetic evidence for involvement of B-lymphocytes in acquired idiopathic sideroblastic anemia. *Blood* 70:1003, 1982.

58. Nakagawa T, Saitoh S, Imoto S, et al: Multiple point mutation of N-ras and K-ras oncogenes in myelodysplastic syndrome and acute myelogenous leukemia. *Oncology* 49:114, 1992.

59. VanKamp H, DePijper C, Verlaan-de Vries M, et al: Longitudinal analysis of point mutations of the N-ras protooncogene in patients with myelodysplasia using archival blood smears. *Blood* 79:1266, 1992.

60. Paquette RL, Landau EM, Pierre RV, et al: N-ras mutations are associated with poor prognosis and increased risk of leukemia in myelodysplastic syndrome. *Blood* 82:590, 1993.

61. Bartram CR: Molecular genetic aspects of myelodysplastic syndromes. *Semin Hematol* 33:139, 1996.

62. Parker J, Mufti GJ: Ras and myelodysplasia: Lessons from the last decade. *Semin Hematol* 33:206, 1996.

63. Padua RA, Guinn BA, Al-Sabah AI, et al: RAS, FMS and p53 mutations and poor clinical outcome in myelodysplasias: A 10-year follow-up. *Leukemia* 12:887, 1998.

64. Plata E, Viniou N, Abazis D, et al: Cytogenetic analysis and RAS mutations in primary myelodysplastic syndromes. *Cancer Genet Cytogenet* 111:124, 1999.

65. Quesnel B, Guillerm G, Vereecque R, et al: Methylation of the p15 (INK4b) gene in myelodysplastic syndromes is frequent and acquired during disease progression. *Blood* 91:2985, 1998.

66. Miyazato A, Ueno S, Ohmine K, et al: Identification of myelodysplastic syndrome-specific genes by DNA microarray analysis with purified hematopoietic stem cell fraction. *Blood* 98:422, 2001.

67. Fadilah SAW, Cheong SK, Roslan H, et al: *GATA-1* and *GATA-2* gene expression is related to the severity of dysplasia in myelodysplastic syndrome. *Leukemia* 16:1563, 2002.

68. Gattermann N: Mitochondrial DNA mutations in the hematopoietic system. *Leukemia* 18:18, 2003.

69. Greenberg PL: Apoptosis and its role in the myelodysplastic syndromes: Implications for disease natural history and treatment. *Leuk Res* 22:1123, 1998.

70. Van de Loosdrecht AA, Vellenga E: Myelodysplasia and apoptosis. *Med Oncol* 17:16, 2000.

71. Huh YO, Jilani I, Estey E, et al: More cell death in refractory anemia with excess blasts in transformation than in acute myeloid leukemia. *Leukemia* 16:2249, 2002.

72. Raza A, Alvi S, Broady-Robinson L, et al: Cell cycle kinetic studies in 68 patients with myelodysplastic syndromes following intravenous iodo- and/or bromodeoxyuridine. *Exp Hematol* 25:530, 1997.

73. Gersuk GM, Beckham C, Loken MR, et al: A role for tumour necrosis factor-alpha, Fas and Fas-ligand in marrow failure associated with myelodysplastic syndrome. *Br J Haematol* 103:176, 1998.

74. Mundle SD, Ali A, Cartlidge JD, et al: Evidence for involvement of tumor necrosis factor-alpha in apoptotic death of bone marrow cells in myelodysplastic syndromes. *Am J Hematol* 60:36, 1999.

75. Parker JE, Fishlock KL, Mijovic A, et al: "Low-risk" myelodysplastic syndrome is associated with excessive apoptosis and an increased ratio of pro-versus anti-apoptotic bcl-2-related proteins. *Br J Haematol* 103:1075, 1998.

76. Amin HM, Jilani I, Estey EH, et al: Increased apoptosis in bone marrow B lymphocytes but not T lymphocytes in myelodysplastic syndrome. *Blood* 102:1866, 2003.

77. Baumann I, Scheid C, Koref MS, et al: Autologous lymphocytes inhibit hemopoiesis in long-term culture in patients with myelodysplastic syndrome. *Exp Hematol* 30:1045, 2002.

78. Moldrem J, Jiang Y, Stetler-Stevenson M, et al: Haematologic response of patients with myelodysplastic syndrome to antithymocyte globulin is associated with a loss of lymphocyte-mediated inhibition of CFU-GM and alterations in T cell receptor Vβ profiles. *Br J Haematol* 102:1314, 1998.

79. Epperson D, Nakamura R, Saunthararajah Y, et al: Oligoclonal T cell expansion in myelodysplastic syndrome: Evidence for an autoimmune process. *Leuk Res* 25:1075, 2001.

80. Rosenfeld C, List A: A hypothesis for the pathogenesis of myelodysplastic syndromes: Implications for new therapies. *Leukemia* 14:2, 2000.

81. Bagby GC: The preleukemic syndrome (hematopoietic dysplasia). *Blood Rev* 2:194, 1988.

82. Noel P, Solberg LA Jr: Myelodysplastic syndromes: Pathogenesis, diagnosis and treatment. *Crit Rev Oncol Hematol* 12:193, 1992.

83. Ahmad YH, Kiehl R, Papac RJ: Myelodysplasia. The clinical spectrum of 51 patients. *Cancer* 76:869, 1995.

84. Hebbar M, Hebbar-Savean K, Fenaux P: Systemic diseases in myelodysplastic syndromes. *Rev Med Intern* 16:897, 1995.

85. Saif MW, Hopkins JL, Gore SD: Autoimmune phenomena in patients with myelodysplastic syndromes and chronic myelomonocytic leukemia. *Leuk Lymphoma* 43:2409, 2002.

86. de la Chapelle A, Lahtinen R: Monosomy 7 predisposes to diabetes insipidus in leukaemia and myelodysplastic syndrome. *Eur J Haematol* 39:404, 1987.

87. Nakamura F, Kishimoto Y, Handa T, et al: Diabetes insipidus manifesting hypodipsic hypernatremia and dehydration. *Am J Hematol* 75:213, 2004.

88. Soppi E, Nousiainen T, Seppa A, et al: Acute febrile neutrophilic dermatosis (Sweet's syndrome) in association with myelodysplastic syndromes: A report of three cases and a review of the literature. *Br J Haematol* 73:43, 1989.

89. Arbetter KR, Hubbard KW, Markovic SN, et al: Case of granulocyte colony-stimulating factor-induced Sweet's syndrome. *Am J Hematol* 61:126, 1999.

90. Avi I, Rosenbaum H, Levy Y, Rowe J: Myelodysplastic syndrome and associated skin lesions: A review of the literature. *Leuk Res* 23:323, 1999.

91. Weber RFA, Geraedts JPM, Kerkhofs H, Leeksma CHW: The preleukemic syndrome. *Acta Med Scand* 207:391, 1980.

92. Ohno E, Ohtsuka E, Watanabe K, et al: Behcet's disease associated with myelodysplastic syndromes. A case report and a review of the literature. *Cancer* 79:262, 1997.

93. Komatsuda A, Miura I, Ohtani H, et al: Crescentic glomerulonephritis accompanied by myeloperoxidase-antineutrophil cytoplasmic antibodies in a patient having myelodysplastic syndrome with trisomy 7. *Am J Kidney Dis* 31:336, 1998.

94. Saitoh T, Murakami H, Uchiumi H, et al: Myelodysplastic syndromes with nephrotic syndrome. *Am J Hematol* 60:200, 1999.

95. Harewood GC, Loftus EV Jr, Tefferi A, et al: Concurrent inflammatory bowel disease and myelodysplastic syndromes. *Inflamm Bowel Dis* 5: 98, 1999.

96. Lesprit P, Piette AM, Baumeloub B, et al: Panniculitis and myelodysplasia: Report of 2 cases. 2:500, 1993.

97. Saif MW, Hopkins JL, Gore SD: Autoimmune phenomena in patients with myelodysplastic syndromes and chronic myelomonocytic leukemia. *Leuk Lymphoma* 43:2083, 2002.

98. Clark RE, Payne HE, Jacobs A: Primary myelodysplastic syndrome and cancer. *Br Med J* 294:937, 1987.

99. Sans-Sabrafen J, Buxó-Costa J, Woessner S, et al: Myelodysplastic syndromes and malignant solid tumors. *Am J Hematol* 41:1, 1992.

100. Florensa L, Vallespi T, Woessner S, et al: Incidence and characteristics of lymphoid malignancies in untreated myelodysplastic syndromes. *Leuk Lymphoma* 23:609, 1996

101. Park S, Merlat A, Guesnu M, et al: Pure red cell aplasia associated with myelodysplastic syndromes. *Leukemia* 14:1709, 2000.

102. Choi JW, Kim Y, Fujino M, Ito M: Significance of fetal hemoglobin-containing erythroblasts (F blasts) and the F blast/F cell ratio in myelodysplastic syndromes. *Leukemia* 19:1478, 2002.

103. Kornberg A, Goldfarb A: Preleukemia manifested by hemolytic anemia with pyruvate-kinase deficiency. *Arch Intern Med* 146:785, 1986.

104. Harris JW, Koscick R, Lazarus HM, et al: Leukemia arising out of paroxysmal nocturnal hemoglobinuria. *Leuk Lymphoma* 32:401, 1999.

105. Lopez M, Bonnet-Gajdos M, Reviron M, et al: Acute leukemia augured before clinical signs by blood group antigen abnormalities and low levels of A and H blood group transferase activities in erythrocytes. *Br J Haematol* 63:535, 1986.

106. Anagnou NP, Ley TJ, Chesbro B, et al: Acquired α-thalassemia in preleukemia is due to decreased expression of all four α-globin genes. *Proc Natl Acad Sci U S A* 80:6051, 1983.

107. Helder J, Deisseroth A: S1 nuclease analysis of α-globin gene expression in preleukemic patients with acquired hemoglobin H disease after transfer to mouse erythroleukemia cells. *Proc Natl Acad Sci U S A* 84: 2387, 1987.

108. Steensma DP, Higgs DR, Fisher CA, Gibbons RJ: Acquired somatic *ATRX* mutations in myelodysplastic syndrome associated with α-thalassemia (ATMDS) convey a more severe hematological phenotype than germline *ATRX* mutations. *Blood* 103:2019, 2004.

109. Group Française de Morphologie Hématologique: French registry of acute leukemia and myelodysplastic syndromes. *Cancer* 60:1385, 1987.

110. Economopoulos T, Stathakis N, Maragoyannis Z, et al: Myelodysplastic syndrome. Clinical significance of monocyte concentration, degree of blastic infiltration and ring sideroblasts. *Acta Haematol* 65:97, 1981.

111. Shetty VT, Mundle SD, Raza A: Pseudo Pelger-Huët anomaly in myelodysplastic syndrome: Hyposegmented or apoptotic neutrophil? *Blood* 98:1273, 2001.

112. Langenhuijsen MM: Neutrophils with ring-shaped nuclei in myeloproliferative disease. *Br J Haematol* 58:227, 1984.

113. Clark RE, Smith SA, Jacobs A: Mycloid surface antigen abnormalities in myelodysplasia: Relation to prognosis and modification by 13-cis retinoic acid. *J Clin Pathol* 40:652, 1987.

114. Cech P, Markert M, Perrin LH: Partial myeloperoxidase deficiency in preleukemia. *Blut* 47:21, 1983.

115. Schofield KP, Stone PCW, Kelsey P, et al: Quantitative cytochemistry of blood neutrophils in myelodysplastic syndromes and chronic granulocytic leukaemia. *Cell Biochem Funct* 1:92, 1983.

116. Elghetany MT, Peterson B, MacCallum J, et al: Deficiency of neutrophilic granule membrane glycoproteins in the myelodysplastic syndromes: A common deficiency in 216 patients studied by the Cancer and Leukemia Group B. *Leuk Res* 21:801, 1997.

117. Ruutu P: Granulocyte function in myelodysplastic syndromes. *Scand J Haematol* 36(suppl 45):66, 1986.

118. Prodan M, Tulissi P, Perticarari S, et al: Flow cytometric assay for the evaluation of phagocytosis and oxidative burst of polymorphonuclear leukocytes and monocytes in myelodysplastic disorders. *Haematologica* 80:212, 1995.

119. Piva E, De Toni S, Caenazzo A, et al: Neutrophil NADPH oxidase activity in chronic myeloproliferative and myelodysplastic diseases by microscopic and photometric assays. *Acta Haematol* 94:16, 1995.

120. Carulli G, Sbrana S, Minnucci S, et al: Actin polymerization in neutrophils from patients affected by myelodysplastic syndromes—A flow cytometric study. *Leuk Res* 21:513, 1997.

121. Nakaseko C, Asai T, Wakita H, et al: Signaling defect in FMLP-induced neutrophil respiratory burst in myelodysplastic syndromes. *Br J Haematol* 95:482, 1996.

122. Pamphilon DH, Aparicio SR, Roberts BE, et al: The myelodysplastic syndromes—A study of haemostatic function and platelet ultrastructure. *Scand J Haematol* 33:486, 1984.

123. Payne CM, Glasser L: An ultrastructural morphometric analysis of platelet grant and fusion granules. *Blood* 67:299, 1986.

124. Rasi V, Lintula R: Platelet-function in the myelodysplastic syndromes. *Scand J Haematol* 36(suppl 45):71, 1986.

125. Hamblin TJ: Immunological abnormalities in myelodysplastic syndromes. *Semin Hematol* 33:150, 1996.

126. Anderson RW, Volsky DJ, Greenberg B, et al: Lymphocyte abnormalities in preleukemia: I. Decreased NK activity, anomalous immunoregulatory cell subsets and deficient EBV receptors. *Leuk Res* 7:389, 1983.

127. Kerndrup G, Meyer K, Ellegaard J, Hokland P: Natural killer (NK)-cell activity and antibody-dependent cellular cytotoxicity (ADCC) in primary preleukemic syndrome. *Leuk Res* 8:239, 1984.

128. Takagi S, Kitagawa S, Takeda A, et al: Natural killer–interferon system in patients with preleukaemic states. *Br J Haematol* 58:71, 1984.

129. Volsky DJ, Anderson RW: Deficiency in Epstein-Barr virus receptors on B lymphocytes of preleukemia patients. *Cancer Res* 43:3923, 1983.

130. Knox SJ, Greenberg BR, Anderson RW, Rosenblatt LS: Studies of T lymphocytes in preleukemic disorders and acute nonlymphocytic leukemia: In vitro radiosensitivity, mitogenic responsiveness, colony formation, and enumeration of lymphocytic subpopulations. *Blood* 61:449, 1983.

131. Baumann MA, Milson TJ, Patrick CW, et al: Immunoregulatory abnormalities in myelodysplastic disorders. *Am J Hematol* 22:17, 1986.

132. Economopoulos T, Economidou J, Giannopoulos G, et al: Immune abnormalities in myelodysplastic syndromes. *J Clin Pathol* 38:908, 1985.

133. Mufti GJ, Figes A, Hamblin TJ, et al: Immunological abnormalities in myelodysplastic syndromes. *Br J Haematol* 63:143, 1986.

134. Gatto S, Ball G, Onida F, et al: Contribution of β-2 microglobulin levels to the prognostic stratification of survival in patients with myelodysplastic syndrome (MDS). *Blood* 102:1622, 2003.

135. Takagi S, Tanaka O, Miura Y: Magnetic resonance imaging of femoral marrow in patients with myelodysplastic syndromes or leukemia. *Blood* 86:316, 1995.

136. Tricot G, DeWolf-Peeters C, Vlietinck R, Verwilghen RL: The importance of bone marrow biopsy in myelodysplastic disorders. *Bibl Hematol* 50:31, 1984.

137. Frisch B, Bartol R: Bone marrow histology in myelodysplastic syndromes. *Scand J Haematol* 36(suppl 45):21, 1986.

138. Delacretaz F, Schmidt PM, Piguet D, et al: Histopathology and myelodysplastic syndromes: The FAB classification (proposals) applied to bone marrow biopsy. *Am J Clin Pathol* 87:180, 1987.

139. Fohlmeister I, Fischer R, Modder B, et al: Aplastic anemia and hypocellular myelodysplastic syndrome. *J Clin Pathol* 38:1218, 1985.

140. Kuriyama K, Tomonaga M, Matsuo T, et al: Diagnostic significance of pseudo Pelger Huët anomalies and micro-megakaryocytes in myelodysplastic syndrome. *Br J Haematol* 63:665, 1986.

141. Tricot G, DeWolf-Peeters C, Vlietinck R, Verwilghen RL: Bone marrow histology in myelodysplastic syndromes. II. Prognostic value of ALIP in MDS. *Br J Haematol* 58:217, 1984.

142. Mangi MH, Mufti GJ: Primary myelodysplastic syndromes: Diagnostic and prognostic significance of immunohistochemical assessment of bone marrow biopsies. *Blood* 79:198, 1992.

143. Bellamy WT, Richter L, Sirjani D, et al: Vascular endothelial cell growth factor (VEGF) is an autocrine promoter of abnormal localized immature precursors (ALIP) and leukemia progenitor formation in myelodysplastic syndromes. *Blood* 97:1427, 2001.

144. Matsushima T, Handa H, Yokohama A, et al: Prevalence and clinical characteristics of myelodysplastic syndrome with bone marrow eosinophilia or basophilia. *Blood* 101:3386, 2003.

145. Smith WB, Ablin A, Goodman JR, Brecher J: Atypical megakaryocytes in the preleukemic phase of AML. *Blood* 42:535, 1973.

146. Queisser W, Queisser U, Ansmann M, et al: Megakaryocyte polyploidization in acute leukemia and preleukemia. *Br J Haematol* 28:261, 1974.

147. Bartl R, Frisch B, Baumgart R: Morphologic classification of the myelodysplastic syndromes (MDS): Combined utilization of bone marrow aspirates and trephine biopsies. *Leuk Res* 16:15, 1992.

148. Maschek H, Georgii A, Kaloutsi V, et al: Myelofibrosis in primary myelodysplastic syndromes: A retrospective study of 352 patients. *Eur J Haematol* l48:208, 1992.

149. Moehler TM, Ho AD, Goldschmidt H, Barlogie B: Angiogenesis in hematological malignancies. *Crit Rev Oncol Hematol* 45:227, 2003.

150. Ribatti D, Polimeno G, Vacca A, et al: Correlation of bone marrow angiogenesis and mast cells with tryptase activity in myelodysplastic syndromes. *Leukemia* 16:1680, 2002.

151. Greenberg PL: Biologic and clinical implications of marrow culture studies in the myelodysplastic syndromes. *Semin Hematol* 33:163, 1996.

152. Chui DHK, Clarke BJ: Abnormal erythroid progenitor cells in human preleukemia. *Blood* 60:362, 1982.

153. Senn JS, Messner HA, Pinkerton PH, et al: Peripheral blood blast cell progenitors in human preleukemia. *Blood* 59:106, 1982.

154. Juvonen E, Partanen S, Knuutila S, Ruutu T: Megakaryocyte colony formation by bone marrow progenitors in myelodysplastic syndrome. *Br J Haematol* 63:331, 1986.

155. Lidbeck J: In vitro colony and cluster growth haemopoietic dysplasia (the preleukaemic syndrome): I. Clinical correlations. *Scand J Haematol* 24:412, 1980.

156. Raymakers R, DeWitte T, Joziasse J, et al: In vitro growth pattern and differentiation predict for progression of myelodysplastic syndromes to acute nonlymphocytic leukemia. *Br J Haematol* 78:35, 1991.

157. Konwalinka G, Peschel C, Schmalzl F, et al: CFU-GM assay, cytochemical and electron microscopic studies in agar in patients with preleukemia syndrome and aplastic anemia. *Int J Cell Cloning* 3:367, 1985.

158. Cambier N, Baruchel A, Schlageter MH, et al: Chronic myelomonocytic leukemia: From biology to therapy. *Hematol Cell Ther* 39:41, 1997.

159. Aul C, Gatterman N, Schneider W: Comparison of in vitro growth characteristics of blast cell progenitors (CFU-BL) in patients with myelodysplastic syndromes and acute myeloid leukemia. *Blood* 80:625, 1992.

160. Flores-Figueroa E, Gutierrez-Espindola G, Guerrero-Rivera S, et al: Hematopoietic progenitor cells from patients with myelodysplastic syndromes: In vitro colony growth and long-term proliferation. *Leuk Res* 23:385, 1999.

161. Sato T, Kim S, Selleri C, et al: Measurement of secondary colony formation after 5 weeks in long-term cultures in patients with myelodysplastic syndrome. *Leukemia* 12:1187, 1998.

162. Aizawa S, Nakano M, Iwase O, et al: Bone marrow stroma from refractory anemia of myelodysplastic syndrome is defective in its ability to support normal CD34-positive cell proliferation and differentiation in vitro. *Leuk Res* 23:239, 1999.

163. Janowska-Wieczorek A, Bilch AR, Jacobs A: Increased circulating colony-stimulating factor-1 in patients with preleukemia, leukemia, and lymphoid malignancies. *Blood* 77:1796, 1991.

164. Verhoef GEG, DeSchouder P, Ceuppens JL: Measurement of serum cytokine levels in patients with myelodysplastic syndromes. *Leukemia* 6:1268, 1992.

165. Bowen D, Yancik S, Bennett L, et al: Serum stem cell factor concentration in patients with myelodysplastic syndromes. *Br J Haematol* 85: 63, 1993.

166. Zwierzina H, Anderson JE, Rollinger-Holzinger I, et al: Endogenous FLT-3 ligand serum levels are associated with disease stage in patients with myelodysplastic syndromes. *Leukemia* 13:553, 1999.

167. Tamura H, Ogata K, Luo S, et al: Plasma thrombopoietin (TPO) levels and expression of TPO receptor on platelets in patients with myelodysplastic syndromes. *Br J Haematol* 103:778, 1998.

168. De Greef GE, Hagemeijer A: Molecular and cytogenetic abnormalities in acute myeloid leukemia and myelodysplastic syndromes. *Baillières Clin Haematol* 9:1, 1996.

169. Fenaux P, Morel P, Lai JL: Cytogenetics of myelodysplastic syndromes. *Semin Hematol* 33:127, 1996.

170. Mecucci C, La Starza R: Cytogenetics of myelodysplastic syndromes. *Forum* 9:4, 1999.

171. Solé F, Espinet B, Sanz GF, et al: Incidence, characterization and prognostic significance of chromosomal abnormalities in 640 patients with primary myelodysplastic syndromes. *Br J Haematol* 108:346, 2000.

172. Estey E, Trujillo JM, Cork A, et al: AML-associated cytogenetic abnormalities inv ((16), del (16), t(8;21)) in patients with myelodysplastic syndromes. *Hematol Pathol* 6:43, 1992.

173. Block AW, Carroll AJ, Hagemeijer A, et al: Rare recurring balanced chromosome abnormalities in therapy-related myelodysplastic syndromes and acute leukemia. *Genes Chromosomes Cancer* 33:401, 2002.

174. Rossi G, Pelizzari AM, Bellotti D, et al: Cytogenetic analogy between myelodysplastic syndrome and acute myeloid leukemia of elderly patients. *Leukemia* 14:636, 2000.

175. Pedersen-Bjergaard J, Pedersen M, Roulston D, Philip P: Different genetic pathways in leukemogenesis for patients presenting with therapy-related myelodysplasia and therapy-related acute myeloid leukemia. *Blood* 86:3542, 1995.

176. Zhang L, Rothman N, Wang Y, et al: Increased aneusomy and long arm deletion of chromosomes 5 and 7 in the lymphocytes of Chinese workers exposed to benzene. *Carcinogenesis* 19:1955, 1998.

177. Olney HJ, Le Beau MM: The cytogenetics and molecular biology of myelodysplastic syndromes, in *The Myelodysplastic Syndromes*, edited by JM Bennett, p 89. Marcel Dekker, New York, 2002.

178. Xie D, Hofmann W-K, Mori N, et al: Allelotype analysis of the myelodysplastic syndrome. *Leukemia* 14:805, 2000.

179. Hoffman W-K, De Vos S, Komor M, et al: Characterization of gene expression of CD34+ cells from normal and myelodysplastic bone marrow. *Blood* 100:3553, 2002.

180. Boultwood J, Lewis S, Wainscoat JS, et al: The 5q- syndrome. *Blood* 84:3253, 1994.

181. Washington LT, Doherty D, Glassman A, et al: Myeloid disorders with deletion 5q as the sole karyotypic abnormality: The clinical spectrum and pathological spectrum. *Leuk Lymphoma* 43:761, 2002.

182. Van den Berghe H, Michaux L: 5q-, twenty-five years later: A synopsis. *Cancer Genet Cytogenet* 94:1, 1997.

183. Bigoni R, Cuneo A, Milani R, et al: Multilineage involvement in the 5q- syndrome: A fluorescent in situ hybridization study on bone marrow smears. *Haematologica* 86:375, 2001.

184. Anderson K, Arvidsson I, Jacobsson B, Hast R: Fluorescence in situ hybridization for the study of cell lineage involvement in myelodysplastic syndromes with chromosome 5 anomalies. *Cancer Genet Cytogenet* 136:101, 2002.

185. Jaju RJ, Jones M, Boultwood J, et al: Combined immunophenotyping and FISH identifies the involvement of B-C cells in 5q- syndrome. *Genes Chromosomes Cancer* 29:276, 2000.

186. Nilsson L, Astrand-Grundastrom I, Arvidsson I, et al: Isolation and characterization of hematopoietic progenitor/stem cells in 5q-deleted myelodysplastic syndromes: Evidence for involvement at the hematopoietic stem cell level. *Blood* 96:2012, 2000.

187. Cermak J, Michalova K, Brezinova J, Zemanova Z: A prognostic impact of separation of refractory cytopenia with multilineage dysplasia and 5q- syndrome from refractory anemia in primary myelodysplastic syndrome. *Leuk Res* 27:221, 2003.

188. Giagounidis AAN, Germing U, Haase S, et al: Clinical, morphological, cytogenetics, and prognostic features of patients with myelodysplastic syndrome and del(5q) including band q31. *Leukemia* 18:113, 2004.

189. Washington LT, Dherty D, Glassman A, et al: Myeloid disorders with deletion of 5q as sole karyotypic abnormality: The clinical and pathological spectrum. *Leuk Lymphoma* 43:761, 2002.

190. Lessard M, Herry A, Berthou C, et al: FISH investigation of 5q and 7q deletions in MDS/AML reveals hidden translocations, insertions and fragmentations of the same chromosomes. *Leuk Res* 22:303, 1998.

191. Boultwood J, Fidler C, Strickson AJ, et al: Narrowing and genomic annotation of the commonly deleted region of the 5q- syndrome. *Blood* 99:4638, 2002.

192. Bernstein R, Philip P, Ueshima Y: Fourth international workshop on chromosomes in leukemia 1982. Abnormalities of chromosome 7 resulting in monosomy 7 or in deletion of the long arm (7q-): Review of translocations, breakpoints, and associated abnormalities. *Cancer Genet Cytogenet* 11:300, 1984.

193. Michiels JJ, Mallios-Zorbala H, Prins MEF, et al: Simple monosomy 7 and myelodysplastic syndrome in thirteen patients without previous cytostatic treatment. *Br J Haematol* 64:425, 1986.

194. Pasquali F, Bernasconi P, Cosalone R, et al: Pathogenetic significance of "pure" monosomy 7 in myeloproliferative disorders. Analysis of 14 cases. *Hum Genet* 62:40, 1982.

195. Kardos G, Baumann I, Passmore SJ, et al: Refractory anemia in childhood: A retrospective analysis of 67 patients with particular reference to monosomy 7. *Blood* 102:1997, 2003.

196. Brozek I, Babinska M, Kardas I, et al: Cytogenetic analysis and clinical significance of chromosome 7 aberrations in acute leukemia. *J Appl Genet* 44:401, 2003.

197. Dohner K, Brown J, Hehmann U, et al: Molecular cytogenetic characterization of a critical region in bands 7q35-q36 commonly deleted in malignant myeloid disorders. *Blood* 92:4031, 1998.

198. Sessarego M, Fugazza G, Gobbi M, et al: Complex structural involvement of chromosome 7 in primary myelodysplastic syndromes determined by fluorescence in situ hybridization. *Cancer Genet Cytogenet* 106:110, 1998.

199. Hayashi Y, Egushi M, Sugita K, et al: Cytogenetic findings and clinical features in acute leukemia and transient myeloproliferation disorder in Down's syndrome. *Blood* 72:15, 1988.

200. Berger R, LeConiat M, Schaison G: Chromosome abnormalities in bone marrow of Fanconi anemia patients. *Cancer Genet Cytogenet* 65:47, 1993.

201. Minelli A, Maserati E, Giudici G, et al: Familial partial monosomy 7 and myelodysplasia: Different parental origin of monosomy 7 suggests action of a mutator gene. *Cancer Genet Cytogenet* 124:147, 2001.

202. Smadja N, Krulik M, DeGramont A, et al: Translocation 1;7 in preleukemic states. *Cancer Genet Cytogenet* 18:189, 1985.

203. Woloschak GF, Dewald GW, Gahn RS, et al: Amplification of RNA and DNA specific for erb B in unbalanced 1;7 chromosomal translocation associated with myelodysplastic syndrome. *J Cell Biochem* 32:23, 1986.

204. Ueda H, Tashiro S, Kojima S, et al: Instability of chromosome 7 in colony forming cells of patients with aplastic anemia. *Int J Hematol* 70: 13, 1999.

205. Kaito K, Kobayashi M, Katayama T, et al: Long-term administration of G-CSF for aplastic anemia is closely related too the early evolution of monosomy 7 MDS in adults. *Br J Haematol* 103:297, 1998.

206. Bjorkman SE: Chronic refractory anemia with sideroblastic bone marrow. A study of four cases. *Blood* 11:250, 1956.

207. Kushner JP, Lee GR, Wintrobe MM, et al: Idiopathic refractory sideroblastic anemia. *Medicine* 50:139, 1971.

208. Chang KL, O'Donnell MR, Slovak ML, et al: Primary myelodysplasia occurring in adults under 50 years old: A clinicopathologic study of 52 patients. *Leukemia* 16:623, 2002.

209. Kardos G, Veerman AJ, De Waal FC, et al: Familial sideroblastic anemia with emergence of monosomy 5 and myelodysplastic syndrome. *Med Pediatr Oncol* 26:54, 1996.

210. Garand R, Gardars J, Bizet M, et al: Heterogeneity of acquired idiopathic sideroblastic anemia (AISA). *Leuk Res* 16:463, 1992.

211. Bowen DT, Jacobs A: Primary acquired sideroblastic erythropoiesis in non-anaemic and minimally anaemic subjects. *J Clin Pathol* 42:56, 1989.

212. Antilla P, Thalainen J, Salo A, et al: Idiopathic macrocytic anaemia in the aged: Molecular and cytogenetic findings. *Br J Haematol* 90:797, 1995.

213. Steensma DP, Dewald GW, Hodnfield JM, et al: Clonal cytogenetic abnormalities in bone marrow specimens without clear morphologic evidence of dysplasia: A form fruste of myelodysplasia? *Leuk Res* 27:235, 2003.

214. Yoshida Y, Oguma S, Tohyama K, et al: Diagnostic and biological significance of sideroblastic erythropoiesis in the myelodysplastic syndromes. *Int J Hematol* 67:137, 1998.

215. Beris PH, Graf J, Miescher PA: Primary acquired sideroblastic and primary acquired refractory anemia. *Semin Hematol* 20:101, 1983.

216. Mecucci C, Van Orshoven A, Vermaelen K, et al: 11 q-chromosome is associated with abnormal iron stores in myelodysplastic syndromes. *Cancer Genet Cytogenet* 27:39, 1987.

217. Parlier V, Van Melle G, Beris PH, et al: Hematological, clinical, and cytogenetic analysis in 109 in patients with primary myelodysplastic syndrome. *Cancer Genet Cytogenet* 78:219, 1994.

218. Berrebi A, Bruck R, Shtalrid M, Chemke J: Philadelphia chromosome in idiopathic acquired sideroblastic anemia. *Acta Haematol* 72:343, 1984.

219. Carroll AJ, Poon M-C, Robinson NC, Christ WM: Sideroblastic anemia associated with thrombocytosis and a chromosome 3 abnormality. *Cancer Genet Cytogenet* 22:183, 1986.

220. Bennett DD, Stanley WS, Johnson CB: Combined phenotypic and genotypic analysis of ringed sideroblasts in acquired idiopathic sideroblastic anemia. *Acta Haematol* 73:235, 1985.

221. DeWald GW, Brecher M, Travis LB, Stupea PJ: Twenty-six patients with hematologic disorders and X-chromosome abnormalities. *Cancer Genet Cytogenet* 42:173, 1989.

222. Chabannori G, Molina L, Pegouri-Bandelier B, et al: A review of 76 patients with myelodysplastic syndromes treated with danazol. *Cancer* 73:3073, 1994.

223. Musto P, Catalano L, Andriani A, et al: Recombinant erythropoietin for refractory anemia with ring sideroblasts. *Hematologia* 77:185, 1992.

224. Hellstrom-Lindberg E, Ahlgren T, Beguin Y, et al: Treatment of anemia in myelodysplastic syndromes with granulocyte colony-stimulating factor plus erythropoietin: Results from a randomized phase II study and long-term follow-up of 71 patients. *Blood* 92:68, 1998.

225. Cazzola M, Barosi G, Gobbi PG, et al: Natural history of idiopathic refractory sideroblastic anemia. *Blood* 71:305, 1988.

226. Cartwright GE, Edwards CG, Skolnick MH, Amos BD: Association of HLA-linked hemochromatosis with idiopathic refractory sideroblastic anemia. *J Clin Invest* 65:980, 1980.

227. Beris P, Samii K, Darbellay R, et al: Iron overload in patients with sideroblastic anaemia is not related to the presence of the haemochromatosis Cys282Tyr and His63Asp mutations. *Br J Haematol* 104:97, 1999.

228. Weintraub LR, Conrad ME, Crosby WH: Iron-loading anemia. Treatment with repeated phlebotomy and pyridoxine. *N Engl J Med* 175:169, 1966.

229. French TJ, Jacobs P: Sideroblastic anemia associated with iron overload treated by repeated phlebotomy. *S Afr Med J* 50:594, 1976.

230. Jensen PD, Heickendorff L, Pedersen B, et al: The effect of iron chelation on haemopoiesis in MDS patients with transfusional iron overload. *Br J Haematol* 94:288, 1996.

231. Lewy RI, Kansu E, Gabuzda T: Leukemia in patients with acquired idiopathic sideroblastic anemia. *Am J Hematol* 6:323, 1979.

232. Cheng DS, Kushner JP, Wintrobe MM: Idiopathic refractory sideroblastic anemia. Incidence and risk factors for leukemic transformation. *Cancer* 44:724, 1979.

233. Hast R, Reizenstein P: Sideroblastic anemia and development of leukemia. *Blut* 42:203, 1981.

234. Streeter RR, Presant CA, Reinhard E: Prognostic significance of thrombocytosis in idiopathic sideroblastic anemia. *Blood* 50:427, 1977.

235. Barton JC, Conrad ME, Parmley R: Acute lymphoblastic leukemia in idiopathic refractory sideroblastic anemia. *Am J Hematol* 9:109, 1980.

236. Cazzola M, Barosi G, Gobbi PG: Natural history of idiopathic refractory sideroblastic anemia. *Blood* 71:305, 1988.

237. Gattermann N, Aul C, Schneider W: Two types of acquired idiopathic sideroblastic anemia (AISA). *Br J Haematol* 74:45, 1990.

238. Greenberg P, Cox C, LeBeau MM, et al: International scoring system for evaluating prognosis in myelodysplastic syndromes. *Blood* 89:2079, 1997.

239. Maes B, Meeus P, Michaux L, et al: Application of the International Prognostic Scoring System for myelodysplastic syndromes. *Ann Oncol* 10:825, 1999.

240. Rosati S, Mick R, Xu F, et al: Refractory cytopenia with multilineage dysplasia: Further characterization of an "unclassifiable" myelodysplastic syndrome. *Leukemia* 10:20, 1996.

241. Matsuda A, Jinnai I, Yagasaki F, et al: Refractory anemia with severe dysplasia: Clinical significance of morphological features in refractory anemia. *Leukemia* 12:482, 1998.

242. Vallespi T, Imbert M, Meccuci C, et al: Diagnosis, classification, and cytogenetics of myelodysplastic syndromes. *Haematologia* 83:258, 1998.

243. Zon LI, Arkin C, Groopman JE: Haematologic manifestations of the human immune deficiency virus (HIV). *Br J Haematol* 66:251, 1987.

244. Thiele J, Zirbas TK, Bertsch HP, et al: AIDS-related bone marrow lesions—Myelodysplastic features or predominant inflammatory-reactive changes (HIV-myelopathy)? A comparative morphometric study by immunohistochemistry with special emphasis on apoptosis and PCNA-labeling. *Anal Cell Path* 11:141, 1996.

245. Haznedar R: Pancytopenia with hypercellular bone marrow as a possible paraneoplastic syndrome. *Am J Hematol* 19:205, 1985.

246. List AF, Brasfield F, Heaton R, et al: Stimulation of hematopoiesis by amifostine in patients with myelodysplastic syndrome. *Blood* 90:3364, 1997.

247. Freifeld A, Marchigiani D, Walsh T, et al: A double-blind comparison of empirical oral and intravenous antibiotic therapy for low-risk febrile patients with neutropenia during cancer chemotherapy. *N Engl J Med* 341:305, 1999.

248. Malik IA, Moid I, Aziz Z, et al: A randomized comparison of fluconazole with amphotericin B as empiric anti-fungal agents in cancer patients with prolonged fever and neutropenia. *Am J Med* 105:478, 1998.

249. Bagby GC, Gabourel JD, Linman JW: Glucocorticoid therapy in the preleukemic syndrome. *Ann Intern Med* 92:55, 1980.

250. Watts EJ, Majer RV, Grun PJ: Hyperfibrotic myelodysplasia: A report of three cases showing haematologic remission following treatment with prednisone. *Br J Haematol* 78:120, 1991.

251. Schuster MW: Will cytokines alter the treatment of myelodysplastic syndrome? *Am J Med Sci* 305:72, 1993.

252. Schouten HC, Vallenga E, Van Rhinen DJ, et al: Recombinant human erythropoietin in patients with myelodysplastic syndromes. *Leukemia* 5:432, 1991.

253. Stein RS, Abels RI, Krantz SB: Pharmacologic doses of recombinant human erythropoietin in the treatment of myelodysplastic syndromes. *Blood* 78:1658, 1991.

254. Rafanelli D, Grossi A, Longo G, et al: Recombinant human erythropoietin for treatment of myelodysplastic syndromes. *Leukemia* 6:323, 1992.

255. Willemze R, VanderLaly N, Zwierzina H, et al: A randomized phase I/II multicenter study of recombinant human granulocyte-macrophage colony-stimulating factor (GM-CSF) therapy for patients with myelodysplastic syndromes and a relatively low risk of acute leukemia. *Ann Hematol* 64:173, 1992.

256. Gradisher WJ, LeBeau MM, O'Laughlin R, et al: Clinical and cytogenetic responses to granulocyte-macrophage colony-stimulating factor in therapy-related myelodysplasia. *Blood* 80:2463, 1992.

257. Bessho M, Itho Y, Kataumi S: A hematologic remission by clonal hematopoiesis after treatment with recombinant human granulocyte-macrophage colony-stimulating factor and erythropoietin in a patient with therapy-related myelodysplastic syndrome. *Leuk Res* 16:123, 1992.

258. Negrin RS, Haeuber DH, Nagler A, et al: Maintenance treatment of patients with myelodysplastic syndromes using recombinant human granulocyte colony-stimulating factor. *Blood* 76:36, 1990.

259. Yoshida Y, Hirashima K, Asano S: A phase II trial of recombinant human granulocyte colony-stimulating factor in the myelodysplastic syndromes. *Br J Haematol* 78:378, 1991.

260. Ganser A, Seipelt G, Lindemann A, et al: Effects of recombinant human interleukin-3 in patients with myelodysplastic syndromes. *Blood* 76:455, 1990.

261. Ganser A, Hoelzer D: Clinical use of hematopoietic growth factors in the myelodysplastic syndromes. *Semin Hematol* 33:186, 1996.

262. Meyerson HJ, Farhi DC, Rosenthal NS: Transient increase in blasts mimicking acute leukemia and progressing myelodysplasia in patients receiving growth factor [comments]. *Am J Clin Pathol* 109:675, 1998.

263. Jonasova A, Neuwirtova R, Cermak J, et al: Cyclosporin A therapy in hypoplastic MDS patients and certain refractory anaemias without hypoplastic bone marrow. *Br J Haematol* 100:304, 1998.

264. Molldrem JJ, Jiang YZ, Stetler-Stevenson M, et al: Haematological response of patients with myelodysplastic syndrome to antithymocyte globulin is associated with a loss of lymphocyte-mediated inhibition of CFU-GM and alterations in T-cell receptor V-beta profiles. *Br J Haematol* 102:1314, 1998.

265. Coiffier B, Adeleine P, Viala JJ, et al: Dysmyelopoietic syndromes: A search for prognostic factors in 193 patients. *Cancer* 52:83, 1983.

266. Garcia S, Sanz MA, Amigo V, et al: Prognostic factors in chronic myelodysplastic syndromes: A multivariate analysis in 107 cases. *Am J Hematol* 27:163, 1988.

267. Dunkley SM, Manoharan A, Kwan YL: Myelodysplastic syndromes:
Prognostic significance of multilineage dysplasia in patients with refractory anemia or refractory anemia with ringed sideroblasts. *Blood* 99:
3870, 2002.

268. Joseph AS, Cinkotal KI, Hunt L, Geary CG: Natural history of smoldering leukemia. *Br J Cancer* 46:160, 1982.

269. Greenberg PL: The smoldering myeloid leukemic states: Clinical and
biological features. *Blood* 61:1035, 1983.

270. Maddox A-M, Keating MJ, Smith TL, et al: Prognostic factors for survival of 194 patients with low infiltrate leukemia. *Leuk Res* 10:995,
1986.

271. Najean Y, Pecking A: Refractory anemia with excess of myeloblasts in
the bone marrow. A clinical trial of androgens in 90 cases. *Br J Haematol* 37:23, 1977.

272. Lavessi AM, Maiolo AT, Chiorboli O, Mozzana R: The bone marrow
karyotype in seventeen cases of refractory anemia with excess blasts
(RAEB). *Ann Genet* 26:220, 1983.

273. Foucar K, Langdon RM II, Armitage JO, et al: Myelodysplastic syndromes. A clinical and pathologic analysis of 109 cases. *Cancer* 56:553,
1985.

274. Hiddemann W, Jahns-Streubel G, Verbeek W, et al: Intensive therapy
for high-risk myelodysplastic syndromes and the biological significance
of karyotype abnormalities. *Leuk Res* 22(suppl 1):S23, 1998.

275. Invernizzi R, Pecci A, Rossi G, et al: Idarubicin and cytosine arabinoside
in the induction and maintenance therapy of high-risk myelodysplastic
syndromes. *Haematologica* 82:660, 1997.

276. Kuriya S, Murai K, Miyairi Y, et al: A combination chemotherapy with
low doses of cytarabine and etoposide for high risk myelodysplastic
syndromes and their leukemic stage. A pilot study. *Cancer* 78:422, 1996.

277. Estey EH: Incorporating new modalities into guidelines. Topotecan for
myelodysplastic syndromes. *Oncology* 12:81, 1998.

278. Estey EH, Thall PF, Pierce S, et al: Randomized phase II study of fludarabine + cytosine arabinoside + idarubicin +/− all-*trans* retinoic
acid +/− granulocyte colony-stimulating factor in poor prognosis newly
diagnosed acute myeloid leukemia and myelodysplastic syndrome.
Blood 93:2478, 1999.

279. Sanz GF, Sanz MA: Progress in intensive chemotherapy for high-risk
myelodysplastic syndromes. *Forum* 9:63, 1999.

280. Cheson BD: Standard and low-dose chemotherapy for the treatment of
myelodysplastic syndromes. *Leuk Res* 22(suppl 1):S17, 1998.

281. Silverman LR, Holland JF, Weinberg RS, et al: Effects of treatment with
5-azacytidine on the in vivo and in vitro hematopoiesis in patients with
myelodysplastic syndromes. *Leukemia* 7(suppl 1):21, 1993.

282. Kornblith AB, Herndon JE II, Silverman EP, et al: Impact of azacytidine
on the quality of life of patients with myelodysplastic syndrome treated
in a randomized phase III trial. *J Clin Oncol* 15:2441, 2002.

283. Gassmann W, Schmitz N, Loffler H, De Witte T: Intensive chemotherapy and bone marrow transplantation for myelodysplastic syndromes.
Semin Hematol 33:196, 1996.

284. Appelbaum FR, Anderson J: Allogeneic bone marrow transplantation
for myelodysplastic syndrome: Outcomes analysis according to IPSS
score. *Leukemia* 12(suppl 1):S25, 1998.

285. Runde V, De Witte T, Arnold R, et al: Bone marrow transplantation
from HLA-identical siblings as first-line treatment in patients with myelodysplastic syndromes: Early transplantation is associated with improved outcome. Chronic Leukemia Working Party of the European
Group for Blood and Marrow Transplantation. *Bone Marrow Transplant*
21:255, 1998.

286. Wattel E, Solary E, Leleu X, et al: A prospective study of autologous
bone marrow or peripheral blood stem cell transplantation after intensive

chemotherapy in myelodysplastic syndromes. Groupe Francais des
Myelodysplasies. Group Ouest-Est d'etude des Leucemies aigues myeloides. *Leukemia* 13:524, 1999.

287. Estey E, Keating M, Pierce S, et al: Application of the International
Scoring System for myelodysplasia to M.D. Anderson patients. *Blood*
90:2843, 1997.

288. National Comprehensive Cancer Network: Myelodysplastic syndromes.
J Natl Compr Cancer Net 1:456, 2003.

289. Alessandrino EP, Amadori S, Bardsi G, et al: Evidence and consensus-
based practice guidelines for the therapy of primary myelodysplastic
syndromes: A statement from the Italian Society of Hematology. *Haematologica* 87:1286, 2002.

290. Bowen D, Culligan D, Jowitt S, et al: Guidelines for diagnosis and therapy
of the myelodysplastic syndromes. *Br J Haematol* 120:187, 2003.

291. Cheson BD: Standard and low-dose chemotherapy for the treatment of
myelodysplastic syndromes. *Leuk Res* 22:s17, 1998.

292. Erba HP: Recent progress in the treatment of myelodysplastic syndrome
in adult patients. *Curr Opin Oncol* 15:1, 2003.

293. Jansen AJ, Essink-Bot ML, Beckers EA, et al: Quality of life measurement in patients with transfusion-dependent myelodysplastic syndromes. *Br J Haematol* 121:270, 2003.

294. Wandt H, Ehninger G, Gallmeier WM: New strategies for prophylactic
platelet transfusion in patients with hematologic diseases. *Oncologist* 6:
446, 2001.

295. Zeigler ZR: Effects of epsilon aminocaproic acid on primary hemostasis.
Haemostasis 21:313, 1991.

296. Goy A, Belanger C, Casadevall N, et al: High doses of intravenous
recombinant erythropoietin for the treatment of anemia in myelodysplastic syndrome. *Br J Haematol* 84:232, 1993.

297. Vadhan-Raj S, Keating M, LeMaistre A, et al: Effects of recombinant
human granulocyte-macrophage colony-stimulating factor in patients
with myelodysplastic syndromes. *N Engl J Med* 317:1545, 1987.

298. Thompson JA, Gilliland DG, Prchal JT, et al: Effect of recombinant
human erythropoietin combined with granulocyte/macrophage colony-
stimulating factor in the treatment of patients with myelodysplastic syndrome. *Blood* 95:1175, 2000.

299. Verhoef G, VandDenBerghe HV, Boogaerts M: Cytogenetic effects on
cells derived from patients with myelodysplastic syndromes during treatment with hemopoietic growth factors. *Leukemia* 6:766, 1992.

300. Tohyama K, Ohmori S, Michishita M: Effects of recombinant G-CSF
and GM-CSF on in vitro differentiation of the blast cells of RAEB and
RAEB-T. *Eur J Haematol* 42:348, 1989.

301. Ferrero D, Bruno B, Pregno P, et al: Combined differentiating therapy
for myelodysplastic syndromes: A phase II study. *Leuk Res* 20:867,
1996.

302. Hofmann WK, Ganser A, Seipelt G, et al: Treatment of patients with
low-risk myelodysplastic syndromes using a combination of all-trans
retinoic acid, interferon alpha, and granulocyte colony-stimulating factor. *Ann Hematol* 78:125, 1999.

303. Gordon MS: Advances in supportive case of myelodysplastic syndromes. *Semin Hematol* 36:21, 1999.

304. Rigolin GM, Porta MD, Bigoni R, et al: RHuEpo administration in patients with low-risk myelodysplastic syndromes: Evaluation of erythroid
precursors' response by fluorescence in situ hybridization on May-Grun-
wald-Giemsa-stained bone marrow samples. *Br J Haematol* 119:652,
2002.

305. Wallvik J, Stenke L, Bernell P, et al: Serum erythropoietin (EPO) levels
correlate with survival and independently predict response to EPO treatment in patients with myelodysplastic syndromes. *Eur J Haematol* 68:
180, 2002.

306. Musto P, Falcone A, Sanpaolo G, et al: Efficacy of a single, weekly
dose of recombinant erythropoietin in myelodysplastic syndromes. *Br J
Haematol* 122:269, 2003.

307. Terpos E, Mougiou A, Kouraklis A, et al: Prolonged administration of erythropoietin increases erythroid response rate in myelodysplastic syndromes: A phase II trail in 281 patients. *Br J Haematol* 118:174, 2002.

308. Thompson JA, Gillilland DG, Prchal JT, et al: Effect of recombinant human erythropoietin combined with granulocyte/macrophage colony-stimulating factor in the treatment of patients with myelodysplastic syndrome. *Blood* 95:1175, 2000.

309. Stein RS: The role of erythropoietin in the anemia of myelodysplastic syndrome. *Clin Lymphoma* 1:S36, 2003.

310. Hellstrom-Lindberg E, Gulbrandsen N, Lindberg G, et al: A validated decision model for treating the anaemia of myelodysplastic syndromes with erythropoietin + granulocyte colony-stimulating factor: Significant effects on quality of life. *Br J Haematol* 120:1037, 2003.

311. Chuncharunee S, Intragumtornchai T, Chaimongkol B, et al: Treatment of myelodysplastic syndrome with low-dose human granulocyte colony-stimulating factor: A multicenter study. *Int J Hematol* 74:144, 2001.

312. O'Malley DP, Whalen M, Banks PM: Spontaneous splenic rupture with fatal outcome following G-CSF administration for myelodysplastic syndrome. *Am J Hematol* 73:294, 2003.

313. Sultana TA, Harada H, Ito K, et al: Expression and functional analysis of granulocyte colony-stimulating factor receptors on CD34++ cells in patients with myelodysplastic syndrome (MDS) and MDS-acute myeloid leukaemia. *Br J Haematol* 212:63, 2003.

314. Nimubona S, Grulois I, Bernard M, et al: Complete remission in hypoplastic acute myeloid leukemia induced by G-CSF without chemotherapy: Report on three cases. *Leukemia* 16:1871, 2002.

315. Cesaro S, Chinello P, De Silvestro G, et al: Granulocyte transfusions from G-CSF-stimulated donors for the treatment of severe infections in neutropenic pediatric patients with onco-hematological diseases. *Support Care Cancer* 11:101, 2003.

316. Kizaki M, Miyakawa Y, Ideda Y: Long-term administration of pegylated recombinant human megakaryocyte growth and development factor dramatically improved cytopenias in a patient with myelodysplastic syndrome. *Br J Haematol* 122:764, 2003.

317. Hellström-Lindberg E, Robért K-H, Gahrton G, et al: A predictive model for the clinical response to low dose ARA-C: A study of 102 patients with myelodysplastic syndromes and acute leukemia. *Br J Haematol* 81:503, 1992.

318. Ganser A, Seipelt G, Eder M, et al: Treatment of myelodysplastic syndromes with cytokines and cytotoxic drugs. *Semin Oncol* 19:95, 1992.

319. Kochenderfer JH, Kobayashi S, Wieder ED, et al: Loss of T-lymphocyte clonal dominance in patients with myelodysplastic syndrome responsive to immunosuppression. *Blood* 100:3639, 2002.

320. Aivado M, Rong A, Stadler M: Favourable response to antithymocyte or antilymphocyte globulin in low-risk myelodysplastic syndrome patients with a 'non-clonal' pattern of X-chromosome inactivation in bone marrow cells. *Eur J Haematol* 68:210, 2002.

321. Selleri C, Maciejewski JP, Catalano L: Effects of cyclosporine on hematopoietic and immune functions in patients with hypoplastic myelodysplasia: In vitro and in vivo studies. *Cancer* 95:1911, 2002.

322. Yazji S, Giles FJ, Tsimberidou A-M, et al: Antithymocyte globulin (ATG)-based therapy in patients with myelodysplastic syndromes. *Leukemia* 17:2101, 2003.

323. Molldrem JJ, Leufer E, Bahceci E, et al: Antithymocyte globulin for treatment of the bone marrow failure associated with myelodysplastic syndromes. *Ann Intern Med* 137:156, 2002.

324. Killick SB, Mufti G, Cavenagh JD, et al: A pilot study of antithymocyte globulin (ATG) in the treatment of patients with 'low-risk' myelodysplasia. *Br J Haematol* 120:679, 2003.

325. Saunthararajah Y, Nakamura R, Nam JM, et al: HLA-DR15 (DR2) is over represented in myelodysplastic syndrome and aplastic anemia and predicts a response to immunosuppression in myelodysplastic syndrome. *Blood* 100:1570, 2002.

326. Saunthararajah Y, Nakamura R, Wesley R, et al: A simple method to predict response to immunosuppressive therapy in patients with myelodysplastic syndrome. *Blood* 102:3025, 2003.

327. Shimamoto T, Iguchi T, Ando K, et al: Successful treatment with cyclosporin A for myelodysplastic syndrome with erythroid hypoplasia associated with T-cell receptor gene rearrangements. *Br J Haematol* 114:358, 2001.

328. Steensma DP, Dispenzieri A, Moore B, et al: Antithymocyte globulin has limited efficacy and substantial toxicity in unselected anemic patients with myelodysplastic syndrome. *Blood* 101:2156, 2003.

329. Atoyebi W, Bywater L, Rawlings L, et al: Treatment of myelodysplasia with oral cyclosporin. *Clin Lab Haematol* 24:211, 2002.

330. Park SJ, Han CW, Lee JH, et al: Cyclosporine A in the treatment of a patient with immune thrombocytopenia accompanied by myelodysplastic syndrome and nephritic syndrome. 110:36, 2003.

331. Yamada T, Tsurumi H, Kasahara S, et al: Immunosuppressive therapy for myelodysplastic syndrome: Efficacy of methylprednisolone pulse therapy with or without cyclosporin A. *J Cancer Res Clin Oncol* 129:485, 2003.

332. Lin JT, Wang WS, Yen CC, et al: Myelodysplastic syndrome complicated by autoimmune hemolytic anemia: Remission of refractory anemia following mycophenolate mofetil. *Ann Hematol* 81:723, 2002.

333. Oka Y, Tsuboi A, Murakami M, et al: Wilms tumor gene peptide-based immunotherapy for patients with overt leukemia from myelodysplastic syndrome (MDS) or MDS with myelofibrosis. *Int J Hematol* 78:56, 2003.

334. Leone G, Teofili L, Voso MT: DNA methylation and demethylating drugs in myelodysplastic syndromes and secondary leukemias. *Haematologica* 87:1324, 2002.

335. Lopez-Karpovitch X, Barrales-Benitez O, Flores M, Piedras J: Effect of azacytidine in the release of leukemia inhibitory factor, oncostatin m, interleukin (IL)-6, and IL-11 by mononuclear cells of patients with refractory anemia. *Cytokine* 20:154, 2002.

336. Gryn J, Zeigler ZR, Shadduck RK, et al: Treatment of myelodysplastic syndromes with 5-azacytidine. 26:893, 2002.

337. Lubbert M, Wijermans P, Kunzmann R, et al: Cytogenetic responses in high-risk myelodysplastic syndrome following low-dose treatment with the DNA methylation inhibitor 5-aza-2'-deoxycytidine. *Br J Haematol* 114:349, 2001.

338. Daskalakis M, Nguyen TT, Nguyen C, et al: Demethylation of a hypermethylated P15/INK4B gene in patients with myelodysplastic syndrome by 5-Aza-2'-deoxycytidine (decitabine) treatment. *Blood* 100:2957, 2002.

339. Sigalotti L, Altomonte M, Colizzi F, et al: Correspondence: 5-Aza-2'-deoxycytidine (decitabine) treatment of hematopoietic malignancies: A multimechanism therapeutic approach? *Blood* 101:4644, 2003.

340. Gore SD, Weng LJ, Zhai S, et al: Impact of the putative differentiating agent sodium phenylbutyrate on myelodysplastic syndromes and acute myeloid leukemia. *Clin Cancer Res* 7:2330, 2001.

341. Ogata K, Yamada T, Ito T, et al: Low-dose etoposide: A potential therapy for myelodysplastic syndromes. *Br J Haematol* 82:354, 1992;287.

342. Robak T, Szmigielska-Kaplon A, Urbanska-Rys H, et al: Efficacy and toxicity of low-dose melphalan in myelodysplastic syndromes and acute myeloid leukemia with multilineage dysplasia. *Neoplasma* 50:172, 2003.

343. Mario AD, Pagano L, Mele L, et al: Use of gemcitabine (GEM) in advanced myelodysplastic syndromes. *Ann Oncol* 12:1494, 2001.

344. Ribrag V, Suzan F, Ravoet C, et al: Phase II trial of CPT-11 in myelodysplastic syndromes with excess of marrow blasts. *Leukemia* 17:319, 2003.

345. Giles FJ, Faderl S, Thomas DA, et al: Randomizing phase I/II study of troxacitabine combined with cytarabine, idarubicin, or topotecan in patients with refractory myeloid leukemias. *J Clin Oncol* 21:1050, 2003.

346. Bouabdallah R, Lefrere F, Rose C, et al: A phase II trial of induction and consolidation therapy of acute myeloid leukemia with weekly oral idarubicin alone in poor risk elderly patients. *Leukemia* 13:1491, 1999.

347. Raza A, Meyer P, Dutt D, et al: Thalidomide produces transfusion independence in long-standing refractory anemias of patients with myelodysplastic syndromes. *Blood* 98:958, 2001.

348. Strupp C, Germing U, Aivado M, et al: Thalidomide for the treatment of patients with myelodysplastic syndromes. *Leukemia* 16:1, 2002.

349. Bertolini F, Mingrone W, Alietti A, et al: Thalidomide in multiple myeloma, myelodysplastic syndromes and histiocytosis. Analysis of clinical results and of surrogate angiogenesis markers. *Ann Oncol* 12:1333, 2001.

350. Tsirigotis P, Venetis E, Rontogianni D, et al: Thalidomide in the treatment of myelodysplastic syndrome with fibrosis. *Leuk Res* 26:965, 2002.

351. Steurer M, Sudmeier I, Stauder R, Gastl G: Thromboembolic events in patients with myelodysplastic syndrome receiving thalidomide in combination with darbepoietin-alpha. *Br J Haematol* 121:101, 2003.

352. List AF, Kurtin S, Glinsmann-Gibson B, et al: Efficacy and safety of CC-5013 for treatment of anemia in patients with myelodysplastic syndromes (MDS). *Blood* 102:184a, 2003.

353. Giles FJ, Stopeck AT, Silverman LR, et al: SU5416, a small molecule tyrosine kinase receptor inhibitor, has biologic activity in patients with refractory acute myeloid leukemia or myelodysplastic syndromes. *Blood* 102:795, 2003.

354. List, AF: New approaches to the treatment of myelodysplasia. *The Oncologist* 7(suppl 1):39, 2002.

355. Invernizzi R, Pecci A, Travaglino E, et al: Clinical and biological effects of treatment with amifostine in myelodyplastic syndromes. *Br J Haematol* 118:246, 2002.

356. Garcia-Manero G, Faderl S, Giles F, et al: A phase I study of idarubicin dose escalation with amifostine and high-dose cytarabine in patients with relapsed acute myelogenous leukemia and myelodysplastic syndromes. *Haematologica* 87:804, 2002.

357. Deeg HJ, Gotlib J, Beckham C, et al: Soluble TNF receptor fusion protein (etanercept) for the treatment of myelodysplastic syndrome: A pilot study. *Leukemia* 16:162, 2002.

358. Rosenfeld C, Bedell C: Pilot study of recombinant human soluble tumor necrosis factor receptor (TNFR:Fc) in patients with low risk myelodysplasia syndrome. *Leuk Res* 26:721, 2002.

359. Maciejewski JP, Risitano Am, Sloand EM, et al: A pilot study of the recombinant soluble human tumour necrosis factor receptor (p75)-Fc fusion protein in patients with myelodysplastic syndrome. *Br J Haematol* 117:119, 2002.

360. Stasi R, Amadori S: Infliximab chimaeric anti-tumour necrosis factor alpha monoclonal antibody treatment for patients with myelodysplastic syndromes. *Br J Haematol* 116:334, 2002.

361. Chan G, DiVenuti G, Miller K: Danazol for the treatment of thrombocytopenia in patients with myelodysplastic syndrome. *Am J Hematol* 71:166, 2002.

362. Sadek I, Zayed E, Hayne O, Fernandez L: Prolonged complete remission of myelodysplastic syndrome treated with danazol, retinoic acid and low-dose prednisone. *Am J Hematol* 64:306, 2000.

363. Nagler A, Rikilis I, Tatarsky I, Fabian I: Effect of 1,25-dihydroxyvitamin D₃ and 13-*cis*-retinoic acid on in vitro hematopoiesis in the myelodysplastic syndromes. *J Lab Clin Med* 110:237, 1987.

364. Rowinsky EK, Conley BA, Jones RJ, et al: Hexamethylene bisacetamide in myelodysplastic syndrome: Effect of five-day exposure to maximal therapeutic concentrations. *Leukemia* 6:526, 1992.

365. List AF: Hematopoietic stimulation by amifostine and sodium phenylbutyrate: What is the potential in MDS? *Leuk Res* 22(suppl 1):S7, 1998.

366. Hast R, Lauren SAL, Reizenstein P: Absent clinical effects of retinoic acid and isotretinoin treatment on the myelodysplastic syndrome. *Hematol Oncol* 7:297, 1989.

367. Ohno R, Naoe T, Hirano M, et al: Treatment of myelodysplastic syndromes with all-trans retinoic acid. *Blood* 81:1152, 1993.

368. Hofmann WK, Ganser A, Seipelt G, et al: Treatment of patients with low-risk myelodysplastic syndromes using a combination of all-trans retinoic acid, interferon alpha, and granulocyte colony-stimulating factor. *Ann Hematol* 78:125, 1999.

369. Richard C, Mazo E, Cuadrado MA, et al: Treatment of myelodysplastic syndrome with 1,25-dihydroxyvitamin D₃. *Am J Med* 23:175, 1986.

370. Motomura S, Kanamori H, Maruta A, et al: The effect of 1-hydroxyvitamin D₃ for prolongation of leukemic transformation-free survival in myelodysplastic syndromes. *Am J Hematol* 38:67, 1991.

371. Yoshida Y: Japanese experience in the treatment of myelodysplastic syndromes. *Hematol Oncol Clin North Am* 6:673, 1992.

372. Paquette RL, Koeffler HP: Differentiation therapy. *Hematol Oncol Clin North Am* 6:687, 1992.

373. DeRosa L, Montuoro A, DeLaurenzi A: Therapy of "high risk" myelodysplastic syndromes with an association of low-dose ara-c, retinoic acid, and 1,25-dihydroxyvitamin D₃. *Biomed Pharmacother* 46:211, 1992.

374. Andreeff M, Stone R, Michaeli J, et al: Hexamethylene bisacetamide in myelodysplastic syndrome and acute myelogenous leukemia: A phase II clinical trial with a differentiation-inducing agent. *Blood* 80:2604, 1992.

375. Raza A, Qawi H, Lisak L, et al: Patients with myelodysplastic syndromes benefit from palliative therapy with amifostine, pentoxifylline, and ciprofloxacin with or without dexamethasone. *Blood* 95:1580, 2000.

376. Miller WH Jr: Molecular targets of arsenic trioxide in malignant cells. *Oncologist* 7(suppl 1):14, 2002.

377. Slack JL, Waxman S, Tricot G, et al: Advances in the management of acute promyelocytic leukemia and other hematologic malignancies with arsenic trioxide. *Oncologist* 7(suppl 1):1, 2002.

378. List A, Beran M, DiPersio J, Slack J, et al: Opportunities for Trisenox® (arsenic trioxide in the treatment of myelodysplastic syndromes. *Leukemia* 17:1499, 2003.

379. Nand S, Ellis T, Messmore H, et al: Phase II trial of recombinant human interferon-α in myelodysplastic syndromes. *Leukemia* 6:220, 1992.

380. Maerevoet M, Van Den Neste E, Delannoy A, et al: Limited activity of mini-dose interferon alpha-2a in the treatment of myelodysplastic syndrome. *Leuk Lymphoma* 21:519, 1996.

381. Petti MC, Latagliata R, Avvisati G, et al: Treatment of high-risk myelodysplastic syndromes with lymphoblastoid alpha interferon. *Br J Haematol* 95:364, 1996.

382. Toze CL, Barnett MJ, Klingeman H-G: Response of therapy-related myelodysplasia to low-dose interleukin-2. *Leukemia* 7:463, 1993.

383. Nand S, Stock W, Stiff P, et al: A phase II trial of interleukin-2 in myelodysplastic syndromes. *Br J Haematol* 101:205, 1998.

384. Cortes J, Giles F, O'Brien S, et al: Results of imatinib mesylate therapy in patients with refractory or recurrent acute myeloid leukemia, high-risk myelodysplastic syndrome, and myeloproliferative disorders. *Cancer* 97:2760, 2003.

385. Drummond MW, Lush CJ, Vickers MA, et al: Imatinib mesylate-induced molecular remission of Philadelphia chromosome-positive myelodysplastic syndrome. *Leukemia* 17:463, 2003.

386. Crump M: Inhibition of raf kinase in the treatment of acute myeloid leukemia. *Curr Pharm Des* 8:2243, 2002.

387. Kurzrock R, Kantarjian H, Cortes J: Farnesyltransferase inhibitor, R11577, in myelodysplastic syndrome: Clinical and biological activities in the Phase 1 setting. *Blood* 102:4527, 2003.

388. Xia Z, Tan MM, Wong WW, et al: Blocking protein geranylgeranylation is essential for lovastatin-induced apoptosis of human acute myeloid leukemia cells. *Leukemia* 15:1398, 2001.

389. Sawyers CL: Finding the next Gleevec: FLT3 targeted kinase inhibitor therapy for acute myeloid leukemia. *Cancer Cell* 1:413, 2002.

390. Beran M: Intensive chemotherapy for patients with high-risk myelodysplastic syndrome. *Int J Hematol* 72:139, 2000.

391. Cortes J, Kantarjian H, Albitar M, et al: A randomized trial of liposomal daunorubicin and cytarabine versus liposomal daunorubicin and topotecan with or without thalidomide as initial therapy for patients with poor prognosis acute myelogenous leukemia or myelodysplastic syndrome. *Cancer* 97:1234, 2003.

392. Estey EH, Thall PF, Cortes JE, et al: Comparison of idarubicin + ara-C-, and fludarabine + ara-C-, topotecan + ara-C-based regimens in treatment of newly diagnosed acute myeloid leukemia, refractory anemia with excess blasts in transformation, or refractory anemia with excess blasts. *Blood* 98:3575, 2001.

393. De la Rubia J, Regadera A, Martin G, et al: FLAG-IDA regimen (fludarabine, cytarabine, idarubicin and G-CSF) in the treatment of patients with high-risk myeloid malignancies. *Leuk Res* 26:725, 2002.

394. Voutsadakis IA: Gemtuzumab ozogamicin (CMA-676, Mylotarg) for the treatment of CD33+ acute myeloid leukemia. *Anticancer Drugs* 13:685, 2002.

395. Cohen AD, Luger SM, Sickles C, et al: Gemtuzumab ozogamicin (Mylotarg) monotherapy for relapsed AML after hematopoietic stem cell transplantation: Efficacy and incidence of hepatic veno-occlusive disease. *Bone Marrow Transplant* 30:23, 2002.

396. Deeg HG, Shulman HM, Anderson JE, et al: Allogeneic and syngeneic marrow transplantation for myelodysplastic syndrome in patients 55 to 66 years of age. *Blood* 95:1188, 2000.

397. Anderson JE, Appelbaum FR, Schoch G, et al: Allogeneic marrow transplantation for myelodysplastic syndrome with advanced disease morphology: A phase II study of busulfan, cyclophosphamide, and total-body irradiation and analysis of prognostic factors. *J Clin Oncol* 14:220, 1996.

398. Demuynck H, Delforge M, Verhoef GE, et al: Feasibility of peripheral blood progenitor cell harvest and transplantation in patients with poor-risk myelodysplastic syndromes. *Br J Haematol* 92:351, 1996.

399. De Witte T, Van Biezen A, Hermans J, et al: Autologous bone marrow transplantation for patients with myelodysplastic syndrome (MDS) or acute myeloid leukemia following MDS. Chronic and Acute Leukemia Working Parties of the European Group for Blood and Marrow Transplantation. *Blood* 90:3853, 1997.

400. Woolfrey AE, Gooley TA, Sievers EL, et al: Bone marrow transplantation for children less than 2 years of age with acute myelogenous leukemia or myelodysplastic syndrome. *Blood* 92:3546, 1998.

401. Arnold R, De Witte T, Van Biezen A, et al: Unrelated bone marrow transplantation in patients with myelodysplastic syndromes and secondary acute myeloid leukemia: An EBMT survey. European Blood and Marrow Transplantation Group. *Bone Marrow Transplant* 21:1213, 1998.

402. Nevill TJ, Fung HC, Shepherd JD, et al: Cytogenetic abnormalities in primary myelodysplastic syndrome are highly predictive of outcome after allogeneic bone marrow transplantation. *Blood* 92:1910, 1998.

403. Sierra J, Perez WS, Rozman C, et al: Bone marrow transplantation from HLA-identical siblings as treatment for myelodysplasia. *Blood* 100:1997, 2002.

404. Guardiola P, Runder V, Bacigalupo A, et al: Retrospective comparison of bone marrow and granulocyte colony-stimulating factor-mobilized peripheral blood progenitor cells for allogeneic stem cell transplantation using HLA identical sibling donors in myelodysplastic syndromes. *Blood* 99:4370, 2002.

405. Castro-Malaspina H, Harris RE, Gajewski J, et al: Unrelated donor marrow transplantation for myelodysplastic syndromes: Outcome analysis in 510 transplants facilitated by the National Marrow Donor Program. *Blood* 99:1943, 2002.

406. Ooi J, Iseki T, Nagayama H, et al: Unrelated cord blood transplantation for adult patients with myelodysplastic syndrome-related secondary acute myeloid leukaemia. *Br J Haematol* 114:834, 2001.

407. Benesch M, Deeg HJ: Hematopoietic cell transplantation for adult patients with myelodysplastic syndromes and myeloproliferative disorders. *Mayo Clin Proc* 78:981, 2003.

408. Luger S, Sacks N: Bone marrow transplantation for myelodysplastic syndrome—Who? when? and which? *Bone Marrow Transplant* 30:199, 2002.

409. Taussig Dc, Davies AJ, Cavenagh JD: Durable remissions of myelodysplastic syndrome and acute myeloid leukemia after reduced-intensity allografting. *J Clin Oncol* 21:3060, 2003.

410. Mielcarek M, Storb R: Non-myeloablative hematopoietic cell transplantation as immunotherapy for hematologic malignancies. *Cancer Treat Rev* 29:283, 2003.

411. Kroger N, Schetelig J, Zabelina T, et al: A fludarabine-based dose-reduced conditioning regimen followed by allogeneic stem cell transplantation from related or unrelated donors in patients with myelodysplastic syndrome. *Bone Marrow Transplant* 28:643, 2001.

412. Parker JE, Shafi T, Pagliuca A, et al: Allogeneic stem cell transplantation in the myelodysplastic syndromes: Interim results of outcomes following reduced-intense conditioning compared with standard preparative regimens. *Br J Haematol* 119:144, 2002.

413. Testoni N, Lemoli RM, Martinelli G, et al: Autologous peripheral blood stem cell transplantation in acute myeloblastic leukaemia and myelodysplastic syndrome patients: Evaluation of tumour cell contamination of leukapheresis by cytogenetic and molecular methods. *Bone Marrow Transplant* 22:1065, 1998.

414. Wattel E, Solary E, Leleu X, et al: A prospective study of autologous bone marrow or peripheral blood stem cell transplantation after intensive chemotherapy in myelodysplastic syndromes. Groupe Francais des Myelodysplasies. Group Ouest-Est d'etude des Leucemies aigues myeloides. *Leukemia* 13:524, 1999.

415. Oosterveld M, Suciu S, Verhoef G, et al: The presence of an HLA-identical sibling donor has no impact on outcome of patients with high-risk MDS or secondary AML (sAML) treated with intensive chemotherapy followed by transplantation: Results of a prospective study of the EORTC, EBMT, SAKK, and GIMEMEA Leukemia Groups (EORTC study 06921). *Leukemia* 17:859, 2003.

416. De Witte T, Suciu S, Verhoef G, et al: Intensive chemotherapy followed by allogeneic or autologous stem cell transplantation for patients with myelodysplastic syndromes (MDSs) and acute myeloid leukemia following MDS. *Blood* 17:859, 2003.

417. De Witte T, Pikkemaat F, Hermans J, et al: Genotypically nonidentical related donors for transplantation of patients with myelodysplastic syndromes: Comparison with unrelated donor transplantation and autologous stem cell transplantation. *Leukemia* 15:1878, 2001.

418. Sanz GF, Sanz MA, Vallespi T, et al: Two regression models and a scoring system for predicting survival and planning treatment in myelodysplastic syndromes: A multivariate analysis of prognostic factors in 370 patients. *Blood* 74:395, 1989.

419. Ganser A, Hoelzer D: Clinical course of myelodysplastic syndromes. *Hematol Oncol Clin North Am* 6:607, 1992.

420. White AD, Culligan DJ, Hoy TG, Jacobs A: Extended cytogenetic follow-up of patients with myelodysplastic syndrome (MDS). *Br J Haematol* 81:499, 1992.

421. Mufti GJ: A guide to risk assessment in the primary myelodysplastic syndrome. *Hematol Oncol Clin North Am* 6:587, 1992.

422. Pfeilstocker M, Reisner R, Nosslinger T, et al: Cross validation of prognostic scores in myelodysplastic syndromes on 386 patients from a single institution confirms importance of cytogenetics. *Br J Haematol* 106:455, 1999.

423. Greenberg PL, Sanz GF, Sanz MA: Prognostic scoring systems for risk assessment in myelodysplastic syndromes. *Forum* 9:17, 1999.

424. Maes B, Meeus P, Michaux L, et al: Application of the International Prognostic Scoring System for myelodysplastic syndromes. *J Oncol* 10:825, 1999.

425. Brown ER, Heerma NA, Tricot G: Spontaneous remission in myelodysplastic syndrome. *Cancer Genet Cytogenet* 46:125, 1990.

426. Minke DM, Colon-Otero G, Cockerill KJ, et al: Refractory thrombocytopenia: A myelodysplastic syndrome that may mimic immune thrombocytopenic purpura. *Am J Clin Pathol* 98:502, 1992.

427. Hoffman R: Acquired pure amegakaryocytic thrombocytopenia purpura. *Semin Hematol* 28:303, 1991.

428. Welte K, Boxer LA: Severe chronic neutropenia: Pathophysiology and therapy. *Semin Hematol* 34:267, 1997.

429. Rosen RB, Kang SJ: Congenital agranulocytosis terminating in acute myelomonocytic leukemia. *J Pediatr* 94:406, 1979.

430. Smith OP, Hann IM, Chessells JM, et al: Haematological abnormalities in Shwachman-Diamond syndrome. *Br J Haematol* 94:279, 1996.

431. Pearson HA, Lobel JS, Kocoshis SA, et al: A new syndrome of refractory sideroblastic anemia with vacuolization of marrow precursors and exocrine pancreatic dysfunction. *J Pediatr* 95:976, 1979.

432. Orlandi E, Alessandrino EP, Caldera D, Bernasconi C: Adult leukemia after aplastic anemia: Report of 8 cases, *Acta Haematol* 79:174, 1988.

433. DePlanque MM, Bacigalupo A, Wüsch A, et al: Long-term follow up of severe aplastic anemia patients treated with antithymocyte globulin. *Br J Haematol* 73:121, 1989.

434. Dunn DE, Tanawattanacharoen P, Boccuni P, et al: Paroxysmal nocturnal hemoglobinuria cells in patients with bone marrow failure syndromes. *Ann Intern Med* 131:401, 1999.

435. Doyle JA, Ginsburg WW: Eosinophilic fasciitis. *Med Clin North Am* 73:1157, 1989.

436. Lakhanpal S, Ginsburg WW, Michet CJ, et al: Eosinophilic fasciitis: Clinical spectrum and therapeutic response in 52 cases. *Semin Arthritis Rheum* 17:221, 1988.

437. Naschitz JE, Boss JH, Misselevich I, et al: The fasciitis-panniculitis syndromes. Clinical and pathologic features. *Medicine* 75:6, 1996.

438. Kim SW, Rice L, Champlin R, Udden MM: Aplastic anemia in eosinophilic fasciitis: Response to immunotherapy and marrow transplantation. *Haematologia* 28:131, 1997.

439. Brusamolino E, Isernia P, Alessandrino EP, et al: Terminal deoxynucleotidyl transferase–positive acute leukemias evolving from a myelodysplastic syndrome. *Am J Hematol* 20:187, 1985.

440. Berneman ZN, Van Bockstaele D, DeMeyer P, et al: A myelodysplastic syndrome preceding acute lymphoblastic leukemia. *Br J Haematol* 60:353, 1985.

441. Ascensao JL, Kay NE, Wright JJ, et al: Lymphoblastic transformation of myelodysplastic syndrome. *Am J Hematol* 22:431, 1986.

442. Bonati A, Delia D, Starcich R: Progression of a myelodysplastic syndrome to pre-B-acute lymphoblastic leukaemia with unusual phenotype. *Br J Haematol* 64:487, 1986.

443. Dayton MA, VanBesien K, Tricot G, et al: Preleukemic state preceding adult acute lymphoblastic leukemia. *Am J Med* 89:657, 1990.

444. Escudier SM, Albitar M, Robertson LE, et al: Acute lymphoblastic leukemia following preleukemic syndromes in adults. *Leukemia* 10:473, 1996.

445. Saarinen UM, Wegelius R: Preleukemic syndrome in children. Report of four cases and review of literature. *Am J Pediatr Hematol Oncol* 6:137, 1984.

446. Breatnach F, Chessells JM, Greaves MF: The aplastic presentation of childhood leukemia: A feature of common ALL. *Br J Haematol* 49:387, 1981.

447. Klingemann H-G, Storb R, Sanders J, et al: Acute lymphoblastic leukaemia after bone marrow transplantation for aplastic anaemia. *Br J Haematol* 63:47, 1986.

448. Nakamori Y, Takahashi M, Moriyama Y, et al: The aplastic presentation of adult acute lymphoblastic leukaemia. *Br J Haematol* 62:782, 1986.

449. Homans AC, Cohen JL, Barker BE, Marzur EM: Aplastic presentation of acute lymphoblastic leukemia: Evidence for cellular inhibition of normal hematopoietic progenitors. *Am J Pediatr Hematol Oncol* 11:456, 1989.

450. DeAlarcon P, Miller M, Stuart MJ: Erythroid hypoplasia: An unusual presentation of childhood leukemia. *Am J Dis Child* 132:763, 1978.

451. Reid MM, Summerfield GP: Distinction between aleukaemic prodrome of childhood acute lymphoblastic leukaemia and aplastic anemia. *J Clin Pathol* 45:697, 1992.

452. MacSween JM, Langley GR: Light-chain disease and sideroblastic anemia–preleukemic chronic granulocytic leukemia. *Can Med Assoc J* 106:995, 1972.

453. Trachida L, Palutke M, Poylik MD, Prasad AS: Primary acquired sideroblastic anemia preceding monoclonal gammopathy and malignant lymphoma. *Am J Med* 55:559, 1973.

454. Papayannis AG, Stathakis NE, Kyrkou K, et al: Primary acquired sideroblastic anemia associated with chronic lymphocytic leukemia. *Br J Haematol* 28:125, 1974.

455. Berkowitz LR, Ross DW, Orringe EP: Hairy cell leukemia with acquired dyserythropoiesis. *JAMA* 140:554, 1980.

456. Catovsky D, Shaw MT, Hoffbrand AV, Dacie JV: Sideroblastic anemia and its association with leukemia and myelomatosis. A report of five cases. *Br J Haematol* 20:385, 1971.

457. Dahlke MA, Nowell PC: Chromosomal abnormalities and dyserythropoiesis in the preleukaemic phase of multiple myeloma. *Br J Haematol* 31:111, 1975.

458. Meckenstock G, Bonatsch CH, Heyll A, et al: T-cell receptor α/δ expressing acute leukemia emerging from sideroblastic anemia: Morphologic, immunological, and cytogenetic features. *Leuk Res* 16:379, 1992.

459. Khaleeli M, Keane WM, Lee GR: Sideroblastic anemia in multiple myeloma. A preleukemic change. *Blood* 41:17, 1973.

460. Greenberg BR, Miller C, Cardoff RD, et al: Concurrent development of preleukaemic lymphoproliferative and plasma cell disorders. *Br J Haematol* 53:125, 1983.

461. Copplestone JA, Mufti GJ, Hamblin TJ, Oscier DG: Immunological abnormalities in myelodysplastic syndromes. *Br J Haematol* 63:149, 1986.

462. Casadevall N, Durieux P, Dubois S, et al: Health, economic, and quality of life effects of erythropoietin and granulocyte colony-stimulating factor for the treatment of myelodysplastic syndromes. *Blood* 104:321, 2004.

ACUTE MYELOGENOUS LEUKEMIA

JANE L. LIESVELD
MARSHALL A. LICHTMAN

Acute myelogenous leukemia (AML) is the result of a sequence of somatic mutations in a multipotential primitive cell or in some cases a more differentiated progenitor cell. Exposure to very high doses of radiation, chronic exposure to benzene, and, perhaps, chronic inhalation of tobacco smoke increase the incidence of the disease. A small but increasing proportion of cases develop after a patient with lymphoma or a nonhematologic cancer is exposed to intensive chemotherapy, especially with alkylating agents or topoisomerase II inhibitors. The mutant hematopoietic cell gains a growth and/or survival advantage in relationship to the normal pool of stem cells. As the progeny of this mutant, now leukemic, multipotential cell proliferates to form approximately 10 billion or more cells, normal hematopoiesis is inhibited, and normal red cell, neutrophil, and platelet blood levels fall. The resultant anemia leads to weakness, exertional limitations, and pallor; the thrombocytopenia to spontaneous hemorrhage, usually in the skin; and the neutropenia and monocytopenia to poor wound healing and minor infections. Severe infection usually does not occur at diagnosis but will if the disease progresses because of lack of treatment or if chemotherapy intensifies the decrease of neutrophil and monocyte blood cell levels. The diagnosis is made by measurement of blood cell counts and examination of blood and marrow cells and is based on identification of leukemic blast cells in the marrow and blood. The diagnosis of AML specifically is confirmed by identification of myeloperoxidase activity in blast cells and by identifying characteristic cluster of differentiation (CD) antigens on the blast cells (e.g., CD13, CD33). The leukemic stem cell is capable of imperfect differentiation and maturation. The clone may contain cells that have the morphologic or immunophenotypic features of erythroblasts, megakaryocytes, monocytes, eosinophils, or rarely basophils in addition to myeloblasts or promyelocytes. When one cell line is sufficiently dominant, the leukemia may be referred to as acute erythroblastic, acute megakaryocytic, acute monocytic, and so on. Certain cytogenetic alterations are more frequent and include t(8;21), t(15;17), inversion 16, trisomy 8, and deletions of all or part of chromosome 5 or 7. A translocation involving chromosome 17 at the site of the retinoic acid receptor alpha (RAR-α) gene is uniquely associated with acute promyelocytic leukemia. AML usually is treated with cytarabine and an anthracycline antibiotic, although other drugs may be added or substituted in poor-prognosis, refractory, or relapsed patients. The exception to this approach is the treatment of acute promyelocytic leukemia with all-*trans*-retinoic acid and an anthracycline antibiotic. High-dose chemotherapy and either autologous stem cell infusion or allogeneic stem cell transplantation may be used in an effort to treat relapse or patients at high risk to relapse after chemotherapy treatment. The probability of remission ranges from approximately 80 percent in children to less than 25 percent in octogenarians. The probability for cure decreases from approximately 40 percent in children to virtually zero in octogenarians.

DEFINITION AND HISTORY

Acute myelogenous leukemia (AML) is a clonal, malignant disease of hematopoietic tissue that is characterized by (1) accumulation of abnormal (leukemic) blast cells, principally in the marrow, and (2) impaired production of normal blood cells. Thus, the leukemic cell infiltration in marrow is accompanied, nearly invariably, by anemia and thrombocytopenia. The absolute neutrophil count may be low or normal, depending on the total white cell count.

The first well-documented case of acute leukemia is attributed to Friedreich,[1] but Ebstein[2] was the first to use the term *acute leukämie* in 1889. This work led to the general appreciation of the clinical distinctions between AML and chronic myelogenous leukemia (CML).[3] In 1878, Neumann,[4] who proposed that marrow was the site of blood cell production, first suggested that leukemia originated in the marrow and used the term *myelogene* (myelogenous) leukemia. The availability of polychromatic stains, as a result of the work of Ehrlich,[5] the description of the myeloblast and myelocyte by Naegeli,[6] and the earliest appreciation of the common origin of red cells and leukocytes by Hirschfield[7] laid the foundation for our current understanding of the disease.

Although Theodor Boveri proposed a critical role for chromosomal abnormalities in the development of cancer in 1914, a series of technical developments in the 1950s was needed to permit informed examination of the chromosomes of cancer cells. Thereafter, the discovery that a G group chromosome was short, consistently, in CML (Philadelphia chromosome) supported the concept that chromosome abnormalities may be specifically linked to a cancer phenotype. This finding was followed by the introduction of banding of chromosomes, which enhanced the identification of individual chromosomes and the point at which they break in the formation of a translocation or deletion. This technologic advance unleashed the power of cancer cytogenetics and initiated an era of leukemia study based not solely on the appearance of cells under the microscope (phenotype) but also by their chromosomal or genic abnormality (genotype).[8] The completion of the major phase of the human genome project further enhanced the specificity of the identification of gene alterations.[9] These advances permitted (1) more precise understanding of the molecular pathology of specific leukemia subtypes, (2) improvement of diagnostic and prognostic methods for the study of AML, and (3) identification of molecular targets for therapy.

The introduction to the clinic by Holland, Ellison, and colleagues[10] of arabinosyl cytosine (cytarabine) in the late 1960s as the first potent drug for treatment of AML, followed by their introduction of the combination of 7 days of cytosine arabinoside and 3 days of daunomycin in the early 1970s (the "7 and 3 regimen")[11] opened the era of effective therapy for AML. This drug combination or its congeners remains the mainstay of treatment 3 decades later. The description of allogeneic marrow (stem cell) transplantation as a curative therapy for AML by Thomas and colleagues[12] in 1977 ushered in the era of stem cell transplantation as a modality to cure eligible patients with AML.

ETIOLOGY AND PATHOGENESIS

ENVIRONMENTAL FACTORS

Table 87-1 lists the major conditions that predispose to subsequent development of AML. Only three well-documented environmental factors are established causal agents: high-dose external low-linear energy transfer radiation exposure,[13,14] chronic benzene exposure,[15-18] and chemotherapeutic agents.[19-24] Most patients have not been exposed to an antecedent causative factor. Exposure to high linear energy transfer radiation from α-emitting radioisotopes such as thorium dioxide

TABLE 87-1 CONDITIONS PEDISPOSING TO DEVELOPMENT OF ACUTE MYELOGENOUS LEUKEMIA

Environmental Factors
Radiation[13,14,25]
Benzene[15-18]
Alkylating agents and other cytotoxic drugs[19-24]
Tobacco smoke[27,28]
Acquired Diseases
Clonal myeloid diseases
  Chronic myelogenous leukemia (Chap. 88)
  Idiopathic myelofibrosis (Chap. 89)
  Primary thrombocythemia (Chap. 111)
  Polycythemia vera (Chap. 56)
  Clonal cytopenias (Chap. 86)
  Paroxysmal nocturnal hemoglobinuria (Chap. 38)
Other hematopoietic disorders
  Aplastic anemia (Chap. 33)
  Eosinophilic fasciitis (Chap. 86)
  Myeloma[31,32]
Inherited Conditions
Sibling with AML[36-38]
Amegakaryocytic thrombocytopenia, congenital[39,40]
Ataxia-pancytopenia[41,42]
Bloom syndrome[43,44]
Congenital agranulocytosis (Kostmann syndrome)[45-48]
Diamond-Blackfan syndrome[49,50]
Down syndrome[51,52]
Dubowitz syndrome[53]
Dyskeratosis congenita[54,55]
Pure (nonsyndromic) familial AML[56]
Familial platelet disorder[57,58]
Fanconi anemia[59,60]
Naxos syndrome[61]
Neurofibromatosis 1[62,63]
Noonan syndrome[64,65]
Poland syndrome[66]
Rothmund-Thomson syndrome[67,68]
Seckel syndrome[69]
Shwachman syndrome[70-72]
Werner syndrome (progeria)[73-75]
Wolf-Hirschhorn syndrome[76]
WT syndrome[77]

increases the risk of AML.[25] Case control studies have sometimes found a relationship between AML and organic solvents, petroleum products, radon exposure, pesticides, and herbicides, but these data have not reached the level of the strong association that exists for benzene, high-dose external irradiation, and certain chemotherapeutic agents.[26] The predominance of studies, but not all, has suggested an association between cigarette smoking and AML.[27,28] Maternal alcohol use has been associated with AML in infancy.[29]

EVOLUTION FROM A CHRONIC CLONAL HEMOPATHY

AML may develop from the progression of other clonal disorders of a multipotential hematopoietic cell, including CML, polycythemia vera, idiopathic myelofibrosis, primary thrombocythemia, and clonal sideroblastic anemia or oligoblastic myelogenous leukemia (see Table 87-1). Clonal progression can occur spontaneously, although with a different probability of occurrence in each chronic disorder (see Chap. 85). The frequency of clonal progression to AML is enhanced by radiation or chemotherapy in patients with polycythemia vera (see Chap. 56) or essential thrombocythemia (see Chap. 111).[23,30]

PREDISPOSING DISEASES

Patients who develop AML may have an antecedent predisposing nonmyeloid disease, such as aplastic anemia (polyclonal T cell disorder), myeloma (monoclonal B cell disorder),[31,32] or, rarely, AIDS (HIV-induced polyclonal T cell disorder).[33] An association between immune thyroid diseases and familial polyendocrine disorder and AML has been suggested.[34,35] A number of inherited conditions carry an increased risk of AML (see Table 87-1).[36-77] In the inherited syndromes, at least three pathogenetic types of gene alterations are represented: (1) DNA repair defects, e.g., Fanconi anemia, (2) susceptibility genes favoring a second mutation, e.g., familial platelet syndrome, (3) tumor suppressor defects, e.g., dyskeratosis congenita, and (4) unknown mechanisms, e.g., ataxia-pancytopenia (see Chap. 33 and reference 46 for further details of each pathogenetic condition).

MOLECULAR PATHOGENESIS

AML results from a series of somatic mutations in either a hematopoietic multipotential cell or, occasionally, a more differentiated, lineage-restricted progenitor cell.[78] Some cases of monocytic leukemia, promyelocytic leukemia, and AML in younger individuals more likely arise in a progenitor cell with lineage restrictions (progenitor cell leukemia).[78-82] Other morphologic phenotypes and older patients likely have disease that originates in a primitive multipotential cell.[78] In the latter case, all blood cell lineages can be derived from the leukemic stem cell because it retains the ability for some degree of differentiation and maturation (see Chap. 85).

Somatic mutation results from a chromosomal translocation in the majority of patients.[83] The translocation results in rearrangement of a critical region of a protooncogene. Fusion of portions of two genes usually does not prevent the processes of transcription and translation; thus, the fusion gene encodes a fusion protein that, because of its abnormal structure, disrupts a normal cell pathway and predisposes to a malignant transformation of the cell. The mutant protein product often is a transcription factor or element in the transcription pathway that disrupts the regulatory sequences controlling growth rate or survival of blood cell progenitors and differentiation and maturation.[83-85] Examples of genes often mutated are core binding factor, retinoic acid receptor (RAR), HOX family, MLL, and others. Core binding factor has two subunits: CBF-β and AML1. Approximately 10 percent of AML cases have translocations involving one or the other of these latter two genes, although the percentage varies depending on the patient's age at onset. In patients younger than 50 years, the frequency is approximately 20 percent. In patients older than 50 years, the frequency is approximately 6 percent. Core binding factor activates genes involved in myeloid and lymphoid differentiation and maturation. These primary mutations are not sufficient to cause AML. Additional activating mutations, for example, in hematopoietic tyrosine kinases FLT3 and Kit or in N-*ras* and K-*ras*, are required to induce a proliferative advantage in the affected primitive cell.[85] Other protooncogene mutations occur in leukemic cells involving *FES, FOS, GATA-1, JUN B, MPL, MYC*, p53, *PU.1, RB, WT1, WNT*, and other genes.[86–95] Their interaction with loss-of-function mutations in hematopoietic transcription factors probably causes the acute leukemia phenotype characterized by disordered proliferation, programmed cell death, differentiation, and maturation.[85] A minimum of two classes of genes has been proposed: class I gene mutations, e.g., *AML1*, which lead to a proliferation and survival advantage to the cells in the clone, and class II gene mutations, e.g., core binding factor, which interacts with the class I mutation, conferring severely disturbed differentiation and maturation patterns on the mutated cell and fostering the evolution of a classic AML phenotype.[85] Because the mutant stem or early progenitor cell can proliferate and retains the capability to differentiate, a wide variety of phenotypes can emerge from a leukemic transformation.

FLT3 encodes a tyrosine kinase receptor in normal myeloid and lymphoid progenitors. Internal tandem duplications of *FLT3* on chromosome 13 occurs in approximately one fourth to one third of adult AML cases but occur more frequently in cases of AML with normal cytogenetic patterns, monocytic phenotype, and *PML-RAR-α* or *DEK-CAN* translocations. The *FLT3-ITD* mutation confers a poor prognosis if the ratio of mutant to wild-type expression is high.[96,97] Hypermethylation of the death-associated protein kinase has been observed in approximately 25 percent of AML cases and is twice as prevalent in cases of AML following cytotoxic therapy. Deletions of all or part of a chromosome (e.g., chromosome 5, 7, or 9) or additional chromosomes (such as trisomy 4, 8, or 13) are common cytogenetic abnormalities (see Chap. 10), although the specific causative oncogenes or tumor suppressor genes in these latter circumstances have not been defined. Deletions in chromosomes 5 and 7 and complex cytogenetics abnormalities are increased in frequency in older patients and cases of AML following cytotoxic therapy compared to *de novo* cases.[98] Because the genes residing on the undeleted homologous segment of chromosome 5 are not mutated, an epigenetic lesion, such as hypermethylation of a gene allelic to one on the deleted segment on chromosome 5, may result in the leukemogenic event.

In acute promyelocytic leukemia, *PML-RAR-α* fusion protein represses retinoic acid-inducible genes, which prevent appropriate maturation of promyelocytes. The induced disruption, which involves corepressor–histone deacetylase complexes, results in the leukemic phenotype (see "Acute Promyelocytic Leukemia" below).[99,100]

MODE OF INHERITANCE

In most cases, little evidence is seen for a strong influence of genetic factors. The identical twin of a child with acute leukemia has a heightened risk of developing the disease. However, the risk appears to be related to intraplacental metastasis and thus falls to the risk of a nonidentical sibling after the first few years of life.[101,102] The risk of AML in a nonidentical sibling in the United States is elevated, perhaps twofold to threefold compared to the risk of AML in unrelated American children of European descent younger than 15 years.[101,103] Clusters of AML cases in families have been documented, but their frequency is rare.[56] Clusters of AML in unrelated persons in a community are uncommon and, when investigated, usually prove to be a chance occurrence.

EPIDEMIOLOGY

AML is the predominant form of leukemia during the neonatal period but represents a small proportion of cases during childhood and adolescence. Approximately 11,000 new cases of AML occur annually, representing approximately 35 percent of the annual new cases of leukemia in the United States. Approximately 8000 patients with AML in the United States die each year as a result of the disease. The mortality rate from AML is approximately 0.5 per 100,000 persons younger than 10 years and increases progressively until the rate reaches approximately 20 per 100,000 persons in their 90s. The exception to this exponential age-related increase in incidence is APL, which does not change in incidence with age over the human life span.[104]

AML accounts for 15 to 20 percent of the acute leukemias in children and 80 percent of the acute leukemias in adults. It is slightly more common in males. Little difference in incidence is seen between individuals of African or European descent at any age. A somewhat lower incidence is seen in persons of Asian descent. An increase in the frequency of AML is seen in Jews, especially those of Eastern European descent. Acute promyelocytic variant of AML is somewhat more frequent in persons of Spanish descent.[105,106]

CLASSIFICATION

Variants of AML can be identified by morphologic features of blood films using polychromatic stains and histochemical reactions,[107] monoclonal antibodies against surface markers,[107–112] or by the presence of specific chromosome translocations.[113] The epitopes on the progenitor cells of several phenotypic variants overlap, and several monoclonal antibodies are required to make specific distinctions among cell types (Table 87-2; see also "Morphologic Variants of Acute Myelogenous Leukemia" below and Table 87-4). Correlation between morphologic and immunologic phenotyping of AML is poor. However, poor correlation is expected because the former method is more subjective, given to observer variation, and is based on qualitative factors, whereas the latter method, which characterizes surface molecular features, is more accurate and reproducible. The correlation is improved only somewhat if morphology and histochemistry are coupled.[114] Gene expression profiling is in its infancy as a classification technique for AML but may prove to be more specific and informative than current methods.[115,116] The outcome will depend on the simplification and automation of such techniques, and the availability of drugs that make such distinctions in the prognostic category of practical utility. Chapter 85 contains the classification of morphologic variants of AML (see Table 85-1 and Fig. 85-2). The need to consider functional markers for drug resistance, such as *MDR* expression, has been proposed to separate more responsive from less responsive AML. However, a cogent argument has been made that, for practical purposes, a classification that initially considers morphologic phenotype and immunophenotype is

TABLE 87-2 IMMUNOLOGIC PHENOTYPES OF AML

	USUALLY POSITIVE
Myeloblastic	CD11, CD13, CD15, CD33, CD117, HLA-DR
Myelomonocytic	CD11, CD13, CD14, CD15, CD32, CD33, HLA-DR
Erythroblastic	Glycophorin, spectrin, ABH antigens, carbonic anhydrase I, HLA-DR
Promyelocytic	CD11, CD13, CD15, CD33
Monocytic	CD11, CD13, CD14, CD33, HLA-DR
Megakaryoblastic	CD34, CD41, CD42, CD61, von Willebrand factor

NOTE: Chapter 14 provides the definition of the antigen that represents a cluster of differentiation (CD).

advisable. Cytogenetics, molecular genetics, gene expression profiling, *MDR* expression, and other considerations can be layered on as available and necessary.[117] This method avoids the problems of the World Health Organization (WHO) classification (see Chap. 85), which has included epiphenomenology based on little justification and overlapping (redundant) cytogenetic and morphologic entries.

CLINICAL FEATURES

SIGNS AND SYMPTOMS

GENERAL

Signs and symptoms that signal the onset of AML include pallor, fatigue, weakness, palpitations, and dyspnea on exertion. The signs and symptoms reflect the development of anemia; however, weakness, loss of sense of well-being, and fatigue on exertion can be out of proportion to the severity of anemia.[118–122]

Easy bruising, petechiae, epistaxis, gingival bleeding, conjunctival hemorrhages, and prolonged bleeding from skin injuries reflect thrombocytopenia and are frequent early manifestations of the disease. Very infrequently, gastrointestinal, genitourinary, bronchopulmonary, or central nervous system (CNS) bleeding occurs at the onset of disease.

Pustules or other minor pyogenic infections of the skin and of minor cuts or wounds are most common. Major infections, such as sinusitis, pneumonia, pyelonephritis, and meningitis, are uncommon presenting features of the disease, partly because absolute neutrophil counts less than $500/\mu l$ (0.5×10^9/liter) are uncommon until chemotherapy starts. With intensification of neutropenia and monocytopenia after chemotherapy, major bacterial, fungal, or viral infections become frequent. Anorexia and weight loss are frequent findings. Fever is present in many patients at the time of diagnosis.[121,123–125] Palpable splenomegaly or hepatomegaly occurs in approximately one third of patients.[118,119,122] Lymphadenopathy is extremely uncommon,[122,126,127] except in the monocytic variant of AML.[128]

SPECIFIC ORGAN SYSTEM INVOLVEMENT

Leukemic blast cells circulate and enter most tissues in small numbers.[129] Occasionally, biopsy or autopsy uncovers marked aggregates or infiltrates of leukemic cells. Collections of such cells may cause functional disturbances. Extramedullary involvement is most common in monocytic or myelomonocytic leukemia.

Skin involvement may be of three types: nonspecific lesions, leukemia cutis, or granulocytic (myeloid) sarcoma of skin and subcutis.[130–135] Nonspecific lesions include macules, papules, vesicles, pyoderma gangrenosum, vasculitis,[136–138] neutrophilic dermatitis (Sweet syndrome),[139] cutis vertices gyrata,[140] and erythema multiforme or nodosum.[130,131] Skin involvement preceding marrow and blood involvement is rare.[135,141]

Sensory organ involvement is very unusual, but retinal, choroidal, iridial, and optic nerve infiltration can occur.[142] Otitis externa and interna, inner ear hemorrhage, and mastoid tumors with seventh nerve involvement may be presenting signs.[143–145]

The *gastrointestinal tract* may be involved at any point, but functional disturbances are unusual.[146,147] The mouth, colon, and anal canal are sites of involvement that most commonly lead to symptoms. Oral manifestations may prompt the patient to visit the dentist. Gingival or periodontal infiltration and dental abscesses may lead to an extraction, followed by prolonged bleeding of an infected tooth socket.[148] Ileotyphlitis (enterocolitis), a necrotizing inflammatory lesion involving the terminal ileum, cecum, and ascending colon, can be a presenting syndrome or occur during treatment.[149–151] Fever, abdominal pain, bloody diarrhea, or ileus may be present and occasionally mimic appendicitis. Intestinal perforation, an inflammatory mass, and associated infection with enteric gram-negative bacilli or clostridial species often

are associated with a fatal outcome. Isolated involvement of the gastrointestinal tract is rare.[152,153] Proctitis, especially common in the monocytic variant of AML, can be a presenting sign or a vexing problem during periods of severe granulocytopenia and diarrhea.[146]

The *respiratory tract* can be involved by infiltrates or tumors, leading to laryngeal obstruction, parenchymal infiltrates, alveolar septal infiltration, or pleural seeding. Each of these events can result in severe symptoms and radiologic findings.[154–158]

Cardiac involvement is frequent but rarely causes symptoms. Symptomatic pericardial infiltrates, transmural ventricular infiltrates with hemorrhage, and endocardial foci with associated intracavitary thrombi can occasionally cause heart failure, arrhythmia, and death.[159] Infiltration of the conducting system or valve leaflets or myocardial infarction has occurred.[160]

The *urogenital system* can be affected. The kidneys are infiltrated with leukemic cells in a high proportion of cases, but functional abnormalities are rare. Hemorrhage in the pelvis or collecting system is frequent.[161,162] Cases of vulvar, bladder neck, prostatic, or testicular involvement have been described.[163–165]

Osteoarticular symptoms may occur. Bone pain, joint pain, and bone necrosis can occur, and rarely arthritis with effusion is present.[166] Crystal-induced arthritis of either calcium pyrophosphate dihydrate (pseudogout) or monosodium urate (gout) may be responsible for the synovitis in some cases.[167]

Central or peripheral *nervous system* involvement by infiltration of leukemic cells is very uncommon, although meningeal involvement is an important consideration in the treatment of the monocytic type of AML.[168,169] An association of CNS involvement and diabetes insipidus in AML with monosomy 7[170] and inversion of chromosome 16[171,172] has been reported.

MYELOID (GRANULOCYTIC) SARCOMA

Myeloid sarcoma (also known as granulocytic sarcoma, chloroma, myeloblastoma, monocytoma) is a tumor composed of myeloblasts, monoblasts, or megakaryocytes.[173–178] The tumors may occur as extramedullary masses without evidence of leukemia in blood or marrow, so-called non-leukemic myeloid sarcomas, or in association with AML. When the tumors appear as isolated lesions, they very frequently are diagnosed as extranodal lymphoma because they look like lymphoid cells on biopsy.[175] They may be found in virtually any location, including the skin; orbit; paranasal sinuses; bone; chest wall; breast; gastrointestinal, respiratory, or genitourinary tract; central or peripheral nervous system; or lymph nodes. The tumors originally were called *chloromas* because of the green color imparted by the high concentration of the enzyme myeloperoxidase present in myelogenous leukemic cells. Biopsy specimens are positive for chloracetate esterase, lysozyme, myeloperoxidase, and cluster of differentiation (CD) markers of myeloid cells. When myeloid sarcomas are the initial manifestation of AML, the appearance of the disease in the blood and marrow may follow weeks or months later. Abnormalities in chromosome 8 are the most frequent cytogenetic disturbance in nonleukemic sarcomas.[178] Systemic chemotherapy, rather than local therapy, should be used for treatment, although the outcome in such cases usually is poor.[178,179] Patients having AML with t(8;21) have a propensity to develop extramedullary leukemia,[180–183] and such patients with myeloid sarcomas have a poorer outcome after treatment.[180,182]

LABORATORY FEATURES

BLOOD CELL FINDINGS

Anemia is a constant feature.[118–122] Red cell life span may be mildly shortened, but the principal cause of anemia is inadequate production of red cells. The reticulocyte count usually is between 0.5 and 2.0

percent. Occasionally patients have rapid destruction of autologous and transfused red cells as a result of an unknown mechanism (milieu hemolysis). The presence of red cell autoantibodies (positive Coombs test) is very uncommon and may be nonspecific (anti-C_3), perhaps related to circulating immune complexes. Red cell morphology is mildly abnormal, with exaggerated variation in cell size and occasional poikilocytes. Nucleated red cells or stippled erythrocytes may be present. Less often, extreme abnormalities of red cell size, shape, and hemoglobin content occur, but these changes are seen more often in oligoblastic myelogenous leukemia (see Chap. 86).

Thrombocytopenia is nearly always present at the time of diagnosis. The mechanism of thrombocytopenia is a combination of inadequate production and decreased survival of platelets. More than half of patients have a platelet count less than 50,000/μl (50 × 10⁹/liter) at the time of diagnosis.[184] Giant platelets and poorly granulated platelets with functional abnormalities can occur.[185] Defects in platelet aggregation and 5-hydroxytryptamine release are frequent.[185]

The total leukocyte count is less than 5000/μl (5 × 10⁹/liter) in approximately half of patients at the time of diagnosis.[118–122] The absolute neutrophil count is less than 1000/μl (1 × 10⁹/liter) in more than half of cases at diagnosis.[118–122] Patients with very elevated total leukocyte counts have a low proportion of mature neutrophils but may have a normal absolute neutrophil count. Hypersegmented, hyposegmented, and hypogranular mature neutrophils may be present. Cytochemical abnormalities of blood neutrophils include low or absent myeloperoxidase or low alkaline phosphatase activity.[186] Defects in phagocytosis or microbial killing are common.[187]

Myeloblasts almost always are present in the blood but may be infrequent in leukopenic patients. Diligent search may uncover the myeloblasts, or examination of a white cell concentrate (buffy coat) may permit their identification. Classic leukemic blast cells are agranular, but mixtures of immature cells, including agranular and slightly granular cells ranging up to overt progranulocytes, can occur. Auer rods are elliptical cytoplasmic inclusions approximately 1.5 μm long and 0.5 μm wide that derive from azurophilic granules (see Chap. 59). The inclusions are present in the blast cells of approximately 15 percent of cases. When present, the inclusions are found in only a small percentage of blast cells when examined with polychrome stains.[107,188] An exception is acute promyelocytic leukemia (APL), in which a high proportion of cells have Auer rods and some have multiple (bundles) of rods. This finding can be dramatic if peroxidase stain is used to highlight the Auer rods.

MARROW FINDINGS

MORPHOLOGY

The marrow always contains leukemic blast cells. From 3 to 95 percent of marrow cells are blasts at the time of diagnosis or relapse (see Color Plates XVI and XVII). The WHO has invoked an arbitrary breakpoint of 20 percent of marrow nucleated cells being blast cells to distinguish polyblastic AML (>20% blasts) from oligoblastic myelogenous leukemia (<20% blasts).[118–122,188] The latter situation is referred to as refractory anemia with excess blasts, a myelodysplastic syndrome (see Chap. 86). Myeloblasts are distinguished from lymphoblasts by any of three pathognomonic features: reactivity with specific histochemical stains; Auer rods in the cells; or reactivity with a panel of monoclonal antibodies against epitopes present on myeloblasts (e.g., CD13, CD33). Leukemic myeloblasts give positive histochemical reactions for peroxidase, Sudan black B, or naphthyl AS-D-chloroacetate esterase stains. Auer rods can be found in the marrow blast cells in approximately one sixth of cases. Blast cells express granulocytic or monocytic surface antigens. They typically do not express either lymphoid surface markers or membrane or cytoplasmic immunoglobulin. No immunoglobulin gene rearrangement or T lymphocyte receptor

gene rearrangement is evident with molecular probes (see "Hybrid and Mixed Leukemias" below). In a proportion of otherwise typical cases of AML, the cells may contain terminal deoxynucleotidyl transferase (TdT).[189,190] Variations in marrow findings are discussed further below in "Morphologic Variants of Acute Myelogenous Leukemia." Normal erythropoiesis, megakaryocytopoiesis, and granulopoiesis are decreased or absent in the marrow aspirate. The biopsy may contain residual islands of erythroblasts or megakaryocytes. Dysmorphic changes in hematopoietic cells, including very small or large erythroblasts with nuclear fragmentation or binucleation or delayed nuclear condensation; small or monolobed megakaryocytes; or hypogranulated, bilobed, or monolobed neutrophils, may occur in 30 to 50 percent of patients with de novo AML.[191] Marrow reticulin fibrosis is common but usually is slight to moderate except in cases of megakaryoblastic leukemia, in which intense fibrosis is the rule.[192] Increased blood vessel density (angiogenesis) has been demonstrated in the marrow of patients with AML compared to normal subjects.[193,194] Various angiogenic factors, including vascular endothelial growth factor (VEGF), basic fibroblast growth factor, angiogenin, and angiopoietin-1, are increased. VEGF detected histochemically in human marrow is closely correlated with the prevalence of leukemic myeloblasts in the various AML subtypes.[195]

MARROW CELL CULTURE

Progenitor cells for granulocytes, monocytes and macrophages, or both granulocytes and macrophages form colonies when normal marrow cells are grown in a viscous medium with a source of growth factors. Marrow cells from patients with AML have heterogeneous growth patterns. The marrow of approximately 85 percent of patients does not have colony-forming cells, but the marrow of 60 percent of patients has cells capable of forming small clusters (4–40 cells) in vitro. Approximately 15 percent of patients retain colony-forming cells but often in reduced numbers and with abnormal maturation patterns.[196,197] Restoration of colony-forming cells in the marrow of treated patients often precedes morphologic evidence of remission.[198] The correlation of pretreatment marrow colonial growth pattern in vitro with the outcome of intensive chemotherapy is not sufficiently strong to use growth pattern as a prognostic variable.[199]

CYTOGENETIC FEATURES

An abnormal number (aneuploidy) or structure (pseudodiploidy) of chromosomes or both are readily evident in approximately 75 percent of cases.[200–203] The most prevalent abnormalities are trisomy 8, monosomy 7, monosomy 21, trisomy 21, and loss of an X or Y chromosome. However, almost any chromosome can be rearranged, added, or lost. In cases of AML following chemotherapy or radiotherapy, loss of part or all of chromosome 5 is a common feature,[204–206] as are the cytogenetic findings noted above for AML, occurring de novo. Table 87-3 lists the most frequent abnormalities and translocations seen in AML (see Chap. 10). The translocations 8;21, 15;17, and inversion 16 confer a more favorable outcome on average. Deletion of all or part of chromosomes 5 and 7 or the presence of complex changes confers an unfavorable prognosis. Other abnormalities (e.g., normal karyotype, +8, 11q23) generally confer an intermediate prognosis.[200–202]

PLASMA CHEMICAL FINDINGS

Prior to treatment, mild to moderate increases in serum uric acid and lactic dehydrogenase levels are frequent. Both levels are higher in myelomonocytic and monocytic AML than in other AML phenotypes.[121,122] Occasional patients have very elevated uric acid levels, which usually occur after chemotherapy if proper precautions are not taken (e.g., hypouricosuric agents and hydration therapy).[224] Abnormalities of sodium, potassium, calcium, or hydrogen ion concentration are infrequent and usually mild.[225,226] Severe hyponatremia associated

TABLE 87-3   CLINICAL CORRELATES OF FREQUENT CYTOGENETIC ABNORMALITIES OBSERVED IN AML

CHROMOSOME ABNORMALITY	GENES AFFECTED	CLINICAL CORRELATION
Loss or Gain of Chromosome	Not defined	Frequent in patients with AML occurring *de novo* and in patients with history of chemical, drug, or radiation exposure and/or previous hematologic disease.[200,201,204,205]
Deletions of part or all of chromosome 5 or 7		
Trisomy 8	Not defined	Very common abnormality in acute myeloblastic leukemia. Poor prognosis, often a secondary change.[201,207]
Translocation		
t(8;21) (q22;q22)	*AML1(RUNX1) –ETO*	Present in ~8% of patients <50 years and in 3% of patients >50 years with AML[206]; associated with loss of Y in males or loss of X in females in more than half the cases. Present in ~40% of myelomonocytic phenotype. High frequency of myeloid sarcomas.[180–183]
t(15;17) (q31; q22)	*PML-RAR-α*	Represents ~6% of cases of AML.[206] Translocation involving chromosome 17, t(15;17), (11;17), or t(5;17) is present in most cases of promyelocytic leukemia.[99,100,208,209]
t(9;11); (p22; q23)	*ALL1 (MLL)–AF9*	Present in ~7% of cases of AML.[210–214] Associated with monocytic leukemia.[211–212] 11q23 translocations in 60% of infants with AML and carries poor prognosis. Rearranges *ALL1 (MLL)* gene.[210–214] Many translocation partners (~20) for 11q23 translocation.[213–216]
t(9;22) (q34; q22)	*BCR–ABL*	Present in ~3% of patients with AML[217,218] (see Chap. 88).
Inversion		
Inv (16)	*CBF-βMYH11*	Present in ~8% of patients <50 years and in ~3% of patients >50 years of age with AML[206]; may be in the form of t(16;16); associated with increased marrow eosinophils; predisposition to cervical lymphadenopathy,[219] better response to therapy.[220–223]

with inappropriate antidiuretic hormone secretion has occurred at presentation.[225,226] Severe hypernatremia as a consequence of diabetes insipidus can be an initial event.[227] Hypokalemia is a more frequent finding at presentation and is related to kaliuresis, although the reason for the proximal renal tubular dysfunction is unclear.[225,226,228] The hypokalemia can be severe and often is worsened by the effects of treatment, especially use of kaliuretic antibiotics.[228] Factitious elevations in serum potassium levels have been reported in patients with hyperleukocytosis as a result of leakage from white cells *in vitro*.[229,230] Factitious hypoglycemia and spurious hypoxia from the effects of high blast cell counts can occur.[227,231]

Hypercalcemia can occur. The pathogenesis probably is multifactorial,[232] but cases with increased ectopic parathormone-like activity in the plasma have been described.[233] Severe lactic acidosis prior to treatment has been reported.[225,234,235] Hypophosphatemia as a result of phosphate uptake by leukemic cells can occur.[236] Ectopic adrenocorticotropic hormone secretion,[237] circulating immune complexes,[238] and abnormal concentrations of coagulation factors or their inhibitors[239] may be present.

Although prothrombin and partial thromboplastin times usually are normal or near normal, abnormal concentrations of coagulation factors are frequent. Elevations of platelet factor 4 and thromboxane B_2 occur often.[240] Decreases in $α_2$-antiplasmin, protein C, and antithrombin III levels are frequent[240] and may be associated with venous thrombosis.[241] Acute promyelocytic and acute monocytic leukemia are associated with hypofibrinogenemia and other indicators of activation of coagulation or fibrinolysis[242] (see "Morphologic Variants of Acute Myelogenous Leukemia" below).

The levels of the shed form of L-selectin[243] and anticardiolipin antibodies[244] in plasma frequently are elevated. The levels of soluble VEGF receptor-1 (VEGFR-1) and VEGFR-2 are elevated in the plasma of patients with AML. The ratio of soluble VEGFR-1 to VEGF correlates with greater leukemic blast cell burden and with less favorable outcome.[245]

SPECIAL CLINICAL FEATURES

HYPERLEUKOCYTOSIS

Approximately 5 percent of patients with AML develop signs or symptoms attributable to a markedly elevated blood blast cell count, usually

greater than $100 × 10^9$/liter[246] (see Chap. 85). The circulations of the CNS, lungs, and penis are most sensitive to the effects of leukostasis. Intracerebral hemorrhage from vascular occlusion, invasion, and disruption, sometimes complicated by thrombocytopenia and vascular insufficiency, sometimes with hemorrhage, are the most virulent manifestations of the syndrome.[247–251] Dizziness, stupor, dyspnea, and priapism may occur.[246–251] Diabetes insipidus is another association.[252,253] A high early mortality in patients with AML correlates with hyperleukocytosis greater than $100 × 10^9$/liter.[249–251] Chemotherapy in hyperleukocytic patients may lead to a pulmonary leukostatic syndrome, presumably from the effects of rigid, effete blast cells or the discharge of large amounts of cell contents and resultant cell aggregation or other effects.[254–256] Larger-vessel vascular occlusion as a result of white thrombi or masses of leukemic cells is very rare.[257–261]

HYPOPLASTIC LEUKEMIA

Approximately 10 percent of patients with AML present with a syndrome that includes pancytopenia, often with inapparent blood blast cells, and absence of hepatic, splenic, or lymph nodal enlargement.[262–264] Approximately 75 percent of these patients are men older than 50 years. Marrow biopsy is hypocellular, which is the unusual feature of the syndrome, but leukemic blast cells are evident and present in a proportion of 15 to 90 percent of marrow cells. Response to intensive chemotherapeutic treatment, often with low-dose cytarabine because of the patients' very high median age, has been relatively good, and 3-year survival rates are approximately the same as the rates of other age-matched patients.[265]

OLIGOBLASTIC (SMOLDERING) LEUKEMIA

In approximately 10 percent of cases, usually in patients older than 50 years, myelogenous leukemia is manifested by anemia and often thrombocytopenia. The leukocyte count may be low, normal, or increased, and a small proportion of blast cells are present in the blood (0–15%) and marrow (3–20%). Such cases have been referred to as *oligoblastic myelogenous leukemia* or *smoldering leukemia*[266–268] or classified as a myelodysplastic syndrome, particularly refractory anemia with excess blasts. The clinical course of the untreated disease can be protracted. The disease has a high morbidity and mortality from infection and hemorrhage and can evolve into overt (polyblastic)

AML. The smoldering or oligoblastic leukemias historically have been grouped with the clonal cytopenias as part of the myelodysplastic syndromes (refractory anemia with excess blasts); thus, the diagnosis and treatment of these variants are discussed in Chapter 86. Biologically and clinically, the disorders in this subset of the myelodysplastic syndrome with blast cell proportions in the marrow above normal are leukemias, not dysplasias, but they have a slower rate of progression than polyblastic myelogenous leukemia. Dysmorphogenesis of red cells, neutrophils, and platelets is more frequent and more striking than in the average case of polyblastic AML (see Chap. 86), but such dysmorphogenesis also occurs in polyblastic leukemia.[191]

NEONATAL MYELOPROLIFERATION AND LEUKEMIA

Four myeloproliferative syndromes related to AML have been identified in the neonate: transient myeloproliferative disorder, transient leukemia, congenital leukemia, and neonatal leukemia.

Transient myeloproliferative disease (TMD) can be present at birth or occur shortly thereafter in approximately 10 percent of infants with Down syndrome.[269–273] The leukocyte count is markedly elevated, blast cells are present in the blood and marrow, and anemia and thrombocytopenia may be present, but the latter are not constant findings. The liver and spleen may be enlarged. Results of cytogenetic studies and marrow cell culture studies are normal, except for trisomy 21, which is characteristic of Down syndrome. The blast cells usually have the phenotype of megakaryocytes. In contrast to congenital leukemia, the elevated white cell and blast cell counts often disappear over a period of weeks to months. In some cases, an additional cytogenetic abnormality is present, which disappears after regression of the myeloproliferative syndrome, suggesting a reversible clonal disorder (transient leukemia) that is replaced by normal hematopoiesis. The presence of trisomy chromosome 21 is essential for the disease as judged by three observations: the trisomy occurs in (1) the TMD clone of patients with constitutional trisomy chromosome 21, (2) the TMD clone in patients with Down syndrome with a cell mosaic pattern of trisomy 21, and (3) phenotypically normal infants without constitutional trisomy 21, but with TMD, in whom only the TMD clone carries trisomy 21. In the latter case, trisomy 21 disappears with resolution of the myeloproliferation.[274] Candidate oncogenes on chromosome 21 include *FPDMM*, *AML1(CBF-β)*, and *IFNAR*, among others.[274] *GATA-1* mutations have been found in nearly all patients with TMD and in acute megakaryocytic leukemia in Down patients.[275] The TMD syndrome may disappear, only to be followed shortly thereafter by acute leukemia, predominantly AML, but occasionally acute lymphocytic leukemia (ALL). One hypothesis for TMD is that the disorder originates in a primitive cell of fetal hepatic hematopoiesis. The cell involutes and is replaced with marrow stem cells. Approximately 25 percent of newborns with Down syndrome and transient leukemia develop acute megakaryocytic leukemia in the first 4 years of life.[276–278] Fatalities are associated with TMD. Very-low-dose cytarabine has been suggested for those patients with severe hepatic fibrosis, very high white cell counts, or hydrops fetalis.[274] TMD cells in these infants are very sensitive to cytarabine.[279,280]

Myelogenous leukemia in patients with Down syndrome often has a megakaryoblastic or erythroid phenotype and may have an interstitial deletion of chromosome 21.[271,272,281,282] The response rate of infants with Down syndrome and AML to chemotherapy has been very high over several years of followup and better than the response of patients without Down syndrome.[276,280,283,284] ALL may occur, and the response to therapy is similar to the response of patients without Down syndrome of the same age. Most solid tumors occur less frequently in Down syndrome patients.[279] Congenital or neonatal leukemia can occur in infants without Down syndrome, but this rare syndrome occurs

more than 10 times less frequently than in newborns with Down syndrome.[281,282] Leukocytosis, blood and marrow blast cells, hepatosplenomegaly, thrombocytopenia, purpura, anemia, and skin infiltrates are usual. The disease has been diagnosed prenatally. Cytogenetic abnormalities can occur and mark the leukemic clone.[282,285,286] Monocytic leukemia and t(4;11) are the most common phenotype and karyotype.[286–288] A case of vertical (transplacental) transmission of acute monocytic leukemia from mother to son has been reported.[289]

Infants who are normal at birth but develop AML in the first few weeks of life (neonatal leukemia) often display pallor, inadequate food intake, insufficient weight gain, diarrhea, and lethargy. The presence of a cytogenetic abnormality on band q23 of chromosome 11 is a very poor prognostic sign. Most infants with congenital or neonatal leukemia do not survive for more than a few weeks or months. Because treatment has been largely ineffective, observation to ascertain if TMD or a transient leukemia is present has been recommended if the clinical picture is unclear.[290]

HYBRID AND MIXED LEUKEMIAS

HYBRID LEUKEMIAS

Although coincidental myeloid and lymphoid clonal diseases have been reported for more than 30 years, the availability of techniques to identify surface antigens with monoclonal antibodies, immunoglobulin gene and T lymphocyte receptor gene rearrangements with molecular methods, and chromosome translocations by chromosome banding cytogenetic techniques has led to the appreciation of several types of hybrid acute leukemia.[291–299]

In bilineal (interlineal) acute leukemias, a proportion of cells (>10%) have lymphoid and myeloid markers; *interlineal* here refers to lymphocytic and hematopoietic gene expression. Bilineal (biphenotypic) leukemias are heterogeneous. Some patients have cells with both lymphoid and myeloid markers (chimeric), whereas other patients have cells with either lymphoid or myeloid markers but evidence that all the cells are part of the same malignant clone (mosaic). The bilineal leukemias may be synchronous (lymphoid and myeloid cells are present simultaneously) or asynchronous (in which lymphoid cells are succeeded by myeloid cells or vice versa), but evidence exists for their origin from the same clone.

Cases of biphenotypic leukemia that are morphologically or cytochemically indicative of myelogenous leukemia have been referred to as LY+AML; the cases that are more indicative of lymphocytic leukemia are referred to as MY+ALL. As a group, interlineal hybrid leukemias treated with current regimens respond to therapy at approximately the same rate as AML cases without lymphoid markers.[291] Some observers suggest altering drug regimens, depending on the balance between lymphoid and myeloid biochemical (drug-response) patterns.[300]

Acute leukemias may be intralineal hybrids in that the blast cells have markers for two or more myeloid lineages (e.g., erythroid, granulocytic, and megakaryocytic) or, in the case of lymphocytic leukemias, both immunoglobulin gene rearrangement (B lymphocyte type) and T cell receptor gene rearrangement (T lymphocyte type).

MYELOID–NATURAL KILLER CELL HYBRIDS AND T(8;13) MYELOID–LYMPHOID LEUKEMIAS

Although most hybrid leukemias share myeloid and either B or T lymphocyte markers, two notable syndromes are associated with hybrid leukemias: (1) the myeloid leukemia and natural killer cell hybrid (CD56+, CD7+, CD13, CD33+)[301–306] and (2) the lymphoma, eosinophilia, and t(8;13) myeloid leukemia hybrid.[307,308] Signs of lymphoma, such as mediastinal or other lymphadenopathy and extranodal lymphoid tumor, are mixed with findings compatible with AML in both syndromes. The morphology of the myeloid–natural killer cell leukemia often simulates APL, with hypergranular cytoplasm present but abnormality of chromosome 17 absent. The hybrids can appear *de novo* or after relapse of a lymphoma, T cell leukemia, or blast crisis of CML. The hybrid leukemias usually have a poor prognosis.

Hybrid leukemias may result from either lineage infidelity caused by genetic misprogramming[301] or promiscuous gene expression, which occurs transiently in the differentiation of normal pluripotential hematopoietic stem cells. In the case of promiscuity, persistence of the transient normal event is thought to be present because of the block in differentiation that occurs.[295,296] Genetic misprogramming (infidelity) could result from rearrangements of the DNA sequences that control the transcription of genes designating differentiation antigens.[309]

MIXED LEUKEMIAS

In these cases, lymphoid and myeloid cells are present simultaneously but are derived from separate clones, or sequential myeloid and lymphoid leukemia are present but the two lineages are derived from separate clones.

MEDIASTINAL GERM CELL TUMORS AND ACUTE MYELOGENOUS LEUKEMIA

An unusual but significant concordance has been reported between mediastinal germ cell tumors and AML, especially the megakaryoblastic variant.[310–314] Mediastinal tumors are rare variants of germ cell tumors. The latter ordinarily occur as testicular teratomas and seminomas in men or as ovarian teratomas in women. They are thought to be derived from yolk sac cells that failed to migrate.[313,314] AML is a hematopoietic stem cell tumor derived from a cell type that is present in the yolk sac. Cytogenetic studies are compatible with a clonal relationship (identity) of mediastinal germ cells and myelogenous leukemia cells.[311,312] Apparently, hematopoietic lineage genes are predisposed to expression in extragonadal (mediastinal) germ cell tumors. Recent use of etoposide, platinum, and related cytotoxic drugs for treatment of mediastinal germ cell tumors may induce secondary AML in a predisposed cell population.

MORPHOLOGIC VARIANTS OF ACUTE MYELOGENOUS LEUKEMIA

Morphologic variants of AML (Table 87-4) may occur *de novo* or may be the manifestation of clonal evolution from essential thrombocythemia, idiopathic myelofibrosis, CML, or other chronic clonal myeloid disorders. For example, every phenotypic variant of AML can occur as the blast crisis of CML (see Chap. 88).

MYELOBLASTIC LEUKEMIA

The designation *acute myeloblastic leukemia* came into existence in the second decade of the 20th century,[4] following the specific description of the myeloblast.[6] Approximately 30 percent of AML cases have the features of acute myeloblastic leukemia, a variant in which the leukemic myeloblast is the predominant cell in the marrow (see Color Plates XVI-1–3). Acute myeloblastic leukemia has been divided into two forms, designated *M0* and *M1* in the French-American-British (FAB) classification, which converts the descriptive term for a leukemic phenotype into a number. In either type, little evidence of maturation of myeloblasts exists, and the marrow is replaced by a monotonous population of blasts. In acute myeloblastic leukemia (M0), the patient's age distribution, presenting white cell count, and cytogenetic abnormalities are not distinctive. The blasts are nonreactive when stained for myeloperoxidase activity, and Auer rods are not seen. The blasts react with antibodies to myeloperoxidase and anti-

bodies to CD13, CD33, and CD34. Human leukocyte antigen (HLA)-DR is positive in most patients. Occasional cases require *in situ* hybridization to identify the myeloperoxidase gene[315] or genomic profiling for early myeloid-associated genes.[316] Abnormal and unfavorable karyotypes (e.g., 5q-,7q-) and higher expression of the multidrug resistance glycoprotein (p170) are more frequent. This phenotypic variant has a poor prognosis.[317–320] In the other type of myeloblastic leukemia, designated *M1*, myeloblasts are present in the blood and compose more than 70 percent of marrow cells. Less than 15 percent of marrow cells are promyelocytes and myelocytes. Auer rods may be present in occasional blasts, but azurophilic granules are not evident in the blasts by light microscopy (see Color Plate XVI-2). At least 3 percent, but usually a much higher percentage, of the blast cells have a positive reaction when stained for peroxidase or with Sudan black or react with monoclonal antibodies specific to myeloblasts, such as CD33. This morphologic subtype is denoted as M1 in the FAB classification.

In many cases of myeloblastic leukemia, more prominent granulocytic maturation is evident (FAB type *M2*). This variant is present in approximately 25 percent of AML cases; thus, myeloblastic leukemia with or without maturation composes more than 50 percent of AML cases. Blasts usually constitute at least 20 percent of the marrow cells. Auer rods may be present in blast cells. Promyelocytes, myelocytes, and segmented neutrophils, the latter often with the acquired Pelger-Hüet anomaly, may constitute 30 to 60 percent of marrow granulocytes. The anomaly is reflected in bilobed or monolobed neutrophils. Histochemical and surface markers of blast cells are typical of myeloblastic leukemia, and monocytic markers are absent or infrequent. A translocation between chromosomes 8 and 21 t(8;21)(q22; q22), often concomitant with loss of the Y chromosome in men or loss of an X chromosome in women, has been associated with the phenotype and occurs in younger patients (average age approximately 30).[321–323] Patients whose cells contain t(8;21) are prone to granulocytic sarcoma.[180,183]

MYELOMONOCYTIC LEUKEMIA

The ability of AML to express cells of the monocytic and granulocytic lineages was first highlighted in the early 1900s by Naegeli. Later, Downey proposed the eponym *Naegeli type* for myelomonocytic leukemia.[324] Approximately 20 percent of patients with AML present with this variant, and they more likely have extramedullary infiltrates in gingiva, skin, or CNS than patients with acute myeloblastic leukemia (see "Myeloid [Granulocytic] Sarcoma" above).[325] A mixture of myeloblasts and monoblasts is found in the blood and marrow. More than 30 percent of marrow cells are a mixed population of myeloblasts, which react with peroxidase or chloracetate esterase, and monoblasts, which react with fluoride-inhibitable nonspecific esterase. More than 20 percent of cells are monoblasts or promonocytes in blood and marrow. In some cases, individual cells react with monocytic and granulocytic histochemical stains.[326] Serum and urinary lysozyme levels are increased in most cases. This variant of AML is referred to as *M4* in the FAB classification. Translocations involving chromosome 3 have been associated with this phenotype.[327]

The proportion of marrow eosinophils[328] or basophils[329] may be increased. A particular variant of myelomonocytic leukemia has increased numbers of marrow eosinophils (10–50%), Auer rods in blast cells, and inversion or rearrangement of chromosome 16.[220–223] The eosinophils are abnormally large, and the eosinophilic myelocytes contain large basophilic granules. Macrophages with ingested Charcot-Leyden crystals may be present. This phenotypic variant of AML has been designated *M4Eo* in the FAB classification. Although this variant has an increased risk of CNS involvement, it carries a more favorable

TABLE 87-4 MORPHOLOGIC VARIANTS OF AML

VARIANT	CYTOLOGIC FEATURES	SPECIAL CLINICAL FEATURES	SPECIAL LABORATORY FEATURES
Acute myeloblastic leukemia (M0, M1, M2)	1. Myeloblasts are usually large; nuclear cytoplasmic ratio 1:1. Cytoplasm usually contains granules and occasionally Auer bodies. Nucleus shows fine reticular pattern and distinct nucleoli.	1. Most common in adults, and most frequent variety in infants.	1. Chromosomes +8, 5, 7, common.
	2. Blast cells are sudanophilic. They are positive for myeloperoxidase and chloroacetate esterase, negative for nonspecific esterase, and negative or diffusely positive for PAS (no clumps or blocks).	2. Three morphologic-cytochemical types (M0, M1, M2)	2. M0 type blast cells positive with antibody to myeloperoxidase and anti-CD34 and CD13 or CD33 coexpression. *AML1* mutations in ~25%.
	3. Electron microscopy shows primary cytoplasmic granules.		3. M1 expresses CD13 and CD33. Positive for myeloperoxidase by cytochemistry.
			4. (M2) AML with maturation often associated with t(8;21) karyotype.
Acute promyelocytic leukemia (M3, M3v)	1. Leukemic cells resemble promyelocytes. They have large atypical primary granules and a kidney-shaped nucleus. Branched or adherent Auer rods are common.	1. Usually in adults.	1. Cell contains t(15;17) or other translocation involving chromosome 17 (*RAR-α* gene).
	2. Peroxidase stain intensely positive.	2. Hypofibrinogenemia and hemorrhage common.	2. Cells are HLA-DR negative.
	3. A variant has microgranules (M3v), otherwise the same course and prognosis.	3. Leukemic cells mature in response to all-*trans*-retinoic acid.	
Acute myelomonocytic leukemia (M4, M4Eo)	1. Both myeloblastic and monoblastic leukemic cells in blood and marrow.	1. Similar to myeloblastic leukemia but with more frequent extramedullary disease.	1. Eosinophilic variant has inversion or translocation of chromosome 16.
	2. Peroxidase-, Sudan-, chloroacetate esterase-, and nonspecific esterase-positive cells.	2. Mildly elevated serum and urine lysozyme.	
	3. M4Eo variant has marrow eosinophilia.		
Acute monocytic leukemia (M5)	1. Leukemia cells are large; nuclear cytoplasmic ratio lower than myeloblast. Cytoplasm contains fine granules. Auer rods are rare. Nucleus is convoluted and may contain large nucleoli.	1. Seen in children or young adults.	1. t(4;11) common in infants.
	2. Nonspecific esterase-positive inhibited by NaF; Sudan-, peroxidase-, and chloroacetate esterase-negative. PAS occurs in granules, blocks.	2. Gum, CNS, lymph node, and extramedullary infiltrations are common.	2. Rearrangement of q11;q23 very frequent.
		3. DIC occurs.	
		4. Plasma and urine lysozyme elevated.	
		5. Hyperleukocytosis common.	
Acute erythroleukemia (M6)	1. Abnormal erythroblasts are in abundance initially in marrow and often in blood. Later the morphologic findings may be indistinguishable from those of AML.	1. Pancytopenia common at diagnosis.	1. Cells reactive with antihemoglobin antibody. Erythroblasts usually are strongly PAS and CD71-positive, express ABH blood group antigens, and react with antihemoglobin antibody.
			2. Cells reactive with anti–Rc-84 (antihuman erythroleukemia cell-line antigen).
Acute megakaryocytic leukemia (M7)	1. Small blasts with pale agranular cytoplasm and cytoplasmic blebs. May mimic lymphoblasts of medium to larger size.	1. Usually presents with pancytopenia.	1. Antigens of von Willebrand factor, and glycoprotein Ib (CD42), IIb/IIIa (CD41), IIIa (CD61) on blast cells.
		2. Markedly elevated serum lactic dehydrogenase levels.	2. Platelet peroxidase positive.
		3. Marrow aspirates are usually "dry taps" because of the invariable presence of myelofibrosis.	
		4. Common phenotype in the AML of Down syndrome.	

NOTE: Parentheses indicate FAB designation. NaF, sodium flouride; DIC, disseminated intravascular coagulation.

prognosis than the average case of AML. Fluorescence *in situ* hybridization (FISH) is a more accurate method for detection of cryptic 16q22 gene rearrangements and is useful in conjunction with conventional cytogenetics for patients with M4Eo AML. A variant of acute myelomonocytic leukemia has an increased number of marrow basophils and a translocation involving chromosomes 6 and 9, t(6;9)(p23; q34).[330] The variant occurs at a younger age, has a poor prognosis, and has a tendency to trilineage dysmorphogenesis and ringed sideroblasts.[331]

ERYTHROLEUKEMIA

Prominence of erythroid cell proliferation in AML cases was noted by Copelli[332] and DiGuglielmo[333] in the early 20th century. Moeschlin[334] used the term *erythroleukemia*. Dameshek[335] suggested the name *DiGuglielmo syndrome* and dissected the disorder into three phases depending on the decreasing prevalence of dysmorphic erythroblasts and the reciprocal increasing prevalence of myeloblasts. Erythroleukemia makes up approximately 5 percent of AML cases and is referred to as *M6* in the FAB classification.[336] Familial erythroleukemia has been described.[337,338]

Anemia and thrombocytopenia are present in nearly all cases. Some patients may have elevated total leukocyte counts. The red cells show marked anisocytosis, poikilocytosis, anisochromia, and basophilic stippling. Nucleated red cells are present in the blood. The marrow erythroblasts are extremely abnormal, with giant multinucleate forms, nuclear budding, and nuclear fragmentation (see Color Plate XVI-7,8 and Color Plate XVII-3–5). Cytogenetic abnormalities are present in approximately two thirds of patients. In the earlier stage or in the less severe form of the disease, so-called erythremic myelosis, granulopoiesis, and thrombopoiesis may be only mildly abnormal. This phase, dominated morphologically by bizarre dysmorphia of erythroblasts, can be protracted but eventually evolves into a dimorphic phase in which myeloblasts are more prominent; severe neutropenia and thrombocytopenia develop; and the patient progresses to *erythroleukemia*. The disease may evolve further into polyblastic AML.[339–342]

During the erythremic myelosis and erythroleukemia stages, erythropoiesis is markedly ineffective. However, some normal influences remain because hypertransfusion decreases both erythropoietin levels and the amount of abnormal erythropoiesis.[343] Spontaneous growth of leukemic erythroid clonogenic cells is a feature of the disease.[344] Periodic acid–Schiff (PAS)-positive erythroblasts are evident in almost all cases.[339,342] The frequency of erythroblastic leukemia is increased if methods for detecting erythroid differentiation more sensitive than light microscopy are used. These cell features include glycophorin A, spectrin, carbonic anhydrase I, ABH blood group antigens, or other antigens that occur on early erythroid progenitors.[345–347] Antihemoglobin antibody and antihuman erythroleukemic cell line antibody often are positive.[340]

Erythremic myelosis can have an indolent course and may be managed for a time without intensive chemotherapy. Treatment is warranted in patients with erythroleukemia, and the results are approximately the same as with other phenotypes in patients of similar age.[342] The more predominant the erythroid component and the lower the proportion of myeloblasts, the better the response to therapy.[345]

PROMYELOCYTIC LEUKEMIA

The association of an exaggerated hemorrhagic syndrome with certain leukemias was described by French hematologists in 1949.[348] In 1957, Hillstad[349] bestowed the appellation *promyelocytic leukemia* upon this morphologic-clinical subtype of AML. This variant, which is called *M3* in the FAB classification, occurs at any age and constitutes approximately 10 percent of AML cases.[208,209,350,351] This subtype of AML occurs with greater than expected frequency among Latinos from Europe and South and Central America[105,106] and among patients with an increased body mass index.[352] Unlike all other major variants of AML, which increase in incidence exponentially with age, the incidence of APL is constant over the human life span.[104] Hemorrhagic manifestations are prominent including hemoptysis, hematuria, vaginal bleeding, melena, hematemesis, and pulmonary and intracranial bleeding, as well as the more typical skin and mucous membrane bleeding. In severely leukopenic patients, blasts may not be evident in the blood. Moderately severe thrombocytopenia $<50 \times 10^9/$liter is present in most cases. The marrow contains few agranular blast cells and some blast-like cells with scant granules. The dominant cells are promyelocytes, which comprise 30 to 90 percent of marrow cells Color Plate XVI-5 and Color Plate XVII-1,2). Auer rods and cells with multiple Auer rods (1 to 10 percent) are present in nearly every case. Promyelocytes with bundles of Auer rods have been referred to as *faggot cells*. Leukemic promyelocytes stain intensely with myeloperoxidase and Sudan black and express CD 9, CD13, and CD33 but not CD34 or HLA-DR.[208,209,350,351]

A variant type of promyelocytic leukemia is referred to as *microgranular (M3v* in the FAB nomenclature).[353–356] Microgranular cases represent approximately 20 percent of patients with promyelocytic leukemia. The leukemic cells may mimic promonocytes with convoluted or lobulated nuclei. Auer rods may be present but are less evident. The majority of the leukemic cells contain azurophilic granules that are so small they are not visible by light microscopy, but the peroxidase stain usually is strongly positive. Typical hypergranulated promyelocytes usually are present on careful inspection. The total white cell count often is highly elevated, and severe coagulopathy is prominent in microgranular cases.[354] Rarely the cells contain eosinophilic or basophilic granules, but t(15;17) is present, and the response to all-*trans*-retinoic acid (ATRA) persists,[357–359] although the basophilic variant can be virulent.[360]

A translocation between chromosome 17 and another chromosome is present in almost all cases of APL and in the acute promyelocytic transformation of CML; it is not found in other AML variants. The t(15;17) is the most frequent ($>95\%$), but variant translocations between chromosome 5 or 11 and 17, isochromosome 17, and other less common variants have been described.[99,208,350,361,362] In some cases, cytogenetic analysis is inadequate, and Southern blot analysis is required to identify the rearrangement of the *RAR-α* gene. A functional distinction is that t(15;17), *PML-RAR-α* fusion, and t(5:17), *NPM-RAR-α* fusion, confer retinoid therapy responsiveness, whereas t(11; 17), *PLZF-RAR-α* fusion, usually is retinoid resistant. In cells with t(11;17), Auer rods are absent and CD56 expression usually is present, offering some clinical variables to provoke special molecular investigations.[363] This resistance may not always be present.[364]

The breakpoint on chromosome 17 is within the gene for the RAR-α, and the breakpoint on chromosome 15 is within the locus of a gene originally referred to as *MYL* and renamed *PML*.[208,365] The gene encodes a unique transcription factor. The translocation results in two new chimeric or fusion genes: *RAR-α-PML*, which is actively transcribed in APL, and *PML-RAR-α*, which also is transcribed and may account for the aberrancy in hematopoiesis. The *PML-RAR-α* gene has two isoforms that produce a short and a long type fusion mRNA, respectively.[366] Patients with the short isoform may have a worse outcome than those with the longer form. Polymerase chain reaction (PCR) for the mRNA of the fusion gene can be used to identify residual cells during remission and may predict relapse. The *PML-RAR-α* transgene can reproduce the disease in mice,[367] although in some models a superimposed *FLT3* mutation is required to express the disease.[100] *FLT3* mutations are frequently found in human disease, especially in the hypogranular variant.[99]

A propensity to hemorrhage is a striking feature of this subtype. The prothrombin and partial thromboplastin times are prolonged, and the plasma fibrinogen level is decreased in most cases. The disturbance in coagulation first was thought to principally result from intravascular coagulation initiated by procoagulant released from the granules of the leukemic promyelocytes. Elevated thrombin–antithrombin complexes, prothrombin fragment 1 + 2, and fibrinopeptide A plasma levels support the supposition. Increased levels of fibrinogen–fibrin degradation products, D-dimer, and evidence of plasminogen activation indicate fibrinolysis.[368–370] Furthermore, decreased levels of plasminogen, increased expression of annexin II on the leukemic cells,[371] and reports of responses to tranexamic acid support a role for fibrinolysis in the bleeding in APL.[372] Release of nonspecific proteases may further contribute to fibrinogenolysis.

Although APL responded to chemotherapy regimens for AML, especially those containing an anthracycline antibiotic such as daunomycin or rubidazone,[373] the cytologic pattern of response in the marrow often was paradoxical.[374–377] Persistence of leukemic promyelocytes preceded remission in the absence of further therapy, whereas induction of marrow cell hypoplasia was classically considered a requirement for remission in patients with AML. Generally, if leukemic blast cells persist after therapy for AML, relapse ensues unless hypoplasia is induced by more cytotoxic therapy. The unusual pattern of response in APL was put into context by reports of successful treatment with isomers of retinoic acid, an agent that leads to maturation of leukemic promyelocytes *in vitro*.[377] In 1988, the success of ATRA in remission induction was reported[378,379] and confirmed.[208,209] Relapse occurs invariably, however, so chemotherapy regimens also are required. Use of ATRA has decreased the risk of early hemorrhagic complications and death and has enhanced the long-term response to chemotherapy. Despite the improvement in therapy, approximately 10 percent of patients die during remission induction, most of hemorrhage. The prolonged remissions of patients with promyelocytic leukemia has been marred in approximately 1 to 5 percent of cases by the later appearance of oligoblastic leukemia with deletions of all or part of chromosome 5 or 7 and no evidence of involvement of chromosome 17, compatible with a myelogenous leukemia secondary to therapy.[380,381] The approach to therapy and outcome is discussed in the "Therapy, Course, and Prognosis" Section below.

MONOCYTIC LEUKEMIA

Monocytic leukemia was first reported by Reschad and Schilling-Torgau[382] in 1913. Approximately 8 percent of patients with AML present with monocytic leukemia, which is referred to as *M5* in the FAB classification. Patients with monocytic leukemia have a higher prevalence (50%) of extramedullary tumors in the skin, gingiva, eyes, larynx, lung, rectum and anal canal, bladder, lymph nodes, meninges, CNS, or other sites than do other phenotypes (<5%). Hepatomegaly and splenomegaly are more frequent in monocytic leukemia.[128,383–385]

The total leukocyte count is higher in a larger proportion of patients, and hyperleukocytosis occurs more frequently (approximately 35%) than in other variants.[386–388] The blood cells may be largely monoblasts or more mature-appearing promonocytes and monocytes. When the blood contains more mature monocytic cells, the marrow contains a lower proportion of blast cells, approximately 25 to 50 percent. When the blood monocytes are largely blast cells, the marrow contains approximately 50 to 90 percent blasts (see Color Plate XVI-4). In nearly all cases 10 to 90 percent of monocytic cells react for nonspecific esterase stains, α-naphthyl acetate esterase, and naphthol AS-D acetate esterase; in a cytochemical or chemoluminescence assay; or with monoclonal antibodies against monocyte surface antigens, especially CD14. Immunoreactivity of cells for lysozyme is characteristic. Serum and urine lysozyme levels are elevated in most patients. Serum lactic dehydrogenase and β_2-microglobulin concentrations are increased in greater than 80 percent of patients.[389] Plasminogen activator inhibitor-2 is present in the plasma and the cells of a high proportion of patients.[390] Auer rods are absent when monoblasts dominate but are present frequently in cases where promonocytes and monocytes are prevalent in blood and marrow. Leukemic monocytes have Fc receptors and can ingest and kill microorganisms in some cases.[391,392]

An association between translocations involving chromosome 11, especially region 11q23, and monocytic leukemia is present.[210–212] In particular, t(9;11) is found in leukemic monocytes.[213,214,385,386] In t(9;11) the β_1-interferon gene is translocated to chromosome 11, and the protooncogene *ETS*-1 is translocated to chromosome 9 adjacent to the α-interferon gene. The latter juxtaposition may be important in the pathogenesis of monocytic leukemia.[393]

The expression of *FOS* is closely correlated with monocytic maturation of cells in myelomonocytic and monocytic leukemia and in normal monocytopoiesis.[394,395] Absence or markedly decreased expression of the retinoblastoma gene growth suppressor product (p105) is present in approximately half of patients with monocytic leukemia. Patients express a more dramatic phenotype.[396] A variant of acute monocytic leukemia in which the leukemic cells have monocytoid features and are positive for early and late monocytic lineage antigens and for terminal deoxynucleotidyl transferase activity often occurs after prior radiotherapy or chemotherapy and is relatively resistant to treatment.[397] A syndrome of acute monoblastic leukemia with t(8;16), resulting in *MOZ-CBP* fusion gene, is characterized by mildly granular promonocytes (simulating hypogranular promyelocytes), intense phagocytosis of red cells, erythroblast, and sometimes neutrophils and platelets in blood and marrow, simulating macrophagic hemophagocytic syndrome, intravascular coagulation or primary fibrinolysis, and a high frequency of extramedullary disease.[398]

The management of monocytic leukemia is complicated by a greater incidence of CNS or meningeal disease either at the time of diagnosis or as a form of relapse during remission. Thus, examination of cerebrospinal fluid should be performed even in the absence of symptoms.[128,385,386] Some therapists recommend prophylactic intrathecal therapy with methotrexate or cytosine arabinoside for patients who enter remission.

Rare cases of dendritic cell or Langerhans cell phenotype have been described[399,400] (see Chap. 72). Uncommon cases of histiocytic sarcoma are the tissue or extramedullary variant of monocytic leukemia[401,402] (see Chap. 72). The outcome of treatment, once thought to be less favorable than with other forms of AML, was comparable to the outcome of other subtypes.[403]

MEGAKARYOBLASTIC LEUKEMIA

In 1963, Szur and Lewis[404] reported patients with pancytopenia, low percentages of blast cells, and intense myelofibrosis but an absence of teardrop red cells, splenomegaly, leukocytosis, and thrombocytosis, the usual features of idiopathic myelofibrosis. They designated the syndrome *malignant myelosclerosis*.[404] Reports of similar cases ensued, with some investigators referring to the syndrome as *acute myelofibrosis*.[405] The development of methods to phenotype megakaryoblasts indicated the cases were variants of AML rather than of myelofibrosis and have been designated *acute megakaryocytic* or *acute megakaryoblastic leukemia*.[280,406,407] This leukemia is referred to as *M7* in the FAB classification. The prevalence of this phenotype is approximately 5 percent of all AML cases if appropriate cell markers are used in the diagnosis and is at least twice that frequency in childhood AML.[408,409] The syndrome is an especially prevalent variant of AML that develops in patients with Down syndrome[284,410] or mediastinal germ cell tumors.[310–314]

Leukemic megakaryoblasts and promegakaryocytes can be difficult to identify by light microscopy using polychrome staining. However, with experience, heightened suspicion can be engendered by blasts with abundant budding cytoplasm or blasts having a lymphoid appearance, especially if the marrow cannot be aspirated because of intense myelofibrosis, which is evident on the marrow biopsy. Initially high-resolution histochemistry for platelet peroxidase and identification of the demarcation membrane system using transmission electron microscopy were required for diagnosis. Now antibodies to von Willebrand factor or to glycoprotein Ib (CD42), IIb/IIIa (CD41), or IIIa (CD61) can be used to identify very primitive megakaryocytic cells.[406,407] A small proportion of megakaryoblasts may be present in other cases of AML, but in megakaryocytic leukemia they are the prominent or the dominant leukemic cells. Moreover, the other key features of the syndrome usually are present, especially severe myelofibrosis.[408]

Patients usually present with pallor, weakness, excessive bleeding and anemia, and leukopenia. Lymphadenopathy or hepatosplenomegaly is uncommon at the time of diagnosis. High leukocyte and blood blast cell counts may be present initially or may develop later. The platelet count may be normal or elevated in many patients at the time of presentation. Marrow aspiration often is unsuccessful ("dry tap") because of extensive marrow fibrosis in most cases. The marrow biopsy contains small blast cells, large blast cells, or a combination of both. The former have a high nuclear to cytoplasmic ratio, have dense chromatin with distinct nucleoli, and resemble lymphoblasts. Cases have been mistaken for ALL. The larger blasts may have some features of maturing megakaryocytes with agranular cytoplasm with cytoplasmic protrusions, clusters of platelet-like structures, or shedding of cytoplasmic blebs. The blast cells are peroxidase negative and tend to aggregate. Confirmation of their megakaryoblastic maturation requires immunocytologic studies of the presence of von Willebrand factor and the immunoreactivity to CD41, CD42, or CD61. The more mature megakaryocytes stain with PAS reagent, contain sodium fluoride-inhibitable nonspecific esterase, and fail to react for α-naphthylbutyrate esterase.

The serum lactic acid dehydrogenase level frequently is strikingly increased and has an isomorphic pattern unlike that seen with other myeloproliferative disorders. Complex chromosome aberrations are common.[411] An association of megakaryoblastic leukemia in infants with t(1;22)(p13;q13) has been reported.[411–414] Abnormalities of chromosome 3 have been linked to clonal hemopathies expressing a prominent megakaryocytic phenotype.[415,416] Progression of idiopathic myelofibrosis or essential thrombocythemia to AML may have the phenotype of acute megakaryocytic leukemia. Paradoxically, in children with Down syndrome the disease can be treated with modified doses of chemotherapy, with a very high remission rate and long-term event-free survival.[417,418] The result is thought to be related to the exquisite sensitivity of the leukemic cells to drug-induced apoptosis,[419] whereas the results in children without Down syndrome or in adults are poor.[420,421]

EOSINOPHILIC LEUKEMIA

Acute eosinophilic leukemia is rare. Increased eosinophils in the marrow but not in the blood is a variant of acute myelomonocytic leukemia and inversion 16 or other abnormalities of chromosome 16 but is not considered an acute eosinophilic leukemia.[220–223] First described in 1912,[422] acute eosinophilic leukemia is a distinct entity that can arise de novo as AML, with 50 to 80 percent of eosinophilic cells in the blood and marrow.[423–425] A specific histochemical reaction, cyanide-resistant peroxidase, permits identification of leukemic blast cells with eosinophilic differentiation and diagnosis of acute eosinoblastic leukemia in some cases of AML with few identifiable eosinophils in blood or marrow.[426] Eosinophilia, not part of the malignant clone, may be a feature of occasional patients with AML, an uncommon reactive phenomenon. In many cases, idiopathic eosinophilia (hypereosinophilic syndrome) is a monoclonal disorder representing a spectrum of more indolent chronic or subacute eosinophilic leukemia to more progressive acute leukemia[427] (see Chaps. 62 and 88). Acute eosinophilic leukemia may develop in patients having the chronic form of a hypereosinophilic syndrome. Overexpression of Wilms tumor gene expression has been proposed as a means of distinguishing acute eosinophilic leukemia from a polyclonal, reactive eosinophilia.[428]

Patients with acute eosinophilic leukemia have a propensity for developing bronchospastic signs and heart failure from endomyocardial fibrosis. Hepatomegaly and splenomegaly are more common than in other variants of AML. Response to treatment is approximately the same as in other types of AML.[426]

BASOPHILIC AND MAST CELL LEUKEMIA

First described in 1906,[429] basophilic differentiation as a feature of AML is a rare event. Most cases of basophilic leukemia evolve from the chronic phase of CML,[430] but de novo acute basophilic leukemia, in which the cells do not contain the Philadelphia chromosome, does occur.[431–436] The cells stain with toluidine blue, and the basophilic granules can be most striking in myelocytes. In some cases of acute myelomonocytic leukemia associated with t(6;9)(p23;q34), basophils may be increased in the marrow but not in the blood. Because CML with t(9;22)(q34;q11) has the same breakpoint (q34) on chromosome 9 as AML with t(6;9) and both diseases are strongly associated with marrow basophilia, a gene(s) at the breakpoint on chromosome 9 may influence basophilopoiesis.[330]

The blood leukocyte count usually is elevated, and proportions of the cells are basophils. The marrow is cellular with a high proportion of blasts and early and late basophilic myelocytes. Special staining with toluidine blue or Astra blue often is necessary to distinguish basophilic from neutrophilic promyelocytes and myelocytes. Immunophenotyping may show myeloid markers (CD33, CD13) that are not specific. Presence of CD9, CD25, or both is characteristic of basophilic differentiation. Cells may have granules with ultrastructural features of basophils and mast cells.[434] Electron microscopy can be useful in identifying basophilic granules in cases where no granules are evident by light microscopy and the phenotype simulates M0.[434] Basophilic leukemia can be confused with promyelocytic leukemia if the basophilic early myelocytes are mistaken for promyelocytes.[437] On the contrary, promyelocytic leukemia may have basophilic maturation and can be mistaken for basophilic leukemia. However, if the cells contain t(15;17), the disease should respond to ATRA and an anthracycline antibiotic.[354,357,358] Prolonged clotting time, intravascular coagulation, and hemorrhage are uncommon presenting features in patients with basophilic leukemia but are common in patients with promyelocytic leukemia. Urticaria and elevated blood histamine levels occur in patients with basophilic leukemia. Rare cases of a chronic course in BCR-ABL–negative basophilic leukemia preceding the onset of rapid progression have occurred.[438] Treatment for acute (Ph-negative) basophilic leukemia is similar to that for other variants of AML.

Mast cell leukemia is a rare manifestation of systemic mast cell disease[439] (see Chap. 63). It can be related to a mutation of the KIT gene.[440] The leukemic mast cells are CD117 (KIT) positive, tryptase positive and myeloperoxidase negative, and CD25 negative.[441] In some cases, electron microscopy of the granule-containing cells may aid in distinguishing basophils from mast cells (see Chap. 63). Extensive, apparently reactive mast cell tissue infiltrations may be provoked by cytokines during the course of AML.[442,443]

HISTIOCYTIC AND DENDRITIC CELL LEUKEMIA

Chapter 72 discusses histiocytic and dendritic cell leukemia.

DIFFERENTIAL DIAGNOSIS

Acute leukemia in infants with Down syndrome should be differentiated from TMD (see "Neonatal Myeloproliferation and Leukemia" above). In adults, the term *pseudoleukemia* has been applied to circumstances that mimic the marrow appearance of promyelocytic leukemia. Recovery from drug-induced or *Pseudomonas aeruginosa*–induced agranulocytosis is characterized by a striking cohort of promyelocytes in the marrow, which upon inspection of the marrow aspirate or biopsy mimics promyelocytic leukemia.[444–446]

In pseudoleukemia, the platelet count may be normal; the degree of leukopenia often is more profound ($<1.0 \times 10^9$/liter) than usually seen in AML[444,445]; promyelocytes contain a prominent paranuclear clear (Golgi) zone not covered with granules; and promyelocytes do not have Auer rods.[446–448] Similar reactions have been reported after granulocyte colony stimulating factor (G-CSF) administration.[449] In patients suspected of having pseudoleukemia, observation for a few days usually clarifies the significance of the marrow appearance, because progressive maturation to segmented neutrophils normalizes the marrow and leads to an increased blood neutrophil count.

In patients with hypoplastic marrows, careful examination of specimens is required to distinguish among aplastic anemia, hypoplastic acute leukemia,[262–264] and hypoplastic oligoblastic leukemia.[450] Leukemic blast cells are evident in the marrow in hypoplastic leukemia, and islands of dysmorphic cells, especially megakaryocytes, are present in hypoplastic oligoblastic leukemia.

Leukemoid reactions and nonleukemic pancytopenias can be distinguished from AML by the absence of leukemic blast cells in the blood or marrow.[451,452] In older children and adults, myeloblasts usually do not constitute more than 2 percent of marrow cells except in patients with leukemia, and the proportion of blast cells usually decreases in the marrow with neutrophilic leukemoid reactions.

THERAPY, COURSE, AND PROGNOSIS

OVERVIEW OF TREATMENT PLAN

The usual treatment of AML includes an initial program termed the *induction* phase. Induction may involve the simultaneous use of multiple agents or a planned sequence of therapy called *timed sequential treatment*. Once a remission is obtained, further treatment usually is indicated to preserve the remission state. The treatment can consist of cytotoxic chemotherapy, stem cell transplantation, or low-dose maintenance therapy, depending upon patient performance status and risk factors. If relapse occurs, treatment options may include different chemotherapy regimens, allogeneic stem cell transplantation, or other investigational regimens.

DECISION TO TREAT

Most patients with AML should be advised to undergo treatment promptly after diagnosis. Although remission rates are lower in older patients, a significant proportion enter remission. Occasionally, very elderly patients refuse treatment or are so ill from unrelated illnesses that treatment may be unreasonable. Age per se is not a contraindication to treatment, and septuagenarians and octogenarians can enter sustained remissions. Treatment can be tailored to the decreased tolerance of older patients, some of whom have a smoldering course (see "Treatment of Older Patients" below). Associated problems, such as hemorrhagic manifestations, severe anemia, or infections, should be treated in parallel. Because remission is necessary to eliminate associated problems, delays in induction chemotherapy treatments usually are detrimental in the long run.

PREPARATION OF THE PATIENT

Orientation of the patient and the family should provide them with an understanding of the disease, the treatment planned, and the adverse effects of treatment. Most patients and their families will be focused upon their new diagnosis of leukemia and the induction chemotherapy treatment phase, but most also want information about prognosis and long-term treatment plans. Because most patients will enter a complete remission and because some patients can expect to have long-term disease-free survival after completion of their treatment regimen, cautious optimism is appropriate in younger patients.

Pretreatment laboratory examination should include blood cell counts, cytochemistry analysis and immunophenotyping of leukemic cells from blood or marrow, marrow examination including cytogenetic and molecular analyses, blood chemistry studies, chest x-ray films, electrocardiogram, and determination of partial thromboplastin and prothrombin times. More extensive evaluation of coagulation factors should be made if (1) clotting times are abnormal, (2) bleeding is exaggerated for the level of the platelet count, or (3) acute promyelocytic or monocytic leukemia is the phenotype. Early HLA typing is useful so that compatible platelet products can be provided if alloimmunization (see Chap. 132) occurs and for patients who will become marrow transplant candidates (see Chap. 22). *Herpes simplex* virus and cytomegalovirus serotyping may be helpful. HIV and hepatitis serology is indicated in certain patients, and patients should have a baseline cardiac scan to determine ejection fraction prior to administration of an anthracycline agent.

A tunneled central venous catheter should be placed. This access to the circulation facilitates administration of chemotherapy, blood components, antibiotics, and other intravenous fluids and medications. It also permits sampling blood for analysis without patient discomfort or concern about venous access. Meticulous skin care at the catheter exit site is required to minimize tunnel infections. Central venous catheters have become a major source of infection during neutropenia, especially with gram-positive organisms.[452]

Therapy for hyperuricemia is required if (1) the pretreatment uric acid level is greater than 7.0 mg/dl (0.4 mmol/liter), (2) the marrow is packed with blast cells, or (3) the blood blast cell count is moderately or markedly elevated. Allopurinol 300 mg/day orally should be given. Allopurinol can cause allergic dermatitis and should not be used if the uric acid level is less than 7 mg/dl and the total white cell count is less than approximately 20,000/μl (20 $\times$ 10^9/liter), as long as hydration is adequate and urine flow is high ($>$150 ml/hour). The dermatitis may appear when antibiotics are instituted. This concurrence may confound the decision to continue antibiotics. Thus, allopurinol should be discontinued after the risk of acute hyperuricosuria or tumor lysis has passed (usually 4–7 days). Recombinant urate oxidase can be used to prevent tumor lysis syndrome. This preparation, although costly, can reduce plasma urate levels by 86 percent within 4 hours of the first drug dose. It is well tolerated, and the recommended dose of rasburicase is 0.2 mg/kg daily for 5 to 7 days, although lower doses have been utilized.[453]

Attention to decreasing pathogen exposure by assiduous hand washing and meticulous care of catheter and intravenous sites is important, especially when the total neutrophil count is less than 500/μl (0.5 $\times$ 10^9/liter). Care of the patient in *a single room* is advisable to provide privacy during periods of intensive care and to help decrease the risk of exogenously acquired infection until the neutrophil count recovers. Unwashed fruits and vegetables and certain forms of marijuana are thought to be sources of pathogenic microorganisms and should be prohibited during the neutropenic period [<500/μl [<0.5 × 10^9/liter]).

REMISSION-INDUCTION THERAPY

PRINCIPLES

The cytotoxic therapy of AML rests on two tenets: (1) two competing populations of cells are present in marrow—a normal polyclonal and a leukemic monoclonal population; and (2) profound suppression of the leukemic cells to the point they are inapparent in the marrow aspirate and biopsy is required to permit restoration of polyclonal hematopoiesis.[454,455] Although these two principles hold in most cases, two deviations from these guidelines are (1) the predisposition of patients with APL to enter remission despite cellular posttherapy marrows[456,457] and (2) the occasional presence of monoclonal hematopoiesis in some cases of AML during remission (see "Results of Treatment" below).

The goal of induction therapy in AML is achievement of complete remission (<2% blasts in the marrow), a neutrophil count greater than 1000/μL, and a platelet count greater than 100,000/μL. An International Working Group for Diagnosis, Standardization of Response Criteria, Treatment Outcomes, and Reporting Standards has redefined outcomes in an effort to standardize reporting of and comparison of data.[458] Other treatment guidelines have been recently published.[459,460] Most adults enter remission with standard induction therapy, but for patients with high-risk disease, consideration can be given to an experimental approach. How durable a complete remission will be attained in an individual patient often is difficult to predict at diagnosis. Gene expression profiling can separate some patients into prognostic groups that may indicate patients with a high risk of not responding to standard approaches.[115,116]

CYTOTOXIC REGIMENS

Anthracycline Antibiotic or Anthraquinone and Cytarabine

Current standard induction treatment for AML involves drug regimens with two or more agents, which include an anthracycline antibiotic or anthraquinone and cytarabine.[461–464] Remission rates in the studies cited range from approximately 55 to 90 percent in adult subjects, depending on the composition of the population treated (Table 87-5). The two most important variables are the age of the patients and the proportion of patients with therapy-induced leukemia or an antecedent clonal myeloid disease. In the studies listed in Table 87-5, the median age of the patient populations was much younger (30s to 50s) than the population of AML patients at large (65–70 years); thus the results cannot be generalized (see "Treatment of Older Patients" below). A combination of anthracycline and cytarabine has been the standard induction therapy since 1973.[11] A now classic, standard induction reg-

TABLE 87-5   REMISSION INDUCTION FOR AML: COMBINATION OF CYTOSINE ARABINOSIDE AND ANTHRACYCLINE ANTIBIOTIC

	DOSE AND SCHEDULE					
CYTARABINE	ANTHRACYCLINE ANTIBIOTIC ± ANOTHER AGENT	NO. OF PATIENTS	AGE RANGE (YEARS) (MEDIAN)	COMPLETE REMISSIONS (%)	YEAR OF REPORT	REFERENCE
200 mg/m² , days 1–7	DNR 60 mg/m², days 1–3	200	16–60 (45)	72	2004	1035
200 mg/m², days 1–7	DNR 60 mg/m², days 1–3 Cladribine 5 mg/m², days 1–5	200	16–60 (45)	69	2004	1035
200 mg/m² twice per day for 10 days (Some in this report received FLAG-Ida vs. H-DAT)	DNR 50 mg/m², days 1, 3, 5 Thioguanine 100 mg/m² twice per day, days 10–20 Gemtuzumab ozogamicin 3 mg/m², day 1	64	18-59 (46.5)	91	2003	478
3 g/m² every 12 h for 8 doses	60 mg/m² DNR daily for 2 days	122	Adults	80	2000	472
100 mg/m² daily for 7 days (2 courses always given)	IDA 12 mg/m² daily for 3 days	153	NR	63	2000	464
2 g/m² every 12 h for 5 days	IDA 5 mg/m² daily for 5 days Etoposide 100 mg/m² daily for 5 days (bid discontinued because of toxicity)	128	15–64 (34)	72	1999	473
3 g/m² every 12 h for 5 days	Mitoxantrone 80 mg/m² (total) Etoposide 150 mg/m² for 3 days	45	<60 (NR)	80	1995	474
3 g/m² every 12 h, days 1, 3, 5, 7	DNR 50 mg/m² for 3 days Etoposide 75 mg/m² for 7 days	101	15–60 (45)	71	1996	471
100 mg/m² continuous infusion daily for 7 days	DNR 50 mg/m² for 3 days Etoposide 75 mg/m² for 7 days	102	15–60 (39)	74	1996	471
500 mg/m² by continuous infusion, days 1–3, 8–10	Mitoxantrone 12 mg/m² for 3 days Etoposide 200 mg/m² IV, days 8–10	133	15–70 (43)	60	1996	475
100 mg/m² daily for 7 days	DNR 45 mg/m² for 3 days	113	NR (55)	59	1992	461
100 mg/m² daily for 7 days	IDA 13 mg/m² for 3 days	101	NR (56)	70	1992	461

The reader is advised to consult the original reports for details of induction and ancillary therapy and consolidation or continuation therapy, which may vary from protocol to protocol. DNR = daunorubicin; FLAG, fludarabine, cytarabine, and granulocyte colony-stimulating factor; H-DAT, hydroxydaunorubicin, cytarabine, thioguanine. IDA = idarubicin; NR = not reported.

imen is cytarabine 100 mg/m² daily by continuous infusion on days 1 through 7 and daunorubicin at 45 mg/m² on days 1 through 3, the so-called "7 and 3 regimen." Dose or schedule modulation of the anthracycline or cytarabine, addition of other agents such as etoposide, in various schedules of administration, represent attempts to improve upon results obtained with standard therapy.[465]

Idarubicin versus Daunomycin Development of drug resistance is reduced with idarubicin relative to other anthracyclines. Idarubicin does not induce P-glycoprotein expression but daunorubicin, doxorubicin, and epirubicin do.[466] Idarubicin 12 mg/m² gives better complete remission rates in younger adults than does daunorubicin 45 mg/m², each given for 3 days. Amsacrine, aclarubicin, and mitoxantrone give improved results over standard-dose daunorubicin. In older adults, mitoxantrone may reduce cardiotoxicity.[467] Higher doses of daunorubicin may yield higher complete response rates,[468] but such use has not been examined in a randomized trial nor has the safety been definitely established. Dexrazoxane may be given during induction to reduce the risk of cardiotoxicity in patients at higher than usual risk because of a history of coronary artery disease or congestive heart failure.[469] *In vitro*, dexrazoxane in combination with various anthracyclines has demonstrated synergistic cytotoxic responses in AML cell lines.[470]

High-Dose versus Standard-Dose Cytarabine High-dose cytarabine does not increase complete remission rates and increases toxicity compared to conventional doses, especially in older patients (for doses of these regimens, see "Postremission Maintenance Therapy/Intensive Consolidation Therapy" below). Patients receiving high-dose cytarabine have more leukopenia, thrombocytopenia, gastrointestinal distress, and eye toxicity. Disease-free survival is better than that achieved with standard therapy, leading some investigators to suggest use of high-dose therapy for induction in patients younger than 50 years.[471] Complete remission rates of greater than 60 percent have been noted with high-dose cytarabine in patients with poor-risk cytogenetics.[472,473]

Timed Sequential Therapy and Other Drugs Timed sequential therapy, which uses agents in a scheduled sequence rather than concurrently, with addition of etoposide may prolong remission duration.[474,475] Timed sequential chemotherapy combining mitoxantrone on days 1 to 3, etoposide on days 8 to 10, and cytarabine on days 1 to 3 and 8 to 10 resulted in a complete remission in 60 percent of patients but a toxic death in 9 percent of patients. Median disease-free survival was 9 months[474] or slightly longer.[476] Adding ATRA,[477] gemtuzumab ozogamicin,[478] cyclosporine,[479] or thalidomide[480] to induction regimens or substituting fludarabine or topotecan for an anthracycline[481] has not improved results significantly. Thus, the practice guidelines for AML, other than promyelocytic leukemia, recommend standard-dose cytarabine plus anthracycline treatment.[460]

Hematopoietic Cytokines to Enhance Chemotherapy G-CSF and granulocyte-monocyte colony stimulating factor (GM-CSF), when used in untreated leukemia, can increase the percentage of leukemic cells in the DNA synthetic phase, resulting in blast population expansion during short-term administration of G-CSF. This process could render the cells more sensitive to simultaneous chemotherapy, but clinical benefit from growth factor priming has not been observed[482,483] despite an increased ratio of intracellular cytosine arabinoside triphosphate to deoxycytidine-5′-triphosphate and enhanced cytarabine incorporation into the DNA of AML blasts.[483] Remission rates or overall survival did not differ among adult patients who received cytarabine plus idarubicin or cytarabine plus amsacrine with or without G-CSF given concurrently, but relapse rates decreased in patients who received G-CSF.[484] Similar negative results occurred with GM-CSF.[482] Thus, these growth factors are not useful as enhancers of chemotherapy. However, complete remissions have occurred in hypoplastic AML after G-CSF treatment without chemotherapy.[485]

Duration of Induction Therapy Patients who have persistent leukemia after the first course of induction chemotherapy generally are given a second similar course. The patient's long-term outcome is worse if two courses of treatment are required even if a complete remission is achieved. Approximately 40 percent of patients with persistent AML after one course of induction therapy have a complete remission after a second course,[486] and disease-free survival at 5 years is approximately 10 percent. In some European centers, two courses of induction chemotherapy are given routinely, but impact on remission rates or overall survival remains uncertain.[487] The longer the time to remission after the first induction therapy, the shorter the duration of disease-free survival.[488,489] High-risk cytogenetic abnormalities, antecedent hematologic disorders, and other poor prognostic factors can be used to assign nonresponders to an experimental chemotherapy regimen designed to treat refractory disease, rather than repeating induction therapy.

SPECIAL CONSIDERATIONS DURING INDUCTION THERAPY

Hyperleukocytosis Patients with blast counts greater than 100,000/μl (100 × 10⁹/liter) require prompt treatment to prevent the most serious complications of hyperleukocytosis: intracranial hemorrhage or pulmonary insufficiency. Hydration should be administered promptly to maintain urine flow greater than 100 ml/hour/m². Cytoreduction therapy can be initiated with hydroxyurea 1.5 to 2.5 g orally every 6 hours (total dose 6–10 g/day) for approximately 36 hours. Appropriate remission induction therapy should be initiated. Simultaneous leukapheresis can decrease blast cell concentration by approximately 30 percent within several hours,[246] without contributing to uric acid release. Leukapheresis may improve acute disturbances resulting from the vascular effects of blast cells, but the procedure may not alter the long-term outcome.[490–492] Inhaled nitric oxide reportedly improves hypoxemia related to hyperleukocytosis.[493]

Antibiotic Therapy Pancytopenia is worsened or induced shortly after treatment is instituted. Absolute neutrophil counts less than 200/μl (0.2 × 10⁹/liter) are expected and are a sign of effective drug action. The patient often becomes febrile (>38°C [100.4°F]), often with associated rigors. Cultures of urine, blood, nasopharynx, and, if available, sputum should be obtained. Because the inflammatory response is blunted by severe neutropenia and monocytopenia, evidence of exudates on physical examination or radiographic studies may be minimal or absent. Antibiotics should be started immediately after cultures are obtained.[494] Chapter 20 describes antibiotic usage in the setting of induction chemotherapy. Infections remain a major cause of therapy-associated morbidity and mortality.[495,496] Gram-positive bacterial isolates now outnumber gram-negative isolates.[492]

Some centers use prophylactic antibacterial, antifungal, and/or antiviral antibiotics, whereas other centers do not. Antifungal prophylaxis can consist of low-dose amphotericin, fluconazole, itraconazole, or voriconazole.[497,498] Acyclovir, valacyclovir, or famciclovir prophylaxis during remission-induction therapy of patients with AML does not affect the duration of fever or the need for antibiotics. The incidence of bacteremia is not reduced, but acute oral infections are less severe.[499] Liposomal amphotericin has less infusion-related toxicity and less nephrotoxicity when used in patients with fever and neutropenia[500] but is more expensive to administer than is conventional amphotericin. The caspofungins and azoles are available for treatment of established fungal infections.[501] Some centers utilize outpatient supportive therapy immediately after induction therapy in adult AML. One approach is use of cotrimoxazole, itraconazole, or fluconazole administered orally until the granulocyte count is greater than 1000/μl, and every-other-day platelet transfusions until the count is greater than 20,000/μl.[502] Some induction regimens, such as so-called FLANG (fludarabine, cytosine arabinoside, Novantrone, and G-CSF), reportedly require fewer hospital days than conventional induction regimens.[503]

Hematopoietic Growth Factors to Treat Cytopenias Cytokine therapy as an adjunctive treatment for AML remains controversial.[504] Although GM-CSF and G-CSF accelerate neutrophil recovery, neither GM-CSF nor G-CSF reproducibly decreases major morbidity or mortality. However, one study has shown decreased mortality from fungal infections in older patients.[505] Use of cytokines during periods of cytopenia following induction therapy is safe, and nearly all trials have shown a modestly reduced duration of severe neutropenia with a variable effect on the incidence of severe infections, antibiotic usage, and duration of hospital stays. Although no increase in relapse has been noted when growth factors are started after completion of chemotherapy, no consistent enhancement of remission, event-free survival, or overall survival has been noted.[506] Therefore, the cost effectiveness of growth factor usage has come into question.

Component Transfusion Therapy Red cell transfusions should be used to keep the hematocrit level greater than 25 ml/dl, or higher in special cases (e.g., symptomatic coronary artery disease) (see Chap. 131). Platelet transfusions should be used for hemorrhagic manifestations related to thrombocytopenia and prophylactically if necessary to maintain the platelet count between $5000/\mu l$ (5×10^9/liter) and $10,000/\mu l$ (10×10^9/liter).[507] Patients without coagulation abnormalities, anticoagulant use, sepsis, or other complications usually can maintain hemostasis with platelet counts of 5000 to $10,000/\mu l$ ($5-10 \times 10^9$/liter). Initially, random donor platelets can be used, although single-donor platelets or HLA-matched platelets may be preferable products and should be tried if random-donor platelets do not raise the platelet count significantly (see Chap. 132).

All red cell and platelet products should be depleted of leukocytes, and all products, including granulocytes for transfusions, should be irradiated to prevent transfusion-associated graft-versus-host disease (GVHD) in this immunosuppressed population (see Chap. 132). This step is particularly important if allogeneic marrow transplantation is being considered. The benefit of using cytomegalovirus-negative blood products compared to leukodepletion to prevent virus transmission in patients who are not virus carriers is unsettled.[508]

Granulocyte transfusion should not be used prophylactically for neutropenia but can be used in patients with high fever, rigors, and bacteremia unresponsive to antibiotics, with fungal infections, or with septic shock (see Chap. 25). G-CSF administration to a volunteer donor increases neutrophil yield fourfold and results in posttransfusion blood neutrophil increments for more than 24 hours after transfusion.[509] G-CSF administration may be warranted for treatment of major fungal infections (see Chap. 20).

Jehovah's Witnesses or others who refuse blood product support can survive tailored chemotherapy.[510] In general, phlebotomy is minimized, and antifibrinolytics, hematinics, and growth factors are utilized to support such patients during severe cytopenias.

Therapy for Hypofibrinogenemic Hemorrhage Patients with evidence of intravascular coagulation (see Chap. 121) or exaggerated primary fibrinolysis (see Chap. 127) should be considered for platelet and fresh-frozen plasma administration before antileukemic therapy is started. If the findings are equivocal, patients should be monitored closely with measurements of fibrinogen levels, fibrin(ogen) degradation products, D-dimer assay, and coagulation times. Intravascular coagulation or primary fibrinolysis may occur in patients with APL and acute monocytic leukemia but also may occur in occasional patients with acute myeloblastic leukemia with Auer rods.

Management of Central Nervous System Disease CNS disease occurs in approximately one in 50 cases at presentation.[511] Prophylactic therapy usually is not indicated, but examination of the spinal fluid

after remission should be considered in (1) monocytic subtypes,[386] (2) cases with extramedullary disease, (3) the inversion 16[172] and t(8; 21)[180,183] genotypes, (4) CD7- and CD56-positive (neural cell adhesion molecule) immunophenotypes,[512] and (5) patients who present with very high blast counts. In these situations, the risk of meningeal leukemia or a brain myeloid sarcoma is heightened. Treatment of meningeal leukemia can include high-dose cytarabine (which penetrates the blood–brain barrier), intrathecal methotrexate, intrathecal cytarabine, cranial radiation, or chemoradiation in combination.[511] Systemic relapse commonly follows relapse in the meninges, and concurrent systemic treatment usually is indicated. Long-term success is unusual unless allogeneic stem cell transplantation is possible. Unless the patient has neurologic symptoms, lumbar puncture generally is deferred until blood blasts have cleared. No consensus exists on a trigger for platelet transfusion in adults with AML undergoing lumbar puncture, but a platelet count less than $20,000/\mu L$ (20×10^9/liter) has been proposed.[513]

Management of Nonleukemic Myeloid Sarcoma Some patients present with myeloid (granulocytic) sarcomas without evidence of leukemia in the blood or marrow (see "Myeloid [Granulocytic] Sarcoma" above). Myeloid sarcoma may be the presenting finding in approximately 2 percent of patients with AML. Such patients should receive intensive AML induction therapy. Intensive therapy results in a longer nonleukemic period than patients who have undergone surgical resection or resection followed by local irradiation.[179] Median relapse-free survival is 12 months after AML-type chemotherapy. Patients with trisomy 8 have poorer survival rates.[178]

POSTREMISSION MAINTENANCE THERAPY

CYTOTOXIC THERAPY

General Considerations Postremission therapy is intended to prolong remission duration and overall survival, but no consensus exists regarding the best approach. Postremission chemotherapy that does not produce profound prolonged cytopenias, closely simulating intensive induction therapy, has produced on average only slight prolongation of remission or life. Regimens that fall between these intensities have been used, with equivocal results. Intensive consolidation therapy after remission results in a somewhat longer remission duration and, more significantly, a subset of patients who have a remission of more than 3 years. The issue of postremission therapy and its impact is complicated by the large proportion of patients with AML who are older than 60 years and the limits of tolerance to intensive therapy in the later decades of life. In addition, a very small pool of leukemic stem cells sustains the process, and elimination of these cells may require approaches other than intensive chemotherapy, especially in adults.

Several randomized trials have studied whether AML patients in first remission should receive consolidation chemotherapy alone, autologous transplantation, or allogeneic marrow transplantation, with no consensus. Allogeneic transplantation was compared to autologous transplantation using unpurged marrow and two courses of intensive chemotherapy in 623 patients who had a complete remission after induction chemotherapy.[514] Disease-free survival was 53 percent at 4 years for those receiving allogeneic marrow, 48 percent for those receiving autologous transplantation, and 30 percent for patients receiving intensive chemotherapy. Overall survival after complete remission was similar in all three groups because patients who relapsed after chemotherapy could be rescued with marrow transplantation. No significant difference in the 4-year disease-free survival between allogeneic marrow transplant (42 percent) and other types of intensive postremission therapy (40 percent) has been found.[515] In one study, a reduced relapse rate in patients receiving autografts but no benefit in disease-free or overall survival was found.[516] In a randomized study, the three postremission treatment groups all had comparable survival.[517] In another study, only patients younger than 15 to 35 years with poor-risk cytogenetics had improved disease-free survival if they had a sibling donor and underwent allogeneic transplantation (43.5% vs. 18.5% at 4 years).[518] Thus, in several studies, the early mortality after allogeneic transplantation and the chemotherapy-induced remissions in patients who relapse following autologous marrow transplantation or chemotherapy have led to comparable overall survival rates. However, leukemia-free survival was greater after allogeneic transplantation.[519] When quality of life was measured for patients in complete remission for 1 to 7 years, those treated with chemotherapy had the highest quality of life and those undergoing allogeneic stem cell transplant the lowest.[520]

The decision to utilize autologous or allogeneic stem cell transplantation or high-dose cytarabine alone for consolidation is individualized based on the patient's age and other prognostic factors, such as high-risk cytogenetic findings and antecedent hematologic disease.[460] Patients with good-risk cytogenetics should receive four cycles of high-dose cytarabine. Patients with poor-risk cytogenetics should be considered for allogeneic or autologous stem cell transplantation after one or two cycles of high-dose cytarabine.

Intensive Consolidation Therapy   For patients who do not receive high-dose chemotherapy with autologous or allogeneic transplantation in first remission, consolidation chemotherapy regimens containing high-dose cytarabine provide better results than intermediate-dose cytarabine,[521,522] but these regimens are not universally accepted.[523] Patients who have ablative allogeneic stem cell transplantation do not require high-dose cytarabine.[524] Patients with t(8;21) have particularly favorable responses to repetitive cycles of high-dose cytarabine. In patients who received three or more cycles, a relapse rate of only 19 percent was seen.[525]

Other regimens, such as those containing gemtuzumab ozogamicin and fludarabine, have been used in postremission therapy.[526] Long-term disease-free survival at 5 years generally is approximately 30 percent when two to four cytarabine-containing regimens are administered.[527,528] Most centers utilize four cycles of 3 g/m² twice daily on days 1, 3, and 5, providing six doses per cycle. The optimal number of cycles for this therapy is not known.[529] High-dose cytarabine can be administered at a dose of 3 g/m² in a 1- to 3- hour intravenous infusion every 12 hours for up to 6 days (12 doses), but this regimen now is rarely utilized because of its toxicity. High-dose cytarabine frequently causes conjunctivitis and photophobia, and glucocorticoid eye drops are usually used every 6 h until 24 h after the last dose of the drug.[530] Cerebellar function abnormalities also may occur, and these require cessation of drug administration. A one hour duration infusion of high-dose or reduced dose (e.g., 2 g/m²) cytarabine may decrease the likelihood of severe cerebellar toxicity.[530] Older patients and patients with renal insufficiency require dose attenuation (i.e., to 2 g/m²).[531]

Additional Maintenance Therapy   Various forms of less intensive maintenance chemotherapy have been attempted after completion of intensive consolidation chemotherapy. Many of the regimens consist of monthly chemotherapy, for example, low-dose 6-thioguanine or cytarabine. Although improved disease-free survival was noted in some studies, no improvement in overall survival has been demonstrated in most studies.[532] Other forms of maintenance therapy, such as interleukin-2, interleukin-2 plus histamine, and induction chemotherapy drugs used at lower doses, have been examined without prolongation of survival. Low-dose interleukin-2 alone has not been found beneficial. Leukemic dendritic cell vaccination, generated *ex vivo* from myelomonocytic leukemic cells, is one of several approaches being tested as maintenance therapy.[533,534]

AUTOLOGOUS STEM CELL INFUSION AFTER ABLATIVE CHEMOTHERAPY OR CHEMORADIOTHERAPY FOR CONSOLIDATION

Removal and cryopreservation of postremission marrow or collection of mobilized blood stem cells from patients with AML and reinfusion of these products following intensive chemotherapy and/or radiotherapy is a form of postremission therapy[535,536] (see Chap. 22). Autologous marrow or blood stem cell rescue can be used in patients with AML who achieve a remission, do not have a compatible stem cell donor, and are up to age 70 years, potentially tripling the proportion of patients amenable to this form of treatment compared to patients who meet the donor and age requirements for ablative allogeneic stem cell transplantation.

Various preparative regimens for autologous transplantation in AML have been utilized,[537] such as busulfan-cyclophosphamide, busulfan-etoposide-cytarabine, high-dose cytarabine-mitoxantrone plus total body irradiation, melphalan plus total body irradiation, and cyclophosphamide plus total body irradiation. A disease-free survival rate of approximately 40 percent at 3 years is average after such regimens in the age range treated.[538,539] Long-term disease-free survival can occur in patients who undergo this treatment for AML in second remission.[540] Patients older than 50 years have inferior outcomes, but no strict upper age limit for this procedure has been determined.[541] Administration of two or more courses of consolidation chemotherapy prior to harvest and transplant is associated with decreased relapse rates and improved disease-free survival. A marrow nucleated cell dose greater than 2×10^8/kg improves disease-free survival.[542] Chemotherapy agents such as 4-hydroperoxycyclophosphamide have been utilized for purging residual leukemic cells,[543,544] and antisense agents reportedly diminish leukemic cell contamination.[545] Use of marrow grafts purged of residual leukemia cells has not significantly improved upon results obtained with unpurged marrow in many studies, suggesting that low proportions of leukemic stem cells may not transplant easily or that they do not survive the freeze–thaw cycle to which autologous marrow is subjected as well as normal stem cells do.[546] In addition, residual leukemia in the patient may contribute to relapse. Thus, the possible benefits of marrow purging remain controversial (see Chap. 22). In long-term cultures from patients newly diagnosed with AML, normal progenitors can be detected, and their numbers are increased by *in vitro* culture with cytokines.[547] In oligoblastic leukemia (myelodysplasia), secondary AML, and therapy-related AML, leukapheresis products obtained after chemotherapy and growth factor treatment contain normal progenitors,[548] indicating mobilized stem cells may be relatively free of leukemic counterparts even in the absence of *ex vivo* purging.[549] Whether use of mobilized blood versus marrow stem cells improves long-term outcomes has not been determined,[549] but early indications are that early mortality may be decreased using blood stem cells.[550] Mobilized progenitor cells can be collected after high-dose cytarabine plus G-CSF or after G-CSF alone.[551]

CHEMORADIOTHERAPY PLUS ALLOGENEIC STEM CELL TRANSPLANTATION FOR CONSOLIDATION THERAPY

General Considerations   Utilization of allogeneic stem cell transplantation for AML is increasing in Europe and the United States.[552] No strict upper age limit for transplantation exists,[553] but many centers use age 60 or 65 years for transplants following ablation of hematopoiesis and 70 years for transplants not following ablation of hematopoiesis (nonmyeloablative transplants). Decisions to proceed to allogeneic transplant should be individualized, and feasibility depends on (1) the availability of a suitable donor, (2) the recipient's age and health status, and (3) whether AML is in remission.

For ablative transplants, the patient is prepared with a regimen that includes total-body irradiation and/or high-dose chemotherapy, after which the donor stem cells are infused by vein. Patients given allogeneic blood stem cells have more rapid hematopoietic reconstitution than patients given marrow stem cells.[554] Chapter 22 describes the indications, procedure, and preparative regimens for stem cell transplantation. With standard-risk leukemia, blood and marrow appear to be equivalent sources for allografting.[555] Engraftment is quicker, but chronic GVHD may be more frequent when blood stem cells are utilized, and longer followup is needed to determine the ultimate effects of blood versus marrow allografts when the donor is a matched sibling.[556] G-CSF–primed donor marrow stem cells may result in less GVHD compared with G-CSF–mobilized blood stem cells.[557] In general, no single preparative regimen is superior for patients with AML in first remission.[558] In one study, cyclophosphamide (Cytoxan) and total-body irradiation lowered relapse risk, but overall results were comparable to conditioning with chemotherapy alone.[559] Postremission consolidation with cytarabine before allogeneic transplantation for AML in first remission does not improve outcome compared with immediate transplant after successful induction.[560]

Related Donors When matched-sibling transplantation is performed for AML in first remission, approximately half of patients have a disease-free survival of 4 years. Small series utilizing T cell depletion have reported 4-year disease-free survival of 65 percent.[561] Leukemia relapses occur in approximately 20 percent of patients who receive an allogeneic transplant.[557] However, compared to age-matched siblings, the overall death rate from other malignancies was higher.[562] Patients who are alive with good performance status 3 years after transplant have excellent prospects of long-term survival.[563] In the posttransplant period, approximately one third of patients die of severe GVHD, opportunistic infection, or interstitial pneumonitis. Marrow transplantation therapy is superior to chemotherapy in that the proportion of subjects who have leukemia relapse is lower, but whether marrow transplantation provides an advantage in overall survival at 3 years is uncertain.[562] The outlook for long-term survival is improved if the AML is in remission prior to transplant, grade III to IV acute GVHD does not occur, and chronic GVHD is low grade.[563–565]

In an attempt to decrease the relapse rate after stem cell transplantation for advanced acute leukemia, ^{131}I-labeled anti-CD45 antibody to deliver radiation to leukemic cells, followed by a standard transplant preparative regimen, has been utilized. Nine of 13 patients with AML were disease free 8 to 41 months after transplant. With this regimen, more radiation can be delivered to hematopoietic tissues compared with liver, lung, or kidney, which may improve the efficacy of marrow transplantation.[566]

Unrelated Donors Approximately 70 percent of all patients with AML are older than 50 years, and the current mean family size in the United States is slightly more than two children per family. Thus, only approximately 10 to 15 percent of subjects with AML are within the age range and have a sibling donor for marrow transplantation. The ability to extend the proportion of patients who can be transplanted has led to histocompatible, unrelated donors or HLA type-mismatched sibling or parent donor transplants.[567] Molecular matching of class I and II HLA alleles adds to the clinical success of unrelated donor transplants but makes finding a donor more difficult.[568] Treatment of high-risk acute leukemia with T cell–depleted stem cells from related donors with one mismatched HLA haplotype with standard conditioning regimens has been successful, with an acceptable incidence of GVHD. However, infectious complications were high.[569] HLA-matched or HLA-mismatched cord blood stem cells can be used in adults with acute leukemia but generally not for patients in first remission.[570,571] In adults, the numbers of progenitor cells available in a single cord product can be limiting.

Nonmyeloablative Transplantation Patients who based upon comorbidities or performance status are deemed too old or too ill to undergo a myeloablative stem cell transplantation may be offered a reduced intensity transplant procedure, provided a suitable donor is available. This type of transplant relies upon graft versus malignancy as primary therapy.[572–574] Uses of this modality have been reported, some specific to AML and some including a variety of hematologic malignancies.[575,576] These regimens have moderate hematologic and nonhematologic toxicity and often can be performed on an outpatient basis. Engraftment and establishment of complete donor chimerism are successful in most patients. GVHD rates have been variable, and the ultimate risk of acute and chronic GVHD with these regimens is unclear. A variety of low-intensity regimens have been proposed.[577] In AML in first remission, the 1-year progression-free survival is approximately 55 percent.[578,579] The role this treatment approach eventually will have in the treatment of AML remains to be defined, and controlled trials with longer followup are needed to answer this question. Nonmyeloablative conditioning with unrelated donors has been utilized successfully.[580,581]

Use of Transplant in Relapsed Patients Some form of allograft usually is recommended for patients in early first relapse or second remission, because long-term survival with chemotherapy alone is improbable, whereas histocompatible sibling transplants have a 25 percent survival rate. However, when transplantation was compared to chemotherapy for AML in second remission, the 3-year probability of event-free survival was 17 percent with chemotherapy and 16 percent with transplant. Patients younger than 30 years who were in remission for at least 1 year fared best.[582] Patients with extramedullary sites of leukemia more likely have extramedullary sites of relapse after allogeneic bone marrow transplantation.[583]

Patients with AML who relapse after allogeneic marrow transplantation can have a long-term remission if they undergo retransplantation.[584] The mechanism of benefit of marrow transplantation was thought to result from high-dose ablative chemoradiotherapy followed by marrow "rescue." The increased relapse rate of AML in patients transplanted with marrow from identical twins, compared to nonidentical siblings, or transplanted with T lymphocyte–depleted marrow has indicated an immunologic effect of donor lymphocytes may determine the results of transplantation. This immunologic response, referred to as *graft-versus-leukemia reaction*, may play a role in preventing leukemia relapses.[585]

Donor Leukocyte Infusion In an attempt to enhance graft-versus-leukemia effects, adoptive immunotherapy with donor mononuclear cell infusions is sometimes utilized to treat relapse of leukemia after allografting.[586,587] These infusions have been successful in only a minority of patients with AML, but given the high mortality associated with alternative procedures such as second transplants, the infusions are a reasonable approach for patients who relapse after allogeneic transplant.[588] GVHD and marrow aplasia are the major complications of this form of treatment.[589] The graft-versus-leukemia reaction is thought to be directed against minor histocompatibility antigens on the cell surface of hematopoietic cells, but reactions against leukemia-specific antigens are possible. Relapses after donor leukocyte infusions for recurring acute leukemia have a higher probability of being extramedullary.[590] Donor lymphocyte infusions are most effective in early relapses and in the presence of chronic GVHD induction.[591] Some patients also enter a new remission upon withdrawal of immune suppression. Patients who enter remission by donor lymphocyte infusion or cessation of immune suppressive agents have a better survival than those who entered remission with chemotherapy alone or after a second transplant.[592] Unrelated donor leukocyte infusions can be used to treat relapsed leukemia after unrelated donor stem cell transplantation.[593] Approximately 40 percent of AML patients enter remission with this treatment. G-CSF has been used as an alternative to donor leukocyte infusions after AML relapse posttransplant.[594] Donor blood stem cells can be combined with chemotherapy for early relapse of AML after allogeneic stem cell transplantation.[595]

Adjunct Therapy with Interleukin-2 and Vaccines Interleukin-2 has been used to modulate natural killer and T cell activity after both autologous and allogeneic transplantation. The efficacy of this approach has not yet been determined.[596] Minor histocompatibility antigens restricted to hematopoietic cells are an ideal target for antileukemic immune responses. Modification of leukemic cells to express costimulatory molecules identical to professional antigen-presenting cells to generate cytotoxic T lymphocyte responses against myeloid leukemia cells may be possible.[597] Irradiated B7.1-transduced primary AML cells can be used as therapeutic vaccines in murine AML.[598] B7.1 is the ligand for the T cell costimulatory molecules CD28 and CTLA-4. Dendritic cells derived *in vitro* from AML cells also can be utilized to stimulate leukemia-specific cytolytic activity in autologous or allogeneic lymphocytes.[533]

Recurrent Leukemia in Donor Cells or New Leukemia in Recipient Cells Recurrence of AML in donor cells has been reported in patients who received marrow transplants from healthy siblings. These recurrences in donor cells occurred in approximately one in 18 relapsed patients who received marrow from a donor of the opposite sex.[599] A similar frequency of relapsed AML is observed in recipient cells but with a different clonal cytogenetic abnormality, suggesting a "new" leukemia.[599] The frequencies are dependent on the sensitivity and specificity of cytogenetic techniques, which have been challenged. AML developing in a stem cell recipient but of donor cell origin long after transplant has been documented in rare cases.[600,601]

TREATMENT OF RELAPSED OR REFRACTORY PATIENTS

CHEMOTHERAPY

Patients who relapse after remission-induction and postinduction therapy have a decreased probability of entering a subsequent remission, and the duration of any remission that occurs is shorter. In patients who relapse more than 1 year after the first remission, the original remission-induction regimen can be readministered or a combination salvage chemotherapy regimen can be administered. One regimen includes high-dose cytosine arabinoside without or with another agent such as mitoxantrone, amsacrine, or etoposide. Table 87-6 lists other chemotherapy regimens for refractory patients.

Refractory leukemia is defined as leukemia that does not respond to initial induction chemotherapy with cytarabine and an anthracycline antibiotic or anthraquinone. Patients with refractory disease are more likely to have disease with adverse cytogenetic findings, a history of antecedent clonal myeloid disease, adverse immunophenotypic features, and expression of multidrug resistance (MDR).[602,603]

Relapsed leukemia is leukemia that recurs following a remission. The duration of remission greatly affects the patient's prognosis and response to additional treatment. The wide range of response rates may not only reflect the regimen used but may also reflect variability in patient selection, age, and other prognostic factors.[603–605]

Chemotherapy regimens can be divided into cytarabine-based, noncytarabine-based, and timed sequential therapy with growth factors and cytotoxic drugs. Table 87-6 lists the response rates; the duration of response usually is measured in months. The duration of response is difficult to define because many patients go on to other therapies, including stem cell transplantation.

Chemomodulation with drugs, such as the cyclosporine analogue PSC-833, can impede the MDR pump *in vitro*. Use of the latter agent necessitates a two-thirds reduction in mitoxantrone and etoposide doses.[606] MDR has been addressed in a regimen using liposomal daunorubicin and cyclosporine to overcome reduced activity of gemtuzumab ozogamicin and cytarabine in refractory AML[607] (see "Modulation of Drug Resistance" below).

Results from second remission-induction therapy are better in younger patients and in those with longer first remissions, longer durations since last chemotherapy, and better general health. The probability of a second remission is approximately 50 percent in younger subjects (15–60 years) and approximately 25 percent in older patients (60–80 years), but the duration of remission nearly always is much shorter than the first remission. An eventual fatal outcome is nearly certain unless allogeneic stem cell transplantation can be performed. Rare patients may have a third (or more) relapse followed by a remission when treated with cytotoxic drugs, but each remission is shorter than the preceding one and usually is measured in weeks. For those who have favorable or normal karyotype, long second remission, and no previous stem cell transplant, intensive chemotherapy can be useful.[608] In one study, approximately 17 percent of 124 patients had a second remission duration at least 2 months longer than the first remission.[609] In patients in relapse treated with the sequential high-dose cytosine arabinoside and mitoxantrone (S-HAM) regimen, the duration of the first remission was the only factor associated with a successful outcome, and unfavorable karyotype was the only factor related to duration of survival.[610] Patients who relapse less than 1 year from remission should be treated with investigational agents, whereas patients who relapse more than 1 year later may benefit from standard reinduction therapy.[611] No standard chemotherapy regimen provides durable remission of AML patients who relapse[612] (see Table 87-6).

ALLOGENEIC STEM CELL TRANSPLANTATION

Allogeneic stem cell transplantation may be the only means to induce a sustained remission in patients with AML who do not enter remission with cytotoxic drug therapy or who relapse after a first remission. Approximately 25 percent of patients with refractory or relapsed AML have a sustained remission of at least 3 years.[630] Transplant-related mortality at 3 years is approximately 50 percent. Relapse rates are higher after sibling than matched-unrelated transplantation.[631,632] If a histocompatible donor is available and the patient is younger than 50 years, stem cell transplantation can be as successful if it is performed when the patient is in early relapse compared with second remission.[633]

OTHER TREATMENT MODALITIES

CHEMOTHERAPY

Several newer chemotherapeutic agents are being examined for treatment of AML. The anthracycline antibiotic WP744 may overcome drug resistance in MDR-positive cells.[634] Troxacitabine, an isomer of cytarabine, has entered into phase I and II trials in AML and has been combined with cytarabine, idarubicin, or topotecan.[635,636] Temozolomide[637] and clofarabine,[638] a nucleoside analogue, induced responses in refractory or relapsed acute leukemias. High-dose hydroxyurea can result in remission in 42 percent of patients with poor-risk leukemias when given at a dosage of 100 mg/kg/day until marrow aplasia occurs or for a maximum of 30 days.[639]

Methylation of DNA at critical sites in cells can cause transcriptional inactivation of genes or chromosomal instability. In AML, aberrant methylation, especially preferential methylation of chromosome 11, has been described.[640] These genes are *in vivo* targets for demethylating agents such as 5-azacytidine or decitibine.[641] Decitabine, a potent hypomethylating agent, can result in maturation and growth arrest of AML cells. It may have synergism with interferons and retinoids. It has effects as a single agent, and in combination with anthracyclines has resulted in response rates of 30 to 50 percent.[642,643] Histone deacetylase inhibitors can restore retinoic acid-dependent transcriptional activation and maturation in AML blasts.[644] Depsipeptide

TABLE 87-6 EXAMPLES OF CHEMOTHERAPY USED FOR RELAPSED OR REFRACTORY PATIENTS

REGIMEN	NO. OF PATIENTS	COMPLETE REMISSION (%) (MEDIAN DURATION)	YEAR	REFERENCE
Fludarabine 25 mg/m², days 1–5 Gemcitabine 10 mg/m²/min for 15 hours	18	16%	2003	629
Gemtuzumab ozogamicin 6 mg/m² IV, days 1 and 13 Idarubicin 12 mg/m², days 2 – 4 Cytarabine 1.5 g/m², days 2–5	15	21% (27 weeks)	2003	628
Mitroxantrone 12 mg/m², days 1–3 Cytarabine 500 mg/m², days 1–3 Followed by (at count recovery) Etoposide 200 mg/m², days 1–3 Cytarabine 500 mg/m², days 1–3	66	36% (5 months)	2003	626
Cladrabine 5 mg/m², days 1–5 Cytarabine 2 g/m², days 1–5 2 h after 2-CdA G-CSF 10 µg/kg/day, days 1–5	58	50% (29% disease-free at 1 year)	2003	625
Fludarabine 30 mg/m², days 1–5 Cytarabine 2 g/m², days 1–5 Idarubicin 10/m² days 1–3 G-CSF 5 µg/kg/day, day +6 until neutrophil recovery	46	52% (13 months)	2003	624
Gemtuzumab ozogamicin 9 mg/m², day 1 Cytarabine 1 g/m² over 2 h, days 1–5 Topotecan 1.25 mg/m², days 1–5	17	12% (8.2 weeks)	2002	627
Gemtuzumab ozogamicin 9 mg/m², days 1 and 15	43	9% 5% CRp	2002	619
Idarubicin, 12mg/m2, IV bolus, days 1–3 Cytarabine, 1g/m2, IV over 2 h, every 12 hours, days 1–5; Topotecan, 1.25mg/m2, IV over 24 h, days 1–5.	27	52%	2001	623
Liposomal daunorubicin (escalating doses), + Cytarabine 2 g/m² IV for 4 days by continuous infusion	62	29%	2001	620
Cytarabine 0.5 g/m² every 12 h for 12 doses days 1 to 6+ Mitoxantrone 5 mg/m² IV, days 1–5	47	62% (112days)	2000	621
Carboplatin 200 mg/m²/day by continuous infusion days 3 to 7+ Idarubicin or mitoxantrone 12 mg/m²/day, days 1–3	53	28% (60 days)	1999	622
Carboplatin 300 mg/m² per day for 5 days continuous infusion Cytarabine 500 mg/m² for 3 days	31	29	1999	617
Mitoxantrone 4 mg/m², days 1–3 Etoposide 40 mg/m², days 1–3 Cytarabine 1 g/m², days 1–3, ± PSC-833	37	32	1999	613
Cyclophosphamide 1 g/m², days 1–3 Etoposide 200 mg/m², days 1–3 Carboplatin 150 mg/m² continuous infusion, days 1–3 Cytarabine 1 g/m², days 1–3	25	12	1998	618
Cladrabine 0.1 mg/kg/day for 7 days continuous infusion plus or minus Daunorubicin 50 mg/m², days 5–7	19	0*	1998	615
Topotecan 4.75 mg/m², days 1–5 Cytarabine 1 g/m², days 1–5	53	4†	1997	616
Fludarabine 30 mg/m², days 1–5 Cytarabine 2 g/m², days 1–5± Idarubicin 12 mg/m², days 1–3 G-CSF 400 µg/m² daily until complete remission	85	66	1995	614

* 100% of treated patients had improvement.
† 39% of treated patients had improvement.
CRp, complete remission except for platelet recovery.
NOTE: The reader is advised to consult the original reference for details of chemotherapy regimen administration.

can promote histone acetylation and gene transcription in AML1/ETO-positive leukemic cells.[645]

GROWTH FACTORS AND RECEPTOR TARGETS

A ricin fusion toxin attached to human GM-CSF[646] and a diphtheria toxin attached to GM-CSF to form a fusion protein are toxic to AML cells.[647] GM-CSF can alter the cellular metabolism of cytarabine and fludarabine in AML patients.[648] A diphtheria toxin IL-3 fusion protein is cytotoxic for blasts that express high-affinity interleukin-3 receptor,[649] and progenitor cells from patients with CD87+ urokinase receptor are sensitive to a diphtheria-toxin-urokinase fusion protein.[650]

ANTIBODIES TO CD33

The CD33 antigen is expressed on approximately 90 percent of AML blasts but is not expressed by the pluripotent hematopoietic stem cell; thus, it is a target for antibody-mediated destruction of AML blasts. Gemtuzumab ozogamicin is a recombinant humanized anti-CD33 monoclonal immunoglobulin (Ig)G4 antibody conjugated to the cytotoxin calicheamicin.[651,652] The conjugated antibody is rapidly internalized and causes subsequent apoptosis.[653] Gemtuzumab ozogamicin administered to AML patients with CD33+ blast cells in untreated first relapse at a dose of 9 mg/m² twice, 14 days apart, produced complete remission in 16 percent of patients and complete remission with incomplete platelet recovery in an another 14 percent of patients.[654] It has been approved by the US Food and Drug Administration for use in patients older than 65 years.[655–657] This agent produces myelosuppression and is associated with an infusional syndrome that can be minimized with glucocorticoids.[658] It does not cause alopecia or mucositis. Hyperbilirubinemia and transaminase elevations can occur. Although it results in similar survival rates as standard chemotherapy reinduction, its use was associated with fewer days of hospitalization.[659] In patients who relapsed between 3 to 11 months, gemtuzumab ozogamicin resulted in higher remission rates compared to regimens containing high-dose cytarabine in different trials. However, in patients who had prolonged first remissions of greater than 19 months, cytarabine resulted in superior remission rates.[660] Prior gemtuzumab ozogamicin exposure may increase the risk of venoocclusive disease in patients who later undergo myeloablative allogeneic stem cell transplant procedures.[661,662]

HuM195, another anti-CD33 antibody, has been utilized in patients with AML with minimal residual disease. It has been conjugated to iodine-131, yttrium-90, and bismuth-213 to deliver radiation to sites of leukemic involvement.[663] Antibodies to CD45 and to CD66 in a radioconjugated form are being studied for advanced AML.[664]

THERAPIES TARGETED TO SIGNAL TRANSDUCTION MEDIATORS

Tyrosine Kinase Inhibitors *FLT3 Inhibitors.* Constitutively activating *FLT3* receptor mutations have been found in approximately 30 percent of patients with AML. Several small-molecule *FLT3* tyrosine kinase inhibitors have been described, including PKC412,[665] CT83518,[666] CEP-701,[667] and SU5416.[668] These agents inhibit *FLT3-ITD* phosphorylation, induce apoptosis *in vitro*, and have efficacy in mouse models of human leukemia. Targeted inhibition of *FLT3* can overcome blockade of myeloid differentiation.[669] These agents are in phase I and II trials, in which they have induced a decline in blood blast cells.[670]

KIT Tyrosine Kinase Inhibitors. Imatinib mesylate. Activation of the Kit tyrosine kinase by somatic mutation has been documented in a minority of AML cases. Paracrine or autocrine activation of *KIT* may occur in AML cells.[671] In culture systems, KIT ligand (stem cell factor) independent, KIT phosphorylation usually is not detected, suggesting that imatinib mesylate has only limited activity.[672] Imatinib mesylate

also inhibits the activity of the proteins platelet-derived growth factor receptor (PDGF-R) and mutant tyrosine kinase (BCR-ABL). Imatinib mesylate has induced a complete remission of refractory secondary AML,[673] but this is an uncommon situation.[674]

Other Tyrosine Kinase Inhibitors. AG1296 is a tyrosine kinase inhibitor of the tryphostin class that inhibits wild-type FLT3, PDGFR, and KIT receptors.[675] SU5416, a small-molecule inhibitor of phosphorylation of VEGFR-1 and VEGFR-2, of *KIT*, and of FLT3 expression has induced one remission and seven cases of improvement among 43 patients treated. Its effect was thought to be primarily antiangigogenic, based upon response correlation with VEGF mRNA levels.[676]

Other Inhibitors of Signal Transduction and Apoptosis Pathways
Small-molecule mitogen-activated protein kinase kinase (MEK) inhibitors inhibit growth and survival of AML cell lines and primary samples of AML cells *in vitro* by blocking constitutive activation of the mitogen-activated protein kinase. These or similar inhibitors may have future therapeutic promise, but no trials have yet been reported.[677]

Many malignancies overexpress antiapoptotic proteins, such as Bcl-2 and Bcl-x_L.[678] Antisense agents to Bcl-2 mRNA in combination with chemotherapy are being tested in patients with AML.[679] The 18-merphosphorothioate Bcl-2 antisense molecule G3139 (Genasense) has been combined with fludarabine, arabinosyl cytosine, and G-CSF (FLAG) therapy. It down-regulates its target Bcl-2.[679] CDDO-Me, a triterpenoid, *in vitro* induces apoptosis and differentiation in AML cells through activation of caspase-8 and caspase-3 and induction of mitochondrial cytochrome *c* release.[680] It can facilitate the maturation of cells by ATRA; down-regulate FLIP, an antagonist of caspase-8; and result in tumor necrosis factor (TNF)-related apoptosis-inducing ligand (TRAIL)-induced apoptosis via a TNF-family death pathway.[681] These agents may have activity in AML.[681] The cyclin-dependent kinase inhibitor flavopiridol potentiates apoptosis in AML cells,[682] and it has entered trials of timed sequential therapy in AML.[683] The proteasome inhibitor bortezomib (PS-341) for use in AML is being studied.[684]

Prenylation Inhibitors *Farnesyltransferase Inhibitors.* Mutation or activation of *RAS* has been seen in the cells of approximately 15 percent of AML patients. Because posttranslational processing by farnesyltransferase is necessary for RAS translocation to the cell membrane, inhibitors of this enzyme are postulated to inhibit RAS activity.[685] These inhibitors also affect processing of numerous other proteins, and often their effects may be independent of *RAS* mutation or activation. Several farnesyltransferase inhibitors are being studied as inhibitors of AML cell growth (BMS-214662, L-778,123, R-115777 (Tipifarnib) and SCH66336 (Lonafarnib).[686–688] In a phase I trial of R115777 in adults with refractory and relapsed AML, clinical responses occurred in 10 of 34 evaluable patients, including two complete remissions. Further trials in untreated AML/MDS patients are ongoing.[689]

Geranylgeranyltransferase-1 Inhibitors. Because many proteins subject to farnesylation also undergo geranylgeranylation, geranylgeranyltransferase-1 inhibitors may have activity in AML and may explain resistance to farnesyl transferase inhibitor monotherapy in patients with AML.[690] Several of these inhibitors are being screened. The statins inhibit geranylation, and cases of responses of AML to lovastatin have been reported.[691] Simvastatin in an additive fashion with cytarabine inhibits AML cell lines.[692] Other studies have suggested the statins may mediate antileukemic effects independent of Ras/Rho prenylation through blockade of cholesterol responses to cellular injury.[693]

MATURATION THERAPIES

A stable benzoic derivative of retinoic acid induces maturation of promyelocytic leukemic cells. It is 10- to 100-fold more potent than

ATRA.[694] Several analogues of vitamin D inhibit AML cells by inducing inhibition of cyclin-dependent kinases.[695] *WAF-1* is induced by vitamin D analogues. When WAF-1 is combined with retinoids, maturation of leukemic cells is observed.[696] In general, AML cells have not responded to retinoids. Single-strand conformational polymorphism analysis and DNA sequencing of leukemic cells from AML other than APL have not found mutations of RAR-α.[697] Nevertheless, combinations of retinoids, growth factors, and chemotherapeutic agents are being examined for therapeutic potential in AML.[698] Leukemias with 11q, -5, and -7 chromosome abnormalities have high telomerase activity, and this activity can be inhibited by maturation-inducing agents.[699] In one study, addition of ATRA to chemotherapy did not improve patient outcome but did result in a 25 percent increase in apoptosis in AML marrow cells *in vitro*.[700] ATRA has induced a complete remission in a patient with acute myelomonocytic leukemia.[701] A novel retinoid (3-Cl-AHPC/MM002) has been found that induces apoptosis in ATRA-resistant leukemia cell lines.[702] Arsenic trioxide (As$_2$O$_3$) induces apoptosis and cytotoxic effects in blasts from patients with AML other than APL, and it is not influenced by permeability glycoprotein (P-gp) expression.[703] Cyclooxygenase-2 inhibitors can suppress proliferation and differentiation in leukemia cell lines.[704]

ANTIANGIOGENESIS AGENTS

Amifostine has cytoprotective effects and some antiangiogenesic potential. It can lead to a complete remission in AML.[705] When 13 patients were treated with thalidomide up to 400 mg/day, seven patients required premature withdrawal from the medication, and four patients had some hematologic improvement.[706] Declining basic fibroblast growth factor levels were found in the responding patients. In a phase II study of SU5416, a small-molecule inhibitor of VEGFR-2, no remissions were seen, and only two of 32 patients being treated improved.[707]

MODULATION OF DRUG RESISTANCE

Numerous mechanisms of drug resistance occur in AML,[708,709] and several attempts to overcome this resistance have been instituted. P-gp, MDR protein-1 (MRP-1), and breast cancer resistance protein (BCRP) expression all have been found in AML.[710] P-gp expression is correlated with decreased rates and shorter duration of remission.[711] Homozygous *MDR-1* gene expression, which encodes P-gp, is associated with shorter relapse-free intervals and poor survival rates and does not vary between diagnosis and relapse in paired samples.[712] PSC-833 has been utilized to modulate P-gp and has been combined with daunorubicin[713] and with mitoxantrone, etoposide, and cytarabine.[714] PSC-833 reduces the clearance of etoposide and mitoxantrone. Idarubicin does not appear to be as affected by P-gp expression.[715] In a phase II study of PSC-833 in previously untreated older patients with AML, considerable early toxicity was noted with the addition of PSC-833 to daunorubicin, etoposide, and cytarabine.[716,717] In a randomized study, addition of cyclosporine A to infusional daunorubicin reduced drug resistance, prolonged remission duration, and improved overall survival. Whether this response resulted entirely from drug efflux modulation or from other immune modulatory effects of cyclosporine was not determined.[718] The FLAG regimen is beneficial for P glycoprotein–positive AML compared with standard anthracycline and cytarabine.[719] AML cells may be protected from cytotoxic agents by high glutathione and γ-glutamylcysteine synthetase levels.[720] Quinine has been examined as a modulator of MDR in a phase III trial. Its addition did not improve survival, but it did improve remission rates in a subgroup of patients demonstrating functional drug resistance as measured by rhodamine-123 efflux.[721]

OTHER IMMUNOTHERAPY APPROACHES

Targeting of a B7-1 (CD30) IgG fusion protein to AML blasts increases their costimulatory and proliferative activity for autologous T cells, an approach that may augment T cell antileukemic activity,[722] given that autologous T cells can mediate antileukemic reactivity.[723] Culture of AML blasts up-regulates costimulatory molecules.[724] Other approaches to generating autologous T cell antileukemic activity include vaccination with AML-specific peptides, immunization with AML blasts exhibiting dendritic cell phenotype and function,[725,726] and pulsing normal dendritic cells with AML-specific peptide sequences.[727] Natural killer cells may mediate antileukemia effects.[728] Low doses of interleukin-2 have been used in the maintenance phase of AML, and some patients have remained on this regimen for 10 or more years without significant side effects.[729] Wilms tumor gene *WT1* is expressed on AML blasts, and a WT1 vaccine may elicit cytotoxic T cell responses against this protein.[730] Other proteins against which such humoral responses have been elicited include minor HLA antigens and proteinase-3.[731]

SPECIAL THERAPEUTIC CONSIDERATIONS

ACUTE PROMYELOCYTIC LEUKEMIA

Induction Treatment ATRA has become a standard component of induction therapy for APL. Used alone, ATRA can induce a short-term remission in at least 80 percent of patients.[732] However, ATRA is combined with an anthracycline such as idarubicin during induction treatment.[733,734] Idarubicin by itself can induce remission in approximately 75 percent of patients.[735] A typical induction regimen for APL is ATRA 45 mg/m^2 daily in divided doses with idarubicin 12 mg/m^2 daily for 4 days. Although cytarabine has been largely abandoned as part of induction, some studies have shown a high degree of efficacy of high-dose cytarabine combined with ATRA.[736] Older patients generally tolerate a combination of ATRA and an anthracycline.[737] Combinations of gemtuzumab ozogamicin are being examined for their effectiveness in APL induction therapy.[738] The combination of ATRA and As$_2$O$_3$ results in more rapid remissions and lower PML-RAR-α transcript levels than after either agent alone.[739] Despite the high remission rates and frequency of long-term event-free survival achieved in this disease, controversies remain regarding therapy for APL because of the 10 percent early death rate, with most patients suffering fatal hemorrhages.[740]

All-*trans*-Retinoic Acid *Dose and Mechanism of Action.* ATRA, an analogue of vitamin A, has been used to initiate the therapy of APL since 1987. The drug is administered in a total dose of 25 to 45 mg/m^2 per day given in two oral doses, with the lower doses equally as effective and less toxic.[741] The drug induces complete remissions in approximately 80 percent of previously untreated patients.[742–746] *In vitro*, ATRA is 10 times more potent in inducing maturation of leukemic promyelocytes to neutrophils than 13-*cis*-retinoic acid, the other naturally occurring isomer.[747] ATRA induces maturation of the leukemic cells and the suppression of the malignant clone, resulting in a switch to polyclonal hematopoiesis and a remission in most cases.[748–750] ATRA may induce synthesis of a protein that selectively degrades PML-RAR-α. ATRA can overcome the recruitment of histone deacetylase activity by the *PML-RAR-α* fusion gene through interference with a nuclear corepressor.[751] Signal transducer and activator of transcription factor STAT-1 is induced and activated by ATRA. Promyelocytic leukemia cells with PML-RAR-α break-fusion sites in *PML* exon 6 have decreased *in vitro* responsiveness to ATRA.[752] The t(11;17) variant of APL in which the promyelocytic leukemia zinc finger (*PLZF*) gene is fused to *RAR-α* does not respond to ATRA.[753] Other types of AML have not responded to ATRA therapy. ATRA is beneficial in APL during the induction and maintenance phases of disease,[754] and improved outcome with ATRA appears to be maintained long term, with 5-year disease survival rates of 75 to 80 percent.[755,756] Additional cytogenetic changes do not influence treatment outcomes with ATRA plus anthracyclines,[757] and ATRA induction can result in favorable long-term results without blood product support.[758]

Toxic Effects. ATRA therapy is associated with dryness of the skin and lips, occasionally leading to mild exfoliation, nausea, headache, arthralgias, and bone pain. The white cell count may rise dramatically in the first week or two of therapy. Serum glutamic-pyruvate transaminase and triglyceride concentrations often increase. Leukemic promyelocytes disappear from the blood in 2 to 4 weeks, and a normal marrow aspirate may be obtained in 4 to 10 weeks. Anemia improves gradually. The majority of patients become PML-RAR-α negative by PCR after the second consolidation therapy in conjunction with ATRA.[759] ATRA has been used successfully to treat promyelocytic leukemia diagnosed during pregnancy.[760,761] ATRA has been used from week 3 of gestation but may result in fetal malformations when it is used during the first trimester.[762]

A rapid increase in the total blood leukocyte count to as high as 80,000/μl (80 $\times$ 10^9/liter) in the first several weeks of therapy, referred to as *retinoic acid syndrome*, is a potential cause of early death during therapy.[763–766] The median time of onset is 11 days, but the syndrome can occur up to 47 days after therapy starts.[765] Two approaches to treatment of this phenomenon have been suggested: early use of cytotoxic chemotherapy[767,768] and glucocorticoid administration.[769,770] The syndrome consists of fever, weight gain, dependent edema, pleural or pericardial effusion, and bouts of hypotension. Respiratory distress is the key feature. In fatal cases, pulmonary interstitial infiltration with maturing granulocytes is prominent. Once respiratory distress is evident, the patient should receive dexamethasone 10 mg intravenously every 12 hours for several days. Because the syndrome may occur at relatively low total white cell counts and its onset is unpredictable, high-dose glucocorticoid therapy should be instituted if respiratory symptoms develop even in the absence of pulmonary infiltrates or an elevated white cell count.[765,768] ATRA can be continued or resumed with glucocorticoids or with concurrent cytotoxic chemotherapy, but the syndrome may recur.[765] It is not observed during maintenance therapy.

Treatment of Coagulopathy Reducing the risk of early death from hemorrhage as a result of the coagulopathy accompanying APL requires use of fresh-frozen plasma, platelet replacement, and fibrinogen replacement.[368,369,771] Heparin treatment often was utilized during induction chemotherapy to prevent onset of disseminated intravascular coagulopathy during treatment in the past but rarely is used now.[772] ATRA may have some corrective effect on coagulation disorders in promyelocytic leukemia.[773] However, the reduction of early fatal hemorrhages has not been significant with ATRA utilized early during treatment. Paradoxically, hypercoagulable clotting tendency may occur in patients during the first months of ATRA therapy.[748]

Chemotherapy Induction of remission with ATRA is followed by relapse in weeks to months unless intensive chemotherapy is used concomitantly.[456,744,745] At relapse, cells show high levels of a cytosolic retinoic-acid-binding protein not detected prior to ATRA therapy.[751] The mechanism of retinoid resistance in leukemic cells may involve cytochrome P450 and P-gp because of induction of various enzymes that may alter ATRA metabolism.[774] ATRA, whether administered as part of induction therapy or as maintenance therapy, confers a disease-free survival advantage. More than 70 percent of patients receiving ATRA at any point were in continuous remission at 2.5 years versus less than 20 percent of patients who never received ATRA.[763] The

acquired *in vivo* resistance that occurs rapidly to ATRA as a single agent requires consolidation of ATRA-induced complete remission with intensive chemotherapy using an anthracycline antibiotic. Customary treatment today involves simultaneous administration of ATRA and an anthracycline antibiotic. Some therapists have returned to combining an anthracycline antibiotic with cytarabine in an effort to decrease CNS relapse. Maintenance therapy with ATRA alone or with the combination of ATRA, mercaptopurine, or methotrexate has been recommended.[733] This therapy has not been examined in a randomized trial of ATRA dosing and scheduling, but ATRA usually is given in an interrupted fashion.

Arsenic Trioxide As$_2$O$_3$ can be useful for patients who relapse.[775–778] As$_2$O$_3$ can trigger apoptosis of promyelocytic leukemia cells at high concentrations and maturation at low concentrations. The presence of PML-RAR-α is important for the response.[777] Apoptosis may occur through induction of activation of caspase-1 and caspase-3 after changes in the mitochondrial membrane potential with increase in H$_2$O$_2$.[779–781] It also may function through nuclear factor-κB (NF-κB) inhibition.[782] As$_2$O$_3$ given at 0.06 to 0.12 mg/kg body weight per day until leukemic cells were eliminated from the marrow induced remission within 12 to 89 days in 11 of 12 patients.[781] Marrow depression did not occur. Rash, light-headedness, fatigue, and musculoskeletal pain were the main side effects. As$_2$O$_3$ can be combined with idarubicin in relapsed patients; it also has been utilized with ATRA.[783–785] A retinoic-acid-like syndrome has been described in patients with APL treated with As$_2$O$_3$.[786] Torsades de pointes has been described with As$_2$O$_3$ use,[787] and monitoring of QTc intervals is recommended.[788]

Other Treatments for Relapsed Disease Conventional chemotherapy can be effective after relapse. Patients younger than 60 years should be considered for allogeneic or autologous transplantation after they have achieved a second remission or for allogeneic transplantation if a second remission cannot be induced.[789] Other treatments for patients in relapse include ATRA if relapse occurs more than 12 months after treatment,[790] As$_2$O$_3$ as described above, and gemtuzumab ozogamicin. Transplantation generally is not recommended for patients with promyelocytic leukemia in first remission given overall good response durations after standard treatments. Allogeneic stem cell transplant is best utilized in advanced APL, especially in patients with persistent disease by PCR.[791] The outcome of autologous stem cell transplant in second complete remission is excellent if the stem cells used are negative for PML-RAR-α.[762] A direct comparison of autologous transplant, allogeneic transplant, and arsenic or ATRA with standard chemotherapy has not been studied in patients with APL in a second remission after relapse.[792] Many cases of extramedullary relapse in APL have been reported.[793] Many of the relapses occur in patients who received ATRA and who initially were diagnosed with hyperleukocytosis,[794] and many of the patients are in marrow remission. Myelodysplastic syndrome can occur in patients in remission with APL, usually 24 months after diagnosis of APL. The complication results from a second (drug-induced) clonal disease in long-term responders.[795–797] Cases of therapy-related APL have been described.[798]

SECONDARY LEUKEMIA

Secondary leukemias arise after a myelodysplastic syndrome or after treatment of another malignancy with cytotoxic chemotherapy or radiation. Secondary AML responds more poorly to chemotherapy and stem cell transplantation than does *de novo* AML. Secondary AML accounts for approximately 15 percent of all AML cases, although this percentage is increasing.[799,800] The leukemogenic risk of treatment regimens depends on the agents used. Development of agents with lower risk of inducing AML is important.[801]

EFFECT OF TOPOISOMERASE II INHIBITORS

Exposure to topoisomerase II inhibitors can lead to AML with *MLL* gene rearrangements on chromosome 11q32.[802] Inversion 16 is an uncommon aberration in secondary AML and, like balanced translocations of chromosome bands 11q32, 21q22, and t(15;17), are associated with prior chemotherapy with topoisomerase II inhibitors when they are seen in the setting of treatment-induced leukemias. The site of breakpoints within the *MYH*11 gene involved in inversion 16 may vary between therapy-induced AML and AML *de novo*.[803] The latency period for development of AML after topoisomerase II inhibitors is approximately 2 years. No relationship with higher cumulative dose or genetic predisposition has been identified.[804] Even the use of low-dose or oral etoposide can be associated with development of secondary AML.

EFFECT OF ALKYLATING AGENTS AND CISPLATIN

Alkylating agents cause secondary AML often preceded by myelodysplasia. The mean latency period after onset of treatment is approximately 6 years. Deletions of all or part of chromosome 5 or 7 are the most common cytogenetic changes. The risk is related to cumulative alkylating agent dose. Germ-line aberrancies of NFI and p53 may increase the risk of AML. Cisplatin used for treatment of ovarian cancer increases the risk of secondary leukemia.[805]

OTHER CYTOTOXIC AGENTS

Other drugs that may increase the risk of secondary leukemias include low-dose weekly methotrexate for rheumatoid arthritis,[806] etanercept therapy,[807] growth hormone administration,[808] and G-CSF given to patients with congenital but not idiopathic or cyclic neutropenia.[809] In the latter case, a cause-and-effect relationship between MDS/AML and G-CSF therapy was not established. Improved survival with G-CSF may allow expression of an underlying leukemic predisposition.

Patients with APL in remission may develop a new oligoblastic leukemia, presumably secondary to therapy.[810] Series of children with treatment-related myelodysplasia or AML have the same latency period as do adults treated with alkylating agents or topoisomerase II inhibitors for AML.[811] Breast cancer patients receiving doxorubicin and cyclophosphamide regimens of such intensity that they required G-CSF support had increased rates of posttherapy AML. Breast and prostate radiotherapy are associated with an increased risk of AML.[812–814] In patients with non-Hodgkin lymphoma, up to 10 percent of patients treated with either conventional chemotherapy or high-dose therapy may develop secondary AML within 10 years.[815] Secondary leukemia is seen after autologous marrow or blood stem cell transplants involving high-dose chemotherapy and/or radiotherapy. In a study of 83 patients after autografting, 12 had nonclonal cytogenetic abnormalities and 10 had clonal abnormalities, five of whom developed secondary AML. Onset occurred 12 to 48 months after autografting. The relative contribution of the underlying disease and conditioning therapy is uncertain.[816] Clonality analysis utilizing X chromosome usage, based on methylation of the human androgen receptor locus in cell samples in patients with lymphoma, found a clonal marrow cell population 6 months after autologous transplantation at a time when no morphologic or clinical evidence of AML was present. AML appeared later in some patients.[817] More than 10 percent of patients with non-Hodgkin lymphoma who underwent stem cell rescue after total body irradiation and cyclophosphamide developed AML at a median followup of 6 years.[818] Using a triple FISH assay to detect loss of chromosomal material from 5q31, 7q22, or 13q14, abnormal cells were detected before high-dose therapy was given to non-Hodgkin lymphoma patients.[819] Thus, some patients are at increased risk for developing secondary AML based on pretreatment chromosome studies.

Secondary leukemia generally is treated similar to *de novo* leukemia. However, given the lower response rates and remission dura-

tions of secondary leukemia, patients can be treated in clinical trials examining new therapies or treated initially with chemotherapy regimens used for refractory disease.[820–823] Some patients may benefit from early stem cell transplantation.[824] Although patients may have a response rate of approximately 50 percent, most soon relapse, and long-term survival is approximately 10 percent.[825] Secondary AML more often has unfavorable cytogenetic features compared to *de novo* leukemia.[826]

TREATMENT OF OLDER PATIENTS

BIOLOGIC FEATURES

Approximately 60 percent of patients with AML are older than 60 years at the time of diagnosis.[827] The disease in this patient age group is less responsive to therapy, and this age group has a higher proportion of patients who have oligoblastic leukemia (MDS); an antecedent clonal myeloid disease; prior chemotherapy for cancer of the breast, ovary, or another site; and comorbid conditions, which decrease the tolerance to intensive chemotherapy programs. The AML cells of elderly patients often have more CD34+ expression, suggesting origin from a more primitive multipotential stem cell. This finding is thought to contribute to longer duration of postchemotherapy aplasia and to the increased risk of induction deaths in this age group.[828] Patients older than 55 years also have a high frequency of unfavorable cytogenetic findings (32%) and higher *MDR1* expression (71%) and functional drug efflux (58%).[829]

CHEMOTHERAPY

The therapist and patient determine whether a standard regimen, a standard regimen with dose reductions, or a special regimen is used.[830–832] Decisions based on chronologic age should be supplanted by measurements of cognitive, neurologic, and physical fitness used by geriatricians to evaluate the wisdom of considering intensive treatment.[833] In patients older than 60 years who are fit and otherwise are considered good candidates, standard two-drug therapy can be used. Remission rates of approximately 35 percent can be achieved. Chemotherapy has been combined with growth factor support to accelerate neutrophil recovery in older patients.[834] In a study in which patients older than 55 years were randomized to receive either placebo or G-CSF after induction therapy, no reduction in the duration of hospitalization, survival prolongation, or costs of supportive care was noted.[835] In previously untreated elderly patients with AML, mitoxantrone induction therapy produces a slightly higher remission rate than does daunorubicin but has no significant effect on remission duration and survival.[836,837] In a prospective randomized trial of idarubicin compared to daunorubicin in combination chemotherapy for AML in patients aged 55 to 65 years, idarubicin resulted in higher remission rates.[838] Oral idarubicin alone has been used with success.[839]

Attenuated standard regimens can be used in older patients. An example of an attenuated regimen is cytarabine 100 mg/m^2 subcutaneously every 12 hours for 10 doses on days 1 through 5 and daunorubicin 30 mg/m^2 intravenously on days 1 through 3 of treatment. One induction regimen is not superior to another in older patients with AML. Outcomes achieved with cytarabine and daunorubicin are comparable to results with mitoxantrone and etoposide.[840] Other regimens for elderly patients include lower total doses of idarubicin, etoposide, and cytarabine (DIVA regimen).[841] Addition of PSC833 to mitoxantrone and etoposide was well tolerated, but a reduction in chemotherapy dose was required to avoid undue toxicity.[842]

AUTOLOGOUS STEM CELL INFUSION

Autologous stem cell transplantation has been used in fit patients older than 60 years.[843] The incidence of relapse is lower when marrow stem cells are used compared to blood stem cells.

POSTREMISSION THERAPY IN OLDER PATIENTS

No consensus exists regarding the best regimen or the number of treatment cycles for postremission therapy in older adults. Regardless of the consolidation regimen, the duration of the leukemia-free survival is longer with high-dose cytarabine and autologous stem cell transplantation, just as it is in younger patients,[843] but fewer older patients can tolerate this therapy. High-dose cytarabine can be used in older adults with AML, but usually at a reduced dose.[844] Older patients treated with attenuated high-dose cytarabine at 750 mg/m² intravenously for 12 doses and then consolidated with four to six doses had an approximately 50 percent remission rate with a median duration of remission of 326 days.[845] Fifty-one percent of 110 patients older than 60 years had a 9-month median remission duration when consolidated with high-dose cytarabine.[846] Older patients are at higher risk for relapse despite successfully completing intensive consolidation therapy, regardless of whether other adverse prognostic features are present. Cytarabine as maintenance therapy may prolong disease-free survival but does not improve overall survival.[847]

Patients older than 80 years do not tolerate treatments well. Remission rates are approximately 30 percent, but the median survival of treated patients is approximately 1 month. Less than 10 percent of patients survive for 1 year.[848]

In summary, treatment options in older patients include (1) no treatment, (2) supportive care, (3) palliative low-dose chemotherapy, (4) attenuated induction chemotherapy, or (5) high-dose chemotherapy regimens. Lower-dose regimens are toxic and can lead to severe cytopenias. Use of colony stimulating factors permit more older patients to tolerate full-dose induction therapy. The Medical Research Council of the United Kingdom observed remission rates of 80 percent in children, 70 percent in adults younger than 50 years, 68 percent in adults 50 to 59 years old, 53 percent in adults 60 to 69 years old, 39 percent in adults 70 to 75 years old, and 22 percent in adults older than 75 years.[849] In one study of patients older than 60 years, the 2-, 5-, and 10-year survivals were 22, 11, and 8 percent, respectively.[850,851] The older patients who remain free of leukemia beyond 1 year have a reasonable quality of life.[852] The National Cancer Institute 5-year relative survival rates for patients with AML are 5 percent for adults aged 65 to 74 years and 2 percent for adults aged 75 years and older.[820]

TREATMENT OF PREGNANT PATIENTS

Leukemia (AML, ALL, CML) is the second most common malignancy of women in the childbearing age group and is expected to occur in approximately one in 75,000 to 100,000 pregnancies.[853,854] No systematic studies of the effects of leukemia on pregnancy or delivery, the effects of the leukemia or its treatment on the fetus, or the postnatal development of the offspring exposed *in utero* to maternal chemotherapy have been performed. Folic acid inhibitors, purine, pyrimidine, or retinoid analogues given during the first trimester of pregnancy increase the probability of major congenital malformations.

Leukapheresis might be useful in the first trimester, when chemotherapy poses a high risk to the embryo. Intensive chemotherapy given to women in the second and third trimesters of pregnancy does not present an inordinate risk to fetal or neonatal development,[855–858] although increased premature delivery, higher perinatal mortality, and lower birth-weight for gestational age are observed, especially if the fetus is exposed to chemotherapy.

Newborn infants may be transiently cytopenic if the mother receives chemotherapy at the time of delivery. ATRA has been used successfully to treat promyelocytic leukemia during pregnancy.[762,857] Development of the newborn usually is normal after intensive chemotherapy for AML.[853,855,856] Vaginal delivery should be used whenever possible. Pregnant women with AML who enter remission have little difficulty with childbirth or postparturition. The remission rates are approximately the rates expected for the age group, and long-term remissions occur with current therapy. Leukemic infiltrates can be found on the maternal side of the placenta but usually not in the villi. One case of maternal-to-fetal transmission of AML has been documented.[858] Transmission of AML from one identical twin to another through a shared placental circulation accounts for the dual occurrence in twins in the first several years of life.[101]

TREATMENT OF CHILDREN

AML represents approximately 15 percent of the acute leukemias in children (younger than 20 years) or approximately 500 children per year. APL is treated as in adults, with ATRA and an anthracycline antibiotic. In other phenotypes of AML, intensive treatment—including initial therapy with cytarabine and daunomycin or doxorubicin and a third drug such as mitoxantrone or 6-thioguanine, followed by intensive multidrug consolidation therapy including agents such as danorubicin, cytarabine, 6-thioguanine, etoposide, and intrathecal cytarabine—has resulted in remission in approximately 80 percent of children and 5-year relapse-free remissions in approximately 50 percent of treated children.[859–864] Most of the children are considered cured.

Monocytic leukemia and hyperleukocytic [>100,000/μl [>100 × 10⁹/liter]) myelogenous leukemia are unfavorable phenotypes. In children, *FLT3* internal tandem duplication mutations are approximately half as common (15%) as in adults (30%) but are a very poor prognostic indicator.[865] Therapy can be adjusted for children based on the presence of poor prognostic variables, which include age younger than 2 years or older than 10 years; abnormalities of chromosome 3, 5, or 7; complex karyotypes; *FLT3* mutations; elevated white cell count (>50,000/μl [50 × 10⁹/liter]); male gender; and, perhaps, most importantly, because it reflects the effect of all factors, the presence of greater than 15 percent blast cells in the marrow examined 14 days after onset of treatment.[864–867] The presence of residual blast cells detected by flow cytometry after induction therapy is a very poor prognostic finding.[868] The duration of first remission predicts the subsequent remission rate and long-term survival in children with relapse.

Autologous stem cell transplantation has not improved outcome compared to current intensive chemotherapy treatment regimens.[869] Allogeneic stem cell transplantation from a histocompatible sibling should be considered in children in first remission with a donor and poor prognostic indicators or in children who relapse.[863,869] Children younger than 2 years previously had a very poor prognosis. They tend to present with myelomonocytic or monocytic leukemia with high blast counts and CNS involvement. The t(9;11) abnormality has a more favorable prognosis. Intensive multidrug regimens have resulted in 3-year survivals approaching 70 percent of all infants treated. Thus, most infants can be successfully treated with intensive chemotherapy or allogeneic stem cell transplantation.[870,871] Cord blood may be a suitable graft option for children with AML who lack an acceptably matched unrelated marrow donor.[872]

Growth failure, neurocognitive abnormalities, endocrine deficiencies, and cardiac abnormalities are found in children treated at a young age.[873] A second malignancy in cured children is approximately 10-fold greater than expected in a matched population by age.[874] Indefinite followup of children in remission or believed to be cured is important to assess developmental and intellectual progress and to evaluate long-term adverse events.

NONHEMATOPOIETIC ADVERSE EFFECTS OF TREATMENT

SKIN RASHES

More than 50 percent of patients with AML develop skin lesions during remission-induction or remission-consolidation therapy. The rash may be on the trunk and extremities. The rash usually is maculopapular initially but can become hemorrhagic in patients who have thrombocytopenia. Allopurinol, trimethoprim-sulfamethoxazole, and other β-lactam antibiotics are commonly implicated causes. Use of multiple drugs enhances the probability of skin reactivity of patients.[875] Cytostatic therapy coupled with the effects of leukemia predisposes patients to an increased frequency of allergic dermatitis.

CARDIAC TOXICITY

Alterations in cardiac function, especially left ventricular and intraventricular septal diastolic wall motion abnormalities, occur frequently in patients after they are exposed to the anthracycline antibiotics, daunorubicin, or doxorubicin.[876,877] The risk of serious cardiac effects is correlated with increasing dose of anthracycline antibiotic, increasing patient age, and presence of underlying heart disease. Adverse effects include electrocardiographic changes, such as prolonged QT interval, myocarditis, pericarditis, myocardial infarction, and congestive heart failure. The incidence of congestive heart failure is dose related and ranges from approximately 5 percent at doses of 550 mg/m^2 to greater than 30 percent at doses of 600 mg/m^2. Chapter 19 discusses the toxicity further. The effects are dose related, and the frequency and long-term sequelae increase as anthracycline dose increases. However, even lower doses of these agents exert negative effects on cardiac myocytes. Measurement of heart wall behavior, valvular competence, and ejection fraction by ultrasound can assist in assessing the risk of proceeding with anthracycline treatment in patients with or without pretreatment heart disease.[876,877] In younger patients, transient abnormalities, although frequent, often improve after therapy is completed. Increased long-term remissions in children and younger adults have led to an increase in serious ventricular and valvular disturbances years after therapy in some patients. Periodic evaluation of cardiac status by ultrasound should be undertaken in long-term survivors.[878] Cardiomyopathy and heart failure can occur 10 to 15 years after therapy. Two approaches that may ameliorate the cardiomyopathic effect of anthracycline antibiotics are the use of these agents in liposome encapsulated preparations[879] and the use of dexrazoxane. Either approach may reduce the cardiotoxicity of anthracycline antibiotics.[880]

HEPATITIS

Hepatitis may occur in multiply transfused patients and usually is mild, but persistent hepatitis can develop. Persistent elevation in serum transaminases occurring after initiation of chemotherapy in patients with AML usually results from blood transfusion-transmitted hepatitis. Hepatitis caused by type A virus is nearly nonexistent early in the course of AML. Cases of type B hepatitis can occur infrequently in patients who are B virus carriers and in whom chemotherapy and transient immunosuppression reactivate the virus.[881,882] These rare cases of fibrosing cholestatic hepatitis can be fulminant. Screening blood products for hepatitis virus C has markedly decreased the risk of hepatitis C.[883] Reactivation of carriers of the C virus after chemotherapy is unusual.[884]

SYSTEMIC CANDIDIASIS SYNDROME

Although microbial sepsis is a common complication of AML treatment, chronic systemic candidiasis syndrome has become of special concern.[885–887] Protracted posttherapy neutropenia, severe mucositis, colonization with Candida, and use of high-dose cytarabine are frequent antecedents of the syndrome.[888] The syndrome is manifested by fever, abdominal pain, and hepatomegaly. Increased serum alkaline phosphatase activity often is noted. Abdominal ultrasound, computed tomography, and magnetic resonance imaging show characteristic hepatic lesions: circular areas of decreased attenuation of liver and often spleen, kidney, lung, or paraspinal muscles by imaging.[889] Ultrasound

reveals multiple hypoechogenic areas with a bull's-eye appearance. Laparoscopic-guided liver biopsy reveals yellow nodules on the liver surface, which on microscopic examination are large granulomas with Candida and pseudohyphae. Cure of this infection is possible with long-term (2–10 months) amphotericin B, supplemented with fluconazole or itraconazole.[890] Measurement of serial serum Candida antigen titers can lead to an early diagnosis of systemic candidiasis and early use of antifungal drugs only in patients at high risk for disseminated candidiasis.[891]

NEUTROPENIC TYPHLITIS

Necrotizing inflammation of the cecum with secondary infection can occur in patients with acute leukemia on intensive chemotherapy.[892,893] Right lower abdominal pain and fever can simulate appendicitis. The diagnosis can be confirmed by sonography or computerized tomographic scanning in which a characteristic mucosal thickening and polypoid appearance are evident.[894,895] Management includes bowel rest, nasogastric suction, parenteral nutrition, and antibiotics. In the absence of resolution, right hemicolectomy should be considered but is a last resort in neutropenic patients.[896]

THROMBOTIC THROMBOCYTOPENIC PURPURA

This syndrome has been reported in patients with solid tumors treated with cisplatin, bleomycin, vinca alkaloids, or mitomycin C. It also has been reported in patients in remission of AML during consolidation chemotherapy[897] (see Chap. 124).

FERTILITY AND GONADAL FUNCTION

Patients treated for AML and especially patients undergoing conditioning for allogeneic stem cell transplantation have decreased gonadal function.[897–901] Men may develop oligospermia. Women may develop ovarian dysfunction and very high gonadotropin levels. Men recover gonadal function more often and sooner than do women. Recovery of ovarian function in women is partly dependent on a younger age at the time of treatment. Women in remission following treatment for AML with allogeneic transplantation can become pregnant and deliver healthy infants.[902,903] Histologic studies of the testes show marked suppression of spermatogenesis as a function of duration of treatment for AML and not of the specific agents used or the patient's age. Residual spermatogenesis in intensively treated patients enables recovery of reproductive function in males.[904] Males receiving intensive daunorubicin, cytosine arabinoside, or 6-thioguanine treatment for AML have conceived children during therapy.[905] Banking of sperm or experimental cryopreservation of ova can be attempted prior to institution of cytotoxic therapy but often is not logistically possible or successful in patients with AML who are acutely ill at presentation and require urgent chemotherapy.[899]

COURSE AND PROGNOSIS

RESULTS OF TREATMENT

Remission rates have improved dramatically, but remission, 5-year survival, and cure rates are most dependent on the patient's age when AML occurs.[852,906] Initial remission rates now approach 90 percent in children, 70 percent in young adults, 50 percent in middle-aged subjects, and 25 percent in the elderly. Within age groups, remission is related to other variables such as cytogenetic risk category and expression of MDR genes in leukemic cells, but these variables also are correlated with age at onset. For example, the more favorable cytogenetic patterns t(8;21), t(15;17), Inv16, or t(16;16) are present in approximately 30 percent of patients between 10 and 39 years old, 15 percent of patients between 40 and 59 years old, and 5 percent of

TABLE 87-7 FREQUENCY OF CYTOGENETIC FINDINGS WITH A MORE
FAVORABLE PROGNOSIS BY AGE GROUP

AGE (YEARS)	# CASES STUDIED	t(8;21) (NO. CASES)	t(15;17) (NO. CASES)	INV16/ t(16;16) (NO. CASES)	TOTAL (NO. CASES)	FAVORABLE KARYO- TYPES%
10–39	307	27	38	33	98	32
40–59	584	36	28	28	92	16
60–69	579	18	24	21	63	11
70–79	381	5	7	5	17	4.5
>80	45	1	2	0	3	6.6
Total	1896	87	99	87	273	22

These observations were made in Germany by Claudia Schock and colleagues and kindly provided to the authors. (see also Schock C, et al. *Blood* 98:3500, 2001).

patients 60 to 90 years old (Table 87-7).[852] Other factors, such as AML evolving from a prior clonal myeloid disease or developing as a result of cytotoxic treatment for another cancer or immune disorder, can decrease the expected remission and survival rates for the age group. Age-related comorbid conditions may limit the appropriateness or tolerance of intensive therapy, decreasing the opportunity for remission. The expected increase in the proportion of old and old-old individuals in the population may decrease remission rates and their duration unless counteracting improvements in treatment approaches are developed.

CLONAL REMISSIONS

A small proportion of patients who enter remission have apparently normal hematopoiesis supported by a single clone rather than the expected polyclonal hematopoiesis.[876–879] Evidence points to this clone being a preleukemic cell rather than a normal stem cell.[907–910] This finding is in keeping with previous hypotheses about the possible patterns of remission and relapse in AML[911–914] and has implications for minimal residual disease detection.

SPONTANEOUS REMISSIONS

Spontaneous disappearance of AML has been reported for more than 100 years; however, most cases reported before 1960 had poor documentation of the diagnosis. Bona fide cases of AML patients who entered complete remission, usually after or concurrent with an infection, occur but are very rare.[915–917] The occurrence of spontaneous remission with infection is consistent with the observation that the antibody response to *Pseudomonas* vaccine[918] correlates with improved probability of chemotherapy-induced remission. Spontaneous remissions often are short lived but have lasted up to 3 years in adults and more than 9 years in children.[919] A particularly notable case of remission for more than 60 years has been documented following "treatment" prior to the introduction of chemotherapeutic drugs. The regimen included arsenic.[920]

LONG-TERM SURVIVAL

Prior to the introduction of chemotherapy for AML 50 years ago, the median survival of patients was approximately 6 weeks,[921] the 1-year survival was approximately 3 percent, and longer survival occurred in less than 1 percent of patients. Five-year survival rates of patients in the United States from 1995 to 2000, based on the Surveillance, Epidemiology, and End-Results Program of the National Cancer Institute, are approximately 45 percent for patients younger than 45 years, 26 percent for patients 45 to 54 years old, 17 percent for patients 55 to 64 years old, 6.0 percent for patients 65 to 74 years old, and 2.0 percent for patients older than 75 years at the time of diagnosis (Table 87-8).[852] Considering that the median age at disease onset is approximately 65 to 70 years and that 75 percent of patients are older than 45 years, the overall median survival is approximately 11 months. A study of the cost of care of older AML patients using Medicare data found that in adults older than 65 years diagnosed between 1991 and 1996, the median survival was 2 months and the 2-year survival was 6 percent.[922] Better survival has been reported for younger patients who have received allogeneic marrow transplantation in first remission, but the confidence limits for remission duration and survival are overlapping for drug-treated and drug- and transplantation-treated groups, and the proportion of AML patients receiving transplantation is very small.[906,923–926]

Relapse (or a new leukemic event) in long-term survivors occurring as late as 8 years after remission has been reported in adults[919,920] and after more than 16 years in children.[919,920] Relapse in long-term survivors nearly always occurs in the marrow in adults and usually in the marrow in children, with occasional childhood cases of CNS or gonadal relapses occurring initially, followed by relapse in the marrow.[924] Studies of long-term survivors of AML have shown that most can return to work and that, at a median followup of 9 years, no increased risk of secondary invasive cancer or secondary AML has occurred.[925,926] An exception to this finding is the occasional report of myelodysplasia in long-term survivors of APL. Health-related quality of life in long-term survivors appears to recover completely as related to physical, psychological, and emotional well-being, but continued sexual dysfunction has been reported.[927] The quality of life at the time of diagnosis and during the course of therapy usually is poor.[927,928]

FEATURES INFLUENCING OUTCOME OF THERAPY IN ACUTE MYELOGENOUS LEUKEMIA

Numerous features are related to outcome of AML treatment. Even with multivariate analysis, dissecting which features are themselves important or are associations that segregate with another prognostic factor is difficult (Table 87-9).

Determining useful prognostic variables in patients with AML is imprecise because negative prognostic factors may be eliminated by better treatment protocols. Moreover, several prognostic factors are significant only when AML is stratified by age or by morphologic phenotype. Conflicting findings are common among studies. In addition, although a prognostic variable may be correlated significantly with a favorable outcome, the lack of a very strong statistical correlation with the outcome of treatment makes the variable's presence or absence of little prognostic value in an individual patient. If a stem cell donor is available, unfavorable prognostic factors could influence the therapist to use allogeneic stem cell transplantation as a means of

TABLE 87-8 ACUTE MYELOGENOUS LEUKEMIA: FIVE-YEAR SURVIVAL
RATES (1995–2000)

AGE (YEARS)	ACUTE MYELOGENOUS LEUKEMIA
<45	44.9
45–54	26.5
55–64	16.6
65–74	5.3
>75	2.3
<65	32.7
>65	3.8

Rates expressed as number of cases per 100.
Data from SEER Cancer Statistics. 5-year survival rates.
Table XIII-10. National Cancer Institute, Washington, D.C.
Available at http://seer.cancer.gov.

TABLE 87-9 PROGNOSTIC FACTORS IN ACUTE MYELOGENOUS LEUKEMIA

Better Prognosis Than Average of All Patients

Early blast clearance during remission induction therapy[929]

Leukemic cells contain t(8;21), t(15;17), inv(16) t(16;16), trisomy 21[200,202,930]

Absence of exaggerated dysmyelopoiesis[931]

Residual normal metaphases admixed with clonal cytogenetic abnormalities[932]

High telomerase activity levels[933]

Low levels of TdT expression by flow cytometry (<5%) (predicts for longer remission)[934]

High bax expression[935] and high Bax/Bcl-2 ratios indicating spontaneous apoptosis[936]

High expression of CD11b, an integrin[937]

Absence of VLA-4 expression on AML blasts[938]

High levels of caspase-3[939]

Mutant CEBPA (CCAAT-enhancer binding protein A) expression[1036]

Poorer Prognosis Than Average of All Patients

Older age: Age at the time of diagnosis has the greatest impact on the probability of remission and on duration of survival. Children in the first 15 years of life, exclusive of the neonatal period, have the highest rate of remission and longest relapse-free remission; patients >60 years have only half the chance of a young adult to enter remission and less likelihood of a long relapse-free remission.[820] There is a gradient of poor response to treatment through adulthood, with the largest decrease after the sixth decade of life.[849]

Unfavorable karyotypes: The cytogenetic pattern of leukemic blast cells influences outcome, but the relationship is complex.[200-202] The presence of 5-, 7-, 5q-, 7q- or of exaggerated hyperdiploidy (>47 chromosomes), trisomy 8, t(6;9), trisomy 11, and multiple chromosomal abnormalities in leukemic cells are poor prognostic signs.

Multidrug resistance phenotype: Leukemic cells expressing P-glycoprotein, a unidirectional drug efflux pump, encoded by the *MDR1*.[940] Expression of this gene product can result in decreased accumulation of anthracyclines, amsacrine, mitoxantrone, and etoposide. Expression of P-glycoprotein does not influence outcome of treatment, but if rhodamine-123 efflux also is increased, relapse is more common.[941-944] Frequently observed in AML cells after relapse. Associated with CD34 expression and chromosome 7 abnormalities.[943] Alternative non-*MDR1*-mediated drug efflux mechanisms are important also.[944-947] *MDR1* expression is low in favorable prognosis subtypes of AML.[948]

Prior clonal hemopathy: Chemotherapy or radiotherapy remission rates are one third to one half that of *de novo* AML in the same age group. Remission duration is shorter with remissions >3 years very uncommon.[949-950] AML developing from the clonal hemopathy may relapse as a smoldering leukemia. It then reverts to AML but can be treated with remissions lasting several years.[951-955]

Higher white cell count: Count >30,000/μl (30 × 10^9 /liter) or a blast cell count >15,000/μl (>15 × 10^9 /liter).[956-957]

Very low platelet count (<30,000/μl [<30 × 10^9/liter]).[957]

High lactic dehydrogenase.[958]

High stem cell mobilizing capacity during complete remission predicts for relapse risk.[959]

Another medical disorder: extreme obesity, diabetes mellitus, chronic renal disease.

Low serum albumin or prealbumin.

Need for intubation or ventilator support during induction therapy.[960]

Autonomous clonal growth of leukemic blast cells.[961]

High Bcl-2 expression.[962]

High Mcl-1 expression: Elevated at the time of leukemic relapse. Suggests prognostic importance or that chemotherapeutic regimen selects for leukemia cells with elevated levels of apoptosis inhibitors.[963]

Low expression of retinoblastoma gene.[964]

High levels of WAF/Cip1 protein: This is a regulator at the G1 checkpoint of cell cycle.[965]

High CD34 expression: High CD34 antigen expression often in AML subtypes M0, M1, and M4.[966] Remission rate of 61 vs. to 88 percent in AML not expressing CD34. Correlation is stronger between high-intensity expression of CD34 and lower remission rate.[966,967] CD34 expression in APL.[968]

GATA-1 expression.[969]

Neural cell adhesion molecule (CD56) expression.[970]

Elevated soluble L-selectin: Seen especially in extramedullary disease.[971]

Higher expression of interleukin-1β gene.[972]

Low *FMS* expression.[972]

Expression of the thrombopoietin receptor (c-*MPL*) mRNA.[973]

FLT3 mutations.[96,97,865]

Elevated expression of IL-3Rα.[974]

MLL tandem duplications[975] and 11p23/MLL abnormalities.[976]

CD56 expression in APL.[977] High incidence of CNS involvement, especially with CD7 expression.[978]

P15 methylation[979]

Microsatellite instability[980] (may not be independent of age and t-AML).

AC133 expression (shorter remissions and disease-free survival).[981]

Constitutive activity of signal transducer and activator of transcription 3 protein (shorter disease-free survival)[982]

BAALC gene expression.[983]

High S-phase activity in cells surviving after 7 days of induction.[984]

High EVI1 expression.[985]

Factors with No or Uncertain Prognostic Findings

Complex karyotype or secondary aberrations in patients with t(8;21), inv(16) t(16;16), or t(9;11)[986]

Myeloid antigens: CD11b expression may be predictive of shorter survival.[987]

Detection of the WT1 (Wilms tumor) transcript.[956]

FLT3-ITD or Asp835 mutations.[989]

Levels of initiator caspases.[990]

Persistent thrombocytopenia after remission induction.[991]

Lung resistance protein: Functional test is needed to assess activity.[992] Expression may predict poor outcome in *de novo* AML.[946,993]

remission maintenance in patients entering remission. The impact of prognostic factors may change in patients treated with allogeneic stem cell transplantation compared with conventional cytotoxic treatment.[994,995]

DETECTION OF MINIMAL RESIDUAL DISEASE

GENERAL CONSIDERATIONS

The tumor cell burden in acute leukemia is approximately one trillion (10^{12}) cells. Apparent marrow aplasia followed by restitution of normal hematopoiesis can occur with at least a three log reduction in leukemic cell numbers, which represents a residual tumor cell burden of approximately one billion cells. Intensification therapy is intended to decrease further the residual cell numbers. With the advent of specific monoclonal antibodies for leukemic cell antigens and FISH coupled with flow cytometry and DNA amplification by PCR, residual leukemic cell populations at or below the level of one billion cells, which are undetectable by light microscopy of stained marrow films, can be quantified.[996] When real-time PCR is used to quantify PML-RAR-α, AML1/ETO, or CBF-β/MYH11, risk for treatment failure can be determined by the levels of the fusion gene at diagnosis and after the first 3 to 4 months of therapy.[997] Sampling remains an important problem because marrow aspiration contains approximately one ten-thousandth of the marrow cell population, and variation among sites of aspiration is well documented. In addition, the markers of the leukemic cell used for detection can change during the course of the disease. For example, persistence of circulating cells containing t(8;21) in patients with AML in long-term remission has been established using PCR.[998]

Marrow examinations are not needed in the majority of AML patients in first complete remission.[999] Cytogenetic followup usually is not helpful. Emergence of a karyotypically unrelated clone of AML cells, especially containing chromosome 7, can occur. Studies using multiparameter flow cytometry to identify leukemic cells by aberrant antigen expression have a high positive predictive value with regard to the incidence of relapse.[1000] Detection of residual disease in AML patients using double immunologic marker analysis for terminal deoxynucleotidyl transferase and myeloid CD antigens can be useful because these two markers are expressed on leukemic cells in the majority of AML patients. These findings are rare in normal marrow cells.[1001,1002] In other cases, aberrant combinations of surface antigens[1001,1003] or increased expression of various surface antigens such as CD34 are seen.[1004] Immunophenotype may change at relapse and has implications for minimal disease detection.[1005] Other methods for detecting minimal residual disease include magnetic resonance imaging; fluorescence DNA in FISH[1006,1007]; reverse transcriptase (RT)-PCR to detect amplification of abnormal fusion genes such as t(15;17), t(8;21), inversion 16, and 11q23; and DNA PCR for mutations in the Ras coding regions.[996] Quantitative assessment of WT1 expression[1008] can be used for MDR monitoring. Real-time quantitative PCR can be used to quantitate MDR more precisely than other methods, but this test requires standardized criteria and is not widely available clinically.[1009]

DETECTING INVERSION 16

Minimal residual disease in acute myelomonocytic leukemia with inversion 16 can be detected by nested PCR with allele-specific amplifications (CBF-β on 16q and MYH11 on 16p).[1010–1013] This fusion transcript occurs not only in the majority of cases of acute myelomonocytic leukemia with marrow eosinophilia (M4Eo) but also in 10 percent of acute myelomonocytic leukemia M4 without eosinophilic abnormalities, a much higher incidence than suggested by the sporadic reports of chromosome 16 abnormalities in AML. Additional screening by either RT-PCR or FISH should be performed in patients with acute

myelomonocytic leukemia, regardless of morphologic features, to evaluate the prognostic usefulness of this fusion transcript in minimal disease detection.[1014] Following completion of chemotherapy (induction and consolidation), patients who had a CBF-β/MYH11 fusion transcript copy number greater than 10 had a shorter remission duration and higher risk for relapse than patients with copy number less than 10.[1013] Evidence indicates transcript ratios of samples may have utility in establishing thresholds for curability and for relapse risk in standard clinical complete remission states in the future.[1015]

DETECTING t(8;21)

Translocation 8;21 is one of the most common translocations in AML, especially in younger patients (see Table 87-7). This translocation fuses the AML1 gene on chromosome 21p to ETO on chromosome 8p to produce the fusion gene.[1016–1019] The fusion has been detected in the majority of patients in remission. One study found its persistence in all patients with t(8;21) after chemotherapy or autologous marrow transplantation.[1020–1022] Using PCR measurement, AML1/ETO was found in patients in complete remission for 12 to 150 months but not in patients who received allogeneic marrow transplantation. The PGK allele, used as a tracking marker, was identical to that detected in the leukemic blasts from the time of initial diagnosis, confirming the persistence and reappearance of leukemic cells from the same clone.[1022] This marker may persist after allogeneic marrow transplantation but is compatible with continued remission.[1023] Quantitation of the amount of the fusion transcript during remission may be more predictive of cure or relapse than a simple qualitative assessment.[1024,1025] Real-time quantitative RT-PCR can be used for this purpose.[1021] Quantitative RT-PCR can predict relapse up to 4 months before clinical onset.[1026] Serial RT-PCR quantification of cases with residual t(8;21) indicates at least 0.1 fg of AML1/ETO competitor dose is present before cytogenetic relapse occurs.[1027] Both ETO and AML1 are expressed in normal CD34+ progenitors.[1028] Blood can be used as an alternative to marrow for quantitating AML1/ETO transcripts.[1029]

DETECTING t(15;17)

Unlike AML with the fusion transcript t(8;21), in APL the t(15;17) fusion transcript usually disappears after intensive therapy.[1030] At least one in 100,000 cells with the PML-RAR-α transcript can be detected by RT-PCR.[1030] FISH also can be used.[1031] Molecular monitoring has enabled treatment to achieve a molecular remission (negative RT-PCR).[1032] Nested PCR can be used to determine the need for additional treatment at the end of consolidation, to determine the advisability of autologous stem cell transplantation in second remission, and to predict relapse after transplantation.[1033] Real-time quantitative RT-PCR may improve the predictive value of MDR assessment and aid in laboratory standardization.[1034]

The technology to detect minimal residual disease has increased in sensitivity and availability. Detection of minimal residual disease to determine a patient's treatment or prognosis remains an evolving area of investigation.

REFERENCES

1. Friedreich N: Ein neuer Fall von Leukämie. *Arch Pathol* 12:37, 1857.
2. Ebstein W: Ueber die acute Leukämie und Pseudoleukämie. *Dtsch Arch Klin Med* 44:343, 1889.
3. Fraenkel A: Ueber acute Leukämie. *Dtsch Med Wochenschr* 21:639, 1895.
4. Neumann E: Ueber myelogene leukäemie. *Berl Klin Wochenschr* 15:69, 1878.
5. Ehrlich P: *Farbenanolytische Untersuchungen zur Histologie und Klinik des Blutes.* Berlin, Hirschwald, 1891.

6. Naegeli O: Ueber rothes Knochenmark und Myeloblasten. *Dtsch Med Wochenschr* 26:287, 1900.

7. Hirschfield H: Zur Kenntnis der Histogenese der granulirten Knochenmarkzellen. *Arch Pathol* 153:335, 1898.

8. Hsu TC: *Human and Mammalian Cytogenetics: An Historical Perspective*, Springer-Verlag, New York, 1979.

9. Subramanian G, Adams MD, Venter JC, Broder S: Implications of the human genome for understanding human biology and medicine. *JAMA* 286:2296, 2001.

10. Ellison RR, Holland JF, Weil M, et al: Arabinosyl cytosine: A useful agent in the treatment of acute leukemia in adults. *Blood* 33:507, 1968.

11. Yates JW, Wallace HJ, Ellison RR, Holland JF: Cytosine arabinoside and daunorubicin therapy in acute non-lymphocytic leukemia. *Cancer Chemother Rep* 52:485, 1973.

12. Thomas ED, Buckner CD, Banaji M, et al: One hundred patients with acute leukemia treated by chemotherapy, total body irradiation, and allogeneic bone marrow transplantation. *Blood* 49:511, 1977.

13. Kato H, Schull WJ: Studies on mortality of A-bomb survivors, report 7. Mortality, 1950–1978. Part I. Cancer mortality. *Radiat Res* 90:395, 1982.

14. Moloney WC: Radiogenic leukemia revisited. *Blood* 70:905, 1987.

15. Snyder R: Benzene and leukemia. *Crit Rev Toxicol* 32:155, 2002.

16. Schattner AR, Nicholich MJ, Bird MG: Determination of leukemogenic benzene exposure concentrations. *Risk Anal* 16:833, 1996.

17. Smith MT, Zhang L, Wang Y, et al: Increased translocations and aneusomy in chromosomes 8 and 21 among workers exposed to benzene. *Cancer Res* 58:2176, 1998.

18. Yin S-N, Hayes RB, Linet MS, et al: A cohort study of cancer among benzene-exposed workers in China: Overall results. *Am J Indust Med* 29:227, 1996.

19. Levine EG, Bloomfield CD: Leukemias and myelodysplastic syndromes secondary to drugs, radiation, and environmental exposure. *Semin Oncol* 19:47, 1992.

20. Thirman MJ, Larson RA: Therapy-related myeloid leukemia. *Hematol Oncol Clin North Am* 10:293, 1996.

21. Pui CH, Relling MV, Behn FG, et al: L-asparaginases may potentiate the leukemogenic effect of the epipodophyllotoxins. *Leukemia* 9:1680, 1995.

22. Travis LB, Holowty EF, Bergfeldt K, et al: Risk of leukemia after platinum-based chemotherapy for ovarian cancer. *N Engl J Med* 340:351, 1999.

23. Sterkers Y, Preudhomme C, Lai J-L, et al: Acute myeloid leukemia and essential thrombocythemia treated with hydroxyurea: High proportion of cases with 17p deletion. *Blood* 91:616, 1998.

24. Van Leeuwen FE: Risk of acute myelogenous leukemia and myelodysplasia following cancer treatment. *Baillieres Clin Haematol* 9:57, 1996.

25. Visfeldt J, Anderson M: Pathoanatomical aspects of malignant haematological disorders among Danish patients exposed to thorium dioxide. *APMIS* 103:29, 1995.

26. Rodella S, Ciccone G, Rege-Cambrin G, et al: Cytogenetics and occupational exposures in acute nonlymphocytic leukemia and myelodysplastic syndrome. *Scand J Work Environ Health* 19:369, 1993.

27. Brownson RC, Novotny TE, Perry MC: Cigarette smoking and adult leukemia: A meta-analysis. *Arch Intern Med* 153:469, 1993.

28. Sandler DP, Shore DL, Anderson JR, et al: Cigarette smoking and risk of acute leukemia: Associations with morphology and cytogenetic abnormalities in bone marrow. *J Natl Cancer Inst* 85:1994, 1993.

29. Shu X-O, Ross JA, Pendergrass TW, et al: Parental alcohol consumption, cigarette smoking and risk of infant leukemia. *J Natl Cancer Inst* 88:24, 1996.

30. Najean Y, Rain J-D: Treatment of polycythemia vera. *Blood* 89:2319, 1997.

31. Wiernik P: Leukemias and plasma cell myeloma. *Cancer Chemother Biol Response Modif* 17:390, 1997

32. Luca DC, Almanaseer IY: Simultaneous presentation of multiple myeloma and acute monocytic leukemia. *Arch Pathol Lab Med* 127:1506, 2003.

33. Peters BS, Matthews J, Gompels M, et al: Acute myeloblastic leukemia in AIDS. *AIDS* 4:367, 1990.

34. Moskowitz C, Dutcher JP, Wiernik PH: Association of thyroid disease with acute leukemia. *Am J Hematol* 39:102, 1992.

35. Willems E, Valdes-Socin H, Betea D, et al: Association of acute leukemia and autoimmune polyendocrine syndrome in two kindreds. *Leukemia* 17:1912, 2003.

36. Lichtenstein P, Holm NV, Verkasalo PK, et al: Environmental and hereditable factors in causation of cancer. *N Engl J Med* 78, 200.

37. Risch N: The genetic epidemiology of cancer. Interpreting family and twin studies and their implications for molecular genetic approaches. *Cancer Epidemiol Biomark Prev* 10:733, 2001.

38. Hemminki K, Vaittinen P, Dong C, Easton D: Sibling risks in cancer: Clues to recessive or X-linked genes? *Br J Cancer* 84:388, 2001.

39. Germeshausen M, Ballmaier M, Welte K: Implications of mutations in hematopoietic growth factor receptor genes in congenital cytopenias. *Ann N Y Acad Sci* 938:305, 2001.

40. Tonelli R, Scardovi AL, Pession A, et al: Compound heterozygosity for two different amino-acid substitution mutations in the thrombopoietin receptor (c-mpl gene) in congenital amegakaryocytic thrombocytopenia (CAMT). *Hum Genet* 107:225, 2000.

41. Li FP, Hecht F, Kaiser-McCaw B, et al: Ataxia-pancytopenia: Syndrome of cerebellar ataxia, hypoplastic anemia, monosomy 7, and acute myelogenous leukemia. *Cancer Genet Cytogenet* 4:189, 1981.

42. Gonzales-del Angel A, Cervera M, Gomez L, et al: Ataxia-pancytopenia syndrome. *Am J Med Genet* 90:252, 2000.

43. German J: Bloom's syndrome: Incidence, age of onset, and types of leukemia in the Bloom's syndrome registry, in *Genetics in Hematologic Disorders*, edited by CS Bartsocas, D Loukopoulos, p 241. Hemisphere, Washington, 1992.

44. Poppe B, Van Limbergen H, Van Roy N, et al: Chromosomal aberrations in Bloom syndrome patients with myeloid malignancies. *Cancer Genet Cytogenet* 128:39, 2001.

45. Freedman MH, Alter BP: Risk of myelodysplastic syndrome and acute myeloid leukemia in congenital neutropenia. *Semin Hematol* 39:128, 2002.

46. Aprikyan AA, Kutyavin T, Stein S, et al: Cellular and Molecular abnormalities in severe congenital neutropenia predisposing to leukemia. *Exp Hematol* 31:372, 2003.

47. Zeidler C, Welte K: Kostmann syndrome and severe congenital neutropenia. *Semin Hematol* 39:82, 2002.

48. Carlsson G, Fasth A: Infantile genetic agranulocytosis, morbus Kostmann: Presentation of six cases from the original "Kostmann family" and a review. *Acta Paediatr* 90:757, 2001.

49. Janov AJ, Leong T, Nathan DG, Guinan EC: Diamond-Blackfan anemia: Natural history and sequelae of treatment. *Medicine* 75:77, 1996.

50. Vlachos A, Klein G, Lipton J: The Blackfan-Diamond anemia registry: Tool for investigating the epidemiology and biology of Diamond-Blackfan anemia. *Pediatr Hematol Oncol* 23:377, 2001.

51. Crentzig U, Ritter J, Vormoor J, et al: Myelodyplasia and acute myelogenous leukemia in Down's syndrome. *Leukemia* 10:1677, 1996.

52. Hasle H: Pattern of malignant disorders in individuals with Down syndrome. *Lancet Oncol* 2:429, 2001.

53. Andrade-Machado R, Machado-Rojas A, De la Toree-Santos ME: Dubowitz syndrome, polymiosits, and aleucemic myeloblastic leukemia. A new association. *Rev Neurol* 35:500, 2001.

54. Marrone A, Mason PJ: Dyskeratosis congenita. *Cell Mol Life Sci* 60:507, 2003

55. Mason PJ: Stem cells, telomerase and dyskeratosis congenita. *Bioessays* 25:126, 2003.

56. Segel GB, Lichtman MA: Familial (inherited) leukemia, lymphoma, and myeloma. *Blood Cells Mol Dis* 32:246, 2004.

57. Michaud J, Wu F, Osato M, et al: In vitro analysis of known and novel RUNX1/AML1 mutations in dominant familial platelet disorder with predisposition to acute myelogenous leukemia: Implications for mechanisms of pathogenesis. *Blood* 99:1364, 2002.

58. Buijs A, Poddighe P, Van Wijk R, et al: A novel CBFA2 single-nucleotide mutation in familial platelet disorder with propensity to develop myeloid malignancies. *Blood* 98:2856, 2001.

59. Rosenberg PS, Greene MH, Alter BP: Cancer incidence in persons with Fanconi anemia. *Blood* 101:822, 2003.

60. Alter BP: Cancer in Fanconi anemia. *Cancer* 97:425, 2003.

61. Polychronopoulou S, Tsatsopoulou A, Papadhimitriou SI, et al: Myelodysplasia and Naxos disease: A novel pathogenetic association? *Leukemia* 16:2335, 2002.

62. Kratz CP, Antonietti L, Shannon KM, et al: Acute myeloid leukemia associated with t(8;21) or trisomy 8 in children with neurofibromatosis type 1. *Pediatr Hematol Oncol* 25:343, 2003.

63. Lurgaespada DA, Brannan CI, Shaughnessy JD, et al: The neurofibromatosic type 1 (NF1) tumor suppressor gene and myeloid leukemia. *Curr Top Microbiol Immunol* 211:233, 1996.

64. Bader-Meunier B, Tchernia G, Miélot F, et al: Occurrence of myeloproliferative disorder in patients with Noonan Syndrome. *J Pediatr* 130:885, 1997.

65. Tartaglia M, Niemeyer CM, Fragale A, et al: Somatic mutations in PTPN11 in juvenile myelomonocytic leukemia, myelodysplastic syndromes and acute myeloid leukemia. *Nat Genet* 34:148, 2003.

66. Fokin AA, Robicsek F: Poland's syndrome revisited. *Ann Thorac Surg* 74:2218, 2002.

67. Pianigiani E, DeAloe G, Andreassi A, et al: Rothmund-Thomson syndrome (Thomson type) and myelodysplasia. *Ped Dermatol* 18:422, 2001.

68. Duker NJ: Chromosome breakage syndromes and cancer. *Am J Med Genet* 115:125, 2002.

69. Hayani A, Suarez CR, Molnar Z, et al: Acute myeloid leukemia in a patient with Seckel syndrome. *J Med Genet* 31:148, 1994.

70. Boocock GR, Morrison JA, Popovic M, et al: Mutations in SBDS are associated with Shwachman-Diamond syndrome. *Nat Genet* 33:97, 2003.

71. Dror Y, Freedman MH: Shwachman-Diamond syndrome. *Br J Haematol* 118:701, 2002.

72. Mitsui T, Kawakami T, Sendo D, et al: Successful unrelated donor bone marrow transplantation for Shwachman-Diamond syndrome with leukemia. *Int J Hematol* 79:189, 2004.

73. Yamada T, Tsurumi H, Murakami N, et al: Werner's syndrome developing acute megakaryoblastic leukemia with der(1;7). *Jpn J Clin Hematol* 38:28, 1997.

74. Tao LC, Stecker E, Gardner HA: Werner's syndrome and acute myeloid leukemia. *CMAJ* 105:951, 1971.

75. Epstein CJ, Martin GM, Schultz AL, Motulsky AG: Werner's syndrome. *Medicine* 45:177, 1996.

76. Sharathkumar A, Kirby M, Freedman M, et al: Malignant hematological disorders in children with Wolf-Hirschhorn syndrome. *Am J Med Genet* 119A:194, 2003.

77. Gonzales CH, Durkin-Stamm MV, Geimer NF, et al: The WT-syndrome—A "new" autosomal dominant pleiotropic trait of radial/ulnar hypoplasia with high risk of bone marrow failure and/or leukemia. *Birth Defects* 13:31, 1977.

78. Fialkow PH, Singer JW, Adamson JW, et al: Acute nonlymphocytic leukemia. Heterogeneity of stem cell origin. *Blood* 57:1068, 1991.

79. Ferraris AM, Broccia G, Meloni T, et al: Clonal origin of cells restricted to monocytic differentiation in acute nonlymphocytic leukemia. *Blood* 64:817, 1984.

80. Greaves MF: Stem cell origins of leukaemia and curability. *Br J Cancer* 67:413, 1993.

81. Turhan AG, Lemoire FB, Debert C, et al: Highly purified primitive hematopoietic stem cells are PML-RARA negative and generate nonclonal progenitors in acute promyelocytic leukemia. *Blood* 85:2154, 1995.

82. Van Lom K, Hagenmeijer A, Vandekerckhove F, et al: Clonality analysis of hematopoietic cell lineages in acute myeloid leukemia and translocation (8;21): Only myeloid cells are part of malignant clone. *Leukemia* 11:202, 1997.

83. Look AT: Oncogene transcription factors in human acute leukemias. *Science* 278:1059, 1997.

84. Tenen DG, Hromas R, Licht JD, Dong-Er Z: Transcription factors, normal myeloid development, and leukemia. *Blood* 90:489, 1997.

85. Kelly LM, Gilliland DG: Genetics of myeloid leukemias. *Annu Rev Genomics Hum Genet* 3:179, 2002.

86. Adams JM, Cosy S: Oncogene cooperation in leukaemogenesis. *Cancer Surv* 15:119, 1992.

87. Bashey A, Gill R, Levi S, et al: Mutational activation of the N-ras oncogene assessed in primary clonogenic culture of acute myeloid leukemia (AML): Implications for the role of N-ras mutation in AML pathogenesis. *Blood* 79:981, 1992.

88. Preisler HD, Kinniburgh AJ, Wei-Dong G, Khan S: Expression of the protooncogenes *c-myc, c-fos,* and *c-fms* in acute myelocytic leukemia at diagnosis and in remission. *Cancer Res* 47:874, 1987.

89. Buesco-Ramos DE, Yang Y, De Leon E: The human MDM-2 oncogene is overexposed in leukemia. *Blood* 82:2617, 1993.

90. Mori N, Hidai H, Yokota J, et al: Mutations of the p53 gene in myelodysplastic syndrome and overt leukaemia. *Leuk Res* 19:869, 1995.

91. Wiede R, Parviz B, Pflüger K-H, et al: The role of decreased retinoblastoma protein expression in acute myelomonocytic and monoblastic leukemias. *Leuk Lymphoma* 17:135, 1995.

92. Ridge SA, Worwood M, Oscier D, et al: FMS mutations in myelodysplastic, leukemic and normal subjects. *Proc Natl Acad Sci U S A* 87:1377, 1990.

93. Menssen HD, Renki HJ, Rodeck U, et al: Presence of Wilm's tumor gene (wt1) transcripts and the WT1 nuclear protein on the majority of human acute leukemias. *Leukemia* 9:1060, 1995.

94. Wellman CL, Whittaker MH: The molecular biology of acute myeloid leukemia. *Clin Lab Med* 10:769, 1990.

95. Vigon I, Dreyfus F, Melle J, et al: Expression of the c-mpl protooncogene in human hematologic malignancies. *Blood* 82:877, 1993.

96. Libura M, Asnafi V, Delabesse E, et al: *FLT3* and *MLL* intragenic abnormalities in AML reflect a common category of genotoxic stress. *Blood* 1902:2198, 2003.

97. Levis M, Small D: FLT3: It does matter in leukemia. *Leukemia* 17:1738, 2003.

98. Mauritzson N, Albin M, Rylander L, et al: Pooled analysis of clinical and cytogenetic features in treatment-related and de novo adult acute myeloid leukemia and myelodysplastic syndromes based on consecutive series of 761 patients analyzed 1976-1993 and on 5098 unselected cases reported in the literature 1974-2001. *Leukemia* 16:2366, 2002.

99. Grimwade D, Enver T: Acute promyelocytic leukemia: Where does it stem from? *Leukemia* 18:375, 2004.

100. Lutz PG, Moog-Lutz C, Cayre YE: Signaling revisited in acute promyelocytic leukemia. *Leukemia* 16:1933, 2002.

101. Greaves MF, Maia AT, Wiemels JL, Ford AM: Leukemia in twins: Lessons in natural history. *Blood* 102:2321, 2003.

102. Wiemels JL, Xiao Z, Buffler PA, et al: In utero origin of of t(8;21) AML1-ETO translocation in childhood acute leukemia. *Blood* 99:3801, 2002.

103. Groves FD, Linet MS, Devesa SS: Epidemiology of leukemia, in *Leukemia*, 6th ed, edited by ES Henderson, TA Lister, MF Greaves, p 145. WB Saunders, New York, 1986.

104. Vickers M, Jackson G, Taylor P: The incidence of acute promyelocytic leukemia appears constant over most of a human lifespan, implying only one rate limiting mutation. *Leukemia* 14:727, 2000.

105. Dover BD, Preston-Martin S, Chang E, et al: High frequency of acute promyelocytic leukemia among Latinos with acute myeloid leukemia. *Blood* 87:308, 1996.

106. Otero JC, Santillana S, Fereyros G: High frequency of acute promyelocytic leukemia among Latinos with acute myeloid leukemias. *Blood* 88:377, 1996.

107. Stanley M, McKenna RW, Ellinger G, Brunning RD: Classification of 358 cases of acute myeloid leukemia by FAB criteria: Analysis of clinical and morphologic features, in *Chronic and Acute Leukemias in Adults*, edited by CD Bloomfield, p 147. Martinus Nijhoff, Boston, 1985.

108. Scott CS, Den Ottolander GJ, Swirsky D, et al: Recommended procedures for the classification of acute leukaemias. *Leuk Lymphoma* 11:37, 1993.

109. Jennings CD, Foon KA: Recent advances in flow cytometry: Application to the diagnosis of hematologic malignancy. *Blood* 90:2863, 1997.

110. Cassanovas RD, Campos L, Mugneret F, et al: Immunophenotypic patterns and cytogenetic anomalies in acute non-lymphoblastic leukemia subtypes: A prospective study of 432 patients. *Leukemia* 12:34, 1998.

111. Del Vecchio L, Di Noto R, Lo Pardo C, et al: Immunological classification of acute leukemias: Comments on the EGIL proposals. *Leukemia* 10:1832, 1996.

112. Paietta E: Classification of acute leukemias: Proposals for the immunological classification of acute leukemias. *Leukemia* 9:2147, 1995.

113. De Greef GE, Hagemeiger A: Molecular and cytogenetic abnormalities in acute myeloid leukemia and myelodysplastic syndromes. *Baillieres Clin Haematol* 9:1, 1996.

114. Kheiri SA, MacKerrell T, Bonagura VR, et al: Flow cytometry with or without cytochemistry for the diagnosis of acute leukemias? *Cytometry* 34:82, 1998.

115. Valik PJM, Verhaak RGW, Beijin A, et al: Prognostically useful gene-expression profiles in acute myeloid leukemia. *N Engl J Med* 350:1617 2004.

116. Bullinger L, Dohner K, Bair E, et al: Use of gene-expression profiling to identify prognostic subclasses in adult acute myeloid leukemia. *N Engl J Med* 350:1605, 2004

117. Head DR: Revised classification of acute myeloid leukemia. *Leukemia* 10:1826, 1996.

118. Boggs DR, Wintrobe MM, Cartwright GE: The acute leukemias. Analysis of 322 cases and review of the literature. *Medicine* 41:163, 1962.

119. Roath S, Isräels MCG, Wilkinson JF: The acute leukemias: A study of 580 patients. *Q J Med* 33:256, 1964.

120. Choi S-I, Simone JV: Acute non-lymphocytic leukemia in 171 children. *Med Pediatr Oncol* 2:119, 1976.

121. Chessels JM, O'Calloghan U, Hardisty RM: Acute myeloid leukaemia in childhood: Clinical features and prognosis. *Br J Haematol* 63:555, 1986.

122. Burns CP, Armitage JO, Frey AL, et al: Analysis of presenting features of adult leukemia. *Cancer* 47:2460, 1981.

123. Goodall PT, Vosti KL: Fever in acute myelogenous leukemia. *Arch Intern Med* 135:1197, 1975.

124. Burke PJ, Braine HG, Rothbun HK, Owens AH: The clinical significance and management of fever in acute myelocytic leukemia. *Johns Hopkins Med J* 139:1, 1976.

125. Chang JC: How to differentiate neoplastic fever from infectious fever in patients with cancer. Usefulness of the naproxen test. *Heart Lung* 16:122, 1987.

126. Gollard RP, Robbins BA, Piro L, Saven A: Acute myelogenous leukemia presenting with bulky lymphadenopathy. *Acta Haematol* 95:129, 1996.

127. Davey DD, Fourcar K, Burns CP, Goekin JA: Acute myelocytic leukemia manifested by prominent generalized lymphadenopathy. *Am J Hematol* 21:89, 1986.

128. Tobelem G, Jacquillat C, Chastang C, et al: Acute monoblastic leukemia: A clinical and biologic study of 74 cases. *Blood* 55:71, 1980.

129. Okano K, Ezumi K, Uda M, et al: Histopathological studies on the mode of leukemic infiltration in various organs. *Med J Osaka Univ* 14:125, 1963.

130. Kaiserling E, Horny H-P, Geerts M-L, Schmid U: Skin involvement in myelogenous leukemia. Morphologic and immunophenotypic heterogeneity of skin infiltrates. *Mod Pathol* 7:771, 1994.

131. Longacre TA, Smoller BR: Leukemia cutis: Analysis of 50 biopsy-proven cases with an emphasis on occurrences in myelodysplastic syndromes. *Am J Clin Pathol* 100:276, 1993.

132. Shaikh BS, Frantz E, Lookingbill DP: Histologically proven leukemia cutis carries a poor prognosis in acute nonlymphocytic leukemia. *Cutis* 39:57, 1987.

133. Sipp N, Radaszkiemicz T, Meijer CJLM, et al: Specific skin manifestations in acute leukemia with monocytic differentiation. *Cancer* 71:124, 1993.

134. Baer MR, Barcos M, Farrell H, et al: Acute myelogenous leukemia in leukemia cutis. *Cancer* 63:2192, 1989.

135. Long JC, Mihm MC: Multiple granulocytic tumors of the skin: Report of six cases of myelogenous leukemia with initial manifestations in the skin. *Cancer* 39:2004, 1977.

136. Bourantas K, Malamou-Mitsi V, Christou L, et al: Cutaneous vasculitis as the initial manifestation in acute myelomonocytic leukemia. *Ann Intern Med* 121:942, 1994.

137. Sheps M, Shapero H, Ramsay C: Bullous pyoderma gangrenosum and acute leukemia. *Arch Dermatol* 114:1842, 1978.

138. Lewis SJ, Poh-Fitzpatrick MB, Walther RR: A typical pyoderma gangrenosum with leukemia. *JAMA* 239:935, 1978.

139. Cho K-H, Han K-H, Sim S-W, et al: Neutophilic dermatoses associated with myeloid malignancy. *Clin Exp Dermatol* 22:269, 1997.

140. Cheson BD, Christensen RM: Cutis verticis gyrata: Unusual chloromatous disease in acute myelogenous leukemia. *Am J Hematol* 8:415, 1980.

141. Muller CP, Ziegler A, Steinke B, et al: Myelosarcomatosis of the skin preceding leukemic generalization of acute myelomonocytic leukemia. *Blut* 58:165, 1987.

142. Kincaid MC, Green WR: Ocular and orbital involvement in leukemia. *Surv Ophthalmol* 27:211, 1983.

143. Paparella MM, Berlinger NT, Oda M: Otological manifestations of leukemia. *Laryngoscope* 83:1510, 1973.

144. Bertrand Y, Lefrère J-J, L'Evergren G, et al: Acute myeloblastic leukemia presenting as apparent acute otitis media. *Am J Hematol* 27:136, 1988.

145. Shiknecht HF, Igarashi M, Chasin WD: Inner ear hemorrhage in leukemia. *Laryngoscope* 75:662, 1965.

146. Dewar GJ, Lim C-NH, Michalyshyn B, Akabutu J: Gastrointestinal complications in patients with acute and chronic leukemia. *Can J Surg* 24:67, 1981.

147. Hunter TB, Bjelland JC: Gastrointestinal complications of leukemia and its treatment. *AJR Am J Roentgenol* 142:513, 1984.

148. Duffy JH, Driscoll EJ: Oral manifestations of leukemia. *Oral Surg* 11:484, 1958.

149. Ahsan N, Schen-Chih, JS, John DD: Acute iliotyphlitis as presenting manifestation of acute myelogenous leukemia. *Am J Clin Pathol* 89:407, 1988.

150. Rodgers B, Seibert JJ: Unusual combination of an appendicolith in a leukemic patient with typhlitis-ultrasound diagnosis. *J Clin Ultrasound* 18:141, 1990.

151. Abramson SJ, Berdon WE, Baker DH: Childhood typhlitis: Its increas-

ing association with acute myelogenous leukemia. *Radiology* 146:61, 1983.

152. Roy J, Vercellotti G, Fenderson M, et al: Isolated relapse of acute myelogenous leukemia presenting as a gastric ulcer. *Am J Hematol* 37:270, 1991.

153. Thompson BC, Feczko PJ, Mezwa DG: Dysphagia caused by acute leukemia infiltration of the esophagus. *Am J Radiol* 155:654, 1990.

154. Ti M, Villafuerte R, Chase PH, Dosik H: Acute leukemia presenting as laryngeal obstruction. *Cancer* 34:427, 1974.

155. Bodey GP, Powell RD, Hersh EM, et al: Pulmonary complications of acute leukemia. *Cancer* 19:781, 1966.

156. Maile CW, Moore AV, Ulreich S, Putnam CE: Chest radiographic-pathologic correlation in adult leukemia patients. *Invest Radiol* 18:495, 1983.

157. Armstrong P, Dyer R, Alford BA, O'Hara M: Leukemic pulmonary infiltrates. Rapid development mimicking pulmonary edema. *AJR Am J Roentgenol* 135:373, 1980.

158. Wu KK, Burns CP: Leukemic pleural infiltrates during bone marrow remission of acute myelocytic leukemia. *Cancer* 33:1179, 1974.

159. Roberts WC, Bodey GP, Wertlake PT: The heart in acute leukemia. A study of 420 autopsy cases. *Am J Cardiol* 21:388, 1968.

160. Lisker SA, Finkelstein D, Brody JI, Beizer LH: Myocardial infarction in acute leukemia. *Arch Intern Med* 119:332, 1967.

161. Norris NH, Weiner J: The renal lesions in leukemia. *Am J Med Sci* 241:512, 1961.

162. Uno Y: Histopathological study of leukemic cell infiltration in the kidney. *Med J Osaka Univ* 18:185, 1967.

163. Russo A, Basquez E, Russo G, Schilvio G: Testicular relapse in acute myelogenous leukemia after 3 1/2 years of complete remission. *Acta Haematol* 65:131, 1981.

164. Quien ET, Wallach B, Sandhaus L, et al: Primary extramedullary leukemia of the prostate. *Am J Hematol* 53:267, 1996.

165. Vanden Broecke R, Van Droogenbroek J, Dhont M: Vulvovaginal manifestations of acute myeloblastic leukemia. *Obstet Gynecol* 88:735, 1996.

166. Marsh WL, Byland DJ, Heath VC, Anderson MJ: Osteoarticular and pulmonary manifestations of acute leukemia. *Cancer* 57:385, 1986.

167. Weinberger A, Schumacher R, Schimmer BM, et al: Arthritis in acute leukemia. *Arch Intern Med* 141:1183, 1981.

168. Pavlovsky S, Eppinger-Helft M, Murill FS: Factors that influence the appearance of central nervous system leukemia. *Blood* 42:935, 1973.

169. Meyer RJ, Ferreira PP, Cuttner J, et al: Central nervous system involvement at presentation in acute granulocytic leukemia. *Am J Med* 68:691, 1980.

170. Castagnola C, Morra E, Bernasconi P, et al: Acute myeloid leukemia and diabetes insipidus: Results in five patients. *Acta Haematol* 93:1, 1995.

171. Holmes R, Keating MJ, Cork A, et al: A unique pattern of central nervous system leukemia in acute myelomonocytic leukemia associated with inv (16) (p13;q32). *Blood* 65:1071, 1985.

172. Glass JP, VanTassel P, Keating MJ, et al: Central nervous system complications of a newly recognized subtype of leukemia: AMML with a pencentric inversion of chromosome 16. *Neurology* 38:639, 1987.

173. Neiman RS, Barcos M, Berard C, et al: Granulocytic sarcoma: A clinicopathologic study of 61 biopsied cases. *Cancer* 48:426, 1981.

174. Byrd JC, Edenfield WJ, Shields DJ, Dawson NA: Extramedullary myeloid cell tumors in acute nonlymphocytic leukemia. A clinical review. *J Clin Oncol* 13:1800, 1995.

175. Menasce LP, Banerjee SS, Becket E, Harris M: Extramedullary myeloid tumor (granulocytic sarcoma) is often misdiagnosed. A study of 26 cases. *Histopathology* 34:391, 1999.

176. Audouin J, Comperat E, Le Tourneau A, et al: Myeloid sarcoma: Clinical and morphologic criteria useful for diagnosis. *Int J Surg Pathol* 11:271, 2003.

177. Hernandez JA, Navarro JT, Rozman M, et al: Primary myeloid sarcoma of the gynecologic tract: A report of two cases progressing to acute leukemia. *Leuk Lymphoma* 43:2151, 2002.

178. Tsimberidou AM, Kantarjian HM, Estey E, et al: Outcome in patients with nonleukemic granulocytic sarcoma treated with chemotherapy with or without radiotherapy. *Leukemia* 17:1100, 2003.

179. Yamauchi K, Yasuda M: Comparison of nonleukenic granulocytic sarcoma. *Cancer* 94:1739, 2002.

180. Byrd JC, Weiss RB, Arthur DC, et al: Extramedullary leukemia adversely affects hematologic complete remission rate and overall survival in patients with t(8;21) (q22;q22): Results from Cancer and Leukemia Group B 8461. *J Clin Oncol* 15:466, 1997.

181. Andrieu V, Radford-Weill I, Troussand X, et al: Molecular detection of t(8;21)/AML1-ETO in AML M1/M2: Correlation with cytogenetics, morphology and immunophenotype. *Br J Haematol* 92:855, 1996.

182. Rege K, Swansbury GJ, Atra AA, et al: Disease features in acute myeloid leukemia with t(8;21)(q22;q22). Influence of age, secondary karyotypic abnormalities, CD19 status, and extramedullary leukemia. *Leuk Lymphoma* 40:67, 2000.

183. Nguyen S, Leblanc T, Fenaux P, et al: A white blood cell index as the main prognostic factor in t(8;21) acute myeloid leukemia (AML): A survey of 161 cases from the French AML intergroup. *Blood* 99:3517, 2002.

184. Rowe JM: Clinical and laboratory features of the myeloid and lymphoid leukemias. *Am J Med Technol* 49:103, 1983.

185. Woodcock BE, Cooper PC, Brown PR, et al: The platelet defect in acute myeloid leukemia. *J Clin Pathol* 37:1339, 1984.

186. Hofmann W-K, Stauch M, Höffken K: Impaired granulocytic function in patients with acute leukaemia: Only partial normalization after successful remission-inducing treatment. *Clin Res Clin Oncol* 124:113, 1998.

187. Suda T, Onai T, Maekawa T: Studies on abnormal polymorphonuclear neutrophils in acute myelogenous leukemia. *Am J Hematol* 15:45, 1983.

188. Glick AD, Paniker K, Flexner JM, et al: Acute leukemia of adults: Ultrastructural, cytochemical, and histological observations in 100 cases. *Am J Pathol* 73:459, 1980.

189. San Miguel JF, Conzalez M, Canizo MC, et al: TdT activity in acute myeloid leukemias defined by monoclonal antibodies. *Am J Hematol* 23:9, 1986.

190. Kaplan SS, Penchansky L, Krause JR, et al: Simultaneous evaluation of terminal deoxynucleotidyl transferase and myeloperoxidase in acute leukemias using an immunocytochemical method. *Am J Clin Pathol* 87:732, 1987.

191. Kahl C, Florschütz A, Müller G, et al: Prognostic significance of dysplastic features of hematopoiesis in patients with de novo acute myelogenous leukemia. *Ann Hematol* 75:91, 1997.

192. Manoharan A, Horsley R, Pitney WR: The reticulin content of bone marrow in acute leukemia in adults. *Br J Haematol* 43:185, 1979.

193. Moehler TM, Ho AD, Goldschmidt H, Barlogie B: Angiogenesis in hematologic malignancies. *Crit Rev Oncol Hematol* 45:227, 2003.

194. Albitar M: Angiogenesis in acute myeloid leukemia and myelodysplastic syndrome. *Acta Haematol* 106:170, 2001.

195. Ghannadan M, Wimazal F, Simonitsch I, et al: Immunohistochemical detection of VEGF in the bone marrow of patients with acute myeloid leukemia. Correlation between VEGF expression and the FAB category. *Am J Clin Pathol* 119:663, 2003.

196. Moore MAS, Spitzer G, Williams N, et al: Agar culture studies in 127 cases of untreated acute leukemia: The prognostic value of reclassification of leukemia according to in vitro growth characteristics. *Blood* 44:1, 1974.

197. Knudtzon S: In vitro culture of leukaemic cells from 81 patients with acute leukemia. *Scand J Haematol* 18:377, 1977.

198. Spitzer G, Dicke KA, McCredre KB, Barlogie B: The early detection of remission in acute myelogenous leukaemia by in vitro cultures. Br J Haematol 35:411, 1977.
199. Goldberg J, Tice D, Nelson DA, Gottliev AJ: Predictive value of in vitro colony and cluster formation in acute nonlymphocytic leukemia. Am J Med Sci 277:81, 1979.
200. Mrózek K, Heinonen K, De la Chapelle A, Bloomfield C: Clinical significance of cytogenetics in acute myeloid leukemia. Semin Oncol 24:17, 1997.
201. Schoch C, Haferlach T, Haase D, et al: Patients with de novo acute myeoid leukaemia and complex karyotype aberrations show a poor prognosis despite intensive treatment: A study of 90 patients. Br J Haematol 112:118, 2001.
202. Weltermann A, Fonatsch C, Haas OA, et al: Impact of cytogenetics on the prognosis of adults with de novo AML in first relapse. Leukemia 18:293, 2004.
203. Martinez-Climent JA, Lane NJ, Rubin CM, et al: Clinical and prognostic significance of chromosomal abnormalities in childhood acute myeloid leukemia de novo. Leukemia 9:95, 1995.
204. Pedersen-Bjergaard J, Philip P: Chromosome characteristics of therapy-related acute nonlymphocytic leukemia and preleukemia: Possible implications for pathogenesis of the disease. Leuk Res 11:315, 1987.
205. Zaccarea A, Alimena G, Baccarani M, et al: Cytogenetic analyses in 89 patients with secondary hematologic disorders: Results of a cooperative study. Cancer Genet Cytogenet 26:65, 1987.
206. Schoch C, Kern W, Krawitz P, et al: Dependence of age-specific incidence of acute myeloid leukemia on karyotype. Blood 98:3500, 2002.
207. Byrd JC, Lawrence D, Arthur DC, et al: Patients with isolated trisomy 8 in acute myeloid leukemia are not cured with cytarabine-based chemotherapy: Results from Cancer and Leukemia Group B 8461. Clin Cancer Res 4:1235, 1998.
208. Melnick A, Licht J: Deconstructing a disease, RARa, its fusion partners, and their roles in the pathogenesis of acute promyelocytic leukemia. Blood 93:3167, 1999.
209. LoCoco F, Diverio D, Falini B, et al: Genetic diagnosis and molecular monitoring in the management of acute promyelocytic leukemia. Blood 94:12, 1999.
210. Mrózek K, Heinonen K, Lawrence D, et al: Adult patients with de novo acute myeloid leukemia and t(9;11) (p22;q23) have a superior outcome to patients with other translocations involving band 11q23: A Cancer and Leukemia Group B study. Blood 90:4532, 1997
211. Poirel H, Rack K, Dalbesse E, et al: Incidence and characterization of MLL gene (11q23) rearrangements in acute myeloid leukemia M1 and M5. Blood 87:2496, 1996.
212. Schoch C, Schnittger S, Klaus M, et al: AML with 11q23/MLL abnormalities as defined by the WHO classification: Incidence, partner chromosomes, FAB subtype, age distribution, and prognostic impact in an unselected series of 1897 cytogenetically analyzed AML cases. Blood 102:2395, 2003.
213. Swansbury GJ, Slater R, Bain BJ, et al: Hematologic malignancies with t(9;11) (p21-22; q23)—A laboratory and clinical study of 125 cases. Leukemia 12:792, 1998.
214. Huret JL, Dessen P, Bernheim A, et al: An atlas on chromosomes in hematological malignancies. Example 11q23 and MLL. Leukemia 15:987, 2001.
215. Scholl C, Breitinger H, Schlenk RF, et al: Development of a real-time RT-PCR assay for the quantification of the most frequent MLL/AF9 fusion types resulting from translocation t(9;11)(p22;q23) in acute myeloid leukemia. Genes Chromosomes Cancer 38:274, 2003.
216. Strissel PL, Strick R, Tomek RJ, et al: DNA structural properties of AF9 are similar to MLL and could act as recombination hot spots resulting in MLL/AF9 translocations and leukemogenesis. Hum Mol Genet 9:1671, 2000.
217. Kurzock R, Shtalrid M, Talpaz M, et al: Expression of c-abl in Philadelphia-positive acute myelogenous leukemia. Blood 70:1584, 1987.
218. Tien H-F, Wang C-W, Chuang S-M, et al: Characterization of Philadelphia-chromosome-positive acute leukemia by clinical, cytochemical, and gene analysis. Leukemia 6:907, 1992.
219. Billstrom R, Ahlgren T, Bekassy AN, et al: Acute myeloid leukemia with inv(16)(p13q22): involvement of cervical lymph nodes and tonsils is common and may be a negative prognostic sign. Am J Hematol 71:15, 2002.
220. Kundu M, Liu PP: Function of the inv 16 fusion gene CBFB-MYH11. Curr Opin Hematol 8:201, 2001.
221. Delauney J, Ve3y N, Leblanc T, et al: Prognosis of Inv 16/t(16;16) acute myeloid leukemia (AML): A survey of 110 cases from the French AML Intergroup. Blood 102:462, 2003.
222. Poirel H, Radford-Weiss I, Rack K, et al: Detection of the chromosome 16 CBFβ-MYH11 fusion transcript in myelomonocytic leukemias. Blood 85:1313, 1995.
223. Haferlach T, Winkemann M, Löffler H, et al: The abnormal eosinophils are part of the leukemic cell population in acute myelomonocytic leukemia with abnormal eosinophils (AML M4 Eo) and carry pericentric inversion 16: A combination of May-Grünwald-Giemsa a staining and fluorescence in situ hybridization. Blood 87:2459, 1996.
224. Kjellstrand CM, Campbell DC, Von Hartitzsch B, Buselmeier TJ: Hyperuricemic acute renal failure. Arch Intern Med 133:349, 1974.
225. O'Regan S, Carson S, Chesney RW, Drummond KN: Electrolyte and acid-base disturbances in the management of leukemia. Blood 49:345, 1977.
226. Mir MA, Delamore IW: Metabolic disorders in acute myeloid leukaemia. Br J Haematol 40:79, 1978.
227. Bergman GE, Baluarte HJ, Naiman JL: Diabetes insipidus as a presenting manifestation of acute myelogenous leukemia. J Pediatr 88:355, 1976.
228. Mir MA, Brabin B, Tang OT, et al: Hypokalemia in acute myeloid leukaemia. Ann Intern Med 82:54, 1975.
229. Salomon J: Spurious hypoglycemia and hyperkalemia in myelomonocytic leukemia. Am J Med Sci 267:359, 1974.
230. Bellevue R, Disik H, Speigel G, Gussoff BD: Pseudohyperkalemia and extreme leukocytosis. J Lab Clin Med 85:660, 1975.
231. Fox MJ, Brody JS, Weintraub LR, et al: Leukocyte larceny: A cause of spurious hypoxia. Am J Med 67:742, 1979.
232. Palva IP, Salokannel SJ: Hypercalcemia in acute leukemia. Blut 24:209, 1972.
233. Zidar BL, Shadduck RK, Winkelstein A, et al: Acute myeloblastic leukemia and hypercalcemia. N Engl J Med 295:692, 1976.
234. Roth GJ, Poite D: Chronic lactic acidosis and acute leukemia. Arch Intern Med 125:317, 1970.
235. Wainer RA, Wiernik PH, Thompson WL: Metabolic and therapeutic studies of a patient with acute leukemia and severe lactic acidosis of prolonged duration. Am J Med 55:255, 1973.
236. Zamkoff KW, Kirshner JJ: Marked hypophosphatemia associated with acute myelomonocytic leukemia. Arch Intern Med 140:1523, 1980.
237. Pflüger K-H, Gramse M, Gropp C, Havemann K: Ectopic ACTH production with autoantibody formation in a patient with acute myeloblastic leukemia. N Engl J Med 305:1632, 1981.
238. Carpenter NA, Fiere DM, Schuh D, et al: Circulating immune complexes and the prognosis of acute myeloid leukemia. N Engl J Med 307:1174, 1982.
239. Bratt G, Bromback M, Paul C, et al: Factors and inhibitors of blood coagulation and fibrinolysis in acute nonlymphoblastic leukaemia. Scand J Haematol 34:332, 1985.
240. Reddy VB, Kowal-Vern A, Hoppensteadt DA, et al: Global and molecular hemostatic markers in acute myeloid leukemia. Am J Clin Pathol 94:397, 1990.

241. Tsumita Y, Matsushima T, Uchiumi H, et al: Acute myeloid leukemia accompanied by multiple thrombophlebitis. *Intern Med* 36:595, 1997.

242. Weltermann A, Pabinger I, Geiseler K, et al: Hypofibrinogenemia in non-M3 acute myeloid leukemia. Incidence, clinical and laboratory characteristics and prognosis. *Leukemia* 12:1182, 1998.

243. Spertini O, Callegari P, Cordey A-S, et al: High levels of the shed form of L-selectin are present in patients with acute leukemia and inhibit blast cell adhesion to activated endothelium. *Blood* 84:1249, 1994.

244. Lossos IS, Bogomolski-Yahalom V, Matzner Y: Anticardiolipin antibodies in acute myeloid leukemia: Prevalence and significance. *Am J Hematol* 57:139, 1998.

245. Wierzbowska A, Robak T, Wrzesien-Kus A, et al: Circulating VEGF and its soluble receptors sVEGFR-1 and sVEGFR-2 in patients with acute leukemia. *Eur Cytokine Netw* 14:149, 2003.

246. Lichtman MA, Heal J, Rowe JM: Hyperleukocytic leukaemia: Rheological and clinical features and management. *Baillieres Clin Hematol* 1:725, 1987.

247. Nowacki P, Zdziarska B, Fryze C, Urasinski I: Co-existence of thrombocytopenia and hyperleukocytosis ("critical period") as a risk factor of haemorrhage into the central nervous system in patients with acute leukaemias. *Haematologia* 31:347, 2002.

248. Wurthner JU, Kohler G, Behringer D, et al: Leukostasis followed by hemorrhage complicating the initiation of chemotherapy in patients with acute myeloid leukemia and hyperleukocytosis: A clinicopathologic report of four cases. *Cancer* 85:368,1999.

249. Ventura GJ, Hester JP, Smith TL, Keating MJ: Acute myeloblastic leukemia with hyperleukocytosis: Risk factors for early mortality in induction. *Am J Hematol* 27:34, 1988.

250. Dutcher J, Schiffer CA, Wiernik PH: Hyperleukocytosis in adult acute nonlymphocytic leukemia: Impact on remission rate, duration, and survival. *J Clin Oncol* 5:1364, 1987.

251. VanBuchem MA, Te Velde J, Willemze R, Spaander PJ: Leucostasis, an underestimated cause of death in leukaemia. *Blut* 56:39, 1988.

252. Dilek I, Uysal A, Demirer T, et al: Acute myeloblastic leukemia associated with hyperleukocytosis and diabetes insipidus. *Leuk Lymphoma* 30:657, 1998.

253. Lavabre-Bertrand T, Bourquard P, Chiesa J, et al: Diabetes insipidus revealing acute myelogenous leukaemia with a high platelet count, monosomy 7 and abnormalities of chromosome 3: A new entity? *Eur J Haematol* 66:66, 2001.

254. Nagler A, Brenner B, Zuckerman E, et al: Acute respiratory failure in hyperleukocytic acute myeloid leukemia. *Am J Hematol* 27:65, 1988.

255. Von Eyben FE, Siddiqui MZ, Spanosi G: High-voltage irradiation and hydroxyurea for pulmonary leukostasis in acute myelomonocytic leukemia. *Acta Haematol* 77:180, 1987.

256. Azoulay E, Fieux F, Moreau D, et al: Acute monocytic leukemia presenting as respiratory failure. *Am J Respir Crit Care Med* 167:1329, 2003.

257. Koote AMM, Thompson J, Bruijn JA: Acute myelocytic leukemia with acute aortic occlusion as presenting symptoms. *Acta Hematol* 75:120, 1986.

258. Foss R, Haddad M, Zaizov R, et al: Recurrent peripheral arterial occlusion by leukemic cells sedimentation in acute promyelocytic leukemia. *J Pediatr Surg* 27:665, 1992.

259. Mataix R, Gómez-Casares MT, Campo C, et al: Acute leg ischaemia as a presentation of hyperleukocytosis syndrome in acute myeloid leukaemia. *Am J Hematol* 51:250, 1996.

260. Murray JC, Dorfman SR, Brandt ML, Dreyer ZE: Renal venous thrombosis complicating acute myeloid leukemia in the hyperleukocytosis. *J Pediatr Hematol Oncol* 18:327, 1996.

261. Cohen Y, Amir G, Da'as N, et al: Acute myocardial infarction as the presenting symptom of acute myeloblastic leukemia with extreme hyperleukocytosis. *Am J Hematol* 71:47, 2002.

262. Berdeaux DH, Glosser L, Serokmann R: Hypoplastic acute leukemia. Review of 70 cases with multivariate regression analysis. *Hematol Oncol* 4:291, 1986.

263. Tuzuner N, Cox C, Rowe JM, Bennett JM: Hypocellular acute leukemia. *Hematol Pathol* 9:195, 1995.

264. Nagai K, Kohno T, Chen Y-X, et al: Diagnostic criteria for hypocellular acute leukemia. *Leuk Res* 7:563, 1996.

265. Iwakiri R, Ohta M, Mikoshiba M, et al: Prognosis of elderly patients with acute myelogenous leukemia: Analysis of 126 AML cases. *Int J Hematol* 75:45, 2002.

266. Barlogie B, Johnston DA, Keating M, et al: Evolution of oligoleukemia. *Cancer* 53:2115, 1984.

267. Maddox A-M, Keating MJ, Smith TL, et al: Prognostic factors for survival of 194 patients with low infiltrate leukemia. *Leuk Res* 10:995, 1986.

268. Niissler V, Sauer H, Pelka-Fleischer R, et al: Clinical, biochemical and cytokinetic parameters for distinguishing smouldering and rapidly proliferating variants of acute leukaemia. *Eur J Haematol* 45:19, 1990.

269. Yumura-Yagi K, Hara J, Talva A, Kawa-Ha K: Phenotypic characteristics of acute megakaryocytic leukemia and transient myelopoiesis. *Leuk Lymphoma* 13:393, 1994.

270. Bhatt S, Schreck R, Graham JM, et al: Transient leukemia with trisomy 21. *Am J Med Genet* 58:310, 1995.

271. Litz CE, Davies S, Brunning RD, et al: Acute leukemia and the transient myeloproliferative disorder associated with Down syndrome: Morphologic immunophenotypic and cytogenetic manifestations. *Leukemia* 9:1432, 1999.

272. Ito E, Kasai M, Hayashi Y, et al: Expression of erythroid-specific genes in acute megakaryoblastic leukaemia and transient myeloproliferative disorder in Down syndrome. *Br J Haematol* 90:607, 1995.

273. Kurukashi H, Junichi H, Keiko Y, et al: Monoclonal nature of transient abnormal myelopoiesis in Down's syndrome. *Blood* 77:1161, 1991.

274. Gamis AS, Hilden J: Transient myeloproliferative disorder. *J Pediatr Hematol Oncol* 241:2, 2002.

275. Gurbuxani S, Vyas P, Crispino JD: Recent insights into the mechanism of myeloid leukemogenesis in Down syndrome. *Blood* 103:399, 2004.

276. Zipursky A, Poon A, Doyle J: Leukemia in Down syndrome: A review. *Pediatr Hematol Oncol* 9:139, 1992.

277. Creutzig U, Ritter J, Vormoor J, et al: Myelodysplasia and acute myelogenous leukemia in Down's syndrome. *Leukemia* 10:1677, 1996.

278. Avet-Loiseau H, Mechinaud F, Harousseau J-L: Clonal hematologic disorders in Down syndrome. *J Pediatr Hematol Oncol* 17:19, 1995.

279. Taub J, Huang X, Ge Y, et al: Cystathionine-beta-synthase cDNA transfection alters sensitivity and metabolism of 1-beta-D-arabinofuranosylcytosine in CCRF-CEM leukemic cells in vitro and in vivo: A model of leukemia in Down syndrome. *Cancer Res* 60:6421, 2000.

280. Lange BJ, Kobrinsky N, Barnard DR, et al: Distinctive demography, biology, and outcome of acute myeloid leukemia and myelodysplastic syndrome in children with Down syndrome: Childrens Cancer Group Studies 2861 and 2891. *Blood* 91:608, 1998.

281. McCoy JP Jr, Overton WR: Immunophenotyping of congenital leukemia. *Cytometry* 22:85, 1995.

282. Kempski HM, Chessells JM, Reeves BR: Deletions of chromosome 21 restricted to the leukemia cells of children with Down syndrome and leukemia. *Leukemia* 11:1973, 1997.

283. Ravindranath Y, Abella E, Kruscher JP, et al: Acute myeloid leukemia (AML) in Down's syndrome is highly responsive to chemotherapy: Experience on Pediatric Oncology Group AML Study 8498. *Blood* 80:2210, 1992.

284. Pui C-H, Kane JR, Crist WM: Biology and treatment of infant leukemias. *Leukemia* 9:762, 1995.

285. Lampert F, Harbott J, Ritterbach J: Cytogenetic findings in acute leukaemias of infants. *Br J Cancer* 66(suppl XVII):S20, 1992.

286. Nagasaka M, Maeda S, Maeda H, et al: Four cases of t(4;11) acute leukemia and its myelomonocytic nature in infants. *Blood* 61:1174, 1983.

287. Hunger SP, Cleary ML: What significance should we attribute to the detection of MLL fusion transcripts? *Blood* 92:709, 1998.

288. Bresters D, Reus AC, Veerman AJ, et al: Congenital leukaemia: The Dutch experience and review of the literature. *Br J Haematol* 7:513, 2002.

289. Osada S, Horibe K, Oiwa K, et al: A case of infantile acute monocytic leukemia caused by vertical transmission of the mother's leukemic cells. *Cancer* 65:1146, 1990.

290. Lampkin BC, Peipon JJ, Price JK, et al: Spontaneous remission of presumed congenital acute nonlymphoblastic leukemia (ANLL) in a karyotypically normal neonate. *Am J Pediatr Hematol Oncol* 7:346, 1985.

291. Lauria F, Raspadori D, Ventura MA, et al: The presence of lymphoid-associated antigens in adult acute myeloid leukemia is devoid of prognostic relevance. *Stem Cells* 13:428, 1995.

292. Carbonell F, Swansbury J, Min T, et al: Cytogenetic findings in acute biphenotypic leukaemia. *Leukemia* 10:1283, 1996.

293. Gagnon GA, Childs CC, LeMaistre A, et al: Molecular heterogeneity in acute leukemia lineage switch. *Blood* 74:2088, 1989.

294. Greaves MF, Chan LC: Mixed lineage leukemia: The implication for hemopoietic differentiation [letter]. *Blood* 68:598, 1986.

295. Greaves MF, Chan LC, Furley AJW, et al: Lineage promiscuity in hemopoietic differentiation and leukemia. *Blood* 67:1, 1986.

296. Schmidt CA, Przybylski GK: What can we learn from leukemia as for the process of lineage commitment in hematopoiesis? *Int Rev Immunol* 20:107, 2001.

297. Neame PB, Soamboonsrup P, Browman G, et al: Simultaneous or sequential expression of lymphoid and myeloid phenotypes in acute leukemia. *Blood* 65:142, 1985.

298. Scott CS, Vulliamy T, Catovsky D, et al: DNA genotypic conservation during phenotypic switch from T-cell acute lymphoblastic leukaemia to acute myeloblastic leukaemia. *Leuk Lymphoma* 1:21, 1989.

299. Jensen AW, Hokland M, Jorgensen H, et al: Solitary expression of CD 7 among T-cell antigens in acute myeloid leukemia. *Blood* 78:1291, 1991.

300. Ferra F, DelVecchio L: Clinical relevance of acute mixed-lineage leukemia. *Blood* 79:2799, 1992.

301. Miwa H, Nakase K, Kita K: Biological characteristics of CD7(+) acute leukemia. *Leuk Lymphoma* 21:239, 1996.

302. Suzuki R, Yamamoto K, Seto M, et al: CD7+ and CD56+ myeloid/natural killer cell precursor acute leukemia: A distinct hematolymphoid disease entity. *Blood* 90:2417, 1997.

303. Scott AA, Head DR, Kropecky KJ, et al: HLA-DR−, CD33+, CD56+, CD16− myeloid/natural killer cell acute leukemia. *Blood* 84:244, 1994.

304. Paietta E, Gallagher RE, Wiernik PH: Myeloid/natural killer cell acute leukemia. *Blood* 84:2824, 1994.

305. Lee PS, Lin CN, Liu C, et al: Acute leukemia with myeloid, B-, and natural killer cell differentiation. *Arch Pathol Lab Med* 127:E93, 2003.

306. Handa H, Motohashi S, Isozumi K, et al: CD7+ and CD56+ myeloid/natural killer cell precursor acute leukemia treated with idarubicin and cytosine arabinoside. *Acta Haematol* 108:47, 2002.

307. Inhorn RC, Aster JC, Roach SA, et al: A syndrome of lymphoblastic lymphoma, eosinophilia, and myeloid hyperplasia malignancy associated with t(8;13) (p11;q11): Description of a distinctive clinical entity. *Blood* 85:1881, 1995.

308. Still IH, Chernova O, Hurd D, et al: Molecular characterization of the t(8;13) (p11;q12) translocation associated with an atypical myeloproliferative disorder: Evidence for three discrete loci involved in myeloid leukemias on 8 p11. *Blood* 90:3136, 1997.

309. Mirro J, Kitchingman GR, Williams DL, Murphy SB: Mixed lineage leukemia: The implication for hemopoietic differentiation [letter]. *Blood* 68:597, 1986.

310. Ladanyi M, Samaniego F, Reuter VE, et al: Cytogenetic and immunohistochemical evidence for the germ cell origin of a subset of acute leukemias associated with mediastinal germ cell tumors. *J Natl Cancer Inst* 82:221, 1990.

311. DeMent, CR, Roth BJ, Heerema N, et al: Hematologic neoplasia associated with primary mediastinal germ-cell tumors. *Hum Pathol* 21:699, 1990.

312. Nichols CR, Roth BJ, Heerema N, et al: Hematologic neoplasia associated with primary mediastinal germ-cell tumors. *N Engl J Med* 322:1425, 1990.

313. Kiffer JD, Sandeman TF: Primary malignant mediastinal germ cell tumors: A study of eleven cases and a review of the literature. *Int J Radiat Oncol Biol Phys* 17:835, 1990.

314. Nichols CR: Mediastinal germ cell tumors: Clinical features and biologic correlates. *Chest* 99:472, 1991.

315. Miyazato H, Sono H, Nasiki Y, et al: Detection of myeloperoxidase gene expression by in situ hybridization in a case of granulocytic sarcoma associated with AML-M0. *Leukemia* 14:1797, 2001.

316. Testa U, Torelli GF, Riccioni R, et al: Human acute stem cell leukemia with multilineage differentiation potential via cascade activation of growth factor receptors. *Blood* 99:4534, 2002.

317. Cuneo A, Ferrant A, Michaux JL, et al: Cytogenetic profile of minimally differentiated (FAB M0) acute myeloid leukemia: Correlation with clinicobiologic findings. *Blood* 85:3688, 1995.

318. Venditti A, Del Poeta G, Buccisano F, et al: Minimally differentiated acute myeloid leukemia (AML M0): Comparison of 25 cases with other French-American-British subtypes. *Blood* 89:621, 1997.

319. Villamor N, Zarco M-A, Rozman M, et al: Acute myeloblastic leukemia with minimal myeloid differentiation: Phenotypical and ultrastructural characteristics. *Leukemia* 12:1071, 1998.

320. Roumier C, Eclache V, Imbert M, et al: M0 AML, clinical and biologic features of the disease, including *AML1* gene mutations. *Blood* 101:1277, 2003.

321. Maruyami F, Stass SA, Estey EH, et al: Detection of AML1/ETO fusion transcript as a tool for diagnosing t(8;21) positive acute myelogenous leukemia. *Leukemia* 8:40, 1994.

322. Schoch C, Haase D, Haferlach T, et al: Fifty-one patients with acute myeloid leukemia and translocation t(8;21) (q22; q22): An additional deletion in 9q is an adverse prognostic factor. *Leukemia* 10:1288, 1996.

323. Wang J, Wang M, Liu JM: Transformation properties of the ETO gene, fusion partner in t(8;21) leukemias. *Cancer Res* 57:2951, 1997.

324. Watkins CH, Hall BE: Monocytic leukemia of the Naegeli and Schilling types. *Am J Clin Pathol* 10:387, 1940.

325. Huhn D, Twardzik L: Acute myelomonocytic leukemia and the French-American-British classification. *Acta Haematol* 69:36, 1983.

326. Scott CS, Morgan M, Limbert HJ, et al: Cytochemical, immunological and ANAE-isoenzyme studies in acute myelomonocytic leukaemia: A study of 39 cases. *Scand J Haematol* 35:284, 1985.

327. Bloomfield CD, Garson OM, Knuutila S, De la Chapelle A: t(1;3)(p36; q21) in acute nonlymphocytic leukemia: A new cytogenetic-clinicopathologic association. *Blood* 66:1409, 1985.

328. Creictzig U, Niederbiermann G, Kitter J, et al: Prognostic significance of eosinophilia in acute myelomonocytic leukemia in relation to induction treatment. *Haematol Blood Transf* 33:226, 1990.

329. Hoyle CF, Sherrington PD, Fischer P, Hayhoe FGT: Basophils in acute leukemia. *J Clin Pathol* 42:785, 1989.

330. Pearson MG, Vardiman JW, LeBeau MM, et al: Increased numbers of marrow basophils may be associated with t(6;9) in ANLL. *Am J Hematol* 18:393, 1985.

331. Alsabeh R, Byrnes RK, Slovak ML, Arber DA: Acute myeloid leukemia with t(6;9) (p23;q34): Association with myelodysplasia, basophilia, and initial CD34 negative phenotype. *Am J Clin Pathol* 107:430, 1997.

332. Copelli M: Di una emopatia sistemizzata rappresentata da una iperplasia eritroblastica (eritromatosis). *Path Riv Quindicin* 4:460, 1912.

333. DiGuglielmo G: Richerche di hematologia: I. Una casa di eritroleucemia. *Folia Med* 13:386, 1917.

334. Moeschlin S: Erythroblastosen, erythroleukemien und erythroblastamien. *Folia Haematol (Frankf)* 64:262, 1940.

335. Dameshek W: The Di Guglielmo syndrome. *Blood* 13:192, 1940.

336. Fouillard L, Labopin M, Gorin N-C, et al: Hematopoietic stem cell transplantation for de novo erythroleukemia: A study of the European Group for Blood and Marrow Transplantation (EBMT). *Blood* 100: 3135, 2002.

337. Novick Y, Marino P, Makower DF, Wiernik PH: Familial erythroleukemia: A distinct clinical and genetic type of familial leukemia. *Leuk Lymphoma* 80:395, 1998.

338. Lee EJ, Schiffer CA, Misawa S, Testa JR: Clinical and cytogenetic features of familial erythroleukaemia. *Br J Haematol* 65:313, 1987.

339. Cuneo A, VanOrshoven A, Michaux JL, et al: Morphologic, immunologic and cytogenetic studies in erythroleukemia: Evidence for multilineage involvement and identification of two distinct cytogeneticclinicopathologic types. *Br J Haematol* 75:346, 1990.

340. Goldberg SL, Noel P, Klumpp TR, Dewald GW: The erythroid leukemias. *Am J Clin Oncol* 21:42, 1998.

341. Olopade OI, Thangavelu M, Larson RA, et al: Clinical, morphologic, and cytogenetic characteristics of 26 patients with acute erythroblastic leukemia. *Blood* 80:2873, 1992.

342. Davey FR, Abraham N Jr, Bronetto VL, et al: Morphologic characteristics of erythroleukemia (Acute myeloid leukemia; FAB-M6): A CALGB study. *Am J Hematol* 49:29, 1995.

343. Adamson JW, Finch CA: Erythropoietin and the regulation of erythropoiesis in diGuglielmo's syndrome. *Blood* 36:590, 1970.

344. Mitjavila MT, Villeval JL, Cramer P, et al: Effects of granulocytemacrophage colony-stimulating factor and erythropoietin on leukemic erythroid colony formation in human early erythroblastic leukemias. *Blood* 70:965, 1987.

345. Mazella FM, Kowel-Vern A, Shrit MA, et al: Acute erythroleukemia evaluation of 48 cases with reference to classification, cell proliferation, cytogenetics, and prognosis. *Am J Clin Pathol* 110:590, 1998.

346. Breton-Gorius J: Phenotypes of blasts in acute erythroblastic and megakaryoblastic leukemia—A review. *Keio J Med* 36:23, 1987.

347. Peterson BA, Levine EG: Uncommon subtypes of acute nonlymphocytic leukemia: Clinical features and management of FAB M5, M6 and M7. *Semin Oncol* 14:425, 1987.

348. Croizat P, Favre-Gilly J: Les aspects du syndrome hémorrhagiue des leucémies. *Sang* 20:417, 1949.

349. Hillstad LK: Acute promyleocytic leukemia. *Acta Med Scand* 159:189, 1957.

350. LoCoco F, Nervi C, Avvisati G, Mandelli F: Acute promyelocytic leukemia: A curable disease. *Leukemia* 12:1866, 1998.

351. Avvisati G, Lo Coco F, Mandelli F: Acute promyelocytic leukemia: Clinical and morphological features and prognostic factors. *Semin Hematol* 38:4, 2001.

352. Estey E, Thall P, Kantarjian H, et al: Association between increased body mass index and a diagnosis of acute promyelocytic leukemia in patients with acute myeloid leukemia. *Leukemia* 11:1661, 1997.

353. Golomb HM, Rowley JD, Vardiman J, et al: "Microgranular" acute promyelocytic leukemia: A distinct clinical, ultrastructural, and cytogenetic entity. *Blood* 55:253, 1980.

354. McKenna RW, Parkin J, Bloomfield C, et al: Acute promyelocytic leukaemia: A study of 39 cases with identification of a hyperbasophilic microgranular variant. *Br J Haematol* 50:201, 1982.

355. Rovelli A, Biondi A, Rajnoldi AC, et al: Microgranular variant of acute promyelocytic leukemia in children. *J Clin Oncol* 10:1413, 1992.

356. Castoldi GL, Liso V, Speechia G, Thomasi P: Acute promyelocytic leukemia: Morphological aspects. *Leukemia* 8(suppl 2):S27, 1994.

357. Umeda M, Nojima Z, Yamaguchi R, et al: Two cases of acute promyelocytic leukemia with marked basophilia—A variant type of APL with the capability of differentiating into basophilis. *Rinsho Ketsveki* 28:2004, 1987.

358. Gotoh H, Murakani S, Oku N, et al: Translocation t(15;17) and t(9;14) (q34;q22) in a case of acute promyelocytic leukemia with increased number of basophils. *Cancer Genet Cytogenet* 36:103, 1988.

359. Yu R-Q, Huang W, Chen S-J, et al: A case of acute eosinophilic granulocytic leukemia with PML-RAR alpha fusion gene expression and response to all-*trans*-retinoic acid. *Leukemia* 11:609, 1997.

360. Invernizzi R, Iannone AM, Bernuzzi S, et al: Acute promyelocytic leukemia toluidine blue subtype. *Leuk Lymphoma* 18(suppl 1):57, 1995.

361. Rowley JD, Golomb HM, Dogherty C: 15/17 translocation, a consistent chromosomal change in acute promyelocytic leukaemia. *Lancet* 1:549, 1977.

362. Lavau C, Dejean A: The t(15;17) translocation in acute promyelocytic leukemia. *Leukemia* 8:1615, 1994.

363. Sainty D, Liso V, Cantu-Rajnoldi A, et al: A new morphologic classification system for acute promelocytic leukemia distinguishes cases with underlying PLZF/RARA gene rearrangements. *Blood* 96:1287, 2000.

364. Petti MC, Fazi F, Gentile M, et al: Complete remission through blast differentiation in PLZF/RARα-positive acute promyelocytic leukemia: In vitro and in vivo studies. *Blood* 100:1065, 2002.

365. DeThé H, Chomienne C, Lanotte M, et al: The t(15;17) translocation of acute promyelocytic leukaemia fuses the retinoic acid receptor α-gene to a novel transcribed locus. *Nature* 347:558, 1990.

366. Huang W, Sun G-L, Li X-S, et al: Acute promyelocytic leukemia: Clinical relevance of two major PML-RARα isoforms and detection of minimal residual disease by retrotranscriptase/polymerase chain reaction to predict relapse. *Blood* 82:1264, 1993.

367. Rego EM, Pandolfi PP: Analysis of molecular genetics of acute promyelocytic leukemia in mouse models. *Semin Hematol* 38:54, 2001.

368. Dombret H, Scrobohaci ML, Ghorra P, et al: Coagulation disorder associated with acute promyelocytic leukemia: Correct effect of all-*trans* retinoic acid. *Leukemia* 7:2, 1993.

369. Tallman MS, Kwaan HC: Reassessing the hemostatic disorder associated with acute promyelocytic leukemia. *Blood* 79:543, 1992.

370. Barbui T, Finazzi G, Falanga A: The impact of all-*trans* retinoic acid on the coagulopathy of acute promyelocytic leukemia. *Blood* 91:3093, 1998.

371. Menell JS, Cesarman GM, Jacovina ATet al: Annexin II and bleeding in acute promyelocytic leukemia. *N Engl J Med* 340:994, 1999.

372. Avvisati G, Ten Cate JW, Büller H, Mandelli F: Tranexamic acid for control of haemorrhage in patients with acute promyelocyte leukaemia. *Lancet* ii:122, 1989.

373. Fenaux P, Tertian G, Castaigne S, et al: A randomized trial of amsacrine and rubidasone on 39 patients with acute promyelocytic leukemia. *J Clin Oncol* 9:1556, 1991.

374. Craddock CG, Crandall BF, Como R: Restoration of effective hemopoiesis preceding suppression of leukemia clone in myeloblastic leukemia. *Am J Med* 59:737, 1975.

375. Amato R, Kantarjian H, Walter R, Keating M: Rebound peripheral blastosis with subsequent remission during induction in a patient with acute promyelocytic leukemia. *Cancer* 61:650, 1988.

376. Stone RM, Maguire M, Goldberg MA, et al: Complete remission in acute promyelocytic leukemia despite persistence of abnormal marrow promyelocytes during induction therapy: Experience in 34 patients. *Blood* 71:690, 1988.

377. Breitman TR, Collins SJ, Keene BR: Terminal differentiation of human promyelocytic leukemic cells in primary culture in response to retinoic acid. *Blood* 57:1000, 1981.

378. Huang ME, Ye YC, Chen SR, et al: Use of all-*trans* retinoic acid in the treatment of acute promyelocytic leukemia. *Blood* 72:567, 1988.

379. Wu X, Wang X, Qen X, et al: Four years experience with treatment of all-*trans* retinoic acid in acute promyelocytic leukemia. *Am J Hematol* 43:183, 1993.

380. Lobe I, Regal-Huguet FR, Vekhoff A, et al: Myelodysplastic syndrome after acute promyelocytic leukemia: The European APLK group experience. *Leukemia* 17:1600, 2003.

381. Garcia-Manero G, Kantarjian HM, Kornblau S, Estey E: Therapy-related myelodysplastic syndrome or acute myelogenous leukemia in patients with acute promyelocytic leukemia. *Leukemia* 17:1888, 2002.

382. Reschad H, Schilling-Torgau V: Ueber eine neue Leukämie durch echte Uebergangsformen (Splenozyten-leukämie) und ihre Bedeutung für die Selbstständigkeit dieser Zellen. *Münch Med Wochenschr* 60: 1981, 1913.

383. Straus DJ, Mertelsmann R, Koziner B, et al: The acute monocytic leukemias. *Medicine* 59:409, 1980.

384. Janvier M, Tobelem G, Daniel MT, et al: Acute monoblastic leukaemia. Clinical, biological data and survival in 45 cases. *Scand J Haematol* 32:385, 1984.

385. Finaux P, Vanhaesbroucke C, Estienne MH, et al: Acute monocytic leukaemia in adults: Treatment and prognosis in 99 cases. *Br J Haematol* 75:41, 1990.

386. Fung H, Shepard JD, Naiman SC, et al: Acute monocytic leukemia: A single institution experience. *Leuk Lymphoma* 19:259, 1995.

387. Cuttner J, Conjalka MS, Reilly M, et al: Association of monocyte leukemia in patients with extreme leukocytosis. *Am J Med* 69:555, 1980.

388. Jourdan E, Dombret H, Glaisner S, et al: Unexpected high incidence of intracranial subdural haematoma during intensive chemotherapy for acute myeloid leukaemia with a monoblastic component. *Br J Haematol* 89:527, 1995.

389. Scott CS, Stark AN, Limbert HJ, et al: Diagnostic and prognostic factors in acute monocytic leukemia: An analysis of 51 cases. *Br J Haematol* 69:247, 1988.

390. Scherrer A, Kruithof EKO, Grob J-P: Plasminogen activator inhibitor-2 in patients with monocytic leukemia. *Leukemia* 5:479, 1991.

391. Van Furth R, Van Zwet TL: Cytochemical, functional, and proliferative characteristics of promonocytes and monocytes from patients with monocytic leukemia. *Blood* 62:298, 1983.

392. Van Furth R, Leijh PCJ, Van Zwet TL, Van den Barselaar MT: Phagocytic and intracellular killing by peripheral blood monocytes of patients with monocytic leukemia. *Blood* 59:1234, 1982.

393. Diaz MO, LeBeau MM, Pitha P, Rowley JD: Interferon and *c-est*-1 genes in the translocation (9;11)(p22;q23) in human acute monocytic leukemia. *Science* 231:265, 1986.

394. Mavilo F, Testa U, Sposi NM, et al: Selective expression of *fos* protooncogene in human acute myelomonocytic and monocytic leukemias: A molecular marker of terminal differentiation. *Blood* 69:160, 1987.

395. Pinto A, Colletta G, DeVecchio L, et al: *c-fos* oncogene expression in human hemopoietic malignancies is restricted to acute leukemias with monocytic phenotype and to subsets of B cell leukemias. *Blood* 70: 1450, 1987.

396. Weide R, Parviz B, Pflüger K-H, Haveman K: Altered expression of the human retinoblastoma gene in monocytic leukaemias. *Br J Haematol* 83:428, 1993.

397. Cuttner J, Seremetis S, Najfield V, et al: TdT-positive acute leukemia with monocytoid characteristics: Clinical, cytochemical, cytogenetic, and immunologic findings. *Blood* 64:237, 1984.

398. Sun T, Wu E: Acute monoblastic leukemia with t(8;16): A distinct clinicopathologic entity. *Am J Hematol* 66:207, 2001.

399. Santiago-Schwarz F, Coppock DL, Hindenburg A, Kern J: Identification of a malignant counterpart of the monocytic-dendritic cell progenitor in acute myeloid leukemia. *Blood* 84:3054, 1994.

400. Pileri SA, Grogan TM, Harris NL, et al: Tumors of histiocytes and accessory dendritic cells: An immunohistochemical approach to classi-

401. fication from the International Lymphoma Study Group based on 61 cases. *Histopathology* 41:1, 2002.

401. Elghetany MT: True histiocytic lymphoma: Is it an entitity? *Leukemia* 11:762, 1997.

402. Esteve J, Rozman M, Campo E, et al: Leukemia after true histiocytic lymphoma: Another type of acute monocytic leukemia with histiocytic differentiation (AML-M5c). *Leukemia* 9:1389, 1995.

403. Tallman MS, Kim HT, Paietta E, et al: Acute monocytic leukemia (French-American-British classification M5) does not have a worse prognosis than other subtypes of acute myeloid leukemia: Report from the Eastern Cooperative Group. *J Clin Oncol* 22:1276, 2004.

404. Lewis SM, Szur L: Malignant myelosclerosis. *Br Med J* 2:472, 1963.

405. Bergsman KL, VanSlyck EJ: Acute myelofibrosis. *Ann Intern Med* 74: 232, 1971.

406. Huang MJ, Li CY, Nichols WL, et al: Acute leukemia with megakaryocytic differentiation. A study of twelve cases identified immunocytochemically. *Blood* 64:427, 1984.

407. Gassman W, Löffler H: Acute megakaryoblastic leukemia. *Leuk Lymphoma* 18:69, 1995.

408. Cripe LD, Hromas R: Malignant disorders of megakaryocytes. *Semin Hematol* 35:200, 1998.

409. Paredes-Aguilera R, Romero-Guzman L, Lopez-Santiago N, Trejo RA: Biological, clinical, and hematological features of acute megakaryoblastic leukemia in children. *Am J Hematol* 73:71, 2003.

410. Zipursky A, Brown E, Christensen H, et al: Leukemia and/or myeloproliferative syndrome in neonates with Down syndrome. *Semin Perinatol* 21:97, 1997.

411. Dastugue N, Lafage-Pochitaloff M, Pages MP, et al: Cytogenetic profile of childhood and adult megakaryoblastic leukemia (M7): A study of the Groupe Francais de Cytogenetique Hematologique (GFCH). *Blood* 100:618, 2002.

412. Carroll A, Civin C, Schneider N, et al: The t(1;22)(p13;q13) is nonrandom and restricted to infants with acute megakaryoblastic leukemia: A pediatric oncology group study. *Blood* 78:748, 1991.

413. Duchayne F, Fenneteau O, Pages MP, et al: Acute megakaryoblastic leukaemia: A national clinical and biological study of adult and childhood cases by the Group Francais d'Hematologie Cellulaire (GFHC). *Leuk Lymphoma* 44:49, 2003.

414. Bernstein J, Dastugue N, Haas OA, et al: Nineteen cases of the t(1; 22)(p13;q13) acute megakaryoblastic leukaemia of infants/children and a review of 39 cases: Report from a t(1;22) study group. *Leukemia* 14:216, 2000.

415. Cuneo A, Mecucci C, Kerim S, et al: Multipotent stem cell involvement in megakaryoblastic leukemia: Cytologic and cytogenetic evidence in 15 patients. *Blood* 74:1781, 1989.

416. Dhyashiki K, Ohyashiki JH, Hojo H, et al: Cytogenetic findings in adult acute leukemia in myeloproliferative disorders with an involvement of megakaryocytic lineage. *Cancer* 65:940, 1990.

417. Kojima S, Sako M, Kato K, et al: An effective chemotherapeutic regimen for acute myeloid leukemia and myelodysplastic syndrome in children with Down's syndrome. *Leukemia* 14:786, 2000.

418. Athale UH, Razzouk BI, Raimondi SC, et al: Biology and outcome of childhood acute megakaryoblastic leukemia: A single institution's experience. *Blood* 97:3727, 2001.

419. Yamada S, Hongo T, Okada S, et al: Distinctive multidrug sensitivity and outcome of acute erythroblastic and megakaryoblastic leukemia in children with Down syndrome. *Int J Hematol* 74:428, 2001.

420. Tallman MS, Neuberg D, Bennett JM, et al: Acute megakaryocytic leukemia: The Eastern Cooperative Group experience. *Blood* 96:2405, 2000.

421. Pagano L, Pulsoni A, Vignetti M, et al: Acute megakaryoblastic leukemia: Experience of GIMEMA trial. *Leukemia* 16:1622, 2002.

422. Stillman RG: A case of myeloid leukemia with predominance of eosinophilic cells. *Med Rec* 81:594, 1912.

423. Harrington DS, Peterson C, Ness M, et al: Acute myelogenous leukemia with eosinophilic differentiation. *Am J Clin Pathol* 90:464, 1988.

424. Kueck DD, Smith RE, Parkin J, et al: Eosinophilic leukemia. A myeloproliferative disorder distinct from the hypereosinophilic syndrome. *Hematol Pathol* 5:195, 1991.

425. Sanada I, Asou N, Kajima S, et al: Acute myelogenous leukemia (FAB M1) associated with t(5;16) and eosinophilia. *Cancer Genet Cytogenet* 43:139, 1989.

426. Gabbas AG, Li CF: Acute non-lymphocytic leukemia with eosinophilic differentiation. *Am J Hematol* 21:29, 1986.

427. Brito-Babapulle F: Clonal eosinophilic disorders and the hypereosinophilic syndrome. *Blood Rev* 11:129, 1997.

428. Menssen HD, Renkl H-J, Rieder H, et al: Distinction of eosinophilic leukaemia from idiopathic hypereosinophilic syndrome by analysis of Wilms tumor gene expression. *Br J Haematol* 101:325, 1998.

429. Joachim G: Über mastzellenleukämien. *Dtsch Arch Klin Med* 87:437, 1906.

430. Goh KO, Anderson FW: Cytogenetic studies in basophilic chronic myelocytic leukemia. *Arch Pathol Lab Med* 193:288, 1979.

431. Shvidel L, Shaft D, Stark B, et al: Acute basophilic leukaemia: Eight unsuspected new cases diagnosed by electron microscopy. *Br J Haematol* 120:774, 2003.

432. Yokohama A, Tsukamoto N, Hatsumi N, et al: Acute basophilic leukemia lacking basophil-specific antigens: The importance of cytokine receptor expression in differential diagnosis. *Int J Hematol* 75:309, 2002.

433. Kubota M, Akiyama Y, Tabata Y, et al: Acute nonlymphocytic leukemia with basophilic differentiation and t(9;11)(p22;q23) in a child. *Am J Hematol* 31:133, 1989.

434. Mezger J, Permanetter W, Gerhartz H, et al: Philadelphia chromosome-negative acute hematopoietic malignancy: Ultrastructural, cytochemical, and immunocytochemical evidence of mast cell and basophil differentiation. *Leuk Res* 14:169, 1990.

435. Duchayne E, Demur C, Rubie H, et al: Diagnosis of acute basophilic leukemia. *Leuk Lymphoma* 32:269, 1999.

436. Petersen LC, Parken JL, Arthur DC, Brunning RD: Acute basophilic leukemia. *Hematopathology* 96:160, 1991.

437. Kubonishi I, Fijishita M, Niiya K, et al: Basophilic differentiation in acute promyelocytic leukaemia. *Acta Haematol Jpn* 48:1390, 1985.

438. Pardanani AD, Morice WG, Hoyer JD, Tefferi A: Chronic basophilic leukemia: A distinct clinico-pathologic entity. *Eur J Haematol* 71:18, 2003.

439. Travis WD, Li C-Y, Hoaglan HC, et al: Mast cell leukemia. Report of a case and review of the literature. *Mayo Clin Proc* 61:957, 1986.

440. Beghini A, Cairoli R, Morra E, Larizza L: In vivo differentiation of mast cells from acute myeloid leukemia blasts carrying a novel activating ligand-independent c-Kit mutation. *Blood Cells Mold Dis* 24:262, 1998.

441. Sperr WR, Horny HP, Lechner K, Valent P: Clinical and biological diversity of leukemias occurring in patients with mastocytosis. *Leuk Lymphoma* 37:473, 2000.

442. Fukuda T, Kakihara T, Kamishima T, et al: Leukemic cell membrane from acute myelogenous leukemias with massive mast cell infiltration has a mast cell differentiation activity under culture condition containing interleukin 3. *Leuk Res* 18:749, 1994.

443. Valent P, Sperr WR, Samorapoompichit P, et al: Myelomastocytic overlap syndromes: Biology, criteria, and relationship to mastocytosis. *Leuk Res* 25:595, 2001.

444. Levine PH, Weintraub LR: Pseudoleukemia during recovery from dapsone-induced agranulocytosis. *Ann Intern Med* 68:1060, 1968.

445. Sanal SM, Campbell EW, Bowdler AJ, Brat PJ: Pseudoleukemia. *Postgrad Med* 65:143, 1979.

446. Dreskin SC, Iberti TJ, Watson-Williams EJ: Pseudoleukemia due to infection. *J Med* 14:147, 1983.

447. Lanham GR, Dahl GV, Billings FT, Stass SA: *Pseudomonas aeruginosa* infection with marrow suppression simulating acute promyelocytic leukemia. *Am J Clin Pathol* 80:404, 1983.

448. Orchard PJ, Moffet HL, Hafez R, Sondel PM: Pseudomonas sepsis simulating acute promyelocytic leukemia. *Pediatr Infect Dis J* 7:66, 1988.

449. Reykdal S, Sham R, Phatak P, Kouides P: Pseudoleukemia following the use of G-CSF. *Am J Hematol* 49:258, 1995.

450. Innes DJ, Hess CE, Bertholf MF, Wade P: Promyelocyte morphology: Differentiation of acute promyelocytic leukemia from benign myeloid proliferations. *Am J Clin Pathol* 88:725, 1987.

451. Ahmed MAM: Promyelocytic leukaemoid reaction: An atypical presentation of mycobacterial infection. *Acta Haematol* 85:143, 1991.

452. Karthaus M, Doellmann T, Klimasch T, et al: Central venous catheter infections in patients with acute leukemia. *Chemotherapy* 48:154, 2002.

453. Hummel M, Duchheidt D, Reiter S, et al: Successful treatment of hyperuricemia with low doses of recombinant urate oxidase in four patients with hematologic malignancy and tumor lysis syndrome. *Leukemia* 17:2542, 2003.

454. LoCoco F, Pelicci PG, D'Adamo F, et al: Polyclonal hematopoietic reconstitution in leukemia patients in remission after suppression of specific gene rearrangements. *Blood* 82:606, 1993.

455. Lichtman MA: The stem cell in the pathogenesis and treatment of myelogenous leukemia. *Leukemia* 15:1489, 2001.

456. Petti MC, Avvisati G, Amadori S, et al: Acute promyelocytic leukemia: Clinical aspects and results of treatment in 62 patients. *Haematologica* 72:151, 1987.

457. Sanz MA, Jarque I, Martin G, et al: Acute promyelocytic leukemia. *Cancer* 6:7, 1988.

458. Cheson BD, Bennett JM, Kopecky KJ, et al: Revised recommendations of the International Working Group for Diagnosis, Standards for Therapeutic Trials in Acute Myeloid Leukemia. *J Clin Oncol* 21:4642, 2003.

459. Fey MF: ESMO minimum clinical recommendations for diagnosis, treatment and follow-up of acute myeloblastic leukemia (AML) in adult patients. *Ann Oncol* 14:1161, 2003.

460. The NCCN acute myeloid leukemia clinical practice guideline in oncology. *J Natl Comprehensive Cancer Network.* 1:510, 2003.

461. Wiernik PH, Banks PLC, Case DC Jr, et al: Cytarabine plus idarubicin or daunorubicin as induction and consolidation therapy for previously untreated adult patients with acute myeloid leukemia. *Blood* 79:313, 1992.

462. Berman E, Heller G, Santorsa J, et al: Results of a randomized trial comparing idarubicin and cytosine arabinoside with daunorubicin and cytosine arabinoside in adult patients in the newly diagnosed acute myelogenous leukemia. *Blood* 77:1666, 1991.

463. Phillips GL, Reece DE, Shepard JD, et al: High-dose cytarabine and daunorubicin induction and postremission chemotherapy for the treatment of acute myelogenous leukemia in adults. *Blood* 77:1429, 1991.

464. Flasshove M, Meusers P, Schutte J, et al: Long-term survival after induction therapy with idarubicin and cytosine arabinoside for de novo acute myeloid leukemia. *Ann Hematol* 79:533, 2000.

465. Rowe JM: What is the best induction regimen for acute myelogenous leukemia? *Leukemia* 12(suppl 1):516, 1998.

466. Hargrave RM, Davey MW, Davey RA, Kidman AD: Development of drug resistance in reduced idarubicin relative to other anthracyclines. *Anticancer Drugs* 6:432, 1995.

467. Feldman EJ: High-dose mitoxantrone in acute leukaemia: New York Medical College experience. *Eur J Cancer Care* 6:27, 1997.

468. Usui N, Dobashi N, Kobayashi T, et al: Role of daunorubicin in the induction therapy for adult acute myeloid leukemia. *J Clin Oncol* 16:2086, 1998.

469. Woodlock TJ, Lifton R, DiSalle M: Coincident acute myelogenous leukemia and ischemic heart disease: Use of the cardioprotectant dexrazoxane during induction chemotherapy. *Am J Hematol* 59:246, 1998.

470. Pearlman M, Jendiroba D, Pagliaro L, et al. Dexrazoxane in combination with anthracyclines lead to a synergistic cytotoxic response in acute myelogenous leukemia cell lines. *Leuk Res* 27:617, 2003.

471. Bishop JF, Matthews JP, Young GA, et al: A randomized study of high-dose cytarabine in induction in acute myeloid leukemia. *Blood* 87:1710, 1996.

472. Stein AS, O'Donnell MR, Slovak ML, et al: High-dose cytosine arabinoside and daunorubicin induction therapy for adult patients with de novo non M3 acute myelogenous leukemia: Impact of cytogenetics on achieving a complete remission. *Leukemia* 14:1191, 2000.

473. Mehta J, Powles R, Treleaven J, et al: The impact of karyotype on remission rates in adult patients with de novo acute myeloid leukemia receiving high-dose cytarabine-based induction chemotherapy. *Leuk Lymphoma* 34:553, 1999.

474. Archimbaud E, Thomas X, Leblond V, et al: Timed sequential chemotherapy for previously treated patients with acute myeloid leukemia: Long-term follow-up of the etoposide, mitoxantrone, and cytarabine-86 trial. *J Clin Oncol* 13:11, 1995.

475. Archimbaud E, Leblond V, Fenaux P, et al: Timed sequential chemotherapy for advanced acute myeloid leukemia. *Hematol Cell Ther* 38:161, 1996.

476. He XY, Pohlman B, Lichtin A, et al: Timed-sequential chemotherapy with concomitant granulocyte colony-stimulating factor for newly diagnosed de novo acute myelogenous leukemia. *Leukemia* 17:1078, 2003.

477. Bolanos-Meade J, Karp JE, Guo C, et al: Timed sequential therapy of acute myelogenous leukemia in adults: A phase II study of retinoids in combination with the sequential administration of cytosine arabinsode, idarubicin and etoposide. *Leuk Res* 27:313, 2003.

478. Kell WJ, Burnett AK, Chopra R, et al: A feasibility study of simultaneous administration of gemtuzumab ozogamicin with intensive chemotherapy in induction and consolidation in younger patients with acute myeloid leukemia. *Blood* 102:4277, 2003.

479. Tsimberidou A, Estey E, Cortes J, et al: Gemtuzumab, fludarabine, cytarabine, and cyclosporine in patients with newly diagnosed acute myelogenous leukemia of high risk myelodysplastic syndromes. *Cancer* 97:1481, 2003.

480. Cortes J, Kantarjian H, Albitar M, et al: A randomized trial of liposomal daunorubicin and cytarabine versus liposomal daunorubicin and topotecan with or without thalidomide as initial therapy for patients with poor prognosis acute myelogenous leukemia or myelodysplastic syndrome. *Cancer* 97:1234, 2003.

481. Estey EH, Thall PF, Cortes JE, et al: Comparison of idarubicin + ara-C, and topotecan + ara-C-, and topotecan + ara-C-based regimens in treatment of newly diagnosed acute myeloid leukemia, refractory anemia with excess blasts in transformation, or refractory anemia with excess blasts. *Blood* 98:3575, 2001.

482. Rowe JM, Neuberg D, Friedenberg W, et al: A phase 3 study of three induction regimens and of priming with GM-CSF in older adults with acute myeloid leukemia: A trial by the Eastern Cooperative Oncology Group. *Blood* 103:479, 2004.

483. Ganser A, Heil G: Use of hematopoietic growth factors in the treatment of acute myelogenous leukemia. *Curr Opin Hematol* 4:191, 1997.

484. Lowenberg B, Van Putten W, Theobald M, et al: Effect of priming with granulocyte colony-stimulating factor on the outcome of chemotherapy for acute myeloid leukemia. *N Engl J Med* 348:743, 2003.

485. Nimubona S, Grulois I, Bernard M, et al: Complete remission in hypoplastic acute myeloid leukemia induced by G-CSF without chemotherapy: Report on three cases. *Leukemia* 16:1872, 2002.

486. Schlenk RF, Benner A, Hartmann F, et al: Risk-adapted postremission therapy in acute myeloid leukemia: Results of the German multicenter AML HD93 treatment trial. *Leuk Res* 17:1521, 2003.

487. Anderlini P, Ghaddar HM, Smith TL, et al: Factors predicting complete remission and subsequent disease-free survival after a second course of induction therapy in patients with acute myelogenous leukemia resistant to the first. *Leukemia* 10:964, 1996.

488. Estey EH, Shen Yu, Thall PF: Effect of time to complete remission on subsequent survival and disease-free survival time in AML, RAEB-t, and RAEB. *Blood* 95:72, 2000.

489. Kern W, Scoch C, Haferlach T, et al: Multivariate analysis of prognostic factors in patients with refractory and relapsed acute myeloid leukemia. *Leukemia* 14:226, 2000.

490. Thiebaut A, Thomas X, Belhabri A, et al: Impact of pre-induction therapy leukapheresis on treatment outcome in adult acute myelogenous leukemia presenting with hyperleukocytosis. *Ann Hematol* 79:501, 2000.

491. Giles FJ, Shen Y, Kantarjian HM, et al: Leukapheresis reduces early mortality in patients with acute myeloid leukemia with high white cell counts but does not improve long-term survival. *Leuk Lymphoma* 42:67, 2001.

492. Porcu P, Farag S, Marucci G, et al: Leukoreduction for acute leukemia. *Ther Apher* 6:15, 2002.

493. Schmidt JE, Tamburro RF, Sillos EM, et al: Pathophysiology-directed therapy for acute hypoxemic respiratory failure in acute myeloid leukemia with hyperleukocytosis. *J Pediatr Hematol Oncol* 25:569, 2003.

494. Hughes WT, Armstrong D, Bodey GP, et al: 1997 guidelines for the use of antimicrobial agents in neutropenic patients with unexplained fever. Infectious Diseases Society of America. *Clin Infect Dis* 25:551, 1997.

495. Lehrenbecher T, Varig D, Kaiser J, et al: Infectious complications in pediatric acute myeloid leukemia: Analysis of the prospective multi-institutional clinical trial AML-BFM 93. *Leukemia* 18:72, 2004.

496. Jagarlamidi R, Kumar L, Kochupillai V, et al: Infections in acute leukemia: An analysis of 240 febrile episodes. *Med Oncol* 17:111, 2000.

497. Uzun O, Anaissie EJ: Antifungal prophylaxis in patients with hematologic malignancies: A reappraisal. *Blood* 86:2063, 1995.

498. Glasmacher A, Molitor E, Hahn C, et al: Antifungal prophylaxis with itraconazole in neutropenic patients with acute leukaemia. *Leukemia* 12:1338, 1998.

499. Bergmann OJ, Mogensen SC, Ellermann-Eriksen S, Ellegaard J: Acyclovir prophylaxis and fever during remission-induction therapy of patients with acute myeloid leukemia: A randomized, double-blind, placebo-controlled trial. *J Clin Oncol* 15:2269, 1997.

500. Walsh TJ, Finberg RW, Arndt C, et al: Liposomal amphotericin B for empirical therapy in patients with persistent fever and neutropenia. National Institute of Allergy and Infectious Disease Mycoses Study Group. *N Engl J Med* 340:764, 1999.

501. Marr KA: New approaches to invasive fungal infections. *Curr Opin Hematol* 10:445, 2003.

502. Ruiz-Arguelles GJ, Apreza-Molina MG, Aleman-Hoey DD, et al: Outpatient supportive therapy after induction to remission therapy in adult acute myelogenous leukaemia (AML) is feasible: A multicentre study. *Eur J Haematol* 54:18, 1995.

503. Clavio M, Quintino S, Masoudi B, et al: Cost of de novo acute myeloid leukemia induction therapy in adults: Analysis of EORTC-GIEMEMA AML10 and FLANG regimens. *J Exp Clin Cancer Res* 20:165, 2001.

504. Schiffer CA: Hematopoietic growth factors and the future of therapeutic research in acute myeloid leukemia. *N Engl J Med* 349:727, 2003.

505. Rowe J, Anderson JW, Mazza JJ, et al: A randomized placebo-controlled phase III study of granulocyte-macrophage colony-stimulating factor in adult patients (>55 to 70 years of age) with acute myelogenous leukemia: A study of the Eastern Cooperative Oncology Group (E1490). *Blood* 86:457, 1995.

506. Hoelzer D, Seipelt G: Granulocyte colony-stimulating factor and granulocyte-macrophage colony-stimulating factor in the treatment of myeloid leukemia. *Curr Opin Hematol* 2:196, 1995.

507. Beutler E: Platelet transfusions: The 20,000/μl trigger. *Blood* 81:1441, 1993.

508. Dumont LJ, Luka J, VandenBroeke T, et al: The effect of leukocyte-reduction method on the amount of human cytomegalovirus in blood products. A comparison of apheresis and filtration methods. *Blood* 97:3640, 2001.

509. Schiffer CA: Granulocyte transfusion therapy. *Curr Opin Hematol* 6:3, 1999.

510. Cullis JO, Duncombe AS, Dudley JM, et al: Acute leukaemia in Jehovah's Witnesses. *Br J Haematol* 100:664, 1998.

511. Castagnola C, Nozza A, Corso A, Bernasconi C: The value of combination therapy in adult acute myeloid leukemia with central nervous system involvement. *Haematologia* 82:577, 1997.

512. Hatano Y, Miura I, Horiuchi T, et al: Cerebellar myeloblastoma formation in CD7-positive, neural cell adhesion molecule (CD56)-positive acute myelogenous leukemia (M1). *Ann Hematol* 75:125, 1997.

513. Vavricka SR, Walter RB, Irani S, et al: Safety of lumbar puncture for adults with acute leukemia and restrictive prophylactic platelet transfusion. *Ann Hematol* 82:570, 2003.

514. Zittoun RA, Madelli F, Willemze R, et al: Autologous or allogeneic bone marrow transplantation compared with intensive chemotherapy in acute myelogenous leukemia. European Organization for Research and Treatment of Cancer (EORTC) and the Gruppo Italiano Malattie Ematologiche Maligne dell-Adulto (GIMEMA) Leukemia Cooperative Groups. *N Engl J Med* 332:217, 1995.

515. Harousseau JL, Cahn JY, Pignon B, et al: Comparison of autologous bone marrow transplantation and intensive chemotherapy as postremission therapy in adult acute myeloid leukemia. The Group Ouest Est Leucemies Aigues Myeloblastiques (GOELAM). *Blood* 90:2978, 1997.

516. Cassileth PA, Harrington DP, Appelbaum FR, et al: Chemotherapy compared with autologous or allogeneic bone marrow transplantation in the management of acute myeloid leukemia in first remission. *N Engl J Med* 339:1649, 1998.

517. Tsimberidou AM, Stavroyinni N, Viniou N, et al: Comparison of allogeneic stem cell transplantation, high-dose cytarabine, and autologous peripheral stem cell transplantation as postremission treatment in patients with de novo acute myelogenous leukemia. *Cancer* 97:1721, 2003.

518. Suciu S, Mandelli F, De Witte T, et al: Allogeneic compared with autologous stem cell transplantation in the treatment of patients younger than 46 years with acute myeloid leukemia (AML) in first complete remission (CR1): An intention-to-treat analysis of the EORTC/GIMEMAAML-10 trial. *Blood* 102:1232, 2003.

519. Gale RP, Buchner T, Zhang MF, et al: HLA-identical sibling bone marrow transplants vs chemotherapy for acute myelogenous leukemia in first remission. *Leukemia* 10:1687, 1996.

520. Zittoun R, Suciu S, Watson M, et al: Quality of life in patients with acute myelogenous leukemia in prolonged first complete remission after bone marrow transplantation (allogeneic or autologous) or chemotherapy: A cross-sectional study of the EORTC-GIMEMA AML 8A trial. *Bone Marrow Transplant* 20:307, 1997.

521. Shpilberg O, Haddad N, Sofer O, et al: Postremission therapy with two different dose regimens of cytarabine in adults with acute myelogenous leukemia. *Leuk Res* 19:893, 1995.

522. Heil G, Mitrou PS, Hoeizer D, et al: High-dose cytosine arabinoside and daunorubicin postremission therapy in adults with de novo acute myeloid leukemia. Long-term follow-up of a prospective multicenter trial. *Ann Hematol* 71:219, 1995.

523. Rowe JM: Uncertainties in the standard care of acute myelogenous leukemia. *Leukemia* 15:677, 2001.

524. Cahn JY, Labopin M, Sierra J, et al. No impact of high-dose cytarabine on the outcome of patients transplanted for acute myeloblastic leukemia in first remission. Acute Leukemia Working Party of the European Group for Blood and Marrow Transplantation (EBMT). *Br J Haematol* 110:308, 2000.

525. Byrd JC, Dodge RK, Carroll A, et al: Patients with t(8;21) (q22) and acute myeloid leukemia have superior failure-free and overall survival when repetitive cycles of high-dose cytarabine are administered. *J Clin Oncol* 17:3767, 1999.

526. Tsimberidou AM, Estey E, Cortes JE, et al: Mylotarg, fludarabine, cytarabine (ara-C), and cyclosporine (MFAC) regimen as post-remission therapy in acute myelogenous leukemia. *Cancer Chemother Pharmacol* 52:449, 2003.

527. Schiller G: Dose-intensive treatment of acute myelogenous leukemia: Improved survival [letter, comment]. *J Clin Oncol* 13:1828, 1995.

528. Mayer RJ, Davis RB, Schiffer CA, et al: Intensive postremission chemotherapy in adults with acute myeloid leukemia. Cancer and Leukemia Group B. *N Engl J Med* 331:896, 1994.

529. Elonen E, Almqvist A, Hanninen A, et al: Comparison between four and eight cycles of intensive chemotherapy in adult acute myeloid leukemia: A randomized trial of the Finnish Leukemia Group. *Leukemia* 12:1041, 1998.

530. Graves T, Hooks MA: Drug-induced toxicities associated with high-dose cytosine arabinoside infusions. *Pharmacotherapy* 9:23, 1989.

531. Smith GA, Damon LE, Rugo HS, et al: High-dose cytarabine dose modification reduces the incidence of neurotoxicity in patients with renal insufficiency. *J Clin Oncol* 15:833, 1997.

532. Hewlett J, Kopecky KJ, Head D, et al: A prospective evaluation of the roles of allogeneic marrow transplantation and low-dose monthly maintenance chemotherapy in the treatment of adult acute myelogenous leukemia (AML): A Southwest Oncology Group study. *Leukemia* 9:562, 1995.

533. Choudhury A, Toubert A, Sutaria S, et al: Human leukemia-derived dendritic cells: Ex vivo development of specific antileukemic cytotoxicity. *Crit Rev Immunol* 18:121, 1998.

534. Choudhury BA, Liang JC, Thomas EK, et al: Dendritic cells derived in vitro from acute myelogenous leukemia cells stimulate autologous, antileukemic T-cell responses. *Blood* 93:780, 1999.

535. Gorin NC, Aegerter P, Auvert B, et al: Autologous bone marrow transplantation for acute myelocytic leukemia in first remission: A European survey of the role of marrow purging. *Blood* 75:1606, 1990.

536. Bruserud O, Ernst P: High dose ara-C combined with autologous peripheral blood stem cell transplantation in the treatment of acute myelogenous leukemia: The question is still not answered. *Stem Cells* 18:459, 2000.

537. Gorin NC: Autologous stem cell transplantation in acute myelocytic leukemia. *Blood* 92:1073, 1998.

538. Schiller G, Lee M, Miller T, et al: Transplantation of autologous peripheral blood progenitor cells procured after high-dose cytarabine-based consolidation chemotherapy for adults with acute myelogenous leukemia in first remission. *Leukemia* 11:1533, 1997.

539. Gondo H, Harada M, Miyamoto T, et al: Autologous peripheral blood stem cell transplantation for acute myelogenous leukemia. *Bone Marrow Transplant* 20:821, 1997.

540. Meloni G, Vignetti M, Avvisati G, et al: BAVC regimen and autograft for acute myelogenous leukemia in second complete remission. *Bone Marrow Transplant* 18:693, 1996.

541. Kusnierz-Glaz CR, Schlegel PG, Wong RM, et al: Influence of age on the outcome of 500 autologous bone marrow transplant procedures for hematologic malignancies. *J Clin Oncol* 15:18, 1997.

542. Mehta J, Powles R, Singhal S, et al: Autologous bone marrow transplantation for acute myeloid leukemia in first remission: Identification of modifiable prognostic factors. *Bone Marrow Transplant* 16:499, 1995.

543. Miller CB, Rowlings PA, Zhang MJ, et al: The effect of graft purging with 4-hydroperoxycyclophosphamie in autologous bone marrow transplantation or acute myelogenous leukemia. *Exp Hematol* 29:1336, 2001.

544. Abdallah A, Egerer G, Weberf-Nordt RM, et al: Long-term outcome in acute myelogenous leukemia autografted with mafosfamide-purged

marrow in a single institution: Adverse events and incidence of secondary myelodysplasia. *Bone Marrow Transplant* 30:15, 2002.

545. Bishop MR, Jackson JD, Tarantolo SR, et al: Ex vivo treatment of bone marrow with phosphorothioate oligonucleotide OL(l) p53 for autologous transplantation in acute myelogenous leukemia and myelodysplastic syndrome. *J Hematother* 6:441, 1997.

546. To LB, Haylock DN, Thorp D, et al: The optimization of collection of peripheral blood stem cells for autotransplantation in acute myeloid leukaemia. *Bone Marrow Transplant* 4:41, 1989.

547. Hogge DE, Ailles LE, Gerhard B: Cytokine responsiveness of primitive progenitors in acute myelogenous leukemia. *Leukemia* 11:2220, 1997.

548. Carella AM, Dejana A, Lerma E, et al: In vivo mobilization of karyotypically normal peripheral blood progenitor cells in high-risk MDS, secondary or therapy-related acute myelogenous leukaemia. *Br J Haematol* 95:127, 1996.

549. Mehta J, Powles R, Horton C et al: Factors affecting engraftment and hematopoietic recovery after unpurged autografting in acute leukemia. *Bone Marrow Transplant* 18:319, 1996.

550. Collison EA, Lashkari A, Malone R, et al: Long-term outcome of autologous transplantation of peripheral blood progenitor cells as postremission management of adult acute myelogenous leukemia in first complete remission. *Leukemia* 17:2183, 2003.

551. Voog E, Le QH, Philip I, et al: Autologous transplantation in acute myeloid leukemia: Peripheral blood stem cell harvest after mobilization in steady state by granulocyte colony-stimulating factor alone. *Ann Hematol* 80:584, 2001.

552. Gratwohl S, Bslfomero H, Honisberger B, et al: Current trends in hematopoietic stem cell transplantation in Europe. *Blood* 100:2374, 2002.

553. Popplewell LL, Forman SJ: Is there an upper age limit for bone marrow transplantation? *Bone Marrow Transplant* 29:277, 2002.

554. Lemoli RM, Bandini G, Leopardi G, et al: Allogeneic peripheral blood stem cell transplantation in patients with early-phase hematologic malignancy: A retrospective comparison of short-term outcome with bone marrow transplantation. *Haematologica* 83:48, 1998.

555. Gorin NC, Labopin M, Rocha V, et al: Marrow versus peripheral blood for geno-identical allogeneic stem cell transplantation in acute myelocytic leukemia: Influence of dose and stem cell source shows better outcome with rich marrow. *Blood* 102:3043, 2003.

556. Champlin RE, Schmitz N, Horowitz MM, et al: Blood stem cells compared with bone marrow as a source of hematopoietic cells for allogeneic transplantation. IBMTR Histocompatibility and Stem Cell Sources Working Committee and the European Group for Blood and Marrow Transplantation (EBMT). *Blood* 95:3702, 2000.

557. Morton J, Hutchins C, Durrant S: Granulocyte-colony-stimulating factor (G-CSF)-primed allogeneic bone marrow: Significantly less graft-versus-host disease and comparable engraftment to G-CSF-mobilized peripheral blood stem cells. *Blood* 98:3186, 2001.

558. Applebaum FR: Is there a best transplant conditioning regimen for acute myeloid leukemia? *Leukemia* 14:497, 2000.

559. Litzow MR, Perez WS, Klein JP, et al: Comparison of outcome following allogeneic bone marrow transplantation with cyclophosphamide-total body irradiation versus busulphan-cyclophosphamide conditioning regimens for acute myelogeneous leukaemia in first remission. *Br J Haematol* 119:1115, 2002.

560. Tallman MS, Rowlings PA, Milone G, et al: Effect of postremission chemotherapy before human leukocyte antigen-identical sibling transplantation for acute myelogenous leukemia in first complete remission. *Blood* 96:1254, 2000.

561. Soiffer RJ, Fairclough D, Robertson M, et al: CD6-depleted allogeneic bone marrow transplantation for acute leukemia in first complete remission. *Blood* 89:3039, 1997.

562. Messner HA: Long-term outcome of allogeneic transplants in acute myeloid leukemia. *Leukemia* 16:751, 2002.

563. Mehta J, Powles R, Treleaven J, et al: Long-term follow-up of patients undergoing allogeneic bone marrow transplantation for acute myeloid leukemia in first complete remission after cyclophosphamide-total body irradiation and cyclosporine. *Bone Marrow Transplant* 18:741, 1996.

564. Robin M, Guardiola P, Dombret H, et al: Allogeneic bone marrow transplantation for acute myeloblastic leukaemic in remission: Risk factors for long-term morbidity and mortality. *Bone Marrow Transplant* 31:877, 2003.

565. Greinex HT, Nachbaur D, Krieger O, et al: Factors affecting long-term outcome after allogeneic haematopoietic stem cell transplantation for acute myelogenous leukaemia: A retrospective study of 172 adult patients reported to the Austrian Stem Cell Transplant Registry. *Br J Haematol* 117:914, 2002.

566. Matthews DC, Appelbaum FR, Eary JF, et al: Development of a marrow transplant regimen for acute leukemia using targeted hematopoietic irradiation delivered by ^{131}I-labeled anti-CD45 antibody, combined with cyclophosphamide and total body irradiation. *Blood* 85:1122, 1995.

567. Petersdorf EW, Gooley TA, Anasefti C, et al: Optimizing outcome after unrelated marrow transplantation by comprehensive matching of HLA class I and 11 alleles in the donor and recipient. *Blood* 92:3515, 1998.

568. Sasazuki T, Juji T, Morishima Y, et al. Effect of matching of class I HLA alleles on clinical outcome after transplantation of hematopoietic stem cells from an unrelated donor. Japan Marrow Donor Program. *N Eng J Med* 339:1177, 1998.

569. Aversa F, Tabilio A, Velardi A, et al: Treatment of high-risk acute leukemia with T-cell-depleted stem cells from related donors with one fully mismatched HLA haplotype. *N Engl J Med* 339:1186, 1998.

570. Ooi J, Iseki T, Takahashi S, et al: Unrelated cord blood transplantation for adult patients with de novo acute myeloid leukemia. *Blood* 103:489, 2004.

571. Michel G, Rocha V, Chevret S, et al: Unrelated cord blood transplantation for childhood acute myeloid leukemia: A Eurocord Group Analysis. *Blood* 102:4290, 2003.

572. Champlin R, Khouri I, Kornblau S, et. al. Allogeneic hematopoietic transplantation as adoptive immunotherapy. Induction of graft-versus-malignancy as primary therapy. *Hematol Oncol Clin North Am* 13:1041, 1999.

573. Wong R, Giralt SG, Martin T, et al: Reduced-intensity conditioning for unrelated donor hematopoietic stem cell transplantation as treatment for myeloid malignancies in patients older than 55 years. *Blood* 102:3052, 2003.

574. Storb R: Mixed allogeneic chimerism and graft-versus-leukemia effects in acute myeloid leukemia. *Leukemia* 16:753, 2002.

575. McSweeney PA, Hiederwieser D, Shizuru JA, et al: Hematopoietic cell transplantation in older patients with hematologic malignancies: Replacing high-dose cytotoxic therapy with graft-versus-tumor effects. *Blood* 97:3390, 2001.

576. Corradini P, Tarella C, Olivieri A, et al: Reduced-intensity conditioning followed by allografting of hematopoietic cells can produce clinical and molecular remissions in patients with poor-risk hematologic malignancies. *Blood* 99:75, 2002.

577. Schlenk RF, Hartmann F, Hensel M, et al: Less intense conditioning with fludarabine, cyclophosphamide, idarubicin and etoposide (FCIE) followed by allogeneic unselected peripheral blood stem cell transplantation in elderly patients with leukemia. *Leukemia* 16:581, 2002.

578. Massenkeil G, Nagy M, Lawang M, et al: Reduced intensity conditioning and prophylactic DLI can cure patients with high-risk acute leukaemia if complete donor chimerism can be achieved. *Bone Marrow Transplant* 31:339, 2003.

579. Giralt S, Anagnastopoulos A, Shahjahanan M, Champlin R: Nonablative stem cell transplantation for older patients with acute leukemias and myelodysplastic syndromes. *Semin Hematol* 39:57, 2002.

580. Maris MB, Niederwieser D, Sandmaier BM, et al: HLA-matched unre-

lated donor hematopoietic cell transplantation after nonmyeloablative conditioning for patients with hematologic malignancies. *Blood* 102: 2021, 2003.

581. Chakraverly R, Peggs K, Chopra R, et al: Limiting transplantation-related mortality following unrelated donor stem cell transplantation by using a nonmyeloablative conditioning regimen. *Blood* 99:1071, 2002.

582. Gale RP, Horowitz MM, Rees JK, et al: Chemotherapy versus transplants for acute myelogenous leukemia in second remission. *Leukemia* 10:13, 1996.

583. Michel G, Boulad F, Small TN, et al: Risk of extramedullary relapse following allogeneic bone marrow transplantation for acute myelogenous leukemia with leukemia cutis. *Bone Marrow Transplant* 20:107, 1997.

584. Blau IW, Basara N, Bischoff M, et al: Second allogeneic hematopoietic stem cell transplantation as treatment for leukemia relapsing following a first transplant. *Bone Marrow Transplant* 25:41, 2000.

585. Shlomchik WD, Emerson SG: The immunobiology of T cell therapies for leukemias. *Acta Haematol* 96:189, 1996.

586. Porter DL, Roth MS, Lee SJ, et al: Adoptive immunotherapy with donor mononuclear cell infusions to treat relapse of acute leukemia or myelodysplasia after allogeneic bone marrow transplantation. *Bone Marrow Transplant* 18:975, 1996.

587. Porter DL: Donor leukocyte infusions in acute myelogenous leukemia. *Leukemia* 17:1035, 2003.

588. Greinix NT: DLI or second transplant. *Ann Hematol* 81:S34, 2002.

589. Van Rhee F, Kolb HJ: Donor leukocyte transfusions for leukemic relapse. *Curr Opin Hematol* 2:423, 1995.

590. Berthou C, Leglise MC, Herry A, et al: Extramedullary relapse after favorable molecular response to donor leukocyte infusions for recurring acute leukemia. *Leukemia* 12:1676, 1998.

591. Carlens S, Remberger M, Aschan J, Ringden O: The role of disease stage in the response to donor lymphocyte infusions as treatment for leukemic relapse. *Biol Blood Marrow Transplant* 7:31, 2001.

592. Keil F, Prinz E, Kalhs P, et al: Treatment of leukemic relapse after allogeneic stem cell transplantation with cytotoreductive chemotherapy and/or second transplants. *Leukemia* 15:355, 2001.

593. Porter DL, Collins RH, Hardy C, et al: Treatment of relapsed leukemia after unrelated donor marrow transplantation with unrelated donor leukocyte infusions. *Blood* 95:1214, 2000.

594. Bishop MR, Tarantolo SR, Pavletic ZS, et al: Filgrastim as an alternative to donor leukocyte infusion for relapse after allogeneic stem-cell transplantation *J Clin Oncol* 18:2269, 2000.

595. Trenschel R, Bernier M, Stryckmans P, et al: Complete remission following donor PBSC after low-dose cytarabine chemotherapy for early relapse of acute myelogenous leukemia after allogeneic stem cell transplantation. *Bone Marrow Transplant* 19:381, 1997.

596. Goodman M, Cabral L, Cassileth P: Interleukin-2 and leukemia. *Leukemia* 12:1671, 1998.

597. Falkenburg JH, Smit WM, Willemze R: Cytotoxic T-lymphocyte (CTL) responses against acute or chronic myeloid leukemia. *Immunol Rev* 157:223, 1997.

598. Dunussi-Joannopoulos K, Krenger W, Weinstein HJ, et al: CD8+ T cells activated during the course of murine acute myelogenous leukemia elicit therapeutic responses to late B7 vaccines after cytoreductive treatment. *Blood* 89:2915, 1997.

599. Boyd CN, Ramberg RC, Thomas ED: The incidence of recurrence of leukemia in donor cells after allogeneic bone marrow transplantation. *Leuk Res* 6:833, 1982.

600. Cooley LD, Sears DA, Udden MN, et al: Donor cell leukemia: Report of a case occurring 11 years after allogeneic bone marrow transplantation and review of the literature. *Am J Hematol* 63:46, 2000.

601. Minden MD, Messner HA, Blech A: Origin of leukemic relapse after bone marrow transplantation detected by restriction fragment length polymorphism. *J Clin Invest* 75:91, 1985.

602. Schiller GJ: Treatment of resistant disease. *Leukemia* 12(suppl I):S20, 1998.

603. Estey E: Treatment of refractory AML. *Leukemia* 10:932, 1996.

604. Estey E, Kornblau S, Pierce S, et al: A stratification system for evaluating and selecting therapies in patients with relapsed or primary refractory acute myelogenous leukemia. *Blood* 88:756, 1996.

605. Estey E, Thall P, David C: Design and analysis of trials of salvage therapy in acute myelogenous leukemia. *Cancer Chemother Pharmacol* 40:S9, 1997.

606. Kornblau SM, Estry E, Madden T, et al: Phase I study of mitoxantrone plus etopside with multidrug blockade by SDZ PSC-833 in relapsed or refractory acute myelogenous leukemia. *J Clin Oncol* 15:1796, 1997.

607. Appostolidou E, Cortes J, Tsimberidou A, et al: Pilot study of gemtuzumab ozogamicin, liposomal daunorubicin, cytarabine and cyclosporine regimen in patients with refractory acute myelogenous leukemia. *Leuk Res* 27:887, 2003.

608. Stolser B, Knobl P, Fonatsch C, et al: Prognosis of patients with second relapse of acute myeloid leukemia. *Leukemia* 14:2059, 2000.

609. Lee S, Tallman MS, Oken MM, et al: Duration of second complete remission compared with first complete remission in patients with acute myeloid leukemia. *Leukemia* 14:1345, 2000.

610. Kern W, Schoch C, Haferlach T, et al: Multivariate analysis of prognostic factors in patients with refractory and relapsed acute myeloid leukemia undergoing sequential high-dose cytosine arabinoside and mitoxantrone (S-HAM) salvage therapy: Relevance of cytogenetic abnormalities. *Leukemia* 14:226, 2000.

611. Estey EH: Treatment of relapsed and refractory acute myelogenous leukemia. *Leukemia* 14:476, 2000.

612. Leopold LH, Willemze R: The treatment of acute myeloid leukemia in first relapse. A comprehensive review of the literature. *Leuk Lymphoma* 43:1715, 2002.

613. Advani R, Saba HI, Tallman MS, et al: Treatment of refractory and relapsed acute myelogenous leukemia with combination chemotherapy plus the multidrug resistance modulator PSC 833 (Valspodar). *Blood* 93:787, 1999.

614. Estey EH, Kantarjian HM, O'Brien, et al: High remission rate, short remission duration in patients with refractory anemia with excess blasts (RAEB) in transformation (RAEB-t) given acute myelogenous leukemia (AML)-type chemotherapy in combination with granulocyte-CSF (G-CSF). *Cytokines Mol Ther* 1:21, 1995.

615. Van Den Neste E, Martiat P, Mineur P, et al: 2-Chlorodeoxyadenosine with or without daunorubicin in relapsed or refractory acute myeloid leukemia. *Ann Hematol* 76:19, 1998.

616. Seiter K, Feldman EJ, Halicka HD, et al: Phase I clinical and laboratory evaluation of topotecan and cytarabine in patients with acute leukemia. *J Clin Oncol* 15:44, 1997.

617. Larrea L, Martinez JA, Sanz GF, et al: Carboplatin plus cytarabine in the treatment of high-risk acute myeloblastic leukemia. *Leukemia* 13: 161, 1999.

618. Kornblau SM, Kantarjian H, O'Brien S, et al: CEAC-cyclophosphamide, etoposide, carboplatinin and cytosine arabinoside: A new salvage regimen for relapsed or refractory acute myelogenous leukemia. *Leuk Lymphoma* 28:371, 1998.

619. Roboz GJ, Knovich MA, Bayer RL, et al: Efficacy and safety of gemtuzumab ozogamicin in patients with poor-prognosis acute myeloid leukemia. *Leuk Lymphoma* 43:1951, 2002.

620. Cortes J, Estey E, O'Brien S, et al: High-dose lipososmal daunorubicin and high-dose cytarabine combination in patients with refractory or relapsed acute myelogenous leukemia. *Cancer* 92:7, 2001.

621. Sternberg DW, Aird W, Neuberg D, et al: Treatment of patients with recurrent and primary refractory acute myelogenous leukemia using mixtoantrone and intermediate-dose cytarabine: A pharmacologically based regimen. *Cancer* 88:2037, 2000.

622. Belhabri A, Thomas X, Troncy J, et al: Continuous-infusion carboplatin in combination with idarubicin or mitoxantrone for high-risk acute myeloid leukemia: A randomised phase II study. *Leuk Lymphoma* 36: 45, 1999.

623. Lee, ST, Jang JH, Suh HC, et al: Idarubicin, cytarabine, and topotecan in patients with refractory or relapsed acute myelogenous leukemia and high-risk myelodysplastic syndrome. *Am J Hematol* 68:237, 2001.

624. Pastore D, Specchia G, Carluccio P, et al: FLAG-IDA in the treatment of refractory/relapsed acute myeloid leukemia: Single-center experience. *Ann Hematol* 82:231, 2003.

625. Wrzesien-Kus A, Robak T, Lech-Maranda E, et al: A multicenter, open, non-comparative, phase II study of the combination of cladribine (2-chlorodeoxyadenosine), cytarabine, and G-CSF as induction therapy in refractory acute myeloid leukemia: A report of the Polish Adult Leukemia Group (PALG). *Eur J Haematol* 71:155, 2003.

626. Revesz D, Chelghoum Y, Le QH, et al: Salvage by timed sequential chemotherapy in primary resistant acute myeloid leukemia: Analysis of prognostic factors. *Ann Hematol* 82:684, 2003.

627. Cortes J, Tsimberidou AM, Alvarez R, et al: Mylotarg combined with topotecan and cytarabine in patients with refractory acute myelogenous leukemia. *Cancer Chemother Pharmacol* 50:497, 2002.

628. Alvarado Y, Tsimberidou A, Kantarjian H, et al: Pilot study of Mylotarg, idarubicin and cytarabine combination regimen in patients with primary resistant or relapsed acute myeloid leukemia. *Cancer Chemother Pharmacol* 51:87, 2003.

629. Rizzieri DA, Ibom VK, Moore JO, et al: Phase I evaluation of prolonged-infusion gemcitabine with fludarabine for relapsed or refractory acute myelogenous leukemia. *Clin Cancer Res* 9:663, 2003.

630. Greinix HT, Keil F, Brugger SA, et al: Long-term leukemia-free survival after allogeneic marrow transplantation in patients with acute myelogenous leukemia. *Ann Hematol* 72:53, 1996.

631. Appelbaum FR: Hematopoietic cell transplantation beyond first remission. *Leukemia* 16:157, 2002.

632. Singhal S, Powles R, Henslee-Downey PJ, et al: Allogeneic transplantation from HLA-matched sibling or partially HLA-missmatched related donors for primary refractory acute leukemia. *Bone Marrow Transplant* 29:291, 2002.

633. Biggs JC, Horowitz MM, Gale RP, et al: Bone marrow transplants may cure patients with acute leukemia never achieving remission with chemotherapy. *Blood* 80:1090, 1992.

634. Faderl S, Estrov Z, Kantarjian HM, et al: WP744, a novel anthracycline with enhanced proapoptotic and antileukemic activity. *Anticancer Res* 21:3777, 2001.

635. Giles FJ, Faderl S, Thomas DA, et al: Randomized phase I/II study of troxacitabine combined with cytarabine, idarubicin, or topotecan in patients with refractory myeloid leukemias. *J Clin Oncol* 21:1050, 2003.

636. Bouufard DY, Jolivet J, Leblond L, et al: Complementary antineoplastic activity of the cytosine and nucleoside analogues troxacitabine (Troxatyl) and cytarabine in human leukemia cells. *Cancer Chemother Pharmacol* 52:497, 2003.

637. Seiter K, Liu D, Loughran T, et al: Phase I study of temozolomide in relapsed/refractory acute leukemia. *J Clin Oncol* 20:3249, 2002.

638. Kantarjian H, Gandhi V, Cortes J, et al: Phase 2 clinical and pharmacologic study of clofarabine in patients with refractory or relapsed acute leukemia. *Blood* 102:2379, 2003.

639. Petti MC, Tafuri A, Latagliata R, et al: High-dose hydroxyurea in the treatment of poor-risk myeloid leukemia. *Ann Hematol* 82:476, 2003.

640. Rush LJ, Dai Z, Smiraglia DJ, et al: Novel methylation targets in de novo acute myeloid leukemia with prevalence of chromosome 11 loci. *Blood* 97:3226, 2001.

641. Lubbert M, Wijermans PW, Jones PA, Hellstrom-Lindberg E: Multiple hypermethylated genes are potential in vivo targets of demethylating agents [response]. *Blood* 101:4645, 2003.

642. Kantarjian HM, O'Brien SM, Estey E, et al: Decitabine studies in chronic and acute myelogenous leukemia. *Leukemia* 11(suppl 1):S35, 1997.

643. Schwartsmann G, Fernandes MS, Schaan MD, et al: Decitabine (5-Aza-2'-deoxycytidine; DAC) plus daunorubicin as a first line treatment in patients with acute myeloid leukemia: Preliminary observations. *Leukemia* 11(suppl 1):S28, 1997.

644. Ferrara EF, Fazi F, Bianchini A, et al: Histone deacetylase-targeted treatment restores retinoic acid signaling and differentiation in acute myeloid leukemia. *Cancer Res* 61:2, 2001.

645. Klisovic MI, Maghraby EA, Parthun MR, et al: Depsipeptide (FR 901228) promotes histone acetylation, gene transcription, apoptosis and its activity is enhanced by DNA methyltransferase inhibitors in AML1/ETO-positive leukemic cells. *Leukemia* 17:350, 2003.

646. Burbage C, Tagge EP, Harris B, et al: Ricin fusion toxin targeted to the human granulocyte-macrophage colony stimulating factor receptor is selectively toxic to acute myeloid leukemia cells. *Leuk Res* 21:681, 1997.

647. Hogge DE, Willman CL, Kreitman RJ, et al: Malignant progenitors from patients with acute myelogenous leukemia are sensitive to a diphtheria toxin-granulocyte-macrophage colony-stimulating factor fusion protein. *Blood* 92:589, 1998.

648. Gandhi V, Estey E, Du M, et al: Modulation of the cellular metabolism of cytarabine and fludarabine by granulocyte-colony-stimulating factor during therapy of acute myelogenous leukemia. *Clin Cancer Res* 1: 169, 1995.

649. Alexander RL, Ramage J, Jucera GL, et al: High affinity interleukin-3 receptor expression on blasts from patients with acute myelogenous leukemia correlates with cytotoxicity of a diphtheria toxin/IL-3 fusion protein. *Leuk Res* 25:875, 2001.

650. Frankel AE, Beran M, Hogge DE, et al: Malignant progenitors from patients with CD87+ acute myelogenous leukemia are sensitive to a diphtheria toxin-urokinase fusion protein. *Exp Hematol* 30:1316, 2002.

651. Larson RA: Current use and future development of gemtuzumab ozogamicin. *Semin Hematol* 38:24, 2001.

652. McGavin JK, Spencer CM: Gemtuzumab ozogamicin. *Drugs* 61:1317, 2001.

653. Van DerVelden VH, Te Marvelde JG, Hoogeveen PG, et al: Targeting of the CD33-calicheamicin immunoconjugate Mylotarg (CMA-676) in acute myeloid leukemia: In vivo and in vitro saturation and internalization by leukemic and normal myeloid cells. *Blood* 97:3197, 2001.

654. Larson RA, Boogaerts M, Estey E, et al: Antibody-targeted chemotherapy of older patients with acute myeloid leukemia in first relapse using Mylotarg (gemtuzumab ozogamicin). *Leukemia* 16:1627, 2002.

655. Bross PF, Beitz J, Chen G, et al: Approval summary: Gemtuzumab ozogamicin in relapsed acute myeloid leukemia. *Clin Cancer Res* 8: 300, 2002.

656. Berger MS, Leopold LH, Dowell JA, et al: Licensure of gemtuzumab ozogamicin for the treatment of selected patients 60 years of age or older with acute myeloid leukemia in first relapse. *Invest New Drugs* 20:395, 2002.

657. Sievers EL, Linenberger M: Mylotarg: Antibody-targeted chemotherapy comes of age. *Curr Opin Oncol* 13:522, 2001.

658. Giles FJ, Cortes JE, Halliburton TA, et al: Intravenous corticosteroids to reduce gemtuzumab ozogamicin infusion reactions. *Ann Pharmacother* 37:1182, 2003.

659. Lang K, Menzin J, Earle CC, Mallick R: Outcomes in patients treated with gemtuzumab ozogamicin for relapsed acute myelogenous leukemia. *Am J Health Syst Pharm* 59:941, 2002.

660. Leopold LH, Berger MS, Cheng S-C, et al: Comparative efficacy and safety of Gemtuzumab ozogamicin monotherapy and high-dose cytarabine combination therapy in patients with acute myeloid leukemia in first relapse. *Clin Adv Hematol Oncol* 1:220, 2003.

661. Wadleigh M, Richardson PG, Zahrieh D, et al: Prior gemtuzumab ozogamicin exposure significantly increases the risk of veno-occlusive disease in patients who undergo myeloablative allogeneic stem cell transplantation. *Blood* 102:1578, 2003.

662. Wadleigh M, Richardson PG, Zahrieh D, et al: Prior gemtuzumab ozogamicin exposure significantly increases the risk of veno-occlusive disease in patients who undergo myeloablative allogeneic stem cell transplantation. *Blood* 102:1578, 2003.

663. Jurcic JG: Antibody therapy for residual disease in acute myelogenous leukemia. *Crit Rev Oncol Hematol* 38:37, 2001.

664. Nemecek ER, Matthews DC: Antibody-based therapy of human leukemia. *Curr Opin Hematol* 9:316, 2002.

665. Weisberg E, Boulton C, Kelly LM, et al: Inhibition of mutant FLT3 receptors in leukemia cells by the small molecule tyrosine kinase inhibitor PKC412. *Cancer Cell* 1:433, 2002.

666. Kelly LM, Yu JC, Boulton CL, et al: CT53518, a novel selective FLT3 antagonist for the treatment of acute myelogenous leukemia (AML). *Cancer Cell* 1:421, 2002.

667. Levis M, Allebach J, Tse KF, et al: A FLT3-targeted tyrosine kinase inhibitor is cytotoxic to leukemia cells in vitro and in vivo. *Blood* 99:3885, 2002.

668. Spiekermann K, Dirschinger RJ, Schwab R, et al: The protein tyrosine kinase inhibitor SU5614 inhibits FLT3 and induces growth arrest and apoptosis in AML-derived cell lines expressing a constitutively activated FLT3. *Blood* 101:1494, 2003.

669. Zheng R, Friedman AD, Small D: Targeted inhibition of FLT3 overcomes the block to myeloid differentiation in 32Dc13 cells caused by expression of FLT3/ITD mutations. *Blood* 100:4154, 2002.

670. Stone RM, De Angelo DJ, Klimek V, et al: Patients with acute myeloid leukemia and an activating mutation in FLT3 respond to a small molecule FLT3 tyrosine kinase inhibitor. *Blood* 105:54, 2005.

671. Heinrich MC, Blanke CD, Druker BJ, Corless CL: Inhibition of KIT tyrosine kinase activity: A novel molecular approach to the treatment of KIT-positive malignancies. *J Clin Oncol* 20:1692, 2002.

672. Scappini B, Onida F, Kantarjian HM, et al: Effects of signal transduction inhibitor 571 in acute myelogenous leukemia cells. *Clin Cancer Res* 7:3884, 2001.

673. Kindler T, Breitenbuecher F, Marx A, et al: Sustained complete hematologic remission after administration of the tyrosine kinase inhibitor imatinib mesylate in a patient with refractory, secondary AML. *Blood* 101:2960, 2003.

674. Kindler T, Breitenbuecher F, Marx A, et al: Efficacy and safety of imatinib in adult patients with C-kit-positive acute myeloid leukemia. *Blood* 103:3644, 2004.

675. Tse K-F, Allebach J, Levis M, et al: Inhibition of the transforming activity of FLT3 internal tandem duplication mutants from AML patients by a tyrosine kinase inhibitor. *Leukemia* 16:2027, 2002.

676. Fiedler W, Mesters R, Tinnefeld H, et al: A phase 2 clinical study of SU5416 in patients with refractory acute myeloid leukemia. *Blood* 102:2763, 2003.

677. Milella M, Kornblau SM, Estrov Z, et al: Therapeutic targeting of the MEK/MAPK signal transduction module in acute myeloid leukemia. *J Clin Invest* 108:851, 2001.

678. Shangary S, Johnson DE: Recent advances in the development of anticancer agents targeting cell death inhibitors in the Bcl-2 protein family. *Leukemia* 17:1470, 2003.

679. Marucci G, Byrd JC, Dai G, et al: Phase 1 and pharmacodynamic studies of G3139, a Bcl-2 antisense oligonucleotide, in combination with chemotherapy in refractory or relapsed acute leukemia. *Blood* 101:425, 2003.

680. Konopleva M, Tsao T, Ruvolo P, et al: Novel triterpenoid CDDO-Me is a potent inducer of apoptosis and differentiation in acute myelogenous leukemia. *Blood* 99:326, 2002.

681. Suh WS, Kim YS, Schimmer AD, et al: Synthetic triterpenoids activate a pathway for apoptosis in AML cells involving downregulation of FLIP and sensitization of TRAIL. *Leukemia* 17:2122, 2003.

682. Rosato RR, Almenara JA, Cartree L, et al: The cyclin-dependent kinase inhibitor flavopiridol disrupts sodium butyrate-induced p21WAF1/CIP1 expression and maturation while reciprocally potentiating apoptosis in human leukemia cells. *Mol Cancer Ther* 1:253, 2002.

683. Karp JE, Ross DD, Yang W, et al: Timed sequential therapy of acute leukemia with flavopiridol: In vitro model for a phase I clinical trial. *Clin Cancer Res* 9:307, 2003.

684. Dai Y, Rahmani M, Grant S: Proteasome inhibitors potentiate leukemic cell apoptosis induced by the cyclin-dependent kinase inhibitor flavopiridol through a SAPK/JNK- and NF-kappaB-dependent process. *Oncogene* 22:7108, 2003.

685. Le DT, Shannon KM: Ras processing as a therapeutic target in hematologic malignancies. *Curr Opin Hematol* 9:308, 2002.

686. Morgan MA, Ganser A, Reuter CWM: Therapeutic efficacy of prenylation inhibitors in the treatment of myeloid leukemia. *Leukemia* 17:1482, 2003.

687. Kurzrock R, Cortes J, Kantarjian H: Clinical development of farnesyltransferase inhibitors in leukemias and myelodysplastic syndrome. *Semin Hematol* 39:20, 2002.

688. Brunner TB, Hahn SM, Gupta AK, et al: Farnesyltransferase inhibitors: An overview of the results of preclinical and clinical investigations. *Cancer Res* 63:5656, 2003.

689. Karp JE, Lancet JE, Kaufmann SH, et al: Clinical and biologic activity of the farnesyltransferase inhibitor R115777 in adults with refractory and relapsed acute leukemias: A phase I clinical-laboratory correlative trial. *Blood* 97:3361, 2001.

690. Morgan MA, Wegner J, Aydilek E, et al: Synergistic cytotoxic effects in myeloid leukemia cells upon cotreatment with farnesyltransferase and geranylgeranyl transferase-1 inhibitors. *Leukemia* 17:1508, 2003.

691. Minden MD, Dimitroulakos J, Nohynek D, Penn LZ: Lovastatin induced control of blast cell growth in an elderly patient with acute myeloblastic leukemia. *Leuk Lymphoma* 40:659, 2001.

692. Lishner M, Bar-Sef A, Elis A, Fabian I: Effect of simvastatin alone and in combination with cytosine arabinoside on the proliferation of myeloid leukemia cell lines. *J Invest Med* 49:319, 2001.

693. Li HY, Appelbaum FR, Willman CL, et al: Cholesterol-modulating agents kill acute myeloid leukemia cells and sensitize them to therapeutics by blocking adaptive cholesterol responses. *Blood* 101:3628, 2003.

694. Gianni M, Li Calzi M, Terao M, et al: AM580, a stable benzoic derivative of retinoic acid, has powerful and selective cyto-differentiating effects on acute promyelocytic leukemia cells. *Blood* 87:1520, 1996.

695. Munker R, Kobayashi T, Eistner E, et al: A new series of vitamin D analogs is highly active for clonal inhibition, differentiation, and induction of WAF1 in myeloid leukemia. *Blood* 88:2201, 1996.

696. Munker R, Zhang W, Elstner E, Koeffler HP: Vitamin D analogs, leukemia and WAF1. *Leuk Lymphoma* 31:279, 1998.

697. Morosetti R, Grignani F, Liberatore C, et al: Infrequent alterations of the RAR alpha gene in acute myelogenous leukemias, retinoic acid–resistant acute promyelocytic leukemias, myelodysplastic syndromes, and cell lines. *Blood* 87:4399, 1996.

698. Usuki K, Kitazume K, Endo M, et al: Combination therapy with granulocyte colony-stimulating factor, all-*trans* retinoic acid, and low-dose cytotoxic drugs for acute myelogenous leukemia. *Intern Med* 34:1186, 1995.

699. Zhang W, Piatyszek MA, Kobayashi T, et al: Telomerase activity in human acute myelogenous leukemia: Inhibition of telomerase activity by differentiation-inducing agents. *Clin Cancer Res* 2:799, 1996.

700. Seiter K, Feldman EJ, Dorota Halicka H, et al: Clinical and laboratory evaluation of all-trans retinoic acid modulation of chemotherapy in patients with acute myelogenous leukaemia. *Br J Haematol* 108:40, 2000.

701. Chen Z, Wang Y, Wang W, et al: All-trans retinoic acid as a single agent induces complete remission in a patient with acute leukemia of M2a subtype. *Chin Med J* 115:58, 2002.

702. Zhang Y, Dawson MI, Ning Y, et al: Induction of apoptosis in retinoid-refractory acute myelogenous leukemia by a novel AHPN analog. *Blood* 102:3743, 2003.

703. Lehman S, Bengtzen S, Paul A, et al: Effects of arsenic trioxide (As2O3) on leukemic cells from patients with non-M3 acute myelogenous leukemia: Studies of cytotoxicity, apoptosis and the pattern of resistance. *Eur J Haematol* 66:357, 2001.

704. Nakanishi Y, Kamijo R, Takizawa K, et al: Inhibitors of cyclooxygenase-2 (COX-2) suppressed the proliferation and differentiation of human leukaemic cell lines. *Eur J Cancer* 37:1570, 2001.

705. Ozturk A, Orhan B, Turken O, et al: Acute myeloblastic leukemia achieving complete remission with amifostine alone. *Leuk Lymphoma* 43:451, 2002.

706. Steins MB, Padro T, Bieker R, et al: Efficacy and safety of thalidomide in patients with acute myeloid leukemia. *Blood* 99:834, 2002.

707. Giles FJ, Cooper MA, Silverman L, et al: Phase II study of SU5416—a small-molecule, vascular endothelial growth factor tyrosine-kinase receptor inhibitor—in patients with refractory myeloproliferative diseases. *Cancer* 97:1920, 2003.

708. Andreeff M, Konopleva M: Mechanisms of drug resistance in AML. *Cancer Treat Res* 112:237, 2002.

709. Soneveld P: Multidrug resistance in haematological malignancies. *J Intern Med* 247:521, 2000.

710. Van der Kolk DM, De Vries EG, Muller M, Vellenga E: The role of drug efflux pumps in acute myeloid leukemia. *Leuk Lymphoma* 43:685, 2002.

711. Tothova E, Elbertova A, Fricova M, et al: P-glycoprotein expression in adult acute myeloid leukemia: Correlation with induction treatment outcome. *Neoplasma* 48:393, 2001.

712. Van den Heuvel-Eibrink MM, Wiemer EAC, DeBoevere MJ, et al: MDR1 gene-related clonal selection and P-glycoprotein function and expression in relapsed or refractory acute myeloid leukemia. *Blood* 97:3605, 2001.

713. Sonneveld P, Burnett A, Vossebeld P, et al: Dose-finding study of valspodar (PSC 833) with daunorubicin and cytarabine to reverse multidrug resistance in elderly patients with previously untreated acute myeloid leukemia. *Hematol J* 1:411, 2000.

714. Visani G, Milligan D, Leoni F, et al: Combined action of PSC 833 (Valspodar), a novel MDR reversing agent, with mitoxantrone, etoposide and cytarabine in poor-prognosis acute myeloid leukemia. *Leukemia* 15:764, 2001.

715. Tsimberidou AM, Paterakis G, Androutsos G, et al: Evaluation of the clinical relevance of the expression and function of P-glycoprotein, multidrug resistance protein and lung resistance protein in patients with primary acute myelogenous leukemia. *Leuk Res* 26:143, 2002.

716. Baer MR, George SL, Dodge RK, et al: Phase 3 study of the multidrug resistance modulator PSC-833 in previously untreated patients 60 years of age or older with acute myeloid leukemia: Cancer and Leukemia Group B Study 9720. *Blood* 100:1224, 2002.

717. Larson RA: Is modulation of multidrug resistance a viable strategy for acute myeloid leukemia? *Leukemia* 17:488, 2003.

718. List AF, Kopecky KJ, Willman CL, et al: Benefit of cyclosporine modulation of drug resistance in patients with poor-risk acute myeloid leukemia: A Southwest Oncology Group study. *Blood* 98:3212, 2001.

719. Higashi Y, Turzanski J, Pallis M, Russell NH: Contrasting in vitro effects for the combination of fludarabine, cytosine arabinoside (Ara-C) and granulocyte colony-stimulating factor (FLAG) compared with daunorubicin and Ara-C in P-glycoprotein-positive and P-glycoprotein-negative acute myeloblastic leukaemia. *Br J Haematol* 111:565, 2000.

720. Slitonen T, Alaruikka P, Mantymaa P, et al: Protection of acute myeloblastic leukemia cells against apoptotic cell death by high glutathione

721. and gamma-glutamylcysteine synthetase levels during etoposide-induced oxidative stress. *Ann Oncol* 10:1361, 1999.

721. Solary E, Drenou B, Campos L, et al: Quinine as a multidrug resistance inhibitor: A phase 3 multicentric randomized study in adult de novo acute myelogenous leukemia. *Blood* 102:1202, 2003.

722. Notter M, Willinger T, Erben U, Thiel E: Targeting of a B7-1 (CD80) immunoglobulin G fusion protein to acute myeloid leukemia blasts increases their costimulatory activity for autologous remission T cells. *Blood* 97:3138, 2001.

723. Brouwer RE, Zwinderman KH, Kluin-Nelemans HC, et al: Expression and induction of costimulatory and adhesion molecules on acute myeloid leukemic cells: Implications for adoptive immunotherapy. *Exp Hematol* 28:161, 2000.

724. Claxton D, Choudhury A: Potential for therapy with AML-derived dendritic cells. *Leukemia* 15:668, 2001.

725. Woiciechowsky A, Regn S, Kolb H-J, Roskrow M: Leukemic dendritic cells generated in the presence of FLT3 ligand have the capacity to stimulate an autologous leukemia-specfic cytotoxic T cell response from patients with acute myeloid leukemia. *Leukemia* 15:246, 2001.

726. Stripecke R, Levine AM, Pullarkat V, Cardoso AA: Immunotherapy with acute leukemia cells modified into antigen-presenting cells: Ex vivo culture and gene transfer methods. *Leukemia* 16:1974, 2002.

727. Galea-Lauri J, Darling D, Mufti G, et al: Eliciting cytotoxic T lymphocytes against acute myeloid leukemia-derived antigens: Evaluation of dendritic cell-leukemia cell hybrids and other antigen-loading strategies for dendritic cell-based vaccination. *Cancer Immunol Immunother* 51:299, 2002.

728. Cooper MA, Caligiuri MA: Immunologic manipulation in AML: From bench to bedside. *Leukemia* 16:736, 2002.

729. Meloni G, Trisolini SM, Capria S, et al: How long can we give interleukin-2? Clinical and immunological evaluation of AML patients after 10 or more years of IL2 administration. *Leukemia* 16:2016, 2002.

730. Elisseeva OA, Oka Y, Tsuboi A, et al: Humoral immune responses against Wilms tumor gene WT1 product in patients with hematopoietic malignancies. *Blood* 99:3272, 2002.

731. Molldrem J: Immune therapy of AML. *Cytotherapy* 4:437, 2002.

732. Ohno R, Asou N, Ohnishi K: Treatment of acute promyelocytic leukemia: Strategy toward further increase of cure. *Leukemia* 17:1454, 2003.

733. Sanz MA, Martin G, Gonzalez M, et al: Risk-adapted treatment of acute promyelocytic leukemia with all-trans-retinoic acid and anthracycline monochemotherapy: A multicenter study by the PETHEMA. *Blood* 103:1237, 2004.

734. Estey E, Thall PF, Pierce S, et al: Treatment of newly diagnosed acute promyelocytic leukemia without cytarabine. *J Clin Oncol* 15:483, 1997.

735. Avvisati G, Petti MC, Lo-Coco F, et al: Induction therapy with idarubicin alone significantly influences event-free survival duration in patients with newly diagnosed hypergranular acute promyelocytic leukemia: Final results of the GIMEMA randomized study LAP 0389 with 7 years of minimal follow-up. *Blood* 100:3141, 2002.

736. Lengfelder E, Reichert A, Schoch C, et al: Double induction strategy including high dose cytarbine in combination with all-trans retinoic acid: Effects in patients with newly diagnosed acute promyelocytic leukemia. German AML Cooperative Group. *Leukemia* 14:1362, 2000.

737. Mandelli F, Latagliata R, Avvisati G, et al: Treatment of elderly patients (> or =60 years) with newly diagnosed acute promyelocytic leukemia. Results of the Italian multicenter group GIMEMA with ATRA and idarubicin (AIDA) protocols. *Leukemia* 17:1085, 2003.

738. Estey EH, Giles FJ, Beran M, et al: Experience with gemtuzumab ozogamycin ("mylotarg") and all-trans retinoic acid in untreated acute promyelocytic leukemia. *Blood* 99:4222, 2002.

739. Shen Z-X, Shi Z-Z, Fang J, et al: All-*trans* retinoic acid/As2O3 combination yields a high quality remission and survival in newly diagnosed acute promyelocytic leukemia. *Proc Natl Acad Sci U S A* 10:1073, 2004.

740. Tallman MS, Rowe JM: Long-term follow-up and potential for cure in acute promyelocytic leukaemia. *Best Pract Res Clin Haematol* 16:535, 2003.

741. Castaigne S, Lefebvre P, Chomienne C, et al: Effectiveness and pharmacokinetics of low-dose all-*trans* retinoic acid (25 mg/m²) in acute promyelocytic leukemia. *Blood* 82:3560, 1993.

742. Castaigne S, Chomienne C, Daniel MT, et al: All-*trans* retinoic acid as differentiating therapy for acute promyelocytic leukemia: I. Clinical results. *Blood* 76:1704, 1990.

743. Tallman MS, Andersen JW, Schiffer CA, et al: All-*trans*-retinoic acid in acute promyelocytic leukemia. *N Engl J Med* 337:1021, 1997.

744. Warrell RP Jr, Frankel SR, Miller WH Jr, et al: Differentiation therapy of acute promyelocytic leukemia with tretinoin (all-*trans*-retinoic acid). *N Engl J Med* 324:1385, 1991.

745. White KL, Wiley JS, Frost T, et al: All-*trans* retinoic acid in the treatment of acute promyelocytic leukemia. *Aust N Z J Med* 22:449, 1992.

746. White KL, Wiley JS, Frost T, et al: All-trans retinoic acid in the treatment of acute promyelocytic leukemia. *Blood* 76:1710, 1992.

747. Chomienne C, Ballerini P, Balitrans N, et al: All-*trans* retinoic acid in acute promyelocytic leukemia: II. In vitro studies: Structure-function relationship. *Blood* 76:1710, 1990.

748. Degos L: Is acute promyelocytic leukemia a curable disease? Treatment strategy for a long-term survival. *Leukemia* 8:911, 1994.

749. Head D, Kopecky KJ, Weick J, et al: Effect of aggressive daunomycin therapy on survival in acute promyelocytic leukemia. *Blood* 86:1717, 1995.

750. Gianni M, Terao M, Fortino L, et al: Stat 1 is induced and activated by all-*trans* retinoic acid in acute promyelocytic leukemia cells. *Blood* 89:1001, 1997.

751. Degos L, Dombret H, Chomienne C, et al: All-*trans*-retinoic acid as a differentiating agent in the treatment of acute promyelocytic leukemia. *Blood* 85:2643, 1995.

752. Gallagher RE, Li YP, Rao S, et al: Characterization of acute promyelocytic leukemia cases with PML-RAR alpha break/fusion sites in PML exon 6: identification of a subgroup with decreased in vitro responsiveness to all-*trans* retinoic acid. *Blood* 86:1540, 1995.

753. Licht JD, Chomienne C, Goy A, et al: Clinical and molecular characterization of a rare syndrome of acute promyelocytic leukemia associated with translocation (11;17). *Blood* 85:1083, 1995.

754. Jansen JH, De Ridder MC, Geertsma WM, et al: Complete remission of t(11;17) positive acute promyelocytic leukemia induced by all-*trans* retinoic acid and granulocyte colony-stimulating factor. *Blood* 94:39, 1999.

755. Tallman MS, Andersen JW, Schiffer CA, et al: All-trans retinoic acid in acute promyelocytic leukemia: Long-term outcome and prognostic factor analysis from the North American Intergroup protocol. *Blood* 100:4298, 2002.

756. Fenaux P, Chevret S, Guerci A, et al: Long-term follow-up confirms the benefit of all-trans retinoic acid in acute promyelocytic leukemia. European APL group. *Leukemia* 14:1371, 2000.

757. Hernandez JM, Martin G, Gutierrez MC, et al: Additional cytogenetic changes do not influence the outcome of patients with newly diagnosed acute promyelocytic leukemia treated with an ATRA plus anthracyclin based protocol. A report of the Spanish group PETHEMA. *Haematologica* 86:807, 2001.

758. Kennedy GA, Marlton P, Cobcroft R, Gill D: Molecular remission without blood product support using all-trans retinoic acid (ATRA) induction and combined arsenic trioxide/ATRA consolidation in a Jehovah's Witness with de novo acute promyelocytic leukemia. *Br J Haematol* 111:1103, 2000.

759. Martinelli G, Ottaviani E, Testoni N, et al: Disappearance of PML/RAR alpha acute promyelocytic leukemia associated transcript during consolidation chemotherapy. *Haematologica* 83:985, 1998.

760. Incerpi MH, Miller DA, Posen R, Byrne JD: All-*trans* retinoic acid for the treatment of acute promyelocytic leukemia in pregnancy. *Obstet Gynecol* 89:826, 1997.

761. Fadilah SA, Hatta AZ, Keng CS, et al: Successful treatment of acute promyelocytic leukemia in pregnancy with all-trans retinoic acid. *Leukemia* 15:1665, 2001.

762. Carridice D, Austin N, Bayston K, Ganly PS: Successful treatment of acute promyelocytic leukaemia during pregnancy. *Clin Lab Hematol* 24:307, 2002.

763. Tallman MS, Andersen JW, Schiffer CA, et al: Clinical description of 44 patients with acute promyelocytic leukemia who developed the retinoic acid syndrome. *Blood* 95:90, 2000.

764. Larsen RS, Tallman MS. Retinoic acid syndrome: Manifestations, pathogenesis, and treatment. *Best Pract Res Clin Hematol* 16:453, 2003.

765. Tallman MS, Andersen JW, Schiffer CA, et al: Clinical description of 44 patients with acute promyelocytic leukemia who developed the retinoic acid syndrome. *Blood* 95:90, 2000.

766. Fenaux P, Chomienne C, Degas L: All-*trans* retinoic acid and chemotherapy in the treatment of acute promyelocytic leukemia. *Semin Hematol* 38:13, 2001.

767. Frankel SR, Eardley A, Lauwers G, et al: The "retinoic acid syndrome" in acute promyelocytic leukemia. *Ann Intern Med* 117:292, 1992.

768. De Botton S, Dombret H, Sanz M, et al: Incidence, clinical features, and outcome of all trans-retinoic acid syndrome in 413 cases of newly diagnosed acute promyelocytic leukemia. The European APL Group. *Blood* 92:2712, 1998.

769. Azlin ZA, Ahmed T: Cure in acute promyelocytic leukemia—Now more readily achievable with less toxic therapy. *Blood* 79:2492, 1992.

770. Tallman MS: Retinoic acid syndrome: A problem of the past? *Leukemia* 16:160, 2002.

771. Falanga A, Barbui T: Coagulopathy of acute promyelocytic leukemia. *Acta Haematol* 106:43, 2001.

772. Goldberg MA, Ginsburg D, Mayer RJ, et al: Is heparin administration necessary during induction chemotherapy for patients with acute promyelocytic leukemia? *Blood* 69:187, 1987.

773. Visani G, Gugliotta L, Tosi P, et al: All-trans retinoic acid significantly reduces the incidence of early hemorrhagic death during induction therapy of acute promyelocytic leukemia. *Eur J Haematol* 64:139, 2000.

774. Kizaki M, Ueno H, Yamazoe Y, et al: Mechanisms of retinoid resistance in leukemic cells: Possible role of cytochrome P450 and P-glycoprotein. *Blood* 87:725, 1996.

775. Chen Z, Chen G-Q, Shen Z-X, et al: Treatment of acute promyelocytic leukemia with arsenic compounds: In vitro and in vivo studies. *Semin Hematol* 38:26, 2001.

776. Zhang TD, Chen GQ, Wang ZG, et al: Arsenic trioxide, a therapeutic agent for APL. *Oncogene* 20:7146, 2001.

777. Soignet SL, Frankel SE, Douer D, et al: United States multicenter study of arsenic trioxide in relapsed acute promyelocytic leukemia. *J Clin Oncol* 19:3852, 2001.

778. Dombret H, Fenaux P, Soignet SL, Tallman MS: Established practice in the treatment of patients with acute promyelocytic leukemia and the introduction of arsenic trioxide as a novel therapy. *Semin Hematol* 39:8, 2002.

779. Chen GQ, Shi XG, Tang W, et al: Use of arsenic trioxide (As₂O₃) in the treatment of acute promyelocytic leukemia (APL): 1. As₂O₃ exerts dose-dependent dual effects on APL cells. *Blood* 89:3345, 1997.

780. Jing Y, Dai J, Chalmers-Redman RME, et al: Arsenic trioxide selectively induces acute promyelocytic leukemia cell apoptosis via a hydrogen peroxide-dependent pathway. *Blood* 94:2102, 1999.

781. Soignet SL, Maslak P, Wang ZG, et al: Complete remission after treatment of acute promyelocytic leukemia with arsenic trioxide. *N Engl J Med* 339:1341, 1998.

782. Mathas S, Lietz A, Janz M, et al: Inhibition of NF-kappaB essentially contributes to arsenic-induced apoptosis. *Blood* 102:1028, 2003.

783. Kwong YL, Au WY, Chim CS, et al: Arsenic trioxide- and idarubicin-induced remissions in relapsed acute promyelocytic leukaemia: Clinicopathological and molecular features of a pilot study. *Am J Hematol* 66:274, 2001.

784. Au WY, Chim CS, Lie AK, et al: Combined arsenic trioxide and all-trans retinoic acid treatment for acute promyelocytic leukaemia recurring from previous relapses successfully treated using arsenic trioxide. *Br J Haematol* 117:130, 2002.

785. Raffoux E, Rousselot P, Poupon J, et al: Combined treatment with arsenic trioxide and all-trans-retinoic acid in patients with relapsed acute promyelocytic leukemia. *J Clin Oncol* 21:2326, 2003.

786. Comacho LH, Soignet SL, Chanel S, et al: Leukocytosis and the retinoic acid syndrome in patients with acute promyelocytic leukemia treated with arsenic trioxide. *J Clin Oncol* 18:2620, 2000.

787. Unnikrishnan D, Dutcher JP, Varshneya N, et al: Torsades de pointes in 3 patients with leukemia treated with arsenic trioxide. *Blood* 97:1514, 2001.

788. Zhou J, Meng R, Li X, et al: The effect of arsenic trioxide on QT interval prolongation during APL therapy. *Chin Med J* 116:1764, 2003.

789. Estey EH: Treatment options for relapsed acute promyelocytic leukaemia. *Best Pract Res Clin Haematol* 16:521, 2003.

790. Tallman MS, Nabhan C, Feusner JH, Rowe JM: Acute promyelocytic leukemia: Evolving therapeutic strategies. *Blood* 99:759, 2002.

791. Lo-Coco F, Romano A, Mengarelli A, et al: Allogeneic stem cell transplantation for advanced acute promyelocytic leukemia: Results in patients treated in second molecular remission or with molecularly persistent disease. *Leukemia* 17:1930, 2003.

792. Nabhan C, Mehta J, Tallman MS: The role of bone marrow transplantation in acute promyelocytic leukemia. *Bone Marrow Transplant* 28:219, 2001.

793. Colvic N, Bogdanovic A, Miljic P, et al: Central nervous system relapse in acute promyelocytic leukemia. *Am J Hematol* 71:60-2002.

794. Sanz MA, Larrea L, Sanz G, et al: Cutaneous promyelocytic sarcoma at sites of vascular access and marrow aspiration. A characteristic localization of chloromas in acute promyelocytic leukemia? *Haematologica* 85:758, 2000.

795. Latagliata R, Petti MC, Fenu S, et al: Therapy-related myelodysplastic syndrome-acute myelogenous leukemia in patients treated for acute promyelocytic leukemia: An emerging problem. *Blood* 99:822, 2002.

796. Lobe I, Rigal-Huguet F, Vekhoff A, et al: Myelodysplastic syndrome after acute promyelocytic leukemia: The European APL group. *Leukemia* 17:1600, 2003.

797. Garcia-Manero G, Kantarjian HM, Kornblau S, Estey E: Therapy-related myelodysplastic syndrome or acute myelogenous leukemia in patients with acute promyelocytic leukemia (APL). *Leukemia* 16:1888, 2002.

798. Beaumont M, Sanz M, Carli PM, et al: Therapy-related acute promyelocytic leukemia. *J Clin Oncol* 21:2123, 2003.

799. Smith MA, McCaffrey RP, Karp JE: The secondary leukemias: Challenges and research directions. *J Natl Cancer Inst* 88:407, 1996.

800. Smith MA, Rubinstein L, Anderson JR, et al: Secondary leukemia or myelodysplastic syndrome after treatment with epipodophyllotoxins. *J Clin Oncol* 17:569, 1999.

801. Ng A, Taylor GM, Eden OB: Treatment-related leukaemia: A clinical and scientific challenge. *Cancer Treat Rev* 26:377, 2000.

802. Super HJ, McCabe NR, Thirman MJ, et al: Rearrangements of the MLL gene in therapy-related acute myeloid leukemia in patients previously treated with agents targeting DNA-topoisomerase 11. *Blood* 82:3705, 1993.

803. Dissing M, Le Beau MM, Pedersen-Bjergaard J: Inversion of chromosome 16 and uncommon rearrangements of the CBFB and MYHI1 genes in therapy-related acute myeloid leukemia: Rare events related to DNA-topoisomerase II inhibitors? *J Clin Oncol* 16:1890, 1998.

804. Felix CA: Secondary leukemias induced by topoisomerase-targeted drugs. *Biochim Biophys Acta* 1400:233, 1998.

805. Pogliani EM, Pioltelli P, Russini F, et al: Acute leukemia following cisplatin for ovarian cancer [letter]. *Hematologica* 72:184, 1987.

806. Kolte B, Baer AN, Sait SN, et al: Acute myeloid leukemia in the setting of low dose weekly methotrexate therapy for rheumatoid arthritis. *Leuk Lymphoma* 42:371, 2001.

807. Bakland G, Nossent H: Acute myelogenous leukemia following etanercept therapy. *Rheumatology (Oxford)* 42:900, 2003.

808. Aktan M, Tanakol R, Nalcaci M, Dincol G: Leukemia in a patient treated with growth hormone. *Endocr J* 47:471, 2000.

809. Freedman MH, Bonilla MA, Fier C, et al: Myelodysplasia syndrome and acute myeloid leukemia in patients with congenital neutropenia receiving G-CSF therapy. *Blood* 96:429, 2000.

810. Andersen MK, Pedersen-Bjergaard J: Therapy-related MDS and AML in acute promyelocytic leukemia. *Blood* 100:1928, 2002.

811. Barnard DR, Lange B, Alonzo TA, et al: Acute myeloid leukemia and myelodysplastic syndrome in children treated for cancer: Comparison with primary presentation. *Blood* 100:427, 2002.

812. Smith RE, Bryant J, DeCillis A, et al: Acute myeloid leukemia and myelodysplastic syndrome after doxorubicin-cyclophosphamide adjuvant therapy for operable breast cancer: The National Surgical Adjuvant Breast and Bowel Project Experience. *J Clin Oncol* 21:1195, 2003.

813. Weldon CB, Jaffe BM, Kahn MJ: Therapy-induced leukemias and myelodysplastic syndromes after breast cancer treatment: An under-emphasized clinical problem. *Am Surg Oncol* 9:717, 2002.

814. Gershkevitsh E, Rosenberg I, Dearnaley DP, Trott KR: Bone marrow doses and leukemia risk in radiotherapy of prostate cancer. *Radiother Oncol* 53:189, 1999.

815. Armitage JO, Carbone PP, Connors JM, et al: Treatment-related myelodysplasia and acute leukemia in non-Hodgkin's lymphoma. *J Clin Oncol* 21:897, 2003.

816. Lambertenghi Deliliers G, Annaloro C, Pozzoli E, et al: Cytogenetic and myelodysplastic alterations after autologous hemopoietic stem cell transplantation. *Leuk Res* 23:291, 1999.

817. Legare RD, Gribben JG, Maragh M, et al: Prediction of therapy-related acute myelogenous leukemia (AML) and myelodysplastic syndrome (MDS) after autologous bone marrow transplant (ABMT) for lymphoma. *Am J Hematol* 56:45, 1997.

818. Micallef IN, Lillington DM, Apostolidis J, et al: Therapy-related myelodysplasia and secondary acute myelogenous leukemia after high-dose therapy with autologous hematopoietic progenitor-cell support for lymphoid malignancies. *J Clin Oncol* 18:847, 2000.

819. Lillington DM, Micallef IN, Carpenter E, et al: Detection of chromosome abnormalities pre-high-dose treatment in patients developing therapy-related myelodysplasia and secondary acute myelogenous leukemia after treatment for non-Hodgkin's lymphoma. *J Clin Oncol* 19:2472, 2001.

820. Amadori S, Picardi A, Fazi P, et al: A phase 11 study of VP-16, intermediate-dose Ara-C and carboplatin (VAC) in advanced acute myelogenous leukemia and blastic chronic myelogenous leukemia. *Leukemia* 10:766, 1996.

821. De Witte T, Suciu S, Peetermans M, et al: Intensive chemotherapy for poor prognosis myelodysplasia (MDS) and secondary acute myeloid leukemia (SAML) following MDS of more than 6 months duration. A pilot study by the Leukemia Cooperative Group of the European Organisation for Research and Treatment in Cancer (EORTC-LCG). *Leukemia* 9:1805, 1995.

822. Tobal K, Newton J, Macheta M, et al: Molecular quantitation of minimal residual disease in acute myeloid leukemia with t(8;21) can identify patients in durable remission and predict relapse. *Blood* 95:815, 2000.

823. Estey EH: Treatment of acute myelogenous leukemia and myelodysplastic syndromes. *Semin Hematol* 32:132, 1995.

824. Witherspoon RP, Deeg HJ, Storer B, et al: Hematopoietic stem-cell transplantation for treatment-related leukemia or myelodysplasia. *J Clin Oncol* 19:2134, 2001.

825. Rowe JM: Therapy of secondary leukemia. *Leukemia* 16:748, 2002.

826. Rosenfield C, Kantarjian H: Is myelodysplastic related acute myelogenous leukemia a distinct entity from de novo acute myelogenous leukemia? Potential for targeted therapies. *Leuk Lymphoma* 41:493, 2001.

827. Brincker H: Estimate of overall treatment results in acute nonlymphocytic leukemia based on age-specific rates of incidence and complete remission. *Cancer Treat Rep* 69:5, 1985.

828. Pinto A, Zulian GB, Archimbaud E: Acute myelogenous leukaemia. *Crit Rev Oncol Hematol* 27:161, 1998.

829. Leith CP, Kopecky KJ, Godwin J, et al: Acute myeloid leukemia in the elderly: Assessment of multidrug resistance (MDR1) and cytogenetics distinguishes biologic subgroups with remarkably distinct responses to standard chemotherapy. A Southwest Oncology Group study. *Blood* 89:3323, 1997.

830. Champlin RE, Gajewski TL, Golde DW: Treatment of acute myelogenous leukemia in the elderly. *Semin Oncol* 16:51, 1989.

831. Ballester O, Moscinski LC, Morris D, Balducci L: Acute myelogenous leukemia in the elderly. *J Am Geriatr Soc* 40:277, 1992.

832. Copplestone JA, Prentice AG: Acute myeloblastic leukaemia in the elderly. *Leukemia Res* 12:617, 1988.

833. Balducci L: Geriatric oncology. *Crit Rev Oncol Hematol* 46:211, 2003.

834. Kalaycio M, Pohlman B, Elson P, et al: Chemotherapy for acute myelogenous leukemia in the elderly with cytarabine, mitoxanthrone, and granulocyte-macrophage colony-stimulating factor. *Am J Clin Oncol* 24:58, 2001.

835. Bennett CL, Hynes D, Godwin J, et al: Economic analysis of granulocyte colony stimulating factor as adjunct therapy for older patients with acute myelogenous leukemia (AML): Estimates from a Southwest Oncology Group clinical trial. *Cancer Invest* 19:603, 2001.

836. Lowenberg B, Suciu S, Archimbaud E, et al: Mitoxantrone versus daunorubicin in induction-consolidation chemotherapy—The value of low-dose cytarabine for maintenance of remission, and an assessment of prognostic factors in acute myeloid leukemia in the elderly: Final report. European Organization for the Research and Treatment of Cancer and the Dutch-Belgian Hemato-Oncology Cooperative Hovon Group. *J Clin Oncol* 16:872, 1998.

837. Lowenberg B, Suciu S, Archimbaud E, et al: Use of recombinant GM-CSF during and after remission induction chemotherapy in patients aged 61 years and older with acute myeloid leukemia: Final report of AML-11, a phase III randomized study of the Leukemia Cooperative Group of European Organisation for the Research and Treatment of Cancer and the Dutch Belgian Hemato-Oncology Cooperative Group. *Blood* 90:2952, 1997.

838. Reiffers J, Huguet F, Stoppa AM, et al: A prospective randomized trial of idarubicin vs daunorubicin in combination chemotherapy for acute myelogenous leukemia of the age group 55 to 75. *Leukemia* 10:389, 1996.

839. Harousseau JF, Rigal-Huguet F, Hurteloup P, et al: Treatment of acute myeloid leukemia in elderly patients with oral idarubicin as a single agent. *Eur J Haematol* 42:182, 1989.

840. Anderson JE, Kopecky KJ, Willman CL, et al: Outcome after induction chemotherapy for older patients with acute myeloid leukemia is not improved with mitoxantrone and etoposide compared to cytarabine and daunorubicin: A Southwest Oncology Group study. *Blood* 100:3869, 2002.

841. Hartman F, Jacobs G, Gotto H, et al: Cytosine arabinoside, idarubicin and divided dose etoposide for the treatment of acute myeloid leukemia in elderly patients. *Leuk Lymphoma* 42:347, 2001.

842. Chauncey TR, Rankin C, Anderson JE, et al: A phase I study of induction chemotherapy for older patients with newly diagnosed acute myeloid leukemia (AML) using mitoxantrone, etoposide, and the MDR modulator PSC 833: A Southwest Oncology Group study 9617. *Leuk Res* 24:567, 2000.

843. Schiller GJ: Postremission therapy of acute myeloid leukemia in older adults. *Leukemia* 10(suppl 1):S18, 1996.

844. Herzig RH: High-dose ara-C in older adults with acute leukemia. *Leukemia* 10 (suppl 1):S10, 1996.

845. Letendre L, Noel P, Litzow MR, et al: Treatment of acute myelogenous leukemia in the older patient with attenuated high-dose ara-C. *Am J Clin Oncol* 21:142, 1998.

846. Schiller G, Lee M: Long-term outcome of high-dose cytarabine-based consolidation chemotherapy for older patients with acute myelogenous leukemia. *Leuk Lymphoma* 25:111, 1997.

847. Lowenberg B: Post-remission treatment of acute myelogenous leukemia. *N Engl J Med* 332:260, 1995.

848. DeLima M, Ghaddar H, Pierce S, Estey E: Treatment of newly-diagnosed acute myelogenous leukaemia in patients aged 80 years and above. *Br J Haematol* 93:89, 1996.

849. Johnson PR, Yin JA: Prognostic factors in elderly patients with acute myeloid leukaemia. *Leuk Lymphoma* 16:51, 1994.

850. Oberg G, Killander A, Bjoreman M, et al: Long-term follow-up of patients > or =60 yr old with acute myeloid leukaemia. *Eur J Haematol* 68:376, 2002.

851. Stone RM: The difficult problem of acute myeloid leukemia in the older adult. *CA Cancer J Clin* 52:363, 2002.

852. Lichtman MA, Rowe JM: The relationship of patient age to the pathobiology of the clonal myeloid disease. *Semin Oncol* 31:185, 2004.

853. Renosos EE, Shepard FA, Messner HA, et al: Acute leukemia during pregnancy: The Toronto Leukemia Study Group Experience with long-term follow-up of children exposed in utero to chemotherapeutic agents. *J Clin Oncol* 5:1098, 1987.

854. Caligiuri MA, Mayer RJ: Pregnancy and leukemia. *Semin Oncol* 16:388, 1989.

855. Aviles A, Neri N: Hematological malignancies and pregnancy: A final report of 84 children who received chemotherapy in utero. *Clin Lymphoma* 2:173, 2001.

856. Greenlund LJ, Letendre L, Tefferi A: Acute leukemia during pregnancy: A single institutional experience with 17 cases. *Leuk Lymphoma* 41:571, 2001.

857. Lipovsky MM, Biesma DH, Christiaens GC, Petersen EJ: Successful treatment of acute promyelocytic leukaemia with all-*trans* retinoic acid during late pregnancy. *Br J Haematol* 94:669, 1996.

858. Osada S, Horibe K, Oiwa K, et al: A case of infantile acute monocytic leukemia caused by vertical transmission of the mother's leukemic cells. *Cancer* 65:1146, 1990.

859. Stevens RF, Hann IM, Wheatley K, Gray RG: Marked improvements in outcome with chemotherapy alone in paediatric acute myeloid leukemia: Results of United Kingdom Medical Research Council's 10th AML trial. MRC Childhood Leukaemia Working Party. *Br J Haematol* 101:130, 1998.

860. Gregory J, Arceci R: Acute myeloid leukemia in children: A review of risk factors and recent trials. *Cancer Invest* 20:1027, 2002.

861. Clark JJ, Smith FO, Arceci RJ: Update in childhood myeloid leukemia: Recent developments in the molecular basis of disease and novel therapies. *Curr Opin Hematol* 10:31, 2002.

862. Creutzig U, Ritter J, Zimmerman M, et al: Improved treatment results in high-risk pediatric acute myeloid leukemia patients after intensification with high-dose cytarabine and mitoxantrone: Results of study acute myeloid leukemia-Berrlin-Frankfort-Muenster 93. *J Clin Oncol* 19:2705, 2001.

863. Arceci RJ: Progress and controversies in the treatment of pediatric acute myelogenous leukemia. *Curr Opin Hematol* 9:353, 2002.

864. Webb DKH, Harrison G, Stevens RF, et al: Relationships between age

1232

PART IX MALIGNANT DISEASES

at diagnosis, clinical featuures, and outome of therapy in children in the Medical Research Council AML 10 and 12 trials for acute myeloid leukemia. *Blood* 98:1714, 2001.

865. Zwaan CM, Meshinchi S, Radich JP, et al: FLT3 internal tandem duplication in 234 children with acute myeloid leukemia: Prognostic significance and relation to cellular drug resistance. *Blood* 102:2387, 2002.

866. Wheatley K, Burnett AK, Goldstone AH, et al: A simple robust, validated and highly predictive index for the determination of risk-directed therapy in acute myeloid leukaemia derived from the MRC AML 10 trial. *Br J Haematol* 107:69, 1999.

867. Wells RJ, Arthur DC, Srivastava A, et al: Prognostic variables in newly diagnosed children and adolescents with acute myeloid leukemia. *Leukemia* 16:601, 2002.

868. Sievers EL, Lange BJ, Alonzo TA, et al: Immunophenotypic evidence of leukemia after induction therapy predicts relapse: Results from a prospective Children's Cancer Group study of 252 patients with acute myeloid leukemia. *Blood* 101:3398, 2003.

869. Woods WG, Neudorf S, Gold S, et al: A comparison of allogeneic bone marrow transplantaion, autologous bone marrow transplantation, and aggressive chemotherapy in children with acute myeloid leukemia in remission: A report from the Children's Cancer Group. *Blood* 97:56, 2001.

870. Kawasaki H, Isoyama K, Eguchi M, et al: Superior outcome of infant acute myeloid leukemia with intensive chemotherapy: Results of the Japan Infant Leukemia Study Group. *Blood* 98:3589, 2001.

871. Chessels JM, Harrison CJ, Kempski H, et al: Clinical features, cytogenetics, and outcome in acute lymphoblastic and myeloid leukemia of infancy: Report from the MRC Childhood Leukemia working party. *Leukemia* 16:776, 2002.

872. Rocha V, Cornish J, Sievers EL, et al: Comparison of outcomes of unrelated bone marrow and umbilical cord blood transplants in children with acute leukemia. *Blood* 97:2962, 2001.

873. Leung W, Hudson MM, Strickland DK, et al: Late effects of treatment in survivors of childhood acute myeloid leukemia. *J Clin Oncol* 18:3273, 2000.

874. Leung W, Ribiero RC, Hudson MM, et al: Second malignancy after treatment of childhood acute myeloid leukemia. *Leukemia* 15:41, 2001.

875. Verhagen C, Stalpers LJA, DePauw BE, Haanen C: Drug-induced skin reactions in patients with acute non-lymphocytic leukaemia. *Eur J Haematol* 38:225, 1987.

876. Kapusta L, Groot-Loonen J, Thijssen JM, et al: Regional cardiac wall motion abnormalities during and shortly after anthracyclines therapy. *Med Pediatr Oncol* 41:426, 2003.

877. Benvenuto GM, Ometto R, Fontanelli A, et al: Chemotherapy-related cardiotoxicity: New diagnostic and preventive strategies. *Ital Heart J* 4:655, 2003.

878. Dietz B, Van der Hem KG: Late-onset cardiotoxicity of chemotherapy and radiotherapy. *Neth J Med* 61:228, 2003.

879. Theodoulou M, Hudis C: Cardiac profiles of liposomal anthracyclines: Greater cardiac safety versus conventional doxorubicin? *Cancer* 100:2052, 2004.

880. Swain SM, Vici P: The current and future role of dexrazoxane as a cardioprotectant in anthracycline treatment: Expert panel review. *J Cancer Res Clin Oncol* 130:1, 2004.

881. Kojima H, Abei M, Takei N, et al: Fatal reactivation of hepatitis B virus following cytotoxic chemotherapy for acute myelogenous leukemia: Fibrosing cholestatic hepatitis. *Eur J Haematol* 69:101, 2002.

882. Ishiga K, Kawatani T, Suou T, et al: Fulminant hepatitis type B after chemotherapy in a serologically negative hepatitis B virus carrier with acute myelogenous leukemia. *Int J Hematol* 73:115, 2001.

883. Bianco E, Marcucci F, Mele A, et al: Italian Multi-Center case-control study. Prevalence of hepatitis C virus infection in lymphoproliferative diseases other than B-cell non-Hodgkin's lymphoma, and in myeloproliferative diseases: An Italian Multi-Center case-control study. *Haematologica* 89:70, 2004.

884. Zuckerman E, Zuckerman T, Douer D, et al: Liver dysfunction in patients infected with hepatitis C virus undergoing chemotherapy for hematologic malignancies. *Cancer* 15:1224, 1998.

885. von Eiff M, Essink M, Roos N, et al: Hepatosplenic candidiasis, a late manifestation of Candida septicemia in neutropenic patients with haematologic malignancies. *Blut* 60:242, 1990.

886. Blade J, Lopez-Guillermo A, Rozman C, et al: Chronic systemic candidiasis in acute leukemia. *Ann Hematol* 64:240, 1992.

887. Roozrokh HC, Stahlfeld KR: Disseminated hepatic candidiasis. *J Am Coll Surg* 194:231, 2002.

888. Sallah S, Wan JY, Nguyen NP, et al: Analysis of factors related to the occurrence of chronic disseminated candidiasis in patients with acute leukemia in a non-bone marrow transplant setting: A follow-up study. *Cancer* 15:1349, 2001.

889. Colovic M, Lazarevic V, Colovic R, et al: Hepatosplenic candidiasis after neutropenic phase of acute leukaemia. *Med Oncol* 16:139, 1999.

890. Sallah S, Semelka R, Kelekis N, et al: Diagnosis and monitoring response to treatment of hepatosplenic candidiasis in patients with acute leukemia using magnetic resonance imaging. *Acta Haematol* 100:77, 1998.

891. Iwasaki H, Misaki H, Nakamura T, Ueda T: Surveillance of the serum Candida antigen titer for initiation of antifungal therapy after postremission chemotherapy in patients with acute leukemia. *Int J Hematol* 71:266, 2000.

892. Blijlevens NM, Donnelly JP, De Pauw BE: Mucosal barrier injury: Biology, pathology, clinical counterparts and consequences of intensive treatment for haematological malignancy: An overview. *Bone Marrow Transplant* 25:1269, 2000.

893. Clark R: Neutropenic colitis (typhlitis). *Cancer Control* 2:522, 1995.

894. Teefey SA, Montana MA, Goldfogel GA, Shuman WP: Sonographic diagnosis of neutropenic typhlitis. *AJR Am J Roentgenol* 149:731.

895. Keidan RD, Fanning J, Gatenby RA, Weese JL: Recurrent typhlitis. A disease resulting from aggressive chemotherapy. *Dis Colon Rectum* 32:206, 1989.

896. Byrnes JJ, Baqueriro H, Gonzalez M, Henseley GT: Thrombotic thrombocytopenic purpura subsequent to acute myelogenous leukemia chemotherapy. *Am J Hematol* 21:299, 1986.

897. Mertens AC, Ramsay NK, Kouris S, Neglia JP: Patterns of gonadal dysfunction following bone marrow transplantation. *Bone Marrow Transplant* 22:345, 1998.

898. Tauchmanova L, Selleri C, De Rosa G, et al: Gonadal status in reproductive age women after haematopoietic stem cell transplantation for haematological malignancies. *Hum Reprod* 18:1410, 2003.

899. Blumenfeld Z, Avivi I, Ritter M, Rowe JM: Preservation of fertility and ovarian function and minimizing chemotherapy-induced gonadotoxicity in young women. *Soc Gynecol Investig* 6:229, 1999.

900. Lopez Andreu JA, Fernandez PJ, et al: Persistent altered spermatogenesis in long-term childhood cancer survivors. *Pediatr Hematol Oncol* 17:21, 2000.

901. Relander T, Cavallin-Stahl E, Garwicz S, et al: Gonadal and sexual function in men treated for childhood cancer. *Med Pediatr Oncol* 35:52, 2000.

902. Hinterberger-Fischer M, Kier P, Kalhs P, et al: Fertility, pregnancies and offspring complications after bone marrow transplantation. *Bone Marrow Transplant* 7:5, 1991.

903. Giri N, Vowels MR, Barr AL, Mameghan H: Successful pregnancy after total body irradiation and bone marrow transplantation for acute leukaemia. *Bone Marrow Transplant* 10:93, 1992.

904. Maguire LC, Dick FR, Sherman BM: The effects of anti-leukemic therapy on gonadal histology in adult males. *Cancer* 48:1967, 1981.

905. Matthews JH, Wood JK: Male fertility during chemotherapy for acute leukemia. *N Engl J Med* 303:1235, 1980.

906. Wahlin A, Markevarn B, Gololeva I, et al: Improved outcome in adult acute myeloid leukemia is almost entirely restricted to young patients and associated stem cell transplantation. *Eur J Hematol* 68:54, 2002.

907. Fialkow PJ, Singer JW, Roskind WH, et al: Clonal development, stem cell differentiation and the nature of clinical remissions in acute non-lymphocytic leukemia: Studies of patients heterozygous for glucose-6-phosphate dehydrogenase. *N Engl J Med* 317:468, 1987.

908. Bartram CR, Ludwig W-D, Hiddemann W, et al: Acute myeloid leukemia: Analysis of *ras* gene mutations and clonality defined by polymorphic X-linked loci. *Leukemia* 3:247, 1989.

909. Fialkow PJ, Janssen JWG, Bartram CR: Clonal remissions in acute nonlymphocytic leukemia: Evidence for a multistep pathogenesis of the malignancy. *Blood* 77:1415, 1991.

910. Busque L, Gilliland DG: Clonal evolution in acute myeloid leukemia. *Blood* 82:337, 1993.

911. Gale RE, Wheadon H, Goldstone AH, et al: Frequency of clonal remission in acute myeloid leukaemia. *Lancet* 341:138, 1993.

912. Killman S-A: Acute leukemia: Development, remission/relapse pattern, relationship between normal and leukaemic haemopoiesis, and the "sleeper-to-feeder" stem cell hypothesis. *Baillieres Clin Haematol* 4:577, 1991.

913. Kudoh S, Asou H, Kyo T, et al: Emergence of karyotypically unrelated clone in remission of de novo acute myeloblastic leukaemias. *Br J Haematol* 89:531, 1995.

914. Jinnai 1, Nagai K, Yoshida S, et al: Incidence and characteristics of clonal hematopoiesis in remission of acute myeloid leukemia in relation to morphological dysplasia. *Leukemia* 9:1756, 1995.

915. Robert EE: Spontaneous complete remission in acute promyelocytic leukemia. *N Y State J Med* 86:662, 1985.

916. Takue Y, Culbert SJ, Van Eys J, et al: Spontaneous cure of end-stage acute nonlymphocytic leukemia complicated with chloroma (granulocytic sarcoma). *Cancer* 58:1101, 1986.

917. Jehn UW, Mempel MA: Spontaneous remission of acute myeloid leukemia. *Blut* 52:165, 1986.

918. Passe S, Miké V, Mertelsmann R, et al: Acute nonlymphoblastic leukemia: Prognostic factors in adults with long-term follow-up. *Cancer* 50:1462, 1982.

919. Evansen SA, Stavem P: Long-term survival in acute leukemia. *Acta Med Scand* 219:79, 1986.

920. Grunwald HW: The cure of acute myeloblastic leukemia in adults. *JAMA* 247:1698, 1982.

921. MacMahon B, Forman D: Variations in the duration of survival of patients with acute leukemia. *Blood* 12:683, 1957.

922. Menzin J, Lang K, Earle C, et al: The outcomes and costs of acute myeloid leukemia among the elderly. *Arch Intern Med* 162:1597, 2002.

923. Burnett AK: Transplantation in first remission of acute myeloid leukemia. *N Engl J Med* 339:1698, 1998.

924. Burnett AK, Goldstone AH, Stevens RM, et al: Randomised comparison of addition of autologous bone-marrow transplantation to intensive chemotherapy for acute myeloid leukaemia in first remission: Results of MRC AML 10 trial. U.K. Medical Research Council Adult and Children's Leukaemia Working Parties. *Lancet* 351:700, 1998.

925. Clift RA, Buckner CD: Marrow transplantation for acute myeloid leukemia. *Cancer Invest* 16:53, 1998.

926. Gale RP, Butturini A: Transplants for acute myelogenous leukemia. *Cancer Invest* 16:66, 1998.

927. Redaelli A, Stephens JM, Brandt S, et al: Short- and long-term effects of acute myeloid leukemia on patient health-related quality of life. *Cancer Treat Rev* 30:103, 2004.

928. Hsu C, Wang JD, Hwang JS, et al: Survival-weighted health profile for long-term survivors of acute myelogenous leukemia. *Qual Life Res* 12:519, 2003.

929. Kern W, Haferlach T, Schoch C, et al: Early blast clearance by remission induction therapy is a major independent prognostic factor for both achievement of complete remission and long-term outcome in acute myeloid leukemia: Data from the German AML Cooperative Group (AMLCG) 1992 Trial. *Blood* 101:64, 2003.

930. Cortes JE, Kantarjian H, O'Brien S, et al: Clinical and prognostic significance of trisomy 21 in adult patients with acute myelogenous leukemia and myelodysplastic syndromes. *Leukemia* 9:115, 1995.

931. Buchner T, Heinecke A: The role of prognostic factors in acute myeloid leukemia. *Leukemia* 10(suppl 1):S28, 1996.

932. Ghaddar HM, Pierce S, Reed P, Estey EH: Prognostic value of residual normal metaphases in acute myelogenous leukemia patients presenting with abnormal karyotype. *Leukemia* 9:779, 1995.

933. Seol JG, Kim ES, Park WH, et al: Telomerase activity in acute myelogenous leukaemia: Clinical and biological implications. *Br J Haematol* 100:156, 1998.

934. Huh Y, Smith TL, Collins P, et al: Terminal deoxynucleotidyl transferase expression in acute myelogenous leukemia and myelodysplasia as determined by flow cytometry. *Leuk Lymphoma* 37:319, 2000.

935. Del Poeta G, Venditti A, Del Principe MI, et al: Amount of spontaneous apoptosis detected by Bax/Bcl-2 ratio predicts outcome in acute myeloid leukemia (AML). *Blood* 101:2125, 2003.

936. Ong YL, McMullin MF, Bailie KE, et al: High bax expression is a good prognostic indicator in acute myeloid leukaemia. *Br J Haematol* 111:182, 2000.

937. Amirghofran Z, Zakerinia M, Shamseddin A: Significant association between expression of the CD11b surface molecule and favorable outcome for patients with acute myeloblastic leukemia. *Int J Hematol* 73:502, 2001.

938. Matsunaga T, Takemoto N, Sato T, et al: Interaction between leukemic-cell VLA-4 and stromal fibronectin is a decisive factor for minimal residual disease of acute myelogenous leukemia. *Nat Med* 9:1158, 2003.

939. Estrov Z, Thall PF, Talpaz M, et al: Caspase 2 and caspase 3 protein levels as predictors of survival in acute myelogenous leukemia. *Blood* 92:3090, 1998.

940. Paietta E: Classical multidrug resistance in acute myeloid leukaemia. *Med Oncol* 14:53, 1997.

941. Ino T, Miyazaki H, Isogai M, et al: Expression of P-glycoprotein in de novo acute myelogenous leukemia at initial diagnosis: Results of molecular and functional assays and correlation with treatment outcome. *Leukemia* 8:1492, 1994.

942. Hart SM, Ganeshaguru K, Hoffbrand AV: Expression of the multidrug resistance-associated protein (MRP) in acute leukaemia. *Leukemia* 8:2163, 1994.

943. Guerci A, Merlin JL, Missoum N, et al: Predictive value for treatment outcome in acute myeloid leukemia of cellular daunorubicin accumulation and P-glycoprotein expression simultaneously determined by flow cytometry. *Blood* 85:2147, 1995.

944. Leith CP, Chen IM, Kopecky KJ, et al: Correlation of multidrug resistance (MDR1) protein expression with functional dye/drug efflux in acute myeloid leukemia by multiparameter flow cytometry: Identification of discordant MDR/efflux+ and MDR1+/efflux- cases. *Blood* 86:2329, 1995.

945. Kohler T, Eller J, Leiblein S, et al: Mechanisms responsible for therapy resistance of acute myelogenous leukemia (AML). *Int J Clin Pharmacol Ther* 36:97, 1998.

946. Filipits M, Stranzl T, Pohl G, et al: Drug resistance factors in acute myeloid leukemia: A comparative analysis. *Leukemia* 14:68, 2000.

947. Massaad-Massade L, Ribrag V, Marie JP, et al: Glutathione system, topoisomerase II level and multidrug resistance phenotype in acute myelogenous leukemia before treatment and at relapse. *Anticancer Res* 17:4647, 1997.

948. Drach D, Zhao S, Drach J, Andreeff M: Low incidence of MDR1 ex-

pression in acute promyelocytic leukaemia. *Br J Haematol* 90:369, 1995.

949. Hoyle CF, DeBastos M, Wheatley K, et al: AML associated with previous cytotoxic therapy, MDS or myeloproliferative disorders: Results from the MRC's 9th AML trial. *Br J Haematol* 72:45, 1989.

950. DeWitte T, Muus P, DePauw B, Haanen C: Intensive antileukemic treatment of patients younger than 65 years with myelodysplastic syndromes and secondary acute myelogenous leukemia. *Cancer* 66:831, 1990.

951. Brito-Babapulle F, Catovsky D, Galton DAG: Clinical and laboratory features of de novo acute myeloid leukaemia with trilineage myelodysplasia. *Br J Haematol* 66:445, 1987.

952. Brito-Babapulle F, Catovsky D, Galton DAG: Myelodysplastic relapse of de novo acute myeloid leukaemia with trilineage myelodysplasia. *Br J Haematol* 68:411, 1988.

953. Rosenthal NS, Farhi DC: Dysmegakaryopoiesis resembling acute megakaryoblastic leukemia in treated acute myeloid leukemia. *Am J Clin Pathol* 95:556, 1991.

954. Layton DM, Ireland RM, Mufti GJ, Bellingham AJ: Myelodysplastic relapse of de novo AML: A heterogenous entity. *Leukemia Res* 11: 1055, 1987.

955. Jowitt SN, Yin JAL, Saunders MJ: Relapsed myelodysplastic clone differs from acute onset clone as shown by X-linked DNA polymorphism patterns in a patient with acute myeloid leukemia. *Blood* 82:613, 1993.

956. O'Brien S, Kantarjian HM, Keating M, et al: Association of granulocytosis with poor prognosis in patients with acute myelogenous leukemia and translocation of chromosomes 8 and 21. *J Clin Oncol* 7: 1081, 1989.

957. Krykowski E, Polkowska-Kulesza E, Robak T, et al: Analysis of prognostic factors in acute leukemias in adults. *Haematol Blood Transf* 30: 369, 1987.

958. Bernard P, Reiffers J, LaComb F, et al: A stage classification for prognosis in adult acute myelogenous leukaemia based upon patient's age, bone marrow karyotype, and clinical features. *Scand J Haematol* 32: 429, 1984.

959. Keating S, Suciu S, De Witte T, et al: The stem cell mobilizing capacity of patients with acute myeloid leukemia in complete remission correlates with relapse risk: Results of the EORTC-GIMEMA AML-10 trial. *Leukemia* 17:60, 2003.

960. Tremblay LN, Hyland RH, Schouten BD, Hanly PJ: Survival of acute myelogenous leukemia patients requiring intubation/ventilatory support. *Clin Invest Med* 18:19, 1995.

961. Hunter AE, Rogers SY, Roberts IAG, et al: Autonomous growth of blast cells is associated with reduced survival in acute myeloblastic leukemia. *Blood* 82:399, 1993.

962. Campos L, Rouault JP, Sabido O, et al: High expression of bcl-2 protein in acute myeloid leukemia cells is associated with poor response to chemotherapy. *Blood* 81:3091, 1993.

963. Kaufmann SH, Karp JE, Svingen PA, et al: Elevated expression of the apoptotic regulator Mcl-1 at the time of leukemic relapse. *Blood* 91: 991, 1998.

964. Zhang W, Xu HJ, Kornblau SM, et al: Growth-factor stimulation reveals two mechanisms of retinoblastoma gene inactivation in human myelogenous leukemia cells. *Leuk Lymphoma* 16:191, 1995.

965. Zhang W, Kornblau SM, Kobayashi T, et al: High levels of constitutive WAFl/Cipl protein are associated with chemoresistance in acute myelogenous leukemia. *Clin Cancer Res* 1:1051, 1995.

966. Raspadori D, Lauria F, Ventura MA, et al: Incidence and prognostic relevance of CD34 expression in acute myeloblastic leukemia: Analysis of 141 cases. *Leuk Res* 21:603, 1997.

967. Dalal Bi, Wu V, Barnett MJ, et al: Induction failure in de novo acute myelogenous leukemia is associated with expression of high levels of CD34 antigen by the leukemic blasts. *Leuk Lymphoma* 26:299, 1997.

968. Lee JJ, Cho D, Chung IJ, et al: CD34 expression is associated with poor clinical outcome in patients with acute promyelocytic leukemia. *Am J Hematol* 73:149, 2003.

969. Shimamoto T, Ohyashiki K, Ohyashiki JH, et al: The expression pattern of erythrocyte/megakaryocyte-related transcription factors GATA-1 and the stem cell leukemia gene correlates with hematopoietic differentiation and is associated with outcome of acute myeloid leukemia. *Blood* 86:3173, 1995.

970. Baer MR, Stewart CC, Lawrence D, et al: Expression of the neural cell adhesion molecule CD56 is associated with short remission duration and survival in acute myeloid leukemia with t(8;21)(q22;q22). *Blood* 90:1643, 1997.

971. Extermann M, Bacchi M, Monai N, et al: Relationship between cleaved L-selectin levels and the outcome of acute myeloid leukemia. *Blood* 92:3115, 1998.

972. Raza A, Preisler HD, Li YQ, et al: Biologic characteristics of newly diagnosed poor prognosis acute myelogenous leukemia. *Am J Hematol* 42:359, 1993.

973. Wetzler M, Baer MR, Bernstein SH, et al: Expression of c-mpl MRNA, the receptor for thrombopoietin, in acute myeloid leukemia blasts identifies a group of patients with poor response to intensive chemotherapy. *J Clin Oncol* 15:2262, 1997.

974. Testa U, Riccioni R, Militi S, et al: Elevated expression of IL-3Ralpha in acute myelogenous leukemia is associated with enhanced blast proliferation, increased cellularity, and poor prognosis. *Blood* 100:2980, 2002.

975. Schnittger S, Kinkelin U, Schoch C, et al: Screening for MLL tandem duplication in 387 unselected patients with AML identify a prognostically unfavorable subset of AML. *Leukemia* 14:796, 2000.

976. Schoch C, Schnittger S, Klaus M, et al: AML with 11q23/MLL abnormalities as defined by the WHO classification: Incidence, partner chromosomes, FAB subtype, age distribution, and prognostic impact in an unselected series of 1897 cytogenetically analyzed AML cases. *Blood* 102:2395, 2003.

977. Di Bono E, Sartori R, Zambello R, et al: Prognostic significance of CD56 antigen expresssion in acute myeloid leukemia. *Haematologica* 87:250, 2002.

978. Kahl C, Florschutz A, Jentsch-Ullrich K, et al: Primary intracranial manifestation of CD7/CD56-positive acute myelogenous leukemia. *Onkologie* 23:580, 2000.

979. Chim CS, Liang R, Tam CY, Kwong YL: Methylation of p15 and p16 genes in acute promyelocytic leukemia: Potential diagnostic and prognostic significance. *J Clin Oncol* 19:2033, 2001.

980. Das-Gupta EP, Seedhouse CH, Russell NH: Microsatellite instability occurs in defined subsets of patients with acute myeloblastic leukaemia. *Br J Haematol* 114:307, 2001.

981. Lee ST, Jang JH, Min YH, et al: AC133 antigen as a prognostic factor in acute leukemia. *Leuk Res* 25:757, 2001.

982. Benekle M, Xia Z, Donohue KA, et al: Constitutive activity of signal transducer and activator of transcription 3 protein in acute myeloid leukemia blasts is associated with short disease-free survival. *Blood* 99:252, 2002.

983. Baldus CD, Tanner SM, Ruppert AS, et al: *BAALC* expression predicts clinical outcome of de novo acyte myeloid leukemia patients with normal cytogenetics. *Blood* 102:1613, 2003.

984. Smith MA, Luxton RW, Pallister CJ, Smith JG: A novel predictive model of outcome in de novo AML based on S-phase activity and proliferative response of blast cells to haemopoietic growth factors. *Leuk Res* 26:345, 2002.

985. Van Doorn-Khosrovani, Erpelinck C, Van Putten WLJ, et al: High *EVI1* expression predicts poor survival in acute myeloid leukemia *Blood* 101:837, 2003.

986. Byrd JC, Mrozek K, Dodge RK, et al: Pretreatment cytogenetic abnormalities are predictive of induction success, cumulative incidence of

relapse, and overall survival in adult patients with de novo acute my-eloid leukemia: Results from Cancer and Leukemia Group B (CALGB 8461). *Blood* 100:4325, 2002.

987. Bradstock K, Matthews J, Benson E, et al: Prognostic value of im-munophenotyping in acute myeloid leukemia. Australian Leukaemia Study Group. *Blood* 84:1220, 1994.

988. Gaiger A, Schmid D, Heinze G, et al: Detection of the WT1 transcript by RT-PCR in complete remission has no prognostic relevance in de novo acute myeloid leukemia. *Leukemia* 12:1886, 1998.

989. Shih LY, Kuo MC, Liang DC, et al: Internal tandem duplication and Asp835 mutations of the FMS-like tyrosine kinase 3 (FLT3) gene in acute promyelocytic leukemia. *Cancer* 98:1206, 2003.

990. Svingen PA, Karp JE, Krajewski S, et al: Evaluation of Apaf-1 and procaspases-2, -3, -7, -8, and -9 as potential prognostic markers in acute leukemia. *Blood* 96:3922, 2000.

991. Heckman KD, Weiner GJ, Burns CP: Persistent thrombocytopenia dur-ing remission in acute leukemia does not preclude long-term disease-free survival. *Am J Hematol* 71:236, 2002.

992. Legrand O, Simonin G, Zittoun R, Marie JP: Lung resistance protein (LRP) gene expression in adult acute myeloid leukemia: A critical eval-uation by three techniques. *Leukemia* 12:1367, 1998.

993. Filipits M, Pohl G, Stranzl T, et al: Expression of the lung resistance protein predicts poor outcome in de novo acute myeloid leukemia. *Blood* 91:1508, 1998.

994. Gale RP, Horowitz MM, Weiner RS, et al: Impact of cytogenetic ab-normalities on outcome of bone marrow transplants in acute myelog-enous leukemia in first remission. *Bone Marrow Transplant* 16:203, 1995.

995. Zapatero A, Martin de Vidales C, Pinar B, et al: Prognostic factors affecting leukemia relapse after allogeneic BMT conditioned with cy-clophosphamide and fractionated TBI. *Bone Marrow Transplant* 18:591, 1996.

996. Sievers EL, Loken MR: Detection of minimal residual disease in acute myelogenous leukemia. *J Pediatr Hematol Oncol* 17:123, 1995.

997. Schnittger S, Weisser M, Schoch C, et al: New score predicting for prognosis in PML-RARA+, AML1-ETO+, or CBFBMYH11+ acute myeloid leukemia based on quantification of fusion transcripts. *Blood* 102:2746, 2003.

998. Nucifora G, Larson RA, Rowley JD: Persistence of the 8;21 translo-cation in patients with acute myeloid leukemia type M2 in long-term remission. *Blood* 82:712, 1993.

999. Estey E, Pierce S: Routine bone marrow exam during first remission of acute myeloid leukemia. *Blood* 87:3899, 1996.

1000. Campana D, Coustan-Smith E: Detection of minimal residual disease in acute leukemia by flow cytometry. *Cytometry* 38:139, 1999.

1001. Adriaansen HJ, Jacobs BC, Kappers-Klunne MC, et al: Detection of residual disease in AML patients by use of double immunological marker analysis for terminal deoxynucleotidyl transferase and myeloid markers. *Leukemia* 7:472, 1993.

1002. Reading CL, Estey EH, Huh YO, et al: Expression of unusual immu-nophenotype combinations in acute myelogenous leukemia. *Blood* 81:3083, 1993.

1003. Kita K, Miwa H, Nakase K, et al: Clinical importance of CD7 expres-sion in acute myelocytic leukemia. The Japan Cooperative Group of Leukemia/Lymphoma. *Blood* 81:2399, 1993.

1004. Porwit-MacDonald A, Janossy G, Ivory K, et al: Leukemia-associated changes identified by quantitative flow cytometry: IV. CD34 overex-pression in acute myelogenous leukemia M2 with t(8;21). *Blood* 87:1162, 1996.

1005. Baer MR, Stewart CC, Dodge RK, et al: High frequency of immuno-phenotype changes in acute myeloid leukemia at relapse: Implications for residual disease detection (Cancer and Leukemia Group B Study 8361). *Blood* 97:3574, 2001.

1006. Arkesteijn GJ, Erpelinck SL, Martens AC, et al: The use of FISH with chromosome specific repetitive DNA probes for the follow-up of leu-kemia patients. Correlations and discrepancies with bone marrow cy-tology. *Cancer Genet Cytogenet* 88:69;1996.

1007. Engel H, Drach J, Keyhani A, et al: Quantitation of minimal residual disease in acute myelogenous leukemia and myelodysplastic syn-dromes in complete remission by molecular cytogenetics of prognitor cells. *Leukemia* 13:568, 1999.

1008. Cilloni D, Gottardi E, De Micheli D, et al: Quantitative assessment of WT1 expression by real time quantitative PCR may be a useful tool for monitoring minimal residual disease in acute leukemia patients. *Leukemia* 16:2115, 2002.

1009. Van der Velden VHJ, Hochhaus A, Gazzaniga G, et al: Detection of minimal residual disease in hematologic malignancies by real-time quantitative PCR: Principles, approaches, and laboratory aspects. *Leu-kemia* 17:1013, 2003.

1010. Hebert J, Cayuela JM, Daniel MT, et al: Detection of minimal residual disease in acute myelomonocytic leukemia with abnormal marrow eo-sinophils by nested polymerase chain reaction with allele specific am-plification. *Blood* 84:2291, 1994.

1011. Laczika K, Novak M, Hilgarth B, et al: Competitive CBFbeta/MYH11 reverse-transcriptase polymerase chain reaction for quantitative as-sessment of minimal residual disease during postremission therapy in acute myeloid leukemia with inversion(16): a pilot study. *J Clin Oncol* 16:1519, 1998.

1012. Costello R, Sainty D, Blaise D, et al: Prognosis value of residual dis-ease monitoring by polymerase chain reaction in patients with CBF beta/MYH11-positive acute myeloblastic leukemia. *Blood* 89:2222, 1997.

1013. Marucci G, Caligiuri MA, Dohner H, et al: Quantification of CBFbeta/MYH11 fusion transcript by real time RT-PCR in patients with INV(16) acute myeloid leukemia. *Leukemia* 15:1072, 2001.

1014. Poirel H, Radford-Weiss I, Rack K, et al: Detection of the chromosome 16 CBF beta-MYH11 fusion transcript in myelomonocytic leukemias. *Blood* 85:1313, 1995.

1015. Buonamici S, Ottaviani E, Testoni N, et al: Real-time quantitation of minimal residual disease in inv(16)-positive acute myeloid leukemia may indicate risk for clinical relapse and may identify patients in a curable state. *Blood* 99:443, 2002.

1016. Erickson P, Gao J, Chank K-S, et al: Identification of breakpoints in t(8;21) acute myelogenous leukemia and isolation of a fusion tran-script, AML 1/ETO with similarity to *Drosophila* segmentation gene, runt. *Blood* 80:1825, 1992.

1017. Nucifora G, Birn DJ, Erickson P, et al: Detection of DNA rearrange-ments in the AML1 and ETO loci and of an AML 1/ETO fusion mRNA in patients with t(8;21) acute myeloid leukemia. *Blood* 81:1573, 1993.

1018. Maseki N, Miyoshi H, Shimuzu K, et al: The 8;21 chromosome trans-location in acute myeloid leukemia is always detectable by molecular analysis using AML 1. *Blood* 81:1573, 1993.

1019. Inokuchi K, Lwakiri R, Futaki M, et al: Minimal residual disease in acute myelogenous leukemia with PML/RAR alpha or AML1/ETO mRNA and phenotypic analysis of possible T and natural killer cells in bone marrow. *Leuk Lymphoma* 29:553, 1998.

1020. Kusec R, Laczika K, Knobl P, et al: AML1/ETO fusion mRNA can be detected in remission blood samples of all patients with t(8;21) acute myeloid leukemia after chemotherapy or autologous bone marrow transplantation. *Leukemia* 8:735, 1994.

1021. Marcucci G, Livak KJ, Bi W, et al: Detection of minimal residual disease in patients with AML1/ETO-associated acute myeloid leuke-mia using a novel quantitative reverse transcription polymerase chain reaction assay. *Leukemia* 12:1482, 1998.

1022. Miyamoto T, Nagafuji K, Akashi K, et al: Persistence of multipotent progenitors expressing AML1/ETO transcripts in long-term remission patients with t(8;21) acute myelogenous leukemia. *Blood* 87:4789, 1996.

1023. Jurlander J, Caligiuri MA, Ruutu T, et al: Persistence of the AML1/ETO fusion transcript in patients treated with allogeneic bone marrow transplantation for t(8;21) leukemia. *Blood* 88:2183, 1996.

1024. Miyamoto T, Nagafuji K, Harada M, et al: Quantitative analysis of AML1/ETO transcripts in peripheral blood stem cell harvests from patients with t(8;21) acute myelogenous leukaemia. *Br J Haematol* 91: 132, 1995.

1025. Miyamoto T, Nagafuji K, Harada M, Niho Y: Significance of quantitative analysis of AML1/ETO transcripts in peripheral blood stem cells from t(8;21) acute myelogenous leukemia. *Leuk Lymphoma* 25:69, 1997.

1026. Tobal K, Liu Yin JA: Molecular monitoring of minimal residual disease in acute myeloblastic leukemia with t(8;21) by RT-PCR. *Leuk Lymphoma* 31:115, 1998.

1027. Muto A, Mori S, Matsushita H, et al: Serial quantification of minimal residual disease of t(8;21) acute myelogenous leukaemia with RT-competitive PCR assay. *Br J Haematol* 95:85, 1996.

1028. Erickson PF, Dessev G, Lasher RS, et al: ETO and AML1 phosphoproteins are expressed in CD34+ hematopoietic progenitors: Implications for t(8;21) leukemogenesis and monitoring residual disease. *Blood* 88:1813, 1996.

1029. Tobal K, Newton J, Macheta M, et al: Molecular quantitation of minimal residual disease in acute myeloid leukemia with t(8;21) can identify patients in durable remission and predict clinical relapse. *Blood* 95:815, 2000.

1030. Takatsuki H, Umemura T, Sadamura S, et al: Detection of minimal residual disease by reverse transcriptase polymerase chain reaction for the PML/RAR alpha fusion MRNA: A study in patients with acute promyelocytic leukemia following peripheral stem cell transplantation. *Leukemia* 9:889, 1995.

1031. Zhao L, Chang KS, Estey EH, et al: Detection of residual leukemic cells in patients with acute promyelocytic leukemia by the fluorescence in situ hybridization method: Potential for predicting relapse. *Blood* 85:495, 1995.

1032. Grimwade D, Lo Coco F: Acute promyelocytic leukemia: A model for the role of molecular diagnosis and residual disease monitoring in a directing treatment approach in acute myeloid leukemia. *Leukemia* 16: 1959, 2002.

1033. Lo Coco F, Breccia M, Diverio D: The importance of molecular monitoring in acute promyelocytic leukaemia. *Best Pract Res Clin Haematol* 16:503, 2003.

1034. Tobal K, Moore H, Macheta M, Liu Yin JA: Monitoring minimal residual diease and preducting relapse in APL by quantitating *PML-RARα* transcripts with a sensitive competitive RT-PCR method. *Leukemia* 15:1060, 2001.

1035. Holowiecki J, Grosicki S, Robak T, et al: Addition of cladribine todaunomycin and cytarabine increases remission rate after a single course of induction treatment in acute myeloid leukemia. Multicenter phase III study. *Leukemia* 18:989, 2004.

1036. Frehling S, Schlenk RF, Stolze I, et al: CEBPA mutation in younger adults with acute myeloid leukemia and normal cytogenetics: Prognostic relevance and analysis of cooperating mutations. *J Clin Oncol* 22:624, 2004.

CHRONIC MYELOGENOUS LEUKEMIA AND RELATED DISORDERS

MARSHALL A. LICHTMAN

JANE L. LIESVELD

The chronic myelogenous leukemias (CMLs) include *BCR* rearrangement-positive CML, chronic myelomonocytic leukemia, juvenile myelomonocytic leukemia, chronic neutrophilic leukemia, chronic monocytic leukemia, and chronic eosinophilic leukemia. The term *chronic*, in contrast to *acute*, once had prognostic implications. However, although the terms remain useful for nosology, they no longer reflect an invariable difference in prognosis. For example, acute myelogenous leukemia in children and young adults has higher remission and cure rates than juvenile or chronic myelomonocytic leukemia in children or adults, respectively.

BCR rearrangement-positive CML presents with anemia, exaggerated granulocytosis, a large proportion of mature neutrophils, absolute basophilia, normal or elevated platelet counts, and, frequently, splenomegaly. The marrow is very hypercellular, and marrow cells contain the Philadelphia chromosome in approximately 90 percent of cases by cytogenetic analysis. A rearrangement of the *BCR* gene on chromosome 22 is present in approximately 95 percent of cases by molecular diagnostic analysis. The disease usually responds to imatinib mesylate, a specific tyrosine kinase inhibitor, and median survival has been extended to beyond 6 years. Allogeneic stem cell transplantation can cure the disease, especially if the transplantation is applied early in the chronic phase. The effect of stem cell transplantation is related in part to a robust graft-versus-leukemia effect, engendered by donor T lymphocytes.

Acronyms and abbreviations that appear in this chapter include: AGP, α_1-acid glycoprotein; ALL, acute lymphocytic leukemia; BCR, breakpoint cluster region; CFU-GM, colony forming unit–granulocyte-monocyte; CLL, chronic lymphocytic leukemia; CML, chronic myelogenous leukemia; CMML, chronic myelomonocytic leukemia; DLI, donor lymphocyte infusion; FISH, fluorescence *in situ* hybridization; G-CSF, granulocyte colony stimulating factor; GM-CSF, granulocyte-monocyte colony stimulating factor; GTP, guanosine triphosphate; GTPase, guanosine triphosphatase; GVHD, graft-versus-host disease; HLA, human leukocyte antigen; HPRT, hypoxanthine phosphoribosyltransferase; hsp, heat shock protein; HUMARA, human androgen receptor assay; IFN, interferon; IL, interleukin; JAK, Janus-associated kinase; LTC-IC, long-term culture-initiating cells; MCP, monocyte chemotactic protein; MDS, myelodysplastic syndrome; MIP, macrophage inflammatory protein; mRNA, messenger RNA; NF-κB, nuclear factor-κB; *NF1*, neurofibromatosis tumor suppressor gene; NK, natural killer; NOD, nonobese diabetic; PCR, polymerase chain reaction; PDGF, platelet-derived growth factor; PDGFR, platelet-derived growth factor receptor; Ph, Philadelphia chromosome; PI3K, phosphatidylinositol-3′-kinase; Rb, retinoblastoma; RT-PCR, reverse transcriptase polymerase chain reaction; SCID, severe combined immunodeficiency; STAT, signal transducer and activator of transcription; TBI, total body irradiation; TdT, terminal deoxynucleotidyl transferase; TGF, transforming growth factor; VEGF, vascular endothelial growth factor; WT, Wilms tumor.

The chronic phase usually is followed by an accelerated phase that often terminates in acute leukemia (blast crisis), at which point therapy with imatinib mesylate and other agents may induce a remission in a proportion of patients, but median survival is measured in months. Blast crisis results in a myelogenous leukemic phenotype in 75 percent of cases and a lymphoblastic leukemic phenotype in approximately 25 percent of cases.

Ph-chromosome–positive acute myeloblastic leukemia may appear *de novo* in approximately 1 percent of cases of AML, and Ph-chromosome–positive acute lymphocytic leukemia (ALL) may occur *de novo* in approximately 20 percent of cases of adult ALL and approximately 5 percent of childhood ALL cases. In Ph-chromosome–positive ALL, the translocation between chromosomes 9 and 22 results in the fusion gene encoding a mutant tyrosine kinase oncoprotein that may be identical in size to that in classic CML, 210 kDa, in approximately one third of cases. A smaller mutant tyrosine kinase, 190 kDa, is encoded in approximately two thirds of cases. In children, the cells in approximately 90 percent of cases contain a 190-kDa mutant tyrosine kinase. These acute leukemias may reflect (1) the presentation of CML in acute blastic transformation without a preceding chronic phase or (2) *de novo* cases resulting from a *BCR-ABL* mutation occurring in a different hematopoietic cell from the event in CML or with as yet unidentified modifying gene alterations.

Chronic myelomonocytic leukemia has variable presenting features. Anemia may be accompanied by mildly or moderately elevated leukocyte counts; an elevated total monocyte count; a low, normal, or elevated platelet count; and sometimes splenomegaly. Although cytogenetic abnormalities may be present, there is no specific genetic marker of the disease. In a small proportion of cases, a translocation involving the platelet-derived growth factor receptor (PDGFR)-β gene is associated with eosinophilia and responsiveness to imatinib mesylate. Juvenile myelomonocytic leukemia occurs in infancy or very early childhood. Anemia, thrombocytopenia, and leukocytosis with monocytosis are usual. The disease is refractory to treatment and, even with current maximal therapy and stem cell rescue, cures are uncommon.

Chronic neutrophilic leukemia presents with mild anemia and exaggerated neutrophilia, with very few immature cells in the blood. Splenomegaly is common. The disease usually occurs after age 60 years and is refractory to current treatment approaches. Chronic and juvenile myelomonocytic leukemia and chronic neutrophilic leukemia have a propensity to evolve into acute myelogenous leukemia. Prior to that time, morbidity and mortality are related to infection, hemorrhage, or complicating medical conditions.

Chronic eosinophilic leukemia represents the major subset of the hypereosinophilic syndrome. It is a clonal disorder with a striking absolute eosinophilia, often neurologic and cardiac manifestations secondary to toxic effects of eosinophil granules, and sometimes a translocation involving the PDGFR-α gene that encodes a mutant tyrosine kinase imparting sensitivity to imatinib mesylate.

DEFINITION AND HISTORY

Chronic myelogenous leukemia (CML) is a pluripotential stem cell disease characterized by anemia, extreme blood granulocytosis and granulocytic immaturity, basophilia, often thrombocytosis, and splenomegaly. The hematopoietic cells contain a reciprocal translocation between chromosomes 9 and 22 in more than 90 percent of patients, which leads to an overtly foreshortened long arm of one of the chromosome pair 22 (i.e., 22, 22q–) referred to as the *Philadelphia (Ph) chromosome*. A rearrangement of the breakpoint cluster region, a segment of the long arm of chromosome 22, defines this form of CML and is present even in the 10 percent of patients without an overt 22q– abnormality. The disease has a very high propensity to evolve into an accelerated phase and/or a rapidly progressive phase resembling acute leukemia, which is very refractory to therapy.

In 1845, Bennett[1] in Scotland and Virchow[2] in Germany reported descriptions of patients with splenic enlargement, severe anemia, and enormous concentrations of leukocytes in their blood at autopsy. Bennett initially favored an extreme pyemia as the explanation, but Virchow argued against suppuration as a cause. Additional cases were reported by Craige[3] and others, and in 1847 Virchow[4] introduced the designation *weisses Blut* and *leukämie* (leukemia). In 1878, Neumann[5] proposed that the marrow not only was the site of normal blood cell production but also was the site from which leukemia originated and used the term *myelogene* (myelogenous) leukemia. Subsequent observations amplified the clinical and laboratory features of the disease, but few fundamental insights were gained until the discovery by Nowell and Hungerford,[6] who reported in 1960 that two patients with the disease had an apparent loss of the long arm of chromosome 21 or 22, an abnormality that was quickly confirmed[7-9] and designated the Philadelphia chromosome.[7] This observation led to a new approach to diagnosis, a marker to study the pathogenesis of the disease, and a focus for future studies of the molecular pathology of the disease. The availability of more sensitive banding techniques to define the structure of chromosomes[10,11] led to the discovery by Rowley[12] that the apparent lost chromosomal material on chromosome 22 was part of a reciprocal translocation between chromosomes 9 and 22. The discovery that the cellular oncogene *ABL* on chromosome number 9 and a segment of chromosome 22, the breakpoint cluster region BCR, fuse as a result of the translocation has provided a basis for the study of the molecular cause of the disease.[13,14] The appreciation that the fusion gene encoded a constitutively active tyrosine kinase that was capable of inducing the disease in mice established the fusion gene as the proximate cause of the malignant transformation. The search for, identification of, and clinical development of a small molecule inhibitor of the mutant kinase has provided a specific agent, imatinib mesylate, with which to inhibit the molecule that incites the disease[15] (see "Etiology and Pathogenesis" below).

EPIDEMIOLOGY

CML accounts for approximately 15 percent of all cases of leukemia or approximately 4600 new cases per year. The disease occurs more often in men than in women (ratio 1.5:1.0) but has similar manifestations and a similar course in both sexes. The age-adjusted incidence rate in the United States is approximately 2.0 per 100,000 persons for men and approximately 1.1 per 100,000 persons for women. The incidence around the world varies by a factor of approximately twofold. The lowest incidence is in Sweden and China (approximately 0.7 per 100,000 persons), and the highest incidence is in Switzerland and the United States (approximately 1.7 per 100,000 persons).[16] Approximately 1600 individuals die of CML annually in the United States, which represents an age-adjusted death rate of approximately 0.9 per 100,000 population per year. The age-specific incidence rate for CML in the United States increases exponentially with age, from approximately 0.5 per 100,000 persons younger than 20 years to a rate of approximately 11.0 per 100,000 octogenarians per year. The mortality rate for CML increases with age, from less than 0.1 per 100,000 population between ages 0 and 14 years to approximately 1.0 per 100,000

in the mid-40s population to over 8.0 per 100,000 in octogenarians per year. Although CML occurs in children and adolescents, less than 10 percent of all cases occur in subjects between 5 and 20 years old. CML represents approximately 3 percent of all childhood leukemias. There is no concordance of the disease between identical twins. A preliminary report indicates that the frequency of the phase I cytochrome P450 (CPY) polymorphism CYP1A1*2A is underrepresented in CML patients compared to controls.[17]

ETIOLOGY AND PATHOGENESIS

ENVIRONMENTAL LEUKEMOGENS

Exposure to very high doses of ionizing radiation can increase the occurrence of CML above the expected frequency in comparable populations. Three major populations, the Japanese exposed to the radiation released by the atomic bomb detonations at Nagasaki and Hiroshima,[18] British patients with ankylosing spondylitis treated with spine irradiation,[19,20] and women with uterine cervical carcinoma who required radiation therapy,[21] had a frequency of CML (as well as acute leukemia) significantly above the frequency expected in comparable unexposed groups. The median latent period was approximately 4 years in irradiated spondylitics, among whom approximately 20 percent of the leukemia cases were CML; 9 years in the uterine cervical cancer patients, of whom approximately 30 percent had CML; and 11 years in the Japanese survivors of the atomic bombs, of whom approximately 30 percent of the leukemia patients had CML.[22] Chemical leukemogens, such as benzene and alkylating agents, have not been identified as causative agents of CML, although they are well established to produce a dose-dependent increase in acute myelogenous leukemia.[23] DNA topoisomerase II inhibitors may be an exception, as they have been found to have a propensity to induce t(9;22)-positive leukemia.[24]

Multiple occurrences of CML in families are rare. One exception to the absence of a familial pattern has been reported,[25] but overall the evidence for inheritance of germline susceptibility genes as a causative factor is virtually nonexistent compared, for example, to chronic lymphocytic leukemia (CLL).[26]

ORIGIN FROM A STEM CELL CLONE

CML results from the malignant transformation of a single stem cell. The disease is acquired (somatic mutation), given that the identical twin of patients with CML and the offspring of mothers with the disease neither carry the Ph chromosome nor develop the disease.[27] The origin of CML from a single hematopoietic stem cell is supported by the following lines of evidence:

1. Involvement of erythropoiesis, neutrophilopoiesis, eosinophilopoiesis, basophilopoiesis, monocytopoiesis, and thrombopoiesis in chronic phase CML[28]
2. Presence of the Ph chromosome (22q–) in erythroblasts; neutrophilic, eosinophilic, and basophilic granulocytes; macrophages; and megakaryocytes[29]
3. Presence of a single glucose-6-phosphate dehydrogenase isoenzyme in red cells, neutrophils, eosinophils, basophils, monocytes, and platelets, but not in fibroblasts or other somatic cells in women with CML who are heterozygotes for isoenzymes A and B[30-32]
4. Presence of the Ph translocation only on a structurally anomalous chromosome 9 or 22 of each chromosome pair in every cell analyzed in occasional patients with a structurally dissimilar 9 or 22 chromosome within the pair[33-35]
5. Presence of the Ph chromosome in one but not the other cell lineage of patients who are a mosaic for sex chromosomes, as in

Turner syndrome (45X/46XX)[36] and Klinefelter syndrome (46XY/47XXY)[37]

6. Molecular studies showing variation in the breakpoint of chromosome 22 among different patients with CML but precisely the same breakpoint among cells within a single patient with CML[38,39]

7. Combined DNA hybridization-methylation analysis of women who have restriction fragment length polymorphisms at the X-linked locus for hypoxanthine phosphoribosyltransferase (HPRT), which enables distinction of the two alleles of the HPRT gene in heterozygous females, coupled with methylation-sensitive restriction enzyme cleavage patterns, which permits delineation of whether cells contain either the maternally derived or the paternally derived copy of the gene[40]

The foregoing observations place the parent cell of the clone at least at the level of the hematopoietic stem cell.

PLURIPOTENTIAL VERSUS HEMATOPOIETIC STEM CELL LESION

Some patients in chronic phase CML have lymphocytes that are derived from the primordial malignant cell. Evidence for this finding includes the following: a single isoenzyme for glucose-6-phosphate dehydrogenase has been found in some T and B lymphocytes in women with CML who are heterozygous for isoenzymes A and B[41]; blood cells from patients with CML induced to proliferate with Epstein-Barr virus (presumptive B lymphocytes) are of the same glucose-6-phosphate dehydrogenase isoenzyme type, have cytoplasmic immunoglobulin heavy and light chains, and contain the Ph chromosome[42]; blood lymphocytes stimulated with B lymphocyte mitogens contain the Ph chromosome[43,44]; purified B lymphocytes from the blood in chronic phase CML contain an abnormal, elongated phosphoprotein coded for by the chimeric gene resulting from the t(9;22)[45]; and fluorescence in situ hybridization (FISH) has detected the BCR-ABL fusion gene in approximately 25 percent of B lymphocytes in some but not all patients in chronic phase.[46,47] These findings suggest that B lymphocytes are derived from the malignant clone, placing the lesion closer to, if not in, the pluripotential stem cell.[41-45] Almost all studies find that the B lymphocyte pool is a mosaic, containing both Ph-chromosome– and BCR-ABL–positive cells and Ph-chromosome– or BCR-ABL–negative cells. Results of studies examining the derivation of T lymphocytes from the malignant clone are more ambiguous but indicate that T lymphocytes are derived from the malignant clone in some but not most patients.[41,43,48-57] Natural killer (NK) cells isolated from patients with chronic phase CML do not contain the BCR-ABL.[58] It is possible that myelopoiesis is invariably clonal and lymphopoiesis is an unpredictable mosaic derived largely from normal residual stem cells. This conclusion is supported by the finding that progenitors of T, B, and NK lymphocytes contain the Ph chromosome and BCR-ABL, but most B cell and all T cell progenitors derived from the leukemic clone undergo apoptosis, leaving unaffected cells in the blood.[59-62]

The cell in which the mutation occurs may be even more primitive in that some endothelial cells generated in vitro express the BCR-ABL fusion gene, as do some cells in the patient's vascular endothelium.[63]

ETIOLOGIC ROLE OF THE PH CHROMOSOME

Early studies indicated that the Ph chromosome may appear after the initial leukemogenic event.[64-67] Patients with CML have developed the Ph chromosome during the course of the disease, have experienced periods of the disease when the Ph chromosome disappeared,[68] or have had Ph-chromosome–positive and Ph-chromosome–negative cells concurrently.[69-73]

Nearly all, if not all, patients with CML have an abnormality of chromosome 22 at a molecular level (BCR rearrangement). Thus, earlier studies indicating an absence of a Ph chromosome were not a valid measure of the normality of chromosome 22. The molecular abnormality in CML involving the ABL gene on chromosome 9 and the BCR gene on chromosome 22 has been established as being the proximate cause of the chronic phase of the disease (see "Molecular Pathology" below).

COEXISTENCE OF NORMAL STEM CELLS

Most, if not all, patients with CML have hematopoietic stem cells that, after treatment[74-76] or culture in vitro,[77-79] use of special cell isolation techniques,[80,81] or use of cell transfer to nonobese diabetic (NOD)/severe combined immunodeficiency (SCID) mice[82] do not have the Ph chromosome[83,84] or the BCR-ABL fusion gene.[85-89] The switch to Ph-chromosome–negative cells in vitro is associated with a loss of monoclonal glucose-6-phosphate dehydrogenase isoenzyme patterns, indicating the persistence and reemergence of normal polyclonal hematopoiesis rather than reversion to a Ph-chromosome–negative clone.[90] In confirmation, BCR–ABL–, CD34+, human leukocyte antigen (HLA)-DR– cells isolated from women with early phase CML are polyclonal using the human androgen receptor assay (HUMARA) to assess X chromosome inactivation patterns.[91] Very primitive hematopoietic cells, the so-called long-term culture-initiating cells (LTC-ICs), are present in Ph-chromosome–negative cytapheresis samples collected during early recovery after chemotherapy for CML.[92] These LTC-ICs are most commonly present when samples are collected within 3 months of diagnosis.[93] Variable levels of BCR-ABL–negative progenitors are found in the CD34+DR– population, but low levels are found in the CD34+CD38– population.[89,94] Preprogenitors for the CD34+DR– cells are predominantly BCR-ABL–negative in both marrow and blood at diagnosis.[95] However, some cells with surface marker characteristics of very primitive normal hematopoietic cells do express the BCR-ABL gene.[96] Both normal and leukemic SCID-repopulating cells coexist in the marrow and blood from CML patients in chronic phase, whereas only leukemic SCID-repopulating cells are detected in blast crisis.[97,98]

PROGENITOR CELL CHARACTERISTICS

PROGENITOR CELL DYSFUNCTION

The leukemic transformation resulting from the BCR-ABL fusion oncogene is maintained by a relatively small number of BCR-ABL stem cells that favor differentiation to self-renewal.[99] This predisposition to differentiation and progenitor cell expansion is mediated by an autocrine interleukin (IL)-3–granulocyte colony stimulating factor (G-CSF) loop.[99] The earliest progenitors have the capacity to undergo marked expansion of erythroid, granulocytic, and megakaryocytic cell populations and have a decreased sensitivity to regulation.[99-101] This expansion is especially dramatic in the more mature progenitor cell compartment.[99,102] The proliferative capacity of individual granulocytic progenitors is decreased compared to normal cells. Thus, the progenitor cell population in marrow and blood expands proportionately more than the increase in granulopoiesis.[103,104] Moreover, the progenitors have buoyant density that is lighter than that of their normal counterparts but similar to that of hepatic fetal granulopoietic progenitors, suggesting an oncofetal pattern.[103] The marked expansion of the total blood granulocyte pool results from a total expansion of granulopoiesis,[102,105] with a minor contribution from prolonged intravascular circulation time.[106] BCR-ABL reduces growth factor dependence of progenitor cells.

Erythroid progenitors are expanded, erythroid precursor maturation is blocked at the basophilic erythroblast stage, and the extent of erythropoiesis is inversely proportional to the total white cell count.[107]

PROGENITOR CELL CHARACTERIZATION

Phenotypic differences of stem and progenitor cells in CML patients compared to normal subjects have been identified.[108] For example, a greater proportion of the circulating leukemic colony forming unit–granulocyte-monocytes (CFU-GMs) express high levels of the adhesion receptor CD44[109] and low levels of L-selectin[110] in contrast to normal cells. Leukemic CD34+ cells overexpress the P glycoprotein that determines the multidrug resistance phenotype.[111]

BCR-ABL–positive progenitors survive less well in long-term culture than do their normal counterparts. Leukemic CFU-GM colonies, unlike normal colonies, decrease in long-term cultures that are deficient in KIT ligand,[112] whereas their proliferation is favored in the presence of KIT ligand.[113] Macrophage inflammatory protein (MIP)-1α does not inhibit growth factor-mediated proliferation of CD34+ cells from CML patients as it does CD34+ cells from normal subjects, even though the MIP-1α receptor is expressed.[114] Another chemokine, monocyte chemotactic protein (MCP)-1, unlike MIP-1α, is an endogenous chemokine that cooperates with transforming growth factor beta (TGF-β) to inhibit the cycling of primitive normal but not CML progenitors in long-term human marrow cultures.[115] Leukemic progenitors are less sensitive than normal progenitors to the antiproliferative effects of TGF-β.[116]

EFFECTS OF BCR-ABL ON CELL ADHESION

Primitive progenitors and blast colony forming cells from patients with CML have decreased adherence to marrow stromal cells.[117,118] This defect is normalized if stromal cells are treated with interferon (IFN)-α.[118,119] As a result, BCR-ABL–negative progenitors are enriched in the adherent fraction of circulating CD34+ cells in chronic phase CML patients. The most primitive BCR-ABL–positive cells in the blood of patients with CML differ from their normal counterparts. They are increased in frequency and are activated, such that signals that block cell mitosis are bypassed.[120]

Ph-chromosome–positive colony forming cells adhere less to fibronectin (and to marrow stroma) than do their normal counterparts. Adhesion is fostered as a result of restoration of cooperation between activated β₁ integrins and the altered epitopes of CD44.[121–123] CML granulocytes have reduced and altered binding to P-selectin because of modification in the CD15 antigens.[124] BCR-ABL–induced defects in integrin function may underlie the abnormal circulation and proliferation of progenitors[125,126] because growth signaling can occur through the fibronectin receptor.[127] IFN-α restores normal integrin-mediated inhibition of hematopoietic progenitor proliferation by the marrow microenvironment.[128]

BCR-ABL–encoded fusion protein p210BCR–ABL binds to actin, and several cytoskeletal proteins are thereby phosphorylated. The p210BCR–ABL interacts with actin filaments through an actin-binding domain. BCR-ABL transfection is associated with increased spontaneous motility, membrane ruffling, formation of long actin extensions (filopodia), and accelerated rate of protrusion and retraction of pseudopodia on fibronectin-coated surfaces. IFN-α treatment slowly converts the abnormal motility phenotype of BCR-ABL–transformed cells toward normal.[129] Integrins regulate the c-ABL–encoded tyrosine kinase activity and its cytoplasmic-nuclear transport.[130] The p210BCR–ABL abrogates the anchorage requirement but not the growth factor requirement for proliferation.[131]

In normal cells exposed to IL-3, paxillin tyrosine residues are phosphorylated. In cells transformed by p210BCR–ABL, the tyrosines of paxillin, vinculin, p125FAK, talin, and tensin are constitutively phosphorylated. Pseudopodia enriched in focal adhesion proteins[131,132] are present in cells expressing p210BCR–ABL.

The sum of evidence suggests that defects in adhesion (contact and anchoring) of CML primitive cells remove them from their controlling signals normally received from microenvironmental cells via cytokine messages. These signals retain the balance among cell survival, cell death, cell proliferation, and cell differentiation. Inappropriate phosphorylation of cytoskeletal proteins, possibly independent of tyrosine kinase, is thought to be the key factor in disturbed integrin function of CML cells.

MOLECULAR PATHOLOGY

Ph CHROMOSOME

The genic disturbance became evident with the knowledge that CML was derived from a primitive cell containing a 22q– abnormality.[6,11] The abnormal chromosome contained only 60 percent of the DNA in other G-group chromosomes.[133] Cytogenetic analysis indicated the G-group chromosome involved was different from the extra G-group chromosome in Down syndrome, which had been assigned number 21. Thus, the former was assigned number 22—even though it proved to be slightly longer than the chromosome involved in Down syndrome.[11,134] The Paris Conference on Nomenclature decided not to undo the concept that Down syndrome is trisomy 21 and assigned the Ph chromosome and its normal counterpart, 22.[135] Using quinacrine (Q) and Giemsa (G) banding, Rowley[12] reported in 1973 that the material missing from chromosome 22 was not lost (deleted) from the cell but was translocated to the distal portion of the long arm of chromosome 9. The amount of material translocated to chromosome 9 was approximately equivalent to that lost from 22, and the translocation was predicted to be balanced.[12] Moreover, the breaks were localized to band 34 on the long arm of 9 and band 11 on the long arm of 22. Therefore, the classic Ph chromosome is t(9;22)(q34;q11), abbreviated t(Ph) (Fig. 88-1). The Ph chromosome can develop on either the maternal or the paternal member of the pair.[136]

MUTATION OF ABL AND BCR GENES

Mutations of the ABL gene on chromosome 9 and of the BCR gene on chromosome 22 are central to the development of CML (Fig. 88-2).[137–139]

In 1982, the human cellular homologue ABL of the transforming sequence of the Abelson murine leukemia virus was localized to human chromosome 9.[140] In 1983, ABL was shown to be on the segment of chromosome 9 that is translocated to chromosome 22[141] by demonstrating reaction to hybridization probes for ABL only in somatic cell hybrids of human CML cells containing 22q– but not those containing 9q+. ABL is closely homologous to the viral oncogene v-abl, which is the cell-transforming portion of the gene. This gene can induce malignant transformation of cells in culture and can induce leukemia in susceptible mice.[142]

The ABL gene is rearranged and amplified in cell lines from patients with CML.[143] Cell lines and fresh isolates of CML cells contain an abnormal, elongated 8-kb RNA transcript,[144–147] which is transcribed from the new chimeric gene produced by the fusion of the 5′ portion of the BCR gene left on chromosome 22 with the 3′ portion of the ABL gene translocated from chromosome 9[141] (Fig. 88-3). The fusion messenger RNA (mRNA) leads to the translation of a unique tyrosine phosphoprotein kinase of 210 kDa (p210BCR–ABL), which can phosphorylate tyrosine residues on cellular proteins similar to the action of the v-abl protein product.[148–152] The anomalous tyrosine kinase is difficult to identify in chronic phase cells because of inhibitors in granulocytes[152]; molecular variants reflect variations in the breakpoint on chromosome 22.[153]

The *ABL* locus contains at least two alleles, one having a 500-bp deletion.[154] In normal cells, the *ABL* protooncogene codes for a tyrosine kinase of molecular weight 145,000, which is translated only in trace quantities and lacks any *in vitro* kinase activity.[149] The fusion product expressed by the *BCR-ABL* gene is hypothesized to lead to malignant transformation because of the abnormally regulated phosphorylating activity of the chimeric tyrosine protein kinase.[150,151,155,156] Construction of *BCR-ABL* fusion genes indicated that *BCR* sequences could also activate a microfilament-binding function, but the tyrosine kinase and microfilament-binding functions were not linked. Nevertheless, tyrosine kinase modification of actin filament function has been proposed as a step in leukemogenesis.[157]

P210^BCR-ABL FUSION PROTEIN

The breakpoints on chromosome 9 are not narrowly clustered, ranging from approximately 15 to more than 40 kb upstream from the most proximate region (first exon) of the *ABL* gene.[140,141,158] The breakpoints on chromosome 22 occur over a very short, approximately 5 to 6 kb, stretch of DNA referred to as the breakpoint cluster region (M-*bcr*),[159,160] which is part of a much longer breakpoint cluster region gene, *BCR*[161,162] (see Fig. 88-3). Three main breakpoint cluster regions have been characterized on chromosome 22: major (M-*bcr*), minor (m-*bcr*), and micro (μ-*bcr*). They encode a p210, p190, and p230 fusion protein, respectively (see Fig. 88-2). The overwhelming majority of CML patients have a *BCR-ABL* fusion gene that encodes a fusion protein of 210 kDa (p210^BCR-ABL) and for which mRNA transcripts have a b3a2 or a b2a2 fusion junction[163] (see Fig. 88-2). A *BCR-ABL* with an e1a2 type of junction has been identified in approximately 50 percent of the Ph-chromosome–positive acute lymphoblastic leukemia cases (see "Ph-Chromosome–Positive Acute Leukemia" below) and results in the production of a *BCR-ABL* protein of 190 kDa (p190^BCR-ABL). Almost all CML cases at diagnosis that encode a p210^BCR-ABL also express *BCR-ABL* transcripts for p190.[164] The biologic or clinical significance of these dual transcripts is not known. Transgenic mice expressing p210^BCR-ABL develop acute lymphoblastic leukemia in the founder mice, but all transgenic progeny have a myeloproliferative disorder resembling CML.[165]

The *BCR* gene encodes a 160-kDa serine-threonine kinase, which, when it oligomerizes, autophosphorylates and transphosphorylates several protein substrates.[166] Aberrant methylation of the M-*bcr* in CML occurs.[163] The first exon sequences of the *BCR* gene potentiate the tyrosine kinase of *ABL* when they fuse as a result of the translocation.[167] The central portion of *BCR* has homology to *DBL*, a gene involved in the control of cell division after the S phase of the cell cycle. The C-terminus of *BCR* has a guanosine triphosphatase (GTPase)-activating protein for p21^rac, a member of the *RAS* family of guanosine triphosphate (GTP)-binding proteins.[168] A reciprocal hybrid gene *ABL-BCR* is formed on chromosome 9q+ when *BCR-ABL* fuses on chromosome 22. The *ABL-BCR* fusion gene actively transcribes in most patients with CML.[169]

Variations in breakpoints involving smaller stretches of chromosome 9 and rearrangements outside the M-*bcr* of chromosome 22 can

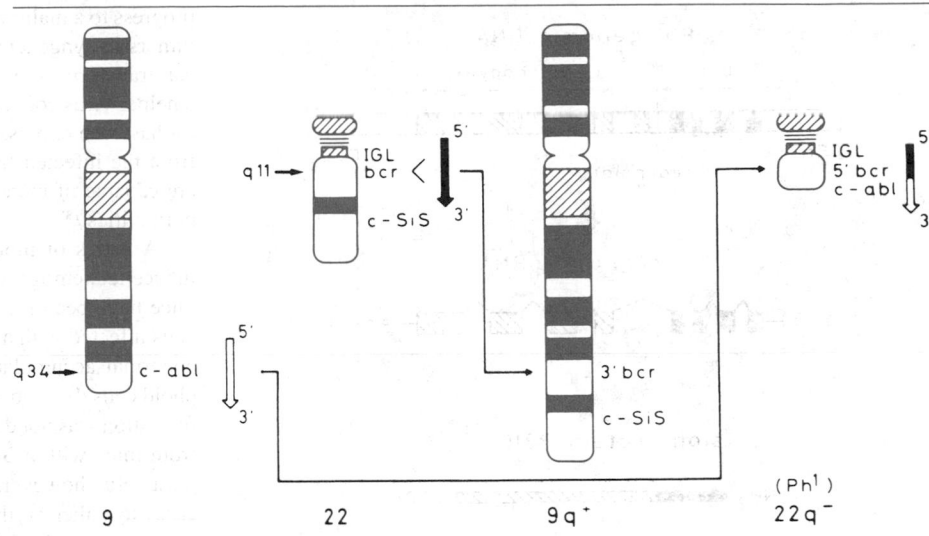

FIGURE 88-1   Schematic diagram of normal chromosome 9 showing the *ABL* gene between band q34 and qter of chromosome 22, which has the *BCR* and *SIS* genes between band q11 and qter. The t(9;22) is shown on the *right*. The *ABL* from chromosome 9 is transposed to the chromosome 22 M-*bcr* sequences, and the terminal portion of chromosome 22 is transposed to the long arm of chromosome 9. The 22q– is the Ph chromosome. bcr, breakpoint cluster region; c-SiS, cellular homologue of the viral simian sarcoma virus-transforming gene; IgL, gene for immunoglobulin light chains. (From De Klein A: Oncogene activation by chromosomal rearrangement in chronic myelocytic leukemia. *Mutat Res* 186:161, 1987, with permission.)

occur.[39] In a few cases of CML with no evident elongation of chromosome 9, molecular probes have shown that *ABL* still is translocated to chromosome 22.[170] In occasional patients with Ph-chromosome-positive CML, the break in chromosome 22 is outside the M-*bcr*, and

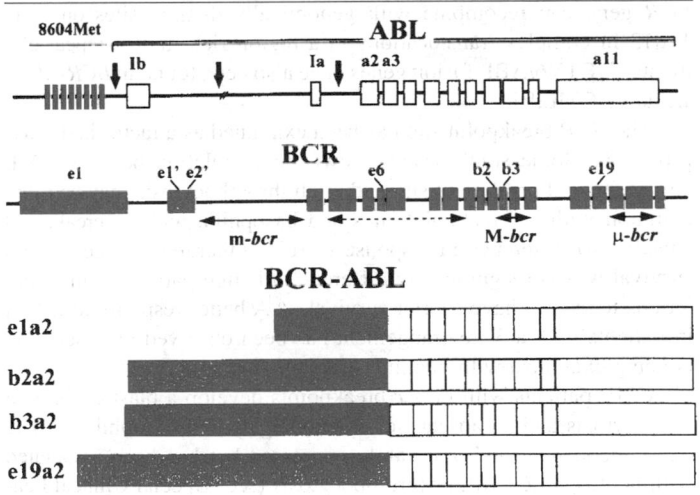

FIGURE 88-2   Schematic representation of the normal *ABL* and *BCR* genes and of the *BCR-ABL* fusion transcripts. In the *upper panel* of the diagram, the possible breakpoint positions in *ABL* are marked by *vertical arrows*. Note the position immediately upstream of the *ABL* locus of the 8604Met gene, for which the function is unknown. The *BCR* gene contains 25 exons, including first (e1') and second (e2') exons. The positions of the three breakpoint cluster regions, m-*bcr*, M-*bcr*, and μ-*bcr*, are shown. The *lower panel* of the figure shows the structure of the *BCR-ABL* messenger RNA fusion transcripts. Breakpoints in μ-*bcr* result in *BCR-ABL* transcripts with an e19a2 junction. *b* and *e* represent the breakpoint in *ABL*. The associated number designates the exon (location) at which the break occurs in each gene. (From ref. 179, with permission.)

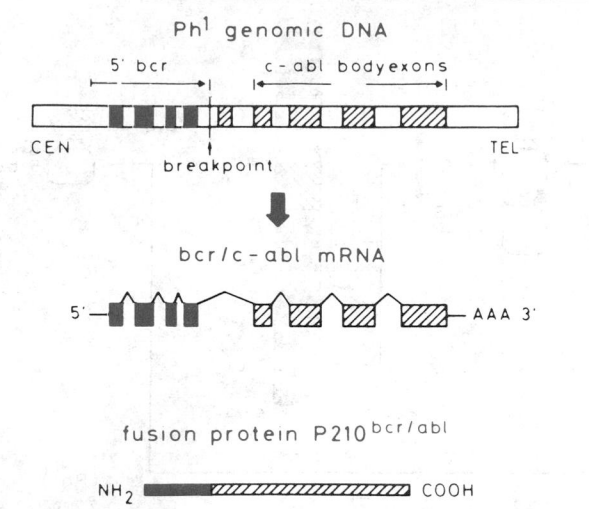

FIGURE 88-3 Molecular effects of the Ph chromosome translocation t(9;22)(q34;q11). The *upper panel* shows the physically joined 5′ *BCR* and the 3′ *ABL* regions on chromosome 22. The exons are *solid* (from chromosome 22, *BCR*) and *hatched* (from chromosome 9, *ABL*). The *middle panel* depicts transcription of chimeric messenger RNA. The *lower panel* shows the translated fusion protein with the amino-terminus derived from the *BCR* of chromosome 22 and the carboxy-terminus from the *ABL* of chromosome 9. (From De Klein A: Oncogene activation by chromosomal rearrangement in chronic myelocytic leukemia. *Mutat Res* 186:161, 1987, with permission.)

transcription of a fusion RNA of the usual type fails or a fusion RNA is transcribed that does not hybridize with the classic M-*bcr* cDNA probe.[171]

In cases in which the Ph chromosome is not found, *BCR-ABL* still may be located on chromosome 9 (a masked Ph chromosome).[172] The *BCR* gene can recombine with genomically distinct sites on band 11q13 in complex translocations in a region rich in Alu repeat elements.[173] ETV6/ABL fusion genes have also been found in *BCR-ABL*–negative CML.[174]

The *BCR* breakpoint site has been examined as a factor in disease prognosis. Some studies have shown no correlation between CML chronicity and breakpoint site, although thrombocytosis may be more common with 3′ breakpoint sites and basophilia with 5′ breakpoint sites.[175] No difference in response to IFN-α therapy was noted, and survival was not significantly different, although patients with 3′ deletions tended to have shorter survival.[176] A better response to IFN-α in patients with a 3′ rearrangement has been observed by others and is being examined with imatinib mesylate therapy.[177]

CML patients with m-*bcr* breakpoints develop a blast crisis with monocytosis and an absence of splenomegaly and basophilia.[178] The p230 encoded by μ-*bcr* is rarely expressed but has been associated with neutrophilic CML or thrombocytosis (see "Special Clinical Features" below). Other rare breakpoints have been described.[179] For example, a case with a 12-bp insert between BCR1 and ABL1 resulted in a *BCR-ABL*–negative (false-negative), Ph-chromosome–positive CML with thrombocythemia.[180] Another novel *BCR-ABL* fusion gene (e6a2) in a patient with Ph-chromosome–negative CML encoded an oncoprotein of 185 kDa.[181] Typical CML has also been associated with an e19a2 junction *BCR-ABL* transcript.[182]

Experimental support for the hypothesis that p210[bcr-abl] tyrosine phosphoprotein kinase is transforming is provided by a retroviral gene transfer system that permits expression of the protein. Mouse marrow cells transfected with *BCR-ABL* develop clonal outgrowths of immature cells expressing the p210[BCR-ABL] tyrosine kinase. Some clones

progress to a malignant phenotype, can be transplanted, and can induce tumors in syngeneic mice.[183] Similar studies suggest the p210[BCR-ABL] can transform 3T3 murine fibroblasts if the *gag* gene sequence from a helper virus cooperates.[184] The *BCR-ABL* gene from a retroviral vector has been expressed in an IL-3–dependent cell line. Clones derived from the infected line transform over months to IL-3 independency, are capable of increased proliferation, and develop chromosomal abnormalities.[185]

A series of mouse models in which the *BCR-ABL* was used to induce leukemogenesis have been described.[186–194] Lethally irradiated mice have been reconstituted with marrow enriched for cycling stem cells infected with a *BCR-ABL*–bearing retrovirus. Fatal diseases with abnormal accumulations of macrophagic, erythroid, mast, and lymphoid cells develop.[185] Classic CML did not occur, and complete transformation was not documented. The cell lines from spleen and marrow from mice with a *BCR-ABL* retrovirus infection were predominantly mast cells; however, these cell lines spontaneously switched in some cases to either erythroid and megakaryocytic, erythroid, or granulocytic lineages displaying maturation. They were transplantable (transformed) and contained the same proviral inserts as the original mast cell line.[195] Murine marrow also has been infected with a retrovirus encoding p210[BCR-ABL] and transplanted into irradiated syngeneic recipients.[186] Although several types of hematologic malignancies developed, a syndrome mimicking human CML also occurred. Mice transgenic for a p190[BCR-ABL] develop an acute lymphocytic leukemia (ALL)-lymphoma syndrome,[187] resembling human Ph-chromosome–positive ALL. When a p210[BCR-ABL] transcript is introduced into a mouse germ line (one-cell fertilized eggs), the p210 founder and progeny transgenic animals developed leukemia of B or T lymphoid or of myeloid origin after a relatively long latency period. In contrast, p190–transgenic mice exclusively developed leukemia of B cell origin, with a relatively short period of latency. This finding was believed to be consistent with the apparent indolence of human CML during the chronic phase.[188] When transgenic mice express p210[BCR-ABL], the transgenes develop ALL, whereas the progeny develop a myeloproliferative disorder.[189]

Mouse models remain important for exploring the pathogenesis of the acute and chronic BCR-ABL mediated leukemias *in vivo* and in examining the potential effects of new drugs targeted at BCR-ABL.[196]

BCR-ABL IN HEALTHY SUBJECTS

BCR-ABL fusion genes can be found in the leukocytes of some normal individuals using a two-step reverse transcriptase polymerase chain reaction assay. Thus, while *BCR-ABL* may be expressed relatively frequently in hematopoietic cells, only infrequently do the cells acquire the additional changes necessary to produce leukemia.[197]

BCR-ABL AND SIGNAL TRANSDUCTION

The tyrosine phosphoprotein kinase activity of the p210[BCR-ABL] has been causally linked to the development of Ph-chromosome–positive leukemia in man.[198–209] The p210[BCR-ABL] interacts with several components of signal transduction pathways[202,203,210] and binds and/or phosphorylates more than 20 cellular proteins in its role as an oncoprotein.[203] A subunit of phosphatidylinositol-3′-kinase (PI3K) associates with p210[BCR-ABL]; this interaction is required for the proliferation of *BCR-ABL*–dependent cell lines and primary CML cells. Wortmannin, a nonspecific inhibitor of the p110 subunit of the kinase, inhibits growth of these cells.[204]

The pathways and interactions invoked by BCR-ABL acting on mitogen-activated protein kinases are multiple and complex.[211,212]

An RAF-encoded serine-threonine kinase activity is regulated by p210[BCR-ABL]. Down-regulation of RAF expression inhibits both

BCR-ABL–dependent growth of CML cells and growth factor–dependent proliferation of normal hematopoietic progenitors.[205]

The efficiency of cell transformation by *BCR-ABL* is affected by an adaptor protein that can interrelate tyrosine kinase signals to RAS. The p210[BCR–ABL] also activates multiple alternative pathways of RAS.[206] PI3K is constitutively activated by BCR-ABL, generates inositol lipids, and is dysregulated by the down-regulation by BCR-ABL of polyinositol phosphates tumor suppressors, such as PTEN and SHIP1.[210] Figure 88-4 demonstrates interaction of p210[bcr–abl] with various mediators of signal transduction.

Reactive oxygen species are increased in BCR-ABL–transformed cells and may act as a second messenger to modulate enzymes regulated by the redox equilibrium. An increase in these reactive oxygen products is postulated to play a role in the acquisition of additional mutations as a result of production of reactive oxygen species through the chronic phase, contributing to the progression to accelerated phase.[210,213]

The adaptor molecule CRKL is a major *in vivo* substrate for p210[BCR–ABL], and it acts to relate p210[BCR–ABL] to downstream effectors. CRKL is a linker protein that has homology to the v-*crk* oncogene product. Antibodies to CRKL immunoprecipitate paxillin, a focal adhesion protein[207] that is phosphorylated by p210[BCR–ABL]. The p210[BCR–ABL] may be physically linked to paxillin by CRKL. CRKL binds to CBL, an oncogene product that induces B cell and myeloid leukemias in mice.[208] The Src homology 3 domains of CRKL do not bind to CBL, but they do bind

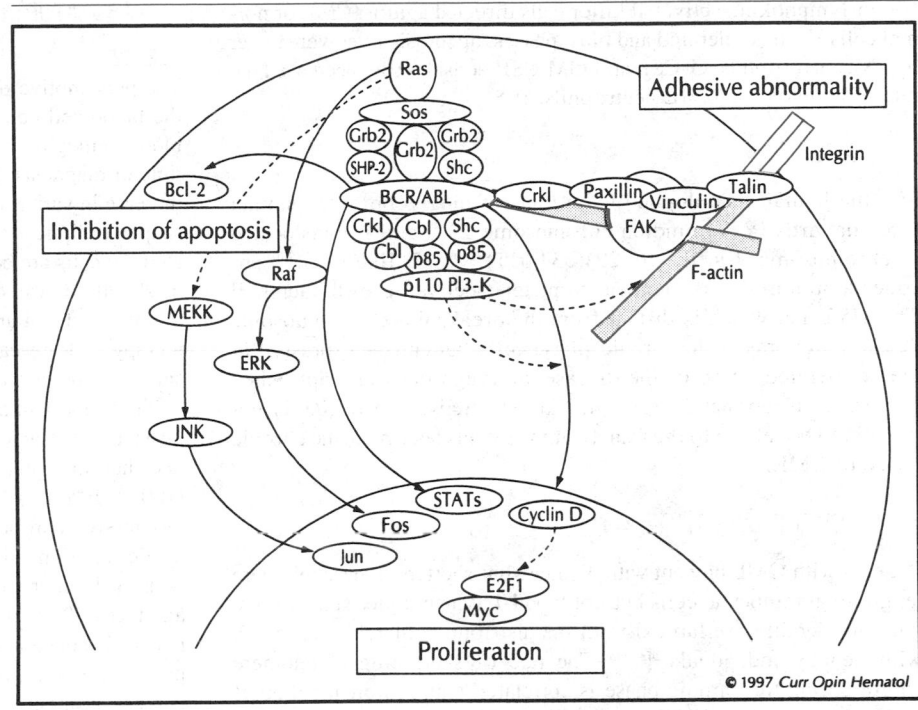

FIGURE 88-4 Major intracellular signaling events associated with *BCR/ABL*. Constitutive activation of ABL protein tyrosine kinase (PTK) induces phosphorylation of the tyrosine moiety of various substrates, including autophosphorylation of *BCR/ABL* and complex formation of *BCR/ABL* with adaptor proteins. This process subsequently activates multiple intracellular signaling pathways, including *RAS* activation and phosphatidylinositol-3′-kinase (PI3-K) activation pathways. *BCR/ABL* also activates the c-MYC pathway, which involves *ABL*-SH2 domain. *BCR/ABL* inhibits apoptosis, possibly in part through up-regulation of Bcl-2, and alters cellular adhesive properties, possibly by interacting with focal adhesion proteins and the actin cytomatrix. *Broken lines* indicate hypothetical pathways. ERK, extracellular signal-regulated kinase; FAK, focal adhesion kinase; JNK, Jun N-terminal kinase; MEKK, MEK kinase; Sos, Son-of-sevenless; STAT, signal transducer and activator of transcription. (From Gotoh A, Broxmeyer HE: The function of BCR/ABL and related proto-oncogenes. *Curr Opin Hematol* 4:3, 1997, with permission.)

BCR-ABL. Therefore, CRKL mediates the oncogenic signal of *BCR-ABL* to CBL. The p120[CBL] and the adaptor proteins CRKL and c-CRK also link c-abl, p190[BCR–ABL], and p210[BCR–ABL] to the PI3K pathway.[209] The p120[CBL] also coprecipitates with the p85 subunit of PI3K, CRKL, and c-CRK. The p210[BCR–ABL] may, therefore, induce the formation of multimeric complexes of signaling proteins.[214] These complexes contain paxillin and talin and may explain some of the adhesive defects of CML cells.[215]

Hef2 also binds to CRKL in leukemic tissues of p190[BCR–ABL] transgenic mice. Hef2 is involved in the integrin signaling pathway[216] and encodes a protein that accelerates GTP hydrolysis of RAS-encoded proteins and neurofibromin. The latter negatively regulates granulocyte-monocyte colony stimulating factor (GM-CSF) signaling through RAS in hematopoietic cells.[217] P62[DOK], a constitutively tyrosine-phosphorylated, p120[RAS] GAP-associated protein, which is rapidly tyrosine-phosphorylated upon activation of the c-*kit* receptor,[218] is also associated with ABL.[219]

Nuclear factor (NF)-κB activation is also required for p210[BCR–ABL]-mediated transformation.[220] Expression of p210[BCR–ABL] leads to activation of NF-κB–dependent transcription via nuclear translocation.[221]

Cell lines that express p210[BCR–ABL] also demonstrate constitutive activation of Janus-associated kinases (JAKs) and signal transducers and activators of transcription (STATs), usually STAT5.[222] STAT5 is also activated in primary mouse bone marrow cells acutely transformed by the *BCR-ABL*[223]; p210[BCR–ABL] coimmunoprecipitates with

and constitutively phosphorylates the common β-subunit of the IL-3 and GM-CSF receptors and JAK2.[224] Both *ABL* and *BCR* are also multifunctional regulators of the GTP-binding protein family Rho[225,226] and the growth factor–binding protein Grb2, which links tyrosine kinases to RAS and forms a complex with *BCR-ABL* and the nucleotide exchange factor Sos that leads to activation of *RAS*.[227]

The p210[BCR–ABL] also activates Jun kinase and requires Jun for transformation.[228] In some CML cell lines, p210[BCR–ABL] is associated with the retinoblastoma (Rb) protein.[229] Loss of the neurofibromatosis (*NF1*) tumor suppressor gene, a RAS GTPase activating protein, also is sufficient to produce a myeloproliferative syndrome in mice akin to human CML resulting from RAS-mediated hypersensitivity to GM-CSF.[230]

EFFECTS OF BCR-ABL ON APOPTOSIS

Whether p210[bcr–abl] influences the expansion of the malignant clone in CML by inhibiting apoptosis is uncertain. In one study, the survival of normal and CML progenitors was the same after *in vitro* incubation in serum-deprived conditions and after treatment with X-irradiation or glucocorticoids.[231] P210[BCR–ABL] inhibits apoptosis by delaying the G₂/M transition of the cell cycle after DNA damage.[232] The p210[BCR–ABL] also may exert an antiapoptotic effect in factor-dependent hematopoietic cells.[233,234]

P210[BCR–ABL] does not prevent apoptotic death induced by human

NK or lymphokine-activated killer cells directed against CML or normal cells.[235] In accelerated and blast phases, apoptosis rates were lower in CML neutrophils. G-CSF and GM-CSF considerably decreased the rate of apoptosis in CML neutrophils.[236]

SIS GENE

SIS, the human homologue of the transforming gene of the simian sarcoma virus,[237] is found on chromosome 22[238] and is translocated to chromosome 9 in the t(9;22)(q34;q11).[239] SIS, like v-sis,[240] encodes a protein that is identical to platelet-derived growth factor.[241] The SIS gene, which is distant from the breakpoint on chromosome 22, is not expressed in chronic phase cells but can be expressed in the accelerated phase of the disease, although the transcript, when expressed, is normal in size (4.0 kb).[242] Activation of SIS is not thought to be related to the transforming events leading to the chronic phase of CML.

TELOMERE LENGTH

Patients with CML present with a somewhat shortened mean telomere length in granulocytic cells but not blood T lymphocytes at diagnosis, but considerable overlap exists in the distribution of telomere length with healthy individuals.[243–245] The rate of shortening of telomere length during the chronic phase is correlated with a more rapid onset of accelerated phase.[243,245] A further significant decrease in telomere length occurs in the accelerated phase of CML. Telomerase activity is increased in the accelerated phase.[246] When therapy permits restoration of Ph-negative cells in the blood, these cells have telomere length comparable to that in matched healthy controls.[247]

CLINICAL FEATURES

SIGNS AND SYMPTOMS

In the 70 percent of patients who are symptomatic at diagnosis, the most frequent complaints include easy fatigability, loss of sense of well-being, decreased tolerance to exertion, anorexia, abdominal discomfort, and early satiety (related to splenic enlargement), weight loss, and excessive sweating.[248–250] The symptoms are vague, nonspecific, and gradual in onset (weeks to months). A physical examination may detect pallor and splenomegaly. The latter was present in approximately 90 percent of patients at diagnosis, but with medical care being sought earlier, the presence of splenomegaly at the time of diagnosis is decreasing in frequency.[249] Sternal tenderness, especially the lower portion, is common; occasionally, patients notice it themselves.

Uncommon presenting symptoms include those of dramatic hypermetabolism (night sweats, heat intolerance, weight loss) simulating thyrotoxicosis; acute gouty arthritis, presumably related in part to hyperuricemia; priapism, tinnitus, or stupor from the leukostasis associated with greatly exaggerated blood leukocyte count elevations[251–253]; left upper quadrant and left shoulder pain as a consequence of splenic infarction and perisplenitis; vasopressin-responsive diabetes insipidus[254,255]; and acne urticata associated with hyperhistaminemia.[256] Acute febrile neutrophilic dermatosis (Sweet syndrome), a perivascular infiltrate of neutrophils in the dermis, can occur. Fever accompanied by painful maculonodular violaceous lesions on the trunk, arms, legs, and face are characteristic.[257,258] Spontaneous rupture of the spleen is a rare event.[259,260] Digital necrosis has been reported as a rare paraneoplastic event.[261,262]

In an increasing proportion of patients, the disease is discovered, coincidentally, when blood cell counts are measured at a "routine" medical examination.

LABORATORY FINDINGS

BLOOD

The presumptive diagnosis of CML can be made from the results of the blood cell counts and examination of the blood film.[28,248,249] The blood hemoglobin concentration is decreased in most patients at the time of diagnosis. Red cells usually are only slightly altered, with an increase in variation from small to large size and only occasional misshapen (elliptical or irregular) erythrocytes. Small numbers of nucleated red cells are commonly present. The reticulocyte count is normal or slightly elevated, but clinically significant hemolysis is rare.[248,263] A positive direct antiglobulin test may develop in patients during IFN therapy.[264] Rare cases of mild erythrocytosis[265,266] or erythroid aplasia[267,268] have been documented.

The total leukocyte count is always elevated at the time of diagnosis and is nearly always greater than $25,000/\mu l$ (25×10^9/liter); at least half the patients have total white counts greater than $100,000/\mu l$ (100×10^9/liter)[28,248,249] (Fig. 88-5). The total leukocyte count rises progressively in untreated patients. Rare patients may have dramatic cyclic variations in white cell counts as much as an order of magnitude with cycle intervals of approximately 60 days.[269,270] Granulocytes at all stages of development are present in the blood and are generally normal in appearance (see Color Plates XIX-1–6). The mean blast cell prevalence is approximately 3 percent but can range from 0 to 10 percent; progranulocyte prevalence is approximately 4 percent; myelocytes, metamyelocytes, and bands account for approximately 40 percent; and segmented neutrophils account for approximately 35 percent of total leukocytes (Table 88-1). Hypersegmented neutrophils are commonly present.

Neutrophil alkaline phosphatase activity is low or absent in more than 90 percent of patients with CML.[271–273] The mRNA for alkaline phosphatase is undetectable in neutrophils of patients with CML.[274] The activity increases toward or to normal in the presence of intense inflammation or infection and when the total leukocytic count is decreased to or near normal with treatment.[273,275] CML neutrophils regain alkaline phosphatase activity after infusion into leukopenic recipients, suggesting the effect of regulators or factors extrinsic to the neutrophils.[276] In vitro, a monocyte-derived soluble mediator is capable of inducing increased alkaline phosphatase activity in neutrophils from CML patients.[277] Neutrophil alkaline phosphate is decreased sporadically in a variety of disorders and conditions[278] but is decreased markedly and consistently in paroxysmal nocturnal he-

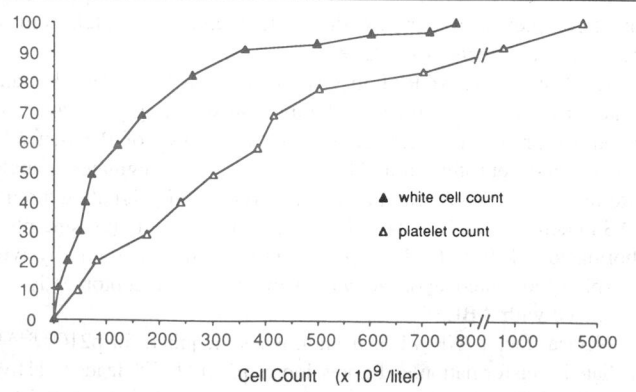

FIGURE 88-5 Total white cell count and platelet count of 90 patients with CML at the time of diagnosis. The cumulative percent of patients is on the *ordinate*, and the cell count is on the *abscissa*. Fifty percent of patients had a white cell count greater than 100×10^9/liter and a platelet count greater than approximately 300×10^9/liter at the time of diagnosis.

TABLE 88-1   BLOOD WHITE CELL DIFFERENTIAL COUNT AT THE TIME OF
DIAGNOSIS IN 90 CASES OF CHRONIC MYELOGENOUS
LEUKEMIA

	PERCENT OF TOTAL LEUKOCYTES (MEAN VALUES)
Myeloblasts	3
Promyelocytes	4
Myelocytes	12
Metamyelocytes	7
Band forms	14
Segmented forms	38
Basophils	3
Eosinophils	2
Nucleated red cells	0.5
Monocytes	8
Lymphocytes	8

SOURCE: University of Rochester Medical Center.
NOTE: In these 90 patients, the mean hematocrit was 31 ml/dl, mean total white cell count was 160×10^9/liter, and mean platelet count was 442×10^9/liter at the time of diagnosis.

moglobinuria,[278] in hypophosphatasia,[279] in approximately one fourth of patients with idiopathic myelofibrosis, and in patients using androgens. Neutrophil alkaline phosphatase is increased in polycythemia vera, in 25 percent of patients with idiopathic myelofibrosis, in pregnant women, and in subjects with inflammatory disorders or infections.

The proportion of eosinophils usually is not increased, but the absolute eosinophil count nearly always is increased. Rarely, eosinophils are so prominent that they dominate the granulocytic cells and lead to the designation *Ph-positive eosinophilic CML*. An absolute increase in the basophil concentration is present in almost all patients, and this finding can be useful in preliminary consideration of the differential diagnosis.[28,280] Basophilic progenitor cells are increased in the blood.[281] The proportion of basophils usually is not greater than 10 to 15 percent during the chronic phase but may, in rare patients, represent 30 to 80 percent of the total leukocyte count during chronic phase and lead to the designation of Ph-chromosome–positive basophilic CML.[282] Unlike mastocytosis, hyperhistaminemia usually is not associated with elevated basophil counts. Cases of exaggerated basophilia and disabling pruritus, urticaria, and gastric hyperacidity have occurred, associated with enormous increases (several hundred-fold) of blood histamine concentration.[283,284] Granules of basophils in patients with CML, unlike normal basophils, contain mast cell α-tryptase.[285] Granulocytes containing both eosinophilic and basophilic granules are commonly present.[286]

The total absolute lymphocyte count is increased (mean approximately 15×10^9/liter) in patients with CML at the time of diagnosis[287] as a result of the balanced increase in T helper and T suppressor cells.[288] B lymphocytes are not increased.[288] T lymphocytes also are increased in the spleen.[289] NK cell activity is defective in CML patients as a result of decreased maturation of these cells *in vivo*[290,291] and perhaps increased apoptosis.[292] The absolute number of circulating NK cells is decreased in patients with CML. The CD56 bright subset is particularly decreased. These cells are reduced more as CML progresses, and they respond less to stimuli that recruit clonogenic NK cells compared to NK cells from normal subjects.[293]

The platelet count is elevated in approximately 50 percent of patients at the time of diagnosis and is normal in most of the rest.[294] The platelet count may increase during the course of the chronic phase. Platelet counts greater than 1,000,000/μl (1000×10^9/liter) are not unusual, and platelet counts as high as 5,000,000 to 7,000,000/μl ($5000–7000 \times 10^9$/liter) have occurred. Thrombohemorrhagic com-

plications of thrombocytosis are infrequent. Occasionally, the platelet count may be below normal at the time of diagnosis, but this finding usually signals an impending progression to the accelerated phase of the disease (see "Accelerated Phase and Blast Crisis of CML" below).

Functional abnormalities of neutrophils (adhesion, emigration, phagocytosis) are mild; are compensated for by high neutrophil concentrations; and do not predispose patients in chronic phase to infections by either usual or opportunistic organisms.[295–297] Platelet dysfunction can occur but is not associated with spontaneous or exaggerated bleeding. A decrease in the second wave of epinephrine-induced platelet aggregation is the most common abnormality and is associated with a deficiency of adenine nucleotides in the storage pool.[298,299]

MARROW

Morphology   The marrow is markedly hypercellular, and hematopoietic tissue takes up 75 to 90 percent of the marrow volume, with fat markedly reduced.[300,301] Granulopoiesis is dominant, with a granulocytic to erythroid ratio between 10:1 and 30:1 rather than the normal 2:1 to 4:1. Erythropoiesis usually is decreased, and megakaryocytes are normal or increased in number. Eosinophils and basophils may be increased, usually in proportion to their increase in the blood. Mitotic figures are increased in number. Uncommonly a juxtamembrane domain mutant of *KIT* coincides with *BCR-ABL* in CML.[302] A rare report of marrow mastocytosis has been explained by a *KIT* mutation as an additional genetic abnormality.[303] Macrophages that mimic Gaucher cells in appearance are sometimes seen (see Color Plate IX-6). This finding is a result of the inability of normal cellular glucocerebrosidase activity to degrade the increased glucocerebroside load associated with markedly increased cell turnover.[304] Macrophages also can become engorged with lipids, which, when oxidized and polymerized, yield ceroid pigment. This pigment imparts a granular and bluish cast to the cells after polychrome staining; such cells have been referred to as *sea-blue histiocytes*[304] (see Color Plate IX-9).

Collagen type III, which takes the silver impregnation stain, is commonly increased at the time of diagnosis (reticulin fibrosis), is strikingly increased in nearly half the patients,[305] and is correlated with the proportion of megakaryocytes in the marrow.[306,307] Increased fibrosis also is correlated with larger spleen size, more severe anemia, and a higher proportion of marrow and blood blast cells.

The marrows of CML patients have a mean doubling of microvessel density compared to healthy controls and have more angiogenesis in marrow than other forms of leukemia.[308,309] This increased marrow vascularity decreases to normal after treatment.[310]

The marrow cells of approximately 50 percent of patients express cancer testis antigens, especially those encoded by *HAGE* genes.[311]

Progenitor Cell Growth   Cells that form colonies of neutrophils and macrophages or eosinophils (CFUs) are increased in the marrow and blood. The increase in CFUs in marrow is approximately 20-fold normal and in blood approximately 500-fold normal. The CFUs are of lighter buoyant density than those in normal marrow.[94] More primitive progenitors that can initiate long-term cultures of hematopoiesis also are markedly increased.[312] Spontaneous blood-derived granulocyte-macrophage colony growth is common, although CFUs also respond to growth factor stimulation.[104]

Cytogenetics   The marrow and nucleated blood cells of more than 90 percent of patients with clinical and laboratory signs that fall within the criteria for the diagnosis of CML contain the Ph chromosome, t(9;22)(q34;q11). The chromosome is present in all blood cell lineages (erythroblasts, granulocytes, monocytes, megakaryocytes, T and B cell progenitors) but is not present in the majority of

Reciprocal translocation

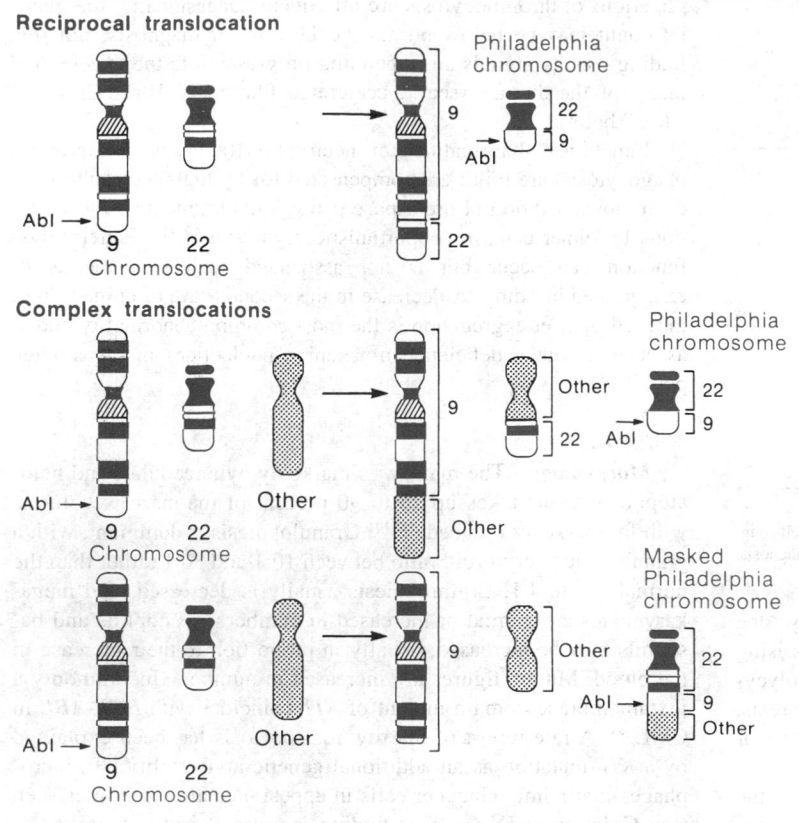

Complex translocations

FIGURE 88-6 Translocations involved in chronic myelogenous leukemia. The positions of the *ABL* gene in each of the chromosomes before and after the translocation are noted. The origin of the chromosomal segments in each of the translocated chromosomes is indicated by a *bracket* on the side of the chromosome. (From Rosson D, Reddy EP: Activation of the abl oncogene and its involvement in chromosomal translocations in human leukemia. *Mutat Res* 195:231, 1988, with permission.)

blood B lymphocytes or in most T lymphocytes.[48,50] Approximately 70 percent of patients in the chronic phase have the classic Ph chromosome in their cells.[313] The remaining 20 percent also have a missing Y chromosome [t(Ph),-Y]; an additional C-group chromosome, usually number 8 [t(Ph),+8]; an additional chromosome 22q– but without the 9q+ [t(Ph), 22q–]; or t(Ph) plus either another stable translocation or another minor clone.[74] These variations have not been shown to affect the duration of the chronic phase. Deletion of the Y chromosome occurs in approximately 10 percent of healthy men older than 60 years.[314,315]

Variant Ph chromosome translocations occur in approximately 5 percent of subjects with CML and involve complex rearrangements (three chromosomes), and every chromosome except the Y chromosome can be involved.[316–320] The Ph chromosome, that is, 22q–, is present, but the gross exchange of chromosomal material involves a chromosome other than 9 (simple variant) or involves exchange of material among chromosomes 9 and 22 and a third or more chromosomes (complex variant) (Fig. 88-6). High-resolution techniques have indicated that 9q34-qter is transposed to 22q11 in simple and in complex translocations.[321,322] Thus, the fusion of 9q34 with 22q11 seems to occur in the cells of most patients with CML.[323] Complex translocations involving chromosome 3 have been notable.[323–325] In rare cases, a reciprocal translocation with a chromosome other than 9 to chromosome 22 is larger than usual, and the posttranslocation shortening of the long arms of 22 is not apparent. This circumstance has been referred to as a *masked Ph chromosome* or *masked translocation* be-

cause the 22q– is not evident by microscopic examination,[326,327] although t(9;22) may occur as judged by banding techniques or molecular probes.[328]

Approximately 10 percent of patients have a deletion of the derivative 9 chromosome adjacent to the chromosome breakpoint. Although this deletion is thought to be an important factor in resistance to drug effects with IFN, it does not appear to be as significant with the introduction of imatinib.[211]

Molecular Probes In a small proportion of patients with a clinical disease analogous to CML, cytogenetic studies do not disclose a classic, variant, or masked Ph chromosome. In these cases, use of a panel of restriction enzymes and Southern blot analyses with a molecular probe for the breakpoint cluster region on chromosome 22 nearly always detects rearrangement of fragments. This finding has led to the conclusion that almost all cases of CML have an abnormality of the long arm of chromosome number 22 (*BCR* rearrangement).[329–333] Ph-chromosome–negative CML cells with *BCR* rearrangement can express the p210[bcr–abl], and such patients have a clinical course similar to Ph-chromosome–positive CML.[329,334–337]

The ability to identify the molecular consequences of the t(9;22), that is, *BCR* rearrangement, mRNA transcripts of the mutant fusion gene, and the p210[bcr–abl], has resulted in diagnostic tests supplementary to cytogenetic analysis.[333] These tests include Southern blot analysis of *BCR* rearrangement,[335–339] polymerase chain reaction (PCR) amplification of the abnormal mRNA,[340] and a less complex variation on the latter, a hybridization protection assay.[341]

Southern blot analysis of the DNA extracted from samples of blood cells should be correlated with marrow cytogenetic analysis. Some occasional discordant cases in which Southern blot analysis does not detect *BCR* gene rearrangement but the marrow cells have Ph-chromosome–positive metaphases can occur. Thus, marrow cytogenetic analysis should be performed if patients achieve a complete disappearance of *BCR*-rearranged cells by Southern blot to avoid overestimating the degree of response.[342]

PCR can achieve a sensitivity of one positive cell in approximately 500,000 to one million cells. This extreme sensitivity requires special care in analysis and the inclusion of negative controls.[343–346] Immunodiagnosis of CML by identification of the p210[bcr–abl] also is possible. This tumor-specific protein for CML is unique, based on the amino acids at the junction between the *ABL* and *BCR* sequences. Oligopeptides corresponding to the junctional amino acids have been synthesized and used as antigens[347–350] to develop specific antibodies to the p210[bcr–abl].

A multicolor FISH method to detect the *BCR-ABL* fusion in patients with CML is a rapid and sensitive alternative to Southern blot and PCR-dependent methods.[351] For diagnostic purposes, FISH is simple, accurate, and sensitive and can detect the various molecular fusions (e.g., b2a2, b3a2, e1a2).[352–356] Interphase FISH is faster and more sensitive than cytogenetics in identifying the Ph chromosome. If the concentration of CML cells is very low, interphase FISH may not detect *BCR-ABL*, so it has limited use for detecting minimal residual disease.[357] Hypermetaphase FISH allows analysis of up to 500 metaphases per sample in less than 1 hour. Several factors influence the false-positive and false-negative rates of FISH identification of *BCR-ABL*, including definition of a fusion signal, nuclear size, and the genomic position of the ABL breakpoint.[358] Double BCR-ABL fusion signals (double-fusion [D]-FISH) have been proposed as being more accurate than the fusion signal used in dual color (single-fusion) S-FISH, because in the latter case a small percentage of the normal BCR and ABL signals overlap.[359]

The frequency of cytogenetic analysis can be reduced if patients are monitored by molecular methods such as quantitative Southern blotting, FISH, quantitative Western blotting, or competitive reverse transcriptase (RT)-PCR. Molecular analyses can be performed on blood samples and therefore are much easier to use than cytogenetic analysis of marrow cell metaphases. Southern blotting, Western blotting, and FISH are quantifiable. Quantitative RT-PCR is the method of choice for monitoring patients for residual disease or reappearance of disease after marrow transplantation. Competitive PCR can detect reappearance of or increasing levels of RNA bcr-abl transcripts prior to clinical relapse in patients after transplantation.[360-362]

CHEMICAL ABNORMALITIES

Uric Acid An increased production of uric acid with hyperuricemia and hyperuricosuria occurs in untreated CML.[363] Uric acid excretion often is two to three times normal in patients with CML. If aggressive therapy leads to rapid cell lysis, excretion of the additional purine load may produce urinary tract blockage from uric acid precipitates. Formation of urinary urate stones is common in patients with CML, and some patients with latent gout may develop acute gouty arthritis or uric acid nephropathy.[364] The likelihood of complications from urate overproduction is greatly increased by starvation, acidosis, renal disease, or diuretic drug therapy.

Serum Vitamin B_{12}-Binding Proteins and Vitamin B_{12} Neutrophils contain vitamin B_{12}-binding proteins, including transcobalamin I and III (syn: R-type B_{12}-binding protein or cobalophilin).[365-368] Patients with myeloproliferative diseases have an increased serum level of B_{12}-binding capacity, and the source of the protein is principally mature neutrophilic granulocytes.[365,366] The increase in transcobalamin level and the resultant increase in vitamin B_{12} concentration are particularly notable in CML, although any increase in the number of neutrophilic granulocytes, as in leukemoid reactions, can be accompanied by an increase in serum B_{12}-binding protein levels and vitamin B_{12} concentration.[368] The serum B_{12} level in CML patients is increased on average to more than 10 times normal.[369] The increase is proportional to the total leukocyte count in untreated patients and falls toward normal levels with treatment, although increased B_{12} levels commonly persist even after the white cell count is lowered to near normal with therapy.

Pernicious anemia and CML may rarely coexist. In this situation, the tissues are vitamin B_{12} deficient, but the serum vitamin B_{12} level may be normal because of the elevated level of transcobalamin I, a binder with a very high affinity for vitamin B_{12}.[369]

Serum Lactic Dehydrogenase, Potassium, Calcium, and Cholesterol The level of serum lactic acid dehydrogenase (LDH) is elevated in CML.[370] Pseudohyperkalemia resulting from the release of potassium from white cells during clotting[371] and spurious hypoxemia or pseudohypoglycemia from in vitro utilization of oxygen or glucose by granulocytes can occur. Hypercalcemia[372] or hypokalemia[373] has occurred during the chronic phase of the disease, but such complications are very rare until the disorder transforms to acute leukemia. Elevated serum and urinary lysozyme levels are features of leukemia with greater monocytic components and are not features of CML.[374] Serum cholesterol is decreased in patients with CML,[375,376] and the severity of the decrease is correlated with shortened duration of patient survival.[376]

Serum Angiogenic Factors Angiogenin, endoglin (CD105), vascular endothelial growth factor (VEGF), β-fibroblast growth factor, and hepatocyte growth factor are increased strikingly in the serum of CML patients.[309,377,378]

SPECIAL CLINICAL FEATURES

BCR-ABL—POSITIVE THROMBOCYTHEMIA

Two syndromes—thrombocythemia with the Ph chromosome and BCR-ABL rearrangement or thrombocythemia without a Ph chromosome but with the BCR-ABL rearrangement—may precede the overt signs of CML or its accelerated phase.[379-385] In general, the disease closely mimics classic thrombocythemia initially: marked platelet elevation, extreme megakaryocytic hyperplasia, normal or mildly elevated white cell count, no or very slight myeloid immaturity in the blood, and minimal anemia. Minor bleeding, such as epistaxis, erythromelalgia, or signs of thrombosis such as cerebral or limb ischemia, occasionally may be present.[386] In some cases, the absolute basophil count is mildly elevated. Using immunostaining, Ph+ thrombocythemia is proposed to be distinctive from Ph− thrombocythemia by small megakaryocytes in the former and large clusters of megakaryocytes in the latter.[386] However, this distinction was not found in other studies,[387] would have to be validated, and would be difficult to use as a discriminator. In two studies, approximately 5 percent of patients with apparent essential thrombocythemia had a Ph chromosome.[381,388] In another study, two of 121 patients with essential thrombocythemia had BCR-ABL transcripts, and one of these patients also had a Ph chromosome in the marrow cells.[389] However, in another study, four of 32 patients with thrombocythemia had low levels of BCR-ABL transcripts in blood cells.[390] Approximately one in 20 patients with CML present with the features of essential thrombocythemia.[382,383] Evolution to blast crisis may occur.[380,391,392] Thus, the frequency of Ph-chromosome–negative, BCR-ABL–positive thrombocythemia ranges from approximately 1.6 to 13 percent of patients, which may reflect in part the range of sensitivity of the detection method.[388-390,393,394]

NEUTROPHILIC CML

A rare variant of BCR-ABL–positive CML has been described in which the elevated white cell count is composed principally of mature neutrophils.[395,396] The white cell count is lower on average (30,000–50,000/μl) at the time of diagnosis than is the case with classic CML (100,000–200,000/μl). Moreover, patients with neutrophilic CML usually do not have basophilia, notable myeloid immaturity in the blood, prominent splenomegaly, or low leukocyte alkaline phosphatase scores. The cells of these patients have the Ph chromosome but have an unusual BCR-ABL fusion gene in that the breakpoint in the BCR gene is between exons 19 and 20. This breakpoint location results in fusion of most of the BCR gene with ABL (e19a2 type BCR-ABL), which leads to a larger fusion protein (230 kDa) compared to the fusion protein in classic CML (210 kDa) (see Fig. 88-2). This correlation between genotype and phenotype was not observed in all cases.[397] This variant usually has an indolent course, which may be the result of very low levels of mRNA for p230 and the undetectable or barely detectable p230 protein in cells.[398]

MINOR-BCR BREAKPOINT—POSITIVE CML

A very small number of patients with Ph-chromosome–positive myeloproliferative disease had the breakpoint on the BCR gene in the first intron (m-bcr), resulting in a 190-kDa fusion protein instead of the classic 210-kDa protein observed in patients with CML (see Fig. 88-2). The m-bcr molecular lesion is similar to that observed in approximately 60 percent of patients with BCR rearrangement-positive ALL. In patients with m-bcr CML, monocytes are more prominent, the white cell count is lower on average, and basophilia and splenomegaly are less prominent than in disease with classic BCR breakpoint (M-bcr).

The few reported cases had a short interval before either myeloid or lymphoid blast transformation developed.[399,400]

HYPERLEUKOCYTOSIS

Approximately 15 percent of patients present with symptoms or signs referable to leukostasis as a result of the intravascular flow-impeding effects of white cell counts greater than $300,000/\mu l$ ($300 \times 10^9/$ liter).[251] Hyperleukocytosis is more prevalent in children with Ph-chromosome–positive CML.[252] The effects of total leukocyte counts from 300,000 to $800,000/\mu l$ ($300–800 \times 10^9/$liter) include impaired circulation of the lung, central nervous system, special sensory organs, and penis, resulting in some combination of tachypnea, dyspnea, cyanosis, dizziness, slurred speech, delirium, stupor, visual blurring, diplopia, retinal vein distention, retinal hemorrhages, papilledema, tinnitus, impaired hearing, or priapism.[253] Such symptoms or signs usually respond to the rapidly decreased white cell count by a combination of leukapheresis and hydroxyurea therapy.

CONCURRENCE OF LYMPHOID MALIGNANCIES

CML has an association with lymphoproliferation that can take four principal forms. (1) Patients may develop CML years after irradiation treatment of non-Hodgkin or Hodgkin lymphoma. (2) Approximately one third of CML patients enter the accelerated phase of the disease by evolution and dedifferentiation of the CML clone into one that supports lymphoblastic proliferation (acute lymphoblastic transformation). (3) Patients may have concurrent lymphoproliferative or plasmacytic malignancies and CML. Lymphoma or lymphoblastic leukemia,[401–407] essential monoclonal gammopathy,[408,409] myeloma,[410–412] or Waldenström macroglobulinemia[413] have occurred in association with CML. Several cases of CML emergence in patients with established CLL have been reported.[414–416] A few patients have presented with simultaneous occurrence of the two diseases.[417,418] A single case of lymphocytic leukemoid reaction simulating CLL that regressed as CML emerged has been reported.[419] In some cases, the CLL lymphocytes did not contain the Ph chromosome whereas the CML cells did, suggesting the presence of two independent clonal disorders.[414,415,420,421] In other cases, the Ph chromosome was present in the myeloid and lymphoid cells, indicating a common origin.[418] (4) Patients may present with Ph-chromosome–positive acute lymphoblastic leukemia and, following chemotherapy-induced remission, develop the features of typical CML.[419]

DIFFERENTIAL DIAGNOSIS

DISEASES MIMICKING CML

The diagnosis of CML is made based on the characteristic granulocytosis, white cell differential count, increased absolute basophil count, and splenomegaly coupled with the presence of the Ph chromosome or its variants (90% of patients) or a *BCR* rearrangement on chromosome 22 (>95% of patients).

Patients with other chronic hematopoietic stem cell diseases, such as polycythemia vera, primary thrombocythemia, or idiopathic myelofibrosis, only occasionally have closely overlapping features. For example, the total white cell count is greater than $30 \times 10^9/$liter in more than 90 percent of patients with CML and increases inexorably over weeks or months of observation, whereas the total white cell count is less than $30 \times 10^9/$liter in more than 90 percent of patients with the three other classic chronic clonal myeloid diseases and usually does not change significantly over months to years. Polycythemia vera is associated with increased red cell mass and hemo-

globin concentration and displays clinical signs of plethora; CML does not have these features. Patients with idiopathic myelofibrosis invariably have marked teardrop poikilocytes and other severe red cell shape, size, and chromicity changes and prominent nucleated red cells in the blood; CML rarely has these features. Patients with primary thrombocythemia have a platelet count greater than 750,000/ μl ($750 \times 10^9/$liter) and usually only mild neutrophilia; the latter white cell findings distinguish it from the small proportion (10%) of CML patients with platelet counts greater than $750,000/\mu l$ ($750 \times 10^9/$liter) at the time of diagnosis. In addition, patients with the clinical features of polycythemia vera or idiopathic myelofibrosis do not have the Ph chromosome or *BCR* rearrangement in their blood and marrow cells, except in extremely rare cases. A very small proportion of patients with apparent essential thrombocythemia have BCR-ABL transcripts in their marrow and blood cells and occasionally a Ph chromosome and may represent an atypical initial phase of CML. (see "*BCR-ABL*–Positive Thrombocythemia" above).

Increased awareness of the features of related disorders, such as chronic myelomonocytic leukemia (CMML) and chronic neutrophilic leukemia, and an appreciation that elderly patients are prone to atypical clonal myeloid diseases have minimized the inappropriate diagnosis of Ph-chromosome–negative CML, which should be avoided unless the clinical features are characteristic of classic CML and a masked Ph chromosome or *BCR* rearrangement is not found.

Reactive leukocytosis can occur with absolute neutrophil counts of 30,000 to $100,000/\mu l$ ($30–100 \times 10^9/$liter). Usually these leukemoid reactions occur in the setting of an overt inflammatory disease (e.g., pancreatitis), cancer (e.g., lung), or infection (pneumococcal pneumonia). If the incitant is not apparent, the absence of granulocytic immaturity, basophilia, splenomegaly, and decreased neutrophil alkaline phosphatase activity argue against CML. The absence of a cytogenetic or molecular abnormality in chromosome 22 virtually eliminates classic CML as a consideration.

The precise diagnosis of CML is helpful in estimating the patient's prognosis, the choice of drugs for treatment, and the timing of special therapies, such as allogeneic stem cell transplantation.

PH-CHROMOSOME—POSITIVE CHRONIC HEMATOPOIETIC STEM CELL DISEASES

The Ph chromosome has been found rarely in patients with apparent polycythemia vera,[29,422] polycythemia vera that later evolves into Ph-chromosome–positive CML,[423–425] idiopathic myelofibrosis,[426,427] and a myelodysplastic syndrome (MDS).[428,429] Molecular studies to determine the presence of the *BCR-ABL* were not performed in cases reported before 1985. Primary (essential) thrombocythemia with a Ph chromosome and/or *BCR-ABL* rearrangement in blood cells was discussed earlier (see "Special Clinical Features" above).

THERAPY

GENERAL CONSIDERATIONS

Hyperuricemia and hyperuricosuria are frequent features of CML at diagnosis or in relapse.[430] The need for treatment of hyperuricemia is a function of the elevated pretreatment serum uric acid concentration, blood white cell concentration, spleen size, and dose of chemotherapy planned. If these variables suggest a high risk for a significant amount of cell lysis, allopurinol 300 mg/day orally and adequate hydration to maintain a good urine flow should be instituted prior to chemotherapy. Allopurinol is associated with a high frequency of allergic skin reactions and should be discontinued after the blood leukocyte count and spleen size are decreased and the risk of exaggerated cell lysis has passed. If hyperuricemia is extreme, alkalinization of urine can be achieved with sodium bicarbonate, and rasburicase can be administered.[431] Rasburicase is a recombinant urate oxidase that converts uric acid to allantoin. Rasburicase, unlike allopurinol, reduces the uric acid pool very rapidly, does not result in the accumulation of xanthine or hypoxanthine, and does not require alkalinization of urine facilitating phosphate excretion.[1089] Although the manufacturer recommends a dose every day for five days, several reports have indicated that one injection will produce a rapid and sustained decrease in serum uric acid, profoundly decreasing the cost of therapy.[1090] Another alternative is to use allopurinol for a few days after one injection of rasburicase. A dose of 0.2 mg/kg of ideal body weight of rasburicase intravenously has been used.[1091]

Previously, treatment of CML was confined to allogeneic stem cell transplantation, IFN-α–based regimens, and other conventional chemotherapy agents such as busulfan and hydroxyurea. The availability of imatinib mesylate (Gleevec™, Glivec™, formerly known as STI571), an inhibitor of the BCR-ABL tyrosine kinase, has rapidly altered the approach to treatment of CML.[432]

INITIAL CYTOREDUCTION THERAPY

Imatinib mesylate (imatinib) now is utilized as initial therapy in almost all patients with CML presenting in the chronic phase. In cases where the white cell count is markedly elevated, hydroxyurea can be used prior to or in conjunction with imatinib. If rapid cytoreduction is required because of signs of the hyperleukocytic syndrome, leukapheresis and hydroxyurea often are combined.

LEUKAPHERESIS
Leukapheresis can control CML only temporarily. For this reason, it is rarely used in chronic phase CML and is useful in only two types of patients: the hyperleukocytic patient in whom rapid cytoreduction can reverse symptoms and signs of leukostasis (e.g., stupor, hypoxia, tinnitus, papilledema, priapism)[251 253] and the pregnant patient with CML who can be controlled by leukapheresis treatment without chemotherapy either during the early months of pregnancy when chemotherapy poses a higher risk to the fetus or, in some cases, throughout the pregnancy.[433,434] Because of the large body burden of leukocytes in marrow, blood, and spleen and the high proliferative rate in CML, leukocyte reduction by apheresis is less efficient than in other types of leukemias.[251,253] Leukapheresis reduces the burden of tumor cells subject to chemotherapeutically induced cytolysis and thus the production and the excretion of uric acid. In hyperleukocytic nonpregnant patients, leukapheresis is best used in conjunction with hydroxyurea to ensure rapid and optimal reduction in white cell count.

HYDROXYUREA
Hydroxyurea 1 to 6 g/day orally, depending on the height of the white cell count, can be used to initiate elective therapy.[435] Urgent treatment of extraordinary total white cell counts may require higher doses. The dose of hydroxyurea should be decreased as the total white cell count decreases and usually is given at 1 to 2 g/day when the total white cell count reaches 20,000/μl (20 $\times$ 10^9/liter). The drug should be temporarily discontinued if the white cell count drops below 5000/μl (5 $\times$ 10^9/liter). If hydroxyurea is being used in combination with imatinib, the hydroxyurea usually is tapered and discontinued once a hematologic response to imatinib is observed.

ANAGRELIDE
Anagrelide can be utilized for platelet reduction in patients who present with elevated platelet counts. In patients who still have significant thrombocythemia after imatinib mesylate is initiated, the com-

bination of imatinib and anagrelide was safe and was associated with an 89 percent complete hematologic response rate.[436]

IMATINIB MESYLATE
Because BCR-ABL tyrosine kinase activity is essential to the transforming function of BCR-ABL, inhibition of the kinase should inhibit CML cells. Imatinib is a 2-phenylaminopyrimidine derivative that entered clinical trials in 1998 as STI571 (formerly CGP57148).[437–441] Imatinib inhibits the Abelson tyrosine kinase because its binding causes the kinase to adopt an inactive conformation in which a centrally located "activation loop" is not phosphorylated.[442] It also inhibits the tyrosine kinase encoded by *KIT* and platelet-derived growth factor receptor (*PDGFR*)-α/β.[443] Figure 88-7 illustrates imatinib's mechanism of action. Imatinib mesylate preferentially reduces the capacity for amplification of granulocyte/macrophage progenitors from CML patients[444] and inhibits the growth of primitive malignant progenitors through reversal of abnormally increased proliferation without an increase in apoptosis.[445]

Imatinib received Food and Drug Administration approval on May 10, 2001 and now is the standard initial therapy for CML.[446] The tablet and capsule forms of imatinib are bioequivalent.[447] Phase I and II studies had demonstrated the efficacy of imatinib in patients previously treated with IFN or in patients in the accelerated phase of the disease; subsequently, the approval was expanded to initial therapy of CML.[448] In general, imatinib has resulted in major cytogenetic responses in 55 percent of patients previously treated with IFN and complete cytogenetic responses in 74 percent of newly diagnosed patients. Molecular remissions rarely occur in patients previously treated with IFN, but approximately 4 percent of newly diagnosed patients have complete molecular responses with greater than 4.5 log reduction in BCR-ABL/ABL transcript ratio as measured by quantitative PCR methods.[441,449] Imatinib appears to provide a survival advantage for patients previously treated with IFN. In newly diagnosed patients, the length of followup is too short to make quantitative estimates, but (1) the tolerance of optimal doses in older patients as compared to IFN, (2) the higher rate of cytogenetic response compared to IFN, and (3) the response of IFN-refractory patients suggest that overall survival will be improved with imatinib as compared to IFN.

Results of Clinical Trials with Imatinib Mesylate   *Results in patients previously treated with IFN.*   When imatinib was administered orally to 83 patients with CML in the chronic phase who did not have cytogenetic responses to IFN therapy, no minimal toxic dose was noted, and complete hematologic remissions were noted at doses of 300 mg/day or higher, usually in the first 4 weeks of therapy. Some complete cytogenetic responses were noted.[450] Nausea, myalgias, edema, and diarrhea were the main side effects and usually were only grade 1 to 2 in intensity. In a later phase II trial in which 532 patients with late chronic phase CML who failed to respond to IFN were treated with imatinib 400 mg/day, major cytogenetic responses were noted in 60 percent of patients and hematologic responses in 95 percent. Only 2 percent of patients discontinued treatment because of adverse effects.[451] Among patients treated with imatinib after IFN failure, those with no cytogenetic response had worse survival than those who continued receiving IFN, but those with some degree of cytogenetic response after 6 months had better survival than controls when switched to imatinib therapy.[452] In another series in which patients previously treated with IFN were treated in the late chronic phase, 44 percent had a complete cytogenetic response that was maintained for 2 years in 75 percent of patients. Most patients with a complete cytogenetic response had a greater than 2 log decrease in BCR-ABL transcript level. In a retrospective series comparing survival in cases of IFN failure treated with imatinib to an historical experience with other therapies, cyto-

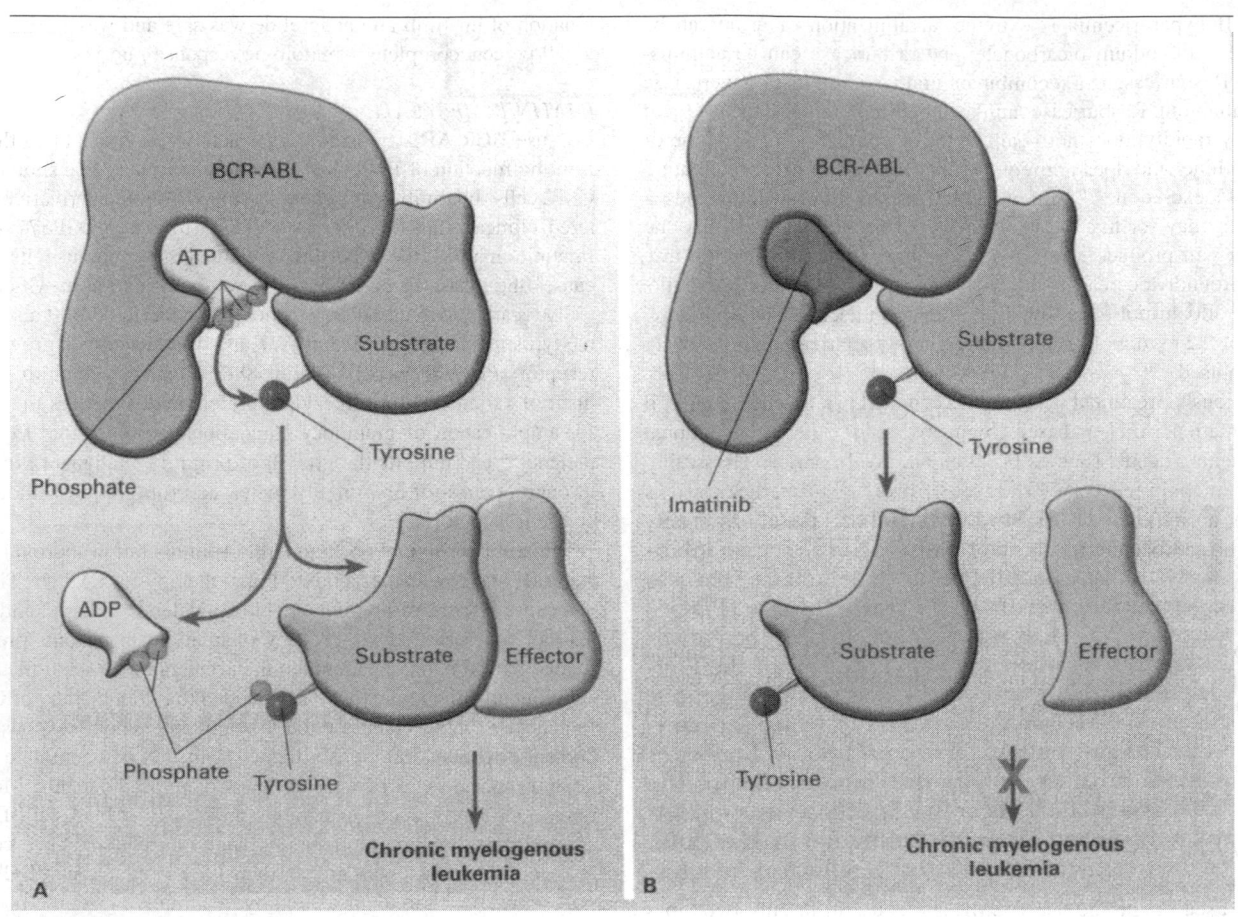

FIGURE 88-7   *(A)* BCR-ABL oncoprotein with a molecule of ATP in the kinase pocket. The substrate is activated by phosphorylation of one of its tyrosine residues. It then can activate other downstream effector molecules. When imatinib mesylate occupies the kinase pocket *(B)*, the action of BCR-ABL is inhibited, preventing phosphorylation of its substrate. (From Savage DG, Antman KH: Imatinib mesylate—a new oral targeted therapy. *N Engl J Med* 346:683, 2002, with permission.)

genetic complete response rates were 62 percent versus 19 percent, and imatinib therapy was a significant independent favorable prognostic factor for survival.[453]

Results of imatinib as initial treatment.   In 50 patients with early chronic phase CML, imatinib 400 mg/day resulted in a major hematologic response in 49 patients, major cytogenetic response in 90 percent, and complete response in 72 percent. A higher incidence of complete and major cytogenetic responses was noted at 8 months compared to expected rates with IFN.[454] In the so-called IRIS trial (Randomized Study of IFN and STI571), 1106 newly diagnosed patients with CML were randomized to treatment with imatinib 400 mg/day or standard IFN doses (5 million units/m²/day) plus low-dose cytarabine. Crossover was allowed. At 18 months of observation, the complete cytogenetic response rate was 76 percent of patients receiving imatinib and 14.5 percent of patients receiving IFN plus low-dose cytarabine. The absence of progression also was better for imatinib (97% vs. 92% with IFN). Many crossovers occurred because of IFN intolerance. No survival differences could be demonstrated, largely because of crossover rescues by imatinib.[455,456] In concurrent quality-of-life analysis, a clear advantage was present for imatinib compared to IFN.[457]

When blood from patients who had complete cytogenetic remission in the IRIS trial was monitored, the levels of BCR-ABL transcripts after 12 months of treatment were decreased by at least 3 logs in 57 percent of patients in the imatinib group but in only 24 percent of patients randomized to the group given IFN plus cytarabine.[458] For

patients who had a complete cytogenetic response and a reduction in transcript levels of at least 3 logs at 12 months, the probability of remaining progression free was 100 percent at 24 months versus 85 percent for patients not in complete cytogenetic response. Imatinib improves survival in patients with newly diagnosed CML in the chronic phase compared to IFN based on historic data.[459] Table 88-2 summarizes the imatinib response at different phases of CML: chronic, accelerated, and blast crisis.

Use of higher daily imatinib doses.   Most patients treated with imatinib 400 mg/day have molecular evidence of residual disease. In 114 patients with newly diagnosed chronic phase CML treated with imatinib 800 mg/day administered in two 400-mg doses approximately q12h, 90 percent had complete cytogenetic responses and 96 percent had major responses (<35% Ph-chromosome–positive metaphases). At a median of 15 months, no patients had progressed and 63 percent showed blood BCR-ABL/ABL percentage ratios of less than 0.05 percent: 28 percent of patients had undetectable BCR-ABL blood levels.[460] High-dose imatinib (800 mg/day) induced complete cytogenetic responses in most patients in the chronic phase who are refractory to IFN, and molecular remissions also occurred.[461] Other investigators have noted only transient benefit from increasing imatinib dose in patients who have not achieved a complete cytogenetic remission while taking conventional doses.[462] The question of whether dose escalation would overcome drug resistance in patients refractory to standard doses also has been examined.[463] Sixty-five percent of patients who did not have a significant hematologic response or who relapsed while receiving imatinib at a dose of 300 or 400 mg/day had a complete or partial hematologic response with higher doses, but few cytogenetic responses were seen. For patients with cytogenetic resistance, 56 percent entered complete or partial cytogenetic responses with higher doses. The responses to higher doses of imatinib in patients lacking a hematologic or cytogenetic response at standard doses usually are transient.[464]

Use of imatinib in patients with variant chromosomal translocations or breakpoints. Patients with variant Ph chromosome translocations have a similar prognosis to that in patients with classic Ph chromosome translocations treated with imatinib.[465] Patients with the b2a3 (e13a3) p210 *BCR-ABL* translocation respond well to imatinib, with similar rates of complete cytogenetic remission.[466] A trend to lower response rates has been noted in patients with deletion of derivative chromosome 9 treated with IFN, but this effect is less apparent with imatinib therapy.[467]

Response to imatinib based on age. In children with CML or Ph-chromosome–positive leukemias and refractory or recurrent disease treated with imatinib 260 to 570 mg/m², 10 of 12 patients with CML in the chronic phase entered complete cytogenetic remission. Responses also were seen in Ph-positive ALL. Weight gain was the most common side effect of imatinib, and marked interpatient variability in imatinib pharmacokinetics was noted.[468]

In a series of 49 patients older than 60 years, similar cytogenetic response rates and survival rates were noted compared to younger patients in the late chronic phase who were treated concurrently, suggesting that age is not a factor in response.[469]

Side effects and special treatment considerations. Imatinib is well tolerated compared with other treatment options in CML, especially IFN. Most adverse effects are manageable and seldom require permanent cessation of therapy. Reduction to subtherapeutic doses is not recommended.[470] The main side effects noted with imatinib have included superficial edema, nausea, muscle cramps, rash, fatigue, and diarrhea.[470,471] Elevated transaminases can occur, and myclosuppression can occur commonly, but more often in IFN-refractory patients than in newly diagnosed patients. The severe periorbital edema occasionally observed is postulated to be related to PDGF and KIT expression by dermal dendrocytes. Surgical decompression of the severe edema has been required rarely.[472] Although no effects on spermatogenesis have been reported, women should be cautioned regarding potential teratogenicity.[472]

Uncommon side effects include severe tumor lysis in the accelerated phase,[473] splenic rupture,[474] cerebral edema and visual disturbances resulting from retinal edema,[475] *Varicella zoster* infection,[476] gynecomastia,[477] and immune-mediated hemolytic anemia.[478]

Cutaneous reactions with imatinib therapy occur in 7 to 21 percent of patients.[479] Except for severe reactions (5%), such as Stevens-Johnson syndrome, exfoliative dermatitis, and erythema multiforme, cutaneous reactions rarely require permanent discontinuation of therapy. With milder reactions, concomitant glucocorticoid therapy or brief discontinuation with gradual reintroduction at a lower dose and then a gradual increase in dose can be accomplished successfully.[480,481] With very mild cases, ongoing treatment with antihistamine or other symptomatic therapy may be successful. Sweet syndrome with CML cell infiltration has been reported at the time of molecular remission in blood.[482] Imatinib effects on skin and hair pigmentation, probably related to KIT binding, have been reported. These effects include hair repigmentation[483] and hypopigmentation of the skin.[484]

TABLE 88-2   RESPONSE TO IMATINAB MESYLATE IN STAGES OF DISEASE

TREATMENT GROUP	COMPLETE HEMATOLOGIC RESPONSE* (%)	MAJOR CYTOGENETIC RESPONSE† (%)	COMPLETE CYTOGENETIC RESPONSE‡ (%)	COMPLETE MOLECULAR RESPONSE¶ (%)
Chronic phase	96	83 (96)	68 (90)	7 (28)
Accelerated phase	34	24	17	—
Blast crisis	8	16	7	—
Interferon failure	95	60	41	—

Numbers represent best response to imatinib mesylate 400 mg/day. Numbers in parentheses represent results with imatinib mesylate 800 mg/day at 18 months in chronic phase patients.[461] Results derived from Refs. 456 and 461.
*Complete hematologic response requires white cell count <10 × 10⁹/liter, platelet count <450 × 10⁹/liter, no immature myeloid cells in the blood, and disappearance of all signs and symptoms related to leukemia (including palpable splenomegaly) lasting for at least 4 weeks.
†Major cytogenetic response is <35% Ph-chromosome–positive cells by cytogenetic analysis of marrow cells.
‡Complete cytogenetic response is no Ph-chromosome–positive cells by standard cytogenetic analysis.
¶Major molecular response usually is defined as BCR-ABL/ABL value <0.05%. Complete molecular response is an undetectable BCR-ABL levels (usually by nested RT-PCR techniques).

Myelosuppression is rarely noted in patients with gastrointestinal stromal tumors treated with imatinib but is common in CML patients, especially at treatment onset when the CML clone accounts for most of the hematopoiesis. Dose reductions to less than 300 mg/day are not recommended for myelosuppression. Doses can be held until blood counts recover. G-CSF and GM-CSF have been reported to successfully prevent or treat neutropenia.[485,486] IL-11 may improve the thrombocytopenia associated with imatinib,[487] but platelet transfusion more commonly is used for severe thrombocytopenia. Patients with chronic cytopenias who receive imatinib have inferior responses. For example, 31 percent of patients without thrombocytopenia had a complete cytogenetic response compared to no patients with thrombocytopenia.[488] Myelosuppression is an independent adverse factor for achieving cytogenetic responses with imatinib.[489]

Extramedullary blast crisis has been treated with imatinib,[490] but the central nervous system is a sanctuary for leukemic cells in mice, nonhuman primates, and presumably humans.[491,492] No significant clinical responses to imatinib have been noted in patients with AML, MDS, atypical CML, or CMML without *PDGFR* or *KIT* mutations.[493]

Other effects of imatinib. Imatinib has been found to cause regression of marrow fibrosis.[494] It reverses VEGF secretion in CML,[495] and it may reverse marrow angiogenesis.[496] It may reduce marrow cellularity and normalize morphologic features regardless of cytogenetic response.[497] Early, quiescent Ph-chromosome–positive cells (CD34+Lin−) have been demonstrated to be insensitive to imatinib *in vitro*.[498]

Defining a response to imatinib. Defining what constitutes a meaningful response to imatinib has led to some controversy. The median BCR-ABL levels for imatinib-treated patients continue to decrease and have not reached a plateau by 24 months. The incidence of progression in imatinib-treated patients, defined by hematologic, cytogenetic, or quantitative PCR criteria, was higher in patients who failed to achieve a 2 log reduction in blood BCR-ABL levels by 6 months of therapy.[499] It has also been proposed that failure to achieve at least a minor cytogenetic remission after 3 months and the development of neutropenia during that time predict a lack of response.[500] Another proposal for adequate imatinib response[501] defines a hematologic response as normalization of all blood cell counts within 3 months and attainment of a complete cytogenetic response at any time up to 18 months (no Ph-chromosome–positive cells upon examination of 30 metaphases). Attainment of a minor cytogenetic response (less than 35% Ph-chromosome–negative metaphases) by 6 months or a major cytogenetic response (greater than 65% Ph-chromosome–negative metaphases) by 12 months is considered a potential response. Loss of response is defined as loss of a complete hematologic or complete cytogenetic response, an increase of 30 or more percentage points in the number of Ph-chromosome–positive metaphases examined at 3-month intervals, development of new cytogenetic abnormalities, or an increase in the BCR-ABL/ABL ratio of 1 log or more on serial RT-PCR testing or into the range associated with metaphase positivity. Patients who have 100 percent Ph-chromosome–positive disease after 6 months of therapy have a minimal chance of later achieving cytogenetic responses and may be offered allogeneic transplantation, if applicable.[502]

Stopping imatinib therapy. Limited data on the advisability of stopping imatinib after attainment of a complete molecular remission or a sustained cytogenetic remission have been published. A spontaneous reversion of blast crisis to the chronic phase upon discontinuation of imatinib has been reported.[503] Two patients in whom imatinib was discontinued because of neutropenia immediately developed blast crisis and additional chromosomal changes, which emerged during withdrawal.[504] In two other patients in whom imatinib was stopped because of a fever, a sustained cytogenetic response was noted up to 15 months later.[505,506] It is advisable to maintain treatment indefinitely or until the criteria for cessation, if any, can be established in clinical trials.

Secondary chromosomal changes with imatinib. Clonal abnormalities in cells lacking a detectable Ph chromosome or *BCR-ABL* rearrangements have been detected in patients undergoing imatinib therapy who previously were treated with IFN.[507,508] These cytogenetic changes were noted in seven patients at a median of 13 months of imatinib therapy, and trisomy 8 was the most frequent abnormality. All of these patients had major cytogenetic responses to imatinib.[507] These findings have prompted the suggestion that all patients taking imatinib undergo routine cytogenetic testing. In some patients, clonal evolution may be related to imatinib resistance.[509] Information regarding the impact of specific additional cytogenetic abnormalities is limited. Clonal abnormalities may be present in up to 10 percent of patients taking imatinib.[510] Some of these cases may be associated with an MDS, especially in those patients with previous exposure to cytarabine and idarubicin. The antiproliferative effect of imatinib may allow restoration of a polyclonal hematopoiesis in complete cytogenetic remission, which might favor the manifestation of a Ph-chromosome–negative disorder.[511] Some investigators have found that, with the possible exception of +8, +Ph, and i(17), additional chromosomal abnormalities at diagnosis are not associated with an inferior outcome.[512,513] In contrast, another group found that development of trisomy 8 in patients taking imatinib, while associated with pancytopenia, did not result in signs of disease progression. In a series of 34 CML patients who developed Ph-chromosome–negative clones while taking imatinib, the most common abnormalities were trisomy 8 and monosomy 7. In 11 of these patients, no archival evidence of these clones was present before imatinib therapy was initiated, and none of the patients developed myelodysplasia.[514] Cytogenetic clonal evolution may not be an important impediment to achieving a major or complete cytogenetic response with imatinib but is an independent poor prognostic factor for survival of patients in chronic and accelerated phases of CML.[515] One case of a fatal MDS during imatinib therapy and emergence of a complex Ph-chromosome–negative clone has been reported, but this case was complicated because an allogeneic transplant had been performed before imatinib therapy.[516]

Development of imatinib resistance. The development of resistance to imatinib is not surprising.[517–521] Its specificity and "snug fit" into the ABL kinase pocket provide the ideal circumstances for resistance.[522] Even in patients with complete cytogenetic response, malignant progenitors at the LTC-IC stage persist, and complete molecular responses are rare.[523] Although more than 95 percent of patients in stable chronic phase continue with major cytogenetic responses after 18 months of imatinib treatment, patients with Ph-chromosome–pos-

itive ALL and patients in the accelerated or blast crisis phase develop rapid resistance to therapy. Several potential mechanisms of resistance include *BCR-ABL* amplification in the presence of imatinib,[524–526] P-glycoprotein–mediated drug efflux,[527,528] altered drug metabolism,[521] acquisition of BCR-ABL–independent signaling characteristics,[526] and point mutations in the ABL kinase domain that alter imatinib binding. Endogenous α_1-acid glycoprotein (AGP) binds to imatinib with high affinity, reducing its distribution into tissues and cells. Increased AGP levels could reduce free plasma levels of imatinib, and displacement of imatinib with an agent that competes for AGP binding, such as erythromycin, could reduce total blood levels.[520,529] This mechanism usually is not considered important in clinical settings. Mutations in the ABL kinase domain may predate imatinib treatment,[530] and several BCR-ABL kinase domain mutants associated with imatinib resistance remain sensitive to the drug, suggesting a need for characterization before a resistant phenotype can be attributed to the given mutation.[531] Some of these mutations may lie outside the kinase domain.

Of these mechanisms, amplified gene expression and increased BCR-ABL protein expression are most often reported in resistant patients.[532] In addition, more than 30 distinct point mutations have been reported. The mutations most associated with resistance have been Thr315Le, Gly250Glu, Glu255Lys, and Thr253His substitutions. Few of the described mutations directly affect binding.[520,533] Mutations in the ATP phosphate-binding loop (P-loop) are most closely associated with a poor prognosis,[534] and these P-loop mutations predict for disease progression.

Dose escalation, combination therapy, and treatment interruption have been proposed as means to overcome drug resistance.[535] Combination therapy from the outset,[535] as in HIV therapy, also has been proposed to prevent development of resistance. It may be possible to use gene expression profiles in the future to predict the clinical effectiveness of imatinib for CML treatment, thereby allowing individualized therapy from the outset.[536]

Combination therapies. Combination therapies with imatinib can be used to improve upon response rates or to overcome resistance. Improved response rates ideally would translate into complete molecular remissions. In patients who did not respond to IFN in the chronic phase or for patients in blast crisis, improved results may result in achievement of a major cytogenetic response.[537] Agents that have been proposed for use in combination to improve response rates have included IFN-α, cytarabine, daunorubicin, homoharringtonine, multi-agent chemotherapy, arsenic trioxide, and decitabine, with some supporting *in vitro* data.[538–543] The combination of imatinib and hydroxyurea has been shown to have some antagonistic effects *in vitro*, but no evidence of these effects *in vivo* has been reported.[544]

In a phase II trial, imatinib and cytarabine were combined for CML treatment in the chronic phase, with administration of imatinib 400 mg/day and cytarabine 20 mg/m²/day via subcutaneous injections on days 15 to 28 of each cycle. In the trial, hematologic toxicity was common, and complete cytogenetic remission was 83 percent. All patients achieved a complete hematologic response.[545] When cytarabine 20 mg/m²/day was combined with imatinib in untreated patients with chronic phase CML for 14 of every 28 days for 12 months, results were good, but whether this result will impact survival is not known.[546] Combining imatinib with chemotherapeutic agents is more myelosuppressive, and final effects on response rates and survival have yet to be determined.[547]

Other combinations proposed to overcome imatinib resistance. Several inhibitors of other signal transduction mediators involved in the downstream effects of BCR-ABL have been proposed for use in imatinib-resistant CML. These inhibitors include the JAK2 inhibitor AG490,[548] the SRC kinase inhibitors, mTOR inhibitors, such as rapamycin,[549] the proteasome inhibitor bortezomib,[550,551] histone deacetylators,[552] PI3K or MEK inhibitors, such as wortmannin and LY294002,[553] and inhibitors of prenylation of RAS-related proteins downstream of BCR-ABL. These agents include the bisphosphonate zolendrate[554] and farnesyltransferase inhibitors.[555,556] The farnesyltransferase inhibitors SCH66336 and R115777 have shown some activity in CML.[557-560]

Because resistance to imatinib occurs through selection for tumor cells harboring BCR-ABL kinase domain point mutations that interfere with drug binding, a new orally bioavailable ABL kinase inhibitor, BMS-354825, with increased potency relative to imatinib and which demonstrates activity against most BCR-ABL mutants tested, is now under development.[561] In a phase I trial in 29 patients with imatinib-resistant chronic phase CML, all patients who received greater than 35 mg/day had hematologic responses.[1084] This inhibitor has activity against LYN kinase, a SHC kinase family member; activity has also been demonstrated in accelerated phase and blast crisis of the disease, which progressed on imatinib[1085] To overcome the resistance caused by mutants in the Gly-rich loops or the Thr315Le mutant, it may be necessary to develop an inhibitor that targets a different conformation of ABL or that does not rely upon the Thr315 area. A compound that inhibits the BCR-ABL kinase outside the ATP-binding site has been described to be active in CML cell lines carrying binding-site mutations and in mice carrying human CML cells.[1086] PD180970 also may be such an inhibitor.[520] Another imatinib congener, AMN107, which has approximately 20 times the potency of imatinib and has effects against some imatinib-resistant cells, is entering a phase I trial. In patients with imatinib-resistant accelerated phase, chronic phase, or Ph+acute lymphoblastic leukemia, therapeutic responses have been documented with these newer agents.[1087,1088]

Imatinib resistance often is associated with restored activation of the BCR-ABL signal transduction pathway, suggesting that BCR-ABL remains a valid target to overcome resistance in these cases.[562] BCR-ABL point mutations isolated from patients with imatinib-resistant CML remain sensitive to inhibitors of the BCR-ABL chaperone heat shock protein (hsp)90, such as geldanamycin.[563] Many of these agents have not yet entered clinical trials. Some are being used in conjunction with imatinib in resistant cases.

Disease prognosis and monitoring during imatinib therapy. Among patients started on imatinib in the chronic phase after prior IFN therapy, an 11 percent relapse rate was noted at 12 months. Only an elevated platelet count and clonal evolution were significant factors predicting hematologic relapse.[564] The absence of a major cytogenetic response within the first 6 months also was associated with hematologic relapse. Early reduction of BCR-ABL mRNA transcript levels predicted cytogenetic response in chronic phase CML patients treated with imatinib after they did not respond to IFN.[565] The ratio of blood BCR-ABL/ABL transcripts at 2 months correlated with eventual cytogenetic response at 6 months. All IFN-pretreated patients had evidence of residual disease with the limited followup available. In another study, low levels of residual disease in patients taking imatinib after IFN therapy were consistent with continuous remission. In patients with complete cytogenetic remission, hypermetaphase FISH and RT-PCR demonstrated residual BCR-ABL−positive cells. Ratios of blood BCR-ABL/ABL transcripts less than 0.1 percent were associated with continuous remission.[537] At time of best response, the median ratio of BCR-ABL/ABL transcripts was 2.1 percent in patients with relapse and 0.075 percent in patients with ongoing remission.[537] Others have also found that high levels of transcripts measured by RT-PCR are associated with short time to relapse.[566] Most have advocated that conventional karyotyping remain the standard of evaluation for treatment response.[567] In multivariate analysis, the cytogenetic response at 3 months was the only independent parameter predictive of major cyto-

genetic response at 6 months and progression-free survival at 2 years.[567]

For patients previously not treated with IFN, at study entry BCR-ABL expression in cytogenetic responders and nonresponders was similar. BCR-ABL expression became significantly different 3 months after treatment and became increasingly different between responders and nonresponders with continued therapy at 6, 9, and 12 months.[568]

One recommended mode of monitoring patients undergoing imatinib therapy is measuring blood counts at least once per month and obtaining marrow samples every 6 months until a complete cytogenetic remission is obtained.[569] Thereafter, marrow samples are obtained yearly to monitor for other clonal abnormalities. Quantitative RT-PCR is performed every 3 months on blood or marrow. A threefold increase in the level of BCR-ABL reactivity, confirmed on a repeat sample at least 1 month later, suggests a loss of response to treatment. In patients who do not have a complete hematologic response at 3 months or a major cytogenetic response after 6 to 12 months, other therapeutic options are considered.[570] The IRIS study also indicates that the molecular response after 2 to 3 months of therapy is a strong predictor of clinical and cytogenetic response.[565] Sequencing the BCR-ABL kinase domain can reveal emergence of resistant clones but is not yet widely available.[571]

Summary of imatinib effects on survival. Imatinib was first utilized for CML treatment in June 1998. Although it has completely altered the treatment approach to CML, its widespread use has raised many unanswered questions. In the past, a cytogenetic response to IFN has been utilized as an important surrogate marker of survival.[572] The extent to which this measure can be generalized to imatinib is uncertain. The IRIS study, for example, will require long-term followup, but speed and durability of hematologic response, degree of cytogenetic response, and degree of molecular response will be utilized as surrogate endpoints.[573,574] The durability of cytogenetic and molecular responses in the face of persistent minimal residual disease during imatinib therapy will require further followup of larger numbers of patients, especially because greater than 95 percent of cases will have molecular evidence of disease at 2 years.[574] Evidence indicates that approximately 20 percent of patients treated with higher doses may achieve molecular remissions.[575]

Use of imatinib has complicated the decision of when to recommend allogeneic stem cell transplantation.[576] Imatinib trials have a 95 percent progression-free survival at 24 months but usually have evidence of ongoing molecular disease. Because stem cell transplantation is associated with high toxicity and mortality rates, deciding when and for whom to utilize this modality while responses to imatinib are ongoing can be difficult. For patients who lose or never achieve imatinib response and for whom an acceptable donor is available, allogeneic stem cell transplantation becomes a goal of treatment.[577] This category generally includes those patients eligible for allogeneic transplantation who have not attained a major cytogenetic response at 1 year.[515]

INTERFERON-α

Treatment with IFN offers a survival advantage compared to treatment with hydroxyurea or busulfan alone.[578-582] A randomized comparison of IFN and hydroxyurea with hydroxyurea monotherapy for CML showed a long-term survival advantage of the combination, and survival was superior to that seen with IFN alone.[583] The achievement of a complete cytogenetic response with IFN was associated with a 30 percent 10-year survival rate. Most of the benefits of IFN are associated with lower-risk prognostic groups and are seen in patients who achieve a hematologic response in 3 to 6 months, major cytogenetic response in 1 year, and complete cytogenetic response thereafter.[546,584] A complete cytogenetic response with IFN is uncommon (13%), but 10-year survival rates are approximately 70 percent and are related to the low-risk profiles according to European and Sokal prognostic scoring systems, with 89 percent probability of survival in low-risk groups at 10 years.[585] Cytogenetic responses to IFN are stable and durable.[584] Approximately 50 percent of complete responders become long-term survivors. The biologic and molecular actions of IFN are not well understood. Expression of the IFN-α2c receptor at diagnosis has been associated with cytogenetic responses,[586] and expression of SOCS3 confers resistance to IFN through suppression of cytokine signaling proteins.[587] In addition to the common toxicities of fatigue, low-grade fever, weight loss, liver function test abnormalities, hematologic changes, and neuropsychiatric symptoms, IFN is associated with autoimmune changes in approximately 30 percent of patients,[588] more commonly in females, in patients undergoing longer treatment periods, and primarily in patients with higher response rates.

Most studies have shown no benefit of high-dose IFN compared with low-dose IFN for chronic phase CML (5 million units/m^2/day vs. 3 million units/m^2 five times per week).[589] Low-dose IFN minimizes toxicity and cost. Pegylated IFN, which has a longer half-life, can be administered as a once per week injection at 6 μg/kg/week.[590] Dose-limiting toxicities are neurotoxicity, thrombocytopenia, fatigue, and liver dysfunction. In later studies, 4.5 μg/kg was proposed as the optimal dose because of the toxicity at higher doses. Pegylated IFN plus low-dose cytosine arabinoside administered weekly is effective but has significant toxicity in patients with CML.[591]

When IFN is combined with cytarabine, IFN has more toxicity and only a small survival benefit.[592] In a phase II study of IFN, 86 patients received IFN plus cytarabine 500 mg/day for 14 days per month. A complete hematologic response was noted in 78 percent of previously untreated patients, but many patients stopped treatment because of side effects.[593] Intermittent IFN and cytarabine schedules have also been proposed.[594] Another study compared IFN plus cytarabine to IFN plus hydroxyurea in newly diagnosed CML patients.[595] Response rates were the same, but more toxicity was noted in the hydroxyurea group. IFN utilization before allogeneic stem cell transplantation does not affect outcome adversely provided IFN is discontinued at least 90 days before the procedure.[596] IFN has also been proposed as an immune stimulant to consolidate imatinib remissions because additive effects have been noted.[597]

USE OF OTHER CHEMOTHERAPEUTIC AGENTS IN CHRONIC PHASE

Hydroxyurea The major side effect of hydroxyurea is an extension of its pharmacologic effect, that is, reversible suppression of hematopoiesis, often with megaloblastic erythropoiesis. The median survival of patients with CML treated with hydroxyurea alone is approximately 5 years. Studies with high-dose hydroxyurea indicate that marrow metaphase cells in some patients lose the Ph chromosome either partially or completely after such therapy.[598] The drug may be very useful in patients of advanced age, in patients with comorbid conditions, and in patients in whom imatinib and IFN cannot be tolerated or are ineffective. Hydroxyurea often is utilized for initial cytoreduction. Chronic use of hydroxyurea has been associated with leg ulcers.[599]

Cytarabine Daily infusion of low-dose cytarabine (15–30 mg/m^2/day) by a portable pump in outpatients has resulted in control of the disease and a partial decrease or complete absence of metaphase cells containing the Ph chromosome.[600] Combinations of hydroxyurea, IFN-α, and cytarabine also can be used.[601] For example, IFN-α2b combined with cytarabine (20 mg/m^2/day for 10 days per month) in the chronic phase was associated with a greater proportion of major cytogenetic response at 12 months after randomization and with greater survival prolongation than was IFN alone.[602] Toxicities with these drug combinations are greater.

Busulfan Once the mainstay of treatment for the chronic phase, busulfan usage now is rare.[603] It is used primarily as part of the preparative regimen for allografting or autografting. Busulfan has fallen out of favor in the treatment of chronic disease because of the inferior survival rates when compared to hydroxyurea and its negative effects on the results of allogeneic stem cell transplantion.[591] It still may be used occasionally in older patients who do not tolerate imatinib or in patients with hypersensitivity reactions to hydroxyurea, such as fever or pneumonitis.[604]

Homoharringtonine Homoharringtonine, a plant alkaloid, can induce responses, including cytogenetic responses, in patients in the late chronic phase.[605] Homoharringtonine also has been utilized in combination with IFN and cytarabine.[540]

Other Cytotoxic Agents Several other chemotherapeutic agents can control the chronic phase of the disease, notably dibromomannitol.[606] Although a wide variety of other agents have been used, including melphalan, cyclophosphamide, 6-mercaptopurine, 6-thioguanine, demecolcine, and uracil mustard, they are largely inferior to hydroxyurea with regard to the proportion of patients who respond well to them.[607] Troxacitabine, when used in untreated or imatinib-resistant CML or CML in blastic phase, resulted in responses in four of 31 cases. Combination treatments have been proposed.[608]

Intensive multidrug regimens have been used in an attempt to eradicate the Ph-chromosome–positive clone and lead to prolongation of remission or cure of the disease. This approach has not significantly increased survival.[609] All-*trans*-retinoic acid and 13-*cis*-retinoic acid also may play roles in management.[610]

Anagrelide Anagrelide has been utilized to treat markedly elevated platelet counts in CML, especially in the presence of thrombosis or bleeding. This agent acts directly to decrease megakaryocyte mass, and it can lead to a precipitous fall in platelet counts.[436] Anagrelide can be combined safely with imatinib.

TREATMENT OF CHRONIC PHASE CML DURING PREGNANCY

Treatment of chronic phase CML during pregnancy is sometimes needed to prevent placental insufficiency from hyperleukocytosis. Imatinib use is not recommended during pregnancy. Hydroxyurea has the lowest mutageneic potential among the cytotoxic agents.[611] IFN can also be safely used during pregnancy. Eight patients treated with IFN from the first trimester have been described,[612] and each of these pregnancies resulted in normal babies, except for one infant with mild thrombocytopenia. All babies had normal growth.[612] Leukapheresis in the first trimester (or longer) also can be used to avoid fetal drug exposure in the first months of pregnancy (see "Leukapheresis" above).

ANTISENSE OLIGODEOXYNUCLEOTIDES

Gene target-selective destruction of cells containing the *BCR-ABL* fusion gene is a theoretical possibility and has been studied *in vitro*. This approach to therapy is highly specific, but several important issues remain to be resolved regarding delivery of these agents *in vivo*.[613,614]

Ribozymes targeting BCR/ABL mRNA have been utilized as anti-CML treatment,[615,616] and most of these approaches probably will have the most utility for *in vitro* purging of CML marrow cells before autotransplantation.[617,618]

IMMUNOTHERAPY

Several antigens have been proposed as targets of immune therapy for CML. These antigens include BCR/ABL itself, PR1, Wilms tumor protein-1 (WT1), minor histocompatibility antigens, CML-66, CML-28, and survivin.[619,620] Other targets are VEGF and hsp90.[621] A BCR-ABL fusion peptide, used as a vaccine, can elicit a specific T cell immune response.[622] CML-derived dendritic cells can process and present endogenous BCR-ABL fusion proteins to CD4+ T lymphocytes in an HLA class II–restricted antigen presentation.[623] Autologous *in vitro* cultured leukemic dendritic cells also have been used as a vaccination in CML patients.[624] Oncogenic transformation by BCR-ABL may increase the susceptibility of leukemic progenitors to NK cell cytotoxicity.[625] Immunization with GM-CSF–producing tumor vaccines is being studied in CML[626] to enhance a vaccine antitumor effect.

RADIOTHERAPY

Splenic irradiation may be useful occasionally in subjects who have entered the accelerated or advanced chronic phase and are troubled with extreme splenomegaly with splenic pain, perisplenitis, and encroachment of the spleen on the gastrointestinal tract.[627] Splenic irradiation may palliate symptoms for a short time.[628]

Radiotherapy may be useful for extramedullary tumors, which may occur occasionally in bone or soft tissue during the late chronic or accelerated phase.

SPLENECTOMY

Splenectomy does not prolong the chronic phase of CML, delay the onset of the accelerated phase, enhance sensitivity to standard or intensive chemotherapy, or prolong survival of patients.[629] In carefully selected patients with symptomatic thrombocytopenia unresponsive to chemotherapy, mechanical discomfort, hypercatabolic symptoms, and portal hypertension, splenectomy may be useful. Postoperative morbidity from infection, thrombosis, or hemorrhage has been high, with mortality rates up to 10 percent reported.[630] Splenectomy does not decrease recurrence of disease after therapy. Splenectomy performed before allografting has not been found to influence the severity of graft-versus-host disease (GVHD) or survival after allogeneic stem cell transplantation.[631] Splenectomy may reverse poor graft function after allogeneic transplantation, but hyposplenism may trigger or worsen chronic extensive GVHD, leading to increased morbidity and mortality.[632]

HIGH-DOSE CHEMOTHERAPY WITH AUTOLOGOUS STEM CELL INFUSION

Ph-chromosome–negative stem cells are present in most patients with CML at the time of diagnosis. Techniques that use these cells to reconstitute hematopoiesis after high-dose therapy have been developed.[633] Ph-chromosome–negative progenitors can be mobilized with G-CSF and collected from the blood of patients who have responded to prior treatment with IFN or imatinib.[634] Such cells also can be collected after recovery from chemotherapy regimens, such as after idarubicin and cytarabine, followed by G-CSF stimulation.[633] G-CSF was used for at least 4 days while imatinib treatment was continued for stem cell mobilization in 58 patients with a complete cytogenetic response. The cells were collected in two cytapheresis procedures in 74 percent of patients, and the cells of 84 percent of those cytapheresis products were negative for the Ph chromosome.[635]

In another series, stem cells were mobilized in 32 patients in complete cytogenetic remission after imatinib, with uninterrupted imatinib therapy in 50 percent of patients and with imatinib temporarily withheld in approximately 50 percent. Blood levels of BCR/ABL were not changed by the use of G-CSF.[636] In yet another series, 13 of 15 patients were successfully mobilized with G-CSF while receiving imatinib, and 28 percent of stem cell harvests were negative for BCR-ABL mRNA. No change in blood BCR-ABL transcript level was noted after stem cell mobilization as assessed by RT-PCR.[637]

BCR-ABL–negative primitive myeloid cells can be selected for autografting early in the chronic phase.[638] Patients autografted with Ph-chromosome–negative progenitors after myeloablative conditioning regimens may have long-term remissions in some cases.[639,640] As yet no evidence indicates this approach prolongs survival.[641] In one series of autografting, 53 patients had a cytogenetic response, and overall survival ranged from 8 to 40 months.[642] In another series, autografting followed by IFN resulted in a 55 percent survival at 10 years.[643] No series of patients autografted with cells mobilized while they were receiving imatinib have been reported, but imatinib can be effective and safe in chronic phase CML patients who have previously undergone autografting,[644] although increased hematologic toxicity was noted.

In addition to positive selection of Ph-chromosome–negative progenitors, based on their lack of HLA-DR expression,[645] negative selection by purging of BCR-ABL–positive progenitors *in vitro* can be used. These approaches have included treatment of cell suspensions with IFN, specific T cell subsets, NK cells,[646] antisense oligonucleotides,[647] ribozymes,[648] various inhibitors of signal transduction pathways, such as genistein,[649] or an inhibitor of the ABL tyrosine kinase.[650] *In vitro* culture of CML marrow favors outgrowth of normal progenitors and offers a means of depleting leukemic progenitors.[651] When such techniques have been used to select cells for autografting, most patients have relapsed.[652] No randomized trials demonstrating that marrow purged of BCR-ABL–positive progenitors improves remission rates or duration of survival compared with autografts without purging have been conducted.

Dendritic cells that possess the Ph chromosome and induce CD8+ cytotoxic T cells specific for leukemia cells can be isolated from CML patients.[653] The ability to identify CML-specific T cells after transplant has not been uniform, however.[654] Such cells could be utilized in a state of minimal disease after autologous stem cell transplantation to achieve a specific anti-CML effect.

ALLOGENEIC AND SYNGENEIC STEM CELL TRANSPLANTATION

Patients in the chronic phase of CML who are younger than 65 years and who have an identical twin[655] or a histocompatible sibling[656,657] or who are younger than 55 years with access to a histocompatible, unrelated donor[658] can be transplanted after intensive therapy, usually with cyclophosphamide and fractionated total body irradiation (TBI) or a combination of busulfan and cyclophosphamide. With nonmyeloablative or so-called "reduced-intensity" conditioning regimens, older patients and those with comorbidities can undergo successful allografting.

ALLOGRAFTING

Stem cell transplantation from HLA-compatible siblings results in engraftment and an actual or projected long-term survival in 45 to 70 percent of recipients.[659–661] In patients older than 50 years, survival rates are slightly less at 5 years. The risk of CML relapse is approximately 20 percent, with a plateau of relapse at 5 to 7 years. Transplanted T lymphocytes, especially if activated by a (mild) GVHD, may be an important factor in preventing leukemic relapse. This phenomenon, referred to as *graft-versus-leukemia reaction*, is thought to suppress the leukemic process through T cell-mediated cytotoxicity.[656] The beneficial effect of the graft-versus-leukemia phenomena may be present in blast crisis[662] and in chronic phase.[663,664] Graft failure is rare in properly conditioned patients in the chronic phase. The majority of survivors have no evidence of residual leukemia cells.[665]

The best outcomes are seen in younger patients when the transplant is performed within 1 year of diagnosis.[666,667] In a large series of 314 children who underwent allografting for CML in chronic phase, the overall survival rate at 3 years was 75 percent, and the disease-free survival rate was 63 percent.[668] Choice of pretransplant conditioning does not appear to have an impact on outcome, but previous treatment with busulfan has a negative impact.[669] Busulfan plus cyclophosphamide and TBI plus cyclophosphamide conditioning regimens have similar probabilities of success in CML.[670,671] Busulfan now can be administered as an intravenous preparation and as a single daily dose.[672] When targeted steady-state busulfan levels are utilized, a 3-year survival rate of 86 percent and a disease-free survival rate of 78 percent with no age effect noted could be achieved.[673] IFN does not increase the probability of treatment failure.[674,675]

In the first 18 months after diagnosis of CML, mortality was higher in patients who had received a stem cell transplant than in the cohort treated without transplants. Between 18 to 56 months, mortality was similar in the two groups. After 56 months, the mortality was lower in the patients who were transplanted.[676] Survival after 7 years was 48 percent with transplant and 32 percent with hydroxyurea or IFN treatment.[676] Comparable analyses using a cohort of imatinib-treated patients are needed. The quality of life of surviving patients may not return to normal but continues to improve after transplantation.[661] The relative benefit of marrow compared to mobilized blood stem cells as the source of the allograft has not been established.[677,678] Mobilized blood stem cells engraft more rapidly but may be associated with more chronic GVHD.

For younger patients who do not have a histocompatible sibling, an unrelated donor or a mismatched family member as a source of stem cells is feasible. The toxicity of this procedure is greater than that of an HLA-identical sibling donor transplant. Five-year disease-free survival is approximately 40 percent.[679] Younger patients with cytomegalovirus-seronegative donors who are matched at the HLA-DRB1 allele by molecular methods fare better.[680] When class I HLA genes are typed with molecular methods, an improvement in matching and better outcomes using unrelated donors are expected. When matched-unrelated donor and sibling donor transplants were compared, unrelated donor transplants had increased risk of graft failure and acute GVHD but only a slightly poorer survival and disease-free survival. For patients who survived to 1 year, only a slightly inferior disease-free survival was observed.[681] The rate of extensive chronic GVHD is up to 60 percent with unrelated donor transplants, but 63 percent disease-free survival in younger CML chronic phase patients has been reported.[682] No evidence has been found for an independent adverse effect of IFN on outcome of unrelated donor transplants in the first chronic phase.[683] Cord blood stem cell transplantation from an unrelated donor has also been used in adults with CML.[684]

The major causes of a stem cell allograft failure in CML include conditioning regimen-related toxicity, GVHD, and relapse of leukemia. Prophylaxis of GVHD may include various methods of T cell depletion *in vitro* or *in vivo* and prevention of the reaction with cyclosporine or tacrolimus and methotrexate. Glucocorticoids are the mainstay of treatment for established GVHD. The risk of leukemia relapse is higher if the allograft is depleted of T cells *in vitro*. Using non–T cell-depleted grafts, the 5-year relapse rate is approximately 20 percent and in unrelated donor transplants is 3 percent.[685] Use of unrelated stem cell allografts compensates for the reduced graft-versus-leukemia activity associated with T cell depletion in patients transplanted in the chronic phase.[686] Patients who have grade I initial acute GVHD with subsequent limited chronic GVHD have the best overall survival.[687] Higher grades of acute GVHD and extensive chronic GVHD have a negative impact on survival. Disease status after allografting can be monitored with cytogenetic studies, PCR, or FISH analysis. A positive PCR assay 3 months after allogeneic transplantation has not been found to correlate with an increased risk of relapse compared with PCR-negative patients. A positive assay at 6 months and beyond is

associated with subsequent relapse. In one series, 42 percent of patients with a positive PCR assay at 6 to 12 months relapsed versus 3 percent with a negative assay.[688] Paradoxically, patients who remain *BCR-ABL* positive more than 36 months after transplant have little propensity for relapse.[688] Serial quantitative RT-PCR analysis of blood specimens has been proposed to distinguish patients destined to relapse.[689] Patients who remain in remission have undetectable, low, or falling BCR-ABL levels on sequential analysis. After 6 to 9 months, these levels are undetectable in most cases. Recognition of relapse at the molecular level may allow for early therapeutic intervention. Graft-versus-leukemia effect may suppress minimal residual disease after allogeneic stem cell transplantation.[690]

Infection with cytomegalovirus, fungi, herpes simplex virus, or herpes zoster virus can cause severe morbidity and early posttransplantation mortality, but these causes of death have decreased in frequency. Poorly controlled GVHD is the major cause of early posttransplantation mortality. The early posttransplantation mortality of approximately 25 percent has stimulated studies that define the optimal time of transplantation in chronic phase by considering variables such as age, percent blood blasts, spleen size, likelihood of remaining in chronic phase for a prolonged period, and probability of successful marrow transplantation in the accelerated phase.[691]

Stem cell transplantation can eradicate the Ph-chromosome–carrying clone and has led to apparent cure of some patients.[692] In the past, some advocated that stem cell transplantation be undertaken during the first year of the chronic phase if a histocompatible sibling or identical twin donor was available.[693] The frequency of cytogenetic remissions with imatinib therapy has altered these recommendations, which remain in flux based on the patient's age, initial response to imatinib, and type of donor available.[694] These recommendations can be formulated only once the following are known: whether imatinib can induce durable molecular remissions, whether imatinib can prolong survival compared with other treatments, and whether imatinib can "cure" CML patients.[695] Individual patient preferences are a major factor in the decision to move to an allograft. Imatinib may result in better disease status before transplant and therefore might improve transplant results, but the ultimate effect of imatinib on allografting remains unknown.[696] Allografting continues to play a prominent role in the treatment of patients with suboptimal imatinib responses and remains the treatment of choice in accelerated phase and blast crisis.

NONMYELOABLATIVE ALLOGENEIC TRANSPLANTS

Nonablative regimens have been developed in an attempt to expand the indication for allogeneic transplantation to older patients. These regimens rely on immunosuppressive therapy to allow engraftment of cells that potentially will generate a graft-versus-leukemia effect. These procedures in general have been associated with acceptable degrees of engraftment, less mortality, similar rates of GVHD, and possible durable effects on persistent or recurrent disease. In the European experience, this type of transplant was associated with a 1-year survival rate of 65 percent.[697] In another series of nonmyeloablative stem cell transplants for CML, 21 of 24 patients were alive at a median followup of 42 months. The probability of survival at 5 years was 85 percent.[698] Conditioning regimens include fludarabine and busulfan,[698,699] TBI and fludarabine, and TBI and cyclophosphamide, but no prospective randomized trials comparing regimens or comparing ablative and nonmyeloablative transplant approaches have been conducted.[698,700,701] In one case, imatinib given concurrently with nonmyeloablative stem cell transplantation did not compromise engraftment and resulted in a cytogenetic remission in a patient with CML in blast crisis.[702] Most nonablative CML transplant patients have T cell mixed chimerism, whereas the majority of cases have granulocyte and dendritic cell lineages of donor origin.[703]

USE OF IMATINIB MESYLATE AFTER STEM CELL TRANSPLANT

Complete cytogenetic remissions with imatinib treatment occur in patients who relapse after allografting and after donor lymphocyte infusion (DLI) fails to give a response, including reports of a molecular response.[704] Complete responses after imatinib therapy have been noted in advanced CML persisting after stem cell transplant.[705] In another series, 45 percent of relapsed patients had a complete cytogenetic response with durability up to 28 months and without significant GVHD.[706] In a series of 28 adults with relapse after allogeneic stem cell transplantation who received imatinib, the response rate was 74 percent, and the complete cytogenetic remission rate was 35 percent. Five patients had recurrence of GVHD, and 13 had previous DLI infusions.[704] In some patients, decreased neutrophil and platelet counts necessitated imatinib dose adjustment. Imatinib may be started posttransplant prior to hematologic relapse in patients who have minimal residual disease by PCR.[706] In one series, imatinib was able to generate complete molecular remissions in 26 percent of chronic phase patients after allografting, with full donor chimerism usually observed.[707]

IMMUNOTHERAPY: ADOPTIVE CELL THERAPY FOR POSTTRANSPLANT RELAPSE

Substantial evidence indicates the effectiveness of allografting in CML does not result solely from the eradication of the leukemic clone with high-dose chemoradiotherapy conditioning regimens but also from adoptive immunotherapy provided by lymphocytes in the allograft, the graft-versus-leukemia effect.[662] This phenomenon has been recreated to produce a therapeutic response by infusing the lymphocytes from the stem cell donor after a relapse following allogeneic stem cell transplantation.[708,709] The overall response rate to DLI is approximately 75 percent. The response rate is higher when this approach is used early after detecting a relapse by PCR[710] compared to use after a hematologic or cytogenetic relapse. Patients with a short interval between transplant and DLI have a higher probability of response than patients with longer intervals. Responses are the same with related versus unrelated donors.[711] Some patients show a very rapid decline of BCR-ABL transcript levels (<6 months after DLI), whereas other patients demonstrate PCR negativity only over a longer period.[712] The responses to DLI can be durable.[713] Molecular responses can occur in up to two thirds of patients.[714] This approach may prevent the need for high-dose cytotoxic chemotherapy that would accompany a second transplant procedure.[715] DLI increases activation markers on T and NK cells and results in increased IL-1 and IFN production.[716]

The main toxicities of DLI have been the induction of GVHD and myelosuppression. Attempts to diminish these toxicities have included use of CD8-depleted donor leukocyte infusions and infusion of smaller numbers of T cells.[717,718] Lower initial cell dose has been associated with less myelosuppression, the same response rate, better survival, and less DLI-related mortality, leading to suggestions that the initial dose should not exceed 0.2×10^8 mononuclear cells/kg.[719] The recommended initial doses are lower in matched unrelated donors. Donor lymphocytes can also be transfected with vectors containing the herpes simplex virus genome in a replication defective form. If GVHD occurs, the lymphocytes can be eradicated with systemic ganciclovir treatment. The ultimate utility of such approaches is still unmeasured.[720] IFN after DLI may improve responses.[721,722]

Methods for administering more specific immune effector cells have been sought. BCR-ABL–specific T cells with marked cytotoxic activity against CML cells can be generated and amplified from the blood of a normal donor.[723,724] HLA-DR1–restricted BCR-ABL (b3a2)-specific, CD4-positive T lymphocytes respond to dendritic cells pulsed with BCR-ABL (b3a2)-peptide and antigen-presenting cells ex-posed to BCR-ABL (b3a2)-containing cell lysates.[725] Peptides derived from the whole sequence of BCR-ABL bind to several class I molecules, allowing specific induction of human cytotoxic T lymphocytes.[726,727] Whether such cells utilized in adoptive immunotherapy will be more effective than donor leukocytes in preventing or treating relapse is not known. Complete remissions of accelerated phase CML by treatment with leukemia-reactive cytotoxic T lymphocytes administered at 5-week intervals have been described. These lines were generated from the allogeneic donor and expanded in vitro to generate cytotoxic T lymphocyte lines.[728]

COURSE AND PROGNOSIS

Several large studies of treatment during the 1970s and early 1980s reported similar survival rates of patients with CML treated with standard chemotherapy, that is, busulfan or hydroxyurea, during the chronic phase.[729–737] Median survival ranged from 39 to 47 months, the 5-year survival rate was approximately 25 to 35 percent of patients, and the 8-year survival rate was 8 to 17 percent of patients. A large randomized study comparing hydroxyurea to busulfan showed a significant prolongation of chronic phase with hydroxyurea[603] and a further prolongation with IFN therapy. Occasional patients have remained in the chronic phase from 10 to 25 years.[738–745] The Surveillance, Epidemiology and End Results Program of the National Cancer Institute provides global statistics based on cancer registries in the United States. Table 88-3 provides the 5-year survival rates from these observations. The data are from the pre-imatinib mesylate period. At the time of diagnosis, the variables most closely associated with duration of chronic phase and thus survival are percent blasts in the blood, liver and spleen size, and total basophil plus eosinophil count. Using these variables in large numbers of patients, the population segregates into three risk groups: better risk, with a median survival of approximately 5.0 years; intermediate risk, with a median survival of 3.5 years; and poor risk, with a median survival of 2.5 years.[746–748] In the better-risk group, 40 percent are alive at 7 years; in the poor-risk group, 10 percent or fewer are alive at 7 years. These figures are based on large numbers of patients treated principally with busulfan. Treatment of chronic phase by hydroxyurea and then by IFN has extended the median survival by approximately 18 months with the former and approximately 36 months, with the latter in patients treated with these agents. Generalizations to all patients with CML based on those studies is not possible because many patients, especially those older than 65 years, cannot tolerate optimal doses of IFN. Thus, the results are for the select group of patients who remain on treatment with those agents. The median survivals also may be further improved by imatinib treatment. One projection indicates the median survival for all patients will exceed 15 years.[1092]

Prognostic indices may be useful in interpreting the results of therapy and may have a major role in deciding the timing of allogeneic

TABLE 88-3 CHRONIC MYELOGENOUS LEUKEMIA: FIVE-YEAR RELATIVE SURVIVAL RATES (1992–1998)

AGE (YEARS)	PERCENT OF PATIENTS
<45	49.2
45–54	45.1
55–64	34.9
65–74	27.6
>75	15.8

SOURCE: Data from Surveillance, Epidemiology, End Results Cancer Statistics, 5-Year Survival Rates, Table XIII-10, National Cancer Institute, Washington, DC. Available at www.seer.cancer.gov.

stem cell transplantation.[691,749] However, the indices may not have sufficient specificity and sensitivity for application to a single patient. Studies linking the precise (3') location of the breakpoint in the *BCR* gene with shortened duration of chronic phase[750] have not been confirmed.[751] Most patients die as a result of conversion from the chronic to the accelerated phase of the disease.[752] Very rare spontaneous remissions of CML have been reported,[753,754] but the disease may recur.[755]

Several other ancillary factors have been associated with poor prognosis in CML. These factors include marrow angiogenesis and marrow fibrosis,[756] telomere length shortening,[757] cellular VEGF expression,[758] large deletions at the t(9;22) breakpoint,[759] derivative chromosome 9 deletions,[760,761] increased marrow fiber content and reduction of medullary erythropoiesis,[762] higher CD7 expression by CD34-positive cells,[763] absence of cadherin 13 expression,[764] and persistence of malignant hematopoietic progenitors in CML in complete cytogenetic remission after imatinib.[523] Deletion of the 5' abl region on der(9), present in approximately 9 percent of patients with CML, occurs at the time of formation of the t(9;22) translocation and may be associated with a slightly worse prognosis.[765] The prognosis may not be worse with imatinib therapy. The type of BCR breakpoint (5' or 3') does not affect the course of chronic phase CML.[751,766] CML that occurs after treatment of other cancers appears to have comparable clinical and survival characteristics as *de novo* CML.[767]

Several prognostic scales have been proposed in CML, including the Sokal and Hasford systems for patients at the time of diagnosis and the European Bone Marrow Transplantation Consortium Risk Score for patients undergoing allogeneic stem cell transplantation,[768] in which performance status is added to the five original variables. The Hasford score, which includes age, spleen size, blast cell count, basophil and eosinophil count, and platelet count, has been validated with good discrimination for survival.[769] The Sokal score was developed much earlier during the busulfan era of treatment and was less accurate in patients treated with IFN. A simple prognostic scale that includes donor type, stage of disease at time of transplantation, age of recipient, sex of donor and recipient, and interval between diagnosis and transplant has been proposed to predict outcome of allogeneic stem cell transplant.[770] These prognostic scales require revalidation given the dramatic impact of conversion to universal imatinib therapy. Low neutrophil count and poor cytogenetic response at 3 months of imatinib therapy may predict a poor overall outcome,[771] but this observation requires validation.[772] Cytogenetic response as a surrogate marker for survival appears to be useful in patients undergoing imatinib therapy.[773]

DETECTION OF MINIMAL RESIDUAL DISEASE

Detection of minimal residual disease by molecular probes makes possible the identification of approximately one cell in 1,000,000 that is derived from the CML clone.[774] Techniques used to monitor residual disease have been reviewed.[775,776] PCR permits observation of the regression of subclinical disease following therapy, persistence of subclinical disease following therapy, or progression of subclinical disease prior to the disease becoming overt and is critical for monitoring responses to CML treatment.[777,778] The stable persistence of subclinical disease does not invariably predict early relapse.[779,780]

The risk of misinterpreting negative results of RT-PCR is increased when very small numbers of transcripts are present.[775] The dilution threshold for reproducible amplification is 250,000 cells. mRNA$^{BCR-ABL}$ can also be detected in single progenitor colonies after culture.[781] A good correlation has been found between the proportion of Ph-chromosome–positive metaphase cells and levels of mRNA$^{BCR-ABL}$, and no difference in the levels of the fusion mRNA

was found between Ph-chromosome–positive and Ph-chromosome–negative, *BCR-ABL*–positive patients.[782–784]

Through utilization of quantitative PCR, an increase of mRNA$^{BCR-ABL}$ expression has been found to precede disease progression. This increase was detected up to 16 months before laboratory or clinical parameters showed phenotypic transformation of the malignant clone.[785] The technique of detecting minimal residual disease is highly sensitive but is subject to false-positive reactions. Nested, competitive RT-PCR is more sensitive than RT-PCR, but RT-PCR, when normalized for the total ABL transcripts, can be used to monitor CML patients during therapy.[786]

Interphase FISH may have a false-positive rate of 5 to 10 percent.[787] FISH is not standardized, but a large number of cells can be rapidly analyzed (100–500). With D-FISH probes, which flank the breakpoints of the *BCR* and *ABL* genes, the false-positive rate is only approximately 0.2 percent.[787] Fixation, specimen preparation, and hybridization conditions may account for differing false-positive ranges and scoring criteria.[788] In patients treated with imatinib, FISH for *BCR-ABL* on interphase blood neutrophils but not unselected white cells correlates with marrow cytogenetics in CML patients treated with imatinib.[789] Although quantitative RT-PCR might be the most useful assay for minimal residual disease, FISH and RT-PCR can be useful complementary techniques.[790] Negative results with quantitative RT-PCR should be confirmed with nested PCR.[787]

For patients undergoing allogeneic stem cell transplantation, the kinetics of minimal residual disease in either standard or nonmyeloablative transplants differ. Reduced-intensity transplants had minimal residual disease. BCR-ABL/ABL ratios were 0.2 percent versus 0.01 percent in transplant patients with traditional conditioning regimens in the first 3 months. By 12 months, however, 20 percent of patients who received standard transplants and 50 percent of patients who received reduced-intensity transplants had reached a level less than 0.01 percent, supporting the concept of different kinetics of disease eradication between the two transplant modalities.[703] Patients who relapse after allografting have reappearance and/or rising levels of BCR-ABL transcripts.[791] Use of quantitative RT-PCR early (3–5 months) after stem cell transplant can project long-term outcomes.[792] When RT-PCR was negative, the 3-year risk of relapse was 16.7 percent; when RT-PCR was positive at a ratio of less than 0.02 percent, the relapse rate was 42.9 percent; and when RT-PCR was positive at a level greater than 0.02 percent, the relapse rate was 86.5 percent. Another group found that detection of blood BCR-ABL at 18 or more months after transplantation was associated with a 19.2 hazard risk of relapse and that patients who had a positive test result but failed to relapse generally had only one positive test result at a low copy number.[793] Performance of qualitative PCR at regular intervals after allogeneic transplant (every 2–4 months in the first year and every 6 months thereafter) has been recommended (Table 88-4). If the PCR results are persistently positive or become positive, quantitative PCR should be performed at monthly or shorter intervals. Molecular relapse is defined as a 10-fold increase of PCR positivity without any signs of cytogenetic relapse.[794]

TABLE 88-4 SUGGESTED MONITORING OF PATIENTS IN CHRONIC PHASE UNDERGOING IMATINIB MESYLATE THERAPY

1. At 3, 6, 9, and 12 months after initiating therapy, perform FISH on blood cells and qPCR for BCR-ABL transcripts if available.
2. At 12 months, obtain marrow for cytogenetics.
3. Thereafter, monitor every 4 months with FISH and qPCR on blood cells.
4. Continue yearly marrow examination of marrow cytogenetics to identify clonal evolution.

FISH = fluorescence *in situ* hybridization; qPCR = quantitative polymerase chain reaction.
SOURCE: Based in part on ref. 569.

Detection of increasing recipient chimerism by FISH for the male chromosome in sex-mismatched donor recipient pairs or variable number of tandem repeats after allogeneic transplant or after DLI infusion also is usually associated with a relapse.[795,796]

Imatinib is associated with a rapid decrease in BCR-ABL transcript levels. Nested PCR transcript levels parallel cytogenetic response, and imatinib is superior to IFN or cytarabine in terms of the speed and degree of molecular responses, but residual disease is rarely eliminated.[797] When quantitative RT-PCR is utilized in patients undergoing imatinib therapy, almost all patients have evidence of residual disease.[798,799] Disadvantages of quantitative RT-PCR in monitoring imatinib response include lack of standardization, inability to detect clonal evolution, and current lack of widespread availability.[787]

ACCELERATED PHASE AND BLAST CRISIS OF CML

DEFINITION

In most cases of CML, the patient's disease eventually changes to a more aggressive, more symptomatic and troublesome phase, which is poorly responsive to therapy that formerly controlled the chronic phase. The failure of therapy to restore or maintain near-normal red cell and white cell counts, increased spleen size, increased numbers of marrow blasts and blood basophils, loss of the sense of well-being, and appearance of extramedullary tumors are the most consistent clinical hallmarks of the metamorphosis of the chronic to the accelerated phase of CML. The most objective findings are a blood blast percentage greater than 10, a platelet count less than $100,000/\mu l$ (100×10^9/liter), blood basophils greater than 20 percent, and new clonal cytogenetic abnormalities accompanying the Philadelphia chromosome.[800]

The terminology used has included *accelerated phase*, *acute phase*, *acute transformation*, or, in its most dramatic expression, *blast crisis*, but the metamorphosis, which can be acute, that is, myeloblastic or lymphoblastic crisis, often is more gradual and manifested by severe dysmorphic hematopoiesis, refractory splenomegaly, and extramedullary tumor masses, hence the preference for *transformation* or *accelerated phase* to describe this transition from a controllable to a poorly controlled malignancy. Blast crisis is the most severe manifestation of the accelerated phase and can occur abruptly or after a period of worsening disease.

PATHOGENESIS

Progression of chronic phase to accelerated phase is marked by an increase in BCR-ABL expression.[801,802] Superimposed on the increased transcription of mRNA[BCR-ABL] are additional cytogenetic abnormalities that are added to the persistent Ph chromosome in approximately 50 to 65 percent of patients.[800,802–805] In lymphoid blast crisis, acquisition of p16/ARF mutations occurs in approximately 50 percent of cases and RB gene mutations in approximately 20 percent of cases. In myeloid blast crisis, approximately 25% of cases have cells containing a p53 mutation.[806] The possible role of loss of p53 function in fostering transformation of a human chronic phase CML clone has been demonstrated in transgenic mice in which p53 function was abrogated.[807] p51/p63 is a member of the p53 gene family that is not mutated in chronic phase but is mutated in approximately 8 percent of patients in blast crisis.[808]

Progression of the clone to a more malignant clone is reflected in a more disordered growth and maturation pattern of progenitor cells in culture, ultimately mimicking the growth failure of acute leukemia,[803] and in increased morphologic and functional abnormalities of blood cells,[809,810] eventuating in a block in maturation and replacement of blood and marrow by blast cells. Thus, the accelerated phase of the

disease results from an evolution of the clone that supported the chronic phase to a much higher degree of malignancy.

Approximately 65 percent of patients have cytogenetic abnormalities in addition to the Ph chromosome. A double Ph chromosome, trisomy 8, and isochromosome 17p are the secondary changes most commonly seen.[806,811] Because the frequency of trisomy 8 was greater after treatment with busulfan compared to hydroxyurea, the frequency of secondary chromosomal changes may be quite different after imatinib mesylate therapy.[806] Clonal instability has also been found in cases of lymphoid blast crisis. Clones distinct from those identified later may be detected before overt lymphoid transformation. Identification of these abortive clones suggests clonal instability before the onset of transformation, which might have prognostic value.[812] FISH has been used to determine which cells have secondary cytogenetic abnormalities, and these cells often are not the blast cells. This finding suggests that some chromosomal abnormalities merely denote genomic instability.[813] The abnormal mRNA and protein product p210[BCR-ABL] are present in the marrow and blood cells of patients who have transformed to acute leukemia.[814–816] Although the breakpoint site on M-bcr was thought to be correlated with the time of the onset of the accelerated phase,[816] subsequent studies have not indicated a correlation between length of chronic phase and the specific site of the BCR-ABL fusion.[817] Rare cases have had deletion of the BCR-ABL fusion gene, loss of transcription of the message, and loss of expression of the p210 tyrosine kinase after transformation, the latter finding suggesting the abnormal protein kinase may not play a unique role in sustaining the acute state.[818] In contrast, the response, albeit temporary, to imatinib indicates that the *mutant BCR-ABL* product plays some role at this stage of the disease.

Numerous molecular changes identified in the cells of patients with acute transformation that might contribute to the increased malignant behavior of the CML clone, including activation of the N-RAS gene,[819,820] rearrangement of the p53 gene,[820–823] hypermethylation of the calcitonin gene,[824] and methylation of the ABL1 gene,[825] have been described. One series found p53 mutations in 17 percent of blast crisis patients. An association between the failure of CML cells to express the retinoblastoma gene product and acute blast crisis with a megakaryoblastic phenotype has been reported.[826] Homozygous deletions of the p16 tumor suppressor gene have been associated with lymphoid transformation of CML,[827] but such deletions have not been seen in the chronic phase and in myeloid blast crisis. p16 is also known as the *cyclin-dependent kinase 4 inhibitor gene* and is located on chromosome 9p21.[828,829] This gene inhibits the kinase CDK-4, which regulates a cell cycle checkpoint prior to commitment to DNA synthesis. The WT gene on chromosome 11p13 encodes a zinc finger motif-containing transcription factor found in CML patients only after progression to blast crisis.[830] Overexpression of the EVI-1 gene has also been found in CML blast crisis.[831,832] Microsatellite instability has not been found to be involved with progression to blast crisis.[833] BCL-2, c-MYC, and various other genes have also been implicated in the evolution of CML.[834–837]

CLINICAL FEATURES

The features that signal the conversion of the chronic to the accelerated phase include unexplained fever, bone pain, weakness, night sweats, weight loss, loss of sense of well-being, arthralgias, and left upper quadrant pain related to splenic enlargement or infarcts. These features may occur weeks in advance of laboratory evidence of the accelerated phase. Localized or diffuse lymphadenopathy or enlarging masses in extralymphatic and extramedullary sites containing Ph-chromosome–positive myeloblasts or lymphoblasts may develop. A poor response of blood cell counts and splenic enlargement despite previously effective therapy may be evident.[800,806,838-840] Symptoms caused by histamine excess in basophilic crisis can be present.[841]

Several of these changes may occur in series or in parallel. The time of onset of transformation and the appearance of a blastic crisis and its clinical expression are unpredictable.

LABORATORY FEATURES

BLOOD FINDINGS[806,838-840]

Anemia may worsen and be associated with increasing poikilocytosis, anisocytosis, and anisochromia. The number of nucleated red cells in the blood may increase. These red cell changes may be accentuated further if advancing marrow fibrosis is a feature of the disease.

The total leukocyte count may fall without treatment. The proportion of blasts increases to greater than 10 percent in blood and marrow in the accelerated phase and when blast crisis ensues represents 20 to 90 percent of the cells. Myelocytes decrease in number. Hyposegmented neutrophils (Pelger-Huët cells) may become evident. Basophils increase and represent 20 to 80 percent of the total blood leukocytes. A decrease of the platelet count to less than $100,000/\mu l$ ($<100 \times 10^9$/liter) develops. Giant platelets, micromegakaryocytes, and megakaryocyte fragments may enter the blood. Decreased progenitor cell growth in culture is present, akin to that in acute leukemia.

MARROW FINDINGS[806,838-840]

The marrow findings are widely variable. Marked dysmorphic changes in one, two, or three of the major cell lineages; an increase in blast count to greater than 10 percent, marrow morphology simulating subacute myelomonocytic leukemia; or, in the extreme, florid blastic transformation with blast counts greater than 30 percent can occur. Reticulin fibers may increase, and occasionally severe reticulin and collagen fibrosis develop. Additional clonal cytogenetic abnormalities develop in as many as half the patients in accelerated phase (see "Cytogenetic Studies" below).

EXTRAMEDULLARY BLAST CRISIS

A variety of symptoms or signs may occur as a result of the specific effects of new extramedullary blastic tumors, referred to as *extramedullary blast crisis*.[842-845] Extramedullary blast crisis is the first manifestation of accelerated phase in approximately 10 percent of patients with CML. Lymph nodes,[843,845] serosal surfaces,[846,847] skin and soft tissue,[842-845] breast,[845,848] gastrointestinal or genitourinary tract,[843,845] bone,[843,845,849-852] and central nervous system[845,853-855] are among the principal areas involved. Isolated or diffuse lymphadenopathy may occur. Bone involvement may lead to severe pain, tenderness, and changes on x-ray films. Central nervous system involvement usually is meningeal and may be preceded by headache, vomiting, stupor, cranial nerve palsies, and papilledema and is associated with an increase in cells, protein, and the presence of blasts in the spinal fluid.[845,853-855]

Appropriate histochemical and immunologic tests are required to determine if the extramedullary disease is composed of phenotypic myeloblasts or lymphoblasts. Because the tumor cells may have features of lymphoma cells, the terms *myeloid* or *granulocytic sarcoma*, *chloroma*, and *myeloblastoma* can be misnomers, and the term *extramedullary blast crisis* is used for this circumstance in CML.[854,856-858] The lymphoblasts, like the myeloblasts, are Ph chromosome positive. A combination of morphology, histochemistry (e.g., peroxidase, lysozyme), terminal transferase assay, and monoclonal antibodies specific for lymphoid or myeloid cells can be used to classify the extramedullary blast cells. Older reports (1930s–1960s) of concurrent lymphoma and CML probably were, in many cases, examples of extramedullary lymphoblast crisis in lymph nodes or other sites.

MARROW BLAST CRISIS

Approximately half of patients with CML enter the accelerated phase by developing acute leukemia. The onset of blast crisis can develop from days[859-861] to decades after diagnosis of CML. The signs and symptoms may include fever, hemorrhage, bone pain, and lymphadenopathy.[800,859-861] The morphology of the acute leukemia usually is myeloblastic or myelomonocytic.[800,862] A substantial proportion of myeloid leukemia in this setting may not have myeloperoxidase demonstrable by cytochemistry.[863] The proportion of cases classified as erythroblastic leukemia is approximately 10 percent based on morphologic features[864] but may be as high as 20 percent if expression of glycophorin-A is used as the determinant.[865] Occasional cases have megakaryoblastic transformation.[826,866] These cases may be difficult to identify by light microscopy because the megakaryoblasts may be mistaken for lymphoid cells or undifferentiated blasts. Myelofibrosis is a feature of this variant. Antiplatelet glycoprotein antibodies and other monoclonal antiplatelet antibodies now are available as reagents to identify megakaryoblasts without the need for ultrastructural studies.[866] Promyelocytic[867-869] and eosinophilic[870] blast crises also can occur. Basophilic leukemia is a known variant of CML.[871] Patients with promyelocytic crisis often have t(15;17) in addition to the Ph chromosome, and some have presented with disseminated intravascular coagulation.[872]

CML may transform into acute lymphoblastic leukemia in approximately 30 percent of CML patients in blastic crisis.[800,873-877] The lymphoid cells generally express terminal deoxynucleotidyl transferase (TdT)[873,874] and are of the B cell lineage,[877-879] as judged by antiimmunoglobulin staining. TdT is a DNA polymerase that adds deoxynucleoside monophosphates from triphosphate substrates to single-stranded DNA by end addition, differing in the latter respect from replicative polymerases.[880] The enzyme is present in normal immature thymocytes and in the blast cells of nearly all patients with acute lymphoblastic leukemia. Rare patients have blasts with a T lymphocyte phenotype.[856,857,881-883] Some cases are biphenotypic; the blasts have both lymphoid and myeloid markers.[862,884-886] Some cases may have myeloperoxidase activity in blast cells and express CD33 or CD13. Myeloid to lymphoid clonal succession following autologous transplantation in the second chronic phase has been described.[887] Patients with lymphoid blast crisis seldom have an intermediate accelerated phase, have less splenomegaly and basophilia, and usually have a higher degree of marrow blast infiltration. Remission rate and survival are somewhat longer in cases of lymphoid compared to myeloid blast crisis.[888]

CYTOGENETIC STUDIES

Most large studies have shown four principal changes in patients' cells prior to, or during, the accelerated phase: additional 22q−, isochromosome 17, trisomy 8, and trisomy 19.[889-891] In addition, a large number of other chromosome abnormalities have been described.[892-896] In one study, 63 percent of 73 blast crisis patients had secondary cytogenetic abnormalities. These abnormalities were more common in myeloid blast crisis and were associated with shorter remission.[812] The changes may be features of myeloid blast crisis compared to lymphoid crisis.[890,894] Some abnormalities, such as inv16, have been associated with early transformation to AML.[891,894,897] A significant proportion (50%) of patients in the accelerated phase or blast crisis have no additional cytogenetic abnormalities beyond t(9;22)(q34;q11) after banding and multicolor FISH analysis.[896] In cases where the blastic transformation is in extramedullary sites, such as lymph nodes or spleen, the additional cytogenetic abnormalities may be in the cells at those sites but not in cells in the blood or marrow.[898]

TREATMENT

Optimal treatment today, aimed at cure, is allogeneic stem cell transplantation if the patient is eligible because of his/her age and donor availability.

CHEMOTHERAPY

The treatment approach is predicated on the phenotype of the blast cells in CML patients with blast crisis. In patients with myeloid phenotypes, the approach has been similar to that used for acute myelogenous leukemia: combinations of an anthracycline antibiotic, such as idarubicin or daunorubicin, with high-dose cytosine arabinoside and sometimes etoposide.[899] Because this approach produces few remissions that are of short duration (median survival approximately 6 months), a variety of other drug combinations incorporating 5-azacytidine, busulfan, cladribine, fludarabine, clofarabine, high-dose cytosine, arabinoside, decitabine, etoposide, farnesyl transferase inhibitors, hydroxyurea, methotrexate, mitoxantrone, plicamycin, tiazofurin, or troxacitabine have been used, but with no significant improvement in outcome.[900]

In patients with lymphoid phenotypes, vincristine sulfate 1.4 mg/m^2 (not to exceed 2 mg/dose) given intravenously once per week and prednisone 60 mg/m^2/day given orally have been the mainstay of treatment. A minimum of two cycles of treatment (2 weeks) should be given to judge responsivity. Approximately one third of patients with lymphoid blast transformation will reenter the chronic phase after such treatment. However, because only about one third of patients have lymphoid blasts, this number represents a remission rate of only approximately 10 percent of patients who enter blast crisis using this approach. Some relapsed patients become TdT negative (myeloblastic relapse). However, even if relapsed patients remain TdT positive, they are not likely to respond to a second treatment. Some therapists argue for a more intensive induction regimen for patients with lymphoblastic crisis, akin to regimens for *de novo* adult ALL or high-risk childhood ALL, and report somewhat better results: higher remission rates and longer remissions. The benefit of such an intensive approach has been small because remission durations have been modest. TdT-positive, CD10 (CALLA)-positive lymphoblasts may be the lymphoblast phenotype most responsive to vincristine and prednisone.[876]

IMATINIB MESYLATE THERAPY

The introduction of imatinib mesylate 300 to 1000 mg/day used alone has produced a proportion of improved responses, such that complete hematologic remissions can occur in approximately 20 percent of patients in blast crisis.[900–902] However, complete cytogenetic responses are uncommon (approximately one in 15 cases). Compared to historical controls of various combinations of chemotherapy, imatinib mesylate used alone results in comparable outcomes (6-month median survival in blast crisis).[900,901] Patients who enter a second chronic phase with therapy fare better than patients who do not. In one retrospective analysis of patients treated with chemotherapy, imatinib mesylate, and autologous transplantation in various combinations, patients entering a second chronic phase had a median survival of 12 months; patients who did not had a median survival of 6 months.[903] However, the median age of this group of patients was 39 years, which is approximately 30 years younger on average than that of the affected population at large.

Imatinib mesylate 600 mg/day administered in the accelerated phase has resulted in approximately 30 percent of patients achieving a complete hematologic response and 15 percent achieving a complete cytogenetic response, with two thirds of patients alive at 12 months.[800]

ALLOGENEIC STEM CELL TRANSPLANTATION

Stem cell transplantation from a histocompatible twin or sibling has been used in some patients after entry into the blastic phase. Occasional patients have had long-term survival. The 3-year survival rate is approximately 15 to 20 percent,[904–906] unlike transplantation in the chronic phase, in which the 3-year survival rate is 50 to 60 percent. However, for patients who present in blast crisis, who develop blast crisis in the first year of the chronic phase, or who delay transplantation for other reasons, transplantation remains the best hope for long-term survival if a histocompatible donor is available.[904,905] Relapse of accelerated phase after allogeneic stem cell transplantation has responded to infusion of donor, *in vitro*-selected, cytotoxic T lymphocytes.[907]

AUTOLOGOUS STEM CELL TRANSPLANTATION

Autografting in the accelerated phase or blast crisis, either with stem cells collected during chronic phase or with mobilized Ph-chromosome–negative progenitor cells collected upon cell rebound after intensive chemotherapy, has resulted in apparent prolonged remission in some patients.[908] Whether Ph-chromosome–negative cells collected during imatinib therapy have the same potential is unknown.

SPLENECTOMY

Splenectomy may be performed for palliation of painful splenic infarctions or hemorrhage. However, the complication rates are high, and the procedure performed in this setting should be avoided if possible.[909]

COURSE AND PROGNOSIS

The accelerated phase of CML generally is very poorly responsive or refractory to treatment and is a morbid state that can be fatal in weeks to months in all but a few patients who undergo a successful stem cell transplant from a histocompatible donor. Patients with myeloid blast crisis have a median survival of approximately 6 months, whereas patients with lymphoid blast crisis have a median survival of approximately 12 months.[900–903] In the earliest study of imatinib mesylate in blast crisis, patients with myeloblastic crisis had a longer median survival (5.5 months) than patients with lymphoid blast crisis plus Ph-chromosome–positive ALL (3 months). The results are so poor that these minor differences are not consequential. The median survival after evidence of clonal evolution in patients in the chronic phase is approximately 15 months. Poorer survival was seen with abnormalities of chromosome 17, other superimposed translocations, or a high percentage of abnormal metaphases.[910] Severe cytopenias from repeated courses of cytotoxic therapy contribute to infections, hemorrhage, and organ dysfunction, especially liver and kidney dysfunction. Opportunistic infections with herpes viruses, cytomegalovirus, or fungi often supervene. The addition of imatinib mesylate therapy has made only a small difference in long-term outcome, although formal studies of combinations of chemotherapy and imatinib mesylate at a higher dose (600 mg/day) have not been completed.

RELATED CLONAL MYELOID DISEASES WITHOUT THE PH CHROMOSOME (TABLE 88-5)

CHRONIC MYELOMONOCYTIC LEUKEMIA

This leukemia is part of the spectrum of clonal myeloid diseases that may have findings that simulate CML. In the past, when rigorous criteria for the diagnosis of CML were not applied, CMML was among a heterogenous group of related diseases that sometimes were referred

TABLE 88-5 TYPES OF CHRONIC MYELOGENOUS LEUKEMIA

TYPE OF CHRONIC MYELOGENOUS LEUKEMIA	MOLECULAR GENETICS	MAJOR CLINICAL FEATURES	FURTHER DETAILS
BCR rearrangement-positive chronic myelogenous leukemia	>95% p210 BCR-ABL; <5% p190 or p230	Splenomegaly in 85% of cases; WBC >25,000/μl; blood blasts <5%; Ph chromosome in 90% of cases; BCR gene rearrangement in 100% of cases	Page 1244
BCR rearrangement-negative chronic myelogenous leukemia	Various cytogenetic changes	Clinical findings similar to BCR rearrangement-positive CML or CMML; Ph chromosome and BCR-ABL fusion gene absent	Page 1266
Chronic myelomonocytic leukemia	Various cytogenetic abnormalities	Anemia, monocytosis >1000/μl; blood blasts <10%; increased plasma and urine lysozyme; BCR rearrangement absent; uncommon cases with PDGFR-β mutation respond to imatinib	Page 1261
Chronic eosinophilic leukemia	Various cytogenetic abnormalities	Blood eosinophil count >1500/μl; cardiac and neurologic manifestations common; a proportion of cases have PDGFR-α mutations and are responsive to imatinib mesylate	Page 1263
Chronic monocytic leukemia	Various cytogenetic changes	Proportion of monocytes elevated; very rare form of leukemia	Page 1264
Juvenile myelomonocytic leukemia	Various cytogenetic changes	Infants and children <4 years; eczematoid or maculopapular rash; anemia and thrombocytopenia; increased HgF in 70% of cases; neurofibromatosis in 10% of cases; BCR rearrangement absent	Page 1265
Chronic neutrophilic leukemia	Various cytogenetic changes	Neutrophilia >20,000/μl; splenomegaly >90% of cases; no blood blasts; platelets >100,000/μl; 75% of cases have normal cytogenetics; BCR rearrangement absent	Page 1266

to as *Ph-chromosome–negative CML*. These diseases share the feature of originating in the clonal expansion of a primitive multipotential hematopoietic cell.[911]

EPIDEMIOLOGY

Most patients with CMML are older than 50 years, and approximately 75 percent of patients are older than 60 years at the time of diagnosis. The median age at diagnosis is approximately 70 years. Occasional cases have been reported in older children and younger adults. Men are affected somewhat more frequently than women (approximately 1.4:1).[912,913]

CLINICAL FINDINGS

Signs and Symptoms The onset usually is insidious, and weakness, infection, or exaggerated bleeding may bring patients to medical attention.[912,913] Hepatomegaly and splenomegaly occur in approximately 50 percent of patients. Leukemia cutis occurs in a small proportion of patients and usually has a monocytic phenotype: CD45, CD68, and lysozyme positive by immunostaining.[914] Immune manifestations, such as vasculitis, pyoderma gangrenosum, immune cytopenias, and connective tissue diseases, may occur in coincidence with CMML.[915]

Blood and Marrow Findings The disease is characterized by anemia and blood monocytosis greater than 1,000/μl (1 × 10^9/liter).[916] The white cell count may be slightly decreased, normal, or moderately elevated. Occasional patients may have hyperleukocytosis with total white cell counts of 250,000 to 300,000/μl (250–300 × 10^9/liter) associated with respiratory insufficiency resulting from pulmonary leukostasis.[917] Immature granulocytes may be present in the blood. Blood myeloblasts may be absent or, when present, do not exceed 10 percent of total white cells. Most patients have thrombocytopenia, but normal or elevated platelet counts may occur. Eosinophilia may be so prominent in occasional cases that the designation *chronic eosinophilic leukemia* may be appropriate.[912,913,918]

The marrow is hypercellular as a result of granulomonocytic hyperplasia; the dominant cells are early myelocytes. The proportion of progranulocytes is increased. Promonocytes also are increased in number. Distinction between poorly granulated myelocytes and promonocytes with primary granules can be difficult. Macronormoblasts and hypersegmented or hyposegmented (Pelger-Huët) neutrophils are frequent. Despite thrombocytopenia, megakaryocytes usually are present in the marrow. Microvessel density is increased in the marrow, and myelomonocytic cells contain cytoplasmic mRNA for VEGF and membrane VEGF receptors.[919,920] *In vitro* colony studies suggest that autocrine stimulation of cell growth by VEGF may occur. "Spontaneous" cluster/colony growth of granulocyte-monocyte colony forming cells occurs *in vitro*. The latter may result from autocrine or paracrine production of GM-CSF, based on anti–GM-CSF inhibition of colony growth.[921]

Cytogenetic Findings Patients with CMML have an approximately 35 percent frequency of chromosomal abnormalities. Monosomy 7 and trisomy 8 are the most prevalent findings. Approximately 35 percent of patients have point mutations of the *K-RAS* or *N-RAS* gene. The *RAS* gene also may be involved in the transforming events. Abnormal methylation of p15^{INK4B} is a common finding in CMML.[922] Translocation between the gene *PDGFR-β* on chromosome 5(q33) and four partner genes—*TEL* at 12(p13), *HIP-1* at 7(q11.2), *H4* at 10(q22), and Rabaptin-5 at 17(p13)—occur in a very small proportion of patients (approximately 3–4%).[912,923-926] This mutation juxtaposes the gene encoding the PDGFR-β with a partner gene, which results in the encoding of a mutant tyrosine kinase that is constitutively activated and sensitive to inhibition by imatinib mesylate[927] (see "Treatment" below). The cases with *PDGFR-β* translocations are more likely to be accompanied by eosinophilia than are cases with other cytogenetic abnormalities.

Serum and Urine Findings Plasma and urine lysozyme concentrations nearly always are elevated. Plasma levels of VEGF, hepatocyte growth factor, and tumor necrosis factor alpha are elevated. Serum B$_{12}$, β_2-microglobulin, and LDH levels often are elevated.[912,913]

TREATMENT

Treatment of most patients with CMML has been unsatisfactory, and remissions of any duration are uncommon. The age and performance status of the patient are considered in determining the intensity of treatment. Cytarabine, either standard or low-dose, etoposide, hydroxyurea, and other approaches used for the oligoblastic myelogenous leukemias have been attempted, but with little success (see Chap. 86). Decitabine and 5-azacytidine have been useful in a small proportion of patients.[912,913] Unfortunately, although a particular approach may confer significant benefit in a small proportion of cases, determining which patients will respond is not possible, except by trial and error. An exception is the patient with a translocation involving PDGFR-β, which itself occurs in only a small percentage of patients. In the case of PDGFR-β fusion genes with several of the partner genes, imatinib mesylate 400 mg/day has resulted in normal blood counts, cytogenetic remissions, and, occasionally, molecular remission.[922–924,928,929] These fortunate patients probably will benefit from this treatment, as evidenced by prolonged remissions and survival, compared to other drug options, but the number of patients and duration of followup do not permit quantitative estimates at this point. Allogeneic stem cell transplantation is an option for the small proportion of younger patients with an appropriate matched-related or unrelated donor.[930]

COURSE AND PROGNOSIS

Median survival in CMML is approximately 12 months, with a range from approximately 1 to more than 60 months. Approximately 20 percent of patients progress to frank AML. Arbitrary stratification of CMML into types 1 and 2 based on the height of the blast count has been proposed, but distinguishing patients by whether they have 8 or 12 percent blasts on a marrow examination is useless for patient care. It is well established that blast percentage usually is a significant correlate with outcome in any patient with a clonal myeloid disease, and this factor among several others should guide therapy. Clusters of prognostic variables have been used to stratify patients into risk groups for survival duration. In general, the severity of the anemia and the height of the blast percentage are the most important. Other variables that may confer a shorter life expectancy are height of the absolute lymphocyte count, high spontaneous rates of myelomonocytic colony growth, higher total leukocyte counts, higher LDH level, and larger spleen size.[931–933] Unfortunately, at this time, unless the patient is a candidate for imatinib therapy or stem cell transplantation, few options will result in long-term therapeutic effects.

CHRONIC EOSINOPHILIC LEUKEMIA

HISTORY AND DEFINITION

The recognition of eosinophilic lineage prominence in myelogenous leukemia dates to a case published in 1912.[934] In 1968, the term *hypereosinophilic syndrome* was introduced to encompass a group of disorders with (1) prolonged exaggerated eosinophilia without an apparent cause, (2) frequent cardiac and neurologic tissue damage, (3) a poor or transient response to therapy, and (4) a progressive course and a high fatality rate. Shortly thereafter, Benvenisti and Ultmann[935] presented five cases of eosinophilic leukemia and reviewed the literature regarding that phenotypic designation. In 1975, Chusid and colleagues[936] described 14 cases of hypereosinophilic syndrome, highlighted the frequency of secondary cardiac and neurologic disorders, and suggested the existence of a continuum of manifestations. Because some cases had clonal cytogenetic abnormalities and hematologic findings compatible with a clonal myeloid disease, the presence of eosinophilic leukemia was suspected in this apparently heterogeneous group of patients.

The relationship of blood eosinophilia to clonal myeloid diseases is complex because the former can be reactive or represent acute eosinophilic leukemia, chronic eosinophilic leukemia, or eosinophilia associated with a different category of disease, such as BCR-ABL–positive CML, idiopathic myelofibrosis, oligoblastic leukemia (MDS), or mastocytosis.[937] Chronic eosinophilic leukemia is a BCR-ABL–negative, clonal myeloid disease with a striking eosinophilia in the blood and marrow, often with clonal cytogenetic abnormalities that have features including, when present, cytogenetic findings that usually distinguish chronic eosinophilic leukemia from other clonal myeloid diseases that may have an associated eosinophilia, such as CMML. The phenotype of the eosinophilic variant of the latter overlaps somewhat with that of chronic eosinophilic leukemia, although the fusion gene associated with CMML involves the PDGFR-β (see "Chronic Myelomonocytic Leukemia" above), whereas in chronic eosinophilic leukemia the cytogenetic findings are different and in some cases involve PDGFR-α. This definition of chronic eosinophilic leukemia recognizes that, at the margins, classification may be arbitrary.

SIGNS AND SYMPTOMS

Fever, cough, weakness, easy fatigability, dyspnea, abdominal pain, maculopapular rash, cardiac symptoms and signs of heart failure, and a variety of neurologic manifestations ranging from peripheral neuropathy to cerebral encephalomalacia may occur, ranging from mild to severe in expression. Splenomegaly often is evident.

LABORATORY FINDINGS

Eosinophilia is a constant finding. Anemia usually but not always is present at the time of presentation. The leukocyte count may be high-normal or more often elevated. Platelet counts often are normal or mildly decreased. The marrow shows myelocytic and eosinophilic hyperplasia and occasionally Charcot-Leyden crystals. Mast cells may be increased. Megakaryocytes usually are present but may appear dysmorphic. Reticular fibrosis is common. Immunophenotyping and PCR does not show evidence of either a clonal T cell population or T cell receptor rearrangement. Pulmonary function studies may provide evidence of fibrotic (restrictive) lung disease. Echocardiography may detect mural thrombi, thickening (fibrosis) of the ventricular wall, valvular dysfunction from papillary muscle, and chordae fibrosis. Magnetic resonance imaging can detect subendocardial fibrosis, thickening of ventricles, and markedly reduced ventricular lumen volume. Serum IgE, vitamin B_{12}, and tryptase levels usually are elevated. Skin biopsy of lesions uncovers intense eosinophilic infiltrates. Neural or brain biopsy may disclose eosinophilic infiltrates, often perivascular, with microthrombi, axonal degeneration, and gliosis.

Cytogenetic Findings   A wide array of cytogenetic findings have been reported in cases of chronic eosinophilic leukemia.[938] Notable translocations include a high frequency of translocations involving chromosome 5, t(1;5), t(2;5), t(5;12), t(6;11), 8p11, trisomy 8, and numerous others infrequently. Chromosome 5 often is translocated at the site of the PDGFR-β gene, and the phenotype usually is more compatible with CMML with eosinophilia. Chromosome 5 from band q31-35 contains several genes relevant to eosinophilopoiesis, including those encoding IL-5, IL-3, GM-CSF, and PDGFR-β. A cryptic interstitial deletion on chromosome 4(q12;q12) results in the fusion gene FIL1L1-PDGFR-α and in a phenotype of chronic eosinophilic leukemia, which is of particular note because, like the PDGFR-β mutations in CMML with eosinophilia, of a near-universal response to treatment with imatinib mesylate.[938–941]

SERUM TRYPTASE LEVEL ELEVATION VERSUS NORMAL

The elevation of serum tryptase level (>11.5 ng/ml) has been used to distinguish a subset of patients who (1) are male, (2) have marrows that are intensely hypercellular with a higher proportion of immature eosinophils and with dysmorphic mast cells with a CD117−CD25+CD2− genotype and phenotype (distinguishing these cells from classic mastocytosis, which are CD117+CD25+CD2+), (3) have dramatically higher serum B_{12} and IgE levels, (4) are more prone to restrictive pulmonary disease and endomyocardial fibrosis, (5) have the FIP1L1-PDGFR-α fusion gene, and (6) are responsive to imatinib mesylate.[941] Patients with normal serum tryptase levels are more prone to obstructive pulmonary restrictive disease, eosinophilic dermatitis, and gastrointestinal complaints.

DIFFERENTIAL DIAGNOSIS

Eosinophilia can occur for many reasons (see Chap. 62). The first step is to identify signs that may point to a clonal myeloid disease. These signs include anemia, thrombocytopenia, splenomegaly, immature eosinophils in the marrow examination, evidence of dysmorphic cells in blood or marrow, for example, atypical megakaryocytes or dysmorphic mast cells, cardiac or pulmonary manifestations, which may occur secondary to chronic eosinophilic leukemia, and markedly elevated serum tryptase or vitamin B_{12} level. The former signs, especially in the aggregate, are highly suggestive, but the presence of a cytogenetic abnormality in myeloid cells is diagnostic of a clonal myeloid disease (leukemia). If the latter is not evident, PCR and/or flow cytometry to search for a clonal T lymphocyte abnormality should be performed. Whether the eosinophilic leukemia is typical or represents an eosinophilia with idiopathic myelofibrosis, CMML, or MDS is in some ways less important than if it has a mutation that is imatinib mesylate sensitive (e.g., PDGFR mutation).

THERAPY

Patients (nearly always men) whose cells display a FIL1L1-PDGFR-α have a very high probability of responding to imatinib mesylate at a dose of 100 to 400 mg/day.[939–942] The tyrosine kinase activity of this fusion protein is two orders of magnitude more sensitive to imatinib than that of BCR-ABL. However, because not all patients taking 400 mg/day achieve a molecular remission, and that goal may be more likely to result in long-term remission, the dose recommended for initial therapy remains at 400 mg/day with PCR monitoring. Dose adjustment upward if molecular remission is not achieved can be considered. Unlike the case in CML, patients with significant side effects when taking imatinib mesylate 400 mg/day have a high probability of having a very good response at lower doses if downward adjustments are necessary.

In patients with eosinophilic leukemia without an imatinib mesylate-sensitive mutation or in patients who become resistant to imatinib mesylate and who are progressing, ablative or nonablative allogeneic stem cell transplantation can be considered if they are in an acceptable age range and have access to a matched-related or matched-unrelated donor.[943,944]

In imatinib mesylate-insensitive patients without the option of transplantation, empirical treatment with glucocorticoids, hydroxyurea, or anti-IL5[945,946] to decrease eosinophil counts and mute the progress of eosinophil-mediated cutaneous, cardiac, pulmonary, and neurologic tissue damage should be considered. This approach may relieve symptoms for a time but is temporizing if therapy with drugs that might be effective in inhibiting clonal expansion or evolution is not effective (e.g., cytarabine, anthracycline antibiotic, etoposide).

COURSE AND PROGNOSIS

If chronic eosinophilic leukemia is not imatinib sensitive, the long-term outlook is one of probable progressive cardiac and neurologic disability. Transformation to acute eosinophilic or myelogenous leukemia can occur. Allogeneic stem cell transplantation is potentially curative. In imatinib-sensitive cases, hematologic normalization, reversal of marrow fibrosis and mastocytosis, resolution of skin lesions, normalization of spleen size, and restoration of well-being occurs in the great preponderance of cases. Cardiac, neurologic, or pulmonary changes usually cannot be reversed but should be stabilized. The long-term outlook with imatinib mesylate therapy is uncertain. However, imatinib likely will decisively and dramatically improve survival compared to other prior therapy and should greatly improve the prognosis of patients with a molecular target for the drug.

CHRONIC BASOPHILIC LEUKEMIA

This type of clinical disorder in which the patient has marrow and blood basophilia and other findings compatible with a clonal myeloid disease without evidence of the Ph chromosome or BCR-ABL is rare. One report of such a syndrome occurring in four patients, culled from all hospitalized patients in that institution over a 25-year observation period, has been published.[1083] In all cases, the marrow was intensely hypercellular in the three major lineages. Dysmorphic megakaryocytes were evident. Basophilia in marrow and blood was striking, although eosinophilia and increased mast cells also were noted, with each alteration in two of the patients. The clinical effects of basophilic mediator release were evident in two patients. One patient evolved to AML; the other recovered after allogeneic transplantation. The cases had very similar findings, leading to the suggestion they represented Ph-negative chronic basophilic leukemia.

CHRONIC MONOCYTIC LEUKEMIA

HISTORY

In 1937, Osgood[947] reviewed his experience with monocytic leukemia and included a case that probably represented the rare disorder chronic monocytic leukemia. In 1981, approximately 28 bona fide cases had been reported, five cases were added, and the characteristics were reviewed.[948]

CLINICAL FINDINGS

Patients range in age from 30 to 80 years. Males are affected more frequently than females. Fever, fatigue, and left upper quadrant pain are the most common complaints. Splenomegaly and hepatomegaly are nearly constant findings.[948–950]

LABORATORY FINDINGS

Anemia is mild. Anisocytosis and poikilocytosis usually are present. The leukocyte count usually is normal or low but can be elevated in a minority of patients. The percentage of monocytes is increased, but the absolute monocyte count often is normal, ranging from 300 to 1500/μl (0.3–1.5 × 10⁹/liter), or mildly elevated. Occasional patients have more striking monocyte counts. The platelet count may be normal or decreased. Rare nucleated red cells may be present in the blood. The monocytes in the blood contain α-naphthol acetate esterase, tartrate-sensitive acid phosphatase, fluoride-sensitive naphthol AS-D acetate esterase, and peroxidase as judged by histochemical tests. The marrow is cellular, often without an increase in monocytes. The Ph chromosome is absent. The leukemic cells are similar to mature monocytes with abundant cytoplasm. Erythrophagocytosis or thrombocytophagocytosis by monocytes may be seen.

The disease often is not recognized because the total white cell count, monocyte count, and number of marrow monocytes may not be elevated until the spleen is removed, usually for diagnostic purposes.[948] Following splenectomy, a gradual leukocytosis of 3000 to 100,000/μl (3–100 × 10⁹/liter) may develop.[948] The absolute monocyte count increases dramatically, often from less than 1000/μl (1 × 10⁹/liter) to as high as 75,000/μl (75 × 10⁹/liter). The marrow may contain more than 50 percent mature monocytes following splenectomy.

The spleen is enlarged (300–2500 g). The red pulp is infiltrated with mononuclear cells, often obliterating sinus lumens. Erythrophagocytosis by the mononuclear cells frequently is evident. Liver biopsy may show a mononuclear infiltrate in the sinusoids. Although clinical lymph node enlargement is rare, lymph node biopsies show striking infiltration by leukemic monocytes.

COURSE, PROGNOSIS, AND TREATMENT

Median survival is approximately 25 months. Patients often die of septicemia[948–950] or acute monocytic leukemia.[951,952] Therapy has not been studied systematically, but neither intensive combination chemotherapy nor glucocorticoids have changed the course of the disease.

JUVENILE MYELOMONOCYTIC LEUKEMIA

EPIDEMIOLOGY

Ph-chromosome–positive, adult-type CML occurring in children younger than 15 years composes approximately 3 percent of childhood leukemias and approximately 10 percent of all cases of CML.[953] Although CML occurs in children of all ages, it is rare in children younger than 5 years. With the exception of a propensity to present with higher total leukocyte counts and with leukostatic signs or symptoms, CML in children has the typical manifestations and course of the disorder seen in adults.

A disorder different from adult-type CML, designated *juvenile myelomonocytic leukemia* (juvenile CML), represents approximately 1.5 percent of childhood leukemias. It occurs most often in infants and children younger than 4 years and is similar in some respects to adult subacute or chronic myelomonocytic leukemia because the two diseases share a prominent monocytic component in the leukemic cell population.[954–956]

PATHOGENESIS

This disorder is a clonal myeloid disease that originates in an early hematopoietic multipotential cell. Evidence indicates this cell may be pluripotential (myeloid-lymphoid) in some cases and myeloid in others.[957–960] *RAS* mutations in hematopoietic cells are present in approximately 20 percent of patients.[961] Approximately one of 10 patients with juvenile myelomonocytic leukemia have mutations of *NF1* and manifest type 1 neurofibromatosis. This frequency is approximately 400 times the expected occurrence in a comparable pediatric population.[962–964] The linkage between neurofibromin, the protein encoded by the *NF1* gene, guanosine triphosphatase activity proteins, and the activation state of *RAS*-encoded proteins has led to a postulated sequence of events that may be triggered by the extraordinarily heightened sensitivity of the colony-forming cells in the marrow and blood of infants with the disease to the proliferative effects of GM-CSF. The latter initiates signal transduction from the cell membrane to the nucleus via *RAS* protein activation.[965,966] Mutations in the *PTPN11* gene have been found in approximately one third of children with juvenile CML, and the mutations in *NF1*, *RAS*, and *PTPN11* usually do not coincide.[960,966] However, they each may act through a common pathway. *PTPN11* encodes SHP-2, a nonreceptor tyrosine kinase, which is an upstream regulator of RAS; thus, all three mutations can contribute to deregulation of RAS signaling. As an aside, children with Noonan syndrome, which is characterized by short stature, dysmorphic facies, skeletal abnormalities, and cardiac defects, have a germ-cell mutation of *PTPN1*. These children may have a transient disorder that closely mimics juvenile myelomonocytic leukemia.[966]

CLINICAL FINDINGS

Symptoms and Signs Infants present with failure to thrive, and children present with malaise, fever, persistent infections, and exaggerated skin, oral, or nasal bleeding. Hepatomegaly can occur. Splenomegaly, sometimes massive, is present in almost all cases. Lymphadenopathy is frequent.[954,955] More than half of the patients have eczematoid or maculopapular skin lesions[967] and xanthomatous lesions, and multiple *café au lait* spots (neurofibromatosis) may occur.[955] The xanthomas may be the earliest signs of neurofibromatosis.[954,955]

Laboratory Findings Anemia, thrombocytopenia, and mild to moderate leukocytosis are common. The leukocyte count usually is greater than 10,000/μl (10 $\times$ 10^9/liter) The blood has an increased monocyte concentration of 1000 to 100,000/μl (1–100 $\times$ 10^9/liter), immature granulocytes including a small percentage of blast cells, and nucleated red cells. Fetal hemoglobin concentration is increased in approximately two thirds of the patients. The marrow aspirate is hypercellular as a result of granulocytic hyperplasia; the number of erythroblasts and of megakaryocytes usually are decreased. Monocytic cells are increased. Leukemic blast cells are present in modest proportions of less than 20 percent.

Cell culture of blood and marrow shows a striking preponderance of monocytic progenitors, even in the absence of overt monocytosis in the marrow.[968,969] Granulocyte-monocyte colony forming cells show a marked tendency to spontaneous growth if adherent (monocytic) cells are not depleted from culture.[969] The effect is mediated by a release of large quantities of GM-CSF by monocytes in culture.[970]

Although clonal chromosome abnormalities have been found in some cases,[971] the cytogenetic abnormalities have no consistent pattern, and more than half of the patients have normal karyotypes. The Ph chromosome is not present.[971–973] The phenotype of monosomy 7 syndrome overlaps with juvenile myelomonocytic leukemia, and this cytogenetic abnormality is present in approximately 15 percent of patients.[954]

COURSE, PROGNOSIS, AND TREATMENT

The median survival of patients with juvenile CML has been less than 2 years.[954,955] Younger children (younger than 2 years) are more likely to have a protracted course.[955] The disease has been refractory to most chemotherapy. In a study of nine patients, four of whom were treated with a five- or six-drug intensive regimen, remissions were 11 to more than 27 months, compared with untreated or lightly treated patients, four of whom died within 7 months.[974] Even in the treated patients, complete suppression of the disease did not occur, and treatment protocols to induce and sustain remissions were lacking.[969] A program of cytosine arabinoside, etoposide, vincristine, and isotretinoin resulted in a highly favorable response in five children treated. Three patients relapsed and were treated with cytarabine by infusion and subcutaneously and with etoposide. All patients were alive, and the range of survival at the time of publication was 8 to 89 months, with a median survival of 27 months. The resistance of these cells to currently available therapy is gruesomely highlighted by the sense of success in prolonging the life of infants and young children by a few years. Intensive therapy can control disease, but curative chemotherapy has been elusive.[975] The inclusion of isotretinoin was based on a prior report of responsiveness to the drug used alone; however, this observation has not been confirmed.[976] The GM-CSF antagonist E21R, inhibitors of *RAF-1* gene expression, blockers of RAS protein farnesylation, and angiogenesis inhibitors are among other drug approaches to the disease being studied.[956,977]

Allogeneic stem cell transplantation is an important approach to therapy and may provide the best chance of long-term survival in selected children.[978,979] Hence, a rapid search for a matched-unrelated donor is important in patients without matched sibling donors. Transplantation from a histocompatible sibling or matched-unrelated donor resulted in an event-free survival at 4 years of 54 percent in one study of 27 patients who used a variety of conditioning regimens. A cytogenetic abnormality, such as monosomy 7, was a dismal prognostic finding in that study, and children transplanted before age 1 year had better results than did older children.[978] DLI has placed a posttransplantation patient in relapse into remission.[980]

A minority of patients have a smoldering course for 2 to 4 years. Thereafter, the disease usually rapidly progresses, and patients die of infection or hemorrhage. Occasional patients have a very long survival (>10 years) despite persistence of abnormal blood counts and splenomegaly, independent of the type or intensity of therapy. Some children convert to a full-blown acute myelogenous leukemia with a rapidly fatal outcome. Cases of juvenile myelomonocytic leukemia may be associated with transformation to acute lymphoblastic leukemia.[981]

CHRONIC NEUTROPHILIC LEUKEMIA

HISTORY, PATHOGENESIS, AND EPIDEMIOLOGY

In 1920, Tuohey[982] described the first recorded case of an unusual sustained neutrophilia with splenomegaly without fever, inflammation, cancer, or other cause of a leukemoid reaction. Use of X-chromosome–linked polymorphic genes in blood cells and FISH of chromosome abnormalities have been indicative of a clonal myeloid disorder.[983–985] Some cases may arise in the hematopoietic multipotential cell, others in a neutrophil progenitor cell[983–987] (see Chap. 85). Evidence points to defective apoptotic signals accounting, in part, for the striking accumulation of segmented neutrophils in the blood.[988] The median age at onset is approximately 65 years. Younger patients may be affected.[989] Like almost all the clonal myeloid diseases, men are affected more frequently than are women.

CLINICAL FEATURES

Symptoms and Signs Patients may complain of weakness, anorexia, weight loss, abdominal pain, and easy bruising. Symptoms and signs of gouty arthritis occur in approximately one third of cases. The spleen is enlarged in almost all cases, and the liver frequently is enlarged. Lymphadenopathy is very infrequent.[987] A hemorrhagic tendency is present in some patients.

Laboratory Findings Although some patients have a normal hemoglobin concentration at the time of presentation, most have mild to moderate anemia on presentation. The reticulocyte count usually is between 0.5 and 3.0 percent. The platelet count rarely is less than 125,000/μl (125 × 10⁹/liter) and usually is normal. Coagulation times are normal. The total leukocyte count usually is between 25,000 and 75,000/μl (25 and 75 × 10⁹/liter) in most cases and only rarely is less than 20,000/μl (20 × 10⁹/liter) or exceeds 100,000/μl (100 × 10⁹/liter). Neutrophils compose 85 to 95 percent of the white cells. Although segmented cells usually dominate, occasional cases have a high proportion of band forms. Very infrequent metamyelocytes, myelocytes, and nucleated red cells may be present in occasional patients. Basophil and eosinophil counts are not increased. Blasts nearly always are absent from the blood. Neutrophil alkaline phosphatase activity is increased in almost all cases.

The marrow invariably shows granulocytic hyperplasia with myeloid:erythroid (M:E) ratios as high as 10:1. Myeloblasts are not overtly increased in number (0.5–3.0 percent). Megakaryocytes are either normal or slightly increased in number and have normal distribution and morphology. Erythropoiesis usually is mildly decreased. Unlike CML, reticulin fibrosis is unusual. A few cases with dysplastic features in the marrow (acquired Pelger-Hüet anomaly, erythroid, dysplasia, micromegakaryocytes) have been reported. By definition, the Ph chromosome, *BCR* gene rearrangements, and *BCR-ABL* transcripts

are absent.[989–992] Most patients have normal karyotypes, but approximately 25 percent of patients have nonrandom abnormalities of chromosomes.[992] Deletions of chromosome 20q and trisomy 21 or 9 are the most common abnormalities. Serum vitamin B$_{12}$-binding protein and vitamin B$_{12}$ levels both are markedly increased above normal. Serum uric acid concentration is increased, and serum lactic dehydrogenase activity may be increased.

Almost every case examined postmortem had liver and splenic enlargement. Portal hepatic and splenic red pulp infiltrates of neutrophils or islands of extramedullary hematopoiesis with immature myeloid cells and megakaryocytes are characteristic.

DIFFERENTIAL DIAGNOSIS

Most leukemoid reactions are associated with an obvious underlying cause, such as pancreatitis, carcinoma, connective tissue disease, smokers neutrophilia, or bacterial infection. The leukocyte alkaline phosphatase level usually is markedly elevated in chronic neutrophilic leukemia and markedly decreased in CML. More to the point, molecular studies identifying *BCR* gene rearrangement or the presence of *BCR-ABL* transcripts should distinguish chronic neutrophilic leukemia (*BCR-ABL* negative) from neutrophilic CML (*BCR-ABL* positive) (see "Special Clinical Features" above). In the latter case, more than half of the patients have thrombocytosis and megakaryocytic hyperplasia, which are uncharacteristic of chronic neutrophilic leukemia.

TREATMENT

No systematic studies of treatment have been reported. Although hydroxyurea, IFN-α, or cytarabine may decrease the white count and spleen size, long-term benefit is unusual.[989–992] Intensive therapy has led to early posttreatment deaths. Allogeneic stem cell transplantation in eligible patients may be curative.[993]

COURSE AND PROGNOSIS

The disease is fatal, with a median survival of approximately 2.5 years and a range of 0.5 to 6 years.[989–992] A case of spontaneous remission has been reported. The prognosis is considerably worse than the prognosis for CML despite the prevalence of mature neutrophils and the paucity of blasts. Causes of death have included (1) intracranial hemorrhage, sometimes in the presence of adequate platelet counts and coagulation times, suggesting a vascular infiltrative process; (2) severe infection; (3) transformation to acute myelogenous leukemia; and (4) the toxic effects of intensive therapy. The disease usually afflicts older subjects, and cardiac, pulmonary, and vascular diseases contribute to a fatal outcome.

A remarkable frequency of concordant essential monoclonal gammopathy or myeloma has been described.[985,994–1002] In two cases, the extreme neutrophilia proved to be a polyclonal response to a plasma cell disorder.[985,1003] Chronic neutrophilic leukemia has evolved from polycythemia vera or oligoblastic leukemia,[1004–1008] supporting its relationship to the clonal hemopathies.[985,1009,1010]

PH-CHROMOSOME—NEGATIVE OR *BCR* REARRANGEMENT-NEGATIVE CML

An ever-diminishing proportion of patients with clinical manifestations within the limits usually applied to the diagnosis of CML have neither a Ph chromosome (classic, variant, or masked) nor evidence of rearrangement within the M-*bcr* on chromosome 22. This circumstance represents true Ph-chromosome–negative CML, perhaps better referred to as *BCR* rearrangement-negative CML. The literature describing Ph-chromosome–negative CML prior to 1987 is difficult to evaluate because many cases were not studied carefully for masked or variant translocations and for *BCR* gene rearrangement. Ph-chromosome–negative CML is a clonal disease[911] that has the propensity for lymphoid and myeloid transformation.[1011,1012]

Although most cases of *BCR* rearrangement-negative CML are closer in manifestations to CMML,[913,914,1013–1016] a few residual cases are difficult to distinguish from classic CML.[1017–1021] In the latter group, absence of acute blast transformation as a terminal event has been observed. As the disease progresses, the patient develops severe cytopenias.[1018] Some patients have transposition of *ABL* to chromosome 22 but not the classic translocation. In such cases, including TEL-ABL translocations, transient responses to imatinib mesylate have been observed.[1022]

Uncommon cases of coexisting BCR– and BCR+ clones have been described. and the basis for such cases is in dispute.[1023] One proposed explanation is that this case is an example of "field carcinogenesis" in which multiple clones coexist.[1023] An alternative explanation is that these cases represent the dual progeny of a single unstable clone.[1024] The long-term survival of patients with CML may permit the emergence of a drug-induced or spontaneous second malignancy, and in the former it may be notably associated with imatinib mesylate (see "Secondary Chromosomal Changes with Imatinib" under "Chronic Myelogenous Leukemia, Initial Cytoreduction Therapy," above).[1025–1027]

PH-CHROMOSOME–POSITIVE ACUTE LEUKEMIA

MYELOGENOUS

Approximately 1 percent of patients with acute myelogenous leukemias have the Ph chromosome t(9;22)(q34;q11) in a significant proportion (10–100 percent) of leukemic blast cells.[1028–1030] The blast cells have surface antigens, such as CD13 and CD33, characteristic of myeloid leukemias.[1031,1032] One interpretation of the concurrence of AML with t(9;22) is that it represents CML presenting in myeloid blast crisis.[1033–1035] The arguments in favor of this proposal are the following. (1) Blast crisis may occur within days after diagnosis of Ph-chromosome–positive CML. (2) Cases can present with additional cytogenetic changes comparable to CML in blast crisis.[1032,1035] (3) Marked hepatosplenomegaly, uncharacteristic of AML, may be present.[1034,1035] (4) Platelet counts may be normal, and basophils exhibit intermittent increases.[1033,1035] (5) A long prodromal period of weakness and weight loss may occur, and some features of CML, such as granulocytosis, can appear after treatment with chemotherapy.[1036] (6) Ph-chromosome–positive AML has a very poor prognosis, as in myeloid blast crisis of CML. (7) The breakpoint on chromosome 22 in the M-*bcr* may be typical of CML, and the product of the fusion *BCR-ABL* gene is a p210 tyrosine kinase identical to that in classic CML.[1032,1034–1040] (8) Occasional cases express p210 and p190 tyrosine kinases, now known to be features of CML.[1040] (9) Some patients enter a remission by converting to a phenotype analogous to chronic phase CML.[451] An alternative view has been promulgated because (1) cases of Ph-chromosome–positive AML can be a mosaic (normal and abnormal karyotypes),[1032] (2) the Ph chromosome may appear later in the course of the disease,[1041] (3) additional chromosomal abnormalities often are different from those seen in the myeloblastic crisis of CML,[1032,1042,1043] and (4) in some cases, the *BCR-ABL* is not encoding a p210 but a p190 mutant tyrosine kinase,[1029,1037,1039,1040,1044] the former being characteristic of CML. Moreover, Ph-chromosome–positive AML has developed following Ph-chromosome–negative oligoblastic leukemia.[1029,1045,1046] Many cases of Ph-chromosome–positive acute leukemia are myeloid-lymphoid hybrids.[1028,1030,1032,1047] Thus, Ph-chromosome–positive AML comes in two varieties: one with a break in M-*BCR* of chromosome 22 with a p210 product, which could be considered analogous to acute blast crisis of CML, and one with a mo-

lecular pathology such that the oncogene product is a p190 protein (m-*BCR*) that could be considered a *de novo* case.

LYMPHOCYTIC

Approximately 3 percent of cases of childhood ALL[1048–1050] and 20 percent of cases of adult ALL[1046,1051] cells contain the Ph chromosome. In children, the clinical and laboratory findings are similar whether or not the lymphoblasts contain the Ph chromosome. However, the prognosis is worse for those with the Ph chromosome, with lower frequencies of remission, shorter remission duration, and less chance of cure with chemotherapy (see Chap. 91).[1050,1051] Remission rates and median survivals also are significantly lower in adults with ALL and the Ph chromosome (see Chap. 91).

Molecular studies of the chromosomes and cells of patients with ALL indicate the disease is heterogeneous. Approximately 20 percent of adults with Ph-chromosome–positive ALL have the t(9;22)(q34; q11) with a *BCR-ABL* fusion gene that codes for and expresses the p210[BCR-ABL] tyrosine kinase.[1052–1071] The leukemic cells of 70 percent of adults with Ph-chromosome–positive ALL and approximately 90 percent of children with the disease have a rearrangement of the *BCR* gene that involves sequences outside the M-*bcr*. In these cases, the mutation encodes a p190[BCR-ABL] product that also is a constitutively activated tyrosine kinase.[1056,1072,1073] The p210[BCR-ABL]-positive adult ALL patients may revert to CML after intensive chemotherapy, whereas ALL patients, whose cells encode a p190[BCR-ABL] mutant tyrosine kinase, if they enter remission do so with reappearance of normal hematopoiesis. The former group of Ph-chromosome–positive ALL is thought to represent presentation of CML in lymphocytic blast crisis; the latter group of Ph-chromosome–positive ALL may represent *de novo* ALL.[1074,1075] The somatic mutation, however, appears to involve a cell that can differentiate into all hematopoietic lineages.[1076] Children with Ph-chromosome–positive ALL have a very high frequency of accompanying cytogenetic abnormalities, including especially loss of chromosome 7, loss of segments of 7p or 9p, hypodiploidy, and a second Ph chromosome.[1073] Patients with ALL with the BCR rearrangement restricted to lymphoid cells have a more favorable prognosis than those with BCR rearrangement present in myeloid and lymphoid cells.[1077,1078]

Phenotyping of blast cells with panels of antibodies to surface antigens, histochemical reactions, and gene rearrangement probes indicates Ph-chromosome–positive leukemias also may be biphenotypic (lymphoid and myeloid lineage) and heterogenous at the site in the *BCR* gene where rearrangements occur.[1078]

MANAGEMENT OF PH-CHROMOSOME –POSITIVE ACUTE LEUKEMIA

This cytogenetic variant of acute leukemia is characterized by extraordinary drug resistance. Although imatinib mesylate doses of 600 to 800 mg/day are expected to produce a hematologic remission in a very small proportion of patients with Ph-chromosome–positive AML, based on the response in patients with CML who go on to a myeloid blast crisis, no formal studies of *de novo* Ph-chromosome–positive AML responses to imatinib mesylate have been performed. In myeloid blast crisis, the uncommon full hematologic response (blood and marrow) usually is short lived, measured in weeks or a few months. This outcome also seems to be the case when therapy with other drugs (e.g., cytarabine, etoposide, anthracycline antibiotics) is included. Occasional cases in which chemotherapy has induced remission in Ph-chromosome–positive AML and imatinib mesylate has appeared to help induce and sustain the remission have been reported.[1079] Thus, in Ph-chromosome–positive AML, a matched-related or matched-unrelated donor stem cell transplant should be considered if the patient is younger than 50 years. This approach may have the highest probability of a long-term remission.

In children with Philadelphia-chromosome–positive ALL, intensive chemotherapy can result in a 5-year event-free survival of approximately 25 percent.[1073] Adults with Philadelphia-chromosome–positive ALL who are in relapse have infrequent (10%) complete hematologic responses (blood and marrow) to imatinib mesylate therapy 400 to 600 mg/day, and the responses usually are short lived (weeks).[1080] The drug has produced remissions in patients with Philadelphia-chromosome–positive ALL who relapse after allogeneic transplantation.[1081] Development of resistance to imatinib mesylate in Philadelphia-chromosome–positive leukemias other than CML usually is rapid. In adults and children with Philadelphia-chromosome–positive ALL, use of allogenic stem cell transplantation is an important modality for attempting to induce long-term remissions.[1051] A high-dose chemotherapy regimen of cyclophosphamide, vincristine, adriamycin, and dexamethasone plus imatinib mesylate has resulted in remissions approaching 2 years in a small proportion of patients with Philadelphia-chromosome–positive ALL.[1082]

REFERENCES

1. Bennett JH: Case of hypertrophy of the spleen and liver, in which death took place from suppuration of the blood. *Edinburgh Med Surg J* 64:313, 1845.
2. Virchow R: Weisses blut. *Froieps Notizen* 36:151, 1845.
3. Craige D: Case of disease of the spleen in which death took place in consequence of the presence of purulent matter in the blood. *Edinburgh Med Surg J* 64:400, 1845.
4. Virchow R: *Die leukaemie in gesammelte abhandlungen zur wissenschaftlichen medizin.* Meidinger, Frankfort, 1865.
5. Neumann E: Ueber myelogene leukämie. *Berl Klin Wochenschr* 15:69, 1878.
6. Nowell PC, Hungerford DA: A minute chromosome in human chronic granulocytic leukemia. *J Natl Cancer Inst* 25:85, 1960.
7. Baike AG, Court Brown WM, Buckton KE, et al: A possible specific chromosome abnormality in human chronic myeloid leukemia. *Nature* 188:1165, 1960.
8. Nowell PC, Hungerford DA: Chromosome studies in human leukemia: II. Chronic granulocytic leukemia. *J Natl Cancer Inst* 27:1013, 1961.
9. Tough IM, Court Brown WM, Buckton KE, et al: Cytogenetic studies in chronic leukemia and acute leukemia associated with mongolism. *Lancet* 1:411, 1961.
10. Caspersson T, Zech L, Johansson C, Modest EJ: Identification of human chromosomes by DNA binding fluorescent agents. *Chromosoma* 30:215, 1970.
11. Caspersson T, Gahrton G, Lindsten J, Zech L: Identification of the Philadelphia chromosome as a number 22 by quinacrine mustard fluorescence analysis. *Exp Cell Res* 63:238, 1970.
12. Rowley JD: A new consistent abnormality in chronic myelogenous leukemia identified by quinacrine fluorescence and Giemsa staining. *Nature* 243:290, 1973.
13. de Klein A, Van Kessel AG, Grosveld G, et al: A cellular oncogene is translocated to the Philadelphia chromosome in chronic myelocytic leukemia. *Nature* 300:765, 1982.
14. Bartram CR, de Klein A, Hagemeijer A, et al: Translocation of c-abl oncogene correlates with the presence of a Philadelphia chromosome in chronic myelocytic leukemia. *Nature* 306:277, 1983.
15. Drucker BJ, Tamura S, Buchdunger E, et al: Effects of a selective inhibitor of the ABL tyrosine kinase in the growth of BCR-ABL positive cells. *Nat Med* 2:561, 1996.
16. Redaelli A, Bell C, Casagrande J, et al: Clinical and epidemiologic burden of chronic myelogenous leukemia. *Expert Rev Anticancer Ther* 4:85, 2004.
17. Löffler H, Bergman J, Huchhaus A, et al: Reduced risk for chronic myelogenous leukemia in individuals with cytochrome P-450 gene polymorphism CYP1A1*2A. *Blood* 98:3874, 2001.
18. Ichimaru M, Ichimaru T, Belsky JL: Incidence of leukemia in atomic bomb survivors belonging to a fixed cohort in Hiroshima and Nagasaki 1950–1971. *J Radiat Res (Tokyo)* 19:262, 1978.
19. Court Brown WM, Doll R: Adult leukemia: Trends in mortality in relation to etiology. *Br Med J* 1:1063, 1959.
20. Court Brown WM, Doll R: Adult leukemia. *Br Med J* 1:1753, 1960.
21. Boice JD Jr, Day NE, Anderson A, et al: Second cancers following radiation treatment for cervical cancer. *J Natl Cancer Inst* 74:955, 1985.
22. Maloney WC: Radiation leukemia revisited. *Blood* 70:905, 1987.
23. Hayes RB, Yin S, Rothman N, et al: Benzene and lymphohematopoietic malignancies in China. *J Tox Environ Health* 61:419, 2000
24. Pederson-Bjergaard J, Bondum-Nielsen K, Karle H, Johansson B: Chemotherapy-related and late-occuring Philadelphia chromosome in AML, ALL, and CML. Similar events related to treatment with DNA topoisomerase II inhibitors? *Leukemia* 11:1571, 1997.
25. Tokuhata GK, Neely CL, Williams DL: Chronic myelocytic leukemia in identical twins and a sibling. *Blood* 31:216, 1968.
26. Segel GB, Lichtman MA: Familial (inherited) leukemia, lymphoma, and myeloma. *Blood Cells Mol Dis* 32:246, 2004.
27. Whang-Peng J, Knutsen T: Chromosomal abnormalities, in *Chronic Granulocytic Leukaemia*, edited by MT Shaw, p 49. Praeger, East Sussex, UK, 1982.
28. Spiers ASD, Bain BJ, Turner JE: The peripheral blood in chronic granulocytic leukemia: A study of 50 untreated Philadelphia positive cases. *Scand J Haematol* 18:25, 1977.
29. Sandberg AA: The leukemias: The Philadelphia chromosome, in *The Chromosomes in Human Cancer and Leukemia*, 2nd ed, p 183. Elsevier, New York, 1990.
30. Fialkow PJ, Garther SM, Yoshida A: Clonal origin of chronic myelocytic leukemia in men. *Proc Natl Acad Sci U S A* 58:1468, 1967.
31. Fialkow PJ, Jacobsen RJ, Papayannopoulou T: Chronic myelocytic leukemia: Clonal origin in a stem cell common to granulocyte, erythrocyte, platelet, and monocyte/macrophage. *Am J Med* 63:125, 1977.
32. Koeffler HP, Levine AM, Sparkes LM, Sparkes RS: Chronic myelocytic leukemia: Eosinophils involved in the malignant clone. *Blood* 55:1063, 1980.
33. Hayata I, Kakati S, Sandberg AA: On the monoclonal origin of chronic myelocytic leukemia. *Proc Jpn Acad* 30:351, 1974.
34. Lawler SD, O'Malley F, Lobb DS: Chromosome banding studies in Philadelphia chromosome positive myeloid leukemia. *Scand J Haematol* 17:17, 1976.
35. Harrison CJ, Chang J, Johnson D, et al: Chromosomal evidence of a common stem cell in acute lymphoblastic leukemia and chronic granulocytic leukemia. *Cancer Genet Cytogenet* 13:331, 1984.
36. Chaganti RSK, Bailey RB, Jhanwar SC, et al: Chronic myelogenous leukemia in the monosomic cell line of a fertile Turner syndrome mosaic (45,X/46,XX). *Cancer Genet Cytogenet* 5:215, 1982.
37. Fitzgerald PH, Pickering AF, Eiby JR: Clonal origin of the Philadelphia chromosome and chronic leukemia. *Br J Haematol* 21:473, 1971.
38. Groffen J, Stephenson JR, Heisterkamp N, et al: Philadelphia chromosomal breakpoints are clustered within a limited region, bcr, on chromosome 22. *Cell* 36:93, 1984.
39. Leibowitz D, Schaefer-Rego K, Popenoe DW, et al: Variable breakpoints on the Philadelphia chromosome in chronic myelogenous leukemia. *Blood* 66:243, 1985.

40. Yoffe G, Chinault AG, Talpaz M, et al: Clonal nature of Philadelphia chromosome positive and negative chronic myelogenous leukemia by DNA hybridization analysis. *Exp Hematol* 15:725, 1987.

41. Fialkow PJ, Denman AM, Jacobsen RJ, Lowenthal MN: Chronic myelocytic leukemia. Origin of some lymphocytes from leukemic stem cells. *J Clin Invest* 62:815, 1978.

42. Martin PJ, Najfeld V, Hansen JA, et al: Involvement of the B-lymphoid system in chronic myelogenous leukaemia. *Nature* 287:49, 1980.

43. Boggs DR: Hematopoietic stem cell theory in relation to possible lymphoblastic conversion in chronic myeloid leukemia. *Blood* 44:449, 1974.

44. Bernheim A, Berger R, Preud'homme JL, et al: Philadelphia chromosome positive blood B lymphocytes in chronic myelocytic leukemia. *Leuk Res* 5:331, 1981.

45. Collins S, Coleman H, Groudine M: Expression of bcr and bcr-abl fusion transcripts in normal and leukemic cells. *Mol Cell Biol* 7:2870, 1987.

46. Al-Amin A, Lennartz K, Runde V, et al: Frequency of clonal B lymphocytes in chronic myelogenous leukemia evaluated by fluorescence in situ hybridization. *Cancer Genet Cytogenet* 104:45, 1998.

47. Torlakovic E, Litz CE, McClure JS, Brunning RD: Direct detection of the Philadelphia chromosome in CD20-positive lymphocytes in chronic myelogenous leukemia by tri-color immunophenotyping/FISH. *Leukemia* 8:1940, 1994.

48. Kearney L, Orchard KH, Hibbin JA, Goldman JM: T-cell cytogenetics in chronic granulocytic leukemia. *Lancet* 1:858, 1981.

49. Nogueira-Costa R, Spitzer G, Cock A, Trijillo JM: E rosette-positive agar colonies containing the Philadelphia chromosome in chronic myeloid leukemia. *Scand J Haematol* 34.184, 1985.

50. Bartram CR, Raghavachar A, Anger B, et al: T lymphocytes lack rearrangement of the bcr gene in Philadelphia chromosome-positive chronic myelogenous leukemia. *Blood* 69:1682, 1985.

51. Fauser AA, Kanz L, Bross KJ, et al: T cells and probably B cells arise from the malignant clone in chronic myelogenous leukemia. *J Clin Invest* 75:1080, 1985.

52. Nitta M, Kato Y, Strife A, et al: Incidence of the B and T lymphocyte lineages in chronic myelogenous leukemia. *Blood* 66:1053, 1985.

53. Aniad S, Dajee D, Willem P, Bezwoda WR: Lack of involvement of T-lymphocytes in the leukaemic population during prolonged chronic phase of Philadelphia chromosome positive chronic myeloid leukaemia. *Leuk Lymphoma* 10:217, 1993.

54. Tsukamoto N, Karasawa M, Maehara T, et al: The majority of T lymphocytes are polyclonal during the chronic phase of chronic myelogenous leukemia. *Ann Hematol* 72:61, 1996.

55. Garicochea B, Chase A, Lazaridou A, Goldman JM: T lymphocytes in chronic myelogenous leukaemia (CML). *Leukemia* 8:1197, 1994.

56. Jonas D, Lubbert M, Kawasaki ES, et al: Clonal analysis of bcr-abl rearrangement in T lymphocytes from patients in the chronic myelogenous leukemia. *Blood* 79:1017, 1992.

57. Haferlach T, Winkemann M, Nickening C, et al: Which components are involved in Philadelphia-chromosome-positive chronic leukemia? *Br J Haematol* 97:99, 1997.

58. Verfaillie C, Miller W, Kay N, McClave P: Adherent lymphokine-activated killer cells in chronic myelogenous leukemia: A benign cell population with potent cytotoxic activity. *Blood* 74:793, 1989.

59. Takahashi N, Miura I, Saitoh K, Miura AB: Lineage involvement of stem cells bearing the Philadelphia chromosome in chronic myeloid leukemia in the chronic phase as shown by a combination of fluorescence-activated cell sorting and fluorescence in situ hybridization. *Blood* 92:4758, 1998.

60. Muñoz L, Bellido M, Sierra J, Nomdedéu JF: Flow cytometric detection of B cell abnormal maturation in chronic myeloid leukemia. *Leukemia* 14:339, 2000.

61. Miura A: Progress in laboratory medicine in chronic myeloid leukemia. *Jap J Clin Pathol* 46:1226, 1998.

62. Muñoz L, Bellido M, Sierra J, Nomdedéu JF: Flow cytometric detection of B cell abnormal maturation in chronic myeloid leukemia. *Leukemia* 14:339, 1999.

63. Gunsilius E, Duba H-C, Petzer AL, et al: Evidence from a leukaemia model for maintenance of vascular endothelium by bone-marrow-derived endothelial cells. *Lancet* 355:1688, 2000.

64. Fialkow PJ, Martin PJ, Najfeld V, et al: Evidence for a multistep pathogenesis of chronic myelogenous leukemia. *Blood* 58:158, 1981.

65. Lisker R, Casas L, Mutchinick O, et al: Late-appearing Philadelphia chromosome in two patients with chronic myelogenous leukemia. *Blood* 56:812, 1980.

66. Kamada N, Uchino H: Chronologic sequence in appearance of clinical and laboratory findings characteristic of chronic myelogenous leukemia. *Blood* 51:843, 1978.

67. Smadja N, Krulik M, DeGramont A, et al: Acquisition of a Philadelphia chromosome concomitant with transformation of a refractory anemia into an acute leukemia. *Cancer* 55:1477, 1985.

68. Fegan C, Morgan G, Whittaker JA: Spontaneous remission in a patient with chronic myeloid leukaemia. *Br J Haematol* 72:594, 1989.

69. Brandt L, Mitelman F, Panani A, Lenner HC: Extremely long duration of chronic myeloid leukaemia with Ph¹ negative and Ph¹ positive bone marrow cells. *Scand J Haematol* 16:321, 1976.

70. Hagemeijer A, Smith EME, Lowenberg B, Abels J: Chronic myeloid leukemia with permanent disappearance of the Ph¹ chromosome and development of new clonal subpopulations. *Blood* 53:1, 1979.

71. Singer JN, Arlin ZA, Najfeld V, et al: Restoration of nonclonal hematopoiesis in chronic myelogenous leukemia (CML) following a chemotherapy induced loss of the Ph¹ chromosome. *Blood* 56:356, 1980.

72. Sokal JE: Significance of Ph¹-negative marrow cells in Ph¹ positive chronic granulocytic leukemia. *Blood* 56:1072, 1980.

73. Smadja N, Krulik M, Audebert AA, et al: Spontaneous regression of cytogenetic and haematologic anomalies in Ph¹-positive chronic myelogenous leukaemia. *Br J Haematol* 63:257, 1986.

74. Goldman JM, Kearney L, Pittman S, et al: Hemopoietic stem cell grafting for chronic granulocytic leukemia. *Exp Hematol* 10:76, 1982.

75. Reiffers J, Vezon G, David B, et al: Philadelphia negative cells in a patient treated with autografting for Ph¹ positive chronic granulocytic leukaemia in transformation. *Br J Haematol* 55:382, 1983.

76. Reiffers J, Broustet A, Goldman JM: Philadelphia chromosome-negative progenitors in chronic granulocytic leukemia. *N Engl J Med* 309:1460, 1983.

77. Coulombel L, Kalousek DK, Eaves CJ, et al: Long-term marrow culture reveals chromosomally normal hemopoietic progenitor cells in patients with Philadelphia chromosome-positive chronic myelogenous leukemia. *N Engl J Med* 308:1493, 1983.

78. Degliantoni G, Mangori L, Rizzoli V: In vitro restoration of polyclonal hematopoiesis in a chronic myelogenous leukemia after in vitro treatment with 4-hydroperoxy-cyclophosphamide. *Blood* 65:753, 1985.

79. Barnett MJ, Eaves CJ, Phillips GL, et al: Successful autografting in chronic myeloid leukemia after maintenance of marrow in culture. *Bone Marrow Transplant* 4:345, 1989.

80. Verfaillie CM, Miller WJ, Boylan K, McGlave PB: Selection of benign primitive hematopoietic progenitors in chronic myelogenous leukemia on the basis of HLA-DR antigen expression. *Blood* 79:1003, 1992.

81. Leemhuis T, Leibowitz D, Cox G, et al: Identification of BCR/ABL-negative primitive hematopoietic progenitor cells within chronic myeloid leukemia marrow. *Blood* 81:801, 1993.

82. Wang JCY, Lapidot T, Cashman JD, et al: High level engraftment of NOD/SCID mice by primitive normal and leukemic hemopoietic cells

from patients with chronic myeloid leukemia in chronic phase. *Blood* 91:2406, 1998.

83. Dunbar CE, Stewart FM: Separating the wheat from the chaff: Selection of benign hematopoietic cells in chronic myeloid leukemia. *Blood* 79:1107, 1992.

84. Strife A, Clarkson B: Biology of chronic myelogenous leukemia: Is discordant maturation the primary defect? *Semin Hematol* 25:1, 1988.

85. Heinzinger M, Waller CF, Rosentiel A, et al: Quality of IL-3 and G-CSF-mobilized peripheral blood stem cells in patients with early chronic phase CML. *Leukemia* 12:333, 1998.

86. Verfaillie CM, Bhatia R, Miller W, et al: BCR/ABL-negative primitive progenitors suitable for transplantation can be selected from the marrow of most early-chronic phase but not accelerated-phase chronic myelogenous leukemia patients. *Blood* 87:4770, 1996.

87. Grand FH, Marley SB, Chase A, et al: BCR/ABL-negative progenitors are enriched in the adherent fraction of CD34+ cells circulating in the blood of chronic phase chronic myeloid leukemia patients. *Leukemia* 11:1486, 1997.

88. Carella AM, Podesta M, Frassoni R, et al: Collection of "normal" blood repopulating cells during early hemopoietic recovery after intensive conventional chemotherapy in chronic myelogenous leukemia. *Bone Marrow Transplant* 12:267, 1993.

89. Guyootat D, Wahabi K, Viallet A, et al: Selection of BCR/ABL-negative stem cells from marrow or blood of patients with chronic myeloid leukemia. *Leukemia* 13:991, 1999.

90. Hogge DE, Coulumbel L, Kalousek D, et al: Nonclonal hemopoietic progenitors in a G6PD heterozygote with chronic myelogenous leukemia revealed after long-term marrow culture. *Am J Hematol* 24:389, 1987.

91. Deforge M, Boogaerts MA, McGlave PB, Verfaillie CM: BCR/ABL-CD34+HLA-DR- progenitor cells in early phase, but not in more advanced phases, of chronic myelogenous leukemia are polyclonal. *Blood* 93:284, 1999.

92. Van den Berg D, Wessman M, Murray L, et al: Leukemic burden in subpopulations of CD34+ cells isolated from the mobilized peripheral blood of alpha-interferon-resistant or -intolerant patients with chronic myeloid leukemia. *Blood* 87:4348, 1996.

93. Podesta M, Piaggio G, Frassoni F, et al: Very primitive hemopoietic cells (LTC-IC) are present in Philadelphia negative cytaphereses collected during early recovery after chemotherapy for chronic myeloid leukemia (CML). *Bone Marrow Transplant* 16:549, 1995.

94. Kirk JA, Reems JA, Roecklein BA, et al: Benign marrow progenitors are enriched in the CD34+/HLA-DRlo population but not in the CD34+/CD38lo population in chronic myeloid leukemia: An analysis using interphase fluorescence in situ hybridization. *Blood* 86:737, 1995.

95. Lewis ID, Haylock DN, Moore S, et al: Peripheral blood is a source of BCR-ABL-negative pre-progenitors in early chronic phase chronic myeloid leukemia. *Leukemia* 11:581, 1997.

96. Maguer-Satta V, Petzer AL, Eaves AC, Eaves CJ: BCR-ABL expression in different subpopulations of functionally characterized Ph+ CD34+ cells from patients with chronic myeloid leukemia. *Blood* 88:1796, 1996.

97. Sirard C, Lapidot T, Vormoor J, et al: Normal and leukemia SCID-repopulating cells (SRC) coexist in the bone marrow and peripheral blood from CML patients in chronic phase, whereas leukemic SRC are detected in blast crisis. *Blood* 87:1539, 1996.

98. Dazzi F, Capelli D, Hasserjian R, et al: The kinetics and extent of engraftment of chronic myelogenous leukemia cells in nonobese diabetic/severe combined immunodeficiency mice reflect the phase of the donor's disease: An in vivo model for chronic myelogenous leukemia biology. *Blood* 92:1390, 1998.

99. Holyoake TL, Jiang X, Drummond MW, et al: Elucidating critical mechanisms of deregulated stem cell turnover in the chronic phase of chronic myelogenous leukemia. *Leukemia* 16:549, 2002.

100. Eaves C, Cashman J, Eaves A: Defective regulation of leukemic hematopoiesis in chronic myeloid leukemia. *Leuk Res* 22:1085, 1998.

101. Clarkson BD, Strife A, Wisniewski D, et al: New understanding of the pathogenesis of CML: A prototype of early neoplasia. *Leukemia* 11:1404, 1997.

102. Bedi A, Zehnbauer BA, Collector MI, et al: BCR-ABL gene rearrangement and expression of primitive hematopoietic progenitors in chronic myeloid leukemia. *Blood* 81:2898, 1993.

103. Moore MA: In vitro culture studies in chronic granulocytic leukaemia. *Clin Haematol* 6:97, 1977.

104. Siitonen T, Zheng A, Savolainen E-R, Koistinen P: Spontaneous granulocyte-macrophage colony growth by peripheral blood mononuclear cells in myeloproliferative disorders. *Leuk Res* 20:187, 1996.

105. Eaves CJ, Eaves AC: Cell culture studies in CML. *Baillieres Clin Haematol* 1:931, 1987.

106. Galbraith PR, Abu-Zahra HT: Granulopoiesis in chronic granulocytic leukemia. *Br J Haematol* 22:135, 1972.

107. Sjögren U, Brandt L: Composition and mitotic activity of the erythropoietic part of the bone marrow in chronic myeloid leukaemia. *Scand J Haematol* 12:18, 1974.

108. Verfaillie CM: Stem cells in chronic myelogenous leukemia. *Hematol Oncol Clin North Am* 11:1079, 1997.

109. Ghaffari S, Dougherty GJ, Lansdorp PM, et al: Differentiation-associated changes in CD44 isoform expression during normal hematopoiesis and their alteration in chronic myeloid leukemia. *Blood* 86:2976, 1995.

110. Kawaishi K, Kimura A, Katch O, et al: Decreased L-selectin expression in CD34-positive cells from patients with chronic myelocytic leukaemia. *Br J Haematol* 93:367, 1996.

111. Turkina AG, Baryshnikov AY, Sedyakhina NP, et al: Studies of P-glycoprotein in chronic myelogenous leukaemia patients: Expression, activity and correlations with CD34 antigen. *Br J Haematol* 92:88, 1996.

112. Agarwal R, Doren S, Hicks B, Dunbar CE: Long-term culture of chronic myelogenous leukemia marrow cells on stem cell factor-deficient stroma favors benign progenitors. *Blood* 85:1306, 1995.

113. Moore S, Haylock DN, Levesque J-P, et al: Stem cell factor as a single agent induces selective proliferation of the Philadelphia chromosome positive fraction of chronic myeloid leukemia CD34+ cells. *Blood* 92:2461, 1998.

114. Chasty RC, Lucas GS, Owen-Lynch PJ, et al: Macrophage inflammatory protein-1 alpha receptors are present on cells enriched for CD34 expression from patients with chronic myeloid leukemia. *Blood* 86:4270, 1995.

115. Cashman JD, Eaves CJ, Sarris AH, Eaves AC: MCP-1, not MIP-1α, is the endogenous chemokine that cooperates with TGF-β to inhibit the cycling of primitive normal but not leukemic (CML) progenitors in long-term human marrow cultures. *Blood* 92:2338, 1998.

116. Murohashi I, Endho K, Nishida S, et al: Differential effects of TGF-beta 1 on normal and leukemic human hematopoietic cell proliferation. *Exp Hematol* 23:970, 1995.

117. Gordon MY, Dowding C, Riley G, et al: Altered adhesive interactions with marrow stroma of haematopoietic progenitor cells in chronic myeloid leukaemia. *Nature* 328:342, 1987.

118. Dowding C, Guo A-P, Osterholz J, et al: Interferon-α overrides the deficient adhesion of chronic myeloid leukemia primitive progenitor cells to bone marrow stromal cells. *Blood* 78:499, 1991.

119. Bhatia R, Wayner EA, McGlave PB, Verfaillie CM: Interferon-α restores normal adhesion of chronic myelogenous leukemia hematopoietic progenitors to bone marrow stroma by correcting impaired β1 integrin receptor function. *J Clin Invest* 94:384, 1994.

120. Verfaillie CM: Stem cells in chronic myelogenous leukemia. *Hematol Oncol Clin North Am* 11:1079, 1997.

121. Bhatia R, Munthe HA, Verfaillie CM: Tyrphostin AG957, a tyrosine kinase inhibitor with anti-BCR/ABL tyrosine activity restores β1 integrin-mediated adhesion and inhibiting signaling in chronic myelogenous leukemia hematopoietic progenitors. *Leukemia* 12:1708, 1998.

122. Lundell BI, McCarthy JB, Kovach NL, Verfaillie CM: Activation of beta1 integrins on CML progenitors reveals cooperation between beta1 integrins and CD44 in the regulation of adhesion and proliferation. *Leukemia* 11:822, 1997.

123. Ghaffari S, Dougherty GJ, Eaves AC, Eaves CJ: Altered patterns of CD44 epitope expression in human chronic and acute myeloid leukemia. *Leukemia* 10:1773, 1996.

124. Vijayan KV, Advani SH, Zingde SM: Chronic myeloid leukemic granulocytes exhibit reduced and altered binding to P-selectin; modification in the CD15 antigens and sialylation. *Leuk Res* 21:59, 1997.

125. Deininger MW, Vieira S, Mendiola R, et al: BCR-ABL tyrosine kinase activity regulates the expression of multiple genes implicated in the pathogenesis of chronic myeloid leukemia. *Cancer Res* 60:2049, 2000.

126. Verfaillie CM, Hurley R, Lundell BI, et al: Integrin-mediated regulation of hematopoiesis: Do BCR/ABL-induced defects in integrin function underlie the abnormal circulation and proliferation of CML progenitors? *Acta Haematol* 29:40, 1997.

127. Symington BE: Growth signalling through the alpha 5 beta 1 fibronectin receptor. *Biochem Biophys Res Commun* 208:126, 1995.

128. Bhatia R, McCarthy JB, Verfaillie CM: Interferon-alpha restores normal beta 1 integrin-mediated inhibition of hematopoietic progenitor proliferation by the marrow microenvironment in chronic myelogenous leukemia. *Blood* 87:3883, 1996.

129. Salgia R, Li JL, Ewaniuk DS, et al: BCR/ABL induces multiple abnormalities of cytoskeletal function. *J Clin Invest* 100:46, 1997.

130. Lewis JM, Baskaran R, Taagepera S, et al: Integrin regulation of c-ABL tyrosine kinase activity and cytoplasmic-nuclear transport. *Proc Natl Acad Sci U S A* 93:15174, 1996.

131. Renshaw MW, McWhirter JR, Wang JY: The human leukemia oncogene bcr-abl abrogates the anchorage requirement but not the growth factor requirement for proliferation. *Mol Cell Biol* 15:1286, 1995.

132. Salgia R, Brunkhorst B, Pisick E, et al: Increased tyrosine phosphorylation of focal adhesion proteins in myeloid cell lines expressing p210BCR/ABL. *Oncogene* 11:1149, 1995.

133. Rudkin GT, Hungerford DA, Nowell PC: DNA content of chromosome Ph¹ and chromosome 21 in human chronic granulocytic leukemia. *Science* 144:1229, 1964.

134. O'Riordan ML, Robinson JA, Buckton KE, Evans HJ: Distinguishing between the chromosome involved in Down's syndrome (trisomy 21) and chronic myeloid leukaemia (Ph¹) by fluorescence. *Nature* 230:167, 1971.

135. Lawler SD: The cytogenetics of chronic granulocytic leukemia. *Clin Haematol* 6:55, 1977.

136. Melo JV, Yan XH, Diamond J, Goldman JM: Balanced parental contribution to the ABL component of the BCR-ABL gene in chronic myeloid leukemia. *Leukemia* 9:734, 1995.

137. Chissoe SL, Bodenteich A, Wang YF, et al: Sequence and analysis of the human ABL gene, the BCR gene, and regions involved in the Philadelphia chromosomal translocation. *Genomics* 27:67, 1995.

138. Melo JV, Deininger MW: Biology of chronic myelogenous leukemia-signaling pathways of initiation and transformation. *Hematol Oncol Clin North Am* 18:545, 2004.

139. Daley GQ, Ben Neriah Y: Implicating the bcr/abl gene in the pathogenesis of Philadelphia chromosome-positive human leukemia. *Adv Cancer Res* 57:151, 1991.

140. Heisterkamp N, Groffen J, Stephenson JR, et al: Chromosomal localization of human cellular homologues of two viral oncogenes. *Nature* 299:747, 1982.

141. Heisterkamp N, Stephenson JR, Groffen J, et al: Localization of the c-abl oncogene adjacent to a translocation breakpoint in chronic myelocytic leukemia. *Nature* 306:239, 1983.

142. Konopka JB, Witte ON: Activation of the abl oncogene in murine and human leukemias. *Biochem Biophys Acta* 823:1, 1985.

143. Collins SJ, Groudine MT: Rearrangements and amplification of c-abl sequences in the human chronic myelogenous leukemia cell line K562. *Proc Natl Acad Sci U S A* 80:4813, 1983.

144. Canaani E, Gale RP, Steiner-Seltz D, et al: Altered transcription of an oncogene in chronic myelocytic leukemia. *Lancet* 1:593, 1984.

145. Gale RP, Canaani E: An 8 kilobase abl RNA transcript in chronic myelogenous leukemia. *Proc Natl Acad Sci U S A* 81:5648, 1984.

146. Collins SJ, Kubonishi I, Miyoshi I, Groudine MT: Altered transcription of the c-abl oncogene in K562 and other chronic myelogenous leukemia cells. *Science* 225:72, 1984.

147. Leibowitz D, Cubbon RM, Bank A: Increased expression of a novel c-abl related RNA in K562 cells. *Blood* 65:526, 1985.

148. Konopka JB, Watanabe SM, Witte ON: An alteration of the human c-abl protein in K562 leukemia cells unmasks associated tyrosine kinase activity. *Cell* 37:1035, 1984.

149. Konopka JB, Watanabe SM, Singer JW, et al: Cell lines and clinical isolates derived from Ph¹-positive chronic myelogenous leukemia patients express c-abl proteins with a common structural alteration. *Proc Natl Acad Sci U S A* 82:1810, 1985.

150. Stam K, Heisterkamp N, Grosveld G, et al: Evidence of a new chimeric bcr/c-abl mRNA in patients with chronic myelocytic leukemia and the Philadelphia chromosome. *N Engl J Med* 313:1429, 1985.

151. Ben-Neriah Y, Daley GQ, Mes-Masson A-M, et al: The chronic myelogenous leukemia-specific P210 protein is the product of the bcr/abl hybrid gene. *Science* 233:212, 1985.

152. Maxwell SA, Kurzrock R, Parson SJ, et al: Analysis of P210bcr-abl tyrosine protein kinase activity in various subtypes of Philadelphia chromosome-positive cells from chronic myelogenous leukemia patients. *Cancer Res* 47:1731, 1987.

153. Kurzrock R, Kloetzer WS, Talpaz M, et al: Identification of molecular variants of P210bcr-abl in chronic myelogenous leukemia. *Blood* 70:233, 1987.

154. Xu DQ, Galibert F: Restriction fragment length polymorphism caused by a deletion within the human c-abl gene (ABL). *Proc Natl Acad Sci U S A* 83:3447, 1986.

155. Popenoe DW, Schaefer-Rego K, Mears JC, et al: Frequent and extensive deletion during the 9,22 translocation in CML. *Blood* 68:1123, 1986.

156. Shtivelman E, Gale RP, Dreazen O, et al: bcr-abl RNA in patients with chronic granulocytic leukemia. *Blood* 69:971, 1987.

157. McWhirter JR, Wang JJ: Activation of tyrosine kinase and microfilament-binding functions of c-abl by bcr sequences in bcr/abl fusion proteins. *Mol Cell Biol* 11:1553, 1991.

158. Bernards A, Rubin CM, Westbrook CA, et al: The first intron in the human c-abl gene is at least 200 kilobases long and is the target for translocations in chronic myelogenous leukemia. *Mol Cell Biol* 7:3231, 1987.

159. Eisenberg A, Silver R, Soper L, et al: The location of breakpoints within the breakpoint cluster region (bcr) of chromosome 22 in chronic myeloid leukemia. *Leukemia* 2:642, 1988.

160. Collins SJ: Breakpoints on chromosomes 9 and 22 in Philadelphia chromosome-positive chronic myelogenous leukemia. *J Clin Invest* 78:1392, 1986.

161. Heisterkamp N, Stam K, Groffen J, et al: Structural organization of the bcr gene and its role in the Ph¹ translocation. *Nature* 315:758, 1985.

162. Gao L-M, Goldman J: Long-range mapping of the normal BCR gene. *Leukemia* 5:555, 1991.

163. Melo JV: BCR-ABL gene variants. *Baillieres Clin Haematol* 10:203, 1997.

164. Saglio G, Pane F, Gottardi E, et al: Consistent amounts of acute leukemia-associated P190BCR/ABL transcripts are expressed by chronic myelogenous leukemia patients at diagnosis. *Blood* 87:1075, 1996.

165. Honda H, Oda H, Suzuki T, et al: Development of acute lymphoblastic leukemia and myeloproliferative disorder in transgenic mice expressing p210bcr/abl: A novel transgenic model for human Ph1-positive leukemias. *Blood* 91:2067, 1998.

166. Maru Y, Witte ON: The BCR gene encodes a novel serine/threonine kinase activity within a single exon. *Cell* 67:459, 1991.

167. Muller AJ, Young JC, Pendergast A-M, et al: BCR first exon sequences specifically activate the BCR/ABL tyrosine kinase oncogene of Philadelphia chromosome-positive human leukemia. *Mol Cell Biol* 11:1785, 1991.

168. Diekmann D, Brill S, Garrett MD, et al: BCR encodes a GTPase-activating protein for p21^{rac}. *Nature* 351:400, 1991.

169. Melo JV, Gordon DE, Goldman JM: The ABL-BCR fusion gene is expressed in chronic myeloid leukemia. *Blood* 81:158, 1993.

170. Bartram CR, de Klein A, Hagemeijer A, et al: Translocation of the human c-abl oncogene correlates with the presence of a Philadelphia chromosome in chronic myelocytic leukaemia. *Nature* 306:277, 1983.

171. Selleri L, Narni F, Emilia G, et al: Philadelphia-positive chronic myeloid leukemia with a chromosome 22 breakpoint outside the breakpoint cluster region. *Blood* 70:1659, 1987.

172. Mohamed AN, Koppitch F, Varterasian M, et al: BCR/ABL fusion located on chromosome 9 in chronic myeloid leukemia with a masked Ph chromosome. *Genes Chromosomes Cancer* 13:133, 1995.

173. Morris C, Jeffs A, Smith T, et al: BCR gene recombines with genomically distinct sites on band 11Q13 in complex BCR-ABL translocations of chronic myeloid leukemia. *Oncogene* 12:677, 1996.

174. Andreasson P, Johansson B, Carlsson M, et al: BCR/ABL-negative chronic myeloid leukemia with ETV6/ABL fusion. *Genes Chromosomes Cancer* 20:299, 1997.

175. Rozman C, Urbano-Ispizua A, Cervantes F, et al: Analysis of the clinical relevance of the breakpoint location within M-BCR and the type of chimeric mRNA in chronic myelogenous leukemia. *Leukemia* 9:1104, 1995.

176. Verschraegen CF, Kantarjian HM, Hirsch-Ginsberg C, et al: The breakpoint cluster region site in patients with Philadelphia chromosome-positive chronic myelogenous leukemia. Clinical, laboratory, and prognostic correlations. *Cancer* 76:992, 1995.

177. Zaccaria A, Martinelli G, Testoni N, et al: Does the type of BCR/ABL junction predict the survival of patients with Ph1-positive chronic myeloid leukemia? *Leuk Lymphoma* 16:231, 1995.

178. Ohno T, Hada S, Sugiyama T, et al: Chronic myeloid leukemia with minor bcr breakpoint developed hybrid type of blast crisis. *Am J Hematol* 57:320, 1998.

179. Melo JV: The diversity of BCR-ABL fusion proteins and their relationship to leukemia phenotype. *Blood* 88:2375, 1996.

180. Rubinstein R, Purves LR: A novel BCR-ABL rearrangement in a Philadelphia chromosome-positive chronic myelogenous leukaemia variant with thrombocythaemia. *Leukemia* 12:230, 1998.

181. Hochhaus A, Reither A, Skladny H, et al: A novel BCR-ABL fusion gene (e6a2) in a patient with Philadelphia chromosome-negative chronic myelogenous leukemia. *Blood* 88:2236, 1996.

182. Briz M, Vilches C, Cabrera R, et al: Typical chronic myelogenous leukemia with e19a2 junction BCR/ABL transcript. *Blood* 90:5024, 1997.

183. McLaughlin J, Chianese E, Witte ON: In vitro transformation of immature hemopoietic cells by P210 bcr/abl oncogene product of the Philadelphia chromosome. *Proc Natl Acad Sci U S A* 84:6558, 1987.

184. Daley GQ, McLaughlin J, Witte ON, Baltimore D: The CML-specific P210 bcr/abl protein, unlike v-abl, does not transform NIH/3T3 fibroblasts. *Science* 237:532, 1987.

185. Elefanty AG, Hariharan IK, Cory S: *Bcr-abl*, the hallmark of chronic myeloid leukaemia in man, induces multiple haemopoietic neoplasms in mice. *EMBO J* 9:1069, 1990.

186. Daley GQ, VanEtten RA, Baltimore D: Induction of chronic myelogenous leukemia in mice by the p210$^{bcr/abl}$ gene of the Philadelphia chromosome. *Science* 247:824, 1990.

187. Voncken JW, Morris C, Pattengale P, et al: Clonal development and karyotype evolution during leukemogenesis of BCR/ABL transgenic mice. *Blood* 79:1029, 1992.

188. Gishizky ML, Johnson-White J, Witte O: Efficient transplantation of BCR-ABL-induced chronic myelogenous leukemia-like syndrome in mice. *Proc Natl Acad Sci U S A* 90:3755, 1993.

189. Daley GQ: Animal models of BCR/ABL-induced leukemias. *Leuk Lymphoma* 11:57, 1993.

190. Voncken JW, Kaartinen V, Pattengale PK, et al: BCR/ABL P210 and P190 cause distinct leukemia in transgeneic mice. *Blood* 86:4603, 1995.

191. Honda H, Oda H, Suzuki T, et al: Development of acute lymphoblastic leukemia and myeloproliferative disorder in transgenic mice expressing p210bcr/abl: A novel transgenic model for human Ph1-positive leukemias. *Blood* 91:2067, 1998.

192. Pear WS, Miller JP, Xu L, et al: Efficient and rapid induction of a chronic myelogenous leukemia-like myeloproliferative disease in mice receiving P210 bcr/abl-transduced bone marrow. *Blood* 92:3780, 1998.

193. Honda M, Ohno S, Takahashi T, et al: Establishment, characterization, and chromosomal analysis of new leukemic cell lines derived from MT/p210/bcr/abl transgenic mice. *Exp Hematol* 26:188, 1998.

194. Zhang X, Ren R: Bcr-Abl efficiency induces in a myeloproliferative disease and production of excess interleukin-3 and granulocyte-macrophage colony-stimulating factor in mice: A novel model for chronic myelogenous leukemia. *Blood* 92:3829, 1998.

195. Elefanty AG, Corsy S: *Bcr-abl*-induced cell lines can switch from mast cell to erythroid or myeloid differentiation in vitro. *Blood* 79:1271, 1992.

196. Van Etten RA: Pathogenesis and treatment of Ph+ leukemia: Recent insights from mouse models. *Curr Opin Hematol* 8:224, 2001.

197. Bose S, Deininger M, Goora-Tybor J, et al: The presence of typical and atypical BCR-ABL fusion genes in leukocytes of normal individuals: Biological significance and implications for the assessment of minimal residual disease. *Blood* 92:3362, 1998.

198. Hirai HS, Tanaka M, Azuma Y, et al: Transforming genes in human leukemia cells. *Blood* 66:1371, 1985.

199. Clarkson BD, Strife A, Wisniewski D, et al: New understanding of the pathogenesis of CML: A prototype of early neoplasia. *Leukemia* 11:1404, 1997.

200. Verfaillie CM: Chronic myelogenous leukemia: From pathogenesis to therapy. *J Hematother* 8:3, 1999.

201. Pasternak G, Hochhaus A, Schultheis B, Hehlmann R: Chronic myelogenous leukemia: Molecular and cellular aspects. *J Cancer Res Clin Oncol* 124:643, 1998.

202. Gotoh A, Broxmeyer HE: The function of BCR/ABL and related proto-oncogenes. *Curr Opin Hematol* 4:3, 1997.

203. Sattler M, Salgia R: Activation of hematopoietic growth factor signal transduction pathways by the human oncogene BCR/ABL. *Cytokine Growth Factor Rev* 8:63, 1997.

204. Skorski T, Kanakaraj P, Nieborowska-Skorska M, et al: Phosphatidylinositol-3 kinase activity is regulated by BCR/ABL and is required for the growth of Philadelphia chromosome-positive cells. *Blood* 86:726, 1995.

205. Skorski T, Nieborowska-Skorska M, Szczylik C, et al: C-RAF-1 serine/threonine kinase is required in BCR/ABL-dependent and normal hematopoiesis. *Cancer Res* 55:2275, 1995.

206. Goga A, McLaughlin J, Afar DE, et al: Alternative signals to RAS for hematopoietic transformation by the BCR-ABL oncogene. *Cell* 82:981, 1995.

207. Salgia R, Uemura N, Okuda K, et al: CRKL links p210BCR/ABL with paxillin in chronic myelogenous leukemia cells. *J Biol Chem* 270:29145, 1995.

208. De Jong R, ten Hoeve J, Heisterkamp N, Groffen J: Crkl is complexed with tyrosine-phosphorylated Cbl in Ph-positive leukemia. *J Biol Chem* 270:21468, 1995.

209. Salgia R, Pisick E, Sattler M, et al: P130CAS forms a signalling complex with the adapter protein CRKL in hematopoietic cells transformed by the BCR/ABL oncogene. *J Biol Chem* 271:25198, 1996.

210. Sattler M, Griffin JD: Molecular mechanisms of transformation by the *BCR-ABL* oncogene. *Sem Hematol* 40:4, 2003.

211. Melo JV, Deininger MWN: Biology of chronic myelogenous-signaling pathways of initiation and transformation. *Hematol Clin North Am* 18:545, 2004.

212. Wong S, Witte ON: The BCR-ABL story: Bench to bedside and back. *Annu Rev Immunol* 22:247, 2004.

213. Sattler M, Verma S, Shrinkhande G, et al: The BCR/ABL tyrosine kinase induces production of reactive species in hematopoietic cells. *J Biol Chem* 275:24273, 2000.

214. Sattler M, Salgia R, Okuda K, et al: The proto-oncogene product p120^{CBL} and the adaptor proteins CRKL and c-CR link c-ABL, p190BCR/ABL and p210BCR/ABL to the phosphatidylinositol-3; kinase pathway. *Oncogene* 12:832, 1996.

215. Salgia R, Sattler M, Pisick E, et al: P210BCR/ABL induces formation of complexes containing focal adhesion proteins and the protooncogene product p120c-CBL. *Exp Hematol* 24:310, 1996.

216. De Jong R, van Wijk A, Haataja L, et al: BCR/ABL-induced leukemogenesis causes phosphorylation of Hef2 and its association with Crkl. *J Biol Chem* 272:32649, 1997.

217. Bollag G, Clapp DW, Shih S, et al: Loss of NF1 results in activation of the Ras signaling pathway and leads to aberrant growth in haematopoietic cells. *Nat Genet* 12:144, 1996.

218. Carpino N, Wisniewski D, Strife A, et al: P62dok: A constitutively tyrosine-phosphorylated, GAP-associated protein in chronic myelogneous leukemia progenitor cells. *Cell* 88:197, 1997.

219. Yamanashi Y, Baltimore D: Identification of the Abl- and ras GAP-associated 62 kDa protein as a docking protein, Dok. *Cell* 88:205, 1997.

220. Reuther JY, Reuther GW, Cortez D, et al: A requirement for NF-kappaB activation in BCR/ABL-mediated transformation. *Genes Dev* 1:12:968, 1998.

221. LaMontagne KR, Flint AJ, Franza BR, et al: Protein tyrosine phosphatase 1B antagonizes signalling by oncoprotein tyrosine kinase p210 bcr/abl in vivo. *Mol Cell Biol* 18:2965, 1998.

222. Chai SK, Nichols GL, Rothman P: Constitutive activation of JAKs and STATs in BCR-abl-expressing cell lines and peripheral blood cells derived from leukemic patients. *J Immunol* 159:4720, 1997.

223. Shuai K, Halpern J, ten Hoeve J, et al: Constitutive activation of STAT5 by the BCR-ABL oncogene in chronic myelogenous leukemia. *Oncogene* 13:247, 1996.

224. Wilson-Rawls J, Xie S, Liu J, et al: P210 Bcr-Abl interacts with the interleukin 3 receptor beta (c) subunit and constitutively induces its tyrosine phosphorylation. *Cancer Res* 56:3426, 1996.

225. Chuang TH, Xu X, Kaartinen V, et al: Abl and Bcr are multifunctional regulators of the Rho GTP-binding protein family. *Proc Natl Acad Sci U S A* 92:10282, 1995.

226. Afar DE, Witte O: Characterization of breakpoint cluster region kinase and SH2-binding activites. *Methods Enzymol* 256:125, 1995.

227. Gishizky ML, Cortez D, Pendergast AM: Mutant forms of growth factor-binding protein-2 reverse BCR-ABL-induced transformation. *Proc Natl Acad Sci U S A* 92:10889, 1995.

228. Raitano AB, Halpern JR, Hambuch TM, Sawyers CL: The Bcr-Abl leukemia oncogene activates Jun kinase and requires Jun for transformation. *Proc Natl Acad Sci U S A* 92:11746, 1995.

229. Miyamura T, Nishimura J, Yufu Y, Nawata H: Interaction of BCR-ABL with the retinoblastoma protein in Philadelphia chromosome-positive cell lines. *Int J Hematol* 67:115, 1997.

230. Largaespada DA, Brannan CI, Jenkins NA, Copeland NG: NF1 deficiency causes Ras-mediated granulocyte/macrophage colony stimulating factor hypersensitivity and chronic myeloid leukaemia. *Nat Genet* 12:137, 1996.

231. Amos TA, Lewis JL, Grand FH, et al: Apoptosis in chronic myeloid leukaemia: Normal responses by progenitor cells to growth factor deprivation, X-irradiation and glucocorticoids. *Br J Haematol* 91:387, 1995.

232. Bedi A, Barber JP, Bedi GC, et al: BCR-ABL-mediated inhibition of apoptosis with delay of G2/M transition after DNA damage: A mechanism of resistance to multiple anticancer agents. *Blood* 86:1148, 1995.

233. Amarante-Mendes GP, Naekyung KC, Liu L, et al: Bcr-Abl exerts its antiapoptotic effect against diverse apoptotic stimuli through blockage of mitochondrial release of cytochrome C and activation of caspase-3. *Blood* 92:1700, 1998.

234. Maguer-Satta V, Burl S, Liu L, et al: BCR-ABL accelerates C2-ceramide-induced apoptosis. *Oncogene* 16:237, 1998.

235. Pierson BA, Miller JS: CD56+bright and CD56+dim natural killer cells in patients with chronic myelogenous leukemia progressively decrease in number, respond less to stimuli that recruit clonogenic natural killer cells, and exhibit decreased proliferation on a per cell basis. *Blood* 88:2279, 1996.

236. Gissinger H, Kurzrock R, Wetzler M, et al: Apoptosis in chronic myelogenous leukemia: Studies of stage-specific differences. *Leuk Lymphoma* 25:121, 1997.

237. Doolittle RF, Hienkapiller MW, Hood LE, et al: Simian sarcoma virus oncogene, v-sis, is derived from the gene (or genes) encoding a platelet-derived growth factor. *Science* 221:275, 1983.

238. Dalla-Favera R, Gallo RC, Giallongo A, Croce C: Chromosomal localization of the human homolog (c-sis) of the simian sarcoma virus onc gene. *Science* 218:686, 1982.

239. Bartram CR, de Klein A, Hagemeijer A, et al: Localization of the human c-sis oncogene in Ph^1 positive and Ph^1 negative chronic myelocytic leukemia by in situ hybridization. *Blood* 63:223, 1984.

240. Waterfield MD, Scarce GT, Whittle N, et al: Platelet derived growth factor is structurally related to the putative transforming protein P28sis of simian sarcoma virus. *Nature* 304:35, 1983.

241. Joseph SF, Ratner L, Clark MF, et al: Transforming potential of human c-sis nucleotide sequences encoding platelet derived growth factor. *Science* 225:636, 1984.

242. Romero P, Blick M, Talpaz M, et al: C-sis and c-abl expression in chronic myelogenous leukemia and other hematologic malignancies. *Blood* 67:839, 1986.

243. Boultwood J, Peniket A, Watkins F, et al: Telomere length shortening in chronic myelogenous leukemia is associated with reduced time to accelerated phase. *Blood* 96:358, 2000.

244. Terasaki Y, Okamura H, Ohtake S, Nakao S: Accelerated telomere length shortening in granulocytes: A diagnostic marker for myeloproliferative diseases. *Exp Hematol* 30:1399, 2002.

245. Drummond MW, Lennard A, Brummendorf TH, Holyoake TL: Telomere shortening correlates with prognostic score at diagnosis and proceeds rapidly during progression of chronic myeloid leukemia. *Leuk Lymphoma* 45:1775, 2004.

246. Ohyashiki K, Ohyashiki JH, Iwama H, et al: Telomerase activity and cytogenetic changes in chronic myeloid leukemia with disease progression. *Leukemia* 11:190, 1997.

247. Brümmendorf TH, Ersöz I, Hartmann U, et al: Telomere length in peripheral blood granulocytes reflects response to treatment with imatinib in patients with chronic myeloid leukemia. *Blood* 101:375, 2003.

248. Thompson RB, Stainsby D: The clinical and haematological features of chronic granulocytic leukaemia in the chronic phase, in *Chronic Granulocytic Leukaemia*, edited by MT Shaw, p 137. Praeger, East Sussex, UK, 1982.

249. Cortes JE, Talpaz M, Kantarkian H: Chronic myelogenous leukemia: A review. *Am J Med* 100:555, 1996.

250. Goldman JM: Chronic myeloid leukemia. *Curr Opin Hematol* 4:277, 1997.

251. Lichtman MA, Rowe JM: Hyperleukocytic leukemias: Rheological, clinical and therapeutic considerations. *Blood* 60:279, 1982.

252. Rowe JM, Lichtman MA: Hyperleukocytosis and leukostasis: Common features of childhood chronic myelogenous leukemia. *Blood* 63:1230, 1984.

253. Lichtman MA, Heal J, Rowe JM: Hyperleukocytic leukaemia. *Baillieres Clin Haematol* 1:725, 1987.

254. Ungaro PC, Gonzalez JJ, Werk EE, MacKay JC: Chronic myelogenous leukemia presenting clinically as diabetes insipidus. *N C Med J* 45:640, 1984.

255. Juan D, Hsu S-D, Hunter J: Case report of vasopressin-responsive diabetes insipidus associated with chronic myelogenous leukemia. *Cancer* 56:1468, 1985.

256. Brydon J, Lucky PA, Duffy T: Acne urticaria associated with chronic myelogenous leukemia. *Cancer* 56:2083, 1985.

257. Cohen PR, Talpaz M, Kurzrock R: Malignancy-associated Sweet's syndrome: A review of the world's literature. *J Clin Oncol* 6:1887, 1988.

258. López JLB, Fonseca E, Mauso F: Sweet's syndrome during the chronic phase of chronic myeloid leukemia. *Acta Haematol* 84:207, 1990.

259. Nestok BR, Goldstein JD, Lipkovic P: Splenic rupture as a cause of sudden death in undiagnosed chronic myelogenous leukemia. *Am J Forensic Med Pathol* 9:241, 1988.

260. Giagounidis AAN, Burk M, Meckenstock G, et al: Pathological rupture of the spleen in hematologic malignancies. *Ann Hematol* 73:297, 1996.

261. Hild DH, Myers TJ: Hyperviscosity in chronic granulocytic leukemia. *Cancer* 46:1418, 1980.

262. D'Hondt L, Guillaume TH, Hemblit Y, Symann M: Digital necrosis associated with chronic myeloid leukemia. *Acta Clin Belg* 52:49, 1997.

263. Arbaje YM, Betran G: Chronic myelogenous leukemia complicated by autoimmune hemolytic anemia. *Am J Med* 88:197, 1990.

264. Steegman JL, Pinilla I, Requena MJ, et al: The direct antiglobulin test is frequently positive in chronic myeloid leukemia patients treated with interferon-α. *Transfusion* 37:446, 1997.

265. Hoppin EC, Lewis JP: Polycythemia rubra vera progressing to Ph¹-positive chronic myelogenous leukemia. *Ann Intern Med* 83:820, 1975.

266. Shenkenberg TD, Waddell CC, Rice L: Erythrocytosis and marked leukocytosis in overlapping myeloproliferative diseases. *South Med J* 75:868, 1982.

267. Haas O, Hinterberger W, Morz R: Pure red cell aplasia as possible early manifestation of chronic myeloid leukemia. *Am J Hematol* 27:20, 1986.

268. Mijovic A, Rolovic Z, Novak A, et al: Chronic myeloid leukemia associated with pure red cell aplasia and terminating in promyelocytic transformation. *Am J Hematol* 31:128, 1989.

269. Inbal A, Aktein E, Barak I, Meytes D: Cyclic leukocytosis and long survival in chronic myeloid leukemia. *Acta Haematol* 69:353, 1983.

270. Umemura T, Hirata J, Kaneko S, et al: Periodic appearance of erythropoietin-independent erythropoiesis in chronic myelogenous leukemia with cyclic oscillation. *Acta Haematol* 76:230, 1986.

271. Mitus WJ, Kiossoglou KA: Leukocyte alkaline phosphatase in myeloproliferative syndrome. *Ann N Y Acad Sci* 155:976, 1968.

272. DePalma L, Delgado P, Werner M: Diagnostic discrimination and cost-effective assay strategy for leukocyte alkaline phosphate. *Clin Chim Acta* 6:83, 1996.

273. Pedersen F: Functional and biochemical phenotype in relation to cellular age of differentiated neutrophils in chronic myeloid leukemia. *Br J Haematol* 51:339, 1982.

274. Rambaldi A, Terao M, Bettoni S, et al: Differences in the expression of alkaline phosphatase in mRNA in chronic myelogenous leukemia and paroxysmal nocturnal hemoglobinuria polymorphonuclear leukocytes. *Blood* 73:1113, 1989.

275. Perillie PE: Studies of the changes in leukocyte alkaline phosphatase following pyrogen stimulation in chronic granulocytic leukemia. *Blood* 29:401, 1967.

276. Rustin GJS, Goldman JM, McCarthy D, et al: An extracellular factor controls neutrophil alkaline phosphatase in chronic granulocytic leukemia. *Br J Haematol* 45:381, 1980.

277. Matsuo T: In vitro modulation of alkaline phosphatase activity in neutrophils from patients with chronic myelogenous leukemia by monocyte-derived activity. *Blood* 67:492, 1986.

278. Tanaka KR, Valentine WN, Fredricks RE: Diseases or clinical conditions associated with low leukocyte alkaline phosphatase. *N Engl J Med* 262:912, 1960.

279. Stinson RA, McPhee J, Lewanczk R, Dinwoodie A: Neutrophil alkaline phosphatase in hypophosphatasia. *N Engl J Med* 312:1642, 1985.

280. Kamada N, Uchino H: Chronologic sequence in appearance of clinical and laboratory findings characteristic of chronic myelocytic leukemia. *Blood* 51:843, 1978.

281. Denberg JA, Wilson WEC, Goodacre R, Brenenstock J: Chronic myeloid leukemia—Evidence for basophil differentiation and histamine synthesis from cultured peripheral blood cells. *Br J Haematol* 45:13, 1980.

282. Goh K-O, Anderson FW: Cytogenetic studies in basophilic chronic myelocytic leukemia. *Arch Pathol Lab Med* 103:288, 1979.

283. Youman JD, Taddeini L, Cooper T: Histamine excess symptoms in basophilic chronic granulocytic leukemia. *Arch Intern Med* 131:560, 1973.

284. Rosenthal S, Schwartz JH, Canellos GP: Basophilic chronic granulocytic leukemia with hyperhistaminemia. *Br J Haematol* 36:367, 1977.

285. Samorapoompichit P, Kiener HP, Schernthaner G-H, et al: Detection of tryptase in cytoplasmic granules of basophils in patients with chronic myeloid leukemia and other myeloid neoplasms. *Blood* 98:2580, 2001.

286. Weil SC, Hrisinko MA: A hybrid eosinophilic-basophilic granulocyte in chronic granulocytic leukemia. *Am J Clin Pathol* 87:66, 1987.

287. Velardi A, Rambotti P, Cernetti C, et al: Monoclonal antibody defined T-cell phenotypes and phytohemagglutinin reactivity of E-rosette forming circulating lymphocytes from untreated chronic myelocyte leukemia patients. *Cancer* 53:913, 1984.

288. Dowding C, Th'ng KH, Goldman JM, Galton DAG: Increased T-lymphocyte numbers in chronic granulocytic leukemia before treatment. *Exp Hematol* 12:811, 1984.

289. Kaur J, Catovsky D, Spiers ASD, Galton DAG: Increase of T-lymphocytes in the spleen in chronic granulocytic leukaemia. *Lancet* 1:834, 1974.

290. Fujimiya Y, Bakke A, Chang WC, et al: Natural killer-cell immunodeficiency in patients with chronic myelogenous leukemia. *Int J Cancer* 37:639, 1986.

291. Fujimiya Y, Chang WC, Bakke A, et al: Natural killer cell immunodeficiency in patients with chronic myelogenous leukemia. *Cancer Immunol Immunother* 24:213, 1987.

292. Mellqvist U-H, Hansson M, Brune M, et al: Natural killer cell dysfunction and apoptosis induced by chronic myelogenous leukemia cells: Role of reactive oxygen species and regulation by histamine. *Blood* 96:1961, 2000.

293. Pierson BA, Miller JS: The role of autologous natural killer cells in chronic myelogenous leukemia. *Leukemia* 11:1404, 1997.

294. Mason JE, DeVita VT, Canellos GP: Thrombocytosis in chronic granulocytic leukemia: Incidence and clinical significance. *Blood* 44:483, 1974.

295. Pederson B: Kinetics and cell function, in *Chronic Granulocytic Leukaemia*, edited by MT Shaw, p 93. Praeger, East Sussex, UK, 1982.

296. Radhika V, Thennarasu S, Naik NR, et al: Granulocytes from chronic myeloid leukemia (CML) patients show differential response to different chemoattractants. *Am J Hematol* 52:155, 1996.

297. Kasimir-Bauer S, Ottinger H, Brittinger G, König W: Philadelphia chromosome-positive chronic myelogenous leukemia: Functional defects in circulating mature neutrophils of untreated and interferon-α-treated patients. *Exp Hematol* 22:426, 1994.

298. Adams T, Schultz L, Goldberg L: Platelet function abnormalities in the myeloproliferative disorders. *Scand J Haematol* 13:215, 1974.

299. Gerrard JM, Stoddard SF, Shapiro RS, et al: Platelet storage pool deficiency and prostaglandin synthesis in chronic granulocytic leukaemia. *Br J Haematol* 40:597, 1978.

300. Knox WF, Bhavani M, Davson J, Geary CG: Histological classification of chronic granulocytic leukaemia. *Clin Lab Haematol* 6:171, 1984.

301. Lorand-Metze I, Vassalo J, Souza CA: Histological and cytological heterogeneity of bone marrow in Philadelphia-positive chronic myelogenous leukaemia at diagnosis. *Br J Haematol* 67:45, 1987.

302. Inokuchi K, Yamaguchi H, Tarusawa M, et al: Abnormality of c-kit oncoprotein in certain patients with chronic myelogenous leukaemia—Potential clinical significance. *Leukemia* 16:170, 2002.

303. Cairoli R, Grillo G, Beghini A, et al: Chronic myelogenous leukemia with acquired c-kit activating mutation and transient bone marrow mastocytosis. *Hematol J* 5:273, 2004.

304. Kelsey PR, Geary CG: Sea-blue histiocytes and Gaucher's cells in bone marrow of patients with chronic myeloid leukaemia. *J Clin Path* 41:960, 1988.

305. Dezmezian R, Kantarjian HM, Keating MJ, et al: The relevance of reticulin stain-measured fibrosis at diagnosis in chronic myelogenous leukemia. *Cancer* 59:1739, 1987.

306. Ghosh K, Varma N, Varma S, Dash S: Cellular composition and reticulin fibrosis in chronic myeloid leukaemia. *Indian J Cancer* 25:128, 1988.

307. Buhr T, Choritz H, Georgü A: The impact of megakaryocyte proliferation for the evolution of myelofibrosis. *Virchows Archiv* 420:473, 1992.

308. Korkolopoulou P, Viniou N, Kavantzas N, et al: Clinicopathologic correlations of bone marrow angiogenesis in chronic myeloid leukemia: A morphometric study. *Leukemia* 17:89, 2003.

309. Aguayo A, Kantarjian H, Manshouri T, et al: Angiogenesis in acute and chronic leukemias and myelodysplastic syndromes. *Blood* 96:2240, 2000.

310. Rumpel M, Friedrich T, Deininger MWN: Imatinib normalizes bone marrow vascularity in patients with chronic myeloid leukemia in first chronic phase. *Blood* 101:4641, 2003.

311. Adams SP, Sahota SS, Mijovic A, et al: Frequent expression of HAGE in presentation chronic myeloid leukemias. *Leukemia* 16:2238, 2002.

312. Udomsakdi C, Eaves CJ, Lansdorp PM, Eaves AC: Phenotypic heterogeneity of primitive leukemic hematopoietic cells in patients with chronic myeloid leukemia. *Blood* 80:2522, 1992.

313. Huret JL: Complex translocations, simple variant translocation and Ph-negative cases in chronic myelogenous leukaemia. *Hum Genet* 85:565, 1990.

314. Sakurai M, Sandberg AA: The chromosomes and causation of human cancer and leukemia: XVIII. The missing Y in acute myeloblastic leukemia (AML) and Ph1-positive chronic myelocytic leukemia. *Cancer* 38:762, 1976.

315. Berger R, Bernheim A: Y chromosome loss in leukemias. *Cancer Genet Cytogenet* 1:1, 1979.

316. Ishihara T, Sasaki M, Oshimura M, et al: A summary of cytogenetic studies on 534 cases of chronic myelogenous leukemia in Japan. *Cancer Genet Cytogenet* 9:81, 1983.

317. Mitelman F: Catalogue of chromosomal aberrations in cancer. *Cytogenet Cell Genet* 36:9, 1983.

318. Heim S, Billstrom R, Kristoffersson U, et al: Variant Ph translocations in chronic myeloid leukemia. *Cancer Genet Cytogenet* 18:215, 1985.

319. Bartram CR, Anger B, Carbonell F, Kleihauer E: Involvement of chromosome 9 in variant Ph1 translocation. *Leuk Res* 9:1133, 1985.

320. Morris CM, Rosman I, Archer SA, et al: A cytogenetic and molecular analysis of five variant Philadelphia translocations in chronic myeloid leukemia. *Cancer Genet Cytogenet* 35:179, 1988.

321. Teyssier JR, Bartram CR, DeVille J, et al: C-abl oncogene and chromosome 22 "bcr" juxtaposition in chronic myelogenous leukemia. *N Engl J Med* 312:1393, 1985.

322. Hagemeijer A, Bartram CR, Smith EME, et al: Is the chromosomal region 9q34 always involved in variants of the Ph1 translocation? *Cancer Genet Cytogenet* 13:1, 1984.

323. DeBraikeleer M, Chiu H-K, Fiser J, Gardner HA: A further case of Philadelphia chromosome-positive chronic myeloid leukemia with t(3;9;22). *Cancer Genet Cytogenet* 35:279, 1988.

324. Latoge-Pochitaloff-Huvalé M, Sainty D, Adriaansen HJ, et al: Translocation (3;21) in Philadelphia positive chronic myeloid leukemia. *Leukemia* 3:554, 1989.

325. Thompson PW, Whittaker JA: Translocation 3;21 in Philadelphia chromosome positive chronic myeloid leukemia at diagnosis. *Cancer* 39:143, 1989.

326. Engel E, McGee BJ, Flexner JM, et al: Philadelphia chromosome (Ph1) translocation in an apparently Ph1 negative, minus G22, case of chronic myeloid leukemia. *N Engl J Med* 291:154, 1974.

327. Verma RS, Dosik H: "Masked" Ph1 chromosome in chronic myelogenous leukaemia (CML). *Blut* 50:129, 1985.

328. Hagemeijer A, de Klein A, Godde-Salz E, et al: Translocation of c-abl to "masked" Ph in chronic myeloid leukemia. *Cancer Genet Cytogenet* 18:95, 1985.

329. Melo JV: The diversity of BCR-ABL fusion proteins and their relationship to leukemic phenotype. *Blood* 88:2375, 1996.

330. O'Brien S, Thall PR, Siciliano MJ: Cytogenetics of chronic myeloid leukemia. *Baillieres Clin Haematol* 10:259, 1997.

331. Bartram CR, Carbonell F: bcr rearrangement in Ph-negative CML. *Cancer Genet Cytogenet* 21:183, 1986.

332. Bartram CR: Rearrangement of bcr and c-abl sequences in Ph-positive acute leukemias and Ph-negative CML—An update. *Curr Stud Hematol Blood Transfus* 31:160, 1987.

333. Ganesan TS, Rassool F, Guo A-P, et al: Rearrangement of the bcr gene in Philadelphia-chromosome negative chronic myeloid leukemia. *Curr Stud Hematol Blood Transfus* 31:153, 1987.

334. Wiedemann LM, Karhi K, Chan LC: Similar molecular alterations occur in related leukemias with and without the Philadelphia chromosome. *Curr Stud Hematol Blood Transfus* 31:149, 1987.

335. Benn P, Loper L, Eisenberg A, et al: Utility of molecular genetic analysis of bcr rearrangement in the diagnosis of chronic myeloid leukemia. *Cancer Genet Cytogenet* 29:1, 1987.

336. Epner DE, Koeffler AP: Molecular genetic advances in chronic myelogenous leukemia. *Ann Intern Med* 113:3, 1990.

337. Dubé I, Dixon J, Beckett T, et al: Location of breakpoints within the major breakpoint cluster region (bcr) in 33 patients with *bcr* rearrangement-positive chronic myeloid leukemia with complex or absent Philadelphia chromosomes. *Genes Chromosomes Cancer* 1:106, 1989.

338. Morris C, Heisterkamp N, Kennedy MA, et al: Ph-negative chronic myeloid leukemia: Molecular analysis of ABL insertion into M-BCR on chromosome 22. *Blood* 76:1812, 1990.

339. Blennerhassett GT, Furth ME, Anderson A, et al: Clinical evaluation of DNA probe assay for the Philadelphia (Ph¹) translocation in chronic myelogenous leukemia. *Leukemia* 2:648, 1988.

340. Lange W, Snyder DS, Castro R, et al: Detection by enzymatic amplification of bcr-abl mRNA in peripheral blood and bone marrow cells of patients with chronic myelogenous leukemia. *Blood* 73:1735, 1989.

341. Dhingra K, Talpaz M, Riggs MC, et al: Hybridization protection assay: A rapid, sensitive, and specific method for detection of Philadelphia chromosome-positive leukemias. *Blood* 77:238, 1991.

342. Gaiger A, Henn T, Horth E, et al: Increase of bcr-abl chimeric mRNA expression in tumor cells of patients with chronic myeloid leukemia precedes disease progression. *Blood* 86:2371, 1995.

343. Stock W, Westbrook CA, Peterson B, et al: Value of molcular monitoring during the treatment of chronic myeloid leukemia: A Cancer and Leukemia Group B study. *J Clin Oncol* 15:26, 1997.

344. Frenoy N, Chabli A, Sol D, et al: Application of a new protocol for nested PCR to the detection of minimal residual bcr/abl transcripts. *Leukemia* 8:1411, 1994.

345. Melo JV, Yan XH, Diamond J, et al: Reverse transcription/polymerase chain reaction (RT/PCR) amplification of very small numbers of transcripts: The risk in misinterpreting negative results. *Leukemia* 10:1217, 1996.

346. Lin F, Chase A, Bunget J, et al: Correlation between the proportion of Philadelphia chromosome-positive metaphase cells and levels of BCR-ABL mRNA in chronic myeloid leukaemia. *Genes Chromosomes Cancer* 13:110, 1995.

347. VanDenderen J, Hermans A, Meeuwsen T, et al: Antibody recognition of the tumor-specific bcr-abl joining region in chronic myeloid leukemia. *J Exp Med* 169:87, 1989.

348. Hagemeyer A, vanderPlas DC, Solkarman D, et al: The Philadelphia translocation in CML and ALL: Recent investigations, new detection methods. *Nouv Rev Fr Hematol* 32:83, 1990.

349. Maxwell SA, Kurzrock R, Parsons SJ, et al: Analysis of p210 bcr-abl tyrosine protein kinase activity in various subtypes of Philadelphia chromosome-positive cells from chronic myelogenous leukemia patients. *Cancer Res* 47:1731, 1987.

350. Guo JQ, Lian JY, Xian YM, et al: BCR-ABL protein expression in peripheral blood cells of chronic myelogenous leukemia patients undergoing therapy. *Blood* 83:3629, 1994.

351. Dewald GW, Schad CR, Christensen ER, et al: The application of in situ fluorescent hybridization to detect M bcr/abl fusion in variant Ph chromosomes in CML and ALL. *Cancer Genet Cytogenet* 71:7, 1993.

352. Cox MC, Maffei L, Buffolino S, et al: A comparative analysis of FISH, RT-PCR, and cytogenetics for the diagnosis of bcr-abl-positive leukemias. *Am J Clin Pathol* 109:24, 1998.

353. Sinclair PB, Green AR, Grace C, Nacheva EP: Improved sensitivity of BCR-ABL detection: A triple-probe three-color fluorescence in situ hybridization system. *Blood* 90:1395, 1997.

354. Acar H, Stewart J, Boyd E, Connor MJ: Identification of variant translocations in chronic myeloid leukemia by fluorescence in situ hybridization. *Cancer Genet Cytogenet* 93:115, 1997.

355. Schoch C, Schnittger S, Bursch S, et al: Comparison of chromosome banding analysis, interphase- and hypermetaphase-FISH, qualitative and quantitative PCR for diagnosis and for follow-up in chronic myeloid leukemia: A study of 350 cases. *Leukemia* 16:53, 2002.

356. Yanagi M, Shinjo K, Takeshita A, et al: Simple and reliably sensitive diagnosis and monitoring of Philadelphia chromosome-positive cells in chronic myeloid leukemia by interphase fluorescence in situ hybridization of peripheral blood cells. *Leukemia* 13:542, 1999.

357. Werner M, Ewig M, Nasarek A, et al: Value of fluorescence in situ hybridization for detecting the bcr/abl gene fusion in interphase cells of routine bone marrow specimens. *Diagn Mol Pathol* 6:282, 1997.

358. Chase A, Grand F, Zhang JG, et al: Factors influencing the false positive and negative rates of BCR-ABL fluorescence in situ hybridization. *Genes Chromosomes Cancer* 18:246, 1997.

359. Pelz AF, Kroning H, Franke A, Wieacker P: High reliability and sensitivity of the BCR/ABL1 D-FISH test for the detection of BCR/ABL rearrangements. *Ann Hematol* 81:147, 2002.

360. Hochhaus A, Reiter A, Skladny H, et al: Molecular monitoring of residual disease in chronic myelogenous leukemia patients after therapy. *Recent Results Cancer Res* 144:36, 1998.

361. Wells SJ, Phillips CN, Winton EF, Farhi DC: Reverse transcriptase-polymerase chain reaction for bcr-abl fusion in chronic myelogenous leukemia. *Am J Clin Pathol* 105:756, 1996.

362. Cox MC, Maffei L, Buffolino S, et al: A comparative analysis of FISH, RT-PCR, and cytogenetics for the diagnosis of bcr-abl-positive leukemias. *Am J Clin Pathol* 109:24, 1998.

363. Krackoff IH: Studies of uric acid biosynthesis in the chronic leukemias. *Arthritis Rheum* 8:772, 1965.

364. Vogler WR, Bain JA, Huguley CM Jr, et al: Metabolic and therapeutic effects of allopurinol in patients with leukemia and gout. *Am J Med* 40:548, 1966.

365. Zittoun J, Marquet J, Zittoun R: The intracellular content of the three cobalamins at various stages of normal and leukaemic myeloid cell development. *Br J Haematol* 31:299, 1975.

366. Zittoun J, Zittoun R, Marquet J, Sultan C: The three transcobalamins in myeloproliferative disorders and acute leukemia. *Br J Haematol* 31:287, 1975.

367. Rosner F, Schreiber ZA: Serum vitamin B$_{12}$ and vitamin B$_{12}$ binding capacity in chronic myelogenous leukemia and other disorders. *Am J Med Sci* 263:473, 1972.

368. Sternman U-H: Intrinsic factor and the B$_{12}$ binding proteins. *Clin Haematol* 5:473, 1976.

369. Corcino JJ, Zalusky R, Greenberg M, Herbert V: Coexistence of pernicious anaemia and chronic myeloid leukaemia: An experiment of nature involving vitamin B$_{12}$ metabolism. *Br J Haematol* 20:511, 1971.

370. Gomez GA, Sokal JE, Walsh D: Prognostic features at diagnosis of chronic myelocytic leukemia. *Cancer* 47:2470, 1981.

371. Bellevue R, Dosik H, Spergel G, Gussoff BD: Pseudohyperkalemia and extreme leukocytosis. *J Lab Clin Med* 85:660, 1975.

372. Ballard HS, Marcus AJ: Hypercalcemia in chronic myelogenous leukemia. *N Engl J Med* 282:663, 1970.

373. Evans JJ, Bozdech MJ: Hypokalemia in nonblastic chronic myelogenous leukemia. *Arch Intern Med* 141:786, 1981.

374. Perillie PE, Finch SC: Muramidase studies in Philadelphia-chromosome-positive and chromosome-negative chronic granulocytic leukemia. *N Engl J Med* 283:456, 1970.

375. Gilbert HS, Ginsberg H: Hypocholesterolemia as a manifestation of disease activity in chronic myeloid leukemia. *Cancer* 51:1428, 1983.

376. Muller CP, Wagner AN, Maucher C, Steinke B: Hypocholesterolemia, an unfavorable feature of prognostic value in chronic myeloid leukemia. *Eur J Haematol* 43:235, 1989.

377. Musolino C, Alonci A, Bellomo G, et al: Levels of soluble angiogenin in chronic myeloid malignancies. *Eur J Haematol* 72:416, 2004.

378. Calabro L, Fonsatti E, Bellomo G, et al: Differential levels of soluble endoglin (CD105) in myeloid malignancies. *J Cell Physiol* 194:171, 2003.

379. Morris CM, Fitzgerald PH, Hollings PE, et al: Essential thrombozcythemia and the Philadelphia chromosome. *Br J Haematol* 70:13, 1988.

380. Stoll DB, Peterson P, Exten R, et al: Clinical presentation and natural history of patients with essential thrombocythemia and the Philadelphia chromosome. *Am J Hematol* 27:77, 1988.

381. Sessarego M, Defferrari R, Dejana AM, et al: Cytogenetic analysis in essential thrombocythemia at diagnosis and at transformation. *Cancer Genet Cytogenet* 43:57, 1989.

382. Pajor L, Kereskai L, Zsdral K, et al: Philadelphia chromosome and/or bcr-abl mRNA-positive primary thrombocytosis: morphometric evidence for the transition from essential thrombocythemia to chronic myeloid leukaemia type myeloproliferation. *Histopathology* 42:53, 2003.

383. Blickstein D, Aviram A, Luboshitz J, et al: BCR-ABL transcripts in bone marrow aspirates of Philadelphia-negative essential thrombocythemia patients: Clinical presentation. *Blood* 90:2768, 1997.

384. Cervantes F, Colomer D, Vives-Corrons JL, et al: Chronic myeloid leukemia of thrombocythemic onset: A CML subtype with distinct hematological and molecular features. *Leukemia* 10:1241, 1996.

385. Martiat P, Ifrah N, Rassool F, et al: Molecular analysis of Philadelphia positive essential thrombocythemia. *Leukemia* 3:563, 1989.

386. Michiels JJ, Berneman Z, Schroyens W, et al: Philadelphia (Ph) chromosome–positive thrombocythemia without features of chronic myeloid leukemia in peripheral blood; natural history and diagnostic differentiation from Ph-negative essential thrombocythemia. *Ann Hematol* 83:504, 2004.

387. Blickstein D, Aviram A, Luboshitz J, et al: BCR-ABC transcripts in bone marrow aspirates of Philadelphia-negative essential thrombocythemia patients; clinical presentation. *Blood* 90:2768, 1997.

388. Pajor L, Kereskai L, Zsdral K, et al: Philadelphia chromosome and/or bcr-abl mRNA positive primary thrombocytosis: Morphometric evidence for the transition from essential thrombocythaemia to chronic myeloid leukaemia type of myeloproliferation. *Histopathology* 42:53, 2003.

389. Damaj G, delabesse E, Le Bihan C, et al: Typical essential thrombocythaemia does not express bcr abelson fusion transcript. *Br J Haematol* 116:812, 2002.

390. Hsu H-C, Tan L-Y, Au L-C, et al: Detection of bcr-abl gene expression at a low level in blood cells of some patients with essential thrombocythemia. *J Lab Clin Med* 143:125, 2004.

391. Paietta E, Rosen N, Roberts M, et al: Philadelphia chromosome positive essential thrombocythemia evolving into lymphoid blast crisis. *Cancer Genet Cytogenet* 25:227, 1987.

392. Michiels JJ, Prins ME, Hagermeijer A, et al: Philadelphia chromosome-positive thrombocythemia and megakaryoblast leukemia. *Am J Clin Pathol* 88:645, 1987.

393. Kwong YL, Chiu EK, Liang RH, et al: Essential thrombocythemia with BCR/ABL rearrangement. *Cancer Genet Cytogenet* 89:74, 1996.

394. Marasca R, Luppi M, Zucchini P, et al: Might essential thrombocythemia carry Ph anomaly? *Blood* 91:3084, 1998.

395. Sanadi I, Yamamoto S, Ogata M, et al: Detection of the Philadelphia chromosome in chronic neutrophilic leukemia. *Jpn J Clin Oncol* 15:553, 1985.

396. Christopoulus C, Kottoris K, Mikraki V, Anevlavis E: Presence of bcr/abl rearrangement in a patient with chronic neutrophilic leukaemia. *J Clin Pathol* 49:1013, 1996.

397. Pane F, Frigeri F, Sindina M, et al: Neutrophilic-chronic myeloid leukemia: A distinct disease with a specific molecular marker (BCR/ABL with C3/A2 junction). *Blood* 88:2410, 1996.

398. Verstovsek S, Lin H, Kantarjian H, et al: Neutrophilic-chronic myeloid leukemia: Low levels of p230 BCR/ABL mRNA and undetectable BCR/ABL protein may predict an indolent course. *Cancer* 94:2416, 2002.

399. Saglio G, Guerrasio A, Rosso C, et al: New type of BCR/ABL junction in Philadelphia chromosome-positive chronic myelogenous leukemia. *Blood* 87:1075, 1996.

400. Ohno T, Hada S, Sugiyama T, et al: Chronic myeloid leukemia with minor-bcr breakpoint developed hybrid type of blast crisis. *Am J Hematol* 57:320, 1998.

401. Knowles DM: Thymoma and chronic myelogenous leukemia. *Cancer* 38:414, 1976.

402. Vannier JP, Bizet M, Bastard C, et al: Simultaneous occurrence of a T-cell lymphoma and a chronic myelogenous leukemia with an unusual karyotype. *Leuk Res* 8:647, 1984.

403. Djulbegovi B, Hadley T, Yen F: Occurrence of high-grade T-cell lymphoma in a patient with Philadelphia chromosome-negative chronic myelogenous leukemia with breakpoint cluster region rearrangement. *Am J Hematol* 36:63, 1991.

404. Tittley P, Trempe JM, van der Jagt R, et al: Occurrence of T-cell lymphoma in a patient with Philadelphia chromosome-positive chronic myelogenous leukemia with rearrangements of BCR and TCR-β genes in the lymph nodes. *Am J Hematol* 42:229, 1993.

405. Hornstein P, Nordenson I, Wahlin A: Philadelphia chromosome negative acute lymphoblastic leukemia preceding Philadelphia positive chronic myelogenous leukemia. *Cancer Genet Cytogenet* 39:147, 1989.

406. Ichinohasama R, Miura I, Takahashi N, et al: Ph-negative non-Hodgkin's lymphoma occurring in chronic phase of Ph-positive chronic myelogenous leukemia is defined as a genetically different neoplasm from extramedullary localized blast crisis: Report of two cases and review of the literature. *Leukemia* 14:169, 2000.

407. Rodler E, Welborn J, Hatcher S, et al: Blastic mantle cell lymphoma developing concurrently in a patient with chronic myelogenous leukemia and a review of the literature. *Am J Hematol* 75:231, 2004.

408. Naparstek Y, Zlotnick A, Polliack A: Coexistent chronic myeloid leukemia and IgA monoclonal gammopathy: Report of a case and review of the literature. *Am J Med Sci* 292:111, 1980.

409. Shoenfeld Y, Berliner S, Ayalone A, et al: Monoclonal gammopathy in patients with chronic and acute myeloid leukemia. *Cancer* 54:280, 1984.

410. Tanaka M, Kimura R, Matsutani A, et al: Coexistence of chronic myelogenous leukemia and multiple myeloma. *Acta Haematol* 99:221, 1998.

411. Schwartzmeier JD, Shehata M, Ackermann J, et al: Simultaneous occurrence of chronic myeloid leukemia and multiple myeloma: Evaluation by FISH analysis and in vitro expansion of bone marrow cells. *Leukemia* 17:1426, 2003.

412. Nitta M, Tsuboi K, Yamashita S, et al: Multiple myeloma preceding development of chronic myelogenous leukemia. *Int J Hematol* 69:170, 1999.

413. Vitali C, Bombardieri S, Spremolla G: Chronic myeloid leukemia in Waldenström's macroglobulinemia. *Arch Intern Med* 141:1349, 1981.

414. Whang-Peng J, Gralnick HR, Johnson RE, et al: Chronic granulocytic leukemia (CGL) during the course of chronic lymphocytic leukemia (CLL): Correlation of blood, marrow, and spleen morphology and cytogenetics. *Blood* 43:333, 1974.

415. Schrieber ZA, Axelrod MR, Abebe LS: Coexistence of chronic myelogenous leukemia and chronic lymphocytic leukemia. *Cancer* 54:697, 1984.

416. Specchia G, Buquicchio C, Albano F, et al: Non-treatment-related chronic myeloid leukemia as a second malignancy. *Leuk Res* 28:115, 2004.

417. Esteve J, Cervantes F, Rives S, et al: Simultaneous occcurrence of B-cell chronic lymphocytic leukemia and chronic myeloid leukemia with

further evolution to lymphoic blast status. *Haematologica* 82:596, 1997.

418. Leoni F, Ferrini PR, Castoldi GL, et al: Simultaneous occurrence of chronic granulocytic leukemia and chronic lymphoid leukemia. *Haematologia* 72:253, 1987.

419. Faguet GB, Little T, Agee JF, Garver FA: Chronic lymphatic leukemia evolving into chronic myelocytic leukemia. *Cancer* 52:1647, 1983.

420. Crescenzi B, Sacchi S, Marasca R, et al: Distinct genomic events in the myeloid and lymphoid lineages in simultaneous presentation of chronic myeloid leukemia and B-chronic lymphocytic leukemia. *Leukemia* 16:955, 2002.

421. Mansat-De Mas V, Regal-Huguet F, Cassar G, et al: Chronic myeloid leukemia associated with B-cell chronic lymphocytic leukemia: Evidence of two separate clones as shown by combined cell-sorting and fluorescence in situ hybridization. *Leuk Lymphoma* 44:867, 2003.

422. Jantunen E, Nousiainen T: Ph-positive chronic myelogenous leukemia evolving after polycythemia vera. *Am J Hematol* 37:212, 1991.

423. Hoppen EC, Lewis JP: Polycythemia rubra vera progressing to Ph-positive chronic myelogenous leukemia. *Ann Intern Med* 83:820, 1975.

424. Haq AU: Transformation of polycythemia vera to Ph-positive chronic myelogenous leukemia. *Am J Hematol* 356:110, 1990.

425. Roth AD, Oral A, Przepiorka D, et al: Chronic myelogenous leukemia and acute lymphoblastic leukemia occurring in the course of polycythemia vera. *Am J Hematol* 43:123, 1993.

426. Foviester RH, Louro JM: Philadelphia chromosome abnormality in angiogenic myeloid metaplasia. *Ann Intern Med* 64:622, 1966.

427. Nowell PC, Kant JA, Finan JB, et al: Marrow fibrosis associated with a Philadelphia chromosome. *Cancer Genet Cytogenet* 59:89, 1992.

428. Roth DG, Richman CM, Rowley JD: Chronic myelodysplastic syndrome (preleukemia) with the Philadelphia chromosome. *Blood* 56:262, 1980.

429. Berrebi A, Bruck R, Shtalrid M, Chemke J: Philadelphia chromosome in idiopathic acquired sideroblastic anemia. *Acta Haematol* 72:343, 1984.

430. Hande K: Hyperuricemia, uric acid nephropathy and the tumor lysis syndrome, in *Renal Complications of Neoplasia*, edited by TD McKinney, p 134. Praeger, New York, 1986.

431. Navolanic PM, Pui CH, Larson RA, et al: Elitek-rasburicase: An effective means to prevent and treat hyperuricemia associated with tumor lysis syndrome, a Meeting Report, Dallas, TX, January, 2002.

432. Stone RM: Optimizing treatment of chronic myeloid leukemia: A rational approach. *Oncologist* 9:259, 2004.

433. Bazatbashi MS, Smith MR, Karanes C, et al: Successful management of Ph chromosome chronic myelogenous leukemia with leukapheresis during pregnancy. *Am J Hematol* 38:235, 1991.

434. Strobl FJ, Voelkerding KY, Smith EP: Management of chronic myeloid leukemia during pregnancy with leukapheresis. *J Clin Apheresis* 14:42, 1999.

435. Kennedy BJ: The evolution of hydroxyurea therapy in chronic myelogenous leukemia. *Semin Oncol* 19(suppl 9):21, 1992.

436. Tsimberidou AM, Colburn DE, Welch MA, et al: Anagrelide and imatinib mesylate combination therapy in patients with chronic myeloproliferative disorders. *Cancer Chemother Pharmacol* 52:229, 2003.

437. Sawyers CL: Tyrosine kinase inhibitors in chronic myeloid leukemia. *Cancer J* 5:63, 1999.

438. Lerma E, Wang T, Fujii T, et al: Development of kinase inhibitors, in *Chronic Myeloid Leukemia—Biology and Treatment*, edited by GQ Daley, CJ Eaves, JM Goldman, R Hehlmann, AM Carello, p 493. Martin Dunitz Ltd., London, UK, 2001.

439. Jahagirdar BN, Miller JS, Shet A, Verfaillie CM: Novel therapies for chronic myelogenous leukemia. *Exp Hematol* 29:543, 2001.

440. Mughal TI, Goldman JM: Chronic myeloid leukemia: Current status and controversies. *Oncology* 18:837, 2004.

441. Goldman JM, Melo JV: Chronic myeloid leukemia—Advances in biology and new approaches to treatment. *N Engl J Med* 349:1451, 2003.

442. Schindler T, Bornmann W, Pellicena P, et al: Structural mechanism for ST1-571 inhibition of abelson tyrosine kinase. *Science* 289:1938, 2000.

443. Buchdunger E, Cioffi CL, Law N, et al: Abl protein-tyrosine kinase inhibitor ST1571 inhibits in vitro signal transduction mediated by c-kit and platelet-derived growth factor receptors. *J Pharmacol Exp Ther* 295:139, 2000.

444. Marley SB, Deininger MWN, Davidson RJ, et al: The tyrosine kinase inhibitor STI571, like interferon-α, preferentially reduces the capacity for amplification of granulocyte-macrophage progenitors from patients with chronic myeloid leukemia. *Exp Hematol* 28:551, 2000.

445. Holtz MS, Slovak ML, Zhang F, et al: Imatinib meylate (STI571) inhibits growth of primitive malignant progenitors in chronic myelogenous leukemia through reversal of abnormally increased proliferation. *Blood* 99:3792, 2002.

446. O'Brien SG, Guilhot F, Larson RA, et al: A new standard treatment for chronic myelogenous leukemia. *N Engl J Med* 348:994, 2003.

447. Nikolova Z, Peng B, Hubert M, et al: Bioequivalence, safety, and tolerability of imatinib tablets compared with capsules. *Cancer Chemother Pharmacol* 53:433, 2004.

448. Cohen MH, Moses ML, Pazdur R: Gleevec for the treatment of chronic myelogenous leukemia: U.S. Food and Drug Administration regulatory mechanisms, accelerated approval, and orphan drug status. *Oncologist* 7:390, 2002.

449. Mughal TI, Yong A, Szydlo RM, et al: Molecular studies in patients with chronic myeloid leukemia in remission 5 years after allogeneic stem cell transplant define the risk of subsequent relapse. *Br J Haematol* 115:569, 2001.

450. Druker B: Signal transduction inhibition: Results from Phase I clinical trials in chronic myeloid leukemia. *Sem Hematol* 38:9, 2001.

451. Kantarjian H, Sawyers C, Hochhaus A, et al: Hematologic and cytogenetic responses to imatinib mesylate in chronic myelogenous leukemia. *N Engl J Med* 346:645, 2002.

452. Marin D, Marktel S, Szydlo R, et al: Survival of patients with chronic-phase chronic myeloid leukemia on imatinib after failure on interferon alfa. *Lancet* 362:617, 2003.

453. Kantarjian H, O'Brien S, Cortes J, et al: Survival advantage with imatinib mesylate therapy in chronic-phase chronic myelogenous leukemia (CML-CP) after IFN-α failure in the late CML-CP, comparison with historical controls. *Clin Cancer Res* 10:68, 2004.

454. Kantarjian HM, Cortes JE, O'Brien S, et al: Imatinib mesylate therapy in newly diagnosed patients with Philadelphia chromosome-positive chronic myelogenous leukemia: High incidence of early complete and major cytogenetic responses. *Blood* 101:97, 2003.

455. O'Brien SG, Guilhot F, Larson RA, et al: Imatinib compared with interferon and low-dose cytarabine for newly diagnosed chronic-phase chronic myeloid leukemia. *N Engl J Med* 348:994, 2003.

456. Druker BJ: Imatinib alone and in combination for chronic myeloid leukemia. *Semin Hematol* 40:50, 2003.

457. Hahn EA, Glendenning GA: Quality of life on imatinib. *Semin Hematol* 40:31, 2003.

458. Hughes TP, Kaeda J, Branford S, et al: Frequency of major molecular responses to imatinib or interferon alfa plus cytarabine in newly diagnosed chronic myeloid leukemia. *N Engl J Med* 349:1423, 2003.

459. Kantarjian HM, O'Brien S, Cortes J, et al: Imatinib mesylate therapy improves survival in patients with newly diagnosed Philadelphia chromosome-positive chronic myelogenous leukemia in chronic phase. Comparison with historic data. *Cancer* 98:2636, 2003.

460. Kantarjian H, Talpaz M, O'Brien S, et al: High-dose imatinib mesylate therapy in newly diagnosed Philadelphia chromosome-positive chronic phase chronic myeloid leukemia. *Blood* 103:2873, 2004.

461. Cortes J, Giles F, O'Brien S, et al: Result of high-dose imatinib mesylate in patients with Philadelphia chromosome-positive chronic myeloid leukemia after failure of interferon-alpha. *Blood* 102:83, 2003.

462. Marin D, Goldman JM, Olavarria E, Apperley JF: Transient benefit only from increasing the imatinib dose in CML patients who do not achieve complete cytogenetic remissions on conventional doses. *Blood* 102:2702, 2003.

463. Kantarjian HM, Talpaz M, O'Brien S, et al: Dose escalation of imatinib mesylate can overcome resistance to standard-dose therapy in patients with chronic myelogenous leukemia. *Blood* 101:473, 2003.

464. Zonder JA, Pemberton P, Brandt H, et al: The effect of dose increase of imatinib mesylate in patients with chronic or accelerated phase chronic myelogenous leukemia with inadequate hematologic or cytogenetic response to initial treatment. *Clin Cancer Res* 9:2092, 2003.

465. El-Zimaity MM, Kantarjian H, Talpaz M, et al: Results of imatinib mesylate therapy in chronic myelogenous leukaemia with variant Philadelphia chromosome. *Br J Haematol* 125:187, 2004.

466. Synder DS, McMahon R, Cohen SR, Slovak ML: Chronic myeloid leukemia with an e13a3 BCR-ABL fusion: Benign course responsive to imatinib with an RT-PCR advisory. *Am J Hematol* 75:92, 2004.

467. Quintas-Cardama A, Kantarjian H, Talpaz M, et al: Deletion of chromosome 9 has no prognostic impact on patients with chronic myeloid leukemia treated with imatinib mesylate. *Blood* 102:184a, 2003.

468. Champagne MA, Capdeville R, Krailo M, et al: Imatinib mesylate (STI571) for treatment of children with Philadelphia chromosome-positive leukemia: Results from a Children's Oncology Group phase I study. *Blood* 104:2655, 2004.

469. Cortes J, Talpaz M, O'Brien S, et al: Effects of age on prognosis with imatinib mesylate therapy for patients with Philadelphia chromosome positive chronic myelogenous leukemia. *Cancer* 98:1105, 2003.

470. Guilhot F. Indications for imatinib mesylate therapy and clinical management. *Oncologist* 9:271, 2004.

471. Hensley ML, Ford JM: Imatinib treatment: Specific issues related to safety, fertility, and pregnancy. *Semin Hematol* 40:21, 2003.

472. Esmaeli B, Prieto VG, Butler CE, et al: Severe periorbital edema secondary to STI571 (Gleevec). *Cancer* 95:881, 2002.

473. Vora A, Bhutani M, Sharma A, Raina V: Severe tumor lysis syndrome during treatment with STI 571 in a patient with chronic myelogenous leukemia accelerated phase. *Ann Oncol* 13:1833, 2002.

474. Elliott MA, Mesa RA, Tefferi A: Adverse events after imatinib mesylate therapy. *N Engl J Med* 346:712, 2002.

475. Kusumi E, Arakawa A, Kami M, et al: Visual disturbance due to retinal edema as a complication of imatinib. *Leukemia* 18:1138, 2004.

476. Mattiuzzi GN, Cortes JE, Talpaz M, et al: Development of Varicella-Zoster virus infection in patients with chronic myelogenous leukemia treated with imatinib mesylate. *Clin Cancer Res* 9:976, 2003.

477. Gambacorti-Passerini C, Tornaghi L, Cavagnini F, et al: Gynaecomastia in men with chronic myeloid leukaemia after imatinib. *Lancet* 361:1954, 2003.

478. Novaretti MCZ, Fonseca GHH, Conchon M, et al: First case of immune-mediated haemolytic anaemia associated with imatinib mesylate. *Eur J Haematol* 71:455, 2003.

479. Sanchez-Gonzalez B, Pascual-Ramirez JC, Fernandez-Abellian P, et al: Severe skin reaction to imatinib in a case of Philadelphia-positive acute lymphoblastic leukemia. *Blood* 101:2446, 2003.

480. Drummond A, Micallef-Eynaud P, Douglas WS, et al: A spectrum of skin reactions caused by the tyrosine kinase inhibitor imatinib mesylate (STI 571, Glivec). *Br J Haematol* 120:911, 2003.

481. Rule SAJ, O'Brien SG, Crossman LC: Managing cutaneous reactions to imatinib therapy. *Blood* 100:3434, 2002.

482. Liu D, Seiter K, Mathews T, et al: Sweet's syndrome with CML cell infiltration of the skin in a patient with chronic-phase CML while taking imatinib mesylate. *Leuk Res* 28SI:S61, 2004.

483. Etienne G, Cony-Makhoul P, Mahon FX: Imatinib mesylate and gray hair. *N Engl J Med* 346:645, 2002.

484. Tjao AS, Kantarjian H, Cortes J, et al: Imatinib mesylate causes hypopigmentation in the skin. *Cancer* 98:2483, 2003.

485. Marin D, Marktel S, Foot N, et al: Granulocyte colony-stimulating factor reverses cytopenia and may permit cytogenetic responses in patients with chronic myeloid leukemia treated with imatinib mesylate. *Haematologica* 88:227, 2003.

486. Quintas-Cardama A, Kantarjian H, O'Brien S, et al: Granulocyte-colony-stimulating factor (filgrastim) may overcome imatinib-induced neutropenia in patients with chronic-phase chronic myelogenous leukemia. *Cancer* 100:2592, 2004.

487. Ault P, Kantarjian H, Welch MA, et al: Interleukin 11 may improve thrombocytopenia associated with imatinib mesylate therapy in chronic myelogenous leukemia. *Leuk Res* 28:613, 2004.

488. van Deventer HW, Hall MD, Orlowski RZ, et al: Clinical course of thrombocytopenia in patients treated with imatinib mesylate for accelerated phase chronic myelogenous leukemia. *Am J Hematol* 71:184, 2002.

489. Sneed TB, Kantarjian HM, Talpaz M, et al: The significance of myelosuppression during therapy with imatinib mesylate in patients with chronic myelogenous leukemia in chronic phase. *Cancer* 100:116, 2004.

490. Naito K, Mori T, Miyazaki K, et al: Successful treatment of extramedullary blast crisis of chronic myelogenous leukemia with imatinib mesylate (STI571). *Intern Med* 42:740, 2003.

491. Neville K, Parise RA, Thompson P, et al: Plasma and cerebrospinal fluid pharmacokinetics of imatinib after administration to nonhuman primates. *Clin Cancer Res* 10:2525, 2004.

492. Wolff N, Richardson JA, Egorin M, Ilaria RL Jr: The CNS is a sanctuary for leukemic cells in mice receiving imatinib mesylate for Bcr/Abl-induced leukemia. *Blood* 101:5010, 2003.

493. Cortes J, Giles F, O'Brien S, et al: Results of imatinib mesylate therapy in patients with refractory or recurrent acute myeloid leukemia, high-risk myelodysplastic syndrome, and myeloproliferative disorders. *Cancer* 97:2760, 2003.

494. Beham-Schmid C, Apfelbeck U, Sill H, et al: Treatment of chronic myelogenous leukemia with the tyrosine kinase inhibitor STI571 results in marked regression of bone marrow fibrosis. *Blood* 99:381, 2002.

495. Ebos JM, Tran J, Master Z, et al: Imatinib mesylate (STI-571) reduces the Bcr-Abl-mediated vascular endothelial growth factor secretion in chronic myelogenous leukemia. *Mol Cancer Res* 1:89, 2002.

496. Kvasnicka HM, Thiele J, Staib P, et al: Reversal of bone marrow angiogenesis in chronic myeloid leukemia following imatinib mesylate (STI571) therapy. *Blood* 103:3549, 2004.

497. Hasserjian RP, Boecklin F, Parker S, et al: STI571 (imatinib mesylate) reduces bone marrow cellularity and normalizes morphologic features irrespective of cytogenetic response. *Am J Clin Pathol* 117:360, 2002.

498. Graham SM, Jorgensen HG, Allan E, et al: Primitive, quiescent, Philadelphia-positive stem cells from patients with chronic myeloid leukemia are insensitive to STI571 in vitro. *Blood* 99:319, 2002.

499. Branford S, Rudzki Z, Harper A, et al: Imatinib produces significantly superior molecular responses compared to interferon alfa plus cytarabine in patients with newly diagnosed chronic myeloid leukemia in chronic phase. *Leukemia* 17:2401, 2003.

500. Rosti G, Martinelli G, Bassi S, et al: Molecular response to imatinib in late chronic-phase chronic myeloid leukemia. *Blood* 103:2284 2004.

501. Goldman JM, Marin D: Management decisions in chronic myeloid leukemia. *Semin Hematol* 40:97, 2003.

502. Kantarjian H, Talpaz M, O'Brien S, et al: Prediction of initial cytogenetic response for subsequent major and complete cytogenetic response to imatinib mesylate therapy in patients with Philadelphia chro-

mosome-positive chronic myelogenous leukemia. *Cancer* 98:1776, 2003.

503. Liu NM, O'Brien S. Spontaneous reversion from blast to chronic phase after withdrawal of imatinib mesylate in a patient with chronic myelogenous leukemia. *Leuk Lymphoma* 43:2413, 2002.

504. Higashi T, Tsukada J, Kato C, et al: Imatinib mesylate-sensitive blast crisis immediately after discontinuation of imatinib mesylate therapy in chronic myelogenous leukemia: Report of two cases. *Am J Hematol* 76:275, 2004.

505. Ghanima W, Kahrs J, Dahl TG 3rd, Tjonnfjord GE: Sustained cytogenetic response after discontinuation of imatinib mesylate in a patient with chronic myeloid leukaemia. *Eur J Haematol* 72:441, 2004.

506. Cortes J, O'Brien S, Kantarjian H: Discontinuation of imatinib therapy after achieving a molecular response. *Blood* 104:2204, 2004.

507. O'Dwyer ME, Gatter KM, Loriaux M, et al: Demonstration of Philadelphia chromosome negative abnormal clones in patients with chronic myelogenous leukemia during major cytogenetic responses induced by imatinib mesylate. *Leukemia* 17:481, 2003.

508. Guilbert-Douet N, Morel F, LeBris M-J, et al: Clonal chromosomal abnormalities in the Philadelphia chromosome negative cells of chronic myeloid leukemia patients treated with imatinib. *Leukemia* 18:1140, 2004.

509. Deininger MWN: Cytogenetic studies in patients on imatinib. *Semin Hematol* 40:50, 2003.

510. Bumm T, Muller C, Al-Ali K, et al: Emergence of clonal cytogenetic abnormalities in Ph-cells in some CML patients in cytogenetic remission to imatinib but restoration of polyclonal hematopoiesis in the majority. *Blood* 101:1941, 2003.

511. Goldberg SL, Medan RA, Rowley SD, et al: Myelodysplastic subclones in chronic myeloid leukemia: Implications for imatinib mesylate therapy. *Blood* 101:781, 2003.

512. Farag SS, Ruppert AS, Mrozek K, et al: Prognostic significance of additional cytogenetic abnormalities in newly diagnosed patients with Philadelphia chromosome-positive chronic myelogenous leukemia treated with interferon-α: A Cancer and Leukemia Group B study. *Int J Oncol* 25:143, 2004.

513. Andersen MK, Pedersen-Bjergaard J, Kjeldsen I, et al: Clonal Ph-negative hematopoiesis in CML after therapy with imatinib mesylate is frequently characterized by trisomy 8. *Leukemia* 16:1390, 2002.

514. Terre C, Eclache V, Rousselot P, et al: Report of 34 patients with clonal chromosomal abnormalities in Philadelphia-negative cells during imatinib treatment of Philadelphia-positive chronic myeloid leukemia. *Leukemia* 18:1340, 2004.

515. Cortes JE, Talpaz M, Giles F, et al: Prognostic significance of cytogenetic clonal evolution in patients with chronic myelogenous leukemia on imatinib mesylate therapy. *Blood* 101:3794, 2003.

516. Chee YL, Vickers MA, Stevenson D, et al: Fatal myelodysplastic syndrome developing during therapy with imatinib mesylate and characterised by the emergence of complex Philadelphia negative clones. *Leukemia* 17:634, 2003.

517. Nimmanapalli R, O'Bryan E, Huang M, et al: Molecular characterization and sensitivity of STI-571 (imatinib mesylate, Gleevec)-resistant, Bcr-Abl-positive, human acute leukemia cells to SRC kinase inhibitor PD180970 and 17-allylamino-17-demethoxygeldanamycin. *Cancer Res* 62:5761, 2002.

518. Paterson SC, Smith KD, Holyoake TL, Jorgensen HG: Is there a cloud in the silver lining for imatinib? *Br J Cancer* 88:983, 2003.

519. Hochhaus A, La Rosse P: Imatinib therapy in chronic myelogenous leukemia: Strategies to avoid and overcome resistance. *Leukemia* 18:1320, 2004.

520. Cowan-Jacob SW, Guez V, Fendrich G, et al: Imatinib (STI571) resistance in chronic myelogenous leukemia: Molecular basis of the underlying mechanism and potential strategies for treatment. *Mini Rev Med Chem* 4:285, 2004.

521. Weisberg E, Griffin JD: Resistance to imatinib (Glivec): Update on clinical mechanisms. *Drug Resist Update* 6:231, 2003.

522. Melo JV: Resistance to imatinib mesylate in CML: All BCR-ABL mutations "are created equal but some are more equal than others." *Blood* 101:4231, 2003.

523. Bhatia R, Holtz M, Niu N, et al: Persistence of malignant hematopoietic progenitors in chronic myelogenous leukemia patients in complete cytogenetic remission following imatinib mesylate treatment. *Blood* 101:4701, 2003.

524. le Coutre P, Tassi E, Varella-Garcia M, et al: Induction of resistance to the Abelson inhibitor STI571 in human leukemic cells through gene amplification. *Blood* 95:1758, 2000.

525. Campbell LJ, Patsouris C, Rayeroux KC, et al: BCR/ABL amplification in chronic myelocytic leukemia blast crisis following imatinib mesylate administration. *Cancer Genet Cytogenet* 139:30, 2002.

526. Donato NJ, Wu JY, Stapley J, et al: BCR-ABL independence and LYN kinase overexpression in chronic myelogenous leukemia cells selected for resistance to STI571. *Blood* 101:690, 2003.

527. Illmer T, Schaich M, Platzbecker U, et al: P-glycoprotein-mediated drug efflux is a resistance mechanism of chronic myelogenous leukemia cells to treatment with imatinib mesylate. *Leukemia* 18:401, 2004.

528. Mahon FX, Belloc F, Lagarde V, et al: MDR1 gene overexpression confers resistance to imatinib mesylate in leukemia cell line models. *Blood* 101:2368, 2003.

529. Gambacorti-Passerini C, Barni R, le Coutre P, et al: Role of alphal acid glycoprotein in the in vivo resistance of human BCR-ABL(+) leukemic cells to the abl inhibitor STI571. *J Natl Cancer Inst* 92:1641, 2000.

530. Roche-Lestienne C, Preudhomme C: Mutations in the ABL kinase domain pre-exist the onset of imatinib treatment. *Semin Hematol* 21:80, 2003.

531. Corbin AS, LaRosee P, Stoffregen EP, et al: Several Bcr-Abl kinase domain mutants associated with imatinib mesylate resistance remain sensitive to imatinib. *Blood* 101:4611, 2003.

532. Hochhaus A, Kreil S, Corbin AS, et al: Molecular and chromosomal mechanisms of resistance to imatinib (STI571) therapy. *Leukemia* 16:2190, 2002.

533. Miething C, Mugler C, Grundler R, et al: Phosphorylation of tyrosine 393 in the kinase domain of Bcr-Abl influences the sensitivity towards imatinib in vivo. *Leukemia* 17:1695, 2003.

534. Branford S, Rudzki Z, Walsh S, et al: Detection of BRC-ABL mutations in patients with CML treated with imatinib is virtually always accompanied by clinical resistance, and mutations in the ATP phosphate-binding loop (P-loop) are associated with a poor prognosis. *Blood* 102:276, 2003.

535. Hochhaus A: Cytogenetic and molecular mechanisms of resistance to imatinib. *Semin Hematol* 40:69, 2003.

536. Ohno R, Nakamura Y: Prediction of response to imatinib by cDNA microarray analysis. *Semin Hematol* 40:42, 2003.

537. Paschka P, Muller MC, Merx K, et al: Molecular monitoring of response to imabinib (Glivec) in CML patients pretreated with interferon alpha. Low levels of residual disease are associated with continuous remission. *Leukemia* 17:1687, 2003.

538. Tipping AJ, Mahon FX, Zafirides G, et al: Drug responses of imatinib mesylate-resistant cells: Synergism of imatinib with other chemotherapeutic drugs. *Leukemia* 16:2349, 2002.

539. Tipping AJ, Melo JV: Imatinib mesylate in combination with other chemotherapeutic drugs: In vitro studies. *Semin Hematol* 40:83, 2003.

540. Kantarjian HM, Talpaz M, Smith TL, et al: Homoharringtonine and low-dose cytarabine in the management of late chronic-phase chronic myelogenous leukemia. *J Clin Oncol* 18:3513, 2000.

541. O'Dwyer ME, La Rosee P, Nimmanapalli R, et al: Recent advances in Philadelphia chromosome-positive malignancies: The potential role of arsenic trioxide. *Semin Hematol* 39:18, 2002.

542. Kantarjian HM, O'Brien S, Corteo J, et al: Results of decitabine (5-aza-2'deoxycytidine) therapy in 130 patients with chronic myelogenous leukemia. *Cancer* 98:522, 2003.

543. Issa JP, Garcia-Manero G, Giles FJ, et al: Phase 1 study of low-dose prolonged exposure schedules of the hypomethylating agent 5-aza-2'-deoxycytidine (decitabine) in hematopoietic malignancies. *Blood* 103:1635, 2004.

544. Thiesing JT, Ohno-Jones S, Kolibaba KS, Druker BJ: Efficacy of STI571, an Abl tyrosine kinase inhibitor, in conjunction with other antileukemic agents against Bcr-Abl-positive cells. *Blood* 96:3195, 2000.

545. Gardembas M, Rousselot P, Tulliez M, et al: Results of a prospective phase 2 study combining imatinib mesylate and cytarabine for the treatment of Philadelphia-positive patients with chronic myelogenous leukemia in chronic phase. *Blood* 102:4298, 2003.

546. Guilhot F, Gardembas M, Rousselot P, et al: Imatinib in combination with cytarabine for the treatment of Philadelphia-positive chronic myelogenous leukemia chronic-phase patients: Rationale and design of phase I/II trials. *Semin Hematol* 40:92, 2003.

547. Chand M, Thakuri M, Keung YK: Imatinib mesylate associated with delayed hematopoietic recovery after concomitant chemotherapy. *Leukemia* 18:886, 2004.

548. Sun X, Layton JE, Elefanty A, Lieschke GJ: Comparison of effects of the thyrosine kinase inhibitors AG957, AG490, and STI571 on BCR-ABL-expressing cells, demonstrating synergy between AG490 and STI571. *Blood* 97:2008, 2001.

549. Mohi MG, Boulton C, Gu TL, et al: Combination of rapamycin and protein tyrosine kinase (PTK) inhibitors for the treatment of leukemias caused by oncogenic PTKs. *Proc Natl Acad Sci U S A* 101:3130, 2004.

550. Gatto S, Scappini B, Pham L, et al: The proteasome inhibitor PS-341 inhibits growth and induces apoptosis in Bcr/Abl-positive cell lines sensitive and resistant to imatinib mesylate. *Haematologica* 88:853, 2003.

551. Dai Y, Rahmani M, Pei XY, et al: Bortezomib and flabopiridol interact synergistically to induce apoptosis in chronic myeloid leukemia cells resistant to imatinib mesylate through both Bcr/Abl-dependent and -independent mechanisms. *Blood* 104:509, 2004.

552. Yu C, Rahmani M, Conrad D, et al: The proteasome inhibitor bortezomib interacts synergistically with histone deacetylase inhibitors to induce apoptosis in Bcr/Abl+ cells sensitive and resistant to STI571. *Blood* 102:3765, 2003.

553. Chu S, Holtz M, Gupta M, Bhatia R: BCR/ABL kinase inhibition by imatinib mesylate enhances MAP kinase activity in chronic myelogenous leukemia CD34+ cells. *Blood* 103:3167, 2004.

554. Kuroda J, Kimura S, Segawa H, et al: The third-generation bisphosphonate zoledronate synergistically augments the anti-Ph+ leukemia activity of imatinib mesylate. *Blood* 102:2229, 2003.

555. Keating A: Chronic myeloid leukemia: Current therapies and the potential role of farnesyltransferase inhibitors. *Semin Hematol* 39:11, 2002.

556. Daley GQ: Towards combination target-directed chemotherapy for chronic myeloid leukemia: Role of farnesyl transferase inhibitors. *Semin Hematol* 40:11, 2003.

557. Nakajima A, Tauchi T, Sumi M, et al: Efficacy of SCH66336, a farnesyl transferase inhibitor, in conjunction with imatinib against BCR-ABL-positive cells. *Mol Cancer Ther* 2:219, 2003.

558. Hoover RR, Mahon FX, Melo JV, Daley GQ: Overcoming STI571 resistance with the farnesyl transferase inhibitor SCH66336. *Blood* 100:1068, 2002.

559. Druker BJ: Overcoming resistance to imatinib by combining targeted agents. *Mol Cancer Ther* 2:225, 2003.

560. Cortes J, Albitar M, Thomas D, et al: Efficacy of the farnesyl transferase inhibitor R115777 in chronic myeloid leukemia and other hematologic malignancies. *Blood* 101:1692, 2003.

561. Shah NP, Nicoll JM, Nagar B, et al: Multiple BCR-ABL kinase domain mutations confer polyclonal resistance to the tyrosine kinase inhibitor imatinib (STI571) in chronic phase and blast crisis chronic myeloid leukemia. *Cancer Cell* 2:117, 2002.

562. Sawyers CL, Hochhaus A, Feldman E, et al: Imatinib induces hematologic and cytogenetic responses in patients with chronic myelogenous leukemia in myeloid blast crisis: Results of a phase II study. *Blood* 99:3530, 2002.

563. Gorre ME, Ellwood-Yen K, Chiosis G, et al: BCR-ABL point mutants isolated from patients with imatinib mesylate-resistant chronic myeloid leukemia remain sensitive to inhibitors of the BCR-ABL chaperone heat shock protein 90. *Blood* 100:3041, 2002.

564. O'Dwyer M: Multifaceted approach to the treatment of Bcr-Abl-positive leukemias. *Oncologist* 7:30, 2002.

565. Merx K, Muller MC, Kreil S, et al: Early reduction of BCR-ABL mRNA transcript levels predicts cytogenetic response in chronic phase CML patients treated with imatinib after failure of interferon alpha. *Leukemia* 16:1579, 2002.

566. Scheuring UJ, Pfeifer H, Wassmann B, et al: Serial minimal residual disease (MRD) analysis as a predictor of response duration in Philadelphia-positive acute lymphoblastic leukemia (Ph+ALL) during imatinib treatment. *Leukemia* 17:1722, 2003.

567. Lange T, Bumm T, Otto S, et al: Quantitative reverse transcription polymerase chain reaction should not replace conventional cytogenetics for monitoring patients with chronic myeloid leukemia during early phase of imatinib therapy. *Haematologica* 89:49, 2004.

568. Wu CJ, Neuberg D, Chillemi A, et al: Quantitative monitoring of BCR/ABL transcript during STI-571 therapy. *Leuk Lymphoma* 43:2281, 2002.

569. Druker BJ: Imatinib as a paradigm of targeted therapies. *J Clin Oncol* 21:239, 2003.

570. Druker BJ: STI571 (Gleevec™) as a paradigm for cancer therapy. *Trends Mol Med* 8:S14, 2002.

571. Hughes T, Branford S: Molecular monitoring of chronic myeloid leukemia. *Semin Hematol* 40:62, 2003.

572. Rosti G, Testoni N, Martinelli G, Baccarani M: The cytogenetic response as a surrogate marker of survival. *Semin Hematol* 40:56, 2003.

573. Carella AM: Questioning the aim of CML therapy in the era of Imatinib? *Leukemia* 17:1199, 2003.

574. DeAngelo DJ, Ritz J: Imatinib therapy for patients with chronic myelogenous leukemia: Are patients living longer? *Clin Cancer Res* 10:1, 2004.

575. Cortes JE, Talpaz M, O'Brien S, et al: High rates of major cytogenetic response in patients with newly diagnosed chronic myeloid leukemia (CML) in early chronic phase treated with imatinib at 400 mg or 800 mg daily. *Blood* 100:95a, 2002.

576. Goldman JM, Marin D, Olavarria E, Apperley JF: Clinical decisions for chronic myeloid leukemia in the imatinib era. *Semin Hematol* 40:98, 2003.

577. Goldman JM: Chronic myeloid leukemia—Still a few questions. *Exp Hematol* 32:2, 2004.

578. Kantarjian HM, Smith TL, O'Brien S, et al: Prolonged survival in chronic myelogenous leukemia after cytogenetic response to interferon-alpha therapy. *Ann Intern Med* 122:254, 1995.

579. Chronic Myeloid Leukemia Trialist's Collaborative Group: Interferon alfa versus chemotherapy for chronic myeloid leukemia: A meta-analysis of seven randomized trials. *J Natl Cancer Inst* 89:1616, 1997.

580. Ohnishi K, Tomonagu M, Kamada N, et al: A long-term follow-up of a randomized trial comparing interferon-α with busulfan for chronic myelogenous leukemia. *Leuk Res* 22:779, 1998.

581. The Italian Cooperative Study Group on Chronic Myeloid Leukemia: Long-term follow-up of the Italian trial of interferon-α vs. conventional chemotherapy in chronic myeloid leukemia. *Blood* 92:1541, 1998.

582. Silver RT, Woolf SH, Hehlmann R, et al: An evidence-based analysis of the effect of busulfan, hydroxyurea, interferon, and allogeneic bone marrow transplantation in treating the chronic phase of chronic myeloid leukemia: Developed for the American Society of Hematology. *Blood* 94:1517, 1999.

583. Hehlmann R, Berger U, Pfirrmann M, et al: Randomized comparison of interferon alpha and hydroxyurea with hydroxyurea monotherapy in chronic myeloid leukemia (CML-Study II): Prolongation of survival by the combination of interferon alpha and hydroxyurea. *Leukemia* 17:1529, 2003.

584. Baccarani M, Russo D, Rosti G, Martinelli G: Interferon-alpha for chronic myeloid leukemia. *Semin Hematol* 40:22, 2003.

585. Bonifazi F, Bandini G, Rondelli D, et al: Reduced incidence of GVHD without increase in relapse with low-dose rabbit ATG in the preparative regimen for unrelated bone marrow transplants in CML. *Bone Marrow Transplant* 32:237, 2003.

586. Barthe C, Mahon F-X, Gharbi M-J, et al: Expression of interferon-α (IFN-α) receptor 2c at diagnosis is associated with cytogenetic response in IFN-α-treated chronic myeloid leukemia. *Blood* 97:3568, 2001.

587. Sakati I, Takeuchi K, Yamauchi H, et al: Constitutive expression of SOCS3 confers resistance to IFN-α in chronic myelogenous leukemia cells. *Blood* 100:2926, 2002.

588. Steegmann JL, Requena MJ, Martin-Tegueira P, et al: High incidence of autoimmune alterations in chronic myeloid leukemia patients treated with interferon-α. *Am J Hematol* 72:170, 2003.

589. Kluin-Nelemans HC, Buck G, Le Cessie S, et al: Randomized comparison of low-dose versus high-dose interferon-alfa in chronic myeloid leukemia: Prospective collaboration of 3 joint trials by the MRC and HOVON groups. *Blood* 103:4408, 2004.

590. Michallet M, Maloisel F, Delain M, et al: Pegylated recombinant interferon alpha-2b vs recombinant interferon alpha-2b for the initial treatment of chronic-phase chronic myelogenous leukemia: A phase III study. *Leukemia* 18:309, 2004.

591. Garcia-Manero G, Talpaz M, Giles FJ, et al: Treatment of Philadelphia chromosome-positive chronic myelogenous leukemia with weekly polyethylene glycol formulation of interferon-alpha-2b and low-dose cytosine arabinoside. *Cancer* 97:3010, 2003.

592. Lindauer M, Fischer T: Interferon-alpha combined with cytarabine in chronic myelogenous leukemia—Clinical benefits. *Leuk Lymphoma* 41:523, 2001.

593. Rosti G, Bonifazi F, Trabacchi E, et al: A phase II study of α-interferon and oral arabinosyl cytosine (YNK01) in chronic myeloid leukemia. *Leukemia* 17:554, 2003.

594. Silver TR, Peterson BL, Szatrowski TP, et al: Treatment of the chronic phase of chronic myeloid leukemia with an intermittent schedule of recombinant interferon alfa-2b and cytarabine: Results from CALGB study 5013. *Leuk Lymphoma* 44:39, 2003.

595. Kuhr T, Burgstaller S, Apfelbeck U, et al: A randomized study comparing interferon (IFN alpha) plus low-dose cytarabine and interferon plus hydroxyurea (HU) in early chronic-phase chronic myeloid leukemia (CML). *Leuk Res* 27:405, 2003.

596. Hehlmann R, Hochhaus A, Kolb H-J, et al: Interferon-α before allogeneic bone marrow transplantation in chronic myelogenous leukemia does not affect outcome adversely, provided it is discontinued at least 90 days before the procedure. *Blood* 94:3668, 1999.

597. Talpaz M: Interferon-alfa-based treatment of chronic myeloid leukemia and implications of signal transduction inhibition. *Semin Hematol* 38:22, 2001.

598. Kolitz JE, Kempin SF, Schluger A, et al: A phase II trial of high-dose hydroxyurea in chronic myelogenous leukemia. *Semin Oncol* 19:27, 1992.

599. Abhyankar D, Shende C, Saikia T, Advani SH: Hydroxyurea induced leg ulcers. *J Assoc Physicians India* 48:926, 2000.

600. Robertson MJ, Tantravaki R, Griffin JD, et al: Hematologic remission and cytogenetic improvement after treatment of stable phase chronic myelogenous leukemia with continuous infusion low-dose cytosine arabinoside. *Am J Hematol* 43:95, 1993.

601. Giulhot F, Dreyfus B, Brizard A, et al: Cytogenetic remission in chronic myelogenous leukemia using interferon alpha-2a and hydroxyurea with or without low-dose cytosine arabinoside. *Leuk Lymphoma* 4:49, 1991.

602. Guilhot F, Chastang C, Michallet M, et al: Interferon alfa-2b combined with cytarabine versus interferon alone in chronic myelogenous leukemia. *N Engl J Med* 337:223, 1997.

603. Hehlmann R, Heimpel H, Hasford J, et al: Randomized comparison of busulfan and hydroyxurea in chronic myelogenous leukemia: Prolongation of survival by hydroxyurea. *Blood* 82:398, 1993.

604. Sandhu HS, Barnes PJ, Hernandez P: Hydroxyurea-induced hypersensitivity pneumonitis: A case report and literature review. *Can Respir J* 7:491, 2000.

605. O'Brien S, Kantarjian H, Keating M, et al: Homoharringtonine therapy induces responses in patients with chronic myelogenous leukemia in late chronic phase. *Blood* 86:3322, 1995.

606. Dibromomannitol Cooperative Study Group: Survival of chronic myeloid leukemia patients treated by dibromomannitol. *Eur J Cancer* 9:583, 1973.

607. Talpaz M, Kantarjian HM, Kurzrock T, Gutterman J: The therapy of chronic myelogenous leukemia: Chemotherapy and interferons. *Semin Hematol* 25:62, 1988.

608. Giles FJ, Feldman EJ, Roboz GJ, et al: Phase II study of troxacitabine, a novel dioxolane nucleoside analog, in patients with untreated or imatinib mesylate-resistant chronic myelogenous leukemia in blastic phase. *Leuk Res* 27:1091, 2003.

609. Clarkson B: Chronic myelogenous leukemia: Is aggressive treatment indicated? *J Clin Oncol* 3:135, 1985.

610. Cortes J, Kantarjian H, O'Brien S, et al: A pilot study of all-trans retinoic acid in patients with Philadelphia chromosome-positive chronic myelogenous leukemia. *Leukemia* 11:929, 1997.

611. Fadilah SA, Ahmad-Zailani R, Soon-Keng C, Norlaila M: Successful treatment of chronic myeloid leukemia during pregnancy with hydroxyurea. *Leukemia* 16:1202, 2002.

612. Mubarek AA, Kakil IR, Al-Homsi U, et al: Normal outcome of pregnancy in chronic myeloid leukemia treated with interferon-alpha in 1st trimester: Report of 3 cases and review of the literature. *Am J Hematol* 69:115, 2002.

613. Clark RE: Antisense therapeutics in chronic myeloid leukaemia: The promise, the progress, and the problems. *Leukemia* 14:347, 2000.

614. Gerwitz AM: Antisense oligonucleotide therapeutics for human leukemia. *Crit Rev Oncol* 8:93, 1997.

615. James HA: The potential application of ribozymes for the treatment of hematological disorders. *J Leuk Biol* 66:361, 1999.

616. Mendoza-Maldonado R, Zentilin L, Fanin R, Giacca M: Purging of chronic myelogenous leukemia cells by retrovirally expressed anti-bcr-abl ribozymes with specific cellular compartmentalization. *Cancer Gene Ther* 9:71, 2002.

617. Cotter FE: Antisense oligonucleotides for haematological malignancies. *Haematologica* 84:19, 1999.

618. Verfaillie CM, McIvor S, Zhao RCH: Gene therapy for chronic myelogenous leukemia. *Mol Med Today* 5:359, 1999.

619. Clark RE, Dodi A, Hill SC, et al: Direct evidence that leukemic cells present HLA-associated immunogenic peptides derived from the BCR-ABL b3a2 fusion protein. *Blood* 98:2887, 2001.

620. Schwartz J, Pinilla-Ibarz J, Yuan RR, Scheinberg DA: Novel targeted and immunotherapeutic strategies in chronic myeloid leukemia. *Semin Hematol* 40:87, 2003.

621. Nossner E, Gastpar R, Milani V, et al: Tumor-derived heat shock protein 90 peptide complexes are cross-presented by human dendritic cells. *J Immunol* 169:5424, 2002.

622. Pinilla-Ibarz J, Cathcart K, Korontsvit T, et al: Vaccination of patients with chronic myelogenous leukemia with bcr-abl oncogene breakpoint fusion peptides generates specific immune responses. *Blood* 95:1781, 2000.

623. Yasukawa M, Ohminami H, Kojima K, et al: HLA class II-restricted antigen presentation of endogenous bcr-abl fusion protein by chronic myelogenous leukemia-derived dendritic cells to CD4+ T lymphocytes. *Blood* 98:1498, 2001.

624. Ossenkoppele GJ, Stam AG, Westers TM, et al: Vaccination of chronic myeloid leukemia patients with autologous in vitro cultured leukemic dendritic cells. *Leukemia* 17:1424, 2003.

625. Baron F, Turhan AG, Giron-Michel J, et al: Leukemic target susceptibility to natural killer cytotoxicity: Relationship with BCR-ABL expression. *Blood* 99:2107, 2002.

626. Borrello I, Sotomayor EM, Rattis F-M, et al: Sustaining the graft-versus-tumor effect through posttransplant immunization with granulocyte-macrophage colony-stimulating factor (GM-CSF)-producing tumor vaccines. *Blood* 95:3011, 2000.

627. Wagner H, McKeough PG, Desforges J, Madoc-Jones H: Splenic irradiation in the treatment of patients with chronic myelogenous leukemia or myelofibrosis and myeloid metaplasia. *Cancer* 58:1204, 1986.

628. McFarland JT, Kuzma C, Millard FE, Johnstone PA: Palliative irradiation of the spleen. *Am J Clin Oncol* 26:178, 2003.

629. The Italian Cooperative Study Group on Chronic Myeloid Leukemia: Results of a prospective randomized trial of early splenectomy in chronic myeloid leukemia. *Cancer* 54:333, 1984.

630. Mesa RA, Elliott MA, Tefferi A: Splenectomy in chronic myeloid leukemia and myelofibrosis with myeloid metaplasia. *Blood Rev* 14:121, 2000.

631. Kalhs P, Schwarzinger I, Anderson G, et al: A retrospective analysis of the long-term effect of splenectomy on late infections, graft-versus-host disease, relapse, and survival after allogeneic marrow transplantation for chronic myelogenous leukemia. *Blood* 86:2028, 1995.

632. Rodrigues CA, Fermino FA, Vasconcelos Y, De Oliveira JS: Refractory chronic GVHD emerging after splenectomy in a marrow transplant recipient with accelerated phase CML. *Bone Marrow Transplant* 32:333, 2003.

633. Goldman J: Autologous stem-cell transplantation for chronic myelogenous leukemia. *Semin Hematol* 30:53, 1993.

634. Talpaz M, Kantarjian H, Liang J, et al: Percentage of Philadelphia chromosome (Ph)-negative and Ph-positive cells found after autologous transplantation for chronic myelogenous leukemia depends on percentage of diploid cells induced by conventional dose chemotherapy before collection of autologous cells. *Blood* 85:3257, 1995.

635. Drummond MW, Marin D, Clark RE, et al: Mobilization of Ph chromosome-negative peripheral blood stem cells in chronic myeloid leukemia patients with imatinib mesylate-induced complete cytogenetic remission. *Br J Haematol* 123:479, 2003.

636. Hui CH, Goh KY, White D, et al: Successful peripheral blood stem cell mobilisation with filgrastim in patients with chronic myeloid leukaemia achieving complete cytogenetic response with imatinib, without increasing disease burden as measured by quantitative real-time PCR. *Leukemia* 17:821, 2003.

637. Kreuzer KA, Kluhs C, Baskaynak G, et al: Filgrastim-induced stem cell mobilization in chronic myeloid leukaemia patients during imatinib therapy: Safety, feasibility and evidence for an efficient in vivo purging. *Br J Haematol* 124:195, 2004.

638. Bhatia R, Verfaillie CM: Autografting for chronic myelogenous leukemia. *Curr Opin Hematol* 2:436, 1995.

639. Kantarjian HM, Talpaz M, Hester J, et al: Collection of peripheral-blood diploid cells from chronic myelogenous leukemia patients early in the recovery phase from myelosuppression induced by intensive-dose chemotherapy. *J Clin Oncol* 18:553, 1995.

640. Carella AJ, Cunningham I, Benvenuto E, et al: Mobilization and transplantation of Philadelphia-negative peripheral blood progenitor cells early in chronic myelogenous leukemia. *J Clin Oncol* 15:1575, 1997.

641. Reiffers J, Mahon FX, Boiron JM, et al: Autografting in chronic myeloid leukemia: An overview. *Leukemia* 10:385, 1996.

642. Lauta VM: Chronic myelogenous leukemia: Elements of conventional chemotherapy and an overview of autografting in the treatment of the chronic phase. *Med Oncol* 20:95, 2003.

643. Meloni G, Capria S, Vignetti M, et al: Ten-year follow-up of a single center prospective trial of unmanipulated peripheral blood stem cell autograft and interferon-alpha in early phase chronic myeloid leukemia. *Haematologica* 86:596, 2001.

644. Cervantes F, Hernandez-Boluda JC, Odriozola J, et al: Imatinib mesylate (STI571) treatment in patients with chronic-phase chronic myelogenous leukaemia previously submitted to autologous stem cell transplantation. *Br J Haematol* 120:500, 2003.

645. Verfaillie CM, Bhatia R, Steinbuch M, et al: Comparative analysis of autografting in chronic myelogenous leukemia: Effects of priming regimen and marrow or blood origin of stem cells. *Blood* 92:1820, 1998.

646. Scheffold C, Brandt K, Johnston V, et al: Potential of autologous immunologic effector cells for bone marrow purging in patients with chronic myeloid leukemia. *Bone Marrow Transplant* 15:33, 1995.

647. De Fabritiis P, Petti MC, Montefusco E, et al: BCR-ABL antisense oligodeoxynucleotide in vitro purging and autologous bone marrow transplantation for patients with chronic myelogenous leukemia in advanced phase. *Blood* 91:3156, 1998.

648. Wright LA, Milliken S, Biggs JC, Kearney P: Ex vivo effects associated with the expression of a bcr-abl-specific ribozyme in a CML cell line. *Antisense Nucleic Acid Drug Dev* 8:15, 1998.

649. Carlo-Stella C, Dotti G, Mangoni L, et al: Selection of myeloid progenitors lacking BCR/ABL in chronic myelogenous leukemia patients after in vitro treatments with the tyrosine kinase inhibitor genistein. *Blood* 88:3091, 1996.

650. Druker BH, Tamura S, Buchdunger E, et al: Effects of a selective inhibitor of the Abl tyrosine kinase on the growth of Bcr-Abl positive cells. *Nat Med* 2:561, 1996.

651. Fogli M, Amabile M, Martinelli G, et al: Selective expansion of normal haemopoietic progenitors from chronic myelogenous leukemia marrow. *Br J Haematol* 101:119, 1998.

652. Coutinho LH, Chang J, Brereta ML, et al: Autografting in Philadelphia (Ph)+ chronic myeloid leukemia using cultured marrow: An update of a pilot study. *Bone Marrow Transplant* 19:969, 1997.

653. Eibl B, Ebner S, Duba C, et al: Dendritic cells generated from blood precursors of chronic myelogenous leukemia patients carry the Philadelphia translocation and can induce a CML-specific primary cytotoxic T-cell response. *Genes Chromosomes Cancer* 20:215, 1997.

654. Lewalle P, Hensel N, Guimaraes A, et al: Helper and cytotoxic lymphocyte responses to chronic myeloid leukemia: Implications for adoptive immunotherapy with T cells. *Br J Haematol* 92:587, 1996.

655. Thomas ED, Clift RA, Fefer A, et al: Marrow transplantation for the treatment of chronic myelogenous leukemia. *Ann Intern Med* 104:155, 1986.

656. Apperley JF: Hematopoietic stem cell transplantation in chronic my-eloid leukemia. *Curr Opin Hematol* 5:445, 1998.

657. Cooperative Study Group on Chromosomes in Transplanted Patients: Cytogenetic follow-up of 100 patients submitted to bone marrow transplantation for Philadelphia chromosome-positive chronic myeloid leukemia. *Eur J Haematol* 40:50, 1988.

658. McGlave P, Bartoch G, Anasetti C, et al: Unrelated donor marrow transplantation therapy for chronic myelogenous leukemia. *Blood* 81:543, 1993.

659. Goldman J: Implications of imatinib mesylate for hematopoietic stem cell transplantation. *Semin Hematol* 38:28, 2001.

660. Barrett J: Allogeneic stem cell transplantation for chronic myeloid leukemia. *Semin Hematol* 40:59, 2003.

661. Messner HA, Curtis JE, Lipton JL, et al: Three decades of allogeneic bone marrow transplants at the Princess Margaret Hospital. *Clin Transplant* p289, 1999.

662. Sullivan KM: Marrow transplantation for disorders of hematopoiesis. *Leukemia* 7:1098, 1993.

663. Horowitz MM, Gale RP, Sondell PM, et al: Graft-versus-leukemia reaction after bone marrow transplantation. *Blood* 75:555, 1990.

664. Antin JH: Graft-versus-leukemia: No longer an epiphenomenon. *Blood* 82:2273, 1993.

665. Van Rhee F, Szydlo RM, Hermans J, et al: Long-term results after allogeneic bone marrow transplantation for chronic myelogenous leukemia in chronic phase: A report from the Chronic Leukemia Working Party of the European Groups for Blood and Marrow Transplantation. *Bone Marrow Transplant* 20:553, 1997.

666. Lee SJ, Kuntz KM, Horowitz MM, et al: Unrelated donor bone marrow transplantation for chronic myelogenous leukemia; a decision analysis. *Ann Intern Med* 127:1080, 1997.

667. Enright H, Daniels K, Arthur DC, et al: Related donor marrow transplant for chronic myeloid leukemia: Patients' characteristics predictive of outcome. *Bone Marrow Transplant* 17:537m, 1996.

668. Cwynarski K, Roberts IA, Iacobelli S, et al: Stem cell transplantation for chronic myeloid leukemia in children. *Blood* 102:1224, 2003.

669. Goldman JM, Szydlo R, Horowitz MM, et al: Choice of pretransplant treatment and timing of transplants for chronic myelogenous leukemia in chronic phase. *Blood* 82:2235, 1993.

670. Socie G, Clift RA, Blaise D, et al: Busulfan plus cyclophosphamide compared with total-body irradiation plus cyclophosphamide before marrow transplantation for myeloid leukemia: Long-term follow-up of 4 randomized studies. *Blood* 98:3569, 2001.

671. Kroger N, Zabelina T, Kruger W, et al: Comparison of total body irradiation vs busulfan in combination with cyclophosphamide as conditioning for unrelated stem cell transplantation in CML patients. *Bone Marrow Transplant* 27:349, 2001.

672. Fernandez HF, Tran HT, Albrecht F, et al: Evaluation of safety and pharmacokinetics of administering intravenous busulfan in a twice-daily or daily schedule to patients with advanced hematologic malignant disease undergoing stem cell transplantation. *Biol Blood Marrow Transplant* 8:486, 2002.

673. Radich JP, Gooley T, Bensinger W, et al: HLA-matched related hematopoietic cell transplantation for chronic-phase CML using a targeted busulfan and cyclophosphamide preparative regimen. *Blood* 102:31, 2003.

674. Tomas JF, Lopez-Lorenzo JL, Requena MJ, et al: Absence of influence of prior treatments with interferon on the outcome of allogeneic bone marrow transplantation for chronic myeloid leukemia. *Bone Marrow Transplant* 22:47, 1998.

675. Giralt S, Szydlo R, Goldman JM, et al: Effect of short-term interferon therapy on the outcome of subsequent HLA-identical sibling bone marrow transplantation for chronic myelogenous leukemia: An analysis from the International Bone Marrow Transplant Registry. *Blood* 95:410, 2000.

676. Gale RP, Hehlmann R, Zhang MJ, et al: Survival with bone marrow transplantation versus hydroxyurea or interferon for chronic myelogenous leukemia. *Blood* 91:1810, 1998.

677. Byrne JL, Stainer C, Hyde H, et al: Low incidence of acute graft-versus-host disease and recurrent leukaemia in patients undergoing allogeneic haemopoietic stem cell transplantation from sibling donors with methotrexate and dose-monitored cyclosporin A prophylaxis. *Bone Marrow Transplant* 22:541, 1988.

678. Goldman J, Apperley J, Kanfer E, et al: Imatinib or transplant for chronic myeloid leukemia? *Lancet* 362:172, 2003.

679. Szydlo R, Goldman JM, Klein JP, et al: Results of allogeneic bone marrow transplants using donors other than HLA-identical siblings. *J Clin Oncol* 15:1767, 1997.

680. Petersdorf EW, Longton GM, Anasetti C, et al: The significance of HLA-DRBI matching on clinical outcome after HLA-A band DR identical unrelated donor transplantation. *Blood* 86:1606, 1995.

681. Weisdorf DJ, Anasetti C, Antin JH, et al: Allogeneic bone marrow transplantation for chronic myelogenous leukemia: Comparative analysis of unrelated versus matched sibling donor transplantation. *Blood* 99:1971, 2002.

682. McGlave PB, Ou Shu X, Wen W, et al: Unrelated donor marrow transplantation for chronic myelogenous leukemia: 9 years' experience of the National Marrow Donor Program. *Blood* 95:2219, 2000.

683. Lee SJ, Klein JP, Anasetti C, et al: The effect of pretransplant interferon therapy on the outcome of unrelated donor hematopoietic stem cell transplantation for patients with chronic myelogenous leukemia in first choice phase. *Blood* 98:3205, 2001.

684. Laporte JP, Gorin NC, Rubinstein P, et al: Cord-blood transplantation from an unrelated donor in an adult with chronic myelogenous leukemia. *N Engl J Med* 335:167, 1997.

685. Enright H, Davies SM, DeFor T, et al: Relapse after non-T cell depleted allogeneic bone marrow transplantation for chronic myelogenous leukemia: Early transplant, use of an unrelated donor and chronic graft-versus-host disease are protective. *Blood* 88:714, 1996.

686. Hessner MJ, Endean DJ, Casper JT, et al: Use of unrelated marrow grafts compensates for reduced graft-versus-leukemia reactivity after T-cell-depleted allogeneic marrow transplantation for chronic myelogenous leukemia. *Blood* 86:3987, 1995.

687. Gratwohl A, Brand R, Apperley J, et al: Graft-versus-host disease and outcome in HLA-identical sibling transplantations for chronic myeloid leukemia. *Blood* 100:3877, 2002.

688. Radich JP, Gehly G, Gooley T, et al: Polymerase chain reaction detection of the BCR-ABL fusion transcript after allogeneic marrow transplantation for chronic myeloid leukemia: Results and implications in 346 patients. *Blood* 85:2632, 1995.

689. Goldman JM: Therapeutic strategies for chronic myeloid leukemia in chronic (stable) phase. *Semin Hematol* 40:10, 2003.

690. Okamoto R, Harano H, Matsuzaki M, et al: Predicting relapse of chronic myelogenous leukemia after allogeneic bone marrow transplantation by BCR/ABL mRNA and DNA fingerprinting. *Am J Clin Path* 104:510, 1995.

691. Segel GB, Simon W, Lichtman MA: Variables influencing the timing of marrow transplantation in patients with chronic myelogenous leukemia. *Blood* 68:1055, 1986.

692. Champlin RE, Goldman JM, Gale RP: Bone marrow transplantation in chronic myelogenous leukemia. *Semin Hematol* 25:74, 1988.

693. Thomas ED, Clift RA: Indications for marrow transplantation in chronic myelogenous leukemia. *Blood* 73:861, 1989.

694. Goldman JM, Druker BJ: Chronic myeloid leukemia: Current treatment options. *Blood* 98:2039, 2001.

695. Goldman JM, Melo JV: Targeting the BCR-ABL tyrosine kinase in chronic myeloid leukemia. *N Engl J Med* 44:1084, 2001.

696. Shimoni A, Kroger N, Zander AR, et al: Imatinib mesylate (STI571)

in preparation for allogeneic hematopoietic stem cell transplantation and donor lymphocyte infusions in patients with Philadelphia-positive acute leukemias. *Leukemia* 17:290, 2003.

697. Garcia-Manero G, Talpaz M, Kantarjian HM: Current therapy of chronic myelogenous leukemia. *Intern Med* 41:254, 2002.

698. Or R, Shapira MY, Resnick I, et al: Nonmyeloablative allogeneic stem cell transplantation for the treatment of chronic myeloid leukemia in first chronic phase. *Blood* 101:441, 2003.

699. Bornhauser M, Kiehl M, Siegert W, et al: Dose-reduced conditioning for allografting in 44 patients with chronic myeloid leukaemia: A retrospective analysis. *Br J Haematol* 115:119, 2001.

700. Das M, Saikia TK, Advani SH, et al: Use of a reduced-intensity conditioning regimen for allogeneic transplantation in patients with chronic myeloid leukemia. *Bone Marrow Transplant* 32:125, 2003.

701. Feinstein L, Storb R: Reducing transplant toxicity. *Curr Opin Hematol* 8:342, 2001.

702. Koh LP, Hwang WY, Chuah CT, et al: Imatinib mesylate (STI-571) given concurrently with nonmyeloablative stem cell transplantation did not compromise engraftment and resulted in cytogenetic remission in a patient with chronic myeloid leukemia in blast crisis. *Bone Marrow Transplant* 31:305, 2003.

703. Uzunel M, Mattsson J, Brune M, et al: Kinetics of minimal residual disease and chimerism in patients with chronic myeloid leukemia after nonmyeloablative conditioning and allogeneic stem cell transplantation. *Blood* 101:469, 2003.

704. McCann SR: Molecular response to imatinib mesylate following relapse after allogeneic SCT for CML. *Blood* 101:1200, 2003.

705. Vandenberghe P, Boeckx N, Ronsyn E, et al: Imatinib mesylate induces durable complete remission of advanced CML persisting after allogeneic bone marrow transplantation. *Leukemia* 17:458, 2003.

706. Ullmann AJ, Hess G, Kolbe K, et al: Current results on the use of imatinib mesylate in patients with relapsed Philadelphia chromosome positive leukemia after allogeneic or syngeneic hematopoietic stem cell transplantation. *Keio J Med* 52:182, 2003.

707. Olavarria E, Craddock C, Dazzi F, et al: Imatinib mesylate (STI571) in the treatment of relapse of chronic myeloid leukemia after allogeneic stem cell transplantation. *Blood* 99:3861, 2002.

708. Kolb HJ, Mittermuller J, Clemm CH, et al: Donor leukocyte transfusions for treatment of recurrent chronic myelogenous leukemia in marrow transplant patients. *Blood* 76:2462, 1990.

709. Dazzi F, Szydlo RM, Goldman JM: Donor lymphocyte infusion for relapse of chronic myeloid leukemia after allogeneic stem cell transplant: Where we now stand. *Exp Hematol* 27:1477, 1999.

710. Van Rhee F, Lin F, Cullis JO, et al: Relapse of chronic myeloid leukemia after allogeneic bone marrow transplant: The case of giving donor leukocyte transfusions before the onset of hematologic relapse. *Blood* 83:3377, 1994.

711. Leis J, Porter DL: Unrelated donor leukocyte infusions to treat relapse after unrelated donor bone marrow transplantation. *Leuk Lymphoma* 43:9, 2002.

712. Dazzi F, Goldman J: Donor lymphocyte infusions. *Curr Opin Hematol* 6:394, 1999.

713. Dazzi F, Szydlo RM, Cross NCP, et al: Durability of responses following donor lymphocyte infusions for patients who relapse after allogeneic stem cell transplantation for chronic myeloid leukemia. *Blood* 96:2712, 2000.

714. Dazzi F: Monitoring of minimal residual disease after allografting: A requirement to guide DLI treatment. *Ann Hematol* 81:S29, 2002.

715. Soiffer RJ, Alyea EP, Ritz J: Immunomodulatory effects of donor lymphocyte infusions following allogeneic bone marrow transplantation. *J Clin Apheresis* 10:139, 1995.

716. Castro FA, Palma PVB, Morais FR, Voltarelli JC: Immunological effects of donor lymphocyte infusion in patients with chronic myeloge-

nous leukemia relapsing after bone marrow transplantation. *Braz J Med Biol Res* 37:201, 2004.

717. Makinnon S: Donor leukocyte infusions. *Baillieres Clin Haematol* 10: 357, 1997.

718. Giralt S, Hester J, Huh T, et al: CD8-depleted donor lymphocyte infusion as treatment for relapsed chronic myelogenous leukemia after allogeneic bone marrow transplantation. *Blood* 86:4337, 1995.

719. Guglielma C, Arcese W, Dazzi F, et al: Donor lymphocyte infusion for relapsed chronic myelogenous leukemia: Prognostic relevance of the initial cell dose. *Blood* 100:397, 2002.

720. Verzeletti S, Bonini C, Marktel S, et al: Herpes simplex virus thymidine kinase gene transfer for controlled graft-versus-host disease and graft-versus-leukemia: Clinical follow-up and improved new vectors. *Hum Gene Ther* 9:2243, 1998.

721. Maravcova J, Nadvornikova S, Zmekova V, et al: Molecular monitoring of responses to DLI and DLI + IFN treatment of post-SCT relapse in patients with CML. *Leuk Res* 27:719, 2003.

722. Vela-Ojeda J, Garcia-Ruiz Esparza MA, Reyes-Maldonado E, et al: Donor lymphocyte infusions for relapse of chronic myeloid leukemia after allogeneic stem cell transplantation: Prognostic significance of the dose of CD3$^+$ and CD4$^+$ lymphocytes. *Ann Hematol* 83:295, 2004.

723. Nieda M, Nicol A, Kikuchi A, et al: Dendritic cells stimulate the expansion of BRC-ABL-specific CD8+ T cells with cytotoxic activity against leukemic cells from patients with chronic myeloid leukemia. *Blood* 92:977, 1998.

724. Smit WM, Rijnbeek M, van Bergen CA, et al: Generation of dendritic cells expressing BCR-ABL from CD34-positive chronic myeloid leukemia precursor cells. *Hum Immunol* 53:216, 1997.

725. Mannering SI, McKenzie JL, Fearnley DB, Hart DN: HLA-DRI-restricted BCR-ABL (b3a2)-specific CD4+ T lymphocytes respond to dendritic cells pulsed with b3a2 peptide and antigen-presenting cells exposed to b3a2 containing cell lysates. *Blood* 90:2990, 1997.

726. ten Bosch GJA, Kessler JH, Joosten AM, et al: A BCR-ABL oncoprotein p210b2a2 fusion region sequence is recognized by HLA-DR2a restricted cytotoxic T lymphocytes and presented by HLA-DR matched cells transfected with an li(b2a2) construct. *Blood* 94:1038, 1999.

727. Greco G, Fruci D, Accapezzato D, et al: Two bcr-abl junction peptides bind HLA-A3 molecules and allow specific induction of human cytotoxic T lymphocytes. *Leukemia* 10:693, 1996.

728. Falkenburg JHF, Wafelman AR, Joosten P, et al: Complete remission of accelerated phase chronic myeloid leukemia by treatment with leukemia-reactive cytotoxic T lymphocytes. *Blood* 94:1201, 1999.

729. Kardinal CG, Bateman JR, Weiner J: Chronic myeloid leukemia. Review of 356 cases. *Arch Intern Med* 136:305, 1976.

730. Tura S, Baccarini M, Corbelli G: Staging of chronic myeloid leukemia. *Br J Haematol* 47:105, 1981.

731. Gomez GA, Sokal JE, Walsh D: Prognostic features at diagnosis of chronic myelogenous leukemia. *Cancer* 47:2470, 1981.

732. Cervantes F, Rozman C: A multivariate analysis of prognostic factors in chronic myeloid leukemia. *Blood* 60:1298, 1982.

733. Sokal JE, Cox EB, Baccarani M, et al: Prognostic discrimination in "good-risk" chronic granulocytic leukemia. *Blood* 63:789, 1984.

734. Sokal JE, Baccarini M, Tura S, et al: Prognostic discrimination among younger patients with chronic granulocytic leukemia: Relevance to bone marrow transplantation. *Blood* 66:1352, 1985.

735. Kantarjian HM, Keating MJ, Walters RS, et al: Clinical and prognostic features of Philadelphia chromosome-negative chronic myelogenous leukemia. *Cancer* 58:2023, 1986.

736. Sokal JE, Baccarini M, Russo D, Tura S: Staging and prognosis in chronic myelogenous leukemia. *Semin Hematol* 25:49, 1988.

737. Kantarjian HM, Keating MK, Smith TL, et al: Proposal for a single synthesis prognostic staging system in chronic myelogenous leukemia. *Am J Med* 88:1, 1990.

738. Dreazen I, Berman M, Gaoe RP: Molecular abnormalities of *bcr* and *c-abl* in chronic myelogenous leukemia associated with a long chronic phase. *Blood* 71:797, 1988.

739. Nowell PC, Jackson L, Weiss A, Kurzrock P: Historical communication: Philadelphia positive chronic myelogenous leukemia followed for 27 years. *Cancer Genet Cytogenet* 34:57, 1988.

740. Selleir L, Emilia G, Temperani P, et al: Philadelphia-positive chronic myelogenous leukemia with typical *bcr/abl* molecular features and atypical, prolonged survival. *Leukemia* 3:538, 1989.

741. Birnie GD, MacKenzie ED, Goyns MH, Pollock A: Sequestration of Philadelphia chromosome-positive cells in the bone marrow of a chronic myeloid leukemia patient in very prolonged remission. *Leukemia* 4:452, 1990.

742. Lamy TH, Dauriac C, Le Prise PY: Long-term survival in chronic granulocytic leukemia. *Br J Haematol* 73:279, 1989.

743. Johansson B, Martens F, Fioretos T, et al: Remarkably long survival of a patient with Ph1-positive chronic myeloid leukemia and 5/bcr rearrangement. *Leukemia* 4:448, 1990.

744. Singer CRJ, McDonald GA, Douglas AS: Twenty-five year survival of chronic granulocytic leukemia with spontaneous karyotype conversion. *Br J Haematol* 57:309, 1984.

745. Wodzinski MA, Potter AM, Lawence ACK: Prolonged survival in chronic granulocytic leukemia associated with loss of the Philadelphia chromosome. *Br J Haematol* 71:296, 1989.

746. Kantarjian HM, Smith TL, McCredie KB, et al: Chronic myelogenous leukemia: A multivariate analysis of the associations of patient characteristics and therapy with survival. *Blood* 66:1326, 1985.

747. Kantarjian HM, Talpaz M: Treatment of chronic myelogenous leukemia. *Hematology* 14:105, 1991.

748. Baccarini M, Russo D, Zuffa E, et al: The prognosis of chronic myeloid leukemia. *Bone Marrow Transplant* 1:126, 1989.

749. Simon W, Segel GB, Lichtman MA: Upper and lower time limits in the decision to recommend marrow transplantation for patients with chronic myelogenous leukemia. *Br J Haematol* 70:31, 1988.

750. Grossman A, Silver RT, Arlin Z, et al: Fine mapping of chromosome 22 breakpoints within the breakpoint cluster region (bcr) implies a role for bcr exon 3 in determining disease duration in chronic myeloid leukemia. *Am J Hum Genet* 45:729, 1989.

751. Morris SW, Daniel L, Ahmed CMI, et al: Relationship of bcr breakpoint to chronic phase duration, survival, and blast crisis lineage in chronic myelogenous leukemia patients presenting in early chronic phase. *Blood* 75:2035, 1990.

752. Giralt S, Kantarjian H, Talpaz M: The natural history of chronic myelogenous leukemia in the interferon era. *Semin Hematol* 32:152, 1995.

753. Smadja N, Krulik M, Audebert AA, et al: Spontaneous regression of cytogenetic and hematologic anomalies in Ph1-positive chronic myelogenous leukemia. *Br J Haematol* 63:257, 1986.

754. Musashi M, Abe S, Yamada T, et al: Spontaneous remission in a patient with chronic myelogenous leukemia. *N Engl J Med* 336:337, 1997.

755. Provan AB, Smith AG: Re-emergence of Philadelphia chromosome positive clone on a patient with previous spontaneous remission of chronic myeloid leukemia. *Leukemia* 9:1600, 1995.

756. Korkolopoulou P, Viniou N, Kavantzas N, et al: Clinicopathologic correlations of bone marrow angiogenesis in chronic myeloid leukemia: A morphometric study. *Leukemia* 17L:89, 2003.

757. Boultwood J, Peniket A, Watkins F, et al: Telomere length shortening in chronic myelogenous leukemia is associated with reduced time to accelerated phase. *Blood* 96:358, 2000.

758. Verstovsek S, Kantarjian H, Manshouri T, et al: Prognostic significance of cellular vascular endothelial growth factor expression in chronic phase chronic myeloid leukemia. *Blood* 99:2265, 2002.

759. Sinclair PB, Nacheva EP, Leversha M, et al: Large deletions at the t(9;22) breakpoint are common and may identify a poor-prognosis subgroup of patients with chronic myeloid leukemia. *Blood* 95:738, 2000.

760. Huntly BJP, Reid AG, Bench AJ, et al: Deletions of the derivative chromosome 9 occur at the time of the Philadelphia translocation and provide a powerful and independent prognostic indicator in chronic myeloid leukemia. *Blood* 98:1732, 2001.

761. Cohen N, Rozenfeld-Granot G, Hardan I, et al: Subgroup of patients with Philadelphia-positive chronic myelogenous leukemia characterized by a deletion of 9q proximal to ABL gene: Expression profiling, resistance to interferon therapy, and poor prognosis. *Cancer Genet Cytogenet* 128:114, 2001.

762. Kvasnicka HM, Thiele J, Schmitt-Graeff A, et al: Prognostic impact of bone marrow erythropoietic precursor cells and myelofibrosis at diagnosis of Ph^{1+} chronic myelogenous leukaemia—A multicentre study on 495 patients. *Br J Haematol* 112:727, 2001.

763. Normann AP, Egeland T, Madshus IH, et al: CD7 expression by CD34+ cells in CML patients, of prognostic significance? *Eur J Haematol* 71:266, 2003.

764. Roman-Gomez J, Castillejo JA, Jimenez A, et al: Cadherin-13, a mediator of calcium-dependent cell-cell adhesion, is silenced by methylation in chronic myeloid leukemia and correlates with pretreatment risk profile and cytogenetic response to interferon alfa. *J Clin Oncol* 21:1472, 2003.

765. Morel F, Ka C, Le Bris MJ, et al: Deletion of the 5'ABL region in Philadelphia chromosome positive chronic myeloid leukemia: Frequency, origin and prognosis. *Leuk Lymphoma* 44:1333, 2003.

766. Prejzner W: Relationship of the BCR gene breakpoint and the type of BCR/ABL transcript to clinical course, prognostic indexes and survival in patients with chronic myeloid leukemia. *Med Sci Monit* 8:193, 2002.

767. Bauduer F, Ducout L, Dastugue N, Marolleau JP: Chronic myeloid leukemia as a secondary neoplasm after anti-cancer radiotherapy: A report of three cases and a brief review of the literature. *Leuk Lymphoma* 43:1057, 2002.

768. Passweg JR, Walker I, Sobocinski KA, et al: Validation and extension of the EBMT Risk Score for patients with chronic myeloid leukemia (CML) receiving allogeneic haematopoietic stem cell transplants. *Br J Haematol* 125:613, 2004.

769. Hasford J, Pfirrmann M, Hehlmann R, et al: Prognosis and prognostic factors for patients with chronic myeloid leukemia: Nontransplant therapy. *Semin Hematol* 40:4, 2003.

770. Qazilbash MH, Devetten MP, Abraham J, et al: Utility of a prognostic scoring system for allogeneic stem cell transplantation in patients with chronic myeloid leukemia. *Acta Haematol* 109:119, 2003.

771. Marin D, Marktel S, Bua M, et al: Prognostic factors for patients with chronic myeloid leukemia in chronic phase treated with imatinib mesylate after failure of interferon alfa. *Leukemia* 17:1448, 2003.

772. Kantarjian HM, O'Brien S, Cortes JE, et al: Complete cytogenetic and molecular responses to interferon-alpha-based therapy for chronic myelogenous leukemia are associated with excellent long-term prognosis. *Cancer* 97:1033, 2003.

773. Rosti G, Martinelli G, Bassi S, et al: Molecular response to imatinib in late chronic-phase chronic myeloid leukemia. *Blood* 103:2284, 2004.

774. Yee K, Anglin P, Keating A: Molecular approaches to the detection and monitoring of chronic myeloid leukemia: Theory and practice. *Blood Rev* 13:105, 1999.

775. Kaeda J, Chase A, Goldman JM: Cytogenetic and molecular monitoring of residual disease in chronic myeloid leukaemia. *Acta Haematol* 107:64, 2002.

776. Hughes T, Branford S: Molecular monitoring of chronic myeloid leukemia. *Semin Hematol* 40:62, 2003.

777. Lowenberg B: Minimal residual disease in chronic myeloid leukemia. *N Engl J Med* 349:1399, 2003.

778. Gabert J: Detection of recurrent translocations using real time PCR; assessment of the technique for diagnosis and detection of minimal residual disease. *Haematologica* 84:107, 1999.

779. Negrin RS, Blume KG: The use of polymerase chain reaction for the detection of minimal residual malignant disease. *Blood* 78:255, 1991.

780. Lee M-S, Kantarjian H, Talpaz M, et al: Detection of minimal residual disease by polymerase chain reaction in Philadelphia chromosome-positive chronic myelogenous leukemia following interferon therapy. *Blood* 79:1920, 1992.

781. Schulze E, Krahl R, Thalmeier K, Helbig W: Detection of bcr-abl mRNA in single progenitor colonies from patients with chronic myeloid leukemia by PCR: Comparison with cytogenetics and PCR from uncultured cells. *Exp Hematol* 23:1649, 1995.

782. Lin F, Chase A, Bungey J, et al: Correlation between the proportion of Philadelphia chromosome-positive metaphase cells and levels of BCR-ABL mRNA in chronic myeloid leukaemia. *Genes Chromosomes Cancer* 13:110, 1995.

783. Thompson JD, Brodsky I, Yunis JJ: Molecular quantification of residual disease in chronic myelogenous leukemia after bone marrow transplantation. *Blood* 79:1629, 1992.

784. Lin F, Chase A, Bungey J, et al: Correlation between the proportion of Philadelphia chromosome-positive metaphase cells and levels of BCR-ABL mRNA in chronic myeloid leukaemia. *Genes Chromosomes Cancer* 18:110, 1995.

785. Gaiger A, Henn T, Horth E, et al: Increase of bcr-abl chimeric mRNA expression in tumor cells of patients with chronic myeloid leukemia precedes disease progression. *Blood* 86:2371, 1995.

786. Guo JQ, Lin H, Kantarjian H, et al: Comparison of competitive-nested PCR and real-time PCR in detecting BCR-ABL fusion transcripts in chronic myeloid leukemia patients. *Leukemia* 16:2447, 2002.

787. O'Dwyer ME: How to monitor patients with chronic myelogenous leukemia. *UNCCN* 1:513, 2003.

788. Cohen N, Novikov I, Hardan I, et al: Standardization criteria for the detection of BCR/ABL fusion in interphase nuclei of chronic myelogenous leukemia patients by fluorescence in situ hybridization. *Cancer Genet Cytogenet* 123:102, 2000.

789. Rheinhold U, Hennig E, Leiblein S, et al: FISH for BCR-ABL on interphases of peripheral blood neutrophils but not of unselected white cells correlates with bone marrow cytogenetics in CML patients treated with imatinib. *Leukemia* 17:1925, 2003.

790. Kim YJ, Kim DW, Lee S, et al: Comprehensive comparison of FISH, RT-PCR, and RQ-PCR for monitoring the BCR-ABL gene after hematopoietic stem cell transplantation in CML. *Eur J Haematol* 68:272, 2002.

791. Hochhaus A, Weisser A, LaRosee P, et al: Detection and quantification of residual disease in chronic myelogenous leukemia. *Leukemia* 14:998, 2000.

792. Olavarria E, Kanfer E, Szydlo R, et al: Early detection of *BCR-ABL* transcripts by quantitative reverse transcriptase-polymerase chain reaction predicts outcome after allogeneic stem cell transplantation for chronic myeloid leukemia. *Blood* 97:1560, 2001.

793. Radich JP, Gooley T, Bryant E, et al: The significance of *bcr-abl* molecular detection in chronic myeloid leukemia patients "late" 18 months or more after transplantation. *Blood* 98:1701, 2001.

794. Lion T: Minimal residual disease. *Curr Opin Hematol* 6:406, 1999.

795. Thiele J, Wickenhauser C, Kvasnicka HM, et al: Mixed chimerism of bone marow CD34+ progenitor cells (genotyping, bcr/abl analysis) after allogeneic transplantation for chronic myelogenous leukemia. *Transplantation* 74:982, 2002.

796. Serrano J, Roman J, Sanchez J, et al. Molecular analysis of lineage-specific chimerism and minimal residual disease by RT-PCR of p210 (BCR-ABL) and p190 (BCR-ABL) after allogeneic bone marrow transplantation for chronic myeloid leukemia: Increasing mixed myeloid

chimerism and p190 (BCR-ABL) detection precede cytogenetic relapse. *Blood* 15:2659, 2000.

797. Muller MC, Gattermann N, Lahaye T, et al: Dynamics of BCR-ABL mRNA expression in first-line therapy of chronic myelogenous leukemia patients with imatinib or interferon alpha/ara-C. *Leukemia* 17:2392, 2003.

798. Hochhaus A: Minimal residual disease in chronic myeloid leukaemia patients. *Best Pract Res Clin Haematol* 15:159, 2002.

799. Lin F, Drummond M, O'Brien S, et al: Molecular monitoring in chronic myeloid leukemia patients who achieve complete cytogenetic remission on imatinib. *Blood* 102:1143, 2003.

800. Giles FJ, Cortes JE, Kantarjian HM, O'Brien S: Accelerated and blastic phase of chronic myelogenous leukemia. *Hematol Oncol Clin North Am* 18:753, 2004.

801. Gaiger A, Henn T, Horth E, et al: Increase of bcr/abl chimeric mRNA expression in tumor cells of patients with chronic myeloid leukemia precedes disease progression. *Blood* 86:2371, 1995.

802. Elmaaglacli AH, Beelen DW, Opalka B, et al: The amount of BCR/ABL fusion transcripts detected by real-time quantitative polymerase chain reaction method in patients with Philadelphia chromosome positive chronic myeloid leukemia disease stages correlates with the disease stages. *Ann Hematol* 79:424, 2000.

803. Lowenberg B, Hagemeijer A, Swart K, Abels J: Serial follow-up of patients with chronic myeloid leukemia (CML) with combined cytogenetic and colony culture methods. *Exp Hematol* 10:123, 1982.

804. Haas OA, Schwarzmeier JD, Nachera E, et al: Investigations on karyotype evolution in patients with chronic myeloid leukemia (CML). *Blut* 48:33, 1984.

805. Swolin B, Weinfeld A, Westin J, et al: Karyotypic evolution in Ph-positive chronic myeloid leukemia in relation to management and disease progression. *Cancer Genet Cytogenet* 18:65, 1985.

806. Cortes J, O'Dwyer ME: Clonal evolution in chronic myelogenous leukemia. *Hematol Oncol Clin North Am* 18:671, 2004.

807. Honda H, Ushijima K, Oda H, et al: Acquired loss of p53 induces blast transformation in p210bcr/abl expressing hematopoietic cells: A transgenic study for blast crisis in human CML. *Blood* 95:1144, 2000.

808. Yamaguchi H, Inokuchi K, Sakuma Y, Dan K: Mutation of p51/p63 gene is associated with blast crisis in chronic myelogenous leukemia. *Leukemia* 15:1729, 2001.

809. Coiffier B, Byron PA, Flere D, et al: Chronic granulocytic leukemia: Early detection of metamorphosis with "in vitro" culture of granulocytic progenitors. *Biomedicine* 33:96, 1980.

810. Todd MB, Waldron JA, Jennings TA, et al: Loss of myeloid differentiation antigens precedes blastic transformation in chronic myelogenous leukemia. *Blood* 70:122, 1987.

811. Grinesshammer M, Heinze B, Bangerter M, et al: Karyotype abnormalities and their clinical significance in blast crisis of chronic myeloid leukemia. *J Mol Med* 75:8836, 1997.

812. Spencer A, Vulliamy T, Kaeda J, et al: Clonal instability preceding lymphoid blastic transformation of chronic myeloid leukemia. *Leukemia* 11:195, 1997.

813. Anastasi J, Feng J, LeBeau MM, et al: The relationship between secondary chromosomal abnormalities and blast transformation in chronic myelogenous leukemia. *Leukemia* 9:628, 1995.

814. Bartram CR, de Klein A, Hagemeijer A, et al: Additional C-abl/bcr rearrangements in a CML patient exhibiting two Ph¹ chromosomes during blast crisis. *Leuk Res* 10:221, 1986.

815. Collins SJ, Grudine MT: Chronic myelogenous leukemia: Amplification of a rearranged c-abl oncogene in both chronic phase and blast crisis. *Blood* 69:893, 1987.

816. Schaefer-Rego K, Dudik H, Popenoe D, et al: CML patients in blast crisis have breakpoints localized to a specific region of the bcr. *Blood* 70:448, 1987.

817. Mills KI, Benn P, Birnie GD: Does the breakpoint within the major breakpoint region (M-bcr) influence the duration of the chronic phase in chronic myeloid leukemia? An analytical comparison of current literature. *Blood* 78:1155, 1991.

818. Bartram CR, Janssen JWG, Becher R, et al: Persistence of chronic myelocytic leukemia despite deletion of rearranged bcr/c-abl sequences in blast crisis. *J Exp Med* 164:1389, 1986.

819. Okabe M, Matsushima S: Philadelphia chromosome-positive leukemia: Molecular analysis of *bcr* and *abl* genes and transforming genes. *Acta Haematol Jpn* 51:1471, 1988.

820. Ahuja H, Bar-Eli M, Arlin Z, et al: The spectrum of molecular alterations in the evolution of chronic myelocytic leukemia. *J Clin Invest* 87:2042, 1991.

821. Kelman Z, Prokocimer M, Peller S, et al: Rearrangements in the p53 gene in Philadelphia chromosome positive chronic myelogenous leukemia. *Blood* 74:2318, 1989.

822. Mashal R, Shtalrid M, Talpaz M, et al: Rearrangement and expression of p53 in the chronic phase and blast crisis of chronic myelocytic leukemia. *Blood* 75:180, 1990.

823. Guinn BA, Mello KI: P53 mutations, methylation and genomic instability in the progression of chronic myeloid leukemia. *Leuk Lymphoma* 26:241, 1997.

824. Malinen T, Palotie A, Pakkala S, et al: Acceleration of chronic myeloid leukemia correlates with calcitonin gene methylation. *Blood* 77:2435, 1991.

825. Asimakopoolos FA, Shteper PJ, Krichevsky S, et al: *ABL1* methylation is a distinct molecular event associated with clonal evolution of chronic myeloid leukemia. *Blood* 94:2452, 1999.

826. Towatari M, Adachi K, Kato H, Saito H: Absence of the human retinoblastoma gene product in the megakaryoblastic crisis of chronic myelogenous leukemia. *Blood* 78:2178, 1991.

827. Sill H, Goldman JM, Cross NC: Homozygous deletions of the p16 tumor-suppressor gene are associated with lymphoid transformation of chronic myeloid leukemia. *Blood* 85:2013, 1995.

828. Hernandez-Boluda J-C, Cervantes F, Colomer D, et al: Genomic p16 abnormalities in the progression of chronic myeloid leukemia into blast crisis. *Exp Hematol* 31:204, 2003.

829. Serra A, Gottardi E, Della Ragione F, et al: Involvement at the cyclin-dependent kinase-4 inhibitor (CDKN2) gene in the pathogenesis of lymphoid blast crisis of chronic myelogenous leukaemia. *Br J Haematol* 91:625, 1995.

830. Menssen HD, Renki JMJ, Rodeck U, et al: Presence of Wilms' tumor gene (wt1) transcripts and the WT1 nuclear protein in the majority of human acute leukemias. *Leukemia* 9:1060, 1995.

831. Mitarri K, Ogawa S, Tanaka T, et al: Generation of the AML1-EVI-1 fusion gene in the t(3;21) (q26;q22) causes blastic crisis in chronic myelocytic leukemia. *EMBO J* 13:504, 1994.

832. Carapeti M, Goldman JM, Cross NC: Overexpression of EV-1 in blast crisis of chronic myeloid leukemia. *Leukemia* 10:1561, 1996.

833. Mori N, Takeuchi S, Tasaka T, et al: Absence of microsatellite instability during the progression of chronic myelocytic leukemia. *Leukemia* 11:151, 1997.

834. Handa H, Hegde UP, Kuteninikov VM, et al: Bcl-2 and c-myc expressions, cell cycle kinetics and apoptosis during the progression of chronic myelogenous leukemia from diagnosis to blastic phase. *Leuk Res* 21:479, 1997.

835. Daheron L, Salmeron S, Patri S, et al: Identification of several genes differentially expressed during progression of chronic myelogenous leukemia. *Leukemia* 12:326, 1998.

836. Foti A, Ahuja HG, Allen SL, et al: Correlation between molecular and clinical events in the evolution of chronic myelocytic leukemia to blast crisis. *Blood* 77:2441, 1991.

837. Mori N, Morosetti R, Loe S, et al: Allelotype analysis in the evolution of chronic myelocytic leukemia. *Blood* 90:2010, 1997.

838. Spiers ASD: Metamorphosis of chronic granulocytic leukemia: Diagnosis, classification and management. *Br J Haematol* 49:1, 1979.

839. Grignani F: Chronic myelogenous leukemia. CRC Critical Review. *Oncol Hematol* 4:31, 1985.

840. Matsuo T, Tomonaga M, Kuriyama K, et al: Prognostic significance of the morphological dysplastic changes in chronic myelogenous leukemia. *Leuk Res* 10:331, 1986.

841. Ishii N, Murakami H, Matsushima T, et al: Histamine excess symptoms in basophilic crisis of chronic myelogenous leukemia. *J Med* 26:235, 1995.

842. Specchia G, Palumbo G, Pastore D, et al: Extramedullary blast crisis in chronic myeloid leukemia. *Leuk Res* 20:905, 1996.

843. Inveradi D, Lazzarino M, Morra E, et al: Extramedullary disease in Ph-positive chronic myelogenous leukemia: Frequency, clinical features, prognostic significance. *Haematologica* 75:146, 1990.

844. Jacknow J, Fizzera G, Gajl-Peczalska K, et al: Extramedullary presentation of the blast crisis of chronic myelogenous leukemia. *Br J Haematol* 61:225, 1985.

845. Terjanian T, Kantarjian H, Keating M, et al: Clinical and prognostic features of patients with Philadelphia chromosome-positive chronic myelogenous leukemia and extramedullary disease. *Cancer* 59:297, 1987.

846. Miksanek T, Reyes CV, Semkuo Z, Molnar ZJ: Granulocytic sarcoma of the peritoneum. *CA Cancer J Clin* 33:40, 1983.

847. Jones TI: Pleural blast crisis in chronic myelogenous leukemia. *Am J Hematol* 44:75, 1993.

848. Pascoe HR: Tumors composed of immature granulocytes occurring in the breast in chronic granulocytic leukemia. *Cancer* 25:697, 1970.

849. Chabner BA, Haskell CM, Canellos GP: Destructive bone lesions in chronic granulocytic leukemia. *Medicine* 48:401, 1969.

850. Licht A, Many N, Rachmilewitz EA: Myelofibrosis, osteolytic bone lesions and hypercalcemia in chronic myeloid leukemia. *Acta Haematol* 49:182, 1973.

851. Lee CH, Morris TCM: Bone marrow necrosis and extramedullary myeloid tumor necrosis in aggressive chronic myeloid leukemia. *Pathology* 11:551, 1979.

852. Asarro S, Sato N, Ueshima Y, et al: Localized blastoma preceding blastic transformation in Ph¹-positive chronic myelogenous leukemia. *Scand J Haematol* 25:251, 1980.

853. Ohyashiki K, Ito H: Characterization of extramedullary tumors in a case of Ph-positive chronic myelogenous leukemia. *Cancer Genet Cytogenet* 15:119, 1985.

854. Sun T, Susin M, Koduru P, et al: Extramedullary blast crisis in chronic myelogenous leukemia. *Cancer* 68:605, 1991.

855. Saikia TK, Dhabhar B, Iyer RS, et al: High incidence of meningeal leukemia in lymphoid blast crisis of chronic myelogenous leukemia. *Am J Hematol* 43:10, 1993.

856. Falini B, Tabilio A, Pelicci PG, et al: T-cell receptor B-chain gene rearrangement in a case of Ph¹-positive chronic myeloid leukaemia blast crisis. *Br J Haematol* 62:776, 1986.

857. Giannone L, Whitlock JA, Kinney MC, et al: Use of the BCR probe to demonstrate extramedullary recurrence of CML with a T cell lymphoid phenotype following bone marrow transplantation. *Bone Marrow Transplant* 3:631, 1988.

858. Ohyashiki J, Ohyashiki K, Shimizu H, et al: Testicular tumor as the first manifestation of B-lymphoid blastic crisis in a case of Ph-positive chronic myelogenous leukemia. *Am J Hematol* 29:164, 1988.

859. Rosenthal S, Canellos GP, DeVita VT, Gralnick HR: Characteristics of blast crisis in chronic granulocytic leukemia. *Blood* 49:705, 1977.

860. Barton JC, Conrad ME: Current status of blastic transformation in chronic myelogenous leukemia. *Am J Hematol* 4:281, 1978.

861. Peterson LC, Bloomfield CD, Brunning RD: Blast crisis as an initial or terminal manifestation of chronic myeloid leukemia. *Am J Med* 60:209, 1976.

862. Bettelheim P, Lutz D, Majdic O, et al: Cell lineage heterogeneity in blast crisis of chronic myeloid leukaemia. *Br J Haematol* 59:395, 1985.

863. Nair C, Chopra M, Shinde S, et al: Immunophenotype and ultrastructural studies in blast crisis of chronic myeloid leukemia. *Leuk Lymphoma* 19:309, 1995.

864. Rosenthal S, Canellos GP, Gralnick HR: Erythroblastic transformation of chronic granulocytic leukemia. *Am J Med* 63:116, 1977.

865. Ekblom M, Borgstrom G, von Willebrand E, et al: Erythroid blast crisis in chronic myelogenous leukemia. *Blood* 62:591, 1983.

866. Lingg G, Schmalzl F, Breton-Gorius J, et al: Megakaryoblastic micromegakaryocytic crisis in chronic myeloid leukemia. *Blut* 51:275, 1985.

867. Castaigne S, Berger R, Jolly V, et al: Promyelocytic blast crisis of chronic myelocytic leukemia with both t(9;22) and t(15;17) in M3 cells. *Cancer* 54:2409, 1984.

868. Berger R, Bernheim A, Daniel MT, Flandrin G: T(15;17) in a promyelocytic form of chronic myeloid leukemia blastic crisis. *Cancer Genet Cytogenet* 8:149, 1983.

869. Misawa S, Lee E, Schiffer CA, et al: Association of translocation (15;17) with malignant proliferation of promyelocytes in acute leukemia and chronic myelogenous leukemia in blast crisis. *Blood* 67:270, 1986.

870. Marinone G, Rossi G, Verzura P: Eosinophilic blast crisis in a case of chronic myeloid leukaemia. *Br J Haematol* 55:251, 1983.

871. Goh K-O, Anderson FW: Cytogenetic studies in basophilic chronic myelocytic leukemia. *Arch Pathol Lab Med* 103:288, 1979.

872. Rosenthal NS, Knapp D, Farhi DC: Promyelocytic blast crisis of chronic myelogenous leukemia. A rare subtype associated with disseminated intravascular coagulation. *Am J Clin Pathol* 103:185, 1995.

873. Lemes A, Gomez Casares MT, de la Iglesia S, et al: P190 BCR-ABL rearrangement in chronic myeloid leukemia and acute lymphoblastic leukemia. *Cancer Genet Cytogenet* 113:100, 1999.

874. Bertazzoni U, Brusamolino E, Isernia P, et al: Diagnostic significance of terminal transferase and adenosine deaminase in acute and chronic myeloid leukemia. *Blood* 60:685, 1982.

875. Schuh AC, Sutherland DR, Horsfall W, et al: Chronic myeloid leukemia arising in a progenitor common to T cells and myeloid cells. *Leukemia* 4:631, 1990.

876. Uike N, Takeichi N, Kimura N, et al: Dual arrangement of immunoglobulin and T-cell receptor genes in blast crisis of CML. *Eur J Haematol* 42:460, 1989.

877. Greaves MF, Verbi W, Reeves, BR, et al: "Pre-B" phenotypes in blast crisis of Ph¹ positive CML: Evidence for a pluripotential stem cell "target." *Leuk Res* 3:181, 1979.

878. Bakhshi A, Minowada J, Arnold A, et al: Lymphoid blast crisis of chronic myelogenous leukemia represents stages in the development of B-cell precursors. *N Engl J Med* 309:826, 1983.

879. Griffin JD, Todd RF, Ritz J, et al: Differentiation patterns in the blastic phase of chronic myeloid leukemia. *Blood* 61:85, 1983.

880. Bollum FJ: Terminal deoxynucleotidyl transferase, in *The Enzymes*, edited by RD Boyer, p 145. Academic, New York, 1974.

881. Dorfman DM, Longtine JA, Fox EA, et al: T-cell blast crisis in chronic myelogenous leukemia. *Am J Clin Pathol* 107:168, 1997.

882. Allouche M, Bourinbaiar A, Georgoulias V, et al: T-cell lineage involvement in lymphoid blast crisis of chronic myeloid leukemia. *Blood* 66:1155, 1985.

883. Gramatzki M, Bartram CR, Muller D, et al: Early T-cell differentiated chronic myeloid leukemia blast crisis with rearrangement of the breakpoint cluster region but not of the T-cell receptor beta chain genes. *Blood* 69:1082, 1987.

884. Dastugue N, Kuhlein E, Duchayne E, et al: T(14:14)(q11;q32) in biphenotypic blastic phase of chronic myeloid leukemia. *Blood* 68:949, 1986.

885. Kuriyama K, Tomonaga M, Yao E, et al: Dual expression of lymphoid/ basophil markers on single blast cells transformed from chronic myeloid leukemia. *Leuk Res* 10:1015, 1986.

886. Yasukawa M, Iwamasa K, Kawamura S, et al: Phenotypic and genotypic analysis of chronic myelogenous leukaemia with T lymphoblastic and megakaryoblastic mixed crisis. *Br J Haematol* 66:331, 1987.

887. Spencer A, Vulliamy T, Chase A, et al: Myeloid to lymphoid clonal suppression following autologous transplantation in second chronic phase of chronic myeloid leukemia. *Leukemia* 9:2138, 1995.

888. Cervantes F, Villamor N, Esteve J, et al: "Lymphoid" blast crisis of chronic myeloid leukaemia is associated with distinct clinicohaematological features. *Br J Haematol* 100:123, 1998.

889. Stoll C, Oberline F: Non-random clonal evolution in 45 cases of chronic myeloid leukemia. *Leuk Res* 46:61, 1980.

890. Sandberg AA: The cytogenetics of chronic myelocytic leukemia (CML): Chronic phase and blastic crisis. *Cancer Genet Cytogenet* 1: 217, 1980.

891. Myint H, Ross FM, Hall JL, et al: Early transformation to acute myeloblastic leukaemia with the acquisition of inv(16) in Ph positive chronic granulocytic leukaemia. *Leuk Res* 21:473, 1997.

892. Sandberg AA: Chronic myelocytic leukemia, in *The Chromosomes in Human Cancer and Leukemia*, 2nd ed, p 465. Elsevier North Holland, New York, 1990.

893. Mitani K, Miyazono K, Urabe A, Takaku F: Karyotypic changes during the course of blastic crisis of chronic myelogenous leukemia. *Cancer Genet Cytogenet* 39:299, 1989.

894. Diez-Martin JL, DeWald GW, Pierre RV, et al: Possible cytogenetic distinction between lymphoid and myeloid blast crisis in chronic granulocytic leukemia. *Am J Hematol* 27:194, 1988.

895. Feinstein E, Cimino G, Gale RP, Canaani E: Initiation and progression of chronic myelogenous leukemia. *Leukemia* 6(suppl 1):37, 1992.

896. Brizard F, Cividin M, Villalva C, et al: Comparison of M-FISH and conventional cytogenetic analysis in accelerated and acute phases of CML. *Leuk Res* 28:345, 2004.

897. Heim S, Christensen EB, Fioretos T, et al: Acute myelomonocytic leukemia with inv(16) (p13q22) complicating Philadelphia chromosome positive chronic myeloid leukemia. *Cancer Genet Cytogenet* 59:35, 1992.

898. Hogge DE, Misawa S, Testa JR, et al: Unusual karyotypic changes and B-cell involvement in a case of lymph node blast crisis of chronic myelogenous leukemia. *Blood* 64:123, 1984.

899. Barone S, Baer MR, Sait SNJ, et al: High-dose cytosine arabinoside and idarubicin treatment of chronic myeloid leukemia in myeloid blast crisis. *Am J Hematol* 67:119, 2001.

900. Kantarjian HM, Cortes J, O'Brien S, et al: Imatinib mesylate (STI571) therapy for Philadelphia chromosome–positive chronic myelogenous leukemia in blast phase. *Blood* 99:3547, 2002.

901. Cortes J, Kantarjian H: Advanced-phase chronic myeloid leukemia. *Semin Hematol* 40:79, 2003.

902. Druker BJ, Sawyers CL, Kantarjian H, et al: Activity of a specific inhibitor of the BCR-ABL tyrosine kinase in the blast crisis of chronic myeloid leukemia and acute lymphoblastic leukemia with the Philadelphia chromosome. *N Engl J Med* 344:1038, 2001.

903. Wadhwa J, Szydio RM, Apperley J, et al: Factors affecting duration of survival after onset of blastic transformation of chronic myeloid leukemia. *Blood* 99:2304, 2002.

904. Champlain R, Ho W, Arenson E, Gale RP: Allogeneic bone marrow transplantation for chronic myelogenous leukemia in chronic or accelerated phase. *Blood* 60:1038, 1982.

905. McGlave PB, Kim TH, Hard DD, et al: Successful allogeneic bone-marrow transplantation for patients in the accelerated phase of chronic granulocytic leukaemia. *Lancet* 2:625, 1982.

906. Martin PJ, Clift RA, Fisher LD, et al: HLA-identical marrow transplantation during accelerated-phase chronic myelogenous leukemia: Analysis of survival and remission duration. *Blood* 77:1978, 1988.

907. Falkenberg JHF, Wafelman AR, Joosten P, et al: Complete remission of accelerated phase chronic myeloid leukemia by treatment with leukemia-reactive cytotoxic T lymphocytes. *Blood* 94:1201, 1999

908. Carella AM, Gaozza E, Raffo MR, et al: Therapy of acute phase chronic myelogenous leukemia with intensive chemotherapy, blood cell autotransplant and cyclosporin A. *Leukemia* 5:517, 1991.

909. Bouvet M, Babiera GV, Termuhlen PM, et al: Splenectomy in the accelerated or blastic phase of chronic myelogenous leukemia: A single-institution 25-year experience. *Surgery* 122:20, 1997.

910. Majiis A, Smith TL, Talpaz M, et al: Signficance of cytogenetic clonal evolution in chronic myelogenous leukemia. *J Clin Oncol* 14:196, 1996.

911. Fialkow PJ, Jacobsen RJ, Singer JW, et al: Philadelphia chromosome (Ph¹)-negative chronic myelogenous leukemia (CML): A clonal disease with origin in a multipotent stem cell. *Blood* 56:70, 1980.

912. Cortes J: CMML: A biologically distinct disease. *Curr Hematol Rep* 2:202, 2003.

913. Onida F, Beran M: Chronic myelomonocytic leukemia: Myeloproliferative variant. *Curr Hematol Rep* 3:218, 2004.

914. McCollum A, Bigelow CL, Elkins SL, et al: Unusual skin lesions in chronic myelomonocytic leukemia. *Southern Med J* 96:681, 2003.

915. Saif MW, Hopkins JL, Gore SD: Autoimmune phenomena in patients with myelodysplastic syndromes and chronic myelomonocytic leukemia. *Leuk Lymphoma* 43:2083, 2002.

916. Cambier N, Baruchel A, Schlageter MH, et al: Chronic myelomonocytic leukemia: From biology to therapy. *Hematol Cell Ther* 39:41, 1997.

917. Stemmler J, Wittman GW, Hacker U, Heinemann V: Leukapheresis in chronic myelomonocytic leukemia with leukostasis syndrome: Elevated serum lactate levels as an early sign of microcirculation failure. *Leuk Lymphoma* 43:1427, 2002.

918. Bain BJ: Hypereosinophilia. *Curr Opin Hematol* 7:21, 2000.

919. Aguayo A, Kantarjian H, Manshouri T, et al: Angiogenesis in acute and chronic leukemias and myelodysplastic syndromes. *Blood* 96:2240, 2000.

920. Bellemy WI, Richter L, Sirjani D, et al: Vascular endothelial cell growth factor in autocrine promoter of abnormal localized precursors and leukemia progenitor formation in myelodysplastic syndromes. *Blood* 97:1427, 2001.

921. Ramshaw HS, Bardy PG, Lee MA, Lopez AQF: Chronic myelomonocytic leukemia requires granulocytic-macrophage colony-stimulating factor for growth in vitro and in vivo. *Exp Hematol* 30:1124, 2002.

922. Tessema M, Länger F, Dingemann J, et al: Aberrant methylation and impaired expression of the p14INK4B cell cycle regulatory gene in chronic myelomonocytic leukemia (CMML). *Leukemia* 17:910, 2003.

923. Magnusson MK, Meade KE, Nakamura R, et al: Activity of STI571 in chronic myelomonocytic leukemia with a platelet-derived growth factor B receptor fusion oncogene. *Blood* 100:1088, 2002.

924. Apperley JF, Gardembas M, Melo JV, et al: Response to imatinib mesylate in patients with chronic myeloproliferative diseases with rearrangements of the platelet-derived growth factor receptor beta. *N Engl J Med* 347:481, 2002.

925. Wessels JW, Fibbe WE, van der Keur D, et al: T(5;12)(q31;p12): A clinical entity with features of both myeloid leukemia and chronic myelomonocytic leukemia. *Cancer Genet Cytogenet* 65:7, 1993.

926. Golub TR, Barker GF, Love HM, Gilliland DG: Fusion of PDGF receptor β to a novel *ets*-like gen, *tel*, in chronic myelomonocytic leukemia with t(5;12) chromosomal translocation. *Cell* 77:307, 1994.

927. Cross NCP, Reiter A: Tyrosine kinase genes in chronic myeloproliferative diseases. *Leukemia* 16:1207, 2002.

928. Gunby RH, Cazzaniga G, Tassi E, et al: Sensitivity to imatinib but low frequency of the TEL/PDGFRβ fusion protein in chronic myelomonocytic leukemia. *Haematologica* 88:408, 2003.

929. Pitini V, Arrigo C, Teti D, et al: Response to STI571 in chronic myelomonocytic leukemia with platelet derived growth factor beta receptor involvement: A new case report. *Haematologica* 88:ECR18, 2003.

930. Kröger N, Zabelina T, Guardiola P, et al: Allogeneic stem cell transplantation of adult chronic myelomonocytic leukemia. *Br J Haematol* 118:67, 2002.

931. Onida F, Kantarjian HM, Smith TL, et al: Prognostic factors and scoring systems in chronic myelomonocytic leukemia: A prospective analysis of 213 patients. *Blood* 99:840, 2002.

932. Germing U, Strupp C, Alvado M, Gattermann N: New prognostic parameters for chronic myelomonocytic leukemia? *Blood* 100:731, 2002.

933. Sagaster V, Ohler L, Berer A, et al: High spontaneous colony growth in chronic myelomonocytic leukemia correlates with increased disease activity and is a novel prognostic factor for predicting short survival. *Ann Hematol* 83:9, 2004.

934. Stillman RG: A case of myeloid leukemia with predominance of eosinophil cells. *Med Rec* 81:594, 1912.

935. Benvenisti DS, Ultmann JE: Eosinophilic leukemia. *Ann Intern Med* 71:731, 1969.

936. Chusid MJ, Dale D, West BG, Wolff SM: The hypereosinophilic syndrome: analysis of fourteen cases with a review of the literature. *Medicine* 54:1, 1975.

937. Brito-Babapulle F: The eosinophilias: Including the idiopathic hypereosinophilic syndrome. *Br J Haematol* 121:203, 2003

938. Bain BJ: Cytogenetic and molecular genetic aspects of eosinophilic leukemia. *Br J Haematol* 122:173, 2003.

939. Gotlib J, Cools J, Malone JM III, et al: The FIP1L1-PDGFRA fusion tyrosine kinase in hypereosinophilic syndrome and chronic eosinophilic leukemia: Implications for diagnosis, classification, and management. *Blood* 103:2879, 2004.

940. Vandenberghe P, Wlodarska I, Michaux L, et al: Clinical and molecular features of *FIP1L1-PDFGRA* (+) chronic eosinophilic leukemia. *Leukemia* 18:734, 2004.

941. Klion AD, Noel P, Akin C, et al: Elevated serum tryptase levels identify a subset of patients with a myeloproliferative variant of idiopathic hypereosinophilic syndrome associated with tissue fibrosis, poor prognosis, and imatinib responsiveness. *Blood* 101:4660, 2003.

942. Salem Z, Zalloua PA, Chehal A, et al: Effective treatment of hypereosinophilic syndrome with imatinib mesylate. *Hematol J* 4:410, 2003.

943. Esteva-Lorenzo FJ, Meehan KR, Spitzer TR, Mazumder A: Allogeneic bone marrow transplantation in a patient with hypereosinophilic syndrome. *Am J Hematol* 51:164, 1996.

944. Juvonen E, Volin L, Koponen A, Ruutu T: Allogeneic blood stem cell transplantation following non-myeloablative conditioning for hypereosinophilic syndrome. *Bone Marrow Transplant* 29:457, 2002.

945. Plotz S-G, Simon H-U, Darsow U, et al: Use of anti-interleukin-5 antibody in the hypereosinophilic syndrome with eosinophilic dermatitis. *N Engl J Med* 349:2334, 2003.

946. Klion AD, Law MA, Noel P, et al: Safety and efficacy of the monoclonal anti-interleukin-5 antibody SCHJ55700 in the treatment of patients with hypereosinophilic syndrome. *Blood* 103:2939, 2004.

947. Osgood EE: Monocytic leukemia. Report of six cases and review of one hundred and twenty-seven cases. *Arch Intern Med* 59:931, 1937.

948. Bearman RM, Kjeldsberg CR, Pangalis GA, et al: Chronic monocytic leukemia in adults. *Cancer* 48:2239, 1981.

949. Beattie JW, Seal RME, Crowther KV: Chronic monocytic leukemia. *Q J Med* 20:131, 1951.

950. Sinn CW, Dick FW: Monocytic leukemia. *Am J Med* 20:588, 1956.

951. Rodgers GM, Carrera CJ, Ries CA, Bainton DF: Blastic transformation of a well differentiated monocytic leukemia. Changes in cytochemical and cell surface markers. *Leuk Res* 6:613, 1982.

952. Wahlin A, Nordenson I, Roos G: Chronic monocytic leukemia terminating in blastic transformation. *Blut* 53:405, 1986.

953. Castro-Malaspina H, Schaison G, Brier J, et al: Philadelphia chromosome positive chronic myelocytic leukemia in children: Survival and prognostic factors. *Cancer* 51:721, 1983.

954. Arico M, Biondi A, Pui C-H: Juvenile myelomonocytic leukemia. *Blood* 90:479, 1997.

955. Neimeyer CM, Arico M, Basso A, et al: Chronic myelomonocytic leukemia in childhood. *Blood* 89:3535, 1997.

956. Niemeyer CM, Kratz C: Juvenile myelomonocytic leukemia. *Curr Oncol Rep* 5:510, 2003.

957. Busque L, Gilliland DG, Prchal JT, et al: Clonality in juvenile chronic myelogenous leukemia. *Blood* 85:21, 1995.

958. Cooper LJN, Shannon KM, Loken MR, et al: Evidence that juvenile chronic myelomonocytic leukemia can arise from a pluripotential stem cell. *Blood* 96:2310, 2000.

959. Flotho C, Valcamonica S, Mach-Pascual S, et al: *RAS* mutations and clonality analysis in children with juvenile myelomonocytic leukemia (JMML). *Leukemia* 13:32, 1999.

960. Guilbert-Douet N, Morel F, Le Bris M-J, et al: Somatic *PTPN11* mutation with a heterogeneous clonal origin in children with juvenile myelomonocytic leukemia. *Leukemia* 18:1142, 2004.

961. Miyauchi J, Asada M, Sasaki M, et al: Mutations of the N-*ras* gene in juvenile chronic myelogenous leukemia. *Blood* 83:2248, 1994.

962. Bader JL, Miller RW: Neurofibromatosis and childhood leukemia. *J Pediatr* 92:925, 1978.

963. Brodeur GM: The NF1 gene in myelopoiesis and childhood myelodysplastic syndrome. *N Engl J Med* 330:637, 1994.

964. Shannon KM: Loss of normal NF1 allele from the bone marrow of children with type 1 neurofibromatosis and malignant myeloid disorders. *N Engl J Med* 330:597, 1994.

965. Bollag G: Loss of NF1 results in activation of RAS signaling pathway and leads to aberrant growth in haematopoietic cells. *Nat Genet* 12:137, 1996.

966. Tartaglia M, Niemeyer CM, Fragale A, et al: Somatic mutations in PTPN11 in juvenile myelomonocytic leukemia, myelodysplastic syndrome and acute myeloid leukemia. *Nat Genet* 34:148, 2003.

967. Owen G, Lewis IJ, Morgan M, et al: Prognostic factors in juvenile chronic granulocytic leukaemia. *Br J Cancer* 66(suppl XVIII):S68, 1992.

968. Estrov Z, Grunberger T, Chan HSL, Freedman MH: Juvenile chronic myelogenous leukemia. Characterization of the disease using cell cultures. *Blood* 67:1382, 1986.

969. Estrov Z, Dube ID, Chan HSL, Freedman MH: Residual juvenile chronic myelogenous leukemia cells detected in peripheral blood during clinical remission. *Blood* 70:1466, 1987.

970. Emanuel PD, Bates LJ, Zhu S-W, et al: The role of monocyte-derived hemopoietic growth factors in the regulation of myeloproliferation in juvenile chronic myelogenous leukemia. *Exp Hematol* 19:1017, 1991.

971. Morerio C, Acquila M, Rosanda C, et al: HCMOGT-1 is a novel fusion partner to *PDGFRB* in juvenile myelomonocytic leukemia with t(5;17)(q33;p11.2). *Cancer Res* 64:2649, 2004.

972. Inoue S, Ravindranath Y, Thompson RI, et al: Cytogenetics of juvenile type chronic granulocytic leukemia. *Cancer* 39:2017, 1977.

973. Brodeur GM, Dow LW, Williams DL: Cytogenetic features of juvenile chronic myelogenous leukemia. *Blood* 53:812, 1979.

974. Chan HSL, Estrov Z, Weitzman SS, Freedman MH: The value of intensive combination chemotherapy for juvenile chronic myelogenous leukemia. *J Clin Oncol* 5:1960, 1987.

975. Kang HJ, Shin HY, Choi HS, Ahn HS: Novel regimen for the treatment of juvenile myelomonocytic leukemia (JMML). *Leuk Res* 28:167, 2004.

976. Pui CH, Arico M: Isotretinoin for juvenile chronic myelogenous leukemia. *N Engl J Med* 332:1520, 1995.

977. Bernard F, Thomas C, Emile JF, et al: Transient hematologic and clinical effects of E21R in a child with end-stage juvenile myelomonocytic leukemia. *Blood* 99:2615, 2002.

978. Locatelli F, Niemeyer C, Angelucci E, et al: Allogeneic bone marrow transplantation for chronic myelomonocytic leukemia in childhood. *J Clin Oncol* 15:556, 1997.

979. Manabe A, Okamura J, Yumura-Yagi K, et al: Allogeneic hematopoietic stem cell transplantation for 27 children with juvenile myelomonocytic leukemia diagnosed based on the criteria of the International JMML Working Group. *Leukemia* 16:645, 2002.

980. Worth A, Rao K, Webb D, et al: Successful treatment of juvenile myelomonocytic leukemia relapsing after stem cell transplantation using donor lymphocyte infusion. *Blood* 101:1713, 2003.

981. Scrideli CA, Baruffi MR, Rogatto SR, et al: B lineage acute lymphoblastic leukemia transformation in a child with juvenile myelomonocytic leukemia, type 1 neurofibromatosis and monosomy of chromosome 7. Possible implications in the leukemogenesis. *Leuk Res* 27:371, 2003.

982. Tuohey EL: A case of splenomegaly with polymorphonuclear neutrophil hyperleukocytosis. *Am J Med Sci* 160:18, 1920.

983. Froberg MK, Brunning RD, Dorion P, et al: Demonstration of clonality in neutrophils using FISH in a case of chronic neutrophilic leukemia. *Leukemia* 12:623, 1998.

984. Böhm J, Schaefer HE: Chronic neutrophilic leukemia: 14 new cases of an uncommon myeloproliferative disorder. *J Clin Pathol* 55:862, 2002.

985. Standen GR, Steers FJ, Jones L: Clonality in chronic neutrophilic leukemia associated with myeloma: Analysis using the X-linked probe M27β. *J Clin Pathol* 46:297, 1993.

986. Bohm J, Kock S, Schaefer HE, Fisch P: Evidence of clonality in chronic neutrophilic leukaemia. *J Clin Pathol* 56:292, 2003.

987. Yanagisawa K, Ohminami H, Sato M, et al: Neoplastic involvement of granulocytic lineage, not granulocytic-monocytic, monocytic, or erythrocytic lineage, in a patient with chronic neutrophilic leukemia. *Am J Hematol* 57:221, 1998.

988. Hasegawa T, Suzuki K, Sakamoto C, et al: Expression of the inhibitor of apoptosis (IAP) family members in human neutrophils: Up-regulation of cIAP2 in chronic neutrophilic leukemia. *Blood* 101:1164, 2003.

989. Hasle H, Olesen G, Kerndrup G, et al: Chronic neutrophilic leukaemia in adolescence and young adulthood. *Br J Haematol* 94:628, 1996.

990. Elliott MA, Dewald GW, Tefferi A, Hanson CA: Chronic neutrophilic leukemia (CNL): a clinical and pathological entity. *Leukemia* 15:35, 2001.

991. Reilly JT: Chronic neutrophilic leukaemia: A distinct clinical entity? *Br J Haematol* 116:10, 2002.

992. Elliott MA: Chronic neutrophilic leukemia. *Curr Hematol Rep* 3:210, 2004.

993. Piliotis E, Kutas G, Lipton JH: Allogeneic bone marrow transplantation in the management of chronic neutrophilic leukemia. *Leuk Lymphoma* 43:2051, 2002.

994. Ito T, Kojima H, Otani K, et al: Chronic neutrophilic leukemia associated with monoclonal gammopathy of undetermined significance. *Acta Haematol* 95:140, 1996.

995. Vorobiof DA, Benjamin A, Kaplan H, Dvilansky A: Chronic granulocytic leukemia, neutrophilic type with paraproteinemia (IgA type K). *Acta Haematol* 60:316, 1978.

996. Carcassonne Y, Gastaut JA, Sebahoun G, Gratecos N: Découverte simultanée chez un même malade d'un myélome, d'une leucémie granuleuse (à polynucléaires neutrophils) et d'une maladie de Paget. *Nouv Rev Fr Hematol* 18:240, 1977.

997. Franchi F, Seminara P, Gruinchi G: Chronic neutrophilic leukemia and myeloma. Report on long survival. *Tumori* 70:105, 1984.

998. Lewis MJ, Oelbaum MH, Coleman M, Allen S: An association between chronic neutrophilic leukaemia and multiple myeloma with a study of cobalamin-binding proteins. *Br J Haematol* 63:173, 1986.

999. Rovira M, Cervantes F, Namdedeu B, Rozman C: Chronic neutrophilic leukaemia preceding for seven years the development of multiple myeloma. *Acta Haematol* 3:94, 1990.

1000. Standen GR, Jasani B, Wagstaff M, Wardrop CAJ: Chronic neutrophilic leukemia and multiple myeloma. *Cancer* 66:162, 1990.

1001. Nagai M, Oda S, Iwamoto M, et al: Granulocyte-colony stimulating factor concentrates in a patient with plasma cell dyscrasia and clinical features of chronic neutrophilic leukaemia. *J Clin Pathol* 49:858, 1996.

1002. Dinçol G, Nalçaci M, Dogan O, et al: Coexistence of chronic neutrophilic leukemia with multiple myeloma. *Leuk Lymphoma* 43:649, 2002.

1003. Masini L, Salvarani C, Macchioni P, et al: Chronic neutrophilic leukemia (CNL) with karyotype abnormalities associated with plasma cell dyscrasia. *Haematologica* 77:277, 1992.

1004. Pascucci M, Dorion P, Makary A, Froberg MK: Chronic neutrophilic leukemia evolving from the myelodysplastic syndrome. *Acta Haematol* 98:163, 1997.

1005. Takamatsu Y, Kondo S, Inoue M, Tamura K: Chronic neutrophilic leukemia with dysplastic features mimicking myelodysplastic syndrome. *Int J Hematol* 63:65, 1996.

1006. Higuchi T, Oba R, Endo M, et al: Transition of polycythemia vera to chronic neutrophilic leukemia. *Leuk Lymphoma* 33:203, 1999.

1007. Billio A, Venturi R, Morello E, et al: Chronic neutrophilic leukemia evolving from polycythemia vera with multiple chromosome rearrangements: A case report. *Haematologica* 86:1225, 2001.

1008. Foa P, Iurlo A, Saglio G, et al: Chronic neutrophilic leukemia associated with polycythemia vera. *Br J Haematol* 78:286, 1991.

1009. Higuchi T, Oba R, Endo M, et al: Transition of polycythemia vera to chronic neutrophilic leukemia. *Leuk Lymphoma* 33:203, 1999.

1010. Iurlo A, Foa P, Mailo AT, et al: Polycythemia vera terminating in chronic neutrophilic leukemia. *Am J Hematol* 35:139, 1990.

1011. Soda H, Kuriyama K, Tomonaga M, et al: Lymphoid crisis with T-cell phenotypes in a patient with Philadelphia chromosome negative chronic myeloid leukemia. *Br J Haematol* 59:671, 1985.

1012. Kessler JF, Grogan TM, Greenberg BR: Philadelphia-chromosome-negative chronic myelogenous leukemia with lymphoid stem cell blastic transformation. *Am J Hematol* 18:201, 1985.

1013. Dobrovic A, Morley AA, Seshadri R, Januszewicz EH: Molecular diagnosis of Philadelphia negative CML using the polymerase chain reaction and DNA analysis: Clinical features and course of M-bcr negative and M-bcr positive CML. *Leukemia* 5:187, 1990.

1014. Martiat P, Michaux JL, Rodhain J, et al: Philadelphia-negative (Ph−) chronic myeloid leukemia (CML): Comparison with Ph+ CML and chronic myelomonocytic leukemia. *Blood* 78:205, 1991.

1015. VanderPlas DC, Grosveld G, Hagemeijer A: Review of clinical, cytogenetic, and molecular aspects of Ph-negative CML. *Cancer Genet Cytogenet* 52:143, 1991.

1016. Galton DA: Haematological differences between chronic granulocytic leukemia, atypical chronic myeloid leukaemia and chronic myelomonocytic leukaemia. *Leuk Lymphoma* 7:343, 1992.

1017. Kato Y, Sawada H, Tashima M et al: Heterogeneous features of Ph-negative CML—Possible existence of Ph-negative, bcr-rearrangement-negative CML. *Acta Haematol* 52:1004, 1989.

1018. Kurzrock R, Kantarjian HM, Shtalrid M, et al: Philadelphia chromosome-negative chronic myelogenous leukemia without breakpoint cluster region rearrangement: A chronic myeloid leukemia with a distinct clinical course. *Blood* 75:445, 1990.

1019. Costello R, Sainty D, LaFage-Pochitaloff M, Gabert J: Clinical and biological aspects of Philadelphia-negative/BCR-negative chronic myeloid leukemia. *Leuk Lymphoma* 25:225, 1997.

1020. Kurzrock R, Bueso-Ramos CE, Kantarjian H, et al: BCR rearrangement-negative chronic myelogenous leukemia revisited. *J Clin Oncol* 19:2915, 2001.

1021. Onida F, Ball G, Kantarjian HM, et al: Characteristics and outcome of patients with Philadelphia chromosome negative, bcr/abl negative chronic myelogenous leukemia. *Cancer* 95:1673, 2002.

1022. O'Brien SG, Viera SA, Connors S, et al: Transient response to imatinib mesylate (STI571) in a patient with ETV6-ABL t(9;12) translocation. *Blood* 99:3465, 2002.

1023. Mauro MJ, Loriaux M, Deininger MW: Ph-positive and −negative myeloproliferative syndromes may coexist. *Leukemia* 18:1305, 2004.

1024. Raskind WH, Ferraris AM, Najfeld V, et al: Further evidence for the existence of a clonal Ph-negative stage in some cases of Ph-positive chronic myelocytic leukemia. *Leukemia* 18:1305, 2004.

1025. Chee YL, Vickers MA, Stevenson D, et al: Fatal myelodysplastic syndrome developing during therapy with imatinib mesylate and characterized by the emergence of complex Philadelphia negative clones. *Leukemia* 17:634, 2003.

1026. Meeus P, Demuynck H, Martiat P, et al: Sustained clonal karyotype abnormalities in the Philadelphia chromosome negative cells of CML patients successfully treated with imatinib. *Leukemia* 17:465, 2003.

1027. Bumm T, Muller C, Al Ali HK, et al: Emergence of clonal cytogenetic abnormalities in Ph-cells in some CML patients in cytogenetic remission to imatinib but restoration of polyclonal hematopoiesis in the majority. *Blood* 101:1941, 2001.

1028. Paietta E, Racevskis J, Bennett JM, et al: Biologic heterogeneity in Philadelphia chromosome-positive acute leukemia with myeloid morphology. *Leukemia* 12:1881, 1998.

1029. Keung YK, Beaty M, Powell BL, et al: Philadelphia chromosome positive myelodysplastic syndrome and acute myeloid leukemia—Retrospective study and review of literature. *Leuk Res* 28:579, 2004.

1030. Saikevych IA, Kerrigan DP, McConnell TS, et al: Multiparameter analysis of acute mixed lineage leukemia: Correlation of a B/myeloid immunophenotype and immunoglobulin and T-cell receptor gene rearrangements with the presence of the Philadelphia chromosome translocation in acute leukemias with myeloid morphology. *Leukemia* 5:373, 1991.

1031. Neuman MP, deSolas I, Parkin JL, et al: Monoclonal antibody study of Philadelphia chromosome-positive blastic leukemias using the alkaline phosphatase anti-alkaline phosphatase (APAAP) technique. *Am J Clin Pathol* 85:564, 1986.

1032. Cuneo A, Ferrant A, Michaux JL, et al: Philadelphia chromosome-positive acute myeloid leukemia: Cytoimmunologic and cytogenetic features. *Haematologica* 81:423, 1996.

1033. Bornstein RS, Nesbit M, Kennedy BJ: Chronic myelogenous leukemia presenting in blast crisis. *Cancer* 30:939, 1972.

1034. Peterson LC, Bloomfield CD, Brunning RD: Blast crisis as an initial or terminal manifestation of chronic myeloid leukemia. *Am J Med* 60:209, 1976.

1035. Worm A-M, Pedersen-Bjergaard J: Chronic myelocytic leukemia presenting in blast transformation. *Scand J Haematol* 18:288, 1977.

1036. Kantarjian HM, Talpaz M, Chingra K, et al: Significance of the p210 versus p190 molecular abnormalities in adults with Philadelphia chromosome-positive acute leukemia. *Blood* 78:2411, 1991.

1037. Chen SJ, Flandrin G, Daniel M-T, et al: Philadelphia-positive acute leukemia: Lineage promiscuity and inconsistently rearranged breakpoint cluster region. *Leukemia* 2:261, 1988.

1038. Price CM, Rasool F, Shirji MKK, et al: Rearrangement of the breakpoint cluster region and expression of p210 BCR-ABL in a "masked" Philadelphia chromosome-positive acute myeloid leukemia. *Blood* 72:1829, 1988.

1039. Westbrook CA, Hooberman AL, Spino C, et al: Clinical significance of the BCR-ABL fusion gene in adult acute lymphoblastic leukemia: A Cancer and Leukemia Group B study. *Blood* 80:2983, 1992.

1040. Lim LC, Heng KK, Vellupillai M, et al: Molecular and phenotypic spectrum of de novo Philadelphia positive acute leukemia. *Int J Mol Med* 4:665, 1999.

1041. Vandenberghe E, Martiat P, Baens M, et al: Megakaryoblastic leukemia with an N-ras mutation and late acquisition of a Philadelphia chromosome. *Leukemia* 5:683, 1991.

1042. Helenglass G, Testa JR, Schiffer CA: Philadelphia chromosome-positive acute leukemia. *Am J Hematol* 25:311, 1987.

1043. Mecucci C, Noens L, Aventin A, et al: Philadelphia-positive acute myelomonocytic leukemia with inversion of chromosome 16 and eosinobasophils. *Am J Hematol* 27:69, 1988.

1044. Kurzrock R, Shtalrid M, Talpaz M, et al: Expression of c-abl in Philadelphia-positive acute myelogenous leukemia. *Blood* 70:1584, 1987.

1045. Smadja N, Krulik M, DeGramont A, et al: Acquisition of Philadelphia chromosome concomitant with transformation of a refractory anemia into acute leukemia. *Cancer* 55:1477, 1985.

1046. Primo D, Tabernero MD, Rasillo A, et al: Patterns of BCR/ABL gene rearrangements by interphase fluorescence in situ hybridization (FISH) in BCR/ABL+ leukemia: Incidence and underlying genetic abnormalities. *Leukemia* 17:1124, 2003.

1047. LoCoco F, Basso G, DiCello PF, et al: Molecular characterization of Ph¹+ hybrid acute leukemia. *Leuk Res* 13:1061, 1989.

1048. Ribeiro RC, Abromowitch M, Raimondi SC, et al: Clinical and biologic hallmarks of the Philadelphia chromosome in childhood acute lymphoblastic leukemia. *Blood* 70:948, 1987.

1049. Christ N, Carroll A, Shuster J, et al: Philadelphia chromosome positive childhood acute lymphoblastic leukemia: Clinical and cytogenetic characteristics and treatment outcome. *Blood* 76:489, 1990.

1050. Pui C-H, Crist WM, Look AT: Biology and clinical significance of cytogenetic abnormalities in childhood acute lymphoblastic leukemia. *Blood* 76:1449, 1990.

1051. Forman SJ, O'Donnell MR, Nademanee DS, et al: Bone marrow transplantation for patients with Philadelphia chromosome-positive acute lymphoblastic leukemia. *Blood* 70:587, 1987.

1052. Houot R, Tavernier E, Le QH, et al: Philadelphia chromosome-positive acute lymphoblastic leukemia in the elderly: prognostic factors and treatment outcome. *Hematology* 9:369, 2004.

1053. Bacher U, Haferlach T, Hiddemann W, et al: Additional clonal abnormalities in Philadelphia-positive ALL and CML demonstrate a different cytogenetic pattern at diagnosis and follow different pathways at progression. *Cancer Genet Cytogenet* 157:53, 2005.

1054. Pane F, Cimino G, Izzo B, et al: Significant reduction of the hybrid BCR/ABL transcripts after induction and consolidation therapy is a powerful predictor of treatment response in adult Philadelphia-positive acute lymphoblastic leukemia. *Leukemia.* 19:628, 2005.

1055. Erikson J, Griffin CA, Ar-Rushdi A, et al: Heterogeneity of chromosome 22 breakpoint in Philadelphia positive acute lymphoblastic leukemia. *Proc Natl Acad Sci U S A* 83:1807, 1986.

1056. Chan LC, Karhi KK, Rayter SI, et al: A novel abl protein expressed in Philadelphia chromosome positive acute lymphoblastic leukaemia. *Nature* 325:635, 1987.

1057. Kurzrock R, Shtalrid M, Romero P, et al: A novel c-abl protein product in Philadelphia-positive acute lymphoblastic leukemia. *Nature* 325:631, 1987.

1058. Dreazen O, Klisak I, Jones G, et al: Multiple molecular abnormalities in Ph¹ chromosome positive acute lymphoblastic leukaemia. *Br J Haematol* 67:319, 1987.

1059. Clark SS, Crist WM, Witte ON: Molecular pathogenesis of Ph-positive leukemias. *Ann Rev Med* 40:113, 1989.

1060. Schaefer-Rego K, Arlin Z, Shapiro LG, et al: Molecular heterogeneity of adult Philadelphia chromosome-positive ALL. *Cancer Res* 48:866, 1988.

1061. Hermans A, Heisterkamp N, vonLindern M, et al: Unique fusion of bcr and c-abl genes in Philadelphia chromosome positive acute lymphoblastic leukemia. *Cell* 51:33, 1987.

1062. Clark SS, McLaughlin J, Crist WM, et al: Unique forms of the abl tyrosine kinase distinguish Ph¹-positive ALL. *Science* 235:85, 1987.

1063. Chen SJ, Chen Z, Hillion J, et al: Ph1-positive, bcr-negative acute leukemias: Clustering of breakpoints on chromosome 22 in the 3′end of the BCR gene first intron. *Blood* 73:1312, 1989.

1064. Rubin CM, Carrino JJ, Dickler MN, et al: Heterogeneity of genomic fusion of *BCR* and *ABL* in Philadelphia chromosome-positive acute lymphoblastic leukemia. *Proc Natl Acad Sci U S A* 85:2795, 1988.

1065. Hooberman AL, Rubin CM, Barton KP, Westerbrook CA: Detection of the Philadelphia chromosome in acute lymphoblastic leukemia by pulsed-field gel electrophoresis. *Blood* 74:1101, 1989.

1066. Dow LW, Tachibana N, Raimondi SC, et al: Comparative biochemical and cytogenetic studies of childhood acute lymphoblastic leukemia with the Philadelphia chromosome and other 22q11 variants. *Blood* 73:1291, 1989.

1067. Seckler-Walker LM, Cooke HMG, Browett PJ, et al: Variable Philadelphia breakpoints and potential lineage restriction of bcr rearrangements in acute lymphoblastic leukemia. *Blood* 72:784, 1988.

1068. Hermans A, Gow J, Selleri L, et al: *Bcr-abl* oncogene activation in Philadelphia chromosome-positive acute lymphoblastic leukemia. *Leukemia* 2:628, 1988.

1069. Melo JV, Gordon DE, Tuszynski A, et al: Expression of the ABL-BCR fusion gene in Philadelphia-positive acute lymphoblastic leukemia. *Blood* 81:2488, 1993.

1070. Suryanarayan K, Hunger SP, Kohler S, et al: Consistent involvement of the BCR gene by 9;22 breakpoints in pediatric acute leukemias. *Blood* 77:324, 1991.

1071. Saglio G, Pane F, Martinelli G, Guerrasio A: BCR/ABL rearrangement and leukemia phenotype. *Leukemia* 13(suppl 1):s96, 1999.

1072. Clark SS, McLaughlin J, Timmons M, et al: Expression of a distinctive BCR-ABL oncogene in Ph¹-positive acute lymphocytic leukemia (ALL). *Science* 239:775, 1988.

1073. Heerema NA, Harbott J, Galimberti S, et al: Secondary cytogenetic aberrations in childhood Philadelphia chromosome positive acute lymphoblastic leukemia are nonrandom and may be associated with outcome. *Leukemia* 18:693, 2004.

1074. de Klein A, Hagemeijer A, Bartram CR, et al: Bcr rearrangement and translocation of the c-abl oncogene in Philadelphia positive acute lymphoblastic leukemia. *Blood* 68:1369, 1986.

1075. Anastasi J, Feng J, Dickstein JI, et al: Lineage involvement by BCR/ABL in Ph+ lymphoblastic leukemias: Chronic myelogenous leukemia presenting in lymphoid blast phase vs Ph+ acute lymphoblastc leukemia. *Leukemia* 10:795, 1996.

1076. Schenk TM, Keyhani A, Bottcher S, et al: Multilineage involvement of Philadelphia chromosome positive acute lymphoblastic leukemia. *Leukemia* 12:666, 1998.

1077. Secker-Walker LM, Craig JM: Prognostic implications of breakpoint and lineage heterogeneity in Philadelphia-positive acute lymphoblastic leukemia: A review. *Leukemia* 7:147, 1993.

1078. Hirsch-Ginsberg C, Childs C, Chang K-S, et al: Phenotypic and molecular heterogeneity in Philadelphia chromosome-positive acute leukemia. *Blood* 71:186, 1988.

1079. Viniou NA, Vassilakopoulos TP, Giakoumi X, et al: Ida-FLAG plus imatinib mesylate-induced remission with chemoresistant Ph1+ acute myeloid leukemia. *Eur J Hematol* 72:58, 2004.

1080. Ottmann OG, Druker BJ, Sawyers CL, et al: A phase 2 study of imatinib in patients with relapsed or refractory Philadelphia-positive acute lymphoid leukemias. *Blood* 100:1965, 2002.

1081. Hoelzer D, Gokbuget N, Ottmann GG: Targeted-therapies in the treatment of Philadelphia-positive acute lymphoblastic leukemia. *Semin Hematol* 39(suppl 3):32, 2002.

1082. Thomas DA, Faderl S, Cortes J, et al: Treatment of Philadelphia-positive acute lymphocytic leukemia with hyper-CVAD and imatinib mesylate. *Blood* 103:4396, 2004.

1083. Ardanani AD, Morice WG, Hoyer JD, Tefferi A: Chronic basophilic leukemia: A distinct clinical entity. *Eur J Hematol* 71:18, 2003.

1084. Sawyers CL, Shah NP, Kantarjian HM, et al: Hematologic and cytogenetic responses in imatinib –resistant chronic phase chronic myeloid leukemia patients treated with dual SRC/ABL kinase inhibitor BMS-354825: Results fronm a Phase I dose escalation study. *Blood* 104:4a, 2004.

1085. Talpaz M, Kantarjian H, Shah NP, et al: Hematologic and cytogenetic responses in imatinib-resistant accelerated and blast phase chronic-myeloid leukemia (CML) patients treated with dual SRC/ABL kinase inhibitor BMS-354825: Results from a phase I escalation study. *Blood* 104:10a, 2004.

1086. Gumireddy K, Baker SJ, Cosenza SC, et al: A non-ATP-competitive inhibitor of BCR-ABL overrides imatinib resistance. *Proc Natl Acad Sci U S A* 102:1992, 2005.

1087. Giles F, Kantarjian H, Weissman B, et al: A phase I/II study of AMN107, a novel aminopyrimidine inhibitor of Bcr-Abl, on a continuous daily dosing schedule in adult patients (pts) with imatinib-resistant advanced phase chronic myeloid leukemia (CML) or relapsed/refractory Philadelphia chromosome (Ph+) acute lymphocytic leukemia (ALL). *Blood* 104:10a, 2004

1088. Weisberg E, Manley PW, Breitenstein W, et al: Characterization of AMN107, a selective inhibitor of native and mutant Bcr-Abl. *Cancer Cell* 7:129, 2005.

1089. Jeha S, Pui CH: Recombinant urate oxidase (rasburicase) in the prophylaxis and treatment of tumor lysis syndrome. *Contrib Nephrol* 147:69, 2005.

1090. Liu CY, Sims-McCallum RP, Schiffer CA: A single dose of rasburicase is sufficient for the treatment of hyperuricemia in patients receiving chemotherapy. *Leuk Res* 29:463, 2005.

1091. Arnold TM, Reuter JP, Delman BS, Shanholtz CB: Use of single-dose rasburicase in an obese female. *Ann Pharmacother* 38:1428, 2004.

1092. Hasford J, Pfirrmann M, Hockhaus A: How long will chronic myeloid leukemia patients treated with imatinib live? *Leukemia* 19:497, 2005.

IDIOPATHIC MYELOFIBROSIS (MYELOFIBROSIS WITH MYELOID METAPLASIA)

MARSHALL A. LICHTMAN

Idiopathic myelofibrosis is one of several disorders in the spectrum of clonal myeloid diseases, malignant diseases that originate in the clonal expansion of a single neoplastic hematopoietic multipotential cell. It is characterized by anemia, mild neutrophilia, thrombocytosis, and splenomegaly. Immature myeloid and erythroid precursors, teardrop-shaped erythrocytes, and large platelets are constant features of the blood film. The marrow has increased reticulin fibers and, often later, collagen fibrosis. This reactive, polyclonal fibroplasia is the result of cytokines released locally by the numerous abnormal megakaryocytes. The disease may be complicated by portal hypertension as a result of very large splenic blood flow and loss of compliance of hepatic vessels and by fibrohematopoietic tumors that can develop in any tissue and lead to symptoms by compression of vital structures. Treatment may include hydroxyurea for thrombocytosis and massive splenomegaly, red cell transfusions for severe anemia, local irradiation of fibrohematopoietic tumors or of the spleen, and splenectomy. Portosystemic shunt surgery may be required for gastroesophageal variceal bleeding. The disease may remain indolent for years or may progress rapidly by further deterioration in hematopoiesis, by massive splenic enlargement and its sequelae, or by transformation to acute myelogenous leukemia. Overall median survival is approximately 5 years.

DEFINITION AND HISTORY

Idiopathic myelofibrosis is a chronic clonal myeloid disorder characterized by (1) anemia, (2) splenomegaly, (3) immature granulocytes, CD34+ cells, erythroblasts, and teardrop-shaped red cells in the blood, (4) marrow fibrosis, and (5) osteosclerosis. The disorder originally was described by Heuck[1] in 1879 under the title "Two Cases of Leukemia and Peculiar Blood and Bone Marrow Findings." In his monograph, Silverstein[2] traces the history of the concepts set forth during the first half of the 20th century to explain the pathogenesis of this disease, including its origin in the marrow, the appearance of extramedullary hematopoiesis, and the relationship of fibrosis to hematopoietic changes. More than 30 designations for the disease have been proposed or used, and different designations are preferred in different countries.[3] *Myelofibrosis with myeloid metaplasia* and *idiopathic myelofibrosis* currently are the two most frequently used terms for the disease. *Ag-*

nogenic myeloid metaplasia was the most frequent in the past but has been replaced by the two terms noted above. No designation has been formulated that accommodates the five key phenomena of (1) a clonal (neoplastic) hematopoietic multipotential cell abnormality, (2) dominant neoplastic megakaryocytopoiesis, (3) a propensity to extramedullary fibrohematopoietic tumors, (4) an intense reactive, polyclonal marrow fibrosis, and (5) osteosclerosis.[4]

EPIDEMIOLOGY

INCIDENCE

AGE AND SEX

Idiopathic myelofibrosis characteristically occurs after age 50 years.[2,4–12] The median age at diagnosis is approximately 65 years,[4,8–10] but the disease can occur from the neonatal period to the ninth decade of life.[2,8,10,13–15] Its occurrence in children usually is in the first 3 years of life.[15–17] In young and middle-aged adults, the disease has the characteristics it has in older subjects, although the proportion of indolent cases may be higher.[13,15,18] In infants, the disorder can mimic the classic disease or show certain features but not others, such as hepatosplenomegaly.[14] In adults, the disease occurs with about equal frequency in men and women.[4,8–12] In young children, girls are afflicted with the disease twice as frequently as boys.[14] Like all clonal myeloid diseases,[19] idiopathic myelofibrosis rarely can cluster in families, suggesting transmission of an unidentified predisposition gene.[20,21] The incidence of the disease is approximately 0.5 cases per 100,000 population per year in Northern European countries.[22–24] A United States county survey reported an incidence of 1.5 case per 100,00 population per year and a median age of onset of 67 years. The latter result is in keeping with several reports based on case series (see above in this section).[25]

ETIOLOGY AND PATHOGENESIS

ANIMAL MODELS

Marrow fibrosis associated with compromise of intramedullary hematopoiesis and development of ectopic foci of hemopoiesis have been induced in animals by chemicals, such as lead acetate and saponin, after infection with the Rauscher rat leukemia and S37 sarcoma viruses, and by high doses of estrogens.[2] Animals injected with marrow extracts, antimarrow serum, or egg albumin have developed marrow fibrosis and splenic hematopoiesis.[2] These observations, along with reports of myelofibrosis in patients with lupus erythematosus, have suggested the possibility of immunologic-mediated hyperplasia of marrow connective tissue[2] (see "Immune Manifestations" below). These forms of myelofibrosis are different from the monoclonal stem cell disease considered in this chapter and do not replicate the pathogenesis of the human disease, which is the result of somatic mutations in an hematopoietic multipotential cell.

More realistic animal models followed the derivation of the myeloproliferative leukemia virus, carrying the oncogene v-*mpl*, which in mice produced a syndrome having features of a mixed idiopathic myelofibrotic–polycythemic disorder.[26] The availability of v-*mpl* led to the isolation of the thrombopoietin receptor and its ligand thrombopoietin.[27] Later models of myelofibrosis and osteosclerosis, mimicking some of the important features of human idiopathic myelofibrosis, were induced in mice by retroviral-mediated overexpression of thrombopoietin.[28,29] The concomitant high levels of fibroplastic factors (transforming growth factor [TGF]-β_1 and platelet-derived growth factor [PDGF]) resulted in intense fibrosis. The disease was cured by murine hematopoietic stem cell transplantation.[28]

A syndrome in mice that results from the GATA-1 (low) mutation also leads to a phenotype that closely simulates human myelofibrosis.

The mice gradually develop anemia, teardrop poikilocytes, myeloid immaturity, marrow fibrosis, extramedullary hematopoiesis, and overexpression of profibrotic cytokines in marrow.[430]

EXOGENOUS FACTORS

Exposure to benzene[30–32] or very-high-dose ionizing radiation[33,34] preceded the development of idiopathic myelofibrosis in a very small proportion of patients with the disease. The former incitant, in exposures greater than 20 ppm·years, is strongly associated with causation of acute myelogenous leukemia (AML). The latter incitant is a well-established environmental cause of AML and chronic myelogenous leukemia (CML) (see Chaps. 87 and 88).

CLONAL HEMOPATHY

The disease arises from the neoplastic transformation of a single hematopoietic multipotential cell, a conclusion derived from studies in women with idiopathic myelofibrosis who also were heterozygous for isotypes A and B of G-6-PD.[35,36] Although the nonhematopoietic tissues of these patients expressed both isotypes, each patient had blood cells with only one G-6-PD isotype. The findings strongly imply the blood cells of each patient arose from only one transformed stem cell. Furthermore, chromosome studies of colonies of hematopoietic progenitor cells in idiopathic myelofibrosis established that the same clonal cytogenetic abnormality is present in erythroblasts, neutrophils, macrophages, basophils, and megakaryocytes.[37] These studies were confirmed by (1) examining X-linked restriction fragment length polymorphisms in women with idiopathic myelofibrosis with heterozygosity for X chromosome-linked genes[38,39] and (2) verifying the presence of a mutation of codon 12 of the N-ras gene in five blood cell lineages of a patient with the disease.[40,41] Lymphocyte derivation from the clone has been noted using mutation in codon 12 of the ras gene as the marker.[40] Using FISH analysis, T and B lymphocytes were found to be derived from clonal expansion of a multipotential hematopoietic cell in three of four patients with idiopathic myelofibrosis with a 13q- or 20q- clonal cytogenetic abnormality.[42] Studies of X chromosome inactivation patterns is complicated by the high prevalence of skewing in normal older woman, making the test less useful in subtle cases of suspected chronic clonal myeloproliferation.[43,44]

ONCOGENES

Isolated findings in individual patients have included retinoblastoma gene mutation or overexpression, ras mutations in approximately one in 20 patients studied and two patients with mutations in c-kit.[45] Mutational analysis of the class III receptor tyrosine kinase genes c-kit, c-fms, and flt3 in 40 to 60 patients with idiopathic myelofibrosis found only two mutation in c-fms, which are of uncertain significance.[45]

HMGA2, a gene on chromosome 12, normally is not expressed in humans and is implicated in uncommon mesenchymal tumors. HMGA2 was expressed in 12 of 12 patients with idiopathic myelofibrosis studied, implying that expression of this gene in myeloid cells plays a role in the disease.[431]

A dominant, gain-of-function mutation in a gene (JAK2) residing on the short arm of chromosome 9, which encodes the JAK2 tyrosine kinase, is present in about 35 to 50 percent of patients with idiopathic myelofibrosis, in about 60 to 80 percent of patients with polycythemia vera (see Chap. 56), and in about 35 percent of patients with essential thrombocythemia see (Chap. 111), but is absent in healthy individuals.[436–438] In patients with myelofibrosis with the mutation, about three quarters are heterozygous and about one quarter are homozygous. The latter state appears to result from allelic duplication, not loss of an allele. It is not yet known how this mutation (JAK2 V617F) links the

three diseases nor if there is an explanation for the dramatically different phenotype and expected survival of the patients with polycythemia and myelofibrosis. Clearly, other factors are operating to account for the diverse phenotypes and the absence of the mutation in a high proportion of patients. The development of an inhibitor of the tyrosine kinase as a potential therapeutic agent would provide important insights into the functional role of the constitutive activation of JAK2 in these disorders.

DYSFUNCTION OF HEMATOPOIESIS

Myeloproliferation usually is the dominant marrow abnormality in the granulocytic and megakaryocytic lineages resulting in intensely cellular marrows and mild to moderate blood granulocytosis and thrombocytosis. Ineffective or hypoplastic hematopoiesis, resulting from exaggerated apoptosis of very early precursors, can be present initially or emerge later as the dominant pathogenetic process, leading to granulocytopenia and/or thrombocytopenia. Anemia is a frequent finding and results from a combination of decreased erythropoiesis, shortened red cell survival, and the effects of splenomegaly on the distribution of red cells in the circulation. Hemolysis can be a prominent factor in some cases. Megakaryocytosis and intense dysmorphogenesis of megakaryocytes are nearly constant features of the disease. Even in intensely fibrotic marrows with severe decreases in erythroid and granulocytic precursors, clusters of megakaryocytes are easily found interspersed between collagen bundles. The term "megakaryocytic myelosis," one of the many synonymous terms for the disease, catches the constancy of this finding. The dominance of megakaryopoiesis may relate to the average fivefold overexpression of FKBP51 in megakaryocytes in idiopathic myelofibrosis. The gene increases resistance to apoptosis, possibly by an effect through the calcineurin pathway.[46] The disease has all the hallmarks of chronic megakaryocytic leukemia. Although elevated levels of thrombopoietin (and interleukin [IL]-6 and IL-11) are found in the serum of patients with idiopathic myelofibrosis, its etiologic role in the human disease is unresolved.[47] A marked increase in thrombopoietin receptors, c-mpl, is observed on the platelets and megakaryocytes of a proportion of patients with idiopathic myelofibrosis.[48] Expression of the polycythemia rubra vera gene PRV-1, also is increased on neutrophils in some patients with the disease.[49,50] The latter group may include patients whose disease is evolving from polycythemia vera to myelofibrosis. Clinical trials may show these epigenetic markers to be of utility in diagnosis when they are made more widely available. Despite the animal models of thrombopoietin-induced myeloproliferation and osteomyelofibrosis and the apparent abnormality of c-mpl receptor sites on human megakaryocytes, autonomous megakaryocyte growth characteristic of human idiopathic myelofibrosis marrow in culture has not been associated with either an autocrine effect of MPL ligand (thrombopoietin) or of a mutation in c-mpl.

FIBROPLASIA

Four of the five major types of collagen[51] are present in normal marrow: type I in bone, type III in blood vessels, and types IV and V in basement membranes. The fine reticulin fibers that are visible after silver impregnation of normal marrow principally are type III collagen. They do not stain with trichrome dyes. The thicker collagen fibers principally are type I collagen and stain with trichrome dyes but do not impregnate with silver. The amount of fine fibrous network in normal marrow that is stained by silver impregnation techniques[52] increases in the marrow of virtually all patients with idiopathic myelofibrosis[53] (Table 89-1). The fibrous network contains collagen and occasionally progresses to include thick collagen bands that are evident with trichrome stains. Collagen types I, III, IV, and V are increased in

TABLE 89-1   FIBROPLASIA IN IDIOPATHIC MYELOFIBROSIS

Marrow Stroma

Increased amount of

Total collagen (hydroxyproline)[54,58]

Type I collagen[54–56,60]

Type III collagen[54–56,60]

Type III procollagen[55–58,60,61]

Type IV collagen[55,62,63]

Laminin[55,62,64]

Fibronectin[65,66]

Tenascin[67]

Vitronectin[68]

Microenvironment TGF-β,[69] bFGF,[69] and substance P[70]

Plasma

Increased concentration of

Prolylhydroxylase[71]

C-terminal peptide of procollagen type I[57]

N-terminal peptide of procollagen type III[56,59,72,73]

Type IV collagen[56,64]

Laminin[56,64]

Fibronectin[66]

Hyaluronan[74]

myelofibrosis, but type III collagen is increased uniformly and preferentially.[54–57] The latter occurrence accounts for the increased plasma concentration of procollagen III amino terminal peptide, a component of collagen type III, which is cleaved during collagen biosynthesis.[56,58,59] Serum prolyl-hydroxylase and marrow and plasma fibronectin also increases in patients with idiopathic myelofibrosis or myelofibrosis from other causes.[55,56]

Marrow fibrosis in idiopathic myelofibrosis is most closely correlated with increased dysmorphic megakaryocytes in the marrow. Even densely fibrotic marrow with little residual granulopoiesis or erythropoiesis usually has numerous megakaryocytes scattered throughout the fibrotic areas.[53,59,75] The increased pathologic emperipolesis of neutrophils in megakaryocytes, evident in human idiopathic myelofibrosis and in mouse models, suggests this may be an additional mechanism of α-granule injury and release of TGF-β and PDGF.[76] Animal models also indicate that marrow monocytes and macrophages may play a subsidiary role in the induction of fibrosis.[76–78] Secretion of PDGF, bFGF, and TGF-β from monocytes that are part of the clone have the potential to act as myeloproliferative growth factors and profibrotic cytokines.[69]

The increased content of marrow collagen types I and III results from release of fibroblast growth factors, which include PDGF,[79,80] epidermal growth factor,[81] endothelial cell growth factor,[81] TGF-β,[68,82,83] and bFGF,[68,84] each of which is present in megakaryocyte α-granules. Other factors, such as tumor necrosis factor alpha, IL-1α, and IL-1β, which can be released from marrow cells, also can stimulate fibroblasts.[85,86] Platelet factor 4, also derived from megakaryocytes, inhibits collagenase and could contribute to collagen accumulation,[75] although studies showing a poor correlation between plasma platelet factor 4 concentration and marrow fibrosis have dampened enthusiasm for the role of this factor.[87] Substance P, a peptide that acts as a neurotransmitter and a modulator of immune and hematopoietic functions, is increased in the fibrotic marrow and colocalizes with fibronectin. It is angiogenic and is a fibroblast mitogen.[69] Its precise role in the complex interactions among fibroblasts, cytokines, and matrix protein deposition is not clear. The high urinary excretion of platelet-derived calmodulin, a putative fibroblast growth factor, in patients with myelofibrosis has

added this compound to the array of factors that may contribute to the fibroplasia.[85] The plasma level of matrix metalloprotein III is decreased and the level of tissue inhibitor of metalloproteinase is increased in patients with idiopathic myelofibrosis.[88] This combination of alterations could contribute to matrix deposition. The pathogenetic role of released growth factors in fibroplasia is incompletely understood. Generalizations from *in vitro* experiments or correlation between two variables provide only a limited perspective. For example, TGF-β can stimulate or inhibit fibroblast growth, depending on the repertoire of other growth factors in the environment.[82,83]

Fibroplasia is associated with an increase in the number and size of marrow sinuses,[53,89] the number of endothelial cells,[90] an increase in vascular volume in the marrow,[91] and an increase in blood flow through the marrow.[62,92] These processes are responsible for the increase in marrow collagen types IV and V and laminin synthesized by endothelial cells in the marrow of patients.[81]

The fibroblastic proliferation in marrow is not an intrinsic part of the abnormal clonal expansion of hematoiesis.[93] In cases of idiopathic myelofibrosis in which G-6-PD isoenzyme studies or chromosome karyotyping establish monoclonal growth of hematopoietic cells, marrow fibroblasts contain both G-6-PD isoenzymes and do not share the clonal chromosome abnormality.[94] The findings strongly imply that the fibroblasts differentiate from a primordial cell different from the hematopoietic stem cell and that their proliferation and enhanced collagen synthesis is a secondary result of abnormal hematopoiesis.

EXTRAMEDULLARY HEMATOPOIESIS

Extramedullary hemopoiesis is consistently present in liver and spleen, where it contributes to organ enlargement.[4–6] Escape of progenitor cells from marrow and their lodgment in other organs may contribute to extramedullary blood cell formation. Reversion of the liver and spleen to their fetal hematopoietic functions is not considered a major factor in extramedullary hematopoiesis, and quantitatively significant, effective hemopoiesis does not occur outside of the marrow (see "Fibrohematopoietic Extramedullary Tumors" below).

CLINICAL FEATURES

PRESENTING SYMPTOMS

About one fourth of patients are asymptomatic at the time of diagnosis; the disease is detected by medical examination for an unrelated reason. In symptomatic patients, fatigue, weakness, shortness of breath, and palpitations are nonspecific but frequent complaints.[5–9] Weight loss is common, but anorexia is less so and night sweats occur infrequently. A dragging sensation in the left upper abdomen caused by an enlarged spleen or early satiety from encroachment of the spleen on the stomach may occur. Severe left upper quadrant or left shoulder pain can occur from splenic infarction and perisplenitis. Patients may report unexpected bleeding. Occasionally, bone pain is prominent, especially in the lower extremities. Fever, weight loss, night sweats, and bone pain are more frequent later in the course of the disease.

PRESENTING SIGNS

Hepatomegaly is detectable in two thirds of patients, and splenomegaly is present on palpation or imaging studies in almost all patients at the time of diagnosis.[5–9] The spleen is mildly enlarged in one fourth, moderately enlarged in half, and massively enlarged in approximately one fourth of patients. Muscle wasting, peripheral edema, and purpura are present infrequently. Bone tenderness may be present. The latter signs may develop in a larger proportion of patients over the course of the disease. As with most diseases, splenomegaly tends to be identified earlier and with less advanced signs because of increased availability of medical care.

Neutrophilic dermatosis, a syndrome that closely mimics the raised and tender plaques of Sweet syndrome, may occur.[95–97] It can be the presenting or a significant complicating feature and can progress to bullae or pyoderma gangrenosum.[95,98] The dermatopathology of neutrophilic dermatosis is different from leukemia cutis and is unrelated to infection or vasculitis. The predominant lesion is an intense polymorphonuclear neutrophilic infiltrate.

Skin infiltrates related to hematopoietic cells (leukemia cutis) are uncommon.[99] These cutaneous lesions may have myeloid cells with giant cells carrying CD61 markers characteristic of megakaryocytes.[100,101]

SPECIAL CLINICAL FEATURES

PREFIBROTIC IDIOPATHIC MYELOFIBROSIS

The presenting findings of the clonal myeloid diseases are changing because of more and earlier access to health care in industrialized countries (Table 89-2). A subset of patients with idiopathic myelofibrosis present without reticulin fibrosis in the marrow.[102,103] Blood hemoglobin may be normal and white cell count mildly elevated. The classic findings of frequent teardrop red cells, myelocytes, and nucleated red cells in the blood film and palpable splenomegaly often are absent. Thrombocytosis is a nearly constant finding. Essential thrombocythemia is closely simulated, but observation eventually shows evolution to idiopathic myelofibrosis. If noticeable teardrop red cells are present, splenomegaly is evident, or white cell counts are greater than $25,000/\mu l$ (25×10^9/liter), suspicion of prefibrotic myelofibrosis should be raised. The most important distinction is the nature of the megakaryocytic expansion.[104] In idiopathic myelofibrosis, bizarre changes are evident with wide variation in megakaryocyte size from very small to giant size cells. Nuclear lobulation is abnormal, with bulky multilobulation, hypolobulation, and free megakaryocyte nuclei in the marrow spaces. In essential thrombocythemia, megakaryocytes are seen but not the severe dysmorphia observed in myelofibrosis. The prefibrotic disease usually evolves into fully developed myelofibrosis over a period of years.

FIBROHEMATOPOIETIC EXTRAMEDULLARY TUMORS

The appearance of symptoms or signs leading to (1) identification of a mass on imaging regardless of location, (2) appearance of signs or symptoms of an effusion in the thorax or abdomen, (3) unexpected neurologic sign, or (4) another finding that appears unexpected in a patient with idiopathic fibrosis should be considered a fibrohematopoietic tumor(s) until proven otherwise. Foci of hematopoiesis may become clinically apparent as fibrohematopoietic tumors in the adrenal glands,[105,106] renal parenchyma,[107–109] and lymph nodes.[110–112] Tumors composed of hematopoietic tissue, sometimes with intense fibrosis, can develop in the bowel,[113–116] breast,[117–119] liver[120,121] lungs,[122–124] mediastinum,[122] pleura and mesentery,[122,125,126] skin,[127,128] synovium,[129] thymus,[122] thyroid,[130] thorax,[131] prostate,[132] spleen,[133] or urinary tract.[131,134–137]

Extramedullary hematopoiesis in the intracranial or intraspinal epidural space can lead to serious neurologic complications, including subdural hemorrhage,[138] delirium,[139,140] increased intracranial pressure,[140] orbital apex syndrome,[141] papilledema,[142] cerebral tumor,[143] coma,[144] motor and sensory impairment,[145,146] spinal cord compression,[146,147] and limb paralysis.[145,146] Intraspinal myelography,[146–148] computed axial tomography,[138,140,144–150] positron emission tomogra-

phy after ^{52}Fe infusion,[139] and magnetic resonance imaging[151,152] each has been used to define the location and nature of the masses.

Hematopoietic foci on serosal surfaces can produce effusions, sometimes massive, in the thorax,[131,153] abdomen,[125,126,154,155] and pericardial space.[156–159] The effusion fluid often contains megakaryocytes, immature granulocytes, and occasionally erythroblasts.[160–162] Splenectomy is sometimes followed by extramedullary hematopoietic tumors in soft tissues,[163] in body cavities, or on serosal surfaces,[162] perhaps as a result of an increase in circulating hematopoietic progenitors[164] and loss of the filtration function of the spleen. In rare cases, extramedullary soft tissue megakaryoblastic tumors simulate the myeloid sarcomas of other types of myelogenous leukemia.[165,166]

PORTAL HYPERTENSION AND VARICES AND PULMONARY HYPERTENSION

In patients with idiopathic myelofibrosis, there can be a massive increase in splenoportal blood flow and a decrease in hepatic vascular compliance or the presence of hepatic vein thrombosis, either of which can result in severe portal hypertension, ascites, esophageal and gastric varices, intraluminal gastrointestinal bleeding, and hepatic encephalopathy.[167–169] The hepatic venous pressure gradient, normally less than 6 torr, is markedly elevated.[170]

Perisinusoidal fibrosis,[171–173] collagen bundles in the spaces of Disse,[172] perisinusoidal fibroplasia,[171–174] and foci of hematopoietic cells[172,175] each appears to contribute to the decreased sinusoidal compliance. Portal vein thrombosis is a complication of idiopathic myelofibrosis and occasionally precedes disease onset.[176]

Rarely, portal hypertension is accompanied by pulmonary hypertension and may result from pulmonary fibrosis[124] or hydrodynamic factors.[177] Pulmonary hypertension may be the principal problem and can be secondary to megakaryocytopoiesis with fibrosis.[178,179] Contrariwise, secondary myelofibrosis with polyclonal hematopoiesis and normal blood CD34 cell concentrations frequently occurs in patients with primary pulmonary hypertension.[432]

IMMUNE MANIFESTATIONS

Abnormalities of humoral immune mechanisms have been observed in up to half of patients with idiopathic myelofibrosis.[180–185] The array of immune products and events reported includes anti–red cell antibodies,[184,186,187] antiplatelet antibodies,[188,189] antinuclear antibodies,[180,181,185] elevated plasma soluble IL-2 receptor,[190] anti-Gal (galactosidic determinants) antibodies,[191] anti–γ-globulins,[180,182,185]

TABLE 89-2   DIAGNOSTIC FINDINGS IN IDIOPATHIC MYELOFIBROSIS

Prefibrotic Stage
- Anemia may be absent or mild
- Leukocytosis may be absent or slight
- Thrombocythemia very frequent
- *BCR-ABL* fusion gene absent
- Cellular marrow with mild increase in granulopoiesis; clusters of very dysmorphic megakaryocytes and megakaryocytic nuclei; no to very slight increase in reticular fibers on silver stain
- Palpable splenomegaly infrequent
- Absent or slight anisopoikilocytosis including teardrop red cells

Fully Developed Stage
- Diffuse marrow reticular fibrosis plus or minus collagen fibrosis
- *BCR-ABL* fusion gene absent
- Splenomegaly
- Anisopoikilocytosis with teardrop red cells in every oil immersion field
- Immature myeloid cells in blood
- Erythroblasts in blood
- Marrow usually hypercellular but invariably has clusters of highly dysmorphic megakaryocytes and megakaryocyte bare nuclei regardless of overall marrow cellularity

antiphospholipid antibodies,[185,192] antitissue or organ-specific antibodies,[182,184] circulating immune complexes,[185,193-195] as well as complement activation,[185,196] immune complex deposition,[187] interstitial immunoglobulin deposition,[182] increased numbers of marrow plasmacytoid lymphocytes,[182,193] and development of amyloidosis.[194,197] Occasional reports of myelofibrosis associated with lupus erythematosus,[198-203] vasculitis,[204] polyarteritis nodosa,[185,205] ulcerative colitis,[206] scleroderma,[207] biliary cirrhosis,[208] Sjögren syndrome,[209] and acute reversible myelofibrosis responsive to glucocorticoids[210] have raised the possibility that immune mechanisms play a role in the development of marrow fibrosis in some circumstances.

BONE CHANGES

A large proportion of patients have osteosclerosis at diagnosis or develop osteosclerosis during the course of the disease,[7-11,211-214] as reflected by increased bone density on imaging studies and histomorphometric analysis of a bone biopsy[212-217] (Table 89-3). The proximal femur and humerus, pelvis, vertebrae, ribs, and skull may be involved. Magnetic resonance imaging (MRI) can uncover evidence of new bone formation and periosteal thickening. Lumbar spine dual-energy x-ray absorption studies and quantitative computed tomography provide evidence for increased bone formation, bone thickening, and higher proportions of cancellous and of woven bone.[217,218] Osteolytic lesions are rare[219] and may reflect a myeloid sarcoma.[220] Periostitis, although infrequent, can lead to debilitating bone pain.[221]

LABORATORY FEATURES

BLOOD CELL COUNTS AND MORPHOLOGY

The range of values for blood cell counts at the time of diagnosis is very broad. Normocytic–normochromic anemia is present in most, but not all, patients[4-12,222-225] (see Table 89-2). Mean hemoglobin concentration in a series of patients at diagnosis is approximately 9.0 to 12.0 g/dl (range 4–20 g/dl).[4-12,224,225] Anisocytosis and poikilocytosis are a constant finding. In all cases, teardrop-shaped red cells (dacrocytes) are present in sufficient number to be found in every oil-immersion field (Fig. 89-1). Nucleated red cells are present in the blood film of most patients and average 2 percent of nucleated cells (range 0–30%). The percentage of reticulocytes is mildly increased but may vary widely in a given case. Anemia may be worsened by expansion of plasma volume and a higher than normal proportion of the red cell volume in an enlarged spleen. Ineffective erythropoiesis can result in a decrease in red cell mass.[222] Erythroid hypoplasia is present in many patients.[226,227] In some patients, hemolysis may be prominent, and polychromatophilia and very elevated reticulocyte counts can occur.[223,224] The antiglobulin (Coombs) test usually is negative, but red

TABLE 89-3 SERUM, URINE, AND BONE CHANGES REFLECTING OSTEOSCLEROSIS[217,218]

- Increased serum alkaline phosphatase
- Increased serum bone GLA-protein
- Increased serum carboxytelopeptidase
- Increased urinary deoxypyridinoline
- Increased bone density by dual-energy x-ray absorption
- Increased bone density by quantitative computed tomography
- Histomorphometry
    - Increased percentage of cancellous bone volume to tissue volume
    - Increased bone formation and resorption (high turnover)
    - Increased trabecular plate thickness
    - Increased percentage of woven bone volume
    - Increased percentage of fibrous area
    - No evidence of mineralization defect

cell autoantibodies can develop and lead to immune-mediated hemolysis,[185,186,228] which rarely has been the presenting finding of the disease.[187] Occasional patients have a positive acid hemolysis and sucrose hemolysis test, reflecting a concurrent clone of cells consistent with paroxysmal nocturnal hemoglobinuria.[229] Acquired hemoglobin H disease, coincident with typical white cells and platelet changes of myelofibrosis, can occur[230] and results in hemolysis, hypochromic–microcytic red cells, marked poikilocytosis, and hemoglobin H inclusions that stain with brilliant cresyl blue. Red cell aplasia, in association with myelofibrosis, has been observed.[225,231]

The total white cell count usually is mildly elevated as a result of granulocytosis.[4-12] The mean total blood white cell count was 10 to 14 $\times 10^9$/liter in four large studies. The range of white cell counts was 0.4 to 237 $\times 10^9$/liter at the time of diagnosis.[4-11,223,224] Myelocytes and promyelocytes are present in small proportions in most patients, and a low proportion of blast cells (0.5–2%) may be found in the blood film. The blood blast cells range from 0 to 20 percent at the time of diagnosis. In patients with blast counts at the high end, which is unusual at presentation, the disease has converged with AML. Hypersegmentation, hyposegmentation (acquired Pelger-Huët anomaly), and abnormal granulation of neutrophils may be present.[4-12] Neutrophil alkaline phosphatase scores may be elevated (25% of patients) or decreased (25% of patients).[232] The percentage of basophils may be slightly increased.[224] Neutropenia is present in approximately 20 percent of patients at the time of diagnosis.[4-12]

The mean platelet count in patient series can range from 175 to 580 $\times 10^9$/liter at the time of diagnosis. Individual counts can range from 15.0 to 3215 $\times 10^9$/liter.[4-12,223,224] The platelet count is elevated in approximately 40 percent of patients.[224] Mild to moderate thrombocytopenia is present in approximately one third of patients at the time of diagnosis. Giant platelets and abnormal platelet granulation are characteristic features of the disease.

Approximately 10 percent of patients present with pancytopenia because of severe impairment of hematopoiesis affecting each cell lineage, coupled with sequestration in a massively enlarged spleen. Pancytopenia usually is associated with intense marrow fibrosis.

Increased concentrations of pluripotential,[233,234] granulocytic,[235,236] monocytic,[236] erythroid,[237] and megakaryocytic[238] progenitor cells are present in the blood of patients as measured by clonogenic assays in semisolid cultures. The frequency of hematopoietic progenitor cells in the blood is correlated with the extent of marrow reticular fiber density.[238] Megakaryocytes also are present in the systemic venous blood.[239] An increase in blood CD34+ cells is very characteristic of idiopathic myelofibrosis, and the concentration of these cells lends weight to the diagnosis. The height of the CD34+ cell count is correlated with the extent of disease and disease progression. Greater than 15 $\times 10^6$/liter blood CD34+ cells is virtually diagnostic of idiopathic myelofibrosis, and patients with greater than 300 $\times 10^6$/liter CD34+ cells have more rapid progression of disease than patients with fewer CD34+ cells.[234]

Mild lymphocytopenia resulting from decreased CD3+, CD4+, CD8+, and CD3-/CD56+ T cells is the rule.[240]

FUNCTIONAL ABNORMALITIES OF BLOOD CELLS

The neutrophils of some patients have impaired phagocytosis, oxygen consumption, nitroblue tetrazolium reduction, and hydrogen peroxide generation, and decreased myeloperoxidase[241,242] and glutathione reductase activities.[242] CD34+ cells have impaired in vitro differentiation to natural killer cells, which appear to be related to a dysregulation in control of IL-15.[243]

Bleeding time can be prolonged out of proportion to the platelet count.[244,245] Platelet abnormalities include impaired aggregation in re-

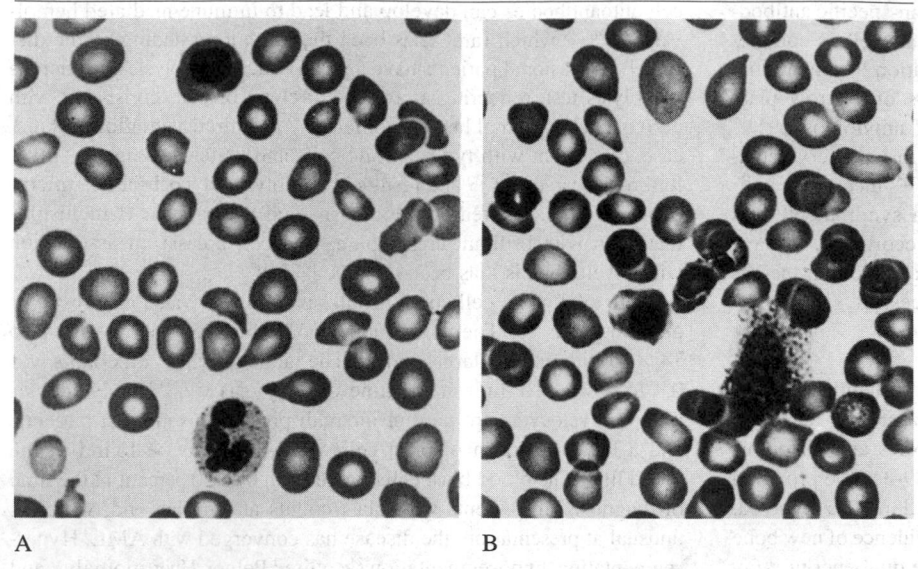

FIGURE 89-1   Blood films from two patients with idiopathic myelofibrosis. *(A)* Characteristic teardrop poikilocytes, a nucleated red cell, and a segmented neutrophil are evident. *(B)* Teardrop red cells, a nucleated red cell, and a promyelocyte are present.

sponse to epinephrine, depletion of dense granule adenosine diphosphate content,[246] decreased platelet lipoxygenase pathway activity,[247] and others.[248,249] Correlation of bleeding or thrombosis with platelet functional abnormalities is weak.[248,249] The lupus anticoagulant has been present but rarely.[192]

MARROW EXAMINATION

MORPHOLOGY
Marrow aspiration often is unsuccessful because of the fibrosis.[4–12,53,54] The marrow biopsy specimen usually is cellular and shows granulocytic and megakaryocytic hyperplasia.[4–12,223,224] Erythroid cells may be decreased, normal, or increased in number. Hematoxylin and eosin stains of the biopsy specimen may show slight collagen fibrosis, but occasionally the fibrosis is extreme. Silver stain usually shows an increase in reticulin fibers, and in half of patients a striking increase in reticulin fibers is seen.[224] In intensely fibrotic marrows, cellularity may be decreased but megakaryocytes usually remain evident.[224] Giant megakaryocytes and micromegakaryocytes, abnormal nuclear lobulation, and naked megakaryocyte nuclei are present.[4–12,250] Thrombopoietin receptors are decreased on megakaryocytes and platelets.[48] Granulocytes may show hyperlobulation and hypolobulation of the nucleus, acquired Pelger-Huët anomaly, nuclear blebs, and nuclear–cytoplasmic maturation asynchrony.[251] Dilated marrow sinusoids are common. Intrasinusoidal, immature hematopoietic cells, and megakaryocytes are present.[53] As a reflection of the high blood flow to marrow-bearing bone and the widened sinusoidal system, microvessel density is significantly increased in approximately 70 percent of patients.[252] Histomorphometric analysis of bone marrow biopsies permit detection of osteosclerosis but imaging is more widely available (see below).[212,214,215]

CYTOGENETIC FINDINGS
Chromosome abnormalities of hematopoietic cells are evident in approximately 40 to 60 percent of patients at the time of diagnosis.[253–258] The most frequent findings are partial trisomy 1q, interstitial deletion of a segment of the long arm of chromosome 13, del 13 (q13q21), which bears the retinoblastoma gene,[41,254–256,259] del 20q, and trisomy 8.[260] Involvement of chromosome 5, 7, 9, 13, 20, or 21 occurs with

heightened frequency.[260] Abnormality of chromosome 12 resulting from several translocations or deletion or inversion occurs in approximately 3 percent of patients.[261] Aneuploidy as a result of monosomy or trisomy is common. Pseudodiploidy, manifested by partial deletions and translocations, occurs. Patients with typical idiopathic myelofibrosis very rarely had the Ph chromosome in their marrow cells.[262] With increasing knowledge of the chromosomes commonly affected, interphase FISH of blood cells is used to look for prevalent abnormalities, compensating for the technical difficulties of harvesting cell suspensions given intense marrow fibrosis.[259] Clonal chromosomal abnormalities found in hematopoietic cells have not been observed in fibroblasts.[94]

MAGNETIC RESONANCE IMAGING
Marrow fibrosis alters the hyperintensity of T1-weighted images that normally results from marrow fat. As cellularity and fibrosis progress, hypointensity of T1-weighted and T2-weighted images develops. MRI does not distinguish between idiopathic myelofibrosis and secondary causes of fibrosis,[213,263,264] but the clinical distinctions usually are very evident from the results of prior physical, blood, and marrow examinations. Patchy or diffuse osteosclerosis is a common finding, as are "sandwich vertebrae," so called because of marked radiodensity of superior and inferior margins of the vertebral body. MRI can identify the uncommon periosteal reactions that usually occur in the distal femur, proximal tibia, or ankle. The reactions represent expansion of marrow cellularity into normally inactive regions of long bones or extramedullary space-occupying lesions of fibrohematopoietic tissue.[213] The findings of sodium fluoride (^{18}F) positron emission tomography can be virtually specific for osteosclerosis of idiopathic myelofibrosis.[265]

PLASMA AND URINE CHEMICAL CHANGES
Serum levels of uric acid, lactic dehydrogenase, bilirubin, alkaline phosphatase, and high-density lipoprotein frequently are elevated.[4–12] Serum levels of albumin and cholesterol frequently are decreased.[266] Hypocalcemia[267] or hypercalcemia[268] may occur. Plasma levels of thrombopoietin and IL-6 are elevated but do not correlate with either platelet or megakaryocyte mass.[269,270] Elevated thrombopoietin is not explained by increased marrow hematopoietic or stromal cell production.[271] Serum soluble IL-2 receptor[272] and serum vascular endothelial growth factor[273] levels are increased. Urinary excretion of calmodulin is approximately three times normal.[85] The serum contains evidence of increased collagen (see Table 89-1) and bone (see Table 89-2) synthesis.

DIFFERENTIAL DIAGNOSIS
CML (see Chap. 88) should be considered in the differential diagnosis of idiopathic myelofibrosis. In CML, the white cell count is greater than 30×10^9/liter (30,000/μl) in almost all patients and greater than 100×10^9/liter (100,000/μl) in half of patients. In myelofibrosis, the white cell count usually is less than 30×10^9/l (30,000/μl) at the time of diagnosis. In CML, red cell shape usually is normal or slightly perturbed. In myelofibrosis, teardrop poikilocytes are present in every oil-immersion field and exaggerated anisocytosis and anisochromia are often prominent. The marrow in CML shows intense granulocytic hyperplasia, with almost

100 percent cellularity and usually no or very slight fibrosis.[274] In myelofibrosis, the marrow has mildly increased cellularity or is hypocellular, with moderate to marked fibrosis. Occasionally, patients with CML develop intense marrow fibrosis and dysmorphic blood cell changes that make distinction between the two diseases difficult.[274] However, the Ph chromosome or the *BCR-ABL* fusion gene is present in CML and absent in idiopathic myelofibrosis. Most cases are readily separable based on the aforementioned distinctions.

Patients with idiopathic myelofibrosis may have pancytopenia or bicytopenia and in that respect mimic patients with oligoblastic leukemia (myelodysplasia [MDS]; see Chap. 86). Contrariwise, patients with oligoblastic leukemia may rarely have intense fibrosis.[275] Prominent splenomegaly is expected in patients with idiopathic myelofibrosis but not in patients with oligoblastic leukemia, which helps to distinguish the former from the latter patients. The absence of a high frequency of teardrop-shaped red cells, nucleated red cells, and striking aniso-poikilocytosis mitigates against idiopathic myelofibrosis.

Because some patients with idiopathic myelofibrosis have platelet counts greater than 600,000 × 10⁹/liter, the diagnosis of primary thrombocythemia may be considered. The aniso-poikilocytosis, nucleated red cells, and myeloid immaturity in the blood film characteristic of myelofibrosis are not present in patients with thrombocythemia. Marrow fibrosis usually is insignificant in thrombocythemia, and splenic enlargement often is absent or slight. For these reasons, a clear distinction usually exists between the two disorders.[224,276] The prefibrotic phase of idiopathic myelofibrosis may mimic essential thrombocythemia, but the more prominent splenomegaly and the more disordered megakaryopoiesis can be used to distinguish the two entities, as does careful observation of disease evolution.[277]

Hairy cell leukemia (see Chap. 93), when associated with shape abnormalities of red cells, pancytopenia, splenomegaly, and fibrotic marrow, can closely mimic idiopathic myelofibrosis.[275,278] Usually, careful scrutiny of the blood and marrow by microscopy, histochemistry, and cell immunophenotype shows evidence of the abnormal mononuclear (hairy) cells characterizing the disease.

Hepatic disease can be associated with cytopenias and splenomegaly, although the specific blood and marrow findings usually make the distinction with idiopathic myelofibrosis obvious. In a review of 170 cases of splenomegaly in a county hospital, hepatic disease was the second most common cause of massive splenomegaly after idiopathic myelofibrosis.[279]

Primary autoimmune myelofibrosis is characterized by intense marrow fibrosis and an increase in marrow polyclonal T and B lymphocytes.[280] Serologic or clinical evidence of lupus erythematosus or other connective tissue diseases is absent, giving primary autoimmune myelofibrosis a definitive diagnostic niche. Cytopenias that occur may be immune mediated (e.g., immune hemolytic disease), and the blood cell findings (poikiloanisocytosis, nucleated red cells, myeloid immaturity) characteristic of idiopathic myelofibrosis usually are absent. The marrow may be cellular with increased megakaryocytes, but strikingly dysmorphic megakaryocytopoiesis is absent. Splenomegaly, a nearly constant feature of idiopathic myelofibrosis, usually is absent. Polyclonal hyperglobulinemia may be present.

Metastatic carcinoma, especially derived from carcinoma of breast or prostate tumors[281-286] or disseminated mycobacterial infection,[287,288] can induce reactive marrow fibrosis and occasionally simulate idiopathic myelofibrosis. Demonstration of metastatic carcinoma cells or mycobacteria in the marrow indicates the etiology. Other disorders reported with secondary myelofibrosis include mastocytosis,[289-292] angioimmunoblastic lymphadenopathy,[293] angiosarcoma,[294] lymphoma,[295-297] multiple myeloma,[298-303] renal osteodystrophy,[304] hypertrophic osteoarthropathy,[305] gray platelet syndrome,[306] systemic lupus erythematosus,[198-201] polyarteritis nodosa,[204] hypereosinophilic syndrome,[307,308] kala azar,[309] idiopathic thrombocytopenic purpura,[310] thrombotic thrombocytopenic purpura,[311] tretinoin administration,[312] neuroblastoma,[313] giant lymph node hyperplasia,[314] vitamin D deficiency rickets,[315-318] Langerhans cell histiocytosis,[319] acute promyelocytic leukemia,[320,321] and malignant histiocytosis.[322] Correction or amelioration of the primary disorder can lead to disappearance of the marrow fibrosis.

Lymphoma,[323,324] chronic lymphocytic leukemia,[325,326] hairy cell leukemia,[327] macroglobulinemia,[328] amyloidosis,[194,197] myeloma,[329,330] malignant teratoma,[331] and essential monoclonal gammopathy[332] reportedly coincide with idiopathic myelofibrosis.

TRANSITIONS TO AND FROM MYELOFIBROSIS AMONG CLONAL HEMOPATHIES

All clonal hematopoietic diseases (AML, CML, oligoblastic leukemia [MDS], lymphomas) may have increased marrow reticulin fibers but only infrequently have collagen fibrosis.[333] Acute megakaryoblastic leukemia is accompanied by intense marrow fibrosis (see Chap. 87). Approximately 15 percent of patients with polycythemia vera, whether treated by phlebotomy, alkylating agents, or ³²P, develop a clinical state indistinguishable from idiopathic myelofibrosis during 20 years of observation[334-336] (see Chap. 56). Essential thrombocythemia may evolve into a myelofibrotic stage, estimated to occur in approximately 7 percent of cases. This estimate is complicated by the question of whether some cases of essential thrombocythemia actually are very early (prefibrotic) idiopathic myelofibrosis.[277] Sideroblastic anemia has progressed to idiopathic myelofibrosis.[337] Rarely, idiopathic myelofibrosis reverts to polycythemia vera, with disappearance of marrow fibrosis.[338-340]

THERAPY

DECISION TO TREAT

A significant proportion (approximately 30%) of asymptomatic patients remain stable for years and do not require specific treatment. Symptomatic anemia, thrombocytopenia, and splenomegaly are the principal initial reasons for therapy.

ANDROGENS AND GLUCOCORTICOIDS

Severe anemia may improve with androgen therapy in some patients.[341-343] Testosterone, oxymetholone, and fluoxymesterone have been used but have virilizing effects. In addition, they have the potential for hepatic injury and other side effects. Danazol 600 to 800 mg/day orally for up to six months can be used. The drug is tapered to the minimum effective dose or discontinued if no significant response occurs.[343] Improvement may be limited to a decreased frequency of red cell transfusion. Androgens often are used after splenectomy if anemia returns and requires transfusion of red cells. Patients undergoing androgen therapy should have periodic assessment of liver size by physical examination, measurement of liver function tests, and, if appropriate, ultrasound imaging to detect liver injury (e.g., peliosis) or tumors.[344] Patients with significant hemolytic anemia may benefit from glucocorticoid therapy. Prednisone 25 mg/m²/day orally can be tried. If tolerated, the dose can be continued for 1 to 2 months and then tapered gradually. In children, high-dose glucocorticoid therapy reportedly ameliorates marrow fibrosis and improves hematopoiesis.[345,346]

RECOMBINANT HUMAN ERYTHROPOIETIN

Serum erythropoietin levels are appropriate to the severity of anemia in patients with myelofibrosis.[347] Use of erythropoietin for treatment of anemia has been largely unsuccessful.[348–350] Although one study suggested some benefit, evaluation of treatment was complicated by concomitant interferon therapy.[351]

DRUG THERAPY

A variety of drugs have been used for treatment of massive splenomegaly, thrombocytosis, or constitutional symptoms.

HYDROXYUREA

Hydroxyurea has become the most commonly used and preferred agent. [352–354] Hydroxyurea can decrease the size of the spleen and liver, decrease or eliminate constitutional symptoms of night sweats or weight loss, and lead to an increase in hemoglobin concentration, a decrease of elevated platelet counts, and occasionally a decrease in the degree of marrow fibrosis. Patients with myelofibrosis often do not have the marrow tolerance to chemotherapy of patients with other chronic myeloproliferative diseases. Hydroxyurea can be administered in doses of 0.5 to 1.0 g/day or 1.0 to 2.0 g orally two to three times per week, depending on the level of pretreatment blood cell counts. Patients should be evaluated for dose adjustment at least every week for 1 month and, if appropriate, extended to every 2 weeks for 2 months. Thereafter, monthly evaluation of dose may be appropriate. Although alkylating agents, especially busulfan and other cytotoxic agents, have been used successfully, they have largely been replaced by hydroxyurea. Use of alkylating agents has resurfaced with the suggestion that melphalan may be useful as first-line therapy.[355]

CYTARABINE

Ascites resulting from peritoneal hematopoietic implants has been treated with intraperitoneal cavity cytarabine.[356] Intrasplenic cytarabine administered via a splenic artery catheter has resulted in significant improvement in a patient.[357]

THALIDOMIDE

Thalidomide is poorly tolerated at optimal doses of approximately 800 mg/day. Most patients receive about half that amount and are tapered to the lowest effective dose. One study of 14 patients found the drug was not beneficial and had high toxicity rates.[358] A second study found some decrease in spleen size and improvement in blood hemoglobin and platelet counts in a minority of patients receiving up to 600 mg/day.[359,434] In subsequent studies, lower doses of thalidomide (50 mg/day) coupled with prednisone were more tolerable and resulted in improvement of anemia and thrombocytopenia in about half of patients, with sustained improvement in some patients after treatment was stopped.[433]

CYCLOSPORINE, ETANERCEPT, IMATINIB MESYLATE, AND TIPIFARNIB

Cyclosporine has been used to achieve a serum level of 100 to 200 ng/ml in severely anemic patients with evidence of immune abnormalities (positive Coombs test, antinuclear antibodies).[360] Three of six patients responded with an increased hemoglobin concentration. Cyclosporine has been used with apparent success in a single patient with myelofibrosis and red cell aplasia.[361]

Tumor necrosis factor alpha has been proposed as a target to inhibit its possible effects in the pathogenesis of idiopathic myelofibrosis.[362] Of 20 patients treated with soluble tumor necrosis factor alpha receptor, 12 had improvement in constitutional symptoms (fever, night sweats, fatigue, weight loss), and four had improved blood counts and decreased spleen size.[363]

Imatinib mesylate for treatment of myelofibrosis has been examined on empirical grounds and has been largely ineffective in influencing the disease course.[364] Modest doses have not been well tolerated, and responses have been infrequent and insubstantial.

The farnesyl transferase inhibitor tipifarnib is not well tolerated. Although it may decrease spleen size, it has shown no advantages over hydroxyurea.

INTRAVENOUS IMMUNOGLOBULIN

Although autoimmune or systemic lupus erythematosus-related myelofibrosis has responded to glucocorticoids or intravenous immune globulin[200,203] and a variety of fibrotic disorders occasionally respond,[428] idiopathic myelofibrosis does not have a sustained response to such therapy because the fundamental lesion is the hematopoietic stem cell neoplasm, severe megakaryocytic dysmorphia, and cytokine release with resultant fibrogenesis and osteogenesis.

INTERFERONS

Interferon-α and interferon-γ act synergistically to inhibit myeloproliferation.[365] The former has been used extensively for treatment of CML (see Chap. 88). Interferon-α has not been used extensively in idiopathic myelofibrosis but has been useful for treatment of splenic enlargement, bone pain, and thrombocytosis in selected patients.[366] Trials comparing interferon therapy with hydroxyurea or other therapy have not been reported.[367] Hydroxyurea is easier to use and has less frequent side effects than interferon.

BISPHOSPHONATES

Debilitating bone pain can be a vexing problem in some patients with osteosclerosis and periostitis. Dramatic improvement in bone pain and hematopoiesis after etidronate 6 mg/kg/day on alternate months[368] or clodronate 30 mg/kg/day for several months, during which marked improvement was still present 33 months later,[369] highlight the potential usefulness of this family of drugs.

RADIOTHERAPY

Radiotherapy can be useful for patients with idiopathic myelofibrosis in several situations. For example, in the presence of (1) severe splenic pain (splenic infarctions) or (2) massive splenic enlargement with contraindication to splenectomy (e.g., thrombocytosis),[370–372] repeated doses of 0.5 to 2 Gy to the spleen can ameliorate the pain.[373] Other situations in which radiation may be useful are (3) ascites resulting from myeloid metaplasia of the peritoneum,[374] (4) focal areas of severe bone pain (periostitis or the osteolysis of a myeloid sarcoma,[221,375] and (5) extramedullary fibrohematopoietic tumors,[110] especially of the epidural space.[148] Low-dose radiation to the liver for symptomatic hepatomegaly and ascites provides only short-term relief.[376] Low-dose radiotherapy to the lung has been used successfully to palliate the effects of pulmonary hypertension thought to result from extensive extramedullary hematopoiesis in the organ. Low-dose radiotherapy has relieved signs of respiratory insufficiency, especially hypoxemia.[179]

SPLENECTOMY

Splenectomy has been important in the management of idiopathic myelofibrosis.[377–381] The major indications for splenectomy include (1) painful enlarged spleen, (2) excessive transfusion requirements or refractory hemolytic anemia, (3) severe thrombocytopenia, and (4) portal hypertension.

Patients who have a prolonged bleeding time or coagulation times are at serious risk for hemorrhage with surgery and should not undergo the procedure unless the abnormalities can be corrected by platelet transfusion and factor replacement therapy. Evidence of low-grade intravascular coagulation, such as elevated D-dimer levels, may require prophylactic heparin therapy and platelet transfusion should excessive bleeding occur. In one series of 223 patients who underwent splenectomy, the basis for the procedure included transfusion-dependent anemia in 45 percent, symptomatic splenomegaly in 39 percent, portal hypertension in 11 percent, and severe thrombocytopenia in 5 percent.[379]

Removal of the spleen in patients with idiopathic myelofibrosis may be difficult. Usually the spleen is adherent to neighboring serosal surfaces and structures and has numerous collateral vessels and very dilated splenoportal arteries and veins. Immediate postoperative mortality is a function of surgical experience and skill and of the rapidity of recognition of postoperative complications. In experienced hands, perioperative mortality is approximately 10 percent. Postoperative morbidity from hemorrhage, subphrenic hematoma, subphrenic abscess, injury to the tail of the pancreas, pancreatic fistulas, or portal vein stump thrombosis occurs in approximately 30 percent of patients. Later, postoperative changes include liver enlargement,[379,382] extramedullary hematopoietic tumors,[159,163] and a decrease in teardrop-shaped red cells.[383] Blast transformation occurs in approximately 15 percent of patients after splenectomy.[379] Postoperative liver enlargement and thrombocytosis have responded to treatment with cladribine.[384] Anagrelide may be useful for exaggerated thrombocytosis (see Chap. 111). The morbidity and mortality from splenectomy and the modest extension of life have led to increasing conservatism regarding its use.[379,385] However, splenectomy can improve the state of patients who are selected carefully and in a timely fashion.

Among 91 patients who underwent subtotal splenectomy preserving the upper pole of the spleen and its blood supply, five had idiopathic myelofibrosis. No surgical mortality occurred, but details of outcome were not reported.[386]

PORTAL-SYSTEMIC VASCULAR SHUNT SURGERY

Circulatory dynamic studies are performed at the time of surgery in patients undergoing operation for portal hypertension and bleeding varices or refractory ascites. In patients in whom the hepatic wedge pressure elevations result from markedly increased blood flow from the spleen to the liver, the preferred treatment procedure for portal hypertension is splenectomy. In patients who have portal hypertension resulting from intrahepatic block or hepatic vein thrombosis and have a hepatic venous pressure gradient well above the upper limits of normal (6 torr), a splenorenal shunt can be performed[387] or, to avoid abdominal surgery, a transjugular intrahepatic portosystemic shunt can be used.[388,389] Variceal sclerotherapy or variceal ligation has been used to treat bleeding varices resulting from portal hypertension.[179]

MARROW CURETTAGE, COLLAGEN SYNTHESIS INHIBITORS, VITAMIN D CONGENERS, IMMUNOGLOBULINS, AND CYCLOSPORINES

Several experimental forms of therapy have been used in a small number of patients. Hematologic remission has been described in one case of myelofibrosis treated by bilateral iliac crest marrow curettage.[390]

Investigative approaches to the disease include use of agents that prevent collagen formation, such as monoamine oxidase inhibitors and lysyl aldehyde chelators such as dehydroproline.[391]

1,25-Dihydroxyvitamin D therapy was associated with improvement of patients with myelofibrosis, although hypercalcemia and hypophosphatemia may prevent continued use.[392] The mechanism of action could relate to a profound antiproliferative effect of 1,25-dihydroxyvitamin D on megakaryocytes, which are the putative source of most of the fibroblast activation factors. No benefit was seen with administration of this

vitamin D analogue in two other reports.[393,394] 1,25-Dihydroxycholecalciferol reportedly ameliorates myelofibrosis.[395] Single cases of improved hematopoiesis and decreased osteosclerosis after intravenous immune globulin[396,428] and sustained improvement in anemia after cyclosporine[397] have been reported.

STEM CELL TRANSPLANTATION

Marrow transplantation therapy has been used increasingly in younger patients with a poor prognosis (e.g., severe anemia and leukopenia or exaggerated leukocytosis) who have a histocompatible sibling.[398–402] Patients engraft at a rate similar to the rate of patients with hematologic diseases without marrow fibrosis[400] (see Chap. 22). Although splenectomy increases the rapidity of neutrophil recovery, the procedure has very high risk. Overall, patients splenectomized before transplant do not fare better than patients not splenectomized.[429]

A study of 66 patients found a markedly different outcome in patients transplanted when they were younger than 45 years (62% 5-year survival) compared with patients who were transplanted when they were older than 45 years (14% 5-year survival). In that analysis, osteosclerosis and prior total body radiation was associated with more severe acute graft-versus-host disease.[403,404] Better results in older patients were described in a brief report. In this latter report of more than 50 patients transplanted, the 23 patients who were older than 45 years had a 3-year disease-free survival of 63 percent and a 5-year disease-free survival of 50 percent.[405] Donor lymphocyte infusion in two patients who had lost donor dominance of hematopoiesis and a return of myelofibrosis resulted in regression of fibrosis and return to normal hematopoiesis for at least 6 and 20 months, respectively, at the time of reporting.[406,407]

The option of nonmyeloablative transplantation in older patients was tested on four patients aged 48 to 58 years. The patients were treated with fludarabine and melphalan and given granulocyte colony stimulating factor (G-CSF) mobilized blood stem cells from a human leukocyte antigen–compatible sibling. All four had rapid engraftment of neutrophils and platelets, stable full-donor chimerism, significantly reduced splenic size and marrow fibrosis, and normal marrow cellularity.[408] Similar results from nonmyeloablative transplantation were achieved in a study of four patients.[409,435] Autologous blood stem cells mobilized with G-CSF and administered after busulfan conditioning to 21 patients with idiopathic myelofibrosis aged 45 to 75 years produced clinical benefit, including improved erythropoiesis, improved platelet counts, and decreased splenic size in a plurality of patients. The 2-year actuarial survival rate was 61 percent.[410]

COURSE AND PROGNOSIS

The rate of disease progression has been associated with at least 13 variables measured at the time of diagnosis. Shorter survival has been associated with older age, male gender, severity of anemia, severity of thrombocytopenia, exaggerated leukocytosis or leukopenia, proportion of blast cells in the blood, proportion of CD34+ cells in the blood, a decreased proliferating cell nuclear antigen index and a decreased apoptotic index by in situ end labeling, degree of liver enlargement, extent of marrow fibrosis, abnormal clonal cytogenetic abnormalities, postsplenectomy spleen histology, and constitutional symptoms of fever, sweating, or weight loss at the time of diagnosis. Each retrospective study has found a different subset of these factors to be significant prognostic factors. The most consistent predictive variables appear to be advanced age, severity of anemia, and clonal cytogenetic abnormality at the time of diagnosis, each of which represents a poor prognostic indicator.[4,8–10,12,233,234,256,411–414]

The median survival of all patients with idiopathic myelofibrosis is approximately 5 years from the time of diagnosis.[411] The 5-year survival is approximately 40 percent of the survival expected for healthy age- and sex-matched controls.[415] Retrospective analysis of prognostic variables permits stratification of patients into slowly progressive and rapidly progressive cohorts.[223,412]

The major causes of death are infection, hemorrhage, postsplenectomy mortality, and acute leukemic transformation.[416–419] Acute leukemia occasionally is preceded by the development of myeloid sarcomas.[220,377,420] Evolution of the disease to acute lymphocytic leukemia or lymphoma may occur.[421,422] An increased risk of progression to leukemia has been reported in splenectomized patients.[423] Rare spontaneous remissions of apparent idiopathic myelofibrosis have been documented.[424,425]

Idiopathic myelofibrosis in infants and children has a more varied pathobiology than in adults. Patients have been followed for decades without requiring significant treatment,[426] and spontaneous remission has been described.[427] Because of its variable course, conservative management may be appropriate while the course of the disease is followed.

REFERENCES

1. Heuck G: Zwei Fälle von Leukämie mit eigenthümlichem Blut-resp Knochenmarksbefund. *Virchows Arch (Pathol Anat)* 78:475, 1879.
2. Silverstein MN: *Agnogenic Myeloid Metaplasia*. Publishing Science, Boston, 1975.
3. Heller EL, Lewisohn MG, Palin WE: Aleukemic myelosis, chronic non-leukemic myelosis, agnogenic myeloid metaplasia, osteosclerosis, leukoerythroblastic anemia, and synonymous designations. *Am J Pathol* 23: 327, 1947.
4. Barosi G: Myelofibrosis with myeloid metaplasia. *Hematol Clin North Am* 17:1211, 2003.
5. Ward HP, Block MH: The natural history of agnogenic myeloid metaplasia (AMM) and a critical evaluation of its relationship with myeloproliferative syndrome. *Medicine* 50:357, 1971.
6. Varki A, Lottenberg R, Griffith R, et al: The syndrome of idiopathic myelofibrosis. *Medicine* 62:353, 1983.
7. Barosi G: Myelofibrosis with myeloid metaplasia. *Hematol Oncol Clin North Am* 17:1211, 2003.
8. Okamura T, Kinukawa N, Niho Y, Mizoguichi H: Primary chronic myelofibrosis: Clinical and prognostic evaluation in 336 Japanese patients. *Int J Hematol* 73:194, 2001.
9. Cervantes F, Pereira A, Esteve J, et al: Idiopathic myelofibrosis: Initial features, evolutionary pattern and survival in a series of 106 patients. *Med Clin North Am* 109:651, 1997.
10. Dupriez B, Morel P, Demory JL, et al: Prognostic factors in agnogenic myeloid metaplasia: A report on 195 cases with a new scoring system. *Blood* 88:1013, 1996.
11. Rupoli S, DaLio L, Sisti S, et al: Primary myelofibrosis: A detailed analysis of the clinicopathologic variables influencing survival. *Ann Hematol* 68:205, 1994.
12. Ozen S, Ferhanoglu B, Senocak M, Tüzüner N: Idiopathic myelofibrosis (agnogenic myeloid metaplasia). *Leuk Res* 21:125, 1997.
13. Shalev O, Goldfarb A, Ariel I, et al: Myelofibrosis in young adults. *Acta Haematol* 70:396, 1983.
14. Sekhar M, Prentice HG, Poyat U, et al: Idiopathic myelofibrosis in children. *Br J Haematol* 93:394, 1996.
15. Cervantes F, Barosi G, Demory JL, et al: Myelofibrosis with myeloid metaplasia in young individuals: Disease characteristics, prognostic factors and identification of risk groups. *Br J Haematol* 102:684, 1998.
16. Cohn SL, Cohn RA, Chou P, et al: Infantile myelofibrosis with nephromegaly secondary to myeloid metaplasia. *Clin Pediatr* 30:59, 1991.
17. Mallouh AA, Sa'di AR: Agnogenic myeloid metaplasia in children. *Am J Dis Child* 146:965, 1992.
18. Cervantes F, Barosi G, Hernández-Boluda J-C, et al: Myelofibrosis with myeloid metaplasia in adult individuals 30 years old or younger: Presenting features, evolution and survival. *Eur J Haematol* 66:324, 2001.
19. Segel GB, Lichtman MA: Familial (inherited) leukemia, lymphoma, and myeloma. *Blood Cells Mol Dis* 32:246, 2004.
20. Kaufman S, Briere J, Bernard J: Familial myeloproliferative syndromes: Study of 6 families and review of literature. *Nouv Rev Fr Hematol* 20: 1, 1978.
21. Péres-Encinas M, Bello JL, Perez-Crespo S, et al: Familial myeloproliferative syndrome. *Am J Hematol* 46:225, 1994.
22. Kutty J, Ridell B: Epidemiology of the myeloproliferative disorders: Essential thrombocythaemia, polycythemia vera, and idiopathic myelofibrosis. *Pathol Biol* 49:164, 2001.
23. McNally RJ, Rowland D, Roman E, Cartwright RA: Age and sex distributions of haematological malignancies in the U.K. *Hematol Oncol* 15:173, 1997.
24. Ridell B, Carneskog J, Wedel H, et al: Incidence of chronic myeloproliferative disorders in the city of Gotesborg, Sweden 1983–1992. *Eur J Haematol* 65:267, 2000.
25. Mesa RA, Silverstein MN, Jacobsen SJ, et al: Population-based incidence and survival figures in essential thrombocythemia and agnogenic myeloid metaplasia: An Olmstead County Study 1976–1995. *Am J Hematol* 61:10, 1999.
26. Wendling F, Varlet P, Charon M, Tambourin P: MPLV: A retrovirus complex inducing an acute myeloproliferative leukemic disorder in adult mice. *Virology* 149:242, 1986.
27. Kaushansky K: Thrombopoietin. *N Engl J Med* 339:746, 1998.
28. Yan X-Q, Lacey D, Hill D, et al: A model of myelofibrosis and osteosclerosis in mice induced by overexpressing thrombopoietin (mpl ligand). *Blood* 88:402, 1996.
29. Villeval JL, Cohen-Solal K, Tuliez M, et al: High thrombopoietin production by hematopoietic cells induces a fatal myeloproliferative syndrome in mice. *Blood* 90:4396, 1997.
30. Aksoy M, Erdem S, Dincol G: Two rare complications of chronic benzene poisoning: Myeloid metaplasia and paroxysmal nocturnal hemoglobinuria. *Blut* 30:255, 1975.
31. Hu H: Benzene-associated myelofibrosis. *Ann Intern Med* 106:171, 1987.
32. Tondel M, Perrson B, Carstensen J: Myelofibrosis and benzene exposure. *Occup Med* 45:31, 1995.
33. Anderson RE, Hoshino T, Yamamoto T: Myelofibrosis with myeloid metaplasia in survivors of the atomic bomb in Hiroshima. *Ann Intern Med* 60:1, 1964.
34. Dungworth DL, Goldman M, Switzer JW, et al: Development of a myeloproliferative disorder in beagles continuously exposed to ^{90}Sr. *Blood* 34:610, 1969.
35. Jacobson RS, Salo A, Fialkow PS: Agnogenic myeloid metaplasia: A clonal proliferation of hematopoietic stem cells with secondary myelofibrosis. *Blood* 51:189, 1978.
36. Kahn A, Bernard JF, Cottreau D, et al: A deficient G-6-PD variant with hemizygous expression in blood cells of a woman with primary myelofibrosis. *Humangenetik* 30:41, 1975.
37. Sato Y, Suda T, Suda J, et al: Multilineage expression of haemopoietic precursors with an abnormal clone in idiopathic myelofibrosis. *Br J Haematol* 64:657, 1986.
38. Kreipe H, Jaquet K, Falgner J, et al: Clonal granulocytes and bone marrow cells in the cellular phase of agnogenic myeloid metaplasia. *Blood* 78:1814, 1991.
39. Tsukamoto N, Morita K, Maehara T, et al: Clonality in chronic myeloproliferative disorders defined by X-chromosome linked probes. *Br J Haematol* 86:253, 1994.

40. Buschle M, Janssen JWG, Drexler H, et al: Evidence for pluripotent stem cell origin of idiopathic myelofibrosis: Clonal analysis of a case characterized by a N-ras gene mutation. *Leukemia* 2:658, 1988.

41. Lebowitz P, Papac R, Ghosh PK: Impaired retinoblastoma susceptibility (Rb) gene expression in agnogenic myeloid metaplasia. *Blood* 76(suppl 1):236A, 1990.

42. Reeder TL, Bailey RJ, Dewald GW, Tefferi A: Both B and T lymphocytes may be clonally involved in myelofibrosis with myeloid metaplasia. *Blood* 101:1981, 2003.

43. Mitterbauer G, Winkler K, Gisslinger H, et al: Clonality analysis using X-chromosome inactivation at the human androgen receptor gene (*HUMARA*). *Am J Clin Pathol* 112:93, 1999.

44. Gale RE, Fielding AK, Harrison CN, Linch DC: Acquired skewing of X-chromosome inactivation patterns in myeloid cells of the elderly suggests stochastic clonal loss with age. *Br J Haematol* 98:512, 1997.

45. Abu-Duhier FM, Goodeve AC, Care RS, et al: Mutational analysis of class III receptor tyrosine kinases (C-KIT, C-FMS, FLT3) in idiopathic myelofibrosis. *Br J Haematol* 120:464, 2003.

46. Giraudier S, Chagraoui H, Komura E, et al: Overexpression of FKBP51 in idiopathic myelofibrosis regulates the growth factor independence of megakaryocyte progenitors. *Blood* 100:2932, 2002.

47. Wang JC, Chen C, Lou LH, et al: Blood thrombopoietin, IL-6, and IL-11 levels in patients with agnogenic myeloid metaplasia. *Leukemia* 11:1827, 1997.

48. Moliterno AR, Hankins WD, Spivak JL: Impaired expression of the thrombopoietin receptor by patients with polycythemia vera. *N Engl J Med* 338:572, 1998.

49. Temerinac S, Klippel S, Strunck E, et al: Cloning of PRV-1, a novel member of the uPAR receptor superfamily, which is overexpressed in polycythemia rubra vera. *Blood* 95:2569, 2000.

50. Liu E, Jelinek J, Pastore YD, et al: Discrimination of polycythemia and thrombocytoses by novel, simple, accurate clonality assays and comparison of PRV-1 expression and BFU-E response to erythropoietin. *Blood* 101.3294, 2003.

51. Prockop DJ, Kivirikko KI, Tuderman L, et al: The biosynthesis of collagen and its disorders. *N Engl J Med* 301:13, 1979.

52. Bauermeister DE: Quantitation of bone marrow reticulin: A normal range. *Am J Clin Pathol* 56:24, 1971.

53. Ivànyi JL, Mahunka M, Papp A, Telek B: Prognostic significance of bone marrow reticulum fibers in idiopathic myelofibrosis: Evolution of clinicopathological parameters in a scoring system. *Haematologica* 26:75, 1994.

54. McCarthy DM: Annotation: Fibrosis of the bone marrow: Content and causes. *Br J Haematol* 59:1, 1985.

55. Apaja-Sarkkinen M, Autio-Harmainen H, Alavaikko M, et al: Immunohistochemical study of basement membrane proteins and type III procollagen in myelofibrosis. *Br J Haematol* 63:571, 1986.

56. Hasselbalch H, Junker P, Lisse I, et al: Serum markers for type IV collagen and type III procollagen in the myelofibrosis-osteomyelosclerosis syndrome and other chronic myeloproliferative disorders. *Am J Hematol* 23:101, 1986.

57. Reilly JT: Pathogenesis of idiopathic myelofibrosis: Role of growth factors. *J Clin Pathol* 45:461, 1992.

58. Charron D, Robert L, Couty MC, Binet JL: Biochemical and histological analysis of bone marrow collagen in myelofibrosis. *Br J Haematol* 41:151, 1979.

59. Podolak-Dawidziak M, Wróbel T, Jelen M: Serum concentration of the amino terminal peptide of type III procollagen (PIIINP) in patients with myeloproliferative disorders (MPD). *Pol Arch Med Wewn* 99:24, 1998.

60. Gay S, Gay RE, Prohal JT: Immunohistological studies of bone marrow collagen, in *Myelofibrosis and the Biology of Connective Tissue*, edited by P Berk, H Castro-Malaspina, LR Wasserman, p 291. Alan R. Liss, New York, 1984.

61. Hasselbalch H, Junker P, Horslev-Patersen K, et al: Procollagen type III amino-terminal peptide in serum in idiopathic myelofibrosis and allied conditions. *Am J Hematol* 33:18, 1990.

62. Reilly JT, Nash JRG, Mackie MJ, McVerry BA: Endothelial cell proliferation in myelofibrosis. *Br J Haematol* 60:625, 1985.

63. Baglin TP, Crocker MA, Timmins A, et al: Bone marrow hypervascularity in patients with myelofibrosis identified by infrared thermography. *Clin Lab Haematol* 13:341, 1991.

64. Dolan G, Forrest P, Eastham J, et al: Serum laminin, procollagen terminal peptide III and thrombocyte platelet derived growth factor concentrations in idiopathic myelofibrosis. *Br J Haematol* 77(suppl 1):73, 1991.

65. Reilly JT, Nash JRG, Mackie MJ, McVerry BA: Immunoenzymatic detection of fibronectin in normal and pathological haemopoietic tissue. *Br J Haematol* 59:497, 1985.

66. Hasselbalch H, Clemmensen I: Plasma fibronectin in idiopathic myelofibrosis and related chronic myeloproliferative disorders. *Scand J Clin Lab Invest* 47:429, 1987.

67. Soini Y, Kamel D, Apaja-Sarkkinen M, et al: Tenascin immunoreactivity in normal and pathological bone marrow. *J Clin Pathol* 46:218, 1993.

68. Reilly JT, Nash JRG: Vitronectin (serum spreading factor): Its localization in normal and fibrotic tissue. *J Clin Pathol* 41:1269, 1988.

69. Le Bousse-Kerdilès MC, Martyré MC, et al: Involvement of the fibrogenic cytokines, TGF-β and bFGF, in the pathogenesis of idiopathic myelofibrosis. *Pathol Biol* 49:153, 2001.

70. Rameshwar P, Oh IIS, Yook C, Chang VT: Substance P fibronectin cytokine interactions in myeloproliferative disorders with bone marrow fibrosis. *Acta Haematol* 109:1, 2003.

71. Wang JC, Wong C, Kao WW: Immunoreactive prolylhydroxylase in patients with primary and secondary myelofibrosis. *Br J Haematol* 65:171, 1987.

72. Barosi G, Costa A, Liberato LN, et al: Serum procollagen III peptide level correlates with disease activity in myelofibrosis with myeloid metaplasia. *Br J Haematol* 72:16, 1989.

73. Hochweiss S, Fruchtman S, Hahn EG, et al: Increased serum procollagen III amino-terminal peptide in myelofibrosis. *Am J Hematol* 15:343, 1983.

74. Hasselbalch H, Junker P, Lisse I, et al: Circulating hyaluronan in the myelofibrosis/osteomyelosclerosis syndrome and other myeloproliferative disorders. *Am J Hematol* 36:1, 1991.

75. Thiele J, Kvasnicka HM, Fischer R, Diehl V: Clinicopathological impact of the interactivity between megakaryocytes and myeloid stroma in chronic myeloproliferative disorders: A concise update. *Leuk Lymphoma* 24:463, 1997.

76. Schmitt A, Drouin A, Masse J-M, et al: Polymorphonuclear neutrophil and megakaryocyte mutual involvement in myelofibrosis pathogenesis. *Leuk Lymphoma* 43:719, 2002.

77. Frey BM, Rafii S, Teterson M, et al: Adenovector-mediated expression of human thrombopoietin cDNA in immune-compromised mice: Insights into the pathophysiology of osteomyelofibrosis. *J Immunol* 160:691, 1998.

78. Rameshwar P, Chang VT, Thacker UF, Gascón P: Systemic transforming growth factor-beta in patients with bone marrow fibrosis-pathophysiological implications. *Am J Hematol* 59:133, 1998.

79. Rosenfeld M, Keating A, Bowen-Pope BF, et al: Responsiveness of the in vitro hematopoietic microenvironment to platelet-derived growth factor. *Leuk Res* 9:427, 1985.

80. Bernabei PA, Arcangeli A, Casini M, et al: Platelet-derived growth factor(s) mitogenic activity in patients with myeloproliferative disease. *Br J Haematol* 63:353, 1986.

81. Thiele J, Rompick V, Wagner S, Fischer R: Vascular architecture and collagen type IV in primary myelofibrosis and polycythemia vera. *Br J Haematol* 80:227, 1992.

82. Johnston JB, Dalal BI, Israels SJ, et al: Deposition of transforming growth factor-β in the marrow in myelofibrosis, and the intracellular localization and secretion of TGF-β by leukemic cells. *Am J Clin Pathol* 103:574, 1995.

83. Martré M-C: TGF-β and megakaryocytes in the pathogenesis of myelofibrosis in myeloproliferative disorders. *Leuk Lymphoma* 20:39, 1995.

84. Martré M-C, LeBousse-Kerdiles M-C, Romquin N, et al: Elevated levels of basic fibroblast growth factor in megakaryocytes and platelets from patients with idiopathic myelofibrosis. *Br J Haematol* 97:441, 1997.

85. Dalley A, Smith JM, Reilly JT, MacNeil S: Investigation of calmodulin and basic fibroblast growth factor (bFGF) in idiopathic myelofibrosis: Evidence for a role of extracellular calmodulin in fibroblast proliferation. *Br J Haematol* 93:856, 1996.

86. Nathan C: Secretory products of macrophages. *J Clin Invest* 79:319, 1987.

87. Burstein SA, Malpass TW, Yee E, et al: Platelet factor-4 excretion in myeloproliferative disease: Implication for the aetiology of myelofibrosis. *Br J Haematol* 57:383, 1984.

88. Wang JC, Novetsky A, Chen C, et al: Plasm matrix metalloproteinase and tissue inhibitor of metalloproteinase in patients with agnogenic myeloid metaplasia or idiopathic primary myelofibrosis. *Br J Haematol* 119:709, 2002.

89. Kvasnica HM, Thiele J, Amend T, Fischer R: Three-dimensional reconstruction of histologic structures in human bone marrow from serial sections of trephine biopsies. *Anal Quant Cytol Histol* 16:159, 1994.

90. Reilly JT, Nash JR, Mackie MJ, et al: Endothelial cell proliferation in myelofibrosis. *Br J Haematol* 60:625, 1985.

91. Charbord P: Increased vascularity of bone marrow in myelofibrosis. *Br J Haematol* 62:595, 1986.

92. VanDyke D, Anger HO, Parker H, et al: Markedly increased bone blood flow in myelofibrosis. *J Nucl Med* 12:506, 1971.

93. Hotta T, Utsumi M, Katoh T, et al: Granulocytic and stromal progenitors in the bone marrow of patient with primary myelofibrosis. *Scand J Haematol* 34:251, 1985.

94. Greenberg BR, Woo L, Veomett JC, et al: Cytogenetics of bone marrow fibroblastic cells in idiopathic chronic myelofibrosis. *Br J Haematol* 66:487, 1987.

95. Caughman W, Stern R, Haynes H: Neutrophilic dermatosis of myeloproliferative disorders: Atypical forms of pyoderma gangrenosum and Sweet's syndrome associated with myeloproliferative disorders. *J Am Acad Dermatol* 9:751, 1983.

96. Gibson LE, Dicken CH, Flach DB: Neutrophilic dermatoses and myeloproliferative disease: Report of two cases. *Mayo Clin Proc* 60:735, 1985.

97. Su WPD, Alegre VA, White WL: Myelofibrosis discovered after diagnosis of Sweet's syndrome. *Int J Dermatol* 29:201, 1990.

98. Kanel KT, Kroboth FJ, Swartz WM: Pyoderma gangrenosum with myelofibrosis. *Am J Med* 82:1031, 1987.

99. Loewy G, Matthew A, Distenfeld A: Skin manifestations of agnogenic myeloid metaplasia. *Am J Hematol* 45:167, 1994.

100. Patel BM, Perniciaro C, Gertz MA: Cutaneous extramedullary hematopoiesis. *J Acad Dermatol* 32:805, 1995.

101. Rogalski C, Paasch U, Friedrich T, et al: Cutaneous extramedullary hematopoiesis in idiopathic myelofibrosis. *Int J Dermatol* 41:883, 2002.

102. Thiele J, Kvasnicka HM, Zankovich R, Diehl V: Early-stage idiopathic (primary) myelofibrosis-current issues of diagnostic features. *Leuk Lymphoma* 43:1035, 2002.

103. Buhr T, Büsche G, Choritz H, et al: Evolution of myelofibrosis in chronic idiopathic myelofibrosis as evidenced in sequential bone marrow biopsy specimens. *Am J Clin Pathol* 119:152, 2003.

104. Thiele J, Kvasnicka HM: Chronic myeloproliferative disorders with thrombocythemia comparative study of two classification systems (PSSG, WHO) on 839 patients. *Ann Hematol* 82:148, 2003.

105. King BF, Kopecky KK, Baker MK, et al: Extramedullary hematopoiesis in the adrenal glands: CT characteristics. *J Comput Assist Tomogr* 11:342, 1987.

106. Wat NM, Tse KK, Chan FL, Lam KS: Adrenal extramedullary hematopoiesis. *Br J Haematol* 100:725, 1998.

107. Woodward N, Ancliffe P, Griffiths MH, Cohen S: Renal myelofibrosis: An unusual cause of renal impairment. *Nephrol Dial Transplant* 15:257, 2000.

108. Schunuelle P, Waldherr R, Lehmann KJ, et al: Idiopathic myelofibrosis with extramedullary hematopoiesis in the kidneys. *Clin Nephrol* 52:256, 1999.

109. Holt SG, Field P, Carmichael P, et al: Extramedullary haemopoiesis in the renal parenchyma as a cause of acute renal failure in myelofibrosis. *Nephrol Dial Transplant* 10:1438, 1995.

110. Shaver RW, Close FC: Extramedullary hemopoiesis in myeloid metaplasia. *Am J Radiol* 137:874, 1981.

111. Williams ME, Innes DJ, Hutchison WT, et al: Extramedullary hematopoiesis: A cause of severe generalized lymphadenopathy in agnogenic myeloid metaplasia. *Arch Intern Med* 145:1308, 1985.

112. Fianza A, Alberici E, Toretta L: Rapidly growing extramedullary hemopoiesis in lymph nodes. *Haematologica* 86:784, 2001.

113. Sharma BK, Pounder RE, Cruse JP, et al: Extramedullary haemopoiesis in the small bowel. *Gut* 27:873, 1986.

114. MacKinnon S, McNicol AM, Lee FD, et al: Myelofibrosis complicated by intestinal extramedullary haemopoiesis and acute small bowel obstruction. *J Clin Pathol* 39:677, 1986.

115. Soloman D, Goodman H, Jacobs P: Rectal stenosis due to extramedullary hematopoiesis. *Clin Radiol* 49:726, 1994.

116. Sunderland K, Barratt J, Pidcock M: Extramedullary hemopoiesis arising in the gut mimicking carcinoma of the cecum. *Pathology* 26:62, 1994.

117. Brooks JJ, Krugman DT, Danjanor I: Myeloid metaplasia presenting as a breast mass. *Am J Surg Pathol* 4:281, 1980.

118. Martinelli G, Santini D, Bazzocchi F, et al: Myeloid metaplasia of the breast: A lesion which clinically mimics carcinoma. *Virchows Arch* 401:203, 1983.

119. Zonderland HM, Michiels JJ, Ten Kate FJW: Mammographic and sonographic demonstration of extramedullary hematopoiesis of the breast. *Clin Radiol* 44:64, 1991.

120. Navarro M, Crespo C, Pérez L, et al: Massive intrahepatic extramedullary hematopoiesis in myelofibrosis. *Abdom Imaging* 25:184, 2000.

121. Gil-Fernández JJ, Martinez-Chamorro C, Tomás JF: A giant hepatic mass of myeloid metaplasia in a patient without myelofibrosis. *Haematologica* 86:445, 2001.

122. Yusen RD, Kollef MH: Acute respiratory failure due to extramedullary hematopoiesis. *Chest* 108:1170, 1995.

123. Asakura S, Colby T: Agnogenic myeloid metaplasia with extramedullary hemopoiesis and fibrosis in the lung. *Chest* 105:1866, 1994.

124. García-Manero G, Schuster S, Patrick H, Martinez J: Pulmonary hypertension in patients with myelofibrosis secondary to myeloproliferative diseases. *Am J Hematol* 60:130, 1999.

125. Yang X, Bhuiya T, Esposito M: Sclerosing extramedullary tumor. *Ann Diag Pathol* 6:183, 2002.

126. Oren I, Goldman A, Haddad N, et al: Ascites and pleural effusion a secondary to extramedullary hematopoiesis. *Am J Med Sci* 318:286, 1999.

127. Pierard GE: Cutaneous hematopoiesis and myelofibrosis. *Ann Pathol* 7:73, 1987.

128. Mizoguchi M, Kawa Y, Minami T, et al: Cutaneous extramedullary hematopoiesis in myelofibrosis. *J Am Acad Dermatol* 22:351, 1990.

129. Heinicke MH, Zarrabi MH, Gorevic PD: Arthritis due to synovial involvement by extramedullary haematopoiesis in myelofibrosis with myeloid metaplasia. *Ann Rheum Dis* 42:196, 1983.

130. Leoni F, Fabbri R, Pascarella A, et al: Extramedullary hematopoiesis in thyroid multinodular goiter preceding clinical evidence of agnogenic myeloid metaplasia. *Histopathology* 28:559, 1996.

131. Kwak H-S, Lee J-M: CT findings of extramedullary hematopoiesis in the thorax, liver, and kidneys in a patient with myelofibrosis. *J Korean Med Sci* 15:460, 2000.

132. Humphrey PA, Vollmer RT: Extramedullary hematopoiesis in the prostate. *Am J Surg Pathol* 15:486, 1991.

133. Macumber C, Young GAR, Selby WS: Myelofibrosis presenting as splenic tumor. *Digest Dis Sci* 44:1817, 1999.

134. Balogh K, O'Hara CJ: Myeloid metaplasia masquerading as a urethral caruncle. *J Urol* 135:789, 1986.

135. Oesterling JE, Keating JP, Leroy AJ, et al: Idiopathic myelofibrosis with myeloid metaplasia involving the renal pelvis, ureters and bladder. *J Urol* 147:1360, 1992.

136. Gryspeerdt S, Oyen R, Van Hoe L, et al: Extramedullary hematopoiesis encasing the pelvicalyceal system. *Ann Hematol* 71:53, 1995.

137. Perazella MA, Buller GK: Nephrotic syndrome associated with agnogenic myeloid metaplasia. *Am J Nephrol* 14:223, 1994.

138. Brown JA, Gomez-Leon G: Subdural hemorrhage secondary to extramedullary hematopoiesis in postpolycythemic myeloid metaplasia. *Neurosurgery* 14:588, 1984.

139. Cornfield DB, Shipkin P, Alluvia A, et al: Intracranial myeloid metaplasia: Diagnosis by CT and Fe52 scans and treatment by cranial irradiation. *Am J Hematol* 15:273, 1983.

140. Lundh B, Brandt L, Cronqvist S, et al: Intracranial myeloid metaplasia in myelofibrosis. *Scand J Haematol* 28:91, 1982.

141. Pless M, Rizzo JFIII,Shang J: Orbital apex syndrome: A rare presentation of extramedullary hematopoiesis. *J Neurooncol* 57:37, 2002.

142. Cameron WR, Ronnert M, Brun A: Extramedullary hematopoiesis of CNS in postpolycythemic myeloid metaplasia. *N Engl J Med* 305:765, 1981.

143. Chan SWW, Datta NN, Thomas TMM, Chan KW: Intracranial chloroma in myelofibrosis. *Surg Neurol* 59:55, 2003.

144. Ligumski M, Polliack A, Benbassat J: Metaplasia of the central nervous system in patients with myelofibrosis and agnogenic myeloid metaplasia. *Am J Med Sci* 275:99, 1979.

145. Stahl SM, Ellinger G, Baringer JR: Progressive myelopathy due to extramedullary hematopoiesis. *Ann Neurol* 5:485, 1979.

146. Cook G, Sharp RA: Spinal cord compression due to extramedullary haemopoiesis in myelofibrosis. *J Clin Pathol* 47:464, 1994.

147. Horwood E, Dowson H, Gupta R, et al: Myelofibrosis presenting as spinal cord compression. *J Clin Pathol* 56:154, 2003.

148. Price F, Bell H: Spinal cord compression due to extramedullary hematopoiesis: Successful treatment in a patient with long-standing myelofibrosis. *JAMA* 253:2876, 1985.

149. Ohtsubo M, Hayaski K, Fukushima T, et al: Intracranial extramedullary haematopoiesis in postpolycythemia myelofibrosis. *Br J Radiol* 67:299, 1994.

150. Urman M, O'Sullivan RA, Nugent RA, Lentle BC: Intracranial extramedullary hematopoiesis. *Clin Nucl Med* 16:431, 1991.

151. Lanir A, Aghai E, Simon JS, et al: MR imaging in myelofibrosis. *J Comput Assist Tomogr* 10:634, 1986.

152. Koch BL, Bisset GS, Bisset RR, Zimmer MB: Intracranial extramedullary hematopoiesis: MR findings with pathologic correlation. *AJR Am J Roentgenol* 162:1419, 1994.

153. Bartlett RP, Greipp PR, Tefferi A, et al: Extramedullary hematopoiesis manifesting as a symptomatic pleural effusion. *Mayo Clin Proc* 70:1165, 1995.

154. Knobel B, Melamud E, Virage I, Meytes D: Ectopic medullary hematopoiesis as a cause of ascites in agnogenic myeloid metaplasia. *Acta Haematol* 89:104, 1993.

155. Lioté F, Yeni P, Teillet-Thiebaud F, et al: Ascites revealing peritoneal and hepatic extramedullary hematopoiesis with peliosis in agnogenic myeloid metaplasia. *Am J Med* 90:111, 1991.

156. Vilaseca J, Arnau JM, Tallada N, et al: Agnogenic myeloid metaplasia presenting as massive pericardial effusion due to extramedullary hematopoiesis. *Acta Haematol (Basel)* 73:239, 1985.

157. Haedersdal C, Hasselbalch H, Devantier A, et al: Pericardial haematopoiesis with tamponade in myelofibrosis. *Scand J Haematol* 34:270, 1985.

158. Imam TH, Doll DC: Acute cardiac tamponade associated with pericardial extramedullary hematopoieses in agnogenic myeloid metaplasia. *Acta Haematol* 98:42, 1997.

159. Nagler A, Brenner B, Argov S, et al: Postsplenectomy pericardial effusion in two patients with myeloid metaplasia. *Arch Intern Med* 146:600, 1986.

160. Pedio G, Krause M, Jansova I: Megakaryocytes in ascitic fluid in a case of agnogenic myeloid metaplasia [letter]. *Acta Cytol* 29:89, 1985.

161. Silverman JF: Extramedullary hematopoietic ascitic fluid cytology in myelofibrosis. *Am J Clin Pathol* 84:125, 1985.

162. Stephenson RW, Britt DA, Schumann GB: Primary cytodiagnosis of peritoneal extramedullary hematopoiesis. *Diag Cytopathol* 2:241, 1986.

163. Hocking WG, Lazar GS, Lipsett JA, et al: Cutaneous extramedullary hematopoiesis following splenectomy for idiopathic myelofibrosis. *Am J Med* 76:956, 1984.

164. Partanen S, Ruutu T, Jubonen E, et al: Effect of splenectomy on circulating haematopoietic progenitors in myelofibrosis. *Scand J Haematol* 37:87, 1986.

165. Hirose Y, Masaki Y, Shimoyama K, et al: Granulocytic sarcoma of megakaryoblastic differentiation in the lymph nodes terminating as acute megakaryocytic leukemia in a case of chronic idiopathic myelofibrosis persisting 16 years. *Eur J Haematol* 67:194, 2001.

166. Chan ACL, Kwong Y-L, Lam CCK: Granulocytic sarcoma megakaryoblastic differentiation complicating chronic idiopathic myelofibrosis. *Hum Pathol* 27:417, 1996.

167. Oishi N, Swisher SN, Stormont JM, et al: Portal hypertension in myeloid metaplasia. *Arch Surg* 81:80, 1960.

168. Rosenbaum DL, Murphy GW, Swisher SN: Hemodynamic studies of the portal circulation in myeloid metaplasia. *Am J Med* 41:360, 1966.

169. Jacobs P, Maze S, Tayob F, et al: Myelofibrosis, splenomegaly, and portal hypertension. *Acta Haematol* 74:45, 1985.

170. Dubois A, Dauzat M, Pignodel C, et al: Portal hypertension in lymphoproliferative and myeloproliferative disorders: Hemodynamic and histological correlations. *Hepatology* 17:246, 1993.

171. Degott C, Carpon JP, Bettan L, et al: Myeloid metaplasia, perisinusoidal fibrosis, and nodular regenerative hyperplasia of the liver. *Liver* 5:276, 1985.

172. Bioulac-Sage P, Roux D, Quinton A, et al: Ultrastructure of sinusoids in patients with agnogenic myeloid metaplasia. *J Submicrosc Cytol* 18:815, 1986.

173. Roux D, Merlio JP, Quinton A, et al: Agnogenic myeloid metaplasia, portal hypertension and sinusoidal abnormalities. *Gastroenterology* 92:1067, 1987.

174. Tsao MS: Hepatic sinusoidal fibrosis in agnogenic myeloid metaplasia. *Am J Clin Pathol* 91:302, 1989.

175. Pereira A, Bruguera M, Cervantes F, Rozman C: Liver involvement at diagnosis of primary myelofibrosis: A clinicopathological study of twenty-two cases. *Eur J Haematol* 40:355, 1988.

176. Valla d, Casadevall N, Huisse MG, et al: Etiology of portal vein thrombosis in adults. *Gastroenterology* 94:1063, 1988.

177. Lee W-C, Lin H-C, Tsay S-H, et al: Esophageal variceal ligation for esophageal variceal hemorrhage in a patient with portal and primary pulmonary hypertension complicating myelofibrosis. *Dig Dis Sci* 46:915, 2001.

178. Yusen RD, Kollef MH: Acute respiratory failure due to extramedullary hematopoiesis. *Chest* 108:1170, 1995.

179. Steensma DP, Hook CC, Stafford SL, Tefferi A: Low-dose, single fraction, whole-lung radiotherapy for pulmonary hypertension associated with myelofibrosis and myeloid metaplasia. *Br J Haematol* 118:813, 2002.

180. Boivin P, Bernard JF, Hakim J, et al: Anomalies immunitaires au cours de splenomegalies myeloides myelosclerose. *Acta Haematol (Basel)* 51: 91, 1974.

181. Lang JM, Oberling F, Mayer S, et al: Autoimmunity in primary myelofibrosis. *Biomedicine* 25:39, 1976.

182. Barge J, Slabodshy-Brousse N, Bernard JF: Histoimmunology of myelofibrosis: A study of 100 cases. *Biomedicine* 29:73, 1978.

183. Vellenga E, Mulder N, The T, et al: A study of the cellular and humoral immune response in patients with myelofibrosis. *Clin Lab Haematol* 4: 239, 1982.

184. Rondeau E, Solal-Celigny P, Dhermy D, et al: Immune disorders in agnogenic myeloid metaplasia: Relations to myelofibrosis. *Br J Haematol* 53:467, 1983.

185. Gordon B: Immunological abnormalities in myelofibrosis. *Prog Clin Biol Res* 154:455, 1984.

186. Khumbananda M, Horowitz HI, Eyster ME: Coombs' positive hemolytic anemia in myelofibrosis with myeloid metaplasia. *Am J Med Sci* 258:89, 1969.

187. Mohite U, Pathare A, Al Kindi S, et al: Autoimmune haemolytic anemia as the presenting manifestation of agnogenic myeloid metaplasia. *Haematologica* 32:495, 2002.

188. Schreiber ZA: Immune thrombocytopenia in postpolythemic myelofibrosis. *Am J Hematol* 54:146, 1997.

189. Seelen MAJ, De Meijer PHEM, Posthuma EF, Meinders AE: Myelofibrosis and thrombocytopenic purpura. *Ann Hematol* 75:129, 1997.

190. Wang JC, Wang A: Plasma soluble interleukin-2 receptor in patients with primary myelofibrosis. *Br J Haematol* 86:380, 1994.

191. Leoni P, Rupoli S, Salvi A, et al: Antibodies against terminal galactosyl alpha(1–3) galactose epitopes in patients with idiopathic myelofibrosis. *Br J Haematol* 85:313, 1993.

192. Bernhardt B, Valleta M: Lupus anticoagulant in myelofibrosis. *Am J Med Sci* 272:229, 1976.

193. Cappio FC, Vigliani R, Novarino A, et al: Idiopathic myelofibrosis: A possible role for immune-complexes in the pathogenesis of bone marrow fibrosis. *Br J Haematol* 49:17, 1981.

194. Akikusa B, Komatsu T, Kondo Y, et al: Amyloidosis complicating idiopathic myelofibrosis. *Arch Pathol Lab Med* 111:525, 1987.

195. Hasselbalch H, Nielsen H, Berild D, et al: Circulating immune complexes in myelofibrosis. *Scand J Haematol* 34:177, 1985.

196. Gordon BR, Coleman M, Kohen P, et al: Immunologic abnormalities in myelofibrosis with activation of the complement system. *Blood* 58:904, 1981.

197. Ferhanoglu B, Erzin Y, Baslar Z, Tüzüner HAN: Secondary amyloidosis in the course of idiopathic myelofibrosis. *Leuk Res* 21:897, 1997.

198. El Mouzan MI, Ahmed MAM, Saleh MAF, et al: Myelofibrosis and pancytopenia in systemic lupus erythematosus. *Am J Med* 81:935, 1986.

199. Matsouka CH, Lioouris J, Andrianokis A: Systemic lupus erythematosus and myelofibrosis. *Clin Rheumatol* 8:402, 1989.

200. Paquette RL, Meshkinpour A, Rosen PJ: Autoimmune myelofibrosis. A steroid-responsive cause of bone marrow fibrosis associated with systemic lupus erythematosus. *Medicine* 73:145, 1994.

201. Ramakrishna R, Kyle PW, Day PJ, Mansharan A: Evan's syndrome, myelofibrosis and systemic lupus erythematosus: Role of procollagens in myelofibrosis. *Pathology* 27:255, 1995.

202. Kiss E, Gál I, Simkovics E, et al: Myelofibrosis in systemic lupus erythematosus. *Leuk Lymphoma* 39:661, 2000.

203. Aharon A, Levy Y, Bar-Dayan Y, et al: Successful treatment of early secondary myelofibrosis in SLE with IVIG. *Lupus* 6:408, 1997.

204. Von Knorring J, Selroos OW, Wegelius O: Myeloid metaplasia in disseminated vascular disease. *Acta Med Scand* 195:137, 1974.

205. Connelly TJ, Abruzzo JL, Schwab RH: Agnogenic myeloid metaplasia with polyarteritis. *J Rheumatol* 9:954, 1982.

206. Arellano-Rodrigo E, Esteve J, Giné E, et al: Idiopathic myelofibrosis associated with ulcerative colitis. *Leuk Lymphoma* 43:1481, 2002.

207. Ben-Chetrit E, Gross DJ, Ikon E, et al: The association between autoimmunity and agnogenic myeloid metaplasia. *Scand J Haematol* 31:410, 1983.

208. Hernández-Beluda JC, Jiménez M, Rosiñol L, Cervantes F: Idiopathic myelofibrosis associated with primary biliary cirrhosis. *Leuk Lymphoma* 43:673, 2002.

209. Marie I, Levesque H, Cailleux N, et al: An uncommon association: Sjogren syndrome and autoimmune myelofibrosis. *Rheumatology* 38:370, 1999.

210. Hasselbalch H, Jans H, Nielsen PL: A distinct subtype of idiopathic myelofibrosis with bone marrow features mimicking hairy cell leukemia: Evidence of an autoimmune pathogenesis. *Am J Hematol* 25:225, 1987.

211. Thiele J, Chen Y-S, Kvasnicka H-M, et al: Evolution of fibro-osteosclerotic bone marrow lesions in primary (idiopathic) osteomyelofibrosis—A histomorphometric study on sequential trephine biopsies. *Leuk Lymphoma* 14:163, 1994.

212. Thiele J, Hoeppner B, Zankovich R, Fischer R: Histomorphometry of bone marrow biopsies in primary osteomyelofibrosis-sclerosis (agnogenic myeloid metaplasia): Correlation between clinical and morphological features. *Virchows Arch* 415:191, 1989.

213. Guermazi A, De Kerviler E, Cazals-Hatem D, et al: Imaging findings in myelofibrosis. *Eur J Radiol* 9:1366, 1999.

214. Thiele J, Kvasnicka HM, Fischer R: Histochemistry and morphometry on bone marrow biopsies in chronic myeloproliferative disorders: Aids to diagnosis and classification. *Ann Hematol* 78:496, 1999.

215. Poulsen LW, Melsen F, Bendix KA: Histomorphometric study of haematologic disorders with respect to marrow fibrosis and osteosclerosis. *Acta Path Microbiol Immunol Scand* 106:495, 1998.

216. Coindre JM, Reiffers J, Goussot JF, et al: Histomorphometric analysis of sclerotic bone from idiopathic myeloid metaplasia. *J Pathol* 144:163, 1984.

217. Diamond T, Smith A, Schnier R, Manoharan A: Syndrome of myelofibrosis and osteosclerosis: A series of case reports and review of the literature. *Bone* 3:498, 2002.

218. Parfitt AM, Drezner MK, Glorieux FH, et al: Bone histomorphometry: Standardization of nomenclature, symbols, and units. *J Bone Miner Res* 2:595, 1987.

219. Cassi E, DePaoli A, Tosi A, et al: Pure osteolytic lesions in myelofibrosis: Report of 2 cases. *Haematologica* 70:178, 1985.

220. Fayemi AO, Gerber MA, Cohen I, et al: Myeloid sarcoma. *Cancer* 32: 253, 1973.

221. Yu JS, Greenway G, Resnick D: Myelofibrosis associated with prominent periosteal bone apposition. *Clin Imaging* 18:89, 1994.

222. Barosi G, Cazzoli M, Frassoni F: Erythropoiesis in myelofibrosis with myeloid metaplasia: Recognition of different classes of patients by erythrokinetics. *Br J Haematol* 48:263, 1981.

223. Barosi G, Berzuinic C, Liberato LN, et al: A prognostic classification of myelofibrosis with myeloid metaplasia. *Br J Haematol* 70:397, 1988.

224. Thiele J, Kvasnicka H-M, Werden C, et al: Idiopathic primary osteomyelofibrosis. *Leuk Lymphoma* 22:303, 1996.

225. Njoku OS, Lewis SM, Catovsky D, et al: Anaemia in myelofibrosis: Its value in prognosis. *Br J Haematol* 54:79, 1983.

226. Howarth JE, Waters HM, Hyde K, Geary CG: Detection of erythroid hypoplasia in myelofibrosis using erythrokinetic studies. *J Clin Pathol* 42:1250, 1989.

227. Thiele J, Windecker R, Kvasnicka HM, et al: Erythropoiesis in primary (idiopathic) osteomyelofibrosis. *Am J Hematol* 46:36, 1994.

228. Bird GW, Wingham J, Richardson SG: Myelofibrosis, autoimmune haemolytic anaemia and Tn-polyagglutinability. *Haematologica* 18:99, 1985.

229. Kuo CY, VanVoolen GA, Morrison AN: Primary and secondary myelofibrosis: Its relationship to the PNH-like defect. *Blood* 40:875, 1972.

230. Veer A, Kosciolek BA, Bauman AW, et al: Acquired hemoglobin H disease in idiopathic myelofibrosis. *Am J Hematol* 6:199, 1979.

231. Barosi G, Baraldi A, Cassola M, et al: Red cell aplasia in myelofibrosis with myeloid metaplasia. *Cancer* 52:1290, 1983.

232. Silverstein MN, Elveback LR: Leukocyte alkaline phosphatase in agnogenic myeloid metaplasia. *Am J Clin Pathol* 61:307, 1974.

233. Douer D, Fabian I, Cline MJ: Circulation pluripotent haemopoietic cells in patients with myeloproliferative disorders. *Br J Haematol* 54:373, 1983.

234. Barosi G, Viarengo G, Pecci A, et al: Diagnostic and clinical relevance of the number of circulating CD34+ cells in myelofibrosis with myeloid metaplasia. *Blood* 98:3249, 2001.

235. Partanen S, Ruutu T, Vuopio P: Circulating haematopoietic progenitors in myelofibrosis. *Scand J Haematol* 29:325, 1982.

236. Wang JC, Cheung CP, Ahmed F, et al: Circulating granulocyte and macrophage progenitor cells in primary and secondary myelofibrosis. *Br J Haematol* 54:301, 1983.

237. Kornberg A, Fibach E, Treves A, et al: Circulating erythroid progenitors in patients with "spent" polycythaemia vera and myelofibrosis with myeloid metaplasia. *Br J Haematol* 52:573, 1982.

238. Čolović MD, Wiernik PH, Janković GM, et al: Circulating haematopoietic progenitor cells in primary and secondary myelofibrosis: Relation to collagen and reticulin fibrosis. *Eur J Haematol* 62:155, 1999.

239. Tinggaard-Pedersen N, Laursen B: Megakaryocytes in cubital venous blood in patients with chronic myeloproliferative diseases. *Scand J Haematol* 30:50, 1983.

240. Cervantes F, Hernandez-Boluda JC, Villamor N, et al: Assessment of peripheral blood lymphocyte subsets in idiopathic myelofibrosis. *Eur J Haematol* 65:104, 2000.

241. Marquetty C, Labro Bryskier MT, Perianin A, et al: Impaired metabolic activity of phagocytosis neutrophils in agnogenic osteomyelofibrosis with splenomegaly. *Am J Med* 16:243, 1984.

242. Perianin A, Labro-Bryskier MT, Marquetty C, et al: Glutathione reductase and nitroblue tetrazolium reduction deficiencies in neutrophils of patients with primary idiopathic myelofibrosis. *Clin Exp Immunol* 57:244, 1984.

243. Briard D, Brouty-Boye D, Giron-Michel J et al: Impaired NK cell differentiation of blood-derived CD34+ progenitors from patients with myeloid metaplasia with myelofibrosis. *Clin Immunol* 106:201, 2003.

244. Murphy S, Davis JL, Walsh PN, et al: Template bleeding time and clinical hemorrhage in myeloproliferative disease. *Arch Intern Med* 138:1251, 1978.

245. Malpass TW, Savage B, Hanson SR, et al: Correlation between bleeding time and depletion of platelet dense granule ADP in patients with myelodysplastic and myeloproliferative disorders. *J Lab Clin Med* 103:894, 1984.

246. Cunietti E, Gandini R, Marcaro G, et al: Defective platelet aggregation and increased platelet turnover in patients with myelofibrosis and other myeloproliferative diseases. *Scand J Haematol* 26:339, 1981.

247. Schafer AL: Deficiency of platelet lipoxygenase activity in myeloproliferative disorders. *N Engl J Med* 306:381, 1982.

248. Shafer AL: Bleeding and thrombosis in the myeloproliferative disorders. *Blood* 64:1, 1984.

249. Barbui T, Cortelazzo S, Viero P, et al: Thrombohaemorrhagic complications in 101 cases of myeloproliferative disorders: Relationship to platelet number and function. *Eur J Cancer Clin Oncol* 19:1593, 1983.

250. Thiele J, Lorenzen J, Manich B, et al: Apoptosis (programmed cell death) in idiopathic (primary) osteo-/myelofibrosis. *Acta Haematol* 97:137, 1997.

251. Thiele J, Holgado S, Choritz H, et al: Chronic megakaryocyte-granulocytic myelosis—An electron microscope study including freeze-fracture. *Virchows Arch A* 375:129, 1977.

252. Mesa RA, Hanson CA, Rajkumar SV, et al: Evaluation and clinical correlations of bone marrow angiogenesis in myelofibrosis with myeloid metaplasia. *Blood* 15:3374, 2000.

253. Miller JB, Testa JR, Lindgren V, et al: The patterns and clinical significance of karyotypic abnormalities in patients with idiopathic polycythemic myelofibrosis. *Cancer* 55:582, 1985.

254. Damor JL, Dupriez B, Fenaux P, et al: Cytogenetic studies and their prognostic significance in agnogenic myeloid metaplasia. *Blood* 72:855, 1988.

255. Nakamura H, Sadamori N, Mine M, et al: Effects of short-term liquid culture of peripheral blood mononuclear cells with recombinant human granulocyte or granulocyte-macrophage colony-stimulating factor in cytogenetic studies of myelofibrosis with myeloid metaplasia. *Leukemia* 6:853, 1992.

256. Reilly JT, Snowden JA, Spearing RL, et al: Cytogenetic abnormalities and their prognostic significance in idiopathic myelofibrosis. *Br J Haematol* 98:96, 1997.

257. Tefferi A, Mesa RA, Schroeder G, et al: Cytogenetic findings and their clinical relevance in myelofibrosis with myeloid metaplasia. *Br J Haematol* 113:763, 2001.

258. Tefferi A, Meyer RG, Wyatt WA, et al: Comparison of peripheral blood interphase cytogenetics with bone marrow karyotype analysis in myelofibrosis with myeloid metaplasia. *Br J Haematol* 115:316, 2001.

259. Sinclair EJ, Forrest EC, Reilly JT, et al: Fluorescence in situ hybridization analysis of 25 cases of idiopathic myelofibrosis and two cases of secondary idiopathic: Monoallelic loss of RB1, D13S319 and D13S25 loci associated with cytogenetic deletion and translocation involving 13q14. *Br J Haematol* 113:365, 2001.

260. Reilly JT: Cytogenetic and molecular genetic aspects of idiopathic myelofibrosis. *Acta Haematol* 108:113, 2002.

261. Andrieux J, Demory JL, Morel P, et al: Frequency of structural abnormalities of the long arm of chromosome 12 in myelofibrosis with myeloid metaplasia. *Cancer Genet Cytogenet* 137:68, 2002.

262. Forrester RH, Louro JM: Philadelphia chromosome abnormality in agnogenic myeloid metaplasia. *Ann Intern Med* 64:622, 1966.

263. Weda F, Takashima T, Suzuki M, Kadoya M: MR diagnosis of myelofibrosis *Radiat Med* 12:135, 1994.

264. Amano Y, Onda M, Amano M, Kumazaki T: Magnetic resonance imaging of myelofibrosis. STIR and gadolinium-enhanced MR images. *Clin Imaging* 21:264, 1997.

265. Schirrmeister H, Bommer M, Buck A, Reske SN: The bone scan ion osteosclerosis. *J Bone Miner Res* 16:2361, 2001.

266. Gilbert HS, Ginsberg H, Fagerstrom R, Brown WV: Characterization of hypocholesterolemia in myeloproliferative diseases. *Am J Med* 71:595, 1981.

267. Naggar L, Jaeger P, Burckhardt P, et al: Hypocalcemia and myelofibrosis: An unrecognized association. *Schweiz Med Wochenschr* 116:1771, 1986.

268. Voss A, Schmidt K, Hasselbalch H, Junker P: Hypercalcemia in idiopathic myelofibrosis. *Am J Hematol* 39:231, 1992.

269. Wang JC, Chen C, Lou L-H, Mora M: Blood thrombopoietin, IL-6 and IL-11 levels in patients with agnogenic myeloid metaplasia. *Leukemia* 11:1827, 1997.

270. Elliott MA, Yoon S-Y, Kao P, et al: Simultaneous measurement of serum thrombopoietin and expression of megakaryocyte c-MPL with clin-

ical and laboratory correlates for myelofibrosis with myeloid metaplasia. *Eur J Haematol* 68:175, 2002.

271. Wang JC, Hashmi G: Elevated thrombopoietin levels in patients with myelofibrosis may not be due to enhanced production of thrombopoietin by bone marrow. *Leuk Res* 27:13, 2003.

272. Wang J, Wang A: Plasma soluble interleukin-2 receptor in patients with primary myelofibrosis. *Br J Haematol* 86:180, 1994.

273. DiRaimondo F, Azzaro MP, Palumbo GA, et al: Elevated vascular endothelial growth factor (VEGF) serum levels in idiopathic myelofibrosis. *Leukemia* 15:976, 2001.

274. Dekmezian R, Kantarjian HM, Heating MJ, et al: The relevance of reticulin stain-measured fibrosis at diagnosis in chronic myelogenous leukemia. *Cancer* 59:1739, 1987.

275. Steensma DP, Hanson C, Letendre L, Teffari A: Myelodysplasia with fibrosis: A distinct entity? *Leuk Res* 25:829, 2001.

276. Thiele J, Zankovich R, Steinberg T, et al: Primary (essential) thrombocythemia versus initial hyperplastic stages of agnogenic myeloid metaplasia with thrombocytosis. *Acta Haematol* 81:192, 1989.

277. Thiele J, Kvasnicka HM, Zancovich R, Diehl V: Relevance of bone marrow features in the differential diagnosis between essential thrombocythemia and early stage idiopathic myelofibrosis. *Haematologica* 85:1126, 2000.

278. Hasselbach H, Jans H, Nielsen PL: A distinct subtype of idiopathic myelofibrosis with bone marrow features mimicking hairy cell leukemia. Evidence of an autoimmune pathogenesis. *Am J Hematol* 25:225, 1979.

279. O'Reilly RA: Splenomegaly at a United States County Hospital: Diagnostic evaluation of 170 patients. *Am J Med Sci* 312:160, 1996.

280. Pullarkat V, Bass RD, Gong JZ, et al: Primary autoimmune myelofibrosis: Definition of a distinct clinicopathologic syndrome. *Am J Hematol* 72:8, 2003.

281. Fortunato A, Mazzone A, Ricevuti G: Myelofibrosis caused by cancer: Presentation of a clinical case with a very difficult diagnosis. *Minerva Med* 76:1051, 1985.

282. Yablonski-Peretz T, Sulkes A, Polliack A, et al: Secondary myelofibrosis with metastatic breast cancer simulating agnogenic myeloid metaplasia: Report of a case and review of the literature. *Med Pediatr Oncol* 13:92, 1985.

283. Ishimura J, Fukushi M: Scintigraphic evaluation of secondary myelofibrosis associated with prostatic cancer before hormonal therapy. *Clin Nucl Med* 15:330, 1990.

284. Smart HE, Canney PA, Kerr DJ: Myelofibrosis associated with metastatic seminoma. *Clin Oncol* 4:132, 1992.

285. Takahashi T, Akihama T, Yamaguchi A, et al: Lysozyme secreting tumor: A case of gastric cancer associated with myelofibrosis due to disseminated bone marrow metastasis. *Jpn J Med* 26:58, 1987.

286. Rubins JM: The role of myelofibrosis in malignant leukoerythroblastosis. *Cancer* 51:308, 1983.

287. Hashim MSK, Kordofani AYA, El Dabi MA: Tuberculosis and myelofibrosis in children. *Ann Trop Paediatr* 17:61, 1997.

288. Viallard J-F, Parrens M, Boiron J-M, et al: Reversible myelofibrosis induced by tuberculosis. *Clin Infect Dis* 34:1641, 2002.

289. Sawers AH, Davson J, Braganza J, et al: Systemic mastocytosis, myelofibrosis and portal hypertension. *J Clin Pathol* 35:617, 1982.

290. Reisberg IR, Oyakawa S: Mastocytosis with malabsorption, myelofibrosis, and massive ascites. *Am J Gastroenterol* 82:54, 1987.

291. Kanbe N, Kurosawa M, Nagata H, et al: Production of fibrogenic cytokines by cord blood-derived cultured human mast cells. *J Allergy Clin Immunol* 106:S85, 2000.

292. Berton A, Levi-Schaffer F, Emonard H, et al: Activation of fibroblasts in collagen lattices by mast cell extracts: A model of fibrosis. *Clin Exp Allergy* 30:485, 2000.

293. Brenner B, Green J, Rosenbaum H, et al: Severe pancytopenia due to marked marrow fibrosis associated with angioimmunoblastic lymphadenopathy. *Acta Haematol* 74:43, 1985.

294. Varma N, Vaiphei K, Varma S: Angiosarcoma presenting with leucoerythroblastic anaemia bone marrow fibrosis and massive splenomegaly. *Br J Haematol* 110:503, 2000.

295. Meckenstock G, Wehmeier A, Schaefer HE, et al: Lymphoid myelofibrosis associated with high grade B cell lymphoma of the liver. *Leuk Lymphoma* 26:197, 1997.

296. Abe Y, Ohshima K, Shiratsuchi M, et al: Cytotoxic T-cell lymphoma presenting as secondary myelofibrosis with high levels of PDGF and TGF-β. *Eur J Haematol* 66:210, 2001.

297. Weirich G, Sandherr M, Fellbaum C, et al: Molecular evidence of bone marrow involvement in advanced case of T$\gamma\delta$ lymphoma with secondary myelofibrosis. *Human Pathol* 29:761, 1998.

298. Vandermolen L, Rice L, Lynch EL: Plasma cell dyscrasia with marrow fibrosis. *Am J Med* 79:297, 1985.

299. Humphrey CA, Morris TCM: The intimate relationship of myelofibrosis and myeloma: Effect of therapy. *Br J Haematol* 73:269, 1989.

300. Patterson KG, Treleavan JG, Zuiable A: Marrow fibrosis in myeloma: Improvement by alkylating agent therapy. *Clin Lab Haematol* 18:221, 1988.

301. Murayama T, Matsui T, Hayaski Y, et al: Plasma cell leukemia with myelofibrosis. *Ann Hematol* 69:151, 1994.

302. Schmidt U, Ruwe M, Leder LD: Multiple myeloma with bone marrow biopsy features simulating concomitant chronic idiopathic myelofibrosis. *Nouv Rev Fr Hematol* 37:159, 1995.

303. Abildgaard N, Bendix-Hanse K, Kristensen JE, et al: Bone marrow fibrosis and disease activity in multiple myeloma monitored by the autoterminal propeptide of procollagen III in serum. *Br J Haematol* 99:641, 1997.

304. Nomura S, Ogawa Y, Osawa G, et al: Myelofibrosis secondary to renal osteodystrophy. *Nephron* 72:683, 1996.

305. Fontenay-Roupie M, Dupuy E, Berrou E, et al: Increased proliferation of bone-marrow-derived fibroblasts in primary hypertropic osteoarthropy with severe myelofibrosis. *Blood* 85:3229, 1995.

306. Jantunen E, Hänninen A, Naukkarinen A, et al: Gray platelet syndrome with splenomegaly and signs of extramedullary hematopoiesis. *Am J Hematol* 46:218, 1994.

307. Sadoun A, Lacotte L, Delwail V, et al: Allogeneic bone marrow transplantation for hypereosinophilic syndrome with advanced myelofibrosis. *Bone Marrow Transplant* 19:741, 1997.

308. Vasquez L, Caballero D, Del Cañizo C, et al: Allogeneic peripheral blood cell transplantation for hypereosinophilic syndrome with myelofibrosis. *Bone Marrow Transplant* 25:217, 2000.

309. Filho FDR, Ferreira VDA, Mendes FDO, et al: Bone marrow fibrosis (pseudo-myelofibrosis) in kala-azar. *Rev Soc Bras Med Trop* 33:363, 2000.

310. Seelen MAJ, De Meijer PHEM, Posthuma EFM, Meinders AE: Myelofibrosis and idiopathic thrombocytopenic purpura. *Ann Hematol* 75:129, 1997.

311. Chang JC, Naqvi T: Thrombotic thrombocytopenic purpura associated with bone marrow metastasis and secondary myelofibrosis in cancer. *Oncologist* 8:375, 2003.

312. Hatake K, Ohtsuki T, Uwai M, et al: Tretinoin induces bone marrow collagenous fibrosis in acute promyelocytic leukemia. *Br J Haematol* 93:646, 1996.

313. Labotka RJ, Morgan RR: Myelofibrosis with neuroblastoma. *Med Pediatr Oncol* 10:21, 1982.

314. Karcher DS, Pearson CE, Butler WM, et al: Giant lymph node hyperplasia involving the thymus with associated nephrotic syndrome and myelofibrosis. *Am J Clin Pathol* 77:100, 1982.

315. Walka MM, Daümling S, Hadorn HB, et al: Vitamin D dependent rickets type II with myelofibrosis and immune dysfunction. *Eur J Pediatr* 114: 213, 1989.

316. Al-Eissa YA, Al-Mashhadami SA: Myelofibrosis in severe combined immunodeficiency due to vitamin D deficiency rickets. *Acta Haematol* 92:160, 1994.

317. Atiq M, Fadoo Z, Naz F, et al: Myelofibrosis in severe vitamin D deficiency rickets. *J Pak Med Assoc* 49:174, 1999.

318. Stéphan JL, Galambrun C, Dutour A, Freycon F: Myelofibrosis: An unusual presentation of vitamin D-deficient rickets. *Eur J Pediatr* 158: 828, 1999.

319. Sartoris DJ, Resnick D: Myelofibrosis arising in treated histiocytosis X. *Eur Pediatr* 144:200, 1985.

320. Fukuno K, Tsurumi H, Yoshikawa T, et al: A variant of acute promyelocytic leukemia with marked myelofibrosis. *Int J Hematol* 74:322, 2001.

321. Mori A, Wada H, Okada M, et al: Acute promyelocytic leukemia with marrow fibrosis at initial presentation. Possible involvement of transforming growth factor-β1. *Acta Haematol* 103:220, 2000.

322. Shah-Reddy I, Subramanian L, Narang S: Myelofibrosis and true histiocytic lymphoma. *Tumor* 71:509, 1985.

323. Jennings WH, Li CY, Kiely JM: Concomitant myelofibrosis with agnogenic myeloid metaplasia and malignant lymphoma. *Mayo Clin Proc* 58:617, 1983.

324. Epstein RJ, Joshua DE, Kronenberg H: Idiopathic myelofibrosis complicated by lymphoma: Report of two cases. *Acta Haematol* 73:40, 1985.

325. Kaufman S, Iuclea S, Reif R: Idiopathic myelofibrosis complicated by chronic lymphatic leukaemia. *Clin Lab Haematol* 9:81, 1987.

326. Nieto LH, Sanchez JMR, Arguelles HA, et al: A case of chronic lymphocytic leukemia overwhelmed by rapidly progressive idiopathic myelofibrosis. *Haematologica* 85:973, 2000.

327. Subramanian VP, Gomez GA, Han T, et al: Coexistence of myeloid metaplasia with myelofibrosis and hairy-cell leukemia. *Arch Intern Med* 145:164, 1985.

328. Ji SQ, Zhu M, Wang YZ: Primary macroglobulinemia with myelofibrosis: Report of a case. *Chin Med J* 100:83, 1987.

329. Humphrey CA, Morris TCM: The intimate relationship of myelofibrosis and myeloma. *Br J Haematol* 73:269, 1989.

330. Meerkin D, Ashkenazi Y, Gottschalk-Sabag S, Hershko C: Plasma cell dyscrasia with myelofibrosis. *Cancer* 73:625, 1994.

331. Kakkar N, Vashishta RK, Banerjee AK, et al: Primary pulmonary malignant teratoma with yolk sac element associated with hematologic neoplasia. *Respiration* 63:52, 1996.

332. Berner Y, Berrebi A: Myeloproliferative disorders and nonmyelomatous paraprotein: A study of five patients and review of the literature. *Isr J Med Sci* 22:109, 1986.

333. Ellis JT, Peterson P: Myelofibrosis in the myeloproliferative disorders. *Prog Clin Biol Res* 154:19, 1984.

334. Najean Y, Rain JD, Dresch C, et al: Risk of leukaemia, carcinoma and myelofibrosis in ^{32}P- or chemotherapy-treated patients with polycythaemia vera. *Leuk Lymphoma* 22(suppl 1):111, 1996.

335. Najean Y, Rain JD: Treatment of polycythemia vera: Use of ^{32}P alone or in combination with maintenance therapy using hydroxyurea in 461 patients greater than 65 years of age. *Blood* 89:2319, 1997.

336. Randi ML, Barbone E, Fabris F, et al: Post-polycythemia myeloid metaplasia. *J Med* 25:363, 1994.

337. Lukowicz DF, Myers TJ, Grasso JA, et al: Sideroblastic anemia terminating in myelofibrosis. *Am J Hematol* 13:253, 1982.

338. Hasselbalch H, Berild D: Transition of myelofibrosis to polycythaemia vera. *Scand J Haematol* 30:161, 1983.

339. Talarico L, Wolf BC, Kumar A, Weintraub LR: Reversal of bone marrow fibrosis and subsequent development of polycythemia vera

340. Palphilon DH, Creamer P, Keeling DH, et al: Restoration of active haemopoiesis in a patient with myelofibrosis and subsequent termination in acute myeloblastic leukaemia: Case report and review of the literature. *Eur J Haematol* 38:279, 1987.

341. Chabannon C, Pegourie B, Sotto JJ, Hallard D: Clinical and hematological improvement in a patient receiving danazol therapy for myelofibrosis with myeloid metaplasia. *Nouv Rev Fr Hematol* 32:165, 1990.

342. Lévy V, Bourgarit A, Delmer A, et al: Treatment of agnogenic myeloid metaplasia with danazol. *Am J Hematol* 53:239, 1996.

343. Cervantes F, Hernández-Boluda J-C, Alverz A, et al: Danazol treatment of idiopathic myelofibrosis with severe anemia. *Haematologica* 85:595, 2000.

344. Makdisi WJ, Cherian R, Vanveldhuizen PJ, et al: Fatal peliosis of the liver and spleen in a patient with agnogenic myeloid metaplasia treated with danazol. *Am J Gastroenterol* 90:317, 1995.

345. Ozsoylu S, Ruacan S: High dose intravenous corticosteroid treatment in childhood idiopathic myelofibrosis. *Acta Haematol* 75:49, 1986.

346. Cetingül N, Yener E, Oztop S, et al: Agnogenic myeloid metaplasia in childhood: A report of two cases and efficiency of intravenous high dose methylprednisolone treatment. *Acta Pediatr Jpn* 36:697, 1994.

347. Barois G, Liberato LN, Guarnone R: Serum erythropoietin in patients with myeloid metaplasia. *Br J Haematol* 83:365, 1993.

348. Rodrigues JN, Martino ML, Muniz R, Prados D: Recombinant human erythropoietin for the treatment of anemia in myelofibrosis with myeloid metaplasia. *Am J Hematol* 39:435, 1994.

349. Tefferi A, Silverstein MN: Recombinant human erythropoietin therapy in patients with myelofibrosis with myeloid metaplasia. *Br J Haematol* 86:893, 1994.

350. Rodriguez JN, Martino ML, Diéguez JC, Prados D: rHuEPO for the treatment of anemia in myelofibrosis with myeloid metaplasia. Experience in 6 patients and meta-analytical approach. *Haematologica* 83:616, 1998.

351. Hasselbalch HC, Clausen NT, Jensen BA: Successful treatment of anemia in idiopathic myelofibrosis with recombinant human erythropoietin. *Am J Hematol* 70:92, 2002.

352. Lofvenberg E, Wahlin A: Management of polycythaemia vera, essential thrombocythaemia and myelofibrosis with hydroxyurea. *Eur J Haematol* 41:375, 1988.

353. Lofvenberg E, Wahlin A, Roos G, Ost A: Reversal of myelofibrosis by hydroxyurea. *Eur J Haematol* 44:33, 1990.

354. Manoharan A: Management of myelofibrosis with intermittent hydroxyurea. *Br J Haematol* 71:252, 1991.

355. Petti MC, Latagliata R, Spadea T, et al: Melphalan treatment in patients with myelofibrosis with myeloid metaplasia. *Br J Haematol* 116:576, 2002.

356. Stahl RL, Hoppstein L, Davidson TG: Intraperitoneal chemotherapy with cytosine arabinoside in agnogenic myelofibrosis with myeloid metaplasia and ascites due to peritoneal extramedullary hematopoiesis. *Am J Hematol* 43:156, 1993.

357. Camba L, Aldrighetti L, Ciceri F, et al: Locoregional intrasplenic chemotherapy for hypersplenism in myelofibrosis. *Br J Haematol* 114: 638, 2001.

358. Merup M, Kutti J, Birgerård G, et al: Negligible clinical effects of thalidomide in patient with myelofibrosis with myeloid metaplasia. *Med Oncol* 19:79, 2002.

359. Piccaluga PP, Visani G, Pileri SA, et al: Clinical efficacy and antiangiogenic activity of thalidomide in myelofibrosis with myeloid metaplasia. A pilot study. *Leukemia* 16:1609, 2002.

360. Centanara E, Guarone R, Ippoliti G, Barosi G: Cyclosporine-A in severe refractory anemia of myelofibrosis with myeloid metaplasia: A preliminary report. *Haematologica* 83:622, 1998.

in patients with myeloproliferative disorders. *Am J Hematol* 30:248, 1989.

361. Nemoto Y, Tsutani H, Imamura S, et al: Successful treatment of acquired myelofibrosis with pure red cell aplasia. *Br J Haematol* 104:420, 1999.

362. Tsimberidou A-M, Giles FJ: TNF-α targeted therapeutic approaches in patients with hematologic malignancies. *Expert Rev Anticancer Ther* 2:277, 2002.

363. Steensma DP, Mesa RA, Li C-Y, et al: Etanercept, a soluble tumor necrosis factor receptor, palliates constitutional symptoms in patients with myelofibrosis with myeloid metaplasia: Results of a pilot study. *Blood* 99:2252, 2002.

364. Tefferi A, Mesa RA, Gray LA, et al: Phase 2 trial of imatinib mesylate in myelofibrosis with myeloid metaplasia. *Blood* 99:3854, 2002.

365. Carlo-Stella C, Cazzola M, Gasner A, et al: Effects of recombinant alpha and gamma interferons on the in vitro growth of circulating hematopoietic progenitors from patients with myelofibrosis and myeloid metaplasia. *Blood* 70:1014, 1987.

366. Sacchi S: The role of α-interferon in essential thrombocythaemia, polycythaema vera and myelofibrosis with myeloid metaplasia (MMM): A concise update. *Leuk Lymphoma* 19:13, 1995.

367. Bachleitner-Hofmann T, Gisslinger H: The role of interferon-α in the treatment of idiopathic myelofibrosis. *Ann Hematol* 78:533, 1999.

368. Sivera P, Cesano L, Guerrasio A, et al: Clinical and hematological improvement induced by etidronate in a patient with idiopathic myelofibrosis and osteosclerosis. *Br J Haematol* 86:397, 1994.

369. Froom P, Elmalah I, Braester A, et al: Clodronate in myelofibrosis: A case report. *Am J Med Sci* 323:115, 2002.

370. Greenberger JS, Chaffey JT, Rosenthal DS, et al: Irradiation for control of hypersplenism and painful splenomegaly in myeloid metaplasia. *Int J Radiat Oncol Biol Phys* 2:1083, 1977.

371. Parmentier C, Charbord P, Tibi M, et al: Splenic irradiation in myelofibrosis, clinical findings and ferrokinetics. *Int J Radiat Oncol Biol Phys* 2:1075, 1977.

372. Wagner H Jr, McKeough PG, Desforges J, et al: Splenic irradiation in the treatment of patients with chronic myelogenous leukemia or myelofibrosis with myeloid metaplasia. *Cancer* 58:1204, 1986.

373. Elliott MA, Tefferi A: Splenic irradiation in myelofibrosis with myeloid metaplasia: A review. *Blood Rev* 13:163, 1999.

374. Jacobs P, Wood L, Robson S: Refractory ascites in the chronic myeloproliferative syndrome. *Am J Hematol* 37:128, 1991.

375. Jacobs P, Sellars S: Granulocytic sarcoma preceding leukaemic transformation in myelofibrosis. *Postgrad Med J* 61:1069, 1985.

376. Teffari A, Jimenez T, Gray LA, et al: Radiation therapy for symptomatic hepatomegaly in myelofibrosis with myeloid metaplasia. *Eur J Haematol* 66:37, 2001.

377. Benbassat J, Penchas S, Ligumski M: Splenectomy in patients with agnogenic myeloid metaplasia: An analysis of 321 published cases. *Br J Haematol* 42:207, 1979.

378. Brenner B, Nagler A, Tatarsky I, Häsmonai M: Splenectomy in agnogenic myeloid metaplasia and post-polycythemic myeloid metaplasia. *Arch Intern Med* 148:2501, 1988.

379. Tefferi A, Mesa RA, Nagorney DM, et al: Splenectomy in myelofibrosis with myeloid metaplasia: A single institution experience with 223 patients. *Blood* 95:2226, 2000.

380. Lafaye F, Rain JD, Clot P, Najean Y: Risks and benefits of splenectomy in myelofibrosis: Analysis of 39 cases. *Nouv Rev Fr Hematol* 36:359, 1994.

381. Tefferi A, Mesa RA, Nagorney DM, et al: Splenectomy in myelofibrosis with myeloid metaplasia. *Blood* 95:2226, 2000.

382. Towell BL, Levine SP: Massive hepatomegaly following splenectomy for myeloid metaplasia: Case report and review of the literature. *Am J Med* 82:371, 1987.

383. DiBella NJ, Silverstein MN, Hoagland HC: Effect of splenectomy on teardrop-shaped erythrocytes in agnogenic myeloid metaplasia. *Arch Intern Med* 137:380, 1977.

384. Tefferi A, Silverstein MN, Li CY: 2-chlorodeoxyadenosine treatment after splenectomy in patients who have myelofibrosis with myeloid metaplasia. *Br J Haematol* 99:352, 1997.

385. Benbassat J, Gilon D, Penchas S: The choice between splenectomy and medical treatment in patients with advanced agnogenic myeloid metaplasia. *Am J Hematol* 33:128, 1990.

386. Petroianu A, Da Silva RG, Simal CJ, et al: Late postoperative follow-up of patients submitted to subtotal splenectomy. *Am Surg* 63:735, 1997.

387. Tefferi A, Barrett SM, Silverstein NM, Nagorney DM: Outcome of portal-systemic shunt surgery for portal hypertension associated with intrahepatic obstruction in patients with agnogenic myeloid metaplasia. *Am J Hematol* 46:325, 1994.

388. Angermayr B, Cejna M, Schoder M, et al: Transjugular intrahepatic portosystemic shunt for treatment of portal hypertension due to extramedullary hematopoiesis in idiopathic myelofibrosis. *Blood* 99:4246, 2002.

389. Belohlavek J, Schwarz J, Jirásek A, et al: Idiopathic myelofibrosis complicated by portal hypertension treated with a transjugular intrahepatic portosystemic shunt (TIPS). *Wien Klin Wochenschr* 113:208, 2001.

390. Matzner Y, Polliack A: Bone marrow curettage in myelodysplastic disorders: A stimulus for regeneration in disturbed hematopoiesis. *JAMA* 246:1926, 1981.

391. Fruchtman SM: Therapeutic implications of collagen metabolism in myelofibrosis. *Prog Clin Biol Res* 154:467, 1984.

392. Petrini M, Cecconi N, Azzara A, et al: 1,25-dihydroxy-vitamin D on the treatment of idiopathic myelofibrosis. *Br J Haematol* 62:399, 1986.

393. Richard C, Mazzora F, Iriondo A, et al: The usefulness of 1,25-dihydroxy-vitamin in the treatment of idiopathic myelofibrosis. *Br J Haematol* 62:399, 1986.

394. Eugster C, Brun-del-Re GP, Bucher U: The role of 1,25-dihydroxy-vitamin D_3(1,25(OH)$_2$D$_3$) in the treatment of idiopathic myelofibrosis [letter]. *Br J Haematol* 65:381, 1987.

395. Arlet P, Nicodeme R, Adoue D, et al: Clinical evidence for 1-dihydroxycholecalciferol action in myelofibrosis [letter]. *Lancet* 1:1013, 1984.

396. Rewald E, De las Mercedes Francischetti: Combining interferon-alpha2b (IFN) and intravenous immunoglobulins IgG, IgM and IgA (IVIG) in rapid progressive myelofibrosis (MF) with trisomy 1 [letter]. *Am J Hematol* 54:340, 1997.

397. Pietrasanta D, Clavio M, Vallebella E, et al: Long-lasting effect of cyclosporin-A on anemia associated with idiopathic myelofibrosis. *Haematologica* 82:458, 1997.

398. Singhal S, Powles R, Treleaven J, et al: Allogeneic bone marrow transplantation for primary myelofibrosis. *Bone Marrow Transplant* 16:743, 1995.

399. Guardiola P, Anderson JE, Bandini G, et al: Allogeneic bone marrow transplantation for agnogenic myeloid metaplasia. *Blood* 93:2831, 1999.

400. Przepiorka D, Giralt S, Khour I, et al: Allogeneic marrow transplantation for myeloproliferative disorders other than chronic myelogenous leukemia: Review of forty cases. *Am J Hematol* 7:24, 1998.

401. McCarty JM: Transplant strategies for idiopathic myelofibrosis. *Semin Hematol* 41(suppl 3):23, 2004.

402. Mittal P, Saliba RM, Giralt SA, et al: Allogeneic transplantation: A therapeutic option for myelofibrosis, chronic myelomonocytic leukemia, and Philadelphia-negative BCR-ABL-negative chronic myelogenous leukemia. *Bone Marrow Transplant* 33:1005,2004.

403. Guardiola P, Anderson JE, Bandini G, et al: Allogeneic stem cell transplantation for agnogenic myeloid metaplasia: A European Group for Blood and Marrow Transplantation, Société Française de Greffe de Moelle, Gruppo Italiano per il Trapianto Midollo Osseo, and Fred Hutchinson Cancer Center Collaborative Study. *Blood* 93:2831, 1999.

404. Guardiola P: Myelofibrosis with myeloid metaplasia. *N Engl J Med* 343: 659, 2000.

405. Deeg HJ, Appelbaum FR: Stem-cell transplantation for myelofibrosis. *N Engl J Med* 334:775, 2001.

406. Byrne JL, Beshti H, Clark D, et al: Induction of remission after donor leucocyte infusion for the treatment of relapsed chronic idiopathic myelofibrosis following allogeneic transplantation: Evidence for a "graft vs. myelofibrosis" effect. *Br J Haematol* 108:430, 2000.

407. Cervantes F, Rovira M, Urbano-Ispizua A,et al: Complete remission of idiopathic myelofibrosis following donor lymphocyte infusion after failure of allogeneic transplantation: Demonstration of a graft-versus-myelofibrosis effect. *Bone Marrow Transplant* 26:697, 2000.

408. Devine SM, Hoffman R, Verma A, et al: Allogeneic blood cell transplantation following reduced-intensity conditioning is effective therapy for older patients with myelofibrosis with myeloid metaplasia. *Blood* 99: 2255, 2002.

409. Hessling J, Kroger N, Werner M, et al: Dose-reduced conditioning regimen followed by allogeneic stem cell transplantation in patients with myelofibrosis with myeloid metaplasia. *Br J Haematol* 119:769, 2002.

410. Anderson JE, Tefferi A, Craig F, et al: Myeloablation and autologous peripheral blood stem cell rescue results in hematologic and clinical responses in patients with myeloid metaplasia with myelofibrosis. *Blood* 98:586, 2001.

411. Visini G, Finelli C, Castelli U, et al: Myelofibrosis with myeloid metaplasia: Clinical and haematological parameters predicting survival in a series of 133 patients. *Br J Haematol* 75:4, 1990.

412. Cervantes F: Prognostic and current practice in treatment of myelofibrosis and myeloid metaplasia: An update anno 2000. *Pathol Biol* 49: 148, 2001.

413. Mesa RA, Li C-Y, Schroeder G, Tefferi A: Clinical correlates of splenic histology and splenic karyotype in myelofibrosis with myeloid metaplasia. *Blood* 97:3665, 2001.

414. Kvasnicka HM, Thiele J, Regn C, et al: Prognostic impact of apoptosis and proliferation in idiopathic (primary) myelofibrosis. *Ann Hematol* 78: 65, 1999.

415. Rozman C, Giralt M, Feliu E, et al: Life expectancy of patients with chronic non-leukemic myeloproliferative disorders. *Cancer* 67:2658, 1991.

416. Silverstein MN, Brown AL, Linman JW: Idiopathic myeloid metaplasia, its evolution into acute leukemia. *Arch Intern Med* 132:709, 1973.

417. Marcus RE, Hibbin JA, Matutes E, et al: Megakaryoblastic transformation of myelofibrosis with expression of the c-*sis* oncogene. *Am J Hematol* 36:186, 1986.

418. Hernandez JM, SanMiguel JF, Gonzalez M, et al: Development of acute leukaemia after idiopathic myelofibrosis. *J Clin Pathol* 45:427, 1992.

419. Mesa R, Silverstein MN, Jacobsen SJ, et al: Population-based incidence and survival figures in essential thrombocythemia and agnogenic myeloid metaplasia: An Olmstead County Study 1976–1995. *Am J Hematol* 61:10, 1999.

420. Chan ACL, Kwong Y-L, Lam CCK: Granulocytic sarcoma of megakaryoblastic differentiation complicating chronic idiopathic myelofibrosis. *Hum Pathol* 27:417, 1996.

421. Polliack A, Prokocimer M, Matzner Y, et al: Lymphoblastic leukemic transformation (lymphoblastic crisis) in myelofibrosis and myeloid metaplasia. *Am J Hematol* 9:211, 1980.

422. Yinon A, Kopolovic J, Dollberg L, Hershko C: Evolution of malignant lymphoma in agnogenic myeloid metaplasia. *Oncology* 45:373, 1988.

423. Barosi G, Ambrosetti A, Centra A: Splenectomy and risk of blast transformation in myelofibrosis with myeloid metaplasia. *Blood* 91:3630, 1998.

424. Shreiner DP: Spontaneous hematologic remission in agnogenic myeloid metaplasia. *Am J Med* 60:1014, 1976.

425. Rani MV, Shreiner DP: Spontaneous "remission" of agnogenic myeloid metaplasia and termination in acute myeloid leukemia. *Arch Intern Med* 141:1481, 1981.

426. Altura RA, Heady DR, Wang WC: Long-term survival of infants with idiopathic myelofibrosis. *Br J Haematol* 109:459, 2000.

427. Sah A, Minford A, Parapia LA: Spontaneous remission of juvenile idiopathic myelofibrosis. *Br J Haematol* 112:1083, 2001.

428. Amital H, Rewald E, Levy Y, et al: Fibrosis regression induced by intravenous gammaglobulin treatment. *Ann Rheum Dis* 62:175, 2003.

429. Li Z, Deeg HJ: Pros and cons of splenectomy in patients with myelofibrosis undergoing stem cell transplantation. *Leukemia* 15:465, 2001.

430. Vannucchi AM, Bianchi L, Cellai C, et al: Development of myelofibrosis in mice genetically impaired for GATA-1 expression (GATA-1(low) mice). *Blood* 100:1123 2002.

431. Andrieux J, Demory JL, Dupriez B, et al: Dysregulation and overexpression of HMGA2 in myelofibrosis with myeloid metaplasia. *Genes Chromosomes Cancer* 39:82, 2004.

432. Popat U, Frost A, Liu EL, et al: Myelofibrosis is frequently seen in patients with primary pulmonary hypertension and is associated with polyclonal hematopoiesis and normal CD34 count. *Blood* 102:919A 2003.

433. Mesa RA, Lliott MA, Schroeder G, Tefferi A: Durable responses to thalidomide-based drug therapy for myelofibrosis with myeloid metaplasia. *Mayo Clin Proc* 79:883, 2004.

434. Strupp C, Germing U, Scherer A, et al: Thalidomide for treatment of idiopathic myelofibrosis. *Eur J Haematol* 72:52, 2004.

435. Greyz N, Miller WE, Andrey J, Masson J: Long-term remission of myelofibrosis following nonmyeloablative allogenic peripheral blood progenitor cell transplantation in older age. *Bone Marrow Transp* 34:833, 2004.

436. Kralovics R, Passamonti F, Buser AS, et al: A gain-of-function mutation of JAK2 in myeloproliferative disorders. *N Engl J Med* 352:1779, 2005.

437. Levine RL, Wadleigh M, Cools J, et al: Activating mutation in the tyrosine kinase JAK2 in polycythemia vera, essential thrombocythemia, and myeloid metaplasia with myelofibrosis. *Cancer Cell* 7:387, 2005.

438. Baxter EJ, Scott LM, Campbell PJ, et al: Acquired mutation of the tyrosine kinase JAK2 in human myeloproliferative disorders. *Lancet* 365: 1054, 2005.

CLASSIFICATION OF MALIGNANT LYMPHOID DISORDERS

THOMAS J. KIPPS

> This chapter outlines the category of neoplastic or preneoplastic lymphocyte and plasma cell disorders. It introduces a framework for evaluating neoplastic lymphocyte and plasma cell disorders, outlines clinical syndromes associated with such disorders, and presents a road map to the chapters in the text that discuss each of these disorders in greater detail. Chapter 80 outlines the diseases caused by nonneoplastic disorders of lymphocytes and plasma cells.

CLASSIFICATION

Lymphocyte malignancies compose a wide spectrum of different morphologic and clinical syndromes (Table 90-1). Lymphocyte neoplasms can originate from cells that are at a stage prior to T and B lymphocyte differentiation from a primitive stem cell or from cells at stages of maturation after stem cell differentiation. Thus, acute lymphocytic leukemias arise from a primitive lymphoid stem cell that may give rise to cells with either B or T cell phenotypes (see Chap. 91). On the other hand, chronic lymphocytic leukemia arises from a more differentiated B lymphocyte progenitor (see Chap. 92) and myeloma from progenitors at even later stages of B lymphocyte maturation (see Chap. 100). Variability in expression of a lymphopoietic stem cell disorder may result in the spectrum of lymphocytic diseases, such as a B lymphocyte or T lymphocyte lymphoma (see Chap. 96), and different types of diseases, such as hairy cell leukemia (see Chap. 93), prolymphocytic leukemia (see Chap. 92), natural killer cell large granular lymphocytic leukemia (see Chap. 94), or plasmacytoma (see Chap. 100).

Hodgkin lymphoma also generally is derived from a neoplastic B cell that has highly mutated immunoglobulin genes that no longer are expressed into protein.

To provide a unified international basis for clinical and investigative work in this field, the International Lymphoma Study Group proposed a classification termed the revised European-American lymphoma (REAL) classification (see Chap. 96),[1] which was modified in 2001 by the World Health Organization (WHO).[2] The REAL/WHO classification scheme makes use of the pathologic, immunophenotypic, genetic, and clinical features of a given lymphocyte tumor to delineate them into separate disease entities (see Table 90-1).[3] For some of these

entities, the neoplastic lymphocytes have distinctive cytogenetic abnormalities, which can be identified using molecular techniques that increasingly are being used in clinical pathology laboratories.[4,5]

The REAL/WHO classification recognizes a basic distinction between lymphocyte predominance Hodgkin lymphoma and classic Hodgkin lymphoma, reflecting the differences in clinical presentation and behavior, morphology, phenotype, and molecular features (see Chap. 97).[2] Studies have identified features that can be used to distinguish classic Hodgkin lymphoma from anaplastic large cell lymphoma and, to a lesser extent, between lymphocyte predominant Hodgkin lymphoma and T cell rich, large B cell lymphoma.

CLINICAL BEHAVIOR

Lymphomas of similar histology can have widely different spectra of associated clinical symptoms and clinical aggressiveness, making impossible the categorization of lymphoma tumors using a generic grading system based on morphology alone. For example, the neoplastic cells in mantle cell lymphoma appear smaller and more differentiated than those of anaplastic large cell lymphomas. However, the validation studies for the REAL classification revealed that patients with mantle cell lymphoma or anaplastic large cell lymphomas have a 5-year survival rate of less than 30 percent or 80 percent, respectively.[6,7] Generally, T cell lymphomas/leukemias have a more aggressive clinical behavior than B cell lymphomas of comparable histology. The tendency for more aggressive disease also applies to lymphoid tumors derived from natural killer cells. A helpful distinction is to divide the lymphoid tumors into one of two categories, namely, indolent lymphomas versus aggressive lymphomas, based upon on the characteristics of the disease at the time of presentation and the patients' life expectancy if the disease is left untreated.[8,9] Clinical studies have verified that the different disease categories defined in the REAL/WHO classification each can be segregated into one or the other of these two major categories (Tables 90-2 and 90-3).[6] Analyses of gene expression patterns using microarray technology have allowed for identification of subcategories within some of the disease categories defined by the REAL/WHO classification that have different tendencies for disease progression, survival, and/or response rates to standard therapies (see Chap. 95).[10-16]

ASSOCIATED CLINICAL SYNDROMES

ABNORMAL PRODUCTION OF IMMUNOGLOBULIN

When B lymphocytes undergo neoplastic transformation and clonal proliferation, they can secrete monoclonal proteins inappropriately (see Chap. 98). If the monoclonal protein is immunoglobulin (Ig)M, IgA, or a member of certain subclasses of IgG (e.g., namely IgG$_3$), its presence may increase the viscosity of the blood, impairing blood flow through the microcirculation (see Chaps. 100 and 102). This process may be impeded further by the associated erythrocyte to erythrocyte aggregation (pathologic rouleaux) that often occurs in blood with a high concentration of immunoglobulin protein. Collectively, this situation may result in the hyperviscosity syndrome, manifested clinically by headache, dizziness, diplopia, stupor, retinal venous engorgement, or frank coma (see Chap. 102).[17,18]

Monoclonal immunoglobulin proteins also can interact with cell surfaces and impair granulocyte or platelet function, or they can interact with coagulation proteins to impair their function in hemostasis. Excessive excretion of immunoglobulin light chains can lead to several types of renal tubular dysfunction and renal insufficiency (see Chap. 100). IgM deposited in glomerular tufts also can lead to renal disease (see Chap. 102). Cryoglobulins (or immunoglobulins that precipitate at temperatures below 37°C) can result in Raynaud syndrome, skin

---

Acronyms and abbreviations that appear in this chapter include: α/β TCR, T cell receptor genes encoding the α- and β-chains of the T cell receptor (see Chap. 78); *ALK*, gene encoding anaplastic lymphoma kinase; cIg, cytoplasmic immunoglobulin; EBV, Epstein-Barr virus; γ/δ TCR, T cell receptor genes encoding the γ- and δ-chains of the T cell receptor (see Chap. 78); HL, Hodgkin lymphoma; HTLV-1, human T cell leukemia virus type 1; Ig, immunoglobulin; IgR, immunoglobulin gene rearrangement; IL, interleukin; MALT, mucosa-associated lymphoid tissue; *MUM1*, gene encoding multiple myeloma oncogene 1; *NPM*, gene encoding nucleophosmin; POEMS, polyneuropathy, organomegaly, endocrinopathy, monoclonal gammopathy, and skin changes; REAL, revised European-American lymphoma; R-S, Reed-Sternberg; sIg, surface immunoglobulin (see Chap. 77); sIgD, surface IgD; sIgM, surface IgM; TAL1, gene encoding T cell acute leukemia-1; TCR, T cell receptor; WHO, World Health Organization.

TABLE 90-1 REVISED EUROPEAN-AMERICAN LYMPHOMA (REAL) CLASSIFICATION

LYMPHOCYTE NEOPLASM	MORPHOLOGY	PHENOTYPE*	GENOTYPE†
B-Cell Neoplasms			
Precursor B Cell Neoplasms			
Lymphoblastic leukemia (see Chap. 91)	Medium to large cells with finely stippled chromatin and scant cytoplasm	TdT+, sIg−, CD10, CD13+/−, CD19, CD34+/−, CD33+/−, CD79a	t(1;19), t(9;22), and 11q13-defects associated with poor prognosis
Lymphoblastic lymphoma (see Chap. 96)	Large cells with high nuclear to cytoplasmic ratio	See above	See above
Mature B cell neoplasms			
Leukemias			
Chronic lymphocytic leukemia (see Chap. 92)	Small cells with round, dense nuclei	Dull sIg, CD5, CD10−, CD19, dull CD20, CD23, CD38+/−	IgR, trisomy 12 (~30%), del at 13q14 (~50%), 11q− (15%)
Prolymphocytic leukemia (see Chap. 92)	≥55% prolymphocytes	Bright sIg, CD5+/−, CD19, CD22	IgR, trisomy 12 (~30%)
Hairy cell leukemia (see Chap. 93)	Small cells with cytoplasmic projections	Dull sIg, CD5+/−, CD10−, CD19, CD20, CD103	IgR
Lymphomas (see Chap. 96)			
Small lymphocytic lymphoma	Small round cells	Dull sIg, CD5, CD19, dull CD20, CD23	IgR, trisomy 12 (~30%), del at 13q14 (~40%), 11q− (~15%)
Lymphoplasmacytoid lymphoma	Small cells with plasmacytoid features	Dull cIg, CD5−, CD10−, CD19, CD20+/−	IgR, t(9;14)(p13;q32) (~50%) involving *PAX5*
Mantle cell lymphoma	Small- to medium-sized cells	sIgM/IgD, CD5, CD10−, CD19, CD20, CD23−	IgR, t(11;14)(q13;q32) (~70%), involving *BCL1*
Follicular lymphoma (follicle center lymphoma)	Small, medium, or large cells with cleaved nuclei	sIg, CD5−, CD10, CD19, bright CD20, CD23+/−	IgR, t(14;18)(q32;q21) (~85%) involving *BCL2*
Marginal zone B cell lymphoma	Small or large monocytoid cells	sIgM+, sIgD−, cIg (~50%), CD5−, CD11c+/−, CD19, CD20, CD23−, CD43+/−	IgR, commonly with trisomy 3 and/or t(11;18)(q21;q21) involving *API2*, *MLT*, or t(1;14)(p22;q32) involving *BCL10*
Mucosa-associated lymphoid tissue (MALT) type	See above	See above	See above
Nodal type	See above	See above	See above
Splenic marginal zone B cell lymphoma	Small to large monocytoid and/or villous lymphocytes	sIgM+, sIgD−, CD5+/−, CD19, CD20, CD23−	IgR
Diffuse large B cell lymphoma	Large, irregular cells that can resemble centroblasts, immunoblasts, multilobate cells, or even RS-like cells	sIgM+, sIgD+/−, CD5+/−, CD10+/−, CD19, CD20	IgR, 3q27 abnormalities and/or t(3;14)(q27;q32) involving *BCL6* (~40%) or t(14,18)(q32;q210) (~25%) involving *BCL2*
Primary mediastinal large B cell lymphoma	Same as above	sIg−, CD5−, CD19, CD20, CD22	Same as above
Burkitt lymphoma	Medium-sized, round cells with abundant cytoplasm	sIgM+, CD5−, CD10, CD19, CD20, CD23−	t(8;14)(q24;q32), t(2;8)(q11;q24), or t(8;22)(q24;q11), involving Ig loci and *C-MYC* at 8q24
Burkitt-like lymphoma	Medium-sized, round cells with abundant cytoplasm	Same as above except sIg−, cIg+/−, and CD10−	Same as above except ~30% have BCL−2 rearrangements
Plasma cell neoplasms			
Plasma cell myeloma (see Chap. 100)	Plasma cells with occasional plasmablasts	cIg, CD5−, CD19, CD20−, CD22, CD38, CD56	IgR, commonly with complex karyotypes and/or t(6;14)(p25;q32) involving *MUM1*
Plasma cell leukemia	Plasmablastic cells with prominent nucleoli	Same as above	Same as above
Plasma cell lymphoma	Plasma cells	Same as above	Same as above
Waldenström macroglobulinemia (see Chap. 102)	Plasmacytoid cells	CD5+/−, CD10+/−, CD19, CD20, CD22, CD38+/−	IgR, complex karyotypes common
Hodgkin Lymphoma (HL) (see Chap. 97)			
Nodular Lymphocyte Predominant HL	"Popcorn cells" with nuclei resembling those of centroblasts	CD19, CD20, CD22, CD45, CD79a, CD15−, and rarely CD30+/−	IgR with high-level expression of *BCL6*
Classic HL			
Nodular sclerosis HL	R-S cells and lacunar cells dispersed in reactive lymphoid nodules	R-S cells typically are CD15+, CD20+/−, CD30+, CD45−, CD79a−	R-S cells generally express *PAX5* and *MUM1*, variable expression of *BCL6*, and have IgR without functional Ig
Lymphocyte-rich HL	Few R-S cells with occasional "popcorn" appearance dispersed in lymphoid nodules	Same as above	Same as above

TABLE 90-1 REVISED EUROPEAN-AMERICAN LYMPHOMA (REAL) CLASSIFICATION (*Continued*)

LYMPHOCYTE NEOPLASM	MORPHOLOGY	PHENOTYPE*	GENOTYPE†
Hodgkin Lymphoma (*Continued*)			
Mixed cellularity HL	R-S cells dispersed among plasma cells, epithelioid histiocytes, eosinophils, and T cells	R-S cells typically are CD15+, CD20+/−, CD30+, CD45−, CD79a−	R-S cells generally express *PAX5* and *MUM1*, variable expression of *BCL6*, and have IgR without functional Ig
Lymphocyte-depleted HL	Prominent numbers of R-S cells with effacement of the nodal structure	Same as above	Same as above
T Cell Neoplasms			
Precursor T Cell Neoplasms			
Acute lymphoblastic leukemia (see Chap. 91)	Medium to large cells with finely stippled chromatin and scant cytoplasm	CD2+/−, cytoplasmic CD3, CD5+/−, CD7, CD10+/−, CD4+/CD8+ or CD4−/CD8−	Abnormalities in TCR loci at 14q11 (TCR-α), 7q34 (TCR-β), or 7p15 (TCR-γ), and/or t(1;14)(p32-34; q11) involving *TAL1*
Lymphoblastic lymphoma (see Chap. 96)	Same as above	Same as above	Same as above
Mature T Cell Neoplasms			
Leukemias			
T cell prolymphocytic leukemia	Small cells with prominent nucleoli and abundant cytoplasm	TdT−, CD2, CD3, CD5, CD7, CD4+/CD8− is more common than CD4−/CD8+	α/β TCR rearrangement, inv14(q11; q32) (~75%)
T cell large granular lymphocytic leukemia (see Chap. 94)	Abundant cytoplasm and azurophilic granules	TdT−, CD2, CD3, CD8, CD16+/−, CD56−, CD57+/−	α/β TCR rearrangement
Lymphomas (see Chap. 96)			
T cell lymphoma, nasal and nasal-type ("angiocentric lymphoma")	Angiocentric and angiodestructive growth	CD2, CD3+/−, CD5+/−, CD56, cytoplasmic CD3	TCR rearrangements variable, EBV present
Cutaneous T cell lymphoma	Small to large cells with cerebriform nuclei	TdT−, CD2, CD3, CD4, CD5, CD7+/−, CD25−	α/β TCR rearrangement
Mycosis fungoides	Same as above	Same as above	Same as above
Sézary syndrome	Same as above	Same as above	Same as above
Angioimmunoblastic T cell lymphoma	Small immunoblasts with pale-staining or clear cells		α/β TCR rearrangement with rare incomplete IgR, trisomy 3 or 5 noted
Peripheral T cell lymphoma (unspecified)	Highly variable	CD2, CD3, CD5, CD7−, CD4 > CD8 > CD4/CD8	α/β TCR rearrangement often with incomplete IgR
Subcutaneous panniculitic T cell lymphoma	Medium-sized atypical cells with irregular nuclei and hyperchromasia	CD2, CD3, CD5, CD7−, CD4, or CD8	α/β TCR rearrangement
Intestinal T cell lymphoma	Small to large atypical lymphocytes	CD2, CD3, CD5, CD7−, CD4−/CD8− or CD4−/CD8+, CD103	β TCR rearrangement
Hepatosplenic γ/δ T cell lymphoma	Small to medium-size cells with condensed chromatin and round nuclei	CD2, CD3, CD4−, CD5, CD7−, CD8+/−	γ/δ TCR rearrangement, isochromosome 7q
Adult T cell lymphoma	Highly variable with multilobed nuclei	CD2, CD3, CD5, CD7−, CD25, CD4 >> CD8	α/β TCR rearrangement and integrated HTLV-1
Anaplastic large-cell lymphoma	Large blastic pleomorphic cells with "horseshoe"-shaped nuclei, prominent nucleoli, and abundant basophilic cytoplasm	TdT−, CD2, CD3, CD5, CD7+/−, CD25+/−, CD30, CD45+/−	TCR rearrangement, t(2;5)(p23;q35) resulting in nucleophosmin–anaplastic lymphoma kinase fusion protein (*NPM, ALK*)
Primary cutaneous CD30-positive lymphoma	Anaplastic large cells as above in cutaneous nodules	TdT−, CD2, CD3, CD5, CD7+/−, CD25+/−, CD30	TCR rearrangement, without t(2; 5)(p23;q35)
Natural Killer Cell Neoplasms			
Large granular lymphocytic leukemia (see Chap. 94)	Abundant cytoplasm and azurophilic granules	TdT−, CD2, CD3−, CD8+/−, CD16, CD56, CD57+/−	No TCR rearrangement
Aggressive natural killer cell leukemia	Same as above	Same as above	No TCR rearrangement, EBV present
Natural killer cell lymphoma, nasal and nasal-type ("angiocentric lymphoma")	Angiocentric and angiodestructive growth	CD2, CD5+/−, CD56, cytoplasmic CD3	No TCR rearrangement, EBV present

* The immunohistochemical and surface antigen phenotypes that typically are found for neoplastic cells of a given disorder are listed. If a CD antigen is indicated (see Chap. 14), then most of the neoplastic cells express that particular surface protein that is expressed by most tumor cells. CD antigens that have a minus sign "−" suffix are characteristically not expressed by the neoplastic cells of that disease entity. CD antigens that have a +/− sign suffix are not expressed by the neoplastic cells of all patients with that entity or are expressed at low or variable levels on the tumor cells.
† The common genetic features associated with a given type of neoplasm are indicated. The numbers in parentheses provide the approximate proportion of cases that have the defined phenotype or genetic abnormality.

ulcerations, purpura, digital infarction, and gangrene (see Chap. 52). These manifestations result from immune complex formation, complement activation, and precipitation of cryoglobulins in cutaneous blood vessels. Finally, excessive production of monoclonal immunoglobulin or immunoglobulin fragments in plasma cell myeloma (see Chap. 100) or heavy-chain disease (see Chap. 103) may lead to formation of amyloid, resulting in primary amyloidosis (see Chap. 101).

Production of autoreactive antibodies spontaneously or in relationship to a B lymphocyte neoplasia may lead to autoimmune hemolytic anemia (see Chap. 52), autoimmune thrombocytopenia (see Chap. 110), or, rarely, autoimmune neutropenia (see Chap. 65). Autoantibodies directed against tissues are implicated in the etiopathogenesis of diseases such as autoimmune thyroiditis, adrenalitis, encephalitis, and conditions involving other organ involvement. Peripheral neuropathies as a result of demyelinization can occur in patients with monoclonal immunoglobulin (see Chaps. 100 and 102). The neural injury often is related to antibody activity against myelin-associated glycoproteins or absorption by nerve tissue. Rarely, the polyneuropathy is associated with organomegaly, endocrinopathy, a monoclonal protein, and skin chains or with the polyneuropathy, organomegaly, endocrinopathy, monoclonal gammopathy, and skin changes (POEMS) syndrome (see Chap. 100).

MARROW AND OTHER TISSUE INFILTRATION

Well-differentiated malignant B lymphocytes, such as those found in the early stages of chronic lymphocytic leukemia or macroglobulinemia, may infiltrate the marrow extensively, causing minimal impairment of hemopoiesis. Eventually, however, further infiltration of marrow by malignant B lymphocytes can suppress normal hemopoiesis, resulting in varying combinations of anemia, granulocytopenia, and/or thrombocytopenia (see Chap. 92). Malignant B lymphocyte proliferation or infiltration may result in any combination of splenomegaly and lymphadenopathy of either superficial or deep lymph nodes. Many B cell lymphomas tend to involve isolated lymph node groups (see Chaps. 96 and 97), whereas B cell chronic lymphocytic leukemia and most low-grade lymphomas tend to involve many superficial and deep lymph node-bearing areas and the spleen (see Chaps. 92 and 96). Prolymphocytic leukemia and hairy cell leukemia, two uncommon B lymphocyte malignancies, are prone to infiltrate the marrow and spleen, sometimes causing massive enlargement of the latter (see Chaps. 92 and 93).

LYMPHOKINE-INDUCED DISORDERS

In addition to the consequences of monoclonal immunoglobulin and tumor proliferation, some lymphocyte malignancies may elaborate cytokines that contribute to the disease morbidity. Patients with cutaneous T cell lymphomas have elevated plasma levels of Th2-type associated cytokines (see Chap. 78), which may account for the relatively high incidence of eosinophilia and eosinophilic pneumonia observed in patients with this disease.[19] In addition, the neoplastic plasma cells in myeloma may secrete interleukin (IL)-1, a cytokine that can stimulate osteoclast proliferation and activity leading to extensive osteolysis, severe bone pain, and pathologic fractures (see Chap. 100).[20] In addition, IL-1 may stimulate production of antidiuretic hormone and contribute to a syndrome of inappropriate secretion of antidiuretic hormone.[21] Dysregulated extrarenal production of calcitriol, the active metabolite of vitamin D, appears to underlie the hypercalcemia associated with Hodgkin lymphoma and other lymphomas (see Chaps. 96 and 97).[22]

SYSTEMIC SYMPTOMS

Large-cell lymphoma, poorly differentiated lymphoma, and Hodgkin lymphoma frequently are associated with fever, night sweats, weight loss, and anorexia (see Chaps. 96 and 97). Patients with lymphomas or Hodgkin lymphoma have an increased incidence of localized or disseminated herpes zoster, and 10 percent or more of these patients may be affected at some time during the course of their illness. Pruritus is common in Hodgkin lymphoma, and its severity parallels disease activity. Systemic symptoms may be present in Hodgkin lymphoma in the absence of obvious, bulky lymph node or splenic tumors, whereas in well-differentiated small-cell lymphomas, such as chronic lymphocytic leukemia and Waldenström macroglobulinemia, fever, night sweats, and significant weight loss are uncommon despite generalized lymphadenopathy and splenomegaly. Rather, fever in patients with chronic lymphocytic leukemia or macroglobulinemia usually is secondary to infectious disease.

METABOLIC SIGNS

Lymphocytic malignancies are associated with the most dramatic metabolic disturbances associated with cancers (see Chap. 96). Some lymphomas and lymphocytic leukemias may have an extremely high proliferative rate, a high death fraction of cells, and, therefore, an enormous turnover of nucleoproteins, sometimes causing hyperuricemia and extreme hyperuricosuria. Burkitt lymphoma or acute lymphocytic leukemia is particularly likely to cause an extreme degree of hyperuricemia, sometimes leading to renal failure prior to cytotoxic therapy. Also, because these and other lymphocytic malignancies are sensitive to cytotoxic drugs and glucocorticoids, cytotoxic therapy may cause extreme hyperuricemia, hyperuricosuria, hyperkalemia, and hyperphosphatemia.[23] This has been called the *tumor lysis syndrome*. Precipitation of uric acid in the renal tubules and collecting system can lead to acute obstructive nephropathy and renal failure unless precautions are taken, such as pretreatment with allopurinol, hydration, and alkalization of the urine.

Hypercalcemia and calciuria are common complications of myeloma because of osteolysis. Hypercalcemia also may occur during the course of lymphomas (see Chap. 96) or plasma cell myeloma (see Chap. 100). This situation may be caused by several mechanisms, including tumor cell production of IL-1, ectopic parathyroid hormone elaboration, excessive bone resorption, and impaired bone formation.[20]

EXTRANODAL INVOLVEMENT

T cell leukemias and lymphomas, in addition to causing lymph node and spleen enlargement, may involve the skin, mediastinum, or central nervous system. As the name implies, cutaneous T cell lymphomas have malignant cells that home to the skin, sometimes producing a severe desquamating erythroderma in Sézary syndrome, small (<2 cm) subcutaneous nodules in primary cutaneous CD30-positive lymphoma, or a variety of nodular infiltrative lesions in mycosis fungoides (see Chap. 96). T cell acute lymphocytic leukemia and lymphoblastic lymphoma frequently cause mediastinal enlargement (see Chap. 96). These diseases frequently involve the leptomeninges and other structures that are transverse to the subarachnoid space, such as the cranial and peripheral nerves.

B cell lymphomas frequently may involve the salivary glands, endocrine glands, joints, heart, lung, kidney, bowel, bone, and, less frequently, other extranodal sites. These diseases may begin as an extranodal tumor, or the tumor may develop during the course of the disease. Marginal zone B cell lymphoma of mucosa-associated lymphoid tissue (MALT) type frequently involves the stomach and salivary glands, although the disease may be encountered in any extranodal site distinguished by the presence of a columnar or cuboidal epithelium.

REFERENCES

1. Harris NL, Jaffe ES, Stein H, et al: A revised European-American classification of lymphoid neoplasms: A proposal from the International Lymphoma Study Group. *Blood* 84:1361, 1994.
2. Chan JK: The new World Health Organization classification of lymphomas: The past, the present, and the future. *Hematol Oncol* 19:129, 2001.
3. Segal GH, Kjeldsberg CR: Practical lymphoma diagnosis: An approach to using the information organized in the REAL proposal. Revised European-American lymphoid neoplasm. *Anat Pathol* 3:147, 1998.
4. Spagnolo DV, Ellis DW, Juneja S, et al: The role of molecular studies in lymphoma diagnosis: A review. *Pathology* 36:19, 2004.
5. Strauchen JA: Immunophenotypic and molecular studies in the diagnosis and classification of malignant lymphoma. *Cancer Invest* 22:138, 2004.
6. A clinical evaluation of the International Lymphoma Study Group classification of non-Hodgkin's lymphoma. The Non-Hodgkin's Lymphoma Classification Project. *Blood* 89:3909, 1997.
7. Fisher RI, Miller TP, Grogan TM: New REAL clinical entities. *Cancer J Sci Am* 4(suppl 2):S5, 1998.
8. Pileri SA, Ascani S, Sabattini E, et al: The pathologist's view point. Part I—Indolent lymphomas. *Haematologica* 85:1291, 2000.
9. Pileri SA, Ascani S, Sabattini E, et al: The pathologist's view point. Part II—Aggressive lymphomas. *Haematologica* 85:1308, 2000.
10. Alizadeh AA, Eisen MB, Davis RE, et al: Distinct types of diffuse large B-cell lymphoma identified by gene expression profiling. *Nature* 403:503, 2000.
11. Rosenwald A, Alizadeh AA, Widhopf G, et al: Relation of gene expression phenotype to immunoglobulin mutation genotype in B cell chronic lymphocytic leukemia. *J Exp Med* 194:1639, 2001.
12. Davis RE, Staudt LM: Molecular diagnosis of lymphoid malignancies by gene expression profiling. *Curr Opin Hematol* 9:333, 2002.
13. Pileri SA, Ascani S, Leoncini L, et al: Hodgkin's lymphoma: The pathologist's viewpoint. *J Clin Pathol* 55:162, 2002.
14. Copur MS, Ledakis P, Bolton M: Molecular profiling of lymphoma. *N Engl J Med* 347:1376, 2002.
15. Lossos IS, Czerwinski DK, Alizadeh AA, et al: Prediction of survival in diffuse large-B-cell lymphoma based on the expression of six genes. *N Engl J Med* 350:1828, 2004.
16. Ramaswamy S: Translating cancer genomics into clinical oncology. *N Engl J Med* 350:1814, 2004.
17. Kwaan HC, Bongu A: The hyperviscosity syndromes. *Semin Thromb Hemost* 25:199, 1999.
18. Kyle RA: Clinical aspects of multiple myeloma and related disorders including amyloidosis. *Pathol Biol (Paris)* 47:148, 1999.
19. Hirshberg B, Kramer MR, Lotem M, et al: Chronic eosinophilic pneumonia associated with cutaneous T-cell lymphoma. *Am J Hematol* 60:143, 1999.
20. Roodman GD: Mechanisms of bone lesions in multiple myeloma and lymphoma. *Cancer* 80:1557, 1997.
21. Chubachi A, Miura I, Hatano Y, et al: Syndrome of inappropriate secretion of antidiuretic hormone in patients with lymphoma-associated hemophagocytic syndrome. *Ann Hematol* 70:53, 1995.
22. Seymour JF, Gagel RF: Calcitriol: The major humoral mediator of hypercalcemia in Hodgkin's disease and non-Hodgkin's lymphomas. *Blood* 82:1383, 1993.
23. Lorigan PC, Woodings PL, Morgenstern GR, Scarffe JH: Tumour lysis syndrome, case report and review of the literature. *Ann Oncol* 7:631, 1996.

ACUTE LYMPHOBLASTIC LEUKEMIA

CHING-HON PUI

Acute lymphoblastic leukemia (ALL) is a malignant disorder that originates in a single B or T lymphocyte progenitor. Proliferation and accumulation of blast cells in the marrow result in suppression of hematopoiesis and, thereafter, anemia, thrombocytopenia, and neutropenia. Lymphoblasts can accumulate in various extramedullary sites, especially the meninges, gonads, thymus, liver, spleen, and lymph nodes. The disease is most common in children but can be seen in individuals of any age. ALL has many subtypes and can be classified by immunologic, cytogenetic, and molecular genetic methods. These methods can identify biologic subtypes requiring treatment approaches that differ in their use of specific drugs or drug combinations, dosages of drug, or duration of treatment required to achieve optimal results. For example, cases of childhood ALL having a hyperdiploid karyotype respond well to extended treatment with methotrexate and mercaptopurine, whereas cases having adverse genetic changes, such as the BCR-ABL fusion, benefit from intensive treatment that includes transplantation of allogeneic hematopoietic stem cells. The relative lack of therapeutic success in adult ALL is partly related to a high frequency of cases having unfavorable genetic abnormalities. Nearly 80 percent of children and 40 percent of adults can expect long-term, leukemia-free survival—and probable cure—with contemporary treatment. Currently, emphasis is placed not only on improving the cure rate but also on improving quality of life by preventing acute and late complications, such as second malignancies, cardiotoxicity, or endocrinopathy that may result from antileukemic treatment.

DEFINITION AND HISTORY

Acute lymphoblastic leukemia (ALL) is a neoplastic disease that results from multistep somatic mutations in a single lymphoid progenitor cell at one of several discrete stages of development. The immunophenotype of leukemic cells at diagnosis reflects the level of differentiation achieved by the dominant clone. The clonal origin of ALL has been established by cytogenetic analysis and by analysis of restriction fragments in female patients who are heterozygous for polymorphic X chromosome–linked genes. In these patients, both alleles are expressed in normal cells, but only a single active parental allele is expressed in leukemic lymphoblasts. Also, analysis of rearrangements of T cell receptor or immunoglobulin genes has documented the monoclonal nature of the disease.[1] Leukemic cells divide more slowly and require more time to synthesize DNA than do normal hem-

atopoietic counterparts.[2] However, leukemic cells accumulate relentlessly because of their altered response to growth and antigrowth signals. They compete successfully with normal hematopoietic cells, resulting in anemia, thrombocytopenia, and neutropenia.[3,4] At diagnosis, leukemic cells not only have replaced normal marrow cells but also have disseminated to various extramedullary sites.

Velpeau[5] is generally credited with the earliest report of leukemia in 1827. Virchow,[6] Bennett,[7] and Craigie[8] recognized the condition as a distinct entity by 1845. In 1847, Virchow coined the term *leukemia*, applying it to two distinct types of the disease—splenic and lymphatic—that could be distinguished from each other based on splenomegaly and enlarged lymph nodes and on the morphologic similarities of the leukemic cells to those normally found in these organs.[9] Ehrlich's introduction of staining methods in 1891 allowed further distinction of leukemia subtypes.[10] Splenic and myelogenous leukemias soon were recognized as the same disease. By 1913, leukemia could be classified as acute or chronic, and as lymphatic or myelogenous.[11] The greater prevalence of ALL in children, especially those aged 1 to 5 years, was recognized in 1917.[12]

Shortly after leukemia was recognized as a discrete disease entity, physicians began using chemicals as palliative therapy. The first advance was the use of a 4-amino antimetabolite of folic acid (aminopterin), prompted by Farber's observation that folic acid might have accelerated the proliferation of leukemic cells. Strikingly, for the first time, complete clinical and hematologic remissions that lasted for several months were seen in children.[13] A year after the report of aminopterin-induced clinical remissions, a newly isolated adrenocorticotrophic hormone was reported to induce prompt though brief remissions in patients with leukemia.[14] Almost concurrently, Elion and colleagues[15] synthesized antimetabolites that interfere with synthesis of purine and pyrimidine. Their findings led to the introduction of mercaptopurine, 6-thioguanine, and allopurinol into clinical use. From 1950 to 1960, many new antileukemic agents and occasional cures were introduced. A "total therapy" approach, devised by Pinkel and colleagues at St. Jude Children's Research Hospital in 1962, consisted of four treatment phases: remission induction, intensification or consolidation, therapy for subclinical central nervous system (CNS) leukemia (or preventive meningeal treatment), and prolonged continuation therapy. By the early 1970s, as many as 50 percent of children could be cured by this innovative strategy.[16] During the same period, a better understanding of the genetics of human histocompatibility and wider use of human leukocyte antigen (HLA) typing culminated in the successful use of bone marrow transplantation for treatment of children in whom leukemia relapsed.[17] Eventually ALL was recognized as a broad term encompassing a heterogeneous group of diseases—clinically, immunologically, and genetically[18,19]—setting the stage for risk-directed therapy.

Treatment of ALL has progressed incrementally, beginning with the development of effective therapy for CNS disease, followed by intensification of early treatment, especially for patients at high risk of relapse. The current cure rates of nearly 80 percent for children (Fig. 91-1) and 40 percent for adults attest to the steady progress made in treating this disease.[4,20] Advances in the molecular classification of ALL—through use of DNA microarrays coupled with methods assessing the functional significance of newly identified genes— almost certainly will lead to the identification of new targets for specific treatment.[4] A clear precedent is the development of imatinib mesylate, which targets leukemias with the BCR-ABL fusion.[21]

ETIOLOGY AND PATHOGENESIS

Initiation and progression of ALL is driven by successive mutations that alter cellular functions, including an enhanced ability of self-renewal, a subversion of control of normal proliferation, a block in dif-

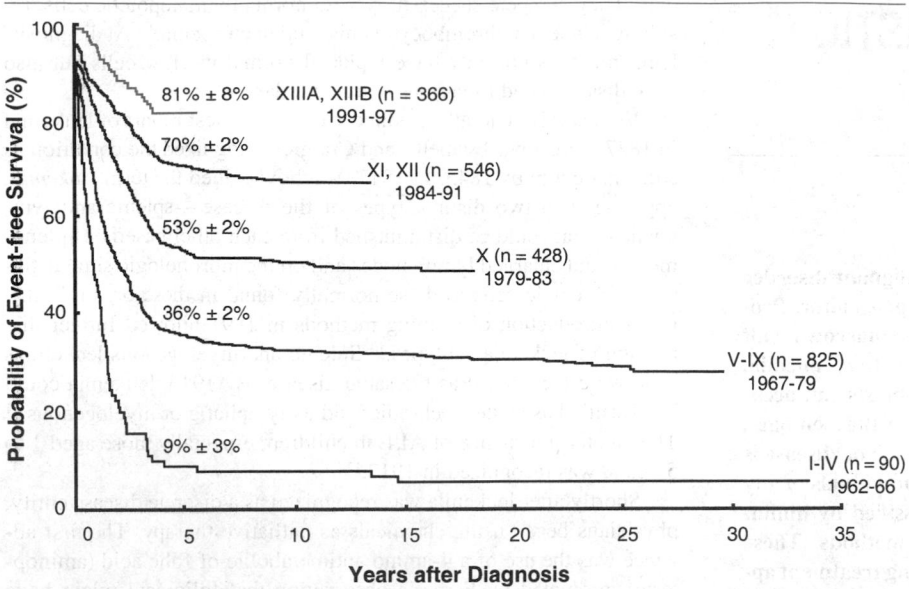

FIGURE 91-1   Kaplan-Meier analysis of event-free survival for 2255 children with ALL treated in 13 consecutive total therapy studies at St. Jude Children's Research Hospital. Early intensification of systemic and intrathecal chemotherapy in the 1990s has boosted the event-free survival estimate to 81% ± 8% (SE). (From CH Pui and WE Evans,[20] with permission.)

ferentiation, and an increased resistance to death signals (apoptosis).[3,4] Environmental agents, such as ionizing radiation and chemical mutagens, have been implicated in the induction of ALL in some patients. However, in most cases, no etiologic factors are discernible. In the favored theory, leukemogenesis reflects the interaction between host pharmacogenetics (susceptibility) and environmental factors, a model that requires confirmation in well-designed population and molecular epidemiologic studies.

INCIDENCE

Almost 4000 cases of ALL are diagnosed annually in the United States.[22] This number represents approximately 12 percent of all cases of leukemias diagnosed in the United States; 60 percent of all cases are in persons younger than 20 years. ALL is the most common malignancy diagnosed in patients younger than 15 years, accounting for 23 percent of all cancers and 76 percent of all leukemias in this age group. Only 20 percent of adult acute leukemias are ALL. Age-specific incidence patterns are characterized by a peak between the ages of 2 and 4 years, followed by falling rates during later childhood, adolescence, and young adulthood (Fig. 91-2).[23] Incidence rises again in the sixth decade and reaches a second, smaller peak in the elderly. The sharp incidence peak of ALL during early childhood has been observed only since the 1930s in the United Kingdom and the United States.[24] In the United States, the peak first appeared in children of European descent and subsequently was seen in children of African descent in the 1960s. The age peak is absent in many developing or underdeveloped countries, suggesting a leukemogenic contribution from factors associated with industrialization. Except for a slight predominance for females in infancy,[25] ALL affects males of European descent more often than females in all age groups. The frequency distribution is similar among those of African descent.[22] In most age groups, the incidence of ALL is higher in those of European descent than in those of African descent, especially among children aged 2 to 3 years.

The incidence of ALL differs substantially in different geographic areas. Rates are higher among populations in Northern and Western

Europe, North America, and Oceania, with lower rates in Asian and African populations.[26] In Europe, the highest rates of ALL among males are found in Spain and the highest rates among females in Denmark. In the United States, the highest rates for both sexes are among Latinos in Los Angeles. A survey by the Surveillance, Epidemiology, and End Results Program indicated that from 1973 to 1995, the age-adjusted incidence of childhood ALL in the United States increased from 2.7 to 3.3 cases per 100,000 persons aged 0 to 14 years. However, changes in diagnostic specificity from the mid-1970s to later eras, resulting in the recognition of not-otherwise-specified forms of lymphoid leukemia as ALL, could account partly for the apparent increase in incidence.[27]

RISK FACTORS

GENETIC SYNDROMES
The precise pathogenetic events leading to the development of ALL are unknown. Only a minority (5%) of cases are associated with inherited, predisposing genetic syndromes. Children with Down syndrome have a 10 to 30 times greater risk of leukemia; acute megakaryoblastic leukemia predominates in patients younger than 3 years, and ALL is predominant in older age groups. In cases of Down syndrome, B cell precursor ALL is more likely, with leukemic cells lacking both favorable and adverse genetic abnormalities.[28] Autosomal recessive genetic diseases associated with increased chromosomal fragility and a predisposition to ALL include ataxia-telangiectasia, Nijmegen breakage syndrome, and Bloom syndrome.[29] Patients with ataxia-telangiectasia have a 70 times greater risk of leukemia and a 250 times greater risk of lymphoma, particularly of the T cell phenotype.[30] The causative gene, termed *ATM* (ataxia-telangiectasia mutated), encodes a protein involved in DNA repair, regulation of cell proliferation, and apoptosis. Laboratory studies supporting the diagnosis of ataxia-telangiectasia include an elevated serum concentration of α-fetoprotein, presence of characteristic chromosomal aberrations, absent or reduced intranuclear serine protein kinase ATM, and increased *in vitro* radiosensitivity.[31] A high prevalence of germline truncating and missense *ATM* gene alterations in children with sporadic T cell ALL suggests a pathogenetic role of *ATM* in lymphoid malignancies.[30] Although impaired immune surveillance contributes to the increased risk of Epstein-Barr virus–related malignancies in patients with acquired immunodeficiencies, no compelling evidence indicates defective immunity contributes to the predisposition to ALL in patients with ataxia-telangiectasia or other congenital immunodeficiency syndromes.

ENVIRONMENTAL FACTORS
In utero (but not postnatal) exposure to diagnostic x-rays confers a slightly increased risk of ALL, which correlates positively with the number of exposures.[32] The evidence is weak for an association between the development of ALL and nuclear fallout; exposure to occupational, natural terrestrial, or cosmic ionizing radiation exposure; or paternal radiation exposure prior to conception. Exposure to low-energy electromagnetic fields produced by a residential power supply and appliances has been largely excluded as an instigating factor in the development of childhood ALL.[4] Although meta-analyses sug-

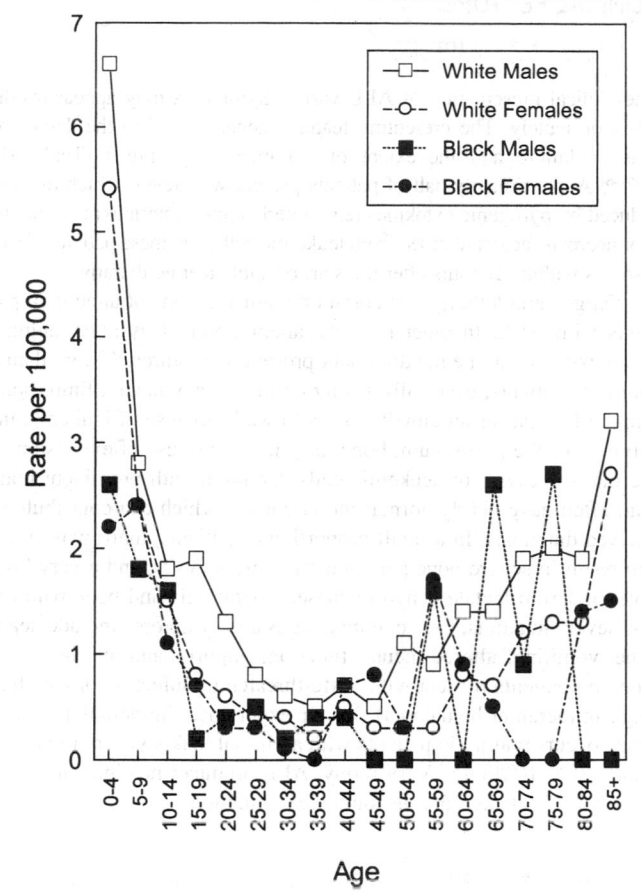

FIGURE 91-2   Age-specific incidence rates for ALL by race and sex. (From SEER data, 1991–1995.[23])

gested a significantly increased risk of leukemia at the highest exposure level,[33] even if the association is real, the proportion of population exposed to such a high level is extremely small (only approximately 1% of leukemias were in this category); thus, the attributable risk is negligible. Pesticide exposure (occupational or home use) and parental cigarette smoking before or during pregnancy have been suggested causes of childhood ALL. Administration of vitamin K to neonates, maternal alcohol consumption during pregnancy, and increased consumption of dietary nitrites also have been suggested causes. However, each of these associations is controversial, and most have been refuted after careful, controlled investigation. An increased incidence of ALL has been reported among women whose drinking water was contaminated with trichloroethylene and among smokers older than 60 years.[24] Both findings require confirmation.

HOST PHARMACOGENETICS

Study findings suggest multiple, subtle genetic polymorphisms of xenobiotic-metabolizing enzymes may interact with environmental, dietary, maternal, and other external factors, thus affecting the development of ALL.[4] For example, various inactivating polymorphisms of detoxifying enzymes (e.g., glutathione S-transferase, reduced nicotinamide adenine dinucleotide phosphate, quinone oxidoreductase) are associated with the development of ALL.[34,35] Low-penetrance polymorphisms of folate-metabolizing enzymes also are associated with the development of ALL. Polymorphic variants of methylenetetrahydrofolate reductase, which catalyzes the reduction of 5,10-methylenetetrahydrofolate to 5-methyltetrahydrofo-

late (the predominant circulating form of folate), are linked to a decreased risk of ALL in adults[36] and children.[37] The protective effect may result from the greater availability of 5,10-methylenetetrahydrofolate and thymidine pools and to an increased fidelity of DNA synthesis. Polymorphisms of two other folate-related genes—serine hydroxymethyltransferase and thymidylate synthase—are associated with a decreased risk of ALL in adults.[38] A role for folate pathways in susceptibility to ALL is suggested by an association between folate supplementation and a decreased risk of ALL in children.[39] However, all these associations must be confirmed by larger studies with careful attention to ethnic and geographic diversity in the frequency of polymorphisms.

IN UTERO DEVELOPMENT OF ALL

Retrospective identification of leukemia-specific fusion genes (e.g., MLL-AF4, TEL-AML1) in the neonatal blood spots and development of concordant leukemia in identical twins indicate some leukemias have a prenatal origin.[40,41] In identical twins with the t(4;11)/MLL-AF4, the concordance rate is nearly 100 percent, and the latency period is short (a few weeks to a few months). These findings suggest this fusion alone either is leukemogenic or requires only a small number of cooperative mutations to cause leukemia. By contrast, the lower concordance rate in twins with the TEL-AML1 fusion or T cell phenotype and the longer postnatal latency period suggest additional postnatal events are required for leukemic transformation.[40] This theory is supported by the identification of rare cells expressing TEL-AML1 fusion transcripts in approximately 1 percent of cord blood samples from newborns, a frequency 100 times higher than the incidence of ALL defined by this fusion transcript.[41] Hyperdiploid ALL, another common subtype of childhood ALL, also appears to arise before birth but requires postnatal events for full malignant transformation.[42] Some researchers believe "delayed" exposures to common infections at a time of increased lymphoid cell proliferation serve as the postnatal instigating events.[41,43] This theory is supported by a higher frequency of childhood ALL in industrialized compared to developing countries and in locations where large numbers of infected and uninfected persons come into contact with each other.[41,43] However, clearly not all childhood cases develop in utero. For example, t(1;19)/E2A-PBX1 ALL appears to have a postnatal origin in most cases.[44] Cases of adult ALL most certainly arise over a protracted time.

ACQUIRED GENETIC CHANGES

In almost all cases of ALL, lymphoblasts have acquired genetic changes, three fourths of which have prognostic and therapeutic relevance (Table 91-1).[4] Changes include abnormalities in the number (ploidy) and structure of chromosomes. The latter comprise translocations (the most frequent abnormality), inversions, deletions, point mutations, and amplifications (see Chap. 10). Although the frequency of particular genetic subtypes differs between childhood and adult cases, the general mechanisms underlying the induction are similar. Mechanisms include aberrant expression of oncoproteins and chromosomal translocations that generate fusion genes encoding transcription factors or active kinases.[4,41,45]

Primary genetic rearrangement by itself is not sufficient to induce overt leukemia. Cooperative mutations are necessary for leukemic transformation and include genetic and epigenetic changes in key growth regulatory pathways, such as those controlled by p53 and by the tumor suppressor RB (retinoblastoma protein) and its related family members p107 and p130. The principal role of RB is controlling entry into the cell cycle.[46] In its hypophosphorylated state, RB inhibits the ability of the E2F family of transcription factors to

TABLE 91-1   FREQUENCIES OF COMMON GENETIC ABERRATIONS IN CHILDHOOD AND ADULT ALL

ABNORMALITY	CHILDREN	ADULTS
Hyperdiploidy (>50 chromosomes)	23–26%	6–7%
Hypodiploidy (<45 chromosomes)	1%	2%
t(1;19)(q23;p13.3)	3% in white, 11% in black	2–3%
t(9;22)(q34;q11.2)	3%	25–30%
t(4;11)(q21;q23)	2%	3–7%
t(8;14)(q23;q32.3)	2%	4%
TEL-AML1 fusion	20–25%	0–3%
HOX11L2 overexpression[a]	2–3%	1%
LYL1 overexpression[a]	1.5%	2.5%
TAL1 overexpression[a]	3–7%	12%
HOX11 overexpression[a]	0.7%	8%
MLL-ENL fusion	0.3%	0.5%
Abnormal 9p	7–11%	6–30%
Abnormal 12p	7–9%	4–6%
del(7p)/del(7q)/monosomy 7	4%	6–11%
+8	2%	10–12%

[a]Abnormalities found in T cell ALL.

transcribe the genes necessary for entry into the S phase. Mitogenic signals induce the formation of active cyclin D–dependent kinase complexes, which together with cyclin E–cdk2, phosphorylate RB and thereby abrogate the ability of RB to inhibit cell proliferation. The activity of cyclin D–dependent kinases in turn is inhibited by the INK4 proteins (e.g., p16^{INK4a}, p15^{INK4b}), thereby preventing phosphorylation of RB. Inactivating mutations or deletions of RB are rare in ALL, but functional inactivation of the RB pathway through deletion or epigenetic silencing of p16^{INK4a} and p15^{INK4b} occurs in nearly all cases of childhood T cell ALL, in a small proportion of childhood B lineage ALL, and in adult T cell ALL.[47,48]

Like *RB*, the *TP53* gene, which encodes the transcription factor p53, itself is rarely altered in ALL; however, components of the p53 pathway are frequently mutated in ALL. The p53 protein functions as a sensor of aberrant cellular changes. Its activation results in either cell cycle arrest or apoptosis, depending on the cellular context.[49] The activity of p53 is negatively regulated in part by its induction of HDM2, which binds to p53 and induces its degradation. HDM2, in turn, is inhibited by the tumor suppressor p14^{ARF}. Deletion or transcriptional silencing of p14^{ARF}, overexpression of HDM2, and silencing of the p53 transcriptional target p21^{CIP1} are common events in ALL.[50,51] Interestingly, p14^{ARF} and p16^{INK4a} are encoded by alternative reading frames in the same genetic locus,[52] and the high frequency of homozygous deletions of both gene products suggests that alterations of the p53 and RB pathways collaborate in leukemogenesis.[4]

Gene expression profiling with DNA microarrays, a robust technique that allows simultaneous analysis of the expression of thousands of genes, not only allows accurate identification of known phenotypic and genotypic subtypes of ALL but also provides insights into their underlying pathobiology.[45,53,54] Microarray analysis allows nearly all T cell cases to be grouped according to multistep oncogenic pathways.[45] Gene expression studies also show that overexpression of flt3, a receptor tyrosine kinase important for development of hematopoietic stem cells, is a secondary event in almost all cases with either *MLL* rearrangements or hyperdiploidy.[53–55] The finding has provided an impetus for clinical testing of flt3 inhibitors. Finally, microarray analysis has identified gene expression profiles having prognostic or therapeutic relevance and may lead to the identification of targets for specific treatment.[54–58]

CLINICAL FEATURES

SIGNS AND SYMPTOMS

The clinical presentation of ALL varies. Symptoms may appear insidiously or acutely. The presenting features generally reflect the degree of marrow failure and the extent of extramedullary spread (Table 91-2).[59–64] Approximately half of patients present with fever, which often is induced by pyrogenic cytokines (e.g., interleukin-1, interleukin-6, and tumor necrosis factor) released from leukemic cells.[65] In these patients, fever resolves within 72 hours after the start of antileukemic therapy.

Fatigue and lethargy are common manifestations of anemia in patients with ALL. In older patients, anemia-related dyspnea, angina, and dizziness may be the dominant presenting features.[63] More than a fourth of patients, especially young children, may have a limp, bone pain, arthralgia, or an unwillingness to walk because of leukemic infiltration of the periosteum, bone, or joint or because of expansion of the marrow cavity by leukemic cells. Children with prominent bone pain often have nearly normal blood counts, which can contribute to delayed diagnosis. In a small proportion of patients, marrow necrosis can result in severe bone pain and tenderness, fever, and a very high level of serum lactate dehydrogenase.[66] Arthralgia and bone pain are less severe in adults. Less common signs and symptoms include headache, vomiting, altered mental function, oliguria, and anuria. Occasionally, patients present with a life-threatening infection or bleeding (e.g., intracranial hematoma). In our experience, intracranial hemorrhage occurs mainly in patients with an initial leukocyte count greater than 400×10^9/liter.[67] Very rarely, ALL produces no signs or symptoms and is detected during routine examination.

TABLE 91-2   PRESENTING CLINICAL FEATURES IN CHILDREN AND ADULTS WITH ACUTE LYMPHOBLASTIC LEUKEMIA

FEATURE	PERCENT OF TOTAL	
	CHILDREN	ADULT
Age (years)		
<1	3	—
1–9	77	—
10–19	20	—
20–39	—	55
40–59	—	36
≥60	—	9
Male	55	62
Symptoms		
Fever	57	33–56
Fatigue	50	?
Bleeding	43	33
Bone or joint pain	25	25
Lymphadenopathy		
None	30	51
Marked (>3 cm)	15	11
Hepatomegaly		
None	34	65
Marked (below umbilicus)	17	?
Splenomegaly		
None	41	56
Marked (below umbilicus)	17	?
Mediastinal mass	8	15
CNS leukemia	3	8
Testicular leukemia	1	0.3

SOURCE: Data presented in Pui and Crist,[59] McKenna and Baehner,[60] Reiter et al.,[61] and Chessells et al.,[62] for childhood ALL; and in Chessells et al.,[62] Hoelzer,[63] and Larson et al.,[64] for adult ALL.

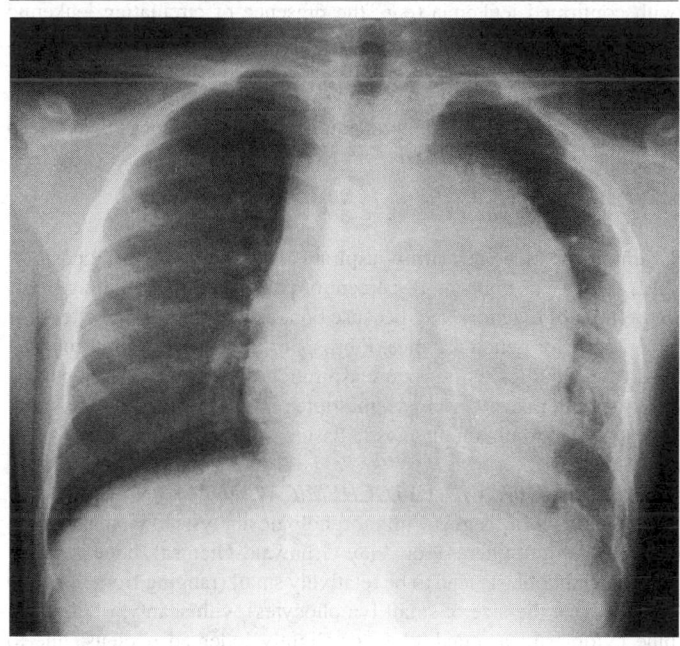

FIGURE 91-3   Chest x-ray film of a 12-year-old black male with T cell ALL and an anterior mediastinal mass.

PHYSICAL FINDINGS

Among the frequently evident findings are pallor, petechiae, and ecchymosis in the skin and mucous membranes and bone tenderness as a result of leukemic infiltration or hemorrhage that stretches the periosteum. Liver, spleen, and lymph nodes are the most common sites of extramedullary involvement, and the degree of organomegaly is more pronounced in children than in adults. An anterior mediastinal (thymic) mass is present in 7 to 10 percent of childhood cases and 15 percent of adult cases (Fig. 91-3). A bulky, anterior mediastinal mass can compress the great vessels and trachea and possibly lead to the superior vena cava syndrome or the superior mediastinal syndrome.[68] Patients with this syndrome present with cough, dyspnea, orthopnea, dysphagia, stridor, cyanosis, facial edema, increased intracranial pressure, and sometimes syncope. Such patients tolerate anesthesia poorly.

Painless enlargement of the scrotum can be a sign of a testicular leukemia or hydrocele, the latter resulting from lymphatic obstruction. Both conditions can be readily diagnosed by ultrasonography. Overt testicular disease is relatively rare, generally seen in infants or patients with T cell leukemia with hyperleukocytosis, and does not require radiation therapy.[69] Other uncommon presenting features include ocular involvement (leukemic infiltration of the orbit, optic nerve, retina, iris, cornea, or conjunctiva), subcutaneous nodules (leukemia cutis), enlarged salivary glands (Mikulicz syndrome), cranial nerve palsy, and priapism (resulting from leukostasis of the corpora cavernosa and dorsal veins or sacral nerve involvement). Epidural spinal cord compression at presentation is a rare but serious finding that requires immediate treatment to prevent permanent paraparesis or paraplegia. In some pediatric patients, infiltration of tonsils, adenoids, appendix, or mesenteric lymph nodes leads to surgical intervention before leukemia is diagnosed.

LABORATORY FEATURES

Anemia, neutropenia, and thrombocytopenia are common in patients with newly diagnosed ALL. The severity reflects the degree of marrow replacement by leukemic lymphoblasts (Table 91-3).[59–64] Presenting leukocyte counts range widely, from 0.1 to 1500 × 10⁹/liter (median 10–12 × 10⁹/liter). Hyperleukocytosis (>100 × 10⁹/liter) is seen in 10 to 16 percent of patients. Profound neutropenia (<0.5 × 10⁹/liter) is found in 20 to 40 percent of patients, rendering them at high risk for infection. Most patients have circulating leukemic blast cells. Hypereosinophilia, generally reactive, may precede the diagnosis of ALL by several months.[70] Some patients, principally male, have ALL with the t(5;14)(q31;q32) chromosomal abnormality and a hypereosinophilic syndrome (pulmonary infiltration, cardiomegaly, and congestive heart failure). These patients often do not have circulating leukemic blasts or other cytopenias and have a relatively low percentage of blasts in the bone marrow.[71] Activation of the interleukin-3 gene on chromosome 5 by the enhancer element of the immunoglobulin heavy-chain gene on chromosome 14 is thought to play a central role in leukemogenesis and the associated eosinophilia in these cases.[71] In patients with anemia, a strong inverse relationship exists between the hemoglobin level and age at diagnosis.[62] Occasionally, a child with ALL has a hemoglobin level as low as 1 g/dl.

Decreased platelet counts often are seen at diagnosis (median, 48–52 × 10⁹/liter). This finding differs from immune thrombocytopenia because the decreased platelet counts almost always are accompanied by anemia, leukocyte abnormalities, or both.[72] Severe bleeding is uncommon, even when platelet counts are as low as 20 × 10⁹/liter, provided infection and fever are absent.[73] Occasional patients, principally male, present with thrombocytosis (>400 × 10⁹/liter).[74] Pancytopenia followed by a period of spontaneous hematopoietic recovery may precede the diagnosis of ALL in rare cases.[75] Coagulopathy, usually mild, can be seen in 3 to 5 percent of patients, most of whom have T cell ALL, and is only rarely associated with clinical bleeding.[63,76] The level of serum lactate dehydrogenase is increased in most patients with ALL and is well correlated with the size of the leukemic infiltrate.[77] Increased levels of serum uric acid are common in patients with a large leukemic cell burden, a finding that reflects an increased rate of purine catabolism. Patients with massive renal involvement can have in-

TABLE 91-3   PRESENTING LABORATORY FEATURES IN CHILDREN AND ADULTS WITH ACUTE LYMPHOBLASTIC LEUKEMIA

FEATURE	PERCENT OF TOTAL	
	CHILDREN	ADULTS
Leukocyte count (× 10⁹/liter)		
<10	50	41
10–49	31	31
50–99	9	12
>100	10	16
Hemoglobin concentration (g/dl)		
<8	52	28
8–10	28	26
>10	20	46
Platelet count (× 10⁹/liter)		
<50	48	52
50–100	20	22
>100	32	26
Leukemic blasts in marrow (%)		
<90	19	29
>90	81	71
Leukemic blasts in blood		
Present	84	92
Absent	16	8

SOURCE: Data presented in Pui and Crist,[59] McKenna and Baehner,[60] Reiter et al.,[61] and Chessells et al.[62] for childhood ALL; and in Chessells et al.,[62] Hoelzer,[63] and Larson et al.[64] for adult ALL.

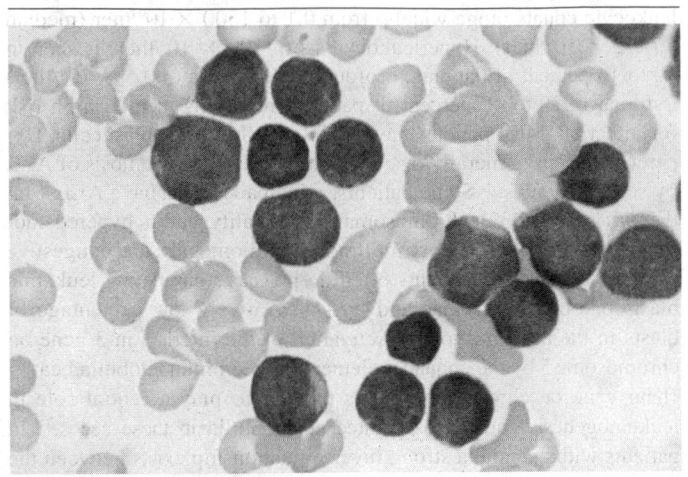

FIGURE 91-4   Typical lymphoblasts with scanty cytoplasm, regular nuclear shape, fine chromatin, and indistinct nucleoli (Wright-Giemsa stain; magnification ×1000).

creased levels of creatinine, urea nitrogen, uric acid, and phosphorus. Occasionally, patients with T cell ALL present with acute renal failure, despite a relatively small leukemic infiltrate.[78] Rarely, patients present with hypercalcemia resulting from release of parathyroid hormone-like protein from lymphoblasts and leukemic infiltration of bone.[79] Liver dysfunction as a result of leukemic infiltration occurs in 10 to 20 percent of patients, usually is mild, and has no important clinical or prognostic consequences.[59] Serum immunoglobulin levels (mostly IgA and IgM classes) are modestly decreased in approximately one third of children with ALL. The reduction reflects the decreased number and impaired function of normal lymphocytes.[80] Urinalysis may show microscopic hematuria and the presence of uric acid crystals.

Chest radiography is needed to detect enlargement of the thymus or mediastinal nodes, with or without pleural effusion (see Fig. 91-3). Although bony abnormalities, such as metaphyseal banding, periosteal reactions, osteolysis, osteosclerosis, and osteopenia, can be found in 50 percent of patients, especially children with low leukocyte counts at presentation,[81] skeletal roentgenography is not necessary for case management. Spinal roentgenography is useful in patients with suspected vertebral collapse.

Examination of the cerebrospinal fluid (CSF) is an essential diagnostic procedure. Leukemic blasts can be identified in as many as one third of pediatric patients at diagnosis of ALL; most of these patients lack neurologic symptoms.[82] Traditionally, CNS leukemia is defined by the presence of at least five leukocytes per microliter of CSF (with leukemic blast cells apparent in a cytocentrifuged sample) or by the presence of cranial nerve palsies. However, with the omission of prophylactic cranial irradiation in contemporary clinical trials, the presence of any leukemic blast cells in the CSF is associated with increased risk of CNS relapse and is an indication to intensify intrathecal therapy.[83] Different opinions exist regarding when the first lumbar puncture should be performed. Many leukemia therapists perform the procedure at diagnosis but do not instill chemotherapeutic agents intrathecally in the event a second diagnostic test is needed to verify the presence of leukemic cells. Others delay the examination because of concern that circulating leukemic cells from the peripheral blood will "seed" the CNS. Two studies have shown that contamination of the CSF by leukemic cells as a result of traumatic lumbar puncture at diagnosis is associated with an inferior treatment outcome in children with ALL.[84,85] In view of this finding, intrathecal therapy is administered immediately after the diagnostic lumbar puncture in all patients

with confirmed leukemia (e.g., the presence of circulating leukemic cells) at St. Jude Children's Research Hospital. The risk of traumatic lumbar puncture can be decreased by administering platelet transfusions to thrombocytopenic patients and by having the most experienced clinician perform the procedure after the patient is under deep sedation or general anesthesia.[83,86]

DIAGNOSIS AND CELL CLASSIFICATION

Examination of bone marrow aspirate is preferable for diagnosis of ALL because as many as 10 percent of patients lack circulating blasts at the time of diagnosis and because bone marrow cells are better than blood cells for genetic studies. Fibrosis or tightly packed marrow can lead to difficulties with marrow aspiration that necessitate biopsy. In patients with marrow necrosis, multiple marrow aspirations are sometimes needed to obtain diagnostic tissue.

MORPHOLOGIC AND CYTOCHEMICAL ANALYSIS

Diagnosis of ALL begins with morphologic analysis of Romanowsky-stained (Wright-Giemsa or May-Grünwald-Giemsa) bone marrow films. Lymphoblasts tend to be relatively small (ranging from the same size to twice the size of small lymphocytes) with scanty, often light-blue cytoplasm; a round, cleft, or slightly indented nucleus; fine to slightly coarse and clumped chromatin; and inconspicuous nucleoli (Fig. 91-4). In some cases, the lymphoblasts are large, with prominent nucleoli, moderate amounts of cytoplasm, and an admixture of smaller blasts (Fig. 91-5). Cytoplasmic granules are found in the lymphoblasts of some patients with ALL (Fig. 91-6). The granules usually are amphophilic (which stain fuchsia), readily distinguishable from the primary myeloid granules (which stain deep purple), and demonstrated to be mitochondria in some cases by electron microscopy. B cell blasts in ALL are characterized by intensely basophilic cytoplasm, regular cellular features, prominent nucleoli, and cytoplasmic vacuolation (Fig. 91-7).

Analysis of only a Romanowsky-stained film is not sufficient to differentiate ALL and acute myelogenous leukemia. The cytochemical stains needed to discriminate between the two leukemias are the Sudan black stain and the stains for myeloperoxidase and the nonspecific esterases, including α-naphthyl butyrate and α-naphthyl acetate esterase. Stains for these esterases generally do not react with leukemic lymphoblasts. Occasionally, a low level of myeloperoxidase is detected in bone marrow samples from ALL patients because of the

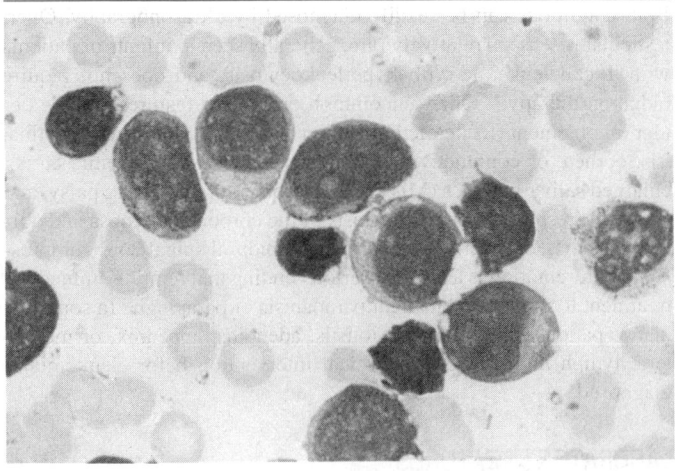

FIGURE 91-5   ALL with large blasts showing prominent nucleoli, moderate amounts of cytoplasm, and an admixture of smaller blasts (Wright-Giemsa stain; magnification ×1000).

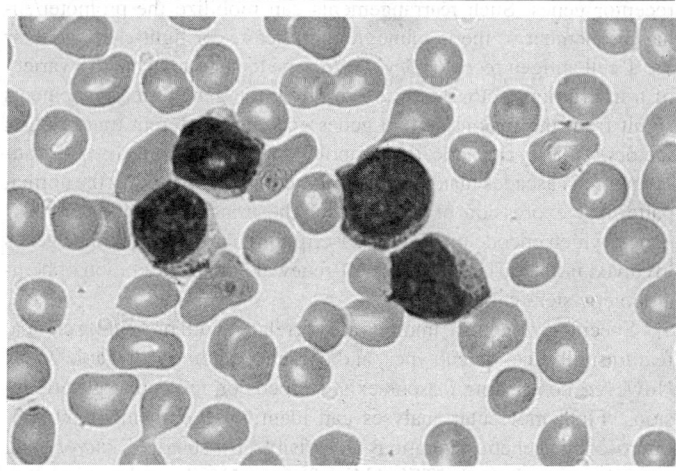

FIGURE 91-6 ALL with cytoplasmic granules. Fuchsia granules are present in the cytoplasm of many blasts. Such granules may lead to a misdiagnosis of acute myeloid leukemia; however, the granules are negative for myeloperoxidase and myeloid-pattern Sudan black B staining (Wright-Giemsa stain; magnification ×1000).

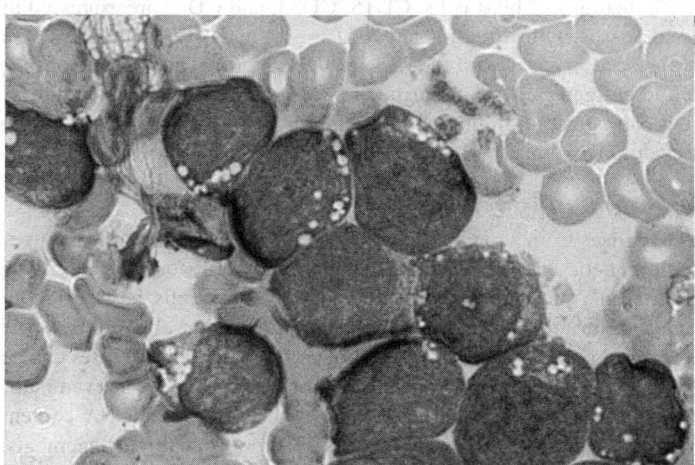

FIGURE 91-7 Mature B cell ALL lymphoblasts. The blasts are characterized by intensely basophilic cytoplasm, regular cellular features, and cytoplasmic vacuolation (Wright-Giemsa stain; magnification ×1000).

presence of residual normal myeloid precursors. Staining with periodic acid–Schiff reagent is positive in more than 70 percent of ALL cases, whereas acid phosphatase reactivity can be demonstrated in approximately 70 percent of cases with a T cell immunophenotype. However, neither stain reacts exclusively with leukemic lymphoid cells.

IMMUNOLOGIC CLASSIFICATION

Because leukemic lymphoblasts lack specific morphologic and cytochemical features, immunophenotyping is an essential part of the diagnostic evaluation. The antibodies that distinguish clusters of differentiation (CD) groups recognize the same cellular antigen but not necessarily the same epitope (see Chap. 14). Most leukocyte antigens lack specificity; hence, a panel of antibodies is needed to establish the diagnosis and to distinguish among the different immunologic subclasses of leukemic cells. The panel used at St. Jude Children's Research Hospital includes antibodies to at least one highly sensitive marker (CD19 for B lineage cells, CD7 for T lineage cells, and CD13 or CD33 for myeloid cells) and antibodies to a highly specific marker (cytoplasmic CD79a for B-lineage cells, cytoplasmic CD3 for T line-

age cells, and cytoplasmic myeloperoxidase for myeloid cells).[20] These analysis methods enable a firm diagnosis in 99 percent of cases.

Although ALL can be further subclassified according to the recognized steps of normal maturation within the B lineage (early pre-B, pre-B, transitional pre-B, and mature B) or T lineage (early, mid, and late thymocyte) pathways, the only distinctions of therapeutic importance are those between T cell, mature B, and other B lineage (B cell precursor) immunophenotypes.[20] In some studies, cases of B cell precursor ALL were subdivided into CD10-positive (so-called common ALL) and CD10-negative (pre-pre-B, pro-B, or CD10-negative B cell precursor) leukemias, whereas cases of T lineage ALL were further classified as pre-T (or pro-T) and mature T cell leukemias.[87,88] Despite their prognostic implications, these refined categories of ALL have not been used in treatment assignment. Table 91-4 summarizes the salient presenting features of six recognized immunologic subtypes of ALL.

Myeloid-associated antigens may be expressed on otherwise typical lymphoblasts. Because of differences in monoclonal antibodies and immunophenotyping techniques, the frequencies of myeloid-associated antigen expression range from 5 to 30 percent in childhood cases and from 10 to 50 percent in adult cases.[64,89] The pattern of myeloid-associated antigen expression is correlated with certain ge-

TABLE 91-4 PRESENTING FEATURES ACCORDING TO IMMUNOLOGIC SUBTYPE

SUBTYPE	TYPICAL MARKERS	CHILDHOOD (%)	ADULT (%)	ASSOCIATED FEATURES
B cell precursor	CD19+, CD22+, CD79a+, cIg±, sIgµ−, HLA-DR+			
Pre-pre-B	CD10−	5	11	Infant or adult age group, high leukocyte count, initial CNS leukemia, pseudodiploidy, *MLL* rearrangement, unfavorable prognosis
Early pre-B	CD10+	63	52	Favorable age group (1–9 years), low leukocyte count, hyperdiploidy (>50 chromosomes)
Pre-B	CD10±, cIg+	16	9	High leukocyte count, black race, pseudodiploidy
B cell	CD19+, CD22+, CD79a+, cIg+, sIgµ+, sIgκ+ or sIgλ+	3	4	Male predominance, initial CNS leukemia, abdominal masses, often renal involvement
T lineage	CD7+, cCD3+			
T cell	CD2+, CD1±, CD4±, CD8±, HLA-DR−, TdT±	12	18	Male predominance, hyperleukocytosis, extramedullary disease
Pre-T	CD2−, CD1−, CD4−, CD8−, HLA-DR±, TdT+	1	6	Male predominance, hyperleukocytosis, extramedullary disease, unfavorable prognosis

cCD3, cytoplasmic CD3; cIg, cytoplasmic immunoglobulin; CNS, central nervous system; sIg, surface immunoglobulin; TdT, terminal deoxynucleotidyl transferase.

netic features of blast cells. CD15, CD33, and CD65 are expressed in ALL cases with a rearranged *MLL* gene, and CD13 and CD33 are expressed in cases with the *TEL-AML1* fusion.[89] The presence of myeloid antigens lacks significance in contemporary treatment programs but can be useful in immunologic monitoring of patients for minimal residual leukemia.[90]

GENETIC CLASSIFICATION

ALL arises from a lymphopoietic progenitor cell having sustained specific genetic damage that leads to malignant transformation and proliferation. Thus, genetic classification of blast cells is expected to yield more relevant biologic information than that obtained by other means. Approximately 75 percent of adult and childhood cases can be readily classified into prognostically or therapeutically relevant subgroups based on the modal chromosome number (or DNA content estimated by flow cytometry), specific chromosomal rearrangements, and molecular genetic changes.[4,20,45,58,91-93] Table 91-5 summarizes the prominent clinical and biologic features of cases with the most common genetic abnormalities.

Two ploidy groups (hyperdiploidy >50 chromosomes and hypodiploidy <45 chromosomes) have clinical relevance. Hyperdiploidy, which is seen in approximately 25 percent of childhood cases and 6 to 7 percent of adult cases, is associated with a favorable prognosis that may reflect an increased cellular accumulation of methotrexate and its polyglutamates, an increased sensitivity to therapeutic antimetabolites, and a marked propensity of these cells to undergo apoptosis.[94-96] By contrast, hypodiploidy is associated with an exceptionally poor prognosis.[91,93,97,98] Flow cytometric determination of cellular DNA content is a useful adjunct to cytogenetic analysis because it is automated, rapid, and inexpensive, and its measurements are not affected by the mitotic index of the cell population; results can be obtained in almost all cases. Flow cytometric studies can sometimes identify a small but drug-resistant subpopulation of near-haploid cells that may have been missed by standard cytogenetic analysis.[97]

Phenotype-specific reciprocal translocations are the most biologically and clinically significant karyotypic changes in ALL. Some translocations identified in cases of B cell and T cell ALL arise from mistakes in the normal recombination mechanisms that generate antigen receptor genes. Such rearrangements can mobilize the promoter/enhancer element of the immunoglobulin heavy- or light-chain gene or the T cell antigen receptor β/γ or α/δ gene to sites adjacent to a variety of transcription factor genes. More often, the genetic rearrangements result from the fusions of two genes encoding different transcription factors.[4] These chimeric transcription factors activate diverse transcriptional cascades that, at least partly, converge to modify the normal pattern of expression of members of the important family of *HOX* genes, which encode the HOX transcription factors that regulate genes involved in the differentiation, self-renewal, and proliferation of hematopoietic stem cells.[4]

Specific cytogenetic findings are correlated with presenting clinical features, blast cell phenotypes, and clinical outcome (see Table 91-5). However, compelling reasons exist to focus on molecular genetic lesions. First, molecular analyses can identify several important submicroscopic genetic alterations not visible by standard karyotyping procedures, such as the *TEL-AML1* fusion, *AML1* amplification, and deletions of tumor suppressor genes.[4,99,100] Second, cases with clinically important genetic rearrangements can be missed because of technical errors (e.g., karyotyping residual normal metaphase cells rather than leukemic metaphase cells). Hence, fluorescence *in situ* hybridization (FISH) and reverse transcriptase polymerase chain reaction (RT-PCR) assays are used frequently. Genetic expression profiling studies have classified T cell ALL cases into several distinct genetic subgroups: *HOX11L2*, *LYL1* plus *LMO2*, *TAL1* plus *LMO1* or *LMO2*, *HOX11*, and *MLL-ENL*. The last two subgroups are associated with a favorable outcome.[45,58] Notably, the chromosomal abnormalities in most cases in the *HOX11* subgroup cannot be identified by conventional cytogenetic or molecular genetic methods.

DIFFERENTIAL DIAGNOSIS

The initial manifestations of ALL can mimic a variety of disorders. The acute onset of petechiae, ecchymoses, and bleeding can suggest idiopathic thrombocytopenic purpura. The latter disorder often is associated with a recent viral infection, large platelets in blood films, normal hemoglobin concentration, and absence of leukocyte abnormalities in blood or marrow. Patients with ALL or aplastic anemia can

---

TABLE 91-5 CLINICAL AND BIOLOGIC FEATURES ASSOCIATED WITH THE MOST COMMON GENETIC SUBTYPES OF ACUTE LYMPHOBLASTIC LEUKEMIA

SUBTYPE	ASSOCIATED FEATURES	ESTIMATED EVENT-FREE SURVIVAL (%) CHILDREN	ADULTS
Hyperdiploidy (>50 chromosomes)	Predominant B cell precursor phenotype; low leukocyte count; favorable age group (1–9 years) and prognosis in children	85–90 at 5 years	30–50 at 5 years
Hypodiploidy (<45 chromosomes)	Predominant B cell precursor phenotype; increased leukocyte count; poor prognosis	30–40 at 3 years	10–20 at 3 years
TEL-AML1 fusion	CD13±/CD33± B cell precursor phenotype; pseudodiploidy; age 1–9 years; favorable prognosis	85–90 at 5 years	Unknown
t(1;19)(q23;p13.3) with *E2A-PBX1* fusion	CD10±/CD20−/CD34− pre-B phenotype; pseudodiploidy; increased leukocyte count; black race; CNS leukemia; prognosis depends on treatment	75–90 at 5 years	20–40 at 3 years
t(9;22)(q34;q11.2) with *BCR-ABL* fusion	Predominant B cell precursor phenotype; older age; increased leukocyte count; dismal outcome in adults and in children with poor early response to induction or with leukocyte counts >50 × 10⁹/liter; improved prognosis with transplant from a matched related donor	20–40 at 5 years	<10 at 3 years
t(4;11)(q21;23) with *MLL-AF4* fusion	CD10±/CD15±/CD33±/CD65± B cell precursor phenotype; infant and older adult age groups; hyperleukocytosis; CNS leukemia; dismal outcome	10–35 at 5 years	10–20 at 3 years
t(8;14)(q24;q32.3)	B cell phenotype; L3 morphology; male predominance; bulky extramedullary disease; favorable prognosis with short-term intensive chemotherapy including high-dose methotrexate, cytarabine, and cyclophosphamide	75–85 at 5 years	50–55 at 4 years
HOX11 overexpression	CD10+ T cell phenotype; favorable prognosis with chemotherapy alone	90 at 5 years	80 at 3 years

SOURCE: Data presented in Pui et al.,[4] Secker-Walker et al.,[91] Faderl et al.,[92] and Mrózek et al.[93]

present with pancytopenia and complications associated with marrow failure. However, in aplastic anemia, hepatosplenomegaly and lymphadenopathy are rare, and the skeletal changes associated with leukemia are absent. The results of bone marrow aspiration or biopsy usually distinguish between the two diseases, although the diagnosis can be difficult in a patient who has hypocellular marrow that is later replaced by lymphoblasts. In one study, transient pancytopenia preceded ALL in 2 percent of all pediatric cases.[75] During the preleukemic phase in these patients, PCR analysis demonstrated monoclonality. This finding suggests hypoplasia resulted from inhibition of normal hematopoiesis by leukemic cells.[101] ALL should be considered in the differential diagnosis of patients with hypereosinophilia, which can be a presenting feature of leukemia or can precede its diagnosis by several months.[70]

Infectious mononucleosis and other viral infections, especially those associated with thrombocytopenia or hemolytic anemia, can be confused with leukemia. Detection of reactive lymphocytes or serologic evidence of Epstein-Barr virus infection helps establish the diagnosis. Patients with acute infectious lymphocytosis, pertussis or parapertussis can have marked lymphocytosis. However, even when leukocyte counts are as high as 50×10^9/liter, the affected cells are mature lymphocytes rather than lymphoblasts. Bone pain, arthralgia, and occasionally arthritis mimic juvenile rheumatoid arthritis, rheumatic fever, other collagen diseases, or osteomyelitis. Bone marrow should be examined if glucocorticoid treatment is planned for presumed rheumatoid diseases.

In children, ALL should be distinguished from small round cell tumors involving the bone marrow, including neuroblastoma, rhabdomyosarcoma, and retinoblastoma. Generally, in patients with solid tumors, a primary lesion may be found by standard diagnostic studies. Disseminated tumor cells often present in characteristic aggregates, and immunophenotypic characteristics of lymphoblasts are absent.

THERAPY

SUPPORTIVE CARE

Optimal management of patients with ALL requires careful attention to supportive care, including immediate treatment or prevention of metabolic and infectious complications (see Chap. 20) and rational use of blood products. Other important supportive care measures, such as use of indwelling catheters, amelioration of nausea and vomiting, pain control, and continuous psychosocial support for the patient and family, are essential.

METABOLIC COMPLICATIONS

Hyperuricemia and hyperphosphatemia with secondary hypocalcemia are frequently encountered at diagnosis, even before chemotherapy is initiated, especially in patients with B cell or T cell ALL or B cell precursor leukemia with high leukemic cell burden. Patients should be given intravenous fluids; allopurinol or rasburicase (recombinant urate oxidase) to treat hyperuricemia; and a phosphate binder, such as aluminum hydroxide, calcium carbonate (if the serum calcium concentration is low), or sevelamer to treat hyperphosphatemia. By inhibiting de novo purine synthesis in leukemic blast cells, allopurinol can reduce the peripheral blast cell count before chemotherapy.[102] Allopurinol can decrease both the anabolism and catabolism of mercaptopurine by depleting intracellular phosphoribosyl pyrophosphate and by inhibiting xanthine oxidase.[103] If mercaptopurine and allopurinol are given together orally, the dosage of mercaptopurine generally must be reduced. Allopurinol can cause skin rashes but seldom causes severe allergic reactions.

Rasburicase breaks down uric acid to allantoin, a readily excreted metabolite that is five to 10 times more soluble than uric acid. Ras-

buricase is more effective than allopurinol, and it facilitates phosphorus excretion, partly because of rasburicase's potent uricolytic effect (which obviates the need to alkalinize urine) and partly because of improved renal function with its use.[104,105] However, rasburicase is contraindicated in patients with glucose-6-dehydrogenase deficiency because hydrogen peroxide, a by-product of uric acid breakdown, can cause methemoglobinemia or hemolytic anemia.

HYPERLEUKOCYTOSIS

For patients with extreme leukocytosis (leukocyte count $>400 \times 10^9$/liter), either leukapheresis or exchange transfusion (in small children) can be used to reduce the burden of leukemic cells. In theory, either treatment should reduce the complications associated with leukostasis, but the short- and long-term benefits of the procedures are questionable.[106,107] Emergency cranial irradiation, once advocated by some leukemia therapists, probably has no role in the treatment of these patients.[106] Preinduction therapy with low-dose glucocorticoids, with addition of vincristine and cyclophosphamide in cases of B cell ALL, is a favored means of ameliorating hyperleukocytosis. Pioneered by French investigators, this method, when used in conjunction with urate oxidase, has largely eliminated tumor lysis syndrome and the need for hemodialysis in patients with B cell ALL.[108]

INFECTION CONTROL

Infections are common in febrile patients with newly diagnosed ALL. Therefore, any patient presenting with fever, especially patients with neutropenia, should be given broad-spectrum antibiotics until infection is excluded. Remission induction therapy can increase susceptibility to infection by exacerbating myelosuppression, immunosuppression, and mucosal breakdown. At least 50 percent of patients undergoing induction therapy experience infections. Special precautions should be taken to reduce the risk of infection during this critical phase of treatment, including reverse protective isolation and air filtration; elimination of contact with people with infections; refraining from eating certain food products, such as raw cheese, uncooked vegetables, or unpeeled fruits; and use of antiseptic mouthwash or sitz baths, especially for patients with mucositis. Administration of granulocyte colony stimulating factor can hasten recovery from neutropenia and reduce the complications of intensive chemotherapy but does not improve the event-free survival rate for children or adults.[109,110] One study suggested growth factor increased the risk of therapy-related acute myeloid leukemia in the context of epipodophyllotoxin-based therapy.[111] Use of early intensification of therapy, especially in combination with dexamethasone, apparently has resulted in an increased risk of disseminated fungal infection.[100] Chapter 20 addresses diagnosis and treatment of fungal and viral infections.

Usually, all patients with ALL are given trimethoprim-sulfamethoxazole, 2 to 3 days per week, as prophylactic therapy for *Pneumocystis carinii (Pneumocytis jiroveci)* pneumonia.[112] Prophylaxis is started after 2 weeks of remission induction and continues until 6 weeks after completion of all chemotherapy. Alternative treatments for patients who cannot tolerate trimethoprim-sulfamethoxazole include aerosolized pentamidine, dapsone, and atovaquone.[113–115] Live virus vaccine should not be administered during immunosuppressive therapy. Siblings and other children who have frequent contact with patients can receive routine immunizations, including inactivated poliomyelitis vaccine. Susceptible patients exposed to varicella virus should receive zoster immunoglobulin within 96 hours of exposure. Such treatment usually prevents or modifies the clinical manifestations of varicella.

HEMATOLOGIC SUPPORT

ALL or its treatment can lead to thrombocytopenia. Hemorrhagic manifestations are common but usually are limited to the skin and mucous membranes. Although rare, bleeding in the CNS, lungs, or gastrointestinal tract can be life threatening. Patients with extremely high leukocyte counts ($>400 \times 10^9$/liter) at diagnosis are more likely to develop such complications.[67] Coagulopathy attributable to disseminated intravascular coagulation, hepatic dysfunction, or chemotherapy usually is mild.[63,76] Patients receiving induction treatment, including L-asparaginase and a glucocorticoid, generally are in a hypercoagulable state.[116,117] Platelet transfusions should be given therapeutically for overt bleeding and may be indicated when platelet counts are less than 10×10^9/liter.[118] Children generally do not have active bleeding during remission induction therapy with prednisone, vincristine, and L-asparaginase, even when platelet counts are less than 10×10^9/liter. A higher threshold for prophylactic platelet transfusions should be considered for active toddlers and patients with fever or infection. Transfusion of packed red cells is indicated in patients with anemia and marrow suppression but should be delayed until the leukocyte count is reduced in patients with extreme hyperleukocytosis.[67] Transfusion should be given slowly in patients with profound but chronic anemia to prevent development of congestive heart failure. Granulocyte transfusions are needed only rarely for patients with absolute neutropenia and documented gram-negative septicemia or disseminated fungal infection, which responds poorly to antimicrobial treatment. All blood products should be irradiated to prevent graft-versus-host disease.

ANTILEUKEMIC THERAPY

Because ALL is a heterogeneous disease with many distinct subtypes, a uniform approach to therapy is not appropriate. Assessing the probability of relapse is necessary to avert undertreatment or overtreatment. No consensus exists on the risk criteria and the terminology for defining prognostic subgroups. Usually, childhood ALL cases are divided into standard-risk, high- (intermediate- or average-) risk, and very-high risk groups, although the US Children's Oncology Group advocates four categories, including low risk to accommodate patients with a very low risk of relapse.[90] Adult cases are generally divided into two risk groups. B cell ALL and often infant ALL are considered special subgroups of ALL that require different treatment.

B CELL ALL

The most effective contemporary treatment regimens for B cell ALL are drug combinations that include cyclophosphamide given over a relatively short time (3–6 months). The first major breakthrough in this disease was reported by French investigators, who achieved a 68 percent event-free survival rate in their LMB84 study featuring high-dose cyclophosphamide, high-dose methotrexate, vincristine, doxorubicin, and conventional doses of cytarabine.[108] In the LMB89 study, the same group reported a cure rate of 87 percent, which was achieved by using increased doses of methotrexate (to 8 g/m² per dose) and cytarabine (3 g/m² per dose) and by adding etoposide for patients with a large leukemic cell burden.[119] This achievement established a standard against which other trials now are assessed. Successful treatments also have been developed by the Berlin-Frankfurt-Münster consortium, which uses a multiagent regimen that incorporates fractionated cyclophosphamide, high-dose methotrexate (5 g/m² per dose), etoposide, ifosfamide, and cytarabine (2 g/m² per dose).[120] The former Pediatric Oncology Group study developed an effective regimen consisting of fractionated doses of cyclophosphamide, vincristine, and doxorubicin, the administration of which is alternated with that of high-dose methotrexate and cytarabine.[121] Whether etoposide or ifosfamide contributed to the improved results requires further study.

Effective CNS therapy is an essential component of successful regimens for B cell ALL and generally consists of methotrexate and cytarabine administered both systematically and intrathecally.

Whether cranial irradiation should be used in therapy for CNS leukemia is controversial. Although cranial irradiation was a component of a very successful French regimen,[119] cranial irradiation was not included in other successful protocols, and the French group has excluded it from their current trial. B cell ALL rarely, if ever, recurs after the first year; therefore, prolonged continuation therapy is not necessary.

The treatment approach used for childhood ALL has been applied to B cell ALL in adults, yielding promising results in several trials.[122–124] A cure rate of approximately 50 percent has been achieved for adult patients, including those with initial CNS leukemia. Some investigators recommend reduced doses of methotrexate and cytarabine for adults older than 60 years to reduce toxicity.[123] Because of its demonstrated efficacy in B cell non-Hodgkin lymphoma,[125] rituximab (anti-CD20) has been incorporated in some front-line clinical trials for B cell ALL.

B CELL PRECURSOR AND T CELL ALL

Treatment for leukemias affecting the B cell precursor and T cell lineages consists of three standard phases: remission induction, intensification (consolidation), and prolonged continuation therapy. CNS-directed therapy, which overlaps other treatments, is started early and is given for different lengths of time, depending on the patient's risk of relapse and the intensity of the primary systemic regimen.

Remission Induction The first goal of therapy for patients with leukemia is inducing a complete remission and restore normal hematopoiesis. The induction regimen invariably includes a glucocorticoid (prednisone, prednisolone, or dexamethasone), vincristine, and L-asparaginase for children or an anthracycline for adults.[90,126,127] Children with high- or very-high-risk ALL and nearly all young adults with ALL receive all four drugs during remission induction in contemporary clinical trials. Improvements in chemotherapy and supportive care have resulted in complete remission rates of approximately 98 percent for children and approximately 85 percent for adults. When a complete clinical remission is induced, patients have various degrees of residual leukemia, and some can still have as many as 10 billion leukemic cells.[128] Because the extent of residual disease is well correlated with long-term outcome,[128–131] the concept of a "molecular" or "immunologic" remission, defined as leukemic involvement of less than 0.01 percent of nucleated marrow cells,[128] is beginning to supplant the traditional perception of remission, which is based solely on morphologic criteria of blast cells.

Attempts have been made to intensify induction therapy based on the premise that more rapid and complete reduction of the leukemic cell burden forestalls the development of drug resistance. However, results of several studies have suggested intensive therapy is unnecessary for children with standard-risk ALL, provided patients receive postinduction intensification therapy.[132,133] Intensive induction can lead to increased early morbidity and mortality.[134,135] More intensive induction regimens with additional cyclophosphamide, high-dose cytarabine, or high-dose anthracycline also have been tested in adults with ALL and have yielded no clear benefit,[136–138] partly because of the low tolerance of adults to drug toxicity.

Perhaps because of its increased penetration into the CNS and its longer half-life,[139] dexamethasone, when used in induction and continuation therapy, provides better control of systemic and CNS disease than does prednisone in children with ALL.[140] Three forms of L-asparaginase, each with a different pharmacokinetic profile, are available: one derived from *Erwinia chrysanthemi*, another prepared from *Escherichia coli*, and a third made of a polyethylene glycol form of the *E. coli* product (pegaspargase).[141] The dosages of the three preparations are based on their half-lives. Pegaspargase, which has the longest half-life, usually is administered at 2500 IU/m² every other week for two doses in cases of newly diagnosed ALL. By contrast, the *Erwinia* preparation, which has the shortest half-life, is administered at 20,000 IU/m² three times per week for six to 12 doses. The doses of *E. coli* L-asparaginase range from 6000 to 10,000 IU/m², administered two to three times per week for six to 12 doses. In one randomized trial, the clinical outcome of patients treated with L-asparaginase derived from *E. coli* was better than the outcome of patients treated with the *Erwinia* preparation given at the same dosage.[142] Different preparations of the *E. coli* enzyme have different pharmacologic and pharmacokinetic properties.[143] These differences mandate dosage adjustment to avoid excessive toxicity.[134,144] A study showed that antibodies to *E. coli* asparaginase cross-reacted with pegaspargase, and use of the latter form of asparaginase at the recommended dose was not very effective in patients who had previously received *E. coli* asparaginase, regardless of clinical hypersensitivity.[145] Intramuscular administration causes less frequent and less severe hypersensitivity reaction than intravenous injection of L-asparaginase. Of the various anthracyclines (daunorubicin, doxorubicin, and mitoxantrone) given to adults with ALL, none has proved superior to any other[146,147]; however, daunorubicin is used most commonly.

Intensification (Consolidation) Therapy When normal hematopoiesis is restored, patients in remission become candidates for intensification therapy. Such treatment, administered shortly after remission induction, refers to high doses of multiple agents not used during the induction phase or to readministration of the induction regimen. More commonly used regimens for childhood ALL include high-dose methotrexate with or without mercaptopurine,[148,149] high-dose L-asparaginase given for an extended period,[150,151] or a combination of dexamethasone, vincristine, L-asparaginase, and doxorubicin, followed by thioguanine, cytarabine, and cyclophosphamide.[122,148] This phase of therapy has improved outcome, even of patients with low-risk ALL.[152] A very high dose of methotrexate (5 g/m²) appears to improve the treatment outcome of patients with T cell ALL.[148,153] This finding is consistent with data indicating T lineage blast cells accumulate methotrexate polyglutamates (active metabolites of the parent compound) less avidly than do B cell precursors[94]; therefore, higher serum levels of the drug are needed for an adequate therapeutic effect.[154] The conventional dose of methotrexate (1 g/m²) may be too low for many patients with B cell precursor ALL.[149] To this end, our study showed that among B lineage ALL, blasts with either *TEL-AML1* or *E2A-PBX1* gene fusion accumulate significantly lower methotrexate polyglutamates compared to those with hyperdiploidy or other genetic abnormalities.[155] This finding suggested patients with *TEL-AML1* or *E2A-PBX1* gene fusion benefit from a higher dose of methotrexate.

The value of intensification treatment is less certain in adults with ALL. In two randomized trials, high doses of cytarabine and daunorubicin, which had been effective against acute myelogenous leukemia, did not result in a clinical outcome that was better than the outcome achieved without these agents.[156,157] In another randomized trial, prolonged (4-month) consolidation therapy with methotrexate, cytarabine, thioguanine, cyclophosphamide, and L-asparaginase yielded essentially the same leukemia-free survival rate as did short (1-month) consolidation therapy with cyclophosphamide and L-asparaginase.[158] These results notwithstanding, patient outcomes in several nonrandomized studies strongly suggest a benefit from intensive consolidation therapy, especially in young adults.[159–161] In cases of T cell ALL, the benefit is derived from cyclophosphamide and cytarabine. In other cases of standard-risk and high-risk ALL, the benefit is derived from high-dose cytarabine.[159,160] More striking perhaps is the markedly improved results in two German multicenter trials using high-dose cytarabine, mitoxantrone, and allogeneic hematopoietic stem cell transplantation in cases bearing the t(4;11),

which generally confers a dismal outcome.[162] By inhibiting the BCR-ABL fusion protein and other constituently active tyrosine kinases, imatinib mesylate has induced or consolidated remission of Philadelphia chromosome/BCR-ABL–positive ALL.[163,164] Several ongoing studies are testing its toxicity and efficacy in combination with chemotherapy in children and adults with this genetic subtype of ALL.

Continuation Therapy Excluding cases of mature B cell leukemia, children with ALL require prolonged continuation therapy for reasons that are poorly understood. Perhaps long-term drug exposure or the host immune system is needed to kill residual, slowly dividing leukemic cells or to suppress their growth and thus allow programmed cell death to occur. Attempts to shorten the duration of moderately intensive chemotherapy to 12 to 18 months or less have resulted in inferior overall event-free survival rates in childhood ALL,[165] although apparently two thirds of patients could be cured with only 12 months of treatment.[166] However, which subgroups of childhood ALL can be cured with abbreviated therapy is unclear. In a meta-analysis of 42 trials, a third year of continuation therapy reduced the likelihood of relapse during the third year, but no advantage to prolonging treatment beyond 3 years was observed.[167] Several studies have demonstrated that the third year of continuation therapy benefits boys but not girls.[168–170] Hence, many studies discontinue all therapy for girls whose ALL remains in remission for 2 to 2.5 years and for boys whose ALL remains in remission for 3 years. Whether adults with ALL require prolonged continuation therapy is unclear. In two trials of postremission treatment given for 5 to 10 months, the median duration of remission ranged from 9 to 12 months.[146,157] These poor results may reflect inadequate treatment for remission induction or for consolidation therapy. In most adult trials, continuation therapy is given for 2 years.

A combination of methotrexate administered weekly and mercaptopurine administered daily constitutes the usual continuation regimen for children with ALL. Accumulation of higher intracellular concentrations of the active metabolites of methotrexate and mercaptopurine and administration of this combination to the limits of tolerance (as indicated by low leukocyte counts) have been associated with improved clinical outcome.[171–174] In one study, the dose intensity of mercaptopurine was the most important pharmacologic factor influencing treatment outcome.[175] However, overzealous use of mercaptopurine is counterproductive, as such use results in neutropenia and interruption of chemotherapy, reducing overall dose intensity. The effect of mercaptopurine is better when the drug is administered in the evening.[176] Mercaptopurine should not be given with milk or milk products containing xanthine oxidase, which can degrade the drug.[177] Although the merits of oral and parenteral administration of methotrexate continue to be debated, the latter route circumvents problems of decreased bioavailability and poor compliance, especially in adolescents.[178] Prolonged oral administration of methotrexate in divided doses has proved inferior to intermittent intravenous infusions at higher doses.[179] By contrast, mercaptopurine is most effective when it is given orally on a daily basis; weekly intravenous administration at a higher dose is ineffective.[140,151,180,181] Antimetabolite treatment should not be withheld because of isolated increases of liver enzymes, because such liver function abnormalities are tolerable and reversible.[182]

A few patients (1/300) have an inherited homozygous deficiency of thiopurine *S*-methyltransferase, the enzyme that catalyzes the *S*-methylation (inactivation) of 6-mercaptopurine. In these patients, standard doses of mercaptopurine have potentially fatal hematologic side effects. The drug should be given in much smaller doses (e.g., 10-fold reduction).[183] Approximately 10 percent of affected patients are heterozygous for the enzyme deficiency and have intermediate levels of thiopurine methyltransferase.[184] This subgroup can be treated safely with only moderate reductions in mercaptopurine dosage and appears to have better clinical outcomes than do patients with the homozygous wild-type phenotype. Importantly, patients with this enzyme deficiency are at risk for therapy-related leukemia and radiation-related brain tumor.[185,186] Whether reducing the mercaptopurine dosage reduces the risk of therapy-related leukemia in these patients is unknown. Identification of the genetic basis of this autosomal codominant trait has enabled molecular diagnosis in these cases.[187] To this end, emphasis has been placed on the study of inherited differences in drug metabolism and disposition resulting from genetic polymorphisms in drug-metabolizing enzymes and in drug transporters, receptors, and targets.[4,188,189] Ultimately, therapy can be designed according to the genetic constitution of the host and the leukemic cells.

Intermittent pulses of vincristine and a glucocorticoid improve the efficacy of antimetabolite-based continuation regimens[167] and have been widely adopted in the treatment of childhood ALL. Another integral component of many protocols is reinduction therapy introduced relatively soon after the first remission. This treatment, which relies on the same drugs used during the initial phase of induction therapy, has improved outcomes for children and adults with ALL.[132,159] Prolonged intensification that includes a second reinduction phase during continuation treatment may further improve the outcome of patients with standard- or high-risk ALL.[150,190] In the latter study, additional pulses of vincristine and prednisone after reinduction treatment did not improve outcome.[190] This result suggests the benefit of double-delayed intensification resulted from either the increased dose intensity of other agents such as asparaginase or anthracycline or the timing or scheduling of the intensification regimen. The finding also suggests steroid and vincristine pulses may not be needed after reinduction therapy.

Therapy of the CNS   The CNS is a common sanctuary for leukemic cells and requires presymptomatic therapy. In the 1970s, the cornerstone of ALL therapy was cranial irradiation (2400 cGy) plus methotrexate administered intrathecally after complete remission was induced. Concern that cranial irradiation could cause second cancer, late neurocognitive deficits, and endocrinopathy stimulated efforts to replace cranial irradiation with early intensification of intrathecal and systemic chemotherapy. This approach has lowered rates of CNS relapse to less than 5 percent in several pediatric and adult studies.[82,161,191,192]

Whether certain groups of patients would still benefit from cranial irradiation is unclear. In one retrospective study, children with T cell ALL and leukocyte counts less than 100×10^9/liter had similar outcomes whether or not cranial irradiation was performed. However, among patients with T cell ALL and higher leukocyte counts, those who received radiation therapy had significantly better long-term responses than patients who received intrathecal therapy exclusively.[193] These results are not conclusive because the systemic chemotherapy differed between the two groups and may have been more effective in the patients who were irradiated. Nonetheless, in the context of effective systemic chemotherapy, a radiation dose as low as 1200 cGy appears to provide adequate protection against CNS relapse, even in high-risk patients (e.g., those with T cell ALL and leukocyte counts $>100 \times 10^9$/liter).[148] We contend that with effective systemic and intrathecal therapy, the need for cranial irradiation can be eliminated in all patients by adhering to the following guidelines.[83] First, traumatic lumbar puncture, which could adversely affect outcome, should be avoided.[84,85] The diagnostic lumbar puncture should be performed by an experienced clinician while the patient is immobile under general anesthesia or deep sedation. Platelets should be administered to patients with thrombocytopenia (i.e., platelet

count $<100 \times 10^9$/liter) and circulating leukemic cells. Second, intrathecal therapy should coincide with the diagnostic lumbar puncture and should be intensified in patients with any amount of identifiable leukemic cells in their CSF and in patients who experience traumatic lumbar puncture or have other high-risk features.[83] Third, patients should remain in a prone position for at least 30 minutes after the procedure.

Allogeneic Stem Cell Transplantation   Hematopoietic stem cell transplantation during first remission remains controversial. In adult ALL, long-term event-free survival rates range from 30 to 40 percent with chemotherapy alone and from 40 to 60 percent with allogeneic transplantation.[126,194–196] However, interpretation of these results is difficult because the proportions of patients in similar risk groups differed among studies, as did the criteria for patient selection. Even so, results of both the adult and pediatric studies suggest allogeneic transplantation benefits some high-risk patients.[194–198] Because of their unfavorable prognosis, patients with the Philadelphia chromosome or those with a poor initial response to induction therapy commonly undergo allogeneic stem cell transplantation during the first remission.[126,196–199] Allogeneic transplantation appeared to improve the outcome of adults with the t(4;11)[162] but not that of children with the same genotype.[200] The indications for transplantation in first remission should be reevaluated as chemotherapy and transplantation continue to improve.

COURSE AND PROGNOSIS

RELAPSE

Relapse is defined as the reappearance of leukemic cells at any site in the body. Most relapses occur during treatment or within the first 2 years after its completion, although initial relapses have been observed 10 or more years after diagnosis.[201] Molecular studies suggest that, in some cases with the *TEL-AML1* fusion, subsequent mutations of the residual preleukemic clone that were not eradicated during initial treatment account for the "late relapse."[202] The marrow remains the most common site of relapse in ALL. Anemia, leukocytosis, leukopenia, thrombocytopenia, enlargement of the liver or spleen, bone pain, fever, or a sudden decrease in tolerance to chemotherapy may signal the onset of marrow relapse. In some contemporary programs of childhood ALL treatment, the rates of CNS and testicular relapse have decreased to 2 percent or less.[151,192,203] Leukemic relapse occasionally occurs at other extramedullary sites, including the eye, ear, ovary, uterus, bone, muscle, tonsil, kidney, mediastinum, pleura, and paranasal sinus.[204]

Marrow relapse, with or without extramedullary involvement, portends a poor outcome for most patients. Factors indicating an especially poor prognosis include relapse while on therapy or after a short initial remission, T cell immunophenotype, the presence of the Philadelphia chromosome, and an isolated hematologic relapse.[205–209] Prolonged second remissions (>3 years) can be achieved with chemotherapy in as many as half of patients with late relapses (i.e., >6 months after cessation of therapy) but in only approximately 10 percent of those with early relapse.[205,207,210] In patients who develop hematologic relapse while on therapy or shortly thereafter, allogeneic hematopoietic stem cell transplantation is the treatment of choice.[211–215] Autologous transplantation as postinduction treatment offers no substantial advantage over chemotherapy.[216,217] For patients without histocompatible related donors, transplantation of stem cells from cord blood or marrow from matched unrelated donors has yielded encouraging results.[218–220] Umbilical cord blood offers a transplant option that does not require the same degree of histocompatibility as do procedures that rely on peripheral blood or marrow stem cells from children or adults.[221,222] Whether the lower risk of graft-versus-host disease associated with cord blood transplants will lead to an increased risk of relapse as a result of reduced graft-versus-leukemia effect is uncertain. Transplantation with large doses of T cell–depleted hematopoietic stem cells from haploidentical donors has resulted in a disease-free survival rate that compares favorably with the results of patients who receive transplants from matched unrelated donors.[223] Outcome may be further improved by a new strategy using a reduced intensity of conditioning regimen and selection of donor-derived alloreactive natural killer cells for haploidentical transplantation.[100,224] For patients with ALL relapses after allogeneic transplantation, a second transplant or donor T lymphocyte infusion occasionally results in sustained remission.[225] For patients who receive only chemotherapy, a second course of CNS-directed treatment is needed to prevent subsequent CNS relapse.[226]

Although extramedullary relapse is frequently an isolated clinical finding, most if not all occurrences are associated with minimal residual disease in the marrow.[227,228] Hence, patients with extramedullary relapse require intensive systemic treatment to prevent subsequent hematologic relapse. The efficacy of retrieval therapy in children with an isolated CNS relapse depends partly on whether the relapse occurs during or after completion of treatment and partly on whether CNS irradiation was previously performed. Intensive chemotherapy and CNS irradiation are expected to achieve long-term second remissions in at least half of the previously unirradiated patients with ALL relapses after completion of therapy.[229,230] For patients in whom relapse develops during therapy and who had previously undergone cranial irradiation, the remission rate generally does not exceed 30 percent.[229–231] Adults with isolated CNS relapse fare much more poorly than children. Some investigators have selected hematopoietic stem cell transplantation as a treatment option for these high-risk cases.[217,231] However, no firm evidence indicates an advantage of either autologous or allogeneic transplantation over intensive chemotherapy.

One third of patients with early testicular relapse and two thirds with late testicular recurrence became long-term survivors after salvage chemotherapy and bilateral testicular irradiation.[232–235] Whether this experience can be extrapolated to patients who have received contemporary intensive treatment is uncertain, especially because testicular relapse has become a rare event. In one study, some patients with late isolated testicular relapses were successfully treated with chemotherapy that included very high-dose methotrexate, without the addition of radiation therapy.[236] The optimal treatment and prognosis for patients with relapse at unusual extramedullary sites also are unclear. However, the same principles that apply to the clinical management of CNS or testicular relapse probably apply to this subgroup.

TREATMENT SEQUELAE

Despite the increasing intensity of curative treatment for childhood ALL, judicious use of supportive care has reduced the rate of early death from 8 percent in the early 1970s to less than 3 percent in the 1990s.[20] However, the death rate among elderly patients receiving remission induction therapy can be as high as 30 percent because of increased hematologic and nonhematologic toxicities (e.g., hepatotoxicity and cardiotoxicity).[63] This poor tolerance of chemotherapy and consequent reduction of dose intensity largely account for the generally poor clinical outcome in elderly patients.

Table 91-6 summarizes common side effects associated with antileukemic therapy. Hyperglycemia develops in 10 percent of children during induction therapy with prednisone, vincristine, and L-asparaginase; in some cases, short-term insulin treatment is required. Adoles-

cent age, obesity, a family history of diabetes mellitus, and Down syndrome are associated with increased susceptibility to hyperglycemia.[237] This induction regimen can cause a hypercoagulable state[238] leading to cerebral thromboses, peripheral vein thromboses, or both, in as many as 5 percent of patients. Cerebral thrombosis should be distinguished from transient ischemic lesions, which are associated with acute hypertension and severe constipation. These lesions are located at the watershed areas between the major cerebral arteries and generally are reversible.[239] Cerebral thrombosis can be readily distinguished from transient ischemic lesions by magnetic resonance imaging or computed tomography (Fig. 91-8). Occasionally, cerebral thrombosis may not be apparent by diagnostic imaging until a few days after the onset of symptoms and signs.

Emphasis on the intensive use of methotrexate and glucocorticoids has led to an increased frequency of neurotoxicity[240–242] and aseptic necrosis of bone,[243–245] underscoring the need for judicious use of even seemingly benign agents. For example, methotrexate given in divided doses of 25 mg/m² every 6 hours four times daily in four weekly courses can result in acute neurologic toxicity if subsequent leucovorin treatment is inadequate.[240] Many long-term survivors of childhood ALL, especially those who received high cumulative doses of glucocorticoid or methotrexate or cranial irradiation, have developed severe osteoporosis.[246,247] Such development highlights the need for early identification of bone lesions and the introduction of therapy to prevent fractures.

Treatment with anthracyclines can produce severe cardiomyopathy, especially when anthracyclines are given in high cumulative and peak doses to young girls.[248,249] Prolonged infusion did not appear to reduce late cardiotoxicity compared to bolus administration.[250] The existence of a safe cumulative dose of anthracycline is controversial.[251] In one study, dexrazoxane prevented or reduced anthracycline-induced cardiotoxicity without interfering with antileukemic activity.[252] Cranial irradiation has been implicated as the cause of numerous late sequelae in children, including second cancer, neurocognitive deficits, and endocrine abnormalities that can lead to obesity, short stature, precocious puberty, and osteoporosis.[20] In general, these complications are seen in girls more often than in boys and in young children more often than in older children. Our long-term followup study of 10-year event-free survivors revealed a 20 percent cumulative risk of second neoplasms at 30 years from start of treatment among patients who had received cranial irradiation. The result was a higher-than-average mortality rate.[253] Patients who had been irradiated also had a high unemployment rate and, among women, a low marital rate. Many children with profound deficiencies of growth hormone are receiving hormone replacement therapy, which permits attainment of acceptable final heights without an increased chance of relapse.[254] However, in one study, growth hormone replacement therapy was associated with a slight increase in second malignancy within the previous site of radiation.[255]

The most devastating complication is the development of brain tumors and acute myelogenous leukemia. Children who undergo cranial irradiation at age 6 years or younger are most susceptible to development of brain tumors.[256] Intensive use of antimetabolites before and during cranial irradiation also increases the risk of brain tumor.[186] The median latency period for high-grade brain tumor is 9 years and is 20 years for low-grade tumors (e.g., meningioma).[253,256]

Acute myelogenous leukemia has been linked to intensive treatment with the epipodophyllotoxins (teniposide and etoposide). The risk of disease apparently depends on treatment schedule, concomitant use of other agents (e.g., L-asparaginase, alkylating agents, perhaps antimetabolites), and host pharmacogenetics.[185,257] The long-term survival rate for patients with this complication is very low, even when the patients undergo allogeneic stem cell transplantation.[185] No evi-

TABLE 91-6   SIDE EFFECTS ASSOCIATED WITH ANTILEUKEMIC THERAPY

TREATMENT	ACUTE COMPLICATIONS	DELAYED COMPLICATIONS
Prednisone (or prednisolone)	Hyperglycemia, hypertension, changes in mood or behavior, acne, increased appetite, weight gain, peptic ulcer, hepatomegaly, myopathy	Avascular necrosis of bone, osteopenia, growth retardation
Dexamethasone	Same as prednisone, except for increased changes in mood or behavior and myopathy but less salt retention	Same as prednisone
Vincristine	Peripheral neuropathy, constipation, chemical cellulitis, seizures, hair loss	None
Daunorubicin, idarubicin, doxorubicin, or epirubicin	Nausea and vomiting, hair loss, mucositis, bone marrow suppression, chemical cellulitis, increased skin pigmentation, hair loss	Cardiomyopathy (with high cumulative dose)
L-Asparaginase	Nausea and vomiting, allergic reactions (manifested as rashes, bronchospasm, severe pain at intramuscular injection site), hyperglycemia, pancreatitis, liver dysfunction, thrombosis, encephalopathy	None
Mercaptopurine	Nausea and vomiting, mucositis, bone marrow suppression, solar dermatitis, liver dysfunction: increased hematologic toxicity in persons lacking thiopurine methyltransferase	Osteoporosis (long-term use), acute myeloid leukemia in persons with thiopurine methyltransferase deficiency
Methotrexate	Nausea and vomiting, liver dysfunction, bone marrow suppression, mucositis (resulting from high-dose treatment), solar dermatitis	Leukoencephalopathy, osteopenia (resulting from long-term use)
Etoposide, teniposide	Nausea and vomiting, hair loss, mucositis, bone marrow suppression, allergic reactions (bronchospasm, urticaria, angioedema, hypotension)	Acute myeloid leukemia
Cytarabine	Nausea and vomiting, fever, skin rashes, mucositis, bone marrow suppression, liver dysfunction, conjunctivitis (resulting from high-dose treatment)	Decreased fertility (with high cumulative dose)
Cyclophosphamide	Nausea and vomiting, hemorrhagic cystitis, bone marrow suppression, syndrome of inappropriate secretion of antidiuretic hormone, hair loss	Bladder cancer or acute myeloid leukemia (rare), decreased fertility (with high cumulative dose)
Intrathecal methotrexate	Headache, fever, seizure, bone marrow suppression, mucositis (in patients with renal dysfunction)	? Encephalopathy or myelopathy (with high cumulative dose)
Brain irradiation	Hair loss, postirradiation somnolence syndrome (6–10 weeks after treatment)	Seizure, mineralizing microangiopathy, growth hormone deficiency, thyroid dysfunction, obesity, osteopenia, brain tumors, basal cell carcinoma, parotid gland carcinoma, hair loss, cataract (rare), dental abnormalities

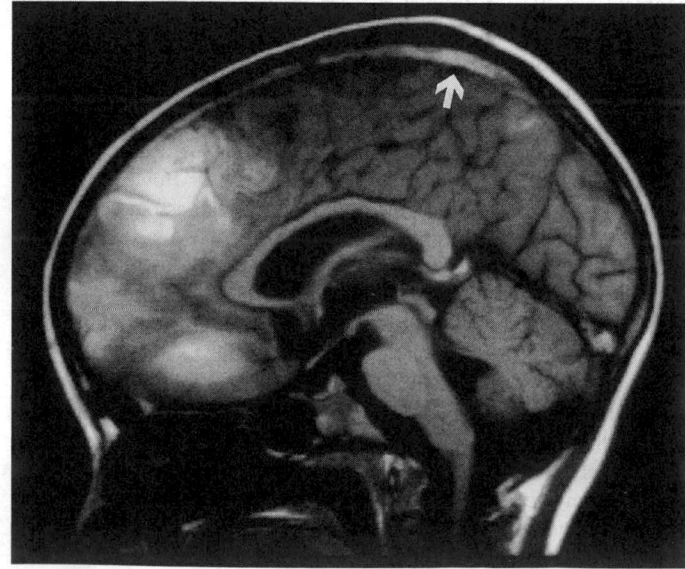

FIGURE 91-8   T1-weighted magnetic resonance image without contrast demonstrates a clot in the superior sagittal sinus (arrow) and several frontal lobe hematomas.

dence indicates an increased incidence of cancer or birth defects among the offspring of adult survivors of childhood ALL.[258–260]

PROGNOSTIC FACTORS

The cornerstone of the modern therapeutic approach to childhood ALL has been careful assessment of the risk of relapse so that only high-risk or very-high-risk patients are treated with intensive therapy. Less toxic treatments (usually antimetabolites) are reserved for low-risk or standard-risk patients. By contrast, almost all adult patients are candidates for intensive therapy. Of the many variables that influence prognosis, treatment is the most important.[261] Some of the factors that emerged as useful prognostic indicators have disappeared as treatment has improved; others have shown predictive strength in one or several trials but not in others. For example, T cell and B cell ALL, once associated with a very poor prognosis, now have long-term response rates of 70 to 85 percent in children[119,120,148,150,151,192] and 50 to 60 percent in adults[122,123,126,127] as a result of effective intensive chemotherapy.

Age and leukocyte count continue to be used for risk classification in almost every pediatric clinical trial involving B cell precursor ALL. In a workshop sponsored by the US National Cancer Institute, participants agreed on a presenting age between 1 and 9 years and a leukocyte count of less than 50×10^9/liter as the minimal criteria for low-risk ALL.[262] These criteria apply only to B cell precursor ALL and not to T cell ALL. Among adults, the outcome of therapy worsens with increasing age and leukocyte count. Age younger than 30 years and leukocyte count less than 30×10^9/liter are considered favorable prognostic indicators.[126,127,156,263,264] However, no clear guidelines exist for assigning prognostic value to particular increments of age or leukocyte numbers. In general, age younger than 60 years is considered a practical guide for selecting candidates who might benefit from intensive therapy, including allogeneic transplantation. Any decision to begin aggressive treatment in patients older than 60 years must be weighed against the risk of increased morbidity and mortality.

Male sex has long been recognized as an adverse prognostic factor in childhood ALL[265,266] but has less influence in adult ALL. Its prognostic significance was abolished in a number of childhood studies in which overall outcome was improved.[151,192,203] Black race continues to confer a poor outcome in the national clinical trials[267-269] but has had no prognostic significance in our single-institution study.[203] This finding is attributed to the equal access to effective treatment regimens at our institution and to the use of stringent risk criteria.

Primary genetic abnormalities have important prognostic significance. Hyperdiploidy (>50 chromosomes) and *TEL-AML1* fusion—seen primarily in children aged 1 to 9 years—are associated with a favorable prognosis.[20] *MLL* rearrangements, which occur in 70 to 80 percent of infants younger than 1 year and in 10 percent of adults, and Philadelphia chromosome with BCR-ABL fusion, which is found in 3 percent of children but in 25 to 30 percent of adult patients, confer a poor outcome.[4] Interestingly, a marked influence of age on the prognosis of genetic subtypes of ALL is observed. For example, Philadelphia chromosome-positive ALL is associated with a poor prognosis in adolescents but a relatively favorable outcome in children 1 to 9 years old who have a low leukocyte count at presentation.[199] Adults with this type of ALL have a dismal prognosis.[126,127] Among patients with *MLL*-rearranged ALL, infants younger than 1 year fare considerably worse than older children.[200,270] The basis of these differences may be related to some combination of secondary genetic events, the development stage of the target cell undergoing malignant transformation, and the pharmacogenetics or pharmacokinetic features of the patient.

A useful adjunct in risk assessment is the response to early treatment, as measured by the rate of clearance of leukemic cells from the blood or marrow with the use of flow cytometric detection of aberrant immunophenotype or analysis by PCR of clonal antigen–receptor gene rearrangements.[129-131] This measure accounts for the drug sensitivity or resistance of leukemic cells and the pharmacodynamics of the drugs, which is affected by the pharmacogenetics of the host. Because tandem application of flow cytometry and PCR has allowed study of minimal residual disease in almost all patients,[128] this factor now is included in the risk classification system at St. Jude (Table 91-7). The expectation is that alteration of treatment intensity according to the level of minimal residual disease will improve the long-term outcome

of patients with ALL. The level of minimal residual leukemia is also a strong predictor of treatment outcome in patients at the time of second remission.[271] Patients with T cell ALL can be monitored by analysis of blood samples instead of bone marrow aspirates because both sources yield comparable levels of residual leukemia.[272]

TABLE 91-7 RISK CLASSIFICATION SYSTEM IN ST. JUDE TOTAL THERAPY STUDY XV

RISK GROUP	FEATURE
Standard	B cell precursor phenotype in patients aged 1–9 years with a presenting leukocyte count $<50 \times 10^9$/liter, *TEL-AML1* fusion, or hyperdiploidy (>50 chromosomes or DNA index >1.16)
	Must not have CNS leukemia (CNS-3 status), testicular leukemia, t(9;22), t(1;19), rearranged *MLL* gene, hypodiploidy, or $\geq 0.01\%$ leukemia cells in marrow after 6-week remission induction
High	T cell ALL and all cases of B cell precursor ALL that do not meet the criteria for standard or very-high-risk ALL
Very high	t(9;22)/*BCR-ABL*, initial induction failure, or $\geq 1\%$ leukemic cells in bone marrow after 6-week remission induction

REFERENCES

1. Gale RE, Wainscoat JS: Clonal analysis using X-linked DNA polymorphisms. *Br J Haematol* 85:2, 1993.

2. Saunders EF, Lampkin BC, Mauer AM: Variation of proliferative activity in leukemic cell populations of patients with acute leukemia. *J Clin Invest* 46:1356, 1967.

3. Gilliland DG, Tallman MS. Focus on acute leukemia. *Cancer Cell* 1: 417, 2002.

4. Pui C-H, Relling MV, Downing JR. Acute lymphoblastic leukemia. *N Engl J Med* 350:49-62, 2004.

5. Velpeau A: Sur la resorption du pus et sur l'alteration du sang dans les maladies, Clinique de persection nenemant. Premier observation. *Rev Med* 26:216, 1827.

6. Virchow R: Weisses blut. *Notiz Geg Natur Heilk* 36:152, 1845.

7. Bennett JH: Case of hypertrophy of the spleen and liver in which death took place from suppuration of the blood. *Edinburgh Med Surg J* 64: 413, 1845.

8. Craigie D: Case of disease of the spleen, in which death took place in consequence of the presence of purulent matter in the blood. *Edinburgh Med Surg J* 64:400, 1845.

9. Virchow R: Weisses Blut und Milztumoren. Part II. Med Z, 1847, 16, 9. *Virchows Arch Path Anat Physiol* 1:565, 1847.

10. Ehrlich P: Farbenanalytische untersuchungen zur histologie und klinik des blutes. *Berl Hirschwald* 137, 1891.

11. Reschad H, Schilling-Torgau V: Ueber eine neue Leukämie durch echte Uebergangsformen (Splenozytenleuämie) und ihre bedeutung für dies, selbständigkeit dieser Zellen. *Munchener Med Wochenschr* 60:1981, 1913.

12. Ward G: The infective theory of acute leukemia. *Br J Child Dis* 14:10, 1917.

13. Farber S, Diamond LK, Mercer RD, et al: Temporary remissions in acute leukemia in children produced by folic acid antagonist, 4-aminopteroyl-glumatic acid (aminopterin). *N Engl J Med* 238:787, 1948.

14. Farber S: The effect of ACTH in acute leukemia in childhood, in *Proceedings of the First Clinical Conference on the Use of ACTH*, edited by JR Mote, p 325. Blakiston, Philadelphia, 1950.

15. Elion GB, Hitchings GH, Vanderwerff H: Antagonists of nucleic acid derivatives; purines. *J Biol Chem* 192:505, 1951.

16. Pinkel D, Hernandez K, Borella L, et al: Drug dosage and remission duration in childhood lymphocytic leukemia. *Cancer* 27:247, 1971.

17. Thomas ED, Buckner CD, Rudolph RH, et al: Allogeneic marrow grafting for hematological malignancy using HLA-matched donor-recipient pairs. *Blood* 38:267, 1971.

18. Sen L, Borella L: Clinical importance of lymphoblasts with T markers in childhood acute leukemia. *N Engl J Med* 292:828, 1975.

19. Williams DL, Look AT, Melvin SL, et al: New chromosomal translocations correlate with specific immunophenotypes of childhood acute lymphoblastic leukemia. *Cell* 36:101, 1984.

20. Pui CH, Evans WE: Acute lymphoblastic leukemia. *N Engl J Med* 339: 605, 1998.

21. Wassmann B, Pfeifer H, Scheuring UJ, et al: Early prediction of response in patients with relapsed or refractory Philadelphia chromosome-positive acute lymphoblastic leukemia (Ph+ ALL) treated with imatinib. *Blood* 103;1495, 2004.

22. Jemal A, Tiwari RC, Murray T, et al: Cancer statistics, 2004. *CA Cancer J Clin* 54:8, 2004.

23. *SEER Cancer Statistics Review, 1973–1995.* National Cancer Institute, Bethesda, 1998.

24. Sandler DP, Ross JA: Epidemiology of acute leukemia in children and adults. *Semin Oncol* 24:3, 1997.

25. Biondi A, Cimino G, Pieters R, Pui CH: Biological and therapeutic aspects of infant leukemia. *Blood* 96:24, 2000.

26. Parkin DM, Muir CS, Whelan SL, et al: *Cancer Incidence in Five Continents,* vol 6, no 120. IARC Scientific Publication, Lyon, 1992.

27. Pui C-H: Acute leukemia in children. *Curr Opin Hematol* 3:249, 1996.

28. Pui C-H, Raimondi SC, Borowitz MJ, et al: Immunophenotypes and karyotypes of leukemic cells in children with Down syndrome and acute lymphoblastic leukemia. *J Clin Oncol* 11:1361, 1993.

29. Vanasse GJ, Concannon P, Willerford DM: Regulated genomic instability and neoplasia in the lymphoid lineage. *Blood* 94:3997, 1999.

30. Liberzon E, Avigad S, Stark B, et al: Germ-line ATM gene alterations are associated with susceptibility to sporadic T-cell acute lymphoblastic leukemia in children. *Genes Chromosomes Cancer* 39:161, 2004.

31. Sun X, Becker-Catania SG, Chen HH, et al: Early diagnosis of ataxia-telangiectasia using radiosensitivity testing. *J Pediatr* 140:724, 2002.

32. Doll R, Wakeford R: Risk of childhood cancer from fetal irradiation. *Br J Radiol* 70:130,1997.

33. Ahlbom A, Day N, Feychting M, et al. A pooled analysis of magnetic fields and childhood leukaemia. *Br J Cancer* 83:692, 2000.

34. Davies SM, Bhatia S, Ross JA, et al: Glutathione S-transferase genotypes, genetic susceptibility, and outcome of therapy in childhood acute lymphoblastic leukemia. *Blood* 100:67, 2002.

35. Smith MT, Wang Y, Skibola CF, et al: Low NAD(P)H:quinone oxidoreductase activity is associated with increased risk of leukemia with MLL translocations in infants and children. *Blood* 100:4590, 2002.

36. Skibola CF, Smith MT, Krane E, et al: Polymorphisms in the methylenetetrahydrofolate reductase gene are associated with susceptibility to acute leukemia in adults. *Proc Natl Acad Sci U S A* 96:12810, 1999.

37. Wiemels JL, Smith RN, Taylor GM, et al: Methylenetetrahydrofolate reductase (MTHFR) polymorphisms and risk of molecularly defined subtypes of childhood acute leukemia. *Proc Natl Acad Sci U S A* 98: 4004, 2001.

38. Skibola CF, Smith MT, Hubbard A, et al: Polymorphisms in the thymidylate synthase and serine hydroxymethyltransferase genes and risk of adult acute lymphocytic leukemia. *Blood* 99:3786, 2002.

39. Thompson JR, Gerald PF, Willoughby ML, Armstrong BK: Maternal folate supplementation in pregnancy and protection against acute lymphoblastic leukaemia in childhood: A case-control study. *Lancet* 358: 1935, 2001.

40. Greaves MF, Maia AT, Wiemels JL, Ford AM: Leukemia in twins: Lessons in natural history. *Blood* 102:2321, 2003.

41. Greaves MF, Wiemels J: Origins of chromosome translocations in childhood leukaemia. *Nat Rev Cancer* 3:639, 2003.

42. Maia AT, Tussiwand R, Cazzaniga G, et al: Identification of preleukemic precursors of hyperdiploid acute lymphoblastic leukemia in cord blood. *Genes Chromosomes Cancer* 40:38, 2004.

43. Kinlen LJ: High-contact paternal occupations, infection and childhood leukaemia: Five studies of unusual population mixing of adults. *Br J Cancer* 76:1539,1997

44. Wiemels JL, Leonard BC, Wang Y, et al: Site-specific translocation and evidence of postnatal origin of the t(1;19) E2A-PBX1 fusion in childhood acute lymphoblastic leukemia. *Proc Natl Acad Sci U S A* 99:15101, 2002.

45. Ferrando AA, Look AT: Gene expression profiling in T-cell acute lymphoblastic leukemia. *Semin Hematol* 40:274-80, 2003.

46. Sherr CJ, McCormick F: The RB and p53 pathways in cancer. *Cancer Cell* 2:103, 2002.

47. Omura-Minamisawa M, Diccianni MB, Batova A, et al: Universal inactivation of both p16 and p15 but not downstream components is an essential event in the pathogenesis of T-cell acute lymphoblastic leukemia. *Clin Cancer Res* 6:1219, 2000.

48. Stock W, Tsai T, Golden C, et al: Cell cycle regulatory gene abnormalities are important determinants of leukemogenesis and disease biology in adult acute lymphoblastic leukemia. *Blood* 95:2364, 2000.

49. Vousden KH, Lu X: Live or let die: The cell's response to p53. *Nat Rev Cancer* 2:594, 2002.

50. Calero Moreno TM, Gustafsson G, Garwicz S, et al: Deletion of the Ink4-locus (the p16ink4a, p14ARF and p15ink4b genes) predicts relapse in children with ALL treated according to the Nordic protocols NOPHO-86 and NOPHO-92. *Leukemia* 16:2037, 2002.

51. Roman-Gomez J, Castillejo JA, Jimenez A, et al: 5' CpG island hypermethylation is associated with transcriptional silencing of the p21(C1P1/WAF1/SDI1) gene and confers poor prognosis in acute lymphoblastic leukemia. *Blood* 99:2291, 2002.

52. Sherr CJ. The INK4a/ARF network in tumour suppression. *Nat Rev Mol Cell Biol* 2:731, 2001.

53. Armstrong SA, Staunton JE, Silverman LB, et al: MLL translocations specify a distinct gene expression profile that distinguishes a unique leukemia. *Nat Genet* 30:41, 2002.

54. Yeoh EJ, Ross ME, Shurtleff SA, et al: Classification, subtype discovery, and prediction of outcome in pediatric acute lymphoblastic leukemia by gene expression profiling. *Cancer Cell* 1:133, 2002.

55. Armstrong SA, Kung AL, Mabon ME, et al: Inhibition of FLT3 in MLL: Validation of a therapeutic target identified by gene expression based classification. *Cancer Cell* 3:173, 2003.

56. Cheok MH, Yang W, Pui CH, et al: Treatment-specific changes in gene expression discriminate in vivo drug response in human leukemia cells. *Nat Genet* 34:85, 2003.

57. Holleman A, Cheok MH, Den Boer ML, et al: Gene-expression patterns in drug-resistant acute lymphoblastic leukemia cells and response to treatment. *N Engl J Med* 351:533, 2004.

58. Ferrando AA, Neuberg DS, Dodge RK, et al: Prognostic importance of TLX1 (HOX11) oncogene expression in adults with T-cell acute lymphoblastic leukaemia. *Lancet* 363:535, 2004.

59. Pui C-H, Crist WM: Acute lymphoblastic leukemia, in *Childhood Leukemia,* edited by C-H Pui, p 288. Cambridge University Press, New York, 1999.

60. McKenna SM, Baehner RL: Diagnosis and treatment of childhood acute lymphoblastic leukemia, in *Neoplastic Diseases of the Blood,* 3rd ed, edited by PH Wiernik, GP Canellos, JP Dutcher, RA Kyle, p 271. Churchill Livingstone, New York, 1996.

61. Reiter A, Schrappe M, Ludwig WD, et al: Chemotherapy in 998 unselected childhood acute lymphoblastic leukemia patients. Results and conclusions of the multicenter trial ALL-BFM 86. *Blood* 84:3122, 1994.

62. Chessells JM, Hall E, Prentice HG, et al: The impact of age on outcome in lymphoblastic leukemia; MRC UKALL X and XA compared: A report from the MRC Paediatric and Adult Working Parties. *Leukemia* 12: 463, 1998.

63. Hoelzer DF: Diagnosis and treatment of adult acute lymphoblastic leukemia, in *Neoplastic Diseases of the Blood,* 3rd ed, edited by PH Wiernik, GP Canellos, JP Dutcher, RA Kyle, p 295. Churchill Livingstone, New York, 1996.

64. Larson LA, Dodge RK, Burns CP, et al: A five-drug remission induction regimen with intensive consolidation for adults with acute lymphoblastic leukemia: Cancer and Leukemia Group B study 8811. *Blood* 85:2025, 1995.

65. Dinarello CA, Bunn PA Jr: Fever. *Semin Oncol* 24:288, 1997.

66. Pui C-H, Stass S, Green A: Bone marrow necrosis in children with malignant disease. *Cancer* 56:1522, 1985.

67. Lowe EJ, Pui C-H, Hancock ML, et al: Early complications in children with acute lymphoblastic leukemia presenting with hyperleukocytosis. *Pediatr Blood Cancer* 45:10, 2005.

68. Ingram L, Rivera GK, Shapiro DN: Superior vena cava syndrome associated with childhood malignancy: Analysis of 24 cases. *Med Pediatr Oncol* 18:476, 1990.

69. Gajjar A, Ribeiro RC, Mahmoud HH, et al: Overt testicular disease at diagnosis is associated with high risk features and a poor prognosis in patients with childhood acute lymphoblastic leukemia. *Cancer* 78:2437, 1996.

70. Brito-Babapulla F: The esoinophils, including the idiopathic hypereosinophilic syndrome. *Br J Haematol* 121:203, 2003.

71. Huang MS, Hasserjian: Case 19-2004: A 12-year-od boy with fatigue and eosinophilia. *N Engl J Med* 350:2604, 2004.

72. Dubansky AS, Boyett JM, Falletta J, et al: Isolated thrombocytopenia in children with acute lymphoblastic leukemia: A rare event in a Pediatric Oncology Group study. *Pediatrics* 84:1068, 1989.

73. Beutler E: Platelet transfusions: The 20,000/μL trigger. *Blood* 81:1411, 1993.

74. Blatt J, Penchansky L, Horn M: Thrombocytosis as a presenting feature of acute lymphoblastic leukemia in childhood. *Am J Hematol* 31:46, 1989.

75. Hasle H, Heim S, Schroeder H, et al: Transient pancytopenia preceding acute lymphoblastic leukemia (pre-ALL). *Leukemia* 9:605, 1995.

76. Ribeiro RC, Pui CH: The clinical and biological correlates of coagulopathy in children with acute leukemia. *J Clin Oncol* 4:1212, 1986.

77. Pui C-H, Dodge RK, Dahl GV, et al: Serum lactic dehydrogenase level has prognostic value in childhood acute lymphoblastic leukemia. *Blood* 66:778, 1985.

78. Jones DP, Stapleton FB, Kalwinsky D, et al: Renal dysfunction and hyperuricemia at presentation and relapse of acute lymphoblastic leukemia. *Med Pediatr Oncol* 18:283, 1990.

79. McKay C, Furman WL: Hypercalcemia complicating childhood malignancies. *Cancer* 72:256, 1993.

80. Welch JC, Lilleyman JS: Immunoglobulin concentrations in untreated lymphoblastic leukemia. *Pediatr Hematol Oncol* 12:545, 1995.

81. Müller HL, Horwitz AE, Kühl J: Acute lymphoblastic leukemia with severe skeletal involvement: A subset of childhood leukemia with a good prognosis. *Pediatr Hematol Oncol* 15:121, 1998.

82. Pui CH, Mahmoud HH, Rivera GK, et al: Early intensification of intrathecal chemotherapy virtually eliminates central nervous system relapse in children with acute lymphoblastic leukemia. *Blood* 92:411, 1998.

83. Pui C-H: Toward optimal central nervous system-directed treatment in childhood acute lymphoblastic leukemia. *J Clin Oncol* 21:179, 2003.

84. Gajjar A, Harrison PL, Sandlund JT, et al: Traumatic lumbar puncture at diagnosis adversely affects outcome in childhood acute lymphoblastic leukemia. *Blood* 96:3381, 2000.

85. Bürger B, Zimmermann M, Mann G, et al: Diagnostic cerebrospinal fluid (CSF) examination in children with acute lymphoblastic leukemia (ALL): Significance of low leukocyte counts with blasts or traumatic lumbar puncture. *J Clin Oncol* 21:184, 2003.

86. Howard SC, Gajjar AJ, Cheng C, et al: Risk factors for traumatic and bloody lumbar puncture in children with acute lymphoblastic leukemia. *JAMA* 288:2001, 2002.

87. Béné MC, Bernier M, Castoldi G, et al: Impact of immunophenotyping on management of acute leukemias. *Haematologica* 84:1024, 1999.

88. Ludwig WD, Reiter A, Löffler H, et al: Immunophenotypic features of childhood and adult acute lymphoblastic leukemia (ALL): Experience of the German multicentre trials ALL-BFM and GMALL. *Leuk Lymphoma* 13:71, 1994.

89. Pui CH, Rubnitz JE, Hancock ML, et al: Reappraisal of the clinical and biologic significance of myeloid-associated antigen expression in childhood acute lymphoblastic leukemia. *J Clin Oncol* 16:3768, 1998.

90. Pui C-H, Campana D, Evans WE: Childhood acute lymphoblastic leukemia—current status and future perspectives. *Lancet Oncol* 2:597, 2001.

91. Secker-Walker LM, Prentice HG, Durrant J, et al: Cytogenetics adds independent prognostic information in adults with acute lymphoblastic leukaemia on MRC trial UKALL XA. *Br J Haematol* 96:601, 1997.

92. Faderl S, Jeha S, Kantarjian HM: The biology and therapy of adult lymphoblastic leukemia. *Cancer* 98:1337, 2003.

93. Mrózek K, Heerema NA, Bloomfield CD: Cytogenetics in acute leukemia. *Blood Reviews* 18:115, 2004.

94. Synold TW, Relling MV, Boyett JM, et al: Blast cell methotrexate-polyglutamate accumulation in vivo differs by lineage, ploidy, and methotrexate dose in acute lymphoblastic leukemia. *J Clin Invest* 94:1996, 1994.

95. Kaspers GJL, Smets LA, Pieters R, et al: Favorable prognosis of hyperdiploid common acute lymphoblastic leukemia may be explained by sensitivity to antimetabolites and other drugs: Results of an in vitro study. *Blood* 85:751, 1995.

96. Ito C, Kumagai M, Manabe A, et al: Hyperdiploid acute lymphoblastic leukemia with 51 to 65 chromosomes: A distinct biological entity with a marked propensity to undergo apoptosis. *Blood* 93:315, 1999.

97. Pui CH, Carroll AJ, Raimondi SC, et al: Clinical presentation, karyotypic characterization, and treatment outcome of childhood acute lymphoblastic leukemia with a near-haploid or hypodiploid <45 line. *Blood* 75:1170, 1990.

98. Harrison CJ, Moorman AV, Broadfield ZJ, et al: Three distinct subgroups of hypodiploidy in acute lymphoblastic leukaemia. *Br J Haematol* 125:552, 2004.

99. Robinson HM, Broadfield ZJ, Cheung KL, et al: Amplication of AML1 in acute lymphoblastic leukemia is associated with a poor outcome. *Leukemia* 17:2249, 2003.

100. Pui CH, Schrappe M, Masera G, et al: Ponte di Legno Working Group: Statement on the right of children with leukemia to have full access to essential treatment and report on the Sixth International Childhood Acute Lymphoblastic Leukemia Workshop. *Leukemia* 18:1043, 2004.

101. Morely AA, Brisco MJ, Rice M, et al: Leukaemia presenting as marrow hypoplasia: Molecular detection of the leukaemic clone at the time of initial presentation. *Br J Haematol* 98:940, 1997.

102. Masson E, Synold TW, Relling MV, et al: Allopurinol inhibits de novo purine synthesis in lymphoblasts of children with acute lymphoblastic leukemia. *Leukemia* 10:56, 1996.

103. Keuzenkamp-Jansen CW, De Abrue RA, Bökkerink JPM, et al: Metabolism of intravenously administered high-dose 6-mercaptopurine with and without allopurinol treatment in patients with non-Hodgkin lymphoma. *J Pediatr Hematol Oncol* 18:145, 1996.

104. Pui C-H, Mahmoud HH, Wiley JM, et al: Recombinant urate oxidase for the prophylaxis or treatment of hyperuricaemia in patients with leukaemia or lymphoma. *J Clin Oncol* 19:697, 2001.

105. Goldman SC, Holcenberg JS, Finklestein JZ, et al: A randomised comparison between rasburicase and allopurinol in children with lymphoma or leukaemia at high risk for tumor lysis. *Blood* 97:2998, 2001.

106. Nelson SC, Bruggers CS, Kurtzberg J, Friedman HS: Management of leukemic hyperleukocytosis with hydration, urinary alkalinization, allopurinol. Are cranial irradiation and invasive cytoreduction necessary? *Am J Pediatr Hematol Oncol* 15:351, 1993.

107. Basade M, Dhar AK, Kulkarni SS, et al: Rapid cytoreduction in childhood leukemic hyperleukocytosis by conservative therapy. *Med Pediatr Oncol* 25:204, 1995.

108. Patte C, Philip T, Rodary C, et al: High survival rate in advanced-stage B-cell lymphomas and leukemias without CNS involvement with a short intensive polychemotherapy: Results from the French Pediatric Oncology Society of a randomized trial of 216 children. *J Clin Oncol* 9:123, 1991.

109. Pui CH, Boyett JM, Hughes WT, et al: Human granulocyte colony-stimulating factor after induction chemotherapy in children with acute lymphoblastic leukemia. *N Engl J Med* 336:1781, 1997.

110. Larson RA, Dodge RK, Linker CA, et al: A randomized controlled trial of filgrastim during remission induction and consolidation chemotherapy for adults with acute lymphoblastic leukemia: CALGB study 9111. *Blood* 92:1556, 1998.

111. Relling MV, Boyett JM, Blanco JG, et al: Granulocyte-colony stimulating factor and the risk of secondary myeloid malignancy. *Blood* 101: 3862, 2003.

112. Hughes WT, Rivera GK, Schell MJ, et al: Successful intermittent chemoprophylaxis for *Pneumocystis carinii* pneumonitis. *N Engl J Med* 316:1627, 1987.

113. Weinthal J, Frost JD, Briones G, Cairo MS: Successful *Pneumocystis carinii* pneumonia prophylaxis using aerosolized pentamidine in children with acute leukemia. *J Clin Oncol* 12:136, 1994.

114. Pui CH, Hughes WT, Evans WE, Crist WM: Prevention of *Pneumocystis carinii* pneumonia in children with cancer. *J Clin Oncol* 12:1522, 1994.

115. Hughes W, Leoung G, Kramer F, et al: Comparison of atovaquone (566C80) with trimethoprim-sulfamethoxazole to treat *Pneumocystis carinii* pneumonia in patients with AIDS. *N Engl J Med* 328:1521, 1993.

116. Pui CH, Jackson CW, Chesney C, et al: Sequential changes in platelet function and coagulation in leukemic children treated with L-asparaginase, prednisone, vincristine. *J Clin Oncol* 1:380, 1983.

117. Mitchell L, Hoogendoorn H, Giles AR, et al: Increased endogenous thrombin generation in children with acute lymphoblastic leukemia: Risk of thrombotic complications in asparaginase-induced antithrombin III deficiency. *Blood* 83:386, 1994.

118. Heckman KD, Weiner GJ, Davis CS, et al: Randomized study of prophylactic platelet transfusion threshold during induction therapy for adult acute leukemia: 10,000/μL versus 20,000/μL. *J Clin Oncol* 15: 1143, 1997.

119. Patte C, Auperin A, Michon J, et al: The Société Francaise d=Oncologie Pédiatrique LMB89 protocol: Highly effective multiagent chemotherapy tailored to the tumor burden and initial response in 561 unselected children with B-cell lymphomas and L3 leukemia. *Blood* 97:3370, 2001.

120. Reiter A, Schrappe M, Tiemann M, et al: Improved treatment results in childhood B-cell neoplasms with tailored intensification of therapy: A report of the Berlin-Frankfurt-Münster group trial NHL-BFM90. *Blood* 94:3294, 1999.

121. Bowman W, Shuster JJ, Cook B, et al: Improved survival for children with B-cell acute lymphoblastic leukemia and stage IV small non-cleaved-cell lymphoma: A pediatric oncology group study. *J Clin Oncol* 14:1252, 1996.

122. Hoelzer D, Ludwig WD, Thiel E, et al: Improved outcome in adult B-cell acute lymphoblastic leukemia. *Blood* 87:495, 1996.

123. Soussain C, Patte C, Ostronoff M, et al: Small noncleaved cell lymphoma and leukemia in adults: A retrospective study of 65 adults treated with the LMB pediatric protocols. *Blood* 85:664, 1995.

124. Thomas DA, Cortes J, O'Brien S, et al: Hyper-CVAD program in Burkitt's-type adult acute lymphoblastic leukemia. *J Clin Oncol* 17:2461, 1999.

125. Coiffier B, Lepage E, Briere J, et al: CHOP chemotherapy plus rituximab compared with CHOP alone in elderly patients with diffuse large-B-cell lymphoma. *N Engl J Med* 346:235, 2002.

126. Hoelzer D, Gökbuget N, Ottmann O, et al: Acute lymphoblastic leukemia, in *Hematology 2002 American Society of Hematology Education Program Book*, p 162. 2002.

127. Kebriaei P, Larson RA: Progress and challenges in the therapy of adult acute lymphoblastic leukemia. *Curr Opin Hematol* 10:284, 2003.

128. Pui CH, Campana D: New definition of remission in childhood acute lymphoblastic leukemia. *Leukemia* 14:783, 2000.

129. Szczepański T, Orfão A, van der Velden VHJ, et al: Minimal residual disease in leukaemia patients. *Lancet Oncol* 2:409, 2001.

130. Vidriales MB, Pérez JJ, López-Berges MC, et al: Minimal residual dis-

131. Campana D: Determination of minimal residual disease in leukaemia patients. *Br J Haematol* 121:823, 2003.

132. Gaynon PS, Trigg ME, Heerema NA, et al: Children's Cancer Group trials in childhood acute lymphoblastic leukemia: 1983–1995. *Leukemia* 14:2223, 2000.

133. Harms DO, Janka-Schaub GE: Co-operative study group for childhood acute lymphoblastic leukemia (COALL): Long-term follow-up trials 82, 85, 89 and 92. *Leukemia* 14:2234, 2000.

134. Liang DC, Hung IJ, Yang CP, et al: Unexpected mortality from the use of *E. coli* L-asparaginase during remission induction therapy for childhood acute lymphoblastic leukemia: A report from the Taiwan Pediatric Oncology Group. *Leukemia* 13:155, 1999.

135. Hurwitz CA, Silverman LB, Schorin MA, et al: Substituting dexamethasone for prednisone complicates remission induction in children with acute lymphoblastic leukemia. *Cancer* 88:1964, 2000.

136. Annino L, Vegna ML, Camera A, et al: Treatment of adult acute lymphoblastic leukemia (ALL): Long-term follow-up of the GIMEMA ALL 0288 randomized study. *Blood* 99:863, 2002.

137. Hallböök H, Simonsson B, Ahlgren T, et al: High-dose cytarabine in upfront therapy for adult patients with acute lymphoblastic leukaemia. *Br J Haematol* 118:748, 2002.

138. Takeuchi J, Kyo T, Naito K, et al: Induction therapy by frequent administration of doxorubicin with four other drugs, followed by intensive consolidation and maintenance therapy for adult acute lymphoblastic leukemia: The JALSG-ALL93 study. *Leukemia* 16:1259, 2002.

139. Balis FM, Lester CM, Chrousos GP, et al: Differences in cerebrospinal fluid penetration of corticosteroids: Possible relationship to the prevention of meningeal leukemia. *J Clin Oncol* 5:202, 1987.

140. Bostrom BC, Sensel MR, Sather HN, et al. Dexamethasone versus prednisone and daily oral versus weekly intravenous mercaptopurine for patients with standard-risk acute lymphoblastic leukemia: A report from the Children's Cancer Group. *Blood* 101:3809, 2003.

141. Asselin BL, Whitin JC, Coppola DJ, et al: Comparative pharmacokinetic studies of three asparaginase preparations. *J Clin Oncol* 11:1780, 1993.

142. Duval M, Suciu S, Ferster A, et al: Comparison of *Escherichia coli*-asparaginase with *Erwinia*-asparaginase in the treatment of childhood lymphoid malignancies: Results of a randomized European Organisation for Research and Treatment of Cancer—Children's Leukemia Group phase 3 trial. *Blood* 99:2734, 2002.

143. Vieira Pinheiro JP, Boos J: The best way to use asparaginase in childhood acute lymphoblastic leukaemia—Still to be defined? *Br J Haematol* 125:177, 2004.

144. Ahlke E, Nowak-Göttl U, Schulze-Westhoff P, et al: Dose reduction of asparaginase under pharmacokinetic and pharmacodynamic control during induction therapy in children with acute lymphoblastic leukaemia. *Br J Haematol* 96:675, 1997.

145. Hak LJ, Relling MV, Cheng C, et al: Asparaginase pharmacodynamics differ by formulation among children with newly diagnosed acute lymphoblastic leukemia. *Leukemia* 18:1072, 2004.

146. Cuttner J, Mick R, Budman DR, et al: Phase III trial of brief intensive treatment of adult acute lymphocytic leukemia comparing daunorubicin and mitoxantrone: A CALGB study. *Leukemia* 5:425, 1991.

147. Fiére D, Lepage E, Sebban C, et al: Adult acute lymphoblastic leukemia: A multicentric randomized trial testing bone marrow transplantation as postremission therapy. *J Clin Oncol* 11:1990, 1993.

148. Schrappe M, Reiter A, Ludwig WD, et al: Improved outcome in childhood acute lymphoblastic leukemia despite reduced use of anthracyclines and cranial radiotherapy: Results of trial ALL-BFM 90. *Blood* 95:3310, 2000.

149. Evans WE, Relling MV, Rodman JH, et al: Conventional compared with

individualized chemotherapy for childhood acute lymphoblastic leuke-mia. *N Engl J Med* 338:499, 1998.

150. Nachman JB, Sather HN, Sensel MG, et al: Augmented post-induction therapy for children with high-risk acute lymphoblastic leukemia and a slow response to initial therapy. *N Engl J Med* 338:1663, 1998.

151. Silverman LB, Gelber RD, Dalton VK, et al: Improved outcome for children with acute lymphoblastic leukemia: Results of Dana-Farber Consortium Protocol 91-01. *Blood* 97:1211, 2001.

152. Chessells JM, Bailey C, Richards SM: Intensification of treatment and survival in all children with lymphoblastic leukaemia: Results of UK Medical Research Council Trial UKALL X. *Lancet* 345:143, 1995.

153. Pui CH, Sallan S, Relling MV, et al: International Childhood Acute Lymphoblastic Leukemia Workshop: Sausalito, CA, 30 November–1 December 2000. *Leukemia* 15:707, 2001.

154. Galpin AJ, Schuetz JD, Masson E, et al: Differences in folylpolygluta-mate synthetase and dihydrofolate reductase expression in human B-lineage versus T-lineage leukemic lymphoblast: Mechanisms for lineage differences in methotrexate polyglutamylation and cytotoxicity. *Mol Pharm* 52:155, 1997.

155. Kager L, Cheok M, Yang W, et al: Folate pathway gene expression differs in subtypes of acute lymphoblastic leukemia and influences meth-otrexate pharmacodynamics. *J Clin Invest* 115:110, 2005.

156. Ellison RR, Mick R, Cuttner J, et al: The effects of postinduction inten-sification treatment with cytarabine and daunorubicin in adult acute lym-phocytic leukemia: A prospective randomized clinical trial by Cancer and Leukemia Group B. *J Clin Oncol* 9:2002, 1991.

157. Cassileth PA, Anderson JW, Bennett JM, et al: Adult acute lymphocytic leukemia: The Eastern Cooperative Oncology Group experience. *Leu-kemia* 6(suppl 2):178, 1992.

158. Stryckmans P, DeWitte TH, Marie JP, et al: Therapy of adult ALL: Overview of 2 successive EORTC studies: (ALL-2 & ALL-3). *Leukemia* 6(suppl 2):199, 1992.

159. Hoelzer D, Gökbuget N: New approaches in acute lymphoblastic leu-kemia in adults: Where do we go? *Semin Oncol* 27:540, 2000.

160. Durrant JJ, Prentice HG, Richards SM: Intensification of treatment for adults with acute lymphoblastic leukaemia: Results of U.K. Medical Re-search Council randomized trial UKALL XA. *Br J Haematol* 99:84, 1997.

161. Kantarjian HM, Thomas D, O'Brien S, et al: Long-term follow-up re-sults of hyperfractionated cyclophosphamide, vincristine, doxorubicin, and dexamethasone (Hyper-CVAD), or dose-intensive regimen, in adult acute lymphocytic leukemia. *Cancer* 101:2788, 2004.

162. Ludwig WD, Rieder H, Bartram CR, et al: Immunophenotypic and geno-typic features, clinical characteristics, and treatment outcome of adult pro-B acute lymphoblastic leukemia: Results of the German multicenter trials GMALL 03/87 and 04/89. *Blood* 92:1898, 1998.

163. Lee S, Kim DW, Kim YJ, et al: Minimal residual disease-based role of imatinib as a first-line interim therapy prior to allogeneic stem cell trans-plantation in Philadelphia chromosome-positive acute lymphoblastic leukemia. *Blood* 102:3068, 2003.

164. Thomas DA, Faderl S, Cortes J, et al: Treatment of Philadelphia chro-mosome-positive acute lymphoblastic leukemia with hyper-CVAD and imatinib mesylate. *Blood* 103:4396, 2004.

165. Riehm H, Gadner H, Henze G, et al: Results and significance of six randomized trials in four consecutive ALL-BFM studies. *Haematol Blood Transfus* 33:439, 1990.

166. Toyoda Y, Manabe A, Tsuchida M, et al: Six months of maintenance chemotherapy after intensified treatment for acute lymphoblastic leu-kemia of childhood. *J Clin Oncol* 18:1508, 2000.

167. Childhood ALL Collaborative Group: Duration and intensity of main-tenance chemotherapy in acute lymphoblastic leukaemia: Overview of 42 trials involving 12,000 randomised children. *Lancet* 347:1783, 1996.

168. Sather H, Miller D, Nesbit M, et al: Differences in prognosis for boys and girls with acute lymphoblastic leukaemia. *Lancet* i:741, 1981.

169. The Medical Research Council's Working Party on Leukaemia in Child-hood: Duration of chemotherapy-in-childhood acute lymphoblastic leu-kaemia. *Med Pediatr Oncol* 10:511, 1982.

170. Trigg ME, Sather H, Coccia P, et al: Duration of maintenance therapy for childhood acute lymphoblastic leukemia. *Proc ASCO* 12:324a, 1993.

171. Lennard L, Lilleyman JS, Loon JV, Weinshilboum RM: Genetic vari-ation in response to 6-mercaptopurine for childhood acute lymphoblastic leukaemia. *Lancet* 336:225, 1990.

172. Whitehead VM, Vuchich MJ, Lauer SJ, et al: Accumulation of high levels of methotrexate polyglutamates in lymphoblasts from children with hyperdiploid (>50 chromosomes) B-lineage acute lymphoblastic leukemia: A Pediatric Oncology Group Study. *Blood* 80:1316, 1992.

173. Schmiegelow K, Schràder H, Gustafsson G, et al: Risk of relapse in childhood acute lymphoblastic leukemia is related to RBC methotrexate and mercaptopurine metabolites during maintenance chemotherapy. *J Clin Oncol* 13:345, 1995.

174. Chessells JM, Harrison G, Lilleyman JS, et al: Continuing (maintenance) therapy in lymphoblastic leukaemia: Lessons from MRC UKALL X. *Br J Haematol* 98:945, 1997.

175. Relling MV, Hancock ML, Boyett JM, et al: Prognostic importance of 6-mercaptopurine dose intensity in acute lymphoblastic leukemia. *Blood* 93:2817, 1999.

176. Schmiegelow K, Glomstein A, Kristinsson J, et al: Impact of morning versus evening schedule for oral methotrexate and 6-mercaptopurine on relapse risk for children with acute lymphoblastic leukemia. *J Pediatr Hematol Oncol* 19:102, 1997.

177. Rivard GE, Lin KT, Leclerc JM, David M: Milk could decrease the bioavailability of 6-mercaptopurine. *Am J Pediatr Hematol Oncol* 11: 402, 1989.

178. Lancaster D, Lennard L, Lilleyman JS: Profile of non-compliance in lymphoblastic leukaemia. *Arch Dis Child* 76:365, 1997.

179. Mahoney DH, Shuster J, Nitschke R, et al: Intermediate-dose intrave-nous methotrexate with intravenous mercaptopurine is superior to re-petitive low-dose oral methotrexate with intravenous mercaptopurine for children with lower risk B-lineage acute lymphoblastic leukemia: A Pe-diatric Oncology Group Phase III trial. *J Clin Oncol* 16:246, 1998.

180. Vilmer E, Suciu S, Ferster A, et al: Long-term results of three random-ized trials (58831, 58832, 58881) in childhood acute lymphoblastic leu-kemia: A CLCG-EORTC report. *Leukemia* 14:2257, 2000.

181. Kamps WA, Bökkerink JPM, Hakvoort-Cammel FGAJ, et al: BFM-oriented treatment for children with acute lymphoblastic leukemia with-out cranial irradiation and treatment reduction for standard risk patients: Results of DCLSG protocol ALL-8 (1991-1996). *Leukemia* 16:1099, 2002.

182. Farrow AC, Buchanan GR, Zwiener RJ, et al: Serum aminotransferase elevation during and following treatment of childhood acute lympho-blastic leukemia. *J Clin Oncol* 15:1560, 1997.

183. Evans WE, Horner M, Chu YQ, et al: Altered mercaptopurine metab-olism, toxic effects, and dosage requirement in a thiopurine methyltrans-ferase-deficient child with acute lymphocytic leukemia. *J Pediatr* 119: 985, 1991.

184. Relling MV, Hancock ML, Rivera GK, et al: Mercaptopurine therapy intolerance and heterozygosity at the thiopurine S-methyltransferase gene locus. *J Natl Cancer Inst* 91:2001, 1999.

185. Pui CH, Relling MV: Topoisomerase II inhibitor-related acute myeloid leukaemia. *Br J Haematol* 109:13, 2000.

186. Relling MV, Rubnitz JE, Rivera GK, et al: High incidence of secondary brain tumors after radiotherapy and antimetabolites. *Lancet* 354:34, 1999.

187. Yates CR, Krynetski EY, Loennechen T, et al: Molecular diagnosis of thiopurine S-methyltransferase deficiency: Genetic basis for azathio-prine and mercaptopurine intolerance. *Ann Intern Med* 126:608, 1997.

188. Relling MV, Dervieux T: Pharmacogenetics and cancer therapy. *Nat Rev Cancer* 1:99, 2001.

189. Evans WE, Relling MV: Moving towards individualized medicine with pharmacogenomics. *Nature* 429:464, 2004.

190. Lange BJ, Bostrom BC, Cherlow JM, et al: Double-delayed intensification improves event-free survival for children with intermediate-risk acute lymphoblastic leukemia: A report from the Children's Cancer Group. *Blood* 99:825, 2002.

191. Conter V, Aricò M, Valsecchi MG, et al: Extended intrathecal methotrexate may replace cranial irradiation for prevention of CNS relapse in children with intermediate-risk acute lymphoblastic leukemia treated with Berlin-Frankfurt-Münster-based intensive chemotherapy. *J Clin Oncol* 13:2497, 1995.

192. Pui CH, Sandlund JT, Pei D, et al: Improved outcome for children with acute lymphoblastic leukemia: Results of Total Therapy Study XIIB at St. Jude Children's Research Hospital. *Blood* 104:2690, 2004.

193. Conter V, Schrappe M, Aricò M, et al: Role of cranial radiotherapy for childhood T-cell acute lymphoblastic leukemia with high WBC count and good response to prednisone. *J Clin Oncol* 15:2786, 1997.

194. Hunault M, Harousseau JL, Delain M, et al: Better outcome of adult acute lymphoblastic leukemia after early genoidentical allogeneic bone marrow transplantation (BMT) than after late high-dose therapy and autologous BMT: a GOELAMS trial. *Blood* 104:3028, 2004.

195. Thomas X, Boiron JM, Huguet F, et al: Outcome of treatment in adults with acute lymphoblastic leukemia: Analysis of the LALA-94 trial. *J Clin Oncol* 22:4075, 2004.

196. Kiehl M, Kraut L, Schwerdtfeger R, et al: Outcome of allogeneic hematopoietic stem-cell transplantation in adult patients with acute lymphoblastic leukemia: no difference in related compared with unrelated transplant in first complete remission. *J Clin Oncol* 22:2816, 2004.

197. Chessells JM, Bailey C, Wheeler K, Richards SM: Bone marrow transplantation for high-risk childhood lymphoblastic leukaemia in first remission: Experience in MRC UKALL X. *Lancet* 340:565, 1992.

198. Marks DI, Bird JM, Cornish JM, et al: Unrelated donor bone marrow transplantation for children and adolescents with Philadelphia-positive acute lymphoblastic leukemia. *J Clin Oncol* 16:931, 1998.

199. Aricò M, Valsecchi MG, Camitta B, et al: Outcome of treatment in children with Philadelphia chromosome-positive acute lymphoblastic leukemia. *N Engl J Med* 342:998, 2000.

200. Pui CH, Gaynon PS, Boyett JM, et al: Outcome of treatment in childhood acute lymphoblastic leukaemia with rearrangements of the 11q23 chromosomal region. *Lancet* 359:1909, 2002.

201. Vora A, Frost L, Goodeve A, et al: Late relapsing childhood lymphoblastic leukaemia. *Blood* 92:2334, 1998.

202. Konrad M, Metzler M, Panzer S, et al: Late relapse evolve from slow-responding subclones in t(12;21)-positive acute lymphoblastic leukemia: Evidence for the persistence of a preleukemic clone. *Blood* 101:3635, 2003.

203. Pui CH, Sandlund JT, Pei D, et al: Results of therapy for acute lymphoblastic leukemia in black and white children. *JAMA* 290:2001, 2003.

204. Bunin NJ, Pui CH, Hustu HO, Rivera GK: Unusual extramedullary relapses in children with acute lymphoblastic leukemia. *J Pediatr* 109:665, 1986.

205. Rivera GK, Zhou Y, Hancock ML, et al: Bone marrow recurrence after initial intensive treatment for childhood acute lymphoblastic leukemia. *Cancer* 103:368, 2005.

206. Beyermann B, Adams HP, Henze G: Philadelphia chromosome in relapsed childhood acute lymphoblastic leukemia: A matched-pair analysis. *J Clin Oncol* 15:2231, 1997.

207. Gaynon PS, Qu RP, Chappell RJ, et al: Survival after relapse in childhood acute lymphoblastic leukemia. Impact of site and time to first relapse— The Children's Cancer Group experience. *Cancer* 82:1387, 1998.

208. Guglielmi C, Cordone I, Boecklin F, et al: Immunophenotype of adult and childhood acute lymphoblastic leukemia: Changes at first relapse and clinico-prognostic implications. *Leukemia* 11:1501, 1997.

209. Chessells JM, Veys P, Kempski H, et al: Long-term follow-up of relapsed childhood acute lymphoblastic leukaemia. *Br J Haematol* 123:396, 2003.

210. Sadowitz PD, Smith SD, Shuster J, et al: Treatment of late bone marrow relapse in children with acute lymphoblastic leukemia: A Pediatric Oncology Group study. *Blood* 81:602, 1993.

211. Barrett AJ, Horowitz MM, Pollock BH, et al: Bone marrow transplants form HLA-identical siblings as compared with chemotherapy for children with acute lymphoblastic leukemia in a second remission. *N Engl J Med* 331:1253, 1994.

212. Martino R, Bellido M, Brunet S, et al: Allogeneic or autologous stem cell transplantation following salvage chemotherapy for adults with refractory or relapsed acute lymphoblastic leukemia. *Bone Marrow Transplant* 21:1023, 1998.

213. Boulad F, Steinherz P, Reyes B, et al: Allogeneic bone marrow transplantation versus chemotherapy for the treatment of childhood acute lymphoblastic leukemia in second remission: A single-institution study. *J Clin Oncol* 17:197, 1999.

214. Zecca M, Pession A, Messina C, et al: Total body irradiation, thiotepa, and cyclophosphamide as a conditioning regimen for children with acute lymphoblastic leukemia in first or second remission undergoing bone marrow transplantation with HLA-identical siblings. *J Clin Oncol* 17:1838, 1999.

215. Schroeder H, Gustafsson G, Saarinen-Pihkala UM, et al: Allogeneic bone marrow transplantation in second remission of childhood acute lymphoblastic leukemia: A population-based case control study from the Nordic countries. *Bone Marrow Transplant* 23:555, 1999.

216. Borgmann A, Schmid H, Hartmann R, et al: Autologous bone-marrow transplants compared with chemotherapy for children with acute lymphoblastic leukaemia in a second remission: A matched-pair analysis. *Lancet* 346:873, 1995.

217. Weisdorf DJ, Billett AL, Hannan P, et al: Autologous versus unrelated donor allogeneic marrow transplantation for acute lymphoblastic leukemia. *Blood* 90:2962, 1997.

218. Laughlin MJ, Eapen M, Rubinstein P, et al: Outcomes after transplantation of cord blood or bone marrow from unrelated donors in adults with leukemia. *N Engl J Med* 351:2265, 2004.

219. Rocha V, Labopin M, Sanz G, et al: Transplants of umbilical-cord blood or bone marrow from unrelated donors in adults with acute leukemia. *N Engl J Med* 351:2276, 2004.

220. Borgmann A, von Stackelberg A, Hartmann R, et al: Unrelated donor stem cell transplantation compared with chemotherapy for children with acute lymphoblastic leukemia in a second remission: A matched-pair analysis. *Blood* 101:3835, 2003.

221. Rocha V, Cornish J, Sievers EL, et al: Comparison of outcomes of unrelated bone marrow and umbilical cord blood transplants in children with acute leukemia. *Blood* 97:2962, 2001.

222. Grewal SS, Barker JN, Davies SM, Wagner JE: Unrelated donor hematopoietic cell transplantation: Marrow or umbilical cord blood? *Blood* 101:4233, 2003.

223. Aversa F, Tabilio A, Veldardi A, et al: Treatment of high-risk acute leukemia with T-cell depleted stem cells from related donors with one fully mismatched HLA haplotype. *N Engl J Med* 339:1186, 1998.

224. Leung W, Iyengar R, Turner V, et al: Determinants of antileukemia effects of allogeneic NK cells. *J Immunol* 172:644, 2004.

225. Bosi A, Laszlo D, Labopin M, et al: Second allogeneic bone marrow transplantation in acute leukemia: Results of a survey by the European Cooperative Group for Blood and Marrow Transplantation. *J Clin Oncol* 19:3675, 2001.

226. Bührer C, Hartmann R, Fengler R, et al: Importance of effective central nervous system therapy in isolated bone marrow relapse of childhood acute lymphoblastic leukemia. *Blood* 83:3468, 1994.

227. Neale GAM, Pui CH, Mahmoud HH, et al: Molecular evidence for minimal residual bone marrow disease in children with "isolated" extramedullary relapse of T-cell acute lymphoblastic leukemia. *Leukemia* 8: 768, 1994.

228. Lal A, Kwan E, Al Mahr M, et al: Molecular detection of acute lymphoblastic leukaemia in boys with testicular relapse. *J Clin Pathol Mol Pathol* 51:277, 1998.

229. Ribeiro RC, Rivera GK, Hudson M, et al: An intensive re-treatment protocol for children with an isolated CNS relapse of acute lymphoblastic leukemia. *J Clin Oncol* 13:333, 1995.

230. Ritchey AK, Pollock BH, Lauer SJ, et al: Improved survival of children with isolated CNS relapse of acute lymphoblastic leukemia: A Pediatric Oncology Group study. *J Clin Oncol* 17:3745, 1999.

231. Messina C, Valsecchi MG, Aricò M, et al: Autologous bone marrow transplantation for treatment of isolated central nervous system relapse of childhood acute lymphoblastic leukemia. *Bone Marrow Transplant* 21:9, 1998.

232. Buchanan GR, Boyett JM, Pollock BH, et al: Improved treatment results in boys with overt testicular relapse during or shortly after initial therapy for acute lymphoblastic leukemia: A Pediatric Oncology Group study. *Cancer* 68:48, 1991.

233. Wofford MM, Smith SD, Shuster JJ, et al: Treatment of occult or late overt testicular relapse in children with acute lymphoblastic leukemia: A Pediatric Oncology Group study. *J Clin Oncol* 10:624, 1992.

234. Finklestein JZ, Miller DR, Feusner J, et al: Treatment of overt isolated testicular relapse in children on therapy for acute lymphoblastic leukemia. A report from the Children's Cancer Group. *Cancer* 73:219, 1994.

235. Grundy RG, Leiper AD, Stanhope R, Chessells JM: Survival and endocrine outcome after testicular relapse in acute lymphoblastic leukaemia. *Arch Dis Child* 76:190, 1997.

236. Van den Berg H, Langeveld NE, Veenhof CHN, Behrendt H: Treatment of isolated testicular recurrence of acute lymphoblastic leukemia without radiotherapy. Report from the Dutch Late Effects Study Group. *Cancer* 79:2257, 1997.

237. Pui CH, Burghen GA, Bowman WP, Aur RJA: Risk factors for hyperglycemia in children with leukemia receiving L-asparaginase and prednisone. *J Pediatr* 99:46, 1981.

238. Pui CH, Chesney CM, Weed J, Jackson CW: Altered von Willebrand factor molecule in children with thrombosis following asparaginase-prednisone-vincristine therapy for leukemia. *J Clin Oncol* 3:1266, 1985.

239. Pihko H, Tyni T, Virkola K, et al: Transient ischemic cerebral lesions during induction chemotherapy for acute lymphoblastic leukemia. *J Pediatr* 123:718, 1993.

240. Winick NJ, Bowman WP, Kamen BA, et al: Unexpected acute neurologic toxicity in the treatment of children with acute lymphoblastic leukemia. *J Natl Cancer Inst* 84:252, 1992.

241. Mahoney DH, Shuster JJ, Nitschke R, et al: Acute neurotoxicity in children with B-precursor acute lymphoid leukemia: An association with intermediate-dose intravenous methotrexate and intrathecal triple therapy—A Pediatric Oncology Group study. *J Clin Oncol* 16:1712, 1998.

242. Rubnitz JE, Relling MV, Harrison PL, et al: Transient encephalopathy following high-dose methotrexate treatment in childhood acute lymphoblastic leukemia. *Leukemia* 12:1176, 1998.

243. Mattano LA, Sather HN, Trigg ME, Nachman JB: Osteonecrosis as a complication of treating acute lymphoblastic leukemia in children: A report from the Children's Cancer Group. *J Clin Oncol* 18:3262, 2000.

244. Strauss AJ, Su JT, Dalton VM, et al: Bony morbidity in children treated for acute lymphoblastic leukemia. *J Clin Oncol* 19:3066, 2001.

245. Ribeiro RC, Fletcher BD, Kennedy W, et al: Magnetic resonance imaging detection of avascular necrosis of the bone in children receiving intensive prednisone therapy for acute lymphoblastic leukemia or non-Hodgkin lymphoma. *Leukemia* 15:891, 2001.

246. Kaste SC, Jones-Wallace D, Rose SR, et al: Bone mineral decrements in survivors of childhood acute lymphoblastic leukemia: Frequency of occurrence and risk factors for their development. *Leukemia* 15:728, 2001.

247. Mandel K, Atkinson S, Barr RD, Pencharz P: Skeletal morbidity in childhood acute lymphoblastic leukemia. *J Clin Oncol* 22:1215, 2004.

248. Lipshultz SE, Lipsitz SR, Mone SM, et al: Female sex and higher drug dose as risk factors for late cardiotoxic effects of doxorubicin therapy for childhood cancer. *N Engl J Med* 332:1738, 1995.

249. Grenier MA, Lipshultz SE: Epidemiology of anthracycline cardiotoxicity in children and adults. *Semin Oncol* 25:72, 1998.

250. Levitt GA, Dorup I, Sorensen K, Sullivan I: Does anthracycline administration by infusion in children affect late cardiotoxicity? *Br J Haematol* 124:463, 2004.

251. Nysom K, Holm K, Lipsitz SR, et al: Relationship between cumulative anthracycline dose and late cardiotoxicity in childhood acute lymphoblastic leukemia. *J Clin Oncol* 16:545, 1998.

252. Lipshultz SE, Rifai N, Dalton VM, et al: The effect of dexrazoxane on myocardial injury in doxorubicin-treated children with acute lymphoblastic leukemia. *N Engl J Med* 351:145, 2004.

253. Pui CH, Cheng C, Leung W, et al: Extended follow-up of long-term survivors of childhood acute lymphoblastic leukemia. *N Engl J Med* 349: 640, 2003.

254. Leung W, Rose SR, Zhou Y, et al: Outcomes of growth hormone replacement therapy in survivors of childhood acute lymphoblastic leukemia. *J Clin Oncol* 20:2959, 2002.

255. Sklar CA, Mertens AC, Mitby P, et al: Risk of disease recurrence and second neoplasms in survivors of childhood cancer treated with growth hormone: A report from the Childhood Cancer Survivor Study. *J Clin Endocrinol Metab* 87:3136, 2002.

256. Walter AW, Hancock ML, Pui CH, et al: Secondary brain tumors in children treated for acute lymphoblastic leukemia at St. Jude Children's Research Hospital. *J Clin Oncol* 16:3761, 1998.

257. Pui CH, Ribeiro RC, Hancock ML, et al: Acute myeloid leukemia in children treated with epipodophyllotoxins for acute lymphoblastic leukemia. *N Engl J Med* 325:1682, 1991.

258. Hawkins MM, Draper GJ, Winter DL: Cancer in the offspring of survivors of childhood leukaemia and non-Hodgkin lymphomas. *Br J Cancer* 71:1335, 1995.

259. Kenney LB, Nicholson HS, Brasseux C, et al: Birth defects in offspring of adult survivors of childhood acute lymphoblastic leukemia. A Children's Cancer Group/National Institutes of Health Report. *Cancer* 78: 169, 1996.

260. Sankila R, Olsen JH, Anderson H, et al: Risk of cancer among offspring of childhood-cancer survivors. *N Engl J Med* 338:1339, 1998.

261. Pui C-H, Crist WM: Biology and treatment of acute lymphoblastic leukemia. *J Pediatr* 124:491, 1994.

262. Smith M, Arthur D, Camitta B, et al: Uniform approach to risk classification and treatment assignment for children with acute lymphoblastic leukemia. *J Clin Oncol* 14:18, 1996.

263. Taylor PRA, Reid MM, Bown N, et al: Acute lymphoblastic leukemia in patients aged 60 years and over: A population-based study of incidence and outcome. *Blood* 80:1813, 1992.

264. Boucheix C, David B, Sebban C, et al: Immunophenotype of adult acute lymphoblastic leukemia, clinical parameters, and outcome: An analysis of a prospective trial including 562 tested patients (LALA87). *Blood* 84: 1603, 1994.

265. Chessells JM, Richards SM, Bailey CC, et al: Gender and treatment outcome in childhood lymphoblastic leukaemia: Report from the MRC UKALL trials. *Br J Haematol* 89:364, 1995.

266. Shuster JJ, Wacker P, Pullen J, et al: Prognostic significance of sex in childhood B-precursor acute lymphoblastic leukemia: A Pediatric Oncology Group Study. *J Clin Oncol* 16:2854, 1998.

267. Pollock BH, DeBaun MR, Camitta BM, et al: Racial differences in the survival of childhood B-precursor acute lymphoblastic leukemia: A Pediatric Oncology Group Study. *J Clin Oncol* 18:813, 2000.

268. Bhatia S, Sather HN, Heerema NA, et al: Racial and ethnic differences in survival of children with acute lymphoblastic leukemia. *Blood* 100:1957, 2002.

269. Kadan-Lottick NS, Ness KK, Bhatia S, Gurney JG: Survival variability by race and ethnicity in childhood acute lymphoblastic leukemia. *JAMA* 290:2008, 2003.

270. Pui C-H, Chessells JM, Camitta B, et al. Clinical heterogeneity in childhood acute lymphoblastic leukemia with 11q23 rearrangements. *Leukemia* 17:700, 2003.

271. Coustan-Smith E, Gajjar A, Hijiya N, et al: Clinical significance of minimal residual disease in childhood acute lymphoblastic leukemia after first relapse. *Leukemia* 18:499, 2004.

272. Coustan-Smith E, Sancho J, Hancock ML, et al: Use of peripheral blood instead of bone marrow to monitor residual disease in children with acute lymphoblastic leukemia. *Blood* 100:2399, 2002.

CHAPTER 92

CHRONIC LYMPHOCYTIC LEUKEMIA AND RELATED DISEASES

THOMAS J. KIPPS

Chronic lymphocytic leukemia (CLL) is a neoplastic disease characterized by the accumulation of small mature-appearing CD5+ B lymphocytes in the blood, marrow, and lymphoid tissues. The causes of this disease are unknown, although genetic factors likely contribute to its development. The leukemic cells from over 50 percent of CLL patients can be found to have clonal chromosomal abnormalities, of which del 13q14-23.1 is the most common chromosomal abnormality in CLL, followed in order by trisomy 12, del 11q22.3-q23.1, del 6q21-q23, and 14q abnormalities. Mutations of the p53 tumor suppressor gene at 17p13.1 are uncommon except in advanced disease. Assessing for clinical stage and various prognostic markers can be useful for deciding when to initiate therapy. Treatment with chlorambucil, with or without prednisone, had been the mainstay of initial treatment, but several studies have confirmed the higher activity of deoxyadenosine analogues such as fludarabine in this disease. New drug combinations, monoclonal antibodies, autologous and allogeneic stem cell transplantation, new agents, and gene therapy are being evaluated because there still are no established cures. This chapter also discusses prolymphocytic leukemia, which can be of B or T cell origin. The latter includes cases that formerly were designated T cell CLL. Although B cell prolymphocytic leukemia can evolve from preexisting cases of CLL, it has many distinctive features including a more adverse clinical outcome. Treatments for B cell prolymphocytic leukemia are similar to those used in CLL, but the response rates are lower and of shorter duration. Similarly, T cell prolymphocytic leukemia is more aggressive than CLL. Rearrangements and mutations in the ataxia-telangiectasia mutated gene and in T cell leukemia-1 and related genes apparently contribute to the pathogenesis of T cell prolymphocytic leuke-mia. Approximately one third of patients have cutaneous involvement causing erythroderma. Treatment with deoxyadenosine analogues appears effective in a subset of patients with this disease. Investigations of new agents, stem cell transplantation, and/or monoclonal antibodies, such as alemtuzumab, are ongoing because no established cures exist for T cell prolymphocytic leukemia.

DEFINITION AND HISTORY

Chronic lymphocytic leukemia (CLL) is a neoplastic disease characterized by the accumulation of small, mature-appearing lymphocytes in the blood, marrow, and lymphoid tissues. CLL has an average incidence of 2.7 persons per 100,000 in the United States and ranges from less than 1 to 5.5 per 100,000 persons worldwide.[1] The risk of developing CLL increases progressively with age and is 2.8 times higher for older men than for older women.[2] Because of its relative indolence, this disease accounts for approximately 0.8 percent of all cancers and nearly 30 percent of all leukemias at any point in time. It is the most common adult leukemia in western societies. Generally, the neoplastic lymphocytes are of the B cell lineage. In less than 2 percent of cases, however, the neoplastic cells are of T cell origin and are considered under the heading T cell prolymphocytic leukemia (PLL).

The first descriptions of patients with CLL were published in the early 10th century.[3–5] In the 1840s, Virchow[5–7] described two forms of chronic leukemia, probably corresponding to CLL and chronic myelogenous leukemia. Patients with the former were noted to have mild-to-moderate splenic enlargement, lymphadenopathy, and large numbers of small agranular cells in the blood that resembled those found in enlarged lymph nodes.[6] Virchow considered this type of leukemia to be principally related to disease of the lymph nodes rather than of the spleen. In 1893, Kundrat[8] introduced the term *lymphosarcoma* to describe an indolent disease that affected lymph nodes. Histochemical staining techniques introduced by Ehrlich[9] at the turn of the century made it possible for pathologists to distinguish between myeloid and lymphocytic leukemias. These methods enabled Türk[10] in 1903 to establish a relationship of the leukemic cells in CLL to those in lymphosarcoma. He proposed the term *lymphomatoses* to describe several lymphoproliferative disorders including CLL. Because of its indolent nature, CLL was considered a "benign" lymphomatosis.

In 1924, Minot and Isaacs[11] described the natural history of 98 patients with CLL, challenging the notion that CLL was a "benign" process. These investigators noted that although γ-radiation could reduce lymph node enlargement or splenomegaly, it apparently did not prolong survival. Radioactive phosphorus later was found effective in reducing lymph node swelling.[12] However, this finding was of limited therapeutic value because of the marrow toxicity of radioactive phosphorus and its inability to reverse disease-related cytopenias or to improve survival.[12] In 1954, Tivey[13] reported the survival data of 685 patients with CLL, observing that the median survival time was approximately 3 years from the onset of symptoms related to CLL. Soon thereafter, alkylating agents,[14] and later glucocorticoids,[15] were found to be effective therapy for CLL. These agents became the mainstays of treatment.

In 1967, Dameshek[16] hypothesized that CLL was an accumulative disease of immunologically incompetent lymphocytes. In the early 1970s, the leukemic cells from most cases of CLL were found to express surface immunoglobulin (Ig), indicating that the neoplastic cells were of B cell origin.[17] Subsequent studies demonstrated that the CLL cells of female patients heterozygous for glucose-6-phosphate dehydrogenase (G-6-PD) expressed only one G-6-PD allele,[18] indicating that the leukemia cells arose from a single B cell clone. Consistent

Acronyms and abbreviations that appear in this chapter include: *ARLTS1*, ADP ribosylation factor-like tumor suppressor gene-1; ATLL, adult T cell leukemia/lymphoma; *ATM* gene, ataxia-telangiectasia mutated gene; BCL, B cell leukemia; cADPR, cyclic ADP ribose; CAP, cyclophosphamide, doxorubicin, prednisone without vincristine; CGH, comparative genomic hybridization; CHOP, cyclophosphamide, doxorubicin, vincristine, prednisone; CLL, chronic lymphocytic leukemia; CTL, cytotoxic T lymphocytes; CVP, cyclophosphamide, vincristine, prednisone; DiSC, differential staining cytotoxicity; EBV, Epstein-Barr virus; FAB, French-American-British; FISH, fluorescence *in situ* hybridization; GM-CSF, granulocyte-macrophage colony stimulating factor; G-6-PD, glucose-6-phosphate dehydrogenase; HCV, hepatitis virus type C; HTLV, human T lymphotropic virus; HTLV-I+, human T lymphotropic virus type I-positive; Ig, immunoglobulin; IgV$_H$, immunoglobulin heavy-chain variable region; MRD, minimal residual disease; PCR, polymerase chain reaction; PLL, prolymphocytic leukemia; *RB* gene, retinoblastoma gene; SDF, stromal cell-derived factor; SMZL, splenic marginal zone B cell lymphoma; TCL, T cell leukemia; TGF, transforming growth factor; TNF, tumor necrosis factor; TRAP, tartrate-resistant isozyme 5 of acid phosphatase; V$_H$ gene, heavy-chain variable-region gene; YAC, yeast artificial chromosome; ZAP-70, zeta-associated protein of 70 kDa.

with this notion, the CLL cells from any one patient were found to express only one type of Ig light chain[19] and idiotype,[20–22] indicating their uniformity in the expression of Ig.

A clinical staging system for patients with CLL introduced by Rai et al.[23] in 1975 delineated the adverse implication of anemia or thrombocytopenia on patient survival. In 1999, patients with leukemia cells that express unmutated Ig variable-region genes were recognized in general to have more aggressive disease than patients whose leukemia cells use mutated antibody genes.[24,25] Nevertheless, gene expression analyses revealed that the leukemia cells of patients with CLL share a common distinctive gene expression profile regardless of Ig mutation status and that only a handful of genes were differentially expressed between these two subtypes.[26,27]

In the late 1980s, purine analogues, such as fludarabine and 2-chlorodeoxyadenosine (cladribine), were found to be effective for treatment of CLL. In the late 1990s, Campath-1H (alemtuzumab) was approved for use in patients with refractory disease. New treatment modalities are being examined, including passive or active immunotherapy or ablative chemotherapy with marrow transplantation, because the disease still is not considered curable.

ETIOLOGY AND PATHOGENESIS

ENVIRONMENTAL FACTORS

No single environmental risk factor has been found to be predictive for CLL. One study noted an increase in CLL in some rural communities, suggesting that an environmental agent(s) associated with farming plays a role.[28] However, other studies found that the incidence of CLL apparently was not associated with exposure to pesticides, sunlight, ionizing radiation, or known carcinogens.[29–34] One study found an increased incidence in CLL among persons exposed to agent orange.[35] Also, a few studies noted an increase in CLL among persons chronically exposed to electromagnetic fields.[36–38] However, whether this association reflects a causal relationship is controversial.

Some studies found a relatively high prevalence of infection with type C hepatitis virus (HCV) in patients with CLL compared with that of the general population,[39,40] suggesting a possible pathogenic role. However, CLL has been found prevalent in certain populations with a negligible incidence of HCV infection,[41] and patients may develop CLL who do not have any trace of exposure to HCV,[42] indicating that infection with HCV is not necessary for development of leukemia. CLL cells are resistant to infection with Epstein-Barr virus (EBV), except in unusual cases,[43] making it unlikely that EBV plays a pathogenic role.

The incidence of CLL in men is twice that in women.[44] One retrospective study of women noted a nonsignificant trend toward reduced risk of this leukemia with increasing parity, prompting speculation that pregnancy lowers the risk for CLL.[45] However, hormones have not been demonstrated to play any role in the development of this disease. Moreover, the use of hormone replacement therapy for postmenopausal symptoms in women apparently does not influence the relative risk for developing CLL.[46]

HEREDITARY FACTORS

Genetic factors apparently contribute to the development of CLL. Although CLL is the most common adult leukemia in western societies, it is relatively rare in Asia. In the United States, the annual incidence of CLL is 3.9 per 100,000 for males and 2.0 per 100,000 for females.[44] However, in Korea, the estimated incidence of this disease is only 1.5 percent of this rate.[47] Similarly, B cell CLL is relatively uncommon in China and is rare in Japan,[48–50] accounting for less than 6 percent of all leukemias in Japan.[51] A very low incidence of B cell CLL is noted even among Japanese immigrants to the United States.[48,52] Likewise, the incidence of CLL in Israel is significantly higher among European immigrants than among those from Africa or Asia.[53]

Although most cases of CLL are sporadic, multiple cases of leukemia may be found within a single family. Families having multiple members with CLL have been reported.[54–60] First-degree relatives of patients with CLL are more than three times at risk for having the disorder or other lymphoid neoplasms than is the general population.[57] Afflicted individuals within such families often present at a younger age than patients with sporadic CLL, suggesting that genetic factors in familial CLL contribute to early leukemogenesis.[61,62]

The genetic factors that contribute to the increased incidence of CLL in certain families are unknown. No association between human leukocyte antigen (HLA) haplotype and disease susceptibility is apparent.[63] One study noted that the leukemic cells of affected family members often expressed Ig heavy-chain variable-region (IgV$_H$) genes of the same IgV$_H$ gene subgroup.[64] However, each patient's leukemia cells have distinctive IgV$_H$ gene rearrangements,[58,64] even those of monozygous twins,[65] indicating they originate from disparate somatic events.

CYTOGENESIS

The leukemic cells of most patients express pan-B cell surface antigens, such as CD19 and CD20 (see Chap. 14), indicating they are derived from the B lymphocyte lineage (see Chap. 76). The level at which the CD20 antigen is expressed, however, is substantially lower than that found on normal circulating B cells.[66,67] CLL B cells also express CD27,[68] a member of the tumor necrosis factor receptor family that also is distinctively expressed on memory B cells.[69]

Studies using gene microarray analyses have provided evidence for the notion that CLL cells are derived from memory-type B cells. Regardless of whether CLL cells use unmutated or mutated Ig genes, they share common expression levels of many genes and have gene expression profiles that are distinct from those of other B cell malignancies, normal nonmalignant adult blood B cells, or even neonatal core blood B cells that coexpress CD5.[26,27] Furthermore, the gene expression patterns observed in CLL appear to be most compatible with that of antigen-experienced, nonnaive B cells typically found within the marginal zone of the spleen.[27] Studies performed in mice made transgenic for the Ig genes that frequently are expressed in CLL suggest that expression of certain Igs may drive differentiation of B cells into cells that can populate the splenic marginal zone.[70] Coupled with the noted restriction in the repertoire of Igs expressed in this disease, mounting evidence implicates the antigen-experienced, memory-type B cell as the normal, nonmalignant counterpart to the CLL B cell.

IMMUNOGLOBULIN EXPRESSION

The leukemic cells from more than 90 percent of patients express low levels of monoclonal surface Ig with either κ or λ light chains. Sixty percent of cases express κ light chains; the other 40 percent express λ light chains.[71–73] Of the heavy-chain isotypes, more than half have surface IgM and IgD (55%), one fourth IgM exclusive of IgD, and approximately 7 percent have Ig isotypes other than IgM or IgD (usually IgG or IgA). Less than 5 percent of cases express IgD without detectable IgM. Both IgM and IgM/IgD expressing CLL frequently express cross-reactive idiotypes (see Chap. 77) that commonly are found on IgM autoantibodies.[74]

The Igs expressed in B cell CLL often have reactivity for self-antigens, most notably for the constant region of human IgG.[75] An important feature of these autoantibodies is their "polyreactivity," or binding activity for two or more seemingly disparate self-antigens. Because of this finding, several investigators have used the term *nat-*

ural autoantibodies to describe these autoantibodies. Such polyreactivity is a characteristic of some antibodies produced by early immature B cells,[76] which subsequently are deleted or experience further Ig gene rearrangements and/or mutation. Despite their apparent lack of specificity, such autoantibodies are dependent upon selected Ig gene rearrangements and selected pairing of Ig heavy and light chains,[77–79] indicating that polyreactivity is a selected binding specificity.

The Ig expressed by CLL B cells may play a role in leukemogenesis.[80–82] For example, an allele of V_H1-69, called *51p1*, is expressed at high frequency and without somatic mutation in CLL (see Chap. 77).[83] Moreover, CLL B cells that express 51p1 have restricted use of certain amino acid sequences within the third complementarity determining region that are not commonly observed in nonmalignant B cells, including normal B cells that use the 51p1 allele of V_H1-69 (see Chap. 77).[84–86] This restriction is not a feature of polyreactive antibodies per se or of antibodies expressed by B cells during fetal development.[78,87] Furthermore, nonrandom pairing appears to occur between certain Ig heavy chains and light chains encoded by particular Ig light-chain variable regions. One striking example of this restriction is the noted pairing between Ig heavy chains encoded by V_H1-69, D3-16, and J_H3 with light chains encoded by one κ light-chain variable-region gene, designated A27. This antibody is expressed by leukemia cells of approximately 1.3 percent of all patients with CLL.[88] As such, there apparently is strong selection in this disease for expression of Igs with a certain binding activity, conceivably for some self-antigen(s) or environmental antigen(s). Because Igs constitute an important receptor governing the proliferation, survival, or death of B cells (see Chap. 76), it is conceivable that the Igs expressed in CLL play a critical role in the early expansion or survival of the nascent leukemia cell clone.

ESSENTIAL MONOCLONAL B CELL LYMPHOCYTOSIS

Studies using sensitive flow cytometry have found populations of B cells with the phenotype of CLL cells in the blood of healthy individuals.[89,90] These cells coexpress CD5 and CD19 with dull coexpression CD20 and CD79b (see Chap. 14). Evaluation of first-degree relatives of CLL patients revealed that 14 percent (8/59) of healthy individuals with two or more affected family members had circulating B cells with these "CLL B cell" characteristics.[89] The detection of such cells in the blood of healthy control subjects was significantly less frequent, suggesting that genetic factors contribute to the relative abundance of these cells in the blood.

Conceivably, an excess of cells with these characteristics could presage development of CLL. Evaluation of the Ig genes used by such B cells from any one subject revealed evidence for oligoclonal (and in some cases monoclonal) gene rearrangements (see Chap. 77), suggesting an apparent excess of B cells belonging to one or a few different clones. Such clonal expansions of B cells were found more frequently in men than in women (with a male-to-female ratio of nearly 2:1) and more common in people ages 60 to 89 years than in younger adults. Because these demographics correspond to the noted predominance of CLL in men and the aged, these clonal B cell expansions are speculated to represent cell populations that potentially could evolve into CLL. The noted frequency of finding such cells in the blood of healthy control subjects appears surprisingly high, with 3.5 percent of tested subjects older than 40 years (n = 910) having detectable blood lymphocytes with such characteristics.[90] At this time, it is uncertain whether persons who have detectable clonal B cell populations are at increased risk for developing CLL. Because the cause and clinical significance of such clonal, blood B cell expansions are unknown, this condition may be termed *essential monoclonal B cell lymphocytosis*. Similar to patients with essential monoclonal gam-

mopathy who have an increased risk for developing plasma cell myeloma (see Chaps. 99 and 100), patients with essential monoclonal B cell lymphocytosis also may have an increased risk for developing CLL than the general population.[91]

ANIMAL MODELS OF CLL

Mice made transgenic for the human T cell leukemia-1 *(TCL1)* gene under the control of a tissue-specific μ Ig enhancer (Eμ-TCL1) develop clonal B cell expansions that are similar to those observed in patients with essential monoclonal B cell lymphocytosis.[92] These animals develop detectable clonal expansions of CD5+ B cell populations in the peritoneum at age 2 months that become evident in the spleen by age 3 to 5 months and then in the marrow by age 5 to 8 months. Elder mice eventually develop a CLL-like disease, with each animal developing a monoclonal outgrowth of B cells that share many features with the leukemia B cells of patients with CLL, including coexpression of CD5, low-level surface Ig, pan-B cell surface antigens, and high-level expression of *TCL1*.[92,93] These cells infiltrate the blood and secondary lymphoid tissues, causing lymphocytosis, splenomegaly, and lymphadenopathy. The pathology of involved lymph nodes appears similar to that of patients with CLL. Similarly, transgenic mice with B cells that overexpress BCL-2 and a mutant tumor necrosis factor (TNF) receptor-associated factor (TRAF2) also appear to develop a lymphoproliferative disease that resembles CLL.[94]

On the other hand, mice made transgenic for *TCL1* using different tissue-specific promoters/enhancers develop other types of lymphoid malignancies.[95,96] As such, overexpression of the *TCL1* gene per se does not cause CLL. Rather, overexpression of *TCL1* by B cells at particular stages of development, combined with other factors, such as stimulation via surface Ig receptors and/or secondary mutations, appears to be required for development of a monoclonal B cell leukemia that resembles CLL.

CYTOGENETIC ABNORMALITIES

Detection of chromosomal abnormalities initially was hampered by the inability to induce leukemic cell proliferation. These cells generally do not grow spontaneously in cell culture and are much more refractory to activation by mitogens or to transformation by EBV than normal B cells.[16,97] As such, the normal karyotypes noted in some samples could reflect an outgrowth of normal bystander lymphocytes.

Using Q-banding and/or G-banding techniques (see Chap. 10) and improved methods for inducing leukemia cell proliferation *in vitro*, the leukemic cells from approximately half of all CLL patients are found to have clonal chromosomal abnormalities.[98–101] Interphase cytogenetics using fluorescence *in situ* hybridization (FISH) has increased the sensitivity for detecting translocations, deletions, or chromosome trisomy.[102–104] Using these techniques, del 13q14-23.1 is the most common chromosomal abnormality in CLL, followed in order by trisomy 12, del 11q22.3-q23.1, del 6q21-q23, deletions at 17p13.1 typically involving deletions/mutations of the *TP53* (also known as p53) tumor suppressor gene,[103,105,106] and 14q abnormalities. Deletions or duplications account for most of the observed genetic defects, as chromosomal translocations are rarely observed in CLL in the absence of *ex vivo* stimulation.[107] New techniques, including use of comparative genomic hybridization (CGH), amplotyping by arbitrarily primed polymerase chain reaction (PCR), or microsatellite allelotyping, can be combined with FISH for detecting additional genetic abnormalities in CLL.[108,109]

CHROMOSOME 13 ANOMALIES

Deletions on the long arm of chromosome 13 are the most common genetic abnormality in CLL, occurring in approximately half of all

CLL cases. These deletions generally occur in the absence of detectable chromosome translocations. Nevertheless, CLL cells with translocations often are noted to have translocations involving the long arm of chromosome 13 with any one of several different chromosomes.[110] Because these translocations generally result in deletions at 13q14, deletions at 13q14 may be the contributing genetic lesion rather than translocation per se.

Deletions in the long arm of chromosome 13 typically occur at 13q14.3 in a region that is telomeric to the retinoblastoma gene *RB1* and centromeric to and including the D13S25 marker.[111–115] Several genes are present in this region, including *DLEU1, DLEU2, RFP2, KCNRG, DLEU6, DLEU7,* and *DLEU8.*[116,117] A highly conserved alternative first exon of the *LEU2* gene, which originates within a G+C region in the vicinity of the D13S272 marker, gives rise to a transcript encoding a new member of the ras superfamily, designated *ARLTS1* (ADP ribosylation factor-like tumor suppressor gene-1).[116] This gene may function like a tumor suppressor gene in CLL and in other types of cancer, such as those involving the colon or breast.[691]

Also found in this region that frequently is deleted in CLL are genes encoding microRNA genes, namely, *miR15* and *miR16.*[118] These miR genes belong to a large family of highly conserved noncoding genes scattered throughout the genome. miRs are transcribed as short hairpin precursors (approximately 70 nt) and are processed into active 21- to 22-nt RNAs by Dicer, a ribonuclease that recognizes target mRNAs via base pairing interactions. These active miRNAs may play an important role in the regulation of temporal and tissue-specific gene expression. Detailed deletion and expression analysis revealed that *miR15* and *miR16* are located within a 30-kb region of loss in CLL, and that both genes are deleted or down-regulated in the majority (approximately 68%) of CLL cases.[118] As such, loss of *miR15* and/or *miR16* may contribute to leukemogenesis and account for the frequent deletions that are observed at 13q14.3 in CLL.

CHROMOSOME 12 ANOMALIES

Ten to thirty percent of all patients have CLL cells with trisomy 12 either as the sole genetic abnormality or in combination with other chromosomal abnormalities.[119–121] It appears that the leukemia cells with trisomy 12 have duplicated one chromosome 12 while retaining the other homologue.[122] As such, this genetic lesion apparently is not recessive, as would be the case for the loss of a tumor suppressor gene, but rather provides for a gene dosage effect. Studies on partial trisomy 12 are consistent with this notion, suggesting that trisomy 12 reflects a gene dosage effect of some genes located between 12q13 and 12q22.[119] For unclear reasons, cases with trisomy 12 more frequently are found to have above-average leukemia cell surface expression of CD25,[123] CD38,[104] and/or CD79b,[124] even though the genes encoding these surface antigens are not located on chromosome 12 (see Chap. 14).

Trisomy 12 may be a secondary event that occurs within an established leukemic clone or preleukemic B cell.[125] Leukemia cells with trisomy 12 often have complex karyotypic abnormalities and atypical and/or prolymphocytic morphology.[104,107,112,119,124,126–128] Furthermore, this abnormality often may be detected in only a subset of the leukemia cells from any one patient.[129,130] Trisomy 12 may not be detectable at diagnosis but is more commonly seen in the leukemia cells of patients with advanced disease or Richter transformation.[98,131–133] Finally, studies suggest that the leukemia cell subset with trisomy 12 may expand during disease progression.[111] Collectively, these studies suggest that trisomy 12 is not a primary factor in leukemogenesis but is acquired during disease evolution.

CHROMOSOME 11 ANOMALIES

Approximately 10 to 20 percent of patients may have leukemia cells with deletions in the long arm of chromosome 11, termed *11q−.*[134–136]

These patients tend to be younger (less than 55 years) and to have more aggressive disease than those without such genetic changes.[135] Furthermore, the leukemia cells of such patients may express lower levels of surface CD11a/CD18, CD11c/CD18, CD31, CD48, and CD58 than CLL cells from patients without 11q−, arguing that such cells may have a distinctive biology.[137]

Deletions on chromosome 11 commonly cluster between 11q14-24, particularly at 11q22.3-q23.1, in a region defined by yeast artificial chromosome (YAC) clones 801e11, 975h6, and 755b11.[134,135] An important gene found within this region is the ataxia-telangiectasia mutated *(ATM)* gene. Upon DNA damage, the normal gene product of *ATM* plays an important role in the activation of the tumor suppressor gene product p53, which induces cell cycle arrest and DNA repair or cell death[138] and is required for leukemia cell sensitivity to many anticancer drugs commonly used for treatment of CLL (e.g., chlorambucil, fludarabine monophosphate). The *ATM* gene often is found lost through deletion or mutation in leukemia cells of patients with relatively aggressive disease that is resistant to many standard therapies.[134,135,139–142] Some CLL patients carry one defective copy of this gene in the germ-line DNA, suggesting that mutations in *ATM* are involved in the pathogenesis of aggressive CLL.[140,143]

CHROMOSOME 6 ANOMALIES

Another recurring chromosome abnormality involves the short arm of chromosome 6, but the altered genes have not been identified.[112] The abnormalities on chromosome 6 typically involve deletions at 6q23, but they also can involve deletions at 6q25-27 and/or 6q21.[144–148] Patients with abnormalities between 6q21 and 6q24 generally have higher proportions of blood prolymphocytes, higher than average expression of CD38, and more aggressive disease than patients with normal cytogenetics or isolated deletions at 13q14.3.[149]

The leukemia cells of several patients have been found to harbor deletions in the long arm of chromosome 6 at 6p24-25, which also have been associated with atypical leukemia cell morphology.[150] However, the frequency of such deletions appears much less than that of deletions in and around 6q23.

CHROMOSOME 17 ANOMALIES

Interphase FISH can detect deletions in the short arm of chromosome 17 at 17p13.1 in approximately 10 percent of all patients.[128] The critical gene in the region that typically is deleted is *TP53.* *TP53* encodes p53, a 53-kDa nuclear phosphoprotein that plays an important role in the induction of proteins responsible for cell cycle arrest and apoptosis of cells damaged by genotoxic stress, such as that affected by ionizing radiation.[151] The leukemia cells harboring deletions at 17p13.1 often have allelic loss of *TP53* and/or single-base inactivating mutations in the highly conserved exon 5, 7, or 8 of the retained *TP53* allele.[152]

Patients who have CLL cells with 17p− and/or *TP53* mutations generally have more advanced disease, a higher leukemia cell proliferative rate, a shorter survival, and greater resistance to first-line therapy.[153–157] Moreover, leukemia cell deletions and/or mutations of *TP53* constitute an independent marker for poor survival.[158] The proportions of leukemia cells that harbor deletions at 17p13.1 in any one patient may increase over time, particularly following treatment with standard therapies.[159] Also, the neoplastic cells from nearly half of the patients with Richter transformation or B cell PLL may have inactivating mutations in *TP53.*[159,160] As such, it appears that *TP53* gene mutations are acquired during the course of the disease and result in leukemic cells that have enhanced resistance to standard anticancer drugs and ionizing radiation.[153]

CHROMOSOME 14 ANOMALIES

Located on chromosome 14, at band 14q32, are the genes encoding the Ig heavy chain (see Chap. 77). This band frequently is the site of translocations in B cell malignancies, with breakpoints often occurring within or near the Ig heavy-chain J segment minigenes or the Ig heavy-chain isotype switch regions.[161] Band q11.2 of chromosome 14 also contains genes encoding the α-chain and the δ-chain of the human T cell receptor (see Chap. 78). Leukemic cells with inversions of chromosome 14, inv(14)(q11q32) most often are derived from the T cell lineage and express T cell differentiation antigens.[162–164] These lesions are common in T cell PLL. Translocations at either of these loci are postulated to reflect an aberrant Ig or T cell receptor gene rearrangement that in turn activates a protooncogene located on the other chromosome involved in the translocation.

t(14;18) Rarely, the leukemic cells in B cell CLL can have t(14; 18) translocations that more commonly are found in low-grade nodular B cell lymphomas (see Chap. 96).[165,166] This translocation juxtaposes the Ig heavy-chain genes with *BCL-2*.

t(14;19)(q32;q13.1) Although an initial report of t(14;19) translocations in CLL found this translocation in three of 30 cases,[167] cytogenetic analyses of 4487 patients with indolent lymphoproliferative diseases, including those with CLL, revealed only six cases had t(14; 19).[168] Only 23 CLL cases having t(14;19) have been reported to date. Such translocations generally involve the isotype switch regions of IgA on chromosome 14 and result in increased transcription of *BCL-3*, a gene near the breakpoint on chromosome 19 that encodes a protein of the IκB family of transcription factors.[168,169] There is a striking association of t(14;19) with trisomy 12. The presence of this and other CLL-associated features argues that patients with t(14;19) do not have a lymphoproliferative disease distinct from that of CLL. Rather, t(14; 19) may be an acquired cytogenetic abnormality that occurs during the evolution of preexisting CLL.

t(11;14)(q13;q32) Translocations involving chromosome 14, at band 14q32, and chromosome 11, at band 11q13, or t(11;14)(q13;q32) first were described in CLL.[170–173] The translocation juxtaposes the heavy-chain Ig genes with a protooncogene, designated *BCL-1* (B cell leukemia-1),[173,174] which subsequently was identified as *PRAD1*, a gene encoding cyclin D1.[175,176] Overexpression of *PRAD1* can contribute to cell transformation[177] and may play a role in the development of some cases of B cell CLL.[177] However, among lymphoid malignancies, the highest incidence of t(11;14) and/or *PRAD1* overexpression is noted in mantle zone cell lymphoma.[178–182] Because the neoplastic B cells of mantle cell lymphoma can share many phenotypic features with the leukemic B cells in CLL (see Chaps. 90 and 96), cases of CLL that previously were thought to have t(11;14)(q13;q32) instead may have represented the leukemic phase of mantle cell lymphoma.[180,181,183–185]

CHROMOSOME 18 ANOMALIES

Approximately 5 percent of CLL patients may have leukemic cells that have aberrant Ig gene rearrangements with the *BCL-2* located on the long arm of chromosome 18 at 18q21.[165,166,186] In contrast to *BCL-2* gene rearrangements in nodular B cell lymphomas, the rearrangements in B cell CLL generally occur at breakpoints in the 5′ end of the *BCL-2* gene and involve the κ or λ Ig light-chain genes on chromosome 2 or 22, respectively.[186] Independent of *BCL-2* gene rearrangement, however, the leukemic cells from nearly all patients with B cell CLL express high levels of the Bcl-2 protein that are comparable to that noted for lymphoma cells carrying the t(14;18)(q32;q21) translocation.[187,188] This is associated with hypomethylation of the *BCL-2* locus.[189] Using pulse-field gel electrophoresis to examine for *BCL-2* gene rearrangements in DNA fragments of 50,000 to 10,000 kb, one study found that each of nine CLL cases had somatic rearrangements that would not have been detected by conventional techniques.[190] This finding suggests that the presence of previously undetected genetic abnormalities in CLL involving chromosome 18 that may be responsible for the high-level expression of *BCL-2*.

LEUKEMIA CELL ACCUMULATION

GROWTH KINETICS

In the spleen, proliferation of CLL cells apparently occurs preferentially in the white pulp zones, even in cases in which both the white and red pulp are extensively infiltrated.[191] However, CLL cells in the blood incorporate extremely low amounts of ^{3}H-thymidine *in vitro*[192] and are mainly in the G_0 stage of the cell cycle, as assessed by flow cytometry.[193] Because most CLL cells are not proliferating, the life span of CLL lymphocytes appears long. Consistent with this finding, human CLL B cells can survive for many weeks after transfer into mice with severe combined immune deficiency.[194] Studies of patients who ingested heavy water to evaluate the growth kinetics of CLL cells *in vivo*, however, revealed that the leukemic cells of each patient had birth rates ranging from 0.1 percent to greater than 1.0 percent of the entire clone per day.[195] Such high leukemia cell birth rates were noted even in patients with apparently stable blood lymphocyte counts. This finding conflicts with the notion that CLL is a static disease. Instead, the finding suggests that the blood lymphocyte count for any one patient is defined by a more dynamic process in which leukemia cells are generated and die at appreciable rates.

"PROLIFERATION CENTERS"

The lymph nodes of patients with CLL characteristically are diffusely infiltrated with monomorphic, small, round lymphocytes that efface the normal node architecture. There can be small clusters of prolymphocyte-appearing cells that form aggregates called *proliferation centers* or *pseudofollicles* that are scattered through the lymph node. The cells in such pseudofollicles appear distinctive in that they express relatively high levels of CD20 and other B cell surface antigens.[196] One study failed to find leukemia cells with the distinctive surface antigen phenotype of "proliferation center" B cells in the blood of patients with CLL.[197] The abundance of proliferation centers varies between the lymph nodes of different patients.[198] However, the relative number of "pseudofollicles" does not have a clear relationship with the extent of lymphocytosis, stage, prior treatment history, or tendency toward progression.[197–199] As such, it may be speculative to call such pseudofollicles "proliferation centers," implying that they contain a subset of proliferating leukemia cells that contribute to disease progression. Another possibility is that such pseudofollicles represent small collections of nonmalignant lymphocytes and accessory cells that are engaged in immune responses to antigen.

RESISTANCE TO APOPTOSIS

CLL cells appear relatively resistant to programmed cell death, or apoptosis (see Chap. 11). CLL B cells express high levels of the antiapoptotic protein Bcl-2.[200] In addition, the neoplastic B cells of patients with CLL also characteristically express high levels of other antiapoptotic proteins, such as Bcl-x$_L$, Mcl-1, and Bag-1[201] and low levels of the proapoptotic protein Bax or Bcl-x$_s$.[202] Bcl-2 and Bax proteins form homodimers and heterodimers that influence the susceptibility to apoptosis.[203,204] Moreover, the relative ratio of Bcl-2 and/or Bcl-x$_L$ to Bax in leukemia cells appears to be related to their resistance to drugs *in vitro*[205–208] and possibly also *in vivo*.

The sensitivity of CLL cells to undergoing spontaneous or drug-induced apoptosis may be influenced by the leukemia cell microenvironment. CLL cells often undergo apoptosis *in vitro* under culture conditions that can support the survival and growth of human B cell lines. However, CLL B cells can survive for long periods *ex vivo* when cultured with marrow stromal cells.[209,210] Similarly, CLL cells can survive for protracted periods *in vitro* when cultured with *nurselike cells*,[211] which are nonleukemic accessory cells that can differentiate from CD14+ blood mononuclear cells when cocultured with CLL B cells.[212] Cells with the distinctive phenotype and morphology of nurselike cells can be found in the secondary lymphoid tissues of patients with CLL,[212] where they presumably function to inhibit apoptosis of leukemia cells *in vivo*. Follicular dendritic cells also may protect CLL cells from undergoing cell death.[213] The ability of marrow stromal cells, nurselike cells, or follicular dendritic cells to inhibit spontaneous apoptosis of CLL cells apparently requires cell–cell contact but may involve several distinctive ligand–receptor interactions.

CHRONIC LYMPHOCYTIC LEUKEMIA CELL TRAFFICKING

CLL cells recirculate from the blood through secondary lymphoid tissues and back into the systemic circulation in response to certain chemokines, such as stromal cell-derived factor (SDF)-1α, CCL21, and/or CCL19.[214] CLL cells have receptors for such chemokines and can manifest chemotaxis toward a chemokine gradient.[215–217] Production of chemokines such as SDF-1α by nurselike cells (NLC) could recruit leukemia cells from the blood into secondary lymphoid tissues, where the leukemia cells in turn could receive survival stimuli from NLC and other stroma elements. Moreover, production of SDF-1α by marrow stromal cells could account for the accumulation of leukemia cells in the marrow, which invariably is infiltrated by leukemia cells in untreated patients with CLL.

Because chemokine receptors are down-modulated in response to the relevant chemokine, leukemia cells within lymphoid compartments potentially could be replaced by newly arriving leukemia cells and then reenter the systemic circulation. The leukemia cells in the blood that fail to reenter such protective compartments might undergo spontaneous cell death and account for the appearance of "smudge" cells that typically are found in the blood smears of patients with this disease. Furthermore, the relative number and activity of such stromal elements might be a limiting factor governing tumor progression, particularly during early stages of the disease when the interdependency of leukemia cells with accessory cells seems most apparent.

IMMUNOLOGIC DEFECTS

IMMUNE DEFICIENCY

Patients with CLL typically develop immune deficiency.[218] Over time patients experience progressive decline in serum Ig levels, resulting in hypogammaglobulinemia. In addition, patients may develop low complement levels,[219] functional defects in bystander T cells,[220] altered leukemia cell expression of major histocompatibility complex antigens,[221,222] and impaired granulocytic function.[223] The immune deficiency associated with CLL often is compounded by the immune suppressive effects of CLL therapy.[224] As such, CLL patients have an increased risk for opportunistic infections and recurrent virus infection, such as those caused by herpes zoster[225,226] or cytomegalovirus.[227] Furthermore, patients with CLL have a higher risk for skin cancers, such as squamous cell carcinoma and basal cell carcinoma, than age-matched controls.[228]

The leukemia cells themselves may contribute to the immunodeficiency noted in patients with the disease. Leukemia B cells elaborate immune suppressive cytokines, such as transforming growth factor (TGF)-β,[229,230] and release soluble surface molecules, such as CD27,[68,231,232] that can interfere with cognate intercellular interactions required for immune activation. High levels of TGF-β also may account for the reversal in the ratio of CD4 to CD8 T cells that often is noted in patients with CLL.[233] CLL B cells have little stimulatory activity in autologous or even allogeneic mixed lymphocyte culture.[234,235] Important accessory molecules required for cognate B cell–T cell interactions, such as CD80 (see Chaps. 14 and 78), are absent or present at low levels on the leukemic cell surface. As such, the phenotype of the leukemia cells makes them poor antigen-presenting cells but possible effective inducers of T cell anergy (see Chap. 78).

CLL B cells are effective in down-modulating expression of the CD40-ligand (CD154), a surface glycoprotein that ordinarily is expressed on CD4+ T cells following immune activation.[236,237] Because CD154 plays a critical role in the development of an immune response (reviewed by Grewal and Flavell[238]), such down-modulation may be responsible for the immune deficiency acquired in CLL. Given the role of CD154 in T cell induction of Ig class switching, this acquired functional defect in CD154 may account for the acquired deficiency of CLL patients to produce IgG of each of the various subclasses.[239]

The acquired immune deficiency of patients with CLL has features in common with that of persons with inherited functional defects in the gene encoding CD154 and/or other inherited immune deficiencies (see Chap. 82). These shared features include the frequent development of intermittent and intercurrent systemic autoimmunity despite profound immune deficiency. Patients with congenital lack of CD154 or other immune deficiencies frequently develop autoimmune hemolytic anemia (see Chap. 52) or immune thrombocytopenic purpura (see Chap. 110).[240,241] These also are the most common autoimmune diseases that develop in patients with CLL.[242,243]

AUTOIMMUNITY

Patients with CLL are prone to developing systemic autoimmune disease. The most common autoimmune disorders result from autoantibodies that are directed against hematopoietic cell antigens, such as those found on red blood cells or platelets,[242,243] although other types of autoimmune disorder also appear more common among CLL patients than in the general population.[244–246] In some cases, the autoantibody might be produced by the neoplastic B cell clone,[247] but most often the autoantibodies are produced by bystander nonneoplastic B cells,[74] reflecting a disease-associated dysregulation in humoral immune tolerance to self-antigens. Patients with CLL also may develop pure red blood cell aplasia[248] or neutropenia[242] secondary to the development of autoantibodies against marrow hematopoietic progenitor cells. Although patients with rheumatoid arthritis reportedly have an increased prevalence of CLL compared to that of the general population,[249] CLL patients in general do not appear to have an increased incidence of pathologic autoimmunity other than that directed against hematopoietic cells.[242,243] As such, the mechanism(s) accounting for the development of autoimmunity may be similar to those involved in development of autoimmune hemolytic anemia or immune thrombocytopenia in patients with certain inherited immune deficiency disorders.[241]

CLINICAL FEATURES

PATIENT POPULATION

At diagnosis, most patients are older than 60 years and 90 percent are older than 50 years. Moreover, the median age at diagnosis is 64 to 70 years.[1] The disease is rare in persons younger than 25 years. There is a 2:1 male to female incidence and prevalence of CLL.

GENERAL SYMPTOMS

More than 25 percent of patients are asymptomatic at diagnosis. Such patients generally are detected because of the discovery of nontender lymphadenopathy or an unexplained absolute lymphocytosis. Otherwise, patients may have only mild symptoms of reduced exercise tolerance, fatigue, or malaise. Patients may experience such symptoms even when they apparently lack major organ involvement or anemia. Because of the advanced age of the affected population, patients sometimes present with an exacerbation of another underlying medical condition, such as pulmonary, cerebrovascular, or coronary artery disease.

Some cases present with chronic rhinitis secondary to nasal involvement of CLL cells.[250] In rare cases, patients present with a sensorimotor polyneuropathy associated with IgM antibody to various gangliosides.[99] For unknown reasons, patients may note exaggerated responses to insect bites, particularly to those of mosquitoes.[251,252]

Patients who present with more advanced disease may experience involuntary weight loss, recurrent infections, bleeding secondary to thrombocytopenia, and/or symptomatic anemia. Patients also might experience night sweats and/or low-grade fevers (the so-called *B symptoms*). However, disease-related fevers greater than 38.5° C are uncommon and should prompt evaluation for complicating infectious disease. Patients with CLL are more prone to viral or bacterial infections secondary to impaired T cell immunity or hypogammaglobulinemia, respectively.

LYMPHADENOPATHY

Nearly 80 percent of all CLL patients have nontender lymphadenopathy at diagnosis, most commonly involving the cervical, supraclavicular, or axillary lymph nodes. Lymph node enlargement ranges from minimal to massive, the latter potentially causing local disfiguration or organ dysfunction. Some patients develop symptoms of upper airway obstruction because of oral-pharyngeal lymphadenopathy. However, it is unusual for the lymphadenopathy in CLL to cause obstruction of vascular or lymphatic channels. Lymphedema of the upper extremities is rare, even in the setting of massive axillary and cervical adenopathy. Superior vena cava obstruction is so uncommon that it should alert the clinician to the possibility of a secondary pulmonary neoplasm. Computerized axial tomography of the abdomen can detect intraabdominal lymph node enlargement in a large number of patients. However, such information has yet to be incorporated into clinical staging schemes. Large mesenteric or abdominal adenopathy rarely can cause lower extremity edema secondary to compression of the inferior vena cava. Occasionally, large retroperitoneal adenopathy can result in ureteral obstruction and hydronephrosis. Rarely, patients develop periportal lymph node enlargement that results in biliary tract obstruction. Some patients may experience acute, painful swelling in previously nontender, chronically enlarged lymph nodes secondary to acute lymphadenitis resulting from infection with herpes simplex virus.[253,254]

SPLENOMEGALY AND HEPATOMEGALY

Approximately half of all CLL patients present with mild to moderate splenomegaly. Occasionally, this condition causes symptoms of early satiety and/or abdominal fullness. Sometimes, splenic enlargement results in hypersplenism, contributing to anemia and thrombocytopenia. However, in CLL such cytopenias are more commonly secondary to extensive marrow involvement with CLL and/or intermittent expression of autoantibodies.[242,255–258] Less frequently, patients develop hepatomegaly secondary to leukemic cell infiltration of the liver. Derangement of hepatic function secondary to visceral involvement usually is mild, and cholestatic jaundice is unusual in the absence of nodal disease causing biliary tract obstruction.

EXTRANODAL INVOLVEMENT

Organ infiltration with leukemic cells is frequently detected at autopsy but is not commonly symptomatic. For example, leukemic cell infiltration of the renal parenchyma can be detected in more than half of all patients examined postmortem. However, CLL only rarely is associated with impaired renal function. Leukemic cell infiltration, however, may become symptomatic when it develops in certain locations, such as in the retro-orbit, where it can produce proptosis. Lymph tissue also may develop in the scalp, subconjunctivae, prostate, gonads, or pharynx, the latter sometimes causing symptoms of upper airway obstruction. Infiltration of the pericardium by leukemia cells can produce a constrictive pericarditis[259] or result in cardiac tamponade.[260]

Occasionally, the leukemic cells infiltrate the lung parenchyma, producing nodular or miliary pulmonary infiltrates that can be detected on chest x-ray film. This finding may be associated with pulmonary function test abnormalities. The respiratory tract mucosa also may be involved. Leukemic infiltration of the pleura may result in hemorrhagic or chylous pleural effusions.[261–263]

The gastrointestinal tract may be infiltrated with leukemic cells, causing abnormal mucosal thickening. This condition may result in ulceration, gastrointestinal bleeding, or malabsorption. The latter may cause dietary deficiencies of essential nutrients, such as folate. The finding of iron deficiency should alert the physician to evaluate for gastrointestinal bleeding from mucosal ulcerations or secondary gastrointestinal malignancy.

Leukemic cell infiltration of the central nervous system is unusual but may produce headache, meningitis, cranial nerve palsy, obtundation, or coma.[264] The development of neurologic changes in CLL, however, may be caused by infections with unusual organisms, including fungi, *Cryptococcus neoformans*, *Listeria monocytogenes*, or other pathogens that generally only afflict an immune compromised host.

LABORATORY FEATURES

BLOOD FINDINGS

The diagnosis of CLL requires a sustained monoclonal lymphocytosis greater than $5000/\mu l$ (5×10^9/liter). At diagnosis, the absolute lymphocyte count generally exceeds $10,000/\mu l$ (10×10^9/liter) and sometimes is greater than $100,000/\mu l$ (100×10^9/liter). Morphologically, the leukemic cells generally appear similar to normal resting lymphocytes. Typically these cells have scanty, bluish cytoplasm upon Wright-Giemsa staining, moderately condensed and mature-appearing nuclei, and a mean cell volume (MCV) of 170 fl (see Color Plates XX-4 and XX-5). A few cells can have prominent nucleoli. During the preparation of the blood film, many CLL lymphocytes apparently are disrupted and appear as smudge cells. Leukemic leukocytosis in excess of $800,000/\mu l$ (800×10^9/liter) may produce blood hyperviscosity.

Patients with CLL may develop anemia secondary to leukemic marrow infiltration, the myelosuppressive effect of chemotherapy and inhibiting cytokines, autoimmunity directed against red cell antigens (see Chap. 52), hypersplenism (see Chap. 55), and/or a poor nutritional status that leads to deficiency of folic acid, vitamin B_{12}, or iron (see Chaps. 39 and 40). The nature of the blood findings vary depending on the factor(s) responsible for the anemia.

Most typically, the red cells are normocytic and normochromic. Approximately 15 percent of patients present with normocytic anemia. In the setting of extreme lymphocytosis, the packed red cell volume may be overestimated unless care is taken to exclude from the measurement the expanded buffy coat containing the leukemic cells. Approximately 20 percent of all CLL patients have a positive Coombs test at some time during their disease because of production of IgG anti-red cell autoantibodies by bystander nonleukemic B cells. Autoimmune hemolytic anemia, however, develops in only approximately 8 percent of CLL patients.

During the most advanced disease stage, patients have thrombocytopenia because of marrow replacement and hypersplenism. At any stage, however, patients can develop immune thrombocytopenia because of antiplatelet antibodies. Generally, the platelet morphology is not remarkable.

MARROW FINDINGS

The marrow invariably is infiltrated with leukemic cells. There are four patterns of marrow involvement (Fig. 92-1).[265–267] In approximately one third of patients, the marrow has an interstitial, or lacy, pattern that is associated with a better prognosis and/or early-stage disease. Approximately 10 percent of patients present with a nodular pattern of marrow involvement, and approximately 25 percent have a mixed nodular-interstitial pattern. These patterns also are associated with a better prognosis. One fourth of patients present with extensive marrow replacement, producing a diffuse pattern that is associated with advanced clinical stage and/or more aggressive disease.[267,268]

LYMPH NODE FINDINGS

The lymph node architecture typically is effaced by a diffuse infiltration of small lymphocytes that have the same morphology as that of the circulating leukemic cells. The node histology is similar to that of low-grade small lymphocytic lymphoma (see Color Plates XXII-9 and 10). As the disease progresses, the nodes may coalesce and form large fixed masses. In rare cases, the lymph node contains a few scattered cells that have the morphology and phenotype of Reed-Sternberg cells typically seen in Hodgkin disease (see Color Plate XXII-32 and see Chap. 97).[269]

IMMUNOLOGIC STUDIES

Several tests are recommended as part of the laboratory evaluation of patients with CLL. Lymphocyte surface immunologic markers can determine monoclonality and the presence of CLL-type lymphocytes. The direct Coombs test can uncover patients who have or are at risk for an immune hemolytic anemia. Measurement of serum Ig quantifies the depression of IgG, IgA, and IgM that predisposes to infection. Skin tests with PPD and other recall antigens can detect anergy. The frequency of the concomitant T cell functional defect increases in advanced stages of CLL.

Flow cytometric analyses can evaluate leukemic cells for expression of B cell or T cell differentiation antigens, surface Ig, and κ or λ

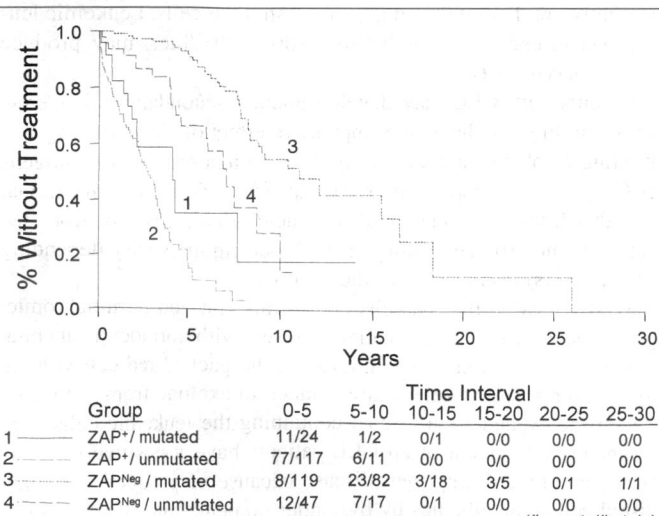

FIGURE 92-1   Relationship between ZAP-70 and IgV$_H$ mutational status and time from diagnosis to initial therapy. Kaplan-Meier curves depict the proportion of untreated patients over time from diagnosis of different groups of cases segregated with respect to IgV$_H$ mutational status and whether they did (ZAP+) or did not (ZAP^{Neg}) express ZAP-70. (Adapted from LZ Rassenti, L Huynh, TL Toy, et al.,[331] with permission.)

light chains. Such studies can distinguish B cell CLL not only from T cell leukemias but also from other B cell leukemias that otherwise mimic B cell CLL (Table 92-1). Examples of useful markers for this purpose are CD5, CD10, CD11c, CD19, CD20, CD22, CD23, CD25, CD38, and CD103 (see Chap. 14).[73,270–273]

CLL cells typically are CD5+, CD10−, CD19+, CD20 (dull), CD23+, CD103−, have weak expression of surface Ig, and have weak or absent expression of membrane CD22 and CD79b. The latter marker identifies an extracellular epitope of the B cell receptor beta chain (see Chap. 77). FMC7, a monoclonal antibody that binds an epitope of CD20 formed when this surface antigen is present at high density,[274] typically does not react with CLL cells, reflecting the low-level expression of CD20 by the leukemia cells of most patients with CLL. Because low-level expression of CD20 is a distinctive characteristic of CLL cells, FMC7 still is used to discriminate CLL from other B cell malignancies.[275]

Cytoplasmic Ig can be detected in CLL B cells and may be a valuable adjunct in B cell phenotyping.[276] Compared to normal cells, CLL B cells have a lower density of surface but a higher content of cytoplasmic Ig. Rarely, intracytoplasmic inclusions of crystalloid Ig have been seen. More than three fourths of patients with CLL may have excess light chains in the Golgi complex and the cisternae of the rough endoplasmic reticulum.[277–279]

SERUM IMMUNOGLOBULINS

The most common finding on serum protein electrophoreses is hypogammaglobulinemia. Nearly three fourths of all B cell CLL patients develop severe hypogammaglobulinemia during the course of their disease. Reduction in the serum levels of IgM precedes that of IgG and IgA. The degree of hypogammaglobulinemia correlates loosely with clinical stage, and virtually all patients with advanced disease have decreased concentrations of serum Ig.

However, 5 percent of patients have a serum monoclonal Ig paraprotein. The serum paraprotein generally is the same type as that present on the leukemic cell surface. When the concentration of IgM paraprotein is high, hyperviscosity may ensue, and the clinical picture can be confused with that of Waldenström macroglobulinemia (see Chap. 102). In some cases, defective and/or unbalanced Ig chain synthesis by the leukemic B cell clone results in μ heavy-chain disease and/or Ig light-chain proteinuria (see Chap. 103). The latter can be detected on urine immunoelectrophoresis (see Chap. 98).

When high-resolution agarose gel electrophoresis is combined with immunofixation, small paraprotein spikes can be identified in the sera or urine samples of nearly two thirds of all patients.[19,280–282] These paraprotein spikes generally have Ig heavy chains that belong to isotypes other than those expressed by the leukemic B cell clone.[19]

DIFFERENTIAL DIAGNOSIS

Chapter 81 discusses the differential diagnosis of lymphocytosis. Lymphocytosis can occur in persons infected with various viruses, *Bordetella pertussis*, or *Toxoplasma gondii* (see Chap. 81). However, the patients who usually encounter such illness generally are much younger than patients with CLL. Also, in contrast to the reactive lymphocytosis that occurs in response to these infections, the lymphocytosis of patients with CLL is persistent and monoclonal. The latter characteristic is important in distinguishing CLL from unusual cases of persistent polyclonal lymphocytosis of B cells that sometimes can masquerade as B cell CLL.[283,284] Flow cytometric analyses of blood mononuclear cells generally can differentiate among reactive lymphocytosis, polyclonal B cell lymphocytosis, and monoclonal lymphocytosis secondary to lymphoproliferative disease.[285]

PROLYMPHOCYTIC LEUKEMIA

PLL is a subacute variant of CLL in which more than half of the blood leukemic cells are large lymphocytes, termed *prolymphocytes*. These cells can be distinguished from the leukemic cells in CLL by size and morphology.[286] Prolymphocytes measure 10 to 15 μm in diameter, whereas CLL cells generally are the size of small resting lymphocytes (7–10 μm in diameter). Also, prolymphocytes in the blood or marrow have round or indented nuclei, each possessing a single prominent thick-rimmed nucleolus and chromatin that is denser than that of a lymphoblast but less dense than that of a typical mature lymphocyte or a CLL B cell (see Color Plate XX-5). The cytoplasm generally is pale blue and agranular, except for occasional intracytoplasmic inclusions that are visible by electron, and sometimes light, microscopy.[287] By scanning electron microscopy, these prolymphocytes often have more surface microvilli than do leukemic cells from patients with B cell CLL. They may involve lymph nodes, generally producing a pseudonodular pattern of infiltration that is distinct from that of the diffuse pattern typical of CLL.[288] In contrast to the leukemic B cells in CLL, prolymphocytes typically express high levels of surface Ig and stain brightly with SN8, a monoclonal antibody specific for CD79b (see Chaps. 14 and 77).[289,290] The neoplastic cells in PLL typically have low expression of CD5 relative to that observed on CLL cells.[291] Table 92-1 lists these and other features that distinguish CLL from PLL. Other features of this disease are discussed in the main section on prolymphocytic leukemia.

HAIRY CELL LEUKEMIA

Table 92-1 lists the clinical and laboratory features that assist in distinguishing CLL from hairy cell leukemia and its variants, hairy cell leukemia variant, and splenic lymphoma with villous lymphocytes.[292] Chapter 93 discusses these diseases.

The neoplastic B cells in hairy cell leukemia are larger than CLL cells (MCV 400 fl) and have more abundant cytoplasm, often with fine filamentous "hairy" projections (see Color Plate XX-7). These cells are strongly positive for tartrate-resistant isozyme 5 of acid phosphatase (TRAP) activity. In contrast to CLL B cells, the neoplastic cells in hairy cell leukemia express high levels of CD11c, the α^X chain of the β_2-integrins, and CD103, the α^E subunit of the β_7-integrins (see Chap. 93).

LYMPHOMAS

Lymphomas can have circulating neoplastic cells, sometimes producing a blood lymphocytosis that may be mistaken for CLL. Chapter 96 discusses the lymphomas. Those lymphomas that most closely can resemble B cell CLL are discussed here.

SMALL LYMPHOCYTIC LYMPHOMA

Low-grade small lymphocytic B cell lymphoma is closely related to B cell CLL in biology and clinical features. The neoplastic cells in small lymphocytic lymphoma with blood involvement are the same morphologically as the leukemic cells in CLL. Moreover, the histology of the involved lymph nodes in CLL and small lymphocytic lymphoma are indistinguishable.[293] Similar to the B cells in CLL, the neoplastic B cells in small lymphocytic lymphoma frequently express Igs that bear autoantibody-associated cross-reactive idiotypes and are encoded

by nonmutated Ig genes.[71,294] Finally, the neoplastic B cells in both diseases express many of the same surface antigens, including CD5.[295] For these reasons, the distinction between these diseases is primarily clinical in that CLL invariably is associated with a blood lymphocytosis (>4000 lymphocytes/μl), whereas small lymphocytic lymphoma invariably is associated with lymph node involvement. Also, although patients with CLL invariably have marrow lymphocytosis, the marrow in small lymphocytic lymphoma is not necessarily involved. When the marrow is involved, the pattern in small lymphocytic lymphoma typically is nodular, rather than interstitial or diffuse.[267] Chapter 96 discusses this disorder further.

MANTLE CELL LYMPHOMA

Mantle cell lymphoma (previously called *centrocytic lymphoma, mantle zone lymphoma*, or *intermediate lymphoma*) in the Working Formulation is an intermediate-grade B cell lymphoma (see Chaps. 90, 95, and 96). In contrast to the diffuse lymph node involvement typical in CLL, the histology of lymph nodes in mantle cell lymphoma typically is one of reactive germinal centers surrounded by well-defined, expanded mantle zones of monoclonal B cells.[296] However, heavily involved lymph nodes may lose this architecture and appear diffusely infiltrated, assuming histology similar to that of involved lymph nodes in CLL.

The neoplastic B cells in mantle cell lymphoma express many of the same surface antigens as do CLL B cells, including CD5 (see Table 92-1). However, in contrast to CLL B cells, mantle cell lymphoma cells generally do not express CD23. Mantle cell lymphoma cells also tend to express higher levels of CD79a and CD79b than do CLL cells.[291,297]

In contrast to CLL cells, mantle cell lymphoma often have t(11;14) translocations involving *BCL-1* and Ig heavy-chain gene complex, resulting in overexpression of cyclin D1.[298,299] The *BCL-1* rearrangements of mantle cell lymphoma can be detected via FISH analyses of the neoplastic cells.[300]

SPLENIC MARGINAL ZONE LYMPHOMA

Splenic marginal zone lymphoma (SMZL) is an indolent lymphoproliferative disease that accounts for approximately 1 percent of all lymphomas (see Chap. 96). Patients with SMZL typically present with marked splenomegaly and often have a moderate lymphocytosis of monoclonal B cells that appear as atypical "villous lymphocytes."[301,302] As such, this disorder commonly is called *splenic lymphoma with villous lymphocytes*. The neoplastic B cells in this disease have a mature B cell phenotype and frequently express IgM and IgD but typically

TABLE 92-1 IMMUNOPHENOTYPE OF CHRONIC B CELL LEUKEMIAS/LYMPHOMAS

DISEASE ENTITY	sIg	CD5	CD10	CD11c	CD19	CD20	CD22	CD23	CD25	CD103
Chronic lymphocytic leukemia	+/−	++	−	−/+	+	+/−	−/+	++	−/+	−
Prolymphocytic leukemia	++	+	−	−/+	+	+/−	+	+/−	−	−
Hairy cell leukemia	+/−	−/+	−	++	+	+	++	−/+	+	++
Mantle cell lymphoma	+	++	−	−	+	+	+	−/+	−	−
Splenic marginal zone lymphoma	+	−/+	−/+	+	+	+	+/−	−/+	−	−
Lymphoplasmacytoid lymphoma	+/−	−/+	−	−	+	+/−	+/−	−/+	+/−	−
Follicular center lymphoma	+	−	+	−	+	++	+	−/+	−	−

− = Leukemia cells do not express the surface antigen; + = leukemia cells from most cases express the surface antigen; +/− = low-level expression; −/+ = most cases either do not express the antigen or express it at very low levels; ++ = high-level expression of the surface antigen in nearly all cases.
sIg = surface immunoglobulin.

lack expression of CD23, CD43, CD10, Bcl-6, and cyclin D1 (see Table 92-1). In contrast to CLL, which has moderate expression of CD5 and weak or negative expression of CD79b, the neoplastic B cells in SMZL have weak or negative expression of CD5 and moderate expression of CD79b.[291,303] Genetic studies have revealed abnormalities in a number of chromosomes; however, 7q31-33 allelic loss appears to be characteristic.[304] The loss of 7q31 spans from 7q31.33 to 7q33 located between sequence tagged site markers SHGC-3275 and D7S725, a region distinct from that commonly deleted in myelodysplastic disease or acute myeloid leukemia (see Chaps. 86 and 87).

Histologically, the spleen in SMZL is characterized by a nodular infiltrate based on preexisting white pulp but also involving the red pulp. Within the white pulp, the infiltrate has a biphasic morphology comprising an inner zone of small lymphocytes and a peripheral (marginal) zone of larger lymphoid cells. Usually the splenic lymph nodes and marrow are also involved by a vaguely nodular infiltrate having similar characteristics. On the other hand, the spleen in CLL typically has diffuse effacement of white pulp architecture and lacks readily identifiable marginal zones.[305]

LYMPHOMAS OF FOLLICULAR CENTER CELL ORIGIN

Low-grade lymphomas of follicular center cell origin also can involve the blood. Often marked adenopathy and occasionally massive splenomegaly are present. The leukemic cells are small and typically have cleaved nuclei with well-delineated nucleoli. Follicular center small cleaved cell lymphomas frequently express the CD10 (CALLA) antigen. In contrast to CLL, these cells often express high levels of surface Ig and generally express neither mouse rosette receptors nor the CD5 antigen (see Table 92-1). The cells are FMC7 positive. Biopsy of a lymph node confirms nodular or diffuse small cleaved cell (poorly differentiated lymphocytic) lymphoma. Chapter 96 discusses these diseases.

LYMPHOPLASMACYTIC LEUKEMIAS

Plasmacytoid lymphocytes can be seen on the blood films and are always present in the marrow of patients with Waldenström macroglobulinemia (see Chap. 102). These cells have abundant, often basophilic, cytoplasm with mature lymphoid nuclei. By flow cytometric analysis these cells express pan-B lymphocyte surface antigens CD19, CD20, and CD24 (see Chap. 14) and are monoclonal as defined by Ig light-chain expression. Similar to CLL B cells, these cells often express CD5 and CD11b. However, they can be distinguished from CLL cells by their expression of the CD10 (CALLA) and/or CD9 antigens and by their lymphoplasmacytic morphology (see Chaps. 90 and 95).

Patients with plasma cell myeloma may develop plasma cell leukemia. The leukemic cells can be distinguished from those in B cell CLL by their plasmacytic morphology, their expression of CD38, PCA-1, CD56, and CD85, and their low-level or lack of expression of CD19, CD20, CD24, CD72, and HLA-DR (see Table 92-1). Chapter 100 discusses plasma cell myeloma.

T CELL CHRONIC LYMPHOPROLIFERATIVE DISORDERS

T cell variants of CLL constitute a heterogeneous group of disorders that must be distinguished from B cell CLL. T cell chronic lymphoproliferative diseases are much less common. Several have counterparts in the various B cell leukemias and are discussed in other chapters, including T cell PLL (discussed below in "T cell Prolymphocytic Leukemia") and T cell lymphoma (see Chap. 96). A subset of large granular lymphocytic leukemias represents another T cell chronic leukemia (discussed in Chap. 94).

These diseases can be distinguished from lymphoproliferative disorders of B cells or natural killer cells by immunophenotype. The leukemic cells from all T cell malignancies lack expression of monoclonal surface Ig or B cell restricted surface differentiation antigens, such as CD19 or CD20 (see Chap. 14), and they generally lack Ig light-chain gene rearrangements (see Chap. 77). Characteristically, chronic T cell leukemias have rearrangement and expression of the genes encoding the T cell receptor for antigen (see Chap. 78) and express the CD3 surface antigens (see Chaps. 14 and 78). The latter is a property exclusive to lymphocytes of the T cell lineage and can be used to distinguish large granular lymphocytic leukemia of T cell versus natural killer cell origin (see Chap. 94).

THERAPY, COURSE, AND PROGNOSIS

CLINICAL STAGING

Because wide variability exists in the rate of disease progression and the incidence of disease-related complications among patients with CLL, the life expectancies of patients with newly diagnosed CLL can vary tremendously. Staging helps to define prognosis and to decide when to initiate therapy.

Two major staging systems have been developed, each with established value in helping to predict survival.[306] The first widely used system was introduced by Rai et al.[23] in 1975. This staging system designated five clinical stages using Roman numerals 0 through IV. Patients in stages 0 and I have a favorable prognosis, whereas patients in stages III and IV have a relatively short survival (Table 92-2). The prognosis of patients in stage II is intermediate. Although confirmed to have useful predictive value,[307] the number of stages was considered excessive by some investigators. Accordingly, in 1981, Binet et al.[308] proposed a three-stage classification system that considered the total lymphoid mass. The most advanced stage, stage C, describes all patients who have anemia and/or thrombocytopenia resulting from impaired marrow function (Table 92-3). The remaining patients are divided into stage A or B, based upon the number of enlarged lymphoid areas (of which there are five: cervical, axillary, or inguinofemoral lymph node, liver, spleen). Patients in group A have fewer than three areas of lymphoid enlargement; patients in group B have three or more areas of lymphoid enlargement (Table 92-3). Most physicians use either the Binet or the Rai staging system. Generally, disease progression follows a stepwise pattern from earlier to later stages.

In 1987, Rai[309] reorganized his original staging system into three categories: low-risk (stage 0), intermediate-risk (stages I and II), and high-risk (stages III and IV) patients. Low-risk patients have a projected median survival of greater than 150 months (see Table 92-2). In contrast, intermediate- and high-risk patients have median survivals of approximately 90 months and 19 months, respectively. Both the

TABLE 92-2 RAI CLINICAL STAGING SYSTEM

REVISED STAGING SYSTEM	ORIGINAL STAGING SYSTEM	CLINICAL FEATURES AT DIAGNOSIS	MEDIAN SURVIVAL (MONTHS)
Low risk	0	Blood and marrow lymphocytosis	>150
	I	Lymphocytosis and enlarged lymph nodes	101
Intermediate risk	II	Lymphocytosis and enlarged spleen and/or liver	>71
High risk	III	Lymphocytosis and anemia (hemoglobin <11 g/dl)	19
	IV	Lymphocytosis and thrombocytopenia (platelets <100,000/μl)	19

TABLE 92-3 BINET CLINICAL STAGING SYSTEM

STAGE	CLINICAL FEATURES AT DIAGNOSIS	MEDIAN SURVIVAL (YEARS)
A	Blood and marrow lymphocytosis and <3 areas* of palpable lymphoid tissue enlargement	>7
B	Blood and marrow lymphocytosis and ≥3 areas of palpable lymphoid tissue enlargement	<5
C	Same as B with anemia (hemoglobin <11 g/dl in men or <10 g/dl in women) or thrombocytopenia (platelets <100,000/μl)	<2

* An area is defined as the cervical, axillary, or inguinofemoral lymph nodes, or the liver and spleen. The liver and spleen together count as one area, as do the right and left cervical lymph nodes. However, bilateral enlargement of the axillary lymph nodes or the inguinofemoral lymph nodes each counts as two areas. Thus, the number of enlarged lymphoid areas can range from one to five.

Binet classification and the modified Rai classification have proven utility in helping to access disease outcome.[309] Despite the advent of new prognostic markers, these staging systems still have independent prognostic value.[310]

OTHER PROGNOSTIC INDICATORS

In addition to the widely accepted staging systems of Rai and Binet, additional indicators can help identify high risk patients who may benefit from closer follow-up. With the exception of a short lymphocyte doubling time, standard guidelines have yet to incorporate these parameters into decision making of when to initiate therapy (Table 92-4).[311] This awaits the outcome of clinical trials to determine the value of early treatment based on these parameters in lieu of standard treatment indications.

LEUKEMIC CELL DOUBLING TIME
CLL B cells generally do not have a high mitotic index and express low levels of the cyclin-dependent kinase inhibitor p27^{kip1} (p27), a protein that ordinarily increases as a cell progresses into S phase. However, some patients have leukemia cells that express relatively high levels of p27.[312] Such patients may have shorter blood lymphocyte doubling times and survival than average patients with CLL.

Patients whose lymphocyte counts double within 1 year have progressive disease, whereas those with stable counts represent a good-risk population. Independent of stage, the median survival for patients with a doubling time less than 12 months is significantly shorter than that of patients who had leukemia cell doubling times of more than 1 year.[313,314]

IMMUNOGLOBULIN GENE MUTATION STATUS
CLL B cells can be segregated into at least two groups that differ with regard to the extent to which their expressed IgV$_H$ genes have undergone somatic mutation.[85,315] About half of all cases have leukemia cells that express nonmutated IgV$_H$ genes; the rest express IgV$_H$ genes with levels of base substitutions that distinguish them from their germ-line counterparts. As such, the latter resemble more the cases of CLL that express IgA or IgG.[316–319] The extent to which IgV$_H$ genes are mutated does not vary within any one leukemia cell population,[320] even when examined over a period of years.[321] As such, it appears certain that leukemia cells that express mutated Ig genes do not evolve from cases that originally expressed unmutated Ig genes.

The mutational status of the Ig genes expressed by CLL cells can be used to segregate patients into two subsets that have significantly different tendencies for disease progression.[24,25] CLL cells that express nonmutated IgV$_H$ genes may have trisomy 12 and atypical morphology

more often than those that expressed mutated IgV$_H$ genes, which in turn more frequently tend to have abnormalities involving 13q14.[322] Furthermore, patients with leukemia cells that express unmutated IgV$_H$ genes have a greater tendency for disease progression than those who have leukemia cells that express IgV$_H$ genes with less than 98 percent nucleic acid sequence homology with their germ-line counterparts,[24,25] an observation confirmed by subsequent studies.[323–327]

One noted exception to this finding appears to be patients who have leukemia cells that use a particular immunoglobulin gene designated IgV$_H$ 3-21. This gene frequently has somatic mutations when expressed by CLL B cells. However, patients who have CLL cells that use a mutated IgV$_H$ 3-21 gene apparently have a risk for aggressive disease similar to that of patients who have leukemia cells that express unmutated IgV$_H$ genes.[81]

ZETA-ASSOCIATED PROTEIN OF 70 KILODALTONS (ZAP-70)
CLL cells that use unmutated IgV$_H$ genes can be distinguished from those that express mutated IgV$_H$ genes through the differential expression of a relatively small subset of genes.[26,27] One of these genes encodes the zeta-associated protein of 70 kDa (ZAP-70). ZAP-70 is a 70-kDa cytoplasmic protein tyrosine kinase that ordinarily is expressed only in natural killer cells and T cells, in which it originally was identified as being able to associate with CD247, the CD3 ζ-chain of the T cell receptor complex (see Chaps. 14 and 78). In contrast to CLL cells that have mutated Ig receptors, CLL cells that use unmutated IgV$_H$ genes express ZAP-70 RNA.[26] Subsequent studies found that CLL B cells that had unmutated V$_H$ genes generally expressed levels of ZAP-70 protein that were comparable to those expressed by normal blood T cells.[328,329] In contrast, CLL B cells that expressed mutated IgV$_H$ genes generally do not express detectable levels of ZAP-70 protein. As such, leukemia cell expression of ZAP-70 can be used as a surrogate marker for Ig mutational status,[329,330] which can segregate patients that have significantly different tendencies for disease progression.

Using sensitive flow cytometric techniques, the distribution of ZAP-70 expression levels by different leukemia populations does not define two discrete subsets. For this reason, it is necessary to define "positive" cases based upon whether they have 20 percent or more labeled leukemia cells with a fluorescence intensity that is above a defined fluorescence threshold for "positive" cells,[329] a cutoff that has apparent clinical significance.[331] This threshold can vary depending upon the background fluorescence intensities of the isotype control-stained leukemia cells and the relative brightness of the fluorochrome-conjugated anti–ZAP-70 monoclonal antibody.

Although CLL cells that express unmutated IgV$_H$ genes generally also express ZAP-70, this is not always the case. Conversely, some CLL cells have ZAP-70 despite expressing mutated IgV$_H$ genes. In one large multiinstitution study,[331] patients with ZAP-70–positive CLL cells had median time from diagnosis to initial therapy of 2.8 years if the leukemia cells expressed unmutated IgV$_H$ genes and 4.2

TABLE 92-4 INDICATIONS FOR THERAPY IN CHRONIC LYMPHOCYTIC LEUKEMIA

Anemia

Thrombocytopenia

Disease-related symptoms

Markedly enlarged or painful spleen

Symptomatic lymphadenopathy

Blood lymphocyte count doubling time <6 months

Prolymphocytic transformation

Richter transformation

years if their leukemia cells express mutated IgV$_H$ genes (see Fig. 92-1). These two subgroups were not significantly different. However, the median time from diagnosis to initial treatment in each of these groups was significantly shorter than the time in patients with ZAP-70–negative CLL cells who had either mutated or unmutated IgV$_H$ genes ($p < 0.001$). The median time from diagnosis to initial therapy among patients who did not have ZAP-70 was 11.0 years in those with mutated IgV$_H$ genes and 7.1 years in those with unmutated IgV$_H$ genes ($p < 0.001$). As such, it appears that expression of ZAP-70 may be a stronger predictor of the need for early treatment in patients with CLL than is IgV$_H$ mutation status.

CD38

The leukemia cells of patients with aggressive disease often express CD38, a surface protein that can synthesize cyclic ADP ribose (c-ADPR) from nicotinamide adenine dinucleotide and hydrolyze c-ADPR to ADP ribose[25] (see Chap. 14). Several studies corroborated the notion that CD38 is an indicator of relatively poor prognosis,[325,332-334] even independent of clinical stage.[323] However, one study concluded that CD38 did not have prognostic significance in a multivariate analysis of other commonly used staging criteria, except in early-stage patients.[335] Confounding this issue further is the observation that patients with CD38-negative leukemia cells might later be found to have leukemia cells that express this surface antigen, suggesting that expression of CD38 is a secondary event in CLL associated with disease evolution.[333] However, another study of more than 160 patients who were sampled on two separate occasions at intervals ranging from 4 to 40 months found that the expression level of CD38 varied by less than 10 percent between the first and second sample.[336] Even so, some studies did not observe an invariant association between expression of CD38 and tendency toward disease progression[337] or between readily identifiable subgroups based on surface antigen phenotype.[338]

The controversy regarding use of CD38 as a prognostic indicator in part could result from differences in the technique used for distinguishing cases considered "positive" versus "negative" for CD38. As with ZAP-70, the distribution of CD38 expression levels on different leukemia populations does not define two discrete subsets.[339] For this reason, it is necessary to define "positive" cases based upon whether they have 30 percent or more labeled leukemia cells with a fluorescence intensity that is above a defined threshold for "positive" cells. This threshold can vary depending upon the background fluorescence intensities of the isotype control-stained leukemia cells and the relative brightness of the fluorochrome-conjugated anti-CD38 monoclonal antibody.

CYTOGENETICS

Survival of patients with abnormal karyotypes is significantly shorter than that of comparably staged patients with normal karyotypes.[340-342] Multiple abnormalities in association with trisomy 12 carry a worse prognosis than trisomy 12 alone.[340,343,344] However, patients who have trisomy 12 as the only cytogenetic abnormality fare worse than those with a normal karyotype or those with isolated abnormalities involving 13q14.[345,346] Patients who have structural abnormalities of chromosome 14 or 6 or deletions of 11q also generally have a more adverse clinical course than those with a normal karyotype.[135,342,347] The prognostic effect of 11q deletion on survival is most apparent for patients younger than 55 years. Deletions of 17p, commonly associated with defects in *TP53*, also are associated with adverse prognosis.[157,342]

SERUM FACTORS

If patients have normal renal function, several serum protein levels become elevated in patients with aggressive disease. Moreover, the relative level of each of these proteins correlates with the kinetics of tumor progression and/or tumor burden. For this reason, potential prognostic value can be obtained by measuring the relative serum levels of β$_2$-microglobulin,[348-350] thymidine kinase,[350,351] soluble CD23,[348,352-354] soluble vascular cell adhesion molecule-1,[355] or soluble CD27.[231,356] Lactate dehydrogenase also is generally elevated in patients with aggressive disease and in nearly all patients with Richter transformation.[357,358] On the other hand, progressive disease more typically is associated with a greater suppression of T cell function and a more marked decline in serum IgA.[359] Hypercalcemia is rare in patients with CLL[360] and may indicate Richter transformation[361,362] (see "Richter Transformation" below).

However, it should be recognized that certain treatments, diseases, or renal dysfunction could affect the relative level of each of these factors, compromising their potential use as predictive markers. This is evident, for example, in patients treated with granulocyte-macrophage colony-stimulating factor (GM-CSF).[363] GM-CSF may increase the serum levels of β$_2$-microglobulin and thymidine kinase independent of disease progression.[364]

MARROW HISTOLOGY

Biopsy can reveal characteristic patterns of marrow infiltration, defined as nodular, interstitial, mixed, or diffuse (Fig. 92-2).[365,366] A diffuse replacement of the marrow is associated with a worse prognosis than is a nodular or interstitial pattern.[265-267,348] The marrow biopsy is more reliable than is the aspirate in distinguishing patients with favorable disease (nodular and/or interstitial) versus nonfavorable disease (diffuse) independent of clinical stage.[365] In addition, marrow biopsy appears more sensitive than the aspirate in detecting marrow infiltration of leukemia cells.[367] However, both the aspirate and biopsy appear to have independent prognostic value.[365,368] As such, evaluation of the marrow is considered desirable, especially for patients prior to therapy.[311]

INDICATIONS FOR THERAPY

No proven cures exist for CLL. Moreover, treatment of early-stage patients with chemotherapy does not appear to offer any survival advantage over that achieved with conservative management.[369] However, for certain patients therapy can reduce morbidity and/or improve survival significantly.

Table 92-4 lists the criteria recommended for deciding when to initiate treatment (Table 92-4).[311] Generally, an elevated blood lymphocyte count by itself is not an indication for therapy. Complications from extreme lymphocytosis, such as leukostasis, are rare in patients with nonprolymphocytic CLL who have blood lymphocyte counts less than 800,000/μl.[370] Also, minor or moderate lymphadenopathy in the absence of other indications usually is not treated. Lymphadenopathy that causes functional disturbances should be treated. Such disturbances include pain caused by nerve impingement from nodal encroachment; obstruction of the small bowel, ureter, or upper airway; or extreme adenopathy causing cosmetic disfigurement.

Newly diagnosed patients without the criteria listed in Table 92-4 should be followed closely for the next several months. During followup examinations, the hemogram should be monitored to access the rate of increase in the lymphocyte count and to evaluate for anemia or thrombocytopenia. Thereafter, patients with early-stage disease and good prognostic features should be followed at 2- to 6-month intervals without chemotherapy.

When the decision is made to initiate treatment, the objectives for therapy should be defined. Once the reasons for initiating chemotherapy are resolved, then treatment should be stopped, as no evidence indicates that continued maintenance therapy improves survival.

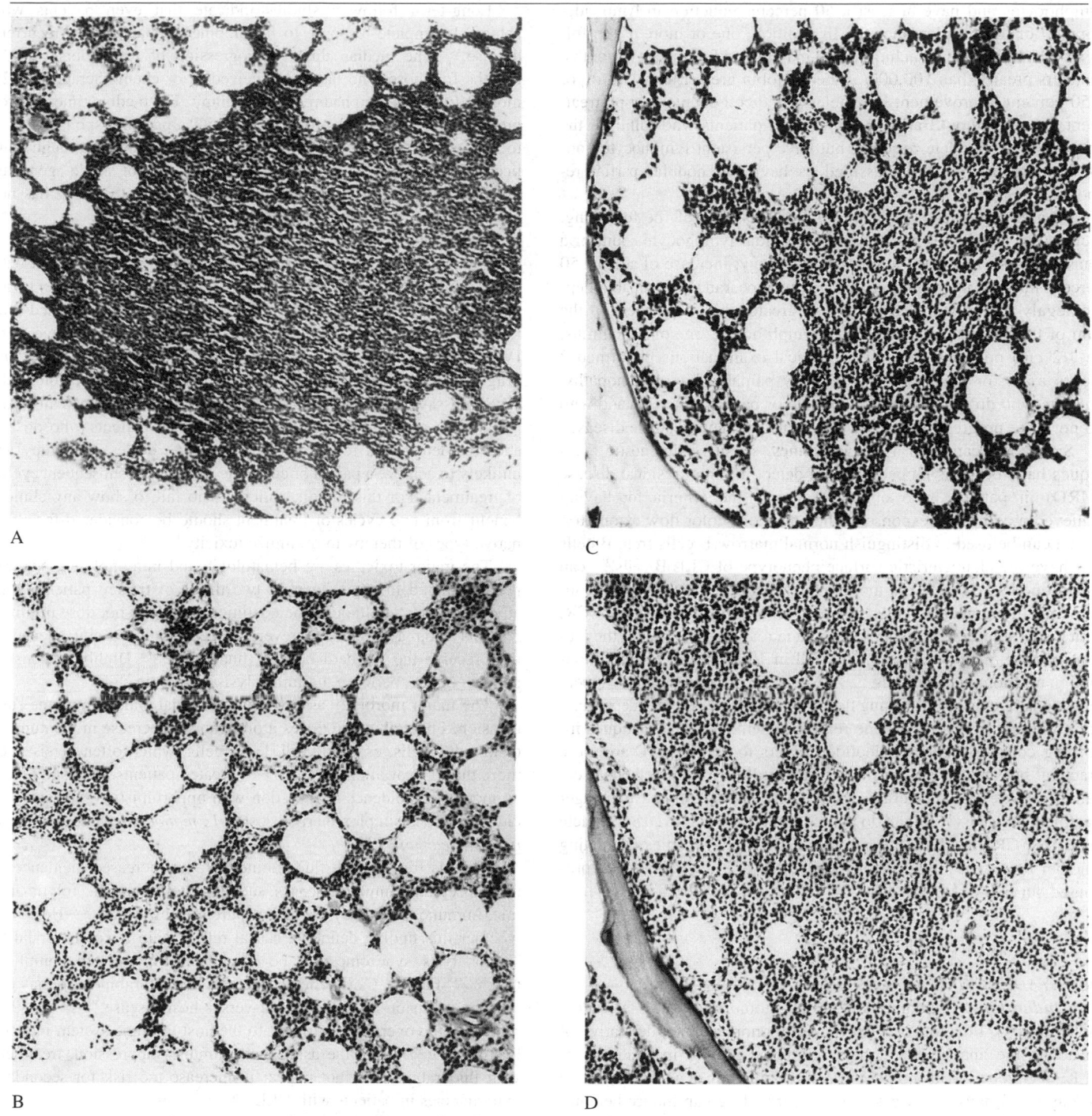

FIGURE 92-2 Photomicrographs of marrow sections demonstrating (A) nodular, (B) interstitial, (C) mixed nodular and interstitial, and (D) diffuse patterns of infiltration. (From GA Pangalis, PA Roussou, C Kittas, et al.,[266] with permission.)

Independent of the criteria listed in Table 92-4, patients who develop autoimmune hemolytic anemia (see Chap. 52), immune thrombocytopenia (see Chap. 110), or other pathologic autoimmune process warrant therapy appropriate for the autoimmune disease.

EVALUATING THE RESPONSE TO THERAPY

In 1996, a National Cancer Institute-sponsored Working Group recommended criteria with which to describe the response to therapy in CLL.[311] The definition of a complete response is largely clinical rather than biologic. A patient has a complete response when he/she becomes free of clinical disease for at least 2 months. The patient must maintain a normal complete blood, with at least 1500 neutrophils, 100,000 platelets, and fewer than 4000 lymphocytes per microliter of blood. The hemoglobin must be greater than 11 g/dl without requiring red cell transfusion. In addition, the patient must lack constitutional symptoms, hepatosplenomegaly, or detectable adenopathy. Finally, the marrow must contain fewer than 30 percent lymphocytes and lack lymphocyte nodules.

For a patient to classify as having a partial response, he/she must experience at least a 50 percent reduction in the number of blood lymphocytes and have at least a 50 percent reduction in lymphadenopathy or hepatosplenomegaly. In addition, one or more of the following criteria must be achieved and maintained for at least 2 months: platelets greater than $100,000/\mu l$, hemoglobin greater than 11 g/dl, or a 50 percent improvement in platelet or red cell counts over pretreatment values without transfusions. Treated patients who fulfill all the criteria for a complete response but have persistent lymphocyte nodules in the marrow are classified as having a nodular partial response.[311]

Progressive disease is defined by at least one of the following: increase of at least 50 percent in the absolute lymphocyte count or a transformation to a more aggressive histology; increase of at least 50 percent in liver or spleen size or the new appearance of palpable hepatomegaly or splenomegaly; increase greater than 50 percent in the sum of the products of at least two lymph nodes (one of which must be >2 cm) on two consecutive physical examinations performed 2 weeks apart; or the appearance of new palpable lymphadenopathy. Patients who do not achieve a complete or partial remission and who do not have progressive disease are defined as having stable disease.

Since publication of 1996 guidelines, sensitive diagnostic techniques have been developed that can detect minimal residual disease (MRD) in patients who otherwise satisfy the criteria for having achieved a complete response to therapy. Four-color flow cytometry, which can be used to distinguish normal marrow B cells from B cells that have the characteristic surface phenotype of CLL B cells,[371] can detect one leukemia cell in more greater than 10,000 to 100,000 nonleukemia mononuclear cells in blood or marrow specimens. PCR, which can amplify the distinctive Ig gene rearrangement(s) of the leukemia clone, may detect one CLL cell in 100,000 to 1,000,000 nonmalignant mononuclear cells.[372] As such, PCR-based methods appear more sensitive than those using flow cytometry but can vary depending upon the nature of the Ig gene rearrangement. Newer techniques involving consensus oligonucleotide primers to detect MRD are more practical but appear less sensitive.[373] Regardless of the methods used, patients who experience eradication of MRD apparently have a longer treatment-free survival than do patients who have achieved a complete response (CR) but have persistent MRD.[80,372,374] Studies evaluating whether treatment intended to eradicate MRD is associated with prolonged survival are in progress.

SINGLE-AGENT THERAPY

DEOXYADENOSINE ANALOGUES

Fludarabine Fludarabine (9-β-D-arabinofuranosyl-2-fluoradenine [F-ara-A], Fludara) is a fluorinated monophosphate derivative of an adenosine analogue that has significant activity in treatment of CLL.[375] Given as a 30-minute intravenous infusion at a dose of 25 mg/m^2/day for 5 days at 4-week intervals, this drug can induce hematologic complete and partial responses in a high percentage of patients.[80] An oral form of fludarabine that may have comparable activity has been developed.[376,377]

Multicenter trials typically have observed overall response rates to parenteral fludarabine of approximately 45 percent, including 10 percent with complete responses, in previously treated patients. Furthermore, overall response rates of approximately 70 percent, including 38 percent with complete responses, are achieved when fludarabine is given as front-line therapy.[378–381] Fludarabine, as a single agent, appears more effective in CLL than some combination chemotherapy regimens, such as CAP (cyclophosphamide 750 mg/m^2 and doxorubicin 50 mg/m^2 on day 1, prednisone 50 mg/m^2/ day on days 1–5).[382] Moreover, remission duration appears significantly longer in patients achieving a response with fludarabine than in those responding to such combination regimens.

Long-term followup studies indicate that even patients who achieved complete response to fludarabine ultimately have recurrent disease.[381] The median time to progression of responders was 33 months for those who had not received prior chemotherapy and 21 months for those who had received therapy. The median times to progression were 27 months for patients with a partial response and 30 to 37 months for those achieving a complete response. Although multicenter clinical trials have confirmed the activity of single-agent fludarabine in CLL,[378–380] treatment of patients with this drug has not been shown to improve overall survival.

Approximately one third of patients who have not received prior therapy and nearly half of those who are refractory to treatment with chlorambucil will not achieve even a partial response to treatment with fludarabine. Logistic regression analysis in one study identified four factors associated with poorer response to fludarabine: Rai stage III to IV disease, prior therapy, older age, and low albumin levels.[383] *In vitro* drug sensitivity testing using a differential staining cytotoxicity (DiSC) assay may have predictive value in identifying patients with fludarabine response disease.[384,385] In addition, patients who do not show evidence of a response to the first two cycles of therapy are unlikely to achieve a partial or complete response to subsequent cycles of treatment. For this reason, patients who fail to show any clinical benefit from two cycles of treatment should be considered for alternative types of therapy to minimize toxicity.

The major toxicities are hematologic and immunologic. Neutropenia is noted in approximately two thirds of treated patients with advanced disease, although the condition usually is not dose limiting. Patients also may experience reversible neurologic toxicity, even after they receive the standard dose of fludarabine.[386] Highly responsive patients may experience the tumor lysis syndrome.[387,388]

The major morbidity associated with fludarabine is immune suppression. Fludarabine produces a pronounced decrease in the number of blood T cells, especially CD4+ T cells, which often persists for more than 1 year after therapy.[389,390] Treated patients apparently have an increased incidence of infection with opportunistic organisms, including herpes simplex, herpes zoster, *L. monocytogenes*, and *Pneumocystis carinii*.[383,390,391]

Patients treated with fludarabine have an increased incidence of new-onset autoimmune diseases, such as autoimmune hemolytic anemia, immune thrombocytopenia, or pure red cell aplasia.[392] However, whether this finding defines a causal relationship is controversial.[393] Tumor lysis syndrome can be another therapy-related complication.[387,388] Finally, CLL patients treated with fludarabine also may develop transfusion-associated graft-versus-host disease,[394,395] possibly reflecting the overall impairment to the host immune system induced by the drug. Despite the associated immune suppression, treatment with fludarabine does not appear to increase the risk for secondary malignancies in patients with CLL.[396]

Cladribine Cladribine (2-chlorodeoxyadenosine) is another deoxyadenosine analogue that has activity in CLL.[397] Different dosage schedules or administration routes have proved effective, although the response rates do not appear to be better than those achieved with fludarabine. Monthly courses of cladribine given via intravenous infusion over 2 hours at 0.12 mg/kg/day for 5 consecutive days has resulted in overall response rates of approximately 40 to 60 percent in patients who previously were treated with alkylating agents.[398] Higher overall response rates are observed in previously nontreated patients. Although one study found that patients refractory to fludarabine still could respond to cladribine,[399] subsequent studies found that patients with advanced CLL refractory to fludarabine therapy were not likely to benefit from treatment with cladribine.[400]

Cladribine also appears effective when administered orally.[401] Overall response rates of 75 percent were noted in previously nontreated CLL patients given cladribine at 10 mg/m²/day for 5 consecutive days of each 28-day course[402] or 10 mg/m²/day orally for 3 consecutive days for each 21-day course.[401]

Treatment with cladribine has not been shown to prolong survival. The median duration of partial remissions is approximately 9 months, and nonresponding patients have a relatively short median survival of approximately 4 months. DiSC assays[384] reportedly have predictive value in assessing a given patient's potential response to therapy.[403] However, the most evident predictor of a good response was a rapid decrease of blood lymphocyte counts following the first course of therapy. As with fludarabine, patients who fail to show any clinical benefit from two cycles of cladribine should be considered for alternative types of therapy to minimize toxicity.

The toxicities of treatment with cladribine are similar to those with fludarabine. Thrombocytopenia is a common dose-limiting toxicity, as is general myelosuppression. As with fludarabine, treated patients experience long-lasting reductions in the levels of blood T cells and have impaired cellular immunity to viral infections. Systemic fungal infections and opportunistic infections are a common cause of morbidity and mortality. In rare cases, patients treated with cladribine experience tumor lysis syndrome.[404]

Pentostatin Pentostatin (deoxycoformycin, Nipent) is a purine analogue synthesized by *Streptomyces antibioticus* that is structurally related to adenosine.[405] This drug inhibits adenosine deaminase, an enzyme important in lymphocyte purine metabolism (see Chap. 68). Pentostatin generally is administered intravenously at a dosage of 4 mg/m²/week for 3 weeks, then 4 mg/m² every other week for 6 weeks and once per month for 6 months.[406] Alternative dosing regimens using pentostatin 2 mg/m²/day for 5 days every 28 days, with the dosage adjusted up or down by 0.5 mg/m² in subsequent cycles based on activity or hematologic toxicity, have been associated with improved response rates.[407] Studies using pentostatin in combination with other antileukemia agents are ongoing because of speculation that this drug has less myelotoxicity than other purine analogues.[408]

ALKYLATING AGENTS

Chlorambucil Since its introduction in 1952, chlorambucil (Leukeran) has been the main alkylating agent used for CLL. Although chlorambucil is useful in palliative therapy for advanced-stage disease, it does not appear to improve survival and should not be used for asymptomatic patients with early-stage disease.[409]

Given orally, chlorambucil generally is well tolerated, without the side effects that sometimes may be seen with other alkylating agents, such as cystitis, alopecia, or gastrointestinal distress. Some sparing of the myeloid and megakaryocytic series occurs. Generally patients are started on a daily oral dose of 2 to 4 mg, which can be advanced to 6 to 8 mg/day if the patient does not experience intolerable hematologic toxicity. Alternatively, patients can be treated intermittently with a total oral dose of approximately 0.4 to 0.7 mg/kg. This dose can be given on day 1 or divided into four equal daily doses and given on days 1 through 4. The cycle is repeated every 2 to 4 weeks, depending on the time to marrow recovery. Pulse chlorambucil is as effective as continuous administration and is less myelotoxic.[410] Complete response rates of 15 percent and partial response rates of 65 percent are common.[411]

Use of high-dose chlorambucil in patients with advanced-stage CLL has been studied.[412] Chlorambucil was given for less than 6 months at a fixed dose of 15 mg/day until the patient achieved a complete response or grade 3 toxicity. This treatment was noted in one single-institution study to result in a higher complete and partial response rate (89.5 percent) than that achieved with cyclophosphamide, doxorubicin, vincristine, and prednisone (CHOP; i.e., six monthly cycles of doxorubicin at 25 mg/m² on day 1, vincristine 1 mg/m² on day

1, cyclophosphamide 30 mg/m² per day, and prednisone 40 mg/m² per day on days 1–5). However, significant myelotoxicity was observed.

Cyclophosphamide Cyclophosphamide is as active as chlorambucil in CLL.[413] Patients can be started on daily oral doses of 50 to 100 mg. Alternatively, patients can be treated intermittently with 500 to 750 mg/m² given intravenously or orally every 3 to 4 weeks, depending on the time to marrow recovery. Because intermittent or daily oral cyclophosphamide predisposes to hemorrhagic cystitis, it should be taken as a single dose in the morning rather than at bedtime. Patients should be encouraged to drink at least 2 to 3 liters of fluid per day.

Bendamustine Bendamustine is an alkylating agent with apparent activity in CLL.[414] When used as a salvage treatment in patients with relapsed or refractory, heavily pretreated CLL, bendamustine 100 mg/m² (days 1 and 2) was effective in inducing complete hematologic remission in six of 21 patients, and another eight patients achieved a partial hematologic remission.[415] In another study, bendamustine was administered daily for 5 days per cycle at 60 mg/m² to patients with indolent lymphoma, including CLL, who previously had been treated with standard chemotherapy. Nearly three fourths of the CLL patients treated at intervals of 4 to 6 weeks achieved partial or complete responses; the median survival time was 32 months.[416] Similar to other alkylating agents, the main treatment-limiting toxicities are hematologic.

GLUCOCORTICOIDS

Glucocorticoids are effective as single agents in CLL, especially for patients with autoimmune hemolytic anemia or immune thrombocytopenia (see Chaps. 52 and 110). Even for nonautoimmune manifestations, prednisone as a single agent can control the disease temporarily in approximately 10 percent of patients.[410] Generally, prednisone is given orally at a dose of 40 to 60 mg/day for 1 week and then tapered and stopped after another week. Thereafter, prednisone 60 mg/day is given every month for 5 days.

Partial responses may be achieved by treatment with intravenous high-dose methylprednisolone at 1 g/m²/day for 5 days at monthly intervals for 7 months.[417] This treatment has apparent activity even in patients with CLL lacking functional p53.[418] Concomitant therapy with H_2 antagonists and prophylactic antibiotics can reduce the rate of treatment-related complications, which include fluid retention, hyperglycemia, and immune suppression.

OTHER AGENTS

Cytosine Arabinoside High-dose cytosine arabinoside has modest activity in advanced-stage CLL.[419] It is administered intravenously at a dosage of 3 g/m² delivered over 2 hours. This dosage can be repeated one to three times every 12 hours to complete one cycle.

Etoposide Patients who did not respond to alkylator-based chemotherapy have been noted to achieve partial responses lasting 2 to 18 months with oral etoposide.[420] Etoposide was administered as a single drug at a dosage of 50 mg/m² per day for 21 days in a 28-day cycle. Myelosuppression was the most common and serious dose-limiting effect.

Mitoxantrone Mitoxantrone, a topoisomerase II inhibitor, may have activity in CLL.[421] Most clinical studies have used mitoxantrone 6 to 10 mg/m² on day 1 of each cycle in combination with other antileukemia agents, such as cyclophosphamide and/or fludarabine,[422,423] cladribine,[424–426] bendamustine,[427] and/or rituximab.[426,428]

MONOCLONAL ANTIBODIES

Alemtuzumab Alemtuzumab (Campath-1H) is humanized monoclonal antibody-specific human CD52 that has been approved by the US Food and Drug Administration for treatment of patients with CLL that is refractory to commonly used drugs, such as chlorambucil and/or fludarabine (Fludara).[429] This antibody binds to a glycosyl phos-phatidylinositol-anchored surface protein found on most lymphocytes (see Chap. 14), including CLL B cells, and can induce complement-mediated and antibody-dependent cellular cytotoxicity.[430–432] In the seminal phase II study, patients with disease refractory to chemotherapy were given intravenous infusions of 30 mg CAMPATH-1H three times per week for 12 weeks.[433] Of the 29 patients who received the therapy, 38 percent experienced a partial remission and 4 percent achieved a complete remission, with median response duration of 12 months.

Similar thrice weekly dosing regimens have been used for subsequent studies.[434] Patients typically are given successively increasing doses of 1, 3, 10, and then 30 mg per injection to mitigate the infusional reactions of fever, chills, and/or rash, which generally are more pronounced during the initial administrations of this antibody. Grade 4 neutropenia is not uncommon but is not an indication to discontinue treatment. Also, alemtuzumab reduces the absolute numbers of blood natural killer cells and T lymphocytes to levels that are less than 25 percent of pretreatment values for more than 9 months following treatment.[435] As such, treated patients have an increased susceptibility to opportunistic infections (especially cytomegalovirus).[430,433,436,437]

Nevertheless, following 8 to 12 weeks of therapy, alemtuzumab is able to induce response rates of approximately 40 percent in heavily pretreated patients and/or more than 80 percent in symptomatic, previously untreated patients.[437] Clinicians should be cautious of prematurely terminating treatment at 4 to 6 weeks in patients whose disease responds to treatment. Although resolution of lymphocytosis occurs early in most patients, the marrow likely is not clear of disease during the first several weeks of treatment. Also, although this monoclonal antibody has significant activity against leukemia cells in the blood and marrow, it appears less effective in clearing cells in secondary lymphoid tissues,[438] where they might be protected from apoptosis by nurselike cells and other stromal elements. Of particular interest, this antibody appears capable of clearing leukemia cells that lack functional p53,[439] which typically are resistant to standard antileukemia drugs. For this reason, strategies incorporating use of alemtuzumab for treatment of patients with MRD following chemotherapy are being evaluated for their capacity to provide more effective therapy for patients with the disease.[371]

To mitigate the problems associated with intravenous alemtuzumab, such as fever, chills, and/or rash, alemtuzumab also has been administered subcutaneously at 30 mg three times per week for 6 or more weeks.[430] Although partial remissions were achieved, the duration of the response to alemtuzumab by either route is relatively short. Nevertheless, alemtuzumab may be of value in eradicating residual disease prior to autologous transplantation in patients with persistent disease after chemotherapy.[374,433,440]

Rituximab   Rituximab (Rituxan) is a monoclonal antibody specific for CD20 that initially was found effective for treatment of follicular lymphoma. Infusion of this rituximab at 375 mg/m^2/week for 4 weeks can induce responses in nearly half of patients treated with relapsed follicular lymphoma.[441,442]

Although CD20 is expressed at low levels by CLL B cells relative to the cells in follicular lymphoma, several clinical trials have demonstrated this monoclonal antibody has a therapeutic benefit in patients with CLL. When used as a single agent at the standard dose of four weekly injections of 375 mg/m^2, rituximab generally can induce only partial responses in less than one third of symptomatic patients.[443,444] Higher response rates may be achieved at higher doses. In one study, thrice weekly infusions of 375 mg/m^2 induced overall response rates of 45 percent in patients previously treated with chemotherapy.[445] In another study, response correlated with dose: 22 percent for patients treated with 500 to 825 mg/m^2, 43 percent for those treated with 1000

to 1500 mg/m^2, and 75 percent for those treated with the highest dose of 2250 mg/m^2.[446] These higher doses may be able to overcome soluble inhibitors to the CD20 monoclonal antibody that are found in the sera of most patients with CLL.[446,447] Nevertheless, the responses observed with even high doses of single-agent rituximab generally are only partial, limited mainly to the lymph nodes, and typically are associated with median times to disease progression of less than 8 months.[446]

Toxicity with the first dose (375 mg/m^2) can be as high as 94 percent of patients, but typically is only grade 1 or 2, predominantly fever and chills.[446] In rare instances, patients have experienced tumor lysis syndrome.[448] More commonly, patients experience a decline in the blood neutrophil count following treatment, sometimes resulting in neutropenia.[449] Finally, patients with leukemia cell counts exceeding 50×10^9/liter at the time of initial treatment may experience a cytokine release syndrome thought to result in part to release of TNF-α or interleukin-6.[450] Such patients experience fever, chills, nausea, vomiting, hypotension, and/or dyspnea during the initial infusion of rituximab. When severe, signs of mild disseminated intravascular coagulation may be evident within 12 hours after initiation of treatment (see Chap. 122). The severity of and risk for infusion-related reactions abate with successive infusions. Problems related to the initial treatment can be mitigated by slowing the infusion rate and splitting the first dose, giving 100 mg rituximab on the first day and then the remainder of the 375 mg/m^2 dose on day 2.

Other Biologic Agents   Other biologic agents for passive immune therapy of CLL are being evaluated. These include monoclonal antibodies or immunotoxins specific for other antigens expressed by CLL cells (e.g., CD23 [IDEC-152], HLA-DR determinants (Hu1D10), and even CD25 [denileukin diftitox, OTAK]).[451] Radiolabeled monoclonal antibodies, such as ibritumomab tiuxetan (Zevalin), also are being evaluated for their capacity to provide a therapeutic benefit. The use of radiolabeled monoclonal antibodies, however, is handicapped by the invariable infiltration of the marrow by CLL cells, making stem cell toxicity a significant concern.

COMBINATION THERAPY

CHLORAMBUCIL AND PREDNISONE

The standard regimen for treating patients who warrant the initiation of chemotherapy has been the combination of oral chlorambucil and prednisone. Each cycle consists of chlorambucil 0.4 to 0.7 mg/kg on day 1, with prednisone 80 mg/day on days 1 through 5. This course is repeated every 2 to 4 weeks, depending on the time to marrow recovery. The dosage of chlorambucil can be divided and given over 2 days. It is raised or lowered based upon the response and degree of myelosuppression. When the white cell count declines below 10,000/μl, the dose of chlorambucil should be reduced to maintain the white cell count between 5000/μl and 10,000/μl. The addition of prednisone to chlorambucil may provide a therapeutic advantage over chlorambucil alone.[411] However, later studies have challenged this notion.[452,453] Nevertheless, responses to the combination of chlorambucil and prednisone occur in approximately 80 percent (complete remissions in 15% plus partial remissions in 65%) of patients.[410,454–456] However, this regimen appears less active than other combination therapy regimens that include newer agents, such as the deoxyadenosine analogues and monoclonal antibodies.

FLUDARABINE-CONTAINING REGIMENS

Fludarabine/Cyclophosphamide   Combinations of fludarabine 20 to 30 mg/m^2/day for 3 days and cyclophosphamide 200 to 300 mg/m^2/day for 3 days given every 28 days can result in favorable clinical responses in extensively pretreated patients.[457] The daily administration of fludarabine 25 to 30 mg/m^2 for 3 days and cyclophosphamide

300 mg/m² for 3 days induced complete responses after four to six courses in 30 to 35 percent in previously untreated patients,[458-461] complete response rates that appear higher than those achieved using single-agent fludarabine.[462] The main complications of this regimen are related to immune suppression and myelosuppression, which can be dose limiting and severe, particularly in heavily pretreated patients. For this reason, fludarabine most commonly is given for 3 days per 28-day cycle at only 25 mg/m² along with cyclophosphamide at 250 mg/m².

Fludarabine/Cyclophosphamide/Rituximab Treatment with rituximab concomitant with fludarabine and cyclophosphamide appears highly effective. When given at 375 mg/m² on day 1 of course 1 and then at 500 mg/m² on day 1 of courses 2 through 6, rituximab when used with fludarabine/cyclophosphamide induced complete responses in 25 percent and overall responses in 73 percent of previously treated patients.[463] Moreover, 32 percent of the patients who achieved a complete response did not have evidence of MRD in the marrow by molecular testing. Higher response rates are observed in previously untreated patients. In one single-institution study of 224 patients, the complete response rate was 70 percent, the nodular partial response rate 10 percent, and the partial response rate 15 percent, for an overall response rate of 95 percent.[464] As with the fludarabine/cyclophosphamide regimen, the major toxicity was related to myelosuppression, with grade 3 to 4 neutropenia occurring during 52 percent of the courses in previously untreated patients.

Fludarabine/Rituximab Combined treatment with rituximab and standard doses of fludarabine generally appears well tolerated and more effective than treatment with single-agent fludarabine. In one study, previously untreated patients were given fludarabine at standard doses of 25 mg/m² on days 1 through 5, 29 through 33, 57 through 61, and 85 through 89, with rituximab 375 mg/m² on days 57, 85, 113, and 151. The overall response rate was 85 percent, with greater than 25 percent achieving a complete response.[465] In a larger multiinstitution study, previously untreated patients were randomized to receive six monthly courses of fludarabine followed 2 months later by rituximab consolidation therapy or six courses of fludarabine concurrently with rituximab.[466] Overall and complete responses were higher in the latter group, which received more rituximab. Patients in this group achieved a complete response rate of 47 percent and overall response rates of 90 percent. The toxicities of treatment were similar to those noted for patients treated with single-agent fludarabine. In multivariate analyses controlling for pretreatment characteristics, long-term follow-up of patients who received fludarabine and rituximab revealed that this group had a significantly better progression-free survival and overall survival than patients treated with fludarabine alone.[467]

Fludarabine/Mitoxantrone-Containing Regimens Treatment with fludarabine 30 mg/m² on days 1 through 3 of a 28-day cycle with mitoxantrone 10 mg/m² on the first day of each cycle has achieved overall response rates of 80 percent in previously nontreated patients and 60 percent in patients who were refractory to therapy with alkylating agents.[457] Subsequent study yielded response rates were 83 percent in previously untreated patients, 87 percent in patients previously treated with alkylating agents, 50 percent in patients whose disease was not refractory to fludarabine at the start of therapy, and 25 percent in patients whose disease was refractory to fludarabine.[423] Of note, only 20 percent of previously untreated patients who received this regimen achieved a complete response, a response rate that appeared not significantly different from that of single-agent fludarabine. Given this finding, use of this regimen does not appear to have a significant advantage over fludarabine alone.

The regimen of fludarabine 25 mg/m² given on days 1 through 3 of a 28-day cycle with cyclophosphamide 200 mg/m² on days 1 through 3 and mitoxantrone 10 mg/m² on the first day of each cycle

yielded complete responses of 50 percent (and overall responses of 78%) after a median of three cycles in patients who had relapsed or who were resistant to standard therapy.[422] Use of this regimen as salvage therapy is under investigation. Myelosuppression is the major dose-limiting toxicity.

Fludarabine/Cisplatin Cisplatin 100 mg/m² administered via continuous intravenous infusion over 4 days has been used in combination with fludarabine 30 mg/m² administered via bolus intravenous infusion on days 3 and 4 of a 28-day cycle.[468] These two drugs, alone or in combination with cytosine arabinoside 500 mg/m² on day 4 of the cycle, did not appear to offer significant benefit over that of single-agent fludarabine for treatment of patients refractory to alkylating agents. Its use as a salvage regimen is under investigation. Myelosuppression is the major dose-limiting toxicity.

Fludarabine/Prednisone Concomitant use of prednisone with fludarabine does not improve the response rate; rather, it increases the risk for opportunistic infection, resulting in poorer outcome than use of fludarabine alone.[381,383] Because of this finding, fludarabine/prednisone combinations are not recommended for patients with CLL.

Fludarabine/Chlorambucil Fludarabine has been used in combination with chlorambucil.[469] Chlorambucil 15 or 20 mg/m² was given orally on day 1, and fludarabine 10, 15, or 20 mg/m² was administered intravenously on days 1 to 5 every 28 days. With chlorambucil 15 mg/m² given on day 1, the maximum tolerated dose for fludarabine was 20 mg/m². Although responses were observed, treatment with this combination has not been shown to be significantly better than that with fludarabine alone.[469]

PENTOSTATIN-CONTAINING REGIMENS

Evaluation of the combination of pentostatin (Nipent) and cyclophosphamide in clinical trials involving relatively small numbers of patients suggest that this regimen may be effective in CLL. Treatment with pentostatin 4 mg/m² and cyclophosphamide 600 mg/m² given on day 1 of each 21-day course achieved complete and overall response rates of 17 percent and 74 percent, respectively, in fludarabine-refractory patients.[470]

Patients with symptomatic or progressive CLL received pentostatin 2 to 4 mg/m² on day 1 of the cycle with oral chlorambucil 30 mg/m² and prednisone 80 mg/day on days 1 through 5 of each 14-day cycle in one multiinstitution trial.[408] Patients who had no prior treatment or were insensitive first relapse achieved complete and overall response rates of 45 percent and 7 percent, respectively. In addition to myelosuppression, severe (grade 3+) infections were observed in 31 percent of treated patients, suggesting that this regimen is particularly immunosuppressive.

The activity of pentostatin or pentostatin and cyclophosphamide may be enhanced by coadministration of rituximab.[471] This option is undergoing evaluation.

CLADRIBINE-CONTAINING REGIMENS

The response to cladribine in combination with cyclophosphamide and prednisone has been evaluated in patients with CLL.[472] Patients received cladribine 0.1 mg/kg/day as a subcutaneous bolus injection on days 1 to 3, with intravenous cyclophosphamide 500 mg/m² on day 1 and oral prednisone 40 mg/m² on days 1 through 5 of a 28-day cycle for a maximum of six cycles. Overall response rates of 88 percent were observed, with four patients achieving a complete clinical and hematologic response and 12 achieving a partial response. In another phase II study, 27 previously untreated patients with CLL received six cycles of intravenous cyclophosphamide 1 g/m² plus oral prednisone 100 mg/m²/day for 5 days, followed by two to six cycles of 2-chlorodeoxyadenosine 5 mg/m²/day for 5 days.[473] This regimen yielded complete and overall response rates of 33 percent and 96 percent, respectively. The major toxicity was related myelosuppression.

Response rates to three courses of cladribine 4 mg/m²/day and cyclophosphamide 350 mg/m²/day for 3 days every 4 weeks in patients with refractory or recurrent CLL appeared inferior to the rates achieved in comparable patients treated with the combination of fludarabine and cyclophosphamide.[474] However, in another study, response rates comparable to that of fludarabine and cyclophosphamide (e.g., complete responses in 30% and overall responses in >80%) were observed in previously untreated patients treated with three to six courses of cladribine 0.12 mg/kg for 3 consecutive days and cyclophosphamide 650 mg/m² on day 1 of each 4-week course.[475] Addition of mitoxantrone to this regimen did not appear to enhance response rates in either previously untreated or refractory patients.[424] Unfortunately, randomized trials are lacking.

CYCLOPHOSPHAMIDE, VINCRISTINE, AND PREDNISONE

The combination of cyclophosphamide, vincristine, and prednisone (CVP) is effective in previously untreated patients and in some patients with refractory CLL.[476] The dosages are cyclophosphamide 300 to 400 mg/m²/day orally for 5 days, vincristine 1 to 2 mg intravenously on day 1, and prednisone 40 mg/m²/day orally for 5 days. The cycle is repeated every 3 to 4 weeks. Approximately 25 percent of patients achieve a complete remission, and approximately 50 percent obtain a partial remission when treated with this regimen.[476] No differences were noted in response rates or survival of CLL patients treated in randomized trials with either CVP versus chlorambucil and prednisone[456] or chlorambucil alone.[477]

Patients previously treated with chlorambucil and prednisone may respond to CVP. Prolonged therapy over a 12- to 18-month period may prolong survival.[454] In one series, patients in Rai stages III and IV had a median survival of 4.2 years following 18 months of therapy, with the median survival of complete responders greater than 60 months. This finding can be compared historically with the 19-month median survival reported in the mid-1970s for patients in stages III and IV.[23] However, treatment with CVP does not appear to offer advantages over treatment with deoxyadenosine analogues such as fludarabine.

CYCLOPHOSPHAMIDE, DOXORUBICIN, VINCRISTINE, AND PREDNISONE

The addition of doxorubicin to CVP chemotherapy (CHOP) has been evaluated in patients with advanced CLL.[478] These patients were treated with CVP; half also received doxorubicin 25 mg/m² on day 1. Adding doxorubicin to the chemotherapeutic regimen increased the median survival from less than 2 years to more than 4 years in one study. However, the mean survival of patients treated with CHOP was similar to that of patients who received CVP over an 18-month period. Vincristine does not appear to add substantially to the CHOP regimen. In a randomized multicenter clinical trial, patients with stage B or stage C CLL were treated with CHOP or with cyclophosphamide, doxorubicin, and prednisone without vincristine (CAP). The rates of partial response and overall response were 64 and 75 percent for the CHOP-treated patients and 65 and 72 percent for the CAP-treated patients, respectively.[478] However, these response rates compare unfavorably with the response of a third group of comparably staged CLL patients who were treated only with fludarabine; this group in the same study achieved partial or overall response rates of 75 and 94 percent, respectively. This finding is consistent with other studies showing that fludarabine appears more effective as a single agent in CLL than these combination regimens.[479]

SPLENECTOMY

Splenectomy may ameliorate the cytopenias associated with advanced-stage CLL, particularly thrombocytopenia.[480–482] In one study, patients who underwent splenectomy for thrombocytopenia and/or anemia had a trend toward improved 3-year actuarial survival ($31 \pm 9\%$) over matched subjects who did not undergo splenectomy ($12 \pm 7\%$).[481] Preoperative performance status appeared to be the best predictor of perioperative and postoperative survival. Laparoscopic and hand-assisted laparoscopic surgery can be used to remove enlarged spleens[483,484] or accessory spleens,[485] thereby reducing the blood loss and required length of hospitalization from that required for standard splenectomy.

RADIATION THERAPY

Systemic irradiation was the first therapeutic modality used in CLL that resulted in some degree of patient improvement.[11] However, the therapeutic benefit was short lived and often resulted in severe marrow suppression.[486]

Irradiation remains a useful technique for localized treatment to ameliorate symptoms resulting from nerve impingement, vital organ compromise, painful bone lesions, or bulky disfigurement. Delivery of 20 Gy in divided doses can result in rapid shrinkage of lymph nodes or masses.

Splenic irradiation is useful in patients with painful splenomegaly,[487] especially in patients considered poor candidates for surgical splenectomy.[488] Patients may experience systemic improvement after splenic irradiation, possibly because of irradiation of leukemic cells circulating through the spleen. However, the low rate of response and the short remission duration argue that splenic irradiation should be combined with other therapeutic approaches.[489]

Endolymphatic radiotherapy[490] and extracorporeal irradiation of blood[491] appear to provide limited improvement in lymphocyte counts but do not appear to improve patient survival. Extracorporeal photochemotherapy also has been attempted for B cell CLL but was found to be ineffective.[492]

LEUKAPHERESIS

Intensive leukapheresis may reduce organomegaly and improve hemoglobin and platelet levels.[493] The measure has been advocated for patients with marrow failure who are refractory to standard therapy.[494] In addition, leukapheresis has been used successfully to treat patients with extreme lymphocytosis to ameliorate clinical symptoms associated with leukostasis and lower the risk for incurring adverse reactions to subsequent antileukemia therapy.[495]

SUPPORTIVE MEASURES

Platelet transfusions may be required for patients with active bleeding who have drug- or disease-related thrombocytopenia (see Chap. 132). Similarly, patients with symptomatic anemia resulting from autoimmune hemolytic anemia (see Chap. 52) or leukemia cell infiltration of the marrow may require transfusions with leukocyte-depleted pack red blood cells (see Chap. 131). Use of recombinant erythropoietin may obviate or reduce the frequency of blood transfusions.

ERYTHROPOIETIN

Treatment of patients who acquire anemia as a disease-related complication may benefit from treatment with recombinant human erythropoietin.[496–499] The patients most likely to improve are those with relatively low levels of erythropoietin.[500] Nevertheless, patients with normal erythropoietin levels and anemia secondary to leukemia cell infiltration of the marrow still may benefit from treatment, starting with thrice weekly injections of epoetin alfa (Procrit or Epogen) at 150 IU/kg or weekly injections of darbepoetin alfa (Aranesp) 0.45 μg/kg. Response requires maintenance therapy to maintain hemoglobin levels at or above 12 g/dl.[501] Patients who do not respond after 4 to 6 weeks of therapy may respond to increased doses of erythropoietin. Those not responding to this increased dose after 4 weeks likely will not benefit from continued erythropoietin therapy.

INVESTIGATIONAL THERAPIES

HEMATOPOIETIC STEM CELL TRANSPLANTATION

Autologous Stem Cell Transplantation Several studies have examined the benefit of high-dose chemotherapy with stem cell rescue in patients with CLL (see Chap. 22). Complicating autologous stem cell transplantation is the high probability that stem cell collections are contaminated with CLL cells, even in patients who have been treated to MRD.[502–504] This finding prompted investigation into more effective purging techniques for removing unwanted leukemia cells prior to transplantation. Nevertheless, a few studies with small numbers of patients showed that complete clinical responses can be achieved in CLL.[505–507] However, long-term followup of treated patients have provided little evidence of a plateau in the survival curves, suggesting that, at best, autologous stem cell transplantation only prolongs disease-free survival.[508]

Allogeneic Stem Cell Transplantation Transplantation with allogeneic stem cells is being evaluated for younger patients with poor-prognosis CLL.[372,509–513] Treatment-related morbidity rates in some series have been high, occurring in approximately half the treated patients.[510] Autologous transplantation requires elimination of leukemia cells that invariably are found in the marrow following conventional treatments. Aggressive treatment may eradicate the leukemia cells to levels that cannot be detected using molecular techniques sensitive for clonal Ig gene rearrangements.[372] Patients who relapse following allogeneic marrow transplantation may respond to infusions of donor leukocytes, demonstrating the effectiveness of a graft-versus-leukemia effect.[512,513] Collectively, these studies provide encouraging evidence that transplantation may be curative in a subset of patients with CLL.[514]

Nonmyeloablative Allogeneic Stem Cell Transplantation Because patients who receive allogeneic cells appear to benefit from a graft-versus-leukemia response, several groups are investigating the use of nonmyeloablative allogeneic stem cell transplantation for patients with CLL refractory to standard therapy.[515–519] Patients are treated with moderate conditioning regimens, such as low-dose total body irradiation or fludarabine–cyclophosphamide combinations, prior to receiving allogeneic stem cells. Generally, complete chimerism, as well as best response, is not achieved immediately posttransplant but may require more than 3 months to develop. Initial treatment-related mortality is lower than that observed for patients treated with standard allogeneic stem cell transplantation, although patients still have a high risk for serious morbidity or mortality secondary to chronic graft-versus-host disease (see Chap. 22). This risk appears to increase following donor leukocyte infusion. Nevertheless, patients with refractory CLL can experience eradication of MRD several weeks following transplant, providing evidence for a graft-versus-leukemia effect.[517–519]

ACTIVE IMMUNE THERAPY AND GENE THERAPY

Cellular vaccines involving the leukemia cell that is modified to enhance its capacity to induce an immune response or dendritic cells pulsed with putative leukemia-associated antigens are under investigation.[520–522] Another strategy is to modify the leukemia cell through transduction of an adenovirus encoding the ligand for CD40 (CD154)

(see Chap. 26). Ligation of CD40 can induce CLL cells to express immune costimulatory molecules that are required for stimulation of allogeneic or autologous T cells. Because CLL cells stimulated in this fashion can induce generation of autologous cytotoxic T cells,[232] methods for ligating CD40 have been incorporated into strategies for treating the disease. Treatment of patients with autologous leukemia cells transduced with Ad-CD154 showed promising results in a phase I clinical study.[523]

DISEASE COMPLICATIONS

INFECTION

Infection is a major cause of morbidity and mortality in CLL.[224,524] Patients generally develop worsening hypogammaglobulinemia and often have an impaired antibody response to microbes and hypogammaglobulinemia, making these patients highly susceptible to recurrent infection. *Streptococcus pneumoniae, Staphylococcus aureus, Streptococcus pyogenes, Escherichia coli,* and the herpes zoster-varicella virus account for most infections. The lungs, skin, and urinary tract are the sites most frequently affected.[524] Fungal, mycobacterial, and cryptococcal infections are uncommon. However, patients treated with purine analogues, such as fludarabine, apparently have an increased incidence of infection with other opportunistic organisms, including herpes simplex, cytomegalovirus, herpes zoster, *Listeria monocytogenes, P. carinii,* and mycobacteria.[383,390,391,525,526] Multivariate analysis identified that disease activity and prior therapy are stronger risk factors than hypogammaglobulinemia for developing serious infections.[527]

Infections usually respond well to antibiotics in CLL patients with early-stage disease. However, at later stages, the response is less satisfactory and more often associated with systemic complications. For such patients antibiotics often must be administered for prolonged periods to eradicate soft tissue or urinary tract infection. Patients can be immunized with nonviable vaccines, such as those used to immunize patients against influenza or *S. pneumoniae.* However, the response to immunization often is poor. Use of live vaccines is contraindicated because of the risk that the attenuated agent will be virulent in the immunocompromised host.

Patients with advanced-stage disease, hypogammaglobulinemia, and low levels of specific antibodies to pneumococcal capsular polysaccharide appear to be at greatest risk for severe or multiple infections.[528,529] Immunoglobulin deficiency is the factor that correlates best with the frequency, severity, and pattern of infection.[524] For this reason, investigators have examined the benefit of treating patients who have severe hypogammaglobulinemia associated with recurrent infections with intravenous γ-globulin 240 to 400 mg/kg every 3 to 4 weeks. Treated patients may experience a decreased frequency of bacterial infections,[530] even when given the lower dose of 240 mg/kg every 4 weeks.[531]

Many of the treatments for CLL are immune suppressive and can enhance the risk for opportunistic infections. Patients treated with alemtuzumab can experience reactivation of cytomegalovirus, which can be treated effectively by oral gancyclovir.[227] Patients treated with deoxyadenosine analogues such as fludarabine have a higher risk for complications related to virus infections, such as those caused by herpes zoster.[532] To mitigate this problem, some treatment regimens incorporate use of oral acyclovir at 400 mg twice daily for patients undergoing therapy.[533]

SYSTEMIC AUTOIMMUNE DISEASE

CLL patients have an increased risk of autoimmune disease.[534] Prednisone at a dosage of 1 mg/kg/day is used to treat autoimmune hemolytic anemia or immune thrombocytopenia and can be tapered slowly to the minimum dosage necessary. Case reports suggest that rituximab may be effective in patients refractory to glucocorticoids.[535] Chapters 52 and 110 discuss these diseases and various treatment regimens for refractory disease. For CLL patients who develop pure red cell aplasia presumed secondary to pathogenic autoantibodies, the combination of cyclosporine and prednisone appears superior to prednisone alone.[536]

SECOND MALIGNANCIES

Patients with CLL are at increased risk for second malignancies.[524,537–539] The most frequent second tumors are melanoma, soft tissue sarcoma, and colorectal, lung, and basal cell skin carcinoma. Patients with CLL also apparently experience higher recurrence rates of basal cell carcinoma after Mohs surgery than does the general population.[540] Multiple myeloma occurs at 10 times the expected rate in patients with CLL[541] but evidently does not arise from the same malignant B cell clone.[542–544] Both untreated and treated CLL patients can develop acute myelogenous leukemia or myelodysplastic syndrome.[545,546] The concurrence of acute myeloid leukemia (AML) or myelodysplastic syndrome (MDS) and untreated CLL may represent two separate disease processes. Nucleoside analogues do not appear to enhance the risk for secondary malignancies.[396] However, for some patients, alkylating agents may contribute to the development of second malignancy. In one large multicenter trial, patients with stage A CLL who were treated with intermittent chlorambucil had a poorer survival than a matched control group of untreated CLL patients, in part because they experienced a higher incidence of epithelial neoplasms.[547]

RICHTER TRANSFORMATION

DEFINITION AND HISTORY

In 1928, Maurice N. Richter[548] described an aggressive lymphoma that developed in a patient with CLL. Now described as Richter transformation, this transition from an indolent leukemia to an aggressive, large B cell, high-grade lymphoma can occur at any time during the course of CLL, occurring in approximately 3 percent of all patients at a median interval of 2 years following the initial diagnosis of CLL.[358,549,550]

ETIOLOGY AND PATHOGENESIS

Nucleic acid sequence analyses of the Ig genes expressed by the original leukemic cells and the high-grade lymphomas of patients with Richter transformation demonstrated that such lymphomas can arise from the original CLL clone.[551,552] Although such lymphomas are suggested to primarily derive from CLL cells that express unmutated Ig genes,[553] CLL cells that express mutated Ig genes also may develop into aggressive lymphomas that express clonally related Ig genes.[550,551] In approximately one fourth of all cases of apparent Richter transformation, however, the lymphoma cells use Ig genes that are distinct from those of the original CLL clone.[552–555] Conceivably, some of these cases may represent cases of coincident B cell malignancies that develop in patients with preexisting CLL.[556,557]

The chromosomal abnormalities in the lymphoma cells of patients with Richter transformation typically are complex and commonly include del 8p, del 9p, del 11q (11q23), 12+, del 13q, 14q+, del 17p, del 20,[131,159,358,550,558,559] and/or translocations involving chromosome 12.[558,560] Trisomy 12 and chromosome 11 abnormalities are more frequent in patients with Richter transformation than in the overall population of patients with CLL. In some cases the lymphoma cells have inactivating mutations or deletions in the p53 tumor suppressor gene, the *ATM* gene, p16INK4A, the *RB* gene, or p21, increased copy number of c-*myc*, and/or loss or decreased expression of p27 or a-*myb*.[133,559]

In some cases the lymphoma cells have microsatellite instability that was not seen in the original leukemia cell population.[561] One case had a 12q13 translocation with chromosome 6 involving the high-mobility group (nonhistone chromosomal) protein isoform I-C (*HMGI-C*) gene, which was expressed by the large-cell lymphoma cell.[560] These genetic lesions often are not found in the original leukemia clone even when the lymphoma cells share expression of the same Ig genes, suggesting that such changes are acquired as secondary/tertiary events in disease evolution.[558,559]

CLINICAL AND LABORATORY FEATURES

The most common clinical and laboratory features associated with Richter transformation (with their respective incidence indicated in parentheses) include (1) elevation of serum lactate dehydrogenase (82%), (2) rapid lymph node enlargement (64%), (3) systemic symptoms of fever and/or weight loss (59%), (4) monoclonal gammopathy on serum protein electrophoresis (44%), and (5) extranodal disease (41%).[358] Patients also may have abdominal symptoms resulting from increasing hepatosplenomegaly or neurologic disorders secondary to central nervous system involvement.[562–564] Occasional patients present with an extranodal mass lesion.[565–567] Patients with Richter transformation often have bulky retroperitoneal adenopathy and massive splenomegaly.

Not all patients with CLL and rapid lymph node enlargement have Richter transformation. Infection with herpes simplex virus can cause acute lymphadenitis.[568] Excisional lymph node biopsy of affected lymph nodes demonstrates zonal necrosis because of herpes simplex infection that can be distinguished from the large cell lymphoma of patients with Richter transformation. Such patients usually respond well to appropriate antiviral therapy.

For this reason, the diagnosis of Richter transformation generally requires lymph node or marrow biopsy. Involved lymph nodes typically are effaced by large immunoblastic cells with abundant basophilic cytoplasm and irregular nuclei with prominent nucleoli.[293] The typical morphology is similar to that of diffuse large B cell lymphoma, immunoblastic variant, according to the World Health Organization classification (see Chap. 90).[569] However, descriptions of the lymphoma cells in tissue vary from this finding to that of a diffuse and monotonous collection of centroblasts or centroblasts intermingled with immunoblasts, similar to what the REAL classification currently describes as diffuse large B cell lymphoma, centroblastic variant.[550] In rare cases, plasmablastic lymphoma cells predominate.[570] Regardless of the histology, the lymphoma cells in Richter transformation typically lack or have weak expression of CD5 and/or IgD, even cases that are clonally related to an original CLL clone that expresses these surface antigens.

Occasional cases of Richter transformation have histology resembling that of Hodgkin lymphoma (see Chap. 97), termed *Richter syndrome with Hodgkin disease features*.[571–580] These cases account for less than one fifth of all cases of Richter transformation, occurring in approximately 0.5 percent of all patients with CLL.[133,314] In such cases the involved lymph nodes have histologic and immunostaining features of Hodgkin disease (see Chap. 97), including typical Hodgkin/Reed-Sternberg cells that may express CD15 and/or CD30. Studies on the expressed Ig genes using single-cell PCR techniques found that Hodgkin/Reed-Sternberg cells were derived from the same clone as the CLL cells in two of three cases examined.[581] In contrast, another similar study found that the Hodgkin/Reed-Sternberg cells in two cases had Ig gene rearrangements distinct from those of the original CLL clone.[580] Nevertheless, other studies suggest that the Hodgkin/Reed-Sternberg cells in most cases may be derived from the original CLL clone.[574] Infection with EBV is implicated as playing a possible pathogenic role in those cases where the Hodgkin/Reed-Sternberg cells are not related to the original CLL clone.[572,580] Such cases have been argued to represent a possible complication of therapy with purine analogues or other agents that may impair immune surveillance.[577,578,580]

THERAPY, COURSE, AND PROGNOSIS

Regimens similar to those used to treat high-grade lymphomas, such as diffuse large cell lymphoma, commonly are used to treat patients with Richter syndrome (see Chap. 96). Although occasional patients have achieved long-term remissions following intensive multiagent chemotherapy,[564] most patients at best achieve only a partial remission and have a very poor prognosis. Various combination therapies are under investigation,[582] including regimens incorporating fludarabine, cytarabine, cyclophosphamide, cisplatin,[583] or fractionated cyclophosphamide, vincristine, liposomal daunorubicin, and dexamethasone (hyper-CVXD) plus rituximab and GM-CSF alternating with methotrexate and cytarabine plus rituximab and GM-CSF.[584]

Patients with apparent Richter syndrome with characteristics similar to those of Hodgkin disease may respond favorably to therapy for Hodgkin lymphoma[579] (see Chap. 97). However, most patients with such characteristics have refractory disease and a clinical course similar to that of patients with classic Richter transformation.[573] Overall, patients with Richter transformation have median survival of 5 months from diagnosis.[358]

CHRONIC LYMPHOCYTIC LEUKEMIA /PROLYMPHOCYTIC LEUKEMIA AND PROLYMPHOCYTIC TRANSFORMATION

In nearly 15 percent of B cell CLL patients, the population of leukemic cells consists of a mixture of small lymphocytes and prolymphocytes, the latter cell type accounting for 10 to 50 percent of the lymphoid cells.[585,586] These patients have been termed to have CLL/PLL, although this term is not in frequent use. These patients have a degree of lymphadenopathy and age distribution similar to that of patients with CLL but more pronounced splenomegaly. In 80 percent of CLL/PLL cases, the proportion of prolymphocytes remains stable, and survival does not differ from that of CLL patients with comparable clinical-stage disease.[587] Such patients generally do not have blood prolymphocyte counts greater than 15,000/μl or massive splenomegaly.

The remaining patients with CLL/PLL undergo a prolymphocytic transformation. This transformation is characterized by a decrease in the proportion of leukemic cells able to form rosettes with mouse erythrocytes, increases in the proportions of blood lymphocytes with prolymphocyte morphology and immunophenotype, and progressive splenomegaly. One study noted the leukemic cells in transformation apparently acquired the t(6;12) translocation that commonly is associated with PLL.[588] Patients with this transformation respond poorly to chemotherapy, and survival is limited. In one study, the mean survival of patients after transformation to PLL was 9 months.[589]

ACUTE LYMPHOBLASTIC LEUKEMIA

Very rarely, patients with B cell CLL develop acute lymphoblastic leukemia.[590] Studies of a few of the dozen cases reported indicate that the acute leukemia can arise from the same B cell clone as that of the CLL cells.[591–594] Blastic transformation has been associated with a sevenfold to eightfold increase in the expression of c-myc and Ig genes.[594] Leukemic blast cells generally express terminal deoxynucleotidyl transferase and high levels of surface Ig and HLA-DR.

PROGNOSIS

No established cures exist for CLL, and spontaneous remissions are extremely rare.[595,596] Nevertheless, the prognosis can vary substantially among different patients, depending upon clinical stage and the pres-

ence or absence of disease features that have been associated with disease progression and/or a more adverse clinical outcome (see "Clinical Staging" above). Studies suggest that newer treatment regimens, incorporating agents such as fludarabine and rituximab, may improve the length of survival.[467]

Patient age had been argued to be an independent prognostic factor.[345,357,597,598] Overall, the 5-year survival rate in the United States is 83 percent for those younger than 65 years and 68 percent for those older than 65 years.[1] However, a large study from the US National Cancer Data Base revealed that the 5-year relative survival was 69.5 percent, 72.2 percent, 63.1 percent, and 41.7 percent for age groups under 40, 40 to 59, 60 to 79, and 80+ years, respectively, indicating that the 5-year survival does not vary significantly among these different age groups.[2] As such, it appears that CLL, and not comorbid disease, caused the greatest percentage of deaths, even among the aged.

Another study also found that younger and older patients have a similar overall median survival probability but had different distributions of causes of deaths.[314] CLL-unrelated deaths and secondary malignancies predominated in the older age group, whereas the direct effects of leukemia were prevalent in the younger age group. At diagnosis, younger and older patients displayed a similar distribution of clinical features, except for a significantly higher male-to-female ratio in younger patients (2.85 vs. 1.29; $p < 0.0001$). Both groups had an elevated rate of second malignancies (8.3% vs. 10.7%), whereas the occurrence of Richter syndrome was significantly higher in younger patients (5.9% vs. 1.2%; $p < 0.00001$). Two subsets of young CLL patients with a different prognostic outcome could be identified. One group, comprising 40 percent of patients younger than 55 years, had long-lasting stable disease without treatment and an actuarial survival probability of 94 percent at 12 years from diagnosis. The remaining patients had progressive disease and a median survival probability of 5 years after therapy.[314] A key feature of patients with the more adverse prognosis is evidence of disease progression.[599]

B CELL PROLYMPHOCYTIC LEUKEMIA

HISTORY AND DEFINITION

B cell PLL is a clinical and morphologic variant of CLL that first was described as a distinct entity in 1973.[600] It is a subacute lymphoid leukemia with an incidence that is approximately 10 percent that of CLL. The diagnosis of PLL requires that at least 55 percent of the circulating leukemic lymphocytes have a prolymphocytic morphology.[585] Such cells are larger than resting lymphocytes and have a high nucleocytoplasmic ratio, a basophilic cytoplasm devoid of granules, moderately condensed chromatin, and a single prominent nucleolus. In 80 percent of such cases, the prolymphocytes are neoplastic B cells,[601] whereas the remaining cases are derived from mature T cells.

ETIOLOGY AND PATHOGENESIS

The etiology is unknown. There is a 4:1 male to female predominance, suggesting that males are much more susceptible to developing this disease. Also, B cell PLL can evolve from B cell CLL.[586] As such, factors that contribute to the pathogenesis or progression of CLL may operate in B cell PLL.

CYTOGENETICS

The karyotype of the leukemia cells from many patients displays the 14q+ abnormality.[602] Trisomy 12 is another recurrent abnormality.[603,604] Deletions of the long arm of chromosome 6 (6q−) and rearrangement affecting chromosomes 1 and 12 are observed occasionally. One study observed a t(6;12)(q15;p13) chromosomal anomaly in several independent cases, leading the investigators to postulate that this anomaly is distinctive for a subset of patients with PLL.[588] The (2;13)(q35;q14) translocation that commonly is associated with pediatric rhabdomyosarcoma has been identified.[605]

The most common abnormalities identified using cytogenetics and FISH analysis is deletion 13q14 (46%), trisomy 12 (21%), and 14q32 rearrangements (21%).[606] Loss of heterozygosity at 17p13.3 associated with inactivating mutations in the *TP53* gene is observed in as many as three fourths of the cases examined.[154,607,608] The high frequency of p53 mutations in B cell PLL is in marked contrast to that observed in B cell CLL and may explain the relative resistance of this disease to therapy. In addition, some cases of B cell PLL have t(2;8) translocations involving the c-*myc* gene that are similar to those observed in Burkitt lymphoma (see Chap. 96).[609] Such mutations may account for the aggressive clinical course of PLL relative to that of B cell CLL.

CYTOGENESIS

B cell PLL is derived from mature B cells that have undergone Ig gene rearrangement (see Chap. 76). These cells invariably have monoclonal Ig gene rearrangements and express many of the same B cell surface antigens, as do leukemic cells in CLL. In many cases, the disease may evolve from preexistent CLL. The Igs expressed by PLL cells frequently bear autoantibody-associated cross-reactive idiotypes, suggesting a biased use of Ig variable region genes similar to that of leukemic cells in B cell CLL.[610] However, sequence analyses indicate the PLL cells from at least half of the patients express nonmutated variable region genes, whereas the remaining cases express mutated variable region genes.[611] The presence of such somatic mutations suggests that the B cell PLL cells from at least some individuals are derived from a postgerminal center B cell (see Chaps. 5 and 77).

CLINICAL FEATURES

More than 50 percent of patients are older than 70 years at diagnosis. Presenting symptoms include fatigue, weakness, weight loss, an acquired bleeding tendency, or early satiety with abdominal discomfort because of splenomegaly. Splenomegaly is massive in nearly two thirds of patients. The liver may be enlarged. Nevertheless, patients typically have minimal palpable lymphadenopathy.

In rare cases, patients present with leukemic meningitis,[612,613] leukemic pleural effusion,[614] or malignant ascites.[615] A few patients develop cardiopulmonary complications because of leukostasis associated with extreme leukocytosis.[616]

LABORATORY FEATURES

More than three fourths of patients have blood lymphocyte counts greater than 100,000/μl.[288,295] The marrow commonly is infiltrated diffusely with neoplastic prolymphocytes. At autopsy, these cells are found to have infiltrated most other organs.[603] At presentation, patients commonly have a normochromic and normocytic anemia, with blood hemoglobin less than 11 g/dl and/or blood platelet counts less than 100,000/μl. As in CLL, patients commonly have hypogammaglobulinemia.[617] However, many patients have a monoclonal gammopathy on serum protein electrophoresis.

PLL B cells express B cell differentiation antigens similar to those of B cell CLL. However, expression of CD5 is variable.[585] Even in cases that evolved from CD5+ CLL B cells, the leukemia cells have low to negligible expression of CD5 (see Table 92-1). Also, in contrast to CLL B cells, PLL cells generally express very high levels of surface Ig, usually IgM with or without IgD[618] and react strongly with the antibody FMC7. In addition, PLL cells generally express high levels of CD22 and often are negative for CD23. Finally, in contrast to CLL B cells, PLL B cells generally stain brightly with SN8, a monoclonal antibody specific for CD79b (see Chaps. 14 and 77).[289,290]

THERAPY, COURSE, AND PROGNOSIS

At presentation, patients commonly have advanced-stage disease that requires treatment. Most patients present with prominent splenomegaly and hyperleukocytosis and have rapid progression soon after diagnosis. Nevertheless, some patients may have a more indolent course.[619] As such, the indications for therapy are similar to those used for patients with CLL. These indications include disease-related symptoms, symptomatic splenomegaly, progressive marrow failure, or a blood prolymphocyte count greater than 200,000/μl.

Treatments for patients with PLL are similar to those for patients with CLL. Alkylating agents similar to those used in CLL are commonly used. However, chlorambucil or cyclophosphamide, in combination with prednisone and/or vincristine, typically yield response rates of less than 20 percent.[585] Treatment with high-dose glucocorticoids appears less effective for patients with PLL than for those with CLL.[417] Partial and complete responses have been observed in approximately half the patients treated with intensive combination chemotherapy regimens similar to those used for treatment of high-grade lymphomas (see Chap. 96), such as CHOP. Unfortunately, responses are relatively short lasting. Although occasional patients respond to salvage regimens,[620,621] the long-term survival is generally poor. Use of rituximab for treatment of PLL appears promising.[622]

The deoxyadenosine analogues are active in this disease. Cladribine 0.1 mg/kg/day for 7 days by continuous infusion every 28 to 35 days has been noted to induce complete and partial remission in approximately half of patients with *de novo* B cell PLL.[623–625] Similarly, fludarabine 30 mg/m² over 30 minutes daily for 5 days every 4 weeks produced complete and partial remissions in nearly 40 percent of patients treated.[626] In another study, the response rates to fludarabine were similar to the rates noted for B cell CLL.[627] Rapid response to fludarabine may be complicated by the tumor lysis syndrome.[628,629] Pentostatin also appears effective, although less so than fludarabine. Twenty patients with PLL were treated with pentostatin (2'deoxycoformycin) at a dosage of 4 mg/m² intravenously once per week for 3 weeks, then every other week for three doses. The major hematologic toxicity of this regimen was thrombocytopenia. Although 45 percent achieved a partial remission, no patients achieved a complete response. The median duration of remission was 9 months. Patients with B cell PLL had a higher rate of response and duration of remission (12 months) than those with disease of T cell origin.[630] However, pentostatin also has some activity in T cell PLL.[631]

Splenectomy may ameliorate symptoms, but only transiently.[480] Splenic irradiation, with 10 to 16 Gy delivered in divided doses to the splenic bed, has been advocated as a primary therapy for this disease,[632,633] especially for symptomatic patients who are considered poor candidates for chemotherapy and/or splenectomy.[634]

Case reports indicate that interferon-α can be effective in inducing cytoreduction in PLL.[635–637] One case of a patient who achieved a 5-year survival following a complete response to interferon-α following splenic irradiation has been reported.[638] However, generally interferon-α appears less effective than chemotherapy. Spontaneous remissions are extremely rare.[639]

T CELL PROLYMPHOCYTIC LEUKEMIA

DEFINITION AND HISTORY

In 1989, the French-American-British (FAB) Cooperative Group distinguished five subgroups of T cell leukemia, namely, T cell CLL, T cell PLL, human T lymphotropic virus type I-positive (HTLV-I+), adult T cell leukemia/lymphoma, and Sézary syndrome.[640] When a new entity called *large granular lymphocytic leukemia* was defined (see Chap. 94), the existence of T cell CLL as a distinct entity became a topic of debate.[641–644] Because of this finding, the World Organization commissioned a panel of experts to draft a new classification of the hematologic neoplasms.[645] At a meeting in November 1997, the panel proposed a categorization of peripheral T cell neoplasms that largely was based on the Revised European-American Lymphoma (REAL) classification (see Chap. 90).[646] However, because of its aggressive clinical behavior, T cell CLL was reclassified under the heading of T cell PLL, without regard to subtle differences in morphology.[647] Even together they account for less than 5 percent of all chronic lymphoid leukemias.

ETIOLOGY AND PATHOGENESIS

The etiology is not established. There is a 3:2 male-to-female predominance, suggesting that males are more susceptible to developing the disease. In contrast to the relatively low incidence of B cell CLL in Japan, the incidence of T cell PLL is five to six times higher in the southern islands of Japan than in western societies.[51]

Infection with HTLV-I has been speculated to play a role in the development of at least some cases of T cell PLL. Evidence for HTLV-I can be found in the leukemia cells of patients with T cell PLL, suggesting a causal relationship.[648] However, another study of 36 patients with T cell PLL from an area that was nonendemic for HTLV-I failed to reveal any evidence of HTLV-I or human T lymphotropic virus type II DNA or transcripts in the leukemia cells.[649] As such, the association of HTLV-I and T cell PLL cells may be coincidental in areas with high rates of HTLV-I infection. Alternatively, multiple mechanisms may be involved in leukemogenesis, some involving HTLV-I in endemic areas.[648]

Consistent with this hypothesis, the cytogenetic features of T cell PLL appear to vary, depending upon the patient population studied. In the United States and Europe, inv(14q), del(11q), translocations involving 11q23, i(8q), trisomy 8q, and rearranged Xq28 are the most common nonrandom chromosomal abnormalities in T cell PLL.[650–653] Moreover, abnormalities of the short arm of chromosome 12 (12p) and/or chromosome 5 (5p) and deletions at 13q14.3 are often observed.[653–655] In contrast, chromosome 14 and 8 abnormalities are infrequently noted in the T cell PLL cells of Japanese patients,[656] suggesting that T cell PLL is a heterogeneous disorder.

GENETICS
Use of CGH to detect chromosomal imbalances in T cell PLL of patients in Europe found that the chromosomal regions most often overrepresented were 8q (75%), 5p (62%), and 14q (37%), as well as 6p and 21 (both 25%).[653] On the other hand, chromosomal regions most often underrepresented were 8p and 11q (75%), 13q (37%), and 6q, 7q, 16q, 17p, and 17q (25%). Less common cytogenetic rearrangements are der⁶(X;6) (p14;q25), der¹³(13;14)(q22;q11),t(5;13)(q34; p11), r¹⁷ (p13q21), and t(17;20)(q21;q13).[657]

The alterations on chromosomes 5, 6, 8, 11, 13, 14, 17, and/or 21 apparently cluster into discrete regions that may contain genes that are deleted or amplified during leukemogenesis or disease progression. For example, the loss of genetic material on the short arm of chromosome 8 (8p) apparently clusters into two regions. The first region is telomeric to YAC 899e2, which contains the fibroblast growth factor receptor 1 gene and appears to cluster within a 1.5-Mb YAC 807a2. The second region is more centromeric, with breakpoints on either side of YAC 806e9, flanked by YAC 940f10 distally and YAC 910d7 proximally, the latter containing the *MOZ* gene.[651] Furthermore, the deletions on the long arm of chromosome 13 (13q) most commonly involve deletion of D13S25 at 13q14.3.[655] Deletions on the short arm of chromosome 17 (17p) typically involve 17p13.1 with deletion of the *TP53* (also known as p53) tumor suppressor gene.[658] The regions

on chromosomes 11 and 14 involve genes at 11q22.3-23.1 and 14q32.1, respectively, which apparently are altered in most cases of T cell PLL (see "Ataxia-Telangiectasia Mutated Gene" and T Cell Leukemia-1 and Related Genes" below).[659,660]

Ataxia-Telangiectasia Mutated Gene Patients with ataxia-telangiectasia are at high risk for developing T cell PLL. Ataxia-telangiectasia is an autosomal recessive disorder characterized by cerebellar ataxia, oculocutaneous telangiectasia, immune deficiency, genome instability, and predisposition to malignancies, particularly T cell neoplasms. *ATM*, the responsible gene, maps to chromosomal region 11q22.3-23.1, is 150 kb in length, consists of 66 exons, and encodes a nuclear phosphoprotein of approximately 350 kDa.[138] Patients with ataxia-telangiectasia frequently develop clonal expansions of T cells that often progress to T cell PLL, suggesting that *ATM* is a predisposing factor. Furthermore, inactivating mutations in *ATM* frequently are observed in both alleles of T cell PLL cells from patients who do not have ataxia-telangiectasia.[661–663] Moreover, *ATM* mutations appear associated with T cell PLL and are infrequent in other T cell malignancies, such as T cell ALL.[664] These findings suggest that *ATM* functions as a tumor suppressor gene in T cell PLL.

T Cell Leukemia-1 and Related Genes Studies of t(X;14)(q28; q11) chromosomal rearrangements in T cell PLL have implicated the two genes *MTCP1* and *TCL1* in the pathogenesis of this disease.[650,665–667] These genes encode two homologous proteins, designated p13 (MTCP1) and p14 (TCL1), with highly similar tertiary structure[668] that often are dysregulated in T cell PLL. In addition, clonal T cell expansions similar to that of T cell PLL that develop in patients with ataxia-telangiectasia also frequently have aberrant expression of these genes and/or harbor translocations involving the 14q32.1 or Xq28 regions, where *TCL1* and *MTCP1* are located.[669] Mice transgenic for *MTCP1* under the control of CD2 regulatory elements spontaneously develop T cell leukemias that share many features with T cell PLL.[670] Similarly, mice transgenic for *TCL1* under transcriptional control of a T cell specific promoter developed T cell leukemias very similar in histology and biology to T cell PLL.[95] As such, the proteins encoded by these genes may play an important role in the pathogenesis of this disease.

CLINICAL FEATURES

Presenting symptoms include fatigue, weakness, weight loss, and early satiety with abdominal discomfort because of splenomegaly.[641,644,671] On presentation, patients generally have blood lymphocyte counts greater than $10 \times 10^3/\mu l$, marrow infiltration, and splenomegaly. In contrast to B cell PLL, lymphadenopathy is a common finding in T cell PLL.

Approximately one third of patients have cutaneous involvement on the torso, arms, and face, which generally is present at the time of diagnosis.[672] Skin manifestations include a diffuse infiltrated erythema, infiltration localized to the face and ears, nodules, and erythroderma, producing a nonscaling, papular, nonpruritic rash. Some cases present with a cutaneous infiltration mimicking a cellulitis that is resistant to antibiotic therapy.[673] Occasional cases present with primary ocular findings, such as panuveitis.[674]

LABORATORY FEATURES

Biopsy of erythematous skin lesions generally shows a perivascular or periappendageal dermal infiltrate of lymphoid cells with a prolymphocytic morphology.[672] Neoplastic T cells invariably can be found infiltrating the marrow, often in an interstitial pattern, with varying degrees of involvement.

The leukemia cells express the T cell differentiation antigens CD2, CD3, CD5, and CD7, but not CD1, HLA-DR, or terminal transferase, reflecting a mature T cell phenotype (see Chaps. 14 and 77). In more than 75 percent of cases the leukemia cells have a helper T cell phenotype as they express CD4 but not CD8.[675] Approximately 15 percent of cases have leukemia cells that express CD8 but not CD4.[641,647,676] In less than 10 percent of cases, the leukemic T cells express both CD4 and CD8,[677] a less mature phenotype implying derivation from a more primitive T cell (see Chaps. 5 and 76). Monoclonal gene rearrangements in the genes encoding the α- and β-chains of the T cell receptor can be detected in the leukemia cell genomic DNA (see Chap. 78).

DIFFERENTIAL DIAGNOSIS

The lymphocytosis of T cell PLL can be distinguished readily from that of the B cell leukemias by immunophenotypic analyses (see "Differential Diagnosis" for CLL above).

POLYCLONAL T CELL LYMPHOCYTOSIS
T cell PLL should be distinguished from other lymphoproliferative processes that can present with T cell lymphocytosis (see Chap. 81), such as the reactive T cell lymphocytosis that can occur in infectious mononucleosis (see Chap. 84). Lymphocytosis resulting from polyclonal T cell expansion generally consists of both CD4+CD8− and CD4−CD8+ T cells and lacks clonal T cell receptor gene rearrangements (see Chap. 78). Southern analyses for T cell receptor gene rearrangements or evaluation for expression of T cell receptor variable region genes can help distinguish T cell PLL from this entity.

LARGE GRANULAR LYMPHOCYTIC LEUKEMIA
The leukemic cells in this disorder have the distinctive morphology of large granular lymphocytes (see Chaps. 90 and 94). These cells have abundant cytoplasm that contains many azurophilic granules. Two major subtypes are defined. In the more common type, the leukemic cells are derived from the T cell lineage and generally express the CD3 surface antigen. This disorder formerly was called Tγ-CLL. In the other subtype, the leukemic cells are derived from natural killer cells and lack expression of CD3. Chapter 94 discusses these diseases.

ADULT T CELL LEUKEMIA/LYMPHOMA
Adult T cell leukemia/lymphoma is endemic to the southwest of Japan and the Caribbean region. Most patients have lymphadenopathy, hypercalcemia, and high white blood cell counts. Skin involvement, lytic bone lesions, and hepatomegaly are common. The leukemic cells have polylobed or convoluted nuclei. The diagnosis can be confirmed by demonstration of antibodies to HTLV-I. It is an aggressive disorder with short survival (discussed in Chap. 96).

MYCOSIS FUNGOIDES AND SÉZARY SYNDROME
Cutaneous T cell lymphomas (Sézary syndrome and mycosis fungoides) have a helper CD4+ T cell phenotype and often have blood involvement. Chapter 96 discusses this disease.

Sézary cell leukemia is a mature T cell leukemia with characteristic cerebriform nuclei, whereas Sézary syndrome involves a mature T cell lymphoma with a similar nuclear morphology. However, the distinction between T cell PLL and Sézary cell leukemia is not straightforward. The leukemia cells in either disease can have similar immune phenotypes and cytogenetic abnormalities.[678] Moreover, clinical manifestations are similar, as is the overall clinical course. This finding has led some investigators to consider Sézary cell leukemia as a variant form of T cell PLL.[678,679]

T CELL CHRONIC LYMPHOCYTIC LEUKEMIA
The major feature distinguishing T cell CLL from T cell PLL was the morphology of the leukemia cells.[644] However, because T cell CLL

and T cell PLL share so many other clinical and laboratory features, the distinction of T cell CLL as a separate entity currently is not considered to be of clinical use. Instead, more attention should be given to distinguishing T cell PLL with the usual CD4+CD8− phenotype from exceptional cases of T cell PLL/T cell CLL that have a CD4−CD8+ phenotype, generally lack prolymphocytic morphology, and have an even more aggressive clinical course than typical T cell PLL.[647,676]

THERAPY

The disease is aggressive and generally refractory to conventional alkylator-based chemotherapy, with a median survival of approximately 7.5 months.[641]

Treatment with deoxyadenosine analogues yields higher response rates, although whether these drugs provide a survival benefit has not been determined. Two articles describe treatment of T cell PLL with cladribine.[680,681] Pentostatin 4 mg/m^2 given intravenously weekly for the first 4 weeks and then every 2 weeks until maximal responses was effective in inducing complete or partial responses in about half of patients with T cell PLL.[631]

Patients with extensive cutaneous involvement may benefit from treatments that commonly are used for mycosis fungoides, such as topical corticosteroids, mechlorethamine, carmustine, ultraviolet light B, psoralen plus ultraviolet A, or total skin electron beam therapy.[682] Chapter 96 discusses these treatments. However, systemic therapy is warranted for patients with T cell PLL, and this situation generally obviates local therapy.

The humanized monoclonal antibody alemtuzumab (Campath-1H) binds to the CD52 antigen, a glycosyl phosphatidylinositol-anchored glycoprotein that is expressed on T cell PLL cells.[683] Clinical trials have found that alemtuzumab induced responses in more than two thirds of heavily pretreated relapsed/refractory patients with T cell PLL.[684] Alemtuzumab is particularly effective in clearing malignant lymphocytes from the blood and marrow. In some cases, treatment results in loss of expression of CD52 by leukemic T cell population.[685] The major toxicity relates to problems of immune suppression, increasing the susceptibility to opportunistic infections and reactivation of viruses. These complications can be minimized by careful monitoring and use of prophylactic antimicrobial therapy.[684]

Treatment of patients with T cell PLL with high-dose chemoradiotherapy and allogeneic stem cell transplantation from HLA-matched sibling donors has resulted in anecdotal success.[686,687]

COURSE AND PROGNOSIS

In one large study, median survival was 3 years for patients with PLL and 8 years for those with CLL.[587] Patients with T cell PLL, however, may have an even poorer prognosis than those with B cell PLL and have a median survival of only approximately 7 months.[688,689] However, some patients may experience an initial indolent clinical course with stable moderate leukocytosis.[690] In addition, how these survival times may be affected by the advent of monoclonal antibody therapy and other new modalities of treatment for this disease is uncertain.

REFERENCES

1. Redaelli A, Laskin BL, Stephens JM, et al: The clinical and epidemiological burden of chronic lymphocytic leukaemia. *Eur J Cancer Care (Engl)* 13:279, 2004.
2. Diehl LF, Karnell LH, Menck HR: The American College of Surgeons Commission on Cancer and the American Cancer Society. The National Cancer Data Base report on age, gender, treatment, and outcomes of patients with chronic lymphocytic leukemia. *Cancer* 86:2684, 1999.

3. Velpeau A: Sur la resorption du pusuaet sur l'alteration du sang dans les maladies clinique de persection nenemant. Premier observation. *Rev Med* 2:216, 1827.

4. Fuller H: Particulars of a case in which enormous enlargement of the spleen and liver, together with dilation of all the blood vessels of the body, were found coincident with a peculiarly altered condition of the blood. *Lancet* 2:43, 1846.

5. Virchow R: Weisses Blut. *Froriep's Notizen* 36:151, 1845.

6. Virchow R: Weisses Blut und Milztumoren: I. *Med Z* 15:157, 1846.

7. Virchow R: Weisses Blut und Milztumoren: II. *Med Z* 16:9, 1847.

8. Kundrat H: Über Lympho-Sarkomatosis. *Wien Med Wochenschr* 6:211, 1893.

9. Ehrlich P: *Farbenanalytische Untersuchungen zur Histologie und Klinik des Blutes.* Hirschwald, Berlin, 1891.

10. Türk W: Ein System der Lymphomatosen. *Wien Kinische Wochenschr* 16:1073, 1903.

11. Minot GR, Isaacs R: Lymphatic leukemia; age incidence, duration and benefit derived from irradiation. *Boston Med Surg* 191:1, 1924.

12. Reinhard EH, Neely CL, Samples DM: Radioactive phosphorus in the treatment of chronic leukemias: Long term results over a period of 15 years. *Ann Intern Med* 50:942, 1959.

13. Tivey H: The prognosis for survival in chronic granulocytic and lymphocytic leukemia. *AJR Am J Roentgenol* 72:68, 1954.

14. Galton DAG, Isreals LG, Nabarro JDN, et al: Clinical trials of p(di-2-chloroethylamino)-phenybutyric acid (CD 1348) in malignant lymphoma. *Br Med J* 2:1172, 1955.

15. Shaw RK, Boggs DR, Silberman HR, et al: A study of prednisone therapy in chronic lymphocytic leukemia. *Blood* 17:182, 1961.

16. Dameshek W: Chronic lymphocytic leukemia—An accumulative disease of immunologically incompetent lymphocytes. *Blood* 29(suppl): 566, 1967.

17. Rubin AD, Schultz E: Surface immunoglobulins on lymphocytes in leukemia. *N Engl J Med* 287:989, 1972.

18. Fialkow PJ, Najfeld V, Reddy AL, et al: Chronic lymphocytic leukaemia: Clonal origin in a committed B-lymphocyte progenitor. *Lancet* 2: 444, 1978.

19. Preud'homme JL, Seligmann M: Surface bound immunoglobulins as a cell marker in human lymphoproliferative diseases. *Blood* 40:777, 1972.

20. Salsano F, Froland SS, Natvig JB, Michaelsen TE: Same idiotype of B-lymphocyte membrane IgD and IgM. Formal evidence for monoclonality of chronic lymphocytic leukemia cells. *Scand J Immunol* 3:841, 1974.

21. Fu SM, Winchester RJ, Feizi T, et al: Idiotypic specificity of surface immunoglobulin and the maturation of leukemic bone-marrow-derived lymphocytes. *Proc Natl Acad Sci U S A* 71:4487, 1974.

22. Schroer KR, Briles DE, Van Boxel JA, Davie JM: Idiotypic uniformity of cell surface immunoglobulin in chronic lymphocytic leukemia. Evidence for monoclonal proliferation. *J Exp Med* 140:1416, 1974.

23. Rai KR, Sawitsky A, Cronkite EP, et al: Clinical staging of chronic lymphocytic leukemia. *Blood* 46:219, 1975.

24. Hamblin TJ, Davis Z, Gardiner A, et al: Unmutated Ig V(H) genes are associated with a more aggressive form of chronic lymphocytic leukemia. *Blood* 94:1848, 1999.

25. Damle RN, Wasil T, Fais F, et al: Ig V gene mutation status and CD38 expression as novel prognostic indicators in chronic lymphocytic leukemia. *Blood* 94:1840, 1999.

26. Rosenwald A, Alizadeh AA, Widhopf G, et al: Relation of gene expression phenotype to immunoglobulin mutation genotype in B cell chronic lymphocytic leukemia. *J Exp Med* 194:1639, 2001.

27. Klein U, Tu Y, Stolovitzky GA, et al: Gene expression profiling of B cell chronic lymphocytic leukemia reveals a homogeneous phenotype related to memory B cells. *J Exp Med* 194:1625, 2001.

28. Waterhouse D, Carman WJ, Schottenfeld D, et al: Cancer incidence in the rural community of Tecumseh, Michigan: A pattern of increased lymphopoietic neoplasms. *Cancer* 77:763, 1996.

29. Cronkite EP: An historical account of clinical investigations on chronic lymphocytic leukemia in the Medical Research Center, Brookhaven National Laboratory. *Blood Cells* 12:285, 1987.

30. Zahm SH, Weisenburger DD, Babbitt PA, et al: Use of hair coloring products and the risk of lymphoma, multiple myeloma, and chronic lymphocytic leukemia [comments]. *Am J Public Health* 82:990, 1992.

31. Inskip PD, Kleinerman RA, Stovall M, et al: Leukemia, lymphoma, and multiple myeloma after pelvic radiotherapy for benign disease. *Radiat Res* 135:108, 1993.

32. Neugut AI, Ahsan H, Robinson E, Ennis RD: Bladder carcinoma and other second malignancies after radiotherapy for prostate carcinoma. *Cancer* 79:1600, 1997.

33. Rushton L, Romaniuk H: A case-control study to investigate the risk of leukaemia associated with exposure to benzene in petroleum marketing and distribution workers in the United Kingdom. *Occup Environ Med* 54:152, 1997.

34. Adami J, Gridley G, Nyren O, et al: Sunlight and non-Hodgkin's lymphoma: A population-based cohort study in Sweden. *Int J Cancer* 80: 641, 1999.

35. Marwick C: Link found between Agent Orange and chronic lymphocytic leukaemia. *BMJ* 326:242, 2003.

36. Floderus B, Persson T, Stenlund C, et al: Occupational exposure to electromagnetic fields in relation to leukemia and brain tumors: A case-control study in Sweden. *Cancer Causes Control* 4:465, 1993.

37. Stone R: Polarized debate. EMFs and cancer [news]. *Science* 258:1724, 1992.

38. Feychting M, Forssen U, Floderus B: Occupational and residential magnetic field exposure and leukemia and central nervous system tumors. *Epidemiology* 8:384, 1997.

39. La Civita L, Zignego AL, Monti M, et al: Type C hepatitis and chronic lymphocytic leukaemia. *Eur J Cancer* 32A:1819, 1996.

40. Bianco E, Marcucci F, Mele A, et al: Prevalence of hepatitis C virus infection in lymphoproliferative diseases other than B-cell non-Hodgkin's lymphoma, and in myeloproliferative diseases: An Italian Multi Center case-control study. *Haematologica* 89:70, 2004.

41. McColl MD, Singer IO, Tait RC, et al: The role of hepatitis C virus in the aetiology of non-Hodgkin's lymphoma—A regional association? *Leuk Lymphoma* 26:127, 1997.

42. Luppi M, Grazia Ferrari M, Bonaccorsi G, et al: Hepatitis C virus infection in subsets of neoplastic lymphoproliferations not associated with cryoglobulinemia. *Leukemia* 10:351, 1996.

43. Avila-Carino J, Lewin N, Tomita Y, et al: B-CLL cells with unusual properties. *Int J Cancer* 70:1, 1997.

44. Cartwright RA, Gurney KA, Moorman AV: Sex ratios and the risks of haematological malignancies. *Br J Haematol* 118:1071, 2002.

45. Adami HO, Tsaih S, Lambe M, et al: Pregnancy and risk of non-Hodgkin's lymphoma: A prospective study. *Int J Cancer* 70:155, 1997.

46. Cerhan JR, Vachon CM, Habermann TM, et al: Hormone replacement therapy and risk of non-Hodgkin lymphoma and chronic lymphocytic leukemia. *Cancer Epidemiol Biomarkers Prev* 11:1466, 2002.

47. Ahn YO, Koo HH, Park BJ, et al: Incidence estimation of leukemia among Koreans. *J Korean Med Sci* 6:299, 1991.

48. Haenszel W, Kurihara M: Studies of Japanese migrants: I. Mortality from cancer and other diseases among Japanese in the United States. *J Natl Cancer Inst* 40:43, 1968.

49. Nishiyama H, Mokuno J, Inoue T: Relative frequency and mortality rate of various types of leukemia in Japan. *Gann* 60:71, 1969.

50. Zheng W, Linet MS, Shu XO, et al: Prior medical conditions and the risk of adult leukemia in Shanghai, People's Republic of China. *Cancer Causes Control* 4:361, 1993.

51. Tamura K, Sawada H, Izumi Y, et al: Chronic lymphocytic leukemia (CLL) is rare, but the proportion of T-CLL is high in Japan. *Eur J Haematol* 67:152, 2001.

52. Yanagihara ET, Blaisdell RK, Hayashi T, Lukes RJ: Malignant lymphoma in Hawaii-Japanese: A retrospective morphologic survey. *Hematol Oncol* 7:219, 1989.

53. Bartal A, Bentwich Z, Manny N, Izak G: Ethnical and clinical aspects of chronic lymphocytic leukemia in Israel: A survey on 288 patients. *Acta Haematol* 60:161, 1978.

54. Gunz FW: The epidemiology and genetics of the chronic leukaemias. *Clin Haematol* 6:3, 1977.

55. Conley CL, Misiti J, Laster AJ: Genetic factors predisposing to chronic lymphocytic leukemia and to autoimmune disease. *Medicine (Baltimore)* 59:323, 1980.

56. Linet MS, Van Natta ML, Brookmeyer R, et al: Familial cancer history and chronic lymphocytic leukemia. A case-control study. *Am J Epidemiol* 130:655, 1989.

57. Cuttner J: Increased incidence of hematologic malignancies in first-degree relatives of patients with chronic lymphocytic leukemia. *Cancer Invest* 10:103, 1992.

58. Shah AR, Maeda K, Deegan MJ, et al: A clinicopathologic study of familial chronic lymphocytic leukemia. *Am J Clin Pathol* 97:184, 1992.

59. Yuille MR, Houlston RS, Catovsky D: Anticipation in familial chronic lymphocytic leukaemia. *Leukemia* 12:1696, 1998.

60. Goldin LR, Pfeiffer RM, Li X, Hemminki K: Familial risk of lymphoproliferative tumors in families of patients with chronic lymphocytic leukemia: Results from the Swedish Family-Cancer Database. *Blood* 104:1850, 2004.

61. Yuille MR, Matutes E, Marossy A, et al: Familial chronic lymphocytic leukaemia: A survey and review of published studies. *Br J Haematol* 109:794, 2000.

62. Rawstron A, Hillmen P, Houlston R: Clonal lymphocytes in persons without known chronic lymphocytic leukemia (CLL): Implications of recent findings in family members of CLL patients. *Semin Hematol* 41:192, 2004.

63. Jones HP, Whittaker JA: Chronic lymphatic leukaemia: An investigation of HLA antigen frequencies and white cell differential counts in patients, relatives and controls. *Leuk Res* 15:543, 1991.

64. Shen A, Humphries C, Tucker P, Blattner F: Human heavy-chain variable region gene family nonrandomly rearranged in familial chronic lymphocytic leukemia. *Proc Natl Acad Sci U S A* 84:8563, 1987.

65. Brok-Simoni F, Rechavi G, Katzir N, Ben-Bassat I: Chronic lymphocytic leukaemia in twin sisters: Monozygous but not identical [letter]. *Lancet* 1:329, 1987.

66. Marti GE, Faguet G, Bertin P, et al: CD20 and CD5 expression in B-chronic lymphocytic leukemia. *Ann N Y Acad Sci* 651:480, 1992.

67. Almasri NM, Duque RE, Iturraspe J, et al: Reduced expression of CD20 antigen as a characteristic marker for chronic lymphocytic leukemia. *Am J Hematol* 40:259, 1992.

68. Ranheim EA, Cantwell MJ, Kipps TJ: Expression of CD27 and its ligand, CD70, on chronic lymphocytic leukemia B cells. *Blood* 85:3556, 1995.

69. Weller S, Braun MC, Tan BK, et al: Human blood IgM "memory" B cells are circulating splenic marginal zone B cells harboring a prediversified immunoglobulin repertoire. *Blood* 104:3647, 2004.

70. Widhopf GF 2nd, Brinson DC, Kipps TJ, Tighe H: Transgenic expression of a human polyreactive Ig expressed in chronic lymphocytic leukemia generates memory-type B cells that respond to nonspecific immune activation. *J Immunol* 172:2092, 2004.

71. Kipps TJ, Robbins BA, Tefferi A, et al: CD5-positive B-cell malignancies frequently express cross-reactive idiotypes associated with IgM autoantibodies. *Am J Pathol* 136:809, 1990.

72. Geisler CH, Larsen JK, Hansen NE, et al: Prognostic importance of flow cytometric immunophenotyping of 540 consecutive patients with B-cell chronic lymphocytic leukemia. *Blood* 78:1795, 1991.

73. Legac E, Chastang C, Binet JL, et al: Proposals for a phenotypic classification of B-chronic lymphocytic leukemia, relationship with prognostic factors. *Leuk Lymphoma* 5S:53, 1991.

74. Kipps TJ, Carson DA: Autoantibodies in chronic lymphocytic leukemia and related systemic autoimmune diseases. *Blood* 81:2475, 1993.

75. Caligaris-Cappio F: B-chronic lymphocytic leukemia: A malignancy of anti-self B cells. *Blood* 87:2615, 1996.

76. Wardemann H, Yurasov S, Schaefer A, et al: Predominant autoantibody production by early human B cell precursors. *Science* 301:1374, 2003.

77. Martin T, Duffy SF, Carson DA, Kipps TJ: Evidence for somatic selection of natural autoantibodies. *J Exp Med* 175:983, 1992.

78. Martin T, Crouzier R, Weber JC, et al: Structure-function studies on a polyreactive (natural) autoantibody. Polyreactivity is dependent on somatically generated sequences in the third complementarity-determining region of the antibody heavy chain. *J Immunol* 152:5988, 1994.

79. Wardemann H, Hammersen J, Nussenzweig MC: Human autoantibody silencing by immunoglobulin light chains. *J Exp Med* 200:191, 2004.

80. Keating MJ, Chiorazzi N, Messmer B, et al: Biology and treatment of chronic lymphocytic leukemia. *Hematology (Am Soc Hematol Educ Program)*:153, 2003.

81. Tobin G, Soderberg O, Thunberg U, Rosenquist R: V(H)3-21 gene usage in chronic lymphocytic leukemia—Characterization of a new subgroup with distinct molecular features and poor survival. *Leuk Lymphoma* 45:221, 2004.

82. Messmer BT, Albesiano E, Efremov DG, et al: Multiple distinct sets of stereotyped antigen receptors indicate a role for antigen in promoting chronic lymphocytic leukemia. *J Exp Med* 200:519, 2004.

83. Kipps TJ, Tomhave E, Pratt LF, et al: Developmentally restricted immunoglobulin heavy chain variable region gene expressed at high frequency in chronic lymphocytic leukemia. *Proc Natl Acad Sci U S A* 86:5913, 1989.

84. Johnson TA, Rassenti LZ, Kipps TJ: Ig VH1 genes expressed in B cell chronic lymphocytic leukemia exhibit distinctive molecular features. *J Immunol* 158:235, 1997.

85. Fais F, Ghiotto F, Hashimoto S, et al: Chronic lymphocytic leukemia B cells express restricted sets of mutated and unmutated antigen receptors. *J Clin Invest* 102:1515, 1998.

86. Potter KN, Orchard J, Critchley E, et al: Features of the overexpressed V1-69 genes in the unmutated subset of chronic lymphocytic leukemia are distinct from those in the healthy elderly repertoire. *Blood* 101:3082, 2003.

87. Schroeder HW Jr, Mortari F, Shiokawa S, et al: Developmental regulation of the human antibody repertoire. *Ann N Y Acad Sci* 764:242, 1995.

88. Widhopf GF 2nd, Rassenti LZ, Toy TL, et al: Chronic lymphocytic leukemia B cells of more than 1% of patients express virtually identical immunoglobulins. *Blood* 104:2499, 2004.

89. Rawstron AC, Yuille MR, Fuller J, et al: Inherited predisposition to CLL is detectable as subclinical monoclonal B-lymphocyte expansion. *Blood* 100:2289, 2002.

90. Rawstron AC, Green MJ, Kuzmicki A, et al: Monoclonal B lymphocytes with the characteristics of "indolent" chronic lymphocytic leukemia are present in 3.5% of adults with normal blood counts. *Blood* 100:635, 2002.

91. Caporaso N, Marti GE, Goldin L: Perspectives on familial chronic lymphocytic leukemia: Genes and the environment. *Semin Hematol* 41:201, 2004.

92. Bichi R, Shinton SA, Martin ES, et al: Human chronic lymphocytic leukemia modeled in mouse by targeted TCL1 expression. *Proc Natl Acad Sci U S A* 99:6955, 2002.

93. Yuille MR, Condie A, Stone EM, et al: TCL1 is activated by chromosomal rearrangement or by hypomethylation. *Genes Chromosomes Cancer* 30:336, 2001.

94. Zapata JM, Krajewska M, Morse HC 3rd, et al: TNF receptor-associated factor (TRAF) domain and Bcl-2 cooperate to induce small B cell lymphoma/chronic lymphocytic leukemia in transgenic mice. *Proc Natl Acad Sci U S A* 101:16600, 2004.

95. Virgilio L, Lazzeri C, Bichi R, et al: Deregulated expression of TCL1 causes T cell leukemia in mice. *Proc Natl Acad Sci U S A* 95:3885, 1998.

96. Hoyer KK, French SW, Turner DE, et al: Dysregulated TCL1 promotes multiple classes of mature B cell lymphoma. *Proc Natl Acad Sci U S A* 99:14392, 2002.

97. Rickinson AB, Finerty S, Epstein MA: Interaction of Epstein-Barr virus with leukaemic B cells in vitro: I. Abortive infection and rare cell line establishment from chronic lymphocytic leukaemic cells. *Clin Exp Immunol* 50:347, 1982.

98. Sole F, Woessner S, Perez-Losada A, et al: Cytogenetic studies in seventy-six cases of B-chronic lymphoproliferative disorders. *Cancer Genet Cytogenet* 93:160, 1997.

99. Hilgenfeld E, Padilla-Nash H, Schrock E, Ried T: Analysis of B-cell neoplasias by spectral karyotyping (SKY). *Curr Top Microbiol Immunol* 246:169, 1999.

100. Morgan R, Chen Z, Richkind K, et al: PHA/IL2: An efficient mitogen cocktail for cytogenetic studies of non-Hodgkin lymphoma and chronic lymphocytic leukemia. *Cancer Genet Cytogenet* 109:134, 1999.

101. Buhmann R, Kurzeder C, Rehklau J, et al: CD40L stimulation enhances the ability of conventional metaphase cytogenetics to detect chromosome aberrations in B-cell chronic lymphocytic leukaemia cells. *Br J Haematol* 118:968, 2002.

102. Tanaka K, Arif M, Eguchi M, et al: Interphase fluorescence in situ hybridization overcomes pitfalls of G-banding analysis with special reference to underestimation of chromosomal aberration rates. *Cancer Genet Cytogenet* 115:32, 1999.

103. Chena C, Arrossagaray G, Scolnik M, et al: Interphase cytogenetic analysis in Argentinean B-cell chronic lymphocytic leukemia patients: Association of trisomy 12 and del(13q14). *Cancer Genet Cytogenet* 146:154, 2003.

104. Goorha S, Glenn MJ, Drozd-Borysiuk E, Chen Z: A set of commercially available fluorescent in-situ hybridization probes efficiently detects cytogenetic abnormalities in patients with chronic lymphocytic leukemia. *Genet Med* 6:48, 2004.

105. Döhner H, Stilgenbauer S, Dohner K, et al: Chromosome aberrations in B-cell chronic lymphocytic leukemia: Reassessment based on molecular cytogenetic analysis. *J Mol Med* 77:266, 1999.

106. Barnabas N, Shurafa M, Van Dyke DL, et al: Significance of p53 mutations in patients with chronic lymphocytic leukemia: A sequential study of 30 patients. *Cancer* 91:285, 2001.

107. Sen F, Lai R, Albitar M: Chronic lymphocytic leukemia with t(14;18) and trisomy 12. *Arch Pathol Lab Med* 126:1543, 2002.

108. Odero MD, Soto JL, Matutes E, et al: Comparative genomic hybridization and amplotyping by arbitrarily primed PCR in stage A B-CLL. *Cancer Genet Cytogenet* 130:8, 2001.

109. Novak U, Tobler A, Fey MF: Allelotyping in B-cell chronic lymphocytic leukemia (B-CLL). *Leuk Lymphoma* 45:887, 2004.

110. Gardiner AC, Corcoran MM, Oscier DG: Cytogenetic, fluorescence in situ hybridisation, and clinical evaluation of translocations with concomitant deletion at 13q14 in chronic lymphocytic leukaemia. *Genes Chromosomes Cancer* 20:73, 1997.

111. Garcia-Marco JA, Price CM, Catovsky D: Interphase cytogenetics in chronic lymphocytic leukemia. *Cancer Genet Cytogenet* 94:52, 1997.

112. Crossen PE: Genes and chromosomes in chronic B-cell leukemia. *Cancer Genet Cytogenet* 94:44, 1997.

113. Bouyge-Moreau I, Rondeau G, Avet-Loiseau H, et al: Construction of a 780-kb PAC, BAC, and cosmid contig encompassing the minimal critical deletion involved in B cell chronic lymphocytic leukemia at 13q14.3. *Genomics* 46:183, 1997.

114. Corcoran MM, Rasool O, Liu Y, et al: Detailed molecular delineation of 13q14.3 loss in B-cell chronic lymphocytic leukemia. *Blood* 91:1382, 1998.

115. Stilgenbauer S, Nickolenko J, Wilhelm J, et al: Expressed sequences as candidates for a novel tumor suppressor gene at band 13q14 in B-cell chronic lymphocytic leukemia and mantle cell lymphoma. *Oncogene* 16:1891, 1998.

116. Bullrich F, Fujii H, Calin G, et al: Characterization of the 13q14 tumor suppressor locus in CLL: Identification of ALT1, an alternative splice variant of the LEU2 gene. *Cancer Res* 61:6640, 2001.

117. Mabuchi H, Fujii H, Calin G, et al: Cloning and characterization of CLLD6, CLLD7, and CLLD8, novel candidate genes for leukemogenesis at chromosome 13q14, a region commonly deleted in B-cell chronic lymphocytic leukemia. *Cancer Res* 61:2870, 2001.

118. Calin GA, Dumitru CD, Shimizu M, et al: Frequent deletions and downregulation of micro-RNA genes miR15 and miR16 at 13q14 in chronic lymphocytic leukemia. *Proc Natl Acad Sci U S A* 99:15524, 2002.

119. Dierlamm J, Michaux L, Criel A, et al: Genetic abnormalities in chronic lymphocytic leukemia and their clinical and prognostic implications. *Cancer Genet Cytogenet* 94:27, 1997.

120. Hjalmar V, Kimby E, Matutes E, et al: Trisomy 12 and lymphoplasmacytoid lymphocytes in chronic leukemic B-cell disorders. *Haematologica* 83:602, 1998.

121. Acar H, Connor MJ: Detection of trisomy 12 and centromeric alterations in CLL by interphase- and metaphase-FISH. *Cancer Genet Cytogenet* 100:148, 1998.

122. Einhorn S, Burvall K, Juliusson G, et al: Molecular analyses of chromosome 12 in chronic lymphocytic leukemia. *Leukemia* 3:871, 1989.

123. Hjalmar V, Hast R, Kimby E: Cell surface expression of CD25, CD54, and CD95 on B- and T-cells in chronic lymphocytic leukaemia in relation to trisomy 12, atypical morphology and clinical course. *Eur J Haematol* 68:127, 2002.

124. Schlette E, Medeiros LJ, Keating M, Lai R: CD79b expression in chronic lymphocytic leukemia. Association with trisomy 12 and atypical immunophenotype. *Arch Pathol Lab Med* 127:561, 2003.

125. Matutes E: Trisomy 12 in chronic lymphocytic leukaemia. *Leuk Res* 20:375, 1996.

126. Woessner S, Sole F, Perez-Losada A, et al: Trisomy 12 is a rare cytogenetic finding in typical chronic lymphocytic leukaemia. *Leuk Res* 20:369, 1996.

127. Matutes E, Oscier D, Garcia-Marco J, et al: Trisomy 12 defines a group of CLL with atypical morphology: Correlation between cytogenetic, clinical and laboratory features in 544 patients. *Br J Haematol* 92:382, 1996.

128. Amiel A, Arbov L, Manor Y, et al: Monoallelic p53 deletion in chronic lymphocytic leukemia detected by interphase cytogenetics. *Cancer Genet Cytogenet* 97:97, 1997.

129. Garcia-Marco J, Matutes E, Morilla R, et al: Trisomy 12 in B-cell chronic lymphocytic leukaemia: Assessment of lineage restriction by simultaneous analysis of immunophenotype and genotype in interphase cells by fluorescence in situ hybridization. *Br J Haematol* 87:44, 1994.

130. Mould S, Gardiner A, Corcoran M, Oscier DG: Trisomy 12 and structural abnormalities of 13q14 occurring in the same clone in chronic lymphocytic leukaemia. *Br J Haematol* 92:389, 1996.

131. Brynes RK, McCourty A, Sun NC, Koo CH: Trisomy 12 in Richter's transformation of chronic lymphocytic leukemia. *Am J Clin Pathol* 104:199, 1995.

132. Shahidi H, Leslie WT, Wool NL, Gregory SA: Transformation of chronic lymphocytic leukemia to immunoblastic lymphoma (Richter's syndrome). *Med Pediatr Oncol* 29:146, 1997.

133. Tsimberidou AM, Keating MJ: Richter syndrome. *Cancer* 103:216, 2004.
134. Stilgenbauer S, Liebisch P, James MR, et al: Molecular cytogenetic delineation of a novel critical genomic region in chromosome bands 11q22.3-923.1 in lymphoproliferative disorders. *Proc Natl Acad Sci U S A* 93:11837, 1996.
135. Döhner H, Stilgenbauer S, James MR, et al: 11q deletions identify a new subset of B-cell chronic lymphocytic leukemia characterized by extensive nodal involvement and inferior prognosis. *Blood* 89:2516, 1997.
136. Karhu R, Knuutila S, Kallioniemi OP, et al: Frequent loss of the 11q14-24 region in chronic lymphocytic leukemia: A study by comparative genomic hybridization. Tampere CLL Group. *Genes Chromosomes Cancer* 19:286, 1997.
137. Sembries S, Pahl H, Stilgenbauer S, et al: Reduced expression of adhesion molecules and cell signaling receptors by chronic lymphocytic leukemia cells with 11q deletion. *Blood* 93:624, 1999.
138. Lavin MF, Khanna KK: ATM: The protein encoded by the gene mutated in the radiosensitive syndrome ataxia-telangiectasia. *Int J Radiat Biol* 75:1201, 1999.
139. Starostik P, Manshouri T, O'Brien S, et al: Deficiency of the ATM protein expression defines an aggressive subgroup of B-cell chronic lymphocytic leukemia. *Cancer Res* 58:4552, 1998.
140. Bullrich F, Rasio D, Kitada S, et al: ATM mutations in B-cell chronic lymphocytic leukemia. *Cancer Res* 59:24, 1999.
141. Bevan S, Yuille MR, Marossy A, et al: Ataxia telangiectasia gene mutations and chronic lymphocytic leukaemia. *Lancet* 353:753, 1999.
142. Eclache V, Caulet-Maugendre S, Poirel HA, et al: Cryptic deletion involving the ATM locus at 11q22.3 approximately q23.1 in B-cell chronic lymphocytic leukemia and related disorders. *Cancer Genet Cytogenet* 152:72, 2004.
143. Stankovic T, Weber P, Stewart G, et al: Inactivation of ataxia telangiectasia mutated gene in B-cell chronic lymphocytic leukaemia. *Lancet* 353:26, 1999.
144. Offit K, Louie DC, Parsa NZ, et al: Clinical and morphologic features of B-cell small lymphocytic lymphoma with del(6)(q21q23). *Blood* 83:2611, 1994.
145. Glassman AB, Harper-Allen EA, Hayes KJ, et al: Chromosome 6 abnormalities associated with prolymphocytic acceleration in chronic lymphocytic leukemia. *Ann Clin Lab Sci* 28:24, 1998.
146. Finn WG, Kay NE, Kroft SH, et al: Secondary abnormalities of chromosome 6q in B-cell chronic lymphocytic leukemia: A sequential study of karyotypic instability in 51 patients. *Am J Hematol* 59:223, 1998.
147. Amiel A, Mulchanov I, Elis A, et al: Deletion of 6q27 in chronic lymphocytic leukemia and multiple myeloma detected by fluorescence in situ hybridization. *Cancer Genet Cytogenet* 112:53, 1999.
148. Fink SR, Paternoster SF, Smoley SA, et al: Fluorescent-labeled DNA probes applied to novel biological aspects of B-cell chronic lymphocytic leukemia. *Leuk Res* 29:253, 2005.
149. Cuneo A, Rigolin GM, Bigoni R, et al: Chronic lymphocytic leukemia with 6q− shows distinct hematological features and intermediate prognosis. *Leukemia* 18:476, 2004.
150. Cuneo A, Roberti MG, Bigoni R, et al: Four novel non-random chromosome rearrangements in B-cell chronic lymphocytic leukaemia: 6p24-25 and 12p12-13 translocations, 4q21 anomalies and monosomy 21. *Br J Haematol* 108:559, 2000.
151. Coates PJ, Lorimore SA, Wright EG: Cell and tissue responses to genotoxic stress. *J Pathol* 205:221, 2005.
152. Thornton PD, Gruszka-Westwood AM, Hamoudi RA, et al: Characterisation of TP53 abnormalities in chronic lymphocytic leukaemia. *Hematol J* 5:47, 2004.
153. el Rouby S, Thomas A, Costin D, et al: P53 gene mutation in B-cell chronic lymphocytic leukemia is associated with drug resistance and is independent of MDR1/MDR3 gene expression. *Blood* 82:3452, 1993.
154. Lens D, De Schouwer PJ, Hamoudi RA, et al: P53 abnormalities in B-cell prolymphocytic leukemia. *Blood* 89:2015, 1997.
155. Cordone I, Masi S, Mauro FR, et al: P53 expression in B-cell chronic lymphocytic leukemia: A marker of disease progression and poor prognosis. *Blood* 91:4342, 1998.
156. Callet-Bauchu E, Salles G, Gazzo S, et al: Translocations involving the short arm of chromosome 17 in chronic B-lymphoid disorders: Frequent occurrence of dicentric rearrangements and possible association with adverse outcome. *Leukemia* 13:460, 1999.
157. Shaw GR, Kronberger DL: TP53 deletions but not trisomy 12 are adverse in B-cell lymphoproliferative disorders. *Cancer Genet Cytogenet* 119:146, 2000.
158. Byrd JC, Stilgenbauer S, Flinn IW: Chronic lymphocytic leukemia. *Hematology (Am Soc Hematol Educ Program)*:163, 2004.
159. Bea S, Lopez-Guillermo A, Ribas M, et al: Genetic imbalances in progressed B-cell chronic lymphocytic leukemia and transformed large-cell lymphoma (Richter's syndrome). *Am J Pathol* 161:957, 2002.
160. Gaidano G, Ballerini P, Gong JZ, et al: P53 mutations in human lymphoid malignancies: Association with Burkitt lymphoma and chronic lymphocytic leukemia. *Proc Natl Acad Sci U S A* 88:5413, 1991.
161. Croce CM: Molecular biology of lymphomas. *Semin Oncol* 20:31, 1993.
162. Zech L, Gahrton G, Hammarstrom L, et al: Inversion of chromosome 14 marks human T-cell chronic lymphocytic leukaemia. *Nature* 308:858, 1984.
163. Hecht F, Morgan R, Hecht BK, Smith SD: Common region on chromosome 14 in T-cell leukemia and lymphoma. *Science* 226:1445, 1984.
164. Larramendy ML, Peltomaki P, Salonen E, Knuutila S: Chromosomal abnormality limited to T4 lymphocytes in a patient with T-cell chronic lymphocytic leukaemia. *Eur J Haematol* 45:52, 1990.
165. Jonveaux P, Hillion J, Bennaceur AL, et al: T(14;18) and bcl-2 gene rearrangement in a B-chronic lymphocytic leukaemia. *Br J Haematol* 81:620, 1992.
166. Raghoebier S, van Krieken JH, Kluin-Nelemans JC, et al: Oncogene rearrangements in chronic B-cell leukemia. *Blood* 77:1560, 1991.
167. Ueshima Y, Bird ML, Vardiman JW, Rowley JD: A 14;19 translocation in B-cell chronic lymphocytic leukemia: A new recurring chromosome aberration. *Int J Cancer* 36:287, 1985.
168. Michaux L, Mecucci C, Stul M, et al: BCL3 rearrangement and t(14;19)(q32;q13) in lymphoproliferative disorders. *Genes Chromosomes Cancer* 15:38, 1996.
169. McKeithan TW, Takimoto GS, Ohno H, et al: BCL3 rearrangements and t(14;19) in chronic lymphocytic leukemia and other B-cell malignancies: A molecular and cytogenetic study. *Genes Chromosomes Cancer* 20:64, 1997.
170. Crossen PE: Cytogenetic and molecular changes in chronic B-cell leukemia. *Cancer Genet Cytogenet* 43:143, 1989.
171. Pittman S, Catovsky D: Prognostic significance of chromosome abnormalities in chronic lymphocytic leukaemia. *Br J Haematol* 58:649, 1984.
172. Meeker TC, Grimaldi JC, O'Rourke R, et al: An additional breakpoint region in the BCL-1 locus associated with the t(11;14)(q13;q32) translocation of B-lymphocytic malignancy. *Blood* 74:1801, 1989.
173. Erikson J, Finan J, Tsujimoto Y, et al: The chromosome 14 breakpoint in neoplastic B cells with the t(11;14) translocation involves the immunoglobulin heavy chain locus. *Proc Natl Acad Sci U S A* 81:4144, 1984.
174. Davey MP, Bertness V, Nakahara K, et al: Juxtaposition of the T-cell receptor alpha-chain locus (14q11) and a region (14q32) of potential importance in leukemogenesis by a 14;14 translocation in a patient with T-cell chronic lymphocytic leukemia and ataxia-telangiectasia. *Proc Natl Acad Sci U S A* 85:9287, 1988.
175. Motokura T, Bloom T, Kim HG, et al: A novel cyclin encoded by a bcl1-linked candidate oncogene [comments]. *Nature* 350:512, 1991.

176. Seto M, Yamamoto K, Iida S, et al: Gene rearrangement and overexpression of PRAD1 in lymphoid malignancy with t(11;14)(q13;q32) translocation. *Oncogene* 7:1401, 1992.

177. Hinds PW, Dowdy SF, Eaton EN, et al: Function of a human cyclin gene as an oncogene. *Proc Natl Acad Sci U S A* 91:709, 1994.

178. Rimokh R, Berger F, Cornillet P, et al: Break in the BCL1 locus is closely associated with intermediate lymphocytic lymphoma subtype. *Genes Chromosomes Cancer* 2:223, 1990.

179. Ambinder RF, Griffin CA: Biology of the lymphomas: Cytogenetics, molecular biology, and virology. *Curr Opin Oncol* 3:806, 1991.

180. Brito-Babapulle V, Ellis J, Matutes E, et al: Translocation t(11;14)(q13; q32) in chronic lymphoid disorders. *Genes Chromosomes Cancer* 5:158, 1992.

181. Williams ME, Swerdlow SH, Rosenberg CL, Arnold A: Characterization of chromosome 11 translocation breakpoints at the bcl-1 and PRAD1 loci in centrocytic lymphoma. *Cancer Res* 52:5541s, 1992.

182. Swerdlow SH, Saboorian MH, Pelstring RJ, Williams ME: Centrocytic lymphoma: A morphometric study with comparison to other small cleaved follicular center cell lymphomas and genotypic correlates. *Am J Pathol* 142:329, 1993.

183. Einhorn S, Meeker T, Juliusson G, et al: No evidence of trisomy 12 or t(11;14) by molecular genetic techniques in chronic lymphocytic leukemia cells with a normal karyotype. *Cancer Genet Cytogenet* 48:183, 1990.

184. Rechavi G, Katzir N, Brok-Simoni F, et al: A search for bcl1, bcl2, and c-myc oncogene rearrangements in chronic lymphocytic leukemia. *Leukemia* 3:57, 1989.

185. Newman RA, Peterson B, Davey FR, et al: Phenotypic markers and BCL-1 gene rearrangements in B-cell chronic lymphocytic leukemia: A Cancer and Leukemia Group B study. *Blood* 82:1239, 1993.

186. Adachi M, Tefferi A, Greipp PR, et al: Preferential linkage of bcl-2 to immunoglobulin light chain gene in chronic lymphocytic leukemia. *J Exp Med* 171:559, 1990.

187. Schena M, Larsson LG, Gottardi D, et al: Growth- and differentiation-associated expression of bcl-2 in B-chronic lymphocytic leukemia cells. *Blood* 79:2981, 1992.

188. Pezzella F, Tse AG, Cordell JL, et al: Expression of the bcl-2 oncogene protein is not specific for the 14;18 chromosomal translocation. *Am J Pathol* 137:225, 1990.

189. Hanada M, Delia D, Aiello A, et al: Bcl-2 gene hypomethylation and high-level expression in B-cell chronic lymphocytic leukemia. *Blood* 82: 1820, 1993.

190. Laytragoon-Lewin N, Kashuba V, Mellstedt H, Klein G: Bcl-2 rearrangement detected by pulsed-field gel electrophoresis (PFGF) in B-chronic lymphocytic leukemia (CLL) cells. *Int J Cancer* 76:909, 1998.

191. Lampert IA, Wotherspoon A, Van Noorden S, Hasserjian RP: High expression of CD23 in the proliferation centers of chronic lymphocytic leukemia in lymph nodes and spleen. *Hum Pathol* 30:648, 1999.

192. Zimmerman TS, Godwin HA, Perry S: Studies of leukocyte kinetics in chronic lymphocytic leukemia. *Blood* 31:277, 1968.

193. Andreeff M, Darzynkiewicz Z, Sharpless TK, et al: Discrimination of human leukemia subtypes by flow cytometric analysis of cellular DNA and RNA. *Blood* 55:282, 1980.

194. Kobayashi R, Picchio G, Kirven M, et al: Transfer of human chronic lymphocytic leukemia to mice with severe combined immune deficiency. *Leuk Res* 16:1013, 1992.

195. Messmer BT, Messmer D, Allen SL, et al: In vivo measurements document the dynamic cellular kinetics of chronic lymphocytic leukemia B cells. *J Clin Invest* 115:755, 2005.

196. Naresh KN: Proliferation center cells in the lymph nodes of B-cell chronic lymphatic leukemia express relatively higher levels of CD20. *Hum Pathol* 31:775, 2000.

197. Asplund SL, McKenna RW, Howard MS, Kroft SH: Immunophenotype does not correlate with lymph node histology in chronic lymphocytic leukemia/small lymphocytic lymphoma. *Am J Surg Pathol* 26:624, 2002.

198. Ben-Ezra J, Burke JS, Swartz WG, et al: Small lymphocytic lymphoma: A clinicopathologic analysis of 268 cases. *Blood* 73:579, 1989.

199. Gupta D, Lim MS, Medeiros LJ, Elenitoba-Johnson KS: Small lymphocytic lymphoma with perifollicular, marginal zone, or interfollicular distribution. *Mod Pathol* 13:1161, 2000.

200. Schimmer AD, Munk-Pedersen I, Minden MD, Reed JC: Bcl-2 and apoptosis in chronic lymphocytic leukemia. *Curr Treat Options Oncol* 4:211, 2003.

201. Kitada S, Andersen J, Akar S, et al: Expression of apoptosis-regulating proteins in chronic lymphocytic leukemia: Correlations with In vitro and In vivo chemoresponses. *Blood* 91:3379, 1998.

202. Gottardi D, Alfarano A, De Leo AM, et al: In leukemic CD5+ B cells the expression of BCL-2 gene family is shifted toward protection from apoptosis. *Br J Haematol* 94:612, 1996.

203. Korsmeyer SJ: Bcl-2 initiates a new category of oncogenes: Regulators of cell death. *Blood* 80:879, 1992.

204. Coulie PG: Human tumour antigens recognized by T cells: New perspectives for anti-cancer vaccines? *Mol Med Today* 3:261, 1997.

205. McConkey DJ, Chandra J, Wright S, et al: Apoptosis sensitivity in chronic lymphocytic leukemia is determined by endogenous endonuclease content and relative expression of BCL-2 and BAX. *J Immunol* 156: 2624, 1996.

206. Pepper C, Bentley P, Hoy T: Regulation of clinical chemoresistance by bcl-2 and bax oncoproteins in B-cell chronic lymphocytic leukaemia. *Br J Haematol* 95:513, 1996.

207. Aguilar Santelises M, Rottenberg ME, Lewin N, et al: Bcl-2, Bax and p53 expression in B-CLL in relation to in vitro survival and clinical progression. *Int J Cancer* 69:114, 1996.

208. Thomas A, El Rouby S, Reed JC, et al: Drug-induced apoptosis in B-cell chronic lymphocytic leukemia: Relationship between p53 gene mutation and bcl-2/bax proteins in drug resistance. *Oncogene* 12:1055, 1996.

209. Panayiotidis P, Jones D, Ganeshaguru K, et al: Human bone marrow stromal cells prevent apoptosis and support the survival of chronic lymphocytic leukaemia cells in vitro. *Br J Haematol* 92:97, 1996.

210. Lagneaux L, Delforge A, Bron D, et al: Chronic lymphocytic leukemic B cells but not normal B cells are rescued from apoptosis by contact with normal bone marrow stromal cells. *Blood* 91:2387, 1998.

211. Burger JA, Tsukada N, Burger M, et al: Blood-derived nurse-like cells protect chronic lymphocytic leukemia B cells from spontaneous apoptosis through stromal cell-derived factor-1. *Blood* 96:2655, 2000.

212. Tsukada N, Burger JA, Zvaifler NJ, Kipps TJ: Distinctive features of "nurselike" cells that differentiate in the context of chronic lymphocytic leukemia. *Blood* 99:1030, 2002.

213. Pedersen IM, Kitada S, Leoni LM, et al: Protection of CLL B cells by a follicular dendritic cell line is dependent on induction of Mcl-1. *Blood* 100:1795, 2002.

214. Burger JA, Kipps TJ: Chemokine receptors and stromal cells in the homing and homeostasis of chronic lymphocytic leukemia B cells. *Leuk Lymphoma* 43:461, 2002.

215. Burger JA, Burger M, Kipps TJ: Chronic lymphocytic leukemia B cells express functional CXCR4 chemokine receptors that mediate spontaneous migration beneath bone marrow stromal cells. *Blood* 94:3658, 1999.

216. Trentin L, Agostini C, Facco M, et al: The chemokine receptor CXCR3 is expressed on malignant B cells and mediates chemotaxis. *J Clin Invest* 104:115, 1999.

217. Till KJ, Lin K, Zuzel M, Cawley JC: The chemokine receptor CCR7 and alpha4 integrin are important for migration of chronic lymphocytic leukemia cells into lymph nodes. *Blood* 99:2977, 2002.

218. Winkelstein A, Jordan PS: Immune deficiencies in chronic lymphocytic leukemia and multiple myeloma. *Clin Rev Allergy* 10:39, 1992.

219. Schlesinger M, Broman I, Lugassy G: The complement system is defective in chronic lymphatic leukemia patients and in their healthy relatives. *Leukemia* 10:1509, 1996.

220. Rossi E, Matutes E, Morilla R, et al: Zeta chain and CD28 are poorly expressed on T lymphocytes from chronic lymphocytic leukemia. *Leukemia* 10:494, 1996.

221. Veenstra H, Jacobs P, Dowdle EB: Abnormal association between invariant chain and HLA class II alpha and beta chains in chronic lymphocytic leukemia. *Cell Immunol* 171:68, 1996.

222. Nuckel H, Rebmann V, Durig J, et al: HLA-G expression is associated with an unfavorable outcome and immunodeficiency in chronic lymphocytic leukemia. *Blood* 105:1694, 2005.

223. Itala M, Vainio O, Remes K: Functional abnormalities in granulocytes predict susceptibility to bacterial infections in chronic lymphocytic leukaemia. *Eur J Haematol* 57:46, 1996.

224. Tsiodras S, Samonis G, Keating MJ, Kontoyiannis DP: Infection and immunity in chronic lymphocytic leukemia. *Mayo Clin Proc* 75:1039, 2000.

225. Bower JH, Hammack JE, McDonnell SK, Tefferi A: The neurologic complications of B-cell chronic lymphocytic leukemia. *Neurology* 48:407, 1997.

226. Hermouet S, Sutton CA, Rose TM, et al: Qualitative and quantitative analysis of human herpesviruses in chronic and acute B cell lymphocytic leukemia and in multiple myeloma. *Leukemia* 17:185, 2003.

227. Laurenti L, Piccioni P, Cattani P, et al: Cytomegalovirus reactivation during alemtuzumab therapy for chronic lymphocytic leukemia: Incidence and treatment with oral ganciclovir. *Haematologica* 89:1248, 2004.

228. Levi F, Randimbison L, Te VC, La Vecchia C: Non-Hodgkin's lymphomas, chronic lymphocytic leukaemias and skin cancers. *Br J Cancer* 74:1847, 1996.

229. Lotz M, Ranheim E, Kipps TJ: Transforming growth factor beta as endogenous growth inhibitor of chronic lymphocytic leukemia B cells. *J Exp Med* 179:999, 1994.

230. Lagneaux L, Delforge A, Bron D, et al: Heterogenous response of B lymphocytes to transforming growth factor-beta in B-cell chronic lymphocytic leukaemia: Correlation with the expression of TGF-beta receptors. *Br J Haematol* 97:612, 1997.

231. van Oers MH, Pals ST, Evers LM, et al: Expression and release of CD27 in human B-cell malignancies. *Blood* 82:3430, 1993.

232. Kato K, Cantwell MJ, Sharma S, Kipps TJ: Gene transfer of CD40-ligand induces autologous immune recognition of chronic lymphocytic leukemia B cells. *J Clin Invest* 101:1133, 1998.

233. Matutes E, Wechsler A, Gomez R, et al: Unusual T-cell phenotype in advanced B-chronic lymphocytic leukaemia. *Br J Haematol* 49:635, 1981.

234. Fu SM, Chiorazzi N, Kunkel HG: Differentiation capacity and other properties of the leukemic cells of chronic lymphocytic leukemia. *Immunol Rev* 48:23, 1979.

235. Ranheim EA, Kipps TJ: Activated T cells induce expression of B7/BB1 on normal or leukemic B cells through a CD40-dependent signal. *J Exp Med* 177:925, 1993.

236. Cantwell M, Hua T, Pappas J, Kipps TJ: Acquired CD40-ligand deficiency in chronic lymphocytic leukemia. *Nat Med* 3:984, 1997.

237. Kneitz C, Goller M, Wilhelm M, et al: Inhibition of T cell/B cell interaction by B-CLL cells. *Leukemia* 13:98, 1999.

238. Grewal IS, Flavell RA: The CD40 ligand. At the center of the immune universe? *Immunol Res* 16:59, 1997.

239. Lacombe C, Gombert J, Dreyfus B, et al: Heterogeneity of serum IgG subclass deficiencies in B chronic lymphocytic leukemia. *Clin Immunol* 90:128, 1999.

240. Martin-Villa JM, Corell A, Ramos-Amador JT, et al: Higher incidence of autoantibodies in X-linked chronic granulomatous disease carriers: Random X-chromosome inactivation may be related to autoimmunity. *Autoimmunity* 31:261, 1999.

241. Etzioni A: Immune deficiency and autoimmunity. *Autoimmun Rev* 2:364, 2003.

242. Hamblin TJ, Oscier DG, Young BJ: Autoimmunity in chronic lymphocytic leukaemia. *J Clin Pathol* 39:713, 1986.

243. Duhrsen U, Augener W, Zwingers T, Brittinger G: Spectrum and frequency of autoimmune derangements in lymphoproliferative disorders: Analysis of 637 cases and comparison with myeloproliferative diseases. *Br J Haematol* 67:235, 1987.

244. Hill PA, Firkin F, Dwyer KM, et al: Membranoproliferative glomerulonephritis in association with chronic lymphocytic leukaemia: A report of three cases. *Pathology* 34:138, 2002.

245. Rosado MF, Morgenszternn D, Abdullah S, et al: Chronic lymphocytic leukemia-associated nephrotic syndrome caused by focal segmental glomerulosclerosis. *Am J Hematol* 77:205, 2004.

246. Ziakas PD, Giannouli S, Psimenou E, et al: Membranous glomerulonephritis in chronic lymphocytic leukemia. *Am J Hematol* 76:271, 2004.

247. Ruzickova S, Pruss A, Odendahl M, et al: Chronic lymphocytic leukemia preceded by cold agglutinin disease: Intraclonal immunoglobulin light-chain diversity in V(H)4-34 expressing single leukemic B cells. *Blood* 100:3419, 2002.

248. Bhavnani M: Cyclosporin A treatment of pure red cell aplasia associated with B-CLL [letter, comment]. *Br J Haematol* 79:137, 1991.

249. Taylor HG, Nixon N, Sheeran TP, Dawes PT: Rheumatoid arthritis and chronic lymphatic leukaemia. *Clin Exp Rheumatol* 7:529, 1989.

250. Amir R, Dowdy YG, Goldberg AN: Chronic rhinitis: A manifestation of chronic lymphocytic leukemia. *Am J Otolaryngol* 20:328, 1999.

251. Weed RI: Exaggerated delayed hypersensitivity to mosquito bites in chronic lymphocytic leukemia. *Blood* 26:257, 1965.

252. Barzilai A, Shpiro D, Goldberg I, et al: Insect bite-like reaction in patients with hematologic malignant neoplasms. *Arch Dermatol* 135:1503, 1999.

253. Higgins JP, Warnke RA: Herpes lymphadenitis in association with chronic lymphocytic leukemia. *Cancer* 86:1210, 1999.

254. Mariette X, Molina JM, Asli B, Brouet JC: A patient with chronic lymphoid leukemia and recurrent necrotic herpetic lymphadenitis. *Am J Med* 107:403, 1999.

255. Rustagi PK, Han T, Ziolkowski L, et al: Granulocyte antibodies in leukaemic chronic lymphoproliferative disorders. *Br J Haematol* 66:461, 1987.

256. Lischner M, Prokocimer M, Zolberg A, Shaklai M: Autoimmunity in chronic lymphocytic leukaemia. *Postgrad Med J* 64:590, 1988.

257. Chablani AT, Badakere SS, Bhatia HM: Incidence of antibodies to nuclear antigens, platelets & circulating immune complexes in leukaemias. *Indian J Med Res* 88:348, 1988.

258. Koerner TA, Weinfeld HM, Bullard LS, Williams LC: Antibodies against platelet glycosphingolipids: Detection in serum by quantitative HPTLC-autoradiography and association with autoimmune and alloimmune processes. *Blood* 74:274, 1989.

259. Habboush HW, Dhundee J, Okati DA, Davies AG: Constrictive pericarditis in B cell chronic lymphatic leukaemia. *Clin Lab Haematol* 18:117, 1996.

260. Giannini O, Schonenberger-Berzins R: Fulminant cardiac tamponade in chronic lymphocytic leukaemia. *Ann Oncol* 8:1168, 1997.

261. Sivakumaran M, Qureshi H, Chapman CS: Chylous effusions in CLL. *Leuk Lymphoma* 18:365, 1995.

262. Zeidman A, Yarmolovsky A, Djaldetti M, Mittelman M: Hemorrhagic pleural effusion as a complication of chronic lymphocytic leukemia. *Haematologia (Budap)* 26:173, 1995.

263. Miyahara M, Shimamoto Y, Sano M, et al: Immunoglobulin gene re-

arrangement in T-cell-rich reactive pleural effusion of a patient with B-cell chronic lymphocytic leukemia. *Acta Haematol* 96:41, 1996.

264. Elliott MA, Letendre L, Li CY, et al: Chronic lymphocytic leukaemia with symptomatic diffuse central nervous system infiltration responding to therapy with systemic fludarabine. *Br J Haematol* 104:689, 1999.

265. Montserrat E, Marques-Pereira JP, Gallart MT, Rozman C: Bone marrow histopathologic patterns and immunologic findings in B-chronic lymphocytic leukemia. *Cancer* 54:447, 1984.

266. Pangalis GA, Roussou PA, Kittas C, et al: Patterns of bone marrow involvement in chronic lymphocytic leukemia and small lymphocytic (well differentiated) non-Hodgkin's lymphoma. Its clinical significance in relation to their differential diagnosis and prognosis. *Cancer* 54:702, 1984.

267. Pangalis GA, Boussiotis VA, Kittas C: Malignant disorders of small lymphocytes. Small lymphocytic lymphoma, lymphoplasmacytic lymphoma, and chronic lymphocytic leukemia: Their clinical and laboratory relationship. *Am J Clin Pathol* 99:402, 1993.

268. Pangalis GA, Roussou PA, Kittas C, et al: B-chronic lymphocytic leukemia. Prognostic implication of bone marrow histology in 120 patients experience from a single hematology unit. *Cancer* 59:767, 1987.

269. Kanzler H, Küppers R, Helmes S, et al: Hodgkin and Reed-Sternberg-like cells in B-cell chronic lymphocytic leukemia represent the outgrowth of single germinal-center B-cell-derived clones: Potential precursors of Hodgkin and Reed-Sternberg cells in Hodgkin's disease. *Blood* 95:1023, 2000.

270. Baldini L, Cro L, Cortelezzi A, et al: Immunophenotypes in "classical" B-cell chronic lymphocytic leukemia. Correlation with normal cellular counterpart and clinical findings. *Cancer* 66:1738, 1990.

271. Sarfati M, Fournier S, Christoffersen M, Biron G: Expression of CD23 antigen and its regulation by IL-4 in chronic lymphocytic leukemia. *Leuk Res* 14:47, 1990.

272. Batata A, Shen B: Immunophenotyping of subtypes of B-chronic (mature) lymphoid leukemia. A study of 242 cases. *Cancer* 70:2436, 1992.

273. De Rossi G, Zarcone D, Mauro F, et al: Adhesion molecule expression on B-cell chronic lymphocytic leukemia cells: Malignant cell phenotypes define distinct disease subsets. *Blood* 81:2679, 1993.

274. Serke S, Schwaner I, Yordanova M, et al: Monoclonal antibody FMC7 detects a conformational epitope on the CD20 molecule: Evidence from phenotyping after rituxan therapy and transfectant cell analyses. *Cytometry* 46:98, 2001.

275. Delgado J, Matutes E, Morilla AM, et al: Diagnostic significance of CD20 and FMC7 expression in B-cell disorders. *Am J Clin Pathol* 120:754, 2003.

276. Pianezze G, Gentilini I, Casini M, et al: Cytoplasmic immunoglobulins in chronic lymphocytic leukemia B cells. *Blood* 69:1011, 1987.

277. Yasuda N, Kanoh T, Shirakawa S, Uchino H: Intracellular immunoglobulin in lymphocytes from patients with chronic lymphocytic leukemia: An immunoelectron microscopic study. *Leuk Res* 6:659, 1982.

278. Newell DG, Hannam-Harris A, Karpas A, Smith JL: The differential ultrastructural localization of immunoglobulin heavy and light chains in human haematopoietic cell lines. *Br J Haematol* 50:445, 1982.

279. Newell DG, Harris AH, Smith JL: The ultrastructural localization of immunoglobulin in chronic lymphocytic lymphoma cells: Changes in light and heavy chain distribution induced by mitogen stimulation. *Blood* 61:511, 1983.

280. Deegan MJ, Abraham JP, Sawdyk M, Van Slyck EJ: High incidence of monoclonal proteins in the serum and urine of chronic lymphocytic leukemia patients. *Blood* 64:1207, 1984.

281. Sinclair D, Dagg JH, Dewar AE, et al: The incidence, clonal origin and secretory nature of serum paraproteins in chronic lymphocytic leukaemia. *Br J Haematol* 64:725, 1986.

282. Pangalis GA, Moutsopoulos HM, Papadopoulos NM, et al: Monoclonal and oligoclonal immunoglobulins in the serum of patients with B-chronic lymphocytic leukemia. *Acta Haematol* 80:23, 1988.

283. Gordon DS, Jones BM, Browning SW, et al: Persistent polyclonal lymphocytosis of B lymphocytes. *N Engl J Med* 307:232, 1982.

284. Wilkinson LS, Tang A, Gjedsted A: Marked lymphocytosis suggesting chronic lymphocytic leukemia in three patients with hyposplenism. *Am J Med* 75:1053, 1983.

285. Batata A, Shen B: Diagnostic value of clonality of surface immunoglobulin light and heavy chains in malignant lymphoproliferative disorders. *Am J Hematol* 43:265, 1993.

286. Melo JV, Wardle J, Chetty M, et al: The relationship between chronic lymphocytic leukaemia and prolymphocytic leukaemia: III. Evaluation of cell size by morphology and volume measurements. *Br J Haematol* 64:469, 1986.

287. Robinson DS, Melo JV, Andrews C, et al: Intracytoplasmic inclusions in B prolymphocytic leukaemia: Ultrastructural, cytochemical, and immunological studies. *J Clin Pathol* 38:897, 1985.

288. Bearman RM, Pangalis GA, Rappaport H: Prolymphocytic leukemia: Clinical, histopathological, and cytochemical observations. *Cancer* 42:2360, 1978.

289. Moreau EJ, Matutes E, A'Hern RP, et al: Improvement of the chronic lymphocytic leukemia scoring system with the monoclonal antibody SN8 (CD79b). *Am J Clin Pathol* 108:378, 1997.

290. Zomas AP, Matutes E, Morilla R, et al: Expression of the immunoglobulin-associated protein B29 in B cell disorders with the monoclonal antibody SN8 (CD79b). *Leukemia* 10:1966, 1996.

291. Cabezudo E, Carrara P, Morilla R, Matutes E: Quantitative analysis of CD79b, CD5, and CD19 in mature B-cell lymphoproliferative disorders. *Haematologica* 84:413, 1999.

292. Matutes E, Morilla R, Owusu-Ankomah K, et al: The immunophenotype of splenic lymphoma with villous lymphocytes and its relevance to the differential diagnosis with other B-cell disorders. *Blood* 83:1558, 1994.

293. Dick FR, Maca RD: The lymph node in chronic lymphocytic leukemia. *Cancer* 41:283, 1978.

294. Pratt LF, Rassenti L, Larrick J, et al: Immunoglobulin gene expression in small lymphocytic lymphoma with little or no somatic hypermutation. *J Immunol* 143:699, 1989.

295. Medeiros LJ, Strickler JG, Picker LJ, et al: "Well-differentiated" lymphocytic neoplasms. Immunologic findings correlated with clinical presentation and morphologic features. *Am J Pathol* 129:523, 1987.

296. Ellison DJ, Turner RR, van Antwerp R, et al: High-grade mantle zone lymphoma. *Cancer* 60:2717, 1987.

297. Bell PB, Rooney N, Bosanquet AG: CD79a detected by ZL7.4 separates chronic lymphocytic leukemia from mantle cell lymphoma in the leukemic phase. *Cytometry* 38:102, 1999.

298. Elnenaei MO, Jadayel DM, Matutes E, et al: Cyclin D1 by flow cytometry as a useful tool in the diagnosis of B-cell malignancies. *Leuk Res* 25:115, 2001.

299. Ruchlemer R, Parry-Jones N, Brito-Babapulle V, et al: B-prolymphocytic leukaemia with t(11;14) revisited: A splenomegalic form of mantle cell lymphoma evolving with leukaemia. *Br J Haematol* 125:330, 2004.

300. Matutes E, Carrara P, Coignet L, et al: FISH analysis for BCL-1 rearrangements and trisomy 12 helps the diagnosis of atypical B cell leukaemias. *Leukemia* 13:1721, 1999.

301. Dogan A, Isaacson PG: Splenic marginal zone lymphoma. *Semin Diagn Pathol* 20:121, 2003.

302. Franco V, Florena AM, Iannitto E: Splenic marginal zone lymphoma. *Blood* 101:2464, 2003.

303. Giannouli S, Paterakis G, Ziakas PD, et al: Splenic marginal zone lymphomas with peripheral CD5 expression. *Haematologica* 89:113, 2004.

304. Andersen CL, Gruszka-Westwood A, Ostergaard M, et al: A narrow deletion of 7q is common to HCL, and SMZL, but not CLL. *Eur J Haematol* 72:390, 2004.

305. Kansal R, Ross CW, Singleton TP, et al: Histopathologic features of

splenic small B-cell lymphomas. A study of 42 cases with a definitive diagnosis by the World Health Organization classification. *Am J Clin Pathol* 120:335, 2003.

306. Skinnider LF, Tan L, Schmidt J, Armitage G: Chronic lymphocytic leukemia. A review of 745 cases and assessment of clinical staging. *Cancer* 50:2951, 1982.

307. Phillips EA, Kempin S, Passe S, et al: Prognostic factors in chronic lymphocytic leukaemia and their implications for therapy. *Clin Haematol* 6:203, 1977.

308. Binet JL, Auquier A, Dighiero G, et al: A new prognostic classification of chronic lymphocytic leukemia derived from a multivariate survival analysis. *Cancer* 48:198, 1981.

309. Rai KR: A critical analysis of staging in CLL, in *Chronic Lymphocytic Leukemia: Recent Progress and Future Direction*, edited by RP Gale, KR Rai, p 253. Alan R Liss, New York, 1987.

310. Vasconcelos Y, Davi F, Levy V, et al: Binet's staging system and VH genes are independent but complementary prognostic indicators in chronic lymphocytic leukemia. *J Clin Oncol* 21:3928, 2003.

311. Cheson BD, Bennett JM, Grever M, et al: National Cancer Institute-sponsored Working Group guidelines for chronic lymphocytic leukemia: Revised guidelines for diagnosis and treatment. *Blood* 87:4990, 1996.

312. Vrhovac R, Delmer A, Tang R, et al: Prognostic significance of the cell cycle inhibitor p27Kip1 in chronic B-cell lymphocytic leukemia. *Blood* 91:4694, 1998.

313. Montserrat E, Sanchez-Bisono J, Vinolas N, Rozman C: Lymphocyte doubling time in chronic lymphocytic leukaemia: Analysis of its prognostic significance. *Br J Haematol* 62:567, 1986.

314. Mauro FR, Foa R, Giannarelli D, et al: Clinical characteristics and outcome of young chronic lymphocytic leukemia patients: A single institution study of 204 cases. *Blood* 94:448, 1999.

315. Schroeder HW Jr, Dighiero G: The pathogenesis of chronic lymphocytic leukemia: Analysis of the antibody repertoire. *Immunol Today* 15:288, 1994.

316. Friedman DF, Moore JS, Erikson J, et al: Variable region gene analysis of an isotype-switched (IgA) variant of chronic lymphocytic leukemia. *Blood* 80:2287, 1992.

317. Ebeling SB, Schutte ME, Logtenberg T: Molecular analysis of VH and VL regions expressed in IgG-bearing chronic lymphocytic leukemia (CLL): Further evidence that CLL is a heterogeneous group of tumors. *Blood* 82:1626, 1993.

318. Hashimoto S, Dono M, Wakai M, et al: Somatic diversification and selection of immunoglobulin heavy and light chain variable region genes in IgG+ CD5+ chronic lymphocytic leukemia B cells. *J Exp Med* 181:1507, 1995.

319. Matolcsy A, Casali P, Nador RG, et al: Molecular characterization of IgA- and/or IgG-switched chronic lymphocytic leukemia B cells. *Blood* 89:1732, 1997.

320. Kipps TJ, Tomhave E, Chen PP, Carson DA: Autoantibody-associated kappa light chain variable region gene expressed in chronic lymphocytic leukemia with little or no somatic mutation. Implications for etiology and immunotherapy. *J Exp Med* 167:840, 1988.

321. Schettino EW, Cerutti A, Chiorazzi N, Casali P: Lack of intraclonal diversification in Ig heavy and light chain V region genes expressed by CD5+IgM+ chronic lymphocytic leukemia B cells: A multiple time point analysis. *J Immunol* 160:820, 1998.

322. Oscier DG, Thompsett A, Zhu D, Stevenson FK: Differential rates of somatic hypermutation in V(H) genes among subsets of chronic lymphocytic leukemia defined by chromosomal abnormalities. *Blood* 89:4153, 1997.

323. Hamblin TJ, Orchard JA, Ibbotson RE, et al: CD38 expression and immunoglobulin variable region mutations are independent prognostic variables in chronic lymphocytic leukemia, but CD38 expression may vary during the course of the disease. *Blood* 99:1023, 2002.

324. Kröber A, Seiler T, Benner A, et al: V(H) mutation status, CD38 expression level, genomic aberrations, and survival in chronic lymphocytic leukemia. *Blood* 100:1410, 2002.

325. Lin K, Sherrington PD, Dennis M, et al: Relationship between p53 dysfunction, CD38 expression, and IgV(H) mutation in chronic lymphocytic leukemia. *Blood* 100:1404, 2002.

326. Oscier DG, Gardiner AC, Mould SJ, et al: Multivariate analysis of prognostic factors in CLL: Clinical stage, IGVH gene mutational status, and loss or mutation of the p53 gene are independent prognostic factors. *Blood* 100:1177, 2002.

327. Stilgenbauer S, Bullinger L, Lichter P, Döhner H: Genetics of chronic lymphocytic leukemia: Genomic aberrations and V(H) gene mutation status in pathogenesis and clinical course. *Leukemia* 16:993, 2002.

328. Chen L, Widhopf G, Huynh L, et al: Expression of ZAP-70 is associated with increased B-cell receptor signaling in chronic lymphocytic leukemia. *Blood* 100:4609, 2002.

329. Crespo M, Bosch F, Villamor N, et al: ZAP-70 expression as a surrogate for immunoglobulin-variable-region mutations in chronic lymphocytic leukemia. *N Engl J Med* 348:1764, 2003.

330. Wiestner A, Rosenwald A, Barry TS, et al: ZAP-70 expression identifies a chronic lymphocytic leukemia subtype with unmutated immunoglobulin genes, inferior clinical outcome, and distinct gene expression profile. *Blood* 101:4944, 2003.

331. Rassenti LZ, Huynh L, Toy TL, et al: ZAP-70 compared with immunoglobulin heavy-chain gene mutation status as a predictor of disease progression in chronic lymphocytic leukemia. *N Engl J Med* 351:893, 2004.

332. Dürig J, Naschar M, Schmucker U, et al: CD38 expression is an important prognostic marker in chronic lymphocytic leukaemia. *Leukemia* 16:30, 2002.

333. Chevallier P, Penther D, Avet-Loiseau H, et al: CD38 expression and secondary 17p deletion are important prognostic factors in chronic lymphocytic leukaemia. *Br J Haematol* 116:142, 2002.

334. Morabito F, Mangiola M, Stelitano C, et al: Peripheral blood CD38 expression predicts time to progression in B-cell chronic lymphocytic leukemia after first-line therapy with high-dose chlorambucil. *Haematologica* 87:217, 2002.

335. Domingo-Domenech E, Domingo-Claros A, Gonzalez-Barca E, et al: CD38 expression in B-chronic lymphocytic leukemia: Association with clinical presentation and outcome in 155 patients. *Haematologica* 87:1021, 2002.

336. D'Arena G, Nunziata G, Coppola G, et al: CD38 expression does not change in B-cell chronic lymphocytic leukemia. *Blood* 100:3052, 2002.

337. Thunberg U, Johnson A, Roos G, et al: CD38 expression is a poor predictor for VH gene mutational status and prognosis in chronic lymphocytic leukemia. *Blood* 97:1892, 2001.

338. Hulkkonen J, Vilpo L, Hurme M, Vilpo J: Surface antigen expression in chronic lymphocytic leukemia: Clustering analysis, interrelationships and effects of chromosomal abnormalities. *Leukemia* 16:178, 2002.

339. Degan M, Rupolo M, Bo MD, et al: Mutational status of IgVH genes consistent with antigen-driven selection but not percent of mutations has prognostic impact in B-cell chronic lymphocytic leukemia. *Clin Lymphoma* 5:123, 2004.

340. Han T, Henderson ES, Emrich LJ, Sandberg AA: Prognostic significance of karyotypic abnormalities in B cell chronic lymphocytic leukemia: An update. *Semin Hematol* 24:257, 1987.

341. Escudier SM, Pereira-Leahy JM, Drach JW, et al: Fluorescent in situ hybridization and cytogenetic studies of trisomy 12 in chronic lymphocytic leukemia. *Blood* 81:2702, 1993.

342. Döhner H, Stilgenbauer S, Benner A, et al: Genomic aberrations and survival in chronic lymphocytic leukemia. *N Engl J Med* 343:1910, 2000.

343. Juliusson G, Robert KH, Ost A, et al: Prognostic information from cyto-

genetic analysis in chronic B-lymphocytic leukemia and leukemic immunocytoma. *Blood* 65:134, 1985.

344. Tefferi A, Bartholmai BJ, Witzig TE, et al: Clinical correlations of immunophenotypic variations and the presence of trisomy 12 in B-cell chronic lymphocytic leukemia. *Cancer Genet Cytogenet* 95:173, 1997.

345. Juliusson G, Oscier DG, Fitchett M, et al: Prognostic subgroups in B-cell chronic lymphocytic leukemia defined by specific chromosomal abnormalities. *N Engl J Med* 323:720, 1990.

346. Montserrat E, Bosch F, Rozman C: B-cell chronic lymphocytic leukemia: Recent progress in biology, diagnosis, and therapy. *Ann Oncol* 8(suppl 1):93, 1997.

347. Oscier DG, Stevens J, Hamblin TJ, et al: Correlation of chromosome abnormalities with laboratory features and clinical course in B-cell chronic lymphocytic leukaemia. *Br J Haematol* 76:352, 1990.

348. Molica S, Levato D, Cascavilla N, et al: Clinico-prognostic implications of simultaneous increased serum levels of soluble CD23 and beta2-microglobulin in B-cell chronic lymphocytic leukemia. *Eur J Haematol* 62:117, 1999.

349. Spati B, Child JA, Kerruish SM, Cooper EH: Behaviour of serum beta 2-microglobulin and acute phase reactant proteins in chronic lymphocytic leukaemia. A multicentre study. *Acta Haematol* 64:79, 1980.

350. Hallek M, Langenmayer I, Nerl C, et al: Elevated serum thymidine kinase levels identify a subgroup at high risk of disease progression in early, nonsmoldering chronic lymphocytic leukemia. *Blood* 93:1732, 1999.

351. Magnac C, Porcher R, Davi F, et al: Predictive value of serum thymidine kinase level for Ig-V mutational status in B-CLL. *Leukemia* 17:133, 2003.

352. Sarfati M, Chevret S, Chastang C, et al: Prognostic importance of serum soluble CD23 level in chronic lymphocytic leukemia. *Blood* 88:4259, 1996.

353. Knauf WU, Ehlers B, Mohr B, et al: Prognostic impact of the serum levels of soluble CD23 in B-cell chronic lymphocytic leukemia. *Blood* 89:4241, 1997.

354. Schwarzmeier JD, Shehata M, Hilgarth M, et al: The role of soluble CD23 in distinguishing stable and progressive forms of B-chronic lymphocytic leukemia. *Leuk Lymphoma* 43:549, 2002.

355. Christiansen I, Sundstrom C, Totterman TH: Elevated serum levels of soluble vascular cell adhesion molecule-1 (sVCAM-1) closely reflect tumour burden in chronic B-lymphocytic leukaemia. *Br J Haematol* 103:1129, 1998.

356. Molica S, Vitelli G, Levato D, et al: CD27 in B-cell chronic lymphocytic leukemia. Cellular expression, serum release and correlation with other soluble molecules belonging to nerve growth factor receptors (NGFr) superfamily. *Haematologica* 83:398, 1998.

357. Lee JS, Dixon DO, Kantarjian HM, et al: Prognosis of chronic lymphocytic leukemia: A multivariate regression analysis of 325 untreated patients. *Blood* 69:929, 1987.

358. Robertson LE, Pugh W, O'Brien S, et al: Richter's syndrome: A report on 39 patients. *J Clin Oncol* 11:1985, 1993.

359. Everaus H, Luik E, Lehtmaa J: Active and indolent chronic lymphocytic leukaemia—Immune and hormonal peculiarities. *Cancer Immunol Immunother* 45:109, 1997.

360. Vlasveld LT, Pauwels P, Ermens AA, et al: Parathyroid hormone-related protein (PTH-rP)-associated hypercalcemia in a patient with an atypical chronic lymphocytic leukemia. *Neth J Med* 54:21, 1999.

361. Beaudreuil J, Lortholary O, Martin A, et al: Hypercalcemia may indicate Richter's syndrome: Report of four cases and review. *Cancer* 79:1211, 1997.

362. Schoevaerdts D, Mineur P, Hennaux V, Sibille C: Hypercalcemia, chronic lymphocytic leukemia and multiple myeloma: Uncommon association. *Acta Clin Belg* 54:217, 1999.

363. de Nully Brown P, Hansen MM: GM-CSF treatment in patients with B-chronic lymphocytic leukemia. *Leuk Lymphoma* 32:365, 1999.

364. Itala M, Pelliniemi TT, Remes K: GM-CSF raises serum levels of beta 2-microglobulin and thymidine kinase in patients with chronic lymphocytic leukaemia. *Br J Haematol* 94:129, 1996.

365. Montserrat E, Villamor N, Reverter JC, et al: Bone marrow assessment in B-cell chronic lymphocytic leukaemia: Aspirate or biopsy? A comparative study in 258 patients. *Br J Haematol* 93:111, 1996.

366. Geisler CH, Hou-Jensen K, Jensen OM, et al: The bone-marrow infiltration pattern in B-cell chronic lymphocytic leukemia is not an important prognostic factor. Danish CLL Study Group. *Eur J Haematol* 57:292, 1996.

367. Sah SP, Matutes E, Wotherspoon AC, et al: A comparison of flow cytometry, bone marrow biopsy, and bone marrow aspirates in the detection of lymphoid infiltration in B cell disorders. *J Clin Pathol* 56:129, 2003.

368. Jarque I, Larrea L, Gomis F, et al: Bone marrow assessment in B-cell chronic lymphocytic leukaemia: Aspirate or biopsy? *Br J Haematol* 95:754, 1996.

369. Chemotherapeutic options in chronic lymphocytic leukemia: A meta-analysis of the randomized trials. CLL Trialists' Collaborative Group. *J Natl Cancer Inst* 91:861, 1999.

370. Lichtman MA, Rowe JM: Hyperleukocytic leukemias: Rheological, clinical, and therapeutic considerations. *Blood* 60:279, 1982.

371. Rawstron AC, Kennedy B, Evans PA, et al: Quantitation of minimal disease levels in chronic lymphocytic leukemia using a sensitive flow cytometric assay improves the prediction of outcome and can be used to optimize therapy. *Blood* 98:29, 2001.

372. Provan D, Bartlett-Pandite L, Zwicky C, et al: Eradication of polymerase chain reaction-detectable chronic lymphocytic leukemia cells is associated with improved outcome after bone marrow transplantation. *Blood* 88:2228, 1996.

373. Bottcher S, Ritgen M, Pott C, et al: Comparative analysis of minimal residual disease detection using four-color flow cytometry, consensus IgH-PCR, and quantitative IgH PCR in CLL after allogeneic and autologous stem cell transplantation. *Leukemia* 18:1637, 2004.

374. Moreton P, Kennedy B, Lucas G, et al: Eradication of minimal residual disease in B-cell chronic lymphocytic leukemia after alemtuzumab therapy is associated with prolonged survival. *J Clin Oncol* 23:2971, 2005.

375. Keating MJ, O'Brien S, Plunkett W, et al: Fludarabine phosphate: A new active agent in hematologic malignancies. *Semin Hematol* 31:28, 1994.

376. Boogaerts MA, van Hoof A, Catovsky D, et al: Activity of oral fludarabine phosphate in previously treated chronic lymphocytic leukemia. *J Clin Oncol* 19:4252, 2001.

377. Rossi JF, van Hoof A, de Boeck K, et al: Efficacy and safety of oral fludarabine phosphate in previously untreated patients with chronic lymphocytic leukemia. *J Clin Oncol* 22:1260, 2004.

378. Gjedde SB, Hansen MM: Salvage therapy with fludarabine in patients with progressive B-chronic lymphocytic leukemia. *Leuk Lymphoma* 21:317, 1996.

379. Angelopoulou MA, Poziopoulos C, Boussiotis VA, et al: Fludarabine monophosphate in refractory B-chronic lymphocytic leukemia: Maintenance may be significant to sustain response. *Leuk Lymphoma* 21:321, 1996.

380. Sorensen JM, Vena DA, Fallavollita A, et al: Treatment of refractory chronic lymphocytic leukemia with fludarabine phosphate via the group C protocol mechanism of the National Cancer Institute: Five-year follow-up report. *J Clin Oncol* 15:458, 1997.

381. Keating MJ, O'Brien S, Lerner S, et al: Long-term follow-up of patients with chronic lymphocytic leukemia (CLL) receiving fludarabine regimens as initial therapy. *Blood* 92:1165, 1998.

382. Johnson S, Smith AG, Loffler H, et al: Multicentre prospective randomised trial of fludarabine versus cyclophosphamide, doxorubicin, and prednisone (CAP) for treatment of advanced-stage chronic lymphocytic

leukaemia. The French Cooperative Group on CLL. *Lancet* 347:1432, 1996.

383. O'Brien S, Kantarjian H, Beran M, et al: Results of fludarabine and prednisone therapy in 264 patients with chronic lymphocytic leukemia with multivariate analysis-derived prognostic model for response to treatment. *Blood* 82:1695, 1993.

384. Mason JM, Drummond MF, Bosanquet AG, Sheldon TA: The DiSC assay. A cost-effective guide to treatment for chronic lymphocytic leukemia? *Int J Technol Assess Health Care* 15:173, 1999.

385. Bosanquet AG, Johnson SA, Richards SM: Prognosis for fludarabine therapy of chronic lymphocytic leukaemia based on ex vivo drug response by DiSC assay. *Br J Haematol* 106:71, 1999.

386. Cohen RB, Abdallah JM, Gray JR, Foss F: Reversible neurologic toxicity in patients treated with standard-dose fludarabine phosphate for mycosis fungoides and chronic lymphocytic leukemia [comments]. *Ann Intern Med* 118:114, 1993.

387. Ramachandran A, Majumdar G: Acute tumour lysis syndrome after oral fludarabine in a patient with chronic lymphocytic leukaemia. *Hematol J* 5:528, 2004.

388. Hussain K, Mazza JJ, Clouse LH: Tumor lysis syndrome (TLS) following fludarabine therapy for chronic lymphocytic leukemia (CLL): Case report and review of the literature. *Am J Hematol* 72:212, 2003.

389. Wijermans PW, Gerrits WB, Haak HL: Severe immunodeficiency in patients treated with fludarabine monophosphate. *Eur J Haematol* 50:292, 1993.

390. Anaissie E, Kontoyiannis DP, Kantarjian H, et al: Listeriosis in patients with chronic lymphocytic leukemia who were treated with fludarabine and prednisone. *Ann Intern Med* 117:466, 1992.

391. Bergmann L, Fenchel K, Jahn B, et al: Immunosuppressive effects and clinical response of fludarabine in refractory chronic lymphocytic leukemia. *Ann Oncol* 4:371, 1993.

392. Hamblin TJ, Orchard JA, Myint H, Oscier DG: Fludarabine and hemolytic anemia in chronic lymphocytic leukemia. *J Clin Oncol* 16:3209, 1998.

393. Keating MJ: Chronic lymphocytic leukemia. *Semin Oncol* 26:107, 1999.

394. Briz M, Cabrera R, Sanjuan I, et al: Diagnosis of transfusion-associated graft-versus-host disease by polymerase chain reaction in fludarabine-treated B-chronic lymphocytic leukaemia. *Br J Haematol* 91:409, 1995.

395. Briones J, Pereira A, Alcorta I: Transfusion-associated graft-versus-host disease (TA-GVHD) in fludarabine-treated patients: Is it time to irradiate blood component? *Br J Haematol* 93:739, 1996.

396. Cheson BD, Vena DA, Barrett J, Freidlin B: Second malignancies as a consequence of nucleoside analog therapy for chronic lymphoid leukemias. *J Clin Oncol* 17:2454, 1999.

397. Robak T: The place of cladribine in the treatment of chronic lymphocytic leukemia: A 10-year experience in Poland. *Ann Hematol* 84:63, 2005.

398. Robak T, Blasinka-Morawiec M, Krykowski E, et al: Intermittent 2-hour intravenous infusions of 2-chlorodeoxyadenosine in the treatment of 110 patients with refractory or previously untreated B-cell chronic lymphocytic leukemia. *Leuk Lymphoma* 22:509, 1996.

399. Juliusson G, Elmhorn-Rosenborg A, Liliemark J: Response to 2-chlorodeoxyadenosine in patients with B-cell chronic lymphocytic leukemia resistant to fludarabine [comments]. *N Engl J Med* 327:1056, 1992.

400. Byrd JC, Peterson B, Piro L, et al: A phase II study of cladribine treatment for fludarabine refractory B cell chronic lymphocytic leukemia: Results from CALGB Study 9211. *Leukemia* 17:323, 2003.

401. Karlsson K, Stromberg M, Liliemark J, et al: Oral cladribine for B-cell chronic lymphocytic leukaemia: Report of a phase II trial with a 3-d, 3-weekly schedule in untreated and pretreated patients, and a long-term follow-up of 126 previously untreated patients. *Br J Haematol* 116:538, 2002.

402. Juliusson G, Christiansen I, Hansen MM, et al: Oral cladribine as pri-

mary therapy for patients with B-cell chronic lymphocytic leukemia. *J Clin Oncol* 14:2160, 1996.

403. Bosanquet AG, Copplestone JA, Johnson SA, et al: Response to cladribine in previously treated patients with chronic lymphocytic leukaemia identified by ex vivo assessment of drug sensitivity by DiSC assay. *Br J Haematol* 106:474, 1999.

404. Anchisi S, Zulian GB, Dietrich PY, Alberto P: Cladribine and tumour lysis syndrome. *Eur J Cancer* 31A:131, 1995.

405. Dillman RO: A new chemotherapeutic agent: Deoxycoformycin (pentostatin). *Semin Hematol* 31:16, 1994.

406. Dillman RO: Pentostatin (Nipent) in the treatment of chronic lymphocyte leukemia and hairy cell leukemia. *Expert Rev Anticancer Ther* 4:27, 2004.

407. Johnson SA, Catovsky D, Child JA, et al: Phase I/II evaluation of pentostatin (2'-deoxycoformycin) in a five day schedule for the treatment of relapsed/refractory B-cell chronic lymphocytic leukaemia. *Invest New Drugs* 16:155, 1998.

408. Oken MM, Lee S, Kay NE, et al: Pentostatin, chlorambucil and prednisone therapy for B-chronic lymphocytic leukemia: A phase I/II study by the Eastern Cooperative Oncology Group study E1488. *Leuk Lymphoma* 45:79, 2004.

409. Dighiero G, Maloum K, Desablens B, et al: Chlorambucil in indolent chronic lymphocytic leukemia. French Cooperative Group on Chronic Lymphocytic Leukemia. *N Engl J Med* 338:1506, 1998.

410. Sawitsky A, Rai KR, Glidewell O, Silver RT: Comparison of daily versus intermittent chlorambucil and prednisone therapy in the treatment of patients with chronic lymphocytic leukemia. *Blood* 50:1049, 1977.

411. Han T, Ezdinli EZ, Shimaoka K, Desai DV: Chlorambucil vs. combined chlorambucil-corticosteroid therapy in chronic lymphocytic leukemia. *Cancer* 31:502, 1973.

412. Jaksic B, Brugiatelli M, Krc I, et al: High dose chlorambucil versus Binet's modified cyclophosphamide, doxorubicin, vincristine, and prednisone regimen in the treatment of patients with advanced B-cell chronic lymphocytic leukemia. Results of an international multicenter randomized trial. International Society for Chemo-Immunotherapy, Vienna. *Cancer* 79:2107, 1997.

413. Huguley CMJ: Treatment of chronic lymphocytic leukemia. *Cancer Treat Rev* 4:261, 1977.

414. Kath R, Blumenstengel K, Fricke HJ, Hoffken K: Bendamustine monotherapy in advanced and refractory chronic lymphocytic leukemia. *J Cancer Res Clin Oncol* 127:48, 2001.

415. Aivado M, Schulte K, Henze L, et al: Bendamustine in the treatment of chronic lymphocytic leukemia: Results and future perspectives. *Semin Oncol* 29:19, 2002.

416. Bremer K: High rates of long-lasting remissions after 5-day bendamustine chemotherapy cycles in pre-treated low-grade non-Hodgkin's-lymphomas. *J Cancer Res Clin Oncol* 128:603, 2002.

417. Thornton PD, Hamblin M, Treleaven JG, et al: High dose methyl prednisolone in refractory chronic lymphocytic leukaemia. *Leuk Lymphoma* 34:167, 1999.

418. Thornton PD, Matutes E, Bosanquet AG, et al: High dose methylprednisolone can induce remissions in CLL patients with p53 abnormalities. *Ann Hematol* 82:759, 2003.

419. Robertson LE, Hall R, Keating MJ, et al: High-dose cytosine arabinoside in chronic lymphocytic leukemia: A clinical and pharmacologic analysis. *Leuk Lymphoma* 10:43, 1993.

420. Shaklai S, Bairey O, Blickstein D, et al: Severe myelotoxicity of oral etoposide in heavily pretreated patients with non-Hodgkin's lymphoma or chronic lymphatic leukemia. *Cancer* 77:2313, 1996.

421. Bellosillo B, Colomer D, Pons G, Gil J: Mitoxantrone, a topoisomerase II inhibitor, induces apoptosis of B-chronic lymphocytic leukaemia cells. *Br J Haematol* 100:142, 1998.

422. Bosch F, Ferrer A, Lopez-Guillermo A, et al: Fludarabine, cyclophos-

phamide and mitoxantrone in the treatment of resistant or relapsed chronic lymphocytic leukaemia. *Br J Haematol* 119:976, 2002.

423. Tsimberidou AM, Keating MJ, Giles FJ, et al: Fludarabine and mitoxantrone for patients with chronic lymphocytic leukemia. *Cancer* 100:2583, 2004.

424. Robak T, Blonski JZ, Kasznicki M, et al: Cladribine combined with cyclophosphamide and mitoxantrone as front-line therapy in chronic lymphocytic leukemia. *Leukemia* 15:1510, 2001.

425. Rogalinska M, Blonski JZ, Hanausek M, et al: 2-Chlorodeoxyadenosine alone and in combination with cyclophosphamide and mitoxantrone induce apoptosis in B chronic lymphocytic leukemia cells in vivo. *Cancer Detect Prev* 28:433, 2004.

426. Emmanouilides C, Territo M, Menco H, et al: Mitoxantrone-cyclophosphamide-rituximab: An effective and safe combination for indolent NHL. *Hematol Oncol* 21:99, 2003.

427. Koppler H, Heymanns J, Pandorf A, Weide R: Bendamustine plus mitoxantrone—A new effective treatment for advanced chronic lymphocytic leukaemia: Results of a phase I/II study. *Leuk Lymphoma* 45:911, 2004.

428. Weide R, Pandorf A, Heymanns J, Koppler H: Bendamustine/mitoxantrone/rituximab (BMR): A very effective, well tolerated outpatient chemoimmunotherapy for relapsed and refractory CD20-positive indolent malignancies. Final results of a pilot study. *Leuk Lymphoma* 45:2445, 2004.

429. Rai KR, Freter CE, Mercier RJ, et al: Alemtuzumab in previously treated chronic lymphocytic leukemia patients who also had received fludarabine. *J Clin Oncol* 20:3891, 2002.

430. Bowen AL, Zomas A, Emmett E, et al: Subcutaneous CAMPATH-1H in fludarabine-resistant/relapsed chronic lymphocytic and B-prolymphocytic leukaemia. *Br J Haematol* 96:617, 1997.

431. Osterborg A, Fassas AS, Anagnostopoulos A, et al: Humanized CD52 monoclonal antibody Campath-1H as first-line treatment in chronic lymphocytic leukaemia. *Br J Haematol* 93:151, 1996.

432. Hale G, Dyer MJ, Clark MR, et al: Remission induction in non-Hodgkin lymphoma with reshaped human monoclonal antibody CAMPATH-1H. *Lancet* 2:1394, 1988.

433. Osterborg A, Dyer MJ, Bunjes D, et al: Phase II multicenter study of human CD52 antibody in previously treated chronic lymphocytic leukemia. European Study Group of CAMPATH-1H Treatment in Chronic Lymphocytic Leukemia. *J Clin Oncol* 15:1567, 1997.

434. Keating M, Coutre S, Rai K, et al: Management guidelines for use of alemtuzumab in B-cell chronic lymphocytic leukemia. *Clin Lymphoma* 4:220, 2004.

435. Lundin J, Porwit-MacDonald A, Rossmann ED, et al: Cellular immune reconstitution after subcutaneous alemtuzumab (anti-CD52 monoclonal antibody, CAMPATH-1H) treatment as first-line therapy for B-cell chronic lymphocytic leukaemia. *Leukemia* 18:484, 2004.

436. Kennedy B, Hillmen P: Immunological effects and safe administration of alemtuzumab (MabCampath) in advanced B-cLL. *Med Oncol* 19(suppl):S49, 2002.

437. Robak T: Alemtuzumab in the treatment of chronic lymphocytic leukemia. *BioDrugs* 19:9, 2005.

438. Osterborg A, Mellstedt H, Keating M: Clinical effects of alemtuzumab (Campath-1H) in B-cell chronic lymphocytic leukemia. *Med Oncol* 19(suppl):S21, 2002.

439. Stilgenbauer S, Döhner H: Campath-1H-induced complete remission of chronic lymphocytic leukemia despite p53 gene mutation and resistance to chemotherapy. *N Engl J Med* 347:452, 2002.

440. Dyer MJ, Kelsey SM, Mackay HJ, et al: In vivo "purging" of residual disease in CLL with Campath-1H. *Br J Haematol* 97:669, 1997.

441. Maloney DG, Grillo-Lopez AJ, White CA, et al: IDEC-C2B8 (Rituximab) anti-CD20 monoclonal antibody therapy in patients with relapsed low-grade non-Hodgkin's lymphoma. *Blood* 90:2188, 1997.

442. McLaughlin P, Grillo-Lopez AJ, Link BK, et al: Rituximab chimeric anti-CD20 monoclonal antibody therapy for relapsed indolent lymphoma: Half of patients respond to a four-dose treatment program. *J Clin Oncol* 16:2825, 1998.

443. Itala M, Geisler CH, Kimby E, et al: Standard-dose anti-CD20 antibody rituximab has efficacy in chronic lymphocytic leukaemia: Results from a Nordic multicentre study. *Eur J Haematol* 69:129, 2002.

444. Hainsworth JD, Litchy S, Barton JH, et al: Single-agent rituximab as first-line and maintenance treatment for patients with chronic lymphocytic leukemia or small lymphocytic lymphoma: A phase II trial of the Minnie Pearl Cancer Research Network. *J Clin Oncol* 21:1746, 2003.

445. Byrd JC, Murphy T, Howard RS, et al: Rituximab using a thrice weekly dosing schedule in B-cell chronic lymphocytic leukemia and small lymphocytic lymphoma demonstrates clinical activity and acceptable toxicity. *J Clin Oncol* 19:2153, 2001.

446. O'Brien SM, Kantarjian H, Thomas DA, et al: Rituximab dose-escalation trial in chronic lymphocytic leukemia. *J Clin Oncol* 19:2165, 2001.

447. Manshouri T, Do KA, Wang X, et al: Circulating CD20 is detectable in the plasma of patients with chronic lymphocytic leukemia and is of prognostic significance. *Blood* 101:2507, 2003.

448. Yang H, Rosove MH, Figlin RA: Tumor lysis syndrome occurring after the administration of rituximab in lymphoproliferative disorders: High-grade non-Hodgkin's lymphoma and chronic lymphocytic leukemia. *Am J Hematol* 62:247, 1999.

449. Voog E, Morschhauser F, Solal-Celigny P: Neutropenia in patients treated with rituximab. *N Engl J Med* 348:2691, 2003.

450. Winkler U, Jensen M, Manzke O, et al: Cytokine-release syndrome in patients with B-cell chronic lymphocytic leukemia and high lymphocyte counts after treatment with an anti CD20 monoclonal antibody (rituximab, IDEC-C2B8). *Blood* 94:2217, 1999.

451. Frankel AE, Fleming DR, Powell BL, Gartenhaus R: DAB389IL2 (ONTAK) fusion protein therapy of chronic lymphocytic leukaemia. *Expert Opin Biol Ther* 3:179, 2003.

452. Catovsky D, Richards S, Fooks J, Hamblin TJ: CLL Trials in the United Kingdom. *Leuk Lymphoma* 5(suppl):105, 1991.

453. Montserrat E, Fontanilles M, Estapé J: Treatment of chronic lymphocytic leukemia: A preliminary report of Spanish (Pethema) trials. *Leuk Lymphoma* 5(suppl):89, 1991.

454. Keller JW, Knospe WH, Raney M, et al: Treatment of chronic lymphocytic leukemia using chlorambucil and prednisone with or without cycle-active consolidation chemotherapy. A Southeastern Cancer Study Group Trial. *Cancer* 58:1185, 1986.

455. Montserrat E, Alcala A, Alonso C, et al: A randomized trial comparing chlorambucil plus prednisone vs cyclophosphamide, melphalan, and prednisone in the treatment of chronic lymphocytic leukemia stages B and C. *Nouv Rev Fr Hematol* 30:429, 1988.

456. Raphael B, Andersen JW, Silber R, et al: Comparison of chlorambucil and prednisone versus cyclophosphamide, vincristine, and prednisone as initial treatment for chronic lymphocytic leukemia: Long-term follow-up of an Eastern Cooperative Oncology Group randomized clinical trial. *J Clin Oncol* 9:770, 1991.

457. O'Brien S, Kantarjian H, Beran M, et al: Fludarabine and granulocyte colony-stimulating factor (G-CSF) in patients with chronic lymphocytic leukemia. *Leukemia* 11:1631, 1997.

458. O'Brien SM, Kantarjian HM, Cortes J, et al: Results of the fludarabine and cyclophosphamide combination regimen in chronic lymphocytic leukemia. *J Clin Oncol* 19:1414, 2001.

459. Schmitt B, Wendtner CM, Bergmann M, et al: Fludarabine combination therapy for the treatment of chronic lymphocytic leukemia. *Clin Lymphoma* 3:26, 2002.

460. Tothova E, Kafkova A, Fricova M, et al: Fludarabine combined with cyclophosphamide is highly effective in the treatment of chronic lymphocytic leukemia. *Neoplasma* 50:433, 2003.

461. Tam CS, Wolf MM, Januszewicz EH, et al: Fludarabine and cyclophosphamide using an attenuated dose schedule is a highly effective regimen for patients with indolent lymphoid malignancies. *Cancer* 100: 2181, 2004.

462. Rai KR, Peterson BL, Appelbaum FR, et al: Fludarabine compared with chlorambucil as primary therapy for chronic lymphocytic leukemia. *N Engl J Med* 343:1750, 2000.

463. Wierda W, O'Brien S, Wen S, et al: Chemoimmunotherapy with fludarabine, cyclophosphamide, and rituximab for relapsed and refractory chronic lymphocytic leukemia. *J Clin Oncol* epub March 4, 2005.

464. Keating MJ, O'Brien S, Albitar M, et al: Early results of a chemoimmunotherapy regimen of fludarabine, cyclophosphamide, and rituximab as initial therapy for chronic lymphocytic leukemia. *J Clin Oncol* epub March 4, 2005.

465. Schulz H, Klein SK, Rehwald U, et al: Phase 2 study of a combined immunochemotherapy using rituximab and fludarabine in patients with chronic lymphocytic leukemia. *Blood* 100:3115, 2002.

466. Byrd JC, Peterson BL, Morrison VA, et al: Randomized phase 2 study of fludarabine with concurrent versus sequential treatment with rituximab in symptomatic, untreated patients with B-cell chronic lymphocytic leukemia: Results from Cancer and Leukemia Group B 9712 (CALGB 9712). *Blood* 101:6, 2003.

467. Byrd JC, Rai K, Peterson BL, et al: Addition of rituximab to fludarabine may prolong progression-free survival and overall survival in patients with previously untreated chronic lymphocytic leukemia: An updated retrospective comparative analysis of CALGB 9712 and CALGB 9011. *Blood* 105:49, 2005.

468. Giles FJ, O'Brien SM, Santini V, et al: Sequential *cis*-platinum and fludarabine with or without arabinosyl cytosine in patients failing prior fludarabine therapy for chronic lymphocytic leukemia: A phase II study. *Leuk Lymphoma* 36:57, 1999.

469. Elias L, Stock-Novack D, Head DR, et al: A phase I trial of combination fludarabine monophosphate and chlorambucil in chronic lymphocytic leukemia: A Southwest Oncology Group study. *Leukemia* 7:361, 1993.

470. Weiss MA, Maslak PG, Jurcic JG, et al: Pentostatin and cyclophosphamide: An effective new regimen in previously treated patients with chronic lymphocytic leukemia. *J Clin Oncol* 21:1278, 2003.

471. Tsiara SN, Kapsali HD, Chaidos A, et al: Treatment of resistant/relapsing chronic lymphocytic leukemia with a combination regimen containing deoxycoformycin and rituximab. *Acta Haematol* 111:185, 2004.

472. Laurencet FM, Zulian GB, Guetty-Alberto M, et al: Cladribine with cyclophosphamide and prednisone in the management of low-grade lymphoproliferative malignancies. *Br J Cancer* 79:1215, 1999.

473. Tefferi A, Li CY, Reeder CB, et al: A phase II study of sequential combination chemotherapy with cyclophosphamide, prednisone, and 2-chlorodeoxyadenosine in previously untreated patients with chronic lymphocytic leukemia. *Leukemia* 15:1171, 2001.

474. Montillo M, Tedeschi A, O'Brien S, et al: Phase II study of cladribine and cyclophosphamide in patients with chronic lymphocytic leukemia and prolymphocytic leukemia. *Cancer* 97:114, 2003.

475. Robak T, Blonski JZ, Kasznicki M, et al: Cladribine combined with cyclophosphamide is highly effective in the treatment of chronic lymphocytic leukemia. *Hematol J* 3:244, 2002.

476. Oken MM, Kaplan ME: Combination chemotherapy with cyclophosphamide, vincristine, and prednisone in the treatment of refractory chronic lymphocytic leukemia. *Cancer Treat Rep* 63:441, 1979.

477. The French Cooperative Group on Chronic Lymphocytic Leukemia: A randomized clinical trial of chlorambucil versus COP in stage B chronic lymphocytic leukemia. *Blood* 75:1422, 1990.

478. French Cooperative Group: Prognostic and therapeutic advances in CLL management: The experience of the French Cooperative Group. French Cooperative Group on Chronic Lymphocytic Leukemia. *Semin Hematol* 24:275, 1987.

479. Friedenberg WR, Anderson J, Wolf BC, et al: Modified vincristine, doxorubicin, and dexamethasone regimen in the treatment of resistant or relapsed chronic lymphocytic leukemia. An Eastern Cooperative Oncology Group study. *Cancer* 71:2983, 1993.

480. Coad JE, Matutes E, Catovsky D: Splenectomy in lymphoproliferative disorders: A report on 70 cases and review of the literature. *Leuk Lymphoma* 10:245, 1993.

481. Seymour JF, Cusack JD, Lerner SA, et al: Case/control study of the role of splenectomy in chronic lymphocytic leukemia. *J Clin Oncol* 15:52, 1997.

482. Ruchlemer R, Wotherspoon AC, Thompson JN, et al: Splenectomy in mantle cell lymphoma with leukaemia: A comparison with chronic lymphocytic leukaemia. *Br J Haematol* 118:952, 2002.

483. Hill J, Walsh RM, McHam S, et al: Laparoscopic splenectomy for autoimmune hemolytic anemia in patients with chronic lymphocytic leukemia: A case series and review of the literature. *Am J Hematol* 75:134, 2004.

484. Smith L, Luna G, Merg AR, et al: Laparoscopic splenectomy for treatment of splenomegaly. *Am J Surg* 187:618, 2004.

485. Velanovich V, Shurafa M: Laparoscopic excision of accessory spleen. *Am J Surg* 180:62, 2000.

486. Rubin P, Bennett JM, Begg C, et al: The comparison of total body irradiation vs chlorambucil and prednisone for remission induction of active chronic lymphocytic leukemia: An ECOG study. Part I: Total body irradiation-response and toxicity. *Int J Radiat Oncol Biol Phys* 7: 1623, 1981.

487. Byhardt RW, Brace KC, Wiernik PH: The role of splenic irradiation in chronic lymphocytic leukemia. *Cancer* 35:1621, 1975.

488. Aabo K, Walbom-Jorgensen S: Spleen irradiation in chronic lymphocytic leukemia (CLL): Palliation in patients unfit for splenectomy. *Am J Hematol* 19:177, 1985.

489. Chisesi T, Capnist G, Dal Fior S: Splenic irradiation in chronic lymphocytic leukemia. *Eur J Haematol* 46:202, 1991.

490. Chiappa S, Bonadonna G, Uslenghi C, et al: The role of endolymphatic radiotherapy in the treatment of chronic lymphatic leukaemia. *Br J Cancer* 20:480, 1966.

491. Chanana AD, Cronkite EP, Rai KR: The role of extracorporeal irradiation of blood in treatment of leukemia. *Int J Radiat Oncol Biol Phys* 1: 539, 1976.

492. Wieselthier JS, Rothstein TL, Yu TL, et al: Inefficacy of extracorporeal photochemotherapy in the treatment of B-cell chronic lymphocytic leukemia: Preliminary results. *Am J Hematol* 41:123, 1992.

493. Marti GE, Folks T, Longo DL, Klein H: Therapeutic cytapheresis in chronic lymphocytic leukemia. *J Clin Apheresis* 1:243, 1983.

494. Cooper IA, Ding JC, Adams PB, et al: Intensive leukapheresis in the management of cytopenias in patients with chronic lymphocytic leukaemia (CLL) and lymphocytic lymphoma. *Am J Hematol* 6:387, 1979.

495. Cukierman T, Gatt ME, Libster D, et al: Chronic lymphocytic leukemia presenting with extreme hyperleukocytosis and thrombosis of the common femoral vein. *Leuk Lymphoma* 43:1865, 2002.

496. Osterborg A, Brandberg Y, Molostova V, et al: Randomized, double-blind, placebo-controlled trial of recombinant human erythropoietin, epoetin Beta, in hematologic malignancies. *J Clin Oncol* 20:2486, 2002.

497. Ludwig H, Rai K, Blade J, et al: Management of disease-related anemia in patients with multiple myeloma or chronic lymphocytic leukemia: Epoetin treatment recommendations. *Hematol J* 3:121, 2002.

498. Straus DJ: Epoetin alfa as a supportive measure in hematologic malignancies. *Semin Hematol* 39:25, 2002.

499. Pangalis GA, Siakantaris MP, Angelopoulou MK, et al: Downstaging Rai stage III B-chronic lymphocytic leukemia patients with the administration of recombinant human erythropoietin. *Haematologica* 87:500, 2002.

500. Mauro FR, Gentile M, Foa R: Erythropoietin and chronic lymphocytic leukemia. *Rev Clin Exp Hematol* 1(suppl):21, 2002.

501. Siakantaris MP, Angelopoulou MK, Vassilakopoulos TP, et al: Correction of disease related anaemia of B-chronic lymphoproliferative disorders by recombinant human erythropoietin: Maintenance is necessary to sustain response. *Leuk Lymphoma* 40:141, 2000.

502. Gribben JG, Neuberg D, Barber M, et al: Detection of residual lymphoma cells by polymerase chain reaction in peripheral blood is significantly less predictive for relapse than detection in bone marrow. *Blood* 83:3800, 1994.

503. Gahn B, Schafer C, Neef J, et al: Detection of trisomy 12 and Rb-deletion in CD34+ cells of patients with B-cell chronic lymphocytic leukemia. *Blood* 89:4275, 1997.

504. Gahn B, Schafer C, Neef J, et al: Detection of trisomy 12 in CD34+ progenitor cells in a patient with B-cell chronic lymphocytic leukemia by fluorescence in situ hybridization. *Ann Oncol* 8(suppl 2):55, 1997.

505. Dreger P, von Neuhoff N, Kuse R, et al: Early stem cell transplantation for chronic lymphocytic leukaemia: A chance for cure? *Br J Cancer* 77:2291, 1998.

506. Pavletic ZS, Bierman PJ, Vose JM, et al: High incidence of relapse after autologous stem-cell transplantation for B-cell chronic lymphocytic leukemia or small lymphocytic lymphoma. *Ann Oncol* 9:1023, 1998.

507. Sutton L, Maloum K, Gonzalez H, et al: Autologous hematopoietic stem cell transplantation as salvage treatment for advanced B cell chronic lymphocytic leukemia. *Leukemia* 12:1699, 1998.

508. Paneesha S, Milligan DW: Stem cell transplantation for chronic lymphocytic leukaemia. *Br J Haematol* 128:145, 2005.

509. Khouri I, Champlin R: Allogenic bone marrow transplantation in chronic lymphocytic leukemia. *Ann Intern Med* 125:780, 1996.

510. Michallet M, Archimbaud E, Bandini G, et al: HLA-identical sibling bone marrow transplantation in younger patients with chronic lymphocytic leukemia. European Group for Blood and Marrow Transplantation and the International Bone Marrow Transplant Registry. *Ann Intern Med* 124:311, 1996.

511. Mehta J, Powles R, Singhal S, et al: T cell-depleted allogeneic bone marrow transplantation from a partially HLA-mismatched unrelated donor for progressive chronic lymphocytic leukemia and fludarabine-induced bone marrow failure. *Bone Marrow Transplant* 17:881, 1996.

512. Mehta J, Powles R, Singhal S, et al: Clinical and hematologic response of chronic lymphocytic and prolymphocytic leukemia persisting after allogeneic bone marrow transplantation with the onset of acute graft-versus-host disease: Possible role of graft-versus-leukemia. *Bone Marrow Transplant* 17:371, 1996.

513. Rondon G, Giralt S, Huh Y, et al: Graft-versus-leukemia effect after allogeneic bone marrow transplantation for chronic lymphocytic leukemia. *Bone Marrow Transplant* 18:669, 1996.

514. Doney KC, Chauncey T, Appelbaum FR: Allogeneic related donor hematopoietic stem cell transplantation for treatment of chronic lymphocytic leukemia. *Bone Marrow Transplant* 29:817, 2002.

515. van Besien K, Keralavarma B, Devine S, Stock W: Allogeneic and autologous transplantation for chronic lymphocytic leukemia. *Leukemia* 15:1317, 2001.

516. Maloney DG, Sandmaier BM, Mackinnon S, Shizuru JA: Non-myeloablative transplantation. *Hematology (Am Soc Hematol Educ Program)*:392, 2002.

517. Schetelig J, Thiede C, Bornhauser M, et al: Evidence of a graft-versus-leukemia effect in chronic lymphocytic leukemia after reduced-intensity conditioning and allogeneic stem-cell transplantation: The Cooperative German Transplant Study Group. *J Clin Oncol* 21:2747, 2003.

518. Dreger P, Brand R, Hansz J, et al: Treatment-related mortality and graft-versus-leukemia activity after allogeneic stem cell transplantation for chronic lymphocytic leukemia using intensity-reduced conditioning. *Leukemia* 17:841, 2003.

519. Khouri IF, Lee MS, Saliba RM, et al: Nonablative allogeneic stem cell transplantation for chronic lymphocytic leukemia: Impact of rituximab on immunomodulation and survival. *Exp Hematol* 32:28, 2004.

520. Wahl U, Nossner E, Kronenberger K, et al: Vaccination against B-cell chronic lymphocytic leukemia with trioma cells: Preclinical evaluation. *Clin Cancer Res* 9:4240, 2003.

521. Kokhaei P, Rezvany MR, Virving L, et al: Dendritic cells loaded with apoptotic tumour cells induce a stronger T-cell response than dendritic cell-tumour hybrids in B-CLL. *Leukemia* 17:894, 2003.

522. Reichardt VL, Brossart P: DC-based immunotherapy of B-cell malignancies. *Cytotherapy* 6:62, 2004.

523. Wierda WG, Cantwell MJ, Woods SJ, et al: CD40-ligand (CD154) gene therapy for chronic lymphocytic leukemia. *Blood* 96:2917, 2000.

524. Robertson TI: Complications and causes of death in B cell chronic lymphocytic leukaemia: A long term study of 105 patients. *Aust N Z J Med* 20:44, 1990.

525. Morra E, Nosari A, Montillo M: Infectious complications in chronic lymphocytic leukaemia. *Hematol Cell Ther* 41:145, 1999.

526. Vavricka SR, Halter J, Hechelhammer L, Himmelmann A: Pneumocystis carinii pneumonia in chronic lymphocytic leukaemia. *Postgrad Med J* 80:236, 2004.

527. Hensel M, Kornacker M, Yammeni S, et al: Disease activity and pretreatment, rather than hypogammaglobulinaemia, are major risk factors for infectious complications in patients with chronic lymphocytic leukaemia. *Br J Haematol* 122:600, 2003.

528. Griffiths H, Lea J, Bunch C, et al: Predictors of infection in chronic lymphocytic leukaemia (CLL). *Clin Exp Immunol* 89:374, 1992.

529. Itala M, Helenius H, Nikoskelainen J, Remes K: Infections and serum IgG levels in patients with chronic lymphocytic leukemia. *Eur J Haematol* 48:266, 1992.

530. Intravenous immunoglobulin for the prevention of infection in chronic lymphocytic leukemia. A randomized, controlled clinical trial. Cooperative Group for the Study of Immunoglobulin in Chronic Lymphocytic Leukemia. *N Engl J Med* 319:902, 1988.

531. Egerer G, Hensel M, Ho AD: Infectious complications in chronic lymphoid malignancy. *Curr Treat Options Oncol* 2:237, 2001.

532. Perkins JG, Flynn JM, Howard RS, Byrd JC: Frequency and type of serious infections in fludarabine-refractory B-cell chronic lymphocytic leukemia and small lymphocytic lymphoma: Implications for clinical trials in this patient population. *Cancer* 94:2033, 2002.

533. Wierda WG: Immunologic monitoring in chronic lymphocytic leukemia. *Curr Oncol Rep* 5:419, 2003.

534. Ward JH: Autoimmunity in chronic lymphocytic leukemia. *Curr Treat Options Oncol* 2:253, 2001.

535. Paydas S: Fludarabine-induced hemolytic anemia: Successful treatment by rituximab. *Hematol J* 5:81, 2004.

536. Chikkappa G, Pasquale D, Zarrabi MH, et al: Cyclosporine and prednisone therapy for pure red cell aplasia in patients with chronic lymphocytic leukemia. *Am J Hematol* 41:5, 1992.

537. Greene MH, Hoover RN, Fraumeni JFJ: Subsequent cancer in patients with chronic lymphocytic leukemia—A possible immunologic mechanism. *J Natl Cancer Inst* 61:337, 1978.

538. Quaglino D, Lusvarghi E, Piccinini L, et al: The association between chronic lymphocytic leukaemia and a solid tumor: A survey study of 258 cases of chronic lymphocytic leukaemia covering an eleven year period. *Haematologica* 61:456, 1976.

539. Kyasa MJ, Hazlett L, Parrish RS, et al: Veterans with chronic lymphocytic leukemia/small lymphocytic lymphoma (CLL/SLL) have a markedly increased rate of second malignancy, which is the most common cause of death. *Leuk Lymphoma* 45:507, 2004.

540. Mehrany K, Weenig RH, Pittelkow MR, et al: High recurrence rates of Basal cell carcinoma after mohs surgery in patients with chronic lymphocytic leukemia. *Arch Dermatol* 140:985, 2004.

541. Quaglino D, Paterlini P, De Pasquale A, et al: Association of chronic lymphocytic leukaemia and multiple myeloma: Report of a case and review of the literature. *Haematologica* 67:576, 1982.

542. Hoffman KD, Rudders RA: Multiple myeloma and chronic lymphocytic leukemia in a single individual. *Arch Intern Med* 137:232, 1977.

543. Jeha MT, Hamblin TJ, Smith JL: Coincident chronic lymphocytic leukemia and osteosclerotic multiple myeloma. *Blood* 57:617, 1981.

544. Pedersen-Bjergaard J, Petersen HD, Thomsen M, et al: Chronic lymphocytic leukaemia with subsequent development of multiple myeloma. Evidence of two B-lymphocyte clones and of myeloma-induced suppression of secretion of an M-component and of normal immunoglobulins. *Scand J Haematol* 21:256, 1978.

545. Lai R, Arber DA, Brynes RK, et al: Untreated chronic lymphocytic leukemia concurrent with or followed by acute myelogenous leukemia or myelodysplastic syndrome. A report of five cases and review of the literature. *Am J Clin Pathol* 111:373, 1999.

546. Coso D, Costello R, Cohen-Valensi R, et al: Acute myeloid leukemia and myelodysplasia in patients with chronic lymphocytic leukemia receiving fludarabine as initial therapy. *Ann Oncol* 10:362, 1999.

547. Effects of chlorambucil and therapeutic decision in initial forms of chronic lymphocytic leukemia (stage A): Results of a randomized clinical trial on 612 patients. The French Cooperative Group on Chronic Lymphocytic Leukemia. *Blood* 75:1414, 1990.

548. Richter MN: Generalized reticular cell sarcoma of lymph nodes associated with lymphatic leukemia. *Am J Pathol* 4:285, 1928.

549. Long JC, Aisenberg AC: Richter's syndrome. A terminal complication of chronic lymphocytic leukemia with distinct clinicopathologic features. *Am J Clin Pathol* 63:786, 1975.

550. Nakamura N, Abe M: Richter syndrome in B-cell chronic lymphocytic leukemia. *Pathol Int* 53:195, 2003.

551. Cherepakhin V, Baird SM, Meisenholder GW, Kipps TJ: Common clonal origin of chronic lymphocytic leukemia and high-grade lymphoma of Richter's syndrome. *Blood* 82:3141, 1993.

552. Bessudo A, Kipps TJ: Origin of high-grade lymphomas in Richter syndrome. *Leuk Lymphoma* 18:367, 1995.

553. Timar B, Fulop Z, Csernus B, et al: Relationship between the mutational status of VH genes and pathogenesis of diffuse large B-cell lymphoma in Richter's syndrome. *Leukemia* 18:326, 2004.

554. Matolcsy A, Inghirami G, Knowles DM: Molecular genetic demonstration of the diverse evolution of Richter's syndrome (chronic lymphocytic leukemia and subsequent large cell lymphoma). *Blood* 83:1363, 1994.

555. Nakamura N, Kuze T, Hashimoto Y, et al: Analysis of the immunoglobulin heavy chain gene of secondary diffuse large B-cell lymphoma that subsequently developed in four cases with B-cell chronic lymphocytic leukemia or lymphoplasmacytoid lymphoma (Richter syndrome). *Pathol Int* 50:636, 2000.

556. Ratnavel RC, Dunn-Walters DK, Boursier L, et al: B-cell lymphoma associated with chronic lymphatic leukaemia: Two cases with contrasting aggressive and indolent behaviour. *Br J Dermatol* 140:708, 1999.

557. Kaufmann H, Ackermann J, Nosslinger T, et al: Absence of clonal chromosomal relationship between concomitant B-CLL and multiple myeloma—A report on two cases. *Ann Hematol* 80:474, 2001.

558. Chena C, Cerretini R, Noriega MF, et al: Cytogenetic, FISH, and molecular studies in a case of B-cell chronic lymphocytic leukemia with karyotypic evolution. *Eur J Haematol* 69:309, 2002.

559. Lee JN, Giles F, Huh YO, et al: Molecular differences between small and large cells in patients with chronic lymphocytic leukemia. *Eur J Haematol* 71:235, 2003.

560. Santulli B, Kazmierczak B, Napolitano R, et al: A 12q13 translocation involving the HMGI-C gene in Richter transformation of a chronic lymphocytic leukemia. *Cancer Genet Cytogenet* 119:70, 2000.

561. Fulop Z, Csernus B, Timar B, et al: Microsatellite instability and hMLH1 promoter hypermethylation in Richter's transformation of chronic lymphocytic leukemia. *Leukemia* 17:411, 2003.

562. Foucar K, Rydell RE: Richter's syndrome in chronic lymphocytic leukemia. *Cancer* 46:118, 1980.

563. Trump DL, Mann RB, Phelps R, et al: Richter's syndrome: Diffuse histiocytic lymphoma in patients with chronic lymphocytic leukemia. A report of five cases and review of the literature. *Am J Med* 68:539, 1980.

564. Harousseau JL, Flandrin G, Tricot G, et al: Malignant lymphoma supervening in chronic lymphocytic leukemia and related disorders. Richter's syndrome: A study of 25 cases. *Cancer* 48:1302, 1981.

565. Milkowski DA, Worley BD, Morris MJ: Richter's transformation presenting as an obstructing endobronchial lesion. *Chest* 116:832, 1999.

566. Fernandez-Suntay JP, Gragoudas ES, Ferry JA, et al: High-grade uveal B-cell lymphoma as the initial feature in Richter syndrome. *Arch Ophthalmol* 120:1383, 2002.

567. Robak T, Gora-Tybor J, Tybor K, et al: Richter's syndrome in the brain first manifested as an ischaemic stroke. *Leuk Lymphoma* 45:1261, 2004.

568. Joseph L, Scott MA, Schichman SA, Zent CS: Localized herpes simplex lymphadenitis mimicking large-cell (Richter's) transformation of chronic lymphocytic leukemia/small lymphocytic lymphoma. *Am J Hematol* 68:287, 2001.

569. Harris NL, Jaffe ES, Diebold J, et al: Lymphoma classification—From controversy to consensus: The REAL and WHO Classification of lymphoid neoplasms. *Ann Oncol* 11(suppl 1):3, 2000.

570. Robak T, Urbanska-Rys H, Strzelecka B, et al: Plasmablastic lymphoma in a patient with chronic lymphocytic leukemia heavily pretreated with cladribine (2-CdA): An unusual variant of Richter's syndrome. *Eur J Haematol* 67:322, 2001.

571. Brecher M, Banks PM: Hodgkin's disease variant of Richter's syndrome. Report of eight cases. *Am J Clin Pathol* 93:333, 1990.

572. Rubin D, Hudnall SD, Aisenberg A, et al: Richter's transformation of chronic lymphocytic leukemia with Hodgkin's-like cells is associated with Epstein-Barr virus infection. *Mod Pathol* 7:91, 1994.

573. Giles FJ, O'Brien SM, Keating MJ: Chronic lymphocytic leukemia in (Richter's) transformation. *Semin Oncol* 25:117, 1998.

574. Pescarmona E, Pignoloni P, Mauro FR, et al: Hodgkin/Reed-Sternberg cells and Hodgkin's disease in patients with B-cell chronic lymphocytic leukaemia: An immunohistological, molecular and clinical study of four cases suggesting a heterogeneous pathogenetic background. *Virchows Arch* 437:129, 2000.

575. O'Sullivan MJ, Kaleem Z, Bolger MJ, et al: Composite prolymphocytoid and Hodgkin transformation of chronic lymphocytic leukemia. *Arch Pathol Lab Med* 124:907, 2000.

576. Isikdogan A, Ayyildiz O, Buyukbayram H, Muftuoglu E: Hodgkin's disease variant of Richter's transformation: A case report. *Med Oncol* 19:109, 2002.

577. Robak T, Szmigielska-Kaplon A, Smolewski P, et al: Hodgkin's type of Richter's syndrome in familial chronic lymphocytic leukemia treated with cladribine and cyclophosphamide. *Leuk Lymphoma* 44:859, 2003.

578. Nemets A, Ben Dor D, Barry T, et al: Variant Richter's syndrome: A rare case of classical Hodgkin's lymphoma developing in a patient with chronic lymphocytic leukemia treated with fludarabine. *Leuk Lymphoma* 44:2151, 2003.

579. Alliot C, Tabuteau S, Desablens B: Hodgkin's disease variant of Richter's syndrome: Complete remission of the both malignancies after 14 years. *Hematology* 8:229, 2003.

580. De Leval L, Vivario M, De Prijck B, et al: Distinct clonal origin in two cases of Hodgkin's lymphoma variant of Richter's syndrome associated with EBV infection. *Am J Surg Pathol* 28:679, 2004.

581. Ohno T, Smir BN, Weisenburger DD, et al: Origin of the Hodgkin/Reed-Sternberg cells in chronic lymphocytic leukemia with "Hodgkin's transformation". *Blood* 91:1757, 1998.

582. Tsimberidou AM, Keating MJ: Richter syndrome: Biology, incidence, and therapeutic strategies. *Cancer* 103:216, 2005.

583. Tsimberidou AM, O'Brien SM, Cortes JE, et al: Phase II study of fludarabine, cytarabine (Ara-C), cyclophosphamide, cisplatin and GM-CSF (FACPGM) in patients with Richter's syndrome or refractory lymphoproliferative disorders. *Leuk Lymphoma* 43:767, 2002.

584. Tsimberidou AM, Kantarjian HM, Cortes J, et al: Fractionated cyclophosphamide, vincristine, liposomal daunorubicin, and dexamethasone plus rituximab and granulocyte-macrophage-colony stimulating factor (GM-CSF) alternating with methotrexate and cytarabine plus rituximab and GM-CSF in patients with Richter syndrome or fludarabine-refractory chronic lymphocytic leukemia. *Cancer* 97:1711, 2003.

585. Melo JV, Catovsky D, Galton DA: The relationship between chronic lymphocytic leukaemia and prolymphocytic leukaemia: I. Clinical and laboratory features of 300 patients and characterization of an intermediate group. *Br J Haematol* 63:377, 1986.

586. Melo JV, Catovsky D, Galton DA: The relationship between chronic lymphocytic leukaemia and prolymphocytic leukaemia: II. Patterns of evolution of 'prolymphocytoid' transformation. *Br J Haematol* 64:77, 1986.

587. Melo JV, Catovsky D, Gregory WM, Galton DA: The relationship between chronic lymphocytic leukaemia and prolymphocytic leukaemia: IV. Analysis of survival and prognostic features. *Br J Haematol* 65:23, 1987.

588. Sadamori N, Han T, Minowada J, et al: Possible specific chromosome change in prolymphocytic leukemia. *Blood* 62:729, 1983.

589. Ghani AM, Krause JR, Brody JP: Prolymphocytic transformation of chronic lymphocytic leukemia. A report of three cases and review of the literature. *Cancer* 57:75, 1986.

590. Zarrabi MH, Grunwald HW, Rosner F: Chronic lymphocytic leukemia terminating in acute leukemia. *Arch Intern Med* 137:1059, 1977.

591. Brouet JC, Preud'homme JL, Seligmann M, Bernard J: Blast cells with monoclonal surface immunoglobulin in two cases of acute blast crisis supervening on chronic lymphocytic leukemia. *Br Med J* 4:23, 1973.

592. McPhedran P, Heath CWJ: Acute leukemia occurring during chronic lymphocytic leukemia. *Blood* 35:7, 1970.

593. Frenkel EP, Ligler FS, Graham MS, et al: Acute lymphocytic leukemic transformation of chronic lymphocytic leukemia: Substantiation by flow cytometry. *Am J Hematol* 10:391, 1981.

594. Torelli UL, Torelli GM, Emilia G, et al: Simultaneously increased expression of the c-myc and mu chain genes in the acute blastic transformation of a chronic lymphocytic leukemia. *Br J Haematol* 65:165, 1987.

595. Buchi G, Termine G, Zappala C, et al: Spontaneous complete remission of CLL. Report of a case studied with monoclonal antibodies. *Acta Haematol* 70:198, 1983.

596. Bernard M, Drenou B, Pangault C, et al: Spontaneous phenotypic and molecular blood remission in a case of chronic lymphocytic leukemia. *Br J Haematol* 107:213, 1999.

597. Mandelli F, De Rossi G, Mancini P, et al: Prognosis in chronic lymphocytic leukemia: A retrospective multicentric study from the GIMEMA group. *J Clin Oncol* 5:398, 1987.

598. Jaksic B, Vitale B, Hauptmann E, et al: The roles of age and sex in the prognosis of chronic leukaemias. A study of 373 cases. *Br J Cancer* 64:345, 1991.

599. Molica S, Levato D, Dattilo A: Natural history of early chronic lymphocytic leukemia. A single institution study with emphasis on the impact of disease-progression on overall survival. *Haematologica* 84:1094, 1999.

600. Catovsky D, Galetto J, Okos A, et al: Prolymphocytic leukaemia of B and T cell type. *Lancet* 2:232, 1973.

601. Katayama I, Aiba M, Pechet L, et al: B-lineage prolymphocytic leukemia as a distinct clinicopathologic entity. *Am J Pathol* 99:399, 1980.

602. Pittman S, Catovsky D: Chromosome abnormalities in B-cell prolymphocytic leukemia: A study of nine cases. *Cancer Genet Cytogenet* 9:355, 1983.

603. Stone RM: Prolymphocytic Leukemia. *Hematol Oncol Clin North Am* 4:457, 1990.

604. Sole F, Woessner S, Espinet B, et al: Cytogenetic abnormalities in three patients with B-cell prolymphocytic leukemia. *Cancer Genet Cytogenet* 103:43, 1998.

605. Adami F, Sancetta R, Trentin L, et al: The pediatric rhabdomyosarcoma translocation (2;13)(q35;q14) in B-prolymphocytic leukemia [letter]. *Leukemia* 7:1676, 1993.

606. Aoun P, Blair HE, Smith LM, et al: Fluorescence in situ hybridization detection of cytogenetic abnormalities in B-cell chronic lymphocytic leukemia/small lymphocytic lymphoma. *Leuk Lymphoma* 45:1595, 2004.

607. De Angeli C, Cuneo A, Aguiari G, et al: 5' region and exon 7 mutations of the TP53 gene in two cases of B-cell prolymphocytic leukemia. *Cancer Genet Cytogenet* 107:137, 1998.

608. Bacher U, Kern W, Schoch C, et al: Discrimination of chronic lymphocytic leukemia (CLL) and CLL/PL by cytomorphology can clearly be correlated to specific genetic markers as investigated by interphase fluorescence in situ hybridization (FISH). *Ann Hematol* 83:349, 2004.

609. Lens D, Coignet LJ, Brito-Babapulle V, et al: B cell prolymphocytic leukaemia (B-PLL) with complex karyotype and concurrent abnormalities of the p53 and c-MYC gene. *Leukemia* 13:873, 1999.

610. Shokri F, Mageed RA, Richardson P, Jefferis R: Immunophenotypic and idiotypic characterisation of the leukaemic B-cells from patients with prolymphocytic leukaemia: Evidence for a selective expression of immunoglobulin variable region (IGV) gene products. *Leuk Res* 17:669, 1993.

611. Davi F, Maloum K, Michel A, et al: High frequency of somatic mutations in the VH genes expressed in prolymphocytic leukemia. *Blood* 88:3953, 1996.

612. Hoffman MA, Valderrama E, Fuchs A, et al: Leukemic meningitis in B-cell prolymphocytic leukemia. A clinical, pathologic, and ultrastructural case study and a review of the literature. *Cancer* 75:1100, 1995.

613. Pastor E, Grau E, Real E, et al: Leukemic meningitis in a patient with B-cell prolymphocytic leukemia. *Haematologica* 82:511, 1997.

614. Andrieu V, Encaoua R, Carbon C, et al: Leukemic pleural effusion in B-cell prolymphocytic leukemia. *Hematol Cell Ther* 40:275, 1998.

615. Shimoni A, Shvidel L, Shtalrid M, et al: Prolymphocytic transformation of B-chronic lymphocytic leukemia presenting as malignant ascites and pleural effusion. *Am J Hematol* 59:316, 1998.

616. Dietrich PY, Pedraza E, Casiraghi O, et al: Cardiac arrest due to leucostasis in a case of prolymphocytic leukaemia. *Br J Haematol* 78:122, 1991.

617. Takenaka T, Nakamine H, Nishihara T, et al: Prolymphocytic leukemia with IgM hypogammaglobulinemia. *Am J Clin Pathol* 80:237, 1983.

618. Caligaris-Cappio F, Janossy G: Surface markers in chronic lymphoid leukemias of B cell type. *Semin Hematol* 22:1, 1985.

619. Shvidel L, Shtalrid M, Bassous L, et al: B-cell prolymphocytic leukemia: A survey of 35 patients emphasizing heterogeneity, prognostic factors and evidence for a group with an indolent course. *Leuk Lymphoma* 33:169, 1999.

620. Lambertenghi-Deliliers G, Maiolo AT, Annaloro C, et al: Complete remission in prolymphocytic leukemia with 4-demethoxydaunorubicin and arabinosyl cytosine. *Cancer* 54:199, 1984.

621. Swift JF, Wold HG, Gandara DR, et al: Prolymphocytic leukemia. Serial responses to therapy. *Cancer* 54:978, 1984.

622. Mourad YA, Taher A, Chehal A, Shamseddine A: Successful treatment of B-cell prolymphocytic leukemia with monoclonal anti-CD20 antibody. *Ann Hematol*, 83:319, 2003.

623. Barton K, Larson RA, O'Brien S, Ratain MJ: Rapid response of B-cell

prolymphocytic leukemia to 2-chlorodeoxyadenosine [letter]. *J Clin Oncol* 10:1821, 1992.

624. Saven A, Lee T, Schlutz M, et al: Major activity of cladribine in patients with de novo B-cell prolymphocytic leukemia. *J Clin Oncol* 15:37, 1997.

625. Lorand-Metze I, Oliveira GB, Aranha FJ: Treatment of prolymphocytic leukemia with cladribine. *Ann Hematol* 76:85, 1998.

626. Kantarjian HM, Childs C, O'Brien S, et al: Efficacy of fludarabine, a new adenine nucleoside analogue, in patients with prolymphocytic leukemia and the prolymphocytoid variant of chronic lymphocytic leukemia. *Am J Med* 90:223, 1991.

627. List AF, Kummet TD, Adams JD, Chun HG: Tumor lysis syndrome complicating treatment of chronic lymphocytic leukemia with fludarabine phosphate. *Am J Med* 89:388, 1990.

628. Smith RE, Stoiber TR: Acute tumor lysis syndrome in prolymphocytic leukemia. *Am J Med* 88:547, 1990.

629. Cannon LM, Spilove L, Rhodes R, et al: Acute tumor lysis syndrome complicating fludarabine treatment of prolymphocytic leukemia. *Conn Med* 57:651, 1993.

630. Döhner H, Ho AD, Thaler J, et al: Pentostatin in prolymphocytic leukemia: Phase II trial of the European Organization for Research and Treatment of Cancer Leukemia Cooperative Study Group. *J Natl Cancer Inst* 85:658, 1993.

631. Dearden C, Matutes E, Catovsky D: Deoxycoformycin in the treatment of mature T-cell leukaemias. *Br J Cancer* 64:903, 1991.

632. Muncunill J, Villa S, Domingo A, et al: Splenic irradiation as primary therapy for prolymphocytic leukaemia. *Br J Haematol* 76:305, 1990.

633. Yamamoto K, Hamaguchi H, Nagata K, et al: Splenic irradiation for prolymphocytic leukemia: Is it preferable as an initial treatment or not? *Jpn J Clin Oncol* 28:267, 1998.

634. Singh AK, Bates T, Wetherley-Mein G: A preliminary study of low-dose splenic irradiation for the treatment of chronic lymphocytic and prolymphocytic leukaemias. *Scand J Haematol* 37:50, 1986.

635. Terashima T, Ohtake K, Ogawa T: Prolymphocytic leukemia treated with natural and recombinant alpha-interferon. *Am J Hematol* 35:56, 1990.

636. Delannoy A, Balligand JL, Ledant T: Interferon and B-cell prolymphocytic leukaemia [letter]. *Br J Haematol* 66:579, 1987.

637. Jacobs P, Le Roux I, Wood L, Bolding E: Interferon response in B-cell prolymphocytic leukemia [letter]. *Br J Haematol* 65:375, 1987.

638. Vivaldi P, Garuti R, Rubertelli M, Mazzon C: Prolymphocytic leukemia: A very satisfactory response to treatment with recombinant interferon alpha. *Haematologica* 77:169, 1992.

639. Blecher TE: "Spontaneous" complete remission in a case of prolymphocytic leukemia [letter]. *Br J Haematol* 63:395, 1986.

640. Bennett JM, Catovsky D, Daniel MT, et al: Proposals for the classification of chronic (mature) B and T lymphoid leukaemias. French-American-British (FAB) Cooperative Group. *J Clin Pathol* 42:567, 1989.

641. Matutes E, Brito-Babapulle V, Swansbury J, et al: Clinical and laboratory features of 78 cases of T-prolymphocytic leukemia. *Blood* 78:3269, 1991.

642. Matutes E, Catovsky D: CLL should be used only for the disease with B-cell phenotype [letter, comment]. *Leukemia* 7:917, 1993.

643. Foon KA, Gale RP: Is there a T-cell form of chronic lymphocytic leukemia? [editorial, comments]. *Leukemia* 6:867, 1992.

644. Hoyer JD, Ross CW, Li CY, et al: True T-cell chronic lymphocytic leukemia: A morphologic and immunophenotypic study of 25 cases. *Blood* 86:1163, 1995.

645. Pileri SA, Milani M, Fraternali-Orcioni G, Sabattini E: From the REAL. Classification to the upcoming WHO scheme: A step toward universal categorization of lymphoma entities? *Ann Oncol* 9:607, 1998.

646. Harris NL, Jaffe ES, Stein H, et al: A revised European-American classification of lymphoid neoplasms: A proposal from the International Lymphoma Study Group. *Blood* 84:1361, 1994.

647. Ascani S, Leoni P, Fraternali Orcioni G, et al: T-cell prolymphocytic leukaemia: Does the expression of CD8+ phenotype justify the identification of a new subtype? Description of two cases and review of the literature. *Ann Oncol* 10:649, 1999.

648. Kojima K, Sawada T, Ikezoe T, et al: Defective human T-lymphotrophic virus type I provirus in T-cell prolymphocytic leukaemia. *Br J Haematol* 105:376, 1999.

649. Pawson R, Schulz TF, Matutes E, Catovsky D: The human T-cell lymphotropic viruses types I/II are not involved in T prolymphocytic leukemia and large granular lymphocytic leukemia. *Leukemia* 11:1305, 1997.

650. Maljaei SH, Brito-Babapulle V, Hiorns LR, Catovsky D: Abnormalities of chromosomes 8, 11, 14, and X in T-prolymphocytic leukemia studied by fluorescence in situ hybridization. *Cancer Genet Cytogenet* 103:110, 1998.

651. Sorour A, Brito-Babapulle V, Smedley D, et al: Unusual breakpoint distribution of 8p abnormalities in T-prolymphocytic leukemia: A study with YACS mapping to 8p11-p12. *Cancer Genet Cytogenet* 121:128, 2000.

652. Pekarsky Y, Hallas C, Croce CM: Molecular basis of mature T-cell leukemia. *JAMA* 286:2308, 2001.

653. Costa D, Queralt R, Aymerich M, et al: High levels of chromosomal imbalances in typical and small-cell variants of T-cell prolymphocytic leukemia. *Cancer Genet Cytogenet* 147:36, 2003.

654. Salomon-Nguyen F, Brizard F, Le Coniat M, et al: Abnormalities of the short arm of chromosome 12 in T cell prolymphocytic leukemia. *Leukemia* 12:972, 1998.

655. Brito-Babapulle V, Baou M, Matutes E, et al: Deletions of D13S25, D13S319 and RB-1 mapping to 13q14.3 in T-cell prolymphocytic leukaemia. *Br J Haematol* 114:327, 2001.

656. Kojima K, Kobayashi H, Imoto S, et al: 14q11 abnormality and trisomy 8q are not common in Japanese T-cell prolymphocytic leukemia. *Int J Hematol* 68:291, 1998.

657. Zver S, Kokalj Vokac N, Zagradisnik B, et al: T cell prolymphocytic leukemia with new chromosome rearrangements. *Acta Haematol* 111:168, 2004.

658. Brito-Babapulle V, Hamoudi R, Matutes E, et al: P53 allele deletion and protein accumulation occurs in the absence of p53 gene mutation in T-prolymphocytic leukaemia and Sezary syndrome. *Br J Haematol* 110:180, 2000.

659. Bradshaw PS, Condie A, Matutes E, et al: Breakpoints in the ataxia telangiectasia gene arise at the RGYW somatic hypermutation motif. *Oncogene* 21:483, 2002.

660. Croce CM, Isobe M, Palumbo A, et al: Gene for alpha-chain of human T-cell receptor: Location on chromosome 14 region involved in T-cell neoplasms. *Science* 227:1044, 1985.

661. Stilgenbauer S, Schaffner C, Litterst A, et al: Biallelic mutations in the ATM gene in T-prolymphocytic leukemia. *Nat Med* 3:1155, 1997.

662. Yuille MA, Coignet LJ, Abraham SM, et al: ATM is usually rearranged in T-cell prolymphocytic leukaemia. *Oncogene* 16:789, 1998.

663. Stoppa-Lyonnet D, Soulier J, Lauge A, et al: Inactivation of the ATM gene in T-cell prolymphocytic leukemias. *Blood* 91:3920, 1998.

664. Luo L, Lu FM, Hart S, et al: Ataxia-telangiectasia and T-cell leukemias: No evidence for somatic ATM mutation in sporadic T-ALL or for hypermethylation of the ATM-NPAT/E14 bidirectional promoter in T-PLL. *Cancer Res* 58:2293, 1998.

665. Madani A, Choukroun V, Soulier J, et al: Expression of p13MTCP1 is restricted to mature T-cell proliferations with t(X;14) translocations. *Blood* 87:1923, 1996.

666. Gritti C, Choukroun V, Soulier J, et al: Alternative origin of p13MTCP1-encoding transcripts in mature T-cell proliferations with t(X;14) translocations. *Oncogene* 15:1329, 1997.

667. De Schouwer PJ, Dyer MJ, Brito-Babapulle VB, et al: T-cell prolym-

phocytic leukaemia: Antigen receptor gene rearrangement and a novel mode of MTCP1 B1 activation. *Br J Haematol* 110:831, 2000.

668. Hoh F, Yang YS, Guignard L, et al: Crystal structure of p14TCL1, an oncogene product involved in T-cell prolymphocytic leukemia, reveals a novel beta-barrel topology. *Structure* 6:147, 1998.

669. Thick J, Metcalfe JA, Mak YF, et al: Expression of either the TCL1 oncogene, or transcripts from its homologue MTCP1/c6.1B, in leukaemic and non-leukaemic T cells from ataxia telangiectasia patients. *Oncogene* 12:379, 1996.

670. Gritti C, Dastot H, Soulier J, et al: Transgenic mice for MTCP1 develop T-cell prolymphocytic leukemia. *Blood* 92:368, 1998.

671. Matutes E, Catovsky D: Similarities between T-cell chronic lymphocytic leukemia and the small-cell variant of T-prolymphocytic leukaemia. *Blood* 87:3520, 1996.

672. Mallett RB, Matutes E, Catovsky D, et al: Cutaneous infiltration in T-cell prolymphocytic leukaemia. *Br J Dermatol* 132:263, 1995.

673. Serra A, Estrach MT, Marti R, et al: Cutaneous involvement as the first manifestation in a case of T-cell prolymphocytic leukaemia. *Acta Derm Venereol* 78:198, 1998.

674. Dhar-Munshi S, Alton P, Ayliffe WH: Masquerade syndrome: T-cell prolymphocytic leukemia presenting as panuveitis. *Am J Ophthalmol* 132:275, 2001.

675. Catovsky D, Wechsler A, Matutes E, et al: The membrane phenotype of T-prolymphocytic leukaemia. *Scand J Haematol* 29:398, 1982.

676. Hui PK, Feller AC, Pileri S, et al: New aggressive variant of suppressor/cytotoxic T CLL. *Am J Clin Pathol* 87:55, 1987.

677. Kluin-Nelemans HC, Gmelig-Meyling FH, Kootte AM, et al: T-cell prolymphocytic leukemia with an unusual phenotype CD4+ CD8+. *Cancer* 60:794, 1987.

678. Brito-Babapulle V, Maljaie SH, Matutes E, et al: Relationship of T leukaemias with cerebriform nuclei to T-prolymphocytic leukaemia: A cytogenetic analysis with in situ hybridization. *Br J Haematol* 96:724, 1997.

679. Pawson R, Matutes E, Brito-Babapulle V, et al: Sezary cell leukaemia: A distinct T cell disorder or a variant form of T prolymphocytic leukaemia? *Leukemia* 11:1009, 1997.

680. Uike N, Choi I, Tokoro A, et al: Adult T-cell leukemia-lymphoma successfully treated with 2-chlorodeoxyadenosine. *Intern Med* 37.411, 1998.

681. Palomera L, Domingo JM, Agullo JA, Soledad Romero M: Complete remission in T-cell prolymphocytic leukemia with 2-chlorodeoxyadenosine. *J Clin Oncol* 13:1284, 1995.

682. Zackheim HS: Cutaneous T cell lymphoma: Update of treatment. *Dermatology* 199:102, 1999.

683. Ravandi F, O'Brien S: Alemtuzumab. *Expert Rev Anticancer Ther* 5:39, 2005.

684. Dearden C: Alemtuzumab in peripheral T-cell malignancies. *Cancer Biother Radiopharm* 19:391, 2004.

685. Birhiray RE, Shaw G, Guldan S, et al: Phenotypic transformation of CD52(pos) to CD52(neg) leukemic T cells as a mechanism for resistance to CAMPATH-1H. *Leukemia* 16:861, 2002.

686. Collins RH, Pineiro LA, Agura ED, Fay JW: Treatment of T prolymphocytic leukemia with allogeneic bone marrow transplantation. *Bone Marrow Transplant* 21:627, 1998.

687. Murase K, Matsunaga T, Sato T, et al: Allogeneic bone marrow transplantation in a patient with T-prolymphocytic leukemia with small-intestinal involvement. *Int J Clin Oncol* 8:391, 2003.

688. Tsai LM, Tsai CC, Hyde TP, et al: T-cell prolymphocytic leukemia with helper-cell phenotype and a review of the literature. *Cancer* 54:463, 1984.

689. Pawson R, Richardson DS, Pagliuca A, et al: Adult T-cell leukemia/lymphoma in London: Clinical experience of 21 cases. *Leuk Lymphoma* 31:177, 1998.

690. Garand R, Goasguen J, Brizard A, et al: Indolent course as a relatively frequent presentation in T-prolymphocytic leukaemia. Groupe Francais d'Hematologie Cellulaire. *Br J Haematol* 103:488, 1998.

691. Calin GA, Trapasso F, Shimizu M, et al: Familial cancer associated with a polymorphism in ARLTS1. *N Engl J Med* 352:1667, 2005.

HAIRY CELL LEUKEMIA

ALAN SAVEN

Hairy cell leukemia is an uncommon neoplastic disorder of B lymphocytes that afflicts principally middle-aged men. The patient usually presents with pancytopenia. Absolute neutropenia and monocytopenia are nearly constant features. The blood and marrow biopsy contain hairy cells, which are lymphocytes that have prominent cytoplasmic projections, and give the disease its name. Splenomegaly, sometimes massive, is a nearly constant feature. The liver and abdominal lymph nodes may be enlarged. The immunophenotypes of the hairy cells, CD11c+, CD19+, CD20+, CD22+, CD25+, and CD103+, confirm the diagnosis. Disease complications include standard or opportunistic infections. Approximately 10 percent of patients may not require immediate treatment. For patients requiring treatment, cladribine is the drug of choice because of the very high complete remission rate and prolonged duration of remission in many patients. Pentostatin also has activity in this disease. Interferon-α, rituximab anti-CD22 recombinant immunotoxin (BL22), or splenectomy can be useful in selected patients unresponsive to cladribine or pentostatin. The patient with hairy cell leukemia can expect a very long duration of survival with current therapy. The 5-year event-free survival rate after treatment is approximately 90 percent of patients initially treated with cladribine.

DEFINITION AND HISTORY

Hairy cell leukemia (HCL) is a rare chronic lymphoproliferative disorder characterized by circulating B lymphocytes that display prominent cytoplasmic projections. The neoplastic B cells infiltrate the marrow and spleen in a characteristic way. Afflicted individuals often are elderly males who present with pancytopenia, splenomegaly, or recurrent serious infections. In 1958, Bouroncle and colleagues[1] recognized the disorder as a distinct clinicopathologic entity and referred to it as *leukemic reticuloendotheliosis*.

EPIDEMIOLOGY

HCL is thought to account for 2 to 3 percent of all adult leukemias in the United States, with 600 new patients diagnosed annually. HCL is predominantly a disease of middle-aged males with a median age at presentation of 52 years. The disease has not been described in children or teenagers. The disease occurs at a 4:1 male to female predominance, with Ashkenazi Jewish males being more frequently affected.

ETIOLOGY AND PATHOGENESIS

Prior exposure to radiation and organic solvents reportedly is more frequent among HCL patients.[2,3] Some investigators have speculated

on an etiologic role for the Epstein-Barr virus in the development of HCL,[4] but the proposal has been disputed.[5] When cytogenetic analyses were performed in 30 patients with HCL, chromosome 5 was involved in clonal aberrations in 12 (40%) patients, most commonly as trisomy 5 or pericentric inversions and interstitial deletions involving band 5q13.[6]

The normal function and precise site of origin in lymphocytic ontogeny of the hairy cell remain unknown, although many characteristics of this elusive cell have been described.[7] Hairy cells represent clonal expansions of mature B cells with phenotypic features of activation.[8] The leading candidates for the normal counterpart of the neoplastic hairy cell is the monocytoid (or marginal zone) B cell. These two cells share morphologic and immunophenotypic similarities. They also express PCA-1 antigen, an early plasma cell marker.[9] However, unlike monocytoid B cells, hairy cells are tartrate-resistant acid phosphatase (TRAP) positive. They appear to lack tight linkage between any normal reactive cell type as seen in benign monocytoid B cell proliferations.

Some investigators, using B-ly7 and CD11c antibodies, identified a small population of normal B lymphocytes that could be the normal counterpart of the hairy cell.[10] In addition, hairy B cell lymphoproliferative disorder—a polyclonal, nonneoplastic proliferation of hairy cells closely resembling HCL–Japanese variant—has been described.[11] Nevertheless, the normal counterpart remains elusive possibly because it is extremely rare or because cells with the classic features of hairy cells exist only after neoplastic transformation.[8]

Hairy cells secrete cytokines, such as tumor necrosis factor alpha, that may contribute to the impaired hematopoiesis seen in the disease by reducing the number of erythroid colony forming units.[12] Macrophage colony stimulating factor induces hairy cell motility.[13] Specific integrin receptors $\alpha_v\beta_3$ responsible for hairy cell motile behavior have been identified.[14]

CLINICAL FEATURES

The diagnostic triad of HCL consists of pancytopenia, splenomegaly, and circulating hairy cells. Pancytopenia occurs in 50 percent of patients; the remaining half usually have a combination of cytopenias.[15] On initial presentation, 25 percent of patients present with fatigue and weakness, 25 percent with easy bruising from thrombocytopenia or opportunistic infections from leukopenia, 25 percent with early satiety or abdominal fullness from splenomegaly, and 25 percent with an incidental finding of splenomegaly or abnormal blood counts on routine examination for an unrelated condition.[16,17]

Splenomegaly, which may be massive, is found in 90 percent of patients.[18,19] Hepatomegaly is rarely a significant finding. Palpable peripheral lymphadenopathy is distinctly uncommon and when found usually is localized. However, since the routine use of computerized axial tomography scans in the evaluation of patients with lymphoproliferative disorders, significant internal adenopathy can be demonstrated in up to one third of patients with HCL.[20,21] In 3 percent of patients, the disease manifests as painful bony lesions, most commonly involving the proximal femur.[22]

At initial diagnosis, up to 30 percent of HCL patients have an absolute neutrophil count less than 0.5×10^9/L, and most demonstrate monocytopenia.[23] These cytopenias predispose patients to infection from a wide variety of typical and opportunistic organisms. Impaired interferon-α production by blood mononuclear cells may predispose patients with HCL to intracellular infections by compromising their cellular immunity.[24] Organisms encountered in febrile HCL patients include *Mycobacterium kansasii* (accounting for 5–10% of mycobacterial disease in this population), *Pneumocystis carinii*, aspergillus, histoplasma, cryptococcus, *Toxoplasma gondii*.[25] Other laboratory abnormalities include liver function test abnormalities in 19 percent,

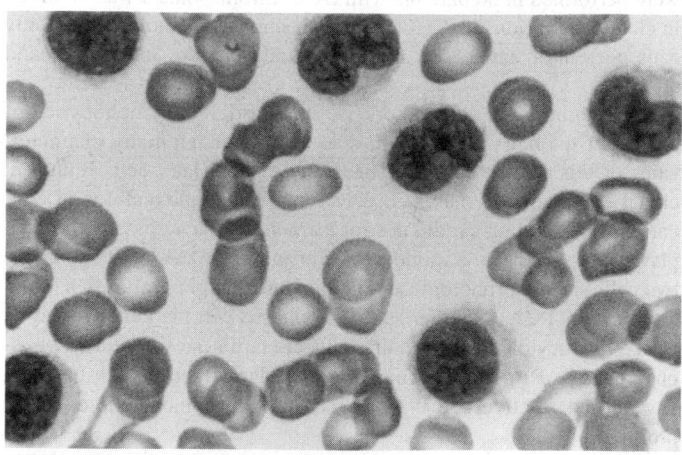

FIGURE 93-1 Blood smear. Hairy cells are small to medium in size, have oval nuclei with finely clumped chromatin, and demonstrate abundant cytoplasm with frayed margins. The cytoplasm has a textured appearance from lamellar arrays of rough endoplasmic reticulum but is agranular (Wright Giemsa stain, ×1000).

azotemia in 27 percent, and hypergammaglobulinemia, possibly monoclonal, in 18 percent.[26] Hypogammaglobulinemia is rare, unlike the case of chronic lymphocytic leukemia. Unusual manifestations include cutaneous vasculitis, leukocytoclastic angiitis, erythema nodosum, and Raynaud phenomenon.[26] Hypocholesterolemia, mainly resulting from a low concentration of low-density lipoprotein cholesterol, is a frequent finding in advanced HCL but reverts to normal after successful treatment.[27,28]

LABORATORY FEATURES

BLOOD

Patients usually present with anemia, thrombocytopenia, and leukopenia. Occasional patients have elevated leukocyte counts as a result of circulating hairy cells. More than 80 percent of patients have absolute neutropenia and monocytopenia.[29–32] Hairy cells are mononu-

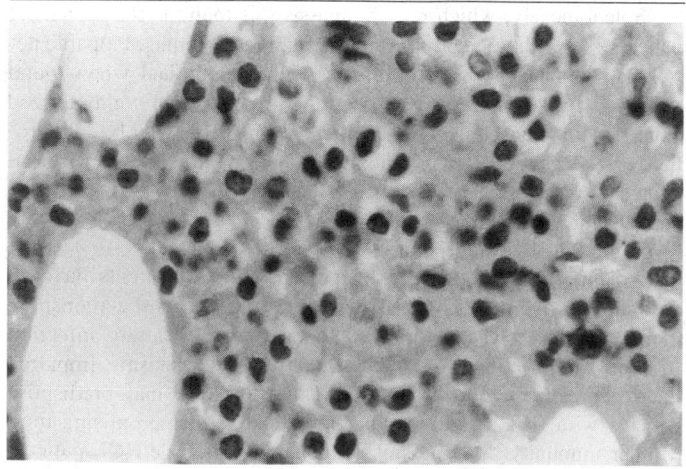

FIGURE 93-2 Histologic section. Diffuse infiltration by a monotonous population of small lymphoid cells having an abundant rim of pale cytoplasm that imparts a well-spaced appearance to the centrally located nuclei, often called a "fried-egg" appearance (hematoxylin and eosin stain, ×400).

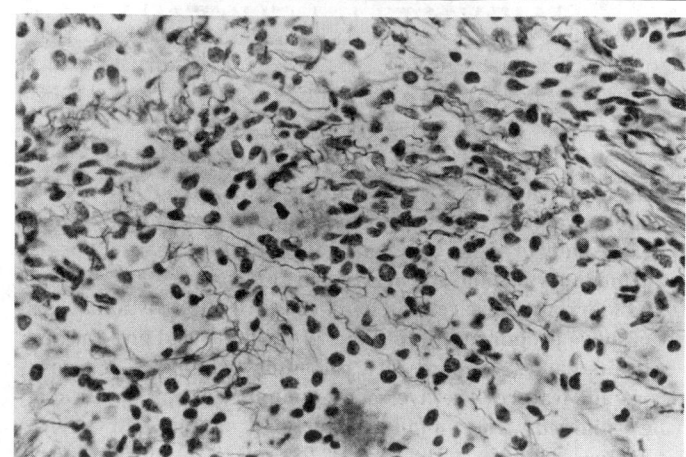

FIGURE 93-3 Marrow biopsy. Extensive diffuse deposition of fibronectin seen as a dense network of black staining fibers associated with infiltration by HCL (silver stain, ×100).

clear cells with eccentric or central nuclei.[29] Nuclear morphology is variable: round, ovoid, reniform, or convoluted. Nuclear forms tend to have a reticular chromatin pattern. Hairy cells have variable amounts of cytoplasm that is blue–gray in appearance, exhibiting thin cytoplasmic projections (Fig. 93-1).

MARROW

The marrow biopsy usually demonstrates hairy cell infiltrates, which may be patchy or difficult to discern in some patients. Marrow involvement may be diffuse or focal. The most subtle pattern of HCL infiltration is a hypocellular marrow with scant infiltration by hairy cells admixed with residual hematopoietic tissue.[30,33] The hairy cells in the marrow aspirate tend to have a slightly coarser reticular chromatin-staining pattern than the hairy cells found in the blood. Hairy cells have monotonous round, oval, or spindle-spaced nuclei that are separated by abundant quantities of pale-staining cytoplasm in a fine fibrillar network. The separation of individual hairy cells is characteristic and referred to as the "fried-egg" appearance (Fig. 93-2). Because of marked marrow reticulin fibrosis, the marrow frequently is difficult or impossible to aspirate (Fig. 93-3). Hairy cells synthesize and assemble a fibronectin matrix that likely contributes to the marrow fibrosis characteristic of the disease.[34] Hairy cells express CD44, a nonintegrin receptor, that may be responsible for hairy cell homing to the glycosaminoglycan and hyaluronan tissue matrix present in the marrow, the engagement of which stimulates fibronectin synthesis, with resultant fibrosis.[35]

SPLEEN, LIVER, AND LYMPH NODES

The spleen usually is enlarged, with a median weight of 1300 g.[36] On section, the spleen has a dark-red, smooth surface. On light microscopy, the hairy cells involve the splenic red pulp. Later, the white pulp atrophies and is replaced. Red cell lakes, which are blood-filled spaces lined by hairy cells that have disrupted the normal sinus architecture, are characteristic.[37] These blood-filled spaces sometimes are referred to as *pseudosinuses*.

Hepatic infiltration is both sinusoidal and portal.[37] Lymph node involvement is marked by both sinusoidal and interstitial involvement.[38]

CYTOCHEMISTRY

The hairy cell cytoplasm usually stains strongly positive for TRAP. Isoenzyme 5 acid phosphatase, present in the hairy cell cytoplasm, resists decolorization by tartrate.[39,40] TRAP staining of peripheral blood buffy coat smears are positive in 90 percent of cases.[39] Weak to moderate TRAP staining may occur in other diseases, including prolymphocytic leukemia and lymphoma.[41]

ELECTRON MICROSCOPY

Electron microscopy occasionally helps establish the diagnosis of HCL.[42] In HCL, electron microscopy shows circumferential cytoplasmic projections with fewer and blunter microvilli than seen in splenic lymphoma with circulating B lymphocytes in which the projections tend to be more polarized at one end of the cell.[43,44] Ribosomal lamella complexes can be found in the cytoplasm of hairy cells by transmission electron microscopy in 50 percent of patients.[39] This cytoplasmic inclusion is a cylindrical structure composed of a central hollow space and an outer sheath of multiple parallel lamellae, with ribosomal-like granules in the interlamellar space.[45] These complexes also have been described in other lymphoproliferative disorders.[46]

IMMUNOPHENOTYPIC PROFILE

Hairy cells, being mature B cells, express the pan B cell antigens CD19, CD20, and CD22, but not CD21, an antigen lost in the later stages of B cell development.[47–49] Most distinctively, hairy cells express high levels of CD11c, CD22, CD25, and CD103.[10] The CD11c antigen, the 150-kDa α-chain of the 150/95 β_2-integrin that ordinarily is expressed on monocytes and neutrophils,[10,50] stains very potently, with an intensity 30-fold greater than chronic lymphocytic leukemia.[51]

HCL was the first B cell lymphoproliferative disorder identified that expressed CD25, the interleukin (IL)-2 receptor. Serum levels of soluble IL-2 receptor are elevated in HCL patients and correlate with disease activity following treatment.[52] CD103 (Bly-7) has the greatest sensitivity and specificity for HCL. It represents the α^E subunit of the $\alpha^E\beta_7$ integrin, known as the human mucosal lymphocyte-1 antigen, which is thought to be involved in lymphocyte homing and adhesion.[53–55] CD45-PECy5 (clone J33) also may be useful for detecting HCL.[56]

CD22 is expressed more intensely on hairy cells than in other B cell chronic lymphoproliferative disorders. CD22 stains 50 times more intensely in HCL than in chronic lymphocytic leukemia, in which only weak expression is seen.[57] Weak expression of CD10 (the CALLA antigen) is seen in 26 percent of cases, and weak expression of CD5 is seen in 5 percent of cases. CD5 is the anomalous T cell antigen strongly expressed on chronic lymphocytic leukemia cells.[58]

Multiparameter two-color immunofluorescence analysis is especially useful for identifying hairy cells because the analysis permits identification of cells coexpressing CD11c, CD25, and CD103 antigens with a pan B cell antigen such as CD19, CD20, or CD22.[57] Using flow cytometry to examine blood lymphocytes, 92 percent of 161 patients with HCL had identifiable circulating hairy cells, in some patients representing less than 1 percent of lymphocytes. In contrast, careful morphologic evaluation of blood lymphocytes revealed hairy cells in only 80 percent of patients.[57]

IMMUNOHISTOCHEMISTRY

Immunohistochemistry performed on marrow biopsy samples can help aid in the diagnosis of HCL and is useful for detecting minimal resid-

TABLE 93-1   DIFFERENTIAL DIAGNOSIS OF HAIRY CELL LEUKEMIA

PARAMETERS	HCL	HCL–VARIANT	SPLENIC LYMPHOMA WITH VILLOUS LYMPHOCYTES
Blood			
Morphology			
Nuclear shape	Ovoid, reniform	Round	Round
Chromatin	Reticular ± nucleolus	Coarse with central nucleolus	Coarse ± nucleolus
Cytoplasm	Blue–gray, abundant	Blue–gray, abundant	Basophilic, scant to moderate
Monocytopenia	+	−	−
TRAP stain	+++	±	±
Aspirated marrow	−	+	+
Splenic involvement	Red pulp	Red pulp	White pulp
Flow cytometry			
CD22	+++	++	++
CD11c	+++	++	+
CD25	++	−	±
CD103	++	±	−

ual disease following systemic therapies. Most monoclonal antibodies used to detect circulating hairy cells in the blood, including anti-CD103 antibodies, require the marrow be processed by frozen section because the antigens are destroyed by fixation and standard processing.[59] In contrast, the CD20 antibody (L26) and another monoclonal antibody (DBA.44) can be used to stain hairy cells in routinely processed paraffin sections of the marrow.[60–62] L26 staining is membranous and accentuates the ruffled, abundant cytoplasm of hairy cells, whereas DBA.44, an undefined antigen, stains in both a cytoplasmic granular and a membranous pattern.

DIFFERENTIAL DIAGNOSIS

HCL must be considered in the differential diagnosis of any disorder resulting in cytopenias and splenomegaly (Table 93-1).

Hairy cell leukemia variant is a unique clinicopathologic entity representing a hybrid between prolymphocytic leukemia and HCL. The nucleus most closely resembles a prolymphocyte and the cytoplasm a hairy cell.[63] Hairy cell variant cells generally have higher nuclear to cytoplasmic ratios, more highly condensed chromatin, and more conspicuous central nucleoli than seen in classic HCL.[64] Afflicted individuals who present with massive splenomegaly frequently are in the leukemia phase, and results of TRAP staining are either negative or only very weakly positive. The circulating cells in HCL–variant usually are CD25-negative and CD103-negative. In a *blastic* variant of HCL, patients have massive splenomegaly, peripheral adenopathy, and cytopenias.[65] The cells are positive with TRAP staining and negative for myeloperoxidase. A newer entity, *hairy B cell lymphoproliferative disorder*, has been described in Japan.[12] In this disease, patients have splenomegaly without lymphadenopathy. They have persistent lymphocytosis (consisting of abnormal lymphocytes with long microvilli) that is polyclonal, CD25-negative, and only weakly TRAP stain-positive.

Splenic lymphoma with circulating villous lymphocytes, a marginal zone lymphoma, is a closely related disorder that can be difficult to distinguish from HCL. Like patients with HCL, patients can present with massive splenomegaly without lymphadenopathy. However, unlike HCL, lymphocytosis is more common.[66] In this disorder, the lymphocytes have more basophilic cytoplasm, and the cytoplasmic projections tend to be polar and more subtle.[67] Circulating plasmacytoid cells are frequently noted.[43] TRAP staining is either negative or very weakly positive.[39,68] Immunophenotypic analysis identifies cells with strong staining for CD11c but frequently are CD103-negative. Monocytopenia is absent. Sections of spleen show predominant involvement in the white pulp resembling a low-grade lymphoma.[66]

B cell prolymphocytic leukemia may be confused with HCL. Both disorders generally occur in elderly men with prominent splenomegaly. B cell prolymphocytic leukemia lymphocytes are only focally TRAP-positive, whereas HCL and HCL–variant demonstrate strongly positive TRAP staining. In B cell prolymphocytic leukemia, white blood cell counts are higher and are CD11c-negative.[69]

THERAPY

TREATMENT INDICATIONS

Ninety percent of patients with HCL require treatment at presentation or sometime during the course of the disease. Standard hematologic parameters for initiating therapy in HCL include anemia (hemoglobulin <8–10 g/dl), thrombocytopenia (platelet count <50–100 × 10⁹/liter), or neutropenia (absolute neutrophil count <0.5–1.0 × 10⁹/liter), especially when associated with recurrent, serious infections. Other less common indications for initiating treatment are symptomatic splenomegaly, leukocytosis with a high proportion of hairy cells (white blood cell count >20 × 10⁹/liter), bulky or painful lymphadenopathy, vasculitis, or bony involvement.

PURINE ANALOGUES

In 1972, Giblett and colleagues[70] made the seminal observation that one third of children with severe combined immunodeficiency syndrome were deficient in the purine catabolic enzyme adenosine deaminase. Adenosine deaminase catalyzes the irreversible deamination of adenosine to inosine and of 2′-deoxyadenosine to 2′-deoxyinosine. Cohen and investigators[71] reported that the intracellular accumulation of deoxyadenosine triphosphate was responsible for the lymphopenia seen in severe combined immune deficiency. Later, Carson and colleagues[72] reported that 2-chlorodeoxyadenosine (cladribine), a chlorine-substituted purine deoxynucleoside, was the most potent among a panel of substituted purine analogues screened for *in vitro* toxicity.

PENTOSTATIN (2′-DEOXYCOFORMYCIN)

Pentostatin is a natural product of *Streptomyces antibioticus* that irreversibly binds to adenosine deaminase. Pentostatin was first shown to have activity in a single patient with HCL in 1984.[73] In the Intergroup Study, which was organized by the National Cancer Institute and reported in 1995, 313 patients with HCL were randomized to either interferon–α-2A 3 mU/m² subcutaneously three times per week or pentostatin 4 mg/m² intravenously every 2 weeks.[74] Of 159 patients randomized to interferon, 17 (11%) achieved a complete response and 43 (27%) a partial response; the overall response rate was 38 percent. Of the 154 patients randomized to pentostatin, 117 (76%) achieved a complete response and four (3%) a partial response; the overall response rate was 79 percent. Response rates were significantly higher and relapse-free survival was significantly longer for patients who received pentostatin than interferon. The crossover design of the study complicated assessment of differences in overall survival. A long-term followup study of 241 HCL patients who received pentostatin in the Intergroup Study revealed that of 154 patients treated with interferon as initial therapy, 87 crossed over to receive pentostatin after the patients did not respond to initial therapy.[75] The median duration of followup was 9.3 years. The estimated 5- and 10-year survival rates for all patients were 90 percent and 81 percent, respectively. Survival curves for patients initially treated with pentostatin and then crossed

over were similar. The mortality rate and incidence of second malignancies were not higher than expected in the general population. Table 93-2 summarizes the response rates of several pentostatin clinical trials.

Pentostatin-induced toxicities include fever, nausea, vomiting, photosensitivity, and keratoconjunctivitis.[76,77] Severe myelosuppression may occur soon after initiation of pentostatin therapy, especially in patients with preexisting myelosuppression.[78,79] Severe infections, including disseminated herpes zoster, *Escherichia coli*, *Haemophilus influenzae*, pneumococcus, and fungal infections, were observed early after initiation of pentostatin.[77] Pentostatin is best not given to patients with active and uncontrolled infections, a poor performance status, or impaired renal function.[80] Pentostatin is strongly immunosuppressive.[81] During pentostatin therapy and for at least 1 year thereafter, CD4 and CD8 lymphocytes can decrease to levels less than 200 cells/ml.

The standard dose of pentostatin for patients with HCL is 4 mg/m² every other week for 3 to 6 months until maximum response is achieved.

CLADRIBINE (2-CHLORODEOXYADENOSINE)

In 1990, investigators at Scripps Clinic, La Jolla, California, first reported on 12 patients with HCL treated with a single 7-day course of cladribine administered at 0.1 mg/kg/day by continuous intravenous infusion.[82] Of the 12 patients, 11 achieved a complete response and one a partial response. Other investigators have reported similar results (see Table 93-2).

Long-term followup of 349 evaluable patients who had received cladribine[83] revealed 319 (91%) achieved complete responses and 22 (7%) partial responses; the overall response rate was 98 percent. The overall median duration of response followup was 52 months. Ninety

TABLE 93-2 INTERFERON AND PURINE NUCLEOSIDE ANALOGUE TREATMENT RESULTS IN HAIRY CELL LEUKEMIA

INVESTIGATORS	NO. OF PATIENTS	RESPONDERS (%) COMPLETE	PARTIAL	MINOR OR NONE
Interferon				
Quesada et al.[93]	30	9	17	4
Foon et al.[114]	14	1	12	1
Rai et al.[115]	25	7	6	12
Golomb et al.[116]	195	7	152	36
Grever et al.[117]	159	17	43	99
Total	423	41 (10%)	230 (54%)	152 (36%)
Purine Nucleoside Analogues				
A. Pentostatin				
Cassileth et al.[78]	50	32	10	8
Kraut et al.[118]	23	20	1	2
Ho et al.[79]	33	11	15	7
Grem et al.[119]	66	37	15	14
Grever et al.[117]	154	117	4	33
Dearden et al.[108]	165	135	25	5
Total	491	352 (72%)	70 (14%)	69 (14%)
B. Cladribine				
Saven et al.[83]	349	319	22	8
Estey et al.[120]	46	36	5	5
Juliusson et al.[121]	16	12	0	4
Hoffman et al.[122]	49	37	12	0
Tallman et al.[123]	50	40	9	1
Dearden et al.[108]	45	38	7	0
Total	555	482 (87%)	55 (10%)	18 (3%)

patients (26%) relapsed at a median of 29 months. The time to treatment failure rate for all 341 responders was 19 percent at 48 months, 16 percent for complete responders, and 54 percent for partial responders. The proportion of patients, if any, who will be cured is not clear because no plateau is evident on the time to treatment failure curve. Also, 25 to 50 percent of patients in morphologic complete remission after cladribine have minimal residual disease detected by immunohistochemical stains of marrow biopsies.[84,85] Of 53 evaluable patients treated with cladribine at first relapse, 33 (62%) achieved complete responses and 14 (26%) achieved partial responses. Thus, patients who relapse can be successfully re-treated with cladribine. A followup study of 207 assessable patients with at least 7 years of followup after cladribine treatment[86] revealed[196] (95%) achieved complete responses and 11 (5%) partial responses after a single course of cladribine. The median first-response duration for all responders was 98 months. Seventy-six patients (37%) experienced relapse after the first course of cladribine. The median time to first relapse for all responders was 42 months. The overall survival rate was 97 percent at 108 months. Forty-seven patients developed 58 second malignancies. The ratio of observed to expected second malignancies was 2.03 (95% confidence interval, 1.49–2.71) (see Table 93-2).

Fever is the principal toxicity of cladribine therapy in HCL, occurring in 42 percent of patients treated. Fever is related to the disappearance of hairy cells and appears most marked in patients with the greatest pretreatment HCL burden, manifested principally as splenomegaly. Documented infections unrelated to a peripherally inserted central catheter device used to deliver the cladribine are uncommon. Dermatomal herpes zoster is the most frequently reported late infection.[83] Like pentostatin, 2-chlorodeoxyadenosine also is immunosuppressive.[87] In one study, a tendency toward restoration of CD4 cells was observed at 6 and 12 months,[88] whereas other studies showed more profound and long-lasting CD4 lymphocytopenia.[89]

Thus, cladribine has emerged as the treatment of choice for HCL given that single courses of cladribine induce long-lasting complete responses in the vast majority of patients following only a single 7-day infusion, relapse rates for complete responders are low, and patients who relapse can be successfully re-treated with cladribine. The recommended dose of cladribine is 0.1 mg/kg/day by continuous intravenous infusion for 7 days. Successful administration of subcutaneous[90] and oral cladribine[91] and a weekly intravenous administration schema[92] have been reported.

INTERFERON

Quesada and colleagues[93] first reported on the successful use of partially purified human α-interferon (leukocyte) in patients with HCL in 1984. In 1986, use of recombinant interferon–α-2B interferon (Intron® A, Schering Corporation, Kenilworth, NY, USA), at 2 mU/m² for 12 months was reported in 64 patients with HCL.[94] In the study, three (5%) patients achieved a complete response and 45 (70%) a partial response. Twelve months of interferon-α therapy is optimal because a longer duration of treatment does not increase response rates or lower relapse rates but increases toxicity.[95,96] Recombinant interferon–α-2A (Roferon®, Hoffmann-La Roche, Nutley, NJ, USA), which has a cysteine residue at position 23 (α-2B has an arginine residue), induced similar response rates when administered to 30 patients with HCL.[97] Median time to treatment failure after discontinuation of interferon was 18 to 25 months.[98] The standard dose recommendation for interferon–α-2B is 2 mU/m² administered subcutaneously three times per week for 12 months. The standard dose recommendation for interferon–α-2A is 3 mU/m² subcutaneously given daily for 6 months and then decreased to three times per week for an additional 6 months.

Table 93-2 summarizes the response rates of several interferon clinical trials.

The most common side effect of interferon is a flu-like syndrome consisting of fever, myalgias, and malaise. Acetaminophen often ameliorates these symptoms, and tachyphylaxis frequently develops over time. An unexpectedly high incidence of second neoplasms in patients after treatment of HCL with interferon–α-2B has been reported.[99] Of 69 patients followed for a median of 91 months, 13 patients (19%) developed a second neoplasm; six were of hematopoietic origin and seven were adenocarcinomas.

Although interferon-α is an active agent against HCL, it does not induce the same high complete response rates seen with the purine nucleoside analogues. Accordingly, use of interferon-α for treatment of HCL should be reserved for patients who have active infections and thus cannot undergo purine nucleoside analogue therapy given their associated T cell immunosuppression[25,87] and for patients who have not responded to previous systemic therapy with a purine nucleoside analogue.[100]

RITUXIMAB

Because hairy cells brightly express the B cell antigen CD20, rituximab (Rituxan, Biogen Idec, Cambridge, MA, USA), a chimeric humanized mouse anti-CD20 monoclonal antibody, represented a rational therapeutic approach. Twenty-four HCL patients who relapsed after treatment with cladribine using rituximab at 375 mg/m² intravenously for 4 weeks were treated.[101] Of the 24 patients, three (13%) achieved complete remissions and three (13%) partial responses. The principal toxicity was culture-negative febrile neutropenia. At a median followup of 14.6 months, two responders had relapsed. In another study, 15 patients with relapsed or refractory HCL after nucleoside analogues were treated with rituximab at 375 mg/m² weekly for 8 weeks.[102] Of the 15 patients, eight (53%) achieved complete responses, and four (26%) achieved partial responses. Of the 12 responders followed for a median of 32 months, five patients progressed. Toxicity was minimal. Rituximab might have a role in HCL patients who relapse after cladribine therapy with a response duration of fewer than 18 months and who demonstrate a significantly hypoplastic marrow or a prior severe opportunistic infection.

ANTI-CD22 RECOMBINANT IMMUNOTOXIN BL22

Recombinant immunotoxin BL22 is effective for treatment of HCL resistant to cladribine.[103,104] BL22 contains the variable domain of an anti-CD22 monoclonal antibody fused to a fragment of a *Pseudomonas* exotoxin. Of 16 patients resistant to cladribine, 11 achieved a complete remission and two had a partial remission with BL22, for an overall response rate of 81 percent. During a median followup of 16 months, three of the 11 complete responders relapsed. Two of the 16 patients developed a reversible hemolytic–uremic syndrome. Although BL22 is an exciting new targeted approach, the results should be interpreted cautiously given the potentially life-threatening nature of this toxicity.

SPLENECTOMY

Splenectomy was the first standard treatment modality regularly used for treatment of HCL because splenectomy rapidly reverses peripheral cytopenias. Ninety percent of patients improve in at least one hematologic parameter, and 40 to 60 percent achieve normalization of blood counts.[105,106] Thrombocytopenia reverses in 75 percent of patients, usually within days of splenectomy. Splenic size alone is not always predictive of response to splenectomy.[36,107] The present indications for splenectomy use are active and uncontrolled infections; thrombocytopenic bleeding; massive, painful, and/or ruptured splenomegaly; and patients who have failed systemic therapies including a purine analogue.

RELAPSES AFTER PURINE ANALOGUE THERAPY

In the absence of prospective, randomized clinical trial results in this HCL patient population, the following treatment algorithm is suggested.[101] Patients are re-treated at relapse only when they demonstrate significant cytopenias, as defined in the "Treatment Indications" section above. For patients who achieve a prior cladribine-induced response of greater than 18 months' duration, a repeat course of cladribine generally is recommended because re-treatment with cladribine in these patients results in an 88 percent response rate.[83] Second courses of cladribine within a 12-month interval are avoided to prevent the potential for cumulative myelotoxicity. Pentostatin also is a therapeutic alternative in this patient cohort.[108] Nonpurine analogue therapy is recommended for HCL patients who relapse after prior cladribine with a response duration of less than 18 months and who have a significantly hypoplastic marrow or a previous severe opportunistic infection. In these patients, splenectomy, interferon, and rituximab are reasonable therapeutic options.

IRRADIATION

Lytic bone lesions, especially in the proximal femur, can be managed with low-dose irradiation at 1500 to 3000 rads.[109,110]

GRANULOCYTE COLONY STIMULATING FACTOR

The first use of recombinant granulocyte colony stimulating factor (G-CSF) in HCL patients was reported in 1988.[111] Because cladribine treatment of HCL is complicated by neutropenic fever in 42 percent of patients, investigators at Scripps Clinic treated 35 HCL patients (with comparison to 105 historic controls) with priming G-CSF followed by cladribine and then G-CSF again to determine if G-CSF would reduce neutropenia and febrile episodes.[112] Although G-CSF regularly increased the absolute neutrophil count in patients with HCL and shortened the duration of severe neutropenia after cladribine, the percentage of febrile patients, number of febrile days, and frequency of admissions for antibiotics were not statistically different in the two groups. Thus, the routine adjunctive use of G-CSF with cladribine for treatment of HCL is not recommended. However, the therapy does have a role in the treatment of actively infected HCL patients.

COURSE AND PROGNOSIS

Ten percent of patients, usually elderly males with smaller sized spleens, normal blood counts, and a lower HCL burden, may be observed for protracted intervals because they generally do not require treatment.[113] Prior to the successful application of interferon and purine nucleoside analogues in the treatment of HCL, patients with HCL had median survivals of only 53 months.[113] Now with purine nucleoside analogue therapy, overall survival rates greater than 95 percent at 4 years have been reported.[83] Regardless of the curative potential of purine nucleoside analogue therapy, patients with HCL now can anticipate long survival. Newer treatment options include rituximab and BL22 immunotoxin. The development of purine nucleoside analogues based on an enhanced understanding of the biochemical pathways of purine metabolism, as exemplified by children with lymphopenia and adenosine deaminase deficiency, provided the rational basis for clinical development of these agents and serves as the paradigm for rational drug design.

ACKNOWLEDGMENT

The author thanks Robert W. Sharpe, MD, Division of Hematopathology, Department of Pathology, Scripps Clinic, La Jolla, California, USA, for providing the pathologic materials shown in Figures 93-1, 93-2, and 93-3.

REFERENCES

1. Bouroncle BA, Wiseman BK, Doan CA: Leukemic reticuloendotheliosis. *Blood* 13:609, 1958.
2. Oleske D, Golomb HM, Farber MD, Levy PS: A case-control inquiry into the etiology of hairy cell leukemia. *Am J Epidemiol* 121:675, 1985.
3. Stewart DJ, Keating MJ: Radiation exposure as a possible etiologic factor in hairy cell leukemia. *Cancer* 46:1577, 1980.
4. Wolf BC, Martin AW, Neiman RS, et al: The detection of Epstein-Barr virus in hairy cell leukemia cells by *in situ* hybridization. *Am J Clin Pathol* 136:717, 1990.
5. Chang KL, Chen YY, Weiss LM: Lack of evidence of Epstein-Barr virus in hairy cell leukemia and monocytoid B-cell lymphoma. *Hum Pathol* 24:58, 1993.
6. Haglund U, Juliusson G, Stellan B, Gahrton G: Hairy cell leukemia is characterized by clonal chromosome abnormalities clustered to specific regions. *Blood* 83:2637, 1994.
7. Goodman GR, Bethel KJ, Saven A: Hairy cell leukemia: An update. *Curr Opin Hematol* 10:258, 2003.
8. Burthem J, Zuzel M, Cawley JC: What is the nature of the hairy cell and why should we be interested [annotation]? *Br J Haematol* 97:511, 1997.
9. Anderson KC, Boyd AW, Fisher DC, et al: Hairy cell leukemia: A tumor of pre-plasma cells. *Blood* 65:620, 1985.
10. Visser L, Shaw A, Slupsky J, et al: Monoclonal antibodies reactive with hairy cell leukemia. *Blood* 74:320, 1989.
11. Machii T, Yamaguchi M, Inoue R, et al: Polyclonal B-cell lymphocytosis with features resembling hairy cell leukemia-Japanese variant. *Blood* 89:2008, 1997.
12. Lindemann A, Ludwig WD, Oster W: High-level secretion of tumor necrosis factor-alpha contributes to hematopoietic failure in hairy cell leukemia. *Blood* 73:880, 1989.
13. Burthem J, Baker PK, Hunt JA, Cawley JC: The function of c-fms in hairy-cell leukemia: Macrophage colony-stimulating factor stimulates hairy-cell movement. *Blood* 83:1381, 1994.
14. Burthem J, Baker PK, Cawley JC: Hairy cell interactions with extracellular matrix: Expression of specific integrin receptors and their role in the cell's response to specific adhesive proteins. *Blood* 84:873, 1994.
15. Turner A, Kjeldsberg CR: Hairy cell leukemia: A review. *Medicine (Baltimore)* 57:477, 1978.
16. Flandrin G, Sigaux F, Sebahoun G, Bouffette P: Hairy cell leukemia: Clinical presentation and follow-up of 211 patients. *Semin Oncol* 11:458, 1984.
17. Catovsky D: Hairy cell leukemia and prolymphocytic leukemia. *Clin Haematol* 6:245, 1977.
18. Katayama I, Finkel HE: Leukemic reticuloendotheliosis. A clinicopathologic study with review of the literature. *Am J Med* 57:115, 1974.
19. Golomb HM: Hairy cell leukemia. An unusual lymphoproliferative disease: A study of 24 patients. *Cancer* 42:946, 1978.
20. Hakimian D, Tallman MS, Hogan DK, et al: Prospective evaluation of internal adenopathy in a cohort of 43 patients with hairy cell leukemia. *J Clin Oncol* 12:268, 1994.
21. Mercieca J, Matutes E, Moskovic E: Massive abdominal lymphadenopathy in hairy cell leukaemia: A report of 12 cases. *Br J Haematol* 82:547, 1992.
22. Quesada JR, Keating MJ, Libshitz HI, Llamas L: Bone involvement in hairy cell leukemia. *Am J Med* 74:228, 1983.

23. Goyette RE: Hairy cell leukemia, in *Hematology: A Comprehensive Guide to the Diagnosis and Treatment of Blood Disorders*, edited by RE Goyette, p 576. PMIC, Los Angeles, 1997.

24. Siegal FP, Shodell M, Shah K, et al: Impaired interferon alpha response in hairy cell leukemia is corrected by therapy with 2-chloro-2'-deoxy-adenosine: Implications for susceptibility to opportunistic infections. *Leukemia* 8:1474, 1994.

25. Kraut EH, Neff JC, Bouroncle BA, et al: Immunosuppressive effects of pentostatin. *J Clin Oncol* 8:848, 1990.

26. Dorsey JK, Penick GD: The association of hairy cell leukemia with unusual immunologic disorders. *Arch Intern Med* 142:902, 1982.

27. Juliusson G, Vitols S, Liliemark J: Mechanisms behind hypocholesterolaemia in hairy cell leukaemia. *BMJ* 310:27, 1995.

28. Juliusson G, Vitols S, Liliemark J: Disease-related hypocholesterolemia in patients with hairy cell leukemia. *Cancer* 76:423, 1995.

29. Bartl R, Frisch B, Hill W: Marrow histology in hairy cell leukemia. *Am J Clin Pathol* 79:531, 1983.

30. Burke JS: The value of the bone-marrow biopsy in the diagnosis of hairy cell leukemia. *J Clin Pathol* 70:876, 1978.

31. Naeim F, Jacobs AD: Marrow changes in patients with hairy cell leukemia treated by recombinant alpha-2 interferon. *Hum Pathol* 16:1200, 1985.

32. Ratain MJ, Golomb HM, Bardawil RG: Durability of responses to interferon alfa-2b in advanced hairy cell leukemia. *Blood* 69:872, 1987.

33. Barton J: Tumor-lysis syndrome nonhematopoietic neoplasms. *Cancer* 64:738, 1989.

34. Burthem J, Cawley JC: The marrow fibrosis of hairy-cell leukemia is caused by the synthesis and assembly of a fibronectin matrix by the hairy cells. *Blood* 83:497, 1994.

35. Aziz KA, Till KJ, Zuzel M, Cawley JC: Involvement of CD44-hyaluronan interaction in malignant cell homing and fibronectin synthesis in hairy cell leukemia. *Blood* 96:3161, 2000.

36. Golomb HM, Vardiman JW: Response to splenectomy in 65 patients with hairy cell leukemia: An evaluation of spleen weight and marrow involvement. *Blood* 61:349, 1983.

37. Nanba K, Soban EJ, Bowling MC, Berard CW: Splenic pseudosinuses and hepatic angiomatous lesions: Distinctive features of hairy cell leukemia. *Am J Clin Pathol* 67:415, 1977.

38. Vardiman JW, Golomb HM: Autopsy findings in hairy cell leukemia. *Semin Oncol* 11:370, 1984.

39. Yam LT, Janckila AJ, Li CY, Lam WKW: Cytochemistry of tartrate-resistant acid phosphatase: Fifteen years' experience. *Leukemia* 1:285, 1987.

40. Li CY, Yam LT, Lam KW: Studies of acid phosphatase isoenzymes in human leukocytes: Demonstration of isoenzyme specificity. *J Histochem Cytochem* 18:901, 1970.

41. Drexler HG, Gaedicke G, Minowade J: Isoenzyme studies in human leukemia-lymphoma cell lines: II. Acid phosphatase. *Leuk Res* 9:537, 1985.

42. Katayama I, Li CY, Yam LT: Ultrastructural characteristics of the "hairy cells" of leukemic reticuloendotheliosis. *Am J Pathol* 361:370, 1972.

43. Melo JV, Robinson DS, Gregory C, Catovsky D: Splenic B cell lymphoma with "villous" lymphocytes in the peripheral blood: A disorder distinct from hairy cell leukemia. *Leukemia* 1:294, 1987.

44. Catovsky D, O'Brien M, Melo JV, et al: Hairy cell leukemia variant: An intermediate disease between hairy cell leukemia and B prolymphocytic leukemia. *Semin Oncol* 11:362, 1984.

45. Rosner MC, Golomb HM: Ribosome-lamella complex in hairy cell leukemia. Ultrastructure and distribution. *Lab Invest* 42:236, 1980.

46. Brunning RD, Parkin J: Ribosome-lamella complexes in neoplastic hematopoietic cells. *Am J Pathol* 79:565, 1975.

47. Korsmeyer SJ, Greene WC, Cossman J, et al: Rearrangement and expression of immunoglobulin genes and expression of Tac antigen in hairy cell leukemia. *Proc Natl Acad Sci U S A* 80:4522, 1983.

48. Hsu S, Yang K, Jaffe ES: Hairy cell leukemia: A B-cell neoplasm with a unique antigenic phenotype. *Am J Clin Pathol* 80:421, 1983.

49. Falini B, Schwarting R, Erber W, et al: The differential diagnosis of hairy cell leukemia with a panel of monoclonal antibodies. *Am J Clin Pathol* 83:289, 1985.

50. Schwarting R, Stein H, Wang CY: The monoclonal antibodies alpha S-HCL-1 (alpha Leu-14) and alpha S-HCL-3 (alpha Leu-M5) allow the diagnosis of hairy cell leukemia. *Blood* 65:974, 1985.

51. Hanson CA, Gribbin TE, Schnitzer B, et al: CD11c (LEU-M5) expression characterizes a B-cell chronic lymphoproliferative disorder with features of both chronic lymphocytic leukemia and hairy cell leukemia. *Blood* 76:2360, 1990.

52. Steis RG, Marcon L, Clark J, et al: Serum soluble IL-2 receptor as a tumor marker in patients with hairy cell leukemia. *Blood* 77:1304, 1988.

53. Micklem KJ, Dong Y, Willis A, et al: HML-1 antigen on mucosa-associated T cells, activated cells, and hairy leukemic cells is a new integrin containing the b7 subunit. *Am J Clin Pathol* 139:1297, 1991.

54. Flenghi L, Spinozzi F, Stein H, et al: A new monoclonal antibody directed against a trimeric molecule (150 kDa, 125 kDa, 105 kDa) associated with hairy cell leukemia. *Br J Haematol* 76:451, 1990.

55. Cepek KL, Parker CM, Madara JL, Brenner MB: Integrin alpha E beta F mediates adhesion of T lymphocytes to epithelial cell. *J Immunol* 150:3459, 1993.

56. Tytherleigh L, Taparia M, Leahy MF: Detection of hairy cell leukaemia in blood and marrow using multidimensional flow cytometry with CD45-PECy5 and SS gating. *Clin Lab Haematol* 23:385, 2001.

57. Robbins BA, Ellison DJ, Spinosa JC, et al: Diagnostic application of two-color flow cytometry in 161 cases of hairy cell leukemia. *Blood* 82:1277, 1993.

58. Linde GA, Hammarstrom L, Persson MAA, et al: Virus-specific antibody activity of different subclasses of immunoglobulins G and A in cytomegalovirus infections. *Infect Immun* 42:237, 1983.

59. Thaler J, Denz H, Dietze O, et al: Immunohistological assessment of marrow biopsies from patients with hairy cell leukemia: Changes following treatment with alpha-2-interferon and deoxycoformycin. *Leuk Res* 13:377, 1989.

60. Stroup R, Sheibani K: Antigenic phenotypes of hairy cell leukemia and monocytoid B-cell lymphoma. An immunohistochemical evaluation of 66 cases. *Hum Pathol* 23:172, 1992.

61. Al Saati T, Caspar S, Brousset P, et al: Production of anti-B monoclonal antibodies (DBB.42, DBA.44, DNA.7, and DND.53) reactive on paraffin-embedded tissues with a new B-lymphoma cell line grafted into athymic nude mice. *Blood* 74:2476, 1989.

62. Hounieu H, Chittal SM, al Saati T, et al: Hairy cell leukemia. Diagnosis of marrow involvement in paraffin-embedded sections with monoclonal antibody DBA.44. *Am J Clin Pathol* 98:26, 1992.

63. Sainati L, Matutes E, Mulligan S, et al: A variant form of hairy cell leukemia resistant to alpha-interferon: Clinical and phenotype characteristics of 17 patients. *Blood* 76:157, 1990.

64. Cawley JC, Burns GF, Hayhoe RGH: A chronic lymphoproliferative disorder with distinctive features: A distinct variant of hairy cell leukemia. *Leuk Res* 4:547, 1980.

65. Diez-Martin JL, Li CY, Banks PM: Blastic variant of hairy cell leukemia. *Am J Clin Pathol* 87:576, 1987.

66. Sun T, Susin M, Brody J: Splenic lymphoma with circulating villous lymphocytes: Report of seven cases and review of the literature. *Am J Clin Pathol* 45:39, 1994.

67. Hanson CA, Ward PC, Schnitzer B: A multilobular variant of hairy cell leukemia with morphologic similarities to T-cell lymphoma. *Am J Surg Pathol* 13:671, 1989.

68. Yam LT, Li CY, Lam KW: Tartrate-resistant acid phosphatase isoenzyme in the reticulum cells of leukemic reticuloendotheliosis. *N Engl J Med* 284:357, 1971.

69. Slovak ML, Weiss LM, Nathwan BN: Cytogenetic studies of composite lymphomas: Monocytoid B-cell lymphoma and other B-cell non-Hodgkin's lymphomas. *Hum Pathol* 24:1086, 1993.

70. Giblett ER, Anderson JE, Cohen F, et al: Adenosine deaminase deficiency in two patients with severely impaired cellular immunity. *Lancet* 2:1067, 1972.

71. Cohen A, Hirshhorn R, Horowitz SD, et al: Deoxyadenosine triphosphate as a potentially toxic metabolite in adenosine deaminase deficiency. *Proc Natl Acad Sci U S A* 75:472, 1978.

72. Carson DA, Wasson DB, Kaye J, et al: Deoxycytidine kinase-mediated toxicity of deoxyadenosine analogs toward malignant human lymphoblasts in vitro and toward murine L1210 leukemia in vivo. *Proc Natl Acad Sci U S A* 77:6865, 1980.

73. Spiers ASD, Parekh SJ: Complete remission in hairy cell leukemia achieved with pentostatin. *Lancet* 1:1080, 1984.

74. Grever M, Kopecky K, Foular K: Randomization comparison of pentostatin versus interferon alpha-2a in previously untreated patients with hairy cell leukemia. *J Clin Oncol* 13:974, 1995.

75. Flinn IW, Kopecky KJ, Foucar MK, et al: Long-term follow-up of remission duration, mortality, and second malignancies in hairy cell leukemia patients treated with pentostatin. *Blood* 96:2981, 2000.

76. Spiers ASD, Parekh SJ, Bishop MB: Hairy cell leukemia: Induction of complete remission with pentostatin (2'-deoxycoformycin). *J Clin Oncol* 2:1336, 1984.

77. Johnston JB, Glazer RI, Pugh L, Israels LG: The treatment of hairy cell leukemia with 2'-deoxycoformycin. *Br J Haematol* 63:525, 1986.

78. Cassileth PA, Cheuvant B, Spiers ASD, et al: Pentostatin induces durable remissions in hairy cell leukemia. *J Clin Oncol* 9:243, 1991.

79. Ho AD, Thaler J, Stryckmans P, et al: Pentostatin in refractory chronic lymphocytic leukemia: A phase II trial of the European Organization for Research and Treatment of Cancer. *J Natl Cancer Inst* 82:1416, 1990.

80. Spiers ASD, Moore D, Cassileth PA, et al: Remissions in hairy cell leukemia with pentostatin (2'-deoxycoformycin). *N Engl J Med* 316:825, 1987.

81. Urba WJ, Baseler MW, Kopp WC, et al: Deoxycoformycin-induced immunosuppression in patients with hairy cell leukemia. *Blood* 73:38, 1989.

82. Piro LD, Carrera CJ, Carson DA, Beutler E: Lasting remissions in hairy cell leukemia induced by a single infusion of 2-chlorodeoxyadenosine. *N Engl J Med* 322:1117, 1990.

83. Saven A, Burian C, Koziol JA, Piro LD: Long-term follow-up of patients with hairy cell leukemia after cladribine treatment. *Blood* 92:1918, 1998.

84. Hakimian D, Tallman MS, Kiley C, Peterson LA: Detection of minimal residual disease by immunostaining of marrow biopsies after 2-chlorodeoxyadenosine for hairy cell leukemia. *Blood* 82:1798, 1993.

85. Ellison DJ, Sharpe RW, Robbins BA, et al: Immunomorphologic analysis of marrow biopsies after treatment with 2-chlorodeoxyadenosine for hairy cell leukemia. *Blood* 84:4310, 1994.

86. Goodman GR, Burian C, Koziol JA, Saven A: Extended follow-up of patients with hairy cell leukemia after treatment with cladribine. *J Clin Oncol* 21:891, 2003.

87. Juliusson G, Lenkei R, Liliemark J: Flow cytometry of blood and marrow cells from patients with hairy cell leukemia: Phenotype of hairy cells and lymphocyte subsets after treatment with 2-chlorodeoxyadenosine. *Blood* 83:3672, 1994.

88. Carrera CJ, Piro LD, Saven A, et al: Restoration of lymphocyte subsets following 2-chlorodeoxyadenosine remission induction in hairy cell leukemia [abstract]. *Blood* 76(suppl 1):260a, 1990.

89. Seymour J, Kurzrock R, Freireich EJ, Estey EH: 2-Chlorodeoxyadenosine induces durable remissions and prolonged suppression of CD4+ lymphocyte counts in patients with hairy cell leukemia. *Blood* 83:2906, 1994.

90. Juliusson G, Heldal D, Hippe E, et al: Subcutaneous injections of 2-chlorodeoxyadenosine for symptomatic hairy cell leukemia. *J Clin Oncol* 13:989, 1995.

91. Juliusson G, Christiansen I, Hansen MM, et al: Oral cladribine as primary therapy for patients with B-cell chronic lymphocytic leukemia. *J Clin Oncol* 14:2160, 1996.

92. Lauria F, Bocchia M, Marotta G, et al: Weekly administration of 2-chlorodeoxyadenosine in patients with hairy cell leukemia: A new treatment schedule effective and safer in preventing infectious complications [letter]. *Blood* 89:1838, 1998.

93. Quesada JR, Reuben J, Manning JT, et al: Alpha-interferon for induction of remission in hairy cell leukemia. *N Engl J Med* 310:15, 1984.

94. Golomb HM, Jacobs A, Fefer A, et al: Alpha-2 interferon therapy of hairy cell leukemia: A multicenter study of 64 patients. *J Clin Oncol* 4:900, 1986.

95. Golomb HM, Ratain MJ, Fefer A, et al: Randomized study of the duration of treatment with interferon alfa-2b in patients with hairy cell leukemia. *J Natl Cancer Inst* 80:369, 1988.

96. Berman E, Heller G, Kempin S, et al: Incidence of response and long-term follow-up in patients with hairy cell leukemia with recombinant alpha-2a. *Blood* 75:839, 1990.

97. Quesada JR, Hersh EM, Manning J, et al: Treatment of hairy cell leukemia with recombinant alpha-interferon. *Blood* 68:493, 1986.

98. Ratain MJ, Golomb HM, Vardiman JW, et al: Relapse after interferon alpha-2b therapy for hairy cell leukemia: Analysis of diagnostic variables. *J Clin Oncol* 6:1714, 1988.

99. Kampmeier P, Spielberger R, Dickstein J, et al: Increased incidence of second neoplasms in patients treated with interferon a-2b for hairy cell leukemia: A clinicopathologic assessment. *Blood* 83:2931, 1994.

100. Seymour JF, Estey EH, Keating MJ, Kurzrock R: Response to interferon-a in patients with hairy cell leukemia relapsing after treatment with 2-chlorodeoxyadenosine. *Leukemia* 9:929, 1995.

101. Nieva J, Bethel K, Saven A: Phase 2 study of rituximab in the treatment of cladribine-failed patients with hairy cell leukemia. *Blood* 102:810, 2003.

102. Thomas DA, O'Brian S, Bueso-Ramos C, et al: Rituximab in relapsed or refractory hairy cell leukemia. *Blood* 102:3906, 2003.

103. Kreitman RS, Wilson WH, Robbins D, et al: Responses in refractory hairy cell leukemia to a recombinant immunotoxin. *Blood* 94:3340, 1999.

104. Kreitman RJ, Wilson WH, Bergeron K, et al: Efficacy of the anti-CD22 recombinant immunotoxin BL22 in chemotherapy-resistant hairy-cell leukemia. *N Engl J Med* 345:241, 2001.

105. Mintz U, Golomb HM: Splenectomy as initial therapy in twenty-six patients with leukemic reticuloendotheliosis (hairy cell leukemia). *Cancer Res* 39:2366, 1979.

106. Jansen J, Hermans J: Splenectomy in hairy cell leukemia: A retrospective multicenter analysis. *Cancer* 47:2066, 1981.

107. Lewis SM, Catovsky D, Hows JM, Ardalan B: Splenic red cell pooling in hairy cell leukemia. *Br J Haematol* 35:351, 1977.

108. Dearden CE, Matutes E, Hilditch BL, et al: Long-term follow-up of patients with hairy cell leukemia after treatment with pentostatin or cladribine. *Br J Haematol* 106:515, 1999.

109. Lembersky BC, Ratain MJ, Golomb HM: Skeletal complications in hairy cell leukemia: Diagnosis and therapy. *J Clin Oncol* 6:1280, 1988.

110. Arkel YS, Lake-Lewin D, Sarapoulous AA, Berman E: Bone lesions in hairy cell leukemia. *Cancer* 53:2401, 1984.

111. Glaspy JA, Baldwin GC, Robertson PA, et al: Therapy for neutropenia in hairy cell leukemia with recombinant human granulocyte colony-stimulating factor. *Ann Intern Med* 109:789, 1988.

112. Saven A, Burian C, Adusumalli J, Koziol JA: Filgrastim for cladribine-induced neutropenic fever in patients with hairy cell leukemia. *Blood* 93:2471, 1999.

113. Golomb HM, Catovsky D, Golde DW: Hairy cell leukemia: A clinical review of 71 cases. *Ann Intern Med* 89:677, 1978.
114. Foon KA, Maluish AE, Abrams PG, et al: Recombinant leukocyte alpha interferon therapy for advanced hairy cell leukemia. Therapeutic and immunologic results. *Am J Med* 80:351, 1986.
115. Rai K, Mick R, Ozer H, et al: Alpha-interferon therapy in untreated active hairy cell leukemia: A Cancer and Leukemia Group B (CALGB) study [abstract]. *Proc Am Soc Clin Oncol* 6:159, 1987.
116. Golomb H, Fefer A, Golde D, et al: Update of a multi-institutional study of 195 patients (pts) with hairy cell leukemia (HCL) treated with interferon alfa-2b (IFN) [abstract]. *Proc Am Soc Clin Oncol* 6:215, 1990.
117. Grever M, Kopecky K, Foucar MK, et al: Randomized comparison of pentostatin versus interferon alfa-2a in previously untreated patients with hairy cell leukemia: An Intergroup Study. *J Clin Oncol* 13:974, 1995.
118. Kraut EH, Bouroncle BA, Grever MR: Pentostatin in the treatment of advanced hairy cell leukemia. *J Clin Oncol* 7:168, 1989.
119. Grem J, King S, Cheson B, et al: Pentostatin in hairy cell leukemia: Treatment by the special exception mechanism. *J Natl Cancer Inst* 81:448, 1989.
120. Estey EM, Kurzrock R, Kantarjian HM, et al: Treatment of hairy cell leukemia with 2-chlorodeoxyadenosine (2-CdA). *Blood* 79:882, 1992.
121. Juliusson G, Liliemark J: Rapid recovery from cytopenia in hairy cell leukemia after treatment with 2-chloro-2'-deoxyadenosine (CdA): Relation to opportunistic infections. *Blood* 79:888, 1992.
122. Hoffman MA, Janson D, Rose E, Rai KR: Treatment of hairy cell leukemia with cladribine: Response, toxicity and long-term follow-up. *J Clin Oncol* 15:1138, 1997.
123. Tallman MS, Hakimian D, Rademaker AW, et al: Relapse of hairy cell leukemia after 2-chlorodeoxyadenosine: Long-term follow-up of the Northwestern University experience. *Blood* 88:1954, 1996.

LARGE GRANULAR LYMPHOCYTIC LEUKEMIA

THOMAS P. LOUGHRAN

MARSHALL E. KADIN

Clonal diseases of larger granular lymphocytes (LGL) can arise from either T cells or natural killer (NK) cells. Although T-LGL and NK-LGL cells have a similar morphology, they have distinctive surface antigen phenotypes and represent two discrete diseases with different clinical features and clinical outcomes. T-LGL leukemia is defined as a clonal proliferation of CD3+ LGL; NK-LGL leukemia is defined as a clonal proliferation of CD3− LGL. The clinical presentation of NK-LGL leukemia is different from that of T-LGL leukemia. Patients with NK-LGL leukemia usually are younger, more often have systemic B symptoms, and typically have more massive hepatosplenomegaly. Lymphadenopathy and gastrointestinal tract involvement are common. Examination of the blood film is important in making the diagnosis of T-LGL leukemia because approximately 25 percent of patients do not have an increased total lymphocyte count. Most patients with T-LGL leukemia have chronic neutropenia, and approximately half have neutrophil counts less than $500/\mu l$ (5×10^8/liter). In contrast, less than one fifth of patients with NK-LGL have severe neutropenia. Anemia is observed in 50 percent and 100 percent of cases of T-LGL and NK-LGL leukemia, respectively. Patients with T-LGL leukemia frequently have humoral immune abnormalities, such as elevated rheumatoid factor, and red cell aplasia may occur. Morbidity and mortality usually result as consequences of neutropenia. In contrast to the chronic course of T-LGL leukemia, NK-LGL leukemia has an acute presentation and poor clinical outcome. Most patients die within 2 months of diagnosis from disseminated disease with multiorgan failure despite aggressive combination chemotherapy.[19] Patients with chronic NK lymphocytosis usually do not require treatment.

DEFINITION AND HISTORY

A clinical syndrome of chronic neutropenia associated with increased numbers of circulating larger granular lymphocytes (LGL) was described in 1977.[1] Clonal cytogenetic abnormalities established its neoplastic nature, and the term *LGL leukemia* was introduced.[2] Other terms used include *Tγ-lymphoproliferative disease*[3] and *lymphoproliferative disease of granular lymphocytes*.[4]

LGLs compose 10 to 15 percent of normal blood mononuclear cells and may be of either CD3− (natural killer [NK] cell) or CD3+ (T cell) lineage. LGL leukemia is of two types: *T-LGL leukemia* and *NK-LGL leukemia*, reflecting different cellular origins.[5,6] T-LGL leukemia is defined as a clonal proliferation of CD3+ LGL; NK-LGL

leukemia is defined as a clonal proliferation of CD3− LGL. T cell receptor gene rearrangement studies are useful for confirming the clonality of T-LGL leukemia.[7] NK cell leukemia also is a clonal disease, as demonstrated by cytogenetics.[8] However, NK cells and NK cell leukemia lack convenient clonal markers, such as antigen receptor gene rearrangements.

ETIOLOGY AND PATHOGENESIS

The etiology of T-LGL leukemia is unknown. Infection with human T cell leukemia virus (HTLV)-II has been detected in two patients.[9] However, most patients are not infected with prototypical members of this retroviral family, including HTLV-I, HTLV-II, or bovine leukemia virus (BLV).[10] Nevertheless, serologic findings show frequent reactivity to the BA-21 epitope of the p21e *env* protein of HTLV-I, suggesting that a cellular or retroviral protein with homology to BA-21 may be important in pathogenesis.[9] Epstein-Barr virus infection has been implicated in the pathogenesis of NK-LGL leukemia.[11] Leukemic LGL show many characteristics of antigen-activated cytotoxic T lymphocytes (CTLs), suggesting that an initial step in LGL expansion is an antigen-driven mechanism. Microarray studies confirm an activated CTL origin showing constitutive overexpression of serine or cysteine proteases, perforin, and caspase 8 in leukemic LGL.[12] Normal CTLs are regulated through apoptosis. Dysregulated apoptosis is a characteristic finding in LGL leukemia and is thought to underlie the pathogenesis of the disease. Leukemic LGL constitutively express high levels of Fas (CD95) and Fas ligand (CD178) yet are resistant to Fas-mediated death.[13] Defective apoptosis, therefore, may contribute to extended cell survival of leukemic LGL.[14] Several survival pathways are activated in LGL leukemia. Inhibition of Fas apoptotic signaling by soluble Fas decoy receptors has been observed.[15] Constitutive signal transducer and activator of transcription (STAT)-3 signaling leading to enhanced expression of Mcl-1 is another possible mechanism leading to apoptotic resistance.[16] Disease manifestations such as neutropenia are related, at least in part, to circulating Fas ligand in these patients.[17]

CLINICAL FEATURES

Table 94-1 summarizes the clinical features of T-LGL leukemia. Rheumatoid arthritis may be a prominent feature of LGL leukemia, sometimes resulting in a clinical picture resembling that of Felty syndrome (see Chap. 65).[18] The clinical presentation of NK-LGL leukemia is different from that of T-LGL leukemia. Patients with NK-LGL leukemia usually are younger, more often have systemic B symptoms, and typically have more massive hepatosplenomegaly. Lymphadenopathy and gastrointestinal tract involvement are common.[19]

LABORATORY FEATURES

HEMATOLOGIC FINDINGS

Examination of the blood film is important in making the diagnosis of T-LGL leukemia because approximately 25 percent of patients do not

TABLE 94-1 CLINICAL FEATURES OF CD3+ LGL LEUKEMIA*

FEATURE	CASES (%)
Recurrent infections	20–40
B symptoms	20–30
Splenomegaly	20–50
Hepatomegaly	1–23
Lymphadenopathy	1–3

* Data on two series of 128 and 68 patients.[5,33]
SOURCE: Lamy T, Loughran TP Jr: Large granular lymphocyte leukemia. *Cancer Control* 5:25, 1998, with permission.

have an increased total lymphocyte count.[6] LGL can be identified by morphology, although immunophenotyping is necessary to distinguish whether the LGLs are of T cell or NK cell lineage. The median LGL count of patients with T-LGL leukemia, however, is $4200/\mu l$ (4.2×10^9/liter). Patients with NK-LGL leukemia generally have much higher LGL counts, sometimes exceeding $50,000/\mu l$ (5.0×10^{10}/liter).

Most patients (84%) with T-LGL leukemia have chronic neutropenia, and approximately half (48%) have neutrophil counts less than $500/\mu l$ (5×10^8/liter).[6] In contrast, less than one fifth (18%) of patients with NK-LGL have severe neutropenia.[6] Anemia is observed in 50 percent and 100 percent of cases of T-LGL and NK-LGL leukemia, respectively. Pure red cell aplasia (see Chap. 34) and Coombs positive hemolytic anemia (see Chap. 52) are seen with T-LGL leukemia.[5,6] Indeed, LGL leukemia is the most commonly associated disease in patients with pure red cell aplasia.[20] Thrombocytopenia and coagulopathy are features of NK-LGL leukemia.[6] Moderate thrombocytopenia occurring with T-LGL leukemia can resemble idiopathic thrombocytopenic purpura (see Chap. 110).[2]

IMMUNOPHENOTYPING

Immunophenotyping can distinguish T-LGL leukemia from NK-LGL leukemia. T-leukemic LGL usually are CD3+, CD4−, CD8+, CD16+, CD56−, CD57+, and often human leukocyte antigen (HLA)-DR+. Less commonly, leukemic LGLs coexpress CD4 and CD8.[21] Leukemic T-LGL usually express the T-cell receptor (TCR) $\alpha\beta+$ heterodimer, although cases with similar clinical features have been described that express the $\gamma\delta$ TCR heterodimer.[22] NK-leukemic LGL usually are CD3−, CD4−, CD8−, CD16+, CD56+, and CD57−.[19]

IMMUNE ABNORMALITIES

Patients with T-LGL leukemia frequently have humoral immune abnormalities, including positive tests for rheumatoid factor or antinuclear antibodies, polyclonal hypergammaglobulinemia, circulating immune complexes, and antineutrophil antibodies (Table 94-2). These patients also may have defects in cellular immunity, such as diminished NK activity.[2] Immune function has not been evaluated in most patients with NK-LGL leukemia.

HISTOPATHOLOGIC FEATURES

T-LGL leukemia invariably affects the spleen, where the major findings are leukemic cell infiltration of the red pulp cords and sinuses, plasma cell hyperplasia, and prominent germinal centers.[2,23] Liver sinusoids and portal areas are infiltrated by LGL. The marrow biopsy may contain nodules of B lymphocytes and scattered LGL, which are better seen in the aspirate. Granulocyte maturation arrest and pure red cell aplasia have been observed. Lymph nodes usually are not involved

but can have expanded paracortical areas containing plasma cells and LGL.

DIFFERENTIAL DIAGNOSIS

The diagnosis of T-LGL leukemia should be considered in patients with chronic or cyclic neutropenia[24] or in patients with pure red cell aplasia or rheumatoid arthritis who have increased concentrations of LGL cells. Cytomegalovirus or HIV infection can lead to a mildly increased concentration of LGL cells. However, the LGLs are not monoclonal.[25] Some patients may have elevated numbers of CD3− LGL but lack the clinical features of NK-LGL leukemia and have a chronic clinical course.[26] An initial study using X-linked probes suggested that these patients have polyclonal expansion of LGL.[27] More recently, NK cells from such patients have been recognized to express a restricted killer immunoglobulin-like receptor (KIR) phenotype of activating receptors. This finding is in contrast to the diversified KIR repertoire seen in normal NK cells (see Chap. 79).[28,29] This restricted KIR phenotype suggests a clonal origin and may have diagnostic utility. Of interest, sera from these patients with chronic NK lymphocytosis also have frequent reactivity to BA-21.[30]

THERAPY, COURSE, AND PROGNOSIS

Morbidity and mortality usually result as consequences of neutropenia.[6] Optimum treatment for correction of neutropenia is not defined. Treatment with oral low-dose methotrexate, cyclosporine, or oral cyclophosphamide has been efficacious in small series.[31–33] In one series, HLA-DR4 genotype predicted hematologic response to cyclosporine.[34] Clinical improvement is associated with reductions in plasma levels of Fas ligand.[17] A report of four patients treated with fludarabine monophosphate indicated that each achieved a therapeutic benefit.[35] Treatment with glucocorticoids has ameliorated the neutropenia of some patients. However, neutropenia generally recurs as the medication is tapered. Splenectomy is also of limited benefit. Experience with recombinant growth factors is limited.[36,37] Single-agent chemotherapy with prednisone, cyclophosphamide, or chlorambucil is effective in correcting pure red cell aplasia associated with T-LGL leukemia.[6] In contrast to the chronic course of T-LGL leukemia, NK-LGL leukemia has an acute presentation and poor clinical outcome. Most patients die within 2 months of diagnosis from disseminated disease with multiorgan failure despite aggressive combination chemotherapy.[19] Patients with chronic NK lymphocytosis usually do not require treatment.

A registry has been formed to better define the natural history of LGL leukemia. Clinical trials are also being administered through the registry. For more information, the registry can be contacted at *tloughran_psu.edu*.

TABLE 94-2   SEROLOGIC FINDINGS IN CD3+ LGL LEUKEMIA*

FEATURE	CASES (%)
Rheumatoid factor	60
Antinuclear antibody	40
Polyclonal hypergammaglobulinemia	10–40
Monoclonal gammopathy	8
Circulating immune complexes	55
Antineutrophil antibody	40
Positive Coombs test	15

* Data from two series of 128 and 68 patients. [5,33]
SOURCE: Lamy T, Loughran TP Jr: Large granular lymphocyte leukemia. *Cancer Control* 5:25, 1998, with permission.

REFERENCES

1. McKenna RW, Parkin J, Kersey JH, et al: Chronic lymphoproliferative disorder with unusual clinical, morphologic, ultrastructural and membrane surface marker characteristics. *Am J Med* 62:588, 1977.

2. Loughran TP Jr, Kadin ME, Starkebaum G, et al: Leukemia of large granular lymphocytes: Association with clonal chromosomal abnormalities and auto-immune neutropenia, thrombocytopenia and hemolytic anemia. *Ann Intern Med* 102:169, 1985.

3. Reynolds CW, Foon KA: Tγ Lymphoproliferative disease and related disorders in humans and experimental animals. A review of the clinical, cellular, and functional characteristics. *Blood* 64:1146, 1984.

4. Semenzato G, Pandolfi F, Chisesi T, et al: The lymphoproliferative disease of granular lymphocytes. A heterogeneous disorder ranging from indolent to aggressive conditions. *Cancer* 60:2971, 1987.

5. Loughran TP Jr: Clonal diseases of large granular lymphocytes. *Blood* 82:1, 1993.

6. Lamy T, Loughran TP Jr: Clinical features of LGL leukemia. *Semin Hematol* 40:185, 2003.

7. Rambaldi A, Pelicci P-G, Allavena P, et al: T cell receptor β chain gene rearrangements in lymphoproliferative disorders of large granular lymphocytes/natural killer cells. *J Exp Med* 162:2156, 1985.

8. Taniwaki M, Tagawa S, Nishigaki H, et al: Chromosomal abnormalities define clonal proliferation in CD3-large granular lymphocyte leukemia. *Am J Hematol* 33:32, 1990.

9. Loughran TP Jr, Hadlock KG, Perzova R, et al: Epitope mapping of HTLV envelope seroreactivity in LGL leukemia. *Br J Haematol* 101:318, 1998.

10. Perzova RN, Loughran TP Jr, Dube S, et al: Lack of BLV and PTLV DNA sequences in the majority of patients with large granular lymphocyte leukaemia. *Br J Haematol* 109:64, 2000.

11. Kawa-Ha K, Ishihara S, Ninomiya T, et al: CD3-negative lymphoproliferative disease of granular lymphocytes containing Epstein-Barr viral DNA. *J Clin Invest* 84:51, 1989.

12. Kothapalli R, Bailey R, Kusmartseva I, et al: Constitutive expression of cytotoxic proteases and down-regulation of protease inhibitors in LGL leukemia. *Int J Oncol* 22:33, 2003.

13. Lamy T, Liu JH, Landowski TH, et al: Dysregulation of CD95/CD95 ligand-apoptotic pathway in CD95+ LGL leukemia. *Blood* 92:4771, 1998.

14. Epling-Burnette PK, Loughran TP Jr: Survival signals in leukemic large granular lymphocytes. *Semin Hematol* 40:213, 2003.

15. Liu JH, Wei S, Lamy T, et al: Blockade of Fas-dependent apoptosis by soluble Fas in LGL leukemia. *Blood* 100:1449, 2002.

16. Epling-Burnette PK, Liu JH, Catlett-Falcone R, et al: Inhibition of STAT3 signaling leads to apoptosis of leukemic large granular lymphocytes and decreased Mcl-1 expression. *J Clin Investig* 107:3, 351, 2001.

17. Liu JH, Wei S, Lamy T, et al: Chronic neutropenia mediated by Fas ligand. *Blood* 95:3119, 2000.

18. Loughran TP Jr, Starkebaum G, Kidd P, Neiman P: Clonal proliferation of large granular lymphocytes in rheumatoid arthritis. *Arthritis Rheum* 31:31, 1988.

19. Cheung MM, Chan JK, Wong KF: Natural killer cell neoplasms: A distinctive group of highly aggressive lymphomas/leukemias. *Semin Hematol* 40:221, 2003.

20. Lacy MQ, Kurtin PJ, Tefferi A, et al: Pure red cell aplasia: Association with large granular lymphocyte leukemia and the prognostic value of cytogenetic abnormalities. *Blood* 87:3000, 1996.

21. Lima M, Almeida J, dos Anjos Teixeira M, et al: TCR$\alpha\beta^+$/CD4$^+$ large granular lymphocytosis, a new clonal T-cell lymphoprliferative disorder. *Am J Pathol* 163:763, 2003.

22. Foroni L, Matutes E, Foldi J, et al: T-cell leukemias with rearrangement of the γ but not β T-cell receptor genes. *Blood* 71:356, 1988.

23. Agnarsson BA, Loughran TP Jr, Starkebaum G, Kadin ME: The pathology of large granular lymphocyte leukemia. *Hum Pathol* 20:643, 1989.

24. Loughran TP Jr, Hammond WP: Adult onset cyclic neutropenia is a "benign" neoplasm associated with clonal proliferation of large granular lymphocytes. *J Exp Med* 164:2089, 1986.

25. Zambello R, Trentin L, Agostini C, et al: Persistent polyclonal lymphocytosis in HIV-1 infected patients. *Blood* 81:3015, 1993.

26. Tefferi A, Li CY, Witzig TE, et al: Chronic natural killer cell lymphocytosis: A descriptive clinical study. *Blood* 84:2721, 1994.

27. Nash R, McSweeney P, Zambello R, et al: Clonal studies of CD3-negative lymphoproliferative disease of granular lymphocytes. *Blood* 81:2363, 1993.

28. Zambello R, Falco M, Della Chiesa M, et al: Expression and function of KIR and natural cytotoxicity receptors in NK-type lymphoproliferative diseases of granular lymphocytes. *Blood* 102:1797, 2003.

29. Epling-Burnette PK, Painter JS, Chaurasia P, et al: Dysregulated NK receptor expression in patients with lymphoproliferative disease of granular lymphocytes. *Blood* 103:3431, 2004.

30. Loughran TP Jr, Hadlock KG, Yang Q, et al: Seroreactivity to an envelope protein of human T-cell leukemia/lymphoma virus in patients with CD3-(NK) lymphoproliferative disease of granular lymphocytes. *Blood* 90:1977, 1997.

31. Loughran TP Jr, Kidd PG, Starkebaum G: Treatment of large granular lymphocyte leukemia with oral low dose methotrexate. *Blood* 84:2164, 1994.

32. Sood R, Stewart CC, Aplan PD, et al: Neutropenia associated with T-cell large granular lymphocyte leukemia: Long-term response to cyclosporine therapy despite persistence of abnormal cells. *Blood* 91:3372, 1998.

33. Dhodapkar MU, Li CY, Lust JA, et al: Clinical spectrum of clonal proliferations of T-large granular lymphocytes: A T-cell clonopathy of undetermined significance? *Blood* 84:1620, 1994.

34. Battiwalla M, Melenhorst J, Saunthararajah Y, et al: HLA-DR4 predicts haematological response to cyclosporine in T-cell large granular lymphocyte lymphoproliferative disorders. *Br J Haematol* 123:449, 2003.

35. Sternberg A, Eagleton H, Pillai N, et al: Neutropenia and anaemia associated with T-cell large granular lymphocyte leukaemia responds to fludarabine with minimal toxicity. *Br J Haematol* 120:699, 2003.

36. Thomssen C, Nissen C, Gratwohl A, et al: Agranulocytosis associated with T-gamma-lymphocytosis: No improvement of peripheral blood granulocyte count with human-recombinant granulocyte-macrophage colony-stimulating factor (GM-CSF). *Br J Haematol* 71:157, 1989.

37. Kaneko T, Ogawa Y, Hirata Y, et al: Agranulocytosis associated with granular lymphocyte leukaemia: Improvement of peripheral blood granulocyte count with human recombinant granulocyte colony-stimulating factor (G-CSF). *Br J Haematol* 74:121, 1990.

PATHOLOGY OF LYMPHOMAS

RANDY D. GASCOYNE

BRIAN F. SKINNIDER

The World Health Organization (WHO) classification of lymphoid neoplasms has gained worldwide acceptance by pathologists and oncologists. The classification identifies three major categories of lymphoid malignancies: B cell neoplasms, T and natural killer (NK) cell neoplasms, and Hodgkin lymphoma. Two major categories are identified within the B cell and T/NK cell neoplasms: precursor neoplasms and peripheral or mature neoplasms. Unlike previous lymphoma classifications, the WHO classification does not group different lymphomas by clinical outcome or histologic grade. It recognizes that each disease has distinctive clinical features and responses to treatment that may correlate with histologic grade or gene expression patterns. The WHO classification recognizes that several of the diseases it describes are heterogenous and likely include two or more distinct diseases that cannot be identified based on current data. The classification remains open to incorporate new data as they become available. One source of new data for classifying lymphoma is the study of gene expression profiling by cDNA microarray technology, which is providing new insights into the classification of diseases such as diffuse large B cell lymphoma and chronic lymphocytic leukemia. Proteomics approaches will add texture to the molecular taxonomy of lymphoma classification.

HISTORICAL ASPECTS OF LYMPHOMA CLASSIFICATION

The classification of malignant lymphoma has been fraught with controversy during much of the 20th century, with much needed consensus reached during the past decade. A detailed discussion of the history of lymphoma classification is beyond the scope of this chapter and can be found elsewhere.[1]

From Thomas Hodgkin's description in 1832 of what became known as Hodgkin disease[2] to the first half of the 20th century, several types of lymphomas with distinctive morphologic and clinical features were described using a variety of terms, including lymphoma, lymphosarcoma, reticulum cell sarcoma, and giant follicular lymphoma.[1] However, many of the terms were not used uniformly, resulting in significant misunderstanding, particularly between pathologists and clinicians. Starting in the 1930s, several attempts were made to classify lymphomas and provide some uniformity of diagnosis. Classifications

included the American Registry of Pathology classification based on morphologic and clinical features in 1934[3] and the Gall and Mallory classification in 1942[4] based primarily on morphologic features. These classifications culminated in the Rappaport classification, initially published in 1956, which divided lymphomas based on growth pattern, cell type, and stage of differentiation.[5,6] Most importantly, this classification demonstrated clinical relevance, showing that lymphomas with a nodular pattern had a better prognosis than diffuse lymphomas.

In the 1960s and 1970s, an explosion of studies on the immune system had a profound effect on our understanding of lymphocyte biology and had a consequent effect on our understanding of malignant lymphomas, which represent tumors of the lymphoid system. Normal lymphocytes now could be classified into distinct lineages (B, T, and natural killer [NK]), which could be determined by expression of lineage-specific surface antigens and eventually by genetic analysis of B and T cell receptors.[7,8] Several new lymphoma classification schemes were developed to incorporate the new immunologic data, the most important being the Kiel classification[9] (used primarily in Europe) and the Lukes and Collins classification[10] (used primarily in North America). By the 1970s, at least five classification schemes were widely used in different parts of the world. At the same time, clinical studies were beginning to show that some patients with aggressive lymphomas could be cured with combination chemotherapy.[11] Oncologists needed to interpret results of clinical trials performed in different institutions, a situation made difficult by the use of different classification schemes that were not easily translated among themselves.

The problem was addressed by the United States National Cancer Institute, which convened a large group of investigators to determine which classification scheme was best at predicting clinical outcome of lymphoma. None of the classification schemes was identified as predicting clinical outcome better than the other schemes. Therefore, pathologists were advised to continue using one of the six classification schemes studied, and a "Working Formulation" was developed so that oncologists could translate clinical data derived in different institutions using different classification schemes.[12] Lymphomas were divided into 10 categories based solely on morphologic features. To help clinicians deal with a large number of lymphoma subtypes, the lymphomas were further grouped into three clinical prognostic groups (clinical grades). Although the Working Formulation was not intended to be a stand-alone classification scheme, it was used as such by many institutions, particularly in North America.

However, increasing phenotypic and genotypic data were further defining several distinctive lymphoma subtypes. The Working Formulation lumped different lymphomas into broad categories that were obscuring the distinctive features of the newly described entities. The Working Formulation categories were based solely on morphologic features and were not able to incorporate new immunologic and molecular genetic data that were recognizing new types of lymphomas, including mantle cell lymphomas, marginal zone lymphomas, and peripheral T cell lymphomas.

In the 1980s and 1990s, several new lymphoma entities based on new immunologic and molecular genetic data were identified. Although attempts were made to incorporate these new entities into the existing classification schemes,[13] problems with uniformity between different institutions persisted. A desire to eliminate the continued confusion ultimately led to a new approach to lymphoma classification proposed by the International Lymphoma Study Group that used all available information, including morphology, immunophenotype, genetic and clinical features, to define a list of distinctive entities that could be uniformly diagnosed by hematopathologists. The proposal was published in 1994 and was known as the Revised European–American Lymphoma (REAL) classification.[14] The REAL classification identified "real" diseases that hematopathologists were recognizing in their daily practice. The authors also attempted to correlate lymphoma classification to normal lymphocyte biology by postulating a cell of origin for each lymphoma. Importantly, this classification identified entities that had distinctive clinical features and could be reproducibly diagnosed by expert hematopathologists.[15]

WORLD HEALTH ORGANIZATION CLASSIFICATION

In the late 1990s, a new World Health Organization (WHO) classification for lymphoproliferative disorders was being developed, based on the REAL classification. Published in 2001, the WHO classification represented a consensus between an international group of more than 50 experienced hematopathologists, including contributions from a clinical advisory committee of hematologists and oncologists experienced in treating lymphomas.[16] The WHO classification (Table 95-1) identified three major categories: B cell neoplasms, T and NK cell neoplasms, and Hodgkin lymphoma. The first two categories were further divided into precursor neoplasms and peripheral or mature neoplasms.

Similar to the REAL classification, distinctive lymphoma entities were identified based upon a combination of morphologic, immunophenotypic, genetic, and clinical features. Several entities were acknowledged as remaining heterogeneous (such as diffuse large B cell lymphoma and peripheral T cell lymphoma, unspecified), and the classification retains flexibility so that new data that further identify distinct diseases within these entities can be incorporated. In distinction from the Working Formulation, lymphomas were not classified based on clinical outcome. The WHO classification agreed that each type of lymphoma that was identified by pathologic and clinical features could have a spectrum of clinical aggressiveness, and that lumping distinct entities into groups based on clinical outcome would inhibit the development of targeted therapeutic approaches. Therefore, the WHO classification represents a complete change from the Working Formulation, with the emphasis on pathologic classification rather than classification based on survival characteristics.

Genome-wide expression studies have been instrumental in further delineating distinctive subtypes of lymphomas of clinical relevance. Using cDNA microarray technology, the expression of thousands of genes at the mRNA level can be studied simultaneously and compared to other tumor samples.[17] The technique is quickly proving to be a very promising approach to further classifying lymphomas. Such studies have (1) defined more than one distinct entity in what was previously characterized as a morphologically homogeneous entity, (2) identified distinct gene expression patterns that each encompasses a disease that may demonstrate morphologic heterogeneity, and (3) identified new surface molecules and signaling pathways that could provide targets for new therapeutic approaches. The impact of the new gene expression profiles is detailed in the sections on separate lymphomas below.

As in the REAL classification, the WHO classification attempts to correlate each lymphoma to normal lymphocyte biology by postulating a cell of origin for each neoplasm. This correlation is particularly well suited for B cell lymphomas in which several distinct stages of normal B cell development can be identified (Fig. 95-1A) but is not as satisfying for T and NK neoplasms. Briefly, B cell development begins in the marrow with precursor B lymphoblasts that differentiate into naive B cells that circulate in the blood. The lymph node is the primary site where B cells encounter antigen, where naive B cells colonize primary follicles and in mantle zones of secondary follicles (see Color Plates XXII-1–5). Upon antigen stimulation, these cells undergo blast transformation and enter the germinal center reaction in the late primary immune response and the secondary immune response. In the germinal center, cells down-regulate *bcl*-2 and initially transform into intermediate-sized cells (follicular B blasts), then into large centro-

TABLE 95-1   WHO CLASSIFICATION OF LYMPHOID NEOPLASMS

B Cell Neoplasms
Precursor B cell neoplasm
    Precursor B lymphoblastic leukemia/lymphoma
Mature B cell neoplasms
    Predominantly disseminated/leukemic neoplasms
        Chronic lymphocytic leukemia/small lymphocytic lymphoma
        B cell prolymphocytic leukemia
        Lymphoplasmacytic lymphoma/Waldenström macroglobulinemia
        Splenic marginal zone lymphoma
        Hairy cell leukemia
        Plasma cell neoplasms
            Plasma cell myeloma
            Plasmacytoma
            Monoclonal immunoglobulin deposition disease
            Heavy chain diseases
    Primary extranodal neoplasm
        Extranodal marginal zone B cell lymphoma (MALT lymphoma)
        Mediastinal (thymic) large B cell lymphoma
        Intravascular large B cell lymphoma
        Primary effusion lymphoma
        Lymphomatoid granulomatosis
    Predominantly nodal neoplasms
        Nodal marginal zone B cell lymphoma
        Follicular lymphoma
        Mantle cell lymphoma
        Diffuse large B cell lymphoma
        Burkitt lymphoma/leukemia

T Cell Neoplasms
Precursor T cell neoplasm
    Precursor T lymphoblastic leukemia/lymphoma
Mature T cell neoplasms
    Predominantly disseminated/leukemic neoplasms
        T cell prolymphocytic leukemia
        T cell large granular lymphocytic leukemia
        Aggressive NK cell leukemia
        Adult T cell leukemia/lymphoma
    Primary extranodal neoplasms
        Extranodal NK/T cell lymphoma, nasal type
        Enteropathy-type T cell lymphoma
        Hepatosplenic T cell lymphoma
        Subcutaneous panniculitis-like T cell lymphoma
        Blastic NK cell lymphoma
        Mycosis fungoides/Sézary syndrome
        Primary cutaneous CD-30 positive T cell lymphoproliferative disorders
    Predominantly nodal neoplasms
        Angioimmunoblastic T cell lymphoma
        Peripheral T cell lymphoma, unspecified
        Anaplastic large cell lymphoma
Hodgkin Lymphoma
Nodular lymphocyte predominant Hodgkin lymphoma
Classic Hodgkin lymphoma
    Nodular sclerosis Hodgkin lymphoma
    Mixed cellularity Hodgkin lymphoma
    Lymphocyte-rich classic Hodgkin lymphoma
    Lymphocyte-depleted Hodgkin lymphoma

blasts, and finally into small centrocytes (see Color Plates XXII-6 and 7).[18] Cells that survive the germinal center up-regulate *bcl*-2 and either differentiate into short-lived plasma cells through an immunoblast stage or differentiate into memory cells that populate follicular marginal zones or recirculate in the blood. Several B cell lymphomas can be correlated with these stages of development (Fig. 95-1*B*) and are mentioned in the sections on separate lymphomas below.

PRACTICAL CONSIDERATIONS IN THE DIAGNOSIS OF LYMPHOMA

Determining a benign from malignant lymphoid infiltrate often can be difficult because malignant lymphocytes in many lymphomas closely resemble their benign counterparts. Therefore, diagnosis commonly rests on demonstrating a combination of an abnormal architectural pattern, an abnormal immunophenotype, and evidence of lymphoid monoclonality. As a result, several ancillary special studies have become instrumental in the diagnosis and classification of lymphoma, requiring special handling of the biopsy material (Table 95-2). Whenever a diagnosis of lymphoma is considered clinically, the surgeon should perform an open biopsy of the largest involved lymph node. The lymph node should be removed intact whenever possible, because assessment of architecture is extremely important in the diagnosis and classification of lymphomas. The lymph node should be sent immediately to the pathology laboratory in the fresh state, at which time the pathologist allocates the tissue for fixation for routine histology and for special studies.

Automated flow cytometry on single-cell suspensions prepared from tissue samples is extremely helpful in demonstrating B cell clonality by surface light-chain restriction. It also determines the expression pattern of surface markers helpful in subclassifying lymphomas, particularly lymphomas of small B cells.[19] Frozen-section immunohistochemistry also can be used to demonstrate surface light-chain restriction. A wide variety of antibodies that can be used on formalin-fixed tissue now are available, allowing accurate diagnosis and subclassification of lymphoma in most cases.[20]

Molecular genetic techniques to determine B or T cell monoclonality or lymphoma-specific chromosomal translocations include polymerase chain reaction (PCR), Southern blot, fluorescence *in situ* hybridization (FISH), and cytogenetic analysis.[21] Although PCR and FISH now can be performed on formalin-fixed tissue, interpretable results might not be obtained because of DNA degradation caused by fixation. These tests are optimally performed on fresh tissue. Results from molecular genetic testing should be interpreted in conjunction with the morphologic and immunophenotypic data, as some benign reactive lymphoid proliferations show evidence of lymphoid monoclonality.[22]

The diagnosis of lymphoma has become more complex than the diagnosis of other malignancies because diagnosis of lymphoma rests on correlation of morphologic features with immunophenotype and genetic data in many cases. Because of the complexity of diagnosis and the relative infrequency of lymphoma in general pathology practice, a second review by a hematopathologist with expertise in lymphoma pathology is recommended. The second review can have a significant impact on the clinical management of patients.[23]

Whereas open biopsy of an involved lymph node is the most useful diagnostic procedure, core needle biopsies and fine needle aspiration can play a role in limited situations. Core needle biopsy might be helpful in the diagnosis of deep-seated disease in the abdomen or retroperitoneum, and the patient may avoid a laparotomy. However, a

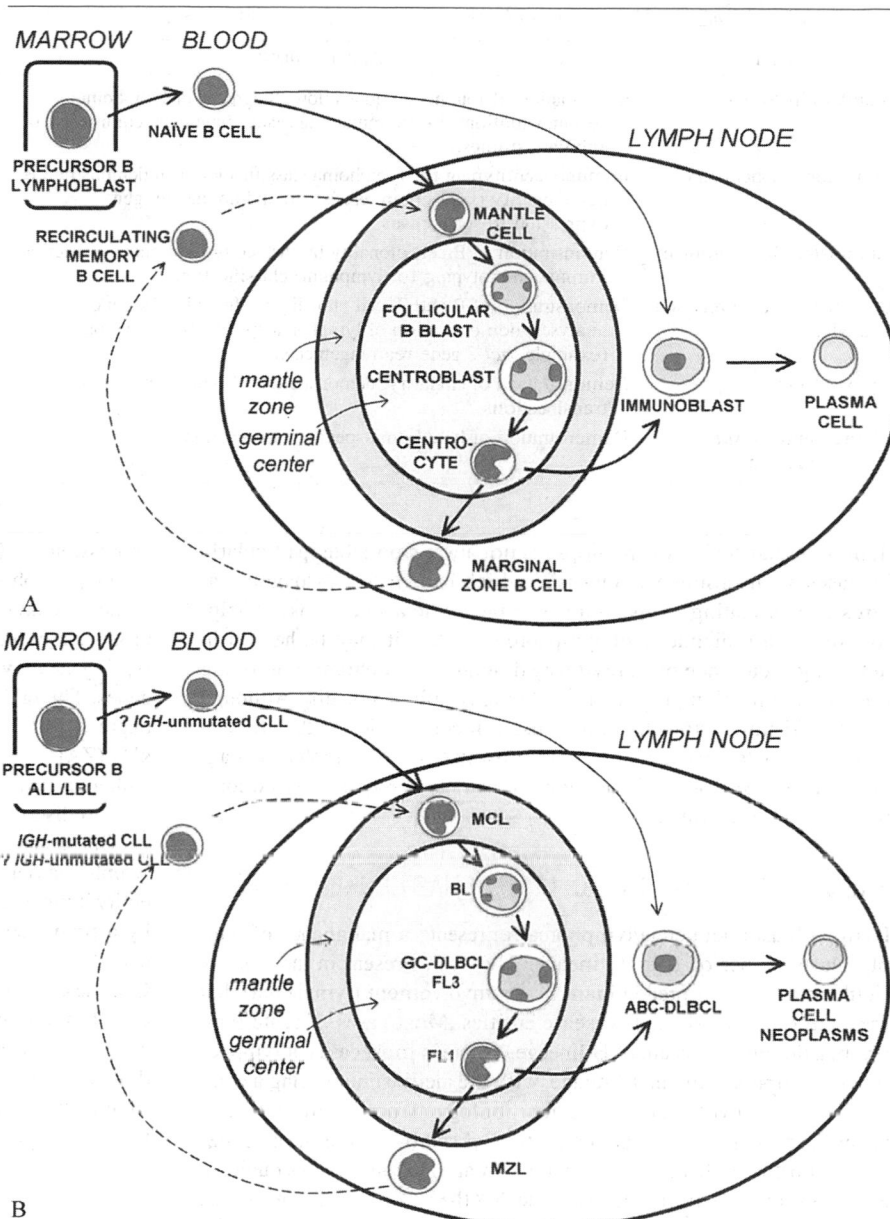

FIGURE 95-1 Stages of B cell development *(A)* correlated with postulated cell of origin of B cell neoplasms *(B)*. *(A)* Precursor B lymphoblasts in the marrow differentiate into mature B cells that circulate in blood and colonize mantle zones of lymphoid follicles. Upon antigen stimulation, the cells can differentiate directly into immunoblasts (early primary immune response) or enter the germinal center reaction (late primary and secondary immune responses). In the germinal center, cells undergo blast transformation and progress to form large centroblasts, followed by small centrocytes. These cells differentiate into either antibody-secreting plasma cells through an immunoblast stage or memory B cells that can recirculate or localize to the marginal zones of lymphoid follicles. *(B)* B cell neoplasms correlate with different stages of development. ALL/LBL, acute lymphoblastic leukemia/lymphoblastic lymphoma; CLL, chronic lymphocytic leukemia; MCL, mantle cell lymphoma; BL, Burkitt lymphoma; GC-DLBCL, germinal center type diffuse large B cell lymphoma; FL3, follicular lymphoma, grade 3; FL1, follicular lymphoma, grade 1; MZL, marginal zone lymphoma; ABC-DLBCL, activated B cell type diffuse large B cell lymphoma.

TABLE 95-2   STANDARD AND ANCILLARY STUDIES FOR LYMPHOMA DIAGNOSIS

METHOD	APPLICATIONS	TYPE OF TISSUE NEEDED
Standard histology	Examination of routine sections allows diagnosis of lymphoma in certain situations. In the remaining cases, diagnosis requires use of ancillary studies.	Formalin-fixed
Immunohistochemistry	Immunophenotyping for lymphoma classification; can demonstrate B cell clonality (light-chain restriction) and unique antigen expression in some cases	Formalin-fixed
Automated flow cytometry	Demonstration of B cell clonality by surface Ig light-chain restriction; immunophenotyping for lymphoma classification	Fresh tissue (single cell suspensions)
Polymerase chain reaction analysis	Demonstration of B and T cell clonality by Ig and TCR gene analyses; demonstration of lymphoma specific translocations (example, *bcl-2* gene rearrangements)	Frozen tissue; can be performed on paraffin tissue but may not yield amplifiable DNA in some cases
Cytogenetics	Demonstration of clonality; demonstration of lymphoma-specific translocations	Sterile fresh tissue
Fluorescence *in situ* hybridization	Demonstration of lymphoma-specific translocations	Fresh tissue; can be performed on paraffin tissue but yield is variable

definitive diagnosis by core biopsy is not always possible (particularly in cases with prominent sclerosis, which can distort cytologic features), necessitating an open biopsy. Fine needle aspiration is not helpful in primary diagnosis of lymphoma,[24,25] but it may be helpful in detecting recurrence of a previously diagnosed lymphoma or in ruling out a nonhematolymphoid lesion causing lymphadenopathy. Although automated flow cytometry can be used in conjunction with cytologic examination to provide additional information for lymphoma diagnosis and classification, tissue biopsy generally is required before commencement of therapy.

PRECURSOR B AND T CELL LYMPHOMAS/LEUKEMIAS

Lymphoblastic leukemia/lymphoma represents a malignancy of lymphoblasts, either of B or T lineage. They can present in the marrow (leukemia) or with predominant tissue involvement (lymphoma), but they are considered single disease entities. Most cases of acute lymphoblastic leukemias are of B lineage, whereas most cases of lymphoblastic lymphoma are of T lineage, with the mediastinum being a common site of involvement. The morphologic features are the same regardless of site or lineage, consisting of small- to intermediate-size cells with finely dispersed nuclear chromatin, inconspicuous nucleoli, and scant cytoplasm (see Color Plate XXII-8). Assessment of lineage and distinction from minimally differentiated acute myeloid leukemia require immunophenotypic data and may require molecular genetic analysis of B and T cell receptors. Lymphoblastic neoplasms are distinguished from other lymphomas by the expression of terminal deoxynucleotide transferase, which is specifically expressed at the lymphoblast stage of development.

MATURE B CELL NON-HODGKIN LYMPHOMAS

CHRONIC LYMPHOCYTIC LEUKEMIA/SMALL LYMPHOCYTIC LYMPHOMA

Chronic lymphocytic leukemia is a neoplasm of mature B lymphocytes characterized by blood and marrow involvement and commonly associated with lymph node involvement (see Chap. 92). Small lymphocytic lymphoma is the nonleukemic form of the disease (see Chaps. 92 and 96). Lymph nodes involved by chronic lymphocytic leukemia show a diffuse infiltrate of small mature lymphocytes admixed with prolymphocytes and para-immunoblasts, which characteristically form ill-defined nodules known as *proliferation* or *growth centers* (see Color Plates XXII-9 and 10). The B cells have a characteristic immunophenotype, demonstrating CD5 and CD23 expression and dim

expression of CD20 and clonal light chain. Studies have divided chronic lymphocytic leukemia into two distinct subtypes with distinct clinical behavior (see Chap. 92). The type with the more favorable prognosis expresses mutated immunoglobulin variable region genes (IgV genes), whereas the other subtype expresses unmutated IgV genes. The IgV gene mutation status is reflected in differences in gene expression.[26,27] The gene encoding the zeta-associated protein of 70 kDa (ZAP-70) is one of these genes, which generally is expressed by leukemia cells that express unmutated IgV genes and hence can be used to discriminate between the two subtypes.[28]

Some cases of chronic lymphocytic leukemia/small lymphocytic lymphoma demonstrate plasmacytic features but are distinct from an entity known as *lymphoplasmacytic lymphoma*, which is characterized by a prominent component of plasmacytic lymphocytes and plasma cells (see Color Plate XXII-11). These cases typically do not express CD5, less often involve blood, and often are associated with a monoclonal immunoglobulin (Ig)M serum protein that can cause hyperviscosity or cryoglobulinemia (Waldenström macroglobulinemia). Although lymphoplasmacytic lymphoma has been suggested to be frequently associated with the cytogenetic alteration t(9;14)(p13;q32), the true frequency of this association remains controversial.

MANTLE CELL LYMPHOMA

Mantle cell lymphoma most commonly involves lymph nodes, but it can involve extranodal sites, including the gastrointestinal tract, as a clinical variant known as *lymphomatous polyposis* (see Color Plate XXII-12). It typically is composed of a uniform population of small lymphocytes with cleaved nuclei and a virtual absence of large transformed cells (see Color Plate XXII-13).[29,30] It most commonly has a diffuse growth pattern, but it can show a nodular or, more rarely, a mantle zone pattern (see Color Plate XXII-14). The postulated cell of origin is the B cell of the inner mantle zone. The lymphoma cells coexpress CD5, as does chronic lymphocytic leukemia, but mantle cell lymphoma can be distinguished by lack of CD23 expression and expression of cyclin D1 (see Color Plate XXII-15). Cyclin D1 expression results from the chromosomal translocation t(11;14)(q13;q32) characteristic of mantle cell lymphoma. Although many pathologists would not diagnose mantle cell lymphoma without evidence of t(11;14) or cyclin D1 expression, gene expression data have demonstrated a subset of mantle cell lymphomas that are cyclin D1−negative.[31] Overall, patients with mantle cell lymphoma have a median survival of approximately 3 years, but gene expression data that determined tumor cell proliferation were able to identify patient subsets that differed in median survival by more than 5 years[31] (see Chap. 96).

FOLLICULAR LYMPHOMA

Follicular lymphoma is a proliferation of cells that correspond to normal germinal center cells[32] retaining expression of germinal center markers (bcl-6, CD10) and demonstrates a follicular architecture (see Color Plate XXII-16) imparted by nodular aggregates of CD21-positive follicular dendritic cells. Follicular lymphomas are composed of a variable mixture of centrocytes (small cleaved cells) and centroblasts (large noncleaved cells). They can be divided into three grades (grades 1–3) based on the number of centroblasts present. The most common is grade 1 (<5 centroblasts per high-power microscopic field), previously known as *follicular small cleaved cell lymphoma* (see Color Plate XXII-17). Grade 3 follicular lymphoma (>15 centroblasts per high-power microscopic field) can be further divided into grade 3A (mixture of centroblasts and centrocytes) (see Color Plate XXII-18) and grade 3B (solid sheets of centroblasts). Data have shown some molecular genetic differences between 3A and 3B cases, but further study is required because no significant clinical impact has been demonstrated.[33–35] Follicular lymphoma can have an accompanying diffuse component, and identification of a diffuse area of large cells (diffuse large B cell lymphoma) indicates transformation to a more aggressive disease. Approximately 90 percent of follicular lymphoma demonstrate the t(14;18)(q32;q21) involving rearrangement of the bcl-2 gene, leading to the constitutive expression of the antiapoptotic Bcl-2 protein. Although Bcl-2 protein expression does not help distinguish follicular lymphoma from other lymphomas, it is a helpful feature in distinguishing it from reactive follicles that are Bcl-2–negative (see Color Plate XXII-19).

MARGINAL ZONE B CELL LYMPHOMAS

Marginal zone lymphomas are characterized by a proliferation of small lymphocytes, commonly with abundant pale cytoplasm (called *monocytoid B cells)* and plasmacytic features. The postulated cell of origin of these lymphomas is the postgerminal center B cell of the marginal zone at various anatomic sites. Marginal zone lymphomas can be divided into three distinct types based on site of presentation: (1) extranodal marginal zone lymphomas of mucosa-associated lymphoid tissue (MALT), (2) splenic marginal zone lymphomas,[36] and (3) nodal marginal zone lymphomas (see Color Plate XXII-20).[37] This classification is supported by distinctive cytogenetic abnormalities in each entity. Extranodal lymphomas of the MALT type are the most common and arise in mucosal sites subject to long-standing chronic inflammation (see Color Plate XXII-21), including chronic infection, the prototypical example being chronic *Helicobacter pylori* infection of the stomach.[38] At early stages of development, many of these lymphomas respond to treatment with antibiotics to eradicate *H. pylori*, whereas later changes, including cases with chromosomal translocations activating genes involved in nuclear factor-κB (NF-κB) signaling,[39] lead to antigen-independent growth (see Chap. 96).

DIFFUSE LARGE B CELL LYMPHOMA

Diffuse large B cell lymphoma is characterized by a diffuse infiltrate of large atypical B cells that can resemble centroblasts or immunoblasts (see Color Plates XXII-22 and 23). In several earlier classification schemes, diffuse large B cell lymphomas were divided into centroblastic and immunoblastic, but this categorization was not advocated by the REAL or WHO classifications because of poor intraobserver and interobserver reproducibility.

Gene expression data have shown that diffuse large B cell lymphoma is a heterogeneous entity consisting of at least three entities having distinct gene expression profiles: (1) cases with an expression profile similar to germinal center B cells (GCB), (2) cases expressing genes typical of activated B cells (ABC), and (3) cases with a different pattern referred to as "unclassifiable" that are neither GCB-type nor ABC-type (see Color Plate XXII-39).[40–42] Importantly, clinical differences were apparent, with GCB-type cases having a significantly better prognosis compared to the other two types, even when clinical prognostic markers are considered (see Chap. 96). Gene expression profiling has identified potential therapeutic targets, indicating the ABC-type shows a pattern of NF-κB activation that plays a role in the proliferation and survival of the cells.[43] This finding may provide novel therapeutic targets for these lymphomas. Although global gene expression profiling performed in a routine manner currently is not possible, division of diffuse large B cell lymphoma into clinically distinct groups may be determined by the expression profile of a limited number of genes using routine immunohistochemistry,[44] thus allowing the method to be performed in routine histopathology laboratories.

Mediastinal large B cell lymphoma is a distinct subtype of diffuse large B cell lymphoma that has been separately identified in the WHO classification.[45] Patients with mediastinal lymphomas typically are younger than those with conventional diffuse large B cell lymphomas, with presentation in the mediastinum. The histology shows large cells with abundant cytoplasm associated with diffuse fibrosis (see Color Plate XXII-24). Gene expression studies have demonstrated an expression profile, distinct from conventional diffuse large B cell lymphoma, that shares some features with classic Hodgkin lymphoma (see Color Plate XXII-40).[46,47]

BURKITT LYMPHOMA

Burkitt lymphoma is a highly aggressive lymphoma characterized histologically by a diffuse infiltrate of intermediate-size cells with a high mitotic rate. The lymphomas commonly have a significant spontaneous cell death (apoptosis), which results in a "starry sky" appearance caused by numerous macrophages that have engulfed the apoptotic debris (known as *tingible body macrophages*) (see Color Plates XXII-25 and 26). The postulated cell of origin is the early follicular B blast cell of the germinal center. Virtually all cases of Burkitt lymphoma are characterized by chromosomal translocations involving the *myc* gene on chromosome 8. The *myc* gene most commonly is translocated to the *IG* heavy-chain gene on chromosome 14, resulting in t(8;14)(q24;q32), but it also can involve the light-chain genes on chromosomes 2p12 (κ) and 22q11 (λ). A diagnosis of Burkitt lymphoma can be suggested based on morphologic examination alone but should be supported by immunophenotypic data (positive for CD20, CD10, and bcl-6; negative for bcl-2; growth fraction near 100% as determined by Ki-67 stain) and confirmed by molecular testing for *myc* translocations whenever possible.

In the WHO classification, the terms "Burkitt-like lymphoma" and "atypical Burkitt lymphoma" are used interchangeably for cases with cytologic features not typical of Burkitt lymphoma but with proven or strong presumptive evidence of a *myc* translocation. However, some pathologists use the term "Burkitt-like lymphoma" as described in the REAL classification to describe lymphomas with cytologic features lying between diffuse large B cell lymphoma and Burkitt lymphoma, with a very high growth fraction, but no evidence of a *myc* translocation (corresponding to small noncleaved non-Burkitt lymphomas in the Working Formulation).[48,49]

MATURE T CELL AND NK CELL NON-HODGKIN LYMPHOMAS

T cells and NK cells share several immunophenotypic and functional features; therefore, these neoplasms are grouped together in the WHO classification. These lymphomas make up 10 to 15 percent of non-Hodgkin lymphomas in Western countries, with a higher incidence in

Asia. The two most common types of mature T cell lymphoma in adults are (1) peripheral T cell lymphoma (PTCL), unspecified, and (2) angioimmunoblastic T cell lymphoma. Anaplastic large cell lymphoma (ALCL) represents a unique subtype of T cell lymphoma particularly common in children.

PTCLs typically grow in a diffuse pattern that effaces normal nodal architecture or, more rarely, show expansion of the interfollicular areas. They show a diverse cytologic spectrum, with most cases showing a mixture of large- to intermediate-size cells and occasional cases showing predominantly small cells (see Color Plates XXII-27 and 28). Cell type has no prognostic relevance. A reactive background consisting of eosinophils, plasma cells, and macrophages may be present, in which case the diagnosis of Hodgkin lymphoma may be entertained. Immunophenotypic data cannot prove clonality as in B cell lymphomas, but evidence of an aberrant T cell phenotype supports a diagnosis of T cell lymphoma. Molecular techniques to demonstrate clonal rearrangement of T cell receptor genes can be helpful in confirming the diagnosis. No specific chromosomal abnormalities have been identified. As currently defined, PTCL is a heterogeneous entity that can be further classified in the future based on gene expression patterns. Angioimmunoblastic T cell lymphoma is uncommon and typically presents with systemic symptoms and polyclonal hypergammaglobulinemia.

ALCL can show significant morphologic variability but typically is composed of large pleomorphic cells characterized by the presence of "hallmark" cells with horseshoe- or kidney-shaped nuclei and a perinuclear eosinophilic region (see Color Plate XXII-29).[50] Early involvement of lymph nodes can be limited to the sinuses, with obliteration of nodal architecture in later stages. ALCL is characterized by uniform, strong expression of CD30 (see Color Plate XXII-30). The majority of cases express one or more T cell antigens and demonstrate clonal T cell receptor gene rearrangement.[50] A minority of cases show no evidence of T cell lineage. Such cases are classified as "null cell" type. Anaplastic lymphoma kinase (ALK) is expressed in a variable proportion of cases (see Color Plate XXII-31), predominantly in children and adolescents, and results from chromosomal translocations involving the *alk* gene on chromosome 2p23, the most common translocation being the t(2;5)(p23;q35) involving the nucleophosmin gene on chromosome 5.[51] ALK expression has been associated with a favorable prognosis compared to ALK-negative ALCL cases.[52] ALK-positive ALCL is a good example of a disease in which a molecular marker (ALK expression) defines a single pathologic entity with distinctive clinical features that could not be identified by morphology or other immunophenotypic features.[53] ALK-negative cases of ALCL are more closely related to PTCL, unspecified.

Other types of mature T/NK cell lymphomas are uncommon and include enteropathy-type T cell lymphoma (an aggressive T cell lymphoma typically arising in the small bowel from a background of celiac disease) and extranodal NK/T cell lymphoma, nasal type (an aggressive Epstein-Barr virus [EBV]-associated neoplasm commonly involving the nasal cavity). A detailed description of these specific lymphoma subtypes is beyond the scope of this chapter and can be found in the WHO classification.[16]

HODGKIN LYMPHOMA

Hodgkin lymphoma consists of two distinct clinicopathologic entities: *classic Hodgkin lymphoma* (including four subtypes) and *nodular lymphocyte predominant Hodgkin lymphoma* (see Chap. 97).

CLASSIC HODGKIN LYMPHOMA

The neoplastic cell of classic Hodgkin lymphoma is the Reed-Sternberg cell, first described more than 100 years ago.[54,55] It is a large cell with two or more nuclei or nuclear lobes, each of which contains a large eosinophilic nucleolus (see Color Plate XXII-32). The presence of Reed-Sternberg cells alone is insufficient for a diagnosis of Hodgkin lymphoma, because cells with similar morphology can be seen in a variety of non-Hodgkin lymphomas and benign reactive conditions.[56] For a diagnosis of Hodgkin lymphoma, diagnostic Reed-Sternberg cells must be found in an appropriate background consisting of a variable polymorphous reactive infiltrate of inflammatory and accessory cells.[57]

Reed-Sternberg cells are derived from B cells in the vast majority of cases of classic Hodgkin lymphoma, as determined by clonal rearrangement of *IG* heavy-chain genes.[58] However, Reed-Sternberg cells have lost most of their B lineage antigens, including expression of *IG*. Reed-Sternberg cells express CD30 in almost all cases of classic Hodgkin lymphoma and express CD15 in the majority (see Color Plates XXII-33 and 34).[57] They typically are negative for CD45 (leukocyte common antigen) and positive for B cell marker CD20 in 20 to 40 percent of cases, usually of variable intensity in a minority of cells. Classic Hodgkin lymphoma is associated with EBV in 20 to 40 percent of cases and is thought to play a role in the pathogenesis of these cases.[59] Reed-Sternberg cells express many cytokines and several members of the tumor necrosis factor receptor family (e.g., CD40, CD30).[60] The cytokines are thought to play a role in the recruitment of reactive infiltrate and to contribute to Reed-Sternberg cell proliferation and survival. The tumor necrosis factor receptor family members can be activated by ligands expressed by the surrounding reactive infiltrate, leading to proliferation and survival.

The most common subtype of classic Hodgkin lymphoma is the nodular sclerosis variant. The variant is characterized by the presence of broad collagen bands dividing the tumor into nodules and by the presence of "lacunar" cells, mononuclear Reed-Sternberg variants that typically show retraction artifact so that the cells appear to be in lacunae (see Color Plate XXII-35). These cells are found within a reactive infiltrate that typically includes prominent eosinophils and lymphocytes. Different grading schemes have been proposed for nodular sclerosis Hodgkin lymphoma, but no prognostic relevance is clear.[61,62]

The second most common subtype is the mixed cellularity variant, which is characterized by Reed-Sternberg cells in a mixed inflammatory background without the broad collagen bands seen in nodular sclerosis (see Color Plate XXII-36). Mixed cellularity cases are more commonly associated with EBV compared to the nodular sclerosis variant.

The lymphocyte-rich and lymphocyte-depleted subtypes of classic Hodgkin lymphoma are the least common, each representing approximately 5 percent of all cases. The lymphocyte-rich variant has a small number of Reed-Sternberg cells in a background of small lymphocytes with absent or rare eosinophils and neutrophils, typically in a nodular pattern. It is easily confused with nodular lymphocyte predominant Hodgkin lymphoma, so immunohistochemical stains to determine the immunophenotype of the Reed-Sternberg cells is required to make the distinction.[63,64] It can rarely have a diffuse growth pattern.

In the past, the lymphocyte-depleted variant had been divided into reticular and diffuse fibrosis types. The diffuse fibrosis variant is characterized by a hypocellular infiltrate with prominent diffuse nonbirefringent sclerosis accompanied by rare Reed-Sternberg cells and a minor reactive inflammatory component. The reticular variant showed an increased number of large atypical cells, commonly with bizarre multinucleated cells, with a minor reactive component. It now is recognized that the vast majority of these cases are cases of ALCL or diffuse large B cell lymphomas, and as such the diagnosis of the reticular variant of lymphocyte-depleted Hodgkin lymphoma is rare and should be made only in the presence of definitive supportive immunophenotypic data.

NODULAR LYMPHOCYTE-PREDOMINANT HODGKIN LYMPHOMA

Nodular lymphocyte-predominant Hodgkin lymphoma has several pathologic and clinical features that are distinct from classic Hodgkin lymphoma.[65] This variant previously was called *lymphocytic and/or histiocytic (L&H) predominance Hodgkin disease* in the Lukes and Butler classification. The malignant population has retained this terminology and is called the *L&H cell*. L&H cells are large cells with a single nucleus that contains multilobated or folded features. They often are referred to as "popcorn" cells because they resemble popped kernels of corn (see Color Plate XXII-37). Nucleoli typically are smaller than the nucleoli seen in classic Reed-Sternberg cells. They differ from Reed-Sternberg cells in classic Hodgkin lymphoma in that they retain expression of CD45 and B-lineage markers (CD20, Ig) and are negative for CD15 and CD30 (see Color Plate XXII-38).[66] As the name implies, the cells have a complete or partial nodular architectural pattern with a background consisting primarily of lymphocytes. Histiocytes are also a common feature, but neutrophils and eosinophils are absent or rare.

REFERENCES

1. Magrath IT: Historical perspective: The evolution of modern concepts of biology and management, in *The Non-Hodgkin's Lymphomas*, 2nd ed, edited by IT Magrath, p 47. Arnold, London, 1997.
2. Hodgkin T: On some morbid appearances of the absorbent glands and spleen. *Trans Med Soc Lond* 17:68, 1832.
3. Callendar GR: Tumors and tumor-like conditions of the lymphocyte, the myelocyte, the erythrocyte, and the reticulum cell. *Am J Pathol* 10:443, 1934.
4. Gall EA, Mallory TB: Malignant lymphoma: A clinicopathologic survey of 618 cases. *Am J Pathol* 18:381, 1942.
5. Rappaport H, Winter W, Hicks E: Follicular lymphoma: A re-evaluation of its position in the scheme of malignant lymphoma, based on a survey of 253 cases. *Cancer* 9:792, 1956.
6. Rappaport H: *Tumors of the Hematopoietic System, Fasc 8*. Armed Forces Institute of Pathology, Washington, 1966.
7. Arnold A, Cossman J, Bakhshi A, et al: Immunoglobulin-gene rearrangements as unique clonal markers in human lymphoid neoplasms. *N Engl J Med* 309:1593, 1983.
8. Aisenberg AC, Krontiris TG, Mak TW, Wilkes BM: Rearrangement of the gene for the beta chain of the T-cell receptor in T-cell chronic lymphocytic leukemia and related disorders. *N Engl J Med* 313:529, 1985.
9. Gerard-Marchant R, Hamlin I, Lennert K, et al: Classification of non-Hodgkin's lymphoma. *Lancet* ii:406, 1974.
10. Lukes RJ, Collins RD: Immunologic characterization of human malignant lymphomas. *Cancer* 34(suppl 4):1488, 1974.
11. Schein PS, Chabner BA, Canellos GP, et al: Potential for prolonged disease-free survival following combination chemotherapy of non-Hodgkin's lymphoma. *Blood* 43:181, 1974.
12. National Cancer Institute sponsored study of classifications of non-Hodgkin's lymphomas: Summary and description of a working formulation for clinical usage. The Non-Hodgkin's Lymphoma Pathologic Classification Project. *Cancer* 49:2112, 1982.
13. Stansfeld AG, Diebold J, Noel H, et al: Updated Kiel classification for lymphomas. *Lancet* 1:292, 1988.
14. Harris NL, Jaffe ES, Stein H, et al: A revised European-American classification of lymphoid neoplasms: A proposal from the International Lymphoma Study Group. *Blood* 84:1361, 1994.
15. A clinical evaluation of the International Lymphoma Study Group classification of non-Hodgkin's lymphoma. By the Non-Hodgkin's Lymphoma Classification Project. *Blood* 89:3909, 1997.
16. Jaffe ES, Harris NL, Stein H, Vardiman JW: *Pathology and Genetics of Tumours of Haematopoietic and Lymphoid Tissues*. IARC Press, Lyon, 2001.
17. Liang P, Pardee AB: Analyzing differential gene expression in cancer. *Nat Rev Cancer* 3:869, 2003.
18. MacLennan IC: Germinal centers. *Annu Rev Immunol* 12:117, 1994.
19. Jennings CD, Foon KA: Recent advances in flow cytometry: Application to the diagnosis of hematologic malignancy. *Blood* 90:2863, 1997.
20. Frizzera G, Wu CD, Inghirami G: The usefulness of immunophenotypic and genotypic studies in the diagnosis and classification of hematopoietic and lymphoid neoplasms. An update. *Am J Clin Pathol* 111(suppl 1):S13, 1999.
21. Mauvieux L, Macintyre EA: Practical role of molecular diagnostics in non-Hodgkin's lymphomas. *Baillieres Clin Haematol* 9:653, 1996.
22. Collins RD: Is clonality equivalent to malignancy: Specifically, is immunoglobulin gene rearrangement diagnostic of malignant lymphoma? *Hum Pathol* 28:757, 1997.
23. Lester JF, Dojcinov SD, Attanoos RL, et al: The clinical impact of expert pathological review on lymphoma management: A regional experience. *Br J Haematol* 123:463, 2003.
24. Hajdu SI, Melamed MR: Limitations of aspiration cytology in the diagnosis of primary neoplasms. *Acta Cytol* 28:337, 1984.
25. Pontifex AH, Haley L: Fine-needle aspiration cytology in lymphomas and related disorders. *Diagn Cytopathol* 5:432, 1989.
26. Klein U, Tu Y, Stolovitzky GA, et al: Gene expression profiling of B cell chronic lymphocytic leukemia reveals a homogeneous phenotype related to memory B cells. *J Exp Med* 194:1625, 2001.
27. Rosenwald A, Alizadeh AA, Widhopf G, et al: Relation of gene expression phenotype to immunoglobulin mutation genotype in B cell chronic lymphocytic leukemia. *J Exp Med* 194:1639, 2001.
28. Wiestner A, Rosenwald A, Barry TS, et al: ZAP-70 expression identifies a chronic lymphocytic leukemia subtype with unmutated immunoglobulin genes, inferior clinical outcome, and distinct gene expression profile. *Blood* 101:4944, 2003.
29. Weisenburger DD, Armitage JO: Mantle cell lymphoma: An entity comes of age. *Blood* 87:4483, 1996.
30. Argatoff LH, Connors JM, Klasa RJ, et al: Mantle cell lymphoma: A clinicopathologic study of 80 cases. *Blood* 89:2067, 1997.
31. Rosenwald A, Wright G, Wiestner A, et al: The proliferation gene expression signature is a quantitative integrator of oncogenic events that predicts survival in mantle cell lymphoma. *Cancer Cell* 3:185, 2003.
32. Jaffe ES, Shevach EM, Frank MM, et al: Nodular lymphoma: Evidence for origin from follicular B lymphocytes. *N Engl J Med* 290:813, 1974.
33. Bosga-Bouwer AG, van Imhoff GW, Boonstra R, et al: Follicular lymphoma grade 3B includes 3 cytogenetically defined subgroups with primary t(14;18) 3q27, or other translocations: t(14;18) and 3q27 are mutually exclusive. *Blood* 101:1149, 2003.
34. Hans CP, Weisenburger DD, Vose JM, et al: A significant diffuse component predicts for inferior survival in grade 3 follicular lymphoma, but cytologic subtypes do not predict survival. *Blood* 101:2363, 2003.
35. Ott G, Katzenberger T, Lohr A, et al: Cytomorphologic, immunohistochemical, and cytogenetic profiles of follicular lymphoma: 2 types of follicular lymphoma grade 3. *Blood* 99:3806, 2002.
36. Thieblemont C, Felman P, Callet-Bauchu E, et al: Splenic marginal-zone lymphoma: A distinct clinical and pathological entity. *Lancet Oncol* 4:95, 2003.
37. Nathwani BN, Drachenberg MR, Hernandez AM, et al: Nodal monocytoid B-cell lymphoma (nodal marginal-zone B-cell lymphoma). *Semin Hematol* 36:128, 1999.
38. Zucca E, Bertoni F, Roggero E, Cavalli F: The gastric marginal zone B-cell lymphoma of MALT type. *Blood* 96:410, 2000.
39. Bertoni F, Cotter FE, Zucca E: Molecular genetics of extranodal marginal zone (MALT-type) B-cell lymphoma. *Leuk Lymphoma* 35:57, 1999.

40. Alizadeh AA, Eisen MB, Davis RE, et al: Distinct types of diffuse large B-cell lymphoma identified by gene expression profiling. *Nature* 403:503, 2000.

41. Rosenwald A, Wright G, Chan WC, et al: The use of molecular profiling to predict survival after chemotherapy for diffuse large-B-cell lymphoma. *N Engl J Med* 346:1937, 2002.

42. Wright G, Tan B, Rosenwald A, et al: A gene expression-based method to diagnose clinically distinct subgroups of diffuse large B cell lymphoma. *Proc Natl Acad Sci U S A* 100:9991, 2003.

43. Davis RE, Brown KD, Siebenlist U, Staudt LM: Constitutive nuclear factor kappaB activity is required for survival of activated B cell-like diffuse large B cell lymphoma cells. *J Exp Med* 194:1861, 2001.

44. Hans CP, Weisenburger DD, Greiner TC, et al: Confirmation of the molecular classification of diffuse large B-cell lymphoma by immunohistochemistry using a tissue microarray. *Blood* 103:275, 2004.

45. van Besien K, Kelta M, Bahaguna P: Primary mediastinal B-cell lymphoma: A review of pathology and management. *J Clin Oncol* 19:1855, 2001.

46. Rosenwald A, Wright G, Leroy K, et al: Molecular diagnosis of primary mediastinal B cell lymphoma identifies a clinically favorable subgroup of diffuse large B cell lymphoma related to Hodgkin lymphoma. *J Exp Med* 198:851, 2003.

47. Savage KJ, Monti S, Kutok JL, et al: The molecular signature of mediastinal large B-cell lymphoma differs from that of other diffuse large B-cell lymphomas and shares features with classical Hodgkin lymphoma. *Blood* 102:3871, 2003.

48. Yano T, van Krieken JH, Magrath IT, et al: Histogenetic correlations between subcategories of small noncleaved cell lymphomas. *Blood* 79:1282, 1992.

49. Macpherson N, Lesack D, Klasa R, et al: Small noncleaved, non-Burkitt's (Burkitt-like) lymphoma: Cytogenetics predict outcome and reflect clinical presentation. *J Clin Oncol* 17:1558, 1999.

50. Stein H, Foss HD, Durkop H, et al: CD30(+) anaplastic large cell lymphoma: A review of its histopathologic, genetic, and clinical features. *Blood* 96:3681, 2000.

51. Duyster J, Bai RY, Morris SW: Translocations involving anaplastic lymphoma kinase (ALK). *Oncogene* 20:5623, 2001.

52. Gascoyne RD, Aoun P, Wu D, et al: Prognostic significance of anaplastic lymphoma kinase (ALK) protein expression in adults with anaplastic large cell lymphoma. *Blood* 93:3913, 1999.

53. Benharroch D, Meguerian-Bedoyan Z, Lamant L, et al: ALK-positive lymphoma: A single disease with a broad spectrum of morphology. *Blood* 91:2076, 1998.

54. Sternberg C: Uber eine Eigenartige unter dem Bilde der Pseudoleukamie verlaufende Tuberculose des lymphatischen Apparates. *Z Heilk* 19:21, 1898.

55. Reed DM: On the pathologic changes in Hodgkin's disease, with especial reference to its relation to tuberculosis. *Johns Hopkins Hosp Rep* 10:133, 1902.

56. Strum SB, Park JK, Rappaport H: Observation of cells resembling Sternberg-Reed cells in conditions other than Hodgkin's disease. *Cancer* 26:176, 1970.

57. Harris NL: Hodgkin's disease: Classification and differential diagnosis. *Mod Pathol* 12:159, 1999.

58. Kuppers R, Rajewsky K: The origin of Hodgkin and Reed/Sternberg cells in Hodgkin's disease. *Annu Rev Immunol* 16:471, 1998.

59. Jarrett RF, MacKenzie J: Epstein-Barr virus and other candidate viruses in the pathogenesis of Hodgkin's disease. *Semin Hematol* 36:260, 1999.

60. Skinnider BF, Mak TW: The role of cytokines in classical Hodgkin lymphoma. *Blood* 99:4283, 2002.

61. MacLennan KA, Bennett MH, Tu A, et al: Relationship of histopathologic features to survival and relapse in nodular sclerosing Hodgkin's disease. A study of 1659 patients. *Cancer* 64:1686, 1989.

62. Ferry JA, Linggood RM, Convery KM, et al: Hodgkin disease, nodular sclerosis type. Implications of histologic subclassification. *Cancer* 71:457, 1993.

63. von Wasielewski R, Werner M, Fischer R, et al: Lymphocyte-predominant Hodgkin's disease. An immunohistochemical analysis of 208 reviewed Hodgkin's disease cases from the German Hodgkin Study Group. *Am J Pathol* 150:793, 1997.

64. Anagnostopoulos I, Hansmann ML, Franssila K, et al: European Task Force on Lymphoma project on lymphocyte predominance Hodgkin disease: Histologic and immunohistologic analysis of submitted cases reveals 2 types of Hodgkin disease with a nodular growth pattern and abundant lymphocytes. *Blood* 96:1889, 2000.

65. Mason DY, Banks PM, Chan J, et al: Nodular lymphocyte predominance Hodgkin's disease. A distinct clinicopathological entity. *Am J Surg Pathol* 18:526, 1994.

66. Chan WC: Cellular origin of nodular lymphocyte-predominant Hodgkin's lymphoma: Immunophenotypic and molecular studies. *Semin Hematol* 36:242, 1999.

THE NON-HODGKIN LYMPHOMAS

KENNETH A. FOON
IRENE GHOBRIAL
LARISA J. GESKIN
SAMUEL A. JACOBS

The lymphomas are a heterogeneous group of clonal (neoplastic) diseases that share the single characteristic of arising as the result of a somatic mutation(s) in a lymphocyte progenitor. The progeny of the affected cell usually carry the phenotype of a B, T, or natural killer cell as judged by immunophenotyping or gene rearrangement studies. Any site of the lymphatic system can be the primary site of origin of the disorder, including lymph nodes, gut-associated lymphatic tissue, skin, or spleen. Any organ, such as the thyroid, lung, bone, brain, or gonads, can be involved either by spread from lymphatic sites or as a manifestation of primary extranodal disease. Classification of the subtypes of disease has been difficult, but newer systems couple immunologic phenotype with histopathologic and cytologic features to arrive at subtype definitions. By convention,

lymphocytic malignancies principally involving the marrow (and blood) are referred to as *lymphocytic leukemia*, whereas those originating in any other lymphoid site are referred to as *lymphoma*. In the former case, lymphoid sites may be involved secondarily; in the latter case, the marrow may be involved secondarily. Diagnosis of lymphoma usually is made by histologic examination of a biopsy specimen, supplemented by lymphoma cell immunophenotyping, cytogenetic evaluation for chromosome translocation sites or another abnormality, molecular analysis for clonal origin, and gene expression analysis where appropriate. Patients often undergo procedures that may involve high-resolution imaging studies, other tissue biopsies, and blood chemical studies to determine the extent (stage) of the disease. Treatment depends on the type of lymphoma and the distribution of disease. Combinations of drugs often are required for optimal treatment. Monoclonal antibody treatment as an addition to multidrug therapy is useful in some subtypes. Radiotherapy may be useful for localized disease. Autologous or allogeneic stem cell transplantation may be used as treatment in eligible patients.

Acronyms and abbreviations that appear in this chapter include: ABVD, doxorubicin, bleomycin, vinblastine, dacarbazine; ACVBP, doxorubicin, cyclophosphamide, vindesine, bleomycin, prednisone; ALCL, anaplastic large cell lymphoma; ALK, anaplastic large cell lymphoma tyrosine kinase; CDE, cyclophosphamide, doxorubicin, etoposide; CHOP, cyclophosphamide, doxorubicin, vincristine, prednisone; CHOPE, CHOP plus etoposide; CLA, cutaneous lymphocyte antigen; CLL, chronic lymphocytic leukemia; CNOP, cyclophosphamide, mitoxantrone, vincristine, prednisone; CNS, central nervous system; CT, computed tomography; CTCL, cutaneous T cell lymphoma; CVP, cyclophosphamide, vincristine, prednisone; CytaBOM, cytarabine, bleomycin, vincristine, methotrexate (with leucovorin rescue); DHAP, dexamethasone, high-dose cytarabine, cisplatin; DLBCL, diffuse large B cell lymphoma; EBV, Epstein-Barr virus; EPOCH, etoposide, prednisone, vincristine, cyclophosphamide, doxorubicin; ESHAP, etoposide, methylprednisolone, cytarabine, cisplatin; FCM, fludarabine, cyclophosphamide, mitoxantrone; FDG, fluoro-2-deoxyglucose; HAART, highly active antiretroviral therapy; HAMA, human antimouse antibodies; HHV, human herpes virus; HTLV, human T cell leukemia/lymphoma (lymphotropic) virus; hyper-CVAD, hyperfractionated cyclophosphamide, doxorubicin, vincristine, dexamethasone; ICE, ifosfamide, carboplatin, etoposide; Ig, immunoglobulin; IL, interleukin; KLH, keyhole limpet hemocyanin; KSHV, Kaposi sarcoma-associated herpes virus; LAK, lymphokine-activated killer; LDH, lactate dehydrogenase; MACOP-B, high-dose methotrexate, doxorubicin, cyclophosphamide, vincristine, prednisone, bleomycin; MALT, mucosa-associated lymphoid tissue; m-BACOD, moderate-dose methotrexate, bleomycin, doxorubicin, cyclophosphamide, vincristine, dexamethasone; MESA, myoepithelial sialadenitis; MF, mycosis fungoides; M-FEPA, methotrexate, vindesine, cyclophosphamide, prednisolone, doxorubicin; MOPP, mechlorethamine, vincristine, procarbazine, prednisone; MRI, magnetic resonance imaging; NHL, non-Hodgkin lymphoma; NK, natural killer; NPM, nucleophosmin; PCR, polymerase chain reaction; PET, positron emission tomography; ProMACE, prednisone, methotrexate, doxorubicin, cyclophosphamide, etoposide; PTGC, progressive transformation of germinal centers; PTLD, posttransplant lymphoproliferative disorder; PUVA, psoralen with ultraviolet radiation of the A spectrum; R-CHOP, rituximab plus CHOP; REAL, revised European-American lymphoma; SDT, skin-directed therapy; SLL, small lymphocytic lymphoma; SLVL, splenic lymphoma with villous lymphocytes; TCR, T cell receptor; Th2, T helper type 2; UVA, ultraviolet radiation of the A spectrum; UVB, ultraviolet radiation of the B spectrum; VEPA, vincristine, cyclophosphamide, prednisolone, doxorubicin; VEPA-B, vincristine, cyclophosphamide, prednisolone, doxorubicin, bleomycin; VEPA-M, vincristine, cyclophosphamide, prednisolone, doxorubicin, methotrexate; VEPP-B, vincristine, etoposide, procarbazine, prednisolone, bleomycin; WHO, World Health Organization.

DEFINITION AND HISTORY

Lymphomas are a heterogeneous group of malignancies of B cells, T cells, and rarely natural killer (NK) cells that usually originate in the lymph nodes, but they may originate in any organ of the body. Lymphoma previously was referred to as *reticulum cell sarcoma, lymphosarcoma*, or *giant follicular lymphoma*.[1-5] In 1966, Rappaport[6] published a classification system based on the patterns of lymphoma cell growth, size, and shape that attempted to correlate morphology with clinical outcome. The classification proved to have some inaccuracies, such as the term *histiocytic* to describe tumors of large transformed lymphocytes that were not derived from the monocyte-macrophage lineage. Nonetheless, the Rappaport classification was an important milestone and became the most widely used classification in the United States. In 1974, Lukes and Collins proposed another classification system, which incorporated morphology with immunologic subtype, that was endorsed by the Committee on Nomenclature.[7] Another scheme, the Kiel classification, had been more popular in Europe.[8] In 1982, a Working Formulation sponsored by the National Cancer Institute attempted to reconcile the large number of competing classifications then in use.[9] The Working Formulation was clinically useful and gained wide popularity. However, with advances in our understanding of the immune system, particularly the use of monoclonal antibodies for subtyping lymphoid cells, and with increasing molecular and genetic advances, a new classification schema became necessary. In 1994, a revised European-American classification of lymphoid neoplasm (REAL) was proposed by the International Lymphoma Study Group.[10] (See Chap. 90.) This group distinguished three major categories of lymphoid malignancies, which included B cell, T cell, and Hodgkin lymphoma. Lymphomas were defined by current morphologic, immunologic, and genetic techniques. Many of the lymphomas were associated with distinct clinical presentations, and cases that did not fit into defined entities were left unclassified. Further subclassification[11] divided each of the B and T cell lineages into (1) indolent lymphomas (low risk), (2) aggressive lymphomas (intermediate risk), and (3) very aggressive lymphomas (high risk). A collaborative project of the European Association for Haematopathology and the Society for Hematopathology began in 1995 to revise the REAL classification. In 2001 they published the World Health Organization (WHO) classification of Tumors of the Haematopoietic and Lymphoid Tissues that is used in this chapter and represents the current worldwide consensus classification of malignancies that arise in a lymphocyte. Table 96-1

A. B cell lymphomas (~88%)
 1. Diffuse large B cell lymphomas (30%)
 2. Follicular lymphoma (25%)
 3. Mucosa-associated lymphatic tissue (MALT) lymphoma (7.5%)
 4. Small lymphocytic lymphoma–chronic lymphocytic leukemia (7.0%)
 5. Mantle cell lymphoma (6.0%)
 6. Mediastinal (thymic) large B cell lymphoma (2.5%)
 7. Lymphoplasmacytic lymphoma–Waldenström macroglobulinemia (<2%)
 8. Nodal marginal zone B cell lymphoma (<2%)
 9. Splenic marginal zone lymphoma (<1%)
 10. Extranodal marginal zone B cell lymphoma (<1%)
 11. Intravascular large B cell lymphoma (<1%)
 12. Primary effusion lymphoma (<1%)
 13. Burkitt lymphoma–Burkitt leukemia (2.5%)
 14. Lymphomatoid granulomatosis (<1%)
B. T and NK cell lymphomas (~12%)
 1. Extranodal T or NK lymphoma
 2. Cutaneous T cell lymphoma (Sézary syndrome and mycosis fungoides)
 3. Anaplastic cell lymphoma
 4. Angioimmunoblastic T cell lymphoma
C. Immunodeficiency-associated lymphoproliferative disorders (see Table 96-18 for inherited diseases associated with immunodeficiencies and lymphoma)

SOURCE: This table is modified from information presented in the *World Health Organization Classification of Tumors: Pathology and Genetics of Tumors of Hematopoietic and Lymphoid Tissues.*[286] The parenthetical percentages are approximate but give some sense of the relative distribution of subtypes.

presents a précis of this classification. Chapter 95 discusses the detailed WHO classification.

EPIDEMIOLOGY

Approximately 54,000 new cases of non-Hodgkin lymphoma (NHL) are projected to be diagnosed and approximately 19,500 persons in the United States are expected to die of lymphoma in 2004.[12] This number represents approximately 4 percent of cancer incidence and approximately 4 percent of all cancer-related deaths. The incidence of lymphoma has increased dramatically in the last half of the 20th century.[13,14] This increase has affected men and women, all age groups, and most histologic types. It has been documented in industrialized countries in Europe and in the United States. The increase preceded the appearance of AIDS, but the latter has added to the effect somewhat in the last 15 years.[15] The increased incidence, which was approximately 3 to 4 percent per year, slowed to approximately 1 percent in the late 1990s, but the mortality rate continues to increase significantly.

Farming has been a constant association with higher lymphoma incidence, and although other occupations have been identified, farming seems to be the most consistent.[16,17]

Variations in racial incidence, histology, and immunologic subtypes are found throughout the world. Lymphoma is more common in males than females and in Americans of European descent than in Americans of African descent. A lower incidence of follicular lymphoma is observed in China and Japan.[18] The United States has a higher incidence of all lymphomas than does Japan, whereas the incidence of extranodal lymphoma is higher in Japan.[19] The incidence peaks in preadolescence, but generally the incidence increases logarithmically with age.[20] Burkitt lymphoma (BL) occurs most fre-

quently in tropical Africa, whereas T cell leukemia/lymphoma is most common in southwest Japan and the Caribbean basin.[21] Cutaneous T cell lymphoma (CTCL) is an uncommon malignancy in the United States, with approximately 1000 new cases reported per year.[22] The average annual adjusted mortality rate is approximately 400 to 500 deaths per year.

ETIOLOGY AND PATHOGENESIS

ENVIRONMENTAL FACTORS

An increased incidence of lymphoma has been observed, especially among farmers and gardeners.[15,16,23] Although several other industrial exposures have been implicated, none has reached a level of scientific certainty. The increased incidence in agricultural workers may be attributed to exposure to a variety of agents, including organochlorines, organophosphates, and phenoxyacid herbicides.[15–17,24–26] Large-scale studies are underway at the National Cancer Institute to examine possible environmental causal relationships to lymphoma incidence. Small but significant increases in lymphoma have been associated with radiation exposure.[27] Increased lymphomas were reported in survivors of the atomic bombing in Hiroshima who were exposed to at least 10 Gy.[28,29] An increased incidence of lymphomas also has been reported for individuals radiated for ankylosing spondylitis.[30] Patients with Hodgkin lymphoma who were treated with radiation therapy and chemotherapy have an increased incidence of NHL.

INFECTIOUS AGENTS

The most compelling evidence for a viral etiology of lymphoma is adult T cell leukemia/lymphoma (see Chap. 91). A C-type RNA tumor virus, isolated from patients, has been designated *human T cell leukemia/lymphoma virus I* (HTLV-I).[31] HTLV-I is an acquired retrovirus that is not related to other known animal retroviruses. HTLV-I can immortalize lymphoid cells in culture and induce malignancy in an infected human host. Incidence of infection with HTLV-I in endemic areas is very high, yet few of these infected patients develop adult T cell leukemia/lymphoma. HTLV-I also leads to a neurologic disorder called *tropical spastic paraparesis.*[32] Host determinants affect transformation of lymphocytes by HTLV-I and may be genetic factors.[33] Development of adult T cell leukemia/lymphoma is associated with infection by the human T cell leukemia virus I.[34] Serum specimens from Japanese patients with adult T cell leukemia/lymphoma are positive for HTLV-I, as are serum samples from adult T cell leukemia/lymphoma patients in the Caribbean, where adult T cell leukemia/lymphoma is endemic.[34] The highest prevalence of adult T cell leukemia/lymphoma in Japan is in the southern island of Kyushi, where 10 to 15 percent of the population has antibody to HTLV-I.[35] On the Japanese islands where adult T cell leukemia/lymphoma is rare, the rate is less than 1 percent. These and additional data from the Caribbean, the southeastern United States, South America, and Africa indicate that adult T cell leukemia/lymphoma clusters in regions where HTLV-I is prevalent.[34,35] How these regions are linked is not known. One hypothesis is that HTLV-I was brought to the Americas from Africa by the slave trade and then to the southern islands of Japan by trade with Japan and Africa.[34,35]

Host susceptibility, a shared environmental exposure, or both contribute to HTLV-I infection. The prevalence of HTLV-I antibodies in close family members is three to four times higher than in the corresponding normal population.[36,37] In some instances, cell cultures of antibody-positive, clinically normal patients yield HTLV-I isolates.[37] Blood donors are routinely screened for antibodies to HTLV-I to prevent transmission by this route.

Some B cell lymphomas may be caused by Epstein-Barr virus (EBV) (see Chap. 84). EBV is a DNA virus in the herpes virus family that first was described in cultured lymphoblasts from patients with African BL.[38] EBV binds to the CD21 antigen (also the receptor for the C3d component of complement) on B lymphocytes.[39] It is capable of transforming B lymphocytes into lymphoblastoid cells that may proliferate perpetually in cell culture.[40] EBV is present in greater than 95 percent of cases of endemic BL and in approximately 20 percent of cases of nonendemic BL.[41,42] Malaria is holoendemic in regions where endemic BL exists.[43] A three-step process in the development of this lymphoma has been proposed.[44,45] (1) EBV initiates a polyclonal proliferation of B cells; (2) malaria stimulates further the proliferating B cells; and (3) the transforming B cells incur specific reciprocal translocations of chromosome 8 with chromosome 2, 14, or 22, resulting in a clonal expansion of B lymphocytes.

Helicobacter pylori can cause mucosa-associated lymphoid tissue (MALT) lymphomas of the stomach and probably causes some of the higher-grade lymphomas, either from transformation of a MALT or *de novo* large cell lymphoma.[46–48] This spiral gram-negative bacillus is the first bacterium demonstrated to cause a human neoplasm.

IMMUNOSUPPRESSION

A variety of types of immunosuppressed individuals develop lymphoma. AIDS-related lymphoma is discussed later in this chapter (see also Chap. 83). Individuals who are immunosuppressed by drugs following organ transplantation have abnormalities ranging from benign proliferations of EBV-infected polyclonal B cells to aggressive malignant lymphoma.[49,50] Extranodal involvement is extremely common in posttransplant lymphomas. The incidence and rapidity of lymphomas have increased with the introduction of immunosuppressive agents such as cyclosporine and OKT3 (murine monoclonal anti-CD3).[50,51] The incidence of lymphomas also has increased in recipients of mismatched T cell-depleted marrow stem cell grafts. Individuals with inherited or acquired immunodeficiency also have B cell lymphomas that are caused by EBV.[52,53] The X-linked lymphoproliferative syndrome is an example of a genetic defect in immunoregulation that leads to the inability to generate an active anti-EBV immune response[54] (see Chap. 84 and "Disorders That Predispose to Lymphoma" below).

CHROMOSOMAL ABNORMALITIES

Chromosomal abnormalities are common in lymphomas (see Chap. 10). Approximately 85 percent of follicle center lymphomas carry the chromosomal translocation t(14;18)(q32;q21) in which the *bcl-2* oncogene on chromosome 18q21 is brought in continuity with the immunoglobulin (Ig) heavy-chain loci on 14q32.[55] The expression of the BCL-2 protein is increased.[56] The accumulation of the BCL-2 protein permits accumulation of long-lived centrocytes, as BCL-2 protein inhibits programmed cell depth (apoptosis), leading to a longer cell life (see Chap. 11).[57] The *bcl-2* rearrangement can be detected by both Southern blot hybridization and the polymerase chain reaction (PCR). In BL, the common genetic abnormality is the translocation of the c-*myc* oncogene from chromosome 8 to either the Ig heavy-chain region on chromosome 14, t(8;14)(q24;q32) or, less commonly, the κ region on chromosome 2, t(2;8)(p13;q24) or the λ region on chromosome 22, t(8;22)(q24;q11). In the African endemic cases, the breakpoint on chromosome 14 includes the heavy-chain joining region, suggesting translocation occurs before complete Ig gene rearrangement in an early B cell. In nonendemic cases, the translocation involves the Ig heavy-chain switch region,

suggesting translocation occurs at a later stage of B cell development.[58] EBV genomes are demonstrated in the tumor cells in most of the African cases, in approximately one third of the cases associated with AIDS[59,60] but less frequently in non-African, nonimmune-deficient cases.[41] The translocation t(2;5)(p23;q35) of anaplastic large cell lymphoma (ALCL) involves the nucleophosmin *(NPM)* gene at 5p35 and the anaplastic large cell lymphoma tyrosine kinase *(ALK)* gene at 2p23,[61] leading to expression of the novel fusion protein p80.[62] This translocation has been identified in approximately 50 percent of systemic cases and may be higher in children with ALCL.[63,64] The t(2;5) translocation is not common in primary cutaneous ALCL.[65] Several cytogenetic abnormalities have been reported in adult T cell leukemia/lymphoma cells. The most common abnormalities are trisomy, or partial trisomy, of 3q, 6q, 14q, and inv.[19] Less common cytogenetic abnormalities include loss of the X chromosome, 7(9;21), 5p, 2q+, 17q+, and trisomy 18.[66,67] In some studies, survival correlates with karyotype abnormalities.

CLINICAL FEATURES

HISTORY AND PHYSICAL EXAMINATION

A complete history and physical examination are important to provide evidence for extranodal disease or a functional disturbance of an organ system. It is important to ascertain whether the patient suspected of having lymphoma has night sweats, fever, or metabolic wasting resulting in loss of more than 10 percent of body weight within the preceding 6 months. The presence of such "B" symptoms has unfavorable prognostic significance.

An examination should be made of all lymph node areas. Involved nodes typically are nontender, firm, and rubbery. The throat should be examined for involvement of the oropharyngeal lymphoid tissue (Waldeyer ring). The aggressive lymphomas more likely involve extranodal sites, such as the skin and central nervous system (CNS) (see "Extranodal Lymphoma" below). Liver and spleen size should be assessed.

STAGING

Table 96-2 lists the staging procedures that can be used. Generally, staging laparotomy is not indicated. Surgery may be indicated to definitively treat low-grade lymphomas of the gastrointestinal tract and for diagnosis of extranodal or nodal disease confined to the abdomen.

TABLE 96-2   STAGING PROCEDURES FOR LYMPHOMA

Initial studies
  History and physical examination
  Biopsy specimen
    Pathologic diagnosis
    Flow cytometry
    Immunohistochemistry
    Cytogenetic analysis
  CT/PET scans of neck, chest, abdomen, and pelvis
Additional studies
  Immunoglobulin and T cell receptor gene rearrangement studies
  Polymerase chain reaction for Bcl-1 and Bcl-2
  Ultrasonography and MRI to clarify abnormalities
  CT scan or MRI of brain if neurologic signs or symptoms
  Analysis of cerebrospinal fluid if neurologic signs or symptoms
  Gastrointestinal studies if Waldeyer ring involvement

CT, computed tomography; MRI, magnetic resonance imaging; PET, positron emission tomography.

TABLE 96-3   ANN ARBOR STAGING SYSTEM

Stage I*	Restricted to one lymph node-bearing area
Stage II*	Two or more areas of nodal involvement on one side of the diaphragm
Stage III*	Lymphatic involvement on both sides of the diaphragm
Stage IV	Liver, marrow, or other extensive extranodal disease
Symptom status A	Absence of fevers, sweats, or weight loss
Symptom status B	Unexplained fevers >38°C, drenching night sweats, weight loss of >10% of body weight in the preceding 6 months
Clinical stage	Assigned stage based only on history, physical findings, and laboratory and imaging studies
Pathologic stage	Assigned stage based only on areas of biopsy-proven involvement
Substage E	Localized, extranodal disease

*The spleen is considered nodal.

The role of surgery for large intraabdominal masses (>10 cm) is controversial and is not routinely recommended.

The Ann Arbor staging classification (Table 96-3) is not optimal for staging lymphoma[52] but still is considered the gold standard and impacts patient survival. The staging system was created for Hodgkin lymphoma, which spreads by contiguity from lymph node areas rather than hematogenously as does lymphoma[68] (see Chap. 97). For this reason, more than 80 percent of patients with low-grade lymphoma and more than 50 percent of patients with intermediate- or high-grade lymphoma present with stage III or IV disease. However, staging is critically important for patients who are truly in stages I and II and are treated by potentially curative radiation therapy if they have low-risk follicle center lymphomas or by a combination of radiation therapy and limited cycles of chemotherapy if they have an intermediate- or high-risk lymphoma.

INTERNATIONAL PROGNOSTIC INDEX

In 1993, a model was proposed to assign a prognosis to patients with aggressive NHL undergoing treatment with doxorubicin-containing chemotherapeutic regimens termed the *International Prognostic Index* (IPI).[69,70] The model used clinical data including (1) tumor stage, (2) serum lactate dehydrogenase (LDH) level, (3) number of extranodal disease sites involved, (4) performance status, and (5) patient age. This model resulted in the IPI, which is used to forecast the behavior of aggressive lymphoma (Table 96-4). For patients younger than 60 years, an age-adjusted IPI has been proposed in which all the factors of the IPI are used, except for age and presence of extranodal sites. The 5-year survival rates for patients 60 years or younger with IPI scores of 0, 1, 2, and 3 were 83, 69, 46, and 32 percent, respectively (Table 96-5 and Figure 96-1).[69]

EXTRANODAL LYMPHOMA

Lymphomas involving extranodal sites most commonly occur simultaneously with nodal involvement, either at the time of diagnosis or sometime during the course of the disease. Extranodal involvement that occurs as the only evidence of lymphoma is referred to as *primary extranodal lymphoma*.

CENTRAL NERVOUS SYSTEM

Between 5 and 10 percent of patients with nodal presentation of lymphoma may develop CNS involvement.[71] These patients have a high incidence of marrow involvement and typically have aggressive histology. Epidural, testes,[72] and paranasal sinus[73] involvement commonly is associated with CNS disease. CNS presentation may include

spinal cord compression, leptomeningeal spread, and/or intracerebral mass lesions. Spinal cord compression typically presents with back pain, followed by extremity weakness, paresis, and paralysis. Leptomeningeal spread may present with cranial nerve palsies and signs of meningeal irritation. Intracerebral mass lesions may present with headaches, lethargy, papilledema, focal neurologic signs, or seizures.

Primary lymphomas originating in and confined to the brain[74] or spinal cord[75] are rare. They almost always have an aggressive histology. Intracerebral tumors have increased dramatically in recent years because of the association with AIDS-related aggressive lymphomas (see Chap. 83). Progressive multifocal leukoencephalopathy occurs as a result of polyoma virus infection in the brain. It is characterized by demyelination and typically is fatal.[76] Paraneoplastic neurologic syndromes such as myasthenia gravis, cerebellar degeneration, peripheral neuropathies, and transverse myelopathy also may be associated with lymphomas.[77]

EYE

The most common presentation of ocular lesions is the periorbital soft tissues, particularly the conjunctival mucosal surfaces and the area surrounding the lacrimal gland.[78] These lesions typically are low risk and commonly have the histology of a MALT or follicle center lymphoma. The preferred therapy is radiation ranging from 25 to 30 Gy, which is curative in the majority of patients.[79] Anecdotal reports of responses to rituximab or rituximab post-radiation suggest that rituximab will have a therapeutic role in these low-grade lymphomas involving the eye. Bilateral involvement, particularly with MALT lymphomas, may be seen. In the rare situation where large cell lymphoma involves the periorbital soft tissue, treatment follows the overall clinical picture.

Intraocular lymphomas are a rare presentation of lymphoma of the eye.[80] Most cases are B cell large cell lymphomas, but they often have a unique indolent pattern. The diagnosis is established by a vitrectomy. There is an approximately 50 percent chance that the disease will be bilateral. Also, the disease frequently is associated with brain or leptomeningeal involvement. The mainstay of therapy is radiation, but most patients experience relapse within the eye or brain. Chemotherapeutic agents typically do not penetrate the eye or brain. Most patients are offered palliation with radiation and glucocorticoids, but recurrence is typical. These tumors behave much like large B cell lymphomas of the brain, and consideration of more aggressive therapy is reasonable.

PARANASAL SINUSES

Lymphomas may involve the frontal, maxillary, ethmoid, and sphenoid sinuses. These lymphomas typically involve bone and present with pain, upper airway obstruction, rhinorrhea, facial swelling, or

TABLE 96-4   INTERNATIONAL PROGNOSTIC FACTOR INDEX FOR NON-HODGKIN LYMPHOMA

RISK FACTORS
Age >60 years
Serum LDH greater than twice normal
Performance status ≥2
Stage III or IV
Extranodal involvement at >1 site

Each factor accounts for one point, for a total score that ranges from 0 to 5. For patients <61 years, the age-adjusted index includes all variables except for age and number of extranodal sites.
LDH, lactic dehydrogenase.
SOURCE: Adapted from reference 69.

epistaxis. Periorbital tumors may present with proptosis, visual loss, or diplopia. These lymphomas typically are large cell lymphomas.[81] Following staging, treatment is planned in three phases, which include systemic, local, and prophylaxis therapy to prevent spread to the CNS.[78] With localized disease, three cycles of chemotherapy are recommended, followed by involved-field radiation. For more advanced disease, six to eight cycles of chemotherapy are recommended. Following standard therapy, six doses of intrathecal chemotherapy over 3 weeks are recommended because of the high incidence of CNS disease. Using this three-step approach to management, the majority of patients are cured.[78]

SKIN

Cutaneous T cell lymphoma includes all of the T cell lymphomas with skin involvement, including mycosis fungoides, adult T cell leukemia/lymphoma, anaplastic large cell lymphoma, and others. However, any lymphoma may secondarily infiltrate the skin. The lesions typically are reddish-purplish[82] nodules and are more common with aggressive lymphomas; however, low-grade lymphoma also may infiltrate the skin. Primary extranodal involvement of the skin is rarely seen in B cell lymphomas and may have a more favorable prognosis.[83]

LUNG

Pulmonary involvement is not common at diagnosis but may be seen with progressive disease.[84] This finding typically is associated with lymphatic spread of tumor from hilar and mediastinal nodes. It may be seen in approximately 20 percent of cases at presentation. Primary lymphomas of the lung are rare and typically have a low-grade histology.[85] Pleural effusions are common, occurring in approximately 25 percent of patients secondary to either central lymphatic obstruction or pleural seeding.

GASTROINTESTINAL TRACT

Approximately 15 percent of patients with nodal disease also have gastrointestinal involvement, and nearly half of patients have disease at autopsy.[86] Patients may present with anorexia, nausea, vomiting, an abdominal mass, or pain. Adjacent mesenteric nodes may be involved and may contribute to the symptoms.[87] Intestinal involvement may be multifocal and may be associated with disease in the Waldeyer ring. The histologic pattern usually is that of an aggressive lymphoma.[88] Ascites typically develops late in the disease. Primary involvement of the gastrointestinal tract is seen in approximately 5 percent of cases. The most frequent site of primary gastrointestinal lymphoma is the stomach, followed by the small intestine, rectum, and colon.[89] Lymphoma of the stomach typically causes dyspeptic symptoms and sometimes anorexia or early satiety. Hemorrhage is unusual but

suggests a high-grade lymphoma. Diagnosis typically is made by gastroscopic biopsy. At gastroscopy, mild to severe gastritis is common. Multiple biopsies are important for obtaining adequate material to determine the presence of *H. pylori*. MALT lymphoma is common, but diffuse large B cell lymphoma (DLBCL) also may arise *de novo* or

TABLE 96-5   OUTCOME ACCORDING TO RISK GROUP DEFINED BY THE INTERNATIONAL PROGNOSTIC INDEX

INTERNATIONAL INDEX	NO. OF RISK FACTORS	COMPLETE RESPONSE RATE (%)	RELAPSE-FREE SURVIVAL (%)		SURVIVAL (%)	
Age-adjusted International Prognostic Index, Patients >60 years						
			2-Year	*5-Year*	*2-Year*	*5-Year*
Low	0 or 1	87	79	70	84	73
Low-intermediate	2	67	66	50	66	51
High-intermediate	3	55	59	49	54	43
High	4 or 5	44	58	40	34	26
Age-adjusted International Index, Patients <61 years						
			2-Year	*5-Year*	*2-Year*	*5-Year*
Low	0	92	88	86	90	83
Low-intermediate	1	78	74	66	79	69
High-intermediate	2	57	62	53	59	46
High	3	46	61	58	37	32

SOURCE: Adapted from reference 69.

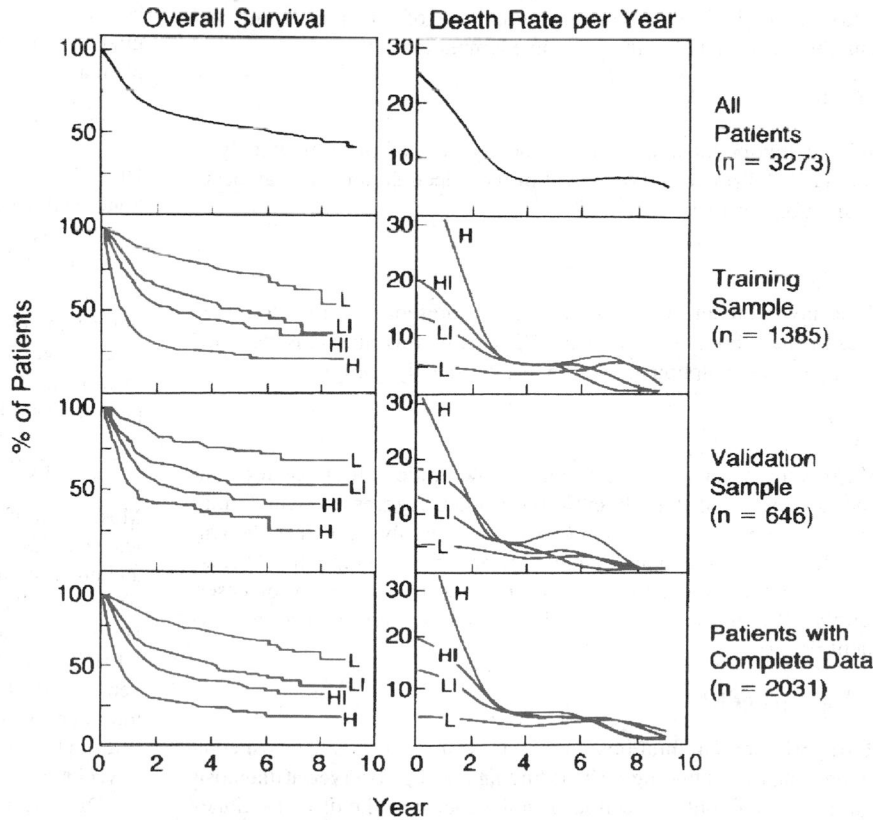

FIGURE 96-1   *(Left panels)* Kaplan-Meier survival curves for the four risk groups. *(Right panels)* Death rates during the study period. Only 2031 of the 3273 patients had sufficient relevant information for classification according to the international index. H, high risk; HI, high-intermediate risk, L, low risk, LI, low-intermediate risk.

may be found in the background of a MALT lymphoma. If both histologies are present, the treatment should be directed at the large cell lymphoma.[90–93]

TESTICULAR LYMPHOMA

Lymphoma at this site typically presents as a painless enlargement of the testis in an older man.[94,95] It usually is a DLBCL. At presentation, two thirds of cases are localized to the testicle or to the testicle and pelvic or abdominal lymph nodes. In the remaining cases, the testicle is one site of metastatic involvement in patients with widespread disease. After orchiectomy has established the diagnosis, patients are staged with a special focus on the remaining testicle. If sonography of the remaining testicle demonstrates a solid mass, it should be assumed to be lymphoma. Patients presenting with testicular lymphoma have a poorer prognosis compared to patients with other DLBCLs.[96] Many patients experience relapse in either the CNS or the opposite testicle.[93] Low-dose radiation to the contralateral testis is recommended, and CNS prophylaxis with high-dose methotrexate after systemic cyclophosphamide, doxorubicin, vincristine, and prednisone (CHOP) or rituximab plus CHOP (R-CHOP) chemotherapy should be considered.[97,98]

LIVER

Hepatic involvement secondary to infiltration of the portal tract is more common in patients with low-risk lymphoma,[99,100] whereas hepatic mass lesions are seen more commonly in patients with aggressive lymphomas.[101] Liver involvement may not be associated with spleen involvement, as typically is seen in Hodgkin disease.[102] Hepatomegaly and jaundice occur in approximately one third of patients during the course of their disease. Primary lymphoma of the liver is rare and usually is associated with aggressive lymphomas.[103]

SPLEEN

Splenic involvement is found in nearly half of patients with lymphoma.[99,100] Primary involvement of the spleen is rare and may occur in all subtypes of lymphoma.[104]

BONE

Bone involvement in patients with nodal presentation is uncommon, as is primary bone involvement.[102] Typically, this finding is restricted to aggressive lymphoma, and the lesions usually are lytic.[105]

MARROW

Marrow involvement is common in low-grade follicle center lymphomas and small lymphocytic lymphoma. Aggressive lymphomas that commonly are associated with marrow involvement include lymphoblastic lymphoma and small noncleaved cell lymphoma. Diffuse large cell lymphoma involves the marrow in 10 percent of cases. Rarely, the marrow is the primary site of lymphoma involvement.[106–108]

GENITOURINARY

Retroperitoneal urethral obstruction by lymph nodes is the most common urinary tract finding.[109] This finding may be observed at diagnosis but more commonly is seen later in the course of the disease. Kidney involvement is common as noted at autopsy, but it rarely causes overt disease. An unusual clinical manifestation is enlarged kidneys, grossly involved with lymphoma; however, this manifestation rarely occurs at presentation. The nephritic syndrome is unusual and may result from renal vein occlusion, glomerulonephritis, or minimal change glomer-

ulopathy. Glomerulopathy is more commonly associated with Hodgkin disease. Lymphomas involving the prostate,[110] testes,[94–98] or ovary[111] are uncommon and typically have aggressive histology and clinical behavior.

OVARIAN OR BREAST

These two sites of lymphoma may relapse in the CNS.[111–113] Therefore, CHOP (or R-CHOP) chemotherapy plus CNS prophylaxis with high-dose intravenous methotrexate with leucovorin rescue is often used. Intrathecal methotrexate can be given but does not prevent intracerebral recurrence.

OTHER SITES

Clinical disease related to cardiac involvement by lymphoma is unusual. However, cardiac involvement may be found at autopsy in 20 percent of cases.[101,114] Other uncommon sites of involvement include the salivary glands,[115] adrenals,[116] and thyroid.[117] Thyroid lymphoma usually is associated with Hashimoto thyroiditis.

DIFFUSE LARGE B CELL LYMPHOMA

DEFINITION

DLBCL is a heterogeneous group of aggressive lymphomas of large transformed B cells. The postulated normal cell counterpart is a proliferating B-centroblast or immunoblast. Gene expression studies indicate DLBCL has at least three subtypes, of which two are principal variants, one derived from germinal center B cells and the other from postgerminal center activated B cells (see "Etiology and Pathogenesis" below).[118] DLBCL can arise *de novo* or may transform from a low-grade lymphoma, such as small B cell lymphoma or follicular lymphoma.

EPIDEMIOLOGY

DLBCL is the most common histologic subtype of NHL in the United States and represents approximately 30 percent of all NHL[119,120] (Table 96-6). It also is the most frequently occurring lymphoma in most parts of the world.[121] The incidence of DLBCL has increased steadily in the second half of the 20th century in most industrialized countries. The most common presentation is in middle-aged and older persons; the median age at diagnosis is 64 years It is more common in men than in women (Table 96-6) and is more common in Americans of European descent than in Americans of African descent.[122]

ETIOLOGY AND PATHOGENESIS

Most cases of DLBCL have no apparent etiology. EBV is associated with DLBCL in posttransplant lymphoproliferative disorders (PTLD) and other immunodeficiency states or in CNS lymphoma. Human herpes virus (HHV)-8 is associated with pleural effusion lymphomas.[123] Hepatitis C has been linked to NHL, but its role in the etiology of DLBCL is not firmly established.[122] Other risk factors for NHL include personal and family history of NHL, primary immunosuppression, autoimmune disorders, organ transplantation, and occupational exposures to toxins, including organochlorine, organophosphate, and phenoxyacid compounds in pesticides and herbicides.[122]

DLBCL is a molecularly heterogeneous disease with multiple complex chromosomal translocations and genetic abnormalities as identified by cytogenetics and gene expression profiling. The disease is derived from B cells that have undergone somatic mutation in the Ig genes in the lymph node germinal center. The *bcl-6* gene rearrangements may be specific for DLBCL.[124] Approximately 40 percent of

TABLE 96-6   SOME FEATURES OF NON-HODGKIN LYMPHOMA

Type of NHL	Frequency Among All NHLs (%)	Median Age at Diagnosis (Years)	Frequency of Stage III and IV Presentation (%)	IPI 4–5	Frequency of Extranodal Involvement (%)	Frequency of Marrow Involvement (%)
DLBCL	31	64	46	19	71*	16
Follicular	22	59	67	7	64	42
MALT	5	60	33	8	98	14
Mantle	6	63	80	23	81	64
Mediastinal DLBCL	2	37	34	11	56	3

The frequency of occurrence of lymphoma subtypes differs slightly from the WHO estimates given in Table 96-1.
* The frequency of 71% for extranodal disease in DLBCL in this study exceeded the usual value of ~40%.
DLBCL, diffuse large B cell lymphoma; IPI, International Prognostic Index; NHL, non-Hodgkin lymphoma.
SOURCE: Adapted from reference 736.

DLBCLs in immunocompetent hosts and approximately 20 percent of HIV-related cases display bcl-6 rearrangements.[125–127]

Chromosomal translocations involving band 3q27 lead to a truncated bcl-6 gene within its 5' flanking region. This situation commonly occurs within the first exon or first intron, leading to complete removal or truncation of the promoter sequences; the coding sequence is left intact.[183] In a small number of cases, the breakpoint is not located in the immediate proximity of the bcl-6 gene. Increased expression of bcl-6 occurs from a process termed *promoter substitution* by which heterologous promoters are juxtaposed to the bcl-6 coding domain. This process occurs through reciprocal translocations between 3q27 and chromosomal partner sites, including 14q32 (IgH), 2p11 (Igκ), and 22q11 (Igλ).[128,129]

The Bcl-6 protein mediates the specific binding of several transcription factors to DNA. It also may be involved in induction of germinal center-associated functions, given that it is expressed in germinal center B cells but not in plasma cells. Therefore, down-regulation of bcl-6 may be necessary for terminal differentiation of B cells to plasma cells and to memory B cells.[130]

Approximately 30 percent of DLBCLs have the t(14;18) translocation involving the Ig heavy-chain gene and bcl-2. The bcl-2 gene rearrangements may occur in DLBCL in two conditions, a transformation of a previous follicular lymphoma or in DLBCL with a germinal center gene expression profile. The presence of p53 mutation in combination with bcl-2 denotes that the tumor is derived from a histologic transformation of a previous follicular lymphoma.[131] The bcl-2 rearrangement is not necessary for expression of Bcl-2 protein. From 25 to 80 percent of DLBCLs in various studies express Bcl-2 protein. The bcl-2 gene rearrangement is associated with nodal and disseminated disease.

Mutations in the variable region of the Ig genes normally allow antibody diversity in germinal center B cells. However, aberrant somatic hypermutation occurs in more than 50 percent of cases of DLBCL.[132] This alteration targets multiple loci, including the protooncogenes PIM1, MYC, RhoH/TTF (ARHH), and PAX5.[132] The c-myc gene rearrangement occurs in 5 to 15 percent of patients with DLBCL.

The heterogeneity of DLBCL is evident from the gene expression profile of patients' lymphoma cells.[118] At least three distinct genetic types can be identified. The most common type, which occurs in 40 percent of cases, is associated with rearrangements of bcl-6 in the absence of other known genetic lesions. The second type involves activation of bcl-2.[133] Cases with neither bcl-2 or bcl-6 rearrangements compose the third genetic group of DLBCL. These genetic subgroups have prognostic relevance because the presence of bcl-2 confers a poorer prognosis,[134] whereas the presence of bcl-6 denotes a better prognosis.[118,135–137]

CLINICAL FEATURES

SIGNS AND SYMPTOMS

DLBCL usually appears in the lymph nodes in the neck or abdomen. The typical presentation is of a rapidly enlarging lymph node or an abdominal mass. B symptoms (drenching night sweats, fever, weight loss) are observed in approximately 30 percent of patients.

Extranodal disease occurs in approximately 40 percent of patients, most commonly involving the gastrointestinal tract.[138,139] Other sites that may be affected include the testis, bone, thyroid, salivary glands, skin, liver, breast, nasal cavity, paranasal sinuses, and CNS.

Unusual symptoms and presentations may occur with some subtypes of DLBCL, such as intravascular large B cell lymphoma, which may present with unexplained fever, or pleural cavity lymphoma, which may present with pleural effusions.

DISEASE STAGE

Staging is based on the Ann Arbor staging system (see Table 96-3). Approximately 25 percent of patients present with early localized disease (stage I). Approximately 25 percent of patients present with stage II disease, whereas approximately 45 percent of patients have disseminated disease (stage IV) at presentation (see Table 96-6). Bulky disease with a mass larger than 10 cm occurs in approximately 25 percent of patients. Stage IV disease is defined by the presence of two or more extranodal sites, diffuse disseminated disease in visceral organs, or marrow involvement.[139] Marrow involvement occurs in approximately 15 percent of patients. Discordant disease in which the marrow is involved by a low-grade lymphoma and not by the DLBCL may occur. It is not associated with a poorer prognosis but increases the risk of late relapse. CNS dissemination may occur after testicular or paranasal sinuses involvement.[140] Elevated LDH level and marrow involvement are other factors associated with CNS involvement.[140] Patients at high risk for CNS dissemination should undergo an examination of spinal fluid for cells and protein content. Patients with involvement of the Waldeyer ring have an increased risk of gastrointestinal lymphoma.

CELL IMMUNOPHENOTYPE

The malignant cells have surface monoclonal Ig of either κ or λ light-chain type. The most commonly expressed surface whole Ig is IgM. Less commonly, the cells are negative for surface Ig.[141] The lymphoma cells generally express the pan B cell antigens, CD19, CD20, CD22, PAX5, and CD79a. They also express CD45 and, less commonly, CD10 or CD5.[142,143] The CD5+ lymphomas may be more aggressive with a worse prognosis.[144] The cells undergo Ig variable-region gene rearrangement and are commonly somatically mutated. Isotype switch variants may occur.[145] Adhesion molecules such as LFA-1 (CD16/CD18) and CD44 are expressed in 50 to 75 percent of DLBCL. CD44 is expressed in highly aggressive subsets of DLBCL and is associated with disseminated disease and a poor prognosis.[146]

COURSE AND PROGNOSIS

The 5-year survival of patients with DLBCL ranges from approximately 25 to 75 percent, depending on the prognostic factors present at diagnosis. Long-term disease-free survival occurs in approximately 40 percent of patients. Several prognostic factors that correlate with poor prognosis have been described.

INTERNATIONAL PROGNOSTIC INDICATOR
Tumor stage, serum LDH level, number of extranodal sites involved, performance status, and patient age are strong determinants of prognosis (see Table 96-4). In this group of patients, the probability of a 5-year survival ranges from 0.73 to 0.26 for a score from 0 through 5. In patients who are diagnosed when they are 60 years or younger, age and presence of extranodal disease are excluded from the prognostic variables. Table 96-5 lists the effect of the prognostic indicators. In the latter group of patients, the probability of a 5-year survival ranges from 0.83 to 0.32 for a score from 0 through 3.

GENE EXPRESSION PROFILES
Specific patterns of gene expression can delineate groups of patients with DLBCL who may differ in their response to therapy and prognosis (Figure 96-2, see Color Plate XXII-39).[136,137] Six genes identified by gene expression analysis and detected by quantitative real-time PCR can identify three prognostic groups in patients with DLBCL (Figure 96-3).[147,148] The six genes that were used in this model occur in the germinal center B cell signature (LMO2, BCL6), activated B cell signature (BCL2, CCND2, SCYA3), and lymph-node signature (FN1). In this study, expression of LMO2, BCL6, and FN1 correlated with prolonged survival, whereas expression of BCL2, CCND2, and SCYA3 correlated with short survival.

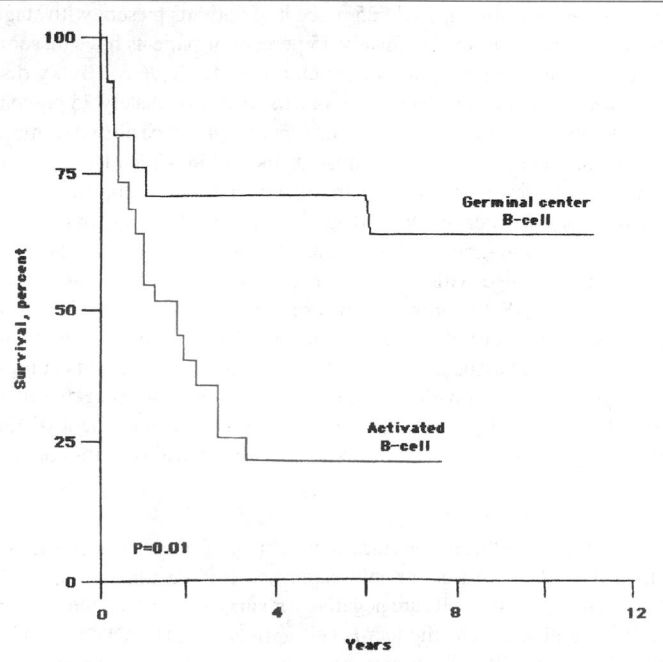

FIGURE 96-2   Overall survival in a group of patients with diffuse large B cell lymphoma whose cell of origin was determined by gene expression profiling. Survival of patients with diffuse large B cell lymphoma whose malignant cells were thought to arise from a germinal center B cell was significantly better than in patients whose cell of origin arose from activated B cells.

OTHER PROGNOSTIC FACTORS
Patients with an elevated β_2-microglobulin level and high serum LDH have a poor prognosis, with a 26 percent survival compared to 81 percent in patients without elevation of these markers.[149] Approximately 70 percent of DLBCL cases are of germinal center origin, as demonstrated by Bcl-6 protein overexpression. Patients with a germinal center B cells pattern have a more favorable prognosis than do patients with the postgerminal center gene expression pattern.[135] The bcl-2 gene rearrangement or Bcl-2 protein expression has been associated with a poor prognosis.[134] Survivin, a member of the inhibitor of apoptosis gene family, is not expressed in normal tissue but is expressed in 60 percent of patients with DLBCL and is associated with a poor prognosis.[150] Overexpression of the Ki-67 proliferation-associated antigen using flow cytometry is a poor prognostic sign.[151] The high number of infiltrating CD4+ T cells in DLBCL is associated with a better prognosis.[152] However, T cell-rich, B cell lymphoma is not a favorable phenotype. Cyclin D3 expression, p53 gene mutation, and expression of serum vascular endothelial growth factor or cytokines such as interleukin (IL)-2, IL-10, and IL-6 have been associated with a poor prognosis.

In a prospective study, 64 percent of 26 patients who had a negative ^{18}F-fluoro-2-deoxyglucose (FDG) positron emission tomography (PET) scan after two cycles of CHOP did not have disease progression, whereas 25 percent of the patients who had a positive PET scan progressed.[153] Abnormal ^{18}F-FDG uptake predicted a lower rate of progression-free and overall survival in a retrospective study of 60 patients undergoing high-dose chemotherapy and hematopoietic stem cell transplantation.[154]

Patients with poor prognostic factors are at high risk for relapse after standard therapy. Relapse usually occurs within the first 2 to 3 years after diagnosis but is rare after 4 years of diagnosis.[155,156] Patients who relapse after a disease-free interval of greater than 4 years may achieve a second complete remission 60 percent of the time. The tumor in patients with relapsed disease may show features of germinal center B cells and have the identical clonal markers as the initial tumor.[157] Patients with poor prognostic factors may be candidates for aggressive initial therapy.[139,158] However, this approach is not considered the standard of care.[159]

THERAPY

GENERAL CONSIDERATIONS
DLBCL is potentially curable with combination chemotherapy. The dose administered during the first 12 weeks of therapy determines survival; therefore, reduction of chemotherapy doses should be avoided if at all possible. Before therapy is instituted, several factors should be considered, including the patient's clinical stage, symptoms, and IPI. In addition, response should be evaluated according to the defined criteria. Other considerations, such as the patient's age and comorbid conditions, are important before a therapeutic intervention is selected. Future trials and therapies can be individualized according to subgroups of DLBCL based on gene expression patterns.

EARLY-STAGE DIFFUSE LARGE B CELL LYMPHOMA
Localized disease occurs in approximately 25 percent of patients. In the early 1980s, the standard of care was radiation therapy.[160] Historically, the 5-year disease-free survival with radiation therapy in stage I disease was 50 percent and in stage II disease was approximately 20 percent. Combining chemotherapy with radiation therapy improved the outcome.[161–166] The addition of chemotherapy resulted in improved control of disseminated and of local sites. Chemotherapy is given prior to radiation therapy.

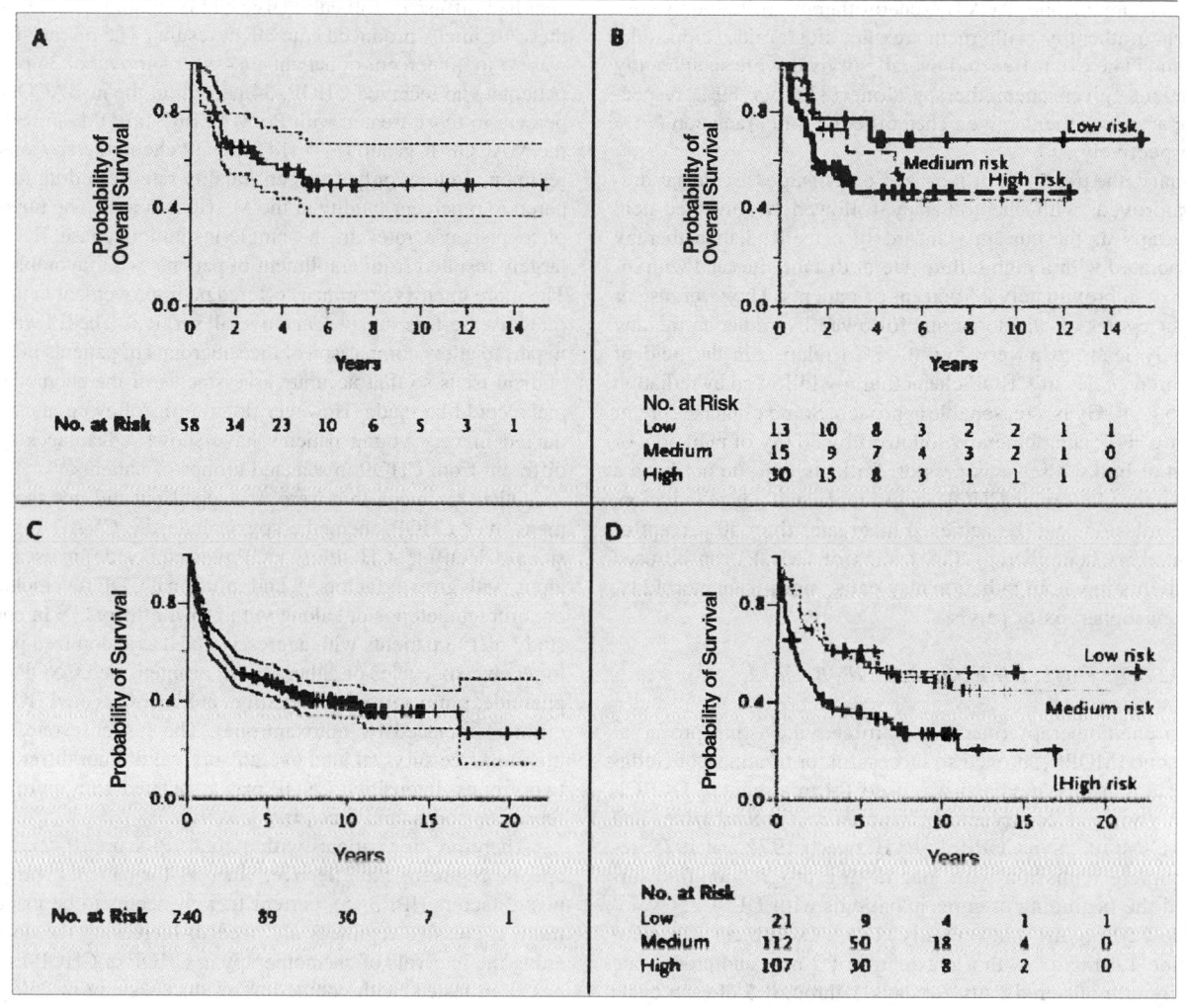

FIGURE 96-3   *(A)* Kaplan-Meier estimates of overall survival in all 58 patients with diffuse large B cell lymphoma (DLBCL) reported by Shipp and colleagues.[136] *(B)* Kaplan-Meier estimates of overall survival in the 58 patients after subdivision into three groups (low, medium, and high risk of death) based on the six-gene model for prediction. *Dotted lines* represent 95% confidence intervals. According to log likelihood estimates, $P = .02$ for the model as a continuous variable and $P = .31$ for the model as a class. *(C, D)* Similar analyses of the data on the 240 patients with DLBCL reported by Rosenwald and colleagues.[158] $P < .001$ for the model based on a continuous variable and for the model based on the three discrete groups shown in the figure.

The role of chemotherapy alone has been studied in several randomized trials.[167–169] A study of localized aggressive NHL randomly assigned 401 patients with stage I and nonbulky stage II disease to receive either eight cycles of CHOP chemotherapy or three cycles of CHOP plus involved-field radiotherapy.[167,168] The 5-year overall and progression-free survival rates of the patients treated with the combined modality were significantly better (82% and 76%, respectively) compared to patients treated with chemotherapy alone (74% and 67%). These benefits were demonstrated largely in patients older than 60 years. Cardiac toxicity and other life-threatening toxicity were much higher in patients treated with chemotherapy alone. A subanalysis using modified IPI criteria showed that patients with poor risk factors had a worse overall survival.

In a trial involving 365 patients with bulky stage I (mediastinal or retroperitoneal mass, or a mass >10 cm), stage IE, stage II, or stage IIE disease, patients were randomized to receive either eight cycles of CHOP alone or eight cycles of CHOP with involved-field radiation.[169] Patients in complete remission received 30 Gy of involved-field radiation or no therapy. Patients with partial remission received 40 Gy to the involved field and radiation to the contiguous noninvolved

regions. Although the detailed results of this study have not yet been published, the 5-year overall survival was 84 percent in the patients receiving combined therapy compared to 70 percent for patients who received chemotherapy alone. The 5-year disease-free survival was 73 percent versus 58 percent, respectively. At 10 years, the overall survival was not significantly different between the two groups, but the disease-free survival was different (57% and 46%, respectively). Patients with poor prognostic factors were more likely to develop recurrent lymphoma.

Two additional European trials were performed.[170,171] In one study, 518 patients older than 60 years with an IPI score of 0 were randomized to four cycles of CHOP with or without radiation therapy (40 Gy to local disease). The 5-year event-free survival was 69 percent in the patients treated with CHOP compared to 64 percent in the patients treated with CHOP plus radiation therapy. The overall survival did not differ between the two groups. However, patients older than 70 years had an improved overall survival with chemotherapy alone. The second study randomized 631 patients with low-risk localized aggressive lymphoma to three cycles of CHOP followed by 30 to 40 Gy of involved-field radiation or doxorubicin, cyclophosphamide, vindesine, bleomycin, and prednisone (ACVBP) chemotherapy followed by consolidation chemotherapy with methotrexate, ifosfamide, etoposide, and cytarabine. The event-free and overall survival were significantly better in patients given chemotherapy alone (83% vs. 89%, respectively) compared to patients given chemotherapy plus radiation (74% vs. 80%, respectively).

In summary, the treatment of localized early-stage disease has dramatically improved, with chemotherapy followed by involved-field radiation therapy as the current standard of care. Radiation therapy alone is associated with a high failure rate at distant sites and with in-field relapse in approximately 20 percent of patients. However, use of three to eight cycles of chemotherapy followed by radiation therapy of 35 to 45Gy leads to a very low (0–7%) relapse in the field of radiation. Three cycles of CHOP chemotherapy followed by radiation therapy of 35 to 40 Gy is a reasonable approach. Some clinicians prefer six cycles of CHOP chemotherapy followed by 30 Gy of radiation, or 36 Gy if initial bulky disease is present. Patients who do not have a complete response following CHOP should receive 40 Gy of radiation, as durable remissions can be achieved in greater than 50 percent of these patients.[172] Chemotherapy (six cycles of CHOP) can be used alone for patients in whom radiation may cause significant morbidity, as in the oronasopharynx or pelvis.

DISSEMINATED-STAGE DIFFUSE LARGE B CELL LYMPHOMA

Combination chemotherapy (mechlorethamine, vincristine, procarbazine, prednisone [MOPP]) proved so successful for treatment of Hodgkin lymphoma that this approach was used for treatment of DLBCL with CHOP and cyclophosphamide, vincristine, procarbazine, and prednisone (C-MOPP, syn.COPP).[173,174] Between 1972 and 1975, reports of complete remission with long-lasting progression-free survival marked the beginning of cures in patients with DLBCL. Cyclophosphamide 750 mg/m^2 intravenously (IV), doxorubicin 50 mg/m^2 IV, vincristine 1.4 mg/m^2 with a maximum of 2 mg, and prednisone 100 mg orally administered daily for days 1 through 5 of each cycle (CHOP) became the most popular regimen in the United States for treatment of DLBCL (Table 96-7). Cycles are repeated every 21 days. CHOP has been administered in other modified regimens with a day 1 and day 8 schedule and variable doses of prednisone. Patients receive four to six cycles, and those who achieve complete remission subsequently receive two more cycles. Most complete responders achieve durable relapse-free survival, depending on the prognostic factors.

Based on the success of CHOP chemotherapy, several combination chemotherapy regimens were developed. Many showed dramatic improvement in the response rates in phase II clinical trials, with up to 80 percent complete remissions and 60 percent disease-free survival.[175,176] Phase II trials of m-BACOD (moderate-dose methotrexate, bleomycin, doxorubicin, cyclophosphamide, vincristine, dexamethasone), ProMACE (prednisone, methotrexate, doxorubicin, cyclophosphamide, etoposide)/CytaBOM (cytarabine, bleomycin, vincristine, methotrexate), and MACOP-B (high-dose methotrexate, doxorubicin, cyclophosphamide, vincristine, prednisone, bleomycin) showed superior responses compared to the results with CHOP chemotherapy.[177] However, the significant responses that were demonstrated in single institutional studies could not be repeated in multiinstitutional studies and were not as significant when reanalyzed after 2 years of observation. A prospective randomized study that compared m-BACOD with CHOP showed no difference in the complete remission rates, disease-free survival, or overall survival.[178] Because of these conflicting data, a four-arm phase III study was conducted and enrolled patients in a randomized prospective trial comparing CHOP, m-BACOD, MACOP-B, and ProMACE/CytaBOM.[155] This landmark trial enrolled 897 patients with intermediate- or high-grade NHL, of whom 85 per-

cent had diffuse or follicular large cell lymphoma. In the trial, each of these regimens produced equivalent results. The disease-free survival was 35 to 40 percent of patients: a 4-year survival of 36 percent in the patients who received CHOP, 34 percent in the m-BACOD group, 45 percent in those treated with ProMACE/CytaBOM, and 39 percent in the MACOP-B group (P = .14). CHOP chemotherapy was the safest regimen, with an only 1 percent fatality rate from drug toxicity compared to 6 percent fatality in the MACOP-B arm. The improved complete response rates in the single-institution phase II clinical trial largely resulted from enrollment of patients with favorable IPI scores. The more intensive regimens offered no improvement in the remission rate, disease-free survival, and overall survival. The IPI was developed in part to allow comparison of the subgroups of patients in the different clinical trials so that accurate assessments of the chemotherapy regimens could be made. However, long-term followup and studies conducted in very young patients have shown advantages to regimens different from CHOP in selected groups of patients.[179]

Other regimens that were developed but did not show improvement over CHOP chemotherapy include the CVAD regimen (infusional CHOP),[180] CHOPE (CHOP plus etoposide) in escalating doses along with growth factors,[181] and infusional CDE (cyclophosphamide, doxorubicin, etoposide) along with growth factors.[182] In one phase III study of 143 patients with aggressive NHL, randomized patients were to receive six cycles of either CHOP or intensified CNOP (cyclophosphamide, mitoxantrone, vincristine, prednisone, i.e., CHOP with doxorubicin replaced by mitoxantrone). The response rate, 5-year progression-free survival, and overall survival did not differ between the two groups. Intensified CNOP was associated with more leukopenia, febrile episodes, and secondary leukemia.[183]

Therefore, for patients with a good IPI score (0–2), current therapeutic regimens are effective, whereas for patients with poor prognostic factors (IPI 3–5), current therapy seems to be inadequate and more aggressive regimens are needed. Increasing the dose or shortening the intervals of chemotherapy in CHOP or CHOP-like regimens has been tested, with conflicting results. A study of 250 patients receiving a CHOP-like regimen that substituted epirubicin for doxorubicin compared standard-dose to intensive-dose therapy with growth factor support. This study showed no advantage of the higher-dose therapy over standard CHOP therapy.[184] Shortening the interval of therapy has been studied by using CHOP with cycle intervals of 14 days compared to the standard 21 days. The study also included two other patient groups: CHOPE at 14-day and 21-day intervals.[185] All patients received radiation therapy to bulky lymphatic masses. The study failed to show a significant difference between the 14-day interval compared to the 21-day interval. Randomized, phase II trials should study newer regimens against CHOP, which is still the standard of care.

CHOP chemotherapy is the standard of care in patients with DLBCL (Figure 96-4). Two cycles should be followed by assessment of clinical response. The optimum number of cycles has not been studied in randomized trials. Most responding patients attain a complete clinical remission following three to four cycles of CHOP; therefore, use of six cycles is reasonable in most patients. Despite the lack of data from randomized studies in patients younger than 60 years, R-CHOP is commonly used by clinicians for all patients with DLBCL.

CHEMOTHERAPY IN PATIENTS OLDER THAN 60 YEARS

More than half of patients diagnosed with DLBCL are older than 60 years. Although many of these patients are as healthy as younger adults and may be treated in a similar fashion as young patients, some older patients either are too frail or are not willing to accept highly aggressive therapeutic interventions. Patients older than 60 years with a low or low-intermediate IPI have worse relapse-free and overall survival

TABLE 96-7 COMBINATION CHEMOTHERAPY FOR INTERMEDIATE-GRADE AND HIGH-GRADE LYMPHOMA

REGIMEN	DOSE	ROUTE	DAYS OF TREATMENT	INTERVAL BETWEEN TREATMENT CYCLES (DAYS)
CHOP				
Cyclophosphamide	750 mg/m²	IV	1	21
Doxorubicin	50 mg/m²	IV	1	
Vincristine	1.4 mg/m²	IV	1	
Prednisone	100 mg/day	PO	1–5	
COP-BLAM				
Cyclophosphamide	400 mg/m²	IV	1	21
Doxorubicin	40 mg/m²	IV	1	
Vincristine	1 mg/m²	IV	1	
Procarbazine	100 mg/m²	PO	1–10	
Prednisone	40 mg/m²	PO	1–10	
Bleomycin	15 mg/m²	IV	14	
ProMACE/CytaBOM				
Cyclophosphamide	650 mg/m²	IV	1	21
Doxorubicin	25 mg/m²	IV	1	
Etoposide	120 mg/m²	IV	1	
Cytarabine	300 mg/m²	IV	8	
Bleomycin	5 mg/m²	IV	8	
Vincristine	1.4 mg/m²	IV	8	
Methotrexate	120 mg/m²	IV	8	
Leucovorin	25 mg/m²	PO	9 (q6h × 4)	
Prednisone	60 mg/m²	PO	1–14	
Cotrimoxazole	2 PO bid			
MACOP-B				
Methotrexate	400 mg/m²	IV	8, 36, 64	One 12-week cycle
Leucovorin	15 mg/m²	PO (q6h × 6)	9, 37, 65	
Doxorubicin	50 mg/m²	IV	1, 15, 29, 43, 57, 71	
Vincristine	1.4 mg/m²	IV	8, 22, 36, 50, 64, 78	
Bleomycin	10 mg/m²	IV	22, 50, 78	
Prednisone	75 mg/m²	PO	1–84 (tapered over days 70–84)	
Cotrimoxazole	2 PO bid			
m-BACOD				
Methotrexate	200 mg/m²	IV	8, 15	21
Leucovorin	10 mg/m²	PO (q6h × 6)	9, 16	
Bleomycin	4 mg/m²	IV	1	
Doxorubicin	45 mg/m²	IV	1	
Cyclophosphamide	600 mg/m²	IV	1	
Vincristine	1 mg/m²	IV	1	
Dexamethasone	6 mg/m²	PO	1–5	
ESHAP (for relapsed lymphoma)				
Etoposide	40 mg/m²	IV/2 h	1–4	21
Methylprednisone	500 mg/m²	IV	1–4	
Cytarabine	2 mg/m²	IV/3 h	5	
Cisplatin	25 mg/m²	CIV	1–4	
DHAP (for relapsed lymphoma)				
Dexamethasone	40 mg/m²	PO or IV	1–4	21
Cisplatin	100 mg/m²	CIV	1	
Cytarabine	2 mg/m²	IV/q12h × 2	2	
ICE (for relapsed lymphoma)				
Ifosfamide	5000 mg/m²	IV (24 h)	1 (day 2)	14
Mesna	5000 mg/m²	IV	1 (day 2)	
Carboplatin	AUC = 5 (maximum 800 mg)	IV	1 (day 2)	
Etoposide	100 mg/m²	IV	1–3	
Neulasta	6 mg	SQ	1 (day 4)	

AUC, area under the curve; BID, two times per day; CIV, continuous intravenous infusion; IV, intravenously; PO, by mouth; SQ, subcutaneously.

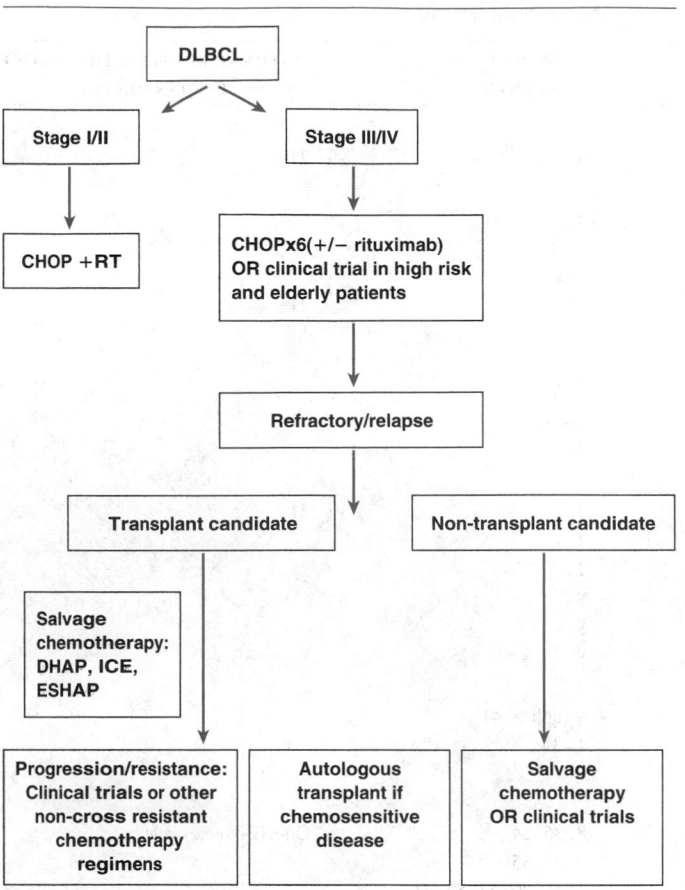

FIGURE 96-4   Approach to the treatment of diffuse large B cell lymphoma (DLBCL). (See Table 96-7 for drugs and doses of multidrug regimens CHOP, DHAP, ICE, and ESHAP.)

rates than younger patients. This status may result from the less aggressive therapeutic interventions often administered in frail patients or from comorbid diseases (e.g., diabetes, renal, pulmonary, cardiac disease).[186] Death may result from unrelated comorbid conditions or treatment-related complications. Therefore, several studies have attempted to modify therapy specifically for older patients.[187,188]

In an attempt to decrease the toxicity of chemotherapy in elderly patients, a randomized trial compared standard CHOP to weekly CHOP in which the dose of CHOP chemotherapy was divided into thirds and each dose was given once per week for 3 weeks, rather than one dose given every 3 weeks.[189] Patients who received the weekly dose had no difference in rates of complete response and progression-free survival, but they had a worse overall survival compared to the group that received standard CHOP therapy. The German High-Grade NHL Study Group showed that older patients might benefit from treatment with a higher dose of CHOP chemotherapy.[190,191] In a randomized trial of six cycles of standard CHOP (CHOP-21) compared to six cycles of CHOP given every 2 weeks (CHOP-14) along with growth factor support and radiotherapy to bulky disease, the complete response rate was 63 percent versus 77 percent for CHOP-21 and CHOP-14, respectively. In patients with elevated serum LDH, the complete response was 49 percent versus 70 percent, respectively. In the older patients, addition of etoposide did not improve the response rate.[191] This result contrasts with the results of the same study in younger patients, in whom the addition of etoposide (CHOPE) resulted in an improved response rate. Several studies have compared treatment with CHOP to treatment with an

alternative regimen substituting mitoxantrone for doxorubicin.[192–194] These studies indicted that treatment with CHOP was superior. A Scandinavian study randomized 455 patients to treatment with CHOP versus CNOP plus or minus growth factor support. The complete remission rate (60% vs. 43%), time to treatment failure, and overall survival rate were higher in patients treated with the CHOP regimen.[194] These results were similar to a Dutch study that demonstrated the complete remission rate (49% vs. 31%) and the 3-year overall survival rate (42% vs. 26%) were higher in patients treated with CHOP.[193] Therefore, the current recommendations are to give CHOP chemotherapy with growth factor support to help minimize the potential deleterious effects of the intensity of therapy.[194–196]

A randomized trial compared CHOP chemotherapy to CHOP in combination with rituximab in older patients.[197] The study randomized 399 patients with a median age of 69 years (range 60–80 years) with previously untreated DLBCL to either eight cycles of standard CHOP or to the same regimen plus rituximab 375 mg/m² on day 1 of each of the eight cycles of CHOP (CHOP-R). Complete response rates in the CHOP-R–treated versus CHOP-treated group were 76 percent and 63 percent, respectively. The 2-year overall survival was 70 percent and 57 percent, respectively. In the patients with a low-risk age-adjusted IPI, the 1-year event-free survival was 81 percent and 57 percent for the CHOP-R–treated and CHOP-treated groups, respectively. In the patients with high-risk disease (two or three adverse factors), the median event-free survival was 18 and 10 months for the CHOP-R–treated and CHOP-treated groups, respectively. Patients with Bcl-2–positive DLBCL, who may be more chemotherapy resistant, may benefit more from the addition of rituximab to the CHOP regimen than do patients with Bcl-2 negative DLBCL. One intergroup phase III trial compared treatment with CHOP versus treatment with R-CHOP, with a second randomization to receive maintenance rituximab or observation in patients 60 years or older with DLBCL.[198] Rituximab 375 mg/m² was given at on days −7 and −3 and two days before cycles 3, 5, and 7. A second study randomized CHOP-treated patients in remission to receive randomized observation versus maintenance therapy with rituximab 375 mg/m² given at weekly times four, repeated every 6 months times four. Five hundred forty patients who had completed induction and 348 who had completed maintenance therapy were evaluable. High-risk patients with IPI scores of 4 and 5 were present in equal proportions in each group (26% in the R-CHOP–treated group and 23% in the CHOP-treated group). The overall response rates did not differ between the R-CHOP and CHOP treatment groups (77% vs. 76%, respectively). The time to treatment failure favored the R-CHOP group, with no difference in overall survival at 2.7-year followup. The time to treatment failure also favored the rituximab maintenance arm, with no difference in overall survival. The addition of rituximab to induction with CHOP chemotherapy did not influence the overall response rate but significantly prolonged time to treatment failure. Maintenance with rituximab significantly prolonged time to treatment failure in patients who were induced with CHOP chemotherapy alone. Therefore, rituximab therapy may lead to a significant overall and event-free survival in elderly patients.

HIGH-DOSE CHEMOTHERAPY AND AUTOLOGOUS HEMATOPOIETIC STEM CELL TRANSPLANTATION

Several studies have examined the role of high-dose therapy followed by autologous transplantation as a consolidation therapy in patients with DLBCL.[199–202] In one early study, 14 patients with poor prognosis received autologous stem cell transplantation in first complete or partial remission, and the outcome was compared to that of historical control groups.[203] Patients who received the high-dose therapy had an overall median survival of 49 months compared to 5 months for patients who received therapy and an autologous transplant after relapse. Several phase II trials of autologous transplant in patients with poor prognosis then were conducted and demonstrated 60 to 80 percent progression-free survival with low rates of mortality.[204–207]

Randomized trials of autologous stem cell transplantation in patients with poor prognosis showed conflicting results. A group of 541 patients in remission after first induction chemotherapy was randomized to receive either high-dose chemotherapy followed by autologous transplantation or sequential conventional chemotherapy. The study demonstrated no survival advantage for autologous transplantation. However, patients who had an intermediate-high or a high age-adjusted IPI showed an improved overall and disease-free survival with autologous transplantation. This finding led to the next study in which 397 consecutive patients younger than 60 years with aggressive NHL and two to three adverse factors in the age-adjusted IPI were randomized to treatment with either the five-drug standard chemotherapy regimen ACVBP or a shortened treatment program with three cycles of chemotherapy followed by high-dose chemotherapy and autologous transplant.[208] The patients who received the latter treatment had an overall survival rate that was inferior to that of patients who received standard therapy. Another study randomized patients to either five cycles of CHOPE chemotherapy with involved-field radiotherapy or a shortened three-course treatment followed by high-dose chemotherapy and autologous transplantation and radiation therapy.[209] No difference in the overall survival rates was found between the high-dose chemotherapy and autologous transplant group and the patients treated with conventional chemotherapy. Other studies have shown an event-free and disease-free survival advantage in patients with poor prognostic factors who were treated with autologous transplantation versus standard therapy.[210] However, these studies did not show an improved rate of overall survival in the autologous stem cell transplantation group. Because of these conflicting data, high-dose chemotherapy and autologous stem cell transplant is not recommended for all patients with newly diagnosed DLBCL; only a subgroup of patients with poor prognostic features may benefit from such aggressive therapy. Abbreviated courses of chemotherapy prior to transplantation are not beneficial, and patients should receive a full course of standard chemotherapy and achieve a maximum response prior to transplantation. A consortium of cooperative oncology groups is evaluating the relative benefit of treatment with eight cycles of CHOP chemotherapy followed by high-dose chemotherapy and autologous transplant at relapse versus treatment with six cycles of CHOP chemotherapy followed by high-dose chemotherapy and autologous transplant in first remission for patients with high-risk DLBCL.[211] Future subtype classifications of DLBCL by gene expression profiling may help identify patients who may benefit from such aggressive therapeutic interventions.

THERAPY FOR EXTRANODAL DISEASE VARIANTS

Most cases of DLBCL are treated in a similar fashion; however, special therapeutic considerations exist for patients in whom the primary site of disease is in the following organs.

Testicular Lymphoma Patients who present with testicular lymphoma have a poorer prognosis compared to those with other DLBCL types.[96] Many patients relapse either in the CNS or in the opposite testicle.[97] The testicle involved with lymphoma usually is surgically excised either for diagnosis or prior to systemic chemotherapy. Low-dose radiation to the contralateral testis is recommended, and CNS prophylaxis with high-dose methotrexate after systemic CHOP (or R-CHOP) chemotherapy should be considered.[96–98]

Ovarian or Breast Lymphoma These two sites of lymphomas may relapse in the CNS.[112,113] Therefore, CHOP chemotherapy plus CNS prophylaxis with intrathecal methotrexate, cytarabine, or high-

dose intravenous methotrexate with leucovorin rescue usually is recommended.

Marrow Involvement with Diffuse Large B Cell Lymphoma Patients who present with a discordant lymphoma (low-grade lymphoma in the marrow with a systemic aggressive lymphoma) are not at a higher risk for CNS relapse.[212] However, patients having marrow involvement with DLBCL have a higher relapse rate at sites that raise the risk of spread to the CNS.[213] Patients with marrow involvement who receive CNS prophylaxis after systemic chemotherapy may have a better 5-year recurrence-free survival compared to patients without CNS prophylaxis.[214–216] Although CNS prophylaxis is controversial, such patients should undergo examination of the spinal fluid following chemotherapy to search for CNS involvement.

Lymphoma During Pregnancy Reports of therapeutic interventions in pregnant patients with lymphoma are limited. Patients with supradiaphragmatic stage I disease may be considered for localized radiotherapy as a temporary measure until the second trimester, when chemotherapy holds less risk for the fetus.[217] If the patient presents with advanced disease in the first trimester, then therapeutic abortion may be considered in order to treat the mother optimally. Limited data are available to guide therapy of aggressive lymphoma occurring during pregnancy. CHOP chemotherapy has been administered to patients after the first trimester, with survival of the fetus.[218] The prognosis of patients who receive optimal chemotherapy is similar to that of non-pregnant patients.[219]

AIDS-Related Diffuse Large B Cell Lymphoma (see Chap. 83) Several studies were conducted prior to the use of highly active antiretroviral therapy (HAART). The investigations included a study of patients treated with a low-dose modified m-BACOD regimen who achieved 64 percent median complete response rate.[220] A randomized study of 192 patients then was conducted that compared the outcome of patients treated with standard-dose M-BACOD to that of patients treated with low-dose M-BACOD. The disease-free survival was longer for patients in the low-dose chemotherapy group, but the overall survival was similar for the two groups of patients.[221]

With the advent of HAART, a retrospective study was performed that compared the outcome in patients treated with CHOP plus HAART versus that of patients treated with CHOP alone.[222] The response rate and median overall survival rate of patients who received HAART plus CHOP chemotherapy were significantly better than the rates of patients treated with chemotherapy alone. A phase III study of HIV patients with DLBCL found that the addition of rituximab to CHOP did not improve survival but was associated with increased incidence of neutropenic infections and treatment-related deaths.[223] Therapy with CDE has been studied in 40 patients, 15 of whom also received HAART.[224] The median complete response rate for the entire group was only 10 percent, with a median survival of 10 months for the responding patients. A study of 39 newly diagnosed patients with AIDS-related lymphoma using a dose-adjusted infusional etoposide, prednisone, vincristine, cyclophosphamide, and doxorubicin (EPOCH) regimen resulted in complete remission in 74 percent of patients and disease-free survival in 73 percent.[225]

HAART should be continued during chemotherapy, with the exception of the EPOCH regimen.[225,226] The goal is to reach an undetectable HIV load. The combination of HAART with chemotherapy does not affect the metabolism of these drugs and leads to improved response rate and overall survival and a decreased incidence of opportunistic infections.[227,228]

The role of high-dose chemotherapy and autologous stem cell transplantation for NHL in the patient with HIV infection is currently being studied in the AIDS malignancy consortium. The challenge with such an approach is the baseline cellular immunodeficiency and the limited marrow reserve of these patients. Seven of nine patients who received high-dose chemotherapy and autologous transplantation and who had undetectable viral loads on HAART remained in complete remission 19 months after transplantation.[229]

Recurrent and Refractory Diffuse Large B Cell Lymphoma

Advances in the treatment of DLBCL have resulted in many complete remissions with long-term disease-free survival. However, as many as 40 to 50 percent of patients with advanced disease may not attain remission with the current treatment regimens. Therefore, many patients need additional therapy. Most relapsed or refractory patients are treated with combination chemotherapy, with response rates ranging from 48 to 78 percent. Some of these multidrug regimens include dexamethasone, cytarabine, and cisplatin (DHAP); etoposide, methylprednisolone, cytarabine, and cisplatin (ESHAP); ifosfamide, carboplatin, and etoposide (ICE), and EPOCH. Several of these regimens use continuous infusion to overcome drug resistance. Single agents such as etoposide,[230] cisplatin,[231] and mitoxantrone[232] may benefit 20 to 30 percent of patients. Several new agents that may be promising in patients with relapsed or refractory DLBCL include liposomal daunorubicin, gemcitabine, paclitaxel, topotecan, and combinations of these agents.[233,234] However, most patients do not attain long-term disease-free survival with these regimens. One of the most useful measures of the likelihood of response to therapy after relapse is the length of the prior remission. This relationship was demonstrated in a trial in which patients who relapsed less than 12 months from the time of initial diagnosis had an overall response rate of 40 percent compared to 69 percent in patients who relapsed after 12 months from the initial time of diagnosis.

Many of the multidrug regimens are used as cytoreductive regimens prior to high-dose chemotherapy with autologous stem cell transplantation. Chemotherapy followed by high-dose chemotherapy with autologous stem cell transplantation has resulted in complete remissions in patients with relapsed or refractory DLBCL. One trial demonstrated that high-dose chemotherapy with autologous transplantation improves overall and disease-free survival compared to conventional chemotherapy. In this multicenter trial, patients with relapsed DLBCL received two cycles of DHAP, and, if they were responsive, were randomly assigned to receive either DHAP for four additional cycles or high-dose chemotherapy followed by autologous transplantation. The patients who received high-dose chemotherapy followed by autologous transplantation had a 46 percent event-free survival at a median followup of 5 years compared to 12 percent in patients given conventional chemotherapy. The overall survival was 53 percent in the group treated with high-dose chemotherapy followed by autologous transplantation compared to 32 percent in the group treated with conventional chemotherapy. The most significant prognostic factor in patients undergoing autologous transplant was the chemosensitivity of the disease. Patients who had refractory disease prior to transplant had only a 10 to 20 percent probability of disease-free survival, whereas patients with chemosensitive disease had a 30 to 50 percent probability of long-term disease-free survival.

Allogeneic stem cell transplantation was compared to autologous transplantation in patients with relapsed lymphoma. Relapse rates were lower in the allogeneic transplant group, although the overall survival did not differ between the two groups. However, the mortality related to therapy in patients receiving an allogeneic transplant ranged from 20 to 50 percent. This mortality rate principally resulted from the complications of graft-versus-host disease. As yet, experience using nonmyeloablative allogeneic transplantation is limited.

Radioimmunotherapy has been shown to be less effective in aggressive lymphomas compared to follicular lymphoma. In phase I and II trials in patients with relapsed refractory NHL, the overall response rate was 83 percent in patients with low-grade or transformed NHL compared to 41 percent in patients with intermediate-grade NHL. Cur-

rent trials are studying the role of radioimmunotherapy as part of the conditioning regimen prior to autologous transplantation and in combination with chemotherapy.

In summary, patients with relapsed disease should undergo multidrug chemotherapy. If chemosensitivity is demonstrated and no contraindications are present, autologous stem cell transplantation should be performed.

DIFFUSE LARGE B CELL LYMPHOMA SUBTYPES

DLBCL has several distinct clinical subtypes. The uncommon subtypes include primary mediastinal (thymic) large B cell lymphoma, intravascular large B cell lymphoma, T cell histiocytic-rich large B cell lymphoma, lymphomatoid granulomatosis, and primary effusion lymphoma.

Primary Mediastinal Large B Cell Lymphoma Histopathology.

This subtype was described in 1980 and is recognized in the REAL and WHO classifications as a distinct entity.[235–237] It is an aggressive lymphoma that more commonly affects young women.[238] It is believed to arise from thymic medullary B cells. The lymphoma cell cytoplasm often has a clear appearance and may be misdiagnosed on biopsy as clear cell carcinomas or gastrointestinal signet ring carcinoma.[239] Nuclear pleomorphism in the lymphoma cells may resemble anaplastic carcinoma or sarcoma.[239] Another feature that mimics carcinoma and sometimes seminoma is the presence of thick connective tissue that forms compartments of epithelial-like solid nests in the tumor. This sclerosing stroma occurs in a significant proportion of patients and is termed *mediastinal large B cell lymphoma with sclerosis*.

Immunohistochemistry usually is helpful in the diagnosis and distinguishes mediastinal large B cell lymphoma from Hodgkin lymphoma, as the former lacks the CD30 and CD15 antigens characteristic of the latter, and it expresses the B cell-associated antigens CD19, CD20, CD22, and CD79a.[239] Other markers that can distinguish this lymphoma from sarcomas, melanoma, thymoma, and seminoma include the melanocytic marker HMB-45, keratin, and placental leukocyte alkaline phosphatase. Rarely, ALCLs present primarily in the mediastinum with the characteristic immunophenotype L26, CD3+, dot-like paranuclear staining with CD30 (Ki-1) antigen, and epithelial membrane antigen positivity.[240]

Clinical features. The clinical presentation usually is a locally invasive anterior mediastinal mass that may lead to airway obstruction and superior vena cava syndrome in approximately 40 percent of patients.[241] Distant spread is infrequent. The prognosis of patients with mediastinal large cell lymphoma was poor[242]; however, use of CHOP chemotherapy followed by radiation has resulted in a 5-year survival of 65 percent.[242] Most relapses occur within the first 2 years of diagnosis. Poor prognostic factors include pleural effusion, extrathoracic involvement, and bulky mediastinal masses.[242]

Treatment. These lymphomas are unusually aggressive. CHOP chemotherapy followed by radiation results in complete response rates ranging from 50 to 80 percent.[243] CHOP and other multidrug regimens achieve similar response rates.[244] In phase II trials, results of high-dose therapy followed by autologous stem cell transplantation have been better than results of conventional chemotherapy.[244,245] The role of adjuvant radiation therapy after chemotherapy is debated. Some physicians report excellent results with chemotherapy alone.[246] However, other studies have indicated the addition of radiation therapy is of pivotal importance and increases complete responses.[247] Therefore, radiation may be useful, especially in patients with bulky disease. Use of FDG-PET may guide the selection of patients who may require the addition of radiation therapy after chemotherapy. Computed tomography (CT) scans may show residual abnormalities in the mediastinum, even after a complete remission. Patients who relapse may be candidates for high-dose therapy and autologous stem cell transplantation. This approach results in a 5-year disease-free survival of 55 percent compared to only 35 percent in patients with the other large cell lymphomas.[248]

Intravascular Large B Cell Lymphoma *Clinical findings.* Intravascular lymphoma is a rare form of lymphoma in which the malignant cells proliferate in small blood vessels without forming masses.[249] Other terms for this lymphoma include *intravascular lymphomatosis, angiotropic large cell lymphoma,* and *malignant angioendotheliomatosis.* The tumor cells are rarely detected in the circulation, the cerebrospinal fluid, or the marrow.[250] It usually involves the small vessels of the CNS, kidneys, lungs, skin, or other organ. Therefore, patients present with systemic symptoms and with symptoms related to organ dysfunction secondary to occlusion of the small vessels with the malignant cells. Fever, skin rash, and neurologic symptoms are common presentations.[251] An aggressive variant of this disease has been described in Asia, where the neurologic and skin symptoms are not prominent, but fever, anemia, thrombocytopenia, hepatosplenomegaly, and hemophagocytic syndrome occur.[252] The diagnosis usually presents a challenge because biopsies of lymph node and marrow fail to detect the malignant cells. Biopsy of skin lesions or even random biopsy of uninvolved skin often detects the malignant cells in the small vessels.[253]

Treatment. Many patients achieve a complete remission with conventional multidrug chemotherapy, such as CHOP, if treated in a timely fashion.[251]

T Cell Histiocyte-Rich Large B Cell Lymphoma This form of lymphoma resembles lymphocyte predominance or mixed cellularity Hodgkin lymphoma with a prominent background of reactive T cells and histiocytes.[254] However, unlike Hodgkin lymphoma, patients have a poor prognosis and present with disseminated disease with liver and spleen involvement. The poor survival is the result of widespread disease at diagnosis given that, matched for IPI to other types of DLBCL, the prognosis is similar.[255,256]

Treatment. Treatment is the same as that used for DLBCL.

Lymphomatoid Granulomatosis *Clinical findings.* This variant is an EBV-positive DLBCL that presents with extensive necrosis and a T cell-rich background.[257,258] The infiltrates can be both angiocentric and angioinvasive. This lymphoma is not related to nasal angiocentric lymphoma, although the infiltrates may have a similar appearance. The clinical presentation and course are different between the two entities. The usual clinical presentation of lymphomatoid granulomatosis is of extranodal disease in the lungs, CNS, and kidneys.

Treatment. Patients are treated with CHOP chemotherapy in a similar fashion as patients with other DLBCL. Interferon-α-2b reportedly has been effective in some patients.[259]

Primary Effusion Lymphoma Primary effusion lymphoma or body cavity lymphoma is a rare lymphoma that is principally encountered as an AIDS-related disorder.[260] It usually occurs with more advanced HIV infection and a low CD4 lymphocyte count (<100 cells/μl). It also may occur in non–HIV-infected patients and may rarely occur in other immunosuppressed patients, as in the setting of cardiac transplantation.[261] The lymphoma cells infiltrate the peritoneal, pleural, and pericardial spaces. Other sites that may be involved include the joint spaces and rarely the meninges.[260] The malignant cells contain the genomic material of HHV-8, also called *Kaposi sarcoma-associated herpes virus (KSHV).*[260–262] The EBV genome may also be identified in the tumor tissue, but its role in the pathogenesis of this lymphoma is not defined.[263] Samples of effusions are positive for the lymphoma cells, which exhibit morphologic features of immunoblastic diffuse large cell lymphoma and anaplastic lymphoma.[260] The tumor rarely spreads beyond the serosal surfaces.[260]

Treatment. Few data regarding the optimal therapy of these lymphomas are available. Local radiation therapy to the body cavity may be used and, if not successful, then multiagent chemotherapy, such as CHOP, may be used.[264] In patients with AIDS, concomitant administration of HAART is important.

Posttransplant Lymphoproliferative Disorder *Clinical findings.* PTLD represents one of the most serious complications of chronic immunosuppression related to organ transplantation and allogeneic hematopoietic stem cell transplantation.[265] The incidence is approximately 1 percent in solid organ transplant recipients, which is 30 to 50 times higher than the incidence of lymphoproliferative diseases in the immunocompetent general population.[266] The major risk factors that have been identified to date include the presence of EBV antibodies in the transplant recipient, development of cytomegalovirus antibodies in the recipient, and intensity of immunosuppressive regimens used.[267–269] The EBV plays a critical role in the pathogenesis of PTLD, and the genome of the virus can be detected in the cells of the majority of cases.[270] However, in approximately 20 to 30 percent of cases, the tissue is negative for virus.[271] PTLD may occur early after transplantation (within 1 year) or at a later time. Early PTLD usually is virus positive, whereas late PTLD may be virus negative. Several pathologic categories of PTLD include plasmacytic hyperplasia, polymorphic lymphoproliferation, and monomorphic lymphoma.[270] The monoclonal PTLD represents a malignant proliferation with cytogenetic abnormalities and Ig gene rearrangements. DLBCL, immunoblastic lymphoma, and BL are the most common presentations of monoclonal PTLD. T cell lymphoma, Hodgkin lymphoma, and plasma cell neoplasms are less common.[272]

Extranodal disease occurs in greater than 50 percent of the patients and most commonly involves the gastrointestinal tract.[273] Involvement of the grafted organ occurs in approximately 30 percent of patients and may lead to organ damage and fatal complications.[274] The incidence of CNS involvement is high, occurring in approximately 20 to 25 percent of patients.[275]

Treatment. Management of PTLD is not uniform. A wide variety of approaches, including immunosuppression reduction, antiviral therapy, interferon, chemotherapy, radiation, and rituximab therapy, have been reported. If feasible, reduction of immunosuppression is the first step in the treatment of these patients. Many cases of polyclonal PTLD may resolve completely with a reduction in immunosuppressive therapy.[276] Patients with late PTLD and more aggressive monoclonal PTLD are less likely to respond.[277] Rituximab has shown promising results in the treatment of CD20+ PTLD.[278–280] Other therapies include multiagent chemotherapy used for aggressive PTLD. Cellular therapy with EBV-specific cytotoxic T lymphocytes has been successful in PTLD following allogeneic stem cell transplantation and currently is under investigation in patients with PTLD following solid organ transplantation.[281–283]

Prognosis. Results of treatment are largely based upon case reports and retrospective studies. The largest study published to date of 61 patients from two transplant centers reported that a performance score of at least 2, the number of sites involved (one vs. more than one), primary CNS localization, a T cell origin, monoclonality, absence of evidence of EBV infection, and treatment with chemotherapy are poor prognostic factors of overall survival.[284] The overall survival rates ranged from 25 to 50 percent in most reported series.

FOLLICULAR LYMPHOMA

DEFINITION

Follicular lymphoma is a neoplasm of a follicle center B cell that is composed of a mixture of cleaved follicle center cells (centrocytes) and large noncleaved follicle center cells (centroblasts). Diffuse areas in lymph nodes may be present and, in fact, may even predominate, but follicles exist. Sclerosis may be seen in diffuse areas. The WHO classification proposes the term *follicular lymphoma, grades I, II, and III*, to distinguish predominantly small, mixed small and large, and large cell patterns, respectively. Grades I and II are treated similarly, whereas grade III disease is treated as is DLBCL.

EPIDEMIOLOGY AND INCIDENCE

Follicular lymphoma, with an annual incidence of 15,000 persons in the United States, accounts for approximately 30 percent of adult NHL in the United States and approximately 20 percent worldwide.[285] The incidence is lower in Americans of African descent than in Americans of European descent and is even lower in Asians and in underdeveloped countries.[286] The median age at diagnosis is 59 years, and the male to female ratio is 1:1.7.[287] Approximately 85 percent of follicular lymphomas in the United States are associated with the t(14:18)(q32; q21) translocation. This chromosomal translocation deregulates the expression of the *bcl*-2 gene product that functions in preventing programmed cell death.[288] A lower incidence of *bcl*-2 translocation is observed in Asians afflicted with follicular lymphoma than in individuals from the United States or Western Europe.[289]

CLINICAL FEATURES

Patients typically present with painless superficial adenopathy and less frequently with vague abdominal complaints from a large abdominal mass. Approximately 10 percent of patients present with B symptoms. The disease usually is widespread at presentation, with involvement of multiple lymph node-bearing sites, liver, and spleen. Marrow biopsy is positive in 40 percent of patients at diagnosis.[290] CNS disease is rare. The disease has a relatively long natural history; the 5-year survival is 70 percent, and the 5-year progression-free survival is 40 percent. Late relapses may occur; thus, whether any subset of patients is cured of the disease is unclear.

Staging of follicular lymphoma usually is accomplished by CT imaging and histologic examination of the marrow biopsy. FDG-PET now is used in many centers for the initial evaluation and monitoring of patients with lymphoma.[153,154] In a series of 42 follicular lymphoma patients, FDG-PET was positive at initial evaluation in 41 patients. However, its use in posttreatment evaluation for complete response after therapy has limitations, given that seven of 28 patients with a negative PET scan had a positive marrow biopsy.[291,292]

LABORATORY FEATURES

MORPHOLOGY AND IMMUNOPHENOTYPE

Follicular lymphoma has a predominantly follicular lymph node pattern, however, the neoplastic follicles are distorted and efface nodal architecture. Interfollicular involvement with neoplastic cells and diffuse areas with sclerosis may be present.[290] Approximately 30 percent of follicular lymphoma cases transform into DLBCL with a more aggressive clinical course. The majority of these cases continue to have a follicular immunophenotype. The WHO has developed a three-grade system of classifying follicular lymphomas according to the proportion of centroblasts detected microscopically:[290] grade 1 lymphomas have 0–5 centroblasts, grade 2 lymphomas have 6–15 centroblasts, and grade 3 lymphomas have greater than 15 centroblasts per high-power microscopic field. Because grade 1 and 2 lymphomas generally follow an indolent course, these lower grades should be distinguished from a grade 3 follicular lymphoma, which typically is treated like a DLBCL.[290]

The lymphoma cells usually express monoclonal surface Ig, are positive for *bcl*-2 and CD10, and express the B cell surface antigens

CD19, CD20, CD22, and CD79a but do not express CD5, CD23, CD11c, or CD43. The presence of *bcl*-6 gene rearrangement in follicular lymphoma may indicate a higher risk of transformation into aggressive lymphoma.

CYTOGENETICS

Cytogenetic abnormalities occur in almost 100 percent of cases of follicular lymphoma. The most common is the *bcl*-2 rearrangement. This translocation results in the juxtaposition of the *bcl*-2 gene on band q21 of chromosome 18 with the Ig heavy chain joining the locus on band 32 of chromosome 14. Similar to other translocations involving chromosome 14, this situation brings DNA segments containing protooncogenes into close proximity to Ig genes.[291] The Ig enhancer element results in amplified expression of the translocated gene product and, thus, overexpression of Bcl-2 protein.[291] Quantitative real-time PCR assays on blood and marrow can determine the number of t(14;18)-expressing cells and may be useful in predicting the outcome of therapy.[292]

THERAPY, COURSE, AND PROGNOSIS

RADIOTHERAPY

Patients with stage I or II disease represent fewer than 30 percent of all cases. These patients are treated with involved-field radiation therapy alone. No evidence indicates adjuvant chemotherapy in this setting improves survival or diminishes the risk for recurrent disease. A retrospective review of 177 patients with stage I and stage II disease with either follicular lymphomas grade I or II uncovered a median survival of 14 years following radiation therapy as a single modality.[293] Most patients received either involved-field or extended-field radiation therapy ranging from 35 to 50 Gy. Approximately 50 percent of the patients were relapse free at 5 to 10 years. Only five of 47 patients who reached 10 years without relapse subsequently developed recurrence.

OBSERVATION ONLY

Patients who present with follicular lymphoma, particularly grades I and II, may have an indolent course with no firm evidence that their disease can be cured. Thus, a "watch and wait" approach is often used for patients with stage III or IV disease who do not have symptomatic bulky masses, B symptoms, major organ dysfunction, or serosal effusions. Some untreated patients have spontaneous remissions and are spared chemotherapy. The reported median survival of "watch and wait" patients was more than 7 years in one study[294] and 4 years in another study.[295] In another trial, patients were randomized to a watch and wait approach until symptomatic or administered immediate combination chemotherapy with ProMACE/MOPP followed by total nodal irradiation.[296] The overall survival rates for the two groups were similar. However, the number of complete remissions and the disease-free survival rates were longer in the patients treated with combined modality therapy.

SINGLE-AGENT CHEMOTHERAPY

Responses to single-agent therapy such as chlorambucil or a nucleoside (Table 96-8) range from 75 to 90 percent of patients.[297–303] All patients eventually relapse.

COMBINATION CHEMOTHERAPY

In randomized trials, single-agent alkylating therapy was compared to treatment with cyclophosphamide, vincristine, and prednisone (CVP). Patients treated with CVP had more complete responses and shorter median time to complete response than patients treated with single-agent therapy but did not have significantly longer overall survival rates.[297,299,300,304–307] Similarly, intensive combination regimens including doxorubicin also demonstrated excellent responses for patients

TABLE 96-8 SINGLE AND COMBINATION AGENTS USED TO TREAT GRADE I AND II FOLLICULAR LYMPHOMA

Agent(s)	Dose	Route	Days(s) of Treatment	Repeat Cycle at Day
Single agents				
Chlorambucil	0.08–0.12 mg/kg	PO	Daily	
	or 0.4–1.0 mg/kg	PO	1	28
Cyclophosphamide	50–100 mg/m²	PO	Daily	
	or 300 mg/m²	PO	1–5	28
Fludarabine	25 mg/m²/day	IV	1–5	28
Pentostatin	4 mg/m²	IV	1	14
Cladribine	0.1 mg/kg/day	IV (continuous)	1–7	28
	or 0.14 mg/kg/day	IV (2 h)	1–5	28
Rituximab	375 mg/m²/day	IV	1, 8, 15, 22	
Combination therapy				
CVP				
Cyclophosphamide	400 mg/m²	PO	1–5	21
Vincristine	1.4 mg/m² (maximum 2 mg)	IV	1	
Prednisone	100 mg/m²	PO	1–5	
COPP				
Cyclophosphamide	400–650 mg/m²	IV	1, 8	28
Vincristine	1.4 mg/m² (maximum 2 mg)	IV	1, 8	
Procarbazine	100 mg/m²	PO	1–14	
Prednisone	40 mg/m²	PO	1–14	
CHOP				
Cyclophosphamide	750 mg/m²	IV	1	21
Doxorubicin	50 mg/m²	IV	1	
Vincristine	1.4 mg/m²	IV	1	
Prednisone	100 mg	PO	1–5	
FND				
Fludarabine	25 mg/m²	IV	1–3	28
Mitoxantrone	10 mg/m²	IV	1	
Dexamethasone	20 mg	IV or PO	1–5	
CF				
Cyclophosphamide	600–1000 mg/m²	IV	1	
Fludarabine	20 mg/m²	IV	1–5	21–28
F CNOP				
Fludarabine	25 mg/m²	IV	1–5	28
Cyclophosphamide	750 mg/m²	IV	1	
Mitoxantrone	12 mg/m²	IV	1	
Vincristine	1.4 mg/m² (maximum 2 mg)	IV	1	
Prednisone	100 mg	PO	1	

with follicular lymphoma, but no evidence indicates such treatment prolongs survival[308–311] (see "Observation Alone" above).

Approximately 90 percent of relapsed follicular lymphoma patients responded to fludarabine, mitoxantrone, and dexamethasone, with 50 percent complete responses.[312] Twenty-seven of 27 previously untreated follicular lymphoma patients responded to a combination of cyclophosphamide and fludarabine, with greater than 90 percent complete responses.[313] Similar responses were reported with three courses of full-dose fludarabine followed by six to eight courses of CNOP, with 96 percent responses and 65 percent complete responses.[314] In patients with multiple recurrences, four of six patients responded to the proteasome inhibitor bortezomib.[315]

RITUXIMAB THERAPY
Rituximab, an anti-CD20 human–mouse chimeric monoclonal antibody, has been approved by the US Food and Drug Administration as

a second-line treatment option for treatment of follicular lymphoma.[316,317] Response rates of 50 percent following a dose of 375 mg/m² given weekly for 4 weeks to previously treated patients have been reported. The majority of responses were partial responses; the complete response rate was only 6 percent. The median time to progression was 13 months after a response. Using an extended 8-week schedule of rituximab in 35 evaluable patients, the overall response rate was 60 percent; the complete response rate was 14 percent, and the median time to progression was approximately 19 months.[318] In a study of 38 patients with follicular lymphoma who received rituximab as initial and maintenance therapy, administered in courses every 6 months, the overall response rate was 76 percent, with a complete response rate of 37 percent and a median progression-free survival of 34 months[319,320] (Table 96-9). Preliminary studies with several other monoclonal antibodies, including anti-CD22, anti-CD80, and HU1D10, showed safety and efficacy in patients with follicular lymphoma.[321]

TABLE 96-9   RITUXIMAB MONOTHERAPY IN PATIENTS WITH FOLLICULAR AND LOW-GRADE LYMPHOMA

DISEASE	NO. OF PATIENTS	PRIOR THERAPY	DOSE LEVEL OF RITUXIMAB	DOSES OF RITUXIMAB	COMPLETE RESPONSE (% OF PATIENTS)	TOTAL RESPONSE (% OF PATIENTS)	MEDIAN DURATION OF RESPONSE (MONTHS)	REFERENCE
LGL	33	Yes	375 mg/m²	4	9 (6)	15%	13	317
FL	118					60%		
Bulky LGL	9	Yes	375 mg/m²	4	0	0	8.1	373
Bulky FL	22				1 (4)	12 (55)		
FL	30	Yes	375 mg/m²	4	5 (17)	14 (47)	6.7	374
LGL	22	No	375 mg/m²	4*	22 (37)	15 (70)	34	319,320
FL	38					29 (76)		
FL	50	No	375 mg/m²	4	13 (26)	37 (73)	NA	318
LGL	7	Yes	375 mg/m²	8	5 (14)	1 (14)	19.4+	375
FL	29					20(69)		
FL	17	Yes	375 mg/m²	6	8 (47)	13 (76)	N/A	376

* This protocol included maintenance rituximab at 6-month intervals in responders.
FL, follicular lymphoma; LGL, low-grade lymphoma; NA, not available.

RITUXIMAB PLUS CHEMOTHERAPY

A number of studies combining rituximab with chemotherapy have reported high overall and complete response rates. In a phase II study of patients with follicular lymphoma treated with six infusions of rituximab and six cycles of CHOP therapy, 30 of 31 patients responded with median response duration greater than 64 months. Seven of eight patients in whom Bcl-2 was detected in blood and/or marrow cells before treatment became Bcl-2 negative by PCR measurement after completion of therapy[291] (Table 96-10). The serial pattern of detection of the t(14;18) translocation in blood and marrow may have an important correlation with clinical outcome. Patients who never became PCR negative had a high risk of relapse in contrast to patients who were persistently PCR negative.

MONOCLONAL ANTIBODY CONJUGATED TO A RADIOISOTOPE

Anti-CD20 radioimmunoconjugates, which chelate the isotopes ^{131}Iodine (^{131}I) and ^{90}Yttrium (^{90}Y) to murine monoclonal antibodies, have been approved by the US Food and Drug Administration for treatment of refractory low-grade lymphoma. Radioimmunoconjugates are an attractive therapeutic option for lymphomas because (1) they have an inherent sensitivity to radiotherapy, (2) their local emission of ionizing radiation by radiolabeled antibodies may kill cells with or without the target antigen in close proximity to the bound antibody, and (3) penetrating radiation may obviate the problem of limited antibody penetration into bulky, poorly vascularized tumors. Several trials have demonstrated excellent responses in patients with

follicular lymphoma who relapsed after chemotherapy and in patients refractory to rituximab.

A multicenter phase II study of ^{131}I-labeled tositumomab in patients with chemotherapy-relapsed or refractory follicular lymphoma found an overall response rate of 57 percent, with a median duration of response of 10 months.[322] In a randomized study comparing ^{90}Y-labeled ibritumomab tiuxetan to rituximab in patients with chemotherapy-refractory follicular lymphoma, the overall response rates were 86 percent and 55 percent, respectively.[323] In a small randomized trial, ^{131}I-radiolabeled tositumomab was compared with unlabeled tositumomab. The response rate was higher in the group that received the radiolabeled form (55% vs. 33%).[324]

Because rituximab therapy is widely used to treat patients with follicular lymphoma, determination of the efficacy of radiolabeled antibody in rituximab refractory patients was important. ^{131}I-labeled tositumomab and ^{90}Y-labeled ibritumomab both had a therapeutic effect in patients refractory to rituximab, with response rates of 70 percent and 74 percent, respectively.[325,326] Furthermore, in 76 previously untreated patients with follicular lymphoma who received ^{131}I-labeled tositumomab, the overall response rate and complete response rate were 97 percent and 63 percent, respectively, with a progression-free survival at 3 years of 68 percent[327] (Table 96-11). In a phase II trial of CHOP followed by ^{131}I-labeled tositumomab, the overall response rate was 90 percent, with 67 percent achieving a complete response. Moreover, 57 percent of patients had improved remission status after receiving ^{131}I-labeled tositumomab.[328]

The major toxicity with both radiolabeled antibodies is myelosup-

TABLE 96-10   RITUXIMAB COMBINATION THERAPY IN PATIENTS WITH FOLLICULAR AND LOW-GRADE LYMPHOMA

DISEASE	NO. OF PATIENTS	PRIOR THERAPY	COMBINATION THERAPY	COMPLETE RESPONDERS (% OF PATIENTS)	TOTAL RESPONDERS (% OF PATIENTS)	MEDIAN DURATION OF RESPONSE (MONTHS)	REFERENCE
FL	20	Yes	Interleukin-2 + rituximab	1 (5)	11 (55)	13	353
LGL	64	Yes	Interferon-α + rituximab	21 (33)	45 (70)	19	372
LGL/FL	36	No	FM → rituximab	13 (36)	29 (80)	NA	378
FL	24	No	CHOP + rituximab	16 (67)	24 (100)	27.8+	379

CHOP, cyclophosphamide, doxorubicin, vincristine, prednisone; FL, follicular lymphoma; FM, fludarabine plus mitoxantrone; LGL, low-grade lymphoma; NA, not available.

TABLE 96-11 RADIOIMMUNOTHERAPY IN PATIENTS WITH FOLLICULAR AND LOW-GRADE LYMPHOMA

DISEASE (NO.)	NO. OF PATIENTS	PRIOR CHEMOTHERAPY	PRIOR RITUXIMAB	LABEL ON RIT	COMPLETE RESPONSE No. (%)	ANY RESPONSE (%)	DURATION OF RESPONSE (MONTHS)	REFERENCE
FL	76	No	No	[131]Iodine	48 (63)	74 (97)	NA	327
LGL (2)	57	Yes	Yes	[90]Yttrium	8 (14)	40 (70)	6.4	325
FL (54)	57	Yes	Yes	[90]Yttrium	8 (14)	40 (70)	6.4	325
TL (1)	57	Yes	Yes	[90]Yttrium	8 (14)	40 (70)	6.4	325
FL (55)	73	Yes	No	[90]Yttrium	22 (30)	47 (86)	14.2	323
LGL (9)	73	Yes	No	[90]Yttrium	20 (30)	6 (67)	14.2	323
TL (9)	73	Yes	No	[90]Yttrium	20 (30)	5 (56)	14.2	323
LGL/FL (37)	47	Yes	No	[131]Iodine	15 (32)	27 (57)	9.9	322
TL (10)	47	Yes	No	[131]Iodine	15 (32)	27 (57)	9.9	322
FL								
Grade I	82	Yes	Mixed	[90]Yttrium	N/A	69 (84)	>11.7	330
Grade II	57	Yes	Mixed	[90]Yttrium	N/A	47 (82)	8.2	330
Grade III	13	Yes	Mixed	[90]Yttrium	N/A	10 (77)	8.1	330

FL, follicular lymphoma; LGL, low-grade lymphoma; NA, not available; RIT, radioimmunotherapy; TL, transformed B cell lymphoma.

pression.[329] The hematologic toxicity tends to occur 5 to 7 weeks after treatment and may take 2 to 4 weeks for recovery.[329] Growth factor administration and red cell and platelet transfusions are required in approximately 20 percent of patients.[379] These agents are murine antibodies. Thus, human antimouse antibodies (HAMA) may be detected in the serum of approximately 1 percent of patients treated with ^{90}Y-labeled ibritumomab[330] and 10 percent of patients treated with ^{131}I-labeled tositumomab.[326] However, in a small study of previously untreated patients who received ^{131}I-labeled tositumomab, HAMA were detected in 65 percent of patients.[327] Certain murine antibody-based assays, such as prostate-specific antigen, may be unreliable in HAMA-positive patients. A major long-term concern with both radiolabeled antibody formulations is the potential for occurrence of myelodysplasia and acute leukemia as late toxic effects. To date, approximately 3 percent of treated patients have developed this complication, which is the frequency of these secondary leukemias in lymphoma patients receiving intensive chemotherapy. Another delayed toxicity of ^{131}I-labeled tositumomab is hypothyroidism, which may occur in a small number of patients despite pretreatment with potassium iodide (see Table 96-11).

HEMATOPOIETIC STEM CELL TRANSPLANTATION

Autologous or allogeneic stem cell transplantation is an additional therapeutic approach for patients with recurrent follicular lymphoma. Similar survival outcomes are reported for autologous and allogeneic transplantation, although allogeneic transplant has a much higher incidence of treatment-related death, whereas autologous transplant has a higher incidence of disease recurrence. In one large retrospective study of 113 follicular lymphoma patients who received allografts, the 3-year probability of disease-free survival was 49 percent.[331] Allografts should be considered for younger patients with follicular lymphoma who do not have an initial conventional chemotherapy-induced complete remission.

Autografts are used more frequently than allografts because they do not have the stringent age restrictions and donor requirements of allografts. Some investigators have used monoclonal antibodies specific for B cell surface antigens for *ex vivo* "purging" of tumor cells from autologous marrow. In one study, detection of residual lymphoma by PCR for the *bcl-2* oncogene rearrangement in the purged marrow proved to be the most important predictor of early relapse following transplantation.[332] Several investigators failed to show benefit from purging in low-grade lymphoma; however, large ran-

domized studies have not been reported.[333–335] Unfortunately, although high-dose therapy may prolong disease-free survival, no definitive evidence to date indicates high-dose therapy prolongs overall survival compared with conventional approaches. No evidence indicates that blood stem cells are superior to marrow stem cells, that regimens that include total body irradiation are superior to drug regimens, or that the outcome of patients with follicular lymphoma, grade II (mixed cellularity) is superior to that of patients with grade I (small cleaved cell) disease.[333]

INTENSIVE MULTIDRUG CHEMOTHERAPY PLUS EARLY AUTOLOGOUS TRANSPLANTATION

An aggressive approach to follicular lymphoma is high-dose chemotherapy and autologous stem cell transplantation in first remission. In one study, 83 patients with previously untreated follicular lymphoma were treated with anthracycline-based chemotherapy, and 77 were eligible for stem cell transplantation.[336] Forty-three patients entered complete remission at a median followup of 45 months. The 3-year estimated disease-free survival was 63 percent, and the overall survival at 3 years was 89 percent. Patient whose marrow was PCR negative after purging had a significantly longer freedom from recurrence than patients who were PCR positive. The overall survival of patients treated with high-dose chemotherapy and autologous stem cell transplantation in first remission is similar to delayed transplantation, with no clear evidence that long-term outcomes are improved.[337,338]

INTERFERON-α THERAPY

High-dose interferon-α is active in heavily pretreated patients with follicular lymphoma.[339,340] Based on these results, studies were designed to determine the role of interferon-α both in the induction phase of treatment and in maintenance therapy. A number of phase III trials were designed to address these issues. Two of four trials included doxorubicin-based regimens, one included CVP, and one had cyclophosphamide as a single agent.[341–345] These studies included relatively low doses of interferon given intermittently, ranging from 2 to 6 million U/m². In one of the studies, disease-free and overall survival were improved.[341] In two studies, an increased remission duration was observed, without an improvement in overall survival.[342–344] A fourth study demonstrated interferon had no impact on remission or survival.[345] Five large randomized trials evaluated interferon-α as postinduction therapy.[342,346–349] Patients were randomized to relatively low doses of interferon-α given three times per week following chemotherapy (2–5 million U/m²). The duration of remission was improved in three of the five trials, but whether overall survival was impacted was not clear. These studies demonstrated interferon-α activity in follicular lymphoma, but a survival benefit after its use was not clear.

INTERLEUKIN-2 THERAPY

IL-2 has been used to treat patients with low-grade lymphoma. In one study, IL-2 and exogenous lymphokine-activated killer (LAK) cells had no effect in patients with advanced low-grade or intermediate-grade lymphoma.[350] In another study, IL-2, alone or in combination with interferon-α, also demonstrated no therapeutic effect in patients with lymphoma.[351] A subsequent study that used higher doses of IL-2 with exogenous LAK cells observed objective responses in three of six patients with low-grade lymphoma.[352] Because IL-2 increases effector cell number, 20 patients were treated with low-dose IL-2 and rituximab, with 11 responses observed. All patients had expansion of CD56+ and CD8+ cells and increased eosinophil counts. Despite increases in effector cells, the toxicity of the rituximab infusions was no worse than expected.[353] However, considering the toxicity and modest activity of IL-2 combinations, envisioning a major role for IL-2 in the treatment of this disease is difficult.

ANTIIDIOTYPE THERAPY

Antibody Therapy B cell malignancies are clonal. Thus, all cells within the tumor express Ig with the same variable-region structure that can be recognized uniquely by antiidiotype antibodies. Therefore, an antiidiotype antibody raised against a patient's tumor cells may recognize a "tumor-specific" antigen. Infusion of murine monoclonal antiidiotype antibodies, combined with interferon-α, chlorambucil, or antibody alone, has yielded response rates of approximately 50 percent in patients with advanced follicular lymphoma.[354–356] Several problems with antiidiotype antibody therapy have been identified, including the high cost of generating custom-made antibodies for each patient's tumor and the fact that idiotype variants within the tumor may be selected during treatment. These variants may be unresponsive to later therapy with the original antiidiotype antibodies.[357]

Vaccine Therapy The idiotypic protein coupled to keyhole limpet hemocyanin (KLH) and combined with an immunologic adjuvant generates specific immune responses in approximately 50 percent of patients treated.[358] Clinical outcome improves in patients who generate a specific immune response against the idiotype.[359,360]

Autologous dendritic cells pulsed *ex vivo* with tumor-specific idiotype (Id) protein produced a measurable response in eight of 10 patients with follicular lymphoma who had relapsed or had residual disease after chemotherapy. They developed a cellular immune responses measured by T cell proliferation, and four of the eight patients had clinical responses. Among 18 additional patients with residual disease in first remission after chemotherapy who received the vaccine, four had further objective responses. Two patients had tumor shrinkage after Id-KLH booster vaccination.[361,362]

IMMUNOTOXIN THERAPY

Monoclonal antibody specific for tumor-associated antigens may be conjugated to toxins, generating immunotoxins. Such immunotoxins may directly deliver toxin to the tumor cells. The most common toxin used in clinical studies is ricin. Ricin is a heterodimeric protein that inhibits protein synthesis by the action of its cytotoxic A-chain. The A-chain is linked covalently to a B-chain that binds galactose, a sugar found in the glycoproteins of almost all mammalian cells. Removing or chemically blocking the B-chain eliminates the cell-binding activity of ricin. Conjugating this modified ricin to monoclonal antibody al-

lows for specific delivery of the toxic A-chain to cells recognized by the monoclonal antibody. Clinical trials with antibody conjugated to either ricin A-chain or using the whole ricin with the B-chain chemically blocked have resulted in a modest responses in patients with follicular lymphoma.[363–365]

COURSE AND PROGNOSIS

The IPI for aggressive lymphomas[366] has been applied retrospectively to follicular lymphomas and is predictive of overall and progression-free survival. Follicular lymphoma, all grades, with a low IPI (0 or 1) has a 5-year overall survival of 84 percent and progression-free survival of 55 percent in contrast to a high IPI (4 or 5) with a 5-year overall survival of 17 percent and progression-free survival of 6 percent (Figure 96-5). Other predictive models have identified patients at different risks of failure with similar results.[367] Controversy exists over whether cases classified as follicular mixed cell type may be curable with aggressive therapy, whereas the small cleaved cell variant is not curable with such therapy. The proportion of the tumor that has a follicular pattern also is correlated with prognosis.[368,369] Purely diffuse cases are very rare and appear to have the worst prognosis.[370]

Patients with grade I and II follicular lymphomas are treated in a similar fashion and have a similar outcome. Grade III follicular lymphomas are more aggressive than the small cleaved or mixed small and large cleaved lymphomas and represent 10 percent of the total cases. They more commonly present with localized disease, compared to grade I and II lymphomas. However, despite the early clinical stage at diagnosis, in some series they have the least favorable prognosis of the follicular lymphomas. Patients with follicular lymphoma relapse over time and frequently undergo transformation to an aggressive DLBCL. As the transformation occurs, the follicular pattern gives way to a diffuse pattern, and the fraction of tumor cells that are large cleaved or noncleaved increases. The growth fraction increases with the number of large cells in the tumor. This transformation is associated with a change in clinical course that leads to therapy-resistant disease. Associated with the morphologic transformation of follicular lymphoma is an accumulation of genetic alterations that probably underlie the transformation process.[371,372]

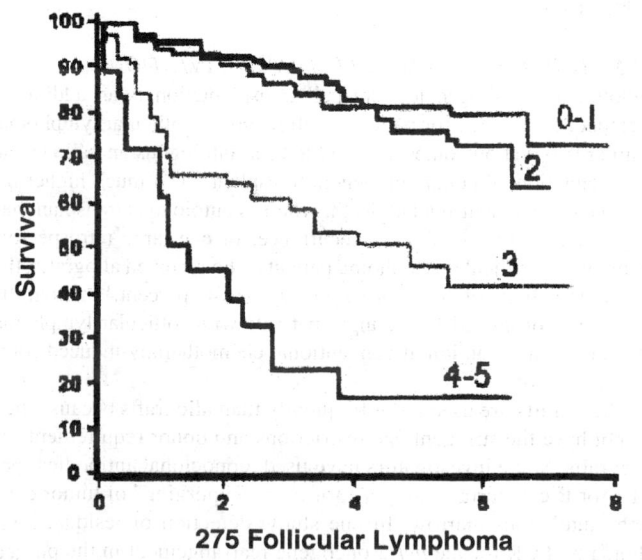

FIGURE 96-5 Overall survival of patients with follicular lymphoma by International Prognostic Index (IPI) score. (See Table 96-4 for definition of IPI.)

MARGINAL ZONE B CELL LYMPHOMA

DEFINITION

Marginal zone lymphomas are distinct B cell neoplasms with variable clinical presentations.[290] The clinicopathologic entities include (1) extranodal marginal zone MALT lymphoma, (2) nodal marginal zone lymphoma, and (3) splenic marginal zone lymphoma.[286] MALT lymphomas account for approximately 7.5 percent, nodal marginal zone accounts for less than 2 percent, and splenic marginal zone lymphoma for less than 1 percent of NHL cases (see Table 96-1).[286]

CELLULAR CHARACTERISTICS

Morphologically, marginal zone B cells have small to medium size, irregular nuclei with dispersed chromatin, and inconspicuous nucleoli resembling centrocytes. The immunophenotypes of nodal marginal zone lymphoma and extranodal marginal zone lymphoma are similar and distinguishable from other small lymphocytic lymphomas. The lymphoma cells in MALT and nodal marginal zone lymphoma are mature B cells, with intense surface membrane Ig, IgM greater than IgG, whereas splenic zone lymphoma is typically IgD positive.[380] The B cell-associated antigen profiles are similar in the three entities: a CD19+CD20+CD22+CD5−CD10−CD23−CD11c− phenotype.[381] Abnormal karyotypes are common, often with rearrangements of chromosome 1p and numerical abnormalities of chromosomes 3 and 7.[382] Trisomy 3 and the t(11;18)(q21lq21) translocation are observed at variable frequencies, depending upon the subtype of marginal zone lymphoma.[383] Transformation to DLBCL may occur.

EXTRANODAL MARGINAL ZONE LYMPHOMA OF MUCOSA-ASSOCIATED LYMPHOID TISSUE

CLINICAL FEATURES

The most common site of MALT lymphoma is the stomach, although primary involvement may occur at many other sites, including small intestine, lung, salivary gland, thyroid, skin, and other soft tissues.[384–389] Because most MALT lymphomas arise at sites normally devoid of lymphoid tissue, often a preceding inflammatory or autoimmune condition, such as Sjögren syndrome, Hashimoto thyroiditis, or, in the case of gastric MALT lymphoma, infection with *H. pylori*, which is found in the stomach in approximately 85 percent of cases, occurs.[390] The association of gastric MALT lymphoma with *H. pylori* is further strengthened by *in vitro* studies demonstrating stimulation of lymphocyte growth in cultures exposed to *H. pylori*.[388]

TREATMENT

Appropriate antibiotic therapy (Table 96-12) has an *H. pylori* eradication rate of approximately 90 percent and results in regression of gastric MALT lymphoma[11,14] in approximately 75 percent of cases, with a complete response rate of approximately 50 percent.[388,390–393] Not all responses are durable, and careful endoscopic followup is required for several years.[394–396]

Factors that suggest resistance to antibiotic therapy include invasion beyond the submucosa and translocations t(11:18) and t(1:14).[397] Patients who do not respond or have only a partial response to antibiotic therapy may be considered for surgery or radiotherapy.[398,399] Because gastric MALT lymphoma is multifocal, the surgical procedure is a total gastrectomy with its associated complications. The excellent results achieved with involved-field radiation, including a complete response rate greater than 95 percent and failure-free survival at 4 years of 89 percent, indicate the approach is very effective.[399] Dissemination occurs in one third of cases, often in other extranodal sites after long disease-free intervals.

TABLE 96-12 REGIMENS FOR TREATMENT OF *HELICOBACTER PYLORI*

DRUG	DOSAGE	FREQUENCY
Omeprazole	20 mg	bid × 14 days
Amoxicillin	1000 mg	bid × 14 days
Clarithromycin	500 mg	bid × 14 days
Omeprazole	20 mg	bid × 14 days
Metronidazole	500 mg	bid × 14 days
Clarithromycin	500 mg	bid × 14 days
Bismuth subsalicylate	525 mg	qid × 14 days
Metronidazole	500 mg	qid × 14 days
Tetracycline	500 mg	qid × 14 days
H₂-antagonist		bid × 28 days

Chemotherapy has not been studied sufficiently in MALT lymphoma. A phase II study of 24 patients reported a complete response rate of 75 percent with continuous monotherapy with either cyclophosphamide or chlorambucil.[400] In another phase II study of chemotherapy-naive patients (19 with gastric and seven with extragastric MALT lymphoma), cladribine was administered for 5 days every 4 weeks for six cycles. Twenty-one assessable patients achieved a complete response, with 24 patients alive at median followup of 32 months.[401] Rituximab also has been evaluated in a phase II study of both untreated and chemotherapy-relapsed patients, including 14 with gastric and 20 with extragastric MALT lymphoma. In the chemotherapy-naive and patients who relapsed after chemotherapy, the overall response rate was 85 percent and 45 percent, respectively, and the complete response rate was 48 percent and 36 percent, respectively.[402,403]

NODAL MARGINAL ZONE MONOCYTOID B CELL LYMPHOMA

CLINICAL FEATURES

The morphologic and immunophenotypic features of nodal marginal zone lymphoma are similar to the features of MALT lymphoma. However, the t(11:18) translocation and trisomy 3 associated with extranodal marginal zone lymphoma are uncommon in nodal marginal zone lymphoma.[388,404] In a retrospective analysis of a small series of patients with nodal marginal zone lymphoma, the median age was between 55 and 60 years, approximately 70 percent of patients had advanced disease, and approximately 30 percent had marrow involvement at presentation.

TREATMENT

No standard chemotherapy regimen exists. Nodal marginal zone lymphoma is responsive to chemotherapy, with a complete response rate of approximately 70 percent in some series, but time to progression is only 1.3 years.[404,405] The 5-year and overall survival of patients with MALT lymphoma with an IPI score of 0 to 3 are significantly greater than the rates of patients with nodal marginal zone lymphoma.[404] Use of rituximab in nodal marginal zone lymphoma has not been adequately evaluated. Retrospective series indicate transformation to large cell lymphoma occurs less frequently in nodal marginal zone lymphoma than in MALT lymphoma.[404,405]

SPLENIC MARGINAL ZONE LYMPHOMA WITH OR WITHOUT VILLOUS LYMPHOCYTES

CLINICAL FEATURES

Splenic marginal zone lymphoma is morphologically and clinically distinct from extranodal MALT lymphomas and nodal marginal zone B cell lymphomas.[380,406,407] In splenic marginal zone lymphoma, small round lymphocytes are present in the mantle and marginal zones of the splenic white pulp, usually with a central residual germinal center, and infiltrate the red pulp.[286] The malignant cells range from small lymphocytes in the mantle zone to larger cells with irregular nuclei and pale cytoplasm in the marginal zones.[286] Overlap exists between this entity and splenic lymphoma with villous lymphocytes (SLVL).[406]

A significant proportion of patients have B symptoms and abdominal discomfort from splenomegaly at the time of presentation. Patients typically have marrow and blood involvement, usually without superficial lymphadenopathy. Autoimmune disorders may herald the diagnosis. A small M component may be present. The immunophenotype is identical to MALT and nodal marginal zone lymphomas. However, analysis of cytogenetics shows allelic loss of chromosome 7q21-31 in up to 40 percent of cases.[408] Trisomy 3 occurs in 17 percent of cases of splenic marginal zone lymphoma, but the t(11;18) translocation has not been described.[286]

TREATMENT

Because splenic marginal zone lymphoma may often follow an indolent course with an overall 5-year survival rate of 80 percent, asymptomatic patients can be followed with a conservative "watch and wait" approach. In symptomatic patients, splenectomy is the treatment of choice. After splenectomy, many patients have improvement of cytopenias and disappearance of atypical circulating cells.[409,410] If the patient does not respond to splenectomy or progresses, single-agent or combination chemotherapy with or without rituximab can be used.[411–413] Seven of nine patients with hepatitis C virus infection and SLVL treated with interferon-α achieved a complete response after loss of detectable viral RNA; another patient achieved a complete response with the addition of ribavirin.[414] Testing for hepatitis C virus infection should be performed in patients diagnosed with splenic lymphoma.

MANTLE CELL LYMPHOMA

DEFINITION AND HISTORY

In the Working Formulation for clinical usage,[415] mantle cell lymphoma was classified with the low-grade lymphomas. However, mantle cell lymphoma now is recognized as having a distinctive histologic appearance, phenotypic profile, and characteristic chromosomal translocation t(11;14) involving the gene encoding the cell cycle regulatory protein cyclin D1 and Ig heavy-chain (IgH) genes. In the WHO classification, mantle cell lymphoma is described as a distinct entity.[289]

EPIDEMIOLOGY AND INCIDENCE

Mantle cell lymphoma composes approximately 6 percent of all lymphomas and 10 percent of neoplasms previously identified as low- to intermediate-grade NHL. The median age at diagnosis is between 60 and 65 years. Most patients present with advanced stage disease. A male predominance of approximately 3:1 is observed.[416–421]

CLINICAL FINDINGS

SIGNS AND SYMPTOMS

Mantle cell lymphoma usually is widespread at diagnosis (stage III or IV), involving lymph nodes, spleen, Waldeyer ring, and marrow.[422] Extranodal sites also may be involved. The disease may present in an extranodal site, especially the gastrointestinal tract (lymphomatous polyposis), in a minority of patients. Less common extranodal sites include skin, breast, and CNS. Prominent blood lymphocytosis may be a feature.

HISTOPATHOLOGY, MORPHOLOGY, AND IMMUNOPHENOTYPE

In mantle cell lymphoma, the lymph nodes typically exhibit effacement by a monomorphic lymphoid proliferation, typically composed of small to medium lymphocytes with irregular or "cleaved" nuclei, most closely resembling centrocytes.[416] Hyalinized small vessels are typically seen. The nuclei have inconspicuous nucleoli. This lymphoma has either a vaguely nodular or diffuse pattern of lymph node histopathology or, rarely, a follicular growth pattern. Some cases involve the mantle zone of reactive follicles, but a purely mantle zone pattern occurs only rarely. A small proportion of cases have larger nuclei with more dispersed chromatin, referred to as the *blastic* variant, in which the lymphoma cells resemble lymphoblasts with pleomorphism, an increased nuclear size, and prominent nucleoli. The blastoid variants have a worse prognosis than the classic form.[289]

The immunophenotype has some similarities to chronic lymphocytic leukemia (CLL) or small lymphocytic lymphoma (SLL) in that the lymphoma cells express surface IgM and IgD, the B cell-associated antigens CD19 and CD20, and CD5.[423,424] The κ and λ light-chain ratio is reversed in mantle cell lymphoma because approximately 60 percent of cases express monoclonal λ light chains. The intensity of staining for B cell antigens and Ig is greater in mantle cell lymphoma than in CLL or SLL. In contrast to CLL or SLL, mantle cell lymphoma cells express CD22 but not CD23 or CD11c and usually are CD10 and Bcl-6 negative; all cases of mantle cell lymphoma are Bcl-2 positive and almost all cases express cyclin D1.

CYTOGENETIC FEATURES

The chromosomal translocation t(11;14)(q13;q32), which involves the cyclin D1 genes (e.g., *CCND1, PRAD1, bcl-1*) on chromosome 11 and the Ig heavy-chain locus on chromosome 14, occurs in approximately 70 percent of cases.[425–431] This situation results in overexpression of the gene known as *CCND1*, which encodes cyclin D1, a cell cycle protein that is not normally expressed in lymphoid cells. Almost all cases show overexpression of cyclin D1 mRNA.[432]

TREATMENT

MULTIDRUG THERAPY

Mantle cell lymphoma is responsive to chemotherapy, but no data indicate mantle cell lymphoma is curable with chemotherapy regimens.[433–436] A randomized study of 63 patients found that CVP compared with CHOP treatment resulted in similar overall response rates of 84 percent and 89 percent, with no significant difference in relapse-free (10 vs. 7 months) or overall (32 vs. 37 months) survival.[155] However, retrospective analyses suggest anthracycline-containing regimens improve outcome in some patients.[434]

In a series of patients receiving sequential therapy with CHOP followed by DHAP, a complete response was observed in two of 28 patients after CHOP, with a complete response in an additional 21 of 25 patients after DHAP. Twenty-three of the 25 patients then received high-dose chemotherapy with autologous blood stem cell transplantation. The event-free and overall survival at 3 years was 83 percent and 90 percent, respectively.[437] A group of 25 untreated patients with mantle cell lymphoma received induction therapy with four cycles of hyper-cyclophosphamide, vincristine, doxorubicin, and dexamethasone (hyper-CVAD) alternated with high-dose methotrexate and cytarabine. After induction, most patients received high-dose chemotherapy with either autologous or allogeneic transplantation. The event-free and overall survival at 3 years was 72 percent and 92 percent, respectively.[438]

MULTIDRUG THERAPY PLUS RITUXIMAB

In a phase II trial, 40 previously untreated patients were treated with six cycles of rituximab and CHOP, with an overall response rate of 95 percent and a complete response rate of 55 percent. The progression-free survival was only 16.6 months, and even attainment of a molecular complete response did not indicate a prolonged progression-free survival.[439] A small randomized study compared rituximab plus fludarabine, cyclophosphamide, and mitoxantrone (FCM) to FCM in relapsed mantle cell lymphoma. The complete (35% vs. 0%) and overall (62% vs. 43%) response rate favored the combination of rituximab and chemotherapy.[440] In a subset analysis, a statistically significant longer overall survival in the rituximab-chemotherapy arm was observed.[440]

Combining rituximab with hyper-CVAD and alternating high-dose methotrexate and cytarabine, 26 of 29 patients entered a complete response after six cycles of therapy, with a median followup of 8 months. The relapse rate was similar to the rate observed in patients receiving an autologous transplant.[441]

RITUXIMAB PLUS THALIDOMIDE

In a phase II study, the combination of rituximab plus thalidomide was evaluated for toxicity and efficacy in mantle cell patients who relapsed or did not respond to CHOP or CHOP-like chemotherapy. The rationale for this combination was that the tumor microenvironment may play a significant role in the growth and survival of malignant B cells and that this combination would target both the tumor cells and the microenvironment. Rituximab was given in the standard dose of 375 mg/m^2 weekly for 4 weeks while thalidomide was started at a dose of 100 mg/day, and escalated to 400 mg/day as tolerated and maintained until the disease progressed. This combination produced an objective response of 81 percent (13/16 patients), with the median time to progression of 20 months.[442,443]

SINGLE-AGENT RITUXIMAB, FLUDARABINE, BORTEZOMIB

Several studies have evaluated single-agent rituximab in mantle cell lymphoma in previously untreated and relapsed patients.[444,445] The overall response rate ranged from 22 to 38 percent, with a complete response rate from 0 to 16 percent. Of interest, the response rate was similar in the treated and untreated groups of patients, with a median duration of response of 1.2 years and no difference in response duration between complete responders and partial responders.[445]

In small phase II studies, purine analogues either as a single agent such as fludarabine or in combination therapy have shown encouraging overall response rates but did not demonstrate significant differences in survival between complete and partial responders.[446–450]

The proteasome inhibitor bortezomib has entered phase II trials of patients with relapsed mantle cell lymphoma. The preliminary results look promising, with 11 of 21 evaluable patients responding, including three complete responders.[451]

RADIOIMMUNOTHERAPY PLUS CHEMOTHERAPY

High-dose myeloablative radioimmunotherapy has been used alone and in combination with high-dose chemotherapy in relapsed mantle cell lymphoma. Seven patients with relapsed mantle cell lymphoma, all of whom had received CHOP or CHOP-like regimens as first-line therapy and had relapsed after high-dose chemotherapy with autologous stem cell transplantation, were treated with a myeloablative dose of ^{131}I-labeled rituximab. Six patients achieved a complete response; five patients are still in complete response at a median followup of 25 months. Sixteen patients with relapsed mantle cell lymphoma with a median of three prior regimens received ^{131}I-labeled tositumomab at a median dose of 510 mCi and 8 to 13 days later received high-dose etoposide and cyclophosphamide with autologous stem cell infu-

sion.[452] Twelve patients had no progression of lymphoma 6 to 57 months after treatment, with overall survival and progression-free survival at 3 years estimated to be 93 percent and 61 percent, respectively.[453]

COURSE AND PROGNOSIS

The disease course is aggressive, and no convincing evidence from any studies indicate chemotherapy is curative. Median survival is 3 to 5 years. The overall response rate of 524 patients with mantle cell lymphoma treated with conventional chemotherapy in 12 trials was 84 percent; 46 percent of treated patients achieved objective complete responses.[421] The median progression-free survival was 20 months in these patients, and the median overall survival was 36 months. The IPI has been applied retrospectively to a series of patients with mantle cell lymphoma and was of limited value because of widely overlapping survival curves among prognostic groups.[422] However, in a series of patients undergoing high-dose chemotherapy and autologous stem cell transplant, molecular remission was a strong prognostic factor predicting progression-free survival.[432]

BURKITT LYMPHOMA

BL is one of the highly aggressive NHLs. It was the first tumor to be etiologically associated with (1) a virus, specifically EBV, (2) a specific chromosomal translocation involving chromosome 8, and (3) one of the first cancers shown to be curable by chemotherapy alone. It presents in three clinically distinct forms: endemic, sporadic, and immunodeficiency associated.[454]

PATHOGENESIS

BL is characterized by monomorphic medium-size cells with round nuclei, multiple nucleoli, and basophilic cytoplasm.[455] The normal counterpart of malignant cells most likely is activated germinal center B cells. The malignant cells are characterized by a translocation between the long arm of chromosome 8, the site of the *myc* protooncogene (8q24), and one of three translocation partners: (1) the Ig heavy-chain region on chromosome 14, (2) the κ light-chain locus on chromosome 2, or (3) the λ light-chain locus on chromosome 22.[348] In a tumor with *myc* deregulation, 100 percent of viable cells should be in cycle and should express Ki-67.[456]

HISTOPATHOLOGY, CELL MORPHOLOGY, AND IMMUNOPHENOTYPE

Burkitt cells have a very high proliferative rate and frequent mitotic figures. These cells are characterized by a high rate of spontaneous apoptosis leading to the characteristic "starry sky" pattern in marrow and lymph nodes, a monomorphic diffuse background of lymphoma cells, and are interspersed with reactive macrophages engulfing cellular debris (see Color Plate XXII-25). BL cells express the B cell antigens CD19, CD20, CD22, and CD79a, and CD10, HLA-DR, and CD43.[357] They lack CD5 and CD23. They lack Bcl-2 but show nuclear staining for Bcl-6 protein (overexpression independent of a *bcl*-6 gene rearrangement).[457,458] In EBV-positive endemic cases, CD21 (the EBV receptor) is expressed and is negative in most EBV-negative nonendemic BL cases.

In HIV-infected individuals, a variant of BL with plasmacytoid appearance may be present and shares features with classic BL and DLBCL. Atypical BL implies that the diagnosis of BL is favored, but the morphology has minimal atypical features and may reflect artifacts of tissue fixation and processing.[459] The term *Burkitt-like lymphoma* is reserved for cases that are between classic BL and DLBCL. These cases have different immunophenotypic and molecular characteristics than classic BL. The *bcl-2* translocation may be present in these cases. A small number of DLBCL cases have a *myc* translocation. If these cases resemble DLBCL morphologically and have a low proliferation fraction, they should be classified as DLBCL.[460]

CLINICAL FEATURES

BL may present in three distinct forms: endemic (African), sporadic, and immunodeficiency associated. These forms differ in their epidemiology, clinical presentation, and genetic features. The nonendemic cases also may have a leukemic presentation.

The endemic (African) form often presents as a jaw or facial bone tumor. It may spread to extranodal sites, especially to the marrow and meninges. Almost all cases are EBV positive. The nonendemic or American form presents as an abdominal mass in approximately 65 percent of cases, often with ascites.[460] Extranodal sites, such as the kidneys, gonads, breast, marrow, and CNS, also may be involved. Involvement of the marrow and CNS is much more common in the nonendemic form. Patients with more than 25 percent marrow involvement with malignant cells usually are referred to as having *acute Burkitt cell leukemia*. In addition, in contrast to the endemic form, only 15 percent of the nonendemic cases are EBV positive.

Immunodeficiency-related cases often involve the lymph nodes and are associated with EBV in 30 percent of the cases. Staging using the system modified for childhood BL may be better than the usual Ann Arbor system, given that BL is largely an extranodal lymphoma.[461]

TREATMENT

BL is a highly aggressive tumor; however, therapy with multiagent chemotherapeutic programs results in excellent long-term remission rates and survival of up to 85 percent of children. Applying the same chemotherapy regimens to adults has shown dramatically improved response rates.[462–464] Risk stratification allows patients with limited disease to be treated with less intensive therapy than more advanced cases and still achieve very high responses. Patients with limited stage disease have an excellent prognosis, with greater than 90 percent cure rates. These patients should not be undertreated. Patients with extensive disease can achieve 80 percent long-term survival. The regimens include seven to nine drugs used over a short period. These drugs include cyclophosphamide, methotrexate, vincristine, prednisone, high-dose methotrexate, high-dose cytarabine, etoposide, and sometimes ifosfamide.[465–467] CNS prophylaxis is given in almost all patients with BL. The only exception are patients with minimal disease, such as those with stage I disease not in proximity to the CNS. Intrathecal methotrexate, with or without intravenous methotrexate and cytarabine, is the mainstay of CNS prophylactic therapy. Radiation therapy does not play a role in the treatment of BL, and use of radiation therapy for limited stage diseases is of no additional benefit.[468]

Shorter durations of chemotherapy (i.e., 6 months) are as good as 18 months of treatment in patients with BL.[465] Other studies have shown a dramatically improved response with use of four cycles of chemotherapy as opposed to 15 cycles.[465] BL has a high proliferative rate, so subsequent chemotherapy cycles should be started as soon as hematologic recovery occurs. Waiting for a fixed period between cycles may lead to regrowth of resistant tumor between cycles. Intensive therapy may be used in children and young adults. Older patients who cannot tolerate these intense regimens may be treated with dose modifications or may require newer strategies such as monoclonal antibodies or radioimmunotherapy. No advantage of autologous stem cell transplantation in patients with BL has been observed.[469]

Patients who relapse tend to have highly resistant disease. These patients can be re-treated with chemotherapy and allogeneic stem cell transplantation because autologous transplantation is not beneficial in these patients.[470] Use of ifosfamide, as in the ICE combination regimen, may be useful for re-treatment, especially if ifosfamide was not used in the initial therapy. Standard therapy for BL, even for older adults, must be more aggressive than CHOP chemotherapy and should include adequate CNS prophylaxis.

ADULT T CELL LEUKEMIA/LYMPHOMA

Adult T cell leukemia/lymphoma is a lymphoproliferative syndrome first described in Japan in 1977 and later identified in the United States, the Caribbean, and other countries.[35,471–474] It is characterized by pleomorphic neoplastic cells with membrane features of mature helper T lymphocytes and can present as a leukemia with blood and marrow involvement or as a lymphoma with extramedullary lymphatic tissue involvement. In most cases, marrow, blood, and lymph node involvement is present initially or develops during the disease course.

EPIDEMIOLOGY

The highest prevalence of HTLV-I infections and the highest incidence of adult T cell leukemia/lymphoma are observed in Southwestern Japan. HTLV-I also is found in the Caribbean, tropical Africa, and South America. The risk of developing adult T cell leukemia/lymphoma among HTLV-I carriers is approximately 2.5 percent.[475] The mean age of patients with adult T cell leukemia/lymphoma is 58 years in Japan and 45 years outside of Japan. HTLV-I infection is more common in females. It is transmitted by sexual and blood-borne routes. A decreased carrier incidence of HTLV-I is observed among younger blood donors.

CLINICAL FINDINGS

Patients with adult T cell leukemia/lymphoma have varied clinical presentations, including an aggressive acute syndrome with leukemia, a lymphoma without lymphocytosis, a chronic process with a modest leukemia phase, and a smoldering condition.[476] Presenting features include lymphadenopathy, hepatomegaly, splenomegaly, cutaneous infiltration, hypercalcemia (with or without lytic bone lesions), and interstitial pulmonary infiltrate.

Onset of symptoms typically is acute, with rapidly developing cutaneous lesions, hypercalcemia, or both.[477] The appearance of skin lesions is variable. Some patients have discrete tumors, whereas others have confluent smaller nodules. Some patients present with plaques, papules, nonspecific erythematous patches, or erythroderma. Cutaneous involvement occurs in approximately two thirds of patients. Focal epidermal infiltration with lymphoma cells or Pautrier microabscesses is seen in most patients with cutaneous involvement. Pautrier microabscesses were thought to be pathognomonic of mycosis fungoides (MF), but they also can be found in patients with adult T cell leukemia/lymphoma. The cutaneous presentation of HTLV-I infection can be similar to that of MF but is variable and inconsistent. Furthermore, serologic studies in most cases of MF show no antibodies to the structural proteins of HTLV-I. However, in some studies the majority of CTCL patients carried the Tax sequence of HTLV-I (which encodes the regulatory protein p40^{Tax}),[478] and transfer of their blood monocytes to mice resulted in HTLV-I seroconversion.[479] The significance of this finding is not known, as Tax positivity alone is not sufficient to cause the disease.[480]

Patients with hypercalcemia typically have weakness, lethargy, confusion, polyuria, and polydipsia.

Typical presentation includes an elevated leukocyte count, ranging from 5000 to 100,000/μl (5–100 × 10^9/liter), with circulating malignant lymphocytes.[363,477] Anemia and thrombocytopenia are uncommon at presentation. An important pathologic feature of adult T cell leukemia/lymphoma is the presence of pleomorphic lymphoid cells in the blood. Not all patients have blood involvement at diagnosis, although circulating leukemia cells eventually are identified in most cases.

Adult T cell leukemia/lymphoma cells have moderately condensed nuclear chromatin, inconspicuous nucleoli, and a markedly irregular nuclear contour that divides the nucleus into several lobes. These cells are characteristic of HTLV-I–associated disease and can be distinguished from Sézary cells and cells of other mature and immature T cell malignancies. In approximately 20 percent of cases, nuclear irregularities are less extreme, and the cells may be difficult to distinguish from Sézary cells. The malignant cells typically have the phenotype of mature helper T cells[481] and express the CD2, CD3, and CD4 antigens. They also express CD25, the p55 subunit of the IL-2 receptor. Clonal rearrangements of the T cell receptor (TCR) β-chain are present.[482–485] Leukemia cells reportedly suppress B cell Ig secretion by a complex mechanism involving induction of suppressor cells after activation of normal suppressor cell precursors.[485]

Lymph node enlargement occurs in all patients, although the nodes initially may be small. Many patients have generalized lymphadenopathy, and most have retroperitoneal adenopathy. Hilar adenopathy is common, but a mediastinal mass is rare. The patient's marrow may be infiltrated with leukemia cells. Additional sites of disease include the lung, liver, skin, gastrointestinal tract, and CNS, which can manifest itself as cord myelopathy and spastic paraparesis. In addition, adult T cell leukemia/lymphoma can be associated with several histologic subtypes, including (1) diffuse, poorly differentiated small cell lymphoma, (2) mixed large and small cell lymphoma, and (3) large cell immunoblastic lymphoma. No apparent correlation exists between clinical course and lymph node histopathology.

Opportunistic infections are common in patients with adult T cell leukemia/lymphoma, especially *Pneumocystis carinii* infection and cryptococcal meningitis. Bacterial and other fungal infections also occur frequently.

Radionuclide bone scans of patients with the acute adult T cell leukemia/lymphoma syndrome typically show a diffuse increased uptake throughout the skeleton, most prominent in the joints and skull. These scans are referred to as *super scans* and are unusual in other patients with malignant lymphomas. Isolated lytic bone lesions also may occur. Typically, the serum alkaline phosphatase level is elevated.

Patients with the smoldering type of adult T cell leukemia/lymphoma have an indolent course, if they do not succumb to opportunistic infections.[486] They typically do not have hypercalcemia, and they have a long survival without therapy. Skin lesions are characteristic and occur as erythema, papules, or nodules. The proportion of adult T cell leukemia/lymphoma cells in the blood is low (<5%), with minimal lymphadenopathy, hepatosplenomegaly, and marrow infiltration. Patients have developed aggressive adult T cell leukemia/lymphoma after years of indolent disease. Patients with smoldering adult T cell leukemia/lymphoma are more likely to have a normal karyotype.

TREATMENT

In Japan, a randomized phase III trial of vincristine, cyclophosphamide, prednisolone, and doxorubicin (VEPA) versus VEPA plus methotrexate (VEPA-M)[487,488] resulted in a complete response rate of 37 percent (11/30) in patients treated with VEPA-M and 17 percent (4/24) in patients treated with VEPA. Median survival, however, was 6 months. Another study tested VEPA-plus bleomycin (VEPA-B) versus methotrexate, vindesine, cyclophosphamide, prednisolone, and doxorubicin (M-FEPA) versus vincristine, etoposide, procarbazine, prednisolone, and bleomycin (VEPP-B). The complete response rate ranged from 28 to 43 percent, with an 8-month median survival.[489] A

combination trial of pentostatin, vincristine, doxorubicin, etoposide, and prednisolone resulted in 28 percent complete responses (17/50) and 24 percent (14/60) partial responses. Median survival, however, was only 7.4 months.[490] An eight-drug combination (vincristine, cyclophosphamide, doxorubicin, prednisolone, nimustine, vindesine, etoposide, carboplatin) used in 96 previously untreated patients resulted in a 30 percent complete response rate and a 40 percent partial response rate, with a median survival of 13 months.[491]

Irinotecan hydrochloride produced a 30 percent (5/13) response.[492,493] Encouraging responses have been observed in patients who received passive immunotherapy or radioimmunotherapy using monoclonal antibodies specific for antigens expressed by the neoplastic T cells, such as CD25.[494,495] Other biologic agents, such as interferon-α, have resulted in modest effects.[496,497] Responses to combination therapy with interferon-α and zidovudine have been reported.[498,499] Allogeneic stem cell transplantation in 10 patients resulted in a median disease-free survival of greater than 17 months.[500]

EXTRANODAL NATURAL KILLER/T CELL LYMPHOMA: NASAL TYPE

CLINICAL FINDINGS

Extranodal NK/T cell lymphoma of the nasal type previously was referred to as lethal midline granuloma, malignant granuloma, and a variety of other names. It involves midline facial structures and is an uncommon subtype representing 1.4 percent of total cases of lymphoma.[501–503] The disease rarely affects Americans of European descent but is common in Asian populations and in Native Americans.[504,505] The disease most commonly affects men, with a median age of 50 years.[506,507] The pathology shows a wide variation of small- or medium-size atypical lymphoid cells with vascular invasion and tissue necrosis. This finding led to its previous description as angiocentric immunoproliferative and angiocentric lymphoma.[508] Most cases are EBV positive and express CD56. Other T cell markers, including CD3, are absent.[509–511] Nasal symptoms with obstruction, bleeding, and a nasal mass are characteristic. Invasion into the nasal sinuses, nasopharynx, and other central facial structures with cranial nerve involvement is not uncommon. Systemic dissemination to the skin, gastrointestinal tract, testis, and blood are a late manifestation of the disease.

TREATMENT

Primary disease is treated with combined local radiation therapy and a chemotherapy regimen that includes doxorubicin, with a 50 percent durable remission.[512–514] Patients are monitored with nasal endoscopy to look for local recurrence. Evaluation for EBV antibodies and antigen is also recommended. High-dose chemotherapy with autologous stem cell rescue has been successful in a number of cases.[515,516]

ENTEROPATHY-TYPE T CELL LYMPHOMA

CLINICAL FINDINGS

Enteropathy-type intestinal T cell lymphoma represents less than 1 percent of all cases of lymphoma. This is a disease of adults who often have a history of gluten-sensitive enteropathy (celiac disease) since childhood.[517,518] Some patients have a brief history of celiac disease as adults prior to developing lymphoma. Lack of response to a gluten-free diet typically precedes the onset of lymphoma.[519] Thus, the disease is common in areas with a high incidence of celiac disease. Patients with enteropathy-type intestinal T cell lymphoma often have a long history of celiac disease. The median patient age is 55 years, with a male to female ratio of 3:1. Approximately 25 percent of patients have a prior history of celiac disease.[520]

The disease most commonly involves the jejunum or ileum, but any component of the gastrointestinal track may be involved. Weight loss, diarrhea, nausea, and vomiting often are the presenting symptoms. Abdominal pain and bowel obstruction are common findings.[520] Patients typically present with jejunal or ileal ulcers, which may be multiple and may have perforated. Most patients are diagnosed at surgery. The tumors contain an admixture of small, medium, large, or anaplastic lymphocytes.[518] Immunophenotypically, the cells are CD3 positive, CD7 positive, sometimes CD8 positive, CD4 negative, and CD103 positive. The TCR β genes are rearranged,[521,522] although a minority express the $\gamma\delta$ receptor.[523] The course usually is aggressive; death often occurs secondary to the consequences of intestinal perforation.

TREATMENT

Combination chemotherapy with a doxorubicin-based regimen is commonly recommended; however, many of the patients cannot tolerate chemotherapy. Response rates are approximately 40 percent. Relapses occur at a median interval of 6 months, with a median survival of approximately 1 year.[520]

HEPATOSPLENIC T CELL LYMPHOMA

CLINICAL FINDINGS

Hepatosplenic T cell lymphoma represents less than 1 percent of all lymphomas and was previously described as hepatosplenic $\gamma\delta$ T cell lymphoma. The tumor cells have a sinus or sinusoidal localization in the liver and spleen,[524] with a similar pattern in the marrow. The cells are CD3+ T cells that typically are CD4 and CD8 negative, although CD8 can be positive rarely; CD56 and TCR-δ are positive in the majority of cases.[524] The phenotype is consistent with immature $\gamma\delta$ T cells. The disease typically occurs in young males who present with hepatosplenomegaly but without lymphadenopathy.[525] B symptoms, thrombocytopenia, and elevated serum LDH are common at presentation. Clonal rearrangement of the TCR γ gene is present, and in most cases the lymphoma cells have an isochromosome 7q [I(7)(q10)], which also may be seen in the $\alpha\beta$ variant of this disease.[526–529]

TREATMENT

The majority of patients respond to initial therapy with a doxorubicin-containing multidrug regimen. However, patients typically relapse early and have a 12-month median survival. The role of high-dose therapy with autologous stem cell rescue and other aggressive forms of therapy is not known.

SUBCUTANEOUS PANNICULITIS-LIKE T CELL LYMPHOMA

CLINICAL FINDINGS

Subcutaneous panniculitis-like T cell lymphoma is a rare disorder presenting with subcutaneous nodules that may be painful.[530–532] The lesions have atypical lymphoid cells, and reactive histiocytes infiltrating adipose tissue often associated with necrosis. In most cases, the tumor is composed of CD8+ $\alpha\beta$ T cells, but CD4– $\gamma\delta$ T cells are seen in a minority of cases and tend to be associated with a more aggressive disease. The cells are activated cytotoxic T cells that express TIA-1, granzymes, and perforin genes.

The lesions typically begin in the extremities and may spontaneously regress for a number of years but eventually progress.[530] The lesions may ulcerate, and patients may have systemic symptoms. The hemophagocytic syndrome may be associated with the disease.[531,532]

TREATMENT

Response to combination chemotherapy has been reported but usually is not long-lasting.[530,533–535] Responses to interferon-α, zidovudine, and cyclosporine also have been reported.[533,536,537] Therapy for this disease remains controversial. No curative therapy exists and standard chemotherapy may be effective, but complete responses are rare. Radiation therapy can be used to control local disease.

CUTANEOUS T CELL LYMPHOMA (MYCOSIS FUNGOIDES AND SÉZARY SYNDROME)

DEFINITION AND HISTORY

CTCL is a heterogeneous group of malignant lymphomas that share the propensity for malignant T lymphocytes expressing cutaneous lymphocyte antigen (CLA) to infiltrate the skin. MF is the most common variant of CTCL, representing 50 percent of all cases. Sézary syndrome is an end-stage variant of MF, affecting approximately 5 percent of patients with MF. MF and Sézary syndrome are the most common malignant proliferations of mature memory T lymphocytes of the helper phenotype (CD4+CD45RO+).[538]

In 1806, Baron Jean-Louis Alibert[539] described a patient who presented with skin patches that grew into plaques and mushroom-like tumors and first coined the term *mycosis fungoides*. In 1938, Sézary and Bouvrain[540] described a syndrome of pruritus, generalized exfoliative erythroderma, and abnormal hyperconvoluted lymphoid cells in the blood. Today this condition is referred to as *Sézary syndrome*, a condition seen in a subset of patients with MF.

Prior to the 1970s, cutaneous lymphomas were believed to be cutaneous counterparts of the systemic lymphomas. In 1975, Lutzner and assoiactes[541] suggested the term *cutaneous T cell lymphoma*, recognizing that these cutaneous lymphomas have significant similarities of malignant cell morphology and phenotype and represent separate entities different from their systemic counterpart. This definition has helped to distinguish cutaneous lymphomas from systemic disease; however, it also led to inappropriate use of an umbrella term *CTCL* interchangeably with MF.

EPIDEMIOLOGY

MF is twice as common in males as in females. The median age at diagnosis is 55 years. Americans of African descent have a higher incidence of MF and a poorer prognosis than Americans of European descent. MF occurs least often in Asians and Hispanics. Evidence for a genetic predisposition (germ-line transmission of susceptibility) in patients with CTCL is inconclusive. Approximately 1000 new cases of MF are reported annually, composing approximately 1.5 percent of all lymphomas. The mortality rate is 0.064 per 100,000 persons per year but varies widely according to the stage of disease. Stage I mortality is not different from the mortality of age-matched controls. However, stage IV has a 27 percent 5-year survival and 10 percent 15-year survival.[22,542] Median survival in Sézary syndrome (end-stage MF) is 1.5 years. The mortality rate of MF in the United States has been declining, possibly because of earlier diagnosis of the disease.[543,544]

ETIOLOGY AND PATHOGENESIS

The etiologies of MF and Sézary syndrome are unknown. HTLV-I originally was isolated from patients thought to have CTCL.[31] Seroepidemiologic studies, however, suggest that HTLV-I is associated with adult T cell leukemia/lymphoma.[34] Fewer than 1 percent of patients with CTCL in the United States have serologic evidence for prior infection with HTLV-I. In a series of CTCL patients from Italy, a new retrovirus, called *HTLV-V*, was isolated. The significance of this finding is not clear.[545]

A "persistent antigen stimulation" hypothesis has been proposed as an initial event after MF was observed to be a disease of mature CD4+ memory cells, but the antigen is not known.[546,547] MF also may be viewed as a disease of immune deregulation. Tumor progression is associated with decreased antigen-specific T cell responses and impaired cell-mediated cytotoxicity.[548–550] On the other hand, improved survival is associated with intact cell-mediated immunity.[551] Progression of MF is associated with progressive T helper type 2 (Th2) skewing and increased production of Th2 cytokines.[552,553] This alteration accounts for many of the immune abnormalities associated with advanced MF, such as hypereosinophilia, increased serum IgA and IgE, impaired NK cell function, and impaired cellular immunity.[554] Late-stage MF and Sézary syndrome is associated with declining immunocompetence, resulting severe life-threatening infections, and a high incidence of secondary malignancies. The latter increase is not attributable to prior treatment with carcinogenic agents alone.[555]

CLINICAL FINDINGS

The clinical presentation of MF is highly variable (Table 96-13). Cutaneous manifestations of the disease result from skin infiltration of malignant CLA-positive lymphocytes and depend on the extent of skin involvement. Patients initially may present with "chronic dermatitis" that is resistant to therapy, which can be misdiagnosed as spongiotic dermatitis (so-called eczema), "psoriasis-like dermatitis," or other chronic, nonspecific pruritic dermatoses. In addition, histologically the abnormal atypical infiltrate can be minimal and can be masked by normal inflammatory infiltrates in the skin, or it can be misinterpreted as normal inflammatory infiltrate because of its CD4+ memory phenotype.

Usually MF progresses through distinct stages of skin involvement, ranging from (1) patch to (2) plaque to (3) tumor, but it may never progress or lesions may arise *de novo*. For descriptive purposes, the skin manifestations of MF are divided into patch stage (patch-only disease), plaque stage (both patches and plaques), and tumor stage (more than one tumor present, usually in the context of patches and plaques). A *patch* is defined as a flat lesion with various degrees of erythema and fine scaling; it may be atrophic or poikilodermatous, containing areas of hyperpigmentation, hypopigmentation, atrophy, and telangiectasias. A *plaque* is a sharply demarcated erythematous, brownish, or violaceous lesion of at least 1-mm elevation with a variable amount of scale. Tumors are elevated at least 5 mm above the skin surface and may resemble a plaque or be dome shaped without

TABLE 96-13 VARIANTS OF MYCOSIS

A. Classic mycosis fungoides
B. Clinical variants
   1. Alopecia mucinosa
   2. Folliculotropic
   3. Granulomatous slack skin
   4. Hypopigmented
   5. Pagetoid reticulosis
   6. Pigmented purpura
C. Erythroderma
   1. Sézary syndrome
   2. Erythrodermic mycosis fungoides
   3. Erythrodermic cutaneous T cell lymphoma

significant scaling. Tumors almost universally are present in the setting of preexisting patches and plaques. A rare variant of MF, so-called *MF d'emblee*, is an aggressive form of MF with a poor prognosis, in which tumors of MF arise *de novo* without preexisting patches or plaques.

Distribution of the lesions depends on the clinical stage at presentation. In earlier stages, the lesions have a predilection for folds and non–sun-exposed body areas ("bathing trunk" distribution). In later stages, such as the tumor stage and erythroderma (generalized skin involvement), the lesions can affect the face and other exposed areas. Tumors may be generalized, and ulceration is common. Progression through the stages is variable but commonly occurs over several years.[556] Lesions usually are associated with pruritus, which may range from mild to excruciatingly severe, leading to insomnia, weight loss, depression, and suicidal ideations.

Erythrodermic skin involvement occurs in 5 percent of patients with MF. Manifestations range from very faint to severe, with significant scaling, keratoderma, painful fissures of the hands and feet, nail dystrophy, and nail loss leading to the patient's inability to walk and maintain daily activities. Severely inflamed skin is a breeding ground for bacteria and other pathogens, with resulting fevers, chills, and septicemia. Extremity peripheral edema may be significant in the later stages and lead to cardiovascular compromise.

DIAGNOSIS

The diagnosis usually is established by skin biopsy. Early lesions may show polymorphic infiltrations (containing mixed inflammatory cells) compatible with several benign diseases. Classically, MF lesions show superficial band-like (lichenoid) lymphocytic infiltrate. The lymphocytes may range from small to large, with characteristic convoluted (cerebriform) nuclei. The hallmark of the malignant infiltrate in MF is epidermotropism (presence of lymphocytes in the epidermis without spongiosis). Malignant lymphocytes infiltrate the epidermis, forming epidermal clusters termed *Pautrier microabscesses*. Atypical lymphocytes line up along the dermo-epidermal junction and are surrounded by a halo artifact, which is a feature of early disease.[557] In more advanced stages, the infiltrate is less polymorphic, with a predominance of larger atypical cells extending deeper into the dermis; epidermotropism may be lost. Transformation to large T cell lymphoma (CD30+ or CD30−) may occur and carries a poor prognosis in the setting of MF.[558–560]

Immunophenotyping plays an important role in diagnosis. The cells usually are CD3+CD4+CD45RO+CD8−, a phenotype associated with mature helper-inducer T lymphocytes.[561–563] These cells function as helper T lymphocytes in *in vitro* assays.[564] The CD7 antigen, expressed by more than 85 percent of normal circulating T lymphocytes, may be absent from the circulating Sézary cells.[565] The cells may express T cell activation markers, such as HLA-DR or CD25 (IL-2 receptor) and have loss of CD26 expression.[566,567] Like most malignant T cells, the MF cells stain for acid phosphatase, α-naphthyl acetate esterase, and β-glucuronidase. The cells are generally negative for peroxidase, alkaline phosphatase, and esterase. Periodic acid–Schiff-positive granules are present in some cases. Rearrangement of the TCRVβ gene can be identified. In rare instances, the classic clinical presentation of MF may be associated with an aberrant CD4 phenotype or may have CD4−CD8+ T cell phenotype.[568,569] Cytogenetic abnormalities are not consistently identified, but loss of heterozygosity on 10q and microsatellite instability may be seen in advanced-stage disease.[570] A possible association exists with homozygous deletion of PTEN and CDKN2A, tumor suppressor genes on V10p and 9p chromosomes, respectively. These may be silenced with progression of disease.[571,572]

STAGING

MF is classified according to the widely accepted modified *tumor, node, metastasis, blood (TNMB) classification*, originally adopted in 1975 by the Mycosis Fungoides Cooperative Study Group.[573,574] Cutaneous lesions are classified using the *T staging system* (Table 96-14). The area of the skin and type of the lesions were found to correlate with patient survival and are important prognostic predictors. Prognosis varies according to tumor burden.[525] The presence of tumors (T3) may indicate a worse prognosis than erythroderma (T4).[542]

The extent of extracutaneous disease depends on the extent of skin involvement. In early disease, significant involvement of lymph nodes and blood is unlikely. However, lymphadenopathy is present in approximately half of patients and increases with progressive cutaneous involvement.[576,577] Lymph nodes are assigned *N category* in the TNMB staging of MF (see Table 96-14). CT scans are used to assess pretreatment involvement of intraabdominal lymph nodes.[578–580]

Histopathologic examination of affected lymph nodes may show partial or complete effacement of normal architecture, with a monomorphic infiltrate of MF cells. In most lymph nodes, the architecture is not effaced, and dermatopathic changes with varying numbers of atypical lymphocytes in the T cell paracortical areas of the node are frequently present. Even the presence of dermatopathic changes alone in the lymph nodes carries prognostic significance[556,575] (see Tables 96-14 and 96-15). The current N staging is being reevaluated.[581] Abnormal lymph nodes should be biopsied regardless of the T stage.

Metastatic disease is the most significant prognostic predictor (see Tables 96-14 and 96-15). Patients with visceral involvement that includes liver, spleen, pleura, and lung have a median survival of less than 1 year.[582] Blood involvement may be an important predictor of progression and survival.[583] The number of circulating Sézary cells increases with advancing disease, and the cells are particularly prominent in patients with generalized erythroderma. However, even in early disease, a high frequency of clonal T cells in the blood may be detected using a highly sensitive PCR technique, suggesting that early

TABLE 96-14 TNMB CLASSIFICATION OF MYCOSIS FUNGOIDES

T: Skin

T0: Clinically and/or histopathologically suspect lesions

T1: Limited plaques, papules, or eczematous patches covering <10% of the skin surface

T2: Generalized plaques, papules, or erythematous patches covering 10% of the skin surface

T3: Tumors (≥1)

T4: Generalized erythroderma

N: Lymph nodes

N0: No clinically abnormal peripheral lymph nodes, pathology negative for CTCL

N1: Clinically abnormal peripheral lymph nodes, pathology negative for CTCL

N2: No clinically abnormal peripheral lymph nodes, pathology positive for CTCL

N3: Clinically abnormal peripheral lymph nodes, pathology positive for CTCL

B: Blood

B0: Atypical circulating cells not present (<5%)

B1: Atypical circulating cells present (>5%, minimal blood involvement)

B2: Leukemia (≥1000 cells/μl CD4 to CD8 ratio of 10 or higher, evidence of a T cell clone in the blood)

M: Visceral organs

M0: No visceral organ involvement

M1: Visceral organ involvement

CTCL = cutaneous T cell lymphoma.

TABLE 96-15 STAGING OF MYCOSIS FUNGOIDES

IA	T1	N0	M0
IB	T2	N0	M0
IIA	T1, T2	N1	M0
IIB	T3	N0, N1	M0
III	T4	N0, N1	M0
IVA	T1–T4	N2, N3	M0
IVB	T1–T4	N0–N3	M1

See Table 96-14 for definition of T1–T4, N0–N3, M0–M1.

systemic disease is common.[584] Blood involvement is rated as *B category* in the TNMB staging (see Table 96-14). For staging purposes, the B2 blood rating is equivalent to nodal involvement.[585] The B2 rating is defined as (1) a Sézary cell count of 1000 cells/mm³ or more; (2) a CD4 to CD8 ratio of 10 or higher caused by an increase in circulating T cells and/or an aberrant loss or expression of pan-T cell markers by flow cytometry; (3) increased lymphocyte counts with evidence of a T cell clone in the blood determined by the Southern blot or PCR technique; or (4) a chromosomally abnormal T cell clone. Malignant cells also can be detected using sensitive techniques such as cytogenetics or TCR gene rearrangement studies.[586–590] Patients with blood involvement have a higher likelihood of lymphadenopathy and visceral involvement. Marrow infiltration is infrequently detected by biopsy despite circulating malignant cells; it is identified at autopsy in 30 to 40 percent of cases. The cytologic appearance of the malignant cells in visceral organs is similar to that of the malignant cells in the skin.[591]

In the erythrodermic subset of MF, three T4 subsets can be identified (Table 96-16). In general, Sézary syndrome, considered to be a triad of exfoliative erythroderma, generalized lymphadenopathy, and leukemia, probably has the worst prognosis among the forms of MF.

DIFFERENTIAL DIAGNOSIS

Diagnosis of MF is based on a constellation of findings, which include clinical presentation, skin and lymph node biopsies (if indicated), and blood evaluation. A number of benign dermatoses can mimic MF or Sézary syndrome, and may even have TCR gene rearrangements.[592–595] Such benign conditions include psoriasis and psoriasiform dermatoses (such as pityriasis rubra pilaris, seborrheic dermatitis, contact dermatitis, and eczema), intertrigo, tinea, drug eruptions, and other conditions.

Cutaneous and systemic lymphomas other than MF should be considered in the differential diagnosis. Smoldering adult T cell leukemia/lymphoma has a number of clinical features similar to MF, but it usually can be distinguished by the presence of antibodies to HTLV-I and by other associated findings unusual in MF. However, this distinction may be difficult.[596,597]

TABLE 96-16 CLASSIFICATION OF ERYTHRODERMIC CUTANEOUS T CELL LYMPHOMA

ERYTHRODERMIC SUBSET (T4)	PREEXISTING MF	BLOOD
Sézary syndrome	Rarely	Leukemia: B2
Erythrodermic mycosis fungoides	Always	Normal or minimally abnormal: B0–B1
Erythrodermic cutaneous T cell lymphoma, not otherwise specified	Absent	Normal or minimally abnormal: B0–B1

Pagetoid reticulosis *(Woringer-Kolopp disease)* is a rare skin disorder that consists of solitary or localized cutaneous plaques. It affects young males almost exclusively. It has a benign course, and the prognosis is excellent.[398–600] It is an epidermal process, with the majority of atypical lymphocytes found within hyperplastic epidermis.[601] Although the disease usually is indolent and localized, some patients present with a disseminated form referred to as the *Ketron-Goodman variant.*[602] The histologic findings are similar to those found in Woringer-Kolopp disease, with predominantly epidermal involvement by malignant cells and a poor prognosis.[602] This variant is a disease of an activated T lymphocyte that only occasionally expresses the helper T cell CD4 antigen.[603,604] Like MF, the neoplastic cells have TCR gene rearrangements.

Other variants of CTCL, such as alopecia mucinosa, folliculotropic MF, and adnexatropic CTCL, should be considered in the differential diagnosis. The diagnosis is made by skin biopsy. CD30+ (Ki-1) and CD30– lymphomas can mimic tumors of MF; they present as erythematous or violaceous nodules that ulcerate. The course of CD30+ lymphomas of the skin is unpredictable, but in the majority of cases they carry a favorable prognosis and tend to regress spontaneously. In rare instances, these lymphomas progress to systemic involvement and have the same prognosis as nodal CD30+ lymphomas.[605,606]

THERAPY

A variety of therapeutic modalities produce remissions in most patients with MF. Cure is uncommon and possible only in early disease. In general, MF therapy is divided into (1) skin-directed therapy (SDT) and (2) systemic therapy (Table 96-17). SDT is the mainstream therapy in early disease but can be used only as an adjunct in systemic disease.

SKIN-DIRECTED THERAPY

Topical Glucocorticoids These agents are effective during early stages of MF. They are limited to temporary short-term use because of suppression of collagen synthesis (skin atrophy), striae formation, hypopigmentation, and secondary infections. The class of topical preparation depends on the area and the site of involvement. Ultrapotent topical glucocorticoids should not be used on the face, neck, and intertriginous areas. Topical steroids are rarely used as monotherapy.

TABLE 96-17 THERAPEUTIC OPTION FOR MYCOSIS FUNGOIDES AND SÉZARY SYNDROME

SKIN-DIRECTED THERAPY	SYSTEMIC THERAPY
Topical Therapy	Immunomodulators
• Topical glucocorticoids	• Interferon-α
• Nitrogen mustard (mechlorethamine)	• Extracorporeal photophoresis (ECP)
• Carmustine (BCNU, nitrosourea)	Direct Elimination of Malignant Cells
• Retinoids (bexarotene, tretinoin)	• ONTAK (DAB$_{389}$-Interleukin-2)
• Topical tacrolimus (Protopic)	• Alemtuzumab (Campath)
• Imiquimod (Aldara)	Retinoids
Light Therapy	• Oral bexarotene (Targretin)
• UVB and PUVA	• Acitretin (Soriatane)
• Photodynamic therapy	• Isotretinoin (Accutane)
	Chemotherapy
	(alone and in combinations)
	• Prednisone, methotrexate
	• Cyclophosphamide; chlorambucil
	• Pentostatin, cladribine, fludarabine, other

PUVA, psoralen and ultraviolet radiation of the A spectrum; UVB, ultraviolet radiation of the B spectrum.

Topical Tacrolimus (Protopic). Topical tacrolimus has been approved for use in atopic dermatitis. It is as effective as mid- to low-potency glucocorticoids for use on facial skin and intertriginous areas in patients with MF. A major advantage of tacrolimus compared with steroids is that it does not suppress collagen synthesis and therefore does not cause skin atrophy.[607]

Topical Nitrogen Mustard This drug is used predominantly in patients with early cutaneous stages of disease. In more advanced stages, this approach is used to supplement other therapies. The major advantage of topical therapy is its relative nontoxicity. Disadvantages include the inconvenience of daily application to large areas of skin, allergic reactions in up to half of cases,[608] the potential for development of skin cancer,[609] and the inability to cure the disease. Nitrogen mustard 10 mg diluted in 60 ml of tap water or 60 g of a water-miscible cream or an anhydrous ointment, which may have less allergic sensitization, is administered daily using a cotton swab or small paint brush. Therapy is continued for up to 12 months in responders. Frequency then is reduced to every other day for an additional 1 to 2 years. Therapy is discontinued after 3 years or when cutaneous lesions disappear completely.

Topical Carmustine (BCNU) Carmustine is not currently widely used for treatment of MF because of its severe irritant reactions and its absorption from the skin that results in systemic toxicity. The preparation ranges from 20 to 40 mg percent in petrolatum ointment. It is applied at night and washed off in the morning. Monitoring includes biweekly complete blood counts to identify marrow suppression. Carmustine causes irreversible skin thinning, telangiectasias, and hyperpigmentation.[610]

Topical Retinoids Bexarotene (Targretin) 1 percent gel is the topical retinoid most commonly used for MF. It is a small lipophilic molecule that is related to vitamin A. It readily crosses the cytoplasmic membrane and binds to nuclear receptors (retinoid X receptors), resulting in changes in gene expression mediated through specific intracellular receptors. Complete responses of 20 percent and overall responses of 60 percent are reported.[611,612] It is applied in a thin layer to the patches and plaques twice daily. The major toxicity is irritation at the site. Topical bexarotene is FDA approved for treatment of MF patients who are refractory to at least one other topical therapy. Oral administration of bexarotene is associated with severe birth defects. Considering potential absorption of the drug from the skin surface, bexarotene should not be given to pregnant women.

Phototherapy Several means of phototherapy currently are available for treatment of MF. They include ultraviolet radiation of the A (UVA) and B (UVB) spectra. UVB therapy and narrow-band UVB both are effective in the treatment of early disease (patches and thin plaques). Phototherapy may result in complete clearing of the lesions. Therapy should be instituted at least three times per week. On average, 4 to 6 weeks are required to achieve the response. Maintenance therapy is required after a response occurs and consists of once weekly UVB irradiation for the long term. The main side effects are related to acute burning because of inadequate dosage. The incidence of skin cancers increases slightly when therapy is used long term.[613–615]

Phototherapy involving UVA radiation is used with psoralen and is referred to as *PUVA*. Psoralen is a phototoxic furocoumarin activated by UVA light. In its active form, psoralen bonds covalently and irreversibly to DNA. UVA light penetrates only the upper part of the dermis. Therefore, psoralen activated by UVA light affects cells primarily in the epidermis and papillary dermis. A 60 percent complete remission rate and long-term remissions (>10 years) have been reported with PUVA; patients with generalized erythroderma and tumors have lower response rates than patients with plaques.[616–618] Psoralen usually is given at a dose of 0.6 mg/kg orally, 2 hours before the UVA light therapy. Treatments initially are given three times per week.

Maintenance therapy may be given every 2 to 4 weeks for an indefinite period. Adverse effects of PUVA therapy include mild nausea, pruritus, and sunburn-like changes, with atrophy and dry skin. PUVA is not cross resistant with other treatment modalities. Disadvantages of PUVA therapy are its inability to cure and its expense. Long-term side effects include an increased incidence of skin cancers and melanoma.

Photodynamic therapy is a new type of photochemotherapy that utilizes two properties of porphyrins: their selective accumulation of porphyrins in the tumor (e.g., 5-aminolevulinic acid) and their ability to generate cytotoxic oxygen species at the tumor site after red-light irradiation. 5-Aminolevulinic acid is a natural porphyrin precursor and upon irradiation is converted in the tumor to the highly photoactive endogenous protoporphyrin IX. Red-light irradiation is safe and penetrates deep in the tissue, allowing for treatment of thick tumors. Photodynamic therapy is especially useful in patients with limited skin area involved by few tumors. The main problem with the treatment is that the pain induced during irradiation limits its use for larger areas.[619,620]

Extracorporeal Photopheresis PUVA can be delivered by an extracorporeal technique.[621,622] White cells are collected by leukapheresis, exposed to a photoactivating drug, and irradiated with UVA. The cells then are reinfused into the patient. The effect may be both a direct cytotoxic effect on the tumor cells and an immunologic effect by activating lymphocytes against the tumor cells. Photopheresis typically is administered every 2 to 4 weeks until clearance of disease. Side effects are minimal and may be related to fluid shifts during procedure.

Total Skin Electron Beam Therapy Electron beam therapy penetrates only into the upper dermis. Systemic effects are minimal, and the complete remission rate is 80 percent.[623–625] Twenty percent of patients remain relapse free at 3 years. The relapse rate depends on the stage of the disease, and the relapse usually is short lived (may be as short as 2–3 weeks) in patients with erythroderma or numerous tumors. Typically, treatment is 4 Gy per week to a total dose of 36 Gy in 8 to 9 weeks. The advantage of electron beam therapy is the high frequency of durable complete responses without systemic toxicity. Disadvantages are alopecia, atrophy, edema, dermatitis, and increased risk of cutaneous malignancy. Up to three courses of electron beam therapy can be safely administered when used in a highly fractionated fashion (1 Gy per dose).

Imiquimod (Aldara) Imiquimod is a new topical immunomodulator that is extremely effective in the treatment of condylomata acuminata, actinic keratoses, basal cell carcinomas, keratoacanthomas, and other cutaneous malignancies. The mode of action is not known but is thought to be related to induction of tumor necrosis factor-α and interferons resulting in activation of Th1-type immune response and rejection of cancer or virally infected cells. Several groups reported the effectiveness of imiquimod in early patch MF.[626,627] It should be used three times per week for 3 months. Long-term followup is not available at this time.

SYSTEMIC THERAPY

Interferon-α Interferon-α can be used as a single agent or combined with other systemic therapies. The response rate when interferon-α is used as a monotherapy is 50 to 70 percent at doses beginning at 3 to 5 × 10^6 units/day or three times per week.[628] Toxicity includes acute flu-like symptoms and fatigue.

Monoclonal Antibodies Alemtuzumab (Campath-1H) is a humanized IgG1 monoclonal antibody that targets the CD52 antigen. Response rates of 50 percent in a small cohort of patients have been reported.[629,630]

Recombinant Fusion Proteins Denileukin diftitox (ONTAK) is an IL-2 diphtheria toxin fusion protein. The safety and efficacy of denileukin diftitox in patients with MF was examined in a phase III trial of 71 patients who had not responded to a median of five prior therapies. Denileukin diftitox was administered in two doses: 9 μg/kg/day or 18 μg/kg/day for 5 consecutive days. The overall response rate was 30 percent of patients, with 10 percent of those treated achieving a complete remission.[631] There was no dose-response relationship, but patients with more advanced disease (stage IIB or higher) had a greater likelihood of response at the higher dose ($P = .07$). The median time to response was 6 weeks, and the duration of response in this trial was approximately 7 months.

Side effects are numerous, including a capillary leak syndrome. Other side effects are infection, hepatitis, increased fluid retention, rash, shortness of breath, and flu-like symptoms such as chills, fever, weakness, bone and muscle pain, headache, nausea, and vomiting. Cardiac arrhythmias and thrombotic emergencies have been reported occasionally.

Chemotherapy The largest experience with single-agent chemotherapy is with alkylating agents, including nitrogen mustard 0.4 mg/kg given intravenously every 4 to 6 weeks, cyclophosphamide, or chlorambucil. Response rates of 60 percent, with 15 percent complete remissions, have been reported.[632,633] Similar results are obtained with methotrexate 2.5 to 10 mg/day orally[634]; bleomycin 7.5 to 15 mg intramuscularly given twice weekly; and doxorubicin 60 mg/m² intravenously given once per month.[635,636] Pegylated doxorubicin used in advanced MF has resulted in an overall response of 88 percent.[637] Purine analogues including fludarabine and pentostatin have response rates as high as 50 percent.[638–640] Gemcitabine has a similar response rate.[641] Single-agent therapy does not cure MF. Chemotherapy with a single agent and polychemotherapy result in a higher incidence of transformation to large cell lymphoma, which carries a worse prognosis than the original diagnosis.[642,643] Because responses to therapy are generally higher after combination therapy, single-agent chemotherapy is used rarely. Combination therapy produces objective responses in greater than 80 percent of patients and complete responses in approximately one fourth of cases.[618,644] Duration of remission varies, with a median of approximately 1 year. No long-term disease-free survival has been reported.

Combined Modality Therapy Several multidrug regimens reportedly improve clinical response in patients with MF, including combination of extracorporeal photophoresis with low-dose interferon-α and oral bexarotene; prednisone and fludarabine; and PUVA and oral bexarotene.[624,645]

Because in general MF is an indolent malignancy of T cells with excellent prognosis in early stages, the treatment should be conservative, with skin-directed therapies (nitrogen mustard, topical glucocorticoids, topical bexarotene) combined with light therapy, low-dose interferon, low-dose methotrexate, or other single-agent chemotherapy. The survival of patients treated with aggressive chemotherapy is not different from the survival of patients treated conservatively, but aggressive chemotherapy results in greater toxicity. Because no curative therapy exists, the goal of therapy is to prevent progression to more advanced stages and to preserve the patient's quality of life for as long as possible.

PROGNOSIS

Prognosis largely depends on the stage at presentation. Fifty percent of deaths among patients with MF result from infections. Septicemia and bacterial pneumonia are common; they usually are caused by *Staphylococcus* or *Pseudomonas* and develop from cutaneous lesions.[556] Herpes virus infections occur in up to 10 percent of patients with advanced MF. Progressive MF with widespread visceral involvement late in the course of the disease is the next most common cause of death.

PRIMARY CUTANEOUS ANAPLASTIC LARGE CELL LYMPHOMA

CLINICAL FINDINGS

CD30+ cutaneous lymphoproliferative disorders are the second most common CTCLs after MF and represent approximately 25 percent of CTCL cases.[646] Primary cutaneous ALCL represents a spectrum of CD30+ lymphoproliferative disorders, including lymphomatoid papulosis and primary cutaneous ALCL as its malignant counterpart. It is defined by the presence of skin involvement without evidence of extracutaneous disease for at least 6 months after presentation.[540] Secondary involvement of lymph nodes may not necessarily be associated with a worse prognosis.[541] In some cases, distinction between lymphomatoid papulosis and primary cutaneous ALCL cannot be made because of discrepancy between clinical features and histologic appearance. These cases are referred to as *borderline lesions*, and their classification should take into consideration their clinical behavior and appearance.

Other CD30+ cutaneous lymphoproliferative disorders include large cell transformation of MF, systemic ALCL, cutaneous NK/T cell lymphoma, and Hodgkin lymphoma. Making the distinction among these cases is critical because management and prognosis are significantly different (see "Treatment" below). The descriptive term *anaplastic* could be omitted from the name of this lymphoma because these lymphomas may have an anaplastic, immunoblastic, or pleomorphic cell morphology. Regardless of pathologic type, these CD30+ large cell lymphomas have a similar clinical course, treatment, and prognosis.[646–649]

CD30+ primary cutaneous ALCL can occur at any age, with the peak incidence in patients in their 60s, with a slight male predominance.[650,651] Primary cutaneous ALCL can occur anywhere on the body. The lesions are brownish to violaceous nodules or tumors, ranging in number from solitary (most commonly) to numerous with generalized involvement. They may regress spontaneously. Histopathologically, at least 75 percent of the large cells should express CD30. Most cases are CD4+, with loss of pan-T cell markers CD2, CD3, and CD5. In rare cases, the cells are CD8+CD30+. In contrast to systemic ALCL, primary cutaneous large cell lymphoma is negative for CD15 and epithelial membrane antigen.[652] In addition, primary cutaneous large cell lymphoma usually does not express ALK-1 or the t(2;5) chromosomal translocation.[653,654] Presence of ALK-1 in cutaneous lesions without systemic involvement does not carry a worse prognosis.

LYMPHOMATOID PAPULOSIS

Lymphomatoid papulosis is the benign counterpart of primary cutaneous ALCL. It is characterized by crops of erythematous, dome-shaped papules or nodules that may ulcerate spontaneously. It regresses over a few months with minor sequela such as scarring or atrophy. The three main histologic types of lymphomatoid papulosis are A, B, and C. The infiltrate usually is wedge shaped with ulcer formation. The large atypical cells of type A resemble immunoblasts of Reed-Sternberg cells. These cells are surrounded by neutrophils and eosinophils. Type B cells resemble MF, with lichenoid lymphocytic infiltrate of cells with cerebriform nuclei and some epidermotropism. Type C cells resemble ALCL, with sheets of large CD30+ cells in the infiltrate. The histologic distinction between lymphomatoid papulosis and the corresponding condition may be difficult, and clinical correlation is required.[655] In rare cases, lymphomatoid papulosis evolves into more aggressive primary cutaneous large cell lymphoma. In addition, a higher incidence of lymphoid and nonlymphoid malignancies is observed in patients with lymphomatoid papulosis.[656]

TREATMENT

Lymphomatoid papulosis is extremely responsive to low-dose methotrexate therapy, requiring 10 to 15 mg weekly, with noticeable clinical response within a month. Other treatment options include oral PUVA therapy, retinoids, topical and systemic glucocorticoids, and intralesional and systemic interferon-α.[646,647,655] Treatment of primary cutaneous large cell lymphoma depends on the extent of skin involvement. In cases of solitary lesions, radiotherapy should be the initial treatment modality. A combination of PUVA and interferon-α may be considered. Combination chemotherapy should be reserved for resistant cases.[646,647,657]

ANAPLASTIC LARGE CELL LYMPHOMA

CLINICAL FINDINGS

ALCL, formally referred to as *Ki-1 lymphoma*, now is a recognized entity that accounts for 2 to 8 percent of all lymphomas. The cells from these patients were first noted to react with an anti–Ki-1 antibody (anti-CD30) raised against an antigen on the Reed-Sternberg cells of Hodgkin lymphoma.[658–661] A nonrandom t(2;5) (p23;q35) translocation[662–664] causes fusion of the *NPM* and *ALK* genes.

CD30+ lymphoma cells tend to grow cohesively and invade lymph node sinuses.[665] The morphologic variants are based on the size of the tumor cells and the reactive cells.[666] The "common type," representing most cases, is characterized by large pleomorphic tumor cells. The "small cell variant," representing 5 to 10 percent of cases, has a dominant population of small- to medium-size tumor cells mixed with large anaplastic cells that stain for CD30 and ALK. The "lymphohistiocytic variant," representing 5 to 10 percent of cases, is closely related to the small cell variant and contains small neoplastic cells mixed with large anaplastic cells and a large number of histiocytes.[667–671] The hallmark for all cell types is CD30 expression. Immunostaining for ALK is highly specific for this disease.[670–672] ALCL displays a T or null phenotype, but the null cell type usually expresses cytotoxic molecules such as perforin, granzyme B, and TIA-1 and has rearranged T cell antigen receptor genes, suggesting a T cell origin.[673,674] The B cell variant is no longer classified under CD30+ ALCL.[675] The t(2;5)(p23;q35) chromosome translocation[662–664] causes the *ALK* gene on chromosome 2 to fuse with the *NPM* gene on chromosome 5.[665] This *NPM-ALK* fusion gene encodes the 80-kDa chimeric protein NPM-ALK (p80). *NPM-ALK* is an oncogene that probably causes ALK-positive ALCL. Two signaling cascades involved in cell proliferation and apoptosis are activated by NPM-ALK, and NPM-ALK supports malignant transformation *in vitro* and *in vivo*.[676–680] A small percentage of ALK-positive large cell lymphomas demonstrate *ALK* fusion to a gene partner other than *NPM*, producing variant ALK fusion proteins.[669,670] The cutaneous form of primary CD30+ ALCL is considered a separate entity by the WHO classification.

ALCL is common in children and adolescents and has a bimodal age distribution. It has an aggressive clinical course, frequently presenting with systemic symptoms, advanced disease, and extranodal localization. The T cell phenotype has a higher predilection for cutaneous involvement, with less frequent marrow and extranodal involvement.[681,682] Differences have been reported for the ALK-positive and ALK-negative subtypes. ALK-positive patients tend to be younger and have better performance status, with less likelihood of elevated LDH levels.[683–685] Nodal presentations are common in both groups, but an increased incidence of extranodal involvement is observed in the ALK-negative group.[686] CNS involvement is rare. Approximately 20 percent of patients have morphologic evidence of marrow involvement, but this rate of involvement is higher as determined using immunohisto-chemical techniques, such as anti-CD30 and anti-ALK antibodies.[687] In general, the remission rates and survival are better for ALCL than for other peripheral T cell lymphomas.[681,682] ALK-positive patients have a better prognosis than ALK-negative patients with ALCL, and 90 percent of children with this disease are ALK positive.[671,684–686] CD56 expression has been shown to be a favorable, independent prognostic factor.[686]

TREATMENT

ALCL has a high frequency in children, and a number of intensive chemotherapy regimens have been studied in children.[688–693] Most regimens include doxorubicin. Most adult patients are treated with doxorubicin-based regimens, with complete responses in approximately 70 percent of treated patients and a 5-year survival in approximately 60 percent of patients.[681,682,684,686] Patients randomized to doxorubicin, bleomycin, vinblastine, and dacarbazine (ABVD) or MACOP-B) had equivalent results.[694] Intensive chemotherapy with autologous stem cell rescue has been investigated with good results, but the number of patients studied has been limited.[695–698] The role of allogeneic stem cell transplant has not been evaluated.[699]

PERIPHERAL T CELL LYMPHOMA, UNSPECIFIED

CLINICAL FINDINGS

The peripheral T cell lymphomas that do not fit into any of the currently recognized diseases are designated *peripheral T cell lymphoma, unspecified* and represent approximately 50 percent of the total cases of T cell lymphoma, excluding anaplastic T cell lymphoma.[700] The majority of cases arise in lymph nodes and include mixtures of small and large atypical lymphoid cells, typically with an inflammatory background. Epithelioid histiocytes may be clustered and are called *lymphoepithelioid cell lymphoma*, previously referred to as *Lennert lymphoma*, which now is considered a morphologic variant of peripheral T cell lymphoma, unspecified.[701] The immunophenotype typically is that of a mature T cell expressing either a CD4 or CD8 phenotype. Deletion of any of the pan-T cell antigens is frequently seen. Rearrangements of TCR genes are common, and the most common phenotype is the CD4+ $\alpha\beta$. In general, patients with peripheral T cell lymphoma are considered to have a more aggressive disease than patients with DLBCL. They have a higher incidence of B symptoms, extranodal involvement, elevated LDH level, and stage 4 disease.[700] Although not all studies have consistently reported a poor outcome for patients with T cell lymphoma,[702–705] most data support the concept that peripheral T cell lymphoma has a higher portion of adverse risk factors and overall poor prognosis.[706–711]

TREATMENT

Patients with peripheral T cell lymphoma typically are treated with doxorubicin-containing regimens that can achieve complete remissions and long-term disease-free survival. However, both response rate and survival are lower than the rates in patients with DLBCL.[712–714] Results with high-dose chemotherapy followed by autologous stem cell rescue are similar to the results in patients with DLBCL,[715–717] suggesting an earlier role for stem cell transplantation. Re-treatment therapies have included cyclosporin, pentostatin, retinoids, and denileukin diftitox.[718–721] Responses have been reported, but none of these therapies stands out as a major new breakthrough for treatment of peripheral T cell lymphoma, unspecified.

ANGIOIMMUNOBLASTIC T CELL LYMPHOMA

CLINICAL FINDINGS

Angioimmunoblastic T cell lymphoma represents approximately 1 percent of all cases of lymphoma. Histologically, a loss of lymphoid architecture with a pleomorphic cellular infiltrate and proliferation of small arborizing blood vessels are observed. Angioimmunoblastic lymphadenopathy with dysproteinemia was described in 1974,[722] and it was recognized that many cases evolved into a peripheral T cell lymphoma.[723] Angioimmunoblastic T cell lymphoma now is considered a separate entity. Although it is malignant, angioimmunoblastic T cell lymphoma appears to be a continuum from a more benign to a frankly malignant stage.[724,725]

Patients with this disease typically are elderly and present with B symptoms, generalized lymphadenopathy, skin rash, polyclonal hypergammaglobulinemia, autoimmune disorders including Coombs positive hemolytic anemia, and infection. The median patient age is 65 years, with a male predominance.[726]

The nodal architecture is effaced with an infiltration of small lymphocytes, plasma cells, immunoblasts, histiocytes, and often eosinophils. The malignant cells are CD4+ $\alpha\beta$ T cells with TCR β and γ rearrangements[724,727,728] that may express CD10 and Bcl-6.[729] Scattered EBV+ B cells likely are secondary to the underlying immunodeficiency.[730] Frequent abnormal karyotypes are reported.[731]

Most patients have an unfavorable prognosis supported by an IPI score greater than 2. Differentiating patients with a more "benign" form of the disease, which usually is evidenced by symptoms and signs, is important. Rearranged TCR genes point to the malignant stage.

TREATMENT

Most patients are treated with doxorubicin-based regimens. The complete response rate is similar to the rate of other peripheral T cell lymphomas (approximately 60%). However, some patients benefit from prednisone alone, particularly those patients with a more benign form of the disease.[732,733] Patients have also responded to low-dose methotrexate and cyclosporine.[734,735]

DISORDERS THAT PREDISPOSE TO LYMPHOMA

A number of inherited and acquired diseases increase the probability of lymphoma development in certain individuals compared to healthy individuals of the same age and gender.[736,737] Table 96-18 lists the major inherited disorders predisposing to lymphoma.

Infectious agents that can lead to lymphoma following their entry into the host include EBV, HIV, HTLV-I, and *H. pylori*. These agents were discussed in "Etiology and Pathogenesis: Infectious Agents" above. HIV-related lymphoma can be similar to those types that occur in immunocompetent subjects, such as DLBCL, BL, and Hodgkin lymphoma. Primary effusion lymphoma and plasmablastic lymphoma of the oral cavity are more specifically related to HIV infection, and polymorphic B cell lymphoma can occur as it can in other immunodeficiency states (e.g., posttransplant).[738]

Posttransplant lymphoproliferative disorders result from posttransplantation immunosuppression. Approximately three fourths of these cases are related to EBV infection, but the precise etiology of the remainder is unknown.[739]

Patients given methotrexate for immune disorders, such as psoriasis or arthritis, have an increased likelihood of developing lymphoma.[740]

TABLE 96-18 INHERITED SYNDROMES PREDISPOSING TO LYMPHOMA

SYNDROME	ALTERED GENES		MECHANISM	LEUKEMIA TYPE	REFERENCES
	INHERITANCE	DESCRIPTION			
DNA repair defects					
Ataxia telangiectasia	R	*ATM* homozygotes Dominant-negative missense mutations	Genomic instability Increased translocations in T cells formed at the time of V(D)J recombination	T cell lymphoma, T ALL, T PLL, B cell lymphoma	741, 742
Bloom	R	BLM	Genomic instability	ALL, lymphoma	743, 744
Nijmegen breakage	R	NBS1	Genomic instability Altered telomere maintenance	Lymphoid tumors	745, 746
Tumor suppressor gene defect					
Li-Fraumeni*	D	P53	Defect in tumor suppressor	CLL, ALL, Hodgkin and Burkitt lymphoma	747, 748
Immunodeficiency states					
Common variable immunodeficiency	R and D	Defect in CD40 signaling	Failure of B cell maturation	B cell lymphoma	744, 749, 750
Severe combined immunodeficiency disease (SCID)	R	ADA	Defective T + B cell function	B cell lymphoma	744
Wiskott-Aldrich	X	*WASP*	Signaling and apoptosis	Hodgkin and non-Hodgkin lymphoma	744, 751–754
X-linked immunodeficiency with normal or increased IgM	X	CD40L	CD40 ligand defect on T cell	Hodgkin and non-Hodgkin lymphoma	755, 756
X-linked lymphoproliferative syndrome (XLP)	X	SAP	Defect in immune signaling	EBV-related B cell lymphoma	757
Apoptotic defect					
Autoimmune lymphoproliferative syndrome (ALPS)	D	*APT* (*FAS*)	Germ-line heterozygous *FAS* mutations Defective apoptosis	Lymphoma	758, 759
Unknown defect					
Dubowitz	R	Unknown	Unknown	ALL, lymphoma	760
Poland	D	May not be inherited	Unknown	ALL, lymphoma	761–763
WT	D	Unknown	Unknown	ALL, Castleman disease	764

* Li-Fraumeni or Li-Fraumeni–like syndrome has been described in which a gene other than *p53* is mutation. *hCHK2* in particular has been described as etiologic.[765,766] We have not included these variants in the table because we are uncertain if lymphoma is one of the cancers for which susceptibility is increased.
ALL, acute lymphocytic leukemia; CLL, chronic lymphocytic leukemia; D, dominant; EBV, Epstein Barr virus; R, recessive; T PLL, T prolymphocytic leukemia; X = X-linked.
SOURCE: Modified from Segel and Lichtman.[736]

NONMALIGNANT DISORDERS OF THE LYMPH NODES THAT MIMIC LYMPHOMA

CASTLEMAN DISEASE

Castleman disease, also called angiofollicular lymph node hyperplasia, giant lymph node hyperplasia, or benign lymphoma, is a heterogeneous entity.[767] In the original description, all patients had localized nonmalignant mediastinal lymphadenopathy. Histologically, Castleman disease is an atypical lymphoproliferative disorder not clearly identified as reactive or neoplastic.[768] Localized Castleman disease has a benign clinical course, with complete local surgical excision eliminating systemic systems and only rare local recurrences.[769] Eighty percent of localized cases are hyaline vascular and 20 percent are plasma cell. Most patients with plasma cell histology are children or young adults who present with abdominal or mediastinal masses.

Multicentric Castleman disease[770] typically is of the plasma cell type, although hyaline vascular and mixed cases have been reported.[771,772] It is a systemic illness with diffuse lymphadenopathy and an aggressive and fatal course associated with infections and complications.[773] The disease has been associated with HIV infections and Kaposi sarcoma.[773] HHV-8 also is linked to the pathogenesis and etiology of the disease.[774] Therapy for multicentric Castleman disease has included high-dose glucocorticoids and combination chemotherapy similar to combinations used for treatment of lymphoma.[772,775] Prolonged remissions were seen in three of eight patients treated with chemotherapy as the initial therapy.[776] An association exists between multicentric Castleman disease and POEMS (polyneuropathy, organomegaly, endocrinopathy, monoclonal protein, and skin changes) syndrome (see Chap. 100).[776,777]

KIKUCHI-FUJIMUTO DISEASE

Kikuchi-Fujimuto disease or histiocytic necrotizing lymphadenitis is a benign self-limiting disease of unknown etiology first described in Japan.[778] It is characterized by posterior cervical lymphadenopathy, fever, and leukopenia; spontaneous resolution occurs within months.[779] It has a female predominance and typically affects patients younger than 40 years.[780] Lymphadenopathy occasionally is generalized. The lymph nodes contain a proliferation of histiocytes with focal necrosis, and T cell immunoblasts may be seen. Glucocorticoids have been used for treatment of severe symptoms.

ROSAI-DORFMAN DISEASE

Rosai-Dorfman disease (sinus histiocytosis with massive lymphade-nopathy) is a polyclonal disorder of unknown etiology.[781] The typical patient is a healthy young adult who presents with massive cervical lymphadenopathy, which may be associated with fever, hypergam-maglobulinemia, and an elevated sedimentation rate.[781,782] Forty percent of cases are extranodal, and 75 percent occur in the head and neck region.[782,783] The disease usually is self-limited. Fifty percent of patients have spontaneous resolution; the remaining patients have stable disease. Rare deaths are attributed to immune dysregulation or visceral involvement. Surgery for localized disease and glucocorticoids or single-agent chemotherapy for generalized disease are treatment options.[783,784] The disease is discussed more comprehensively in Chapter 72.

PROGRESSIVE TRANSFORMATION OF GERMINAL CENTERS

Progressive transformation of germinal centers (PTGC) is a benign disorder of unknown etiology.[785] Atypically it is a systematic lymphadenopathy in young adults. Follicular hyperplasia and loss of the defined border between the germinal center and mantle zone are observed,[786] but the overall lymphoid architecture is preserved. The lymph nodes may spontaneously regress or they may remain stable. PTGC may be associated with nodular lymphocyte-predominant Hodgkin lymphoma.[786,787] Therapy is not recommended for PTGC unless it is clearly associated with Hodgkin lymphoma.

INFLAMMATORY PSEUDOTUMOR OF LYMPH NODES

Inflammatory pseudotumor of lymph nodes occurs in young adults who present with enlarged lymph nodes at single or multiple sites; they also may have systemic symptoms.[788,789] Lymph node biopsy reveals inflammatory cells, activated histiocytes, and fibroblasts with blood vessels in a sclerotic stroma with the connective tissue of the lymph node. Inflammatory pseudotumor is believed to represent the end stage of a response to infection, with spontaneous regression in most cases.[788,789]

MYOEPITHELIAL SIALADENITIS

Most salivary gland lymphomas consist of MALT and are thought to arise from a benign or active infiltrate termed *myoepithelial sialadenitis* (MESA).[790,791] MESA is found in Sjögren syndrome and is responsible for salivary gland dysfunction. The transition from reactive MESA to lymphoma is not well understood. Ig gene rearrangements may be identified in benign lesions.[792]

MISCELLANEOUS LYMPHADENOPATHIES

Other causes of lymphadenopathy that occasionally have been confused with lymphoma include infections, autoimmune disorders, and drug hypersensitivity reactions. Among drugs, the most common are anticonvulsants such as phenytoin and carbamazepine,[793] antibiotics such as sulfas and penicillin, aspirin, and allopurinol.[794]

REFERENCES

1. Oberling C: Les reticulosarcomes et les reticuloendotheliosarcomes de la moelle ossue se (sarcomes d'Ewing). *Bull Assoc Fr Etude Cancer* 17: 259, 1928.
2. Roulet F: Das primare Retothelsarkom der Lymphknoten. *Virchows Arch A Pathol Anat Histol* 277:15, 1930.
3. Ewing J: Endothelioma of lymph nodes. *J Med Res* 28:1, 1913.
4. Brill NE, Baehr G, Rosenthal N: Generalized giant lymph follicle hyperplasia of lymph nodes and spleen: A hitherto undescribed type. *JAMA* 84:668, 1925.
5. Symmers D: Follicular lymphadenopathy with splenomegaly: A newly recognized disease of the lymphatic system. *Arch Pathol Lab Med* 3: 816, 1927.
6. Rappaport H: Tumors of the hematopoietic system, in *Atlas of Tumor Pathology*, sec 3, fasc 8, pp 97–161. U.S. Armed Forces Institute of Pathology, Washington, DC, 1966.
7. Lukes RJ, Craver LF, Hall TC, et al: Report of the nomenclature committee. *Cancer Res* 26:1311, 1966.
8. Lennert K, Mohri N, Stein H, Kaiserling E: The histopathology of malignant lymphoma. *Br J Haematol* 31(suppl):193, 1975.
9. The Non-Hodgkin's Lymphoma Pathologic Classification Project: National Cancer Institute sponsored study of classifications of non-Hodgkin's lymphomas: Summary and description of a Working Formulation for clinical usage. *Cancer* 49:2112, 1982.
10. Harris NL, Jaffe ES, Stein H, et al: A revised European-American classification of lymphoid neoplasms: A proposal from the International Lymphoma Study Group. *Blood* 84:1361, 1994.
11. Hiddemann W, Longo DL, Coiffier B, et al: Lymphoma classification—The gap between biology and clinical management is closing. *Blood* 88: 4085, 1996.
12. Cancer Statistics 2004. *CA Cancer J Clin* 54:8, 2004.
13. Cartwright R, Brincker H, Carli PM, et al: The rise in incidence of lymphoma in Europe 1985–1992. *Eur J Cancer* 35:627, 1999.
14. Devesa SS, Fears T: Non-Hodgkin's lymphoma time trends: United States and international data. *Cancer Res* 52(suppl):5432s, 1992.
15. Hardell L, Eriksson M: A case-control study of non-Hodgkin lymphoma and exposure to pesticides. *Cancer* 85:1353, 1999.
16. Osburn S: *Do Pesticides Cause Lymphoma? Research Report*. Lymphoma Foundation of America, Chevy Chase, MD, 2001.
17. Hooper WC, Holman RC, Clarke MJ, Chorba TL: Trends in non-Hodgkin's lymphoma (NHL) and HIV-associated NHL deaths in the United States. *Am J Hematol* 66:159, 2001.
18. Ng CS, Chan JKC, Lo STH, et al: Immunophenotypic analysis of Hodgkin's lymphomas in Chinese. A study of 75 cases in Hong Kong. *Pathology* 18:419, 1986.
19. Kadin ME, Bernard CW, Nanba K, Wakasa H: Lymphoproliferative diseases in Japan and Western countries: Proceedings of United States-Japan seminar. *Hum Pathol* 14:745, 1983.
20. Cutler SJ, Young JL: Third national cancer survey: Incidence data. *Natl Cancer Inst Monogr* 40:1, 1975.
21. Shih L-Y, Liang D-C: Non-Hodgkin's lymphoma in Asia. *Hematol Oncol Clin North Am* 5:983, 1991.
22. Weinstock MA, Horm JW: Population-based estimate of survival and determinants of prognosis in patients with mycosis fungoides. *Cancer* 62:1658, 1988.
23. Pearce NE, Sheppard RA, Smith AH, et al: Non-Hodgkin's lymphoma and farming: An expanded case-control study. *Int J Cancer* 39:155, 1987.
24. Woods JS, Polissar L, Severson RK, et al: Soft tissue sarcoma and non-Hodgkin's lymphoma in relation to phenoxyherbicide and chlorinated phenol exposure in western Washington. *J Natl Cancer Inst* 78:899, 1987.
25. Morrison HI, Wilkins K, Semenel WR, et al: Herbicides and cancer. *J Natl Cancer Inst* 84:1866, 1992.
26. Levin PH, Hoover RN: The emerging epidemic of non-Hodgkin's lymphoma: Current knowledge regarding etiologic factors. *Cancer Res* 52: 54325, 1992.
27. Beebe GW, Kato H, Land C: Studies of the mortality of A-bomb survivors. Mortality and radiation dose 1950–1974. *Radiat Res* 75:138, 1978.

28. Anderson RE, Nishiyama H, Yohei I, et al: Pathogenesis of radiation related leukemia and lymphoma. Speculations based primarily on experience of Hiroshima and Nagasaki. *Lancet* 1:1060, 1972.

29. Miller RW: Delayed radiation effects in atomic bomb survivors. *Science* 166:569, 1969.

30. Court-Brown WM, Doll R: *Leukemia and aplastic anemia in patients irradiated for ankylosing spondylitis. Medical Research Council Special Report Series*, no 295, Her Majesty's Stationery Office, London, 1957.

31. Poiesz BJ, Ruscetti FW, Gazdar AF, et al: Detection and isolation of type C retrovirus particles from fresh and cultured lymphocytes of a patient with cutaneous T-cell lymphoma. *Proc Natl Acad Sci U S A* 77: 7415, 1980.

32. Jacobson S, Raine CS, Mingioli ES, et al: Isolation of an HTLV-I-like retrovirus from patients with tropical spastic paraparesis. *Nature* 331: 540, 1988.

33. Snoda S: Relationship of HTLV-I-related adult T-cell leukemia and HTLV-I-associated myelopathy to distinct HLA haplotypes. *Jikken Igaku* 5:769, 1987.

34. Wong-Staal F, Gallo RC: The family of human T-lymphotropic leukemia viruses: HTLV-I as the cause of adult T cell leukemia and HTLV-III as the cause of acquired immunodeficiency syndrome. *Blood* 65: 253,1985.

35. Blattner WA, Kalyanaraman VS, Robert-Guroff M, et al: The human type-C retrovirus HTLV, in blacks from the Caribbean region, and relationship to adult T-cell leukemia/lymphoma. *Int J Cancer* 30:257, 1982.

36. Robert-Guroff M, Kalyanaraman VS, Blattner WA, et al: Evidence for human T-cell lymphoma-leukemia virus infection of family members of human T cell lymphoma-leukemia virus positive T-cell leukemia-lymphoma patients. *J Exp Med* 157:248, 1983.

37. Sarin PS, Aoki T, Shibata A, et al: High incidence of human type-C retrovirus (HTLV) in family members of a HTLV-positive Japanese T-cell leukemia patient. *Proc Natl Acad Sci U S A* 80:2370, 1983.

38. Epstein MA, Achang BG, Barr YH: Virus particles in cultured lymphoblasts from Burkitt's lymphoma. *Lancet* 1:702, 1964.

39. Nemerow GR, Wolfert R, McNaughton ME, Cooper NR: Identification and characterization of the Epstein-Barr virus receptor on human B-lymphocytes and its relation to the C3d complement receptor (CR2). *J Virol* 55:347, 1985.

40. Henle W, Diehl V, Kohn G, et al: Herpes-type virus and chromosome marker in normal leucocytes after growth with irradiated Burkitt cells. *Science* 157:1064, 1967.

41. Anderson M, Klein G, Ziegler J, Henle W: Association of Epstein-Barr viral genomes with American Burkitt lymphoma. *Nature* 260:357, 1976.

42. Potter M, Mushinski JF: Oncogenes in B neoplasia. *Cancer Invest* 2: 285, 1984.

43. Morrow RH Jr: Epidemiological evidence for the role of falciparum malaria in the pathogenesis of Burkitt's lymphoma, in *Burkitt's Lymphoma: A Human Cancer Model*, edited by G Lenoir, T O'Conor, CLM Olweny, p 177. ARC Scientific, Lyon, France, 1985.

44. Klein G: Lymphoma development in mice and humans: Diversity of initiation is followed by convergent cytogenetic evolution. *Proc Natl Acad Sci U S A* 76:2442, 1979.

45. Klein G: Specific chromosomal translocations and the genesis of B-cell-derived tumors in mice and men. *Cell* 19:311, 1983.

46. Nakamura S, Akazawa K, Yao T, Tsuneyoshi M: A clinicopathologic study of 233 cases with special reference to evaluation with the MIB-1 index. *Cancer* 76:1313, 1995.

47. Isaacson PG, Spencer J: Gastric lymphoma and *Helicobacter pylori. Important Adv Oncol*: p 111, 1996.

48. Nakamura S, Yao T, Aoyagi K, et al: *Helicobacter pylori* and primary gastric lymphoma: A histopathologic and immunohistochemical analysis of 237 patients. *Cancer* 79:3, 1997.

49. Kinlen LJ: Incidence of cancer in rheumatoid arthritis and other disorders after immunosuppressive therapy. *Am J Med* 78(suppl 1A):44, 1985.

50. Penn I: Cancers complicating organ transplantation. *N Engl J Med* 23: 1767, 1990.

51. Swinnen IJ, Costanzo-Nordin MR, Fisher SG, et al: Increased incidence of lymphoproliferative disorder after immunosuppression with the monoclonal antibody OKT3 in cardiac-transplant receipts. *N Engl J Med* 323:1723, 1990.

52. Segel GB, Lichtman MA: Familial (inherited) leukemia, lymphoma, and myeloma. *Blood Cells Mol Dis* 32:246, 2004.

53. Filipovich AH, Mathur D, Kamat T, Shapiro RS: Primary immunodeficiencies: Genetic risk factors for lymphoma. *Cancer Res* 52(suppl): 5465s, 1992.

54. Sullivan JL: Epstein-Barr virus and lymphoproliferative disorders. *Semin Hematol* 25:269, 1988.

55. Ong ST, Le Beau MM: Chromosomal abnormalities and molecular genetics of non-Hodgkin's lymphoma. *Semin Oncol* 25:447, 1998.

56. Korsmeyer SJ: Bcl-2 initiates a new category of oncogenes: Regulators of cell death. *Blood* 80:879, 1992.

57. Hockenbery D, Zutter M, Hickey W, et al: BCL2 protein is topographically restricted in tissues characterized by apoptotic cell death. *Proc Natl Acad Sci U S A* 88:6961, 1991.

58. Neri A, Barriga F, Knowles D, et al: Different regions of the immunoglobulin heavy-chain locus are involved in chromosomal translocations in distinct pathogenetic forms of Burkitt lymphoma. *Proc Natl Acad Sci U S A* 85:2748, 1988.

59. Hamilton-Dutoit S, Pallesen G, Franzmann M, et al: AIDS-related lymphoma. Histopathology, immunophenotype, and association with Epstein-Barr virus as demonstrated by in situ nucleic acid hybridization. *Am J Pathol* 138:149, 1991.

60. Ballerini P, Gaidano G, Gong J, et al: Multiple genetic lesions in AIDS-related non-Hodgkin's lymphoma. *Blood* 81:166, 1993.

61. Filippa DA, Ladanyi M, Wollner N, et al: CD30 (Ki-1)-positive malignant lymphomas: Clinical, immunophenotypic, histologic, and genetic characteristics and differences with Hodgkin's disease. *Blood* 87:2905, 1996.

62. Morris SW, Kirstein MN, Valentine MB, et al: Fusion of a kinase gene, ALK, to a nucleolar protein gene, NPM, in non Hodgkin's lymphoma. *Science* 263:1281, 1994.

63. Lopategui JR, Sun L-H, Chan JKC, et al: Low frequency association of the t(2;5)(p23;q35) chromosomal translocation with CD30+ lymphomas from American and Asian patients. *Am J Pathol* 146:323, 1995.

64. Downing JR, Shurtleff SA, Zielenska M, et al: Molecular detection of the (2;5) translocation of non-Hodgkin's lymphoma by reverse transcriptase polymerase chain reaction. *Blood* 85:3416, 1995.

65. DeCoteau JF, Butmarc JR, Kinney MC, Kadin ME: The t(2;5) chromosomal translocation is not a common feature of primary cutaneous CD30+ lymphoproliferative disorders: Comparison with anaplastic large-cell lymphoma of nodal origin. *Blood* 87:3437, 1996.

66. Sanada I, Tanaka R, Kumagai E, et al: Chromosomal aberrations in adult T-cell leukemia: Relationship to the clinical severity. *Blood* 65:649, 1985.

67. Whang-Peng J, Bunn PA, Knutsen T, et al: Cytogenetic studies in human T-cell lymphoma virus (HTLV)-positive leukemia-lymphoma in the United States. *J Natl Cancer Inst* 74:357, 1985.

68. Carbone PP: Report on the committee on Hodgkin's disease staging classification. *Cancer Res* 31:1860, 1971.

69. A predictive model for aggressive non-Hodgkin's lymphoma. The International Non-Hodgkin's Lymphoma Prognostic Factors Project. *N Engl J Med* 329:987, 1993.

70. A clinical evaluation of the International Lymphoma Study Group classification of Non-Hodgkin's Lymphoma. The Non-Hodgkin's Lymphoma Classification Project. *Blood* 89:3909, 1997.

71. Mackintosh FR, Colby TV, Podosky WJ, et al: Central nervous system involvement in non-Hodgkin's lymphoma: An analysis of 105 cases. *Cancer* 49:586, 1982.

72. Martenson JA Jr, Buskirk SJ, Illstrup DM, et al: Patterns of failure in primary testicular non-Hodgkin's lymphoma. *J Clin Oncol* 6:297, 1988.

73. Frierson HF, Mills SE, Innes DJ: Non-Hodgkin's lymphomas of the sinonasal region: Histologic subtypes and their clinicopathologic features. *Am J Clin Pathol* 81:721, 1984.

74. Pollack IF, Lunsford LD, Flickinger JC, et al: Prognostic factors in the diagnosis and treatment of primary central nervous system lymphomas. *Cancer* 63:939, 1989.

75. Epelbaum R, Haim N, Ben-Shahar M, et al: Non-Hodgkin's lymphoma presenting with spinal epidural involvement. *Cancer* 58:2120, 1986.

76. Richardson EP Jr: Progressive multifocal leukoencephalopathy 30 years later. *N Engl J Med* 318:315, 1988.

77. Henson RA, Urich H: *Cancer and the Nervous System.* Blackwell, Oxford, 1982.

78. Conners JM: Problems in lymphoma management: Special sites of presentation. *Oncology* 12:188, 1998.

79. Esik O, Ikeda H, Mukai K, Kaneko A: A retrospective analysis of different modalities for treatment of primary orbital non-Hodgkin's lymphomas. *Radiother Oncol* 38:13, 1996.

80. Whitcup SM, de Smet MD, Rubin BI, et al: Intraocular lymphoma: Clinical and histopathologic diagnosis. *Ophthalmology* 100:1399, 1993.

81. Abbondanzo SL, Wenig BM: Non-Hodgkin's lymphoma of the sinonasal tract: A clinicopathologic and immunophenotypic study of 120 cases. *Cancer* 75:1281, 1995.

82. Wood GS, Burke JS, Horning S, et al: The immunologic and clinicopathologic heterogeneity of cutaneous lymphomas other than mycosis fungoides. *Blood* 62:464, 1983.

83. Willemze R, Meijer CJLM, Scheffer E, et al: Diffuse large cell lymphomas of follicular center cell origin presenting in the skin: A clinicopathologic and immunologic study of 16 patients. *Am J Pathol* 126:325, 1987.

84. Manoharan A, Pitney WR, Schonnel ME, Bader LV: Intrathoracic manifestations in non-Hodgkin's lymphoma. *Thorax* 34:29, 1979.

85. Kennedy JL, Nasthwani BN, Burke JS, et al: Pulmonary lymphomas and other pulmonary lymphoid lesions: A clinicopathologic and immunologic study of 64 patients. *Cancer* 56:539, 1985.

86. Solidoro A, Salazar F, Flor J, et al: Endoscopic tissue diagnosis of gastric involvement in the staging of non-Hodgkin's lymphoma. *Cancer* 48:1053, 1981.

87. Kim H, Dorfman RF: Morphological studies of 84 untreated patients subjected to laparotomy for the staging of non-Hodgkin's lymphomas. *Cancer* 33:657, 1974.

88. List AF, Greer JP, Cousar JC, et al: Non-Hodgkin's lymphomas of the gastrointestinal tract: An analysis of clinical and pathologic features affecting outcome. *J Clin Oncol* 6:1125, 1988.

89. Haber DA, Mayer RJ: Primary gastrointestinal lymphoma. *Semin Oncol* 15:154, 1988.

90. Shchepotin IB, Evans SR, Shabahang M, et al: Primary non-Hodgkin's lymphoma of the stomach: Three radical modalities of treatment in 75 patients. *Ann Surg Oncol* 3:277, 1996.

91. Rabbi C, Aitini E, Cavazzini G, et al: Stomach preservation in low- and high-grade primary gastric lymphomas: Preliminary results. *Haematologica* 81:15, 1996.

92. Ernst M, Stein H, Ludwig D, et al: Surgical therapy of gastrointestinal non-Hodgkin's lymphomas. *Eur J Surg Oncol* 22:177, 1996.

93. Haim N, Leviov M, Ben-Arieh Y, et al: Intermediate and high-grade gastric non-Hodgkin's lymphoma: A prospective study of non-surgical treatment with primary chemotherapy, with or without radiotherapy. *Leuk Lymphoma* 17:321, 1995.

94. Doll DC, Weiss RB: Malignant lymphoma of the testis. *Am J Med* 81:515, 1986.

95. Touroutoglou N, Dimopoulos MA, Younes A, et al: Testicular lymphoma: Late relapses and poor outcome despite doxorubicin-based therapy. *J Clin Oncol* 13:1361, 1995.

96. Zucca EC, Conconi A, Mughal TI, et al: Patterns of outcome and prognostic factors in primary large-cell lymphoma of the testis in a survey by the International Extranodal Lymphoma Study Group. *J Clin Oncol* 21:20, 2003.

97. Fonseca RH, Habermann TM, Colgan JP, et al: Testicular lymphoma is associated with a high incidence of extranodal recurrence. *Cancer* 88:154, 2000.

98. Visco CM, Medeiros LJ, Mesina OM, et al: Non-Hodgkin's lymphoma affecting the testis: Is it curable with doxorubicin-based therapy? *Clin Lymphoma* 2:40, 2001.

99. Goffinet DR, Castellino RA, Kim H: Staging laparotomies in unselected previously untreated patients with non-Hodgkin's lymphomas. *Cancer* 32:672, 1973.

100. Moran EM, Ultmann JE, Ferguson DJ, et al: Staging laparotomy in non-Hodgkin's lymphoma. *Br J Cancer* 31(suppl II):228, 1975.

101. Risdall R, Hoppe RT, Warnke R: Non-Hodgkin's lymphoma: A study of the evolution of the disease based upon 92 autopsied cases. *Cancer* 44:529, 1979.

102. Rosenberg SA, Diamond HD, Jaslowitz B, et al: Lymphosarcoma: A review of 1269 cases. *Medicine* 40:31, 1961.

103. DeMent SH, Mann RB, Staal SP, et al: Primary lymphomas of the liver: Report of six cases and review of the literature. *Am J Clin Pathol* 88:255, 1987.

104. Kehoe J, Straus DJ: Primary lymphoma of the spleen: Clinical features and outcome after splenectomy. *Cancer* 62:1433, 1988.

105. Clayton F, Butler JJ, Ayala AG, et al: Non-Hodgkin's lymphoma in bone: Pathologic and radiologic features with clinical correlates. *Cancer* 60:2494, 1987.

106. Rosenburg SA: Bone marrow involvement in the non-Hodgkin's lymphomata. *Br J Cancer* 31(suppl II):261, 1975.

107. Stein RS, Ultmann JE, Byrne GE Jr, et al: Bone marrow involvement in non-Hodgkin's lymphoma. *Cancer* 37:629, 1976.

108. Chabner BA, Johnson RE, Young RC, et al: Sequential nonsurgical and surgical staging of non-Hodgkin's lymphoma. *Ann Intern Med* 85:149, 1976.

109. Coggins CH: Renal failure in lymphoma. *Kidney Int* 17:847, 1980.

110. Bostwick DG, Mann RB: Malignant lymphomas involving the prostate: A study of 13 cases. *Cancer* 56:2932, 1985.

111. Paladugu RR, Bearman RM, Rappaport H: Malignant lymphoma with primary manifestation in the gonad. *Cancer* 45:561, 1980.

112. Osborne BR, Robboy SJ: Lymphomas or leukemia presenting as ovarian tumors. An analysis of 42 cases. *Cancer* 52:1933, 1983.

113. Giardini RP, Piccolo C, Rilke F: Primary non-Hodgkin's lymphomas of the female breast. *Cancer* 69:725, 1992.

114. Levitt LJ, Ault KA, Pinkus GS, et al: Pericarditis and early cardiac tamponade as a primary manifestation of lymphosarcoma cell leukemia. *Am J Med* 67:719, 1979.

115. Colby TV, Dorfman RF: Malignant lymphomas involving the salivary glands. *Pathol Annu* 14(pt 2):307, 1979.

116. Harris GJ, Tio FO, Von Hoff DD: Primary adrenal lymphoma. *Cancer* 63:799, 1989.

117. Hamburger JI, Miller JM, Kini SR: Lymphoma of the thyroid. *Ann Intern Med* 99:685, 1983.

118. Alizadeh AA, Eisen MB, Davis RE, et al: Distinct types of diffuse large B-cell lymphoma identified by gene expression profiling. *Nature* 403:503, 2000.

119. Harris N, Jaffe E, Stein H, et al: A revised European-American classification of lymphoid neoplasms: A proposal from the International Lymphoma Study Group. *Blood* 84:1361, 1994.

120. Armitage J, Weisenburger D: New approach to classifying non-Hodgkin's lymphomas: Clinical features of the major histologic subtypes. *J Clin Oncol* 16:2780, 1998.

121. Anderson J, Armitage JO, Weisenburger DD: Epidemiology of the non-Hodgkin's lymphomas: Distributions of the major subtypes differ by geographic locations. Non-Hodgkin's Lymphoma Classification Project. *Ann Oncol* 9:717, 1998.

122. Groves F, Linet MS, Travis LB, Devesa SS: Cancer surveillance series: Non-Hodgkin's lymphoma incidence by histologic subtype in the United States from 1978 through 1995. *J Natl Cancer Inst* 92:1240, 2000.

123. Lyons SL, Liebowitz DN: The roles of human viruses in the pathogenesis of lymphoma. *Semin Oncol* 25:461, 1998.

124. Ye BH, Lista F, Lo Coco F, et al: Alterations of a zinc finger-encoding gene, BCL-6, in diffuse large-cell lymphoma. *Science* 262:747, 1993.

125. Lo Coco F, Ye BH, Lista F, et al: Rearrangements of the BCL6 gene in diffuse large cell non-Hodgkin's lymphoma. *Blood* 83:1757, 1994.

126. Gaidano G, Lo Coco F, Ye BH, et al: Rearrangements of the BCL-6 gene in acquired immunodeficiency syndrome-associated non-Hodgkin's lymphoma: Association with diffuse large-cell subtype. *Blood* 84:397, 1994.

127. Dalla-Favera R, Migliazza A, Chang CC, et al: Molecular pathogenesis of B cell malignancy: The role of BCL-6. *Curr Top Microbiol Immunol* 246:257, 1999.

128. Ye BH, Chiganti S, Chang CC, et al: Chromosomal translocations cause deregulated BCL6 expression by promoter substitution in B cell lymphoma. *EMBO J* 14:6209, 1995.

129. Kaneita YY, Yoshida S, Ishiguro N, et al: Detection of reciprocal fusion 5'-BCL6/partner-3' transcripts in lymphomas exhibiting reciprocal BCL6 translocations. *Br J Haematol* 113:803, 2001.

130. Chang CY, Ye BH, Chaganti RS, Dalla-Favera R: BCL-6, a POZ/zinc-finger protein, is a sequence-specific transcriptional repressor. *Proc Natl Acad Sci U S A* 93:6947, 1996.

131. Lo Coco FG, Gaidano G, Louie DC, et al: P53 mutations are associated with histologic transformation of follicular lymphoma. *Blood* 82:2289, 1993.

132. Pasqualucci L, Neumeistes P, Goossens T, et al: Hypermutation of multiple proto-oncogenes in B-cell diffuse large-cell lymphomas. *Nature* 412:341, 2001.

133. Huang JS, Sanger WG, Greiner TC, et al: The t(14;18) defines a unique subset of diffuse large B-cell lymphoma with a germinal center B-cell gene expression profile. *Blood* 99:2285, 2002.

134. Gascoyne RA, Adomat SA, Krajewski S, et al: Prognostic significance of Bcl-2 protein expression and Bcl-2 gene rearrangement in diffuse aggressive non-Hodgkin's lymphoma. *Blood* 90:244, 1997.

135. Lossos IJ, Jones CD, Warnke R, et al: Expression of a single gene, BCL-6, strongly predicts survival in patients with diffuse large B-cell lymphoma. *Blood* 98:945, 2001.

136. Shipp M, Ross KN, Tamayo P, et al: Diffuse large B-cell lymphoma outcome prediction by gene-expression profiling and supervised machine learning. *Nat Med* 8:68, 2002.

137. Hans C, Weisenburger DD, Greiner TC, et al: Confirmation of the molecular classification of diffuse large B-cell lymphoma by immunohistochemistry using a tissue microarray. *Blood* 103:275, 2004.

138. Aviles AN, Neri N, Huerta-Guzman J: Large bowel lymphoma: An analysis of prognostic factors and therapy in 53 patients. *J Surg Oncol* 80:111, 2002.

139. Parfyani SH, Hoppe RT, Burke JS, et al: Extralymphatic involvement in diffuse non-Hodgkin's lymphoma. *J Clin Oncol* 1:682, 1983.

140. van Besien KH, Ha CS, Murphy S, et al: Risk factors, treatment, and outcome of central nervous system recurrence in adults with intermediate-grade and immunoblastic lymphoma. *Blood* 91:1178, 1998.

141. Doggett R, Wood GS, Horning S, et al: The immunologic characteriza-

tion of 95 nodal and extranodal diffuse large cell lymphomas in 89 patients. *Am J Pathol* 115:245, 1984.

142. Stein H, Lennert K, Feller AC, Mason DY: Immunohistological analysis of human lymphoma: Correlation of histological and immunological categories. *Adv Cancer Res* 42:67, 1984.

143. Doggett R, Wood GS, Horning S, et al: The immunologic characterization of 95 nodal and extranodal diffuse large cell lymphomas in 89 patients. *Am J Pathol* 115:245, 1984.

144. Yamaguchi M, Seto M, Okamoto M, et al: De novo CD5+ diffuse large B-cell lymphoma: A clinicopathologic study of 109 patients. *Blood* 99:815, 2002.

145. Ottensmeier C, Stevenson FK: Isotype switch variants reveal clonally related subpopulations in diffuse large B-cell lymphoma. *Blood* 96:2550, 2000.

146. Stauder R, Eisterer W, Thaler J, Gunthert U: CD44 variant isoforms in non-Hodgkin's lymphoma: A new independent prognostic factor. *Blood* 85:2885, 1995.

147. Alizadeh AA, Elsen M, Davis RE, et al: Distinct types of diffuse large B-cell lymphoma identified by gene expression profiling. *Nature* 403:503, 2000.

148. Lossos I, Czerwinski DK, Alizadeh AA, et al: Prediction of survival in diffuse large-B-cell lymphoma based on the expression of six genes. *N Engl J Med* 350:1828, 2004.

149. Swan FJ, Velasquez WS, Tucker S, et al: A new serologic staging system for large-cell lymphomas based on initial beta 2-microglobulin and lactate dehydrogenase levels. *J Clin Oncol* 7:1518, 1989.

150. Adida C, Haioun C, Gaulard P, et al: Prognostic significance of surviving expression in diffuse large B-cell lymphomas. *Blood* 96:1921, 2000.

151. Croghan T, Lippman SM, Spier CM, et al: Independent prognostic significance of a nuclear proliferation antigen in diffuse large cell lymphomas as determined by the monoclonal antibody Ki-67. *Blood* 71:1157, 1988.

152. Ansell S, Stenson M, Habermann TM, et al: CD4+ T-cell immune response to large B-cell non-Hodgkin's lymphoma predicts patient outcome. *J Clin Oncol* 19:720, 2001.

153. Zijlstra J, Hockstra OS, Raijmakers PG, et al: 18FDG positron emission tomography versus 67Ga scintigraphy as prognostic test during chemotherapy for non-Hodgkin's lymphoma. *Br J Haematol* 123:454, 2003.

154. Spaepen K, Stroobants S, Dupont P, et al: Prognostic value of pretransplantation positron emission tomography using fluorine 18-fluorodeoxyglucose in patients with aggressive lymphoma treated with high-dose chemotherapy and stem cell transplantation. *Blood* 102:53, 2003.

155. Fisher F, Gaynor ER, Dahlberg S, et al: Comparison of a standard regimen (CHOP) with three intensive chemotherapy regimens for advanced non-Hodgkin's lymphoma. *N Engl J Med* 328:1002, 1993.

156. Lee A, Connors JM, Klimo P, et al: Late relapse in patients with diffuse large-cell lymphoma treated with MACOP-B. *J Clin Oncol* 15:1745, 1997.

157. de Jong D, Glas AM, Boerrigter L, et al: Very late relapse in diffuse large B-cell lymphoma represents clonally related disease and is marked by germinal center cell features. *Blood* 102:324, 2003.

158. Rosenwald A, Wright G, Chan WC, et al: The use of molecular profiling to predict survival after chemotherapy for diffuse large-B-cell lymphoma. *N Engl J Med* 346:1937, 2002.

159. Wilson W, Grossbard ML, Pittaluga S, et al: Dose-adjusted EPOCH chemotherapy for untreated large B-cell lymphomas: A pharmacodynamic approach with high efficacy. *Blood* 99:2685, 2002.

160. Chen M, Prosnitz LR, Gonzalez-Serva A, Fischer DB: Results of radiotherapy in control of stage I and II non-Hodgkin's lymphoma. *Cancer* 43:1245, 1979.

161. Longo D, Glatstein E, Duffey PL, et al: Treatment of localized aggressive lymphomas with combination chemotherapy followed by involved-field radiation therapy. *J Clin Oncol* 7:1295, 1989.

162. Tondini C, Zanini M, Lombardi F, et al: Combined modality treatment with primary CHOP chemotherapy followed by locoregional irradiation in stage I or II histologically aggressive non-Hodgkin's lymphomas. *Ann Oncol* 11:720, 1993.

163. Jones S, Miller TP, Connors JM: Long-term follow-up and analysis for prognostic factors for patients with limited-stage diffuse large-cell lymphoma treated with initial chemotherapy with or without adjuvant radiotherapy. *J Clin Oncol* 7:1186, 1989.

164. Vokes E, Ultmann JE, Golomb HM, et al: Long term survival of patients with localized diffuse histiocytic lymphoma. *J Clin Oncol* 3:1309, 1985.

165. Monfardini S, Banfi A, Bonadonna G, et al: Improved five year survival after combined radiotherapy-chemotherapy for stage I-II non-Hodgkin's lymphoma. *Int J Radiat Oncol Biol Phys* 6:125, 1980.

166. Nissen N, Ersboll J, Hansen HS, et al: A randomized study of radiotherapy versus radiotherapy plus chemotherapy in stage I-II non-Hodgkin's lymphomas. *Cancer* 52:1, 1983.

167. Miller T, Dahlberg S, Cassady JR, et al: Chemotherapy alone compared with chemotherapy plus radiotherapy for localized intermediate- and high-grade non-Hodgkin's lymphoma. *N Engl J Med* 339:21, 1998.

168. Miller T, Leblanc M, Spier C, et al: CHOP alone compared to CHOP plus radiotherapy for early stage aggressive non-Hodgkin's lymphomas: Update of the Southwest Oncology Group (SWOG) randomized trial [abstract]. *Blood* 98:724a, 2001.

169. Horning S, Glick JH, Kim K, et al: Final report of E1484: CHOP v CHOP + radiotherapy (RT) for limited stage diffuse aggressive lymphoma. *Blood* 98:724a, 2001.

170. Fillet G, Bonnet C: Radiotherapy is unnecessary in elderly patients with localized aggressive non-Hodgkin's lymphoma: Results of the GELA LNH 93-4 study. *Blood* 100:93a, 2002.

171. Reyes F, Lepage E, Munck JN, et al: Superiority of chemotherapy alone with ACVBP regimen over treatment with three cycles of CHOP plus radiotherapy in low risk localized aggressive lymphoma: The LNH93-1 GELA study. *Blood* 100:93a, 2002.

172. Wilder R, Rodriguez MA, Tucker SL, et al: Radiation therapy after a partial response to CHOP chemotherapy for aggressive lymphomas. *Int J Radiat Oncol Biol Phys* 50:743, 2001.

173. DeVita VT Jr, Canellos GP, Chabner B, et al: Advanced diffuse histiocytic lymphoma, a potentially curable disease. *Lancet* i:248, 1975.

174. Coltman C, Dahlberg S, Jones S, et al: CHOP is curative in thirty percent of patients with large cell lymphoma: A twelve-year Southwest Oncology Group follow-up, in *Advances in Cancer Chemotherapy*, edited by AT Skarin, p 71. Park Row, New York, 1986.

175. Gaynor EU, Ultmann JE, Golomb HM, Sweet DL: Treatment of diffuse histiocytic lymphoma (DHL) with COMLA (cyclophosphamide, oncovin, methotrexate, leucovorin, cytosine arabinoside): A 10-year experience in a single institution. *J Clin Oncol* 3:1596, 1985.

176. Schein PD, DeVita VT Jr, Hubbard S, et al: Bleomycin, adriamycin, cyclophosphamide, vincristine, and prednisone (BACOP) combination chemotherapy in the treatment of advanced diffuse histiocytic lymphoma. *Ann Intern Med* 85:417, 1976.

177. Fisher RD, DeVita VT Jr, Hubbard SM, et al: Diffuse aggressive lymphomas: Increased survival after alternating flexible sequences of proMACE and MOPP chemotherapy. *Ann Intern Med* 98:304, 1983.

178. Gordon L, Harrington D, Andersen J, et al: Comparison of a second-generation combination chemotherapeutic regimen (m-BACOD) with a standard regimen (CHOP) for advanced diffuse non-Hodgkin's lymphoma. *N Engl J Med* 327:1342, 1992.

179. Linch D, Smith P, Hancock BW, et al: A randomized British National Lymphoma Investigation trial of CHOP vs. a weekly multi-agent regimen (PACEBOM) in patients with histologically aggressive non-Hodgkin's lymphoma. *Ann Oncol* 11 (suppl 1):87, 2000.

180. Gaynor ERU, Unger JM, Miller TP, et al: Infusional CHOP chemotherapy (CVAD) with or without chemosensitizers offers no advantage over standard CHOP therapy in the treatment of lymphoma: A Southwest Oncology Group Study. *J Clin Oncol* 19:750, 2001.

181. Bartlett NP, Petroni GR, Parker BA, et al: Dose-escalated cyclophosphamide, doxorubicin, vincristine, prednisone, and etoposide (CHOPE) chemotherapy for patients with diffuse lymphoma: Cancer and Leukemia Group B studies 8852 and 8854. *Cancer* 92:207, 2001.

182. Sparano J, Weller E, Nazeer T, et al: Phase 2 trial of infusional cyclophosphamide, doxorubicin, and etoposide in patients with poor-prognosis, intermediate-grade non-Hodgkin lymphoma: An Eastern Cooperative Oncology Group trial (E3493). *Blood* 100:1634, 2002.

183. Pangalis G, Vassilakopoulos TP, Michalis E, et al: A randomized trial comparing intensified CNOP vs. CHOP in patients with aggressive non-Hodgkin's lymphoma. *Leuk Lymphoma* 44:635, 2003.

184. Wolf M, Mathews J, Stone J, et al: Dose-intensification does not improve outcome in aggressive non-Hodgkin's lymphoma (NHL), report of a randomized trial by the Australian Leukemia and Lymphoma Group. *Blood* 96:832a, 2000.

185. Pfreundschuh M, Truemper L, Schmits R, et al: 2-weekly vs. 3-weekly CHOP with and without etoposide in young patients with low-risk (low LDH) aggressive non-Hodgkin's lymphoma: Results of the completed NHL-B-1 trial of the DSHNHL [abstract]. *Blood* 100:92a, 2002.

186. Goss P: Non-Hodgkin's lymphomas in elderly patients. *Leuk Lymphoma* 10:147, 1993.

187. Zinzani P, Storti S, Zaccaria A, et al: Elderly aggressive-histology non-Hodgkin's lymphoma: First-line VNCOP-B regimen experience on 350 patients. *Blood* 94:33, 1999.

188. Bessell E, Burton GP, Haynes AP, et al: A randomised multicentre trial of modified CHOP versus MCOP in patients aged 65 years and over with aggressive non-Hodgkin's lymphoma. *Ann Oncol* 14:258, 2003.

189. Meyer R, Browman GP, Samosh ML, et al: Randomized phase II comparison of standard CHOP with weekly CHOP in elderly patients with non-Hodgkin's lymphoma. *J Clin Oncol* 13:2386, 1995.

190. Pfreundschuh M, Trumper L, Kloess M, et al: 2-weekly CHOP(CHOP-14): The new standard regimen for patients with aggressive non-Hodgkin's lymphoma (NHL) >60 years of age [abstract]. *Blood* 98:725a, 2001.

191. Wunderlich A, Kloess M, Reiser M, et al: Practicability and acute haematological toxicity of 2- and 3-weekly CHOP and CHOEP chemotherapy for aggressive non-Hodgkin's lymphoma: Results from the NHL-B trial of the German High-Grade Non-Hodgkin's Lymphoma Study Group (DSHNHL). *Ann Oncol* 14:881, 2003.

192. Tirelli U, Errante D, Van Glabbeke M, et al: CHOP is the standard regimen in patients > or = 70 years of age with intermediate-grade and high-grade non-Hodgkin's lymphoma: Results of a randomized study of the European Organization for Research and Treatment of Cancer Lymphoma Cooperative Study Group. *J Clin Oncol* 16:27, 1998.

193. Sonneveld P, de Ridder M, van der Lelie H, et al: Comparison of doxorubicin and mitoxantrone in the treatment of elderly patients with advanced diffuse non-Hodgkin's lymphoma using CHOP versus CNOP chemotherapy. *J Clin Oncol* 13:2530, 1995.

194. Osby E, Hagberg H, Kvaloy S, et al: CHOP is superior to CNOP in elderly patients with aggressive lymphoma while outcome is unaffected by filgrastim treatment: Results of a Nordic Lymphoma Group randomized trial. *Blood* 101:3840, 2003.

195. Sonnen R, Schmidt WP, Kuse R, Schmitz N: Treatment results of aggressive B non-Hodgkin's lymphoma in advanced age considering comorbidity. *Br J Haematol* 119:634, 2002.

196. Morrison V, Picozzi V, Scott S, et al: The impact of age on delivered dose intensity and hospitalizations for febrile neutropenia in patients with intermediate-grade non-Hodgkin's lymphoma receiving initial CHOP chemotherapy: A risk factor analysis. *Clin Lymphoma* 2:47, 2001.

197. Coiffier B, Lepage E, Briere J, et al: CHOP chemotherapy plus rituximab compared with CHOP alone in elderly patients with diffuse large-B-cell lymphoma. *N Engl J Med* 346:235, 2002.

198. Habermann T, Weller E, Morisson V, et al: Phase II trial of rituximab-CHOP (R-CHOP) vs. CHOP with a second randomization to maintenance rituximab (MR) or observation in patients 60 years of age and older with diffuse large B-cell lymphoma (DLBCL). *Blood* 102: 6a, 2003.

199. Santini G, Sslvagno L, Leoni P, et al: VACOP-B versus VACOP-B plus autologous bone marrow transplantation for advanced diffuse non-Hodgkin's lymphoma: Results of a prospective randomized trial by the non-Hodgkin's Lymphoma Cooperative Study Group. *J Clin Oncol* 16: 2796, 1998.

200. Kluin-Nelemans HC, Zagonel V, Anastasopoulou A, et al: Standard chemotherapy with or without high-dose chemotherapy for aggressive non-Hodgkin's lymphoma: Randomized phase III EORTC study. *J Natl Cancer Inst* 93:22, 2001.

201. Verdonck LF, van Putten WL, Hagenbeek A, et al: Comparison of CHOP chemotherapy with autologous bone marrow transplantation for slowly responding patients with aggressive non-Hodgkin's lymphoma. *N Engl J Med* 332:1045, 1995.

202. Haioun C, Lepage E, Gisselbrecht C, et al: Benefit of autologous bone marrow transplantation over sequential chemotherapy in poor-risk aggressive non-Hodgkin's lymphoma: Updated results of the prospective study LNH87-2. Groupe d'Etude des Lymphomes de l'Adulte. *J Clin Oncol* 15:1131, 1997.

203. Gulati S, Shank B, Black P, et al: Autologous bone marrow transplantation for patients with poor-prognosis lymphoma. *J Clin Oncol* 6:1303, 1988.

204. Nademanee A, Molina A, O'Donnell MR, et al: Results of high-dose therapy and autologous bone marrow/stem cell transplantation during remission in poor-risk intermediate- and high-grade lymphoma: International index high and high-intermediate risk group. *Blood* 90:3844, 1997.

205. Cortelazzo S, Rossi A, Bellavita P, et al: Clinical outcome after autologous transplantation in non-Hodgkin's lymphoma patients with high international prognostic index (IPI). *Ann Oncol* 10:427, 1999.

206. Pettengell R, Radford JA, Morgenstern GR, et al: Survival benefit from high-dose therapy with autologous blood progenitor-cell transplantation in poor-prognosis non-Hodgkin's lymphoma. *J Clin Oncol* 14:586, 1996.

207. Freedman A, Takvorian T, Neuberg D, et al: Autologous bone marrow transplantation in poor-prognosis intermediate-grade and high-grade B-cell non-Hodgkin's lymphoma in first remission: A pilot study. *J Clin Oncol* 11:931, 1993.

208. Gisselbrecht C, Lepage E, Molina T, et al: Shortened first-line high-dose chemotherapy for patients with poor-prognosis aggressive lymphoma. *J Clin Oncol* 20:2472, 2002.

209. Kaiser U, Uebelacker I, Abel U, et al: Randomized study to evaluate the use of high-dose therapy as part of primary treatment for "aggressive" lymphoma. *J Clin Oncol* 20:4413, 2002.

210. Haioun C, Lepage E, Gisselbrecht C, et al: Survival benefit of high-dose therapy in poor-risk aggressive non-Hodgkin's lymphoma: Final analysis of the prospective LNH87-2 protocol—A Groupe d'Etude des Lymphomes de l'Adulte study. *J Clin Oncol* 18:3025, 2000.

211. Fisher R: Autologous stem-cell transplantation as a component of initial treatment for poor-risk patients with aggressive non-Hodgkin's lymphoma: Resolved issues versus remaining opportunity. *J Clin Oncol* 20: 4411, 2002.

212. Fisher DJ, Jacobsen JO, Ault KA, Harris NL: Diffuse large cell lymphoma with discordant bone marrow histology. Clinical features and biological implications. *Cancer* 64:1879, 1989.

213. Levitt LD, Dawson DM, Rosenthal DS, Moloney WC: CNS involvement in the non-Hodgkin's lymphomas. *Cancer* 45:545, 1980.

214. Haioun C, Besson C, Lepage E, et al: Incidence and risk factors of central nervous system relapse in histologically aggressive non-Hodgkin's lymphoma uniformly treated and receiving intrathecal central ner-

vous system prophylaxis: A GELA study on 974 patients. Groupe d'Etudes des Lymphomes de l'Adulte. *Ann Oncol* 11:685, 2000.

215. Bos G, van Putten WL, van der Holt B, et al: For which patients with aggressive non-Hodgkin's lymphoma is prophylaxis for central nervous system disease mandatory? Dutch HOVON Group. *Ann Oncol* 9:191, 1998.

216. Tomita N, Kodoma F, Kanamori H, et al: Prophylactic intrathecal methotrexate and hydrocortisone reduces central nervous system recurrence and improves survival in aggressive non-Hodgkin lymphoma. *Cancer* 95:576, 2002.

217. Resnik R: Cancer during pregnancy. *N Engl J Med* 341:120, 1999.

218. Aviles A, Diaz-Maqueo JC, Torras V, et al: Non-Hodgkin's lymphomas and pregnancy: Presentation of 16 cases. *Gynecol Oncol* 37:335, 1990.

219. Zuazu J, Julia A, Sierra J, et al: Pregnancy outcome in hematologic malignancies. *Cancer* 67:703, 1991.

220. Levine A, Wernz JC, Kaplan L, et al: Low-dose chemotherapy with central nervous system prophylaxis and zidovudine maintenance in AIDS-related lymphoma. A prospective multi-institutional trial. *JAMA* 266:84, 1991.

221. Kaplan L, Strauss DJ, Testa MA, et al: Low-dose compared with standard-dose m-BACOD chemotherapy for non-Hodgkin's lymphoma associated with human immunodeficiency virus infection. National Institute of Allergy and Infectious Diseases AIDS Clinical Trials Group. *N Engl J Med* 336:1641, 1997.

222. Navarro J, Ribera JM, Oriol A, et al: Influence of highly active antiretroviral therapy on response to treatment and survival in patients with acquired immunodeficiency syndrome-related non-Hodgkin's lymphoma treated with cyclophosphamide, hydroxydoxorubicin, vincristine and prednisone. *Br J Haematol* 112:909, 2001.

223. Kaplan L, Scadden DT, AIDS Malignancy Consortium: No benefit from rituximab in a randomized phase III trial of CHOP with or without rituximab for patients with HIV-associated non-Hodgkin's lymphoma: AIDS malignancies consortium study 010. *Proc Am Soc Clin Oncol* 22: 564, 2003.

224. Spina M, Vaccher E, Juzbasic S, et al: Human immunodeficiency virus-related non-Hodgkin lymphoma: Activity of infusional cyclophosphamide, doxorubicin, and etoposide as second-line chemotherapy in 40 patients. *Cancer* 92:200, 2001.

225. Little R, Pittaloga S, Grant N, et al: Highly effective treatment of acquired immunodeficiency syndrome-related lymphoma with dose-adjusted EPOCH: Impact of antiretroviral therapy suspension and tumor biology. *Blood* 101:4653, 2003.

226. Ratner L, Redden D, Hamzeh F, et al: Third AIDS Malignancy Conference, Bethesda, MD, Chemotherapy for HIV associated non-Hodgkin's lymphoma in combination with highly active antiretroviral therapy (HAART) is not associated with excessive toxicity [abstract 92]. *AIDS Public Policy J* 21:A34, 1999.

227. Vaccher E, di Gennaro G, Schioppa O, et al: Highly active antiretroviral therapy (HAART) significantly improves disease free survival (DFS) in patients (pts) with HIV-related non-Hodgkin's lymphoma (HIV-NHL) treated with chemotherapy (CT). *Proc Am Soc Clin Oncol* 20:281a, 2001.

228. Thirlwell CS, Sarker D, Stebbing J, Bower M: Acquired immunodeficiency syndrome-related lymphoma in the era of highly active antiretroviral therapy. *Clin Lymphoma* 4:86, 2003.

229. Krishnan A, Molina A, Zaia J, et al: Autologous stem cell transplantation for HIV-associated lymphoma. *Blood* 98:3857, 2001.

230. Schmoll H: Review of etoposide single-agent activity. *Cancer Treat Rev* 9 (suppl):21, 1982.

231. Shipp M, Takvorian RC, Canellos GP: High-dose cytosine arabinoside. Active agent in treatment of non-Hodgkin's lymphoma. *Am J Med* 77: 845, 1984.

232. Bajetta E, Buzzoni R, Valagussa P, Bonadonna G: Mitoxantrone: An

active agent in refractory non-Hodgkin's lymphomas. *Am J Clin Oncol* 11:100, 1988.

233. Savage D, Rule SA, Tighe M, et al: Gemcitabine for relapsed or resistant lymphoma. *Ann Oncol* 11:595, 2000.

234. Tulpule A, Rarick MU, Kolitz J, et al: Liposomal daunorubicin in the treatment of relapsed or refractory non-Hodgkin's lymphoma. *Ann Oncol* 12:457, 2001.

235. Addis BI, Issacsom PG: Large cell lymphoma of the mediastinum: A B-cell tumour of probable thymic origin. *Histopathology* 10:379, 1986.

236. Lamarre LJ, Jacobsen JO, Aisenberg AC, Harris NL: Primary large cell lymphoma of the mediastinum. A histologic and immunophenotypic study of 29 cases. *Am J Surg Pathol* 13:730, 1989.

237. Barth T, Leithauser F, Joos S, et al: Mediastinal (thymic) large B-cell lymphoma: Where do we stand? *Lancet Oncol* 3:229, 2002.

238. Nguyen L, Ha CS, Hess M, et al: The outcome of combined-modality treatments for stage I and II primary large B-cell lymphoma of the mediastinum. *Int J Radiat Oncol Biol Phys* 47:1281, 2000.

239. Perrone T, Frizzera G, Rosai J: Mediastinal diffuse large-cell lymphoma with sclerosis. A clinicopathologic study of 60 cases. *Am J Surg Pathol* 10:176, 1986.

240. Nakagawa A, Nakamura S, Koshikawa T, et al: Clinicopathologic study of primary mediastinal non-lymphoblastic non-Hodgkin's lymphomas among the Japanese. *Acta Pathol Jpn* 43:44, 1993.

241. van Besien K, Kelta M, Bahaguna P: Primary mediastinal B-cell lymphoma: A review of pathology and management. *J Clin Oncol* 19:1855, 2001.

242. Suster S: Primary large-cell lymphomas of the mediastinum. *Semin Diagn Pathol* 16:51, 1999.

243. Jacobson J, Aisenberg AC, Lamarre L, et al: Mediastinal large cell lymphoma. An uncommon subset of adult lymphoma curable with combined modality therapy. *Cancer* 62:1893, 1988.

244. Sehn L, Antin JH, Shulman LN, et al: Primary diffuse large B-cell lymphoma of the mediastinum: Outcome following high-dose chemotherapy and autologous hematopoietic cell transplantation. *Blood* 91:717, 1998.

245. Aisenberg A: Primary large cell lymphoma of the mediastinum. *Semin Oncol* 26:251, 1999.

246. Cazals-Hatem D, Lepage E, Brice P, et al: Primary mediastinal large B-cell lymphoma. A clinicopathologic study of 141 cases compared with 916 nonmediastinal large B-cell lymphomas, a GELA ("Groupe d'Etude des Lymphomes de l'Adulte") study. *Am J Surg Pathol* 20:877, 1996.

247. Zinzani P, Martelli M, Magagnoli M, et al: Treatment and clinical management of primary mediastinal large B-cell lymphoma with sclerosis: MACOP-B regimen and mediastinal radiotherapy monitored by (67)Gallium scan in 50 patients. *Blood* 94:3289, 1999.

248. Popat U, Przepiork D, Champlin R, et al: High-dose chemotherapy for relapsed and refractory diffuse large B-cell lymphoma: Mediastinal localization predicts for a favorable outcome. *J Clin Oncol* 16:63, 1998.

249. Ferry J, Harris NL, Picker LJ, et al: Intravascular lymphomatosis (malignant angioendotheliomatosis). A B-cell neoplasm expressing surface homing receptors. *Mod Pathol* 1:444, 1988.

250. Cobcroft R: Images in haematology. Diagnosis of angiotropic large B-cell lymphoma from a peripheral blood film. *Br J Haematol* 104:429, 1999.

251. DiGiuseppe J, Nelson WG, Seifter EJ, et al: Intravascular lymphomatosis: A clinicopathologic study of 10 cases and assessment of response to chemotherapy. *J Clin Oncol* 12:2573, 1994.

252. Murase T, Nakamura S, Kawauchi K, et al: An Asian variant of intravascular large B-cell lymphoma: Clinical, pathological, and cytogenetic approaches to diffuse large B-cell lymphoma associated with haemophagocytic syndrome. *Br J Haematol* 111:826, 2000.

253. Gill S, Melosky B, Haley L, ChanYan C: Use of random skin biopsy to diagnose intravascular lymphoma presenting as fever of unknown origin. *Am J Med* 114:56, 2003.

254. Delabie J, Vandenberghe E, Kennes C, et al: Histiocyte-rich B-cell lymphoma. A distinct clinicopathologic entity possibly related to lymphocyte predominant Hodgkin's disease, paragranuloma subtype. *Am J Surg Pathol* 16:37, 1992.

255. Achten R, Verhoef G, Vanuytsel L, De Wolf-Peeters C: T-cell/histiocyte-rich large B-cell lymphoma: A distinct clinicopathologic entity. *J Clin Oncol* 20:1269, 2002.

256. Bouabdallah R, Mounier N, Guettier C, et al: T-cell/histiocyte-rich large B-cell lymphomas and classical diffuse large B-cell lymphomas have similar outcome after chemotherapy: A matched-control analysis. *J Clin Oncol* 21:1271, 2003.

257. Guinee DG Jr, Jaffe E, Kingma D, et al: Pulmonary lymphomatoid granulomatosis. Evidence for a proliferation of Epstein-Barr virus infected B-lymphocytes with a prominent T-cell component and vasculitis. *Am J Surg Pathol* 18:753, 1994.

258. Haque A, Myers JL, Hudnall SD, et al: Pulmonary lymphomatoid granulomatosis in acquired immunodeficiency syndrome: Lesions with Epstein-Barr virus infection. *Mod Pathol* 11:347, 1998.

259. Wilson W, Kingma DW, Raffeld M, et al: Association of lymphomatoid granulomatosis with Epstein-Barr viral infection of B lymphocytes and response to interferon-alpha 2b. *Blood* 87:4531, 1996.

260. Nador R, Cesarman E, Chadburn A, et al: Primary effusion lymphoma: A distinct clinicopathologic entity associated with the Kaposi's sarcoma-associated herpes virus. *Blood* 88:645, 1996.

261. Dotti G, Fiovvhi R, Motta T, et al: Primary effusion lymphoma after heart transplantation: A new entity associated with human herpesvirus-8. *Leukemia* 13:664, 1999.

262. Karcher DA, Alkan S: Human herpesvirus-8-associated body cavity-based lymphoma in human immunodeficiency virus-infected patients: A unique B-cell neoplasm. *Hum Pathol* 28:801, 1997.

263. Horenstein M, Nador RG, Chadburn A, et al: Epstein-Barr virus latent gene expression in primary effusion lymphomas containing Kaposi's sarcoma-associated herpesvirus/human herpesvirus-8. *Blood* 90:1186, 1997.

264. Simonelli C, Spina M, Cinelli R, et al: Clinical features and outcome of primary effusion lymphoma in HIV-infected patients: A single-institution study. *J Clin Oncol* 21:3948, 2003.

265. Penn I: Cancers complicating organ transplantation. *N Engl J Med* 323:1767, 1990.

266. Adami J, Gabel H, Lindelof B, et al: Cancer risk following organ transplantation: A nationwide cohort study in Sweden. *Br J Cancer* 89:1221, 2003.

267. Walker R, Paya CV, Marshall WF, et al: Pretransplantation seronegative Epstein-Barr virus status is the primary risk factor for posttransplantation lymphoproliferative disorder in adult heart, lung, and other solid organ transplantations. *J Heart Lung Transplant* 14:214, 1995.

268. Swinnen LC-N, Costanzo-Nordin MR, Fisher SG, et al: Increased incidence of lymphoproliferative disorder after immunosuppression with the monoclonal antibody OKT3 in cardiac-transplant recipients. *N Engl J Med* 323:1723, 1999.

269. Cockfield SP, Preiksaitis JK, Jewell LD, Parfrey NA: Post-transplant lymphoproliferative disorder in renal allograft recipients. Clinical experience and risk factor analysis in a single center. *Transplantation* 56:88, 1993.

270. Hanto D: Classification of Epstein-Barr virus-associated posttransplant lymphoproliferative diseases: Implications for understanding their pathogenesis and developing rational treatment strategies. *Annu Rev Med* 46:381, 1995.

271. Leblond V, Davi F, Charlotte F, et al: Posttransplant lymphoproliferative disorders not associated with Epstein-Barr virus: A distinct entity? *J Clin Oncol* 16:2052, 1998.

272. Leblond V, Sutton L, Dorent R, et al: Lymphoproliferative disorders after organ transplantation: A report of 24 cases observed in a single center. *J Clin Oncol* 13:961, 1995.

273. Nalesnik M, Jaffe R, Starzl TE, et al: The pathology of posttransplant lympho-proliferative disorders occurring in the setting of cyclosporine A-prednisone immunosuppression. *Am J Pathol* 133:173, 1998.

274. Kew CE, Lopez-Ben R, Smith JK, et al: Postransplant lymphoproliferative disorder localized near the allograft in renal transplantation. *Transplantation* 69:809, 2000.

275. Penn IP, Porat G: Central nervous system lymphomas in organ allograft recipients. *Transplantation* 59:240, 1995.

276. Rees L, Thomas A, Amlot PL: Disappearance of an Epstein-Barr virus-positive post-transplant plasmacytoma with reduction of immunosuppression. *Lancet* 352:789, 1998.

277. Tsai DE, Hardy CL, Tomaszewski JE, et al: Reduction in immunosuppression as initial therapy for posttransplant lymphoproliferative disorder: Analysis of prognostic variables and long-term follow-up of 42 adult patients. *Transplantation* 71:1076, 2001.

278. Yang J, Tao Q, Flinn IW, et al: Characterization of Epstein-Barr virus-infected B cells in patients with posttransplantation lymphoproliferative disease: Disappearance after rituximab therapy does not predict clinical response. *Blood* 96:4055, 2000.

279. Cook RC, Connors JM, Gascoyne RD, et al: Treatment of post-transplant lymphoproliferative disease with rituximab monoclonal antibody after lung transplantation. *Lancet* 354:1698, 1999.

280. Zilz ND, Olson LJ, McGregor CG: Treatment of posttransplant lymphoproliferative disorder with monoclonal CD20 antibody (rituximab) after heart transplantation. *J Heart Lung Transplant* 20:770, 2001.

281. Papadopoulos EB, Ladanyi M, Emanuel D, et al: Infusions of donor leukocytes to treat Epstein-Barr virus-associated lymphoproliferative disorders after allogeneic bone marrow transplantation. *N Engl J Med* 330:1185, 1994.

282. O'Reilly RJ, Small TN, Papadopoulos E, et al: Biology and adoptive cell therapy of Epstein-Barr virus-associated lymphoproliferative disorders in recipients of marrow allografts. *Immunol Rev* 157:195, 1997.

283. Haque TT, Taylor C, Wilkie GM, et al: Complete regression of post-transplant lymphoproliferative disease using partially hla-matched Epstein-Barr virus-specific cytotoxic T cells 1. *Transplantation* 72:1399, 2001.

284. Leblond V, Dehedin N, Mamzer-Bruneel MF, et al: Identification of prognostic factors in 61 patients with posttransplantation lymphoproliferative disorders. *J Clin Oncol* 19:772, 2001.

285. Groves FD, Linet MS, Travis LB, Devesa SS: Cancer surveillance series: Non-Hodgkin's lymphoma incidence by histologic subtype in the United States from 1978 through 1995. *J Natl Cancer Inst* 92:1240, 2000.

286. Nathwani BN, Piris MA, Harris NL, et al: Follicular lymphoma, in *World Health Organization Classification of Tumours. Pathology and Genetics of Tumors of Haematopoietic and Lymphoid Tissues,* edited by ES Jaffe, NL Harris, H Stein, JW Vardiman, p 162. IARC Press, Lyon, France, 2001.

287. The Non-Hodgkin's Lymphoma Classification Project: A clinical evaluation of the International Lymphoma Study Group classification of non-Hodgkin's lymphoma. *Blood* 89:3909, 1997.

288. Korsmeyer S: Bcl-2 initiates a new category of oncogenes: Regulators of cell death. *Blood* 80:879, 1992.

289. Biagi JJ, Seymour JF: Insights into the molecular pathogenesis of follicular lymphoma arising from analysis of geographic variation. *Blood* 99:4265, 2002.

290. Harris NL, Jaffe ES, Diebold J, et al: World Health Organization classification of neoplastic diseases of the hematopoietic and lymphoid tissues: Report of the Clinical Advisory Committee meeting—Airlie House, Virginia, November 1997. *J Clin Oncol* 17:3835, 1999.

291. Czuczman MS, Grillo-Lopez AJ, McLaughlin P, et al: Clearing of cells bearing the bcl-2 [t(14;18)] translocation from blood and marrow of

292. patients treated with rituximab alone or in combination with CHOP chemotherapy. *Ann Oncol* 12:109, 2001.

292. Rambaldi A, Lazzari M, Manzoni C, et al: Monitoring of minimal residual disease after CHOP and rituximab in previously untreated patients with follicular lymphoma. *Blood* 99:856, 2002.

293. Manus MPM, Hoppe RT: Is radiotherapy curative for stage I and II low-grade follicular lymphoma? Results of a long-term follow-up study of patients treated at Stanford University. *J Clin Oncol* 14:1282, 1996.

294. Portlock CS, Rosenberg SA: No initial therapy for stage II and IV non-Hodgkin's lymphoma of favorable histologic types. *Ann Intern Med* 90:10, 1979.

295. Straus DJ, Gaynor JJ, Leiberman PH, et al: Non-Hodgkin's lymphomas: Characteristics of long-term survivors following conservative treatment. *Am J Med* 82:247, 1986.

296. Young RC, Longo DL, Glatstein E, et al: The treatment of indolent lymphomas: Watchful waiting vs. aggressive combined modality treatment. *Semin Hematol* 25:11, 1988.

297. Kennedy BJ, Bloomfield CD, Kiang DT, et al: Combination versus successive single agent chemotherapy in lymphocytic lymphoma. *Cancer* 41:23, 1978.

298. Jones SE, Rosenberg SA, Kaplan HS, et al: Non-Hodgkin's lymphomas: II. Single agent chemotherapy. *Cancer* 30:31, 1972.

299. Portlock CS, Rosenberg SA, Glatstein E, Kaplan HS: Treatment of advanced non-Hodgkin's lymphomas with favorable histologies: Preliminary results of a prospective trial. *Blood* 47:747, 1976.

300. Hoppe RT, Kushlan P, Kaplan HS, et al: The treatment of advanced stage favorable histology non-Hodgkin's lymphoma: A preliminary report of randomized trial comparing single agent chemotherapy, combination chemotherapy, and whole body irradiation. *Blood* 58:592, 1981.

301. Hochster HS, Kim K, Green MD, et al: Activity of fludarabine in previously treated non-Hodgkin's low-grade lymphoma: Results of an Eastern Cooperative Oncology Group Study. *J Clin Oncol* 10:28, 1992.

302. Kay AC, Saven A, Carrera CJ, et al: 2-Chlorodeoxyadenosine treatment of low-grade lymphomas. *J Clin Oncol* 10:371, 1992.

303. Duggan DB, Anderson JR, Dillman R, et al: 2 Deoxycoformycin (pentostatin) for refractory non-Hodgkin's lymphoma: A CALGB phase II study. *Med Pediatr Oncol* 18:203, 1990.

304. Lister TA, Cullen MH, Beard MEJ, et al: Comparison of combined and single-agent chemotherapy in non-Hodgkin's lymphoma of favorable histological type. *Brit Med J* 1:533, 1978.

305. Luce JK, Gamble JF, Wilson HE, et al: Combined cyclophosphamide, vincristine and prednisone therapy of malignant lymphoma. *Cancer* 28:306, 1971.

306. Bagley CM Jr, DeVita VT Jr, Berard CW, Canellos GP: Advanced lymphosarcoma: Intensive cyclical combination chemotherapy with cyclophosphamide, vincristine, and prednisone. *Ann Intern Med* 76:227, 1972.

307. Schein PS, Chabner BA, Cannellos GP, et al: Potential for prolonged disease-free survival following combination chemotherapy of non-Hodgkin's lymphoma. *Blood* 43:181, 1974.

308. Peterson BA, Anderson JR, Fizzera G, et al: Nodular mixed lymphoma (NML): A comparative trial of cyclophosphamide (CTX) and cyclophosphamide, adriamycin, vincristine, prednisone, and bleomycin (CAVPB). *Blood* 66:216, 1985.

309. Jones SE, Grozea PN, Metz EN, et al: Improved complete remission rates and survival for patients with large cell lymphoma treated with chemoimmunotherapy. *Cancer* 51:1083, 1983.

310. McLaughlin P, Fuller LM, Velasquez WS, et al: Stage III follicular lymphoma: Durable remissions with a combined chemotherapy-radiotherapy regimen. *J Clin Oncol* 5:587, 1987.

311. Dana BW, Dahlberg S, Nathwani BN, et al: Long-term follow-up of patients with low-grade malignant lymphomas treated with doxorubicin-based chemotherapy or chemoimmunotherapy. *J Clin Oncol* 11:644, 1993.

312. McLaughlin P, Hagemeister FB, Romaguera JE, et al: Fludarabine, mitoxantrone, and dexamethasone: An effective new regimen for indolent lymphoma. *J Clin Oncol* 14:1262, 1996.

313. Hochester H, Oken M, Winter J, et al: Prolonged time to progression (TTP) in patients with low-grade lymphoma (LGL) treated with cyclophosphamide and fludarabine [ECOG 1491]. *Proc Am Soc Clin Oncol* 16:66a, 1998.

314. Nitkin R, LaRocca RV, Bard V, et al: Phase II trial of a sequential therapy with fludarabine, vincristine, and prednisone for low-grade follicular lymphoma. *Am J Hematol* 70:181, 2002.

315. O'Connor OA, Wright J, Moskowitz C, et al: Phase II clinical experience with the proteasome inhibitor bortezomib (formerly PS-341) in patients with indolent lymphomas. *Proc Am Soc Clin Oncol* 22:566, 2003.

316. Maloney DG, Grillo-Lopez AJ, Bodkin DJ, et al: IDEC-C2B8: Results of a phase I multi-dose trial in patients with relapsed non-Hodgkin's lymphoma. *J Clin Oncol* 15:3266, 1997.

317. McLaughlin P, Grillo-Lopez A, Link BK, et al: Rituximab chimeric anti-CD20 monoclonal antibody therapy for relapsed indolent lymphoma: Half of patients respond to a four-dose treatment program. *J Clin Oncol* 16:2825, 1998.

318. Colombat P, Salles G, Brousse N, et al: Rituximab (anti-CD20 monoclonal antibody) as single first-line therapy for patients with follicular lymphoma with a low tumor burden: Clinical and molecular evaluation. *Blood* 97:101, 2001.

319. Hainsworth JD, Litchy S, Burris HA III, et al: Rituximab as first line and maintenance therapy for patients with indolent non-Hodgkin's lymphoma. *J Clin Oncol* 20:4261, 2002.

320. Hainsworth JD, Burris HA III, Morrissey LH, et al: Rituximab monoclonal antibody as initial systemic therapy for patients with low-grade non-Hodgkin lymphoma. *Blood* 95:3052, 2000.

321. Leonard JP, Coleman M, Matthews JC, et al: Epratuzumab (anti-CD22) and rituximab (anti-CD20) combination immunotherapy for non-Hodgkin's lymphoma: Preliminary response data. *Proc Am Soc Clin Oncol* 21:266a, 2002.

322. Vose JM, Wahl RL, Saleh M, et al: Multicenter phase II study of iodine-131 tositumomab for chemotherapy-relapsed/refractory low-grade and transformed low-grade B-cell non-Hodgkin's lymphomas. *J Clin Oncol* 18:1316, 2000.

323. Witzig TE, Gordon LI, Cabanillas F, et al: Randomized controlled trial of yttrium-90-labeled ibritumomab tiuxetan radioimmunotherapy versus rituximab immunotherapy for patients with relapsed or refractory low-grade, follicular, or transformed B-cell non-Hodgkin's lymphoma. *J Clin Oncol* 20:2453, 2002.

324. Davis T, Kaminski M, Leonard J, et al: Results of a randomized study of Bexxar (tositumomab and iodine-131 tositumomab) versus unlabelled tostitumomab in patients with relapsed or refractory low-grade or transformed non-Hodgkin's lymphoma. *Blood* 98:843a, 2001.

325. Witzig TE, Flinn IW, Gordon LI, et al: Treatment with ibritumomab tiuxetan radioimmunotherapy in patients with rituximab-refractory follicular non-Hodgkin's lymphoma. *J Clin Oncol* 20:3262, 2002.

326. Kaminski MS, Zelenetz AD, Press OW, et al: Pivotal study of iodine I 131 tositumomab for chemotherapy refractory low-grade or transformed low-grade B-cell non-Hodgkin's lymphomas. *J Clin Oncol* 19:3918, 2001.

327. Kaminski MS, Tuck M, Regan D, et al: High response rates and durable remissions in patients with previously untreated, advanced-stage, follicular lymphoma treated with tositumomab and iodine I-131 tositumomab (Bexxar®). *Blood* 100:356a, 2002.

328. Press OW, Unger JM, Braziel RM, et al: A phase 2 trial of CHOP chemotherapy followed by tositumomab/iodine I 131 tositumomab for previously untreated follicular non-Hodgkin lymphoma: SWOG S9911. *Blood* 102:1606, 2003.

329. Dillman RO: Radiolabeled anti-CD20 monoclonal antibodies for the treatment of B-cell lymphoma. *J Clin Oncol* 20:3545, 2002.

330. Gordon LI, Witzig T, Molina A, et al: Yttrium 90-labeled ibritumomab tiuxetan radioimmunotherapy produces high response rates and durable remissions in patients with previously treated B-cell lymphoma. *Clin Lymphoma* 5:98, 2004.

331. van Besien K, Sobocinski KA, Rowlings PA, et al: Allogeneic marrow transplantation for low-grade lymphoma. *Blood* 92:1832, 1998.

332. Gribben JG, Freedman AS, Neuberg D, et al: Immunologic purging of marrow assessed by PCR before autologous bone marrow transplantation for B-cell lymphoma. *N Engl J Med* 325:1525, 1991.

333. Bierman PI, Vose JM, Anderson JR, et al: High-dose therapy with autologous hematopoietic rescue for follicular low-grade non-Hodgkin's lymphoma. *J Clin Oncol* 15:445, 1997.

334. Colombat P, Donadio D, Fouillard L, et al: Value of autologous bone marrow transplantation in follicular lymphoma: A France autogreffe retrospective study of 42 patients. *Bone Marrow Transplant* 13:157, 1994.

335. Cervantes F, Shu XO, McGlave PB, et al: Autologous bone marrow transplantation for non-transformed low-grade non-Hodgkin's lymphoma. *Bone Marrow Transplant* 16:387, 1995.

336. Freedman AS, Gribben JG, Neuberg D, et al: High-dose therapy and autologous bone marrow transplantation in patients with follicular lymphoma during first remission. *Blood* 88:2780, 1996.

337. Apostolidis J, Gupta RK, Grenzelias D, et al: High-dose therapy with autologous bone marrow support as consolidation of remission in follicular lymphoma: Long-term clinical and molecular follow-up. *J Clin Oncol* 18:527, 2000.

338. Rohatiner A, Johnson P, Price C, et al: Myeloablative therapy with autologous bone marrow transplantation as consolidation therapy for recurrent follicular lymphoma. *J Clin Oncol* 12:1177, 1994.

339. Foon KA, Sherwin SA, Abrams PG, et al: Treatment of advanced non-Hodgkin's lymphoma with recombinant leukocyte A interferon. *N Engl J Med* 311:1148, 1984.

340. Horning SJ, Merigan TC, Krown SE, et al: Human interferon alpha in malignant lymphoma and Hodgkin's disease. Results of the American Cancer Society trial. *Cancer* 56:1305, 1985.

341. Solal-Celigny P, Lepage E, Brousse N, et al: Doxorubicin-containing regimen with or without interferon alfa-2b for advanced follicular lymphomas: Final analysis of survival and toxicity in the Groupe d'Etude des Lymphomas Folliculaires 86 trial. *J Clin Oncol* 16:2332, 1998.

342. Arranz R, Garcia-Alfonso P, Sobrino P, et al: Role of interferon alfa-2b in the induction and maintenance treatment of low-grade non-Hodgkin's lymphoma: Results from a prospective, multicenter trial with double randomization. *J Clin Oncol* 16:1538, 1998.

343. Smalley RV, Anderson JW, Hawkins MJ, et al: Interferon alfa combined with cytotoxic chemotherapy for patients with non-Hodgkin's lymphoma. *N Engl J Med* 327:1336, 1992.

344. Andersen JW, Smalley RV: Interferon alfa plus chemotherapy for non-Hodgkin's lymphoma: Five-year follow-up [letter]. *N Engl J Med* 329:1821, 1993.

345. Peterson BA, Petroni GR, Oken MM, et al: Cyclophosphamide versus cyclophosphamide plus interferon alpha-2b in follicular low-grade lymphomas: An intergroup phase III trial (CALGB 8691 and EST 7486). *Proc Am Soc Clin Oncol* 16:48a, 1997.

346. Hagenbeck A, Carde P, Meerwaldt JH, et al: Maintenance of remission with human recombinant interferon alfa-2a in patients with stages III and IV low-grade malignant non-Hodgkin's lymphoma. European Organization for Research and Treatment of Cancer Lymphoma Cooperative Group. *J Clin Oncol* 16:41, 1998.

347. Price CG, Rohatiner AZ, Steward W, et al: Interferon alfa-2b in addition to chlorambucil in the treatment of follicular lymphoma: Preliminary results of a randomized trial in progress. *Eur J Cancer* 27:S34, 1991.

348. Unterhalt M, Herman R, Koch P, et al: Long term interferon alpha maintenance prolongs remission duration in advanced low-grade lymphomas

and is related to the efficacy of the initial cytoreductive chemotherapy. *Blood* 88:1801a, 1996.

349. Dana BW, Unter J, Fisher RI: A randomized study of alpha-interferon consolidation in patients with low-grade lymphoma who have responded to PRO-MACE-MOPP (Day 1-8). *Proc Am Soc Clin Oncol* 17:3a, 1998.

350. Bernstein ZP, Vaickus L, Friedman N, et al: Interleukin-2 lymphokine-activated killer cell therapy of non-Hodgkin's lymphoma and Hodgkin's disease. *J Immunother* 10:141, 1991.

351. Duggan DB, Santarelli MT, Zamkoff K, et al: A phase II study of recombinant interleukin-2 with or without recombinant interferon-β in non-Hodgkin's lymphoma. A study of the Cancer and Leukemia Group B. *J Immunother* 12:115, 1992.

352. Weber JS, Yang JC, Topalian SL, et al: The use of interleukin-2 and lymphokine-activated killer cells for the treatment of patients with non-Hodgkin's lymphoma. *J Clin Oncol* 10:33, 1992.

353. Friedberg JW, Neuberg D, Gribben JG, et al: Combination with rituximab and interleukin 2 in patients with relapsed or refractory follicular non-Hodgkin's lymphoma. *Br J Haematol* 117:828, 2002.

354. Meeker TC, Lowder J, Maloney DG, et al: A clinical trial of anti-idiotype therapy of B-cell malignancy. *Blood* 65:1349, 1985.

355. Brown SL, Miller RA, Horning SJ, et al: Treatment of B-cell lymphoma with anti-idiotypic antibodies alone and in combination with alpha interferon. *Blood* 73:651, 1989.

356. Maloney DG, Brown S, Czerwinski DK, et al: Monoclonal anti-idiotype antibody therapy of B-cell lymphoma: The addition of a short course of chemotherapy does not interfere with the antitumor effect nor prevent the emergence of idiotype-negative variant cells. *Blood* 80:1502, 1992.

357. Cleary ML, Meeker TI, Levy S, et al: Clustering of extensive somatic mutations in the variable region of an immunoglobulin heavy chain gene from a human B-cell lymphoma. *Cell* 44:97, 1986.

358. Kwak LW, Campbell MJ, Czerwinski DK, et al: Induction of immune responses in patients with B-cell lymphoma against the surface-immunoglobulin idiotype expressed by their tumors. *N Engl J Med* 327:1209, 1992.

359. Nelson EL, Li X, Hsu FJ, et al: Tumor-specific, cytotoxic T-lymphocyte response after idiotype vaccination for B-cell, non-Hodgkin's lymphoma. *Blood* 88:580, 1996.

360. Hsu FJ, Caspar CB, Czerwinski D, et al: Tumor-specific idiotype vaccines in the treatment of patients with B-cell lymphoma—Long-term results of a clinical trial. *Blood* 89:3129, 1997.

361. Timmerman JM, Czerwinski DK, Davis TA, et al: Idiotype-pulsed dendritic cell vaccination for B-cell lymphoma: Clinical and immune responses in 35 patients. *Blood* 99:1517, 2002.

362. Hsu F, Benike C, Fagnoni F, et al: Vaccination of patients with B cell lymphoma using autologous antigen pulsed dendritic cells. *Nat Med* 2:1038, 1996.

363. Stone MJ, Sausville EA, Fay JW, et al: A phase I study of bolus versus continuous infusion of the anti-CD19 immunotoxin, IgG-HD37-dgA, in patients with B-cell lymphoma. *Blood* 88:1188, 1996.

364. Grossbard ML, Freeman AS, Ritz J, et al: Serotherapy of B-cell neoplasms with anti-B4 blocked ricin: A phase I trial of daily bolus infusion. *Blood* 79:576, 1992.

365. Conry RM, Khazaeli MB, Saleh MN, et al: Phase I trial of an anti-CD19 deglycosylated ricin A chain immunotoxin in non-Hodgkin's lymphoma: Effect of an intensive schedule of administration. *J Immunol* 18:231, 1996.

366. Lopez-Buillermo A, Montserrat E, Bosch F, et al: Applicability of the International Index for Aggressive Lymphomas to patients with low-grade lymphoma. *J Clin Oncol* 12:1343, 1994.

367. Federico M, Vitolo U, Zinzani PL, et al: Prognosis of follicular lymphoma: A predictive model based on a retrospective analysis of 987 cases. *Blood* 95:783, 2000.

368. Warnke R, Kim H, Fuks Z, Dorfman R: The co-existence of nodular and diffuse patterns in nodular non-Hodgkin's lymphomas. *Cancer* 40:1229, 1997.

369. Ezdinli E, Costello W, Kucuk O, Berard C: Effect of the degree of nodularity on the survival of patients with nodular lymphomas. *J Clin Oncol* 5:413, 1987.

370. Brittinger G, Bartels H, Common H, et al: Clinical and prognostic relevance of the Kiel classification of non-Hodgkin's lymphomas: Results of a prospective multicenter study by the Kiel lymphoma study group. *Hematol Oncol* 2:296, 1984.

371. Lossos IS, Levy R: Higher-grade transformation of follicle center lymphoma is associated with somatic mutation of the 5′ encoding regulatory region of the bcl-6 gene. *Blood* 96:635, 2002.

372. Akasaka T, Lossos IS, Levy R: BCL6 gene translocation in follicular lymphoma: A harbinger of eventual transformation to diffuse aggressive lymphoma. *Blood* 102:1443, 2003.

373. Davis TA, White CA, Grillo-Lopez AJ, et al: Single-agent monoclonal antibody efficacy in bulky non-Hodgkin's lymphoma: Results of a phase II trial of rituximab. *J Clin Oncol* 17:1851, 1999.

374. Feuring-Buske M, Kneba M, Unterhalt M, et al: IDEC-C2B8 (rituximab) anti-CD20 antibody treatment in relapsed advanced-stage follicular lymphomas: Results of a phase-II study of the German Low-Grade Lymphoma Study Group. *Ann Hematol* 79:493, 2000.

375. Piro LD, White CA, Grillo-Lopez AJ, et al: Extended rituximab (anti-CD20 monoclonal antibody) therapy for relapsed or refractory low-grade or follicular non-Hodgkin's lymphoma. *Ann Oncol* 10:655, 1999.

376. Aviles A, Leon MI, Diaz-Maqueo JC, et al: Rituximab in the treatment of refractory follicular lymphoma—Six doses are better than four. *J Hematother Stem Cell Res* 10:313, 2001.

377. Sacchi S, Federico M, Vitolo U, et al: Clinical activity and safety of combination immunotherapy with IFN-alpha 2a and rituximab in patients with relapsed low-grade non-Hodgkin's lymphoma. *Haematologica* 86:951, 2001.

378. Gregory SA, Venugopal P, Adler SS, et al: Phase II study of fludarabine phosphate and mitoxantrone followed by anti-CD20 monoclonal antibody in the treatment of patients with newly diagnosed, advanced low-grade non-Hodgkin's lymphoma (LGNHL): Interim results. *Blood* 102:1499a, 2003.

379. Czuczman MS, Grillo-Lopez AJ, White CA, et al: Treatment of patients with low-grade B-cell lymphoma with the combination of chimeric anti-CD20 monoclonal antibody and CHOP chemotherapy. *J Clin Oncol* 17:268, 1999.

380. Mollejo M, Menarguez J, Lloret E, et al: Splenic marginal zone lymphoma: A distinctive type of low-grade B-cell lymphoma. A clinicopathological study of 13 cases. *Am J Surg Pathol* 19:1146, 1995.

381. Jennings CD, Foon KA: Recent advances in flow cytometry: Application to the diagnosis of hematologic malignancy. *Blood* 90:2863, 1997.

382. Wotherspoon AC, Pan LX, Diss TC, Isaacson PG: Cytogenetic study of B-cell lymphoma of mucosa-associated lymphoid tissue. *Cancer Genet Cytogenet* 8:35, 1992.

383. Ott G, Katzenberg T, Greiner A, et al: The t(11;18)(q21;q21) chromosome translocation is a frequent and specific aberration in low-grade but not high-grade malignant non-Hodgkin's lymphomas of the mucosa-associated lymphoid tissue (MALT) type. *Cancer Res* 57:3944, 1997.

384. Isaacson P, Wright DH: Malignant lymphoma of mucosa-associated lymphoid tissue. A distinctive type of B-cell lymphoma. *Cancer* 52:1410, 1983.

385. Isaacson P, Wright DH: Extranodal malignant lymphoma arising from mucosa-associated lymphoid tissue. *Cancer* 53:2515, 1984.

386. Harris NL, Isaacson PG: What are the criteria for distinguishing MALT from non-MALT lymphoma at extranodal sites? *Am J Clin Pathol* 111:S126, 1999.

387. Zucca E, Conconi A, Pedrinis E, et al: Nongastric marginal zone B-cell

lymphoma of mucosa-associated lymphoid tissue. *Blood* 101:2489, 2003.

388. Zucca E, Bertoni F, Roggero E, Cavalli F: The gastric marginal B-cell lymphoma of MALT type. *Blood* 96:410, 2000.

389. Pelstring RJ, Essell JH, Kurtin PJ, et al: Diversity of organ site involvement among malignant lymphomas of mucosa-associated tissues. *Am J Clin Pathol* 96:738, 1991.

390. Parsonnet J, Hansen S, Rodriguez L, et al: Helicobacter pylori and gastric lymphoma. *Gastroenterology* 108:610, 1994.

391. Howden CW, Hunt RH: Guidelines for the management of Helicobacter pylori infection. Ad Hoc Committee on Practice Parameters of the American College of Gastroenterology. *Am J Gastroenterol* 93:2330, 1998.

392. de Jong D, Aleman BMP, Taal BG, Boot H: Controversies and consensus in the diagnosis, work-up and treatment of gastric lymphoma: An international survey. *Ann Oncol* 10:275, 1999.

393. Pinotti G, Zucca E, Roggero E, et al: Clinical features, treatment and outcome in a series of 93 patients with low-grade gastric MALT lymphoma. *Leuk Lymphoma* 26:527, 1997.

394. Hyjek E, Smith WJ, Isaacson PG: Primary B-cell lymphoma of salivary glands and its relationship to myoepithelial sialadenitis. *Hum Pathol* 19: 766, 1988.

395. Sackmann M, Morgner A, Rudolph B, et al: Regression of gastric MALT lymphoma after eradication of Helicobacter pylori is predicted by endosonographic staging. *Gastroenterology* 113:1087, 1997.

396. Pavlick AC, Geres H, Portlock C: Endoscopic ultrasound in the evaluation of gastric small lymphocytic mucosa-associated lymphoid tumors. *J Clin Oncol* 15:1761, 1997.

397. Liu H, Ye H, Ruskone-Fourmestraux A, et al: T(11:18) is a marker for all stage gastric MALT lymphomas that will not respond to *H. pylori* eradication. *Gastroenterology* 122:1286, 2002.

398. Bartlett DL, Karpeh MS Jr, Filippa DA, Brennan MF: Long-term follow-up after curative surgery for early gastric lymphoma. *Ann Surg* 223:53, 1996.

399. Schechter NR, Portlock CS, Yahalom J: Treatment of mucosa-associated lymphoid tissue lymphoma of the stomach with radiation alone. *J Clin Oncol* 16:1916, 1998.

400. Hammel P, Haloun C, Chaumette MT, et al: Efficacy of single-agent chemotherapy in low-grade B-cell mucosa-associated lymphoid tissue lymphoma with prominent gastric expression. *J Clin Oncol* 13:2524, 1995.

401. Jager G, Neumeister P, Brezinshek R, et al: Treatment of extranodal marginal zone B-cell lymphoma of mucosa-associated lymphoid tissue type with cladribine: A phase II study. *J Clin Oncol* 20:3872, 2002.

402. Conconi A, Martinelli G, Thieblemont C, et al: Clinical activity of rituximab in extranodal marginal zone B-cell lymphoma of MALT type. *Blood* 102:2741, 2003.

403. Conconi A, Zucca E, Pedrinis E, et al: Nongastric marginal zone B-cell lymphoma of mucosa-associated lymphoid tissue. *Blood* 101:2489, 2003.

404. Berger F, Felman P, Thieblemont C, et al: Non-MALT marginal zone B-cell lymphomas: A description of clinical presentation and outcome in 124 patients. *Blood* 95:1950, 2000.

405. Nathwani BN, Anderson JR, Armitage JO, et al: Marginal zone B-cell lymphoma: A clinical comparison of nodal and mucosa-associated lymphoid tissue types. *J Clin Oncol* 17:2486, 1999.

406. Troussard X, Valensi F, Duchayne E, et al: Splenic lymphoma with villous lymphocytes: Clinical presentation, biology and prognostic factors in a series of 100 patients. *Br J Haematol* 937:31, 1996.

407. Schmid C, Kirkha N, Diss T, Isaacson PG: Splenic marginal zone cell lymphoma. *Am J Surg Pathol* 16:455, 1992.

408. Mateo M, Manuela M, Villuendas R, et al: 7q31-32 allelic loss is a frequent finding in splenic marginal zone lymphoma. *Am J Pathol* 154: 1583, 1999.

409. Murakami H, Irisawa H, Saitoh T, et al: Immunological abnormalities in splenic marginal zone cell lymphoma. *Am J Hematol* 5:173, 1997.

410. Chacon JI, Mollejo M, Munoz E, et al: Splenic marginal zone lymphoma: Clinical characteristics and prognostic factors in a series of 60 patients. *Blood* 100:1648, 2002.

411. Lefrere F, Hermine O, Belanger C, et al: Fludarabine: An effective treatment in patients with splenic lymphoma with villous lymphocytes. *Leukemia* 14:573, 2000.

412. Lefrere F, Hermine O, Francois S, et al: Lack of efficacy of 2-chlorodeoxyadenosine in the treatment of splenic lymphoma with villous lymphocytes. *Leuk Lymphoma* 10:113, 2000.

413. Czuczman MS: Immunochemotherapy in indolent non-Hodgkin's lymphoma. *Semin Oncol* 29:11, 2002.

414. Hermine O, Lefrere F, Bronowicki JP, et al: Regression of splenic lymphoma with villous lymphocytes after treatment of hepatitis C virus infection. *N Engl J Med* 347:89, 2002.

415. Non-Hodgkin's Lymphoma Pathologic Classification Project: National Cancer Institute sponsored study of classifications of non-Hodgkin's lymphomas: Summary and description of a Working Formulation for clinical usage. *Cancer* 49:2112, 1982.

416. Weisenburger DD, Armitage JO: Mantle cell lymphoma—An entity comes of age. *J Am Soc Hematol* 87:4483, 1996.

417. Hiddemann W, Unterhalt M, Herrmann R, et al: Mantle-cell lymphomas have more widespread disease and a slower response to chemotherapy compared with follicle-center lymphomas: Results of a prospective comparative analysis of the German low-grade lymphoma study group. *J Clin Oncol* 16:1922, 1998.

418. Velders GA, Kluin-Nelemans JC, De Boer CJ, et al: Mantle-cell lymphoma: A population-based clinical study. *J Clin Oncol* 14:1269, 1996.

419. Aratoff LH, Connors JM, Klasa RJ, et al: Mantle cell lymphoma: A clinicopathologic study of 80 cases. *Blood* 89:2067, 1997.

420. Majlis A, Pugh WC, Rodriguez MA, et al: Mantle cell lymphoma: Correlation of clinical outcome and biologic features with three histologic variants. *J Clin Oncol* 15:1664, 1997.

421. Press OW, Grogan TM, Fisher RI: Evaluation and management of mantle cell lymphoma. *Adv Leuk Lymphoma* 6:3, 1996.

422. Hiddemann W, Brittenger G, Tiemann M, et al: Presentation features and clinical course of mantle cell lymphoma—Results of a European survey. *Ann Oncol* 7:22, 1996.

423. Swerdlow SH, Habeshaw JA, Murray LJ, et al: Centrocytic lymphoma. A distinct clinicopathologic and immunologic entity. A multiparameter study of 18 cases at diagnosis and relapse. *Am J Pathol* 113: 181, 1983.

424. Lardelli P, Bookman MA, Sundeen J, et al: Lymphocytic lymphoma of intermediate differentiation. Morphologic and immunophenotypic spectrum and clinical correlations. *Am J Surg Pathol* 14:752, 1990.

425. Segal GH, Masih AS, Fox AC, et al: CD5-expression B-cell non-Hodgkin's lymphomas with bcl-1 gene rearrangement have a relatively homogeneous immunophenotype and are associated with an overall poor prognosis. *Blood* 85:1570, 1995.

426. Medeiros L, van Krieken J, Jaffe E, Raffeldt M: Association of bcl-1 rearrangements with lymphocytic lymphoma of intermediate differentiation. *Blood* 76:2086, 1990.

427. Rimokh R, Berger F, Cornillet P, et al: Break in the BCL 1 locus is closely associated with intermediate lymphocytic lymphoma subtype. *Genes Chrom Cancer* 2:223, 1990.

428. Williams ME, Westermann CD, Swerdlow SH: Genotypic characterization of centrocytic lymphoma: Frequent rearrangement of the chromosome 11 bcl-1 locus. *Blood* 76:1387, 1990.

429. Vandeberghe E, De Wolf-Peeters C, Van den Oord J, et al: Translocation (11;14): A cytogenetic anomaly associated with B-cell lymphomas of non-follicle center cell lineage. *J Pathol* 163:13, 1991.

430. Rosenberg C, Wong E, Petty E, et al: Overexpression of PRAD1, a

candidate BCL 1 breakpoint region oncogene, in centrocytic lymphomas. *Proc Natl Acad Sci U S A* 88:9638, 1991.

431. Williams M, Swerdlow A, Rosenberg C, Arnold A: Characterization of chromosome 11 translocation breakpoints at the bcl-1 and PRAD 1 loci in centrocytic lymphoma. *Cancer Res* 52:5541, 1992.

432. Pott C, Schrader C, Derner N, et al: Molecular remission predicts progression-free survival in mantle cell lymphoma after peripheral blood stem cell transplantation. *Ann Oncol* 69:226a, 2002.

433. Meusers P, Hense J, Brittinger G: Mantle cell lymphoma: Diagnostic criteria, clinical aspects and therapeutic problems. *Leukemia* 11(suppl 2):S60, 1997.

434. Zucca E, Roggero E, Pinotti G, et al: Patterns of survival in mantle cell lymphoma. *Ann Oncol* 6:257, 1995.

435. Vandenberghe E, De Wolf-Peeters C, Vaughan HG, et al: Clinical outcome of 65 cases of mantle cell lymphoma initially treated with non-intensive therapy by the British National Lymphoma Investigation Group. *Br J Haematol* 99:842, 1997.

436. Meusers P, Engelhard M, Bartels H, et al: Multicentre random therapeutic trial for advanced centrocytic lymphoma: Anthracycline does not improve the prognosis. *Hematol Oncol* 7:365, 1989.

437. Lefrè F, Delmer A, Suzan F, et al: Sequential chemotherapy by CHOP and DHAP regimens followed by high-dose therapy with stem cell transplantation induces a high rate of complete response and improves event-free survival in mantle cell lymphoma: A prospective study. *Leukemia* 16:587, 2002.

438. Khouri IF, Ramaguera J, Kantarjian H, et al: Hyper-CVAD and high-dose methotrexate/cytarabine followed by stem-cell transplantation: An active regimen for aggressive mantle-cell lymphoma. *J Clin Oncol* 16:3803, 1998.

439. Howard OM, Gribben JG, Neuberg DS, et al: Rituximab and CHOP induction therapy for newly diagnosed mantle-cell lymphoma: Molecular complete responses are not predictive of progression-free survival. *J Clin Oncol* 20:1288, 2002.

440. Hiddemann W, Dreyling M, German Low Grade Lymphoma Study Group: Rituximab plus chemotherapy in follicular and mantle cell lymphoma. *Semin Oncol* 30(suppl 12):16, 2003.

441. Romaguera JE, Dang NH, Hagemeister FB, et al: Preliminary report of rituximab with intensive chemotherapy for untreated aggressive mantle cell lymphoma (MCL). *Blood* 96:733a, 2000.

442. Drach J, Kaufmann H, Puespoek A, et al: Marked anti-tumor activity of rituximab plus thalidomide in patients with relapsed/resistant mantle cell lymphoma. *Blood* 606a, 2002.

443. Drach J, Kaufman H, Woehrer S, et al: Durable remissions after rituximab plus thalidomide for relapsed/refractory mantle cell lymphoma. *Proc Am Soc Clin Oncol* 23:6583a, 2004.

444. Ghielmini M, Hsu Schmitz S-F, Burki K, et al: The effect of rituximab on patients with follicular and mantle-cell lymphoma. *Ann Oncol* 11:S123, 2000.

445. Foran JM, Rohatiner AZS, Cunningham D, et al: European phase II study of rituximab (chimeric anti-CD20 monoclonal antibody) for patients with newly diagnosed mantle-cell lymphoma and previously treated mantle-cell lymphoma, immunocytoma, and small B-cell lymphocytic lymphoma. *J Clin Oncol* 18:317, 2000.

446. Cohen BJ, Moskowitz C, Straus D, et al: Cyclophosphamide/fludarabine (CF) is active in the treatment of mantle cell lymphoma. *Leuk Lymphoma* 42:1015, 2001.

447. Decaudin D, Bosq J, Tertian G, et al: Phase II trial of fludarabine monophosphate in patients with mantle-cell lymphomas. *J Clin Oncol* 16:579, 1998.

448. Zinzani PL, Magagnoli M, Moretti L, et al: Randomized trial of fludarabine versus fludarabine and idarubicin as frontline treatment in patients with indolent or mantle-cell lymphoma. *J Clin Oncol* 18:773, 2000.

449. Foran JM, Rohatiner AZS, Coiffler B, et al: Multicenter phase II study

450. Rummel MJ, Chow KU, Karakas T, et al: Reduced-dose cladribine (2-CdA) plus mitoxantrone is effective in the treatment of mantle-cell and low-grade non-Hodgkin's lymphoma. *Eur J Cancer* 38:1739, 2002.

451. Goy A, Younes A, McLaughlin B, et al: Update on a phase 2 study of bortezomib in patients with relapsed or refractory indolent or aggressive non-Hodgkin's lymphoma. *Proc Am Soc Clin Oncol* 23:6581a, 2004.

452. Behr TM, Griesinger F, Riggert J, et al: High-dose myeloablative radioimmunotherapy of mantle cell non-Hodgkin lymphoma with the iodine-131-labeled chimeric anti-CD20 antibody C2B8 and autologous stem cell support. *Cancer* 94:1363, 2002.

453. Gopal AK, Rajendran JG, Petersdorf SH, et al: High-dose chemo-radioimmunotherapy with autologous stem cell support for relapsed mantle cell lymphoma. *Blood* 99:3158, 2002.

454. Wright D: What is Burkitt's lymphoma? *J Pathol* 182:125, 1997.

455. Yano T, van Kricken J, Magrath I, et al: Histogenetic correlations between subcategories of small non-cleaved cell lymphomas. *Blood* 79:1282, 1992.

456. Braziel R, Arber DA, Slovak ML, et al: The Burkitt-like lymphomas: A Southwest Oncology Group study delineating phenotypic, genotypic, and clinical features. *Blood* 97:3713, 2001.

457. Garcia C, Weiss LM, Warnke RA: Small noncleaved cell lymphoma: An immunophenotypic study of 18 cases and comparison with large cell lymphoma. *Hum Pathol* 17:454, 1986.

458. Falini B, Fizzotti M, Pileri S, et al: Bcl-6 protein expression in normal and neoplastic lymphoid tissues. *Ann Oncol* 8(suppl):101, 1997.

459. Grogan T, Warnke RA, Kaplan HS: A comparative study of Burkitt's and non-Burkitt's "undifferentiated" malignant lymphoma: Immunologic, cytochemical, ultrastructural, cytologic, histopathologic, clinical and cell culture features. *Cancer* 49:181, 1982.

460. Sweetenham J, Pearce R, Taghipour G, et al: Adult Burkitt's and Burkitt-like non-Hodgkin's lymphoma—Outcome for patients treated with high-dose therapy and autologous stem-cell transplantation in first remission or at relapse: Results from the European Group for Blood and Marrow Transplantation. *J Clin Oncol* 14:2465, 1996.

461. McGrath IT, Janus C, Edwards BK, et al: An effective therapy for both undifferentiated (including Burkitt's) lymphomas and lymphoblastic lymphomas in children and young adults. *Blood* 63:1102, 1984.

462. Soussain C, Patte C, Ostronoff M, et al: Small noncleaved cell lymphoma and leukemia in adults. A retrospective study of 65 adults treated with the LMB pediatric protocols. *Blood* 85:664, 1995.

463. Bishop P, Rao VK, Wilson WH: Burkitt's lymphoma: Molecular pathogenesis and treatment. *Cancer Invest* 18:574, 2000.

464. Cairo M, Sposto R, Perkins SL, et al: Burkitt's and Burkitt-like lymphoma in children and adolescents: A review of the Children's Cancer Group Experience. *Br J Haematol* 120:660, 2003.

465. Magrath I, Adde M, Shad A, et al: Adults and children with small non-cleaved-cell lymphoma have a similar excellent outcome when treated with the same chemotherapy regimen. *J Clin Oncol* 14:925, 1996.

466. Rizzieri D, Johnson JL, Niedzwiecki D, et al: Efficacy and toxicity of brief duration high intensity chemotherapy for small noncleaved cell lymphoma/FAB L3 acute lymphoblastic leukemia: Results of CALGB 9251. *Blood* 96:829a, 2000.

467. Lee E, Pettroni GR, Schiffer CA, et al: Brief-duration high-intensity chemotherapy for patients with small noncleaved-cell lymphoma or FAB L3 acute lymphocytic leukemia: Results of cancer and leukemia group B study 9251. *J Clin Oncol* 19:4014, 2001.

468. Link M, Donaldson SS, Berard CW, et al: Results of treatment of childhood localized non-Hodgkin's lymphoma with combination chemotherapy with or without radiotherapy. *N Engl J Med* 322:1169, 1990.

469. Jost L, Jacky E, Dommann-Scherrer C, et al: Short-term weekly chemo-

therapy followed by high-dose therapy with autologous bone marrow transplantation for lymphoblastic and Burkitt's lymphomas in adult patients. *Ann Oncol* 6:445, 1995.

470. Grigg A, Seymour JF: Graft versus Burkitt's lymphoma effect after allogeneic marrow transplantation. *Leuk Lymphoma* 43:889, 2002.

471. Uchiyama T, Yodoi J, Sagawa K, et al: Adult T-cell leukemia: Clinical and hematologic features of 16 cases. *Blood* 50:481, 1977.

472. Bunn PA, Schechter GP, Jaffe E, et al: Clinical course of retrovirus associated adult T-cell lymphoma in the United States: Staging, evaluation, and management. *N Engl J Med* 309:257, 1983.

473. Catovsky D, Greaves MF, Rose M, et al: Adult T-cell lymphoma/leukemia in blacks from the West Indies. *Lancet* 1:639, 1982.

474. Bunn PA: Clinical features, in T-cell lymphoproliferative syndrome associated with human T-cell leukemia/lymphoma virus. *Ann Intern Med* 100:543, 1984.

475. Tajima K: The 4th nation-wide study of adult T-cell leukemia/lymphoma (ATL) in Japan: Estimates of risk of ATL and its geographical and clinical features. The T- and B-Cell Malignancy Study Group. *Int J Cancer* 45:237, 1990.

476. Shimoyama M: Diagnostic criteria and classification of clinical subtypes of adult T-cell leukemia-lymphoma: A report from the Lymphoma Study Group [1984–1987]. *Br J Haematol* 79:428, 1991.

477. Uchiyama T, Yodoi J, Sagawa K, et al: Adult T-cell leukemia: Clinical and hematologic features of 16 cases. *Blood* 50:481, 1977.

478. Pancake BA, Wassef EH, Zucker-Franklin D: Demonstration of antibodies to human T-cell lymphotropic virus-I tax in patients with the cutaneous T-cell lymphoma, mycosis fungoides, who are seronegative for antibodies to the structural proteins of the virus. *Blood* 88:3004, 1996.

479. Shohat M, Hodak E, Hannig H, et al: Evidence for the cofactor role of human T-cell lymphotropic virus type 1 in mycosis fungoides and Sezary syndrome. *Br J Dermatol* 141:44, 1999.

480. Zucker-Franklin D, Pancake BA: Human T-cell lymphotropic virus type 1 tax among American blood donors. *Clin Diagn Lab Immunol* 5:831, 1998.

481. Waldmann TA, Greene WC, Sarin PS, et al: Functional and phenotypic comparison of human T-cell leukemia/lymphoma virus positive adult T-cell leukemia with human T-cell leukemia/lymphoma virus negative Sezary leukemia, and their distinction using anti-tac. *J Clin Invest* 73:1711, 1984.

482. Flug F, Pelicci PG, Bonetti F, et al: T-cell receptor gene rearrangements as markers of lineage and clonality in T-cell neoplasms. *Proc Natl Acad Sci U S A* 82:3460, 1984.

483. Waldmann TA, David MM, Bongiovanni KF, Korsmeyer SJ: Rearrangements of genes for the antigen receptor on T-cells as markers of lineage and clonality in human lymphoid neoplasms. *N Engl J Med* 313:776, 1985.

484. Bertness V, Lirsch I, Hollis G, et al: T-cell receptor gene arrangements as clinical markers of human T-cell lymphomas. *N Engl J Med* 313:534, 1985.

485. Aisenberg AC, Krontiris TG, Mak TW, Wilkes BM: Rearrangement of the gene for the beta-chain of the T-cell receptor in T-cell chronic lymphocytic leukemia and related disorders. *N Engl J Med* 313:530, 1985.

486. Yamaguchi K, Nishimura H, Kohrogi H, et al: A proposal for smoldering adult T-cell leukemia: A clinicopathologic study of five cases. *Blood* 62:758, 1983.

487. Shimoyama M, Ota K, Kikuchi M, et al: Chemotherapeutic results and prognostic factors of patients with advanced non-Hodgkin's lymphoma treated with VEPA or VEPA-M. *J Clin Oncol* 6:128, 1988.

488. Shimoyama M, Ota K, Kikuchi M, et al: Major prognostic factors of adult patients with advanced T-cell lymphoma/leukemia. *J Clin Oncol* 6:1088, 1998.

489. Tobinai K, Shimoyama M, Minato K, et al: Japan Clinical Oncology Group phase II trial of second-generation "LSG4 protocol" in aggressive T- and B-lymphoma: A new predictive model for T- and B-lymphoma. *Proc Am Soc Clin Oncol* 13:378, 1994.

490. Tsukasaki K, Tobinai K, Shimoyama M, et al: Deoxycoformycin-containing combination chemotherapy for adult T-cell leukemia lymphoma: Japan Clinical Oncology Group study (JCOG9109). *Int J Hematol* 77:164, 2003.

491. Yamada Y, Tomonaga M, Fukuda H, et al: A new G-CSF-supported combination chemotherapy, LSG15, for adult T-cell leukemia-lymphoma (ATL): Japan Clinical Oncology Group (JCOG) Study 9303. *Br J Haematol* 113:375, 2001.

492. Ohno R, Okada K, Masaoka T, et al: An early phase II study of CPT-11: A new derivative of camptothecin for the treatment of leukemia and lymphoma. *J Clin Oncol* 8:1907, 1990.

493. Tsuda H, Takatsuki K, Ohno R, et al: Treatment of adult T-cell leukemia-lymphoma with irinotecan hydrochloride. *Br J Cancer* 70:771, 1994.

494. Waldmann TA, Goldman CK, Bongiovanni KF, et al: Therapy of patients with human T-cell lymphotrophic virus I-induced adult T-cell leukemia with anti-Tac, a monoclonal antibody to the receptor for interleukin-2. *Blood* 72:1805, 1988.

495. Waldmann TA, White JD, Carrasquillo JA, et al: Radioimmunotherapy of interleukin-2R α-expressing adult T-cell leukemia with Yttrium-90-labeled Anti-Tac. *Blood* 86:4063, 1995.

496. Tamura K, Makino S, Araki Y, et al: Recombinant interferon beta and gamma in the treatment of adult T-cell leukemia. *Cancer* 59:1069, 1987.

497. Saigo K, Shiozawa S, Shiozawa K, et al: Alpha-interferon treatment for adult T-cell leukemia: Low levels of circulating alpha-interferon and its clinical effectiveness. *Blut* 56:83, 1988.

498. Gill PS, Harrington W Jr, Kaplan MH, et al: Treatment of adult T-cell leukemia-lymphoma with a combination of interferon alfa and zidovudine. *N Engl J Med* 332:1744, 1995.

499. Hermine O, Bouscary D, Gessain A, et al: Brief report: Treatment of adult T-cell leukemia-lymphoma with zidovudine and interferon alfa. *N Engl J Med* 332:1749, 1995.

500. Utsunomiya A, Miyazaki Y, Takatsuka Y, et al: Improved outcome of adult T cell leukemia/lymphoma with allogeneic hematopoietic stem cell transplantation. *Bone Marrow Transplant* 27:15, 2001.

501. Ho Fc, Choy D, Loke SL, et al: Polymorphic reticulosis and conventional lymphomas of the nose and upper aerodigestive tract: A clinicopathologic study of 70 cases, and immunophenotypic studies of 16 cases. *Hum Pathol* 21:1041, 1990.

502. Chan JK: Natural killer cell neoplasms. *Anat Pathol* 3:77, 1998.

503. Chan JK: Peripheral T-cell and NK-cell neoplasms: An integrated approach to diagnosis. *Mod Pathol* 12:177, 1999.

504. Liang R, Loke SL, Ho FC, et al: Histologic subtypes and survival of Chinese patients with non-Hodgkin's lymphomas. *Cancer* 66:1850, 1990.

505. Quintanilla-Martinez L, Franklin JL, Guerrero I, et al: Histological and immunophenotypic profile of nasal NK/T cell lymphomas from Peru: High prevalence of p53 overexpression. *Hum Pathol* 30:849, 1999.

506. Liang R, Todd D, Chan TK, et al: Nasal lymphoma. A retrospective analysis of 60 cases. *Cancer* 66:2205, 1990.

507. Kato N, Yasukawa K, Onozuka T, et al: Nasal and nasal-type T/NK-cell lymphoma with cutaneous involvement. *J Am Acad Dermatol* 40:850, 1999.

508. Chan JK, Ng CS, Ngan KC, et al: Angiocentric T-cell lymphoma of the skin. An aggressive lymphoma distinct from mycosis fungoides. *Am J Surg Pathol* 12:861, 1988.

509. Chiang AK, Tao Q, Srivastava G, et al: Nasal NK- and T-cell lymphomas share the same type of Epstein-Barr virus latency as nasopharyngeal carcinoma and Hodgkin's disease. *Int J Cancer* 68:285, 1996.

510. Gutierrez MI, Spangler G, Kingma D, et al: Epstein-Barr virus in nasal lymphomas contains multiple ongoing mutations in the EBNA-1 gene. *Blood* 92:600, 1998.

511. Gaal K, Weiss LM, Chen WG, et al: Epstein-Barr virus nuclear antigen (EBNA-1) carboxy-terminal and EBNA-4 sequence polymorphisms in nasal natural killer/T-cell lymphoma in the United States. *Lab Invest* 82: 957, 2002.

512. Liang R, Todd D, Chan TK, et al: Treatment outcome and prognostic factors for primary nasal lymphoma. *J Clin Oncol* 13:666, 1995.

513. Kim GE, Cho JH, Yang WI, et al: Angiocentric lymphoma of the head and neck: Patterns of systemic failure after radiation treatment. *J Clin Oncol* 18:54, 2000.

514. Cheung MM, Chan JK, Lau WH, et al: Primary non-Hodgkin's lymphoma of the nose and nasopharynx: Clinical features, tumor immunophenotype, and treatment outcome in 113 patients. *J Clin Oncol* 16:70, 1998.

515. Liang R, Chen F, Lee CK, et al: Autologous bone marrow transplantation for primary nasal T/NK cell lymphoma. *Bone Marrow Transplant* 19:91, 1997.

516. Nawa Y, Takenaka K, Shinagawa K, et al: Successful treatment of advanced natural killer cell lymphoma with high-dose chemotherapy and syngeneic peripheral blood stem cell transplantation. *Bone Marrow Transplant* 23:1321, 1999.

517. Isaacson P, Spencer J, Connolly C, et al: Malignant histiocytosis of the intestine: A T-cell lymphoma. *Lancet* 2:688, 1985.

518. Harris NL, Jaffe ES, Stein H, et al: A revised European-American classification of lymphoid neoplasms: A proposal from the International Lymphoma Study Group. *Blood* 84:1361, 1994.

519. Trier JS: Celiac sprue. *N Engl J Med* 325:1709, 1991.

520. Gale J, Simmonds PD, Mead GM, et al: Enteropathy-type intestinal T-cell lymphoma: Clinical features and treatment of 31 patients in a single center. *J Clin Oncol* 18:795, 2000.

521. Isaacson PG, O'Connor NT, Spencer J, et al: Malignant histiocytosis of the intestine: A T-cell lymphoma. *Lancet* 2:688, 1985.

522. Murray A, Cuevas EC, Jones DB, et al: Study of the immunohistochemistry and T cell clonality of enteropathy associated T cell lymphoma. *Am J Pathol* 146:509, 1995.

523. Katoh A, Oshima K, Kanda M, et al: Gastrointestinal T cell lymphoma: Predominant cytotoxic phenotypes, including alpha/beta, gamma/delta T cell and natural killer cells. *Leuk Lymphoma* 39:97, 2000.

524. Farcet JP, Gualard P, Marolleau JP, et al: Hepatosplenic T-cell lymphoma: Sinusal/sinusoidal localization of malignant cells expressing the T-cell receptor gamma delta. *Blood* 75:2213, 1990.

525. Weidmann E: Hepatosplenic T cell lymphoma. A review of 45 cases since the first report describing the disease as a distinct lymphoma entity in 1990. *Leukemia* 14:991, 2000.

526. Kanavaros P, Farcet JP, Gaulard P, et al: Recombinative events of the T cell antigen receptor delta gene in peripheral T cell lymphomas. *J Clin Invest* 87:6566, 1991.

527. Alonzozana EL, Stamberg J, Kumar D, et al: Isochromosome 7q: The primary cytogenetic abnormality in hepatosplenic gamma delta T cell lymphoma. *Leukemia* 11:1367, 1997.

528. Jonvaux P, Daniel MT, Martel V, et al: Isochromosome 7q and trisomy 8 are consistent primary, non-random chromosomal abnormalities associated with hepatosplenic T gamma/delta lymphoma. *Leukemia* 10: 1453, 1996.

529. Wang CC, Tien HF, Lin MT, et al: Consistent presence of isochromosome 7q in hepatosplenic T gamma/delta lymphoma: A new cytogenetic-clinicopathologic entity. *Genes Chromosomes Cancer* 12:161, 1995.

530. Go RS, Wester SM: Immunophenotypic and molecular features, clinical outcomes, and prognostic factors associated with subcutaneous panniculitis-like T-cell lymphoma: A systematic analysis of 156 patients reported in the literature. *Cancer* 101:1404, 2004.

531. Paulli M, Berti E: Cutaneous T-cell lymphomas (including rare subtypes). Current concepts: II. *Haematologica* 89:1372, 2004.

532. Takeshita M, Okamura S, Oshiro Y, et al: Clinicopathologic differences between 22 cases of CD56-negative and CD56-positive subcutaneous panniculitis-like lymphoma in Japan. *Hum Pathol* 35:231, 2004.

533. Wang CY, Su WP, Kurtin PJ: Subcutaneous panniculitic T-cell lymphoma. *Int J Dermatol* 35:1, 1996.

534. Matsue K, Itoh M, Tsukuda K, et al: Successful treatment of cytophagic histiocytic panniculitis with modified CHOP-E. Cyclophosphamide, adriamycin, vincristine, prednisone, and etoposide. *Am J Clin Oncol* 17: 470, 1994.

535. Weenig RH, Ng CS, Perniciaro C: Subcutaneous panniculitis-like T-cell lymphoma: An elusive case presenting as lipomembranous panniculitis and a review of 72 cases in the literature. *Am J Dermatol* 23:206, 2001.

536. Papenfuss JS, Aouun P, Bierman PJ, et al: Subcutaneous panniculitis-like T-cell lymphoma: Presentation of 2 cases and observations. *Clin Lymphoma* 3:175, 2002.

537. Salhany KE, Macon WR, Choi JK, et al: Subcutaneous panniculitis-like T-cell lymphoma: Clinicopathologic, immunophenotypic, and genotypic analysis of alpha/beta and gamma/delta subtypes. *Am J Surg Pathol* 22: 881, 1998.

538. Lorincz AL: Cutaneous T-cell lymphoma (mycosis fungoides). *Lancet* 347:871, 1996.

539. Alibert JL: *Description des maladies de la peau observées à l'Hôpital Saint-Louis et exposition des meilleures méthodes suivies pour leur traitement.* Barrois l'aîné et fils, Paris, 1806.

540. Sézary A, Bouvrain Y: Erythrodermie avec présence de cellules monstrueses dans le derme et dans lang circulant. *Bull Soc Fr Dermatol Syphiligr* 45:254, 1938.

541. Lutzner M, Edelson R, Schein P, et al: Cutaneous T-cell lymphomas: The Sezary syndrome, mycosis fungoides, and related disorders. *Ann Intern Med* 83:534, 1975.

542. Kim YH, Liu HL, Mraz-Gernhard S, et al: Long-term outcome of 525 patients with mycosis fungoides and Sezary syndrome: Clinical prognostic factors and risk for disease progression. *Arch Dermatol* 139:857, 2003.

543. Weinstock MA, Reynes JF: The changing survival of patients with mycosis fungoides: A population-based assessment of trends in the United States. *Cancer* 85:208, 1999.

544. Weinstock MA, Gardstein B: Twenty-year trends in the reported incidence of mycosis fungoides and associated mortality. *Am J Public Health* 89:1240, 1999.

545. Fine RM: HTLV-V: A new retrovirus associated with cutaneous T cell lymphoma (mycosis fungoides). *Int J Dermatol* 27:473, 1988.

546. Burg G, Dummer R, Haeffner A: From inflammation to neoplasia: Mycosis fungoides evolves from reactive inflammatory conditions (lymphoid infiltrates) transforming into neoplastic plaques and tumors. *Arch Dermatol* 137:949, 2001.

547. Tan RS, Butterworth CM, McLaughlin H: Mycosis fungoides—A disease of antigen persistence. *Br J Dermatol* 91:607, 1974.

548. Hoppe RT, Medeiros LJ, Warnke RA, Woods GS: CD8-positive tumor-infiltrating lymphocytes influence the long-term survival of patients with mycosis fungoides. *J Am Acad Dermatol* 32:448, 1995.

549. Seo N, Tokura Y, Matsomoto K, et al: Tumour-specific cytotoxic T lymphocyte activity in Th2-type Sezary syndrome: Its enhancement by interferon-gamma (IFN-gamma) and IL-12 and fluctuations in association with disease activity. *Clin Exp Immunol* 112:403, 1998.

550. Yoo EK, Cassin M, Lessin ST, Rook AH: Complete molecular remission during biologic response modifier therapy for Sezary syndrome is associated with enhanced helper T type 1 cytokine production and natural killer cell activity. *J Am Acad Dermatol* 45:208, 2001.

551. Vonderheid EC, Ekgote SK, Kerrigan K, et al: The prognostic significance of delayed hypersensitivity to dinitrochlorobenzene and mechlorethamine hydrochloride in cutaneous T cell lymphoma. *J Invest Dermatol* 110:946, 1998.

552. Dummer R, Geertsen R, Ludwig E: Sezary syndrome, T-helper 2 cytokines and accessory factor-1 (AF-1). *Leuk Lymphoma* 28:515, 1998.

553. Vowels BR, Cassin M, Vonderheid EC, Rook AH: Aberrant cytokine production by Sezary syndrome patients: Cytokine secretion pattern resembles murine Th2 cells. *J Invest Dermatol* 99;90, 1992.

554. Rook AH, Heald P: The immunopathogenesis of cutaneous T-cell lymphoma. *Hematol Oncol Clin North Am* 9:997, 1995.

555. Smoller BR: Risk of secondary cutaneous malignancies in patients with long-standing mycosis fungoides. *J Am Acad Dermatol* 31:295, 1994.

556. Epstein EH Jr, Levin DL, Crot JD Jr, et al: Mycosis fungoides. Survival, prognostic features, response to therapy, and autopsy findings. *Medicine (Baltimore)* 51:61, 1972.

557. Naraghi ZS, Seirati H, Valikhani M, et al: Assessment of histologic criteria in the diagnosis of mycosis fungoides. *Int J Dermatol* 42:45, 2003.

558. Sigel JE, His ED: Immunohistochemical analysis of CD30-positive lymphoproliferative disorders for expression of CD95 and CD95L. *Mod Pathol* 13:446, 2000.

559. Duncan LM: Cutaneous lymphoma. Understanding the new classification schemes. *Dermatol Clin* 17:569, 1999.

560. Liu HL, Hoppert RT, Kohler S, et al: CD30+ cutaneous lymphoproliferative disorders: The Stanford experience in lymphomatoid papulosis and primary cutaneous anaplastic large cell lymphoma. *J Am Acad Dermatol* 49:1049, 2003.

561. Haynes BF, Metzger RS, Minna JD, et al: Phenotypic characterization of cutaneous T-cell lymphoma. Use of monoclonal antibodies to compare with other malignant T cells. *N Engl J Med* 304:1319, 1981.

562. Kung PC, Berger CL, Goldstein G, et al: Cutaneous T cell lymphoma: characterization by monoclonal antibodies.. *Blood* 57:261, 1981.

563. Schroff RW, Foon KA, Billing RJ, Fahey JL: Immunologic classification of lymphocytic leukemias based on monoclonal antibody-defined cell surface antigens. *Blood* 59:207, 1982.

564. Broder S, Edelson RL, Lutzner MA, et al: The Sezary syndrome: A malignant proliferation of helper T cells. *J Clin Invest* 58:1297, 1976.

565. Haynes BF, Hensley LL, Jegasothy BV: Phenotypic characterization of skin-infiltrating T cells in cutaneous T-cell lymphoma: Comparison with benign cutaneous T-cell infiltrates. *Blood* 60:463, 1982.

566. Jones D, Dang NH, Duvic M, et al: Absence of CD26 expression is a useful marker for diagnosis of T-cell lymphoma in peripheral blood. *Am J Clin Pathol* 115:885, 2001.

567. Bernengo MG, Novelli M, Quaglino P, et al: The relevance of the CD4+ CD26− subset in the identification of circulating Sezary cells. *Br J Dermatol* 144:125, 2001.

568. Lu D, Patel KA, Duric M, Jones D: Clinical and pathological spectrum of CD8-positive cutaneous T-cell lymphomas. *J Cutan Pathol* 29:465, 2002.

569. Santucci M, Pimpinelli N, Massid J, et al: Cytotoxic/natural killer cell cutaneous lymphomas. Report of EORTC Cutaneous Lymphoma Task Force Workshop. *Cancer* 97:610, 2003.

570. Scarisbrick JJ, Woolford AJ, Russell-Jones R, Whittaker SJ: Loss of heterozygosity on 10q and microsatellite instability in advanced stages of primary cutaneous T-cell lymphoma and possible association with homozygous deletion of PTEN. *Blood* 95:2937, 2000.

571. Navas IC, Algara P, Mateo M, et al: P16(INK4a) is selectively silenced in the tumoral progression of mycosis fungoides. *Lab Invest* 82:123, 2002.

572. Navas IC, Ortiz-Romero PL, Villuendas R, et al: P16(INK4a) gene alterations are frequent in lesions of mycosis fungoides. *Am J Pathol* 156:1565, 2000.

573. Bunn PA Jr, Lamberg SI: Report of the Committee on Staging and Classification of Cutaneous T-Cell Lymphomas. *Cancer Treat Rep* 63:725, 1979.

574. Lamberg SI, Bunn PA Jr: Cutaneous T-cell lymphomas. Summary of the Mycosis Fungoides Cooperative Group-National Cancer Institute Workshop. *Arch Dermatol* 115:1103, 1979.

575. Bunn PA Jr, Huberman MS, Whang-Peng J, et al: Prospective staging evaluation of patients with cutaneous T-cell lymphomas. Demonstration of a high frequency of extracutaneous dissemination. *Ann Intern Med* 93:223, 1980.

576. Green SB, Byar PR, Lamberg SI: Prognostic variables in mycosis fungoides. *Cancer* 47:2671, 1981.

577. Lamberg SI, Green SB, Byar DP, et al: Clinical staging for cutaneous T-cell lymphoma. *Ann Intern Med* 100:187, 1984.

578. Fuks ZY, Castellino RA, Carmel JA, et al: Lymphography in mycosis fungoides. *Cancer* 34:106, 1974.

579. Hamminga L, Mulder JD, Evans C, et al: Staging lymphography with respect to lymph node histology, treatment, and follow-up in patients with mycosis fungoides. *Cancer* 47:692, 1981.

580. Toro JR, Stoll HL Jr, Stomper PC, Oseroff AR: Prognostic factors and evaluation of mycosis fungoides and Sézary syndrome. *J Am Acad Dermatol* 37:58, 1992.

581. Breneman DL, Ragu US, Breneman JC, et al: Lymph node grading for staging of mycosis fungoides may benefit from examination of multiple excised lymph nodes. *J Am Acad Dermatol* 48:702, 2003.

582. Zackheim HS, Amin S, Kashni-Sabet M, McMillan A: Prognosis in cutaneous T-cell lymphoma by skin stage: Long-term survival in 489 patients. *J Am Acad Dermatol* 40:418, 1999.

583. Scarisbrick JJ, Whittakers S, Evans AV, et al: Prognostic significance of tumor burden in the blood of patients with erythrodermic primary cutaneous T-cell lymphoma. *Blood* 97:624, 2001.

584. Muche JM, Lukowsky A, Asadrullah K, et al: Demonstration of frequent occurrence of clonal T cells in the peripheral blood of patients with primary cutaneous T-cell lymphoma. *Blood* 90:1636, 1997.

585. Vonderheid EC, Bernengo MG, Burg G, et al: Update on erythrodermic cutaneous T-cell lymphoma: Report of the International Society for Cutaneous Lymphomas. *J Am Acad Dermatol* 46:95, 2002.

586. Bergman R: How useful are T-cell receptor gene rearrangement studies as an adjunct to the histopathologic diagnosis of mycosis fungoides? *Am J Dermatopathol* 21:498, 1999.

587. Cherny S, Mraz S, Su L, et al: Heteroduplex analysis of T-cell receptor gamma gene rearrangement as an adjuvant diagnostic tool in skin biopsies for erythroderma. *J Cutan Pathol* 28:351, 2001.

588. Delfau-Larue MH, Dalac S, Lepage E, et al: Prognostic significance of a polymerase chain reaction-detectable dominant T-lymphocyte clone in cutaneous lesions of patients with mycosis fungoides. *Blood* 92:3376, 1998.

589. Poszepczynska-Guigne E, Bagot M, Wechsler J, et al: Minimal residual disease in mycosis fungoides follow-up can be assessed by polymerase chain reaction. *Br J Dermatol* 148:265, 2003.

590. Wood GS, Tung RM, Haeffner AC, et al: Detection of clonal T-cell receptor gamma gene rearrangements in early mycosis fungoides/Sézary syndrome by polymerase chain reaction and denaturing gradient gel electrophoresis (PCR/DGGE). *J Invest Dermatol* 103:34, 1994.

591. Long JC, Mihm MC: Mycosis fungoides with extracutaneous dissemination: A distinct clinicopathologic entity. *Cancer* 34:1745, 1974.

592. Smith DI, Vnencak-Jones CL, Boyd AS: T-lymphocyte clonality in benign lichenoid keratoses. *J Cutan Pathol* 29:623, 2002.

593. Nihal M, Mikkola D, Horrath M, et al: Cutaneous lymphoid hyperplasia: A lymphoproliferative continuum with lymphomatous potential. *Hum Pathol* 34:617, 2003.

594. Holm N, Flaig MJ, Yazdi AS, Sander CA: The value of molecular analysis by PCR in the diagnosis of cutaneous lymphocytic infiltrates. *J Cutan Pathol* 29:447, 2002.

595. Shieh S, Mikkola DL, Wood GS: Differentiation and clonality of

lesional lymphocytes in pityriasis lichenoides chronica. *Arch Dermatol* 137:305, 2001.

596. Zucker-Franklin D: The role of human T cell lymphotropic virus type I tax in the development of cutaneous T cell lymphoma. *Ann N Y Acad Sci* 941:86, 2001.

597. Kikuchi A, Ohata Y, Matsumoto H, et al: Anti-HTLV-1 antibody positive cutaneous T-cell lymphoma. *Cancer* 79:269, 1997.

598. Palmer RA, Keefe M, Slater D, Whittaker SJ: Case 4: Pagetoid reticulosis (Woringer-Kolopp type) or unilesional mycosis fungoides (MF). *Clin Exp Dermatol* 27:345, 2002.

599. Wood GS, Weiss LM, Hu CH, et al: T-cell antigen deficiencies and clonal rearrangements of T-cell receptor genes in pagetoid reticulosis (Woringer-Kolopp disease). *N Engl J Med* 318:164, 1988.

600. Cohen EL: Woringer-Kolopp disease (pagetoid reticulosis). *Clin Exp Dermatol* 3:447, 1978.

601. Scarabello A, Fantini F, Giannetti A, Cerroni L: Localized pagetoid reticulosis (Woringer-Kolopp disease). *Br J Dermatol* 147:806, 2002.

602. Nakada T, Sueki H, Iijima M: Disseminated pagetoid reticulosis (Ketron-Goodman disease): Six-year follow-up. *J Am Acad Dermatol* 47:S183, 2002.

603. Fierro MT, Novelli M, Savoia P, et al: CD45RA+ immunophenotype in mycosis fungoides: Clinical, histological and immunophenotypical features in 22 patients. *J Cutan Pathol* 28:356, 2001.

604. Haghighi B, Smoller BR, LeBoit PE, et al: Pagetoid reticulosis (Woringer-Kolopp disease): An immunophenotypic, molecular, and clinicopathologic study. *Mod Pathol* 13:502, 2000.

605. Bekkenk MW, Vermeer MH, Jansen PM, van Marion AM: Peripheral T-cell lymphomas unspecified presenting in the skin: Analysis of prognostic factors in a group of 82 patients. *Blood* 102:2213, 2003.

606. Bekkenk MW, Geelen FA, van Voorst Vader PC, et al: Primary and secondary cutaneous CD30(+) lymphoproliferative disorders: A report from the Dutch Cutaneous Lymphoma Group on the long-term follow-up data of 219 patients and guidelines for diagnosis and treatment. *Blood* 95:3653, 2000.

607. Reitamo S, Harper J, Bos JD, et al: Tacrolimus ointment does not affect collagen synthesis: Results of a single-center randomized trial. *J Invest Dermatol* 111:396, 1998.

608. Vonderheid EC, Van Scott EJ, Johnson WC, et al: Topical chemotherapy and immunotherapy of mycosis fungoides: Intermediate-term results. *Arch Dermatol* 113:454, 1977.

609. Du Vivier A, Vonderheid EC, Van Scott EJ, Urbach F: Mycosis fungoides, nitrogen mustard and skin cancer. *Br J Dermatol* 99:61, 1978.

610. Zackheim HS, Epstein EH Jr, Grekin DA: Treatment of mycosis fungoides with topical BCNU. *Cancer Treat Rep* 63:623, 1979.

611. Kempf W, Kettelhack N, Duvic M, Burg G: Topical and systemic retinoid therapy for cutaneous T-cell lymphoma. *Hematol Oncol Clin North Am* 17:1405, 2003.

612. Martin AG: Bexarotene gel: A new skin-directed treatment option for cutaneous T-cell lymphomas. *J Drugs Dermatol* 2:155, 2003.

613. Baron ED, Stevens SR: Phototherapy for cutaneous T-cell lymphoma. *Dermatol Ther* 16:303, 2003.

614. Ramsay DL, Lish KM, Yalowitz CB, Soter NA: Ultraviolet-B phototherapy for early-stage cutaneous T-cell lymphoma. *Arch Dermatol* 128:931, 1992.

615. Samson Yashar S, Gielczyk R, Scherschun L, Lim HW: Narrow-band ultraviolet B treatment for vitiligo, pruritus, and inflammatory dermatoses. *Photodermatol Photoimmunol Photomed* 19:164, 2003.

616. Gilchrest BA: Methoxsalen photochemotherapy for mycosis fungoides. *Cancer Treat Rep* 63:663, 1979.

617. Herrmann JJ, Roenigk HH Jr, Hurria A, et al: Treatment of mycosis fungoides with photochemotherapy (PUVA): Long-term follow-up. *J Am Acad Dermatol* 33:234, 1995.

618. Roenigk HH Jr, Kuzel TM, Skoutelis AP, et al: Photochemotherapy

alone or combined with interferon alpha-2a in the treatment of cutaneous T-cell lymphoma. *J Invest Dermatol* 95:198S, 1990.

619. Orenstein A, Haik J, Tamir J, et al: Photodynamic therapy of cutaneous lymphoma using 5-aminolevulinic acid topical application. *Dermatol Surg* 26:765, 2000.

620. Edstrom DW, Porwit A, Ros AM: Photodynamic therapy with topical 5-aminolevulinic acid for mycosis fungoides: Clinical and histological response. *Acta Derm Venereol* 81:184, 2001.

621. Edelson R, Berger C, Gasparro F, et al: Treatment of cutaneous T-cell lymphoma by extracorporeal photochemotherapy. Preliminary results. *N Engl J Med* 316:297, 1987.

622. Knobler R, Girardi M: Extracorporeal photochemoimmunotherapy in cutaneous T cell lymphomas. *Ann N Y Acad Sci* 941:123, 2001.

623. Jones GW, Kacinski BM, Wilson LD, et al: Total skin electron radiation in the management of mycosis fungoides: Consensus of the European Organization for Research and Treatment of Cancer (EORTC) Cutaneous Lymphoma Project Group. *J Am Acad Dermatol* 47:364, 2002.

624. Duvic M, Apisarnthanarax N, Cohen DS, et al: Analysis of long-term outcomes of combined modality therapy for cutaneous T-cell lymphoma. *J Am Acad Dermatol* 49:35, 2003.

625. Hoppe R: Total skin electron beam therapy in the management of mycosis fungoides, in *The Role of High Energy Electrons in the Treatment of Cancer*, edited by MJ Vaeth, p 80. S Karger, Basel, Switzerland, 1991.

626. Do JH, McLaughlin SS, Gaspari AA: Topical imiquimod therapy for cutaneous T-cell lymphoma. *Skinmed* 2:316, 2003.

627. Dummer R, Urosevic M, Kempf W, et al: Imiquimod induces complete clearance of a PUVA-resistant plaque in mycosis fungoides. *Dermatology* 207:116, 2003.

628. Olsen EA: Interferon in the treatment of cutaneous T-cell lymphoma. *Dermatol Ther* 16:311, 2003.

629. Kennedy GA, Seymour JF, Wolf M, et al: Treatment of patients with advanced mycosis fungoides and Sezary syndrome with alemtuzumab. *Eur J Haematol* 71:250, 2003.

630. Lundin J, Hagberg H, Repp R, et al: Phase 2 study of alemtuzumab (anti-CD52 monoclonal antibody) in patients with advanced mycosis fungoides/Sézary syndrome. *Blood* 101:4267, 2003.

631. Olsen E, Duvic M, Frankel A: Pivotal phase III trial of two dose levels of denileukin diftitox for the treatment of cutaneous T-cell lymphoma. *J Clin Oncol* 19:376, 2001.

632. Van Scott EJ, Auerbach R, Clendenning WE: Treatment of mycosis fungoides with cyclophosphamide. *Arch Dermatol* 85:499, 1962.

633. Van Scott EJ, Grekin DA, Kalmanson JD, et al: Frequent low doses of intravenous mechlorethamine for late-stage mycosis fungoides lymphoma. *Cancer* 36:1613, 1975.

634. Zackheim HS, Kashani-Sabet M, Hwang ST: Low-dose methotrexate to treat erythrodermic cutaneous T-cell lymphoma: Results in twenty-nine patients. *J Am Acad Dermatol* 34:626, 1996.

635. Spigel SC, Coltman CA Jr: Therapy of mycosis fungoides with bleomycin. *Cancer* 32:767, 1973.

636. Levi JA, Diggs CH, Wiernik PH: Adriamycin therapy in advanced mycosis fungoides. *Cancer* 39:1967, 1977.

637. Wollina U, Dummer R, Brockmeyer NJ, et al: Multicenter study of pegylated liposomal doxorubicin in patients with cutaneous T-cell lymphoma. *Cancer* 98:993, 2003.

638. Foss FM: Activity of pentostatin (Nipent) in cutaneous T-cell lymphoma: Single-agent and combination studies. *Semin Oncol* 27:58, 2000.

639. Kurzrock R: Therapy of T cell lymphomas with pentostatin. *Ann N Y Acad Sci* 941:200, 2001.

640. Quaglino P, Fierro MT, Rossotto GL, et al: Treatment of advanced mycosis fungoides/Sézary syndrome with fludarabine and potential adjunctive benefit to subsequent extracorporeal photochemotherapy. *Br J Dermatol* 150:327, 2004.

641. Zinzani PL, Baliva G, Magognoli M, et al: Gemcitabine treatment in

pretreated cutaneous T-cell lymphoma: Experience in 44 patients. *J Clin Oncol* 18:2603, 2000.

642. Vonderheid EC: Treatment of cutaneous T cell lymphoma: 2001. Recent results. *Cancer Res* 160:309, 2002.

643. Abd-el-baki J, Demierre MF, Li N, Foss FM: Transformation in mycosis fungoides: The role of methotrexate. *J Cutan Med Surg* 6L:109, 2002.

644. Rosen ST, Foss FM: Chemotherapy for mycosis fungoides and the Sézary syndrome. *Hematol Oncol Clin North Am* 9:1109, 1995.

645. Vonderheid EC: Treatment planning in cutaneous T-cell lymphoma. *Dermatol Ther* 16:276, 2003.

646. Willemze R, Meijer CJ: Primary cutaneous CD30-positive lymphoproliferative disorders. *Hematol Oncol Clin North Am* 17:1319, 2003.

647. Kadin ME, Carpenter D: Systemic and primary cutaneous anaplastic large cell lymphomas. *Semin Hematol* 40:244, 2003.

648. Willemze R, Beljaards RC: Spectrum of primary cutaneous CD30 (Ki-1)-positive lymphoproliferative disorders. A proposal for classification and guidelines for management and treatment. *J Am Acad Dermatol* 28:973, 1993.

649. Bergman R, Marcus-Farber BS, Manov L, et al: Clinicopathologic reassessment of non-mycosis fungoides primary cutaneous lymphomas during 17 years. *Int J Dermatol* 41:735, 2002.

650. Tomaszewski MM, Moad JC, Lupton GP: Primary cutaneous Ki-1(CD30) positive anaplastic large cell lymphoma in childhood. *J Am Acad Dermatol* 40:857, 1999.

651. Bekkenk MW, Geelen FA, van Voorst Vader PC, et al: Primary and secondary cutaneous CD30(+) lymphoproliferative disorders: A report from the Dutch Cutaneous Lymphoma Group on the long-term follow-up data of 219 patients and guidelines for diagnosis and treatment. *Blood* 95:3653, 2000.

652. Gorczyca W, Tsang P, Liu Z, et al: CD30-positive T-cell lymphomas co-expressing CD15: An immunohistochemical analysis. *Int J Oncol* 22:319, 2003.

653. Jaffe ES: Anaplastic large cell lymphoma: The shifting sands of diagnostic hematopathology. *Mod Pathol* 14:219, 2001.

654. DeCoteau JF, Butmarc JR, Kinney MC, Kadin ME: The t(2;5) chromosomal translocation is not a common feature of primary cutaneous CD30+ lymphoproliferative disorders: Comparison with anaplastic large-cell lymphoma of nodal origin. *Blood* 87:3437, 1996.

655. El Shabrawi-Caelen L, Kerl H, Cerroni L: Lymphomatoid papulosis: Reappraisal of clinicopathologic presentation and classification into subtypes A, B, and C. *Arch Dermatol* 140:441, 2004.

656. Wang HH, Myers T, Lach LJ, et al: Increased risk of lymphoid and nonlymphoid malignancies in patients with lymphomatoid papulosis. *Cancer* 86:1240, 1999.

657. Liu HL, Hoppe R, Kohler S, et al: CD30+ cutaneous lymphoproliferative disorders: The Stanford experience in lymphomatoid papulosis and primary cutaneous anaplastic large cell lymphoma. *J Am Acad Dermatol* 49:1049, 2003.

658. Stein H, Mason DY, Gerdes J, et al: The expression of the Hodgkin's disease associated antigen Ki-1 in reactive and neoplastic lymphoid tissue: Evidence that Reed-Sternberg cells and histiocytic malignancies are derived from activated lymphoid cells. *Blood* 66:848, 1985.

659. Agnarsson BA, Kadin ME: Ki-1 positive large cell lymphoma. A morphologic and immunologic study of 19 cases. *Am J Surg Pathol* 12:264, 1988.

660. Delsol G, Al Saati T, Gatter K, et al: Coexpression of epithelial membrane antigen (EMA), Ki-1, and interleukin-2 receptor by anaplastic large cell lymphomas: Diagnostic value in so-called malignant histiocytosis. *Am J Pathol* 130:59, 1988.

661. Schwab U, Stein H, Gerdes J, et al: Production of a monoclonal antibody specific for Hodgkin and Sternberg-Reed cells of Hodgkin's disease and a subset of normal lymphoid cells. *Nature* 299:65, 1982.

662. Rimokh R, Magaud JP, Berger F, et al: A translocation involving a specific breakpoint (q35) on chromosome 5 is characteristic of anaplastic large cell lymphoma ("Ki-1 lymphoma"). *Br J Haematol* 71:31, 1989.

663. Bitter MA, Franklin WA, Larson RA, et al: Morphology in Ki-1 (CD30)-positive non-Hodgkin's lymphoma is correlated with clinical features and the presence of a unique chromosomal abnormality, t(2;5)(p23;q35). *Am J Surg Pathol* 14:305, 1990.

664. Mason DY, Bastard C, Rimokh R, et al: CD30-positive large cell lymphomas ("Ki-1 lymphoma") are associated with a chromosomal translocation involving 5q35. *Br J Haematol* 74:161, 1990.

665. Morris SW, Kirstein MN, Valentine MB, et al: Fusion of a kinase gene, ALK, to a nucleolar protein gene, NPM, in non-hodgkin's lymphoma. *Science* 263:1281, 1994.

666. Kadin ME: Anaplastic large cell lymphoma and its morphological variants. *Cancer Surv* 30:77, 1997.

667. Stein H, Foss HD, Durkop H, et al: CD30(+) anaplastic large cell lymphoma: A review of its histopathologic, genetic, and clinical features. *Blood* 96:3681, 2000.

668. Falini B: Anaplastic large cell lymphoma: Pathological, molecular, and clinical features. *Br J Haematol* 114:741, 2001.

669. Benharroch D, Meguerian-Bedoyan Z, Lamant L, et al: ALK-positive lymphoma: A single disease with a broad spectrum of morphology. *Blood* 91:2076, 1998.

670. Falini B, Bigerna B, Fizzotti M, et al: ALK expression defines a distinct group of T/null lymphomas ("ALK lymphomas") with a wide morphological spectrum. *Am J Pathol* 153:875, 1998.

671. Falini B, Pileri S, Zinzani PL, et al: ALK+ lymphoma: Clinico-pathological findings and outcome. *Blood* 93:2697, 1999.

672. Pulford K, Lamant L, Morris SW, et al: Detection of anaplastic lymphoma kinase (ALK) and nucleolar protein nucleophosmin (NPM)-ALK proteins in normal and neoplastic cells with the monoclonal antibody ALK1. *Blood* 89:1394, 1997.

673. Krenacs L, Wellmann A, Sorbara L, et al: Cytotoxic cell antigen expression in anaplastic large cell lymphomas of T-cell and null-cell type and Hodgkin's disease: Evidence for distinct cellular origin. *Blood* 89:980, 1997.

674. Foss HD, Anagnostopoulos I, Araujo I, et al: Anaplastic large-cell lymphomas of T-cell and null-cell phenotype express cytotoxic molecules. *Blood* 88:4005, 1996.

675. Haralambieva E, Pulford KA, Lamant L, et al: Anaplastic large-cell lymphomas of B-cell phenotype are anaplastic lymphoma kinase (ALK) negative and belong to the spectrum of diffuse large B-cell lymphomas. *Br J Haematol* 109:584, 2001.

676. Kuefer MU, Look AT, Pulford K, et al: Retrovirus-mediated gene transfer of NPM-ALK causes lymphoid malignancy in mice. *Blood* 90:2901, 1997.

677. Duyster J, Bai RY, Morris SW: Translocations involving anaplastic lymphoma kinase (ALK). *Oncogene* 20:5623, 2001.

678. Slupianek A, Nieborowska-Skorska M, Hoser G, et al: Role of phosphatidylinositol 3-kinase-Akt pathway in nucleophosmin/anaplastic lymphoma kinase-mediated lymphomagenesis. *Cancer Res* 61:2194, 2001.

679. Bai RY, Ouyang T, Miething C, at al: Nucleophosmin-anaplastic lymphoma kinase associated with anaplastic large-cell lymphoma activates the phosphatidylinositol 3-kinase/Akt antiapoptotic signaling pathway. *Blood* 96:4319, 2000.

680. Zhang Q, Raghunath PN, Zue L, et al: Multilevel dysregulation of STAT3 activation in anaplastic lymphoma kinase-positive T/null-cell lymphoma. *J Immunol* 168:466, 2002.

681. Tilly H, Gaulard P, Lepage E, et al: Primary anaplastic large-cell lymphoma in adults: Clinical presentation, immunophenotype, and outcome. *Blood* 90:2727, 1997.

682. Gisselbrecht C, Gualard P, Lepage E, et al: Prognostic significance of

T-cell phenotype in aggressive non-Hodgkin's lymphomas. Groupe d'Etudes des Lymphomas de l'Adulte (GELA). *Blood* 92:76, 1998.

683. Falini B, Pulford K, Pucciarini A, et al: Lymphomas expressing ALK fusion protein(s) other than NPM-ALK. *Blood* 94:3509, 1999.

684. Gascoyne RD, Aoun P, Wu D, et al: Prognostic significance of anaplastic lymphoma kinase (ALK) protein expression in adults with anaplastic large cell lymphoma. *Blood* 93:3913, 1999.

685. Shiota M, Nakamura S, Ichinohasama R, et al: Anaplastic large cell lymphomas expressing the novel chimeric protein P80NPM/ALK: A distinct clinicopathologic entity. *Blood* 86:1954, 1995.

686. Suzuki R, Kagami Y, Takeuchi K, et al: Prognostic significance of CD56 expression for ALK-positive and ALK-negative anaplastic large-cell lymphoma of T/null cell phenotype. *Blood* 96:2993, 2000.

687. Fraga M, Brousset P, Schlaifer D, et al: Bone marrow involvement in anaplastic large cell lymphoma. Immunohistochemical detection of minimal disease and its prognostic significance. *Am J Clin Pathol* 103:82, 1995.

688. Brugieres L, Deley MC, Pacquement H, et al: CD30(+) anaplastic large-cell lymphoma in children: Analysis of 82 patients enrolled in two consecutive studies of the French Society of Pediatric Oncology. *Blood* 92:3591, 1998.

689. Seidemann K, Tiemann M, Schrappe M, et al: Short-pulse B-non-Hodgkin lymphoma-type chemotherapy is efficacious treatment for pediatric anaplastic large cell lymphoma: A report of the Berlin-Frankfurt-Munster Group Trial NHL-BFM 90. *Blood* 97:3699, 2001.

690. Reiter A, Schrappe M, Tiemann M, et al: Successful treatment strategy for Ki-1 anaplastic large-cell lymphoma of childhood: A prospective analysis of 62 patients enrolled in three consecutive Berlin-Frankfurt-Munster group studies. *J Clin Oncol* 12:899, 1994.

691. Vecchi V, Burnelli R, Pileri S, et al: Anaplastic large cell lymphoma (Ki-1+/CD30+) in childhood. *Med Pediatr Oncol* 21:402, 1993.

692. Sandlund JT, Pui CH, Santana VM, et al: Clinical features and treatment outcome for children with CD30+ large-cell non-Hodkin's lymphoma. *J Clin Oncol* 12:895, 1994.

693. Anderson JR, Jenkin RD, Wilson JF, et al: Long-term follow-up of patients treated with COMP or LSA2L2 therapy for childhood non-Hodgkin's lymphoma: A report of CCG-551 from the Childrens Cancer Group. *J Clin Oncol* 11:1024, 1993.

694. Zinzani PL, Martelli M, Magagnoli M, et al: Anaplastic large cell lymphoma Hodgkin's-like: A randomized trial of ABVD versus MACOP-B with and without radiation therapy. *Blood* 92:790, 1998.

695. Fanin R, Silvestri F, Geromin A, et al: Primary systemic CD30 (Ki-1)-positive anaplastic large cell lymphoma of the adult: Sequential intensive treatment with the F-MACHOP regimen (+/- radiotherapy) and autologous bone marrow transplantation. *Blood* 87:1243, 1996.

696. Fanin R, Ruiz de Elvira MC, Sperotto A, et al: Autologous stem cell transplantation for T and null cell CD30-positive anaplastic large cell lymphoma: Analysis of 64 adult and paediatric cases reported to the European Group for Blood and Marrow Transplantation (EBMT). *Bone Marrow Transplant* 23:437, 1999.

697. Deconinck E, Lamy T, Foussard C, et al: Autologous stem cell transplantation for anaplastic large-cell lymphomas: Results of a prospective trial. *Br J Haematol* 109:736, 2000.

698. Haioun C, Lepage E, Gisselbrecht C, et al: Survival benefit of high-dose therapy in poor-risk aggressive non-Hodgkin's lymphoma: Final analysis of the prospective LNH87-2 protocol—A groupe d'Etude des lymphomas de l'Adulte study. *J Clin Oncol* 18:3025, 2000.

699. Chakravari V, Kamani NR, Bayever E, et al: Bone marrow transplantation for childhood Ki-1 lymphoma. *J Clin Oncol* 8:657, 1990.

700. Rudiger T, Weisenburger DD, Anderson JR, et al: Peripheral T-cell lymphoma (excluding anaplastic large-cell lymphoma): Results from the Non-Hodgkin's Lymphoma Classification Project. *Ann Oncol* 13:140, 2002.

701. Kim H, Jacobs C, Warnke RA, Dorfman RF: Malignant lymphoma with a high content of epithelioid histiocytes: A distinct clinicopathologic entity and a form of so-called "Lennert's Lymphoma." *Cancer* 41:620, 1978.

702. Kwak LW, Wilson M, Weiss LM, et al: Similar outcome of treatment of B-cell and T-cell diffuse large-cell lymphomas: The Stanford experience. *J Clin Oncol* 9:1426, 1991.

703. Rudders RA, DeLellis RA, Ahl ET Jr, et al: Adult non-Hodgkin's lymphoma. Correlation of cell surface marker phenotype with prognosis, the new Working Formulation, and the Rappaport and Lukes-Collins histomorphologic schemes. *Cancer* 52:2289, 1983.

704. Karakas T, Bergmann L, Stutte HJ, et al: Peripheral T-cell lymphomas respond well to vincristine, adriamycin, cyclophosphamide, prednisone, and etoposide (VACPE) and have a similar outcome as high-grade B-cell lymphomas. *Leuk Lymphoma* 24:121, 1996.

705. Liang R, Todd D, Ho FC: Aggressive non-Hodgkin's lymphoma: T-cell versus B-cell. *Hematol Oncol* 14:1, 1996.

706. Lippman SM, Miller TP, Spier CM, et al: The prognostic significance of the immunophenotype in diffuse large-cell lymphoma: A comparative study of the T-cell and B-cell phenotype. *Blood* 72:436, 1988.

707. Armitage JO, Vose JM, Linder J, et al: Clinical significance of immunophenotype in diffuse aggressive non-Hodgkin's lymphoma. *J Clin Oncol* 7:1783, 1989.

708. Shimizu K, Hamajima N, Ohnishi K, et al: T-cell phenotype is associated with decreased survival in non-Hodgkin's lymphoma. *Jpn J Cancer Res* 80:720, 1989.

709. Shimoyama M, Oyama A, Tajima K, et al: Differences in clinicopathological characteristics and major prognostic factors between B-lymphoma and peripheral T-lymphoma excluding adult T-cell leukemia/lymphoma. *Leuk Lymphoma* 10:335, 1993.

710. Hutchison RE, Fairclough DL, Holt H, et al: Clinical significance of histology and immunophenotype in childhood diffuse large cell lymphoma. *Am J Clin Pathol* 95:787, 1991.

711. Gisselbrecht C, Gaulard P, Lepage E, et al: Prognostic significance of T-cell phenotype in aggressive non-Hodgkin's lymphomas. Groupe d'Etudes des Lymphomes de l'Adulte (GELA). *Blood* 92:76, 1998.

712. Liang R, Todd D, Chan TK, et al: Peripheral T cell lymphoma. *J Clin Oncol* 5:750, 1987.

713. Greer JP, York JC, Cousar JB, et al: Peripheral T-cell lymphoma: A clinicopathologic study of 42 cases. *J Clin Oncol* 2:788, 1984.

714. Coiffier B, Berger F, Bryon PA, et al: T-cell lymphomas: Immunologic, histologic, clinical, and therapeutic analysis of 63 cases. *J Clin Oncol* 6:1584, 1988.

715. Vose JM, Peterson C, Bierman PJ, et al: Comparison of high-dose therapy and autologous bone marrow transplantation for T-cell and B-cell non-Hodgkin's lymphomas. *Blood* 76:424, 1990.

716. Rodriguez J, Munsell M, Yazji S, et al: Impact of high-dose chemotherapy on peripheral T-cell lymphomas. *J Clin Oncol* 19:3766, 2001.

717. Blystad AK, Enblad G, Kvaloy S, et al: High-dose therapy with autologous stem cell transplantation in patients with peripheral T-cell lymphomas. *Bone Marrow Transplant* 27:711, 2001.

718. Cooper DL, Braverman IM, Sarris AH, et al: Cyclosporine treatment of refractory T-cell lymphomas. *Cancer* 71:2335, 1993.

719. Mercieca J, Matutes E, Dearden C, et al: The role of pentostatin in the treatment of T-cell malignancies: Analysis of response rate in 145 patients according to disease subtype. *J Clin Oncol* 12:2588, 1994.

720. Cheng AL, Su IJ, Chen CC, et al: Use of retinoic acids in the treatment of peripheral T-cell lymphoma: A pilot study. *J Clin Oncol* 12:1185, 1994.

721. Dang N, Hagemeister F, Fayad L, et al: Phase II study of denileukin diftitox (ONTAK) for relapsed/refractory B and T-cell non-Hodgkin's lymphoma [abstract]. *Blood* 100:1405, 2002.

722. Frizzera G, Moran EM, Rappaport H: Angio-immunoblastic lymphad-enopathy with dysproteinaemia. *Lancet* 1:1070, 1974.

723. Brice P, Calvo F, d'Agay MF, et al: Peripheral T-cell lymphoma fol-lowing angioimmunoblastic lymphadenopathy. *Nouv Rev Fr Hematol* 29:371, 1987.

724. Willenbrock K, Roers A, Seidl C, et al: Analysis of T-cell subpopula-tions in T-cell non-Hodgkin's lymphoma of angioimmunoblastic lym-phadenopathy with dysproteinemia type by single target gene amplifi-cation of T-cell receptor-beta gene rearrangements. *Am J Pathol* 158:1851, 2001.

725. Smith JL, Hodges E, Quin CT, et al: Frequent T and B cell oligoclones in histologically and immunophenotypically characterized angioimmu-noblastic lymphadenopathy. *Am J Pathol* 156:661, 2000.

726. Siegert W, Agthe A, Greisser H, et al: Treatment of angioimmunoblastic lymphadenopathy (AILD)-type T-cell lymphoma using prednisone with or without the COPLAM/IMVP-16 regimen. A multicenter study. Kiel Lymphoma Study Group. *Ann Intern Med* 117:364, 1992.

727. Weiss LM, Strickler JG, Dorfman RF, et al: Clonal T-cell populations in angioimmunoblastic lymphadenopathy and angioimmunoblastic lym-phadenopathy-like lymphoma. *Am J Pathol* 122:392, 1986.

728. Feller AC, Griesser H, Schilling CV, et al: Clonal gene rearrangement patterns correlate with immunophenotype and clinical parameters in pa-tients with angioimmunoblastic lymphadenopathy. *Am J Pathol* 133:549, 1988.

729. Attygalle A, Al-Jehani R, Diss TC, et al: Neoplastic T cells in angio-immunoblastic T-cell lymphoma express CD10. *Blood* 99:627, 2002.

730. Weiss LM, Jaffe ES, Liu XF, et al: Detection and localization of Epstein-Barr viral genomes in angioimmunoblastic lymphadenopathy and angio-immunoblastic lymphadenopathy-like lymphoma. *Blood* 79:1789, 1992.

731. Schlegelberger B, Zwingers T, Hohenadel K, et al: Significance of cyto-genetic findings for the clinical outcome in patients with T-cell lym-phoma of angioimmunoblastic lymphadenopathy type. *J Clin Oncol* 14:593, 1996.

732. Siegert W, Nerl C, Agthe A, et al: Angioimmunoblastic lymphadenop-athy (AILD)-type T-cell lymphoma: Prognostic impact of clinical ob-servations and laboratory findings at presentation. The Kiel Lymphoma Study Group. *Ann Oncol* 6:659, 1995.

733. Pautier P, Devidas A, Delmer A, et al: Angioimmunoblastic-like T-cell non-Hodgkin's lymphoma: Outcome after chemotherapy in 33 patients and review of the literature. *Leuk Lymphoma* 32:545, 1999.

734. Takemori N, Kodaira J, Toyoshima N, et al: Successful treatment of immunoblastic lymphadenopathy-like T-cell lymphoma with cyclo-sporin A. *Leuk Lymphoma* 35:389, 1999.

735. Quintini G, Iannitto E, Barbera V, et al: Response to low-dose oral methotrexate and prednisone in two patients with angio-immunoblastic lymphadenopathy-type T-cell lymphoma. *Hematol J* 2:393, 2001.

736. Segel GB, Lichtman MA: Familial (inherited) leukemia, lymphoma, and myeloma. An overview. *Blood Cells Mol Dis* 32:246, 2004.

737. Borisch B, Raphael M, Swerdlow SH, Jaffe E: Lymphoproliferative dis-orders associated with primary immune disorders, in *World Health Or-ganization Classification of Tumors: Tumors of Hematopoietic and Lym-phoid Tissue*, edited by ES Jaffe, NL Harrs, H Stein, JW Vardiman, p 257. IARC Press, Lyon, France, 2001.

738. Raphael M, Borisch B, Jaffe ES: Lymphomas associated with infection by the human immunodeficiency virus (HIV), in *World Health Orga-nization Classification of Tumors: Tumors of Hematopoietic and Lym-phoid Tissue*, edited by ES Jaffe, NL Harrs, H Stein, JW Vardiman, p 260. IARC Press, Lyon, France, 2001.

739. Harris NL, Swerdlow SH, Fizzerra G, Knowles DM: Post-transplant lympho-proliferative disorders, in *World Health Organization Classifi-cation of Tumors: Tumors of Hematopoietic and Lymphoid Tissue*, ed-ited by ES Jaffe, NL Harrs, H Stein, JW Vardiman, p 264. IARC Press, Lyon, France, 2001.

740. Harris NL, Swerdlow SH: Methotrexate-associated lymphoproliferative disorders, in *World Health Organization Classification of Tumors: Tu-mors of Hematopoietic and Lymphoid Tissue*, edited by ES Jaffe, NL Harrs, H Stein, JW Vardiman, p 270. IARC Press, Lyon, France, 2001.

741. Taylor AM, Metcalfe JA, Thick J, Mak YF: Leukemia and lymphoma in ataxia telangiectasia. *Blood* 87:423, 1996.

742. Meyn MS: Ataxia-telangiectasia, cancer and the pathology of the ATM gene. *Clin Genet* 55:289, 1999.

743. Taylor AM: Chromosome instability syndromes. *Best Pract Clin Hae-matol* 14:631, 2001.

744. Mueller BU, Pizzo PA: Cancer in children with primary or secondary immunodeficiencies. *J Pediatrics* 126:1, 1995.

745. Siwicki JK, Degerman S, Chrzanowska KH, Roos G: Telomere main-tenance and cell cycle regulation in spontaneously immortalized T-cell lines from Nijmegen breakage syndrome. *Exp Cell Res* 287:178, 2003.

746. Varon R, Reis A, Henze G, et al: Mutations in the Nijmegen syndrome gene (NBS1) in childhood acute lymphoblastic leukemia. *Cancer Res* 61:3570, 2001.

747. Felix CA, D'Amico D, Mitsudomi T, et al: Absence of hereditary p53 mutations in 10 familial leukemia pedigrees. *J Clin Invest* 90:653, 1992.

748. Pepper C, Thomas A, Hoy T, et al: Leukemia and non-leukemic lym-phocytes from patients with Li-Fraumeni syndrome demonstrate loss of p53 function, BCL-2 family dysregulation and intrinsic resistance to conventional chemotherapeutic drugs but not flavopiridol. *Cell Cycle* 2:53, 2003.

749. Cunningham-Rundles C, Bodian C: Common variable immunodefi-ciency: Clinical and immunological features of 248 patients. *Clin Im-munol* 92:34,1999.

750. Farrington M, Grosmaire LS, Nonoyama S, et al: CD40 ligand expres-sion is defective in a subset of patients with common variable immu-nodeficiency. *Proc Natl Acad Sci U S A* 91:1099, 1994.

751. Leverrier Y, Lorenzi R, Blundell MP, et al: Cutting edge: The Wiskott-Aldrich syndrome protein is required for efficient phagocytosis of apop-totic cells. *J Immunol* 166:4831, 2001.

752. Rengan R, Ochs HD: Molecular biology of the Wiskott-Aldrich syn-drome. *Rev Immunogenet* 2:243, 2000.

753. Gilson D, Taylor RE: Long-term survival following non-Hodgkin lymphoma arising in Wiskott-Aldrich syndrome. *Clin Oncol* 11:283, 1999.

754. Perry GS 3rd, Spector BD, Schuman LM, et al: The Wiskott-Aldrich syndrome in the United States and Canada (1892-1979). *J Ped* 97:72, 1980.

755. Allen RC, Armitage RJ, Conley ME, et al: CD40 ligand gene defects responsible for X-linked hyper-IgM syndrome. *Science* 259:990, 1993.

756. Aruffo A, Farrington M, Hollenbaugh D, et al: The CD40 ligand, gp39, is defective in activated T cells from patients with X-linked hyper-IgM syndrome. *Cell* 72:291, 1993.

757. Macginnitie AJ, Geha R: X-linked lymphoproliferative disease: Genetic lesions and clinical consequences. *Curr Allergy Asthma Rep* 2:361, 2002.

758. Strauss SE, Jaffe ES, Puck JM, et al: The development of lymphomas in families with autoimmune lymphoproliferative syndrome with germ-line fas mutations and defective lymphocyte apoptosis. *Blood* 98:194, 2001.

759. Holzelova E, Vonarbourg C, Stolzenberg M-C, et al: Autoimmune lym-phoproliferative syndrome with somatic FAS mutations. *N Engl J Med* 351:1409, 2004.

760. Grobe H: Dubowitz syndrome and acute lymphatic leukemia. *Mon-atsschr Kinderheilkd* 131:467, 1983.

761. Fokin AA, Robicsek F: Poland syndrome revisited. *Ann Thorac Surg* 74:2218, 2002.

762. Parikh PM, Karandikar SM, Koppikar S, et al: Poland syndrome with acute lymphoblastic leukemia in an adult. *Med Pediatr Oncol* 16:290, 1988.

763. Sackey K, Odone V, George SL, Murphy SB: Poland syndrome associated with childhood non-Hodgkin lymphoma. *Am J Dis Child* 138: 600, 1984.

764. Vergin C, Cetingul N, Kavakli K, et al: A patient with WT syndrome and Castleman disease. *Acta Paediatr Jpn* 37:108, 1995.

765. Bell DW, Varley JM, Szydlo TE, et al: Heterozygous germ line hCHK2 mutations in Li-Fraumeni syndrome. *Science* 24:2528, 1999.

766. Varley J: TP53, hChk2, and the Li-Fraumeni syndrome. *Methods Mol Biol* 222:117, 2003.

767. Castleman B, Iverson L, Menendez VP: Localized mediastinal lymph node hyperplasia. *Cancer* 9:822, 1956.

768. Frizzera G: Atypical lymphoproliferative disorders, in *Neoplastic Hematopathology*, edited by DM Knowles, p 454. Williams & Wilkins, Baltimore, 1992.

769. Keller AR, Hochholzer L, Castleman B: Hyaline-vascular and plasma cell types of giant lymph node hyperplasia of the mediastinum and other locations. *Cancer* 29:670, 1972.

770. Gaba AR, Stein RS, Sweet DL, Variakojis D: Multicentric giant lymph node hyperplasia. *Am J Clin Pathol* 69:86, 1978.

771. Frizzera G, Peterson BA, Bayrd ED, Goldman A: A systemic lymphoproliferative disorder with morphologic features of Castleman disease: Clinical findings and clinicopathologic correlations in 15 patients. *J Clin Oncol* 3:1202, 1985.

772. Weisenburger DD, Nathwani BN, Winberg CD, Rappaport H: Multicentric angiofollicular lymph node hyperplasia: A clinicopathologic study of 16 cases. *Hum Pathol* 16:162, 1985.

773. Lachant NA, Sun NC, Leong LA, et al: Multicentric angiofollicular lymph node hyperplasia (Castleman disease) followed by Kaposi sarcoma in two homosexual males with the acquired immunodeficiency syndrome (AIDS). *Am J Clin Pathol* 83:27, 1985.

774. Parravinci C, Corbellino M, Paulli M, et al: Expression of a virus-derived cytokine, KSHV vIL-6, in HIV-seronegative Castleman disease. *Am J Pathol* 151:1517, 1997.

775. Kessler E: Multicentric giant lymph node hyperplasia. A report of seven cases. *Cancer* 56:2446, 1985.

776. Herrada J, Cabanillas F, Rice L, et al: The clinical behavior of localized and multicentric Castleman disease. *Ann Intern Med* 128:657, 1998.

777. Munoz G, Geijo P, Moldenhauer F, et al: Plasmacellular Castleman disease and POEMS syndrome. *Histopathology* 17:172, 1990.

778. Fujimoto Y, Kozima Y, Yamaguchi K: Cervical subacute necrotizing lymphadenitis. A new clinicopathologic agent. *Naika* 20:920, 1972.

779. Lin HC, Su CY, Huang CC, et al: Kikuchi disease: A review and analysis of 61 cases. *Otolaryngol Head Neck Surg* 128:650, 2003.

780. Norris AH, Krasinskas AM, Salhany KE, et al: Kikuchi-Fujimoto disease: A benign cause of fever and lymphadenopathy. *Am J Med* 101: 401, 1996.

781. Rosai J, Dorfman RF: Sinus histiocytosis with massive lymphadenopathy: A newly recognized benign clinicopathologic entity. *Arch Pathol* 87:63, 1969.

782. Foucar E, Rosai J, Dorfman RF: Sinus histiocytosis with massive lymphadenopathy (Rosai-Dorfman disease): Review of the entity. *Semin Diagn Pathol* 7:19, 1990.

783. Kademani D, Patel SG, Prasad ML, et al: Intraoral presentation of Rosai-Dorfman disease: A case report and review of the literature. *Oral Surg Oral Med Oral Pathol Oral Radiol Endod* 93:699, 2002.

784. Pulsoni A, Anghel G, Falcucci P, et al: Treatment of sinus histiocytosis with massive lymphadenopathy (Rosai-Dorfman disease): Report of a case and literature review. *Am J Hematol* 69:67, 2002.

785. Lennert K, Hansmann ML: Progressive transformation of germinal centers: Clinical significance and lymphocytic predominance of Hodgkin's disease—The Kiel experience. *Am J Surg Pathol* 11:149, 1987.

786. Verma A, Stock W, Norohna S, et al: Progressive transformation of germinal centers: Report of 2 cases and review of the literature. *Acta Haematol* 108:33, 2002.

787. Poppema S, Kaiserling E, Lennert K: Hodgkin's disease with lymphocytic predominance, nodular type (nodular paragranuloma) and progressively transformed germinal centers—A cytohistological study. *Histopathology* 3:295, 1979.

788. Perrone T, De Wolf Peeters C, Frizzera G: Inflammatory pseudotumor of lymph nodes: A distinctive pattern of nodal reaction. *Am J Surg Pathol* 12:351, 1988.

789. Davis RE, Warnke RA, Dorfman RF: Inflammatory pseudotumor of lymph nodes: Additional observations and evidence for an inflammatory etiology. *Am J Surg Pathol* 15:744, 1991.

790. Hyjek E, Smith WJ, Isaacson PG: Primary B-cell lymphoma of salivary glands and its relationship to myoepithelial sialadenitis. *Hum Pathol* 19: 766, 1998.

791. Quintana PG, Kapadia SB, Bahler DW, et al: Salivary gland lymphoid infiltrates associated with lymphoepithelial lesions: A clinicopathologic, immunophenotypic, and genotypic study. *Hum Pathol* 28:850, 1997.

792. Fishleder A, Tubbs R, Hesse B, Levine H: Uniform detection of immunoglobulin-gene rearrangement in benign lymphoepithelial lesions. *N Engl J Med* 316:1118, 1987.

793. Saltzstein SL, Ackerman LV: Lymphadenopathy induced by anticonvulsant drugs and mimicking clinically and pathologically malignant lymphomas. *Cancer* 12:164, 1959.

794. Segal GH, Clough JD, Tubbs RR: Autoimmune and iatrogenic causes of lymphadenopathy. *Semin Oncol* 20:611, 1993.

HODGKIN LYMPHOMA

SANDRA J. HORNING

Classic Hodgkin lymphoma, characterized by the Reed-Sternberg cell, is a monoclonal germinal center B cell disorder that does not express antigen receptor but has escaped apoptosis through alternative mechanisms. Morphologic and immunophenotypic features can distinguish five subtypes of Hodgkin lymphoma. Each subtype is spread in a reliable, contiguous manner. [18F]-Fluorodeoxyglucose positron emission tomography has emerged as an effective means for assessing disease and response to treatment. Doxorubicin is a highly active agent in combination with other drugs, and radiotherapy is an effective modality, particularly in combination with chemotherapy and in bulky disease. Hodgkin lymphoma is approached with curative intent as current survival exceeds 85 percent for all stages. High-dose therapy and autologous transplantation are effective for relapsed disease. Consideration for treatment complications that occur years later guides therapy and followup in Hodgkin lymphoma, which disproportionately affects adolescents and young adults. Major treatment challenges include maintenance of high cure rates with less toxic treatment, including integration of biologic therapies.

DEFINITION AND HISTORY

Classic Hodgkin lymphoma is a neoplasm of lymphoid tissue, in most cases derived from germinal center B cells, defined by the presence of the malignant Reed-Sternberg and Hodgkin cells (RS-H) with characteristic immunophenotype and appropriate cellular background.

Acronyms and abbreviations that appear in this chapter include: ABVD, Adriamycin (doxorubicin), bleomycin, vinblastine, dacarbazine; BEACOPP, bleomycin, etoposide, Adriamycin (doxorubicin), cyclophosphamide, vincristine, procarbazine, prednisone; BEAM, bischloroethylnitrosourea (carmustine), etoposide, Ara-C (cytarabine), melphalan; CALGB, Cancer and Acute Leukemia Group B; CBV, cyclophosphamide, bischloroethylnitrosourea (carmustine), etoposide; ChlVPP, chlorambucil, vinblastine, procarbazine, prednisone; COPP, cyclophosphamide, vincristine, procarbazine, prednisone; CT, computed tomography; EBNA1, Epstein-Barr nuclear antigen 1; EBV, Epstein-Barr virus; EBVP, epirubicin, bleomycin, vinblastine, prednisone; EORTC, European Organization for the Research and Treatment of Cancer; ESR, erythrocyte sedimentation rate; FADD, Fas-associated death domain; FDG, fluorodeoxyglucose; FLICE, FADD-like ICE; FLIP, FLICE-like inhibitory protein; GHSG, German Hodgkin Study Group; HLA, human lymphocyte antigen; ICE, IL-1−converting enzyme; IgV$_{H}$, immunoglobulin heavy-chain variable region; IκB, inhibitor of κB; IL, interleukin; L&H, lymphocyte and histiocyte; LMP, latent membrane protein; MAPK, mitogen-activated protein kinase; MOPP, mechlorethamine (nitrogen mustard), Oncovin (vincristine), procarbazine, prednisone; MVPP, nitrogen mustard, vinblastine, procarbazine, prednisone; NCI, National Cancer Institute; NF-κB, nuclear factor-κB; NLPHL, nodular lymphocyte-predominant Hodgkin lymphoma; NSHL, nodular sclerosis Hodgkin lymphoma; PET, positron emission tomography; RANK, receptor activator of NF-κB; RS-H, Reed-Sternberg and Hodgkin; RT, radiation therapy; STAT, signal transducer and activator of transcription; TARC, thymus activation-regulated cytokine; TGF, transforming growth factor; Th, T helper; TNF, tumor necrosis factor; TNFR, tumor necrosis factor receptor; TRAF, TNF receptor-associated factor; TRAIL, TNF receptor apoptosis-inducing ligand; VAPEC-B, vinblastine, doxorubicin, prednisone, etoposide, cyclophosphamide, bleomycin; VBM, vinblastine, bleomycin, methotrexate; XIAP, X-linked inhibitor of apoptosis protein.

Four histologic subtypes of classic Hodgkin lymphoma (nodular sclerosis, mixed cellularity, lymphocyte-rich, and lymphocyte-depleted) are distinguished based on the microscopic appearance and relative proportions of RS-H cells, lymphocytes, and fibrosis. Nodular lymphocyte-predominant subtype represents the other major category of Hodgkin lymphoma that is distinguished by giant cells, which, unlike classic Hodgkin lymphoma, express typical B lineage markers.

HISTORICAL ASPECTS

In his historic 1832 paper entitled "On some morbid appearances of the absorbent glands and spleen," Thomas Hodgkin[1] described the clinical histories and gross postmortem findings of seven cases of the disease that was later to bear his name. In 1856, Samuel Wilks[2] independently described 10 cases of "a peculiar enlargement of the lymphatic glands frequently associated with disease of the spleen," including four of Hodgkin's original cases. Upon discovering Hodgkin's original report, Wilks[3] used the appellation "Hodgkin's disease" in a subsequent series of 15 cases published in 1865.

Thirteen years after Hodgkin's original paper, the first cases of leukemia were described. Cases in which the neoplastic cells remained confined to the lymphatic system were described by Dreschfield[4] in 1892 and Kundrat[5] in 1893; the latter gave the name "lymphosarcoma" to these cases. The description of additional members of the lymphoma-leukemia complex continued throughout the 20th century up to the present time.

Carl Sternberg[6] in 1898 and Dorothy Reed[7] in 1902 are credited with the first definitive and thorough histopathologic descriptions of Hodgkin lymphoma, although a number of investigators from England, Germany, and France previously had recognized the characteristic multinucleated giant cells. In 1926, Fox[8] examined microscopic sections from the gross specimens of three of Hodgkin's original cases preserved in the Gordon Museum of Guy's Hospital in London. Remarkably, the preserved microanatomy allowed him to confirm the histopathologic diagnosis in two of the cases. Jackson and Parker[9] made the first serious effort at the histopathologic classification of Hodgkin lymphoma, correlating their findings with prognosis. A second advance was made in 1966 when Lukes and associates[10] proposed a classification that related well to clinical presentation and course. Their proposal was slightly modified into the Rye classification, in which four histopathologic subtypes were described: lymphocyte-predominant, nodular sclerosis, mixed cellularity, and lymphocyte depleted. In the World Health Organization Classification of Lymphoid Neoplasms, the nodular lymphocyte-predominant subtype is clearly distinguished from classic Hodgkin lymphoma.[11] The "lymphocyte-rich" subtype of classic Hodgkin lymphoma was introduced in this classification (Table 97-1).

In 1950, Peters[12] described a clinical staging system that emphasized the diagnostic evaluation of the anatomic extent of disease. In 1952, Kinmouth[13] introduced lower-extremity lymphangiography, which allowed roentgenologic visualization of the pelvic and retroperitoneal lymph nodes and was found to be far more sensitive than palpation or other radiographic methods. The frequency of unsuspected splenic involvement was revealed in a group of 65 patients

TABLE 97-1   WORLD HEALTH ORGANIZATION CLASSIFICATION OF HODGKIN LYMPHOMA

Nodular lymphocyte-predominant Hodgkin lymphoma
Classic Hodgkin lymphoma
   Lymphocyte-rich
   Nodular sclerosis (grades I and II)
   Mixed cellularity
   Lymphocyte-depleted

subjected to laparotomy and splenectomy with biopsy of splenic hilar, paraaortic, and mesenteric nodes and liver at Stanford University.[14] These diagnostic procedures led to improved understanding of the mode of dissemination of disease and correlated well with prognosis, culminating in the modern concepts of staging codified at the Rye, New York, conference in 1965[15] and further refined at the Workshop on the Staging of Hodgkin Disease in Ann Arbor, Michigan, in 1971.[16]

Pusey[17] in 1902 and Senn[18] in 1903 were the first to report dramatic regressions of lymphadenopathy with the x-rays newly discovered by Roentgen in 1896. Based upon the nearly inevitable appearance of recurrences in untreated areas, Gilbert[19] proposed the systematic treatment of both involved and uninvolved areas in 1939. Peters[12] is given credit for the first demonstration of the curative potential of radiotherapy in her classic 1950 paper. The development of megavoltage radiotherapy (doses >4000 cGy), as reported by Kaplan[20] in 1962, permitted the delivery of tumoricidal doses to almost all lymphoid regions in the body within acceptable limits of normal tissue tolerance.

The chemotherapy of Hodgkin lymphoma originated as a byproduct of the wartime work on the mustard gases.[21,22] Following the initial work with the nitrogen mustards, antimetabolites were synthesized, and a number of alkaloids and antibiotics extracted from various plant, fungal, and microbial sources became available for clinical use. DeVita and colleagues[23] introduced the first highly effective combination chemotherapy MOPP (mechlorethamine [nitrogen mustard], Oncovin [vincristine], procarbazine, prednisone), based on experimental studies indicating the desirability of combining agents with nonoverlapping toxicities. Combination chemotherapy extended the curative potential for Hodgkin lymphoma to advanced disease. The ABVD (Adriamycin [doxorubicin], bleomycin, vinblastine, dacarbazine) regimen introduced by Bonadonna and colleagues[24] represented another major advance. Based on a more favorable safety profile and greater efficacy, ABVD replaced MOPP.

EPIDEMIOLOGY

The incidence of Hodgkin lymphoma in the United States has been stable over the past several decades, with an estimated 7880 cases in 2004.[25] The incidence is higher in men than in women and higher in Americans of European descent than in Americans of African descent.

Hodgkin lymphoma has a bimodal incidence peak at ages 15 to 34 years and over 60 years.[26–29] Three distinct forms of Hodgkin lymphoma have been described: a childhood form (ages 0–14 years), a young adult form (15–34 years), and an older adult form (55–74 years). The nodular sclerosis subtype predominates in young adults, whereas the mixed cellularity subtype is more common in the pediatric population and in older age populations. A male predominance at all ages is noted but is most marked in childhood cases (85%).

An increased risk of Hodgkin lymphoma in the young adult population has been associated with high socioeconomic status.[26,30,31] High intelligence, small family size, single-family dwelling, high educational attainment of patients and their immediate families, and delayed parity in women all have been associated with increased risk. Although associations with occupational exposure and lifestyle factors have been reported, the collective data do not support causal relationships.[29]

The geographic patterns vary for the three major age groups. The incidence of Hodgkin lymphoma is greater in childhood in less developed countries, whereas the incidence peaks in young adulthood and is associated with more favorable histologic subtypes in developed countries.[32] An intermediate picture may be seen in rural areas of developing countries. Together these data suggest a remarkable association between socioeconomic and environmental factors in the incidence of Hodgkin lymphoma.

Epidemiologic similarities between young adult Hodgkin lymphoma and multiple sclerosis have led to the hypothesis that the two diseases have a related etiology. Observations of familial clustering of the two disorders are consistent with shared environmental or constitutional etiologies.[33]

POSSIBLE INFECTIOUS ETIOLOGY

The demographic features have long supported the concept that one or more subtypes of Hodgkin lymphoma have an infectious etiology. In 1966, MacMahon[26] proposed that the first age peak in young adults was infectious in nature, whereas the second peak resulted from causes similar to those for other lymphomas.

Several reports of clustering of Hodgkin lymphoma at the time of diagnosis suggested the possibility of infectious transmission.[34,35] The weaknesses of the retrospective methodology in these studies have been critically assessed, and further statistical analyses indicate the cases likely occurred by chance alone.[32] Some population-based studies have found significant case aggregation (shared exposure) in schools, but these results have been seriously questioned based on the methods used.[36–39]

A threefold increased risk of young adult Hodgkin lymphoma is conferred by a prior history of serologically confirmed infectious mononucleosis.[40–42] Elevated titers of Epstein-Barr virus (EBV), the etiologic agent of infectious mononucleosis, have been reported in people diagnosed with Hodgkin lymphoma. A large population study showed that people who developed Hodgkin lymphoma had abnormally high titers of some anti-EBV antibodies in prediagnostic sera.[43] The epidemiologic features of Hodgkin lymphoma appear to fit a polio model where delayed age at infection leads to an increased risk of young adult disease. In less developed countries, where early infection is probable, childhood Hodgkin lymphoma is more common than young adult disease, whereas the reverse is true in developed countries. A similar pattern of geographic occurrence and age at initial infection also occurs for EBV infection.

EBV genomes have been detected in approximately one third of Hodgkin lymphoma tissues in developed countries, with the highest proportion reported in the mixed cellularity category.[44] Several studies report a high incidence of EBV association (85–100%) in pediatric Hodgkin lymphoma.[45–48] Geographic, ethnic, and racial factors have been implicated in the association of EBV with pediatric Hodgkin lymphoma.[46] A high frequency of EBV within RS-H cells is reported in HIV-infected individuals with Hodgkin lymphoma.[49] The apparent incongruent association of positive EBV-serology with young adult Hodgkin lymphoma, which is predominantly EBV-negative nodular sclerosis subtype, was resolved by two reports of a significantly increased risk of Hodgkin lymphoma after serologically verified infectious mononucleosis limited to EBV-positive cases in young adults.[50,51] The median incubation time was approximately 4.1 years. These data indicate a likely causal association between infectious mononucleosis-related EBV infection and the EBV-positive subgroup of Hodgkin lymphoma in young adults.

GENETIC BASIS

The increased risk among identical but not fraternal twins provides the strongest evidence for a genetic association with Hodgkin lymphoma.[52] Hodgkin lymphoma-prone families, with or without other forms of cancer, have been described in the literature, and an estimated 4.5 percent of cases are familial.[53–55] Standard incidence ratios for age-specific familial risk from the Swedish Cancer Registry were higher for Hodgkin lymphoma (4.8) than for any other neoplasm.[56] Relative risks for familial Hodgkin lymphoma are stronger in individuals younger than 40 years, males, and siblings, and a shared risk with chronic lymphocytic leukemia and non-Hodgkin lymphoma has been described.[57] Examples of cases associated with consanguinity also have been reported.[58,59] The fact that the time interval between diagnoses in affected siblings is shorter than their age differences supports an environmental influence in Hodgkin lymphoma-prone families.[60] The increased incidence in same sex siblings (ninefold) versus opposite sex siblings (fivefold) also supports an environmental influence.[61] In contrast, connubial occurrence in Hodgkin lymphoma is rare.[62] Lack of concordance of EBV association in tissues and serology argues against a viral role in the pathogenesis of familial Hodgkin lymphoma, but other data support this hypothesis.[63,64] In addition to the presentation of both Hodgkin lymphoma and a non-Hodgkin lymphoma in the same individual, both diagnoses have been noted in lymphoma-prone families, favoring a common mechanism of lymphomagenesis.[57,65]

Immunoregulatory genes within or near the major histocompatibility complex that may govern susceptibility to viral infections have been postulated to influence susceptibility to Hodgkin lymphoma.[66] This hypothesis is supported by the demonstration of lifelong, depressed cellular immunity in Hodgkin lymphoma patients and their healthy relatives.[67] Specific human lymphocyte antigen (HLA) regions have been implicated in the etiology of Hodgkin lymphoma, and increased HLA haplotype sharing has been observed among relatives in multiple-case families.[66,68,69] Several studies using molecular techniques have made epidemiologic and prognostic associations between HLA-DP alleles and Hodgkin lymphoma.[70–72] Susceptibility to nodular sclerosis was associated with DRB1*1501, DQB1*0602, and the DQB1*0303 alleles in a case-unrelated control study, and linkage disequilibrium with familial nodular sclerosis Hodgkin lymphoma (NSHL) was demonstrated for the DRB1*1501-DQA1*0102-DQB1*0602 haplotype.[73]

ETIOLOGY AND PATHOGENESIS

Difficulty in characterizing the neoplastic cells, which account for only approximately 1 to 2 percent of the cellular composition, led to controversy regarding the etiology and pathogenesis of Hodgkin lymphoma for more than 150 years. Molecular analyses of single cells facilitated discovery that classic Hodgkin lymphoma, in the large majority of cases, and nodular lymphocyte-predominant are clonal disorders derived from germinal center B cells.[74] The need to survive negative selection in the germinal center, determination of constitutive activity of the transcription factor nuclear factor-κB (NF-κB), and involvement of EBV in a subset of cases led to hypotheses on the means by which RS-H cells undergo malignant transformation. Application of genomic technology may further clarify the molecular changes underlying malignant transformation and cellular proliferation.

ORIGIN OF THE REED-STERNBERG CELL

The histologic diagnosis of Hodgkin lymphoma is based on the recognition of the Reed-Sternberg cell in an appropriate cellular background. The classic Reed-Sternberg cell has a bilobed nucleus with prominent eosinophilic nucleoli separated by a clear space from the thickened nuclear membrane (Figure 97-1, A). Mononuclear variants (Hodgkin cells) have similar nuclear characteristics and may represent Reed-Sternberg cells cut in a plane that shows only one lobe of the nucleus. Reed-Sternberg cells are not pathognomonic for Hodgkin lymphoma; they can be seen in reactive and other neoplastic conditions. Study of the Reed-Sternberg cell has been complicated by the fact that the neoplastic cells are sparsely interspersed among a reactive mixed cell population of lymphocytes, eosinophils, histiocytes, plasma cells, and neutrophils.

IMMUNOHISTOCHEMISTRY AND ANTIGEN RECEPTOR REARRANGEMENTS

Reed-Sternberg cells and their mononuclear variants (RS-H) demonstrate inconsistent lineage-specific antigen expression. Immunohistochemistry defines two major categories of Hodgkin lymphoma. Approximately 85 percent of classic Hodgkin lymphoma (nodular sclerosis and mixed cellularity) patients express the CD30 antigen,[75] a marker of lymphocyte activation (see Chap. 14).[76,77] The majority of RS-H cells in classic Hodgkin lymphoma express the CD15 antigen, which is characteristically expressed in the late stages of granulopoiesis (see Chap. 14).[78,79] However, CD15 expression is not limited to granulocytes and monocytes; it has been identified in activated T cells, cytomegalovirus-infected cells, and nonlymphoid cells.[80–82] Most RS-H cells express the interleukin (IL)-2 receptor (CD25 or Tac), characteristic of activated T cells.[83] A minority of classic Hodgkin lymphomas expresses the B cell antigens CD19 and CD20.[84–86]

The RS-H cells in nodular lymphocyte-predominant, known as *lymphocyte and histiocyte* (L&H) variants, have a unique polylobated, "popcorn" appearance. They consistently express B cell markers such as CD20 and CD45 (leukocyte common antigen) (see Figure 97-1, B).[87] They lack expression of CD15 and have variable expression of CD30.[88] The synthesis of cytoplasmic J-chain and immunoglobulin, expression of Bcl-6 in L&H cells, and light-chain restriction in some cases indicate the germinal center B cell origin of this subtype (see Chap. 77).[89–92]

The category of lymphocyte-rich Hodgkin lymphoma requires immunohistochemistry for diagnosis.[93] In this subtype, the majority of cells are small B lymphocytes, and a nodular or follicular pattern may be seen. The RS-H cells express CD15 and CD30, lack CD45, and may or may not express CD20. Although the morphologic features of the lymphocyte-rich subtype may be confused with nodular lymphocyte-predominant, the immunophenotype of the RS-H cells is that of classic Hodgkin lymphoma. Gene expression studies provide further evidence that these entities are distinct.[94]

The cellular origin of RS-H cells was finally determined through isolation of single cells by micromanipulation of histologic sections and analysis for immunoglobulin variable-gene rearrangements that demonstrated clonality.[74,95] The rearranged immunoglobulin heavy-chain variable region (IgV_H) genes carried a high number of somatic mutations, indicating a germinal center or postgerminal center origin of classic RS-H cells (see Chap. 77).[96–98] However, the mutation pattern did not support a gain in B cell receptor affinity. The precursor of RS-H cells is thought to be a preapoptotic germinal center B cell that escaped negative selection. Rare cases of classic Hodgkin lymphoma with a clonal T cell receptor gene rearrangement have been reported.[99] In contrast, single cell analyses in nodular lymphocyte-predominant demonstrated clonal immunoglobulin gene rearrangements with ongoing mutations, an intraclonal diversity consistent with a germinal center origin of L&H cells.[100–102] The lack of expression of surface immunoglobulin in classic Hodgkin lymphoma distinguishes the disorder from B cell lymphomas. Multiple factors account for this finding, including (1) destructive mutations within the rearranged genes or nonfunctional rearrangements, (2) mutations in the immunoglobulin promoter that prevent binding of transcription factors, and (3) deficiency in immunoglobulin-specific transcription factors.[103] In summary, the RS-H cell in classic Hodgkin lymphoma represents a monoclonal outgrowth of germinal center B cells that do not express antigen receptor but have escaped apoptosis through alternate mechanisms and have acquired growth self-sufficiency (Figure 97-2).

RESISTANCE TO APOPTOSIS

Because RS-H cells harbor crippling IgV_H heavy-chain gene mutations in a substantial proportion of cases and thus lack expression of func-

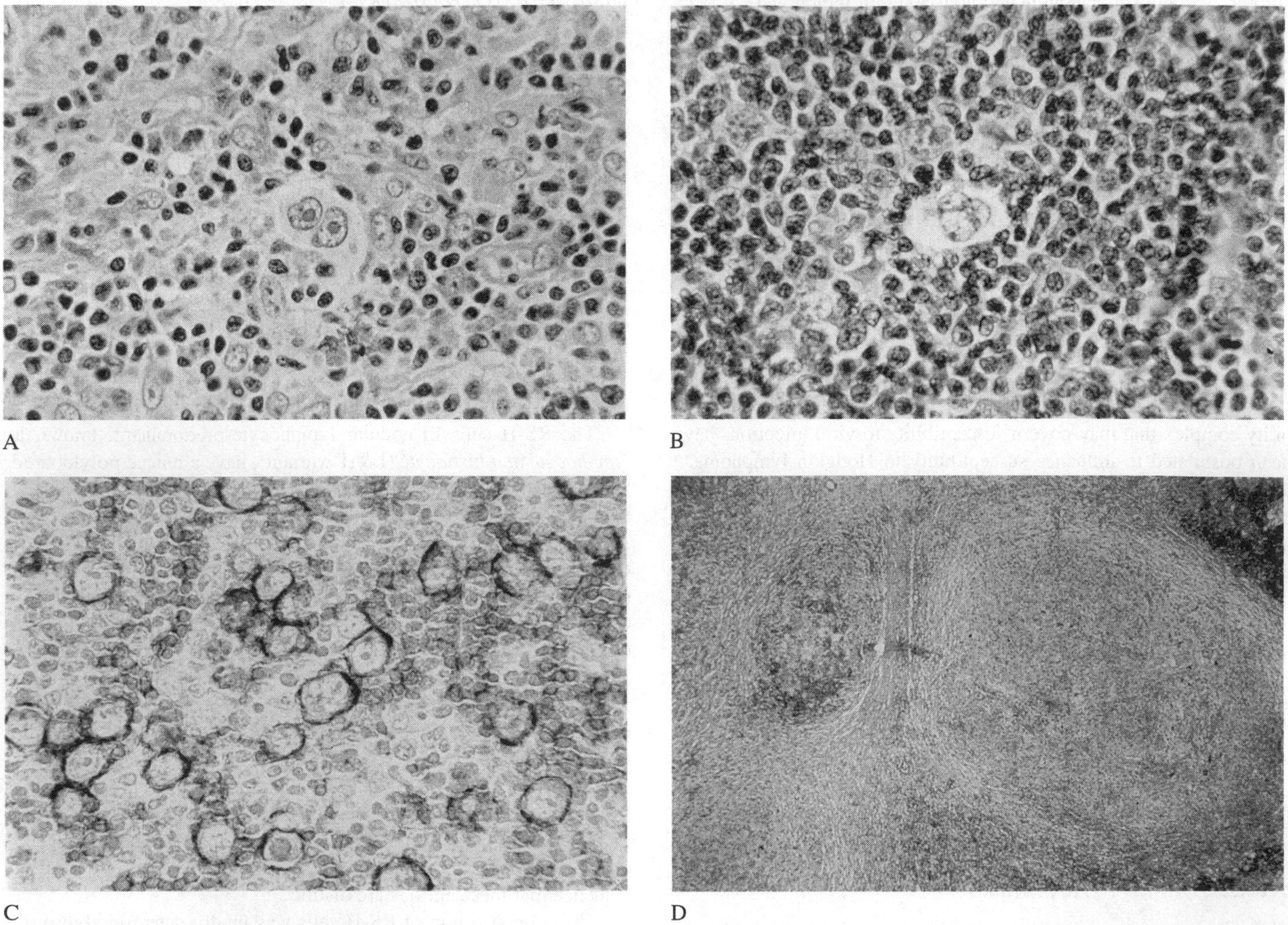

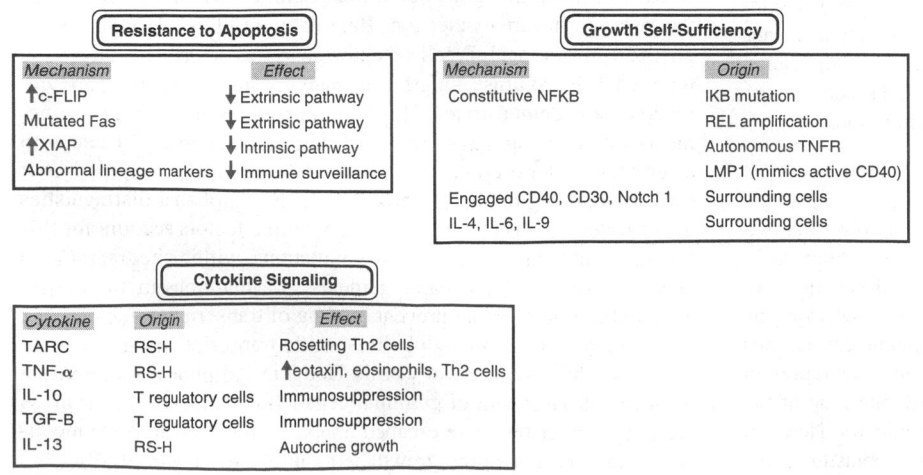

FIGURE 97-1   *(A)* Characteristic Reed-Sternberg cell of Hodgkin disease and surrounding mononuclear variants. *(B)* Lymphocyte and histiocyte (L&H) variant of the nodular form of lymphocyte predominance. (The "histiocyte" actually is a lymphocyte.) Note the multilobulated "popcorn" nucleus and surrounding small lymphocytes. *(C)* Immunoperoxidase staining of the L&H variant of the nodular form of lymphocyte predominance with the L26 antibody directed against a pan-B cell antigen (CD20) outlines the large atypical cells. *(D)* Low-power view of nodular sclerosis showing broad bands of collagen partitioning the lymph node into nodules.

Resistance to Apoptosis

Mechanism	Effect
↑c-FLIP	↓ Extrinsic pathway
Mutated Fas	↓ Extrinsic pathway
↑XIAP	↓ Intrinsic pathway
Abnormal lineage markers	↓ Immune surveillance

Growth Self-Sufficiency

Mechanism	Origin
Constitutive NFKB	IKB mutation
	REL amplification
	Autonomous TNFR
	LMP1 (mimics active CD40)
Engaged CD40, CD30, Notch 1	Surrounding cells
IL-4, IL-6, IL-9	Surrounding cells

Cytokine Signaling

Cytokine	Origin	Effect
TARC	RS-H	Rosetting Th2 cells
TNF-α	RS-H	↑eotaxin, eosinophils, Th2 cells
IL-10	T regulatory cells	Immunosuppression
TGF-B	T regulatory cells	Immunosuppression
IL-13	RS-H	Autocrine growth

FIGURE 97-2   Functions altered in Reed-Sternberg-Hodgkin and surrounding cells, leading to resistance to apoptosis, growth self-sufficiency, and abnormal cytokine signaling. See text for definitions of abbreviations.

tional B cell surface receptors, resistance to apoptosis is of keen interest in the approach to treating Hodgkin lymphoma.[74,104] In the physiologic immune reaction, B cells that express immunoglobulins that do not bind antigens effectively are eliminated by Fas-mediated apoptosis. Fas resistance has been demonstrated in Hodgkin lymphoma cell lines.[105] Resistance is infrequently mediated by mutations in the gene encoding Fas (CD95). Rather, Hodgkin cells express high levels of cellular Fas-associated death domain (FADD)-like IL-1β–converting enzyme (FLICE) inhibitory protein (c-FLIP), an inhibitor of FAS-mediated apoptosis.[106] Evidence for c-FLIP as a protector from Fas-mediated death in RS-H cells is strengthened by the demonstration that down-regulation of c-FLIP by small interfering RNA ribonucleotides is associated with reduced viability of classic Hodgkin lymphoma cells.[107,108] In addition to CD95, expression of c-FLIP interferes with death receptor signaling mediated by cross-linking of the tumor necrosis factor (TNF)-related apoptosis-inducing ligand (TRAIL) receptors 1 and 2, which are expressed by RS-H cells.[108] The signaling pathways responsible for c-FLIP regulation in the absence of B cell receptor signaling in classic Hodgkin lymphoma remain incompletely understood.

The apoptotic pathways of Hodgkin RS-H cells also can be inhibited by the X-linked inhibitor of apoptosis protein (XIAP). XIAP inhibits active caspases. High-level expression of Bcl-2 and Bcl-x_L by RS-H cells also can antagonize Bax-mediated apoptosis at the mitochondrial membrane.[109–111] Another mechanism for resisting apoptosis in Hodgkin lymphoma may be evasion of immunologic surveillance by follicular dendritic cells and T cells resulting from the expression of cell surface molecules specific for other cell types. These markers include CD15 (granulocytes), CD30, perforin (T cells), Notch-1 (T cells), and thymus activation-regulated cytokine ([TARC] dendritic cells).

GROWTH SIGNAL SELF-SUFFICIENCY
The complex autocrine or paracrine interactions between RS-H and bystander cells have long been the subject of inquiry. Observations on primary tissues and several well-characterized Hodgkin cell lines indicate RS-H cells secrete a variety of cytokines that may be responsible for the presence and characteristics of the nonmalignant cells surrounding them. In turn, these reactive cells produce cytokines that can affect RS-H cells and further influence the surrounding cellular milieu. CD40 ligand, IL-4, IL-6, and IL-9 appear to stimulate the growth of RS-H cells.[112]

A common effector mechanism for autonomously active signaling pathways is the nuclear translocation of the heterodimeric NF-κB via binding of specific inflammatory cell surface receptors and initiation of transcription of its target genes. Constitutive nuclear activity of NF-κB has been demonstrated in Hodgkin lymphoma cell lines and subsequently, by immunohistochemistry, in the nuclei of RS-H cells in primary tissues.[109] These observations established an integral role of NF-κB as an effector of transforming events in classic Hodgkin lymphoma, leading to self-sufficiency in growth. Explanations for the constitutive activity of NF-κB include mutations in the inhibitor of κB (IκB),[113] amplification of the NF-κB/REL locus,[114] and autonomous activity of CD30,[115] CD40,[116] receptor activator of NF-κB (RANK),[117] and Notch-1 signaling pathways.[118]

EBV is thought to be an important environmental factor, at least for the subset of EBV-positive cases of young adult Hodgkin lymphoma occurring after infectious mononucleosis. The transforming ability of EBV is mediated through the EBV-encoded genes known as *latent membrane proteins* (LMPs). The expression pattern in RS-H cells of LMP1, LMP2a, and Epstein-Barr nuclear antigen 1 (EBNA1) is characteristic of a latent viral infection (type 2 latency). LMP1 mimics a constitutively active CD40 receptor, which leads to NF-κB activation and up-regulation of antiapoptotic genes in antigen-activated B cells.[119] LMP2a activates survival signals while shutting down B cell receptor expression.[120] Thus, EBV may allow RS-H progenitors to survive negative selection in the germinal center and acquire other attributes in regulatory elements that lead to clonal expansion.

CYTOKINE SIGNALING
The relative amounts of collagen sclerosis and inflammatory cells and the cytology of the malignant RS-H cells define the histologic subtypes of Hodgkin lymphoma. Notably, more than 90 percent of involved Hodgkin lymphoma tissues compose immune cells. Multiple studies have concluded that Hodgkin lymphoma is a tumor with disturbed cytokine production. RS-H cells secrete T helper cell 2 (Th2) cytokines and chemokines such as TARC, which results in rosetting of CD4+ Th2 cells around the malignant cells,[121] and TNF-α, which results in secretion of eotaxin by fibroblasts and consequent attraction of eosinophils and recruitment of Th2 cells.[122] In turn, CD4+CD25+ T cells inhibit the cytotoxic function of T cells via secretion of IL-10 and transforming growth factor (TGF)-β.[123] The Th2 cytokine IL-13 is secreted by RS-H cells and stimulates their growth by an autocrine mechanism.[124] The attracted immune cells provide survival signals to RS-H cells by engaging surface receptors such as Notch-1, CD30, and CD40. Binding of these tumor necrosis factor receptor (TNFR) family members on RS-H cells results in cell proliferation and survival via TNFR-associated factor (TRAF) molecules and the mitogen-activated protein kinase (MAPK) pathway.[125] Cytokine signaling through signal transducer and activator of transcription (STAT) expression is implicated by STAT6 and STAT3 activation in RS-H cells,[126,127] and the latter may further subdue the immune response. In summary, abnormal cytokine signaling contributes to RS-H proliferation and survival and maintains an environment in which an effective host immune response against RS-H cells cannot be mounted.

GENETIC ALTERATIONS
Mutations in the IκB α gene that enable NF-κB to translocate to the nucleus in the absence of stimulatory signals have been reported in EBV-negative and EBV-positive Hodgkin lymphoma.[113] Fas mutations occur in a minority of Hodgkin lymphoma cases.[128,129] Nevertheless, defective Fas signaling may be involved in the pathogenesis of Hodgkin lymphoma. Secondary Fas mutations may cooperate in Hodgkin lymphomagenesis. In addition, inherited Fas mutations, observed in patients with autoimmune lymphoproliferative syndrome, apparently result in a 50-fold increased risk of developing Hodgkin lymphoma.[130]

Mutations in the tumor suppressor p53 or the N-*ras* oncogene typically are not observed. Primary RS-H cells do not demonstrate microsatellite instability but do express the most prominent mismatch repair genes hMSH2 and hMLH1.[131]

Chromosomal instability, however, is characteristic of Hodgkin lymphoma with loss of heterozygosity on 4q, 6p, 9q, and 17p.[132,133] Study of micromanipulated RS-H cells using a genome-wide approach demonstrated recurrent imbalances on 6q25 in 11 of 14 cases.[134] A putative tumor suppressor gene on 6q has been postulated for B cell lymphomas, particularly in the setting of progressed disease. Recurrent gains on chromosome 2p, 9p, and 12q have been associated with amplification of specific genes, providing further evidence of the intrinsic instability of Hodgkin lymphoma.

MOLECULAR PROFILING
Microarray technology has been used to characterize Hodgkin lymphoma cell lines. The gene expression profile of classic Hodgkin lymphoma appears to be related to the activated B cell-like subset of diffuse large B cell lymphoma.[135] Compared with other B cell lymphomas or normal B cell subsets, 45 genes were highly down-regulated and 27 genes were highly up-regulated.[136] Gene expression in Hodgkin cell lines also demonstrated overlap with EBV-transformed lymphoblastoid cell lines.[136] Two independent groups established a close relationship in gene expression among a distinctive clinical subset of non-Hodgkin lymphoma, primary mediastinal large B cell lymphoma, and classic Hodgkin lymphoma.[137,138] These disorders have clinical overlap in their presentation in younger adults, primarily women, with mediastinal adenopathy.

CLINICAL FEATURES

PRESENTING MANIFESTATIONS

HISTORY AND PHYSICAL EXAMINATION

Constitutional symptoms, some of which confer a less favorable prognosis, may accompany the diagnosis of Hodgkin lymphoma. Fever greater than 38°C, drenching night sweats, and weight loss exceeding 10 percent of baseline body weight during the 6 months preceding diagnosis are designated as *B disease*. Fevers usually are low grade and irregular.[139] Rarely, a cyclic pattern of high fevers for 1 to 2 weeks alternating with afebrile periods of similar duration is present at diagnosis. This classic Pel-Ebstein fever is virtually diagnostic.[140,141] Generalized pruritus, often accompanied by marked excoriation, may be present at diagnosis but is not prognostically significant.[142] Pain in the involved lymph nodes immediately after alcohol ingestion is a curious complaint that is nearly specific to Hodgkin lymphoma. It occurs in fewer than 10 percent of patients and has no prognostic significance.[143] The etiology of these symptoms has been the subject of speculation but remains largely unexplained. Patients with extensive intrathoracic disease may present with cough, chest pain, dyspnea, and rarely hemoptysis. Infrequently, patients present with bone pain, including the constellation of back pain accompanied by signs and symptoms of spinal cord compression.

Detection of an unusual mass or swelling in the superficial lymph nodes is the most common presentation of Hodgkin lymphoma. Lymphadenopathy usually is nontender and has a "rubbery" consistency. A diffuse, puffy swelling rather than a discrete mass may be apparent in the supraclavicular, infraclavicular, or anterior chest wall regions. Infrequently, compression of the superior vena cava results in facial swelling and engorgement of the veins in the neck and upper chest. Auscultation of the chest may reveal a pleural effusion. Palpation is an insensitive method for detecting intraabdominal adenopathy or organ enlargement, but examination should be oriented toward the liver, spleen, and upper retroperitoneal area. Although parenchymal or meningeal involvement of the central nervous system is rare, a variety of paraneoplastic syndromes has been described in Hodgkin lymphoma. Patients have presented with signs of progressive multifocal leukoencephalopathy,[144] subacute cerebellar degeneration,[145,146] necrotizing myelopathy,[147] subacute sensory or motor neuropathy,[148] episodic neurologic dysfunction,[149] memory loss,[150] the Guillain-Barré syndrome,[151] and granulomatous angiitis of the central nervous system.[152]

RADIOGRAPHIC FEATURES

Intrathoracic disease is present at diagnosis in two thirds of patients. Mediastinal adenopathy is common in Hodgkin lymphoma, particularly in young women with nodular sclerosis.[153] Although computed tomography (CT) of the chest is standard, a standing chest x-ray film is used to describe mediastinal mass size.[154] Hilar adenopathy, pulmonary parenchymal involvement, pleural effusions, pericardial effusions, and chest wall masses may be appreciated by chest CT; these conditions are more common in the presence of extensive mediastinal disease. CT of the abdomen and pelvis is routinely used in the diagnostic evaluation of Hodgkin lymphoma. Although technologic advances have greatly increased the resolution of this technique and the subsequent detection of celiac, portal, splenic hilar, and mesenteric lymph nodes, the correlation with histologic involvement of the spleen, determined historically by laparotomy staging, has been disappointing.

Whole-body [18F]-fluorodeoxyglucose positron emission tomography (FDG-PET) correlates well with CT evaluation and may demonstrate additional areas of disease, although this information results in few changes in stage or initial therapy.[155,156] FDG-PET imaging can distinguish active residual disease (increased glucose metabolism) from inactive residual tissue, which is a major problem in assessing remission status after treatment. The positive predictive value of FDG-PET scans obtained at therapy end ranged from 25 to 100 percent.[157] False-positive FDG-PET scans can be seen in followup because of thymic hyperplasia, granulomatous disease, or infectious disorders. In addition to evaluation of residual masses, FDG-PET is being incorporated in early response monitoring for risk stratification. Overall, the predictive accuracy of FDG-PET is dependent upon reader expertise and clinical correlation. In situations where false-positive results are more likely, such as previously uninvolved anatomic sites or those without concomitant abnormality on CT scan, tissue biopsy confirmation is recommended. Use of combined CT and FDG-PET technology results in improved anatomic definition of sites with increased signal.

CLINICAL AND PATHOLOGIC CORRELATION

A strong correlation exists among age at onset, anatomic extent of disease, and histologic subtype of Hodgkin lymphoma. Approximately 10 percent of patients present with nodular lymphocyte-predominant Hodgkin lymphoma (NLPHL), which is considered a unique subtype. Progressive transformation of germinal centers may precede or follow NLPHL at other sites.[91,158] The cellular composition is predominantly benign B lymphocytes with or without histiocytes. The characteristic multilobated L&H cells are relatively abundant (see Figure 97-1, *B* and *C*). Patients most commonly present with stage I disease (70%), particularly in the axillae, with a 4:1 male predominance.[159] This subtype has been associated with large cell non-Hodgkin lymphoma as a composite tumor, or the large cell lymphoma may occur at a later date.[160,161] The large cell variant T-cell rich, B cell lymphoma may be difficult to distinguish from NLPHL and may occur concurrently or subsequently.[162]

NSHL is noted for its distinctive histologic features and frequent involvement of the lower cervical, supraclavicular, and mediastinal lymph nodes in adolescents and young adults, particularly females. Approximately 70 percent of patients present with limited-stage disease. Nodular sclerosis constitutes the majority of Hodgkin lymphoma cases, ranging from 40 to 70 percent. One distinguishing histologic feature is the lacunar cell, an RS variant that results from retraction of the cytoplasm of RS-H cells during formalin fixation. Another distinguishing feature is the thickened capsule and fibrous bands that divide the lymphoid tissue into cellular nodules (see Figure 97-1, *D*). NSHL has been subclassified as type I or II based on the frequency of malignant cells and normal lymphocytes. The malignant cells are numerous in the relatively lymphocyte-depleted type II subtype, also referred to as the *syncytial variant*. The clinical and prognostic significance of NSHL subtypes is controversial, with some authors reporting inferior outcomes for type II.[163-165]

Mixed cellularity Hodgkin lymphoma involves both pediatric and older age groups and is more commonly associated with advanced-stage disease, constitutional symptoms, and immunodeficiency. Approximately 30 to 50 percent of patients present with this histology. Classic RS-H cells are easily found amid a cellular background composed of lymphocytes, eosinophils, plasma cells, and histiocytes (see Figure 97-1, *D*). This subtype has been characterized as having a worse prognosis in the historical literature, but the differences have been largely blurred by modern therapy.

The incidence of lymphocyte-depleted Hodgkin lymphoma is much lower than originally reported, because many cases have been reclassified as non-Hodgkin lymphoma.[166] Two subtypes have been described: reticular and diffuse fibrosis. The reticular variant contains abundant pleomorphic neoplastic cells. The more common diffuse fibrosis variant, as the name implies, has a prominent fibroblastic proliferation with few normal lymphocytes. RS-H cells are sparse. The disease presents in the older age group with symptomatic, extensive disease. Peripheral and mediastinal adenopathy is much less common than in other cases of Hodgkin lymphoma.[167] Presentation with fever of unknown origin, jaundice, hepatosplenomegaly, or pancytopenia is not uncommon. This subtype is associated with the acquired immunodeficiency syndrome.

The World Health Organization classification of lymphoma introduced the lymphocyte-rich subtype in 1999 (see Table 97-1). Lymphocyte-rich Hodgkin lymphoma was discovered during an expert pathology review of cases of nodular lymphocyte-predominant.[93] The two subtypes differ subtly on morphologic grounds, but the major difference is that the RS-H cells in lymphocyte-rich Hodgkin lymphoma have a classic immunophenotype. The presenting features are similar, although patients with the lymphocyte-rich subtype tend to be older than patients with NLPHD.[93] A higher rate of multiple relapses and a more favorable prognosis upon relapse are characteristic of patients with NLPHL.

ANATOMIC DISTRIBUTION OF DISEASE

Approximately 60 to 80 percent of clinical presentations are in the cervical nodes, 6 to 20 percent in axillary nodes, and 6 to 12 percent in the inguinal nodes.[139] A minority of patients presents with exclusive subdiaphragmatic disease. In a historical series of 285 consecutive, unselected, untreated patients evaluated at Stanford University, 272 patients underwent staging laparotomy, a surgical diagnostic procedure in which the intraabdominal and pelvic lymph nodes are sampled, the spleen is removed and examined pathologically in thin slices, the liver is biopsied by needle and wedge technique, and the marrow is biopsied. The frequency of splenic involvement at laparotomy in untreated patients averaged 37 percent in 17 published series.[139] Involvement of the spleen was strongly dependent on histologic subtype. Sixty percent of patients of mixed cellularity or lymphocyte-depleted Hodgkin lymphoma had splenic involvement, but only 34 percent of patients with nodular lymphocyte-predominant or nodular sclerosis disease had splenic involvement. Hepatic and bone marrow disease were invariably associated with splenic involvement.

Two different theories, the *contiguity theory* of Rosenberg and Kaplan[168] and the *susceptibility theory* of Smithers,[169] were proposed for the mode of spread of Hodgkin lymphoma. In support of the former theory, most cases of Hodgkin lymphoma appear to spread via lymphatic channels to contiguous lymphatic structures in a predictable, nonrandom pattern. Controversy has surrounded the mode of spread to the spleen, which lacks afferent lymphatics. When four or more lymph node regions were involved, the possibility of spread by hematogenous distribution appeared more likely.[170] Disseminated disease is more common in mixed cellularity and lymphocyte-depleted, consistent with the vascular invasion reported in these subtypes.[171] Whereas the concept of vascular invasion is controversial, it reportedly is more common in the spleen than in lymph nodes and connotes a poor prognosis.[172] Even when the disease spreads beyond the lymphatic system, patterns of association as described by Kaplan and Rosenberg are evident.

STAGING

The extent of Hodgkin lymphoma is classified using the four-stage Ann Arbor classification (Table 97-2).[16] *Clinical stage* refers to the results of physical, radiographic, and laboratory examination, whereas *pathologic stage* refers to the use of additional biopsy procedures. The classification is further characterized by the presence or absence of constitutional symptoms. Extranodal disease, representing extracapsular extension of lymph node disease that could be incorporated in a standard radiotherapy field, is distinguished from disseminated, stage IV disease. The correlation of this staging classification system with prognosis was extensively verified when radiotherapy served as the

TABLE 97-2 ANN ARBOR HODGKIN DISEASE STAGING CLASSIFICATION*

STAGE

I	Involvement of one lymph node region or lymphoid structure
II	Two or more lymph node regions on the same side of the diaphragm
III	Lymph node regions on both sides of the diaphragm
III₁	with splenic hilar, celiac, or portal nodes
IIII₂	with paraaortic, iliac or, inguinal nodes
IV	Involvement of extranodal sites(s) beyond that designated E

MODIFYING FEATURES

A	No symptoms
B	Fever, drenching night sweats, weight loss >10% in 6 months
X	Bulky disease: mediastinal disease >0.33 maximal intrathoracic diameter or >10 cm maximal diameter of a nodal mass
E	Involvement of single, contiguous, or proximal extranodal site
CS	Clinical stage
PS	Pathological stage

principal treatment for all but stage IV disease. Additional prognostic information, such as mediastinal bulk, other bulky nodal masses, and extent of subdiaphragmatic nodal disease, was included in a modification of the Ann Arbor system known as the *Cotswold classification* in 1989.[173]

Prognostic factors and recommended staging procedures for untreated patients have evolved with changes in therapy. Exploratory laparotomy and splenectomy, which historically advanced approximately one third of clinical stage I and II patients to pathologic stage III and IV while reducing fewer than one fourth of clinical stage III patients to pathologic stage I or II, is no longer performed.[174] Prognostic indicators of laparotomy findings have been described.[175] Laparotomy was abandoned because of the superior quality of modern radiologic imaging and the routine use of systemic chemotherapy in early-stage disease, which has replaced wide-field irradiation and, with it, the requirement for precise anatomic definition of disease. CT of the chest, abdomen, and pelvis and FDG-PET provide sensitive delineation of involved sites, except for the spleen and marrow.

Marrow involvement occurs in 5 to 20 percent of new patients and is more common in patients of older age, advanced stage, less favorable histology, or with constitutional symptoms or immunodeficiency. Because the marrow almost never is involved in young asymptomatic patients with favorable clinical presentations (e.g., stages I or II), marrow biopsy may be omitted in routine staging.

LABORATORY FEATURES

Hodgkin lymphoma has no diagnostic laboratory features. A complete blood count may reveal granulocytosis,[176] eosinophilia,[177] lymphocytopenia,[178] thrombocytosis,[179] or anemia.[180] The anemia usually results from chronic disease but in rare instances results from hemolysis secondary to high fever[181] or associated with a positive Coombs test.[182] Thrombocytopenia may occur as a result of marrow involvement, hypersplenism, or an autoimmune mechanism.[183–185] Autoimmune neutropenia has been reported in Hodgkin lymphoma.[186] Cytopenias are particularly common in advanced-stage disease and lymphocyte-depleted histology. Elevation of the erythrocyte sedimentation rate (ESR) is most common in advanced disease and correlates with constitutional symptoms.[187,188] The degree of ESR elevation has been correlated with prognosis, particularly in limited-stage disease.[189] Although nonspecific, it can be useful during followup by heralding recurrent disease. Serum lactate dehydrogenase levels are elevated in 30 to 40 percent of patients at diagnosis.[190,191] The alkaline phosphatase level may be elevated in Hodgkin lymphoma, nonspecifically in limited disease, or in association with involvement of the liver, bone, or marrow in advanced disease.[192] Hypercalcemia is unusual in Hodgkin lymphoma and appears to be secondary to synthesis of increased levels of 1,25-dihydroxyvitamin D by Hodgkin lymphoma tissue.[193] A variety of other abnormalities has been reported, including hypoglycemia[194,195] resulting from an autoantibody to insulin receptors, and inappropriate secretion of antidiuretic hormone.[196]

Anemia, granulocytosis, lymphopenia, and low serum albumin constitute four of seven adverse prognostic factors identified in advanced Hodgkin lymphoma by an international consortium.[197] Similar to the non-Hodgkin lymphomas, serum β_2-microglobulin levels correlate with tumor burden and prognosis in Hodgkin lymphoma.[198] Serum levels of soluble CD30, IL-6, IL-10, or the IL-2 receptor each has been associated with constitutional symptoms and advanced disease.[199–202]

Examination of pleural fluid in Hodgkin lymphoma may reveal transudative, exudative, or chylous properties. Because cytology rarely yields diagnostic RS-H cells, the etiology is most often considered to be one of central lymphatic obstruction. Laboratory abnormalities may be prominent in rare presentations of Hodgkin lymphoma. These findings include abnormal liver function tests associated with marked enlargement of porta hepatis nodes and biliary obstruction or intrahepatic cholestasis.[203] The nephrotic syndrome is a rare presentation of Hodgkin lymphoma.[204]

DIFFERENTIAL DIAGNOSIS

Clinically enlarged lymph nodes may be associated with a variety of infectious, inflammatory, autoimmune, and neoplastic disorders. Biopsy of suspicious adenopathy should be reviewed by an experienced hematopathologist. The differential diagnosis usually is between Hodgkin and a non-Hodgkin lymphoma, sometimes referred to as *gray zone lymphomas*. The syncytial variant of NSHL may be particularly troublesome. Distinction from primary mediastinal B cell lymphoma may be difficult based on clinical and histologic features. New evidence indicates this disorder is genetically akin to classic Hodgkin lymphoma.[137,138] Mixed cellularity Hodgkin lymphoma may demonstrate a spectrum of pattern and cellular and stromal composition and must be distinguished from peripheral T cell lymphoma. A T cell-rich, B cell lymphoma can be difficult to distinguish from NLPHL.[162] Immune markers have proved invaluable for differential diagnosis. Nonneoplastic conditions that may simulate Hodgkin lymphoma include viral infections, particularly infectious mononucleosis. Depleted nodes of any histology may resemble the diffuse fibrosis variant of lymphocyte-depleted, including the depleted phase of lymph nodes from HIV-infected patients. The diagnosis in an extranodal site depends upon the organ involved and whether a diagnosis of Hodgkin lymphoma is known. Diagnostic RS cells are not required in liver and marrow because the foci of involvement are so small. The rare presentations of Hodgkin lymphoma, such as those in the central nervous system or liver or a fever of unknown origin, may lead to an extensive differential diagnosis.

THERAPY

RADIOTHERAPY

The pioneering work of Henry S. Kaplan and his colleagues at Stanford University provided the basis for modern radiotherapy. Hodgkin lymphoma first became a curable neoplasm through the systematic study of the spread of the disease and the use of supervoltage radiotherapy techniques. Kaplan provided evidence for a tumoricidal dose level, and a number of investigators have contributed to the current knowledge regarding the dose-response association.[205,206] This important concept led to the incorporation of high doses that could permanently ablate Hodgkin lymphoma. Modern supervoltage techniques allow administration of high doses of radiation in large volumes with acceptable normal tissue tolerance. This method has the advantage of increased dose depth that spares the skin and sharp beam edges that reduce scatter, minimizing radiating adjacent normal tissue. The modern linear accelerator provides x-rays in the 4- to 8-MeV range. When used alone, radiotherapy doses to involved fields usually ranged from 3500 to 4400 cGy, with prophylactic doses of 3000 to 3500 cGy to uninvolved tissues. Other data suggested that 3000 cGy administered to involved sites may be adequate.[207] Tumor doses of 150 to 200 cGy are given daily five times per week.

The classic regions of radiotherapy used for treatment of Hodgkin lymphoma included the mantle, paraaortic region, and pelvis. The mantle region encompassed the cervical, supraclavicular, infraclavicular, axillary, mediastinal, and hilar nodes. The paraaortic region included the splenic pedicle or the spleen, if still intact. Together, these regions were referred to as *subtotal lymphoid irradiation*. The combination of the paraaortic region and the pelvic region was called an *inverted Y*, and total lymphoid irradiation referred to the combined mantle and inverted Y regions. In the current management of Hodgkin lymphoma, wide-field irradiation is used infrequently. When used, match lines between fields must not overlap to ensure the spinal cord does not receive excessive radiation that can result in myelopathy. Pelvic irradiation requires careful shielding of the testes in men and consideration for oophoropexy plus shielding in premenopausal women.[208,209]

In the setting of combined chemotherapy and radiotherapy, modifications of the mantle field have been made to address adverse consequences of treatment. The axillae and the upper neck are not included in the field. Lung blocks are shaped to ensure adequate irradiation of the tumor volume. The whole heart is not treated unless evidence of pericardial involvement is present. A pericardial block is placed at 1500 cGy and a subcarinal block is placed at 3000 cGy. These modifications and use of radiotherapy after disease reduction with chemotherapy result in less radiation exposure to the neck, female breast, heart, and lungs, all of which should result in fewer late complications. The technical aspects of radiotherapy are extremely important and include use of simulators, individually constructed blocks, detailed patient positioning, careful beam definition, and verification of dose with dosimetry.

CHEMOTHERAPY

From 1942 to 1963, a number of single chemotherapy drugs became available for clinical use.[21,22] Nitrogen mustard, other alkylating agents, the antifols, glucocorticoids, the vinca alkaloids, and procarbazine each was studied in advanced disease. Responses were observed, but no evidence of cure was observed. The first modern combination chemotherapy program was devised by DeVita and colleagues.[23] The MOPP program differed from previous attempts in its curative intent, longer (6-month) treatment program, and introduction of a sliding scale for dose adjustment based upon hematologic toxicity. The national mortality figures for Hodgkin lymphoma decreased by more than 60 percent in the decade following the introduction of MOPP chemotherapy.[210] In the 20-year followup of the original series of 188 advanced stage patients treated with MOPP at the National Cancer Institute (NCI), 54 percent were continuously free of disease.[211]

A number of modifications were made to the original MOPP regimen with the intention of reducing acute toxicity, particularly the neuropathy and nausea and vomiting.[212] Of the MOPP-like regimens, the MVPP (nitrogen mustard, vinblastine, procarbazine, prednisone) regimen, which substitutes vinblastine for vincristine, and the ChlVPP (chlorambucil, vinblastine, procarbazine, prednisone) regimen, which substitutes chlorambucil for nitrogen mustard and vinblastine for vincristine) had comparable efficacy with somewhat improved tolerance.[213,214] Neither the use of maintenance therapy nor the addition of bleomycin improved outcome compared with the original MOPP program administered in full doses.[212,215]

Bonadonna and colleagues developed an important alternative regimen for treatment of Hodgkin lymphoma. ABVD was effective in the treatment of patients who had not responded to MOPP.[216,217] In addition, this regimen has a different toxicity profile from MOPP. ABVD subsequently was used alone, in combination with radiotherapy, and with MOPP in alternating or "hybrid" programs.[218–221]

Multiple alternative chemotherapy regimens have been introduced for treatment of Hodgkin lymphoma. The German Hodgkin Lymphoma Study Group (GHSG) developed the BEACOPP (bleomycin, etoposide, Adriamycin [doxorubicin], cyclophosphamide, vincristine, prednisone, procarbazine) combination, which has been tested in standard and escalated doses.[222] The Stanford group developed the abbreviated 12-week combination Stanford V (doxorubicin, vinblastine, vincristine, bleomycin, nitrogen mustard, etoposide, prednisone).[223] Table 97-3 lists the drugs, doses, and schedules of combination chemotherapy programs effective in the management of Hodgkin lymphoma.

FAVORABLE, LIMITED-STAGE DISEASE

Favorable, limited-stage disease can be defined as asymptomatic stage I or II supradiaphragmatic disease with no bulky sites and none or only one extranodal site. For many years, extended-field (subtotal lymphoid) radiotherapy, usually administered after staging laparotomy, was the treatment of choice for these patients in the United States based on a pivotal clinical trial conducted at Stanford University. In this study, extended-field radiotherapy yielded a highly significant advantage in freedom from relapse over the involved field, and this observation was confirmed in subsequent results from multiple studies.[224] Further, a meta-analysis concluded that more extensive radiotherapy increased the chance of cure by more than 30 percent, although no survival benefit was seen at 10 years.[225] Although highly selected and laparotomy staged, very favorable patients are an exception to the requirement for extended fields. However, radiotherapy is no longer considered standard treatment for classic Hodgkin lymphoma based upon late effects and its inferiority to combined modality treatment. In addition, the description of prognostic factors for the probability of occult disease, improvements in radiographic imaging, and the desire to eliminate staging laparotomy resulted in the current routine use of clinical staging.

The change in the standard treatment for favorable, early-stage disease was compelled by the observation that the overall mortality rate from other causes exceeded deaths resulting from Hodgkin lym-

TABLE 97-3 COMBINATION CHEMOTHERAPY REGIMENS FOR HODGKIN LYMPHOMA

ACRONYM	DRUGS	DOSE	ROUTE	SCHEDULE (DAYS)	INTERVAL BETWEEN CYCLES (DAYS)	REFERENCE
MOPP	Nitrogen mustard	6 mg/m²	IV	1, 8	28	23
	Vincristine*	1.4 mg/m²	IV	1, 8		
	Procarbazine	100 mg/m²	PO	1–14		
	Prednisone	40 mg/m²	PO	1–14†		
ABVD	Adriamycin	25 mg/m²	IV	1, 15	28	24
	Bleomycin	10 U/m²	IV	1, 15		
	Vinblastine	6 mg/m²	IV	1, 15		
	Dacarbazine	375 mg/m²	IV	1, 15		
MOPP/ABVD	Alternate cycles of MOPP and ABVD					218
BEACOPP (escalated)	Bleomycin	10 U/m²	IV	8	21	222
	Etoposide	100 mg/m² (200)	IV	1–3		
	Adriamycin	25 mg/m² (35)	IV	1		
	Cyclophosphamide	650 mg/m² (1250)	IV	1		
	Vincristine*	1.4 mg/m²	IV	8		
	Procarbazine	100 mg/m²	PO	1–7		
	Prednisone	40 mg/m²	PO	1–14		
	G-CSF	(5 μg/kg)	SQ	8+		
Stanford V	Vinblastine	6 mg/m²	IV	Weeks 1, 3, 5, 7, 9, 11		222
	Adriamycin	25 mg/m²	IV	Weeks 1, 3, 5, 7, 9, 11		
	Vincristine*	1.4 mg/m²	IV	Weeks 2, 4, 6, 8, 10		
	Bleomycin	5 U/m²	IV	Weeks 2, 4, 6, 8, 10		
	Nitrogen mustard	6 mg/m²	IV	Weeks 1, 5, 9		
	Etoposide	60 mg/m² × 2	IV	Weeks 3, 7, 11		
	Prednisone	40 mg/m²	PO	Weeks 1–10 taper		
	Granulocyte colony stimulating factor	5 μg/kg	SQ	Upon first delay/reduction × 5 days, odd weeks only		

* Vincristine dose can be capped at 2 mg.　† Prednisone given on cycles 1 and 4 in original report.　Values in parentheses refer to escalated BEACOPP.

phoma at 15 to 20 years.[226] The largest cause of mortality is second cancers related to the extent and possibly the dose of radiotherapy treatment. Thus, interest in reducing or eliminating radiotherapy in limited Hodgkin lymphoma without compromising the therapeutic results has increased. Stanford University investigators first demonstrated that chemotherapy could substitute for extended-field radiotherapy in stage I and II patients. In sequential clinical trials, MOPP and VBM (vinblastine, bleomycin, methotrexate) given as adjuvants to involved-field radiotherapy yielded equivalent or superior results.[224,227] In a subsequent trial, clinically staged patients were randomized to subtotal lymphoid radiotherapy or a combination of limited radiotherapy and VBM, with excellent results in both treatment arms.[228] The European Organization for the Research and Treatment of Cancer (EORTC) randomized patients to six cycles of EBVP (epirubicin, bleomycin, vinblastine, prednisone) plus involved-field radiotherapy or subtotal radiotherapy in selected clinically staged I to IIA patients with favorable prognostic features. At 6 years, the event-free survival in the combined modality arm was 90 percent, significantly higher than radiotherapy alone.[229] Additional studies conducted by the US Intergroup and the GHSG confirmed the superiority of combined modality treatment over wide-field radiotherapy alone.[230,231]

Subsequent clinical trials were designed to determine the optimal number of cycles of chemotherapy and the volume and dose of radiotherapy when the two modalities were used in limited Hodgkin lymphoma. The Milan Tumor Institute described greater than 95 percent disease control with four cycles of ABVD and radiotherapy. In this trial, no advantage of extended-field over involved-field treatment was observed.[232] A GHSG study reached similar conclusions.[233] Excellent preliminary results (91% progression-free survival at 3 years) have been reported by the Manchester group with just 4 weeks of VAPEC-B (vinblastine, doxorubicin, prednisone, etoposide, cyclophosphamide, bleomycin) chemotherapy and limited radiotherapy.[234] An 8-week course of Stanford V and limited-field and dose radiotherapy yielded comparable results in favorable clinical stage I to IIA patients, with 95 percent event-free survival at 8 years reported.[235] A comparison of two versus four cycles of ABVD chemotherapy paired with 20- or 30-Gy radiotherapy was made in a four-arm trial conducted by the GHSG, and final results are awaited. Although these outstanding results with modest therapy are encouraging, the strategy of short-course chemotherapy and involved-field radiotherapy allows omission of mediastinal radiotherapy, a source of considerable morbidity, in just 20 percent of patients. Thus, considerable interest in chemotherapy alone for treatment in limited-stage Hodgkin lymphoma exists.

Historically, MOPP and ChlVPP were studied in pediatric Hodgkin lymphoma, with cures greater than 75 to 80 percent.[236,237] MOPP chemotherapy and subtotal lymphoid irradiation were compared in pathologically staged patients in two prospective randomized trials with disparate outcomes.[238,239] However, these studies generated little enthusiasm because of the undesirable toxicity profile of MOPP. A North American study in which a radiotherapy-containing strategy, based on risk factors, was compared to ABVD alone in selected limited-stage patients has been reported.[240] At 5 years, the progression-free survival significantly favored the radiotherapy-containing approach, but the absolute difference (87% vs 93%) was modest, and no survival differences were observed. A single institution study of ABVD versus ABVD plus radiation therapy (RT) demonstrated no significant difference in the treatment arms, but the trial was relatively underpowered to show treatment difference.[241] Other studies comparing chemotherapy alone with combined modality treatment included limited-stage and advanced-stage patients and both adults and children.[242,243] Together these studies show no or only a modest (<13%) benefit of combined modality treatment compared with ABVD-containing chemotherapy. Longer followup of these studies to include the

impact of late effects and the mature results of low-dose radiotherapy regimens are awaited with interest.

Several subsets of limited-stage patients deserve further mention. Classical stage I Hodgkin lymphoma patients presenting with inguinofemoral disease can be treated with brief chemotherapy and involved-field radiotherapy. More extensive subdiaphragmatic presentations of Hodgkin lymphoma are best managed with a full course of chemotherapy alone or combined modality therapy. Historically, approximately half of patients with masses greater than one third of the chest diameter relapsed after radiotherapy alone and their management is discussed below.[154,244] Similarly, stage I to IIB patients are generally managed with chemotherapy or combined modality. European groups have divided Hodgkin lymphoma patients into early-stage, intermediate-stage, and advanced-stage categories. Their intermediate group is also defined based on treatment outcomes primarily incorporating radiotherapy and include determinants of age, mediastinal mass size, presence of extranodal disease, ESR, and number of involved disease sites.[245]

NLPHL presents as asymptomatic, limited-stage disease in most (approximately 80%) patients.[93] Peripheral lymph nodes in the neck, axilla, or groin are commonly involved as stage IA disease. Because of the low likelihood of occult disease in NLPHL and the tendency for the disease to remain localized for years, regional RT is considered the treatment of choice. The European Task Force on Lymphoma reported a 96 percent complete response rate and 99 percent and 94 percent 8-year disease-specific survival for stage I and II disease, respectively.[93]

LOCALLY EXTENSIVE, LIMITED-STAGE HODGKIN LYMPHOMA

Extensive mediastinal Hodgkin lymphoma frequently is accompanied by extranodal extension to lung, pericardium, and chest wall. Pleural effusions may be seen. Use of combined chemotherapy and radiation (combined modality therapy) results in freedom from relapse in greater than 85 percent of patients. Application of radiotherapy after chemotherapy also reduces radiotherapy exposure to the normal heart and lung tissue. The optimal chemotherapy regimen and its duration, radiation dose, and volume for combined treatment have been the subjects of investigation. In the Milan study of 232 patients treated with subtotal lymphoid irradiation sandwiched between six courses of chemotherapy, the ABVD/RT combination was significantly superior to the MOPP/RT combination, as measured by freedom from progression and survival.[246,247] Subsequently, the Milan group reported the efficacy of four cycles of ABVD and involved-field radiotherapy in stage I to II patients, many of whom had massive mediastinal disease.[232] The 12-week Stanford V program, which includes modified mantle radiotherapy, provided greater than 90 percent durable remissions in patients with massive mediastinal disease.[223] The GHSG compared ABVD/RT with BEACOPP/RT in intermediate Hodgkin lymphoma patients, a proportion of whom had extensive mediastinal disease, and the mature results are awaited with interest. Data are insufficient to determine the efficacy of chemotherapy alone for treatment of bulky mediastinal Hodgkin lymphoma, but historically MOPP chemotherapy alone cured less than half of the patients.[248]

ADVANCED DISEASE

In the past, stage IIIA Hodgkin lymphoma was managed with radiotherapy or combined modality treatment according to the anatomic extent of subdiaphragmatic disease. Currently, all stage III and IV patients are primarily managed with chemotherapy. In the 20-year followup of the original MOPP series, freedom from progression was 54 percent and survival was 48 percent in advanced-stage patients, the majority of whom had IVB disease.[211] Constitutional symptoms, male sex, higher stage, and administration of vincristine lower than the projected rate were prognostic for complete response. Bonadonna and colleagues[219] showed that MOPP alternating with ABVD was superior to MOPP in stage IV patients. Subsequently, the Cancer and Acute Leukemia Group B (CALGB) proved that doxorubicin-containing chemotherapy combinations were superior to MOPP in patients with stages IIIA, IIIB, and IV disease (Table 97-4).[249,250] The failure-free survival rates were similar for ABVD (61%) and MOPP/ABVD (65%), and both were significantly better than the rates achieved with MOPP (50%). In two randomized trials, MOPP and ABV(D) "hybrid" regimens, as detailed in Table 97-3, had efficacy comparable to MOPP alternating with ABVD.[221,251]

A subsequent Intergroup study led by CALGB randomized patients to ABVD alone versus the MOPP/ABV hybrid regimen. The study was stopped early because of excess deaths and second cancers in the hybrid arm. No differences in efficacy were noted, with 63 percent of ABVD patients and 66 percent of hybrid patients failure-free at 5 years, but ABVD emerged as the standard treatment for advanced-stage Hodgkin lymphoma based on a more favorable toxicity profile.[252]

The GHSG developed the BEACOPP regimen based upon mathematical modeling that indicated a moderate increase in chemotherapy dose intensity would result in a significantly increased cure rate. BEACOPP is delivered every 3 weeks and features relatively dose-intense etoposide and cyclophosphamide. The escalated version incorporates even higher doses of these drugs made possible by use of granulocyte colony stimulating factor. Patients with initial tumors that were at least 5 cm or residual radiographic disease received radiotherapy after chemotherapy. Escalated BEACOPP resulted in 87 percent freedom from progression at 5 years, significantly greater than the 76 percent for standard BEACOPP and 69 percent for COPP/ABVD.[222] Survival was superior for escalated BEACOPP compared to COPP/ABVD. The results achieved (cure rates >80%) are the best recorded for a large phase III trial in advanced Hodgkin lymphoma. However, BEACOPP has not been universally accepted as the new standard in advanced Hodgkin lymphoma because of complications of sterility and increased risk for secondary leukemia. The GHSG next sought to reduce the risk of treatment-related morbidity by comparing the combination of four cycles of escalated BEACOPP and four cycles of standard BEACOPP with eight cycles of escalated BEACOPP. Results of this comparative trial are not yet available. An international study currently is comparing the hybrid standard and escalated BEACOPP regimen with ABVD in patients with a high international prognostic score.[253]

Stanford investigators developed an alternative approach to locally extensive and advanced Hodgkin lymphoma, abbreviating the duration of therapy and reducing the cumulative drug doses.[223] The Stanford V regimen was administered over 12 weeks and given in combination with radiotherapy for patients with bulky (≥5 cm) nodal or macroscopic splenic disease. Freedom from progression greater than 85 percent and overall survival greater than 95 percent were reported with this approach in several phase II studies,[223,254,255] but inferior results were observed in a phase III trial in which responses were judged at 8 weeks and radiotherapy was administered per physician preference rather than the original protocol prescription.[256] The Intergroup study in North America is testing ABVD versus the Stanford V chemotherapy and radiotherapy in locally extensive and advanced Hodgkin lymphoma.

TABLE 97-4　RESULTS OF COMBINATION CHEMOTHERAPY FOR ADVANCED HODGKIN DISEASE

GROUP	ACRONYM	NO.	FAILURE-FREE SURVIVAL %	OVERALL SURVIVAL %	FOLLOWUP (YEARS)	REFERENCE
NCL	MOPP	188	54	48	20	211
CALGB	MOPP	123	38	58	10	249,250
	ABVD	115	50	68		
	MOPP/ABVD	123	58	70		
CALGB	MOPP/ABV hybrid	428	66	81	5	252
	ABVD	428	63	82		
GHSG	COPP/ABVD	260	69*	83	5	222
	BEACOPP standard	469	76*	88		
	BEACOPP escalated	466	87*	91		

* Freedom from progression.

Low-dose irradiation as a consolidation to combination chemotherapy was reported as a successful strategy in adults and children in single arm experiences.[257,258] Although several trials showed no significant advantage for low-dose consolidative radiotherapy when compared with chemotherapy alone in randomized trials, these studies were criticized as underpowered.[259–262] In pediatric Hodgkin lymphoma patients in all stages, use of low-dose radiotherapy for patients in complete remission after COPP/ABVD chemotherapy provided an approximately 5 percent benefit in failure-free survival at 3 years.[243] In another study, including both adults and children in all disease stages, radiotherapy after ABVD improved event-free survival by 12 percent at 8 years.[242] The application of 30-Gy, involved-field radiotherapy to patients in complete remission after MOPP/ABV was studied in an adequately powered phase III trial.[263] No significant difference in failure-free survival was observed. Of note, all patients in partial remission received 40 Gy in this study, and their outcome was not different from the outcome in complete remission patients. A large GHSG study randomized patients to observation or consolidative radiotherapy—with the incorporation of a central review panel—following a full course of BEACOPP, with no difference in outcome in preliminary analysis.[264] In summary, these data do not support the routine use of radiotherapy following a full course of chemotherapy in advanced Hodgkin lymphoma. However, the role of this potent treatment in patients with an incomplete response or following a brief course of chemotherapy likely is more significant.

RECURRENT DISEASE

Historically, approximately 70 percent of patients who relapse after radiotherapy alone could be cured with MOPP chemotherapy, although patients with extensive disease at recurrence and constitutional symptoms had a less favorable prognosis.[265,266] The outlook was significantly less favorable for patients who relapsed after chemotherapy alone or combined therapy. In the NCI MOPP experience, the length of prior remission had a significant effect on the ability of patients to respond to subsequent treatment. Relapse-free survival for remissions longer than 1 year was 24 percent at 11 years compared with 11 percent for patients with shorter remissions.[267] Approximately half of the deaths in the group with longer remissions resulted from second cancers and other treatment complications, indicative of the cumulative effects of cancer treatment. The Milan group confirmed the importance of initial remission duration and found equivalent results whether the same regimen, a non–cross-resistant regimen, or an alternating approach was used.[268,269]

High-dose therapy and autologous peripheral blood stem cell transplantation improved the outlook for patients with recurrent Hodgkin lymphoma and now is routinely used in first relapse for most patients. Disease-free survival rates of 50 to 60 percent are expected at 5 years, and transplant-related mortality is less than 5 percent.[270-273] The superiority of transplantation in patients with relapsed Hodgkin lymphoma was established in two randomized trials.[274,275] A variety of high-dose regimens have been used, including BEAM (bischloroethylnitrosourea [carmustine], etoposide, Ara-C [cytarabine], melphalan), CBV (cyclophosphamide, bischloroethylnitrosourea [carmustine], etoposide), and the combination of total-body irradiation, etoposide, and cyclophosphamide. Augmented regimens of CBV and high-dose sequential chemotherapy have been developed to further intensify treatment,[272,276-278] but the superiority of any single regimen has not been definitively established. Several groups have described the prognostic factors for success of transplantation.

The success of allogeneic transplantation in multiply recurrent Hodgkin lymphoma has been limited by significant transplant-related mortality, although long-term disease control has been observed with anecdotal evidence of graft-versus-Hodgkin effect.[279] Early results with nonmyeloablative conditioning regimens appear promising, but more comprehensive study and longer followup are needed to evaluate the success of this approach.[245,280]

The anti-CD20 antibody rituximab is associated with a high response rate but limited durability as a single agent for treatment of NLPHL.[281,282] Monoclonal antibodies directed against the CD30 antigen are well tolerated in classic Hodgkin lymphoma, and phase II trials are in progress.[283,284] Based on the key role of IκB, which is subject to ubiquitination and release of NF-κB, interest exists in the therapeutic potential of the proteosome inhibitor bortezomib in Hodgkin lymphoma. Phase II and combination studies are in progress. Additional drugs with activity in recurrent Hodgkin lymphoma include vinorelbine and gemcitabine.[285-287] Several groups have investigated immunotherapy in the form of cytotoxic T cells directed against EBV proteins.[288] Developing new therapeutics in Hodgkin lymphoma remains challenging because of the efficacy of existing treatments.

COURSE AND PROGNOSIS

The goal of treatment is curing the greatest number of patients with minimal complications. Figure 97-3 illustrates the freedom from progression and overall survival in 256 patients managed at Stanford University from January 1989 to December 2003 with brief chemotherapy and reduced-field and reduced-dose radiotherapy. At 8 years, 97 percent of patients are estimated to be alive and 91 percent are continuously free of disease. Such outstanding results have been achieved by refining the use of radiotherapy and chemotherapy. However, the late effects of treatment for Hodgkin lymphoma remain a concern for cured patients and for a small subset of patients with refractory disease.

CLINICAL PROGNOSTIC FACTORS

A number of complex prognostic factor schemes have been developed for limited Hodgkin lymphoma treated with radiotherapy alone (Table 97-5). Massive mediastinal disease and constitutional symptoms were consistently identified as independent predictors of relapse, whereas only older age was predictive of inferior survival.[154,244,289,290] European and Canadian investigators incorporated gender, age, ESR, number of Ann Arbor disease sites, stage, and histology into stratifications for very favorable, favorable, and unfavorable disease categories.[245,291,292] The EORTC defines three or more nodal sites, ESR greater than 50 in asymptomatic patients, ESR greater than 40 in symptomatic patients, and histology as indicators of intermediate disease, whereas the GHSG designates any one of massive mediastinal disease, extranodal disease, ESR greater than 40, and four or more nodal sites as intermediate disease (Table 97-5). Interpreting the literature in early-stage Hodgkin lymphoma requires consideration of the variable eligibility criteria among different studies. The significance of these factors when newer combined modality treatments are used for limited-stage disease is unknown, but these or other features may emerge as prognostic factors as treatment intensities are reduced.

An international consortium pooled patient data and identified a prognostic score for advanced Hodgkin lymphoma based on seven factors (see Table 97-5)[197]: male sex, age at least 45 years, stage IV, white blood count at least 15,000/μl, lymphocyte count less than 600/μl or <8%, hemoglobin less than 10.5 g/dl, and albumin less than 4 g/dl. The presence of each factor reduced the freedom from progression by approximately 7 percent. Only 7 percent of patients were in the worst prognostic group (5-7 factors), and the freedom from progression in this subset was 42 percent at 5 years. Consensus with regard to prognostic factors promotes uniformity in clinical trial design and provides a rationale for alternative approaches in high-risk subsets. Of note, the superiority of escalated BEACOPP was seen across the spectrum of the international prognostic score, with the major survival gains in poor-risk patients with four or more factors.[222] Outcomes after the Stanford V program were significantly inferior in the small subset of patients with an international prognostic score of 4 or more.[223] The influence of age in Hodgkin lymphoma patients is consistent regardless of tumor burden. Dose reductions explain inferior results in a subset of older patients but outcomes are worse, even when dose of therapy is considered.[293,294] The BEACOPP regimen was associated with unacceptable toxicity and demonstrated no improvement over ABVD for patients older than 65 years.[295]

FDG-PET imaging at completion of treatment provides a high degree of negative predictive value, ranging from 81 to 100 percent. The positive predictive value is more variable but improves with clinical correlation and nuclear medicine expertise. FDG-PET scans obtained early during chemotherapy may be highly predictive of the clinical course. In one study, progression-free survival at 1 year was 92 percent for patients with negative scans compared to 0 percent for patients with positive scans.[296] Functional imaging also is predictive in patients with recurrent disease managed with high-dose therapy and autotransplantation.[297]

Patients with primary progressive Hodgkin lymphoma have the least favorable prognosis.[298] Fortunately, newer treatment

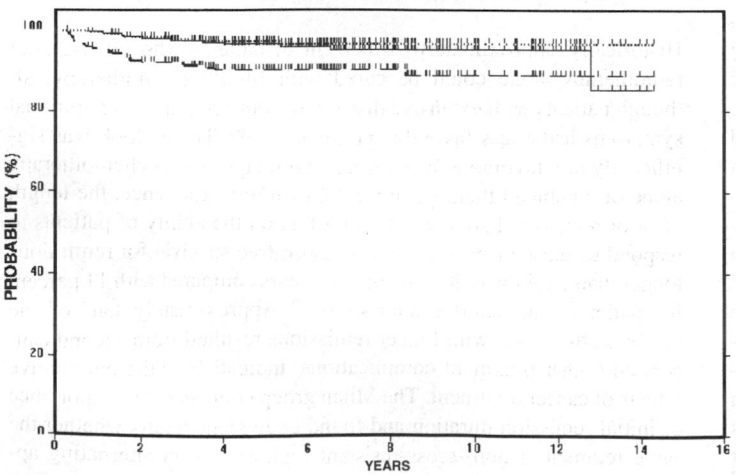

FIGURE 97-3 Survival data for 256 patients treated with brief chemotherapy and radiotherapy at Stanford University from 1989 to 2003. Overall survival (*solid line*) was estimated to be 95 percent, disease-specific survival (*dotted line*) 97 percent, and freedom from progression (*dashed line*) 91 percent at 10 years.

TABLE 97-5   (A) ADVERSE PROGNOSTIC FACTORS FOR LOCALIZED HODGKIN LYMPHOMA

North America*	EORTC	GHSG
Mediastinal mass ratio >0.33	Mediastinal mass ratio >0.35	Mediastinal mass ratio >0.35
Nodal mass >10 cm	Age >50 years	Extranodal disease
B symptoms	>3 nodal regions	>2 nodal regions
	Elevated ESR†	Elevated ESR†

(B) INTERNATIONAL PROGNOSTIC FACTORS FOR ADVANCED HODGKIN LYMPHOMA

Factor	Relative risk
Stage IV	1.26
Male sex	1.35
Age ≥45 years	1.39
Hemoglobin <10.5 g/dl	1.35
WBC ≥15,000/μl	1.41
Lymphocyte count <600/μl or <8%	1.38
Albumin <4 g/dl	1.49

N factors	Population (%)	Freedom from progession at 5 years (%)
0	7	84
1	22	77
2	29	67
3	23	60
4	12	51
5–7	7	42

* Canada and United States.
† Different values applied.
ESR = erythrocyte sedimentation rate; WBC = White blood cell count.

approaches such as BEACOPP have reduced the proportion of patients in this category. Among patients referred for transplantation, sensitivity to standard-dose second-line chemotherapy predicts for better survival. Responding patients had an event-free survival of 60 percent versus 19 percent for patients without a response.[299] Prognostic factors for the success of transplantation include response to initial therapy and time to relapse, stage of disease at relapse, constitutional symptoms at relapse, and response to second-line chemotherapy.[272,276] The international prognostic score also has prognostic significance in the setting of recurrent disease among transplant recipients.[300] The GHSG developed a prognostic score based on time to relapse, anemia, and stage for relapsed disease and a prognostic score based on performance status, age, and attainment of a temporary remission for patients with primary progressive disease.[301,302]

BIOLOGIC PROGNOSTIC MARKERS

Clinical prognostic factors are surrogates for the underlying cellular and molecular biology of Hodgkin lymphoma. Prognostic significance has been ascribed to histopathologic grading of nodular sclerosis, with inconsistent results.[163,165] Aberrations in the typical immunophenotype of classic Hodgkin lymphoma, such as CD20+ or CD15−, have been associated with worse prognoses in some but not all evaluations.[303–305] Likewise, some but not all investigators found Bcl-2 expression was prognostically significant.[306–309] Tissue microarray techniques, which enable study of numerous markers, have been applied to Hodgkin lymphomas.[309] Cell cycle and apoptosis markers may add to clinical prognostic factors. The prognostic significance of EBV association with Hodgkin lymphoma has been studied extensively and indicates that

EBV-positive Hodgkin lymphoma may confer a favorable outcome in younger patients with early-stage disease, but the opposite appears to be the case in older individuals.[310,311] Serum levels of factors, such as soluble CD30, IL-6, IL-10, and the IL-2 receptor, reportedly correlate with constitutional symptoms and advanced disease.[199–202,312] Serum IL-10, which was independent of other clinical prognostic factors in several studies, likely is a measure of immunosuppression.[313–315]

COMPLICATIONS OF TREATMENT

Treatment of Hodgkin lymphoma is associated with important acute and chronic side effects. The acute complications of chemotherapy and radiotherapy may be troublesome but are relatively easily managed. Late treatment effects in the form of sterility, cardiopulmonary disease, and second malignancy are more serious.

Acute leukemia and myelodysplasia were the initial second malignancies observed after successful treatment for Hodgkin lymphoma with MOPP chemotherapy.[316–318] The risk following MOPP was proportional to the cumulative dose of alkylating agents and was associated with recurring abnormalities of chromosomes 5 and 7.[319,320] Actuarial risks of 1 to 10 percent with relative risks greater than 100 have been reported over a 7- to 10-year period. In a multiinstitutional, case-control study of 29,552 Hodgkin lymphoma patients, the relative risk of acute leukemia was increased in patients who received more than six cycles of MOPP chemotherapy, and no increased risk was found with combined radiation and chemotherapy.[319] Acute leukemia may follow treatment of Hodgkin lymphoma with higher doses of etoposide and doxorubicin, as in the BEACOPP regimen.[222] This form of leukemia tends to occur earlier and be associated with balanced translocations of chromosome 11. The risk of acute leukemia is significantly less, although not absent, after ABVD chemotherapy.[252] Prognosis for the response to treatment of secondary leukemia is poor (see Chap. 87).[321]

The relative risk of non-Hodgkin lymphomas is increased after treatment for Hodgkin lymphoma.[322,323] These non-Hodgkin lymphomas typically are diffuse, aggressive B cell lymphomas that may occur early or late after treatment. No clear relationship to the type of primary treatment has been observed. The incidence of secondary lymphoma in a series of 5406 patients treated on GHSG protocols was 0.9 percent. Prognosis was poor, with a 2-year estimated survival rate of 30 percent.[324] Some investigators have considered the non-Hodgkin lymphomas to be a result of the ongoing immunodeficiency, whereas others have suggested a common cell of origin.[325] Diffuse, large B cell lymphoma and its variants are most frequent in NLPHL, where an aggressive approach to treatment should be pursued.[326]

An increased risk of solid cancers after treatment for Hodgkin lymphoma has long been recognized.[323,327,328] The risk is related to radiotherapy exposure, with tumors occurring in-field or at the edges of the radiotherapy field. The overall actuarial risk of second solid cancer malignancy at 15 years was approximately 18 percent.[323] Cancers of the lung, stomach, bone, and soft tissue were observed in a temporal pattern consistent with radiation-induced neoplasms. The latency for developing second cancers is an important consideration. For instance, an increased risk for breast cancer and thyroid cancer was only appreciated when mean followup was 10 or more years.[329–331] Breast cancer is increased in women treated before age 30 years and is markedly increased in children and adolescents.[329,331,332] Cofactors are important for defining the risk of second cancers. For example, breast cancer risk is highest for women treated before age 30 years and for those who continue to have normal menses.[333] Lung cancer risk is greatest among older patients with a history of tobacco use and is increased with greater alkylating agent exposure and with radiotherapy.[334]

Mediastinal radiotherapy is associated with an increased risk of cardiac disease. An increased risk of death from coronary artery disease and acute myocardial infarction has been identified in adults and children.[226,335,336] Other types of cardiac disease often are asymptomatic, including valvular disease, conduction defects, and cardiomyopathy.[337,338] The risks of radiation-related heart disease do not appear to be influenced significantly by the addition of chemotherapy. The onset of increased risk is within 5 to 10 years. Because risk is associated with the dose and volume of radiotherapy and the latency is 5 to 10 plus years, the hazards associated with current lower-dose therapy and smaller fields remain to be assessed.[339]

Approximately 90 percent of males become permanently sterile by six cycles of MOPP chemotherapy.[340] The risk is related to the cumulative dose of alkylating agents such that two to three cycles of MOPP result in azoospermia in approximately 50 percent of patients.[341] Female fertility after MOPP is related to age at treatment and the cumulative alkylating agent dose.[342,343] Women older than 25 years at treatment have an 80 percent probability of sterility following six courses of MOPP. The ABVD combination is associated with temporary amenorrhea and azoospermia, with full recovery noted in 50 to 90 percent of patients.[344,345] Several authors have described pregnancy outcome following treatment for Hodgkin lymphoma. No increase in birth defects or complications of pregnancy has been seen.[343]

Lhermitte sign, a transient complaint of an "electric shock" sensation produced by head flexion, is a common sequela of mantle radiotherapy.[346] An elevated thyroid-stimulating hormone level, with or without a low T3 or T4, is seen in approximately 30 percent of patients following mantle radiotherapy.[330] Rarely, hyperthyroidism, Graves ophthalmopathy, or thyroid neoplasms occur after neck radiotherapy.[330] The incidence of radiation pneumonitis depends on the volume of lung irradiated and the total dose. Symptoms include cough, dyspnea, and fever. Although prospective assessment of pulmonary function demonstrates reduced lung volumes following mantle radiotherapy, recovery is seen in 12 to 24 months, and symptomatic radiation pneumonitis is unusual.[347,348]

Full-dose RT interferes with normal growth and development in children. Current therapy programs use low-dose or no radiotherapy for all stages of disease. Overwhelming sepsis is a rare event in patients who have been splenectomized and treated for Hodgkin lymphoma, particularly children (see Chap. 55).[349,350] Vaccination against encapsulated organisms 10 to 14 days before starting treatment is advised. However, neither vaccines nor antibiotic prophylaxis may provide protection in all cases. Fatigue is commonly reported in Hodgkin lymphoma survivors and has been related to pulmonary function and peak oxygen uptake.[337,351] Psychosocial sequelae of treatment for Hodgkin lymphoma deserve further study.[352] With the high rates of cure currently attained in the management of Hodgkin lymphoma (see Figure 97-3), reduction in late effects and quality of life assume even greater importance.

REFERENCES

1. Hodgkin T: On some morbid appearances of the absorbent glands and spleen. *Med Chir Trans* 17:68, 1832.
2. Wilks S: Cases of lardaceous disease and some allied affections, with remarks. *Guys Hosp Rep* 17:103, 1856.
3. Wilks S: Cases of enlargement of the lymphatic glands and spleen, or Hodgkin's disease, with remarks. *Guys Hosp Rep* 11:56, 1865.
4. Dreschfield J: Clinical lecture on acute Hodgkin's (or pseudoleucocythemia). *BMJ* 1:893, 1892.
5. Kundrat H: Uber Lympho-sarkomatosis. *Wien Wochneschr* 6:211, 1893.
6. Sternberg C: Uber eine eigenartige unter dem Bilde der Pseudoleukamie verlaufende Tuberculose des lymphatischen Appartes. *Z Heilkd* 19:21, 1898.
7. Reed D: On the pathological changes in Hodgkin's disease, with special reference to its relation to tuberculosis. *Johns Hopkins Hosp Rep* 10:133, 1902.
8. Fox H: Remarks on the presentation of microscopial preparations made from some of the original tissue described by Thomas Hodgkin. *Ann Med History* 8:370, 1926.
9. Jackson H, Parker F: *Hodgkin's Disease and Allied Disorders*. Oxford University, New York, 1947.
10. Lukes RJ, Butler JJ, Hicks EB: Natural history of Hodgkin's disease as related to its pathologic picture. *Cancer* 19:317, 1966.
11. Stein H, Delsol G, Pileri SA: Hodgkin lymphoma, in *World Health Organization (WHO) Classification of Tumours—Pathology & Genetics—Tumours of Haematopoietic and Lymphoid Tissues*, edited by ESHN Jaffe, H Stein, J Vardiman, p 237. IARC (International Agency for Research on Cancer), Lyon, 2001.
12. Peters M: A study of survivals in Hodgkin's disease treated radiologically. *Am J Roentgenol* 63:299, 1950.
13. Kinmouth J: Lymphangiography in man: Method of outlining lymphatic trunks and operation. *Clin Sci (Lond)* 11:13, 1952.
14. Glatstein E, Guerney J, Rosenberg S, Kaplan H: The value of laparotomy and splenectomy in the staging of Hodgkin's disease. *Cancer* 24:709, 1969.
15. Rosenberg S: Report of the committee on the staging of Hodgkin's disease. *Cancer Res* 26:1310, 1966.
16. Carbone P, Kaplan H, Musshoff K: Report of the committee on the Hodgkin's disease staging. *Cancer Res* 31:1860, 1971.
17. Pusey W: Cases of sarcoma and of Hodgkin's disease treated by exposures to x-rays: A preliminary report. *JAMA* 38:166, 1902.
18. Senn N: Therapeutical value of roentgen ray in treatment of pseudoleukemia. *N Y Med J* 77:665, 1903.
19. Gilbert R: Radiotherapy in Hodgkin's disease (malignant granulomatosis): Anatomic and clinical foundations, governing principles, results. *Am J Roentgenol* 41:198, 1939.
20. Kaplan H: The radical radiotherapy of regionally localized Hodgkin's disease. *Radiology* 78:553, 1962.
21. Goodman L, Wingtrobe M, Dameshek W: Nitrogen mustard therapy: Use of methyl-bis(β-chloroethyl)amine hydrochloride and tris-(β-chloroethyl)amine hydrochloride for Hodgkin's disease, lymphosarcoma, leukemia, and certain allied and miscellaneous disorders. *JAMA* 132:126, 1946.
22. Jacobson L, Spurr C, Baron EG: Nitrogen mustard therapy: Use of methyl-bis(β-chloroethyl)amine hydrochloride on neoplastic disorders of the hematopoietic system. *JAMA* 132:263, 1946.
23. DeVita V, Serpick A, Carbone P: Combination chemotherapy in the treatment of advanced Hodgkin's disease. *Ann Intern Med* 73:881, 1970.
24. Bonadonna G, Zucali R, Monfardini S, et al: Combination chemotherapy of Hodgkin's disease with adriamycin, bleomycin, vinblastine, and imidazole carboxamide versus MOPP. *Cancer* 36:252, 1975.
25. Landis SH, Murray T, Bolden S, Wingo PA: Cancer statistics 1999. *CA Cancer J Clin* 49:8, 1999.
26. MacMahon B: Epidemiology of Hodgkin's disease. *Cancer Res* 26:1189, 1966.
27. Grufferman S, Duong T, Cole P: Occupation and Hodgkin's disease. *J Natl Cancer Inst* 57:1193, 1976.
28. Stewart SL, King JB, Thompson TD, et al: Cancer mortality surveillance—United States 1990–2000. *MMWR Surveill Summ* 53:1, 2004.
29. Cartwright RA, Watkins G: Epidemiology of Hodgkin's disease: A review. *Hematol Oncol* 22:11, 2004.
30. Gutensohn N, Cole P: Childhood social environment and Hodgkin's disease. *N Engl J Med* 304:135, 1981.

31. Westergaard T, Melbye M, Pedersen JB, et al: Birth order, sibship size and risk of Hodgkin's disease in children and young adults: A population-based study of 31 million person-years. *Int J Cancer* 72:977, 1997.

32. Grufferman S, Delzell E: Epidemiology of Hodgkin's disease. *Epidemiol Rev* 6:76, 1984.

33. Hjalgrim H, Rasmussen S, Rostgaard K, et al: Familial clustering of Hodgkin lymphoma and multiple sclerosis. *J Natl Cancer Inst* 96:780, 2004.

34. Vianna NJ, Greenwald P, Davies JN: Extended epidemic of Hodgkin's disease in high-school students. *Lancet* 1:1209, 1971.

35. Klinger RJ, Minton JP: Case clustering of Hodgkin's disease in a small rural community, with associations among cases. *Lancet* 1:168, 1973.

36. Vianna NJ, Greenwald P, Davies JNP: Epidemiologic evidence for transmission of Hodgkin's disease: The lymphoid tissue barrier. *N Engl J Med* 10:499, 1974.

37. Cuneo JM: Infectious aspects of Hodgkin's disease. *N Engl J Med* 290: 345, 1974.

38. Pike MC, Henderson BE, Casagrande J: Infectious aspects of Hodgkin's disease. *N Engl J Med* 290:341, 1974.

39. Grufferman S, Cole P, Levitan TR: Evidence against transmission of Hodgkin's disease in high schools. *N Engl J Med* 300:1006, 1979.

40. Rosdahl N, Larsen SO, Clemmesen J: Hodgkin's disease in patients with previous infectious mononucleosis: 30 years' experience. *BMJ* 2:253, 1974.

41. Munoz N, Davidson RLJ, Witthoff B: Infectious mononucleosis and Hodgkin's disease. *Int J Cancer* 22:10, 1978.

42. Kvale G, Hoiby EA, Pedersen E: Hodgkin's disease in patients with previous infectious mononucleosis. *Int J Cancer* 23:593, 1979.

43. Mueller N, Evans A, Harris N: Altered antibody titers to Epstein-Barr virus before the diagnosis of Hodgkin's disease. *N Engl J Med* 320:689, 1989.

44. Jarrett RF: Risk factors for Hodgkin's lymphoma by EBV status and significance of detection of EBV genomes in serum of patients with EBV-associated Hodgkin's lymphoma. *Leuk Lymphoma* 44(suppl 3): S27, 2003.

45. Armstrong AA, Alexander FE, Paes RP, et al: Association of Epstein-Barr virus with pediatric Hodgkin's disease. *Am J Pathol* 142:1683, 1993.

46. Ambinder RF, Browning PJ, Lorenzana I, et al: Epstein-Barr virus and childhood Hodgkin's disease in Honduras and the United States. *Blood* 81:462, 1993.

47. Chang KL, Albújar PF, Chen YY, et al: High prevalence of Epstein-Barr virus in the Reed-Sternberg cells of Hodgkin's disease occurring in Peru. *Blood* 81:496, 1993.

48. Weinreb M, Day PJ, Murray PG, et al: Epstein-Barr virus (EBV) and Hodgkin's disease in children: Incidence of EBV latent membrane protein in malignant cells. *J Pathol* 168:365, 1992.

49. Herndier BG, Sanchez HC, Chang KL, et al: High prevalence of Epstein-Barr virus in the Reed-Sternberg cells of HIV-associated Hodgkin's disease. *Am J Pathol* 142:1073, 1993.

50. Hjalgrim H, Askling J, Rostgaard K, et al: Characteristics of Hodgkin's lymphoma after infectious mononucleosis. *N Engl J Med* 349:1324, 2003.

51. Alexander FE, Lawrence DJ, Freeland J, et al: An epidemiologic study of index and family infectious mononucleosis and adult Hodgkin's disease (HD): Evidence for a specific association with EBV+ve HD in young adults. *Int J Cancer* 107:298, 2003.

52. Mack TM, Cozen W, Shibata DK, et al: Concordance for Hodgkin's disease in identical twins suggesting genetic susceptibility to the young-adult form of the disease. *N Engl J Med* 332:413, 1995.

53. Ferraris AM, Racchi O, Rapezzi D, et al: Familial Hodgkin's disease: A disease of young adulthood? *Ann Hematol* 74:131, 1997.

54. Lynch HT, Saldivar VA, Guirgis HA, et al: Familial Hodgkin's disease and associated cancer. A clinical-pathologic study. *Cancer* 38:2033, 1976.

55. Creagan ET, Fraumeni JJ: Familial Hodgkin's disease. *Lancet* 2:547, 1972.

56. Hemminki K, Li X, Czene K: Familial risk of cancer: Data for clinical counseling and cancer genetics. *Int J Cancer* 108:109, 2004.

57. Goldin LR, Pfeiffer RM, Gridley G, et al: Familial aggregation of Hodgkin lymphoma and related tumors. *Cancer* 100:1902, 2004.

58. Abramson JH, Pridan H, Sacks MI, et al: A case-control study of Hodgkin's disease in Israel. *J Natl Cancer Inst* 61:307, 1978.

59. Haim N, Cohen Y, Robinson E: Malignant lymphoma in first-degree blood relatives. *Cancer* 49:197, 1982.

60. Vianna NJ, Davies JN, Polan AK, Wolfgang P: Familial Hodgkin's disease: An environmental and genetic disorder. *Lancet* 2:854, 1974.

61. Grufferman S, Cole P, Smith PG, Lukes RJ: Hodgkin's disease in siblings. *N Engl J Med* 296:248, 1977.

62. Vianna NJ: *Lymphoreticular Malignancies, Epidemiologic and Related Aspects.* University Park, Baltimore, MD, 1975.

63. Lin AY, Kingma DW, Lennette ET, et al: Epstein-Barr virus and familial Hodgkin's disease. *Blood* 88:3160, 1996.

64. Alexander FE, Jarrett RF, Cartwright RA, et al: Epstein-Barr Virus and HLA-DPB1-*0301 in young adult Hodgkin's disease: Evidence for inherited susceptibility to Epstein-Barr Virus in cases that are EBV(+ve). *Cancer Epidemiol Biomarkers Prev* 10:705, 2001.

65. Bjerrum OW, Hasselbalch HC, Drivsholm A, Nissen NI: Non-Hodgkin malignant lymphomas and Hodgkin's disease in first-degree relatives. Evidence for a mutual genetic predisposition? *Scand J Haematol* 36: 398, 1986.

66. Hors J, Dausset J: HLA and susceptibility to Hodgkin's disease. *Immunol Rev* 70:167, 1983.

67. Cimino G, Lo CF, Cartoni C, et al: Immune-deficiency in Hodgkin's disease (HD): A study of patients and healthy relatives in families with multiple cases. *Eur J Cancer Clin Oncol* 24:1595, 1988.

68. Bodmer JG, Tonks S, Oza AM, et al: HLA-DP based resistance to Hodgkin's disease. *Lancet* 1:1455, 1989.

69. Berberich FR, Berberich MS, King MC, et al: Hodgkin's disease susceptibility: Linkage to the HLA locus demonstrated by a new concordance method. *Hum Immunol* 6:207, 1983.

70. Oza AM, Tonks S, Lim J, et al: A clinical and epidemiological study of human leukocyte antigen-DPB alleles in Hodgkin's disease. *Cancer Res* 54:5101, 1994.

71. Tonks S, Oza AM, Lister TA, Bodmer JG: Association of HLA-DPB with Hodgkin's disease. *Lancet* 340:968, 1992.

72. Klitz W, Aldrich CL, Fildes N, et al: Localization of predisposition to Hodgkin disease in the HLA class II region. *Am J Hum Genet* 54:497, 1994.

73. Harty LC, Lin AY, Goldstein AM, et al: HLA-DR, HLA-DQ, and TAP genes in familial Hodgkin disease. *Blood* 99:690, 2002.

74. Küppers R, Rajewsky K, Zhao M, et al: Hodgkin disease: Hodgkin and Reed-Sternberg cells picked from histological sections show clonal immunoglobulin gene rearrangements and appear to be derived from B cells at various stages of development. *Proc Natl Acad Sci U S A* 91: 10962, 1994.

75. Stein H, Mason DY, Gerdes J, et al: The expression of the Hodgkin's disease associated antigen Ki-1 in reactive and neoplastic lymphoid tissue: Evidence that Reed-Sternberg cells and histiocytic malignancies are derived from activated lymphoid cells. *Blood* 66:848, 1985.

76. Miettinen M: CD30 distribution. Immunohistochemical study on formaldehyde-fixed, paraffin-embedded Hodgkin's and non-Hodgkin's lymphomas. *Arch Pathol Lab Med* 116:1197, 1992.

77. Penny RJ, Blaustein JC, Longtine JA, Pinkus GS: Ki-1-positive large cell lymphomas, a heterogenous group of neoplasms. Morphologic, im-

munophenotypic, genotypic, and clinical features of 24 cases. *Cancer* 68:362, 1991.

78. Schienle HW, Stein N, Muller RW: Neutrophil granulocytic cell antigen defined by a monoclonal antibody—Its distribution within normal haemic and non-haemic tissue. *J Clin Pathol* 35:959, 1982.

79. Stein H, Uchánska-Ziegler B, Gerdes J, et al: Hodgkin and Sternberg-Reed cells contain antigens specific to late cells of granulopoiesis. *Int J Cancer* 29:283, 1982.

80. Pinkus GS, Said JW: Leu-M1 immunoreactivity in nonhematopoietic neoplasms and myeloproliferative disorders. An immunoperoxidase study of paraffin sections. *Am J Clin Pathol* 85:278, 1986.

81. Rushin JM, Riordan GP, Heaton RB, et al: Cytomegalovirus-infected cells express Leu-M1 antigen. A potential source of diagnostic error. *Am J Pathol* 136:989, 1990.

82. Swerdlow SH, Wright SA: The spectrum of Leu-M1 staining in lymphoid and hematopoietic proliferations. *Am J Clin Pathol* 85:283, 1986.

83. Hsu SM, Tseng CK, Hsu PL: Expression of p55 (Tac) interleukin-2 receptor (IL-2R), but not p75 IL-2R, in cultured H-RS cells and H-RS cells in tissues. *Am J Pathol* 136:735, 1990.

84. Lauritzen AF, Moller PH, Nedergaard T, et al: Apoptosis-related genes and proteins in Hodgkin's disease. *APMIS* 107:636, 1999.

85. von Wasielewski R, Mengel M, Fischer R, et al: Classical Hodgkin's disease. Clinical impact of the immunophenotype. *Am J Pathol* 151:1123, 1997.

86. Papadimitriou CS, Bai MK, Kotsianti AJ, et al: Phenotype of Hodgkin and Sternberg-Reed cells and expression of CD57 (LEU7) antigen. *Leuk Lymphoma* 20:125, 1995.

87. Pinkus GS, Said JW: Hodgkin's disease, lymphocyte predominance type, nodular—Further evidence for a B cell derivation. L & H variants of Reed-Sternberg cells express L26, a pan B cell marker. *Am J Pathol* 133:211, 1988.

88. Pinkus GS, Said JW: Hodgkin's disease, lymphocyte predominance type, nodular—A distinct entity? Unique staining profile for L&H variants of Reed-Sternberg cells defined by monoclonal antibodies to leukocyte common antigen, granulocyte-specific antigen, and B-cell-specific antigen. *Am J Pathol* 118:1, 1985.

89. Stein H, Hansmann ML, Lennert K, et al: Reed-Sternberg and Hodgkin cells in lymphocyte-predominant Hodgkin's disease of nodular subtype contain J chain. *Am J Clin Pathol* 86:292, 1986.

90. Schmid C, Sargent C, Isaacson PG: L and H cells of nodular lymphocyte predominant Hodgkin's disease show immunoglobulin light-chain restriction. *Am J Pathol* 139:1281, 1991.

91. Poppema S, Kaiserling E, Lennert K: Nodular paragranuloma and progressively transformed germinal centers. Ultrastructural and immunohistologic findings. *Virchows Arch B Cell Pathol* 31:211, 1979.

92. Falini B, Bigerna B, Pasqualucci L, et al: Distinctive expression pattern of the BCL-6 protein in nodular lymphocyte predominance Hodgkin's disease. *Blood* 87:465, 1996.

93. Diehl V, Sextro M, Franklin J, et al: Clinical presentation, course, and prognostic factors in lymphocyte-predominant Hodgkin's disease and lymphocyte-rich classical Hodgkin's disease: Report from the European Task Force on Lymphoma Project on Lymphocyte-Predominant Hodgkin's Disease. *J Clin Oncol* 17:776, 1999.

94. Brauninger A, Wacker HH, Rajewsky K, et al: Typing the histogenetic origin of the tumor cells of lymphocyte-rich classical Hodgkin's lymphoma in relation to tumor cells of classical and lymphocyte-predominance Hodgkin's lymphoma. *Cancer Res* 63:1644, 2003.

95. Küppers R, Roers A, Kanzler H: Molecular single cell studies of normal and transformed lymphocytes. *Cancer Surv* 30:45, 1997.

96. Kanzler H, Küppers R, Hansmann ML, Rajewsky K: Hodgkin and Reed-Sternberg cells in Hodgkin's disease represent the outgrowth of a dominant tumor clone derived from (crippled) germinal center B cells. *J Exp Med* 184:1495, 1996.

97. Bargou RC, Emmerich F, Krappmann D, et al: Constitutive nuclear factor-kappaB-RelA activation is required for proliferation and survival of Hodgkin's disease tumor cells. *J Clin Invest* 100:2961, 1997.

98. Jox A, Zander T, Küppers R, et al: Somatic mutations within the untranslated regions of rearranged Ig genes in a case of classical Hodgkin's disease as a potential cause for the absence of Ig in the lymphoma cells. *Blood* 93:3964, 1999.

99. Muschen M, Rajewsky K, Brauninger A, et al: Rare occurrence of classical Hodgkin's disease as a T cell lymphoma. *J Exp Med* 191:387, 2000.

100. Braeuninger A, Küppers R, Strickler JG, et al: Hodgkin and Reed-Sternberg cells in lymphocyte predominant Hodgkin disease represent clonal populations of germinal center-derived tumor B cells. Erratum: 94(25): 14211. *Proc Natl Acad Sci U S A* 94:9337, 1997.

101. Ohno T, Stribley JA, Wu G, et al: Clonality in nodular lymphocyte-predominant Hodgkin's disease. *N Engl J Med* 337:459, 1997.

102. Marafioti T, Hummel M, Anagnostopoulos I, et al: Origin of nodular lymphocyte-predominant Hodgkin's disease from a clonal expansion of highly mutated germinal-center B cells. *N Engl J Med* 337:453, 1997.

103. Thomas RK, Re D, Wolf J, Diehl V: Part I: Hodgkin's lymphoma—Molecular biology of Hodgkin and Reed-Sternberg cells. *Lancet Oncol* 5:11, 2004.

104. Marafioti T, Hummel M, Foss HD, et al: Hodgkin and Reed-Sternberg cells represent an expansion of a single clone originating from a germinal center B-cell with functional immunoglobulin gene rearrangements but defective immunoglobulin transcription. *Blood* 95:1443, 2000.

105. Re D, Hofmann A, Wolf J, et al: Cultivated H-RS cells are resistant to CD95L-mediated apoptosis despite expression of wild-type CD95. *Exp Hematol* 28:31, 2000.

106. Thomas RK, Kallenborn A, Wickenhauser C, et al: Constitutive expression of c-FLIP in Hodgkin and Reed-Sternberg cells. *Am J Pathol* 160:1521, 2002.

107. Dutton A, O'Neil JD, Milner AE, et al: Expression of the cellular FLICE-inhibitory protein (c-FLIP) protects Hodgkin's lymphoma cells from autonomous Fas-mediated death. *Proc Natl Acad Sci U S A* 101:6611, 2004.

108. Mathas S, Lietz A, Anagnostopoulos I, et al: c-FLIP mediates resistance of Hodgkin and Reed-Sternberg cells to death receptor-induced apoptosis. *J Exp Med* 199:1041, 2004.

109. Garcia JF, Camacho FI, Morente M, et al: Hodgkin and Reed-Sternberg cells harbor alterations in the major tumor suppressor pathways and cell-cycle checkpoints: Analyses using tissue microarrays. *Blood* 101:681, 2003.

110. Kashkar H, Haefs C, Shin H, et al: XIAP-mediated caspase inhibition in Hodgkin's lymphoma-derived B cells. *J Exp Med* 198:341, 2003.

111. Kashkar H, Kronke M, Jurgensmeier JM: Defective Bax activation in Hodgkin B-cell lines confers resistance to staurosporine-induced apoptosis. *Cell Death Differ* 9:750, 2002.

112. Skinnider BF, Mak TW: The role of cytokines in classical Hodgkin lymphoma. *Blood* 99:4283, 2002.

113. Emmerich F, Theurich S, Hummel M, et al: Inactivating I kappa B epsilon mutations in Hodgkin and Reed-Sternberg cells. *J Pathol* 201:413, 2003.

114. Joos S, Menz CK, Wrobel G, et al: Classical Hodgkin lymphoma is characterized by recurrent copy number gains of the short arm of chromosome 2. *Blood* 99:1381, 2002.

115. Horie R, Watanabe T, Morishita Y, et al: Ligand-independent signaling by overexpressed CD30 drives NF-kappaB activation in Hodgkin-Reed-Sternberg cells. *Oncogene* 21:2493, 2002.

116. Annunziata CM, Safiran YJ, Irving SG, et al: Hodgkin disease: Pharmacologic intervention of the CD40-NF kappa B pathway by a protease inhibitor. *Blood* 96:2841, 2000.

117. Fiumara P, Younes A: CD40 ligand (CD154) and tumour necrosis factor-related apoptosis inducing ligand (Apo-2L) in haematological malignancies. *Br J Haematol* 113:265, 2001.

118. Jundt F, Anagnostopoulos I, Forster R, et al: Activated Notch1 signaling promotes tumor cell proliferation and survival in Hodgkin and anaplastic large cell lymphoma. *Blood* 99:3398, 2002.

119. Gires O, Zimber-Strobl U, Gonnella R, et al: Latent membrane protein 1 of Epstein-Barr virus mimics a constitutively active receptor molecule. *EMBO J* 16:6131, 1997.

120. Caldwell RG, Wilson JB, Anderson SJ, Longnecker R: Epstein-Barr virus LMP2A drives B cell development and survival in the absence of normal B cell receptor signals. *Immunity* 9:405, 1998.

121. Maggio E, van den Berg A, Diepstra A, et al: Chemokines, cytokines and their receptors in Hodgkin's lymphoma cell lines and tissues. *Ann Oncol* 13(suppl 1):52, 2002.

122. Jundt F, Anagnostopoulos I, Bommert K, et al: Hodgkin/Reed-Sternberg cells induce fibroblasts to secrete eotaxin, a potent chemoattractant for T cells and eosinophils. *Blood* 94:2065, 1999.

123. Marshall NA, Christie LE, Munro LR, et al: Immunosuppressive regulatory T cells are abundant in the reactive lymphocytes of Hodgkin lymphoma. *Blood* 103:1755, 2004.

124. Kapp U, Yeh WC, Patterson B, et al: Interleukin 13 is secreted by and stimulates the growth of Hodgkin and Reed-Sternberg cells. *J Exp Med* 189:1939, 1999.

125. Zheng B, Fiumara P, Li YV, et al: MEK/ERK pathway is aberrantly active in Hodgkin disease: A signaling pathway shared by CD30, CD40, and RANK that regulates cell proliferation and survival. *Blood* 102:1019, 2003.

126. Kube D, Holtick U, Vockerodt M, et al: STAT3 is constitutively activated in Hodgkin cell lines. *Blood* 98:762, 2001.

127. Skinnider BF, Elia AJ, Gascoyne RD, et al: Signal transducer and activator of transcription 6 is frequently activated in Hodgkin and Reed-Sternberg cells of Hodgkin lymphoma. *Blood* 99:618, 2002.

128. Maggio EM, Van Den Berg A, De Jong D, et al: Low frequency of FAS mutations in Reed-Sternberg cells of Hodgkin's lymphoma. *Am J Pathol* 162:29, 2003.

129. Muschen M, Re D, Brauninger A, et al: Somatic mutations of the CD95 gene in Hodgkin and Reed-Sternberg cells. *Cancer Res* 60:5640, 2000.

130. Straus SE, Jaffe ES, Puck JM, et al: The development of lymphomas in families with autoimmune lymphoproliferative syndrome with germline Fas mutations and defective lymphocyte apoptosis. *Blood* 98:194, 2001.

131. Re D, Zander T, Diehl V, Wolf J: Genetic instability in Hodgkin's lymphoma. *Ann Oncol* 13(suppl 1):19, 2002.

132. Hasse U, Tinguely M, Leibundgut EO, et al: Clonal loss of heterozygosity in microdissected Hodgkin and Reed-Sternberg cells. *J Natl Cancer Inst* 91:1581, 1999.

133. Staratschek-Jox A, Thomas RK, Zander T, et al: Loss of heterozygosity in the Hodgkin-Reed Sternberg cell line L1236. *Br J Cancer* 84:381, 2001.

134. Re D, Starostik P, Massoudi N, et al: Allelic losses on chromosome 6q25 in Hodgkin and Reed Sternberg cells. *Cancer Res* 63:2606, 2003.

135. Alizadeh AA, Eisen MB, Davis RE, et al: Distinct types of diffuse large B-cell lymphoma identified by gene expression profiling. *Nature* 403:503, 2000.

136. Kuppers R, Klein U, Schwering I, et al: Identification of Hodgkin and Reed-Sternberg cell-specific genes by gene expression profiling. *J Clin Invest* 111:529, 2003.

137. Rosenwald A, Wright G, Leroy K, et al: Molecular diagnosis of primary mediastinal B cell lymphoma identifies a clinically favorable subgroup of diffuse large B cell lymphoma related to Hodgkin lymphoma. *J Exp Med* 198:851, 2003.

138. Savage KJ, Monti S, Kutok JL, et al: The molecular signature of mediastinal large B-cell lymphoma differs from that of other diffuse large B-cell lymphomas and shares features with classical Hodgkin lymphoma. *Blood* 102:3871, 2003.

139. Kaplan HS: *Hodgkin's Disease.* Harvard University, Cambridge, MA, 1980.

140. Pel PK: Zur symptomatolgie der sogennanten pseudoleukamie: II. Pseudoleukamie oder chronisches Ruckfallsfieber? *Berlin Klin Wochenschr* 24:844, 1887.

141. Ebstein WV: Das chronische Ruckfallsfieber, eine neu infectionskrankheit. *Berlin Klin Wochenschr* 24:565, 1887.

142. Tubiana M, Attie E, Flamant R, et al: Prognostic factors in 454 cases of Hodgkin's disease. *Cancer Res* 31:1801, 1971.

143. Atkinson K, Austin DE, McElwain TJ, Peckham MJ: Alcohol pain in Hodgkin's disease. *Cancer* 37:895, 1976.

144. Bjerrum OW, Hansen OE: Progressive multifocal leucoencephalopathy in Hodgkin's disease. *Scand J Haematol* 34:442, 1985.

145. Trotter JL, Hendin BA, Osterland CK: Cerebellar degeneration with Hodgkin disease. An immunological study. *Arch Neurol* 33:660, 1976.

146. Greenberg HS: Paraneoplastic cerebellar degeneration. A clinical and CT study. *J Neurooncol* 2:377, 1984.

147. Dansey RD, Hammond TG, Lai K, Bezwoda WR: Subacute myelopathy: An unusual paraneoplastic complication of Hodgkin's disease. *Med Pediatr Oncol Suppl* 16:284, 1988.

148. Sagar HJ, Read DJ: Subacute sensory neuropathy with remission: An association with lymphoma. *J Neurol Neurosurg Psychiatry* 45:83, 1982.

149. Feldmann E, Posner JB: Episodic neurologic dysfunction in patients with Hodgkin's disease. *Arch Neurol* 43:1227, 1986.

150. Carr I: The Ophelia syndrome: Memory loss in Hodgkin's disease. *Lancet* 1:844, 1982.

151. Julien J, Vital C, Aupy G, et al: Guillain-Barré syndrome and Hodgkin's disease—ultrastructural study of a peripheral nerve. *J Neurol Sci* 45:23, 1980.

152. Rewcastle NB, Tom MI: Non-infectious granulomatis angiitis of the nervous system associated with Hodgkin's disease. *J Neurol Neurosurg Psychiatry* 25:51, 1962.

153. Filly R, Bland N, Castellino RA: Radiographic distribution of intrathoracic disease in previously untreated patients with Hodgkin's disease and non-Hodgkin's lymphoma. *Radiology* 120:277, 1976.

154. Mauch P, Gorshein D, Cunningham J, Hellman S: Influence of mediastinal adenopathy on site and frequency of relapse in patients with Hodgkin's disease. *Cancer Treat Rep* 66:809, 1982.

155. Jerusalem G, Warland V, Najjar F, et al: Whole-body 18F-FDG PET for the evaluation of patients with Hodgkin's disease and non-Hodgkin's lymphoma. *Nucl Med Comm* 20:13, 1999.

156. Bangerter M, Moog F, Buchmann I, et al: Whole-body 2-[18F]-fluoro-2-deoxy-D-glucose positron emission tomography (FDG-PET) for accurate staging of Hodgkin's disease. *Ann Oncol* 9:1117, 1998.

157. Meyer RM, Ambinder RF, Stroobants S: Hodgkin's lymphoma: Evolving concepts with implications for practice. In *Hematology 2004*, The Am Soc Hematol Educ Program Book, edited by VC Broudy, N Berliner, RA Larson, LL Leung, p 184. 2004.

158. Burns BF, Colby TV, Dorfman RF: Differential diagnostic features of nodular L & H Hodgkin's disease, including progressive transformation of germinal centers. *Am J Surg Pathol* 8:253, 1984.

159. Hansmann ML, Zwingers T, Boske A, et al: Clinical features of nodular paragranuloma (Hodgkin's disease, lymphocyte predominance type, nodular). *J Cancer Res Clin Oncol* 108:321, 1984.

160. Miettinen M, Franssila KO, Saxen E: Hodgkin's disease, lymphocytic predominance nodular. Increased risk for subsequent non-Hodgkin's lymphomas. *Cancer* 51:2293, 1983.

161. Sundeen JT, Cossman J, Jaffe ES: Lymphocyte predominant Hodgkin's disease nodular subtype with coexistent "large cell lymphoma," Histo-

logical progression or composite malignancy? *Am J Surg Pathol* 12:599, 1988.

162. Rudiger T, Gascoyne RD, Jaffe ES, et al: Workshop on the relationship between nodular lymphocyte predominant Hodgkin's lymphoma and T cell/histiocyte-rich B cell lymphoma. *Ann Oncol* 13(suppl 1):44, 2002.

163. MacLennan KA, Bennett MH, Tu A, et al: Relationship of histopathologic features to survival and relapse in nodular sclerosing Hodgkin's disease. A study of 1,659 patients. *Cancer* 64:1686, 1989.

164. Masih AS, Weisenburger DD, Vose JM, et al: Histologic grade does not predict prognosis in optimally treated, advanced-stage nodular sclerosing Hodgkin's disease. *Cancer* 69:228, 1992.

165. von Wasielewski S, Franklin J, Fischer R, et al: Nodular sclerosing Hodgkin disease: New grading predicts prognosis in intermediate and advanced stages. *Blood* 101:4063, 2003.

166. Kant JA, Hubbard SM, Longo DL, et al: The pathologic and clinical heterogeneity of lymphocyte-depleted Hodgkin's disease. *J Clin Oncol* 4:284, 1986.

167. Neiman RS, Rosen PJ, Lukes RJ: Lymphocyte-depletion Hodgkin's disease. A clinicopathological entity. *N Engl J Med* 288:751, 1973.

168. Rosenberg SA, Kaplan HS: Evidence for an orderly progression in the spread of Hodgkin's disease. *Cancer Res* 26:1225, 1966.

169. Smithers DW: Spread of Hodgkin's disease. *Lancet* 1:1262, 1970.

170. Hutchison GB: Anatomic patterns by histologic type of localized Hodgkin's disease of the upper torso. *Lymphology* 5:1, 1972.

171. Rappaport H, Berard CW, Butler JJ, et al: Report of the Committee on Histopathological Criteria Contributing to Staging of Hodgkin's Disease. *Cancer Res* 31:1864, 1971.

172. Naeim F, Waisman J, Coulson WF: Hodgkin's disease: The significance of vascular invasion. *Cancer* 34:655, 1974.

173. Lister TA, Crowther D, Sutcliffe SB, et al: Report of a committee convened to discuss the evaluation and staging of patients with Hodgkin's disease: Cotswolds meeting. *J Clin Oncol* 7:1630, 1989.

174. Kaplan HS, Dorfman RF, Nelsen TS, Rosenberg SA: Staging laparotomy and splenectomy in Hodgkin's disease: Analysis of indications and patterns of involvement in 285 consecutive, unselected patients. *J Natl Cancer Inst Monogr* 36:291, 1973.

175. Leibenhaut MH, Hoppe RT, Efron B, et al: Prognostic indicators of laparotomy findings in clinical stage I-II supradiaphragmatic Hodgkin's disease. *J Clin Oncol* 7:81, 1989.

176. Simmons AV, Spiers AS, Fayers PM: Haematological and clinical parameters in assessing activity in Hodgkin's disease and other malignant lymphomas. *Q J Med* 42:111, 1973.

177. Tauro GP: Hodgkin's disease associated with raised eosinophil counts. *Med J Aust* 2:604, 1966.

178. MacLennan KA, Hudson BV, Jelliffe AM, et al: The pretreatment peripheral blood lymphocyte count in 1,100 patients with Hodgkin's disease: The prognostic significance and the relationship to the presence of systemic symptoms. *Clin Oncol* 7:333, 1981.

179. Ultmann JE, Cunningham JK, Gellhorn A: The clinical picture of Hodgkin's disease. *Cancer Res* 26:1047, 1966.

180. MacLennan KA, Vaughan HB, Easterling MJ, et al: The presentation haemoglobin level in 1,103 patients with Hodgkin's disease (BNLI report no 21). *Clin Radiol* 34:491, 1983.

181. Storgaard L, Karle H: Fever and haemolysis in Hodgkin's diseases. *Acta Med Scand* 197:311, 1975.

182. Jones SE: Autoimmune disorders and malignant lymphoma. *Cancer* 31:1092, 1973.

183. Sonnenblick M, Kramer R, Hershko C: Corticosteroid responsive immune thrombocytopenia in Hodgkin's disease. *Oncology* 43:349, 1986.

184. Cohen JR: Idiopathic thrombocytopenic purpura in Hodgkin's disease: A rare occurrence of no prognostic significance. *Cancer* 41:743, 1978.

185. Kedar A, Khan AB, Mattern JQ, et al: Autoimmune disorders complicating adolescent Hodgkin's disease. *Cancer* 44:112, 1979.

186. Hunter JD, Logue GL, Joyner JT: Autoimmune neutropenia in Hodgkin's disease. *Arch Intern Med* 142:386, 1982.

187. Le Bourgeois J, Tubiana M: The erythrocyte sedimentation rate as a monitor for relapse in patients with previously treated Hodgkin's disease. *Int J Radiat Oncol Biol Phys* 2:241, 1977.

188. Haybittle JL, Hayhoe FG, Easterling MJ, et al: Review of British National Lymphoma Investigation studies of Hodgkin's disease and development of prognostic index. *Lancet* 1:967, 1985.

189. Tubiana M, Henry-Amar M, van der Werf-Manning B, et al: A multivariate analysis of prognostic factors in early stage Hodgkin's disease. *Int J Radiat Oncol Biol Phys* 11:23, 1985.

190. Schilling RF, McKnight B, Crowley JJ: Prognostic value of serum lactic dehydrogenase level in Hodgkin's disease. *J Lab Clin Med* 99:382, 1982.

191. Friedenberg WR, Gatlin PF, Mazza JJ, et al: Prognostic value of serum lactic dehydrogenase level in Hodgkin's disease. *J Lab Clin Med* 103:489, 1984.

192. Aisenberg AC, Kaplan MM, Rieder SV: Serum alkaline phosphatase at the onset of Hodgkin's disease. *Cancer* 26:318, 1970.

193. Mercier RJ, Thompson JM, Harman GS, Messerschmidt GL: Recurrent hypercalcemia and elevated 1,25-dihydroxyvitamin D levels in Hodgkin's disease. *Am J Med* 84:165, 1988.

194. Braund WJ, Naylor BA, Williamson DH, et al: Autoimmunity to insulin receptor and hypoglycaemia in patient with Hodgkin's disease. *Lancet* 1:237, 1987.

195. Walters EG, Tavare JM, Denton RM, Walters G: Hypoglycaemia due to an insulin-receptor antibody in Hodgkin's disease. *Lancet* 1:241, 1987.

196. Eliakim R, Vertman E, Shinhar E: Syndrome of inappropriate secretion of antidiuretic hormone in Hodgkin's disease. *Am J Med Sci* 291:126, 1986.

197. Hasenclever D, Diehl V: A prognostic score for advanced Hodgkin's disease. International Prognostic Factors Project on Advanced Hodgkin's Disease. *N Engl J Med* 339:1506, 1998.

198. Dimopoulos MA, Cabanillas F, Lee JJ, et al: Prognostic role of serum beta 2-microglobulin in Hodgkin's disease. *J Clin Oncol* 11:1108, 1993.

199. Nadali G, Vinante F, Ambrosetti A, et al: Serum levels of soluble CD30 are elevated in the majority of untreated patients with Hodgkin's disease and correlate with clinical features and prognosis. *J Clin Oncol* 12:793, 1994.

200. Kurzrock R, Redman J, Cabanillas F, et al: Serum interleukin 6 levels are elevated in lymphoma patients and correlate with survival in advanced Hodgkin's disease and with B symptoms. *Cancer Res* 53:2118, 1993.

201. Pizzolo G, Chilosi M, Vinante F, et al: Soluble interleukin-2 receptors in the serum of patients with Hodgkin's disease. *Br J Cancer* 55:427, 1987.

202. Sarris AH, Kliche KO, Pethambaram P, et al: Interleukin-10 levels are often elevated in serum of adults with Hodgkin's disease and are associated with inferior failure-free survival. *Ann Oncol* 10:433, 1999.

203. Lieberman DA: Intrahepatic cholestasis due to Hodgkin's disease. An elusive diagnosis. *J Clin Gastroenterol* 8:304, 1986.

204. Routledge RC, Hann IM, Jones PH: Hodgkin's disease complicated by the nephrotic syndrome. *Cancer* 38:1735, 1976.

205. Kaplan HS: Evidence for a tumoricidal dose level in the radiotherapy of Hodgkin's disease. *Cancer Res* 26:1221, 1966.

206. Vijayakumar S, Myrianthopoulos LC: An updated dose-response analysis in Hodgkin's disease. *Radiother Oncol* 24:1, 1992.

207. Hanks GE, Kinzie JJ, Herring DF, Kramer S: Patterns of care outcome studies in Hodgkin's disease: Results of the national practice and implications for management. *Cancer Treat Rep* 66:805, 1982.

208. Trueblood HW, Enright LP, Ray GR, et al: Preservation of ovarian function in pelvic radiation for Hodgkin's disease. *Arch Surg* 100:236, 1970.

209. Pedrick TJ, Hoppe RT: Recovery of spermatogenesis following pelvic irradiation for Hodgkin's disease. *Int J Radiat Oncol Biol Phys* 12:117, 1986.

210. Feuer EJ, Kessler LG, Baker SG, et al: The impact of breakthrough clinical trials on survival in population based tumor registries. *J Clin Epidemiol* 44:141, 1991.

211. Longo DL, Young RC, Wesley M, et al: Twenty years of MOPP therapy for Hodgkin's disease. *J Clin Oncol* 4:1295, 1986.

212. De Vita VT Jr, Hubbard SM, Longo DL: The chemotherapy of lymphomas: Looking back, moving forward—The Richard and Hinda Rosenthal Foundation award lecture. *Cancer Res* 47:5810, 1987.

213. Sutcliffe SB, Wrigley PF, Peto J, et al: MVPP chemotherapy regimen for advanced Hodgkin's disease. *BMJ* 1:679, 1978.

214. McElwain TJ, Toy J, Smith E, et al: A combination of chlorambucil, vinblastine, procarbazine, and prednisolone for treatment of Hodgkin's disease. *Br J Cancer* 36:276, 1977.

215. Frei E, Luce JK, Gamble JF, et al: Combination chemotherapy in advanced Hodgkin's disease. Induction and maintenance of remission. *Ann Intern Med* 79:376, 1973.

216. Santoro A, Bonadonna G: Prolonged disease-free survival in MOPP-resistant Hodgkin's disease after treatment with adriamycin, bleomycin, vinblastine, and dacarbazine (ABVD). *Cancer Chemother Pharmacol* 2:101, 1979.

217. Santoro A, Bonfante V, Bonadonna G: Salvage chemotherapy with ABVD in MOPP-resistant Hodgkin's disease. *Ann Intern Med* 96:139, 1982.

218. Santoro A, Bonadonna G, Bonfante V, Valagussa P: Alternating drug combinations in the treatment of advanced Hodgkin's disease. *N Engl J Med* 306:770, 1982.

219. Bonadonna G, Valagussa P, Santoro A: Alternating non-cross-resistant combination chemotherapy or MOPP in stage IV Hodgkin's disease. A report of 8-year results. *Ann Intern Med* 104:739, 1986.

220. Klimo P, Connors JM: MOPP/ABV hybrid program: Combination chemotherapy based on early introduction of seven effective drugs for advanced Hodgkin's disease. *J Clin Oncol* 3:1174, 1985.

221. Viviani S, Bonadonna G, Santoro A, et al: Alternating versus hybrid MOPP and ABVD combinations in advanced Hodgkin's disease: Ten-year results. *J Clin Oncol* 14:1421, 1996.

222. Diehl V, Franklin J, Pfreundschuh M, et al: Standard and increased-dose BEACOPP chemotherapy compared with COPP-ABVD for advanced Hodgkin's disease. *N Engl J Med* 348:2386, 2003.

223. Horning SJ, Hoppe RT, Breslin S, et al: Stanford V and radiotherapy for locally extensive and advanced Hodgkin's disease: Mature results of a prospective clinical trial. *J Clin Oncol* 20:630, 2002.

224. Rosenberg SA, Kaplan HS: The evolution and summary results of the Stanford randomized clinical trials of the management of Hodgkin's disease: 1962-1984. *Int J Radiat Oncol Biol Phys* 11:5, 1985.

225. Specht L, Gray RG, Clarke MJ, Peto R: Influence of more extensive radiotherapy and adjuvant chemotherapy on long-term outcome of early-stage Hodgkin's disease: A meta-analysis of 23 randomized trials involving 3,888 patients. International Hodgkin's Disease Collaborative Group. *J Clin Oncol* 16:830, 1998.

226. Hancock SL, Hoppe RT, Horning SJ, Rosenberg SA: Intercurrent death after Hodgkin disease therapy in radiotherapy and adjuvant MOPP trials. *Ann Intern Med* 109:183, 1988.

227. Horning SJ, Hoppe RT, Hancock SL, Rosenberg SA: Vinblastine, bleomycin, and methotrexate: An effective adjuvant in favorable Hodgkin's disease. *J Clin Oncol* 6:1822, 1988.

228. Horning SJ, Hoppe RT, Mason J, et al: Stanford-Kaiser Permanente G1 study for clinical stage I to IIA Hodgkin's disease: Subtotal lymphoid irradiation versus vinblastine, methotrexate, and bleomycin chemotherapy and regional irradiation. *J Clin Oncol* 15:1736, 1997.

229. Noordijk EM, Carde P, Hagenbeek A, et al: Combination of radiotherapy and chemotherapy is advisable in all patients with clinical stage I-II Hodgkin's disease. Six year results of the EORTC-GPMC controlled clinical trials "H7-VF," "H7-F," and "H7-UF" [abstract]. *Int J Radiat Oncol Biol Phys* 77.173, 1997.

230. Press OW, LeBlanc M, Lichter AS, et al: Phase III randomized intergroup trial of subtotal lymphoid irradiation versus doxorubicin, vinblastine, and subtotal lymphoid irradiation for stage IA to IIA Hodgkin's disease. *J Clin Oncol* 19:4238, 2001.

231. Tesch H, Sieber M, Ruffer J, et al: Two cycles ABVD plus radiotherapy is more effective than radiotherapy alone in early stage HD: Interim analysis of the HD7 trial of the GHSG clinic of internal medicine, University of Cologne. *Blood* 92(suppl I):485a, 1998.

232. Bonadonna G, Bonfante V, Viviani S, et al: ABVD plus subtotal nodal versus involved-field radiotherapy in early-stage Hodgkin's disease: Long-term results. *J Clin Oncol* 22:2835, 2004.

233. Engert A, Schiller P, Josting A, et al: Involved-field radiotherapy is equally effective and less toxic compared with extended-field radiotherapy after four cycles of chemotherapy in patients with early-stage unfavorable Hodgkin's lymphoma: Results of the HD8 trial of the German Hodgkin's Lymphoma Study Group. *J Clin Oncol* 21:3601, 2003.

234. Radford JA, Cowan RA, Ryder WDJ, et al: Four weeks of neo-adjuvant chemotherapy significantly reduces the progression rate in patients treated with limited field radiotherapy for clinical stage IA/IIA Hodgkin's disease. Results of a randomized trial [abstract]. *Ann Oncol* 66:21, 1996.

235. Horning SJ, Hoppe RT, Breslin S, et al: Very brief (8 week) chemotherapy and low dose (30 Gy) radiotherapy for limited stage Hodgkin's disease: Preliminary results of the Stanford-Kaiser G4 study of Stanford V + RT. *Blood* 94:387, 1999.

236. Olweny CL, Katongole ME, Kiire C, et al: Childhood Hodgkin's disease in Uganda: A ten year experience. *Cancer* 42:787, 1978.

237. Ekert H, Waters KD, Smith PJ, et al: Treatment with MOPP or ChlVPP chemotherapy only for all stages of childhood Hodgkin's disease. *J Clin Oncol* 6:1845, 1988.

238. Longo DL, Glatstein E, Duffey PL, et al: Radiation therapy versus combination chemotherapy in the treatment of early-stage Hodgkin's disease: Seven-year results of a prospective randomized trial. *J Clin Oncol* 9:906, 1991.

239. Biti GP, Cimino G, Cartoni C, et al: Extended-field radiotherapy is superior to MOPP chemotherapy for the treatment of pathologic stage I-IIA Hodgkin's disease: Eight-year update of an Italian prospective randomized study. *J Clin Oncol* 10:378, 1992.

240. Meyer R, Gospodarowicz M, Connors JM, et al: A randomized phase III comparison of single-modality ABVD with a strategy that includes radiation therapy in patients with early-stage Hodgkin's disease: The HD-6 trial of the National Cancer Institute of Canada Clinical Trials Group (Eastern Cooperative Oncology Group Trial JHD06). *Blood* 101:81a, 2003.

241. Straus DJ, Portlock CS, Qin J, et al: Results of a prospective randomized clinical trial of doxorubicin, bleomycin, vinblastine, and dacarbazine (ABVD) followed by radiation therapy (RT) versus ABVD alone for stages I, II, and IIIA nonbulky Hodgkin disease. *Blood* 104:3483, 2004.

242. Laskar S, Gupta T, Vimal S, et al: Consolidation radiation after complete remission in Hodgkin's disease following six cycles of doxorubicin, bleomycin, vinblastine, and dacarbazine chemotherapy: Is there a need? *J Clin Oncol* 22:62, 2004.

243. Nachman JB, Sposto R, Herzog P, et al: Randomized comparison of low-dose involved-field radiotherapy and no radiotherapy for children with Hodgkin's disease who achieve a complete response to chemotherapy. *J Clin Oncol* 20:3765, 2002.

244. Hoppe RT, Coleman CN, Cox RS, et al: The management of stage I-II Hodgkin's disease with irradiation alone or combined modality therapy: The Stanford experience. *Blood* 59:455, 1982.

245. Diehl V, Stein H, Hummel M, et al: Hodgkin's lymphoma: Biology and treatment strategies for primary, refractory, and relapsed disease. In *Hematology 2003*, Am Soc Hematol Educ Program Book, edited by VC Broudy, JT Prchal, GJ Tricot, p 225. 2003.

246. Santoro A, Bonadonna G, Valagussa P, et al: Long-term results of combined chemotherapy-radiotherapy approach in Hodgkin's disease: Superiority of ABVD plus radiotherapy versus MOPP plus radiotherapy. *J Clin Oncol* 5:27, 1987.

247. Bonfante V, Santoro A, Viviani S, et al: ABVD in the treatment of Hodgkin's disease. *Semin Oncol* 19(2 suppl 5):38, discussion 44, 1992.

248. Longo DL, Russo A, Duffey PL, et al: Treatment of advanced-stage massive mediastinal Hodgkin's disease: The case for combined modality treatment. *J Clin Oncol* 9:227, 1991.

249. Canellos GP, Anderson JR, Propert KJ, et al: Chemotherapy of advanced Hodgkin's disease with MOPP, ABVD, or MOPP alternating with ABVD. *N Engl J Med* 327:1478, 1992.

250. Canellos GP, Niedzwiecki D: Long-term follow-up of Hodgkin's disease trial. *N Engl J Med* 346:1417, 2002.

251. Connors JM, Klimo P, Adams G, et al: Treatment of advanced Hodgkin's disease with chemotherapy—Comparison of MOPP/ABV hybrid regimen with alternating courses of MOPP and ABVD: A report from the National Cancer Institute of Canada clinical trials group. *J Clin Oncol* 15:1638, 1997.

252. Duggan DB, Petroni GR, Johnson JL, et al: Randomized comparison of ABVD and MOPP/ABV hybrid for the treatment of advanced Hodgkin's disease: Report of an intergroup trial. *J Clin Oncol* 21:607, 2003.

253. Hasenclever D, Diehl V: A prognostic score to predict freedom from progression in advanced Hodgkin's disease. *N Engl J Med* 339:1056, 1998.

254. Horning SJ, Williams J, Bartlett NL, et al: Assessment of the Stanford V regimen and consolidative radiotherapy for bulky and advanced Hodgkin's disease: Eastern Cooperative Oncology Group pilot study E1492. *J Clin Oncol* 18:972, 2000.

255. Aversa SM, Salvagno L, Soraru M, et al: Stanford V regimen plus consolidative radiotherapy is an effective therapeutic program for bulky or advanced-stage Hodgkin's disease. *Acta Haematol* 112:141, 2004.

256. Chisesi T, Federico M, Levis A, et al: ABVD versus stanford V versus MEC in unfavourable Hodgkin's lymphoma: Results of a randomised trial. *Ann Oncol* 13(suppl 1):102, 2002.

257. Prosnitz LR, Farber LR, Kapp DS, et al: Combined modality therapy for advanced Hodgkin's disease: 15-year follow-up data. *J Clin Oncol* 6:603, 1988.

258. Donaldson SS, Link MP: Combined modality treatment with low-dose radiation and MOPP chemotherapy for children with Hodgkin's disease. *J Clin Oncol* 5:742, 1987.

259. Meerwaldt JH, Coleman CN, Fischer RI, et al: Role of additional radiotherapy in advanced stages of Hodgkin's disease. *Ann Oncol* 4:83, 1992.

260. Fabian CJ, Mansfield CM, Dahlberg S, et al: Low-dose involved field radiation after chemotherapy in advanced Hodgkin disease. A Southwest Oncology Group randomized study. *Ann Intern Med* 120:903, 1994.

261. Diehl V, Loeffler M, Pfreundschuh M, et al: Further chemotherapy versus low-dose involved-field radiotherapy as consolidation of complete remission after six cycles of alternating chemotherapy in patients with advance Hodgkin's disease. German Hodgkins' Study Group (GHSG). *Ann Oncol* 6:901, 1995.

262. Weiner MA, Leventhal B, Brecher ML, et al: Randomized study of intensive MOPP-ABVD with or without low-dose total-nodal radiation therapy in the treatment of stages IIB, IIIA2, IIIB, and IV Hodgkin's disease in pediatric patients: A Pediatric Oncology Group study. *J Clin Oncol* 15:2769, 1997.

263. Aleman BM, Raemaekers JM, Tirelli U, et al: Involved-field radiotherapy for advanced Hodgkin's lymphoma. *N Engl J Med* 348:2396, 2003.

264. Diehl V, Schiller P, Engert A, et al: Results of the third interim analysis of the HD12 trial of the GHSG: 8 courses of escalated BEACOPP versus 4 baseline courses of BEACOPP with or without additive radiotherapy for advanced stage Hodgkin's lymphoma [abstract]. *Blood* 102:85, 2003.

265. Portlock CS, Rosenberg SA, Glatstein E, Kaplan HS: Impact of salvage treatment on initial relapses in patients with Hodgkin disease, stages I-III. *Blood* 51:825, 1978.

266. Roach MD, Brophy N, Cox R, et al: Prognostic factors for patients relapsing after radiotherapy for early-stage Hodgkin's disease. *J Clin Oncol* 8:623, 1990.

267. Longo DL, Duffey PL, Young RC, et al: Conventional-dose salvage combination chemotherapy in patients relapsing with Hodgkin's disease after combination chemotherapy: The low probability for cure. *J Clin Oncol* 10:210, 1992.

268. Viviani S, Santoro A, Negretti E, et al: Salvage chemotherapy in Hodgkin's disease. Results in patients relapsing more than twelve months after first complete remission. *Ann Oncol* 1:123, 1990.

269. Bonadonna G, Santoro A, Gianni AM, et al: Primary and salvage chemotherapy in advanced Hodgkin's disease: The Milan Cancer Institute experience. *Ann Oncol* 1: 9, 1991.

270. Chopra R, McMillan AK, Linch DC, et al: The place of high-dose BEAM therapy and autologous bone marrow transplantation in poor-risk Hodgkin's disease. A single-center eight-year study of 155 patients. *Blood* 81:1137, 1993.

271. Bierman PJ, Anderson JR, Freeman MB, et al: High-dose chemotherapy followed by autologous hematopoietic rescue for Hodgkin's disease patients following first relapse after chemotherapy. *Ann Oncol* 7:151, 1996.

272. Horning SJ, Chao NJ, Negrin RS, et al: High-dose therapy and autologous hematopoietic progenitor cell transplantation for recurrent or refractory Hodgkin's disease: Analysis of the Stanford University results and prognostic indices. *Blood* 89:801, 1997.

273. Reece DE, Connors JM, Spinelli JJ, et al: Intensive therapy with cyclophosphamide, carmustine, etoposide +/- cisplatin, and autologous bone marrow transplantation for Hodgkin's disease in first relapse after combination chemotherapy. *Blood* 83:1193, 1994.

274. Linch DC, Winfield D, Goldstone AH, et al: Dose intensification with autologous bone-marrow transplantation in relapsed and resistant Hodgkin's disease: Results of a BNLI randomized trial. *Lancet* 341:1051, 1993.

275. Schmitz N, Pfistner B, Sextro M, et al: Aggressive conventional chemotherapy compared with high-dose chemotherapy with autologous haemopoietic stem-cell transplantation for relapsed chemosensitive Hodgkin's disease: A randomized trial. *Lancet* 359:2065, 2002.

276. Nademanee A, O'Donnell MR, Snyder DS, et al: High-dose chemotherapy with or without total body irradiation followed by autologous bone marrow and/or peripheral blood stem cell transplantation for patients with relapsed and refractory Hodgkin's disease: Results in 85 patients with analysis of prognostic factors. *Blood* 85:1381, 1995.

277. Josting A, Rudolph C, Mapara M, et al: Cologne high-dose sequential chemotherapy in relapsed and refractory Hodgkin lymphoma: Results of a large multicenter study of the German Hodgkin Lymphoma Study Group (GHSG). *Ann Oncol* 16:116, 2005.

278. Stiff PJ, Unger JM, Forman SJ, et al: The value of augmented preparative regimens combined with an autologous bone marrow transplant for the management of relapsed or refractory Hodgkin disease: A Southwest Oncology Group phase II trial. *Biol Blood Marrow Transplant* 9: 529, 2003.

279. Sureda A, Schmitz N: Role of allogeneic stem cell transplantation in relapsed or refractory Hodgkin's disease. *Ann Oncol* 13(suppl 1):128, 2002.

280. Schmitz N, Sureda A, Robinson S: Allogeneic transplantation of hematopoietic stem cells after nonmyeloablative conditioning for Hodgkin's disease: Indications and results. *Semin Oncol* 31:27, 2004.

281. Rehwald U, Schulz H, Reiser M, et al: Treatment of relapsed CD20+ Hodgkin lymphoma with the monoclonal antibody rituximab is effective

281. and well tolerated: Results of a phase 2 trial of the German Hodgkin Lymphoma Study Group. *Blood* 101:420, 2003.

282. Ekstrand BC, Lucas JB, Horwitz SM, et al: Rituximab in lymphocyte-predominant Hodgkin disease: Results of a phase 2 trial. *Blood* 101: 4285, 2003.

283. Ansell S, Byrd J, Horwitz SM, et al: Phase I/II study of a fully human anti-CD30 monoclonal antibody (MDX-060) in Hodgkin's disease (HD) and anaplastic large cell lymphoma (ALCL) [abstract]. *Blood* 102:632, 2003.

284. Bartlett NL, Bernstein SH, Leonard JP, et al: Safety, antitumor activity and pharmacokinetics of six weekly doses of SGN-30 (anti-CD30 monoclonal antibody) in patients with refractory or recurrent CD30+ hematologic malignancies. Session Type: Poster Session 561-II [abstract]. *Blood* 102:2390, 2003.

285. Santoro A, Bredenfeld H, Devizzi L, et al: Gemcitabine in the treatment of refractory Hodgkin's disease: Results of a multicenter phase II study. *J Clin Oncol* 18:2615, 2000.

286. Zinzani PL, Bendandi M, Stefoni V, et al: Value of gemcitabine treatment in heavily pretreated Hodgkin's disease patients. *Haematologica* 85:926, 2000.

287. Rule S, Tighe M, Davies S, Johnson S: Vinorelbine in the treatment of lymphoma. *Hematol Oncol* 16:101, 1998.

288. Bollard CM, Aguilar L, Straathof KC, et al: Cytotoxic T lymphocyte therapy for Epstein-Barr virus+ Hodgkin's disease. *J Exp Med* 200: 1623, 2004.

289. Specht L, Nordentoft AM, Cold S, et al: Tumor burden as the most important prognostic factor in early stage Hodgkin's disease. Relations to other prognostic factors and implications for choice of treatment. *Cancer* 61:1719, 1988.

290. Mauch PM: Controversies in the management of early stage Hodgkin's disease. *Blood* 83:318, 1994.

291. Tubiana M, Henry AM, Carde P, et al: Toward comprehensive management tailored to prognostic factors of patients with clinical stages I and II in Hodgkin's disease. The EORTC Lymphoma Group controlled clinical trials: 1964-1987. *Blood* 73:47, 1989.

292. Gospodarowicz MK, Sutcliffe SB, Clark RM, et al: Analysis of supradiaphragmatic clinical stage I and II Hodgkin's disease treated with radiation alone. *Int J Radiat Oncol Biol Phys* 22:859, 1992.

293. Kennedy BJ, Loeb VJ, Peterson V, et al: Survival in Hodgkin's disease by stage and age. *Med Pediatr Oncol Suppl* 20:100, 1992.

294. Enblad G, Glimelius B, Sundstrom C: Treatment outcome in Hodgkin's disease in patients above the age of 60: A population-based study. *Ann Oncol* 2:297, 1991.

295. Ballova V, Ruffer JU, Haverkamp H, et al: A prospectively randomized trial carried out by the German Hodgkin Study Group (GHSG) for elderly patients with advanced Hodgkin's disease comparing BEACOPP baseline and COPP-ABVD (study HD9elderly). *Ann Oncol* 16:124, 2005.

296. Mikhaeel NG, Mainwaring P, Nunan T, Timothy AR: Prognostic value of interim and post treatment FDG-PET scanning in Hodgkin lymphoma. *Ann Oncol* 13(suppl 2):21, 2002.

297. Moskowitz C: An update on the management of relapsed and primary refractory Hodgkin's disease. *Semin Oncol* 31(2 suppl 4):54, 2004.

298. Josting A, Reiser M, Rueffer U, et al: Treatment of primary progressive Hodgkin's and aggressive non-Hodgkin's lymphoma: Is there a chance for cure? *J Clin Oncol* 18:332, 2000.

299. Moskowitz CH, Kewalramani T, Nimer SD, et al: Effectiveness of high dose chemoradiotherapy and autologous stem cell transplantation for patients with biopsy-proven primary refractory Hodgkin's disease. *Br J Haematol* 124:645, 2004.

300. Bierman PJ, Lynch JC, Bociek RG, et al: The International Prognostic Factors Project score for advanced Hodgkin's disease is useful for predicting outcome of autologous hematopoietic stem cell transplantation. *Ann Oncol* 13:1370, 2002.

301. Josting A, Rueffer U, Franklin J, et al: Prognostic factors and treatment outcome in primary progressive Hodgkin lymphoma: A report from the German Hodgkin Lymphoma Study Group. *Blood* 96:1280, 2000.

302. Josting A, Franklin J, May M, et al: New prognostic score based on treatment outcome of patients with relapsed Hodgkin's lymphoma registered in the database of the German Hodgkin's lymphoma study group. *J Clin Oncol* 20:221, 2002.

303. Portlock CS, Donnelly GB, Qin J, et al: Adverse prognostic significance of CD20 positive Reed-Sternberg cells in classical Hodgkin's disease. *Br J Haematol* 125:701, 2004.

304. von Wasielewski R, Mengel M, Fischer R, et al: Classical Hodgkin's disease. Clinical impact of the immunophenotype. *Am J Pathol* 151: 1123, 1997.

305. Tzankov A, Krugmann J, Fend F, et al: Prognostic significance of CD20 expression in classical Hodgkin lymphoma: A clinicopathological study of 119 cases. *Clin Cancer Res* 9:1381, 2003.

306. Brink AA, Oudejans JJ, van den Brule AJ, et al: Low p53 and high bcl-2 expression in Reed-Sternberg cells predicts poor clinical outcome for Hodgkin's disease: Involvement of apoptosis resistance? *Mod Pathol* 11:376, 1998.

307. Rassidakis GZ, Medeiros LJ, Vassilakopoulos TP, et al: BCL-2 expression in Hodgkin and Reed-Sternberg cells of classical Hodgkin disease predicts a poorer prognosis in patients treated with ABVD or equivalent regimens. *Blood* 100:3935, 2002.

308. Vassallo J, Metze K, Traina F, et al: The prognostic relevance of apoptosis-related proteins in classical Hodgkin's lymphomas. *Leuk Lymphoma* 44:483, 2003.

309. Montalban C, Garcia JF, Abraira V, et al: Influence of biologic markers on the outcome of Hodgkin's lymphoma: A study by the Spanish Hodgkin's Lymphoma Study Group. *J Clin Oncol* 22:1664, 2004.

310. Montalban C, Abraira V, Morente M, et al: Epstein-Barr virus latent membrane protein 1 expression has a favorable influence in the outcome of patients with Hodgkin's disease treated with chemotherapy. *Leuk Lymphoma* 39:563, 2000.

311. Glavina-Durdov M, Jakic-Razumovic J, Capkun V, Murray P: Assessment of the prognostic impact of the Epstein-Barr virus-encoded latent membrane protein-1 expression in Hodgkin's disease. *Br J Cancer* 84: 1227, 2001.

312. Pizzolo G, Vinante F, Chilosi M, et al: Serum levels of soluble CD30 molecule (Ki-1 antigen) in Hodgkin's disease: Relationship with disease activity and clinical stage. *Br J Haematol* 75:282, 1990.

313. Viviani S, Notti P, Bonfante V, et al: Elevated pretreatment serum levels of Il-10 are associated with a poor prognosis in Hodgkin's disease, the Milan Cancer Institute experience. *Med Oncol* 17:59, 2000.

314. Bohlen H, Kessler M, Sextro M, et al: Poor clinical outcome of patients with Hodgkin's disease and elevated interleukin-10 serum levels. Clinical significance of interleukin-10 serum levels for Hodgkin's disease. *Ann Hematol* 79:110, 2000.

315. Axdorph U, Sjoberg J, Grimfors G, et al: Biological markers may add to prediction of outcome achieved by the International Prognostic Score in Hodgkin's disease. *Ann Oncol* 11:1405, 2000.

316. Arseneau JC, Sponzo RW, Levin DL, et al: Nonlymphomatous malignant tumors complicating Hodgkin's disease. Possible association with intensive therapy. *N Engl J Med* 287:1119, 1972.

317. Canellos GP, Arseneau JC, DeVita VT, et al: Second malignancies complicating Hodgkin's disease in remission. *Lancet* 1:947, 1975.

318. Coleman CN, Williams CJ, Flint A, et al: Hematologic neoplasia in patients treated for Hodgkin's disease. *N Engl J Med* 297:1249, 1977.

319. Kaldor JM, Day NE, Clarke EA, et al: Leukemia following Hodgkin's disease. *N Engl J Med* 322:7, 1990.

320. Levine EG, Bloomfield CD: Leukemias and myelodysplastic syndromes secondary to drug, radiation, and environmental exposure. *Semin Oncol* 19:47, 1992.

321. Josting A, Wiedenmann S, Franklin J, et al: Secondary myeloid leuke-
     mia and myelodysplastic syndromes in patients treated for Hodgkin's
     disease: A report from the German Hodgkin's Lymphoma Study Group.
     J Clin Oncol 21:3440, 2003.

322. Van LF, Somers R, Taal BG, et al: Increased risk of lung cancer, non-
     Hodgkin's lymphoma, and leukemia following Hodgkin's disease.
     J Clin Oncol 7:1046, 1989.

323. Tucker MA, Coleman CN, Cox RS, et al: Risk of second cancers after
     treatment for Hodgkin's disease. *N Engl J Med* 318:76, 1988.

324. Rueffer U, Josting A, Franklin J, et al: Non-Hodgkin's lymphoma after
     primary Hodgkin's disease in the German Hodgkin's Lymphoma Study
     Group: Incidence, treatment, and prognosis. *J Clin Oncol* 19:2026, 2001.

325. Jaffe ES, Zarate OA, Medeiros LJ: The interrelationship of Hodgkin's
     disease and non-Hodgkin's lymphomas—Lessons learned from com-
     posite and sequential malignancies. *Semin Diagn Pathol* 9:297, 1992.

326. Huang JZ, Weisenburger DD, Vose JM, et al: Diffuse large B-cell lym-
     phoma arising in nodular lymphocyte predominant Hodgkin lymphoma.
     A report of 21 cases from the Nebraska Lymphoma Study Group. *Leuk
     Lymphoma* 44:1903, 2003.

327. Boivin JF, Hutchison GB, Lyden M, et al: Second primary cancers
     following treatment of Hodgkin's disease. *J Natl Cancer Inst* 72:233,
     1984.

328. Henry AM: Second cancers after radiotherapy and chemotherapy for
     early stages of Hodgkin's disease. *J Natl Cancer Inst* 71:911, 1983.

329. Hancock SL, Tucker MA, Hoppe RT: Breast cancer after treatment of
     Hodgkin's disease. *J Natl Cancer Inst* 85:25, 1993.

330. Hancock SL, Cox RS, McDougall IR: Thyroid diseases after treatment
     of Hodgkin's disease. *N Engl J Med* 325:599, 1991.

331. Shapiro CL, Mauch PM: Radiation-associated breast cancer after Hodg-
     kin's disease: Risks and screening in perspective. *J Clin Oncol* 10:1662,
     1992.

332. Bhatia S, Robison LL, Oberlin O, et al: Breast cancer and other second
     neoplasms after childhood Hodgkin's disease. *N Engl J Med* 334:745,
     1996.

333. van Leeuwen FE, Klokman WJ, Stovall M, et al: Roles of radiation dose,
     chemotherapy, and hormonal factors in breast cancer following Hodg-
     kin's disease. *J Natl Cancer Inst* 95:971, 2003.

334. Travis LB, Gospodarowicz M, Curtis RE, et al: Lung cancer following
     chemotherapy and radiotherapy for Hodgkin's disease. *J Natl Cancer
     Inst* 94:182, 2002.

335. Hancock SL, Donaldson SS, Hoppe RT: Cardiac disease following treat-
     ment of Hodgkin's disease in children and adolescents. *J Clin Oncol* 11:
     1208, 1993.

336. Boivin JF, Hutchison GB, Lubin JH, Mauch P: Coronary artery disease
     mortality in patients treated for Hodgkin's disease. *Cancer* 69:1241,
     1992.

337. Adams MJ, Lipsitz SR, Colan SD, et al: Cardiovascular status in long-
     term survivors of Hodgkin's disease treated with chest radiotherapy.
     J Clin Oncol 22:3139, 2004.

338. Heidenreich PA, Hancock SL, Lee BK, et al: Asymptomatic cardiac
     disease following mediastinal irradiation. *J Am Coll Cardiol* 42:743,
     2003.

339. Eriksson F, Gagliardi G, Liedberg A, et al: Long-term cardiac mortality
     following radiation therapy for Hodgkin's disease: Analysis with the
     relative seriality model. *Radiother Oncol* 55:153, 2000.

340. Chapman RM, Sutcliffe SB, Rees LH, et al: Cyclical combination
     chemotherapy and gonadal function. Retrospective study in males. *Lan-
     cet* 1:285, 1979.

341. Da CM, Meistrich ML, Fuller LM, et al: Recovery of spermatogenesis
     after treatment for Hodgkin's disease: Limiting dose of MOPP chemo-
     therapy. *J Clin Oncol* 2:571, 1984.

342. Chapman RM, Sutcliffe SB, Malpas JS: Cytotoxic-induced ovarian fail-
     ure in women with Hodgkin's disease: I. Hormone function. *JAMA* 242:
     1877, 1979.

343. Horning SJ, Hoppe RT, Kaplan HS, Rosenberg SA: Female reproductive
     potential after treatment for Hodgkin's disease. *N Engl J Med* 304:1377,
     1981.

344. Anselmo AP, Cartoni C, Bellantuono P, et al: Risk of infertility in pa-
     tients with Hodgkin's disease treated with ABVD vs. MOPP vs. ABVD/
     MOPP. *Haematologica* 75:155, 1990.

345. Viviani S, Santoro A, Ragni G, et al: Gonadal toxicity after combination
     chemotherapy for Hodgkin's disease. Comparative results of MOPP vs.
     ABVD. *Eur J Cancer Clin Oncol* 21:601, 1985.

346. Carmel RJ, Kaplan HS: Mantle irradiation in Hodgkin's disease. An
     analysis of technique, tumor eradication, and complications. *Cancer* 37:
     2813, 1976.

347. Smith LM, Mendenhall NP, Cicale MJ, et al: Results of a prospective
     study evaluating the effects of mantle irradiation on pulmonary function.
     Int J Radiat Oncol Biol Phys 16:79, 1989.

348. Horning SJ, Adhikari A, Rizk N, et al: Effect of treatment for Hodgkin's
     disease on pulmonary function: Results of a prospective study. *J Clin
     Oncol* 12:297, 1994.

349. Donaldson SS, Kaplan HS: Complications of treatment of Hodgkin's
     disease in children. *Cancer Treat Rep* 66:977, 1982.

350. Rosner F, Zarrabi MH: Late infections following splenectomy in Hodg-
     kin's disease. *Cancer Invest* 1:57, 1983.

351. Knobel H, Havard Loge J, Brit Lund M, et al: Late medical complica-
     tions and fatigue in Hodgkin's disease survivors. *J Clin Oncol* 19:3226,
     2001.

352. Bloom JR, Fobair P, Gritz E, et al: Psychosocial outcomes of cancer: A
     comparative analysis of Hodgkin's disease and testicular cancer. *J Clin
     Oncol* 11:979, 1993.

PLASMA CELL NEOPLASMS: GENERAL CONSIDERATIONS

STEPHEN M. BAIRD

Plasma cell neoplasms are monoclonal tumors of plasma cells and their precursors. It is important to distinguish plasma cell neoplasms from benign conditions that do not require specific therapy. Although monoclonal immunoglobulin protein generally is detected in plasma cell myeloma, other conditions also may result in production of a relative excess of monoclonal immunoglobulin. This chapter summarizes the laboratory studies used to evaluate for monoclonal proteinemia or monoclonal immunoglobulin gene rearrangements. This chapter delineates laboratory features that can be used to distinguish plasma cell myeloma from related conditions that may give rise to an excess of monoclonal immunoglobulin. This chapter provides references to relevant chapters in the textbook that focus on a particular plasma cell or B cell disorder.

DEFINITION AND HISTORY

PLASMA CELL NEOPLASMS

Plasma cell neoplasms are monoclonal expansions of a single late-stage B lymphocyte with the predisposition to mature into plasma cells. All the differentiated cells within the neoplasm produce the same whole immunoglobulin chain or chain fragment. In a given neoplasm, the monoclonal proteins generally have the same heavy-chain class (γ, α, μ, δ, or ε), same light-chain class (κ or λ), and same idiotypes (or antigenic determinants of the immunoglobulin variable regions, see Chap. 77).[1] The neoplastic plasma cells and their precursor small lymphocytes have the same immunoglobulin gene rearrangements and chromosomal anomalies, if any are present.[2-5] Since Henry Bence Jones[6] first discovered what turned out to be monoclonal light chains in the urine of myeloma patients 150 years ago, the monoclonal immunoglobulin molecules (or their constituent chains) produced by plasma cell neoplasms have remained the best examples of tumor-specific antigens in the field of oncology. These proteins usually are called *M* proteins, which at various times in history has stood for *malignant, myeloma,* and now *monoclonal* proteins. Table 98-1 lists the diseases associated with M proteins. Some of the diseases are benign and nonprogressive, whereas some are malignant.

ESSENTIAL MONOCLONAL GAMMOPATHY

The term *benign* must be used cautiously when describing monoclonal gammopathies in patients who do not have overt malignant plasmacytoma or multiple myeloma. Clinical and laboratory features con-

sistent with monoclonal gammopathy are an M protein level less than 2.5 g/dl, few or no monoclonal light chains in the urine, and no anemia or change in serum calcium (Table 98-2). No bony lesions are observed on skeletal surveys, and the plasmacytosis in the marrow, if present, is less than 30 percent.[7,8] The concept that this condition is benign is based on the condition's generally indolent biologic behavior. However, a low but significant percentage of patients with monoclonal gammopathy develop frank B cell malignancies each year.[9-13] For this reason, the term *benign monoclonal gammopathy* largely has been replaced by the term *monoclonal gammopathy of undetermined significance* (MGUS) (see Chap. 99).

CHRONIC COLD AGGLUTININ SYNDROME

Chronic cold agglutinin syndrome is a disease in which elderly patients produce a monoclonal immunoglobulin (Ig)M molecule that binds red blood cells and causes their agglutination at temperatures significantly below 37°C (98.6°F) (see Chap. 52). The syndrome may be seen in patients without other apparent evidence of malignant disease, in patients with lymphoma (see Chap. 96), or in patients with Waldenström macroglobulinemia (see Chap. 102). The apparently benign form of the disease may progress to malignancy.[16,17] The disorder bears no relationship to acute, postinfectious cold agglutinin syndrome, in which the offending immunoglobulins are polyclonal and disappear after the inciting infectious agent is eradicated.

CRYOGLOBULINS

Cryoglobulins are complexes of immunoglobulins that precipitate upon exposure to cold (see Chap. 102). Three classes of cryoglobulins have been recognized for convenience of description. *Type 1 cryoglobulins* are monoclonal IgM, IgG, or IgA molecules. *Type 2 cryoglobulins* are monoclonal immunoglobulins, usually of the IgM class, with antibody activity against other immunoglobulins, usually IgG. An association of type 2 cryoglobulins with hepatitis B and C infection has been reported.[18-20] *Type 3 cryoglobulins* are composed of polyclonal immunoglobulins with antiimmunoglobulin activity. Cryoglobulins may cause a variety of pathologic conditions, all related to the formation of immune complexes and the attendant inflammation and coagulation disorders. They are detected by allowing serum to stand and precipitate or gel at 4°C (39.2°F) for 24 to 72 hours.

TABLE 98-1 DISEASES ASSOCIATED WITH M PROTEINS

DISEASE	REFERENCE
Benign	
Essential monoclonal gammopathy	Chapter 99
Chronic cold agglutinin syndrome	Chapter 52
Transient (after inflammation)	Chapter 99
Transient (after marrow transplant)	Chapter 22
Immunodeficiency (see particularly T cell)	Chapter 83
Neoplastic	
Plasma cell myeloma	Chapter 100
Neoplasms producing γ, α, μ, δ, or ε heavy chains and either κ or λ light chains	
Neoplasms producing only κ or λ light chains	
Neoplasms that do not make detectable immunoglobulin	
Neoplasms causing amyloidosis or light-chain deposition in tissues	Chapter 101
Neoplasms causing dermatologic lesions	
Waldenström macroglobulinemia	Chapter 102
Heavy-chain disease: α, γ, μ, or rarely δ, but no light chains	Chapter 103
Chronic lymphocytic leukemia and related lymphomas	Chapter 92

Acronyms and abbreviations that appear in this chapter include: CSF, cerebrospinal fluid; EBV, Epstein-Barr virus; GM-CSF, granulocyte-monocyte colony stimulating factor; IFN-α, interferon alpha; Ig, immunoglobulin; IL, interleukin; KSHV, Kaposi sarcoma–associated herpesvirus; MGUS, monoclonal gammopathy of undetermined significance; MHC, major histocompatibility complex; TNF, tumor necrosis factor.

TABLE 98-2   SOME BIOLOGIC FEATURES OF MONOCLONAL GAMMOPATHY

	MULTIPLE MYELOMA	MGUS	IMMUNO-DEFICIENCY
Clonal size	Large	Medium	Small
Immunoglobulin production	>25 mg/ml	<25 mg/ml	<2.5 mg/ml
Proliferation	Progressive	Persistent	Transient
Abnormal immunoglobulin structure	Frequent	Rare	Never
Bone destruction	Frequent	Never	Never
Mouse models			
Transformed clone	+	+	−
Transplantable generations	<4	−	
Autonomous growth	+	+?	−
Immortality	+	−	−

SOURCE: Modified from Radl.[14,15]

TRANSIENT M PROTEINS

Transient M proteins occasionally are associated with inflammation (see Chap. 99).[21–23] Monoclonal molecules also have been described in hyperimmunized laboratory animals. They do not progress to malignant disease and are not always high-affinity antibodies to the presumed cause of inflammation or experimental immunogen.

Patients with any of a variety of congenital immunodeficiencies in which the T cell arm of immunity is more affected than the B cell arm may develop transient, low-level monoclonal gammopathies, typically of the IgM class (see Chap. 99). The immunodeficiencies have become apparent with the development of techniques more sensitive for detection of the disorders. Immunodeficient patients receiving marrow transplants frequently exhibit a transient monoclonal gammopathy early in their posttransplant course.[24,25] If the patient or donor is infected with Epstein-Barr virus (EBV), the gammopathy may be oligoclonal and herald the development of a potentially fatal EBV-driven lymphoproliferative disorder.

The incidence of multiple myeloma in individuals older than 25 years is approximately 30 per 100,000. The incidence of monoclonal gammopathy is approximately 100 times as high, and the transient monoclonal gammopathies associated with all the various forms of inflammation and immunodeficiency are approximately 400 times more frequent (see Chaps. 22, 99, and 100). The frequency of all the disorders increases dramatically with age. The monoclonal gammopathies in immunodeficient hosts occur at a much younger age than multiple myeloma or monoclonal gammopathy.

ETIOLOGY AND PATHOGENESIS

GENETIC BACKGROUND

In the mouse, the genetic background of the animal is an important risk factor for developing monoclonal gammopathy or plasmacytomas. Approximately 60 percent of C57BL/Ka mice develop M proteins of the IgM class by age 21 months. Approximately 40 percent of C3H and NZB mice develop M proteins of the IgM class. However, BALB/c and CBA/Kij strains have a very low incidence of spontaneous plasma cell neoplasm. Surprisingly, mice of the BALB/c strain are most susceptible to developing plasmacytomas after repeated intraperitoneal injections of mineral oil. NZB mice also are fairly susceptible to induction of plasmacytomas by this method. However, C57BL/Ka mice are resistant.[14,15,26]

Human families with a high incidence of plasma cell neoplasms have been reported.[27,28] No consistent genetic aberrations have been described in these families. Multiple myeloma occurs more frequently in relatives of patients with the disease than in the general population.[29,30] In the United States, African-Americans have a higher incidence of multiple myeloma than Caucasians.[31] These observations indicate the host's genetic background is an important risk factor for development of plasma cell neoplasms in mammals.

Numerous attempts have been made to induce plasmacytomas that secrete antibodies to specific antigens in BALB/c mice. The animals were hyperimmunized with any one of a variety of antigens in mineral oil. Plasmacytomas arose but almost never made antibodies reactive with the injected antigen.[32] Thus, no relationship between chronic antigenic stimulation and development of plasma cell neoplasms is apparent in these animals. However, this is not the case with Aleutian minks infected with the Aleutian disease virus.[33] Many of these animals develop M proteins consisting of antibodies that bind specifically to the infecting virus. In humans, no consistent relationship is observed between prior inflammatory disease and subsequent development of a plasma cell neoplasm. However, monoclonal gammopathies occur at increased frequency in patients with inflammatory and autoimmune diseases.[21,22,34–36] Although restricted v region genotypes exist in diseases such as chronic lymphocytic leukemia, no evidence indicates their monoclonal antibodies bind to an antigen that stimulates disease development.

CHROMOSOMAL ANOMALIES

Approximately 90 percent of mouse plasmacytomas induced by mineral oil in mice show consistent chromosomal anomalies.[37] In these plasmacytomas, the c-myc gene on mouse chromosome 15 is fused with either the immunoglobulin heavy-chain locus on mouse chromosome 12 or the immunoglobulin κ light-chain locus on mouse chromosome 6.[37,38] The fusion of c-myc with an immunoglobulin heavy- or light-chain locus resembles the typical chromosomal anomalies seen in human Burkitt lymphoma.[39] However, the biologic behaviors of murine plasmacytomas and human Burkitt lymphoma are radically different, and no virus (such as EBV) has been associated with murine or human plasmacytomas.

Certain chromosomal abnormalities in neoplastic cells may be seen repeatedly in patients with multiple myeloma or plasma cell leukemia (late, preterminal stage of multiple myeloma) (see Chap. 100).[40] Additions to the long arm of chromosome 14 (14q$^+$) have been described in 30 to 50 percent of multiple myeloma patients. Often the donated material is from chromosome 11, generating a t(11;14) (q13;q32).[41] Multiple myeloma and plasma cell leukemia cells may have abnormalities of chromosome 1 in approximately 50 to 70 percent of cases. The anomalies are highly variable, and no consistent deletions, additions, or translocations have been found. Finally, rare patients have deletions of chromosome 22 in the region of the immunoglobulin λ light-chain locus. Interestingly, chromosomal anomalies associated with the immunoglobulin κ light-chain region on chromosome 2 have not been described in humans, even though approximately two thirds of M proteins express κ light chains.

Patients with trisomies of chromosomes 6, 9, and 17 tend to have prolonged survival, whereas patients with monosomy 13 (loss of Rb) have shortened survival[42] (see Chap. 100). However, cytogenetic studies normally are not performed on multiple myeloma patients. Because neoplastic plasma cells or their precursors often divide relatively slowly, the inability to find an abnormal karyotype in some biopsy specimens may reflect the fact that only normal hematopoietic cells were induced into metaphase. Therefore, negative results may be false negatives.

CYTOKINES

Interleukin (IL)-6 is a potent stimulator of plasmacytoma growth.[43–47] In cultures of freshly isolated marrow cells from patients with multiple myeloma, IL-6 is produced predominantly by monocytoid cells and fibroblasts. With time in culture, the myeloma cells themselves may produce IL-6, which in turn may stimulate plasma cell growth *in vitro*. IL-6 may play such a role in patients with multiple myeloma. In one study, injected monoclonal antibodies to IL-6 significantly inhibited tumor cell growth *in vivo*.[46] In addition, other cytokines, such as granulocyte-monocyte colony stimulating factor (GM-CSF), IL-3, IL-1, and low-dose interferon alpha (IFN-α), may synergize with IL-6 to stimulate the growth of plasmacytomas. Kaposi sarcoma–associated herpesvirus (KSHV) is found in bone marrow dendritic cells of patients with multiple myeloma and occasionally in patients with MGUS. KSHV-encoded IL-6 is transcribed in these bone marrow dendritic cells.[48] Malignant precursors of myeloma cells appear to adhere to the dendritic cells.[49] Finally, rearrangements of the IL-6 receptor gene in myeloma cells have been described, in at least one case. As the tumor progresses, malignant cells may escape from their dependency on IL-6. None of these studies has related the effects of cytokines to the observed chromosomal anomalies prevalent in multiple myeloma. The gene for IL-1 is on chromosome 2q; IL-3 and GM-CSF are on 5q; IFN-α is on 9p; IFN-γ is on 12q; and IL-6 is on 7p.[41]

The malignant cells of multiple myeloma produce other cytokines that contribute to the pathophysiology of the bone disease, resulting in lytic lesions of bone. The osteolytic lesions weaken the bone matrix and may lead to pathologic fractures. The lesions are produced by osteoclasts that are activated by cytokines released by the malignant plasma cells themselves. Formerly called *osteoclast activating factor*, the factor involved now is thought to be a combination of different cytokines, including IL-1, tumor necrosis factor-alpha (TNF-α), IL-5, TNF-β, and/or IL-6 (see Chap. 100).[50,51]

LABORATORY FEATURES

SURFACE MARKERS

Cell marker studies show a great deal of lineage infidelity in multiple myeloma. Malignant B cells may express both early and late B cell antigens and antigens characteristic of granulocytes, monocytes, or megakaryocytes.[52–54] This finding led some investigators to suggest that the transformed cell of multiple myeloma is really the marrow stem cell. However, lineage infidelity commonly is seen in marker studies of a variety of neoplasms. Such lineage infidelity may reflect dysregulation in the expression of cellular differentiation antigens secondary to malignant transformation. Nonetheless, multiple myeloma probably is not a disease in which the transforming event occurs in mature plasma cells.

Cells resembling small lymphocytes may have the same immunoglobulin gene rearrangements, immunoglobulin idiotypes, and surface antigens as all malignant plasma cells.[52] As such, these neoplasms may be composed of transformed B cells that have retained their abilities to mature into plasma cells. Thus, myeloma contrasts with lymphocytic lymphomas, which usually do not produce significant numbers of plasma cells. This situation may be analogous to the difference between chronic myelogenous leukemia, in which malignant cells may mature into segmented neutrophils, and acute myelogenous leukemia, in which very few do mature into segmented neutrophils (see Chaps. 87 and 88). The spectrum of disorders producing M protein includes tumors of small lymphocytes, such as chronic lymphocytic leukemia and small lymphocytic lymphoma, and tumors of plasmacytoid lymphocytes, such as Waldenström macroglobulinemia. These types of tumor usually produce IgM, whereas plasmacytomas usually produce IgG or IgA.

In lymphoid neoplasms, cells from a single transformed clone can have the morphology of a small lymphocyte, a lymphoblast, or a plasma cell. By convention, a fully mature plasma cell is assumed to be incapable of reentering the cycle of cell division, but this inability has not been demonstrated rigorously in plasma cell neoplasms. In fact, on histologic sections of marrow from multiple myeloma patients, many plasma cells have nuclei with an immature chromatin pattern rather than the highly condensed pattern of normal plasma cells. An increased frequency of binucleate or multinucleate cells also is observed. The abilities to divide and incorporate tritiated thymidine into DNA are criteria that are useful in distinguishing "malignant" from "benign" plasma cell neoplasms.[7,51] These criteria are not routinely used in the clinical laboratory because other, less expensive tests yield similar information. The typical flow cytometry phenotype of multiple myeloma cells is CD45-, HLADR-, CD19-, CD20-, PCA1+, CD38+, CD138+, Ki 67 variable, and monoclonal cytoplasmic Ig+ (γ>α>μ; K>λ).

ZONAL ELECTROPHORESIS

SERUM

The most common screening test for an M protein is serum electrophoresis. In this test, a few microliters of serum are spotted onto a support medium, such as cellulose acetate, that has been equilibrated at a basic pH. When an electric current is applied across the support medium, the proteins in the serum migrate toward the anode at a velocity proportional to the ratio of their negative charge to molecular weight. After a migration period of approximately 30 minutes, depending on the precise conditions, the cellulose acetate is taken up, dried, immersed in a stain that detects proteins, such as ponceau SX or Coomassie blue, and examined by eye or densitometry. Figure 98-1 illustrates the procedure and typical results.

Albumin is the most abundant protein in normal serum. This protein migrates as a sharp peak because, except in rare cases, all albumin molecules have exactly the same amino acid sequence and hence the same electrophoretic mobility. In contrast, the γ-globulins comprise immunoglobulins that have millions of different amino acid sequences

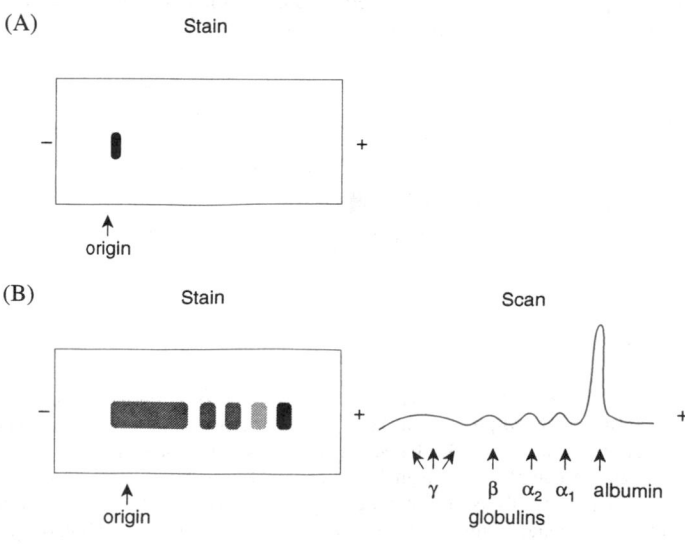

FIGURE 98-1   Normal serum electrophoresis. *(A)* Apply serum to support medium. *(B)* Electrophoretically separate proteins. Stain, observe, and scan.

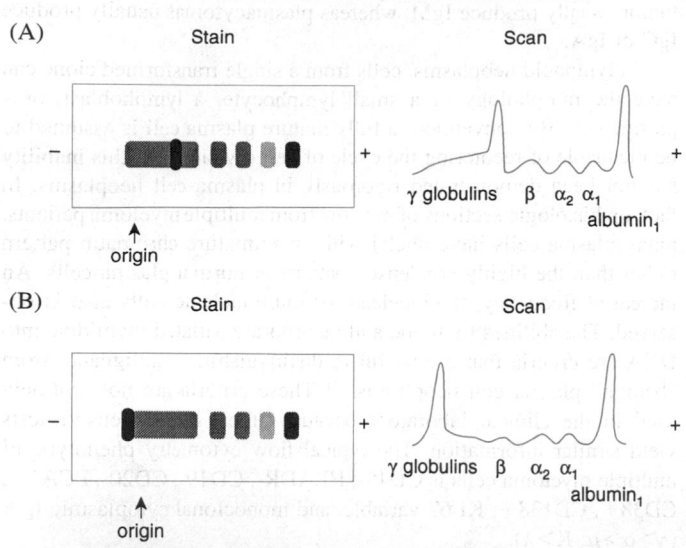

FIGURE 98-2   M protein electrophoresis. *(A)* Fast-moving M protein spike. *(B)* Slow-moving M protein spike.

and varying carbohydrate side chains. Consequently, these proteins migrate in a very broad band that typically contains IgA and IgM in the front (toward the β-globulins) and IgG spread through the entire range of globulins. IgD and IgE normally are secreted at such low levels that they are not detectable by this method. When a plasma cell neoplasm produces an M protein, the electrophoretic pattern is altered (Fig. 98-2).

A monoclonal immunoglobulin protein may migrate anywhere in the globulin region. IgM and IgA M proteins tend to migrate faster than most IgG molecules. Accordingly, the M protein in example 1 of Fig. 98-2 probably is an IgA or IgM, whereas the spike in example 2 probably is an IgG molecule. To distinguish these immunoglobulin classes with certainty requires either immunoelectrophoresis or immunofixation electrophoresis. Figure 98-3 illustrates false monoclonal "immunoglobulins."

SPINAL FLUID AND URINE

Electrophoresis can be performed on concentrated specimens of cerebrospinal fluid (CSF) or urine. Evaluation of CSF allows for detection

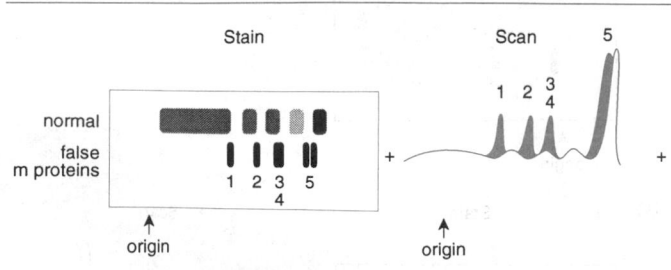

FIGURE 98-3   False M proteins. Band 1 is typical of fibrinogen, which may be confused with M proteins of the IgA or IgM class. If fibrinogen is present, the serum was incompletely clotted or plasma was used. Band 2 is hemoglobin–haptoglobin complexes or high levels of transferrin, which may be seen in intravascular hemolysis or iron deficiency respectively. Band 3/4 may be seen with hyperalphaglobulinemia (one of the acute phase reactants, as is haptoglobin) and with some of the congenital hyperlipoproteinemias. Band 5 is an albumin variant resulting from a rare autosomal trait, bisalbuminemia, or from some drugs, such as penicillin, that bind to albumin and alter its electrophoretic mobility.

of a plasmacytoma secreting M protein in the central nervous system. Evaluation of the urine is useful for detecting excessive and unbalanced synthesis of immunoglobulin molecules. Because proteins larger than albumin (or 67 kDa) normally do not pass through the glomeruli, whole immunoglobulins ordinarily do not pass into the urine. However, free immunoglobulin light chains are only approximately 25 kDa and hence pass freely through the glomerulus. Patients with a circulating M protein who pass whole immunoglobulins in their urine generally have severe renal dysfunction, often because of renal amyloidosis secondary to deposition of immunoglobulin chains in the renal parenchyma.

Free light chains that appear in the urine can be detected by sulfosalicylic acid precipitation, electrophoresis of concentrated urine, immunoelectrophoresis, or immunofixation electrophoresis. The last two techniques also are useful for evaluating whether the immunoglobulin light chains are only κ, only λ, or both. The common urine dipstick relies on bromphenol blue, a dye that binds specifically to albumin.[55] Thus, dipsticks are not reliable screening tools for Bence Jones protein, and sulfosalicylic acid should be used.

Urine electrophoresis is one of the most important tools for diagnosis and followup of patients with plasma cell neoplasms. The neoplastic B cells of many myeloma patients produce excess immunoglobulin light chain or light chain alone. When the amount of immunoglobulin light chain filtered through the glomeruli exceeds the resorption capacity of the proximal tubules, free light chains are excreted into the urine. The amount of light chain excreted in a fixed amount of time often is proportional to the amount of light chain produced, which in turn is proportional to the number of neoplastic plasma cells. Thus, serial measurements of the amount of immunoglobulin light chain excreted over time are a convenient way to follow tumor mass and the effects of therapy.

Measurements of immunoglobulin light chains in urine do not always correlate with the rate of immunoglobulin light-chain production. Immunoglobulin light chains normally are reabsorbed and metabolized in the proximal tubules of the kidney. As renal damage progresses, the amount of light chains excreted in the urine increases, partly because of deteriorating renal function. For this reason, the best estimate of tumor cell mass in a patient with multiple myeloma is by measuring the M protein in serum. However, mutations of tumor cells that cause them to secrete less immunoglobulin, hydration of the patient, and renal disease also may influence the amount of serum M protein, independent of tumor cell burden.

IMMUNOELECTROPHORESIS AND IMMUNOFIXATION ELECTROPHORESIS

Figures 98-4 and 98-5 illustrate the principles of immunoelectrophoresis and immunofixation electrophoresis, respectively. These techniques are useful for identifying the immunoglobulin heavy-chain class and light-chain type in putative M proteins.

Table 98-3 lists several clinical conditions that generally are associated with a serum protein abnormality that can be detected by electrophoresis, immunoelectrophoresis, or immunofixation electrophoresis. These techniques are useful for detecting a variety of serum protein abnormalities other than M proteins.

IMMUNOGLOBULIN GENE REARRANGEMENTS

The most specific means to determine whether a lymphoproliferative disorder is monoclonal is by analyzing immunoglobulin gene rearrangement. In the laboratory, the most *common* technique is flow cytometry, looking for light-chain (κ or λ) restriction on tumor cells. Because B cells rearrange both immunoglobulin heavy- and light-chain genes to produce unique immunoglobulin genes, the detection of non–germ-line DNA immunoglobulin gene fragments following digestion with restriction endonucleases has become a common research technique (see Chap. 77). Genomic DNA isolated from a suspected B cell neoplasm is digested with one or more restriction endonucleases that each cut DNA at specific recognition sequences. If the DNA between the target sites has rearranged to join constant, joining, and variable regions from which a messenger RNA can be transcribed, the DNA will be of a different length compared to that of germ-line sequences or the DNA encoding any other heavy- or light-chain mRNA (see Chap. 77). When the products of digestion are electrophoresed on a sizing gel and then labeled by hybridization with specific DNA probes, monoclonal bands may be identified. This technique is useful for evaluating B cell lymphoproliferative disorders that secrete insufficient amounts of immunoglobulin to be detected in serum. Rearrangement of immunoglobulin heavy-chain genes occurs very early in B cell development and may be detected even in cells that produce no M protein (see Chap. 77). Both monoclonal and oligoclonal rearrangements can be detected by the technique, making it particularly valuable in the diagnosis of lymphoproliferative disorders in immunodeficient hosts, in whom truly oligoclonal, life-threatening lymphoproliferations are now being observed.[56–58]

QUANTITATIVE IMMUNOGLOBULIN ASSAYS

Immunoglobulins in serum, urine, or CSF usually are measured by nephelometry. This technique is based on the observation that antigen–antibody complexes form cloudy precipitates. The precipitates can be detected photoelectrically. Varying dilutions of the fluid in question are incubated with antibodies specific for any one of the different immunoglobulin heavy and light chains. After precipitates form, the amount of precipitate is determined by comparison with standard curves produced by precipitating immunoglobulins of known concentration. This now-automated technique has replaced the slow, labor-intensive, and semiquantitative technique of radial immunodiffusion.

SERUM β_2-MICROGLOBULIN

β_2-Microglobulin is the light chain of class I molecules of the major histocompatibility complex (MHC). Class I molecules are present on essentially all nucleated cells, including lymphocytes and plasma cells. In rapidly dividing cell populations, membrane turnover leads to shedding of many molecules, including class I MHC. Because β_2-microglobulin is not covalently linked to its heavy chain, it is released into the extracellular fluid and the blood. Because its molecular weight is less than 12,000, it is filtered through the normal glomerulus. However, β_2-microglobulin is reabsorbed by normal proximal renal tubules and does not appear in significant quantities in the urine. In patients with plasma cell neoplasms, however, serum β_2-microglobulin levels increase because of increased neoplastic cell turnover. Also, as myeloma protein-induced renal damage occurs, reduced glomerular filtration increases serum β_2-microglobulin levels. Renal tubular dysfunction in-

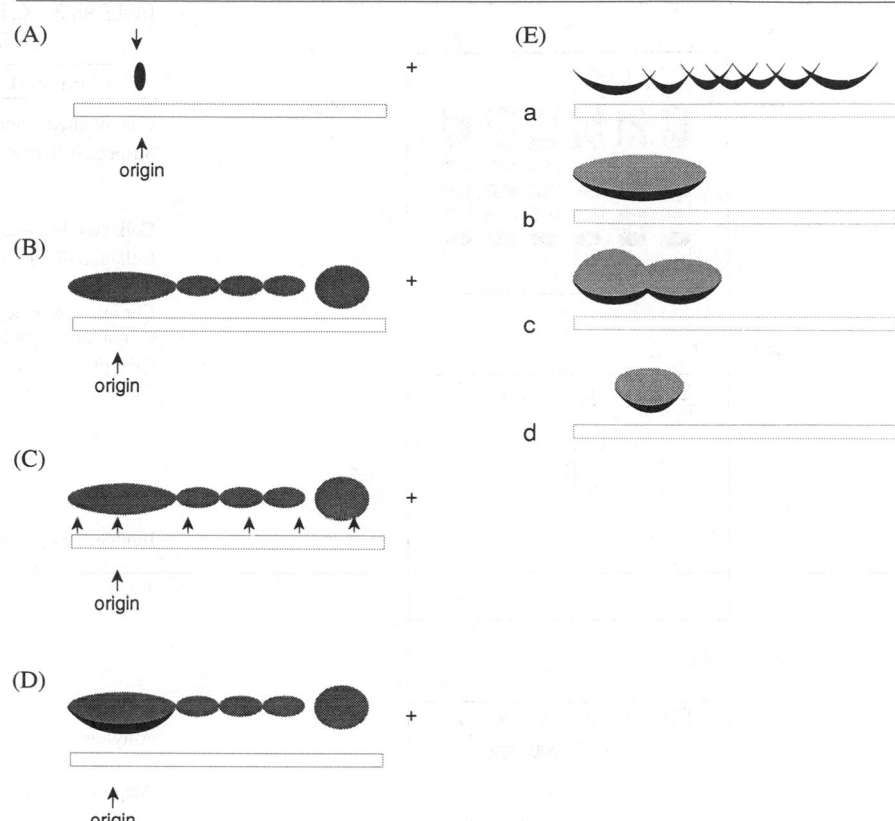

FIGURE 98-4 Immunoelectrophoresis. *(A)* Sample application. A few microliters of serum are placed at the origin in a support medium such as cellulose acetate. *(B)* Electrophoresis. Proteins separate based on the charge-to-weight ratio at a given pH. *(C)* Application of antibody in the trough. Antibody to serum protein diffuses from the trough toward electrophoretically size-separated proteins. *(D)* Formation of precipitin arcs. Precipitate forms where antibody reacts with antigenic serum protein(s). *(E)* Typical patterns. *a*, Antibody to whole serum detects many different proteins. *b*, Typical arc formed by antibody to IgG is very broad. Normal IgG molecules vary in amino acid sequence and hence electrophoretic mobility. The antiserum detects them all, mostly because of its reactivity with immunoglobulin heavy chains. *c*, Anti IgG detecting a monoclonal IgG within a polyclonal background. The monoclonal IgG distorts the smooth arc because of its increased amount relative to that of other IgG species and its unique electrophoretic mobility. *d*, Monoclonal immunoglobulin heavy or light chain with no polyclonal background. The arc is narrower than the polyclonal pattern because of the unique electrophoretic mobility of the monoclonal proteins.

creases serum levels even further. Therefore, serum β_2-microglobulin provides another parameter with which to monitor for neoplastic cell mass, cell turnover, effect on renal function, and response to treatment.[59–62]

SERUM VISCOSITY

Large molecules such as IgM pentamers and IgA dimers can significantly increase serum viscosity. Some IgG molecules, particularly those of the IgG3 subclass, tend to aggregate and increase serum viscosity.[63] *In vivo*, increased serum viscosity can cause sludging of capillary flow and disturbances of vision, other central nervous system abnormalities, and some clotting disorders (see "Waldenström Macroglobulinemia" in Chap. 102). In the laboratory, serum viscosity is measured as resistance to flow through standardized glass tubing compared to distilled water. The test usually is performed at room temperature, which is highly variable. If a patient has cryoglobulins, which aggregate increasingly at temperatures below 37°C (98.6°F), then serum viscosity measurements should be performed at 37°C (98.6°F) to obtain clinically relevant information. The relative vis-

A

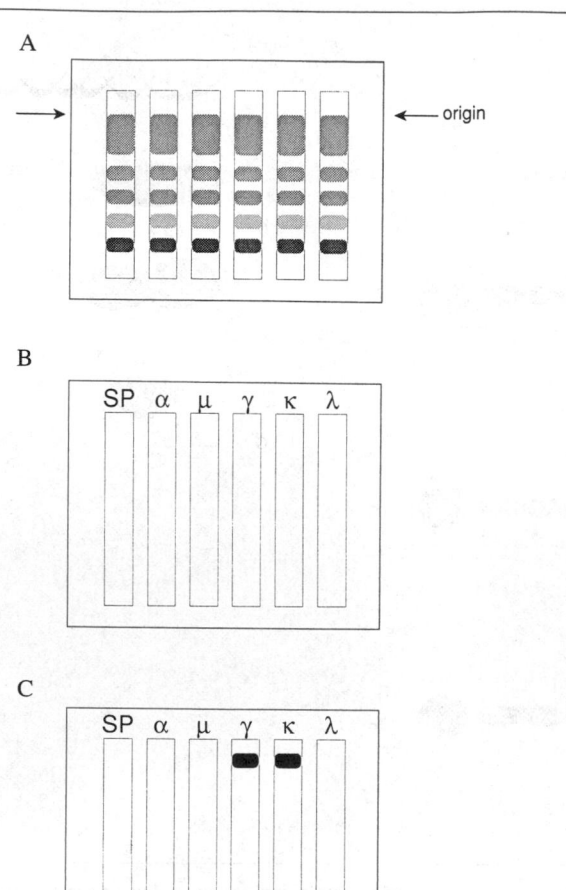

← origin

B

C

FIGURE 98-5 Immunofixation electrophoresis. *(A)* Serum samples are placed in each of several lanes of an agarose gel support medium for protein electrophoresis. *(B)* Overlay each lane with antiserum to a specific immunoglobulin heavy or light chain, typically anti-α, -μ, -γ, -κ, or -λ. Allow precipitation to occur. *(C)* Wash and stain. Only immunoprecipitates remain in the gel. Nonprecipitated proteins wash out. Results show an IgG$_\kappa$ M protein.

cosity of normal serum ranges up to 1.8 times that of water. Patients usually do not experience clinical symptoms with serum viscosities of 4 or less.

AMYLOIDOSIS

The type of amyloidosis associated with plasma cell neoplasms is caused by the deposition of light chains or light-chain fragments in tissues (see Chap. 101). The name *amyloid*, meaning "starch-like," comes from the polysaccharide groups attached to immunoglobulin light- (and heavy-) chain molecules. Amyloid can deposit in any tissue and often has a predilection for packing in and around the walls of small blood vessels. Amyloid is best detected by tissue biopsy, often of the kidney, liver, rectum, oral cavity, heart, or skin. Tissue light-chain deposition has a regular order and binds dyes such as Congo red or thioflavin B.[64] Under polarized light or a fluorescence microscope, the lesions have a characteristic appearance that permits establishing the diagnosis. Amyloidosis may severely impair organ function and is a potentially serious complication of plasma cell neoplasms. Tissue amyloid deposits may interfere with hemostasis and complicate needle biopsies of internal organs.[65]

TABLE 98-3 CLINICAL INDICATIONS FOR ELECTROPHORESIS OF SERUM AND URINE PROTEINS

CLINICAL INDICATION	ABNORMALITY AND INTERPRETATION
Unexplained edema or ascites	Hypoalbuminemia
Suspected liver disease	Hypoalbuminemia frequent; hyperglobulinemia suggests cirrhosis or chronic active hepatitis
Collagen diseases, sarcoidosis	Polyclonal hyperglobulinemia
Collagen diseases, sarcoidosis	Hypogammaglobulinemia or agammaglobulinemia
Chronic lymphocytic leukemia, malignant lymphoma	Hypogammaglobulinemia or, rarely, IgG or IgM M proteins
Unexplained proteinuria	Albumin or a mixture of all serum proteins found with urinary tract infections or the nephrotic syndrome; homogeneous urine proteins that migrate in the globulin region usually indicative of plasma cell neoplasms secreting free light or heavy chains
Evidence of plasma cell myeloma	Serum or urinary monoclonal neoplasms, e.g., bone pain, protein, with reduced normal immunoglobulins, frequent infections, elevated immunoglobulins and sedimentation rate, rouleaux, hypoalbuminemia, proteinuria, hyperviscosity, or osteolytic skeletal lesions
Amyloidosis	Monoclonal serum or urinary proteins frequent
Acquired clotting disorders	M proteins or amyloid bind to some clotting factors, such as I, II, VIII, IX, X, and XI
Acquired neuropathy	M proteins infiltrate peripheral nerves

REFERENCES

1. Kubagawa H, Vogler LB, Capra JD, et al: Studies on the clonal origin of multiple myeloma: Use of individually specific (idiotype) antibodies to trace the oncogenic event to its earliest point of expression in B-cell differentiation. *J Exp Med* 150:792, 1979.

2. Berenson J, Wong R, Kim K, et al: Evidence of peripheral blood B lymphocyte but not T lymphocyte involvement in multiple myeloma. *Blood* 70:1550, 1987.

3. Lindstrom FD, Hardy WR, Eberle BJ, et al: Multiple myeloma and benign monoclonal gammopathy: Differentiation by immunofluorescence of lymphocytes. *Ann Intern Med* 78:837, 1973.

4. Ueshima Y, Rowley JD: Chromosome studies in patients with multiple myeloma and related paraproteinemias, in *Neoplastic Diseases of the Blood*, vol 1, edited by PH Wiernick, GP Canellos, RA Kyle, CA Schiffer, p 499. Churchill Livingstone, New York, 1985.

5. Lewis JP, MacKenzie MR: Non-random chromosome aberrations associated with multiple myeloma. *Hematol Oncol* 2:307, 1984.

6. Bence Jones H: Papers on chemical pathology, lecture 3. *Lancet* 2:269, 1847.

7. Boccadoro M, Gavarotti P, Fossati G, et al: Low plasma cell ³H-thymidine incorporation in monoclonal gammopathy of undetermined significance (MGUS), smouldering myeloma and remission phase myeloma: A reliable indicator of patients not requiring therapy. *Br J Haematol* 58:689, 1984.

8. Kyle RA: "Benign" monoclonal gammopathy: A misnomer? *JAMA* 251: 1849, 1984.

9. Axelsson U, Backmann R, Hallen J: Frequency of pathological proteins (M-components) in 6995 sera from an adult population. *Acta Med Scand* 179:235, 1966.

10. Axelsson U: An eleven-year follow-up on 64 subjects with M-components. *Acta Med Scand* 201:173, 1977.

11. Kyle RA, Greipp PR: Monoclonal gammopathies of undetermined origin, in *Neoplastic Diseases of the Blood*, vol 2, edited by PH Wiernick, GP Canellos, RA Kyle, CA Schiffer, p 653. Churchill Livingstone, New York, 1985.

12. Hallen J: Frequency of "abnormal" serum globulins (M-components) in the aged. *Acta Med Scand* 173:737, 1963.

13. Englisova M, Englis M, Kyral V, et al: Changes of immunoglobulin synthesis in old people. *Exp Gerontol* 3:125, 1968.

14. Radl J, Hollander CF, Van Den Berg P, et al: Idiopathic paraproteinemia: I. Studies in an animal model—The aging C57BL/KaLwRij mouse. *Clin Exp Immunol* 33:395, 1978.

15. Radl J: Age-related monoclonal gammopathies: Clinical lessons from the aging C57BL mouse. *Immunol Today* 11:234, 1990.

16. Frank M, Atkinson JP, Gadek J: Cold agglutinins and cold agglutinin disease. *Annu Rev Med* 28:291, 1977.

17. Crisp D, Pruzanski W: B cell neoplasms with homogeneous cold-reacting antibodies (cold agglutinins). *Am J Med* 72:915, 1982.

18. Brouet J, Clouvel JP, Danon F, et al: Biologic and clinical significance of cryoglobulins: A report of 86 cases. *Am J Med* 57:775, 1974.

19. De Bandt M, Ribard P, Meyer O, et al: Type II IgM monoclonal cryoglobulinemia and hepatitis C virus infection [letter]. *Clin Exp Rheumatol* 9:659, 1991.

20. Gorevic PD, Kassab HJ, Levo Y, et al: Mixed cryoglobulinemia: Clinical aspects and long-term follow-up of 40 patients. *Am J Med* 69:287, 1980.

21. Penny R, Hughes S: Repeated stimulation of the reticuloendothelial system and the development of plasma cell dyscrasias. *Lancet* 1:77, 1970.

22. Rosenblatt J, Hall CA: Plasma-cell dyscrasia followed prolonged stimulation of reticuloendothelial system. *Lancet* 1:301, 1970.

23. Turesson I, Rausing A: Gaucher's disease and benign monoclonal gammopathy. *Acta Med Scand* 197:507, 1975.

24. Fischer AM, Simon F, Le Deist F, et al: Prospective study of the occurrence of monoclonal gammopathies following bone marrow transplantation in young children. *Transplantation* 49:731, 1990.

25. Mitus AJ, Stein R, Rappeport JM, et al: Monoclonal and oligoclonal gammopathy after bone marrow transplantation. *Blood* 74:2764, 1989.

26. Potter M, Pumphrey JG, Bailey DW: Genetics of susceptibility of plasmacytoma induction: I. BALB/c AnN(C), C57BL/6N(B6), C57BL/Ka(BK), (CxB6)F₁, (CxBK)F₁ and CxB recombinant inbred strains. *J Natl Cancer Inst* 54:1413, 1976.

27. Blattner WA: Multiple myeloma and macroglobulinemia, in *Cancer, Epidemiology and Prevention*, edited by D Schottenfeld, JF Fraumeni Jr, p 795. WB Saunders, Philadelphia, 1982.

28. Meijers KAE, Leeuw B, Voormolen-Kalova M: The multiple occurrence of myeloma and asymptomatic paraproteinemia within one family. *Clin Exp Immunol* 12:185, 1972.

29. Williams RC, Erickson JL, Polesky HF, et al: Studies on monoclonal immunoglobulins (M-components) in various kindreds. *Ann Intern Med* 67:309, 1967.

30. Kalff MW, Higmans W: Immunoglobulin analysis in families of macroglobulinemia patients. *Clin Exp Immunol* 5:479, 1969.

31. Potter LM, Blattner WA: Etiology an epidemiology of multiple myeloma and related disorders, in *Neoplastic Diseases of the Blood*, vol 1, edited by PH Wiernick, GP Canellos, RA Kyle, CA Schiffer, p 413. Churchill Livingstone, New York, 1985.

32. Cohn M, Notani G, Rice SA: Characterization of the antibody to the C carbohydrate produced by a transplantable mouse plasmacytoma. *Immunochemistry* 6:111, 1969.

33. Porter DD, Larsen AE, Porter HG: Aleutian disease of mink. *Adv Immunol* 29:261, 1980.

34. Goldenberg GJ, Paraskevas F, Israels LG: The association of rheumatoid arthritis with plasma cell and lymphocytic neoplasms. *Arthritis Rheum* 12:569, 1969.

35. Wegelius O, Skrifvars B: Rheumatoid arthritis terminating in plasmacytoma. *Acta Med Scand* 187:133, 1970.

36. Isomaki HA, Hakulmen T, Joutsenlahti U: Excess risk of lymphomas, leukemias and myelomas in patients with rheumatoid arthritis. *J Chronic Dis* 31:691, 1978.

37. Potter M: Concepts of pathogenesis and experimental models of immunoglobulin-secreting tumors in animals, in *Neoplastic Diseases of the Blood*, vol 1, edited by PH Wiernick, GP Canellos, RA Kyle, CA Schiffer, p 393. Churchill Livingstone, New York, 1985.

38. Mushinski JF, Bauer SR, Potter M, et al: Increased expression of myc and related oncogene RNA characterizes most BALB/c plasmacytomas induced by pristane or Abelson virus. *Proc Natl Acad Sci U S A* 80:1073, 1983.

39. Rowley JD: Human oncogene locations and chromosome aberrations. *Nature* 301:290, 1983.

40. Heim S, Mitelman F: Chronic lymphoproliferative disorders, in *Cancer Cytogenetics*, edited by T Moore, p 175. Alan R. Liss, New York, 1987.

41. Cavanaugh M, Chan HS, Cohen IH, et al: *Regional localization of genes and DNA segments on human chromosomes*: number 5, HGM10, p 26. Howard Hughes Medical Institute and Yale University, 1989.

42. Perez-Simon JA, Garcia-Sanz R, Taberno MD, et al: Prognostic value of numerical chromosome aberrations in multiple myeloma: A FISH analysis of 15 different chromosomes. *Blood* 91:3366, 1998.

43. Klein B, Zhang XG, Jourdan M, et al: Interleukin 6 is the central tumor growth factor in vitro and in vivo in multiple myeloma. *Eur Cytokine Netw* 1:193, 1990.

44. Hirano T: Interleukin 6 (IL-6) and its receptor: Their role in plasma cell neoplasias. *Int J Cell Cloning* 9:166, 1991.

45. Nilsson K, Jernberg H, Pettersson M: IL-6 as a growth factor for human multiple myeloma cells—A short overview. *Curr Top Microbiol Immunol* 166:3, 1990.

46. Klein B, Zhang X-G, Jourdan M, et al: Interleukin-6 is a major myeloma cell growth factor in vitro and in vivo especially in patients with terminal disease. *Curr Top Microbiol Immunol* 166:23, 1990.

47. Suematsu S, Hibi M, Sugita T, et al: Interleukin 6 (IL-6) and its receptor (IL-6R) in myeloma/plasmacytoma. *Curr Top Microbiol Immunol* 166:13, 1990.

48. Retteg MB, Ma HJ, Vescio RA, et al: Kaposi's sarcoma-associated herpesvirus infection of bone marrow-dendritic cells from multiple myeloma patients. *Science* 276:1851, 1997.

49. Vidriales MB, Anderson KC: Adhesion of multiple myeloma cells to the bone marrow microenvironment: Implications for future therapeutic strategies. *Mol Med Today* 2:425, 1996.

50. Lichtenstein A, Berenson J, Norma D, et al: Production of cytokines by bone marrow cells obtained from patients with multiple myeloma. *Blood* 74:1206, 1989.

51. Bataille R, Jourdan M, Zhang X-G, et al: Serum levels of interleukin 6, a potent myeloma cell growth factor, as a reflection of disease severity in plasma cell dyscrasias. *J Clin Invest* 84:2008, 1989.

52. Bergsagel DE: Plasma cell myeloma: Biology and treatment. *Annu Rev Med* 42:167, 1991.

53. Grogan TM, Durie B, Spier CM, et al: Myelomonocytic antigen positive myeloma. *Blood* 73:763, 1989.

54. Epstein J, Xiao H, He X: Markers of multiple hematopoietic lineages in multiple myeloma. *N Engl J Med* 322:664, 1990.

55. Smith JK: The significance of the "protein error" of indicators in the diagnosis of Bence Jones proteinuria. *Acta Haematol* 530:144, 1963.

56. Harnly ME, Swan SH, Holly EA, et al: Temporal trends in the incidence of non-Hodgkin's lymphoma and selected malignancies in a population

with a high incidence of acquired immunodeficiency syndrome (AIDS). *Am J Epidemiol* 128:261, 1988.

57. Cleary ML, Dorfman RF, Sklar J: Failure in immunological control of the virus infection: Post-transplant lymphomas, in *The Epstein-Barr Virus: Recent Advances*, edited by MA Epstein, BG Achong, p 163. Heinemann Medical, London, 1986.

58. Beral V, Peterman T, Berkelman R, et al: AIDS-associated non-Hodgkin lymphoma. *Lancet* 337:805, 1991.

59. Child AJ, Kushwaha MRS: Serum beta 2-microglobulin in lymphoproliferative and myeloproliferative diseases. *Hematol Oncol* 2:391, 1984.

60. Bataille R, Grenier J, Sany J, et al: Beta-2-microglobulin: Optimal use for staging, prognosis and treatment—A prospective study of 160 patients. *Blood* 63:468, 1984.

61. Bataille R, Durie BGM, Grenier J, et al: Prognostic factors and staging in multiple myeloma: A reappraisal. *J Clin Oncol* 4:80, 1986.

62. Cuzik J, Cooper EH, MacLennan ICM: The prognostic value of serum β2 microglobulin compared with other presentation features in myelomatosis. *Br J Cancer* 52:1, 1985.

63. Capra JD, Kunkel HG: Aggregation of γ3 proteins: Relevance to the hyperviscosity syndrome. *J Clin Invest* 49:610, 1970.

64. Franklin EC: Immunopathology of the amyloid diseases. *Hosp Pract* 15: 70, 1980.

65. Kyle RA, Greipp PR: Amyloidosis (AL): Clinical and laboratory features in 229 cases. *Mayo Clin Proc* 58:665, 1983.

ESSENTIAL MONOCLONAL GAMMOPATHIES

MARSHALL A. LICHTMAN

Essential monoclonal gammopathy is defined by two key features: (1) the presence of a monoclonal immunoglobulin in the serum or of monoclonal light chains in the urine and (2) the absence of evidence for an overt or progressive malignancy of B lymphocytes or plasma cells (e.g., lymphoma, myeloma, or amyloidosis). Essential monoclonal gammopathy increases in prevalence from approximately 1 percent in individuals aged 30 years to 10 percent in those 80 years older. The condition has been reported in association with a large variety of disorders, especially nonlymphocytic cancers. These coincidences are thought, in most cases, to be the chance concurrence of conditions that have a high prevalence in older populations. Some cases of essential monoclonal gammopathy are symptomatic because the immunoglobulin can interact with plasma proteins or neural tissue and cause serious dysfunction, for example, an acquired bleeding disorder or incapacitating neuropathies. In such cases, disability may be so great that attempts to remove the immunoglobulin by plasmapheresis and to suppress its production using immune or cytotoxic therapy can be warranted. Because myeloma or lymphoma may be about to emerge at the time the monoclonal immunoglobulin is first detected, periodic evaluation of the patient is required to ascertain if essential monoclonal gammopathy is the appropriate diagnosis. Long-term followup at appropriate intervals is prudent to detect conversion from a stable, asymptomatic condition to a progressive lymphoma or myeloma, which occurs in approximately 1 percent of cases per year. In the absence of a symptomatic gammopathy or evolution to a progressive clonal gammopathy, careful periodic followup is all that is required.

DEFINITION AND HISTORY

The syndrome of essential monoclonal gammopathy has two important characteristics. The first feature is a plasma immunoglobulin (Ig) or urinary Ig light chain that has the molecular features of the product of a single clone of B lymphocytes or plasma cells: homogeneous electrophoretic migration and a single light-chain type. The second feature is the absence of evidence of an overt neoplastic disorder of B lymphocytes or plasma cells, such as lymphoma, myeloma, or amyloidosis.

The observations that Bence Jones proteinuria can precede by many years the clinical signs of multiple myeloma[1] and that hyperglobulinemia without evidence of multiple myeloma can occur in some patients[2] antedated the concept of monoclonal gammopathy as a syndrome. With the more frequent clinical application of zonal electrophoresis of plasma proteins during the 1950s and 1960s, patients were discovered who had a monoclonal Ig either without an associated dis-

ease or with diseases such as nonlymphoid cancers, infections, and inflammatory disorders, which typically are not associated with a monoclonal proliferation of B lymphocytes.[3-10] The presence of a monoclonal protein in plasma or urine is referred to as *essential monoclonal gammopathy* if it is not associated with a disease. More than 30 synonyms for the syndrome have been used, particularly *essential monoclonal gammopathy* and *benign monoclonal gammopathy*.[6] *Monoclonal gammopathy of unknown significance* became fashionable as a designation preferable to *benign monoclonal gammopathy* because some patients progressed to myeloma, macroglobulinemia, amyloidosis, or a B cell lymphoma over decades of observation.[10,11] The term *essential monoclonal gammopathy* seems best, because it neither highlights a benign process nor indicates that the risks of subsequent lymphoma or myeloma are unknown; those risks are widely appreciated. Table 99-1 presents a classification of monoclonal gammopathies.

OCCURRENCE

Monoclonal gammopathy can occur at any age, but it is unusual before puberty, and its frequency increases with age.[12] The frequency of a serum paraprotein using zonal electrophoresis is approximately 1 percent in persons older than 25 years,[4] approximately 3 percent in those older than 70 years,[4,9] and approximately 10 percent in those older than 80 years.[3] A much higher prevalence of monoclonal gammopathy has been reported using more sensitive screening methods, such as isoelectric focusing or immunoblotting.[13,14] The prevalence rate among Americans of African descent is significantly greater than the rates among those of European descent in each age group over 50 years.[15,16] Familial occurrence also has been described.[17,18] An increased incidence of monoclonal gammopathy is associated with several occupational groups, including farmers and industrial workers.[19]

ETIOLOGY AND PATHOGENESIS

Monoclonal gammopathy can be compared with any benign tumor, such as a colonic polyp, which can remain the same size indefinitely or undergo malignant transformation at an unpredictable future time.

Monoclonal gammopathy is caused by the proliferation of a single B lymphocyte, a plasma cell progenitor, leading to a clonal population that reaches a steady state at or below approximately 1×10^{11} cells. At this cell population density, marrow lymphocyte or plasma cell prevalence is indistinguishable from that of normal marrow. IgG and IgA monoclonal gammopathy arise from somatically mutated post switch preplasma cells and may have translocations involving the Ig heavy-chain region on chromosome 14. IgM monoclonal gammopathy arises from a mutated postgerminal center lymphocyte that does not have evidence of isotype switching.[20] Not surprisingly, this situation determines the phenotype of the clonal B lymphocytic diseases that may evolve, principally plasma cell phenotypes of myeloma or plasmacytoma for IgG and IgA and Waldenström macroglobulinemia and lymphomas for IgM monoclonal gammopathies. The expanded clone secretes monoclonal Ig at a rate per cell sufficient for detection by standard tests. The clonal expansion, however, does not cause osteolysis, hypercalcemia, renal insufficiency, inhibit hematopoietic proliferation and maturation, or impair differentiation of polyclonal B lymphocytes to plasma cells. As such, polyclonal Ig synthesis is nor-

TABLE 99-1 TYPES OF MONOCLONAL IMMUNOGLOBULIN SYNTHESIZED BY ABNORMAL CELL CLONE

IgG, IgA, IgM,[6-11] IgE,[27] IgD[28,29]

IgG + IgA, IgG + IgM, IgG + IgA + IgM[30-33]

Monoclonal κ or λ light chain (Bence Jones proteinuria)[10,34]

Acronyms and abbreviations that appear in this chapter include: AIDS, acquired immunodeficiency syndrome; Ig, immunoglobulin; IL, interleukin.

mal, and patients do not necessarily incur an increased risk of infection. The cells in the benign clone do not accumulate further and do not elaborate significant amounts of osteoclast-activating factors that are responsible for bone destruction.

Despite these significant differences from myeloma in the behavior of the neoplastic B cells, cytogenetic abnormalities akin to those seen in myeloma may be present in plasma cells derived from patients with essential monoclonal gammopathy.[20–27] Standard cytogenetic evaluations usually are normal. However, clones containing numerical abnormalities (e.g., trisomy or monosomy) involving chromosomes 3, 7, 11,13, 17, and 18 and translocations involving 14q, the site of the Ig heavy-chain genes, have been identified with fluorescence *in situ* hybridization. The presence of clonal cytogenetics changes may or may not be antecedents to clonal evolution. Although approximately 25 to 30 percent of patients with myeloma have an antecedent period of essential monoclonal gammopathy and presumably undergo clonal evolution to myeloma,[23,26] the presence of clonal cytogenetic abnormalities does not necessarily result in such evolution.[20,25] Gene expression studies of plasma cells isolated from normal marrow and marrow from patients with essential monoclonal gammopathy have identified genes that are differentially underexpressed or overexpressed.[28,29] Expression patterns identified several hundred genes that were significantly different when plasma cells from normal subjects and patients with monoclonal gammopathy were compared.[29]

The C57BL mouse provides a model of benign monoclonal gammopathy. The frequency of monoclonal gammopathy increases with mouse age.[30] The condition can be transferred to either irradiated or nonirradiated mice by marrow or spleen cells.[31] The transfer can be accomplished only during the first four consecutive transplantations, and no effect is seen on the survival of the recipient compared with that of appropriate control subjects. In contrast, if mouse B cell lymphoma or myeloma cells are transplanted into normal mice, the engraftment frequency is higher than that of B cells from mice with benign gammopathy. Passage from the original recipient to a new recipient is unlimited. Progressive disease develops, and survival of recipients is decreased. Thus, an intrinsic difference exists in the growth potential (degree of malignancy) of these two B cell clones.[23] The frequency of monoclonal gammopathy increases with age, but progression to multiple myeloma in the C57BL mouse is a rare event.[32] Studies in transgenic mice and their litter mates replicate the increased incidence of B cell clones and gammopathy with aging.[33]

Occasionally, monoclonal gammopathy occurs from the exaggerated production of natural antibody by a B lymphocyte clone.[34] For example, patients with cold agglutinins may have monoclonal IgM for years. A few monoclonal IgM antibodies act as rheumatoid factors and may form cryoglobulins through complex formation with IgG molecules.

CLINICAL FEATURES

BLOOD CELLS AND MARROW

Blood counts and the marrow examination are normal. Notably anemia is not present and the proportion of plasma cells in marrow is less than 10 percent. Although percent of plasma cells is the most predictive morphologic feature of myeloma, the presence of cytological atypia as judged by overt plasma cell nucleoli is a finding even more characteristic of myeloma.[35] Use of interphase fluorescence *in situ* hybridization has uncovered numerical chromosome abnormalities in the plasma cells of more than 50 percent of subjects. Alterations include trisomy 6 or 9 and monosomy 13 or 17.[25] The role of these clones in the evolution of myeloma awaits longitudinal study because the frequency of these chromosome abnormalities is significantly different

compared to the frequency in patients with myeloma. Quantitative microscopy of marrow microvessels per high-power field using immunohistochemistry indicates microvessel density on average is threefold greater than in normal subjects but far less than in patients with myeloma, although overlap with myeloma is seen.[36]

MONOCLONAL PROTEIN

Characteristically, individuals are detected by the unexpected identification of a monoclonal protein in plasma or urine in the absence of symptoms or signs caused by diseases associated with monoclonal proteins (e.g., anemia, marrow plasmacytosis, lymph node enlargement, plasmacytoma, bone lesions, or amyloid deposits).[6–10,34,37–44]

Some patients have monoclonal proteins with antibody specificity directed against plasma or cell proteins, resulting in symptomatic pathophysiologic effects, such as immune hemolytic anemia,[45] acquired von Willebrand disease,[46,47] immune neutropenia,[48,49] or other functional manifestations (Table 99-2).

Rare patients with essential urinary light-chain excretion and renal disease have been described.[55–57]

NEUROPATHIES

A significant association exists between the occurrence of neuropathies and essential monoclonal gammopathy.[58–61] Approximately 10 percent of patients with idiopathic neuropathy have a monoclonal Ig, a frequency about eight times that of age-adjusted healthy comparison groups.[58–62] The frequency of neuropathy among patients with monoclonal gammopathy varies between 5 and 30 percent, depending on the distribution of Ig class. IgM monoclonal gammopathy has a significantly higher frequency of neuropathy than does IgG or IgA monoclonal gammopathy.[58,59] Monoclonal antibodies, especially IgM, can react with peripheral nerve myelin, specifically with myelin-associated glycoprotein, glycolipids, or sulfatides.[63–68] Although various anti-nerve antibodies are present in approximately 40 percent of patients with neuropathy and IgG monoclonal gammopathy, a similar frequency has been found in such patients without neuropathy.[58,69] Neuropathy in the absence of reactivity of the monoclonal protein with nerve implies other mechanisms also operate to cause nerve damage.[58,60,67] For example, 25 percent of 16 patients with IgG monoclonal gammopathy and neuropathy had polyclonal, not monoclonal, antibodies against neurofilament protein.[67] In addition, a proportion of patients develop a detectable monoclonal protein after the onset of the neuropathy and sometimes years after.[69]

Patients with essential IgM gammopathy and neuropathy can have dysesthesia of the hands and feet, loss of vibration and position sense, atrophy of distal muscles, ataxia, and intention tremor.[65,66,68] The monoclonal antibodies reactive with nerve antigens usually are of the IgM type. Serum often contains antibodies to myelin-associated glycoprotein.[58] In contrast, patients with essential IgG or IgA gammopathy usually have chronic inflammatory demyelinating polyneuropathy, but a minority have sensory axonal or mixed neuropathy.[69–72]

TABLE 99-2 FUNCTIONAL ABNORMALITIES ASSOCIATED WITH ESSENTIAL MONOCLONAL GAMMOPATHY

Plasma protein disturbances

   Antierythrocyte antibodies,[45] acquired von Willebrand disease,[46,47] immune neutropenia,[48,49] cryoglobulinemia,[10] cryofibrinogenemia,[10] acquired C1 esterase inhibitor deficiency (angioedema),[10] acquired antithrombin,[50] insulin antibodies,[51,52] antiacetylcholine receptor antibodies,[53] "antiphospholipid" antibodies[54]

Renal disease[55–57]

Neuropathies[58–75]

The neuropathy may be (1) mild with minor motor and/or sensory signs with or without mild functional impairment, (2) moderately disabling but with full range of activities, or (3) severely disabling, interfering with walking, dressing, and eating.[69] The course may be relapsing and remitting or progressive. Essential IgA gammopathy has been associated with dysautonomia.[73] The presence or absence of antibody to myelin-associated glycoprotein may have an effect on the specific nature of the neuropathic manifestations.[60,65-68]

Demyelinization is reflected in decreased nerve conduction velocity. Axonal loss is reflected in decreased sensory potentials.[60,64,65,70-74] Electromyography may show denervation of muscles.[60,64] Immunofluorescence studies of sural nerve or of skin biopsies may uncover Ig binding to nerve.[60,65] Morphologic studies of nerve biopsies may show decreased or absent myelinated fibers or axonal degeneration.

Six treatment approaches may result in improvement in the neuropathies: (1) glucocorticoids alone, (2) intravenous Ig administration, e.g., 0.4 g/kg body weight per day for 5 days, (3) immunoadsorption of perfused blood with staphylococcal protein A, (4) plasma exchange, e.g., total of 220 ml/kg, administered in four to five treatments, (5) immunosuppressive cytotoxic chemotherapy, such as cyclophosphamide, e.g., 2.5 mg/kg body weight per day, or chlorambucil, e.g., 0.05 mg/kg body weight per day with or without added glucocorticoids, e.g., prednisone 0.5 mg/kg body weight per day, and (6) high-dose cytotoxic therapy with autologous hematopoietic stem cell rescue.[60,68,69,75-82] In some cases, use of plasmapheresis has been followed by cytotoxic therapy in an effort to produce a sustained effect. Plasma exchange has shown benefit in a clinical trial. The other modalities of treatment await such studies.[60] Response rates to each form of therapy are low and duration of response is variable,[60,69,76-81] but some patients, perhaps one in six, obtain significant improvement for prolonged periods.

COINCIDING DISORDERS

Monoclonal gammopathy unrelated to a clinically evident proliferation of B lymphocytes or plasma cells has been observed in association with a wide variety of conditions (Table 99-3).[83-144] Although they are grouped under the designation *monoclonal gammopathy with a coincidental disease*, few such reports have examined whether the coincidence is greater than expected from a control group matched for age and ethnicity, the two variables having the greatest impact on the incidence of monoclonal gammopathy. Non–B cell malignancies, including solid tumors,[3,5,6,119-122] myeloproliferative disorders,[123-127] and non–B cell lymphomas,[128-131] are associated with paraproteinemia. These relationships could result from various factors: (1) patients with an M component have an increased risk of developing cancer, (2) the M component is an antibody against some antigen associated with the cancer, (3) the globulin is the product of cancer cells, or (4) coincidence. The last possibility is favored by one epidemiologic study that found the same frequency of monoclonal gammopathy in a matched control group as in cancer patients.[9] Furthermore, when the monoclonal Ig is associated with a cancer, it usually persists after surgical excision of the tumor.

Chemotherapy, radiotherapy, organ or marrow transplantation,[132-137] and other miscellaneous disorders[5,7,10,16,17,90,91] have been associated with a transient or persistent monoclonal Ig (see Table 99-3).

The high prevalence of monoclonal proteins and associated diseases, especially after age 50 years, indicates some of these associations are coincidental. Thus, although surgical correction of hyperparathyroidism has been associated with disappearance of the plasma monoclonal protein,[101] statistical studies of this disorder suggest a coincidental relationship in most patients.[102] In hematopoietic stem cell

TABLE 99-3 DISORDERS REPORTED IN COINCIDENCE WITH MONOCLONAL GAMMOPATHY

Connective tissue diseases and autoimmune diseases: Crohn disease, Hashimoto thyroiditis, lupus erythematosus, myasthenia gravis, pernicious anemia, polymyalgia rheumatica, psoriatic arthritis, rheumatoid arthritis, scleroderma, Sjögren disease[83-91]

Corneal diseases: pseudo-Kayser-Fleischer ring,[92] corneal gammopathy[93]

Cutaneous diseases: hyperkeratotic spicules, pyoderma gangrenosum (neutrophilic dermatoses), psoriasis, scleromyxedema, Schnitzler syndrome, urticaria[94-100]

Endocrine diseases: hyperparathyroidism[101,102]

Gaucher disease[103,104]

Hepatic disease: cirrhosis,[91] hepatitis,[105,106]

Hereditary spherocytosis[107]

Infectious diseases: bacterial endocarditis, *Corynebacterium* species, cytomegalovirus, human immunodeficiency virus, *Mycobacterium tuberculosis*, purpura fulminans[91,108-112]

Metabolic disease: hyperlipidemia[113]

Neutropenia, chronic[114]

Pituitary macroadenoma [115]

Pregnancy[116]

Pseudomyeloma (severe osteoporosis)[117,118]

Non–B cell or plasma cell neoplasms

Carcinomas: colon, lung, prostate, other[3,5,6,119-122]

Myeloproliferative diseases: acute and chronic myelogenous leukemia, polycythemia vera[123-127]

T cell lymphomas: Sézary syndrome[128-131]

After chemotherapy, radiotherapy, or marrow, kidney, or liver transplantation[132-137]

Miscellaneous diseases[138-140]

Transient, monoclonal, or oligoclonal gammopathies[141-143]

Factitious hyperterremia[144]

---

diseases, some observers have proposed that the paraprotein reflects subtle B cell lineage involvement. In inflammatory, autoimmune, and infectious diseases, the association has been viewed as an unusual expansion of a restricted population of B lymphocytes. Following marrow transplantation, the presence of oligoclonal blood B lymphocyte populations reflects the process of reconstitution of the B cell population.

LABORATORY FEATURES

PLASMA AND URINARY MONOCLONAL IMMUNOGLOBULINS

The monoclonal protein usually is IgG; however, IgM, IgA, IgD, and IgE, urinary light chains, double gammopathy involving IgA and IgG or IgM and IgA, and triple gammopathy can occur (see Table 99-1).[119,145] By definition, no findings other than a plasma or urinary M component are present that permit diagnosis of B lymphocyte or plasma cell malignancy.

In monoclonal gammopathy of the IgG type, the concentration of monoclonal Ig usually is less than 3.0 g/dl. In the IgA or IgM type, the concentration usually is less than 2.5 g/dl.[10,145] However, dramatic exceptions to this rule exist. Occasional patients with essential monoclonal gammopathy have concentrations as high as 6.0 g/dl. Some patients have Bence Jones proteinuria as the sole manifestation of monoclonal gammopathy.[1,10] The amount of urinary light chains excreted occasionally is so large (>1.0 g/day) that renal dysfunction develops.[55]

Most patients with myeloma or macroglobulinemia have significantly depressed non-monoclonal Ig levels. For example, patients with IgG myeloma usually have very low IgA and IgM concentrations and reduced polyclonal IgG level. Patients with monoclonal gammopathy usually have normal polyclonal Ig levels. Any depression of their polyclonal Ig levels usually is not as severe as in myeloma.[10,145,146]

OLIGOCLONAL IMMUNOGLOBULINS

Oligoclonal or monoclonal serum Igs have been detected with high-resolution agarose gel electrophoresis in hospitalized patients with acute phase reactions or polyclonal hyperglobulinemia.[143] Oligoclonal Ig bands are frequently seen in the cerebrospinal fluid and serum of patients with a variety of neurologic conditions, especially in patients with multiple sclerosis when the fluids are analyzed by isoelectric focusing.[147] Patients with acquired immunodeficiency syndrome (AIDS) have B cell activation and aberrancies of B cell regulation. High-resolution electrophoresis indicates most AIDS patients with advanced disease have monoclonal or oligoclonal serum Ig bands. Subjects with AIDS, lymphadenopathy syndrome, or antibody to the human immunodeficiency virus also have oligoclonal or monoclonal Ig bands by standard zonal electrophoresis.[109,110] These monoclonal proteins are IgG.

LYMPHOCYTE AND PLASMA CELL PHENOTYPES

The concentration of plasma cells in the marrow is less than 10 percent, and the incorporation of tritiated thymidine into marrow plasma cells is negligible (<1%) in essential monoclonal gammopathy. Marrow plasma cells in monoclonal gammopathy do not express neural cell adhesion molecule, whereas myeloma cells strongly express this surface protein.[148] Blood T lymphocyte subset levels are normal in monoclonal gammopathy, whereas CD4+ T cell levels are lower and CD8+ T cell levels higher in myeloma and macroglobulinemia.[149–152] Blood B cell concentration is normal in monoclonal gammopathy but often is decreased in myeloma patients. Clonally restricted, idiotype-positive blood B cells are characteristic of myeloma but not of monoclonal gammopathy.[153]

β_2-microglobulin is the light chain of cell surface HLA molecules and normally is present at low concentrations in serum. Its concentration in serum frequently is elevated in myeloma, and the magnitude of the elevation is positively correlated with tumor mass. β_2-microglobulin concentration is not elevated in essential monoclonal gammopathy.[154,155]

The distinction between stable essential monoclonal gammopathy and emerging (so-called larval myeloma) or low-infiltrate myeloma (so-called smoldering myeloma) with a very low tumor burden is blurred at the margins. This finding has not kept investigators from looking for a distinguishing test. More than 35 variables have been studied as an index for discriminating benignity from malignancy (Table 99-4). No single test is sufficiently sensitive and specific to be useful in an individual patient. Periodic examination of the patient is the best method for detecting the emergence of myeloma or a related disease. Measurement of the concentration of the serum monoclonal protein, urinary light chains, serum β_2-microglobulin, and hemoglobin concentration at appropriate intervals is required. The marrow should be reexamined if the monoclonal protein level increases or hemoglobin concentration decreases significantly. Practical methods for measuring bone density would be additional useful measures of stability or progression.

COURSE, PROGNOSIS, AND THERAPY

Longitudinal studies have reported three major patterns of outcome for patients with essential monoclonal gammopathy.[10,194–196] Approximately 25 percent of patients do not progress. In this group, occasional patients experience increases in monoclonal protein concentration of

TABLE 99-4 VARIABLES USED IN AN ATTEMPT TO DISTINGUISH ESSENTIAL MONOCLONAL GAMMOPATHY FROM MYELOMA OR LYMPHOMA

Lymphocytes and Immunoglobulins
  M protein serum concentration[145,146,156–158]
  Igκ light chain[158]
  Light chains in urine[158]
  Polyclonal Ig serum concentration[158]
  β_2-microglobulin or C-reactive protein serum concentration[154,155,157–159]
  Ig-secreting cells in blood[160]
  Idiotype-reactive blood T lymphocytes[161,162]
  CD4-to-CD8 lymphocyte ratio in blood or marrow[151,163–165]
  Clonally restricted B lymphocytes[153,166,167]
  Natural killer cell frequency[168]

Plasma Cells
  Frequency[6,7,9,10,158]
  Morphology[149,169,170]
  MB2 antibody reactivity[171]
  Proliferative index[149,150,159,169]
  Asynchronous replication [172]
  DNA content or interphase fluorescent in situ hybridization[21–23,169]
  Ratio of monoclonal CD19-/CD38+/CD56++ to polyclonal CD19+/CD38++/CD56- cells[173]
  Blood or marrow concentration[10,149,150,158,166]
  J chains[174]
  Acid phosphatase[175]
  Multidrug resistance expression[176]
  CD19 expression[177]
  CD56/neural cell adhesion molecule expression[148,177]
  Proportion of CD19+/CD56- plasma cells in marrow[178]
  5′ Nucleotidase[179]

Bone Integrity
  Magnetic resonance imaging[180,181]
  Dual-energy x-ray absorptiometry[182]
  Histomorphometry[183]
  Urinary pyridinium–collagen complexes[184]

Miscellaneous
  Marrow microvessel density[36]
  Neural cell adhesion molecules[185]
  Serum Il-1β[186]
  Serum IL-6, IL-10, soluble CD16, soluble IL-6 receptor, IL-1β[187–192]
  Serum TGF-β[193]
  Urinary deoxypyridoline excretion rate[193]
  Hemoglobin concentration
  Mononuclear cell E-cadhedrin gene methylation[203]

up to 50 percent of their initial diagnostic value. However, these patients restabilize and do not develop signs of myeloma, macroglobulinemia, amyloidosis, or lymphoproliferative disease. About half of patients die of an unrelated cause. The remaining 25 to 30 percent of patients develop plasmacytoma myeloma, amyloidosis, macroglobulinemia, lymphoma, or chronic lymphocytic leukemia over 2 decades of observation. The latter group of patients continues to increase slowly without reaching a plateau. Evolution to a progressive clonal B cell disorder has been observed more than 25 years after the diagnosis of monoclonal gammopathy. The actuarial risk of progressing to a clonal B cell malignancy for all classes of monoclonal protein is approximately 1 percent per year.[194–197] IgM gammopathy progresses to lymphoma, Waldenström macroglobulinemia, amyloidosis, or chronic lymphocytic leukemia.[204] Although one large study found that IgM monoclonal gammopathy progressed to a progressive clonal lymphoid disorder at a rate of approximately 1.5 percent per year,[198] two other large studies found no significant difference in the rate of progression when patients with IgG or IgM were compared.[199,200] IgG or IgA monoclonal gammopathy evolves principally into myeloma, plasmacytoma, or amyloidosis. Patients with higher percentages of plasma cells in the marrow or higher monoclonal Ig levels at the time of diagnosis evolve to a progressive clonal B lymphocyte disease more rapidly.[199–202] In rare patients, the monoclonal protein appears transiently in relation to a disease (e.g., infection)[141–143] or disappears spontaneously even when not associated with a disease.[3]

Generally, the diagnosis of essential monoclonal gammopathy cannot be made with certainty at the time of the initial evaluation. Periodic reexamination is required to document a stable clinical course. Therapy usually is not required without a confirmed diagnosis of myeloma, macroglobulinemia, amyloidosis, or lymphoma with evidence of progressive disease. Therapy may be indicated, however, if the monoclonal protein interferes with the vital function of a normal plasma or tissue constituent or is associated with a disabling neuropathy.

REFERENCES

1. Prentiss RG Jr: Multiple myeloma with diffuse skeletal involvement: Case report. *Mil Surg* 80:294, 1937.

2. Waldenstrom JG: Incipient myelomatosis or essential hyperglobulinemia with fibrinogenopenia: A new syndrome? *Acta Med Scand* 117: 216, 1944.

3. Hallen J: Frequency of "abnormal serum globulins" (M-components) in the aged. *Acta Med Scand* 173:737, 1963.

4. Axelsson U, Bachmann R, Hallen J: Frequency of pathological proteins (M-components) in 6995 sera from an adult population. *Acta Med Scand* 179:235, 1966.

5. Migliore PJ, Alexanian R: Monoclonal gammopathy in human neoplasia. *Cancer* 21:1127, 1968.

6. Ritzmann SE, Loukes D, Sakai H, et al: Idiopathic (asymptomatic) monoclonal gammopathies. *Arch Intern Med* 135:95, 1975.

7. Amies A, Ko HS, Pruzanski W: M-components: A review of 1242 cases. *Can Med Assoc J* 114:889, 1976.

8. Lindstrom FD, Dahlstrom V: Multiple myeloma or benign monoclonal gammopathy? A study of differential diagnostic criteria in 44 cases. *Clin Immunol Immunopathol* 10:168, 1978.

9. Salerin JP, Vicariot M, Deroff P, et al: Monoclonal gammopathies in the adult population of Finistère, France. *J Clin Pathol* 35:63, 1982.

10. Kyle RA: Monoclonal gammopathy of undetermined significance and solitary myeloma. *Hematol Oncol Clin North Am* 11:71, 1997.

11. Owen RG, Parapia LA, Higginson J, et al: Clinicopathological correlates of IgM paraproteinemias. *Clin Lymphoma* 1:39, 2000.

12. Ligthart GL, Radl J, Corberand JX, et al: Monoclonal gammopathies in human aging: Increased occurrence with age and correlation with health status. *Mech Ageing Dev* 52:235, 1990.

13. Sinclair D, Sheehan T, Parrott DMV, Stott DI: The incidence of monoclonal gammopathy in a population over 45 years old determined by isoelectric focusing. *Br J Haematol* 67:745, 1986.

14. Radl J, Wels J, Hoogeven CM: Immunoblotting with (sub)class specific antibodies reveals a high frequency of monoclonal antibodies in persons thought to be immunodeficient. *Clin Chem* 34:1839, 1988.

15. Schecter GP, Shoff N, Chan C, et al: The frequency of monoclonal gammopathy in black and white veterans in a hospital population, in *Epidemiology and Biology of Multiple Myeloma*, edited by GI Obrams, M Potter, p 93. Springer-Verlag, New York, 1991.

16. Singh J, Dudley AW, Kulig KA: Increased incidence of monoclonal gammopathy of undetermined significance in blacks and its age-related differences with whites on the basis of a study of 397 men and one woman in a hospital setting. *J Lab Clin Med* 116:785, 1990.

17. Bizzaro N, Pasini P: Familial occurrence of multiple myeloma and monoclonal gammopathy of undetermined significance in siblings. *Haematologica* 75:58, 1990.

18. Lynch HT, Sanger WG, Pirruccello S, et al: Familial multiple myeloma: A family study and review of the literature. *J Natl Cancer Inst* 94: 1479, 2001.

19. Pasqualetti P, Collacciani A, Casole R: Risk of monoclonal gammopathy of undetermined significance. *Am J Hematol* 52:217, 1996.

20. Fonesca R, Bailey RJ, Ahmann GJ, et al: Genomic abnormalities in monoclonal gammopathy of undetermined significance. *Blood* 100: 1417, 2002.

21. Zandecki M, Lai JL, Genevieve F, et al: Several cytogenetic subclones may be identified within plasma cells from patients with monoclonal gammopathy of undetermined significance both at diagnosis and during the indolent course of the disease. *Blood* 90:3682, 1997.

22. Avet-Loiseau H, Facon T, Daviet A, et al: 14q32 translocations and monosomy 13 observed in monoclonal gammopathy of undetermined significance delineate a multistep process for the oncogenesis of multiple myeloma. *Cancer Res* 59:4546, 1999.

23. Avet-Loiseau H, Li J-Y, Morineau N: Monosomy 13 is associated with the transition of monoclonal gammopathy of undetermined significance to multiple myeloma. *Blood* 94:2583, 1999.

24. Bernasconi P, Cavigliano PM, Boni M, et al: Long-term follow up with conventional cytogenetics and band 13q14 interphase/metaphase in situ hybridization monitoring in monoclonal gammopathies of undetermined significance. *Br J Haematol* 118:545, 2002.

25. Rasillo A, Tabernero MD, Sanchez ML, et al: Fluorescence in situ hybridization analysis of aneuploidization patterns in monoclonal gammopathy of undetermined significance versus multiple myeloma and plasma cell leukemia. *Cancer* 97:601, 2003.

26. Zojer N, Ludwig H, Fiegi M, et al: Patterns of somatic mutations in VH genes reveal pathways of clonal transformations from MGUS to multiple myeloma. *Blood* 101:4137, 2003.

27. Lloveras E, Sole F, Florensa L, et al: Contribution of cytogenetics and in situ hybridization to the study of monoclonal gammopathy of undetermined significance. *Cancer Genet Cytogenet* 132:25, 2002.

28. Davies FE, Dring AM, Li C, et al: Insights into the multistep transformation of MGUS to myeloma using microarray expression analysis. *Blood* 102:4504, 2003.

29. Zhan F, Hardin J, Kordesmeier B, et al: Global gene expression profiling of multiple myeloma, monoclonal gammopathy of undetermined significance, and normal bone marrow plasma cells. *Blood* 99:1745, 2002.

30. Radl J, Hollander CF: Homogeneous immunoglobulins in sera of mice during aging. *J Immunol* 112:2271, 1974.

31. Radl J, DeGlopper E, Schuit HRE, Zurcher C: Idiopathic paraproteinemia: II. Transplantation of the paraprotein-producing clone from old to young 57B1/KaLwRij mice. *J Immunol* 122:609, 1979.

32. Radl J: Age-related monoclonal gammopathies: Clinical lessons from the aging C57BL mouse. *Immunol Today* 11:234, 1990.

33. van Arkel C, Hopstaken CM, Zurcher C, et al: Monoclonal gammopathies in aging m,x-transgenic mice: Involvement of the B-1 cell lineage. *Eur J Immunol* 27:2436, 1997.

34. George G, Gilburd B, Schoenfeld Y: The emerging concept of pathogenic natural antibodies. *Hum Antibodies* 8:70, 1997.

35. Milla F, Oriol A, Aguilar J, et al: Usefulness and reproducibility of cytomorphic evaluations to differentiate myeloma from monoclonal gammopathies of unknown significance. *Am J Clin Pathol* 115:127, 2001.

36. Rajkumar SV, Mesa RA, Fonesca R, et al: Bone marrow angiogenesis in 400 patients with monoclonal gammopathy of undetermined significance, multiple myeloma, and primary amyloidosis. *Clin Cancer Res* 8: 2210, 2002.

37. Ludwig H, Vormittag W: "Benign" monoclonal Ig E gammopathy. *Br Med J* 281:539, 1980.

38. O'Connor ML, Rice DT, Buss DH, Muss HB: Immunoglobulin D benign monoclonal gammopathy. *Cancer* 68:611, 1991.

39. Kinoshita K, Nagai H, Murate T, et al: Ig D monoclonal gammopathy of undetermined significance. *Int J Hematol* 65:169, 1997.

40. Imhof JW, Balliux RE, Mul NAJ, Poen H: Monoclonal and diclonal gammopathies. *Acta Med Scand* 179(suppl 455):102, 1966.

41. Jensen K, Jensen B, Olesen H: Three M-components in serum from an apparently healthy person. *Scand J Haematol* 4:485, 1967.

42. Kyle RA, Robinson RA, Katzmann JA: The clinical aspects of biclonal gammopathies: Review of 57 cases. *Am J Med* 71:999, 1981.

43. Riddell S, Traczyk Z, Paraskevas F, Israels LG: The double gammopathies: Clinical and immunological studies. *Medicine (Baltimore)* 65: 135, 1986.

44. Kyle RA, Greipp PR: "Idiopathic" Bence-Jones proteinuria. *N Engl J Med* 306:564, 1982.

45. Kay NE, Gordon LI, Douglas SD: Autoimmune hemolytic anemia in association with monoclonal IgM(k) with anti-i-activity. *Am J Med* 64: 845, 1978.

46. Friederich PW, Wever PC, Briet E, et al: Successful treatment with recombinant factor VIIa of therapy-resistant severe bleeding in a patient with acquired von Willebrand disease. *Am J Hematol* 66:292, 2001.

47. Lamboley V, Zabraniecki L, Sie P, et al: Myeloma and monoclonal gammopathy of uncertain significance associated with acquired von Willebrand's syndrome. Seven new cases with a literature review. *Joint Bone Spine* 69:62, 2002.

48. Nocente R, Cammarota G, Gentiloni Silveri N, et al: A case of Sweet's syndrome associated with monoclonal immunoglobulin of IgG-lambda type and p-ANCA positivity. *Panminerva Med* 44:149, 2002.

49. Carrington PA, Walsh SE, Houghton JB: Benign paraproteinemia and immune neutropenia. *Clin Lab Haematol* 2:407, 1989.

50. Gabriel DA, Carr ME, Cook L, Roberts HR: Spontaneous antithrombin in a patient with benign paraprotein. *Am J Hematol* 25:85, 1987.

51. Sluiter WJ, Marrink J, Houwen B: Monoclonal gammopathy with an insulin binding IgG(K) M-component, associated with severe hypoglycaemia. *Br J Haematol* 62:679, 1986.

52. Wasada T, Egueli Y, Takayama S, Yoo K, et al: Insulin autoimmune syndrome associated with benign monoclonal gammopathy. *Diabetes Care* 12:147, 1989.

53. Ahlberg RE, Lefvert AK: Monoclonal gammopathy and antibody activity against the acetylcholine receptor. *Am J Hematol* 29:49, 1988.

54. Disdier P, Swiader L, Aillaud M-F, et al: Ig M monoclonal gammopathy, lymphoid proliferations and lupus anticoagulant. *Am J Med* 102:319, 1997.

55. Maldonado JE, Velosa JA, Kyle RA, et al: Fanconi syndrome in adults: A manifestation of a latent form of myeloma. *Am J Med* 58:354, 1975.

56. Gavarotti P, Fortina F, Costa D, et al: Benign monoclonal gammopathy presenting with severe renal failure. *Scand J Haematol* 36:115, 1986.

57. Maes B, Vanwalleghem J, Kuypers D, et al: IgA antiglomerular basement membrane disease associated with bronchial carcinoma and monoclonal gammopathy. *Am J Kidney Dis* 33:E3, 1999

58. Vital A: Paraproteinemic neuropathies. *Brain Pathol* 11:399, 2001.

59. Kelly JJ: Neuropathies of monoclonal gammopathies of undetermined significance. *Hematol Oncol Clin North Am* 13:1203, 1999.

60. Ropper AH, Gorsin KC: Neuropathies associated with paraproteinemia. *N Engl J Med* 338:1601, 1998.

61. Kissel JT, Mendell JR: Neuropathies associated with monoclonal gammopathies. *Neuromusc Disord* 6:3, 1996.

62. Vallatt JM, Jauberteau MO, Bordessoule D, et al: Link between peripheral neuropathy and monoclonal dysglobulinemia: A study of 66 cases. *J Neurol Sci* 137:124, 1996.

63. Lee KW, Inghirami G, Spatz L, et al: The B-cells that express anti-MAG antibodies in neuropathy and non-malignant IgM monoclonal gammopathy belong to the CD5 subpopulation. *J Neuroimmunol* 31:83, 1991.

64. Cocito D, Durelli L, Isoardo G: Different clinical, electrophysiological and immunological features of CDIP associated with paraproteinemia. *Acta Neurol Scand* 108:274, 2003.

65. Chassande B, Léger J-M, Younes-Chennoufi AB, et al: Peripheral neuropathy associated with IgM monoclonal gammopathy: Correlation between M-protein antibody activity and clinical/electrophysiological features in 40 cases. *Muscle Nerve* 21:55, 1998.

66. Pestronk A, Li F, Bieser BS, et al: Anti-MAG antibodies. *Neurology* 44: 1131, 1994.

67. Stubbs EB Jr, Lawlor MW, Richards MP, et al: Anti-neurofilament antibodies in neuropathy with monoclonal gammopathy of undetermined significance produce experimental motor nerve conduction block. *Acta Neuropathol* 105:109, 2003.

68. Ellie E, Vital A, Steck A, et al: Neuropathy associated with "benign" anti-myelin-associated glycoprotein IgM gammopathy: Clinical, immunological, neurophysiological pathological findings and response to treatment in 33 cases. *J Neurol* 243:34, 1996.

69. Di Troia A, Carpo M, Meucci N, et al: Clinical features and anti-neural reactivity in neuropathy associated with IgG monoclonal gammopathy of undetermined significance. *J Neurol Sci* 164:64, 1999.

70. Gorsin KC, Ropper AH: Axonal neuropathy associated with monoclonal gammopathy of undetermined significance. *J Neurol Neurosurg Psychiatry* 63:163, 1997.

71. Wilson JR, Stittsworth JD Jr, Fisher MA: Electrodiagnostic patterns in MGUS neuropathy. *Electromyogr Clin Neurophysiol* 41:409, 2001.

72. Nicholas G, Maisonobe T, Le Forestier N, et al: Proposed revised electrophysiological criteria for chronic inflammatory demyelinating polyradiculopathy. *Muscle Nerve* 25:26, 2002.

73. Bailey RO, Ritaccio AL, Bishop MB, Wu AY: Benign monoclonal IgAk gammopathy associated with polyneuropathy and dysautonomia. *Acta Neurol Scand* 73:574, 1986.

74. Jonsson V, Schroder HD, Trojaborg W, et al: Autoimmune reactions in patients with M-component and peripheral neuropathy. *J Intern Med* 232:185, 1992.

75. Gorsin KC, Allan G, Ropper AH: Chronic inflammatory demyelinating polyneuropathy: Clinical features and response to treatment in 67 consecutive patients with and without a monoclonal gammopathy. *Neurology* 48:321, 1997.

76. Latov N: Pathogenesis and therapy of neuropathies associated with monoclonal gammopathies. *Ann Neurol* 37(suppl 1):532, 1995.

77. Sghirlanzoni A, Solari A, Ciano C: Chronic inflammatory demyelinating polyradiculopathy: Long-term course and treatment of 60 patients. *Neurol Sci* 21:31, 2000.

78. Kiprov DD, Miller RG: Paraproteinemia associated with demyelinating polyneuropathy or myositis: Treatment with plasmapheresis and immunosuppressive drugs. *Artif Organs* 9:47, 1985.

79. Gorson KC: Clinical features, evaluation, and treatment of patients with polyneuropathy associated with monoclonal gammopathy of undetermined significance (MGUS). *J Clin Apheresis* 14:149, 1999.

80. Blume G, Pestronk A, Goodnough LT: Anti-MAG antibody-associated polyneuropathies: Improvement following immunotherapy with monthly plasma exchange and IV cyclophosphamide. *Neurology* 45: 1577, 1995.

81. Oksenhendler E, Chevret S, Léger JM, et al: Plasma exchange and chlorambucil in polyneuropathy associated with monoclonal IgM gammopathy. *J Neurol Neurosurg Psychiatry* 59:243, 1995.

82. Lee YC, Came N, Schwarer A, Day B: Autologous peripheral blood stem cell transplantation for peripheral neuropathy secondary to monoclonal gammopathy of unknown significance. *Bone Marrow Transplant* 30:53, 2002.

83. Burner E, Swahlen A, Cruchaud A: Nonmalignant monoclonal immunoglobulinemia, pernicious anemia, and gastric carcinoma: A model of immunologic dysfunction. *Am J Med* 60:1019, 1976.

84. Rowland LP, Osserman EF, Scharfman WB, et al: Myasthenia gravis with a myeloma-type gamma-G (IgG) immunoglobulin abnormality. *Am J Med* 46:599, 1969.

85. Ilfeld D, Barzilay J, Vana D, et al: IgG monoclonal gammopathy in four patients with polymyalgia rheumatica (letter). *Ann Rheum Dis* 44:501, 1985.

86. Nanji AA: Monoclonal gammopathy associated with Crohn's disease during treatment with total parenteral nutrition. *J Parenteral Nutr* 9:621, 1985.

87. Wallach D, Carado Y, Foldes C, Cottennot F: Dermatomyositis and monoclonal gammopathy. *Ann Dermatol Venereol* 112:783, 1985.

88. McFadden N, Ree K, Syland E, Larse TE: Scleredema adultorum associated with a monoclonal gammopathy and generalized hyperpigmentation. *Arch Dermatol* 123:629, 1987.

89. Oikarinen A, Ala-Kokko L, Palatsi R, et al: Scleroderma and paraproteinemia. *Arch Dermatol* 123:226, 1987.

90. Johnsson V, Svendsen B, Vostrup S, et al: Multiple autoimmune manifestations in monoclonal gammopathy of undetermined significance and chronic lymphocytic leukemia. *Leukemia* 10:327, 1996.

91. Kyle RA: Monoclonal gammopathy of unknown significance (MGUS). *Ballieres Clin Haematol* 8:761, 1995.

92. Probst LE, Hoffman E, Cherian MG, et al: Ocular copper deposition associated with benign monoclonal gammopathy and hypercupremia. *Cornea* 15: 94, 1996.

93. Secundo W, Seifert P: Monoclonal corneal gammopathy: Topographic considerations. *Ger J Ophthalmol* 5:262, 1996.

94. deKleijn EM, Telgt D, Laan R: Schnitzler's syndrome presenting as fever of unknown origin (FUO): The role of cytokines in its systemic features. *Neth J Med* 51:140, 1997.

95. Puddu P, Cianchini G, Giardelli CR, et al: Schnitzler's syndrome: Report of a new case and review of the literature. *Clin Exp Rheumatol* 15:91, 1997.

96. Wayte JA, Rogers S, Powell FC: Pyoderma gangrenosum, erythema elevatum diutinum and Ig A monoclonal gammopathy. *Australas J Dermatol* 36:21, 1995.

97. Doutre MS, Beylot C, Bioulac P, Bezian JH: Monoclonal IgM and chronic urticaria: Two cases. *Ann Allergy* 58:413, 1987.

98. Samochocki Z, Szudzinski A: Gangrenous pyoderma in monoclonal IgA gammopathy and functional disorders of T lymphocytes. *Przegl Dermatol* 73:409, 1986.

99. Abraham Z, Feuerman EJ: IgA benign monoclonal gammopathy with recurrent self-healing skin tumors. *J Am Acad Dermatol* 21:1303, 1989.

100. Paul C, Fermaud J-P, Flageul B, et al: Hyperkeratotic spicules and monoclonal gammopathy. *J Am Acad Dermatol* 33:346, 1995.

101. Schnur MJ, Appel GB, Bilezikian JP: Primary hyperparathyroidism and benign monoclonal gammopathy. *Arch Intern Med* 137:1201, 1977.

102. Rao DS, Antonelli R, Kane KR, et al: Primary hyperparathyroidism and monoclonal gammopathy. *Henry Ford Hosp Med J* 39:41, 1991.

103. Schoenfeld Y, Berliner S, Pinkhas J, Beutler E: The association of Gaucher's disease and dysproteinemias. *Acta Haematol (Basel)* 64:241, 1980.

104. Brady K, Corash L, Bhargava E: Multiple myeloma arising from monoclonal gammopathy of unknown significance in a patient with Gaucher's disease. *Arch Pathol Lab Med* 121:1108, 1997.

105. Andreone P, Zignego AL, Cursaro C, et al: Prevalence of monoclonal gammopathies in patients with hepatitis C virus infection. *Ann Intern Med* 129:294, 1998.

106. Hamazaaki K, Baba M, Hasegawa H, et al: Chronic hepatitis associated with monoclonal gammopathy of undetermined significance. *Gastroenterol Hepatol* 18:459, 2003.

107. Schafer AL, Miller JB, Lester EP, et al: Monoclonal gammopathy in hereditary spherocytosis: A possible pathogenetic relation. *Ann Intern Med* 88:45, 1978.

108. Danon F, Bussel A, Perol Y: Immunoglobulines monoclonales infections a cytomegalovirus et hémopathies malignes. *Ann Immunol* 128A: 83, 1977.

109. Papadopoulos NM, Lane HC, Costello R, et al: Oligoclonal immunoglobulins in patients with the acquired immunodeficiency syndrome. *Clin Immunol Immunopathol* 35:43, 1985.

110. Heriot K, Hallquist AE, Tomar RH: Paraproteinemia in patients with acquired immunodeficiency syndrome (AIDS) or lymphadenopathy syndrome (LAS). *Clin Chem* 31:1224, 1985.

111. Kouns DM, Marty AM, Sharpe RW: Oligoclonal bands in serum protein electrophoretograms of individuals with human immunodeficiency virus antibodies. *JAMA* 256:2343, 1986.

112. Ong F, Hermans J, Noordik EM, et al: A population-based registry on paraproteinaemia in the Netherlands. *Br J Haematol* 99:914, 1997.

113. Johnston JD, Lumb PJ, Wierzbicki AS: Hyperlipidaemia in association with benign paraproteinemia. *Ann Clin Bichem* 34:697, 1997.

114. Papadaki HA, Eliopoulos DG, Ponticoglou C, Eliopoulos GD: Increased frequency of monoclonal gammopathy of undetermined significance in patients with nonimmune chronic idiopathic neutropenia syndrome. *Int J Hematol* 73:339, 2001.

115. Tucci A, Bonadonna S, Cattaneo C, et al: Transformation of MGUS to overt multiple myeloma: The possible role of pituitary microadenoma secreting high levels of insulin-like growth factor 1 (IGF-1). *Leuk Lymphoma* 44:543, 2003.

116. Chryssikkopoulos A, Dalamaga AL, Hassiakos D: Monoclonal gammopathy of unknown significance in pregnancy. *Clin Exp Obstet Gynecol* 24:31, 1997.

117. Buonocore E, Solmon A, Kerley HE: Pseudomyeloma. *Radiology* 95: 41, 1970.

118. Maldonado JE, Riggs L, Bayrd ED: Pseudomyeloma. *Arch Intern Med* 135:267, 1975.

119. Kyle RA: Monoclonal gammopathy of unknown significance. *Curr Top Microbiol Immunol* 210:375, 1996.

120. Solomon A: Homogeneous (monoclonal) immunoglobulins in cancer. *Am J Med* 63:169, 1977.

121. Colls BM, Lorier MA: Immunocytoma, cancer, and other associations of monoclonal gammopathy: A review of 224 cases. *N Z Med J* 82:221, 1975.

122. Abdul M, Hassein NM: Gammopathy associated with advanced prostate cancer. *Urol Res* 23:185, 1995.

123. Shoenfeld Y, Berliner S, Ayalone A, et al: Monoclonal gammopathy in patients with chronic and acute myeloid leukemia. *Cancer* 54:280, 1984.

124. Berner Y, Berrebi A: Myeloproliferative disorders and nonmyelomatous paraprotein. *Isr J Med Sci* 22:109, 1986.

125. Tosato F, Fossaluzza V, Rossi P, et al: Monoclonal gammopathy of undetermined significance in a case of primary thrombocythemia. *Haematologica (Pavia)* 71:417, 1986.

126. Economopoulos T, Economidou J, Papageorgiou E, et al: Monoclonal gammopathy in chronic myeloproliferative disorders. *Blut* 58:7, 1989.

127. Ito T, Kojima H, Otani K, et al: Chronic neutrophilic leukemia associated with monoclonal gammopathy of unknown significance. *Acta Haematol* 95:140, 1996.

128. Offit K, Macris NT, Hellman G, Rotterdam, HZ: Consecutive lymphoma with monoclonal gammopathy in a married couple. *Cancer* 57:277, 1986.

129. Venencie PY, Winkelmann RK, Puissant A, Kyle RA: Monoclonal gammopathy in Sézary syndrome: Report of three cases and review of the literature. *Arch Dermatol* 120:605, 1984.

130. Kamihira S, Taguchi H, Kinoshita K, Ichimaru M: Monoclonal gammopathy in adult T-cell leukemia/lymphoma: A report of three cases. *Jpn J Clin Oncol* 14:699, 1984.

131. Chisesi I, Capnist G, Barbui T: Two serum IgG M-components of differing light chain types in a case of Hodgkin's disease. *Acta Haematol (Basel)* 55:250, 1976.

132. VanCamp B, Reynaerts PH, Naets JP, Radl J: Transient IgA₁-λ paraproteinemia during treatment of acute myeloblastic leukemia. *Blood* 55: 21, 1980.

133. Hammarstrom L, Smith CIE: Frequent occurrence of monoclonal gammopathies with an imbalanced light-chain ratio following bone marrow transplantation. *Transplantation* 43:447, 1987.

134. Mitus AJ, Stein R, Rappeport JM, et al: Monoclonal and oligoclonal gammopathy after bone marrow transplantation. *Blood* 74:2764, 1989.

135. Passweg J, Thiel G, Bock HA: Monoclonal gammopathy after intense induction immunosuppression in renal transplant patients. *Nephrol Dial Transplant* 11:2461, 1996.

136. Badley AD, Portela DF, Patel R, et al: Development of monoclonal gammopathy precedes the development of Epstein-Barr virus-induced posttransplant lymphoproliferative disorder. *Liver Transplant Surg* 2: 375, 1996.

137. Touchard G, Pasdeloup T, Parpeix J, et al: High prevalence and usual persistence of serum monoclonal immunoglobulins evidenced by sensitive methods in renal transplant recipients. *Nephrol Dial Transplant* 12:1199, 1997.

138. Ho JL, Polde PA, McEniry D, et al: Acquired immunodeficiency syndrome with progressive multifocal leukoencephalopathy and monoclonal B-cell proliferation. *Ann Intern Med* 100:693, 1984.

139. Nagler A, Ben-Arieh Y, Brenner B, et al: Eosinophilic fibrohistiocytic lesion of bone marrow associated with monoclonal gammopathy and osteolytic lesions. *Am J Hematol* 23:277, 1986.

140. Hineman VL, Phyliky RL, Banks PM: Angiofollicular lymph node hyperplasia and peripheral neuropathy: Association with monoclonal gammopathy. *Mayo Clin Proc* 57:379, 1982.

141. Radl J, VandenBerg A: Transitory appearance of homogeneous immunoglobulins—paraproteins—in children with severe combined immunodeficiency before and after transplantation, in *Protides of Biological Fluids*, vol 20, edited by H Peeters, p. 203. Pergamon, Oxford, 1973.

142. DelCarpio J, Espinoza LR, Lauater S, Osterland CK: Transient monoclonal proteins in drug hypersensitivity reactions. *Am J Med* 66:1051, 1979.

143. Keshgegian AA: Prevalence of small monoclonal proteins in the serum of hospitalized patients. *Am Soc Clin Pathol* 77:436, 1982.

144. Bakker AJ, Kothman-Tijkotte MJ: Artifactually high concentration of iron determined in serum from a patient with a monoclonal immunoglobulin. *Clin Chem* 36:1517, 1990.

145. Malacrida V, De-Francesco D, Banfi G, et al: Laboratory investigation of monoclonal gammopathy during 10 years of screening in a general hospital. *J Clin Pathol* 40:793, 1987.

146. Moller-Petersen J, Schmidt EB: Diagnostic value of the concentration of M-component in initial classification of monoclonal gammopathy. *Scand J Haematol* 26:295, 1986.

147. Link H, Kostulas V: Utility of isoelectric focusing of cerebrospinal fluid and serum of agarose evaluated for neurological patients. *Clin Chem* 29: 810, 1983.

148. Ely SA, Knowles DM: Expression of CD56/neural adhesion molecule correlates with the presence of lytic bone lesions in multiple myeloma and distinguishes myeloma from monoclonal gammopathy of undetermined significance and lymphomas with plasmacytoid differentiation. *Am J Pathol* 160:1293, 2002.

149. Greipp PR, Kyle RA: Clinical, morphological and cell kinetic differences among multiple myeloma, monoclonal gammopathy of undetermined significance and smoldering myeloma. *Blood* 62:166, 1983.

150. Boccadoro M, Gavarotti P, Fossati G: Low plasma cell 3(H)-thymidine incorporation in MGUS, smoldering myeloma and remission phase myeloma: Reliable identification of patients not requiring therapy. *Br J Haematol* 58:689, 1984.

151. San Miguel JF, Caballero MD, Gonzalez M: T-cell subpopulations in patients with monoclonal gammopathies: Essential monoclonal gammopathy, multiple myeloma and Waldenstrom macroglobulinemia. *Am J Hematol* 20:267, 1985.

152. Lindstrom FD, Hardy WR, Eberle BJ, Williams RC Jr: Multiple myeloma and benign monoclonal gammopathy: Differentiation by immunofluorescence of lymphocytes. *Ann Intern Med* 78:837, 1973.

153. Billadeau D, Greipp P, Ahmann G, et al: Detection of B-cells clonally related to the tumor population in multiple myeloma and MGUS. *Curr Top Microbiol Immunol* 194:9, 1995.

154. Morrell A, Riesen W: Serum β₂-macroglobulin, serum creatinine and bone marrow plasma cells in benign and malignant monoclonal gammopathy. *Acta Haematol (Basel)* 64:87, 1980.

155. Fine JM, Lambin P, Desjobert H: Serum neopterin and β₂-microglobulin concentrations in monoclonal gammopathies. *Acta Med Scand* 224:179, 1988.

156. Vuckovic J, Ilic A, Knezevic N, et al: Progress in monoclonal gammopathy of undetermined significance. *Br J Haematol* 97:649, 1997.

157. Bataille R: New insights in the clinical biology of multiple myeloma. *Semin Hematol* 34:23, 1997.

158. Baldini L, Guffanti A, Cesana BM, et al: Role of different hematologic variables in defining the risk of malignant transformation in monoclonal gammopathy. *Blood* 87:92, 1996.

159. French M, Fench P, Remy F, et al: Plasma cell proliferation in monoclonal gammopathy: Relations with other biologic variables—Diagnostic and prognostic significance. *Am J Med* 98:60, 1995.

160. Witzig TE, Gonchoroff NJ, Katzmann JA, et al: Peripheral blood B cell labeling indices are a measure of disease activity in patients with monoclonal gammopathies. *J Clin Oncol* 6:1041, 1988.

161. Yi Q, Eriksson I, He W, et al: Idiotype-specific T lymphocytes in monoclonal gammopathies: Evidence for the presence of CD4+ and CD8+ subsets. *Br J Haematol* 96:338, 1997.

162. Yi Q, Osterborg A, Bergenbrant S, et al: Idiotype-reactive T-cell subsets and tumor load in monoclonal gammopathies. *Blood* 86:3043, 1995.

163. Halapi E, Werner A, Wahlstrom J, et al: T cell repertoire in patients with multiple myeloma and monoclonal gammopathy of undetermined significance: Clonal CD8+ T cell expansions are found preferentially in patients with a low tumor burden. *Eur J Immunol* 27:2245, 1997.

164. Corso A, Castelli G, Pagnucco G, et al: Bone marrow T-cell subsets in patients with monoclonal gammopathies: Correlation with clinical stage and disease. *Haematologia* 82:43, 1997.

165. Miguel-Garcia A, Matutes E, Tarin F, et al: Circulating Ki 67 positive lymphocytes in multiple myeloma and benign monoclonal gammopathy. *J Clin Pathol* 48:835, 1995.

166. Billadeau D, Van Ness B, Kimlinger T, et al: Clonal circulation cells are common in plasma cell proliferative disorders: A comparison of monoclonal gammopathy, smoldering myeloma, and active myeloma. *Blood* 88:289, 1996.

167. Isaksson E, Bjockholm M, Holm G, et al: Blood clonal B-cell excess in patients with monoclonal gammopathy of undetermined significance (MGUS): Association with malignant transformation. *Br J Haematol* 92: 71, 1996.

168. Sawanoborj M, Suzuki K, Nakagawa Y, et al: Natural killer cell frequency and serum cytokine levels in monoclonal gammopathies: Correlation of bone marrow granular lymphocytes to prognosis. *Acta Haematol* 98:150, 1997.

169. Leo E, Kropff M, Lindemann A, et al: DNA aneuploidy, increased proliferation and nuclear area of plasma cells in monoclonal gammopathy

of undetermined significance and multiple myeloma. *Anal Quant Cytol Histol* 17:113, 1995.

170. Turesson I: Nucleolar size in benign and malignant plasma cell proliferation. *Acta Med Scand* 197:7, 1975.

171. Dehou MF, Schots R, Lacor P, Arras N, et al: Diagnostic and prognostic value of the MB2 monoclonal antibody in paraffin-embedded bone marrow sections of patients with multiple myeloma and monoclonal gammopathy of undetermined significance. *J Clin Pathol* 94:287, 1990.

172. Amiel A, Kirgner I, Gaber E, et al: Replication pattern in cancer: Asynchronous replication in multiple myeloma and in monoclonal gammopathy. *Cancer Genet Cytogenet* 108:32, 1999.

173. Almeida J, Orfao A, Mateo G, et al: Immunophenotype and DNA content characteristics of plasma cells in multiple myeloma and monoclonal gammopathy of undetermined significance. *Pathol Biol* 47:119, 1999.

174. Yasuda N, Kanoh T, Uchino H: J chain synthesis in human myeloma cells: Light and electron microscopic studies. *Clin Exp Immunol* 40:573, 1980.

175. Cassuto JP, Hammore IC, Pastorelli F, et al: Plasma cell acid phosphatase, a discriminative test for benign and malignant monoclonal gammopathies. *Biomedicine* 27:97, 1977.

176. Sonneveld P, Durie BGM, Lokhorst HM, et al: Analysis of multidrug-resistance (MDR-1) glycoprotein and CD56 expression to separate monoclonal gammopathy from multiple myeloma. *Br J Haematol* 83:63, 1993.

177. Zandecki N, Facon T, Bernard F, et al: CD19 and immunophenotype of bone marrow plasma cells in monoclonal gammopathy of undetermined significance. *J Clin Pathol* 48:548, 1995.

178. Sezer O, Heider U, Zavrski I, Possinger K: Differentiation of monoclonal gammopathy of undetermined significance and multiple myeloma using flow cytometric characteristics of plasma cells. *Haematologica* 86:837, 2001.

179. Majumdar G, Heard SE, Singh AK: Use of cytoplasmic 5-prime nucleotidase for differentiating malignant from benign monoclonal gammopathies. *J Clin Pathol* 43:891, 1990.

180. Van de Berg BC, Michaux L, Lecouvet FE, et al: Nonmyelomatous monoclonal gammopathy: Correlation of bone marrow MR images with laboratory findings and spontaneous clinical outcome. *Radiology* 202:249, 1997.

181. Bellaiche L, Laredo J-D, Lioté F, et al: Magnetic resonance appearance of monoclonal gammopathies of unknown significance and multiple myeloma. *Spine* 22:2551, 1997.

182. Laroche M, Attal M, Pouilles JM, et al: Dual-energy x-ray absorption in patients with multiple myeloma and benign gammopathies. *Clin Exp Rheumatol* 14:108, 1996.

183. Bataille R, Chappard D, Basle M: Quantifiable excess of bone resorption in monoclonal gammopathy is an early symptom of malignancy: A prospective study of 87 bone biopsies. *Blood* 87:4762, 1996.

184. Pecherstorfer M, Seibel MJ, Woitge HW, et al: Bone resorption in multiple myeloma and in monoclonal gammopathy of undetermined significance: Quantification by urinary pyridinium cross-links of collagen. *Blood* 90:3743, 1997.

185. Ong F, Kaiser U, Seelen PJ, et al: Serum neural cell adhesion molecule differentiates multiple myeloma from paraproteinemias due to other causes. *Blood* 87:712, 1996.

186. Lacy MQ, Donovan KA, Heimbach JK, et AL: Comparison of interleukin-1 beta expression by in situ hybridization in monoclonal gammopathy of undetermined significance and multiple myeloma. *Blood* 93:300, 1999.

187. Greco C, Ameglio F, Alvino S, et al: Selection of patients with monoclonal gammopathy of undetermined significance is mandatory for a reliable use of interleukin-6 and other nonspecific multiple myeloma serum markers. *Acta Haematol* 92:1, 1994.

188. Mathiot C, Mary JY, Tartour E, et al: Soluble CD16 (sCD16), a marker of malignancy in individuals with monoclonal gammopathy of undetermined significance (MGUS). *Br J Haematol* 95:660, 1996.

189. Gaillard JP, Bataille R, Brailly H, et al: Increased and highly stable levels of functional soluble interleukin-6 receptor levels in sera of patients with monoclonal gammopathy. *Eur J Immunol* 23:820, 1993.

190. DuVillard L, Guiguet M, Casasnovas R-O, et al: Diagnostic value of serum IL-6 level in monoclonal gammopathies. *Br J Haematol* 89:243, 1995.

191. Cozzolino F, Torcia M, Aldinucci D, et al: Production of interleukin-1 by bone marrow myeloma cells. *Blood* 74:380, 1989.

192. Donovan KA, Lacy MQ, Kline MP, et al: Contrast in cytokine expression between patients with monoclonal gammopathy of undetermined significance or multiple myeloma. *Leukemia* 12:593, 1998.

193. Diamond T, Levy S, Smith A, et al: Non-invasive markers of bone turnover and plasma cytokines differ in osteoporotic patients with multiple myeloma and monoclonal gammopathies of undetermined significance. *Intern Med* 31:272, 2001.

194. Pasqualetti P, Festucci V, Collacciani A, Casale R: The natural history of monoclonal gammopathy of undetermined significance. *Acta Haematol* 97:174, 1997.

195. Gregersen H, Ibsen JS, Mellemkjaer L, et al: Mortality and causes of death in patients with monoclonal gammopathy of undetermined significance. *Br J Haematol* 112:353, 2001.

196. Kyle RA: A long-term study of the prognosis in monoclonal gammopathy of undetermined significance. *N Engl J Med* 346:564, 2002.

197. Pasqualetti P, Casale R: Risk of malignant transformation in patients with monoclonal gammopathy of undetermined significance. *Biomed Pharmacother* 51.74, 1997.

198. Kyle RA, Therneau TM, Rajkumar SV, et al: Long-term follow-up of IgM monoclonal gammopathy of undetermined significance. *Blood* 102:3759, 2003.

199. Gregersen H, Mellemkjaer L, Ibsen JS, et al: The impact of M-component type and immunoglobulin concentration on risk of malignant transformation in patients with monoclonal gammopathy of undetermined significance. *Haematologica* 86:1172, 2001.

200. Montoto S, Rozman K, Rosinol L, et al: Malignant transformation in IgM monoclonal gammopathy of undetermined significance. *Semin Oncol* 30:178, 2003.

201. Van De Donk N, De Weerdt O, Eureling M, et al: Malignant transformation of monoclonal gammopathy of undetermined significance: Cumulative incidence and prognostic factors. *Leuk Lymphoma* 42:609, 2001.

202. Cesana C, Klersy C, Barbarano L, et al: Prognostic factors for malignant transformation in monoclonal gammopathy of undetermined significance and smoldering multiple myeloma. *J Clin Oncol* 15:1625, 2002.

203. Seidl S, Ackerman J, Kaufmann H, et al: DNA methylation analysis identifies the E-cadherin gene as a potential marker of disease progression in patients with monoclonal gammopathy. *Cancer* 100:2598, 2004.

204. Morra E, Cesana C, Klersy C, et al: Clinical characteristics and factors predicting evolution of asymptomatic IgM monoclonal gammopathies and IgM-related disorders. *Leukemia* 18:1512, 2004.

CHAPTER 100

PLASMA CELL MYELOMA

BART BARLOGIE
JOHN SHAUGHNESSY
JOSHUA EPSTEIN
RALPH SANDERSON
ELIAS ANAISSIE
RONALD WALKER
GUIDO TRICOT

Myeloma is a malignancy of late-stage B cells that mature principally into neoplastic plasma cells that generally produce a complete and/or partial (light-chain) monoclonal immunoglobulin protein. Myeloma cells can induce alterations in the marrow microenvironment, which, in turn, provides survival factors that contribute to the resistance of myeloma cells to many anticancer drugs. The disease can cause clinical symptoms via tumor mass effects (cord compression), cytokine production (anemia), bone destruction (pain), protein deposition in visceral organs (kidney, heart), and immunosuppression (infection). Clinical manifestations of myeloma vary as a result of the heterogeneous biology, spanning the entire spectrum from indolent disease to highly aggressive myeloma with extramedullary features. Magnetic resonance imaging has become an important staging tool. Fluorodeoxyglucose positron emission tomography permits functional metabolic imaging of the entire body and, hence, detection of both intramedullary and extramedullary lesions. A high serum level of β_2-microglobulin or C-reactive protein or a plasma cell labeling index generally is associated with a poor prognosis. The presence of abnormal cytogenetics identifies one third of patients with a grave prognosis, even after intensive therapy. Gene expression profiling has identified signaling pathways relevant to the manifestation, progression, or prognosis of the disease. High-dose melphalan, followed by autologous hematopoietic stem cell infusion, has become a standard of care for patients up to age 70 years with symptomatic myeloma. After tandem autotransplants, nearly 50 percent achieve complete remission, and median survival has been extended beyond 6.5 years. Several new agents, such as the immunomodulatory drugs thalidomide and CC-5013 (Revlimid) and the proteasome inhibitor bortezomib (Velcade), have demonstrated activity in advanced or refractory disease. Bisphosphonates and recombinant erythropoietin can help alleviate myeloma-associated bone disease and anemia, respectively.

DEFINITION AND HISTORY

Myeloma is a disease of neoplastic B lymphocytes that invariably mature into plasma cells that synthesize abnormal amounts of immunoglobulin (Ig) or Ig fragments. Clinical manifestations are heterogeneous and include tumor formation, monoclonal Ig production, decreased Ig secretion by normal plasma cells leading to hypogammaglobulinemia, impaired hematopoiesis, osteolytic bone disease, hypercalcemia, and renal dysfunction. Symptoms are caused by tumor mass effects, by cytokines released directly by tumor cells or indirectly by host cells (marrow stroma and bone cells) in response to adhesion of tumor cells, and by the myeloma protein leading to deposition diseases, notably AL (amyoid-light chain) amyloidosis and light-chain deposition disease (LCDD) (see Chap. 101).

Myeloma belongs to a spectrum of disorders referred to as *plasma cell dyscrasias*. These disorders include clinically benign conditions, such as essential monoclonal gammopathy (see Chap. 99); rare and biologically intriguing disorders, such as Castleman disease (see Chap. 96) and α-heavy-chain disease (see Chap. 103); macroglobulinemia (see Chap. 102); solitary plasmacytoma with a high potential for cure when arising in soft tissue; and the most common malignant entity, plasma cell myeloma, a disseminated B cell malignancy that is not curable with conventional-dose chemotherapy. All disorders share plasma cell morphologic features, and most are associated with production of Ig molecules (see Chap. 77). Whereas most plasma cell dyscrasias result from expansion of a single clone of cells, with resultant monoclonal protein secretion, oligoclonal and polyclonal protein abnormalities accompany some conditions, such as Castleman disease or angioimmunoblastic lymphoproliferative disease, now recognized as a T cell lymphoma (see Chap. 96).

EPIDEMIOLOGY

Myeloma accounts for approximately 1 percent of all malignancies and 10 percent of hematologic tumors, representing the second most frequently occurring hematologic malignancy in the United States.[1] At any one time, 50,000 people suffer from myeloma, and approximately 15,000 are diagnosed each year. The median age is approximately 65 years, although occasionally myeloma occurs in the second decade of life.

ENVIRONMENTAL EXPOSURE

Environmental exposure to radiation or chemicals has been associated with an increased incidence of myeloma.[2] Studies of atomic bomb survivors showed an increased incidence of plasma cell myeloma 15 to 20 years after radiation exposure.[3] On the other hand, results of

Acronyms and abbreviations that appear in this chapter include: AML, acute myeloid leukemia; β_2M, β_2-microglobulin; bALP, bone alkaline phosphatase; bFGF, basic fibroblast growth factor; BNP, brain natriuretic protein; BrdU, bromodeoxyuridine; CAM, cell adhesion molecule; CAM-DR, cell adhesion-mediated drug resistance; CR, complete response; CRAB, hypercalcemia, renal failure, anemia, bone lesions; CRP, C-reactive protein; CT, computed tomography; CTx, cytoxan; CVAMP, cyclophosphamide, vincristine, doxorubicin, methylprednisolene; DEX, dexamethasone; DT-PACE, dexamethasone, thalidomide, cisplatin [Platinol], doxorubicin [Adriamycin], cyclophosphamide, etoposide; EFS, event-free survival; FDG, fluorodeoxyglucose; FGF, fibroblast growth factor; FISH, fluorescence *in situ* hybridization; HGF, hepatocyte growth factor; HHV, human herpes virus; HSV, herpes simplex virus; Ig, immunoglobulin; IGF, insulin growth factor; IL, interleukin; ISS, International Staging System; KSHV, Kaposi sarcoma-associated herpes virus; LCDD, light-chain deposition disease; LDH, lactate dehydrogenase; MDR, multidrug resistance gene; MDS, myelodysplastic syndrome; MEL, melphalan; MIP, macrophage inflammatory protein; MP, melphalan-prednisone; MRI, magnetic resonance imaging; MVD, microvessel density; N-CAM, neural cell adhesion molecule; NF-κB, nuclear factor-κB; NTX, N-terminal cross-linking telopeptide of type I collagen; OC, osteocalcin; OPG, osteoprotegerin; OS, overall survival; PBSC, peripheral blood stem cells; PET, positron emission tomography; PR, partial response; RANKL, receptor activator of nuclear factor-κB ligand; STIR, short tau inversion recovery; TBI, total body irradiation; TGF-β, transforming growth factor β; TMP-SMX, trimethoprim-sulfamethoxazole; TNF, tumor necrosis factor; TRAIL, tumor necrosis factor-related apoptosis-inducing ligand; TRACP-5b, tartrate-resistant acid phosphatase isoenzyme 5b; VAD, vincristine, doxorubicin, dexamethasone; VBAD, vincristine, BCNU (carmustine), doxorubicin, dexamethasone; VBAP, vincristine, BCNU (carmustine), Adriamycin, prednisone; VMCB(P), vincristine, melphalan, cyclophosphamide, BCNU (carmustine), predisone; VBMCP, vincristine, carmustine (BCNU), melphalan, cyclophosphamide, prednisone; VEGF, vascular endothelial growth factor; VMCP, vincristine, melphalan, cyclophosphamide, prednisone.

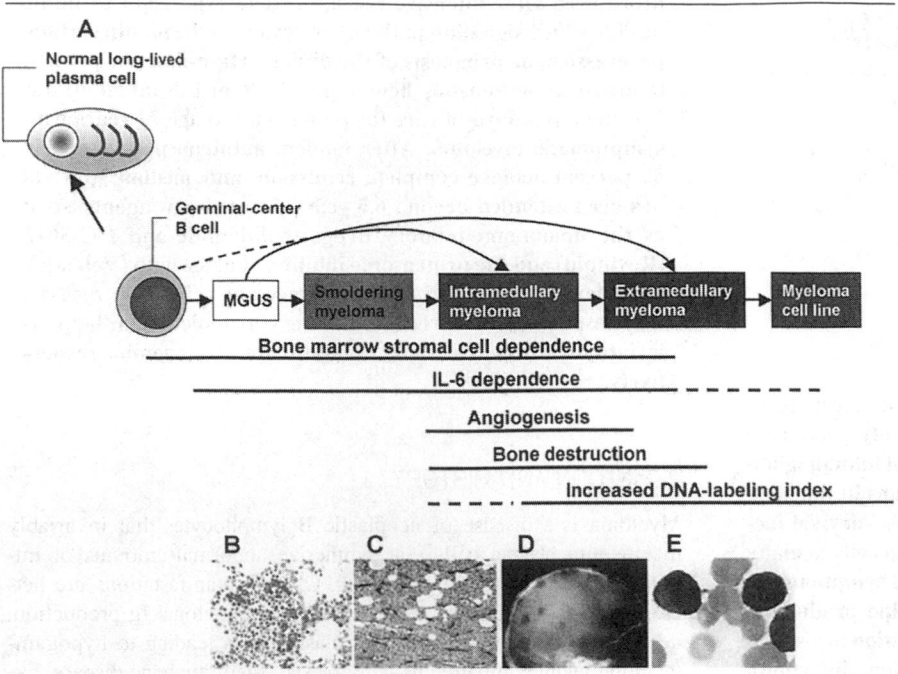

FIGURE 100-1   Stages of myeloma. (A) Myeloma arises from a normal germinal center B cell. At least 30 to 50 percent of malignant myeloma seems to arise from the benign plasma cell neoplasm monoclonal gammopathy. It does not always pass through a period of smoldering myeloma. Initially, myeloma is confined to the marrow (intramedullary), but with time the tumor can acquire the ability to grow in extramedullary locations (e.g., blood, pleural fluid, and skin). Some of these extramedullary myelomas can establish immortalized cell lines *in vitro*. The transition of monoclonal gammopathy to intramedullary myeloma is manifested by increased numbers of myeloma cells at multiple foci and is associated with angiogenesis and osteolytic bone destruction. (B) Low proliferative index in a patient with monoclonal gammopathy. Bright red surface staining for syndecan identifies the plasma cells (10%), none of which stain for the brown nuclear proliferation marker Ki67 (Color Plate XXI-10). (C) Marrow biopsy stained for CD34 identifies endothelial cells *(darker linear areas)* and emphasizes the increased vascularity in myeloma. (D) Skull x-ray film shows the classic "punched out" lytic bone lesions. Although the skull lesions are asymptomatic, extensive vertebral involvement causes compression fractures, resulting in pain and loss of height (average 5 cm by the time of diagnosis). (E) Blood film identifies circulating plasma cells in a patient with plasma cell leukemia. IL, interleukin; MGUS, monoclonal gammopathy of undetermined significance. (From Kuehl and Bergsagel,[31] with permission.)

epidemiologic studies attempting to establish associations between myeloma and certain infections or autoimmune diseases are inconclusive.[4]

Human herpes virus-8 (HHV-8, also called Kaposi sarcoma-associated herpes virus [KSHV]), is involved in the pathogenesis of pleural cavity lymphoma,[5] Kaposi sarcoma,[6] and Castleman disease.[7] Some investigators have identified HHV-8 in marrow dendritic cells of myeloma patients[8–11]; however, these findings have not been confirmed by other investigators.[12–14] Current research focuses on inflammatory alterations of the marrow microenvironment, which may contribute to the transition from essential monoclonal gammopathy to myeloma.[15]

ETIOLOGY AND PATHOGENESIS

The etiology of human myeloma is unknown.[16] Although family clusters have been observed, the incidence is too low to postulate a genetic predisposition.[17,18]

ANIMAL MODELS

Primary human myeloma cells can survive and expand upon injection into fetal human bones implanted into mice with severe combined immunodeficiency (SCID-hu).[19] Several important biologic principles

have been established by studying this model system: (1) mature myeloma cells with a CD138+/CD45− phenotype retain self-renewal and transplantation potential[20]; (2) human myeloma cell growth is restricted to and dependent upon the human bone microenvironment; (3) myeloma growth and development of bone destruction are critically linked; (4) agents targeting components of the marrow microenvironment, such as osteoclasts, osteoblasts, and endothelial cells, can control the growth of myeloma cells[21]; and (5) extramedullary myeloma is no longer dependent upon osteoclasts.[22] Similar findings were observed in the 5T murine myeloma model,[23–25] in which myeloma growth was associated with angiogenesis and depended on osteoclasts.[26–29]

DISEASE EVOLUTION AND GENETIC ALTERATIONS

Although not proven, most cases of symptomatic myeloma evolve from the precursor condition monoclonal gammopathy,[30] which is a stable neoplasm until it undergoes, unpredictably, clonal evolution to myeloma, often through an indolent or smoldering stage. *De novo* myeloma, without a preceding stage of monoclonal gammopathy, has been postulated for a small proportion of patients who develop the disease at a very young age (<30 years).

The presence of somatic hypermutations in the Ig variable-region genes of plasma cells of subjects with monoclonal gammopathy and myeloma strongly suggests that malignant transformation has occurred in a B cell that has undergone differentiations in the germinal center (Figure 100-1).[31–35] Subsequently, myeloma cells home to, survive in, and expand exclusively within the marrow until the late stages of the disease, when extramedullary growth can ensue, at which point long-term human myeloma cell lines can be established.[36,37] The presence of clonotypic cells in the blood, even at diagnosis, underscores the importance of hematogenous spread as a means of disease dissemination.[38–47] Although present at the monoclonal gammopathy stage,[48] intraclonal variation typically is absent in established myeloma.[45,46,49,50]

Interphase fluorescence *in situ* hybridization (FISH)[51,52] and other molecular genetic studies have identified five primary recurrent chromosomal rearrangements involving IgH translocations[32]: 11q13, cyclin D1[53–61]; 4p16.3, fibroblast growth factor (FGF)-R3, and MM SET[62–67]; 6p21, cyclin D3[68]; 16q23, c-MAF[69]; and 20q11, MAF-B,[70] which account for almost 40 percent of all genetic abnormalities seen in myeloma patients, particularly those with nonhyperdiploid cytogenetics.[71] These translocations result from errors in IgH switch recombination during B cell development in germinal centers and have been detected even at the monoclonal gammopathy stage, together with RB-1 deletions.[72–76] Complex unbalanced translocations (c-*myc*) or insertions, often involving multiple chromosomes, represent secondary genetic alterations.[77–81] Mutations of *ras*[78,82–90] or p53[91–98] develop in advanced disease.

Although universally aneuploid according to DNA flow cytometric[99] and interphase FISH analyses,[51] the hypoproliferative nature of

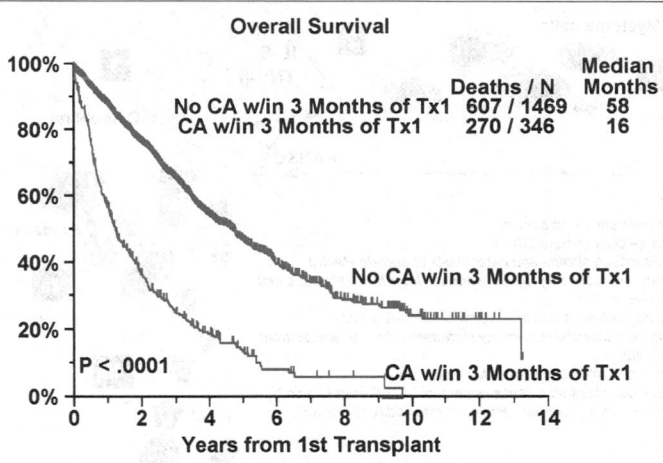

Overall Survival

	Deaths / N	Median Months
No CA w/in 3 Months of Tx1	607 / 1469	58
CA w/in 3 Months of Tx1	270 / 346	16

P < .0001

FIGURE 100 2 Survival by chromosomal abnormalities (CA). In trials of high-dose melphalan-based tandem autotransplants, the presence of metaphase CA in 19 percent of 1815 patients treated identified high-risk disease with short survival.

myeloma[100] and its stromal dependence[101] account for the high frequency (65–70%) of normal diploid metaphase karyotypes (originating in normal hematopoietic cells) observed in untreated patients.[102–105] The remaining third of untreated myeloma patients often have complex cytogenetic abnormalities involving, on average, 11 different chromosomes (Color Plate XXI-13). Although initially thought to represent a major technical shortcoming of standard cytogenetics, the *in vitro* mitotic capacity of myeloma in the absence of a surrounding marrow habitat defines a myeloma entity that is stroma independent, referred to as *malignant myeloma*, and has a very poor prognosis (Figure 100-2).[106]

A major breakthrough in myeloma genetics was the successful application of gene expression profiling of highly purified CD138+ plasma cells (Color Plate XXI-12).[107–112] Myelomatous and normal marrow plasma cells, but not monoclonal gammopathy and myeloma cells, could be readily distinguished.[113] Gene expression levels were linked to additions, deletions, and translocations of genetic material. Primary translocations were associated with so-called spiked gene expression patterns, enabling the detection of cyclin D3 as a newly recognized translocation.[68] In preliminary investigations of 200 patients receiving tandem autotransplants, gene expression profiling identified genes that had prognostic implications that were stronger than those of standard prognostic variables, including cytogenetics.[114] Gene profiling also has been applied to whole marrow biopsies. In the context of paired analysis with CD138+ myeloma plasma cells, the microenvironment signature was observed to be differentially altered in relationship to distinct myeloma genetic entities.[115]

CYTOKINES AND CHEMOKINES

Milestones in myeloma biologic research are linked to the discovery of interleukin (IL)-6 as a myeloma growth and survival factor[116–122] and to the recognition of stromal cell dependence.[34,101,123] A critical cell adhesion-mediated cross-talk exists between myeloma plasma cells (endowed with receptors for a multiplicity of growth-promoting cytokines and chemokines,

especially IL-6,[124] IL-15,[125,126] insulin-like growth factor [IGF]-1,[127] and hepatocyte growth factor [HGF][128]) and various host cell compartments.[129–131] A hallmark of the plasma cell stage of B cell differentiation, CD138 (syndecan-1),[132–135] is shed and often deposited abundantly in the extracellular matrix, trapping growth-promoting and proangiogenic cytokines and thus contributing to myeloma progression and invasion (Color Plate XXI-10). Indeed, soluble syndecan-1 levels are of prognostic importance.[136–139] Growth and survival signals are mediated via PI 3/AKT, STAT 3, RAS/MAPK, and nuclear factor (NF)-κB[140–147] pathways (Figure 100-3). Thus, the myeloma/marrow microenvironment interaction holds important clues to the understanding of disease progression or drug resistance and opens new avenues for novel therapeutic interventions.[148]

BONE METABOLISM

Osteolytic bone lesions are a hallmark of advanced myeloma, eventually developing in 70 to 80 percent of patients. The lesions result from an imbalance of osteoclast and osteoblast number and function.[149] The underlying mechanisms include osteoclast activation through the receptor activation of NF-κB ligand (RANKL)[150] and the macrophage inflammatory protein (MIP)-1α/β chemokine and the IL-3 axes.[151] Expression of RANKL by stromal cells is drastically increased upon contact with myeloma cells, whereas its decoy receptor osteoprotegerin (OPG) is suppressed and additionally inactivated by syndecan-mediated internalization into myeloma plasma cells (Figure 100-4).[152,153] MIP-1α, which originates in myeloma cells,[154,155] directly facilitates maturation of precursor cells into osteoclasts, which are further activated via MIP-1α–induced RANKL expression by stromal cells, resulting in increased bone resorption.[156,157] DKK1 and FRZB, which are expressed and secreted by myeloma cells, interfere with WNT signaling, thus inhibiting osteoblast maturation and aggravating bone destruction.[158]

Some of these pathways can be targeted therapeutically by administration of decoy receptors for RANKL (OPG and RANK-Fc).[152,159] In the SCID-hu model system, administration of these molecules is associated with prevention of osteolytic bone disease and inhibition of myeloma cell growth.[152] Thus, a new paradigm of a strong interdependence between myeloma cells and osteoclasts has emerged, such

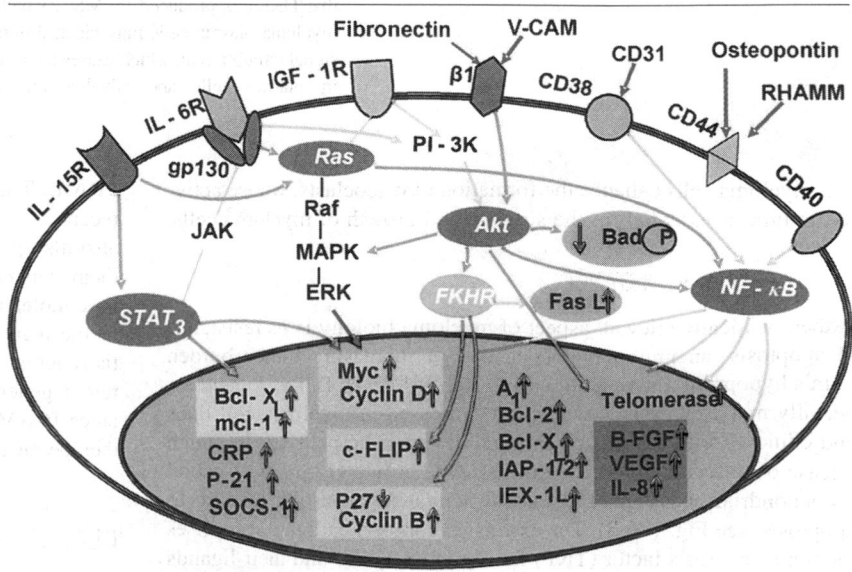

FIGURE 100-3 Microenvironment provides factors that engage receptors present on myeloma cells, which promote their survival and proliferation.

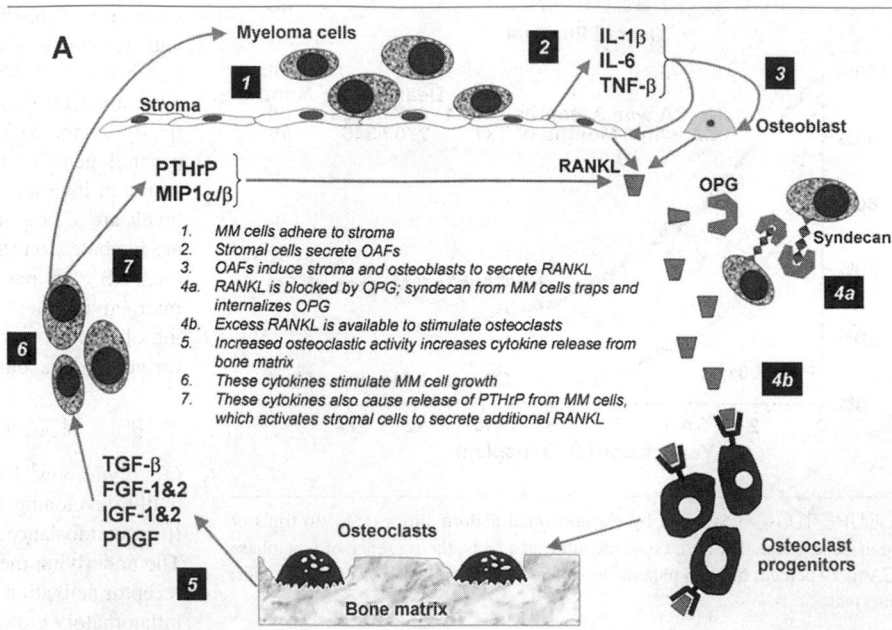

A

Myeloma cells

Stroma

PTHrP
MIP1α/β

IL-1β
IL-6
TNF-β

Osteoblast

RANKL

OPG

Syndecan

1. MM cells adhere to stroma
2. Stromal cells secrete OAFs
3. OAFs induce stroma and osteoblasts to secrete RANKL
4a. RANKL is blocked by OPG; syndecan from MM cells traps and internalizes OPG
4b. Excess RANKL is available to stimulate osteoclasts
5. Increased osteoclastic activity increases cytokine release from bone matrix
6. These cytokines stimulate MM cell growth
7. These cytokines also cause release of PTHrP from MM cells, which activates stromal cells to secrete additional RANKL

TGF-β
FGF-1&2
IGF-1&2
PDGF

Osteoclasts

Bone matrix

Osteoclast progenitors

FIGURE 100-4 Mechanism of bone destruction in myeloma. *(A)* Bone destruction is caused by activation of osteoclasts but also by block of differentiation of mesenchymal precursor cells to mature osteoblasts (modified from Tricot[130]), resulting in increased bone destruction and decreased bone formation. *(B)* New insights have been gained into the role of the microenvironment in multiple myeloma. A model integrates the temporal variation in DKK1 expression into the natural history of a subtype of myeloma that interacts closely with cells of the bone microenvironment. During the earliest stages of myeloma (disease progression is depicted from *left* to *right*), myeloma plasma cells (cells with dark gray nucleus and light gray cytoplasm) grow in a diffuse interstitial pattern and do not exhibit MRI- or x-ray–defined bone lesions. Myeloma plasma cells at this stage do not express DKK1. Mesenchymal stem cells, also termed *marrow stromal cells* (MSC), characterized as STRO-1+, IL-6+, receptor activator of NF-κB ligand (RANKL)+, alkaline phosphatase (ALP)–, express the Wnt receptors FZD and LRP5 and respond to Wnt signal by stabilizing cytoplasmic β-catenin, which in turn translocates to the nucleus where it interacts with latent TCF/LEF transcription factors to induce target genes. This action results in differentiation of MSC into mature bone-mineralizing osteoblasts, characterized as ALP+, osteoprotegerin (OPG)+, STRO-1–, RANKL–, IL-6–. During disease progression, myeloma plasma cells begin synthesizing DKK1. The mechanism by which DKK1 is activated is unknown. Myeloma-derived DKK1, a potent inhibitor of Wnt signaling, binds to the LRP coreceptor upon MSC blocking of Wnt signaling, which results in phosphorylation of β-catenin by GSK3B, followed by ubiquination and degradation by the proteasome. The antagonism of Wnt signaling blocks the terminal differentiation of MSC into osteoblasts. Gregory and colleagues[396] showed that DKK1 is produced by MSC, which induce the cells to reenter the cell cycle. Thus, DKK1 made by myeloma plasma cells may block differentiation and induce proliferation of MSC. Myeloma plasma cells signal through Wnt, which causes their proliferation.[397,398] Whether DKK1 also down-regulates Wnt signaling in plasma cells and whether this action influences myeloma cell proliferation are not clear. *(continued)*

that myeloma cells enhance the formation of osteoclasts, whose activity, in turn, is essential for the survival and growth of myeloma cells.

APOPTOSIS RESISTANCE

A therapeutically relevant aspect of myeloma biology is its resistance to apoptosis, an important mechanism of increasing tumor burden in this hypoproliferative malignancy. Bcl-2,[140,160,161] Bcl-x$_L$,[162] and especially mcl-1,[162] each of which are expressed in myeloma cell lines and clinical isolates, function through the intrinsic pathway in which release of mitochondrial constituents (cytochrome C, SMAC [second mitochondrial activator of caspases] activates caspase-9, leading to apoptosis (see Fig. 106-3). The extrinsic apoptosis pathway comprises the tumor necrosis factor (TNF) family of receptors and their ligands TNF, Fas ligand, and tumor necrosis factor-related apoptosis-inducing ligand (TRAIL). Death receptors 4 and 5, expressed on myeloma cell lines and primary tumor isolates, can be activated upon ligation by

TRAIL. This action can be blocked by expression of TRAIL decoy receptors, such as OPG. Sequestration of OPG by soluble syndecan-1 also may protect myeloma cells from TRAIL activation. A recurring theme emerges where the relative levels of proapoptotic and antiapoptotic molecules, acting in a cell autonomous manner or in the context of the marrow microenvironment, determine the outcome of potentially lethal signals. Thus, the efficacy of treatment is determined by tumor genetic features, so-called cell adhesion-mediated drug resistance (CAM-DR), and by epigenetic changes that can be exploited therapeutically (Figure 100-5).

CLINICAL FEATURES

Patients with myeloma may present with symptoms of anemia, bone pain, pathologic fractures, bleeding tendency, and/or peripheral neuropathy. These signs and symptoms generally result from tumor mass

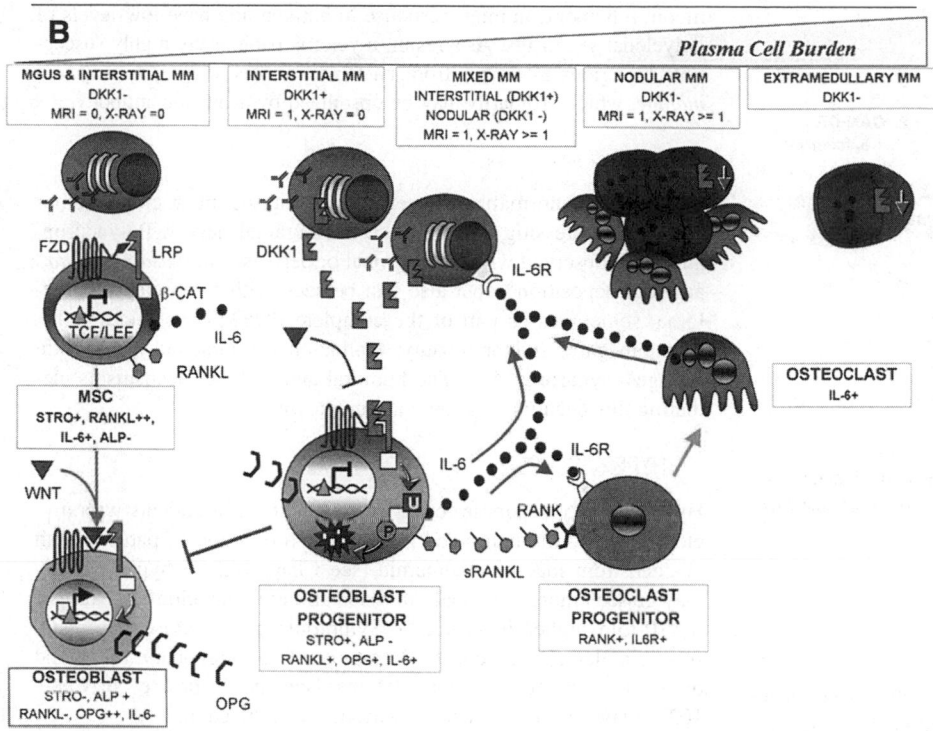

FIGURE 100-4   (CONTINUED)   Osteoblast progenitor cells, but not mature osteoblasts, are a rich source of RANKL,[399] suggesting that DKK1-mediated block of osteoblast differentiation significantly contributes to elevated RANKL in the marrow of myeloma patients. At this stage, plasma cells have an interstitial or mixed interstitial and nodular growth pattern with MRI-defined focal lesions. DKK1 expression can be detected in plasma cells that grow interstitially; however, expression is dramatically reduced or undetectable by immunohistochemistry in cells within focal lesions. During progression, myeloma plasma cells shift from a predominantly interstitial growth pattern (DKK1+) to a nodular pattern, where large sheets of plasma cells (DKK1−) form foci and exhibit aggressive morphologic characteristics (high nuclear to cytoplasmic ratio and prominent nucleoli). Down-regulation of DKK1 expression accompanies the shift from interstitial to nodular growth. The continued and chronic exposure of the bone marrow to elevated DKK1 results in overproduction of RANKL and IL-6 by immature osteoblasts, and MSC result in differentiation of osteoclast progenitors into mature bone-resorbing osteoclasts that also produce IL-6. The loss of mature osteoblasts and the increase in osteoclasts lead to x-ray–detectable lytic bone lesions found exclusively adjacent to nodular plasmacytomas. Down-regulation of DKK1 in plasma cells within these nodules likely results from direct contact with osteoclasts.[400] The molecular means by which osteoclasts extinguish DKK1 expression in myeloma plasma cells is not known. As disease progresses, interstitial growth gives way to a largely nodular growth pattern. In the terminal stages of disease, plasma cell growth is highly proliferative and can become extramedullary. Plasma cells derived from virtually all extramedullary stages of myeloma are DKK1−. FGF, fibroblast growth factor; IGF, insulin-like growth factor; IL, interleukin; MIP, macrophage inflammatory protein; OAF, osteoclast-activating factor; OPG, osteoprotegerin; PDGF, platelet-derived growth factor; PTHrP, parathyroid hormone-related protein; TGF, transforming growth factor; TNF, tumor necrosis factor.

effects or from the proteins or cytokines secreted by tumor cells or normal accessory cells under the influence of tumor cell products (Figure 100-6).

PAIN

Pain suffered by subjects with myeloma frequently results from vertebral compression fractures at sites of osteopenia or, more typically, from lytic bone lesions. These lesions result from excessive osteoclast activation (see above)[124,163,164] and inhibition of compensatory osteoblastic activity.[149] Localized pain can be induced by regional tumor growth toward the spinal cord and nerve roots. Painful mass effects can be provoked by amyloid deposition (see Chap. 101) at various anatomic sites, such as the median nerve sheath, as in amyloid-associated carpal tunnel syndrome.[165]

ANEMIA

Anemia of variable severity affects more than two thirds of patients with myeloma. Overexpression of Fas ligand, MIP-1α, and TRAIL by myeloma cells triggers death signals in immature erythroblasts.[166] Most patients have an inappropriate erythropoietin response for the degree of their anemia, which is further accentuated in the presence of renal failure.[167] The blunted erythropoietin response may result from abundant production of cytokines, such as IL-1 and TNF-β,[168] or increased serum viscosity levels.[169] Overproduction of IL-6 by marrow stroma, normal accessory cells, and/or tumor cells may contribute to the anemia of myeloma. However, possibly because of the thrombopoietic activity of this cytokine,[170] myeloma patients typically do not manifest significant thrombocytopenia in the absence of other factors.

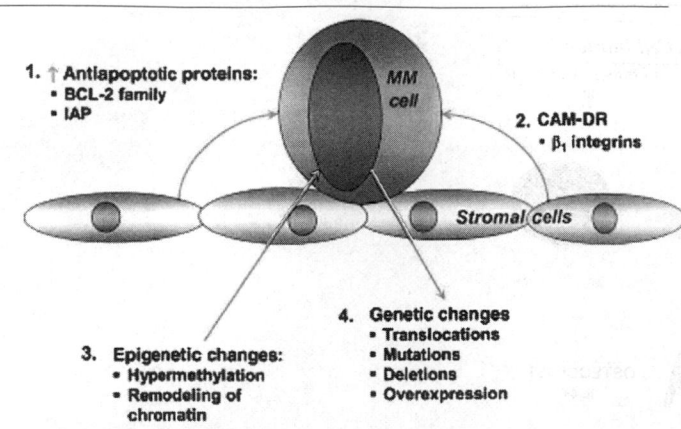

FIGURE 100-5   Multiple mechanisms of drug resistance in myeloma. CAM-DR, cell adhesion-mediated drug resistance; IAP, inhibitors of apoptosis; MM, multiple myeloma.[401]

NEPHROPATHY

Abnormalities of renal function occur when the tubular absorptive capacity for light chains is exhausted, resulting in interstitial nephritis because of light-chain casts.[171,172] The second most common cause of nephropathy is hypercalcemia with hypercalciuria, leading to volume depletion and prerenal azotemia. In addition, hypercalcemia is conducive to calcium deposits in the renal tubules, also producing interstitial nephritis.[173,174] AL amyloidosis associated with light-chain proteinuria usually presents as a nephrotic syndrome but over time can lead to renal failure (see Chap. 101).[175–177] AL amyloidosis is more common in patients with λ light-chain myeloma proteins than in patients with κ light-chain myeloma, especially in those with λ light-chain proteins that have Ig variable regions belonging to the λ VI light-chain subgroup. Probably underestimated, however, is the frequency of Ig LCDD, a disease more commonly associated with κ light-chain myeloma proteins often at barely detectable levels. This condition also leads to impaired glomerular filtration.[177,178]

Tumor cell involvement of the kidneys is uncommon but should be suspected in patients with renal enlargement; however, renal enlargement more often results from AL amyloid (see Chap. 101).[176] A complicating factor in the pathogenesis of renal failure in myeloma includes the frequent use of nonsteroidal antiinflammatory drugs for pain control.[179] Studies using IL-6 transgenic mice that express an IL-6 transgene under the control of the metallothionein-1 promoter indicate that constitutive high-level expression of IL-6 in the liver can induce dysproteinemia and a protracted acute-phase response, leading to renal pathology with features remarkably similar to those observed in human myeloma kidney.[180]

An important reason for renal function impairment is the liberal administration of bisphosphonates, especially when administered rapidly (e.g., less than 2 hours for pamidronate or less than 30 minutes for zoledronic acid). Thus, especially in patients in remission, we advocate review of renal function prior to each cycle of bisphosphonate therapy. Occasionally, nonspecific proteinuria precedes the onset of renal failure.

INFECTIONS

Deficiencies in cellular immune function account for the recurrent infections commonly seen in myeloma.[181–183] The mechanisms underlying this immunodeficiency remain obscure, although myeloma cell expression of transforming growth factor β (TGF-β)[184] and Fas ligand have been implicated.[185] In addition, patients have impaired ability to

mount a humoral immune response to antigen and have low levels of polyclonal serum Igs. As a result, myeloma patients are highly susceptible to serious infections from bacteria, such as *Streptococcus pneumoniae*, which ordinarily may be opsonized by a specific antibody.

NEUROPATHY

Neurologic abnormalities generally are caused by regional tumor growth compressing the spinal cord or cranial nerves. Polyneuropathies are observed with perineuronal or perivascular *(vasa nervorum)* amyloid deposition[165] but also can be seen with osteosclerotic myeloma, sometimes as part of the complete POEMS (*p*olyneuropathy, *o*rganomegaly, *e*ndocrinopathy, *m*onoclonal gammopathy, and *s*kin changes) syndrome.[186,187] The humoral and cellular mechanisms mediating this peculiar syndrome are unknown.

HYPERVISCOSITY

Hyperviscosity occurs in fewer than 10 percent of patients with myeloma.[188–191] Although noted in a higher proportion of patients with Waldenström macroglobulinemia (see Chap. 102),[192] hyperviscosity may be seen more commonly in association with myeloma because of its 10-fold higher incidence.[193] Symptoms of hyperviscosity result from circulatory problems leading to cerebral, pulmonary, renal, and other organ dysfunction (see "Hyperviscosity Syndrome" in Chap. 102). Hyperviscosity often is associated with bleeding.

Although a general correlation exists between clinical symptoms and relative serum viscosity, the relationship between serum Ig levels and symptoms is not consistent among patients. This finding may be related to the different physicochemical properties of each of the classes and subclasses of Ig molecules (see Chap. 77). Because of a greater tendency for IgA to form polymers, patients with IgA myeloma have hyperviscosity more frequently than do patients with IgG myeloma, and almost one fourth of IgA myeloma patients may have features of the hyperviscosity syndrome.[190] Among patients with IgG myeloma, those with tumors expressing Igs of the IgG3 subclass are the most susceptible to developing this syndrome.[194]

BLEEDING AND THROMBOSIS

Bleeding has been reported in 15 percent of patients with IgG myeloma and in more than 30 percent of patients with IgA myeloma.[195,196] The bleeding may result from anoxia and thrombosis in capillary circulation, perivascular amyloid, and/or an acquired coagulopathy,[193] such

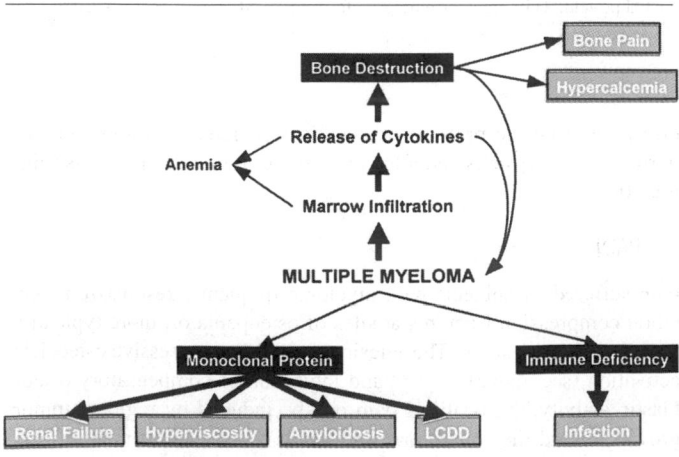

FIGURE 100-6   Disease manifestations in myeloma. LCDD, light-chain deposition disease.

TABLE 100-1 MYELOMA: FREQUENCY OF SIGNS AND SYMPTOMS

Symptoms and Laboratory Features	Frequency (%)
Bone pain (spine, chest, less common in long bones)	65
Weakness and fatigue	50
Anemia	65
Renal insufficiency	20
Hypercalcemia	20
Serum M peak on standard electrophoresis	80
M peak on immunofixation of serum or urine	97
IgG	50
IgA	20
Only light chain	20
Urinary M-protein	75
Marrow plasmacytosis >10%	90

as coagulation factor X deficiency, in the case of primary amyloidosis. Thrombocytopenia, however, is rare in early phases of myeloma, even with extensive marrow involvement.[197]

A new syndrome of thromboembolic disease in myeloma has been linked to the use of thalidomide, especially in combination with doxorubicin.[198] Use of low molecular weight heparin has been an effective means of preventing such complications, especially during the early phases of therapy when a high burden of myeloma cells is present.[198]

EXTRAMEDULLARY DISEASE

Plasma cell leukemia (>2000/μL) is rare at presentation (<1%) but can develop in 5 percent of patients as a terminal disease manifestation.[199–202] Using appropriate tools (CD138+CD45− or DNA/cytoplasmic Ig flow cytometry), low levels of circulating plasma cells can be detected in the majority of patients. Other extramedullary disease manifestations are observed with increasing frequency as the duration of disease control is extended by high-dose melphalan and current therapy. Visceral organ involvement of liver, lymph nodes, spleen, kidneys, breasts, pleura, meninges, and cutaneous sites should be suspected in the presence of elevated serum lactate dehydrogenase (LDH) levels[203,204] and is best confirmed by computed tomography (CT) or, more recently, positron emission tomography (PET) scanning. Such extramedullary disease almost always is accompanied by usually complex cytogenetic abnormalities, a high plasma cell labeling index, and high-grade immunoblastic morphology.[205]

TABLE 100-2 CRITERIA FOR DIAGNOSIS OF PLASMA CELL MYELOMA*

Major Criteria
 Plasmacytomas on tissue biopsy
 Marrow plasmacytosis with >30% plasma cells
 Monoclonal globulin spike on serum electrophoresis >3.5 g/dl for IgG or >2.0 g/dl for IgA; 1.0 g/24 h of κ or λ light-chain excretion on urine electrophoresis in the absence of amyloidosis
Minor Criteria
 Marrow plasmacytosis 10–30%
 Monoclonal globulin spike present but less than the levels defined above
 Lytic bone lesions
 Normal IgM <0.05 g/dl, IgA <0.1 g/dl, or IgG <0.6 g/dl

* The diagnosis of plasma cell myeloma is confirmed when at least one major and one minor criterion or at least *three minor criteria* are documented in *symptomatic* patients with *progressive* disease. The presence of features not specific for the disease supports the diagnosis, particularly if of recent onset: anemia, hypercalcemia, azotemia, bone demineralization, or hypoalbuminemia.

TABLE 100-3 CRITERIA FOR CLASSIFICATION OF MYELOMA*

M-protein in serum and/or urine
Marrow (clonal) plasma cells* or plasmacytoma
Related Organ or Tissue Impairment (ROTI; end-organ damage, including bone lesions)

* If flow cytometry is performed, most plasma cells (>90%) show a "neoplastic" phenotype.
Some patients may have no symptoms but have ROTI (related organ or tissue impairment).
SOURCE: The International Myeloma Working Group. *British Journal of Haematology* 2003;121:749–757 (Table V). © 2003 Mayo Foundation.

LABORATORY FEATURES

The diagnosis of even symptomatic plasma cell myeloma often is delayed by months. Patients may have complaints of persistent back pain following minor trauma or of recurrent infections. Such complaints in the setting of unexplained hyperproteinemia or proteinuria, anemia, renal insufficiency, hypoalbuminemia, dysproteinemia, or marked elevation of the erythrocyte sedimentation rate should prompt laboratory evaluation for plasma cell myeloma (Table 100-1).

Table 100-2 summarizes the commonly accepted diagnostic criteria for myeloma. The International Myeloma Working Group has issued simplified criteria for the classification of myeloma and related disorders (see "Differential Diagnosis" below).[206] For the diagnosis of symptomatic myeloma, neither a minimum serum or urine M-protein level nor a minimal clonal marrow plasmacytosis level was included (Table 100-3).

The most critical criterion of symptomatic disease, and hence initiation of therapy, is evidence of organ or tissue impairment (end-organ damage) manifested by anemia, hypercalcemia, lytic bone lesions, renal insufficiency, hyperviscosity, amyloidosis, or recurrent infections (hypercalcemia, renal failure, anemia, bone lesions [CRAB]; Table 100-4, see Figure 100-6).

INITIAL EVALUATION

Minimal evaluation requirements include evaluation of the hemogram; inspection of the blood film for the presence of rouleaux; performance of a multichemical scan for detection of hypercalcemia, azotemia, or elevated LDH level; serum protein electrophoresis; measurement of urinary protein excretion; and marrow aspiration and biopsy. Radiographic examination should include the axial skeleton (skull, entire spine, pelvis). Table 100-5 summarizes the laboratory tests recommended by the International Myeloma Working Group.

TABLE 100-4 MYELOMA-RELATED ORGAN OR TISSUE IMPAIRMENT RELATED TO THE PLASMA CELL PROLIFERATIVE PROCESS*

• Calcium-induced: serum calcium >0.25 mmol/liter above the upper limit of normal or >2.75 mmol/liter
• Renal insufficiency: creatinine >173 mmol/liter
• Anemia: hemoglobin 2 g/dl below the lower limit of normal or hemoglobin <10 g/dl
• Bone: Lytic lesions or osteoporosis with compression fracture (MRI or CT may clarify)
• Other: Symptomatic hyperviscosity, amyloidosis, recurrent bacterial infections (>2 episodes in 12 months)

* CRAB-calcium-induced, renal insufficiency, anemia, or bone lesions; ROTI-related organ or tissue impairment.
SOURCE: The International Myeloma Working Group. *British Journal of Haematology* 2003;121:749–757 (Table II). © 2003 Mayo Foundation.

TABLE 100-5   STUDIES FOR MYELOMA EVALUATION

History and physical examination
Complete total blood cell and differential counts; examination of blood film
Chemistry screen including calcium and creatinine
Serum protein electrophoresis and immunofixation
Nephelometric quantification of immunoglobulins
Urinalysis and 24-h urine collection for electrophoresis and immunofixation
Marrow aspirate and trephine biopsy (cytogenetics, immunophenotyping, and
   plasma cell labeling index if available)
Radiologic skeletal bone survey including spine, pelvis, skull, humeri and
   femurs; MRI may be helpful
β_2-microglobulin, C-reactive protein, lactate dehydrogenase levels
Measurement of free serum monoclonal light chains if available

SOURCE: The International Myeloma Working Group. *British Journal of Haematology*
2003;121:749–757 (Table IV). © 2003 Mayo Foundation.

HEMATOLOGIC ABNORMALITIES

BLOOD CELL ALTERATIONS

Tumor involvement of the marrow typically causes anemia, the degree
of which appears related to tumor mass. Possibly because of thrombopoietic activity of IL-6, myeloma patients typically do not manifest
significant thrombocytopenia unless the marrow is replaced by myeloma cells. However, thrombocytopenia may develop subsequent to
therapy or from autoimmune mechanisms (such as those accounting
for anemia or factor VIII deficiency[207–209]). Some patients present with
thrombocytosis secondary to hyposplenism because of AL amyloid.

COAGULATION ABNORMALITIES

The antibody portion (fragment antigen-binding [Fab]) of the myeloma
protein may bind to fibrin during clotting and prevent fibrin aggregation. This condition probably represents the most common coagulopathy in patients with myeloma.[210] Factor X deficiency associated with
systemic AL amyloidosis apparently cannot be traced to an inhibitor
in vitro (see Chap. 101).[211]

Hypercoagulable states may result from protein-C deficiency, perhaps as a consequence of monoclonal Igs exhibiting anti-protein C
activity. Lupus anticoagulants also have been reported in association
with myeloma, but they have not been traced to a direct action of the
monoclonal Ig.[212]

MARROW FINDINGS

The marrow shows varying degrees of neoplastic cell replacement. Cytologically, myeloma cells consist predominantly of plasma cells exhibiting varying degrees of immaturity (Color Plates XXI-4, 5, 7, and 11A).
A small number of larger cells with prominent nucleoli and scant cytoplasm usually is present. Such plasmablasts tend to increase with disease progression and may represent the dominant tumor cell population
during the terminal disease phase.[213,214] A trephine biopsy examination
is critical to determine the pattern of marrow involvement, which may
be diffuse, focal, or mixed (Color Plate XXI-11B).[215,216] Osteoclasts often are increased and osteoblasts decreased (Color Plates XV-1, 2, and
3). Amyloid deposition, recognized on Congo red stain, may be diffuse
or focal and sometimes only perivascular. Specialized laboratories can
perform qualitative assessment of microvessel density (MVD) using
CD131 or CD34 monoclonal antibodies (Color Plate XXI-11C).[217,219]
Secondary myelodysplastic changes typically develop after prolonged
treatment with alkylating agents, such as melphalan or nitrosoureas, although a primary myelodysplastic syndrome (MDS) can occur concurrently with myeloma in older patients.[220,221] Pancytopenia in the context
of a hypercellular marrow should prompt cytogenetic and interphase
FISH studies to detect the most commonly encountered chromosome

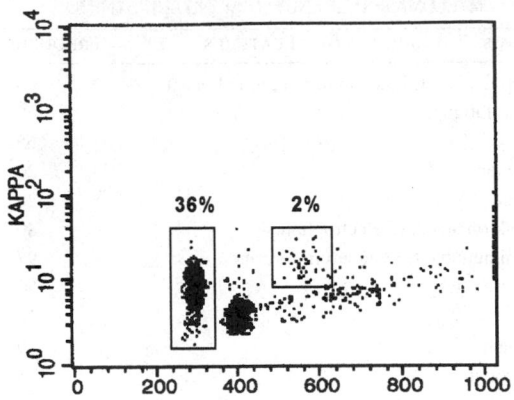

At diagnosis

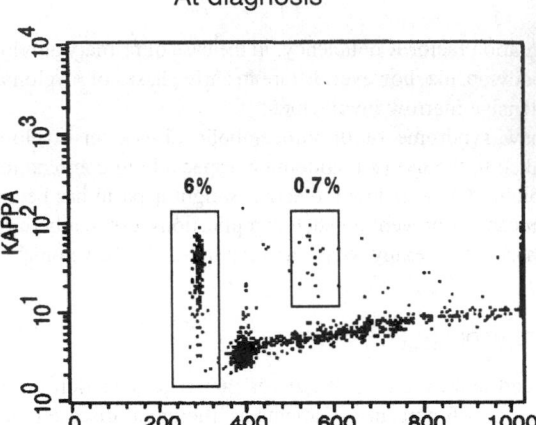

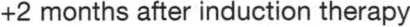

+2 months after induction therapy

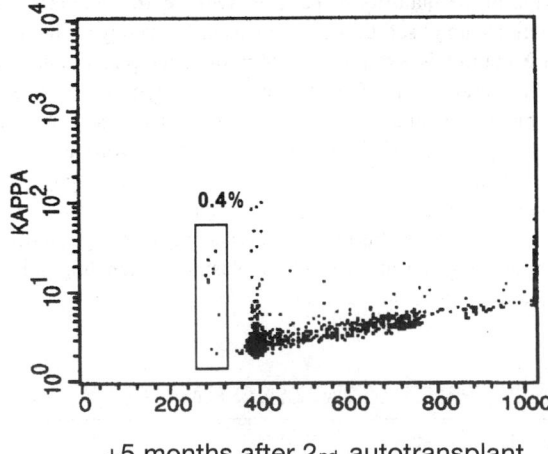

+5 months after 2nd autotransplant

FIGURE 100-7   Flow cytometric analysis of bone marrow nuclear DNA
content (propidium iodide) and cytoplasmic immunoglobulin light-chain content (fluorescein isothiocyanate-conjugated anti-κ monoclonal antibody). Serial
examinations during treatment revealed progressive decrease of hypodiploid κ
light-chain–restricted tumor cell population in marrow.

abnormalities associated with related treatment and MDS: −5, 5q-; −7,
7q-; t(1;7)(q10;p10); +8; del 20q; and involvement of 11q23 or 21q22
in case of treatment-related acute myeloid leukemia (AML) induced by
topoisomerase II-inhibiting cytotoxic agents.

The frequent presence of DNA aneuploidy and universal light-
chain restriction, which is characteristic of myeloma, has been ex-

ploited diagnostically to quantitate marrow involvement by two-parameter flow cytometry, using propidium iodide for nuclear DNA staining and anti-κ and anti-λ light-chain antibodies to label cytoplasmic Ig (Figure 100-7).[222] When applied to blood, DNA/cytoplasmic Ig flow cytometry accurately quantifies the concentration of circulating myeloma cells with high sensitivity (0.1%). Hyperdiploidy can be detected in 70 percent of cases; hypodiploidy associated with primary drug resistance is rare (5–10%).[99,100] The monoclonal nature of tumor cells can be verified by analysis of Ig gene rearrangements in the DNA isolated from neoplastic plasma cells.[223,224] Most laboratories perform flow cytometric studies to detect CD138+CD45− mature plasma cells,[120,225] frequently coexpressing CD56+ (neural cell adhesion molecule [N-CAM]).[226,227] Others have focused on the drug resistance phenotype (multidrug resistance gene [MDR] and LRP).[228–234] Fewer than 20 percent of patients express CD20+[60] or CD117+ (Kit),[235] which have not been effectively targeted by rituximab or imatinib mesylate. Sensitive flow cytometric analysis can be used to quantitate and detect minimal residual disease at a detection level of one residual myeloma cell in approximately 10,000 to 100,000 cells.[236]

CYTOGENETICS

Metaphase cytogenetic studies should be performed routinely to identify the one third of newly diagnosed patients with myeloma cells harboring cytogenetic abnormalities, which confer a poor prognosis, especially in cases of hypodiploidy and chromosome 13 deletions.[205,237–242] In some series, interphase FISH studies were helpful, in discerning deletions in chromosome 13[243–245] or of p53.[92] When performed with metaphase karyotyping, however, FISH-defined deletions in chromosome 13 are not of additional prognostic value (Figure 100-8).[246]

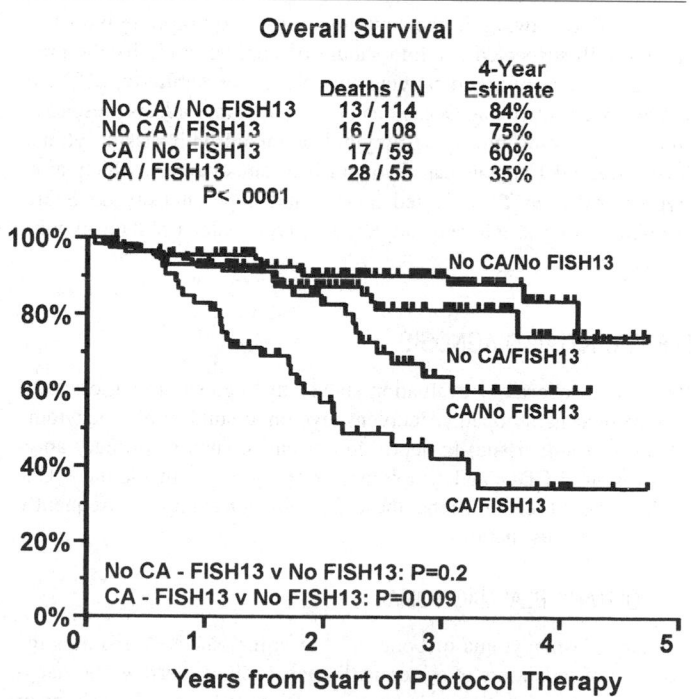

Overall Survival

	Deaths / N	4-Year Estimate
No CA / No FISH13	13 / 114	84%
No CA / FISH13	16 / 108	75%
CA / No FISH13	17 / 59	60%
CA / FISH13	28 / 55	35%

P< .0001

No CA - FISH13 v No FISH13: P=0.2
CA - FISH13 v No FISH13: P=0.009

Years from Start of Protocol Therapy

FIGURE 100-8 Overall survival among newly diagnosed patients treated according to total therapy 2, according to metaphase cytogenetic abnormalities (CA) and interphase fluorescence *in situ* hybridization (FISH)-defined chromosome 13 deletion (FISH13). The 222 patients without CA had similar outcomes whether or not FISH13 was present. By contrast, FISH13 distinguished a high-risk group among the 114 patients with CA.

PLASMA CELL LABELING INDEX

Because mature plasma cells represent the dominant tumor phenotype in most myeloma cases, the proportion of cycling cells typically is exceedingly small.[100,247–250] Thus, the plasma cell labeling index, as determined by tritiated thymidine or bromodeoxyuridine (BrdU) techniques, averages 0.5 percent. Fewer than 5 percent of patients display values greater than 5 percent.[251,252] The BrdU labeling index of marrow and blood has become an important prognostic variable. As values exceed 0.5 percent at diagnosis, the durations of event-free and overall survival are progressively shortened. A major advance in the assessment of myeloma proliferative activity has been the application of multiparameter flow cytometry, which permits more accurate connotation of BrdU-positive light chain-restricted plasma cells and ploidy status.[253]

IMMUNOGLOBULIN M MYELOMA

A rare diagnostic dilemma is an IgM myeloma entity that is distinct from the more common IgM-producing lymphoplasmacytic cell dyscrasia, Waldenström macroglobulinemia (histopathologic diagnosis, immunocytoma).[61,254] Upon examination, plasma cells, rather than the lymphoplasmacytic infiltrate, dominate the marrow of IgM myeloma, whereas mastocytosis is a hallmark of immunocytoma. DNA aneuploidy and the presence of lytic bone lesions support a diagnosis of IgM myeloma. Myeloma, also of the IgM isotype, is resistant to purine analogues, which are effective in Waldenström macroglobulinemia (see Chap. 102).[255,256]

MYELOMA PROTEIN AND OTHER DISEASE-RELATED ABNORMALITIES

Most patients with myeloma secrete a monoclonal Ig that can be detected by immunofixation analysis. The Igs produced by the tumor cells can have unique Ig idiotypes (see Chaps. 77 and 98).[40]

Myeloma protein studies should include serum protein electrophoresis to quantitate the M region (M-peak) in combination with nephelometric quantitation of Ig levels, a 24-hour urine collection to measure urinary protein and, in conjunction with urine electrophoresis, Bence Jones protein, which often is excreted in excess of 1 g/day. Immunofixation of serum and urine is needed to determine the Ig heavy- and light-chain isotypes. Approximately 60 percent of myeloma patients have detectable monoclonal IgG (usually >3.5 g/dl), 20 percent have monoclonal IgA (typically >2 g/dl), and 20 percent have only monoclonal Ig light chains. Excess light-chain proteinuria, however, can accompany IgG, IgA, and, especially, IgD myeloma.

A small proportion of patients have nonsecretory myeloma, in which the neoplastic plasma cells do not produce significant amounts of monoclonal Ig, although most cases still contain readily identifiable cytoplasmic Ig. The introduction of assays to quantitate circulating free κ and free λ light chains has made possible the reclassification of approximately one half to two thirds of patients previously thought to have nonsecretory myeloma.[257] Myelomas producing monoclonal IgD, IgE, IgM, or more than one Ig class are rare. The presence of small serum M-protein concentrations should alert the clinician to the possibility of the IgD myeloma isotype, especially when associated with λ light-chain proteinuria.

Suppression of polyclonal Ig classes is typical of symptomatic myeloma.[183] Even patients with light-chain myeloma, nonsecretory myeloma, or IgD or IgE myeloma often have depressed serum IgG, IgA, and IgM levels. Unlike other myeloma isotypes, IgD myelomas make Igs that more commonly have λ rather than κ light chains.

Serum levels of β_2-microglobulin (β_2M), shed from the surface of myeloma plasma cells, reflect tumor burden.[258–260] Because of its renal mode of excretion, β_2M serum levels are variably elevated in

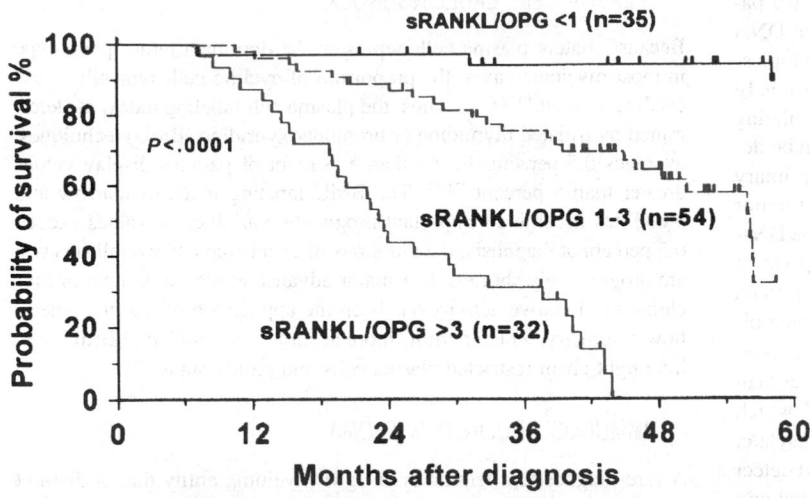

FIGURE 100-9 Probability of survival of myeloma patients using soluble receptor activator of nuclear factor-κB ligand (sRANKL) to osteoprotegerin (OPG) ratio as an independent variable. sRANKL to OPG ratio predicts survival in multiple myeloma. Proposal for a novel prognostic index. (From Terpos et al,[402] with permission.)

the setting of renal failure. β_2M concentrations also can be elevated with viral infections[261,262] and as a result of treatment with interferon.[263] Serum levels of C-reactive protein (CRP) reflect endogenous IL-6 activity and often are increased in cases with hypoalbuminemia because of IL-6–mediated suppression of albumin production by hepatocytes.[264] Elevated serum LDH levels, unrelated to hemolysis or renal failure, or thrombotic thrombocytopenic purpura should prompt appropriate imaging studies to search for extramedullary disease, typically with high-grade features, including cytogenetic abnormalities.[265]

MARKERS OF BONE DISEASE

RANKL and OPG have been associated not only with myeloma bone disease but also with clinical outcome (Figure 100-9),[266] attesting to the close interrelation between myeloma progression and components of the marrow microenvironment, especially hematopoiesis-derived osteoclasts and mesenchymal cell-derived osteoblasts.[267] These bone markers, along with serum levels of tartrate-resistant acid phosphatase isoenzyme 5b (TRACP-5b, a novel resorption marker only produced by activated osteoclasts)[6] and elevated levels of bone collagen degradation products, including the N-terminal cross-linking telopeptide of type I collagen (NTX), can predict early progression of bone disease in myeloma.[268,269] Bone alkaline phosphatase (bALP) and osteocalcin (OC), markers of bone formation, are suppressed in myeloma patients. The s-RANKL/OPG ratio is highly correlated with serum levels of TRACP-5b, IL-6, and β_2M and with urinary excretion of NTX.[266]

IMAGING STUDIES

Radiographic studies of the long bones, skull, and ribs can reveal osteolytic lesions. Detectable osteolytic lesions require at least 30 percent loss of bone mass[270] and, hence, represent an end stage of bone destruction. When seen on CT, vertebral lesions typically involve the marrow space, whereas metastatic disease from other malignancies more often involves the pedicle and the portion of the vertebral body adjacent to the pedicle ("vertebral pedicle sign"[271]) (Figure 100-10, A and B).

Magnetic resonance imaging (MRI) of axial marrow, including head, entire spine, pelvis, and preferably also shoulders and sternum,

detects intramedullary focal disease in approximately 60 to 70 percent of patients at diagnosis, long before the onset of bone destruction (Figure 100-10, C).[272] These lesions are sometimes masked in cases of extensive marrow involvement, resulting in diffuse hyperintensity on short tau inversion recovery (STIR)-weighted images, and are unmasked after a few cycles of effective therapy (Figure 100-10, D). The number of MRI-detectable focal lesions has marked adverse prognostic consequences, second only to the presence of cytogenetic abnormalities (multivariate regression analysis) (Table 100-6 and Figure 100-10, E).[273]

Fluorodeoxyglucose (FDG)-PET whole-body scanning can provide high anatomic detail when performed in the context of CT scanning (Figure 100-10, F–I). Its usefulness is being investigated for predicting response and survival by early therapy-induced FDG suppression, as has been shown in malignant lymphoma. Bone densimetric analysis can establish the need for bisphosphonate administration and should be performed annually.[274]

AMYLOIDOSIS OR LIGHT-CHAIN DEPOSITION DISEASE

Clinical symptoms of congestive heart failure, nephrotic syndrome, malabsorption, coagulopathy, or neuropathy should prompt a careful search for primary amyloidosis. Facial cutaneous and oral mucosal amyloid lesions are readily recognized, as are "raccoon's eyes," resulting from capillary fragility. Cardiac amyloidosis may be associated with low voltage on electrocardiogram, arrhythmias, increased interventricular septal thickness of less than 12 mm, diastolic dysfunction, or speckling on echocardiogram. The value of the brain natriuretic protein (BNP) awaits further investigation.[275] Appropriate biopsy of tissues with suspected amyloid should be applied to clarify the presence and extent of accompanying amyloidosis or, similarly, LCDD in patients with myeloma. Occasionally, primary amyloidosis presents as tumors consisting mostly of amyloid or mixed with plasmacytoma. Typically, MRI signals can distinguish plasmacytomas, which show hypointensity on T1-weighted images and hyperintensity on STIR-weighted images, whereas amyloidoma-type lesions remain hypointense.

DIFFERENTIAL DIAGNOSIS

The initial laboratory evaluation should distinguish among essential monoclonal gammopathy, indolent myeloma; solitary plasmacytoma of bone or soft tissue; Ig deposition diseases, such as primary amyloidosis and LCDD; and symptomatic or progressive myeloma.[276] Clinicians should recognize that these are transition stages and frequently not clear-cut distinctions.

SOLITARY PLASMACYTOMA

Solitary plasmacytoma of bone[277–279] or soft tissue[280,281] requires the absence of indicators of systemic disease, such as marrow plasmacytosis, anemia, and other lytic bone or soft tissue lesions. Histologic or cytologic evidence of monoclonal plasma cell infiltration is required. Approximately 50 percent of patients with solitary plasmacytoma have small levels of M-protein in serum or urine that typically disappear upon institution of effective radiotherapy (40–50 Gy), as shown by immunofixation analysis. Persistence of M-protein may indicate a background of essential monoclonal gammopathy or the presence of

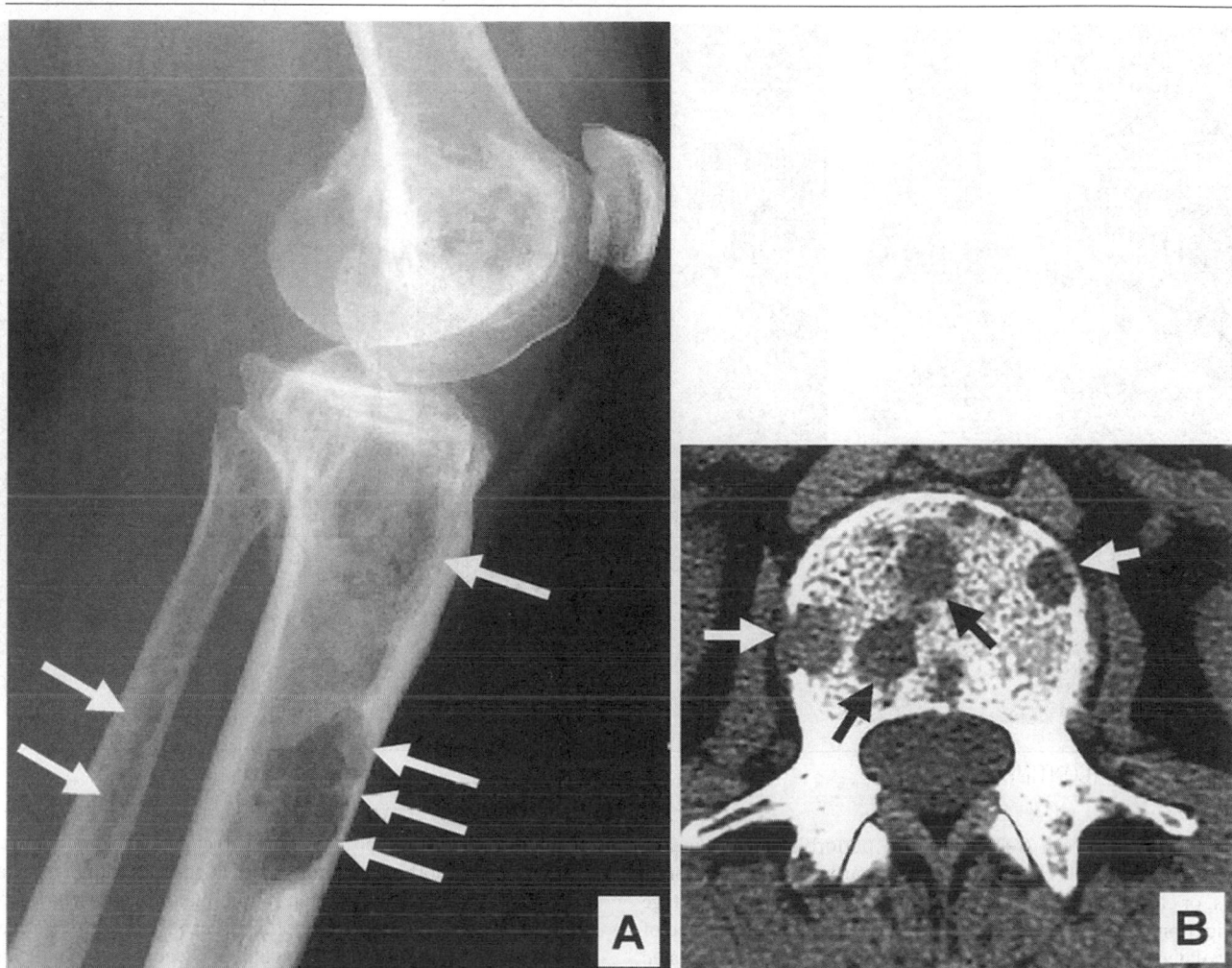

FIGURE 100-10 *(A)* Typical x-ray appearance of focal lytic lesions resulting from multiple myeloma *(arrows)* seen in a lateral view of the tibia and fibula. *(B)* CT scan of a lumbar vertebral body shows involvement of the "red marrow" space of the vertebral body. *(C)* MRI detects intramedullary tumor months before changes are apparent on x-ray film. STIR-weighted MRI *(left)* demonstrates a focal lesion at L3, not seen on a concurrent x-ray series *(center)* but visible 1 year later *(right)*. *(D)* STIR-weighted MRI shows diffuse hyperintensity prior to therapy *(left)*. Seven months after initiation of successful therapy, three focal lesions were unmasked *(right)*. *(E)* Survival after total therapy 2 (see Figure 100-8) is negatively affected not only by cytogenetics (CA) but also by the numbers of MRI-defined focal lesions (FL). *(F)* FDG-PET scan (anterior three-dimensional maximum intensity projection image with attenuation correction) of a patient with multiple myeloma. More than 100 focal (F) lesions and diffuse (D) marrow tumor infiltration are seen. *(G)* FDG-PET "superscan" showing severe skeletal infiltration and involvement of the liver (L), spleen (S), pancreas (P), and other extramedullary sites. Focal bone lesions are seen in the legs. *(H)* MRI STIR image showing hyperintensity in thoracic and lumbar spine. *(I)* FDG-PET scan corresponding to Figure 100-10H. *(continued)*

multifocal lesions. CT is recommended for a more detailed evaluation of early bone disease not recognized on standard roentgenographic examination.[282] MRI and FDG-PET scanning are powerful tools for detecting plasma cell myeloma involving the marrow in a macrofocal fashion or solitary plasmacytoma.[277,283–286] The detection of a solitary MRI lesion (cytologically proven) in the setting of an otherwise benign monoclonal gammopathy changes the diagnosis to solitary plasmacytoma. In contrast to most patients with plasma cell myeloma, patients with solitary plasmacytoma or essential monoclonal gammopathy have normal serum Ig levels.

Multiple solitary plasmacytomas may be seen at the outset as a result of advanced imaging by MRI and PET, or they may develop over time in approximately 5 percent of patients with apparently solitary plasmacytoma (Table 100-7). Results of random marrow examinations should be negative.

AL AMYLOIDOSIS

Primary AL amyloidosis and Ig deposition diseases are best characterized as monoclonal gammopathies with clinical manifestations, because of normal tissue infiltration by these processes, although they can accompany overt myeloma. Additional diagnostic procedures are indicated for patients with lymphadenopathy or hepatosplenomegaly to evaluate for extramedullary disease or protein deposition disease. The diagnosis of AL amyloid (see Chap. 101) often can be made by fine needle aspiration of subcutaneous fat or by biopsy of the rectal mucosa,[287] although we recommend biopsy of the clinically involved tissue. Staining the tissue with Congo red may reveal perivascular amyloid with its classic apple-green birefringence when viewed under polarized light.[288] AL amyloid also may be detectable on marrow biopsy.[177] Amyloidosis should be suspected in patients with macrog-

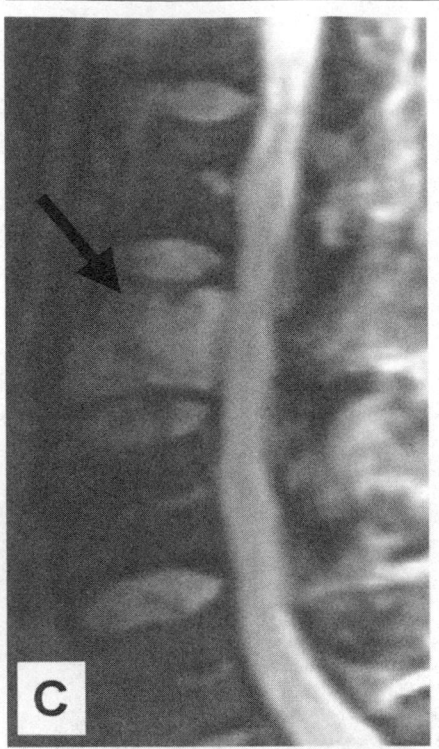
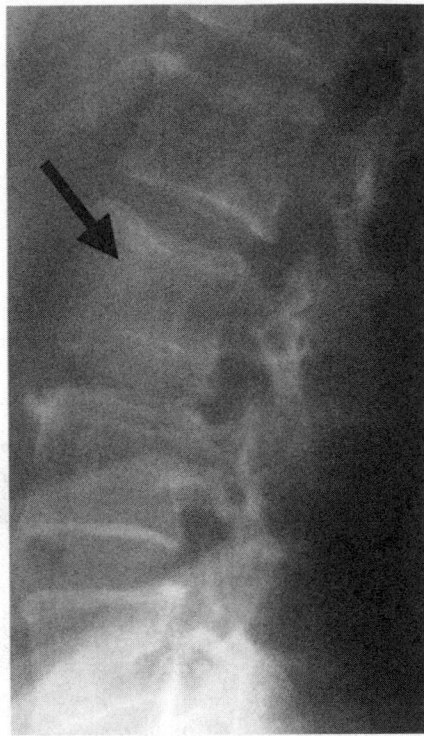
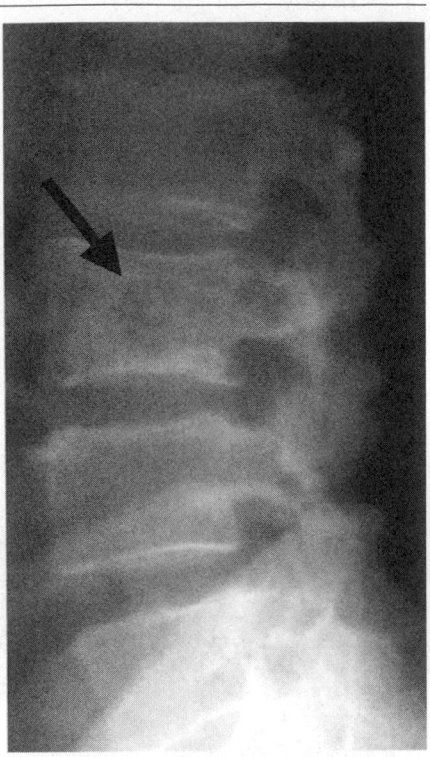

FIGURE 100-10 (CONTINUED)

lossia or "raccoon's eyes" (resulting from periorbital subcutaneous hemorrhages because of vascular fragility), carpal tunnel syndrome, nephrosis, or cardiomegaly associated with arrhythmias or low-voltage and conduction defects on electrocardiogram.[289] Patients suspected of having isolated cardiac amyloid with myeloma should be evaluated via echocardiography.[290] Endomyocardial biopsy may establish the diagnosis. Orthostatic hypotension also should alert the clinician to the possibility of systemic amyloidosis as a result of amyloid deposition in *vasa nervorum* of the autonomic nervous system or in adrenal glands, resulting in hypoadrenalism. Recognizing amyloidosis as a major cause of morbidity and mortality in patients with myeloma may be difficult. Because LCDD can mimic many manifestations of AL amyloidosis but requires immunofluorescence analysis of unfixed tissue, formalin fixation should be avoided whenever protein deposition disease is suspected.

THERAPY, COURSE, AND PROGNOSIS
STAGING AND PROGNOSIS

Once the diagnosis of plasma cell myeloma has been established, tumor staging should be performed (Table 100-8).[291] Studies measuring *in vitro* Ig production by myeloma cells have led to a clinically applicable method for estimating tumor mass.[292] A tumor staging system has been derived using standard laboratory measurements, including hemoglobin concentration, protein levels in serum and urine, presence of hypercalcemia, and extent of bone disease.[291] The Durie-Salmon staging system has remained in use for more than 30 years and has permitted better interpretation of therapeutic trials according to comparably staged patients.

However, because of the interpretation, especially of lytic bone lesions, other variables that are more quantitative and can better assess disease risk have been used for tumor staging. The serum concentration of β_2M currently provides the most reliable and prognostic marker for survival of patients with plasma cell myeloma.[258-260] Additional independent factors include the plasma cell labeling index[100,251] and CRP levels, reflect-

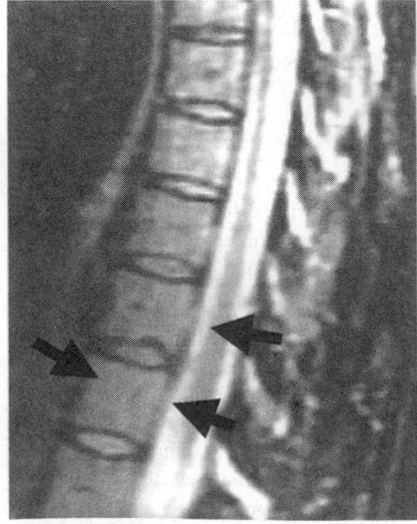
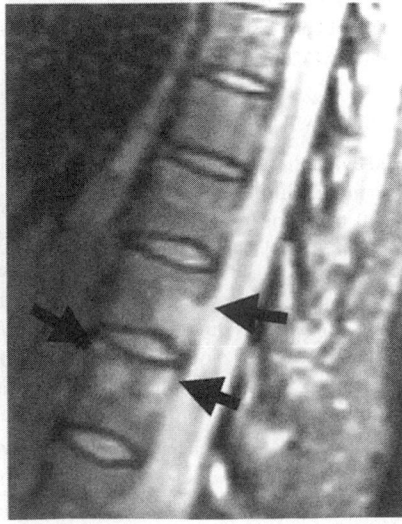

FIGURE 100-10 (CONTINUED)

ing *in vivo* IL-6 activity.[264] Increased IL-6 activity mediates many of the abnormalities encountered in myeloma, including hypoalbuminemia, anemia, and lytic bone disease.[2,293,294] Serum concentrations of syndecan-1, the hallmark of terminal plasma cell differentiation, reflect tumor burden and have been linked to outcome.[134,136–139] The degree of marrow plasmacytosis, as assessed by flow cytometry of DNA and cytoplasmic Ig, obviously reflects tumor burden and hence has prognostic utility.[222] However, this evaluation is compromised by the patchy marrow involvement often observed in this malignancy. Hypodiploidy identifies marked resistance to standard drug regimens and, as a result, is associated with inferior survival.[295]

Cytologically plasmablastic myeloma, present in less than 10 percent of newly diagnosed patients, is an adverse parameter frequently associated with a high plasma cell labeling index,[213,214] a high incidence of extramedullary disease, an elevated serum LDH level,[203,265] and a high incidence of karyotypic anomalies, all recognized to confer poor prognosis independently. In the setting of high-dose therapy, histologic evaluation of marrow biopsy sections identified short event-free and overall survival in the 20 percent of patients presenting with immature morphology (Bartl grade >1) and increased mitotic activity (≥1 per high-power field), regardless of β_2M or CRP level or cytogenetics.[215,216] Increased marrow microvessel density has been associated with poor prognosis.[217,219,296] The major angiogenic factors include vascular endothelial growth factor (VEGF) and basic fibroblast growth factor (bFGF) produced by myeloma cells themselves and by stromal cells in the marrow microenvironment.[218]

The Southwest Oncology Group introduced a staging system based on serum β_2M and albumin. Its predictive power has been confirmed by the International Staging System (ISS), which is based on world-

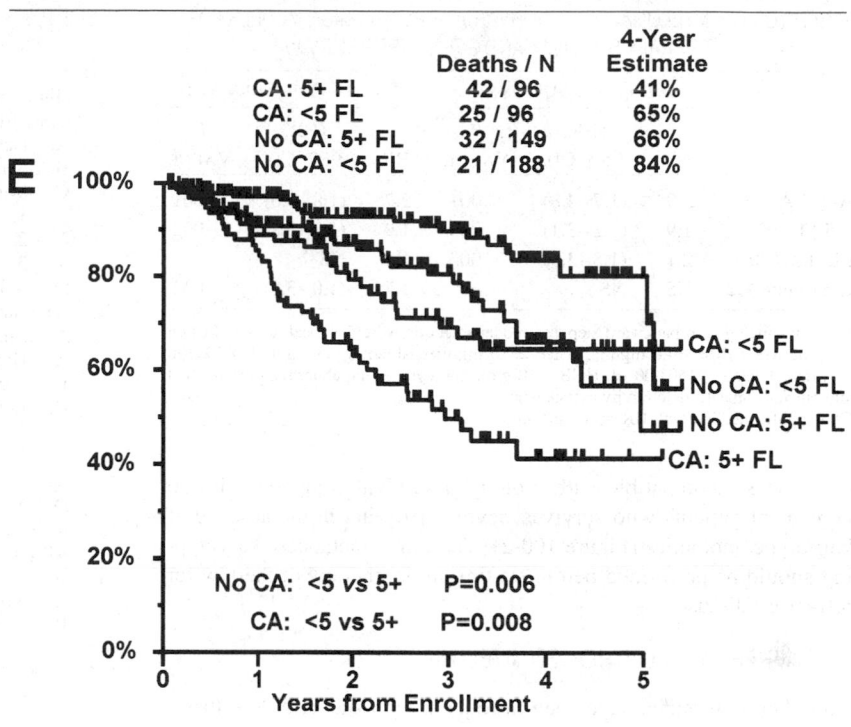

	Deaths / N	4-Year Estimate
CA: 5+ FL	42 / 96	41%
CA: <5 FL	25 / 96	65%
No CA: 5+ FL	32 / 149	66%
No CA: <5 FL	21 / 188	84%

No CA: <5 *vs* 5+   P=0.006
CA: <5 *vs* 5+   P=0.008

FIGURE 100-10   (CONTINUED)

wide submission of data from more than 11,000 patients (Table 100-9 and Figure 100-11). Cytogenetic data were available for only a limited number of patients. When the ISS was evaluated in the context of tandem autotransplants for nearly 900 newly diagnosed patients with concurrent karyotype information, the latter retained independent adverse implications in each of the three ISS stages (Figure 100-12). In fact, when examined in the context of nearly 2000 patients who received tandem melphalan-based autotransplants, abnormal cytoge-

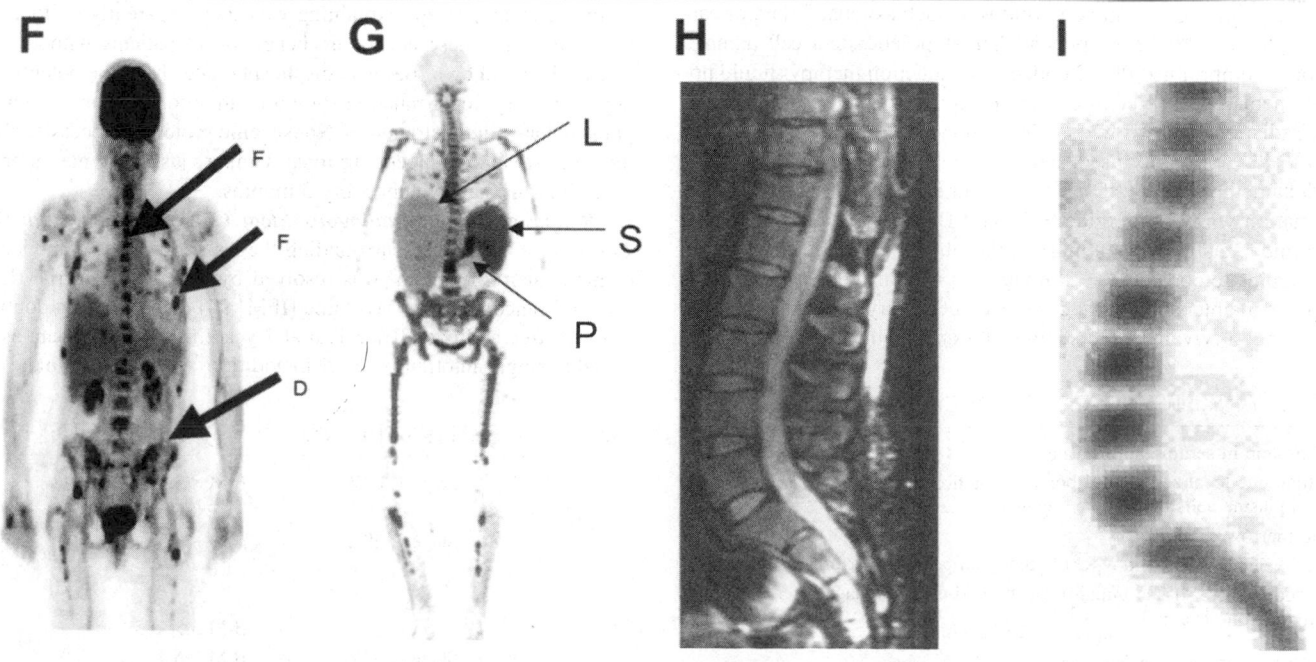

FIGURE 100-10   (CONTINUED)

TABLE 100-6 MYELOMA: COX MULTIVARIATE REGRESSION MODELS FOR OVERALL SURVIVAL AND EVENT-FREE SURVIVAL

	OVERALL SURVIVAL			EVENT-FREE SURVIVAL		
	HR	(HR, 95% CI)	P VALUE	HR	(HR, 95% CI)	P VALUE
Any CA	2.9	(1.7–4.8)	<.001	2.7	(1.8–4.0)	<.001
≥5 FL	1.9	(1.2–3.1)	.008	1.9	(1.3–2.8)	.002
LDH ≥190	2.1	(1.3–3.5)	.003	NS	NS	
Creatinine ≥2	NS	NS		1.7	(1.0–3.0)	.042

Variables included in backward stepwise model selection were 5+ focal lesions (FL) on baseline MRI, β_2M ≥4.0 mg/liter, CRP ≥4.0 mg/liter, albumin <3.5 g/dl, LDH ≥190 IU/liter, platelets <150,000/μl, HGB <10 g/dl, any cytogenetic abnormality (CA), and any chromosome 13 deletion by cytogenetics.
CI = confidence interval; HR = hazard ratio.

netics was incompatible with prolonged survival compared with 20 percent of patients who survived beyond 10 years in the absence of karyotype anomalies (Figure 100-2). Therefore, metaphase karyotyping should be performed before starting initial therapy or therapy for refractory disease.

THERAPY FOR UNTREATED MYELOMA

Complete remissions have been infrequent with standard-dose therapies. According to a meta-analysis,[297] event-free and overall survival were not extended by combination regimens compared to treatment with melphalan and prednisone.[298,299]

AUTOLOGOUS STEM CELL-SUPPORTED HIGH-DOSE THERAPIES

Randomized clinical trials[300,301] and controlled studies[302,303] indicate that high-dose melphalan 200 mg/m² supported by autologous peripheral blood stem cells (PBSC; mobilized with cyclophosphamide or etoposide plus filgrastim or filgrastim alone) can be effective in achieving marked tumor cytoreduction in patients up to age 70 years. Nevertheless, single-agent melphalan 200 mg/m² appears less toxic than conditioning regimens using total body irradiation (TBI).[314] Melphalan dose reduction to 140 or 100 mg/m² may be warranted in older patients or in those with significant comorbidities, such as renal failure or cardiac amyloidosis.[304–313] To prevent hematopoietic stem cell damage that could compromise PBSC collection, induction therapy should not include hematopoietic stem cell-toxic regimens (melphalan, nitrosoureas, radiation to marrow-containing bone sites, such as pelvis and spine).[315,316] Commonly used regimens include vincristine, doxorubicin, dexamethasone (VAD),[317–319] dexamethasone alone[320,321] or in combination with thalidomide,[322,323] and DT-PACE (dexamethasone, thalidomide, cisplatin [Platinol], doxorubicin [Adriamycin], cyclophosphamide, etoposide).[324] Although not conclusively studied, posttransplant maintenance strategies seem necessary to sustain disease control and survival. In the setting of standard therapy, greater glu-

TABLE 100-7 MULTIPLE SOLITARY PLASMACYTOMAS (± RECURRENT)

No M-protein in serum and/or urine*

More than one localized area of bone destruction or extramedullary tumor of clonal plasma cells that may be recurrent

Normal marrow examination

Normal skeletal survey and MRI of spine and pelvis if performed

No related organ or tissue impairment (no end-organ damage other than the localized bone lesions)

* A small M-component may be present.
SOURCE: The International Myeloma Working Group. *British Journal of Haematology* 2003;121:749–757 (Table IX). © 2003 Mayo Foundation.

TABLE 100-8 MYELOMA: ASSESSMENT OF TUMOR MASS (DURIE-SALMON)

I. High tumor mass (stage III) (>1.2 × 10¹²/m²)*
   One of the following abnormalities must be present:
   A. Hemoglobin <8.5 g/dl, hematocrit <25%
   B. Serum calcium >12 mg/dl
   C. Very high serum or urine myeloma protein production rates:
      1. IgG peak >7 g/dl
      2. IgA peak >5 g/dl
      3. Bence Jones protein >12 g/24 h
   D. >3 lytic bone lesions on bone survey (bone scan not acceptable)
II. Low tumor mass (stage I) (<0.6 × 10¹²/m²)*
   All of the following must be present:
   A. Hemoglobin >10.5 g/dl or hematocrit >32%
   B. Serum calcium normal
   C. Low serum myeloma protein production rates:
      1. IgG peak <5 g/dl
      2. IgA peak <3 g/dl
      3. Bence Jones protein <4 g/24 h
   D. No bone lesions or osteoporosis
III. Intermediate tumor mass (stage II) (0.6–1.2 × 10¹²/m²)*
   All patients who do not qualify for high or low tumor mass categories are considered to have intermediate tumor mass.
   A. No renal failure (creatinine ≤2 mg/dl)
   B. Renal failure (creatinine >2 mg/dl)

* Estimated number of neoplastic plasma cells.

cocorticoid dose intensity has been shown to improve event-free and overall survival,[325] which may be further improved by the addition of thalidomide. Although interferon initially appeared promising in standard therapy trials,[326–328] maintaining therapy with interferon failed to extend event-free or overall survival in responders to either standard-dose or high-dose therapy with single autotransplant in a US Intergroup trial.[329]

Bisphosphonate Use Monthly administration of bisphosphonates (pamidronate 90 mg intravenously over 2 hours[330] or zoledronic acid 4 mg over 30 minutes[331]) has become an important adjunct in the management of myeloma bone disease. In addition to their well-documented efficacy in delaying onset and reducing frequency of myeloma-related skeletal events[332,333] by inactivating osteoclasts, these agents induce apoptosis of myeloma cells[8,334] and display immunoregulatory effects, perhaps explaining why they apparently prolong survival. Whether these agents are beneficial in patients without bone disease is not known. Because bisphosphonates have the potential for nephrotoxicity, renal function should be monitored prior to each bisphosphonate administration.[335] Nonspecific proteinuria occasionally is the earliest sign of impending renal damage, justifying measurement of 24-hour urinary protein every 3 months.[313]

Reapplication of Autologous Stem Cell-Supported High-Dose Therapy Controversy surrounding the issue of repeated application of melphalan 200 mg/m² was resolved by a randomized trial (Intergroupe Francophone du Myélome [IFM] 94) demonstrating doubling of event-free and overall survival at 7 years following tandem as opposed to single autotransplant.[336] In addition, when viewed in the con-

TABLE 100-9 MYELOMA: INTERNATIONAL STAGING SYSTEM (ISS)

Stage 1: 28%	β_2M <3.5
	ALB ≥3.5
Stage 2: 39%	β_2M <3.5
	ALB <3.5
	or
	β_2M 3.5–5.5
Stage 3: 33%	β_2M >5.5

ALB = serum albumin in g/dl; β_2M = serum β_2-microglobulin in mg/liter.

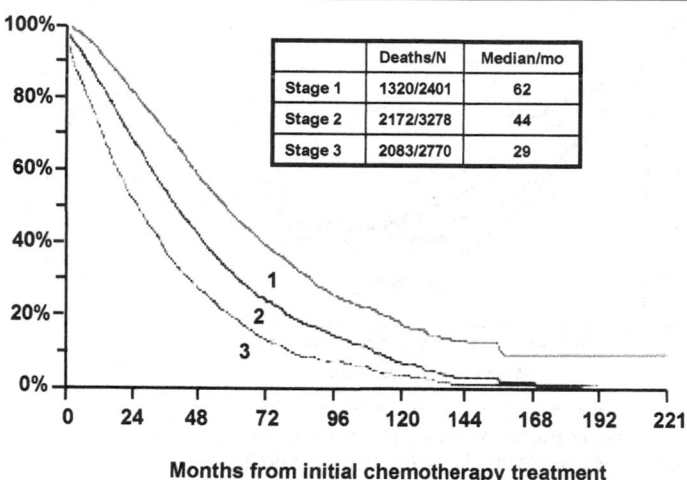

	Deaths/N	Median/mo
Stage 1	1320/2401	62
Stage 2	2172/3278	44
Stage 3	2083/2770	29

Months from initial chemotherapy treatment

FIGURE 100-11 Survival of previously untreated patients with multiple myeloma according to the International Staging System introduced in 2003.[403]

text of Arkansas Total Therapy trials (see below), total therapies 1 and 2 provided superior outcome compared to more intensive remission induction therapy, higher total melphalan dose (400 mg/m²), or post-tandem transplant consolidation or maintenance therapies (Figures 100-13 and 100-14).[313] On the other hand, survival curves for Medical Research Council (MRC) VII (standard therapy vs. single autotransplant with melphalan 200 mg/m²),[301] IFM 90 (standard therapy vs. single autotransplants with melphalan 140 mg/m² + TBI 8 Gy),[300] and SWOG Intergroup trial 9321 (induction VAD followed by VBMCP [vincristine, carmustine (BCNU), melphalan, cyclophosphamide, prednisone] maintenance vs. melphalan 140 mg/m² + TBI 12 Gy) appear highly similar[329] (Tables 100-10 and 100-11).

Allogeneic Stem Cell Transplants The high mortality rate of myeloablative allogeneic transplant regimens declined from 50 percent to 10 to 15 percent when reduced intensity conditioning regimens were applied.[338–344] Follow-up of most studies is too short to determine whether exploitation of the well-recognized graft-versus-myeloma effect translates into more durable disease control than reported with autotransplants.[345–347] We advocate the exploration of mini-allogeneic transplants only in the setting of high-risk myeloma with cytogenetic abnormalities, thus matching the risk of intervention with the risk of the disease. Specifically, standard melphalan (200 mg/m²)-based au-

totransplant (after appropriate induction) is followed within 3 to 4 months by a planned mini-allogeneic transplant with preconditioning regimens of either melphalan 100 mg/m² or TBI 2 Gy with or without fludarabine.

SPECIAL CLINICAL CONSIDERATIONS

RENAL FAILURE AND OLDER AGE

The rapid hematopoietic recovery afforded by mobilized PBSC, which was confirmed in the IFM 94 trial,[336] was critical for the successful administration of melphalan to populations particularly vulnerable to high-dose therapy (high-risk populations), such as patients with renal failure[307,308,348] or those of advanced age (>70 years).[304,305] Mucositis and other extramedullary toxicities commonly encountered in elderly patients receiving the standard high-dose melphalan regimen of 200 mg/m² are seldom seen in patients treated with melphalan 140 mg/m² and, especially 100 mg/m².[306] In such cases, prior cytoreduction can be achieved with relatively noncytotoxic regimens, such as regimens using high-dose dexamethasone either alone or in combination with thalidomide. In the absence of adequate tumor cytoreduction or persistent renal insufficiency of recent onset resulting from presumed cast nephropathy, melphalan dose-adjusted autotransplants should be instituted promptly after PBSC collection with hematopoietic growth factors alone or in combination with intermediate-dose cyclophosphamide (1.5–3.0 g/m²). From 70 to 80 percent of patients can achieve at least 75 percent M-protein reduction, resulting in improvement in 50 percent of patients and normalization of renal function in some cases.[308]

PRIMARY AL AMYLOIDOSIS AND IMMUNOGLOBULIN DEPOSITION DISEASE

Even though their tumor load is very low, patients with primary AL amyloidosis and Ig deposition disease suffer from the consequences of myeloma secretory products, even at relatively modest amounts. The result is damage to kidneys, heart, gastrointestinal tract, liver, spleen, and peripheral and autonomic nerves. All current treatments target the monoclonal plasma cell population. Whereas standard melphalan-prednisone (MP) has been only marginally effective, high-dose dexamethasone pulsing plus interferon, which results in more rapid and profound responses in myeloma, has also shown encouraging results in primary amyloidosis.[349,350] Similar positive results have been obtained with dexamethasone plus melphalan.[351] Although thalidomide may be useful in noncardiac AL amyloidosis, it should be used with caution in the setting of cardiac disease because of its well-rec-

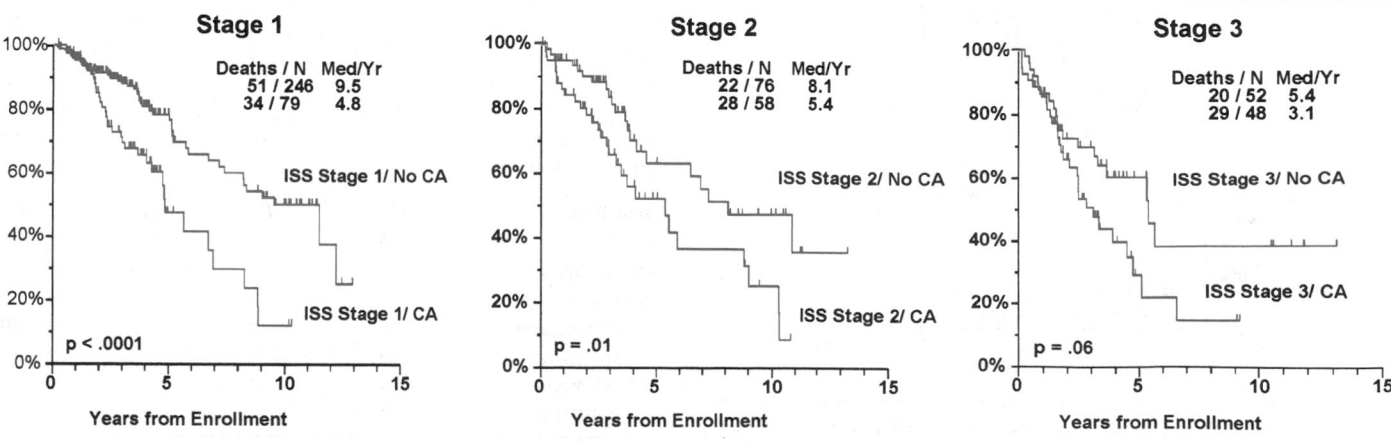

FIGURE 100-12 Survival with total therapies 1 and 2 according to International Staging System (ISS) and cytogenetic abnormalities (CA).

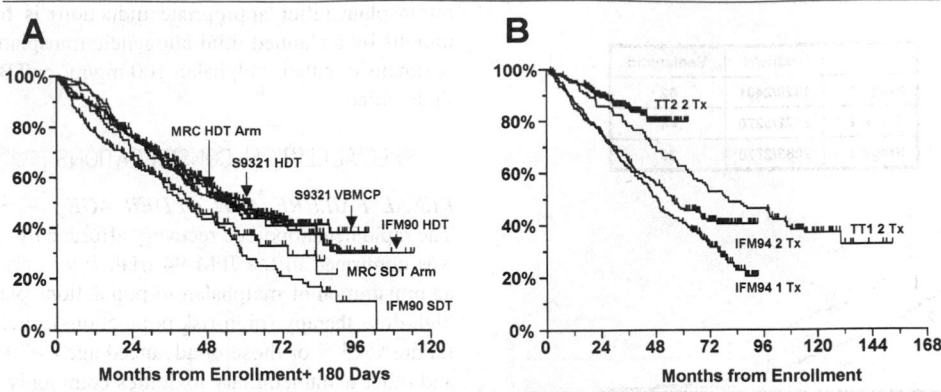

FIGURE 100-13   Total therapy trials provide superior outcome for patients with multiple myeloma. *(A)* Survival comparison of single autotransplant versus standard therapy trials. Medical Research Council (MRC) VII high-dose therapy (HDT) arm applied melphalan 200 mg/m^2 versus standard therapy (SDT) using ABCM (Adriamycin, BCNU, Cytoxan, melphalan). Intergroupe Francophone du Myélome (IFM) 90 trial compared HDT with melphalan 140 mg/m^2 plus total body irradiation (TBI) 8 Gy versus VMCP (vincristine, melphalan, cyclophosphamide, prednisone)/VBAP (vincristine, BCNU [carmustine], Adriamycin, prednisone) in the standard arm. SWOG Intergroup trial 9321 applied 140 mg/m^2 plus 12 Gy in the HDT arm versus VBMCP (vincristine, BCNU [carmustine], melphalan, cyclophosphamide, prednisone) in the standard arm. To account for differences in times of randomization (MRC VII and IFM 90) at enrollment in S9321 after induction with VAD (vincristine, Adriamycin, dexamethasone) for four cycles, data are shown from a joint landmark of 180 days post enrollment. *(B)* Tandem autotransplants (2 Tx) versus single transplant (1 Tx) (IFM 94: 2 Tx melphalan 140 mg/m^2 followed by melphalan 140 mg/m^2 plus TBI 8 Gy, 1 Tx melphalan 140 mg/m^2 plus TBI 8 Gy). Arkansas total therapy programs 1 (TT 1) and 2 (TT 2) both applied tandem transplants (see text for details).

ognized bradycardic effects. The Boston University group has pioneered the use of autologous stem cell-supported high-dose melphalan and has demonstrated end-organ responses, especially in patients achieving complete remission defined by myeloma protein elimination (Figure 100-15).[352] Cardiac amyloid remains the most challenging clinical condition. It currently is addressed with repeated cycles of dose-reduced melphalan (70–100 mg/m^2) and stem cell support to prevent cardiac catastrophes possibly linked to arrhythmias caused by fluid overload or cytokines.[310]

BONE AND EXTRAMEDULLARY PLASMACYTOMAS

Patients with soft tissue solitary plasmacytomas often can be cured with local radiation (at least 4.5 Gy). By contrast, this local treatment

approach fails in the majority of patients with presumed solitary plasmacytomas of bone.[353] The development of myeloma in such patients probably reflects multifocal systemic disease present at the outset, which now might be revealed by MRI[354] and PET scanning using 2-[^{18}F]fluoro-2-deoxy-D-glucose.[355] Prospective trials are needed to determine whether, by applying appropriate staging tools, solitary plasmacytomas of bone truly exist and, if so, if they can be cured by local irradiation.

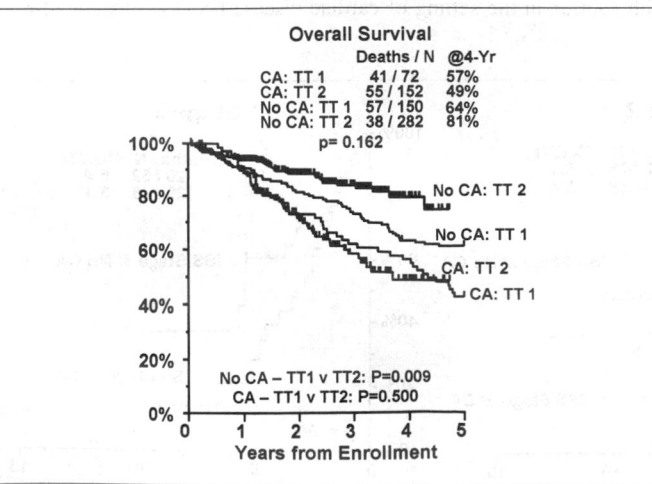

FIGURE 100-14   Superior event-free and overall survival with total therapy 2 (TT 2) versus total therapy 1 (TT 1) in the absence of cytogenetic abnormalities (CA).

TABLE 100-10   MYELOMA: MULTIVARIATE PROGNOSTIC ANALYSIS

	ALL PATIENTS (N = 704)		NO CA (N = 432)	
SURVIVAL	HR	P	HR	P
Overall survival				
Any CA	1.6	<.01	NA	
Total therapy 2	.8	.24	.6	.02
Complete response*	.7	.02	.8	.2
Second transplant*	.5	<.01	.4	<.01
β_2M ≥4 mg/liter	1.5	<.01	1.3	.3
CRP ≥4 mg/liter	1.3	.03	1.7	.01
LDH ≥190 U/liter	1.7	<.01	2.1	<.01
Event-free survival	HR	P	HR	P
Any CA	1.5	<.01	NA	
Total therapy 2	.5	<.01	.4	<.01
Complete response*	.7	<.01	.7	.03
Second transplant*	.6	<.01	.6	.01
β_2M ≥4 mg/liter	1.6	<.01	1.4	.04
CRP ≥4 mg/liter	1.4	.01	1.3	.1
LDH ≥190 U/liter	1.4	.01	1.6	.02

* Time-dependent covariates.
HR, hazard ratio; CA, cytogenetic abnormality; *P*, probability.

TABLE 100-11 SUMMARY OF HIGH-DOSE THERAPY TRIALS IN MYELOMA

AUTHOR	RANDOM-IZATION	REGIMENS	N	AGE (MEAN YEARS)	MEDIAN FOLLOWUP (MONTHS)	% COMPLETE RESPONSE (P)	EVENT-FREE SURVIVAL (MEDIAN MONTHS) (P)	OVERALL SURVIVAL (MEDIAN MONTHS) (P)
Standard-dose Therapy vs. High-dose Therapy								
Attal[a] IFM 90*	Pretreatment	VMCP/VBAP × 18 vs. VMCP/VBAP × 4–6 → CTX + MEL 140 + TBI 8 Gy	100 vs. 100	58 vs. 57	108	14 vs. 38 (<.001)	18 vs. 28 (.01)	44 vs. 57 (20% vs. 35% @ 7 years) (.03)
Child[b] MRC VII*	Pretreatment	ABCM × 4–12 vs. CVAMP × 3 → CTX + MEL 200	200 vs. 201	56 vs. 55	42	8 vs. 44 (<.001)	20 vs. 32 (16% vs. 36% @ 4 years) (<.001)	42 vs. 54 (46% vs. 55% @ 4 years) (.04)
Blade[c] PETHEMA†	Responders to induction	ABCM/VBAD × 12 vs. ABCM/VBAD × 4 → MEL 200	83 vs. 81	56 vs. 56	66	11 vs. 30 (<.002)	34 vs. 43 (NA)	67 vs. 65 (NA)
Single High-dose Transplant vs. Tandem Transplant								
Attal[d] IFM 94*	Pretreatment	VAD × 3–4 → G-CSF → MEL 140 + TBI 8 Gy vs. VAD × 3–4 → G-CSF → MEL 140; MEL 140 + TBI 8 Gy	199 vs. 200	52 vs. 52	75	42 vs. 50 >n-CR (<.1)	25 vs. 30 (10% vs. 20% @ 7 years) (<.03)	48 vs. 58 (21% vs. 42% @ 7 years) (.01)
Cavo[e] BOLOGNA 96	Pretreatment	VAD × 4 → CTX → MEL 200 vs. VAD × 4 → CTX → MEL 200; MEL 120 + Busulfan	110 vs. 110	53 vs. 53	38	21 vs. 24 (NS)	25 vs. 34 (NA) (<.05)	56 vs. 60 (NS)
Fermand[f] MAG 95	Pretreatment	DEX × 2 → CTX → VAD × 3–4 → MEL 140 + VP16 + CTX + TBI 12 Gy vs. DEX × 2 → CTX → VAD × 3–4 → MEL 140; MEL 140 + VP16 + TBI 12 Gy	97 vs. 96	50 vs. 50	53	39 vs. 37 (NS)	31 vs. 33 (NS)	49 vs. 73 (NA) (.14)
Segeren[g] HOVON* (intermediate-dose therapy)	After VAD ± response	VAD × 3–4 → CTX → MEL 70 × 2 vs. VAD × 3–4 → CTX → MEL 70 × 2 → CTX + TBI 9 Gy	129 vs. 132	55 vs. 56	40	14 vs. 28 (.004)	(NA) (15% vs. 29% @ 4 years) (<.03)	(NA)(55% vs. 50% @ 4 years) (<.3)
Standard-dose Therapy vs. Tandem Transplant								
Barlogie[h] SWOG vs. TT I*	Historical controls	VMCB (P)/VBAP (P)/VAD vs. VAD × 2–3 → CTX → EDAP → MEL 200 × 2 (<PR, MEL 140 + TBI 8.5 Gy)	152 vs. 152	52 vs. 52	114	NA vs. 41	16 vs. 37 (5% vs. 15% @ 10 years) (<.0001)	43 vs. 79 (15% vs. 33% @ 10 years) (<.0001)

[a] Attal M, Harousseau JL, Stoppa AM, et al: A prospective, randomized trial of autologous bone marrow transplantation and chemotherapy in multiple myeloma. Intergroupe Francais du Myelome. *N Engl J Med* 335:91-7,1996.

[b] Child JA, Morgan GJ, Davies FE, et al: High-dose chemotherapy with hematopoietic stem-cell rescue for multiple myeloma. *N Engl J Med* 348:1875-83, 2003.

[c] Blade J, Sureda A, Ribera J, et al: High-dose therapy autotransplantation/intensification vs continued conventional chemotherapy in multiple myeloma patients responding to initial treatment chemotherapy. Results of a prospective randomized trial from the Spanish Cooperative Group. *PETHEMA* 98:815a, 2001.

[d] Attal M, Harousseau JL, Facon T, et al., and the InterGroupe Francophone du Myelome. Single versus double autologous stem-cell transplantation for multiple myeloma. *N Engl J Med* 349:2495, 2003. Erratum in *N Engl J Med* 350:2628, 2004.

[e] Cavo M, Tosi P, Zamagni E, et al. The Bologna 96 clinical trial of single versus double PBSC transplantation for previously untreated MM: Results of an interim analysis. In *VIIIth International Myeloma Workshop*. Banff, Canada, 2001.

[f] Fermand JP, Marolleau JP, Alberti C. *Single versus tandem high-dose therapy (HDT) supported with autologous blood stem cell (ABSC) transplantation using unselected or CD-34 enriched ABSC: Preliminary results of a two by two design randomized trial in 230 young patients with multiple myeloma.* In *VIIIth International Myeloma Workshop*. Banff, Canada, 2001.

[g] Segeren CN, Sonneveld P, van der Holt B, et al: Intensive versus double intensie therapy in previously untreated multiple myeloma: A prospective randomized phase III study in 450 patients. In *VIIIth International Myeloma Workshop*. Banff, Canada, 2001.

[h] Barlogie B, Jagannath S, Vesole DH, et al: Superiority of tandem autologous transplantation over standard therapy for previously untreated multiple myeloma. *Blood* 89:789, 1997.

Maintenance = *IFN, †IFN and DEX.

SOURCE: Barlogie B, Shaughnessy JD, Tricot G, et al.,[337] with permission.

CTx, cytoxan; CVAMP, cyclophosphamide, vincristine, doxorubicin, methylprednisolone; DEX, dexamethasone; MEL, melphalan; N, number of patients in each arm of the study; PR, partial response; VBAD, vincristine, BCNU (carmustine), doxorubicin, dexamethasone; VMCB(P), vincristine, melphalan, cyclophosphamide, BCNU (carmustine), prednisone.

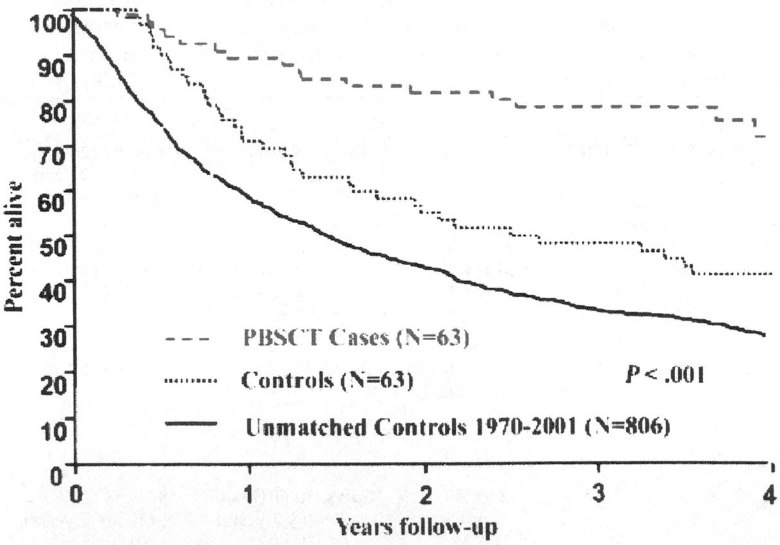

FIGURE 100-15 Survival from initial diagnosis of 932 patients with immunoglobulin light-chain amyloid. Case control comparison ($P < .001$). Cases (n = 63) received peripheral blood stem cell transplantation (PBSCT). Controls (n = 63) did not undergo transplantation. Unmatched cases (n = 806) are included for comparison.[404]

Local radiation, typically administered with high-dose dexamethasone, has a palliative role in the treatment of focal lesions as part of disseminated myeloma. However, especially in newly diagnosed patients, primary systemic therapy controls focal problems, including cord compression, as quickly and effectively as does local radiation in the large majority of patients (Figure 100-16, *A*). Avoiding radiation to major marrow-containing skeletal regions preserves the ability to procure adequate PBSC quantities. In advanced disease, determining whether the source of pain is local tumor growth or vertebral collapse, with bone particles compressing the cord, is critical. In the latter case, surgical intervention is the preferred treatment approach. Vertebroplasty and kyphoplasty have become important adjuncts of disease management, promptly alleviating pain resulting from vertebral collapse (Figure 100-16, *B* and *C*).[356,357]

SMOLDERING MULTIPLE MYELOMA

Patients with smoldering myeloma historically have been followed without therapy.[358–360] Once the diagnosis is established through careful monitoring of disease markers over 2 to 3 months, patients at some institutions have been offered thalidomide plus bisphosphonate therapy.[361] This therapy has shown promising results in terms of delaying the onset of progression to symptomatic disease and, in approximately 20 to 30 percent of patients, inducing mostly partial responses.[362] The Southwest Oncology Group has initiated a trial for patients with smoldering myeloma at

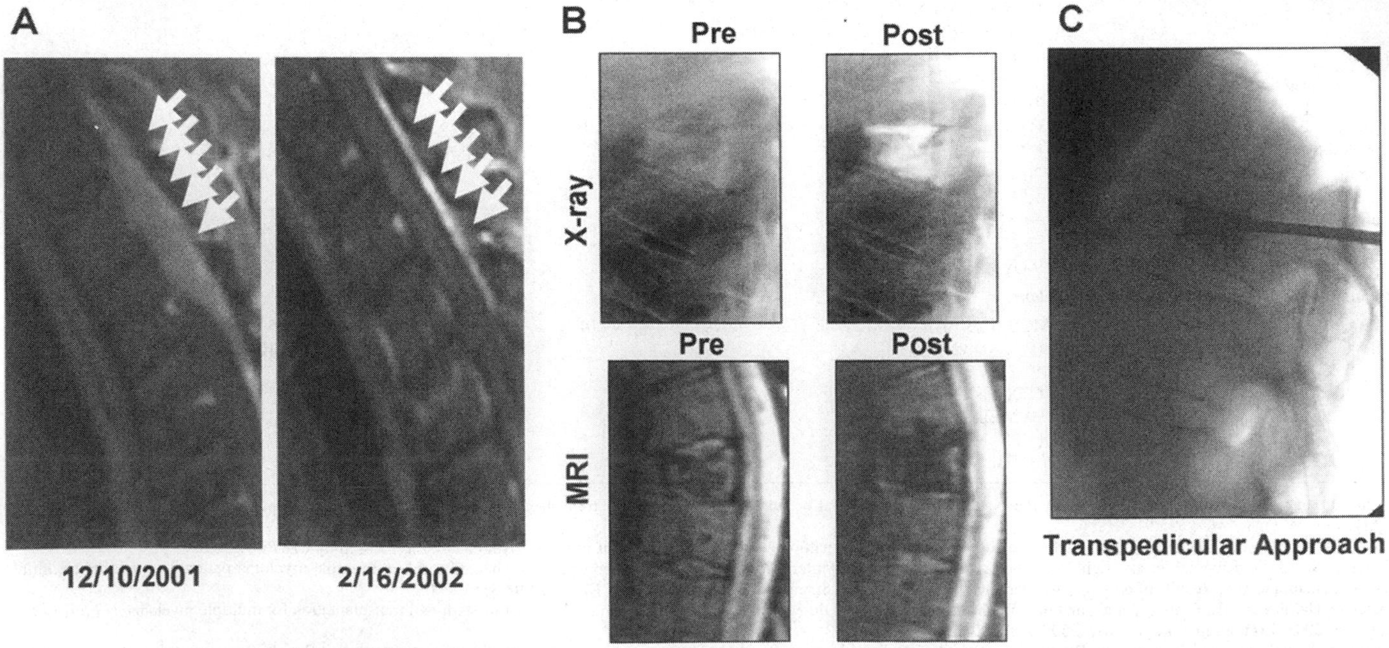

FIGURE 100-16 *(A)* Cord compression detected by MRI. Example of rapid resolution of extensive spinal cord compression as a result of combination chemotherapy with DT-PACE: dexamethasone 40 mg daily × 4, thalidomide 400 mg daily × 4, 4-day continuous intravenous infusions of cisplatin (Platinol) 10 mg/m²/day, doxorubicin (Adriamycin) 10 mg/m²/day, cyclophosphamide 400 mg/m²/day, and etoposide 40 mg/m²/day. Epidural disease from multiple myeloma responds to treatment: Postgadolinium T1-weighted MRI before *(left)* and after *(right)* treatment of epidural disease *(arrows)*. Only a thin "stripe" of enhancing tissue remains after treatment. *(B)* Vertebroplasty for compression fracture. X-ray films *(top)* and STIR-weighted MRI sagittal images *(bottom)* of a compression fracture of T7 before and after vertebroplasty via standard transpedicular approach. *(C)* Immediate and dramatic pain relief, resulting from improved mechanical stability and the neurotoxic effects of polymethylmethacrylate, typically is observed.

high risk for early progression (IgA isotype, Bence Jones excretion >1 g/day, and presence of 1+ lytic lesions), evaluating thalidomide plus dexamethasone plus zoledronic acid. This secondary prevention trial is aimed at disease control through therapeutic cotargeting of myeloma cells and the marrow microenvironment.

MONITORING DISEASE MARKERS FOR DOCUMENTATION OF RESPONSE AND RELAPSE

Many current induction regimens affect tumor cytoreduction rapidly so that M-protein reduction of at least 50 percent is apparent within a few months of therapy. Thus, at least monthly myeloma protein evaluations should be performed during induction. After two to four induction cycles and prior to high-dose melphalan-based autotransplant, the disease is restaged, including marrow examination with cytogenetics and MRI of affected areas to determine whether intramedullary or extramedullary bulk disease has been reduced. Further restaging should be performed prior to a second transplant, which, when considered, should be administered within 2 to 4 months after the first high-dose therapy. Maintenance therapy with dexamethasone, thalidomide, or its combination should be initiated within 3 months of autotransplant. Disease monitoring should be performed at least every 2 months for the first year. Marrow biopsy, including cytogenetic examinations, should be performed at least semiannually and more frequently if cytogenetic abnormalities were documented at diagnosis. MRI examination of previously abnormal sites should be performed every 3 to 6 months.

Complete remission is defined by normalization of marrow aspirate and biopsy morphologically, preferably also by DNA/cytoplasmic Ig flow cytometry, and, in the majority of patients with secretory disease, by the disappearance of monoclonal protein in serum and urine on immunofixation analysis.[363] The persistence of reactivity on immunofixation in the absence of M-protein peaks on standard electrophoresis of serum or urine qualifies as *near-complete remission*. Oligoclonal Igs can be detected by immunofixation analysis, especially after melphalan-based autotransplants. Rather than representing relapse, as suggested by trace M-protein readings on standard electrophoresis, the emergence of Igs different from those secreted by the original myeloma clone reflects recovery of normal B cell function accompanied by recovery of uninvolved Ig levels and clinically is a favorable feature of sustained disease control.[364] MRI-based or PET scan-based definitions of complete response are being evaluated for their capacity to predict event-free and overall survival.

Partial remission requires the reduction of measurable myeloma serum concentration by at least 50 percent and Bence Jones proteinuria by at least 90 percent, or to less than 100 mg/day, with normalization of marrow aspirate and biopsy.

Approximately 5 to 10 percent of patients who present with low-secretory or nonsecretory myeloma will require more frequent marrow and MRI follow-up examinations to document response. Serum free light-chain levels are useful in at least half of patients historically categorized as nonsecretors.

Disease features can change over the course of the disease, which now often spans up to 8 years. With successive relapses, myeloma dedifferentiation occurs not infrequently, resulting in more bizarre myeloma cell morphology in the marrow, loss of previously secreted complete Ig (and switch to only light-chain secretion or "Bence Jones escape"), or complete loss of Ig secretory capacity, often associated with extramedullary spread best signified by increased LDH levels. Occasionally, unexplained anemia or pancytopenia accompanies disappearing myeloma protein markers, necessitating prompt marrow examination to detect fulminant relapse.

THERAPY FOR PREVIOUSLY TREATED MYELOMA

The cardinal questions arising in this setting pertain to the timing of the initial diagnosis, whether the disease was truly symptomatic and progressive, the type of treatment applied, and the degree and duration of response observed. Special attention should be paid to the development of MDS, especially in the context of long-term standard melphalan plus prednisone or nitrosourea combinations such as VBMCP (M$_2$ regimen). Pancytopenia associated with hypercellular marrow and megaloblastic changes should prompt cytogenetic or interphase FISH studies to detect secondary MDS, especially in the presence of only minor marrow plasmacytosis. In case of disease recurrence (on or off treatment) requiring therapy, careful analysis of marrow aspirate and biopsy, including cytogenetics, proliferative markers, and serum LDH level, should be performed. Primary unresponsive disease should be distinguished from untested or resistant relapse.

NEW THERAPEUTIC AGENTS

THALIDOMIDE
When thalidomide's efficacy in advanced and refractory myeloma was first reported in 1999,[365] it represented only the third independently active compound used for treatment of myeloma. Long-term follow-up of 169 patients enrolled in a phase II clinical trial using incremental dosing of thalidomide up to 800 mg/day confirmed the original observation of a partial response rate in approximately one third of patients and extended event-free and overall survival, with cytogenetic abnormalities conferring a poor prognosis (Table 100-12 and Figure 100-17).[366]

A marked *in vivo* synergy between thalidomide and dexamethasone[370] has been confirmed clinically and has prompted evaluation of this combination for response induction prior to and for maintenance therapy after autotransplantations.[322,323] Much remains to be learned about thalidomide dosing and scheduling in different clinical scenarios[371] and the purported mechanisms of its antimyeloma effects.[372]

Thalidomide can be combined with chemotherapy because thalidomide is not myelosuppressive.[367,368] However, peripheral neuropathy is a major treatment-limiting toxicity that affects 50 to 80 percent of patients, the severity and reversibility of which are related to the dose and duration of drug administration.[369] In case of grade 2 neuropathy, dose reduction or suspension of therapy frequently improves or resolves the symptoms. In approximately one third of patients, higher thalidomide doses ($\geq$400 mg) are associated with grade 3 neurotoxicity that sometimes is not readily reversible.

CC-5013
CC-5013 (Revlimid) is an immunomodulatory agent that exhibits almost no sedative effects and only occasionally exhibits neurotoxic side effects. Responses have been reported in one third of patients with advanced or refractory myeloma.[373,374] Many of these patients previously were exposed to thalidomide, although true thalidomide resistance was infrequently established. Unlike thalidomide, CC-5013 causes myelosuppression that, in the setting of compromised marrow reserve because of extensive prior cytotoxic drug exposure, may not be fully reversible. In a phase III trial for advanced myeloma that compared two different schedules of administration (alternating-day schedule of 50 mg for 10 doses vs. daily 25 mg for 20 doses every 28 days), a higher response rate was observed with the 25-mg daily-dose schedule (Table 100-13 and Figure 100-18). Greater than

TABLE 100-12   THALIDOMIDE THERAPY PATIENT CHARACTERISTICS

PARAMETER	PERCENTAGE OF PATIENTS
Age ≥60 years	44
β_2M ≥4 mg/liter	22
Abnormal cytogenetics	66
Deletion 13	37
Prior therapy ≥60 months	20
Prior high-dose therapy	76
>1 cycle	53
No. of patients	169

TABLE 100-13   CC-5013 (REVLIMID) THERAPY: PATIENT CHARACTERISTICS BY TREATMENT ARM

	TREATMENT ARM		
FACTOR	ALL PATIENTS	CONTINUOUS DOSING	SYNCOPATED DOSING
Age ≥ 60 years	42/67 (63%)	25/36 (69%)	17/31 (55%)
β_2M ≥4 mg/liter	30/67 (45%)	16/36 (44%)	14/31 (45%)
LDH ≥190 UI/liter	27/66 (41%)	15/36 (42%)	12/30 (40%)
Cytogenetic abnormalities	41/67 (61%)	23/36 (64%)	18/31 (58%)
CA13	30/67 (45%)	17/36 (47%)	13/31 (42%)
Prior therapy of ≥ 60 months	26/67 (39%)	15/36 (42%)	11/31 (35%)
Prior high-dose therapy	50/67 (75%)	27/36 (75%)	23/31 (74%)
>1 cycle of prior high-dose therapy	33/67 (49%)	18/36 (50%)	15/31 (48%)

n/N (%): n=number with factor for group level; N=number known with or without factor for group level.

grade 2 thrombocytopenia was linked to pretreatment platelet count less than 100,000/μL (100 × 10^9/L), which is a reflection of impaired hematopoietic reserve. Trials have been initiated to evaluate the response to therapy with CC-5013 alone or in combination with dexamethasone.

BORTEZOMIB

The proteasome inhibitor bortezomib (Velcade) represents an entirely new class of agents,[375,376] sometimes with remarkable activity in the treatment of myeloma that is refractory to multiple lines of standard-dose or high-dose regimens (including thalidomide).[377,378] Combination trials of bortezomib with melphalan and pegylated doxorubicin (Doxil; ALZA Pharmaceuticals, Mountain View, CA) are in progress.[379,380]

A combination of bortezomib plus thalidomide was evaluated in 73 patients in a phase I to II fashion.[313] Because of concerns about potential synergistic neurotoxicity among patients previously exposed to thalidomide, the trial called for administration of bortezomib 1.0 mg/m^2 (days 1, 4, 8, and 11, repeated every 21 days) and added thalidomide with a second cycle. Cohorts consisting of at least 10 patients received thalidomide 50 mg, escalated to daily doses of 100, 150, and 200 mg in the absence of grade 3 neurotoxicity. Subsequently, bortezomib was administered at the standard dose of 1.3 mg/m^2 (days 1, 4, 8, and 11), and the same iteration of thalidomide dose escalation was performed. The majority of patients previously had been exposed to high-dose therapy and thalidomide. Nearly half of patients had abnormal cytogenetics. A high response rate in this setting was observed (Table 100-14 and Figure 100-19). A partial response (>50% M-protein reduction in the serum and/or

>90 percent reduction in Bence Jones proteinuria) was obtained in 60 percent of patients at the end of cycle 3 and reached 75 percent by cycle 8. Remarkably, 20 to 30 percent of patients achieved near-complete remission (only immunofixation positive). Response to the combination was independent of prior thalidomide exposure. Event-free survival and overall survival were particularly impressive among the approximately 50 percent of patients who lacked cytogenetic abnormalities prior to study enrollment. Remarkably, no synergistic neurotoxicity was observed.

OTHER THERAPEUTIC AGENTS

Agents under investigation for their potential role in the treatment of myeloma include arsenic trioxide,[381,382] monoclonal antibodies to IL-6[383] and CD20,[384] and farnesyl transferase inhibitors.[385–387] High expression of *kit* in 20 to 40 percent of myeloma patients justifies studies with imatinib mesylate. Research in progress also is targeting unique 14q32 translocations, such as rearrangements involving the FGF receptor-3 gene *(FGF-R3)*, which often is associated with chromosome 13 deletions and a poor prognosis.[388]

DT-PACE REGIMEN FOR HIGH-GRADE RELAPSE

A combination of dexamethasone 40 mg/day for 4 days, thalidomide 400 mg for 4 days, and 4-day continuous intravenous infusions of

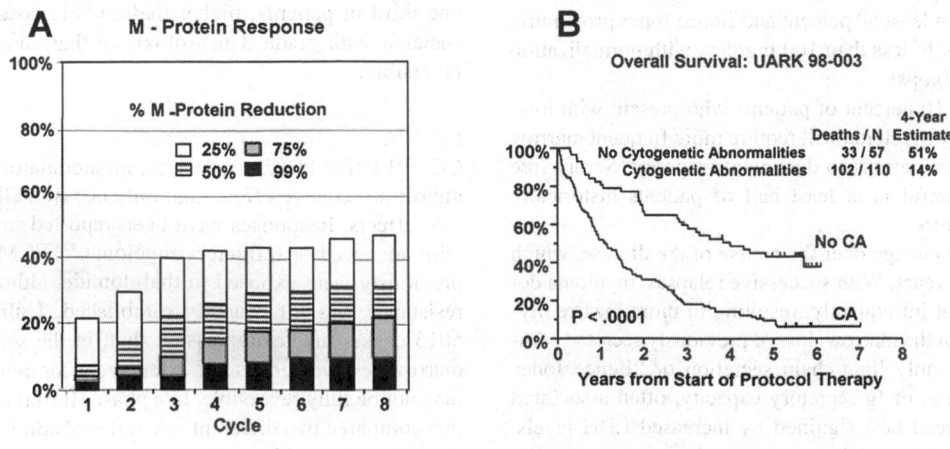

FIGURE 100-17   Thalidomide salvage therapy. *(A)* M-Protein response. *(B)* Overall survival rate. Note inferior outcome in the presence of cytogenetic abnormalities (CA).

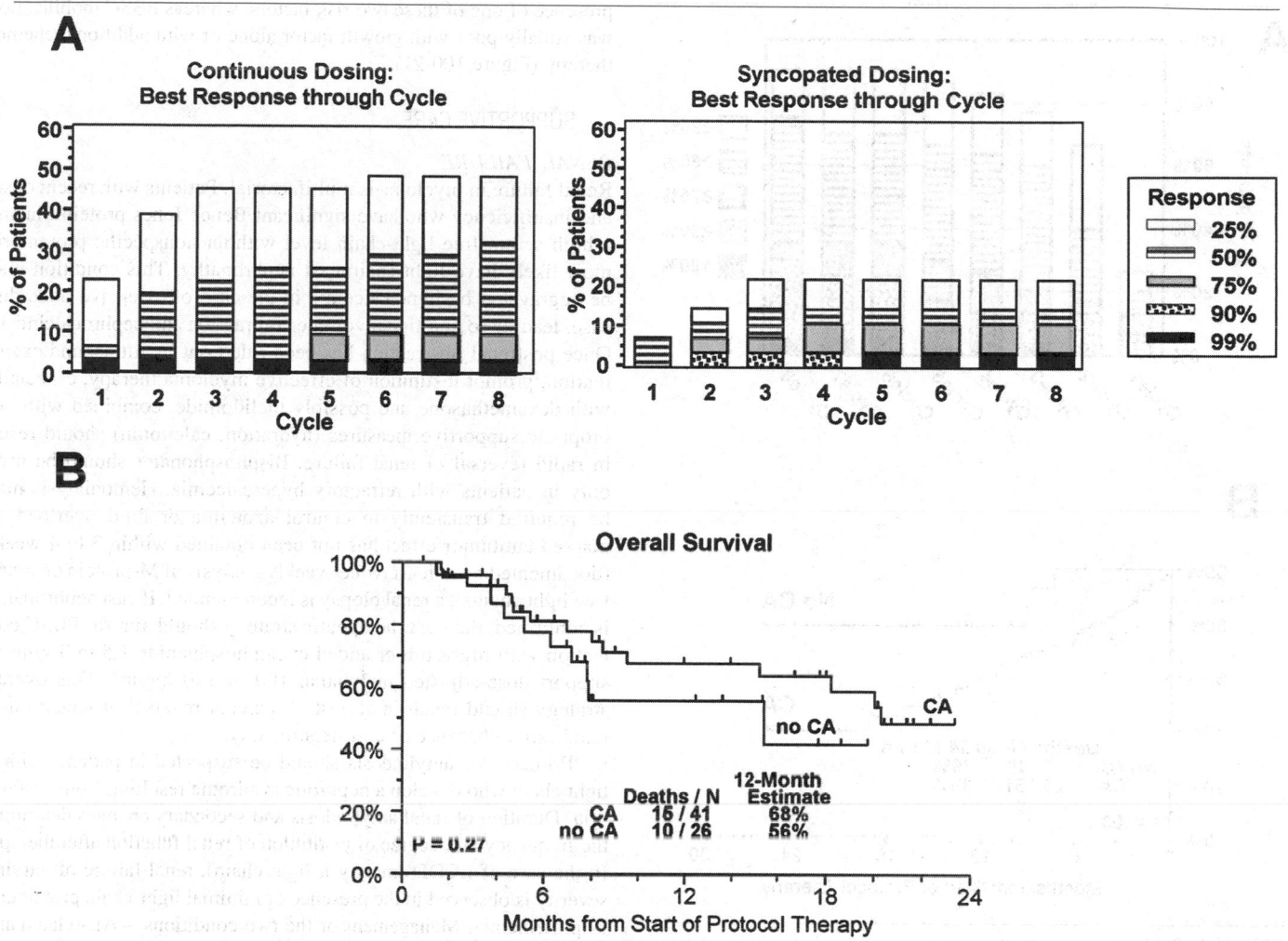

FIGURE 100-18   CC-5013 (Revlimid) salvage therapy using two different dose schedules (see text for details). Patient characteristics are given in Table 100-13. (A) Cumulative response to daily dosing at 25 mg (left) versus 50 mg on alternating days (right). (B) Overall survival. No difference is observed between groups with or without cytogenetic abnormalities (CA).

cisplatin (Platinol) 10 mg/m², doxorubicin (Adriamycin) 10 mg/m², cyclophosphamide 400 mg/m², and etoposide 40 mg/m² (DT-PACE) has been highly effective and well tolerated in the setting of fulminant relapse with cytogenetic abnormalities, high LDH level, and plasmablastic morphology.[324] Gastrointestinal toxicity was uncommon. When DT-PACE was combined with filgrastim and erythropoietin, rapid recovery of hematopoiesis ensued and even permitted

PBSC collection for subsequent stem cell-supported high-dose therapy.

FURTHER HIGH-DOSE THERAPY WITH AUTOLOGOUS STEM CELL SUPPORT

Although initially controversial, most investigators agree that autologous stem cell-supported high-dose melphalan provides more sus-

TABLE 100-14   BORTEZOMIB (VELCADE) + THALIDOMIDE SALVAGE THERAPY: PATIENT CHARACTERISTICS BY COHORT

| PARAMETER | TOTAL | BORTEZOMIB 1.0 MG/M² | | | | BORTEZOMIB 1.3 MG/M² | | |
		THAL 50 MG	THAL 100 MG	THAL 150 MG	THAL 200 MG	THAL 50 MG	THAL 100 MG	THAL 150 MG
No. of patients	73	12	10	10	14	11	10	6
% Age ≥60 years	55	67	60	50	50	55	40	67
% β₂M ≥4 mg/liter	56	75	30	60	62	50	60	50
% LDH ≥250 U/liter	18	8	0	40	29	18	20	0
% Abnormal cytogenetics	45	45	33	78	50	40	44	0
% Prior Rx ≥5 years	37	42	40	40	21	45	40	0
% Prior autotransplant	81	92	100	90	64	73	70	100
% Prior THAL	78	83	90	90	79	73	80	33

β₂M = β₂-microglobulin; LDH = lactate dehydrogenase; THAL = thalidomide.

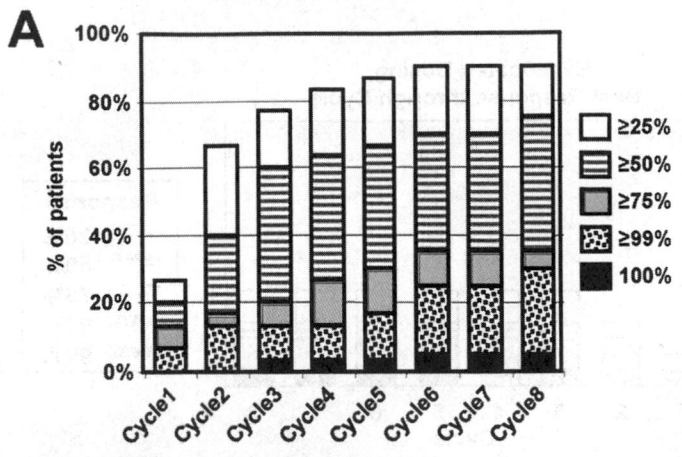

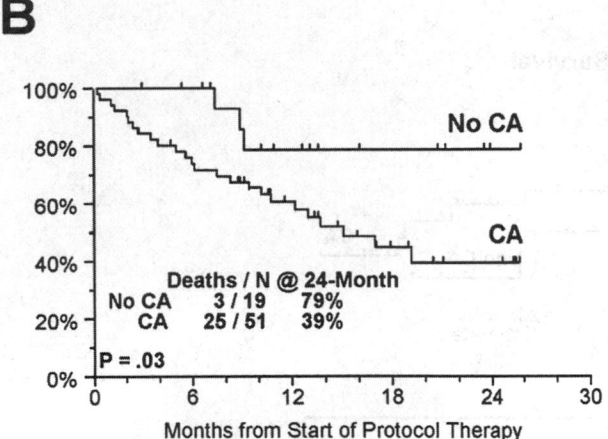

FIGURE 100-19 Bortezomib (Velcade) plus thalidomide salvage therapy (see text for details). Patient characteristics are given in Table 100-14. *(A)* Cumulative incidence of M-protein reduction by level. *(B)* Superior survival is observed in the absence of cytogenetic abnormalities (CA).

tained disease control and survival when it is used up front rather than as salvage therapy for patients who do not respond to standard-dose chemotherapy. A further melphalan-based autotransplant should be considered for consolidation after salvage therapy in patients who derived at least 3 to 4 years of disease control after their initial transplant (Figure 100-20).

CONSIDERATIONS REGARDING AUTOLOGOUS PERIPHERAL BLOOD STEM CELL COLLECTION

Review of nearly 1000 patients whose stem cells were mobilized after administration of growth factor or non–stem cell toxic chemotherapy regimens plus growth factor support identified features that favored collections of at least 2,000,000 CD34 cells/kg/day. These features included platelet counts greater than 200,000/μL (200 × 10^9/liter), prior therapy not exceeding 12 months, use of chemotherapy added to growth factor support, and younger age.[316] Conversely, poor mobilization (<1 million CD34 cells/kg/day) was associated with thrombocytopenia (<200,000/μL), prior therapy exceeding 12 months, use of growth factor alone, and older age. Based on these considerations, the yield was highest at 6,000,000 CD34 cells/kg/day in the absence of platelet and prior treatment risk factors and when chemotherapy was applied, compared to 2 million CD34 cells/kg/day with growth factor alone. A similar advantage for chemotherapy was noted in the

presence of one of these two risk factors, whereas PBSC mobilization was equally poor with growth factor alone or with additional chemotherapy (Figure 100-21).

SUPPORTIVE CARE

RENAL FAILURE

Renal failure in myeloma is multifactorial. Patients with recent onset and insufficiency who have significant Bence Jones proteinuria and a high serum free light-chain level without nonspecific proteinuria most likely have light-chain cast nephropathy. This condition may be aggravated by hypercalcemia in the case of extensive bone disease, leading to additional volume contraction and nephrocalcinosis. Once postrenal obstruction has been ruled out by ultrasound examination, prompt institution of effective myeloma therapy, especially with dexamethasone and possibly thalidomide, combined with appropriate supportive measures (hydration, calcitonin) should result in rapid reversal of renal failure. Bisphosphonates should be used only in patients with refractory hypercalcemia. Hemodialysis may be required transiently to control azotemia or fluid overload. If marked antitumor effect has not been obtained within 3 to 4 weeks (documented by at least twice-weekly analysis of M-protein or serum free light chains), a renal biopsy is recommended. If cast nephropathy is confirmed, the next therapeutic strategy should aim for PBSC collection with filgrastim or added cyclophosphamide 1.5 to 3 g/m^2 to support dose-adjusted melphalan 100 to 140 mg/m^2. This overall strategy should result in almost 90 percent reversal of recent-onset renal failure because of cast nephropathy.

Primary AL amyloidosis should be suspected in patients with λ light chain who develop a nephrotic syndrome resulting from proteinuria. Duration of renal amyloidosis and secondary changes determine the frequency and degree of restitution of renal function after therapy. In the case of LCDD (mostly κ light chain), renal failure of varying severity is observed in the presence of minimal light-chain proteinuria or proteinemia. Management of the two conditions—AL-related and LCDD-related renal failure—should follow the general strategy outlined for cast nephropathy. However, renal function improves more slowly and is less likely to return to normal.

ANEMIA

Recombinant human erythropoietin has been shown to significantly decrease the frequency of transfusion requirements and improve the quality of life of anemic myeloma patients.[389] The impact of treatment is greater in patients with limited prior therapy. Patients with mild anemia (hemoglobin levels 11–12 g/dl) should not be excluded from erythropoietin therapy because the greatest incremental improvement in quality of life appears to occur when hemoglobin increases to 13 g/dl. Anemic patients should receive erythropoietin at doses of 40,000 U/week until hemoglobin levels exceed 13 g/dl. In intensive therapy-based programs, such an approach decreases transfusion requirements and improves quality of life. Darbopoietin at a dose of 200 μg every 2 weeks is equally effective.

BONE PAIN AND HYPERCALCEMIA

Dexamethasone is a potent drug used in the acute management of hypercalcemia, renal failure, and myeloma-related bone pain. It also is used as part of most upfront and salvage regimens. Subcutaneous calcitonin can augment glucocorticoid-induced antihypercalcemic effects. In the absence of renal failure, pamidronate or zoledronic acid provides sustained control of hypercalcemia and some pain relief. In the setting of persistent hypercalcemia (refractory to hydration, dexamethasone, and calcitonin), bisphosphonates are indicated, even in the presence of renal failure, but at reduced dose and infusion rates(e.g., pamidronate 45 mg intravenously over 2–3 hours; zoledronic acid 2 mg intravenously over 30 minutes).

MYELOSUPPRESSION

Hematopoietic growth factors, especially filgrastim, are used mainly in the context of blood stem cell procurement and after transplant. They likely will not facilitate more frequent administration of higher doses of melphalan or other alkylators targeting early hematopoietic progenitor cells. However, they have been shown to alleviate neutropenia associated with intensive stem cell-sparing regimens, such as DT-PACE or single-agent high-dose cyclophosphamide or etoposide.

IMMUNOSUPPRESSION AND INFECTIONS

Defects in B and T cell function are common in patients with symptomatic myeloma. With therapy, additional immune defects may develop, depending on the modality used (glucocorticoids, cytotoxic chemotherapy, autologous or allogeneic stem cell transplantation) and whether or not the patient has renal failure or progressive disease.[390] The cellular immune defects that increase the risk for serious infections are severe neutropenia and depressed CD4 T cell counts. After effective cytoreduction, especially with melphalan-based autotransplants, uninvolved Igs recover promptly within months,[364] whereas CD4+ T cells remain suppressed, sometimes for years.[391] The type and intensity of antineoplastic therapy used and the ensuing immunosuppression and end-organ toxicity (particularly mucositis) dictate the approach to infection management.[390] Preventing infection in the autologous transplant setting relies on infusing sufficiently high doses of CD34+ cells (preferably $\geq 5 \times 10^6$/kg),[391] avoiding TBI,[314] adjusting melphalan dose intensity for renal function[307,308,348] and age,[304,305] and providing effective infection control and antimicrobial prophylaxis.[390,392] Treatment with low-dose acyclovir (400 mg BID) can reduce herpes simplex virus (HSV) reactivation among HSV-seropositive patients. Use of fluoroquinolones and fluconazole can protect against bacterial and yeast infections in high-risk patients. The role of prophylactic hematopoietic growth factors in this setting is unclear. Following recovery, patients may develop infections with herpes zoster virus or *Pneumocystis carinii*, particularly when CD4 and CD8 T cell counts remain low (<400 and <800 cells/μL, respectively) more than 3 months after autotransplant.[393] Prophylaxis with acyclovir and trimethoprim-sulfamethoxazole (TMP-SMX), or alternatives, is recommended. The role of intravenous Igs remains controversial.

Patients undergoing allotransplants are at high risk for developing severe fungal infections, even when nonmyeloablative regimens are used.[392,394,395]

Myeloma patients exhibit a poor antibody response to pneumococcal and influenza vaccines. Whether vaccination will be effective after immune reconstitution among long-term myeloma survivors remains to be determined.

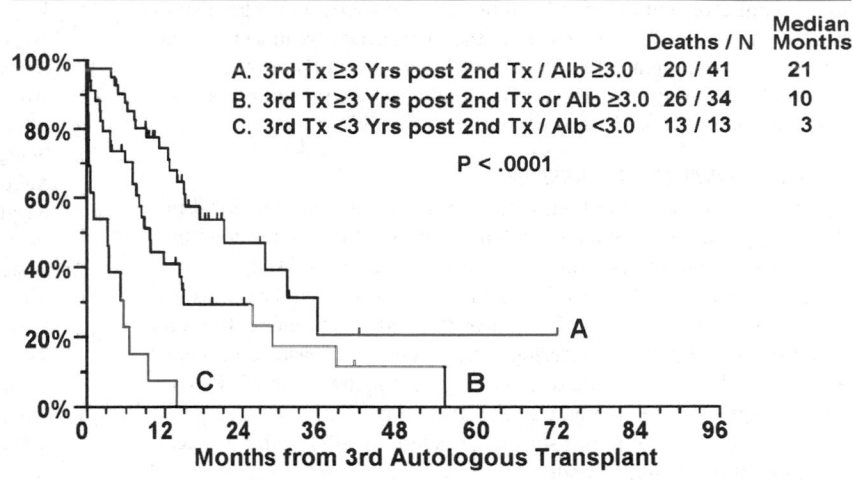

FIGURE 100-20 Salvage (third [3rd]) autotransplant for relapse after tandem autotransplant. Eighty-eight patients received mainly melphalan (200 mg/m²)-based autotransplant for a median of 30 months after a second autotransplant. According to multivariate analysis, a longer time lapse from second transplant (HR 0.8, P = .003) and albumin less than 3.0 g/dl before third transplant (HR 3.3, P < .0001) were independent features associated with survival from third transplant. Greatest benefit was seen among the 41 patients with a transplant 2–transplant 3 interval of at least 3 years and albumin of at least 3.0 g/dl, with progressive survival shortening in the presence of one and two unfavorable features.

HYPERVISCOSITY SYNDROME

This diagnosis is made by measuring serum viscosity or by funduscopic examination, which shows a slow blood flow in often distorted blood vessels. Hyperviscosity can give the clinical and radio-

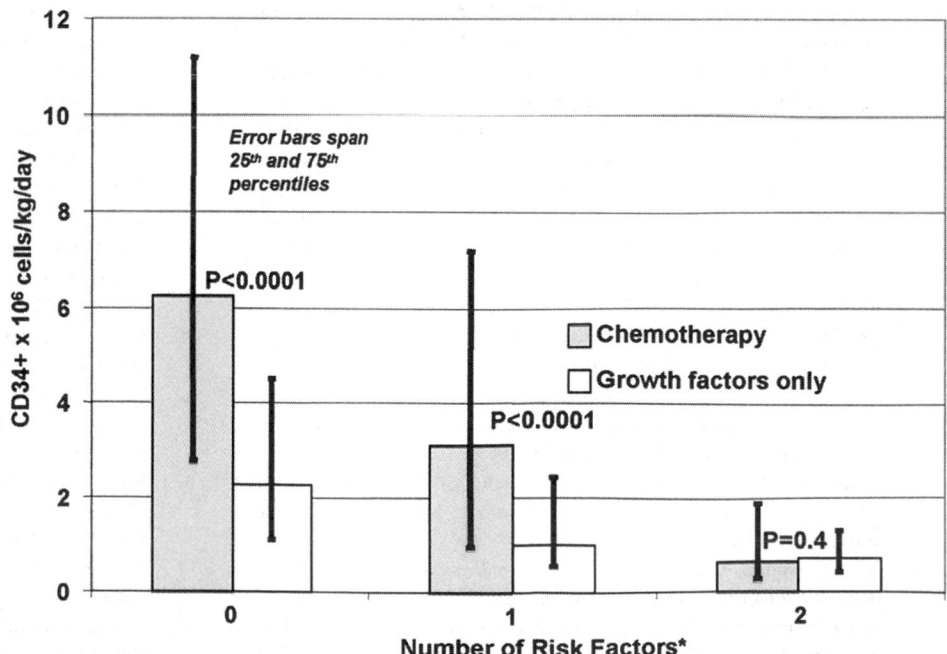

FIGURE 100-21 Comparison of CD34+ cell yields for mobilization with chemotherapy versus growth factors alone, according to the number of risk factors. Each pair of columns shows the median CD34+ cell yield within risk groups 0 and 1 or with both risk factors. The risk factors are platelet counts less than 200 × 10⁹/liter and prior therapy for more than 12 months.[405]

logic picture of pulmonary edema but only worsens with administration of diuretics. Plasmapheresis is the appropriate treatment for patients with symptomatic hyperviscosity, which occurs more often with IgA and IgG3 isotypes. Treatment should be continued until serum viscosity normalizes or clinical symptoms resolve.

SPINAL CORD COMPRESSION

Spinal cord compression traditionally has been treated with local radiotherapy and/or decompressive laminectomy. Although local radiotherapy has curative potential for the management of truly solitary plasmacytoma, its role in palliation must be assessed in the context of long-term management and in light of the underlying cause. In more recently treated patients suffering from systemic disease, chemotherapy that includes high-dose dexamethasone pulsing, as in DT-PACE, has provided remarkable activity. In the absence of symptom relief and given the lack of tumor shrinkage noted on MRI within 1 week, local radiation should be added.

If cord compression results from vertebral collapse without identifiable plasmacytoma on MRI, radiation may not be beneficial, and decompressive laminectomy should be the treatment of choice. Local doses of radiotherapy to the spinal cord should not exceed 30 Gy, and liberal use of local radiation for the management of rib fractures is discouraged.

REFERENCES

1. Bergsagel D: The incidence and epidemiology of plasma cell neoplasms. *Stem Cells* 13(suppl 2):1, 1995.
2. Riedel DA, Pottern LM: The epidemiology of multiple myeloma. *Hematol Oncol Clin North Am* 6:225, 1992.
3. Ichimaru M, Ishimaru T, Mikami M, et al: Multiple myeloma among atomic bomb survivors in Hiroshima and Nagasaki 1950-1976: Relationship to radiation dose absorbed by marrow. *J Natl Cancer Inst* 69:323, 1982.
4. Gramenzi A, Buttino I, D'Avanzo B, et al: Medical history and the risk of multiple myeloma. *Br J Cancer* 63:769, 1991.
5. Said W, Chien K, Takeuchi S, et al: Kaposi sarcoma-associated herpesvirus (KSHV or HHV8) in primary effusion lymphoma: Ultrastructural demonstration of herpesvirus in lymphoma cells. *Blood* 87:4937, 1996.
6. Schalling M, Ekman M, Kaaya EE, et al: A role for a new herpes virus (KSHV) in different forms of Kaposi sarcoma. *Nat Med* 1:707, 1995.
7. Soulier J, Grollet L, Oksenhendler E, et al: Kaposi sarcoma-associated herpesvirus-like DNA sequences in multicentric Castleman disease. *Blood* 86:1276, 1995.
8. Rettig MB, Ma HJ, Vescio RA, et al: Kaposi sarcoma-associated herpesvirus infection of bone marrow dendritic cells from multiple myeloma patients. *Science* 276(5320):1851, 1997.
9. Said JW, Rettig MR, Heppner K, et al: Localization of Kaposi sarcoma-associated herpesvirus in bone marrow biopsy samples from patients with multiple myeloma. *Blood* 90:4278, 1997.
10. Chauhan D, Bharti A, Raje N, et al: Detection of Kaposi sarcoma herpesvirus DNA sequences in multiple myeloma bone marrow stromal cells. *Blood* 93:1482, 1999.
11. Raje N, Gong J, Chauhan D, et al: Bone marrow and peripheral blood dendritic cells from patients with multiple myeloma are phenotypically and functionally normal despite the detection of Kaposi sarcoma herpesvirus gene sequences. *Blood* 93:1487, 1999.
12. Tarte K, Olsen SJ, Yang Lu Z, et al: Clinical-grade functional dendritic cells from patients with multiple myeloma are not infected with Kaposi sarcoma-associated herpesvirus. *Blood* 91:1852, 1998.
13. Yi Q, Ekman M, Anton D, et al: Blood dendritic cells from myeloma patients are not infected with Kaposi sarcoma-associated herpesvirus (KSHV/HHV-8). *Blood* 92:402, 1998.
14. Tisdale JF, Stewart AK, Dickstein B, et al: Molecular and serological examination of the relationship of human herpesvirus 8 to multiple myeloma: Orf 26 sequences in bone marrow stroma are not restricted to myeloma patients and other regions of the genome are not detected. *Blood* 92:2681, 1998.
15. Bourguet CC, Logue EE: Antigenic stimulation and multiple myeloma. A prospective study. *Cancer* 72:2148, 1993.
16. Bataille R, Harousseau JL: Multiple myeloma. *N Engl J Med* 336:1657, 1997.
17. Lynch HT, Sanger WG, Pirruccello S, et al: Familial multiple myeloma: A family study and review of the literature. *J Natl Cancer Inst* 93:1479, 2001.
18. Segel GB, Lichtman MA: Familial (inherited) leukemia, lymphoma, and myeloma: an overview. *Blood Cells Mol Dis* 32:246, 2004.
19. Yaccoby S, Barlogie B, Epstein J: Primary myeloma cells growing in SCID-hu mice: A model for studying the biology and treatment of myeloma and its manifestations. *Blood* 92:2908, 1998.
20. Yaccoby S, Epstein J: The proliferative potential of myeloma plasma cells manifest in the SCID-hu host. *Blood* 94:3576, 1999.
21. Yaccoby S, Johnson CL, Mahaffey SC, et al: Antimyeloma efficacy of thalidomide in the SCID-hu model. *Blood* 100:4162, 2002.
22. Yaccoby S, Pearse RN, Johnson CL, et al: Myeloma interacts with the bone marrow microenvironment to induce osteoclastogenesis and is dependent on osteoclast activity. *Br J Haematol* 116:278, 2002.
23. Radl J: Animal model of human disease. Benign monoclonal gammopathy (idiopathic paraproteinemia). *Am J Pathol* 105:91, 1981.
24. Radl J, Croese JW, Zurcher C, et al: Animal model of human disease. Multiple myeloma. *Am J Pathol* 132:593, 1988.
25. Mundy GR: Mechanisms of bone disease in multiple myeloma, in *Monoclonal Gammapathies III—Clinical Significance and Basic Mechanisms*, edited by J Radl, B van Camp, p. 51. Proceedings of the Third EURAGE Symposium, Brussels, 1991.
26. Vanderkerken K, De Leenheer E, Shipman C, et al: Recombinant osteoprotegerin decreases tumor burden and increases survival in a murine model of multiple myeloma. *Cancer Res* 63:287, 2003.
27. Asosingh K, De Raeve H, Van Riet I, et al: Multiple myeloma tumor progression in the 5T2MM murine model is a multistage and dynamic process of differentiation, proliferation, invasion, and apoptosis. *Blood* 101:3136, 2003.
28. Asosingh K, De Raeve H, Menu E, et al: Angiogenic switch during 5T2MM murine myeloma tumorigenesis: Role of CD45 heterogeneity. *Blood* 103:3131, 2004.
29. Van Valckenborgh E, De Raeve H, Devy L, et al: Murine 5T multiple myeloma cells induce angiogenesis in vitro and in vivo. *Br J Cancer* 86:796, 2002.
30. Kyle RA, Therneau TM, Rajkumar SV, et al: A long-term study of prognosis in monoclonal gammopathy of undetermined significance. *N Engl J Med* 346:564, 2002.
31. Kuehl WM, Bergsagel PL: Multiple myeloma: Evolving genetic events and host interactions. *Nat Rev Cancer* 2:175, 2002.
32. Bergsagel PL, Kuehl WM: Chromosome translocations in multiple myeloma. *Oncogene* 20:5611, 2001.
33. Barlogie B, Epstein J, Selvanayagam P, et al: Plasma cell myeloma—New biological insights and advances in therapy. *Blood* 73:865, 1989.
34. Hallek M, Bergsagel PL, Anderson KC: Multiple myeloma: Increasing evidence for a multistep transformation process. *Blood* 91:3, 1998.
35. MacLennan ICM, Chan EYT: The origin of bone marrow plasma cells, in *Epidemiology and Biology of Multiple Myeloma*, edited by GI Obrams, M Potter, p 129. Springer, Berlin, 1991.
36. Okuno Y, Takahashi T, Suzuki A, et al: Establishment and characterization of four myeloma cell lines which are responsive to interleukin-6 for their growth. *Leukemia* 5:585, 1991.

37. Durie BG, Vela E, Baum V, et al: Establishment of two new myeloma cell lines from bilateral pleural effusions: Evidence for sequential in vivo clonal change. *Blood* 66:548, 1985.

38. Bast EJ, van Camp B, Reynaert P, et al: Idiotypic peripheral blood lymphocytes in monoclonal gammopathy. *Clin Exp Immunol* 47:677, 1982.

39. Berenson J, Wong R, Kim K, et al: Evidence for peripheral blood B lymphocyte but not T lymphocyte involvement in multiple myeloma. *Blood* 70:1550, 1987.

40. Mellstedt H, Holm G, Pettersson D, et al: Idiotype-bearing lymphoid cells in plasma cell neoplasia. *Clin Haematol* 11:65, 1982.

41. Pilarski LM, Jensen GS: Monoclonal circulating B cells in multiple myeloma. A continuously differentiating, possibly invasive, population as defined by expression of CD45 isoforms and adhesion molecules. *Hematol Oncol Clin North Am* 6:297, 1992.

42. Pilarski LM, Mant MJ, Ruether BA: Pre-B cells in peripheral blood of multiple myeloma patients. *Blood* 66:416, 1985.

43. Ruiz Arguelles GJ, Katzmann JA, Greipp PR, et al: Multiple myeloma: Circulating lymphocytes that express plasma cell antigens. *Blood* 64: 352, 1984.

44. Berenson JR, Lichtenstein AK: Clonal rearrangement of immunoglobulin genes in the peripheral blood of multiple myeloma patients. *Br J Haematol* 73:425, 1989.

45. Corradini P, Boccadoro M, Voena C, et al: Evidence for a bone marrow B cell transcribing malignant plasma cell VDJ joined to C mu sequence in immunoglobulin (IgG)- and IgA-secreting multiple myelomas. *J Exp Med* 178:1091, 1993.

46. Billadeau D, Ahmann G, Greipp P, et al: The bone marrow of multiple myeloma patients contains B cell populations at different stages of differentiation that are clonally related to the malignant plasma cell. *J Exp Med* 178:1023, 1993.

47. Chen BJ, Epstein J: Circulating clonal lymphocytes in myeloma constitute a minor subpopulation of B cells. *Blood* 87:1972, 1996.

48. Zandecki M, Lai JL, Genevieve F, et al: Several cytogenetic subclones may be identified within plasma cells from patients with monoclonal gammopathy of undetermined significance, both at diagnosis and during the indolent course of this condition. *Blood* 90:3682, 1997.

49. Bakkus MH, Heirman C, Van Riet I, et al: Evidence that multiple myeloma Ig heavy chain VDJ genes contain somatic mutations but show no intraclonal variation. *Blood* 80:2326, 1992.

50. Vescio RA, Cao J, Hong CH, et al: Myeloma Ig heavy chain V region sequences reveal prior antigenic selection and marked somatic mutation but no intraclonal diversity. *J Immunol* 155:2487, 1995.

51. Zandecki M, Lai JL, Facon T: Multiple myeloma: Almost all patients are cytogenetically abnormal. *Br J Haematol* 94:217, 1996.

52. Tabernero D, San Miguel JF, Garcia-Sanz M, et al: Incidence of chromosome numerical changes in multiple myeloma: Fluorescence in situ hybridization analysis using 15 chromosome-specific probes. *Am J Pathol* 149:153, 1996.

53. Janssen JW, Vaandrager JW, Heuser T, et al: Concurrent activation of a novel putative transforming gene, myeov, and cyclin D1 in a subset of multiple myeloma cell lines with t(11;14)(q13;q32). *Blood* 95:2691, 2000.

54. Vaandrager JW, Kluin P, Schuuring E: The t(11;14) (q13;q32) in multiple myeloma cell line KMS12 has its 11q13 breakpoint 330 kb centromeric from the cyclin D1 gene. *Blood* 89:349, 1997.

55. Meeus P, Stul MS, Mecucci C, et al: Molecular breakpoints of t(11; 14)(q13;q32) in multiple myeloma. *Cancer Genet Cytogenet* 83:25, 1995.

56. Ronchetti D, Finelli P, Richelda R, et al: Molecular analysis of 11q13 breakpoints in multiple myeloma. *Blood* 93:1330, 1999.

57. Raynaud SD, Bekri S, Leroux D, et al: Expanded range of 11q13 breakpoints with differing patterns of cyclin D1 expression in B-cell malignancies. *Genes Chromosomes Cancer* 8:80, 1993.

58. Hoyer JD, Hanson CA, Fonseca R, et al: The (11;14)(q13;q32) translocation in multiple myeloma. A morphologic and immunohistochemical study. *Am J Clin Pathol* 113:831, 2000.

59. Vasef MA, Medeiros LJ, Yospur LS, et al: Cyclin D1 protein in multiple myeloma and plasmacytoma: An immunohistochemical study using fixed, paraffin-embedded tissue sections. *Mod Pathol* 10:927, 1997.

60. Robillard N, Avet-Loiseau H, Garand R, et al: CD20 is associated with a small mature plasma cell morphology and t(11;14) in multiple myeloma. *Blood* 102:1070, 2003.

61. Avet-Loiseau H, Garand R, Lode L, et al: Translocation t(11;14)(q13; q32) is the hallmark of IgM, IgE, and nonsecretory multiple myeloma variants. *Blood* 101:1570, 2003.

62. Chesi M, Nardini E, Lim RS, et al: The t(4;14) translocation in myeloma dysregulates both FGFR3 and a novel gene, MMSET, resulting in IgH/MMSET hybrid transcripts. *Blood* 92:3025, 1998.

63. Richelda R, Ronchetti D, Baldini L, et al: A novel chromosomal translocation t(4,14)(p16.3, q32) in multiple myeloma involves the fibroblast growth-factor receptor 3 gene. *Blood* 90:4062, 1997.

64. Intini D, Baldini L, Fabris S, et al: Analysis of FGFR3 gene mutations in multiple myeloma patients with t(4;14). *Br J Haematol* 114:362, 2001.

65. Chesi M, Brents LA, Ely SA, et al: Activated fibroblast growth factor receptor 3 is an oncogene that contributes to tumor progression in multiple myeloma. *Blood* 97:729, 2001.

66. Ronchetti D, Greco A, Compasso S, et al: Deregulated FGFR3 mutants in multiple myeloma cell lines with t(4;14): Comparative analysis of Y373C, K650E and the novel G384D mutations. *Oncogene* 20(27): 3553, 2001.

67. Perfetti V, Coluccia AM, Intini D, et al: Translocation T(4;14)(p16.3; q32) is a recurrent genetic lesion in primary amyloidosis. *Am J Pathol* 158:1599, 2001.

68. Shaughnessy J Jr, Gabrea A, Qi Y, et al: Cyclin D3 at 6p21 is dysregulated by recurrent chromosomal translocations to immunoglobulin loci in multiple myeloma. *Blood* 98:217, 2001.

69. Chesi M, Bergsagel PL, Shonukan OO, et al: Frequent dysregulation of the c-maf proto-oncogene at 16q23 by translocation to an Ig locus in multiple myeloma. *Blood* 91:4457, 1998.

70. Hanamura I, Iida S, Akano Y, et al: Ectopic expression of MAFB gene in human myeloma cells carrying (14;20)(q32;q11) chromosomal translocations. *Jpn J Cancer Res* 92:638, 2001.

71. Fonseca R, Harrington D, Oken MM, et al: Biological and prognostic significance of interphase fluorescence in situ hybridization detection of chromosome 13 abnormalities (delta13) in multiple myeloma: An eastern cooperative oncology group study. *Cancer Res* 62:715, 2002.

72. Dao DD, Sawyer JR, Epstein J, et al: Deletion of the retinoblastoma gene in multiple myeloma. *Leukemia* 8:1280, 1994.

73. Avet-Loiseau H, Facon T, Daviet A, et al: 14q32 translocations and monosomy 13 observed in monoclonal gammopathy of undetermined significance delineate a multistep process for the oncogenesis of multiple myeloma. Intergroupe Francophone du Myelome. *Cancer Res* 59:4546, 1999.

74. Drach J, Angerler J, Schuster J, et al: Interphase fluorescence in situ hybridization identifies chromosomal abnormalities in plasma cells from patients with monoclonal gammopathy of undetermined significance. *Blood* 86:3915, 1995.

75. Zandecki M, Obein V, Bernardi F, et al: Monoclonal gammopathy of undetermined significance: Chromosome changes are a common finding within bone marrow plasma cells. *Br J Haematol* 90:693, 1995.

76. Rasillo A, Tabernero MD, Sanchez ML, et al: Fluorescence in situ hybridization analysis of aneuploidization patterns in monoclonal gammopathy of undetermined significance versus multiple myeloma and plasma cell leukemia. *Cancer* 97:601, 2003.

77. Greil R, Fasching B, Loidl P, et al: Expression of the c-myc proto-oncogene in multiple myeloma and chronic lymphocytic leukemia: An in situ analysis. *Blood* 78:180, 1991.

78. Ernst TJ, Gazdar A, Ritz J, et al: Identification of a second transforming gene, rasn, in a human multiple myeloma line with a rearranged c-myc allele. *Blood* 72:1163, 1988.

79. Sawyer JR, Lukacs JL, Thomas EL, et al: Multicolour spectral karyotyping identifies new translocations and a recurring pathway for chromosome loss in multiple myeloma. *Br J Haematol* 112:167, 2001.

80. Shou Y, Martelli ML, Gabrea A, et al: Diverse karyotypic abnormalities of the c-myc locus associated with c-myc dysregulation and tumor progression in multiple myeloma. *Proc Natl Acad Sci U S A* 97:228, 2000.

81. Avet-Loiseau H, Gerson F, Magrangeas F, et al: Rearrangements of the c-myc oncogene are present in 15% of primary human multiple myeloma tumors. *Blood* 98:3082, 2001.

82. Neri A, Murphy JP, Cro L, et al: Ras oncogene mutation in multiple myeloma. *J Exp Med* 170:1715, 1989.

83. Paquette RL, Berenson J, Lichtenstein A, et al: Oncogenes in multiple myeloma: Point mutation of N-ras. *Oncogene* 5:1659, 1990.

84. Portier M, Moles JP, Mazars GR, et al: P53 and RAS gene mutations in multiple myeloma. *Oncogene* 7:2539, 1992.

85. Liu P, Leong T, Quam L, et al: Activating mutations of N- and K-ras in multiple myeloma show different clinical associations: Analysis of the Eastern Cooperative Oncology Group Phase III Trial. *Blood* 88:2699, 1996.

86. Bezieau S, Devilder MC, Avet-Loiseau H, et al: High incidence of N and K-Ras activating mutations in multiple myeloma and primary plasma cell leukemia at diagnosis. *Hum Mutat* 18:212, 2001.

87. Bezieau S, Avet-Loiseau H, Moisan JP, et al: Activating Ras mutations in patients with plasma-cell disorders: A reappraisal. *Blood* 100:1101, 2002; author reply 100:1103, 2002.

88. Corradini P, Ladetto M, Voena C, et al: Mutational activation of N- and K-ras oncogenes in plasma cell dyscrasias. *Blood* 81:2708,1993.

89. Matozaki S, Nakagawa T, Nakao Y, et al: RAS gene mutations in multiple myeloma and related monoclonal gammopathies. *Kobe J Med Sci* 37:35, 1991.

90. Crowder C, Kopantzev E, Williams K, et al: An unusual H-Ras mutant isolated from a human multiple myeloma line leads to transformation and factor-independent cell growth. *Oncogene* 22:649, 2003.

91. Neri A, Baldini L, Trecca D, et al: P53 gene mutations in multiple myeloma are associated with advanced forms of malignancy. *Blood* 81:128, 1993.

92. Drach J, Ackermann J, Fritz E, et al: Presence of a p53 gene deletion in patients with multiple myeloma predicts for short survival after conventional-dose chemotherapy. *Blood* 92:802, 1998.

93. Schultheis B, Kramer A, Willer A, et al: Analysis of p73 and p53 gene deletions in multiple myeloma. *Leukemia* 13:2099, 1999.

94. Mazars GR, Portier M, Zhang XG, et al: Mutations of the p53 gene in human myeloma cell lines. *Oncogene* 7:1015, 1992.

95. Corradini P, Inghirami G, Astolfi M, et al: Inactivation of tumor suppressor genes, p53 and Rb1, in plasma cell dyscrasias. *Leukemia* 8:758, 1994.

96. Preudhomme C, Facon T, Zandecki M, et al: Rare occurrence of P53 gene mutations in multiple myeloma. *Br J Haematol* 81:440, 1992.

97. Ackermann J, Meidlinger P, Zojer N, et al: Absence of p53 deletions in bone marrow plasma cells of patients with monoclonal gammopathy of undetermined significance. *Br J Haematol* 103:1161, 1998.

98. Teoh G, Urashima M, Ogata A, et al: MDM2 protein overexpression promotes proliferation and survival of multiple myeloma cells. *Blood* 90:1982, 1997.

99. Latreille J, Barlogie B, Dosik G, et al: Cellular DNA content as a marker of human multiple myeloma. *Blood* 55:403, 1980.

100. Latreille J, Barlogie B, Johnston D, et al: Ploidy and proliferative characteristics in monoclonal gammopathies. *Blood* 59:43, 1982.

101. Caligaris-Cappio F, Bergui L, Gregoretti MG, et al: Role of bone marrow stromal cells in the growth of human multiple myeloma. *Blood* 77:2688, 1991.

102. Dewald GW, Kyle RA, Hicks GA, et al: The clinical significance of cytogenetic studies in 100 patients with multiple myeloma, plasma cell leukemia, or amyloidosis. *Blood* 66:380, 1985.

103. Gould J, Alexanian R, Goodacre A, et al: Plasma cell karyotype in multiple myeloma. *Blood* 71:453, 1988.

104. Sawyer JR, Waldron JA, Jagannath S, et al: Cytogenetic findings in 200 patients with multiple myeloma. *Cancer Genet Cytogenet* 82:41, 1995.

105. Van den Berghe H: Chromosomes in plasma-cell malignancies. *Eur J Haematol* 43(suppl 51):47, 1989.

106. Shaughnessy J, Jacobson J, Sawyer J, et al: Continuous absence of metaphase-defined cytogenetic abnormalities, especially of chromosome 13 and hypodiploidy, ensures long-term survival in multiple myeloma treated with Total Therapy I: Interpretation in the context of global gene expression. *Blood* 101:3849, 2003.

107. Zhan F, Hardin J, Kordsmeier B, et al: Global gene expression profiling of multiple myeloma, monoclonal gammopathy of undetermined significance, and normal bone marrow plasma cells. *Blood* 99:1745, 2002.

108. De Vos J, Couderc G, Tarte K, et al: Identifying intercellular signaling genes expressed in malignant plasma cells by using complementary DNA arrays. *Blood* 98:771, 2001.

109. Tarte K, De Vos J, Thykjaer T, et al: Generation of polyclonal plasmablasts from peripheral blood B cells: A normal counterpart of malignant plasmablasts. *Blood* 100:1113, 2002.

110. Claudio JO, Masih-Khan E, Tang H, et al: A molecular compendium of genes expressed in multiple myeloma. *Blood* 100:2175, 2002.

111. Magrangeas F, Nasser V, Avet-Loiseau H, et al: Gene expression profiling of multiple myeloma reveals molecular portraits in relation to the pathogenesis of the disease. *Blood* 101:4998, 2003.

112. Zhan F, Tian E, Bumm K, et al: Gene expression profiling of human plasma cell differentiation and classification of multiple myeloma based on similarities to distinct stages of late-stage B-cell development. *Blood* 101:1128, 2003.

113. Davies FE, Dring AM, Li C, et al: Insights into the multistep transformation of MGUS to myeloma using microarray expression analysis. *Blood* 102:4504, 2003.

114. Shaughnessy J, Rasmussen E, Zhan F, et al: Gene expression profiling can be used to predict EFS in myeloma patients treated with high dose therapy and tandem stem cell transplant [abstract 662]. *Blood* 102:190a, 2003.

115. Shaughnessy J, Zhan F, Tian E, et al: The non-tumor cell component of myeloma bone marrow is altered and can be used to stratify patient groups: A gene expression profiling study [abstract 823]. *Blood* 102:234a, 2003.

116. Kawano M, Hirano T, Matsuda T, et al: Autocrine generation and requirement of BSF-2/IL-6 for human multiple myelomas. *Nature* 332:83, 1988.

117. Klein B, Zhang XG, Jourdan M, et al: Paracrine rather than autocrine regulation of myeloma-cell growth and differentiation by interleukin-6. *Blood* 73:517, 1989.

118. Caligaris-Cappio F, Bergui L, Gaidano GL, et al: In vitro studies provide evidence that multiple paracrine loops may be operating in multiple myeloma, in *Epidemiology and Biology of Multiple Myeloma*, edited by GI Obrams, M Potter, p 123. Springer, Berlin, 1991.

119. Thomas X, Xiao HQ, Chang R, et al: Circulating B lymphocytes in multiple myeloma patients contain an autocrine IL-6 driven premyeloma cell population. *Curr Top Microbiol Immunol* 182:201, 1992.

120. Hata H, Xiao H, Petrucci MT, et al: Interleukin-6 gene expression in multiple myeloma: A characteristic of immature tumor cells. *Blood* 81: 3357, 1993.

121. Brandt SJ, Bodine DM, Dunbar CE, et al: Dysregulated interleukin 6 expression produces a syndrome resembling Castleman disease in mice. *J Clin Invest* 86:592, 1990.

122. Suematsu S, Matsusaka T, Matsuda T, et al: Generation of plasmacytomas with the chromosomal translocation t(12;15) in interleukin 6 transgenic mice. *Proc Natl Acad Sci U S A* 89:232, 1992.

123. Grigorieva I, Thomas X, Epstein J: The bone marrow stromal environment is a major factor in myeloma cell resistance to dexamethasone. *Exp Hematol* 26:597, 1998.

124. Bataille R, Klein B: The bone-resorbing activity of interleukin-6. *J Bone Miner Res* 6:1143, 1991.

125. Tinhofer I, Marschitz I, Henn T, et al: Expression of functional interleukin-15 receptor and autocrine production of interleukin-15 as mechanisms of tumor propagation in multiple myeloma. *Blood* 95:610, 2000.

126. Hjorth-Hansen H, Waage A, Borset M: Interleukin-15 blocks apoptosis and induces proliferation of the human myeloma cell line OH-2 and freshly isolated myeloma cells. *Br J Haematol* 106:28, 1999.

127. Xu F, Gardner A, Tu Y, et al: Multiple myeloma cells are protected against dexamethasone-induced apoptosis by insulin-like growth factors. *Br J Haematol* 97:429, 1997.

128. Borset M, Hjorth-Hansen H, Seidel C, et al: Hepatocyte growth factor and its receptor c-met in multiple myeloma. *Blood* 88:3998, 1996.

129. Anderson KC: Moving disease biology from the laboratory to the clinic. *Semin Oncol* 29(6 suppl 17):17, 2002.

130. Tricot G: New insights into role of microenvironment in multiple myeloma. *Lancet* 355:248, 2000.

131. Roodman GD: Role of the bone marrow microenvironment in multiple myeloma. *J Bone Miner Res* 17:1921, 2002.

132. Ridley RC, Xiao H, Hata H, et al: Expression of syndecan regulates human myeloma plasma cell adhesion to type I collagen. *Blood* 81:767, 1993.

133. Wijdenes J, Vooijs WC, Clement C, et al: A plasmocyte selective monoclonal antibody (B-B4) recognizes syndecan-1. *Br J Haematol* 94:318, 1996.

134. Dhodapkar MV, Kelly T, Theus A, et al: Elevated levels of shed syndecan-1 correlate with tumour mass and decreased matrix metalloproteinase-9 activity in the serum of patients with multiple myeloma. *Br J Haematol* 99:368, 1997.

135. Dhodapkar MV, Abe E, Theus A, et al: Syndecan-1 is a multifunctional regulator of myeloma pathobiology: Control of tumor cell survival, growth, and bone cell differentiation. *Blood* 91:2679, 1998.

136. Borset M, Hjertner O, Yaccoby S, et al: Syndecan-1 is targeted to the uropods of polarized myeloma cells where it promotes adhesion and sequesters heparin-binding proteins. *Blood* 96:2528, 2000.

137. Aref S, Goda T, El-Sherbiny M: Syndecan-1 in multiple myeloma: Relationship to conventional prognostic factors. *Hematology* 8:221, 2003.

138. Rigolin GM, Tieghi A, Ciccone M, et al: Soluble urokinase-type plasminogen activator receptor (suPAR) as an independent factor predicting worse prognosis and extra-bone marrow involvement in multiple myeloma patients. *Br J Haematol* 120:953, 2003.

139. Seidel C, Sundan A, Hjorth M, et al: Serum syndecan-1: A new independent prognostic marker in multiple myeloma. *Blood* 95:388, 2000.

140. Feinman R, Koury J, Thames M, et al: Role of NF-kappaB in the rescue of multiple myeloma cells from glucocorticoid-induced apoptosis by bcl-2. *Blood* 93:3044, 1999.

141. Qiang YW, Kopantzev E, Rudikoff S: Insulin-like growth factor-I signaling in multiple myeloma: Downstream elements, functional correlates, and pathway cross-talk. *Blood* 99:4138, 2002.

142. Chauhan D, Uchiyama H, Akbarali Y, et al: Multiple myeloma cell adhesion-induced interleukin-6 expression in bone marrow stromal cells involves activation of NF-kappa B. *Blood* 87:1104, 1996.

143. Mitsiades N, Mitsiades CS, Poulaki V, et al: Biologic sequelae of nuclear factor-kappaB blockade in multiple myeloma: Therapeutic applications. *Blood* 99:4079, 2002.

144. Ge NL, Rudikoff S: Insulin-like growth factor I is a dual effector of multiple myeloma cell growth. *Blood* 96:2856, 2000.

145. Kishimoto T, Akira S, Narazaki M, et al: Interleukin-6 family of cytokines and gp130. *Blood* 86:1243, 1995.

146. Hideshima T, Nakamura N, Chauhan D, et al: Biologic sequelae of interleukin-6 induced PI3-K/Akt signaling in multiple myeloma. *Oncogene* 20:5991, 2001.

147. Pene F, Claessens YE, Muller O, et al: Role of the phosphatidylinositol 3-kinase/Akt and mTOR/P70S6-kinase pathways in the proliferation and apoptosis in multiple myeloma. *Oncogene* 21:6587, 2002.

148. Damiano JS, Cress AE, Hazlehurst LA, et al: Cell adhesion mediated drug resistance (CAM-DR): Role of integrins and resistance to apoptosis in human myeloma cell lines. *Blood* 93:1658, 1999.

149. Bataille R, Chappard D, Marcelli C, et al: Mechanisms of bone destruction in multiple myeloma: The importance of an unbalanced process in determining the severity of lytic bone disease. *J Clin Oncol* 7:1909, 1989.

150. Hofbauer LC, Heufelder AE: Osteoprotegerin and its cognate ligand: A new paradigm of osteoclastogenesis. *Eur J Endocrinol* 139:152, 1998.

151. Lee JW, Chung HY, Ehrlich LA, et al: IL-3 expression by myeloma cells increases both osteoclast formation and growth of myeloma cells. *Blood* 103:2308, 2004.

152. Pearse RN, Sordillo EM, Yaccoby S, et al: Multiple myeloma disrupts the TRANCE/osteoprotegerin cytokine axis to trigger bone destruction and promote tumor progression. *Proc Natl Acad Sci U S A* 98:11581, 2001.

153. Standal T, Seidel C, Hjertner O, et al: Osteoprotegerin is bound, internalized, and degraded by multiple myeloma cells. *Blood* 100:3002, 2002.

154. Abe M, Hiura K, Wilde J, et al: Role for macrophage inflammatory protein (MIP)-1alpha and MIP-1beta in the development of osteolytic lesions in multiple myeloma. *Blood* 100:2195, 2002.

155. Choi SJ, Cruz JC, Craig F, et al: Macrophage inflammatory protein 1-alpha is a potential osteoclast stimulatory factor in multiple myeloma. *Blood* 96:671, 2000.

156. Oyajobi BO, Franchin G, Williams PJ, et al: Dual effects of macrophage inflammatory protein-1alpha on osteolysis and tumor burden in the murine 5TGM1 model of myeloma bone disease. *Blood* 102:311, 2003.

157. Han Z, Boyle DL, Chang L, et al: C-Jun N-terminal kinase is required for metalloproteinase expression and joint destruction in inflammatory arthritis. *J Clin Invest* 108:73, 2001.

158. Tian E, Zhan F, Walker R, et al: The role of the Wnt-signaling antagonist DKK1 in the development of osteolytic lesions in multiple myeloma. *N Engl J Med* 349:2483, 2003.

159. Body JJ, Greipp P, Coleman RE, et al: A phase I study of AMGN-0007, a recombinant osteoprotegerin construct, in patients with multiple myeloma or breast carcinoma related bone metastases. *Cancer* 97(suppl 3): 887, 2003.

160. Hamilton MS, Barker HF, Ball J, et al: Normal and neoplastic human plasma cells express bcl-2 antigen. *Leukemia* 5:768, 1991.

161. Pettersson M, Jernberg-Wiklund H, Larsson LG, et al: Expression of the bcl-2 gene in human multiple myeloma cell lines and normal plasma cells. *Blood* 79:495, 1992.

162. Fenton RG: Therapeutic targets, in American Society of Hematology 45th Annual Meeting and Exposition. San Diego, California, 2003.

163. Cozzolino F, Torcia M, Aldinucci D, et al: Production of interleukin-1 by bone marrow myeloma cells. *Blood* 74:380, 1989.

164. Garrett IR, Durie BG, Nedwin GE, et al: Production of lymphotoxin, a bone-resorbing cytokine, by cultured human myeloma cells. *N Engl J Med* 317:526, 1987.

165. Hind CRK, Baltz ML, Pepys MB: Amyloidosis, in *Multiple Myeloma and Other Paraproteinaemias*, edited by IW Delamore, p 234. Churchill Livingstone, Edinburgh, 1986.

166. Silvestris F, Cafforio P, Tucci M, et al: Negative regulation of erythroblast maturation by Fas-L(+)/TRAIL(+) highly malignant plasma cells: A major pathogenetic mechanism of anemia in multiple myeloma. *Blood* 99:1305, 2002.

167. Ludwig H, Pecherstorfer M, Leitgeb C, et al: Recombinant human erythropoietin for the treatment of chronic anemia in multiple myeloma and squamous cell carcinoma. *Stem Cells* 11:348, 1993.

168. Faquin WC, Schneider TJ, Goldberg MA: Effect of inflammatory cytokines on hypoxia-induced erythropoietin production. *Blood* 79:1987, 1992.

169. Singh A, Eckardt KU, Zimmermann A, et al: Increased plasma viscosity as a reason for inappropriate erythropoietin formation. *J Clin Invest* 91:251, 1993.

170. Kerr R, Stirling D, Ludlam CA: Interleukin 6 and haemostasis. *Br J Haematol* 115:3, 2001.

171. Solomon A, Weiss DT: A perspective of plasma cell dyscrasias: Clinical implications of monoclonal light chains in renal disease, in *The Kidney in Plasma Cell Dyscrasias*, edited by G Minetti, G D'Amico, C Ponticelli, p 3. Kluwer, Dordrecht, Netherlands, 1988.

172. Solomon A, Weiss DT, Kattine AA: Nephrotoxic potential of Bence Jones proteins. *N Engl J Med* 324:1845, 1991.

173. Alexanian R, Barlogie B, Dixon D: Renal failure in multiple myeloma. Pathogenesis and prognostic implications. *Arch Intern Med* 150:1693, 1990.

174. Alexanian R, Barlogie B: Implications of renal failure in multiple myeloma, in *The Kidney in Plasma Cell Dyscrasias*, edited by L Minetti, G D'Amico, C Ponticelli, p 260. Kluwer, Dordrecht, Netherlands, 1988.

175. Zucker-Franklin D: Renal amyloidosis: New perspectives, in *The Kidney in Plasma Cell Dyscrasias*, edited by L Minetti, G D'Amico, C Ponticelli, p 45. Kluwer, Dordrecht, Netherlands, 1988.

176. Kyle RA, Greipp PR: Amyloidosis (AL). Clinical and laboratory features in 229 cases. *Mayo Clin Proc* 58:665, 1983.

177. Buxbaum J: Mechanisms of disease: Monoclonal immunoglobulin deposition. Amyloidosis, light chain deposition disease, and light and heavy chain deposition disease. *Hematol Oncol Clin North Am* 6:323, 1992.

178. Gallo G, Buxbaum J: Monoclonal immunoglobulin deposition disease: Immunopathologic aspects of renal involvement, in *The Kidney in Plasma Cell Dyscrasias*, edited by L Minetti, G D'Amico, C Ponticelli, p 171. Kluwer, Dordrecht, Netherlands, 1988.

179. Reeves WB, Foley RJ, Weinman EJ: Nephrotoxicity from nonsteroidal anti-inflammatory drugs. *South Med J* 78:318, 1985.

180. Fattori E, Della Rocca C, Costa P, et al: Development of progressive kidney damage and myeloma kidney in interleukin-6 transgenic mice. *Blood* 83:2570, 1994.

181. Ullrich S, Zolla-Pazner S: Immunoregulatory circuits in myeloma. *Clin Haematol* 11:87, 1982.

182. Jacobson DR, Zolla-Pazner S: Immunosuppression and infection in multiple myeloma. *Semin Oncol* 13:282, 1986.

183. Broder S, Humphrey R, Durm M, et al: Impaired synthesis of polyclonal (nonparaprotein) immunoglobulins by circulating lymphocytes from patients with multiple myeloma: role of suppressor cells. *N Engl J Med* 293:887, 1975.

184. Lynch RG: A role for TGF-beta in the immunodeficiency of malignant plasma cell tumors [abstract], in *Third EURAGE Symposium*. Brussels, Belgium, 1991.

185. Villunger A, Egle A, Marschitz I, et al: Constitutive expression of Fas (Apo-1/CD95) ligand on multiple myeloma cells: A potential mechanism of tumor-induced suppression of immune surveillance. *Blood* 90:12, 1997.

186. Waldenstrom JG, Adner A, Gydell K, et al: Osteosclerotic "plasmocytoma" with polyneuropathy, hypertrichosis, and diabetes. *Acta Med Scand* 203:297, 1978.

187. Miralles GD, O'Fallon JR, Talley NJ: Plasma-cell dyscrasia with polyneuropathy. The spectrum of POEMS syndrome. *N Engl J Med* 327:1919, 1992.

188. Pruzanski W, Watt JG: Serum viscosity and hyperviscosity syndrome in IgG multiple myeloma. Report on 10 patients and a review of the literature. *Ann Intern Med* 77:853, 1972.

189. Preston FE, Cooke KB, Foster ME, et al: Myelomatosis and the hyperviscosity syndrome. *Br J Haematol* 38:517, 1978.

190. Chandy KG, Stockley RA, Leonard RC, et al: Relationship between serum viscosity and intravascular IgA polymer concentration in IgA myeloma. *Clin Exp Immunol* 46:653, 1981.

191. Somer T: Hyperviscosity syndrome in plasma cell dyscrasias. *Adv Microcirculation* 6:1, 1975.

192. Waldenstrom JG: Incipient myelomatosis or "essential" hyperglobulinaemia with fibrinogenopenia—A new syndrome. *Acta Med Scand* 117:216, 1944.

193. Kelsey PR, Delamore IW: Clinical features of multiple myeloma, in *Multiple Myeloma and Other Paraproteinaemias*, edited by IW Delamore, p 117. Churchill Livingstone, Edinburgh, 1986.

194. Capra JD, Kunkel HG: Aggregation of gamma-G3 proteins: Relevance to the hyperviscosity syndrome. *J Clin Invest* 49:610, 1970.

195. Perkins HA, MacKenzie MR, Fudenberg HH: Hemostatic defects in dysproteinemias. *Blood* 35:695, 1970.

196. Lackner H: Hemostatic abnormalities associated with dysproteinemias. *Semin Hematol* 10:125, 1973.

197. Barlogie B, Gale RP: Multiple myeloma and chronic lymphocytic leukemia: Parallels and contrasts. *Am J Med* 93:443, 1992.

198. Zangari M, Siegel E, Barlogie B, et al: Thrombogenic activity of doxorubicin in myeloma patients receiving thalidomide: Implications for therapy. *Blood* 100:1168, 2002.

199. Bichel J, Effersoe P, Gormsen H, et al: Leukemic myelomatosis (plasma cell leukemia): A review with report of four cases. *Acta Radiol* 37:196, 1952.

200. Noel P, Kyle RA: Plasma cell leukemia: An evaluation of response to therapy. *Am J Med* 83:1062, 1987.

201. Garcia-Sanz R, Orfao A, Gonzalez M, et al: Primary plasma cell leukemia: Clinical, immunophenotypic, DNA ploidy, and cytogenetic characteristics. *Blood* 93:1032, 1999.

202. Guikema JE, Vellenga E, Abdulahad WH, et al: CD27-triggering on primary plasma cell leukaemia cells has anti-apoptotic effects involving mitogen activated protein kinases. *Br J Haematol* 124:299, 2004.

203. Barlogie B, Smallwood L, Smith T, et al: High serum levels of lactic dehydrogenase identify a high-grade lymphoma-like myeloma. *Ann Intern Med* 110:521, 1989.

204. Cherng NC, Asal NR, Kuebler JP, et al: Prognostic factors in multiple myeloma. *Cancer* 67:3150, 1991.

205. Fassas AB, Spencer T, Sawyer J, et al: Both hypodiploidy and deletion of chromosome 13 independently confer poor prognosis in multiple myeloma. *Br J Haematol* 118:1041, 2002.

206. Greipp PR, San Miguel JF, Durie BG, et al: A new international staging system for multiple myeloma from the International Myeloma Working Group. *Blood* 102:190a, 2003.

207. Glueck HI, Hong R: A circulating anticoagulant in gamma-1A-multiple myeloma: Its modification by penicillin. *J Clin Invest* 44:1866, 1965.

208. Wenz B, Friedman G: Acquired factor VIII inhibitor in a patient with malignant lymphoma. *Am J Med Sci* 268:295, 1974.

209. Kelsey PR, Leyland MJ: Acquired inhibitor to human factor VIII associated with paraproteinaemia and subsequent development of chronic lymphatic leukaemia. *Br Med J (Clin Res Ed)* 285:174, 1982.

210. Coleman M, Vigliano EM, Weksler ME, et al: Inhibition of fibrin monomer polymerization by lambda myeloma globulins. *Blood* 39:210, 1972.

211. Furie B, Greene E, Furie BC: Syndrome of acquired factor X deficiency and systemic amyloidosis in vivo studies of the metabolic fate of factor X. *N Engl J Med* 297:81, 1977.

212. Kunkel LA: Acquired circulating anticoagulants in malignancy. *Semin Thromb Hemost* 18:416, 1992.

213. Greipp PR, Raymond NM, Kyle RA, et al: Multiple myeloma: Significance of plasmablastic subtype in morphological classification. *Blood* 65:305, 1985.

214. Greipp PR, Leong T, Bennett JM, et al: Plasmablastic morphology—An independent prognostic factor with clinical and laboratory correlates: Eastern Cooperative Oncology Group (ECOG) myeloma trial E9486 report by the ECOG Myeloma Laboratory Group. *Blood* 91:2501, 1998.

215. Bartl R, Frisch B, Fateh-Moghadam A, et al: gHistologic classification and staging of multiple myeloma. A retrospective and prospective study of 674 cases. *Am J Clin Pathol* 87:342, 1987.

216. Waldron J, Jazieh R, Jagannath S, et al: Bone marrow morphology adds critical prognostic information to other standard parameters including cytogenetics among newly diagnosed multiple myeloma patients receiving total therapy. *Blood* 90:90a, 1997.

217. Munshi N, Wilson CS, Penn J, et al: Antiogenesis in newly diagnosed multiple myeloma: Poor prognosis with increased microvessel density (MVD) in bone marrow biopsies. *Blood* 92(suppl 1):98a, 1998.

218. Bellamy WT, Richter L, Frutiger Y, et al: Expression of vascular endothelial growth factor and its receptors in hematopoietic malignancies. *Cancer Res* 59:728, 1999.

219. Kumar S, Fonseca R, Dispenzieri A, et al: Bone marrow angiogenesis in multiple myeloma: Effect of therapy. *Br J Haematol* 119:665, 2002.

220. Govindarajan R, Jagannath S, Flick JT, et al: Preceding standard therapy is the likely cause of MDS after autotransplants for multiple myeloma. *Br J Haematol* 95:349, 1996.

221. Tricot G, Barlogie B, Sawyer J, et al: MM-MDS is a poor prognostic marker for outcome after tandem transplants in multiple myeloma (MM). *Proc Am Soc Clin Oncol* [abstract] 22:567, 2003.

222. Barlogie B, Alexanian R, Pershouse M, et al: Cytoplasmic immunoglobulin content in multiple myeloma. *J Clin Invest* 76:765, 1985.

223. Billadeau D, Quam L, Thomas W, et al: Detection and quantitation of malignant cells in the peripheral blood of multiple myeloma patients. *Blood* 80:1818, 1992.

224. Aubin J, Davi F, Nguyen-Salomon F, et al: Description of a novel FR1 IgH PCR strategy and its comparison with three other strategies for the detection of clonality in B cell malignancies. *Leukemia* 9:471, 1995.

225. Bataille R, Robillard N, Pellat-Deceunynck C, et al: A cellular model for myeloma cell growth and maturation based on an intraclonal CD45 hierarchy. *Immunol Rev* 194:105, 2003.

226. Epstein J: Myeloma phenotype: Clues to disease origin and manifestation. *Hematol Oncol Clin North Am* 6:249, 1992.

227. Van Camp B, Durie BG, Spier C, et al: Plasma cells in multiple myeloma express a natural killer cell-associated antigen: CD56 (NKH-1; Leu-19). *Blood* 76:377, 1990.

228. Epstein J, Xiao HQ, Oba BK: P-glycoprotein expression in plasma-cell myeloma is associated with resistance to VAD. *Blood* 74:913, 1989.

229. Dalton WS, Durie BG, Alberts DS, et al: Characterization of a new drug-resistant human myeloma cell line that expresses P-glycoprotein. *Cancer Res* 46:5125, 1986.

230. Dalton WS, Grogan TM, Meltzer PS, et al: Drug-resistance in multiple myeloma and non-Hodgkin lymphoma: Detection of P-glycoprotein and potential circumvention by addition of verapamil to chemotherapy. *J Clin Oncol* 7:415, 1989.

231. Dalton WS, Grogan TM, Rybski JA, et al: Immunohistochemical detection and quantitation of P-glycoprotein in multiple drug-resistant human myeloma cells: Association with level of drug resistance and drug accumulation. *Blood* 73:7472, 1989.

232. Dalton WS: Detection of multidrug resistance gene expression in multiple myeloma. *Leukemia* 11:1166, 1997.

233. Sonneveld P, Lokhorst HM, Vossebeld P: Drug resistance in multiple myeloma. *Semin Hematol* 34(4 suppl 5):34, 1997.

234. Raaijmakers HG, Izquierdo MA, Lokhorst HM, et al: Lung-resistance-related protein expression is a negative predictive factor for response to conventional low but not to intensified dose alkylating chemotherapy in multiple myeloma. *Blood* 91:1029, 1998.

235. Ocqueteau M, Orfao A, Garcia-Sanz R, et al: Expression of the CD117 antigen (c-Kit) on normal and myelomatous plasma cells. *Br J Haematol* 95:489, 1996.

236. Almeida J, Orfao A, Ocqueteau M, et al: High-sensitive immunophenotyping and DNA ploidy studies for the investigation of minimal residual disease in multiple myeloma. *Br J Haematol* 107:121, 1999.

237. Tricot G, Sawyer JR, Jagannath S, et al: Unique role of cytogenetics in the prognosis of patients with myeloma receiving high-dose therapy and autotransplants. *J Clin Oncol* 15:2659, 1997.

238. Desikan R, Barlogie B, Sawyer J, et al: Results of high-dose therapy for 1,000 patients with multiple myeloma: Durable complete remissions and superior survival in the absence of chromosome 13 abnormalities. *Blood* 95:4008, 2000.

239. Jacobson J, Barlogie B, Shaughnessy J, et al: MDS-type abnormalities within myeloma signature karyotype (MM-MDS): Only 13% 1-year survival despite tandem transplants. *Br J Haematol* 122:430, 2003.

240. Tricot G, Barlogie B, Jagannath S, et al: Poor prognosis in multiple myeloma is associated only with partial or complete deletions of chromosome 13 or abnormalities involving 11q and not with other karyotype abnormalities. *Blood* 86:4250, 1995.

241. Smadja NV, Bastard C, Brigaudeau C, et al: Hypodiploidy is a major prognostic factor in multiple myeloma. *Blood* 98:2229, 2001.

242. Seong C, Delasalle K, Hayes K, et al: Prognostic value of cytogenetics in multiple myeloma. *Br J Haematol* 101:189, 1998.

243. Zojer N, Konigsberg R, Ackermann J, et al: Deletion of 13q14 remains an independent adverse prognostic variable in multiple myeloma despite its frequent detection by interphase fluorescence in situ hybridization. *Blood* 95:1925, 2000.

244. Facon T, Avet-Loiseau H, Guillerm G, et al: Chromosome 13 abnormalities identified by FISH analysis and serum beta2-microglobulin produce a powerful myeloma staging system for patients receiving high-dose therapy. *Blood* 97:1566, 2001.

245. Konigsberg R, Zojer N, Ackermann J, et al: Predictive role of interphase cytogenetics for survival of patients with multiple myeloma. *J Clin Oncol* 18:804, 2000.

246. Shaughnessy J Jr, Tian E, Sawyer J, et al: Prognostic impact of cytogenetic and interphase fluorescence in situ hybridization-defined chromosome 13 deletion in multiple myeloma: Early results of total therapy II. *Br J Haematol* 120:44, 2003.

247. Drewinko B, Alexanian R, Boyer H, et al: The growth fraction of human myeloma cells. *Blood* 57:333, 1981.

248. Durie BG, Salmon SE, Moon TE: Pretreatment tumor mass, cell kinetics, and prognosis in multiple myeloma. *Blood* 55:364, 1980.

249. Greipp PR, Witzig TE, Gonchoroff NJ, et al: Immunofluorescence labeling indices in myeloma and related monoclonal gammopathies. *Mayo Clin Proc* 62:969, 1987.

250. Boccadoro M, Massaia M, Dianzani U, et al: Multiple myeloma: Biological and clinical significance of bone marrow plasma cell labeling index. *Haematologica* 72:171, 1987.

251. Greipp PR, Lust JA, O'Fallon WM, et al: Plasma cell labeling index and beta 2-microglobulin predict survival independent of thymidine kinase and C-reactive protein in multiple myeloma. *Blood* 81:3382, 1993.

252. Witzig TE, Gonchoroff NJ, Katzmann JA, et al: Peripheral blood B cell labeling indices are a measure of disease activity in patients with monoclonal gammopathies. *J Clin Oncol* 6:1041, 1988.

253. San Miguel JF, Garcia-Sanz R, Gonzalez M, et al: A new staging system for multiple myeloma based on the number of S-phase plasma cells. *Blood* 85:448, 1995.

254. Kyle RA, Garton JP: The spectrum of IgM monoclonal gammopathy in 430 cases. *Mayo Clin Proc* 62:719, 1987.

255. Dhodapkar MV, Jacobson JL, Gertz MA, et al: Prognostic factors and response to fludarabine therapy in patients with Waldenstrom macroglobulinemia: Results of United States intergroup trial (Southwest Oncology Group S9003). *Blood* 98:41, 2001.

256. Dimopoulos MA, Panayiotidis P, Moulopoulos LA, et al: Waldenstrom macroglobulinemia: Clinical features, complications, and management. *J Clin Oncol* 18:214, 2000.

257. Bradwell AR, Tang LX, Drayson MT, et al: Immunoassay for detection of free light chains in serum of patients with nonsecretory myeloma [abstract 4901]. *Blood* 96:271b, 2000.

258. Child JA, Norfolk DR, Cooper EH: Serum beta 2-microglobulin in myelomatosis. *Br J Haematol* 63:406, 1986.

259. Garewal H, Durie BG, Kyle RA, et al: Serum beta 2-microglobulin in the initial staging and subsequent monitoring of monoclonal plasma cell disorders. *J Clin Oncol* 2:51, 1984.

260. Bataille R, Grenier J, Sany J: Beta-2-microglobulin in myeloma: Optimal use for staging, prognosis, and treatment—A prospective study of 160 patients. *Blood* 63:468, 1984.

261. Lifson AR, Hessol NA, Buchbinder SP, et al: Serum beta 2-microglobulin and prediction of progression to AIDS in HIV infection. *Lancet* 339:1436, 1992.

262. Grieco MH, Reddy MM, Kothari HB, et al: Elevated beta 2-microglobulin and lysozyme levels in patients with acquired immune deficiency syndrome. *Clin Immunol Immunopathol* 32:174, 1984.

263. Sprague SM, Popovtzer MM: Is beta 2-microglobulin a mediator of bone disease? *Kidney Int* 47:1, 1995.

264. Bataille R, Boccadoro M, Klein B, et al: C-reactive protein and beta-2 microglobulin produce a simple and powerful myeloma staging system. *Blood* 80:733, 1992.

265. Dimopoulos MA, Barlogie B, Smith TL, et al: High serum lactate dehydrogenase level as a marker for drug resistance and short survival in multiple myeloma. *Ann Intern Med* 115:931, 1991.

266. Terpos E, Szydlo R, Apperley JF, et al: Soluble receptor activator of nuclear factor kappaB ligand-osteoprotegerin ratio predicts survival in multiple myeloma: Proposal for a novel prognostic index. *Blood* 102:1064, 2003.

267. Bataille R, Chappard D, Marcelli C, et al: Recruitment of new osteoblasts and osteoclasts is the earliest critical event in the pathogenesis of human multiple myeloma. *J Clin Invest* 88:62, 1991.

268. Sezer O, Heider U, Zavrski I, et al: RANK ligand and osteoprotegerin in myeloma bone disease. *Blood* 101:2094, 2003.

269. Mundy GR: Metastasis to bone: Causes, consequences, and therapeutic opportunities. *Nat Rev Cancer* 2:584, 2002.

270. Resnick D: *Bone and Joint Imaging*, 2nd ed, edited by L Bralow, p 1329. WB Saunders, Philadelphia, 1996.

271. Jacobson HG, Poppel MH, Shapiro JH, et al: The vertebral pedicle sign: A roentgen finding to differentiate metastatic carcinoma from multiple myeloma. *Am J Roentgenol* 80:817, 1958.

272. Angtuaco EJ, Fassas AB, Walker R, et al: Multiple myeloma: Clinical review and diagnostic imaging. *Radiology* 231:11, 2004.

273. Walker RC, Barlogie B, Jacobson J, et al: Prospective evaluation of 460 patients from Total Therapy II—Identification of characteristics on baseline MRI examinations of prognostic significance—Importance of focal lesions in multiple myeloma, in *9th International Multiple Myeloma Workshop*. Salamanca, Spain, 2003.

274. Abildgaard N, Brixen K, Kristensen JE, et al: Assessment of bone involvement in patients with multiple myeloma using bone densitometry. *Eur J Haematol* 57:370, 1996.

275. Palladini G, Campana C, Klersy C, et al: Serum N-terminal probrain natriuretic peptide is a sensitive marker of myocardial dysfunction in AL amyloidosis. *Circulation* 107:2440, 2003.

276. International Myeloma Working Group: Criteria for the classification of monoclonal gammopathies, multiple myeloma, and related disorders: A report of the International Myeloma Working Group. *Br J Haematol* 121:749, 2003.

277. Dimopoulos MA, Moulopoulos A, Delasalle K, et al: Solitary plasmacytoma of bone and asymptomatic multiple myeloma. *Hematol Oncol Clin North Am* 6:359, 1992.

278. Bataille R, Sany J: Solitary myeloma: Clinical and prognostic features of a review of 114 cases. *Cancer* 48:845, 1981.

279. Corwin J, Lindberg RD: Solitary plasmacytoma of bone vs. extramedullary plasmacytoma and their relationship to multiple myeloma. *Cancer* 43:1007, 1979.

280. Knowling MA, Harwood AR, Bergsagel DE: Comparison of extramedullary plasmacytomas with solitary and multiple plasma cell tumors of bone. *J Clin Oncol* 1:255, 1983.

281. Whittaker JA: Solitary plasmacytoma, in *Multiple Myeloma and Other Paraproteinaemias*, edited by IW Delamore, p 193. Churchill Livingstone, New York, 1986.

282. Kyle RA, Schreiman JS, McLeod RA, et al: Computed tomography in diagnosis and management of multiple myeloma and its variants. *Arch Intern Med* 145:1451, 1985.

283. Daffner RH, Lupetin AR, Dash N, et al: MRI in the detection of malignant infiltration of bone marrow. *AJR Am J Roentgenol* 146:353, 1986.

284. Moulopoulos LA, Dimopoulos MA, Weber D, et al: Magnetic resonance imaging in the staging of solitary plasmacytoma of bone. *J Clin Oncol* 11:1311, 1993.

285. Dohner H, Guckel F, Knauf W, et al: Magnetic resonance imaging of bone marrow in lymphoproliferative disorders: Correlation with bone marrow biopsy. *Br J Haematol* 73:12, 1989.

286. Angtuaco E, Jazieh A, Ferris E, et al: Complete remission by MRI (MR-CR) after tandem autotransplants associated with superior survival. *Blood* 92(suppl 1):97a, 1998.

287. Libbey CA, Skinner M, Cohen AS: Use of abdominal fat tissue aspirate in the diagnosis of systemic amyloidosis. *Arch Intern Med* 143:1549, 1983.

288. Cooper JH: A histochemical construct of the amylois fibril, in *Amyloidosis E. A. R. S.*, edited by PA Tribe, p 31. Wright, Bristol, 1983.

289. Ridolfi RL, Bulkley BH, Hutchins GM: The conduction system in cardiac amyloidosis. Clinical and pathologic features of 23 patients. *Am J Med* 62:677, 1977.

290. Hind CR, Gibson DG, Lavender JP, et al: Non-invasive demonstration of cardiac involvement in acquired forms of systemic amyloidosis. *Lancet* 1:1417, 1984.

291. Durie BG, Salmon SE: A clinical staging system for multiple myeloma. Correlation of measured myeloma cell mass with presenting clinical features, response to treatment, and survival. *Cancer* 36:842, 1975.

292. Salmon SE, Smith BA: Immunoglobulin synthesis and total body tumor cell number in IgG multiple myeloma. *J Clin Invest* 49:1114, 1970.

293. Klein B, Bataille R: Cytokine network in human multiple myeloma. *Hematol Oncol Clin North Am* 6:273, 1992.

294. Bataille R, Chappard D, Klein B: Mechanisms of bone lesions in multiple myeloma. *Hematol Oncol Clin North Am* 6:285, 1992.

295. Smith L, Barlogie B, Alexanian R: Biclonal and hypodiploid multiple myeloma. *Am J Med* 80:841, 1986.

296. Rajkumar SV, Kyle RA: Angiogenesis in multiple myeloma. *Semin Oncol* 28:560, 2001.

297. Myeloma Trialists' Collaborative Group: Combination chemotherapy versus melphalan plus prednisone as treatment for multiple myeloma: An overview of 6,633 patients from 27 randomized trials. *J Clin Oncol* 16:3832, 1998.

298. Bergsagel DE, Sprague CC, Austin C, et al: Evaluation of new chemotherapeutic agents in the treatment of multiple myeloma: IV. L-phenylalanine mustard (NC-8806). *Cancer Chemother Rep* 21:87, 1962.

299. Alexanian R, Haut A, Khan AU, et al: Treatment for multiple myeloma. Combination chemotherapy with different melphalan dose regimens. *JAMA* 208:1680, 1969.

300. Attal M, Harousseau JL, Stoppa AM, et al: A prospective, randomized trial of autologous bone marrow transplantation and chemotherapy in multiple myeloma. Intergroupe Francais du Myelome. *N Engl J Med* 335:91, 1996.

301. Child JA, Morgan GJ, Davies FE, et al: High-dose chemotherapy with hematopoietic stem-cell rescue for multiple myeloma. *N Engl J Med* 348:1875, 2003.

302. Barlogie B, Jagannath S, Vesole DH, et al: Superiority of tandem autologous transplantation over standard therapy for previously untreated multiple myeloma. *Blood* 89:789, 1997.

303. Lenhoff S, Hjorth M, Holmberg E, et al: Impact on survival of high-dose therapy with autologous stem cell support in patients younger than 60 years with newly diagnosed multiple myeloma: A population-based study. Nordic Myeloma Study Group. *Blood* 95:7, 2000.

304. Siegel DS, Desikan KR, Mehta J, et al: Age is not a prognostic variable with autotransplants for multiple myeloma. *Blood* 93:51, 1999.

305. Badros A, Barlogie B, Siegel E, et al: Autologous stem cell transplantation in elderly multiple myeloma patients over the age of 70 years. *Br J Haematol* 114:600, 2001.

306. Palumbo A, Triolo S, Argentino C, et al: Dose-intensive melphalan with stem cell support (MEL100) is superior to standard treatment in elderly myeloma patients. *Blood* 94:1248, 1999.

307. Badros A, Barlogie B, Siegel E, et al: Results of autologous stem cell transplant in multiple myeloma patients with renal failure. *Br J Haematol* 114:822, 2001.

308. Lee CK, Barlogie B, Zangari M, et al: Dialysis-dependent renal failure in patients with myeloma can be reversed by high-dose myeloablative therapy and autotransplant. *Blood* 100:431a, 2002.

309. Falk RH, Comenzo RL, Skinner M: The systemic amyloidoses. *N Engl J Med* 337:898, 1997.

310. Kumar S, Lacy M, Dispenzieri A, et al: Peripheral blood stem cell transplantation for primary systemic amyloidosis with cardiac involvement. *Blood* 100:180a, 2002.

311. Skinner M, Sanchorawala V, Seldin DC, et al: High-dose melphalan and autologous stem-cell transplantation in patients with AL amyloidosis: An 8-year study. *Ann Intern Med* 140:85, 2004.

312. Gertz MA, Lacy MQ, Dispenzieri A: Therapy for immunoglobulin light chain amyloidosis: The new and the old. *Blood Rev* 18:17, 2004.

313. Barlogie B, Shaughnessy J, Jacobson J, et al: Improving disease control in myeloma, in *American Society of Hematology 45th Annual Meeting and Exposition*. San Diego, California, 2003.

314. Moreau P, Facon T, Attal M, et al: Comparison of 200 mg/m(2) melphalan and 8 Gy total body irradiation plus 140 mg/m(2) melphalan as conditioning regimens for peripheral blood stem cell transplantation in patients with newly diagnosed multiple myeloma: Final analysis of the Intergroupe Francophone du Myelome 9502 randomized trial. *Blood* 99: 731, 2002.

315. Tricot G, Jagannath S, Vesole D, et al: Peripheral blood stem cell transplants for multiple myeloma: Identification of favorable variables for rapid engraftment in 225 patients. *Blood* 85:588, 1995.

316. Morris CL, Siegel E, Barlogie B, et al: Mobilization of CD34+ cells in elderly patients (>/= 70 years) with multiple myeloma: Influence of age, prior therapy, platelet count and mobilization regimen. *Br J Haematol* 120:413, 2003.

317. Barlogie B, Smith L, Alexanian R: Effective treatment of advanced multiple myeloma refractory to alkylating agents. *N Engl J Med* 310:1353, 1984.

318. Samson D, Gaminara E, Newland A, et al: Infusion of vincristine and doxorubicin with oral dexamethasone as first-line therapy for multiple myeloma. *Lancet* 2:882, 1989.

319. Salmon SE, Crowley JJ, Grogan TM, et al: Combination chemotherapy, glucocorticoids, and interferon alfa in the treatment of multiple myeloma: A Southwest Oncology Group study. *J Clin Oncol* 12:2405, 1994.

320. Alexanian R, Barlogie B, Dixon D: High-dose glucocorticoid treatment of resistant myeloma. *Ann Intern Med* 105:8, 1986.

321. Alexanian R, Dimopoulos MA, Delasalle K, et al: Primary dexamethasone treatment of multiple myeloma. *Blood* 80:887, 1992.

322. Rajkumar SV, Hayman S, Gertz MA, et al: Combination therapy with thalidomide plus dexamethasone for newly diagnosed myeloma. *J Clin Oncol* 20:4319, 2002.

323. Weber D, Rankin K, Gavino M, et al: Thalidomide alone or with dexamethasone for previously untreated multiple myeloma. *J Clin Oncol* 21:16, 2003.

324. Lee CK, Barlogie B, Munshi N, et al: DTPACE: An effective, novel combination chemotherapy with thalidomide for previously treated patients with myeloma. *J Clin Oncol* 21(14):2732, 2003.

325. Berenson J, Crowley J, Barlogie B, et al: Alternate day oral prednisone maintenance therapy improves progression-free and overall survival in multiple myeloma patients. *Blood* 92(suppl 1):318a, 1998.

326. Mandelli F, Avvisati G, Amadori S, et al: Maintenance treatment with recombinant interferon alfa-2b in patients with multiple myeloma responding to conventional induction chemotherapy. *N Engl J Med* 322: 1430, 1990.

327. Ludwig H, Cohen AM, Polliack A, et al: Interferon-alpha for induction and maintenance in multiple myeloma: Results of two multicenter randomized trials and summary of other studies. *Ann Oncol* 6:467, 1995.

328. Salmon SE, Crowley JJ, Balcerzak SP, et al: Interferon versus interferon plus prednisone remission maintenance therapy for multiple myeloma: A Southwest Oncology Group Study. *J Clin Oncol* 16:890, 1998.

329. Barlogie B, Kyle R, Anderson K, et al: Comparable survival in multiple myeloma (MM) with high dose therapy (HDT) employing MRL 140 mg/m2 + TBI 12 by autotransplants versus standard dose therapy with VBMCP and no benefit from interferon (IFN) maintenance: Results of intergroup trial S9321 [abstract 135]. *Blood* 102:42a, 2003.

330. Berenson JR, Lichtenstein A, Porter L, et al: Efficacy of pamidronate in reducing skeletal events in patients with advanced multiple myeloma. Myeloma Aredia Study Group. *N Engl J Med* 334:488, 1996.

331. Berenson JR, Rosen LS, Howell A, et al: Zoledronic acid reduces skeletal-related events in patients with osteolytic metastases. *Cancer* 91: 1191, 2001.

332. Berenson JR: Advances in the biology and treatment of myeloma bone disease. *Semin Oncol* 29(6 suppl 17):11, 2002.

333. Berenson JR, Lichtenstein A, Porter L, et al: Long-term pamidronate treatment of advanced multiple myeloma patients reduces skeletal events. Myeloma Aredia Study Group. *J Clin Oncol* 16:593, 1998.

334. Gordon S, Helfrich MH, Sati HI, et al: Pamidronate causes apoptosis of plasma cells in vivo in patients with multiple myeloma. *Br J Haematol* 119:475, 2002.

335. Berenson JR, Hillner BE, Kyle RA, et al: American Society of Clinical Oncology clinical practice guidelines: The role of bisphosphonates in multiple myeloma. *J Clin Oncol* 20:3719, 2002.

336. Attal M, Harrouseau JL, Facon T, et al: Double autologous transplantation improves survival of multiple myeloma patients: Final analysis of a prospective randomized study of the "Intergroupe Francophone du Myelome" (IFM 94). *Blood* 100:5a, 2002.

337. Barlogie B, Shaughnessy JD, Tricot G, et al: Treatment of multiple myeloma. *Blood* 103:20, 2004.

338. Attal M, Harousseau JL: Randomized trial experience of the Intergroupe Francophone du Myelome. *Semin Hematol* 38:226, 2001.

339. Gahrton G, Tura S, Ljungman P, et al: Allogeneic bone marrow transplantation in multiple myeloma. European Group for Bone Marrow Transplantation. *N Engl J Med* 325:1267, 1991.

340. Bensinger WI, Maloney D, Storb R: Allogeneic hematopoietic cell transplantation for multiple myeloma. *Semin Hematol* 38:243, 2001.

341. Giralt S, Thall PF, Khouri I, et al: Melphalan and purine analog-containing preparative regimens: Reduced-intensity conditioning for patients with hematologic malignancies undergoing allogeneic progenitor cell transplantation. *Blood* 97:631, 2001.

342. Badros A, Barlogie B, Siegel E, et al: Improved outcome of allogeneic transplantation in high-risk multiple myeloma patients after nonmyeloablative conditioning. *J Clin Oncol* 20:1295, 2002.

343. Kroger N, Sayer HG, Schwerdtfeger R, et al: Unrelated stem cell transplantation in multiple myeloma after a reduced-intensity conditioning with pretransplantation antithymocyte globulin is highly effective with low transplantation-related mortality. *Blood* 100:3919, 2002.

344. Lee CK, Badros A, Barlogie B, et al: Prognostic factors in allogeneic transplantation for patients with high-risk multiple myeloma after reduced intensity conditioning. *Exp Hematol* 31:73, 2003.

345. Tricot G, Vesole DH, Jagannath S, et al: Graft-versus-myeloma effect: Proof of principle. *Blood* 87:1196, 1996.

346. Maloney D, Sahebi F, Stockerl-Goldstein KE, et al: Combining an allogeneic grant-vs.-myeloma effect with high-dose autologous stem cell rescue in the treatment of multiple myeloma. *Blood* 99:434a, 2001.

347. Badros A, Barlogie B, Morris C, et al: High response rate in refractory and poor-risk multiple myeloma after allotransplantation using a nonmyeloablative conditioning regimen and donor lymphocyte infusions. *Blood* 97:2574, 2001.

348. San Miguel JF, Lahuerta JJ, Garcia-Sanz R, et al: Are myeloma patients with renal failure candidates for autologous stem cell transplantation? *Hematol J* 1:28, 2000.

349. Dhodapkar MV, Jagannath S, Vesole D, et al: Treatment of AL-amyloidosis with dexamethasone plus alpha interferon. *Leuk Lymphoma* 27:351, 1997.

350. Dhodapkar MV, Jacobson J, Hussein M, et al. High dose dexamethasone (Dex) with maintenance Dex/alpha interferon leads to improved survival in patients with primary systemic amyloidosis: results of US Intergroup Trial Southwest Oncology Group (SWOG) S9628. *Proc Am Soc Clin Oncol* 22:566, 2003 (abstr 2278).

351. Palladini G, Perfetti V, Obici L, et al: Association of melphalan and high-dose dexamethasone is effective and well tolerated in patients with AL (primary) amyloidosis who are ineligible for stem cell transplantation. *Blood* 103:2936, 2004.

352. Dispenzieri A, Kyle RA, Lacy MQ, et al: Superior survival in primary systemic amyloidosis patients undergoing peripheral blood stem cell transplantation: A case-control study. *Blood* 103:3960, 2004.

353. Dimopoulos MA, Moulopoulos LA, Maniatis A, et al: Solitary plasmacytoma of bone and asymptomatic multiple myeloma. *Blood* 96:2037, 2000.

354. Moulopoulos LA, Maris TG, Papanikolaou N, et al: Detection of malignant bone marrow involvement with dynamic contrast-enhanced magnetic resonance imaging. *Ann Oncol* 14:152, 2003.

355. Durie BG, Waxman AD, D'Agnolo A, et al: Whole-body (18)F-FDG PET identifies high-risk myeloma. *J Nucl Med* 43:1457, 2002.

356. Fourney DR, Schomer DF, Nader R, et al: Percutaneous vertebroplasty and kyphoplasty for painful vertebral body fractures in cancer patients. *J Neurosurg* 98(suppl 1):21, 2003.

357. Dudeney S, Lieberman IH, Reinhardt MK, et al: Kyphoplasty in the treatment of osteolytic vertebral compression fractures as a result of multiple myeloma. *J Clin Oncol* 20:2382, 2002.

358. Alexanian R: Localized and indolent myeloma. *Blood* 56:521, 1980.

359. Kyle RA, Greipp PR: Smoldering multiple myeloma. *N Engl J Med* 302:1347, 1980.

360. Dimopoulos MA, Moulopoulos A, Smith T, et al: Risk of disease progression in asymptomatic multiple myeloma. *Am J Med* 94:57, 1993.

361. Dhodapkar MV, Singh J, Mehta J, et al: Anti-myeloma activity of pamidronate in vivo. *Br J Haematol* 103:530, 1998.

362. Weber DM, Dimopoulos MA, Moulopoulos LA, et al: Prognostic features of asymptomatic multiple myeloma. *Br J Haematol* 97:810, 1997.

363. Blade J, Samson D, Reece D, et al: Criteria for evaluating disease response and progression in patients with multiple myeloma treated by high-dose therapy and haemopoietic stem cell transplantation. Myeloma Subcommittee of the EBMT. European Group for Blood and Marrow Transplant. *Br J Haematol* 102:1115, 1998.

364. Zent CS, Wilson CS, Tricot G, et al: Oligoclonal protein bands and Ig isotype switching in multiple myeloma treated with high-dose therapy and hematopoietic cell transplantation. *Blood* 91:3518, 1998.

365. Singhal S, Mehta J, Desikan R, et al: Antitumor activity of thalidomide in refractory multiple myeloma. *N Engl J Med* 341:1565, 1999.

366. Barlogie B, Desikan R, Eddlemon P, et al: Extended survival in advanced and refractory multiple myeloma after single-agent thalidomide: Identification of prognostic factors in a phase 2 study of 169 patients. *Blood* 98:492, 2001.

367. Barlogie B, Tricot G, Anaissie E: Thalidomide in the management of multiple myeloma. *Semin Oncol* 28:577, 2001.

368. Barlogie B, Zangari M, Spencer T, et al: Thalidomide in the management of multiple myeloma. *Semin Hematol* 38:250, 2001.

369. Kumar S, Gertz MA, Dispenzieri A, et al: Response rate, durability of response, and survival after thalidomide therapy for relapsed multiple myeloma. *Mayo Clin Proc* 78:34, 2003.

370. Hideshima T, Anderson KC: Molecular mechanisms of novel therapeutic approaches for multiple myeloma. *Nat Rev Cancer* 2:927, 2002.

371. Durie BG: Low-dose thalidomide in myeloma: Efficacy and biologic significance. *Semin Oncol* 29(6 suppl 17):34, 2002.

372. Anderson KC: Targeted therapy for multiple myeloma. *Semin Hematol* 38:286, 2001.

373. Zangari M, Tricot G, Zeldis J, et al: Results of phase I study of CC-5013 for the treatment of multiple myeloma patients who relapse after high dose chemotherapy. *Blood* 98:775a, 2001.

374. Richardson PG, Schlossman RL, Weller E, et al: Immunomodulatory drug CC-5013 overcomes drug resistance and is well tolerated in patients with relapsed multiple myeloma. *Blood* 100:3063, 2002.

375. Adams J, Palombella VJ, Sausville EA, et al: Proteasome inhibitors: A novel class of potent and effective antitumor agents. *Cancer Res* 59:2615, 1999.

376. Hideshima T, Mitsiades C, Akiyama M, et al: Molecular mechanisms mediating antimyeloma activity of proteasome inhibitor PS-341. *Blood* 101:1530, 2003.

377. Richardson P, Barlogie B, Berenson J, et al: A phase II multicenter study of the proteasome inhibitor bortezomib (VelcadeTM, formally PS-341) in multiple myeloma patients with relapsed/refractory disease. *Blood* 100:104a, 2002.

378. Richardson P, Berenson J, Irwin D, et al: Phase II trial of PS-341, a novel proteasome inhibitor, alone or in combination with dexamethasone, in patients with multiple myeloma who have relapsed following front-line therapy and are refractory to their most recent therapy. *Blood* 98:774a, 2001.

379. Yang HH, Vescio R, Adams J, et al: A phase I/II study of combination treatment with bortezomib and melphalan (Vc+M) in patients with relapsed or refractory multiple myeloma. *Proc Am Soc Clin Oncol* 22:582a, 2001.

380. Ma MH, Yang HH, Parker K, et al: The proteasome inhibitor PS-341 markedly enhances sensitivity of multiple myeloma tumor cells to chemotherapeutic agents. *Clin Cancer Res* 9:1136, 2003.

381. Munshi NC, Tricot G, Desikan R, et al: Clinical activity of arsenic trioxide for the treatment of multiple myeloma. *Leukemia* 16:1835, 2002.

382. Hussein MA: Arsenic trioxide: A new immunomodulatory agent in the management of multiple myeloma. *Med Oncol* 18:239, 2001.

383. Bataille R, Barlogie B, Lu ZY, et al: Biologic effects of anti-interleukin-6 murine monoclonal antibody in advanced multiple myeloma. *Blood* 86:685, 1995.

384. Hussein M, Karam M, McLain D, et al: Biologic and clinical evaluation of Rituxan in the management of newly diagnosed multiple myeloma patients. *Blood* 94:313a, 1999.

385. Hu L, Shi Y, Hsu JH, et al: Downstream effectors of oncogenic ras in multiple myeloma cells. *Blood* 101:3126, 2003.

386. Karp JE, Kaufmann SH, Adjei AA, et al: Current status of clinical trials of farnesyltransferase inhibitors. *Curr Opin Oncol* 13:470, 2001.

387. Mackley P, Shain KH, Dalton WS, et al: Farnesyl transferase inhibitor-R115777 decreases Akt phosphorylation in multiple myeloma cell lines and its apoptotic effects correlate with phosphoAKT expression levels. *Blood* 100:810a, 2002.

388. Fonseca R, Oken MM, Greipp PR: The t(4;14)(p16.3;q32) is strongly associated with chromosome 13 abnormalities in both multiple myeloma and monoclonal gammopathy of undetermined significance. *Blood* 98:1271, 2001.

389. Osterborg A, Brandberg Y, Molostova V, et al: Randomized, double-blind, placebo-controlled trial of recombinant human erythropoietin, epoetin Beta, in hematologic malignancies. *J Clin Oncol* 20:2486, 2002.

390. Nucci M, Anaissie E: Risks and epidemiology of infection after autologous hematopoietic stem cell transplantation, in *Transplant Infections*, edited by R Bowden, P Ljungman, C Paya, p 39. Lippincott Williams & Wilkins, Philadelphia, 2003.

391. Weaver CH, Schwartzberg LS, Hainsworth J, et al: Treatment-related mortality in 1000 consecutive patients receiving high-dose chemotherapy and peripheral blood progenitor cell transplantation in community cancer centers. *Bone Marrow Transplant* 19:671, 1997.

392. Anaissie EJ, Stratton SL, Dignani MC, et al: Pathogenic molds (including Aspergillus species) in hospital water distribution systems: A 3-year prospective study and clinical implications for patients with hematologic malignancies. *Blood* 101:2542, 2003.

393. Offidani M, Corvatta L, Olivieri A, et al: A predictive model of varicella-zoster virus infection after autologous peripheral blood progenitor cell transplantation. *Clin Infect Dis* 32:1414, 2001.

394. Uzun O, Anaissie EJ: Antifungal prophylaxis in patients with hematologic malignancies: A reappraisal. *Blood* 86:2063, 1995.

395. Junghanss C, Marr KA: Infectious risks and outcomes after stem cell transplantation: Are nonmyeloablative transplants changing the picture? *Curr Opin Infect Dis* 15:347, 2002.

396. Gregory CA, Singh H, Prockop DJ: Dkk-1 is required for re-entry into the cell cycle of human adult stem cells from bone marrow stroma (hMSCs). *J Biol Chem* 278:28067, 2004.

397. Qiang W, Yao I, Tosato G, Rudikoff S: Insulin-like growth factor 1 induces migration and invasion of human multiple myeloma cells. *Blood* 103:301, 2004.

398. Derksen PWB, Tjin E, Meijer HP, et al: Illegitimate WNT signaling promotes proliferation of multiple myeloma cells. *Proc Natl Acad Sci U S A* 101:6122, 2004.

399. Farrugia AN, Atkins GJ, To LB, et al: Receptor activator of nuclear factor-kB ligand expression by human myeloma cells mediates osteoclast formation in vitro and correlates with bone destruction in vivo. *Cancer Research* 63:5438, 2003.

400. Yaccoby S, Wezeman M, Henderson A, et al: Mesenchyman stem cells differentiate into osteogenic cells and inhibit a subset of myeloma in vivo. *Blood* 102:210, 2003.

401. Tricot G, van Rhee F, Barlogie B: Treatment advances in multiple myeloma. *Br J Haematol* 125:26, 2004.

402. Terpos E, Szydlo R, Apperley J, et al: Soluble receptor activator of nuclear factor kB ligand-osteoprotegerin ratio predicts survival in multiple myeloma: Proposal for a novel prognostic index. *Blood* 102:1064, 2003.

403. Greipp PR, San Miguel JF, Avet-Loiseau H, et al: Development of an international prognostic index (IPI) for myeloma: Report of the international myeloma working group. *Hematol J* 4:S42, 2003

404. Dispenzieri A, Kyle R, Lacy M, et al: Superior survival in primary systemic amyloidosis patients undergoing peripheral blood stem cell transplantation: A case-control study. *Blood* 103:3960, 2004.

405. Morris C, Siegel E, Barlogie B, et al: Mobilization of CD34+ cells in elderly patients (>70 years) with multiple myeloma: Influence of age, prior therapy, platelet count, and mobilization regimen. *Br J Haematol* 120:413,2003.

THE AMYLOIDOSES

DANIEL R. JACOBSON
DAVID C. SELDIN
JOEL N. BUXBAUM

The amyloidoses are disorders of secondary structure in which a soluble protein secreted from a cell forms insoluble, fibrillar tissue deposits, leading to organ dysfunction. The site and rate of deposition determine the clinical presentation. All amyloid deposits contain a single major fibrillar component and minor nonfibrillar components. To date, 24 different fibril proteins have been isolated from different forms of human amyloidosis; one is immunoglobulin light chain. Light-chain amyloidosis (AL) is caused by a monoclonal plasma cell disorder in which the secreted immunoglobulin, either because of its amino acid sequence or some other structural feature, is predisposed to fibrillogenesis under physiologic conditions. AL is characterized by fatigue, weight loss, purpura, heart failure, proteinuria, renal failure, gastrointestinal dysfunction, neuropathy, and various other symptoms, depending upon the organ(s) involved. Diagnosis of amyloidosis (of any type) is made by biopsy of an affected organ or subcutaneous fat aspiration followed by Congo red staining. In the face of similar clinical features, distinguishing AL from the other systemic amyloidoses, in which AL-specific treatment would be inappropriate, is critical. Chemotherapy reduces the size of the plasma cell clone producing the amyloidogenic light chain and prolongs survival.

SYSTEMIC AMYLOIDOSES

DEFINITION AND HISTORY

The systemic amyloidoses are characterized by the extracellular accumulation of insoluble protein fibrils. Deposits were first identified in autopsy specimens by their homogeneous, eosinophilic appearance in conventional histologic sections stained with hematoxylin and eosin. Subsequently they were shown to bind metachromatic dyes and the dye Congo red, with a characteristic apple-green birefringence when the stained tissues were examined under polarized light. Electron microscopy and x-ray diffraction revealed a fibrillar ultrastructure,

with extensive β-pleated sheet secondary structure. All the amyloidoses possess these staining and ultrastructural properties.

Historically, the amyloidoses were classified according to the clinical or pathologic features of the associated diseases. Secondary amyloidosis accompanied chronic inflammatory processes. Familial amyloidosis was recognized by distinctive clinical manifestations within kindreds. All other types, except the type occurring in association with myeloma, were termed *primary*, in the sense that they were idiopathic. The development of methods for dissolving and fractionating amyloid fibrils extracted from tissues permitted the identification of 24 different proteins as amyloid precursors to date (Table 101-1). Classification now is based on the chemical nature of the fibrillar component of the deposits. Terms such as *primary*, *secondary*, *senile*, *dialysis-associated*, and *myeloma-associated* have been abandoned in favor of the etiologically based, chemical terminology.[1]

All amyloid deposits contain a major (85–95%) fibrillar component, which is soluble in water and buffers of low ionic strength, and nonfibrillar components that are extractable with conventional ionic strength buffers. The nonfibrillar components include the "P" (pentagonal) component, apolipoprotein E, and the heparan sulfate proteoglycan perlecan, which are found in all types of amyloid. Complement components, proteases, and membrane constituents have been demonstrated in some, but not all, tissue deposits. P component composes 5 to 10 percent of the total deposited protein. It is derived from circulating serum amyloid P (SAP) component, which behaves as a typical acute-phase reactant in mice but not in humans. P component has structural homology to C-reactive protein and belongs to the pentraxin group of proteins.[2]

LIGHT-CHAIN AMYLOIDOSIS

RELATIONSHIP TO OTHER PLASMA CELL DYSCRASIAS

Light-chain amyloidosis (AL) is caused by a monoclonal plasma cell disorder. It is related to myeloma (see Chap. 100) and to essential monoclonal gammopathy (see Chap. 99). These disorders can be categorized by the total body burden of monoclonal plasma cells. When the clone is large, diagnostic criteria for myeloma are fulfilled. When the clone is small, with little or no evidence of clinical disease, the diagnosis is essential monoclonal gammopathy. In most patients with a monoclonal plasma cell disorder, whether myeloma or essential monoclonal gammopathy, the secreted monoclonal immunoglobulin (Ig) remains soluble in body fluids. In other cases, the physicochemical characteristics of the Ig light (L) chains or L-chain fragments lead to its deposition as amyloid. From 10 to 20 percent of AL patients fulfill diagnostic criteria for myeloma; the other patients, in effect, have essential monoclonal gammopathy in which the clonal Ig product is amyloidogenic. AL without myeloma previously was called *primary systemic amyloidosis*, a term that should be abandoned in favor of the modern name, which applies whether or not the patient has myeloma. From 10 to 20 percent of myeloma patients develop clinical evidence of AL,[3,4] although additional patients have subclinical deposition. Investigation for AL in the subcutaneous fat, marrow, or involved organs revealed subclinical amyloidosis in 38 percent of newly diagnosed myeloma patients.[5]

In addition to monoclonal gammopathies in which the secreted Ig is found only in the serum and/or urine and those in which tissue amyloid is present, monoclonal protein accumulation in various organs without formation of fibrils occurs. Patients with this condition have nonamyloid monoclonal immunoglobulin deposition disease (MIDD).[6–8] The Ig deposits do not bind Congo red, do not contain P component or other components of amyloid fibrils, and, unlike amyloid deposits, do not possess a fibrillar ultrastructure. The kidneys and heart are the most frequent sites for MIDD.[7] The pathologic diagnosis

TABLE 101-1   MODERN (CHEMICAL) CLASSIFICATION OF HUMAN AMYLOIDOSIS

AMYLOID PROTEIN	PRECURSOR PROTEIN	CLINICAL SYNDROME(S)
AL	Immunoglobulin light chains or light-chain fragments	Plasma cell disorders
AH[26,28,35]	Immunoglobulin heavy chain	Systemic amyloidosis
ATTR[121,125,201–203]	Transthyretin (TTR)	Familial amyloidotic polyneuropathy, familial amyloid cardiomyopathy, senile systemic amyloidosis, isolated vitreous amyloidosis
AA[204,205]	Apo-SAA	Inflammation-associated, acquired or inherited (tumor necrosis factor receptor-associated periodic syndrome [TRAPS], familial Mediterranean fever)
$A\beta_2M$[152,153]	β_2-microglobulin	Dialysis-associated amyloid
AApoAI[157]	Apolipoprotein AI	Familial amyloidosis involving various organs
AApoAII[157]	Apolipoprotein AII	Familial renal amyloidosis
AFib[157]	Fibrinogen α-chain	Familial renal amyloidosis
ALys[157]	Lysozyme	Familial systemic amyloidosis
ACys[158]	Cystatin C	Hereditary cerebral hemorrhage with amyloidosis, Icelandic type
$A\beta$[158]	β-protein precursor	Alzheimer disease; Down syndrome; hereditary cerebral hemorrhage with amyloidosis, Dutch type
APrP[158]	Prion protein	Creutzfeldt-Jakob disease, Gerstmann-Sträussler-Scheinker disease
AGel[163]	Gelsolin	Hereditary corneal amyloidosis
AKer[163]	Keratoepithelin	Hereditary corneal amyloidosis
ALac[163]	Lactoferrin	Hereditary corneal amyloidosis
ACal[160]	Calcitonin	Medullary carcinoma of the thyroid (in multiple endocrine neoplasia)
AIAPP[206]	Amylin (islet amyloid polypeptide)	Insulinoma, type II diabetes mellitus
AANF[159]	Atrial natriuretic factor	Isolated atrial amyloidosis
APro[162]	Prolactin	Pituitary amyloid
ACytokeratin[167]	Keratin	Cutaneous amyloidosis
Abri/ADan[158]	Bri/Dan	Familial British and Danish dementia
AIns[166]	Insulin	Iatrogenic
AMed[164]	Lactadherin	Senile aortic
APin[165]	To be named	Pindborg tumor-associated protein

of nonamyloid MIDD depends upon the identification of non-Congophilic Ig deposits in tissues via immunohistochemistry, using specific anti-H and anti-L sera, and the presence of the characteristic ultrastructural appearance.[6–8] MIDD is probably underdiagnosed because appropriate immunohistochemical staining is not routinely performed.

ETIOLOGY AND PATHOGENESIS

MECHANISMS OF AMYLOID FORMATION

The amyloid precursor proteins are relatively small, with molecular weights between 4000 and 25,000. They do not share any detectable amino acid sequence homology, although the secondary structures of many of the proteins have substantial β-pleated sheet structure. The known exceptions include serum amyloid A (SAA) and PrP^c, which contain little or no β-folding in the precursor despite extensive β-sheet in the deposited fibrils. The clinical amyloidoses are in vivo disorders of secondary protein structure in which the precursor proteins are secreted from the cell in a soluble form, only to become insoluble at some tissue site, ultimately compromising organ function. They represent an extracellular subset of a spectrum of disorders of secondary protein structure. The protein aggregates in the intracellular forms—Parkinson's disease (cytoplasmic) and Huntington's disease (intranuclear)—lack the in vivo amyloid-defining properties.[9,10]

In some cases, the aberrant secondary structure seen in amyloid reflects a hereditary alteration in sequence that predisposes to fibril

formation, as seen in the proteins transthyretin (TTR), lysozyme, fibrinogen, cystatin c, gelsolin, amyloid-β protein precursor (AβPP), and apolipoprotein A1 (ApoA1). In other cases, wild-type molecules are the fibril precursors (TTR, β_2-microglobulin [β_2M], ApoA1). The deposits are primarily extracellular, but fibrillar structures within lysosomes of macrophages and the cisternae of plasma cells in AL marrow have been reported.[11] In the localized forms of amyloidosis, the deposits are close to the site of synthesis of the precursor. In the systemic amyloidoses, the deposits form either locally or at a distance from the precursor-producing cells. AL usually is a systemic disorder, but localized AL may occur in the setting of an apparently confined plasma cell proliferation.

The role of P component and of the other accessory molecules in amyloid deposition is not clear. Although they do not appear to be an absolute requirement for fibril formation, they may stabilize the fibril, protecting it from proteolysis once it is formed, or enhance the transition from prefibril to fibril. In experimental systems, the rate of amyloid deposition is slower in the absence of P component.[12] Intravenously injected purified P component preferentially binds to amyloid deposits. This property has been exploited clinically, using radiolabeled P component, to localize and quantify the total body burden of amyloid.[13,14]

Apolipoprotein E (ApoE) is found in all types of amyloid deposits.[15] One ApoE allele (ApoE4) is strongly associated with Alzheimer disease. ApoE4 has been suggested to also be a risk factor for other forms of amyloidosis, but its association with other amyloidoses is less well supported by the epidemiologic evidence.[16–20] The mechanism of ApoE involvement is not known.

The heparan sulfate proteoglycan perlecan is a basement membrane component intimately associated with all types of tissue amyloid deposits.[21] As with P component and ApoE, its role in amyloidogenesis remains undefined. Compounds known to bind to heparan sulfate proteoglycans, such as anionic sulfonates, decrease fibril deposition in murine models of AA disease and have been suggested as potential therapeutic agents.[22]

In some instances (e.g., uniformly in AA, frequently in AL, and inconsistently, perhaps in a tissue-related manner, in TTR), the amyloid precursors undergo proteolysis, which may enhance the kinetics of folding into a profibrillar structural intermediate. In some of the amyloidoses (e.g., Aβ or AA), a normal proteolytic process may be disturbed, yielding a higher than normal concentration of a profibrillar molecule. Whether tissue deposition is purely physicochemical or depends upon an interaction equivalent to that between ligand and receptor, in which some component of tissue ground substance is the binding target, is not known. When cleavage occurs relative to deposition in cases in which proteolysis is observed also is not known. In AL, Aβ, and amyloidosis related to TTR (ATTR), clinicopathologic and experimental evidence exists for deposition of nonfibrillar, non-Congo Red-binding forms of the same molecules as found in the fibrils.[23–25] Nonfibrillar deposits probably represent a processing or deposition intermediate but could be an alternative form of deposition.

Structure of Immunoglobulin-Related Amyloid Fibrils   Examination by immunofluorescent and immunohistologic techniques and immunogold electron microscopy reveal that tissue AL amyloid deposits contain a single Ig polypeptide chain. In nearly all cases, the deposits consist of monoclonal L chains and/or their derived peptides.[6] Rarely, the deposits contain only H-chain determinants and are classified as heavy-chain amyloidosis (AH) rather than AL.[26–28]

Extraction of L-chain–related amyloid deposits using distilled water or low ionic strength buffers yields fibril subunits composed of L-chain fragments, whole chains, or both. The fragments include the amino-terminus of the light chain and extend into the constant region. Their molecular mass usually is approximately 16,000 Daltons but may be as small as 5000 Daltons.[6] The deposited peptides include constant-region sequences in 90 percent of patients, which enables staining with commercially available anti–L-chain sera specific for constant-region determinants. On the other hand, 10 percent of patients with AL have deposits that lack constant-region sequences and consequently fail to bind either anti-κ or anti-λ antisera. In most cases, the deposits contain complete L chains and L-chain fragments. Complete chains are rarely seen as the sole component of the deposit.[6]

The presence of L-chain fragments as the major component of the deposits suggests a proteolytic origin of the fibril precursor from an intact amyloidogenic L chain, although direct *in vivo* evidence for this hypothesis is lacking. Occasional ultrastructural demonstration of L-chain fibrils within the cisternae of malignant plasma cells or within macrophages supports the role of lysosomal digestion of the precursor to yield fibril.[11] However, such findings also could be explained by phagocytic ingestion of preformed fibrils. One cell culture experiment suggested plasma cell–macrophage interaction in the production of AL fibrils.[29] *In vitro* experiments have shown that lysosomal enzymes can digest L chains to molecules that form fibrils *in vitro*.[30] In other studies, the propensity of a light chain to form amyloid fibrils *in vitro* following protease digestion did not correlate with *in vivo* amyloid formation.[30,31] Marrow cells obtained from all patients with AL synthesize excess L chains, whether or not free L chains are detected in the patients' serum or urine. In some instances, the cells contain L-chain fragments, but the synthetic or degradative origin of the fragments has not been definitively established.[32,33]

In addition to the chemical analysis of deposited AL fibrils, studies of light chains isolated from the serum and/or urine of patients with AL have provided information. In some instances, the fibrils also were available, but in others the L chains were assumed, but not proven, to be identical with the deposited proteins based on the immunohistochemistry. λ AL is approximately two times as prevalent as κ AL,[6,34] even though the normal ratio of λ to κ Igs in the sera of normal adults is 1:2 (see Chap. 77). In contrast, in nonamyloid MIDD, κ chains are the predominant light chain. In instances where H chains were the major amyloid component, chemical analysis revealed that the precursor H chain displayed domain deletions that resulted in polypeptides the size of L chains.[26,35] The heavy chains also were smaller than normal in cases of nonamyloid MIDD containing both H- and L-chain deposition.[36]

Within L-chain classes, not all variable (v) regions have the same fibrillogenic potential. L chains of the $V_{\lambda VI}$ subgroup are the most amyloidogenic. Clonal plasma cell proliferative diseases in which the $V_{\lambda VI}$ gene is expressed almost always are associated with amyloid deposition.[37] Data obtained using molecular probes specific for germline v-region genes suggest that monoclonal L chains of the $V_{\lambda VI}$ class are more likely to be associated with renal disease than with other organ involvement and are less likely to be associated with myeloma.[34] No such pattern has been demonstrated for other germline V genes expressed in amyloid proteins. Among κ V genes, the $V_{\kappa I}$ subgroup is overrepresented among amyloid-forming L chains,[34] whereas some other subclasses appear underrepresented in amyloidosis relative to plasma cell disorders without essential amyloidosis.[6]

Within the v-region families, certain amino acid residues at particular positions in the L-chain sequence seem to render those chains more amyloidogenic. When a combination of such residues is present, the chances that an L chain will be associated with tissue amyloid deposition are increased.[38,39] Other substitutions seem more likely to be associated with the nonfibrillar deposits of MIDD.[40] Another structural feature that appears to predispose to AL deposition is enzymatic glycosylation of the L chain. Whereas 15 percent of human L chains bear sugar residues, almost one third of amyloidogenic L chains are glycosylated.[6] The nature of the contribution of glycosylation to amyloidogenesis is unknown.

DIAGNOSIS

Amyloidosis is diagnosed by demonstration of Congo red–binding material with the characteristic apple-green fluorescence under polarized light in a biopsy specimen. For many years, rectal biopsy was the procedure of choice. Subcutaneous fat aspiration is the first approach to obtaining material for Congo red and immunohistochemical staining.[41–43] The combination of fat aspiration and rectal biopsy identifies 80 to 90 percent of patients later found to have amyloid elsewhere. Other sampling sites include salivary glands, stomach, and marrow (Table 101-2).[44–46] Biopsy of an organ with impaired function, such as kidney or heart, is a high-yield procedure that can help establish the relationship between organ dysfunction and amyloid deposition.

Because the various types of amyloidosis require different approaches to treatment, only determining that a patient has amyloidosis is not adequate. Evidence of clonality of bone marrow plasma cells and/or monoclonal light chains in the serum and/or urine supports the diagnosis of AL. On the other hand, the clinical pictures of different types of amyloidosis often are similar, and distinguishing between AL and other types of amyloidosis may be impossible clinically. In particular, the distinction between AL and cardiac ATTR solely based on clinical features is particularly difficult, because patient age, the pattern of organ involvement, and the consequences of deposition often are similar. For instance, in individuals older than 70 years, a group in which serum monoclonal Ig protein (M-proteins) is common, the most prevalent form of cardiac amyloidosis is TTR derived. Furthermore, AL, TTR, and $\beta_2 M$ amyloidoses all can present as carpal tunnel syndrome or gastrointestinal amyloidosis, but each has a different etiology and requires a different treatment. Thus, the "gold standard" for diagnosis of amyloid type is immunohistochemistry or immunoelectron microscopy of a biopsy specimen using antibodies against the major amyloid fibril precursors.

When cardiac amyloidosis is suspected because of the results of noninvasive cardiac testing, the definitive distinction between AL and ATTR can be made by endomyocardial biopsy, with Congo red staining and immunohistochemical staining of the tissue sample. In a patient with congestive heart failure and noninvasive testing suggestive of amyloidosis, subcutaneous fat aspiration can provide material for definitive diagnosis, avoiding the more invasive endomyocardial biopsy. Without immunohistologic identification of the deposited protein, an incorrect presumptive diagnosis of AL can lead to ineffective and harmful treatment. A technical caveat is that immunohistochemical staining for AL is less robust than staining for other amyloid types so that, in some cases, AL appears not to stain with any specific antiamyloid antibodies. In this setting, the experience of the pathologist in diagnosing amyloidosis is paramount. When immunohistochemistry is not diagnostic, supplementation with biochemical studies of amyloid extracted from tissues can help identify the deposited protein.[47]

TABLE 101-2 BIOPSY DIAGNOSIS OF AMYLOIDOSIS

SITE	SENSITIVITY (%)	ADVANTAGES	DISADVANTAGES
Subcutaneous fat	80–90	No mortality, little morbidity	Insensitive in β_2M and A amyloid associated with familial Mediterranean fever
Rectal mucosa	75–85	Routine processing	Occasional complication (bleeding); must include vessels
Bone marrow	30–40 in AL[46,109]	Can be assessed at same time as presence of multiple myeloma	Not reliable in other than light-chain amyloidosis
Gingiva	15–20	Easily accessible	Insensitive
Stomach	75–85	High sensitivity in single center[44]	Requires endoscopy; sensitivity needs confirmation in other centers
Salivary gland	75	High sensitivity in single center[45]	Needs confirmation in other centers and in broader spectrum of amyloidoses
Involved organ (liver, kidney, lung, heart)	90–100	High sensitivity, high specificity: allows definitive attribution of clinical features to amyloid deposition[52]	Occasional serious complications

CLINICAL FEATURES

GENERAL CLINICAL FEATURES

AL is the most common form of systemic amyloidosis in the United States. In Olmstead County, Minnesota, AL prevalence is approximately one case per 100,000 people.[4] Whether this estimate, which was obtained in a relatively homogeneous northern European-derived population, applies to other ethnic groups is not known.

The clinical picture of patients with AL varies widely. In one large series of AL patients, the median age at diagnosis was 64 years.[4] The most common presenting symptoms are weakness and weight loss, followed by purpura, particularly in loose facial tissue. Prognosis depends upon the pattern of tissue deposition. The kidney is the most frequent site of AL deposits; the heart, peripheral nerves, gastrointestinal tract, and liver also are affected. Any organ can be involved, with symptoms and physical findings reflecting the extent of anatomic compromise. Patients with clinical cardiac involvement have the worst prognosis, whereas patients with signs and symptoms limited to peripheral nerves have the longest survival.[48] Other favorable prognostic features include a low number of clonal plasma cells in the marrow and normal renal function.[49,50]

Initial physical findings include peripheral edema, hepatomegaly, purpura, orthostatic hypotension, peripheral neuropathy, carpal tunnel syndrome, and macroglossia.[4,51,52] Peripheral edema and hypotension may be related to congestive heart failure and/or the nephrotic syndrome. Purpura results from vascular fragility produced by amyloid deposition in the subendothelium of the small blood vessels and may be very prominent in patients with coagulopathy.[53,54] Macroglossia has been less common at the time of initial presentation in later series than in older studies, perhaps because of earlier diagnosis.[4] Occurrence of macroglossia strongly suggests the amyloid is of the AL type because macroglossia has been seen only in AL and occasionally in β_2M amyloid.[55]

The factors leading to the pattern of tissue deposition in a given patient are not known. Amyloid in a particular organ leads to similar clinical consequences regardless of the chemical type. For example, cardiac AL and cardiac TTR amyloidosis produce similar symptoms and findings on electrocardiography and echocardiography, although AL cardiomyopathy typically runs a much more rapid clinical course.[56,57] In a large series from one large amyloidosis referral center,

the median survival following diagnosis of AL was just over 1 year, with fewer than 5 percent of patients surviving 10 years.[58] Patients with cardiac presentation have a median survival of approximately 6 months.[4,48] Renal and cardiac involvement were the most common causes of death before aggressive dialysis was used in patients with renal amyloid; now cardiac deaths predominate.

RENAL INVOLVEMENT

The most common renal manifestation of AL disease is proteinuria. From 30 to 50 percent of AL patients excrete at least 1 g/day of predominantly non–L-chain protein in the urine.[4,51,59] AL also can cause hematuria. Azotemia is a late manifestation of renal AL, but dialysis can stabilize the course of extensive kidney involvement and is an option in patients who develop renal failure.[60] Renal biopsy reveals deposits in the glomerular mesangium and later along the basement membrane. Nonamyloid Ig deposits also are detected by immunohistochemical staining.[7]

CARDIOVASCULAR INVOLVEMENT

AL deposits in the heart occur in the ventricular interstitium and along the conduction system.[61,62] The amyloid causes diastolic dysfunction, congestive heart failure, and arrhythmias, including heart block, premature ventricular contractions, and various tachyarrhythmias.[4,63,64] Deposits in the coronary arteries, usually the smaller intracardiac arterioles, may cause a clinical picture similar to atherosclerotic coronary artery disease.[62,63,65] Interstitial deposition leads to thickening of the ventricular walls without the increased chamber volume that occurs in heart failure arising from hypertension. Late in the course of the disease, the stiff myocardium can yield cardiac catheterization data similar to constrictive pericarditis. Cardiac involvement eventually occurs in more than 75 percent of patients with AL.[59,66] Death results from cardiac deposition with congestive heart failure or arrhythmias in approximately half of AL patients. The actual number may be higher because some patients have undiagnosed terminal arrhythmias.[4]

No noninvasive test is sufficiently sensitive or specific for diagnosing cardiac amyloidosis in all cases. Electrocardiography often shows a low-voltage QRS complex in the limb leads.[67] In some cases, loss of anterior forces suggests anteroseptal infarction that is not confirmed at autopsy.[68] The most useful diagnostic test for cardiac amyloidosis, other than endomyocardial biopsy, is echocardiography, which reveals increased ventricular wall thickness, increased septal thickness, and the appearance of granular "sparkling." The latter finding is neither sensitive nor specific enough to be diagnostic but is suggestive when present. Evaluation of diastolic function by Doppler echocardiography shows impaired ventricular relaxation early with shortened deceleration times later, ultimately showing a pattern much like that of constrictive pericarditis. The ejection fraction is preserved until late in the disease. Other echocardiographic findings include valvular thickening and insufficiency, atrial enlargement, and rarely atrial thrombosis.[69–71] Scanning with radiolabeled P component (currently available only in Europe) is a sensitive noninvasive means of detecting and monitoring the amount of amyloid in many organs.[13] It is not useful for diagnosing cardiac amyloid because the myocardial signal does not stand out from the background created by the label in the intracardiac blood.[13] The combined use of electrocardiography and echocardiography appears to have the most diagnostic value.[72,73]

AL (and other systemic amyloidoses) can lead to severe orthostatic hypotension with restriction of normal activity and syncope.[4] Poor cardiac contractility resulting from myocardial deposition, autonomic neuropathy secondary to amyloid deposits in the peripheral nerves, and impaired arteriolar responsiveness related to endothelial amyloidosis all may contribute. Diuretic treatment of heart failure or the nephrotic syndrome with reduction of intravascular volume also predisposes to symptomatic hypotension.

NEUROLOGIC INVOLVEMENT

Sensorimotor neuropathy, consequent to deposition in peripheral nerves with axonal degeneration of the small nerve fibers, occurs in approximately 20 percent of AL cases. The symmetric sensory impairment and weakness, sometimes accompanied by painless ulcers, is similar to that of diabetic neuropathy.[4] The lower extremities usually are affected more severely than the upper extremities. Diagnosis can be made by sural nerve biopsy, although the actual deposits may be proximal to the sural nerve and not in the biopsy specimen.[74] Cranial neuropathy or various other unusual neuropathies are seen occasionally.[75,76] Autonomic neuropathy, leading to orthostatic hypotension, diarrhea, or impotence, may be incapacitating.[77] The combination of severe peripheral and autonomic neuropathy is a common presentation of familial ATTR, but the patient's age and family history should facilitate an accurate diagnosis.

CARPAL TUNNEL SYNDROME

Carpal tunnel syndrome was the initial presenting finding in 20 percent of AL patients evaluated in a large referral center.[4] Involvement of the carpal ligament is also seen in β_2M amyloid in patients undergoing dialysis and in TTR amyloidosis, with or without a TTR variant.[78,79] Treatment is surgical. At the time of carpal tunnel release, the tissue specimen can be stained with Congo red and immunohistochemistry performed if a definitive diagnosis was not previously established. Amyloidosis is responsible for only a small fraction of symptomatic individuals undergoing surgery for relief of median nerve compression.

GASTROINTESTINAL INVOLVEMENT

All forms of systemic amyloidosis involve the gastrointestinal tract. Most patients with AL have histologic evidence of infiltration of the gut, particularly in the blood vessels, but the deposition is symptomatic in only a minority of patients.[4] Macroglossia can become severe enough to interfere with swallowing and breathing.[80] Gastric AL can cause hematemesis, nausea, and vomiting.[81] Intestinal AL can impair motility and cause hemorrhage, obstruction, constipation, and diarrhea, or alternating constipation and diarrhea.[82–85] Malabsorption from AL is rare.[4,86] AL autonomic neuropathy also contributes to impaired gastrointestinal motility.

Hepatic AL causing hepatomegaly is common and can be associated with intrahepatic cholestasis and an elevated alkaline phosphatase level (and eventually serum bilirubin), although an elevated hepatocellular transaminase level resulting from cell death is rare even when massive amyloidosis is present.[87] Splenomegaly also may develop and usually is asymptomatic,[88] but functional asplenism can produce Howell-Jolly bodies in the peripheral blood. Spontaneous rupture of a massively infiltrated liver or spleen is a surgical emergency.[4,89,90]

RESPIRATORY TRACT INVOLVEMENT

Systemic AL commonly deposits in the respiratory tract, in a nodular or diffuse pattern. Any part of the respiratory tree, from nasopharynx to pulmonary alveoli, may be involved. Involvement often is asymptomatic, although alveolar or diffuse interstitial involvement can cause dyspnea. Chest radiography reveals a reticular nodular pattern or interstitial infiltration.[91–93] Pleural effusions can occur but usually result from local pleural infiltration with amyloid rather than from heart failure.[94]

MUSCULOSKELETAL SYSTEM

AL deposits in the joints may resemble seronegative rheumatoid arthritis.[95,96] Deposits in the glenohumeral articulation may cause localized pain and swelling ("shoulder pad sign").[97] Deposits in skeletal muscle may produce pseudohypertrophy.[98,99] Congophilic fibrils may be seen in the synovial fluid.

BLEEDING

Bleeding may be a severe manifestation of AL or of any of the systemic amyloidoses. Subendothelial deposition results in capillary fragility and mucocutaneous hemorrhage.[105,106] A deficiency in coagulation factor X, secondary to its binding to AL amyloid fibrils, can produce life-threatening bleeding.[53,54,107] Less often, extensive liver involvement leads to decreased levels of other vitamin K-dependent clotting factors.[54]

LOCALIZED LIGHT-CHAIN AMYLOIDOSIS

Localized amyloid deposits, including amyloid masses termed *amyloidomas*, may be found in various sites even in the absence of systemic disease. In some cases, plasma cells have been demonstrated histologically surrounding the deposits. In one case, DNA sequencing revealed that the local plasma cells were producing the deposited L chains.[100] For unknown reasons, the tracheobronchial tree is the most common site of localized AL; it does not progress to systemic disease.[101] Localized AL deposits involving the urinary tract,[100,102] mediastinum, retroperitoneum, and skin, as either plaques or nodules, can occur.[103,104]

MONOCLONAL IMMUNOGLOBULIN DEPOSITION DISEASE

Patients with MIDD without myeloma usually present with proteinuria or the full nephrotic syndrome with nodular glomerulosclerosis and slowly developing renal failure. Tubular deposits and Bence Jones cast nephropathy are seen when MIDD occurs during the course of myeloma. The histology usually is associated with rapidly developing renal failure.[7] As in AL, cardiac involvement can occur. Despite the differences in the intramyocardial distribution of amyloid and MIDD deposits, the physiologic consequences of alterations in relaxation and compliance, distortions in the voltage/mass relationship, diastolic dysfunction, arrhythmias, and congestive heart failure are similar.[108]

LABORATORY FEATURES

MONOCLONAL IMMUNOGLOBULINS AND MARROW FINDINGS

The cardinal laboratory finding in AL and MIDD—a monoclonal immunoglobulin light chain—is detected on routine protein electrophoresis and immunofixation in the serum or concentrated urine of 80 to 90 percent of patients.[4,51,109] A monoclonal protein likely would be detected in all patients with systemic deposition disease if a sufficiently sensitive assay were available.[110] Measurement of serum free light chains is a new clinical assay that is more sensitive than protein electrophoresis and is useful for monitoring disease progression and response to treatment.[111] The concentration of normal immunoglobulins often is decreased, as in myeloma.[51,112] The combination of hypogammaglobulinemia and proteinuria should suggest a diagnosis of AL or MIDD. In contrast, systemic AA usually is associated with polyclonal hyperglobulinemia related to persistent inflammation and increased interleukin (IL)-6 production.

Approximately 40 percent of patients have more than 10 percent plasma cells in the marrow.[4,113] Light-chain immunophenotyping of the marrow cells, even in the absence of increased numbers of plasma cells, usually reveals the distortion in the ratio of κ to λ, reflecting the L-chain type of the amyloid precursor.[114]

COAGULATION SYSTEM ABNORMALITIES

Many clotting abnormalities have been described in AL. Factor X may bind to amyloid fibrils, leading to its rapid clearance from the blood, with consequent prolongation of the prothrombin and partial thromboplastin times.[53] Elevated levels of tissue and urine plasminogen activators and a decreased level of tissue plasminogen activator inhibitor, leading to hyperfibrinolytic states, have been reported.[115]

DIFFERENTIAL DIAGNOSIS

The differential diagnosis of AL includes MIDD or, if a diagnosis of amyloidosis has already been made, non-Ig forms of systemic amyloidosis. Diagnostic confusion in the evaluation of biopsies can be created by the binding of Congo red to collagen. The nonspecific nature of the binding usually can be clarified by immunohistochemical analysis and electron microscopy. Differentiation of AL from other types of amyloidosis usually is made immunohistochemically, although, immunohistochemistry using available antisera against AL is not always positive, and the definitive diagnosis of AL can be difficult even in the hands of an experienced pathologist.

TRANSTHYRETIN AMYLOIDOSIS

Transthyretin (formerly known as *prealbumin*) is a normal serum protein that transports thyroxine and retinol binding protein. The protein consists of four identical subunits of 127 amino acids and contains considerable β-pleated sheet structure. It is synthesized in the liver, choroid plexus, and retina and is regulated independently in the liver and choroids.[116] Hepatic, but not choroid plexus, synthesis is decreased during inflammation and malnutrition. Accordingly, the serum TTR concentration has been used as an indicator of malnutrition in clinical practice.[124]

ATTR resembles AL in that they both affect the peripheral and autonomic nervous systems, heart, and gastrointestinal tract. Renal disease is thought to be less common in ATTR than in AL, although renal disease is well described[117] in patients with ATTR and the V30M TTR variant.

TTR amyloid occurs in two molecular contexts. *Normal-sequence TTR* commonly forms amyloid deposits in the cardiac ventricles, gastrointestinal tract, carpal ligament, and other organs of elderly people.[68,78,118–122] It can be confused with AL because monoclonal serum or urine proteins may be present coincidentally in such patients. *Variant TTRs*, which contain point mutations, form systemic deposits that usually involve the heart and/or peripheral nerves but usually occur at an earlier age. Familial ATTR is confirmed by demonstrating a variant protein in the serum, by tests such as mass spectrometric peptide mapping, and/or by a variant gene shown by polymerase chain reaction and sequencing or restriction analysis.[123]

TTR's involvement in the pathogenesis of amyloidosis was first noted when a mutant molecule (TTR V30M) was found to be the fibril precursor of the amyloid found in the systemic and peripheral nerve deposits in Portuguese patients with familial amyloidotic polyneuropathy (FAP). FAP is characterized by predominant peripheral and autonomic neuropathy and involvement of the heart, gastrointestinal tract, and vitreous.[125,126] The pattern of organ involvement varies among kindreds. The age of onset varies from the teens to beyond 60 years. In the advanced stage of disease, proteinuria, renal failure, lower cranial nerve involvement, decreased salivation, macroglossia, goiter, and neuropathic knee or ankle damage may occur. In the latter stages

of the disease, if the patient has no positive family history, ATTR is most apt to be confused with AL but can be distinguished by its longer, more indolent clinical course.[56]

Other familial amyloid syndromes with different clinical patterns of involvement (predominant upper or lower extremity neuropathy, varying degrees of involvement of the heart, kidneys, GI tract, and eye) have been reported. Some TTR mutations have characteristic clinical findings, but phenotypic variation is seen even with the same mutation.[125,127] When TTR primarily affects the heart, without significant neuropathy, and a TTR mutation is present, the disease is termed *familial amyloid cardiomyopathy* (FAC). More than 80 amyloid-associated mutations throughout the TTR molecule have been described.[128] TTR V30M FAP, and occasionally FAP arising from other mutations, has been treated with liver transplantation to replace the gene encoding the variant TTR with a wild-type gene. This form of therapy has resulted in some clinical improvement, particularly in patients with autonomic neuropathy.[129]

Isolated ventricular amyloid in elderly people, generally without a family history of amyloidosis, originally was called *senile cardiac amyloidosis* (SCA). Although the deposition originally was thought to be incidental, now the deposits appear to be the cause of death in half the cases.[130] Detailed autopsy studies indicated that many patients with SCA also had deposits in the lungs and blood vessels, so the alternative name *senile systemic amyloidosis* (SSA) was proposed. Ventricular TTR deposition has been found at autopsy in 10 to 25 percent of persons older than 80 years. Functional abnormalities, including atrial fibrillation and congestive heart failure, occur in the absence of any anatomically definable cardiac disease other than the amyloid deposits. The TTR deposits in SCA/SSA have wild-type sequence.[131]

Occasional patients present when they are in their 60s to 80s with severe cardiac ATTR but no known family history. Despite the negative family history, some patients had a TTR mutation; thus, they had FAC and not SCA/SSA.[121,132,133] The most common mutation in this age group is a substitution of Ile for Val at position 122, which is carried by 3 to 4 percent of African Americans.[134] Thus, there are over 1 million gene carriers in the United States, with approximately 150,000 persons older than 60 years at risk for cardiac deposition.[121] Distinguishing these patients from those with cardiac AL based on clinical grounds can be difficult.

AMYLOIDOSIS A

Worldwide, amyloid A (AA) is the most common systemic amyloidosis. The AA protein composes the fibril in the amyloid deposition accompanying chronic inflammatory diseases in various settings: (1) infectious (e.g., leprosy, osteomyelitis, tuberculosis); (2) acquired noninfectious inflammatory (e.g., rheumatoid arthritis, Crohn disease); (3) neoplastic (atrial myxoma, renal carcinomas); and (4) inherited (familial Mediterranean fever [FMF], tumor necrosis factor receptor-associated periodic syndrome [TRAPS], Muckle-Wells syndrome, familial cold urticaria, chronic infantile neurologic cutaneous and articular syndrome).

In emerging nations, AA more likely occurs subsequent to untreated or long-standing infections. In contrast, most patients with AA in the United States and Western Europe have an underlying rheumatic disorder, such as rheumatoid arthritis. Even in association with noninfectious inflammatory disease, the incidence of AA varies considerably among countries with apparently similar levels of economic development, suggesting that factors other than the degree of industrialization play a role.

Approximately 70 percent of patients with AA have renal disease (tubular disorders, nephrotic syndrome, and/or renal insufficiency) at the time of diagnosis.[52,135] Renal vein thrombosis may occur, but whether it occurs more frequently in amyloidosis than in nephrotic syndrome from other causes is unclear.[136] Gastrointestinal involvement, hepatomegaly, and splenomegaly are common. Adrenal deposits can be seen, but clinical adrenal insufficiency is rare. Peripheral neuropathy and clinically significant cardiac involvement are rare. For unclear reasons, subcutaneous fat aspiration generally is not useful in patients with AA associated with FMF.[137]

The precursor molecule apoprotein of serum amyloid A (Apo-SAA) circulates in the serum bound to high-density lipoprotein and behaves as an acute-phase reactant. The concentration of SAA in normal serum is barely detectable but with inflammation may increase by two to three orders of magnitude. SAA is involved in the intracellular metabolism of cholesterol by inflammatory cells. Production of Apo-SAA, but not its tissue deposition, is part of the normal inflammatory response.[138] Three SAA genes, two of which have multiple alleles, encode the expressed isoforms of the protein. An SAA pseudogene also exists.[139] SAA1 is the protein predominantly deposited in human AA disease. SAA1 allele frequencies vary in different ethnic groups. These differences may be responsible for the varied incidences of AA observed during the course of inflammatory diseases, as populations vary in their prevalence of amyloidogenic alleles.[140]

Renal AA has been found in association with some tumors, most commonly renal cell carcinoma, Hodgkin disease, and rarely atrial myxomas.[141,142] The relationship may arise secondary to cytokine production by the tumor or by inflammatory cells responding to the tumor.

Differences in the frequency of AA disease have been seen in different ethnic groups. The autosomal recessive disease FMF (a periodic febrile disorder with features of serositis, arthritis, and skin rashes) is associated with high levels of SAA production.[143] The febrile disease is associated with mutations in the pyrin/marenostrin gene, which is expressed in granulocytes. The normal function of the pyrin/marenostrin protein may be to inhibit the inflammatory response, probably by involvement in neutrophil apoptosis. In Armenian kindreds, the frequency of renal amyloidosis is low, whereas in Sephardic Jews, renal involvement is common by age 30 years and ultimately is fatal.[144,145] The ethnic variation may be related to differences in the mutations in each group, variation in other genes controlling the process of amyloidogenesis, or differences in environmental influences in the various populations.[146] Male gender and homozygosity for the α-allele of SAA 1.1 have now been demonstrated to be associated with greater risk for AA occurrence in the context of the same mutation.[147]

In AA associated with FMF, colchicine prophylaxis reduces the frequency and severity of febrile episodes.[148] Elimination of renal amyloidosis in patients who adhere to the thrice-daily colchicine regimen probably results from reduced inflammation rather than an amyloid-specific effect. Colchicine also inhibits experimental AA formation in murine inflammatory models.[149] Because of these observations, colchicine has been used empirically in patients with AA unrelated to FMF, but evidence for its benefit is largely anecdotal.[150]

AA has been described in association with other hereditary periodic febrile disorders. It occurs in approximately 15 percent of patients with familial Hibernian fever, a disorder caused by mutations in tumor necrosis factor receptor superfamily member 1A (TNFRSF1A). In the autosomal dominant Muckle-Wells syndrome, AA deposition accompanies deafness, urticaria, and febrile episodes in 25 percent of patients. Mutations in the CIAS1 gene, which encodes a protein named cryopyrin, are responsible for Muckle-Wells syndrome, familial cold urticaria, and chronic infantile neurologic cutaneous and articular syndrome, although the latter have a much lower frequency of amyloidosis. In each of these disorders, a periodic overexuberant inflammatory response appears to result in prolonged stimulation of SAA production.[151] Other genes (e.g., particular SAA alleles) likely are, but have not yet been demonstrated to be, responsible for the susceptibility

of patients to amyloid deposition in the context of an inability to terminate or suppress inflammation.[147]

β_2-MICROGLOBULIN AMYLOID

Patients undergoing long-term hemodialysis develop carpal tunnel amyloid consisting of β_2M-derived fibrils.[152,153] This type of amyloid primarily involves synovial membranes and causes trigger finger, bone cysts, and destructive spondyloarthropathy. The heart, gastrointestinal tract, liver, lung, prostate, adrenals, and tongue may be involved. β_2M amyloidosis increases with the duration of hemodialysis. It first appears after approximately 5 years and increases to 20 percent at 10 years, 30 to 50 percent at 15 years, and 80 to 100 percent at 20 years, although improvements in dialysis techniques appear to have reduced the occurrence considerably.[154] Deposits also occur in patients treated with continuous ambulatory peritoneal dialysis and reportedly occur in patients with renal failure who have not undergone dialysis. The characteristic x-ray lesions resemble the lytic bone lesions of myeloma (see Chap. 100). These features usually allow the AL and β_2M amyloidoses to be distinguished clinically. The diagnosis should be confirmed by biopsy demonstration of amyloid staining with anti-β_2M antiserum. Subcutaneous fat aspiration usually is not helpful.[155] Kidney transplantation may arrest amyloid progression in patients who develop this syndrome while they are undergoing dialysis treatment.

β_2M, the light-chain component of the major histocompatibility complex, is both excreted and catabolized by the kidney. In renal failure, β_2M accumulates in the serum. Formerly, the pore size of conventional dialysis membranes did not allow filtration of β_2M. Serum levels may reach 30 to 60 times normal in dialysis patients. The introduction of dialysis membranes with a higher clearance of β_2M and greater attention to the quality of water used to prepare the dialysate seem to have reduced the frequency and the morbidity and mortality from this debilitating complication of dialysis. The pathogenesis appears to be more complicated than simple mass action; however, it may involve activation of macrophages by dialysis membranes, inducing these cells to produce more β_2M with nonenzymatic glycation of the protein. It also may involve activation of macrophages via the receptor for advanced glycation end products.[156]

OTHER FORMS OF AMYLOIDOSIS

HEREDITARY RENAL AMYLOIDOSES

The hereditary renal amyloidoses (amyloidosis ApoAI [AApoAI], ApoAII [AApoAII], amyloidosis fibrinogen α-chain [AFib], amyloidosis lysozyme [ALys]) can resemble AL with renal involvement and should be considered when a renal biopsy shows amyloid deposition.[157] The clinical differentiation between the hereditary renal amyloidoses and AL with a dominant renal presentation often is suggested by the family history and immunoglobulin studies. The definitive diagnosis is made by immunohistologic staining of the biopsy material with antibodies specific for the candidate amyloid precursor proteins.

AMYLOIDOSES LOCALIZED TO THE CENTRAL NERVOUS SYSTEM

Little clinical confusion should exist between AL disease and any of the primarily CNS amyloidoses because AL deposits are rarely found in the central nervous system, although they may be found in the cerebral vessels. The primary CNS amyloidoses include amyloidosis cystatin C (ACys); hereditary cerebral hemorrhage with amyloidosis–Icelandic type, in which the precursor is the protease inhibitor cystatin c; the Aβ amyloidoses, including Dutch-type hereditary cerebral hemorrhage with amyloidosis, Alzheimer disease, and Down syndrome;

amyloidosis PrP (APrP), the prionoses including Creutzfeldt-Jakob disease (CJD), Gerstmann-Sträussler-Scheinker (GSS) disease, fatal familial insomnia (FFI), bovine spongiform encephalopathy, kuru, and scrapie in goats and sheep; and Abri/ADan, familial British/Danish dementia.[158]

OTHER LOCALIZED AMYLOIDOSES

Four polypeptide hormones have been defined as the fibril precursors in tissue-specific localized amyloidoses: AANF in isolated atrial amyloid,[159] ACal in medullary carcinoma of the thyroid,[160] AIAPP seen in the pancreatic islets in association with type II diabetes mellitus,[161] and APro from pituitary adenomas.[162] Three proteins—gelsolin, keratoepithelin, and lactoferrin—have been found in fibrils from patients with autosomal dominant corneal amyloidosis.[163] Medin, an integral fragment of lactadherin, which is produced in aortic smooth muscle cell, forms the amyloid seen in the aorta of all elderly humans.[164] A novel protein, as yet unnamed, has been described in the amyloid associated with Pindborg tumors.[165] Insulin has been found in fibrils at the site of insulin injection.[166] Cytokeratin has been found in amyloidosis localized to the skin.[167]

THERAPY, COURSE, AND PROGNOSIS

Potential treatments of any of the amyloidoses in theory can be directed at interfering with any of several pathogenetic processes. Production of the precursor can be reduced or its catabolism enhanced; generation of the profibrillar intermediate can be blocked; interactions between profibrillar molecules yielding the fibril can be inhibited; deposition can be slowed; or deposits can be actively mobilized. At present, standard treatment of AL involves only one of these strategies, that is, reducing production of the monoclonal Ig precursor via chemotherapy or occasionally via radiotherapy or surgery of a localized amyloidogenic plasmacytoma. Equally important are supportive measures that maintain organ function in the absence of specific treatment or while specific therapy is administered.

CHEMOTHERAPY

The rationale for chemotherapy is that AL, like myeloma, is caused by proliferation of a plasma cell clone; therefore, drugs likely to benefit AL patients are the same as those that are useful for myeloma (see Chap. 100). In the past, assessing the response to therapy in AL was more difficult than in myeloma because most patients have small or absent M components on serum protein electrophoresis and modest elevations of marrow plasma cells. The availability of the new quantitative free light-chain assay provides a sensitive method for assessing treatment responses in AL patients. Other consensus criteria for hematologic and organ response are being developed and will be widely used in future clinical trials. Studies of AL therapy require that all cases have a tissue diagnosis of the type of amyloid (e.g., AL vs. ATTR or the hereditary renal amyloidoses).

STANDARD-DOSE CHEMOTHERAPY

The first effective regimen for myeloma treatment was oral melphalan and prednisone. When this regimen was attempted for treatment of AL, several case reports suggested occasional benefit. In the initial randomized studies of melphalan and prednisone versus placebo or colchicine, several patients demonstrated objective responses to chemotherapy. In one study, a trend toward improved survival was seen with chemotherapy; however, statistical significance was not attained.[168] In a subsequent trial, patients were randomized to one of three arms: (1) melphalan and prednisone; (2) melphalan, prednisone, and colchicine; or (3) colchicine alone.[169] Median survival was greater

in the melphalan-prednisone-colchicine and melphalan-prednisone arms (18 and 17 months, respectively) than in the colchicine alone arm (8.5 months). In a second trial, 100 patients were randomized to receive oral melphalan, prednisone, and colchicine, or colchicine alone.[170] Overall survival in the melphalan-prednisone-colchicine group was 12.2 months compared with 6.7 months in the colchicine alone group. The difference did not reach statistical significance ($P = .087$) because of the small sample size and the early deaths of patients with severe cardiac or renal disease in the two treatment arms. Taken together, these studies demonstrated a survival benefit of melphalan and prednisone compared with placebo in AL. Patients with renal involvement and the nephrotic syndrome are most likely to respond to chemotherapy with objective improvement in end-organ damage. Approximately one fourth of this patient group will experience a decrease in proteinuria of at least 50 percent, with most showing a complete disappearance of proteinuria. Functional improvement can occur in nearly any affected organ but is least common in neuropathy.[48,170]

Other regimens used for myeloma have been explored for treatment of AL. In one study, patients were randomized to melphalan and prednisone or a five-drug regimen consisting of vincristine, carmustine, melphalan, cyclophosphamide, and prednisone. Response rates and survival were not different between the two groups.[171] In a phase II trial, high-dose dexamethasone also produced responses in some AL patients, but survival was not superior to the rate expected from treatment with melphalan and prednisone based on historic controls.[172] For patients who respond to chemotherapy, no data defining the optimal duration of treatment are available. In patients with objective improvement in organ function who do not develop toxicity, some investigators have continued chemotherapy for 1 or 2 years.[48,169] When disease initially responds but then progresses when the patient is taken off treatment, chemotherapy—the same or a different regimen—can be resumed. Little information is available on the usefulness of maintenance therapy, mirroring the situation in myeloma.

Melphalan has considerable leukemogenic potential. The actuarial risk for acute myelogenous leukemia in one study of patients with myeloma treated with melphalan was 17 percent at 50 months.[173] In two other studies, 5 percent of patients developed myelodysplasia (including several with chromosomal abnormalities and/or progression to acute myelogenous leukemia) in 3 years of followup.

HIGH-DOSE CHEMOTHERAPY

To improve survival in myeloma patients, studies of "high-dose" chemotherapy followed by autologous marrow or blood stem cell rescue were undertaken. After several phase II trials of high-dose therapy demonstrated favorable response and survival rates in selected patients, two large multicenter randomized phase III trials were undertaken. These trials demonstrated survival benefits for patients treated with high-dose melphalan chemotherapy and autologous stem cell transplantation compared with standard-dose chemotherapy.[174,175]

Following upon the success of myeloma treatment, several centers have used high-dose melphalan chemotherapy and autologous stem cell transplantation for treatment of AL. The first case reports in the early 1990s soon were followed by small case series, larger single-center trials, and the first multicenter trial. The toxicity of transplantation is different for patients with AL amyloidosis compared to patients with other hematologic diseases. The cardiac, renal, neuropathy, gastrointestinal, and coagulation problems seen in AL patients present unique sets of challenges during all phases of treatment, beginning with stem cell mobilization, reinfusions, and postchemotherapy neutropenia.[176] Peritransplant mortality rates are higher than for patients with other hematologic diseases without organ dysfunction and have varied among centers from 10 percent to as high as 40 percent. Successful treatment appears to depend upon the experience of the treating hematologists and the availability of subspecialty consultants familiar with the organ complications. Various formulas are being developed to identify good- and poor-risk patients. All investigators have found that cardiomyopathy increases risk. Multiorgan involvement is a poor prognostic indicator in some studies,[177] as are age and kidney function. However, other investigators have not found outcome to be highly dependent upon age[178] or kidney function; even hemodialysis patients have undergone successful treatment to prevent the development of other organ failure.[179] Given these evolving criteria for treatment and the complexity of managing these patients during high-dose therapy, patients should continue to be referred to experienced centers for evaluation and treatment in appropriate clinical trials.

Despite these challenges, durable hematologic remission and improved organ function occur at a far higher rate than with oral melphalan and prednisone regimens. In the large single-center trials from Boston University Medical Center and the Mayo Clinic, complete hematologic responses (disappearance of marrow plasma cells and serum monoclonal Ig) reportedly occur in 40 percent of evaluable patients[178] and major improvements in hematologic disease or organ function in 50 percent of patients.[180] An Eastern Cooperative Oncology Group multicenter study achieved similar results.[181] Partial responses were difficult to assess in AL amyloidosis because of the small size of the circulating M component in most patients, but the new free light-chain assay allows quantitative measurement of the pathologic light chain. Early results indicate that 87 percent of 67 patients in whom serial free light-chain measurements were obtained had reductions greater than 50 percent.

These hematologic responses are accompanied by significantly improved organ function[178,180,181] and quality of life[182] and are durable in many patients. In addition, the risk of secondary acute myelogenous leukemia appears to be lower after pulse intravenous chemotherapy (only approximately 1% of patients in the study from Boston University Medical Center[178]) compared with the much higher rates seen after prolonged oral melphalan-containing regimens.[173]

Hematologic and organ responses are more frequent, as is life extension. Median survival of treated patients exceeds 4.5 years.[178] In a case-control study, the survival benefit at 4 years for 63 patients treated with transplant protocols compared to 63 matched patients treated in other ways was a remarkable 75 percent (71% vs. 41%).[183] To confirm these results, a randomized multicenter phase III trial comparing transplant to an optimal nontransplant regimen is needed; however, what the nontransplant arm should be is unclear. The ineffectiveness of melphalan and prednisone makes this regimen ethically difficult to recommend to good-risk, transplant-eligible patients. The myeloma trials used vincristine, adriamycin, and dexamethasone (VAD) or other intravenous regimens, other than melphalan and prednisone, in the control arm. For AL, nontransplant regimens that show some promise include nonmyeloablative intravenous doses of melphalan[184] and oral melphalan combined with high-dose dexamethasone rather than prednisone.[185] As these or other regimens are explored and the durability of responses is determined, a suitable randomized trial will be designed.

NOVEL CHEMOTHERAPEUTIC AGENTS FOR LIGHT-CHAIN AMYLOIDOSIS

Newer agents used for treatment of myeloma, such as thalidomide, CC-5013 (Revlimid), and bortezomib, also may be useful for treatment of AL (see Chap. 100). Thalidomide's proposed mechanisms of action include antiangiogenesis and modulation of the tumor microenvironment. In initial studies, patients with AL who received thalidomide developed more severe side effects than the effects observed in other patient populations, including fluid retention with worsening congestive heart failure, neuropathy, and exacerbation of renal dysfunction,

plus side effects seen in other populations (sedation, constipation, deep venous thrombosis, bradycardia), with a response rate of 25 percent.[186,187] Revlimid, a thalidomide analogue anticipated to have fewer side effects, is now in clinical trials. Bortezomib, a proteosome inhibitor postulated to block nuclear factor-κB activation and thereby promote apoptosis, has activity in myeloma but also has toxicity that might limit its use in AL. Trials with this agent in AL are planned.

THERAPY OF LOCALIZED LIGHT-CHAIN AMYLOIDOSIS

Treatment of localized AL (most often in the tracheobronchial tree,[101] lungs,[92] or genitourinary tract[102]) has not been systematically studied. Because progression to systemic disease rarely occurs, chemotherapy is not indicated. Localized radiotherapy, aimed at destroying the local collection of plasma cells producing the AL precursor, can be of clinical benefit.[188] In patients with massive macroglossia, surgical resection has not been effective. Relief can sometimes be achieved with laser techniques, although formal studies of efficacy have not been reported.

PHARMACOLOGIC AGENTS DESIGNED TO BREAK DOWN AMYLOID FIBRILS

The antiamyloid activity of 4-iododoxorubicin (Idox), an anthracycline analogue of doxorubicin, was discovered serendipitously when Idox was being studied as a cytotoxic chemotherapeutic agent for treatment of myeloma. One patient with myeloma and AL began excreting a large amount of light chains into the urine and experienced dramatic clinical improvement within days.[189] Subsequently, five of eight patients treated in a pilot trial responded with clinical improvement, which appeared unrelated to any cytotoxic effect on the plasma cell clone. From 1995 to 1997, Idox was given to another 14 patients in a single-institution study and to 28 patients at other institutions on a compassionate basis. Of these 42 patients, 13 had disease responses, and 15 showed stabilized disease. A phase II trial of Idox for AL found activity in a minority of patients.[190] Responses are transient, and disease typically progressed after a period of months. Other small molecules that offer promise for disruption of fibrils in vivo are under development.[191] A strategy that involves dissolving formed fibrils and decreasing the production of fibrillogenic protein ultimately will likely be most successful; thus, the best use of agents such as Idox likely is in conjunction with chemotherapy.

TREATMENT OF NONAMYLOID MONOCLONAL IMMUNOGLOBULIN DEPOSITION DISEASE

As in AL, once the diagnosis of MIDD is established, determination of whether the patient has myeloma (e.g., serum and urine evaluation for monoclonal protein, bone marrow aspiration and biopsy, skeletal survey) should be made. Regimens effective for myeloma and AL should be used to reduce end-organ damage because MIDD is a similar monoclonal plasma cell disorder. However, no published studies have addressed chemotherapeutic treatment of nonamyloid MIDD in a systematic fashion.

SUPPORTIVE MEASURES

CARDIAC INVOLVEMENT

Diuretics are the mainstay of therapy for congestive heart failure resulting from amyloidosis. Hypotension resulting from a low ejection fraction and/or autonomic neuropathy may limit diuretic use but can be treated with the β-adrenergic agent midodrine or with flucortisone, which are effective in some patients. However, if edema is troubling and hypotension is asymptomatic, use of diuretics can be increased. Use of digoxin and calcium channel blockers must be avoided in both

AL and TTR cardiac amyloidosis because these compounds bind to amyloid fibrils and reportedly increase congestive heart failure and produce arrhythmias.[132,192-195] Pacemakers are useful in some patients with symptomatic bradycardia.[196,197] Atrial and ventricular arrhythmias are common as amyloid cardiomyopathy progresses, and patients are at high risk for sudden death. Arrhythmias can be treated medically, with amiodarone as the first drug of choice. Implantable defibrillators can be considered in some patients but are not always efficacious in the setting of a thickened myocardium and diastolic dysfunction. Cardiac transplants have been performed in a small number of AL patients. This therapy may be lifesaving for patients with severe disease but should be followed by aggressive chemotherapy to reduce production of the amyloidogenic light chain; otherwise, amyloid will recur in the transplanted organ.[198-200]

RENAL INVOLVEMENT

Hemodialysis and peritoneal dialysis are indicated in patients with AL and renal failure.[60] Renal transplantation has been used in patients with amyloidosis. Because AL is a systemic disease and hemodialysis is generally effective, renal transplantation is rarely indicated, except perhaps in occasional patients who have shown particularly good responses to chemotherapy, in whom long survival may be expected. In the absence of effective chemotherapy, reaccumulation of amyloid in the transplanted kidney has been reported.

REFERENCES

1. International Nomenclature Committee on Amyloidosis: Part 1. Nomenclature of amyloid fibril proteins. *Amyloid* 6:63, 1999.
2. Emsley J, White HE, O'Hara BP, et al: Structure of pentameric human serum amyloid P component. *Nature* 367:338, 1994.
3. Ivanyi B: Frequency of light chain deposition nephropathy relative to renal amyloidosis and Bence Jones cast nephropathy in a necropsy study of patients with myeloma. *Arch Pathol Lab Med* 114:986, 1990.
4. Kyle RA, Gertz MA: Primary systemic amyloidosis: Clinical and laboratory features in 474 cases. *Semin Hematol* 32:45, 1995.
5. Desikan KR, Dhodapkar MV, Hough A, et al: Incidence and impact of light chain associated (AL) amyloidosis on the prognosis of patients with multiple myeloma treated with autologous transplantation. *Leuk Lymphoma* 27:315, 1997.
6. Buxbaum J: Mechanisms of disease: Monoclonal immunoglobulin deposition. Amyloidosis, light chain deposition disease, and light and heavy chain deposition disease. *Hematol Oncol Clin North Am* 6:323, 1992.
7. Buxbaum J, Gallo G: Nonamyloidotic monoclonal immunoglobulin deposition disease. Light-chain, heavy-chain, and light- and heavy-chain deposition diseases. *Hematol Oncol Clin North Am* 13:1235, 1999.
8. Montseny JJ, Kleinknecht D, Meyrier A, et al: Long-term outcome according to renal histological lesions in 118 patients with monoclonal gammopathies. *Nephrol Dial Transplant* 13:1438, 1998.
9. Conway KA, Harper JD, Lansbury PT: Accelerated in vitro fibril formation by a mutant alpha synuclein linked to early-onset Parkinson's disease. *Nat Med* 4:1318, 1998.
10. Karpuj MV, Garren H, Slunt H, et al: Transglutaminase aggregates Huntington into nonamyloidogenic polymers, and its enzymatic activity increases in Huntington disease brain nuclei. *Proc Natl Acad Sci U S A* 96:7388, 1999.
11. Ishihara T, Takahashi M, Koga M, et al: Amyloid fibril formation in the rough endoplasmic reticulum of plasma cells from a patient with localized Alambda amyloidosis. *Lab Invest* 64:265, 1991.
12. Botto M, Hawkins PN, Bickerstaff MC, et al: Amyloid deposition is delayed in mice with targeted deletion of the serum amyloid P component gene. *Nat Med* 3:855, 1997.
13. Hawkins PN, Cavender JP, Pepys MB: Evaluation of systemic amyloidosis by scintigraphy with ^{125}I-labeled serum amyloid P component. *N Engl J Med* 323:508, 1990.
14. Pepys MB: Amyloid P component and the diagnosis of amyloidosis. *J Intern Med* 232:519, 1992.
15. Gallo G, Wisniewski T, Choi-Miura N-H, et al: Potential role of apolipoprotein-E in fibrillogenesis. *Am J Pathol* 145:526, 1994.
16. Korpela MM, Lehtimaki T, Mustonen JT, Pasternack A: Prevalence of serum apolipoprotein E4 isoprotein is not increased in rheumatoid arthritis patients with amyloidosis: Comment on article by Hasegawa et al. *Arthritis Rheum* 41:1328, 1998.
17. Gejyo F, Suzuki S, Kimura H, et al: Increased risk of dialysis-related amyloidosis in patients with the apolipoprotein E4 allele. *Amyloid* 4:13, 1997.
18. Hasegawa H, Nishi SI, Ito S, et al: High prevalence of serum apolipoprotein E4 isoprotein in rheumatoid arthritis patients with amyloidosis. *Arthritis Rheum* 39:1728, 1998.
19. Kindy MS, deBeer FC, Markesbery WR, et al: Apolipoprotein E genotypes in AA and AL amyloidoses. *Amyloid* 2:159, 1995.
20. Lovat LB, Booth SE, Booth DR, et al: Apolipoprotein E4 genotype is not a risk factor for systemic AA amyloidosis or familial amyloid polyneuropathy. *Amyloid* 2:163, 1995.
21. Kisilevsky R, Fraser P: Proteoglycans and amyloid fibrillogenesis, in *The Nature and Origin of Amyloid Fibrils*, edited by GR Bock, JA Goode, p 58. John Wiley & Sons, Chichester, 1996.
22. Kisilevsky R, Lemieux LJ, Fraser PE, et al: Arresting amyloidosis in vivo using small molecule anionic sulphonates or sulphates: Implications for Alzheimer's disease. *Nat Med* 1:143, 1995.
23. Teng MH, Yin JY, Vidal R, et al: Amyloid and nonfibrillar deposits in mice transgenic for wild-type human transthyretin: A possible model for senile systemic amyloidosis. *Lab Invest* 81:385, 2001.
24. Gallo G, Picken M, Buxbaum J: Deposits in monoclonal immunoglobulin deposition disease lack amyloid P-component. *Mod Pathol* 1:453, 1988.
25. Tagliavini F, Ghiso J, Timmers W, et al: Coexistence of Alzheimer's amyloid precursor protein and amyloid protein in cerebral vessel walls. *Lab Invest* 62:761, 1990.
26. Eulitz M, Weiss D, Solomon A: Immunoglobulin heavy-chain-associated amyloidosis. *Proc Natl Acad Sci U S A* 87:6542, 1990.
27. Solomon A, Weiss DT, Murphy C: Primary amyloidosis associated with a novel heavy-chain fragment (AH amyloidosis). *Am J Hematol* 45:171, 1994.
28. Copeland JN, Kouides PA, Grieff M, Nadasdy T: Metachronous development of nonamyloidogenic lambda night chain deposition disease and IgG heavy chain amyloidosis in the same patient. *Am J Surg Pathol* 27:1477, 2003.
29. Durie B, Persky B, Soehnlen BJ, et al: Amyloid production in human myeloma stem-cell culture with morphologic evidence of amyloid secretion by associated macrophages. *N Engl J Med* 307:1689, 1982.
30. Epstein WV, Tan M, Wood IS: Formation of "amyloid" fibrils in vitro by action of human kidney lysosomal enzymes on Bence Jones proteins. *J Lab Clin Med* 84:107, 1974.
31. Linke RP, Zucker-Franklin D, Franklin EC: Morphologic, chemical, and immunologic studies of amyloid-like fibrils formed from Bence Jones proteins by proteolysis. *J Immunol* 111:10, 1973.
32. Buxbaum JN, Hurley ME, Chuba JV, Spiro T: Amyloidosis of the AL type. Clinical, morphologic, and biochemical aspects of the response to therapy with alkylating agents and prednisone. *Am J Med* 67:867, 1979.
33. Picken M, Gallo GR, Buxbaum JN, Frangione B: Characterization of renal amyloid derived from the variable region of the lambda light chain subgroup II. *Am J Pathol* 124:82, 1986.
34. Comenzo RL, Wally J, Kica G, et al: Clonal immunoglobulin light chain variable region germline gene use in AL amyloidosis: Association with

dominant amyloid-related organ involvement and survival after stem cell transplantation. *Br J Haematol* 106:744, 1999.

35. Tan SY, Murdoch IE, Sullivan TJ, et al: Primary localized orbital amyloidosis composed of the immunoglobulin gamma heavy chain CH3 domain. *Clin Sci* 87:487, 1994.

36. Moulin B, Deret S, Mariette X, et al: Nodular glomerulosclerosis with deposition of monoclonal immunoglobulin heavy chains lacking CH1. *J Am Soc Nephrol* 10:519, 1998.

37. Solomon A, Frangione B, Franklin EC: Bence Jones proteins and light chains of immunoglobulins. Preferential association of the V lambda VI subgroup of human light chains with amyloidosis AL (lambda). *J Clin Invest* 70:453, 1982.

38. Hurle MR, Helms LR, Li L, et al: A role for destabilizing amino acid replacements in light chain amyloidosis. *Proc Natl Acad Sci U S A* 91: 5446, 1994.

39. Raffen R, Dieckman LJ, Szpunar M, et al: Physicochemical consequences of amino acid variations that contribute to fibril formation by immunoglobulin light chains. *Protein Sci* 8:509, 1999.

40. Gallo G, Goni F, Boctor F, et al: Light chain cardiomyopathy: Structural analysis of the light chain tissue deposits. *Am J Pathol* 148:1397, 1996.

41. Kaplan B, Vidal R, Kumar A, et al: Immunochemical microanalysis of amyloid proteins in fine-needle aspirates of abdominal fat. *Am J Clin Pathol* 112:403, 1999.

42. Gertz MA, Li CY, Shirahama T, Kyle RA: Utility of subcutaneous fat aspiration for the diagnosis of systemic amyloidosis (immunoglobulin light chain). *Arch Intern Med* 148:929, 1988.

43. Ansari-Lari MA, Ali SZ: Fine-needle aspiration of abdominal fat pad for amyloid detection: A clinically useful test? *Diagn Cytopathol* 30: 178, 2004.

44. Yamada M, Hatakeyama S, Tsukagoshi H: Gastrointestinal amyloid deposition in AL (primary or myeloma associated) and AA (secondary) amyloidosis. Diagnostic value of gastric biopsy. *Hum Pathol* 16:1206, 1985.

45. Dupond J, De Wazieres B, Saile R, et al: Systemic amyloidosis in the elderly: Diagnostic value of the test of subcutaneous abdominal fat and the labial salivary glands. Prospective study in 100 aged patients. *Rev Med Interne* 16:314, 1995.

46. Gertz MA, Lacy MQ, Dispenzieri A: Amyloidosis: Recognition, confirmation, prognosis, and therapy. *Mayo Clin Proc* 74:490, 1999.

47. Kaplan B, Martin BM, Livneh A, et al: Biochemical subtyping of amyloid in formalin-fixed tissue samples confirms and supplements immunohistologic data. *Am J Clin Pathol* 121:794, 2004.

48. Gertz MA, Kyle RA, Greipp PR: Response rates and survival in primary systemic amyloidosis. *Blood* 77:257, 1991.

49. Perfetti V, Colli Vignarelli M, Anesi E, et al: The degrees of plasma cell clonality and marrow infiltration adversely influence the prognosis of AL amyloidosis patients. *Haematologica* 84:218, 1999.

50. Kyle RA, Gertz MA, Greipp PR, et al: Long-term survival (10 years or more) in 30 patients with primary amyloidosis. *Blood* 93:1062, 1999.

51. Pruzanski W, Katz A: Clinical and laboratory findings in primary generalized and multiple-myeloma-related amyloidosis. *Can Med Assoc J* 114:906, 1976.

52. Browning MJ, Banks RA, Tribe CR, et al: Ten years' experience of an amyloid clinic—A clinicopathological survey. *Q J Med* 54:213, 1985.

53. Lucas FV, Fishleder AJ, Becker RC, et al: Acquired factor X deficiency in systemic amyloidosis. *Cleve Clin J Med* 54:399, 1987.

54. Gertz MA, Kyle RA: Hepatic amyloidosis (primary [AL], immunoglobulin light chain): The natural history in 80 patients. *Am J Med* 85:73, 1988.

55. Matsuo K, Nakamoto M, Yasunaga C, et al: Dialysis-related amyloidosis of the tongue in long-term hemodialysis patients. *Kidney Int* 52:832, 1997.

56. Olson LJ, Gertz MA, Edwards WD, et al: Senile cardiac amyloidosis with myocardial dysfunction. Diagnosis by endomyocardial biopsy and immunohistochemistry. *N Engl J Med* 317:738, 1987.

57. Moyssakis I, Triposkiadis F, Rallidis L, et al: Echocardiographic features of primary, secondary and familial amyloidosis. *Eur J Clin Invest* 29:484, 1999.

58. Gertz MA, Lacy MQ, Dispenzieri A: Therapy for immunoglobulin light chain amyloidosis: The new and the old. *Blood Rev* 18:17, 2004.

59. Cohen AS: Amyloidosis. *N Engl J Med* 277:522, 574, 1967.

60. Gertz MA, Kyle RA, O'Fallon WM: Dialysis support of patients with primary systemic amyloidosis. *Arch Intern Med* 152:2245, 1992.

61. Ridolfi RL, Bulkley BH, Hutchins GM: The conduction system in cardiac amyloidosis: Clinical and pathologic features of 23 patients. *Am J Med* 62:677, 1977.

62. Arbustini E, Merlini G, Gavazzi A, et al: Cardiac immunocyte-derived (AL) amyloidosis: An endomyocardial biopsy study in 11 patients. *Am Heart J* 130:528, 1995.

63. Roberts WC, Waller BF: Cardiac amyloidosis causing cardiac dysfunction: Analysis of 54 necropsy patients. *Am J Cardiol* 52:137, 1983.

64. Falk RH, Rubinow A, Cohen AS: Cardiac arrhythmias in systemic amyloidosis: Correlation with echocardiographic abnormalities. *J Am Coll Cardiol* 3:107, 1984.

65. Smith RRL, Hutchins GM: Ischemic heart disease secondary to amyloidosis of intramyocardial arteries. *Am J Cardiol* 44:413, 1979.

66. Kyle RA, Gertz MA: Cardiac amyloidosis. *Int J Cardiol* 28:139, 1990.

67. Carroll JD, Gaasch WH, McAdam KPWJ: Amyloid cardiomyopathy: Characterization by a distinctive voltage/mass relationship. *Am J Cardiol* 49:9, 1982.

68. Smith TJ, Kyle RA, Lie JT: Clinical significance of histopathologic patterns of cardiac amyloidosis. *Mayo Clin Proc* 59:547, 1984.

69. Klein AL, Hatle LK, Taliercio CP, et al: Prognostic significance of Doppler measures of diastolic function in cardiac amyloidosis: A Doppler echocardiography study. *Circulation* 83:808, 1991.

70. Cueto-Garcia L, Tajik AJ, Kyle RA, et al: Serial echocardiographic observations in patients with primary systemic amyloidosis: An introduction to the concept of early (asymptomatic) amyloid infiltration of the heart. *Mayo Clin Proc* 59:589, 1984.

71. Tei C, Dujardin KS, Hodge DO, et al: Doppler index combining systolic and diastolic myocardial performance: Clinical value in cardiac amyloidosis. *J Am Coll Cardiol* 28:658, 1996.

72. Simons M, Isner JM: Assessment of relative sensitivities of noninvasive tests for cardiac amyloidosis in documented cardiac amyloidosis. *Am J Cardiol* 68:425, 1992.

73. Swaram CA, Jugdutt BI, Amy RWM, et al: Cardiac amyloidosis: Combined use of two-dimensional echocardiography and electrocardiography in noninvasive screening before biopsy. *Clin Cardiol* 8:511, 1985.

74. Simmons Z, Blaivas M, Aguilera AJ, et al: Low diagnostic yield of sural nerve biopsy in patients with peripheral neuropathy and primary amyloidosis. *J Neurol Sci* 120:60, 1993.

75. Traynor AE, Gertz MA, Kyle RA: Cranial neuropathy associated with primary amyloidosis. *Ann Neurol* 29:451, 1991.

76. Vucic S, Chong PS, Cros D: Atypical presentations of primary amyloid neuropathy. *Muscle Nerve* 28:696, 2003.

77. Nordborg C, Kristensson K, Olsson Y, Sourander P: Involvement of the autonomic nervous system in primary and secondary amyloidosis. *Acta Neurol Scand* 49:31, 1973.

78. Kyle RA, Gertz MA, Linke RP: Amyloid localized to tenosynovium at carpal tunnel release: Immunohistochemical identification of amyloid type. *Am J Clin Pathol* 97:250, 1992.

79. Murakami T, Tachibana S, Endo Y, et al: Familial carpal tunnel syndrome due to amyloidogenic transthyretin His 114 variant. *Neurology* 44:315, 1994.

80. Reinish EI, Raviv M, Srolovitz H, Gornitsky M: Tongue, primary amyloidosis, and multiple myeloma. *Oral Surg Oral Med Oral Pathol* 77: 121, 1994.

81. Menke DM, Kyle RA, Fleming CR, et al: Symptomatic gastric amyloidosis in patients with primary systemic amyloidosis. *Mayo Clin Proc* 68:763, 1993.

82. Brandt K, Cathcart ES, Cohen AS: A clinical analysis of the course and prognosis of forty-two patients with amyloidosis. *Am J Med* 44:955, 1968.

83. Battle WM, Rubin MR, Cohen S, Snape WJ Jr: Gastrointestinal motility dysfunction in amyloidosis. *N Engl J Med* 301:24, 1979.

84. Rubinow A: Esophageal manometry in systemic amyloidosis. A study of 30 patients. *Am J Med* 75:951, 1983.

85. Brandt K, Cathcart ES, Streiff R, Cohen AS: Amyloidosis of the stomach associated with impaired gastric secretion of intrinsic factor and the development of vitamin B_{12} deficiency. *Isr J Med Sci* 4:1005, 1968.

86. Carlson HC, Breen JF: Amyloidosis and plasma cell dyscrasias: Gastrointestinal involvement. *Semin Roentgenol* 21:128, 1986.

87. Park MA, Mueller PS, Kyle RA, et al: Primary (AL) hepatic amyloidosis: Clinical features and natural history in 98 patients. *Medicine (Baltimore)* 82:291, 2003.

88. Gertz MA, Kyle RA: Hepatic amyloidosis: Clinical appraisal in 77 patients. *Hepatology* 25:118, 1997.

89. Gastineau DA, Gertz MA, Rosen CB, Kyle RA: Computed tomography for diagnosis of hepatic rupture in primary systemic amyloidosis. *Am J Hematol* 37:194, 1991.

90. Ooi LLPJ, Lynch SV, Graham DA, Rong RW: Spontaneous liver rupture in amyloidosis. *Surgery* 120:117, 1996.

91. Talbot AR: Laryngeal amyloidosis. *J Laryngol Otol* 104:147, 1990.

92. Utz JP, Swensen SJ, Gertz MA: Pulmonary amyloidosis. The Mayo Clinic experience from 1980 to 1993. *Ann Intern Med* 124:407, 1996.

93. Hui AN, Koss MN, Hochholzer L, Wehunt WD: Amyloidosis presenting in the lower respiratory tract. Clinicopathologic, radiologic, immunohistochemical, and histochemical studies on 48 cases. *Arch Pathol Lab Med* 110:212, 1986.

94. Berk JL, Keane J, Seldin DC, et al: Persistent pleural effusions in primary systemic amyloidosis: Etiology and prognosis. *Chest* 124:969, 2003.

95. Wiernik PH: Amyloid joint disease. *Medicine (Baltimore)* 51:465, 1972.

96. Duna GF, Cash JM: Rheumatic manifestations of dysproteinemias and lymphoproliferative disorders. *Rheum Dis Clin North Am* 22:39, 1996.

97. Katz GA, Peter JB, Pearson CM, Adams WS: The shoulder-pad sign—A diagnostic feature of amyloid arthropathy. *N Engl J Med* 288:354, 1973.

98. Yamada M, Tsukagoshi H, Hatakeyama S: Skeletal muscle amyloid deposition in AL-(primary or myeloma-associated), AA-(secondary), and prealbumin-type amyloidosis. *J Neurol Sci* 85:223, 1988.

99. Santiago RM, Scharnhorst D, Ratkin G, Crouch EC: Respiratory muscle weakness and ventilatory failure in AL amyloidosis with muscular pseudohypertrophy. *Am J Med* 83:175, 1987.

100. Yood RA, Skinner M, Rubinow A, et al: Bleeding manifestations in 100 patients with amyloidosis. *JAMA* 249:1322, 1983.

101. Rapoport M, Yona R, Kaufman S, et al: Unusual bleeding manifestations of amyloidosis in patients with multiple myeloma. *Clin Lab Haematol* 16:349, 1994.

102. Furie B, Voo L, McAdam KP, Furie BC: Mechanism of factor X deficiency in systemic amyloidosis. *N Engl J Med* 304:827, 1981.

103. Hamidi Asl K, Liepnieks JJ, Nakamura M, Benson MD: Organ-specific (localized) synthesis of Ig light chain amyloid. *J Immunol* 162:5556, 1999.

104. O'Regan A, Fenlon HM, Beamis JFJ, et al: Tracheobronchial amyloidosis. The Boston University experience from 1984 to 1999. *Medicine (Baltimore)* 79:69, 2000.

105. Tirzaman O, Wahner-Roedler DL, Malek RS, et al: Primary localized amyloidosis of the urinary bladder: A case series of 31 patients. *Mayo Clin Proc* 75:1264, 2000.

106. Krishnan J, Chu WS, Elrod JP, Frizzera G: Tumoral presentation of amyloidosis (amyloidomas) in soft tissues. A report of 14 cases. *Am J Clin Pathol* 100:135, 1993.

107. Piette WW: Myeloma, paraproteinemias, and the skin. *Med Clin North Am* 70:155, 1986.

108. Buxbaum JN, Genega EM, Lazowski P, et al: Infiltrative nonamyloidotic monoclonal immunoglobulin light chain cardiomyopathy: An underappreciated manifestation of plasma cell dyscrasias. *Cardiology* 93:220, 2000.

109. Kyle RA, Greipp PR: Amyloidosis (AL). Clinical and laboratory features in 229 cases. *Mayo Clin Proc* 58:665, 1983.

110. Perfetti V, Garini P, Vignarelli MC, et al: Diagnostic approach to and follow-up of difficult cases of AL amyloidosis. *Haematologica* 80:409, 1995.

111. Abraham RS, Katzmann JA, Clark RJ, et al: Quantitative analysis of serum free light chains. A new marker for the diagnostic evaluation of primary systemic amyloidosis. *Am J Clin Pathol* 119:274, 2003.

112. Cathcart ES, Ritchie RF, Cohen AS, Brandt K: Immunoglobulins and amyloidosis. An immunologic study of sixty-two patients with biopsy-proved disease. *Am J Med* 52:93, 1972.

113. Wolf BC, Kumar A, Vera JC, Neiman RS: Bone marrow morphology and immunology in systemic amyloidosis. *Am J Clin Pathol* 86:84, 1986.

114. Swan N, Skinner M, O'Hara CJ: Bone marrow core biopsy specimens in AL (primary) amyloidosis. A morphologic and immunohistochemical study of 100 cases. *Am J Clin Pathol* 120:610, 2003.

115. Sane DC, Pizzo SV, Greenberg CS: Elevated urokinase-type plasminogen activator level and bleeding in amyloidosis: Case report and literature review. *Am J Hematol* 31:53, 1989.

116. Yan C, Costa RH, Darnell JE Jr, et al: Distinct positive and negative elements control the limited hepatocyte and choroid plexus expression of transthyretin in transgenic mice. *EMBO J* 9:869, 1990.

117. Lobato L, Beirao I, Guimaraes SM, et al: Familial amyloid polyneuropathy type I (Portuguese): Distribution and characterization of renal amyloid deposits. *Am J Kidney Dis* 31:940, 1998.

118. Pitkänen P, Westermark P, Cornwell GG III: Senile systemic amyloidosis. *Am J Pathol* 117:391, 1984.

119. Cornwell GG III, Westermark P, Natvig JB, Murdoch W: Senile cardiac amyloid: Evidence that fibrils contain a protein immunologically related to prealbumin. *Immunology* 44:447, 1981.

120. Hodkinson HM, Pomerance A: The clinical significance of senile cardiac amyloidosis: A prospective clinico-pathological study. *Q J Med* XLVI: 381, 1977.

121. Jacobson DR, Pastore RD, Yaghoubian R, et al: Variant-sequence transthyretin (isoleucine 122) in late-onset cardiac amyloidosis in black Americans. *N Engl J Med* 336:466, 1997.

122. Rocken C, Saeger W, Linke RP: Gastrointestinal amyloid deposits in old age. *Path Res Pract* 190:641, 1994.

123. Lim A, Prokaeva T, McComb ME, et al: Characterization of transthyretin variants in familial transthyretin amyloidosis by mass spectrometric peptide mapping and DNA sequence analysis. *Anal Chem* 74:741, 2002.

124. Smith FR, Suskind R, Thanangkul O, et al: Plasma vitamin A, retinol-binding protein and prealbumin concentrations in protein-calorie malnutrition: III. Response to varying dietary treatments. *Am J Clin Nutr* 28:732, 1975.

125. Plante-Bordeneuve V, Lalu T, Misrahi M, et al: Genotypic-phenotypic variations in a series of 65 patients with familial amyloid polyneuropathy. *Neurology* 51:708, 1998.

126. Buxbaum JN, Tagoe C: The genetics of the amyloidoses. *Annu Rev Med* 53:543, 2000.

127. Jacobson DR, Buxbaum JN: Genetic aspects of amyloidosis. *Adv Hum Genet* 20:69, 1991.

128. Connors LH, Lim A, Prokaeva T, et al: Tabulation of human transthyretin (TTR) variants 2003. *Amyloid* 10:160, 2003.

129. Herlenius G, Wilczek HE, Larsson M, Ericzon BG: Ten years of international experience with liver transplantation for familial amyloidotic polyneuropathy: Results from the Familial Amyloidotic Polyneuropathy World Transplant Registry. *Transplantation* 77:64, 2004.

130. Lie JT, Hammond H: Pathology of the senescent heart: Anatomic observations on 237 autopsy studies of patients 90 to 105 years old. *Mayo Clin Proc* 63:552, 1988.

131. Gustavsson Å, Jahr H, Tobiassen R, et al: Amyloid fibril composition and transthyretin gene structure in senile systemic amyloidosis. *Lab Invest* 73:703, 1995.

132. Jacobson DR, Ittmann M, Buxbaum JN, et al: Cardiac amyloidosis resulting from transthyretin Ile 122 deposition in African-Americans: Two case reports. *Tex Heart Inst J* 24:45, 1997.

133. Jacobson DR, Pan T, Kyle RA, Buxbaum JN: Transthyretin Ile20, a new variant associated with late-onset cardiac amyloidosis. *Hum Mutat* 9:83, 1997.

134. Jacobson DR, Pastore R, Pool S, et al: Revised transthyretin Ile 122 allele prevalence in African-Americans. *Hum Genet* 98:236, 1996.

135. Helin HJ, Korpela MM, Mustonen JT, Pasternack AI: Renal biopsy findings and clinicopathologic correlations in rheumatoid arthritis. *Arthritis Rheum* 38:242, 1995.

136. Ekelund L: Radiologic findings in renal amyloidosis. *AJR Am J Roentgenol* 129:851, 1977.

137. Tishler M, Pras M, Yaron M: Abdominal fat tissue aspirate in amyloidosis of familial Mediterranean fever. *Clin Exp Rheumatol* 6:395, 1988.

138. Marhaug G, Dowton SB: Serum amyloid A: An acute phase apolipoprotein and precursor of AA amyloid. *Baillieres Clin Rheumatol* 8:553, 1994.

139. International Nomenclature Committee on Amyloidosis. Part 2. Revised nomenclature for serum amyloid A (SAA). *Amyloid* 6:67, 1999.

140. Booth DR, Booth SE, Gillmore JD: SAA1 alleles as risk factors in reactive systemic AA amyloidosis. *Amyloid* 5:262, 1998.

141. Champion M, Richards RL: Amyloidosis in Hodgkin disease: A Scottish survey. *Scot Med J* 24:9, 1979.

142. Dictor M, Hasserius R: Systemic amyloidosis and nonhematologic malignancy in a large autopsy series. *Acta Pathol Microbiol Scand [A]* 89:411, 1981.

143. Samuels J, Aksentijevich I, Torosyan Y, et al: Familial Mediterranean fever at the millennium; clinical spectrum, ancient mutations and a survey of 100 American referrals to the National Institutes of Health. *Medicine* 77:268, 1998.

144. Pras M, Bronshpigel N, Zemer D, Gafni J: Variable incidence of amyloidosis in familial Mediterranean fever among different ethnic groups. *Johns Hopkins Med J* 150:22, 1982.

145. Schwabe AD, Peters RS: Familial Mediterranean fever in Armenians: Analysis of 100 cases. *Medicine* 53:453, 1974.

146. Livneh A, Langevitz P, Shinar Y, et al: MEFV mutation analysis in patients suffering from amyloidosis of familial Mediterranean fever. *Amyloid* 6:1, 1999.

147. Cazeneuve C, Ajrapetyan H, Papin S, et al: Identification of MEFV-independent modifying genetic factors for familial Mediterranean fever. *Am J Hum Genet* 67:1136, 2000.

148. Zemer D, Pras M, Sohar E, et al: Colchicine in the prevention and treatment of the amyloidosis of familial Mediterranean fever. *N Engl J Med* 314:1001, 1986.

149. Shirahama T, Cohen A: Blockage of amyloid induction by colchicine in an animal model. *J Exp Med* 140:1102, 1999.

150. Kagan A, Husar M, Frumkin A, Rapoport J: Reversal of nephrotic syndrome due to AA amyloidosis in psoriatic patients on long-term colchicine treatment. Case report and review of the literature. *Nephron* 82:348, 1999.

151. Hull KM, Drewe E, Aksentijevich I, et al: The TNF receptor-associated periodic syndrome (TRAPS): Emerging concepts of an autoinflammatory disorder. *Medicine (Baltimore)* 81:349, 2002.

152. Winchester JF, Salsberg JA, Levin NW: Beta-2 microglobulin in ESRD: An in-depth review. *Adv Ren Replace Ther* 10:279, 2003.

153. Gejyo F, Narita I: Current clinical and pathogenetic understanding of beta2-m amyloidosis in long-term haemodialysis patients. *Nephrology (Carlton)* 8(suppl 2):S45, 2003.

154. Jimenez RE, Price DA, Pinkus GS, et al: Development of gastrointestinal beta2-microglobulin amyloidosis correlates with time on dialysis. *Am J Surg Pathol* 22:729, 1998.

155. Varga J, Idelson BA, Felson D, et al: Lack of amyloid in abdominal fat aspirates from patients undergoing longterm hemodialysis. *Arch Intern Med* 147:1455, 1987.

156. Miyata T, Inagi R, Lida Y, et al: Involvement of Beta2 microglobulin with advanced glycation end products in the pathogenesis of hemodialysis-associated amyloidosis. *J Clin Invest* 93:521, 1994.

157. Hawkins PN: Hereditary systemic amyloidosis with renal involvement. *J Nephrol* 16:443, 2003.

158. Revesz T, Ghiso J, Lashley T, et al: Cerebral amyloid angiopathies: A pathologic, biochemical, and genetic view. *J Neuropathol Exp Neurol* 62:885, 2003.

159. Looi LM: Isolated atrial amyloidosis: A clinicopathologic study indicating increased prevalence in chronic heart disease. *Hum Pathol* 24:602, 1993.

160. Saad MF, Ordonez NG, Rashid RK, et al: Medullary carcinoma of the thyroid: A study of the clinical features and prognostic factors in 161 patients. *Medicine* 63:319, 1984.

161. Kahn SE, Andrikopoulos S, Verchere CB: Islet amyloid: A long-recognized but underappreciated pathological feature of type 2 diabetes. *Diabetes* 48:241, 1999.

162. Westermark P, Eriksson L, Engstrom U, et al: Prolactin-derived amyloid in the aging pituitary gland. *Am J Pathol* 150:67, 1997.

163. Klintworth GK: The molecular genetics of the corneal dystrophies—Current status. *Front Biosci* 8:d687, 2003.

164. Haggqvist B, Naslund J, Sletten K, et al: Medin: An integral fragment of aortic smooth muscle cell-produced lactadherin forms the most common human amyloid. *Proc Natl Acad Sci U S A* 96:8669, 1999.

165. Solomon A, Murphy CL, Weaver K, et al: Calcifying epithelial odontogenic (Pindborg) tumor-associated amyloid consists of a novel human protein. *J Lab Clin Med* 142:348, 2003.

166. Storkel S, Schneider HM, Muntefering H, Kashiwagi S: Iatrogenic, insulin-dependent, local amyloidosis. *Lab Invest* 48:108, 1983.

167. Chang YT, Liu HN, Wang WJ, et al: A study of cytokeratin profiles in localized cutaneous amyloids. *Arch Dermatol Res* 296:83, 2004.

168. Kyle RA, Greipp PR, Garton JP, Gertz MA: Primary systemic amyloidosis. Comparison of melphalan/prednisone versus colchicine. *Am J Med* 79:708, 1985.

169. Kyle RA, Gertz MA, Greipp PR, et al: A trial of three regimens for primary amyloidosis: Colchicine alone, melphalan and prednisone, and melphalan, prednisone, and colchicine. *N Engl J Med* 336:1202, 1997.

170. Skinner M, Anderson JJ, Simms R, et al: Treatment of 100 patients with primary amyloidosis: A randomized trial of melphalan, prednisone, and colchicine versus colchicine only. *Am J Med* 100:290, 1996.

171. Gertz MA, Lacy MQ, Lust JA, et al: Prospective randomized trial of melphalan and prednisone versus vincristine, carmustine, melphalan, cyclophosphamide, and prednisone in the treatment of primary systemic amyloidosis. *J Clin Oncol* 17:262, 1999.

172. Gertz MA, Lacy MQ, Lust JA, et al: Phase II trial of high-dose dexamethasone for untreated patients with primary systemic amyloidosis. *Med Oncol* 16:104, 1999.

173. Bergsagel DE, Bailey AJ, Langley GR, et al: The chemotherapy on plasma-cell myeloma and the incidence of acute leukemia. *N Engl J Med* 301:743, 1979.

174. Attal M, Harousseau JL, Stoppa AM, et al: A prospective, randomized trial of autologous bone marrow transplantation and chemotherapy in multiple myeloma. Intergroupe Francais du Myelome. *N Engl J Med* 335:91, 1996.

175. Child JA, Morgan GJ, Davies FE, et al: High-dose chemotherapy with hematopoietic stem-cell rescue for multiple myeloma. *N Engl J Med* 348:1875, 2003.

176. Sanchorawala V, Wright DG, Seldin DC, et al: An overview of the use of high-dose melphalan with autologous stem cell transplantation for the treatment of AL amyloidosis. *Bone Marrow Transplant* 28:637, 2001.

177. Comenzo RL, Gertz MA: Autologous stem cell transplantation for primary systemic amyloidosis. *Blood* 99:4276, 2002.

178. Skinner M, Sanchorawala V, Seldin DC, et al: High-dose melphalan and autologous stem-cell transplantation in patients with AL amyloidosis: An 8-year study. *Ann Intern Med* 140:85, 2004.

179. Casserly LF, Fadia A, Sanchorawala V, et al: High-dose intravenous melphalan with autologous stem cell transplantation in AL amyloidosis-associated end-stage renal disease. *Kidney Int* 63:1051, 2003.

180. Gertz MA, Lacy MQ, Dispenzieri A, et al: Stem cell transplantation for the management of primary systemic amyloidosis. *Am J Med* 113:549, 2002.

181. Gertz MA, Blood E, Vesole DH, et al: A multicenter phase 2 trial of stem cell transplantation for immunoglobulin light-chain amyloidosis (E4A97): An Eastern Cooperative Oncology Group Study. *Bone Marrow Transplant* 34:149, 2004.

182. Seldin DC, Anderson JJ, Sanchorawala V, et al: Improvement in quality of life of patients with AL amyloidosis treated with high dose melphalan and autologous stem cell transplantation. *Blood* 104:1888, 2004.

183. Dispenzieri A, Kyle RA, Lacy MQ, et al: Superior survival in primary systemic amyloidosis patients undergoing peripheral blood stem cell transplant: A case control study. *Blood* 103:3960, 2004.

184. Lachmann HJ, Gallimore R, Gillmore JD, et al: Outcome in systemic AL amyloidosis in relation to changes in concentration of circulating free immunoglobulin light chains following chemotherapy. *Br J Haematol* 122:78, 2003.

185. Palladini G, Perfetti V, Obici L, et al: Association of melphalan and high-dose dexamethasone is effective and well tolerated in patients with AL (primary) amyloidosis who are ineligible for stem cell transplantation. *Blood* 103:2936, 2004.

186. Seldin DC, Choufani EB, Dember LM, et al: Tolerability and efficacy of thalidomide for the treatment of patients with light chain-associated (AL) amyloidosis. *Clin Lymphoma* 3:241, 2003.

187. Dispenzieri A, Lacy MQ, Rajkumar SV, et al: Poor tolerance to high doses of thalidomide in patients with primary systemic amyloidosis. *Amyloid* 10:257, 2003.

188. Monroe AT, Walia R, Zlotecki RA, Jantz MA: Tracheobronchial amyloidosis: A case report of successful treatment with external beam radiation therapy. *Chest* 125:784, 2004.

189. Gianni L, Bellotti V, Gianni A, Merlini G: New drug therapy of amyloidoses: Resorption of AL-type deposits with 4'-iodo-4'-deoxydoxorubicin. *Blood* 86:855, 1995.

190. Gertz MA, Lacy MQ, Dispenzieri A, et al: A multicenter phase II trial of 4'-iodo-4'-deoxydoxorubicin (IDOX) in primary amyloidosis (AL). *Amyloid* 9:24, 2002.

191. De Lorenzi E, Giorgetti S, Grossi S, et al: Pharmaceutical strategies against amyloidosis: Old and new drugs in targeting a "protein misfolding disease." *Curr Med Chem* 11:1065, 2004.

192. Gertz MA, Skinner M, Connors LG, et al: Selective binding of nifedipine to amyloid fibrils. *Am J Cardiol* 55:1646, 1985.

193. Gertz MA, Falk RH, Skinner M, et al: Worsening of congestive heart failure in amyloid heart disease treated by calcium channel-blocking agents. *Am J Cardiol* 55:1845, 1985.

194. Griffiths BE, Hughes P, Dowdle R, Stephens MR: Cardiac amyloidosis with asymmetrical septal hypertrophy and deterioration after nifedipine. *Thorax* 37:711, 1982.

195. Rubinow A, Skinner M, Cohen AS: Digoxin sensitivity in amyloid cardiomyopathy. *Circulation* 63:1285, 1981.

196. Mathew V, Olson LJ, Gertz MA, Hayes DL: Symptomatic conduction system disease in cardiac amyloidosis. *Am J Cardiol* 80:1491, 1997.

197. Mathew V, Chaliki H, Nishimura RA: Atrioventricular sequential pacing in cardiac amyloidosis: An acute Doppler echocardiographic and catheterization hemodynamic study. *Clin Cardiol* 20:723, 1997.

198. Hosenpud JD, DeMarco T, Frazier OH, et al: Progression of systemic disease and reduced long-term survival in patients with cardiac amyloidosis undergoing heart transplantation: Follow-up results of a multicenter survey. *Circulation* 84(suppl 3):III338, 1991.

199. Dubrey S, Simms RW, Skinner M, Falk RH: Recurrence of primary (AL) amyloidosis in a transplanted heart with four-year survival. *Am J Cardiol* 76:739, 1995.

200. Pelosi F Jr, Capehart J, Roberts WC: Effectiveness of cardiac transplantation for primary (AL) cardiac amyloidosis. *Am J Cardiol* 79:532, 1997.

201. Barouch FC, Benson MD, Mukai S: Isolated vitreoretinal amyloidosis in the absence of transthyretin mutations. *Arch Ophthalmol* 122:123, 2004.

202. Saraiva MJ: Hereditary transthyretin amyloidosis: Molecular basis and therapeutical strategies. *Expert Rev Mol Med* 2002:1, 2002.

203. Westermark P, Bergstrom J, Solomon A, et al: Transthyretin-derived senile systemic amyloidosis: Clinicopathologic and structural considerations. *Amyloid* 10(suppl 1):48, 2003.

204. Masson C, Simon V, Hoppe E, et al: Tumor necrosis factor receptor-associated periodic syndrome (TRAPS): Definition, semiology, prognosis, pathogenesis, treatment, and place relative to other periodic joint diseases. *Joint Bone Spine* 71:284, 2004.

205. Aringer M: Periodic fever syndromes—A clinical overview. *Acta Med Austriaca* 31:8, 2004.

206. Clark A, Nilsson MR: Islet amyloid: A complication of islet dysfunction or an aetiological factor in type 2 diabetes? *Diabetologia* 47:157, 2004.

MACROGLOBULINEMIA

THOMAS J. KIPPS

Macroglobulinemia is the term describing a serum immuno-globulin (Ig)M concentration above normal levels. Monoclonal macroglobulinemia can occur without clinical findings and be of no health consequence (essential monoclonal macroglobulin-emia), or it can be the product of cells in several B lympho-plasmacytic or lymphocytic malignancies, the most character-istic of which is Waldenström macroglobulinemia. The latter condition usually occurs after age 60 years. The symptoms and signs are a function of lymphocytic infiltration of marrow lead-ing to cytopenias, especially anemia, infiltration of peripheral tissues leading to lymphadenopathy and hepatosplenomegaly, and consequences of IgM in the circulation and deposited in organs. The former may lead to the hyperviscosity syndrome such that patients lose cognitive function because of inadequate cerebral blood flow. The latter can result in specific organ dysfunction such as renal insufficiency. The disease often is in-dolent, and patients may not require treatment for years. Al-kylating drugs, fludarabine, rituximab, thalidomide, glucocor-ticoids, and other agents may produce remissions in patients with progressive disease, but drug therapy is not curative. In the small proportion of eligible patients younger than 50 years, allogeneic stem cell transplantation can be considered. In un-usual circumstances, monoclonal IgM can be associated with a clinical picture closer in phenotype to myeloma (IgM myeloma) or extramedullary plasmacytoma. Chronic lymphocytic leu-kemia and occasionally other small B cell malignancies may be associated with monoclonal macroglobulinemia.

DEFINITION AND HISTORY

The term *macroglobulinemia* describes an increased blood concentra-tion of immunoglobulin (Ig)M. Although the term commonly connotes Waldenström macroglobulin, several other disorders also may be as-sociated with a monoclonal macroglobulin.[1,2] In addition, some con-ditions are associated with increased polyclonal serum IgM protein.[3]

The types of disorders associated with a monoclonal macroglob-ulinemia vary with the study population. Physicians in specialized cen-ters often see macroglobulinemia associated with lymphoplasmacytic and B lymphocyte neoplasms. On the other hand, physicians at pri-mary treatment centers that use serum electrophoresis as a screening test more commonly see patients with essential macroglobulinemia or macroglobulinemia that is not associated with overt lymphoprolifera-tive disease. Of 213 patients with essential macroglobulinemia who had a median per patient followup at the Mayo Clinic of 6.3 years, 6 (3%) developed Waldenström macroglobulinemia, 3 (1%) developed chronic lymphocytic leukemia, 17 (8%) developed B cell lymphoma, and 3 (1%) developed primary amyloidosis.[4] Risk for progression to

lymphoma or a related disorder 10 years after detection of essential macroglobulinemia was 14 percent with an initial monoclonal protein concentration of 0.5 g/dl or less, 26 percent with 1.5 g/dl, 34 percent for 2.0 g/dl, and 41 percent for more than 25 g/dl.[4]

LYMPHOPLASMACYTIC NEOPLASMS

WALDENSTRÖM MACROGLOBULINEMIA

In 1944, Jan Waldenström described two male patients who had fa-tigue, a tendency to bleed from the gums and nasal mucosa, lymphad-enopathy, worsening normochromic anemia, a low serum fibrinogen despite an "excessive sedimentation of the erythrocytes," and an ex-tremely high serum viscosity secondary to a pathologic serum "eu-globulin" (macroglobulin) of approximately 1,000,000 kDa.[5,6] These patients lacked any lytic bone lesions on x-ray film and did not have any typical signs of myeloma, even on postmortem examination. This syndrome, now known as Waldenström macroglobulinemia, is the manifestation of a neoplastic disease in a clone of IgM-producing B cells.

Waldenström macroglobulinemia is an uncommon disease, ac-counting for approximately 6 percent of all B cell lymphoproliferative disorders. It has only one sixth the estimated prevalence of plasma cell myeloma (see Chap. 100). In the United States, the age-adjusted in-cidence rate per one million person-years at risk is 3.4 for men and 1.7 for women.[7] These rates increase sharply with age, from 0.1 for individuals younger than 45 years to 36.3 for men 75 years or older and 16.4 for women 75 years or older. Several web sites maintained by foundations provide information on the clinical features, research, and treatments for patients with the disease (e.g., *www.iwmf.com*, *www.waldenstromsresearch.org*, *www.iwmf.com/athens.htm*).

IgM MYELOMA AND EXTRAMEDULLARY PLASMACYTOMA

Patients with monoclonal macroglobulinemia associated with lytic bone lesions or hypercalcemia may be diagnosed as having IgM my-eloma. The neoplastic plasma cells have a surface phenotype with characteristics overlapping those of Waldenström macroglobulinemia and plasma cell myeloma. Plasma cells of IgM myeloma have high-level expression of cluster of differentiation (CD)38 but weak or negligible expression of CD5, CD10, CD20, CD22, CD23, CD45, HLA DR, FMC7, and surface immunoglobulin.[8] Extramedullary plas-macytomas also can produce monoclonal IgM proteins and have fea-tures in common with plasma cell myeloma. Chapter 100 discusses these conditions.

B LYMPHOCYTIC NEOPLASMS

Patients with low-grade B cell lymphomas or B cell chronic lympho-cytic leukemia can have a monoclonal macroglobulinemia as a result of IgM produced by the neoplastic B cell clone. Chapters 96 and 92, respectively, discuss these diseases.

ESSENTIAL MONOCLONAL MACROGLOBULINEMIA

Patients can have monoclonal macroglobulinemia without associated anemia, lymphadenopathy, hepatosplenomegaly, bone lesions, or ev-idence of disease progression. Patients are classified as having essen-tial monoclonal macroglobulinemia, a subtype of essential monoclonal gammopathy. Patients with essential monoclonal gammopathy are at increased risk for developing plasma cell myeloma or Waldenström macroglobulinemia.[9] Chapter 100 discusses this condition. Should the excess monoclonal IgM protein have binding activity for the "i" or "I" carbohydrate determinant found predominantly on neonatal and adult erythrocytes, respectively, the macroglobulin may agglutinate red cells in the cold. Patients who have hemolytic anemia secondary to the continuous production of such autoantibodies have the cold agglutinin syndrome. Chapter 52 discusses this condition.

Acronyms and abbreviations that appear in this chapter include: CAP, cyclo-phosphamide, doxorubicin, and prednisone; CD, cluster of differentiation, HHV; human herpes virus; hsp, heat shock protein; Ig, immunoglobulin; INF-α, interferon alpha; MAb, monoclonal antibody; PPAR-γ, peroxisome proliferator-activated receptor-gamma; SAHA, suberoylanilide hydroxamic acid.

ETIOLOGY

The etiology of Waldenström macroglobulinemia is unknown. Although the cases of patients developing Waldenström macroglobulinemia years after radiation therapy have been reported,[10] a significant increase in the incidence of this disease has not been noted in persons previously exposed to ionizing radiation or other environmental toxins.[11]

Hepatitis C infection has been associated with development of Waldenström macroglobulinemia.[12] An association between macroglobulinemia and hepatitis C infection was noted in a study of B cell malignancies in Japan that included four patients with Waldenström macroglobulinemia.[13] Another report noted the unusual development of Waldenström macroglobulinemia in five young Americans of African descent (median age 38 years) that was associated with hepatitis C infection and a history of intravenous heroin and cocaine use.[14] The finding that patients with hepatitis C can have an associated macroglobulinemia that resolves after treatment with interferon alpha (IFN-α)[15] suggests a possible relationship between uncontrolled hepatitis C infection and the development of Waldenström macroglobulinemia. However, whether hepatitis C is involved in all or most cases of macroglobulinemia is controversial.[16]

Some investigators have speculated that infection of marrow stromal dendritic cells by human herpesvirus (HHV) type 8, also known as Kaposi sarcoma–associated herpesvirus, might be a key factor in the etiology and pathogenesis of monoclonal gammopathies, including Waldenström macroglobulinemia.[17,18] However, in one survey of 20 patients, only one patient had evidence of HHV-8 in the marrow.[19]

Although Waldenström macroglobulinemia is an uncommon disease, it has been noted in the kindred of certain families[16,20,21] and in monozygotic twins.[22] "Unaffected" family members often have immunologic or serum immunoglobulin abnormalities.[20,23] Moreover, the prevalence of IgM monoclonal gammopathy in first-degree relatives of familial Waldenström macroglobulinemia may be as high as 6.3 percent, representing a 10-fold increase relative to that estimated for the general population.[24] This finding has led some investigators to speculate that genetic factors contribute to the etiopathogenesis of the disease.

Various chromosomal abnormalities have been described in neoplastic cells of patients with Waldenström macroglobulinemia.[25,26] Although karyotype analyses of marrow specimens generally fail to reveal abnormal metaphases, deletions can be detected, particularly in the long arm of chromosome 6 (del(6q)) in the region spanning 6q21-q23.[27–29] Although translocations of t(9;14)(p13;q32) involving the PAX-5 gene have been observed in cases of lymphoplasmacytic lymphoma,[30,31] translocations involving the immunoglobulin genes are rare in Waldenström macroglobulinemia.[29] Also, aneuploidy is less common than in plasma cell myeloma (see Chap. 100) and generally is associated with aggressive clinical disease.[28] Trisomy 12 and deletions at 13q14 are much less frequent than observed in chronic lymphocytic leukemia (see Chap. 92). Deletions of 17p13.1 potentially involving the P53 gene are uncommon at diagnosis but may be acquired during disease progression.[32,33]

PATHOGENESIS

The neoplastic cells in Waldenström macroglobulinemia may be derived from B cells that have differentiated through the germinal center but have yet to undergo immunoglobulin isotype switch recombination.[34] The immunoglobulins produced by such cells are of the IgM class and variable regions encoded by genes that have undergone somatic mutation.[34,35] Little if any intraclonal diversity in the IgM appears to be produced by the neoplastic B cells in Waldenström macroglobulinemia.[34] However, there is some evidence for clonal evolution in the IgM produced by the neoplastic B cell clone,[36] suggesting a role for antigen in the pathogenesis and/or progression of the disease.

The IgM produced by neoplastic B cells causes much of the morbidity associated with Waldenström macroglobulinemia. Blood viscosity increases when the concentration of IgM in the blood rises. High blood viscosity affects platelet function[37] and impairs capillary blood flow, reducing oxygen delivery through the microcirculation.[38] This situation can result in the hyperviscosity syndrome. High blood viscosity also is associated with viscous pancreatic secretions, increasing the risk for developing pancreatitis.[39] In addition, high serum levels of macroglobulins can cause abnormal cerebrovascular permeability, by either a direct toxic effect or viscosity-related ischemia. This situation can lead to infiltration of the cerebral parenchyma by IgM and lymphoplasmacytic cells and, ultimately, focal degeneration of the white matter, resulting in leukoencephalopathy.[40]

Occasionally the monoclonal IgM protein reacts with self-antigens to cause disease.[41,42] For example, the monoclonal IgM may have rheumatoid factor activity or binding activity for the constant region of human IgG.[43] IgM rheumatoid factors can form immune complexes with IgG, especially at low temperatures, leading to complement activation and tissue destruction secondary to immune complex deposition.[44,45] Some patients can develop myopathy associated with monoclonal IgM proteins that react with muscle self-antigens.[46] More often, the IgM protein reacts with red blood cells, particularly at low temperatures, sometimes causing autoimmune hemolytic anemia (see Chap. 52).[47] On rare occasions, the monoclonal IgM reacts with platelets, causing immune thrombocytopenic purpura.[48] Rare cases of paraneoplastic retinopathy that are presumed secondary to reactivity of the monoclonal IgM with proteins in the retinal photoreceptors have been described.[49]

The IgM protein is implicated as a factor contributing to some of the neurologic disorders associated with this disease. Although in most cases the monoclonal IgM protein does not react with any specific antigen,[50] in some patients it reacts with the myelin-associated glycoprotein or other components of peripheral nerve sharing a common carbohydrate determinant with myelin-associated glycoprotein.[51,52] Other patients can have an IgM that reacts with chondroitin sulfate C,[53] myelin basic protein,[54] or nerve glycolipids, such as G_{M1} ganglioside.[55,56] Patients with an IgM reactive with myelin-associated glycoprotein often develop a sensory demyelinating peripheral neuropathy, whereas elevated titers of anti-G_{M1} ganglioside antibodies are associated with lower motor neuron syndromes with multifocal motor conduction block.[56] The severity of neuropathy can be related to the level of monoclonal IgM autoantibody.[57]

If the monoclonal IgM protein precipitates from the serum upon cooling, it is called a cryoglobulin. Cryoglobulins in general are classified as type I (monoclonal), type II (mixed), or type III (polyclonal). Monoclonal IgM proteins of patients with Waldenström macroglobulinemia can be either type I or type II according to whether they form cryoprecipitates by themselves or as an immune complex (usually with polyclonal IgG), respectively. Patients with cryoglobulinemia can develop cold hypersensitivity, particularly if the cryoglobulin precipitates at temperatures higher than 22°C (71.6°F) and is present at blood concentrations greater than 20 g/liter.[58–60]

In some patients, the abnormal monoclonal IgM protein interferes with hemostasis.[58,61] Coating of platelets by the monoclonal IgM protein can produce defects in platelet aggregation secondary to impaired release of platelet factor 3.[62] Also, some monoclonal IgM proteins bind coagulation factors and inhibit coagulation.[63] For example, some IgM proteins bind to fibrin and inhibit fibrin monomer aggregation, resulting in a bulky, gelatinous, transparent clot with impaired clot retraction.[44] When combined with impaired platelet function, this process can produce a bleeding diathesis. Also, monoclonal IgM proteins inhibit factor VIII, factor V, and factor VII.[63] Such IgM proteins can lead to depletion of one or more coagulation factors *in vivo*. Finally, the plasma of Waldenström macroglobulinemia patients can have strong lupus anticoagulant activity if the monoclonal IgM has binding activity for the phosphatidylserine or phosphatidylethanolamine of cephalin.[64]

CLINICAL FEATURES

Patients with Waldenström macroglobulinemia generally are in their 60s or 70s and are a median age of 63 years at diagnosis.[65,66] Although occasionally young adults develop Waldenström macroglobulinemia,[14] less than 3 percent of patients are younger than 40 years. The disease is more common in patients of European descent than in those of African descent and in men.[65,66]

Patients most commonly present with complaints of fatigue, weakness, and weight loss. They also often note episodic bleeding, particularly from the gums and nasal mucosa.[67] Patients also can present with symptoms and signs of the hyperviscosity syndrome.

The most common physical findings are lymphadenopathy and hepatosplenomegaly. Dependent purpura and evidence of bleeding from the mucosal surfaces of the gastrointestinal tract also are common findings. Secondary to serum hyperviscosity, patients often have dilated and tortuous retinal veins and may develop bilateral optic disc swelling.[68]

The physical properties of the IgM paraprotein can produce symptoms. Patients with cryoglobulinemia may complain of cold hypersensitivity, noting that exposure to low temperatures precipitates urticaria, purpura, acral cyanosis, or Raynaud phenomenon.[60] Some patients may have multiple flesh-colored, sometimes pruritic papules on extensor skin surfaces secondary to skin deposition of monoclonal IgM. In some cases, the IgM protein reacts with epidermal basement membrane antigens.[38,42]

Various skin lesions are associated with Waldenström macroglobulinemia. Patients can have purpura, ulcers, or urticarial lesions caused by hyperviscosity of the blood, immune complex-mediated vascular damage, immunoglobulin deposition, or amyloid deposition.[69] In addition, some patients have translucent, flesh-colored papules, resulting from monoclonal IgM deposits. When such deposits occur in the tarsus, the patient can develop eyelid thickening and ptosis.[70] Some patients can develop a bullous dermatosis associated with the monoclonal IgM protein.[71–74] In such cases, deposits of the macroglobulin often can be found lining the subepidermis at the point of separation in the upper dermis, suggesting the monoclonal IgM has an unusual reactivity for skin-associated antigens. Patients with Waldenström macroglobulinemia associated with cryoglobulinemia can develop skin ulcers and/or purplish papules, particularly on exposed areas of the lower extremities.[75] A few patients develop violaceous skin lesions composed of lymphoplasmacytic infiltrates. The latter cutaneous manifestations may be a harbinger that the disease is undergoing transformation to high-grade lymphoma.

Not infrequently, patients develop a peripheral neuropathy. Most commonly, the symptoms are of a slowly progressive, symmetric, and predominantly sensory peripheral neuropathy that affects the legs more severely than the arms.[76] The symptoms can antedate the diagnosis of Waldenström macroglobulinemia by several years and sometimes bear no defined relationship to the duration or severity of the macroglobulinemia, particularly if the monoclonal IgM protein does not react with nerve-associated antigens. Often high serum titers of antibodies to antigens such as myelin-associated glycoprotein are detected.[76]

However, nearly half of macroglobulinemia patients with neuropathy have monoclonal IgM proteins with no detectable reactivity with such nerve components, implying the pathogenesis of macroglobulinemia-associated neuropathy is heterogeneous.

Occasionally, organ-system disease can develop from direct involvement by the neoplastic B cells. Some patients have involvement of the gastrointestinal tract with B cell lymphoma.[77,78] Furthermore, a few patients have endobronchial lesions with direct infiltration of the pulmonary parenchyma by lymphocytes, plasma cells, and amyloid as the primary clinical manifestation of their disease.[79,80] Hilar and mediastinal lymphadenopathy is not uncommon in such settings.

A few patients with Waldenström macroglobulinemia develop features of *POEMS syndrome* (*p*olyneuropathy, *o*rganomegaly, *e*ndocrinopathy, *m*onoclonal gammopathy, and *s*kin changes),[81] a syndrome that more commonly is observed in patients with plasma cell myeloma (see Chap. 100).

THE HYPERVISCOSITY SYNDROME

Waldenström macroglobulinemia patients can develop a hyperviscosity syndrome. Although usually associated with severe macroglobulinemia, the syndrome also is noted occasionally in patients with IgG or IgA myeloma (see Chap. 100).

Symptoms generally do not develop unless the serum viscosity is more than four times that of water.[38] However, plasma viscosity is not a perfect indicator of blood viscosity in the setting of macroglobulinemia, because red cell concentration also is an important determinant of blood viscosity.[82] Headache, possibly secondary to an expanded plasma volume and increased intracranial pressure, is a common early symptom. Patients also may complain of visual blurring. Occasionally, patients have mental status changes, ranging from impaired mentation to frank dementia. Ataxia, nystagmus, vertigo, confusion, disturbances of consciousness progressing to coma, and a diffuse brain syndrome, sometimes designated *coma paraproteinaemicum*, can develop in patients with marked hyperviscosity. Patients with hyperviscosity-induced stroke[83] and dementia[84] who improve following plasmapheresis have been described. Secondary to anemia, an increased blood viscosity, and an expanded plasma volume, these patients can develop symptoms and signs of congestive heart failure.

Funduscopic evaluation may reveal dilatation and segmentation of retinal and conjunctival vessels.[85] This situation gives the retinal veins a "link-sausage" appearance. In addition, these patients often have retinal hemorrhages and sometimes frank papilledema. Less commonly, patients develop central retinal vein occlusion.[86]

LABORATORY FINDINGS

SERUM IMMUNOGLOBULIN AND BLOOD VISCOSITY

By definition, the serum IgM level is elevated in macroglobulinemia. The blood levels of the other immunoglobulin classes usually are normal or depressed. On serum protein electrophoresis, serum IgM usually produces a tall, narrow peak or a dense band that migrates to the γ region of the serum electrophoresis pattern (see Chap. 98). Patients with macroglobulinemia who develop symptoms generally have serum IgM concentrations greater than 30 g/liter.

The IgM usually is a pentamer having a molecular weight of approximately 900,000 (see Chap. 77). Some patients also have a monomeric serum IgM protein of 165,000 molecular weight that diffuses more rapidly in the electrophoresis gel. This situation may create a double ring when the IgM is measured by immunodiffusion (see Chap. 98), causing some laboratories to overestimate the amount of serum IgM.

The immunoglobulins expressed in Waldenström macroglobulin-emia apparently constitute a skewed repertoire. The light chain of the monoclonal IgM is κ in 75 percent of patients.[4] In addition, these immunoglobulins often bear cross-reactive idiotypes that frequently are found on immunoglobulins expressed in chronic lymphocytic leukemia and by mantle zone B cells (see Chap. 92).[87]

Serum viscosity is elevated in most patients, but only 20 percent have symptoms related to hyperviscosity. Patients with a serum viscosity greater than four times that of water may develop the hyperviscosity syndrome. However, higher plasma viscosity can be offset by the anemia that commonly is associated with the disease. For this reason, blood rheology performed on whole blood at $+32°C$ ($+89.6°F$) to $+37°C$ ($+98.6°F$) at low shear rates may be the best indicator of actual blood viscosity.[82]

BLOOD AND MARROW CELLS

Nearly four fifths of patients with Waldenström macroglobulinemia present with a hemoglobin concentration less than 120 g/liter.[4] Leukopenia also can be present at diagnosis, but the platelet count typically is in the normal range.

The anemia usually results from a mildly decreased red cell survival time and impaired erythropoiesis. The erythrocytes usually are normocytic and normochromic. However, the electronically measured mean corpuscular volume can be elevated spuriously because of erythrocyte aggregation. The severity of the anemia often is exaggerated artificially because of expanded plasma volume. This situation results from the increased oncotic pressure of plasma that contains an elevated concentration of IgM protein.[88]

The blood may contain a population of monoclonal B lymphocytes, even in asymptomatic patients.[89,90] By flow cytometric analysis, these cells express pan–B lymphocyte surface antigens CD19, CD20, CD22, and CD24, and monoclonal immunoglobulin bearing either κ or λ light chains.[91] The monoclonal B cells of approximately one fifth of patients also express CD5 and/or CD23 but typically lack expression of CD10, CD11c, and CD103. These B lymphocytes typically express CD27, which commonly also is found on memory-type B cells, and have high-level expression of the anti-apoptotic protein BCL-2.[91] The size of the circulating monoclonal B lymphocyte population correlates with the clinical course of the disease, increasing in patients who do not respond or who progress.

The marrow aspirate often is hypocellular. However, marrow biopsy specimens generally are hypercellular and diffusely infiltrated with lymphocytes, plasmacytoid lymphocytes, and some plasma cells.[92] Similar to the marrow in chronic lymphocytic leukemia (see Chap. 92), different patterns of marrow infiltration are observed. In a retrospective survey of patient marrow specimens, the patterns of lymphocyte infiltration were diffuse (seen in 45%), nodular–interstitial (22%), mixed paratrabecular–nodular (20%), or paratrabecular (13%).[92] Mast cells often are increased in number. The lymphocytes tend to be small, basophilic, and well-differentiated cells, often resembling plasma cells. The neoplastic plasmacytoid cells in Waldenström macroglobulinemia differ from those seen in plasma cell myeloma in that they more often also coexpress CD5, CD20, and/or CD22.[91] Periodic acid–Schiff-positive material (called *Dutcher bodies*) are sometimes seen in lymphoid cells, the interstitium, and blood vessel walls. The lymphocytes, plasmacytoid lymphocytes, and plasma cells express the same monoclonal IgM protein[93] but are of different levels of maturity, consisting of small lymphocytes carrying surface IgM/IgD, IgM plasmacytoid cells with low-level surface IgM, or mature plasma cells with only cytoplasmic IgM.

DISORDERS OF HEMOSTASIS

The clotting abnormality detected most frequently is prolongation of the thrombin time.[44] Less frequently, a patient's plasma has an elevated prothrombin time or activated partial thromboplastin time secondary to depletion of a coagulation factor(s) or to the presence of a lupus anticoagulant.[63,64,94]

Platelet function often is impaired, resulting in a prolonged bleeding time, impaired clot retraction, defective prothrombin consumption, poor thromboplastin generation with the patient's platelets, defective platelet aggregation *in vivo*, and defective platelet adhesion *in vitro*.[37,62,95]

RENAL ABNORMALITIES

Renal insufficiency occurs less frequently in patients with Waldenström macroglobulinemia than in patients with plasma cell myeloma,[96] although the blood urea nitrogen is elevated above 8 mmol/liter (25 mg/dl) in approximately one third of patients.[97,98] The urine of nearly 80 percent of patients has detectable immunoglobulin light chains that apparently are produced by the neoplastic B cell clone.[4,99] However, because the amount of excreted light chain rarely exceeds 2.0 g in 24 hours, its detection generally requires that the urine sample be concentrated prior to zonal electrophoresis or immunoelectrophoresis.

Glomerular lesions occur more frequently in patients with Waldenström macroglobulinemia than in patients with plasma cell myeloma. The IgM protein can precipitate on the endothelial side of the glomerular basement membrane, forming deposits so large that they occlude the glomerular capillaries. Some patients have amyloid deposits in the renal parenchyma and develop renal interstitial infiltrates of lymphocytes and plasma cells that appear similar to those found in the marrow.[98]

Some patients develop a nephrotic syndrome associated with an immune-mediated glomerulonephritis.[100] One patient had monoclonal granular deposits of IgM, IgG, and the third component of complement along the glomerular basement membrane that was associated with a low serum complement level.[101] Another patient had a monoclonal IgM that reacted with glomerular antigens, resulting in deposition of IgM in glomerular and interstitial capillaries.[102]

DIFFERENTIAL DIAGNOSIS

Patients with essential monoclonal macroglobulinemia should be distinguished from those with Waldenström macroglobulinemia or IgM myeloma.[103–105] Table 102-1 presents the clinical and laboratory findings that are helpful in making this distinction. The concentration of monoclonal IgM can vary widely in Waldenström macroglobulinemia, thus not allowing definition of concentration that reliably distinguishes this disorder from essential monoclonal gammopathy or other lymphoproliferative disorders.[66] Nevertheless, in addition to being symptomatic, patients with IgM-producing lymphoplasmacytic neoplasms usually have anemia, a monoclonal IgM protein level greater than 30 g/liter, increased serum viscosity, and symptoms and signs that progress over time. For this reason, patients deemed to have essential monoclonal macroglobulinemia should undergo followup evaluation for evidence of disease progression.

Monoclonal macroglobulinemia can develop in patients with a variety of lymphoid neoplasms. Patients with chronic lymphocytic leukemia generally have monoclonal B cell lymphocytosis greater than $5000/\mu l$ (5×10^9/liter) (see Chap. 92). Patients with lymphoma may be diagnosed by biopsy of a lymph node or other tissue (see Chap.

TABLE 102-1   DISTINCTIONS BETWEEN ESSENTIAL VERSUS
             WALDENSTRÖM MACROGLOBULINEMIA

	ESSENTIAL MACROGLOBULINEMIA	WALDENSTRÖM MACROGLOBULINEMIA
Symptoms	Usually none but may have peripheral neuropathy or cold sensitivity	Fatigue, weight loss, headache, epistaxis, neurologic symptoms, or cold hypersensitivity
Physical findings	Usually none	Hepatosplenomegaly, purpura, lymphadenopathy, Raynaud phenomenon neurologic signs, retinopathy
Laboratory findings		
IgM protein (g/liter)	Usually <30 and stable	Often >30 and increasing
Hemoglobin (g/liter)	Usually >120	<120 in 80% of patients
Serum viscosity	Normal	Increased

96). Lytic skeletal lesions and hypercalcemia indicate the monoclonal macroglobulinemia is secondary to IgM myeloma (see Chap. 100).

Monoclonal IgM gammopathy also is a feature of *Schnitzler syndrome*, an uncommon, generally benign disorder defined by urticaria and monoclonal IgM gammopathy that often is associated with fever of unknown origin, elevated erythrocyte sedimentation rate, and bone pain.[106] However, some patients later develop Waldenström macroglobulinemia.

THERAPY

Waldenström macroglobulinemia is incurable.[105] Therefore, therapy is directed toward prevention and/or palliation of the associated clinical sequelae of macroglobulinemia. Treatment must be individualized based on clinical manifestations, presence or absence of signs or symptoms of hyperviscosity, and the patient's potential for developing toxic side effects of the selected treatment regimen.

Asymptomatic patients may be followed without specific therapy. However, patients should be evaluated periodically for reduced hemoglobin level, increased serum IgM, deteriorating renal function, or other clinical manifestations of the disease, such as hyperviscosity, lymphadenopathy, hepatosplenomegaly, bleeding tendencies, or neurologic changes. Symptomatic patients should receive chemotherapy.[103]

Unfortunately, data recommending one agent over any other for first-line therapy are insufficient. However, the need for rapid disease control, patient age, presence of cytopenias, and potential candidacy for autologous stem cell transplantation should be considered when defining a treatment plan. Exposure to alkylating drugs or nucleoside analogues should be limited in patients considered excellent candidates for autologous stem cell transplantation.[107] Instead, such patients should be considered for treatment with rituximab or other forms of nonmyelotoxic therapy if stem cells have not been previously harvested.

ALKYLATING AGENTS

Chlorambucil is an effective agent and can be considered for first-line therapy.[107] Treatment with chlorambucil 0.1 mg/kg/day or 0.3 mg/kg/day orally for 7 days repeated every 6 weeks provides for objective responses in nearly three fourths of patients, with a median survival of 5.4 years.[108] Alternatively, patients may receive oral high-dose intermittent chlorambucil 0.7 mg/kg on day 1 or 0.2 to 0.3 mg/kg on days 1 through 4. This regimen often is administered with 40 to 60 mg prednisone orally on days 1 through 4. This cycle may be repeated every 21 to 28 days. Monitoring blood cell counts is essential. The initial dose may need to be decreased, depending on platelet and leukocyte counts and the therapeutic response.

The M-2 protocol (carmustine, cyclophosphamide, vincristine, melphalan, and prednisone) also may be effective for patients with this disease. Unfortunately, no randomized trials comparing the effectiveness of treatment for symptomatic macroglobulinemia have been reported. In one institution, 33 patients with symptomatic Waldenström macroglobulinemia received this therapy every 5 weeks for 2 years and every 10 weeks for an additional 1 to 3 years.[109] Responses were observed in 27 patients (81%), of whom 21 (63%) had partial responses and survival ranged from 1 to more than 120 months. In another institution, 34 patients received 7 days of oral melphalan 6 mg/m²/day, cyclophosphamide 125 mg/m²/ day, and prednisone 40 mg/m²/day for 7 days.[110] Courses were repeated every 4 to 6 weeks for a total of 12 courses. Responding patients subsequently received continuous treatment with chlorambucil and prednisone until relapse. Following this regimen, 23 of 31 evaluated patients (74%) responded to induction therapy, and eight (26% of the 31 evaluated patients) achieved a complete remission. Other effective drug combinations include cyclophosphamide, doxorubicin, and prednisone (CAP).[111] However, the response rates and response duration achieved using these combination drug therapies do not appear to be significantly better than those achieved using single-agent chlorambucil. As such, the general recommendation is that combination drug therapies be used only in the context of a clinical trial.[107]

NUCLEOSIDE ANALOGUES

CLADRIBINE (2-CHLORODEOXYADENOSINE)

The adenine nucleoside analogue cladribine is an effective agent and can be considered for first-line therapy or for treatment of disease refractory to alkylating drugs.[107,112] Treatment with this drug as a single agent produces objective response rates of 40 to 90 percent in previously untreated patients and between 30 and 60 percent in previously treated patients, with a median response duration ranging from 8 to 22 months.[113–118] Previously treated patients with disease relapse off therapy generally respond better than those receiving therapy because of an inadequate response to alkylating agents. Patients who are refractory to fludarabine generally do not respond to cladribine,[119] although the converse may not be the case.[120]

Different dosing regimens have proved effective. Most patients receive cladribine as a continuous intravenous infusion at 0.1 mg/kg body weight per day for 7 days.[113–115] This cycle is repeated 1 month later and, in some cases, at monthly intervals thereafter, particularly if the patient does not respond adequately to the first two courses and has not experienced significant myelosuppression. Alternatively, patients can be treated with intravenous cladribine 0.12 to 0.14 mg/kg body weight per day over 2 hours for 5 consecutive days.[117,118] This cycle is repeated at monthly intervals three to five times, again provided the patient does not experience significant drug toxicity or myelosuppression. Cladribine also has been administered as a subcutaneous bolus injection at 0.1 mg/kg body weight per day for 5 days, which is repeated every 4 weeks, yielding response rates comparable to those achieved with continuous intravenous infusion.[121] Unfortunately, few head-to-head comparison studies evaluating the relative efficacy of each of these regimens have been reported,[114] thus not allowing definition of the relative merits of each of the approaches.

Cladribine has been used in combination with cyclophosphamide, prednisone, and/or rituximab for treatment of Waldenström macroglobulinemia.[112,122] In one nonrandomized consecutive study, 90 previously untreated patients each received cladribine alone for 7 days at 0.1 mg/kg/day by continuous infusion (group I), continuous infusion cladribine with oral prednisone at 60 mg/m²/day for 7 days (group II), subcutaneous injections of cladribine at 1.5 mg/m² every 8 hours for 7 days with oral cyclophosphamide at 40 mg/m² twice per day for 7 days (group III), or subcutaneous cladribine and oral cyclophosphamide with weekly intravenous infusions of rituximab at 375 mg/m² for 4 weeks (group IV). Patients in this study generally received a second course of therapy after 4 to 6 weeks. Overall response (complete and partial response) was 94 percent for group I, 60 percent for group II, 84 percent for group III, and 94 percent for group IV. Because the response rates of patients treated with single-agent cladribine appear similar to those of patients treated with multiple agents, combination therapy with cladribine, alkylating drugs, and/or rituximab currently is not recommended except in the context of a clinical trial.[107]

The major toxicity of cladribine is acute myelosuppression and chronic immune suppression secondary to T cell depletion. As such, treated patients have a higher risk of developing common and opportunistic infections.[123,124] One case report described a patient who, following treatment with cladribine, developed Epstein-Barr virus–associated lymphoproliferative disease and lymphoma similar to that seen in posttransplant patients receiving systemic immunosuppressive therapy.[125]

Cases of patients who experienced marked increases in serum IgM following treatment with cladribine believed to be secondary to acute lysis of tumor cells have been reported.[126] For this reason, patients should be monitored for new onset of symptoms or signs of the hyperviscosity syndrome during the initial cycles of therapy. Patients treated with cladribine may develop autoimmune hemolytic anemia weeks to months after therapy.[127]

FLUDARABINE

The adenine nucleoside analogue fludarabine monophosphate also is effective for treatment of Waldenström macroglobulinemia and can be considered for initial therapy or treatment of disease refractory to alkylating drugs.[107] Fludarabine generally is given as a daily intravenous dose of 25 mg/m² for 5 days every 4 weeks unless the patient experiences significant myelotoxicity. Many patients receive up to six courses of treatment, although fewer courses may be effective, yielding response rates of 60 to 80 percent in previously untreated patients and 30 to 50 percent in patients previously treated with alkylating drugs, with a median response duration ranging from 10 to 44 months.[111,128–134] Treatment with fludarabine appears more active in salvage therapy than does combination drug therapy with CAP.[111] Also, some patients who appeared refractory to cladribine had good responses to treatment with fludarabine,[120] although the number of such cases is too small to consider this observation definitive.

Fludarabine has been used in combination with cyclophosphamide to treat patients with Waldenström macroglobulinemia. In one study, patients received intravenous fludarabine at 25 mg/m²/day for 3 days and cyclophosphamide at 250 mg/m² per day for 3 days every 4 weeks over a 16-week period.[135] Over half of the treated patients experienced resolution of all symptoms and a partial response with a median response duration of 24 months. Because the overall response rates with fludarabine and cyclophosphamide do not appear significantly better than the rate observed with fludarabine alone, patients are not recommended for combination drug therapy except in the context of a clinical trial.[107]

The major toxicity of fludarabine is acute myelosuppression and chronic immune suppression similar to that noted for patients treated with cladribine.[136] After treatment with fludarabine, patients are at increased risk for developing opportunistic infections.[137] One case report

described a patient who, following treatment with fludarabine, developed watery diarrhea, nausea, and vomiting secondary to uncontrolled infection with astrovirus that was successfully treated with intravenous immunoglobulin infusions.[138] Treatment-related mortality most commonly is associated with pancytopenia and infection.

MONOCLONAL ANTIBODIES

RITUXIMAB

Rituximab, a primatized monoclonal antibody (MAb) specific for CD20, is an effective agent for treatment of patients with Waldenström macroglobulinemia. Intravenous rituximab administered at the standard dose of 375 mg/m² every week for 4 weeks produces objective response rates ranging from 30 to 75 percent.[139,140] Patients may have a delayed response to therapy, typically achieving maximum benefit approximately 3 months after treatment.[140] The response rate of treatment-naive patients versus that of patients previously treated with alkylating drugs or purine analogues does not appear to be different. Rituximab also may be effective in treating patients with IgM autoantibody-related neuropathies or other autoimmune manifestations.[107,141]

Patients treated with rituximab can experience transient increases in serum monoclonal IgM similar to that observed in some patients treated with the purine analogues.[140] This situation should not necessarily be considered indicative of treatment failure. Instead, attention should be paid to signs or symptoms of the hyperviscosity syndrome in patients during the initial cycles of therapy, particularly those patients with relatively high levels of serum IgM protein prior to therapy. Some patients may experience a delayed proinflammatory syndrome following treatment with rituxan that can resemble early rheumatoid arthritis.[142] The syndrome generally responds well to oral prednisone at 1 mg/kg body weight per day for 1 to 3 days, followed by a rapid taper.

OTHER MABS

Other MAbs are being considered for treatment of Waldenström macroglobulinemia. Although the neoplastic cells in this disease generally express CD52,[143] studies evaluating the clinical activity of CAMPATH-1H (alemtuzumab) in this disease have not been performed. Use of radiolabeled MAb is problematic because of the risk for myelosuppression, particularly in patients with extensive marrow involvement of neoplastic cells.

OTHER AGENTS

GLUCOCORTICOIDS

Glucocorticoids can be useful for treatment of Waldenström macroglobulinemia, particularly in patients with severe pancytopenia who are not candidates for treatment with myelosuppressive drugs.[144,145] In addition, prednisone has been used in combination therapy with other anticancer drugs,[111,122] although the effectiveness of such combinations has not been demonstrated to exceed that of single-agent therapy. Glucocorticoids also can be useful for treating paraneoplastic syndromes that sometimes are observed in patients with Waldenström macroglobulinemia, such as the nephrotic syndrome caused by protein thrombi in the glomerulocapillary lumen[100,146] or paraneoplastic pemphigus.[73]

THALIDOMIDE

Thalidomide, an immune-modulatory and antiangiogenic agent with therapeutic activity in plasma cell myeloma,[147] appears to have activity in Waldenström macroglobulinemia. In one study, 20 patients were given a starting dose of 200 mg daily with dose escalation in 200-mg increments every 14 days as tolerated to a maximum of 600 mg.[148] Five (25%) achieved a partial response within 3 months of therapy, including two patients who previously had been treated with other anticancer drugs. However, the elderly patients in this study poorly tolerated the common adverse effects of thalidomide (e.g., constipation, somnolence, fatigue, mood changes), and few could tolerate treatment at the highest dose or continued therapy beyond 2 months. For this reason, clinical studies are evaluating the capacity of low-dose thalidomide to enhance the activity of other agents when used in combination for treatment of this disease.[149,150] In addition, thalidomide and glucocorticoids are being evaluated for treatment of patients with refractory disease because of the noted activity of this nonmyelotoxic combination in patients with plasma cell myeloma.[151,152]

INVESTIGATIONAL AGENTS

Various agents are being evaluated for their potential utility in the treatment of patients with Waldenström macroglobulinemia.[150,153] The agents include the proteasome inhibitor PS-341,[154,155] antibiotics such as clarithromycin (Biaxin [BXN], Abbott Laboratories, Abbott Park, IL, USA),[149] histone deacetylase inhibitors such as suberoylanilide hydroxamic acid (SAHA),[156,157] the ansamycin family of inhibitors (e.g., geldanamycin and its analogues) of the heat shock protein 90 (hsp90) molecular chaperone,[158] INF-α,[159] and the thiazolidinedione group of peroxisome proliferator-activated receptor-gamma (PPAR-γ) agonists (e.g., ciglitazone or rosiglitazone).[153] These agents, used alone or in combination with other drugs or MAbs, may prove effective in the treatment of this disease.

STEM CELL TRANSPLANTATION

The role of stem cell transplantation in patients with Waldenström macroglobulinemia is not established. A review of 24 published cases of patients treated with high-dose chemotherapy followed by autologous stem cell transplantation revealed that nine achieved a complete response and 14 a partial response, including several with disease refractory to standard therapy.[160] Fewer patients treated with allogeneic stem cell transplantation have been reported.[161,162] The small number of reported patients precludes making any conclusions except that autologous or allogeneic stem cell transplantation is feasible for patients with Waldenström macroglobulinemia and warrants further investigation, particularly for younger patients with aggressive and/or refractory disease.

PLASMAPHERESIS

Patients with symptomatic hyperviscosity should be treated with plasmapheresis.[107] In some cases, plasmapheresis can be used to alleviate the autoimmune pathology resulting from a self-reactive monoclonal IgM protein.[163] Conventional plasma exchange is superior to cascade filtration, in which proteins are removed as a function of their size.[164,165] Daily plasma exchanges of 3000 to 4000 ml with albumin, rather than plasma, are particularly effective in reducing the serum IgM level and serum viscosity.[38,166] This treatment often is initiated concomitantly with chemotherapy to reduce the production of the abnormal monoclonal IgM protein.

RED CELL TRANSFUSIONS

Patients with Waldenström macroglobulinemia may require periodic transfusions of packed red cells because of symptomatic anemia. These patients often have artificially low hemoglobin and hematocrit levels as a result of expanded plasma volume. Consequently, these patients should not receive red cell transfusions simply based on low hemoglobin. Moreover, because of the increased serum viscosity of macroglobulinemia, these patients actually may have reduced capillary blood flow following transfusions of packed red cells because of in-

creased blood viscosity. For this reason, patients with symptomatic hyperviscosity should not be transfused unless therapy is implemented to reduce the serum IgM level. In addition, patients should be monitored for signs of fluid overload or congestive heart failure prior to and during red cell transfusion. Leukocyte-depleted, packed red cells should be administered slowly, at a rate not exceeding 1 unit per 2-hour period.

SPLENECTOMY

Splenectomy is rarely indicated except for management of symptomatic splenomegaly, including painful splenomegaly or hypersplenism that precludes treatment with cytotoxic drugs.[107] Moreover, splenectomy may benefit patients with hypersplenism who have severe cytopenias despite having evidence of adequate myelopoiesis on marrow biopsy. Anecdotal reports of patients with disappearance of monoclonal IgM following splenectomy have been published.[167,168]

COURSE AND PROGNOSIS

Waldenström macroglobulinemia is an indolent disease that generally progresses over a period of years. In the most recent retrospective study, the median survival from diagnosis was 106 months.[169] However, the clinical course is variable. Features associated with poorer prognosis are hemoglobin levels less than 10 g/dl, age greater than 65 years, weight loss, and cryoglobulinemia.[60,169,170] Patients with a worse prognosis have at diagnosis two or more of the features or any one feature associated with low platelet count, splenomegaly, lymphadenopathy, a lymphoplasmacytic infiltrate occupying greater than 50 percent of the marrow, and/or high levels of serum macroglobulin.[92,169] Elevated serum β_2 microglobulin and low serum albumin also are associated with a poorer prognosis. However, marrow histology or plasma cell expression of proliferating cell nuclear antigen does not have an apparent relationship to survival.[92]

Hyperviscosity, anemia, hemorrhage, thrombosis, or infections often are contributory causes of death. Neoplastic lymphocytes may infiltrate the liver, spleen, marrow, lymph nodes, lung, skin, and/or gastrointestinal mucosa. In some patients, the concentration of IgM paraprotein decreases as the tumor burden increases. Further dedifferentiation of the neoplastic cells and loss of their ability to produce IgM protein may explain this effect. This process suggests the neoplastic cells dedifferentiate and lose their ability to produce IgM protein. This situation often is associated with an accelerated deterioration in the clinical course. In some cases, the disease evolves into a high-grade lymphoma with characteristics similar to those of Richter transformation in chronic lymphocytic leukemia.[171,172] In such cases, the patient may develop hypercalcemia or infiltrative skin lesions as an early manifestation of the transformation to high-grade lymphoma.[69,172] Some patients develop acute myelogenous leukemia,[173,174] immunoblastic sarcoma,[175,176] or chronic myelogenous leukemia[177] as a preterminal event. Most of these cases occurred after treatment with alkylating agents.

REFERENCES

1. Baldini L, Guffanti A, Cesana BM, et al: Role of different hematologic variables in defining the risk of malignant transformation in monoclonal gammopathy. *Blood* 87:912, 1996.
2. Herrinton LJ: The epidemiology of monoclonal gammopathy of unknown significance: A review. *Curr Top Microbiol Immunol* 210:389, 1996.
3. Fuleihan RL: The X-linked hyperimmunoglobulin M syndrome. *Semin Hematol* 35:321, 1998.

4. Kyle RA, Therneau TM, Rajkumar V, et al: Long-term follow-up of IgM monoclonal gammopathy of undetermined significance. *Blood* 102: 3759, 2003.

5. Waldenström J: Incipient myelomatosis or "essential" hyperglobulinemia with fibrinogenopenia—A new syndrome? *Acta Med Scand* 117: 216, 1944.

6. Kyle RA, Anderson KC: A tribute to Jan Gosta Waldenström [editorial]. *Blood* 89:4245, 1997.

7. Groves FD, Travis LB, Devesa SS, et al: Waldenström's macroglobulinemia: Incidence patterns in the United States 1988–1994. *Cancer* 82: 1078, 1998.

8. Haghighi B, Yanagihara R, Cornbleet PJ: IgM myeloma: Case report with immunophenotypic profile. *Am J Hematol* 59:302, 1998.

9. Isaksson E, Björkholm M, Holm G, et al: Blood clonal B-cell excess in patients with monoclonal gammopathy of undetermined significance (MGUS): Association with malignant transformation. *Br J Haematol* 92: 71, 1996.

10. Epenetos AA, Rohatiner A, Slevin M, Woothipoom W: Ankylosing spondylitis and Waldenstrom's macroglobulinaemia: A case report. *Clin Oncol* 6:83, 1980.

11. Tepper A, Moss CE: Waldenstrom's macroglobulinemia: Search for occupational exposure. *J Occup Med* 36:133, 1994.

12. Silvestri F, Barillari G, Fanin R, et al: Risk of hepatitis C virus infection, Waldenström's macroglobulinemia, and monoclonal gammopathies [letter, comment]. *Blood* 88:1125, 1996.

13. Izumi T, Sasaki R, Tsunoda S, et al: B cell malignancy and hepatitis C virus infection. *Leukemia* 11(suppl 3):516, 1997.

14. Ahmed S, Shurafa MS, Bishop CR, Varterasian M: Waldenström's macroglobulinemia in young African-American adults. *Am J Hematol* 60: 229, 1999.

15. Schott P, Pott C, Ramadori G, Hartmann H: Hepatitis C virus infection-associated non-cryoglobulinaemic monoclonal IgMkappa gammopathy responsive to interferon-alpha treatment. *J Hepatol* 29:310, 1998.

16. Custodi P, Cerutti A, Cassani P, et al: Familial occurrence of IgMk gammapathy: No involvement of HCV infection [letter]. *Haematologica* 80:484, 1995.

17. Agbalika F, Mariette X, Marolleau JP, et al: Detection of human herpesvirus-8 DNA in bone marrow biopsies from patients with multiple myeloma and Waldenström's macroglobulinemia [letter]. *Blood* 91: 4393, 1998.

18. Mikala G, Xie J, Berencsi G, et al: Human herpesvirus 8 in hematologic diseases. *Pathol Oncol Res* 5:73, 1999.

19. Brousset P, Theriault C, Roda D, et al: Kaposi's sarcoma-associated herpesvirus (KSHV) in bone marrow biopsies of patients with Waldenstrom's macroglobulinaemia. *Br J Haematol* 102:795, 1998.

20. Blattner WA, Garber JE, Mann DL, et al: Waldenstrom's macroglobulinemia and autoimmune disease in a family. *Ann Intern Med* 93:830, 1980.

21. Ogmundsdóttir HM, Jóhannesson GM, Sveinsdóttir S, et al: Familial macroglobulinaemia: Hyperactive B-cells but normal natural killer function [published erratum appears in *Scand J Immunol* 41:650, 1995]. *Scand J Immunol* 40:195, 1994.

22. Fine JM, Muller JY, Rochu D, et al: Waldenstrom's macroglobulinemia in monozygotic twins. *Acta Med Scand* 220:369, 1986.

23. Taleb N, Tohme A, Abi Jirgiss D, et al: Familial macroglobulinemia in a Lebanese family with two sisters presenting Waldenstrom's disease. *Acta Oncol (Madr)* 30:703, 1991.

24. McMaster ML: Familial Waldenstrom's macroglobulinemia. *Semin Oncol* 30:146, 2003.

25. Palka G, Spadano A, Geraci L, et al: Chromosome changes in 19 patients with Waldenstrom's macroglobulinemia. *Cancer Genet Cytogenet* 29: 261, 1987.

26. Calasanz MJ, Cigudosa JC, Odero MD, et al: Cytogenetic analysis of 280 patients with multiple myeloma and related disorders: Primary breakpoints and clinical correlations. *Genes Chromosomes Cancer* 18: 84, 1997.

27. White AD, Clark RE, Jacobs A: Isochromosome (6p) in Waldenstrom's macroglobulinemia. *Cancer Genet Cytogenet* 58:89, 1992.

28. Mansoor A, Medeiros LJ, Weber DM, et al: Cytogenetic findings in lymphoplasmacytic lymphoma/Waldenstrom macroglobulinemia. Chromosomal abnormalities are associated with the polymorphous subtype and an aggressive clinical course. *Am J Clin Pathol* 116:543, 2001.

29. Schop RF, Kuehl WM, Van Wier SA, et al: Waldenstrom macroglobulinemia neoplastic cells lack immunoglobulin heavy chain locus translocations but have frequent 6q deletions. *Blood* 100:2996, 2002.

30. Iida S, Rao PH, Ueda R, et al: Chromosomal rearrangement of the PAX-5 locus in lymphoplasmacytic lymphoma with t(9;14)(p13;q32). *Leuk Lymphoma* 34:25, 1999.

31. Pangalis GA, Angelopoulou MK, Vassilakopoulos TP, et al: B-chronic lymphocytic leukemia, small lymphocytic lymphoma, and lymphoplasmacytic lymphoma, including Waldenström's macroglobulinemia: A clinical, morphologic, and biologic spectrum of similar disorders. *Semin Hematol* 36:104, 1999.

32. Schop RF, Jalal SM, Van Wier SA, et al: Deletions of 17p13.1 and 13q14 are uncommon in Waldenstrom macroglobulinemia clonal cells and mostly seen at the time of disease progression. *Cancer Genet Cytogenet* 132:55, 2002.

33. Chang H, Samiee S, Li D, et al: Analysis of IgH translocations, chromosome 13q14 and 17p13.1(p53) deletions by fluorescence in situ hybridization in Waldenstrom's macroglobulinemia: A single center study of 22 cases. *Leukemia* 18:1160, 2004.

34. Sahota SS, Forconi F, Ottensmeier CH, et al: Typical Waldenstrom macroglobulinemia is derived from a B-cell arrested after cessation of somatic mutation but prior to isotype switch events. *Blood* 100:1505, 2002.

35. Sahota SS, Forconi F, Ottensmeier CH, Stevenson FK: Origins of the malignant clone in typical Waldenstrom's macroglobulinemia. *Semin Oncol* 30:136, 2003.

36. Ciric B, VanKeulen V, Rodriguez M, et al: Clonal evolution in Waldenstrom macroglobulinemia highlights functional role of B-cell receptor. *Blood* 97:321, 2001.

37. van Breugel HF, de Groot PG, Heethaar RM, Sixma JJ: Role of plasma viscosity in platelet adhesion. *Blood* 80:953, 1992.

38. Reinhart WH, Lutolf O, Nydegger UR, et al: Plasmapheresis for hyperviscosity syndrome in macroglobulinemia Waldenstrom and multiple myeloma: Influence on blood rheology and the microcirculation. *J Lab Clin Med* 119:69, 1992.

39. Hertan HI, Pitchumoni CS: Chronic calcific pancreatitis in a patient with Waldenstrom's macroglobulinemia. *Am J Gastroenterol* 86:633, 1991.

40. Scheithauer BW, Rubinstein LJ, Herman MM: Leukoencephalopathy in Waldenstrom's macroglobulinemia. Immunohistochemical and electron microscopic observations. *J Neuropathol Exp Neurol* 43:408, 1984.

41. Waldenstrom JG: Antibody activity of monoclonal immunoglobulins in myeloma, macroglobulinemia and benign gammapathy. *Med Oncol Tumor Pharmacother* 3:135, 1986.

42. Cobb MW, Domloge-Hultsch N, Frame JN, Yancey KB: Waldenstrom macroglobulinemia with an IgM-kappa antiepidermal basement membrane zone antibody. *Arch Dermatol* 128:372, 1992.

43. Artandi SE, Canfield SM, Tao MH, et al: Molecular analysis of IgM rheumatoid factor binding to chimeric IgG. *J Immunol* 146:603, 1991.

44. Coleman M, Vigliano EM, Weksler ME, Nachman RL: Inhibition of fibrin monomer polymerization by lambda myeloma globulins. *Blood* 39:210, 1972.

45. Vital A, Vital C: Immunoelectron identification of endoneurial IgM deposits in four patients with Waldenstrom's macroglobulinemia: A spe-

cific ultrastructural pattern related to the presence of cryoglobulin in one case. *Clin Neuropathol* 12:49, 1993.

46. al-Lozi MT, Pestronk A, Yee WC, Flaris N: Myopathy and paraproteinemia with serum IgM binding to a high-molecular-weight muscle fiber surface protein. *Ann Neurol* 37:41, 1995.

47. Gologan R, Dima I, Butoianu E, et al: Autoimmune hemolytic anemia with warm antibodies complicated with an intercurrent attack of hemolysis with cold agglutinins in a case of Waldenström disease. *Romanian J Intern Med* 34:149, 1996.

48. Varticovski L, Pick AI, Schattner A, Shoenfeld Y: Anti-platelet and anti-DNA IgM in Waldenström macroglobulinemia and ITP. *Am J Hematol* 24:351, 1987.

49. Sen HN, Chan CC, Caruso RC, et al: Waldenstrom's macroglobulinemia-associated retinopathy. *Ophthalmology* 111:535, 2004.

50. Lacroix-Desmazes S, Mouthon L, Pashov A, et al: Analysis of antibody reactivities toward self antigens of IgM of patients with Waldenström's macroglobulinemia. *Int Immunol* 9:1175, 1997.

51. Nobile-Orazio E, Francomano E, Daverio R, et al: Anti-myelin-associated glycoprotein IgM antibody titers in neuropathy associated with macroglobulinemia. *Ann Neurol* 26:543, 1989.

52. Steck AJ: Neurological manifestations of malignant and non-malignant dysglobulinaemias. *J Neurol* 245:634, 1998.

53. Sherman WH, Latov N, Hays AP, et al: Monoclonal IgM kappa antibody precipitating with chondroitin sulfate C from patients with axonal polyneuropathy and epidermolysis. *Neurology* 33:192, 1983.

54. Kira J, Inuzuka T, Hozumi I, et al: A novel monoclonal antibody which reacts with a high molecular weight neuronal cytoplasmic protein and myelin basic protein (MBP) in a patient with macroglobulinemia. *J Neurol Sci* 148:47, 1997.

55. Ilyas AA, Quarles RH, Dalakas MC, Brady RO: Polyneuropathy with monoclonal gammopathy: Glycolipids are frequently antigens for IgM paraproteins. *Proc Natl Acad Sci U S A* 82:6697, 1985.

56. Bosch EP, Smith BE: Peripheral neuropathies associated with monoclonal proteins. *Med Clin North Am* 77:125, 1993.

57. Latov N: Neuropathy, heredity, and monoclonal gammopathy. *Arch Neurol* 57:641, 2000.

58. Lieberman F, Marton LS, Stefansson K: Pattern of reactivity of IgM from the sera of eight patients with IgM monoclonal gammopathy and neuropathy with components of neural tissues: Evidence for interaction with more than one epitope. *Acta Neuropathol (Berl)* 68:196, 1985.

59. Dispenzieri A: Symptomatic cryoglobulinemia. *Curr Treat Options Oncol* 1:105, 2000.

60. Michael AB, Lawes M, Kamalarajan M, et al: Cryoglobulinaemia as an acute presentation of Waldenstrom's macroglobulinaemia. *Br J Haematol* 124:565, 2004.

61. Harbord M, Ivanova S, Akhtar N, Gupta Y: Waldenstrom macroglobulinaemia presenting as bleeding diathesis with paradoxical coagulation of blood samples. *J Accid Emerg Med* 15:331, 1998.

62. Penny R, Castaldi PA, Whitsed HM: Inflammation and haemostasis in paraproteinaemias. *Br J Haematol* 20:35, 1971.

63. Lackner H: Hemostatic abnormalities associated with dysproteinemias. *Semin Hematol* 10:125, 1973.

64. Wisloff F, Michaelsen TE, Godal HC: Monoclonal IgM with lupus anticoagulant activity in a case of Waldenström's macroglobulinaemia. *Eur J Haematol* 38:456, 1987.

65. Dimopoulos MA, Panayiotidis P, Moulopoulos LA, et al: Waldenstrom's macroglobulinemia: Clinical features, complications, and management. *J Clin Oncol* 18:214, 2000.

66. Owen RG, Treon SP, Al-Katib A, et al: Clinicopathological definition of Waldenstrom's macroglobulinemia: Consensus panel recommendations from the Second International Workshop on Waldenstrom's Macroglobulinemia. *Semin Oncol* 30:110, 2003.

67. Bakri K, Haydar AA, Davis J, et al: Waldenstrom's macroglobulinaemia presenting as isolated epistaxis: A common complaint but a rare cause. *Int J Clin Pract* 58:81, 2004.

68. Pinna A, Dore S, Dore F, et al: Bilateral optic disc swelling as the presenting sign of Waldenstrom's macroglobulinaemia. *Acta Ophthalmol Scand* 81:413, 2003.

69. Appenzeller P, Leith CP, Foucar K, et al: Cutaneous Waldenstrom macroglobulinemia in transformation. *Am J Dermatopathol* 21:151, 1999.

70. Klapper SR, Jordan DR, Pelletier C, et al: Ptosis in Waldenström's macroglobulinemia. *Am J Ophthalmol* 126:315, 1998.

71. Whittaker SJ, Bhogal BS, Black MM: Acquired immunobullous disease: A cutaneous manifestation of IgM macroglobulinaemia. *Br J Dermatol* 135:283, 1996.

72. West NY, Fitzpatrick JE, David-Bajar KM, Bennion SD: Waldenström macroglobulinemia-induced bullous dermatosis. *Arch Dermatol* 134:1127, 1998.

73. Becker LR, Bastian BC, Wesselmann U, et al: Paraneoplastic pemphigus treated with dexamethasone/cyclophosphamide pulse therapy. *Eur J Dermatol* 8:551, 1998.

74. Schadlow MB, Anhalt GJ, Sinha AA: Using rituximab (anti-CD20 antibody) in a patient with paraneoplastic pemphigus. *J Drugs Dermatol* 2:564, 2003.

75. Weinberg JM, Ioffreda M, White SM, et al: Purplish papules on the legs. Diagnosis: Type I cryoglobulinemia in association with WM. *Arch Dermatol* 136:1263, 2000.

76. Rudnicki SA, Harik SI, Dhodapkar M, et al: Nervous system dysfunction in Waldenström's macroglobulinemia: Response to treatment. *Neurology* 51:1210, 1998.

77. Rosenthal JA, Curran WJ Jr, Schuster SJ: Waldenström's macroglobulinemia resulting from localized gastric lymphoplasmacytoid lymphoma. *Am J Hematol* 58:244, 1998.

78. Kaila VL, el-Newihi HM, Dreiling BJ, et al: Waldenström's macroglobulinemia of the stomach presenting with upper gastrointestinal hemorrhage. *Gastrointest Endosc* 44:73, 1996.

79. Fadil A, Taylor DE: The lung and Waldenström's macroglobulinemia. *South Med J* 91:681, 1998.

80. Zatloukal P, Bezdícek P, Schimonová M, et al: Waldenström's macroglobulinemia with pulmonary amyloidosis. *Respiration* 65:414, 1998.

81. Pavord SR, Murphy PT, Mitchell VE: POEMS syndrome and Waldenström's macroglobulinaemia. *J Clin Pathol* 49:181, 1996.

82. Persson SU, Larsson H, Odeberg H: How should blood rheology be measured in macroglobulinaemia? *Scand J Clin Lab Invest* 58:669, 1998.

83. Pavy MD, Murphy PL, Virella G: Paraprotein-induced hyperviscosity. A reversible cause of stroke. *Postgrad Med* 68:109, 1980.

84. Mueller J, Hotson JR, Langston JW: Hyperviscosity-induced dementia. *Neurology* 33:101, 1983.

85. Lekhra OP, Sawhney IM, Gupta A, et al: Venous stasis retinopathy in Waldenstrom's macroglobulinemia. *J Assoc Physicians India* 44:61, 1996.

86. Avashia JH, Fath DF: Bilateral central retinal vein occlusion in Waldenstrom's macroglobulinemia. *J Am Optom Assoc* 60:657, 1989.

87. Axelrod O, Silverman GJ, Dev V, et al: Idiotypic cross-reactivity of immunoglobulins expressed in Waldenstrom's macroglobulinemia, chronic lymphocytic leukemia, and mantle zone lymphocytes of secondary B-cell follicles. *Blood* 77:1484, 1991.

88. MacKenzie MR, Fudenberg HH: Macroglobulinemia: An analysis for forty patients. *Blood* 39:874, 1972.

89. Smith BR, Robert NJ, Ault KA: In Waldenstrom's macroglobulinemia the quantity of detectable circulating monoclonal B lymphocytes correlates with clinical course. *Blood* 61:911, 1983.

90. Jensen GS, Andrews EJ, Mant MJ, et al: Transitions in CD45 isoform expression indicate continuous differentiation of a monoclonal CD5+

CD11b+ B lineage in Waldenstrom's macroglobulinemia. *Am J Hematol* 37:20, 1991.

91. San Miguel JF, Vidriales MB, Ocio E, et al: Immunophenotypic analysis of Waldenstrom's macroglobulinemia. *Semin Oncol* 30:187, 2003.

92. Andriko JA, Aguilera NS, Chu WS, et al: Waldenström's macroglobulinemia: A clinicopathologic study of 22 cases. *Cancer* 80:1926, 1997.

93. Pettersson D, Mellstedt H, Holm G: Characterization of the monoclonal blood and bone marrow B lymphocytes in Waldenstrom's macroglobulinaemia. *Scand J Immunol* 11:593, 1980.

94. Krumdieck R, Shaw DR, Huang ST, et al: Hemorrhagic disorder due to an isoniazid-associated acquired factor XIII inhibitor in a patient with Waldenstrom's macroglobulinemia. *Am J Med* 90:639, 1991.

95. Doumenc J, Prost RJ, Samama M, Bousser J: [Anomalies of platelet aggregation during Waldenstrom's disease. (Apropos of 3 cases)] Anomalie de l'agregation plaquettaire au cours de la maladie de Waldenstrom. (A propos de 3 cas.). *Nouv Rev Fr Hematol* 6:734, 1966.

96. Kyle RA: Monoclonal gammopathies and the kidney. *Annu Rev Med* 40:53, 1989.

97. Krajny M, Pruzanski W: Waldenstrom's macroglobulinemia: Review of 45 cases. *CMAJ* 114:899, 1976.

98. Morel-Maroger L, Basch A, Danon F, et al: Pathology of the kidney in Waldenstrom's macroglobulinemia. Study of sixteen cases. *N Engl J Med* 283:123, 1970.

99. Solomon A, Weiss DT, Macy SD, Antonucci RA: Immunocytochemical detection of kappa and lambda light chain V region subgroups in human B-cell malignancies. *Am J Pathol* 137:855, 1990.

100. Harada Y, Ido N, Okada T, et al: Nephrotic syndrome caused by protein thrombi in glomerulocapillary lumen in Waldenstrom's macroglobulinaemia. *Br J Haematol* 110:880, 2000.

101. Martelo OJ, Schultz DR, Pardo V, Perez-Stable E: Immunologically-mediated renal disease in Waldenstrom's macroglobulinemia. *Am J Med* 58:567, 1975.

102. Lindstrom FD, Hed J, Enestrom S: Renal pathology of Waldenstrom's macroglobulinaemia with monoclonal antiglomerular antibodies and nephrotic syndrome. *Clin Exp Immunol* 41:196, 1980.

103. Quaglino D, Di Leonardo G, Pasqualoni E, et al: Therapeutic management of hematological malignancies in elderly patients. Biological and clinical considerations. Part IV: Multiple myeloma and Waldenström's macroglobulinemia. *Aging* 10:5, 1998.

104. Owen RG, Barrans SL, Richards SJ, et al: Waldenstrom macroglobulinemia. Development of diagnostic criteria and identification of prognostic factors. *Am J Clin Pathol* 116:420, 2001.

105. Ghobrial IM, Witzig TE: Waldenstrom macroglobulinemia. *Curr Treat Options Oncol* 5:239, 2004.

106. Lim W, Shumak KH, Reis M, et al: Malignant evolution of Schnitzler's syndrome—Chronic urticaria and IgM monoclonal gammopathy: Report of a new case and review of the literature. *Leuk Lymphoma* 43:181, 2002.

107. Gertz MA, Anagnostopoulos A, Anderson K, et al: Treatment recommendations in Waldenstrom's macroglobulinemia: Consensus panel recommendations from the Second International Workshop on Waldenstrom's Macroglobulinemia. *Semin Oncol* 30:121, 2003.

108. Kyle RA, Greipp PR, Gertz MA, et al: Waldenstrom's macroglobulinaemia: A prospective study comparing daily with intermittent oral chlorambucil. *Br J Haematol* 108:737, 2000.

109. Case DCJ, Ervin TJ, Boyd MA, Redfield DL: Waldenstrom's macroglobulinemia: Long-term results with the M-2 protocol. *Cancer Invest* 9:1, 1991.

110. Petrucci MT, Avvisati G, Tribalto M, et al: Waldenstrom's macroglobulinaemia: Results of a combined oral treatment in 34 newly diagnosed patients. *J Intern Med* 226:443, 1989.

111. Leblond V, Levy V, Maloisel F, et al: Multicenter, randomized comparative trial of fludarabine and the combination of cyclophosphamide-doxorubicin-prednisone in 92 patients with Waldenstrom macroglobulinemia in first relapse or with primary refractory disease. *Blood* 98:2640, 2001.

112. Weber DM, Dimopoulos MA, Delasalle K, et al: 2-Chlorodeoxyadenosine alone and in combination for previously untreated Waldenstrom's macroglobulinemia. *Semin Oncol* 30:243, 2003.

113. Dimopoulos MA, Kantarjian H, Estey E, et al: Treatment of Waldenstrom macroglobulinemia with 2-chlorodeoxyadenosine. *Ann Intern Med* 118:195, 1993.

114. Delannoy A, Ferrant A, Martiat P, et al: 2-Chlorodeoxyadenosine therapy in Waldenstrom's macroglobulinaemia. *Nouv Rev Fr Hematol* 36:317, 1994.

115. Dimopoulos MA, Weber D, Delasalle KB, et al: Treatment of Waldenstrom's macroglobulinemia resistant to standard therapy with 2-chlorodeoxyadenosine: Identification of prognostic factors. *Ann Oncol* 6:49, 1995.

116. Fridrik MA, Jäger G, Baldinger C, et al: First-line treatment of Waldenström's disease with cladribine. Arbeitsgemeinschaft Medikamentöse Tumortherapie. *Ann Hematol* 74:7, 1997.

117. Liu ES, Burian C, Miller WE, Saven A: Bolus administration of cladribine in the treatment of Waldenström macroglobulinaemia. *Br J Haematol* 103:690, 1998.

118. Hellmann A, Lewandowski K, Zaucha JM, et al: Effect of a 2-hour infusion of 2-chlorodeoxyadenosine in the treatment of refractory or previously untreated Waldenstrom's macroglobulinemia. *Eur J Haematol* 63:35, 1999.

119. Dimopoulos MA, Weber DM, Kantarjian H, et al: 2Chlorodeoxyadenosine therapy of patients with Waldenström macroglobulinemia previously treated with fludarabine. *Ann Oncol* 5:288, 1994.

120. Lewandowski K, Halaburda K, Hellmann A: Fludarabine therapy in Waldenstrom's macroglobulinemia patients treated previously with 2-chlorodeoxyadenosine. *Leuk Lymphoma* 43:361, 2002.

121. Betticher DC, Hsu Schmitz SF, Ratschiller D, et al: Cladribine (2-CDA) given as subcutaneous bolus injections is active in pretreated Waldenström's macroglobulinaemia. Swiss Group for Clinical Cancer Research (SAKK). *Br J Haematol* 99:358, 1997.

122. Laurencet FM, Zulian GB, Guetty-Alberto M, et al: Cladribine with cyclophosphamide and prednisone in the management of low-grade lymphoproliferative malignancies. *Br J Cancer* 79:1215, 1999.

123. Van Den Neste E, Delannoy A, Vandercam B, et al: Infectious complications after 2-chlorodeoxyadenosine therapy. *Eur J Haematol* 56:235, 1996.

124. Wong SS, Woo PC, Yuen KY: Candida tropicalis and Penicillium marneffei mixed fungaemia in a patient with Waldenstrom's macroglobulinaemia. *Eur J Clin Microbiol Infect Dis* 20:132, 2001.

125. Niesvizky R, Zhu AX, Louie D, Michaeli J: Epstein-Barr virus-associated lymphoma after treatment of macroglobulinemia with cladribine [letter]. *N Engl J Med* 341:55, 1999.

126. Krishna VM, Carey RW, Bloch KJ: Marked increase in serum IgM during treatment of Waldenstrom's macroglobulinemia with cladribine. *N Engl J Med* 348:2045, 2003.

127. Tetreault SA, Saven A: Delayed onset of autoimmune hemolytic anemia complicating cladribine therapy for Waldenstrom macroglobulinemia. *Leuk Lymphoma* 37:125, 2000.

128. Kantarjian HM, Alexanian R, Koller CA, et al: Fludarabine therapy in macroglobulinemic lymphoma. *Blood* 75:1928, 1990.

129. Dimopoulos MA, O'Brien S, Kantarjian H, et al: Fludarabine therapy in Waldenstrom's macroglobulinemia. *Am J Med* 95:49, 1993.

130. Zinzani PL, Gherlinzoni F, Bendandi M, et al: Fludarabine treatment in resistant Waldenstrom's macroglobulinemia. *Eur J Haematol* 54:120, 1995.

131. O'Brien S, Kantarjian H, Keating MJ: Purine analogs in chronic lymphocytic leukemia and Waldenström's macroglobulinemia. *Ann Oncol* 7(suppl 6):S27, 1996.

132. Foran JM, Rohatiner AZ, Coiffier B, et al: Multicenter phase II study of fludarabine phosphate for patients with newly diagnosed lymphoplasmacytoid lymphoma, Waldenström's macroglobulinemia, and mantle-cell lymphoma. *J Clin Oncol* 17:546, 1999.

133. Thalhammer-Scherrer R, Geissler K, Schwarzinger I, et al: Fludarabine therapy in Waldenstrom's macroglobulinemia. *Ann Hematol* 79:556, 2000.

134. Dhodapkar MV, Jacobson JL, Gertz MA, et al: Prognostic factors and response to fludarabine therapy in patients with Waldenstrom macroglobulinemia: Results of United States intergroup trial (Southwest Oncology Group S9003). *Blood* 98:41, 2001.

135. Dimopoulos MA, Hamilos G, Efstathiou E, et al: Treatment of Waldenstrom's macroglobulinemia with the combination of fludarabine and cyclophosphamide. *Leuk Lymphoma* 44:993, 2003.

136. Leblond V, Choquet S: Fludarabine in Waldenstrom's macroglobulinemia. *Semin Oncol* 30:239, 2003.

137. Costa P, Luzzati R, Nicolato A, et al: Cryptococcal meningitis and intracranial tuberculoma in a patient with Waldenstrom's macroglobulinemia treated with fludarabine. *Leuk Lymphoma* 28:617, 1998.

138. Björkholm M, Celsing F, Runarsson G, Waldenström J: Successful intravenous immunoglobulin therapy for severe and persistent astrovirus gastroenteritis after fludarabine treatment in a patient with Waldenström's macroglobulinemia. *Int J Hematol* 62:117, 1995.

139. Treon SP, Agus DB, Link B, et al: CD20-directed antibody-mediated immunotherapy induces responses and facilitates hematologic recovery in patients with Waldenstrom's macroglobulinemia. *J Immunother* 24: 272, 2001.

140. Dimopoulos MA, Zervas C, Zomas A, et al: Treatment of Waldenstrom's macroglobulinemia with rituximab. *J Clin Oncol* 20:2327, 2002.

141. Pestronk A, Florence J, Miller T, et al: Treatment of IgM antibody associated polyneuropathies using rituximab. *J Neurol Neurosurg Psychiatry* 74:485, 2003.

142. Buda-Okreglak EM, Drabick JJ, Delaney NR: Proinflammatory syndrome mimicking acute rheumatoid arthritis in a patient with Waldenstrom's macroglobulinemia treated with rituximab. *Ann Hematol* 83: 117, 2004.

143. Salisbury JR, Rapson NT, Codd JD, et al: Immunohistochemical analysis of CDw52 antigen expression in non-Hodgkin's lymphomas. *J Clin Pathol* 47:313, 1994.

144. Kondo H, Yokoyama K: IgM myeloma: Different features from multiple myeloma and macroglobulinaemia. *Eur J Haematol* 63:366, 1999.

145. Gertz MA: Waldenstrom's macroglobulinemia: A review of therapy. *Leuk Lymphoma* 43:1517, 2002.

146. Yonemura K, Suzuki T, Sano K, et al: A case with acute renal failure complicated by Waldenstrom's macroglobulinemia and cryoglobulinemia. *Ren Fail* 22:511, 2000.

147. Rajkumar SV, Kyle RA: Thalidomide in the treatment of plasma cell malignancies. *J Clin Oncol* 19:3593, 2001.

148. Dimopoulos MA, Zomas A, Viniou NA, et al: Treatment of Waldenstrom's macroglobulinemia with thalidomide. *J Clin Oncol* 19:3596, 2001.

149. Coleman M, Leonard J, Lyons L, et al: BLT-D (clarithromycin [Biaxin], low-dose thalidomide, and dexamethasone) for the treatment of myeloma and Waldenstrom's macroglobulinemia. *Leuk Lymphoma* 43:1777, 2002.

150. Desikan R, Li Z, Jagannath S: Waldenstrom's macroglobulinaemia: Current therapy and future approaches. *BioDrugs* 16:201, 2002.

151. Myers B, Grimley C, Dolan G: Thalidomide and low-dose dexamethasone in myeloma treatment. *Br J Haematol* 114:245, 2001.

152. Dimopoulos MA, Zervas K, Kouvatseas G, et al: Thalidomide and dexamethasone combination for refractory multiple myeloma. *Ann Oncol* 12:991, 2001.

153. Mitsiades CS, Mitsiades N, Richardson PG, et al: Novel biologically based therapies for Waldenstrom's macroglobulinemia. *Semin Oncol* 30: 309, 2003.

154. Adams J, Kauffman M: Development of the proteasome inhibitor Velcade (Bortezomib). *Cancer Invest* 22:304, 2004.

155. Adams J: The development of proteasome inhibitors as anticancer drugs. *Cancer Cell* 5:417, 2004.

156. Rosato RR, Grant S: Histone deacetylase inhibitors in clinical development. *Expert Opin Investig Drugs* 13:21, 2004.

157. Vigushin DM, Coombes RC: Targeted histone deacetylase inhibition for cancer therapy. *Curr Cancer Drug Targets* 4:205, 2004.

158. Goetz MP, Toft DO, Ames MM, Erlichman C: The Hsp90 chaperone complex as a novel target for cancer therapy. *Ann Oncol* 14:1169, 2003.

159. Vela-Ojeda J, Garcia-Ruiz Esparza MA, Padilla-Gonzalez Y, et al: IFN-alpha as induction and maintenance treatment of patients newly diagnosed with Waldenstrom's macroglobulinemia. *J Interferon Cytokine Res* 22:1013, 2002.

160. Anagnostopoulos A, Giralt S: Stem cell transplantation (SCT) for Waldenstrom's macroglobulinemia (WM). *Bone Marrow Transplant* 29: 943, 2002.

161. Anagnostopoulos A, Aleman A, Giralt S: Autologous and allogeneic stem cell transplantation in Waldenstrom's macroglobulinemia: Review of the literature and future directions. *Semin Oncol* 30:286, 2003.

162. Tournilhac O, Leblond V, Tabrizi R, et al: Transplantation in Waldenstrom's macroglobulinemia—The French experience. *Semin Oncol* 30: 291, 2003.

163. Patel TC, Moore SB, Pineda AA, Witzig TE: Role of plasmapheresis in thrombocytopenic purpura associated with Waldenström's macroglobulinemia. *Mayo Clin Proc* 71:597, 1996.

164. Höffkes HG, Heemann UW, Teschendorf C, et al: Hyperviscosity syndrome: Efficacy and comparison of plasma exchange by plasma separation and cascade filtration in patients with immunocytoma of Waldenström's type. *Clin Nephrol* 43:335, 1995.

165. Clark WF, Rock GA, Buskard N, et al: Therapeutic plasma exchange: An update from the Canadian Apheresis Group. *Ann Intern Med* 131: 453, 1999.

166. Siami GA, Siami FS: Plasmapheresis and paraproteinemia: Cryoprotein-induced diseases, monoclonal gammopathy, Waldenström's macroglobulinemia, hyperviscosity syndrome, multiple myeloma, light chain disease, and amyloidosis. *Ther Apher* 3:8, 1999.

167. Humphrey JS, Conley CL: Durable complete remission of macroglobulinemia after splenectomy: A report of two cases and review of the literature. *Am J Hematol* 48:262, 1995.

168. Takemori N, Hirai K, Onodera R, et al: Durable remission after splenectomy for Waldenstrom's macroglobulinemia with massive splenomegaly in leukemic phase. *Leuk Lymphoma* 26:387, 1997.

169. Dimopoulos MA, Hamilos G, Zervas K, et al: Survival and prognostic factors after initiation of treatment in Waldenstrom's macroglobulinemia. *Ann Oncol* 14:1299, 2003.

170. Gobbi PG, Bettini R, Montecucco C, et al: Study of prognosis in Waldenström's macroglobulinemia: A proposal for a simple binary classification with clinical and investigational utility. *Blood* 83:2939, 1994.

171. Marinella MA, Kim MH, Anderson MM: Waldenstrom's macroglobulinemia transformed into immunoblastic lymphoma presenting with malignant ascites [letter]. *Am J Hematol* 51:249, 1996.

172. Beaudreuil J, Lortholary O, Martin A, et al: Hypercalcemia may indicate Richter's syndrome: Report of four cases and review. *Cancer* 79:1211, 1997.

173. Salberg D, Kurtides S, McKeever WP: Monomyelocytic leukemia in an

untreated case of Waldenstrom macroglobulinemia. *Arch Intern Med* 137:514, 1977.

174. Rodríguez JN, Fernández-Jurado A, Martino ML, Prados D: Waldenström's macroglobulinemia complicated with acute myeloid leukemia. Report of a case and review of the literature [letter]. *Haematologica* 83: 91, 1998.

175. Leonhard SA, Muhleman AF, Hurtubise PE, Martelo OJ: Emergence of immunoblastic sarcoma in Waldenstrom's macroglobulinemia. *Cancer* 45:3102, 1980.

176. Emmerich B, Pemsl M, Wust I, et al: Conversion of an IGM secreting immunocytoma in a high grade malignant lymphoma of immunoblastic type. *Blut* 46:81, 1983.

177. Vitali C, Bombardieri S, Spremolla G: Chronic myeloid leukemia in Waldenstrom's macroglobulinemia. *Arch Intern Med* 141:1349, 1981.

HEAVY-CHAIN DISEASES

JOEL N. BUXBAUM

ALICE ALEXANDER

**The heavy-chain diseases are rare monoclonal B cell prolifer-
ative disorders in which the immunoglobulin product of the
neoplastic cells is a truncated heavy chain unattached to a light
chain. Historically, analysis of the domain structure of the γ
heavy-chain disease proteins provided one of the early clues to
the exon-intron structure of immunoglobulin genes. The aberrant proteins are the products of deletion (and perhaps insertion) events that may have occurred in the transformed B
cell clone during the process of gene rearrangement responsible
for normal immunoglobulin synthesis or possibly while undergoing the hypermutation required for antibody diversification
and affinity maturation in germinal centers. The diagnosis is
established by immunoelectrophoresis or immunofixation of serum, urine, or (in the case of α heavy-chain diseases) secretory
fluids, or by immunohistologic analysis of the proliferating
cells. The heavy-chain diseases behave clinically as B cell lymphomas of varying degrees of aggressiveness. The exception is
α heavy-chain disease. Early in its course, it is a reversible
monoclonal disorder, possibly arising during the response to
one or more infectious agents, and curable by intensive antibiotic treatment. Beyond that stage, its prognosis is variable.
Few definitive data support specific treatment of the lymphomatous forms of any of the heavy-chain diseases.**

DEFINITION AND HISTORY

The heavy-chain diseases (HCDs) are proliferative disorders of B cells
that synthesize and secrete incomplete immunoglobulin (Ig) heavy (H)
chains. These diseases initially were recognized as gammopathies by
the presence of monoclonal proteins in the patients' serum or urine.
The disorders were defined in terms of the production of structurally
aberrant Ig. Because the neoplastic cells displayed plasmacytic features, they were viewed as myeloma variants and were studied for the
insights they could provide into Ig structure. The immunochemical
description of the first HCD protein suggested that the γ chain was
divided into domains. Moreover, it raised the possibility the domains
were encoded by separate genes (or gene segments), an insight recalled
in the first publications describing the actual structure of murine Ig
heavy-chain genes.[1] The original definition, which remains valid for
clinical diagnostic purposes, demanded that patients' sera or urine contain a deleted Ig H chain without a bound L chain.[2,3] Later work demonstrated that heavy-chain molecules with similar structures could be
identified within the neoplastic cells of some cases of so-called nonsecretory myeloma or lymphoma or in tissue deposits that compromised
organ function in heavy-chain or light-chain and heavy-chain deposition disease.[4,5] In some instances, defective Ig light chains could also
be identified.[6] In μ-HCD, despite the absence of Ig light chains in the
serum protein, the μ-fragment–synthesizing cells produce L chains in
the majority of cases. Even in the first case of μ-HCD, intact Ig light
chains were identified in the proliferating cells, but they were not covalently linked to the μ fragment in either the cells or the serum.[7,8]
Although the identification of HCD proteins is still largely consistent
with the original criteria, variations on the theme, detectable by more
precise molecular techniques, have allowed an expanded view of the
circumstances leading to production of the benchmark proteins.

ETIOLOGY AND PATHOGENESIS

The etiology of the HCDs is not known. Some of the factors responsible for this disease may be similar to the factors involved in the
etiology and pathogenesis of plasma cell myeloma or chronic lymphocytic leukemia (CLL). In one instance, an N-*ras* mutation was
found in the bone marrow and a cell line generated from the peripheral
blood of a γ-HCD patient.[9] Chapters 90 and 98 discuss the etiology
of plasmacytic and lymphocytic disorders.

The observations that none of the HCDs resemble plasma cell myeloma or Waldenström macroglobulinemia stimulated investigations
into the nature of the HCD cell and attempts to place it somewhere in
the relatively orderly scheme of B cell differentiation (see Chap. 76).
Although the infiltrates contain plasma cells, the predominant cell is
a lymphocyte, perhaps more precisely reflecting the nature of the tumor stem cell that retains some capacity to mature. Molecular studies
have suggested that these cells most likely arose in germinal centers,
because the Ig gene abnormalities appear to reflect mechanisms that
are associated with the normal process of somatic hypermutation responsible for generating diversity in Ig hypervariable regions.[10,11]

CHRONIC ANTIGENIC STIMULATION

Infection is thought to play the major role in the development of α-
chain disease. The disorder is usually found in nonindustrialized societies in which gastrointestinal infections are common.[12] A causal
relationship between infection and pathogenesis is supported by the
observation that early stages of the disease can be successfully treated
with antibiotics alone (see "Therapy, Course, Prognosis" below).

There is a high frequency of autoimmune disorders preceding or
concurrent with the diagnosis of HCD, particularly of the γ class.[13]
This mode of autoreactive immunostimulation may be related to γ-
HCD pathogenesis in the same fashion as immunostimulatory exposure to gastrointestinal organisms is associated with the development
of α-HCD.

STRUCTURAL ANALYSIS OF DEFECTIVE Ig MOLECULES

DEFECTIVE γ HEAVY CHAINS
Structural analysis of the defective monoclonal γ heavy chains of 23
patients with γ-HCD reveals several characteristic features (Fig. 103-
1A). In two cases, OMM[14] and RIV,[15] cDNA and genomic sequence
data also are available. The proteins usually initiate with a normal
variable (V)-region amino acid sequence. In most cases, the sequence
is short and abruptly interrupted by a large deletion encompassing the
remainder of the V region, although four of the proteins shown in
Figure 103-1A appear to have retained all or most of the V, D, and J
sequences.[16–19] In all γ-HCD proteins, the entire C_H1 domain is also
deleted, with normal sequence resuming at the hinge (or occasionally
the C_H2 domain). No light chains are associated with the defective H
chains, which usually are found in the serum as disulfide-linked dimers.[20]

DEFECTIVE α HEAVY CHAINS
As a group, the α chains of patients with α-HCD have features similar
to those seen in the defective γ chains of the patients with γ-HCD.

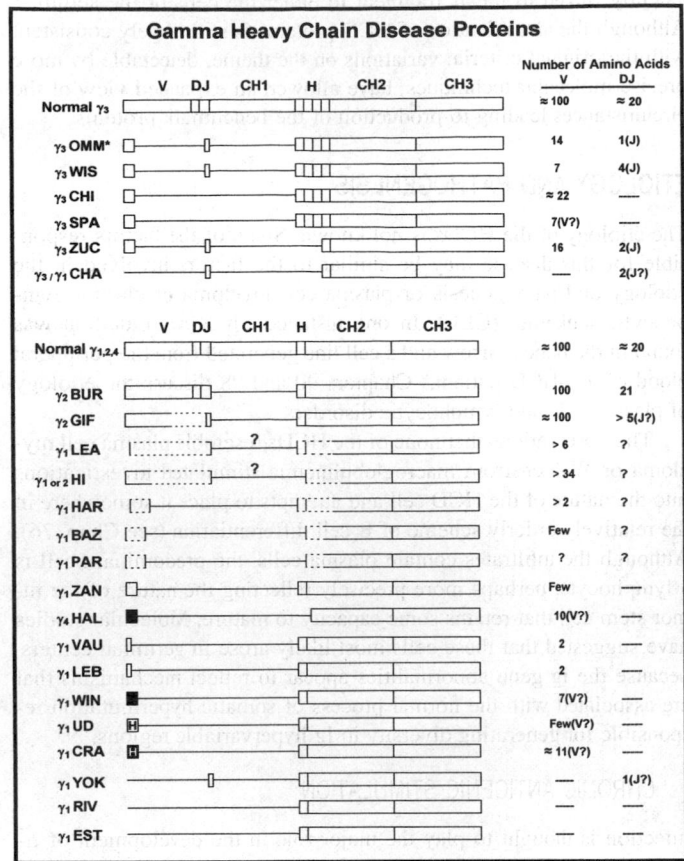

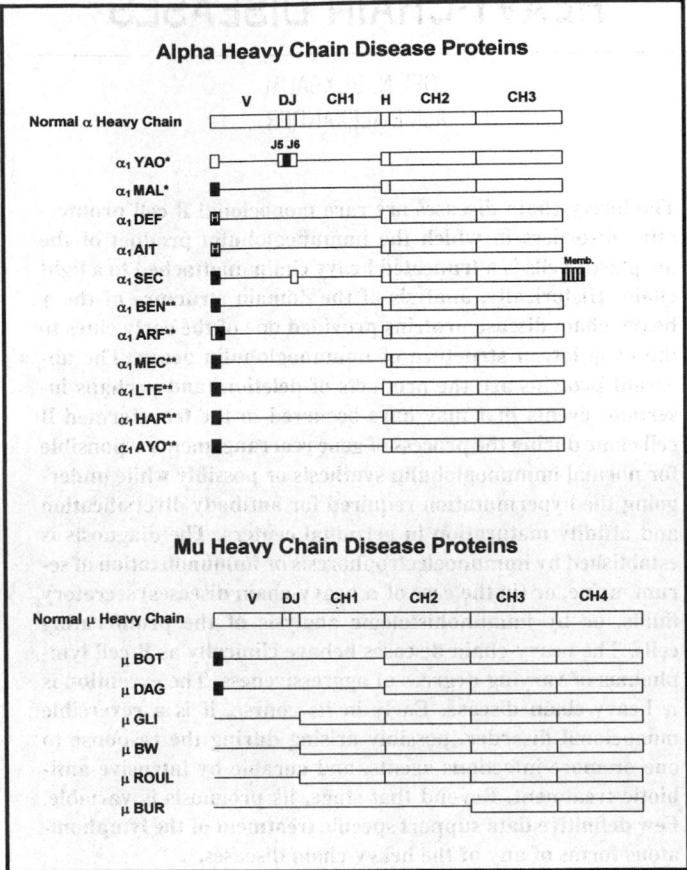

A   **B**

FIGURE 103-1   *(A, B)* *Structures are primary synthetic protein products synthesized by HCD cells. Serum proteins were modified after synthesis and did not contain any amino acids before the hinge. **Structures are deduced amino acid sequences determined by cDNA sequencing. *H* indicates heterogeneous amino acid sequences. ■ indicates unusual amino acid sequences. *Boxes* indicate coding regions. *Lines* indicate deletions. *Dashed lines* indicate likely structures for which sequence data are missing. ? indicates probable missing domain based on molecular weight and partial protein structure analysis. CH1, CH2, CH3, CH4, constant regions of heavy chains; D, diversity segment; H, hinge region; J, joining region; Memb., membrane exon; V, variable region. OMM,[14] WIS,[52] CHI,[53] SPA,[54] ZUC,[55] CHA,[56] γBUR,[16] GIF,[17] LEA,[18] HI,[19] HAR,[18] BAZ,[57] PAR,[58] ZAN,[59] HAL,[60] VAU, LEB,[61] WIN,[26] UD,[62] CRA,[63] YOK,[64] RIV,[15] EST,[65] YAO,[66] MAL,[27] DEF,[67] AIT,[68] SEC,[21] BEN, ARF, MEC, LTE, HAR, AYO,[69] BOT,[70] DAG,[71] GLI,[25] BW,[22] ROUL,[24] μBUR.[72]

These features include deleted V regions, missing C$_H$1 domains, and the absence of associated light chains. In cases where amino acid or nucleotide sequence data are available (see Fig. 103-1*B*), most of the proteins have short, non–Ig-related sequences of unknown origin at the amino-terminus.[21]

Figure 103-2 shows the genomic structures of the genes encoding three α-HCD proteins. As in the γ-HCD genes OMM and RIV, strikingly similar noncontiguous deletions are present in the V/J and switch/C$_H$1 regions of the α heavy-chain genes. The genomic structures show that the non-Ig coding regions actually are part of larger regions containing unusual sequences of varying length, which include noncoding and coding sequences. The inserted regions show no homology to any known sequences, and their mechanism of origin is unclear.

DEFECTIVE μ HEAVY CHAINS

Like the defective heavy chains of patients with the other classes of HCD, the μ-HCD proteins contain large V-region deletions (see Fig. 103-1*B*). In contrast to the other classes, the μ proteins often contain intact constant regions including the C$_H$1 domains.[22]

The gene sequence data are available for only one μ-HCD protein (Fig. 103-2). It encodes a normal μ constant region containing C$_H$1.

The VDJ region is present but has a single base deletion producing a frameshift that generates three stop codons. An inserted stretch of nucleotides immediately 3′ to J destroyed the J donor splice site, causing the cell to splice the 3′ donor site of the leader exon directly to the acceptor of the C$_H$1 domain, eliminating the V-region sequences from the mature mRNA.

IG LIGHT CHAINS

Many patients with μ-HCD also synthesize monoclonal L chains, detectable as Bence-Jones proteins in serum and/or urine. In some cases, immunofluorescence showed that the same cells produced both the light and heavy chains.[23,24] The light chains can associate with the short H chains in the serum but do not form covalent bridges, even in cases where the C$_H$1 domain, which contains the cysteine capable of forming the H-L interchain disulfide bond, is present.[25] Monoclonal Ig light-chain production is rare in patients with γ-HCD or α-HCD, but synthesis of truncated fragments has been noted.[20,26–28]

GENETIC BASIS FOR DEFECTIVE IgS

The structural features of the HCD proteins can be interpreted in terms of our knowledge of Ig gene structure. As expected for secretory proteins, HCD genes encode a leader peptide, which is cleaved from the molecule before secretion. If the HCD gene contains intact V and J splice sites, those regions will be present in the mature mRNA and primary synthetic product, even if they contain extensive deletions, insertions, or other in-frame mutations. If no intact V or J splice sequences are present, the donor splice site of the leader peptide will be joined to the next available splice acceptor site (see Fig. 103-2).

The presence of large deletions in the switch/C_H1 regions of the five γ-HCD and α-HCD genes sequenced to date explain why the corresponding HCD proteins lack C_H1. Because the normal C_H1 acceptor splice site is deleted, the donor splice site of the leader, or J region, is spliced directly to the next available functional splice acceptor site at the beginning of the hinge or C_H2 domain. Other HCD proteins with missing C_H1 domains would be expected to contain similar switch/C_H1 deletions in their DNA. Thus, deletions and mutations of coding regions and splice sites explain why entire domains can be missing from the cytoplasmic mRNA and protein.

Any explanation for the origin of HCD proteins must account for the three main defects in HCD cells: the two noncontiguous deletions in the V/J and switch/C_H1 regions of the heavy chains and the absence of associated light chains. If the HCD abnormalities occur at random, it should be possible to isolate molecules from serum displaying any combination of the three defects. Normal heavy chains unassociated with light chains have never been identified in serum. Biosynthetic studies of Ig-secreting cells have shown that, in the absence of light chains, the C_H1 domain of heavy chains will bind to heavy-chain binding protein (BiP), a heat shock protein inside the cell and undergo degradation rather than secretion.[29] If light chains are present, they will bind to the C_H1 domain of the heavy chain and prevent the attachment to BiP. Four characterized γ-HCD proteins contain C_H1 deletions and appear to have intact VDJ regions.[16–19] In the synthesizing cells, the absence of light chains does not prevent secretion of the aberrant heavy chains because the C_H1 domain is missing. Thus, the proteins cannot bind BiP. γ-HCD and α-HCD proteins containing only the V/J deletion and intact C_H1 domains have not been described. Such proteins might be synthesized but would not be secreted in the absence of L chains because of intracellular binding of BiP by the C_H1 domain. This situation was demonstrated in a study of a nonsecreting myeloma, which did not produce L chains but synthesized heavy chains that lacked the VDJ region and had an intact C_H1 domain.[30] The abnormal H chains were shown to undergo intracellular degradation rather than secretion.

Whether the V/J or switch/C_H1 deletion occurs first in HCD cells is unclear, and whether the first deletion influences the second deletion is not known. Abnormal VDJ recombination, as an initial event, is suggested by the finding of a significant fraction of cells with aberrant joins when normal human peripheral mononuclear cells are exposed to Epstein-Barr virus (EBV).[31] If the cells persist after EBV infection or are generated at some rate throughout life, they could represent potential tumor stem cells. However, deletion of the V region during VDJ joining would render the early B cell unable to synthesize membrane Ig containing a normal antigen-combining site, and such cells could no longer be stimulated by antigen cognate for the original antibody. Because switching is generally considered an antigen-dependent event, and most HCD cells have switched from μ to γ or α, the occurrence of a V-region deletion before switching would require the isotype change to be driven by an antigen-independent mechanism such as cytokine stimulation or a proliferative oncogenic event.

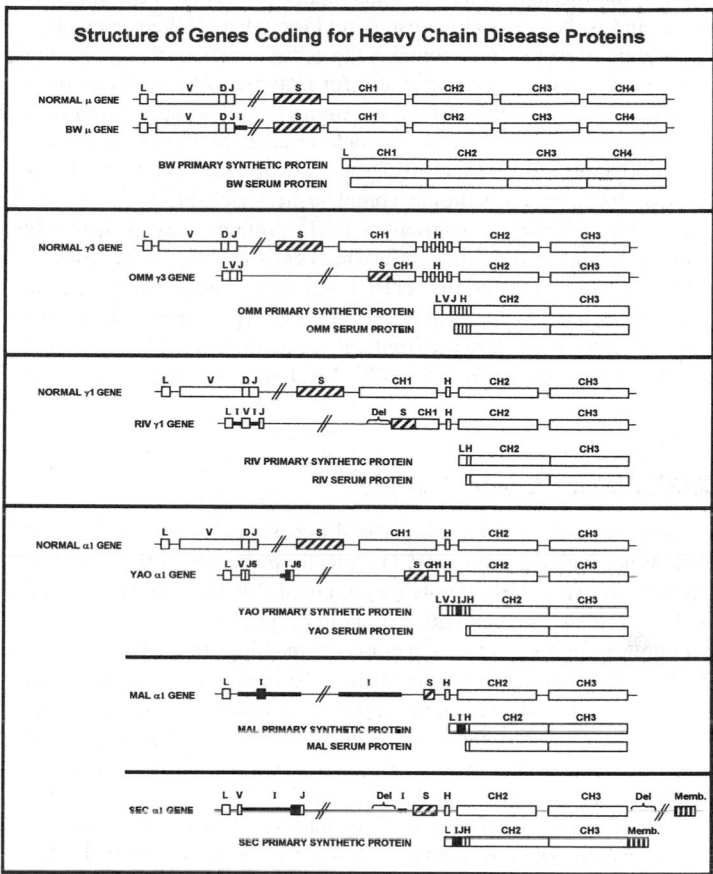

FIGURE 103-2 *Boxes* indicate coding regions. *Hatched box* indicates switch region. ■ indicates inserted coding sequence. ■ indicates inserted noncoding sequence. *Lines* indicate intervening (noncoding) sequences. CH1, CH2, CH3, CH4, constant regions of heavy chains; D, diversity segment; Del, deleted sequence; H, hinge region; I, inserted sequence; J, joining region; L, leader region; Memb., membrane exon; S, switch region; V, variable region. BW,[22] OMM,[14] RIV,[15] YAO,[66] MAL,[27] SEC.[21]

The switch-region deletion as the initial abnormality is suggested by the existence of four γ-HCD proteins (see Fig. 103-1A) that appear to possess intact V regions and switch/C_H1 deletions.[16–19] Alternatively, these molecules may represent a category of HCD proteins arising by a different, independent mechanism, either related to or as a result of oncogenic transformation.

The V-region deletions and insertions in HCD may be a consequence of the normal somatic hypermutation process. During affinity maturation of normal B cells, a process localized to germinal centers, the visible consequences of hypermutation are single base substitutions rather than deletions or insertions. However, a study involving single-cell polymerase chain reaction analysis of normal human lymphocytes showed that deletions and insertions also were common in germinal center-derived B cells undergoing hypermutation but were rare in naive pregerminal center cells.[10,11] The role of this mechanism in the generation of V-region deletions in HCD would be strengthened if the cells synthesizing the abnormal proteins in the patients were shown to carry germinal center markers.

HCD proteins of the γ_3 and α_1 classes are overrepresented relative to their frequency among intact human Ig proteins. The reason for this finding is not known. However, it is noteworthy that the Ig H-chain genes encoding these two heavy chains are arranged in two closely linked clusters in germ-line DNA (see Chap. 77). The first cluster contains the μ/δ pair, followed sequentially by the genes encoding the γ_3, γ_1, and α_1 heavy-chain constant regions, whereas the second cluster, located 3' to the first, contains the genes encoding the γ_2, γ_4, and α_2 constant regions. The preference for isotypes of the first cluster in HCD may be a function of their proximity to μ. Switching from μ to an isotype in the second cluster would require the switching mechanism to operate over greater distances, possibly decreasing the likelihood of forming a functional complete heavy-chain gene. Alternatively, the switch/C_H1 deletion in HCD proteins may prematurely terminate a sequential process, in which cells initially switch from μ to another isotype in the first cluster and then switch again to a gene from the second cluster. Support for this concept comes from studies in which cells were shown to undergo sequential switching, selecting constant-region genes in a 5' to 3' direction under the influence of cytokines.[32]

CLINICAL FEATURES

Initially, each class of HCD appeared to have a characteristic clinical phenotype. Patients with γ-HCD typically presented with a systemic lymphoma, particularly involving lymphoid structures in the head and neck.[33] α-HCD was, and still appears to be, primarily a gut-associated lymphoproliferative state, sometimes responding to antibiotics.[34] μ-HCD was first described as an aberrant form of CLL.[35] Although the original associations were generally correct, time has revealed that the deleted proteins are found in a broader array of clinical contexts. Most interesting has been a number of reports of individuals who had tissue deposits of Igs analogous to AL (amyloid light chain) amyloidosis but not showing the characteristic Congophilia. Most of these deposits have consisted of light chains, but some have shown either heavy-chain antigenic determinants or both heavy-chain and light-chain peptides. Chemical analysis has revealed that the involved heavy-chain proteins displayed deletions similar to those seen in the HCDs. Such patients now have been reported with deposits related to γ, α, or μ chains. The deposits frequently have been renal, but articular and muscle depositions also have been described. Structural studies have demonstrated C_H1 and C_H2 deletions.[4,5]

γ HEAVY-CHAIN DISEASE

From the initial report in 1964 to 1989, almost 100 cases of γ HCD were recorded.[36,37] Since then, approximately 30 additional cases have been reported, 15 from a single referral center, suggesting that knowledge about the clinical aspects of the disorder has been incorporated into the body of medical practice. γ-HCD appears to have the broadest range of clinical presentations among the HCDs.[38] The most common initial symptom complex is systemic, with anemia, weight loss, and fever. In many individuals, detection of lymphadenopathy or splenomegaly triggers further investigation. Some form of lymphoma is the final diagnosis in three fourths of patients.

The waxing and waning lymphadenopathy and palatal and uvular swelling related to the involvement of Waldeyer ring, described in the early cases, are not as frequent as originally believed. Although the features are characteristic, they occur in fewer than 20 percent of γ-HCD patients.

A striking association has been noted of the occurrence of γ-HCD in patients with preexisting or concurrent autoimmune disease.[13] Fully one third of reported patients had some form of immunologically based inflammatory disease, most commonly rheumatoid arthritis. Autoimmune hemolytic anemia, systemic and discoid lupus erythematosus, and Sjögren syndrome also have been seen associated with the disease.

The clinical features of γ-HCD differ from myeloma (Table 103-1; see Chap. 100), as the features of μ-HCD differ from those of

TABLE 103-1   CLINICAL FEATURES OF MYELOMA AND γ HEAVY-CHAIN DISEASE

	MYELOMA	γ HEAVY CHAIN DISEASE
Anemia	Common	Common
Fever	Occasional	Occasional
Frequent infections	Yes	Yes
Lymphadenopathy	No	Yes
Hepatomegaly	Rare	Common
Splenomegaly	Rare	Common
Osteolytic lesions	Common	Very rare
Renal failure (cast nephropathy)	Common	Not reported
Renal amyloidosis	Occasional	Rare

Waldenström disease (Table 103-2; see Chap. 102). Renal disease and osteolytic lesions are far less common in γ-HCD. Renal failure secondary to light-chain (Bence-Jones) proteinuria or AL amyloid is rare because of the lack of production and secretion of Ig light chains (see Chap. 101).

Lymphadenopathy is present in approximately half of cases, splenomegaly is detectable in between half and three fourths, and hepatomegaly occurs in approximately one third. Extralymphoid presentations have been seen in 10 to 15 percent, with cutaneous or thyroid infiltrates specifically reported. In contrast to μ-HCD, only three individuals with γ-HCD proteins had CLL.

α HEAVY-CHAIN DISEASE

Unlike the other HCDs, most cases of α-HCD arise in a characteristic environmental setting. The patients are usually young—in their teens and twenties—and live in nonindustrialized locales with relatively poor sanitation. The disease has been described as "little more than an academic curiosity" in industrialized nations, but it is widely prevalent in developing countries.[12] Thus, the major clinical series and systematic approaches to therapy have been reported from Tunisia, Iran, Pakistan, India, Thailand, South Africa, and Mexico. The index case and the cases in which the structural features of the proteins have been best characterized were individuals of North African origin.

The most common clinical presentation is recurrent or chronic diarrhea with abdominal pain and weight loss because of malabsorption. Fever is common. For a period of time, confusion existed over whether Mediterranean lymphoma with malabsorption and α-HCD were different conditions, primarily because the HCD protein was not found in many of the lymphoma cases. It now is clear that most patients with

TABLE 103-2   CLINICAL FEATURES OF WALDENSTRÖM MICROGLOBULINEMIA AND μ HEAVY-CHAIN DISEASE

	WALDENSTRÖM	μ HEAVY CHAIN DISEASE
Anemia	Common	Common
Fever	Occasional	Occasional
Frequent infections	Yes	Yes
Lymphadenopathy	Yes	Yes
Hepatomegaly	Yes	Yes
Splenomegaly	Yes	Yes
Hyperviscosity	Common	Never
Osteolytic lesions	Rare	20%
Renal failure (cast nephropathy)	Occasional	Rare
Renal amyloidosis	Occasional	Occasional
Peripheral neuropathy	Common	Not yet reported

clinical Mediterranean lymphoma produce the defective IgA proteins at some time in the disease course. In a substantial number of individuals the protein can be found only in the intestinal secretions, whereas in other patients its presence is limited to the cytoplasm of the gut-infiltrating plasma cells. All of these patients now are classified as having immunoproliferative small intestinal disease.[39,40]

In addition to the diarrhea, malabsorption, and weight loss, growth retardation is common, and digital clubbing is present in 33 to 66 percent of patients. Mesenteric lymphadenopathy frequently is manifested as an intestinal mass, but extraabdominal lymphadenopathy is rare. Splenic involvement is unusual. Moderate hepatomegaly occurs in 20 to 25 percent of cases. Ascites is seen occasionally, as is peripheral edema, both a result of hypoalbuminemia.

μ HEAVY-CHAIN DISEASE

Of the major Ig classes, μ-HCD is the least common. Approximately 30 cases have been documented since its original description.[35] More cases likely have been seen but not reported, particularly in the last 10 years. Alternatively, because the clinical picture is not specific, it is possible that additional cases have been diagnosed as CLL or B cell lymphoma and the protein abnormality not recognized. Initially, all the reported cases had a clinical picture consistent with CLL; however, with better diagnostic procedures and a higher index of suspicion, the defining protein abnormality has been noted in a broader range of clinical settings. Currently, it appears that only one third of patients with μ-HCD have CLL. Thorough investigation of serum proteins in more than 150 consecutive patients with CLL failed to identify a single instance of μ-HCD, suggesting that fewer than 1 percent of CLL patients actually have an associated HCD protein.[41] Other clinical presentations varied from myeloma and monoclonal gammopathy of uncertain significance (see Chap. 99) with few or no symptoms (20%) to that of a systemic disease with weight loss, fever, anemia, and chronic infections. Splenomegaly is found in all cases, hepatomegaly in 75%, and peripheral lymphadenopathy in 40 percent of μ-HCD patients. Ten percent of cases were associated with the simultaneous detection of an intact IgM protein in the serum, and another 10 percent had clinical myeloma or extramedullary plasmacytoma.

δ AND ε HEAVY-CHAIN DISEASE

No cases have been reported in which an incomplete ε chain was identified. A single case of δ-HCD has been described in which the patient had the clinical features of myeloma with osteolytic lesions of the skull, marrow plasmacytosis, and acute renal failure. Immunochemical analysis of the serum revealed a polymerized δ fragment, without attached L chains. No sequence data were obtained.[42]

LABORATORY FEATURES

DETECTION OF ABNORMAL IGS

As a rule, neoplastic HCD cells do not produce large amounts of Ig. Hence, the abnormal HCD protein may be difficult to detect. Nevertheless, a combination of electrophoretic, immunoelectrophoretic, and immunofixation techniques can establish the diagnosis.[43] In a minority of cases, the HCD protein is seen as a prominent, discrete, homogeneous band of β electrophoretic mobility on serum or urine electrophoresis. The immunoelectrophoretic pattern, when developed with specific anti–heavy-chain and anti–light-chain antisera, shows an H-chain specific arc, not reacting with either the anti-κ or anti-λ L-chain antisera. This is the rule in proteins of the γ class; however, intact monoclonal IgA or IgM proteins may not react with some anti–L-chain sera, giving the false impression of α-HCD or μ-HCD. This

finding is more common with immunoelectrophoretic than with immunofixation techniques. In those instances, it may be necessary to separate the monoclonal proteins from the serum, treating them with a reducing agent to cleave the interchain disulfide bonds and subjecting them to gel electrophoresis, followed by Western blotting to determine the size of the Ig H-chain polypeptide and the presence of an Ig L chain.

More commonly, the proteins are present in smaller amounts and give heterogeneous patterns on electrophoresis, either because of N-terminal proteolysis or partial digestion of the sugar moieties attached to the H chains. Again, immunoelectrophoresis or immunofixation with development of the patterns with a panel of anti-H and anti-L antibodies can strongly suggest the diagnosis. More detailed, structural analysis can be performed on the isolated, reduced, and alkylated H-chain monomer and can confirm the presence or absence of associated light chains in specialized laboratories.

LABORATORY FEATURES OF γ-HCD

Marrow aspirates or biopsies in γ-HCD show a pleomorphic histology, with lymphocytes, plasma cells, and morphologically intermediate lymphocytoid plasma cells (or plasmacytoid lymphocytes) making up a significant proportion of the infiltrate. In 25 to 30 percent of cases, the marrow is nondiagnostic or normal. Immunophenotyping of the marrow reveals a lymphoid population staining only for the γ chain with no staining for Ig light chains. In some cases where the HCD protein concentration was too low or too electrophoretically heterogeneous to be identified in serum or urine, immunophenotyping was the definitive diagnostic test. In a few patients the analysis revealed more than a single proliferating clone, and in some patients the analysis demonstrated a major population of proliferating T cells and a quantitatively minor B-cell clone producing the γ-HCD protein.

LABORATORY FEATURES OF α-HCD

The techniques described above ("Detection of Abnormal Ig") usually detect a circulating α-HCD protein. Occasionally, the aberrant molecule cannot be seen in the serum, urine, or gastrointestinal secretions. Instead, a population of plasmacytoid cells is found in the intestinal epithelium, lymph nodes, or marrow that stain only for α heavy-chain determinants. In these cases, the typical molecular abnormality of HCD can be identified by analysis of cDNA prepared from mRNA extracted from the α-positive cells.[44]

Serial small bowel biopsies have shown that the early phases of the disease are characterized by dense mucosal and lamina propria infiltration with mature plasma cells producing the monoclonal α-chain fragment.[44] The jejunum is the usual site of involvement with the duodenum and the ileum affected less often. The disease may be patchy, and different areas may be in different stages of development at the same time, requiring biopsies from several sites for accurate staging. As the disease progresses, fewer plasma cells are seen and the dominant cells, still derived from the same clone, are more blastic, with little or no production of the α fragment. At this point, the cells have infiltrated beyond the lamina propria into the muscularis layer. In the latter stage, extensive infiltration of the regional nodes with similar cells occurs. Final pathologic diagnoses have included lymphoma of the low-, intermediate-, or high-grade immunoblastic type, mantle zone lymphoma, or parafollicular B cell lymphoma. Rarely, the tumor cells are seen in the marrow, although the frequency of marrow involvement has not been precisely determined.

Early imaging of the small bowel reveals a pseudopolypoid appearance. When the muscularis is penetrated, a more cobblestone-like picture is seen. In the late stages, tumor masses are defined and surface ulceration is detectable. Definitive diagnosis requires small bowel biopsies from more than one site along the jejunum and the demonstration of the α fragment in the serum, urine, intestinal secretions, or the cells infiltrating the gastrointestinal mucosa. If nodal involvement is seen, mesenteric lymph node biopsy may yield the same findings. The differential diagnosis includes celiac disease, diffuse intestinal giardiasis, Western-type intestinal lymphoma (which is not associated with α-HCD protein production), bacterial overgrowth syndrome, and Whipple disease. Many of the patients have concomitant chronic parasitic or bacterial infections, such as *Helicobacter pylori*. The relevance of the infections to pathogenesis is unclear, although the pathogens contribute to the symptoms and must be treated.

Instances of patients with circulating α-HCD proteins have been found in other clinical contexts in more industrialized parts of the world. A single 3-year-old child with frequent infections, hypogammaglobulinemia, and leukopenia was found to have a defective α chain, but no structural studies were reported.[45] Rare patients in the United States and Japan, with localized (gut) or disseminated Western-type lymphomas, had similar serum proteins.[46] Single individuals with goiter or skin lesions and no detectable systemic disease other than the circulating α-HCD protein have been described. These cases may result from a different mode of pathogenesis than that responsible for the intestinal form of the disease.

LABORATORY FEATURES OF μ-HCD

The marrow is infiltrated with lymphocytes, plasma cells, and prominent plasmacytoid lymphocytes. Although the marrow of almost all of the patients contains the multivacuolated plasma cells described in the index case, the vacuoles are not universally apparent.[23] Their presence has sometimes been the feature suggesting the diagnosis, with subsequent confirmation by immunoelectrophoresis.

Osteolytic lesions or pathologic fractures have been reported in 20 percent of cases, a frequency much closer to that seen in myeloma than in macroglobulinemia.

Urinary excretion of the μ fragment was noted in only two patients; presumably the fragment polymers were too large to be filtered by intact renal glomeruli. Monoclonal L chains have been found in the urine in two thirds of cases. Nonetheless, renal complications, such as cast nephropathy with renal failure and AL amyloidosis, have been infrequent.[47] Ig light chains capable of producing amyloid are found in approximately 12 percent of cases, an incidence that is not significantly different from the incidence in patients with myeloma.

THERAPY, COURSE, AND PROGNOSIS

γ HEAVY-CHAIN DISEASE

The clinical course is variable. Survival from the time of recognition of the protein abnormality has ranged from 1 month to 20 years. Patients presenting with an obvious lymphoma have a more aggressive course. The lymphomas have been treated with a variety of regimens, including splenic or other local irradiation and combinations of chemotherapy, usually including cyclophosphamide or chlorambucil, or vincristine and prednisone. A single case of a complete response to fludarabine after a partial remission with epirubicin, chlorambucil, and prednisone has been reported.[38,48] Some patients with active autoimmune disease have been treated with prednisone. Disappearance of the γ-HCD protein with treatment has not always been predictive of a good overall response.

α HEAVY-CHAIN DISEASE

Since 1965, 10 studies, all including more than 10 patients, have assessed the impact of treatment. The utility of clinical staging was not recognized until the late 1970s, making difficult the interpretation of details of responsiveness prior to that time. Mean survival was approximately 8 months in the absence of a response, and only half the patients responded to any treatment. Later studies have classified patients into those with mucosal infiltration with plasma cells (stage A) and those with deeper infiltration or nodal spread (stages B and C).[49-51] From 25 to 75 percent (depending on the series) of stage A patients treated with antibiotics (usually tetracycline 1–2 g/day for 6–8 months) showed some response. The cumulative response to antibiotic therapy (all studies) was 53 percent, with overall 5-year survival between 29 and 75 percent and 5-year disease-free survival (one study) 43 percent. An occasional stage A patient also received abdominal irradiation. Stage B and C patients were sometimes treated with similar antibiotic regimens and chemotherapy, usually including cyclophosphamide and prednisone (e.g., cyclophosphamide, doxorubicin, vincristine, and prednisone [CHOP]; cyclophosphamide, vincristine, procarbazine, and prednisone [COPP]; bleomycin, Adriamycin, cyclophosphamide, vincristine, and prednisone [BACOP]; see Chap. 96).

μ HEAVY-CHAIN DISEASE

The course is variable, with survival ranging from 1 to 11 months after the appearance of symptoms. No systematic studies of treatment have been reported. A variety of drug protocols have been used, most including alkylating agents (chlorambucil, melphalan, cyclophosphamide), with inconsistent responses. More aggressive approaches possibly will be more effective.

REFERENCES

1. Kataoka T, Yamawaki-Kataoka Y, Yamagishi H, Honjo T: Cloning immunoglobulin gamma 2b chain gene of mouse: Characterization and partial sequence determination. *Proc Natl Acad Sci U S A* 76:4240, 1979.
2. Franklin EC, Lowenstein J, Bigelow B, Meltzer M: Heavy chain disease. *Am J Med* 37:332, 1964.
3. Osserman EF, Takatsuki K: Clinical and immunochemical studies of four cases of heavy (H-gamma-2) chain disease. *Am J Med* 37:351, 1964.
4. Khamlichi AA, Aucouturier P, Preud'homme JL, Cogne M: Structure of abnormal heavy chains in human heavy-chain-deposition disease. *Eur J Biochem* 229:54, 1995.
5. Kambham N, Markowitz GS, Appel GB, et al: Heavy chain deposition disease: The disease spectrum. *Am J Kidney Dis* 33:954, 1999.
6. Matuchansky C, Cogne M, Lemaire M, et al: Nonsecretory alpha-chain disease with immunoproliferative small-intestinal disease. *N Engl J Med* 320:1534, 1989.
7. Ballard HS, Hamilton LM, Marcus AJ, Illes CH: A new variant of heavy-chain disease (mu-chain disease). *N Engl J Med* 282:1060, 1970.
8. Buxbaum J, Franklin EC, Scharff MD: Immunoglobulin M heavy chain disease: Intracellular origin of the mu chain fragment. *Science* 169:770, 1970.
9. Moskovits T, Jacobson DR, Buxbaum J: N-ras oncogene activation in a patient with gamma heavy chain disease. *Am J Hematol* 41:302, 1992.
10. Goossens T, Klein U, Kuppers R: Frequent occurrence of deletions and duplications during somatic hypermutation: Implications for oncogene translocations and heavy chain disease. *Proc Natl Acad Sci U S A* 95:2463, 1998.
11. Klein U, Goossens T, Fischer M, et al: Somatic hypermutation in normal and transformed human B cells. *Immunol Rev* 162:261, 1998.
12. Ryan JC: Premalignant conditions of the small intestine. *Semin Gastrointest Dis* 7:88, 1996.

13. Husby G, Blichfeldt P, Brinch L, et al: Chronic arthritis and gamma heavy chain disease: Coincidence or pathogenic link? *Scand J Rheumatol* 27:257, 1998.

14. Alexander A, Anicito I, Buxbaum J: Gamma heavy chain disease in man. Genomic sequence reveals two noncontiguous deletions in a single gene. *J Clin Invest* 82:1244, 1988.

15. Guglielmi P, Bakhshi A, Cogne M, et al: Multiple genomic defects result in an alternative RNA splice creating a human gamma H chain disease protein. *J Immunol* 141:1762, 1988.

16. Prelli F, Frangione B: Franklin's disease: Ig gamma 2 H chain mutant BUR. *J Immunol* 148:949, 1992.

17. Cooper SM, Franklin EC, Frangione B: Molecular defect in a gamma-2 heavy chain. *Science* 176:187, 1972.

18. Frangione B, Franklin EC, Smithies O: Unusual genes at the aminoterminus of human immunoglobulin variants. *Nature* 273:400, 1978.

19. Terry WD, Ohms J: Implications of heavy chain disease protein sequences for multiple gene theories of immunoglobulin synthesis. *Proc Natl Acad Sci U S A* 66:558, 1970.

20. Teng MH, Rosen S, Gorny MK, et al: Gamma heavy chain disease in man: Independent structural abnormalities and reduced transcription of a functionally rearranged lambda L-chain gene result in the absence of L-chains. *Blood Cells Mol Dis* 26:177, 2000.

21. Cogne M, Preud'homme JL: Gene deletions force nonsecretory alpha-chain disease plasma cells to produce membrane-form alpha-chain only. *J Immunol* 145:2455, 1990.

22. Bakhshi A, Guglielmi P, Siebenlist U, et al: A DNA insertion/deletion necessitates an aberrant RNA splice accounting for a mu heavy chain disease protein. *Proc Natl Acad Sci U S A* 83:2689, 1986.

23. Zucker-Franklin D, Franklin EC: Ultrastructural and immunofluorescence studies of the cells associated with mu-chain disease. *Blood* 37:257, 1971.

24. Cogne M, Aucouturier P, Brizard A, et al: Complete variable region deletion in a mu heavy chain disease protein (ROUL). Correlation with light chain secretion. *Leuk Res* 17:527, 1993.

25. Franklin EC, Frangione B, Prelli F: The defect in mu heavy chain disease protein GLI. *J Immunol* 116:1194, 1976.

26. Hauke G, Schiltz E, Bross KJ, et al: Unusual sequence of immunoglobulin L-chain rearrangements in a gamma heavy chain disease patient. *Scand J Immunol* 36:463, 1992.

27. Tsapis A, Bentaboulet M, Pellet P, et al: The productive gene for alpha-H chain disease protein MAL is highly modified by insertion-deletion processes. *J Immunol* 143:3821, 1989.

28. Cogne M, Bakhshi A, Korsmeyer SJ, Guglielmi P: Gene mutations and alternate RNA splicing result in truncated Ig L chains in human gamma H chain disease. *J Immunol* 141:1738, 1988.

29. Hendershot L, Bole D, Kohler G, Kearney JF: Assembly and secretion of heavy chains that do not associate posttranslationally with immunoglobulin heavy chain-binding protein. *J Cell Biol* 104:761, 1987.

30. Cogne M, Guglielmi P: Exon skipping without splice site mutation accounting for abnormal immunoglobulin chains in nonsecretory human myeloma. *Eur J Immunol* 23:1289, 1993.

31. Brokaw JL, Wetzel SM, Pollok BA: Conserved patterns of somatic mutation and secondary VH gene rearrangement create aberrant Ig-encoding genes in Epstein-Barr virus-transformed and normal human B lymphocytes. *Int Immunol* 4:197, 1992.

32. Petrini J, Shell B, Hummel M, Dunnick W: The immunoglobulin heavy chain switch: Structural features of gamma 1 recombinant switch regions. *J Immunol* 138:1940, 1987.

33. Buxbaum JN: Heavy chain disease in man. *Ric Clin Lab* 6:301, 1976.

34. Rambaud JC, Bognel C, Prost A, et al: Clinico-pathological study of a patient with "Mediterranean" type of abdominal lymphoma and a new type of IgA abnormality ("alpha chain disease"). *Digestion* 1:321, 1968.

35. Franklin EC: Mu-chain disease. *Arch Intern Med* 135:71, 1975.

36. Fermand JP, Brouet JC, Danon F, Seligmann M: Gamma heavy chain "disease": Heterogeneity of the clinicopathologic features. Report of 16 cases and review of the literature. *Medicine (Baltimore)* 68:321, 1989.

37. Kyle RA, Greipp PR, Banks PM: The diverse picture of gamma heavy-chain disease. Report of seven cases and review of literature. *Mayo Clin Proc* 56:439, 1981.

38. Wahner-Roedler DL, Witzig TE, Loehrer LL, Kyle RA: Gamma-heavy chain disease: Review of 23 cases. *Medicine (Baltimore)* 82:236, 2003.

39. Rambaud JC, Halphen M, Galian A, Tsapis A: Immunoproliferative small intestinal disease (IPSID): Relationships with alpha-chain disease and "Mediterranean" lymphomas. *Springer Semin Immunopathol* 12:239, 1990.

40. Martin IG, Aldoori MI: Immunoproliferative small intestinal disease: Mediterranean lymphoma and alpha heavy chain disease. *Br J Surg* 81:20, 1994.

41. Wahner-Roedler DL, Kyle RA: Mu-heavy chain disease: Presentation as a benign monoclonal gammopathy. *Am J Hematol* 40:56, 1992.

42. Vilpo JA, Irjala K, Viljanen MK, et al: Delta-Heavy chain disease. A study of a case. *Clin Immunol Immunopathol* 17:584, 1980.

43. Franklin EC: The heavy chain diseases. *Harvey Lect* 78:1, 1982.

44. Galian A, Lecestre MJ, Scotto J, et al: Pathological study of alpha-chain disease, with special emphasis on evolution. *Cancer* 39:2081, 1977.

45. Faux JA, Crain JD, Rosen FS, Merler E: An alpha heavy chain abnormality in a child with hypogammaglobulinemia. *Clin Immunol Immunopathol* 1:282, 1973.

46. Cohen HJ, Gonzalvo A, Krook J, et al: New presentation of alpha heavy chain disease: North American polypoid gastrointestinal lymphoma. Clinical and cellular studies. *Cancer* 41:1161, 1978.

47. Preud'homme JL, Bauwens M, Dumont G, et al: Cast nephropathy in mu heavy chain disease. *Clin Nephrol* 48:118, 1997.

48. Agrawal S, Abboudi Z, Matutes E, Catovsky D: First report of fludarabine in gamma-heavy chain disease. *Br J Haematol* 88:653, 1994.

49. Akbulut H, Soykan I, Yakaryilmaz F, et al: Five-year results of the treatment of 23 patients with immunoproliferative small intestinal disease: A Turkish experience. *Cancer* 80:8, 1997.

50. Ben Ayed F, Halphen M, Najjar T, et al: Treatment of alpha chain disease. Results of a prospective study in 21 Tunisian patients by the Tunisian-French intestinal Lymphoma Study Group. *Cancer* 63:1251, 1989.

51. Salimi M, Spinelli JJ: Chemotherapy of Mediterranean abdominal lymphoma. Retrospective comparison of chemotherapy protocols in Iranian patients. *Am J Clin Oncol* 19:18, 1996.

52. Frangione B, Rosenwasser E, Prelli F, Franklin EC: Primary structure of human gamma 3 immunoglobulin deletion mutant: Gamma 3 heavy-chain disease protein Wis. *Biochemistry* 19:4304, 1980.

53. Frangione B: A new immunoglobulin variant: Gamma 3 heavy-chain disease protein CHI. *Proc Natl Acad Sci U S A* 73:1552, 1976.

54. Frangione B, Franklin EC: Correlation between fragmented immunoglobulin genes and heavy chain deletion mutants. *Nature* 281:600, 1979.

55. Wolfenstein-Todel C, Frangione B, Prelli F, Franklin EC: The amino acid sequence of "heavy chain disease" protein ZUC. Structure of the Fc fragment of immunoglobulin G3. *Biochem Biophys Res Commun* 71:907, 1976.

56. Arnaud P, Wang AC, Gianazza E, et al: Gamma heavy chain disease protein CHA: Immunological and structural studies. *Mol Immunol* 18:379, 1981.

57. Smith LL, Barton BP, Garver FA, et al: Physicochemical and immunochemical properties of gamma 1 heavy chain disease protein BAZ. *Immunochemistry* 15:323, 1978.

58. Rabin BS, Moon J: Clinical findings in a case of newly defined gamma heavy chain disease protein. *Clin Exp Immunol* 14:563, 1973.

59. Franklin EC, Prelli F, Frangione B: Human heavy chain disease protein WIS: Implications for the organization of immunoglobulin genes. *Proc Natl Acad Sci U S A* 76:452, 1979.

60. Frangione B, Lee L, Haber E, Bloch KJ: Protein Hal: Partial deletion of a "gamma" immunoglobulin gene(s) and apparent reinitiation at an internal AUG codon. *Proc Natl Acad Sci U S A* 70:1073, 1973.

61. Franklin EC, Kyle R, Seligmann M, Frangione B: Correlation of protein structure and immunoglobulin gene organization in the light of two new deleted heavy chain disease proteins. *Mol Immunol* 16:919, 1979.

62. Sala P, Tonutti E, Pizzolitto S, et al: Immunochemical and structural characterization of an IgG1 heavy chain disease. *Ric Clin Lab* 19:59, 1989.

63. Franklin EC, Frangione B: The molecular defect in a protein (CRA) found in gamma-1 heavy chain disease, and its genetic implications. *Proc Natl Acad Sci U S A* 68:187, 1971.

64. Nabeshima Y, Ikenaka T: N- and C-terminal amino acid sequences of a gamma-heavy chain disease protein YOK. *Immunochemistry* 13:245, 1976.

65. Biewenga J, Frangione B, Franklin EC, Van Loghem E: A gamma 1 heavy-chain disease protein (EST) lacking the entire VH and CHl domains. *Scand J Immunol* 11:601, 1980.

66. Bentaboulet M, Mihaesco E, Gendron MC, et al: Genomic alterations in a case of alpha heavy chain disease leading to the generation of composite exons from the JH region. *Eur J Immunol* 19:2093, 1989.

67. Wolfenstein-Todel C, Mihaesco E, Frangione B: "Alpha chain disease" protein def: Internal deletion of a human immunoglobulin A1 heavy chain. *Proc Natl Acad Sci U S A* 71:974, 1974.

68. Wolfenstein-Todel C, Mihaesco E, Frangione B: Variant of a human immunoglobulin: "alpha chain disease" protein AIT. *Biochem Biophys Res Commun* 65:47, 1975.

69. Fakhfakh F, Dellagi K, Ayadi H, et al: Alpha heavy chain disease alpha mRNA contain nucleotide sequences of unknown origins. *Eur J Immunol* 22:3037, 1992.

70. Barnikol-Watanabe S, Mihaesco E, Mihaesco C, et al: The primary structure of mu-chain-disease protein BOT. Peculiar amino-acid sequence of the N-terminal 42 positions. *Hoppe Seylers Z Physiol Chem* 365:105, 1984.

71. Mihaesco C, Ferrara P, Guillemot JC, et al: A new extra sequence at the amino terminal of a mu heavy chain disease protein (DAG). *Mol Immunol* 27:771, 1990.

72. Lebreton JP, Ropartz C, Rousseaus J, et al: Immunochemical and biochemical study of a human Fc mu-like fragment (mu-chain disease). *Eur J Immunol* 5:179, 1975

HEMOSTASIS
AND
THROMBOSIS

MEGAKARYOPOIESIS AND THROMBOPOIESIS

KENNETH KAUSHANSKY

Each day the adult human produces approximately 1×10^{11} platelets, a level of production that can increase 10- to 20-fold in times of increased demand. Production of platelets depends on the proliferation and differentiation of hematopoietic stem and progenitor cells to a cell committed to the megakaryocyte lineage, its maturation to a large, polyploid megakaryocyte, and its final fragmentation into platelets. The external influences that impact megakaryopoiesis and thrombopoiesis are a supportive marrow stroma consisting of endothelial and other cells, matrix glycosaminoglycans, and a family of protein hormones and cytokines, including thrombopoietin, stem cell factor, interleukin-6, interleukin-11, and stromal-cell derived factor-1. The role of the cytokines essential for these processes has been defined, insights into the two most unusual aspects of thrombopoiesis—endomitosis and proplatelet formation—have been gathered, and reagents to specifically modify platelet production have been generated. This chapter focuses on the development of megakaryocytes, their precursors and their progeny, and the hematopoietic growth factors and transcriptionally active molecules that control the survival, proliferation, and differentiation of these cells.

KINETICS OF THROMBOPOIESIS

The circulatory half-life of a platelet is approximately 10 days in humans with normal platelet counts but is somewhat shorter in patients with moderate (7 days) to severe (5 days) thrombocytopenia, as a higher proportion of the total body platelet mass is consumed in the day-to-day function of maintaining vascular integrity.[1] Based on a "normal" level of 200,000 platelets/μl, a blood volume of 5 liters, and a half-life of 10 days, 1×10^{11} platelets per day are produced. If one megakaryocyte produces approximately 1000 platelets, approximately 1×10^8 megakaryocytes are generated in the marrow each day.

Several independent lines of evidence indicate the transit time from megakaryocyte progenitor cell to release of platelets into the circulation ranges from 4 to 7 days. For example, following platelet apheresis, the platelet count falls, recovers substantially by day 4, and completely recovers by day 7.[2] In most physiologic and pathological states the platelet count is inversely related to plasma thrombopoietin levels. For example, liver failure is associated with moderate thrombocytopenia as a result of splenomegaly and thrombopoietin deficiency. Within the first week following orthotopic liver transplantation, the platelet count rises substantially, with kinetics matching those of thrombopoietin infusion.[3,4] These findings indicate expansion of the

megakaryocyte mass takes from 3 to 4 days following a thrombopoietin stimulus in humans and, coupled with the approximate 12 hours required for platelet release,[5] results in a relatively brisk response to thrombocytopenia.

CELLULAR PHYSIOLOGY OF THROMBOPOIESIS

Platelets form by fragmentation of megakaryocyte membrane exvaginations termed *proplatelets*, in a process that consumes nearly the entire cytoplasmic complement of membranes, organelles, granules, and soluble macromolecules. Each megakaryocyte is estimated to give rise to 1000 to 3000 platelets[6,7] before the residual nuclear material is engulfed and eliminated by marrow macrophages.[8] The continuum of megakaryocyte development is arbitrarily divided into four stages. The major criteria differentiating these stages are the quality and quantity of the cytoplasm, and the size, lobulation, and chromatin pattern of the nucleus (Table 104-1).

MEGAKARYOBLAST

Stage I megakaryocytes, also termed *megakaryoblasts*, account for approximately 20 percent of all cells destined to form platelets. These cells in human marrow are 8 to 24 μm in spherical diameter, contain a relatively large, minimally indented nucleus with loosely organized chromatin and multiple nucleoli, and scant basophilic cytoplasm containing a small Golgi complex, a few mitochondria and α-granules, and abundant free ribosomes (Fig. 104-1).

SURFACE ADHESION MOLECULE EXPRESSION

Although elegant experiments clearly demonstrated that the gene for integrin α_{IIb} is expressed as early as the erythroid-megakaryocytic progenitor stage[9] and possibly in the common myeloid progenitor, the cell surface protein becomes demonstrable and functionally important only at the early stages of megakaryocyte development. Integrin $\alpha_{IIb}\beta_3$ is an integral transmembrane protein of two subunits, but only the α-subunit is megakaryocyte lineage specific. Absence of integrin $\alpha_{IIb}\beta_3$ leads to Glanzmann thrombasthenia resulting from failure of the defective platelets to engage fibrinogen and other adhesive ligands during hemostasis (see Chap. 112). Megakaryocytes and platelets contain in their cytoplasmic membranes about twice the amount of integrin $\alpha_{IIb}\beta_3$ as is present on the cell surface. The granule compartment serves as a mobilizable pool that is exteriorized upon platelet activation. During the early and mid stages of megakaryocyte development, the granule content of integrin rises. Moreover, as developing megakaryocytes do not synthesize but contain fibrinogen in their α-granules and cells from patients with Glanzmann thrombasthenia do not, integrin $\alpha_{IIb}\beta_3$ clearly begins to function, at least at the level of fibrinogen binding and uptake, long before platelet formation.

The glycoprotein (Gp) Ib-IX complex is expressed only slightly after the appearance of integrin $\alpha_{IIb}\beta_3$.[10] Although endothelial cells reportedly express GpIb,[11] its levels are very low; otherwise, GpIb is

TABLE 104-1   MATURATION STAGES OF MEGAKARYOCYTES

TERM	SIZE (μM)	MORPHOLOGY
Megakaryoblast (stage I)	>10	Lobed nucleus, basophilic cytoplasm
Basophilic megakaryocyte (stage II)	>20	Horseshoe-shaped nucleus, basophilic cytoplasm, azurophilic granules around centrosome
Granular megakaryocyte (stage III)	>25–50	Large multilobed nucleus, acidophilic cytoplasm, numerous azurophilic granules
Mature megakaryocyte (stage IV)	>25–50	Pyknotic nucleus, groups of 10–12 azurophilic granules

A

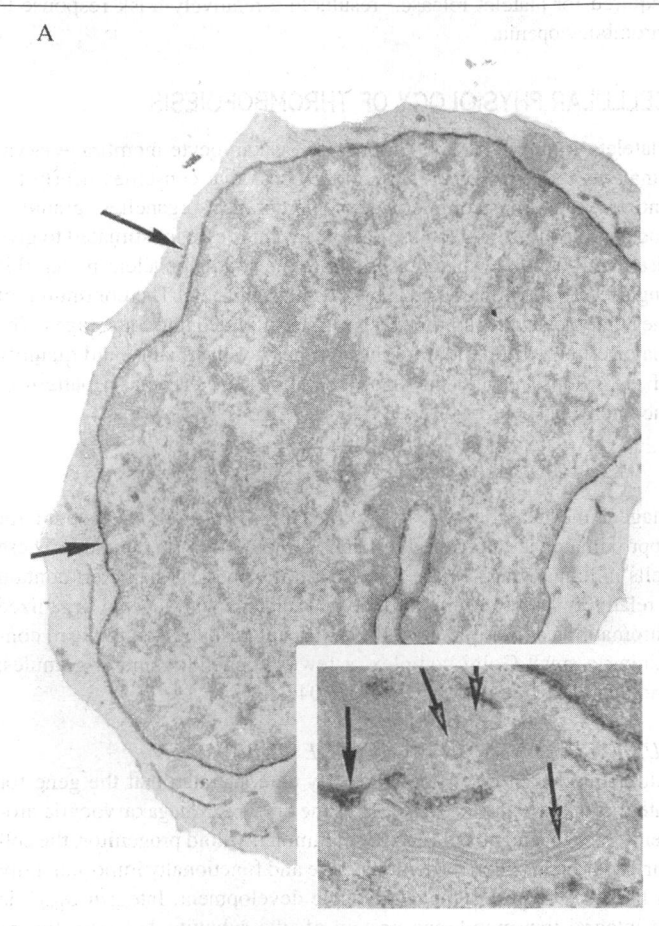

FIGURE 104-1   Electron micrograph of a normal human megakaryoblast stained for platelet peroxidase. The small cell (<9 μm) exhibits dense platelet peroxidase in the perinuclear space and endoplasmic reticulum *(arrows)* (magnification ×12,150). *(Inset)* Enlargement of the Golgi zone. The Golgi saccules and vesicles are devoid of platelet peroxidase *(open arrows)*, whereas the endoplasmic reticulum contains platelet peroxidase activity *(closed arrow)* (magnification ×25,000). (Courtesy of Dr. J. Breton-Gorius.)

a second megakaryocyte-specific protein. Glycoprotein V also is expressed in complex with GpIb and GpIX, in a ratio of 2:2:1 (Ib:IX:V).[12] However, its genetic elimination has little effect on platelet adhesion,[13] and unlike GpIb and GpIX, no mutations of GpV are associated with Bernard-Soulier disease.[14] Therefore, GpV does not appear to be required for the GpIb-V-IX complex to function as a von Willebrand factor receptor. Rather, GpV is a target of thrombin, potentially playing a role in platelet activation.[15]

DEMARCATION MEMBRANES

Another feature of the megakaryoblast is the initial development of demarcation membranes, which begin as invaginations of the plasma membrane and ultimately develop into a highly branched interconnected system of channels that course through the cytoplasm. The demarcation membrane system is in open communication with the extracellular space, based on studies using electron dense tracers.[16] Biochemical analysis indicates the composition of these membranes is very similar to the plasma membrane at each stage of megakaryocyte development. Over the 72 hours required for stage III/IV cells to develop from megakaryoblasts, the demarcation membrane system grows substantially. The purpose of the demarcation membrane system has been disputed for several decades. As the term implies, many be-

lieved the demarcation membrane system acts to compartmentalize the megakaryocyte cytoplasm into "platelet territories," which ultimately fragment into mature platelets along the cleavage planes so formed. In contrast, the current belief is that these membranes provide the material necessary for development of proplatelet processes, structures that form in stage IV megakaryocytes and give rise upon fragmentation to mature platelets. Much work is presently focused on this question.[17]

ENDOMITOSIS

One of the most characteristic features of megakaryocyte development is endomitosis, a unique form of mitosis in which the DNA is repeatedly replicated in the absence of nuclear or cytoplasmic division. The resultant cells are highly polyploid. Endomitosis begins in megakaryoblasts (Fig. 104-2) following the many standard cell divisions required to expand the number of megakaryocytic precursor cells and is completed by the end of stage II megakaryocyte development.[18] During the endomitotic phase, each cycle of DNA synthesis produces an exact doubling of all the chromosomes, resulting in cells containing DNA content from eight to 128 times the normal chromosomal complement in a single, highly lobated nucleus. Although poorly understood for many years, the ability to produce large numbers of normal megakaryocytes in culture has started to shed light on this enigmatic process. Endomitosis is not simply the absence of mitosis but rather consists of recurrent cycles of aborted mitoses.[19] Cell cycle kinetics in endomitotic cells also are unusual, characterized by a short G_1 phase, a relatively normal DNA synthesis phase, a short G_2 phase, and a very short endomitosis phase.[20] During the latter phase, megakaryocytic chromosomes condense, the nuclear membrane breaks down, and mul-

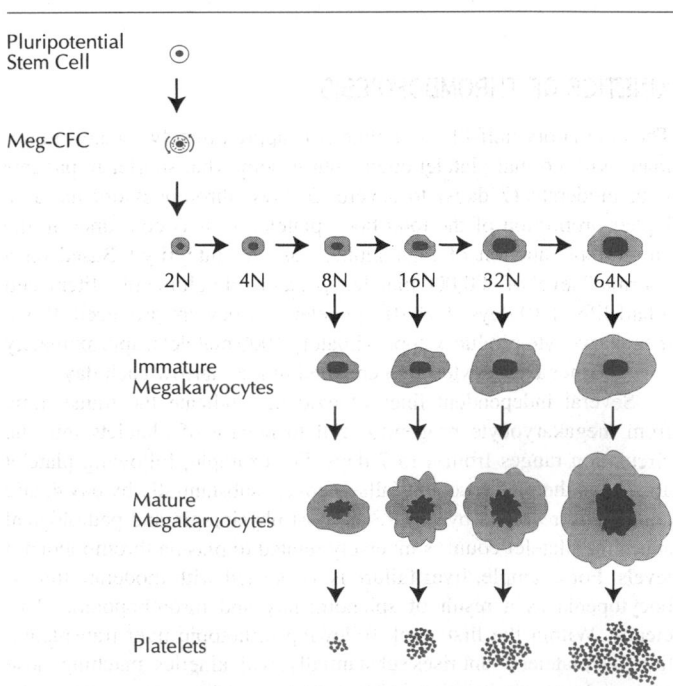

FIGURE 104-2   Origin and development of megakaryocytes. The pluripotential stem cell produces a progenitor committed to megakaryocyte differentiation (colony forming unit–megakaryocyte [CFU-MK]), which can undergo mitosis. Eventually the CFU-MK stops mitosis and enters endomitosis. During endomitosis, neither cytoplasm nor nucleus divides, but DNA replication proceeds and gives rise to immature polyploid progenitors, which then enlarge and mature into morphologically identifiable, mature megakaryocytes that shed platelets. This figure does not necessarily imply that endomitosis and platelet formation are sequential but they can occur simultaneously.

tiple (at advanced stages) mitotic spindles form upon which the replicated chromosomes assemble. However, following initial chromosomal separation, individual chromosomes fail to complete their normal migration to opposite poles of the cell, the spindle dissociates, the nuclear membrane reforms around the entire chromosomal complement, and the cell once again enters G_1 phase.

REGULATION OF GENE EXPRESSION

The promoters for integrin α_{IIb}, GpIb, GpVI, GpIX, and platelet factor-4 genes have been the focus of several studies and are active at the megakaryoblast stage of development. Consensus sequences for both GATA-1 and members of the Ets family of transcription factors (e.g., Fli-1) are present in the 5′ flanking regions of these genes, deletion of which reduces or eliminates reporter gene expression,[21–24] at least in mature hematopoietic cells. MafB also enhances GATA-1 and Ets activity during megakaryoblast differentiation,[25] induced by activation of ERK1/2, one of the primary downstream events of thrombopoietin stimulation.[26]

Another target of GATA-1 in megakaryocytes is polyphosphate-4-phosphatase (P4P), which was first identified by subtraction cloning between normal and GATA-1 knockdown megakaryocytes.[27] One of the unexplained features of megakaryocytes in GATA-1 knockdown mice is that, rather than massive cell death as seen in GATA-1–deficient erythroid progenitors,[28] the aberrantly developing megakaryoblasts in GATA-1 knockdown marrow are highly abundant and proliferate in vitro far greater than control cells.[29] P4P catalyzes hydrolysis of the D-4 position phosphate of $PI_{3,4}P$ and $PI_{3,4,5}P$. These membrane phospholipids are products of phosphoinositol-3-kinase (PI3K) action on membrane phospholipids, and they play an important role in the proliferative and survival response to megakaryocyte growth factors. When reintroduced into the knockdown mice, P4P diminishes the exuberant growth characteristic of the knockdown cells.[27] These findings are similar to the phenotype of cells from PTEN or SHIP knockout mice, enzymes that hydrolyze the D-3 and D-5 positions of $PI_{3,4,5}P$.

Another transcription factor vital for megakaryoblast differentiation is RUNX1 (also termed CBFA2 and AML1), the gene responsible for thrombocytopenia seen in familial platelet disorder/predisposition to acute myelogenous leukemia[30] (see Chap. 110). In this disorder, haploinsufficiency of RUNX1 is associated with thrombocytopenia. As its genetic elimination in mice leads to significant maturation defects in the megakaryocyte lineage,[31] the human disorder almost certainly results from this genetic alteration. During normal megakaryoblast differentiation, RUNX1 levels rise and, conversely, fall during erythroid differentiation. In response to phosphorylation by ERK1/2, RUNX1, in complex with CBFβ and together with GATA-1, induces integrin α_{IIb} and integrin α_2 expression in megakaryoblast-like cells,[32] providing the beginnings of a molecular explanation for megakaryocyte development.

CYTOKINE DEPENDENCY

The cytokines, hormones, and chemokines responsible for survival and proliferation of megakaryoblasts include thrombopoietin, interleukin (IL)-3, stem cell factor (also termed mast cell growth factor, steel factor, and c-kit ligand), and stromal cell-derived factor (SDF)-1. The former is the most critical (for additional details, see the more extensive discussion below in "Hormones and Cytokines"). Genetic elimination of the TPO gene in mice leads to circulating platelet levels approximately 10 percent of normal. Homozygous or complex heterozygous mutation of the gene encoding the thrombopoietin receptor c-Mpl leads to congenital amegakaryocytic thrombocytopenia, in which platelet levels are approximately 10 percent of normal because of a near absence of megakaryocytic progenitors and megakaryoblasts (see Chap. 110). The importance of stem cell factor to megakaryoblast

development is revealed by experimental findings both in vitro and in vivo. Genetic reduction in thrombopoietin or its receptor c-kit leads to a 50 percent reduction in circulating platelet levels.[33] The cytokine acts in synergy with thrombopoietin to enhance megakaryocyte production in semisolid and suspension culture systems.[34] Evidence that IL-3 contributes to megakaryopoiesis is weakest. Genetic elimination of the gene fails to affect platelet counts, even when combined with thrombopoietin deficiency,[35] but the cytokine can induce growth of marrow progenitors into colonies containing immature megakaryocytes in vitro in the absence of thrombopoietin.[36] Finally, the chemokine SDF-1 appears to play a role in megakaryocyte proliferation. In vitro, SDF-1 acts in synergy with thrombopoietin to support the survival and proliferation of megakaryocyte progenitors.[37] The combination of the cell adhesion molecule VCAM-1 and SDF-1 restores megakaryopoiesis in TPO and c-mpl null mice.[38]

SIGNAL TRANSDUCTION

The survival and proliferation of megakaryoblasts depends on at least two thrombopoietin-induced signaling pathways: PI3K and mitogen-activated protein kinase (MAPK) (see Chap. 13). In the presence of chemical inhibitors of PI3K, the favorable effects of thrombopoietin on megakaryocyte progenitor survival and proliferation are eliminated,[39] although constitutively activating this pathway is not sufficient for thrombopoietin-induced growth. MAPK is another important signaling pathway stimulated by thrombopoietin. Using purified marrow megakaryocytic progenitors and model cell lines, several groups showed that inhibition of MAPK blocks megakaryoblast maturation[26,40–42] because of its effect of activating Ets transcription factors.

STAGE II MEGAKARYOCYTES

Stage II megakaryocytes contain a lobulated nucleus and more abundant but less intensely basophilic cytoplasm. Ultrastructurally, the cytoplasm contains more abundant α-granules and organelles. The demarcation membrane system begins to expand at this stage of development. Stage II megakaryocytes measure up to 30 μm in diameter, compose approximately 25 percent of marrow megakaryocytes, and are the stage of development during which endomitosis is most prominent, generating cells displaying ploidy values of 8N to 64N.

ENDOMITOSIS

Whereas megakaryoblasts are generally thought to be able to expand by cell division, at an early stage of their maturation the cells begin to undergo endomitosis, in which cells diverge from the normal cell cycle during mid to late anaphase. Like normally mitotic cells, endomitotic megakaryocytes condense their chromatin into chromosomes, form a spindle, dissolve the nuclear membrane, and assemble the chromosomes on a metaphase plate, then the chromosomes begin to separate during early anaphase. However, rather than the dividing chromosomes migrating to opposite poles of the cell to allow the formation of a cleavage furrow, the chromosomes quickly decondense, the nuclear membrane reforms around the entire chromosomal complement, and the endomitotic cells reenter G_1 and then S phase. A number of attempts to understand this process at the biochemical level have involved leukemic cell lines. Alterations in cyclin B, cdc2, cell cycle kinase inhibitors, and aurora kinases all have been claimed to be responsible for endomitosis.[43–46] Unfortunately, although these hypotheses possibly explain the polyploidy in various leukemic cell lines, the hypotheses have not been substantiated in studies of normal endomitotic megakaryocytes.[19,47,48]

CYTOPLASMIC DEVELOPMENT

Early in megakaryocyte development, the cytoplasm acquires a rich network of microfilaments and microtubules. Toward stages III and IV, the proteins accumulate in the cell periphery, creating an organelle poor peripheral zone. Biochemically, the megakaryocyte cytoskeleton is composed of actin, α-actinin, filamin, nonmuscle myosin (including the product of the *MYH9* gene, mutated in several giant platelet thrombocytopenic syndromes[49,50]; see Chap. 110), β_1 tubulin, talin, and several other actin-binding proteins. Like platelets, megakaryocytes can respond to external stimuli by changing shape, transporting organelles around the cytoplasm, and secreting granules. These functions are dependent on the microfilament and microtubule systems of the cell. In addition, microtubules play a vital role during the later stages of platelet formation.[51]

REGULATION OF GENE EXPRESSION

As discussed earlier, GATA-1 is vital for committing primitive multipotent progenitors to the erythroid/megakaryocyte pathway. However, the transcription factor also is critical later in megakaryopoiesis, for cytoplasmic development. The first convincing evidence that GATA proteins affect megakaryocyte development came from overexpression studies of *GATA-1* in a leukemic cell line, in which the transcription factor led to partial megakaryocytic differentiation.[52] Reduction in *GATA-1* expression also impairs cytoplasmic development in murine megakaryocytes, reducing demarcation membranes and platelet-specific granules.[29]

PLATELET GRANULE FORMATION

Although more prominent in later stages of differentiation, platelet-specific α-granules first begin to form adjacent to the Golgi apparatus as 300- to 500-nm round or oval organelles in stage II megakaryocytes. Three distinct compartments are recognized in α-granules: (1) a central electron dense nucleoid, containing fibrinogen, platelet factor-4, β-thromboglobulin, transforming growth factor (TGF)-β_1, vitronectin, and tissue plasminogen activator-like plasminogen activator; (2) a peripheral zone, containing tubules and von Willebrand factor (arranged much like that seen in endothelial cell Weibel-Palade bodies); and (3) the granule membrane, containing many of the critical platelet receptors for cell rolling (P-selectin), firm adhesion (GpIb-V-IX), and aggregation (integrin $\alpha_{IIb}\beta_3$). Proteins present in α-granules arise from *de novo* MK synthesis (e.g., GpIb-V-IX, GpIV, integrin $\alpha_{IIb}\beta_3$, von Willebrand factor, P-selectin, β-thromboglobulin, platelet-derived growth factor), nonspecific pinocytosis of environmental proteins (albumin and IgG), or cell surface membrane receptor-mediated uptake from the environment (e.g., fibrinogen, fibronectin, factor V).

STAGE III/IV MEGAKARYOCYTES

Continued cytoplasmic maturation characterizes stage III/IV megakaryocyte development. Cells are extremely large (40–60 μm in diameter) and display a low nuclear to cytoplasmic ratio (Fig. 104-3). Cytoplasmic basophilia disappears as cells progress from stage III to IV. The demarcation membrane system gradually replaces the endoplasmic reticulum and Golgi apparatus during the final stages of maturation. The nucleus usually is eccentrically placed. Although the nucleus sometimes appears as several distinct nuclei in biopsy sections, it remains highly lobulated but single at all stages of MK development. In occasional marrow sections, neutrophils or other marrow cells are seen transiting through the cytoplasm of the mature megakaryocyte, a process termed *emperipolesis*, and is of no pathological significance.

PROPLATELET FORMATION

Careful microscopic studies have localized marrow megakaryocytes to the abluminal surface of sinusoidal endothelial cells. In specially prepared specimens, the megakaryocytes can be seen issuing long slender cytoplasmic processes between endothelial cells and into the sinusoidal lumen, structures termed *proplatelet processes* (Fig. 104-4).[53] The processes have been reproduced *in vitro*. The processes consist of a β-tubulin cytoskeleton and highway, transporting organelles and platelet constituents from the megakaryocyte to the terminal projection, the nascent platelet.[17]

MEMBRANE COMPOSITION

Most of the specific characteristics of platelet membranes are present at stages III and IV of megakaryocyte development. Megakaryocyte membrane lipid composition progressively changes through development, achieving approximately four times the content of phospholipids and cholesterol as found in immature cells. Megakaryocytes contain about the same amounts of membrane neutral and phospholipid as platelets but contain relatively more phosphatidylinositol and less phosphatidylserine and arachidonic acid.

REGULATION OF GENE EXPRESSION

One transcription factor that plays an important role in the final stages of megakaryocyte maturation is NF-E2. Initially described as an erythroid-specific, heterodimeric protein belonging to the basic leucine zipper family of transcription factors, NF-E2 is composed of a ubiquitously expressed p18 subunit and a p45 protein present also in megakaryocytes.[54,55] NF-E2 binds to tandem AP-1–like motifs, such as those seen in the second DNAse hypersensitive site of the β-globin locus control region, and is required for β-globin expression.[56] However, genetic elimination of p45 failed to significantly affect erythropoiesis. Rather, p45 deficient mice display prominent alterations in megakaryocyte development and severe thrombocytopenia[57] leading to death from widespread hemorrhage soon after birth. Examination of the animals reveals modest expansion of marrow megakaryocytes but failure of the cells to produce platelets because of defects in cytoplasmic maturation, including substantial reductions in platelet granules and demarcation membranes. Thus, the loss of either GATA-1 or NF-E2 results in failure of late aspects of cellular maturation. As p45 NF-E2 is induced by GATA-1/FOG,[58] the lack of cytoplasmic development in GATA-deficient mice likely is an indirect effect.

Nearly all studies of megakaryopoiesis have focused on the marrow. The final stages of megakaryocyte fragmentation also are proposed to occur in the lung, at least for some cells, a theory based on the finding that platelet levels in pulmonary venous blood exceed those found in the pulmonary artery.[59] Whether this process represents the migration and fragmentation of intact megakaryocytes in the lung or merely the final size reduction of large fragments of megakaryocyte cytoplasm that also are released into the blood is not clear. Some data exist supporting the notion that lung megakaryocytes contribute to blood platelet production.[60] However, in mice administered high doses of thrombopoietin, with platelet counts as high as 4 million/μm^3, neither intact megakaryocytes nor denuded nuclei were found in the lungs of these animals.[61] One study found that canine lungs contain 2.5 megakaryocytes per cm^2.[62] Extrapolation of these data suggest human lungs contain approximately 6000 megakaryocytes, only enough to account for a small proportion (<0.1%) of daily platelet production.

PLATELET FORMATION

Numerous studies have indicated thrombopoietin is the primary regulator of megakaryocyte maturation.[36,63] However, despite the impor-

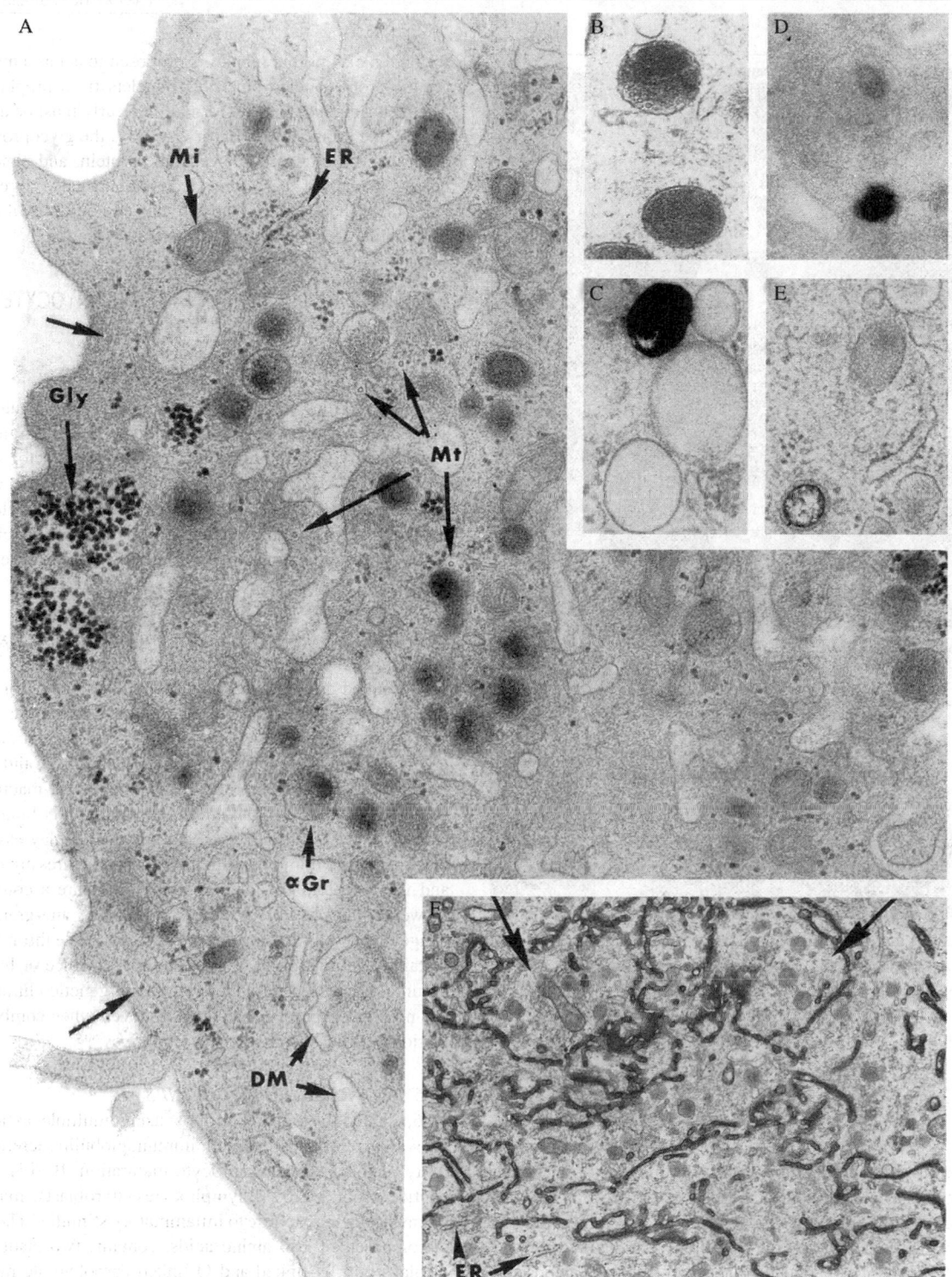

FIGURE 104-3   *(A)* Ultrastructure of the cytoplasm of a mature megakaryocyte. The majority of the granules are α-granules (αGr) exhibiting dense nucleoid. Demarcation membranes (DM) are slightly dilated. Transverse sections of microtubules (Mt) are dispersed. At the periphery, a longitudinal microtubule runs under the cell membrane *(arrows)*. Dense aggregates of glycogen (Gly), small cisternae of endoplasmic reticulum (ER), and free ribosomes are seen (magnification ×30,320). *(B)* Morphology of an α-granule. Dense nucleoid is located at the *top*. In a clear zone at the opposite pole, four transverse sections of tubular structures are adjacent to the granule membrane (magnification ×37,200). *(C)* Dense body can be distinguished from α-granule by the black deposit when calcium is added to the fixative (magnification ×37,200). *(D)* Cytochemical detection of acid phosphatase using β-glycophosphate as substrate and cerium as a trapping agent. Dense cerium–phosphate precipitates are present in lysosomal granules, whereas α-granules are unreactive (magnification ×37,200). *(E)* Microperoxisome visualized using alkaline diaminobenzidine. Note the small size of a reactive granule compared to the α-granule. *(F)* Distribution of a dense tracer filling the lumen of the demarcation membrane system in a maturing megakaryocyte *(arrows)*. In contrast to the demarcation membrane system, which is open to the extracellular space, the endoplasmic reticulum (ER) is not labeled (magnification ×9700). (Courtesy of Dr. Janine Breton-Gorius.)

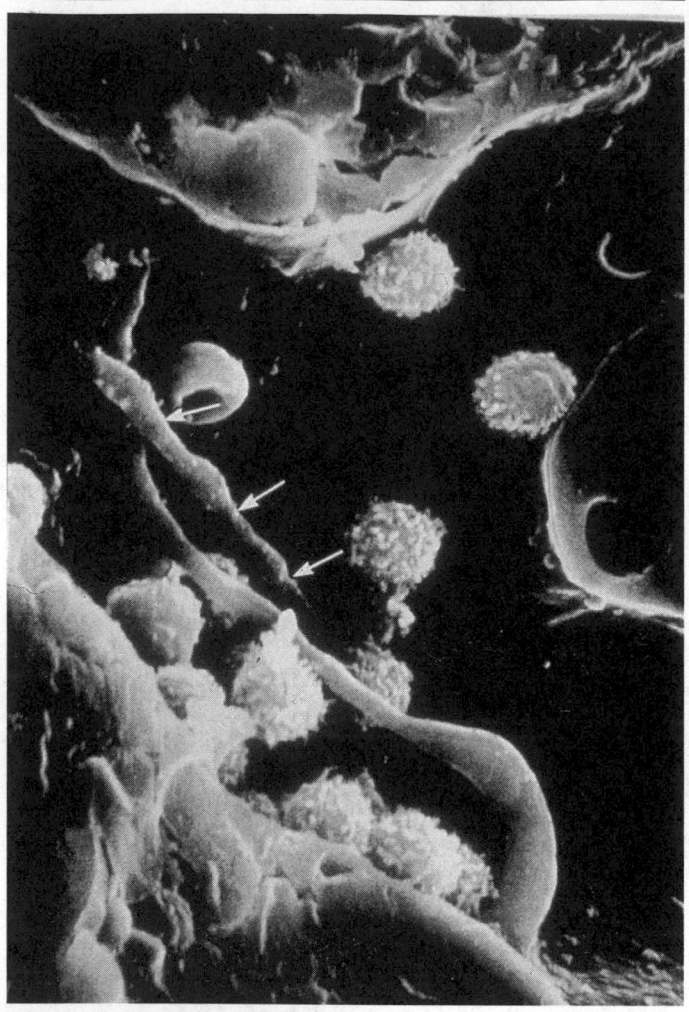

FIGURE 104-4 Megakaryocyte proplatelet processes in the bone marrow sinusoid. Scanning electron micrograph showing the luminal view of the confluence of two bone marrow sinusoids with two proplatelet processes protruding through the lining endothelial cells. One of the processes has intermittent constrictions (arrows), indicating potential sites for platelet formation. Other cells depicted include lymphocytes and erythrocytes (magnification ×3000). (From RP Becker and P De Bruyn,[54] with permission.)

tance of the hormone for generation of fully mature megakaryocytes from which platelets arise, elimination of the cytokine during the final stages of platelet formation is not detrimental.[64] Although proplatelet formation is possible under serum-free conditions,[65] most investigators have reported the presence of plasma and/or an integrin ligand-containing substratum (e.g., fibronectin or vitronectin) stimulates the process substantially.[64,66] These findings suggest external signals probably are required for normal platelet formation. One report suggests the thrombin–antithrombin complex with or without high density lipoprotein particles mediates the favorable effect of plasma on proplatelet formation,[67] although other data suggest prothrombin and its conversion to thrombin by megakaryocytes inhibit the process.[68] Although the cytokine(s) required for this process is not known, activation of protein kinase C-α clearly is necessary for the process to occur.[66]

Platelet formation involves massive reorganization of megakaryocyte cytoskeletal components, including actin and tubulin, during a highly active, motile process in which the termini of the process branch and issue platelets.[5] The size of the individual platelets formed is of interest. Unfortunately, little is known about this aspect of platelet

formation except that tubulin is proposed to act as a measuring device for the proper site to pinch off platelets from proplatelet processes. The mechanism of platelet formation clearly must be affected in some way by the transcription factor GATA-1, the glycoprotein Ib-IX complex, the Wiskott-Aldrich syndrome protein, and platelet myosin, as defects in each of these genes leads to unusually large or small platelets[69] (see Chap. 110). Finally, localized apoptosis likely plays a role in initiating the final stages of platelet formation.[70,71]

EXTRINSIC REGULATION OF MEGAKARYOCYTE PRODUCTION

HORMONES AND CYTOKINES

Several cytokines, first identified using alternate hematopoietic activity assays, affect megakaryocyte development. IL-3, granulocyte-macrophage colony stimulating factor, and stem cell factor support the proliferation of MK progenitors in plasma-containing cultures.[72–74] In 1994, several groups reported the purification and/or cloning of thrombopoietin.[75] This cytokine clearly is the primary regulator of megakaryopoiesis but cannot explain thrombopoiesis in its entirety.

INTERLEUKIN-3

IL-3 is a 25- to 30-kDa protein produced almost exclusively by T lymphocytes.[76] The mature human protein contains 133 amino acids, but N-linked carbohydrate modification accounts for the larger than expected M_r of the cytokine. Granulocyte-macrophage colony stimulating factor is an 18- to 30-kDa protein also produced by T lymphocytes. However, endothelial cells, monocytes, and fibroblasts also produce the protein and, like IL-3, granulocyte-macrophage colony-stimulating factor is highly modified with both N-linked and O-linked carbohydrate.[77] Although the two proteins display essentially no primary sequence homology, their tertiary structures are highly related,[78] and the receptors for the two cytokines share a common subunit.[79] However, the physiologic relevance of IL-3 and granulocyte-macrophage colony stimulating factor for steady-state thrombopoiesis is uncertain. Administration of the cytokines to mice or humans has only minimal effects on thrombopoiesis, and genetic elimination of either has no impact on megakaryopoiesis, even when combined with elimination of other thrombopoietic cytokines.[80,81]

IL-6 AND RELATED CYTOKINES

IL-6, cloned by several groups using multiple assays (hepatocyte growth, myeloma cell growth, immunoglobulin secretion, antiviral activity), enhances megakaryocyte maturation. IL-6 is a 26-kDa polypeptide produced by T lymphocytes, fibroblasts, macrophages, and stromal cells in response to inflammatory stimuli.[82] The mature protein is composed of 184 amino acids, contains two disulfide bonds, and displays both N-linked and O-linked carbohydrate modification. Although IL-6 alone fails to affect in vitro megakaryopoiesis, it augments the number of megakaryocyte colonies obtained in the presence of IL-3 or stem cell factor[83] and exerts primarily a differentiating effect.[84,85] Administration of IL-6 to mice or nonhuman primates or patients results in a modest thrombocytosis.[86–88] These findings suggest IL-6 contributes to megakaryopoiesis in vivo, a conclusion supported by its production by tumor cells in selected cases of paraneoplastic thrombocytosis.[89] However, genetic elimination of the cytokine fails to significantly affect basal platelet production.[90] Evidence suggests the cytokine affects platelet production indirectly[91] by stimulating thrombopoietin production.

IL-6 acts through a heterodimeric receptor, composed of a signaling subunit, termed Gp130, and an affinity converting subunit, termed IL-6Rα. Gp130 also acts as the signaling subunit for several other cytokines, including IL-11 and leukemia inhibitory factor. Therefore, the finding that these cytokines also stimulate megakaryopoiesis in a manner similar to that of IL-6 is not surprising. IL-11 and leukemia inhibitory factor act in synergy with IL-3 or stem cell factor to augment megakaryocyte formation. IL-11 is a 23-kDa polypeptide, initially cloned from a gibbon marrow stromal cell line, whose activity can support the proliferation of an IL-6 responsive myeloma cell line.[92] Leukemia inhibitory factor initially cloned as a *human interleukin* that induced *DA-1* cells to proliferate (hence its alternate name of *HILDA*) or leukemic M1 cells to differentiate.[93] Leukemia inhibitory factor displays a wide range of activities,[94] including (1) inducing the acute phase hepatic response, (2) inducing an adrenergic to cholinergic switch in neurons, (3) inhibiting lipoprotein lipase in adipocytes, and (4) maintaining pluripotentiality in embryonic cells.

Like IL-6, IL-11 and leukemia inhibitory factor enhance MK maturation *in vitro*[95,96] and augment the effects of IL-3 and stem cell factor on primitive hematopoietic cells. Consistent with the *in vitro* findings, administration of either recombinant IL-11 or leukemia inhibitory factor to rodents, nonhuman primates, or humans produces modest thrombocytosis.[97–100] Despite the *in vitro* and *in vivo* findings, genetic elimination of either leukemia inhibitory factor or the IL-11 receptor has no effect on thrombopoiesis,[101] even when combined with elimination of the thrombopoietin receptor.[102]

STEM CELL FACTOR

In contrast to the hematopoietic cytokine family, stem cell factor is more closely related to other hematopoietic proteins that utilize protein tyrosine kinase receptors, such as macrophage colony stimulating factor and the flt-3 ligand.[103] Nevertheless, stem cell factor stimulates megakaryocyte colony growth when used in combination with other cytokines.[104] Moreover, genetic elimination of its receptor *c-kit* reduces megakaryocyte production[105] and the rebound thrombocytosis that occurs following immunosuppressive therapy.[106,107]

Stem cell factor was first identified using several different biologic assays (in addition to this term, the cytokine has been dubbed *c-kit* ligand, mast cell growth factor, and steel factor).[108] Later studies indicate the cytokine acts primarily on primitive cells of the hematopoietic, melanogenic, and germ cell lineages. Stem cell factor is a dimeric protein composed of two identical noncovalently linked polypeptides. The soluble form monomer contains 165 residues,[109] derived by proteolytic cleavage of a membrane-bound splicoform of the molecule.[110] The membrane bound form is more active than the soluble cytokine, as intracellular signaling in response to membrane-bound stem cell factor is prolonged in receptor-bearing cells.[111] Moreover, a naturally occurring mutant allele of the gene (*Sl^d*), which allows production of the soluble but not the membrane-bound form of the cytokine, results in a phenotype nearly identical to deletion of the entire locus,[112] again pointing to the importance of the membrane-bound form present on marrow stromal cells.

FLT-3 LIGAND

The flt ligand initially was identified as a ligand for a novel member of the protein tyrosine kinase family of receptors.[103] This growth factor also affects megakaryocyte formation. Like stem cell factor, to which it is most closely related, flt ligand is found in both soluble and membrane-bound forms, is a noncovalently linked dimer, and affects primarily primitive hematopoietic cells.[113] Although several studies have shown that flt ligand used alone does not support megakaryocyte colony formation, some studies suggest flt ligand works in synergy with other megakaryocyte stimulatory agents to augment the proliferation of megakaryocytic progenitor cells in culture.[114,115] Administration of flt ligand to mice expands the number of marrow and splenic progenitor cells that can give rise to megakaryocytes *in vitro*.[116] However,

genetic elimination of either flt ligand or its receptor does not produce a platelet phenotype.

THROMBOPOIETIN

The term *thrombopoietin* was first coined in 1958 to describe the primary regulator of platelet production.[117] A major impetus to the discovery of thrombopoietin in 1986 was the identification of the myeloproliferative leukemia virus (MPLV), which induces a vast expansion of hematopoietic cells.[118] The responsible viral oncogene was characterized in 1990,[119] and its cellular homologue c-mpl was cloned in 1992.[120] Based on the presence of two copies of the hematopoietic cytokine receptor motif[121] and the ability of a fusion of c-Mpl and the IL-4 receptor to signal in factor dependent cells,[122] *c-mpl* clearly encoded a growth factor receptor, but its ligand was not known. Using three distinct strategies, four separate groups were able to clone cDNA for the corresponding hormone and report their results in 1994 (reviewed in ref. 75). The gene for thrombopoietin encodes a 36-kDa polypeptide,[123] which also is predicted to be extensively posttranslationally modified, resulting in an approximately 50- to 70-kDa protein.

Thrombopoietin bears striking homology to erythropoietin, the primary regulator of erythropoiesis, within the amino-terminal half of the predicted polypeptide. The two proteins are more closely related than any other two cytokines within the hematopoietic cytokine family, sharing 20 percent identical amino acids, an additional 25 percent conservative substitutions, and identical positions of three of the four cysteine residues. Unlike any of the other cytokines in the family, thrombopoietin contains a 181-residue carboxyl-terminal extension, which bears homology to no known proteins. Two functions have been assigned to this region: it prolongs the circulatory half-life of the hormone,[3] and it aids in its secretion from the cells that normally synthesize the hormone.[124]

The biologic activities of thrombopoietin have been demonstrated *in vitro* and *in vivo*, in mice, rats, dogs, nonhuman primates, and man. Incubation of marrow cells with thrombopoietin stimulates megakaryocyte survival and proliferation, alone and in combination with other cytokines.[34] *In vivo*, thrombopoietin stimulates platelet production in a log-linear manner to levels 10-fold higher than baseline[3,61,125] without affecting the peripheral blood red or white cell counts. In addition, because of its affect on hematopoietic stem cells (see Chap. 15), the number of erythroid and myeloid progenitors and mixed myeloid progenitors in marrow and spleen also are increased,[126,127] an effect that is particularly impressive when the hormone is administered following myelosuppressive therapy.[126,128,129] This effect likely results from the synergy between thrombopoietin and the other hematopoietic cytokines circulating at high levels in this condition.

Based on genetic studies, thrombopoietin clearly is the primary regulator of thrombopoiesis. Elimination of the c-mpl or TPO gene leads to profound thrombocytopenia in mice as a result of a greatly reduced number of megakaryocyte progenitors, mature megakaryocytes, and the reduced polyploidy of the remaining megakaryocytes.[130] A similar result occurs in humans. Patients with congenital amegakaryocytic thrombocytopenia (CAMT) display numerous homozygous or mixed heterozygous nonsense or severe missense mutations of the thrombopoietin receptor c-Mpl[131,132] (see Chap. 110). The effect of thrombopoietin on hematopoietic stem cells is particularly revealed by consideration of children with CAMT. Within 5 years of birth, nearly every patient with CAMT develops aplastic anemia as a result of stem cell exhaustion.

The thrombopoietin gene displays an unusual 5′ flanking structure. Unlike the majority of genes that initiate translation of the encoded polypeptide with the first ATG codon present in the mRNA, thrombopoietin translation initiates at the eighth ATG codon located within the third exon of a full-length transcript.[133] Moreover, the eighth ATG is embedded in the short open reading frame of the seventh ATG, a particularly inefficient circumstance for translation initiation.[134] As such, little thrombopoietin protein is produced for any given amount of mRNA. Although this molecular arrangement has no known physiologic consequences, it forms the basis for an unusual form of disease, a disorder of translation efficiency. Four cases of autosomal dominant familial thrombocytosis have been linked to mutations in the region surrounding the initiation codon. In two families, a single mutation in different nucleotides of the intron 3 splice donor sequence results in alternate splicing of the primary thrombopoietin transcript, eliminating the seventh and eighth ATG codons, creating a new amino-terminus by fusing of the fifth open reading frame with the TPO coding sequence. This novel thrombopoietin mRNA is efficiently translated, resulting in supraphysiologic levels of hormone production and nonclonal expansion of thrombopoiesis.[135,136] In another mutant thrombopoietin allele, deletion of a single nucleotide within the seventh open reading frame leads to its fusion with the thrombopoietin coding sequence and now enhanced translation of thrombopoietin from the seventh ATG codon.[137] A fourth mutation has been described within the seventh open reading frame, leading to premature termination of that short peptide, preventing its interference with translation initiation from the usual eighth initiation codon,[138] again enhancing thrombopoietin production (reviewed in ref. 139).

Regulation of thrombopoietin production has received much attention. Experimental induction of immune-mediated thrombocytopenia results in relatively rapid restoration of platelet levels, followed by a brief period of rebound thrombocytosis.[140] In these experimental cases and in most naturally occurring cases of thrombocytopenia, plasma hormone concentrations vary inversely with platelet counts, rising to maximal levels within 24 hours of onset of profound thrombocytopenia.[141] Two nonmutually exclusive models have been advanced to explain these findings. In the first model, thrombopoietin production is constitutive, but its consumption, and hence the level remaining in the blood to affect megakaryopoiesis, is determined by the mass of c-Mpl receptors present on platelets and megakaryocytes accessible to the plasma.[142] In this way, states of thrombocytosis result in increased thrombopoietin consumption (by the expanded platelet mass of c-Mpl receptors), reducing megakaryopoiesis. Conversely, thrombocytopenia reduces peripheral blood thrombopoietin destruction, resulting in elevated blood levels of the hormone that drive megakaryopoiesis and platelet recovery. This model is based on one of the mechanisms regulating macrophage colony stimulating factor levels.[143] The invariable levels of thrombopoietin-specific mRNA present in the liver and kidney of experimental animals and patients with thrombocytopenia or thrombocytosis support this model.[144,145] Moreover, thrombopoietin knockout mice display a gene dosage effect.[146] Platelet levels in heterozygous mice are intermediate between that seen in wild-type and nullizygous animals, suggesting active regulation of the remaining thrombopoietin allele cannot compensate for the mild (60% of normal) thrombocytopenia induced by the loss of one allele.

A second model suggests thrombopoietin expression is a regulated event. Very low platelet levels can induce thrombopoietin-specific mRNA production. Several studies have shown that thrombopoietin mRNA levels are modulated in response to moderate to severe thrombocytopenia, at least in the marrow.[145,147,148] The signal(s) responsible for this form of thrombopoietin regulation is being uncovered. CD40 ligand, platelet-derived growth factor, fibroblast growth factor, TGF-β, platelet factor-4, and thrombospondin modulate thrombopoietin production from marrow stromal cells.[149,150]

The human thrombopoietin gene 5' flanking region lacks a TATA box or CAAT motif and directs transcription initiation at multiple sites over a 50-nucleotide region.[151] Reporter gene analysis in a hepatocyte cell line identified an Ets2 transcription factor-binding motif responsible for high-level expression of the gene. The 5' flanking region also includes SP-1, AP-2, and NF-κB binding sites,[152] although the contribution of these transcription factors to thrombopoietin gene expression, either under steady state or inflammatory conditions, has not been studied.

STROMAL CELL-DERIVED FACTOR-1

Chemokines are members of a rapidly growing class of molecules that play multiple roles in blood cell physiology.[153] Initially defined as substances that induce leukocyte chemotaxis, four classes of the 8- to 12-kDa polypeptides have been recognized, based on the spacing of cysteine residues close to the amino-terminus of the proteins. An equally rapidly growing family of chemokine receptors also has been discovered, classified by the subfamily of chemokines they serve. All chemokine receptors are members of the seven-transmembrane family of receptors that signal through heterotrimeric G proteins.

Most work has been conducted with the CC and CXC subfamilies of chemokines, molecules that display modest inhibitory effects on cell proliferation when used alone and potent effects when used in combination on hematopoietic progenitors at all levels of development.[154] On many levels, the CXC chemokine SDF-1 and its receptor CXCR4 are notable exceptions to the many features shared by most members of the chemokine family. For example, although all the other genes for the known CXC chemokines reside on the long arm of human chromosome 14, *Sdf-1* localizes to the long arm of chromosome 10.[155] Moreover, most chemokine receptors can be activated by multiple ligands. For example, the chemokine MIP-1α can bind and activate CCR1 and CCR5, and IL-8 can bind both CXCR1 and CXCR2.[156] In contrast, as the phenotype of genetic elimination of both CXCR4 and SDF-1 are almost identical,[157,158] CXCR4 appears to be the only receptor for SDF-1, and SDF-1 is the only ligand for CXCR4.

The marrow stroma is the primary source of SDF-1, and most of the cell types known to express CXCR4 are hematopoietic in origin. One of the major phenotypes in SDF-1– or CXCR4-deficient neonatal mice is marrow aplasia, thought to be secondary to failure of perinatal hematopoietic stem cell homing[159] (see Chap. 15). In addition, megakaryocytes display CXCR4[160] and migrate in response to an SDF-1 concentration gradient.[161] Several groups have shown that SDF-1 augments thrombopoietin-induced megakaryocyte growth in suspension culture.[37,160] Later studies have shown the synergy between SDF-1 and other stimuli on megakaryocyte growth extends to cell surface adhesion.[38]

TRANSFORMING GROWTH FACTOR-β

In addition to the many positive regulators of megakaryopoiesis, several substances down-modulate their development. Five isoforms of TGF-β have been identified, all disulfide-linked homodimers each containing 112 residues.[162] Transforming growth factor-β_1 is the predominant type of TGF found in hematopoietic tissues. Platelet α-granules are a particularly rich source of the cytokine. In general, transforming growth factors are inhibitors of hematopoiesis,[163,164] particularly of megakaryocyte development.[165,166] The best understood TGF-β growth inhibitory effects are exerted on cell cycle progression. After binding to one of five receptors, two pathways that block cell cycle progression are activated. pRb is hypophosphorylated,[167] antagonizing the effects of G_1 phase cyclin-dependent kinases, and cell cycle inhibitors including p27 and p15^{INK} are up-regulated, affecting cell cycle progression.[168,169] In contrast to these negative effects of TGF-β on cell proliferation, the cytokine enhances megakaryocyte differentiation.

INTERFERON-α

A second class of cytokines that negatively impact thrombopoiesis are the interferons (IFNs), proteins first defined by their ability to induce an antiviral state in mammalian cells.[170] Biochemical fractionation has revealed three classes of IFNs: IFN-α, a family of 17 distinct but highly homologous molecules; IFN-β, a single molecule more distantly related to the various isoforms of IFN-α; and IFN-γ, a unique molecule that shares functional properties but not structure with the others. IFNs exert profound inhibitory effects on hematopoiesis.[171]

The genes for the IFN-α/β subfamily cluster on the short arm of chromosome 9 and encode 165- to 172-residue polypeptides, of which 35 percent are invariant across the family of IFN-α molecules. IFNs of the α/β type are produced by transcriptional up-regulation in fibroblasts and leukocytes in response to viruses and other infectious agents and to inflammatory cytokines. Once bound to the IFN receptors, a cascade of kinases and intracellular mediators are triggered, initiated by JAK kinases, STAT transcription factors, and p38 MAPK (see Chap. 13), resulting in changes in gene transcription.

IFN-α inhibits megakaryopoiesis, the clinical use of which is responsible for modest to severe thrombocytopenia in a significant number of patients undergoing therapy for chronic viral hepatitis.[172,173] The mechanisms responsible for the inhibitory effect of IFN-α are multifactorial. Some studies suggest a direct inhibitory effect of IFN-α on growth factor-induced proliferation pathways. For example, the cytokine augments double-stranded RNA activated protein kinase activity, inhibiting translation initiation factor-2, implicating reduction of the growth factor-induced protein synthesis necessary for growth factor response.[174] IFN-β induces expression of the cell cycle inhibitor p27^{kip1}, arresting cells in G_0/G_1.[175] Other studies have demonstrated IFN-α induces a SOCS-1-based feedback mechanism that cross-reacts and depresses thrombopoietin signaling.[176] Thus, in addition to the multiple positive mediators of megakaryopoiesis, several cytokines block the process and can lead to thrombocytopenia.

MEGAKARYOCYTE MICROENVIRONMENT

Chapter 4 details the role of the marrow microenvironment in hematopoiesis. This chapter discusses only aspects particularly vital for megakaryocyte growth. The cellular concentration within the marrow is estimated to be 10^9/ml. Therefore, cell–cell and cell–matrix interactions certainly will occur.[177] Marrow stromal cells influence hematopoiesis in a number of ways, perhaps the most prominent through production of several cytokines that positively or negatively affect megakaryocyte growth.[145,178–180] Stromal cells are the origin of a number of extracellular matrix proteins and glycomucins that either directly affect hematopoietic cells or indirectly affect hematopoietic cells by binding growth factors and presenting them in a functional context.[181,182] Stromal cells also bear ligands for Notch proteins, cell surface receptors that are critical mediators of cell fate decisions.[183] Notch and its ligands Delta and Jagged play important roles as regulators of hematopoietic progenitor cell proliferation[184] and play a potential role in influencing the lineage fate choice between erythropoiesis and megakaryopoiesis.[185] Cell–cell interactions mediated by integrins present on hematopoietic cells and counterreceptors on stromal cells are very important for megakaryopoiesis,[186] both by bringing hematopoietic cells into close proximity to stromal cells producing soluble or cell-bound cytokines and more directly by triggering or augmenting intracellular signaling, promoting entry into the cell cycle, and preventing programmed cell death.

THERAPEUTIC MANIPULATION OF THROMBOPOIESIS BY NATURALLY OCCURRING CYTOKINES

Thrombocytopenia is a major clinical problem with multiple origins (see Chap. 110). Primary bone marrow diseases, certain infections, and solid tumors with a high propensity for marrow metastases directly affect platelet production. Nearly all leukemias, advanced lymphomas, and myelomas ultimately cause thrombocytopenia by this mechanism. Hypersplenism or thrombopoietin deficiency leads to platelet sequestration and thrombocytopenia in patients with hepatic failure. Consumptive coagulopathies, initiated by infection, tumors, or severe injury, can be responsible for severe thrombocytopenia. In other patients, autoimmune thrombocytopenia arises during the course of disease or is a primary disease. However, the most common cause of significant thrombocytopenia is the use of potentially curative or palliative chemotherapy or radiation therapy in patients with malignancy. An estimated 300,000+ persons yearly worldwide undergo courses of chemotherapy adequate to produce clinically significant thrombocytopenia. Recovery from the marrow suppressive effects of most chemotherapeutic agents occurs within 1 to 3 weeks following discontinuation of therapy. However, some agents, including mitomycin C or nitrosoureas, may produce prolonged periods of marrow suppression. Tumor- or treatment-related thrombocytopenia often delays much needed additional therapy, may necessitate potentially complicated platelet transfusions (see Chap. 132), and cause significant morbidity and occasional mortality. Given the increased understanding of the humoral basis for megakaryopoiesis and thrombopoiesis, numerous attempts have been made to manipulate these processes for therapeutic benefit.

INTERLEUKIN-11

IL-11 augments the growth of megakaryocytic progenitors in the presence of IL-3[187,188] and acts to promote megakaryocyte maturation rather than proliferation.[189,190] The preclinical effects of IL-11 were evaluated in mice, rats, and subhuman primates and revealed moderate activity in normal animals and following cytoreductive therapy.[98,191,192]

The first clinical trials of IL-11 were reported in abstract form in 1993 and 1994.[193,194] Randomized clinical trials were reported a few years later.[195–197] Most studies reported IL-11 ameliorated drug-induced thrombocytopenia. For example, IL-11 administered to patients with advanced stages of breast cancer undergoing multiple courses of anthracycline-based chemotherapy significantly reduced the need for platelet transfusions by 27 percent. However, use of the drug in patients undergoing autologous stem cell transplantation did not enhance platelet recovery or other indices of hematopoiesis. Although chemical evidence of an acute phase response was noted in many of the patients treated in these studies, the drug was generally well tolerated, although fluid retention has been a significant side effect often necessitating concomitant use of diuretics. IL-11 (oprelvekin) was approved by the Food and Drug Administration in 1998 for use in patients undergoing chemotherapy who have evidence of previous drug-induced thrombocytopenia.

INTERFERON-α

As noted earlier in this chapter (see "Hormones and Cytokines"), IFN suppresses hematopoiesis and thrombopoiesis by multiple mechanisms. As a consequence, IFN-α has been used to reduce platelet counts in patients with many forms of myeloproliferative disease. The first reported clinical trial was performed in patients with a mixture of these disorders. The trial found the mean platelet count decreased significantly from 1050×10^9/L to 340×10^9/L.[198] Long-term therapy with IFN also was shown to be effective and safe.[199]

From these and other studies, IFN (two to five million units 3 times per week) clearly effectively reduces the platelet count toward normal in most patients with myeloproliferative disease. More aggressive regimens (two to six million units daily) result in complete hematologic remissions but with no evidence that the clonal disorder responsible has been affected.[200] Not surprisingly, reduced energy level, weight loss, myalgia, and depression have been consistently reported, forcing discontinuation of the drug in approximately one third of patients taking low to moderate doses of various forms of IFN-α.[201] Of some concern and possibly related to its effects on the immune system, a significant number of patients treated with IFN for thrombocytosis have developed antibodies to the administered drug, with subsequent reduced efficacy.[202]

THROMBOPOIETIN

Clinically, the most important activity of thrombopoietin likely is its effects on megakaryopoiesis, potentially ameliorating the thrombocytopenia that occurs in natural and iatrogenic states of marrow failure. In this regard, a number of promising results in preclinical trials of the cytokine have been reported.[126,128,129,203] In general, in rodent, dog, and nonhuman primates, almost every model of myelosuppression or immune-mediated platelet destruction has responded favorably to parenteral administration of thrombopoietin. In addition to the favorable effects on platelet recovery, many of these studies also reported enhanced recovery or hematopoietic progenitors of all lineages, accelerated recovery of erythrocytes or leukocytes, or both. The only exception to these generally favorable results has been reported in animal models of stem cell transplantation, where negligible to minimal acceleration of blood cell recovery was found, unless the stem cell donor was treated with the hormone.[204,205]

A number of clinical trials in patients with cancer undergoing cytotoxic therapy have been conducted. Results were varied, with the hormone helpful in many patients[206–208] but not in all clinical situations.[209,210] In general, the hormone has been useful in patients administered moderately aggressive chemotherapeutic regimens that produce clinically important thrombocytopenia. However, the hormone has not been helpful in the setting of high-dose, prolonged cytotoxic therapy, as in the treatment of acute myelogenous leukemia, or in stem cell transplantation, unless, as in the animal studies, it is administered to the stem cell donor.[211] Thrombopoietin also reportedly increases platelet levels in patients with immune-mediated thrombocytopenia.[212] The timing of drug administration can significantly impact both the total amount of drug required and its efficacy.[213] For example, administration of one dose of drug before and once following myelosuppressive therapy was as effective as any other multidose regimen. This regimen resulted in significant reductions in nadir platelet counts and the need for platelet transfusion during chemotherapy cycles supplemented with thrombopoietin. Nevertheless, use of a modified form of recombinant thrombopoietin is associated with antibody formation to the drug, which cross-reacts with and neutralizes the native hormone, resulting in thrombocytopenia.[214] Although this effect has not been reported with a nonmodified recombinant thrombopoietin, most efforts using thrombopoietin in patients with thrombocytopenia are focusing on small peptide or organic mimics that bind to and activate the thrombopoietin receptor[215–217] (reviewed in ref. 218), agents that presently are undergoing clinical trials.

REFERENCES

1. Hanson SR, Slichter SJ: Platelet kinetics in patients with bone marrow hypoplasia: Evidence for a fixed platelet requirement. *Blood* 66:1105, 1985.

2. Dettke M, Hlousek M, Kurz M, et al: Increase in endogenous thrombopoietin in healthy donors after automated plateletpheresis. *Transfusion* 38:449, 1998.

3. Harker LA, Marzec UM, Hunt P, et al: Dose-response effects of pegylated human megakaryocyte growth and development factor on platelet production and function in nonhuman primates. *Blood* 88:511, 1996.

4. O'Malley CJ, Rasko JE, Basser RL, et al: Administration of pegylated recombinant human megakaryocyte growth and development factor to humans stimulates the production of functional platelets that show no evidence of in vivo activation. *Blood* 88:3288, 1996.

5. Italiano JE Jr, Lecine P, Shivdasani RA, Hartwig JH: Blood platelets are assembled principally at the ends of proplatelet processes produced by differentiated megakaryocytes. *J Cell Biol* 147:1299, 1999.

6. Harker LA, Finch CA: Thrombokinetics in man. *J Clin Invest* 48:963, 1969.

7. Stenberg PE, Levin J: Mechanisms of platelet production. *Blood Cells* 15:23, 1989.

8. Radley JM, Haller CJ: Fate of senescent megakaryocytes in the bone marrow. *Br J Haematol* 53:277, 1983.

9. Tronik-Le Roux D, Roullot V, Schweitzer A, et al: Suppression of erythro-megakaryocytopoiesis and the induction of reversible thrombocytopenia in mice transgenic for the thymidine kinase gene targeted by the platelet glycoprotein alpha IIb promoter. *J Exp Med* 181:2141, 1995.

10. Debili N, Robin C, Schiavon V, et al: Different expression of CD41 on human lymphoid and myeloid progenitors from adults and neonates. *Blood* 97:2023, 2001.

11. Wu G, Essex DW, Meloni FJ, et al: Human endothelial cells in culture and in vivo express on their surface all four components of the glycoprotein Ib/IX/V complex. *Blood* 90:2660, 1997.

12. Hickey MJ, Hagen FS, Yagi M, Roth GJ: Human platelet glycoprotein V: Characterization of the polypeptide and the related Ib-V-IX receptor system of adhesive, leucine-rich glycoproteins. *Proc Natl Acad Sci U S A* 90:8327, 1993.

13. Kahn ML, Diacovo TG, Bainton DF, et al: Glycoprotein V-deficient platelets have undiminished thrombin responsiveness and do not exhibit a Bernard-Soulier phenotype. *Blood* 94:4112, 1999.

14. Lopez JA, Andrews RK, Afshar-Kharghan V, Berndt MC: Bernard-Soulier syndrome. *Blood* 91:4397, 1998.

15. Ramakrishnan V, DeGuzman F, Bao M, et al: A thrombin receptor function for platelet glycoprotein Ib-IX unmasked by cleavage of glycoprotein V. *Proc Natl Acad Sci U S A* 98:1823, 2001.

16. Breton-Gorius J, Reyes F: Ultrastructure of human bone marrow cell maturation. *Int Rev Cytol* 46:251, 1976.

17. Italiano JE Jr, Shivdasani RA: Megakaryocytes and beyond: The birth of platelets. *J Thromb Haemost* 1:1174, 2003.

18. Ebbe S, Stohlman F Jr: Megakaryocytopoiesis in the rat. *Blood* 26:20, 1965.

19. Vitrat N, Cohen-Solal K, Pique C, et al: Endomitosis of human megakaryocytes are due to abortive mitosis. *Blood* 91:3711, 1998.

20. Odell TT Jr., Reiter RS: Generation cycle of rat megakaryocytes. *Exp Cell Res* 53:321, 1968.

21. Lemarchandel V, Ghysdael J, Mignotte V, et al: GATA and Ets cis-acting sequences mediate megakaryocyte-specific expression. *Mol Cell Biol* 13:668, 1993.

22. Bastian LS, Kwiatkowski BA, Breininger J, et al: Regulation of the megakaryocytic glycoprotein IX promoter by the oncogenic Ets transcription factor Fli-1. *Blood* 93:2637, 1999.

23. Ramachandran B, Surrey S, Schwartz E: Megakaryocyte-specific positive regulatory sequence 5′ to the human PF4 gene. *Exp Hematol* 23:49, 1995.

24. Furihata K, Kunicki TJ: Characterization of human glycoprotein VI gene 5′ regulatory and promoter regions. *Arterioscler Thromb Vasc Biol* 22:1733, 2002.

25. Sevinsky JR, Whalen AM, Ahn NG: Extracellular signal-regulated kinase induces the megakaryocyte GPIIb/CD41 gene through MafB/Kreisler. *Mol Cell Biol* 24:4534, 2004.

26. Rojnuckarin P, Drachman JG, Kaushansky K: Thrombopoietin-induced activation of the mitogen-activated protein kinase (MAPK) pathway in normal megakaryocytes: Role in endomitosis. *Blood* 94:1273, 1999.

27. Vyas P, Norris FA, Joseph R, et al: Inositol polyphosphate 4-phosphatase type I regulates cell growth downstream of transcription factor GATA-1. *Proc Natl Acad Sci U S A* 97:13696, 2000.

28. Pevny L, Simon MC, Robertson E, et al: Erythroid differentiation in chimaeric mice blocked by a targeted mutation in the gene for transcription factor GATA-1. *Nature* 349:257, 1991.

29. Shivdasani RA, Fujiwara Y, McDevitt MA, Orkin SH: A lineage-selective knockout establishes the critical role of transcription factor GATA-1 in megakaryocyte growth and platelet development. *EMBO J* 16:3965, 1997.

30. Song WJ, Sullivan MG, Legare RD, et al: Haploinsufficiency of CBFA2 causes familial thrombocytopenia with propensity to develop acute myelogenous leukaemia. *Nat Genet* 23:166, 1999.

31. Ichikawa M, Asai T, Saito T, et al: AML-1 is required for megakaryocytic maturation and lymphocytic differentiation, but not for maintenance of hematopoietic stem cells in adult hematopoiesis. *Nat Med* 10:299, 2004.

32. Elagib KE, Racke FK, Mogass M, et al: RUNX1 and GATA-1 coexpression and cooperation in megakaryocytic differentiation. *Blood* 101:4333, 2003.

33. Ebbe S, Phalen E, Stohlman F Jr: Abnormalities of megakaryocytes in W-WV mice. *Blood* 42:857, 1973.

34. Broudy VC, Lin NL, Kaushansky K: Thrombopoietin (c-mpl ligand) acts synergistically with erythropoietin, stem cell factor, and interleukin-11 to enhance murine megakaryocyte colony growth and increases megakaryocyte ploidy in vitro. *Blood* 85:1719, 1995.

35. Gainsford T, Roberts AW, Kimura S, et al: Cytokine production and function in c-mpl-deficient mice: No physiologic role for interleukin-3 in residual megakaryocyte and platelet production. *Blood* 91:2745, 1998.

36. Kaushansky K, Broudy VC, Lin N, et al: Thrombopoietin, the Mpl ligand, is essential for full megakaryocyte development. *Proc Natl Acad Sci U S A* 92:3234, 1995.

37. Hodohara K, Fujii N, Yamamoto N, Kaushansky K: Stromal cell-derived factor-1 (SDF-1) acts together with thrombopoietin to enhance the development of megakaryocytic progenitor cells (CFU-MK). *Blood* 95:769, 2000.

38. Avecilla ST, Hattori K, Heissig B, et al: Chemokine-mediated interaction of hematopoietic progenitors with the bone marrow vascular niche is required for thrombopoiesis. *Nat Med* 10:64, 2004.

39. Geddis AE, Fox NE, Kaushansky K: Phosphatidylinositol 3-kinase is necessary but not sufficient for thrombopoietin-induced proliferation in engineered Mpl-bearing cell lines as well as in primary megakaryocytic progenitors. *J Biol Chem* 276:34473, 2001.

40. Miyazaki R, Ogata H, Kobayashi Y: Requirement of thrombopoietin-induced activation of ERK for megakaryocyte differentiation and of p38 for erythroid differentiation. *Ann Hematol* 80:284, 2001.

41. Pettiford SM, Herbst R: The protein tyrosine phosphatase HePTP regulates nuclear translocation of ERK2 and can modulate megakaryocytic differentiation of K562 cells. *Leukemia* 17:366, 2003.

42. Dorsey JF, Cunnick JM, Mane SM, Wu J: Regulation of the Erk2-Elk1 signaling pathway and megakaryocytic differentiation of Bcr-Abl(+) K562 leukemic cells by Gab2. *Blood* 99:1388, 2002.

43. Datta NS, Williams JL, Caldwell J, et al: Novel alterations in CDK1/cyclin B1 kinase complex formation occur during the acquisition of a polyploid DNA content. *Mol Biol Cell* 7:209, 1996.

44. Zhang Y, Nagata Y, Yu G, et al: Aberrant quantity and localization of Aurora-B/AIM-1 and survivin during megakaryocyte polyploidization and the consequences of Aurora-B/AIM-1-deregulated expression. *Blood* 103:3717, 2004.

45. Matsumura I, Tanaka H, Kawasaki A, et al: Increased D-type cyclin expression together with decreased cdc2 activity confers megakaryocytic differentiation of a human thrombopoietin-dependent hematopoietic cell line. *J Biol Chem* 275:5553, 2000.

46. Zhang Y, Wang Z, Ravid K: The cell cycle in polyploid megakaryocytes is associated with reduced activity of cyclin B1-dependent cdc2 kinase. *J Biol Chem* 271:4266, 1996.

47. Carow CE, Fox NE, Kaushansky K: Kinetics of endomitosis in primary murine megakaryocytes. *J Cell Physiol* 188:291, 2001.

48. Geddis AE, Kaushansky K: Megakaryocytes express functional aurora kinase B in endomitosis. *Blood* 104:1017, 2004.

49. Seri M, Cusano R, Gangarossa S, et al: Mutations in MYH9 result in the May-Hegglin anomaly, and Fechtner and Sebastian syndromes. The May-Hegglin/Fechtner Syndrome Consortium. *Nat Genet* 26:103, 2000.

50. Kelley MI, Jawien W, Ortel TL, Korczak JF: Mutation of MYH9, encoding non-muscle myosin heavy chain A, in May-Hegglin anomaly. *Nat Genet* 26:106, 2000.

51. Hartwig J, Italiano J Jr: The birth of the platelet. *J Thromb Haemost* 1:1580, 2003.

52. Visvader JE, Elefanty AG, Strasser A, Adams JM: GATA-1 but not SCL induces megakaryocytic differentiation in an early myeloid line. *EMBO J* 11:4557, 1992.

53. Tavassoli M, Aoki M: Localization of megakaryocytes in the bone marrow. *Blood Cells* 15:3, 1989.

54. Becker RP, De Bruyn P: The transmural passage of blood cells into myeloid sinusoids and the entry of platelets into sinusoidal circulation; a scanning electron microscope investigation. *Am J Anat* 145:183-205, 1975.

55. Andrews NC, Erdjument-Bromage H, Davidson MB, et al: Erythroid transcription factor NF-E2 is a haematopoietic-specific basic-leucine zipper protein. *Nature* 362:722, 1993.

56. Bean TL, Ney PA: Multiple regions of p45 NF-E2 are required for beta-globin gene expression in erythroid cells. *Nucleic Acids Res* 25:2509, 1997.

57. Shivdasani RA, Rosenblatt MF, Zucker-Franklin D, et al: Transcription factor NF-E2 is required for platelet formation independent of the actions of thrombopoietin/MGDF in megakaryocyte development. *Cell* 81:695, 1995.

58. Querfurth E, Schuster M, Kulessa H, et al: Antagonism between C/EBPbeta and FOG in eosinophil lineage commitment of multipotent hematopoietic progenitors. *Genes Dev* 14:2515, 2000.

59. Howell WH DD: The production of blood platelets in the lungs. *J Exp Med* 65:177, 1939.

60. Slater DN, Trowbridge EA, Martin JF: The megakaryocyte in thrombocytopenia: A microscopic study which supports the theory that platelets are produced in the pulmonary circulation. *Thromb Res* 31:163, 1983.

61. Kaushansky K, Lok S, Holly RD, et al: Promotion of megakaryocyte progenitor expansion and differentiation by the c-Mpl ligand thrombopoietin. *Nature* 369:568, 1994.

62. Kaufman RM, Airo R, Pollack S, et al: Origin of pulmonary megakaryocytes. *Blood* 25:767, 1965.

63. Harker LA, Marzec UM, Kelly AB: Effects of Mpl ligands on platelet production and function in nonhuman primates. *Stem Cells* 16(suppl 2):107, 1998.

64. Choi ES, Nichol JL, Hokom MM, et al: Platelets generated in vitro from proplatelet-displaying human megakaryocytes are functional. *Blood* 85:402, 1995.

65. Norol F, Vitrat N, Cramer E, et al: Effects of cytokines on platelet production from blood and marrow CD34+ cells. *Blood* 91:830, 1998.

66. Rojnuckarin P, Kaushansky K: Actin reorganization and proplatelet formation in murine megakaryocytes: The role of protein kinase C alpha. *Blood* 97:154, 2001.

67. Ishida Y, Yano K, Ito T, et al: Purification of proplatelet formation (PPF) stimulating factor: Thrombin/antithrombin III complex stimulates PPF of megakaryocytes in vitro and platelet production in vivo. *Thromb Haemost* 85:349, 2001.

68. Hunt P, Hokom MM, Wiemann B, et al: Megakaryocyte proplatelet-like process formation in vitro is inhibited by serum prothrombin, a process which is blocked by matrix-bound glycosaminoglycans. *Exp Hematol* 21:372, 1993.

69. Geddis AE, Kaushansky K: Inherited thrombocytopenias: Toward a molecular understanding of disorders of platelet production. *Curr Opin Pediatr* 16:15, 2004.

70. Li J, Kuter DJ: The end is just the beginning: Megakaryocyte apoptosis and platelet release. *Int J Hematol* 74:365, 2001.

71. De Botton S, Sabri S, Daugas E, et al: Platelet formation is the consequence of caspase activation within megakaryocytes. *Blood* 100:1310, 2002.

72. Quesenberry PJ, Ihle JN, McGrath E: The effect of interleukin 3 and GM-CSA-2 on megakaryocyte and myeloid clonal colony formation. *Blood* 65:214, 1985.

73. Kaushansky K, O'Hara PJ, Berkner K, et al: Genomic cloning, characterization, and multilineage growth-promoting activity of human granulocyte-macrophage colony-stimulating factor. *Proc Natl Acad Sci U S A* 83:3101, 1986.

74. Briddell RA, Bruno E, Cooper RJ, et al: Effect of c-kit ligand on in vitro human megakaryocytopoiesis. *Blood* 78:2854, 1991.

75. Kaushansky K: Thrombopoietin: The primary regulator of platelet production. *Blood* 86:419, 1995.

76. Yang YC, Ciarletta AB, Temple PA, et al: Human IL-3 (multi-CSF): Identification by expression cloning of a novel hematopoietic growth factor related to murine IL-3. *Cell* 47:3, 1986.

77. Wong GG, Witek JS, Temple PA, et al: Human GM-CSF: Molecular cloning of the complementary DNA and purification of the natural and recombinant proteins. *Science* 228:810, 1985.

78. Feng Y, Klein BK, Vu L, et al: 1H 13C, and 15N NMR resonance assignments, secondary structure, and backbone topology of a variant of human interleukin-3. *Biochemistry* 34:6540, 1995.

79. Lopez AF, Eglinton JM, Gillis D, et al: Reciprocal inhibition of binding between interleukin 3 and granulocyte-macrophage colony-stimulating factor to human eosinophils. *Proc Natl Acad Sci U S A* 86:7022, 1989.

80. Scott CL, Robb L, Mansfield R, et al: Granulocyte-macrophage colony-stimulating factor is not responsible for residual thrombopoiesis in Mpl null mice. *Exp Hematol* 28:1001, 2000.

81. Chen Q, Solar G, Eaton DL, de Sauvage FJ: IL-3 does not contribute to platelet production in c-Mpl-deficient mice. *Stem Cells* 16(suppl 2):31, 1998.

82. Kishimoto T: The biology of interleukin-6. *Blood* 74:1, 1989.

83. Quesenberry PJ, McGrath HE, Williams ME, et al: Multifactor stimulation of megakaryocytopoiesis: Effects of interleukin 6. *Exp Hematol* 19:35, 1991.

84. Williams N, De Giorgio T, Banu N, et al: Recombinant interleukin 6 stimulates immature murine megakaryocytes. *Exp Hematol* 18:69, 1990.

85. Mei RL, Burstein SA: Megakaryocytic maturation in murine long-term bone marrow culture: Role of interleukin-6. *Blood* 78:1438, 1991.

86. Ishibashi T, Kimura H, Shikama Y, et al: Interleukin-6 is a potent thrombopoietic factor in vivo in mice. *Blood* 74:1241, 1989.

87. Asano S, Okano A, Ozawa K, et al: In vivo effects of recombinant human interleukin-6 in primates: Stimulated production of platelets. *Blood* 75:1602, 1990.

88. van Gameren MM, Willemse PH, Mulder NH, et al: Effects of recombinant human interleukin-6 in cancer patients: A phase I–II study. *Blood* 84:1434, 1994.

89. Blay JY, Favrot M, Rossi JF, Wijdenes J: Role of interleukin-6 in paraneoplastic thrombocytosis. *Blood* 82:2261, 1993.

90. Bernad A, Kopf M, Kulbacki R, et al: Interleukin-6 is required in vivo for the regulation of stem cells and committed progenitors of the hematopoietic system. *Immunity* 1:725, 1994.

91. Kaser A, Brandacher G, Steurer W, et al: Interleukin-6 stimulates thrombopoiesis through thrombopoietin: Role in inflammatory thrombocytosis. *Blood* 98:2720, 2001.

92. Du X, Williams DA: Interleukin-11: Review of molecular, cell biology, and clinical use. *Blood* 89:3897, 1997.

93. Gough NM: Molecular genetics of leukemia inhibitory factor (LIF) and its receptor. *Growth Factors* 7:175, 1992.

94. Hilton DJ: LIF: Lots of interesting functions. *Trends Biochem Sci* 17:72, 1992.

95. Debili N, Masse JM, Katz A, et al: Effects of the recombinant hematopoietic growth factors interleukin-3, interleukin-6, stem cell factor, and leukemia inhibitory factor on the megakaryocytic differentiation of CD34+ cells. *Blood* 82:84, 1993.

96. Teramura M, Kobayashi S, Hoshino S, et al: Interleukin-11 enhances human megakaryocytopoiesis in vitro. *Blood* 79:327, 1992.

97. Metcalf D, Nicola NA, Gearing DP: Effects of injected leukemia inhibitory factor on hematopoietic and other tissues in mice. *Blood* 76:50, 1990.

98. Neben TY, Loebelenz J, Hayes L, et al: Recombinant human interleukin-11 stimulates megakaryocytopoiesis and increases peripheral platelets in normal and splenectomized mice. *Blood* 81:901, 1993.

99. Farese AM, Myers LA, MacVittie TJ: Therapeutic efficacy of recombinant human leukemia inhibitory factor in a primate model of radiation-induced marrow aplasia. *Blood* 84:3675, 1994.

100. Gordon MS, McCaskill-Stevens WJ, Battiato LA, et al: A phase I trial of recombinant human interleukin-11 (neumega rhIL-11 growth factor) in women with breast cancer receiving chemotherapy. *Blood* 87:3615, 1996.

101. Nandurkar HH, Robb L, Tarlinton D, et al: Adult mice with targeted mutation of the interleukin-11 receptor (IL11Ra) display normal hematopoiesis. *Blood* 90:2148, 1997.

102. Gainsford T, Nandurkar H, Metcalf D, et al: The residual megakaryocyte and platelet production in c-Mpl-deficient mice is not dependent on the actions of interleukin-6, interleukin-11, or leukemia inhibitory factor. *Blood* 95:528, 2000.

103. Lyman SD, James L, Vanden Bos T, et al: Molecular cloning of a ligand for the flt3/flk-2 tyrosine kinase receptor: A proliferative factor for primitive hematopoietic cells. *Cell* 75:1157, 1993.

104. Avraham H, Vannier E, Cowley S, et al: Effects of the stem cell factor, c-kit ligand, on human megakaryocytic cells. *Blood* 79:365, 1992.

105. Ebbe S, Phalen E, Stohlman F Jr: Abnormalities of megakaryocytes in Sl-Sld mice. *Blood* 42:865, 1973.

106. Arnold J, Ellis S, Radley JM, Williams N: Compensatory mechanisms in platelet production: The response of Sl/Sld mice to 5-fluorouracil. *Exp Hematol* 19:24, 1991.

107. Hunt P, Zsebo KM, Hokom MM, et al: Evidence that stem cell factor is involved in the rebound thrombocytosis that follows 5-fluorouracil treatment. *Blood* 80:904, 1992.

108. Broudy VC: Stem cell factor and hematopoiesis. *Blood* 90:1345, 1997.

109. Langley KE, Bennett LG, Wypych J, et al: Soluble stem cell factor in human serum. *Blood* 81:656, 1993.

110. Cheng HJ, Flanagan JG: Transmembrane kit ligand cleavage does not require a signal in the cytoplasmic domain and occurs at a site dependent on spacing from the membrane. *Mol Biol Cell* 5:943, 1994.

111. Miyazawa K, Williams DA, Gotoh A, et al: Membrane-bound Steel factor induces more persistent tyrosine kinase activation and longer life span of c-kit gene-encoded protein than its soluble form. *Blood* 85:641, 1995.

112. Flanagan JG, Chan DC, Leder P: Transmembrane form of the kit ligand growth factor is determined by alternative splicing and is missing in the Sld mutant. *Cell* 64:1025, 1991.

113. Lyman SD, Jacobsen SE: c-kit ligand and Flt3 ligand: Stem/progenitor cell factors with overlapping yet distinct activities. *Blood* 91:1101, 1998.

114. Ramsfjell V, Borge OJ, Veiby OP, et al: Thrombopoietin, but not erythropoietin, directly stimulates multilineage growth of primitive murine bone marrow progenitor cells in synergy with early acting cytokines: Distinct interactions with the ligands for c-kit and FLT3. *Blood* 88:4481, 1996.

115. Piacibello W, Garetto L, Sanavio F, et al: The effects of human FLT3 ligand on in vitro human megakaryocytopoiesis. *Exp Hematol* 24:340, 1996.

116. Brasel K, McKenna HJ, Morrissey PJ, et al: Hematologic effects of flt3 ligand in vivo in mice. *Blood* 88:2004, 1996.

117. Kelemen E CI, Tanos B: Demonstration and some properties of human thrombopoietin in thrombocythemic sera. *Acta Haematol (Basel)* 20: 350, 1958.

118. Wendling F, Varlet P, Charon M, Tambourin P: MPLV: A retrovirus complex inducing an acute myeloproliferative leukemic disorder in adult mice. *Virology* 149:242, 1986.

119. Souyri M, Vigon I, Penciolelli JF, et al: A putative truncated cytokine receptor gene transduced by the myeloproliferative leukemia virus immortalizes hematopoietic progenitors. *Cell* 63:1137, 1990.

120. Vigon I, Mornon JP, Cocault L, et al: Molecular cloning and characterization of MPL, the human homolog of the v-Mpl oncogene: Identification of a member of the hematopoietic growth factor receptor superfamily. *Proc Natl Acad Sci U S A* 89:5640, 1992.

121. Cosman D: The hematopoietin receptor superfamily. *Cytokine* 5:95, 1993.

122. Skoda RC, Seldin DC, Chiang MK, et al: Murine c Mpl: A member of the hematopoietic growth factor receptor superfamily that transduces a proliferative signal. *EMBO J* 12:2645, 1993.

123. Lok S, Kaushansky K, Holly RD, et al: Cloning and expression of murine thrombopoietin cDNA and stimulation of platelet production in vivo. *Nature* 369:565, 1994.

124. Linden HM, Kaushansky K: The glycan domain of thrombopoietin enhances its secretion. *Biochemistry* 39:3044, 2000.

125. Basser RL, Rasko JE, Clarke K, et al: Thrombopoietic effects of pegylated recombinant human megakaryocyte growth and development factor (PEG-rHuMGDF) in patients with advanced cancer. *Lancet* 348: 1279, 1996.

126. Kaushansky K, Broudy VC, Grossmann A, et al: Thrombopoietin expands erythroid progenitors, increases red cell production, and enhances erythroid recovery after myelosuppressive therapy. *J Clin Invest* 96: 1683, 1995.

127. Farese AM, Hunt P, Boone T, MacVittie TJ: Recombinant human megakaryocyte growth and development factor stimulates thrombocytopoiesis in normal nonhuman primates. *Blood* 86:54, 1995.

128. Akahori H, Shibuya K, Obuchi M, et al: Effect of recombinant human thrombopoietin in nonhuman primates with chemotherapy-induced thrombocytopenia. *Br J Haematol* 94:722, 1996.

129. Neelis KJ, Hartong SC, Egeland T, Thomas GR, et al: The efficacy of single-dose administration of thrombopoietin with coadministration of either granulocyte/macrophage or granulocyte colony-stimulating factor in myelosuppressed rhesus monkeys. *Blood* 90:2565, 1997.

130. Gurney AL, Carver-Moore K, de Sauvage FJ, Moore MW: Thrombocytopenia in c-Mpl-deficient mice. *Science* 265:1445, 1994.

131. van den Oudenrijn S, Bruin M, Folman CC, et al: Mutations in the thrombopoietin receptor, Mpl, in children with congenital amegakaryocytic thrombocytopenia. *Br J Haematol* 110:441, 2000.

132. Ballmaier M, Germeshausen M, Schulze H, et al: c-mpl mutations are the cause of congenital amegakaryocytic thrombocytopenia. *Blood* 97: 139, 2001.

133. Sohma Y, Akahori H, Seki N, et al: Molecular cloning and chromosomal localization of the human thrombopoietin gene. *FEBS Lett* 353:57, 1994.

134. Morris D: *cis*-Acting mRNA structures in gene-specific translational control, in *Post-Transcriptional Gene Regulation*, edited by JB Harford, DR Morris, p 165. Wiley-Liss, New York, 1997.

135. Wiestner A, Schlemper RJ, Van der Maas AP, Skoda RC: An activating splice donor mutation in the thrombopoietin gene causes hereditary thrombocythaemia. *Nat Genet* 18:49, 1998.

136. Jorgensen MJ, Raskind WH, Wolff JF, et al: Familial thrombocytosis associated with overproduction of thrombopoietin due to a novel splice donor site mutation. *Blood* 92:205a, 1998.

137. Kondo T, Okabe M, Sanada M, et al: Familial essential thrombocythemia associated with one-base deletion in the 5'-untranslated region of the thrombopoietin gene. *Blood* 92:1091, 1998.

138. Ghilardi N, Wiestner A, Kikuchi M, et al: Hereditary thrombocythaemia in a Japanese family is caused by a novel point mutation in the thrombopoietin gene. *Br J Haematol* 107:310, 1999.

139. Cazzola M, Skoda RC: Translational pathophysiology: A novel molecular mechanism of human disease. *Blood* 95:3280, 2000.

140. Odell TT Jr, McDonald TP, Detwiler TC: Stimulation of platelet production by serum of platelet-depleted rats. *Proc Soc Exp Biol Med* 108: 428, 1961.

141. Nichol JL, Hokom MM, Hornkohl A, et al: Megakaryocyte growth and development factor. Analyses of in vitro effects on human megakaryopoiesis and endogenous serum levels during chemotherapy-induced thrombocytopenia. *J Clin Invest* 95:2973, 1995.

142. Kuter DJ, Rosenberg RD: The reciprocal relationship of thrombopoietin (c-Mpl ligand) to changes in the platelet mass during busulfan-induced thrombocytopenia in the rabbit. *Blood* 85:2720, 1995.

143. Bartocci A, Mastrogiannis DS, Migliorati G, et al: Macrophages specifically regulate the concentration of their own growth factor in the circulation. *Proc Natl Acad Sci U S A* 84:6179, 1987.

144. Emmons RV, Reid DM, Cohen RL, et al: Human thrombopoietin levels are high when thrombocytopenia is due to megakaryocyte deficiency and low when due to increased platelet destruction. *Blood* 87:4068, 1996.

145. McCarty JM, Sprugel KH, Fox NE, et al: Murine thrombopoietin mRNA levels are modulated by platelet count. *Blood* 86:3668, 1995.

146. de Sauvage FJ, Carver-Moore K, Luoh SM, et al: Physiological regulation of early and late stages of megakaryocytopoiesis by thrombopoietin. *J Exp Med* 183:651, 1996.

147. Sungaran R, Markovic B, Chong BH: Localization and regulation of thrombopoietin mRNa expression in human kidney, liver, bone marrow, and spleen using in situ hybridization. *Blood* 89:101, 1997.

148. Guerriero A, Worford L, Holland HK, et al: Thrombopoietin is synthesized by bone marrow stromal cells. *Blood* 90:3444, 1997.

149. Solanilla A, Dechanet J, El Andaloussi A, et al: CD40-ligand stimulates myelopoiesis by regulating flt3-ligand and thrombopoietin production in bone marrow stromal cells. *Blood* 95:3758, 2000.

150. Sungaran R, Chisholm OT, Markovic B, et al: The role of platelet alpha-granular proteins in the regulation of thrombopoietin messenger RNA expression in human bone marrow stromal cells. *Blood* 95:3094, 2000.

151. Kamura T, Handa H, Hamasaki N, Kitajima S: Characterization of the human thrombopoietin gene promoter. A possible role of an Ets transcription factor, E4TF1/GABP. *J Biol Chem* 272:11361, 1997.

152. Chang MS, McNinch J, Basu R, et al: Cloning and characterization of the human megakaryocyte growth and development factor (MGDF) gene. *J Biol Chem* 270:511, 1995.

153. Rollins BJ: Chemokines. *Blood* 90:909, 1997.

154. Broxmeyer HE, Mantel CR, Aronica SM: Biology and mechanisms of action of synergistically stimulated myeloid progenitor cell proliferation and suppression by chemokines. *Stem Cells* 15(suppl 1):69, discussion 15(suppl 1):78, 1997.

155. Shirozu M, Nakano T, Inazawa J, et al: Structure and chromosomal localization of the human stromal cell-derived factor 1 (SDF1) gene. *Genomics* 28:495, 1995.

156. Luster AD: Chemokines—Chemotactic cytokines that mediate inflammation. *N Engl J Med* 338:436, 1998.

157. Nagasawa T, Hirota S, Tachibana K, et al: Defects of B-cell lymphopoiesis and bone-marrow myelopoiesis in mice lacking the CXC chemokine PBSF/SDF-1. *Nature* 382:635, 1996.

158. Ma Q, Jones D, Borghesani PR, et al: Impaired B-lymphopoiesis, myelopoiesis, and derailed cerebellar neuron migration in CXCR4- and SDF-1-deficient mice. *Proc Natl Acad Sci U S A* 95:9448, 1998.

159. Aiuti A, Webb IJ, Bleul C, et al: The chemokine SDF-1 is a chemoattractant for human CD34+ hematopoietic progenitor cells and provides a new mechanism to explain the mobilization of CD34+ progenitors to peripheral blood. *J Exp Med* 185:111, 1997.

160. Wang JF, Liu ZY, Groopman JE: The alpha-chemokine receptor CXCR4 is expressed on the megakaryocytic lineage from progenitor to platelets and modulates migration and adhesion. *Blood* 92:756, 1998.

161. Hamada T, Mohle R, Hesselgesser J, et al: Transendothelial migration of megakaryocytes in response to stromal cell-derived factor 1 (SDF-1) enhances platelet formation. *J Exp Med* 188:539, 1998.

162. Daopin S, Piez KA, Ogawa Y, Davies DR: Crystal structure of transforming growth factor-beta 2: An unusual fold for the superfamily. *Science* 257:369, 1992.

163. Keller JR, Mantel C, Sing GK, et al: Transforming growth factor beta 1 selectively regulates early murine hematopoietic progenitors and inhibits the growth of IL-3-dependent myeloid leukemia cell lines. *J Exp Med* 168:737, 1988.

164. Dybedal I, Jacobsen SE: Transforming growth factor beta (TGF-beta), a potent inhibitor of erythropoiesis: Neutralizing TGF-beta antibodies show erythropoietin as a potent stimulator of murine burst-forming unit erythroid colony formation in the absence of a burst-promoting activity. *Blood* 86:949, 1995.

165. Ishibashi T, Miller SL, Burstein SA: Type beta transforming growth factor is a potent inhibitor of murine megakaryocytopoiesis in vitro. *Blood* 69:1737, 1987.

166. Kuter DJ, Gminski DM, Rosenberg RD: Transforming growth factor beta inhibits megakaryocyte growth and endomitosis. *Blood* 79:619, 1992.

167. Laiho M, DeCaprio JA, Ludlow JW, et al: Growth inhibition by TGF-beta linked to suppression of retinoblastoma protein phosphorylation. *Cell* 62:175, 1990.

168. Polyak K, Kato JY, Solomon MJ, et al: p27Kip1, a cyclin-Cdk inhibitor, links transforming growth factor-beta and contact inhibition to cell cycle arrest. *Genes Dev* 8:9, 1994.

169. Teofili L, Martini M, Di Mario A, et al: Expression of p15(ink4b) gene during megakaryocytic differentiation of normal and myelodysplastic hematopoietic progenitors. *Blood* 98:495, 2001.

170. Theofilopoulos AN, Baccala R, Beutler B, Kono DH: Type I interferons (/) in immunity and autoimmunity. *Annu Rev Immunol* 23:307, 2005.

171. Broxmeyer HE, Cooper S, Rubin BY, Taylor MW: The synergistic influence of human interferon-gamma and interferon-alpha on suppression of hematopoietic progenitor cells is additive with the enhanced sensitivity of these cells to inhibition by interferons at low oxygen tension in vitro. *J Immunol* 135:2502, 1985.

172. Fattovich G, Giustina G, Favarato S, Ruol A: A survey of adverse events in 11,241 patients with chronic viral hepatitis treated with alfa interferon. *J Hepatol* 24:38, 1996.

173. Dusheiko G: Side effects of alpha interferon in chronic hepatitis C. *Hepatology* 26(suppl 1):112S, 1997.

174. Jaster R, Tschirch E, Bittorf T, Brock J: Interferon-alpha inhibits proliferation of Ba/F3 cells by interfering with interleukin-3 action. *Cell Signal* 11:769, 1999.

175. Kuniyasu H, Yasui W, Kitahara K, et al: Growth inhibitory effect of interferon-beta is associated with the induction of cyclin-dependent kinase inhibitor p27Kip1 in a human gastric carcinoma cell line. *Cell Growth Differ* 8:47, 1997.

176. Wang Q, Miyakawa Y, Fox N, Kaushansky K: Interferon-alpha directly represses megakaryopoiesis by inhibiting thrombopoietin-induced signaling through induction of SOCS-1. *Blood* 96:2093, 2000.

177. Long MW: Blood cell cytoadhesion molecules. *Exp Hematol* 20:288, 1992.

178. Toksoz D, Zsebo KM, Smith KA, et al: Support of human hematopoiesis in long-term bone marrow cultures by murine stromal cells selectively expressing the membrane-bound and secreted forms of the human homolog of the steel gene product, stem cell factor. *Proc Natl Acad Sci U S A* 89:7350, 1992.

179. Yang L, Yang YC: Regulation of interleukin (IL)-11 gene expression in IL-1 induced primate bone marrow stromal cells. *J Biol Chem* 269:32732, 1994.

180. Linenberger ML, Jacobson FW, Bennett LG, et al: Stem cell factor production by human marrow stromal fibroblasts. *Exp Hematol* 23:1104, 1995.

181. Gordon MY, Riley GP, Watt SM, Greaves MF: Compartmentalization of a haematopoietic growth factor (GM-CSF) by glycosaminoglycans in the bone marrow microenvironment. *Nature* 326:403, 1987.

182. Roberts R, Gallagher J, Spooncer E, et al: Heparan sulphate bound growth factors: A mechanism for stromal cell mediated haemopoiesis. *Nature* 332:376, 1988.

183. Artavanis-Tsakonas S, Matsuno K, Fortini ME: Notch signaling. *Science* 268:225, 1995.

184. Karanu FN, Murdoch B, Miyabayashi T, et al: Human homologues of Delta-1 and Delta-4 function as mitogenic regulators of primitive human hematopoietic cells. *Blood* 97:1960, 2001.

185. Lam LT, Ronchini C, Norton J, et al: Suppression of erythroid but not megakaryocytic differentiation of human K562 erythroleukemic cells by notch-1. *J Biol Chem* 275:19676, 2000.

186. Fox NE, Kaushansky K: Engagement of integrin a4b1 enhances thrombopoietin-induced megakaryopoiesis. *Exp Hematol* 33:94, 2005.

187. Bruno E, Briddell RA, Cooper RJ, Hoffman R: Effects of recombinant interleukin 11 on human megakaryocyte progenitor cells. *Exp Hematol* 19:378, 1991.

188. Neben S, Turner K: The biology of interleukin 11. *Stem Cells* 11(suppl 2):156, 1993.

189. Burstein SA, Mei RL, Henthorn J, et al: Leukemia inhibitory factor and interleukin-11 promote maturation of murine and human megakaryocytes in vitro. *J Cell Physiol* 153:305, 1992.

190. Yonemura Y, Kawakita M, Masuda T, et al: Synergistic effects of interleukin 3 and interleukin 11 on murine megakaryopoiesis in serum-free culture. *Exp Hematol* 20:1011, 1992.

191. Yonemura Y, Kawakita M, Masuda T, et al: Effect of recombinant human interleukin-11 on rat megakaryopoiesis and thrombopoiesis in vivo: Comparative study with interleukin-6. *Br J Haematol* 84:16, 1993.

192. Schlerman FJ, Bree AG, Kaviani MD, et al: Thrombopoietic activity of recombinant human interleukin 11 (rHuIL-11) in normal and myelosuppressed nonhuman primates. *Stem Cells* 14:517, 1996.

193. Gordon MS SG, Battiato L, et al: The in vivo effects of subcutaneously (SC) administered recombinant human interleukin-11 (Neumega™ rhIL-

11 growth factor; rhIL-11) in women with breast cancer (BC). *Blood* 82(suppl 1):498a, 1993.

194. Champlin RE MR, Kaye JA, et al: Recombinant human interleukin eleven (rhIL-11) following autologous BMT for breast cancer. *Blood* 84(suppl 1):395a, 1994.

195. Tepler I, Elias L, Smith JW 2nd, et al: A randomized placebo-controlled trial of recombinant human interleukin-11 in cancer patients with severe thrombocytopenia due to chemotherapy. *Blood* 87:3607, 1996.

196. Isaacs C, Robert NJ, Bailey FA, et al: Randomized placebo-controlled study of recombinant human interleukin-11 to prevent chemotherapy-induced thrombocytopenia in patients with breast cancer receiving dose-intensive cyclophosphamide and doxorubicin. *J Clin Oncol* 15:3368, 1997.

197. Vredenburgh JJ, Hussein A, Fisher D, et al: A randomized trial of recombinant human interleukin-11 following autologous bone marrow transplantation with peripheral blood progenitor cell support in patients with breast cancer. *Biol Blood Marrow Transplant* 4:134, 1998.

198. Tichelli A, Gratwohl A, Berger C, et al: Treatment of thrombocytosis in myeloproliferative disorders with interferon alpha-2a. *Blut* 58:15, 1989.

199. Gisslinger H, Ludwig H, Linkesch W, et al: Long-term interferon therapy for thrombocytosis in myeloproliferative diseases. *Lancet* 1:634, 1989.

200. Sacchi S, Gugliotta L, Papineschi F, et al: Alfa-interferon in the treatment of essential thrombocythemia: Clinical results and evaluation of its biological effects on the hematopoietic neoplastic clone. Italian Cooperative Group on ET. *Leukemia* 12:289, 1998.

201. Taylor PC, Dolan G, Ng JP, et al: Efficacy of recombinant interferon-alpha (rIFN-alpha) in polycythaemia vera: A study of 17 patients and an analysis of published data. *Br J Haematol* 92:55, 1996.

202. Tornebohm-Roche E, Merup M, Lockner D, Paul C: Alpha-2a interferon therapy and antibody formation in patients with essential thrombocythemia and polycythemia vera with thrombocytosis. *Am J Hematol* 48:163, 1995.

203. Hokom MM, Lacey D, Kinstler OB, et al: Pegylated megakaryocyte growth and development factor abrogates the lethal thrombocytopenia associated with carboplatin and irradiation in mice. *Blood* 86:4486, 1995.

204. Fibbe WE, Heemskerk DP, Laterveer L, et al: Accelerated reconstitution of platelets and erythrocytes after syngeneic transplantation of bone marrow cells derived from thrombopoietin pretreated donor mice. *Blood* 86:3308, 1995.

205. Molineux G, Hartley C, McElroy P, et al: Megakaryocyte growth and development factor accelerates platelet recovery in peripheral blood progenitor cell transplant recipients. *Blood* 88:366, 1996.

206. Fanucchi M, Glaspy J, Crawford J, et al: Effects of polyethylene glycol-conjugated recombinant human megakaryocyte growth and development factor on platelet counts after chemotherapy for lung cancer. *N Engl J Med* 336:404, 1997.

207. Vadhan-Raj S, Murray LJ, Bueso-Ramos C, et al: Stimulation of megakaryocyte and platelet production by a single dose of recombinant human thrombopoietin in patients with cancer. *Ann Intern Med* 126:673, 1997.

208. Basser RL, Underhill C, Davis I, et al: Enhancement of platelet recovery after myelosuppressive chemotherapy by recombinant human megakaryocyte growth and development factor in patients with advanced cancer. *J Clin Oncol* 18:2852, 2000.

209. Archimbaud E, Ottmann OG, Yin JA, et al: A randomized, double-blind, placebo-controlled study with pegylated recombinant human megakaryocyte growth and development factor (PEG-rHuMGDF) as an adjunct to chemotherapy for adults with de novo acute myeloid leukemia. *Blood* 94:3694, 1999.

210. Bolwell B, Vredenburgh J, Overmoyer B, et al: Phase 1 study of pegylated recombinant human megakaryocyte growth and development factor (PEG-rHuMGDF) in breast cancer patients after autologous peripheral blood progenitor cell (PBPC) transplantation. *Bone Marrow Transplant* 26:141, 2000.

211. Somlo G, Sniecinski I, Ter Veer A, et al: Recombinant human thrombopoietin in combination with granulocyte colony-stimulating factor enhances mobilization of peripheral blood progenitor cells, increases peripheral blood platelet concentration, and accelerates hematopoietic recovery following high-dose chemotherapy. *Blood* 93:2798, 1999.

212. Nomura S, Dan K, Hotta T, et al: Effects of pegylated recombinant human megakaryocyte growth and development factor in patients with idiopathic thrombocytopenic purpura. *Blood* 100:728, 2002.

213. Vadhan-Raj S, Patel S, Bueso-Ramos C, et al: Importance of predosing of recombinant human thrombopoietin to reduce chemotherapy-induced early thrombocytopenia. *J Clin Oncol* 21:3158, 2003.

214. Li J, Yang C, Xia Y, et al: Thrombocytopenia caused by the development of antibodies to thrombopoietin. *Blood* 98:3241, 2001.

215. Kimura T, Kaburaki H, Tsujino T, et al: A non-peptide compound which can mimic the effect of thrombopoietin via c-Mpl. *FEBS Lett* 428:250, 1998.

216. de Serres M, Yeager RL, Dillberger JE, et al: Pharmacokinetics and hematological effects of the PEGylated thrombopoietin peptide mimetic GW395058 in rats and monkeys after intravenous or subcutaneous administration. *Stem Cells* 17:316, 1999.

217. Broudy VC, Lin NL: AMG531 stimulates megakaryopoiesis in vitro by binding to Mpl. *Cytokine* 25:52, 2004.

218. Kaushansky K: Hematopoietic growth factor mimetics. *Ann N Y Acad Sci* 938:131, 2001.

PLATELET MORPHOLOGY, BIOCHEMISTRY, AND FUNCTION

LESLIE V. PARISE

SUSAN S. SMYTH

ARUN S. SHET

BARRY S. COLLER

Platelets are small anucleate cell fragments adapted to adhere to damaged blood vessels, to aggregate one with another, and to facilitate the generation of thrombin. These actions contribute to hemostasis by producing a platelet plug and then reinforcing the plug by the action of thrombin converting fibrinogen to fibrin strands. To accomplish these tasks, platelets have surface receptors that can bind adhesive glycoproteins; these include the glycoprotein Ib/IX/V complex, which supports platelet adhesion by binding von Willebrand factor even under conditions of high shear, and the $\alpha IIb\beta 3$ (GPIIb-IIIa) receptor,

Acronyms and abbreviations that appear in this chapter include: ADMIDAS, adjacent to MIDAS; ADP, adenosine diphosphate; AMP, adenosine monophosphate; AngII, angiotensin II; APP, amyloid precursor protein; ATP, adenosine triphosphate; ATPDase, ATP diphosphohydrolase; ATPase, adenosine triphosphatase; Btk, Bruton tyrosine kinase; cAMP, cyclic adenosine monophosphate; CD40L, CD40 ligand; COX, cyclooxygenase; CTAP, connective tissue-activating peptide; DAG, diacylglycerol; DTS, dense tubular system; EDTA, ethylenediaminetetraacetic acid; EPR, effector cell protease receptor; ERK, extracellular signal-related kinase; FAK, focal adhesion tyrosine kinase; FasL, Fas ligand; FcγRIIA, Fc γ receptor IIA; FcR, Fc receptor; FERM, proteins four point one (4.1), ezrin, radixin, and moesin; FOG, friend of GATA; GDP, guanosine diphosphate; GP, glycoprotein; GPI, glycosyl phosphatidylinositol; GTP, guanosine triphosphate; HLA, human leukocyte antigen; HPS, Hermansky-Pudlak syndrome; 5-HT, serotonin; hTRPC, human canonical transient receptor potential; IAP, integrin-associated protein; ICAM, intracellular adhesion molecule; IL, interleukin; IP$_3$, inositol 1,4,5-trisphosphate; ITAM, immunoreceptor tyrosine-based activation motif; ITIM, immunoreceptor tyrosine-based inhibitory motif; JAM, junctional adhesion molecule; LAMP, lysosomal-associated membrane protein; LAP, latency-associated peptide; LDL, low-density lipoprotein; LIMBS, ligand-induced metal binding site; LPA, lysophosphatidic acid; LTBP, latent TGF-β-binding protein; lysoPC, lysophosphophosphatidylcholine; lysoPLD, lysophospholipase D; MAPK, mitogen-activated protein kinase; MIDAS, metal ion-dependent adhesion site; mRNA, messenger ribonucleic acid; NAP, neutrophil-activating peptide; NMR, nuclear magnetic resonance; NO, nitric oxide; NSF, N-ethylmaleimide sensitive factor; PAF, platelet-activating factor; PAI, plasminogen-activator inhibitor; PAR, protease-activated receptor; PC, phosphatidylcholine; PDE, phosphodiesterase; PDGF, platelet-derived growth factor; PDI, protein disulfide isomerase; PE, phosphatidylethanolamine; PECAM, platelet endothelial cell adhesion molecule; PF4, platelet factor 4; PG, prostaglandin; PH, pleckstrin homology; PI3K, phosphatidylinositol (phosphoinositide)-3-kinase; PIPKI, phosphatidylinositol phosphate kinase type 1γ; PKA, protein kinase A; PKC, protein kinase C; PLA, phospholipase A; PLC, phospholipase C; PNH, paroxysmal nocturnal hemoglobinuria; PPAR, peroxisome proliferator-activated receptor; PSGL, P-selectin glycoprotein ligand; PSI, plexins, semiphorins, integrins; PSP, platelet Sec1 protein; S1P, spingosphine-1-phosphate; SERCA, sarcoplasmic-endoplasmic reticulum calcium ATPase; SHP, Src homology-containing protein tyrosine phosphatase; SNAP, soluble NSF-associated protein; SNARE, SNAP receptor; TGF, transforming growth factor; TLT, TREM-like transcript; TNF, tumor necrosis factor; TP, thromboxaneprostanoid receptor; TREM, triggering receptors express on myeloid cells; TSP, thrombospondin; TXA$_2$, thromboxane A$_2$; u-PAR, urokinase plasminogen activator receptor; VAMP, vesicle-associated membrane protein; VASP, vasodilator-stimulated phosphoprotein; VEGF, vascular endothelial growth factor; vWF, von Willebrand factor; WASP, Wiskott-Aldrich syndrome protein.

which is platelet specific and mediates platelet aggregation by binding fibrinogen and/or von Willebrand factor. Other receptors for adhesive glycoproteins [$\alpha 2\beta 1$ (GPIa-IIa), GPVI, and perhaps others for collagen; $\alpha 5\beta 1$ (GPIc*-IIa) for fibronectin; and $\alpha 6\beta 1$ (GPIc-IIa) for laminin] also contribute to platelet adhesion, but their precise contributions are less well defined. Activated platelets express both surface P-selectin, which mediates interactions with leukocytes, and CD40 ligand, which activates a number of proinflammatory cells, and releases chemokines and a soluble form of CD40 ligand, thus initiating an inflammatory reaction. Platelet coagulant activity results from the exposure of negatively charged phospholipids on the surface of platelets, generation of platelet microparticles, release and activation of platelet factor V, and perhaps exposure of specific receptors for activated coagulation factor. Platelets change shape with activation as a result of a complex reorganization of the platelet membrane skeleton and cytoskeleton. With activation, platelets undergo release of α-granule, dense body, and lysosomal contents. The activation process involves a number of receptors for agonists, such as adenosine diphosphate, epinephrine, thrombin, collagen, thromboxane A$_2$, vasopressin, serotonin, platelet-activating factor, lysophosphatidic acid, sphingosine-1-phosphate, and thrombospondin, and several signal transduction pathways, including phosphoinositide metabolism, arachidonic acid release and conversion into thromboxane A$_2$, and phosphorylation of a number of different target proteins. Increases in intracellular calcium result from, and further contribute to, platelet activation. Platelet activation results in a change in the conformation of the $\alpha IIb\beta 3$ receptor, leading to high-affinity ligand binding and platelet aggregation.

Platelets also act as storehouses for a variety of molecules that affect platelet function, inflammation, vascular tone, fibrinolysis, and wound healing. These agents are actively released upon platelet activation. Other vasoactive and platelet-activating substances are newly synthesized when platelets are activated. Through cooperative biochemical interactions, platelets can communicate with, and are affected by, other blood cells and endothelial cells.

Quantitative and qualitative disorders of platelets produce hemorrhagic diatheses (see Chaps. 110–113). In pathologic states, uncontrolled platelet thrombus formation can lead to vasoocclusion and ischemic necrosis, as, for example, in myocardial infarction and stroke (see Chap. 126). Platelets may also facilitate tumor metastasis.

PLATELET MORPHOLOGY AND BIOCHEMISTRY

LIGHT MICROSCOPIC APPEARANCE

On films made from blood anticoagulated with the strong calcium chelating agent ethylenediaminetetraacetic acid (EDTA) and stained with Wright stain, platelets appear as small bluish-gray, oval to round bodies with several purple-red granules (see Color Plate XIII-1 and Chap. 2). The mean diameter of platelets varies among individuals, ranging from approximately 1.5 to 3.0 μm, approximately one third to one fourth the diameter of erythrocytes. Considerable variability in the size of platelets also exists in a single individual, with occasional platelets in normal blood samples having diameters greater than half the diameter of erythrocytes. Overall, platelet size appears to follow a log normal distribution.[1] When unanticoagulated blood is used to prepare blood films, platelets undergo variable activation and spreading; thus, platelet aggregates are commonly seen. Platelets from such specimens may demonstrate three or four very long and thin processes extending out from the body of the platelet (filopodia), and some platelets may be devoid of granules.

ELECTRON MICROSCOPIC APPEARANCE AND BIOCHEMISTRY

Electron microscopy reveals a fuzzy coat (glycocalix) extending 14 to 20 nm from the platelet surface, which is thought to be composed of membrane glycoproteins, glycolipids, mucopolysaccharides, and adsorbed plasma proteins (Fig. 105-1).[2] Platelets move in an electric field as if they have a net negative surface charge. Sialic acid residues attached to proteins and lipids are major contributors to this negative charge.[3] The electrostatic repulsion created by the negative surface charge may help prevent resting platelets from attaching to each other or to negatively charged endothelial cells.

The surface of the platelet has a number of indentations that are thought to be the openings of the open canalicular system, which is an elaborate channel system composed of invaginations of the plasma membrane that extend throughout the platelet (see Fig. 105-1 and "Membrane Systems" below). The contents of platelet granules can gain access to the outside when the granules fuse with either the plasma membrane or any region of the open canalicular system. Similarly, glycoproteins contained within granule membranes can join the plasma membrane after granule fusion with either the plasma membrane or the open canalicular system.

PLASMA MEMBRANE

The platelet plasma membrane is a trilaminar unit composed of a bilayer of phospholipids in which cholesterol, glycolipids, and glycoproteins are embedded.[2,4] Platelets prepared by the freeze-fracture technique demonstrate more intramembranous particles embedded in the outer platelet membrane leaflet than in the inner leaflet, which is the reverse of findings in erythrocytes. This observation presumably reflects the many external receptors that mediate platelet interactions. The plasma membrane is thought to contain the sodium- and calcium-adenosine triphosphatase (ATPase) pumps that control the intracellular ionic environment of the platelet. Approximately 57 percent of platelet phospholipids are contained in the plasma membrane (Table 105-1). The phospholipids are asymmetrically organized in the plasma membrane. The negatively charged phospholipids are almost exclusively present in the inner leaflet, whereas the others are more evenly distributed.[5] The negatively charged phospholipids, especially phosphatidylserine, are able to accelerate several steps in the coagulation sequence. Therefore, their presence in the inner leaflet of resting platelets, separated from the plasma coagulation factors, is thought to be a control mechanism for preventing inappropriate coagulation.[6,7] During platelet activation induced by select agonists, the aminophospholipids may become exposed on the platelet surface or on the surface of microparticles (see "Platelet Coagulant Activity" below).[6-9]

The phospholipid asymmetry in resting platelets can be maintained by an adenosine triphosphate (ATP)-dependent aminophospholipid translocase that actively moves phosphatidylserine and phosphatidylethanolamine (PE) from the outer to the inner leaflet.[6,10] Interactions of negatively charged phospholipids with cytoskeletal or other cytoplasmic elements also may contribute to the asymmetry.[6,7,11,12]

Lipid rafts are cholesterol- and sphingolipid-rich membrane domains that are important in signaling and intracellular trafficking. Platelets contain lipid rafts rich in the marker proteins flotillin (1 and 2) and stomatin, CD36, CD9, αIIbβ3, and glucose transporter GLUT-3.[13] After platelet activation, glycoprotein VI (GPVI), the Fc γ receptor IIA (FcγRIIA), and the GPIb-IX-V complex join lipid rafts.[14,15] Factor XI binds to lipid rafts and undergoes activation.[16] c-Src,[17] phosphatidic acid, and phosphatidylinositol (phosphoinositide)-3-kinase (PI3K) products also concentrate in rafts.[18,19] The calcium entry channel human canonical transient receptor potential-1 (hTRPC1) also is associated with lipid rafts in platelets and, upon platelet activation, contributes to calcium entry that is regulated by the state of intracellular calcium stores (store-mediated calcium entry).[20]

Table 105-1 outlines the lipid composition of platelet membranes. The enrichment of selected phospholipids with arachidonic acid is striking, furnishing a store of arachidonic acid for release and conversion into thromboxane A_2 (TXA$_2$) (see "Signaling Pathways in Platelet Activation and Aggregation" below).

The glycoproteins in the plasma membrane are discussed in the section on "Membrane Systems" below.

CYTOSKELETAL ELEMENTS

Membrane Skeleton A planar network of thin, elongated spectrin tetramers interconnected by the ends of actin filaments is present immediately below the plasma membrane and the membranes of the open canalicular system (Fig. 105-2).[21,22] Filamin-A (actin-binding protein) can interact with both the transmembrane glycoprotein GPIbα and the actin immediately below the membrane, thus connecting these components to the spectrin network and forming a membrane cytoskeleton that probably stabilizes the membrane's discoid shape. In addition, the association of GPIbα with the membrane skeleton restricts the expansion of the spectrin network and probably helps to organize receptors into linear arrays on the platelet surface, thus enhancing receptor cooperation (Fig. 105-2).[23] Other proteins found in the membrane skeleton include talin, vinculin, dystrophin-related protein, molecules implicated in signal transduction, and several isoenzymes of protein kinase C (PKC) (see section on "Membrane Systems" below).[23] Talin has been implicated in control of αIIbβ3 activation by virtue of binding to the cytoplasmic domains of αIIbβ3 (Fig. 105-3).[24-28] The protein vimentin (M_r 58,000), which is an important component of intermediate filaments, is present in platelets and contributes to the membrane cytoskeleton. When platelets are activated, vitronectin–plasminogen-activator inhibitor-1 (PAI-1) complexes bind to surface vimentin where they are strategically located to inhibit fibrinolysis.[29] With platelet activation, αIIbβ3 and α2β1 also may join the cytoskeleton. Thus, the cytoskeleton may affect whether receptors are free to move in the plane of the membrane and may have a role in moving certain receptors from the surface to the interior of platelets and vice versa via the open canalicular system.[23,30] The membrane skeleton also may be important in platelet spreading after adhesion.

Microtubules The circumferential band of microtubules present below the plasma membrane probably plays an important role in platelet formation from megakaryocytes and contributes to the platelet's discoid shape.[2,31-33] On cross-section, approximately eight to 12 separate hollow structures are observed at the tapered ends of the platelet, but these structures may derive from the multiple windings of a single coil of approximately 100 μm. Microtubules are 25-nm, hollow polarized polymers composed of 13 protofilaments consisting of α,β-tubulin dimers (each M_r 110,000) that associate with several proteins of high molecular weight (microtubule-associated proteins).[22,33,34] Platelets contain four different tubulin isoforms (β_1, β_2, β_4, β_5). β_1 is dominant and is megakaryocyte- and platelet-specific. Targeted gene deletion of β_1-tubulin in mice results in thrombocytopenia and abnormal platelet and microtubule morphology.[33] Approximately 50 to 60 percent of the platelet tubulin is in microtubules, and a dynamic equilibrium exists between the polymerized and free tubulin subunits.[22,35] Motor proteins of the dynein and kinesin families also are associated with microtubules[36] and contribute to the genesis and function of platelets.

Microfilaments The platelet is rich in actin, a protein that can polymerize into microfilamentous bundles (see section on "Platelet Cytoskeleton" below).[21-23] In resting platelets, microfilaments are not

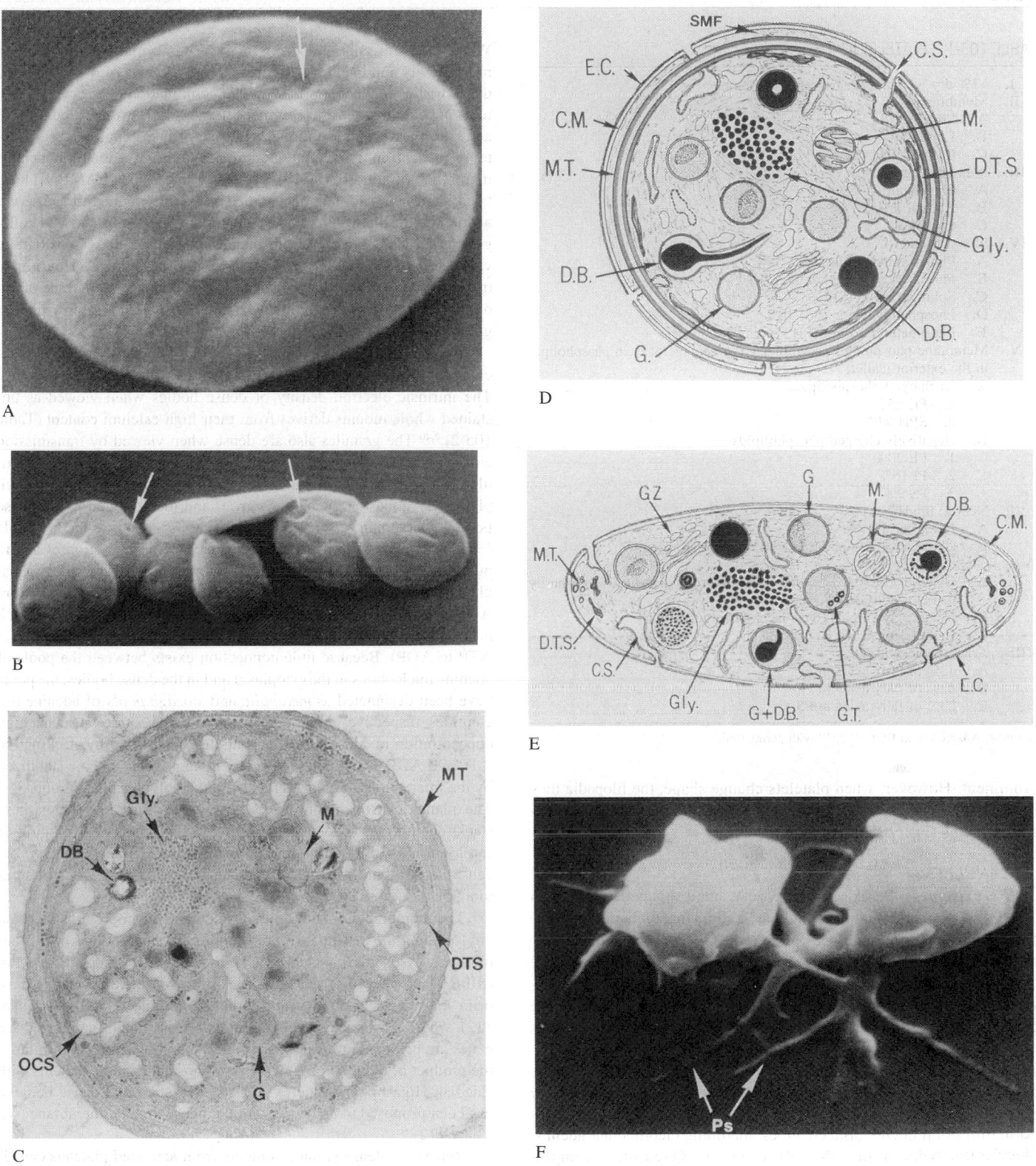

FIGURE 105-1   *(A, B)* Discoid platelets. The lentiform shape of blood platelets is well preserved in samples fixed in glutaraldehyde and critical point dried for study in the scanning electron microscope. The indentations apparent on the otherwise smooth surfaces of the platelets *(arrows)* indicate sites where channels of the open canalicular system communicate with the cell exterior *(A:* ×13,200; *B:* ×35,000). *(C–E)* Ultrastructural features observed in thin sections of discoid platelets cut in the equatorial plane *(C, D)* or cross section *(E)*. Components include the exterior coat (E.C.), trilaminar unit cell membrane (C.M.), and submembrane area containing the specialized filaments (SMF) of the membrane skeleton. The plasma membrane indentations form the walls of the channels of the surface-connected or open canalicular system (C.S. and OCS). The circumferential band of microtubules (M.T.) is seen as a continuous band beneath the plasma membrane on the equatorial section and as small open cylinders at the ends of the platelet on the cross section. Glycogen granules (Gly) are prominent punctate structures in the cytoplasm, and residual Golgi zones (GZ) can be identified. Organelles include mitochondria (M), dense bodies (D.B.), and α-granules (G), many of which have regions of electron density (nucleoids). The dense tubular system (DTS and D.T.S.), the platelet equivalent of the sarcoplasmic reticulum, sequesters calcium *(C:* ×30,000). *(F)* Platelet shape change. Platelets exposed to ADP and then fixed and examined by scanning electron microscopy. The platelets lose their discoid shape and become spiny spheres with long extensions, variably referred to as *filopodia* or *pseudopodia* (Ps) (×17,000). (From JG White,[1218] with permission.)

TABLE 105-1 PLATELET LIPIDS

I. 17% dry weight, primarily in membranes
II. Membranes
   A. Protein 57%
   B. Lipid 35%
   C. Carbohydrate 8%
III. Membrane lipids
   A. Phospholipid 75%
   B. Neutral lipid 20%
   C. Glycolipid 5%
IV. Phospholipids
   A. Phosphatidylcholine (PC) 38%
   B. Phosphatidylethanolamine (PE) 27%
   C. Sphingomyelin (SPH) 17%
   D. Phosphatidylserine (PS) 10%
   E. Phosphatidylinositol (PI) 5%
V. Membrane phospholipid asymmetry (percentage of each phospholipid in the exterior leaflet)
   A. Uncharged phospholipids
     1. PC 45%
     2. SPH 93%
   B. Negatively charged phospholipids
     1. PE 20%
     2. PI 16%
     3. PS 9%
VI. Neutral lipids
   A. Cholesterol 95%
   B. Cholesterol:phospholipid = 0.5 on molar basis
VII. Glycolipids
   A. Gangliosides [0.5% of total lipids; 6% of total sialic acid; primarily hematoside (GM3)]
   B. Neutral glycolipids (64% lactosyl ceramide)
   C. Ceramides (A and B)
VIII. Arachidonic acid (29;4)
   A. 42% of fatty acids in PI
   B. 32% of fatty acids in PE
   C. 23% of fatty acids in PS

SOURCE: Adapted from BS Coller,[1224] with permission.

prominent. However, when platelets change shape, the filopodia they form contain bundles of microfilaments made up of actin and associated proteins (Fig. 105-4).[2,34]

ORGANELLES

Peroxisomes Peroxisomes are very small organelles present in platelets. They are thought to contribute to lipid metabolism, especially plasmalogen synthesis, and may participate in the synthesis of platelet-activating factor (PAF).[37] They contain acyl-CoA dihydroxyacetone phosphate acyltransferase, which catalyzes the first step in the synthesis of ether phospholipids. Deficiencies of this enzymatic activity have been identified in the cerebrorenal Zellweger syndrome, and platelet activity can be used to diagnose the disorder.[38,39]

Mitochondria Platelets contain approximately four to seven mitochondria of relatively small size that are involved in oxidative energy metabolism (see "Platelet Energy Metabolism" below).[40,41] Abnormalities of mitochondrial enzymes, including nicotinamide adenine dinucleotide reduced form (NADH) coenzyme Q reductase (complex I), have been implicated in the pathophysiology of aging and several neurodegenerative disorders, including Alzheimer disease, schizophrenia, and some forms of Parkinson disease. Assays of platelet mitochondrial enzyme levels were used in the studies.[42–47] In addition, hyperglycemia-induced mitochondrial superoxide generation may contribute to the enhanced platelet aggregation observed in diabetes.[48]

Lysosomes Platelets have lysosomal granules that contain acid hydrolases typical for these organelles. Among the enzymes thought to originate from platelet lysosomes are β-glucuronidase, cathepsins, aryl sulfatase, β-hexosaminidase, β-galactosidase, endoglucosidase (heparitinase), β-glycerophosphatase, elastase, and collagenase.[40]

When platelets undergo secretion, lysosomal contents are released more slowly and incompletely than are the contents of α-granules and dense bodies.[49–51] Moreover, a unique combination of exocytosis proteins appears to control lysosomal release,[52] and stronger inducers of activation are required to induce release of lysosomal contents. Proteins present in lysosomal membranes (e.g., lysosomal-associated membrane protein [LAMP]-1, LAMP-2, and CD63 [LAMP-3]) have been identified, and their appearance on the plasma membrane serves as markers of the platelet release reaction.[53,54] The elastase and collagenase activities released from platelet lysosomes may contribute to vascular damage at sites of platelet thrombus formation.[55] Heparitinase may be able to cleave heparin-like molecules from the surface of endothelial cells, and the resulting soluble molecules appear to inhibit growth of smooth muscle cells.[56]

Dense Bodies Platelets contain approximately three to eight electron-dense organelles, 20 to 30 nm in diameter (see Fig. 105-1).[2,57] The intrinsic electron density of dense bodies when viewed as unstained whole mounts derives from their high calcium content (Table 105-2).[2,40] The granules also are dense when viewed by transmission electron microscopy because they are highly osmophilic.[57] Dense granules contain high concentrations of serotonin, which is taken up from plasma by a plasma membrane carrier and then trapped in the dense bodies.[57] Trapping of serotonin may occur as a result of the lower pH (~6.1) maintained in dense granules because of the action of an H^+ pumping ATPase on the dense body membrane.[57] Adenosine diphosphate (ADP) and ATP are highly concentrated in dense bodies.[40] More ADP than ATP is present in the dense bodies (2:3 ATP to ADP), which is the reverse of their relative concentrations in the cytoplasm (8:1 ATP to ADP). Because little connection exists between the pools of adenine nucleotides in the cytoplasm and in the dense bodies, the pools have been designated as *metabolic* and *storage pools* of adenine nucleotides, respectively.[40] Storage of adenine nucleotides at such a high concentration in dense bodies appears to be achieved by stacking the ATP and ADP purine rings vertically in aggregates that are stabilized by the interactions of calcium ions with the polyphosphate groups.[58,59] The planar hydroxyindole rings of serotonin also may enter these stacks, helping to account for the trapping mechanism. Trapping of serotonin must differ from that of adenine nucleotides, however, because dense granule serotonin exchanges readily with external serotonin.[40]

The membrane of dense granules contains glycoproteins that also are found on the plasma membrane and on the membranes of α-granules and lysosomes, including CD36, LAMP-2, CD63, P-selectin, αIIbβ3, and GPIb-IX. Abnormalities of seven different genes have been implicated in Hermansky-Pudlak syndrome (HPS) (see Chap. 112), which is characterized by abnormal dense bodies and thus these genes are presumed to participate in dense body formation. Similarly, the product of the Lyst gene, which is abnormal in some patients with Chediak-Higashi syndrome (who also have abnormal dense bodies), has been proposed to associate with the dense granule membrane (see Chap. 112).[60]

Release of dense granule contents from activated platelets constitutes an important positive feedback mechanism for platelet aggregation because ADP is a potent platelet agonist and serotonin is a weak agonist (see below) (Fig. 105-5). ATP is a partial antagonist of ADP-induced activation. However, because ATP is rapidly catabolized to ADP in plasma ($T_{1/2}$ = 1.5 minutes) and ADP is rapidly catabolized to adenosine monophosphate ([AMP], $T_{1/2}$ = 4 min) and then to adenosine,[40] a platelet inhibitor,[61] predicting the overall effect of ATP release is difficult. Adding to the complexity *in vivo* is the presence of an ecto-ATP diphosphohydrolase (ecto-ATPDase) (CD39) present on endothelial and lymphoid cells, which can metabolize ATP and ADP to AMP and thus probably limits the amount of ADP present.[62] ATP

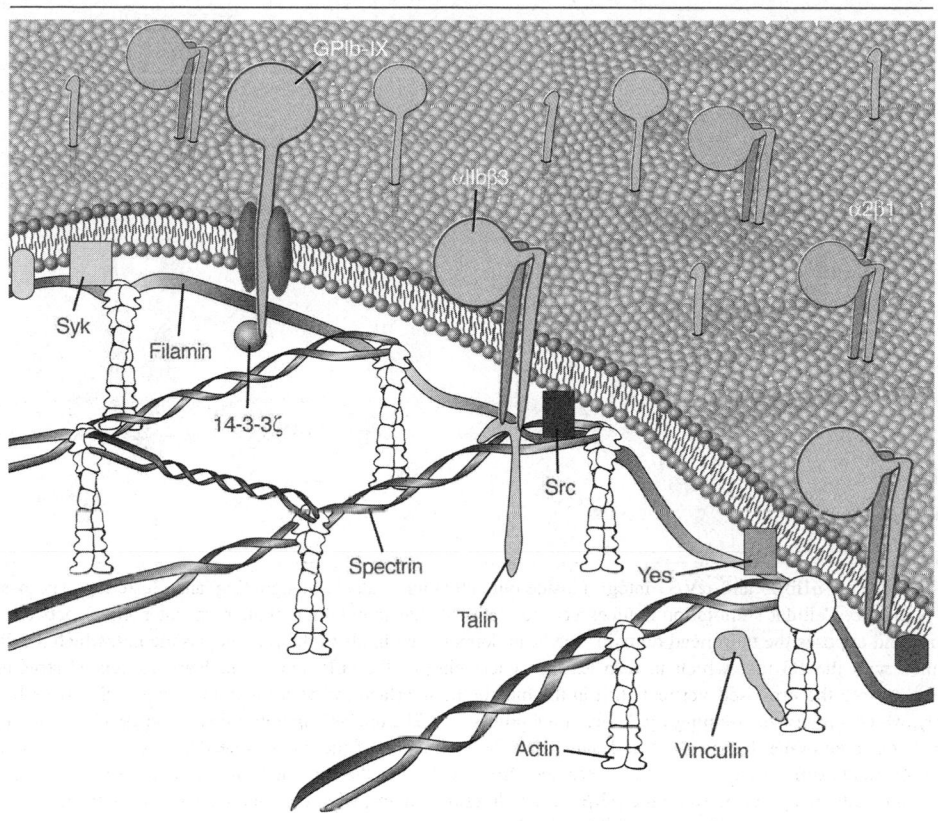

FIGURE 105-2 Diagrammatic depiction of established and hypothetical connections between select platelet transmembrane glycoproteins and the underlying membrane skeleton. Although evidence exists for direct interactions between αIIbβ3 with talin and Src and between GPIbα with 14-3-3ζ and filamin, the remainder of the interactions are only hypothetical and are based on the recovery of proteins in the membrane skeleton fraction of solubilized platelets. (Adapted from JEB Fox,[371] with permission.)

released from platelets also may serve as a high-energy phosphate source for platelet ecto protein kinases, which can phosphorylate several proteins, including GPIV.[63–66]

α-Granules α-Granules are the most abundant granules in platelets, numbering approximately 50 to 80 per platelet.[67,68] They are approximately 200 nm in diameter on cross section. They demonstrate internal variation in electron density, often with an eccentric area of accentuated electron density, termed a *nucleoid*, in which β-thromboglobulin, platelet factor 4 (PF4), and proteoglycans are concentrated (see Figs. 105-1 and 105-6).[2] The more electron-lucent areas contain tubular elements in which von Willebrand factor (vWF), multimerin, and factor V are preferentially localized.[69] Table 105-2 lists some of the most important proteins present in α-granules. Small amounts of virtually all plasma proteins are nonspecifically taken up into α-granules; therefore, the plasma levels of these proteins determine their platelet levels.[70,71] For example, because the α-granule pool of immunoglobulins (Ig) represents the vast majority of platelet Ig, total platelet Ig is much more affected by plasma Ig levels than by changes in surface Ig (see Chap. 110).[70,71]

The platelet-specific proteins PF4 and the β-thromboglobulin family are present in α-granules at concentrations that are approximately 20,000 times higher than their plasma concentrations (when each is expressed as a fraction of total protein in platelets or plasma, respectively; see Table 105-2).[72,73] These M_r 7000 to 11,000 proteins all bind to heparin but with varying affinities. They also share amino acid sequence homology with each other and with other members of the "intercrine-cytokine" family of molecules, such as interleukin (IL)-8 (neutrophil-activating peptide 1 [NAP1]), which are active in inflammation, cell growth, and malignant transformation (Fig. 105-7).[74–76]

PF4 is a CXC chemokine (CXCL4) that does not contain the Glu-Leu-Arg (ELR) conserved sequence (see Fig. 105-7).[77,78] It binds to heparin with high affinity and can neutralize heparin's anticoagulant activity.[72,79–81] PF4 tetramers complex with a proteoglycan carrier.[82,83] Specific PF4 lysine residues (amino acids 61, 62, 65, 66) have been implicated in its binding to heparin, and x-ray crystallography indicates these lysines are on the surface of the PF4 tetramer and interact with negatively charged heparin molecules that wind around this core.[84–86]

After PF4 is released from platelets, it binds to heparin-like molecules on the surface of endothelial cells.[85] Heparin administration can mobilize this endothelial-bound pool of PF4 into the circulation.[85] PF4–heparin complexes and PF4–heparin-like molecule complexes on endothelial cells have been implicated as the target antigens in heparin-induced thrombocytopenia with thrombosis.[87,88] PF4 also binds to hepatocytes, which take up and catabolize PF4.[89] PF4 is a weak neutrophil and fibroblast attractant.[77,90] It inhibits angiogenesis, perhaps through inhibition of endothelial cell proliferation.[91] A large number of other activities have been ascribed to PF4, including histamine release from basophils,[92] inhibition of tumor growth[93] and megakaryocyte maturation,[94,95] reversal of immunosuppression,[90,96] enhancement of fibroblast attachment to substrata,[97] potentiation of platelet aggregation,[98] inhibition of contact activation,[99] and enhancement of both polymorphonuclear leukocyte responsiveness to the activating peptide f-Met-Leu-Phe and monocyte responsiveness to lipopolysaccharide.[100,101]

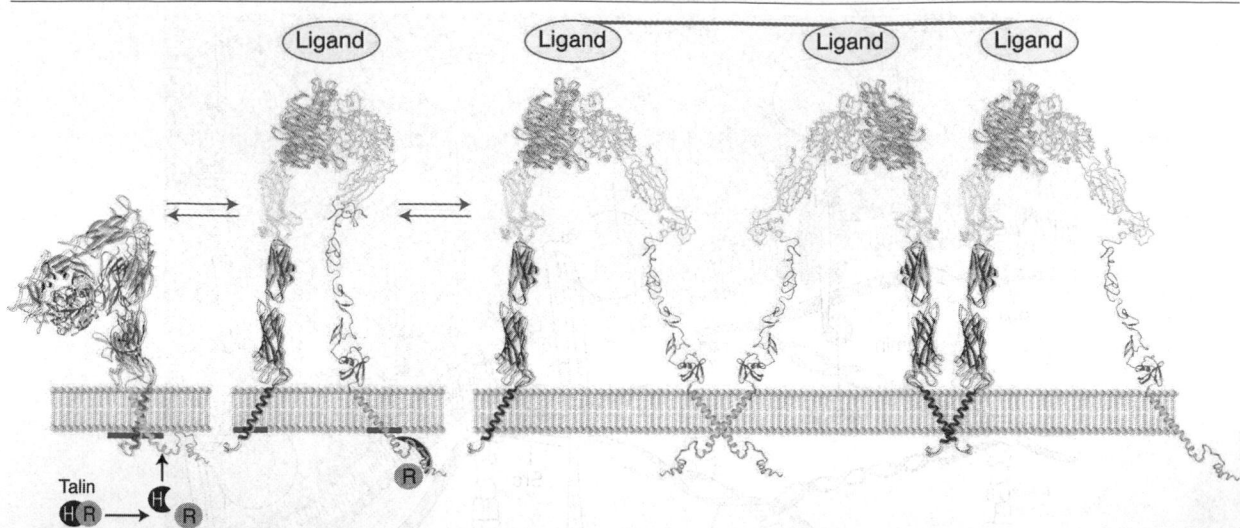

FIGURE 105-3   Model for αIIbβ3 and αVβ3 integrin inside-out activation, outside-in signaling, and clustering. The α-subunit is in *black* and the β-subunit is in *blue*. Cellular stimulation induces a conformational change in talin that alters the interactions between the talin head (H) and rod (R) domains and exposes the talin head domain. The head domain then binds to the β3 cytoplasmic tail, which displaces the α-subunit tail from its complex with the β3 tail, which in turn leads to unclasping of the tails and a membrane-associated structural change of the cytoplasmic face.[26,1176] Note the proposed vertical shift in the membrane interface for both membrane-proximal helices before and after unclasping *(blue bars)*, which suggests a "fanning-out" unclasping process.[1176] The unclasping both initiates the opening of the integrin C-terminal stalks (including the transmembrane domains)[1219] and diminishes the interaction of the integrin headpiece with the stalks. These changes are necessary for the switchblade shift of the extracellular headpiece from the bent to the extended form for high-affinity ligand binding.[504] Ligand binding to the integrin results in a pivot between the β3 βA(I) and hybrid domains, which results in greater leg separation. This conformational change may initiate outside-in signaling. The ligated integrins cluster, possibly via oligomerization of transmembrane domains.[396] The model was generated based on the crystal structures of the αVβ3 extracellular domains[1220] (which was used as the model for the bent integrin in the *left panel*) and the αIIbβ3 headpiece[497] (which was used with the αVβ3 crystal structure to form composites for the *middle and right panels*), and the nuclear magnetic resonance structure of the cytoplasmic domain,[26,1176] with the helices extending to the transmembrane domain. (Adapted from J Qin, O Vinogradova, and EF Plow,[1221] with permission).

The β-thromboglobulin family of proteins are CXC chemokines that contain the conserved Glu-Leu-Arg (ELR) sequence (see Fig. 105-7 and Table 105-2).[77] They include platelet basic protein, low-affinity PF4 (connective tissue-activating peptide [CTAP]-III), β-thromboglobulin, and β-thromboglobulin-F (NAP2, CXCL7).[73,102–104] All of these proteins share the same carboxy-terminus but differ in the length of their amino-termini, presumably because of proteolytic digestion of the parent molecule, platelet basic protein (see Fig. 105-7). These proteins bind to heparin but with lower affinity than PF4; thus, they neutralize heparin less well. Unlike PF4, they are cleared from the circulation by the kidney rather than the liver.[105] CTAP-III is a weak fibroblast mitogen, and β-thromboglobulin is a chemoattractant for fibroblasts.[77] β-thromboglobulin-F NAP2 (CXCL7) binds to CXCR2 and is chemotactic for granulocytes and activates them to undergo endocytosis.[77,78,104] Platelet α-granules also contain additional chemokines (see Table 105-2) that can variably activate leukocytes and platelets.[78]

Table 105-3 lists the biochemistry of the adhesive glycoproteins contained in α-granules and others variably present in plasma and extracellular matrix (see Chap. 117 for fibrinogen and Chap. 118 for vWF). Their relative concentrations in α-granules varies significantly. Their localization in platelet α-granules allows them to achieve high local concentrations when they are released from platelets at the site of vascular injury.

Multimerin comprises a family of disulfide-linked homomultimers, ranging from M_r 450,000 to many millions of daltons in size.[106] The M_r 450,000 multimer is thought to be a trimer of a single subunit of either M_r 167,000[107] or M_r 155,000[106] that is synthesized in megakaryocytes and endothelial cells and stored in the electron-lucent re-

gion of α-granules in platelets and dense-core granules in endothelial cells.[108] It colocalizes with vWF in platelets but not endothelial cells. Although multimerin's multimeric structure is similar to that of vWF, the deduced amino acid sequence of its subunit is not homologous to that of vWF.[106] The prepromultimerin subunit contains 1228 amino acids. It undergoes glycosylation and proteolysis during synthesis. It is composed of a number of domains, including an amino-terminal region that includes an RGD sequence, coiled coil sequences, epidermal growth factor-like domains, and a carboxy-terminal globular head similar to that found in the complement protein C1q. Multimerin binds both factor V and factor Va, and all of the biologically active factor V in platelets is bound to multimerin.[69] With thrombin activation of platelets, factor V separates from multimerin, and the higher molecular weight multimerin multimers bind to platelets. Multimerin does not circulate in plasma at an appreciable concentration, but it may act as an adhesive extracellular matrix protein.

Fibrinogen is concentrated in α-granules, as judged by the ratio of platelets to plasma fibrinogen. Megakaryocytes do not appear to synthesize fibrinogen; rather, it is taken up from plasma by a process that involves the αIIbβ3 receptor.[109] Because fibrinogen molecules that contain altered sequences in the γ-chain are not stored in α-granules, even when the molecules are heterodimeric (i.e., contain one normal and one abnormal γ-chain), uptake possibly requires simultaneous binding of a fibrinogen molecule to two different αIIbβ3 receptors via the γ-chain carboxy-terminal sequence (see "αIIbβ3" below and Chap. 112).[109,110]

The vWF stored in platelet α-granules appears to contribute to hemostasis because in certain pathologic states the stored vWF correlates better with bleeding symptoms than does plasma vWF (see

Chap. 118). vWF is made in megakaryocytes and endothelial cells (see Chaps. 104 and 118). The multimeric structure of platelet vWF is thought to reflect endothelial vWF more nearly than plasma vWF given that higher M_r multimers are present (see Chap. 118).

Fibronectin is present in α-granules, but no clear role of this adhesive protein in platelet function under normal conditions has been identified. However, fibronectin can support platelet thrombus formation in mice that lack both fibrinogen and vWF.[111]

Vitronectin, a molecule that binds readily to glass, also binds to PAI-1, the urokinase plasminogen activator receptor (u-PAR), collagen, and heparin. It forms ternary complexes with serine proteases and serpins in the coagulation and complement systems. It is present in platelets at levels that suggest it is concentrated,[112] but it does not appear to be synthesized in megakaryocytes. The binding of PAI-1 to vitronectin stabilizes PAI-1 in its active conformation, but only the approximately 5 percent of PAI-1 complexed with vitronectin in platelet α-granules has been proposed to be active.[29] Mice deficient in vitronectin have been reported to be protected from, or have a predisposition to develop, thrombosis, depending on the method of thrombosis induction.[113–115]

Thrombospondin (TSP)-1 is unique among the adhesive glycoproteins in blood because it is present almost exclusively inside the platelet.[116–118] It constitutes approximately 20 percent of the released platelet proteins. TSP-1 is synthesized by megakaryocytes, cultured endothelial cells, and other cultured cells.[119,120] Although αIIbβ3, GPIb-IX, αVβ3, proteoglycans, integrin-associated protein ([IAP] CD47), and GPIV (CD36) all have been implicated as receptors for TSP,[121–127] CD47 appears to be most important in initiating platelet activation by TSP (see "Signaling Pathways in Platelet Activation and Aggregation" below).[125,126,128] The phosphorylation state of GPIV (CD36) may affect its ability to bind TSP.[123] TSP contains an Arg-Gly-Asp (RGD) sequence, which may contribute to its binding to platelets, but other regions probably also are involved.[117] The conformation of TSP varies with the calcium concentration of the surrounding environment. TSP can interact with many other adhesive glycoproteins, including fibronectin and fibrinogen,[129–131] and it is a component of the extracellular matrix.[132] TSP appears to stabilize platelet aggregates that are formed.[133] It also may modulate fibrinolysis and activate latent transforming growth factor β (TGF-β) (see below).[134,135]

Platelets contribute approximately 20 percent of the factor V present in whole blood, with nearly all of it in the α-granules.[136–138] Human platelet factor V appears to be taken up from plasma rather than synthesized in megakaryocytes, which is in stark contrast to the situation in mice, and it associates with multimerin when it is stored in α-granules.[139,140] Platelet-derived factor V appears to undergo unique posttranslational modifications and proteolytic activation, resulting in resistance to protein C-catalyzed inactivation.[141–143] Evidence from patients with inhibitors to factor V and deficiencies of plasma and platelet factor V indicate that platelet-derived factor V has

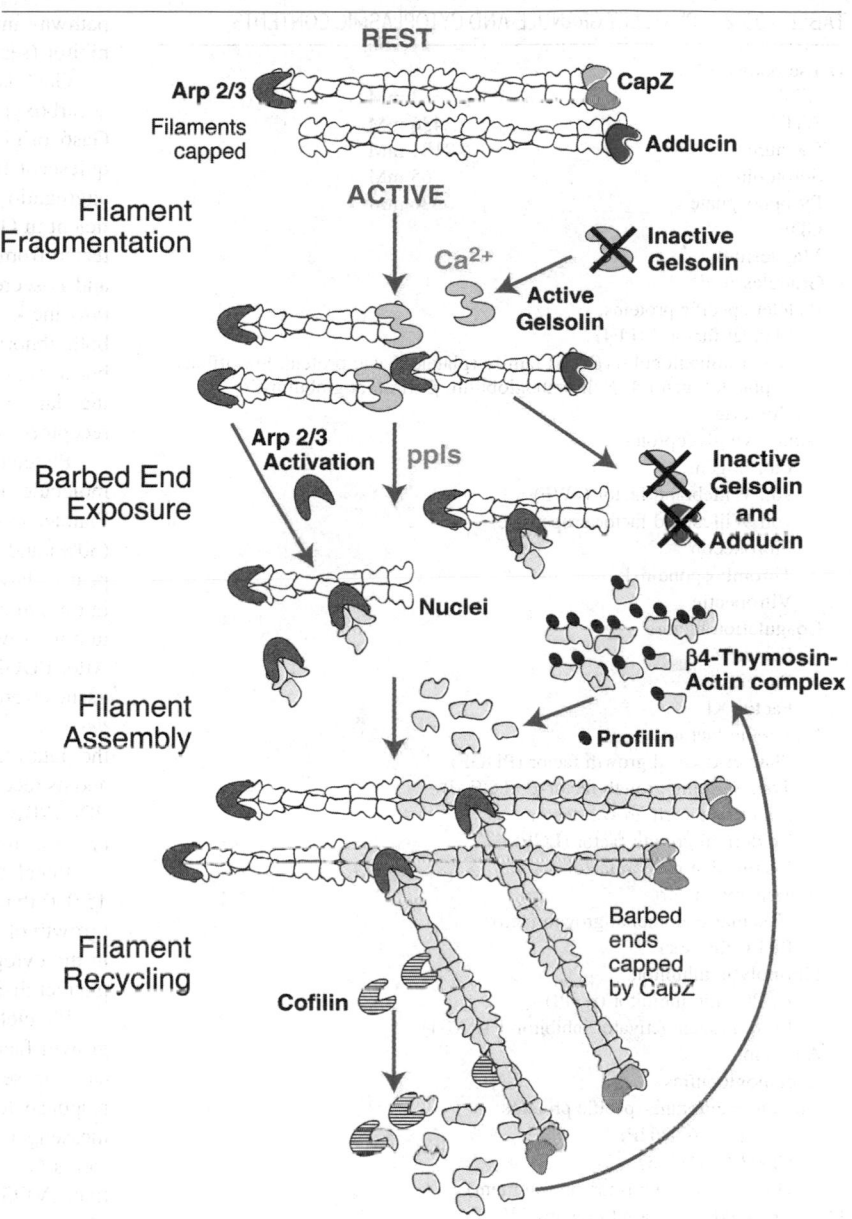

FIGURE 105-4   Control of platelet actin assembly. *(Rest)* Forty percent of the actin in the resting cell is filamentous. The remainder of the actin is soluble and is in a 1:1 complex with β4-thymosin. Filaments are stable because greater than 98 percent are capped on their barbed ends by CapZ and adducin. The actin-related protein complex (Arp 2/3) caps approximately 50 percent of the pointed ends of the filaments. *(Active)* Shape change begins when intracellular calcium concentration rises into the micromolar level and gelsolin becomes active. Gelsolin binds to actin filaments, interdigitates into the filaments, and then severs them. After fragmentation, gelsolin remains bound to the barbed filament end. Assembly of actin begins when capping proteins are dissociated from the barbed ends of the filament fragments by polyphosphoinositides (ppIs) and WASP family proteins, and Arp 2/3 is activated to nucleate *de novo* filaments. Actin monomers, stored in complex with β4-thymosin, are the source of the actin for this polymerization event. Transfer of actin monomers from β4-thymosin to the barbed ends of actin filaments is facilitated by profilin. Once assembly is complete, CapZ recaps the barbed filament ends. (Adapted from JH Hartwig,[22] with permission.)

an important role in hemostasis.[138,144,145] Platelets undergo microvesiculation when activated, and the microvesicles, which are rich in factor V, are potent promoters of coagulation.[146]

Protein S (see Chap. 107), plasminogen activator-1 (see Chap. 127), and α_2-plasmin inhibitor (see Chap. 127) also are contained in α-granules and can be released from platelets. Similarly, tissue factor

TABLE 105-2   PLATELET GRANULE AND CYTOPLASMIC CONTENTS

Dense bodies[1225]
    ADP .... 653 mM
    ATP .... 436 mM
    Calcium .... 2181 mM
    Serotonin .... 65 mM
    Pyrophosphate .... 326 mM
    GDP
    Magnesium
α-Granules[67,71,73]
    Platelet-specific proteins:
        Platelet factor 4 (PF4)
        β-Thromboglobulin (β-TG) family (platelet basic protein, low-affinity platelet factor 4, β-thromboglobulin, β-thromboglobulin-F)
    Multimerin
    Adhesive glycoproteins
        Fibrinogen
        von Willebrand factor (vWF)
        von Willebrand factor propeptide
        Fibronectin
        Thrombospondin-1
        Vitronectin
    Coagulation factors
        Factor V
        Protein S
        Factor XI
    Mitogenic factors
        Platelet-derived growth factor (PDGF)
        Transforming growth factor-β (TGF-β)
        Endothelial cell growth factor
        Epidermal growth factor (EGF)
        Insulin-like growth factor 1
    Angiogenic factors
        Vascular endothelial growth factor
        PF4 (inhibitor)
    Fibrinolytic inhibitors
        α_2-Plasmin inhibitor (α_2-PI)
        Plasminogen-activator inhibitor-1 (PAI-1)
    Albumin
    Immunoglobulins
    Granule membrane-specific proteins
        P-selectin (CD62P)
        CD63 (LAMP-3)
        GMP 33 (thrombospondin fragment)
Other secreted or released proteins[67,73]
    Protease nexin I
    Gas6
    Amyloid β-protein precursor (protease nexin II)
    Tissue factor pathway inhibitor (TFPI)
    Factor XIII
    α_1-Protease inhibitor
    Cl-inhibitor
    High molecular weight kininogen
    α_2-Macroglobulin
    Vascular permeability factor
    Interleukin-1β
    Histidine-rich glycoprotein
Chemokines
    MIP-1α (CCL3)
    RANTES (CCL5)
    MCP-3 (CCL7)
    GRO-α (CXCL1)
    PF4 (CXCL4)
    ENA-78 (CXCL5)
    NAP-2 (CXCL7)
    IL-8 (CXCL8)
    TARC (CCL17)

pathway inhibitor (see Chap. 106), α_1-protease inhibitor, and C-1 inhibitor (see Chap. 107) have also been identified.

Gas6 is an M_r 75,000 vitamin K-dependent protein that contains γ-carboxyglutamic acids and is similar in structure to protein S.[147,148] Gas6 originally was isolated as a growth arrest-specific gene from quiescent fibroblasts but subsequently was found to enhance platelet aggregation and secretion in response to several agonists.[149] Mice deficient in Gas6 have abnormalities in platelet aggregation and are protected from experimental thrombosis.[149] Gas6 is present in α-granules and is secreted with platelet activation. Platelets also express Mer, a tyrosine kinase receptor for Gas6. Mice deficient in Mer demonstrate both abnormalities in platelet aggregation and protection from thrombosis, but not to the same extent as mice deficient in Gas6.[150] Conflicting data exist as to whether platelets also express two other Gas6 receptors, axl and rse, which are in the same family as Mer.[150,151]

Platelet-derived growth factor (PDGF) is a disulfide-linked dimeric molecule of M_r 30,000 that is mitogenic for smooth muscle cells.[152] Platelet α-granules contain a mixture of the homodimer PDGF-BB (30%) and the heterodimer PDGF-AB (70%); the different forms appear to have different functional activities.[153] PDGF may play a role in normal cell proliferation and in the development of atherosclerosis, tumor growth, wound repair, and fibroproliferative responses.[154–156] After PDGF was discovered in platelets and was given its name, other tissues were found to produce the same factor; thus, the name *platelet-derived growth factor* is misleading. PDGF is structurally related to the putative transforming protein p28[sis] of simian sarcoma virus,[157,158] and its receptor is in the tyrosine kinase family.[159] Recombinant human PDGF-BB (becaplermin) is approved as adjunctive therapy for improve healing of foot ulcerations in diabetics.[160]

Platelet-derived endothelial cell growth factor is a protein of M_r 45,000 that stimulates endothelial cell proliferation and angiogenesis (growth of new blood vessels).[161] This protein is thought to be present in the cytoplasm of platelets and thus is released only at the time of platelet disintegration.

Platelets contain high concentrations of vascular endothelial growth factor (VEGF), an important stimulator of angiogenesis, and can release VEGF after stimulation *in vitro* and during the hemostatic response to a bleeding time wound.[162–164] Megakaryocytes express messenger ribonucleic acid (mRNA) encoding the three VEGF isoforms (121, 165, and 189 amino acids),[165] and immunoblot has identified VEGF protein bands of M_r 34,000 and 44,000 in platelets.[166] Platelets and megakaryocytes express the gene transcript for a VEGF receptor termed *KDR*.[167] VEGF-C, another endothelial growth factor structurally related to VEGF, has been identified in platelets.[168] Increased platelet levels of VEGF have been reported in malignancies,[169] and platelet VEGF has been postulated to play a role in tumor growth[170] and proliferative retinopathy in sickle cell disease.[171,172]

Epidermal growth factor has been identified in platelets, but the kinetics of its release upon thrombin or collagen stimulation differs from that of other granule proteins.[173]

Platelets contain the highest levels of all peripheral tissues of amyloid precursor proteins (APP), which contain the self-aggregating 40- to 43-amino-acid residue peptide Aβ that has been strongly implicated in the pathogenesis of Alzheimer disease.[174–176] The isoforms containing the Kunitz protease inhibitor domain (APP 770, APP 751) predominate in platelets. Although synthesized as a membrane protein, platelet APP is cleaved by α-, β-, and γ-secretase activities, producing all of the fragments produced by neurons, including the soluble sAPPα, sAPPβ, and Aβ peptides, and the corresponding remaining C-terminal membrane-associated fragments.[177,178] Calpain can also cleave platelet APP.[179] Approximately 90 percent of platelet APP is soluble and stored in α-granules, but full-length APP surface expression is increased threefold by thrombin stimulation.[180] Platelets are the

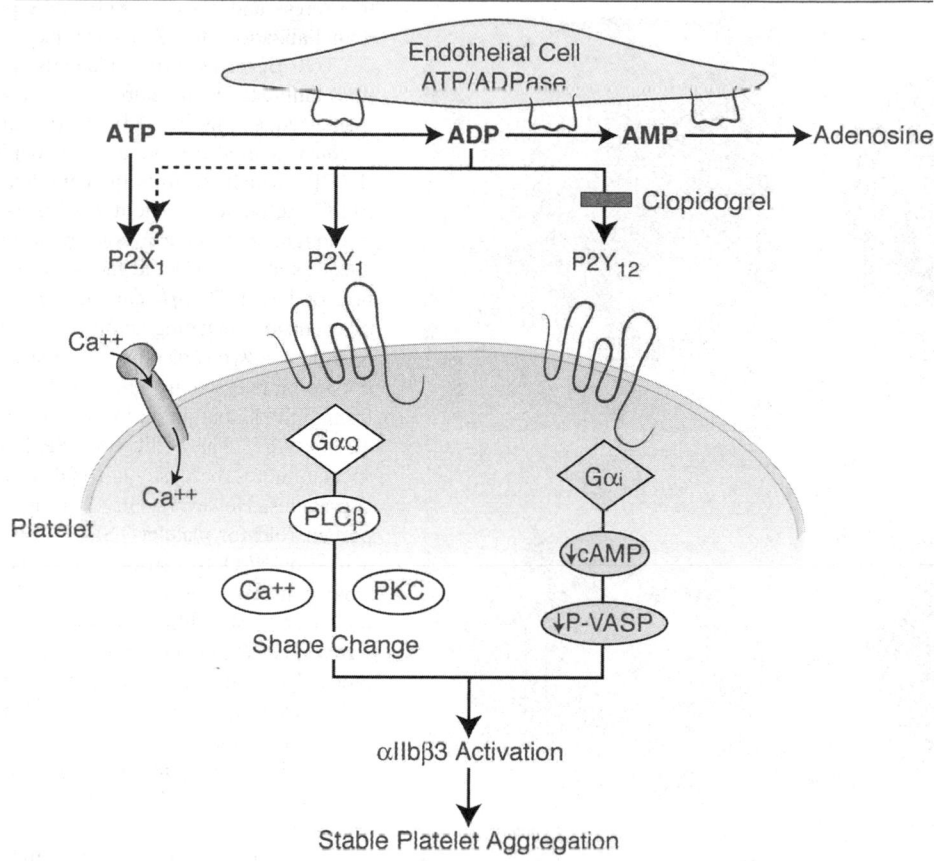

FIGURE 105-5 Platelet purine receptor signaling. ADP acts through two primary G-protein coupled receptors on platelets: $P2Y_1$ and $P2Y_{12}$. The $P2Y_1$ receptor couples to the heterotrimeric GTP-binding protein $G\alpha q$, which in turn activates $PLC\beta$, resulting in elevations in intracellular calcium (Ca^{2+}) and activation of protein kinase C (PKC). The $P2Y_{12}$ receptor couples through the heterotrimeric GTP-binding protein $G\alpha i$ to inhibit adenylyl cyclase and reduce both cAMP and phospho-VASP levels. The actions of ADP at both $P2Y_1$ and $P2Y_{12}$ receptors are required for maximal ADP-induced platelet aggregation. The thienopyridine drugs ticlopidine and clopidogrel are antagonists of the $P2Y_{12}$ receptor and, thereby, partially inhibit ADP-induced platelet aggregation. ATP acts through the $P2X_1$ receptor, which is a ligand-gated calcium channel. Whether ADP can also activate this receptor is unclear. The platelet-activating effects of circulating ATP and ADP are terminated by the ectonucleotidase activity of endothelial cell CD39, which sequentially hydrolyzes the terminal phosphate groups of ATP and ADP to generate AMP. AMP subsequently is converted to adenosine, which inhibits platelet activation via specific G-protein coupled adenosine receptors.

major source of plasma sAPPs and $A\beta$.[177,181] APPs released by platelets are potent inhibitors of factor XIa[182] and IXa.[183,184] They also can inhibit platelet aggregation induced by ADP or epinephrine. In contrast, $A\beta$ appears to enhance ADP-induced platelet aggregation and support platelet adhesion. Plasma $A\beta$ possibly contributes to brain $A\beta$ in Alzheimer disease.[175] Patients with Alzheimer disease reportedly have altered platelet APP metabolism.[185–190]

Factor XIII is present in the cytoplasm of platelets. It differs from plasma factor XIII in having only the "a" subunits (see Chap. 106).[191–194] Platelet factor XIII accounts for approximately 50 percent of total blood factor XIII[191,192] and may contribute to the plasma pool.[195] Upon platelet activation, factor XIII redistributes to the platelet periphery, where it associates with the cytoskeleton and cross-links filamin and vinculin.[196] It also may cross-link thymosin β_4 to fibrin after thrombin stimulation[197] and, in concert with calpain, decrease $\alpha IIb\beta 3$ adhesive function in thrombus formation on collagen.[198] Transglutaminase-mediated conjugation of serotonin to α-granule proteins after platelet stimulation with collagen and thrombin results in the generation of a subpopulation of platelets that are coated with fibrin-

ogen, TSP, factor V, vWF, and fibronectin, either directly through ligand–receptor interactions or through interactions between the serotonin conjugates and platelet surface fibrinogen or TSP (COAT platelets).[199,200]

Platelet α-granules contain a high concentration of TGF-β_1, a 25,000 molecular weight homodimeric protein that promotes the growth of certain cells and inhibits the growth of others.[201] For example, TGF-β can increase thrombopoietin production by bone marrow stromal cells. Thrombopoietin in turn induces megakaryocyte expression of TGF-β receptors, allowing TGF-β to arrest the maturation of megakaryocyte colony forming units.[202] It also induces synthesis of extracellular matrix proteins, PAI-1, and metalloproteinases. It has been implicated in wound healing, malignancy, and tissue fibrosis.[201] In addition, TGF-β_1 reportedly enhances platelet aggregation through a nontranscriptional effect.[203] Migration of endothelial cells is inhibited by TGF-β_1, but it acts as a chemoattractant for monocytes and fibroblasts. TGF-β exists in three isoforms (TGF-β_1, TGF-β_2, TGF-β_3) and has a wide tissue distribution, but platelets contain only TGF-β_1. TGF-β_1 released from platelets can stimulate smooth muscle cells

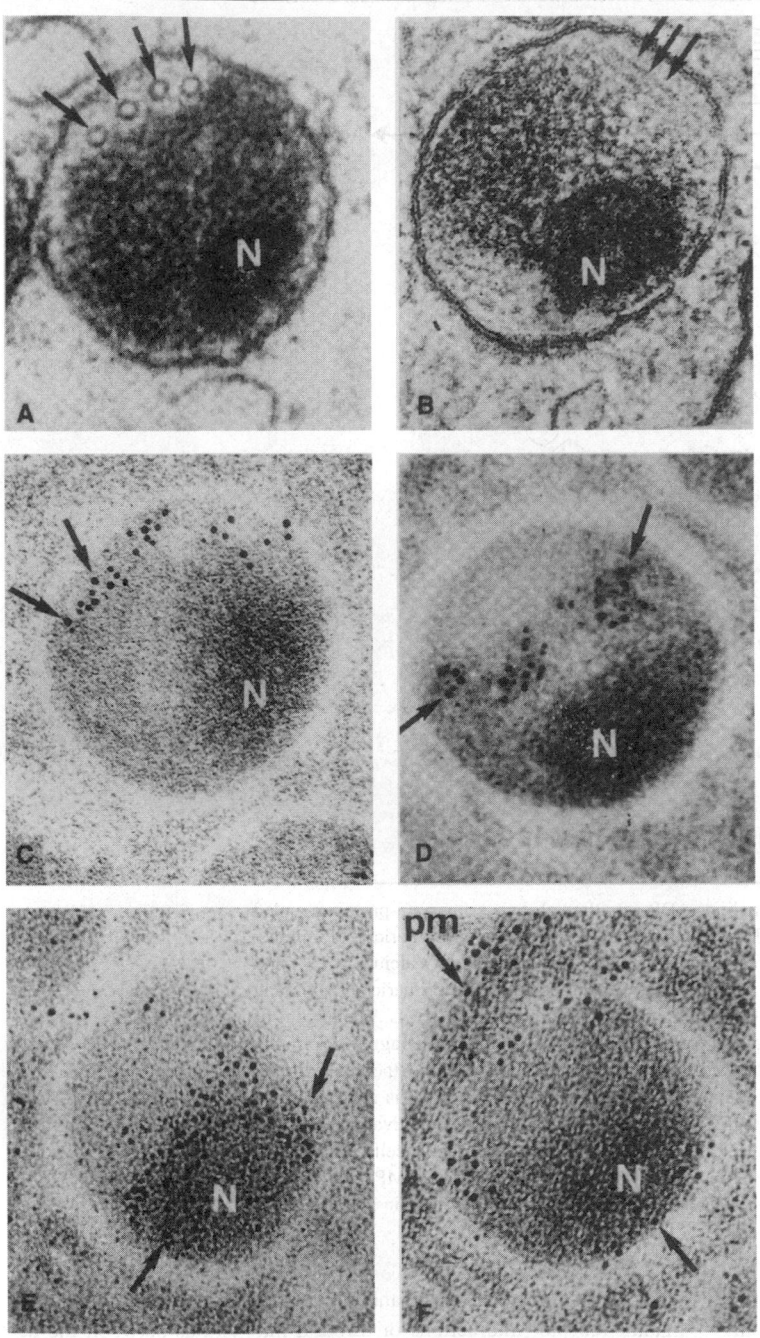

FIGURE 105-6   Compartmentalization within α-granules. Transmission electron micrographs of α-granules. *(A)* Electron-dense nucleoid (N) separated from an electron lucent zone by a zone of intermediary density. The tubular structures (sectioned transversely; *arrows)* represent the location of high molecular weight multimers of von Willebrand factor. *(B)* The tubular structures are sectioned longitudinally *(arrows)* and are similar in appearance to Weibel-Palade bodies in endothelial cells, which also contain von Willebrand factor multimers. *(C)* Immunogold labeling of von Willebrand factor in the tubular area *(arrows).* *(D)* Immunogold labeling of fibrinogen in the intermediary zone *(arrows).* Albumin and growth factors are also found in this region. *(E)* Immunogold staining of β-thromboglobulin in the dense nucleoid. Proteoglycans, platelet factor 4, and other platelet-specific proteins are also localized to this area. *(F)* Immunogold labeling of αIIbβ3 in the α-granule membrane and plasma membrane (pm) (×120,000). (From EM Cramer,[234] with permission.)

to express and release VEGF, thus perhaps supporting reendothelialization after vascular injury.[204]

TGF-β_1 released from platelets is inactive (latent) because it is complexed with a portion of its precursor protein (latency-associated peptide [LAP]). A fraction of LAP is covalently coupled to another protein, the latent TGF-β–binding protein (LTBP), which localizes the complex to the extracellular matrix.[205] Activation of latent TGF-β_1 is a complex process that is thought to involve a conformational change in LAP that alters its ability to shield the active site in TGF-β_1.[205] Activation of latent TGF-β_1 can be achieved by several different mechanisms, including acidification; proteolysis by plasmin, a furin-like enzyme, or other enzymes; interaction with integrin αVβ6; or interaction with TSP-1 or a small peptide derived from TSP-1, but the physiologic activator(s) remains unclear.[135,205,206] The ability of TSP-1 to activate TGFβ_1 is of special interest because both TGF-β_1 and TSP-1 are present in α-granules. However, data from mice do not support an important role for platelet TSP in either TGF-β_1 packaging or activation.[207] Only a small percentage of the TGF-β_1 released from platelets with thrombin stimulation becomes activated, but the amount is sufficient to activate synthesis of PAI-1.[206–208] Active TGF-β can bind to three different cell surface proteins, a proteoglycan (β-glycan), and two serine/threonine kinases.[201,209]

Platelets may release proteins that affect the uptake of oxidized low-density lipoproteins by macrophages, furnishing another potential link between platelet activation and atherosclerosis.[210]

Exosomes   In addition to α-granules, activated platelets release both microparticles (see "Platelet Coagulant Activity" below), which are derived from the plasma membrane, and exosomes, which are the internal membrane vesicles of multivascular bodies and α-granules.[211] Exosomes are smaller than microparticles (40–100 nm vs. 100–1000 nm), enriched in CD63 and tetraspanins (see section below on "Tetraspanins"), and relatively deficient in membrane proteins such as GPIb-IX and platelet endothelial cell adhesion molecule (PECAM)-1. Unlike microparticles, exosomes are not highly procoagulant as judged by their inability to bind prothrombin or factor X, or to present negatively charged phospholipids on their surface. They may, however, contain NAD(P)H oxidase activity, which has the potential to generate reactive oxygen species that contribute to endothelial cell apoptosis in sepsis.[212]

Ribosomes and Messenger RNA   Platelets contain only a relatively small number of ribosomes, have just remnants of a Golgi apparatus (see Fig. 105-1), and have only a small amount of mRNA.[213,214] Because they lack nuclei, they cannot synthesize mRNA. Application of the polymerase chain reaction to platelet mRNA has permitted the molecular biologic analysis of platelet membrane glycoproteins and select plasma proteins that are synthesized in platelets, such as vWF.[215,216] Of note, mRNA for a number of protein transcripts are present on platelet polysomes.[217] Regulated synthesis of new proteins by platelets has been reported after thrombin activation as a result of redistribution of the eukaryotic initiation factor 4E. Signaling produced by ligand engagement of αIIbβ3 appears to be necessary to initiate the process.[218–220] Among the newly translated proteins is pro–IL-Iβ, providing a link between thrombosis and inflammation.[217] Signaling through α2β1 (GPIa-IIa) also can initiate platelet protein synthesis.[219]

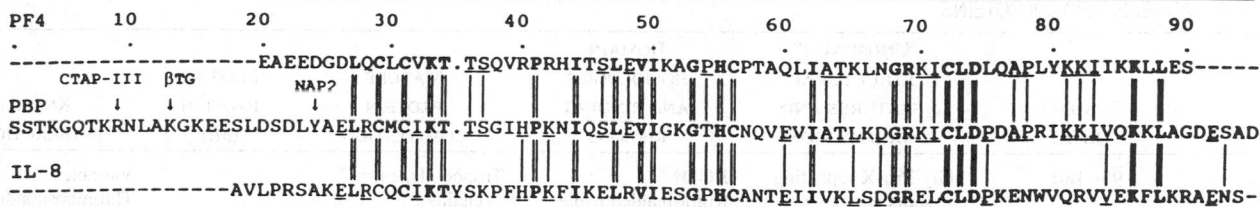

FIGURE 105-7   Comparison of the amino acid sequences of platelet factor 4 (PF4), platelet basic protein (PBP), and interleukin-8/NAP1 (IL-8). *Double vertical lines* indicate identical amino acids in all three sequences. *Single vertical lines* indicate identical amino acids (*underlined*) in two of the three proteins. *Dots* denote artificial breaks inserted to improve alignment. Note that PBP and IL-8 share the ELR sequence (amino acids 26–28 in PBP) conserved in a number of CXC chemokines, but PF4 does not contain this sequence. Cleavage of peptide bond between R9 (*arrow*) and N10 of PBP yields low-affinity PF4 or CTAP III (LA-PF4/CTAP-III). Cleavage of peptide bond between K13 (*arrow*) and G14 yields β-thromboglobulin (βTG). Cleavage of peptide bond between Y24 (*arrow*) and A25 yields β-thromboglobulin fragment or NAP-2 (βTG-F/NAP2). (Adapted from S Niewiarowski, JC Holt, and JJ Cook,[72] with permission.)

MEMBRANE SYSTEMS

Open Canalicular System   The surface-connected open canalicular system is an elaborate series of conduits that begin as indentations of the plasma membrane and course throughout the interior of the platelet (see Fig. 105-1).[2,221] Tracer studies demonstrate that the open canalicular system is contiguous with the exterior of the platelet, even though elements of the open canalicular system may appear as closed vesicles or vacuoles by electron microscopy of sectioned platelets.[2,221,222]

The open canalicular system may serve several functions. It provides a mechanism for entry of external elements into the interior of the platelet. It provides a potential route for the release of granule contents to the outside, eliminating the need for granule fusion with the plasma membrane itself.[222,223] This latter function is especially important because, under most circumstances, platelet granules appear to move to the center of the platelet upon platelet activation rather than to the periphery.[2,224] Controversy remains, however, regarding the relative frequency with which secretion occurs via the open canalicular system versus direct fusion with the plasma membrane.[2,225]

The open canalicular system represents an extensive internal store of membrane. Both filopodia formation and platelet spreading after adhesion require a dramatic increase in surface plasma membrane compared to the plasma membrane of resting platelets. New membrane cannot be synthesized during the short time course of these phenomena. Thus, the membrane of the open canalicular system most likely contributes to the increase in plasma membrane under these conditions. The membranes of α-granules, dense bodies, and, to a lesser extent, lysosomes also may contribute, but only if the stimulus is sufficient to induce the fusion of these organelles with the plasma membrane (release reaction). Finally, the membrane of the open canalicular system may serve as a storage site for plasma membrane glycoproteins under certain circumstances. For example, platelet activation by thrombin can lead to a consistent, selective loss of GPIb-IX from the platelet surface. Electron microscopy indicates the GPIb-IX becomes sequestered in the open canalicular system.[30,226,227] Plasmin may produce a similar phenomenon.[30,228] Platelet activation leads to an increase in surface αIIbβ3, and although much of this αIIbβ3 is thought to derive from α-granule membranes, at least some may come from αIIbβ3 in the membranes of dense bodies and the open canalicular system.[30,229] Similarly, GPVI, the P2Y₁ ADP receptor, the TXA₂ receptor, and perhaps other receptors are present in the open canalicular system and can be recruited to the platelet surface with activation.[230,231]

Dense Tubular System   The dense tubular system (DTS) is a closed-channel network of residual endoplasmic reticulum character-ized histocytochemically by the presence of peroxidase activity.[2,232–234] The channels of the DTS are less extensive than those of the open canalicular system and tend to cluster in regions in close approximation to the open canalicular system.[2] The DTS has been likened to the sarcoplasmic reticulum of muscle because it can sequester ionized calcium and release it when platelets are activated.[235,236] Calreticulin, a calcium-binding protein found in the DTS, probably helps to sequester calcium.[237,238] Release of calcium from the DTS involves the binding of inositol 1,4,5-trisphosphate (IP₃), a messenger molecule formed during signal transduction, to IP₃ type II receptors on the DTS membrane.[239,240] Cyclic AMP inhibits calcium release from the DTS, either by enhancing the calcium pumping mechanism[241] or by inhibiting release induced by IP₃.[242] Nitric oxide (NO) inhibits calcium uptake by the DTS at high concentrations and stimulates uptake at low concentrations by effects on the calcium ATPase(s) sarcoplasmic-endoplasmic reticulum calcium ATPase (SERCA)26 and SERCA3.[243,244] Depletion of intracellular calcium stores activates store-mediated calcium entry into platelets via reversible coupling of IP₃ type II receptors on the DTS membrane and the putative calcium entry channel designated hTRPC1 in the plasma membrane.[20]

The DTS membrane probably is also a major site of prostaglandin and thromboxane synthesis.[236,245] The peroxidase activity used to identify the DTS is an enzymatic component of prostaglandin synthesis.[245,246]

PLATELET PROTEOME AND TRANSCRIPTOME

A number of different approaches have been applied to characterize the proteins expressed by platelets at both the mRNA and protein levels.[247–258] These approaches have included analyses of intact platelets, proteins released from platelets with activation, and platelet proteins modified as a result of activation. Various chromatographic, two-dimensional gel electrophoresis, and mass spectrometric techniques have been used to identify proteins. Microarray and serial analysis of gene expression techniques have been used to detect mRNA. These studies have confirmed previous data regarding synthesis of platelet-specific proteins, identified new proteins that were not previously known to be associated with platelets, characterized posttranslational modifications of proteins associated with platelet activation, and identified the presence of a number of hypothetical proteins in platelets. Although the techniques are still being refined and isolation of pure populations of platelets remains a challenge, these approaches—by analyzing large numbers of proteins and mRNA transcripts—demonstrate their enormous potential for dissecting the molecular mechanisms of platelet function.

TABLE 105-3   ADHESIVE GLYCOPROTEINS

PROTEIN	SUBUNIT (KDA)	UNUSUAL 1° STRUCTURAL FEATURES AND MODIFICATIONS	DOMAIN HOMOLOGIES AND BINDING REGIONS	MATURE PROTEIN COMPOSITION	MATURE PROTEIN (M_r)	KNOWN INTERACTIONS
Collagens	95–180	Gly-Pro-X repeating sequence Hydroxylysine Hydroxyproline	RGD† Right-handed triple helix	Tropocollagen = 3 chains		Variable Thrombospondin
Type I	α1(I) α2(I)		DGEA† vWF C†	[α1(I)]2α2(I) (major component) [α1(I)]$_3$		Fibronectin von Willebrand factor
Type III	α1(III)		vWF C	[α1(III)]3		
Type VI	α1(VI) α2(VI) α3(VI)		3 vWF A† 3 vWFA 12 vWF A	α1(VI) α2(VI) α3(VI)		
von Willebrand factor	220 (2050 amino acids)	Large propeptide (741 amino acids); A, B, C, D, E repeats	αIIbβ3—RGD 1789–1791 A domains GPIb—230–310	Dimer = protomer Multimers of protomers from 2 to ~40 via disulfide bonds	880,000–~20,000,000	Collagen Heparin Factor VIII Fibrin
Fibrinogen	Aα = 63 (625 amino acids) Bβ = 56 (461 amino acids) γ = 47 (427 amino acids)	Alternately spliced γ-chains Phosphorylation of Aα	2 RGDs in Aα (95–97 and 572–574) αVβ3—RGD 572–574 αIIbβ3—C-terminal γ chain dodecamer (400–411)	2 Aα, 2 Bβ, 2 γ via disulfide bonds	340,000	Thrombospondin ?Collagen Staphylococci Factor XIII Thrombn
Vitronectin	1 chain = 75 (458 amino acids) 2 chain = 65+10 via disulfide bonds	Met→Thr polymorphism	RGD Somatomedin B 2 Hemopexin	Same as subunits	75,000 and 65,000+ 10,000	Glass Plastic Heparin Serine protease: serpin complexes PAI-1† u-PAR† Factor XIII
Fibronectin	220 (2355 amino acids)	Type I, II, and III repeats Alternately spliced forms	RGD (1493–1495)	Heterodimer via disulfide bonds	440,000	Fibrin Heparin Collagen DNA Staphylococci
Thrombo-spondin-1	180 (1150 amino acids)		RGD (?functional) VTCG† α1(I) collagen Epidermal growth factor Malaria antigen	Trimer via disulfide bonds	450,000	Calcium Plasminogen Collagen Fibrinogen Histidine-rich glycoprotein Fibronectin Laminin Heparin
Osteopontin	32 (298 amino acids)	Phosphorylation Sulfation	RGD			Hydroxyapatite Plaque components
Laminin	A = 400 B$_1$ = 215 (1765 amino acids) B$_2$ = 205 (1576 amino acids)		YIGSR† RGD (?functional) EGF†	A, B$_1$, B$_2$, via disulfide bonds	850,000	Collagen type IV Nidogen/entactin Osteonectin Heparin sulfate C1q Plasminogen Plasmin
Multimerin	155 or 167	Large prepropeptide (1228 amino acids)	RGD in N-terminal region EGF		450,000–~5,000,000	Factor V

* Assumes 10^{11} platelets per milliliter of packed platelets.

† RDG, arginine-glycine-aspartic acid sequence; vWF A, vWF C, von Willebrand factor A and C repeats; DGEA, VTCG, and YIGSR, other amino acid sequences involved in function EGF-epidermal growth factor; PAI-1-plasminogen activator-1; u-PAR-urokinase plasminogen activator receptor.

Known platelet receptors	Electron microscopic structure	Plasma concentration (μG/ML)	Platelet concentration* (μG/ML)	Ratio platelet/plasma	Sites of synthesis
$\alpha 2\beta 1$ (GPIa-IIa;CD49b/CD29; VLA-2) GPVI GPIV (CD36)?	Tropocollagen = rodlike coil, 15×3000; other forms have variable degrees of fibril formation	—	—	—	Fibroblasts
GPIb (CD42b, c) αIIbβ3 (GPIIb-IIIa; CD41/CD61)	Elliptical, nodular coil, length 5000, but with some 11,000 Å	10	34	3.4	Endothelial cells Megakaryocytes
αIIbβ3 (GPIIb-IIIa; CD41/CD61) αVβ3 (CD51/CD61)	Trinodular, asymmetric; 475-Å diameter	3000	7300	2.4	Hepatocytes
αIIbβ3 (GPIIb-IIIa; CD41/CD61) αVβ3 (CD51/CD61)		350	800	2.3	?Hepatocytes
$\alpha 5\beta 1$ (GPIc*-IIa (CD49e/CD29; VLA-5) αIIbβ3 (GPIIb-IIIa; CD41/CD61)	Extended antiparallel dimeric structure	300	315	1.1	Hepatocytes Fibroblasts ?Endothelial cells Megakaryocytes Monocytes, etc.
GPIV (CD36) αIIbβ3 (GPIIb-IIIa; CD41/CD61)? Integrin-associated protein (CD47)	Three asymmetric dumbbells, joined near smaller globular domains	0.16	4900	30,625	Megakaryocytes Many cultured cells
αVβ3		—	—	—	Bone ?Other cells
$\alpha 6\beta 1$ (GPIc/IIa; CD49f/CD29; VLA-6)	Cross-like structure	—	—	—	Fibroblasts Many other cell types
Unknown	Unknown	—	—	—	Megakaryocytes Endothelial cells

PLATELET PHYSIOLOGY AND BIOCHEMISTRY

OVERVIEW OF PLATELET ADHESION, AGGREGATION, AND PLATELET THROMBUS FORMATION

The hemostatic system is under elaborate control mechanisms lest the response either be inadequate to meet the hemorrhagic challenge or result in inappropriate thrombosis in response to trivial provocation. Evolutionary pressures probably have favored a more active hemostatic system because individuals with more active hemostatic systems were more likely to avoid death from hemorrhage prior to attaining sexual maturity or during childbirth. Our active hemostatic system appears to be less well adapted to our modern age, which is characterized by long life spans and progressive vascular disease, because the deposition of a platelet–fibrin thrombus on a damaged atherosclerotic plaque can lead to myocardial infarction or stroke.

The platelet's major function is to seal openings in the vascular tree. It is appropriate, therefore, that the initiation signal for platelet deposition and activation is exposure of underlying portions of the blood vessel wall that normally are concealed from circulating platelets by an intact endothelial lining (Fig. 105-8 and Table 105-4).[259] Additional parameters that probably control the platelet response are (1) the depth of injury, with deeper damage exposing more platelet-reactive materials and tissue factor (see Chap. 106)[260–263]; (2) the vascular bed, with the blood vessels serving mucocutaneous tissues especially dependent on platelets for hemostasis, in contrast to the vascular beds in muscles and joints, which rely more on the coagulation mechanism; (3) the age of the individual, because the composition of the blood vessel wall probably changes with age; (4) the hematocrit, because increased numbers of erythrocytes enhance platelet interactions with the blood vessel wall by forcing platelets to the periphery of the bloodstream (as the erythrocytes disproportionately occupy the axial region) and imparting radially directed energy to platelets as the erythrocytes engage in flip-flop motions[264,265]; and (5) the speed of blood flow and the size of the blood vessel, which determine the number of platelets passing by in a given time, the amount of time a platelet has to interact with the blood vessel wall or other platelets, the rate of dilution of platelet-activating agents, and the forces tending to pull a platelet from the vessel wall or another platelet (shear rate).[261,264] The vasospastic response that accompanies vascular injury, to which platelets contribute by release of TXA_2 and serotonin, probably plays a key role in decreasing hemorrhage and facilitating platelet and fibrin deposition via its effect on blood flow.

Platelet thrombi appear capable of rapidly recruiting tissue factor from the blood. The tissue factor is associated with small lipid-containing vesicles and may derive from leukocyte membranes that contain P-selectin glycoprotein ligand (PSGL-1), a ligand for the P-selectin expressed on the surface of activated platelets.[266,267] An alternatively spliced form of tissue factor circulating in blood also may associate with platelet thrombi.[268] Some investigators have reported the presence of tissue factor in platelet α-granules that leads to surface expression when platelets are activated, but others have not been able to identify platelet tissue factor.[269] Activated platelets expressing P-selectin also recruit neutrophils and monocytes expressing PSGL-1 (Fig. 105-9). Generation of P-selectin–containing microparticles from platelets and binding of platelets and/or these microparticles to leukocytes can lead to initiation of synthesis and "de-encryption" (or de-cryption) of tissue factor, with the latter resulting in greater tissue factor activity per unit tissue factor antigen.[270] All of these mechanisms may contribute to the initiation of coagulation on the surface of the platelet thrombus.[270–273]

The shear rate differentially affects platelet adhesion to surfaces. vWF-dependent adhesion is most important at higher shear rates, probably because high shear rates cause conformational changes in vWF

and/or platelet GPIb.[265,274–278] Very high shear rates can cause platelets to aggregate via a mechanism that involves vWF binding to GPIb-IX, followed by intracellular signaling leading to activation of $\alpha IIb\beta 3$.[279–282] Platelets contribute more significantly to arterial thrombi than to venous thrombi, perhaps as a result of differences in the shear rates in the different beds.[261]

The subendothelial layer immediately subjacent to the endothelium contains a large number of adhesive proteins (see Table 105-4),[259,261] and the platelet has receptors for many of these proteins (see Tables 105-3 and 105-5). GPIb-IX is a receptor complex that is particularly important in mediating adhesion to vWF immobilized in the subendothelium. This receptor appears to dominate the adhesion process at high shear (see Chap. 118).[277,282] Three different sources of vWF may contribute to the subendothelial vWF: synthesis by endothelial cells, deposition from plasma, or release from platelet α-granules.[277,283] Subendothelial vWF appears to associate with type VI collagen,[284] but it can bind to multiple collagen types. Plasma vWF binds via its A3 domain to types I and III collagens when they are exposed by deep injury in the blood vessel wall.[265,275,278] The interaction between GPIbα and vWF does not in itself cause firm adhesion; rather, it results in tethering and slow translocation, probably because the bonds between vWF and GPIbα not only form rapidly but also dissociate rapidly.[259,275,277] Adhesion initiated by interactions between GPIbα and vWF are stabilized by interactions between vWF and $\alpha IIb\beta 3$.[259,277,285]

The biologic contributions of the interactions between the $\alpha 6\beta 1$ (GPIc-IIa) receptor and laminin, the $\alpha 5\beta 1$ (GPIc*-IIa) receptor and fibronectin, and the $\alpha V\beta 3$ receptor and vitronectin in initiating platelet adhesion remain unknown, but some experimental data support the role of the first two in mice.[286] The $\alpha IIb\beta 3$ integrin can function as an adhesion receptor for immobilized fibrinogen even in the absence of platelet activation,[287,288] but platelet activation is required for $\alpha IIb\beta 3$-mediated adhesion to vWF and fibronectin[288] and for platelet thrombus formation. Platelets may interact directly with exposed collagen via GPVI and $\alpha 2\beta 1$ (GPIa-IIa) or perhaps with one or more of the many other receptors implicated in platelet–collagen interactions (e.g., GPIV, p65).[286,289–300] The density of $\alpha 2\beta 1$ receptors on platelets affects the efficiency of platelet thrombus formation on collagen-coated surfaces.[301–304] In addition, fibrinogen, fibronectin, and vWF, whether released from platelets or circulating in plasma, may bind to collagen. These proteins in turn may interact with platelet $\alpha IIb\beta 3$, $\alpha 5\beta 1$ (GPIc*-IIa), and/or GPIb-IX, completing a sandwich mechanism initiated by collagen exposure.[278,292]

Depending on the vascular bed, available adhesive glycoproteins, and shear conditions, various combinations of platelet receptors, including GPIbα, $\alpha 2\beta 1$ (GPIa-IIa), GPVI, and $\alpha IIb\beta 3$, likely act in concert to transform the tethering and slow translocation of platelets initiated by GPIbα interacting with vWF into stable platelet adhesion.[259,265,277,278,282,295,300,305]

For platelet plug formation to occur, platelets must undergo activation and adhesion. Table 105-6 and Figure 105-10 provide physiologic and pathologic platelet activators, which are divided into strong and weak agents. Most of these activators are released or synthesized at the site of vascular injury, resulting in a local response. In addition, cooperative biochemical interactions between erythrocytes and platelets may enhance platelet activation.[306]

Vascular injury has been speculated to result in release of ADP from erythrocytes, thus leading to platelet activation. Adhesion of platelets to subendothelial structures, particularly vWF at high shear, may itself lead to platelet activation, including generation of TXA_2, release of ADP and serotonin, and activation of $\alpha IIb\beta 3$ receptors on the luminal side of the platelet to their high-affinity ligand-binding states.[277] These positive feedback mechanisms ensure an adequate he-

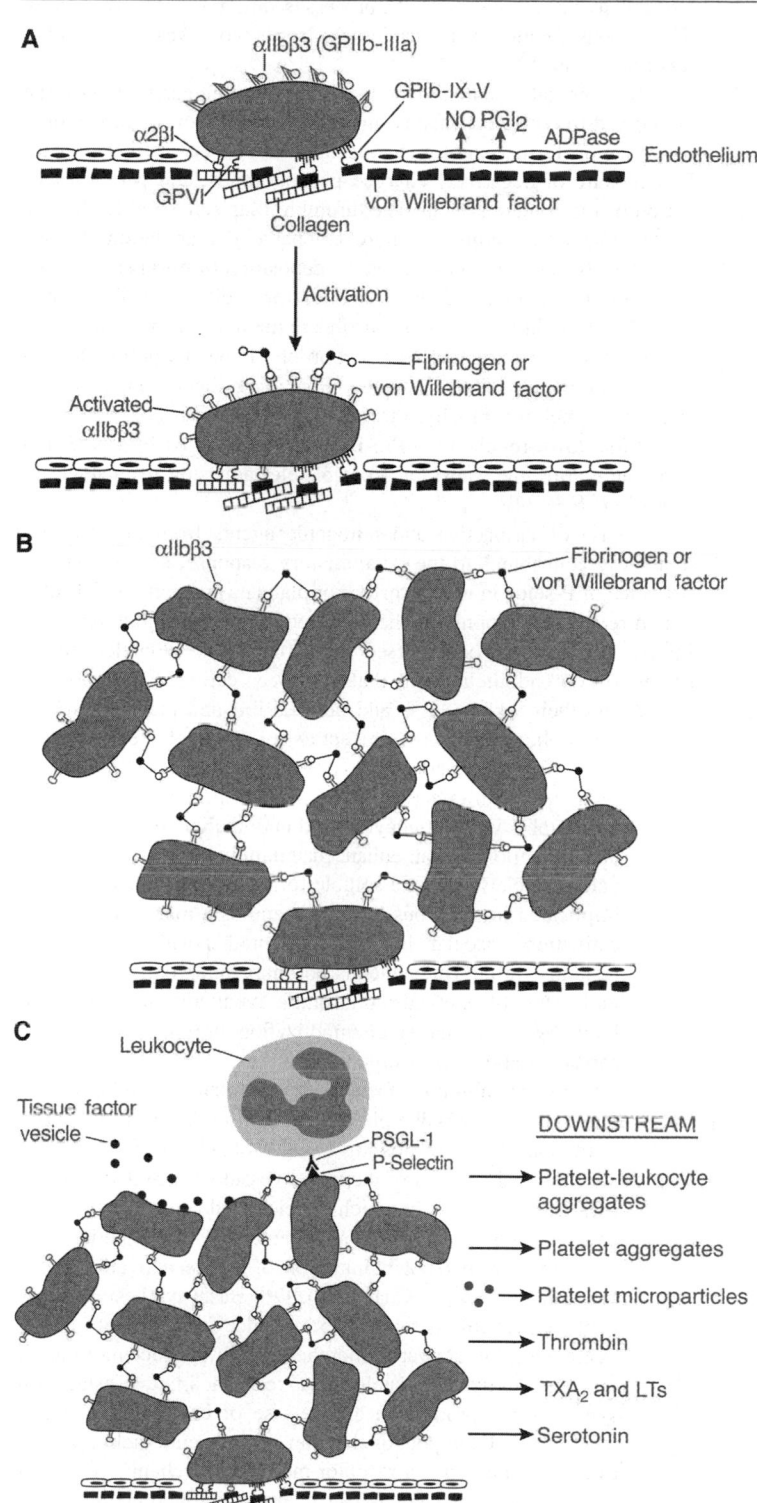

FIGURE 105-8 Platelet adhesion, activation, aggregation, and platelet-leukocyte interactions. *(A)* Endothelial cells limit platelet deposition because they separate platelets from the adhesive proteins in the subendothelial area, produce two inhibitors of platelet function (nitric oxide [NO] and prostacyclin [PGI_2]), and contain a potent ADPase enzyme (CD39) in their membranes that digests ADP released from platelets. Platelet adhesion is initiated by loss of endothelial cells (or, in the case of an atherosclerotic lesion, rupture or erosion of the plaque), which exposes adhesive glycoproteins such as collagen and von Willebrand factor in the subendothelium. Other adhesive glycoproteins probably also are exposed (Table 105-4). In addition, von Willebrand factor and perhaps other adhesive glycoproteins in plasma deposit in the damaged area, in part by binding to collagen. Platelets adhere to the subendothelium via receptors that bind to the adhesive glycoproteins. GPIb binding to von Willebrand factor plays a prominent role, but $\alpha2\beta1$ (GPIa-IIa) and GPVI binding to collagen and other platelet receptors (Table 105-5) probably also play a role. After platelets adhere, they undergo an activation process that leads to a conformational change in $\alpha IIb\beta3$ receptors involving headpiece extension and leg separation (see Fig. 105-3), resulting in their ability to bind with high-affinity select multivalent adhesive proteins, most prominently fibrinogen and von Willebrand factor, including the von Willebrand factor that binds to collagen in the subendothelial area. *(B)* Platelet aggregation occurs when the multivalent adhesive glycoproteins bind simultaneously to $\alpha IIb\beta3$ receptors on two different platelets, resulting in receptor cross-linking. Clustering of the receptors probably also contributes to the stability of the aggregates (not shown). *(C)* After platelets adhere and aggregate, they help to initiate coagulation by binding tissue factor-containing vesicles circulating in the plasma, exposing negatively charged phospholipids on their surface (not shown), releasing platelet factor V (not shown), and releasing procoagulant microparticles. Activated platelets also express P-selectin on their surface, which leads to recruitment of leukocytes via interactions between platelet P-selectin and P-selectin glycoprotein ligand-1 (PSGL-1) expressed on the surface of leukocytes. Other interactions between platelets and leukocytes are detailed in Fig. 105-9. Thrombus formation is a dynamic cyclical process, with platelets repeatedly adhering, aggregating, and then breaking off and embolizing downstream. Platelet–leukocyte aggregates, platelet aggregates, platelet microparticles, thrombin, thromboxane A_2 (TXA_2), leukotrienes (LTs), and serotonin probably all go downstream and affect the microvasculature. Ultimately the vessel either becomes fully occluded or loses its thrombogenic reactivity, that is, it becomes passivated.

mostatic response. Depending on the nature of the surface to which they adhere, platelets also undergo variable spreading reactions and become anchored by a process that at least partially involves $\alpha IIb\beta3$ ligation and clustering, cytoskeletal reorganization, and tyrosine phosphorylation. These reactions also contribute to initiating the release reaction.[307–311] When exposed to collagen, some platelets are first recruited to the surface by platelet–platelet interactions with already adherent platelets and only then adhere to, and spread on, the collagen.[310]

The activated luminal $\alpha IIb\beta3$ receptors on adherent platelets may bind vWF, fibrinogen, or perhaps other adhesive glycoproteins and await interaction with another platelet, which itself may have undergone activation of its $\alpha IIb\beta3$ receptors as a result of exposure to released ADP and TXA_2. Alternatively, a platelet may become activated and bind vWF or fibrinogen while still circulating, in which case the platelet–ligand complex may bind directly to an activated $\alpha IIb\beta3$ receptor on the luminal surface. The binding of adhesive ligands to platelet receptors then repeats itself, resulting in the recruitment of addi-

TABLE 105-4   COMPONENTS OF THE BLOOD VESSEL WALL THAT ARE HEMOSTATICALLY ACTIVE

I. Subendothelium
    von Willebrand factor
    Collagen (types IV, V, VI)
    Fibronectin
    Thrombospondin
    Laminin
    Vitronectin
    Fibrinogen (fibrin)
II. Media
    Collagen (types I, III)
III. Adventitia
    Collagen (types I, III)
    Tissue factor

SOURCE: Adapted from BS Coller,[261] with permission.

tional layers of platelets and ultimately the formation of a hemostatic plug. Intravital videomicroscopy of the mesenteric and cremasteric circulations of mice after endothelial cell damage demonstrates that, at least in these vascular beds, platelet thrombus formation initially is a highly dynamic process, with many platelets depositing but then embolizing. Thrombus growth is relatively slow compared to what would be its growth rate if all of the platelets that deposited remained

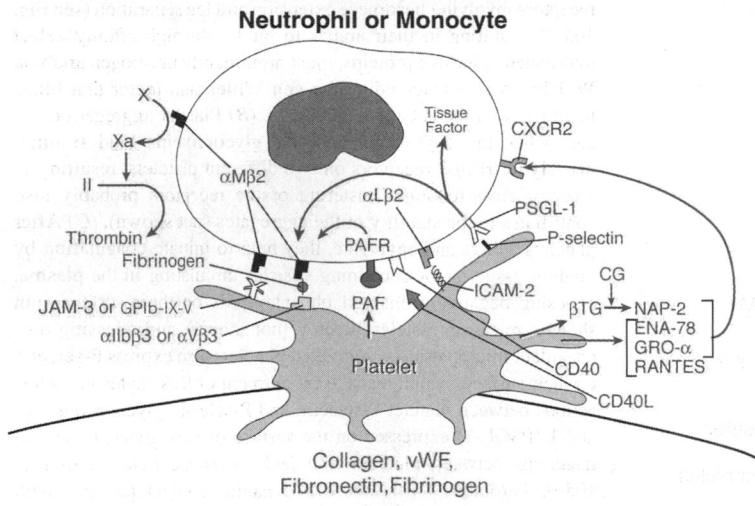

Neutrophil or Monocyte

FIGURE 105-9   Platelet–leukocyte interactions. A number of interactions can occur between platelets and leukocytes, including neutrophils and monocytes. The interaction between platelet P-selectin and leukocyte P-selectin glycoprotein ligand-1 (PSGL-1) probably is the most important initial interaction (and can lead to tissue factor synthesis by monocytes), but fibrinogen binding simultaneously to activated αMβ2 on leukocytes and either αIIbβ3 or αVβ3 on platelets may play a role under certain circumstances. Platelets can release platelet-activating factor (PAF), which can interact with a PAF receptor (PAFR) on leukocytes, leading to αMβ2 activation and binding of fibrinogen and factor X. Leukocyte αMβ2 can also interact with platelet junctional adhesion molecule-3 (JAM-3) or GPIb. Platelets can release chemokines (e.g., ENA-78, GRO-α, and RANTES), and β-thromboglobulin (βTG) released by platelets can be converted by leukocyte cathepsin G (CG) into the potent chemotactic CXC chemokine NAP-2. Some of the chemokines, in turn, activate leukocytes by binding to the chemokine receptor CXCR2. Platelets also contain the potent immune-stimulating molecule CD40 ligand (CD40L), and both express it on the platelet surface and release it into the circulation upon platelet activation. The interaction between thrombospondin and CD36 molecules on both platelets and some leukocytes and the presence of CD40 on platelets are not shown. vWF, von Willebrand factor.

attached to the surface.[312–314] The process is similar in the carotid artery of the mouse, which is a considerably larger blood vessel but still is less than 1 mm.[315]

The aggregated platelets can facilitate thrombin generation by one or more different mechanisms, including recruitment of bloodborne tissue factor, formation of microvesicles, exposure of activated factor V, exposure of negatively charged phospholipids, and perhaps activation of the contact system. The thrombin thus generated further activates platelets, leading to more extensive degranulation. It also activates coagulation and initiates the deposition of fibrin strands that reinforce the platelet and serve as sites for additional vWF deposition.[316] Thrombin may help to consolidate the plug by initiating platelet-mediated clot retraction (see section on "Platelet Contractile Elements and Platelet Shape Change, Spreading, Secretion, and Clot Retraction" below). Finally, thrombin affects the surface membrane receptors, down-regulating GPIb-IX, up-regulating αIIbβ3, and perhaps facilitating the transition from platelet adhesion to platelet aggregation.[30,226,227,317]

Release of vasoactive and mitogenic agents from platelets undoubtedly contributes to the inflammatory response, as does the appearance of P-selectin on the surface of platelets and endothelial cells, which recruits neutrophils to the damaged region (see "Platelet–Leukocyte Interactions" below) (see Fig. 105-9).[318–320] Platelets themselves roll on endothelial cells that have been activated to expose P-selectin on their surface,[320,321] and both GPIbα and platelet PSGL-1 have been implicated as counterreceptors for endothelial cell P-selectin.[282,322,323] Platelets also express CD40 ligand (CD40L) on their surface after activation,[324] which can interact with CD40 on lymphocytes, monocytes, and endothelial cells, leading to cell activation and an enhanced inflammatory response. Activated platelets release a soluble form of CD40L that has been implicated in thrombus formation and as a marker of platelet activation, vascular disease, and a predisposition to develop restenosis after percutaneous coronary intervention.[325–330] Finally, the platelet–fibrin thrombi eventually resolve, most likely by a combination of embolization, fibrinolysis, and macrophage removal of debris.

Several inhibitory factors balance platelet activation and thus prevent excessive platelet deposition (Table 105-7). The dilutional effects of flowing blood probably are most important; thus, alterations of the blood vessel surface that produce local areas of stasis in which platelets and coagulation factors can concentrate are prothrombogenic.[261,264] Endothelial cells can synthesize two potent inhibitors of platelet activation: prostacyclin and NO (see Chap. 108).[331,332] Basal synthesis of prostacyclin probably is too low to influence formation of platelet aggregates, but activated endothelial cells produce more prostacyclin. Activated platelets also can facilitate prostacyclin synthesis via production and release of endoperoxide intermediates and compounds that can activate endothelial prostacyclin production via receptor-mediated mechanisms. In addition, activated platelets can release microparticles that can transfer arachidonic acid to endothelial cells.[333] Thus, prostacyclin may contribute significantly to platelet inhibition at sites of injury. NO, which is synthesized by endothelial cells, is a potent inhibitor of ex vivo platelet adhesion and aggregation. Data from animal models suggest that a deficiency of NO predisposes animals to thrombosis.[332,334,335] NO synthesis probably is enhanced at sites of injury as a result of release from activated platelets, so NO may well contribute to platelet inhibition, especially because it apparently synergizes with prostacyclin.[332,336] Endothelial cells also have CD39, an ecto-ADPase that can digest ATP and ADP to AMP and thus can limit the effects of released ADP (see Fig. 105-5).[62,66] Under certain conditions, leukocytes appear to interact biochemically with platelets to limit platelet activation,[337] but cathepsin G released from activated leukocytes can activate platelets.[338,339]

Because thrombin is such a potent activator of platelets, the control mechanisms that limit thrombin production also can be considered control mechanisms for platelet aggregation (see Chap. 107). Platelets can become desensitized to stimulation by some agonists if they previously were exposed to low concentrations of that agonist (homologous desensitization). In the penumbra of released platelet agonists, some platelets possibly become inhibited by this mechanism.[340–342]

The $\alpha IIb\beta 3$ receptor occupies a central role in determining the extent of platelet aggregation, in part because it is present at an extraordinarily high density on the platelet surface (receptors are probably less than 20 nm apart).[343–346] This high density permits it to rapidly initiate platelet aggregation. On the other hand, the receptor is not in its high-affinity ligand-binding state on resting platelets; rather, it must be activated by agonists, including ADP, serotonin, thrombin, collagen, and TXA$_2$, which are localized to sites of vascular injury.[309,344,345] As a result, platelets can circulate in plasma containing high concentrations of the $\alpha IIb\beta 3$ ligands fibrinogen and vWF without ongoing platelet thrombus formation.

Thus, platelet adhesion is controlled by the exposure of the subendothelium, with the platelet GPIb-IX receptor for immobilized vWF and the $\alpha IIb\beta 3$ receptor for immobilized fibrinogen always competent to interact with these adhesive ligands.[278,287,288,347] In contrast, the ability of $\alpha IIb\beta 3$ to mediate platelet aggregation by binding fluid-phase vWF[348] or fibrinogen[344–346,349] is under the control of an elaborate activation mechanism that limits the response to sites of vascular injury.

The agonists that activate the $\alpha IIb\beta 3$ receptor likely work in combination in vivo. The mixture of agonists present probably changes as the process unfolds, with collagen perhaps more important at the beginning, thrombin more important later on, and the other agonists contributing in varying mixtures throughout. Platelet activation induced by multiple agonists simultaneously is not simply additive; synergistic interactions are well documented.[350,351] Although epinephrine is a relatively weak platelet agonist itself, it probably plays an important role by enhancing the platelet's response to other agonists, including the ability to overcome aspirin-induced inhibition of platelet thrombus formation.[352] Changes in epinephrine levels that can accompany cigarette smoking or vascular collapse, as may occur during myocardial infarction, may have significant effects on platelet thrombus formation.[352–354] Finally, platelets can be activated by shear stresses ex vivo. Although the in vivo significance of this phenomenon remains unknown, it offers another potential link between the blood vessel narrowing produced by atherosclerotic vascular disease and platelet activation.[278,280,281,355]

PLATELET ENERGY METABOLISM

Platelets have sizable stores of glycogen that can often be seen by electron microscopy (see Fig. 105-1). Glycogen can be broken down into glucose-1-phosphate, and platelets can take up glucose from their surrounding medium. Both sources of glucose can be converted to glucose-6-phosphate, which can enter glycolysis or the hexose monophosphate shunt. Platelet glycolysis rates significantly exceed those of erythrocytes and skeletal muscle.[356] Oxidative metabolism probably contributes to energy production in resting platelets, but less than 1 percent of the pyruvic acid produced by glycolysis is estimated to actually enter the citric acid cycle; the remainder terminates in lactate or pyruvate, which leave the platelet.[357] Platelet mitochondria are capable of β-oxidation of fatty acids, but the extent to which this process contributes to energy production is not clear.[358–361] Platelets can ac-

tively metabolize acetate, and this ability has been exploited to improve platelet storage conditions.[361,362] Amino acids may act as energy sources and feed into the citric acid cycle, but the contribution of this process to platelet energy metabolism is uncertain.

As in all cells, ATP consumption by platelets is partially devoted to maintaining ionic and osmotic homeostasis.[363,364] In addition, the continuous polymerization and depolymerization of actin involves conversion of ATP to ADP, which may account for as much as 40 percent of the ATP consumption in resting platelets.[365] The inositol phosphates, which are important in signal transduction, undergo continual dephosphorylation and rephosphorylation. These reactions have been estimated to consume as much as 7 percent of the total ATP produced.[366] Protein phosphorylation also occurs as an ongoing event, but its fractional use of ATP is not clear.

Depleting platelets of the metabolic pool of ATP and ADP decreases their ability to respond to stimuli, but the effect is not uniform. Thus, shape change is only minimally affected, whereas increasingly significant effects on platelet aggregation, α-granule and dense granule secretion, arachidonic acid liberation, and lysosome secretion are observed.[49,50,367,368]

Platelet stimulation is accompanied by a marked increase in both glycolytic activity and oxidative ATP production, perhaps as a result of the abruptly decreased ATP level that occurs with platelet activation or the increased cytoplasmic pH.[359] The increased ATP appears to be utilized, at least in part, in phosphoinositide phosphorylation and protein phosphorylation.

PLATELET CONTRACTILE ELEMENTS AND PLATELET SHAPE CHANGE, SPREADING, SECRETION, AND CLOT RETRACTION

Table 105-8 lists the major components of the platelet contractile system. These elements are thought to contribute to platelet shape change, spreading, secretion, and clot retraction after platelet activation.

PLATELET CYTOSKELETON

The platelet cytoskeleton, namely, the elements that contribute to the maintenance and change of its shape, is operationally defined as proteins that are insoluble in the presence of the nonionic detergent Triton X-100 under defined ionic conditions (see section on "Cytoskeletal Elements" above).[22,23,369–371] The cytoskeleton of resting platelets consists of the membrane skeleton, which lies just beneath the membrane, and a lacy cytoplasmic actin filament network composed of 2000 to 5000 linear actin polymers, which also contains α-actin, filamins (actin-binding proteins) A (X) and B (3), tropomyosin, vinculin, and caldesmon (see Fig. 105-2).[369,372–375] The filamins act as self-associating scaffolding molecules that interact with the cytoplasmic tail of GPIbα, small GTPases, phosphatases, kinases, and actin, thus localizing and concentrating these cytoplasmic proteins near the membrane. The association of filamin with GPIbα compresses the underlying spectrin lattice.[22]

With platelet activation, phosphorylated myosin joins the cytoskeleton, as does talin, and the cytoskeleton becomes an electron-dense mass of bundled filaments.[369,376,377] Platelet membrane glycoproteins $\alpha IIb\beta 3$ and $\alpha 2\beta 1$ also join the cytoskeleton of activated platelets, probably via interaction between actin, vinculin, talin, and the cytoplasmic domains of the membrane glycoproteins.[23,378] Inside-out activation of $\alpha IIb\beta 3$ from its inactive to active conformation has been associated with cytoskeletal changes, particularly the binding of talin to the $\beta 3$ integrin cytoplasmic domain.[24,27,379,380] The focal adhesion tyrosine kinase (FAK) pp125^{FAK} may play a role in the process.[307,381] The tyrosine kinase pp60^{src}, which is abundant in platelets;[381] cortactin, an M_r 85,000 protein that is phosphorylated on tyrosine; and small

TABLE 105-5 IMPORTANT PLATELET SURFACE PROTEINS

Gene Family	Common Name	Platelet Chain Designation	Integrin Designation	VLA† Designation	CD† Designation		Nonreduced M_r		Reduced M_r
Integrins	Fibrinogen receptor	GPIIb-IIIa	αIIbβ3		αIIbβ3-CD41a	αIIb	145,000	αIIbα	125,000
					αIIb-CD41b			αIIbβ	23,000
					β3-CD61	β3	90,000		114,000
	Collagen receptor	GPIa-IIa	α2β1	VLA-2	α2-CD49b	α2	150,000		
					β1-CD29	β1	138,000		148,000
	Fibronectin receptor	GPIc*-IIa	α5β1	VLA-5	α5-CD49e	α5	140,000		
					β1-CD29	β1	138,000		148,000
	Laminin receptor	GPIc-IIa	α6β1	VLA-6	α6-CD49f	α6	140,000		
					β1-CD29	β1	138,000		148,000
	Vitronectin receptor	αV/IIIa	αVβ3		αV-CD51	αV	150,000	αV	125,000
					β3-CD61			αV	25,000
						GPIIIa	90,000		114,000
Leucine-rich repeat glycoproteins	von Willebrand factor receptor	GPIb-IX			Ib/IX-CD42	GPIb	170,000	GPIbα	145,000
					Ibα-CD42b			GPIbβ	22,000
					Ibβ-CD42c				
					IX-CD42a	GPIX	17,000		17,000
		GPV				GPV	82,000		82,000
Immunoglobulin family cell adhesion molecules	PECAM-I				CD31		130,000		
	FcγRII				CD32		40,000		
	HLA Class 1								
	ICAM-2				CD102				59,000
	GPVI						62,000		65,000
	IAP				CD47		50,000		
Selectins	P-Selectin				CD62P		140,000		
	(GMP 140; PADGEM)								
Tetraspanins	p24				CD9		24,000		
					CD63				
	PETA-3				CD151		27,000		
	LAMP-3 (granulophysin)				CD63		53,000		
Miscellaneous	GPIV				CD36		88,000		
	LAMP-1				CD107a		110,000		
	LAMP-2				CD107b		120,000		
	67 kDa Laminin receptor						67,000		
	ADP P2X1 receptor						70,000		
	Leukosialin, sialophorin				CD43		90,000		
Seven transmembrane domain (G-protein linked) receptors (select)	PAR-1						70,000		
	PAR-4								
	Thromboxane A₂ receptor								55,000
	α₂-Adrenergic receptor								64,000
	Vasopressin receptor						125,000		
	ADP P2Y₁ Receptor								
	ADP P2Y₁₂ Receptor								

* Number of leucine-rich repeats.

† VLA = very late antigen; CD = cluster of differentiation, see Chap. 14.

Fib = fibrinogen; Fn = fibronectin; IAP = integrin-associated protein; PSGL-1 = P-selectin glycoprotein ligand-1; Osp = Osteopontin; TSP = thrombospondin; Vn = vitronectin; vWF = von willebrand factor.

Amino Acids	Carbohydrate	Lipid	Phosphorylated	Chromosome	Ligands	Platelet Specific	Function	Molecules on Platelet Surface (S) or Internal (I)
αIIb 1039	+	–	–	17	Fib, vWF	+	Adhesion,	(S) 80,000
β3 762	+	–	+	17	Fn, Vn ?TSP	+	aggregation, protein trafficking	(I) 40,000
α2 1152				5	Collagen	–	Adhesion	(S) 1,000
β1 778				10		–		
α5 1008				12	Fn	–	Adhesion	(S) 1,000
β1 778				10				
α6				2	Laminin	–	Adhesion	(S) 1,000
β3 778				10				
αV 1048				2	Vn, Fib, vWF	–	?Adhesion	(S) 100
					Fn, ?Tsp, Osteopontin		?Protein trafficking	
GPIIIa 762	+	–		17				
GPIbα 610(8)*	+	–		1	vWF, thrombin	+?	Adhesion (high	(S) 25,000
GPIbβ 181(1)*	+	+	–	22		+?	shear), ?thrombin activation	(S) 25,000
GPIX 160(1)*	+	+	+	3		+?		(S) 25,000
GPV 544(15)*	+	+	+	3		+?		(S) 12,500
PECAM-1 738	+	?	+	17	Heparin	–	?Adhesin	(S) 8,000
FcγRII 324	+		+	1	Immune complexes	–	Immune complex binding	(S)~1,000
HLA	+			6	—		Histocompatibility	(S)
ICAM-2 274				17	LFA-1	–	Platelet–leukocyte adhesion	(S) 2,600
GPVI 316	+	–		?	Collagen	+	Activation	(S)~2,000
IAP 287	+			3	TSP	–	Activation	
P-selectin 830	+	+	+	1	Sialyl-Le^x	–	Platelet-leukocyte adhesion	(I) 20,000
					PSGL-1			
CD9 228	+				?	–	Activation	(S) 40,000
CD151 253	+	–	–	11	?	–	Activation	(I)~2,000
LAMP-3 238	+							(I) 10,000
GPIV 471	+		+	7	Collagen, TSP	–	Adhesion	(S) 20,000
LAMP-1 389	+			13	?	–	?	(I) 1,200
LAMP-2 381	+			X	?			
67 kDa ?295				X	Laminin	–	Adhesion	
P2X1 399	+			17	ADP	–	Activation	(S) 13–130
CD43 400	+		+	16	ICAM-1	–	Adhesion	
PAR-1 425				5	Thrombin	–	Activation	(S) ~1,800
PAR-4 385	+		+	19	Thrombin	–	Activation	
TXA$_2$ 343				19	PGH$_2$/ Thromboxane A$_2$	–	Activation	~200
α$_2$-Adrenergic 450				10	Epinephrine	–	Activation	~250
Vasopressin 418				?x	Vasopressin	–	Activation	~75
P2Y1 373	+			3	ADP	–	Activation	
P2Y12 342				3	ADP	+	Activation	

TABLE 105-6   PHYSIOLOGIC AND PATHOLOGIC PLATELET ACTIVATORS

Strong
  Adhesion to collagen and perhaps other elements exposed in normal blood
    vessels after vascular damage
  Adhesion to elements exposed in atherosclerotic blood vessels after plaque
    rupture
  Thrombin
  High concentrations of collagen in vitro
Weak
  ADP
  Epinephrine
  Thromboxane A$_2$/prostaglandin H$_2$
  Serotonin
  Platelet-activating factor
  Vasopressin
  Thrombospondin-1
  Angiotensin
Other
  Shear
  Thrombolytic agents (plasmin)

SOURCE: Adapted from BS Coller,[261] with permission.

GTP-binding proteins such as Rho, Rac, and Cdc42 also may play a role.[21,23,371,382]

Platelets contain calpains, which are calcium-dependent, sulfhydryl-containing, neutral proteases composed of two subunits that preferentially cleave cytoskeletal proteins, particularly filamins and talin.[382,383] Calpains also reportedly cleave the cytoplasmic domain of

TABLE 105-7   FACTORS THAT PREVENT OR INHIBIT PLATELET
ACTIVATION

Flowing blood
Prostacyclin (PGI$_2$)
Nitric oxide (NO)
Endothelial cell CD39 (ATP diphosphohydrolase; ecto-ADPase)
Platelet refractoriness
Leukocyte–platelet interactions*
Inhibitors of thrombin generation and thrombin action

* Both activating and inhibitory interactions.
SOURCE: Adapted from BS Coller,[261] with permission.

β3 and a number of molecules involved in signaling, including kinases and phosphatases (see "Calcium-Dependent Proteases [Calpains]" below). μ-Calpain requires micromolar calcium concentrations, and m-calpain requires millimolar calcium for activation. Calpains have been proposed to be involved in cytoskeletal reorganization upon platelet activation and to specifically enhance binding of ligand to αIIbβ3 via cleavage of the integrin β3 cytoplasmic tail and talin.[27,384–386] Calpains also have been implicated in platelet spreading, microparticle formation, and generation of platelet coagulant activity.[382,387,388] Mice lacking μ-calpain have reduced platelet aggregation and clot retraction but normal bleeding time.[389]

PLATELET SHAPE CHANGE
Platelet shape change occurs in response to many different agonists. It involves loss of the normal platelet discoid shape (diameter ~1.5–2.5 μm, width ~0.5–0.9 μm) and transformation to a spiny sphere

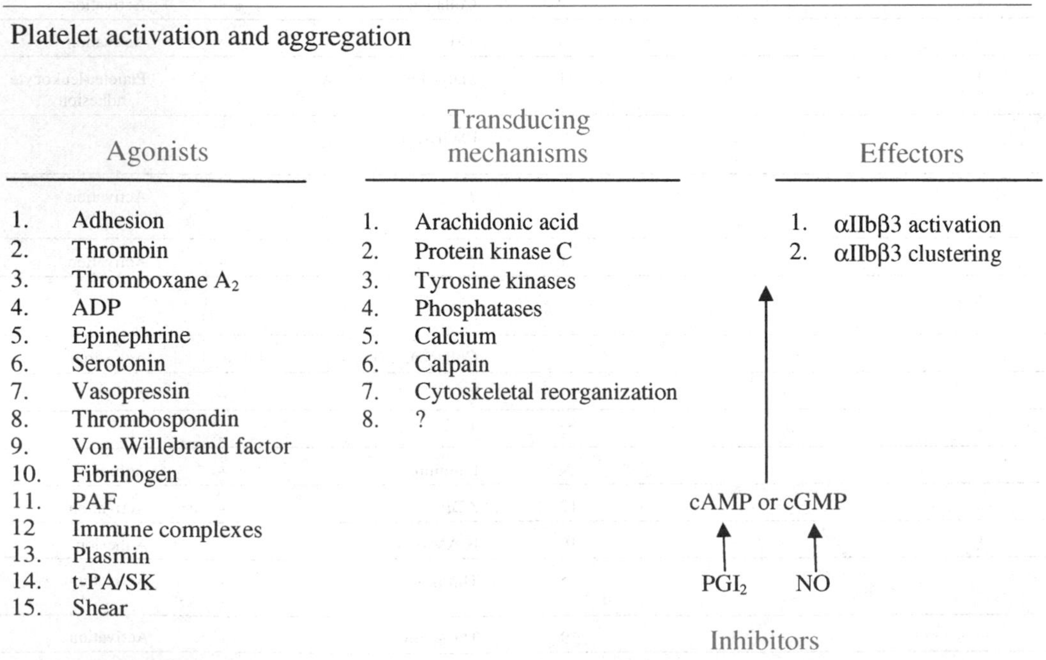

Platelet activation and aggregation

Agonists	Transducing mechanisms	Effectors
1. Adhesion	1. Arachidonic acid	1. αIIbβ3 activation
2. Thrombin	2. Protein kinase C	2. αIIbβ3 clustering
3. Thromboxane A$_2$	3. Tyrosine kinases	
4. ADP	4. Phosphatases	
5. Epinephrine	5. Calcium	
6. Serotonin	6. Calpain	
7. Vasopressin	7. Cytoskeletal reorganization	
8. Thrombospondin	8. ?	
9. Von Willebrand factor		
10. Fibrinogen		
11. PAF		
12 Immune complexes		
13. Plasmin		
14. t-PA/SK		
15. Shear		

cAMP or cGMP

PGI$_2$ NO

Inhibitors

FIGURE 105-10   Platelet activation and aggregation. Many different agents and phenomena can initiate platelet activation, and a select group are listed as agonists. Virtually all of these agonists are released, synthesized, present, or occur at sites of vascular injury, providing both geographic and temporal restriction of the response. These agonists can initiate aggregation either alone or in combination with one or more other agonists. A number of different signal transduction mechanisms have been defined that convert the agonist signal into a change in the conformation of the αIIbβ3 receptor and related changes that result in ligand binding, receptor clustering, and platelet aggregation. A number of additional receptor–ligand interactions reportedly enhance the stability of platelet aggregates.[1222] Two inhibitors produced by endothelial cells, prostacyclin (PGI$_2$) and nitric oxide (NO), inhibit signal transduction via increases in cAMP and cGMP, respectively. PAF, platelet activating factor; SK, streptokinase; t-PA, tissue plasminogen activator.

TABLE 105-8 PLATELET CYTOSKELETAL PROTEINS*

PROTEIN	PROPERTIES
Actin[1226]	$M_r = 42,000$ 20%–30% of total platelet protein (0.55 M; 2×10^6 per platelet) β and γ forms present at a ratio of 5:1 Monomeric actin (G-actin) bound to calcium-ATP (or ADP) Polymerization requires energy (ATP→ADP) and produces F-actin F-actin filaments: two strands of intertwined helices with polarity based on ability to interact with myosin fragment ("pointed" and "barbed" ends) Steady-state polymerization: monomers lost from pointed end while others join barbed end ("treadmilling")
Profilin[1227]	$M_r = 15,200$ Forms 1:1 reversible complex with actin monomer Prevents actin polymerization May help "recharge" actin monomers with ATP
Gelsolin[1228]	$M_r = 81,000$ (5 μM; 2×10^4 per platelet) Binds to barbed end of F-actin filaments Severs actin filaments Facilitates nucleation Produces shorter filaments with gel→sol transformation
Thymosin β_4[370,1229]	$M_r = 5,000$ (0.55 M; 2×10^6 per platelet) Binds actin monomer Inhibits actin polymerization
Tropomyosin[1230]	$M_r = 28,000$; rod shaped dimer of 35 nm length Binds to groove on actin filament (six actins:one tropomyosin) Not all actin filaments have bound tropomyosin
Caldesmon[1231]	$M_r = 80,000$; asymmetric Binds to actin, tropomyosin, myosin, and calmodulin May control actin filament bundling and actomyosin ATPase
Filamin A (X) and B (3) (actin-binding protein)[21-23,371,1232,1233]	Filamin A/B = 10:1 $M_r = 260,000$ subunit; tail-to-tail dimer; elongated 162-nm flexible rod; phosphorylated 2%–3% of platelet protein Binds actin with one actin-binding protein molecule per 14 actin molecules Binds GPIbα cytoplasmic domain and links GPIb-IX to actin Binds small GTPases RalA, Ras, Rho, Cdc42; kinases and phosphatases; exchange factors Trio and Toll Cross-links actin filaments to form a gel Dephosphorylation leads to loss of activity
Talin[27,1234,1235]	$M_r = 235,000$ 3% of platelet protein Binds to $\beta3$ integrin cytoplasmic tail to activate αIIbβ3; also binds vinculin and α-actinin; cleaved and activated by calpain
α-Actinin[1227]	$M_r = 100,000$ and 102,000; dimer Binds actin at 1:10 stoichiometry; binds Ca^{2+} Forms gel with F-actin; cooperates with actin-binding protein; promotes actin polymerization
Vinculin[377,1236,1237]	$M_r = 130,000$ Binds to talin; may link actin to membrane proteins at adhesion sites
Myosin II[1238,1239]	$M_r = 480,000$ ($2 \times 200,000$, $2 \times 20,000$, $2 \times 16,000$) 2%–5% of platelet protein; 325×111-nm filaments Myosin light chain ($M_r = 20,000$); phosphorylated; required for ATPase activity
Myosin light-chain kinase[1240]	$M_r = 105,000$ Phosphorylates myosin light chain and activates actomyosin ATPase leading to contraction
Calmodulin[1241]	$M_r = 17,000$ Binds four calciums and activates myosin light-chain kinase
CapZ[21,22]	$M_r = 36,000$ and 32,000 (5 μM; 2×10^4 per platelet) Heterodimer Binds barbed ends of actin filaments
Cofilin[21,22]	$M_r = 20,000$ Accelerates depolymerization of actin filaments
Fimbrin (L-plastin)	$M_r = 68,000$ Bundles actin filaments Found in microvilli
VASP[21,22]	$M_r = 50,000$ Tetrameric Binds profilin, vinculin, zyxin
GTPases[22,371,382]	Cdc42—filopodia Rho—stress fibers Rac—lamellipods and ruffles Rap1b—$\alpha_{IIb}\beta_3$ control
Tyrosine kinases	pp60[src] pp125[Fak]—αIIbβ3 signaling pp72[syk]—GPVI signaling
Adaptor proteins	14-3-3ζ—binds to GPIbα Pleckstrin—phosphorylated on activation
PI kinases	PI3 kinase PI$_4$P-5 kinase
Spectrin	α,β heterodimers form head to head tetramers Bind to actin filaments
α,γ-Adducins	Cap barbed ends of actin filaments and bind to spectrin Phosphorylated with platelet activation and cleaved by calpain

* See JEB Fox,[371] JL Daniel,[1242] MI Furman et al.,[369] JH Hartwig,[22] and JH Hartwig et al.[21]

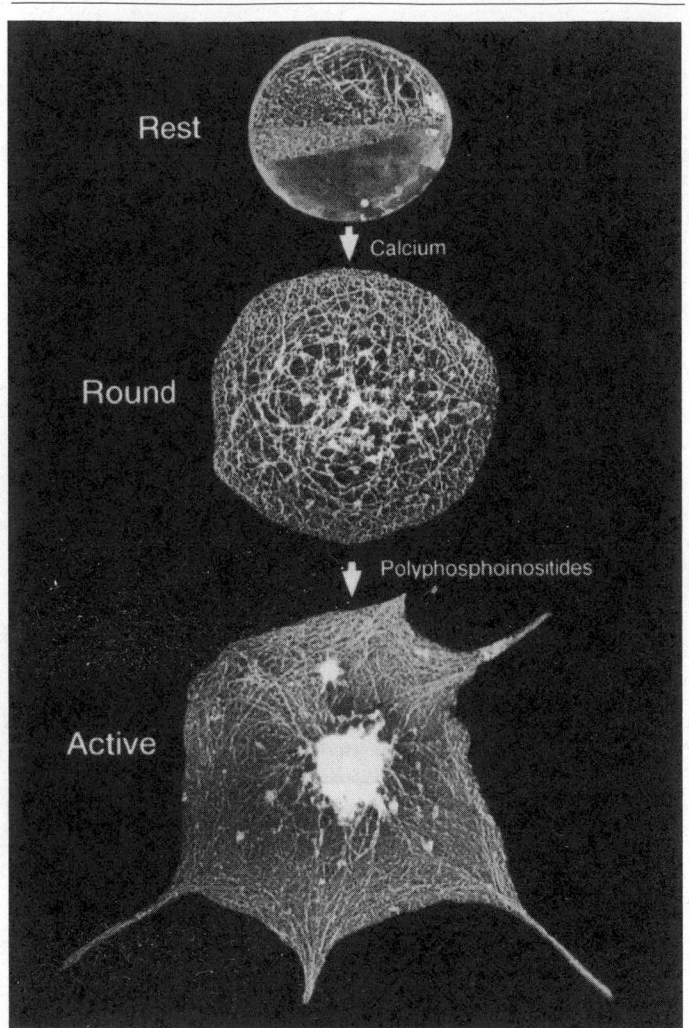

FIGURE 105-11 Control of platelet shape change. Resting platelets are small discs. Platelets convert from discs in two steps. In the first step, a calcium transient activates platelet gelsolin. Gelsolin binds, severs, and caps actin filaments. Fragmentation of endogenous filaments causes the cell to become spherical. In the second step, spherical cells protrude lamellae and filopods. Actin filament assembly drives the protrusion of cellular processes. (Adapted from JH Hartwig et al,[21] with permission.)

thin actin filaments predominate (60%). However, with activation, actin polymerization occurs and monomeric actin decreases to 20 to 40 percent of total actin.[369,371] Actin filaments in resting platelets are relatively stable because their barbed ends (the ends from which they can grow by adding additional actin monomers) are capped with the proteins CapZ and α,γ-adducins (see Fig. 105-4).[21]

The initial step in shape change is marked by the activation of gelsolin that results from a rise in cytoplasmic calcium to micromolar levels. Gelsolin severs existing actin filaments and caps the newly created barbed ends. These actions increase the number of actin filaments by an estimated 10-fold and substitute gelsolin for CapZ and α,γ-adducins as the actin filament capping proteins.[21] Severing of actin filaments that interact with the planar lattice composed of filamin (actin-binding protein), GPIb-IX, and spectrin in the membrane cytoskeleton releases the constraints on the spectrin network. Thus, the membrane skeleton can swell (but not produce filopodia) (see Fig. 105-11) by incorporating into the plasma membrane the membranes from the open canalicular system and later the membranes from the granules that release their contents. Activation of the Arp2/3 complex, which can bind actin on its pointed ends to create new barbed ends, results in a threefold increase in Arp2/3 associated with the cytoskeleton and the generation of new actin polymer nucleation sites.

The protrusive force for filopodia development comes from subsequent actin polymerization on the newly severed actin filaments, including those attached to the plasma membrane. Uncapping of the actin filaments appears to be accomplished by inactivation of gelsolin by phosphoinositides that are produced during platelet activation, including phosphatidylinositol-3,4-bisphosphate ($PI_{3,4}P_2$), $PI_{4,5}P_2$, and $PI_{3,4,5}P_3$.[21] The uncapped actin filaments act as nuclei onto which actin monomers (which are maintained in an available pool by association with thymosin β_4) can assemble. Profilin accelerates actin polymerization by facilitating the transfer of actin from the actin-thymosin-β_4 complex to the barbed ends of the actin filaments. Other proteins that have been implicated in organizing the tips of the filopodia where the actin bundles attach to the plasma membrane are the small GTPase Cdc42, the exchange protein Wiskott-Aldrich syndrome protein (the protein abnormal in Wiskott-Aldrich syndrome), vinculin, vasodilator-stimulated phosphoprotein (VASP), zyxin, and profilin.[238] As the filopodia form, the platelet's granules and organelles move to the center and are surrounded by the microtubule coil, resulting in increased electron density. Activation of myosin II via phosphorylation of myosin light-chain kinase contributes to the inward contractile force by its interaction with the actin fibers.

PLATELET SPREADING AND SURFACE-INDUCED ACTIVATION

After platelets adhere to surfaces, they undergo variable degrees of spreading and activation. The patterns of spreading and activation depend primarily on the protein surface on which they spread, with collagen consistently inducing the most activation.[294,393] Activation can result in release of granule contents and exposure of activated $\alpha IIb\beta3$ receptors on the luminal surface of the platelets, where they are strategically located to bind adhesive glycoprotein ligands that can recruit additional platelets.[394] If the surface density of platelets is sufficient, the platelets can also enter into lateral associations, which appear to depend on activated $\alpha IIb\beta3$.[310] In general, platelet spreading results in the development of broad lamellipodia rather than spike-like filopodia (see Figs. 105-1 and 105-11).[21,382] The different morphologies of platelet spreading reflect differences in the organization of the orthogonal network of actin filaments. In turn, these differences reflect the different signals initiated by the adhesion process. Both phosphoinositides and the small GTPase molecules Rac and Rho appear to be particularly important in this process (Fig. 105-12).[22] Pleckstrin, a platelet protein

with long, thin filopodia extending several micrometers out from the surface, ending in points that are as small as 0.1 μm in diameter (see Figs. 105-1 and 105-11).[2,390] In the aggregometer, the initial decrease in light transmission immediately after adding certain agonists generally has been assumed to be a reflection of platelets undergoing shape change,[391] but this interpretation has been challenged by the suggestion that microaggregation rather than shape change accounts for this phenomenon.[392] Although the reason platelets undergo shape change is unclear, one possibility is that it reduces electrostatic repulsion even without reducing surface charge density. Thus, after changing shape, the tip of a platelet can approach and make contact with a surface or a cell, and the great bulk of the repulsive surface charge now is at a distance.[3]

Actin fibril formation, which is an important component of shape change, is a complex, energy-requiring process that depends on nucleation, polymerization, helix winding, and filament bundling (see Fig. 105-4).[22,369] The proteins listed in Table 105-8 either facilitate or inhibit these processes. In resting platelets, actin monomers and small,

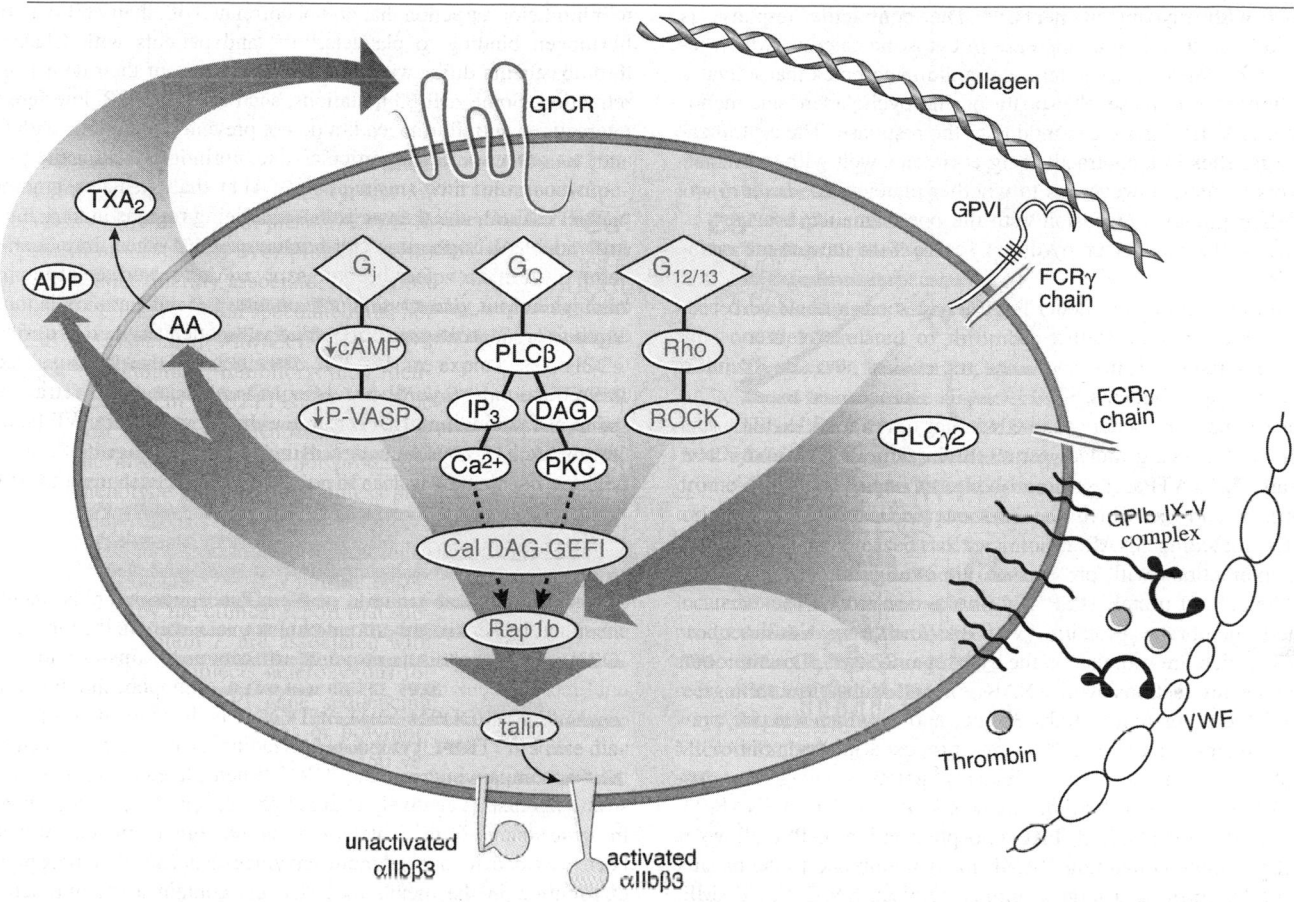

FIGURE 105-12   General scheme of agonist activation of platelets. Agonists stimulate specific platelet receptors, including seven transmembrane-spanning G-protein coupled receptors (GPCR) and receptors, such as the collagen receptor GPVI, coupled to tyrosine kinases. GPCRs activate heterotrimeric G proteins by converting the α-subunit to a GTP-bound state. This action causes the α-subunit and β,γ-subunits to separate and activate downstream effectors. Inhibition of adenylyl cyclase by Gi lowers cAMP levels, which in turn promotes dephosphorylation of downstream targets such as the cytoskeletal regulator protein vasodilator-stimulated phosphoprotein (VASP). Activation of phospholipase $C\beta$ (PLCβ) by Gq results in hydrolysis of membrane phosphatidylinositol bisphosphate (PIP$_2$) to generate diacylglycerol (DAG), an activator of protein kinase C (PKC), and inositol trisphosphate, which increases intracellular calcium (Ca^{2+}) levels. Heterotrimeric G-proteins such as G$_{12/13}$ regulate a pathway that leads to activation of the small GTP-binding protein Rho and its downstream effector Rho kinase (ROCK). The collagen receptor GPVI signals through tyrosine kinases that activate PLCγ2. Adhesive receptors such as the GPIb-IX-V complex, which interacts with von Willebrand factor (vWF) and is acted upon by thrombin, can also elicit intracellular signaling through ill-defined pathways that may include, at least in part, the Fc γ-chain. With platelet activation, dense granules can fuse with the plasma membrane, resulting in the release of ADP and other bioactive molecules, and thromboxane A$_2$ (TXA$_2$) is generated from arachidonic acid. Released ADP and TXA$_2$ reinforce platelet activation by acting through specific GPCRs. Ultimately, platelet activation results in the conversion of the major platelet integrin αIIbβ3 from an inactive to an active state capable of binding large multimeric molecules such as fibrinogen. Although the precise events that lead up to activation of αIIbβ3 are not known, activation of the small GTP-binding protein Rap1b by the calcium- and DAG-sensitive exchange factor Cal DAG-GEF1 appears to be involved. Binding of talin to the cytoplasmic domain of β3 may be one of the final common steps in activation of the integrin.

that is phosphorylated during platelet activation, appears to participate in this process by binding to phosphoinositides and affecting Rac via an exchange factor.[395] Signaling after adhesion results from the assembly of protein complexes on the cytoplasmic surfaces of the receptor(s) involved in the adhesion process. These complexes then initiate local cytoskeletal rearrangements and generation of signaling molecules that probably act throughout the platelet.[219,309]

Membrane glycoproteins are affected by cytoskeletal rearrangements associated with platelet shape change and spreading. Activation of platelets in suspension under certain conditions results in movement of GPIb-IX receptors from the surface of platelets to the open canalicular system.[226,227] With adherent platelets, GPIb internalization is much slower.[238] The initial effect of activation on αIIbβ3 is an increase in receptors on the plasma membranes as the αIIbβ3 receptors in α-granules, and perhaps dense bodies and the open canalicular sys-

tem, join the plasma membrane. After activation, more αIIbβ3 molecules become associated with the cytoskeleton, presumably reflecting the interaction with talin and ligand-induced αIIbβ3 clustering. The association results in the development of protein complexes, including cytoskeletal proteins, on the cytoplasmic surface of the receptor.[27,309,396] When ligand-coated beads are added to adherent platelets and bind to αIIbβ3 receptors, the beads are transported to the center of the platelets, indicating the cytoskeleton can move αIIbβ3 receptors having attached ligand.[397,398]

PLATELET SECRETION

The contractile mechanism involving actin and myosin is thought to mediate granule secretion and clot retraction, but the details remain obscure.[57,369] After the initial platelet shape change, actin becomes organized centrally into thick filamentous masses, where it probably associates with myosin filaments.[369] The contractile response is thought to be initiated by an increase in cytosolic calcium, which results in the formation of a calcium–calmodulin complex that activates myosin light-chain kinase. Phosphatases and cyclic adenosine monophosphate (cAMP) kinase can modulate the response. The centralization of organelles in a contractile ring correlates well with secretion.[2] Controversy exists, however, as to whether platelets secrete the contents of their granules by fusion with the open canalicular system in the center of the platelet or by direct fusion with the plasma membrane.[2,225]

An intricate multistep model for granule secretion has been proposed in which granules tether and dock to the inner leaflet of the plasma membrane and then additional molecular interactions lead to fusion of the lipid bilayers.[52,57,68,399–409] The process is analogous to exocytosis in neurons, where detailed studies have identified important roles for the following molecules: N-ethylmaleimide sensitive factor (NSF), an Mg^{2+}-ATPase; soluble NSF-associated proteins (SNAPs; including α and γ, which can activate NSF); SNAP receptors (SNAREs; including SNAP-23 and syntaxins 2, 4, and 7, which can mediate interactions with proteins on the cytoplasmic face of granules); platelet Sec1 protein (PSP; an orthologue of Munc 18c); vesicle-associated membrane proteins (VAMPs; including VAMP-3 and VAMP-8, which are proteins on the cytoplasmic face of granules that can mediate interactions with SNAREs); and Rabs (low molecular weight GTPases, including Rabs 3b, 6c, and 8, which are phosphorylated on platelet activation).[68] In one proposed model,[68] SNAP-23 on the plasma membrane of unactivated platelets is engaged by syntaxin 4. With activation, NSF disengages syntaxin 4 from SNAP-23, and PSP binds to syntaxin 4. PKC phosphorylation of PSP allows it to join the granule containing VAMP in its membrane to the plasma membrane by forming a large complex between SNAP-23, VAMP, syntaxin 4, PSP, Rab effector, and a phosphorylated Rab in the vesicle membrane. PKC then releases PSP from the complex, allowing the development of a trans-SNARE complex between VAMP, syntaxin 4, and SNAP-23. Calcium then results in the final fusion event. Lipids, particularly PIP_2 and phosphatidic acid, appear to contribute to the process, with PIP_2 hydrolysis both activating PKC and supplying calcium via IP_3.[409]

CLOT RETRACTION

When blood initially clots in the test tube, the fibrin mesh extends throughout, trapping virtually all of the serum in a gel-like state. If platelets are present, within minutes to hours the clot retracts, extruding a very large fraction of the serum.[410] This process is thought to mimic *in vivo* phenomena that result in consolidation of thrombi and perhaps enhancement of wound healing. Clot retraction also has been implicated in decreasing the efficiency of thrombolysis, which may partially account for the resistance of platelet-rich thrombi to fibrinolytic agents.[411] Although the platelet requirement for clot retraction is indisputable and temporal studies strongly incriminate a contractile mechanism involving actin and myosin,[412,413] no model describing the details of the process has gained acceptance.[414] Proposed mechanisms include movement of platelet filopodia along fibrin strands, tugging of fibrin strands by filopodia, and internalization of fibrin by the action of the membrane skeleton.[412–417] Platelet $\alpha IIb\beta3$ is required for clot retraction, as demonstrated by studies of patients with Glanzmann thrombasthenia (see Chap. 112) and studies of normal platelets in the presence of agents that block either the $\alpha IIb\beta3$ receptor[415,418–423] or the fibrinogen γ-chain C-terminal sequence that mediates interactions with the $\alpha IIb\beta3$ receptor.[424] Clot retraction correlates temporally with an $\alpha IIb\beta3$-dependent decrease in protein tyrosine phosphorylation, presumably via activation of one or more phosphatases.[425] Results with $\alpha IIb\beta3$ antagonists demonstrate, however, differences in their ability to inhibit clot retraction that do not correlate with their ability to block fibrinogen binding to platelets,[415,423] and patients with Glanzmann thrombasthenia differ with regard to the extent of their defect in clot retraction. Some $\alpha IIb\beta3$ mutations, such as $\beta3$ L262P, interfere with interactions with fibrinogen but do not prevent interactions with fibrin and clot retraction.[426] Of particular note, fibrinogen lacking the γ-chain C-terminal sequence (residues 400–411) that mediates binding to platelet $\alpha IIb\beta3$, and the two RGD-containing regions in fibrinogen, is still capable of supporting clot retraction.[427,428] When fibrinogen converts to fibrin, new sites become exposed on the surface of the molecule. Therefore, one possible explanation for this paradox is that additional or alternative $\alpha IIb\beta3$ binding sequences in the fibrinogen γ-chain (e.g., residues 316–322, 370–383, or other regions) mediate clot retraction.[429,430] GPIb-IX also may contribute to clot retraction by virtue of the binding of GPIbα to the thrombin and/or vWF bound to the fibrin.[431,432] Thus, although $\alpha IIb\beta3$ is required for clot retraction, the process is not a simple reflection of fibrinogen binding to $\alpha IIb\beta3$.

PLATELET COAGULANT ACTIVITY

In resting platelets, the negatively charged phospholipids, including phosphatidyl serine, are present almost exclusively in the inner leaflet. Among the mechanisms proposed to account for this asymmetry are unidirectional enzymatic movement by an aminophospholipid translocase and/or association between the negatively charged phospholipids and elements in the cytoplasm, including cytoskeletal elements and their accompanying proteins.[10,12,433] When platelets are activated by strong agonists, negatively charged phospholipids are redistributed to the outer leaflet of the platelet plasma membrane, movement that has been ascribed to one or more enzymes that can alter phospholipid distribution in the membrane. Platelets contain a calcium-activated plasma membrane "scramblase" (phospholipid scramblase 1) of predicted molecular weight approximately 35,000 that in model systems reverses the asymmetric distribution of negatively charged phospholipids in membrane bilayers. The role of this enzyme *in vivo* is uncertain because the platelets of mice lacking this enzyme can redistribute their negatively charged phospholipids upon activation.[433–435] A highly homologous enzyme, phospholipid scramblase 3, has also been identified in platelets and other cells, but its role is uncertain.[436] A "floppase" activity, which promotes outward directed lipid transport, has been postulated in platelets, and although the multidrug resistance protein 1 (ABC1) has been suggested to account for this activity in erythrocytes,[437] no specific molecule with this function has yet been identified in platelets.[438] A floppase would also be a candidate for reversing the phospholipid asymmetry with platelet activation. Because platelet activation with strong agonists also results in the formation of microparticles, which are particularly rich in surface-exposed negatively charged phospholipids, the molecular reorganization of the membrane that produces microparticles also may result in surface exposure of negatively charged phospholipids on both the microparticles and the residual platelet membrane. Microparticles also are rich in factor Va and thus actively support thrombin generation.[8,333,439]

Microparticle formation can be induced *in vitro* by activation of platelets with the calcium ionophore A23187, complement C5b-9, the combination of thrombin and collagen, by adding tissue factor to recalcified platelet-rich plasma, or by high shear stress.[333,440–442] Incubation of platelets with sera from patients with heparin-induced thrombocytopenia also can produce microparticles,[443,444] perhaps accounting, in part, for the thrombosis that is sometimes associated with the disorder. Elevations of cytosolic calcium, calpain activation, cytoskeletal reorganization, protein phosphorylation, and phospholipid translocation all have been implicated in microparticle formation. Inhibition of $\alpha IIb\beta3$, and perhaps $\alpha V\beta3$, decreases tissue factor-induced platelet coagulant activity and microparticle formation in the presence or absence of fibrin,[441] whereas inhibition of GPIb inhibits tissue factor-induced microparticle formation only in the presence of fibrin.[442]

The biologic relevance of platelet microparticles is supported by the finding of increased circulating levels of platelet microparticles in patients with activated coagulation and fibrinolysis, diabetes mellitus, sickle cell anemia, human immunodeficiency virus infection, unstable angina, heparin-induced thrombocytopenia with thrombosis, and adult respiratory distress syndrome.[333,445] Microparticles can bind to fibrin thrombi via one or more of the receptors present on their surface, including αIIbβ3, GPIb-IX, P-selectin, and perhaps PSGL-1.[446]

Microparticles bind factors VIII, Va, and Xa, allowing them to form both the tenase and prothrombinase complexes on their surface.[333] They also can bind protein S and facilitate inactivation of factors Va and VIIIa, which could serve an anticoagulant function.[447,448] In addition, microparticles can activate platelets by supplying arachidonic acid. In a similar manner, they can activate endothelial cells and monocytes, resulting in enhanced monocyte attachment to endothelial cells, a potential contributor to atherosclerosis.[333]

Platelet activation leading to increased platelet coagulant activity shares several features with cell apoptosis, including surface exposure of negatively charged phospholipids and membrane blebbing leading to microparticle formation. Platelets contain the apoptosis-related proteins procaspase-3 and procaspase-9, and the caspase activators APAF-1 and cytochrome c.[449-451] Conflicting data exist, however, regarding the relative roles of caspases and calpains in the development of platelet coagulant activity.[449]

Although conflicting data exist on whether resting platelets contain tissue factor, in vivo and ex vivo platelet thrombi can recruit tissue factor from blood by binding leukocyte-derived, tissue factor-containing microparticles or by binding an alternatively spliced, soluble form of tissue factor.[268,271,452-455] The interaction between PSGL-1 on the surface of leukocyte-derived microparticles and P-selectin on the surface of activated platelets appears to play an important role in the binding of microparticles to platelet thrombi.[455] Interactions between platelets and leukocytes, and perhaps leukocyte-derived microparticles, reportedly enhance ("de-encrypt" or decrypt) tissue factor activity.[270]

Incontrovertible evidence exists that platelets accelerate thrombin formation, but the precise mechanisms involved remain controversial.[138,456-459] The effect of platelets on activation of factor X by factors IXa and VIIIa and the activation of prothrombin by factors Xa and Va have been extensively studied.[138,459] Both reactions are accelerated by platelets, most dramatically when the platelets have been activated by thrombin or other agonists. Platelets also can accelerate factor VIII activation by thrombin.[460] Factor VIIIa on platelets likely acts as a binding site for factor IXa, and factor Va on platelets likely acts as a binding site for factor Xa.[461] The effector cell protease receptor (EPR)-1 or a similar molecule may act as another binding site for factor Xa on activated platelets.[462] A separate receptor for factor IXa also may exist on platelets, and only approximately 10 percent of activated platelets have been suggested to expose on average approximately 6000 factor IXa binding sites per platelet.[463] The concept that only a subpopulation of platelets develops a procoagulant phenotype with activation is supported by data from the percentage of activated platelets demonstrating high levels of factors Va and Xa (COAT platelets).[138,199,200,464] Whether factors VIIIa and Va bind to specific receptors on platelets or whether they bind nonspecifically to negatively charged phospholipids, most particularly phosphatidylserine, that join the outer leaflet of the platelet plasma membrane bilayer when platelets are activated remains unclear.[138,433,456,457,461] Assembly of the factor IXa–factor VIIIa–platelet complex increases the catalytic efficiency of factor X activation (k_{cat}/K_m) by a factor of 2.4×10^6.[138] Prothrombin

binds to approximately 20,000 sites on activated platelets with a K_d equal to its plasma concentration ($\sim$0.15 μM).[465] The αIIbβ3 integrins bind prothrombin via an RGD-dependent mechanism and may contribute to localization of prothrombin to the surface of unactivated and activated platelets.[466]

Binding of activated coagulation factors to the surface of platelets appears to protect them from inactivation by inhibitors in plasma and platelets.[138] For example, the presence of platelet microparticles confers resistance to activated protein C in a clotting assay, an observation that has both theoretical and practical implications.[467] The relatively large platelet pool of factor V,[136,468] which appears to be complexed to multimerin,[106] and the ability of platelet proteases to activate it[142,143,469] also probably contribute to platelet coagulant activity. The bleeding diathesis in patients with Quebec platelet syndrome, who have proteolysis of platelet α-granule factor V, supports the potential importance of platelet factor V in normal hemostasis (see Chap. 112), as do studies of another patient with abnormal platelet factor V.[459] Further support comes from data on the hemostatic effectiveness of transfused platelets containing factor V in patients with inhibitors to plasma factor V.[138,145,470]

Evidence supporting the crucial relevance of platelet microparticle formation to platelet coagulant activity has been gathered from observations of patients with significant bleeding diatheses and defects in platelet microparticle formation (Scott syndrome, see Chap. 112).[457,459,471] Platelets from the most intensively studied patient had an impaired ability to accelerate the activation of both factor X and prothrombin. In addition, this patient's platelets exhibited both abnormal factor V binding and exposure of negatively charged phospholipids. In flow chamber studies, her platelets did not support normal fibrin deposition. The defect in microparticle formation appears to be the primary abnormality, given that the patient's erythrocytes also failed to undergo normal vesiculation in response to the calcium ionophore A23187.[457,472] Although an abnormality in the scramblase enzyme was considered a possible cause of this patient's abnormalities, no mutation was identified in phospholipid scramblase 1.[472]

In addition to the platelet's role in accelerating the activation of factor X and prothrombin, other connections exist between platelets and the coagulation system. These connections include (1) the presence of fibrinogen in α-granules and perhaps on the surface of platelets, where it is strategically located for interactions with locally generated thrombin[109,138]; (2) the presence of intracellular vWF and the binding of extracellular vWF to platelets (via GPIb/X and αIIbβ3), with potential colocalization of factor VIII attached to the vWF (see Chap. 118); (3) activation of factor XI by thrombin on the platelet surface,[473,474] with the dimeric structure of factor XI allowing it to interact with both the platelet and factor IX simultaneously[475]; (4) a factor XI-like protein associated with platelet membranes, which may be an alternatively spliced form of factor XI lacking exon V (the level of this factor appears to correlate better with hemorrhagic symptoms than does the level of plasma factor XI[138,476]); (5) the presence of cytoplasmic factor XIII (see Chap. 106); (6) the presence in platelets of inhibitors of coagulation (α_1-protease inhibitor, C-1 inhibitor, tissue factor pathway inhibitor, thrombin inhibitor protease nexin I, and factors IXa and XIa inhibitor protease nexin II or β-amyloid precursor protein)[138,183]; and (7) promotion of factor XII activation by ADP-treated platelets.[138]

PLATELET MEMBRANE GLYCOPROTEINS, PLATELET ADHESION, AND PLATELET AGGREGATION

Platelet membrane glycoproteins mediate the interactions between the platelet and its external environment. Receptors can receive signals from outside the platelet and send signals inside. In addition, receptors can receive signals from inside the platelet that affect their external domains. Platelet glycoprotein receptors are derived from several different receptor families (integrins, leucine-rich glycoproteins, immunoglobulin (Ig) cell adhesion molecules, selectins, quadraspanins, and seven transmembrane domain receptors; see Table 105-5). One member of the integrin family, $\alpha IIb\beta 3$, is essentially unique to platelets, as is GPVI, whereas the leucine-rich glycoproteins GPIb-IX and GPV appear to have highly restricted expression, including primarily platelets and cytokine-activated endothelial cells.[477–479] All of the other receptors are expressed more widely on other cell types.

INTEGRINS

Integrin receptors are heterodimeric complexes composed of an α-subunit containing three or four divalent cation-binding domains and a β-subunit rich in disulfide bonds. Both subunits are transmembrane glycoproteins and are coded by different genes. There are at least 17 α-subunits and eight β-subunits.[343,480,481] Three major families of integrin receptors are recognized based on the β-subunit: β_1, β_2, and β_3. Integrins are widely distributed on different cell types, and each integrin demonstrates unique ligand-binding properties. Integrin receptors mediate interactions between cells and between proteins and cells. They also are involved in protein trafficking in cells. Integrin receptors can transduce messages from outside the cell to inside the cell and from inside the cell to outside the cell.

$\alpha IIb\beta 3$ (GPIIb-IIIa; Fibrinogen Receptor; CD41/CD61) The $\alpha IIb\beta 3$ complex, a member of the $\beta 3$ integrin receptor family, is the dominant platelet receptor. From 80,000 to 100,000 receptors are present on the surface of a resting platelet.[343,344,346,480,482] Another 20,000 to 40,000 receptors are present inside platelets, primarily in α-granule membranes but also in dense bodies and membranes lining the open canalicular system. These receptors are able to join the plasma membrane when platelets are activated and undergo the release reaction.[483–485] On average, $\alpha IIb\beta 3$ receptors are less than 20 nm apart on the platelet surface and thus are among the most densely expressed adhesion/aggregation receptors present on any cell type.

On resting platelets, $\alpha IIb\beta 3$ has low affinity for fibrinogen in solution. However, when platelets are activated with ADP, epinephrine, thrombin, or other agonists, $\alpha IIb\beta 3$ binds fibrinogen with higher affinity (see Fig. 105-3).[344,345,349] The signal transduction mechanisms that mediate activation are discussed in the section "Signaling Pathways in Platelet Activation and Aggregation" below (see Fig. 105-12). Activation induces changes in the $\alpha IIb\beta 3$ receptor itself that are responsible for the change in fibrinogen-binding affinity,[486,487] but changes in the microenvironment surrounding $\alpha IIb\beta 3$ also may be involved. The $\alpha IIb\beta 3$ receptors in α-granules appear to cycle to and from the plasma membrane.[488] This recycling helps to explain the ability of $\alpha IIb\beta 3$ to take up fibrinogen from plasma and transport it to α-granules, where it is concentrated.[109,112]

Data from other integrin receptors led to the identification of a cell recognition sequence composed of Arg-Gly-Asp (RGD) in the ligand fibronectin.[489,490] This same sequence is important in ligand binding to $\alpha V\beta 3$ and $\alpha IIb\beta 3$. Fibrinogen contains one RGD sequence near the carboxyl-terminus of each of the two Aα chains (amino acids 572–574) and another at amino acids 95 to 97.[491] In addition, the carboxyl-terminal 12-amino-acid region of each of the two γ-chains (amino acids 400–411) contains a sequence that includes Lys-Gln-Ala-Gly-Asp-Val, which appears to be the most important in the binding of fibrinogen to platelets.[288,492–494] vWF contains an RGD sequence in its carboxy-terminal domain that mediates binding to $\alpha IIb\beta 3$.[275,278] Small, synthetic peptides containing the RGD or γ-chain sequence inhibit the binding of fibrinogen to platelets, and these observations have been exploited to produce therapeutic agents (tirofiban and eptifibatide) that inhibit platelet thrombus formation (see Chap. 126). Similarly, mono-

clonal antibodies that inhibit binding of ligands to $\alpha IIb\beta 3$ have been developed, including one that has been developed into the antiplatelet drug abciximab (see Chap. 126).

Binding of fibrinogen to $\alpha IIb\beta 3$ appears to be a multistep process.[344] (1) The initial interaction most likely occurs via the γ-chain carboxy-terminal region(s) and is divalent cation dependent.[288,493,494] (2) Subsequent interactions, which may involve exclusion of the divalent cations and internalization of the fibrinogen,[495] render the binding irreversible, even when divalent cations are removed.[496] (3) Binding of fibrinogen induces changes in the receptor that can be recognized by antibodies (ligand-induced binding sites) and probably involves, at least in part, a reorientation between domains in the head region of $\beta 3$, leading to a swingout motion in $\beta 3$ and separation between the leg regions of αIIb and $\beta 3$ (see Fig. 105-3).[497] (4) Binding of fibrinogen to $\alpha IIb\beta 3$ induces changes in fibrinogen (receptor-induced binding sites) that can be recognized by antibodies and may involve exposure of the Aα chain Arg-Gly-Asp-Phe (RGDF) sequence at amino acids 95 to 98.[498,499] (5) Fibrinogen binding induces receptor clustering.[396,500]

By electron microscopy, integrin receptors appear to have a globular head of 8×12 nm and two 18-nm long tails or legs, representing the carboxyl-terminal regions of each subunit, including their hydrophobic transmembrane domains.[501,502] Crystallographic and biochemical data from $\alpha IIb\beta 3$ and crystallographic and electron microscopy data of the related integrin receptor $\alpha V\beta 3$ indicate the unactivated receptors are in a bent conformation and that activation involves both extension of the receptor head and a swingout motion in the β_3 subunit (see Fig. 105-3).[503–509] Thus, the published electron micrographs of $\alpha IIb\beta 3$ probably show the extended (activated) forms of the receptor.

$\alpha IIb\beta 3$ shares the same basic structural features of all integrin receptors (see Table 105-5). The α-subunit αIIb is a transmembrane protein with four characteristic divalent cation-binding sites (Fig. 105-13). The mature protein contains 1008 amino acids,[343,480,510] with one transmembrane domain. During processing, the extracellular domain is cleaved into a heavy chain and a light chain connected by a disulfide bond. The β-subunit $\beta 3$ contains 762 amino acids and is rich in cysteine residues, with a characteristic cysteine-rich region near its transmembrane domain.[343,480,511] The αIIb and $\beta 3$ cytoplasmic tails consist of 20 and 47 amino acids, respectively. The genes encoding αIIb and $\beta 3$ are very close to one another on chromosome 17 at q21.32 but are not so close that they share common regulatory domains.[512,513] Both proteins are synthesized in megakaryocytes and join to form a calcium-dependent, noncovalent complex in the rough endoplasmic reticulum.[480,514] Calnexin probably serves as a chaperone for αIIb,[515] but which chaperone(s) is involved in $\beta 3$ folding and/or $\alpha IIb\beta 3$ complex formation is unclear. The $\alpha IIb\beta 3$ complex subsequently undergoes further processing in the Golgi apparatus, where the carbohydrate structures undergo maturation and the pro-GPIIb molecule is cleaved into its heavy and light chains by furin or a similar enzyme.[480,516,517] Approximately 15 percent of the mass of both αIIb and $\beta 3$ is composed of carbohydrate.[518] The mature $\alpha IIb\beta 3$ complex is transported to the plasma membrane or the membranes of α-granules or dense bodies. If αIIb and $\beta 3$ do not form a proper complex, because of either a structural abnormality or failure to synthesize one of the subunits, the glycoproteins that are synthesized are not transported to the Golgi or expressed on the membrane surface (see Chap. 112). Degradation of αIIb appears to involve retro-translocation from the endoplasmic reticulum into the cytoplasm, ubiquitination, and proteolysis by the megakaryocyte proteasome.[515]

The amino-terminal region of αIIb contains a seven-blade β-propeller domain. Each blade is composed of four β-strands connected by loops (see Fig. 105-13). The propeller interacts with the βA (I-like) domain of $\beta 3$, forming the globular head region observed in electron micrographs. The four calcium ions bound by the propeller domain interact with β hairpin loops in blades 4 to 7, which extend away from the interface with β3. In addition, a unique αIIb cap subdomain is composed of four loops from blades 1 to 3 that are unique to αIIb and contribute to its ligand-binding specificity. A crystal-based tertiary structure is not yet available for the remainder of the extracellular domains of the molecule. However, based on the high level of homology between αIIb and αV, it likely is composed of domains very similar to the thigh and calf domains identified in αVβ3.[506,519] The cytoplasmic domain of αIIb interacts with the cytoplasmic domain of β3. The interaction is important in controlling activation of the αIIbβ3 receptor, but the precise details are incompletely understood (see Fig. 105-3).[346,520–522] The cytoplasmic domain of αIIb has a GFFKR sequence near the membrane that is thought to control inside-out activation of the αIIbβ3 receptors, as mutations or deletions in this region result in the receptor adopting a high affinity for fibrinogen.[346,523–525] The more distal region of the cytoplasmic domain probably adopts an α-helical conformation, followed by a turn and folding back to the α-helix.[26] Disrupting the conformation of this region also results in a constitutively high-affinity receptor.[26,526]

The β3-subunit is composed of a series of domains, but they are not linearly arranged because the first domain (plex-ins, semiphorins, and integrins [PSI]) was subjected to insertion of a hybrid domain, which itself was subjected to insertion of a βA (I-like) domain, a domain homologous to the vWF A domain and integrin I domains, both of which bind ligands (see Fig. 105-13).[503,527] The double insertion in the PSI domain explains the presence of a long-range disulfide bond extending from C13 to C435. Thus, even though the βA domain makes contact with the αIIb propeller (via Arg261 and other residues that interact with two rings of hydrophobic residues in the αIIb "cage"), it does not contain the amino-terminus of the molecule. The PSI domain contains Leu33, which defines PlA1 (HPA-1a) specificity, as opposed to the alloantigen PlA2 (HPA-1b), which is produced by a Pro33 polymorphism. The β3 leg or stalk is composed of four integrin EGF domains that are rich in disulfide bonds. This region interacts with the αIIb stalk region and the globular head in the bent, unactivated receptor, but not in the activated receptor.[503] Consistent with the importance of the integrin EGF domains in receptor activation is the observation that mutations in this area can activate the receptor, as can the binding of monoclonal antibodies.[528–530] Mutating any one of the cysteines in the integrin EGF domains so as to impair the normal disulfide bonding also results in constitutive activation of the receptor.[531] Activation of αIIbβ3 has been proposed to involve breaking and/or reorganizing disulfide bonds.[532] Adding certain reducing agents to platelets can cause activation of αIIbβ3, fibrinogen binding, and platelet aggregation.[532,533] An enzyme capable of catalyzing the breakage of disulfide bonds and exchange of thiol groups and disulfide bonds in proteins (protein disulfide isomerase [PDI]) has been identified on the surface of platelets and in platelet releasates.[532,534,535] Moreover, regions in β3 have the same consensus sequence (CGXC) present in PDI that is thought to mediate disulfide bond breakage and thiol exchange.[536] One model suggests αIIbβ3 can achieve a low level of activation without alterations in disulfide bonds, but maximal activation requires PDI or similar activity along with a source of thiols, such as plasma glutathione or a membrane NAD(P)H oxidoreductase system.[532]

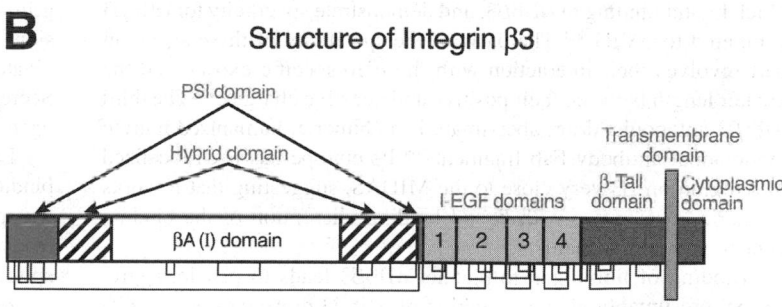

FIGURE 105-13 (A) αIIbβ3 and αVβ3 extracellular domain structure. The α-subunit is composed of an N-terminal β-propeller domain, a thigh domain, and two calf domains. The depicted α-subunit is a composite of the αIIbβ propeller[497] and the remainder from αVβ3.[509] The β3 subunit is composed of a βA(I) domain, a hybrid domain, a pleckstrin, semiphorin, integrin (PSI) domain, four integrin-epidermal growth factor (I-EGF) domains, and a β-terminal domain.[497,509] (B) Domain structure of integrin β3. The N-terminus of β3 is in the PSI domain. Based on structural homology to other proteins, the hybrid domain appears to have been inserted into the PSI domain and the βA(I) domain into the hybrid domain. Note that despite the large number of intervening amino acids, C13 is adjacent to C435 in the PSI domain and thus can be linked by a disulfide bond. (Adapted from T Xiao, J Takagi, BS Coller, et al.,[497] with permission.)

The cytoplasmic domain of β3 contains a sequence (LLITIHD) that is predicted to interact with the αIIb GFFKR region via a salt bridge, and mutations in this region that are predicted to disrupt the interaction result in αIIbβ3 activation.[537] Disruption of the interaction between the cytoplasmic domains of αIIb and β3, most likely as a result of talin binding to β3, has been proposed as an important mechanism of αIIbβ3 activation (see Fig. 105-3).[27,309,380,520–526,538,539] The β3 tail also contains two NXXY motifs, and Y747 and Y759 within these motifs are phosphorylated upon platelet aggregation, thus producing docking sites for signaling molecules. Studies in mice and in recombinant systems demonstrate a role for these sites in clot retraction and platelet aggregate stability.[540,541]

A number of proteins bind to the cytoplasmic domains of αIIb and/or β3, either directly or through interactions with other proteins, including signaling molecules (src, shc, pp125[FAK], paxillin, and integrin-linked kinase, all of which bind to β3), cytoskeletal proteins (skelemin, α-actin, and myosin, which bind to β3, and filamin and talin, which bind to αIIb and/or β3), and other proteins (β3-endonexin and CD98 which bind to β3 and CIB and calreticulin, which bind to αIIb).[346,380,522,539,542–556] These interactions are important in mediating inside-out signaling and outside-in signaling.

The junction between the αIIb propeller and the β3 βA (I-like) domain is the site of ligand binding to αIIbβ3. This region of β3 contains three divalent cation-binding sites: metal ion-dependent adhesion site (MIDAS), adjacent to MIDAS (ADMIDAS), and ligand-induced metal binding site (LIMBS).

Solution of the crystal structure of αVβ3 demonstrated that an RGD peptide bound primarily via interactions between the Arg in the peptide and two Asp residues (D150 and D218) in αV and between the Asp in the peptide and the MIDAS cation.[509] The binding pocket in αIIbβ3 is similar to that of αVβ3, except for the following differences: only one Asp in αIIb (D224) is available to interact with an Arg (or Lys as in the fibrinogen γ-chain peptide), the distance between D224 in αIIb and the MIDAS cation is longer, and a cap subdomain of the αIIb propeller contributes Phe160 to a hydrophobic exosite in combination with Tyr190.[497] As a result, the pocket can selectively bind peptides containing the longer Lys residue (KGD peptides). X-ray crystallography-derived tertiary structures are available for the αIIbβ3 receptor headpiece with the drugs eptifibatide and tirofiban, which are effective antithrombotic agents because of their ability to block ligand binding to αIIbβ3, and demonstrate specificity for αIIbβ3 compared to αVβ3.[503] The basis of the specificity of these agents in part involves their interaction with the αIIb-specific exosite and the greater length between their positive and negative charges.[503] The third αIIbβ3 antagonist drug, abciximab, is a chimeric, humanized murine monoclonal antibody Fab fragment.[505] Its epitope has been localized to a region on β3 very close to the MIDAS, suggesting that it works by steric interference with ligand binding, disruption of the binding pocket, or both mechanisms.[505]

Binding of fibrinogen to platelet αIIbβ3 leads to platelet aggregation, presumably via cross-linking of αIIbβ3 molecules on two different platelets by fibrinogen.[502] The dimeric and relatively rigid structure of fibrinogen and the location of the binding sites at the ends of the γ-chains all are consistent with such a model because the two binding sites on a single fibrinogen molecule probably are more than 45 nm apart. Soon after fibrinogen binds, it can be dissociated from the platelet by chelating the divalent cations, but the binding becomes irreversible within 1 hour.[496] Fibrinogen binding alone is not sufficient for platelet aggregation, but the events necessary after fibrinogen binding, which probably include ligand- and/or cytoskeletal-mediated receptor clustering, are not well understood.[2,496,557,558] After ligands bind to αIIbβ3, "outside-in" signaling through αIIbβ3 can occur, resulting in a number of phosphorylation events, changes in the platelet cytoskeleton, platelet spreading, and even initiation of protein translation.[219,309]

In addition to fibrinogen, several other proteins can bind to αIIbβ3 on activated platelets, including vWF, fibronectin, vitronectin, TSP, and prothrombin.[121,466,559] Each of these proteins contains an RGD sequence in the region implicated in the initial interaction with platelets. There are, however, subtle differences in the binding of each of these ligands with regard to divalent cation preference and competent activating agents.[486] The binding of all of these other ligands also can be inhibited by RGD-containing peptides, indicating a common requirement for the interaction between the RGD sequence in the protein and the RGD-binding site in αIIbβ3.[560,561]

As measured in the aggregometer, platelet aggregation ex vivo depends upon fibrinogen binding to αIIbβ3. Whether fibrinogen is the most important ligand supporting platelet aggregation in vivo is less clear, because studies performed in model systems under flowing conditions indicate vWF is the major ligand at higher shear rates.[348] Even in the aggregometer, vWF can partially substitute for fibrinogen if the fibrinogen concentration is very low.[562] In vivo mice deficient in both vWF and fibrinogen still make platelet thrombi in response to vascular injury, and fibronectin has been implicated in supporting the development of such thrombi.[111,314,563]

In contrast to the requirement for platelet activation in order for platelets to bind soluble fibrinogen (or other adhesive glycoproteins), resting platelets adhere to fibrinogen immobilized on a surface.[287,288] This activation-independent adhesion may result from alterations in the structure of fibrinogen when it is immobilized on a surface.[499,564] Alternatively, it may result from the constant presence of a few αIIbβ3 receptors that are transiently in the proper conformation to bind fibrinogen and the favorable kinetics achieved as a result of the high local density of fibrinogen that accompanies immobilization on a surface.

Fibrinogen and/or fibrin have been identified on the surface of damaged blood vessels; thus, αIIbβ3 may mediate platelet adhesion under those circumstances.[565] In contrast, αIIbβ3 on resting platelets does not mediate adhesion to vWF or fibronectin[288]; however, if platelets are activated, αIIbβ3 can support adhesion to these glycoproteins.[560] In models of platelet accumulation under flowing conditions, αIIbβ3 acts in synergy with GPIb-IX, vWF, and fibrinogen at the apex of thrombi, where shear forces are greatest.[285,300,305] The αIIbβ3 integrin has also been implicated in platelet spreading after adhesion,[308,310,394] and it is necessary for clot retraction (see section on "Platelet Contractile Elements and Platelet Shape Change, Spreading, Secretion, and Clot Retraction," above) and uptake of plasma fibrinogen into platelet α-granules.[109,112]

Less well-defined roles for αIIbβ3 have been suggested in the binding of plasminogen[566] and factor XIIIa[387] to platelets, calcium transport across the platelet membrane,[567–569] IgE binding to platelets leading to parasite cytotoxicity,[570] and interactions with the Borrelia spirochetes causing Lyme disease[571] and the Hantavirus.[572]

α2β1 (GPIa-IIa; Collagen Receptor; VLA-2; CD49b/CD29)

Integrin α2β1 (GPIa-IIa) is widely distributed on different cell types and can mediate adhesion to collagen (see Fig. 105-17).[291–293,573–576] The α2 subunit (GPIa) contains a region of 191 amino acids inserted in the amino-terminal β propeller region (I domain) that is homologous to similar regions in other proteins that are known to interact with collagen, including vWF and cartilage matrix protein.[577] This region has a MIDAS domain, and crystallographic data of the α2I domain in complex with a collagen-related peptide containing the type I collagen sequence GFOGER (where O indicates hydroxyproline) demonstrate that the glutamic acid in the peptide coordinates a magnesium ion in MIDAS.[578–580]

Although a number of early observations suggested that α2β1 was the principal platelet collagen receptor, particularly based on bleeding defects in patients with diminished receptor levels (see Chap. 112),[576,581] GPVI now appears to play a central role in collagen-mediated platelet activation and adhesion (see "Signaling Pathways in Platelet Activation and Aggregation" below). GPVI signaling and perhaps other agonists appear to activate α2β1 and other integrins.[578,582] Thus, following initiation of collagen adhesion and activation mediated by GPVI, α2β1 may promote firm adhesion to collagen, stabilize thrombus growth on collagen, and promote procoagulant activity.[298,583]

The affinity of $\alpha2\beta1$ also may be modulated by alterations in disulfide bonds, as inhibition of platelet protein disulfide isomerase and sulfhydryl blocking agents inhibit $\alpha2\beta1$-mediated platelet adhesion to type I collagen and the related peptide GFOGER.[532,584]

Ligand binding to $\alpha2\beta1$ is enhanced in the presence of magnesium or manganese and is inhibited by calcium. Therefore, the conditions in human blood, where calcium is abundant and magnesium is present at only low levels, do not provide optimal cation concentrations for the receptor's function.[292] Integrin $\alpha2\beta1$ can, however, mediate platelet adhesion to collagen in heparinized blood.[292,293] Regions of collagen type I have been implicated as potential binding sites for $\alpha2\beta1$.[585] The peptide sequences 502 to 516 of collagen type I α_1 chain, containing a Gly-Glu-Arg (GER) sequence, may be of particular importance,[586] but other interactions also may contribute to the interaction.[587] In type III collagen, amino acids 522 to 528 of fragment α_1 (III) CB4 contain a binding region for $\alpha2\beta1$.[588]

At least three alleles for the $\alpha2$ gene differ at nucleotides 807 (T or C) and 1648 (G or A). The 807 substitution does not affect the amino acid sequence, but the 1648 substitution causes a change from Glu to Lys, resulting in the Br^b and Br^a alloantigens (HPA-5a and HPA-5b). Allele 1 (T-G) is present in 39 percent of individuals, allele 2 (C-G) in 53 percent, and allele 3 (C-A) in 7 percent.[302,589] Individuals with allele 1 have higher $\alpha2\beta1$ platelet density than individuals with allele 2; individuals with allele 3 have the lowest density. The density of $\alpha2\beta1$ correlates with platelet deposition on collagen under flow. The association of these polymorphisms with cardiovascular disease morbidity and mortality, including the risk of developing myocardial infarction[590,591] and stroke,[592] has been extensively studied without firm conclusions, although a possible association with cardiovascular risk has been suggested.[593–595]

Integrin $\alpha2\beta1$ probably is linked to the membrane skeleton and is competent to mediate adhesion on resting platelets.[596] Its ligand specificity appears to be determined by the cell on which it is expressed, given that on endothelial cells it functions as a laminin receptor and as a collagen receptor.[597] Engagement of $\alpha2\beta1$[598] can initiate platelet protein synthesis.[219]

$\alpha5\beta1$ (GPIc*-IIa; Fibronectin Receptor; VLA-5; CD49e/CD29)

The $\beta1$ integrin $\alpha5\beta1$ is expressed on a wide variety of cells and mediates adhesion to fibronectin.[489,490] The receptor plays an important role in cell–matrix interactions, and studies of cells other than platelets indicate a role for this receptor in developmental biology and metastasis formation. RGD-containing peptides can inhibit cell adhesion mediated by $\alpha5\beta1$, but other regions in fibronectin probably also contribute. As with other integrin receptors, adhesion depends on the presence of divalent cations. Integrin $\alpha5\beta1$ is competent to mediate adhesion of resting platelets to fibronectin,[599,600] although the physiologic role of this receptor on platelets is not clear. Although $\alpha5\beta1$ may be involved in platelet hemostasis and/or thrombosis, its function primarily may consist of enhancing megakaryocyte binding to marrow matrix, given that it seems to serve this function on other hematopoietic precursors.[601] Integrin $\alpha5\beta1$ is not the only fibronectin receptor on platelets; with appropriate activation, αIIb$\beta3$ also can bind fibronectin.[121]

$\alpha6\beta1$ (GPIc-IIa; Laminin Receptor; VLA-6; CD49f/CD29)

Platelet adhesion to laminin can be mediated by the $\alpha6\beta1$ integrin receptor.[602,603] This adhesion is best demonstrated in the presence of magnesium or manganese; calcium does not support adhesion. This receptor is competent on resting platelets, but its role in platelet physiology is not clear. A molecular weight 67,000 laminin receptor has also been identified on platelets and is present on other cells as well.[604]

$\alpha V\beta3$ (Vitronectin Receptor; CD51/CD61)

The $\alpha V\beta3$ receptor shares the same $\beta3$ subunit as αIIb$\beta3$ (GPIIb-IIIa) (see Figs. 105-3 and 105-13).[481,511] The αV and αIIb subunits have 36 percent sequence

identity.[605] Integrin $\alpha V\beta3$ differs dramatically from αIIb$\beta3$ in its platelet surface density, with only approximately 50 to 100 $\alpha V\beta3$ receptors per platelet.[606] The crystal structure of the external domains of $\alpha V\beta3$ alone and in complex with a peptide containing the RGD cell recognition sequence found in a number of ligands have been solved at high resolution.[509,607] Such RGD peptides inhibit ligand binding to $\alpha V\beta3$. The most important findings were as follows: (1) the receptor adopts a bent conformation in which the globular headpiece composed of the N-terminal β-propeller region of αV and the βA (I-like) domain of $\beta3$ lies near the legs of the αV and $\beta3$ subunits, and (2) the RGD peptide binds to the headpiece, with the Arg (R) making contact with αV and the Asp (D) making contact with the MIDAS domain in $\beta3$. Current evidence suggests that the bent conformation is the inactive one and that activation results in extension of the headpiece and pivoting between the $\beta3$ βA and hybrid domains in association with leg separation.[503,504] The $\alpha V\beta3$ receptor can mediate adhesion to vitronectin, but only in the presence of magnesium or manganese, not calcium.[606] It also can mediate interactions with fibrinogen, vWF, prothrombin, and TSP.[122,608–611] Platelet stimulation can activate $\alpha V\beta3$, analogous to activation of αIIb$\beta3$ and $\alpha2\beta1$. Activated $\alpha V\beta3$ may uniquely mediate adhesion to osteopontin, a protein found in high concentrations in atherosclerotic plaque.[612] The receptor's role in platelet physiology is not defined, but it may contribute to the development of platelet coagulant activity.[441]

The $\alpha V\beta3$ receptor also is present on endothelial cells,[492,610] osteoclasts,[613] smooth muscle cells, and other cells. It has been implicated in bone resorption,[614–616] endothelial–matrix interactions,[492,610] lymphoid cell apoptosis,[617] neovascularization,[618] tumor angiogenesis,[619–623] and intimal hyperplasia after vascular injury.[624–626]

The presence or absence of $\alpha V\beta3$ on the platelets of patients with Glanzmann thrombasthenia can help localize the abnormality to either GPIIb (if $\alpha V\beta3$ is present in normal or increased amounts) or GPIIIa (if $\alpha V\beta3$ is reduced or absent) (see Chap. 112).

$\beta2$ Integrins ($\alpha L\beta2$, $\alpha M\beta2$, $\alpha X\beta2$; CD11a/CD18, CD11b/CD18, CD11c/CD18)

Although $\beta2$ integrins traditionally have been viewed as leukocyte specific, $\alpha L\beta2$ has been detected on the surface of activated human platelets.[627] $\beta2$ integrins have been detected on mouse platelets, and $\beta2$-null mice demonstrate decreased platelet survival and diminished localization of platelets at sites of inflammation.[628,629]

LEUCINE-RICH REPEAT GLYCOPROTEIN RECEPTORS

GPIb/GPIX/GPV (CD42)

GPIb is composed of GPIbα (CD42b) (610 amino acids) disulfide-bonded to GPIbβ (CD42c) (122 amino acids).[274,282,477,630,631] GPIb appears to exist on the surface of platelets in a 1:1 complex with GPIX (160 amino acids) and a 2:1 complex with GPV (Fig. 105-14). The GPIbα gene is on the short arm of chromosome 17, the GPIbβ gene is on the long arm of chromosome 22, and the GPIX gene is on the long arm of chromosome 3.[632–634] The function of GPIX is unknown, but it is required for efficient surface expression of GPIb.[635] GPIb-IX is expressed on megakaryocytes and platelets; controversy exists as to whether GPIb-IX is expressed on endothelial cells, either constitutively or after cytokine activation.[478,479,636–641] The promoters for GPIb-IX lack TATA or CAAT boxes but contain binding sites for the GATA and ETS families of transcription factors, which, along with the expression of the cofactor FOG (Friend of GATA-1), may account for the limited expression of GPIb-IX.[282,642–650]

A genetic polymorphism in GPIbα affects the number of repeating 13 amino acid units (1, 2, 3, or 4) and produces changes in the molecular weight of GPIbα (Fig. 105-15).[651] The two-repeat variant is most common, but considerable ethnic variation in the frequency of the different numbers of repeats exists. This molecular weight polymorphism has been linked to the Sib and Ko alloantigens, which have

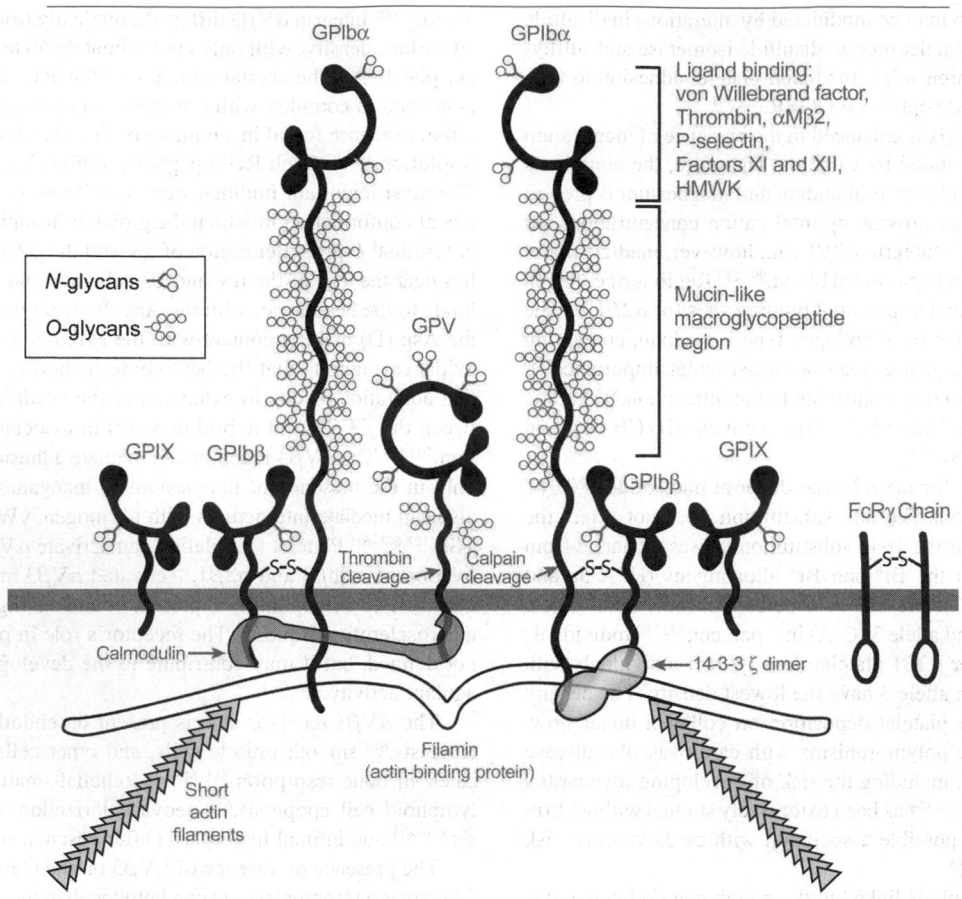

FIGURE 105-14   Schematic representation of the GPIb-IX-V complex and associated proteins. The complex consists of four polypeptide chains, each of which is encoded by its own gene. The arrangement is hypothetical but is based on the stoichiometry of two copies each of GPIbα, GPIbβ, and GPIX for every copy of GPV, and the demonstration that GPV associates predominantly with GPIbα. The N-terminal region of GPIbα can bind a number of different ligands, with von Willebrand factor and thrombin the best characterized and most established as important in platelet physiology. The mucin-like region is very rich in carbohydrate and provides GPIbα with an extended conformation, making it the receptor that probably extends furthest from the surface of the platelet. Thrombin can cleave GPV. A variety of proteins, particularly calpain, can cleave GPIbα near its insertion into the membrane. The cleavage product glycocalicin circulates in plasma. In the cytoplasmic domain, the complex associates with several proteins, including 14-3-3ζ, calmodulin, and filamin (actin-binding protein). It is through the association with the latter protein that the complex is linked to a submembrane structure of short actin filaments known as the platelet membrane skeleton (see Fig. 105-2). The Fc receptor γ-chain (FcRγ chain) probably also is associated with the complex, although the stoichiometry is not established, and may participate in signaling via the GPIb-IX-V complex. HMWK, high molecular weight kininogen. (Adapted from JA Lopez and MC Berndt,[282] with permission).

been localized to a T→M variation at amino acid 145 of GPIbα, with M associated with either three or four repeats and T associated with either one or two repeats (see Chap. 129).[589] Some but not all reports suggest an association between the alleles with the larger number of repeats and vascular disease.[589,652–654] Two other GPIbα polymorphisms have been described: (1) C or T at position −5 from the ATG start codon (RS system) and (2) a nucleotide dimorphism at the third base of the codon for Arg358.[631,655,656] A C at position −5 is present in only 8 to 17 percent of individuals and more closely resembles the sequence surrounding the ATG start codon (Kozak sequence) considered optimal for translation. This polymorphism is associated with higher levels of platelet surface GPIb and may be a risk factor for ischemic vascular disease.[657–665] GPIb has been implicated as a target antigen in autoimmune thrombocytopenia and in quinine- and quinidine-induced thrombocytopenia (see Chap. 110).

GPIbα has a large number of O-linked carbohydrate chains terminating in sialic acid residues,[666] and the latter contribute significantly to the negative charge of the platelet membrane (see Fig. 105-14).[3] Electron micrographic analysis indicates GPIb exists as a long flexible rod (~60 nm) with two globular domains of approximately 9 and 16 nm.[667] Thus, GPIb probably extends much further out from the platelet's surface than does αIIbβ3, which may account for its primacy in platelet adhesion and the increased risk for cardiovascular disease in individuals with longer GPIb molecules because of an increased number of 13 amino acid repeats. The long extension also may make it susceptible to conformational changes induced by shear forces.[477] The extracellular region of GPIbα is readily cleaved by a variety of proteases, including platelet calpains,[668] yielding a soluble fragment named glycocalicin that circulates in normal plasma at 1 to 3 μg/ml.[669] Levels of plasma glycocalicin correlate with platelet production and

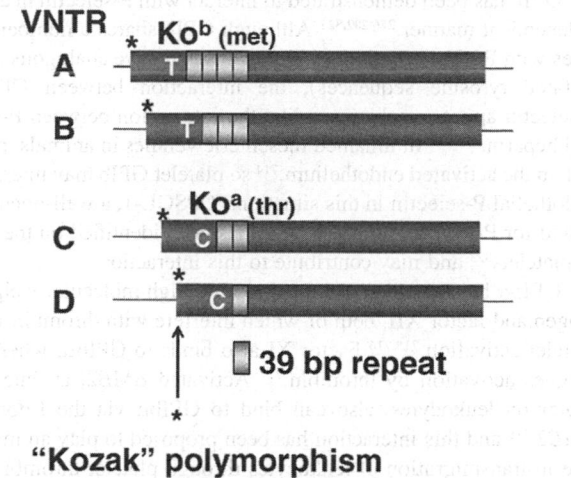

FIGURE 105-15 Polymorphisms of platelet GPIbα. The four alleles of GPIbα have been defined by the variable number of tandem repeats (VNTR), Ko, and Kozak polymorphisms. The four VNTR polymorphisms are defined as A to D, according to the number of 39 base pair repeats (corresponding to 13 amino acid repeats in the protein), which are depicted as *white rectangles*. A has four repeats, B has three repeats, C has two repeats, and D has one repeat. The Ko polymorphism results from a T to C nucleotide substitution that alters the amino acid coding from methionine (met) to threonine (thr). The *asterisk* indicates the location of the nucleotide substitution that generates a sequence that better conforms to the consensus Kozak sequence. (Adapted from PF Bray,[589] with permission.)

thus can be used to differentiate thrombocytopenia resulting from decreased platelet production from thrombocytopenia resulting from increased platelet destruction.[670–676]

GPIbβ and GPIX have free sulfhydryl groups in their cytoplasmic domains that undergo palmitoylation, at least partly, further anchoring these proteins to the membrane.[677,678] The penultimate serine residue at the carboxyl-terminus of GPIbα is phosphorylated, providing an attachment site for the signal-complex protein 14-3-3ζ.[679] Similarly, GPIbβ can undergo phosphorylation of Ser166 in its cytoplasmic domain as a result of protein kinase A (PKA) activation via cAMP, providing another binding site for 14-3-3ζ.[680–682] The cytoplasmic domain of GPIbα connects GPIb to filamin A (actin-binding protein), thus connecting GPIb to the platelet cytoskeleton.[276,596,683] Alterations in the cytoskeleton can affect GPIb functional activity.[684–686] The 14-3-3ζ protein can bind PI3K and has been implicated in GPIb-mediated intracellular signaling that results in αIIbβ3 activation.[276,687] GPIb also appears to be in close proximity to FcγRIIA and the Fc receptor (FcR) γ-chain, two receptors that can initiate signaling via tyrosine phosphorylation of their cytoplasmic immunoreceptor tyrosine-containing activation motifs (ITAM) sequences by Src family kinases and recruitment of the tyrosine kinase syk.[688–691]

GPIbα has eight leucine-rich repeats in the amino-terminal region of its extracellular domain, whereas GPIbβ and GPIX have one each.[274,630,634] These repeats are consensus sequences of 24 amino acids with seven regularly spaced leucines. Well-defined disulfide loop sequences flank the repeats.[477] Similar leucine-rich repeats are present in a variety of other proteins.

The crystal structure of the amino-terminus of GPIbα (amino acid residues 1–305) alone and in complex with the A1 domain of vWF provides important information on the interactions between these proteins (Fig. 105-16). This region of GPIbα adopts a curved shape made up of an amino-terminal β-hairpin flanking sequence (finger) containing a C4-C17 disulfide loop (H1-D18), eight leucine-rich repeats (K19-

W204), a β-switch regulatory loop region (V227-S241), and a C-terminal sulfated anionic region (D269-D287), with Y276, Y278, and Y279 undergoing posttranslation sulfation.[692–694] The vWF-A1 domain interacts with the concave face of GPIbα with two areas of tight interactions, at the amino-terminal β-hairpin + first leucine-rich repeat (with vWF A1 domain loops α1β2, β3α2, and α3β4), and a more extensive interaction at leucine-rich repeats 5 to 8 + the β-switch regulatory loop region (with vWF A1 domain helix α3, loop α3β4, and strand β3). The structure of the vWF A1 domain when not bound to GPIbα differs from that of the bound vWF A1 in that the α1β2 loop protrudes in a way that prevents interaction with GPIbα.[694] This observation and others related to differences in the ability of different-size fragments of vWF and GPIbα to interact indicate other regions of both proteins probably contribute to the binding and activation of the receptor. The crystal structure of GPIbα with the naturally occurring mutation M239V in the β-switch regulatory loop region that results in platelet-type (pseudo-) von Willebrand disease (see Chap. 112) has been obtained[693] and demonstrates a more stable conformation, which probably accounts for the approximately sixfold increase in binding affinity, primarily through an increased association rate (see Fig. 112-4). Other natural and site-directed mutations causing the platelet-type von Willebrand disease pattern of enhanced vWF binding (G233V, V234G, D235V, K237V) also affect the regulatory loop region. A number of Bernard-Soulier syndrome mutations that cause loss of vWF binding to GPIbα localize to the concave face of leucine-rich repeats 5, 6, and 7 (L129P, A156V, and L179del) and to the sides of leucine-rich repeat 2 (C65R and L57P) (see Fig. 112-4).[692]

A molecular model for GPIbβ has been proposed based on homology to the Nogo receptor and GPIbα.[695] Four conserved disulfide bonds are predicted (C1-C7, C5-C14, C68-C93, C70-C116), along with the unpaired C122, which cross-links to GPIbα. The molecule presents a hydrophobic surface that may interact with the hydrophobic face of GPIbα and a more hydrophilic β-sheet face that may participate in vWF binding.

Plasma vWF does not bind to GPIb under static conditions unless the antibiotic ristocetin or the snake venom botrocetin is added. The mechanism by which ristocetin induces vWF binding to GPIb is un-

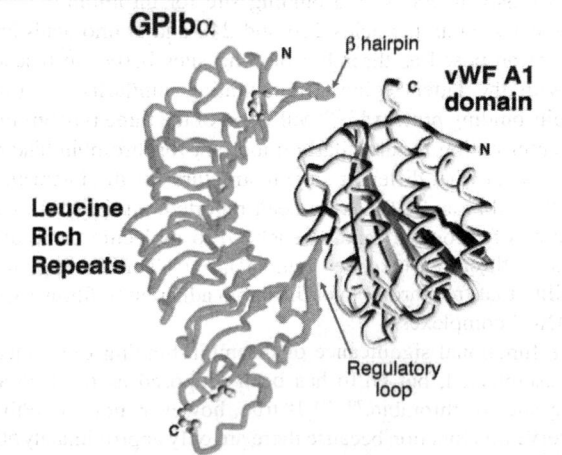

FIGURE 105-16 Structure of the complex between the N-terminus of GPIbα and the A1 domain of von Willebrand factor (vWF). The amino-terminal region of GPIbα folds into a concave surface produced by the leucine-rich repeats, and the A1 domain of von Willebrand factor fits into this structure. Flanking the cysteine-rich repeats in GPIbα are an N-terminal β hairpin region and a C-terminal regulatory loop. The latter is important in controlling access of the von Willebrand factor A1 domain to the GPIb binding site. (Adapted from JJ Dumas, R Kumar, T McDonagh, et al.,[694] with permission).

clear, but effects on vWF and on platelet surface charge have been described, and dimerization of ristocetin molecules also has been implicated.[283,477,696,697] Botrocetin binds to vWF, exposing the site that binds to GPIb.[698] Peptide studies implicate the anionic, sulfated tyrosine region of GPIb as the binding site for botrocetin-treated vWF.[477]

Unlike $\alpha IIb\beta3$, which requires intact, activated platelets to bind to vWF, GPIb-mediated vWF binding does not require platelet activation or even platelet metabolic integrity; in fact, fixed platelets are readily agglutinated in the presence of vWF and either ristocetin or botrocetin.[283] This observation forms the basis of the assay of plasma vWF activity (see Chap. 118).

Platelets adhere to vWF when the latter is immobilized on a surface, even in the absence of ristocetin or botrocetin.[277,283,347,699] Under these circumstances, vWF is believed to undergo a conformational change that allows for direct interactions. However, proposing a change in vWF conformation may not be necessary because the interaction between vWF and GPIb appears to have both high association and dissociation rates, permitting tethering and translocation on a surface coated with a high density of vWF but with minimal interaction in the fluid phase.[275] Similarly, vWF associated with fibrin can interact with platelet GPIb without ristocetin or botrocetin.[316,700] The C1C2 domains of vWF appears to contain a fibrin-binding site.[432]

Shear stress is an important factor in GPIb-mediated adhesion of platelets to immobilized vWF and subendothelial surfaces.[274,277,347,699,701,702] Platelets deficient in GPIb or platelets in which GPIb has been blocked with monoclonal antibodies[347,701] adhere poorly to subendothelial surfaces at all shear rates, but the defect in blood from patients with von Willebrand disease is manifest primarily at higher shear rates.[277,278,347] In a possibly related phenomenon, subjecting platelets to high shear stresses can induce platelet aggregation, which is mediated by vWF binding to GPIb, followed by platelet activation and $\alpha IIb\beta3$-dependent platelet aggregation.[279,281,703] Whether the shear rates generated *in vivo* in stenotic blood vessels are of sufficient magnitude and duration to produce a similar degree of platelet activation is unknown. In addition, whether the effect of shear is acting on GPIb, vWF, or both also is unclear,[274,275,281,477] but shear-induced changes in the structure of vWF, leading to a more extended conformation, have been defined.[704]

GPIb also functions as a binding site for thrombin.[477,705,706] The regions between amino acids 216 and 240 and amino acids 269 and 287 were proposed as thrombin binding sites based on biochemical data, with the latter region demonstrating similarity to hirudin, a thrombin-binding protein.[477,707] Sulfation of the three tyrosine residues in the latter region is particularly important for thrombin binding.[276]

Two somewhat different crystal structures of the interactions between thrombin and GPIb have been reported, but in both cases two molecules of thrombin bind to each GPIb molecule using different regions on thrombin (exosites I and II).[708-710] This finding raises the possibility that free thrombin or thrombin adherent to fibrin can cluster GPIb-IX-V complexes.

The functional significance of thrombin binding to platelet GPIb is not established, but GPIb has been proposed as the high-affinity binding site for thrombin.[705,711] If true, however, not all GPIb molecules serve this function because there are only approximately 50 high-affinity thrombin-binding sites and approximately 25,000 GPIb molecules per platelet.[705,706] One possible explanation is that only the subpopulation of GPIb molecules in lipid rafts function in activating platelets.[15] Platelets lacking GPIb (Bernard-Soulier syndrome) do, in fact, have blunted responses to thrombin (see Chap. 112). In one possible model, binding of thrombin to GPIb facilitates its effect on one or more of the other thrombin receptors, and experimental data support this hypothesis.[712,713]

GPIb has been demonstrated to interact with P-selectin in a cation-independent manner.[276,282,322] Although GPIb shares a number of features with PSGL-1 (both are sialomucins and have analogous anionic/sulfated tyrosine sequences), the interaction between GPIb and P-selectin appears to be more like the interaction between P-selectin and heparin.[276,282] In inflamed mesenteric venules in animals, platelets roll on the activated endothelium,[714] so platelet GPIb may interact with endothelial P-selectin in this situation.[276] PSGL-1, a well-documented ligand for P-selectin on leukocytes, has been identified on the surface of platelets[323] and may contribute to this interaction.

GPIbα has been demonstrated to bind high molecular weight kininogen and factor XII, both of which interfere with thrombin-induced platelet activation.[715,716] Factor XI also binds to GPIbα, where it undergoes activation by thrombin.[717] Activated $\alpha M\beta2$, an integrin receptor on leukocytes, also can bind to GPIbα via the I-domain of $\alpha M\beta2$,[718] and this interaction has been proposed to play an important role in transmigration of leukocytes through platelet thrombi at sites of vascular injury.

Glycoprotein V, the third member of the GPIb-IX-V complex, has a molecular weight of 82,000 and is composed of 544 amino acids, including 15 leucine-rich repeats.[719-722] GPV appears to form a noncovalent complex with GPIb-IX. However, because the number of GPV molecules on the surface of platelets is approximately 50 percent of the number of GPIb and GPIX molecules,[723] the basic unit has been suggested to consist of two GPIb molecules, two GPIX molecules, and one GPV molecule.[282,477,631] GPV is deficient in platelets from patients with Bernard-Soulier syndrome (see Chap. 112), but GPV is not required for surface expression of the GPIb-IX complex.[724] A soluble fragment of molecular weight 69,000 is cleaved from GPV by thrombin, but cleavage does not correlate with thrombin-induced platelet activation.[725] Platelets from mice lacking GPV appear to respond more actively to thrombin and ADP than wild-type mice, raising the possibility that GPV inhibits platelet activation.[726] The platelets from these mice also adhere to immobilized vWF and can bind vWF in the presence of botrocetin, indicating that GPV is not required for interaction between vWF and the GPIb-IX-V complex.[726] Removing a portion of GPV by thrombin proteolysis has been proposed to allow thrombin access to GPIbα, thus facilitating its ability to activate platelets. In support of this model, thrombin's ability to activate platelets does not require proteolytic activity if GPV is absent, suggesting a direct nonproteolytic effect mediated via GPIbα.[727]

IMMUNOGLOBULIN FAMILY OF CELL SURFACE ADHESION RECEPTORS

Platelet Endothelial Cell Adhesion Molecule-1 (CD31) PECAM-1 is a transmembrane glycoprotein of the Ig gene family. It has six Ig-like domains of the C2 group and an M_r of 130,000.[728] In addition to platelets and endothelial cells, PECAM-1 is expressed on monocytes, myeloid cells, and some lymphocyte subsets. Approximately 8000 PECAM-1 molecules are present on the surface of platelets.[729] PECAM promotes homophilic interactions via a homophilic binding domain in the immunoglobin-like repeats. The cytoplasmic tail of PECAM is 118 amino acids in length and contains serine, threonine, and tyrosine phosphorylation sites.

Early studies demonstrated that antibodies that cross-linked PECAM-1 molecules on the platelet surface enhanced platelet adhesion and aggregate formation,[730] suggesting that PECAM-1 could function as a costimulatory agonist, working in concert with platelet $\alpha IIb\beta3$.[730] PECAM has been classified as a member of the immunoreceptor tyrosine-based inhibitory motifs (ITIM) family of inhibitory receptors. Ig-ITIM proteins contain the XYXXL consensus sequence that, upon phosphorylation, recruits and activates phosphatases, such as Src homology-containing protein tyrosine phosphatase (SHP)-1 and SHP-2,[731] via their Src homology 2 (SH2) domains. PECAM contains two ITIM domains and appears to negatively regulate collagen-induced platelet activation mediated by the ITAM-bearing GPVI/FcR γ-chain complex and GPIb-IX-V signaling. Platelets from mice lacking PECAM-1 are hyperresponsive to subthreshold doses of collagen and, compared to wild-type mice, form larger platelet thrombi on vWF and in experimental settings *in vivo*.

In endothelial cells, PECAM-1 is localized to the contact areas between endothelial cells, where it likely is involved in controlling transmigration of leukocytes.[732] It appears to be capable of both homotypic and heterotypic adhesive interactions, with the latter perhaps mediated by glycosaminoglycan interactions with a region in the second Ig domain.[733] An antibody to PECAM-1 decreased neutrophil accumulation and myocardial infarct size in a rat model of ischemia-reperfusion injury.[734]

TREM-Like Transcript-1 TREM-like transcript (TLT)-1 is a receptor whose external domain is homologous to those in the family termed *triggering receptors express on myeloid cells* (TREMs). Like those receptors, it contains a single V-set Ig domain, but its cytoplasmic domain is much longer and carries a canonical ITIM motif capable of becoming phosphorylated and binding SHP-1.[735] The phosphatase then can dephosphorylate signaling molecules, leading to inhibition of platelet activation. PECAM-1 has a similar ability to bind SHP-1. TLT-1 appears to be restricted in expression to platelets and megakaryocytes. It is located primarily in α-granule membranes in unactivated platelets and joins the plasma membrane when platelets are activated.

GPVI GPVI is an M_r 62,000 transmembrane glycoprotein of 316 amino acids (Fig. 105-17).[290] Its extracellular region contains two Ig C2-like domains, and its transmembrane domain contains an Arg residue that is essential for association with the FcR γ-chain. The 51 amino acid cytoplasmic domain contains a proline-rich sequence that binds Src homology 3 (SH3) domains of Src family tyrosine kinases. Signaling through GPVI requires the FcR γ-chain, which becomes phosphorylated by the Src kinases Fyn and/or Lyn to initiate a cascade of intracellular signaling events. (For a discussion of the role of GPVI as a receptor for collagen, see "Signaling Pathways in Platelet Activation and Aggregation" below.) Two alternatively spliced forms and several polymorphisms have been identified for GPVI.

Fc Receptor γ-Chain Platelets contain the FcR γ-chain,[736] which exists as a homodimer of molecular weight 20,000 that physically and functionally associates with GPVI[737] and GPIb-IX[689] (see Figs. 105-12, 105-14, and 105-17). In mouse platelets, the absence of FcR γ-chain results in lack of surface expression of GPVI. The FcR γ-chain and FcγRIIA are the only known platelet proteins with ITAMs. Phosphorylation of the ITAM domain serves to recruit proteins with SH2 domains,[738,739] which are essential for collagen-mediated signaling through the GPVI/FcR γ-chain pathway.[740] The FcR γ-chain also may contribute to GPIb-IX–mediated intracellular signaling after vWF binding.[282,689,691]

Fc γ Receptor IIA (FcγRIIA, CD32) FcγRIIA is a low-affinity Ig receptor of molecular weight 40,000 that is widely distributed on hematopoietic cells. Three different mRNA transcripts (A, B, C) make similar FcγRIIA molecules[741] that are preferentially expressed on dif-

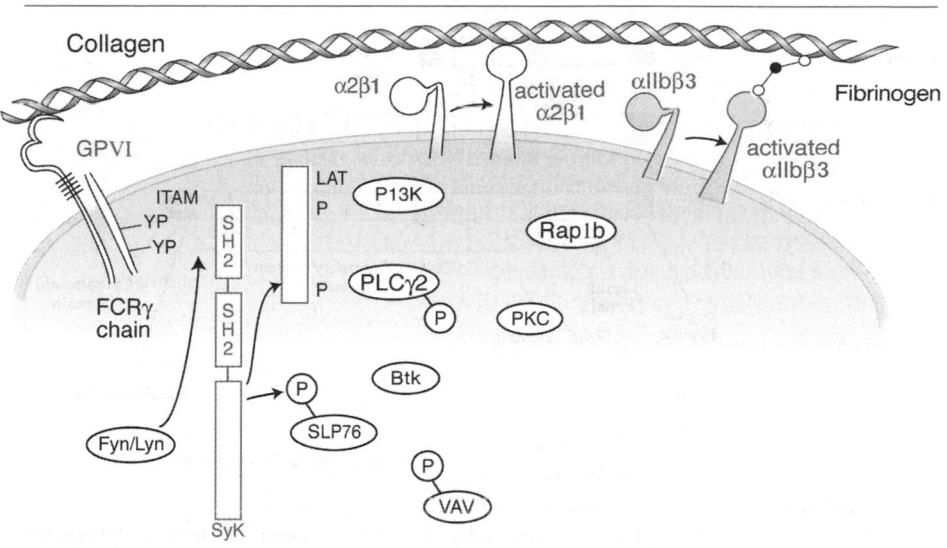

FIGURE 105-17   Collagen activation of platelets. The platelet collagen receptor GPVI is physically and functionally coupled to the ITAM-containing FcRγ chain. Upon collagen binding to GPVI, tyrosine motifs within the FcRγ chain are phosphorylated (P) by the Src family kinase Fyn. This action initiates a chain of events that includes recruitment of the tyrosine kinase Syk, which is phosphorylated and activated by Fyn and Lyn, and phosphorylation of adaptor proteins LAP and SLP76. A signaling cascade activates Bruton tyrosine kinase (BTK), PLCγ2, protein kinase C (PKC), and phosphoinositol-3-kinase (PI3K). Ultimately integrins α2β1 and αIIbβ3 are converted to a high-affinity ("active") state. Activation of α2β1 promotes firm adhesion to collagen and reinforces intracellular signaling pathways.

ferent cells. In addition, the H131R polymorphism within FcγRIIA affects the binding of different IgG subclasses.[742]

FcγRIIA on platelets may bind immune complexes generated in certain diseases.[743,744] It also may provide a second binding site for antibodies that bind to platelets via their antibody-binding site (see "CD9" below). This second interaction potentially can lead to bridging between platelets, with the antibody binding to an antigen on one platelet and an FcγRIIA receptor on another platelet.[745] Another possibility is that antibodies bind to both an antigen and an FcγRIIA on a single platelet. These interactions can lead to platelet activation because cross-linking of FcγRIIA can initiate tyrosine phosphorylation, phosphoinositol metabolism, activation of phospholipase C (PLC)γ2, calcium signaling, and cytoskeletal rearrangements.[746,747] This type of interaction appears to play an important role in heparin-induced thrombocytopenia. FcγRIIA expression on platelets shows considerable variation among individuals (~600–1500 molecules per platelet), and this variation correlates with FcγRIIA-mediated function.[744] Variation in FcγRIIA density may explain individual differences in immune-mediated disorders, such as heparin-induced thrombocytopenia with thrombosis.[748] The H131R polymorphism also may have clinical significance because the R131 allele is associated with increased binding of activation-dependent antibodies to platelets.[749] The homozygous H/H genotype is overrepresented in patients with heparin-induced thrombocytopenia,[750] but the R/R 131 genotype may confer a higher risk of developing thrombosis in patients with heparin-induced thrombocytopenia.[751] The R/R genotype also may be associated with the likelihood of requiring splenectomy in patients with immune thrombocytopenia.[752] FcγRIIA has been suggested to be in close proximity to the GPIb-IX-V complex,[477] and signal transduction that accompanies vWF binding to GPIb may be mediated at least in part through FcγRIIA.[691,753] Cooperation between FcγRIIA and C1q receptor has been reported.[754]

Intracellular Adhesion Molecule-2 (CD102) Intracellular adhesion molecule (ICAM)-2, a member of the Ig family of receptors,

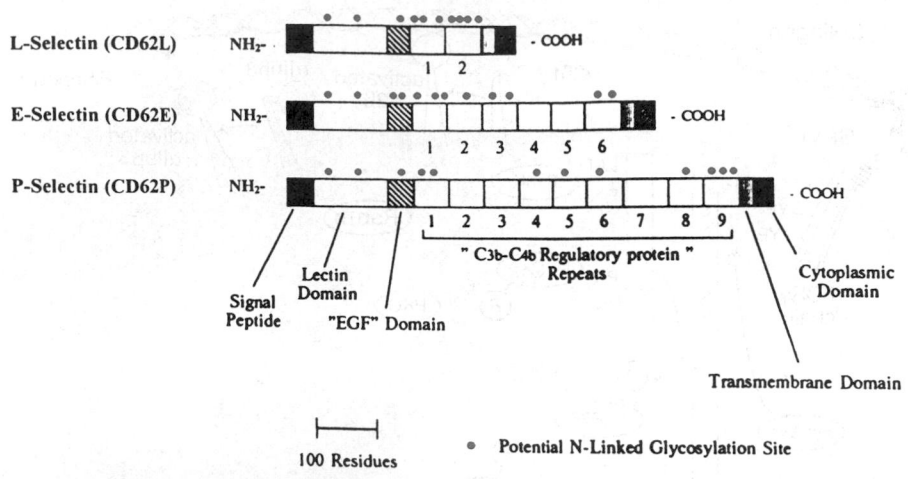

FIGURE 105-18 Structures of the selectins L-selectin (CD62L), E-selectin (CD62E), and P-selectin (CD62P). (Adapted from RP McEver,[1223] with permission.)

is an endothelial cell ligand for the $\beta2$-integrin $\alpha L\beta2$ (LFA-1) on lymphocytes and myeloid cells.[755] Approximately 2600 ICAM-2 molecules are present on platelets, distributed on the membrane surface and open canalicular system.[755] Platelet ICAM-2 may contribute to platelet–leukocyte interactions (see "Platelet–Leukocyte Interactions" below).

Human Leukocyte Antigen Human leukocyte antigen (HLA) class I molecules are expressed on the surface of platelets (for discussion see Chap. 129).

FcεRI Platelets express the high-affinity IgE receptor FcεRI and appear to participate in both defense against parasitic diseases and allergic phenomena.[756,757]

Junctional Adhesion Molecule-1 (F11) Junctional adhesion molecule (JAM)-1 (F11) was identified on platelets by the ability of a monoclonal antibody directed against the receptor to initiate platelet activation via cross-linking to FcγRIIA.[758–761] The protein contains two Ig domains. Although its precise role in platelet physiology is unknown, in endothelial cells it participates in tight junction formation.

Junctional Adhesion Molecule-3 The JAM-3 transmembrane protein has an M_r of 43,000 and 279 amino acids. It contains two C2-type Ig domains in its extracellular domain and three potential tyrosine phosphorylation sites in its cytoplasmic domain.[762] It is expressed on platelets but not granulocytes, monocytes, lymphocytes, or erythrocytes. It shares 32 percent homology with JAM-1. Based on monoclonal antibody binding studies, platelets contain approximately 1600 copies of JAM-3. Platelet JAM-3 acts as a counterreceptor for leukocyte $\alpha M\beta2$ and $\alpha X\beta2$ receptors and contributes to platelet–leukocyte interactions under some conditions.[762] Its precise role in platelet physiology is uncertain.

SELECTINS

P-Selectin (GMP140; PADGEM; CD62P) P-selectin, is an M_r 140,000 glycoprotein present in the membrane of α-granules in resting platelets that joins the plasma membrane when platelets are activated.[318,319,763] Approximately 13,000 P-selectin molecules are detected by antibodies on the surface of activated platelets. Therefore, expression of P-selectin on circulating platelets has been used as an indicator of in vivo activation of platelets.[54,486] It is present in the Weibel-Palade body membranes of endothelial cells and, as in platelets, joins the plasma membrane when endothelial cells are activated.[318,763]

P-selectin has a modular structure in which the amino-terminal region has a calcium-dependent lectin domain that binds carbohydrate-

containing structures. Adjacent to the lectin domain is an epidermal growth factor domain, followed by nine repeats that are homologous to complement regulatory proteins ("sushi" domains), a transmembrane domain, and a cytoplasmic domain (Fig. 105-18).[319,763] The cytoplasmic domain contains serine, threonine, tyrosine, and histidine residues that can be phosphorylated. In addition, a cysteine residue becomes acylated with stearic or palmitic acid. Alternatively spliced forms of P-selectin may be produced in which sushi domains are omitted. The selectin family also includes E-selectin (ELAM-1; CD62E), which is expressed on the surface of activated endothelial cells, and L-selectin (LAM-1; CD62L), which is present on myeloid and lymphoid cells.[764]

Soluble P-selectin is present in plasma from humans and mice. Alternative splicing generates a soluble form of human P-selectin that lacks the transmembrane domain.[765] In mice, a portion of soluble P-selectin is derived from proteolytic cleavage of surface P-selectin by an unidentified protease.[766]

Recognition of ligand by P-selectin requires specific carbohydrate and protein structures. Fucose and sialic acid are important carbohydrate components, with sialyl-3-fucosyl-N-acetyllactosamine (sLe^x; CD15S) a preferred ligand structure.[767–770] Myeloid and tumor cell sulfatides also may act as ligands for P-selectin.[771,772] PSGL-1, a mucin-like transmembrane glycoprotein homodimer (M_r 220,000) expressed on neutrophils, monocytes, lymphocytes, and to a small extent on platelets, is an important ligand for P-selectin.[323,773–775] Both sulfation of tyrosine residues contained in an anionic region and branched fucosylation of O-linked carbohydrates are required for optimal binding to P-selectin.

P-selectin can mediate the attachment of neutrophils and monocytes to platelets and endothelial cells. Thus, neutrophils and monocytes may be recruited to sites of vascular injury where platelets deposit and become activated (see "Platelet–Leukocyte Interactions" below). Platelet P-selectin can recruit procoagulant monocyte-derived microparticles containing both PSGL-1 and tissue factor to growing thrombi in vivo.[455] Binding of P-selectin to PSGL-1 on monocytes can trigger tissue factor synthesis,[776] and infusing a P-selectin chimeric molecule into mice results in generation of procoagulant microparticles.[777] Soluble P-selectin may promote a prothrombotic state in humans by increasing tissue factor-expressing microparticles in plasma. The risk of future cardiovascular events is elevated in apparently healthy women with the highest levels of soluble P-selectin.[778]

In intact blood vessels, the rapid on and off rates of the interactions between PSGL-1 on neutrophils and P-selectin on endothelial cells allow leukocytes to roll on the endothelium, the first step in leukocyte transmigration (see Chap. 68).[779] The rapid up-regulation of P-selectin after endothelial cell activation allows for a quick response. Platelets reportedly roll on activated endothelium, apparently from an interaction between endothelial P-selectin and perhaps either platelet GPIbα[276,714] or platelet PSGL-1.[321,323] Upon their co-release from endothelial Weibel-Palade bodies, P-selectin may tether ultralarge vWF multimers to the surface of activated endothelium and thereby promote GPIbα-mediated platelet rolling.[780]

Genetic and pharmacologic targeting of P-selectin or PSGL-1 in experimental animal models suggests these receptors may modulate thrombolysis, restenosis, deep venous thrombosis, cerebral ischemia and infarction, atherosclerosis, and thrombotic glomerulonephritis (reviewed in ref. 272).

TETRASPANINS

CD9 CD9 is a protein of 228 amino acids that contains four putative transmembrane domains, making it a member of the tetraspanin superfamily.[781,782] CD9 is present on endothelial cells, smooth muscle cells, cultured fibroblasts, some lymphoblasts, eosinophils, basophils, and other cells. CD9 is present at high density on the platelet surface (~40,000 molecules per platelet).[783] It colocalizes with αIIbβ3 on the inner surface of α-granules in resting platelets and on pseudopods of activated platelets.[784] Binding of monoclonal antibodies specific for CD9 to platelets results in platelet aggregation by triggering phosphoinositol metabolism via a mechanism that also requires binding to the platelet FcγRIIA receptor.[785–787] Platelet activation induced by binding of such antibodies requires external calcium and results in an association between CD9 and αIIbβ3.[788]

CD63 (Granulophysin; LAMP-3) CD63, a member of the tetraspanin superfamily of M_r 53,000, appears to be present in both lysosomal and dense granule membranes in platelets.[53,789] CD63 is present in Weibel-Palade bodies in endothelial cells, the lysosomal membranes of a variety of other cells, and the membranes of melanosomes. It joins the surface membrane when platelets are activated, making it a useful marker for platelet activation.[53,54] CD63 appears to be markedly reduced or absent from the dense bodies of patients with Hermansky-Pudlak syndrome,[789] who have oculocutaneous albinism and a defect in platelet dense bodies (see Chap. 112). The amino acid sequence of CD63 has been deduced from cDNA cloning.[790]

CD151 (PETA-3) CD151 is a glycoprotein member of the tetraspanin superfamily of M_r 27,000.[791,792] It is present on platelets, endothelial cells, and many other cells.[793] Antibodies to CD151, like those to CD9, can initiate platelet aggregation by binding to both CD151 and FcγRIIA.[791] The role of CD151 in platelet physiology remains to be firmly established, but it may participate with FcγRIIA as a signal transduction complex.[791] CD151 appears to functionally associate with αIIbβ3 and, in mice, loss of CD151 impairs platelet aggregation and clot retraction.[794]

GLYCOSYL PHOSPHATIDYLINOSITOL-ANCHORED PROTEINS (CD55, CD59, CD109, UROKINASE PLASMINOGEN ACTIVATOR RECEPTOR, PRION PROTEIN)

At least six separate platelet proteins are attached to the membrane through a glycosyl phosphatidylinositol (GPI) link. They include proteins involved in complement regulation (CD55, decay accelerating factor; CD59, membrane inhibitor of reactive lysis)[795]; CD109, an M_r 170,000 protein that carries both ABO oligosaccharides and an alloantigen (Gov) involved in neonatal isoimmune thrombocytopenia[796]; u-PAR, which binds urokinase plasminogen activator and has been implicated in fibrinolysis, platelet adhesion, and platelet survival[797,798]; and an M_r 500,000 protein of unknown identity. Patients with paroxysmal nocturnal hemoglobinuria (PNH) have abnormalities in the GPI anchor and thus variably lack all of the GPI-linked proteins. The diagnosis of PNH can be established by assessing platelet expression of these proteins.[799–801] Patients with PNH reportedly have platelet function abnormalities,[799] raising the possibility that one or more of these proteins has a role in platelet function, but no specific platelet function roles have yet been assigned to the proteins. Of particular interest is the presence of the normal prion protein, which is an M_r 27,000 to 30,000 GPI-linked protein that is both up-regulated and shed from the platelet surface with platelet activation.[802–805] Platelets contain the majority of the prion protein present in normal blood.

TYROSINE KINASE RECEPTORS

Eph Kinases and Ephrin Ligands Eph kinase receptors compose the largest family of cell surface-associated tyrosine kinases, with 14 members identified in mammals. Eph kinases have a conserved structure consisting of an amino-terminal extracellular ephrin-binding domain, two fibronectin type II repeats, and intracellular kinase, sterile α motif (SAM), and PDZ binding domains. A total of eight ephrins have been identified that serve as cell surface ligands for the Eph kinases. In general, Eph A kinases recognize ephrins that contain a GPI anchor (ephrin A family), whereas Eph B kinases bind to ligands with a transmembrane domain (ephrin B family). The Eph receptors and the ephrins appear to signal bidirectionally at sites of cell-to-cell contact. Platelets contain two Eph kinases, EphA4 and EphB1, and ephrin B1.[806] Messenger RNA for ephrinA3 has been detected in platelets, but confirmation of the presence of ephrinA3 protein in platelets is lacking. Forced clustering of either Eph kinases or ephrins in platelets promotes cytoskeletal reorganization, adhesion, granule secretion, and Rap1b activation in concert with other platelet stimuli.[806,807] Thus, Eph kinase–ephrin interactions may stabilize platelet aggregates after platelet–platelet contact has occurred.

Thrombopoietin Receptor (c-Mpl; CD110) The thrombopoietin receptor (M_r 80,000–84,000) is expressed at low levels on platelets (~25–224 per platelet) and binds thrombopoietin with high affinity (K_d ~ 0.50 nM).[808–810] Steady-state plasma levels of thrombopoietin are maintained by platelet and megakaryocyte thrombopoietin binding via the thrombopoietin receptor, with subsequent internalization of the complex and growth factor degradation. Although its major function is to stimulate megakaryocyte growth and maturation (see Chap. 104), thrombopoietin also can sensitize platelets to activation by agonists.[811–816]

Insulin Receptor Platelets express low levels of insulin receptors and respond to insulin stimulation by increasing expression of prostacyclin receptors.[817,818]

MISCELLANEOUS

CD40 Ligand (CD40L; CD154) and CD40 CD40L (CD154) is a trimeric transmembrane protein (M_r 33,000) of the tumor necrosis factor (TNF) family that localizes to α-granules in resting platelets and rapidly appears on the surface of platelets upon activation (see Fig. 105-9). Within minutes to hours of platelet activation, an 18,000-dalton fragment of CD40L is released from the platelet surface by an unidentified metalloproteinase. This soluble form of CD40L circulates as a trimer. The bulk of soluble CD40L in plasma is derived from activated platelets and can serve as a marker for platelet activation *in vivo*. Elevated levels of soluble CD40L are observed in acute coronary syndromes, following percutaneous coronary intervention, in the setting of coronary artery bypass surgery, and in peripheral vascular disease (reviewed in refs. 328 and 819).[327] Moreover, elevated levels of soluble CD40L are associated with recurrent cardiovascular events in the setting of acute coronary syndromes[327,820] and restenosis following percutaneous coronary intervention.[330] CD40L and, to a lesser extent, its counterreceptor CD40 have been implicated in the progression of atherosclerosis in animal models.

The extracellular portion of CD40L binds to CD40, a transmembrane receptor of M_r 48,000 daltons. Approximately 600 to 1000 copies of CD40 are present on both resting and activated platelets.[329] CD40L reportedly initiates platelet activation via binding to CD40,[821] but the functional significance of CD40–CD40L interactions in platelet physiology remains to be determined. CD40L also contains a KGD sequence (RGD in mice) that has been implicated in binding to αIIbβ3. In mice, CD40L–αIIbβ3 interactions appear to stabilize thrombus growth,[329] perhaps by activating receptor mediated signaling.[325] Additionally, αIIbβ3 antagonists block the release of soluble CD40L from activated platelets. Both platelet-associated and soluble CD40L may stimulate CD40-bearing leukocytes to release proinflammatory cytokines. CD40L may inhibit endothelial cell migration after vascular injury.[822] The inhibitory affects of CD40L on reendothelialization may partially explain why elevated levels of soluble CD40L are associated with higher rates of clinical restenosis.[330] Finally, platelet CD40L may modulate adaptive immunity by serving as a costimulatory signal for antigen-presenting cells.[823,824]

GPIV (CD36) GPIV (CD36) is an M_r 88,000 glycoprotein that is highly, but variably, expressed on platelets (~20,000 copies per platelet).[124,825–827] Biochemical data suggest that it may form dimers and multimers.[828] Increased platelet surface expression of GPIV has been described in patients with myeloproliferative disorders.[829] It is present on monocytes, endothelial cells, hematopoietic cell lines, and melanoma cells. It has been proposed as a platelet receptor for TSP[830] and collagen,[831,832] but the functional significance of these interactions remains unclear because individuals who lack GPIV (CD36) on an inherited basis (Nak^a-negative) do not have a bleeding disorder[833] (see Chap. 112). GPIV (CD36) may play a role in the TSP-mediated interaction reported between platelets and sickle erythrocytes[834] and in the binding of *Plasmodium falciparum*–infected erythrocytes to endothelial cells and monocytes.[835] CD36 has been implicated in monocyte binding of oxidized low-density lipoprotein (LDL; scavenger receptor) and myocardial uptake of long-chain fatty acids.[836] It has been implicated in the metabolic syndrome involving hypertension, diabetes, and accelerated atherosclerosis, and in angiogenesis and inflammation.[837–840]

The nucleotide sequence of GPIV cDNA encodes a protein of 471 residues with an M_r of 53,000 and 10 potential N-linked glycosylation sites.[835] It is unusual because it has two putative transmembrane domains and two short cytoplasmic tails. The cytoplasmic regions may associate with intracellular tyrosine kinases of the Src family and undergo phosphorylation.[841] Moreover, the phosphorylation status of the extracellular region of the protein may control its ligand-binding properties,[123] offering a potential explanation for some of the variable results obtained under different conditions.[123,124,842]

LAMP-1 and LAMP-2 (CD107a, CD107b) LAMP-1 and LAMP-2 are lysosome-associated membrane proteins that are approximately 30 percent homologous. They are integral membrane glycoproteins (M_r 110,000 and 120,000, respectively) that are contained within lysosomal membranes.[843] When platelets undergo the release reaction, they join the plasma membrane. Each protein has two extracellular disulfide-bonded loops containing 36 to 38 amino acids. The loops are separated by a region rich in proline and serine that shares homology with the hinge region of IgA. Multiple N-linked glycosylation sites are present on each glycoprotein, and they contain more than 60 percent carbohydrate. Among the carbohydrate residues are polylactosaminoglycans that may possess sLe^x structures, which are thought to interact with selectins (see section above on "Selectins").

C1q Receptors Platelets have several receptors for C1q, an M_r 460,000 glycoprotein composed of six globular domains attached to a short collagen-like triple helix.[844–846] One receptor is for the collagen-like domain (cC1qR, M_r 60,000–67,000 nonreduced and 72,000–75,000 reduced). The second receptor is for the globular domain (gC1qR, M_r 28,000–33,000).[847,848] A third receptor of M_r 126,000 enhances phagocytosis.[849] C1q circulates with C1r and C1s as a calcium-dependent complex, but interaction with immune complexes ultimately leads to dissociation of the complex and release of free C1q, with its collagen-like domain exposed. cC1qR has sequence homology to calreticulin and can modulate platelet–collagen interactions at low collagen concentrations. It may localize immune complexes and, when cross-linked by aggregated C1q, can initiate platelet activation, aggregation, secretion, and expression of platelet coagulant activity.[850] Binding of C1q monomers to platelets inhibits collagen-induced platelet aggregation but has little effect on platelet adhesion to collagen.[851] C1q multimers, however, support platelet adhesion and can induce aggregation via activation of αIIbβ3.[850] C1q can augment platelet ag-

gregation induced by aggregated IgG.[754] gC1qR may self-associate to form a doughnut-shaped ternary complex.[852] In addition to binding C1q, this receptor can bind *Staphylococcus aureus* protein A on endothelial cells, where it functions as a receptor for high molecular weight kininogen.[848] It may, therefore, participate in contact activation.

67-kDa Laminin Receptor An M_r 67,000 protein identified as a laminin receptor on several different cells has been detected on platelets. It can mediate platelet adhesion to laminin under certain conditions.[604] The relative roles of this receptor and the integrin receptor $\alpha 6\beta 1$, which also mediates the interaction between platelets and laminin, are unknown.

GMP-33 (Thrombospondin Amino-Terminal Fragment) An M_r 33,000 α-granule membrane protein was initially identified as an activation-dependent protein that joins the plasma membrane when platelets undergo the release reaction. Approximately 4000 antibody molecules directed against GMP-33 bind to unactivated platelets and 19,000 bind to activated platelets.[853] Subsequent studies identified this antigen as a membrane-associated fragment from the amino-terminus of TSP.[854]

Leukosialin, Sialophorin (CD43) Leukosialin, a glycoprotein of M_r 90,000, may act as a ligand for ICAM-1.[855] It is expressed on myeloid and some lymphoid cells. Abnormalities in leukosialin have been described in Wiskott-Aldrich syndrome (see Chap. 112).

Toll-Like Receptors 1 and 6 Toll-like receptors are involved in innate immunity by virtue of their ability to sense products of protozoa, fungi, viruses, and bacteria, including endotoxin, and then activate intracellular signaling pathways to initiate the inflammatory response.[856] The receptors have been identified in atherosclerotic lesions.[857] Toll-like receptors 1 and 6 have been identified in platelets and in platelet-rich coronary thrombi, but the role of these receptors in platelet function is not established.[858]

Peroxisome Proliferator-Activated Receptors γ Peroxisome proliferator-activated receptors (PPAR) are a nuclear hormone receptor family of ligand-activated transcription factors.[859] PPARγ is one of the three PPAR subtypes and is widely expressed in white adipose tissue, macrophages, B and T lymphocytes, smooth muscle cells, fibroblasts, and endothelial cells. It has been implicated in metabolism, insulin responsiveness, adipocyte differentiation, immune function, and inflammation. PPARγ is present in platelets in a conformation that can bind to DNA, suggesting that an endogenous ligand is present in platelets, perhaps lysophosphatidic acid (LPA).[859] PPARγ agonists decrease thrombin-induced platelet aggregation and release of ATP, thromboxane, and CD40L. Thus, PPARγ appears to downregulate platelet activation.

Fas Ligand Fas ligand (FasL) is a membrane glycoprotein that, like CD40L, belongs to the TNF family of cytokines.[860] Its receptor, Fas (Apo-1, CD95), is expressed on a wide variety of normal and malignant cells. Engagement of Fas by FasL initiates signaling that results in apoptosis, and this process is important in embryonic development, cellular hemostasis, and immune regulation. Resting platelets contain FasL but do not express it on the platelet surface.[860] With activation, platelets both express FasL on their surface and release a soluble form of FasL, analogous to activation-dependent CD40L platelet expression and release. The surface-expressed FasL on platelets is biologically active and can initiate apoptosis. The soluble form of FasL may act as an inhibitor of apoptosis induced by surface-expressed FasL.[860]

PLATELETS AND THROMBOLYSIS

The interactions between platelets and the fibrinolytic system are complex. Table 105-9 contains a partial listing.[861–864] Both profibrinolytic[134,566,865–871] and antifibrinolytic[872–880] effects of platelets have been described, and predicting the net effect is difficult. Because platelet-rich thrombi resist thrombolysis in animal models, the antifibrinolytic effects of platelets appear to predominate *in vivo*.[881]

The effects of fibrinolytic agents on platelets are complex. Considerable evidence indicates that fibrinolytic agents can activate platelets soon after administration,[882-888] via either a direct effect of plasmin,[889-892] perhaps acting on PAR-4,[893] or an indirect effect through the paradoxical generation of thrombin.[863,894-897] Interpretation of the latter studies are complicated by the reported ability of tissue plasminogen activator to release fibrinopeptides from fibrinogen, one of the hallmarks of thrombin activation.[898]

Stimulation of platelets by thrombolytic agents may prolong the time required for reperfusion of blood vessels occluded by thrombi and may contribute to reocclusion after successful reperfusion.[261,861] In animal models and in humans, potent antiplatelet agents can speed reperfusion, abolish reocclusion, and diminish the size of myocardial infarcts.[899-901] However, in large-scale clinical trials, the benefits of combining $\alpha IIb\beta3$ antagonists with fibrinolytic agents in enhancing coronary thrombolysis have been counterbalanced by an increase in major hemorrhage.[902] In experimental models of stroke, paradoxically, early treatment with an $\alpha IIb\beta3$ antagonist reduces the hemorrhage associated with thrombolytic therapy, perhaps by preventing platelet aggregation in the microcirculation and the release of agents that can damage the vasculature and diminish its integrity.[55,903,904]

With prolonged use of thrombolytic agents, inhibition of platelet function may occur via a variety of mechanisms[228,885,888,905-915] that might contribute to some of the hemorrhagic phenomena and prolonged bleeding times observed with this therapy. The inhibition may be caused by the thrombolytic agents making the platelets refractory to further stimulation.

PLATELET—LEUKOCYTE INTERACTIONS, PLATELET-TISSUE FACTOR INTERACTIONS, AND THE ROLE OF PLATELETS IN INFLAMMATION

Leukocytes can bind to activated platelets and in model systems transmigrate through a platelet monolayer (reviewed in ref. 916) (see Fig. 105-9). Animal models and studies of human tissue demonstrate that within hours after vascular injury, leukocytes become enmeshed in platelet thrombi and/or transiently form a monolayer on top of adherent or aggregated platelets.[917,918] The surface association of leukocytes with platelets is transient, lasting less than 1 day. These interactions may be important at sites of vascular injury where leukocytes deposit on adherent and aggregated platelets. Such deposition of leukocytes has been associated with the development of intimal hyperplasia after vascular injury in animal models.[919] By depositing chemokines such as RANTES (CCL5) on activated endothelium[920,921] or by direct interactions with leukocytes,[922] platelets may enhance leukocyte recruitment to inflamed or atherosclerotic endothelium and thereby promote the development and progression of atherosclerosis.

Many mechanisms of platelet—leukocyte interactions have been defined, but the initial interaction appears to be mediated primarily by the interaction between P-selectin (CD62P) expressed on the surface of activated platelets and PSGL-1 on the surface of neutrophils and monocytes.[763,767,923-927] P-selectin—PSGL-1 interactions are characterized by rapid on and off rates that promote tethering and rolling of leukocytes along adherent platelets. These transient interactions are stabilized by subsequent contacts mediated largely by activation of leukocyte $\beta2$ integrins. Platelets can synthesize and release PAF, which can activate leukocyte $\alpha M\beta2$, as can the CXC chemokines released by activated platelets, ENA-78 and GRO-α, and the chemokine NAP-2 produced by the action of leukocyte cathepsin G on β-thromboglobulin secreted by platelets (reviewed in refs. 78 and 928) (see

TABLE 105-9 PLATELETS AND THROMBOLYSIS

Profibrinolytic effects of platelets

Tissue plasminogen activator (t-PA) and single-chain urokinase-type t-PA identified on or in platelets.

Unactivated platelets bind plasminogen, and binding is enhanced by thrombin.

Thrombospondin, a plasminogen-binding protein, is expressed on the surface of platelets after activation.

Activation of plasminogen by t-PA is enhanced by platelets.

Clot lysis is enhanced by platelets in some model systems.

Antifibrinolytic effects of platelets

Plasminogen activator inhibitor-1 and α_2-antiplasmin are present in platelet granules.

Platelets release a protein that stimulates cells to release a fibrinolysis inhibitor.

Platelets contain factor XIII, which can cross-link fibrin, making it resist fibrinolysis, and can cross-link α_2-antiplasmin to fibrin, enhancing its antifibrinolytic effects.

Platelet $\alpha IIb\beta3$ can bind plasma factor XIIIa directly or indirectly, localizing it to the site of thrombus formation.

Platelets facilitate clot retraction, which diminishes the efficiency of fibrinolysis.

Platelet-activating effects of thrombolytic agents

Streptokinase and t-PA activate platelets *in vivo* and *in vitro*.

Plasmin, at high doses, can aggregate platelets.

Thrombolytic agents may paradoxically generate the potent platelet agonist thrombin or release it from thrombi.

Thrombolytic agents may blunt the prostacyclin increase that accompanies acute thrombosis.

Platelet-inhibiting effects of thrombolytic agents

Plasmin, at low doses, can inhibit platelet activation and aggregation.

Platelets can be disaggregated by t-PA by selective lysis of platelet-bound fibrinogen.

Plasmin can cause redistribution and/or cleavage of platelet glycoprotein Ib.

Inhibition of platelet aggregation by the depletion of plasma fibrinogen, if severe, and generation of fibrin(ogen) degradation products.

Proteolysis of plasma von Willebrand factor.

Prolongation of bleeding time.

SOURCE: Adapted from BS Coller, [261] with permission.

Fig. 105-7). Activated $\alpha M\beta2$ on leukocytes can interact with platelet GPIbα[322] and with platelet-bound fibrinogen via a region(s) on the γ-chain (amino acids 190–202[929] and 377–395[930]). TSP may serve as a bridging molecule between GPIV (CD36) receptors, which are expressed on both platelets and mononuclear cells.[931] Platelets have ICAM-2 on their surface, which is a ligand for the leukocyte integrin receptor $\alpha L\beta2$. Although this ligand—receptor interaction appears to have only a minor role in platelet—leukocyte adhesion, it may be more important in leukocyte tethering.[928]

Transcellular metabolism of eicosanoids can result in production of unique products (see Chap. 117), and leukocytes can modify platelet activation.[932] In a complementary fashion, the intimate relationship between leukocytes and platelets allows the latter to contribute to the inflammatory response, including the release of chemokines that can activate leukocytes: PDGF, which can affect fibroblast and smooth muscle cells; TGF-$\beta1$, which both stimulates and inhibits cellular growth; and PF4, which can prime neutrophils and has antiangiogenic activity. Platelets contain FcγIIA receptors that can localize IgG and immune complexes, resulting in complement activation. Finally, platelets express CD40L on their surface after activation, and this molecule can interact with CD40 on leukocytes and endothelial cells, leading to their activation and elaboration of a number of proinflammatory molecules (see "CD40 Ligand [CD40L; CD154] and CD40" above).[324,933,934] Platelet CD40L also promotes procoagulant activity in endothelial cells.[935]

Platelet–leukocyte interactions may be important in the initiation of coagulation and fibrin formation through a P-selectin–dependent pathway. Platelet–leukocyte aggregates facilitate thrombin generation to a greater extent than either platelets or leukocytes alone.[936,937] Coincubation of platelets and leukocytes generates tissue factor activity, partly through P-selectin–PSGL-1 interactions. Induction of tissue factor activity involves both *de novo* protein synthesis and exposure ("de-encryption") of latent tissue factor. The latter may occur by P-selectin–mediated production of tissue factor containing microparticles from leukocytes. Real-time imaging of platelet thrombus formation *in vivo* indicates tissue factor accumulates in growing thrombi before leukocytes become associated with thrombus. Accumulation of tissue factor and fibrin formation at the site of thrombus depends on both platelet P-selectin and PSGL-1. These observations, coupled with the finding of bloodborne tissue factor antigen in circulation,[266] has led to a model in which platelet P-selectin recruits tissue factor-containing leukocyte microparticles to platelet-rich thrombi.[267] In mice, increases in soluble P-selectin levels promote a procoagulant state associated with elevated levels of leukocyte-derived microparticles.[938] A P-selectin–Ig chimeric molecule can increase levels of leukocyte-derived microparticles *in vitro* and normalize the bleeding time in hemophilia A mice.[777]

Several clinical observations support a potential role for platelet–leukocyte interactions in vascular disease, including the presence of circulating platelet–leukocyte aggregates in patients with unstable angina[939] and after coronary artery angioplasty.[940] In the latter situation, the presence of such aggregates appears to confer a worse prognosis for ischemic vascular complications.[940] Circulating platelet–leukocyte aggregates are perhaps the most sensitive indicator of systemic platelet activation, reflecting the expression of P-selectin on the surface of platelets.[941] Analysis of polymorphisms of PSGL-1 involving variable numbers of tandem repeats demonstrated that the longer PSGL-1 molecules were better able to form platelet–leukocyte aggregates and the longer polymorphisms are associated with increased cerebrovascular disease.[653]

SIGNALING PATHWAYS IN PLATELET ACTIVATION AND AGGREGATION

OVERVIEW

Platelets generally circulate in a quiescent state but are poised to be activated in response to a variety of agonists that become available at sites of vascular injury or ruptured atherosclerotic plaques (see Fig. 105-10). A number of different phenomena occur with platelet activation (Table 105-10). Agonists differ in their intrinsic ability to produce these phenomena, and added complexity derives from differences in dose responses to each agonist and the synergistic effects of agonists used in combination. Agonists are diverse (see Table 105-6 and Fig. 105-10) and include small and large soluble molecules, enzymes, and immobilized adhesive glycoproteins. They can be classified as either "strong" or "weak," depending on whether full activation, including the release reaction, can be initiated without the augmenting effect of platelet aggregation itself (see Table 105-6). Low doses of strong agonists behave like weak agonists. Most agonists are released, synthesized, or formed at the site of vascular injury, which undoubtedly serves to localize the response.

Agonists bind to receptors of two general categories: seven transmembrane, G-protein coupled receptors and receptors that can initiate phosphorylation of target proteins (see Fig. 105-12). In both cases, a sequence of signaling events ultimately leads to platelet activation. Physiologic responses of platelets to agonists are listed in Table 105-

TABLE 105-10 PHENOMENA ASSOCIATED WITH PLATELET ACTIVATION

Increased platelet cytosolic calcium

Shape change

Change in $\alpha IIb\beta 3$ to high-affinity ligand-binding conformation(s)

Generation of arachidonic acid metabolites (e.g., thromboxane A_2)

Phosphorylation of select platelet proteins

Platelet aggregation

Induction of platelet coagulant activity

Generation of microparticles that are procoagulant and proinflammatory

Release of α-granule contents

Release of dense granule contents

Release of lysosomal contents

Surface expression of proteins contained in lysosomal membranes

Surface expression of proteins contained in α-granule membranes, e.g., P-selectin

Recruitment of microvesicles containing tissue factor from blood

Recruitment of circulating neutrophils and monocytes via P-selectin

10. Many of the responses lead to activation of the $\alpha IIb\beta 3$ receptor to a high-affinity ligand-binding state and subsequent platelet aggregation. Moreover, binding of ligands to platelets and platelet aggregation itself further propagate signals that are required for stabilization of platelet aggregates and clot retraction. The major agonists, receptors, and signaling pathways involved in the early stages of platelet activation that lead to shape change, granule secretion, and platelet aggregation and the postaggregation signaling events are described in this section.

AGONIST-INDUCED PLATELET ACTIVATION

Many platelet agonists initiate platelet activation by binding to seven transmembrane heterotrimeric, G-protein coupled receptors, such as the $P2Y_1$ ADP receptor (see Figs. 105-5, 105-12, and 105-19). When such receptors are activated, the $G\alpha$ subunit exchanges guanosine diphosphate (GDP) for guanosine triphosphate (GTP) and dissociates from the β,γ complex. The free $G\alpha$ subunit and, in some cases, the β,γ complex can activate some relatively common downstream pathways and initiate positive feedback loops (see Fig. 105-11). Activation of these pathways usually is intertwined. One common pathway involves the activation of one or more isozymes of PLC, leading to phosphoinositide hydrolysis. Three classes of PLC (β, γ, δ), have been described, and multiple isozymes exist within each class.[942] The most well-studied PLCs in platelets include PLCβ and PLCγ2. PLCβ often is activated downstream of the seven transmembrane G-protein coupled, receptor family, whereas PLCγ2 can be activated by phosphorylation on tyrosine, which is a downstream signal from other types of agonist receptors. PLC of either type hydrolyzes phospholipids between the glycerol backbone and the phosphate moiety. The PLCβ class is relatively specific for phosphoinositides, whereas PLCγ also can cleave other types of phospholipids. The hydrolysis of one particular phosphoinositide, phosphatidylinositol-4,5-bisphosphate, by either class of PLC is critical in platelet function because it results in the formation of two important products: IP_3 and diacylglycerol (DAG). IP_3 binds to specific receptors on the dense tubular system, causing a release of intracellular calcium, which is important for activation of a number of signaling enzymes and proteins involved in cytoskeletal reorganization (see section on "Additional Intermediate Signaling Molecules" below), and for platelet granule fusion and the release reaction. DAG binds to PKC and participates in its conversion to an active enzyme. For many agonists, activation of one or more of the multiple isozymes of PKC is an obligatory step in the conversion of $\alpha IIb\beta 3$ to a high-affinity fibrinogen receptor and subsequent platelet aggrega-

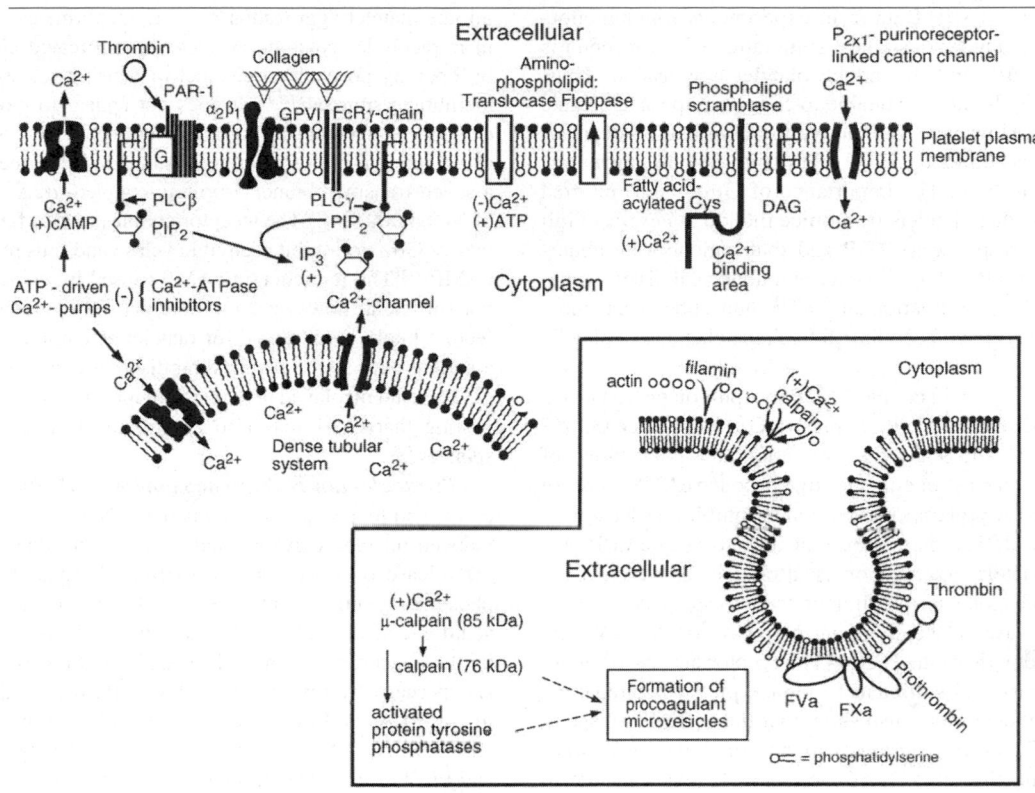

FIGURE 105-19 Schematic representation of platelet calcium homeostasis and the reactions leading to procoagulant expression. Thrombin activates protease-activated receptor-1 (PAR-1), which interacts with G proteins and stimulates phospholipase $C\beta$ (PLCβ) to split phosphatidylinositol-4,5-bisphosphate (PIP$_2$) into 1,2-diacylglycerol (DAG) and inositol-1,4,5-triphosphate (IP$_3$). Collagen binds to the integrin receptor $\alpha 2\beta 1$ (GPIa-IIa) and activates platelets through tyrosine phosphorylation of the Fc receptor γ-chain (FcR γ-chain), which is associated with the membrane glycoprotein GPVI. This action leads to tyrosine phosphorylation and activation of PLCγ2, which, like PLCβ, splits PIP$_2$ and produces IP$_3$. The IP$_3$ opens Ca^{2+} channels in the intracellular membrane system called the *dense tubular system*, which serves as an intracellular Ca^{2+} store. ATP-driven Ca^{2+} pumps, both in dense tubular system membranes and in the plasma membrane, carry Ca^{2+} out of the cytosol by active transport. This process can be inhibited by specific Ca^{2+}-ATPase inhibitors. Further platelet activation via diacylglycerol (DAG) and protein kinase C and activation of phospholipase A$_2$ with formation of thromboxane A$_2$ are not shown. Activation of the phospholipid scramblase by Ca^{2+} ions and a concomitant Ca^{2+}-mediated inhibition of ATP-dependent aminophospholipid translocase that serves to maintain the normal phospholipid asymmetry lead to translocation of negatively charged phosphatidylserine to the outer membrane bilayer. This is a prerequisite for formation of the complexes of coagulation factors on the platelet surface. Ca^{2+}-induced activation of the proteolytic enzyme calpain is important for formation of microvesicles (microparticles). Protein tyrosine phosphatase activities are associated with calpain activation and microvesiculation in an as yet unknown manner. The microparticles express a procoagulant surface. Substances that activate or inhibit the various processes are labeled with plus (+) or minus (−), respectively. FVa, factor Va; FXa, factor Xa. (From NO Solum,[7] with permission.)

tion.[554,943,944] One consequence of PKC activation is the release of ADP from dense granules. Released ADP acts at its own seven transmembrane G-protein coupled receptors to potentiate the action of numerous agonists. The precise mechanism(s) by which PKC causes $\alpha IIb\beta 3$ activation remains unclear.

Activation of a number of receptors leads to activation of phospholipase A$_2$ (PLA$_2$), which releases arachidonic acid from membrane lipid stores. Arachidonic acid is rapidly converted to the prostaglandin (PG) products PGH$_2$ and thromboxane A$_2$ (TXA$_2$), which are themselves potent activators of platelet aggregation (see below).

P2Y$_1$, P2Y$_{12}$, and P2X$_1$ Purine Receptors for ADP and ATP
Platelets express receptors for both ADP and ATP (see Fig. 105-5). Both nucleotides are present in platelet dense granules and are secreted when platelets are activated by adequate concentrations of most, if not all, agonists. Another source of these nucleotides is red blood cells. Damaged red blood cells or those subjected to high shear stress may release ADP and ATP, increasing their local concentrations. ADP is

an especially important physiologic agonist, not only because it can induce platelet aggregation independent of other agonists but because secreted ADP contributes significantly to the full aggregation response induced by many other agonists. This finding has been convincingly demonstrated in experimental systems in which secreted ADP is rapidly degraded or inhibited. Moreover, submaximal concentrations of ADP synergize with other agonists, and this phenomenon has been most well studied with epinephrine (see below). ADP induces or contributes to a variety of responses in platelets: shape change, granule release, TXA$_2$ production, activation of $\alpha IIb\beta 3$, and platelet aggregation.[945] Pharmacologic and cloning and sequencing studies suggest ADP exerts its full effect on platelets through at least two different receptors (P2Y$_1$ and P2Y$_{12}$). These receptors are G-protein coupled and are responsible for most of the physiologic effects of ADP.

The platelet P2Y$_1$ receptor has been cloned and sequenced. Like most heterotrimeric G-protein coupled receptors, it is predicted to span the membrane seven times.[946] Data from experiments with inhibitors of P2Y$_1$ and mice lacking P2Y$_1$ suggest stimulation of this receptor is necessary, but not sufficient, to induce platelet aggregation. Thus, platelets from P2Y$_1$-null mice are unable to change shape or aggregate in response to ADP. However, ADP activation does cause a decrease in cAMP via its effects on P2Y$_{12}$.[947,948] P2Y$_1$ couples to heterotrimeric G-proteins containing Gαq. The importance of Gαq can be inferred from the observation that platelets from mice that do not express Gαq do not aggregate in response to ADP and that patients with abnormalities in Gαq have a bleeding disorder and abnormal platelet function (see Chap. 112).[949] Activation of PLCβ and subsequent phosphoinositide hydrolysis have been linked to shape change and platelet activation.

P2Y$_{12}$, the other G-protein coupled ADP receptor on platelets, also has been cloned and sequenced. It couples to Gαi rather than Gαq[950] (reviewed in refs. 951 and 952). Gαi activation causes inhibition of the adenylyl cyclases, a class of enzymes that produce cAMP. Because cAMP activates type A protein kinases, which inhibit platelet activation by a variety of effects, the notion that inhibition of cAMP production promotes platelet aggregation is attractive. However, a decreased cAMP level alone is insufficient to activate platelets.[953,954] Synergistic effects between the signaling pathways of the P2Y$_1$ and P2Y$_{12}$ receptors (and perhaps the P2X$_1$ ATP receptor discussed below) appear to be necessary and sufficient to induce platelet aggregation. Data from P2Y$_{12}$-deficient mice also show that their platelets respond only weakly to ADP and less vigorously than normal to other agonists such as collagen and thrombin.[955] Studies of P2Y$_{12}$ knockout mice demonstrate that P2Y$_{12}$ contributes to multiple steps during thrombosis, including platelet adhesion and activation, thrombus growth, and thrombus stability.[956]

P2X$_1$, the third purine nucleotide receptor on platelets, is a member of the P2X family of ligand-gated ion channels rather than a G-protein coupled receptor.[957] This receptor is predicted to span the plasma membrane twice and is largely extracellular.[958] Although P2X$_1$ has been described as both an ATP and an ADP receptor, the bulk of current evidence suggests it is an ATP receptor that is antagonized by ADP.[959,960] Because ATP antagonizes the P2Y$_{12}$ receptor, the overall contribution of P2X$_1$, which is stimulated by ATP, to platelet activation is not clear. Nonetheless, ATP is released from platelets upon stimulation with agonists such as collagen,[961] and ATP binding to P2X$_1$ causes a rapid calcium influx.[962] However, a calcium influx induced by stimulation of this receptor alone does not appear to be sufficient to induce platelet shape change or aggregation.[953] However, it does synergize with the P2Y platelet ADP receptors.[962] This synergy likely results from the specific downstream signaling events evoked by ATP stimulation of this receptor, which include calcium influx and extracellular signal-related kinase (ERK) 2 activation.[961] Support for a biologically important role for this receptor comes from data on both mice with targeted deletions of P2X$_1$, which have impaired *in vivo* thrombus formation,[963] and mice that overexpress P2X$_1$, which have a prothrombotic phenotype.[964] A variant of P2X$_1$ P(2X1del), which lacks 17 amino acids, has been described in megakaryocyte-like cell lines,[965] but its functional role is uncertain.[959,960]

Several antiplatelet agents inhibit ADP-induced platelet activation. Thus, metabolites of ticlopidine and clopidogrel inhibit the P2Y$_{12}$ receptor (see Chap. 21), whereas soluble CD39 catabolizes ADP and ATP.[966]

Epinephrine When added to platelet-rich plasma, epinephrine uniquely initiates a first phase of aggregation without first inducing shape change. After a plateau period, a second wave of aggregation occurs. The ability of epinephrine to synergize with other agonists, such as ADP, is well documented, but controversy exists as to whether epinephrine, in the absence of released ADP or TXA$_2$, is sufficient to

initiate platelet aggregation.[967–969] Epinephrine can cause an elevation in intracellular calcium, even in aspirin-treated platelets,[967] possibly by opening an external channel or causing release of calcium from membrane sources.[968,969] It does not appear to mobilize intracellular calcium or generate measurable amounts of IP$_3$. Analysis of the purified epinephrine receptor and its nucleotide sequence identified it as a seven transmembrane, G-protein coupled, α2A adrenergic receptor of M_r 64,000.[970,971] The receptor couples to Gαi family members, primarily Gαz, to inhibit adenylyl cyclase and thus prevent formation of cAMP.[972] The reduction in cAMP caused by epinephrine probably is not sufficient, however, to initiate platelet aggregation, and other effectors likely are required for platelet activation.[973–976] Platelets from a patient with a chronic bleeding disorder contained reduced amounts of Gαi1 and displayed impaired epinephrine-induced aggregation, suggesting that Gαi1 may also contribute to epinephrine-mediated responses.[977]

Prostaglandin H$_2$/Thromboxane A$_2$ The metabolism of arachidonic acid to TXA$_2$ is a fundamental pathway contributing to agonist-induced platelet activation and aggregation. Many agonists stimulate the release of arachidonic acid from phosphatidylcholine (PC) and phosphatidyl ethanolamine (PE) in the plasma membrane.[978] Most arachidonic acid is released by the action of PLA$_2$, but some is released by the concerted actions of PLC and DAG kinase, followed by PLA$_2$ and perhaps by the action of PLC followed by the action of DAG lipase. PLA$_2$ is a cytosolic enzyme, with multiple isoforms in platelets.[979] PLA$_2$ acts on the C2 position of triacylglycerols such as PC and PE, forming free arachidonic acid and the resulting lysophospholipid. PLA$_2$ also converts phosphatidic acid into lysophosphatidic acid (LPA), which is also a platelet agonist. Some PLA$_2$ isozymes are activated by the increase in intracellular platelet calcium that occurs during agonist-stimulated activation, whereas other isozymes are activated in a calcium-independent manner.

Arachidonic acid subsequently is metabolized by prostaglandin H$_2$ synthase-1 (cyclooxygenase-1 [COX-1]) to PGG$_2$ and then to PGH$_2$.[980,981] Thromboxane synthase next converts PGH$_2$ to TXA$_2$, which is spontaneously and rapidly converted to the inactive metabolite TXB$_2$.[982] TXA$_2$ and its precursor PGH$_2$ both can stimulate platelet thromboxane receptors to induce platelet aggregation.[982–984] An inducible cyclo-oxygenase enzyme (COX-2) is present in many cells involved in mediating the inflammatory response and megakaryocytes, but only trace amounts are present in normal platelets.[985,986] COX inhibitors, such as aspirin, inhibit platelet function by inhibiting COX-1 and decreasing TXA$_2$ production.[982] Some patients whose platelets are resistant to aspirin inhibition have been hypothesized to have increased amounts of COX-2, which is not as readily inhibited by aspirin as COX-1.[983]

TXA$_2$ is a potent platelet agonist that exerts its effects via interaction with specific members of the thromboxaneprostanoid receptor (TP) family of G-protein coupled receptors. The two TP isoforms in human platelets (TPα and TPβ) arise from alternative splicing of exon 3 of the TP gene. TPβ, but not TPα, undergoes agonist-induced internalization.[987] Although both TPα and TPβ mRNA can be detected in platelet lysates, TPα appears to be the dominant form.[988] The TXA$_2$ receptor has been localized to the platelet plasma membrane.[989] On sodium dodecyl sulfate-polyacrylamide gel electrophoresis, it migrates as a broad band of apparent M_r 55,000 to 57,000[990,991] because of variability in glycosylation.[988] Pharmacologic studies have suggested the existence of two distinct TXA$_2$ receptor subtypes based on differing affinities for agonist ligands. The low-affinity binding sites may mediate platelet aggregation and granule secretion, whereas the high-affinity sites seem to be associated with platelet shape change.[992] Studies of TP-deficient mice demonstrate this gene locus is responsible for most, if not all, of the biologic effects attributed to TXA$_2$.[993] Bleeding

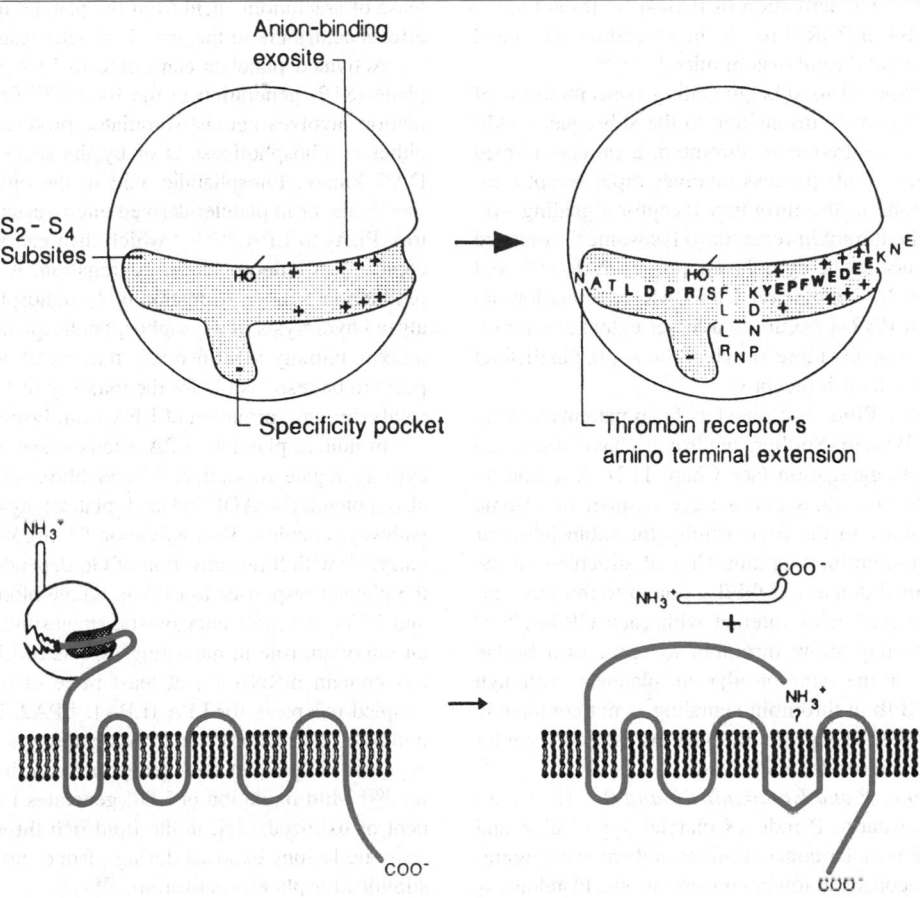

FIGURE 105-20   Model for thrombin–protease activated receptor-1 (PAR-1) interactions. *(Top left)* Thrombin is depicted as a ball with a groove containing its subsites, positively charged anion-binding exosite, and negatively charged pocket that confers ligand binding specificity. The active site serine is depicted by the serine hydroxyl (OH) group. *(Top right)* The receptor's LDPR sequence interacts with thrombin's subsites, the receptor's negatively charged YEPFWEDEE sequence binds to thrombin's anion-binding exosite, and the positively charged loop interacts with the specificity pocket. Thrombin cleaves the receptor between R41 and S42. *(Bottom)* After cleavage, the new amino-terminus acts as a tethered ligand and inserts into the membrane, initiating activation. (From TK Vu, DT Hung, VI Wheaton, et al.,[1008] with permission.)

times in these mice are prolonged, confirming the importance of this pathway in normal hemostasis. Platelet aggregation to collagen, but not ADP, is delayed, demonstrating the importance of TXA_2 production to the collagen response in platelets. TXA_2 pathways activate $G\alpha q$,[949,994] $G\alpha 12$ and $G\alpha 13$,[995,996] $G\alpha 11$,[997] and $G\alpha i2$.[998,999] Activation of $G\alpha q$ is essential for aggregation and secretion, whereas the $G\alpha 12/\alpha 13$ pathways contribute to shape change and aggregation.[1000–1002] At present, whether TP directly couples to $G\alpha i$[1003] or activates this pathway indirectly via released ADP is unclear.[999,1000] A significant portion of PGH_2/TXA_2-induced platelet aggregation actually is mediated by secreted ADP, as ADP scavenger systems inhibit aggregation induced by a stable PGH_2/TXA_2 analogue either partially (30%)[1004] or totally.[1003]

Thrombin   Thrombin is derived from the inactive zymogen prothrombin, which circulates in plasma. When acted upon by the prothrombinase complex (factor Xa, factor Va, Ca^{2+}) assembled on the membrane of activated platelets and other cells, prothrombin is cleaved into thrombin (see Chap. 106),[1005] one of the most potent platelet agonists. The proteolytic activity of thrombin is required for its role as a platelet agonist.[1006] Thrombin activates the protease-activated receptor (PAR)-1, a seven transmembrane G-protein coupled receptor on

platelets and other cells,[1007,1008] by cleaving an extracellular 41-amino-acid peptide from the amino-terminus of the receptor (Fig. 105-20). Removal of this peptide results in a new amino-terminus that acts as a "tethered ligand" by binding to another region of PAR-1 to activate the receptor and initiate signal transduction. Short peptides modeled after the "tethered ligand" region (e.g., SFLLRN) also activate PAR-1 signaling. The 41-amino-acid cleavage product of PAR-1 also can induce platelet aggregation by a poorly defined mechanism.[1009]

Cloning of PAR-1 and gene deletion experiments in mice led to the discovery of additional members of the PAR family.[1010,1011] PAR-1 and PAR-4 are the main thrombin signaling receptors on human platelets; PAR-3 functions as a cofactor on mouse platelets; and PAR-2 is a receptor for trypsin and other proteases. Short peptide sequences that function as selective agonists have been identified for PAR-1 (TFLLR), PAR-2 (SLIGRL), and PAR-4 (AYPGKF). On human platelets, a full response to thrombin requires both PAR-1 and PAR-4.[1011,1012] The receptors display distinct kinetics of activation and desensitization. PAR-1 mediates a substantial portion of thrombin signaling, but PAR-4 contributes at high doses of thrombin.[1012–1015] PAR-3 and PAR-4 serve as thrombin receptors on mouse platelets,[1010] where PAR-4 is the primary signaling system[1016] and PAR-3 functions as a cofactor for the cleavage and activation of PAR-4 by thrombin.[1017] Deficiency of either PAR-4 or PAR-3 results in a bleeding defect and protection from experimental thrombosis in mice.[1016,1018]

When platelets are exposed to subaggregating concentrations of thrombin, they become relatively insensitive to the subsequent addition of an aggregating concentration of thrombin, a process termed *homologous desensitization*. This process involves rapid receptor internalization and alterations in the thrombin receptor signaling systems.[1019] Trafficking of the thrombin receptor to lysosomes is dictated by the amino acid sequence in the cytoplasmic tail of PAR-1[1020] and requires phosphorylation. In comparison with PAR-1, activation-dependent internalization of PAR-4 occurs to a lesser extent and termination of PAR-4 signaling occurs more slowly,[1014] resulting in distinct patterns of signaling through each receptor.

Thrombin can bind to GPIbα, and platelets from patients lacking the GPIb-IX complex (Bernard-Soulier syndrome) have decreased thrombin-induced platelet aggregation (see Chap. 112). A region on GPIbα with three sulfated tyrosines and a large number of anionic amino acids, with homology to the high-affinity thrombin inhibitor hirudin, contains the thrombin-binding site. Crystal structures of the extracellular amino-terminal domain of GPIbα bound to thrombin indicate that two thrombin molecules interact with each GPIbα.[709,710] This bivalent interaction may allow thrombin to serve as a bridge linking GPIbα receptors on the same or adjacent platelets. Although the physiologic role of GPIb in thrombin signaling is not completely established, thrombin binding may promote signaling through receptor multimerization and/or enhanced PAR cleavage.

Tachykinins: Substance P and Endokinins A and B The tachykinin neurotransmitter substance P induces platelet aggregation and the release reaction at micromolar concentrations and enhances aggregation induced by other agonists at lower concentrations. Platelets express two seven transmembrane G-protein coupled receptors for substance P (NK_1 and NK_2), and NK_1 has been implicated in mediating the response to substance P.[1021] In addition, an amidated peptide from the carboxyl-terminus of the related tachykinins endokinins A and B ($GKASQFFGLM-NH_2$) initiates platelet aggregation. Substance P has also been identified in platelets, and platelets secrete substance P when activated.

Chemokine Receptors (CCR1, CCR3, CCR4, CXCR1, CXCR4) Based on monoclonal antibody binding and/or mRNA expression studies, platelets and/or megakaryocytes express the seven transmembrane G-protein coupled chemokine receptors CCR1, CCR3, CCR4, CXCR1, and CXCR4 (reviewed in ref. 78). These receptors may play a role in megakaryopoiesis and platelet production. In addition, a number of chemokines, particularly PF4 (CXCL4), CXCL12, CCL13, and CCL22, have been variably found to either augment platelet activation and aggregation induced by other agonists or actually fully initiate platelet adhesion, activation, and aggregation. Because high concentrations of the chemokines relative to plasma concentrations are required to demonstrate these effects, the role these receptors play in platelet physiology is unclear, but local chemokine levels may be higher in areas of inflammation.

Lipid Mediators: Platelet-Activating Factor, Lysophosphatidic Acid, and Sphingosphine-1-Phosphate PAF (a mixture of 1-*O*-hexadecyl-2-acetyl-sn-glycero-3-phosphocholine and 1-*O*-octadecyl-2-acetyl-sn-glycero-3-phosphocholine[1022]) is a phospholipid ether produced by platelets, leukocytes, and other cells. PAF is a potent platelet agonist and mediator of inflammation. Cellular responses to PAF are mediated by a specific seven transmembrane, G-protein coupled receptor.[1023,1024] PAF induces G-protein–dependent inhibition of adenylyl cyclase and activation of PLC,[1025] which cause phosphoinositol turnover, leading to the activation of PKC and an increase in intracellular Ca^{2+}.[1024] PAF also indirectly activates PLA_2, which causes release of arachidonic acid from the platelet membrane.[1026] All of these effects contribute to the overall platelet response to PAF.

Activated platelets contribute to LPA and spingosphine-1-phosphate (S1P) generation in the blood.[1027] One pathway for LPA formation involves agonist-stimulated production of phosphatidic acid, either by phospholipase D or by the sequential actions of PLC and DAG kinase. Phosphatidic acid in the outer portion of the plasma membrane or in platelet-derived microvesicles is hydrolyzed by secretory PLA_2 to LPA,[1028,1029] which then can act on its extracellular receptor(s) to induce platelet aggregation. A second pathway for LPA production is direct formation by lysophospholipase D (lysoPLD)-catalyzed hydrolysis of a lysophosphophosphatidylcholine (lysoPC). Autotaxin, initially identified as a tumor-cell derived motility factor, appears to be responsible for the majority of lysoPLD activity in serum, catalyzing the formation of LPA from lysoPC.[1030]

In human platelets, LPA elicits shape change,[1031] platelet-monocyte aggregate formation,[1032] and fibronectin-matrix assembly.[1033] It also potentiates ADP-induced platelet aggregation. LPA signaling pathways couple to Rho activation,[1031] Src kinase activity, and calcium entry,[1034] with little activation of Gq-dependent pathways.[1035] Some of the platelet responses to LPA in whole blood are attenuated by $P2Y_1$ and $P2Y_{12}$ receptor antagonists, suggesting that released ADP plays an important role in mediating aspects of LPA's responses.[1034] Platelets contain mRNA for at least three of the four known G-protein coupled receptors for LPA (LPA1, LPA2, LPA3),[1036] but the contribution of the receptors to LPA signaling is not clear. Some evidence suggests the platelet LPA receptor has a distinct pharmacologic profile.[1037] Mild oxidation of LDL generates LPA, and the LPA component of oxidized LDL in the lipid-rich thrombogenic core of atherosclerotic lesions exposed during plaque rupture may be an important stimulus for platelet activation.[1038]

Serotonin Platelets serve as the major serotonin (5-hydroxytryptophan [5-HT]) storage site in the circulation because they have the capacity to take up serotonin actively and store it in dense granules. Release of serotonin from the dense granules during platelet activation may amplify platelet aggregation and granule release. Serotonergic receptors, which are seven transmembrane G-protein coupled receptors, exist in seven main subfamilies ($5\text{-}HT_1$ to $5\text{-}HT_7$).[1039] The receptor that mediates serotonin's effects on platelet function initially was defined as being a $5\text{-}HT_2$ receptor.[1040] However, data now demonstrate it is of the $5\text{-}HT_{2A}$ subtype and that it is essentially identical to the $5\text{-}HT_{2A}$ receptor present in the brain frontal cortex.[1041,1042] The $5\text{-}HT_2$ receptor-blocking compound ketanserin antagonizes serotonin's stimulatory effects on platelets and neurons.[1043] Two naturally occurring amino acid substitutions have been identified in the receptor.[1044] Platelets from patients heterozygous for the H452Y polymorphism have a blunted calcium response when stimulated with serotonin compared to platelets from patients homozygous for H452.[1044] Silent polymorphisms in the $5\text{-}HT_{2A}$ gene (T102C in exon 1 and -1438A/G in the promoter region) have been correlated with nonfatal acute myocardial infarctions and enhanced $5\text{-}HT_{2A}$ receptor-mediated small platelet aggregate formation.[1045] Many studies have been performed correlating platelet serotonin transporter activity and $5\text{-}HT_{2A}$ receptors with a number of neuropsychiatric disorders.[1046–1050] Some concern exists, however, about the correlation between $5\text{-}HT_{2A}$ receptors on platelets and those in the brain.[1051]

Addition of serotonin in micromolar concentrations to platelets *in vitro* causes elevation of intracellular calcium, PLC activation, protein phosphorylation, and mild aggregation.[1052,1053] In whole blood, serotonin itself does not cause platelet aggregation, but it does enhance aggregation induced by ADP and thrombin.[1054] Serotonin released from platelets can cause vasoconstriction of blood vessels that have suffered endothelial damage,[1055] further promoting thrombus formation. Inhibition of serotonin's action has a favorable effect in animal models of thrombosis and vascular damage, but whether the benefit derives from effects on platelet aggregation or vasoconstriction is not clear.[1056]

A role for serotonin in linking procoagulant proteins to activated platelets has been described. Serotonin becomes covalently attached via a transglutaminase-dependent reaction to multiple transglutaminase substrates, including fibrinogen, vWF, TSP, fibronectin, and α_2-antiplasmin. These serotonylated proteins then associate via an unknown receptor to a subpopulation of activated platelets termed *COAT platelets*.[1057] Tissue transglutaminase in platelets can also catalyze the addition of serotonin into the small G-proteins Rab4 and RhoA in a reaction that renders them constitutively active and promotes α-granule secretion.[1058]

Vasopressin Vasopressin interacts with platelets to induce shape change, aggregation, and dense granule release.[1059] These events follow an induced rise in intracellular calcium and PLC activation.[1060] The platelet binding site is classified pharmacologically as a V_1-type receptor,[1061] and radiolabeled vasopressin binds with a K_d of 1 to 10 nM.[1062] Unlike the case with V_2 receptors that activate adenylate cyclase, V_1 receptors appear to activate PLC,[1063] perhaps via coupling through Gαq11.[1064] Fewer than 100 binding sites for vasopressin are present per platelet,[1065] and controversy exists as to whether physiologic concentrations of vasopressin are sufficiently high to activate platelets directly.[1066,1067] Even if vasopressin does not directly activate platelets, it may be able to enhance platelet activation induced by other agonists. Vasopressin V_{1a} receptor antagonists inhibit vasopressin-induced platelet aggregation.[1068]

Angiotensin II Platelets express angiotensin II (AngII) AT1-type receptors.[1069] AngII treatment of platelet-rich plasma results in shape change but not platelet aggregation.[1070,1071] Infusion of AngII into normal volunteers results in platelet activation as assessed by plasma β-thromboglobulin levels and platelet surface expression of P-selectin and fibrinogen binding sites.[1072] Certain AT1 receptor antagonists, such as losartan and irbesartan, also competitively inhibit TXA$_2$ receptors on platelets.[1070,1073,1074] AT1 receptor antagonists also stimulate NO release from isolated platelets.[1075] In hypertensive rats treated with losartan, platelet function appears to be attenuated,[1076] but data in humans on the effects of administering AT1 receptor antagonists are inconsistent.[1077,1078]

Thrombospondin and Integrin-Associated Protein (CD47) TSP, a large disulfide-bonded trimer (subunit M_r 160,000), is both a platelet α-granule protein and an extracellular matrix protein present in the subendothelium. TSP is rapidly released from platelets upon thrombin stimulation. In addition to its role as an adhesive protein, TSP functions as an agonist to stimulate αIIbβ3-mediated platelet aggregation.[1079,1080] Multiple potential TSP receptors are present on platelets, including GPIV (CD36), αIIbβ3, αVβ3, and IAP (CD47). Of these receptors, CD47 is most strongly implicated as the major signaling receptor in response to TSP. CD47 was first discovered as a protein that copurifies with integrins, including αIIbβ3,[1079] αVβ3,[1081] and α2β1.[1082] The sequence of CD47 indicates it has a single Ig-like extracellular domain, five membrane-spanning regions, and a short cytoplasmic tail.[128,1080,1081] CD47 probably generates signals independent of integrins and affects integrin function via downstream effects. CD47 couples physically and functionally to the large G-protein Gαi,[1083] which is notable because all known large G-proteins couple to seven instead of five transmembrane-spanning receptors. Further downstream signaling probably involves the activation of tyrosine kinases, including Syk, Lyn, and p125^{FAK}, as well as PLCγ2.[1079] Studies of mice with targeted deletions of CD47 demonstrate a role for this protein in stimulating platelet adhesion to activated endothelium under low shear rates.[1084]

How other TSP binding sites on platelets contribute to the overall response induced by TSP is not clear. GPIV copurifies with several tyrosine kinases, including Fyn, Lyn, and Yes.[1085] However, whether TSP binding to GPIV activates these kinases and whether they then contribute to the observed platelet response are unknown.

TSP-1 also functions as a reductase for vWF. In α-granules TSP-1 appears to reduce vWF multimer size.[1086,1087] In contrast, TSP-1 also binds to the A3 domain of plasma vWF, where it competes for ADAMTS13 binding, thus slowing the rate of vWF cleavage and favoring large vWF multimers.[1087]

Collagen Upon vascular injury, collagens in the subendothelium are exposed to flowing blood and promote both platelet attachment and activation, thereby contributing to normal hemostasis. Collagen is also thought to be one of the most thrombogenic substances in atherosclerotic plaques and upon plaque rupture is believed to contribute to platelet aggregation and thrombus formation, leading to ischemic damage.[1088] The types of collagen present in the subendothelium include I, III, IV, V, VI, VIII, and XIII,[1089] with types I and III (>95%) the most abundant. Under conditions that mimic physiologic blood flow, platelets adhere tightly to collagen types I, III, and IV, weakly to types VI, VII, and VIII, and not at all to type V. However, under static conditions, platelets can adhere to all of those collagens and to types II and V.[1090]

Collagen-induced platelet activation probably involves multiple receptors, most notably integrin α2β1 (GPIa-IIa) and GPVI (see Fig. 105-17). The I (inserted) domain in the α2 subunit of α2β1 is homologous to a number of collagen-binding domains in other proteins and mediates adhesion of the receptor to collagen. GPVI is an M_r 62,000 glycoprotein from the Ig superfamily[290,1091–1093] that functions in concert with the FcR γ-chain, with the latter initiating intracellular signaling.[1094] The regions of GPVI that interact with collagen and peptide modeled after collagen have been mapped, and lysine 59 on the extracellular surface of GPVI appears critical for this interaction.[1095] Other collagen receptors on platelets include GPIV (CD36)[827] and an M_r 65,000 protein called GP65.[1096] The potential interrelation of all these collagen receptors is unknown, but considerable evidence indicates at least GPVI and α2β1 work in concert, perhaps by assembling intracellular proteins into complexes, because interactions of collagen with both α2β1 and GPVI are required for a full platelet response.[581,1097,1098]

Glycoprotein VI exists in a stable physical complex with the FcR γ-chain, and the FcR γ-chain is absent from GPVI-deficient platelets.[737] The addition of either collagen or an antibody that can cross-link GPVI induces tyrosine phosphorylation of the FcR γ-chain.[737] The kinases contributing to this event probably are Fyn and/or Lyn.[1099] Tyrosine phosphorylation of the ITAM on the FcR γ-chain increases the ITAM's affinity for proteins containing SH2 domains, resulting in the recruitment of such proteins to the FcR γ-chain. The nonreceptor tyrosine kinase Syk contains two adjacent SH2 domains and a tyrosine kinase domain. In platelets from normal mice, Syk physically associates with the FcR γ-chain and becomes phosphorylated and activated after collagen stimulation.[737] In platelets from mice lacking FcR γ-chain, collagen is unable to induce Syk phosphorylation and activation.[1094] Similarly, in platelets lacking GPVI or in platelets in which the α2β1 integrin is blocked, collagen-induced Syk phosphorylation is inhibited, demonstrating that GPVI, α2β1, and Syk all participate in the platelet response to collagen. The β-subunit of the α2β1 receptor also has tyrosines spaced in a manner reminiscent of an ITAM motif; thus, Syk might also associate with this collagen receptor. In addition to Syk,[1100] Src[1101] becomes tyrosine phosphorylated in response to collagen. Although Src is an abundant kinase in platelets, its role in platelet signaling is unclear, because mice lacking Src do not suffer from any obvious bleeding disorder.[1102] Syk, on the other hand, appears to play a critical role in collagen activation of platelets, because platelets from mice lacking Syk do not aggregate or undergo secretion in response to collagen.[1094] Collagen stimulation of platelets also results in tyrosine phosphorylation and activation of PLCγ2,[1103] and activation of this enzyme causes phosphoinositide hydrolysis, leading to αIIbβ3 activation. PLCγ2 activation occurs downstream of Syk, as evidenced by the findings that collagen is unable to activate PLCγ2 in platelets pretreated with a Syk-selective inhibitor[1097] or in platelets from Syk knockout mice.[1094] Whether Syk activates PLCγ2 directly is unknown, but Bruton tyrosine kinase (Btk) might be positioned between Syk and PLCγ2 because patients lacking Btk not only exhibit the B cell deficiency X-linked agammaglobulinemia but also show reduced platelet responsiveness to collagen and diminished phosphorylation of PLCγ2.[1104] Signaling via GPVI also activates the other major collagen receptor α2β1,[1105,1106] perhaps via talin binding to the β1 cytoplasmic domain,[27] elimination of an inhibitory influence of the α2 cytoplasmic domain,[27] and/or extracellular disulfide exchange.[584]

Intermediate events of GPVI signaling involve activation of Rap-1, a small G-protein that has been implicated in integrin activation in platelets and megakaryocytes.[1107] Full GPVI-induced Rap-1 activation appears to involve both release of ADP (acting on the P2Y$_{12}$ ADP receptor) and ADP receptor-independent pathways.[1108] GPVI signaling also results in activation of at least one negative regulator of platelet function, c-CBL, which is tyrosine phosphorylated and activated downstream of Src kinases. Platelets deficient in c-CBL show enhanced aggregation responses in response to GPVI engagement.[1109] Although much of the GPVI-mediated signaling occurs via the associated FcRγ, the cytoplasmic domain of GPVI also contains a highly basic region that binds calmodulin and a proline-rich region that binds Src kinases, which also appear to contribute to GPVI-mediated signaling.[1110]

The α2β1 integrin can also signal in response to collagen, independent of GPVI, and induce phosphorylation and activation of many of the same signaling components attributed to the GPVI-induced signaling cascade, such as Src, Syk, SLP-76, and PLC2. Other components include plasma membrane calcium ATPase and p125^{FAK}.[1111] However, separate studies indicate α2β1 must be in an active conformation in order to participate in this signaling.[1112] Thus, collagen-induced signaling via GPVI appears to activate α2β1, allowing both receptors to participate in the signaling necessary for a full response to collagen.[1112]

The levels of GPVI and α2β1 expressed on platelets vary among individuals, but whether a correlation exists between the levels of expression of each of them is unclear.[1113–1115] The level of expression of these receptors does, however, correlate with the ability of platelets to be stimulated by collagen. GPVI is present on the membranes of the open canalicular system and α-granules, but these pools are not detectable on the surface of resting platelets. These pools merge with the plasma membrane pool in stimulated platelets, increasing the apparent surface expression of GPVI by approximately 60 percent.[1116]

GPIV (CD36) can also bind collagen, and antibodies to GPIV partially inhibit platelet adhesion to collagen.[1117] Currently no evidence indicates that GPIV contributes to collagen-induced signaling in platelets, as platelets from patients lacking GPIV respond normally to collagen.[1118]

Platelets stimulated with collagen exhibit several distinct responses. Whereas elevated cAMP levels normally inhibit platelet aggregation, collagen-stimulated platelets are relatively resistant to inhibition by cAMP.[1119] This finding may be related to the fact that collagen stimulates the PLCγ isotype, which is insensitive to cAMP-mediated inhibition, whereas other agonists such as thrombin stimulate PLCβ, which is inhibited by cAMP. In addition, phosphatase inhibition decreases collagen-induced, but not thrombin-induced or ADP-

induced, platelet aggregation,[1120] suggesting that one or more phosphatases are critical in collagen-induced platelet aggregation.

GPIb-IX-V   The GPIb-IX-V complex promotes the initial interactions of platelets with vWF, particularly under conditions of high shear, resulting in platelet tethering. GPIb-IX-V also can initiate signals that activate the αIIbβ3 receptor, resulting in firm platelet adhesion and aggregation.[282] Some of the first evidence that the GPIb-IX-V complex could serve as a signaling receptor came from studies in which antibodies to αIIbβ3 partially inhibited ristocetin-induced platelet aggregation.[418] Subsequently, ristocetin-mediated interaction of vWF with platelets was observed to cause PIP$_2$ metabolism, activation of PKC, and increased intracellular calcium levels. Likewise, shear forces initiate signaling through the binding of vWF to GPIb-IX-V.[1121] In heterologous systems, such as CHO cells expressing both GPIb-IX and αIIbβ3, occupancy of GPIb-IX by vWF can lead to activation of αIIbβ3.[1122,1123] In platelets, the GPIb-IX-V complex associates with signaling proteins with ITAM motifs, such the FCγRIIA receptor[688] and FcR γ-chain[691]; however, engagement of GPIb-IX-V alone is sufficient to activate αIIbβ3 (see Fig. 105-14).[1124] The signaling pathway triggered by engagement of GPIb-IX-V is incompletely understood but appears to involve activation of Src[1124–1126] and PI3K and recruitment of the adaptor proteins SLP-76 and ADAP (SLAP-130).[1124] The result is activation of PLCγ2,[1127] PKC, and αIIbβ3. Signaling through the GPIb-IX-V complex also causes release of arachidonic acid and generation of TXA$_2$. A cGMP and MAP kinase-dependent pathway for GPIb-IX–mediated activation of αIIbβ3 has been reported.[1128] The GPIb-IX-V complex binds several intracellular proteins, including filamin (an actin-binding protein),[683] calmodulin,[1129] and 14-3-3ζ.[680,1130,1131] Activation of c-RAF by 14-3-3ζ may link GPIb-IX-V signaling to the Raf/MEK/ mitogen-activated protein kinase (MAPK) signaling pathway. Moreover, protein 14-3-3ζ exists as a dimer, which may allow it to bridge and dimerize GPIb molecules.[1130] In CHO cells, clustering of GPIb-IX promotes stable adhesion via αIIbβ3.[1132]

The GPIb-IX-V complex appears to be involved in transmitting at least one cAMP-dependent inhibitory signal. Thus, elevated cAMP, which activates PKA, induces phosphorylation of GPIbβ on serine 166.[682] Elevated cAMP also normally inhibits agonist-induced platelet actin polymerization. However, in platelets from patients with Bernard-Soulier syndrome who lack GPIb-IX-V, actin polymerization proceeds normally after collagen stimulation, even when cAMP is elevated, suggesting that cAMP-mediated phosphorylation of GPIbβ may be required for cAMP-mediated inhibition.[1133]

Glycoprotein V, an M_r 82,000 membrane-spanning protein that is a member of the leucine-rich repeat family and complexes with GPIb-IX, is a substrate for thrombin.[1134] GPV-null platelets display enhanced responses to thrombin,[1135] and GPV-null mice have accelerated thrombus growth in response to vascular injury.[1136] Proteolytically inactive thrombin selectively activates mouse platelets lacking GPV and induces thrombosis in GPV-deficient but not wild-type mice.[727] Together, these observations suggest GPV functions as a negative regulator of thrombin signaling through GPIb-IX, and, in its absence, thrombin may function as a ligand for GPIb-IX.

ADDITIONAL INTERMEDIATE SIGNALING MOLECULES

Calcium   Elevation of intracellular calcium has a multitude of effects on platelet physiology.[976,1137] The concentration of calcium in resting platelets (100–500 nM) is very low compared to the plasma concentration (~2 mM). Exposure of platelets to most agonists is accompanied by a rapid, transient rise in the intracellular free calcium ion concentration to micromolar levels, followed by a quick return to normal resting levels. The cytoplasmic calcium concentration at any given time is a result of the rates of passive influx, active extrusion across the plasma membrane, and both active release and/or uptake of the ion by the DTS, which is a calcium storage depot in platelets analogous to the sarcoplasmic reticulum in muscle. Active calcium extrusion and uptake are mediated by several pumps (see Fig. 105-19). The cytosolic pool of calcium turns over rapidly as a result of a plasma membrane sodium-calcium antiporter, whereas the DTS contains a more slowly exchanging pool of calcium regulated by a calcium-magnesium ATPase (SERCA3), a pump that also appears to be located in the plasma membrane.[1138] During agonist stimulation, most calcium enters the platelet cytosolic compartment through receptor-operated calcium channels (reviewed in ref. 1139) in the plasma membrane. Collagen, for example, causes sodium entry into platelets, which reverses the sodium-calcium antiporter to promote calcium entry, thus contributing to platelet aggregation.[1140] Release of intracellular calcium from the DTS also occurs rapidly in response to agonist stimulation, in large part because of the IP_3 generated as part of the phosphoinositide cycle.[1139,1141] This calcium release occurs in part as a result of calcium channels such as TRPC6 and TRPC1, whose function is controlled by the level of platelet calcium stores.[20,1139] $\alpha IIb\beta 3$ also may participate in calcium entry.[1142]

Elevation of calcium induces numerous downstream events, including activation of calcium-sensitive forms of PLA_2[1143] and PKC[1144]; calmodulin-dependent enzymes such as myosin light-chain kinase, which phosphorylates myosin light chain[1145] and promotes cytoskeletal rearrangements required for platelet shape change; and gelsolin, which facilitates actin severing and rearrangement, secretion, and aggregation. In addition, calcium probably plays a direct role in the membrane fusion events that result in degranulation and the release reaction. Calcium-dependent proteases or calpains also become activated and play an important role in postaggregation events. The calcium-binding protein CIB[1146] binds to the membrane proximal region of αIIb[1147] and contributes to platelet spreading.[311]

Phosphoinositide-3-Kinases The PI3Ks are a family of lipid kinases that phosphorylate the D-3 hydroxyl group of the myoinositol ring of phosphoinositides (reviewed in Zhang et al.[1148] and Rittenhouse[1149]). Class I PI3Ks are heterodimeric protein complexes containing both regulatory and catalytic subunits that utilize phosphatidylinositol (PI), $PI_{4,5}P_2$ as substrates to form PI_3P, $PI_{3,4}P_2$, and $PI_{3,4,5}P_3$, respectively. Platelets contain two isoforms of PI3K, designated class Ia and class Ib, that have distinct subunits and regulatory features. The catalytic subunit of class Ia PI3K is an M_r 110,000 to 120,000 protein. The regulatory subunit p85 (PI3K p85α) has two SH2 domains, a breakpoint cluster region homology domain, a proline-rich region, and a single SH3 domain. Members of this class of PI3K possess intrinsic serine-threonine protein kinase activity in addition to lipid kinase activity. They appear to be regulated, at least in part, by binding of the p85 subunit to tyrosine-phosphorylated proteins. Following platelet activation, PI3K can be coimmunoprecipitated with the tyrosine kinases Src and Syk. Class Ib PI3K (PI3Kγ) has been isolated from platelets and neutrophils and contains the catalytic subunit p110γ, which is activated by the β,γ-subunit of heterodimeric G-proteins. Both isoforms of PI3K appear to associate with the platelet cytoskeleton after agonist activation.

In platelets, 3-phosphorylated phosphoinositides are produced in response to a variety of agonists, including thrombin, TXA_2, LPA, ADP, and collagen, and may mediate early signaling events that precede $\alpha IIb\beta 3$ activation and late events involved in stabilizing fibrinogen binding and platelet aggregation.[1148–1150] Thrombin stimulates rapid accumulation of $PI_{3,4,5}P_3$ and $PI_{3,4}P_2$. The latter requires fibrinogen binding to $\alpha IIb\beta 3$ and calpain activity.[1151] Collagen promotes the association of PI3K p85α via its SH2 domains with tyrosine-phosphorylated forms of FcR γ-chain and the regulatory protein linker-for-activator T (LAT) cells to modulate PI3K.[1152] Platelets from mice

lacking PI3K p85α aggregate normally to ADP, thrombin, U46619, and PMA but display impaired responses to collagen and collagen-related peptide and diminished tyrosine phosphorylation of the PI3K effectors Btk, Tec, Akt, and PLCγ2.[1153] FcγRIIA-induced platelet aggregation requires PI3K activity, which is upstream of PLCγ2 in the pathway.[1154] Platelets also contain PI3Kγ, the second isoform of PI3K. Platelets from mice lacking the PI3Kγ isoform aggregate normally to thrombin and collagen but have impaired responses to ADP. PI3Kγ-deficient mice are protected from ADP-induced thromboembolism.[1155] The mechanism of this effect requires further study.

Many of the biologic actions of PI3K are mediated by their phospholipid products, which bind to specific sequences in proteins. The pleckstrin homology (PH) domains ($\sim$100 amino acids long), present in pleckstrin and other platelet proteins involved in signal transduction, recognize the Akt kinase, PDK, $PI_{3,4}P_2$, $P_{4,5}P_2$, and $PI_{3,4,5}P_3$.[1156] Binding of PI_3 to the amino-terminal PH domain in PLCγ enhances its activity.[1157] $PI_{3,4,5}P_3$ binding to PH domains in Btk[1158] targets Btk to the plasma membrane, where it is further phosphorylated and activated.[1159] PDK is activated by binding $PI_{3,4,5}P_3$ and in turn phosphorylates and activates the serine/threonine kinase Akt.[1160,1161] Akt activation is biphasic, occurring before and after platelet aggregation.[1151] Two isoforms of Akt (Akt1 and Akt2) are present in human platelets.[1162] Deficiency of Akt2 in mice impairs platelet aggregation, secretion, and fibrinogen binding in response to low doses of thrombin and U46619, but has minimal effects on collagen signaling.[1163] Akt2-null mice have normal bleeding times but are protected from experimental thrombosis. Studies of mice lacking Akt have yielded conflicting reports as to the role of the protein in platelet signaling events.[1163,1164]

Small G-Proteins Some members of the Ras superfamily of small GTPases modulate integrin receptor activation. Small GTPases, like their large G-protein counterparts, cycle between a resting GDP-bound state and an active GTP-bound state. In their active state, small GTPases can interact with and activate downstream signaling molecules, thus acting as molecular switches. One small GTPase, R-Ras, activates $\alpha IIb\beta 3$ when both are expressed in CHO cells—cells that normally are unable to activate this integrin by a signal transduction cascade.[1165]

The small G-protein RhoA has an established role in stress fiber formation in nucleated cells.[1166] In platelets, RhoA is required for vinculin-dependent focal adhesion formation in platelets adherent to fibrinogen[1167] but not for $\alpha IIb\beta 3$ activation.[1167]

Rap1 is a small G-protein that is activated in platelets in response to many different agonists.[1108,1168,1169] Experiments with megakaryocytes have demonstrated that overexpression of active Rap1 enhances agonist-induced integrin activation but does not itself activate $\alpha IIb\beta 3$.[1107]

The small G-protein H-Ras may function to suppress integrin activation.[1170] H-Ras in other cells often is part of a pathway involving the serine/threonine kinases Raf, MEK, and MAPK. Whether an H-Ras/Raf/MEK/MAPK pathway is inhibitory in platelets is not entirely clear, however, as a soluble MEK inhibitor attenuates rather than enhances platelet aggregation to low concentrations of collagen and arachidonic acid.[1171] Moreover, H-Ras is activated by platelet agonists,[1172] so the exact role of H-Ras in platelet activation remains to be determined. Based on studies in nucleated cells, PEA-15, a small protein that contains a death effector domain,[1173] may act in concert with an R-Ras dependent pathway to oppose the inhibitory effects of H-Ras on integrin function. Thus, the small G-proteins appear to have the capacity to both up-regulate and down-regulate the activation state of $\alpha IIb\beta 3$.

Calcium-Dependent Proteases (Calpains) After ligand binding, integrin clustering, and platelet aggregation, neutral proteases termed *calpains* become activated by a rise in intracellular calcium.[382] The most important and well-studied class of calpains in platelets are the μ-calpains, which are activated by micromolar concentrations of calcium. m-Calpains, which require millimolar concentrations of calcium for activation, also exist in platelets. Each form of calpain consists of a common M_r 30,000 subunit paired with a catalytic subunit of M_r 80,000. Activated μ-calpains cleave numerous proteins,[382] including filamin (actin-binding protein), integrin β3, SNAP-23, WASP, Btk, cortactin, certain forms of PKC, and talin. Cleavage of talin by calpain *in vitro* enables talin to activate αIIbβ3,[24] but the role of calpain in activation of αIIbβ3 by talin in intact platelets is uncertain. In addition, calpain appears to be upstream of, and able to induce, activation of the small G-proteins Rac and RhoA.[382] These small G-proteins have profound effects on cytoskeletal structure. Rac is involved in lamellipodia formation,[1174] and Rho is linked to stress fiber formation.[1166] Thus, calpains, by their effects on structural and signaling molecules, appear to affect the signaling and cytoskeletal rearrangements that occur following platelet aggregation. Mice deficient in μ-calpain demonstrate abnormal platelet aggregation, decreased clot retraction, and reduced tyrosine phosphorylation of the β3 subunit of αIIbβ3, supporting an important role in platelet function.[389]

INSIDE-OUT ACTIVATION OF αIIBβ3 AND OUTSIDE-IN SIGNALING BY ACTIVATED αIIBβ3

The active state of αIIbβ3 is defined as the conformation that is competent to bind large soluble adhesive proteins such as fibrinogen and vWF with relatively high affinity. Precise regulation of the activation state of αIIbβ3 is essential for maintenance of normal hemostasis, such that αIIbβ3 activation occurs only upon vascular injury. Crystallographic and electron microscopic studies suggest that the extracellular portion of the related integrin αVβ3 is in a bent conformation when inactive and in an extended conformation when activated (see Fig. 105-3).[504,1175] The activation state of αIIbβ3 is controlled by the cytoplasmic domains of this integrin in concert with specific intracellular binding proteins. Thus, under basal conditions, interactions between the cytoplasmic domains of αIIb and β3 maintain the receptor in an inactive state. Interrupting the interactions between the cytoplasmic domains results in long-range conformational changes that convert the extracellular portion of the integrin to an active state.[1176] Current data indicate interactions between regions of the αIIb and β3 cytoplasmic domains closest to the membrane involve salt bridges between acidic and basic amino acid residues of each subunit.[521,525] Mutations that disrupt these interactions result in αIIbβ3 activation.[525] In addition, maintenance of the resting state of αIIb may require a hairpin turn in αIIb such that the acidic carboxyl-terminus of the αIIb cytoplasmic domain folds back on itself to interact with the membrane proximal region.[26] The β3 cytoplasmic tail, carboxyl-terminal to the membrane proximal region that interacts with αIIb, is predicted from nuclear magnetic resonance (NMR) studies to interact via or near its NPLY sequence with the plasma membrane in the resting platelet.[1176] Cytoskeletal restraints appear to further maintain αIIbβ3 in an inactive conformation, as treatment of platelets with low doses of the actin depolymerizing agents activate the integrin.[1177] Upon agonist activation, the cytoskeletal protein talin may play a key role in the conversion of αIIbβ3 and several other integrins to an active conformation.[27] Talin itself can exist in a conformation that is either less or more favorable for binding to β3 at multiple sites. The affinity of talin for αIIb increases in response to $PI_{4,5}P_2$ binding to talin.[1178] $PI_{4,5}P_2$ may be generated locally from phosphatidylinositol via the enzyme phosphatidylinositol phosphate kinase type 1γ (PIPKI), which can bind to talin.[1179,1180] Talin is composed of an M_r 47,000 head domain and an M_r 190,000 rod domain. The head domain contains a FERM domain, named for the proteins four point one (4.1), ezrin, radixin, and moesin,

which promotes specific interactions with cytoplasmic regions of multiple proteins. The F3 region of the FERM domain, which resembles a PTB domain,[1181] interacts with the NPLY region of integrin β3,[1181,1182] likely disrupting its interaction with the membrane.[1176] The binding site on F3 is not available when PIPKI is bound to talin, so presumably any prebound PIPKI is displaced from talin upon talin interaction with β3.[1183] A subsequent interaction of the talin head domain with a more membrane proximal region of β3 is predicted[380] that may disrupt its interaction with αIIb, resulting in αIIbβ3 activation.[1176] In studies of the related integrin LFA-1, in which the technique of fluorescence resonance energy transfer was used to measure precise molecular distances, the integrin cytoplasmic tails appeared to become more distant from one other in response to agonist activation.[538] Moreover, the intramolecular interactions within the αIIb cytoplasmic domain are predicted to be disrupted.[1176] Evidence from NMR studies indicates the active integrin cytoplasmic domains may enter further into the plasma membrane, which could promote long-range conformational changes in αIIbβ3.[1176] The rod-like region of talin also interacts with β3,[1184] and an unknown region of talin interacts with αIIb.[539] Although these interactions may serve to stabilize or subsequently cluster the integrin, their exact roles are unknown. Finally, after the interactions between the αIIb and β3 cytoplasmic domains has occurred, αIIb cytoplasmic domains from adjacent αIIbβ3 receptors have been proposed to form homodimers and β3 cytoplasmic domains to form homotrimers, resulting in stabilization of the activated state and clustering of αIIbβ3 receptors.[396,1185]

Platelet aggregation is commonly described as progressing through two phases, an initial reversible aggregation phase, which often is the response observed with low concentrations of agonists, followed by a stronger, irreversible phase. The irreversible phase of aggregation correlates with TXA_2 production and platelet secretion of ADP. Fibrinogen binding to αIIbβ3 and the platelet-platelet contacts that occur during the initial phase of aggregation initiate specific signal transduction events, resulting in positive feedback loops that promote irreversible aggregation, maintain secretion, and initiate later events such as clot retraction.[541]

Fibrinogen or vWF binding to the extracellular region of αIIbβ3 transmits long-range conformational changes to the integrin cytoplasmic domains, perhaps via a pivot action between the β3 βA (I-like) and hybrid domains[503] that induce signaling from outside the platelet to inside the platelet (outside-in signaling).[526,530] These conformational changes, along with integrin clustering,[500] likely are the bases for outside-in signal transduction through αIIbβ3, perhaps by altering the association of cytoplasmic domains with one another and initiating recruitment of proteins with enzymatic activity to the cytoplasmic tails, forming complexes capable of generating signaling molecules.

One important signaling molecule that is constitutively associated with the β3 cytoplasmic tail is the tyrosine kinase Src.[1186,1187] Src binds to the carboxyl-terminus of the integrin in resting platelets via its SH3 domain independent of its catalytic activity.[1186] This pool of Src in unstimulated platelets appears to exist in a minimally active state, with its activity suppressed in part by the Src regulator Csk, which phosphorylates Src at Tyr 529. Platelet adhesion to fibrinogen increases the Src activity associated with αIIbβ3 in part because of the dissociation of Csk and subsequent dephosphorylation of Src 529.[1187] Full Src activation occurs upon αIIbβ3 clustering and transphosphorylation of Src on Tyr 418. Src activation is required for several subsequent signaling events, such as activation of the tyrosine kinase Syk. Syk, along with Src, is required for platelet spreading on fibrinogen.[1186] Syk binds to unphosphorylated β3 via its amino-terminus.[1188,1189] Some of these events have now been visualized in living platelets.[1190]

When platelets are aggregated in response to one of multiple agonists, the β3 cytoplasmic domain becomes phosphorylated on tyrosine.[540,548] Two sites of potential tyrosine phosphorylation exist on the β3 cytoplasmic domain, and both may be used. Several molecules have been identified that bind specifically to the tyrosine-phosphorylated cytoplasmic domain of β3. A synthetic β3 cytoplasmic domain peptide containing phosphate groups on the two candidate tyrosines binds to the contractile protein myosin,[540] and this interaction may facilitate the transmission of cytoskeletal tension from inside the platelet to outside and thus initiate clot retraction. Recombinant mutated β3 that cannot be phosphorylated is unable to support extensive clot retraction when expressed in a cell line.[540] Other proteins that bind to the diphosphorylated β3 cytoplasmic domain include the adapter proteins SHC,[549] which also become tyrosine phosphorylated during platelet aggregation.[549] Therefore, SHC may link diphosphorylated β3 to the Ras/Raf/MAPK pathway.[549,1191] Mice containing mutated β3 molecules that cannot be phosphorylated exhibit a mild bleeding disorder as evidenced by occasional rebleeding of tail cuts. Moreover, platelets derived from these mice form abnormally loose thrombi when activated by shear forces.[541] Other β3 cytoplasmic domain binding proteins have been described, including skelemin, a member of a family of proteins that regulate myosin,[546] and talin.

Some signaling events that occur downstream of αIIbβ3 require only integrin clustering, whereas other events require clustering, ligand binding, and/or platelet aggregation. For example, the tyrosine kinase Syk becomes activated in response to αIIbβ3 clustering, independent of cytoskeletal assembly, whereas activation of the tyrosine kinase p125[FAK] requires integrin clustering, ligand binding to αIIbβ3, and cytoskeletal assembly.[1192] Activation of Syk downstream of αIIbβ3 leads to phosphorylation of Vav1, a guanine nucleotide exchange factor for Rac, and lamellipodia formation in a cell line. Syk and Vav1 cooperate to activate Jun N-terminal kinase, ERK2, and Akt.[1192] These pathways likely are also involved in postaggregation events in the platelet.

Proteins other than the well-described αIIbβ3 ligands fibrinogen and vWF also induce signaling events via binding to αIIbβ3. One such protein is CD40L, a TNF family member that is expressed on a variety of cells including activated platelets. Platelets are also the major source of a soluble form of CD40L.[326] In addition to binding to its classic receptor CD40, CD40L also binds to αIIbβ3 on platelets and induces signaling events[325] that are required for normal arterial thrombus formation in mice.[329] CD40L may initiate platelet aggregation by binding to CD40 on platelets.[821]

INHIBITORY PATHWAYS IN PLATELETS

Prostaglandins Prostaglandins that inhibit platelet activation include PGE_2 and PGI_2 (also called prostacyclin) (reviewed in refs. 1193 and 1194). In the vasculature, the endothelium produces PGI_2 and PGE_2, which are important for maintaining vascular patency.[1195] Inhibition is initiated by the binding of these PGs to their own specific G-protein coupled receptors. PG receptor occupancy converts the Gα subunit to the GTP-bound active form, which then activates adenylyl cyclase. Adenylyl cyclase catalyzes the formation of cAMP. The exact amount of cAMP present in the cell also is determined by its rate of breakdown by phosphodiesterase (PDE). Therefore, agents that inhibit PDE, such as theophylline, caffeine, and the drug cilostazol, also elevate cAMP levels in platelets and other cells. cAMP then activates PKA, which phosphorylates specific target proteins. PKA inhibits platelet activation by several pathways. One mechanism involves PKA-dependent phosphorylation of VASP (see "Nitric Oxide" below). A separate mechanism involves the phosphorylation and inhibition of Gα13, which couples to the TXA_2 receptor, thus impairing this activation pathway.[1196] Also, PKA phosphorylates GPIbβ on serine 166 and negatively regulates the ability of GPIb to bind vWF.[1197] In addition, PKA may phosphorylate and inhibit the IP_3 receptor, which

would repress agonist-induced intracellular calcium mobilization.[1198] Phosphoinositide metabolism also is affected as the activities of both PLC and PLA_2 are suppressed.[1199] Moreover, PKA also phosphorylates Raf kinase on three sites, which inhibits Raf kinase function in part by inhibiting its binding to the activating protein RasGTP.[1200,1201] Finally, the small G-protein Rap1b, which contributes to αIIbβ3 activation,[1107] is phosphorylated by PKA,[1202] although it appears that this phosphorylation event does not inhibit platelet function[1203] and in fact may contribute to Rap1b activation.[1204]

Nitric Oxide NO is synthesized from L-arginine by NO synthase in endothelial cells, platelets, and other cells. Formation of NO is enhanced at sites of shear stress and by platelet agonists (e.g., thrombin or ADP),[1205] and it readily diffuses into platelets.[1206,1207] Similar to PGI_2 and PGE_2, NO pretreatment of platelets inhibits platelet activation and can reverse platelet aggregation soon after initiation. However, NO works not by elevating cAMP but instead by increasing cGMP.[1208] NO synthase activity in platelets increases during platelet activation, suggesting that NO production is a normal negative feedback mechanism that limits further platelet aggregation. NO and PGI_2 act synergistically to inhibit platelet activation.[1209]

Elevation in intracellular cGMP levels activates cGMP-dependent protein kinase (PKG), whose downstream targets include ERK and the TXA_2 receptor.[1210] In mice, the absence of PKG results in enhanced platelet accumulation along damaged vessels after ischemic injury, supporting an important role for PKG in platelet deposition.[1211] VASP, a member of the proline-rich, actin-regulatory Ena/VASP protein family, is phosphorylated in response to elevations in either cAMP or cGMP,[1212] and both PKA and PKG phosphorylate VASP in vitro.[1213] A role for VASP in inhibition of platelet function was established in studies of VASP-deficient mice. Platelets obtained from the mice display increased P-selectin expression and αIIbβ3 activation in response to agonists,[1214] and platelet adhesion at sites of vascular injury or atherosclerosis is enhanced in VASP-deficient mice.[1215] The enhanced platelet adhesion in VASP-null mice is not corrected by NO, suggesting that VASP is a key negative regulator of platelet function in the cGMP-mediated pathways.

Elevation in intracellular cGMP also can increase cAMP levels via inhibition of PDE activity.[1216] This cross-talk between cGMP- and cAMP-dependent pathways may synergize to contribute to the inhibitory effects of NO on platelet function.

CD39 (ATP Diphosphohydrolase; Ecto-ADPase) Vascular endothelium regulates platelet function by producing prostacyclin and NO and expressing CD39, a plasma membrane-associated ATPDase (ecto-ADPase) that converts extracellular ATP and ADP to AMP (see Fig. 105-5).[66,1217] CD39 limits the platelet-activating effects of ADP released by damaged tissues, red blood cells, and activated platelets. Furthermore, AMP generated by CD39 is degraded by ecto-5′-nucleotidase to adenosine, an inhibitor of ADP-induced platelet activation. CD39 is an M_r 95,000 cell surface glycoprotein expressed on endothelial cells, activated natural killer cells, B cells, and T cells. It contains two putative transmembrane regions separated by an extracellular domain with six glycosylation sites and apyrase-like regions that confer ATPDase activity. A soluble recombinant form of CD39 inhibits platelet aggregation and recruitment in vitro and may have potential as an antithrombotic agent in vivo.[966]

REFERENCES

1. Holme S, Heaton A, Konchuba A, Hartman P: Light scatter and total protein signal distribution of platelets by flow cytometry as parameters of size. *J Lab Clin Med* 112:223, 1988.

2. White JG: Anatomy and structural organization of the platelet, in: *Hemostasis and Thrombosis: Basic Principles and Clinical Practice*, ed-

ited by RW Colman, J Hirsh, VJ Marder, EW Salzman, p 397. JB Lippincott, Philadelphia, 1993.

3. Coller BS: Biochemical and electrostatic considerations in primary platelet aggregation. *Ann N Y Acad Sci* 416:693, 1984.

4. van Joost T, van Ulsen J, Vuzevski VD, et al: Purpuric contact dermatitis to benzoyl peroxide. *J Am Acad Dermatol* 22:359, 1990.

5. Schick PK: Megakaryocyte and platelet lipids, in *Hemostasis and Thrombosis: Basic Principles and Clinical Practice*, edited by RW Colman, J Hirsh, VJ Marder, EW Salzman, p 574. JB Lippincott, Philadelphia, 1993.

6. Heemskerk JW, Bevers EM, Lindhout T: Platelet activation and blood coagulation. *Thromb Haemost* 88:186, 2002.

7. Solum NO: Procoagulant expression in platelets and defects leading to clinical disorders. *Arterioscler Thromb Vasc Biol* 19:2841, 1999.

8. Sims PJ, Faioni EM, Wiedmer T, Shattil SJ: Complement proteins C5b-9 cause release of membrane vesicles from the platelet surface that are enriched in the membrane receptor for coagulation factor Va and express prothrombinase activity. *J Biol Chem* 263:18205, 1988.

9. Sims PJ, Wiedmer T, Esmon CT, et al: Assembly of the platelet prothrombinase complex is linked to vesiculation on the platelet plasma membrane. Studies in Scott syndrome: An isolated defect in platelet procoagulant activity. *J Biol Chem* 264:137, 1989.

10. Bevers EM, Tilly RHJ, Senden JMG, et al: Exposure of endogenous phosphatidylserine at the outer surface of stimulated platelets is reversed by restoration of aminophospholipid translocase activity. *Biochemistry* 28:2382, 1989.

11. Tuszynski GP, Mauco GP, Koshy A, et al: The platelet cytoskeleton contains elements of the prothrombinase complex. *J Biol Chem* 259:6947, 1984.

12. Comfurius P, Bevers EM, Zwaal RFA: The involvement of cytoskeleton in the regulation of transbilayer movement of phospholipids in human blood platelets. *Biochim Biophys Acta* 815:143, 1985.

13. Mairhofer M, Steiner M, Mosgoeller W, et al: Stomatin is a major lipid-raft component of platelet alpha granules. *Blood* 100:897, 2002.

14. Locke D, Chen H, Liu Y, et al: Lipid rafts orchestrate signaling by the platelet receptor glycoprotein VI. *J Biol Chem* 277:18801, 2002.

15. Shrimpton CN, Borthakur G, Larrucea S, et al: Localization of the adhesion receptor glycoprotein Ib-IX-V complex to lipid rafts is required for platelet adhesion and activation. *J Exp Med* 196:1057, 2002.

16. Baglia FA, Shrimpton CN, Lopez JA, Walsh PN: The glycoprotein Ib-IX-V complex mediates localization of factor XI to lipid rafts on the platelet membrane. *J Biol Chem* 278:21744, 2003.

17. Heijnen HF, Van Lier M, Waaijenborg S, et al: Concentration of rafts in platelet filopodia correlates with recruitment of c-Src and CD63 to these domains. *J Thromb Haemost* 1:1161, 2003.

18. Bodin S, Tronchere H, Payrastre B: Lipid rafts are critical membrane domains in blood platelet activation processes. *Biochim Biophys Acta* 1610:247, 2003.

19. Bodin S, Giuriato S, Ragab J, et al: Production of phosphatidylinositol 3,4,5-trisphosphate and phosphatidic acid in platelet rafts: Evidence for a critical role of cholesterol-enriched domains in human platelet activation. *Biochemistry* 40:15290, 2001.

20. Brownlow SL, Harper AG, Harper MT, Sage SO: A role for hTRPC1 and lipid raft domains in store-mediated calcium entry in human platelets. *Cell Calcium* 35:107, 2004.

21. Hartwig JH, Barkalow K, Azim A, Italiano J: The elegant platelet: Signals controlling actin assembly. *Thromb Haemost* 82:392, 1999.

22. Hartwig JH: Platelet structure, in *Platelets*, edited by AD Michelson, p 37. Academic Press, San Diego, 2002.

23. Fox JE: The platelet cytoskeleton. *Thromb Haemost* 70:884, 1993.

24. Yan B, Calderwood DA, Yaspan B, Ginsberg MH: Calpain cleavage promotes talin binding to the beta 3 integrin cytoplasmic domain. *J Biol Chem* 276:28164, 2001.

25. Ulmer TS, Yaspan B, Ginsberg MH, Campbell ID: NMR analysis of structure and dynamics of the cytosolic tails of integrin alpha IIb beta 3 in aqueous solution. *Biochemistry* 40:7498, 2001.

26. Vinogradova O, Velyvis A, Velyviene A, et al: A structural mechanism of integrin alpha(IIb)beta(3) "inside-out" activation as regulated by its cytoplasmic face. *Cell* 110:587, 2002.

27. Tadokoro S, Shattil SJ, Eto K, et al: Talin binding to integrin beta tails: A final common step in integrin activation. *Science* 302:103, 2003.

28. Tremuth L, Kreis S, Melchior C, et al: A fluorescence cell biology approach to map the second integrin-binding site of talin to a 130-amino acid sequence within the rod domain. *J Biol Chem* 279:22258, 2004.

29. Podor TJ, Singh D, Chindemi P, et al: Vimentin exposed on activated platelets and platelet microparticles localizes vitronectin and plasminogen activator inhibitor complexes on their surface. *J Biol Chem* 277:7529, 2002.

30. Nurden P, Heilmann E, Pannocchia A, Nurden AT: Two-way trafficking of membrane glycoproteins on thrombin-activated human platelets. *Semin Hematol* 31:240, 1994.

31. Cramer EM, Norol F, Guichard J, et al: Ultrastructure of platelet formation by human megakaryocytes cultured with the Mpl ligand. *Blood* 89:2336, 1997.

32. Italiano JE Jr, Lecine P, Shivdasani RA, Hartwig JH: Blood platelets are assembled principally at the ends of proplatelet processes produced by differentiated megakaryocytes. *J Cell Biol* 147:1299, 1999.

33. Italiano JE, Hartwig JH: Megakaryocyte development and platelet formation, in *Platelets*, edited by AD Michelson, p 21. Academic Press, San Diego, 2002.

34. Crawford N, Scrutton MC: Biochemistry of the blood platelet, in *Haemostasis and Thrombosis*, edited by AL Bloom, CD Forbes, DP Thomas, EGD Tuddenham, p 89. Churchill Livingstone, England, 1994.

35. Kenney DM, Linck RW: The cytoskeleton of unstimulated blood platelets: Structure and composition of the isolated marginal microtubular band. *J Cell Sci* 78:1, 1985.

36. Sheetz MP: Microtubule motor complexes moving membranous organelles. *Cell Struct Funct* 21:369, 1996.

37. van den Bosch H, de Vet EC, Zomer AW: The role of peroxisomes in ether lipid synthesis. Back to the roots of PAF. *Adv Exp Med Biol* 416:33, 1996.

38. Wanders RJ, van Weringh G, Schrakamp G, et al: Deficiency of acyl-CoA:dihydroxyacetone phosphate acyltransferase in thrombocytes of Zellweger patients: A simple postnatal diagnostic test. *Clin Chim Acta* 151:217, 1985.

39. van den Bosch H, Schrakamp G, Hardeman D, et al: Ether lipid synthesis and its deficiency in peroxisomal disorders. *Biochimie* 75:183, 1993.

40. Holmsen H: Platelet secretion and energy metabolism, in *Hemostasis and Thrombosis: Basic Principles and Clinical Practice*, edited by RW Colman, J Hirsh, VJ Marder, EW Salzman, p 524. JB Lippincott, Philadelphia, 1993.

41. Shuster RC, Rubenstein AJ, Wallace DC: Mitochondrial DNA in anucleate human blood cells. *Biochem Biophys Res Commun* 155:1360, 1988.

42. Schapira AH: Mitochondrial dysfunction in neurodegenerative disorders. *Biochim Biophys Acta* 1366:225, 1998.

43. Lenaz G, Bovina C, Castelluccio C, et al: Mitochondrial complex I defects in aging. *Mol Cell Biochem* 174:329, 1997.

44. Cardoso SM, Proenca MT, Santos S, et al: Cytochrome c oxidase is decreased in Alzheimer's disease platelets. *Neurobiol Aging* 25:105, 2004.

45. Mancuso M, Filosto M, Bosetti F, et al: Decreased platelet cytochrome c oxidase activity is accompanied by increased blood lactate concen-

tration during exercise in patients with Alzheimer disease. *Exp Neurol* 182:421, 2003.

46. Lenaz G, D'Aurelio M, Merlo PM, et al: Mitochondrial bioenergetics in aging. *Biochim Biophys Acta* 1459:397, 2000.

47. Dror N, Klein E, Karry R, et al: State-dependent alterations in mitochondrial complex I activity in platelets: A potential peripheral marker for schizophrenia. *Mol Psychiatry* 7:995, 2002.

48. Yamagishi SI, Edelstein D, Du XL, Brownlee M: Hyperglycemia potentiates collagen-induced platelet activation through mitochondrial superoxide overproduction. *Diabetes* 50:1491, 2001.

49. Holmsen H, Kaplan KL, Dangelmaier CA: Differential energy requirements for platelet responses: A simultaneous study of aggregation, three secretory processes, arachidonate liberation, phosphatidylinositol turnover and phosphatidate production. *Biochem J* 208:9, 1982.

50. Verhoeven AJM, Mommersteeg ME, Akkerman JWN: Quantification of energy consumption in platelets during thrombin-induced aggregation and secretion: Tight coupling between platelet responses and the increment in energy consumption. *Biochem J* 221.777, 1984.

51. Ciferri S, Emiliani C, Guglielmini G, et al: Platelets release their lysosomal content in vivo in humans upon activation. *Thromb Haemost* 83:157, 2000.

52. Chen D, Lemons PP, Schraw T, Whiteheart SW: Molecular mechanisms of platelet exocytosis: Role of SNAP-23 and syntaxin 2 and 4 in lysosome release. *Blood* 96:1782, 2000.

53. Nieuwenhuis HK, van Osterhout JJG, Rozemuller E, et al: Studies with a monoclonal antibody against activated platelets: Evidence that a secreted 53,000 molecular weight lysosome-like granule protein is exposed on the surface of activated platelets in the circulation. *Blood* 70:838, 1987.

54. Abrams C, Shattil SJ: Immunological detection of activated platelets in clinical disorders. *Thromb Haemost* 65:467, 1991.

55. Zhang ZG, Zhang L, Tsang W, et al: Dynamic platelet accumulation at the site of the occluded middle cerebral artery and in downstream microvessels is associated with loss of microvascular integrity after embolic middle cerebral artery occlusion. *Brain Res* 912:181, 2001.

56. Castellot JJ, Favreau LV, Karnovsky MJ, Rosenberg RD: Inhibition of vascular smooth muscle cell growth by endothelial cell derived heparin. Possible role of a platelet endoglucosidase. *J Biol Chem* 257:11256, 1982.

57. McNicol A, Israels SJ: Platelet dense granules: Structure, function and implications for haemostasis. *Thromb Res* 95:1, 1999.

58. Ugurbil K, Holmsen H, Shulman RG: Adenine nucleotide storage pools and secretion in platelets as studied by 31P nuclear magnetic resonance. *Proc Natl Acad Sci U S A* 76:2227, 1979.

59. Ugurbil K, Fukami MH, Holmsen H: 31P-NMR studies of nucleotide and amine storage in the dense granules of pig platelets. *Biochemistry* 23:4097, 1984.

60. Nagle DL, Karim MA, Woolf EA, et al: Identification and mutation analysis of the complete gene for Chediak-Higashi syndrome. *Nat Genet* 14:307, 1996.

61. FitzGerald GA: Dipyridamole. *N Engl J Med* 316:1247, 1987.

62. Marcus AJ, Safier LB, Hajjar KA, et al: Inhibition of platelet function by an aspirin-insensitive endothelial cell ADPase. Thromboregulation by endothelial cells. *J Clin Invest* 88:1690, 1991.

63. Naik UP, Kornecki E, Ehrlich YH: Phosphorylation and dephosphorylation of human platelet surface proteins by an ecto-protein kinase/phosphatase system. *Biochim Biophys Acta* 1092:256, 1991.

64. Kalafatis M, Rand MD, Jenny RJ, et al: Phosphorylation of factor Va and factor VIIIa by activated platelets. *Blood* 81:704, 1993.

65. Hatmi M, Gavaret JM, Elalamy I, et al: Evidence for cAMP-dependent platelet ectoprotein kinase activity that phosphorylates platelet glycoprotein IV (CD36). *J Biol Chem* 271:24776, 1996.

66. Marcus AJ, Broekman MJ, Drosopoulos JH, et al: The endothelial cell ecto-ADPase responsible for inhibition of platelet function is CD39. *J Clin Invest* 99:1351, 1997.

67. Harrison P, Cramer EM: Platelet α granules. *Blood Rev* 7:52, 1993.

68. Reed GL: Platelet secretion, in *Platelets*, edited by AD Michelson, p 181. Academic Press, San Diego, 2002.

69. Hayward CP, Furmaniak-Kazmierczak E, Cieutat AM, et al: Factor V is complexed with multimerin in resting platelet lysates and colocalizes with multimerin in platelet alpha-granules. *J Biol Chem* 270:19217, 1995.

70. George JN: Platelet immunoglobulin G: Its significance for the evaluation of thrombocytopenia and for understanding the origin of alpha-granule protein. *Blood* 76:859, 1990.

71. George JN: Platelet IgG: Measurement, interpretation, and clinical significance. *Prog Hemost Thromb* 10:97, 1991.

72. Niewiarowski S, Holt JC, Cook JJ: Biochemistry and physiology of secreted platelet proteins, in *Hemostasis and Thrombosis: Basic Principles and Clinical Practice*, edited by RW Colman, J Hirsh, VJ Marder, EW Salzman, p 546. JB Lippincott, Philadelphia, 1993.

73. Niewiarowski S: Secreted platelet proteins, in *Haemostasis and Thrombosis*, edited by AL Bloom, CD Forbes, DP Thomas, EGD Tuddenham, p 167. Churchill Livingstone, England, 1994.

74. Kawahara RS, Deuel TF: Platelet-derived growth factor-inducible gene JE is a member of a family of small inducible genes related to platelet factor 4. *J Biol Chem* 264:679, 1989.

75. Brown KD, Zurawski SM, Mosmann TR, Zurawski G: A family of small inducible proteins secreted by leukocytes are members of a new super-family that includes leukocyte and fibroblast-derived inflammatory agents, growth factors, and indicators of various activation processes. *J Immunol* 142:679, 1989.

76. Oppenheim JJ, Zachariae COC, Mukaida N, Matsushima K: Properties of the novel proinflammatory supergene "intercrine" cytokine family. *Annu Rev Immunol* 9:617, 1991.

77. Rollins BJ: Chemokines. *Blood* 90:909, 1997.

78. Gear AR, Camerini D: Platelet chemokines and chemokine receptors: Linking hemostasis, inflammation, and host defense. *Microcirculation* 10:335, 2003.

79. Handin RI, Cohen HJ: Purification and binding properties of human platelet factor 4. *J Biol Chem* 58:731, 1976.

80. Loscalzo J, Melnick B, Handin RI: The interaction of platelet factor 4 and glycosaminoglycans. *Arch Biochem Biophys* 240:446, 1985.

81. Rucinski B, Niewiarowski S, Strzyzewski M, et al: Human platelet factor 4 and its C-terminal peptides: Heparin binding and clearance from the circulation. *Thromb Haemost* 63:493, 1990.

82. Barber AG, Kaser-Glanzmann R, Jakabova M, Luscher EF: Chromatography of chondroitin sulfate proteoglycan carrier for heparin neutralizing activity (platelet factor 4) released from human blood platelets. *Biochim Biophys Acta* 286:312, 1972.

83. Huang SS, Huang JS, Deuel TF: Proteoglycan carrier of human platelet factor 4: Isolation and characterization. *J Biol Chem* 257:11546, 1982.

84. Cowan SW, Bakshi EN, Machim KJ, Isaacs NW: Binding of heparin to human platelet factor 4. *Biochem J* 234:485, 1986.

85. Busch C, Dawes J, Pepper DW, Wasteson A: Binding of platelet factor 4 to cultured human umbilical vein endothelial cells. *Thromb Res* 19:129, 1980.

86. Clore GM, Gronenborn AM: Three-dimensional structures of alpha and beta chemokines. *FASEB J* 9:57, 1995.

87. Visentin GP, Ford SE, Scott JP, Aster RH: Antibodies from patients with heparin-induced thrombocytopenia/thrombosis are specific for platelet factor 4 complexed with heparin or bound to endothelial cells. *J Clin Invest* 93:81, 1994.

88. Warkentin TE: Heparin-induced thrombocytopenia. *Curr Hematol Rep* 1:63, 2002.

89. Rucinski B, Stewart GJ, DeFeo PA, et al: Uptake and processing of human platelet factor 4 by hepatocytes. *Proc Soc Exp Biol Med* 186: 361, 1987.

90. Deuel TF, Senior RM, Change D, et al: Platelet factor 4 is chemotactic for neutrophils and monocytes. *Proc Natl Acad Sci U S A* 78:4854, 1981.

91. Maione TE, Gray GS, Petro J, et al: Inhibition of angiogenesis by recombinant human platelet factor-4 and related peptides. *Science* 247: 77, 1990.

92. Brindley LL, Sweet JM, Goetzl EJ: Stimulation of histamine release from human basophils by human platelet factor 4. *J Clin Invest* 72: 1218, 1983.

93. Yamaguchi K, Ogawa K, Katsube T, et al: Platelet factor 4 gene transfection into tumor cells inhibits angiogenesis, tumor growth and metastasis. *Anticancer Res* 25:847, 2005.

94. Gewirtz AM, Calabretta B, Rucinski B, et al: Inhibition of human megakaryocytopoiesis in vitro by platelet factor 4 and a synthetic C-terminal PF4 peptide. *J Clin Invest* 83:1477, 1989.

95. Han ZC, Sensebe L, Abgrall JF, Briere J: Platelet factor 4 inhibits human megakaryocytopoiesis in vitro. *Blood* 75:1234, 1990.

96. Katz IR, Thorbecke GJ, Bell MK, et al: Protease-induced immunoregulatory activity of platelet factor 4. *Proc Natl Acad Sci U S A* 83:3491, 1986.

97. Beyth RJ, Culp LA: Complementary adhesive responses of human skin fibroblasts to the cell-binding domain of fibronectin and the heparin sulfate-binding protein, platelet factor 4. *Exp Cell Res* 155:537, 1984.

98. Capitanio AM, Niewiarowski S, Rucinski B, et al: Interaction of platelet factor 4 with human platelets. *Biochim Biophys Acta* 839:161, 1985.

99. Dumenco LL, Everson B, Culp LA, Ratnoff OD: Inhibition of the activation of Hageman factor (Factor XII) by platelet factor 4. *J Lab Clin Med* 112:394, 1988.

100. Engstad CS, Lia K, Rekdal O, et al: A novel biological effect of platelet factor 4 (PF4): Enhancement of LPS-induced tissue factor activity in monocytes. *J Leukoc Biol* 58:575, 1995.

101. Aziz KA, Cawley JC, Zuzel M: Platelets prime PMN via released PF4: Mechanism of priming and synergy with GM-CSF. *Br J Haematol* 91: 846, 1995.

102. Castor CW, Miller JW, Walz D: Structural and biological characteristics of connective tissue activating peptide (CTAP III), a major human platelet-derived growth factor. *Proc Natl Acad Sci U S A* 80:765, 1983.

103. Holt JC, Harrie ME, Holt AM, et al: Characterization of human platelet basic protein, a precursor form of low-affinity platelet factor 4 and beta-thromboglobulin. *Biochemistry* 25:1988, 1986.

104. Walz A, Dewald B, von Tscharner V, Baggiolini M: Effects of the neutrophil-activating peptide NAP-2, platelet basic protein, connective tissue-activating peptide III and platelet factor 4 on human neutrophils. *J Exp Med* 170:1745, 1989.

105. Bastl CP, Musial J, Kloczewiak M, et al: Role of kidney in the catabolic clearance of human platelet antiheparin proteins from rat circulation. *Blood* 57:233, 1981.

106. Hayward CP: Multimerin: A bench-to-bedside chronology of a unique platelet and endothelial cell protein—From discovery to function to abnormalities in disease. *Clin Invest Med* 20:176, 1997.

107. Polgar J, Magnenat E, Wells TN, Clemetson KJ: Platelet glycoprotein Ia* is the processed form of multimerin—Isolation and determination of N-terminal sequences of stored and released forms. *Thromb Haemost* 80:645, 1998.

108. Hayward CP, Cramer EM, Song Z, et al: Studies of multimerin in human endothelial cells. *Blood* 91:1304, 1998.

109. Harrison P: Platelet a-granular fibrinogen. *Platelets* 3:1, 1992.

110. Coller BS, Seligsohn U, West SM, et al: Absence of the g-Leu 427 (g') variant in the platelet alpha-granular fibrinogen pool supports the role of glycoprotein IIb/IIIa in mediating fibrinogen uptake in platelets/megakaryocytes. *Blood* 79:3394, 1992.

111. Ni H, Yuen PS, Papalia JM, et al: Plasma fibronectin promotes thrombus growth and stability in injured arterioles. *Proc Natl Acad Sci U S A* 100:2415, 2003.

112. Coller BS, Seligsohn U, West SM, et al: Platelet fibrinogen and vitronectin in Glanzmann thrombasthenia: Evidence consistent with specific roles for glycoprotein IIb/IIIA and $\alpha V\beta 3$ integrins in platelet protein trafficking. *Blood* 78:2603, 1991.

113. Fay WP, Parker AC, Ansari MN, et al: Vitronectin inhibits the thrombotic response to arterial injury in mice. *Blood* 93:1825, 1999.

114. Eitzman DT, Westrick RJ, Nabel EG, Ginsburg D: Plasminogen activator inhibitor-1 and vitronectin promote vascular thrombosis in mice. *Blood* 95:577, 2000.

115. Konstantinides S, Schafer K, Thinnes T, Loskutoff DJ: Plasminogen activator inhibitor-1 and its cofactor vitronectin stabilize arterial thrombi after vascular injury in mice. *Circulation* 103:576, 2001.

116. Baenziger NL, Brodie GN, Majerus PW: A thrombin-sensitive protein of human platelet membranes. *Proc Natl Acad Sci U S A* 68:240, 1971.

117. Lawler J, Hynes RO: The structure of human thrombospondin, an adhesive glycoprotein with multiple calcium-binding sites and homologies with several different proteins. *J Cell Biol* 103:1635, 1986.

118. Adams JC, Lawler J: The thrombospondins. *Int J Biochem Cell Biol* 36:961, 2004.

119. Mosher DF, Doyle MJ, Jaffe EA: Synthesis and secretion of thrombospondin by cultured human endothelial cells. *J Cell Biol* 93:343, 1982.

120. Schwartz BS: Monocyte synthesis of thrombospondin. *J Biol Chem* 264:7512, 1989.

121. Plow EF, McEver RP, Coller BS, et al: Related binding mechanisms for fibrinogen, fibronectin, von Willebrand factor and thrombospondin on thrombin-stimulated human platelets. *Blood* 66:724, 1985.

122. Lawler J, Hynes RO: An integrin receptor on normal and thrombasthenic platelets which binds thrombospondin. *Blood* 74:2022, 1989.

123. Asch AS, Liu I, Briccetti FM, et al: Analysis of CD36 binding domains: Ligand specificity controlled by dephosphorylation of an ectodomain. *Science* 262:1436, 1993.

124. Aiken ML, Ginsberg MH, Byers-Ward V, Plow EF: Effects of OKM5, a monoclonal antibody to glycoprotein IV, on platelet aggregation and thrombospondin surface expression. *Blood* 76:2501, 1990.

125. Chung J, Wang XQ, Lindberg FP, Frazier WA: Thrombospondin-1 acts via IAP/CD47 to synergize with collagen in alpha2beta1-mediated platelet activation. *Blood* 94:642, 1999.

126. Chung J, Gao AG, Frazier WA: Thrombospondin acts via integrin-associated protein to activate the platelet integrin alphaIIbbeta3. *J Biol Chem* 272:14740, 1997.

127. Jurk K, Clemetson KJ, de Groot PG, et al: Thrombospondin-1 mediates platelet adhesion at high shear via glycoprotein Ib (GPIb): An alternative/backup mechanism to von Willebrand factor. *FASEB J* 17:1490, 2003.

128. Gao AG, Lindberg FP, Finn MB, et al: Integrin-associated protein is a receptor for the C-terminal domain of thrombospondin. *J Biol Chem* 271:21, 1996.

129. Leung LLK, Nachman RL: Complex formation of platelet thrombospondin with fibrinogen. *J Clin Invest* 70:542, 1982.

130. Tuszynski GP, Srivastava S, Switalska HI, et al: The interaction of human platelet thrombospondin with fibrinogen. *J Biol Chem* 260: 12240, 1985.

131. Elzie CA, Murphy-Ullrich JE: The N-terminus of thrombospondin: The domain stands apart. *Int J Biochem Cell Biol* 36:1090, 2004.

132. Dardik R, Lahav J: Functional changes in the conformation of thrombospondin-1 during complexation with fibronectin or heparin. *Exp Cell Res* 248:407, 1999.

133. Leung LLK: Role of thrombospondin in platelet aggregation. *J Clin Invest* 74:1764, 1984.

134. Silverstein RL, Leung LLK, Harpel PC, Nachman RL: Complex formation of platelet thrombospondin with plasminogen. *J Clin Invest* 74:1625, 1984.

135. Schultz-Cherry S, Murphy-Ullrich JE: Thrombospondin causes activation of latent transforming growth factor-beta secreted by endothelial cells by a novel mechanism. *J Cell Biol* 122:923, 1993.

136. Tracy PB, Eide LC, Bowie EJW, Mann KG: Radioimmunoassay of factor V in human plasma and platelets. *Blood* 60:59, 1982.

137. Chesney CM, Pifer D, Colman RW: Subcellular localization and secretion of factor V from human platelets. *Proc Natl Acad Sci U S A* 78:5180, 1981.

138. Bouchard BA, Butenas S, Mann KG, et al: Interactions between platelets and the coagulation system, in *Platelets*, edited by AD Michelson, p 229. Academic Press, San Diego, 2002.

139. Camire RM, Pollak ES, Kaushansky K, Tracy PB: Secretable human platelet derived factor V originates from the plasma pool. *Blood* 92:3035, 1998.

140. Yang TL, Pipe SW, Yang A, Ginsburg D: Biosynthetic origin and functional significance of murine platelet factor V. *Blood* 102:2851, 2003.

141. Kane WH, Mruk JS, Majerus PW: Activation of coagulation factor V by a platelet protease. *J Clin Invest* 70:1092, 1982.

142. Tracy PB, Nesheim ME, Mann KG: Proteolytic alterations of factor Va bound to platelets. *J Biol Chem* 662:669, 1983.

143. Gould WR, Silveira JR, Tracy PB: Unique in vivo modifications of coagulation factor V produce a physically and functionally distinct platelet-derived cofactor: Characterization of purified platelet derived factor V/Va. *J Biol Chem* 279:2383, 2004.

144. Tracy PB, Giles AR, Mann KG, et al: Factor V (Quebec): A bleeding diathesis associated with a qualitative platelet factor V deficiency. *J Clin Invest* 74:1221, 1984.

145. Nesheim ME, Nichols WL, Cole TL, et al: Isolation and study of an acquired inhibitor of human coagulation factor V. *J Clin Invest* 405:415, 1986.

146. Bode AP, Sandberg H, Dombrose FA, Lentz BR: Association of factor V activity with membranous vesicles released from human platelets: Requirement for platelet stimulation. *Thromb Res* 39:49, 1985.

147. Manfioletti G, Brancolini C, Avanzi G, Schneider C: The protein encoded by a growth arrest-specific gene (gas6) is a new member of the vitamin K-dependent proteins related to protein S, a negative coregulator in the blood coagulation cascade. *Mol Cell Biol* 13:4976, 1993.

148. Melaragno MG, Fridell YW, Berk BC: The Gas6/Axl system: A novel regulator of vascular cell function. *Trends Cardiovasc Med* 9:250, 1999.

149. Angelillo-Scherrer A, de Frutos P, Aparicio C, et al: Deficiency or inhibition of Gas6 causes platelet dysfunction and protects mice against thrombosis. *Nat Med* 7:215, 2001.

150. Chen C, Li Q, Darrow AL, et al: Mer receptor tyrosine kinase signaling participates in platelet function. *Arterioscler Thromb Vasc Biol* 24:1118, 2004.

151. Angelillo-Scherrer A, et al: Deficiency in one Gas6 receptor (Axl, Sky or Mer) protects mice against thrombosis because of a platelet dysfunction. *Thromb Haemost* 1(suppl 1):OC245, 2003.

152. Deuel TF, Huang SS, Huang JS: Platelet derived growth factor: Purification, characterization and role in normal and abnormal cell growth, in *Biochemistry of Platelets*, edited by DR Phillips, MA Shuman, p 347. Academic Press, London, 1986.

153. Heldin C-H, Westermark B: Platelet-derived growth factor: Three isoforms and two receptor types. *Trends Genet* 5:108, 1989.

154. Ross R: Peptide regulatory factors. Platelet-derived growth factor. *Lancet* 1:1179, 1989.

155. Madtes DK, Raines EW, Ross R: Modulation of local concentrations of platelet-derived growth factor. *Am Rev Respir Dis* 140:1118, 1989.

156. Berk BC, Alexander RW: Vasoactive effects of growth factors. *Biochem Pharmacol* 38:219, 1989.

157. Waterfield MD, Scrace GT, Whittle N, et al: Platelet-derived growth factor is structurally related to the putative transforming protein p28-sis of simian sarcoma virus. *Nature* 304:35, 1983.

158. Doolittle RF, Hunkapiller MW, Hood LE, et al: Simian sarcoma virus onc gene, v-sis, is derived from the gene (or genes) encoding a platelet-derived growth factor. *Science* 21:275, 1983.

159. Williams LT: Signal transduction by the platelet-derived growth factor receptor. *Science* 243:1564, 1989.

160. Nagai MK, Embil JM: Becaplermin: Recombinant platelet derived growth factor, a new treatment for healing diabetic foot ulcers. *Expert Opin Biol Ther* 2:211, 2002.

161. King GL, Buchwald S: Characterization and partial purification of an endothelial cell growth factor from human platelets. *J Clin Invest* 73:392, 1984.

162. Maloney JP, Silliman CC, Ambruso DR, et al: In vitro release of vascular endothelial growth factor during platelet aggregation. *Am J Physiol* 275:H1054, 1998.

163. Weltermann A, Wolzt M, Petersmann K, et al: Large amounts of vascular endothelial growth factor at the site of hemostatic plug formation in vivo. *Arterioscler Thromb Vasc Biol* 19:1757, 1999.

164. Webb NJ, Bottomley MJ, Watson CJ, Brenchley PE: Vascular endothelial growth factor (VEGF) is released from platelets during blood clotting: Implications for measurement of circulating VEGF levels in clinical disease. *Clin Sci (Lond)* 94:395, 1998.

165. Mohle R, Green D, Moore MA, et al: Constitutive production and thrombin-induced release of vascular endothelial growth factor by human megakaryocytes and platelets. *Proc Natl Acad Sci U S A* 94:663, 1997.

166. Amirkhosravi A, Amaya M, Siddiqui F, et al: Blockade of GPIIb/IIIa inhibits the release of vascular endothelial growth factor (VEGF) from tumor cell-activated platelets and experimental metastasis. *Platelets* 10:285, 1999.

167. Katoh O, Tauchi H, Kawaishi K, et al: Expression of the vascular endothelial growth factor (VEGF) receptor gene, KDR, in hematopoietic cells and inhibitory effect of VEGF on apoptotic cell death caused by ionizing radiation. *Cancer Res* 55:5687, 1995.

168. Wartiovaara U, Salven P, Mikkola H, et al: Peripheral blood platelets express VEGF-C and VEGF which are released during platelet activation. *Thromb Haemost* 80:171, 1998.

169. Salven P, Orpana A, Joensuu H: Leukocytes and platelets of patients with cancer contain high levels of vascular endothelial growth factor. *Clin Cancer Res* 5:487, 1999.

170. Verheul HM, Pinedo HM: Tumor growth: A putative role for platelets? *Oncologist* 3:II, 1998.

171. Solovey A, Gui L, Ramakrishnan S, et al: Sickle cell anemia as a possible state of enhanced anti-apoptotic tone: Survival effect of vascular endothelial growth factor on circulating and unanchored endothelial cells. *Blood* 93:3824, 1999.

172. Cao J, Mathews MK, McLeod DS, et al: Angiogenic factors in human proliferative sickle cell retinopathy. *Br J Ophthalmol* 83:838, 1999.

173. Kiuru J, Viinikka L, Myllyla G, et al: Cytoskeleton-dependent release of human platelet epidermal growth factor. *Life Sci* 49:1997, 1991.

174. Bush AI, Martins RN, Rumble B, et al: The amyloid precursor protein of Alzheimer's disease is released by human platelets. *J Biol Chem* 265:15977, 1990.

175. Li Q, Beyreuther K, Masters CL: Alzheimer's disease, in *Platelets*, edited by AD Michelson, p 503. Academic Press, San Diego, 2002.

176. Borroni B, Colciaghi F, Archetti S, et al: Predicting cognitive decline in Alzheimer disease. Role of platelet amyloid precursor protein. *Alzheimer Dis Assoc Disord* 18:32, 2004.

177. Li QX, Whyte S, Tanner JE, et al: Secretion of Alzheimer disease Abeta amyloid peptide by activated human platelets. *Lab Invest* 78: 461, 1998.

178. Li Q, Cappai R, Evin G, et al: Products of the Alzheimer disease amyloid precursor protein generated by b-secretase are present in human platelets, and secreted upon degranulation. *Am J Alzheimers Dis Other Demen* 13:236, 1998.

179. Li QX, Evin G, Small DH, et al: Proteolytic processing of Alzheimer disease beta A4 amyloid precursor protein in human platelets. *J Biol Chem* 270:14140, 1995.

180. Li QX, Berndt MC, Bush AI, et al: Membrane-associated forms of the beta A4 amyloid protein precursor of Alzheimer's disease in human platelet and brain: Surface expression on the activated human platelet. *Blood* 84:133, 1994.

181. Van Nostrand WE, Schmaier AH, Farrow JS, et al: Protease nexin-2/ amyloid beta-protein precursor in blood is a platelet-specific protein. *Biochem Biophys Res Commun* 175:15, 1991.

182. Scandura JM, Zhang Y, Van Nostrand WE, Walsh PN: Progress curve analysis of the kinetics with which blood coagulation factor XIa is inhibited by protease nexin-2. *Biochemistry* 36:412, 1997.

183. Schmaier AH, Dahl LD, Rozemuller AJM, et al: Protease nexin-2/ amyloid b protein precursor. A tight-binding inhibitor of coagulation factor IXa. *J Clin Invest* 92:2540, 1993.

184. Schmaier AH, Dahl LD, Hasan AA, et al: Factor IXa inhibition by protease nexin-2/amyloid beta-protein precursor on phospholipid vesicles and cell membranes. *Biochemistry* 34:1171, 1995.

185. Rosenberg RN, Baskin F, Fosmire JA, et al: Altered amyloid protein processing in platelets of patients with Alzheimer disease. *Arch Neurol* 54:139, 1997.

186. Borroni B, Akkawi N, Martini G, et al: Microvascular damage and platelet abnormalities in early Alzheimer's disease. *J Neurol Sci* 203: 189, 2002.

187. Di Luca M, Pastorino L, Bianchetti A, et al: Differential level of platelet amyloid beta precursor protein isoforms: An early marker for Alzheimer disease. *Arch Neurol* 55:1195, 1998.

188. Baskin F, Rosenberg RN, Iyer L, et al: Platelet APP isoform ratios correlate with declining cognition in AD. *Neurology* 54:1907, 2000.

189. Davies TA, Long HJ, Tibbles HE, et al: Moderate and advanced Alzheimer's patients exhibit platelet activation differences. *Neurobiol Aging* 18:155, 1997.

190. Davies TA, Fine RE, Johnson RJ, et al: Non-age related differences in thrombin responses by platelets from male patients with advanced Alzheimer's disease. *Biochem Biophys Res Commun* 194:537, 1993.

191. McDonagh J, McDonagh RP Jr, Delage JM, Wagner RH: Factor XIII in human plasma and platelets. *J Clin Invest* 48:940, 1969.

192. Devine DV, Bishop PD: Platelet-associated factor XIII in platelet activation, adhesion, and clot stabilization. *Semin Thromb Hemost* 22: 409, 1996.

193. Lorand L, Graham RM: Transglutaminases: Crosslinking enzymes with pleiotropic functions. *Nat Rev Mol Cell Biol* 4:140, 2003.

194. Adany R, Bardos H: Factor XIII subunit A as an intracellular transglutaminase. *Cell Mol Life Sci* 60:1049, 2003.

195. Inbal A, Muszbek L, Lubetsky A, et al: Platelets but not monocytes contribute to the plasma levels of factor XIII subunit A in patients undergoing autologous peripheral blood stem cell transplantation. *Blood Coagul Fibrinolysis* 15:249, 2004.

196. Serrano K, Devine DV: Intracellular factor XIII crosslinks platelet cytoskeletal elements upon platelet activation. *Thromb Haemost* 88:315, 2002.

197. Huff T, Otto AM, Muller CS, et al: Thymosin beta4 is released from human blood platelets and attached by factor XIIIa (transglutaminase) to fibrin and collagen. *FASEB J* 16:691, 2002.

198. Kulkarni S, Jackson SP: Platelet factor XIII and calpain negatively regulate integrin alpha IIbbeta 3 adhesive function and thrombus growth. *J Biol Chem* 279:30697, 2004.

199. Szasz R, Dale GL: Thrombospondin and fibrinogen bind serotonin-derivatized proteins on COAT-platelets. *Blood* 100:2827, 2002.

200. Szasz R, Dale GL: COAT platelets. *Curr Opin Hematol* 10:351, 2003.

201. Shi Y, Massague J: Mechanisms of TGF-beta signaling from cell membrane to the nucleus. *Cell* 113:685, 2003.

202. Sakamaki S, Hirayama Y, Matsunaga T, et al: Transforming growth factor-beta1 (TGF-beta1) induces thrombopoietin from bone marrow stromal cells, which stimulates the expression of TGF-beta receptor on megakaryocytes and, in turn, renders them susceptible to suppression by TGF-beta itself with high specificity. *Blood* 94:1961, 1999.

203. Hoying JB, Yin M, Diebold R, et al: Transforming growth factor beta1 enhances platelet aggregation through a non-transcriptional effect on the fibrinogen receptor. *J Biol Chem* 274:31008, 1999.

204. Kronemann N, Bouloumia A, Bassus S, et al: Aggregating human platelets stimulate expression of vascular endothelial growth factor in cultured vascular smooth muscle cells through a synergistic effect of transforming growth factor-beta(1) and platelet-derived growth factor(AB). *Circulation* 100:855, 1999.

205. Annes JP, Munger JS, Rifkin DB: Making sense of latent TGFbeta activation. *J Cell Sci* 116:217, 2003.

206. Blakytny R, Ludlow A, Martin GE, et al: Latent TGF-beta1 activation by platelets. *J Cell Physiol* 199:67, 2004.

207. Abdelouahed M, Ludlow A, Brunner G, Lawler J: Activation of platelet-transforming growth factor beta-1 in the absence of thrombospondin-1. *J Biol Chem* 275:17933, 2000.

208. Slivka SR, Loskutoff DJ: Platelets stimulate endothelial cells to synthesize type 1 plasminogen activator inhibitor. Evaluation of the role of transforming growth factor beta. *Blood* 77:1013, 1991.

209. Lin HY, Wang XF, Ng-Eaton E, et al: Expression cloning of the TGF-beta type II receptor, a functional transmembrane serine/threonine kinase. *Cell* 68:775, 1992.

210. Fuhrman B, Brook GJ, Aviram M: Proteins derived from platelet alpha granules modulate the uptake of oxidized low density lipoprotein by macrophages. *Biochim Biophys Acta* 1127:15, 1992.

211. Heijnen HF, Schiel AE, Fijnheer R, et al: Activated platelets release two types of membrane vesicles: Microvesicles by surface shedding and exosomes derived from exocytosis of multivesicular bodies and alpha-granules. *Blood* 94:3791, 1999.

212. Janiszewski M, Do Carmo AO, Pedro MA, et al: Platelet-derived exosomes of septic individuals possess proapoptotic NAD(P)H oxidase activity: A novel vascular redox pathway. *Crit Care Med* 32:818, 2004.

213. Ts'ao CH: Rough endoplasmic reticulum and ribosomes in blood platelets. *Scand J Haematol* 8:134, 1971.

214. Booyse FM, Hoveke TP, Rafelson ME Jr: Studies on human platelets: II. Protein synthetic activity of various platelet populations. *Biochim Biophys Acta* 157:660, 1968.

215. Newman PJ, Derbes RS, Aster RH: The human platelet alloantigens, PlA1 and PlA2, are associated with a leucine33/proline33 amino acid polymorphism in membrane glycoprotein IIIa, and are distinguishable by DNA typing. *J Clin Invest* 83:1778, 1989.

216. Ginsburg D, Konkle BA, Gill JC, et al: Molecular basis of human von Willebrand disease: Analysis of platelet von Willebrand factor mRNA. *Proc Natl Acad Sci U S A* 86:3723, 1989.

217. Lindemann S, Tolley ND, Dixon DA, et al: Activated platelets mediate inflammatory signaling by regulated interleukin 1beta synthesis. *J Cell Biol* 154:485, 2001.

218. Weyrich AS, Dixon DA, Pabla R, et al: Signal-dependent translation of a regulatory protein, Bcl-3, in activated human platelets. *Proc Natl Acad Sci U S A* 95:5556, 1998.

219. Pabla R, Weyrich AS, Dixon DA, et al: Integrin-dependent control of translation: Engagement of integrin alphaIIbbeta3 regulates synthesis of proteins in activated human platelets. *J Cell Biol* 144:175, 1999.

220. Lindemann S, Tolley ND, Eyre JR, et al: Integrins regulate the intracellular distribution of eukaryotic initiation factor 4E in platelets. A checkpoint for translational control. *J Biol Chem* 276:33947, 2001.

221. Behnke O: The morphology of blood platelet membrane systems. *Ser Haematol* 3:3, 1970.

222. White JG: Electron microscopic studies of platelet secretion. *Prog Hemost Thromb* 2:49, 1974.

223. Suzuki H, Yamazaki H, Tanoue K: Immunocytochemical studies on co-localization of alpha-granule membrane alphaIIbbeta3 integrin and intragranular fibrinogen of human platelets and their cell-surface expression during the thrombin-induced release reaction. *J Electron Microsc (Tokyo)* 52:183, 2003.

224. Stenberg PE, Shuman MA, Levine SP, Bainton D: Redistribution of α granules and their contents in thrombin-stimulated platelets. *J Cell Biol* 98:748, 1984.

225. Ginsberg MH, Taylor L, Painter RG: The mechanism of thrombin-induced platelet factor 4 secretion. *Blood* 55:661, 1980.

226. George JN, Pickett EB, Saucerman S, et al: Platelet surface glycoproteins. Studies on resting and activated platelets and platelet membrane microparticles in normal subjects, and observations in patients during adult respiratory distress syndrome and cardiac surgery. *J Clin Invest* 78:340, 1986.

227. Michelson AD: Thrombin-induced down-regulation of the platelet membrane glycoprotein Ib-IX complex. *Semin Thromb Hemost* 18:18, 1992.

228. Michelson AD, Barnard MR: Plasmin-induced redistribution of platelet glycoprotein Ib. *Blood* 76:2005, 1990.

229. Suzuki H, Nakamura S, Itoh Y, et al: Immunocytochemical evidence for the translocation of α-granule membrane glycoprotein IIb/IIIa (integrin αIIbβ3) of human platelets to the surface membrane during the release reaction. *Histochemistry* 97:381, 1992.

230. Suzuki H, Murasaki K, Kodama K, Takayama H: Intracellular localization of glycoprotein VI in human platelets and its surface expression upon activation. *Br J Haematol* 121:904, 2003.

231. Nurden P, Poujol C, Winckler J, et al: Immunolocalization of P2Y1 and TPalpha receptors in platelets showed a major pool associated with the membranes of alpha-granules and the open canalicular system. *Blood* 101:1400, 2003.

232. Breton-Gorius J, Guichard J: Ultrastructural localization of peroxidase activity in human platelets and megakaryocytes. *Am J Pathol* 66:277, 1972.

233. White JG: Interaction of membrane systems in blood platelets. *Am J Pathol* 66:295, 1972.

234. Cramer EM: Platelets and megakaryocytes: Anatomy and structural organization, in *Hemostasis and Thrombosis: Basic Principles in Clinical Practice*, edited by RW Colman, J Hirsh, VJ Marder, AW Clowes, JN George, p 411. Lippincott Williams & Wilkins, Philadelphia, 2001.

235. Robblee LS, Shepro D, Belamarich FA: Calcium uptake and associated adenosine triphosphate activity of isolated platelet membranes. *J Gen Physiol* 61:462, 1973.

236. Menashi S, Davis C, Crawford N: Calcium uptake associated with an intracellular membrane fraction prepared from human blood platelets by high-voltage, free-flow electrophoresis. *FEBS Lett* 140:298, 1982.

237. Michalak M, Mariani P, Opas M: Calreticulin, a multifunctional Ca2+ binding chaperone of the endoplasmic reticulum. *Biochem Cell Biol* 76:779, 1998.

238. Hartwig JH: Platelet morphology, in *Thrombosis and Hemorrhage*, edited by J Loscalzo, AI Schafer, p 207. Williams & Wilkins, Baltimore, 1999.

239. Brownlow SL, Sage SO: Rapid agonist-evoked coupling of type II Ins(1,4,5)P3 receptor with human transient receptor potential (h-TRPC1) channels in human platelets. *Biochem J* 375:697, 2003.

240. van Gorp RM, Feijge MA, Vuist WM, et al: Irregular spiking in free calcium concentration in single, human platelets. Regulation by modulation of the inositol trisphosphate receptors. *Eur J Biochem* 269:1543, 2002.

241. Kaser-Glanzmann R, Jakabova M, George JN, Luscher EF: Further characterization of calcium accumulating vesicles from human blood platelets. *Biochim Biophys Acta* 542:357, 1978.

242. Tertyshnikova S, Fein A: Inhibition of inositol 1,4,5-trisphosphate-induced Ca2+ release by cAMP-dependent protein kinase in a living cell. *Proc Natl Acad Sci U S A* 95:1613, 1998.

243. Pernollet MG, Lantoine F, Devynck MA: Nitric oxide inhibits ATP-dependent Ca2+ uptake into platelet membrane vesicles. *Biochem Biophys Res Commun* 222:780, 1996.

244. Teijeiro RG, Silveira JR, Sotelo JR, Benech JC: Calcium efflux from platelet vesicles of the dense tubular system. Analysis of the possible contribution of the Ca2+ pump. *Mol Cell Biochem* 199:7, 1999.

245. Gerrard JM, White JG, Rao GHR, Townsend D: Localization of platelet prostaglandin production in the platelet dense tubular system. *Am J Pathol* 83:283, 1976.

246. Picot D, Loll PJ, Garavito RM: The X-ray crystal structure of the membrane protein prostaglandin H_2 synthase-1. *Nature* 367:243, 1994.

247. Gevaert K, Eggermont L, Demol H, Vandekerckhove J: A fast and convenient MALDI-MS based proteomic approach: Identification of components scaffolded by the actin cytoskeleton of activated human thrombocytes. *J Biotechnol* 78:259, 2000.

248. Marcus K, Immler D, Sternberger J, Meyer HE: Identification of platelet proteins separated by two-dimensional gel electrophoresis and analyzed by matrix assisted laser desorption/ionization-time of flight-mass spectrometry and detection of tyrosine-phosphorylated proteins. *Electrophoresis* 21:2622, 2000.

249. Gravel P, Sanchez JC, Walzer C, et al: Human blood platelet protein map established by two-dimensional polyacrylamide gel electrophoresis. *Electrophoresis* 16:1152, 1995.

250. Maguire PB, Wynne KJ, Harney DF, et al: Identification of the phosphotyrosine proteome from thrombin activated platelets. *Proteomics* 2:642, 2002.

251. Sloane AJ, Duff JL, Wilson NL, et al: High throughput peptide mass fingerprinting and protein macroarray analysis using chemical printing strategies. *Mol Cell Proteomics* 1:490, 2002.

252. Maguire PB, Fitzgerald DJ: Platelet proteomics. *J Thromb Haemost* 1:1593, 2003.

253. Coppinger JA, Cagney G, Toomey S, et al: Characterization of the proteins released from activated platelets leads to localization of novel platelet proteins in human atherosclerotic lesions. *Blood* 103:2096, 2004.

254. Garcia A, Prabhakar S, Hughan S, et al: Differential proteome analysis of TRAP-activated platelets: Involvement of DOK-2 and phosphorylation of RGS proteins. *Blood* 103:2088, 2004.

255. McRedmond JP, Park SD, Reilly DF, et al: Integration of proteomics and genomics in platelets: A profile of platelet proteins and platelet-specific genes. *Mol Cell Proteomics* 3:133, 2004.

256. Garcia A, Prabhakar S, Brock CJ, et al: Extensive analysis of the human platelet proteome by two-dimensional gel electrophoresis and mass spectrometry. *Proteomics* 4:656, 2004.

257. Gnatenko DV, Dunn JJ, McCorkle SR, et al: Transcript profiling of human platelets using microarray and serial analysis of gene expression. *Blood* 101:2285, 2003.

258. Immler D, Gremm D, Kirsch D, et al: Identification of phosphorylated proteins from thrombin-activated human platelets isolated by two-dimensional gel electrophoresis by electrospray ionization-tandem mass

spectrometry (ESI-MS/MS) and liquid chromatography-electrospray ionization-mass spectrometry (LC-ESI-MS). *Electrophoresis* 19:1015, 1998.

259. Ruggeri ZM: Platelets in atherothrombosis. *Nat Med* 8:1227, 2002.

260. Badimon L, Badimon JJ, Turitto VT, et al: Platelet thrombus formation on collagen type I. A model of deep vessel injury. Influence of blood rheology, von Willebrand factor, and blood coagulation. *Circulation* 78:1431, 1988.

261. Coller BS: Platelets in cardiovascular thrombosis and thrombolysis, in *The Heart and Cardiovascular System*, edited by HA Fozzard, RB Jennings, AM Katz, HE Morgan, E Haber, p 219. Raven Press, New York, 1991.

262. Weiss HJ, Turitto VT, Baumgartner HR, et al: Evidence for the presence of tissue factor activity on subendothelium. *Blood* 73:968, 1989.

263. Wilcox JN, Smith KM, Schwartz SM, Gordon D: Localization of tissue factor in the normal vessel wall and in the atherosclerotic plaque. *Proc Natl Acad Sci U S A* 86:2839, 1989.

264. Goldsmith HL, Turitto VT: Rheological aspects of thrombosis and haemostasis: Basic principles and applications. *Thromb Haemost* 55:415, 1986.

265. de Groot PG, Sixma JJ: Perfusion chambers, in *Platelets*, edited by AD Michelson, p 347. Academic Press, San Diego, 2002.

266. Giesen PL, Rauch U, Bohrmann B, et al: Blood-borne tissue factor: Another view of thrombosis. *Proc Natl Acad Sci U S A* 96:2311, 1999.

267. Furie B, Furie BC: Role of platelet P-selectin and microparticle PSGL-1 in thrombus formation. *Trends Mol Med* 10:171, 2004.

268. Bogdanov VY, Balasubramanian V, Hathcock J, et al: Alternatively spliced human tissue factor: A circulating, soluble, thrombogenic protein. *Nat Med* 9:458, 2003.

269. Engelmann B, Luther T, Muller I: Intravascular tissue factor pathway—A model for rapid initiation of coagulation within the blood vessel. *Thromb Haemost* 89:3, 2003.

270. Osterud B: The role of platelets in decrypting monocyte tissue factor. *Semin Hematol* 38:2, 2001.

271. Muller I, Klocke A, Alex M, et al: Intravascular tissue factor initiates coagulation via circulating microvesicles and platelets. *FASEB J* 17: 476, 2003.

272. Cambien B, Wagner DD: A new role in hemostasis for the adhesion receptor P-selectin. *Trends Mol Med* 10:179, 2004.

273. Scholz T, Temmler U, Krause S, et al: Transfer of tissue factor from platelets to monocytes: Role of platelet-derived microvesicles and CD62P. *Thromb Haemost* 88:1033, 2002.

274. Roth GJ: Developing relationships: Arterial platelet adhesion, glycoprotein Ib, and leucine-rich glycoproteins. *Blood* 77:5, 1991.

275. Ruggeri ZM: Structure and function of von Willebrand factor. *Thromb Haemost* 82:576, 1999.

276. Andrews RK, Shen Y, Gardiner EE, et al: The glycoprotein Ib-IX-V complex in platelet adhesion and signaling. *Thromb Haemost* 82:357, 1999.

277. Ruggeri ZM: Von Willebrand factor, platelets and endothelial cell interactions. *J Thromb Haemost* 1:1335, 2003.

278. Savage B, Ruggeri ZM: Platelet thrombus formation in flowing blood, in *Platelets*, edited by AD Michelson, p 215. Academic Press, San Diego, 2002.

279. Moake JL, Turner NA, Stathopoulos NA, et al: Involvement of large plasma von Willebrand factor (vWF) multimers and unusually large vWF forms derived from endothelial cells in shear stress-induced platelet aggregation. *J Clin Invest* 78:1456, 1986.

280. Ikeda Y, Handa M, Kawano K, et al: The role of von Willebrand factor and fibrinogen in platelet aggregation under varying shear stress. *J Clin Invest* 87:1234, 1991.

281. Ruggeri ZM: Mechanisms of shear-induced platelet adhesion and aggregation. *Thromb Haemost* 70:119, 1993.

282. Lopez JA, Berndt MC: The GPIb-IX-V complex, in *Platelets*, edited by AD Michelson, p 85. Academic Press, San Diego, 2002.

283. Coller BS: Platelet von Willebrand factor interactions, in *Platelet Glycoproteins*, edited by J George, D Phillips, A Nurden, p 215. Plenum, New York, 1985.

284. Rand JH, Patel ND, Schwartz E, et al: 150-kD von Willebrand factor binding protein extracted from human vascular subendothelium is type VI collagen. *J Clin Invest* 88:253, 1991.

285. Goto S, Ikeda Y, Saldivar E, Ruggeri ZM: Distinct mechanisms of platelet aggregation as a consequence of different shearing flow conditions. *J Clin Invest* 101:479, 1998.

286. Gruner S, Prostredna M, Schulte V, et al: Multiple integrin-ligand interactions synergize in shear-resistant platelet adhesion at sites of arterial injury in vivo. *Blood* 102:4021, 2003.

287. Coller BS: Interaction of normal, thrombasthenic, and Bernard-Soulier platelets with immobilized fibrinogen: Defective platelet-fibrinogen interaction in thrombasthenia. *Blood* 55:169, 1980.

288. Savage B, Ruggeri ZM: Selective recognition of adhesive sites in surface-bound fibrinogen by glycoprotein IIb-IIIa on nonactivated platelets. *J Biol Chem* 266:11227, 1991.

289. Chiang TM, Rinaldy A, Kang AH: Cloning, characterization, and functional studies of a nonintegrin platelet receptor for type I collagen. *J Clin Invest* 100:514, 1997.

290. Clemetson JM, Polgar J, Magnenat E, et al: The platelet collagen receptor glycoprotein VI is a member of the immunoglobulin superfamily closely related to FcalphaR and the natural killer receptors. *J Biol Chem* 274:29019, 1999.

291. Clemetson KJ: Platelet collagen receptors: A new target for inhibition? *Haemostasis* 29:16, 1999.

292. Coller BS, Beer JH, Scudder LE, Steinberg MH: Collagen-platelet interactions: Evidence for a direct interaction of collagen with platelet GPIa/IIa and an indirect interaction with platelet GPIIb/IIa mediated by adhesive proteins. *Blood* 74:182, 1989.

293. Saelman EU, Nieuwenhuis HK, Hese KM, et al: Platelet adhesion to collagen types I through VIII under conditions of stasis and flow is mediated by GPIa/IIa ($\alpha 2\beta 1$-integrin). *Blood* 83:1244, 1994.

294. Watson SP: Collagen receptor signaling in platelets and megakaryocytes. *Thromb Haemost* 82:376, 1999.

295. Nakamura T, Kambayashi J, Okuma M, Tandon NN: Activation of the GP IIb-IIIa complex induced by platelet adhesion to collagen is mediated by both alpha2beta1 integrin and GP VI. *J Biol Chem* 274: 11897, 1999.

296. Matsuno K, Diaz-Ricart M, Montgomery RR, et al: Inhibition of platelet adhesion to collagen by monoclonal anti-CD36 antibodies. *Br J Haematol* 92:960, 1996.

297. Nieswandt B, Watson SP: Platelet-collagen interaction: Is GPVI the central receptor? *Blood* 102:449, 2003.

298. Kuijpers MJ, Schulte V, Bergmeier W, et al: Complementary roles of glycoprotein VI and alpha2beta1 integrin in collagen-induced thrombus formation in flowing whole blood ex vivo. *FASEB J* 17:685, 2003.

299. Kato K, Kanaji T, Russell S, et al: The contribution of glycoprotein VI to stable platelet adhesion and thrombus formation illustrated by targeted gene deletion. *Blood* 102:1701, 2003.

300. Savage B, Almus-Jacobs F, Ruggeri ZM: Specific synergy of multiple substrate-receptor interactions in platelet thrombus formation under flow. *Cell* 94:657, 1998.

301. Kunicki TJ, Orchekowski R, Annis D, Honda Y: Variability of integrin alpha 2 beta 1 activity on human platelets. *Blood* 82:2693, 1993.

302. Kritzik M, Savage B, Nugent DJ, et al: Nucleotide polymorphisms in the alpha2 gene define multiple alleles that are associated with differences in platelet alpha2 beta1 density. *Blood* 92:2382, 1998.

303. Roest M, Sixma JJ, Wu YP, et al: Platelet adhesion to collagen in healthy volunteers is influenced by variation of both alpha(2)beta(1) density and von Willebrand factor. *Blood* 96:1433, 2000.

304. Henrita VZ, Saelman EU, Schut-Hese KM, et al: Platelet adhesion to collagen type IV under flow conditions. *Blood* 88:3862, 1996.

305. Ruggeri ZM, Dent JA, Saldivar E: Contribution of distinct adhesive interactions to platelet aggregation in flowing blood. *Blood* 94:172, 1999.

306. Santos MT, Valles J, Marcus AJ, et al: Enhancement of platelet reactivity and modulation of eicosanoid production by intact erythrocytes. A new approach to platelet activation and recruitment. *J Clin Invest* 87:571, 1991.

307. Shattil S: Regulation of platelet anchorage and signaling by integrin αIIbβ3. *Thromb Haemost* 70:224, 1993.

308. Weiss HJ, Turitto VT, Baumgartner HR: Further evidence that glycoprotein IIb-IIIa mediates platelet spreading on subendothelium. *Thromb Haemost* 65:202, 1991.

309. Shattil SJ: Signaling through platelet integrin αIIbβ3: Inside-out, outside-in and sideways. *Thromb Haemost* 82:318, 1999.

310. Patel D, Vaananen H, Jirouskova M, et al: The dynamics of GPIIb/IIIa-mediated platelet-platelet interactions in platelet adhesion/thrombus formation on collagen in vitro as revealed by videomicroscopy. *Blood* 101:929, 2003.

311. Naik UP, Naik MU: Association of CIB with GPIIb/IIIa during outside-in signaling is required for platelet spreading on fibrinogen. *Blood* 102:1355, 2003.

312. Denis CC, Methia N, Frenette PS, et al: A mouse model of severe von Willebrand disease: Defects in hemostasis and thrombosis. *Proc Nat Acad Sci U S A* 95:9524, 1998.

313. Celi A, Merrill-Skoloff G, Gross P, et al: Thrombus formation: Direct real-time observation and digital analysis of thrombus assembly in a living mouse by confocal and widefield intravital microscopy. *J Thromb Haemost* 1:60, 2003.

314. Ni H, Denis CV, Subbarao S, et al: Persistence of platelet thrombus formation in arterioles of mice lacking both von Willebrand factor and fibrinogen. *J Clin Invest* 106:385, 2000.

315. Jirouskova M, Chereshnev I, Vaananen H, et al: Antibody blockade or mutation of the fibrinogen gamma-chain C-terminus is more effective in inhibiting murine arterial thrombus formation than complete absence of fibrinogen. *Blood* 103:1995, 2004.

316. Loscalzo J, Inbal A, Handin RI: von Willebrand protein facilitates platelet incorporation into polymerizing fibrin. *J Clin Invest* 78:1112, 1986.

317. Michelson AD, Barnard MR: Thrombin-induced changes in platelet membrane glycoproteins Ib, IX, and IIb-IIIa complex. *Blood* 70:1673, 1987.

318. McEver RP, Beckstead JH, Moore KL, et al: GMP-140, a platelet-granule membrane protein, is also synthesized by vascular endothelial cells and is localized in Weibel-Palade bodies. *J Clin Invest* 84:92, 1989.

319. McEver RP: Properties of GMP-140, an inducible granule membrane protein of platelets and endothelium. *Blood Cells* 16:73, 1990.

320. McEver RP: P-selectin/PSGL-1 and other interactions between platelets, leukocytes, and endothelium, in *Platelets*, edited by AD Michelson, p 139. Academic Press, San Diego, 2002.

321. Frenette PS, Johnson RC, Hynes RO, Wagner DD: Platelets roll on stimulated endothelium in vivo: An interaction mediated by endothelial P-selectin. *Proc Natl Acad Sci U S A* 92:7450, 1995.

322. Romo GM, Dong JF, Schade AJ, et al: The glycoprotein Ib-IX-V complex is a platelet counterreceptor for P-selectin. *J Exp Med* 190:803, 1999.

323. Frenette PS, Denis CV, Weiss L, et al: P-selectin glycoprotein ligand 1 (PSGL-1) is expressed on platelets and can mediate platelet-endothelial interactions in vivo. *J Exp Med* 191:1413, 2000.

324. Henn V, Slupsky JR, Grafe M, et al: CD40 ligand on activated platelets triggers an inflammatory reaction of endothelial cells. *Nature* 391:591, 1998.

325. Prasad KS, Andre P, He M, et al: Soluble CD40 ligand induces beta3 integrin tyrosine phosphorylation and triggers platelet activation by outside-in signaling. *Proc Natl Acad Sci U S A* 100:12367, 2003.

326. Prasad KS, Andre P, Yan Y, Phillips DR: The platelet CD40L/GP IIb-IIIa axis in atherothrombotic disease. *Curr Opin Hematol* 10:356, 2003.

327. Heeschen C, Dimmeler S, Hamm CW, et al: Soluble CD40 ligand in acute coronary syndromes. *N Engl J Med* 348:1104, 2003.

328. Andre P, Nannizzi-Alaimo L, Prasad SK, Phillips DR: Platelet-derived CD40L: The switch-hitting player of cardiovascular disease. *Circulation* 106:896, 2002.

329. Andre P, Prasad KS, Denis CV, et al: CD40L stabilizes arterial thrombi by a beta3 integrin–dependent mechanism. *Nat Med* 8:247, 2002.

330. Cipollone F, Ferri C, Desideri G, et al: Preprocedural level of soluble CD40L is predictive of enhanced inflammatory response and restenosis after coronary angioplasty. *Circulation* 108:2776, 2003.

331. Luscher TF: Platelet-vessel wall interaction: Role of nitric oxide, prostaglandins and endothelins. *Baillieres Clin Haematol* 6:609, 1993.

332. Loscalzo J: Nitric oxide insufficiency, platelet activation, and arterial thrombosis. *Circ Res* 88:756, 2001.

333. Barry OP, FitzGerald GA: Mechanisms of cellular activation by platelet microparticles. *Thromb Haemost* 82:794, 1999.

334. Freedman JE, Loscalzo J, Barnard MR, et al: Nitric oxide released from activated platelets inhibits platelet recruitment. *J Clin Invest* 100:350, 1997.

335. Freedman JE, Sauter R, Battinelli EM, et al: Deficient platelet-derived nitric oxide and enhanced hemostasis in mice lacking the NOSIII gene. *Circ Res* 84:1416, 1999.

336. Smith JA, Henderson AH, Randall MD: Endothelium-derived relaxing factor, prostanoids and endothelins, in *Haemostasis and Thrombosis*, edited by AL Bloom, CD Forbes, DP Thomas, EGD Tuddenham, p 183. Churchill Livingstone, England, 1994.

337. Valles J, Santos MT, Marcus AJE, et al: Down-regulation of human platelet reactivity by neutrophils. Participation of lypoxygenase derivatives and adhesive proteins. *J Clin Invest* 92:1357, 1993.

338. Selak MA: Cathepsin G and thrombin: Evidence for two different platelet receptors. *Biochem J* 297:269, 1994.

339. Molino M, Di Lallo M, Martelli N, et al: Effects of leukocyte-derived cathepsin G on platelet membrane glycoprotein Ib-IX and IIb-IIIa complexes: A comparison with thrombin. *Blood* 82:2442, 1993.

340. Peerschke EI: Ca^{2+} mobilization and fibrinogen binding of platelets refractory to adenosine diphosphate stimulation. *J Lab Clin Med* 106:111, 1985.

341. Murray R, FitzGerald GA: Regulation of thromboxane receptor activation in human platelets. *Proc Natl Acad Sci U S A* 86:124, 1989.

342. Coughlin SR: Protease-activated receptors and platelet function. *Thromb Haemost* 82:353, 1999.

343. Phillips DR, Charo IF, Parise LV, Fitzgerald LA: The platelet membrane glycoprotein IIb-IIIa complex. *Blood* 71:831, 1988.

344. Plow EF, Ginsberg MH: Cellular adhesion: GPIIb-IIIa as a prototypic adhesion receptor. *Prog Hemost Thromb* 9:117, 1989.

345. Peerschke EI: The platelet fibrinogen receptor. *Semin Hematol* 22:241, 1985.

346. Hato T, Ginsberg MH, Shattil SJ: Integrin αIIbβ3, in *Platelets*, edited by AD Michelson, p 105. Academic Press, San Diego, 2002.

347. Sixma JJ: Interaction of blood platelets with the vessel wall, in *Haemostasis and Thrombosis*, edited by AL Bloom, CD Forbes, DP Thomas, EGD Tuddenham, p 259. Churchill Livingstone, England, 1994.

348. Weiss HJ, Hawiger J, Ruggeri ZM, et al: Fibrinogen-independent platelet adhesion and thrombus formation on subendothelium mediated by glycoprotein IIb-IIIa complex at high shear rate. *J Clin Invest* 83:288, 1989.

349. Bennett JS: The platelet-fibrinogen interaction, in *Platelet Membrane Glycoproteins*, edited by JN George, AT Nurden, DR Phillips, p 193. Plenum, New York, 1985.

350. Steen VM, Holmsen H: Synergism between thrombin and epinephrine in human platelets: Different dose-response relationships for aggregation and dense granule secretion. *Thromb Haemost* 54:680, 1985.

351. Ware JA, Smith M, Salzman EW: Synergism of platelet-aggregating agents. Role of elevation of cytoplasmic calcium. *J Clin Invest* 80:267, 1987.

352. Folts JD, Rowe GG: Epinephrine potentiation of in vivo stimuli reverses aspirin inhibition of platelet thrombus formation in stenosed canine coronary arteries. *Thromb Res* 50:507, 1988.

353. Folts JD, Bonebrake FC: The effects of cigarette smoke and nicotine on platelet thrombus formation in stenosed dog coronary arteries: Inhibition with phentolamine. *Circulation* 65:465, 1989.

354. Hjemdahl P, Chronos NA, Wilson DJ, et al: Epinephrine sensitizes human platelets in vivo and in vitro as studied by fibrinogen binding and P-selectin expression. *Arterioscler Thromb* 14:77, 1994.

355. Moake JL, Turner NA, Stathopoulos NA, et al: Shear-induced platelet aggregation can be mediated by vWF released from platelets, as well as by exogenous large or unusually large vWF multimers, requires adenosine diphosphate, and is resistant to aspirin. *Blood* 71:1366, 1988.

356. Karpatkin S, Langer RM: Biochemical energetics of simulated platelet plug formation: Effect of thrombin, adenosine diphosphate, and epinephrine on intra- and extracellular adenine nucleotide kinetics. *J Clin Invest* 47:2158, 1968.

357. Akkerman JWN, Gorter G, Schrama L, Holmsen H: A novel technique for rapid determination of energy consumption in platelets: Determination of different energy consumption associated with three secretory responses. *Biochem J* 210:145, 1983.

358. Akkerman JWN, Holmsen H: Interrelationships among platelet responses: Studies on the burst in protein liberation, lactate production and oxygen uptake during platelet aggregation and Ca++ secretion. *Blood* 57:956, 1981.

359. Akkerman JWN, Verhoeven AJM: Energy metabolism and function, in *Platelet Responses and Metabolism*, edited by H Holmsen, p 69. CRC Press, Boca Raton, 1987.

360. Holmsen H, Farstad M: Energy metabolism, in *Platelet Responses and Metabolism*, edited by H Holmsen, p 245. CRC Press, Boca Raton, 1987.

361. Guppy M, Abas L, Neylon C, et al: Fuel choices by human platelets in human plasma. *Eur J Biochem* 244:161, 1997.

362. Shimizu T, Murphy S: Roles of acetate and phosphate in the successful storage of platelet concentrates prepared with an acetate-containing additive solution. *Transfusion* 33:304, 1993.

363. Simons ER, Greenberg-Sperssky SM: Transmembrane monovalent cation gradients, in *Platelet Responses and Metabolism*, edited by H Holmsen, p 31. CRC Press, Boca Raton, 1987.

364. Dean WL: Structure, function and subcellular localization of a human platelet Ca++-ATPase. *Cell Calcium* 10:289, 1989.

365. Daniel JL, Molish IR, Robkin L, et al: Nucleotide exchange between cytosolic ATP and F-actin-bound ADP may be a major ATP-utilizing process in unstimulated platelets. *Eur J Biochem* 156:677, 1986.

366. Verhoeven AJM, Tysnes O-B, Aarbakke GM, et al: Turnover of the phosphomonoester groups of polyphosphoinositol lipids in unstimulated platelets. *Eur J Biochem* 166:3, 1987.

367. Holmsen H, Kaplan KL, Dangelmaier CA: Differential requirements for platelet responses: A simultaneous study of dense granule, α-granule and acid hydrolase secretion, arachidonate liberation, phosphati-

368. Akkerman JW, Gorter G, Soons H, Holmsen H: Close correlation between platelet responses and adenylate energy charge during transient substrate depletion. *Biochim Biophys Acta* 760:34, 1983.

369. Furman MI, Gardner TM, Goldschmidt-Clermont PJ: Mechanisms of cytoskeletal reorganization during platelet activation. *Thromb Haemost* 70:229, 1993.

370. Nachmias VT, Yoshida K: The cytoskeleton of the blood platelets: A dynamic structure. *Adv Cyclic Nucleotide Res* 2:181, 1999.

371. Fox JEB: Platelet cytoskeleton, in *Hemostasis and Thrombosis: Basic Principles and Clinical Practice*, edited by RW Colman, J Hirsh, VJ Marder, AW Clowes, JN George, p 429. Lippincott Williams & Wilkins, Philadelphia, 2001.

372. Fox JEB, Boyles JK, Reynolds CC, Phillips DR: Actin filament content and organization in unstimulated platelets. *J Cell Biol* 98:1985, 1984.

373. Escolar G, Krumwiede M, White JG: Organization of the actin cytoskeleton of resting and activated platelets in suspension. *Am J Pathol* 123:86, 1986.

374. Gorlin JB, Henske E, Warren ST, et al: Actin-binding protein (ABP-280) filamin gene (FLN) maps telomeric to the color vision locus (R/GCP) and centromeric to G6PD in Xq28. *Genomics* 17:496, 1993.

375. Takafuta T, Wu G, Murphy GF, Shapiro SS: Human beta-filamin is a new protein that interacts with the cytoplasmic tail of glycoprotein Ibalpha. *J Biol Chem* 273:17531, 1998.

376. Nachmias VT: Cytoskeleton of human platelets at rest and after spreading. *J Cell Biol* 86:795, 1980.

377. Gonnella PA, Nachmias VT: Platelet activation and microfilament bundling. *J Biol Chem* 89:146, 1981.

378. Phillips DR, Jennings LK, Edwards HH: Identification of membrane proteins mediating the interaction of human platelets. *J Cell Biol* 86:77, 1980.

379. Bennett JS, Zigmond S, Vilaire G, et al: The platelet cytoskeleton regulates the affinity of the integrin alpha(IIb)beta(3) for fibrinogen. *J Biol Chem* 274:25301, 1999.

380. Patil S, Jedsadayanmata A, Wencel-Drake JD, et al: Identification of a talin-binding site in the integrin beta(3) subunit distinct from the NPLY regulatory motif of post-ligand binding functions. The talin n-terminal head domain interacts with the membrane-proximal region of the beta(3) cytoplasmic tail. *J Biol Chem* 274:28575, 1999.

381. Shattil SJ, Brugge JS: Protein tyrosine phosphorylation and the adhesive functions of platelets. *Curr Opin Cell Biol* 3:869, 1991.

382. Fox JEB: On the role of calpain and Rho proteins in regulating integrin-induced signaling. *Thromb Haemost* 82:391, 1999.

383. Fox JEB, Goll DE, Reynolds CC, Phillips DR: Identification of two proteins (actin-binding protein and P235) that are hydrolyzed by endogenous Ca++-dependent protease during platelet aggregation. *J Biol Chem* 260:1060, 1985.

384. Fox JE, Reynolds CC, Phillips DR: Calcium-dependent proteolysis occurs during platelet aggregation. *J Biol Chem* 258:9973, 1983.

385. Fox JE, Taylor RG, Taffarel M, et al: Evidence that activation of platelet calpain is induced as a consequence of binding of adhesive ligand to the integrin, glycoprotein IIb-IIIa. *J Cell Biol* 120:1501, 1993.

386. Xi X, Bodnar RJ, Li Z, et al: Critical roles for the COOH-terminal NITY and RGT sequences of the integrin beta3 cytoplasmic domain in inside-out and outside-in signaling. *J Cell Biol* 162:329, 2003.

387. Fox JEB, Austin CD, Reynolds CC, et al: Evidence that agonist-induced activation of calpain causes the shedding of procoagulant-containing microvesicles from the membrane of aggregating platelets. *J Biol Chem* 266:13289, 1991.

388. Dachary-Prigent J, Freyssinet J-M, Pasquet J-M, et al: Annexin V as a probe of aminophospholipid exposure and platelet membrane vesic-

ulation: A flow cytometry study showing a role for free sulfhydryl groups. *Blood* 81:2554, 1993.

389. Azam M, Andrabi SS, Sahr KE, et al: Disruption of the mouse mu-calpain gene reveals an essential role in platelet function. *Mol Cell Biol* 21:2213, 2001.

390. Nachmias VT: Platelet and megakaryocyte shape change: Triggered alterations in the cytoskeleton. *Semin Hematol* 20:261, 1983.

391. Maurer-Spurej E, Devine DV: Platelet aggregation is not initiated by platelet shape change. *Lab Invest* 81:1517, 2001.

392. Born GV, Dearnley R, Foulks JG, Sharp DE: Quantification of the morphological reaction of platelets to aggregating agents and of its reversal by aggregation inhibitors. *J Physiol* 280:193, 1978.

393. Heemskerk JW, Vuist WM, Feijge MA, et al: Collagen but not fibrinogen surfaces induce bleb formation, exposure of phosphatidylserine, and procoagulant activity of adherent platelets: Evidence for regulation by protein tyrosine kinase-dependent Ca2+ responses. *Blood* 90:2615, 1997.

394. Coller BS, Kutok JL, Scudder LE, et al: Studies of activated GPIIb/IIIa receptors on the luminal surface of adherent platelets. Paradoxical loss of luminal receptors when platelets adhere to high density fibrinogen. *J Clin Invest* 92:2796, 1993.

395. Ma AD, Abrams CS: Pleckstrin homology domains and phospholipid-induced cytoskeletal reorganization. *Thromb Haemost* 82:399, 1999.

396. Li R, Mitra N, Gratkowski H, et al: Activation of integrin alphaIIbbeta3 by modulation of transmembrane helix associations. *Science* 300:795, 2003.

397. Olorundare OE, Simmons SR, Albrecht RM: Cytochalasin D and E: Effects on fibrinogen receptor movement and cytoskeletal reorganization in fully spread, surface-activated platelets: A correlative light and electron microscopic investigation. *Blood* 79:99, 1992.

398. White JG: Induction of patching and its reversal on surface-activated human platelets. *Br J Haematol* 76:108, 1990.

399. Lemons PP, Chen D, Bernstein AM, et al: Regulated secretion in platelets: Identification of elements of the platelet exocytosis machinery. *Blood* 90:1490, 1997.

400. Karniguian A, Zahraoui A, Tavitian A: Identification of small GTP-binding rab proteins in human platelets: Thrombin-induced phosphorylation of rab3B, rab6, and rab8 proteins. *Proc Natl Acad Sci U S A* 90:7647, 1993.

401. Morimoto T, Ogihara S: ATP is required in platelet serotonin exocytosis for protein phosphorylation and priming of secretory vesicles docked on the plasma membrane. *J Cell Sci* 109(Pt 1):113, 1996.

402. Gerrard JM, Beattie LL, Park J, et al: A role for protein kinase C in the membrane fusion necessary for platelet granule secretion. *Blood* 74:2405, 1989.

403. Augustine GJ, Burns ME, DeBello WM, et al: Exocytosis: Proteins and perturbations. *Annu Rev Pharmacol Toxicol* 36:659, 1996.

404. Reed GL, Houng AK, Fitzgerald ML: Human platelets contain SNARE proteins and a Sec1p homologue that interacts with syntaxin 4 and is phosphorylated after thrombin activation: Implications for platelet secretion. *Blood* 93:2617, 1999.

405. Flaumenhaft R, Croce K, Chen E, et al: Proteins of the exocytotic core complex mediate platelet alpha-granule secretion. Roles of vesicle-associated membrane protein, SNAP-23, and syntaxin 4. *J Biol Chem* 274:2492, 1999.

406. Bernstein AM, Whiteheart SW: Identification of a cellubrevin/vesicle associated membrane protein 3 homologue in human platelets. *Blood* 93:571, 1999.

407. Chen D, Bernstein AM, Lemons PP, Whiteheart SW: Molecular mechanisms of platelet exocytosis: Role of SNAP-23 and syntaxin 2 in dense core granule release. *Blood* 95:921, 2000.

408. Polgar J, Reed GL: A critical role for N-ethylmaleimide-sensitive fusion protein (NSF) in platelet granule secretion. *Blood* 94:1313, 1999.

409. Flaumenhaft R: Molecular basis of platelet granule secretion. *Arterioscler Thromb Vasc Biol* 23:1152, 2003.

410. Budtz-Olsen OE: *Clot Retraction*, Charles Thomas, Springfield, 1951.

411. Kunitada S, FitzGerald GA, Fitzgerald DJ: Inhibition of clot lysis and decreased binding of tissue-type plasminogen activator as a consequence of clot retraction. *Blood* 79:1420, 1992.

412. Pollard TD, Fujiwara K, Handin R, Weiss G: Contractile proteins in platelet activation and contraction. *Ann N Y Acad Sci* 283:218, 1977.

413. Cohen I, Gerrard JM, White JG: Ultrastructure of clots during isometric contraction. *J Cell Biol* 91:775, 1982.

414. Cohen I: The mechanism of clot retraction, in *Platelet Membrane Glycoproteins*, edited by JN George, AT Nurden, DR Phillips, p 299. Plenum Press, New York, 1985.

415. Carr ME Jr, Carr SL, Hantgan RR, Braaten J: Glycoprotein IIb/IIIa blockade inhibits platelet-mediated force development and reduces gel elastic modulus. *Thromb Haemost* 73:499, 1995.

416. Leistikow EA: Platelet internalization in early thrombogenesis. *Semin Thromb Hemost* 22:289, 1996.

417. Morgenstern E, Daub M, Dierichs R: A new model for in vitro clot formation that considers the mode of the fibrin(ogen) contacts to platelets and the arrangement of the platelet cytoskeleton. *Ann N Y Acad Sci* 936:449, 2001.

418. Coller BS, Peerschke EI, Scudder LE, Sullivan CA: A murine monoclonal antibody that completely blocks the binding of fibrinogen to platelets produces a thrombasthenic-like state in normal platelets and binds to glycoproteins IIb and/or IIIa. *J Clin Invest* 72:325, 1983.

419. Collet JP, Montalescot G, Lesty C, Weisel JW: A structural and dynamic investigation of the facilitating effect of glycoprotein IIb/IIIa inhibitors in dissolving platelet-rich clots. *Circ Res* 90:428, 2002.

420. Huang TC, Jordan RE, Hantgan RR, Alevriadou BR: Differential effects of c7E3 Fab on thrombus formation and rt-PA-mediated thrombolysis under flow conditions. *Thromb Res* 102:411, 2001.

421. Braaten JV, Jerome WG, Hantgan RR: Uncoupling fibrin from integrin receptors hastens fibrinolysis at the platelet-fibrin interface. *Blood* 83:982, 1994.

422. Seiffert D, Pedicord DL, Kieras CJ, et al: Regulation of clot retraction by glycoprotein IIb/IIIa antagonists. *Thromb Res* 108:181, 2002.

423. Mousa SA, Khurana S, Forsythe MS: Comparative in vitro efficacy of different platelet glycoprotein IIb/IIIa antagonists on platelet-mediated clot strength induced by tissue factor with use of thromboelastography: Differentiation among glycoprotein IIb/IIIa antagonists. *Arterioscler Thromb Vasc Biol* 20:1162, 2000.

424. Jirouskova M, Smyth SS, Kudryk B, Coller BS: A hamster antibody to the mouse fibrinogen gamma chain inhibits platelet-fibrinogen interactions and FXIIIa-mediated fibrin cross-linking, and facilitates thrombolysis. *Thromb Haemost* 86:1047, 2001.

425. Osdoit S, Rosa JP: Fibrin clot retraction by human platelets correlates with alpha(IIb)beta(3) integrin-dependent protein tyrosine dephosphorylation. *J Biol Chem* 276:6703, 2001.

426. Ward CM, Kestin AS, Newman PJ: A Leu262Pro mutation in the integrin beta(3) subunit results in an alpha(IIb)-beta(3) complex that binds fibrin but not fibrinogen. *Blood* 96:161, 2000.

427. Rooney MM, Farrell DH, van Hemel BM, et al: The contribution of the three hypothesized integrin-binding sites in fibrinogen to platelet-mediated clot retraction. *Blood* 92:2374, 1998.

428. Rooney MM, Parise LV, Lord ST: Dissecting clot retraction and platelet aggregation. Clot retraction does not require an intact fibrinogen gamma chain C terminus. *J Biol Chem* 271:8553, 1996.

429. Podolnikova NP, Yakubenko VP, Volkov GL, et al: Identification of a novel binding site for platelet integrins alpha IIb beta 3 (GPIIbIIIa) and alpha 5 beta 1 in the gamma C-domain of fibrinogen. *J Biol Chem* 278:32251, 2003.

430. Remijn JA, Ijsseldijk MJ, de Groot PG: Role of the fibrinogen gamma-chain sequence gamma316-322 in platelet-mediated clot retraction. *J Thromb Haemost* 1:2245, 2003.

431. Dubois C, Steiner B, Kieffer N, Reigner SC: Thrombin binding to GPIbalpha induces platelet aggregation and fibrin clot retraction supported by resting alphaIIbbeta3 interaction with polymerized fibrin. *Thromb Haemost* 89:853, 2003.

432. Keuren JF, Baruch D, Legendre P, et al: Von Willebrand factor C1C2 domain is involved in platelet adhesion to polymerized fibrin at high shear rate. *Blood* 103:1741, 2004.

433. Bevers EM, Comfurius P, Dekkers DW, Zwaal RF: Lipid translocation across the plasma membrane of mammalian cells. *Biochim Biophys Acta* 1439:317, 1999.

434. Zhou Q, Zhao J, Stout JG, et al: Molecular cloning of human plasma membrane phospholipid scramblase. A protein mediating transbilayer movement of plasma membrane phospholipids. *J Biol Chem* 272:18240, 1997.

435. Zhou Q, Zhao J, Wiedmer T, Sims PJ: Normal hemostasis but defective hematopoietic response to growth factors in mice deficient in phospholipid scramblase 1. *Blood* 99:4030, 2002.

436. Wiedmer T, Zhou Q, Kwok DY, Sims PJ: Identification of the three new members of the phospholipid scramblase gene family. *Biochim Biophys Acta* 1463:244, 2000.

437. Hamon Y, Broccardo C, Chambenoit O, et al: ABC1 promotes engulfment of apoptotic cells and transbilayer redistribution of phosphatidylserine. *Nat Cell Biol* 2:399, 2000.

438. Zwaal RF, Comfurius P, Bevers EM: Scott syndrome, a bleeding disorder caused by defective scrambling of membrane phospholipids. *Biochim Biophys Acta* 1636:119, 2004.

439. Thiagarajan P, Tait JF: Collagen-induced exposure of anionic phospholipid in platelets and platelet-derived microparticles. *J Biol Chem* 266:24302, 1991.

440. Miyazaki Y, Nomura S, Miyake T, et al: High shear stress can initiate both platelet aggregation and shedding of procoagulant containing microparticles. *Blood* 88:3456, 1996.

441. Reverter JC, Beguin S, Kessels H, et al: Inhibition of platelet-mediated, tissue factor-induced thrombin generation by the mouse/human chimeric 7E3 antibody. Potential implications for the effect of c7E3 Fab treatment on acute thrombosis and "clinical restenosis." *J Clin Invest* 98:863, 1996.

442. Beguin S, Kumar R, Keularts I, et al: Fibrin-dependent platelet procoagulant activity requires GPIb receptors and von Willebrand factor. *Blood* 93:564, 1999.

443. Lee DH, Warkentin TE, Denomme GA, et al: A diagnostic test for heparin-induced thrombocytopenia: Detection of platelet microparticles using flow cytometry. *Br J Haematol* 95:724, 1996.

444. Kelton JG: Heparin-induced thrombocytopenia: An overview. *Blood Rev* 16:77, 2002.

445. George JN, Pickett EB, Saucerman S, et al: Platelet surface glycoproteins. Studies on resting and activated platelets and platelet membrane microparticles in normal subjects, and observations in patients during adult respiratory distress syndrome and cardiac surgery. *J Clin Invest* 78:340, 1986.

446. Siljander P, Carpen O, Lassila R: Platelet-derived microparticles associate with fibrin during thrombosis. *Blood* 87:4651, 1996.

447. Dahlback B, Wiedmer T, Sims PJ: Binding of anticoagulant vitamin K-dependent protein S to platelet-derived microparticles. *Biochemistry* 31:12769, 1992.

448. Tans G, Rosing J, Thomassen MC, et al: Comparison of anticoagulant and procoagulant activities of stimulated platelets and platelet-derived microparticles. *Blood* 77:2641, 1991.

449. Shcherbina A, Remold-O'Donnell E: Role of caspase in a subset of human platelet activation responses. *Blood* 93:4222, 1999.

450. Wolf BB, Goldstein JC, Stennicke HR, et al: Calpain functions in a caspase-independent manner to promote apoptosis-like events during platelet activation. *Blood* 94:1683, 1999.

451. Augereau O, Rossignol R, DeGiorgi F, et al: Apoptotic-like mitochondrial events associated to phosphatidylserine exposure in blood platelets induced by local anaesthetics. *Thromb Haemost* 92:104, 2004.

452. Giesen PL, Rauch U, Bohrmann B, et al: Blood-borne tissue factor: Another view of thrombosis. *Proc Natl Acad Sci U S A* 96:2311, 1999.

453. Rauch U, Bonderman D, Bohrmann B, et al: Transfer of tissue factor from leukocytes to platelets is mediated by CD15 and tissue factor. *Blood* 96:170, 2000.

454. Balasubramanian V, Grabowski E, Bini A, Nemerson Y: Platelets, circulating tissue factor, and fibrin colocalize in ex vivo thrombi: Real-time fluorescence images of thrombus formation and propagation under defined flow conditions. *Blood* 100:2787, 2002.

455. Falati S, Liu Q, Gross P, et al: Accumulation of tissue factor into developing thrombi in vivo is dependent upon microparticle P-selectin glycoprotein ligand 1 and platelet P-selectin. *J Exp Med* 197:1585, 2003.

456. Zwaal RFA, Comfurius P, Bevers EM: Platelet procoagulant activity and microvesicle formation. Its putative role of hemostasis and thrombosis. *Biochim Biophys Acta* 1180:1, 1992.

457. Weiss HJ: Scott syndrome—A disorder of platelet coagulant activity. *Semin Hematol* 31:312, 1994.

458. Swords NA, Tracy PB, Mann KG: Intact platelet membranes, not platelet-released microvesicles, support the procoagulant activity of adherent platelets. *Arterioscler Thromb* 13:1613, 1993.

459. Weiss HJ, Lages B: Platelet prothrombinase activity and intracellular calcium responses in patients with storage pool deficiency, glycoprotein IIb-IIIa deficiency, or impaired platelet coagulant activity—A comparison with Scott syndrome. *Blood* 89:1599, 1997.

460. Hultin MB: Modulation of thrombin-mediated activation of factor VIII: C by calcium ions, phospholipid, and platelets. *Blood* 66:53, 1985.

461. Nesheim ME, Furmaniak-Kazmierczak E, Henin C, Cote G: On the existence of platelet receptors for factor V(a) and factor VIII(a). *Thromb Haemost* 70:80, 1993.

462. Bouchard BA, Catcher CS, Thrash BR, et al: Effector cell protease receptor-1, a platelet activation-dependent membrane protein, regulates prothrombinase-catalyzed thrombin generation. *J Biol Chem* 272:9244, 1997.

463. London FS, Marcinkiewicz M, Walsh PN: A subpopulation of platelets responds to thrombin- or SFLLRN-stimulation with binding sites for factor IXa. *J Biol Chem* 279:19854, 2004.

464. Alberio L, Safa O, Clemetson KJ, et al: Surface expression and functional characterization of alpha-granule factor V in human platelets: Effects of ionophore A23187, thrombin, collagen, and convulxin. *Blood* 95:1694, 2000.

465. Scandura JM, Ahmad SS, Walsh PN: A binding site expressed on the surface of activated human platelets is shared by factor X and prothrombin. *Biochemistry* 35:8890, 1996.

466. Byzova TV, Plow EF: Networking in the hemostatic system. Integrin alphaiibbeta3 binds prothrombin and influences its activation. *J Biol Chem* 272:27183, 1997.

467. Taube J, McWilliam N, Luddington R, et al: Activated protein C resistance: Effect of platelet activation, platelet-derived microparticles, and atherogenic lipoproteins. *Blood* 93:3792, 1999.

468. Chiu HC, Schick P, Colman RW: Biosynthesis of coagulation factor V by megakaryocytes. *J Clin Invest* 75:339, 1985.

469. Osterud B, Rapaport SI, Lavine KK: Factor V activity of platelets: Evidence for an activated factor V molecule and for a platelet activator. *Blood* 49:834, 1977.

470. Chediak J, Ashenhurst JB, Garlick I, Desser RK: Successful management of bleeding in a patient with factor V inhibitor by platelet transfusions. *Blood* 56:835, 1980.

471. Toti F, Satta N, Fressinaud E, et al: Scott syndrome, characterized by impaired transmembrane migration of procoagulant phosphatidylserine and hemorrhagic complications, is an inherited disorder. *Blood* 87:1409, 1996.

472. Zhou Q, Sims PJ, Wiedmer T: Expression of proteins controlling transbilayer movement of plasma membrane phospholipids in the B lymphocytes from a patient with Scott syndrome. *Blood* 92:1707, 1998.

473. Baglia FA, Walsh PN: Thrombin-mediated feedback activation of factor XI on the activated platelet surface is preferred over contact activation by factor XIIa or factor XIa. *J Biol Chem* 275:20514, 2000.

474. Oliver JA, Monroe DM, Roberts HR, Hoffman M: Thrombin activates factor XI on activated platelets in the absence of factor XII. *Arterioscler Thromb Vasc Biol* 19:170, 1999.

475. Gailani D, Ho D, Sun MF, et al: Model for a factor IX activation complex on blood platelets: Dimeric conformation of factor XIa is essential. *Blood* 97:3117, 2001.

476. Walsh PN: Platelets and factor XI bypass the contact system of blood coagulation. *Thromb Haemost* 82:234, 1999.

477. Lopez JA: The platelet glycoprotein Ib-IX complex. *Blood Coagul Fibrinolysis* 5:97, 1994.

478. Rajagopalan V, Essex DW, Shapiro SS, Konkle BA: Tumor necrosis factor-alpha modulation of glycoprotein Ib-alpha expression in human endothelial and erythroleukemia cells. *Blood* 80:153, 1992.

479. Wu G, Essex DW, Meloni FJ, et al: Human endothelial cells in culture and in vivo express on their surface all four components of the glycoprotein Ib/IX/V complex. *Blood* 90:2660, 1997.

480. Bennett JS: The molecular biology of platelet membrane proteins. *Semin Hematol* 27:186, 1990.

481. Hynes R: Integrins. Bidirectional, allosteric signaling machines. *Cell* 110:673, 2002.

482. Wagner CL, Mascelli MA, Neblock DS, et al: Analysis of GPIIb/IIIa receptor number by quantification of 7E3 binding to human platelets. *Blood* 88:907, 1996.

483. Woods VL Jr, Wolff LE, Keller DM: Resting platelets contain a substantial centrally located pool of glycoprotein IIb-IIIa complexes which may be accessible to some but not other extracellular proteins. *J Biol Chem* 261:15242, 1986.

484. Cramer ER, Savidge GF, Vainchenker W, et al: A granule pool of glycoprotein IIb-IIIa in normal and pathologic platelets and megakaryocytes. *Blood* 75:1220, 1990.

485. Youssefian T, Masse JM, Rendu F, et al: Platelet and megakaryocyte dense granules contain glycoproteins Ib and IIb-IIIa. *Blood* 89:4047, 1997.

486. Coller BS: Activation-specific platelet antigens, in *Platelet Immunobiology: Molecular and Clinical Aspects*, edited by TJ Kunicki, JN George, p 166. JB Lippincott, Philadelphia, 1989.

487. Sims PJ, Ginsberg MH, Plow EF, Shattil SJ: Effect of platelet activation on the conformation of the plasma membrane glycoprotein IIb-IIIa complex. *J Biol Chem* 266:7345, 1991.

488. Wencel-Drake JD: Plasma membrane GPIIb/IIIa. Evidence for a cycling receptor pool. *Am J Clin Pathol* 136:61, 1990.

489. Hynes RO: Integrins: A family of cell surface receptors. *Cell* 48:549, 1987.

490. Ruoslahti E: Fibronectin and its receptors. *Annu Rev Biochem* 57:375, 1988.

491. Doolittle RF, Watt KWK, Cottrell BA, et al: The amino acid sequence of the alpha-chain of human fibrinogen. *Nature* 280:464, 1979.

492. Cheresh DA, Berliner SA, Vicente V, Ruggeri ZM: Recognition of distinct adhesive sites on fibrinogen by related integrins on platelets and endothelial cells. *Cell* 58:945, 1989.

493. Farrell DH, Thiagarajan P, Chung DW, Davie EW: Role of fibrinogen α and γ chain sites in platelet aggregation. *Proc Natl Acad Sci U S A* 89:10729, 1992.

494. Farrell DH, Thiagarajan P: Binding of recombinant fibrinogen mutants to platelets. *J Biol Chem* 269:226, 1994.

495. Wencel-Drake JD, Boudignon-Proudhon C, Dieter MG, et al: Internalization of bound fibrinogen modulates platelet aggregation. *Blood* 87:602, 1996.

496. Peerschke EIB: Events occurring after thrombin-induced fibrinogen binding to platelets. *Semin Thromb Hemost* 18:34, 1992.

497. Xiao T, Takagi J, Coller BS, et al: Structural basis for allostery in integrins and binding of ligand-mimetic therapeutics. *Nature* 432:59, 2004.

498. Zamarron C, Ginsberg MH, Plow EF: A receptor-induced binding site in fibrinogen elicited by its interaction with platelet membrane glycoprotein IIb-IIIa. *J Biol Chem* 266:17106, 1991.

499. Ugarova TP, Budzynski AZ, Shattil SJ, et al: Conformational changes in fibrinogen elicited by its interaction with platelet membrane glycoprotein GPIIb-IIIa. *J Biol Chem* 268:21080, 1993.

500. Hato T, Pampori N, Shattil SJ: Complementary roles for receptor clustering and conformational change in the adhesive and signaling functions of integrin alphaIIb beta3. *J Cell Biol* 141:1685, 1998.

501. Carrell NA, Fitzgerald LA, Steiner B, et al: Structure of human platelet membrane glycoproteins IIb and IIIa as determined by electron microscopy. *J Biol Chem* 260:1743, 1985.

502. Weisel JW, Nagaswami C, Vilaire G, Bennett JS: Examination of the platelet membrane glycoprotein IIb-IIIa complex and its interaction with fibrinogen and other ligands by electron microscopy. *J Biol Chem* 267:16637, 1992.

503. Xiao T, Takagi J, Coller BS, et al: Structural basis for allostery in integrins and binding of ligand-mimetic therapeutics to the platelet receptor for fibrinogen [unpublished]. 2004.

504. Takagi J, Petre BM, Walz T, Springer TA: Global conformational rearrangements in integrin extracellular domains in outside-in and inside-out signaling. *Cell* 110:599, 2002.

505. Artoni A, Li J, Mitchell B, et al: Integrin β3 regions controlling binding of murine mAb 7E3: Implications for the mechanism of integrin αIIbβ3 activation. *Proc Natl Acad Sci U S A* 101:13114, 2004.

506. Arnaout M, Goodman S, Xiong J: Coming to grips with integrin binding to ligands. *Curr Opin Cell Biol* 14:641, 2002.

507. Arnaout MA: Integrin structure: New twists and turns in dynamic cell adhesion. *Immunol Rev* 186:125, 2002.

508. Xiong JP, Stehle T, Diefenbach B, et al: Crystal structure of the extracellular segment of integrin alpha Vbeta3. *Science* 294:339, 2001.

509. Xiong JP, Stehle T, Zhang R, et al: Crystal structure of the extracellular segment of integrin alpha Vbeta3 in complex with an Arg-Gly-Asp ligand. *Science* 296:151, 2002.

510. Poncz M, Eisman R, Heidenreich R, et al: Structure of the platelet membrane glycoprotein IIb. Homology to the alpha subunits of the vitronectin and fibronectin membrane receptors. *J Biol Chem* 262:8476, 1987.

511. Fitzgerald LA, Steiner B, Rall SC Jr, et al: Protein sequence of endothelial glycoprotein IIIa derived from a cDNA clone. Identity with platelet glycoprotein IIIa and similarity to "integrin." *J Biol Chem* 262:3936, 1987.

512. Bray PF, Barsh G, Rosa JP, et al: Physical linkage of the genes for platelet membrane glycoproteins IIb and IIIa. *Proc Natl Acad Sci U S A* 85:8683, 1988.

513. Thornton MA, Poncz M, Korostishevsky M, et al: The human platelet alphaIIb gene is not closely linked to its integrin partner beta3. *Blood* 94:2039, 1999.

514. Steiner B, Parise LV, Leung B, Phillips DR: Ca^{+2} dependent structural transitions of the platelet glycoprotein IIb-IIIa complex. Preparation of stable glycoprotein IIb and IIIa monomers. *J Biol Chem* 266:14986, 1991.

515. Mitchell B, Li J, Fisher EA, French DL: Modifications of asparagine-linked glycans mark the IIb integrin subunit for endoplasmic reticulum-associated degradation (ERAD): A model for IIb3 quality control [abstract]. *Blood* 102:1036a, 2003.

516. Duperray A, Troesch A, Berthier R, et al: Biosynthesis and assembly of platelet GPIIb-IIIa in human megakaryocytes: Evidence that assembly between pro-GPIIb and GPIIIa is a prerequisite for expression of the complex on the cell surface. *Blood* 74:1603, 1989.

517. O'Toole TE, Loftus JC, Plow EF, et al: Efficient surface expression of platelet GPIIb-IIIa requires both subunits. *Blood* 74:14, 1989.

518. McEver RP, Baenziger JU, Majerus PW: Isolation and structural characterization of the polypeptide subunits of membrane glycoprotein IIb-IIIa from human platelets. *Blood* 59:80, 1982.

519. Xiong JP, Stehle T, Diefenbach B, et al: Crystal structure of the extracellular segment of integrin alpha Vbeta3. *Science* 294:339, 2001.

520. Muir TW, Williams MJ, Ginsberg MH, Kent SB: Design and chemical synthesis of a neoprotein structural model for the cytoplasmic domain of a multisubunit cell-surface receptor: Integrin alpha IIb beta 3 (platelet GPIIb-IIIa). *Biochemistry* 33:7701, 1994.

521. Haas TA, Plow EF: The cytoplasmic domain of alphaIIb beta3. A ternary complex of the integrin alpha and beta subunits and a divalent cation. *J Biol Chem* 271:6017, 1996.

522. Vallar L, Melchior C, Plancon S, et al: Divalent cations differentially regulate integrin alphaIIb cytoplasmic tail binding to beta3 and to calcium- and integrin-binding protein. *J Biol Chem* 274:17257, 1999.

523. O'Toole TE, Mandelman D, Forsyth J, et al: Modulation of the affinity of integrin αIIbβ3 (GPIIb-IIIa) by the cytoplasmic domain of alpha IIb. *Science* 254:845, 1991.

524. O'Toole TE, Katagiri Y, Faull RJ, et al: Integrin cytoplasmic domains mediate inside-out signal transduction. *J Cell Biol* 124:1047, 1994.

525. Hughes PE, Diaz-Gonzalez F, Leong L, et al: Breaking the integrin hinge. A defined structural constraint regulates integrin signaling. *J Biol Chem* 271:6571, 1996.

526. Leisner TM, Wencel-Drake JD, Wang W, Lam SC: Bidirectional transmembrane modulation of integrin alphaIIbbeta3 conformations. *J Biol Chem* 274:12945, 1999.

527. Xiong JP, Stehle T, Goodman SL, Amin AM: A novel adaptation of the integrin PSI domain revealed from its crystal structure. *J Biol Chem* 279:40252, 2004.

528. Kashiwagi H, Tomiyama Y, Tadokoro S, et al: A mutation in the extracellular cysteine-rich repeat region of the beta3 subunit activates integrins alphaIIbbeta3 and alphaVbeta3. *Blood* 93:2559, 1999.

529. Frelinger AL III, Du XP, Plow EF, Ginsberg MH: Monoclonal antibodies to ligand-occupied conformers of integrin alpha IIb beta 3 (glycoprotein IIb-IIIa) alter receptor affinity, specificity, and function. *J Biol Chem* 266:17106, 1991.

530. Du X, Gu M, Weisel JW, et al: Long range propagation of conformational changes in integrin alpha IIb beta 3. *J Biol Chem* 268:23087, 1993.

531. Kamata T, Ambo H, Puzon-McLaughlin W, et al: Critical cysteine residues for regulation of integrin alphaIIbbeta3 are clustered in the epidermal growth factor domains of the beta3 subunit. *Biochem J* 378:1079, 2004.

532. Essex DW: The role of thiols and disulfides in platelet function. *Antioxid Redox Signal* 6:736, 2004.

533. Zucker MB, Masiello NC: Platelet aggregation caused by dithiothreitol. *Thromb Haemost* 51:119, 1984.

534. Chen K, Detwiler TC, Essex DW: Characterization of protein disulphide isomerase released from activated platelets. *Br J Haematol* 90:425, 1995.

535. Essex DW, Chen K, Swiatkowska M: Localization of protein disulfide isomerase to the external surface of the platelet plasma membrane. *Blood* 86:2168, 1995.

536. O'Neill S, Robinson A, Deering A, et al: The platelet integrin alpha IIbbeta 3 has an endogenous thiol isomerase activity. *J Biol Chem* 275:36984, 2000.

537. Hughes PE, O'Toole TE, Ylanne J, et al: The conserved membrane-proximal region of an integrin cytoplasmic domain specifies ligand binding affinity. *J Biol Chem* 270:12411, 1995.

538. Kim M, Carman CV, Springer TA: Bidirectional transmembrane signaling by cytoplasmic domain separation in integrins. *Science* 301:1720, 2003.

539. Knezevic I, Leisner TM, Lam SC: Direct binding of the platelet integrin alphaIIbbeta3 (GPIIb-IIIa) to talin. Evidence that interaction is mediated through the cytoplasmic domains of both alphaIIb and beta3. *J Biol Chem* 271:16416, 1996.

540. Jenkins AL, Nannizzi-Alaimo L, Silver D, et al: Tyrosine phosphorylation of the beta3 cytoplasmic domain mediates integrin-cytoskeletal interactions. *J Biol Chem* 273:13878, 1998.

541. Law DA, DeGuzmann FR, Heiser P, et al: Integrin cytoplasmic tyrosine motif is required for outside-in alphaIIbbeta3 signalling and platelet function. *Nature* 401:808, 1999.

542. Shattil SJ, O'Toole T, Eigenthaler M, et al: Beta 3-endonexin, a novel polypeptide that interacts specifically with the cytoplasmic tail of the integrin beta 3 subunit. *J Cell Biol* 131:807, 1995.

543. Eigenthaler M, Hofferer L, Shattil SJ, Ginsberg MH: A conserved sequence motif in the integrin beta3 cytoplasmic domain is required for its specific interaction with beta3-endonexin. *J Biol Chem* 272:7693, 1997.

544. Calderwood DA, Zent R, Grant R, et al: The talin head domain binds to integrin {beta} subunit cytoplasmic tails and regulates integrin activation. *J Biol Chem* 274:28071, 1999.

545. Zent R, Fenczik CA, Calderwood DA, et al: Class- and splice variant-specific association of CD98 with integrin beta cytoplasmic domains. *J Biol Chem* 275:5059, 2000.

546. Reddy KB, Gascard P, Price MG, et al: Identification of an interaction between the m-band protein skelemin and beta-integrin subunits. Co-localization of a skelemin-like protein with beta1- and beta3-integrins in non-muscle cells. *J Biol Chem* 273:35039, 1998.

547. Calderwood DA, Shattil SJ, Ginsberg MH: Integrins and actin filaments: Reciprocal regulation of cell adhesion and signaling. *J Biol Chem* 275:22607, 2000.

548. Law DA, Nannizzi-Alaimo L, Phillips DR: Outside-in integrin signal transduction. Alpha IIb beta 3-(GP IIb IIIa) tyrosine phosphorylation induced by platelet aggregation. *J Biol Chem* 271:10811, 1996.

549. Cowan KJ, Law DA, Phillips DR: Identification of shc as the primary protein binding to the tyrosine-phosphorylated beta 3 subunit of alpha IIbbeta 3 during outside-in integrin platelet signaling. *J Biol Chem* 275:36423, 2000.

550. Schaller MD, Otey CA, Hildebrand JD, Parsons JT: Focal adhesion kinase and paxillin bind to peptides mimicking beta integrin cytoplasmic domains. *J Cell Biol* 130:1181, 1995.

551. Hannigan GE, Leung-Hagesteijn C, Fitz-Gibbon L, et al: Regulation of cell adhesion and anchorage-dependent growth by a new beta 1-integrin-linked protein kinase. *Nature* 379:91, 1996.

552. Otey CA, Pavalko FM, Burridge K: An interaction between alpha-actinin and the beta 1 integrin subunit in vitro. *J Cell Biol* 111:721, 1990.

553. Naik UP, Patel PM, Parise LV: Identification of a novel calcium-binding protein that interacts with the integrin alphaIIb cytoplasmic domain. *J Biol Chem* 272:4651, 1997.

554. Shock DD, Naik UP, Brittain JE, et al: Calcium-dependent properties of CIB binding to the integrin alphaIIb cytoplasmic domain and translocation to the platelet cytoskeleton. *Biochem J* 342:729, 1999.

555. Leung-Hagesteijn CY, Milankov K, Michalak M, et al: Cell attachment to extracellular matrix substrates is inhibited upon downregulation of

expression of calreticulin, an intracellular integrin alpha-subunit-binding protein. *J Cell Sci* 107(Pt 3):589, 1994.

556. Rojiani MV, Finlay BB, Gray V, Dedhar S: In vitro interaction of a polypeptide homologous to human Ro/SS-A antigen (calreticulin) with a highly conserved amino acid sequence in the cytoplasmic domain of integrin alpha subunits. *Biochemistry* 30:9859, 1991.

557. Heilmann E, Hourdille P, Pruvost A, et al: Thrombin-induced platelet aggregates have a dynamic structure: Time-dependent redistribution of GPIIb/IIIa complexes and secreted adhesive proteins. *Arterioscler Thromb* 11:704, 1991.

558. Isenberg WM, McEver RP, Phillips DR, et al: The platelet fibrinogen receptor: An immunogold-surface replica study of agonist-induced ligand binding and receptor clustering. *J Cell Biol* 104:1655, 1987.

559. Asch E, Podack E: Vitronectin binds to activated human platelets and plays a role in platelet aggregation. *J Clin Invest* 85:1372, 1990.

560. Haverstick DM, Cowan JF, Yamada KM, Santoro SA: Inhibition of platelet adhesion to fibronectin, fibrinogen, and von Willebrand factor substrates by a synthetic tetrapeptide derived from the cell binding domain of fibronectin. *Blood* 66:946, 1985.

561. Plow EF, D'Souza SE, Ginsberg MH: Ligand binding to GPIIb-IIIa: A status report. *Semin Thromb Hemost* 18:324, 1992.

562. Schullek J, Jordan J, Montgomery RR: Interaction of von Willebrand factor with human platelets in the plasma milieu. *J Clin Invest* 73:421, 1984.

563. Ni H, Papalia JM, Degen JL, Wagner DD: Control of thrombus embolization and fibronectin internalization by integrin alpha IIb beta 3 engagement of the fibrinogen gamma chain. *Blood* 102:3609, 2003.

564. Moskowitz KA, Kudryk B, Coller BS: Fibrinogen coating density affects the conformation of immobilized fibrinogen: Implications for platelet adhesion and spreading. *Thromb Haemost* 79:824, 1998.

565. Hatton MW, Moar SL, Richardson M: Deendothelialization in vivo initiates a thrombogenic reaction at the rabbit aorta surface. Correlation of uptake of fibrinogen and antithrombin III with thrombin generation by the exposed subendothelium. *Am J Pathol* 135:499, 1989.

566. Miles LA, Ginsberg MH, White JG, Plow EF: Plasminogen interacts with human platelets through two distinct mechanisms. *J Clin Invest* 77:2001, 1986.

567. Peerschke EI, Grant RA, Zucker MB: Decreased association of 45-calcium with platelets unable to aggregate due to thrombasthenia or prolonged calcium deprivation. *Br J Haematol* 46:247, 1980.

568. Powling MJ, Hardisty RM: Glycoprotein IIb-IIIa complex and Ca++ influx into stimulated platelets. *Blood* 66:731, 1985.

569. Rybak MEM, Renzulli LA: Effect of calcium channel blockers on platelet GPIIb-IIIa as a calcium channel in liposomes: Comparison with effects on the intact platelet. *Thromb Haemost* 67:131, 1991.

570. Ameisen JC, Joseph M, Caen JP, et al: A role for glycoprotein IIb-IIIa complexes in the binding of IgE to human platelets and platelet IgE-dependent cytolytic function. *Br J Haematol* 64:21, 1986.

571. Coburn J, Barthold SW, Leong JM: Diverse Lyme disease spirochetes bind integrin alpha IIb beta 3 on human platelets. *Infect Immun* 62:5559, 1994.

572. Gavrilovskaya IN, Brown EJ, Ginsberg MH, Mackow ER: Cellular entry of hantaviruses which cause hemorrhagic fever with renal syndrome is mediated by beta3 integrins. *J Virol* 73:3951, 1999.

573. Pischel KD, Hemler MD, Huang C, et al: Use of the monoclonal antibody 12F1 to characterize the differentiation antigen VLA-2. *J Immunol* 138:226, 1987.

574. Kunicki DJ, Nugent DJ, Staats SJ, et al: The human fibroblast II extracellular matrix receptor mediates platelet adhesion to collagen and is identical to the platelet glycoprotein Ia-IIa complex. *J Biol Chem* 263:4516, 1988.

575. Staatz WD, Rajpara SM, Wayner EA, et al: The membrane glycoprotein Ia-IIa (VLA-2) complex mediates the Mg++-dependent adhesion of platelets to collagen. *J Cell Biol* 108:1917, 1989.

576. Barnes MJ, Knight CG, Farndale RW: The collagen-platelet interaction. *Curr Opin Hematol* 5:314, 1998.

577. Takada Y, Hemler ME: The primary structure of the VLA-2/collagen receptor a2 subunit (platelet GPIa): Homology to other integrins and the presence of a possible collagen-binding domain. *J Cell Biol* 109:397, 1987.

578. Clemetson KJ: Platelet receptors, in *Platelets*, edited by AD Michelson, p 65. Academic Press, San Diego, 2002.

579. Emsley J, King SL, Bergelson JM, Liddington RC: Crystal structure of the I domain from integrin alpha2beta1. *J Biol Chem* 272:28512, 1997.

580. Emsley J, Knight CG, Farndale RW, et al: Structural basis of collagen recognition by integrin alpha2beta1. *Cell* 101:47, 2000.

581. Nieuwenhuis HK, Akkerman JWN, Houdijk WPM, Sixma JJ: Human blood platelets showing no response to collagen fail to express surface glycoprotein Ia. *Nature* 318:470, 1985.

582. Schoolmeester A, Vanhoorelbeke K, Katsutani S, et al: Monoclonal antibody IAC-1 is specific for activated alpha2beta1 and binds to amino acids 199 to 201 of the integrin alpha2 I-domain. *Blood* 104:390, 2004.

583. He L, Pappan LK, Grenache DG, et al: The contributions of the alpha 2 beta 1 integrin to vascular thrombosis in vivo. *Blood* 102:3652, 2003.

584. Lahav J, Wijnen EM, Hess O, et al: Enzymatically catalyzed disulfide exchange is required for platelet adhesion to collagen via integrin alpha2beta1. *Blood* 102:2085, 2003.

585. Staatz WD, Walsh JJ, Pexton T, Santoro SA: The α2β1 integrin cell surface collagen receptor binds to the α1(I)-CB3 peptide of collagen. *J Biol Chem* 265:4778, 1990.

586. Knight CG, Morton LF, Onley DJ, et al: Identification in collagen type I of an integrin alpha2 beta1-binding site containing an essential GER sequence. *J Biol Chem* 273:33287, 1998.

587. Santoro SA, Walsh JJ, Staatz WD, Baranski KJ: Distinct determinants on collagen support α2β1 integrin-mediated platelet adhesion and platelet activation. *Cell Regul* 2:905, 1991.

588. Verkleij MW, Ijsseldijk MJ, Heijnen-Snyder GJ, et al: Adhesive domains in the collagen III fragment alpha1(III)CB4 that support alpha2b. *Thromb Haemost* 82:1137, 1999.

589. Bray PF: Integrin polymorphisms as risk factors for thrombosis. *Thromb Haemost* 82:337, 1999.

590. Moshfegh K, Wuillemin WA, Redondo M, et al: Association of two silent polymorphisms of platelet glycoprotein Ia/IIa receptor with risk of myocardial infarction: A case-control study. *Lancet* 353:351, 1999.

591. Santoso S, Kunicki TJ, Kroll H, et al: Association of the platelet glycoprotein Ia C807T gene polymorphism with nonfatal myocardial infarction in younger patients. *Blood* 93:2449, 1999.

592. Carlsson LE, Santoso S, Spitzer C, et al: The alpha2 gene coding sequence T807/A873 of the platelet collagen receptor integrin alpha2beta1 might be a genetic risk factor for the development of stroke in younger patients. *Blood* 93:3583, 1999.

593. von Beckerath N, Koch W, Mehilli J, et al: Glycoprotein Ia gene C807T polymorphism and risk for major adverse cardiac events within the first 30 days after coronary artery stenting. *Blood* 95:3297, 2000.

594. Matsubara Y, Murata M, Maruyama T, et al: Association between diabetic retinopathy and genetic variations in alpha2beta1 integrin, a platelet receptor for collagen. *Blood* 95:1560, 2000.

595. Roest M, Banga JD, Grobbee DE, et al: Homozygosity for 807 T polymorphism in alpha(2) subunit of platelet alpha(2)beta(1) is associated with increased risk of cardiovascular mortality in high-risk women. *Circulation* 102:1645, 2000.

596. Fox JEB: Linkage of a membrane skeleton to integral membrane glycoproteins in human platelets. Identification of one of the glycoproteins as glycoprotein Ib. *J Clin Invest* 76:1673, 1985.

597. Elices MJ, Hemler ME: The integrin VLA-2 can be a laminin as well as a collagen receptor. *Proc Natl Acad Sci U S A* 86:9906, 1989.

598. Kirchhofer D, Languinol R, Ruoslahti E, Pierschbacher MD: α2β1 integrins from different cell types show different binding specificities. *J Biol Chem* 265:615, 1990.

599. Piotrowicz RS, Orchekowski RP, Nugent DJ, et al: Glycoprotein Ic-IIa functions as an activation-independent fibronectin receptor on human platelets. *J Cell Biol* 106:1359, 1988.

600. Wayner EA, Carter WG, Piotrowicz RS, Kunicki TJ: The function of multiple extracellular matrix receptors in mediating cell adhesion to extracellular matrix: Preparation of monoclonal antibodies to the fibronectin receptor that specifically inhibit cell adhesion of fibronectin and react with platelet glycoproteins Ic-IIa. *J Cell Biol* 107:1881, 1988.

601. Vuillet-Gaugler MH, Breton-Gorius J, Vainchenker W, et al: Loss of attachment to fibronectin with terminal human erythroid differentiation. *Blood* 75:865, 1990.

602. Sonnenberg A, Modderman PW, Hogervorst F: Laminin receptor on platelets is the integrin VLA-6. *Nature* 336:487, 1988.

603. Hindriks G, Ijsseldijk MJ, Sonnenberg A, et al: Platelet adhesion to laminin: Role of Ca2+ and Mg2+ ions, shear rate, and platelet membrane glycoproteins. *Blood* 79:928, 1992.

604. Tandon NN, Holland EA, Kralisz U, et al: Interaction of human platelets with laminin and identification of the 67 kDa laminin receptor on platelets. *Biochem J* 274:535, 1991.

605. Fitzgerald LA, Poncz M, Steiner B, et al: Comparison of cDNA-derived protein sequences of the human fibronectin and vitronectin receptor alpha-subunits and platelet glycoprotein IIb. *Biochemistry* 26:8158, 1987.

606. Coller BS, Cheresh DA, Asch E, Seligsohn U: Platelet vitronectin receptor expression differentiates Iraqi-Jewish from Arab patients with Glanzmann thrombasthenia in Israel. *Blood* 77:75, 1991.

607. Xiong JP, Stehle T, Diefenbach B, et al: Crystal structure of the extracellular segment of integrin alpha Vbeta3. *Science* 294:339, 2001.

608. Kieffer N, Fitzgerald LA, Wolf D, et al: Adhesive properties of the β3 integrins. Comparison of GPIIb-IIIa and the vitronectin receptor individually expressed in human melanoma cells. *J Cell Biol* 113:451, 1991.

609. Lam SC, Plow EF, D'Souza SE, et al: Isolation and characterization of a platelet membrane protein related to the vitronectin receptor. *J Biol Chem* 264:3742, 1989.

610. Charo IF, Bekeart LS, Phillips DR: Platelet glycoprotein IIb-IIIa-like proteins mediate endothelial cell attachment to adhesive proteins and the extracellular matrix. *J Biol Chem* 262:9935, 1987.

611. Byzova TV, Plow EF: Activation of alphaVbeta3 on vascular cells controls recognition of prothrombin. *J Cell Biol* 143:2081, 1998.

612. Bennett JS, Chan C, Vilaire G, et al: Agonist-activated alphavbeta3 on platelets and lymphocytes binds to the matrix protein osteopontin. *J Biol Chem* 272:8137, 1997.

613. Beckstead JH, Stenberg PE, McEver RP, et al: Immunohistochemical localization of membrane and alpha-granule proteins in human megakaryocytes: Application to plastic-embedded bone marrow biopsy specimens. *Blood* 67:285, 1986.

614. Davies J, Warwick J, Totty N, et al: The osteoclast functional antigen, implicated in the regulation of bone resorption, is biochemically related to the vitronectin receptor. *J Cell Biol* 109:1817, 1989.

615. McHugh KP, Hodivala-Dilke K, Zheng MH, et al: Mice lacking beta3 integrins are osteosclerotic because of dysfunctional osteoclasts. *J Clin Invest* 105:433, 2000.

616. Feng X, Novack DV, Faccio R, et al: A Glanzmann's mutation in beta 3 integrin specifically impairs osteoclast function. *J Clin Invest* 107:1137, 2001.

617. Savill J, Dransfield I, Hogg N, Haslett C: Vitronectin receptor-mediated phagocytosis of cells undergoing apoptosis. *Nature* 343:170, 1990.

618. Brooks PC, Clark RA, Cheresh DA: Requirement of vascular integrin αVβ3 for angiogenesis. *Science* 264:569, 1994.

619. Varner JA, Cheresh DA: Integrins and cancer. *Curr Opin Cell Biol* 8:724, 1996.

620. Trikha M, Zhou Z, Nemeth JA, et al: CNTO 95, a fully human monoclonal antibody that inhibits alphav integrins, has antitumor and antiangiogenic activity in vivo. *Int J Cancer* 110:326, 2004.

621. Ellegala DB, Leong-Poi H, Carpenter JE, et al: Imaging tumor angiogenesis with contrast ultrasound and microbubbles targeted to alpha(v)beta3. *Circulation* 108:336, 2003.

622. Kumar CC: Integrin alpha v beta 3 as a therapeutic target for blocking tumor-induced angiogenesis. *Curr Drug Targets* 4:123, 2003.

623. Kerr JS, Slee AM, Mousa SA: The alpha v integrin antagonists as novel anticancer agents: An update. *Expert Opin Investig Drugs* 11:1765, 2002.

624. Choi ET, Engel L, Callow AD, et al: Inhibition of neointimal hyperplasia by blocking αvβ3 integrin with a small peptide antagonist GpenGRGDSPCA. *J Vasc Surg* 19:125, 1994.

625. Sajid M, Stouffer GA: The role of alpha(v)beta3 integrins in vascular healing. *Thromb Haemost* 87:187, 2002.

626. Stouffer GA, Smyth SS: Effects of thrombin on interactions between beta3-integrins and extracellular matrix in platelets and vascular cells. *Arterioscler Thromb Vasc Biol* 23:1971, 2003.

627. Philippeaux MM, Vesin C, Tacchini-Cottier F, Piguet PF: Activated human platelets express beta2 integrin. *Eur J Haematol* 56:130, 1996.

628. Guo J, Piguet PF: Stimulation of thrombocytopoiesis decreases platelet beta2 but not beta1 or beta3 integrins. *Br J Haematol* 100:712, 1998.

629. Piguet PF, Vesin C, Rochat A: Beta2 integrin modulates platelet caspase activation and life span in mice. *Eur J Cell Biol* 80:171, 2001.

630. Lopez JH, Chung DW, Fujikawa K, et al: The a and b chains of human platelet glycoprotein Ib are both transmembrane proteins containing a leucine-rich amino acid sequence. *Proc Natl Acad Sci U S A* 85:2135, 1988.

631. Lopez JA, Andrews RK, Afshar-Kharghan V, Berndt MC: Bernard-Soulier syndrome. *Blood* 91:4397, 1998.

632. Du X, Beutler L, Ruan C, et al: Glycoprotein Ib and glycoprotein IX are fully complexed in the intact platelet membrane. *Blood* 69:1524, 1987.

633. Hickey MJ, Williams SA, Roth GJ: Human platelet GPIX: An adhesive prototype of leucine-rich glycoproteins with flank-center-flank structures. *Proc Natl Acad Sci U S A* 86:6773, 1989.

634. Hickey MJ, Deaven LL, Roth GJ: Human platelet glycoprotein IX. Characterization of cDNA and localization of the gene to chromosome 3. *FEBS Lett* 274:189, 1991.

635. Lopez JA, Leung B, Reynolds CC, et al: Efficient plasma membrane expression of a functional platelet glycoprotein Ib-IX complex requires the presence of its three subunits. *J Biol Chem* 267:12851, 1992.

636. Sprandio JD, Shapiro SS, Thiagarajan P, McCord S: Cultured human umbilical vein endothelial cells contain a membrane glycoprotein immunologically related to platelet glycoprotein Ib. *Blood* 71:234, 1988.

637. Asch AS, Adelman B, Fujimoto M, Nachman RL: Identification and isolation of a platelet GPIb-like protein in human umbilical vein endothelial cells and bovine aortic smooth muscle cells. *J Clin Invest* 81:1600, 1988.

638. Konkle BA, Shapiro SS, Asch AS, Nachman RL: Cytokine-enhanced expression of glycoprotein Ib alpha in human endothelium. *J Biol Chem* 265:19833, 1990.

639. Bombeli T, Schwartz BR, Harlan JM: Adhesion of activated platelets to endothelial cells: Evidence for a GPIIbIIIa-dependent bridging mechanism and novel roles for endothelial intercellular adhesion molecule 1 (ICAM-1), alphavbeta3 integrin, and GPIbalpha. *J Exp Med* 187:329, 1998.

640. Tan L, Kowalska MA, Romo GM, et al: Identification and characterization of endothelial glycoprotein Ib using viper venom proteins modulating cell adhesion. Blood 93:2605, 1999.

641. Perrault C, Lankhof H, Pidard D, et al: Relative importance of the glycoprotein Ib-binding domain and the RGD sequence of von Willebrand factor for its interaction with endothelial cells. Blood 90:2335, 1997.

642. Uzan G, Prenant M, Prandini MH, et al: Tissue-specific expression of the platelet GPIIb gene. J Biol Chem 266:8932, 1991.

643. Prandini MH, Uzan G, Martin F, et al: Characterization of a specific erythromegakaryocytic enhancer within the glycoprotein IIb promoter. J Biol Chem 267:10370, 1992.

644. Lemarchandel V, Ghysdael J, Mignotte V, et al: GATA and Ets cis-acting sequences mediate megakaryocyte-specific expression. Mol Cell Biol 13:668, 1993.

645. Martin F, Prandini MH, Thevenon D, et al: The transcription factor GATA-1 regulates the promoter activity of the platelet glycoprotein IIb gene. J Biol Chem 268:21606, 1993.

646. Block KL, Poncz M: Platelet glycoprotein IIb gene expression as a model of megakaryocyte-specific expression. Stem Cells 13:135, 1995.

647. Hashimoto Y, Ware J: Identification of essential GATA and Ets binding motifs within the promoter of the platelet glycoprotein Ib alpha gene. J Biol Chem 270:24532, 1995.

648. Bastian LS, Yagi M, Chan C, Roth GJ: Analysis of the megakaryocyte glycoprotein IX promoter identifies positive and negative regulatory domains and functional GATA and Ets sites. J Biol Chem 271:18554, 1996.

649. Tsang AP, Visvader JE, Turner CA, et al: FOG, a multitype zinc finger protein, acts as a cofactor for transcription factor GATA-1 in erythroid and megakaryocytic differentiation. Cell 90:109, 1997.

650. Krause DS, Perkins AS: Gotta find GATA a friend. Nat Med 3:960, 1997.

651. Lopez JA, Ludwig EW, McCarthy BJ: Polymorphism of human glycoprotein Ibα results from a variable number of repeats of a 13-amino acid sequence in the mucin-like macroglycopeptide region. Structure function implications. J Biol Chem 267:10055, 1992.

652. Murata M, Matsubara Y, Kawano K, et al: Coronary artery disease and polymorphisms in a receptor mediating shear stress-dependent platelet activation. Circulation 96:3281, 1997.

653. Gonzalez-Conejero R, Lozano ML, Rivera J, et al: Polymorphisms of platelet membrane glycoprotein Ib associated with arterial thrombotic disease. Blood 92:2771, 1998.

654. Carlsson LE, Greinacher A, Spitzer C, et al: Polymorphisms of the human platelet antigens HPA-1, HPA-2, HPA-3, and HPA-5 on the platelet receptors for fibrinogen (GPIIb/IIIa), von Willebrand factor (GPIb/IX), and collagen (GPIa/IIa) are not correlated with an increased risk for stroke. Stroke 28:1392, 1997.

655. Kaski S, Kekomaki R, Partanen J: Systematic screening for genetic polymorphism in human platelet glycoprotein Ibalpha. Immunogenetics 44:170, 1996.

656. Suzuki K, Hayashi T, Akiba J, et al: StyI polymorphism at nucleotide 1610 in the human platelet glycoprotein Ib alpha gene. Jpn J Hum Genet 41:419, 1996.

657. Afshar-Kharghan V, Li CQ, Khoshnevis-Asl M, Lopez JA: Kozak sequence polymorphism of the glycoprotein (GP) Ibalpha gene is a major determinant of the plasma membrane levels of the platelet GP Ib-IX-V complex. Blood 94:186, 1999.

658. Baker RI, Eikelboom J, Lofthouse E, et al: Platelet glycoprotein Ibalpha Kozak polymorphism is associated with an increased risk of ischemic stroke. Blood 98:36, 2001.

659. Meisel C, Afshar-Kharghan V, Cascorbi I, et al: Role of Kozak sequence polymorphism of platelet glycoprotein Ibalpha as a risk factor for coronary artery disease and catheter interventions. J Am Coll Cardiol 38:1023, 2001.

660. Douglas H, Michaelides K, Gorog DA, et al: Platelet membrane glycoprotein Ibalpha gene -5T/C Kozak sequence polymorphism as an independent risk factor for the occurrence of coronary thrombosis. Heart 87:70, 2002.

661. Kenny D, Muckian C, Fitzgerald DJ, et al: Platelet glycoprotein Ib alpha receptor polymorphisms and recurrent ischaemic events in acute coronary syndrome patients. J Thromb Thrombolysis 13:13, 2002.

662. Rosenberg N, Zivelin A, Chetrit A, et al: Effects of platelet membrane glycoprotein polymorphisms on the risk of myocardial infarction in young males. Isr Med Assoc J 4:411, 2002.

663. Jilma-Stohlawetz P, Homoncik M, Jilma B, et al: Glycoprotein Ib polymorphisms influence platelet plug formation under high shear rates. Br J Haematol 120:652, 2003.

664. Carlsson LE, Lubenow N, Blumentritt C, et al: Platelet receptor and clotting factor polymorphisms as genetic risk factors for thromboembolic complications in heparin-induced thrombocytopenia. Pharmacogenetics 13:253, 2003.

665. Ozelo MC, Origa AF, Aranha FJ, et al: Platelet glycoprotein Iba polymorphisms modulate the risk for myocardial infarction. Thromb Haemost 92:384, 2004.

666. Tsuji T, Tsunehisa S, Watanabe Y, et al: The carbohydrate moiety of human platelet glycocalicin. J Biol Chem 258:6335, 1983.

667. Fox JEB, Aggerbeck LP, Berndt MC: Structure of the glycoprotein Ib-IX complex from platelet membranes. J Biol Chem 263:4882, 1988.

668. Solum NO, Hagen I, Filion-Myklebust C, Staback T: Platelet glycocalicin: Its membrane association in solvent and aqueous media. Biochim Biophys Acta 597:235, 1990.

669. Coller BS, Kalomiris EL, Steinberg M, Scudder LE: Evidence that glycocalicin circulates in normal plasma. J Clin Invest 73:794, 1984.

670. Kurata Y, Hayashi S, Kiyoi T, et al: Diagnostic value of tests for reticulated platelets, plasma glycocalicin, and thrombopoietin levels for discriminating between hyperdestructive and hypoplastic thrombocytopenia. Am J Clin Pathol 115:656, 2001.

671. Steinberg MH, Kelton JG, Coller BS: Plasma glycocalicin. An aid in the classification of thrombocytopenic disorders. N Engl J Med 317:1037, 1987.

672. Kunishima S, Kobayashi S, Takagi A, et al: Rapid detection of plasma glycocalicin by a latex agglutination test. A useful adjunct in the differential diagnosis of thrombocytopenia. Am J Clin Pathol 100:579, 1993.

673. Kunishima S, Kobayashi S, Naoe T: Increased but highly dispersed levels of plasma glycocalicin in patients with disseminated intravascular coagulation. Eur J Haematol 56:173, 1996.

674. Beer JH, Buchi L, Steiner B: Glycocalicin: A new assay—The normal plasma levels and its potential usefulness in selected diseases. Blood 83:691, 1994.

675. Steffan A, Pradella P, Cordiano I, et al: Glycocalicin in the diagnosis and management of immune thrombocytopenia. Eur J Haematol 61:77, 1998.

676. Himmelfarb J, Nelson S, McMonagle E, et al: Elevated plasma glycocalicin levels and decreased ristocetin-induced platelet agglutination in hemodialysis patients. Am J Kidney Dis 32:132, 1998.

677. Kalomiris EL, Coller BS: Thiol-specific probes indicate that the alpha chain of platelet glycoprotein Ib is a transmembrane protein with a reactive endofacial sulfhydryl group. Biochemistry 24:5430, 1985.

678. Muszbek L, Laposata M: Glycoprotein Ib and glycoprotein IX in human platelets are acylated with palmitic acid through thioester linkages. J Biol Chem 264:9716, 1989.

679. Du X, Fox JE, Pei S: Identification of a binding sequence for the 14-3-3 protein within the cytoplasmic domain of the adhesion receptor, platelet glycoprotein Ib alpha. J Biol Chem 271:7362, 1996.

680. Calverley DC, Kavanagh TJ, Roth GJ: Human signaling protein 14-3-3zeta interacts with platelet glycoprotein Ib subunits Ibalpha and Ib-beta. *Blood* 91:1295, 1998.

681. Andrews RK, Harris SJ, McNally T, Berndt MC: Binding of purified 14-3-3 zeta signaling protein to discrete amino acid sequences within the cytoplasmic domain of the platelet membrane glycoprotein Ib-IX-V complex. *Biochemistry* 37:638, 1998.

682. Wardell MR, Reynolds CC, Berndt MC, et al: Platelet glycoprotein Ib beta is phosphorylated on serine 166 by cyclic AMP-dependent protein kinase. *J Biol Chem* 264:15656, 1989.

683. Andrews RK, Fox JE: Identification of a region in the cytoplasmic domain of the platelet membrane glycoprotein Ib-IX complex that binds to purified actin-binding protein. *J Biol Chem* 267:18605, 1992.

684. Coller BS: Inhibition of von Willebrand factor-dependent platelet function by increased platelet cyclic AMP and its prevention by cytoskeleton-disrupting agents. *Blood* 57:846, 1981.

685. Coller BS: Effects of tertiary amine local anesthetics on von Willebrand factor-dependent platelet function: Alteration of membrane reactivity and degradation of GPIb by a calcium-dependent protease(s). *Blood* 248:1355, 1982.

686. Dong JF, Li CQ, Sae-Tung G, et al: The cytoplasmic domain of glycoprotein (GP) Ibalpha constrains the lateral diffusion of the GP Ib-IX complex and modulates von Willebrand factor binding. *Biochemistry* 36:12421, 1997.

687. Munday AD, Berndt MC, Mitchell CA: Phosphoinositide 3-kinase forms a complex with platelet membrane glycoprotein Ib-IX-V complex and 14-3-3zeta. *Blood* 96:577, 2000.

688. Sullam PM, Hyun WC, Szollosi J, et al: Physical proximity and functional interplay of the glycoprotein Ib-IX-V complex and the Fc receptor FcgammaRIIA on the platelet plasma membrane. *J Biol Chem* 273:5331, 1998.

689. Falati S, Edmead CE, Poole AW: Glycoprotein Ib-V-IX, a receptor for von Willebrand factor, couples physically and functionally to the Fc receptor g-chain, Fyn, and Lyn to activate human platelets. *Blood* 94:1648, 1999.

690. Watson SP, Asazuma N, Atkinson B, et al: The role of ITAM- and ITIM-coupled receptors in platelet activation by collagen. *Thromb Haemost* 86:276, 2001.

691. Wu Y, Suzuki-Inoue K, Satoh K, et al: Role of Fc receptor gamma-chain in platelet glycoprotein Ib-mediated signaling. *Blood* 97:3836, 2001.

692. Uff S, Clemetson JM, Harrison T, et al: Crystal structure of the platelet glycoprotein Ib(alpha) N-terminal domain reveals an unmasking mechanism for receptor activation. *J Biol Chem* 277:35657, 2002.

693. Huizinga EG, Tsuji S, Romijn RA, et al: Structures of glycoprotein Ibalpha and its complex with von Willebrand factor A1 domain. *Science* 297:1176, 2002.

694. Dumas JJ, Kumar R, McDonagh T, et al: Crystal structure of the wild-type von Willebrand factor A1-glycoprotein Ibalpha complex reveals conformation differences with a complex bearing von Willebrand disease mutations. *J Biol Chem* 279:23327, 2004.

695. Tang J, Stern-Nezer S, Liu PC, et al: Mutation in the leucine-rich repeat C-flanking region of platelet glycoprotein Ibbeta impairs assembly of von Willebrand factor receptor. *Thromb Haemost* 92:75, 2004.

696. Scott JP, Montgomery RR, Retzinger GS: Dimeric ristocetin flocculates proteins, binds to platelets, and mediates von Willebrand factor-dependent agglutination of platelets. *J Biol Chem* 266:8149, 1991.

697. Berndt MC, Ward CM, Booth WJ, et al: Identification of aspartic acid 514 through glutamic acid 542 as a glycoprotein Ib-IX complex receptor recognition sequence in von Willebrand factor. Mechanism of modulation of von Willebrand factor by ristocetin and botrocetin. *Biochemistry* 31:11144, 1992.

698. Andrews RK, Booth WJ, Gorman JJ, et al: Purification of botrocetin from Bothrops jararaca venom. Analysis of the botrocetin-mediated interaction between von Willebrand factor and the human platelet membrane glycoprotein Ib-IX complex. *Biochemistry* 28:8317, 1989.

699. Olson JD, Zaleski A, Herrmann D, Flood PA: Adhesion of platelets to purified solid-phase von Willebrand factor: Effect of wall shear rate, ADP, thrombin, and ristocetin. *J Lab Clin Med* 114:6, 1989.

700. Parker RI, Gralnick HR: Fibrin monomer induces binding of endogenous vWF to the glycocalicin portion of platelet glycoprotein Ib. *Blood* 70:1589, 1987.

701. Sakariassen KS, Fressinaud E, Grima JP, et al: Role of platelet membrane glycoproteins and von Willebrand factor in adhesion of platelets to subendothelium and collagen. *Ann N Y Acad Sci* 516:52, 1987.

702. Sakariassen KS, Nievelstein PFEM, Coller BS, Sixma JJ: The role of platelet membrane glycoproteins Ib and IIb-IIIa in platelet adherence to human artery subendothelium. *Br J Haematol* 63:681, 1986.

703. Ikeda Y, Murata M, Araki Y, et al: Importance of fibrinogen and platelet membrane glycoprotein IIb/IIIa in shear-induced platelet aggregation. *Thromb Res* 51:157, 1988.

704. Siediecki CA, Lestini BJ, Kottke-Marchant KK, et al: Shear-dependent changes in the three-dimensional structure of human von Willebrand factor. *Blood* 88:2939, 1996.

705. Jamieson GA: The activation of platelets by thrombin: A model for activation by high and moderate affinity receptor pathways. *Prog Clin Biol Res* 283:137, 1988.

706. Ruggeri Z: The platelet glycoprotein Ib-IX complex. *Prog Hemost Thromb* 10:35, 1991.

707. Katagiri Y, Hayashi Y, Yamamoto K, et al: Localization of von Willebrand factor and thrombin-interactive domains in human platelet glycoprotein Ib. *Thromb Haemost* 63:122, 1990.

708. Vanhoorelbeke K, Ulrichts H, Romijn RA, et al: The GPIbalpha-thrombin interaction: Far from crystal clear. *Trends Mol Med* 10:33, 2004.

709. Celikel R, McClintock RA, Roberts JR, et al: Modulation of alpha-thrombin function by distinct interactions with platelet glycoprotein Ibalpha. *Science* 301:218, 2003.

710. Dumas JJ, Kumar R, Seehra J, et al: Crystal structure of the GPIbalpha-thrombin complex essential for platelet aggregation. *Science* 301:222, 2003.

711. Harmon JT, Jamieson GA: The glycocalicin portion of platelet glycoprotein Ib expresses both high and moderate affinity receptor sites of thrombin. A soluble radioreceptor assay for the injection of thrombin with platelets. *J Biol Chem* 261:13224, 1986.

712. Adam F, Verbeuren TJ, Fauchere JL, et al: Thrombin-induced platelet PAR4 activation: Role of glycoprotein Ib and ADP. *J Thromb Haemost* 1:798, 2003.

713. De Candia E, Hall SW, Rutella S, et al: Binding of thrombin to glycoprotein Ib accelerates the hydrolysis of Par-1 on intact platelets. *J Biol Chem* 276:4692, 2001.

714. Frenette PS, Moyna C, Hartwell DW, et al: Platelet-endothelial interactions in inflamed mesenteric venules. *Blood* 91:1318, 1998.

715. Bradford HN, Dela Cadena RA, Kunapuli SP, et al: Human kininogens regulate thrombin binding to platelets through the glycoprotein Ib-IX-V complex. *Blood* 90:1508, 1997.

716. Bradford HN, Pixley RA, Colman RW: Human factor XII binding to the glycoprotein Ib-IX-V complex inhibits thrombin-induced platelet aggregation. *J Biol Chem* 275:22756, 2000.

717. Baglia FA, Badellino KO, Li CQ, et al: Factor XI binding to the platelet glycoprotein Ib-IX-V complex promotes factor XI activation by thrombin. *J Biol Chem* 277:1662, 2002.

718. Simon DI, Chen Z, Xu H, et al: Platelet glycoprotein Iba is a counter-receptor for the leukocyte integrin Mac-1 (CD11b/CD18). *J Exp Med* 192:193, 2000.

719. Berndt MC, Phillips DR: Purification and preliminary physiochemical characterization of human platelet membrane glycoprotein V. *J Biol Chem* 256:59, 1981.

720. Zafar RS, Walz DA: Platelet membrane glycoprotein V: Characterization of the thrombin-sensitive glycoprotein from human platelets. *Thromb Res* 53:31, 1989.

721. Shimomura T, Fujimura K, Maehama S, et al: Rapid purification and characterization of human platelet glycoprotein V: The amino acid sequence contains leucine-rich repetitive modules as in glycoprotein Ib. *Blood* 75:2349, 1990.

722. Lanza F, Morales M, de La Salle C, et al: Cloning and characterization of the gene encoding the human platelet glycoprotein V. A member of the leucine-rich glycoprotein family cleaved during thrombin-induced platelet activation. *J Biol Chem* 268:20801, 1993.

723. Modderman PW, Admiraal LG, Sonnenberg A, von dem Borne AEGKR: Glycoproteins V and Ib-IX form a noncovalent complex in the platelet membrane. *J Biol Chem* 267:364, 1992.

724. Dong JF, Gao S, Lopez JA: Synthesis, assembly, and intracellular transport of the platelet glycoprotein Ib-IX-V complex. *J Biol Chem* 273:31449, 1998.

725. McGowan EB, Ding A, Detwiler TC: Correlation of thrombin-induced glycoprotein V hydrolysis and platelet activation. *J Biol Chem* 258:11243, 1983.

726. Ramakrishnan V, Reeves PS, DeGuzman F, et al: Increased thrombin responsiveness in platelets from mice lacking glycoprotein V. *Proc Natl Acad Sci U S A* 96:13336, 1999.

727. Ramakrishnan V, DeGuzman F, Bao M, et al: A thrombin receptor function for platelet glycoprotein Ib-IX unmasked by cleavage of glycoprotein V. *Proc Natl Acad Sci U S A* 98:1823, 2001.

728. Newman PJ, Berndt MC, Gorski J, et al: PECAM-1 (CD31) cloning and relation to adhesion molecules of the immunoglobulin gene superfamily. *Science* 247:1219, 1990.

729. Metzelaar MJ, Korteweg J, Sixma JJ, Nieuwenhuis HK: Biochemical characterization of PECAM-1 (CD31 antigen) on human platelets. *Thromb Haemost* 66:700, 1991.

730. Varon D, Jackson DE, Shenkman B, et al: Platelet/endothelial cell adhesion molecule-1 serves as a costimulatory agonist receptor that modulates integrin-dependent adhesion and aggregation of human platelets. *Blood* 91:500, 1998.

731. Jackson DE, Ward CM, Wang R, Newman PJ: The protein-tyrosine phosphatase SHP-2 binds platelet/endothelial cell adhesion molecule-1 (PECAM-1) and forms a distinct signaling complex during platelet aggregation. Evidence for a mechanistic link between PECAM-1- and integrin-mediated cellular signaling. *J Biol Chem* 272:6986, 1997.

732. Albelda SM, Muller WA, Buck CA, Newman PJ: Molecular and cellular properties of PECAM-1 (endoCAM/CD31): A novel vascular cell-cell adhesion molecule. *J Cell Biol* 114:1059, 1991.

733. DeLisser HM, Yan HC, Newman PJ, et al: Platelet/endothelial cell adhesion molecule-1 (CD31)-mediated cellular aggregation involves cell surface glycosaminoglycans. *J Biol Chem* 268:16037, 1993.

734. Gumina RJ, el Schultz J, Yao Z, et al: Antibody to platelet/endothelial cell adhesion molecule-1 reduces myocardial infarct size in a rat model of ischemia-reperfusion injury. *Circulation* 94:3327, 1996.

735. Washington AV, Schubert RL, Quigley L, et al: A TREM family member, TLT-1, is found exclusively in the alpha-granules of megakaryocytes and platelets. *Blood* 104:1042, 2004.

736. Gibbins J, Asselin J, Farndale R, et al: Tyrosine phosphorylation of the Fc receptor gamma-chain in collagen-stimulated platelets. *J Biol Chem* 271:18095, 1996.

737. Tsuji M, Ezumi Y, Arai M, Takayama H: A novel association of Fc receptor gamma-chain with glycoprotein VI and their co-expression as a collagen receptor in human platelets. *J Biol Chem* 272:23528, 1997.

738. Reth M: Antigen receptor tail clue. *Nature* 338:383, 1989.

739. Flaswinkel H, Barner M, Reth M: The tyrosine activation motif as a target of protein tyrosine kinases and SH2 domains. *Semin Immunol* 7:21, 1995.

740. Chacko GW, Duchemin AM, Coggeshall KM, et al: Clustering of the platelet Fc gamma receptor induces noncovalent association with the tyrosine kinase p72syk. *J Biol Chem* 269:32435, 1994.

741. Qiu WQ, de Bruin D, Brownstein BH, et al: Organization of the human and mouse low-affinity Fc gamma R genes: Duplication and recombination. *Science* 248:732, 1990.

742. Parren PW, Warmerdam PA, Boeije LC, et al: On the interaction of IgG subclasses with the low affinity Fc gamma RIIa (CD32) on human monocytes, neutrophils, and platelets. Analysis of a functional polymorphism to human IgG2. *J Clin Invest* 90:1537, 1992.

743. Rosenfeld SI, Looney RJ, Leddy JP, et al: Human platelet Fc receptor for immunoglobulin G. Identification as a 40,000-molecular-weight membrane protein shared by monocytes. *J Clin Invest* 76:2317, 1985.

744. Rosenfeld SI, Ryan DH, Looney RJ, et al: Human Fc gamma receptors: Stable inter-donor variation in quantitative expression on platelets correlates with functional responses. *J Immunol* 138:2869, 1987.

745. Anderson GP, van de Winkel JG, Anderson CL: Anti-GPIIb/IIIa (CD41) monoclonal antibody-induced platelet activation requires Fc receptor-dependent cell-cell interaction. *Br J Haematol* 79:75, 1991.

746. Hildreth JE, Derr D, Azorsa DO: Characterization of a novel self-associating Mr 40,000 platelet glycoprotein. *Blood* 77:121, 1991.

747. Gratacap MP, Payrastre B, Viala C, et al: Phosphatidylinositol 3,4,5-trisphosphate-dependent stimulation of phospholipase C gamma2 is an early key event in FcgammaRIIA-mediated activation of human platelets. *J Biol Chem* 273:24314, 1998.

748. Chong BH, Pilgrim RL, Cooley MA, Chesterman CN: Increased expression of platelet IgG Fc receptors in immune heparin-induced thrombocytopenia. *Blood* 81:988, 1993.

749. Chen J, Dong JF, Sun C, et al: Platelet FcgammaRIIA His131Arg polymorphism and platelet function: Antibodies to platelet-bound fibrinogen induce platelet activation. *J Thromb Haemost* 1:355, 2003.

750. Denomme GA, Warkentin TE, Horsewood P, et al: Activation of platelets by sera containing IgG1 heparin-dependent antibodies: An explanation for the predominance of the Fc gammaRIIa "low responder" (his131) gene in patients with heparin-induced thrombocytopenia. *J Lab Clin Med* 130:278, 1997.

751. Carlsson LE, Santoso S, Baurichter G, et al: Heparin-induced thrombocytopenia: New insights into the impact of the FcgammaRIIa-R-H131 polymorphism. *Blood* 92:1526, 1998.

752. Williams Y, Lynch S, McCann S, et al: Correlation of platelet Fc gammaRIIA polymorphism in refractory idiopathic (immune) thrombocytopenic purpura. *Br J Haematol* 101:779, 1998.

753. Torti M, Bertoni A, Canobbio I, et al: Rap1B and Rap2B translocation to the cytoskeleton by von Willebrand factor involves FcgammaII receptor-mediated protein tyrosine phosphorylation. *J Biol Chem* 274:13690, 1999.

754. Peerschke EI, Ghebrehiwet B: C1q augments platelet activation in response to aggregated Ig. *J Immunol* 159:5594, 1997.

755. Diacovo TG, deFougerolles AR, Bainton DF, Springer TA: A functional integrin ligand on the surface of platelets: Intercellular adhesion molecule-2. *J Clin Invest* 94:1243, 1994.

756. Joseph M, Gounni AS, Kusnierz JP, et al: Expression and functions of the high-affinity IgE receptor on human platelets and megakaryocyte precursors. *Eur J Immunol* 27:2212, 1997.

757. Hasegawa S, Pawankar R, Suzuki K, et al: Functional expression of the high affinity receptor for IgE (FcepsilonRI) in human platelets and its intracellular expression in human megakaryocytes. *Blood* 93:2543, 1999.

758. Gupta SK, Pillarisetti K, Ohlstein EH: Platelet agonist F11 receptor is a member of the immunoglobulin superfamily and identical with junc-

tional adhesion molecule (JAM): Regulation of expression in human endothelial cells and macrophages. *IUBMB Life* 50:51, 2000.

759. Naik UP, Naik MU, Eckfeld K, et al: Characterization and chromosomal localization of JAM-1, a platelet receptor for a stimulatory monoclonal antibody. *J Cell Sci* 114:539, 2001.

760. Kornecki E, Walkowiak B, Naik UP, Ehrlich YH: Activation of human platelets by a stimulatory monoclonal antibody. *J Biol Chem* 265:10042, 1990.

761. Sobocka MB, Sobocki T, Banerjee P, et al: Cloning of the human platelet F11 receptor: A cell adhesion molecule member of the immunoglobulin superfamily involved in platelet aggregation. *Blood* 95:2600, 2000.

762. Santoso S, Sachs UJ, Kroll H, et al: The junctional adhesion molecule 3 (JAM-3) on human platelets is a counterreceptor for the leukocyte integrin Mac-1. *J Exp Med* 196:679, 2002.

763. Larsen E, Celi A, Gilbert GE, et al: PADGEM protein: A receptor that mediates the interaction of activated platelets with neutrophils and monocytes. *Cell* 59:305, 1989.

764. Haskard DO: Adhesive proteins, in *Haemostasis and Thrombosis*, edited by AL Bloom, CD Forbes, DP Thomas, EGD Tuddenham, p 233. Churchill Livingstone, England, 1994.

765. Ishiwata N, Takio K, Katayama M, et al: Alternatively spliced isoform of P-selectin is present in vivo as a soluble molecule. *J Biol Chem* 269:23708, 1994.

766. Hartwell DW, Mayadas TN, Berger G, et al: Role of P-selectin cytoplasmic domain in granular targeting in vivo and in early inflammatory responses. *J Cell Biol* 143:1129, 1998.

767. Hamburger SA, McEver RP: GMP-140 mediates adhesion of stimulated platelets to neutrophils. *Blood* 75:550, 1990.

768. Geng JG, Bevilacqua P, Moore KL, et al: Rapid neutrophil adhesion to activated endothelium mediated by GMP-140. *Nature* 343:757, 1990.

769. Handa K, Nudelman ED, Stroud MR, et al: Selectin GMP-140 (CD62; PADGEM) binds to sialosyl-Le(a) and sialosyl-Le(x), and sulfated glycans modulate this binding. *Biochem Biophys Res Commun* 181:1223, 1991.

770. Polley MJ, Phillips ML, Wayner E, et al: CD62 and endothelial cell-leukocyte adhesion molecule I (ELAM-1) recognize the same carbohydrate ligand, sialyl-Lewis^x. *Proc Natl Acad Sci U S A* 88:6224, 1991.

771. Aruffo A, Kolanus W, Walz G, et al: CD62/P-selectin recognition of myeloid and tumor cell sulfatides. *Cell* 67:35, 1991.

772. Stone JP, Wagner DD: P-selectin mediates adhesion of platelets to neuroblastoma and small cell lung cancer. *J Clin Invest* 92:804, 1993.

773. Sako D, Chang XJ, Barone KM, et al: Expression cloning of a functional glycoprotein ligand for P-selectin. *Cell* 75:1179, 1993.

774. Yang J, Furie BC, Furie B: The biology of P-selectin glycoprotein ligand-1: Its role as a selectin counterreceptor in leukocyte-endothelial and leukocyte-platelet interaction. *Thromb Haemost* 81:1, 1999.

775. McEver RP, Cummings RD: Perspectives series: Cell adhesion in vascular biology. Role of PSGL-1 binding to selectins in leukocyte recruitment. *J Clin Invest* 100:485, 1997.

776. Celi A, Pellegrini G, Lorenzet R, et al: P-selectin induces the expression of tissue factor on monocytes. *Proc Natl Acad Sci U S A* 91:8767, 1994.

777. Hrachovinova I, Cambien B, Hafezi-Moghadam A, et al: Interaction of P-selectin and PSGL-1 generates microparticles that correct hemostasis in a mouse model of hemophilia A. *Nat Med* 9:1020, 2003.

778. Ridker PM, Buring JE, Rifai N: Soluble P-selectin and the risk of future cardiovascular events. *Circulation* 103:491, 2001.

779. Mayadas TN, Johnson RC, Rayburn H, et al: Leukocyte rolling and extravasation are severely compromised in P selectin-deficient mice. *Cell* 74:541, 1993.

780. Padilla A, Moake JL, Bernardo A, et al: P-selectin anchors newly released ultralarge von Willebrand factor multimers to the endothelial cell surface. *Blood* 103:2150, 2004.

781. Boucheix C, Benoit P, Frachet P, et al: Molecular cloning of the CD9 antigen. A new family of cell surface proteins. *J Biol Chem* 266:117, 1991.

782. Lanza F, Wolf D, Fox CF, et al: CDNA cloning and expression of platelet p24/CD9. Evidence for a new family of multiple membrane-spanning proteins. *J Biol Chem* 266:10638, 1991.

783. Hato T, Ikeda K, Yasukawa M, et al: Exposure of platelet fibrinogen receptors by a monoclonal antibody to CD9 antigen. *Blood* 72:224, 1988.

784. Brisson C, Azorsa DO, Jennings LK, et al: Co-localization of CD9 and GPIIb-IIIa (alpha IIb beta 3 integrin) on activated platelet pseudopods and alpha-granule membranes. *Histochem J* 29:153, 1997.

785. Jennings LK, Fox CF, Kouns WC, et al: The activation of human platelets mediated by anti-human platelet p24/CD9 monoclonal antibodies. *J Biol Chem* 265:3815, 1990.

786. Hato T, Sumida M, Yasukawa M, et al: Induction of platelet Ca2+ influx and mobilization by a monoclonal antibody to CD9 antigen. *Blood* 75:1087, 1990.

787. Worthington RE, Carroll RC, Boucheix C: Platelet activation by CD9 monoclonal antibodies is mediated by the Fc gamma II receptor. *Br J Haematol* 74:216, 1990.

788. Slupsky JR, Seehafer JG, Tang SC, et al: Evidence that monoclonal antibodies against CD9 antigen induce specific association between CD9 and the platelet glycoprotein IIb-IIIa complex. *J Biol Chem* 264:12289, 1989.

789. Nishibori M, Cham B, McNicol A, et al: The protein CD63 is in platelet dense granules, is deficient in a patient with Hermansky-Pudlak syndrome, and appears identical to granulophysin. *J Clin Invest* 91:1775, 1993.

790. Metzelaar MJ, Wijngaard PL, Peters PJ, et al: CD63 antigen. A novel lysosomal membrane glycoprotein, cloned by a screening procedure for intracellular antigens in eukaryotic cells. *J Biol Chem* 266:3239, 1991.

791. Roberts JJ, Rodgers SE, Drury J, et al: Platelet activation induced by a murine monoclonal antibody directed against a novel tetra-span antigen. *Br J Haematol* 89:853, 1995.

792. Fitter S, Tetaz TJ, Berndt MC, Ashman LK: Molecular cloning of cDNA encoding a novel platelet-endothelial cell tetra-span antigen, PETA-3. *Blood* 86:1348, 1995.

793. Sincock PM, Mayrhofer G, Ashman LK: Localization of the trans-membrane 4 superfamily (TM4SF) member PETA-3 (CD151) in normal human tissues: Comparison with CD9, CD63, and alpha5beta1 integrin. *J Histochem Cytochem* 45:515, 1997.

794. Lau LM, Wee JL, Wright MD, et al: The tetraspanin superfamily member, CD151 regulates outside-in integrin alphaIIbbeta3 signalling and platelet function. *Blood* 104:2368, 2004.

795. Polgar J, Clemetson JM, Gengenbacher D, Clemetson KJ: Additional GPI-anchored glycoproteins on human platelets that are absent or deficient in paroxysmal nocturnal haemoglobinuria. *FEBS Lett* 327:49, 1993.

796. Kelton JG, Smith JW, Horsewood P, et al: ABH antigens on human platelets: Expression on the glycosyl phosphatidylinositol-anchored protein CD109. *J Lab Clin Med* 132:142, 1998.

797. Wohn KD, Kanse SM, Deutsch V, et al: The urokinase-receptor (CD87) is expressed in cells of the megakaryoblastic lineage. *Thromb Haemost* 77:540, 1997.

798. Piguet PF, Vesin C, Da Laperousaz C, Rochat A: Role of plasminogen activators and urokinase receptor in platelet kinetics. *Hematol J* 1:199, 2000.

799. Grunewald M, Grunewald A, Schmid A, et al: The platelet function defect of paroxysmal nocturnal haemoglobinuria. *Platelets* 15:145, 2004.

800. Hernandez-Campo PM, Martin-Ayuso M, Almeida J, et al: Comparative analysis of different flow cytometry-based immunophenotypic methods for the analysis of CD59 and CD55 expression on major peripheral blood cell subsets. *Cytometry* 50:191, 2002.

801. Jin JY, Tooze JA, Marsh JC, Gordon-Smith EC: Glycosylphosphatidylinositol (GPI)-linked protein deficiency on the platelets of patients with aplastic anaemia and paroxysmal nocturnal haemoglobinuria: Two distinct patterns correlating with expression on neutrophils. *Br J Haematol* 96:493, 1997.

802. Holada K, Mondoro TH, Muller J, Vostal JG: Increased expression of phosphatidylinositol-specific phospholipase C resistant prion proteins on the surface of activated platelets. *Br J Haematol* 103:276, 1998.

803. Barclay GR, Hope J, Birkett CR, Turner ML: Distribution of cell-associated prion protein in normal adult blood determined by flow cytometry. *Br J Haematol* 107:804, 1999.

804. Starke R, Cramer E, Harrison P: Expression of cell-associated prion protein on normal human platelets. *Br J Haematol* 110:748, 2000.

805. MacGregor I, Hope J, Barnard G, et al: Application of a time resolved fluoroimmunoassay for the analysis of normal prion protein in human blood and its components. *Vox Sang* 77:88, 1999.

806. Prevost N, Woulfe D, Tanaka T, Brass LF: Interactions between Eph kinases and ephrins provide a mechanism to support platelet aggregation once cell-to-cell contact has occurred. *Proc Natl Acad Sci U S A* 99:9219, 2002.

807. Prevost N, Woulfe DS, Tognolini M, et al: Signaling by ephrinB1 and Eph kinases in platelets promotes Rap1 activation, platelet adhesion, and aggregation via effector pathways that do not require phosphorylation of ephrinB1. *Blood* 103:1348, 2004.

808. Fielder PJ, Hass P, Nagel M, et al: Human platelets as a model for the binding and degradation of thrombopoietin. *Blood* 89:2782, 1997.

809. dem Borne AE, Folman C, Linthorst GE, et al: Thrombopoietin and its receptor: Structure, function and role in the regulation of platelet production. *Baillieres Clin Haematol* 11:409, 1998.

810. Kaushansky K: Thrombopoietin: A tool for understanding thrombopoiesis. *J Thromb Haemost* 1:1587, 2003.

811. Ezumi Y, Takayama H, Okuma M: Thrombopoietin, c-Mpl ligand, induces tyrosine phosphorylation of Tyk2, JAK2, and STAT3, and enhances agonists-induced aggregation in platelets in vitro. *FEBS Lett* 374:48, 1995.

812. Chen J, Herceg-Harjacek L, Groopman JE, Grabarek J: Regulation of platelet activation in vitro by the c-Mpl ligand, thrombopoietin. *Blood* 86:4054, 1995.

813. Kojima H, Hamazaki Y, Nagata Y, et al: Modulation of platelet activation in vitro by thrombopoietin. *Thromb Haemost* 74:1541, 1995.

814. Rodriguez-Linares B, Watson SP: Thrombopoietin potentiates activation of human platelets in association with JAK2 and TYK2 phosphorylation. *Biochem J* 316(Pt 1):93, 1996.

815. Oda A, Miyakawa Y, Druker BJ, et al: Thrombopoietin primes human platelet aggregation induced by shear stress and by multiple agonists. *Blood* 87:4664, 1996.

816. Kubota Y, Arai T, Tanaka T, et al: Thrombopoietin modulates platelet activation in vitro through protein-tyrosine phosphorylation. *Stem Cells* 14:439, 1996.

817. Hajek AS, Joist JH: Platelet insulin receptor. *Methods Enzymol* 215:398, 1992.

818. Kahn NN: Insulin-induced expression of prostacyclin receptors on platelets is mediated through ADP-ribosylation of Gi alpha protein. *Life Sci* 63:2031, 1998.

819. Aukrust P, Damas JK, Solum NO: Soluble CD40 ligand and platelets: Self-perpetuating pathogenic loop in thrombosis and inflammation? *J Am Coll Cardiol* 43:2326, 2004.

820. Varo N, de Lemos JA, Libby P, et al: Soluble CD40L: Risk prediction after acute coronary syndromes. *Circulation* 108:1049, 2003.

821. Inwald DP, McDowall A, Peters MJ, et al: CD40 is constitutively expressed on platelets and provides a novel mechanism for platelet activation. *Circ Res* 92:1041, 2003.

822. Urbich C, Dernbach E, Aicher A, et al: CD40 ligand inhibits endothelial cell migration by increasing production of endothelial reactive oxygen species. *Circulation* 106:981, 2002.

823. Czapiga M, Kirk AD, Lekstrom-Himes J: Platelets deliver costimulatory signals to antigen-presenting cells: A potential bridge between injury and immune activation. *Exp Hematol* 32:135, 2004.

824. Elzey BD, Tian J, Jensen RJ, et al: Platelet-mediated modulation of adaptive immunity. A communication link between innate and adaptive immune compartments. *Immunity* 19:9, 2003.

825. Tandon NN, Lipsky RH, Burgess WH, Jamieson GA: Isolation and characterization of platelet glycoprotein IV (CD36). *J Biol Chem* 264:7570, 1989.

826. Legrand C, Pidard D, Beiso P, et al: Interaction of a monoclonal antibody to glycoprotein IV (CD36) with human platelets and its effect on platelet function. *Platelets* 2:99, 1991.

827. Daviet L, McGregor JL: Vascular biology of CD36: Roles of this new adhesion molecule family in different disease states. *Thromb Haemost* 78:65, 1997.

828. Thorne RF, Meldrum CJ, Harris SJ, et al: CD36 forms covalently associated dimers and multimers in platelets and transfected COS-7 cells. *Biochem Biophys Res Commun* 240:812, 1997.

829. Thibert V, Bellucci S, Cristofari M, et al: Increased platelet CD36 constitutes a common marker in myeloproliferative disorders. *Br J Haematol* 91:618, 1995.

830. Asch AS, Barnwell J, Silverstein RL, Nachman RL: Isolation of the thrombospondin membrane receptor. *J Clin Invest* 79:1054, 1987.

831. Tandon NN, Kralisz U, Jamieson GA: Identification of glycoprotein IV (CD36) as a primary receptor for platelet-collagen adhesion. *J Biol Chem* 264:7576, 1989.

832. Diaz-Ricart M, Tandon NN, Gomez-Ortiz G, et al: Antibodies to CD36 (GPIV) inhibit platelet adhesion to subendothelial surfaces under flow conditions. *Arterioscler Thromb Vasc Biol* 16:883, 1996.

833. Yamamoto N, Ikeda H, Tandon NN, et al: A platelet membrane glycoprotein (GP) deficiency in healthy blood donors: Nak^a-platelets lack detectable GPIV (CD36). *Blood* 76:1698, 1990.

834. Wun T, Paglieroni T, Field CL, et al: Platelet-erythrocyte adhesion in sickle cell disease. *J Investig Med* 47:121, 1999.

835. Oquendo P, Hundt E, Lawler J, Seed B: CD36 directly mediates cytoadherence of *Plasmodium falciparum* infected erythrocytes. *Cell* 58:95, 1989.

836. Nozaki S, Tanaka T, Yamashita S, et al: CD36 mediates long-chain fatty acid transport in human myocardium: Complete myocardial accumulation defect of radiolabeled long-chain fatty acid analog in subjects with CD36 deficiency. *Mol Cell Biochem* 192:129, 1999.

837. Hirano K, Kuwasako T, Nakagawa-Toyama Y, et al: Pathophysiology of human genetic CD36 deficiency. *Trends Cardiovasc Med* 13:136, 2003.

838. Hajjar DP, Gotto AM: Targeting CD36: Modulating inflammation and atherogenesis. *Curr Atheroscler Rep* 5:155, 2003.

839. Pravenec M, Kurtz TW: Genetics of Cd36 and the hypertension metabolic syndrome. *Semin Nephrol* 22:148, 2002.

840. Nicholson AC, Han J, Febbraio M, et al: Role of CD36, the macrophage class B scavenger receptor, in atherosclerosis. *Ann N Y Acad Sci* 947:224, 2001.

841. Huang MM, Bolen JB, Barnwell JW, et al: Membrane glycoprotein IV (CD36) is physically associated with the Fyn, Lyn, and Yes protein-tyrosine kinases in human platelets. *Proc Natl Acad Sci U S A* 88:7844, 1991.

842. Aiken JW, Ginsberg MH, Plow EF: Mechanisms for expression of thrombospondin on the platelet surface. *Semin Thromb Hemost* 13:307, 1987.

843. Silverstein RL, Febbraio M: Identification of lysosome-associated membrane protein-2 as an activation-dependent platelet surface glycoprotein. *Blood* 80:1470, 1992.

844. Peerschke EIB, Ghebrehiwet B: Human blood platelets possess specific binding sites for C1q. *J Immunol* 138:1537, 1987.

845. Peerschke EI, Ghebrehiwet B: Platelet receptors for the complement component C1q: Implications for hemostasis and thrombosis. *Immunobiology* 199:239, 1998.

846. Ghebrehiwet B, Lim BL, Kumar R, et al: GC1q-R/p33, a member of a new class of multifunctional and multicompartmental cellular proteins, is involved in inflammation and infection. *Immunol Rev* 180:65, 2001.

847. Ghebrehiwet B, Lim BL, Peerschke EI, et al: Isolation, cDNA cloning, and overexpression of a 33-kD cell surface glycoprotein that binds to the globular "heads" of C1q. *J Exp Med* 179:1809, 1994.

848. Herwald H, Dedio J, Kellner R, et al: Isolation and characterization of the kininogen-binding protein p33 from endothelial cells. Identity with the gC1q receptor. *J Biol Chem* 271:13040, 1996.

849. Nepomuceno RR, Tenner AJ: C1qRP, the C1q receptor that enhances phagocytosis, is detected specifically in human cells of myeloid lineage, endothelial cells, and platelets. *J Immunol* 160:1929, 1998.

850. Peerschke EI, Reid KB, Ghebrehiwet B: Platelet activation by C1q results in the induction of alpha IIb/beta 3 integrins (GPIIb-IIIa) and the expression of P-selectin and procoagulant activity. *J Exp Med* 178:579, 1993.

851. Peerschke EI, Ghebrehiwet B: Platelet membrane receptors for the complement component C1q. *Semin Hematol* 31:320, 1994.

852. Jiang J, Zhang Y, Krainer AR, Xu RM: Crystal structure of human p32, a doughnut-shaped acidic mitochondrial matrix protein. *Proc Natl Acad Sci U S A* 96:3572, 1999.

853. Metzelaar MJ, Heijnen HF, Sixma JJ, Nieuwenhuis HK: Identification of a 33-Kd protein associated with the alpha-granule membrane (GMP-33) that is expressed on the surface of activated platelets. *Blood* 79:372, 1992.

854. Damas C, Vink T, Nieuwenhuis HK, Sixma JJ: The 33-kDa platelet alpha-granule membrane protein (GMP-33) is an N-terminal proteolytic fragment of thrombospondin. *Thromb Haemost* 86:887, 2001.

855. Rosenstein Y, Park JK, Hahn WC, et al: CD43, a molecule defective in Wiskott-Aldrich syndrome, binds ICAM-1. *Nature* 354:233, 1991.

856. Beutler B: Inferences, questions and possibilities in Toll-like receptor signalling. *Nature* 430:257, 2004.

857. Edfeldt K, Swedenborg J, Hansson GK, Yan ZQ: Expression of toll-like receptors in human atherosclerotic lesions: A possible pathway for plaque activation. *Circulation* 105:1158, 2002.

858. Shiraki R, Inoue N, Kawasaki S, et al: Expression of Toll-like receptors on human platelets. *Thromb Res* 113:379, 2004.

859. Akbiyik F, Ray DM, Gettings KF, et al: Human bone marrow megakaryocytes and platelets express PPARgamma, and PPARgamma agonists blunt platelet release of CD40 ligand and thromboxanes. *Blood* 104:1361, 2004.

860. Ahmad R, Menezes J, Knafo L, Ahmad A: Activated human platelets express Fas-L and induce apoptosis in Fas-positive tumor cells. *J Leukoc Biol* 69:123, 2001.

861. Coller BS: Platelets and thrombolytic therapy. *N Engl J Med* 322:33, 1990.

862. Coller BS: Augmentation of thrombolysis with antiplatelet drugs. Overview. *Coron Artery Dis* 6:911, 1995.

863. Korbut R, Gryglewski RJ: Platelets in fibrinolytic system. *J Physiol Pharmacol* 46:409, 1995.

864. Kolev K, Machovich R: Molecular and cellular modulation of fibrinolysis. *Thromb Haemost* 89:610, 2003.

865. Thorsen S, Brakman P, Astrup T: Influence of platelets on fibrinolysis: A critical review, in *Hematologic Reviews*, edited by JL Ambrole, p 123. Marcel Dekker, New York, 1972.

866. Carroll RC, Radcliffe RD, Taylor FB, Gerrard JM: Plasminogen, plasminogen activator and platelets in the regulation of clot lysis. *J Lab Clin Med* 100:986, 1982.

867. Miles LA, Plow EF: Binding and activation of plasminogen on the platelet surface. *J Biol Chem* 260:4303, 1985.

868. Stricker RB, Wong D, Shiu DT, et al: Activation of plasminogen by tissue plasminogen activator on normal and thrombasthenic platelets: Effects on surface proteins and platelet aggregation. *Blood* 68:275, 1986.

869. Jeanneau C, Sultan Y: Tissue plasminogen activator in human megakaryocytes and platelets: Immunocytochemical localization, immunoblotting and zymographic analysis. *Thromb Haemost* 19:529, 1988.

870. Park S, Harker LA, Marzec UM, Levin EG: Demonstration of single chain urokinase-type plasminogen activator on human platelet membrane. *Blood* 73:1421, 1989.

871. de Haan J, van Oeveren W: Platelets and soluble fibrin promote plasminogen activation causing downregulation of platelet glycoprotein Ib/IX complexes: Protection by aprotinin. *Thromb Res* 92:171, 1998.

872. Plow EF, Collen D: The presence and release of α_2-antiplasmin from human platelets. *Blood* 58:1069, 1981.

873. Smariga PE, Maynard JR: Purification of a platelet protein which stimulates fibrinolytic inhibition and tissue factor in human fibroblasts. *J Biol Chem* 257:11960, 1982.

874. Erickson LA, Ginsberg MH, Loskutoff DJ: Detection and partial characterization of an inhibitor of plasminogen activator in human platelets. *J Clin Invest* 74:1465, 1984.

875. Kruithof EKO, Tran-Thang C, Bachmann F: Studies on the release of plasminogen activator inhibitor from human platelets. *Thromb Haemost* 55:201, 1986.

876. Francis CW, Marder VJ: Rapid formation of large molecular weight alpha-polymers in cross-linked fibrin induced by high factor XIII concentrations: Role of platelet factor XIII. *J Clin Invest* 80:1459, 1987.

877. Fay WP, Eitzman DT, Shapiro AD, et al: Platelets inhibit fibrinolysis in vitro by both plasminogen activator inhibitor-1 dependent and independent mechanisms. *Blood* 83:351, 1994.

878. Cox AD, Devine DV: Factor XIIIa binding to activated platelets is mediated through activation of glycoprotein IIb-IIIa. *Blood* 83:1006, 1994.

879. Kawasaki T, Dewerchin M, Lijnen HR, et al: Vascular release of plasminogen activator inhibitor-1 impairs fibrinolysis during acute arterial thrombosis in mice. *Blood* 96:153, 2000.

880. Binder BR, Christ G, Gruber F, et al: Plasminogen activator inhibitor 1: Physiological and pathophysiological roles. *News Physiol Sci* 17:56, 2002.

881. Jang I-K, Gold HK, Ziskind AA, et al: Differential sensitivity of erythrocyte-rich and platelet-rich arterial thrombi to lysis with recombinant tissue-type plasminogen activator. A possible explanation for resistance to coronary thrombolysis. *Circulation* 79:920, 1989.

882. Ohlstein EH, Storer B, Fujita T, Shebuski RJ: Tissue-type plasminogen activator and streptokinase induce platelet hyperaggregability in the rabbit. *Thromb Res* 46:575, 1987.

883. Fitzgerald DJ, Catella F, Roy L, FitzGerald GA: Marked platelet activation in vivo after intravenous streptokinase in patients with acute myocardial infarction. *Circulation* 77:142, 1988.

884. Shebuski RJ: Principles underlying the use of conjunctive agents with plasminogen activators. *Ann N Y Acad Sci* 667:382, 1992.

885. Rudd MA, George D, Amarante P, et al: Temporal effects of thrombolytic agents on platelet function in vivo and their modulation by prostaglandins. *Circ Res* 67:1175, 1990.

886. Kerins DM, Roy L, FitzGerald GA, Fitzgerald DJ: Platelet and vascular function during coronary thrombolysis with tissue-type plasminogen activator. *Circulation* 80:1718, 1990.

887. Fitzgerald DJ, Wright F, FitzGerald GA: Increased thromboxane biosynthesis during coronary thrombolysis: Evidence that platelet activation and thromboxane A_2 modulate the response to tissue-type plasminogen activator in vivo. *Circ Res* 65:83, 1989.

888. Penny WF, Ware JA: Platelet activation and subsequent inhibition by plasmin and recombinant tissue-type plasminogen activator. *Blood* 79:91, 1992.

889. Niewiarowski S, Senyi AF, Gillies P: Plasmin-induced platelet aggregation and platelet release reaction. *J Clin Invest* 52:1647, 1973.

890. Schafer AI, Maas AK, Ware JA, et al: Platelet protein phosphorylation, elevation of cytostolic calcium, and inositol phospholipid breakdown in platelet activation induced by plasmin. *J Clin Invest* 78:73, 1986.

891. Ervin AL, Peerschke EI: Platelet activation by sustained exposure to low-dose plasmin. *Blood Coagul Fibrinolysis* 12:415, 2001.

892. Ishii Watabe A, Uchida E, Mizuguchi H, Hayakawa T: On the mechanism of plasmin-induced platelet aggregation. Implications of the dual role of granule ADP. *Biochem Pharmacol* 59:1345, 2000.

893. Quinton TM, Kim S, Derian CK, et al: Plasmin-mediated activation of platelets occurs by cleavage of protease-activated receptor 4. *J Biol Chem* 279:18434, 2004.

894. Eisenberg PR, Sherman LA, Jaffe AS: Paradoxic elevation of fibrinopeptide A after streptokinase: Evidence for continued thrombosis despite intense fibrinolysis. *J Am Coll Cardiol* 10:527, 1987.

895. Owen J, Friedman KD, Grossman BA, et al: Thrombolytic therapy with tissue plasminogen activator or streptokinase induces transient thrombin activity. *Blood* 72:616, 1988.

896. Leopold JA, Loscalzo J: Platelet activation by fibrinolytic agents: A potential mechanism for resistance to thrombolysis and reocclusion after successful thrombolysis. *Coron Artery Dis* 6:923, 1995.

897. Szczeklik A: Thrombin generation in myocardial infarction and hypercholesterolemia. Effects of aspirin. *Thromb Haemost* 74:77, 1995.

898. Weitz JI, Cruickshank MK, Though D, et al: Human tissue-type plasminogen activator releases fibrinopeptides A and B from fibrinogen. *J Clin Invest* 82:1700, 1988.

899. Coller BS: Inhibitors of the platelet glycoprotein IIb/IIIa receptor as conjunctive therapy for coronary artery thrombolysis. *Coron Artery Dis* 3:1016, 1992.

900. Eccleston D, Topol EJ: Inhibitors of platelet glycoprotein IIb/IIIa as augmenters of thrombolysis. *Coron Artery Dis* 6:947, 1995.

901. O'Donnell CJ, Jonas MA, Hennekens CH: Aspirin augmentation of the efficacy of thrombolysis. *Coron Artery Dis* 6:936, 1995.

902. Topol EJ: Reperfusion therapy for acute myocardial infarction with fibrinolytic therapy or combination reduced fibrinolytic therapy and platelet glycoprotein IIb/IIIa inhibition: The GUSTO V randomised trial. *Lancet* 357:1905, 2001.

903. Lapchak PA, Araujo DM, Song D, Zivin JA: The nonpeptide glycoprotein IIb/IIIa platelet receptor antagonist SM-20302 reduces tissue plasminogen activator-induced intracerebral hemorrhage after thromboembolic stroke. *Stroke* 33:147, 2002.

904. Zhang L, Zhang ZG, Zhang R, et al: Adjuvant treatment with a glycoprotein IIb/IIIa receptor inhibitor increases the therapeutic window for low-dose tissue plasminogen activator administration in a rat model of embolic stroke. *Circulation* 107:2837, 2003.

905. Kowalski E, Kopec M, Wegrzynowicz A: Influence of fibrinogen degradation products (FDP) on platelet aggregation, adhesiveness and viscous metamorphosis. *Thromb Diath Haemorrh* 10:406, 1963.

906. Schafer AL, Adelman B: Plasmin inhibition of platelet function and of arachidonic acid metabolism. *J Clin Invest* 75:456, 1985.

907. Adelman B, Michelson AD, Loscalzo J, et al: Plasmin effect on platelet glycoprotein Ib-von Willebrand factor interactions. *Blood* 64:32, 1985.

908. Loscalzo J, Vaughan DE: Tissue plasminogen activator promotes platelet disaggregation in plasma. *J Clin Invest* 79:1749, 1987.

909. Schafer AL, Zavoico GB, Loscalzo J, Maas AK: Synergistic inhibition of platelet activation by plasmin and prostaglandin I_2. *Blood* 69:1504, 1987.

910. Adnot S, Ferry N, Nanoune J, Lacombe ML: Plasmin: A possible physiological modulator of human platelet adenylate cyclase system. *Clin Sci* 72:467, 1987.

911. Gimple LW, Gold HK, Leinbach RC, et al: Correlation between template bleeding times and spontaneous bleeding during treatment of acute myocardial infarction with recombinant tissue-type plasminogen activator. *Circulation* 80:581, 1989.

912. Michelson AD, Gore JM, Rybak ME, et al: Effect of in vivo infusion of recombinant tissue-type plasminogen activator on platelet glycoprotein Ib. *Thromb Res* 60:421, 1990.

913. Federici AB, Berkowitz SD, Mannucci PM, et al: Proteolysis of von Willebrand factor in patients undergoing thrombolytic therapy [abstract]. *Circulation* 78(suppl II):120, 1988.

914. Johnstone MT, Andrews T, Ware JA, et al: Bleeding time prolongation with streptokinase and its reduction with 1-desamino-8-D-arginine vasopressin. *Circulation* 82:2142, 1990.

915. Kamat SG, Schafer AI: Antiplatelet effects of fibrinolytic agents: A potential contributor to the hemostatic defect after thrombolysis. *Coron Artery Dis* 6:930, 1995.

916. Coller BS: Binding of abciximab to $\alpha V\beta 3$ and activated $\alpha M\beta 2$ receptors: With a review of platelet-leukocyte interactions. *Thromb Haemost* 82:326, 1999.

917. Farb A, Sangiorgi G, Carter AJ, et al: Pathology of acute and chronic coronary stenting in humans. *Circulation* 99:44, 1999.

918. Merhi Y, Provost P, Chauvet P, et al: Selectin blockade reduces neutrophil interaction with platelets at the site of deep arterial injury by angioplasty in pigs. *Arterioscler Thromb Vasc Biol* 19:372, 1999.

919. Smyth SS, Reis ED, Zhang W, et al: $\beta 3$-integrin-deficient mice, but not P-selectin-deficient mice, develop intimal hyperplasia after vascular injury. *Circulation* 103:2501, 2001.

920. von Hundelshausen P, Weber KS, Huo Y, et al: RANTES deposition by platelets triggers monocyte arrest on inflamed and atherosclerotic endothelium. *Circulation* 103:1772, 2001.

921. Schober A, Manka D, von Hundelshausen P, et al: Deposition of platelet RANTES triggering monocyte recruitment requires P-selectin and is involved in neointima formation after arterial injury. *Circulation* 106:1523, 2002.

922. Huo Y, Schober A, Forlow SB, et al: Circulating activated platelets exacerbate atherosclerosis in mice deficient in apolipoprotein E. *Nat Med* 9:61, 2003.

923. Yeo EL, Sheppard JA, Feuerstein IA: Role of P-selectin and leukocyte activation in polymorphonuclear cell adhesion to surface adherent activated platelets under physiologic shear conditions (an injury vessel wall model). *Blood* 83:2498, 1994.

924. Diacovo TG, Roth SJ, Buccola JM, et al: Neutrophil rolling, arrest, and transmigration across activated, surface-adherent platelets via sequential action of P-selectin and the beta 2-integrin CD11b/CD18. *Blood* 88:146, 1996.

925. Sheikh S, Nash GB: Continuous activation and deactivation of integrin CD11b/CD18 during de novo expression enables rolling neutrophils to immobilize on platelets. *Blood* 87:5040, 1996.

926. Kirchhofer D, Riederer MA, Baumgartner HR: Specific accumulation of circulating monocytes and polymorphonuclear leukocytes on platelet thrombi in a vascular injury model. *Blood* 89:1270, 1997.

927. Konstantopoulos K, Neelamegham S, Burns AR, et al: Venous levels of shear support neutrophil-platelet adhesion and neutrophil aggregation in blood via P-selectin and beta2-integrin. *Circulation* 98:873, 1998.

928. Weber C, Springer TA: Neutrophil accumulation on activated, surface-adherent platelets in flow is mediated by interaction of Mac-1 with fibrinogen bound to alphaIIbbeta3 and stimulated by platelet-activating factor. *J Clin Invest* 100:2085, 1997.

929. Altieri DC, Plescia J, Plow EF: The structural motif glycine 190-valine 202 of the fibrinogen gamma chain interacts with CD11b/CD18 integrin (alpha M beta 2, Mac-1) and promotes leukocyte adhesion. *J Biol Chem* 268:1847, 1993.

930. Ugarova TP, Solovjov DA, Zhang L, et al: Identification of a novel recognition sequence for integrin alphaM beta2 within the gamma-chain of fibrinogen. *J Biol Chem* 273:22519, 1998.

931. Silverstein RL, Asch AS, Nachman RL: Glycoprotein IV mediates thrombospondin-dependent platelet-monocyte and platelet-U937 cell adhesion. *J Clin Invest* 84:546, 1989.

932. Marcus AJ, Safier LB: Thromboregulation: Multicellular modulation of platelet reactivity in hemostasis and thrombosis. *FASEB J* 7:516, 1993.

933. Alderson MR, Armitage RJ, Tough TW, et al: CD40 expression by human monocytes: Regulation by cytokines and activation of monocytes by the ligand for CD40. *J Exp Med* 178:669, 1993.

934. Yellin MJ, Brett J, Baum D, et al: Functional interactions of T cells with endothelial cells: The role of CD40L-CD40-mediated signals. *J Exp Med* 182:1857, 1995.

935. Slupsky JR, Kalbas M, Willuweit A, et al: Activated platelets induce tissue factor expression on human umbilical vein endothelial cells by ligation of CD40. *Thromb Haemost* 80:1008, 1998.

936. Goel MS, Diamond SL: Neutrophil cathepsin G promotes prothrombinase and fibrin formation under flow conditions by activating fibrinogen-adherent platelets. *J Biol Chem* 278:9458, 2003.

937. Goel MS, Diamond SL: Neutrophil enhancement of fibrin deposition under flow through platelet-dependent and -independent mechanisms. *Arterioscler Thromb Vasc Biol* 21:2093, 2001.

938. Andre P, Hartwell D, Hrachovinova I, et al: Pro-coagulant state resulting from high levels of soluble P-selectin in blood. *Proc Natl Acad Sci U S A* 97:13835, 2000.

939. Ott I, Neumann FJ, Gawaz M, et al: Increased neutrophil-platelet adhesion in patients with unstable angina. *Circulation* 94:1239, 1996.

940. Mickelson JK, Lakkis NM, Villarreal-Levy G, et al: Leukocyte activation with platelet adhesion after coronary angioplasty: A mechanism for recurrent disease? *J Am Coll Cardiol* 28:345, 1996.

941. Michelson AD, Barnard MR, Krueger LA, et al: Circulating monocyte-platelet aggregates are a more sensitive marker of in vivo platelet activation than platelet surface P-selectin: Studies in baboons, human coronary intervention, and human acute myocardial infarction. *Circulation* 104:1533, 2001.

942. Pawelczyk T: Isozymes delta of phosphoinositide-specific phospholipase C. *Acta Biochim Pol* 46:91, 1999.

943. Hirata T, Ushikubi F, Kakizuka A, et al: Two thromboxane A2 receptor isoforms in human platelets. Opposite coupling to adenylyl cyclase with different sensitivity to Arg60 to Leu mutation. *J Clin Invest* 97:949, 1996.

944. Murphy CT, Westwick J: Selective inhibition of protein kinase C. Effect on platelet-activating-factor-induced platelet functional responses. *Biochem J* 283:159, 1992.

945. Kunapuli SP: Functional characterization of platelet ADP. *Platelets* 9:343, 1998.

946. Henderson DJ, Elliot DG, Smith GM, et al: Cloning and characterisation of a bovine P2Y receptor. *Biochem Biophys Res Commun* 212:648, 1995.

947. Fabre JE, Nguyen M, Latour A, et al: Decreased platelet aggregation, increased bleeding time and resistance to thromboembolism in P2Y1-deficient mice. *Nat Med* 5:1199, 1999.

948. Leon C, Hechler B, Freund M, et al: Defective platelet aggregation and increased resistance to thrombosis in purinergic P2Y(1) receptor-null mice. *J Clin Invest* 104:1731, 1999.

949. Offermanns S, Toombs CF, Hu YH, Simon MI: Defective platelet activation in G alpha(q)-deficient mice. *Nature* 389:183, 1997.

950. Hollopeter G, Jantzen HM, Vincent D, et al: Identification of the platelet ADP receptor targeted by antithrombotic drugs. *Nature* 409:202, 2001.

951. Conley PB, Delaney SM: Scientific and therapeutic insights into the role of the platelet P2Y12 receptor in thrombosis. *Curr Opin Hematol* 10:333, 2003.

952. Dorsam RT, Kunapuli SP: Central role of the P2Y12 receptor in platelet activation. *J Clin Invest* 113:340, 2004.

953. Jin J, Daniel JL, Kunapuli SP: Molecular basis for ADP-induced platelet activation. II. The P2Y1 receptor mediates ADP-induced intracellular calcium mobilization and shape change in platelets. *J Biol Chem* 273:2030, 1998.

954. Mills DC, Puri R, Hu CJ, et al: Clopidogrel inhibits the binding of ADP analogues to the receptor mediating inhibition of platelet adenylate cyclase. *Arterioscler Thromb* 12:430, 1992.

955. Foster CJ, Prosser DM, Agans JM, et al: Molecular identification and characterization of the platelet ADP receptor targeted by thienopyridine antithrombotic drugs. *J Clin Invest* 107:1591, 2001.

956. Andre P, Delaney SM, LaRocca T, et al: P2Y12 regulates platelet adhesion/activation, thrombus growth, and thrombus stability in injured arteries. *J Clin Invest* 112:398, 2003.

957. MacKenzie AB, Mahaut-Smith MP, Sage SO: Activation of receptor-operated cation channels via P2X1 not P2T purinoceptors in human platelets. *J Biol Chem* 271:2879, 1996.

958. Valera S, Hussy N, Evans RJ, et al: A new class of ligand-gated ion channel defined by P2x receptor for extracellular ATP. *Nature* 371:516, 1994.

959. Oury C, Toth-Zsamboki E, Vermylen J, Hoylaerts MF: Does the P(2X1del) variant lacking 17 amino acids in its extracellular domain represent a relevant functional ion channel in platelets? *Blood* 99:2275, 2002.

960. Vial C, Pitt SJ, Roberts J, et al: Lack of evidence for functional ADP-activated human P2X1 receptors supports a role for ATP during hemostasis and thrombosis. *Blood* 102:3646, 2003.

961. Oury C, Toth-Zsamboki E, Vermylen J, Hoylaerts MF: P2X(1)-mediated activation of extracellular signal-regulated kinase 2 contributes to platelet secretion and aggregation induced by collagen. *Blood* 100:2499, 2002.

962. Vial C, Rolf MG, Mahaut-Smith MP, Evans RJ: A study of P2X1 receptor function in murine megakaryocytes and human platelets reveals synergy with P2Y receptors. *Br J Pharmacol* 135:363, 2002.

963. Hechler B, Lenain N, Marchese P, et al: A role of the fast ATP-gated P2X1 cation channel in thrombosis of small arteries in vivo. *J Exp Med* 198:661, 2003.

964. Oury C, Kuijpers MJ, Toth-Zsamboki E, et al: Overexpression of the platelet P2X1 ion channel in transgenic mice generates a novel prothrombotic phenotype. *Blood* 101:3969, 2003.

965. Greco NJ, Tonon G, Chen W, et al: Novel structurally altered P(2X1) receptor is preferentially activated by adenosine diphosphate in platelets and megakaryocytic cells. *Blood* 98:100, 2001.

966. Gayle RB, Maliszewski CR, Gimpel SD, et al: Inhibition of platelet function by recombinant soluble ecto-ADPase/CD39. *J Clin Invest* 101:1851, 1998.

967. Banga HS, Simons ER, Brass LF, Rittenhouse SE: Activation of phospholipases A and C in human platelets exposed to epinephrine: Role of glycoproteins IIb/IIIa and dual role of epinephrine. *Proc Natl Acad Sci U S A* 83:9197, 1986.

968. Shattil SJ, Budzynski A, Scrutton MC: Epinephrine induces platelet fibrinogen receptor expression, fibrinogen binding, and aggregation in whole blood in the absence of other excitatory agonists. *Blood* 73:150, 1989.

969. Lanza F, Beretz A, Stierle A, et al: Epinephrine potentiates human platelet activation but is not an aggregating agent. *Am J Physiol* 255:1276, 1988.

970. Regan JW, Nakata H, DeMarinis RM, et al: Purification and characterization of the human platelet alpha 2-adrenergic receptor. *J Biol Chem* 261:3894, 1986.

971. Kobilka BK, Matsui H, Kobilka TS, et al: Cloning, sequencing, and expression of the gene coding for the human platelet alpha 2-adrenergic receptor. *Science* 238:650, 1987.

972. Yang J, Wu J, Kowalska MA, et al: Loss of signaling through the G protein, Gz, results in abnormal platelet activation and altered responses to psychoactive drugs. *Proc Natl Acad Sci U S A* 97:9984, 2000.

973. Homcy CJ, Graham RM: Molecular characterization of adrenergic receptors. *Circ Res* 56:635, 1985.

974. Yang J, Wu J, Jiang H, et al: Signaling through Gi family members in platelets. Redundancy and specificity in the regulation of adenylyl cyclase and other effectors. *J Biol Chem* 277:46035, 2002.

975. Haslam RJ, Davidson MM, Fox JE, Lynham JA: Cyclic nucleotides in platelet function. *Thromb Haemost* 40:232, 1978.

976. Salzman EW, Ware JA: Ionized calcium as an intracellular messenger in blood platelets. *Prog Hemost Thromb* 9:177, 1989.

977. Patel YM, Patel K, Rahman S, et al: Evidence for a role for Galphai1 in mediating weak agonist-induced platelet aggregation in human platelets: Reduced Galphai1 expression and defective Gi signaling in the platelets of a patient with a chronic bleeding disorder. *Blood* 101:4828, 2003.

978. Marcus A: Platelet eicosanoid metabolism, in *Hemostasis and Thrombosis: Basic Principles and Clinical Practice*, edited by RW Colman, J Hirsch, VJ Marder, EW Salzman, p 676. JB Lippincott, Philadelphia, 1987.

979. Puri RN: Phospholipase A2: Its role in ADP- and thrombin-induced platelet activation mechanisms. *Int J Biochem Cell Biol* 30:1107, 1998.

980. Crofford LJ: COX-1 and COX-2 tissue expression: Implications and predictions. *J Rheumatol* 24:15, 1997.

981. Warner TD, Mitchell JA: Cyclooxygenases: New forms, new inhibitors, and lessons from the clinic. *FASEB J* 18:790, 2004.

982. Dubois RN, Abramson SB, Crofford L, et al: Cyclooxygenase in biology and disease. *FASEB J* 12:1063, 1998.

983. Smith JB, Willis AL: Aspirin selectively inhibits prostaglandin production in human platelets. *Nat New Biol* 231:235, 1971.

984. Svensson J, Hamberg M, Samuelsson B: On the formation and effects of thromboxane A2 in human platelets. *Acta Physiol Scand* 98:285, 1976.

985. Weber AA, Zimmermann KC, Meyer-Kirchrath J, Schror K: Cyclooxygenase-2 in human platelets as a possible factor in aspirin resistance. *Lancet* 353:900, 1999.

986. Rocca B, Secchiero P, Ciabattoni G, et al: Cyclooxygenase-2 expression is induced during human megakaryopoiesis and characterizes newly formed platelets. *Proc Natl Acad Sci U S A* 99:7634, 2002.

987. Parent JL, Labrecque P, Orsini MJ, Benovic JL: Internalization of the TXA2 receptor alpha and beta isoforms. Role of the differentially spliced cooh terminus in agonist-promoted receptor internalization. *J Biol Chem* 274:8941, 1999.

988. Habib A, FitzGerald GA, Maclouf J: Phosphorylation of the thromboxane receptor alpha, the predominant isoform expressed in human platelets. *J Biol Chem* 274:2645, 1999.

989. Komiotis D, Wencel-Drake JD, Dieter JP, et al: Labeling of human platelet plasma membrane thromboxane A2/prostaglandin H2 receptors using SQB, a novel biotinylated receptor probe. *Biochem Pharmacol* 52:763, 1996.

990. Kim SO, Lim CT, Lam SC, et al: Purification of the human blood platelet thromboxane A2/prostaglandin H2 receptor protein. *Biochem Pharmacol* 43:313, 1992.

991. Ushikubi F, Nakajima M, Hirata M, et al: Purification of the thromboxane A2/prostaglandin H2 receptor from human blood platelets. *J Biol Chem* 264:16496, 1989.

992. Takahara K, Murray R, FitzGerald GA, Fitzgerald DJ: The response to thromboxane A2 analogues in human platelets. Discrimination of two binding sites linked to distinct effector systems. *J Biol Chem* 265:6836, 1990.

993. Thomas DW, Mannon RB, Mannon PJ, et al: Coagulation defects and altered hemodynamic responses in mice lacking receptors for thromboxane A2. *J Clin Invest* 102:1994, 1998.

994. Gabbeta J, Yang X, Kowalska MA, et al: Platelet signal transduction defect with Galpha subunit dysfunction and diminished Galphaq in a patient with abnormal platelet responses. *Proc Natl Acad Sci U S A* 94:8750, 1997.

995. Djellas Y, Manganello JM, Antonakis K, Le Breton GC: Identification of Galpha13 as one of the G-proteins that couple to human platelet thromboxane A2 receptors. *J Biol Chem* 274:14325, 1999.

996. Allan CJ, Higashiura K, Martin M, et al: Characterization of the cloned HEL cell thromboxane A2 receptor: Evidence that the affinity state can be altered by G alpha 13 and G alpha q. *J Pharmacol Exp Ther* 277:1132, 1996.

997. Nakahata N, Miyamoto A, Ohkubo S, et al: Gq/11 communicates with thromboxane A2 receptors in human astrocytoma cells, rabbit astrocytes and human platelets. *Res Commun Mol Pathol Pharmacol* 87:243, 1995.

998. Ushikubi F, Nakamura K, Narumiya S: Functional reconstitution of platelet thromboxane A2 receptors with Gq and Gi2 in phospholipid vesicles. *Mol Pharmacol* 46:808, 1994.

999. Paul BZ, Jin J, Kunapuli SP: Molecular mechanism of thromboxane A(2)-induced platelet aggregation. Essential role for p2t(ac) and alpha(2a) receptors. *J Biol Chem* 274:29108, 1999.

1000. Klages B, Brandt U, Simon MI, et al: Activation of G12/G13 results in shape change and Rho/Rho-kinase-mediated myosin light chain phosphorylation in mouse platelets. *J Cell Biol* 144:745, 1999.

1001. Nieswandt B, Schulte V, Zywietz A, et al: Costimulation of Gi- and G12/G13-mediated signaling pathways induces integrin alpha IIbbeta 3 activation in platelets. *J Biol Chem* 277:39493, 2002.

1002. Dorsam RT, Kim S, Jin J, Kunapuli SP: Coordinated signaling through both G12/13 and G(i) pathways is sufficient to activate GPIIb/IIIa in human platelets. *J Biol Chem* 277:47588, 2002.

1003. Pulcinelli FM, Ashby B, Gazzaniga PP, Daniel JL: Protein kinase C activation is not a key step in ADP-mediated exposure of fibrinogen receptors on human platelets. *FEBS Lett* 364:87, 1995.

1004. Knezevic I, Dieter JP, Le Breton GC: Mechanism of inositol 1,4,5-trisphosphate-induced aggregation in saponin-permeabilized platelets. *J Pharmacol Exp Ther* 260:947, 1992.

1005. Ofosu FA, Liu L, Freedman J: Control mechanisms in thrombin generation. *Semin Thromb Hemost* 22:303, 1996.

1006. Phillips DR: Thrombin interaction with human platelets. Potentiation of thrombin-induced aggregation and release by inactivated thrombin. *Thromb Diath Haemorrh* 32:207, 1974.

1007. Hung DT, Vu TK, Wheaton VI, et al: Cloned platelet thrombin receptor is necessary for thrombin-induced platelet activation. *J Clin Invest* 89:1350, 1992.

1008. Vu TK, Hung DT, Wheaton VI, Coughlin SR: Molecular cloning of a functional thrombin receptor reveals a novel proteolytic mechanism of receptor activation. *Cell* 64:1057, 1991.

1009. Furman MI, Liu L, Benoit SE, et al: The cleaved peptide of the thrombin receptor is a strong platelet agonist. *Proc Natl Acad Sci U S A* 95: 3082, 1998.

1010. Ishihara H, Zeng D, Connolly AJ, et al: Antibodies to protease-activated receptor 3 inhibit activation of mouse platelets by thrombin. *Blood* 91:4152, 1998.

1011. Kahn ML, Zheng YW, Huang W, et al: A dual thrombin receptor system for platelet activation. *Nature* 394:690, 1998.

1012. Kahn ML, Nakanishi-Matsui M, Shapiro MJ, et al: Protease-activated receptors 1 and 4 mediate activation of human platelets by thrombin. *J Clin Invest* 103:879, 1999.

1013. Andrade-Gordon P, Maryanoff BE, Derian CK, et al: Design, synthesis, and biological characterization of a peptide-mimetic antagonist for a tethered-ligand receptor. *Proc Natl Acad Sci U S A* 96:12257, 1999.

1014. Shapiro MJ, Weiss EJ, Faruqi TR, Coughlin SR: Protease-activated receptors 1 and 4 are shut off with distinct kinetics after activation by thrombin. *J Biol Chem* 275:25216, 2000.

1015. Covic L, Gresser AL, Kuliopulos A: Biphasic kinetics of activation and signaling for PAR1 and PAR4 thrombin receptors in platelets. *Biochemistry* 39:5458, 2000.

1016. Sambrano GR, Weiss EJ, Zheng YW, et al: Role of thrombin signalling in platelets in haemostasis and thrombosis. *Nature* 413:74, 2001.

1017. Nakanishi-Matsui M, Zheng YW, Sulciner DJ, et al: PAR3 is a cofactor for PAR4 activation by thrombin. *Nature* 404:609, 2000.

1018. Weiss EJ, Hamilton JR, Lease KE, Coughlin SR: Protection against thrombosis in mice lacking PAR3. *Blood* 100:3240, 2002.

1019. Hoxie JA, Ahuja M, Belmonte E, et al: Internalization and recycling of activated thrombin receptors. *J Biol Chem* 268:13756, 1993.

1020. Trejo J, Coughlin SR: The cytoplasmic tails of protease-activated receptor-1 and substance P receptor specify sorting to lysosomes versus recycling. *J Biol Chem* 274:2216, 1999.

1021. Graham GJ, Stevens JM, Page NM, et al: Tachykinins regulate the function of platelets. *Blood* 104:1058, 2004.

1022. McIntyre TM, Zimmerman GA, Prescott SM: Biologically active oxidized phospholipids. *J Biol Chem* 274:25189, 1999.

1023. Honda Z, Nakamura M, Miki I, et al: Cloning by functional expression of platelet-activating factor receptor from guinea-pig lung. *Nature* 349: 342, 1991.

1024. Nakamura M, Honda Z, Izumi T, et al: Molecular cloning and expression of platelet-activating factor receptor from human leukocytes. *J Biol Chem* 266:20400, 1991.

1025. Carlson SA, Chatterjee TK, Fisher RA: The third intracellular domain of the platelet-activating factor receptor is a critical determinant in receptor coupling to phosphoinositide phospholipase C-activating G proteins. Studies using intracellular domain minigenes and receptor chimeras. *J Biol Chem* 271:23146, 1996.

1026. Chao W, Liu H, Hanahan DJ, Olson MS: Protein tyrosine phosphorylation and regulation of the receptor for platelet-activating factor in rat Kupffer cells. Effect of sodium vanadate. *Biochem J* 288:777, 1992.

1027. Sano T, Baker D, Virag T, et al: Multiple mechanisms linked to platelet activation result in lysophosphatidic acid and sphingosine 1-phosphate generation in blood. *J Biol Chem* 277:21197, 2002.

1028. Fourcade O, Simon MF, Viode C, et al: Secretory phospholipase A2 generates the novel lipid mediator lysophosphatidic acid in membrane microvesicles shed from activated cells. *Cell* 80:919, 1995.

1029. Fourcade O, Le Balle F, Fauvel J, et al: Regulation of secretory type-II phospholipase A2 and of lysophosphatidic acid synthesis. *Adv Enzyme Regul* 38:99, 1998.

1030. Umezu-Goto M, Kishi Y, Taira A, et al: Autotaxin has lysophospholipase D activity leading to tumor cell growth and motility by lysophosphatidic acid production. *J Cell Biol* 158:227, 2002.

1031. Retzer M, Essler M: Lysophosphatidic acid-induced platelet shape change proceeds via Rho/Rho kinase-mediated myosin light-chain and moesin phosphorylation. *Cell Signal* 12:645, 2000.

1032. Haseruck N, Erl W, Pandey D, et al: The plaque lipid lysophosphatidic acid stimulates platelet activation and platelet-monocyte aggregate formation in whole blood: Involvement of P2Y1 and P2Y12 receptors. *Blood* 103:2585, 2004.

1033. Olorundare OE, Peyruchaud O, Albrecht RM, Mosher DF: Assembly of a fibronectin matrix by adherent platelets stimulated by lysophosphatidic acid and other agonists. *Blood* 98:117, 2001.

1034. Maschberger P, Bauer M, Baumann-Siemons J, et al: Mildly oxidized low density lipoprotein rapidly stimulates via activation of the lysophosphatidic acid receptor Src family and Syk tyrosine kinases and Ca2+ influx in human platelets. *J Biol Chem* 275:19159, 2000.

1035. Siess W: Athero- and thrombogenic actions of lysophosphatidic acid and sphingosine-1-phosphate. *Biochim Biophys Acta* 1582:204, 2002.

1036. Motohashi K, Shibata S, Ozaki Y, et al: Identification of lysophospholipid receptors in human platelets: The relation of two agonists, lysophosphatidic acid and sphingosine 1-phosphate. *FEBS Lett* 468:189, 2000.

1037. Hooks SB, Santos WL, Im DS, et al: Lysophosphatidic acid-induced mitogenesis is regulated by lipid phosphate phosphatases and is Edg-receptor independent. *J Biol Chem* 276:4611, 2001.

1038. Siess W, Zangl KJ, Essler M, et al: Lysophosphatidic acid mediates the rapid activation of platelets and endothelial cells by mildly oxidized low density lipoprotein and accumulates in human atherosclerotic lesions. *Proc Natl Acad Sci U S A* 96:6931, 1999.

1039. Hoyer D, Clarke DE, Fozard JR, et al: International Union of Pharmacology classification of receptors for 5-hydroxytryptamine (Serotonin). *Pharmacol Rev* 46:157, 1994.

1040. De Clerck F, Xhonneux B, Leysen J, Janssen PA: Evidence for functional 5-HT2 receptor sites on human blood platelets. *Biochem Pharmacol* 33:2807, 1984.

1041. Cook EH Jr, Fletcher KE, Wainwright M, et al: Primary structure of the human platelet serotonin 5-HT2A receptor: Identify with frontal cortex serotonin 5-HT2A receptor. *J Neurochem* 63:465, 1994.

1042. Roth BL, Willins DL, Kristiansen K, Kroeze WK: 5-Hydroxytryptamine2-family receptors (5-hydroxytryptamine2A, 5-hydroxytryptamine2B, 5-hydroxytryptamine2C): Where structure meets function. *Pharmacol Ther* 79:231, 1998.

1043. Leysen JE, Eens A, Gommeren W, et al: Identification of nonserotonergic [3H]ketanserin binding sites associated with nerve terminals in rat brain and with platelets; relation with release of biogenic amine metabolites induced by ketans. *J Pharmacol Exp Ther* 244:310, 1988.

1044. Ozaki N, Manji H, Lubierman V, et al: A naturally occurring amino acid substitution of the human serotonin 5-HT2A receptor influences amplitude and timing of intracellular calcium mobilization. *J Neurochem* 68:2186, 1997.

1045. Shimizu M, Kanazawa K, Matsuda Y, et al: Serotonin-2A receptor gene polymorphisms are associated with serotonin-induced platelet aggregation. *Thromb Res* 112:137, 2003.

1046. Arora RC, Meltzer HY: Serotonin2 receptor binding in blood platelets of schizophrenic patients. *Psychiatry Res* 47:111, 1993.

1047. Coccaro EF, Kavoussi RJ, Sheline YI, et al: Impulsive aggression in personality disorder correlates with platelet 5-HT2A receptor binding. *Neuropsychopharmacology* 16:211, 1997.

1048. Pandey GN: Altered serotonin function in suicide. Evidence from platelet and neuroendocrine studies. *Ann N Y Acad Sci* 836:182, 1997.

1049. Wolfe BE, Metzger E, Jimerson DC: Research update on serotonin function in bulimia nervosa and anorexia nervosa. *Psychopharmacol Bull* 33:345, 1997.

1050. Tomiyoshi R, Kamei K, Muraoka S, et al: Serotonin-induced platelet intracellular Ca2+ responses in untreated depressed patients and imipramine responders in remission. *Biol Psychiatry* 45:1042, 1999.

1051. Cho R, Kapur S, Du L, Hrdina P: Relationship between central and peripheral serotonin 5-HT2A receptors: A positron emission tomography study in healthy individuals. *Neurosci Lett* 261:139, 1999.

1052. de Chaffoy DC, Leysen JE, De Clerck F, et al: Evidence that phospholipid turnover is the signal transducing system coupled to serotonin-S2 receptor sites. *J Biol Chem* 260:7603, 1985.

1053. Erne P, Pletscher A: Rapid intracellular release of calcium in human platelets by stimulation of 5-HT2-receptors. *Br J Pharmacol* 84:545, 1985.

1054. Li N, Wallen NH, Ladjevardi M, Hjemdahl P: Effects of serotonin on platelet activation in whole blood. *Blood Coagul Fibrinolysis* 8:517, 1997.

1055. Houston DS, Shepherd JT, Vanhoutte PM: Aggregating human platelets cause direct contraction and endothelium-dependent relaxation of isolated canine coronary arteries. Role of serotonin, thromboxane A2, and adenine nucleotides. *J Clin Invest* 78:539, 1986.

1056. Golino P, Ashton J, Glas-Grewaalt P, et al: Mediation or reocclusion by thromboxane A2 and serotonin after thrombolysis with tissue-type plasminogen activator in a canine preparation of coronary thrombosis. *Circulation* 77:678, 1988.

1057. Dale GL, Friese P, Batar P, et al: Stimulated platelets use serotonin to enhance their retention of procoagulant proteins on the cell surface. *Nature* 415:175, 2002.

1058. Walther DJ, Peter JU, Winter S, et al: Serotonylation of small GTPases is a signal transduction pathway that triggers platelet alpha-granule release. *Cell* 115:851, 2003.

1059. Haslam RJ, Rosson GM: Aggregation of human blood platelets by vasopressin. *Am J Physiol* 223:958, 1972.

1060. Pollock WK, MacIntyre DE: Desensitization and antagonism of vasopressin-induced phosphoinositide metabolism and elevation of cytosolic free calcium concentration in human platelets. *Biochem J* 234:67, 1986.

1061. Thomas ME, Osmani AH, Scrutton MC: Some properties of the human platelet vasopressin receptor. *Thromb Res* 32:557, 1983.

1062. Thibonnier M, Roberts JM: Characterization of human platelet vasopressin receptors. *J Clin Invest* 76:1857, 1985.

1063. Siess W, Stifel M, Binder H, Weber PC: Activation of V1-receptors by vasopressin stimulates inositol phospholipid hydrolysis and arachidonate metabolism in human platelets. *Biochem J* 233:83, 1986.

1064. Thibonnier M, Goraya T, Berti-Mattera L: G protein coupling of human platelet V1 vascular vasopressin receptors. *Am J Physiol* 264:C1336, 1993.

1065. Berrettini WH, Post RM, Worthington EK, Casper JB: Human platelet vasopressin receptors. *Life Sci* 30:425, 1982.

1066. Siess W: Molecular mechanisms of platelet activation. *Physiol Rev* 69:58, 1989.

1067. Wun T, Paglieroni T, Lachant NA: Physiologic concentrations of arginine vasopressin activate human platelets in vitro. *Br J Haematol* 92:968, 1996.

1068. Serradeil-Le Gal C, Wagnon J, Valette G, et al: Nonpeptide vasopressin receptor antagonists: Development of selective and orally active V1a, V2 and V1b receptor ligands. *Prog Brain Res* 139:197, 2002.

1069. Crabos M, Bertschin S, Buhler FR, et al: Identification of AT1 receptors on human platelets and decreased angiotensin II binding in hypertension. *J Hypertens Suppl* 11(suppl 5):S230, 1993.

1070. Lopez-Farre A, Sanchez DM, Monton M, et al: Angiotensin II AT(1) receptor antagonists and platelet activation. *Nephrol Dial Transplant* 16(suppl 1):45, 2001.

1071. Jagroop IA, Mikhailidis DP: Angiotensin II can induce and potentiate shape change in human platelets: Effect of losartan. *J Hum Hypertens* 14:581, 2000.

1072. Larsson PT, Schwieler JH, Wallen NH: Platelet activation during angiotensin II infusion in healthy volunteers. *Blood Coagul Fibrinolysis* 11:61, 2000.

1073. Li P, Fukuhara M, Diz DI, et al: Novel angiotensin II AT(1) receptor antagonist irbesartan prevents thromboxane A(2)-induced vasoconstriction in canine coronary arteries and human platelet aggregation. *J Pharmacol Exp Ther* 292:238, 2000.

1074. Monton M, Jimenez A, Nunez A, et al: Comparative effects of angiotensin II AT-1-type receptor antagonists in vitro on human platelet activation. *J Cardiovasc Pharmacol* 35:906, 2000.

1075. Kalinowski L, Matys T, Chabielska E, et al: Angiotensin II AT1 receptor antagonists inhibit platelet adhesion and aggregation by nitric oxide release. *Hypertension* 40:521, 2002.

1076. Jimenez AM, Monton M, Garcia R, et al: Inhibition of platelet activation in stroke-prone spontaneously hypertensive rats: Comparison of losartan, candesartan, and valsartan. *J Cardiovasc Pharmacol* 37:406, 2001.

1077. Owens P, Kelly L, Nallen R, et al: Comparison of antihypertensive and metabolic effects of losartan and losartan in combination with hydrochlorothiazide—A randomized controlled trial. *J Hypertens* 18:339, 2000.

1078. Schieffer B, Bunte C, Witte J, et al: Comparative effects of AT1-antagonism and angiotensin-converting enzyme inhibition on markers of inflammation and platelet aggregation in patients with coronary artery disease. *J Am Coll Cardiol* 44:362, 2004.

1079. Chung J, Gao AG, Frazier WA: Thrombospondin acts via integrin-associated protein to activate the platelet integrin alphaIIbbeta3. *J Biol Chem* 272:14740, 1997.

1080. Dorahy DJ, Thorne RF, Fecondo JV, Burns GF: Stimulation of platelet activation and aggregation by a carboxyl-terminal peptide from thrombospondin binding to the integrin-associated protein receptor. *J Biol Chem* 272:1323, 1997.

1081. Lindberg FP, Gresham HD, Schwarz E, Brown EJ: Molecular cloning of integrin-associated protein: An immunoglobulin family member with multiple membrane-spanning domains implicated in alpha v beta 3-dependent ligand binding. *J Cell Biol* 123:485, 1993.

1082. Wang XQ, Frazier WA: The thrombospondin receptor CD47 (IAP) modulates and associates with alpha2 beta1 integrin in vascular smooth muscle cells. *Mol Biol Cell* 9:865, 1998.

1083. Frazier WA, Gao AG, Dimitry J, et al: The thrombospondin receptor integrin-associated protein (CD47) functionally couples to heterotrimeric Gi. *J Biol Chem* 274:8554, 1999.

1084. Lagadec P, Dejoux O, Ticchioni M, et al: Involvement of a CD47-dependent pathway in platelet adhesion on inflamed vascular endothelium under flow. *Blood* 101:4836, 2003.

1085. Huang MM, Bolen JB, Barnwell JW, et al: Membrane glycoprotein IV (CD36) is physically associated with the Fyn, Lyn, and Yes protein-tyrosine kinases in human platelets. *Proc Natl Acad Sci U S A* 88:7844, 1991.

1086. Pimanda JE, Annis DS, Raftery M, et al: The von Willebrand factor-reducing activity of thrombospondin-1 is located in the calcium-binding/C-terminal sequence and requires a free thiol at position 974. *Blood* 100:2832, 2002.

1087. Pimanda JE, Ganderton T, Maekawa A, et al: Role of thrombospondin-1 in control of von Willebrand factor multimer size in mice. *J Biol Chem* 279:21439, 2004.

1088. van Zanten GH, de Graaf S, Slootweg PJ, et al: Increased platelet deposition on atherosclerotic coronary arteries. *J Clin Invest* 93:615, 1994.

1089. van der Rest M, Garrone R: Collagen family of proteins. *FASEB J* 5:2814, 1991.

1090. Saelman EU, Kehrel B, Hese KM, et al: Platelet adhesion to collagen and endothelial cell matrix under flow conditions is not dependent on platelet glycoprotein IV. *Blood* 83:3240, 1994.

1091. Ichinohe T, Takayama H, Ezumi Y, et al: Collagen-stimulated activation of Syk but not c-Src is severely compromised in human platelets lacking membrane glycoprotein VI. *J Biol Chem* 272:63, 1997.

1092. Ishibashi T, Ichinohe T, Sugiyama T, et al: Functional significance of platelet membrane glycoprotein p62 (GP VI), a putative collagen receptor. *Int J Hematol* 62:107, 1995.

1093. Kehrel B, Wierwille S, Clemetson KJ, et al: Glycoprotein VI is a major collagen receptor for platelet activation: It recognizes the platelet-activating quaternary structure of collagen, whereas CD36, glycoprotein IIb/IIIa, and von Willebrand factor do not. *Blood* 91:491, 1998.

1094. Poole A, Gibbins JM, Turner M, et al: The Fc receptor gamma-chain and the tyrosine kinase Syk are essential for activation of mouse platelets by collagen. *EMBO J* 16:2333, 1997.

1095. Smethurst PA, Joutsi-Korhonen L, O'Connor MN, et al: Identification of the primary collagen-binding surface on human glycoprotein VI by site-directed mutagenesis and by a blocking phage antibody. *Blood* 103:903, 2004.

1096. Chiang TM: Collagen-platelet interaction: Platelet non-integrin receptors. *Histol Histopathol* 14:579, 1999.

1097. Keely PJ, Parise LV: The alpha2beta1 integrin is a necessary co-receptor for collagen-induced activation of Syk and the subsequent phosphorylation of phospholipase Cgamma2 in platelets. *J Biol Chem* 271: 26668, 1996.

1098. Sugiyama T, Okuma M, Ushikubi F, et al: A novel platelet aggregating factor found in a patient with defective collagen-induced platelet aggregation and autoimmune thrombocytopenia. *Blood* 69:1712, 1987.

1099. Briddon SJ, Watson SP: Evidence for the involvement of p59fyn and p53/56lyn in collagen receptor signalling in human platelets. *Biochem J* 338:203, 1999.

1100. Fujii C, Yanagi S, Sada K, et al: Involvement of protein-tyrosine kinase p72syk in collagen-induced signal transduction in platelets. *Eur J Biochem* 226:243, 1994.

1101. Shattil SJ, Ginsberg MH, Brugge JS: Adhesive signaling in platelets. *Curr Opin Cell Biol* 6:695, 1994.

1102. Soriano P, Montgomery C, Geske R, Bradley A: Targeted disruption of the c-src proto-oncogene leads to osteopetrosis in mice. *Cell* 64:693, 1991.

1103. Daniel JL, Dangelmaier C, Smith JB: Evidence for a role for tyrosine phosphorylation of phospholipase Cg2 in collagen-induced platelet cytosolic calcium mobilization. *Biochem J* 302:617, 1994.

1104. Quek LS, Bolen J, Watson SP: A role for Bruton's tyrosine kinase (Btk) in platelet activation by collagen. *Curr Biol* 8:1137, 1998.

1105. Jung SM, Moroi M: Platelet collagen receptor integrin alpha2beta1 activation involves differential participation of ADP-receptor subtypes P2Y1 and P2Y12 but not intracellular calcium change. *Eur J Biochem* 268:3513, 2001.

1106. Wang Z, Leisner TM, Parise LV: Platelet alpha2beta1 integrin activation: Contribution of ligand internalization and the alpha2-cytoplasmic domain. *Blood* 102:1307, 2003.

1107. Bertoni A, Tadokoro S, Eto K, et al: Relationships between Rap1b, affinity modulation of integrin alpha IIbbeta 3, and the actin cytoskeleton. *J Biol Chem* 277:25715, 2002.

1108. Larson MK, Chen H, Kahn ML, et al: Identification of P2Y12-dependent and -independent mechanisms of glycoprotein VI-mediated Rap1 activation in platelets. *Blood* 101:1409, 2003.

1109. Auger JM, Best D, Snell DC, et al: C-Cbl negatively regulates platelet activation by glycoprotein VI. *J Thromb Haemost* 1:2419, 2003.

1110. Locke D, Liu C, Peng X, et al: Fc Rgamma -independent signaling by the platelet collagen receptor glycoprotein VI. *J Biol Chem* 278:15441, 2003.

1111. Inoue O, Suzuki-Inoue K, Dean WL, et al: Integrin alpha2beta1 mediates outside-in regulation of platelet spreading on collagen through activation of Src kinases and PLCgamma2. *J Cell Biol* 160:769, 2003.

1112. Chen H, Kahn ML: Reciprocal signaling by integrin and nonintegrin receptors during collagen activation of platelets. *Mol Cell Biol* 23:4764, 2003.

1113. Best D, Senis YA, Jarvis GE, et al: GPVI levels in platelets: Relationship to platelet function at high shear. *Blood* 102:2811, 2003.

1114. Chen H, Locke D, Liu Y, et al: The platelet receptor GPVI mediates both adhesion and signaling responses to collagen in a receptor density-dependent fashion. *J Biol Chem* 277:3011, 2002.

1115. Furihata K, Clemetson KJ, Deguchi H, Kunicki TJ: Variation in human platelet glycoprotein VI content modulates glycoprotein VI-specific prothrombinase activity. *Arterioscler Thromb Vasc Biol* 21:1857, 2001.

1116. Suzuki H, Murasaki K, Kodama K, Takayama H: Intracellular localization of glycoprotein VI in human platelets and its surface expression upon activation. *Br J Haematol* 121:904, 2003.

1117. Nakamura T, Jamieson GA, Okuma M, et al: Platelet adhesion to type I collagen fibrils: Role of GPVI in divalent cation-dependent and -independent adhesion and thromboxane A2 generation. *J Biol Chem* 273:4338, 1998.

1118. Daniel JL, Dangelmaier C, Strouse R, Smith JB: Collagen induces normal signal transduction in platelets deficient in CD36 (platelet glycoprotein IV). *Thromb Haemost* 71:353, 1994.

1119. Smith JB, Selak MA, Dangelmaier C, Daniel JL: Cytosolic calcium as a second messenger for collagen-induced platelet responses. *Biochem J* 288:925, 1992.

1120. Greenwalt DE, Tandon NN: Platelet shape change and Ca2+ mobilization induced by collagen, but not thrombin or ADP, are inhibited by phenylarsine oxide. *Br J Haematol* 88:830, 1994.

1121. Chow TW, Hellums JD, Moake JL, Kroll MH: Shear stress-induced von Willebrand factor binding to platelet glycoprotein Ib initiates calcium influx associated with aggregation. *Blood* 80:113, 1992.

1122. Gu M, Xi X, Englund GD, et al: Analysis of the roles of 14-3-3 in the platelet glycoprotein Ib-IX-mediated activation of integrin alpha(IIb)beta(3) using a reconstituted mammalian cell expression model. *J Cell Biol* 147:1085, 1999.

1123. Zaffran Y, Meyer SC, Negrescu E, et al: Signaling across the platelet adhesion receptor glycoprotein Ib-IX induces alpha IIbbeta 3 activation both in platelets and a transfected Chinese hamster ovary cell system. *J Biol Chem* 275:16779, 2000.

1124. Kasirer-Friede A, Cozzi MR, Mazzucato M, et al: Signaling through GP Ib-IX-V activates {alpha}IIb{beta}3 independently of other receptors. *Blood* 103:3403, 2004.

1125. Marshall SJ, Asazuma N, Best D, et al: Glycoprotein IIb-IIIa-dependent aggregation by glycoprotein Ibalpha is reinforced by a Src family kinase inhibitor (PP1)-sensitive signalling pathway. *Biochem J* 361: 297, 2002.

1126. Marshall SJ, Senis YA, Auger JM, et al: GPIb-dependent platelet activation is dependent on Src kinases but not MAP kinase or cGMP-dependent kinase. *Blood* 103:2601, 2004.

1127. Mangin P, Yuan Y, Goncalves I, et al: Signaling role for phospholipase C gamma 2 in platelet glycoprotein Ib alpha calcium flux and cytoskeletal reorganization. Involvement of a pathway distinct from FcR gamma chain and Fc gamma RIIA. *J Biol Chem* 278:32880, 2003.

1128. Li Z, Xi X, Gu M, et al: A stimulatory role for cGMP-dependent protein kinase in platelet activation. *Cell* 112:77, 2003.

1129. Andrews RK, Munday AD, Mitchell CA, Berndt MC: Interaction of calmodulin with the cytoplasmic domain of the platelet membrane glycoprotein Ib-IX-V complex. *Blood* 98:681, 2001.

1130. Gu M, Du X: A novel ligand-binding site in the zeta-form 14-3-3 protein recognizing the platelet glycoprotein Ibalpha and distinct from the c-Raf-binding site. *J Biol Chem* 273:33465, 1998.

1131. Du X, Harris SJ, Tetaz TJ, et al: Association of a phospholipase A2(14-3-3 protein) with the platelet glycoprotein Ib-IX complex. *J Biol Chem* 269:18287, 1994.

1132. Kasirer-Friede A, Ware J, Leng L, et al: Lateral clustering of platelet GP Ib-IX complexes leads to up-regulation of the adhesive function of integrin alpha IIbbeta 3. *J Biol Chem* 277:11949, 2002.

1133. Fox JE, Berndt MC: Cyclic AMP-dependent phosphorylation of glycoprotein Ib inhibits collagen-induced polymerization of actin in platelets. *J Biol Chem* 264:9520, 1989.

1134. Phillips DR, Agin PP: Thrombin-induced alterations in the surface structure of the human platelet plasma membrane. *Ser Haematol* 6:292, 1973.

1135. Ramakrishnan V, Reeves PS, DeGuzman F, et al: Increased thrombin responsiveness in platelets from mice lacking glycoprotein V. *Proc Natl Acad Sci U S A* 96:13336, 1999.

1136. Ni H, Ramakrishnan V, Ruggeri ZM, et al: Increased thrombogenesis and embolus formation in mice lacking glycoprotein V. *Blood* 98:368, 2001.

1137. Rink TJ: Cytosolic calcium in platelet activation. *Experientia* 44:97, 1988.

1138. Kovacs T, Felfoldi F, Papp B, et al: All three splice variants of the human sarco/endoplasmic reticulum Ca2+-ATPase 3 gene are translated to proteins: A study of their co-expression in platelets and lymphoid cells. *Biochem J* 358:559, 2001.

1139. Hassock SR, Zhu MX, Trost C, et al: Expression and role of TRPC proteins in human platelets: Evidence that TRPC6 forms the store-independent calcium entry channel. *Blood* 100:2801, 2002.

1140. Roberts DE, McNicol A, Bose R: Mechanism of collagen activation in human platelets. *J Biol Chem* 279:19421, 2004.

1141. Jones GD, Gear AR: Subsecond calcium dynamics in ADP- and thrombin-stimulated platelets: A continuous-flow approach using indo-1. *Blood* 71:1539, 1988.

1142. Rybak ME, Renzulli LA: Effect of calcium channel blockers on platelet GPIIb-IIIa as a calcium channel in liposomes. Comparison with effects on the intact platelet. *Thromb Haemost* 67:131, 1992.

1143. Dessen A, Tang J, Schmidt H, et al: Crystal structure of human cytosolic phospholipase A2 reveals a novel topology and catalytic mechanism. *Cell* 97:349, 1999.

1144. Khan WA, Blobe G, Halpern A, et al: Selective regulation of protein kinase C isoenzymes by oleic acid in human platelets. *J Biol Chem* 268:5063, 1993.

1145. Scholey JM, Taylor KA, Kendrick-Jones J: Regulation of non-muscle myosin assembly by calmodulin-dependent light chain kinase. *Nature* 287:233, 1980.

1146. Naik MU, Naik UP: Calcium- and integrin-binding protein regulates focal adhesion kinase activity during platelet spreading on immobilized fibrinogen. *Blood* 102:3629, 2003.

1147. Barry WT, Boudignon-Proudhon C, Shock DD, et al: Molecular basis of CIB binding to the integrin alpha IIb cytoplasmic domain. *J Biol Chem* 277:28877, 2002.

1148. Zhang J, Zhang J, Shattil SJ, et al: Phosphoinositide 3-kinase gamma and p85/phosphoinositide 3-kinase in platelets. Relative activation by thrombin receptor or beta-phorbol myristate acetate and roles in promoting the ligand-binding function of alphaIIbbeta3 integrin. *J Biol Chem* 271:6265, 1996.

1149. Rittenhouse SE: Phosphoinositide 3-kinase activation and platelet function. *Blood* 88:4401, 1996.

1150. Hartwig JH, Kung S, Kovacsovics T, et al: D3 phosphoinositides and outside-in integrin signaling by glycoprotein IIb-IIIa mediate platelet actin assembly and filopodial extension induced by phorbol 12-myristate 13-acetate. *J Biol Chem* 271:32986, 1996.

1151. Banfic H, Downes CP, Rittenhouse SE: Biphasic activation of PKBalpha/Akt in platelets. Evidence for stimulation both by phosphatidylinositol 3,4-bisphosphate, produced via a novel pathway, and by phosphatidylinositol 3,4,5-trisphosphate. *J Biol Chem* 273:11630, 1998.

1152. Gibbins JM, Briddon S, Shutes A, et al: The p85 subunit of phosphatidylinositol 3-kinase associates with the Fc receptor gamma-chain and linker for activitor of T cells (LAT) in platelets stimulated by collagen and convulxin. *J Biol Chem* 273:34437, 1998.

1153. Watanabe N, Nakajima H, Suzuki H, et al: Functional phenotype of phosphoinositide 3-kinase p85alpha-null platelets characterized by an impaired response to GP VI stimulation. *Blood* 102:541, 2003.

1154. Gratacap MP, Payrastre B, Viala C, et al: Phosphatidylinositol 3,4,5-trisphosphate-dependent stimulation of phospholipase C-gamma2 is an early key event in FcgammaRIIA-mediated activation of human platelets. *J Biol Chem* 273:24314, 1998.

1155. Hirsch E, Bosco O, Tropel P, et al: Resistance to thromboembolism in PI3Kgamma-deficient mice. *FASEB J* 15:2019, 2001.

1156. Leevers SJ, Vanhaesebroeck B, Waterfield MD: Signalling through phosphoinositide 3-kinases: The lipids take centre stage. *Curr Opin Cell Biol* 11:219, 1999.

1157. Bae YS, Cantley LG, Chen CS, et al: Activation of phospholipase C-gamma by phosphatidylinositol 3,4,5-trisphosphate. *J Biol Chem* 273:4465, 1998.

1158. Salim K, Bottomley MJ, Querfurth E, et al: Distinct specificity in the recognition of phosphoinositides by the pleckstrin homology domains of dynamin and Bruton's tyrosine kinase. *EMBO J* 15:6241, 1996.

1159. Li Z, Wahl MI, Eguinoa A, et al: Phosphatidylinositol 3-kinase-gamma activates Bruton's tyrosine kinase in concert with Src family kinases. *Proc Natl Acad Sci U S A* 94:13820, 1997.

1160. Alessi DR, James SR, Downes CP, et al: Characterization of a 3-phosphoinositide-dependent protein kinase which phosphorylates and activates protein kinase Balpha. *Curr Biol* 7:261, 1997.

1161. Stokoe D, Stephens LR, Copeland T, et al: Dual role of phosphatidylinositol-3,4,5-trisphosphate in the activation of protein kinase B. *Science* 277:567, 1997.

1162. Kroner C, Eybrechts K, Akkerman JW: Dual regulation of platelet protein kinase B. *J Biol Chem* 275:27790, 2000.

1163. Woulfe D, Jiang H, Morgans A, et al: Defects in secretion, aggregation, and thrombus formation in platelets from mice lacking Akt2. *J Clin Invest* 113:441, 2004.

1164. Chen J, De S, Damron D, et al: Impaired platelet response to thrombin and collagen in AKT-1 deficient mice. *Blood* 104:1703, 2004.

1165. Zhang Z, Vuori K, Wang H, et al: Integrin activation by R-ras. *Cell* 85:61, 1996.

1166. Ridley AJ, Hall A: The small GTP-binding protein rho regulates the assembly of focal adhesions and actin stress fibers in response to growth factors. *Cell* 70:389, 1992.

1167. Leng L, Kashiwagi H, Ren XD, Shattil SJ: RhoA and the function of platelet integrin alphaIIbbeta3. *Blood* 91:4206, 1998.

1168. Franke B, van Triest M, de Bruijn KM, et al: Sequential regulation of the small GTPase Rap1 in human platelets. *Mol Cell Biol* 20:779, 2000.

1169. Woulfe D, Jiang H, Mortensen R, et al: Activation of Rap1B by G(i) family members in platelets. *J Biol Chem* 277:23382, 2002.

1170. Hughes PE, Renshaw MW, Pfaff M, et al: Suppression of integrin activation: A novel function of a Ras/Raf-initiated MAP kinase pathway. *Cell* 88:521, 1997.

1171. McNicol A, Philpott CL, Shibou TS, Israels SJ: Effects of the mitogen-activated protein (MAP) kinase kinase inhibitor 2-(2'-amino-3'-methoxyphenyl)-oxanaphthalen-4-one (PD98059) on human platelet activation. *Biochem Pharm* 55:1759, 1998.

1172. Shock DD, He K, Wencel-Drake JD, Parise LV: Ras activation in platelets after stimulation of the thrombin receptor, thromboxane A2 receptor or protein kinase C. *Biochem J* 321:525, 1997.

1173. Ramos JW, Kojima TK, Hughes PE, et al: The death effector domain of PEA-15 is involved in its regulation of integrin activation. *J Biol Chem* 273:33897, 1998.

1174. Nobes CD, Hall A: Rho, rac, and cdc42 GTPases regulate the assembly of multimolecular focal complexes associated with actin stress fibers, lamellipodia, and filopodia. *Cell* 81:53, 1995.

1175. Xiong JP, Stehle T, Diefenbach B, et al: Crystal structure of the extracellular segment of integrin alpha Vbeta3. *Science* 294:339, 2001.

1176. Vinogradova O, Vaynberg J, Kong X, et al: Membrane-mediated structural transitions at the cytoplasmic face during integrin activation. *Proc Natl Acad Sci U S A* 101:4094, 2004.

1177. Bennett JS, Zigmond S, Vilaire G, et al: The platelet cytoskeleton regulates the affinity of the integrin alpha(IIb)beta(3) for fibrinogen. *J Biol Chem* 274:25301, 1999.

1178. Martel V, Racaud-Sultan C, Dupe S, et al: Conformation, localization, and integrin binding of talin depend on its interaction with phosphoinositides. *J Biol Chem* 276:21217, 2001.

1179. Di Paolo G, Pellegrini L, Letinic K, et al: Recruitment and regulation of phosphatidylinositol phosphate kinase type 1 gamma by the FERM domain of talin. *Nature* 420:85, 2002.

1180. Ling K, Doughman RL, Firestone AJ, et al: Type I gamma phosphatidylinositol phosphate kinase targets and regulates focal adhesions. *Nature* 420:89, 2002.

1181. Calderwood DA, Yan B, de Pereda JM, et al: The phosphotyrosine binding-like domain of talin activates integrins. *J Biol Chem* 277:21749, 2002.

1182. Garcia-Alvarez B, de Pereda JM, Calderwood DA, et al: Structural determinants of integrin recognition by talin. *Mol Cell* 11:49, 2003.

1183. Ling K, Doughman RL, Iyer VV, et al: Tyrosine phosphorylation of type Igamma phosphatidylinositol phosphate kinase by Src regulates an integrin-talin switch. *J Cell Biol* 163:1339, 2003.

1184. Xing B, Jedsadayanmata A, Lam SC: Localization of an integrin binding site to the C terminus of talin. *J Biol Chem* 276:44373, 2001.

1185. Li R, Babu CR, Lear JD, et al: Oligomerization of the integrin alphaIIbbeta3: Roles of the transmembrane and cytoplasmic domains. *Proc Natl Acad Sci U S A* 98:12462, 2001.

1186. Arias-Salgado EG, Lizano S, Sarkar S, et al: Src kinase activation by direct interaction with the integrin beta cytoplasmic domain. *Proc Natl Acad Sci U S A* 100:13298, 2003.

1187. Obergfell A, Eto K, Mocsai A, et al: Coordinate interactions of Csk, Src, and Syk kinases with [alpha]IIb[beta]3 initiate integrin signaling to the cytoskeleton. *J Cell Biol* 157:265, 2002.

1188. Woodside DG, Obergfell A, Leng L, et al: Activation of Syk protein tyrosine kinase through interaction with integrin beta cytoplasmic domains. *Curr Biol* 11:1799, 2001.

1189. Woodside DG, Obergfell A, Talapatra A, et al: The N-terminal SH2 domains of Syk and ZAP-70 mediate phosphotyrosine-independent binding to integrin beta cytoplasmic domains. *J Biol Chem* 277:39401, 2002.

1190. De Virgilio M, Kiosses WB, Shattil SJ: Proximal, selective, and dynamic interactions between integrin {alpha}IIb{beta}3 and protein tyrosine kinases in living cells. *J Cell Biol* 165:305, 2004.

1191. Kumar G, Wang S, Gupta S, Nel A: The membrane immunoglobulin receptor utilizes a Shc/Grb2/hSOS complex for activation of the mitogen-activated protein kinase cascade in a B-cell line. *Biochem J* 307:215, 1995.

1192. Miranti CK, Leng L, Maschberger P, et al: Identification of a novel integrin signaling pathway involving the kinase Syk and the guanine nucleotide exchange factor Vav1. *Curr Biol* 8:1289, 1998.

1193. Majerus PW: Arachidonate metabolism in vascular disorders. *J Clin Invest* 72:1521, 1983.

1194. Moncada S, Whittle BJ: Biological actions of prostacyclin and its pharmacological use in platelet studies. *Adv Exp Med Biol* 192:337, 1985.

1195. Marcus AJ: The role of lipids in platelet function: With particular reference to the arachidonic acid pathway. *J Lipid Res* 19:793, 1978.

1196. Manganello JM, Huang JS, Kozasa T, et al: Protein kinase A-mediated phosphorylation of the Galpha13 switch I region alters the Galphabetagamma13-G protein-coupled receptor complex and inhibits Rho activation. *J Biol Chem* 278:124, 2003.

1197. Bodnar RJ, Xi X, Li Z, et al: Regulation of glycoprotein Ib-IX-von Willebrand factor interaction by cAMP-dependent protein kinase-mediated phosphorylation at Ser 166 of glycoprotein Ib(beta). *J Biol Chem* 277:47080, 2002.

1198. Cavallini L, Coassin M, Borean A, Alexandre A: Prostacyclin and sodium nitroprusside inhibit the activity of the platelet inositol 1,4,5-trisphosphate receptor and promote its phosphorylation. *J Biol Chem* 271:5545, 1996.

1199. Nishimura T, Yamamoto T, Komuro Y, Hara Y: Antiplatelet functions of a stable prostacyclin analog, SM-10906 are exerted by its inhibitory effect on inositol 1,4,5-trisphosphate production and cytosolic Ca2++ increase in rat platelets stimulated by thrombin. *Thromb Res* 79:307, 1995.

1200. Cook SJ, McCormick F: Inhibition by cAMP of Ras-dependent activation of Raf. *Science* 262:1069, 1993.

1201. Dumaz N, Marais R: Protein kinase A blocks Raf-1 activity by stimulating 14-3-3 binding and blocking Raf-1 interaction with Ras. *J Biol Chem* 278:29819, 2003.

1202. Fischer TH, Collins JH, Gatling MN, White GC: The localization of the cAMP-dependent protein kinase phosphorylation site in the platelet rat protein, rap 1B. *FEBS Lett* 2832:173, 1991.

1203. Siess W, Grunberg B: Phosphorylation of rap1B by protein kinase A is not involved in platelet inhibition by cyclic AMP. *Cell Signal* 5:209, 1993.

1204. Lou L, Urbani J, Ribeiro-Neto F, Altschuler DL: CAMP inhibition of Akt is mediated by activated and phosphorylated Rap1b. *J Biol Chem* 277:32799, 2002.

1205. Luscher TF, Diederich D, Siebenmann R, et al: Difference between endothelium-dependent relaxation in arterial and in venous coronary bypass grafts. *N Engl J Med* 319:462, 1988.

1206. Goretski J, Hollocher TC: Trapping of nitric oxide produced during denitrification by extracellular hemoglobin. *J Biol Chem* 263:2316, 1988.

1207. Loscalzo J, Welch G: Nitric oxide and its role in the cardiovascular system. *Prog Cardiovasc Dis* 38:87, 1995.

1208. Mellion BT, Ignarro LJ, Ohlstein EH, et al: Evidence for the inhibitory role of guanosine 3',5'-monophosphate in ADP-induced human platelet aggregation in the presence of nitric oxide and related vasodilators. *Blood* 57:946, 1981.

1209. Radomski MW, Palmer RM, Moncada S: Modulation of platelet aggregation by an L-arginine-nitric oxide pathway. *Trends Pharmacol Sci* 12:87, 1991.

1210. Wang GR, Zhu Y, Halushka PV, et al: Mechanism of platelet inhibition by nitric oxide: In vivo phosphorylation of thromboxane receptor by cyclic GMP-dependent protein kinase. *Proc Natl Acad Sci U S A* 95:4888, 1998.

1211. Massberg S, Sausbier M, Klatt P, et al: Increased adhesion and aggregation of platelets lacking cyclic guanosine 3',5'-monophosphate kinase I. *J Exp Med* 189:1255, 1999.

1212. Aszodi A, Pfeifer A, Ahmad M, et al: The vasodilator-stimulated phosphoprotein (VASP) is involved in cGMP- and cAMP-mediated inhibition of agonist-induced platelet aggregation, but is dispensable for smooth muscle function. *EMBO J* 18:37, 1999.

1213. Butt E, Abel K, Krieger M, et al: CAMP- and cGMP-dependent protein kinase phosphorylation sites of the focal adhesion vasodilator-stimulated phosphoprotein (VASP) in vitro and in intact human platelets. *J Biol Chem* 269:14509, 1994.

1214. Hauser W, Knobeloch KP, Eigenthaler M, et al: Megakaryocyte hyperplasia and enhanced agonist-induced platelet activation in vasodilator-stimulated phosphoprotein knockout mice. *Proc Natl Acad Sci U S A* 96:8120, 1999.

1215. Massberg S, Gruner S, Konrad I, et al: Enhanced in vivo platelet adhesion in vasodilator-stimulated phosphoprotein (VASP)-deficient mice. *Blood* 103:136, 2004.

1216. Maurice DH, Haslam RJ: Molecular basis of the synergistic inhibition of platelet function by nitrovasodilators and activators of adenylate cyclase: Inhibition of cyclic AMP breakdown by cyclic GMP. *Mol Pharmacol* 37:671, 1990.

1217. Kaczmarek E, Koziak K, Sevigny J, et al: Identification and characterization of CD39/vascular ATP diphosphohydrolase. *J Biol Chem* 271:33116, 1996.

1218. White JG: Platelet ultrastructure, in *Hemostasis and Thrombosis*, edited by AL Bloom, CD Forbes, PT Duncan, EGD Tuddenham, p 49. Churchill Livingstone, Edinburgh, 1994.

1219. Luo BH, Springer TA, Takagi J: A specific interface between integrin transmembrane helices and affinity for ligand. *PLoS Biol* 2:776, 2004.

1220. Xiong JP, Stehle T, Diefenbach B, et al: Crystal structure of the extracellular segment of integrin alphaVbeta3. *Science* 294:339, 2001.

1221. Qin J, Vinogradova O, Plow EF: Integrin bidirectional signaling: A molecular view. *PLoS Biol* 2:726, 2004.

1222. Brass L: Fifty (or more) ways to leave your platelets (in a thrombus). *Arterioscler Thromb Vasc Biol* 24:989, 2004.

1223. McEver RP: Selectins: Novel receptors that mediate leukocyte adhesion during inflammation. *Thromb Haemost* 65:223, 1991.

1224. Coller BS: Disorders of platelets, in *Disorders of Hemostasis*, edited by OD Ratnoff, CD Forbes, p 73. Grune & Stratton, Orlando, 1984.

1225. Holmsen H, Weiss HJ: Secretable storage pools in platelets. *Annu Rev Med* 30:119, 1979.

1226. Pollard TD: Actin. *Curr Opin Cell Biol* 2:33, 1990.

1227. Vandekerckhove J: Actin-binding proteins. *Curr Opin Cell Biol* 2:41, 1990.

1228. Weeds AG, Gooch J, Pope B, Harris HE: Preparation and characterization of pig plasma and platelet gelsolins. *Eur J Biochem* 161:69, 1986.

1229. Weber A, Nachmias VT, Pennise CR, et al: Interaction of thymosin-b-4 with muscle and platelet actin. Implications for actin sequestration in resting platelets. *Biochemistry* 31:6179, 1992.

1230. Smillie LB: Structure and function of tropomyosins from muscle and non-muscle. *Trends Biochem Sci* 4:151, 1981.

1231. Vandekerckhove J: Structural principles of actin-binding proteins. *Curr Opin Cell Biol* 1:15, 1989.

1232. Lind SE, Stossel TP: The microfilament network of the platelet. *Prog Hemost Thromb* 6:63, 1982.

1233. Chen M, Stracher A: In situ phosphorylation of platelet actin-binding protein by cAMP-dependent protein kinase stabilizes it against proteolysis by calpain. *J Biol Chem* 264:14282, 1989.

1234. Beckerle MC, Miller DE, Bertagnolli ME, Locke SJ: Activation-dependent redistribution of the adhesion plaque protein, talin, in intact human platelets. *J Cell Biol* 109:3333, 1989.

1235. O'Halloran T, Beckerle MC, Burridge K: Identification of talin as a major cytoplasmic protein implicated in platelet activation. *Nature* 317:449, 1985.

1236. Koteliansky VE, Gneushev GN, Glukhova MA, et al: Identification and isolation of vinculin from platelets. *FEBS Lett* 165:26, 1984.

1237. Langer B, Gonnella PA, Nachmias VT: A-actinin and vinculin in normal and thrombasthenic platelets. *Blood* 63:606, 1984.

1238. Lucas RC, Rosenberg S, Shafiq S, et al: The isolation and characterization of a cytoskeleton and a contractile apparatus from platelets, in *Protides of Biological Fluids*, edited by H Peeters, p 465. Pergamon Press, New York, 1975.

1239. Wang L-L, Bryan J: Isolation of calcium-dependent platelet proteins that interact with actin. *Cell* 25:637, 1981.

1240. Hathaway DR, Adelstein RS: Human platelet myosin light chain kinase requires the calcium binding protein calmodulin for activity. *Proc Natl Acad Sci U S A* 76:1653, 1979.

1241. Wolff DJ, Brostrom CO: Properties and functions of the calcium-dependent regulator protein. *Adv Cyclic Nucleotide Res* 11:27, 1979.

1242. Daniel JL: Platelet contractile proteins, in *Hemostasis and Thrombosis: Basic Principles and Clinical Practice*, edited by RW Colman, J Hirsh, VJ Marder, EW Salzman, p 557. JB Lippincott, Philadelphia, 1993.

MOLECULAR BIOLOGY AND BIOCHEMISTRY OF THE COAGULATION FACTORS AND PATHWAYS OF HEMOSTASIS

HAROLD R. ROBERTS
DOUGALD M. MONROE III
MAUREANE HOFFMAN

Blood coagulation is a delicately balanced system. When the system functions as it should, the blood is maintained in a fluid state in the vasculature yet rapidly clots to seal an injury. When hemostatic functions fail, hemorrhagic phenomena result. This chapter addresses molecular and biochemical features of the proteins of the coagulation system and how they interact with cells and with one another to provide hemostasis in the living organism. The coagulation factors are grouped as follows: (1) vitamin K–dependent zymogens (prothrombin, factors VII, IX, and X, protein C); (2) soluble cofactors (protein S, factors V and VIII, von Willebrand factor); (3) factor XI and the other "contact" factors; (4) cell-associated cofactors (tissue factor, thrombomodulin); (5) fibrinogen; (6) factor XIII; and (7) plasma coagulation protease inhibitors. Table 106-1 lists the major features of the coagulation factors discussed in this chapter. A model of the coagulation pathway based on our current understanding of cell–cell and cell–protein interactions regulating hemostasis is presented. The scheme emphasizes the importance of cellular localization and plasma protease inhibitors in confining the coagulation reactions to a specific site of injury in hemostasis.

VITAMIN K-DEPENDENT ZYMOGENS (PROTHROMBIN, FACTORS VII, IX, AND X, AND PROTEIN C)

COMMON STRUCTURAL AND FUNCTIONAL FEATURES

The vitamin K–dependent coagulation zymogens are precursors of serine proteases that must be proteolytically activated to express their enzymatic activity. They all share a similar protein domain structure (Fig. 106-1). Each of the mature vitamin K–dependent coagulation zymogen proteins has an amino-terminal γ-carboxy glutamic acid (Gla) domain with nine to 12 Gla residues. This domain is followed by a hydrophobic region. All except prothrombin have two epidermal growth factor (EGF)-like domains, and all have a serine protease domain in their carboxy-terminal regions. Prothrombin has two kringle domains instead of EGF-like domains. Specific functions are associated, at least in part, with specific domains.

In addition to the functional modules found in the mature protein, each vitamin K–dependent factor is synthesized with an amino-terminal signal sequence directing it to the endoplasmic reticulum (ER), followed by a 19- to 25-amino-acid propeptide. The propeptide is recognized by the γ-glutamyl carboxylase that catalyzes carboxylation of glutamic acid residues in the amino-terminal portion of the molecule. Following translocation into the ER, the signal sequence is removed by a microsomal signal peptidase. The propeptide is cleaved following carboxylation before the mature protein is secreted.

The proteins are homologous, and their gene structures are highly similar. The coding regions of the vitamin K–dependent factors are similar in size. However, the intron lengths vary substantially and account for the differences in overall gene size (prothrombin 20 kb, factor VII 13 kb, factor IX 33 kb, factor X 25 kb, protein C 10 kb). Although the cDNA of all the vitamin K–dependent factors has been sequenced, the noncoding regions have been characterized only to varying degrees of detail. The vitamin K–dependent coagulation zymogens are synthesized primarily by the liver, and all have specific regulatory elements that direct liver-specific expression.

In factors VII, IX, and X and proteins C and Z, the introns are located in identical positions in the genes,[1–3] suggesting these enzymes evolved by duplication of a common ancestral precursor gene. The regions of the molecules that constitute "functional" domains tend to be encoded in their entirety by a single exon, that is, the signal peptide by one exon, the propeptide and Gla region by the next exon, etc. This "modular" design suggests how "exon shuffling" could splice together intact functional units of different proteins, giving rise to new proteins with novel properties.

The Gla domain characteristic of vitamin K–dependent factors mediates interaction of the protein with lipid membranes. The Gla domain is named for the modified amino acids found in the first 42 residues of the mature protein. Gla residues are produced by post-translational modification of glutamic acid residues carried out by a specific γ-glutamyl carboxylase[4] in the ER (Fig. 106-2). The propeptide sequence is required for γ-carboxylation and is highly conserved among the vitamin K–dependent factors. Amino acids at positions −18, −17, −16, −15, and −10 are critical for recognition by the carboxylase.[5,6] This carboxylase requires oxygen, carbon dioxide, and the reduced form of vitamin K for its action. For each glutamyl residue that is carboxylated, one molecule of reduced vitamin K is converted to the epoxide form. A separate enzyme complex, the vitamin K epoxide reductase, is required to convert the epoxide form of vitamin K back to the reduced form. The gene for the epoxide reductase has been sequenced[7] and mutations in the gene resulting in warfarin resistance identified.[8] Warfarin inhibits the activity of the vitamin K epoxide reductase and prevents recycling of vitamin K back to the reduced form. Therefore, the effect of warfarin is to inhibit γ-glutamyl carboxylation, resulting in the presence of a heterogeneous population of undercarboxylated forms of the Gla-containing factors in the circulation. These undercarboxylated forms have reduced activity. Because warfarin blocks the epoxide reductase (rather than blocking the carboxylase) and prevents recycling of vitamin K, the effects of warfarin poisoning can be reversed by vitamin K administration. Mutations of the carboxylase can lead to low levels of all of the Gla-containing factors.[9]

Acronyms and abbreviations that appear in this chapter include: AP-1, transcription factor activator protein-1; APC, activated protein C; aPTT, activated partial thromboplastin time; AT, antithrombin; BiP, immunoglobulin-binding protein; bp, base pairs; C/EBP, CCAAT/enhancer binding protein; COAT, collagen and thrombin stimulated; EGF, epidermal growth factor; EPCR, endothelial cell protein C receptor; ER, endoplasmic reticulum; ERGIC, endoplasmic reticulum–Golgi intermediate compartment; Gla, γ-carboxy glutamic acid; HK, high molecular weight kininogen; HNF, hepatic nuclear factor; IL, interleukin; K_d, dissociation constant; LMAN-1, mannose-binding lectin-1 gene product; MCFD-2, multiple coagulation factor deficiency protein-2; MZF-1, myeloid-enriched transcription factor; NF-κB, nuclear factor-κB; PAR, proteolytically activated receptors; PK, prekallikrein; PS, phosphatidylserine; SCR, short consensus repeat; TAFI, thrombin-activatable fibrinolysis inhibitor; TF, tissue factor; TFPI, tissue factor pathway inhibitor; TM, thrombomodulin; vWF, von Willebrand factor; ZPI, protein Z–dependent protease inhibitor.

TABLE 106-1   CHARACTERISTICS OF COAGULATION PROTEINS

	PROTEIN	CONCENTRATION (μg/mL)	PLASMA HALF-LIFE (h)	CHROMOSOME
Zymogens				
Gla	Prothrombin (factor II)	100–150	60–70	11p11-q12
	Factor VII	0.5	3–6	13q34
	Factor IX	4–5	18–24	Xq27.1-q27.2
	Factor X	8–10	30–40	13q34
	Protein C	4–5	6	2q13-q14
non-Gla	Factor XI	5	52	4q32-q35
	Factor XII	30	60	5q33
	Prekallikrein	50	35	4q35
	Factor XIII A chain[a]	10	240	6p24-p25
	Factor XIII B chain[a]	22		1q31-q32.1
	Thrombin activatable fibrinolysis inhibitor (TAFI)	6		13q14
Cofactors				
Soluble	Factor V[b]	5–10	12	1q21-q25
	Factor VIII	0.1–0.2	8–12	Xq28
	vWF	10	12	12p13.2
	Protein S	25	42	3p11.1-q11.2
	Protein Z	2–3	60	13q34
	High molecular weight kininogen	70	150	3q26
Cellular	Tissue factor	—	—	1p21-p22
	Thrombomodulin	—	—	20p12-cen
Structural Protein				
	Fibrinogen	2000–4000	72–120	
	Aα chain			4q23-q32
	Bβ chain			4q23-q32
	γ chain			4q23-q32
Inhibitors	Antithrombin	150–400	72	1q23-q25
	Tissue factor pathway inhibitor	0.1	8	2q31-q32.1
	Protein Z-dependent protease inhibitor	1–1.6		

[a] All of the factor XIII A chain is in complex with factor XIII B chain. Only half of factor XIII B chain is in complex with factor XIII A chain, the rest is free in plasma.

[b] Platelets carry significant amounts of factor XIIIa (roughly half of the total factor XIII activity) and factor V (20% of circulating factor V).

[c] Approximately 60% of the protein S is in complex with C4b binding protein.

The calcium-bound form of the Gla domain is responsible for mediating association with phospholipid membranes. Lipids with negatively charged head groups, primarily phosphatidylserine (PS), are required for this binding. Even in the absence of the appropriate protein cofactor, binding to phospholipids increases the proteolytic activity of Gla-containing proteases. PS is required for activity on synthetic phospholipid membranes. The role of PS in mediating coagulation reactions on cellular membranes, such as platelets, is more complex. PS normally is not exposed on the outer membrane leaflet of cells in contact with flowing blood. Further, activation of cells (particularly platelets) often is accompanied by exposure of PS on the outer leaflet of cell membranes. Because this activation enhances the ability to support coagulation reactions, exposure of PS on the outer surface of cells often is assumed to be sufficient to account for the cell's ability to support coagulation reactions. However, other studies have shown that the level of coagulant activity on cells does not directly correlate with the amount of PS exposure. This result stands in contrast to studies with phospholipid membranes in which the level of coagulant activity is directly related to the amount of PS expressed. Thus, PS exposure may be necessary for cells to support coagulation reactions, but other features, such as cell receptors and/or binding proteins, also are necessary (reviewed in ref. 10).

Very high homology in the amino acid sequence is observed in the first 42 residues of the Gla-containing proteins. This finding implies the three-dimensional structure is highly conserved and few specific interactions are determined by this region. Binding of Gla-containing proteins to phospholipids once was believed to be mediated by calcium ion "bridging" between the Gla residues and the negatively charged phospholipid. This mechanism provided a good explanation for why both calcium and negatively charged phospholipid were required for binding. However, binding of Gla-containing factors to lipid surfaces now is believed to be mediated by membrane insertion of hydrophobic residues present in the first 10 amino acids of the Gla domain. Calcium is essential for this occurrence because calcium binding to the Gla residues induces a dramatic conformational change that exposes the hydrophobic amino acid residues in a "patch" on the surface of the protein that allows the protein to insert into the phospholipid membrane (Fig. 106-3).[11,12]

The striking degree of homology among the Gla domains of the vitamin K–dependent clotting factors suggests the affinity of the calcium–Gla complexes for phospholipids also is very similar. However, this situation is not true. Factors IX and X bind much more strongly to phosphatidylcholine/PS-containing vesicles than does factor VII.[13] The reasons for these marked differences are not clear.

The first EGF domain of the vitamin K–dependent proteins has a calcium ion binding site that does not involve Gla residues but does

FIGURE 106-1 (ON OPPOSITE PAGE)   Comparison of the Gla-containing zymogens. Basic structural elements of the Gla-containing zymogens are shown. Each *circle* is an amino acid. The pre-pro leader sequence contains the signal peptide and elements that direct carboxylation of glutamyl residues. Cleavage of the leader sequence is indicated by a *slight separation* from the mature protein. All have a Gla domain, with the Gla residues indicated by *filled blue circles*. Prothrombin has a finger loop followed by two kringle domains. Factors VII, IX, and X and protein C have epidermal growth factor–like domains. Prothrombin and factors VII and IX circulate as single-chain molecules. Factor X and protein C circulate as two chains that are disulfide linked. All have a catalytic domain that is homologous between the Gla-containing zymogens. The active site residues His, Asp, and Ser are indicated by the *black circles* in the catalytic domain. Cleavages that convert the zymogen to an active enzyme are indicated by the *arrows*. In factors IX and X and protein C, the released activation peptide is indicated by the *gray circles*. After cleavage, all of the molecules are two-chain, disulfide-linked molecules. The disulfide connecting the catalytic domain with the rest of the molecule is shown by the *heavy bond*. All catalytic domains except that of prothrombin remain attached to the Gla domain after activation.

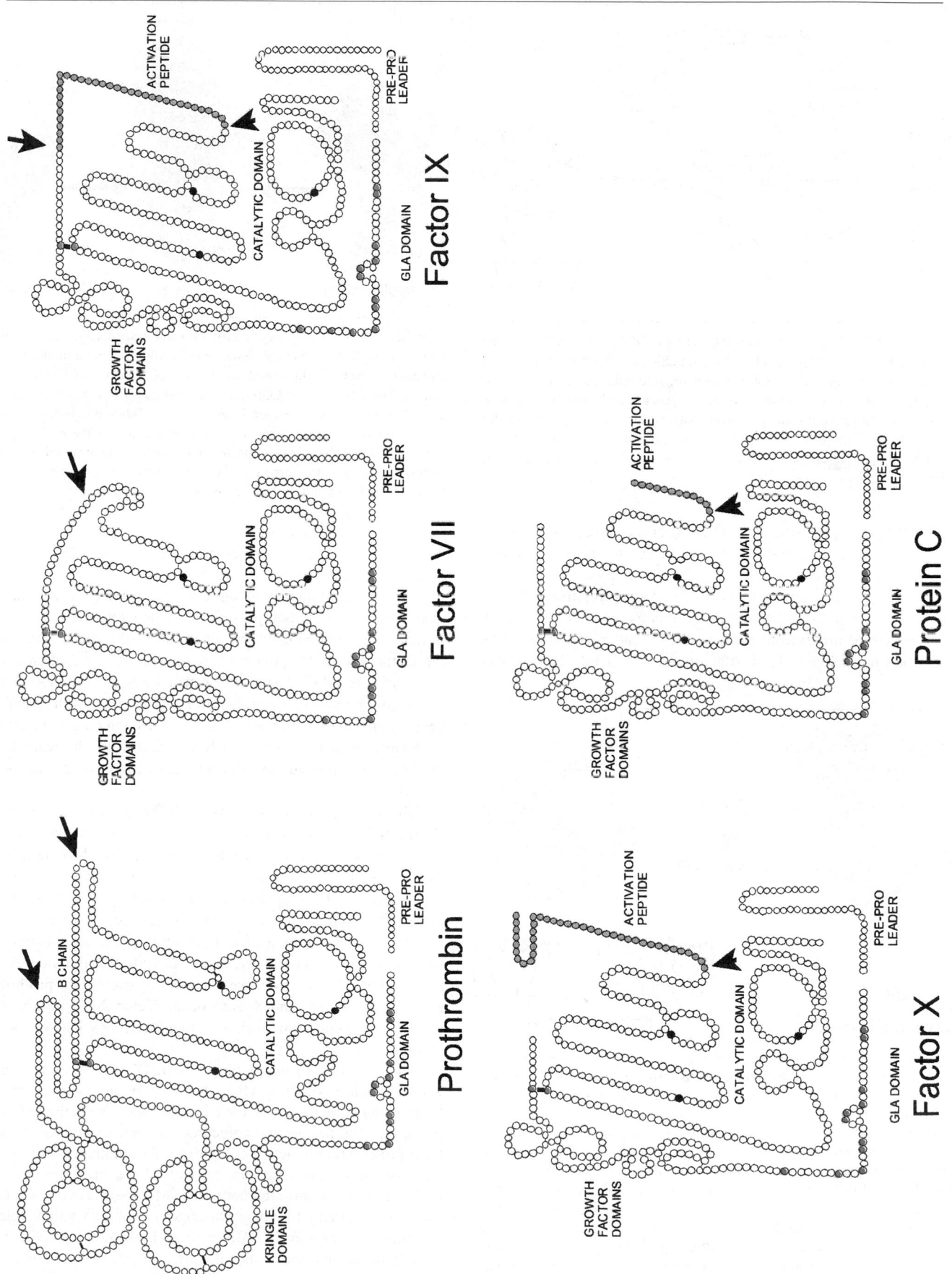

Factor IX

Factor VII

Protein C

Prothrombin

Factor X

ACTIVATION PEPTIDE

PRE-PRO LEADER

CATALYTIC DOMAIN

GLA DOMAIN

GROWTH FACTOR DOMAINS

B CHAIN

KRINGLE DOMAINS

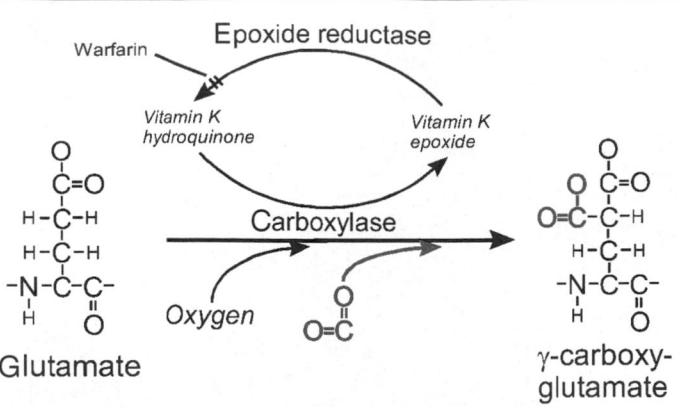

FIGURE 106-2   Vitamin K carboxylase activity. Glutamyl residues are converted to γ-carboxy glutamyl residues by a specific carboxylase. This reaction requires oxygen, carbon dioxide (shown in *blue*), and reduced vitamin K in the form of a hydroquinone. Carbon dioxide is incorporated onto the γ-carbon providing a second carboxylate group on that residue. In the process of this reaction, reduced vitamin K is converted to an epoxide. Reduced vitamin K is recycled by a specific epoxide reductase, a reaction that can be blocked by warfarin.

involve a β-hydroxy aspartic acid. The conserved aspartic acid residue is modified posttranslationally by a β-hydroxylase about which little is known. Binding of calcium to this EGF-1 site appears to be important in activity and probably orients the Gla domain relative to the rest of the molecule. The EGF-1 and EGF-2 domains serve, at least in part, to space the serine protease domain above the lipid membrane surface. Factor VIIa interaction with its cofactor—tissue factor (TF)—is me-

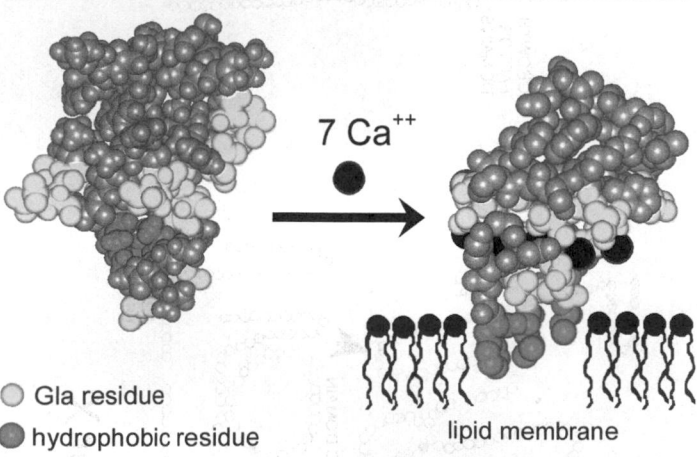

FIGURE 106-3   Calcium ion binding to the Gla domain alters the conformation of the Gla domain. Molecular models of the Gla domain of prothrombin are shown. The calcium-bound form is taken from the x-ray crystal structure of Soriano-Garcia et al.[11] The noncalcium form is modeled from the nuclear magnetic resonance structure of factor X.[12] Each *circle* shows the position of an amino acid. Gla residues are colored *light blue*. Hydrophobic residues believed to be important in membrane insertion are shown in *dark blue* (residues 6, 7, and 9). In the absence of calcium, the negatively charged Gla residues are exposed to the solution, and the hydrophobic residues are buried. Calcium ion binding to Gla residues provides sufficient energy to alter the overall conformation of the Gla domain and expose the hydrophobic residues (residues 6, 7, 9). In this view, only four of the seven bound calcium ions are seen. Insertion of the hydrophobic residues into a membrane is illustrated schematically.

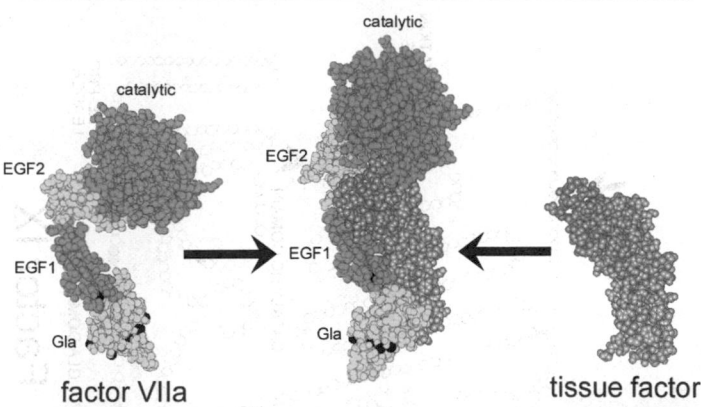

FIGURE 106-4   Complex of factor VIIa and tissue factor. The crystal structure of tissue factor[17] and the tissue factor complex[18] and a model of the free structure of factor VIIa (based on the crystal structure of factor IXa[19]) are shown. The Gla domain, EGF domains, and catalytic domain of factor VIIa are indicated. Calcium ions are shown in *black*. Binding to tissue factor alters the overall structure of factor VIIa. The orientation of the EGF1 domain is identical in factor VIIa in the modeled free structure and in complex with tissue factor. The crystal structure of the complex shows multiple close contacts between tissue factor and multiple domains of factor VIIa.

diated, at least in part, by direct interaction between TF and both EGF domains of factor VIIa (Fig. 106-4).

All of the Gla-containing zymogens undergo activation by cleavage of at least one peptide bond (see Fig. 106-1). Activation is indicated by appending the letter "a" to the end of the name of the factor, except for protein C. Activated protein C often is abbreviated aPC or APC. The cleavage that leads to activation generates a new amino terminal that folds back and interacts with specific residues in the serine protease domain. This interaction changes the conformation of the protein such that the active site residues (His, Ser, Asp) are aligned, and the protease activity of the factor is expressed.

The serine protease domains of all the Gla-containing proteases show a high homology to each other and to chymotrypsin and trypsin. All have trypsin-like activity, with an almost absolute specificity for cleaving arginyl residues. However, unlike trypsin, which shows little specificity beyond cleaving after an arginyl or lysyl residue, the activated coagulation factors have extended substrate specificity pockets, such that only a small number of amino acid sequences are recognized by each activated factor. Despite the high degree of homology between the protease domains of protein C, prothrombin, and factors VII, IX, and X, each of the factors has a highly specific function in coagulation mediated by surface loops that are not highly homologous.

The activated forms of factors VII, IX, and X each associates with a specific cofactor. TF is the cofactor for factor VIIa, factor VIIIa is the cofactor for factor IXa, and factor Va is the cofactor for factor Xa. The factors and cofactors associate on cell membranes to form proteolytically active complexes. Thrombin does not require a cofactor for its procoagulant activity. However, upon association with the cofactor thrombomodulin (TM), its specificity is changed from procoagulant (clotting fibrinogen) to anticoagulant (cleaving and activating protein C). Although each of the proteases has some activity in the absence of its cofactor, association with cofactor dramatically enhances its activity. Table 106-2 lists the enhancement of factor IXa activity by calcium, activated platelets, and the factor VIII cofactor.[14,15] Thus, the physiologic coagulant activity of factors VIIa,

TABLE 106-2 COFACTOR ENHANCEMENT OF FACTOR IXA ACTIVITY

CONDITIONS	RELATIVE RATE
IXa/Ca^{2+}	1
IXa/Ca^{2+}/platelet[a]	150[b]
IXa/Ca^{2+}/VIIIa	250[c]
IXa/Ca^{2+}/platelet[a]/VIIIa	9,000,000[b]

[a] Platelets were activated with thrombin.
[b] Rates are given as k_{cat}/Km and are taken from Rawala-Sheikh et al.[14]
[c] Rates are given as k_{cat}/Km and are taken from Gilbert et al.[15]

IXa, and Xa is expressed only as part of a complete procoagulant complex (Table 106-3). The complexes are sometimes named for their physiologic substrate: the factor IXa/VIIIa complex is termed the "tenase" or "intrinsic tenase" complex, the factor VIIa/TF complex the "extrinsic tenase" complex, and the factor Xa/Va complex the "prothrombinase" complex. The cofactors enhance proteolytic activity by two basic mechanisms: (1) they have binding sites for both substrate and enzyme and bring the two into close proximity; and (2) they associate with the protease and induce a conformational change that enhances enzymatic activity. The structure of the factor VIIa/TF complex has been determined by x-ray crystallography.[16] Figure 106-4 illustrates the projected change in conformation of the factor VIIa molecule when it binds to its cofactor TF.[17–19] The factor IXa/VIIIa and Xa/Va complexes have not been crystallized, but generally similar conformational changes likely occur during formation of these complexes.

PROTHROMBIN (FACTOR II)

PROTEIN STRUCTURE

Like the other vitamin K–dependent zymogens, plasma prothrombin is primarily synthesized in the liver. It circulates as a single-chain zymogen M_r of approximately 72,000, with a plasma half-life of approximately 60 hours. Figure 106-5 shows a schematic representation. Prothrombin has 10 Gla residues. Instead of the EGF region present in most vitamin K–dependent zymogens, prothrombin has two kringle domains. Kringle domains are structures held together by three disulfide bonds that schematically resemble a Danish pastry called a "kringle." The primary function of kringle structures apparently is binding other proteins such as activators, substrates, cofactors, or receptors.[20]

MOLECULAR BIOLOGY

The human prothrombin gene has been localized to chromosome 11, near the centromere.[21] It has been completely sequenced and is composed of 14 exons separated by 13 introns (Fig. 106-6). The 5' flanking region of the prothrombin gene contains the promoter region and two or more cis-acting enhancer sequences. Unlike many other promoters, the promoter region of the prothrombin gene does not contain a TATA box. It has multiple potential sites of transcription initiation extending from 3 to 38 base pairs (bp) upstream from the initial methionine. The site at −31 is the most likely start site. The region between −887 and −875 likely is a binding site for hepatic nuclear factor-1 (HNF-1), a DNA-binding protein that plays a role in liver-specific expression of a number of genes.[22] An additional site in the prothrombin promoter region with non–tissue-specific enhancer activity lies just upstream to the HNF-1 site.

One unusual feature of the prothrombin gene is the presence of many repetitive sequences in its 5' flanking region.[23] Approximately 41 percent of the gene and upstream sequence consists of Alu repeats. The function of these repetitive sequences, if any, is not known.

Several polymorphisms of the prothrombin gene have been described. One of the polymorphisms now is recognized to have important functional consequences. This G to A transition in the 3' untranslated region (20210 G→A) of the prothrombin gene is associated with higher than normal levels of plasma prothrombin.[24] Increased prothrombin levels are associated with an increased risk of thromboembolic phenomena (see Chap. 122).

ACTIVATION AND ACTIVITY

Prothrombin is cleaved by the factor Xa/Va prothrombinase (IIase) complex in two places (Arg271 and Arg320; Fig. 106-7).[11,25–27] The catalytic domain (thrombin; M_r 36,600) is released from the remainder of the molecule (prothrombin fragment 1.2). Because one molecule of prothrombin fragment 1.2 is released for each molecule of thrombin, assays for fragment 1.2 reflect the level of prothrombin activation.

Thrombin cleaves a number of biologically important substrates. It removes fibrinopeptides A and B from fibrinogen to form fibrin monomers that spontaneously polymerize to form a fibrin clot (see Chap. 117). The anion-binding exosite spans residues 387–398 and is involved in binding to fibrinogen, TM, hirudin, heparin cofactor II, and the proteolytically activated thrombin receptors. Interestingly, this region of thrombin is identical in human, bovine, rat, and mouse.[28] In addition to directly clotting fibrinogen, thrombin has a procoagulant effect, participating in positive feedback loops by activating platelets and coagulation factors V, VIII, XI, and XIII.

Thrombin is a potent platelet activator through at least two types of receptors, which include the G protein-linked proteolytically activated receptors PAR-1 and PAR-4 and platelet glycoprotein Ibα (see Chap. 105).

Another function of thrombin is activating a procarboxypeptidase B-like enzyme to its active state, a reaction enhanced by TM. The active carboxypeptidase inhibits plasmin-mediated fibrinolysis by removing carboxy-terminal lysine residues, which facilitate plasminogen binding, from partially degraded fibrin. Thus, the carboxypeptidase has been termed "thrombin-activatable fibrinolysis inhibitor" (TAFI) (see Chap. 127).[29,30]

In addition to its procoagulant activity, thrombin has an anticoagulant function. Thus, thrombin binds to the cofactor TM on endothelial cells, which allows it to activate protein C.[31,32] Thrombin also has growth factor and cytokine-like activities that may play a role in atherosclerosis, wound healing, and inflammation.[33]

The primary plasma inhibitor of thrombin in coagulation is antithrombin (AT). Heparin cofactor II also inhibits thrombin and may serve as an extravascular thrombin inhibitor that regulates the growth factor and cytokine-like activities of thrombin.[33]

TABLE 106-3 PROTEASE/COFACTOR COMPLEXES

ENZYME	COFACTOR	SUBSTRATE	CELLULAR LOCATION
Factor VIIa	Tissue factor	Factor X	Many cells[a]
		Factor IX	
Factor IXa	Factor VIIIa	Factor X	Platelets
Factor Xa	Factor Va	Prothrombin	Platelets[b]
Thrombin	Thrombomodulin	Protein C	Endothelium
Activated protein C	Protein S	Factor Va	Endothelium
		Factor VIIIa	

[a] TF is constitutively expressed on many extravascular cells (e.g., stromal cells, epithelial cells, astrocytes) and induced by inflammatory mediators in many other cells (e.g., monocytes, endothelial cells).
[b] Many other cells have low levels of factor Xa/factor Va activity.

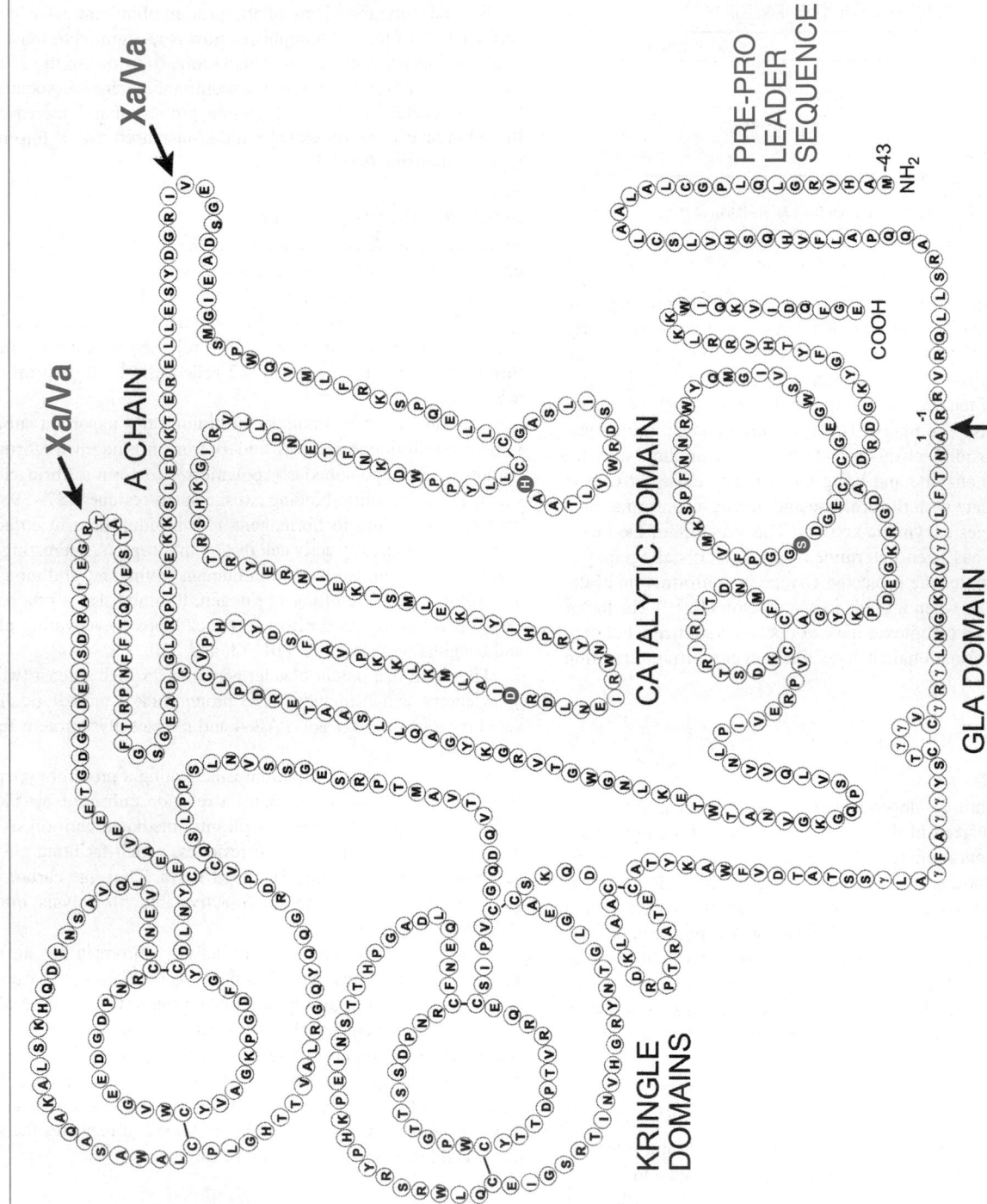

FIGURE 106-5   Domains of prothrombin. Each amino acid in prothrombin is shown. Gla residues are indicated by the symbol γ. The cleavage site to remove the pre-pro leader sequence is indicated by an *arrow*. The active residue sites His, Asp, and Ser are shown by *blue circles*. Cleavage sites for factor Xa/factor Va are shown by *arrows*. Cleavage removes the Gla domain and kringles, leaving thrombin composed of a small A chain disulfide linked to the catalytic domain (B chain).

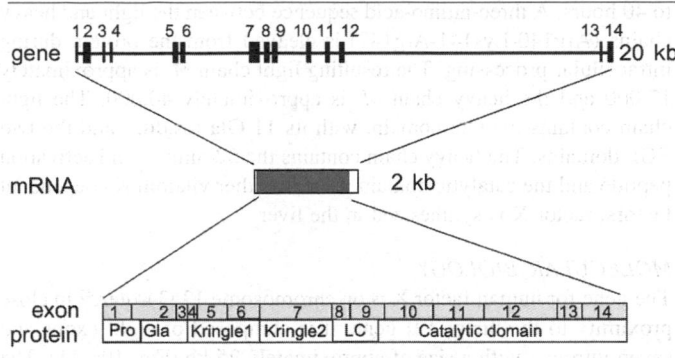

FIGURE 106-6   Relation between gene structure and protein structure in prothrombin. The exons, introns, mRNA, and protein structure are indicated. Promoter elements upstream from exon 1 are not shown but are discussed in the text. The mRNA is 2 kb, with small 5′ and 3′ untranslated regions. Gla, γ-carboxy glutamic acid domain; Kringle1 and Kringle 2, kringle domains; LC, light chain (also called the A chain); Pro, pre-pro leader sequence.

FACTOR VII

PROTEIN STRUCTURE

Factor VII circulates as a single-chain zymogen of M_r 50,000. It has the shortest half-life of the procoagulant factors, approximately 3 to 6 hours (see Table 106-1). Factor VII has 10 Gla residues.

MOLECULAR BIOLOGY

The human factor VII gene is located on chromosome 13, very close to the gene for factor X. The gene consists of eight exons and seven introns, an overall size of approximately 13 kb, and an organization similar to the other vitamin K–dependent factors (Fig. 106-8).[1,2]

The major transcription start site in the factor VII gene is at position −51. Three other minor start sites have been described.[34] A hormone-responsive element and binding sites for the *trans*-acting factors HNF-4 and Sp-1 are present between −233 and −58 in the promoter region of the factor VII gene.

ACTIVATION AND ACTIVITY

Factor VII binds to TF with a dissociation constant (K_d) in the subnanomolar range. Once bound to its cofactor, factor VII can be activated by a number of different proteases that cleave between Arg152 and Ile153. The physiologic activator of factor VII is thought to be factor Xa, although significant autoactivation by factor VIIa can occur.[35] Unlike prothrombin, the catalytic domain of factor VII is linked to the rest of the molecule by a disulfide bond, so no portion is cleaved from the protein (see Fig. 106-1). The factor VIIa/TF complex activates both factors IX and X. It is inhibited by tissue factor pathway inhibitor (TFPI) in complex with factor Xa. It also is inhibited by AT, but only in the presence of heparin.

FACTOR IX

PROTEIN STRUCTURE

Factor IX is synthesized in hepatocytes and circulates as a single-chain zymogen of M_r 57,000, with a plasma half-life of 18 to 24 hours. It has 12 Gla residues. Only approximately 40 percent of factor IX molecules are hydroxylated at aspartic acid 64 in the EGF-1 domain. All the other Gla-containing zymogens have complete hydroxylation of the homologous residues (Fig. 106-9). Factor IX contains N-linked and O-linked carbohydrate moieties found mostly in the activation peptide. In the mature molecule, the tyrosine reside at position 155 is sulfated whereas the serine residue at position 158 is phosphorylated. Factor IX, unlike other vitamin K–dependent factors, binds effectively to collagen IV *in vitro*.[36] The molecule appears to bind to collagen IV *in vivo* and may account for the observation that when factor IX is infused into hemophilia B patients, recovery is only 50 percent of the expected value (see Chap. 115).[37] The physiologic relevance of this observation remains to be precisely determined, but studies sug-

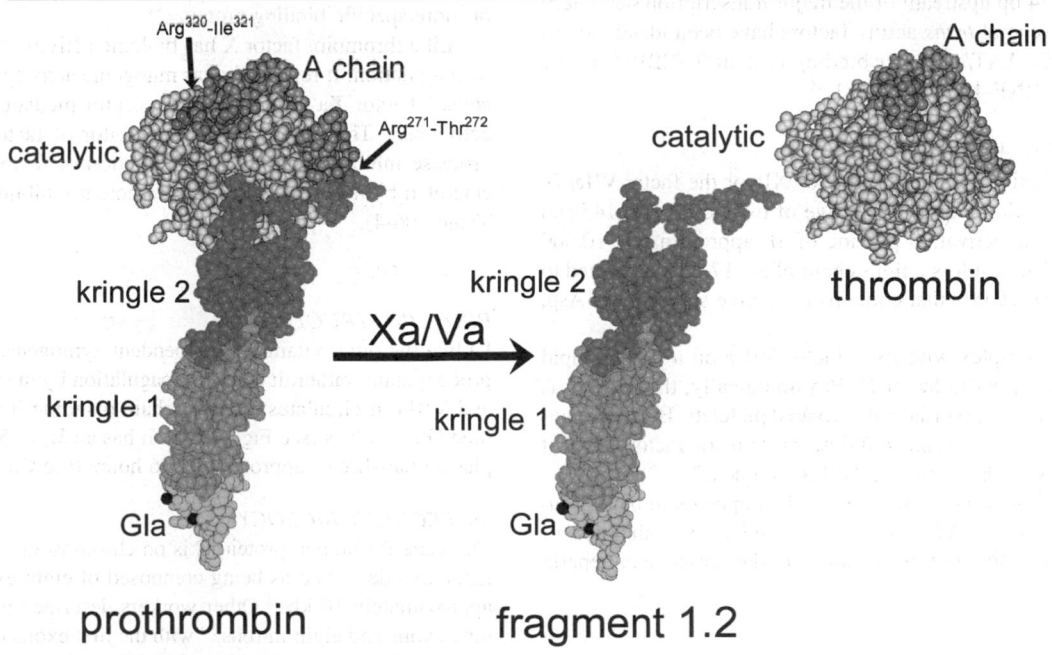

FIGURE 106-7   Activation of prothrombin. Model of prothrombin constructed from four crystal structures is shown.[11,25–27] The Gla domain, both kringle domains, and the catalytic domain (B chain) are shown. Calcium ions are shown in *black*. Cleavage by factor Xa/factor Va releases thrombin from the rest of the molecule, fragment 1.2.

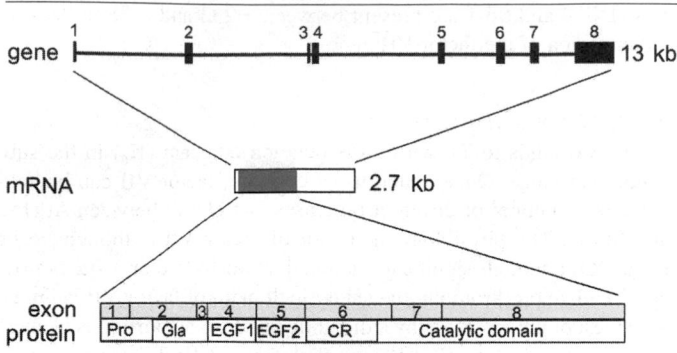

FIGURE 106-8   Relation between gene structure and protein structure in factor VII. The exons, introns, mRNA, and protein structure are indicated. Promoter elements upstream from exon 1 are not shown but are discussed in the text. The mRNA is 2.7 kb, with a small 5′ untranslated region and a relatively large 3′ untranslated region. The site of proteolytic activation is between the connecting region and the catalytic domain. CR, connecting region; EGF epidermal growth factor–like domain; Gla, γ-carboxy glutamic acid domain; Pro, pre-pro leader sequence.

gest factor IX mutants lacking collagen IV binding exhibit a greater recovery.[38]

MOLECULAR BIOLOGY

The gene for factor IX is located on the tip of the long arm of the X chromosome at position Xq27.1-q27.2.[39] Therefore, deficiency of factor IX (hemophilia B) is sex linked. The gene contains eight exons, seven introns, and a long 1.4-kb 3′-untranslated region, for an overall size of 33 kb (Fig. 106-10).

Eight polymorphisms have been described within or flanking the factor IX gene. These polymorphisms can be useful for antenatal diagnosis and carrier detection of hemophilia B by restriction fragment length polymorphism analysis.[40]

The promoter activity of the 5′ untranslated region of the factor IX gene resides 274 bp upstream of the major transcription start site.[41] Binding sites for several *trans*-acting factors have been identified, including sites for CCAAT/enhancer binding protein (C/EBP),[42] D-site binding protein,[43] HNF-4,[44] and HNF-1.[45]

ACTIVATION AND ACTIVITY

Factor IX can be activated by either factor XIa or the factor VIIa/TF complex. Full activation requires cleavage of two bonds (Arg145 and Arg180) releasing an activation peptide of M_r approximately 10,000 (see Fig. 106-9). The result is a light chain of M_r 17,000 connected to a heavy chain of M_r 30,000 that contains the active site residues Asp, His, and Ser.

Factor IXa in complex with its cofactor VIIIa on a phospholipid membrane surface activates factor X. Physiologically, this activity is primarily expressed on the surface of activated platelets. Evidence suggests platelets express a receptor/binding protein for factor IXa that promotes assembly of the factor IXa/VIIIa complex.[46]

The primary plasma inhibitor of factor IXa appears to be AT. Inhibition of factor IXa by AT is slow compared to AT inhibition of thrombin. However, inhibition is enhanced in the presence of heparin (Table 106-4).

FACTOR X

PROTEIN STRUCTURE

Factor X circulates as a two-chain, disulfide-linked zymogen of M_r 59,000 (see Fig. 106-1), with a plasma half-life of approximately 30

to 40 hours. A three-amino-acid sequence between the light and heavy chains (Arg140-Lys141-Arg142) is cleaved from the protein during intracellular processing. The resulting light chain M_r is approximately 17,000 and the heavy chain M_r is approximately 40,000. The light chain contains the Gla domain, with its 11 Gla residues and the two EGF domains. The heavy chain contains the 52-amino-acid activation peptide and the catalytic domain. Like all other vitamin K–dependent factors, factor X is synthesized in the liver.

MOLECULAR BIOLOGY

The gene for human factor X is on chromosome 13q34-qter,[47] in close proximity to the factor VII gene. It is composed of eight exons and seven introns,[1] with a size of approximately 25 kb (Fig. 106-11). The 3′ untranslated region is unusually short—only 10 bp. A number of potentially useful polymorphisms have been identified.[48]

The factor X promoter region has been sequenced and characterized. The region lacks a typical TATA box but contains a CCAAT sequence at −120 to −116. Factor X appears to have multiple start sites of transcription.[49] This finding is consistent with multiple start sites reported for other promoters lacking a TATA box. Like the factor IX gene, a binding site for HNF-4 has been identified.[50] However, unlike the factor IX gene, a binding site for C/EBP is not evident.

ACTIVATION AND ACTIVITY

Factor X can be activated to fully active factor Xaα by factor VIIa/TF or factor IXa/VIIIa by cleavage at the Arg194-Ile195 bond in the heavy chain. Further autocatalytic cleavage near the carboxy-terminus of the heavy chain releases a 19-amino-acid peptide to yield "beta-Xa," which also is enzymatically active.

Factor Xa in complex with factor Va on a phospholipid membrane surface activates prothrombin to thrombin by cleaving two peptide bonds. Factor Xa also may play a physiologic role in activation of factors VII,[51] VIII,[52] and V.[53] Although any membrane surface that expresses anionic phospholipid can support prothrombinase complex assembly, the activated platelet surface is especially well suited for this purpose. Prothrombinase assembly on platelets is not strictly a function of phospholipid composition but is likely coordinated by one or more specific binding proteins.[54]

Like thrombin, factor X has biologic activities not directly related to coagulation. It reportedly has mitogenic activity for smooth muscle cells.[55] Factor Xa also possesses receptor-mediated proinflammatory activities.[56] The primary plasma inhibitor of factor Xa is the serine protease inhibitor (serpin) AT. Inhibition of factor Xa by AT is accelerated by heparin. TFPI is also a potent inhibitor of factor Xa (see Table 106-4).

PROTEIN C

PROTEIN STRUCTURE

Unlike the other vitamin K–dependent zymogens, protein C is not a procoagulant; rather, it controls coagulation by inactivating factors Va and VIIIa. It circulates as a two-chain disulfide-linked zymogen with nine Gla residues (see Fig. 106-1). It has an M_r of 59,000, with a short plasma half-life of approximately 6 hours (see Chap. 107).

MOLECULAR BIOLOGY

The gene for human protein C is on chromosome 2p13-14.[57] It originally was described as being composed of eight exons with a size of approximately 10 kb.[58] Other workers described protein C as having nine exons and eight introns,[59] with the first exon corresponding to the 5′-noncoding region (Fig. 106-12). Thus, the first exon is transcribed from the gene into mRNA but is not translated into protein. The gene structure is very similar to the other vitamin K–dependent factors, with especially close homology to factor IX.

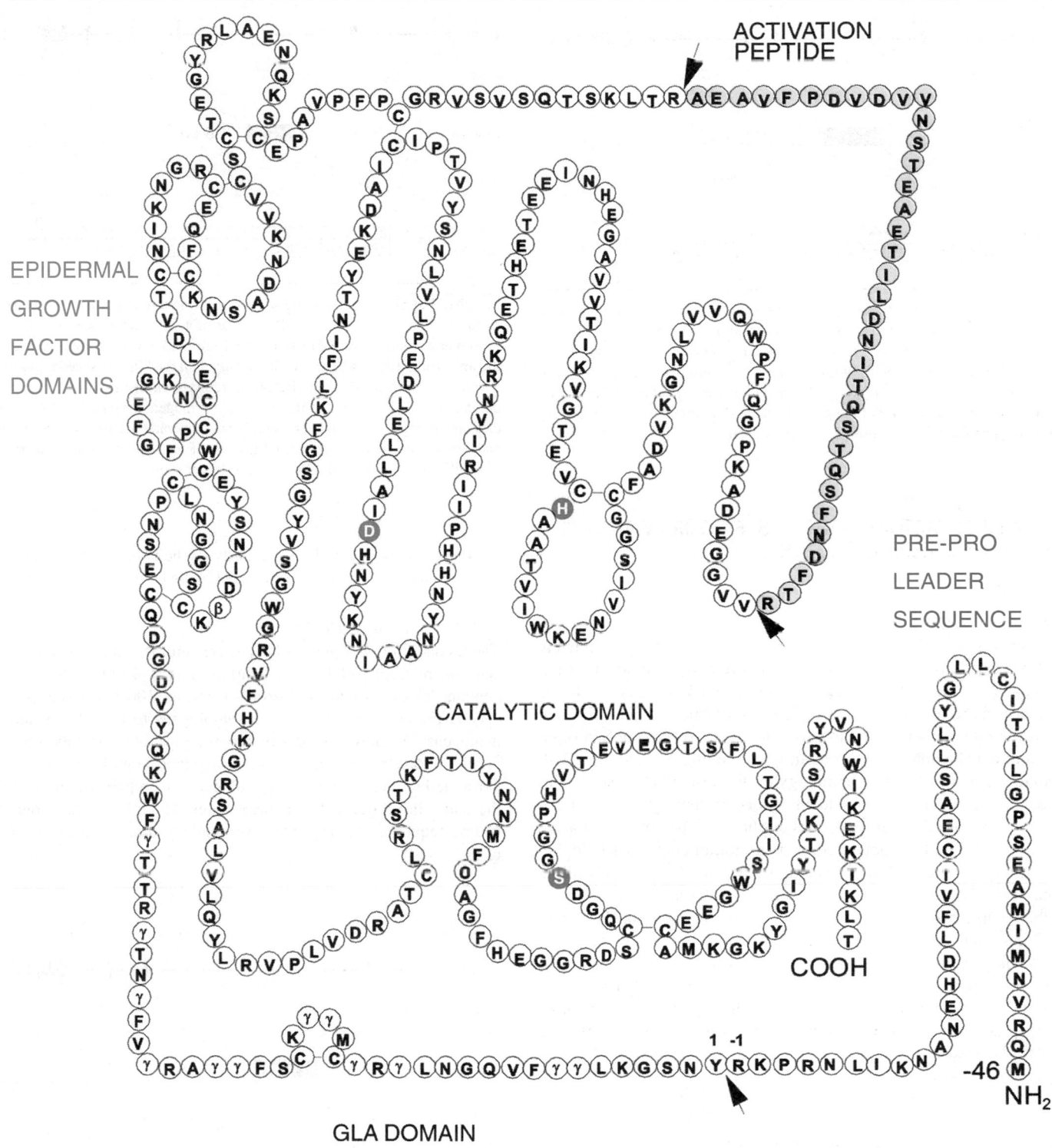

FIGURE 106-9   Domains of factor IX. Each amino acid in factor IX is shown. Gla residues are indicated by the symbol γ. The cleavage site to remove the pre-pro leader sequence is indicated by an *arrow*. The active site residues His, Asp, and Ser are shown by *blue circles*. Cleavage sites for factor XIa and factor VIIa/tissue factor are shown by *arrows*.

ACTIVATION AND ACTIVITY

Protein C is activated by thrombin in complex with the cell surface cofactor TM. A single cleavage at Arg169-Leu170 releases a 12-amino-acid activation peptide leading to APC with M_r of 56,000. Activation of protein C is modulated in part by the endothelial cell protein C receptor (EPCR).[60]

APC in complex with its cofactor protein S proteolytically inactivates factors Va and VIIIa. The APC/protein S complex inactivates factor Va better on endothelial cells than on platelets.[61] Factor V reportedly can act as a cofactor for inactivation of factors Va and VIIIa by APC.[62] The primary inhibitor of APC is the serpin protein C inhibitor, also known as plasminogen activator inhibitor-3.[63]

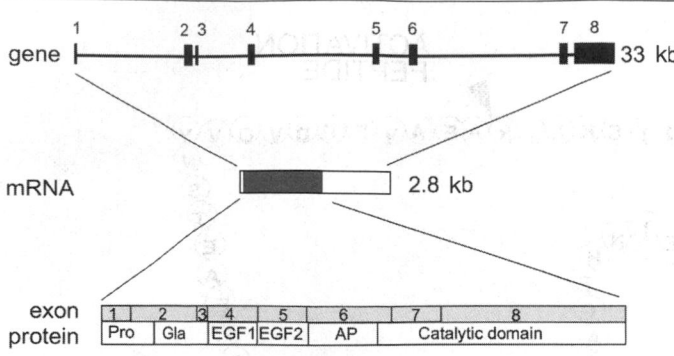

FIGURE 106-10 Relation between gene structure and protein structure in factor IX. The exons, introns, mRNA, and protein structure are as indicated. Promoter elements upstream from exon 1 are not shown but are discussed in the text. The mRNA is 2.8 kb, with a small 5′ untranslated region and a relatively large 3′ untranslated region. AP, activation peptide released after cleavage of two bonds; EGF, epidermal growth factor–like domains; Gla, γ-carboxy glutamic acid domain; Pro, pre-pro leader sequence.

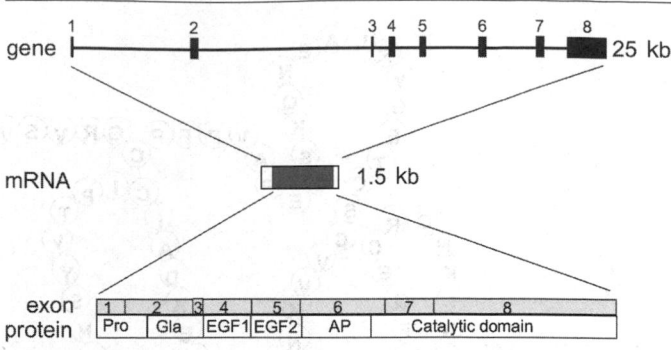

FIGURE 106-11 Relation between gene structure and protein structure in factor X. The exons, introns, mRNA, and protein structure are as indicated. Promoter elements upstream from exon 1 are not shown but are discussed in the text. The mRNA is 1.5 kb, with a relatively large 5′ untranslated region and a small 3′ untranslated region. Before secretion, cleavage in activation peptide domain processes factor X to the two-chain zymogen that circulates. A second cleavage releases the activation peptide and generates factor Xa activity. AP, activation peptide; EGF, epidermal growth factor–like domains; Gla, γ-carboxy glutamic acid domain; Pro, pre-pro leader sequence.

SOLUBLE COFACTORS (PROTEIN S, FACTORS V AND VIII, AND VON WILLEBRAND FACTOR)

PROTEIN S

PROTEIN STRUCTURE

Protein S is a single-chain plasma glycoprotein of M_r approximately 75,000, with a plasma half-life of approximately 42 hours. It is dependent on vitamin K for its synthesis. Protein S contains 11 Gla residues in the amino-terminal region. Its structure is quite different from the Gla-containing zymogens (Fig. 106-13). Protein S is organized into a Gla domain, a thrombin-sensitive finger region, four EGF domains, and a region with homology to steroid-binding proteins. Unlike the other vitamin K–dependent factors, protein S does not contain a serine protease domain, so it does not have the potential to catalyze reactions. Each EGF domain contains a modified amino acid, either β-hydroxyaspartic acid or β-hydroxyasparagine. Protein S circulates both in the free form (~40% of the total amount) and in a form bound to the complement regulatory protein C4b-binding protein. The steroid hormone-binding globulin-like region of protein S is involved in binding to the β-subunit of C4b-binding protein. Like the Gla-containing zymogens, protein S is synthesized with a signal peptide that directs it to the ER and a propeptide that binds to the γ-glutamyl carboxylase. The signal sequence and propeptide are removed before the mature protein is secreted.

Protein S is synthesized primarily by hepatocytes,[64] but also by endothelial cells,[65] megakaryocytes,[66] Leydig cells,[67] and osteoblasts.[68]

MOLECULAR BIOLOGY

The human protein S gene is located on chromosome 3, spanning the centromere from p11.1-q11.2. It is more than 80 kb in length and contains 15 exons and 14 introns[69] (see Fig. 106-13). Exons 1 to 8 encode protein domains that are homologous to the Gla-containing zymogens. The intron–exon structure is typical of the members of this family. Exons 9 to 15 encode protein segments homologous to steroid hormone-binding globulin. A pseudogene of protein S is located on the same chromosome. It is approximately 55 kb in size and contains coding sequences for regions corresponding to amino acids 46–635 of protein S.

TABLE 106-4 CHARACTERIZATION OF TFPI AND AT INHIBITION OF COAGULATION FACTORS

		TIME TO 50% INHIBITION[a]	
INHIBITOR	PROTEASE	−HEPARIN (MIN)	+HEPARIN (MIN)
Antithrombin	Thrombin	1.5	<0.1
	Factor Xa	4	<0.1
	Factor IXa	60	0.6
Tissue factor pathway inhibitor	Factor Xa	0.3	<0.1

[a] Time to 50% inhibition in plasma. *In vivo*, natural glycosaminoglycan molecules on endothelium and other cells accelerate the rate of inhibition.

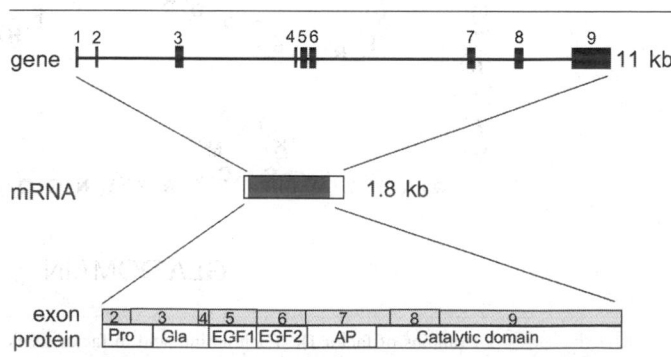

FIGURE 106-12 Relation between gene structure and protein structure in protein C. The exons, introns, mRNA, and protein structure are as indicated. The mRNA is 1.8 kb, with a small 5′ untranslated region coded for by exon 1 and a relatively small 3′ untranslated region. Before secretion, cleavage in the activation peptide domain processes protein C to the two-chain zymogen that circulates. A second cleavage releases the very small activation peptide and generates activated protein C. AP, activation peptide; EGF, epidermal growth factor–like domains; Gla, γ-carboxy glutamic acid domain; Pro, pre-pro leader sequence.

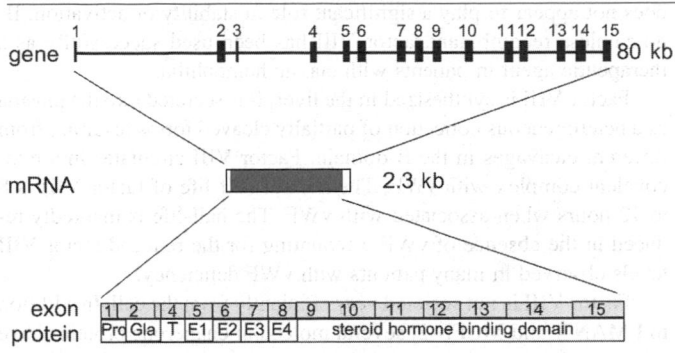

FIGURE 106-13   Relation between gene structure and protein structure in protein S. The exons, introns, mRNA, and protein structure are as indicated. The mRNA is 2.3 kb, with a small 5′ and 3′ untranslated region. E, epidermal growth factor–like domains; Gla, γ-carboxy glutamic acid domain; Pro, pre-pro leader sequence; T, thrombin-sensitive finger region.

ACTIVITY

Protein S serves as a cofactor for cleavage and inactivation of factors Va and VIIIa by APC. It does not require proteolytic activation for its cofactor activity. To serve as a cofactor for APC, protein S must be in the free form rather than bound to C4b-binding protein. Protein S alone has a low level of anticoagulant activity by virtue of its ability to compete with factor Xa for binding to factor Va.[70] This activity is not reduced by binding to C4b-binding protein.[71] Although the C4b-binding protein is an acute phase reactant, its β-subunit, which binds protein S, is not increased in inflammatory states. Therefore, the free protein S concentration is not affected by the acute phase response.

FACTOR V

PROTEIN STRUCTURE

Factors V and VIII are homologous in their gene structures, amino acid sequences, and protein domain structures. They have similar mechanisms of intracellular processing in the ER and Golgi apparatus and defects in these mechanisms can result in combined deficiency of factors V and VIII. The mannose-binding lectin-1 gene product LMAN-1 (also called ERGIC-53) is a protein found in the intermediate compartment of the Golgi apparatus that facilitates secretion of both factor V and factor VIII.[72] Mutations in the LMAN-1 gene lead to a hereditary deficiency of both factors V and VIII[73] that accounts for approximately two thirds of the cases of combined deficiency (see Chap. 116). Analysis of patients without defects in LMAN-1 suggests that mutations of a second protein, multiple coagulation_factor deficiency protein-2 (MCFD-2), also accounts for a number of the cases of combined factor V and VIII deficiency.[74] The gene product of MCDF-2 is a protein of M_r 16,000 localized to the ER–Golgi intermediate compartment (ERGIC) through a direct, calcium-dependent interaction with LMAN-1. The MCFD-2–LMAN-1 complex appears to form a specific cargo receptor for the ER to Golgi transport of selected proteins, including factors V and VIII.

Factor V is a large glycoprotein of M_r approximately 330,000. It has a plasma half-life of approximately 12 hours, with some reports of a half-life up to 36 hours (reviewed in ref. 75). It has the following domain organization: A1-A2-B-A3-C1-C2 (Fig. 106-14). The three A domains have significant homology to the copper-binding plasma protein ceruloplasmin. The C domains have some homology to fat globule proteins. The C2 domain of factor V mediates binding to lipid membranes.[76] The A and C domains of factor V are approximately 40 percent identical to the homologous regions in factor VIII. In contrast, the B domains show little homology between the two proteins and are

not known to be homologous to any other proteins. In factor V, unlike factor VIII, sequences in the B domain appear to be important in promoting its activation by thrombin. The acidic regions of factor V have a high proportion of Asp and Glu residues. These regions are thought to be important in promoting activation, possibly by providing a site of interaction with the anion binding exosite of thrombin.

Factor V shows five potential sites for tyrosine sulfation at residues 696, 698, 1494, 1510, and 1565. Sulfation of factor V also plays a role in factor V activity by enhancing activation by thrombin and by promoting maximal factor Xa activation of prothrombin.[77] Factor V contains N-linked and O-linked carbohydrate moieties, most of which are clustered in the B domain.

MOLECULAR BIOLOGY

The gene for factor V is located on chromosome 1q21 to q25 very close to the genes for the selectin family of leukocyte adhesion molecules. The factor V gene spans approximately 70 kb and consists of 25 exons (see Fig. 106-14). The gene structure is very similar to that of the factor VIII gene, with exon–intron boundaries occurring at exactly the same location in 21 of 24 cases.[78] The mechanisms governing factor V gene transcription and translation are not clear.

ACTIVATION AND ACTIVITY

Factor V circulates in plasma as a single-chain molecule. As much as 20 percent of the circulating factor V pool is found in platelet α-granules. Platelet factor V is heterogeneous because of cleavages in the B domain by calpain and other platelet proteases. Theses cleavages produce a partially activated form of platelet factor V. Activated platelet factor V also is more resistant to inactivation by APC.[61,79] In platelets, but not in plasma, factor V is complexed to a large multimeric protein called *multimerin*.[80] Multimerin has a massive repeating structure. Some of the multimers having molecular weights of several million. Multimerin has structural features suggesting it may mediate adhesive interactions. Although multimerin appears functionally similar to von Willebrand factor (vWF), the two proteins share no structural homology.

Full factor V cofactor activity is achieved only after cleavage at several bonds (Fig. 106-15). Factor V is believed to be primarily activated by thrombin *in vivo*, although it can be activated by factor Xa,[53] and factor Xa appears to be the preferred activator of factor V released from platelet α- granules.[79] Thrombin cleaves factor V at Arg709 and Arg1545, producing a two-chain heterodimeric molecule consisting of

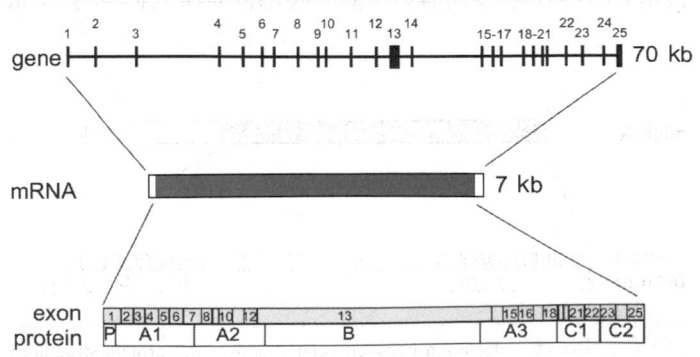

FIGURE 106-14   Relation between gene structure and protein structure in factor V. The exons, introns, mRNA, and protein structure are as indicated. The mRNA is 7 kb, with some 5′ and 3′ untranslated sequence. The A domains have homology to ceruloplasmin. The C domains have homology to fat globule proteins. The B domain is released upon activation and has no significant homology to any other identified protein. P, propeptide leader sequence.

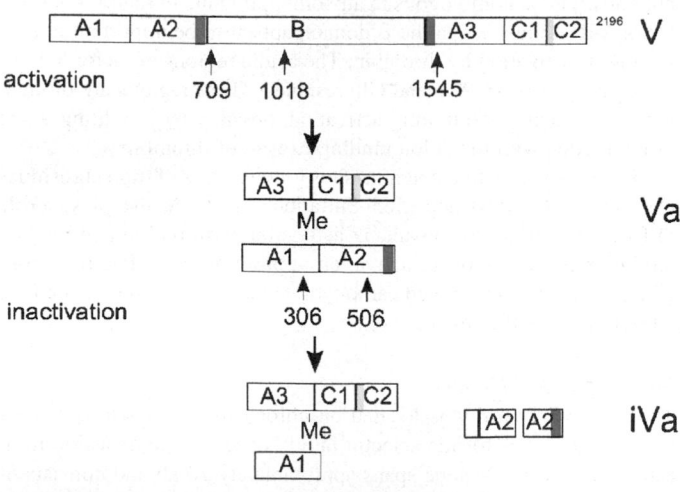

FIGURE 106-15 Activation and inactivation of factor V. For full cofactor activity, factor V must be cleaved by thrombin or factor Xa. The acidic domains, shown in *dark blue*, are believed to bind to the anion binding exosite in thrombin and enhance thrombin activation of factor V. Cleavage of residue 1018 enhances cleavage at residue 1545. Heavy and light chains are held together by noncovalent interactions mediated by metal ions (Me). Membrane binding is mediated through a site in the C2 domain (shown in *light blue*). Cleavage at residues 306 and 506 inactivates factor V by releasing two A2 fragments (iVa).

an A1-A2 heavy chain (M_r 110,000) noncovalently linked through calcium ions with an A3-C1-C2 light chain (M_r 73,000). APC catalyzes inactivation of factor Va by proteolysis of Arg306 and Arg506, resulting in dissociation of the cleaved A2 fragments (Fig. 106-15).[75] A common Arg506Gln mutation in factor V leads to resistance to inactivation by APC (factor V Leiden) and is associated with an increased risk of venous thromboembolism (see Chap. 122).[81]

FACTOR VIII

PROTEIN STRUCTURE

The domain organization of the factor VIII protein is A1-A2-B-A3-C1-C2, like that of factor V (Fig. 106-16). In factor VIII, the B domain

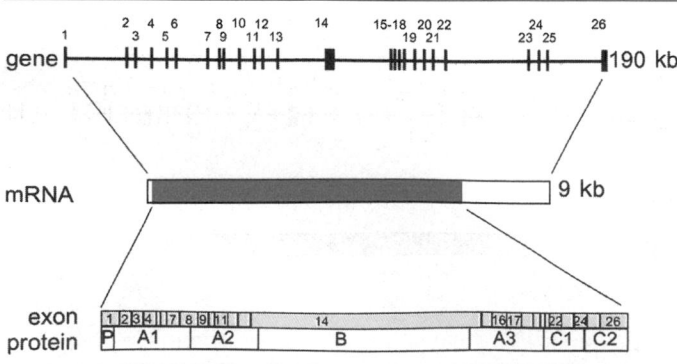

FIGURE 106-16 Relation between gene structure and protein structure in factor VIII. The exons, introns, mRNA, and protein structure are as indicated. Promoter elements upstream from exon 1 are not shown but are discussed in the text. The mRNA is 9 kb, with some 5′ untranslated sequence and a large 3′ untranslated region. The A domains have homology to ceruloplasmin. The C domains have homology to fat globule proteins. The B domain is released upon activation and has no significant homology to any other identified protein. P, propeptide leader sequence.

does not appear to play a significant role in stability or activation. B-domainless recombinant factor VIII has been used successfully as a therapeutic agent in patients with classic hemophilia.

Factor VIII is synthesized in the liver. It is secreted into the plasma as a heterogeneous collection of partially cleaved forms resulting from different cleavages in the B domain. Factor VIII circulates in a non-covalent complex with vWF. The normal half-life of factor VIII is 8 to 12 hours when associated with vWF. The half-life is markedly reduced in the absence of vWF, accounting for the reduced factor VIII levels observed in many patients with vWF deficiency.

Factor VIII is not secreted very efficiently from the cell. In addition to LMAN-1 and MCFD-2, several molecular chaperone proteins have been identified that appear to play a role in regulating transit of the factor VIII protein through secretory and/or degradative pathways. Calnexin and calreticulin are chaperone proteins that preferentially interact with glycoproteins containing monoglucosylated N-linked oligosaccharides. These proteins bind to the heavily glycosylated B domain of factor VIII and enhance both its intracellular degradation and secretion.[82] Factor V associates with calreticulin but not with calnexin. Factor VIII, but not factor V, also interacts through its A1 domain with another chaperone protein, immunoglobulin-binding protein (BiP). Association with BiP appears to enhance the stability of factor VIII but also retards its secretion.[83]

Factor VIII has six tyrosine residues that are modified by sulfation (residues 346, 718, 719, 723, 1664, 1680). Sulfation of these residues is required for optimal activation by thrombin, maximal activity in complex with factor IXa, and maximal affinity of factor VIII for vWF.

The acidic regions of factor VIII appear to promote activation by interacting with the anion-binding exosite of thrombin. In addition, the site for factor VIII binding to vWF is in the acidic domain in the light chain of factor VIII.[84]

MOLECULAR BIOLOGY

The factor VIII gene is located on the X chromosome at q28. Deficiency of factor VIII results in classic sex-linked hemophilia A. The factor VIII gene contains 26 exons (see Fig. 106-16), one more than factor V. Exon 5 of factor V corresponds to exons 5 and 6 of the factor VIII gene.[85] The gene for factor VIII is much larger than the gene for factor V, spanning approximately 190 kb. This finding largely results because six of the introns in the factor VIII gene are much larger than the corresponding introns in the factor V gene. The mRNA for factor VIII is also much larger (9 kb) than that for factor V because of a 1.8-kb 3′-untranslated region in the factor VIII message.

ACTIVATION AND ACTIVITY

Factor VIII is activated by thrombin or factor Xa by cleavages at arginyl residues 372, 740, and 1689 (Fig. 106-17). This process produces a heterotrimeric molecule consisting of A1 and A2 domains noncovalently linked with an A3-C1-C2 light chain through calcium ions. Activation also results in release of factor VIIIa from vWF. The factor VIIIa molecule is thermodynamically unstable. Dissociation of the A2 domain results in spontaneous loss of activity. Factor VIIIa also is inactivated by thrombin or APC through additional cleavages at arginyl residues 336 and 562 (Fig. 106-17).

VON WILLEBRAND FACTOR

Chapter 118 discusses the structure, molecular biology, and activities of vWF in greater detail.

PROTEIN STRUCTURE AND ACTIVITY

vWF is a large multimeric glycoprotein that serves as a carrier for factor VIII and is required for normal platelet adhesion to components of the vessel wall. It is synthesized as a pre-propolypeptide with a 22-

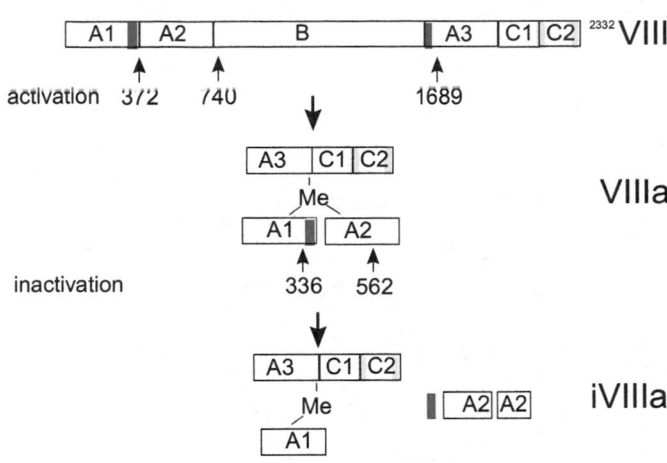

FIGURE 106-17 Activation and inactivation of factor VIII. For full cofactor activity, factor VIII must be cleaved by thrombin or factor Xa. The acidic domains, shown in *dark blue*, are believed to bind to the anion binding exosite in thrombin and enhance thrombin activation of factor VIII. The acidic domain in the A3 domain mediates vWF binding. The chains of factor VIIIa are held together by noncovalent interactions mediated by metal ions (Me). Factor VIIIa is thermodynamically unstable because the A2 domain can spontaneously dissociate from the complex. Membrane binding is mediated through sites in the C2 domain (shown in *light blue*). Cleavages at residues 336 and 562 inactivate factor VIIIa, releasing the A2 fragments (iVIIIa).

amino-acid signal sequence, a 741-amino-acid precursor polypeptide called vWF antigen II, and the mature vWF polypeptide chain.[86] The mature vWF protein contains three A domains, three B domains, two C domains, and four D domains. The A domains are structurally homologous to a family of proteins involved in extracellular matrix or cell adhesive functions.[87] Factor VIII binds to the amino-terminal region of vWF, within the first 272 amino acids of the mature protein subunit.[88] In addition to acting as a carrier for factor VIII, vWF is necessary for normal platelet adhesion and activity (see Chap. 105).

In the ER, the pro-vWF monomers form disulfide-stabilized dimers. The dimers move to the Golgi apparatus, where they assemble into high molecular weight multimers, which also are held together by disulfide bonds. The propeptide is essential for multimerization. The propeptide usually is removed before secretion of the mature vWF multimers. The circulating vWF multimers range in size from M_r approximately 500,000 to greater than 20,000,000.[89] The higher molecular weight multimers are most effective in promoting platelet adhesion. However, all multimers can bind factor VIII and enhance its stability. The plasma half-life of vWF is approximately 12 hours.

MOLECULAR BIOLOGY

The vWF gene is located on chromosome 12 and spans approximately 180 kb. It contains 52 exons.[90] vWF is synthesized only in endothelial cells and megakaryocytes.

FACTOR XI AND THE CONTACT FACTORS

FACTOR XI

PROTEIN STRUCTURE

Factor XI, along with factor XII, high molecular weight kininogen (HK), and prekallikrein (PK), are sometimes referred to as the *contact factors*. Factor XI is a zymogen precursor of a serine protease. Factor XI circulates in complex with the nonenzymatic cofactor HK.

Factor XI is synthesized in the liver. It has a plasma mean half-life of approximately 52 hours. Although factor XI is synthesized as a single chain, it circulates as a homodimer held together by a disulfide bond.[91] Each subunit is M_r approximately 80,000, including approximately 5 percent carbohydrate. Each factor XI subunit contains four repeats of a structural motif called an "apple domain" (Fig. 106-18). Each apple domain contains 90 or 91 amino acids held together by three disulfide bonds. Specific functions have been assigned to the different apple domains within factor XI,[92-95] including sites for binding to HK, prothrombin, platelets, factor IX, thrombin, and factor XIIa.

MOLECULAR BIOLOGY

The human factor XI gene is 23 kb in length and is localized to chromosome 4q32-35.[96] It consists of 15 exons and 14 introns (Fig. 106-19).[97] The gene lacks canonical CAAT and TATA boxes, which may account for the multiple transcription initiation sites that have been identified. Exon 1 encodes a 5′ untranslated region that is transcribed into mRNA but not translated into protein. The signal peptide is encoded in exon 2. Each of the four apple domains is encoded in two exons. The light chain is encoded in five exons, with an organization similar to the homologous proteins PK, tissue plasminogen activator, urokinase, and factor XII. An HNF-4α binding site required for liver-specific expression is located between −375 and −363 bp.[98]

ACTIVATION AND ACTIVITY

Factor XI can be activated by more than one mechanism *in vitro*. *In vitro*, factor XI can be activated by factor XIIa. In the fluid phase and on charged surfaces, thrombin can activate factor XI even in the absence of other contact factors.[99,100] Factor XI also can be activated by thrombin on the surface of activated platelets, and this pathway is perhaps the most likely mechanism of activation *in vivo*.[101] More than one mechanism may operate under certain circumstances, but definitive proof is lacking.

In contrast to the other contact factors, deficiencies of factor XI can lead to excessive bleeding usually related to injury.[102] The bleeding tendency reflects the significant role of factor XI in hemostasis (see Chap. 116).

Activation by either factor XIIa or thrombin results from cleavage of the Arg369-Ile370 bond in the factor XI subunit. This process leads to the presence of two active sites in each factor XIa dimer. Each subunit has a heavy chain containing the apple domains and a light chain containing the catalytic domain (see Fig. 106-18). Both the heavy and light chains interact with the substrate factor IX.[103] Factor XIa activation of factor IX is calcium dependent but does not require any other cofactor. Factor XIa binds with high affinity to activated platelets and can activate factor IX with the same efficiency as unbound factor XIa.[104] Binding to activated platelets could localize factor XIa to the site of clot formation and protect it from plasma protease inhibitors.

Factor XIa is susceptible to inhibition by several plasma protease inhibitors that circulate in high concentrations. The serpin protease nexin-1 has the highest affinity for factor XIa, followed by C1 esterase inhibitor, AT, α_1 protease inhibitor, and α_2 plasmin inhibitor.[105] Platelets also contain tight-binding Kunitz-type inhibitor of factor XIa, protease nexin 2.[106]

FACTOR XII, PK, AND HK

PROTEIN STRUCTURE

Factor XII and PK are zymogen precursors of proteases. PK has four apple domains and is highly homologous to factor XI. Factor XII is homologous to plasminogen activators. HK is a nonenzymatic cofactor that circulates in complex with factor XI and with PK. In addition to

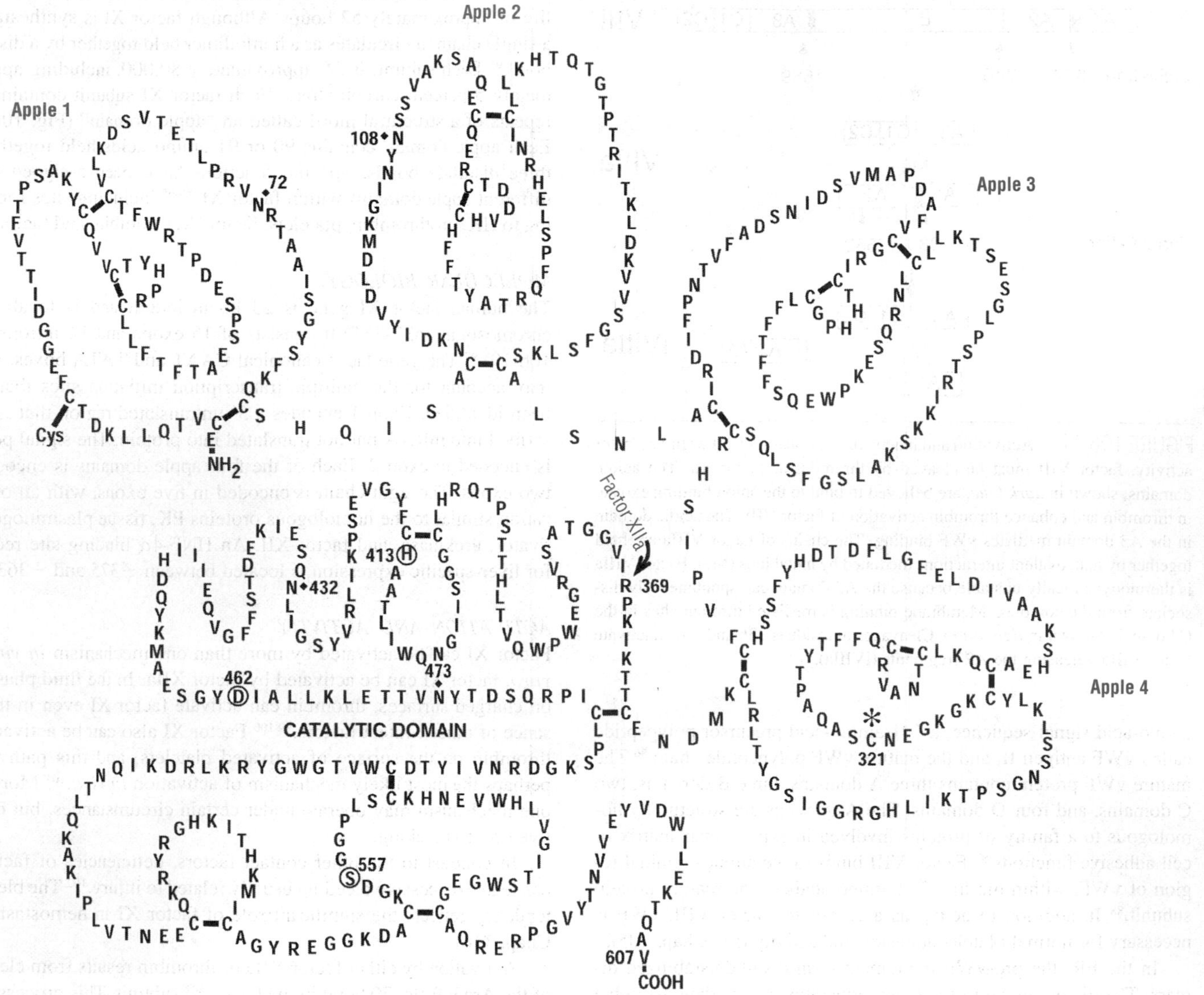

FIGURE 106-18 Domains of factor XI. Each amino acid in circulating factor XI is shown. The disulfide bond that links the factor XI homodimers is indicated by the Cys residue in the first apple domain. The apple domains (A1–A4) are named for their appearance in this type of schematic. The active site residues His, Asp, and Ser residues are *circled*. The cleavage site for factor XIIa is shown by the *arrow*.

its nonenzymatic role in contact activation, HK acts as a thiol protease inhibitor and as an antiadhesive protein. HK is cleaved at two sites by kallikrein to release the bioactive nonapeptide bradykinin, a potent vasodilator. Table 106-1 lists the plasma levels, plasma half-lives, and chromosomal locations of factor XII, PK and HK.[107] All three proteins are synthesized in the liver.

MOLECULAR BIOLOGY

The gene for factor XII is located on chromosome 5q33-qter and spans approximately 12 kb. It contains 14 exons. The intron–exon structure of the gene is similar to the plasminogen activator family of serine proteases. Portions of the gene are homologous to domains found in fibronectin and tissue-type plasminogen activator. The gene for PK is located on chromosome 4q35, close to the factor XI gene, and spans 30 kb. It has 15 exons with 14 introns and is homologous to the factor XI gene.[108] The gene for HK is located on chromosome 3, contains 11 exons, and spans 27 kb. HK and low molecular weight kininogen are produced from the same gene by alternative splicing. Both proteins

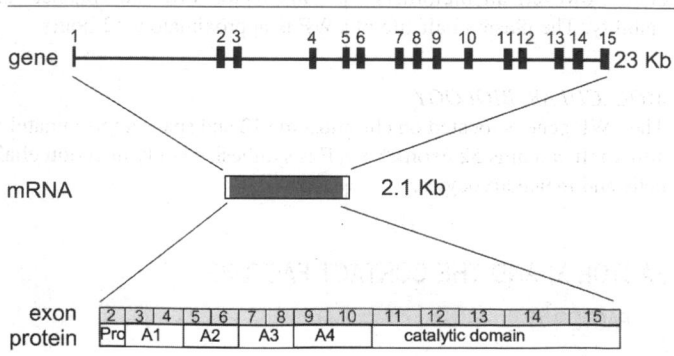

FIGURE 106-19 Relation between gene structure and protein structure in factor XI. The exons, introns, mRNA, and protein structure are as indicated. The mRNA is 2.1 kb, with a small 5′ and 3′ untranslated region. A, apple domains; Pro, pre-pro leader sequence.

serve as precursors to bradykinin, but low molecular weight kininogen has no interaction with the coagulation proteins.

ACTIVATION AND ACTIVITY

Factor XII, HK, and PK are responsible for contact activation of blood coagulation as determined by the activated partial thromboplastin time (aPTT). In this clinical laboratory test, plasma is mixed with a reagent such as glass, kaolin, celite, or ellagic acid, which provides a negatively charged surface. Contact activation involves both protein–protein and protein–surface interactions that lead to activation of factor XII. Factor XIIa activates factor XI, which then activates factor IX. Even though factor XII, HK, and PK are required for a normal aPTT, they do not appear to be required for normal hemostasis. Individuals who are deficient in any of these factors do not have a bleeding tendency, even after significant trauma or surgery. However, factor XII, HK, and PK, along with complement factor C1q, participate in inflammatory responses that involve the blood clotting system, fibrinolysis, and generation of kinins.[109,110]

CELL-ASSOCIATED COFACTORS

TISSUE FACTOR

PROTEIN STRUCTURE

TF is the cellular receptor and cofactor for factor VII and VIIa (see Fig. 106-4). TF is composed of 263 amino acids: a 219-amino-acid extracellular domain, a 23-residue transmembrane portion, and a 21-residue intracytoplasmic domain (Fig. 106-20).[111] A cysteine in the intracytoplasmic domain is linked to a palmityl fatty acid, which down-regulates phosphorylation of the cytoplasmic domain.[112] Many of the coagulation factors share a high degree of homology, but the structure of TF is unique. TF is the only procoagulant protein that is an integral membrane protein. It is homologous to the type 2 cytokine receptors.[113] This family includes the receptors for interleukin (IL)-10, interferon-α, interferon-β, and interferon-γ. The TF molecule has been crystallized. The extracellular domain folds in a manner typical of the cytokine receptor homology unit (see Fig. 106-4).[18,114] These structural features suggest TF is a multifunctional protein with both signal transducing and procoagulant functions.

MOLECULAR BIOLOGY

The human TF gene is located on chromosome 1p21-p22.[115] The DNA sequence of the TF gene consists of six exons and five introns that

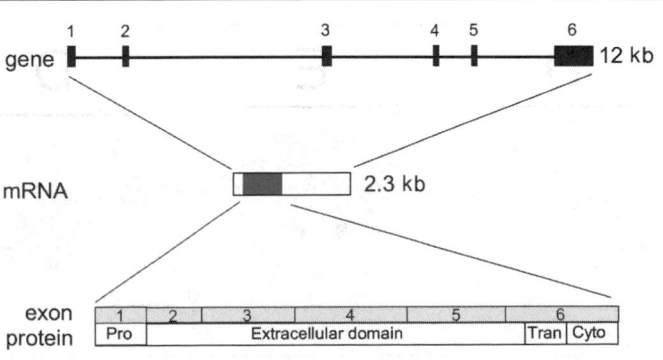

FIGURE 106-20   Relation between gene structure and protein structure in tissue factor. The exons, introns, mRNA, and protein structure are as indicated. The mRNA is 2.3 kb, with 5′ untranslated region and a large 3′ untranslated region. Cyto, cytoplasmic domain; Pro, pre-pro leader sequence; Tran, transmembrane region.

span approximately 12 kb.[116] The first exon codes for the signal peptide; the second through fifth exons encode the extracellular domain. The sixth exon codes for the transmembrane and cytoplasmic domains and a relatively long 3′ untranslated region. An alternatively spliced form of TF that lacks the membrane-anchoring domain has been described.[117] It reportedly is present in the blood and possesses cofactor activity, but its role in hemostasis or thrombosis remains to be clarified.

The initiation site for transcription of the TF gene is well defined. The region with promoter activity is located from −383 to −121 bp relative to the start site.[118] The promoter contains a serum response element with a putative binding site for Sp-1 and a lipopolysaccharide responsive element with transcription factor activator protein AP-1 and nuclear factor (NF)-κB–like sites.

TF is expressed constitutively on many extravascular tissues. TF is not normally expressed by cells in contact with flowing blood, but TF expression can be induced on blood monocytes and vascular endothelial cells by bacterial products, inflammatory cytokines, and engagement of P-selectin glycoprotein ligand-1 on monocytes.[119–122] Expression of intravascular TF may contribute to the procoagulant state associated with inflammation or infection.

ACTIVATION AND ACTIVITY

The factor VIIa/TF complex is thought to be the major physiologic initiator of blood coagulation. TF is normally expressed in the adventitia of blood vessels and by epidermal, stromal, and glial cells.[123,124] Leukocytes, which normally have no TF activity, can express TF when exposed to vessel media or collagen.[125] The process of coagulation is initiated when an injury ruptures a vessel and allows blood to come into contact with extravascular TF. Circulating factor VII bound to TF is rapidly converted to the active protease factor VIIa.[51] The factor VIIa/TF complex can activate factors IX and X.[126]

The binding of factor VIIa to TF enhances its proteolytic activity by almost three orders of magnitude.[127,128] However, unlike binding of factor IXa or Xa to its cofactor, binding of factor VIIa to TF does not strictly require calcium,[129] and the affinity of the interaction is only slightly enhanced by the presence of anionic phospholipid.[130,131] However, cleavage of factor IX or X by factor VIIa/TF is enhanced by anionic phospholipid.[131] This effect results from enhanced binding of the substrate rather than any effect of the phospholipid on the catalytic efficiency of the VIIa/TF complex.

The affinity of factor VIIa binding for TF on cells is very high (20–80 pM). Binding of factor VIIa to TF that is reconstituted into synthetic phospholipid vesicles always results in enhanced factor VIIa proteolytic activity. However, binding of factor VIIa to cellular sources of TF does not always correlate with enhanced enzymatic activity. This finding suggests cells regulate the cofactor activity of TF in a manner that is not reproduced by synthetic phospholipid vesicles.

TF does not require proteolytic activation to express its activity. However, TF apparently occurs in a latent or "encrypted" form,[132,133] that is, TF detected as antigen on the cell surface may not express detectable clotting activity. TF is hypothesized to form dimers that block access to the substrate binding site on TF. Dimerized ("encrypted") TF could still bind factor VII but would be inactive because it could not bind factor IX or X. The physiologic regulators controlling TF encryption are not clear, and whether this is an important regulatory mechanism *in vivo* remains to be determined.

In addition to its role as a cofactor in coagulation, TF is thought to play important roles in cell signaling. The signaling can occur through proteolytic activity of factor VIIa bound to TF[134] and through formation of a VIIa/TF/Xa complex.[135] This cell signaling has been suggested to play important roles in cell migration needed for wound healing, inflammation, and vasculogenesis. The importance of this signaling in vasculogenesis is suggested by the observation that mice in

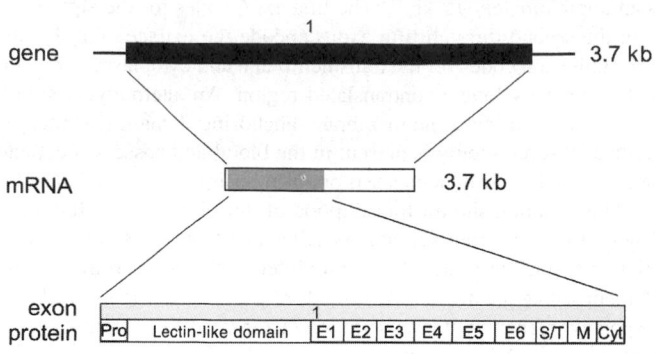

gene   3.7 kb

mRNA   3.7 kb

exon
protein | Pro | Lectin-like domain | E1 | E2 | E3 | E4 | E5 | E6 | S/T | M | Cyt |

FIGURE 106-21   Relation between gene structure and protein structure in thrombomodulin. The thrombomodulin gene has no introns. It covers 3.7 kb on chromosome 20 (p12-centromere). The mRNA is the same size, with a small 5′ untranslated region and a large 3′ untranslated region. Cyt, cytoplasmic domain; E, epidermal growth factor–like domains; M, transmembrane region; Pro, pre-pro leader sequence; S/T, serine- and threonine-rich region.

which the TF gene has been knocked out die during embryonic development, partly because of disorganization of the yolk sac vasculature.[136]

THROMBOMODULIN

PROTEIN STRUCTURE

TM is a transmembrane protein of M_r 78,000.[137] It is the cellular cofactor for thrombin.[138] TM has a leader sequence followed by lectin-like domains homologous to the asialoglycoprotein receptor (Fig. 106-21)[139] but has no known lectin-like activity. Following the lectin-like domain are six EGF-like domains. The fourth, fifth and sixth domains are responsible for thrombin-binding and protein C–activating activities (Fig. 106-21).[140] A serine- and threonine-rich region follows the EGF domains and is the site of O-linked glycosylation. A chondroitin sulfate moiety, which enhances TM anticoagulant activity, is attached to Ser492 in this region.[141] The 23-amino-acid transmembrane domain follows the serine- and threonine-rich region, followed by a short cytoplasmic tail.

MOLECULAR BIOLOGY

The human TM gene is located on chromosome 20p12-cen[142] and spans approximately 3.7 kb. It consists of a single exon (see Fig. 106-21). Intronless genes are uncommon and include rhodopsin, angiogenin, mitochondrial genes, interferon-α, interferon-β, and β-adrenergic receptors. The functional significance of the lack of introns is not known.

ACTIVATION AND ACTIVITY

Thrombin can cleave a number of substrates without a cofactor, such as fibrinogen, factors V and VIII, and the PARs. However, binding to the cofactor TM localizes thrombin to endothelial cell surfaces and induces a conformational change such that its ability to activate protein C is enhanced 1000- to 2000-fold. Thrombin bound to TM no longer activates platelets, does not cleave fibrinogen, and does not activate factor V or factor VIII.[143] Thus, TM changes the activity of thrombin from procoagulant to anticoagulant. TM also enhances the ability of thrombin to activate TAFI.[29]

TM is expressed on the surface of vascular endothelial cells. In conjunction with EPCR-1, TM appears to play a major role in preventing thrombosis on intact endothelium.[144] In mice, knocking out either TM or EPCR-1 creates an embryonically lethal phenotype correlated with increased placental fibrin deposition.[145,146] TM also has

been detected in mesothelial cells,[147] mononuclear phagocytes,[148] squamous epithelium,[149] megakaryocytes, and malignant cells,[31,150] where its function is unknown. The level of TM expression differs among endothelial cells from various sites.[151] Endothelial TM and TF expressions are regulated by inflammatory cytokines in a reciprocal fashion. Thus, thrombosis may be favored at sites of inflammation by concurrent elevation of endothelial TF and depression of endothelial TM.

Protein C inhibitor is an effective inhibitor of the thrombin/TM complex.[152]

FIBRINOGEN

PROTEIN STRUCTURE

When fibrinogen is converted to fibrin, it forms the structural meshwork that consolidates an initial platelet plug into a solid hemostatic clot. The physiologic importance of fibrinogen is underscored by the bleeding diathesis associated with afibrinogenemia[153,154] and some dysfibrinogenemias (see Chap. 117).[155] Other dysfibrinogenemias are associated with thromboembolic disease (database is available at *http://www.geht.org/databaseang/fibrinogen*).[154,156]

Fibrinogen is a dimeric glycoprotein whose dominant form has an M_r of 340,000. It is found in plasma and in platelet α-granules. Each of the two subunits contains three disulfide-linked polypeptide chains[157] referred to as the Aα (M_r 66,500), Bβ (M_r 52,000), and γ (M_r 46,500) chains. Fibrinopeptides A and B are released from the amino-termini of the Aα and Bβ chains by thrombin cleavage of the Arg16-Gly17 and Arg14-Gly15 bonds, respectively.[158] The central globular domain of fibrinogen is called the *E domain*. The E domain includes the disulfide-linked amino-termini of all six polypeptide chains referred to as the *N-terminal disulfide knot*.[159] The E domain is linked by helical, coiled-coil domains to the carboxy-terminal globular domains of the three chains, designated the *D domains*. A trinodular model of fibrinogen structure has been established from the crystal structure of fibrinogen (Fig. 106-22).[160] N-linked glycosylation occurs at Asn364 of the Bβ chain and Asn52 of the γ chain.

In normal individuals, the plasma half-life of fibrinogen is 3 to 5 days.[161] Only a small proportion of the catabolism results from consumption. Plasma fibrinogen is synthesized in the liver. Fibrinogen is an acute phase reactant, and its synthesis can be increased up to 20-fold with a strong inflammatory stimulus.[162,163] IL-6 is an important mediator of increased fibrinogen synthesis during an acute phase re-

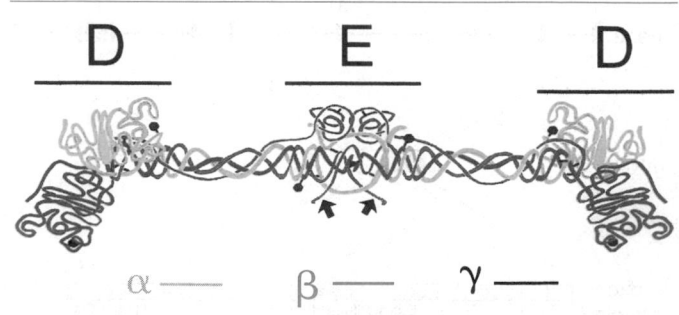

FIGURE 106-22   Structure of fibrinogen. Fibrinogen is a dimer. Each dimer consists of three chains: Aα *(gray)*, Bβ *(dark blue)*, and γ *(black)*. The disulfides linking the two dimers are in the central E domain. The D domains consist primarily of the carboxy-terminal regions of the Bβ and γ chains. The helical region connecting the two domains consists of all three chains intertwined. (Adapted from Côté et al. *Blood* 92:2195, 1998.)

sponse,[164] and IL-6 secretion can be up-regulated by fibrin(ogen) degradation products.

MOLECULAR BIOLOGY

The genes for the three chains of fibrinogen are found within a 50-kb length of DNA on chromosome 4 at q23-q32 (Fig. 106-23).[165] The genes for all three chains have been sequenced. The genomic sequences show a high degree of homology, suggesting they are derived through duplication of a common ancestral gene.[166,167] The homology extends to sites upstream of the gene, suggesting common regulatory elements reside in these areas, thus helping to coordinate synthesis of the three chains.[168]

Studies of tissue-specific expression and acute phase regulation of the mRNA of the fibrinogen chains have revealed some surprises. Expression of the γ-chain is regulated by ubiquitous factors such as SP1, whereas transcription of the Aα and Bβ genes requires the liver-specific factor HNF-1.[169] The Bβ chain promoter contains an IL-6–responsive element[170] that appears to be present in the upstream sequences of the other chains. Because of the differences in the promoter regions of the genes for the three chains, the tissue distribution differs. The highest levels of mRNA for all three chains are found in the liver. However, γ-chain transcripts are found in a number of organs that lack transcripts of the other chains. Messenger RNA for Aα and Bβ is found in the kidney, consistent with the presence of HNF-1 in the kidney.[171]

Because of the presence of fibrinogen in the α-granules of platelets, megakaryocytes initially were presumed to synthesize fibrinogen. However, although some γ-chain transcripts are present in bone marrow precursors, most of the fibrinogen found within platelets appears to be taken up from the plasma by $\alpha_{IIb}\beta_3$-mediated endocytosis (see Chap. 105).[172,173]

ACTIVATION AND ACTIVITY

Thrombin binds to the central domain of fibrinogen[174] and proteolytically releases two fibrinopeptides A (Aα 1-16) and two fibrino-

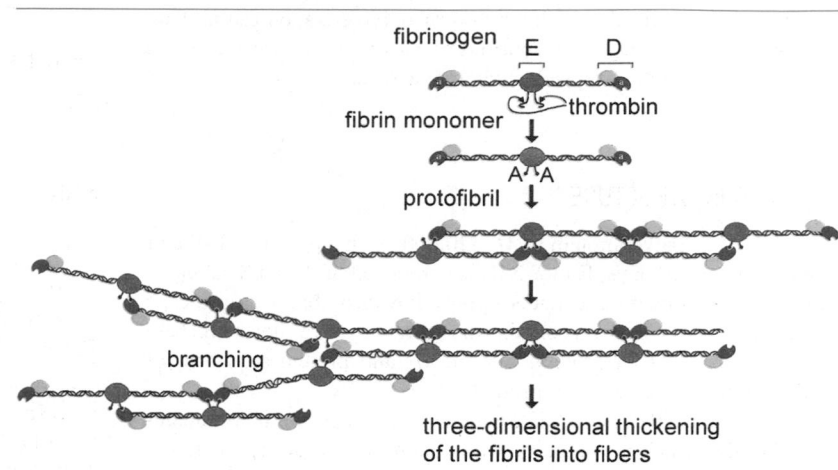

FIGURE 106-24 Cleavage of fibrinogen and polymerization of fibrin. The structure of fibrinogen is indicated schematically. Cleavage sites for fibrinopeptide A by thrombin are shown. Cleavage of the B peptide is not shown in this figure. Release of fibrinopeptide A exposes binding sites in the E domain that match complementary sites in the D domain. Fibrin monomers polymerize by half-staggered overlaps. Polymerization also can lead to branched structures. (Adapted from Côté et al. *Blood* 92:2195, 1998.)

peptides B (Bβ 1-14) from each fibrinogen molecule. Release of fibrinopeptides exposes binding sites in the E domain that have complementary sites in the D domains of other fibrin monomers.[175,176] These complementary binding sites lead to the initial formation of two-stranded protofibrils having a half staggered overlap configuration (Fig. 106-24). Protofibrils then aggregate into thick fibers consisting of 14 to 22 protofibrils that branch into a meshwork of interconnected thick fibers.[177] The half-staggered overlap of the fibrin monomers gives a characteristic cross-banded pattern on electron micrographs.[178] Calcium appears to enhance lateral fiber growth by binding to sites on human fibrinogen.[179,180]

During fibrin monomer polymerization, other plasma proteins also bind to the surface of the developing meshwork. These proteins include elements of the fibrinolytic system and a variety of adhesive proteins including fibronectin, thrombospondin, and vWF. These surface proteins influence the generation, cross-linking, and lysis of fibrin. Fibrin(ogen) also has specific integrin-binding sites essential for platelet binding (for additional details see Chap. 105). The thrombin that initiates fibrin polymerization also activates factor XIII, which stabilizes the fibrin polymer by cross-linking. Factor XIIIa also cross-links other bound proteins, such as plasminogen activator-1, vitronectin, fibronectin, and α2-antiplasmin, to the fibrin network.

Once formed, the fibrin mesh can be degraded by the fibrinolytic system (see Chap. 127). Plasmin cleaves fibrin and fibrinogen in an ordered sequence at arginyl and lysyl bonds, giving rise to a series of soluble degradation products.[181] Plasmin digestion of fibrinogen initially cleaves the Aα polar appendage and the Bβ 1-42 fragment, generating fragment X (M_r 250,000), which still can form a clot, albeit slowly. Further action of plasmin releases a D fragment (M_r 100,000) from fragment X to form fragment Y (M_r 150,000). Fragment Y is further cleaved to form another fragment D and a fragment E (M_r 50,000). Similar fragments are generated during plasmin digestion of cross-linked fibrin, with two exceptions: (1) Bβ 15-42 is released from the des 1-14 Bβ chain of fibrin, and (2) D dimer and other covalently cross-linked degradation products are cleaved from the cross-linked fibrin polymer. Monoclonal antibodies recognizing the fibrin D-dimer fragments can help discriminate fibrin degradation products from fibrinogen degradation products.[182] Although the large X fragment still can polymerize into a weak clot,[183] the smaller Y and D fragments inhibit normal fibrin

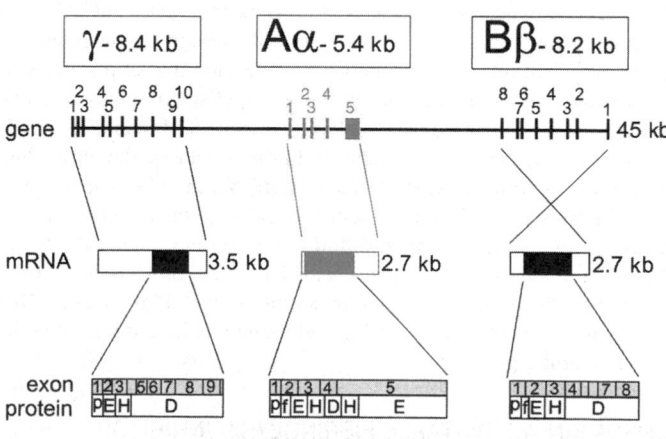

FIGURE 106-23 Relation between gene structure and protein structure in fibrinogen. The exons, introns, mRNA, and protein structure for the three chains of fibrinogen are shown. The Bβ chain is translated in the opposite direction from the Aα and γ chains. D, residues in the D domain; E, residues in the E domain; f, fibrinopeptic residues; H, residues in the helical connecting region; P, pre-pro leader sequence.

monomer polymerization.[184] Inhibition of polymerization can prolong the thrombin time and lead to spuriously low values of fibrinogen when measured by thrombin-dependent clotting assays.

FACTOR XIII

PROTEIN STRUCTURE

Factor XIII is a glycoprotein of M_r 320,000, with a plasma half-life of approximately 10 days. Factor XIII is composed of A and B subunits. It is a protransglutaminase that is activated by thrombin in the presence of calcium.[185] The A chain contains the cysteine active site; the B chain functions as a carrier protein. The cDNA and protein sequences of both subunits have been determined.[186-188]

The factor XIII A chain is a unique member of the transglutaminase family, which is composed of calcium- and thiol-dependent enzymes found in all human tissues and fluids. Factor XIIIa cross-links proteins between the γ-carbon of glutamine in one protein and the ε-amino group of lysine in the other. The A chain contains 731 amino acids with M_r approximately 83,000 (Fig. 106-25).

The B chain is homologous to complement regulatory proteins. It is synthesized as a chain of 661 amino acids starting with a signal peptide. The mature B chain is composed of 641 amino acids,[188] with M_r approximately 76,500, including 8.5 percent carbohydrate. The B chain contains 10 short consensus repeat (SCR) units (also called GP-1 or sushi domains) (Fig. 106-26). Each SCR contains 60 to 70 amino acids, containing four conserved cysteine residues with a characteristic pattern of disulfide bonds.[189] In plasma, the B subunit is present in molar excess over the A component. Thus, all circulating A subunit is bound to B subunit. The B subunit also occurs free in circulation.

In addition to plasma, factor XIII occurs in platelets, monocytes, and monocyte-derived macrophages. The plasma factor is a heterotetramer consisting of paired A and B subunits (A2B2). In platelet and other cells, factor XIII exists as an A2 dimer and lacks the B domain. Monocytes/macrophages can synthesize factor XIII,[190] and the factor XIII found in platelets probably is synthesized by megakaryocytes.[191] Cells of bone marrow origin seem to be the primary site for synthesis of subunit A in plasma factor XIII, but hepatocytes also may contribute.[185] The B subunit of plasma factor XIII is synthesized in the liver.

MOLECULAR BIOLOGY

The factor XIII A chain gene has been localized to chromosome 6 p24-p25.[192] It contains 15 exons and 14 introns and is more than 160 kb

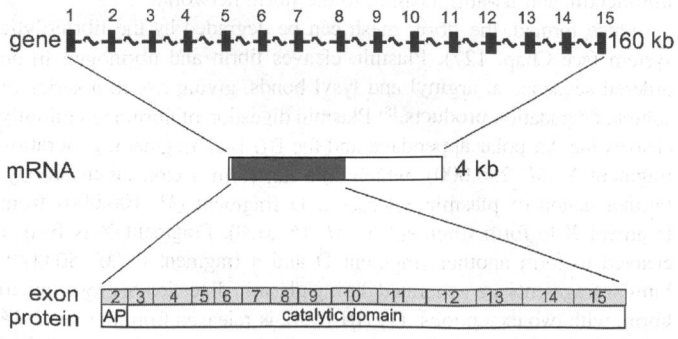

FIGURE 106-25   Relation between gene structure and protein structure in the factor XIII A chain. The exons, mRNA, and protein structure for the factor XIII A chain are shown. The size of the introns in the factor XIII A chain has not been published. The mRNA is 4 kb, with some 5′ untranslated sequence coded in exon 1 and a large 3′ untranslated region. AP, activation peptide.

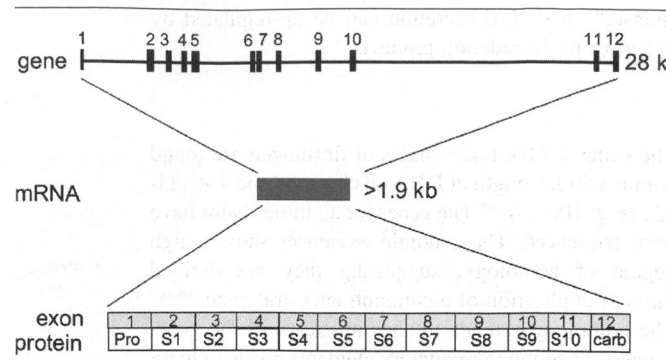

FIGURE 106-26   Relation between gene structure and protein structure in the factor XIII B chain. The exons, introns, mRNA, and protein structure are as indicated. Full-length cDNA has not been isolated, so the size of the mRNA is not known. carb, carboxy-terminal region; Pro, propeptide; S, sushi (SCR) domains.

in size (see Fig. 106-25).[187] The fibrin-binding domain is encoded by exons 2 to 12. The active site, with its reactive thiol at Cys314, is present in exon 7. The structure of the factor XIII A-chain gene is quite similar to that of other transglutaminases; however, it has unique regulatory mechanisms. Transcription is regulated by a myeloid-enriched transcription factor (MZF-1–like protein) and two ubiquitous transcription factors (NF-1 and SP-1).[193] The factor GATA-1 acts as an enhancer, as does Ets-1.[193] The transcription initiation site for the A chain is 76 bp upstream from the first intron/exon boundary.[193]

The factor XIII B chain has been localized to chromosome 1q31-q32.1. It has 12 exons separated by 11 introns and is approximately 28 kb in size (see Fig. 106-26).[186] Each SCR is encoded by a single exon. Regulation of factor XIII B-chain expression is poorly understood. A total of 30 potential start sites are located upstream of the initial methionine.

ACTIVATION AND ACTIVITY

Plasma factor XIII circulates in association with its substrate fibrinogen. The key step in activation of plasma factor XIII is thrombin cleavage of the Arg37-Gly38 bond in the A chain to release an activation peptide of M_r 4500. This process leads to dissociation of the A and B subunits and exposure of the active site on the free A subunits. Cellular factor XIII in platelets becomes activated through a nonproteolytic process. When intracytoplasmic Ca^{2+} is elevated during platelet activation, the zymogen, in the absence of the B chain, assumes an active configuration.[185] The main physiologic function of plasma factor XIIIa is to cross-link the α- and γ-chains of fibrin to stabilize the fibrin plug. A clot forms in the absence of factor XIII, but the clot is inadequate for hemostasis. Additional protein substrates of factor XIIIa include components of the clotting and fibrinolytic system, and multiple adhesive and contractile proteins. Factor XIIIa also protects fibrin from fibrinolysis by cross-linking it to α_2-antiplasmin.[194] Plasma factor XIII also is involved in wound healing and tissue repair, and it is essential to maintaining pregnancy.

THROMBIN ACTIVATABLE FIBRINOLYSIS INHIBITOR

PROTEIN STRUCTURE

TAFI is the zymogen precursor to a zinc-bound metalloprotease. It has been called carboxypeptidase B, R, and U. It has an M_r of 60,000, with 20 percent of the mass consisting of carbohydrate attached to four sites within the first 92 amino acids. In sequence alignments with other members of the carboxypeptidase A family, active site residues (Glu271, Arg125) and zinc-binding residues (His67, Glu70, His196) in TAFI are conserved.

MOLECULAR BIOLOGY

The gene for TAFI has been localized to 13q14. The gene contains 11 exons with 10 introns and spans 48 kb.[195] TAFI is synthesized in the liver. The TAFI promoter has a C/EBP binding site that regulates liver synthesis.[196] The promoter lacks a consensus TATA box, and transcription is initiated from multiple sites. Plasma concentration of TAFI in individuals can vary from four to 15 μg/mL with a strong correlation between plasma levels and polymorphisms in the promoter and 3′ regions.[197]

ACTIVATION AND ACTIVITY

TAFI is activated by cleavage by thrombin and plasmin, a reaction that is accelerated 1000-fold when thrombin is bound to TM. Both enzymes cleave after Arg-92 to give an activated form of M_r 37,000 (TAFIa) with release of the large activation peptide. TAFIa catalyzes removal of carboxy-terminal lysine and arginine residues from fibrin and fibrin cleavage products. These residues are important for binding and activation of plasminogen. Removal of these residues by TAFIa reduces clot-catalyzed formation of plasmin, resulting in decreased clot lysis. TAFIa also may have an anti-inflammatory role because it can efficiently cleave bradykinin. A polymorphism in TAFI is associated with lower blood pressure in individuals homozygous for the polymorphism.[198]

Inhibitors of TAFIa have not been identified; however, the molecule is thermodynamically unstable with a half-life of less than 15 minutes at 37°C.[199]

INHIBITORS

Many protease inhibitors are present in plasma, but the two most specifically involved in inhibition of coagulation factors are TFPI and AT (see Table 106-4). The protein Z/protein Z–dependent protease inhibitor (ZPI) system is emerging as a potentially important regulator of the coagulation system.[200]

Coagulation inhibitors are discussed in detail in Chapter 107.

TISSUE FACTOR PATHWAY INHIBITOR

PROTEIN STRUCTURE AND ACTIVITY

TFPI is a single-chain polypeptide with M_r 34,000 to 40,000, depending on the degree of proteolysis of the carboxy-terminal region. TFPI contains three Kunitz-type protease inhibitor domains. The second Kunitz domain binds and inhibits factor Xa, and this binding is required for the first Kunitz domain to bind and inhibit the factor VIIa/TF complex. The function of the third Kunitz domain is not clear, but it may be involved in binding to glycosaminoglycans. Thus, TFPI is unique among the coagulation protease inhibitors in two respects. First, it has inhibitory sites for both factor Xa and the factor VIIa/TF complex. Second, TFPI cannot inhibit the VIIa/TF complex unless it also has bound factor Xa.[201,202]

The primary site of plasma TFPI synthesis is endothelial cells.[203] The major pool of TFPI is bound to heparan sulfate on the surface of endothelial cells. Most of the remaining TFPI in blood is bound to lipoproteins. Administration of heparin releases the endothelial cell-bound TFPI and raises the plasma level several-fold.[204] A third pool is the alternatively spliced form of TFPI (TFPI-β), which is anchored to endothelial cells via a glycosyl phosphatidylinositol linkage.[205]

TFPI is only present in the plasma at approximately 2.5 nM, compared to AT at approximately 2000 nM. However, its rate of reaction with factor Xa in plasma is similar to that of AT. Therefore, TFPI contributes significantly to inhibition of factor Xa *in vivo*.

MOLECULAR BIOLOGY

The gene for human TFPI is located on chromosome 2q31-q32.1. It has nine exons that span 70 kb. The first two exons code for a 5′ untranslated region, and coding begins at exon 3. No TATA box is present in the promoter region of the TFPI gene. DNA sequences consistent with binding sites for the transcription factors GATA-2, AP-1, and NF-1 are present in the 5′ untranslated region of the TFPI gene. GATA-2 binding is believed to be necessary for constitutive expression of TFPI by endothelial cells.[203]

TFPI is synthesized in two alternatively spliced forms, α and β. TFPI-β lacks the third Kunitz domain and has a unique carboxy-terminal. TFPI-α is the predominant form in circulation. A significant fraction of TFPI-β is linked to the endothelial cells via a glycosyl phosphatidylinositol anchor, but TFPI-β also is found in plasma and has inhibitory activity similar to that of TFPI-α.[206]

ANTITHROMBIN

PROTEIN STRUCTURE AND ACTIVITY

AT is a member of the large family of serpins. These inhibitors act as "suicide" substrates for their target proteases through a surface-exposed structure termed a *reactive site* loop. An amino acid sequence in the reactive site loop of AT is cleaved by the target protease to form a 1:1 covalent complex that blocks the active site of the protease. The primary proteases targeted by AT are thrombin, factor Xa, and factor IXa.[207–209] Inhibition of these proteases is accelerated by heparin or glycosaminoglycans such as heparan sulfate. Factor VIIa is resistant to inhibition by AT unless it is complexed to TF in the presence of heparin or cell surface glycosaminoglycans.[210,211] The protease–serpin complex is cleared from the circulation by receptor-mediated endocytosis in the liver.[212] AT is an important physiologic inhibitor of the blood coagulation proteases because its deficiency leads to a significantly increased risk of thrombosis (see Chap. 122).

MOLECULAR BIOLOGY

The gene for AT is located on chromosome 1 q23-25. The gene has seven exons and spans approximately 13.5 kb. Little is known about transcriptional regulation of AT. The region from −89 to −68 has been implicated in the binding of transcription factors from rat liver,[213] but the specific transcription factors involved are not clear.

PROTEIN Z/PROTEIN Z–DEPENDENT PROTEASE INHIBITOR

PROTEIN STRUCTURE AND ACTIVITY

ZPI is a serine protease inhibitor of M_r 72,000 that inhibits coagulation factor Xa. Its inhibition of factor Xa is enhanced more than 1000-fold in the presence of protein Z, a vitamin K–dependent plasma protein.[214] Protein Z is a plasma glycoprotein of M_r 62,000. Like the other Gla-containing proteins, protein Z consists of a Gla domain, hydrophobic region, and two EGF domains. However, instead of a catalytic domain, the carboxy-terminal region of protein Z contains a domain that, although homologous to the catalytic domain of the other Gla-containing proteins, lacks the His and Ser residues characteristic of the catalytic triad of trypsin-like serine proteases. Thus, protein Z has no protease activity. In normal plasma, which has a molar excess of ZPI over protein Z, all protein Z circulates in complex with ZPI.[215]

The normal role of protein Z/ZPI in the coagulation system is not clear. Protein Z deficiency in a mouse model does not lead to thrombosis but dramatically worsens the thrombotic tendency of mice that simultaneously express the factor V Leiden genotype, a known risk factor for thrombosis.[216]

MOLECULAR BIOLOGY

The chromosomal location of the gene for ZPI is not known. The gene for protein Z is on the long arm of chromosome 13 (q34) in close proximity to the genes for factors X and VII.[3] The gene spans 14 kb and consists of nine exons and eight introns. The intron–exon boundaries are identical to the other Gla-containing coagulation proteins. An alternative exon codes for a unique peptide of 22 amino acids in the pre-pro leader sequence. The gene is transcribed into a 1.6-kb mRNA.

PATHWAYS OF HEMOSTASIS

EARLY MODELS OF COAGULATION

In the 1960s, two groups proposed a model of coagulation that envisaged a sequential series of steps in which activation of one clotting factor led to activation of another clotting factor, finally leading to a burst of thrombin generation.[217,218] Each clotting factor was thought to exist as a proenzyme that could be converted to an active enzyme.

The original cascade models subsequently were modified to include the observation that some procoagulants were cofactors and did not possess enzymatic activity. In addition, the clotting sequences were divided into so-called *extrinsic* and *intrinsic* systems (Fig. 106-27). The extrinsic system consisted of factor VIIa and TF, with the latter viewed as extrinsic to the circulating blood. The factors in the so-called intrinsic system were all viewed as being intravascular. Both pathways could activate factor X, which in complex with its cofactor Va could convert prothrombin to thrombin. Although these earlier concepts of coagulation were extremely valuable, several groups recognized that

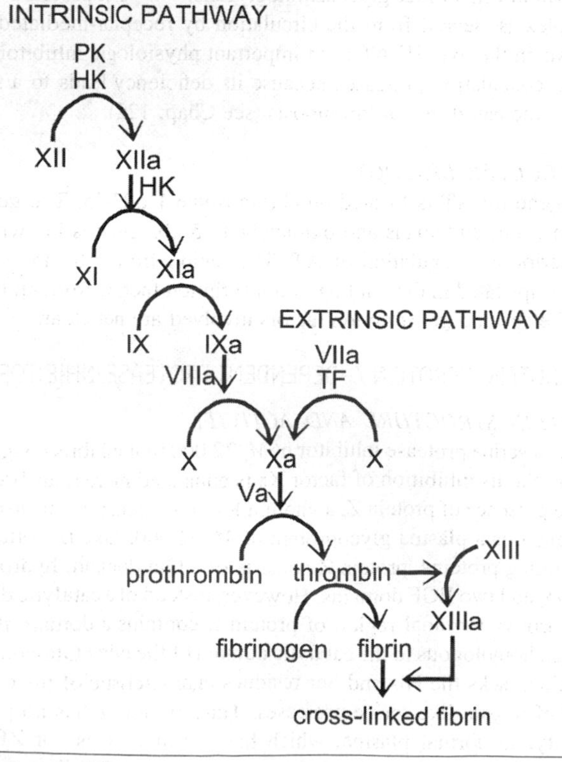

FIGURE 106-27 Cascade model of coagulation. The model shows successive activation of coagulation factors proceeding from the *top* of the schematic to thrombin generation and fibrin formation at the *bottom* of the schematic. The intrinsic and extrinsic pathways are indicated.

the intrinsic and extrinsic systems could not operate independently of one another and that all the clotting factors were somehow interrelated. Only in this way could hemostasis *in vivo* be explained.

REVISION OF THE COAGULATION MODELS

Key observations made by several groups led to revisions of earlier models of coagulation. A major observation was that a complex of factor VIIa/TF activated not only factor X but also factor IX.[126] Other important observations led to the conclusion that the major initiating event in hemostasis *in vivo* was the formation of a factor VIIa/TF complex at the site of injury.[219–221] This conclusion led to the belief that factor VIII and IX deficiency, which resulted in hemophilia A and B, respectively, were abnormalities of the VIIa/TF pathway, even though factors IX and VIII were considered components of the intrinsic system. *In vivo* coagulation was recognized to be regulated by control mechanisms, one of which was the localization of the coagulation reactions to cell surfaces. In addition, earlier and then subsequent observations emphasized the importance of plasma inhibitors of each step of the coagulation process. These inhibitors include TFPI, which inhibits the factor VIIa/TF/Xa complex[202,222]; proteins C and S, which inactivate factors Va and VIIIa[144,223,224]; and AT, which inhibits thrombin and other coagulation proteases.[225]

A CELL-BASED MODEL OF COAGULATION

ROLE OF THE TF-BEARING CELL

The goal of hemostasis is to produce a fibrin clot to seal a site of injury or rupture in the blood vessel wall. This process is initiated when TF-bearing cells are exposed to blood at a site of injury (see Fig. 106-28). TF is anchored to cells via a transmembrane domain and acts as a receptor for plasma factor VII. Once bound to TF, zymogen factor VII is rapidly converted to factor VIIa through mechanisms not yet completely understood but which may involve factor Xa and autoactivation. The resulting factor VIIa/TF complex, localized by cells to the site of injury, catalyzes two important reactions: (1) activation of factor X to factor Xa and (2) activation of factor IX to IXa. Factors Xa and IXa formed on the TF-bearing cells have distinct and separate functions in initiating blood coagulation.[10]

Factor Xa formed on the TF-bearing cell interacts with its cofactor Va to form a prothrombinase complex sufficient to generate a very small amount of thrombin in the vicinity of the TF cells (Fig. 106-28). Although the small amount of thrombin may not be sufficient to clot fibrinogen, it is sufficient to initiate events that "prime" the clotting system for a subsequent burst of thrombin generation. Experiments using a cell-based model have shown that minute amounts of thrombin are formed in the milieu of TF-bearing cells exposed to plasma concentrations of procoagulants, even in the absence of platelets. The small amounts of factor Va required for prothrombinase assembly on the TF-bearing cells are activated by factor Xa[53] or by noncoagulation proteases elaborated by the cells.[226] The small amounts of thrombin generated on the TF-bearing cells are capable of accomplishing the following[101,227]: (1) activating platelets, (2) activating factor V, (3) activating factor VIII and dissociating factor VIII from vWF, and (4) activating factor XI (Fig. 106-29). The activity of the factor Xa formed by the factor VIIa/TF complex is restricted to the TF-bearing cell. Factor Xa, which diffuses off the cell surface, is rapidly inhibited by TFPI or AT.

Unlike factor Xa, the primary site of activity of factor IXa formed by factor VIIa/TF is on activated platelets in close proximity to the TF-bearing cell. Factor IXa can diffuse to adjacent cell surfaces because it is not inhibited by TFPI and is inhibited much more slowly by AT than is factor Xa (see Table 106-4).

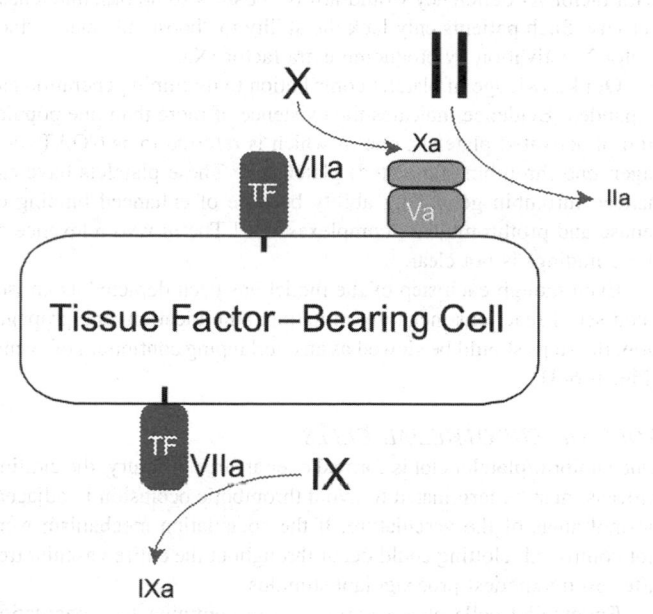

FIGURE 106-28   Role of TF-bearing cells. Factor VIIa bound to tissue factor can activate factors X and IX. Factors Xa and IXa activated by factor VIIa/TF play distinct roles in coagulation. Factor Xa is assembled into a prothrombinase complex on the surface of the tissue factor bearing cell. This process generates a small amount of thrombin.

In addition to the pool of extravascular, cell-anchored TF, a number of reports have documented the presence of TF antigen and active TF protein in the circulation. This TF probably exists largely in association with membrane vesicles that have been shed from the surface of monocytes or endothelial cells.[228,229] Such membrane vesicles can be shed from many cell types, particularly in the setting of inflam-

matory stimuli or during apoptosis. Their presence in the blood has been reported in association with a wide range of inflammatory and prothrombotic states, including atherosclerotic vascular disease, severe infections, and malignancy. However, some circulating TF may be present as the soluble, alternatively spliced variant of the TF protein.[117] The precise role of this circulating TF is not known, but evidence indicates it may initiate or contribute to propagation of thrombotic phenomena.[230,231]

ROLE OF ACTIVATED PLATELETS

Platelets also play a major role in localizing clotting reactions to the site of injury because platelets adhere and aggregate at the same sites where TF is exposed. Platelet localization and activation are mediated by vWF, thrombin, platelet receptors, and vessel wall components such as collagen (see Chap. 105).[232]

Once platelets are activated, cofactors Va and VIIIa are rapidly localized to the platelet membrane surface (see Fig. 106-29). Cofactor binding is mediated in part by exposure of phosphatidyl serine on the platelet membrane, a process resulting from a flip-flop mechanism whereby phosphatidyl serine on the inner leaflet of the membrane bilayer flips to the outside.[233] In addition, the cofactors appear to bind to the platelet surface before binding of the respective enzymes.[234]

Factor IXa formed by the factor VIIa/TF complex binds to the surface of activated platelets (Fig 106-30). Specific receptors on the activated platelets bind factor IXa and promote formation of active factor IXa/VIIIa complexes.[235,236] Once the platelet "tenase" complex is assembled, factor X is recruited from the plasma and is activated to factor Xa on the platelet surface. Factor Xa then associates with factor Va on the surface to generate a burst of thrombin sufficient to clot fibrinogen and form a hemostatic plug (Fig. 106-30). Factor XIII, activated by thrombin, cross-links fibrin and stabilizes the hemostatic

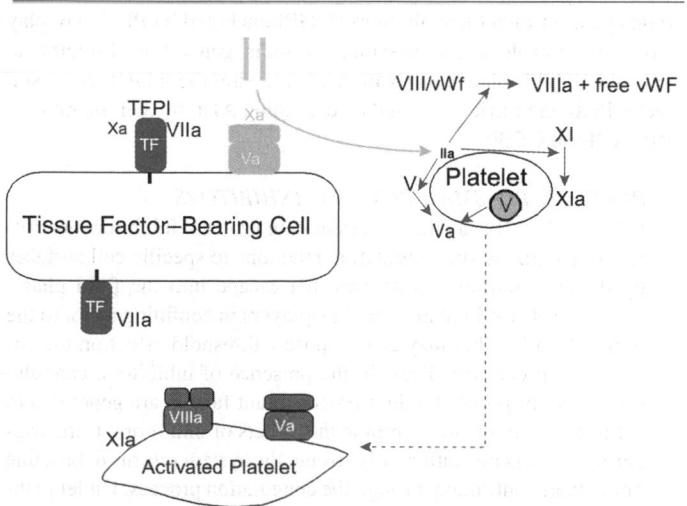

FIGURE 106-29   Role of thrombin generated by TF-bearing cells. After the initial generation of factor Xa on TF-bearing cells, subsequent factor Xa generation is shut down when TFPI reacts with factor Xa to inactivate the factor VIIa/TF complex. The small amount of thrombin generated on the TF-bearing cell (see Fig. 106-28) plays a critical role in priming platelets for subsequent coagulation steps. This thrombin activates platelets, releases factor V from alpha granules, activates factor V, activates factor VIII releasing it from vWF, and activates factor XI.

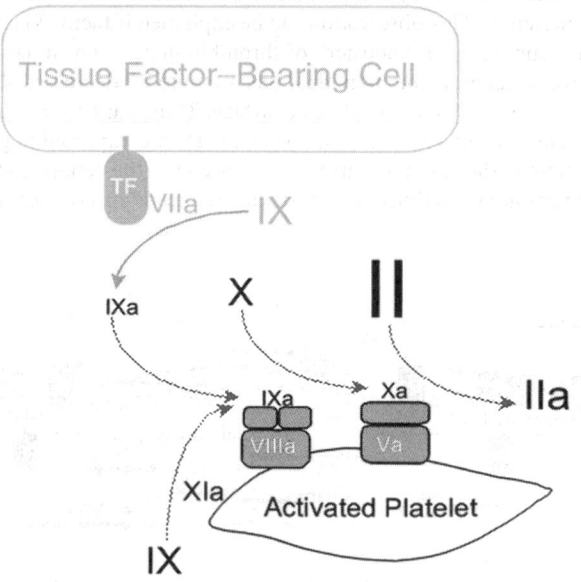

FIGURE 106-30   Role of platelets. Factor IXa, generated on TF-bearing cells, is only slowly inhibited by plasma inhibitors, so it can make its way to the primed platelet surface where it binds to factor VIIIa. Factor IXa activates factor X on the platelet surface. Factor Xa complexes to factor Va and activates prothrombin, leading to the burst of thrombin generation responsible for cleaving fibrinogen. Additional factor IXa is supplied by factor XIa on the platelet surface.

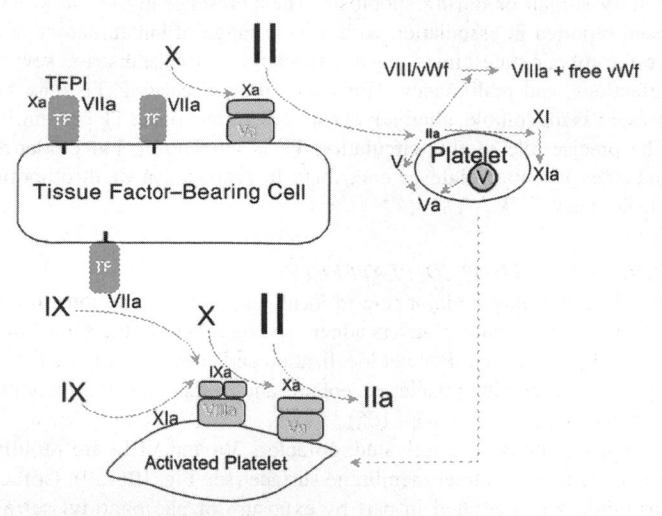

FIGURE 106-31 Cell-based model of hemostasis. The sequence of events—initiation, amplification, and propagation (shown in Figs. 106-28 through 106-30)—is summarized.

plug, rendering it impermeable. Thrombin also activates TAFI, which helps to stabilize the fibrin clot.

Factor XI can bind to platelet surfaces and be activated by thrombin,[101,104,237] bypassing the need for factor XIIa. The platelet-bound factor XIa then activates more factor IX to IXa. Thus, factor XI activation appears to enhance platelet tenase activity and serve as a "booster" mechanism to enhance thrombin generation. The enhanced thrombin generation resulting from the effect of factor XIa probably ensures activation of TAFI.[238]

The role of factor XI in hemostasis has been a point of major interest because even severe factor XI deficiency does not result in a hemorrhagic tendency comparable to that seen in severe factor VIII or IX deficiency. This observation can be explained if factor XI is viewed as an "enhancer" or "booster" of thrombin generation. In factor VIII and IX deficiency, the individual has a markedly decreased ability to generate factor Xa on the platelet surface. Thus, patients with a severe deficiency of either factor VIII or factor IX are expected to generate insufficient thrombin for hemostasis because the tenase and hence prothrombinase activity are markedly reduced. In contrast, patients

with factor XI deficiency would always possess some baseline tenase activity. Such patients only lack the ability to "boost" platelet surface factor X activation by producing extra factor IXa.

Our knowledge of platelet contribution to thrombin generation has expanded. Evidence indicates the existence of more than one population of activated platelets, one of which is referred to as COAT (collagen and thrombin stimulated) platelets.[239] These platelets have enhanced thrombin generating ability because of enhanced binding of tenase and prothrombinase complexes.[240,241] The *in vivo* relevance of these findings is not clear.

Even though each step of the model has been depicted as an isolated set of reactions including initiation, amplification, and propagation, the steps should be viewed as an overlapping continuum of events (Fig. 106-31).

ROLE OF ENDOTHELIAL CELLS

Once a fibrin/platelet clot is formed over an area of injury, the clotting process must be terminated to avoid thrombotic occlusion in adjacent normal areas of the vasculature. If the coagulation mechanism were not controlled, clotting could occur throughout the entire vascular tree after even a modest procoagulant stimulus.

Endothelial cells play a major role in confining the coagulation reactions to a site of injury and preventing clot extension to areas where an intact endothelium is present (see Chap. 108). Endothelial cells have two major types of anticoagulant/antithrombotic activities (Fig. 106-32). The protein C/S/TM system is activated in response to thrombin generation.[61] Some of the thrombin formed during the coagulation process can diffuse away or be swept downstream from a site of injury. When thrombin reaches an intact endothelial cell, it binds to TM on the endothelial surface. The thrombin/TM complex, in conjunction with EPCR, then activates protein C, which binds to its cofactor protein S and inactivates any factor Va or VIIIa that finds its way to the adjacent endothelial cell membrane. This action prevents the generation of additional thrombin in the vasculature. The endothelial cell also possesses other anticoagulant features. The protease inhibitors AT and TFPI are always present bound to heparan sulfates expressed on the endothelial surface, where they can inactivate proteases near an intact endothelium.[242] GPI-anchored TFPI-β may play a role in controlling intravascular thrombin generation. Endothelial cells also inhibit platelet activation by releasing the inhibitors prostacyclin PGI$_2$ and nitric oxide and by degrading ADP by their membrane ecto-ADPase CD39.[243]

ROLE OF PLASMA PROTEASE INHIBITORS

Like cell-based coagulation, circulating protease inhibitors are critical in localizing the coagulation reactions to specific cell surfaces by directly inhibiting proteases that escape into the fluid phase. Plasma protease inhibitors are key players in confining a clot to the proper location, but they also impose a threshold effect on the coagulation process.[244] Thus, in the presence of inhibitors, coagulation does not proceed unless procoagulant factors are generated in sufficient amounts to overcome the effects of inhibitors. If the triggering event is not sufficiently strong, the system returns to baseline rather than continuing through the coagulation process. Under pathologic conditions, the trigger for clotting may be so strong as to overwhelm the control mechanisms and lead to disseminated intravascular coagulation or thrombosis (see Chap. 121).

ROLE OF FIBRINOLYSIS

Once a hemostatic clot forms, some provision must be made for the clot's eventual removal as wound healing occurs. Dissolution of clots is accomplished by the fibrinolytic system (discussed in detail in Chap. 127).

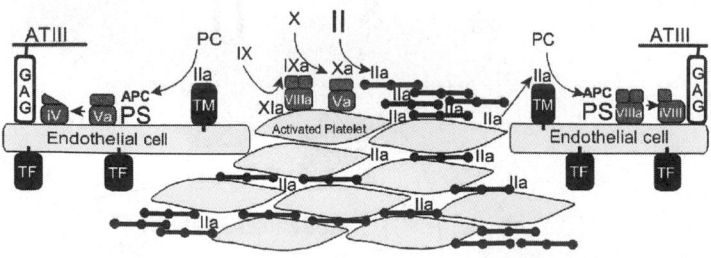

FIGURE 106-32 Role of endothelial cells. Activated coagulation proteins generated on platelets localized to the site of an injury must be confined to the site of injury. Activated coagulation factors that move to an endothelial cell surface are rapidly inhibited by AT associated with glycosaminoglycans (GAG) on the endothelial surface. Thrombin that reaches the endothelial cell surface binds to thrombomodulin (TM). Once bound, thrombin can no longer cleave fibrinogen. Instead, thrombin activates protein C, leading to the formation of activated protein C (APC)/protein S (PS) complexes on the endothelial cell surface. APC/PS on the endothelial cell surface inactivates procoagulant factors on the endothelium (iV, iVIII).

CONCEPT OF BASAL COAGULATION AND ANTICOAGULATION

The coagulation process proceeds only when enough thrombin is generated on or near the TF-bearing cell to trigger activation of platelets and cofactors. Of question, however, is if minute hemostatic plugs are not constantly formed throughout the body to maintain the integrity of the vascular tree. A low level of coagulation factor activation probably occurs at all times.[245] More than 30 years ago, fibrinopeptides were shown to be continuously cleaved from fibrinogen at low levels in normal individuals.[246] Low levels of circulating factor VIIa and of the activation peptides from factors IX and X in the blood of normal individuals have been demonstrated.[247–249] This situation has been called "basal" coagulation and may result from the minor injuries to vessels that occur during normal daily activities, or perhaps when the lower molecular weight coagulation factors percolate through the extravascular spaces. Speculation that circulating TF or microparticles contribute to basal coagulation is tempting, but the role of such microparticles in the coagulation process is not well defined and any potential role in basal coagulation is not demonstrated.

Basal coagulation must be balanced by basal activity of the anticoagulation and fibrinolytic systems. This need is evidenced by the presence of low levels of APC, protein C activation peptide, and tissue plasminogen activator activity in normal individuals.[250]

BLOOD COAGULATION AS A PART OF THE HOST DEFENSE MECHANISM

The process of hemostasis is only a small part of the overall host response to injury. Although different parts of the host response are presented as though they were truly separate processes, coagulation, fibrinolysis, inflammation, the immune response, and wound healing are interrelated parts of the overall response to injury. The close interaction is reflected in the close structural relationships between many proteins of the coagulation and immune/inflammatory systems. For example, TF is structurally analogous to type 2 cytokine receptors.[251] Furthermore, a number of coagulation proteins have multiple diverse activities in the host response to injury. Thrombin not only acts as a procoagulant to clot fibrinogen but also as a growth factor and cytokine that promotes monocyte, fibroblast and endothelial cell influx, and proliferation in an area of recent injury. By generating thrombin, the coagulation process not only stops bleeding in the short term but also sets the stage for removal of damaged tissue and wound healing in the long term.[33] Platelets have multiple roles in the response to injury. They release growth factors and cytokines upon activation, some of which play key roles in wound healing and atherosclerosis. Factor Xa, TF, and fibrinogen fragments similarly seem to have roles as inflammatory mediators and cell growth regulators. In addition, the contact factors (factor XII, PK, HK) may play a role as a bridge between the coagulation reactions and other host defense mechanisms. No doubt the list of multifunctional molecules will grow as understanding of the blood clotting mechanism increases.

REFERENCES

1. Leytus S, Foster D, Kurachi K, Davie E: Gene for human factor X, a blood coagulation factor whose gene organization is essentially identical to that of factor IX and protein C. *Biochemistry* 25:5098, 1986.

2. Yoshitake S, Schach BG, Foster DC, et al: Nucleotide sequence of the gene for human factor IX (antihemophilic factor B). *Biochemistry* 24: 3736, 1985.

3. Fujimaki K, Yamazaki T, Taniwaki M, Ichinose A: The gene for human protein Z is localized to chromosome 13 at band q34 and is coded by eight regular exons and one alternative exon. *Biochemistry* 37:6838, 1998.

4. Wu SM, Cheung WF, Frazier D, Stafford DW: Cloning and expression of the cDNA for human gamma-glutamyl carboxylase. *Science* 254: 1634, 1991.

5. Jorgensen M, Cantor A, Furie B, et al: Recognition site directing vitamin K-dependent γ-carboxylation residues on the propeptide of factor IX. *Cell* 48:185, 1987.

6. Huber P, Schmitz T, Griffin J, et al: Identification of amino acids in the γ-carboxylation recognition site on the propeptide of prothrombin. *J Biol Chem* 265:12467, 1990.

7. Li T, Chang CY, Jin DY, et al: Identification of the gene for vitamin K epoxide reductase. *Nature* 427:541, 2004.

8. Rost S, Fregin A, Ivaskevicius V, et al: Mutations in VKORC1 cause warfarin resistance and multiple coagulation factor deficiency type 2. *Nature* 427:537, 2004.

9. Brenner B, Sánchez-Vega B, Wu SM, et al: A missense mutation in γ-glutamyl carboxylase gene causes combined deficiency of all vitamin K-dependent blood coagulation factors. *Blood* 92:4554, 1998.

10. Monroe DM, Hoffman M, Roberts HR: Platelets and thrombin generation. *Arterioscler Thromb Vasc Biol* 22:1381, 2002.

11. Soriano-Garcia M, Padmanabhan K, De Vos AM, Tulinsky A: The Ca²⁺ ion and membrane binding structure of the Gla domain of Ca-prothrombin fragment 1. *Biochemistry* 31:2554, 1992.

12. Sunnerhagen M, Forsen S, Hoffren AM, et al: Structure of the Ca(2+)-free Gla domain sheds light on membrane binding of blood coagulation proteins. *Nat Struct Biol* 2:504, 1995.

13. Nelsestuen G, Kisiel W, DiScipio RG: Interaction of vitamin K-dependent proteins with membranes. *Biochemistry* 12:2134, 1978.

14. Rawal-Sheikh R, Ahmad SS, Ashby B, Walsh PN: Kinetics of coagulation factor X activation by platelet-bound factor IXa. *Biochemistry* 29: 2606, 1990.

15. Gilbert GE, Arena AA: Partial activation of the factor VIIIa-factor IXa enzyme complex by dihexanoic phosphatidylserine at submicellar concentrations. *Biochemistry* 36:10768, 1997.

16. Kirchhofer D, Guha A, Nemerson Y, et al: Activation of blood coagulation factor VIIa with cleaved tissue factor extracellular domain and crystallization of the active complex. *Proteins* 22:419, 1995.

17. Muller Y, Ultsch M, de Vos A: The crystal structure of the extracellular domain of tissue factor refined to 1.7 Å resolution. *J Molec Biol* 256: 144, 1996.

18. Banner DW, D'Arcy A, Chene C, et al: The crystal structure of the complex of blood coagulation factor VIIa with human soluble tissue factor. *Nature* 380:41, 1996.

19. Brandstetter H, Bauer M, Huber R, et al: X-ray structure of clotting factor IXa: Active site and module structure related to Xase activity and hemophilia B. *Proc Natl Acad Sci U S A* 92:9796, 1995.

20. Patthy L, Trexler M, Vali Z, et al: Kringles: Modules specialized for protein binding. Homology of the gelatin-binding region of fibronectin with the kringle structure of proteases. *FEBS Lett* 171:131, 1984.

21. Royle N, Irwin D, Koschinsky ML, et al: Human genes encoding prothrombin and ceruloplasmin map to 11p11-q12 and 3q21-q24, respectively. *Somat Cell Mol Genet* 13:285, 1987.

22. Chow B-C, Ting V, Tufaro F, MacGillivray R: Characterization of a novel liver-specific enhancer in the human prothrombin gene. *J Biol Chem* 266:18927, 1991.

23. Degen S: The prothrombin gene and its liver-specific expression. *Semin Thromb Hemost* 18:230, 1992.

24. Poort S, Rosendaal F, Bertina R: A common genetic variant in the 3′-untranslated region of the prothrombin gene is associated with elevated plasma prothrombin levels and an increase in venous thrombosis. *Blood* 88:3698, 1996.

25. Bode W, Mayr I, Baumann U, et al: The refined 1.9 Å crystal structure of human alpha-thrombin: Interaction with D-Phe-Pro-Arg chloromethylketone and significance of the Try-Pro-Pro-Trp insertion segment. *EMBO J* 8:3467, 1989.

26. Martin PD, Malkowski MG, Box J, et al: New insights into the regulation of the blood clotting cascade derived from the X-ray crystal structure of bovine meizothrombin des F1 in complex with PPACK. *Structure* 5:1681, 1997.

27. Vijayalakshmi J, Padmanabhan KP, Mann KG, Tulinsky A: The isomorphous structures of prethrombin2, hirugen-, and PPACK-thrombin: Changes accompanying activation and exosite binding to thrombin. *Protein Sci* 3:2254, 1994.

28. Banefield D, MacGillivray R: Partial characterization of vertebrate prothrombin cDNAse: Amplification and sequence analysis of the B chain of thrombin from nine different species. *Proc Natl Acad Sci U S A* 89:2779, 1992.

29. Nesheim M: Fibrinolysis and the plasma carboxypeptidase. *Curr Opin Hematol* 5:309, 1998.

30. Boffa MB, Nesheim ME, Koschinsky ML: Thrombin activatable fibrinolysis inhibitor (TAFI): Molecular genetics of an emerging potential risk factor for thrombotic disorders. *Curr Drug Targets Cardiovasc Haematol Disord* 1:59, 2001.

31. Dittman W, Nelson S: Thrombomodulin, in *Molecular Basis of Thrombosis and Hemostasis*, edited by KA High, HR Roberts, p 425. Marcel Dekker, New York, 1995.

32. Esmon CT: The protein C pathway. *Chest* 124:26S, 2003.

33. Church FC, Hoffman MR: Heparin cofactor II and thrombin: Heparin-binding proteins linking hemostasis and inflammation. *Trends Cardiovasc Med* 4:140, 1994.

34. Pollak E, Hung H, Godin W, et al: Functional characterization of the human factor VII 5'-flanking region. *J Biol Chem* 271:1738, 1996.

35. Pedersen AH, Lund-Hansen T, Bisgaard-Frantzen H, et al: Autoactivation of human recombinant factor VII. *Biochemistry* 28:9331, 1989.

36. Wolberg AS, Stafford DW, Erie DA: Human factor IX binds to specific sites on the collagenous domain of collagen IV. *J Biol Chem* 272:16717, 1997.

37. Cheung WF, van den Born J, Kuhn K, et al: Identification of the endothelial cell binding site for factor IX. *Proc Natl Acad Sci U S A* 93:11068, 1996.

38. Gui T, Lin HF, Jin DY, et al: Circulating and binding characteristics of wild-type factor IX and certain Gla domain mutants in vivo. *Blood* 100:153, 2002.

39. Camerino G, Grzeschik K, Jaye M, et al: Regional localization on the human X chromosome and polymorphism of the coagulation factor IX gene (hemophilia B locus). *Proc Natl Acad Sci U S A* 81:498, 1984.

40. Winship P, Rees D, Alkan M: Detection of polymorphisms at cytosine phosphoguanadine dinucleotides and diagnosis of haemophilia B carriers. *Lancet* 1:631, 1989.

41. High K, Roberts H: Factor IX, in *Molecular Basis of Thrombosis and Hemostasis*, edited by K High, H Roberts, p 215. Marcel Dekker, New York, 1995.

42. Landschulz W, Johnson P, McKnight S: Homologous recognition of a promoter domain common to the MSV LTR and the HSV tk gene. *Cell* 44:565, 1986.

43. Mueller C, Maire P, Schibler U: DBP, a liver-enriched transcriptional activator, is expressed late in ontogeny and its tissue specificity is determined posttranslationally. *Cell* 61:279, 1990.

44. Sladek F, Zhong W, Lai E, Darnell JJ: Liver-enriched transcription factor NHF-4 is a novel member of the steroid hormone receptor superfamily. *Genes Dev* 4:2353, 1990.

45. Paonessa G, Gounari F, Frank R, Cortese R: Purification of a NF1-like DNA-binding protein from rat liver and cloning of the corresponding cDNA. *EMBO J* 7:3115, 1988.

46. Ahmad SS, London FS, Walsh PN: The assembly of the factor X-activating complex on activated human platelets. *J Thromb Haemost* 1:48, 2003.

47. Scambler P, Williamson R: The structural gene for human coagulation factor X is located on chromosome 13q34. *Cytogenet Cell Genet* 39:231, 1985.

48. Watzke H, High K: Factor X, in *Molecular Basis of Thrombosis and Hemostasis*, edited by K High, H Roberts, p 239. Marcel Dekker, New York, 1995.

49. Huang M, Hung H, Stanfield-Oakley S, High K: Characterization of the human coagulation factor X promoter. *J Biol Chem* 267:15440, 1992.

50. Hung H, High K: Liver-enriched transcription factor HNF-4 and ubiquitous factor NF-Y are critical for expression of blood coagulation factor X. *J Biol Chem* 271:2323, 1996.

51. Rao L, Rapaport SI: Activation of factor VII bound to tissue factor: A key early step in the tissue factor pathway of blood coagulation. *Proc Natl Acad Sci U S A* 85:6687, 1988.

52. Neuenschwander PF, Jesty J: Thrombin-activated and factor Xa-activated human factor VIII: Differences in cofactor activity and decay rate. *Arch Biochem Biophys* 296:426, 1992.

53. Monkovic DD, Tracy PB: Activation of human factor V by factor Xa and thrombin. *Biochemistry* 29:1118, 1990.

54. Bouchard BA, Catcher CS, Thrash BR, et al: Effector cell protease receptor-1, a platelet activation-dependent membrane protein, regulates prothrombinase-catalyzed thrombin generation. *J Biol Chem* 272:9244, 1997.

55. Gasic GP, Arenas CP, Gasic TB, Gasic GJ: Coagulation factors X, Xa, and protein S as potent mitogens of cultured aortic smooth muscle cells. *Proc Natl Acad Sci U S A* 89:2317, 1992.

56. Altieri DC, Edgington TS: Identification of effector cell protease receptor-1. A leukocyte-distributed receptor for the serine protease factor Xa. *J Immunol* 145:246, 1990.

57. Patrucchini P, Aiello V, Palazzi P, et al: Sublocalization of the human protein C gene on chromosome 2q13-q14. *Hum Genet* 81:191, 1989.

58. Foster D, Yoshitake S, Davie E: The nucleotide sequence for the gene for human protein C. *Proc Natl Acad Sci U S A* 82:4673, 1985.

59. Plutzky J, Hoskins J, Long G, Crabtree G: Evolution and organization of the human protein C gene. *Proc Natl Acad Sci U S A* 83:546, 1986.

60. Esmon CT: Inflammation and thrombosis. *J Thromb Haemost* 1:1343, 2003.

61. Oliver JA, Monroe DM, Church FC, et al: Activated protein C cleaves factor Va more efficiently on endothelium than on platelet surfaces. *Blood* 100:539, 2002.

62. Shen L, Dahlbäck B: Factor V and protein S as synergistic cofactors to activated protein C in degradation of factor VIIIa. *J Biol Chem* 269:18735, 1994.

63. Cooper S, Church F: PCI: Protein C inhibitor? *Adv Exp Med Biol* 425:45, 1997.

64. Fair D, Marlar R: Biosynthesis and secretion of factor VII, protein C, protein S and the protein inhibitor from a human hepatoma cell line. *Blood* 67:64, 1986.

65. Fair D, Marlar R, Levin E: Human endothelial cells synthesize protein S. *Blood* 67:1168, 1986.

66. Ogura M, Tanabe N, Nishioka J, et al: Biosynthesis and secretion of functional protein S by a human megakaryoblastic cell line. *Blood* 70:301, 1987.

67. Dahlbäck B: Protein S and C4b-binding protein: Components involved in the regulation of the protein C anticoagulant system. *Thromb Haemost* 66:49, 1991.

68. Maillard C, Berruyer M, Serre C, et al: Protein S, a vitamin K-dependent protein, is a bone matrix component synthesized and secreted by osteoblasts. *Endocrinology* 130:1599, 1992.

69. Edenbrandt C-M, Lundvall A, Wydro R, Stenflo J: Molecular analysis of the gene for vitamin K-dependent protein S and its pseudogene: Cloning and partial characterization. *Biochemistry* 29:7861, 1990.

70. Hackeng T, van't Veer C, Meijers J, Bouma B: Human protein S inhibits prothrombinase complex activity on endothelial cells and platelets via direct interactions with factors Va and Xa. *J Biol Chem* 269:21051, 1994.

71. Rezende SM, Simmonds RE, Lane DA: Coagulation, inflammation, and apoptosis: Different roles for protein S and the protein S-C4b binding protein complex. *Blood* 103:1192, 2004.

72. Moussalli M, Pipe S, Nichols W, et al: Mistargeting of the lectin ERGIC-53 to the endoplasmic reticulum impairs the secretion of coagulation factors V and VIII. *Blood* 92:474a, 1998.

73. Nichols W, Seligsohn U, Zivelin A, et al: Mutations in the ER-Golgi intermediate compartment protein ERGIC-53 cause combined deficiency of coagulation factors V and VIII. *Cell* 93:61, 1998.

74. Zhang B, Cunningham MA, Nichols WC, et al: Bleeding due to disruption of a cargo-specific ER-to-Golgi transport complex. *Nat Genet* 34:220, 2003.

75. Ortel T, Keller F, Kane W: Factor V, in *Molecular Basis of Thrombosis and Hemostasis*, edited by KA High, HR Roberts, p 119. Marcel Dekker, New York, 1995.

76. Ortel TL, Quinn-Allen MA, Keller FG, et al: Localization of functionally important epitopes within the second C-type domain of coagulation factor V using recombinant chimeras. *J Biol Chem* 269:15898, 1994.

77. Pittman DD, Tomkinson KN, Michnick D, et al: Posttranslational sulfation of factor V is required for efficient thrombin cleavage and activation and for full procoagulant activity. *Biochemistry* 33:6592, 1994.

78. Cripe L, Moore K, Kane W: Structure of the gene for human factor V. *Biochemistry* 31:3777, 1992.

79. Gould WR, Silveira JR, Tracy PB: Unique in vivo modifications of coagulation factor V produce a physically and functionally distinct platelet-derived cofactor: Characterization of purified platelet-derived factor V/Va. *J Biol Chem* 279:2383, 2004.

80. Hayward C: Multimerin: A bench-to-bedside chronology of a unique platelet and endothelial cell protein—From discovery to function to abnormalities in disease. *Clin Invest Med* 20:176, 1997.

81. Bertina RM, Koeleman BP, Koster T, et al: Mutation in blood coagulation factor V associated with resistance to activated protein C. *Nature* 369:64, 1994.

82. Pipe S, Morris J, Shah J, Kaufman R: Differential interaction of coagulation factor VIII and factor V with protein chaperones calnexin and calreticulin. *J Biol Chem* 273:8537, 1998.

83. Swaroop M, Moussalli M, Pipe S, Kaufman R: Mutagenesis of a potential immunoglobulin-binding protein-binding site enhances secretion of coagulation factor VIII. *J Biol Chem* 272:24121, 1997.

84. Lollar P, Hill-Eubanks E, Parker C: Association of the FVIII light chain with von Willebrand factor. *J Biol Chem* 263:10451, 1988.

85. Gitschier J, Wood W, Goralka T, et al: Characterization of the human factor VIII gene. *Nature* 312:326, 1984.

86. Bonthron D, Handin R, Kaufman R, et al: Structure of pre-pro-von Willebrand factor and its expression in heterologous cells. *Nature* 324:270, 1986.

87. Colombatti A, Bonaldo P: The superfamily of proteins with von Willebrand factor type A-domains: One theme common to components of extracellular matrix, hemostasis, cellular adhesion, and defense mechanisms. *Blood* 77:2305, 1991.

88. Foster P, Fulcher C, Marti T, et al: A major factor VIII binding domain resides within the amino-terminal 272 amino acid residues of von Willebrand factor. *J Biol Chem* 262:8443, 1987.

89. Zimmerman T, Roberts J, Edgington T: Factor VIII-related antigen: Multiple molecular forms in human plasma. *Proc Natl Acad Sci U S A* 72:5121, 1975.

90. Mancuso D, Tuley E, Westfield L, et al: Structure of the gene for human von Willebrand factor. *J Biol Chem* 264:19514, 1989.

91. Fujikawa K, Chung DW: Factor XI, in *Molecular Basis of Thrombosis and Hemostasis*, edited by KA High, HR Roberts, p 257. Marcel Dekker, New York, 1995.

92. Baglia FA, Seaman FS, Walsh PN: The Apple 1 and Apple 4 domains of factor XI act synergistically to promote the surface–mediated activation of factor XI by factor XIIa. *Blood* 85:2078, 1995.

93. Baglia FA, Jameson BA, Walsh PN: Identification and characterization of a binding site for platelets in the Apple 3 domain of coagulation factor XI. *J Biol Chem* 270:6734, 1995.

94. Baglia FA, Jameson BA, Walsh PN: Identification and characterization of a binding site for factor XIIa in the Apple 4 domain of coagulation factor XI. *J Biol Chem* 268:3838, 1993.

95. Baglia FA, Walsh PN: A binding site for thrombin in the apple 1 domain of factor XI. *J Biol Chem* 271:3652, 1996.

96. Kato A, Asaki R, Davie E, Aoki N: Factor XI gene (F11) is located on the distal end of the long arm of chromosome 4. *Cytogenet Cell Genet* 52:77, 1989.

97. Asakai R, Davie E, Chung D: Organization of the gene for human factor XI. *Biochemistry* 26:7221, 1987.

98. Tarumi T, Kravtsov DV, Zhao M, et al: Cloning and characterization of the human factor XI gene promoter: Transcription factor hepatocyte nuclear factor 4alpha (HNF-4alpha) is required for hepatocyte-specific expression of factor XI. *J Biol Chem* 277:18510, 2002.

99. Gailani D, Broze GJ Jr: Factor XI activation in a revised model of blood coagulation. *Science* 253:909, 1991.

100. Naito K, Fujikawa K: Activation of human blood coagulation factor XI independent of factor XII. Factor XI is activated by thrombin and factor XIa in the presence of negatively charged surfaces. *J Biol Chem* 266:7353, 1991.

101. Oliver J, Monroe D, Roberts H, Hoffman M: Thrombin activates factor XI on activated platelets in the absence of factor XII. *Arterioscler Thromb Vasc Biol* 19:170, 1999.

102. Ragni MV, Sinha D, Seaman F, et al: Comparison of bleeding tendency, factor XI coagulant activity, and factor XI antigen in 25 factor XI-deficient kindreds. *Blood* 65:719, 1985.

103. Sinha D, Seaman FS, Walsh PN: Role of calcium ions and the heavy chain of factor XIa in the activation of human coagulation factor IX. *Biochemistry* 26:3768, 1987.

104. Sinha D, Seaman FS, Koshy A, et al: Blood coagulation factor XIa binds specifically to a site on activated human platelets distinct from that for factor XI. *J Clin Invest* 73:1550, 1984.

105. Knauer DJ, Majumdar D, Fong PC, Knauer MF: SERPIN regulation of factor XIa. The novel observation that protease nexin 1 in the presence of heparin is a more potent inhibitor of factor XIa than C1 inhibitor. *J Biol Chem* 275:37340, 2000.

106. Cronlund AL, Walsh PN: A low molecular weight platelet inhibitor of factor XIa: Purification, characterization, and possible role in blood coagulation. *Biochemistry* 31:1685, 1992.

107. Saito H, Kojima T: Factor XII, prekallikrein and high molecular weight kininogen, in *Molecular Basis of Thrombosis and Hemostasis*, edited by KA High, HR Roberts, p 269. Marcel Dekker, New York, 1995.

108. Yu H, Anderson PJ, Freedman BI, et al: Genomic structure of the human plasma prekallikrein gene, identification of allelic variants, and analysis in end-stage renal disease. *Genomics* 69:225, 2000.

109. Colman RW: Biologic activities of the contact factors in vivo—Potentiation of hypotension, inflammation, and fibrinolysis, and inhibition of cell adhesion, angiogenesis and thrombosis. *Thromb Haemost* 82:1568, 1999.

110. Schmaier AH: The plasma kallikrein-kinin system counterbalances the renin-angiotensin system. *J Clin Invest* 109:1007, 2002.

111. Morrissey JH, Fakhrai H, Edgington TS: Molecular cloning of the cDNA

for tissue factor, the cellular receptor for the initiation of the coagulation protease cascade. *Cell* 50:129, 1987.

112. Dorfleutner A, Ruf W: Regulation of tissue factor cytoplasmic domain phosphorylation by palmitoylation. *Blood* 102:3998, 2003.

113. Martin D, Boys C, Ruf W: Tissue factor: Molecular recognition and cofactor function. *FASEB J* 9:852, 1995.

114. Mueller BM: Different roles for plasminogen activators and metalloproteinases in melanoma metastasis. *Curr Top Microbiol Immunol* 213:65, 1996.

115. Kao F-T, Hartz J, Horton R, et al: Regional assignment of human tissue factor gene (F3) to chromosome 1p21-22. *Somat Cell Molec Genet* 14: 407, 1988.

116. Mackman N, Morrissey JH, Fowler B, Edgington TS: Complete sequence of the human tissue factor gene, a highly regulated cellular receptor that initiates the coagulation protease cascade. *Biochemistry* 28: 1755, 1989.

117. Bogdanov VY, Balasubramanian V, Hathcock J, et al: Alternatively spliced human tissue factor: A circulating, soluble, thrombogenic protein. *Nat Med* 9:458, 2003.

118. Mackman N, Fowler B, Edgington TS, Morrissey JH: Functional analysis of the human tissue factor promoter and induction by serum. *Proc Natl Acad Sci U S A* 87:2254, 1990.

119. Gregory SA, Morrissey JH, Edgington TS: Regulation of tissue factor gene expression in the monocyte procoagulant response to endotoxin. *Mol Cell Biol* 9:2752, 1989.

120. Schecter AD, Rollins BJ, Zhang YJ, et al: Tissue factor is induced by monocyte chemoattractant protein-1 in human aortic smooth muscle and THP-1 cells. *J Biol Chem* 272:28568, 1997.

121. Conway EM, Bach R, Rosenberg RD, Konigsberg WH: Tumor necrosis factor enhances expression of tissue factor mRNA in endothelial cells. *Thromb Res* 53:231, 1989.

122. Hoffman M, Cooper S: Thrombin enhances monocyte secretion of tumor necrosis factor and Interleukin-1 beta by two distinct mechanisms. *Blood Cells Mol Dis* 21:156, 1995.

123. Drake TA, Morrissey JH, Edgington TS: Selective cellular expression of tissue factor in human tissues. Implications for disorders of hemostasis and thrombosis. *Am J Pathol* 134:1087, 1989.

124. Eddleston M, de la Torre J, Oldstone M, et al: Astrocytes are the primary source of tissue factor in the murine central nervous system. A role for astrocytes in cerebral hemostasis. *J Clin Invest* 92:349, 1993.

125. Giesen PLA, Rauch U, Bohrmann B, et al: Blood-borne tissue factor: Another view of thrombosis. *Proc Natl Acad Sci U S A* 96:2311, 1999.

126. Østerud B, Rapaport SI: Activation of factor IX by the reaction product of tissue factor and factor VII: Additional pathway for initiating blood coagulation. *Proc Natl Acad Sci U S A* 74:5260, 1977.

127. Shigematsu Y, Miyata T, Higashi S: Expression of human soluble tissue factor in yeast and enzymatic properties of its complex with factor VIIa. *J Biol Chem* 267:21329, 1992.

128. Lawson JH, Butenas S, Mann KG: The evaluation of complex-dependent alterations in human factor VIIa. *J Biol Chem* 267:4834, 1992.

129. Neuenschwander PF, Morrissey JH: Roles of the membrane-interactive regions of factor VIIa-tissue factor. *J Biol Chem* 269:8007, 1994.

130. Neuenschwander PF, Morrissey JH: Deletion of the membrane anchoring region of tissue factor abolishes autoactivation of factor VII but not cofactor function. Analysis of a mutant with a selective deficiency in activity. *J Biol Chem* 267:14477, 1992.

131. Krishnaswamy S, Field KA, Edgington TS, et al: Role of the membrane surface in the activation of human coagulation factor X. *J Biol Chem* 267:26110, 1992.

132. Bach R, Moldow C: Mechanism of tissue factor activation on HL-60 cells. *Blood* 89:3270, 1997.

133. Bach R, Rifkin DB: Expression of tissue factor procoagulant activity:

134. Versteeg HH, Sorensen BB, Slofstra SH, et al: VIIa/tissue factor interaction results in a tissue factor cytoplasmic domain-independent activation of protein synthesis, p70, and p90 S6 kinase phosphorylation. *J Biol Chem* 277:27065, 2002.

135. Riewald M, Ruf W: Mechanistic coupling of protease signaling and initiation of coagulation by tissue factor. *Proc Natl Acad Sci U S A* 98: 7742, 2001.

136. Mackman N: Role of tissue factor in hemostasis, thrombosis, and vascular development. *Arterioscler Thromb Vasc Biol* 24:1015, 2004.

137. Wen D, Dittman W, Ye R, et al: Human thrombomodulin: Complete cDNA sequence and chromosome localization of the gene. *Biochemistry* 26:4350, 1987.

138. Esmon N, Owen W, Esmon C: Isolation of a membrane-bound cofactor for thrombin-catalyzed activation of protein C. *J Biol Chem* 257:859, 1982.

139. Patthy L: Detecting distant homologies of mosaic proteins: Analysis of thrombomodulin, thrombospondin, complement components C9, C8 alpha, C8 beta, vitronectin and plasma cell membrane glycoprotein PC-1. *J Mol Biol* 202:689, 1988.

140. Stearns D, Kurosawa S, Esmon C: Microthrombomodulin. Residues 310-486 from the epidermal growth factor homology domain of rabbit thrombomodulin will accelerate protein C activation. *J Biol Chem* 264: 3352, 1989.

141. Parkinson J, Vlahos C, Yan S, Bang N: Recombinant human thrombomodulin: Regulation of cofactor activity and anticoagulant function by a glycosaminoglycan side chain. *Biochem J* 283:151, 1992.

142. Espinosa R, Sadler J, LeBeau M: Regional localization of the human thrombomodulin gene to 20p12-cen. *Genomics* 5:649, 1989.

143. Esmon C, Esmon N, Hams K: Complex formation between thrombin and thrombomodulin inhibits both thrombin-catalyzed fibrin formation and factor V activation. *J Biol Chem* 257:7944, 1982.

144. Cadroy Y, Diquelou A, Dupouy D, et al: The thrombomodulin/protein C/protein S anticoagulant pathway modulates the thrombogenic properties of the normal resting and stimulated endothelium. *Arterioscler Thromb Vasc Biol* 17:520, 1997.

145. Healy AM, Rayburn HB, Rosenberg RD, Weiler H: Absence of the blood-clotting regulator thrombomodulin causes embryonic lethality in mice before development of a functional cardiovascular system. *Proc Natl Acad Sci U S A* 92:850, 1995.

146. Gu JM, Crawley JT, Ferrell G, et al: Disruption of the endothelial cell protein C receptor gene in mice causes placental thrombosis and early embryonic lethality. *J Biol Chem* 277:43335, 2002.

147. Verhagen HJ, Heijnen-Snyder GJ, Pronk A, et al: Thrombomodulin activity on mesothelial cells: Perspectives for mesothelial cells as an alternative for endothelial cells for cell seeding on vascular grafts. *Br J Haematol* 95:542, 1996.

148. McCachren SS, Diggs J, Weinberg JB, Dittman WA: Thrombomodulin expression by human blood monocytes and by human synovial tissue lining macrophages. *Blood* 78:3128, 1991.

149. Raife TJ, Demetroulis EM, Lentz SR: Regulation of thrombomodulin expression by all-trans retinoic acid and tumor necrosis factor-alpha: Differential responses in keratinocytes and endothelial cells. *Blood* 88: 2043, 1996.

150. Ishii H, Nakana M, Tsubouchi J, et al: Distribution of thrombomodulin in human tissues and characterization of thrombomodulin in plasma. *Acta Haematol Jpn* 51:1218, 1998.

151. Dichek D, Quertermous T: Variability in mRNA levels in HUVECs of different lineage and time in culture. *In Vitro Cell Dev Biol* 25:289, 1989.

152. Rezaie A, Cooper S, Church F, Esmon C: Protein C inhibitor is a potent inhibitor of the thrombin-thrombomodulin complex. *J Biol Chem* 270: 25336, 1995.

Regulation by cytosolic calcium. *Proc Natl Acad Sci U S A* 87:6995, 1990.

153. Neerman-Arbez M: The molecular basis of inherited afibrinogenaemia. *Thromb Haemost* 86:154, 2001.

154. Hanss M, Biot F: A database for human fibrinogen variants. *Ann N Y Acad Sci* 936:89, 2001.

155. Carrell N, McDonagh J: Functional defects in abnormal fibrinogens, in *Fibrinogen: Structural Variants and Interaction*, edited by A Henschen, B Hesse, J McDonagh, T Saldeen, p 155. Walter deGruyter, Berlin, 1985.

156. Egeberg O: Inherited fibrinogen abnormality causing thrombophilia. *Thromb Diath Haemorrh* 17:176, 1967.

157. Gardlund B, Hessel B, Marguerie G, et al: Primary structure of human fibrinogen. Characterization of disulfide-containing cyanogen-bromide fragments. *Eur J Biochem* 77:595, 1977.

158. Blomback B: Studies on the action of thrombotic enzymes on bovine fibrinogen as measured by N-terminal analysis. *Avkiv Kemi* 12:321, 1958.

159. Blomback B, Blomback M, Henschen A, et al: N-terminal disulfide knot of human fibrinogen. *Nature* 218:130, 1968.

160. Doolittle RF: Determining the crystal structure of fibrinogen. *J Thromb Haemost* 2:683, 2004.

161. Collen D, Tytgat C, Claeys H: Metabolism and distribution of fibrinogen I. Fibrinogen turnover in physiological conditions in humans. *Br J Haematol* 22:681, 1972.

162. Reeve K, Franks J: Fibrinogen synthesis, distribution and degradation. *Semin Thromb Hemost* 1:129, 1974.

163. Fuller G, Otto J, Woloski B: The effects of hepatocyte-stimulating factor on fibrinogen biosynthesis in hepatocyte monolayers. *J Cell Biol* 101:1481, 1985.

164. Huber P, Laurent M, Dalmon J: Human β-fibrinogen gene expression. Upstream sequences involved in its tissue specific expression and its dexamethasone and interleukin-6 stimulation. *J Biol Chem* 265:5695, 1990.

165. Chung D, Harris I, Davie E: Nucleotide sequences of the three genes coding for human fibrinogen, in *Advances in Experimental Medicine and Biology*, vol 48, edited by C Liu, S Chien, p 39. Plenum, New York, 1990.

166. Doolittle R: The amino acid sequence of the α-chain of human fibrinogen. *Nature* 280:464, 1979.

167. Kant I, Fornace A, Saxe D: Evolution and organization of the fibrinogen locus on chromosome 4: Gene duplication accompanied by transposition and inversion. *Proc Natl Acad Sci U S A* 82:2344, 1985.

168. Morgan J, Courtois G, Fourel G: Spl, a CAAT binding factor and the adenovirus major late promoter transcription factor interact with functional regions of the gamma-fibrinogen promoter. *Mol Cell Biol* 8:2628, 1988.

169. Courtois G, Morgan J, Campbell L, et al: Interaction of a liver-specific nuclear factor with the fibrinogen and α1 antitrypsin promoters. *Science* 238:688, 1987.

170. Dalmon J, Laurent M, Courtois G: The human β fibrinogen promoter contains a HAF-1 dependent IL-6 responsive element. *Mol Cell Biol* 13:1183, 1993.

171. Haidaris P, Courtney M: Molecular biology and regulation of the fibrinogen gene: Tissue-specific and ubiquitous expression of fibrinogen γ-chain mRNA. *Blood Coagul Fibrinolysis* 1:433, 1990.

172. Handagama PJ, Shuman MA, Bainton DF: In vivo defibrination results in markedly decreased amounts of fibrinogen in rat megakaryocytes and platelets. *Am J Pathol* 137:1393, 1990.

173. Louache F, Debili N, Cramer E, et al: Fibrinogen is not synthesized by human megakaryocytes. *Blood* 77:311, 1991.

174. Vali Z, Scheraga H: Localization of the binding site on fibrin for the secondary binding site of thrombin. *Biochemistry* 27:1956, 1988.

175. Olexa S, Budzynaski A: Evidence for four different polymerization sites involved in human fibrin formation. *Proc Natl Acad Sci U S A* 77:1374, 1980.

176. Kaczmarek E, McDonagh J: Thrombin binding to the Aα, Bβ, and gamma-chains of fibrinogen and to their remnants contained in fragment E. *J Biol Chem* 263:13896, 1988.

177. Weisel I, Phillips G, Cohen C: The structure of fibrinogen and fibrin: II. Architecture of the fibrin clot. *Ann N Y Acad Sci* 408:367, 1983.

178. Hantgan R, Fowler R, Erickson H, Hermans J: Fibrin assembly: A comparison of electron microscopic and light scattering results. *Thromb Haemost* 44:119, 1980.

179. Dang C, Shin C, Bell W: Fibrinogen sialic acid residues are low affinity calcium-binding sites that influence fibrin assembly. *J Biol Chem* 264:15104, 1989.

180. Nieuwenhuizen W, van Ruijven-Vermneer J, Nooijen W: Recalculation of calcium-binding properties of human and rat fibrin(ogen) and their degradation products. *Thromb Res* 22:653, 1981.

181. Marder V, Budzynski A: Degradation products of fibrinogen and cross-linked fibrin: Projected clinical applications. *Thromb Diath Haemorrh* 32:49, 1974.

182. Elms M, Bunce I, Bundesen P, et al: Measurement of cross-linked fibrin degradation products: An immunoassay using monoclonal antibodies. *Thromb Haemost* 50:591, 1983.

183. Hermans J, McDonagh J: Fibrin: Structure and interactions. *Semin Thromb Hemost* 8:11, 1982.

184. Williams J, Hantgan R, Hermanns J, McDonagh J: Characterization of the inhibition of fibrin assembly by fibrinogen fragment D. *Biochemistry* 197:661, 1981.

185. Lai T-S, Greenberg C: Factor XIII, in *Molecular Basis of Thrombosis and Hemostasis*, edited by KA High, HR Roberts, p 287. Marcel Dekker, New York, 1995.

186. Bottenus R, Ichinose A, Davie E: Nucleotide sequence of the gene for the b subunit of human factor XIII. *Biochemistry* 29:11195, 1990.

187. Ichinose A, Davie E: Characterization of the gene for the a subunit of human factor XIII (plasma transglutaminase) a blood coagulation factor. *Proc Natl Acad Sci U S A* 85:5829, 1988.

188. Ichinose A: Amino acid sequence of the b subunit of human factor XIII, a protein composed of ten repetitive segments. *Biochemistry* 25:4633, 1986.

189. Ichinose A, Bottenus R, Davie E: Structure of transglutaminase. *J Biol Chem* 265:13411, 1990.

190. Henricksson P, Becker S, McDonagh J: Identification of intracellular factor XIII in human monocytes and macrophages. *J Clin Invest* 76:528, 1985.

191. McDonagh J, McDonagh R, Deleage J, Wagner R: Factor XIII in human plasma and platelets. *J Clin Invest* 48:940, 1969.

192. Weisberg L, Shiu D, Greenberg C, et al: Localization of the gene for coagulation factor XIII A-chain to chromosome 6 and identification of sites of synthesis. *J Clin Invest* 79:649, 1987.

193. Kida M, Souri M, Yamamoto M, et al: Transcriptional regulation of cell type-specific expression of the TATA-less A subunit gene for human coagulation factor XIII. *J Biol Chem* 274:6138, 1999.

194. Sakata Y, Aoki N: Cross-linking of a$_2$-plasmin inhibitor to fibrin by fibrin-stabilizing factor. *J Clin Invest* 65:290, 1980.

195. Boffa MB, Reid TS, Joo E, et al: Characterization of the gene encoding human TAFI (thrombin-activatable fibrinolysis inhibitor; plasma procarboxypeptidase B). *Biochemistry* 38:6547, 1999.

196. Boffa MB, Hamill JD, Bastajian N, et al: A role for CCAAT/enhancer-binding protein in hepatic expression of thrombin-activable fibrinolysis inhibitor. *J Biol Chem* 277:25329, 2002.

197. Henry M, Aubert H, Morange PE, et al: Identification of polymorphisms in the promoter and the 3′ region of the TAFI gene: Evidence that plasma TAFI antigen levels are strongly genetically controlled. *Blood* 97:2053, 2001.

198. Koschinsky ML, Boffa MB, Nesheim ME, et al: Association of a single nucleotide polymorphism in CPB2 encoding the thrombin-activable fi-

brinolysis inhibitor (TAF1) with blood pressure. *Clin Genet* 60:345, 2001.

199. Schneider M, Boffa M, Stewart R, et al: Two naturally occurring variants of TAFI (Thr-325 and Ile-325) differ substantially with respect to thermal stability and antifibrinolytic activity of the enzyme. *J Biol Chem* 277:1021, 2002.

200. Broze GJ Jr: Protein Z-dependent regulation of coagulation. *Thromb Haemost* 86:8, 2001.

201. Broze GJ Jr, Warren LA, Novotny WF, et al: The lipoprotein-associated coagulation inhibitor that inhibits the factor VII-tissue factor complex also inhibits factor Xa: Insight into its possible mechanism of action. *Blood* 71:335, 1988.

202. Warn-Cramer B, Rao L, Maki S, Rapaport SI: Modifications of extrinsic pathway inhibitor (EPI) and factor Xa that affect their ability to interact and to inhibit factor VIIa/tissue factor: Evidence for a two-step model of inhibition. *Thromb Haemost* 60:453, 1988.

203. Ameri A, Kuppuswamy M, Basu S, Bajaj S: Expression of tissue factor pathway inhibitor by cultured endothelial cells in response to inflammatory mediators. *Blood* 79:3219, 1992.

204. Sandset P, Abildgaard U, Larsen M: Heparin induces release of extrinsic coagulation pathway inhibitor (EPI). *Thromb Res* 50:803, 1988.

205. Zhang J, Piro O, Lu L, Broze GJ Jr.: Glycosyl phosphatidylinositol anchorage of tissue factor pathway inhibitor. *Circulation* 108:623, 2003.

206. Chang J-Y, Monroe DM, Oliver JA, Roberts HR: TFPIβ, a second product from the mouse tissue factor pathway inhibitor (TFPI) gene. *Thromb Haemost* 81:1999.

207. Griffith MJ: Measurement of the heparin enhanced-antithrombin III/thrombin reaction rate in the presence of synthetic substrates. *Thromb Res* 25:245, 1982.

208. Fuchs HE, Trapp HG, Griffith MJ, et al: Regulation of Factor IXa in vitro in human and mouse plasma and in vivo in the mouse. *J Clin Invest* 73:1696, 1984.

209. Sheffield W, Wu Y, Blajchman M: Antithrombin: Structure and function, in *Molecular Basis of Thrombosis and Hemostasis*, edited by KA High, HR Roberts, p 355. Marcel Dekker, New York, 1995.

210. Hamamoto T, Kisiel W: The effect of cell surface glycosaminoglycans (GAGs) on the inactivation of factor VIIa—Tissue factor activity by antithrombin III. *Int J Hematol* 68:67, 1998.

211. Rao LV, Rapaport SI, Hoang AD: Binding of factor VIIa to tissue factor permits rapid antithrombin III/heparin inhibition of factor VIIa. *Blood* 81:2600, 1993.

212. Pizzo S: Serpin receptor 1: A hepatic receptor that mediates the clearance of antithrombin III protease complexes. *Am J Med* 87:10S, 1989.

213. Ochoa A, Brunel F, Mendelson D, et al: Different liver nuclear proteins bind to similar DNA sequences in the 5′ flanking regions of three hepatic genes. *Nucleic Acids Res* 17:116, 1989.

214. Han X, Fiehler R, Broze GJ Jr: Isolation of a protein Z-dependent plasma protease inhibitor. *Proc Natl Acad Sci U S A* 95:9250, 1998.

215. Tabatabai A, Fiehler R, Broze GJ Jr: Protein Z circulates in plasma in a complex with protein Z-dependent protease inhibitor. *Thromb Haemost* 85:655, 2001.

216. Yin ZF, Huang ZF, Cui J, et al: Prothrombotic phenotype of protein Z deficiency. *Proc Natl Acad Sci U S A* 97:6734, 2000.

217. Macfarlane RG: An enzyme cascade in the blood clotting mechanism, and its function as a biological amplifier. *Nature* 202:498, 1964.

218. Davie EW, Ratnoff OD: Waterfall sequence for intrinsic blood clotting. *Science* 145:1310, 1964.

219. Nemerson Y, Esnouf MP: Activation of a proteolytic system by a membrane lipoprotein: Mechanism of action of tissue factor. *Proc Natl Acad Sci U S A* 70:310, 1973.

220. Nemerson Y: The tissue factor pathway of blood coagulation. *Semin Hematol* 29:170, 1992.

221. Repke D, Gemmell CH, Guha A, et al: Hemophilia as a defect of the tissue factor pathway of blood coagulation: Effect of factors VIII and IX on factor X activation in a continuous-flow reactor. *Proc Natl Acad Sci U S A* 87:7623, 1990.

222. Broze GJ Jr, Girard TJ, Novotny WF: Regulation of coagulation by a multivalent Kunitz-type inhibitor. *Biochemistry* 29:7539, 1990.

223. Hockin MF, Kalafatis M, Shatos M, Mann KG: Protein C activation and factor Va inactivation on human umbilical vein endothelial cells. *Arterioscler Thromb Vasc Biol* 17:2765, 1997.

224. Fay PJ, Smudzin TM, Walker FJ: Activated protein C-catalyzed inactivation of human factor VIII and VIIIa. *J Biol Chem* 266:20139, 1991.

225. Pieters J, Willems G, Hemker HC, Lindhout T: Inhibition of factor IXa and factor Xa by antithrombin III/heparin during factor X activation. *J Biol Chem* 263:15313, 1988.

226. Allen DH, Tracy PB: Human coagulation factor V is activated to the functional cofactor by elastase and cathepsin G expressed at the monocyte surface. *J Biol Chem* 270:1408, 1995.

227. Monroe DM, Hoffman M, Roberts HR: Transmission of a procoagulant signal from tissue factor-bearing cells to platelets. *Blood Coagul Fibrinolysis* 7:459, 1996.

228. Mallat Z, Benamer H, Hugel B, et al: Elevated levels of shed membrane microparticles with procoagulant potential in the peripheral circulating blood of patients with acute coronary syndromes. *Circulation* 101:841, 2000.

229. Satta N, Freyssinet JM, Toti F: The significance of human monocyte thrombomodulin during membrane vesiculation and after stimulation by lipopolysaccharide. *Br J Haematol* 96:534, 1997.

230. Balasubramanian V, Vele O, Nemerson Y: Local shear conditions and platelet aggregates regulate the incorporation and activity of circulating tissue factor in ex-vivo thrombi. *Thromb Haemost* 88:822, 2002.

231. Balasubramanian V, Grabowski E, Bini A, Nemerson Y: Platelets, circulating tissue factor, and fibrin colocalize in ex vivo thrombi: Real-time fluorescence images of thrombus formation and propagation under defined flow conditions. *Blood* 100:2787, 2002.

232. Falati S, Gross P, Merrill-Skoloff G, et al: Real-time in vivo imaging of platelets, tissue factor and fibrin during arterial thrombus formation in the mouse. *Nat Med* 8:1175, 2002.

233. Williamson P, Bevers EM, Smeets EF, et al: Continuous analysis of the mechanism of activated transbilayer lipid movement in platelets. *Biochemistry* 34:10448, 1995.

234. Monroe DM, Roberts HR, Hoffman M: Platelet procoagulant complex assembly in a tissue factor-initiated system. *Br J Haematol* 88:364, 1994.

235. Ahmad SS, Rawala-Sheikh R, Walsh PN: Platelet receptor occupancy with factor IXa promotes factor X activation. *J Biol Chem* 264:20012, 1989.

236. Ahmad SS, Rawala-Sheikh R, Ashby B, Walsh PN: Platelet receptor-mediated factor X activation by factor IX. High-affinity factor IXa receptors induced by factor VIII are deficient on platelets in Scott syndrome. *J Clin Invest* 84:824, 1998.

237. Baglia FA, Walsh PN: Prothrombin is a cofactor for the binding of factor XI to the platelet surface and for platelet-mediated factor XI activation by thrombin. *Biochemistry* 37:2271, 1998.

238. von dem Borne PA, Bajzar L, Meijers JC, et al: Thrombin-mediated activation of factor XI results in a thrombin-activatable fibrinolysis inhibitor-dependent inhibition of fibrinolysis. *J Clin Invest* 99:2323, 1997.

239. Alberio L, Safa O, Clemetson KJ, et al: Surface expression and functional characterization of alpha-granule factor V in human platelets: Effects of ionophore A23187, thrombin, collagen, and convulxin. *Blood* 95:1694, 2000.

240. Dale GL, Friese P, Batar P, et al: Stimulated platelets use serotonin to enhance their retention of procoagulant proteins on the cell surface. *Nature* 415:175, 2002.

241. Kempton CL, Hoffman M, Roberts HR, Monroe DM: Platelet heterogeneity: variation in coagulation complexes on platelet subpopulations *Arterioscler Thromb Vasc Biol* 25:861, 2005.

242. de Agostini A, Watkins S, Slayter H, et al: Localization of the anticoagulantly active heparan sulphate proteoglycans in vascular endothelium: Antithrombin binding on cultured endothelial cells and perfused rat aorta. *J Cell Biol* 111:1293, 1990.

243. Marcus AJ, Broekman MJ, Drosopoulos JHF, et al: The endothelial cell ecto-ADPase responsible for inhibition of platelet function is CD39. *J Clin Invest* 99:1351, 1997.

244. Jesty J, Beltrami E, Willems G: Mathematical analysis of a proteolytic positive-feedback loop: Dependence of lag time and enzyme yields on the initial conditions and kinetic parameters. *Biochemistry* 32:6266, 1993.

245. Brakman P, Albrechtsen OK, Astrup T: A comparative study of coagulation and fibrinolysis in blood from normal men and women. *Br J Haematol* 12:74, 1966.

246. Nossel H, Yudelman I, Canfield R: Measurement of fibrinopeptide A in human blood. *J Clin Invest* 54:43, 1974.

247. Bauer KA, Kass BL, Ten Cate H, et al: Factor IX is activated in vivo by the tissue factor mechanism. *Blood* 76:731, 1990.

248. Bauer KA, Kass BL, Ten Cate H, et al: Detection of factor X activation in humans. *Blood* 74:2007, 1989.

249. Morrissey JH: Tissue factor modulation of factor VIIa activity: Use in measuring trace levels of factor VIIa in plasma. *Thromb Haemost* 74:185, 1995.

250. Conard J, Bauer KA, Gruber A, et al: Normalization of markers of coagulation activation with a purified protein C concentrate in adults with homozygous protein C deficiency. *Blood* 82:1159, 1993.

251. Harlos K, Martin DM, O'Brien DP, et al: Crystal structure of the extracellular region of human tissue factor. *Nature* 370:662, 1994.

CHAPTER 107

CONTROL OF COAGULATION REACTIONS

JOHN H. GRIFFIN

The blood coagulation system, like a powerful engine in idling mode, is always active and generating thrombin at very low levels and is poised for explosive generation of thrombin. The requirement for positive feedback activation of clotting factors (e.g., factors V, VIII, XI, and VII) imparts special threshold properties to the blood coagulation pathways, making the coagulant response nonlinearly responsive to stimuli. Analysis of blood coagulation as a threshold system suggests all-or-none responses to various levels of stimuli, depending on the ensemble of reactions that determine up-regulation and down-regulation of thrombin generation. Because of synergies between cellular and humoral anticoagulant mechanisms, the presence of multiple coagulation inhibitors with complementary modes of action prevents massive thrombin generation in the absence of a substantial procoagulant stimulus. This chapter highlights mechanisms that inhibit blood coagulation, with an emphasis on plasma proteins whose defects cause hereditary thrombophilias. The majority of identifiable thrombophilic defects involves the anticoagulant protein C pathway, with protein C at its center and multiple cofactors or effectors including thrombomodulin, endothelial protein C receptor, protein S, high-density lipoprotein, and factor V. The substrates for enzymatic action of activated protein C include the plasma clotting factors Va and VIIIa and protease activated receptor-1 as a key cell-signaling target. Variant factor V containing Gln506 in place of Arg506 (factor V Leiden) causes hereditary activated protein C resistance by impairing the efficiency of the protein C pathway. Plasma protease inhibitors are essential to block coagulation factor proteases. Antithrombin neutralizes all proteases of the intrinsic coagulation pathway, including thrombin and factors Xa, IXa, XIa, and XIIa, in reactions stimulated by physiologic heparan sulfate or pharmacologic heparins. Tissue factor pathway inhibitor neutralizes the extrinsic coagulation pathway factors VIIa and Xa. Other plasma protease inhibitors also can neutralize various coagulation proteases, although the clinical significance of these reactions is less apparent than reactions of heparin-dependent antithrombin or tissue factor pathway inhibitor.

Acronyms and abbreviations that appear in this chapter include: APC, activated protein C; C4BP, C4b-binding protein; DIC, disseminated intravascular coagulation; EGF, epidermal growth factor; EPCR, endothelial cell protein C receptor; EPI, extrinsic pathway inhibitor; Gla, γ-carboxyglutamic acid; HDL, high-density lipoprotein; LACI, lipoprotein-associated coagulation inhibitor; MHC, major histocompatibility complex; NMDA, N-methyl-D-aspartate; PAR, protease-activated receptor; serpin, *serine protease inhibitor*; SHBG, sex hormone-binding globulin; TFPI, tissue factor pathway inhibitor; TM, thrombomodulin; TSR, thrombin-sensitive region; ZPI, protein Z-dependent protease inhibitor.

INTRODUCTION

Control of coagulation reactions is essential for normal hemostasis. As part of the tangled web of host defense systems that respond to vascular injury, the blood coagulation factors (see Chap. 106) act in concert with the endothelium and platelets to generate a protective fibrin-platelet clot, forming a hemostatic plug. Thrombosis occurs when the protective clot is extended beyond its beneficial size, when a clot occurs inappropriately at sites of vascular disease, or when a clot embolizes to other sites in the circulatory bed. For normal hemostasis, both procoagulant and anticoagulant factors must interact with the vascular components and cell surfaces, including the vessel wall (see Chap. 108) and platelets (see Chap. 105). Moreover, the action of the fibrinolytic system must be integrated with coagulation reactions for timely formation and dissolution of blood clots (see Chap. 127).

This chapter highlights the major physiologic mechanisms for down-regulation of blood coagulation reactions and the plasma proteins that inhibit blood coagulation, with an emphasis on those mechanisms whose defects are clinically significant based on insights gleaned from consideration of the hereditary thrombophilias (see Chap. 122). Chapter 106 provides a complete description of blood coagulation factors and hemostatic pathways.

BLOOD COAGULATION PATHWAYS AND THE PROTEIN C PATHWAY

Although more than 40 years have elapsed since the elaboration of the cascade model[1,2] for blood coagulation pathways (see Fig. 106-27), the basic outline of sequential conversions of protease zymogens to active serine proteases still is useful, albeit with important modifications, for representing blood coagulation reactions. The major conceptual advances for procoagulant pathways in the past 2 decades emphasize both positive and negative feedback reactions affecting thrombin generation (Fig. 107-1).

In positive feedback reactions, procoagulant thrombin activates platelets and factors V, VIII, and XI (see Chap. 106).[3-7] Small amounts of thrombin can be generated by trace amounts of tissue factor via the extrinsic pathway. Subsequently, thrombin can activate factors XI, VIII, and V, thereby stimulating each of the steps in the intrinsic pathway and thus amplifying thrombin generation (see Fig. 107-1).

Negative feedback reactions involve the expression of activated protein C (APC) anticoagulant activity that is generated by the protein C cellular pathway[8,9] (Fig. 107-2). The protein C cellular pathway is defined here as involving reactions that generate APC and reactions that mediate the direct effects of APC on cells. The direct effects of APC on cells,[9] which are entirely independent of the action of APC on factors Va and VIIIa, are manifested as antiinflammatory and antiapoptotic activities and as alterations of gene expression profiles (see "Activated Protein C Direct Cellular Activities" below). The direct effects of APC on cells indirectly down-regulate thrombin generation because inflammation and apoptosis contribute to reactions that promote thrombin generation.[9]

For APC generation by the protein C cellular pathway, binding of thrombin to thrombomodulin (TM) converts the bound thrombin from a procoagulant enzyme to an anticoagulant enzyme that converts the protein C zymogen to the anticoagulant serine protease APC (see Fig. 107-1 and 107-2). This surface-dependent reaction is enhanced by the endothelial cell protein C receptor (EPCR) that binds protein C.[8,10,11] In a subsequent negative feedback loop, APC with the aid of its nonenzymatic cofactor protein S inactivates factors Va and VIIIa by highly selective proteolysis, yielding inactive (i) cofactors and factors V_i and VIII_i. Protein S also can directly inhibit factors VIIIa, Xa, and Va.[12-15] Thus, APC and protein S inhibit multiple steps in the intrinsic coagulation pathway.

Blood Coagulation Pathways   Protein C Pathway

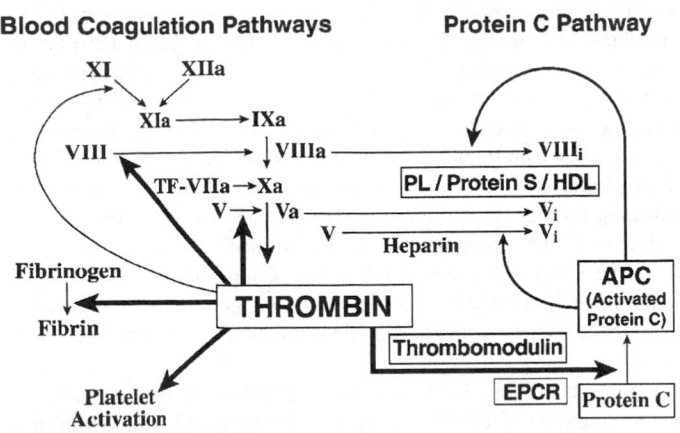

FIGURE 107-1 Blood coagulation pathways and protein C anticoagulant pathway. Thrombin can be either procoagulant *(left)* or anticoagulant *(right)*, depending on cofactors and surfaces. Coagulant thrombin clots fibrinogen and activates platelets and factors V, VIII, XI, and XIII. Conversion of zymogen protein C to anticoagulant activated protein C (APC) by thrombomodulin-bound thrombin is enhanced by endothelial protein C receptor (EPCR). APC with its nonenzymatic cofactor protein S inactivates factors Va and VIIIa by highly selective proteolysis (e.g., at Arg506 and Arg306 in factor Va), yielding inactivated (i) factors V_i and VIII_i. This anticoagulant action may be enhanced by phospholipid (PL) surfaces on platelets, endothelial cells, or their microparticles. HDL can also provide protein S-dependent anticoagulant APC-cofactor activity. Similarly, neutral glycosphingolipids such as glucosylceramide can enhance APC anticoagulant activity. HDL, high-density lipoprotein. (Adapted from JH Griffin,[371] with permission.)

At all steps in the coagulation pathways, each clotting protease can be inhibited by one or more plasma protease inhibitors in reactions stimulated by negatively charged glycosaminoglycans such as heparan sulfate or heparin.[16] Given the highly nonlinear nature of the coagulation pathways with both positive and negative feedback reactions, synergy between the protein C pathway and plasma protease inhibitors is important for regulating thrombin generation.

Coagulation factors are activated physiologically and continuously at a low basal level. Plasma from all normal subjects contains circulating active enzymes, factor VIIa[17] and APC,[18] and various polypeptide fragments generated by the action of clotting proteases, namely, fibrinopeptides,[19,20] prothrombin fragment 1+2,[21] and activation peptides derived from factors IX and X.[22,23] The presence of multiple clotting factors that require positive feedback activation (e.g., factors V, VIII, XI, and VII) imparts special threshold properties to the blood coagulation pathways, making the coagulant response nonlinearly responsive to stimuli. Theoretical analysis of blood coagulation as a threshold system suggests an all-or-none response to various levels of stimulation, depending on the ensemble of activating and inhibitory reactions that defines up-regulation and down-regulation of thrombin generation.[24,25] The coagulation system appears to be active, but idling, and poised for extensive and explosive generation of thrombin. Because of synergy among various cellular and humoral anticoagulant mechanisms that establish a threshold system, the presence of multiple coagulation inhibitors with complementary modes of action prevents massive thrombin generation in the absence of a substantial procoagulant stimulus.

HEREDITARY DEFICIENCIES ASSOCIATED WITH THROMBOTIC DISEASE

Evidence for the physiologic importance of specific factors for controlling coagulation reactions comes from clinical observations and animal model studies. Major identified genetic risk factors for venous thrombosis involve protein structural defects in factor V, protein C, protein S, and antithrombin (see Chap. 122). In addition, gene regulatory defects are associated with thrombotic disease, such as the nt G20210A polymorphism in the prothrombin gene that causes elevated levels of prothrombin and the defects in protein C regulatory elements that decrease protein C expression. Deficiencies of TM also might be associated with increased risk of arterial thrombosis. Association of hereditary abnormalities of EPCR with an increased risk of thrombosis has been suggested but remains controversial.

PROTEIN C PATHWAY COMPONENTS

Figure 107-3 shows schematic representations of the structures of protein C, protein S, TM, and EPCR. These proteins contain multiple domains, each of which may mediate different molecular functions. Tables 106-1 and 107-1 list values for the molecular weight, normal plasma concentration, chromosomal location, and gene structures of these factors. As substrates of APC, factors Va and VIIIa also are participants in the reactions of the anticoagulant protein C pathway. Moreover, certain forms of factor V can act as an APC cofactor for inactivation of factor VIIIa (see section on "Activated Protein C Anticoagulant Cofactors").[26,27]

PROTEIN C

In 1976, Stenflo[28] designated a bovine plasma vitamin K-dependent protein that eluted in the third peak (peak C) from an anion exchange column as bovine "protein C." Protein C was found to be identical to the previously identified anticoagulant factor autoprothrombin II-A.[29] Biochemical studies showed that protein C is a zymogen that can be isolated from either bovine or human plasma and converted to an anticoagulantly active serine protease by the action of thrombin.[30,31]

Protein C is synthesized in the liver as a polypeptide precursor of 461 residues, with a prepropeptide of 42 amino acids that contains the signal for carboxylation of Glu residues by a carboxylase that forms nine γ-carboxyglutamic acid (Gla) residues and secretion of the mature protein.[32–34] The mature glycoprotein of M_r 62,000 contains 419 residues (see Fig. 106-12) and N-linked carbohydrate. The majority of the secreted protein C molecules are cleaved by a furin-like endoprotease that releases Lys156-Arg157 and generates a two-chain zymogen that circulates in plasma at 70 nM (4 μg/ml).[35,36] The heavy and light chains of plasma protein C are covalently linked by a disulfide bond that keeps the serine protease globular domain (residues 170–419) covalently tethered to the N-terminal string of three domains: the Gla domain and the epidermal growth factor-like domains EGF1 and EGF2 (see Fig. 107-3).[32–34,37–39]

The Gla domain of protein C (residues 1–42) and APC is important for a number of functions, including binding to phospholipid-containing membranes, TM, and EPCR; thus, incomplete carboxylation impairs the functional anticoagulant activity of APC.[40–45] The EGF1 domain undergoes an unusual posttranslational modification resulting in β-hydroxyaspartic acid at residue 71, and this modification appears essential for full anticoagulant activity.[46] The two EGF modules in the light chain also may contribute to interactions of APC with protein S and of protein C with TM.

The serine protease domain of protein C is homologous to other trypsin-like proteases. Three-dimensional modeling[47,48] and x-ray crystallographic structures[39] reflect the structural similarity of APC to members of the serine protease family, of which chymotrypsin is the prototype. APC's trypsin-like protease domain exerts its anticoagulant activity by highly specific interactions with factors Va and VIIIa, followed by cleavage at only two Arg-containing peptide bonds (see

"Activated Protein C Anticoagulant Activity" below). These stereo-specific interactions involve both the APC enzymatic active site region and a number of APC residues that are termed *exosites* because they are not located in the immediate vicinity of APC's enzymatic active site. APC exosites are essential for specific recognition of the macromolecular substrates factors Va and VIIIa.[49-55]

PROTEIN C AND ACTIVATED PROTEIN C THERAPY

Purified plasma protein C concentrate has been successfully used to treat patients with thrombotic episodes.[56,57] Recombinant APC (Xigris) reduces all-cause 28-day mortality in patients with severe sepsis.[58] The successful therapy for severe sepsis using APC followed sepsis studies in baboons.[59] Other preclinical studies[60] suggest APC may be useful in multiple settings, including ischemic stroke[61,62] or islet transplantation[63] for diabetes, and have shed light on *in vivo* mechanisms for APC beneficial effects (see "Activated Protein C Direct Cellular Activities").

PROTEIN C GENE

The protein C gene, comprising nine exons and eight introns, is located on chromosome 2q14-21 and spans 11 kb (see Fig. 106-12 and Table 107-1).[64-69] The protein C gene is homologous to the genes for factors VII, IX, and X (see Chap. 106).

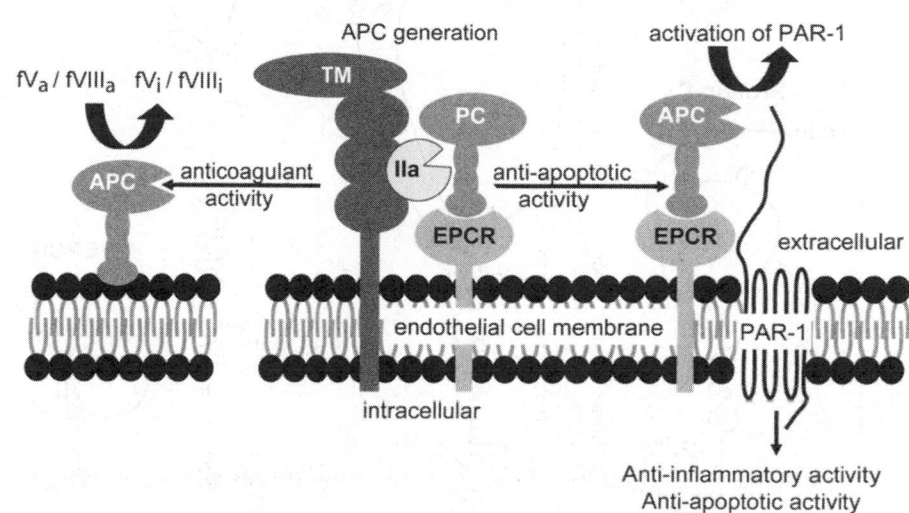

FIGURE 107-2   Activated protein C (APC) anticoagulant activity and the protein C (PC) cellular pathway. On an endothelial surface, APC generation follows binding of PC to endothelial protein C receptor (EPCR), where PC is activated by limited proteolysis by the thrombin–thrombomodulin complex (IIa:TM). This action of thrombin liberates a dodecapeptide (residues 158–169) from PC to generate anticoagulant APC, which exerts its activity by proteolytic inactivation of factors Va and VIIIa on surfaces containing phospholipids, such as cellular or microparticle surfaces. Direct effects of APC on cells are initiated by activation of protease-activated receptor-1 (PAR-1) by EPCR-bound APC. The Gla domain of APC binds to EPCR to allow the protease domain to cleave the extracellular N-terminal tail of PAR-1, which results in generation of antiinflammatory and antiapoptotic activities and alteration of gene expression profiles. (Adapted from LO Mosnier and JH Griffin,[272] with permission.)

PROTEIN C MUTATIONS

Hereditary protein C deficiency associated with thrombosis is caused by numerous mutations, and a database of more than 100 different mutations was published.[70] Based on three-dimensional models of the protease domain of protein C, the structural basis for protein C defects has been rationalized.[48,71,72] Most mutations that cause type I protein C deficiency, characterized by parallel reductions in activity and antigen, involve amino acid residues that form the hydrophobic cores of the two folded globulin-like domains that are characteristic of serine proteases. These mutations destabilize either the process or the product of protein folding, and they result in unstable molecules that are poorly secreted and/or exhibit a very short circulatory half-life. In contrast, most mutations that cause type II defects (reduced activity but normal antigen levels), that is, circulating dysfunctional molecules, involve polar surface residues that do not affect polypeptide folding or thermodynamic stability. These polar residues presumably are involved in protein–protein interactions important for expression of anticoagulant activity.

Severe protein C deficiency resulting from homozygous knockout of the mouse protein C gene showed a similar phenotype as severe human protein C deficiency (see Chap. 122), with perinatal consumptive coagulopathy in the brain and liver and either death or massive thrombosis that occurred *in utero* or shortly after birth.[73]

PROTEIN S

Protein S was first purified from plasma by DiScipio and colleagues,[74,75] who named it *protein S* in honor of Seattle, the city of its discovery. It is a vitamin K-dependent glycoprotein that is synthesized by hepatocytes, neuroblastoma cells, kidney cells, testis, megakaryocytes, and endothelial cells[76-80] and is found in platelet α-granules.[81] Protein S is inducible by interleukin-4 in T cells.[82]

Protein S is synthesized as a precursor protein of 676 amino acids that gives rise to a mature secreted single-chain glycoprotein of 635 residues with three N-linked carbohydrate side chains (see Figs. 106-13 and 107-3).[83-86] Eleven Gla residues in the N-terminal region of mature protein S contribute to Ca^{2+}-mediated binding of the protein to phospholipid membranes. The thrombin-sensitive region (TSR), which includes residues 47 to 72, follows the Gla-domain (see Fig. 107-3). Four EGF modules, each containing one unusual residue of β-hydroxyaspartic acid or β-hydroxyasparagine, have functions that have not been established, although they likely contribute to Ca^{2+} binding.[84,87-89]

The C-terminal region of protein S, the sex hormone-binding globulin (SHBG)-like region (residues 270–635), contains binding sites for C4b-binding protein (C4BP) (see "Activated Protein C-Independent Anticoagulant Activity of Protein S")[90,91] and factors V and Va.[92,93] Thus, different domains of protein S exhibit a number of different binding sites for different plasma proteins.

PROTEIN S GENE

The protein S gene, comprising 15 exons and 14 introns, is located on chromosome 3p11.1-11.2 and spans 80 kb (see Fig. 106-13 and Table 107-1).[68,94-101] The protein S gene has limited homology with other genes for vitamin K-dependent factors in the Gla and EGF domains (see Chap. 106) and notable homology of the region coding for residues 240 to 635 with genes of the SHBG family. Because humans

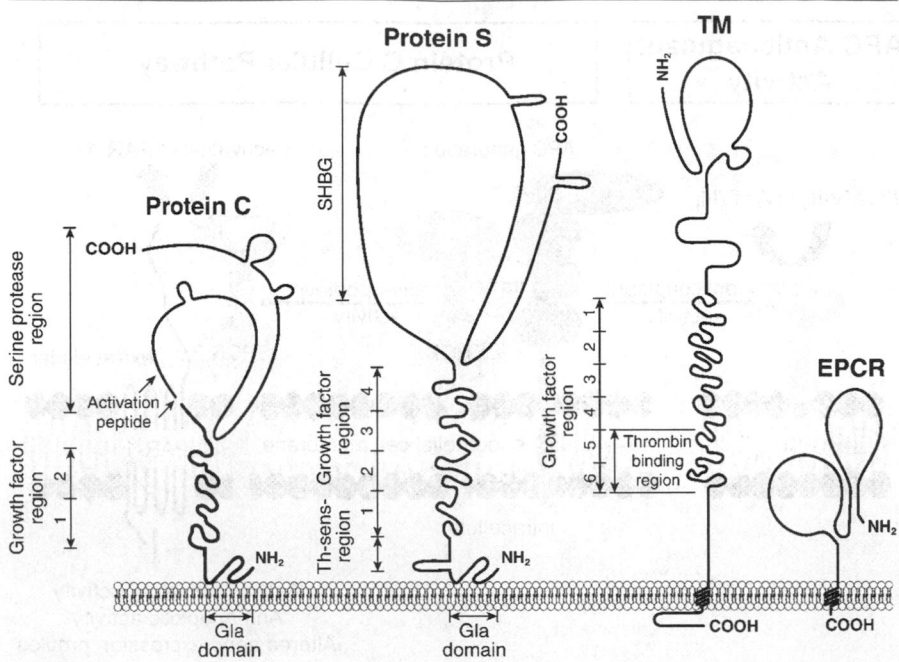

FIGURE 107-3   Membrane-bound protein C, protein S, thrombomodulin (TM), and the endothelial cell protein C receptor (EPCR). Each protein is a multidomain protein that extends above the surface of cell membranes, and different domains mediate different functions of each protein. Protein C and protein S can bind reversibly to phospholipid membranes through their NH₂-terminal domains, which contain 9 or 11 γ-carboxyglutamic acid (Gla) residues that bind four to six Ca²⁺ ions. Thrombomodulin and EPCR are integral membrane proteins that are embedded in cell membranes by a single hydrophobic transmembrane sequence. (Adapted from CT Esmon,[108] with permission.)

harbor a protein S pseudogene that contains several stop codons and is not translated, the normal active gene is designated as *protein S1* or *protein Sα*, and the pseudogene is designated *protein S2* or *protein Sβ*. The pseudogene is 97 percent homologous with the normal gene and is located very close to the normal protein S gene on chromosome 3.

PROTEIN S MUTATIONS
Hereditary protein S deficiency associated with thrombosis is caused by numerous mutations, and a database of more than 100 different mutations was published.[102] One protein S polymorphism present in less than 1 percent of Caucasians causes replacement of Ser460 by Pro and results in absence of N-linked carbohydrate on Asn458 in the

variant, designated *protein S Heerlen*.[103] Although initially controversial, no significant functional consequence of the absence of this carbohydrate or of the presence of Pro460 for protein S functions has been established.

THROMBOMODULIN

TM was discovered and named by Esmon and Owen,[104,105] who demonstrated that endothelial cell surfaces possess a nonenzymatic cofactor that accelerates protein C activation by thrombin. Binding of thrombin to TM converts thrombin from a procoagulant enzyme to an anticoagulant enzyme because TM-bound thrombin loses its normal ability to clot fibrinogen or activate platelets.[106,107] TM is a multidomain transmembrane protein comprising an N-terminal lectin-like domain, six EGF domains, a Ser/Thr-rich region, a single membrane-spanning sequence, and an intracellular C-terminal tail (see Fig. 107-3).[7,108–110] Much is known about structure–function relationships of this protein.[7,108,111–115] EGF domains 4, 5, and 6 are essential for activation of protein C, with the latter two domains binding thrombin and the first domain binding protein C. The mature protein has 557 amino acid residues and variable amounts of N-linked and O-linked carbohydrates that cause variability in molecular size. Glycosaminoglycans, notably chondroitin sulfate, covalently attached to the Ser/Thr-rich region contribute to the functional properties of TM either by enhancing protein C activation by thrombin or by accelerating neutralization of thrombin by protease inhibitors. Modulation of the substrate specificity of thrombin by TM involves conformational changes in thrombin caused by binding of TM.[116]

Low levels of soluble TM circulate in plasma, presumably as a result of limited proteolysis of the protein near its transmembrane cell surface anchor.[117] The functional significance of circulating TM is unknown, although variations in its plasma level arise in different clinical conditions.

THROMBOMODULIN GENE
The TM gene, which lacks introns, is located on chromosome 20p12 and spans 3.7 kb (see Fig. 106-21 and Table 107-1).[110,117–119] Down-

TABLE 107-1   CHARACTERISTICS OF BLOOD COAGULATION REGULATORY MOLECULES

	MOLECULAR WEIGHT (KDA)	PLASMA CONCENTRATION (μG/LITER)	HALF-LIFE (H)	CHROMOSOME	GENE (KB)	EXONS (N)	FUNCTION
Protein C	62	4	6	2q13-14	11	9	Anticoagulant protease
Protein S	75	26	42	3p11.1-11.2	80	15	APC-cofactor coagulation inhibitor
Thrombomodulin	60–105	0.020	ND	20p11.2–cen	3.7	1	Receptor for thrombin/protein C
Endothelial protein C receptor (EPCR)	46	0.098	ND	20q11.2	6	4	Receptor for protein C/APC
Protease activated receptor-1 (PAR-1)	68	—	—	5q13	27	2	G-protein coupled receptor
Antithrombin	58	150	70	1q23-25	14	7	Protease inhibitor
Tissue factor pathway inhibitor (TFPI)	34	0.1	ND	2q31-32.1	85	9	Protease inhibitor
Heparin cofactor II	66	70	60	22q11	16	5	Protease inhibitor

regulation of the TM gene is stimulated by a variety of inflammatory agents, including endotoxin, interleukin-1, and tissue necrosis factor alpha and is up-regulated by retinoic acid.[120] In general, agents that down-regulate TM expression usually up-regulate tissue factor expression in a manner consistent with the general concept that these cellular factors exert opposing activities on the hemostatic balance (see Chap. 106).

THROMBOMODULIN MUTATIONS

TM genetic mutations are not strongly established as clinically significant, but they may be associated with increased risk of arterial thrombosis and myocardial infarction but not venous thrombosis (see Chap. 122).[121–123]

ENDOTHELIAL PROTEIN C RECEPTOR

EPCR that binds both protein C and APC with similar affinities was cloned by Fukudome and Esmon[10] in 1994. Subsequent studies, especially those by Esmon's laboratory, have defined many properties of murine, bovine, and human EPCR.[45,124–134]

The mature EPCR glycoprotein contains 221 amino acid residues and N-linked carbohydrate, giving an Mr of 46,000. EPCR is an integral membrane protein that is homologous to CD1/major histocompatibility complex (MHC) class I molecules. The N-terminus is part of an extracellular domain that is connected to a single transmembrane sequence that is followed by a short Arg-Arg-Cys-COOH cytoplasmic tail (see Fig. 107-3). The cytoplasmic tail can be palmitoylated, and this modification may localize EPCR to caveolae. EPCR binds protein C and APC equally well and appears to bind through their Gla domains. EPCR is mainly located on the surface of large vessels, in contrast to the predominant localization of TM in the microcirculation. EPCR on endothelial surfaces enhances by fivefold the rate of activation of protein C by thrombin–TM (see Fig. 107-2). Based on the homology between EPCR and CD1/MHC class I molecules, a three-dimensional model of EPCR was constructed, allowing speculation about EPCR structure–function relationships.[135] The subsequent three-dimensional structure of EPCR determined by x-ray crystallography confirmed the expected overall folding of the protein, identified the site of binding of the protein C Gla domain, and revealed the presence of a single phospholipid molecule bound in a groove on the surface.[134]

Soluble EPCR is found in normal human plasma at 100 ng/ml. In purified reaction mixtures, soluble EPCR at relatively high levels inhibits the anticoagulant action of APC on factor Va but not the reaction of APC with protease inhibitors.[125,136] Levels of soluble EPCR are increased during disseminated intravascular coagulation (DIC) and in patients with systemic lupus erythematosus, and EPCR increases are not correlated with alterations in circulating TM levels.[137] Because soluble EPCR binds protein C and APC with an affinity similar to the membrane-bound molecule, EPCR has been speculated to bind the protein C and the APC Gla domains without thermodynamically significant contributions from membrane phospholipids, a speculation seemingly confirmed by the crystallographic structure of EPCR.[134]

APC exerts antiinflammatory activity that appears to be independent of its anticoagulant activity (see "Activated Protein C Direct Cellular Activities").[9,58] EPCR in APC–EPCR complexes modulates the biologic activity of APC by shifting its proteolytic specificity from the coagulant factors Va and VIIIa toward protease-activated receptor (PAR)-1 (see Fig. 107-2).

ENDOTHELIAL CELL PROTEIN C RECEPTOR GENE

The EPCR gene, comprising four exons and three introns, is located on chromosome 20q11.2 and spans 6 kb.[138]

PROTEASE ACTIVATED RECEPTOR-1

PAR-1 was discovered as the high-affinity platelet receptor for thrombin.[139] PAR-1 is the prototype of a four-member family of G-protein coupled receptors that share an unusual mechanism of activation, namely activation by proteases.[140–146] Each PAR contains seven transmembrane helical domains and an extracellular N-terminal tail that is cleaved by an activating protease such that the newly generated amino terminus is a tethered ligand that triggers activation of the coupled G-protein. Human platelets use PAR-1 and PAR-3 for activation by thrombin, whereas murine platelets require PAR-3 and PAR-4 but not PAR-1.

PROTEASE ACTIVATED RECEPTOR-1 GENE

PAR-1 contains only two introns, is located on chromosome 5q13 and spans 25 kb (see Table 107-1).[140] Much is known about many factors that can either up-regulate or down-regulate the PAR-1 gene.[140–146]

ACTIVATION OF PROTEIN C

Protein C is converted to an active serine protease following cleavage by thrombin at the Arg169-Leu170 peptide bond in a Ca^{2+}-dependent reaction that liberates a dodecapeptide (residues 158-169) from protein C. This reaction is accelerated by orders of magnitude by TM (see "Thrombomodulin" above).[7,8,30,31]

Proof that thrombin is a physiologic activator of protein C includes the demonstrations that thrombin infusions into baboons generate anticoagulant activity resulting from APC.[147,148] Interestingly, thrombin infusion into hyperlipidemic monkeys with atherosclerosis generated less APC and caused a poorer ex vivo response to APC compared with normolipidemic control monkeys,[149] showing that hyperlipidemia and vascular disease can affect protein C activation.

Proof that TM is a physiologic antithrombotic cofactor comes from studies of mice containing a targeted point mutation in TM that markedly impairs its ability to activate protein C. Mice with a specific Glu to Pro mutation in the loop between EGF4 and EGF5 in TM have a hypercoagulable state, fibrin deposition, and a severely reduced ability to activate protein C.[150,151] However, TM has additional biologic functions, including a critical as yet undefined role in fetal development, because complete knockout of the TM gene is associated with embryonic lethality before development of an intact cardiovascular system.[152] The N-terminal lectin-like domain of TM that is not required for protein C activation plays a key role in normal embryonic development by mechanisms that are not yet clear.[7,153]

Ischemia causes protein C activation in vivo. A brief occlusion of the left anterior descending coronary artery in pigs results in APC generation.[154] During cerebral ischemia in humans undergoing routine endarterectomy, APC increases in venous cerebral blood.[155] Protein C is significantly activated during cardiopulmonary bypass, mainly during the minutes immediately after aortic unclamping in the ischemic vascular beds.[156] Streptokinase therapy for acute myocardial infarction increases circulating APC.[157]

Circulating APC concentration in normal human subjects is highly correlated with circulating levels of protein C zymogen.[158] Based on protein C infusion studies in protein C-deficient subjects, the level of circulating APC is strongly determined by the concentration of protein C.[159]

EPCR is required for normal protein C activation in response to thrombin infusions in experimental animals.[160] EPCR likely contributes to setting the basal levels of circulating APC because in vitro studies of thrombin-dependent protein C activation show that EPCR enhances protein C activation by thrombin–TM.[129] This concept for protein C activation is presented in Fig. 107-2, which schematically indicates activation of EPCR-bound protein C. This model for protein C activation allows EPCR to substitute for negatively charged phospholipids; it also implies that a cellular response to a specific stimulus brings EPCR and TM in close proximity such that protein C activation is enhanced by a specific agonist that itself does not generate thrombin or up-regulate TM (see Fig. 107-2).

TM is abundantly present in the small blood vessels but less so in large vessels, whereas EPCR is more abundant in large vessels than in small vessels.[120] TM levels vary markedly in different tissues,[161] with significant consequences for a variable tendency for fibrin deposition in different organs.[108,150,151] In contrast to an initial report that TM is absent in brain,[162] low levels are expressed in brain,[163–166] and brain-specific activation of protein C in humans occurs during carotid occlusion.[155]

Proteolytic cleavage and activation of protein C can be effected by meizothrombin, plasmin, or factor Xa.[167–170] On the surface of cultured endothelial cells, negatively charged sulfated polysaccharides in the presence of phospholipid vesicles containing phosphatidylethanolamine can enhance the rate of protein C activation by factor Xa to approach the protein C activation rate of thrombin–TM.[170] However, no data yet indicate whether protein C activation by meizothrombin, plasmin, or factor Xa is physiologically relevant.

Protein C activation is stimulated by platelet factor 4. Interestingly, physiologically relevant concentrations of platelet factor 4 stimulate thrombin-dependent APC generation both *in vitro* by cultured endothelial cells and *in vivo* in a primate thrombin infusion model, suggesting platelet factor 4 plays a previously unsuspected physiologic role in enhancing APC generation.[171–173]

ACTIVATED PROTEIN C ACTIVITIES

APC exerts anticoagulant activity. APC also interacts directly with cell receptors, providing antiinflammatory and antiapoptotic activities and altering gene expression profiles (see Fig. 107-2). Both the anticoagulant activity of APC and the direct effects of APC on cells are mediated by different sets of molecular interactions and are clearly physiologic and clinically relevant.

ACTIVATED PROTEIN C ANTICOAGULANT ACTIVITY

Mechanisms for APC's direct anticoagulant activity involve factors V and VIII, the two homologous coagulation cofactors that circulate as inactive molecules and that are converted to active cofactors by limited proteolysis (see Chap. 106 and Figs. 106-15 and 106-17). APC circulates at 40 pM in normal humans, and an inverse correlation exists between fibrinopeptide A and APC levels in healthy nonsmoking adults, suggesting that APC is a significant regulator of basal thrombin activity.[18,174] APC also indirectly exerts anticoagulant effects through its direct effects on cells (see "Activated Protein C Direct Cellular Activities" below).

Factors V and VIII are synthesized as large single-chain precursor coagulation cofactors of M_r 330,000, consisting of three homologous A domains (A1, A2, and A3) and two homologous C domains (C1 and C2) with a very large intervening, nonhomologous domain, designated B domain, which connects the A2 and A3 domains. In factors Va and VIIIa, the A domains form heterotrimeric structures such as ceruloplasmin, whereas the C domains form head-to-tail heterodimeric structures.[27,54,175–180] Activation of factor V is accomplished by limited proteolysis at Arg709, Arg1018, and Arg1545 by thrombin, factor Xa, or other proteases (Fig. 107-4). Cleavage at Arg1545 is the key step for generating factor Va activity because proteolysis releases the B domain that blocks binding of factor Xa to factor Va.[181–184] The various

forms of factor Va (Fig. 107-4) are composed of two polypeptide chains, one bearing the A1-A2 domains and the other bearing the A3-C1-C2 domains. The noncovalent interactions between the two chains are stabilized by Ca^{2+} ions because these chains dissociate in the absence of divalent metal ions. Although generally similar to factor V activation, factor VIII activation (see Fig. 106-17) involves formation of a heterotrimer of polypeptide chains, consisting of A1 domain and A2 domain noncovalently linked with A3-C1-C2 domains through calcium ions. In contrast to heterodimeric factor Va, heterotrimeric factor VIIIa is intrinsically unstable because of spontaneous dissociation of the A2 domain.[185]

FACTORS Va AND VIIIa AS SUBSTRATES FOR ACTIVATED PROTEIN C

Irreversible proteolytic inactivation of factors Va and VIIIa by APC can be accomplished by proteolysis at Arg506 and Arg306 in factor Va and Arg562 and Arg362 in factor VIIIa (see Figs. 106-15, 106-17, and 107-4).[27,179,186–190] Currently, the most common identifiable venous thrombosis risk factor involves a mutation of Arg506 to Gln in factor V (factor V Leiden) that results in APC resistance (see Chap. 122). The complexities of APC-dependent inactivation of factor Va and VIIIa are compounded by the number of different molecular forms of Va and VIIIa that can be generated by limited proteolysis with a variety of proteases and by their differing susceptibilities to APC and to the different APC cofactors. Although some elements of these complexities are clear, many details are not well understood. A poor anticoagulant response, that is, "APC resistance," can be caused by a number of molecular defects in APC cofactors or in APC's substrates.

ACTIVATED PROTEIN C RESISTANCE

APC resistance is defined as an abnormally reduced anticoagulant response of a plasma sample to APC (see Chap. 122) and can be caused by many potential abnormalities in the protein C anticoagulant pathway. Abnormalities include defective APC cofactors, defective APC substrates, or other molecules that interfere with normal functioning of the protein C anticoagulant pathway (e.g., autoantibodies against APC, APC cofactors, or APC substrates).

A report of familial venous thrombosis associated with APC resistance without an identifiable defect in four Swedish families[191] led to an intensive search for a genetic explanation that was soon found to involve replacement of G by A at nucleotide 1691 in exon 10 of the factor V gene, which causes the amino acid replacement of Arg506 by Gln.[192–194] This factor V variant, which arose in a single Caucasian founder approximately 21,000 to 34,000 years ago,[195] is known as *factor V Leiden*. This mutation currently is a common, but not the only, cause of APC resistance.

The molecular mechanism for APC resistance of Gln506-factor V is based on the fact that the variant molecule is inactivated 10 times slower than normal Arg506-factor Va.[27,179,194,196–198] The variant factor Va exhibits only partial resistance to APC because cleavage at Arg306 in factor Va also occurs, causing complete loss of factor Va activity.[199] This finding helps explain why APC resistance resulting from Gln506-factor V is a mild risk factor for venous thrombosis and why a combination of genetic risk factors or a combination of genetic and acquired risk factors for venous thrombosis is found in a significant fraction of symptomatic patients (see Chap. 122). Another possibility to help explain the mild risk of venous thrombosis associated with Gln506-factor V is that factor Va may be inactivated *in vivo* by proteases other than APC that cleave at sites other than residue Arg506.

A factor V haplotype, designated R2, has been associated with mild APC resistance,[200] although the R2 haplotype appears to be a risk factor only when present with a Gln506-factor V allele.[201]

Plasma and recombinant factor V can exist in two biochemically distinct forms, designated *factor V1* and *factor V2*.[202–205] Factor V1 has N-linked carbohydrate on Asn2181, near the phospholipid binding region of the C2 domain, whereas factor V2 has none. Because the N-linked carbohydrate appears to decrease the apparent affinity of factor V1 or Va1 for phospholipid, it reduces the specific clotting activity and susceptibility to APC. Normal plasma contains a mixture of factors V1 and V2. Removal of the carbohydrate attached to factor V increases the rate of inactivation of factor Va by APC, although the clinical significance of this phenomenon is unknown.[206]

APC resistance with no identifiable genetic or acquired abnormalities in patients with venous and arterial thrombosis has been reported.[207–211] Further studies are needed to identify the causes of APC resistance in these patients, and further work is needed to develop and compare various APC resistance assays that have different sensitivities to different physiologic variables or plasma components. For example, APTT-based assays are not equivalently sensitive as are dilute tissue-factor-based assays to plasma high-density lipoprotein (HDL) levels or oral contraceptive use.[212,213] Plasma variables, such as elevated prothrombin levels, may affect the response to APC by inhibiting APC anticoagulant action,[214] although hyperprothrombinemia might also inhibit fibrinolysis.[215]

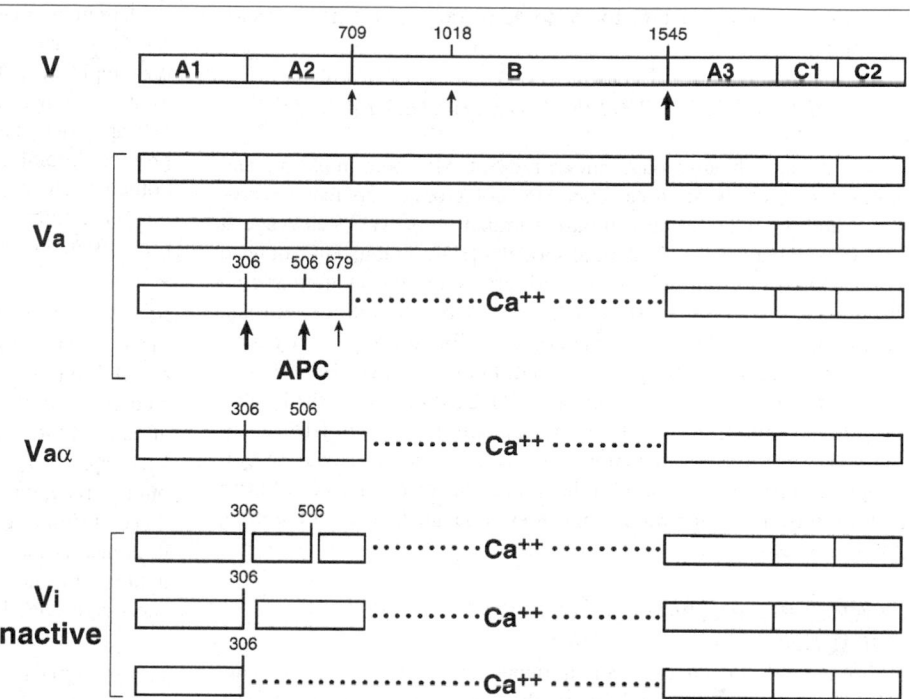

FIGURE 107-4 Proteolytic activation and inactivation of factors V and Va. *Lines* represent polypeptide structures of factor V, active factor Va species, and inactive factor V_i. Activation of factor V by thrombin, factor Xa, or Russell viper venom is associated with cleavages at Arg709, Arg1018, and Arg1545. Inactivation of factor Va by activated protein C (APC) involves cleavages at Arg506, Arg306, and Arg679. If factor Va is cleaved by APC only at Arg506, designated as *factor Vaα*, it exhibits approximately 70 percent procoagulant activity. Cleavage at Arg306 is the most important cleavage for full inactivation of factor Va and is markedly phospholipid dependent and enhanced approximately 20-fold by protein S. Protein S-dependent cleavage at Arg306 by APC is also enhanced by high-density lipoprotein and glucosylceramide. The *bottom line* indicates that dissociation of the A2 domain is associated with inactivation of factor Va. (Based on a scheme kindly provided by Dr. T. Hackeng.)

FUNCTIONAL VARIABILITY IN FORMS OF CLEAVED FACTORS Va AND VIIIa

Proteolytic activation of factors Va and VIIIa by thrombin or factor Xa can generate different forms of each active cofactor that differ in specific activity. For example, factor VIIIa generated by factor Xa has lower specific activity and longer half-life than that generated by thrombin,[185,216] and factor Va generated by cleavage only at Arg709 and Arg1018 (without cleavage at Arg1545) has a lower specific activity than that generated after cleavage at Arg1545.[181–183,217] Factor Va can be cleaved at Arg1765, yielding forms of factor Va with differing specific activities.[184] Factor VIIa–tissue factor complexes can cleave factor V at novel sites to produce a form of factor V that can be destroyed by APC without the requirement for full activation of the factor V cofactor precursor.[218]

ACTIVATED PROTEIN C ANTICOAGULANT COFACTORS

APC anticoagulant activity is enhanced by a number of factors that may be termed *APC anticoagulant cofactors*, which include Ca^{2+} ions, certain but not all phospholipids, protein S, factor V, glycosphingolipids, and HDL.

PHOSPHOLIPIDS AS ACTIVATED PROTEIN C COFACTORS
Certain phospholipids, such as phosphatidylserine, phosphatidylethanolamine, and cardiolipin, enhance the anticoagulant activity of APC. The latter two phospholipids stimulate the APC pathway anticoagulant activities much greater than they stimulate the procoagulant pathway activities.[219–222]

PROTEIN S AS ACTIVATED PROTEIN C COFACTOR
Lane and colleagues[223] reviewed protein S structure and activities. Protein S, as an anticoagulant APC cofactor, forms a 1:1 complex with APC and enhances by 10- to 20-fold the rate of APC's cleavage at Arg306 in factor Va but not the Arg506 cleavage.[199,224] Part of the mechanism for this activity of protein S may be related to its ability to bring the active site of APC closer to the plane of the phospholipid membrane on which the APC–protein S complex is located when the complex is formed.[225,226] Protein S also facilitates the action of APC on factor VIIIa.[227,228] Protein S enhances APC's action, in part at least, by ablating the ability of factor Xa to protect factor Va from APC.[229] The TSR and EGF domains of protein S are implicated in binding APC for expression of anticoagulant activity by the APC–protein S complex.[223,230–235] Cleavage of TSR by thrombin abolishes normal binding of protein S to phospholipid and its APC-cofactor anticoagulant activity.[223,236–239]

FACTOR V AS ACTIVATED PROTEIN C COFACTOR
Factor V apparently can have anticoagulant and procoagulant properties because it enhances the anticoagulant action of APC against factor VIIIa in a reaction in which protein S acts synergistically with factor V.[26,27,240,241] Cleavage of factor V at Arg1545, which optimizes factor Va procoagulant activity, ablates the molecule's anticoagulant cofactor activity. However, when factor V is cleaved at Arg506 by APC, its APC cofactor activity is increased 10-fold. This observation suggests that Gln506-factor V has two potential prothrombotic defects, namely, resistance of the variant factor Va to APC inactivation and

resistance of the variant factor V to activation of its APC cofactor function.[27,241]

HIGH DENSITY LIPOPROTEIN AS ACTIVATED PROTEIN C COFACTOR

HDL enhances the anticoagulant activity of APC both in plasma and in purified reaction mixtures. This APC cofactor activity requires protein S and involves, at least in part, stimulation of APC's cleavage at Arg306 in factor Va.[213] In animal models, HDL inhibits DIC induced by endotoxin infusion in baboons and ferric chloride–induced arterial thrombosis in rats.[242,243] HDL is heterogeneous in both protein and lipid composition. The components responsible for this activity have not been identified, although large HDL but not small HDL possesses APC anticoagulant cofactor activity (JH Griffin, unpublished data). The clinical significance of this anticoagulant property of HDL is unclear. However, venous thrombosis is associated with a pattern of dyslipoproteinemia consistent with the hypothesis that deficiency of large HDL is a risk factor for venous thrombosis (Deguchi et al: *Circulation.* 2005, in press.)

GLYCOSPHINGOLIPIDS AS ACTIVATED PROTEIN C COFACTORS

Although both procoagulant and anticoagulant reactions are markedly enhanced by the presence of negatively charged phospholipid surfaces *in vitro*, certain lipids and lipoproteins selectively enhance anticoagulant reactions in plasma.[244] Plasma glucosylceramide (GlcCer) deficiency is a potential risk factor for venous thrombosis.[245] Functional relationships between the protein C anticoagulant pathway and this neutral glycolipid came from studies showing that depletion or augmentation of GlcCer in normal plasma either reduces or enhances, respectively, the anticoagulant response to APC.[246] Moreover, several glycosphingolipids enhance the anticoagulant response of plasma to APC,[246] and biophysical studies show that GlcCer binds to APC and increases the anticoagulant activity of APC by increasing its affinity for lipid surfaces where anticoagulant reactions can occur.[247] GlcCer is present in plasma, mainly in lipoproteins, at a concentration of approximately 10 μM. However, it is also ubiquitously present in all cells, where it is located in the cytoplasm and on the external leaflet of cellular membrane bilayers clustered in detergent-insoluble microdomains or rafts. Based on these findings, microdomains enriched in neutral glycosphingolipids were hypothesized to serve as "anticoagulant microdomains" because GlcCer would promote APC binding.[247] Furthermore, such glycosphingolipid-enriched domains might mediate other APC-dependent functions, such as APC's direct effects on cells (see "Activated Protein C Direct Cellular Activities" below).

The discovery that neutral glycosphingolipids could affect the anticoagulant APC pathway stimulated further studies on the effects of sphingolipids on coagulation reactions. Sphingosine was discovered to be a potent inhibitor of thrombin generation in plasma and on cell surfaces because it can inhibit interactions between factors Va and Xa.[248]

ACTIVATED PROTEIN C DIRECT CELLULAR ACTIVITIES

In addition to its direct anticoagulant activity involving inactivation of factors Va and VIIIa, APC indirectly exerts anticoagulant and antithrombotic effects by acting directly on cells. As discussed in Chapter 106, coagulation reactions cannot be viewed in the absence of the integrated host defense system, which involves a tangled web of biologic processes involving multiple overlapping and integrated pathways. In particular, inflammation, coagulation, and thrombosis are intertwined *in vivo* via multiple proteases and cell-based mechanisms (see reviews[7–9,249–252]).

Circulating cell-derived microparticles carrying procoagulant tissue factor, and adhesive molecules can promote thrombin formation that might be either hemostatic or pathogenic for thrombosis.[253–259] Many such microparticles arise from apoptosis, especially endothelial cell apoptosis, and these endothelial cell-derived microparticles can promote thrombin generation.[260–269] Hence, because APC inhibits endothelial cell apoptosis,[9,55,63,270–273] APC can indirectly decrease thrombin generation and reduce thrombogenesis *in vivo*. APC also can suppress tissue factor expression on monocytes.[274]

ACTIVATED PROTEIN C AND SEVERE SEPSIS

Strong evidence for the physiologic significance of the direct effects of APC on cells comes from clinical research[58] and animal model studies.[60,62] In the PROWESS trial, recombinant human APC reduced all-cause 28-day relative mortality by 19 percent in patients with severe sepsis.[58] However, two other potent anticoagulants—antithrombin and recombinant tissue factor pathway inhibitor (TFPI)—failed to do so in similar large, multicenter phase III studies.[275,276] A reasonable inference is that APC's direct effects on cells involving antiinflammatory and antiapoptotic activities are invoked to help explain the success of APC in reducing mortality in severe sepsis.

ACTIVATED PROTEIN C EFFECTS ON CELLS AND RELATED ANIMAL MODELS

Animal model studies of APC's neuroprotective effects for ischemic stroke and excitotoxic injury caused by N-methyl-D-aspartate (NMDA) suggest that APC's physiologic effects involve more than its anticoagulant activity, presumably its direct effects on cells.[61,271,277] Neuroprotection by APC in these models was observed at low APC doses that had no effect on fibrin deposition or restoration of blood flow resulting from anticoagulant action. Interestingly, besides direct cytoprotection for brain endothelial cells against ischemic injury, APC can direct protection for neurons against NMDA-induced excitotoxic injury both *in vivo* and *in vitro*.[277] Thus, emerging evidence from animal model studies of brain injury and APC's protective effects supports the hypothesis that APC provides physiologic neuroprotection by acting directly on cells *in vivo*.

CELLULAR RECEPTORS FOR PHYSIOLOGIC EFFECTS OF ACTIVATED PROTEIN C ON CELLS

Receptors and some of the mechanisms responsible for the effects of APC on cells have been clarified.[9] APC can significantly alter the gene expression profile of cultured endothelial cells,[270] and this direct effect of APC on cells requires EPCR and PAR-1.[278] Furthermore, APC's inhibition of staurosporine-induced apoptosis of cultured endothelial cells requires the same two receptors.[272] Evidence clearly demonstrates an *in vivo* role for these two receptors for APC's neuroprotective effects in a murine ischemic stroke model.[271] Both *in vitro* and *in vivo* studies show that the cytoprotective direct effects of APC on neurons subjected to NMDA-induced excitotoxicity required PAR-1 and PAR-3.[277] In baboons, EPCR is required for APC-dependent reduction of mortality in *Escherichia coli*-induced sepsis.[160]

Although few details are known about the intracellular mechanisms for APC's antiinflammatory and antiapoptotic activities, APC clearly has major effects on cells. Some key mechanistic details have become clear. These effects involve extensive alterations in gene expression profiles in a manner suggestive of alterations of nuclear factor-κB–dependent intracellular mechanisms,[63,170,278,279] increases in intracellular Ca^{2+} ion flux,[280] phosphorylation of several key intracellular signaling kinases,[278] and major shifts in the levels of proapoptotic and antiapoptotic factors.[270,271,278] Notably, APC down-regulates the key regulatory transcription factor p53 in stressed cells and reduces up-regulation of the proapoptotic Bax while blunting down-regulation of the antiapoptotic factor Bcl-2, among others.[271,277]

Thus, evidence from *in vivo* and *in vitro* studies strongly supports the scheme for APC direct effects on cells involving EPCR and PAR-1 depicted in Figure 107-2. Future investigations on APC cellular receptors and intracellular mechanisms involved in the protein C cellular pathway likely will provide novel clinical insights with diagnostic and therapeutic potential.

INHIBITION OF ACTIVATED PROTEIN C

APC is a normal component of circulating blood and likely contributes to antithrombotic surveillance mechanisms.[18] Circulating APC levels are determined by the balance between mechanisms for APC generation and mechanisms for APC inhibition and clearance. Determinants of APC generation include (1) protein C zymogen levels, (2) endogenous thrombin generation, and (3) availability of TM and EPCR. Clearance of circulating APC is based on inhibition of APC by protease inhibitors and clearance of APC–inhibitor complexes.[281,282] The major plasma inhibitors of APC include α_1-antitrypsin, protein C inhibitor, and α_2-macroglobulin.[281,283–290]

ACTIVATED PROTEIN C-INDEPENDENT ANTICOAGULANT ACTIVITY OF PROTEIN S

Protein S has both indirect and direct anticoagulant activity.[223] For the former, protein S acts as a nonenzymatic APC cofactor. For the latter, independent of APC, protein S inhibits coagulation reactions by directly binding to procoagulant factors. APC-independent activity of protein S is based on the ability of protein S to inhibit directly the activity of the prothrombinase complex by reversibly binding to factor Va and/or factor Xa.[12–15] Ternary complexes of protein S–factor Va–factor Xa may be formed.[291] TSR and the EGF3 domains of protein S (see Fig. 107-3) likely bind factor Xa, contributing to APC-independent anticoagulant activity.[231,292] Protein S also can bind factor VIIIa and inhibit activation of factor X by factor IXa–factor VIIIa complexes.[293–295]

C4BP is a plasma protein that enhances inactivation of the complement cascade by binding to C4b and promoting proteolytic inactivation of C4b by factor I. C4BP reversibly binds protein S with high affinity,[296–298] and formation of this complex affects some of the anticoagulant activities of protein S.[223] When factor Va is the targeted substrate, the APC cofactor activity of protein S is neutralized by its binding to C4BP.[299,300] However, the association of C4BP with protein S does not ablate its ability to serve as an APC cofactor when the substrate is factor VIIIa or its ability to inhibit the prothrombinase complex. This latter observation is explained by the ability of C4BP to block binding of protein S to factor Va but not to factor Xa. C4BP in plasma is a heteropolymer containing two different kinds of disulfide-linked polypeptides, six or seven α-chains and a single β-chain, with the latter chain responsible for binding protein S.[301–303] Residues 30 to 45 of the β-chain bind to the SHBG domain of protein S.[90,304,305] Because the affinity of protein S for C4BP is so high, the amount of free protein S in plasma is determined by the absolute concentrations of the two proteins, such that the normal concentrations are approximately 240 nM protein S–C4BP complexes and 120 nM free protein S.[298] During an acute phase reaction, the level of C4BP α-chain but not β-chain is increased so that the change in total C4BP does not alter the level of free and bound protein S.[306]

Protein S can protect brain endothelium against ischemic injury in murine stroke models and can protect neurons against NMDA-induced excitotoxic injury.[307] Protein S has direct effects on cells by activating one or more transmembrane receptor tyrosine kinases.[223] Moreover,

protein S promotes clearance of apoptotic cells,[308] and this antiapoptotic activity of protein S might contribute to its antithrombotic activity, as discussed above for the indirect antithrombotic activity of APC acting via its antiapoptotic activity.

INHIBITION OF COAGULATION PROTEASES BY PROTEASE INHIBITORS

Antithrombin, initially designated *antithrombin III*, is the clinically most important inhibitor of clotting factor proteases (see Chap. 122). Antithrombin can neutralize all proteases of the intrinsic coagulation pathway, including thrombin and factors Xa, IXa, XIa, and XIIa, in reactions that are enhanced by heparin and related glycosaminoglycans[16] (see Chap. 106). However, antithrombin does not inhibit the anticoagulant protease APC. TFPI, previously described as *lipoprotein-associated coagulation inhibitor (LACI)*, can neutralize factors VIIa and Xa, proteases of the extrinsic coagulation pathway. In addition, other plasma protease inhibitors can neutralize various coagulation proteases, although the clinical significance of these reactions is less well defined than the reaction of antithrombin with thrombin.

ANTITHROMBIN

Antithrombin is synthesized in the liver and is present in plasma at 150 μg/ml. It is a typical member of the *ser*ine protease *in*hibitor (serpin) superfamily.[309] Based on x-ray crystallographic studies,[310–316] images of serpin–protease complexes in various reaction states have emerged, and the mechanism for the effects of heparin on the reaction of thrombin with antithrombin is reasonably clear.[16,317]

The neutralization of proteases by antithrombin results from a stable enzyme–antithrombin complex that is formed by a molecular mechanism characteristic of inhibitory serpins.[309–317] Following binding of a protease to a "reactive site" loop in a serpin, a single peptide bond in the serpin is cleaved with formation of an acyl-enzyme intermediate via the active site Ser residue. This metastable enzyme–serpin complex either can break apart because of deacylation, or it can form a more stable covalent enzyme–serpin complex. To break apart the enzyme–serpin covalent complex, deacylation liberates the cleaved product and regenerates the active site Ser residue of the protease. However, following cleavage at the reactive site residue, serpins have a remarkable ability to undergo major conformational changes that can distort the protease's active site region and lock the enzyme into the protease–serpin complex in which both the serpin and the protease are essentially deformed.[16,309–317] The dominant structural feature of native serpins is a large five-stranded β-sheet that defines the structure of an ellipsoidal protein. Following cleavage at the reactive residue in the reactive center loop by a protease, this extended loop is able to partially or completely insert itself into the five-stranded β-sheet, forming a very stable six-stranded β-sheet. If this insertion reaction proceeds before deacylation occurs, then the protease remains covalently attached to the reactive center P1 residue through the protease's active site Ser residue, and a stable covalent protease–inhibitor complex with each protein in an altered conformation is formed.[315]

Heparin enhancement of the rate of reaction between antithrombin and thrombin is caused by two distinct effects of heparin, one involving conformational effects on antithrombin and the other involving "approximation" effects on both thrombin and antithrombin.[316,318–321] For the first effect, a particular pentasaccharide within heparin is most potent at causing a conformational change that converts antithrombin from its native state of moderate reactivity to a conformation with relatively high reactivity. This pentasaccharide contains a specific sulfated sequence of glucosamine and iduronic acid residues.[16,318,322,323] When it is present in a large heparin molecule, it accelerates the reaction of antithrombin not only with thrombin but essentially with any target protease. On the other hand, the approximation effect mainly affects its reaction with thrombin and results from the fact that both thrombin and antithrombin have high affinity for heparin. When both thrombin and antithrombin are simultaneously bound to heparin, they encounter each other much more frequently than when they are free in solution, thus increasing the reaction rate. Heparan sulfates also act in this manner. This approximation mechanism is not significant for proteases other than thrombin (e.g., factor Xa) unless the protease has a very high affinity for heparin. A synthetic pentasaccharide comprising these critical five saccharide units was successfully developed to provide the FDA-approved drug Fonda-parinux, which has the property of accelerating reaction of antithrombin with factor Xa by several orders of magnitude while accelerating the reaction with thrombin only several-fold (see Chap. 21). In effect, the synthetic pentasaccharide is a factor Xa inhibitor via the action of antithrombin.

The mature antithrombin polypeptide chain contains 432 amino acid residues after cleavage of a propeptide from a 464-residue precursor.[324] It has four sites for N-linked carbohydrate attachment, one of which (Asn135) is variably glycosylated, giving rise to a β-isoform that has higher affinity for heparin.[325,326] Heparin binding to antithrombin is mediated by a number of positively charged Arg and Lys residues in the N-terminal region of the molecule, including Lys11, Arg13 and Asn45, Arg46, Arg47, Glu113, Lys114, Lys125, and Arg129,[316] whereas the reactive center loop containing the scissile peptide bond at Arg393-Ser394 is near the C-terminus.[316]

ANTITHROMBIN GENE
The antithrombin gene, comprising seven exons and six introns, spans 13.4 kb and is located on chromosome 1q23-25.[327–330]

ANTITHROMBIN MUTATIONS
Hereditary deficiencies of antithrombin are well recognized as risk factors for venous thrombosis (see Chap. 122). More than one hundred different mutations have been reported to be associated with thrombosis. An extensive database of mutations has been published and is available on the World Wide Web at http://www1.imperial.ac.uk/medicine/about/divisions/is/haemo/coag/antithrombin/default.html.[331]

Mutations that cause antithrombin deficiency are scattered throughout the molecule. Molecular defects can be classified as *type I*, characterized by parallel decreases in antigen and activity, or *type II*, characterized by circulating dysfunctional molecules such that plasma has decreased functional activity but normal or near-normal antigen levels. Type II defects are further classified based on whether the dysfunction involves only reactive center defects that can be tested in the absence of heparin, only heparin-binding defects that can be tested only in the presence of heparin, or both of these defects (pleiotropic effects). Reactive center defects carry the largest risk of thrombosis, whereas heparin-binding defects are associated with less risk of venous thrombosis (see Chap. 122). For example, a remarkable variant, designated *antithrombin London*, was described in which the reactive center Arg residue was missing and the molecule had high affinity for heparin, and this mutation was associated with early onset of thrombotic symptoms.[332]

TISSUE FACTOR PATHWAY INHIBITOR

The mature TFPI protein, also known as *lipoprotein-associated coagulation inhibitor* (LACI) or *extrinsic pathway inhibitor* (EPI), has an M_r of 34,000 and contains an acidic N-terminal sequence, three homologous but distinct Kunitz-type protease inhibitor domains, and a C-terminal positively charged basic amino acid sequence.[6,333] Al-

though present at only 100 ng/ml in normal plasma, TFPI is a significant inhibitor of the extrinsic coagulation pathway, which functions synergistically with the protein C pathway and antithrombin to suppress thrombin generation. TFPI is synthesized by endothelial cells and smooth muscle cells.[6,334] More than half of the TFPI in plasma is associated with lipoproteins, especially LDL,[335] and a substantial amount of TFPI is released by endothelial cells when heparin is infused.[336] Multiple forms of TFPI are present in the blood and on the endothelium, not only because of its association with lipoproteins but also because two alternatively spliced forms of TFPI, designated TFPIα and TFPIβ, are present.[337,338] TFPIα is the full-length protein, whereas TFPIβ contains an unrelated sequence that replaces the third Kunitz-type domain. Each form of TFPI, especially TFPIβ, can be covalently modified by addition of phosphatidylinositol that localizes the TFPI to the membrane. The interaction of TFPI with lipoproteins greatly reduces the measurable anticoagulant activity and, when TFPI is bound to cells, lipoprotein (a) inhibits TFPI activity.[339] The C-terminus and the third Kunitz-type domain of TFPIα are required for normal binding to the endothelial surface.[340]

TFPI neutralizes factors Xa and VIIa by a somewhat complicated mechanism (Fig. 107-5).[6,341–344] Initially, the second Kunitz domain of TFPI reacts with and inhibits the active site of factor Xa. Subsequently, this binary complex reacts with factor VIIa in the tissue factor–VIIa complex, forming a quaternary protein complex on a membrane. TFPI can react with factor VIIa in the absence of factor Xa, but at a much slower rate. Interestingly, TFPI can neutralize factor Xa when the enzyme is bound in a prothrombinase complex, that is, in a factor Xa–factor Va–phospholipid complex. Because TFPI requires factor Xa for kinetically favorable reactions with factor VIIa, TFPI does not shut off initiation of the extrinsic pathway by tissue factor until a significant amount of factor Xa is generated. Then TFPI provides negative feedback inhibition of the generation of factor Xa by the VIIa–tissue factor complex.

Animal model studies show that TFPI functions physiologically as an inhibitor of coagulation.[6,341,342] Depletion of TFPI predisposes animals to endotoxin-induced DIC and the generalized Schwarzman reaction, and treatment of animals with TFPI reduces mortality from *E. coli* septic shock. In gene knockout studies, mice carrying complete deficiency of TFPI do not survive beyond the neonatal period and die of hemorrhage with signs of fibrin formation, suggestive of consumptive coagulopathy.[345]

TISSUE FACTOR PATHWAY INHIBITOR GENE
The sequence of TFPI was established from cloning of its cDNA and the TFPI gene, which contains nine exons, spans 85 kb, and is located on chromosome 2q31-32.1.[333,346,347]

TISSUE FACTOR PATHWAY INHIBITOR MUTATIONS
Hereditary abnormalities of TFPI have been suggested to be associated with an increased risk of venous thrombosis.[348,349]

OTHER PROTEASE INHIBITORS

HEPARIN COFACTOR II
Heparin cofactor II, a serpin whose inhibitory activity is enhanced by dermatan sulfate, inhibits thrombin *in vivo* and *in vitro* by an approximation mechanism.[350,351] Several reports have linked heparin cofactor II deficiency to venous thrombosis.[352–354] Interestingly, a severe heparin cofactor II deficiency was reported for an asymptomatic subject.[355]

PROTEIN Z-DEPENDENT PROTEASE INHIBITOR
Protein Z-dependent protease inhibitor (ZPI) is a plasma serpin that inhibits factors Xa and XIa.[356–358] Protein Z, a vitamin K-dependent

protein that contains a Gla-domain, stimulates factor Xa inhibition but not factor XIa inhibition by ZPI. However, heparin augments the rate of reaction between factor XIa and ZPI. Protein Z is homologous to other vitamin K-dependent zymogens but lacks any protease activity because two of the three active site residues typical for serine proteases are altered. In plasma, ZPI is in slight protein molar excess over protein Z with which it can noncovalently associate, and almost all plasma protein Z has been speculated, but not proved, to be associated with ZPI. If ZPI is a physiologic coagulation inhibitor, then deficiency of either protein Z or ZPI is implied to be associated with thrombosis. Knocking out the protein Z gene in a mouse does not produce a thrombotic phenotype in the mouse unless protein Z deficiency coexists with factor V Leiden, in which case the mouse exhibits a hypercoagulable, prothrombotic state.[359] This murine observation is mirrored by the clinical report that subnormal levels of protein Z are associated with venous thrombosis in subjects heterozygous for factor V Leiden.[360] One ZPI gene sequencing study reported that ZPI mutations or polymorphisms were found more frequently in 250 venous thrombosis patients (4.4% of patients) than in 250 control subjects (0.8% of subjects), suggesting that hereditary ZPI defects are associated with venous thrombosis.[361] This hypothesis merits its future investigation.

OTHER MINOR PROTEASE INHIBITORS

Thrombin in plasma can be inhibited not only by antithrombin but also by α_2-macroglobulin,

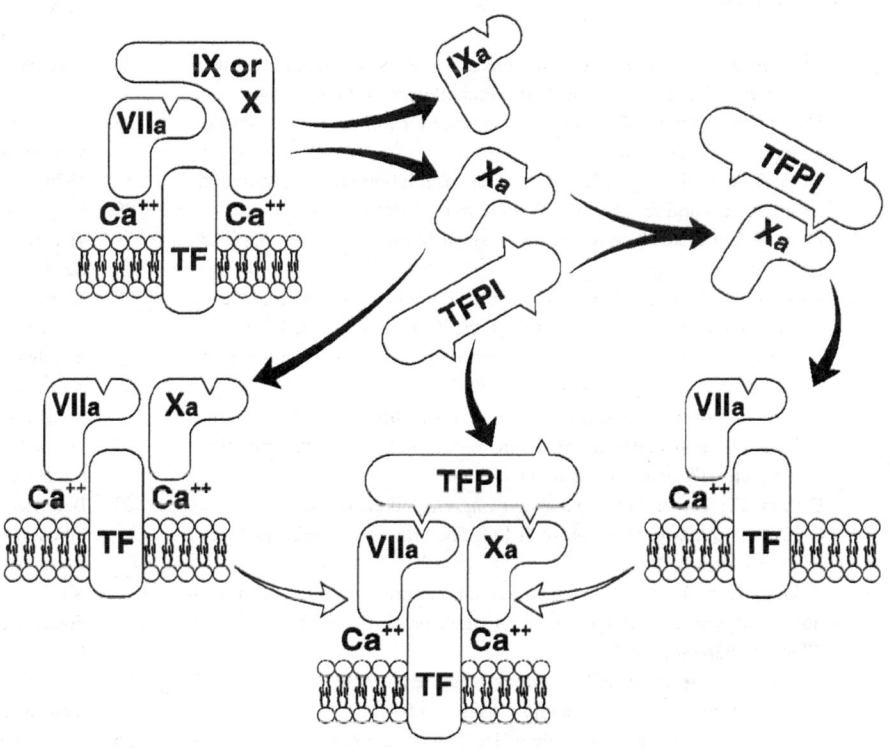

FIGURE 107-5 Feedback inhibition of factor VIIa by tissue factor pathway inhibitor (TFPI) in factor Xa–TFPI complexes. Surface-bound factor VIIa–tissue factor (TF) complexes generate factors IXa and Xa (top left). Free TFPI is a multivalent protease inhibitor containing three Kunitz-type protease inhibitor domains. After factor Xa complexes with and is inhibited by the Kunitz-2 domain of TFPI, the Xa–TFPI complex (right side) can bind to and inhibit a TF–factor VIIa complex, forming a quaternary complex (bottom center). Alternatively, TFPI may combine with a surface-bound ternary complex of TF–VIIa–Xa (bottom left) to form a final quaternary complex (bottom center). (Adapted from GJ Broze Jr,[6] with permission.)

which is an acute phase reactant. No association between defects in bleeding or thrombosis have been associated with this inhibitor. In purified reaction mixtures, protein C inhibitor also efficiently neutralizes thrombin in the presence of TM,[362,363] although no studies have shown this to be a physiologic reaction or that it is associated with thrombosis.

MURINE GENE DELETION STUDIES OF ANTICOAGULANT FACTORS

Genetically modified mice offer unique opportunities to study the regulation of coagulation and thrombosis, and the number of interesting genetically altered mouse strains is rapidly growing, as reviewed by Weiler.[364,365] Complete removal of the functional protein of a gene is invaluable for inferring the essential functional properties of a given gene product. Mutant mice lacking protein C[73] or antithrombin[366] confirm the overwhelming importance of these factors for inhibiting coagulation. The fact that the mouse deficient in protein C resembles the severely deficient infant described in 1983[367] helps to validate the use of genetically altered mice for protein C pathway studies. Complete deletion of the TM[152] or EPCR[368] gene is embryonically lethal for reasons that are not entirely apparent. Some related insights come from genetic manipulations that either alter only part of the TM gene product[150] or allow a very low level of EPCR expression (e.g., 5% of normal levels).[369] Alterations of the TM gene demonstrated that the EGF domains of TM were essential for normal generation of APC by thrombin, as predicted from numerous in vitro functional proteomics

studies.[7,150] Although low levels of EPCR allow mice to survive and reproduce, such mice are useful for probing the functional importance of normal levels of this receptor. Studies showed that normal levels of EPCR are required for normal neuroprotective activities of infused APC.[271]

The availability of a factor V Leiden mouse model in which the murine factor V Arg residue comparable to human factor V Arg506 is replaced by Gln confirms the prothrombotic phenotype of this mutation and permits studies of both genetic and environmental factors that possibly influence the thrombotic phenotype of factor V Leiden.[370]

The embryonic lethality of deleting the TFPI gene is characterized by bleeding that is consistent with consumptive coagulopathy, showing that TFPI functions as a key regulator of coagulation in vivo.[345] The asymptomatic nature of protein Z deficiency is notable, as is the fact that combining this deficiency with the murine prothrombotic factor V Leiden genotype produces a more severe thrombotic phenotype.[359] This finding suggests that protein Z is a mild risk factor for thrombosis that becomes more apparent when combined with another moderate risk factor, supporting the general hypothesis that thrombotic episodes often require the presence of multiple mild to moderate risk factors.

Although directly translating genetic studies of mice to the clinical situation clearly is subject to a number of limitations, the growing availability of genetically modified mice carrying coagulation defects sets the stage for significant advances in understanding the regulation of thrombin generation, coagulation, and thrombosis.

REFERENCES

1. MacFarlane RG: An enzyme cascade in the blood clotting mechanism and its function as a biological amplifier. *Nature* 202:498, 1964.
2. Davie EW, Ratnoff OD: Waterfall sequence for intrinsic blood clotting. *Science* 145:1310, 1964.
3. Davie EW, Fujikawa K, Kisiel W: The coagulation cascade: Initiation, maintenance, and regulation. *Biochemistry* 30:10363, 1991.
4. Furie B, Furie BC: The molecular basis of blood coagulation. *Cell* 53:505, 1988.
5. Lammle B, Griffin JH: Formation of the fibrin clot: The balance of procoagulant and inhibitory factors. *Clin Haematol* 14:281, 1985.
6. Broze GJ Jr: Tissue factor pathway inhibitor and the revised theory of coagulation. *Annu Rev Med* 46:103, 1995.
7. Van de Wouwer M, Collen D, Conway EM: Thrombomodulin-protein C-EPCR system integrated to regulate coagulation and inflammation. *Arterioscler Thromb Vasc Biol* 24:1, 2004.
8. Esmon CT: The protein C pathway. *Chest* 124:26S, 2003.
9. Griffin JH, Zlokovic BV, Mosnier LO: The protein C cellular pathway. *Blood* (in press), 2005.
10. Fukudome K, Esmon CT: Identification, cloning, and regulation of a novel endothelial cell protein C/activated protein C receptor. *J Biol Chem* 269:26486, 1994.
11. Esmon CT: Structure and functions of the endothelial cell protein C receptor. *Crit Care Med* 32(suppl 5):S298, 2004.
12. Mitchell CA, Kelemen SM, Salem HH: The anticoagulant properties of a modified form of protein S. *Thromb Haemost* 60:298, 1988.
13. Heeb MJ, Mesters RM, Tans G, et al: Binding of protein S to factor Va associated with inhibition of prothrombinase that is independent of activated protein C. *J Biol Chem* 268:2872, 1993.
14. Heeb MJ, Rosing J, Bakker HM, et al: Protein S binds to and inhibits factor Xa. *Proc Natl Acad Sci U S A* 91:2728, 1994.
15. Hackeng TM, van't Veer C, Meijers JCM, Bouma BN: Human protein S inhibits prothrombinase complex activity on endothelial cells and platelets via direct interactions with factors Va and Xa. *J Biol Chem* 269:21051, 1994.
16. Huntington JA: Mechanisms of glycosaminoglycan activation of the serpins in hemostasis. *J Thromb Haemost* 1:1535, 2003.
17. Morrissey JH, Macik BG, Neuenschwander PF, Comp PC: Quantitation of activated factor VII levels in plasma using a tissue factor mutant selectively deficient in promoting factor VII activation. *Blood* 81:734, 1993.
18. Gruber A, Griffin JH: Direct detection of activated protein C in blood from human subjects. *Blood* 79:2340, 1992.
19. Nossel HL, Yudelman I, Canfield RE, et al: Measurement of fibrinopeptide A in human blood. *J Clin Invest* 54:43, 1974.
20. Nossel HL: Radioimmunoassay of fibrinopeptides in relation to intravascular coagulation and thrombosis. *N Engl J Med* 295:428, 1976.
21. Bauer KA, Rosenberg RD: The pathophysiology of the prethrombotic state in humans: Insights gained from studies using markers of hemostatic system activation. *Blood* 70:343, 1987.
22. Bauer KA, Kass BL, ten Cate H, et al: Detection of factor X activation in humans. *Blood* 74:2007, 1989.
23. Bauer KA, Kass BL, ten Cate H, et al: Factor IX is activated in vivo by the tissue factor mechanism. *Blood* 76:731, 1990.
24. Jesty J, Beltrami E, Willems G: Mathematical analysis of a proteolytic positive-feedback loop: Dependence of lag time and enzyme yields on the initial conditions and kinetic parameters. *Biochemistry* 32:6266, 1993.
25. Beltrami E, Jesty J: Mathematical analysis of activation thresholds in enzyme-catalyzed positive feedbacks: Application to the feedbacks of blood coagulation. *Proc Natl Acad Sci U S A* 92:8744, 1995.
26. Shen L, Dahlbäck B: Factor V and protein S as synergistic cofactors to

27. Nicolaes GA, Dahlback B: Factor V and thrombotic disease: Description of a Janus-faced protein. *Arterioscler Thromb Vasc Biol* 22:530, 2002.
28. Stenflo JA: A new vitamin K-dependent protein: Purification from bovine plasma and preliminary characterization. *J Biol Chem* 251:355, 1976.
29. Seegers WH, Novoa E, Henry RL, Hassouna HI: Relationship of "new" vitamin K-dependent protein C and "old" autoprothrombin II-A. *Thromb Res* 8:543, 1976.
30. Kisiel W, Canfield WM, Ericsson LH, Davie EW: Anticoagulant properties of bovine plasma protein C following activation by thrombin. *Biochemistry* 16:5824, 1977.
31. Kisiel W: Human plasma protein C. Isolation, characterization and mechanism of activation by α-thrombin. *J Clin Invest* 64:761, 1979.
32. Foster D, Davie EW: Characterization of a cDNA coding for human protein C. *Proc Natl Acad Sci U S A* 81:4766, 1984.
33. Beckmann RJ, Schmidt RJ, Santerre RF, et al: The structure and evolution of a 461 amino acid human protein C precursor and its messenger RNA, based upon the DNA sequence of cloned human liver cDNA's. *Nucleic Acids Res* 13:5233, 1985.
34. Foster DC, Rudinski MS, Schach BG, et al: Propeptide of human protein C is necessary for γ-carboxylation. *Biochemistry* 26:7003, 1987.
35. Heeb MJ, Schwarz HP, White T, et al: Immunoblotting studies of the molecular forms of protein C in plasma. *Thromb Res* 52:33, 1988.
36. Griffin JH, Evatt B, Zimmerman TS, et al: Deficiency of protein C in congenital thrombotic disease. *J Clin Invest* 68:1370, 1981.
37. Fernlund P, Stenflo JA: Amino acid sequence of the light chain of bovine protein C. *J Biol Chem* 257:12170, 1982.
38. Stenflo JA, Fernlund P: Amino acid sequence of the heavy chain of bovine protein C. *J Biol Chem* 257:12180, 1982.
39. Mather T, Oganessyan V, Hof P, et al: The 2.8 Å crystal structure of Gla-domainless activated protein C. *EMBO J* 15:6822, 1996.
40. Kurosawa S, Galvin JB, Esmon NL, Esmon CT: Proteolytic formation and properties of functional domains of thrombomodulin. *J Biol Chem* 262:2206, 1987.
41. Zhang L, Castellino FJ: A gamma-carboxyglutamic acid variant (gamma⁶D, gamma⁷D) of human activated protein C displays greatly reduced activity as an anticoagulant. *Biochemistry* 29:10828, 1990.
42. Zhang L, Castellino FJ: Role of the hexapeptide disulfide loop present in the gamma-carboxyglutamic acid domain of human protein C in its activation properties and in the in vitro anticoagulant activity of activated protein C. *Biochemistry* 30:6696, 1991.
43. Jhingan A, Zhang L, Christiansen WT, Castellino FJ: The activities of recombinant gamma-carboxyglutamic-acid-deficient mutants of activated human protein C toward human coagulation factor Va and factor VIII in purified systems and in plasma. *Biochemistry* 33:1869, 1994.
44. Zhang L, Castellino FJ: The binding energy of human coagulation protein C to acidic phospholipid vesicles contains a major contribution from leucine 5 in the gamma-carboxyglutamic acid domain. *J Biol Chem* 269:3590, 1994.
45. Regan LM, Mollica JS, Rezaie AR, Esmon CT: The interaction between the endothelial cell protein C receptor and protein C is dictated by the gamma-carboxyglutamic acid domain of protein C. *J Biol Chem* 272:26279, 1997.
46. Ohlin AK, Landes G, Bourdon P, et al: Beta-hydroxyaspartic acid in the first epidermal growth factor-like domain of protein C. Its role in Ca²⁺ binding and biological activity. *J Biol Chem* 263:19240, 1988.
47. Fisher CL, Greengard JS, Griffin JH: Models of the serine protease domain of the human antithrombotic plasma factor activated protein C and its zymogen. *Protein Sci* 3:588, 1994.
48. Greengard JS, Fisher CL, Villoutreix B, Griffin JH: Structural basis for type I and type II deficiencies of antithrombotic plasma protein C: Pat-

activated protein C in degradation of factor VIIIa. *J Biol Chem* 269:18735, 1994.

terns revealed by three-dimensional molecular modeling of mutations of the protease domain. *Proteins* 18:367, 1994.

49. Gale AJ, Heeb MJ, Griffin JH: The autolysis loop of activated protein C interacts with factor Va and differentiates between the Arg506 and Arg306 cleavage sites. *Blood* 96:585, 2000.

50. Friedrich U, Nicolaes GA, Villoutreix BO, Dahlback B: Secondary substrate-binding exosite in the serine protease domain of activated protein C important for cleavage at Arg-506 but not at Arg-306 in factor Va. *J Biol Chem* 276:23105, 2001.

51. Rezaie AR: Exosite-dependent regulation of the protein C anticoagulant pathway. *Trends Cardiovasc Med* 13:8, 2003.

52. Gale AJ, Griffin JH: Characterization of a thrombomodulin binding site on protein C and its comparison to an activated protein C binding site for factor Va. *Proteins* 54:433, 2004.

53. Gale AJ, Tsavaler A, Griffin JH: Molecular characterization of an extended binding site for coagulation factor Va in the positive exosite of activated protein C. *J Biol Chem* 277:28836, 2002.

54. Dahlback B, Villoutreix BO: Molecular recognition in the protein C anticoagulant pathway. *J Thromb Haemost* 1:1525, 2003.

55. Mosnier LO, Gale AJ, Yegneswaran S, Griffin JH: Activated protein C variants with normal cytoprotective but reduced anticoagulant activity. *Blood* 104:1740, 2004.

56. Dreyfus M, Magny JF, Bridey F, et al: Treatment of homozygous protein C deficiency and neonatal purpura fulminans with a purified protein C concentrate. *N Engl J Med* 325:1565, 1991.

57. Rivard GE, David M, Farrell C, Schwarz HP: Treatment of purpura fulminans in meningococcemia with protein C concentrate. *J Pediatr* 126:646, 1995.

58. Bernard GR, Vincent JL, Laterre PF, et al: Efficacy and safety of recombinant human activated protein C for severe sepsis. *N Engl J Med* 344:699, 2001.

59. Taylor FB, Chang A, Esmon CT, et al: Protein C prevents the coagulopathic and lethal effects of *Escherichia coli* infusion in the baboon. *J Clin Invest* 79:918, 1987.

60. Griffin JH, Zlokovic BV, Fernandez JA: Activated protein C: Potential therapy for severe sepsis, thrombosis, and stroke. *Semin Hematol* 39:197, 2002.

61. Shibata M, Kumar SR, Amar A, et al: Anti-inflammatory, antithrombotic, and neuroprotective effects of activated protein C in a murine model of focal ischemic stroke. *Circulation* 103:1799, 2001.

62. Griffin JH, Fernandez JA, Liu D, et al: Activated protein C and ischemic stroke. *Crit Care Med* 32:S247, 2004.

63. Contreras JL, Eckstein C, Smyth CA, et al: Activated protein C preserves functional islet mass after intraportal transplantation: A novel link between endothelial cell activation, thrombosis, inflammation, and islet cell death. *Diabetes* 53:2804, 2004.

64. Foster DC, Yoshitake S, Davie EW: The nucleotide sequence of the gene for human protein C. *Proc Natl Acad Sci U S A* 82:4673, 1985.

65. Esmon CT, Fukudome K: Cellular regulation of the protein C pathway. *Semin Cell Biol* 6:259, 1995.

66. Rocchi M, Roncuzzi L, Santamaria R, et al: Mapping through somatic cell hybrids and cDNA probes of protein C to chromosome 2, factor X to chromosome 13, and alpha 1-acid glycoprotein to chromosome 9. *Hum Genet* 74:30, 1986.

67. Kato A, Miura O, Sumi Y, Aoki N: Assignment of the human protein C gene (PROC) to chromosome region 2q14-q21 by in situ hybridization. *Cytogenet Cell Genet* 47:46, 1988.

68. Long GL, Marshall A, Gardner JC, Naylor SL: Genes for human vitamin K-dependent plasma proteins C and S are located on chromosomes 2 and 3, respectively. *Somat Cell Mol Genet* 14:93, 1988.

69. Patracchini P, Aiello V, Palazzi P, et al: Sublocalization of the human protein C gene on chromosome 2q13-q14. *Hum Genet* 81:191, 1989.

70. Reitsma PH, Bernardi F, Doig RG, et al: Protein C deficiency: A database of mutations 1995 update. On behalf of the Subcommittee on Plasma Coagulation Inhibitors of the Scientific and Standardization Committee of the ISTH. *Thromb Haemost* 73:876, 1995.

71. Greengard JS, Griffin JH, Fisher CL: Possible structural implications of 20 mutations in the protein C protease domain. *Thromb Haemost* 72:869, 1994.

72. Wacey AI, Pemberton S, Cooper DN, et al: A molecular model of the serine protease domain of activated protein C: Application to the study of missense mutations causing protein C deficiency. *Br J Haematol* 84:290, 1993.

73. Jalbert LR, Rosen ED, Moons L, et al: Inactivation of the gene for anticoagulant protein C causes lethal perinatal consumptive coagulopathy in mice. *J Clin Invest* 102:1481, 1998.

74. DiScipio RG, Hermodson MA, Yates SG, Davie EW: A comparison of human prothrombin, factor IX (Christmas factor), factor X (Stuart factor), and protein S. *Biochemistry* 16:698, 1977.

75. DiScipio RG, Davie EW: Characterization of protein S, a gamma-carboxyglutamic acid containing protein from bovine and human plasma. *Biochemistry* 18:899, 1979.

76. Fair DS, Marlar RA: Biosynthesis and secretion of factor VII, protein C, protein S, and the protein C inhibitor from a human hepatoma cell line. *Blood* 67:64, 1986.

77. Phillips DJ, Greengard JS, Fernández JA, et al: Protein S, an antithrombotic factor, is synthesized and released by neural tumor cells. *J Neurochem* 61:344, 1993.

78. Stern D, Brett J, Harris K, Nawroth P: Participation of endothelial cells in the protein C-protein S anticoagulant pathway: The synthesis and release of protein S. *J Cell Biol* 102:1971, 1986.

79. Malm J, He XH, Bjartell A, et al: Vitamin K-dependent protein S in Leydig cells of human testis. *Biochem J* 302:845, 1994.

80. Fair DS, Marlar RA, Levin EG: Human endothelial cells synthesize protein S. *Blood* 67:1168, 1986.

81. Schwarz HP, Heeb MJ, Wencel-Drake JD, Griffin JH: Identification and characterization of protein S in human platelets. *Blood* 66:1452, 1985.

82. Smiley ST, Boyer SN, Heeb MJ, et al: Protein S is inducible by interleukin 4 in T cells and inhibits lymphoid cell procoagulant activity. *Proc Natl Acad Sci U S A* 94:11484, 1997.

83. Lundwall A, Dackowski W, Cohen E, et al: Isolation and sequence of the cDNA for human protein S, a regulator of blood coagulation. *Proc Natl Acad Sci U S A* 83:6716, 1986.

84. Dahlbäck B, Lundwall A, Stenflo JA: Primary structure of bovine vitamin K-dependent protein S. *Proc Natl Acad Sci U S A* 83:4199, 1986.

85. Ploos van Amstel HK, van der Zanden L, Reitsma PH, Bertina RM: Human protein S cDNA encodes Phe-16 and Tyr 222 in consensus sequences for the post-translational processing. *FEBS Lett* 222:186, 1987.

86. Hoskins J, Norman DK, Beckmann RJ, Long GL: Cloning and characterization of human liver cDNA encoding a protein S precursor. *Proc Natl Acad Sci U S A* 84:349, 1987.

87. Stenflo JA, Lundwall A, Dahlbäck B: BHydroxyasparagine in domains homologous to the epidermal growth factor precursor in vitamin K-dependent protein S. *Proc Natl Acad Sci U S A* 84:368, 1987.

88. Dahlbäck B, Hildebrand B, Linse S: Novel type of very high affinity calcium-binding sites in β-hydroxy-asparagine-containing epidermal growth factor-like domains in vitamin K-dependent protein S. *J Biol Chem* 265:18481, 1990.

89. Nelson RM, VanDusen WJ, Friedman PA, Long GL: A-Hydroxyaspartic acid and α-hydroxyasparagine residues in recombinant human protein S are not required for anticoagulant cofactor activity or for binding to C4b-binding protein. *J Biol Chem* 266:20586, 1991.

90. Fernández JA, Heeb MJ, Griffin JH: Identification of residues 413–433 of plasma protein S as essential for binding to C4b-binding protein. *J Biol Chem* 268:16788, 1993.

91. Chang GTG, Maas BHA, Ploos van Amstel HK, et al: The carboxy terminal loop of human protein S is involved in the interaction with C4b-binding protein. *Blood* 78(suppl):277a, 1991.

92. Heeb MJ, Kojima Y, Tans G, et al: C-terminal residues 621–635 of protein S are essential for binding to factor Va. *J Biol Chem* 274:36187, 1999.

93. Nyberg P, Dahlback B, Garcia DF: The SHBG-like region of protein S is crucial for factor V-dependent APC-cofactor function. *FEBS Lett* 433: 28, 1998.

94. Ploos van Amstel JK, Van der Zanden AL, Bakker E, et al: Two genes homologous with human protein S cDNA are located on chromosome 3. *Thromb Haemost* 58:982, 1987.

95. Watkins PC, Eddy R, Fukushima Y, et al: The gene for protein S maps near the centromere of human chromosome 3. *Blood* 71:238, 1988.

96. Gershagen S, Fernlund P, Lundwall A: A cDNA coding for human sex hormone binding globulin: Homology to vitamin K-dependent protein S. *FEBS Lett* 220:129, 1987.

97. Baker ME, French FS, Joseph DR: Vitamin K-dependent protein S is similar to rat androgen-binding protein. *Biochem J* 243:293, 1987.

98. Schmidel DK, Tatro AV, Phelps LG, et al: Organization of the human protein S gene. *Biochemistry* 29:7845, 1990.

99. Rapaport SI: Inhibition of factor VIIa/tissue factor-induced blood co-agulation: With particular emphasis upon a factor Xa-dependent inhib-itory mechanism. *Blood* 73:359, 1989.

100. Edenbrandt C-M, Lundwall A, Wydro R, Stenflo JA: Molecular analysis of the gene for vitamin K-dependent protein S and its pseudogene. Clon-ing and partial gene organization. *Biochemistry* 29:7861, 1990.

101. Gershagen S, Fernlund P, Edenbrandt C-M: The genes for SHBG/ABP and the SHBG-like region of vitamin K-dependent protein S have evolved from a common ancestral gene. *J Steroid Biochem Mol Biol* 40: 763, 1991.

102. Gandrille S, Borgel D, Ireland H, et al: Protein S deficiency: A database of mutations. For the Plasma Coagulation Inhibitors Subcommittee of the Scientific and Standardization Committee of the International Soci-ety on Thrombosis and Haemostasis. *Thromb Haemost* 77:1201, 1997.

103. Bertina RM, Ploos van Amstel HK, Van Wijngaarden A, et al: Heerlen polymorphism of protein S, an immunologic polymorphism due to di-morphism of residue 460. *Blood* 76:538, 1990.

104. Esmon CT, Owen WG: Identification of an endothelial cell cofactor for thrombin-catalyzed activation of protein C. *Proc Natl Acad Sci U S A* 78:2249, 1981.

105. Esmon CT, Owen WG: The discovery of thrombomodulin. *J Thromb Haemost* 2:209, 2004.

106. Esmon CT, Esmon NL, Harris KW: Complex formation between throm-bin and thrombomodulin inhibits both thrombin-catalyzed fibrin for-mation and factor V activation. *J Biol Chem* 257:7944, 1982.

107. Esmon NL, Carroll RC, Esmon CT: Thrombomodulin blocks the ability of thrombin to activate platelets. *J Biol Chem* 258:12238, 1983.

108. Esmon CT: The roles of protein C and thrombomodulin in the regulation of blood coagulation. *J Biol Chem* 264:4743, 1989.

109. Jackman RW, Beeler DL, VanDeWater L, Rosenberg RD: Characteriza-tion of a thrombomodulin cDNA reveals structural similarity to the low density lipoprotein receptor. *Proc Natl Acad Sci U S A* 83:8834, 1986.

110. Jackman RW, Beeler DL, Fritze L, et al: Human thrombomodulin gene is intron depleted: Nucleic acid sequences of the cDNA and gene predict protein structure and suggest sites of regulatory control. *Proc Natl Acad Sci U S A* 84:6425, 1987.

111. Sadler JE, Lentz SR, Sheehan JP, et al: Structure-function relationships of the thrombin-thrombomodulin interaction. *Haemostasis* 23(suppl 1): 183, 1993.

112. Ye J, Esmon CT, Johnson AE: The chondroitin sulfate moiety of throm-bomodulin binds a second molecule of thrombin. *J Biol Chem* 268:2373, 1993.

113. Bourin MC, Ohlin AK, Lane DA, et al: Relationship between antico-agulant activities and polyanionic properties of rabbit thrombomodulin. *J Biol Chem* 263:8044, 1988.

114. Nawa K, Sakano K, Fujiwara H, et al: Presence and function of chon-droitin-4-sulfate on recombinant human soluble thrombomodulin. *Biochem Biophys Res Commun* 171:729, 1990.

115. Suzuki K, Hayashi T, Nishioka J, et al: A domain composed of epider-mal growth factor-like structures of human thrombomodulin is essential for thrombin binding and for protein C activation. *J Biol Chem* 264: 4872, 1989.

116. Ye J, Esmon NL, Esmon CT, Johnson AE: The active site of thrombin is altered upon binding to thrombomodulin. *J Biol Chem* 266:23016, 1991.

117. Takano S, Kimura S, Ohdama S, Aoki N: Plasma thrombomodulin in health and diseases. *Blood* 76:2024, 1990.

118. Shirai T, Shiojiri S, Ito H, et al: Gene structure of human thrombo-modulin, a cofactor for thrombin-catalyzed activation of protein C. *J Biochem* 103:281, 1988.

119. Espinosa R III, Sadler JE, Le Beau MM: Regional localization of the human thrombomodulin gene to 20p12-cen. *Genomics* 5:649, 1989.

120. Esmon CT: Cell mediated events that control blood coagulation and vascular injury. *Annu Rev Cell Biol* 9:1, 1993.

121. Norlund L, Holm J, Zoller B, Ohlin AK: A common thrombomodulin amino acid dimorphism is associated with myocardial infarction. *Thromb Haemost* 77:248, 1997.

122. Ireland H, Kunz G, Kyriakoulis K, et al: Thrombomodulin gene muta-tions associated with myocardial infarction. *Circulation* 96:15, 1997.

123. Wu KK: Soluble thrombomodulin and coronary heart disease. *Curr Opin Lipidol* 14:373, 2003.

124. Fukudome K, Esmon CT: Molecular cloning and expression of murine and bovine endothelial cell protein C–activated protein C receptor (EPCR). The structural and functional conservation in human, bovine, and murine EPCR. *J Biol Chem* 270:5571, 1995.

125. Regan LM, Stearns-Kurosawa DJ, Kurosawa S, et al: The endothelial cell protein C receptor. Inhibition of activated protein C anticoagulant function without modulation of reaction with proteinase inhibitors. *J Biol Chem* 271:17499, 1996.

126. Fukudome K, Kurosawa S, Stearns-Kurosawa DJ, et al: The endothelial cell protein C receptor. Cell surface expression and direct ligand binding by the soluble receptor. *J Biol Chem* 271:17491, 1996.

127. Stearns-Kurosawa DJ, Kurosawa S, Mollica JS, et al: The endo-thelial cell protein C receptor augments protein C activation by the thrombin-thrombomodulin complex. *Proc Natl Acad Sci U S A* 93: 10212, 1996.

128. Laszik Z, Mitro A, Taylor FB Jr, et al: Human protein C receptor is present primarily on endothelium of large blood vessels: Implications for the control of the protein C pathway. *Circulation* 96:3633, 1997.

129. Xu J, Esmon NL, Esmon CT: Reconstitution of the human endothelial cell protein C receptor with thrombomodulin in phosphatidylcholine vesicles enhances protein C activation. *J Biol Chem* 274:6704, 1999.

130. Fukudome K, Ye X, Tsuneyoshi N, et al: Activation mechanism of an-ticoagulant protein C in large blood vessels involving the endothelial cell protein C receptor. *J Exp Med* 187:1029, 1998.

131. Liang Z, Rosen ED, Castellino FJ: Nucleotide structure and character-ization of the murine gene encoding the endothelial cell protein C re-ceptor. *Thromb Haemost* 81:585, 1999.

132. Ye X, Fukudome K, Tsuneyoshi N, et al: The endothelial cell protein C receptor (EPCR) functions as a primary receptor for protein C activation on endothelial cells in arteries, veins, and capillaries. *Biochem Biophys Res Commun* 259:671, 1999.

133. Simmonds RE, Lane DA: Structural and functional implications of the intron/exon organization of the human endothelial cell protein C–acti-vated protein C receptor (EPCR) gene: Comparison with the structure

133. of CD1/major histocompatibility complex alpha1 and alpha2 domains. *Blood* 94:632, 1999.

134. Oganesyan V, Oganesyan N, Terzyan S, et al: The crystal structure of the endothelial protein C receptor and a bound phospholipid. *J Biol Chem* 277:24851, 2002.

135. Villoutreix BO, Blom AM, Dahlback B: Structural prediction and analysis of endothelial cell protein C–activated protein C receptor. *Protein Eng Des Sel* 12:833, 1999.

136. Kurosawa S, Stearns-Kurosawa DJ, Hidari N, Esmon CT: Identification of functional endothelial protein C receptor in human plasma. *J Clin Invest* 100:411, 1997.

137. Kurosawa S, Stearns-Kurosawa DJ, Carson CW, et al: Plasma levels of endothelial cell protein C receptor are elevated in patients with sepsis and systemic lupus erythematosus: Lack of correlation with thrombomodulin suggests involvement of different pathological processes [letter]. *Blood* 91:725, 1998.

138. Hayashi T, Nakamura H, Okada A, et al: Organization and chromosomal localization of the human endothelial protein C receptor gene. *Gene* 238:367, 1999.

139. Vu TK, Hung DT, Wheaton VI, Coughlin SR: Molecular cloning of a functional thrombin receptor reveals a novel proteolytic mechanism of receptor activation. *Cell* 64:1057, 1991.

140. Kahn ML, Nakanishi-Matsui M, Shapiro MJ, et al: Protease-activated receptors 1 and 4 mediate activation of human platelets by thrombin. *J Clin Invest* 103:879, 1999.

141. Coughlin SR: Thrombin signalling and protease-activated receptors. *Nature* 407:258, 2000.

142. Macfarlane SR, Seatter MJ, Kanke T, et al: Proteinase-activated receptors. *Pharmacol Rev* 53:245, 2001.

143. Bahou WF: Protease-activated receptors. *Curr Top Dev Biol* 54:343, 2003.

144. Major CD, Santulli RJ, Derian CK, Andrade-Gordon P: Extracellular mediators in atherosclerosis and thrombosis: Lessons from thrombin receptor knockout mice. *Arterioscler Thromb Vasc Biol* 23:931, 2003.

145. Trejo J: Protease-activated receptors: New concepts in regulation of G protein-coupled receptor signalling and trafficking. *J Pharmacol Exp Ther* 307:437, 2003.

146. Nakanishi-Matsui M, Zheng YW, Sulciner DJ, et al: PAR3 is a cofactor for PAR4 activation by thrombin. *Nature* 404:609, 2000.

147. Comp PC, Jacocks RM, Ferrell GL, Esmon CT: Activation of protein C in vivo. *J Clin Invest* 70:127, 1982.

148. Hanson SR, Griffin JH, Harker LA, et al: Antithrombotic effects of thrombin-induced activation of endogenous protein C in primates. *J Clin Invest* 92:2003, 1993.

149. Lentz SR, Fernandez JA, Griffin JH, et al: Impaired anticoagulant response to infusion of thrombin in atherosclerotic monkeys associated with acquired defects in the protein C system. *Arterioscler Thromb Vasc Biol* 19:1744, 1999.

150. Weiler-Guettler H, Christie PD, Beeler DL, et al: A targeted point mutation in thrombomodulin generates viable mice with a prethrombotic state. *J Clin Invest* 101:1983, 1998.

151. Christie PD, Edelberg JM, Picard MH, et al: A murine model of myocardial microvascular thrombosis. *J Clin Invest* 104:533, 1999.

152. Healy AM, Rayburn HB, Rosenberg RD, Weiler H: Absence of the blood-clotting regulator thrombomodulin causes embryonic lethality in mice before development of a functional cardiovascular system. *Proc Natl Acad Sci U S A* 92:850, 1995.

153. Conway EM, Van de Wouwer M, Pollefeyt S, et al: The lectin-like domain of thrombomodulin confers protection from neutrophil-mediated tissue damage by suppressing adhesion molecule expression via nuclear factor kappaB and mitogen-activated protein kinase pathways. *J Exp Med* 196:565, 2002.

154. Snow TR, Deal MT, Dickey DT, Esmon CT: Protein C activation following coronary artery occlusion in the in situ porcine heart. *Circulation* 84:293, 1991.

155. Macko RF, Killewich LA, Fernandez JA, et al: Brain-specific protein C activation during carotid artery occlusion in humans. *Stroke* 30:542, 1999.

156. Petaja J, Pesonen E, Fernandez JA, et al: Cardiopulmonary bypass and activation of antithrombotic plasma protein C. *J Thorac Cardiovasc Surg* 118:422, 1999.

157. Gruber A, Pal A, Kiss RG, et al: Generation of activated protein C during thrombolysis. *Lancet* 342:1275, 1993.

158. Macko RF, Ameriso SF, Gruber A, et al: Impairments of the protein C system and fibrinolysis in infection-associated stroke. *Stroke* 27:2005, 1996.

159. Conard J, Bauer KA, Gruber A, et al: Normalization of markers of coagulation activation with a purified protein C concentrate in adults with homozygous protein C deficiency. *Blood* 82:1159, 1993.

160. Taylor FB Jr, Peer GT, Lockhart MS, et al: Endothelial cell protein C receptor plays an important role in protein C activation in vivo. *Blood* 97:1685, 2001.

161. Bajaj MS, Kuppuswamy MN, Manepalli AN, Bajaj SP: Transcriptional expression of tissue factor pathway inhibitor, thrombomodulin and von Willebrand factor in normal human tissues. *Thromb Haemost* 82:1047, 1999.

162. Ishii H, Salem HH, Bell CE, et al: Thrombomodulin, an endothelial anticoagulant protein, is absent from the human brain. *Blood* 67:362, 1986.

163. Wong VL, Hofman FM, Ishii H, Fisher M: Regional distribution of thrombomodulin in human brain. *Brain Res* 556:1, 1991.

164. Boffa MC, Jackman RW, Peyri N, et al: Thrombomodulin in the central nervous system. *Nouv Rev Fr Hematol* 33:423, 1991.

165. Tran ND, Wong VL, Schreiber SS, et al: Regulation of brain capillary endothelial thrombomodulin mRNA expression. *Stroke* 27:2304, 1996.

166. Wang L, Tran ND, Kittaka M, et al: Thrombomodulin expression in bovine brain capillaries. Anticoagulant function of the blood-brain barrier, regional differences, and regulatory mechanisms. *Arterioscler Thromb Vasc Biol* 17:3139, 1997.

167. Hackeng TM, Tans G, Koppelman SJ, et al: Protein C activation on endothelial cells by prothrombin activation products generated in situ: Meizothrombin is a better protein C activator than α-thrombin. *Biochem J* 319:399, 1996.

168. Varadi K, Philapitsch A, Santa T, Schwarz HP: Activation and inactivation of human protein C by plasmin. *Thromb Haemost* 71:615, 1994.

169. Haley PE, Doyle MF, Mann KG: The activation of bovine protein C by factor Xa. *J Biol Chem* 264:16303, 1989.

170. Rezaie AR: Rapid activation of protein C by factor Xa and thrombin in the presence of polyanionic compounds. *Blood* 91:4572, 1998.

171. Slungaard A, Key NS: Platelet factor 4 stimulates thrombomodulin protein C-activating cofactor activity. A structure-function analysis. *J Biol Chem* 269:25549, 1994.

172. Dudek AZ, Pennell CA, Decker TD, et al: Platelet factor 4 binds to glycanated forms of thrombomodulin and to protein C. A potential mechanism for enhancing generation of activated protein C. *J Biol Chem* 272:31785, 1997.

173. Slungaard A, Fernandez JA, Griffin JH, et al: Platelet factor 4 enhances generation of activated protein C in vitro and in vivo. *Blood* 102:146, 2003.

174. Fernandez JA, Petaja J, Gruber A, Griffin JH: Activated protein C correlates inversely with thrombin levels in resting healthy individuals. *Am J Hematol* 56:29, 1997.

175. Pemberton S, Lindley P, Zaitsev V, et al: A molecular model for the triplicated A domains of human factor VIII based on the crystal structure of human ceruloplasmin. *Blood* 89:2413, 1997.

176. Villoutreix BO, Dahlback B: Structural investigation of the A domains of human blood coagulation factor V by molecular modeling. *Protein Sci* 7:1317, 1998.

177. Pellequer JL, Gale AJ, Griffin JH, Getzoff ED: Homology modeling of factor Va, a cofactor of the prothrombinase complex. *Protein Sci* 7:159, 1998;

178. Pellequer JL, Gale AJ, Griffin JH, Getzoff ED: Homology models of the C domains of blood coagulation factors V and VIII: A proposed membrane binding mode for FV and FVIII C2 domains. *Blood Cell Mol Dis* 24:448, 1998.

179. Mann KG, Kalafatis M: Factor V: A combination of Dr. Jekyll and Mr. Hyde. *Blood* 101:20, 2003.

180. Adams TE, Hockin MF, Mann KG, Everse SJ: The crystal structure of activated protein C-inactivated bovine factor Va: Implications for cofactor function. *Proc Natl Acad Sci U S A* 101:8918, 2004.

181. Camire RM, Kalafatis M, Tracy PB: Proteolysis of factor V by cathepsin G and elastase indicates that cleavage at Arg1545 optimizes cofactor function by facilitating factor Xa binding. *Biochemistry* 37:11896, 1998.

182. Steen M, Dahlback B: Thrombin-mediated proteolysis of factor V resulting in gradual B-domain release and exposure of the factor Xa-binding site. *J Biol Chem* 277:38424, 2002.

183. Toso R, Camire RM: Removal of B-domain sequences from factor V rather than specific proteolysis underlies the mechanism by which cofactor function is realized. *J Biol Chem* 279:21643, 2004.

184. Fay PJ: Regulation of factor VIIIa in the intrinsic factor Xase. *Thromb Haemost* 82:193, 1999.

185. Thorelli E, Kaufman RJ, Dahlbäck B: Cleavage requirements for activation of factor V by factor Xa. *Eur J Biochem* 247:12, 1997.

186. Marlar RA, Kleiss AJ, Griffin JH: Mechanism of action of human activated protein C, a thrombin-dependent anticoagulant enzyme. *Blood* 59:1067, 1982.

187. Suzuki K, Stenflo JA, Dahlbäck B, Teodorsson B: Inactivation of human coagulation factor V by activated protein C. *J Biol Chem* 258:1914, 1983.

188. Fulcher CA, Gardiner JE, Griffin JH, Zimmerman TS: Proteolytic inactivation of activated human factor VIII procoagulant protein by activated protein C and its analogy to factor V. *Blood* 63:486, 1984.

189. Guinto ER, Esmon CT: Loss of prothrombin and of factor Xa-factor Va interactions upon inactivation of factor Va by activated protein C. *J Biol Chem* 259:13986, 1984.

190. Kalafatis M, Rand MD, Mann KG: The mechanism of inactivation of human factor V and human factor Va by activated protein C. *J Biol Chem* 269:31869, 1994.

191. Dahlbäck B, Carlsson M, Svensson PJ: Familial thrombophilia due to a previously unrecognized mechanism characterized by poor anticoagulant response to activated protein C: Prediction of a cofactor to activated protein C. *Proc Natl Acad Sci U S A* 90:1004, 1993.

192. Bertina RM, Koeleman BPC, Koster T, et al: Mutation in blood coagulation factor V associated with resistance to activated protein C. *Nature* 369:64, 1994.

193. Greengard JS, Sun X, Xu X, et al: Activated protein C resistance caused by Arg506Gln mutation in factor Va. *Lancet* 343:1361, 1994.

194. Sun X, Evatt B, Griffin JH: Blood coagulation factor Va abnormality associated with resistance to activated protein C in venous thrombophilia. *Blood* 83:3120, 1994.

195. Zivelin A, Griffin JH, Xi X, et al: A single genetic origin for a common Caucasian risk factor for venous thrombosis. *Blood* 89:397, 1997.

196. Heeb MJ, Kojima Y, Greengard J, Griffin JH: Activated protein C resistance: Molecular mechanisms based on studies using purified Gln506-factor V. *Blood* 85:3405, 1995.

197. Kalafatis M, Bertina RM, Rand MD, Mann KG: Characterization of the molecular defect in factor V^{R506Q}. *J Biol Chem* 270:4053, 1995.

198. Rosing J, Hoekema L, Nicolaes GAF, et al: Effects of protein S and factor Xa on peptide bond cleavages during inactivation of factor Va and factor Va^{R506Q} by activated protein C. *J Biol Chem* 270:27852, 1995.

199. Gale AJ, Xu X, Pellequer JL, et al: Interdomain engineered disulfide bond permitting elucidation of mechanisms of inactivation of coagulation factor Va by activated protein C. *Protein Sci* 11:2091, 2002.

200. Bernardi F, Faioni EM, Castoldi E, et al: A factor V genetic component differing from factor V R506Q contributes to the activated protein C resistance phenotype. *Blood* 90:1552, 1997.

201. Faioni EM, Franchi F, Bucciarelli P, et al: Coinheritance of the HR2 haplotype in the factor V gene confers an increased risk of venous thromboembolism to carriers of factor V R506Q (Factor V Leiden). *Blood* 94:3062, 1999.

202. Rosing J, Bakker H, Thomassen MC, et al: Characterization of two forms of human factor Va with different cofactor activities. *J Biol Chem* 268:21130, 1993.

203. Hoekema L, Nicolaes GA, Hemker HC, et al: Human factor Va1 and factor Va2: Properties in the procoagulant and anticoagulant pathways. *Biochemistry* 36:3331, 1997.

204. Kim SW, Ortel TL, Quinn-Allen MA, et al: Partial glycosylation at asparagine-2181 of the second C-type domain of human factor V modulates assembly of the prothrombinase complex. *Biochemistry* 38:11448, 1999.

205. Nicolaes GA, Villoutreix BO, Dahlback B: Partial glycosylation of Asn2181 in human factor V as a cause of molecular and functional heterogeneity. Modulation of glycosylation efficiency by mutagenesis of the consensus sequence for N-linked glycosylation. *Biochemistry* 38:13584, 1999.

206. Fernández JA, Hackeng TM, Kojima K, Griffin JH: The carbohydrate moiety of factor V modulates inactivation by activated protein C. *Blood* 89:4348, 1997.

207. Fisher M, Fernández JA, Ameriso SF, et al: Activated protein C resistance in ischemic stroke not due to factor V arginine^{506}→glutamine mutation. *Stroke* 27:1163, 1996.

208. Van der Bom JG, Bots ML, Haverkate F, et al: Reduced response to activated protein C is associated with increased risk for cerebrovascular disease. *Ann Intern Med* 125:265, 1996.

209. De Visser MC, Rosendaal FR, Bertina RM: A reduced sensitivity for activated protein C in the absence of factor V Leiden increases the risk of venous thrombosis. *Blood* 93:1271, 1999.

210. Rodeghiero F, Tosetto A: Activated protein C resistance and factor V Leiden mutation are independent risk factors for venous thromboembolism. *Ann Intern Med* 130:643, 1999.

211. Kiechl S, Muigg A, Santer P, et al: Poor response to activated protein C as a prominent risk predictor of advanced atherosclerosis and arterial disease. *Circulation* 99:614, 1999.

212. Griffin JH, Kojima K, Banka CL, et al: High-density lipoprotein enhancement of anticoagulant activities of plasma protein S and activated protein C. *J Clin Invest* 103:219, 1999.

213. Curvers J, Thomassen MC, Nicolaes GA, et al: Acquired APC resistance and oral contraceptives: Differences between two functional tests. *Br J Haematol* 105:88, 1999.

214. Smirnov MD, Safa O, Esmon NL, Esmon CT: Inhibition of activated protein C anticoagulant activity by prothrombin. *Blood* 94:3839, 1999.

215. Colucci M, Binetti BM, Tripodi A, et al: Hyperprothrombinemia associated with prothrombin G20210A mutation inhibits plasma fibrinolysis through a TAFI-mediated mechanism. *Blood* 103:2157, 2004.

216. Neuenschwander P, Jesty J: A comparison of phospholipid and platelets in the activation of human factor VIII by thrombin and factor Xa, and in the activation of factor X. *Blood* 72:1761, 1988.

217. Keller FG, Ortel TL, Quinn-Allen MA, Kane WH: Thrombin-catalyzed activation of recombinant human factor V. *Biochemistry* 34:4118, 1995.

218. Safa O, Morrissey JH, Esmon CT, Esmon NL: Factor VIIa/tissue factor generates a form of factor V with unchanged specific activity, resistance to activation by thrombin, and increased sensitivity to activated protein C. *Biochemistry* 38:1829, 1999.

219. Bakker HM, Tans G, Janssen-Claessen T, et al: The effect of phospholipids, calcium ions and protein S on rate constants of human factor Va inactivation by activated human protein C. *Eur J Biochem* 208:171, 1992.

220. Smirnov MD, Esmon C: Phosphatidylethanolamine incorporation into vesicles selectively enhances factor Va inactivation by activated protein C. *J Biol Chem* 269:816, 1994.

221. Smirnov MD, Triplett DT, Comp PC, et al: On the role of phosphatidylethanolamine in the inhibition of activated protein C activity by antiphospholipid antibodies. *J Clin Invest* 95:309, 1995.

222. Fernández JA, Kojima K, Hackeng TM, Griffin JH: Cardiolipin, a protein C pathway cofactor: Implications for anticardiolipin antibody syndrome. *Thromb Haemost* 73:1392, 1995.

223. Rezende SM, Simmonds RE, Lane DA: Coagulation, inflammation, and apoptosis: Different roles for protein S and the protein S-C4b binding protein complex. *Blood* 103:1192, 2004.

224. Nishioka J, Suzuki K: Inhibition of cofactor activity of protein S by a complex of protein S and C4b-binding protein: Evidence for inactive ternary complex formation between protein S, C4b-binding protein, and activated protein C. *J Biol Chem* 265:9072, 1990.

225. Yegneswaran S, Wood GM, Esmon CT, Johnson AE: Protein S alters the active site location of activated protein C above the membrane surface. A fluorescence resonance energy transfer study of topography. *J Biol Chem* 272:25013, 1997.

226. Yegneswaran S, Smirnov MD, Safa O, et al: Relocating the active site of activated protein C eliminates the need for its protein S cofactor. A fluorescence resonance energy transfer study. *J Biol Chem* 274:5462, 1999.

227. Gardiner JE, McGann MA, Berridge CW, et al: Protein S as a cofactor for activated protein C in plasma and in the inactivation of purified factor VIII:C. *Circulation* 70:205a, 1984.

228. Koedam JA, Meijers JCM, Sixma JJ, Bouma BN: Inactivation of human factor VIII by activated protein C. Cofactor activity of protein S and protective effect of von Willebrand factor. *J Clin Invest* 82:1236, 1988.

229. Solymoss S, Tucker MM, Tracy PB: Kinetics of inactivation of membrane-bound factor Va by activated protein C: Protein S modulates factor Xa protection. *J Biol Chem* 263:14884, 1988.

230. Dahlback B, Hildebrand B, Malm J: Characterization of functionally important domains in human vitamin K-dependent protein S using monoclonal antibodies. *J Biol Chem* 265:8127, 1990.

231. Yegneswaran S, Hackeng T, Johnson AE, Griffin JH: Phospholipid-dependent protein S interaction with factor Xa mediated through the thrombin-sensitive region of protein S. *Thromb Haemost* 82:428, 1999.

232. Leroy-Matheron C, Gouault-Heilmann M, Aiach M, Gandrille S: A mutation of the active protein S gene leading to an EGF1-lacking protein in a family with qualitative (type II) deficiency. *Blood* 91:4608, 1998.

233. He X, Shen L, Villoutreix BO, Dahlback B: Amino acid residues in thrombin-sensitive region and first epidermal growth factor domain of vitamin K-dependent protein S determining specificity of the activated protein C cofactor function. *J Biol Chem* 273:27449, 1998.

234. Stenberg Y, Drakenberg T, Dahlback B, Stenflo J: Characterization of recombinant epidermal growth factor (EGF)-like modules from vitamin-K-dependent protein S expressed in *Spodoptera* cells—the cofactor activity depends on the N-terminal EGF module in human protein S. *Eur J Biochem* 251:558, 1998.

235. He X, Shen L, Dahlbäck B: Expression and functional characterization of chimeras between human and bovine vitamin-K-dependent protein-S-defining modules important for the species specificity of the activated protein C cofactor activity. *Eur J Biochem* 227:433, 1995.

236. Dahlbäck B, Hildebrand B: Degradation of human complement component C4b in the presence of the C4b-binding protein-protein S complex. *Biochem J* 209:857, 1983.

237. Suzuki K, Nishioka J, Hashimoto S: Regulation of activated protein C by thrombin-modified protein S. *J Biochem* 94:699, 1983.

238. Walker FJ: Regulation of vitamin K-dependent protein S: Inactivation by thrombin. *J Biol Chem* 259:10335, 1984.

239. Dahlbäck B, Lundwall A, Stenflo JA: Localization of thrombin cleavage sites in the amino-terminal region of bovine protein S. *J Biol Chem* 261:5111, 1986.

240. Váradi K, Rosing J, Tans G, et al: Factor V enhances the cofactor function of protein S in the APC-mediated inactivation of factor VIII: Influence of the factor V^{R506Q} mutation. *Thromb Haemost* 76:208, 1996.

241. Thorelli E, Kaufman RJ, Dahlback B: Cleavage of factor V at Arg 506 by activated protein C and the expression of anticoagulant activity of factor V. *Blood* 93:2552, 1999.

242. Pajkrt D, Lerch PG, van der Poll T, et al: Differential effects of reconstituted high-density lipoprotein on coagulation, fibrinolysis and platelet activation during human endotoxemia. *Thromb Haemost* 77:303, 1997.

243. Li D, Weng S, Yang B, et al: Inhibition of arterial thrombus formation by ApoA1 Milano. *Arterioscler Thromb Vasc Biol* 19:378, 1999.

244. Griffin JH, Fernandez JA, Deguchi H: Plasma lipoproteins, hemostasis and thrombosis. *Thromb Haemost* 86:386, 2001.

245. Deguchi H, Fernandez JA, Pabinger I, et al: Plasma glucosylceramide deficiency as potential risk factor for venous thrombosis and modulator of anticoagulant protein C pathway. *Blood* 97:1907, 2001.

246. Deguchi H, Fernandez JA, Griffin JH: Neutral glycosphingolipid-dependent inactivation of coagulation factor Va by activated protein C and protein S. *J Biol Chem* 277:8861, 2002.

247. Yegneswaran S, Deguchi H, Griffin JH: Glucosylceramide, a neutral glycosphingolipid anticoagulant cofactor, enhances the interaction of human- and bovine-activated protein C with negatively charged phospholipid vesicles. *J Biol Chem* 278:14614, 2003.

248. Deguchi H, Yegneswaran S, Griffin JH: Sphingolipids as bioactive regulators of thrombin generation. *J Biol Chem* 279:12036, 2004.

249. Esmon CT: Interactions between the innate immune and blood coagulation systems. *Trends Immunol* 25:536, 2004.

250. Levi M, van der Poll T, Buller HR: Bidirectional relation between inflammation and coagulation. *Circulation* 109:2698, 2004.

251. Strukova SM: Role of platelets and serine proteinases in coupling of blood coagulation and inflammation. *Biochemistry (Mosc)* 69:1067, 2004.

252. Pawlinski R, Pedersen B, Erlich J, Mackman N: Role of tissue factor in haemostasis, thrombosis, angiogenesis and inflammation: Lessons from low tissue factor mice. *Thromb Haemost* 92:444, 2004.

253. Giesen PL, Rauch U, Bohrmann B, et al: Blood-borne tissue factor: Another view of thrombosis. *Proc Natl Acad Sci U S A* 96:2311, 1999.

254. Nieuwland R, Berckmans RJ, McGregor S, et al: Cellular origin and procoagulant properties of microparticles in meningococcal sepsis. *Blood* 95:930, 2000.

255. Berckmans RJ, Nieuwland R, Boing AN, et al: Cell-derived microparticles circulate in healthy humans and support low grade thrombin generation. *Thromb Haemost* 85:639, 2001.

256. Joop K, Berckmans RJ, Nieuwland R, et al: Microparticles from patients with multiple organ dysfunction syndrome and sepsis support coagulation through multiple mechanisms. *Thromb Haemost* 85:810, 2001.

257. Freyssinet JM: Cellular microparticles: What are they bad or good for? *J Thromb Haemost* 1:1655, 2003.

258. Shet AS, Aras O, Gupta KMJH, et al: Sickle blood contains tissue factor positive microparticles derived from endothelial cells and monocytes. *Blood* 102:2678, 2003.

259. Chou J, Mackman N, Merrill-Skoloff G, et al: Hematopoietic cell-derived microparticle tissue factor contributes to fibrin formation during thrombus propagation. *Blood* 104:3190, 2004.

260. Casciola-Rosen L, Rosen A, Petri M, Schlissel M: Surface blebs on apoptotic cells are sites of enhanced procoagulant activity: Implications for coagulation events and antigenic spread in systemic lupus erythematosus. *Proc Natl Acad Sci U S A* 93:1624, 1996.

261. Bombeli T, Karsan A, Tait JF, Harlan JM: Apoptotic vascular endothelial cells become procoagulant. *Blood* 89:2429, 1997.

262. Hotchkiss RS, Swanson PE, Freeman BD, et al: Apoptotic cell death in patients with sepsis, shock, and multiple organ dysfunction. *Crit Care Med* 27:1230, 1999.

263. Mallat Z, Benamer H, Hugel B, et al: Elevated levels of shed membrane microparticles with procoagulant potential in the peripheral circulating blood of patients with acute coronary syndromes. *Circulation* 101:841, 2000.

264. Wang J, Weiss I, Svoboda K, Kwaan HC: Thrombogenic role of cells undergoing apoptosis. *Br J Haematol* 115:382, 2001.

265. Jimenez JJ, Jy W, Mauro LM, et al: Endothelial microparticles released in thrombotic thrombocytopenic purpura express von Willebrand factor and markers of endothelial activation. *Br J Haematol* 123:896, 2003.

266. Diamant M, Tushuizen ME, Sturk A, Nieuwland R: Cellular microparticles: New players in the field of vascular disease? *Eur J Clin Invest* 34:392, 2004.

267. Dignat-George F, Camoin-Jau L, Sabatier F, et al: Endothelial microparticles: A potential contribution to the thrombotic complications of the antiphospholipid syndrome. *Thromb Haemost* 91:667, 2004.

268. Horstman LL, Jy W, Jimenez JJ, Ahn YS: Endothelial microparticles as markers of endothelial dysfunction. *Front Biosci* 9:1118, 2004.

269. Morel O, Toti F, Hugel B, Freyssinet JM: Cellular microparticles: A disseminated storage pool of bioactive vascular effectors. *Curr Opin Hematol* 11:156, 2004.

270. Joyce DE, Gelbert L, Ciaccia A, et al: Gene expression profile of antithrombotic protein C defines new mechanisms modulating inflammation and apoptosis. *J Biol Chem* 276:11199, 2001.

271. Cheng T, Liu D, Griffin JH, et al: Activated protein C blocks p53-mediated apoptosis in ischemic human brain endothelium and is neuroprotective. *Nat Med* 9:338, 2003

272. Mosnier LO, Griffin JH: Inhibition of staurosporine-induced apoptosis of endothelial cells by activated protein C requires protease activated receptor-1 and endothelial cell protein C receptor. *Biochem J* 373:65, 2003.

273. Liu D, Cheng T, Guo H, et al: Tissue plasminogen activator neurovascular toxicity is controlled by activated protein C. *Nat Med* 10:1379, 2004.

274. Shu F, Kobayashi H, Fukudome K, et al: Activated protein C suppresses tissue factor expression on U937 cells in the endothelial protein C receptor-dependent manner. *FEBS Lett* 477:208, 2000.

275. Warren BL, Eid A, Singer P, et al: For the KyberSept trial study group. High-dose antithrombin III in severe sepsis: A randomized controlled trial. *JAMA* 286:1869, 2001.

276. Abraham E, Reinhart K, Opal S, et al: For the OPTIMIST trial study group. Efficacy and safety of tifacogin (recombinant tissue factor pathway inhibitor) in severe sepsis: A randomized controlled trail. *JAMA* 290:238, 2003.

277. Guo H, Liu D, Gelbard H, et al: Activated protein C prevents neuronal apoptosis via protease activated receptors 1 and 3. *Neuron* 41:563, 2004.

278. Riewald M, Petrovan RJ, Donner A, et al: Activation of endothelial cell protease activated receptor 1 by the protein C pathway. *Science* 296:1880, 2002.

279. Joyce DE, Grinnell BW: Recombinant human activated protein C attenuates the inflammatory response in endothelium and monocytes by modulating nuclear factor-kappaB. *Crit Care Med* 30:S288, 2002.

280. Domotor E, Benzakour O, Griffin JH, et al: Activated protein C alters cytosolic calcium flux in human brain endothelium via binding to endothelial protein C receptor and activation of Protease Activated Receptor-1. *Blood* 101:4797, 2003.

281. Heeb MJ, Gruber A, Griffin JH: Identification of divalent metal ion-dependent inhibition of activated protein C by α_2-macroglobulin and α_2-antiplasmin in blood and comparisons to inhibition of factor Xa, thrombin, and plasmin. *J Biol Chem* 226:17606, 1991.

282. Okajima K, Koga S, Kaji M, et al: Effect of protein C and activated protein C on coagulation and fibrinolysis in normal human subjects. *Thromb Haemost* 63:48, 1990.

283. Heeb MJ, Griffin JH: Physiologic inhibition of human activated protein C by α_1-antitrypsin. *J Biol Chem* 263:11613, 1988.

284. Heeb MJ, España F, Geiger M, et al: Immunological identity of heparin-dependent plasma and urinary protein C inhibitor and plasminogen activator inhibitor-3. *J Biol Chem* 262:15813, 1987.

285. Heeb MJ, España F, Griffin JH: Inhibition and complexation of activated protein C by two major inhibitors in plasma. *Blood* 73:446, 1989.

286. España F, Vicente V, Tabernero D, et al: Determination of plasma protein C inhibitor and of two activated protein C-inhibitor complexes in normals and in patients with intravascular coagulation and thrombotic disease. *Thromb Res* 59:593, 1990.

287. España F, Gilabert J, Aznar J, et al: Complexes of activated protein C with α_1-antitrypsin in normal pregnancy and in severe preeclampsia. *Am J Obstet Gynecol* 164:1310, 1991.

288. Hoogendoorn H, Nesheim ME, Giles AR: A qualitative and quantitative analysis of the activation and inactivation of protein C in vivo in a primate model. *Blood* 75:2164, 1990.

289. España F, Gruber A, Heeb MJ, et al: In vivo and in vitro complexes of activated protein C with two inhibitors in baboons. *Blood* 77:1754, 1991.

290. Scully MF, Toh CH, Hoogendoorn H, et al: Activation of protein C and its distribution between its inhibitors, protein C inhibitor, α_1-antitrypsin and α_2-macroglobulin, in patients with disseminated intravascular coagulation. *Thromb Haemost* 69:448, 1993.

291. Hayashi T, Nishioka J, Suzuki K: Molecular mechanism of the dysfunction of protein S(Tokushima) (Lys155→Glu) for the regulation of the blood coagulation system. *Biochim Biophys Acta* 1272:159, 1995.

292. Stenberg Y, Muranyi A, Steen C, et al: EGF-like module pair 3-4 in vitamin K-dependent protein S: Modulation of calcium affinity of module 4 by module 3 and interaction with factor X. *J Mol Biol* 293:653, 1999.

293. van't Veer C, Hackeng TM, Biesbroeck D, et al: Increased prothrombin activation in protein S-deficient plasma under flow conditions on endothelial cell matrix: An independent anticoagulant function of protein S in plasma. *Blood* 85:1815, 1995.

294. Koppelman SJ, Hackeng TM, Sixma JJ, Bouma BN: Inhibition of the intrinsic factor X activating complex by protein S: Evidence for a specific binding of protein S to factor VIII. *Blood* 86:1062, 1995.

295. Koppelman SJ, van't Veer C, Sixma JJ, Bouma BN: Synergistic inhibition of the intrinsic factor X activation by protein S and C4b-binding protein. *Blood* 86:2653, 1995.

296. Dahlbäck B: Purification of human C4b-binding protein and formation of its complex with vitamin K-dependent protein S. *Biochem J* 209:847, 1983.

297. Nelson RM, Long GL: Solution-phase equilibrium binding interaction of human protein S with C4b-binding protein. *Biochemistry* 30:2384, 1991.

298. Griffin JH, Gruber A, Fernández JA: Reevaluation of total, free and bound protein S and C4b-binding protein levels in plasma anticoagulated with citrate or hirudin. *Blood* 79:3203, 1992.

299. Comp PC, Nixon RR, Cooper MR, Esmon CT: Familial protein S deficiency is associated with recurrent thrombosis. *J Clin Invest* 74:2082, 1984.

300. Dahlbäck B: Inhibition of the protein Ca cofactor function of human and bovine protein S by C4b-binding protein. *J Biol Chem* 261:12022, 1986.

301. Hillarp A, Dahlbäck B: Novel subunit in C4b-binding protein required for protein S binding. *J Biol Chem* 263:12759, 1988.

302. Hillarp A, Hessing M, Dahlbäck B: Protein S binding in relation to the subunit composition of human C4b-binding protein. *FEBS Lett* 259:53, 1989.

303. Hillarp A, Dahlbäck B: Cloning of cDNA coding for the beta chain of human complement component C4b-binding protein: Sequence homology with the alpha chain. *Proc Natl Acad Sci U S A* 87:1183, 1990.

304. Fernández JA, Griffin JH: A protein S binding site on C4b-binding protein involves β chain residues 31-45. *J Biol Chem* 269:2535, 1994.

305. Fernández JA, Griffin JH, Chang GTG, et al: Involvement of amino acid residues 423-429 of human protein S in binding to C4b-binding protein. *Blood Cell Mol Dis* 24:101, 1998.

306. García de Frutos P, Alim RI, Härdig Y, et al: Differential regulation of α and β chains of C4b-binding protein during acute-phase response resulting in stable plasma levels of free anticoagulant protein S. *Blood* 84:815, 1994.

307. Liu D, Guo H, Griffin JH, et al: Protein S confers neuronal protection during ischemic/hypoxic injury in mice. *Circulation* 107:1791, 2003.

308. Anderson HA, Maylock CA, Williams JA, et al: Serum-derived protein S binds to phosphatidylserine and stimulates the phagocytosis of apoptotic cells. *Nat Immunol* 4:87, 2003.

309. Huber R, Carrell RW: Implications of the three-dimensional structure of α_1-antitrypsin for structure and function of serpins. *Biochemistry* 28:8951, 1989.

310. Schreuder HA, de Boer B, Dijkema R, et al: The intact and cleaved human antithrombin III complex as a model for serpin-proteinase interactions. *Nat Struct Biol* 1:48, 1994.

311. Mourey L, Samama JP, Delarue M, et al: Crystal structure of cleaved bovine antithrombin III at 3.2 Å resolution. *J Mol Biol* 232:223, 1993.

312. Carrell RW, Stein PE, Fermi G, Wardell MR: Biological implications of a 3 Å structure of dimeric antithrombin. *Structure* 2:257, 1994.

313. Whisstock J, Skinner R, Lesk AM: An atlas of serpin conformations. *Trends Biochem Sci* 23:63, 1998.

314. Skinner R, Abrahams JP, Whisstock JC, et al: The 2.6 Å structure of antithrombin indicates a conformational change at the heparin binding site. *J Mol Biol* 266:601, 1997.

315. Huntington JA, Read RJ, Carrell RW: Structure of a serpin-protease complex shows inhibition by deformation. *Nature* 407:923, 2000.

316. Li W, Johnson DJ, Esmon CT, Huntington JA: Structure of the antithrombin-thrombin-heparin ternary complex reveals the antithrombotic mechanism of heparin. *Nat Struct Mol Biol* 11:857, 2004.

317. Quinsey NS, Greedy AL, Bottomley SP, et al: Antithrombin: In control of coagulation. *Int J Biochem Cell Biol* 36:386, 2004.

318. Rosenberg RD, Rosenberg JS: Natural anticoagulant mechanisms. *J Clin Invest* 74:1, 1984.

319. Rosenberg RD, Damus PS: The purification and mechanism of action of human antithrombin-heparin cofactor. *J Biol Chem* 248:6490, 1973.

320. Olson ST, Bjork I, Sheffer R, et al: Role of the antithrombin-binding pentasaccharide in heparin acceleration of antithrombin-proteinase reactions. Resolution of the antithrombin conformational change contribution to heparin rate enhancement. *J Biol Chem* 267:12528, 1992.

321. Gettins PG, Fan B, Crews BC, et al: Transmission of conformational change from the heparin binding site to the reactive center of antithrombin. *Biochemistry* 32:8385, 1993.

322. Choay J, Petitou M, Lormeau JC, et al: Structure-activity relationship in heparin: A synthetic pentasaccharide with high affinity for antithrombin III and eliciting high anti-factor Xa activity. *Biochem Biophys Res Commun* 116:492, 1983.

323. Bourin MC, Lindahl U: Glycosaminoglycans and the regulation of blood coagulation. *Biochem J* 289:313, 1993.

324. Olds RJ, Lane DA, Chowdhury V, et al: Complete nucleotide sequence

of the antithrombin gene: Evidence for homologous recombination causing thrombophilia. *Biochemistry* 32:4216, 1993.

325. Picard V, Ersdal-Badju E, Bock SC: Partial glycosylation of antithrombin III asparagine-135 is caused by the serine in the third position of its N-glycosylation consensus sequence and is responsible for production of the beta-antithrombin III isoform with enhanced heparin affinity. *Biochemistry* 34:8433, 1995.

326. Turko IV, Fan B, Gettins PG: Carbohydrate isoforms of antithrombin variant N135Q with different heparin affinities. *FEBS Lett* 335:9, 1993.

327. Bock SC, Wion KL, Vehar GA, Lawn RM: Cloning and expression of the cDNA for human antithrombin III. *Nucleic Acids Res* 10:8113, 1982.

328. Bock SC, Harris JF, Balazs I, Trent JM: Assignment of the human antithrombin III structural gene to chromosome 1q23-25. *Cytogenet Cell Genet* 39:67, 1985.

329. Chandra T, Stackhouse R, Kidd VJ, Woo SL: Isolation and sequence characterization of a cDNA clone of human antithrombin III. *Proc Natl Acad Sci U S A* 80:1845, 1983.

330. Prochownik EV, Markham AF, Orkin SH: Isolation of a cDNA clone for human antithrombin III. *J Biol Chem* 258:8389, 1983.

331. Lane DA, Bayston T, Olds RJ, et al: Antithrombin mutation database: 2nd (1997) update. For the Plasma Coagulation Inhibitors Subcommittee of the Scientific and Standardization Committee of the International Society on Thrombosis and Haemostasis. *Thromb Haemost* 77:197, 1997.

332. Raja SM, Chhablani N, Swanson R, et al: Deletion of P1 arginine in a novel antithrombin variant (antithrombin London) abolishes inhibitory activity but enhances heparin affinity and is associated with early onset thrombosis. *J Biol Chem* 278:13688, 2003.

333. Wun TC, Kretzmer KK, Girard TJ, et al: Cloning and characterization of a cDNA coding for the lipoprotein-associated coagulation inhibitor shows that it consists of three tandem Kunitz-type inhibitory domains. *J Biol Chem* 263:6001, 1988.

334. Caplice NM, Mueske CS, Kleppe LS, et al: Expression of tissue factor pathway inhibitor in vascular smooth muscle cells and its regulation by growth factors. *Circ Res* 83:1264, 1998.

335. Lesnik P, Vonica A, Guerin M, et al: Anticoagulant activity of tissue factor pathway inhibitor in human plasma is preferentially associated with dense subspecies of LDL and HDL and with Lp(a). *Arterioscler Thromb* 13:1066, 1993.

336. Sandset PM, Abildgaard U, Larsen ML: Heparin induces release of extrinsic coagulation pathway inhibitor (EPI). *Thromb Res* 50:803, 1988.

337. Chang JY, Monroe DM, Oliver JA, Roberts HR: TFPIbeta, a second product from the mouse tissue factor pathway inhibitor (TFPI) gene. *Thromb Haemost* 81:45, 1999.

338. Zhang J, Piro O, Lu L, Broze GJ: Glycosyl phosphatidylinositol anchorage of tissue factor pathway inhibitor. *Circulation* 108:623, 2003.

339. Caplice NM, Panetta C, Peterson TE, et al: Lipoprotein (a) binds and inactivates tissue factor pathway inhibitor: A novel link between lipoproteins and thrombosis. *Blood* 98:2980, 2001.

340. Piro O, Broze GJ Jr: Role for the Kunitz-3 domain of tissue factor pathway inhibitor-alpha in cell surface binding. *Circulation* 110:3567, 2004.

341. Bajaj MS, Birktoft JJ, Steer SA, Bajaj SP: Structure and biology of tissue factor pathway inhibitor. *Thromb Haemost* 86:959, 2001.

342. Kato H: Regulation of functions of vascular wall cells by tissue factor pathway inhibitor: Basic and clinical aspects. *Arterioscler Thromb Vasc Biol* 22:539, 2002.

343. Girard TJ, Warren LA, Novotny WF, et al: Functional significance of the Kunitz-type inhibitory domains of lipoprotein-associated coagulation inhibitor. *Nature* 338:518, 1989.

344. Rao LV, Rapaport SI: Studies of a mechanism inhibiting the initiation of the extrinsic pathway of coagulation. *Blood* 69:645, 1987.

345. Huang ZF, Broze G Jr: Consequences of tissue factor pathway inhibitor gene-disruption in mice. *Thromb Haemost* 78:699, 1997.

346. Van der Logt CP, Reitsma PH, Bertina RM: Intron-exon organization of the human gene coding for the lipoprotein-associated coagulation inhibitor: The factor Xa dependent inhibitor of the extrinsic pathway of coagulation. *Biochemistry* 30:1571, 1991.

347. Girard TJ, Eddy R, Wesselschmidt RL, et al: Structure of the human lipoprotein-associated coagulation inhibitor gene. Intron/exon gene organization and localization of the gene to chromosome 2. *J Biol Chem* 266:5036, 1991.

348. Kleesiek K, Schmidt M, Gotting C, et al: The 536C→T transition in the human tissue factor pathway inhibitor (TFPI) gene is statistically associated with a higher risk for venous thrombosis. *Thromb Haemost* 82:1, 1999.

349. Dahm A, van Hylckama Vlleg A, Bendz B, et al: Low levels of tissue factor pathway inhibitor (TFPI) increase the risk of venous thrombosis. *Blood* 101:4387, 2003.

350. Tollefsen DM, Majerus DW, Blank MK: Heparin cofactor II. Purification and properties of a heparin-dependent inhibitor of thrombin in human plasma. *J Biol Chem* 257:2162, 1982.

351. Andersson TR, Sie P, Pelzer H, et al: Elevated levels of thrombin-heparin cofactor II complex in plasma from patients with disseminated intravascular coagulation. *Thromb Res* 66:591, 1992.

352. Sie P, Dupouy D, Pichon J, Boneu B: Constitutional heparin cofactor II deficiency associated with recurrent thrombosis. *Lancet* 2:415, 1985.

353. Tran TH, Marbet GA, Duckert F: Association of hereditary heparin cofactor II deficiency with thrombosis. *Lancet* 20:413, 1985.

354. Bertina RM, van der Linden IK, Engesser L, et al: Hereditary heparin cofactor II deficiency and the risk of development of thrombosis. *Thromb Haemost* 57:196, 1987.

355. Corral J, Aznar J, Gonzalez-Conejero R, et al: Homozygous deficiency of heparin cofactor II: Relevance of P17 glutamate residue in serpins, relationship with conformational diseases, and role in thrombosis. *Circulation* 110:1303, 2004.

356. Broze GJ: Protein Z dependent regulation of coagulation. *Thromb Haemost* 86:813, 2001.

357. Han X, Huang Z-F, Fiehler R, Broze GJ: The protein Z-dependent protease inhibitor is a serpin. *Biochemistry* 38:11073, 1999.

358. Han X, Fiehler R, Broze GJ: Characterization of the protein Z-dependent protease inhibitor. *Blood* 99:3049, 2000.

359. Yin Z-F, Huang Z-F, Cui J, et al: Prothrombotic phenotype of protein Z deficiency. *Proc Natl Acad Sci U S A* 97:6734, 2000.

360. Kemkes-Matthes B, Nees M, Kuhnel G, et al: Protein Z influences the prothrombotic phenotype in Factor V Leiden patients. *Thromb Res* 106:183, 2002.

361. Water N, Tan T, Ashton F, et al: Mutations within the protein Z-dependent protease inhibitor gene are associated with venous thromboembolic disease: A new form of thrombophilia. *Br J Haematol* 127:190, 2004.

362. Suzuki K, Deyashiki Y, Nishioka J, et al: Characterization of a cDNA for human protein C inhibitor: A new member of the plasma serine protease inhibitor superfamily. *J Biol Chem* 262:611, 1987.

363. Rezaie AR, Cooper ST, Church FC, Esmon CT: Protein C inhibitor is a potent inhibitor of the thrombin-thrombomodulin complex. *J Biol Chem* 270:25336, 1995.

364. Sood R, Weiler H: Embryogenesis and gene targeting of coagulation factors in mice. *Best Pract Res Clin Haematol* 16:169, 2003.

365. Weiler H: Mouse models of thrombosis: Thrombomodulin. *Thromb Haemost* 92:467, 2004.

366. Ishiguro K, Kojima T, Kadomatsu K, et al: Complete antithrombin deficiency in mice results in embryonic lethality. *J Clin Invest* 106:873, 2000.

367. Branson HE, Katz J, Marble R, Griffin JH: Inherited protein C deficiency and coumarin-responsive chronic relapsing purpura fulminans in a newborn infant. *Lancet* 2:1165, 1983.

368. Gu JM, Crawley JT, Ferrell G, et al: Disruption of the endothelial cell protein C receptor gene in mice causes placental thrombosis and early embryonic lethality. *J Biol Chem* 277:43335, 2002.

369. Castellino FJ, Liang Z, Volkir SP, et al: Mice with a severe deficiency of the endothelial protein C receptor gene develop, survive, and reproduce normally, and do not present with enhanced arterial thrombosis after challenge. *Thromb Haemost* 88:462, 2002.

370. Cui J, Eitzman DT, Westrick RJ, et al: Spontaneous thrombosis in mice carrying the factor V Leiden mutation. *Blood* 96:4222, 2000.

371. Griffin JH: The thrombin paradox. *Nature* 378:337, 1995.

VASCULAR FUNCTION IN HEMOSTASIS

KATHERINE A. HAJJAR
NAOMI L. ESMON
AARON J. MARCUS
WILLIAM MULLER

Blood vessels and their constituents are critical for control of hemostasis, thrombosis, and inflammation. Single endothelial cells, which line the entire vascular system from the heart to the smallest capillary, are responsible for maintenance of blood fluidity. They modulate metabolic interchange between the bloodstream and the surrounding tissues. In addition, endothelial cells have the unique capability to express and elaborate thromboregulatory molecules, which act at all stages of the hemostatic process, in response to specific agonists. Proinflammatory leukocyte adhesion molecules, many of which also are prothrombotic, are expressed in response to endothelial cell perturbation and injury. Although normally quiescent, endothelial cells retain the capacity for cell division and migration, processes that initiate new vessel development during angiogenesis. Thromboregulatory molecules orchestrate vascular remodeling events involving endothelial cells, smooth muscle cells, and leukocytes. These responses are essential for tissue growth and repair.

Vascular reactivity is controlled by endothelial cell products that act throughout the hemostatic process (Table 108-1). The products acting at the initial stages interfere with platelet reactivity and with the contractile state of the blood vessel. They include nitric oxide (NO), several eicosanoids, and the ecto-ADPase/cluster of differentiation 39 (CD39). The endothelins, on the other hand, constitute a group of endothelium-derived polypeptides that induce prolonged vasoconstriction. Following modulation of the primary hemostatic plug, later-acting endothelial cell thromboregulators either neutralize thrombin or promote thrombolysis. The thromboregulators include the natural anticoagulant antithrombin (AT), which inhibits thrombin and factor Xa in the presence of endothelial cell heparan proteoglycan cofactors; tissue factor (TF) pathway inhibitor, which blocks factor VII/TF activity; and the thrombomodulin (TM)–protein C system, which inhibits the cofactor activity of factors Va and VIIIa. In addition, the endothelial cell fibrinolytic system, which includes endothelium-derived plasminogen activators, their inhibitors, and their receptors, serves to orchestrate thrombolysis further. Inflammatory thromboregulators include the endothelial cell adhesion molecules, a special class of glycoproteins (GPs) that mediate leukocyte interactions in the inflammatory setting. The inflammatory adhesion molecules include the cell adhesion molecules, the selectins, the junctional adhesion molecules (JAMs), and CD99.

ENDOTHELIAL CELLS AND HEMOSTASIS

The endothelium represents a dynamic interface between flowing blood and the vessel wall. The endothelium is subject to a panoply of physical forces, circulating factors, and cell–cell interactions that create regionally specific phenotypes. The endothelium regulates the fluid state of blood, vascular tone, inflammatory processes, vascular permeability, and vascular fragility. In its basal state, the endothelium is both thromboresistant and profibrinolytic.

In vivo, endothelial cells are highly heterogeneous. They undergo a process whereby they acquire specialized characteristics in response to signals from the local microenvironment. Thus, small and large vessel endothelial cells *in vivo*, and even endothelial cells from different tissues within the same organ, may express distinct patterns of surface molecules, show different membrane specializations such as fenestrae, and have varying synthetic capabilities.

Human umbilical vein endothelial cells, first cultivated in the early 1970s, have served as an informative model in vascular biology. However, we now know that studies based upon such large vessel endothelial cells may be subject to significant limitations. First, cultured

Acronyms and abbreviations that appear in this chapter include: ADP, adenosine diphosphate; APC, activated protein C; apo(a), apolipoprotein(a); AT, antithrombin; cAMP, cyclic adenosine monophosphate; CD, cluster of differentiation; COX, cyclooxygenase; DDAVP, (1-deamino, 8-D-arginine) vasopressin; EDRF, endothelium-derived relaxing factor; EGF, epidermal growth factor; EGF5, epidermal growth factor domain 5; EPCR, endothelial cell protein C receptor; ET-1, endothelin-1; GP, glycoprotein; H_4B, 6R-tetrahydro-L-biopterin; HC, homocysteine; ICAM, intercellular adhesion molecule; IFN, interferon; IL, interleukin; JAM, junctional adhesion molecule; LDL, low-density lipoprotein; LFA, lymphocyte function-associated antigen; Lp(a), lipoprotein(a); Mac, macrophage; MAdCAM, mucosal addressin cell adhesion molecule; MAP, mitogen-activated protein; MAPTAM, bis(2-amino-5-methylphenoxy)ethane-N,N,N′,N′-tetraacetic acid tetraacetoxymethyl ester; MHC, major histocompatibility complex; NF-κB, nuclear factor-κB; NK, natural killer; NO, nitric oxide; NOS, nitric oxide synthase; PAF, platelet-activating factor; PAI, plasminogen activator inhibitor; PAR, protease-activated receptor; PCI, protein C inhibitor; PECAM, platelet endothelial cell adhesion molecule; PG, prostaglandin; PSGL, P-selectin glycoprotein ligand; scu-PA, single-chain urokinase-type plasminogen activator; sEPCR, soluble form of endothelial cell protein C receptor; TAFI, thrombin activatable fibrinolysis inhibitor; TF, tissue factor; TGF, transforming growth factor; TIMP-1, tissue inhibitor of metalloproteinase; TM, thrombomodulin; TNF, tumor necrosis factor; t-PA, tissue plasminogen activator; u-PA, urokinase plasminogen activator; u-PAR, urokinase plasminogen activator receptor; VCAM, vascular cell adhesion molecule; VEGF, vascular endothelial growth factor; VLA, very late antigen; vWF, von Willebrand factor.

TABLE 108-1 ENDOTHELIAL CELL THROMBOREGULATORS

Modulators of Platelet Reactivity
   Nitric oxide (NO)
   Eicosanoids (prostacyclin, PGD_2)
   Endothelial cell ecto-ADPase/CD39
Regulators of Vasoreactivity
   Endothelin
Anticoagulant Systems
   Antithrombin
   Heparan proteoglycans
   Tissue factor pathway inhibitor (TFPI)
   Thrombomodulin-protein C-protein S pathway
Profibrinolytic Agents
   Tissue plasminogen activator-I
   Urokinase
   Plasminogen activator inhibitor
   Urokinase receptor
   Annexin 2
Inflammatory Adhesion Molecules
   CAMs
   Selectins
   JAMs
   CD99

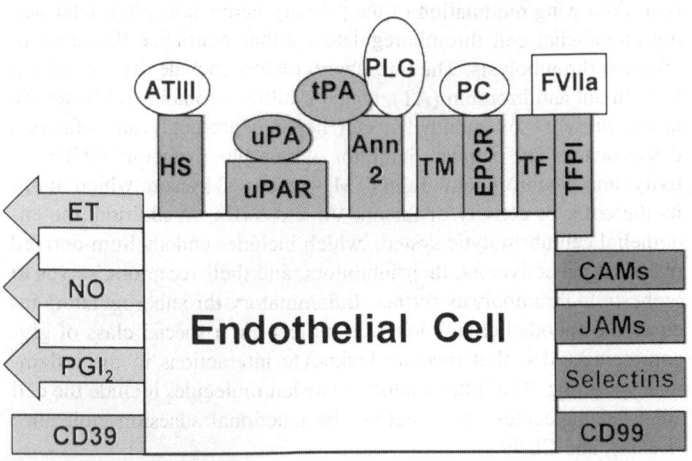

FIGURE 108-1 Schematic depiction of endothelial cell thromboregulatory molecules. Products that are secreted and exert their effects in the fluid phase are represented by *arrows*. Cell surface-associated molecules are shown as *rectangles*. Metabolites synthesized by endothelial cells are *shaded*. Thromboregulators that modulate platelet activation, recruitment, and blood vessel contractility are shown on the *left*. Agents that regulate components of the coagulation cascade and/or fibrinolytic system are located at the *top*. Inflammatory molecules whose expression or activity is directed by inflammatory mediators are shown at the *right*. Ann 2, annexin 2; ATIII, antithrombin III; CAMs, cellular adhesion molecules; CD39, endothelial cell ecto-ADPase/CD39; EPCR, endothelial cell protein C receptor; ET, endothelin; FVIIa, factor VIIa; HS, heparan sulfate; JAMs, junctional adhesion molecules; NO, nitric oxide; PC, protein C; PGI$_2$, prostacyclin; PLG, plasminogen; TF, tissue factor; TFPI, tissue factor pathway inhibitor; TM, thrombomodulin; tPA, tissue plasminogen activator; uPA, urokinase plasminogen activator; uPAR, uPA receptor. These components are discussed further in the text.

endothelial cells exist in an active, replicative mode compared to their *in vitro* counterparts. In addition, cultured endothelial cells tend to lose their specific regional characteristics and revert to a dedifferentiated state with repeated passage. With the introduction of transgenic animal models and more extensive use of primary endothelial cells from different vascular beds, more effective comparisons can be made between *in vivo* and *in vitro* studies.

THROMBOREGULATION BY VASCULAR CELLS

Thromboregulation is defined as a process by which blood or vascular wall cells may interact to modulate thrombus formation. Thromboregulation occurs in the setting of cell proximity or actual contact. It may be cell associated or involve released compounds generated via agonist exposure. Most, if not all, thromboregulatory reactions are biochemical in nature and result in formation of novel biologically active metabolites that could have been synthesized only via interactions between heterogeneous cell types in the vascular compartment. Thromboregulatory systems prevent or reverse platelet accumulation, activation of coagulation factors, and formation of fibrin. They are the

key to maintaining blood fluidity and the antithrombotic process (Fig. 108-1).[1–12]

The physiologic defense systems that render endothelial surfaces thromboresistant and antifibrinolytic can be circumvented by excessive shear stress, mechanical or chemical injury, increased turbulence, and inflammation.[13] Such conditions transform the endothelium into a prothrombotic and antifibrinolytic surface, which also is atherogenic,[13,14] and up-regulate expression of leukocyte and endothelial cell adhesion molecules, TF,[13,14] and eicosanoids. These events commonly occur at the site of the ruptured atherosclerotic plaque in the coronary and cerebrovascular circulation,[9,12] exposing TF to the circulation.[14] Because the eicosanoids (prostaglandin [PG]I$_2$, PGD$_2$), NO, and ecto-ADPase/CD39 operate at very early stages in the hemostatic/thrombotic cascade, they represent attractive targets for therapeutic intervention (Table 108-2).[2,11]

Historically, Virchow[15] suggested that the factors responsible for thrombus formation could be classified into three categories, known as "Virchow's triad." The first category involved alterations in blood flow pattern, the second related to pathologic changes in the intimal surface of the blood vessels, and the third reflected reactivities in blood constituents, even though platelets were not recognized at the time. In retrospect, this ingenious hypothesis was his recognition of thrombosis as a process driven by cell–cell interactions and further modulated by inflammatory mediators. The latter was verified biochemically in 1982.[4,16]

PROSTACYCLIN AS A THROMBOREGULATOR

The discovery of endoperoxides and thromboxanes by Hamburg, Svensson, and Samuelsson[16] in the early 1970s (for which these investigators were awarded the Nobel prize) initiated a new era in platelet biochemistry and physiology. The important implication was that the releasate from activated platelets contained two vasoconstrictors, serotonin and thromboxane. The latter also caused platelet aggregation that operated via adenosine diphosphate (ADP) release.[17] Subsequently, an additional endothelium-derived eicosanoid that caused vasodilatation and inhibition of platelet aggregation was characterized by Moncada and colleagues. This substance initially was named PGX but later was characterized as prostacyclin (PGI$_2$).[18,19]

BIOSYNTHESIS OF PROSTACYCLIN

A broad range of agonists, hormonal, biochemical, or physical (e.g., shear stress) stimulates eicosanoid production in endothelial cells. Upon exposure to stimuli, intracellular calcium levels increase, which in turn activates phospholipases such as A$_2$ and C. The phospholipases catalyze formation of free arachidonate from phospholipids in the cell membrane. Activity of phospholipase A$_2$ is rate limiting for eicosanoid production in certain tissues. The free arachidonate becomes oxygenated and cyclized by the action of the microsomal enzyme PGH synthase 1 (also known as cyclooxygenase [COX]-1). The cyclic endoperoxide PGG$_2$ forms and is quickly reduced to PGH$_2$ via inherent peroxidase activity in COX-1. Endoperoxides are transferred to eicosanoid end products within seconds. The major and most important

TABLE 108-2 EARLY PROTHROMBOTIC AND ANTITHROMBOTIC THROMBOREGULATORS ASSOCIATED WITH HUMAN ENDOTHELIAL CELLS

CLASS	TYPE	SITE OF ACTION	ASPIRIN SENSITIVITY	MODE OF ACTION
Eicosanoids	PGI$_2$, PGD$_2$	Fluid phase autacoid	Sensitive	Elevation of platelet cAMP
Nitrovasodilators	NO	Fluid phase autacoid	Insensitive	Elevation of platelet cGMP
Ecto-nucleotidases	ADPase/CD39	Endothelial cell surface	Insensitive	Enzymatic removal of secreted ADP
Thromboxane	TXA$_2$	Fluid phase vasoconstrictor and platelet agonist	Sensitive	Lowers platelet cAMP
Endothelins	ET-1, ET-2	Fluid phase vasoconstrictor peptide	Insensitive	Direct vasoconstrictor

COX-1 product in endothelial cells is PGI_2, the formation of which is catalyzed by the isomerase PGI synthase. Other endothelial cell isomerases catalyze formation of PGE_2, $PGF_{2\alpha}$, and PGD_2 (Fig. 108-2). PGD_2 acts similarly to PGI_2 on the same receptor. PGI_2 has a half-life of 3 minutes and undergoes chemical hydrolysis to the inactive form 6-keto-$PGF_{1\alpha}$. Synthesis of PGG_2/PGH_2 is common to a variety of tissues, but its subsequent processing is specific for a given tissue. For example, in platelets, thromboxane synthase catalyzes metabolism of PGH_2 to thromboxane A_2.[16,18,19] Platelets and leukocytes also contain cytosolic enzymes that catalyze oxygenation of arachidonate to lipid hydroperoxides, that is, the lipoxygenases. In leukocytes, the hydroxy acids are critical for formation of leukotrienes. In platelets, lipoxygenase products are enhanced by aspirin ingestion.[1,2] Endothelial cells do not synthesize lipoxygenase products. However, endothelial cells take part in production of lipoxygenase products via transcellular metabolism.[20]

TWO ISOFORMS OF PROSTACYCLIN G/H SYNTHASE

When an early response gene from 3T3 fibroblasts was cloned, cDNA was observed to be homologous to COX-1.[21] The existence of two forms of COX—COX-1 (constitutive) and COX-2 (induced as an intermediate early gene in monocytes, macrophages, neutrophils, and endothelial cells)—then became clear.[22] Thus, COX-2 is inducible in endothelial cells by prothrombotic, inflammatory, or mitogenic stimuli. In neutrophils, COX-2 is induced by inflammatory stimuli.[23–31] In any given species, approximately 60 percent homology exists between deduced amino acid sequences. COX-1 contains 576 residues, compared to 587 for COX-2. A C-terminal sequence of 18 amino acids in COX-2 is absent in COX-1. Antibodies directed at this C-terminal sequence can identify COX-2 by Western blot. The catalytic activities of the two COX enzymes are similar, and all amino acids critical for COX-1 activity are conserved in COX-2. The active site in COX-1 is slightly larger than the active site of COX-2, which is important for design of COX inhibitors. COX-2 contains mannose and an additional N-glycosylation site at the 18-amino acid C-terminal sequence. An N-glycosylation site at Asn410 is required for COX-1 folding into its active conformation. The gene for COX-1 is located on chromosome 9 and spans 22 kb of genomic DNA. The gene for COX-2 is located on chromosome 1 and spans 8 kb of genomic DNA. Transcription of COX-2 proceeds via several signaling mechanisms, including cyclic adenosine monophosphate (cAMP)/protein kinase A, protein kinase C, tyrosine kinases, and pathways activated by growth factors, endotoxin, and cytokines.[21–31]

AUTOCOID FUNCTION OF PROSTACYCLIN

Activity of PGI_2 as a vascular smooth muscle relaxant is demonstrable following infusion of the parent molecule or its analogues. The inhibitory action of PGI_2 results from interaction with its receptor on vascular smooth muscle cells and platelets. The biochemical effects of PGI_2 are mediated through G proteins and result in increased intraplatelet concentrations of cAMP.[9] This process leads to abolition of shape change, inhibition of platelet secretion, and impaired binding of von Willebrand factor (vWF) and fibrinogen to the platelet surface. At high shear rates, PGI_2 inhibits platelet adhesion to subendothelium.[9] Because of side effects, utilization of prostacyclin or its analogues as therapeutic agents for occlusive vascular diseases has not been possible.[2]

NITRIC OXIDE

Nitric oxide or nitrogen monoxide (NO) is a colorless gas. In mammals, it is a ubiquitous free radical, synthesized from arginine. NO is a major example of a signaling molecule that crosses the plasma membrane and activates an enzyme intracellularly. It has a half-life of approximately 5 to 10 seconds. NO participates in a wide variety of biologic actions, including neurotransmission, vasodilation, macrophage cytotoxicity, and inhibition of platelet aggregation. NO was the first gas to be characterized as an intracellular messenger. NO represents the action of a molecule that originally was defined as endothelium-derived relaxing factor (EDRF).[32] Furchgott, Ignaro, and Murad received the 1998 Nobel Prize for their discovery of NO as a vasodilator.

Upon release from an activated endothelial cell, NO induces vasodilation, regulates normal vascular tone, and inhibits platelet aggregation. NO overproduction may be involved in the pathogenesis of hypotension that accompanies endotoxin-induced shock. Underproduction or deficiency may result in the intense vasoconstriction observed in the pulmonary circulation of patients with sickle cell anemia.[33] Abnormally low NO levels in the pulmonary circulation may contribute to pulmonary hypertension.[33–36] In vascular endothelial cells, nitric oxide synthase (NOS) catalyzes formation of NO from L-arginine, in the presence of nicotinamide adenine dinucleotide phosphate (NADPH) and oxygen. L-arginine subsequently is converted to citrulline and NO. The endothelial cell isoform of NOS (eNOS or the NOS3 gene product) functions constitutively and is further activated by receptor agonists that elevate intracellular calcium. Major stimuli include ADP, thrombin, bradykinin, and shear stress.[9] Shear forces induce transcriptional activation of the eNOS gene because its promoter contains a shear response consensus

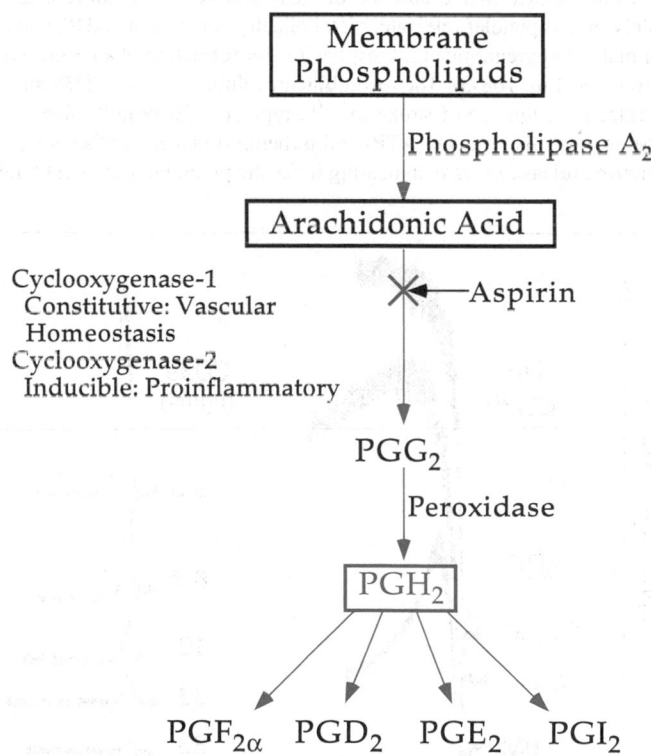

FIGURE 108-2 Oxygenation by cyclooxygenases and transformation of released arachidonate to prostacyclin and other eicosanoids in endothelial cells. This situation is in contrast to platelets, which process arachidonate to thromboxane and 12-hydroxyeicosatraenoic acid (12-HETE). In response to prothrombotic or inflammatory stimuli, the essential fatty acid arachidonate is released from phospholipids in the cell membrane by the enzyme phospholipase A_2 (PLA_2). Regulatory enzymes in this pathway include cyclooxygenase COX-1, which functions mainly in the endoplasmic reticulum, and COX-2, which functions principally in the nucleus. COX-1 and COX-2 catalyze insertion of two molecules of oxygen into free arachidonate to form endoperoxide PGG_2, which then is peroxidized to the endoperoxide PGH_2. The endoperoxides are common precursors to all eicosanoids.[375]

sequence (GAGACC).[9] Acetylcholine released by activated nerve terminals in the vessel wall activates the endothelial cell to produce and release NO. The NO that forms activates guanylate cyclase, thereby generating cyclic GMP. NO becomes oxidized to nitrite and then to nitrate, which is measurable in blood samples. NO in the circulation is rapidly inactivated by erythrocytes.[34–36] Inhalation of NO has a vasodilatory effect on the pulmonary vasculature. In patients with congestive heart failure and pulmonary congestion, NO inhalation decreases pulmonary hypertension and increases pulmonary ventilation.[32,34–42] This NO effect also explains the action of nitroglycerin. An NO donor has been used for many years to treat patients with angina resulting from coronary artery disease.[41]

Importantly, NO production by endothelial cells is impaired in the presence of the thiol-containing amino acid homocysteine (HC). Cynomolgus monkeys with diet-induced hyperhomocysteinemia ($11 \mu M$) demonstrated reduced blood flow in the lower extremity and an impaired response to endothelial cell-dependent vasodilators.[38] Similarly, NO production by endothelial cells *in vitro* is significantly inhibited in the presence of HC, possibly by a mechanism involving impairment of the enzyme glutathione peroxidase.[39,40]

STRUCTURE AND BIOCHEMICAL PROPERTIES OF NOS

Two isoforms of NOS exist. One form is constitutively synthesized and regulated by Ca^{2+} and calmodulin. The second form is cytokine inducible and posttranscriptionally regulated.[34] The inducible and constitutive forms are mainly cytosolic. A membrane-bound constitutive NOS isoform containing a myristoylation consensus sequence has been isolated from bovine aortic endothelial cells.[34] Endothelial NOS is M_r 144,000 and shares 57 percent amino acid sequence identity with neuronal NOS. The cofactor 6R-tetrahydro-L-biopterin (H_4B) participates in inducible and constitutive NOS isoform reactions. H_4B is believed to stabilize the enzyme in a manner allowing for maximum activity of the NOS subunit to which the pterin binds.[34,35] Biologic reactions controlled by NO include vasodilation, regulation of normal vascular tone, and inhibition of platelet aggregation.[41,42]

BLOCKADE OF PLATELET AGGREGATION AND SECRETION BY NO

NO release from endothelial cells blocks platelet activation and secretion in response to agonists such as thrombin. The action of NO is not affected by aspirin. Thus, the activity of NO does not result from participation of endothelial eicosanoids.[42]

In addition to the constitutive isoform of NOS (eNOS, the NOS3 gene product), endothelial cells stimulated by agonists such as cytokines express the inducible form of NO synthase (iNOS), which is the NOS2 gene product. By this mechanism, NO further inhibits platelet reactivity and reduces vessel tone via relaxation of vascular smooth muscle. Biochemically, this process results from NO binding to the heme prosthetic group of guanylyl cyclase. The inhibitory effect of NO on platelet secretion can be monitored by measuring serotonin release or surface expression of P-selectin. The ability of NO to inhibit mobilization of intracellular platelet calcium results in reduced conformational changes in platelet membrane GPIIb-IIIa, a prerequisite for fibrinogen binding and subsequent aggregation. Other effects of NO, such as inhibition of leukocyte adhesion to the endothelial surface, inhibition of smooth muscle migration, and reduction of smooth muscle proliferation, suggest NO secretion into the microenvironment is a major component of the tissue response to vascular injury.[34,35,41]

ENDOTHELIN

In addition to synthesizing two important vasodilators (PGI₂, NO), endothelial cells produce endothelins, which are potent vasoconstric-

tors. The endothelins constitute a group of 21-amino-acid peptides produced in a broad spectrum of cells.[43,44] Endothelin-1 (ET-1) is not stored in cells but forms from the inactive precursor preproendothelin-1. Transcription of the gene encoding preproendothelin-1 is induced by shear stress, hypoxia, or ischemia. Preproendothelin-1 is cleaved by an ET-1–converting enzyme, thereby forming the active peptide. ET-1, which is released from the activated endothelial cell, binds to a G-protein–coupled receptor in smooth muscle. The binding process induces an increased cytosolic calcium concentration, resulting in smooth muscle contraction. When concentrations of other thromboregulators such as NO are decreased, the action of ET-1 may be amplified and result in greater vasoconstriction.[43,44]

ET-1 release has been reported in the hepatorenal syndrome, a form of renal failure occurring in patients with severe liver disease. This disorder is characterized by intense and prolonged renal vasoconstriction. The hypoxia, oxidant injury, and endotoxemia characteristic of end-stage liver disease, probably are agonists for endothelin production. The renal vasoconstriction has been attributed to activation of the sympathetic and renin–angiotensin systems in the kidney.[41,43,44]

ECTO-ADPASE/CD39/NTPDASE 1

Of the three endothelial systems that control platelet reactivity—prostacyclin, NO, and endothelial ecto-ADPase/CD39—only CD39 is an integral membrane component and is substrate activated.[45] It maintains vascular fluidity in the absence of PGI₂ and NO. The enzyme acts solely on the platelet releasate, metabolically neutralizing ADP, a major platelet aggregating agent responsible for formation of an occlusive thrombus (Fig. 108-3). The recombinant, soluble form of CD39 ameliorates the sequelae of stroke in wild-type and CD39 null mice.[1,2,11] The enzyme also reduces ATP- and ischemia-induced cardiac norepinephrine release *in vitro*, indicating it has the potential to prevent fatal

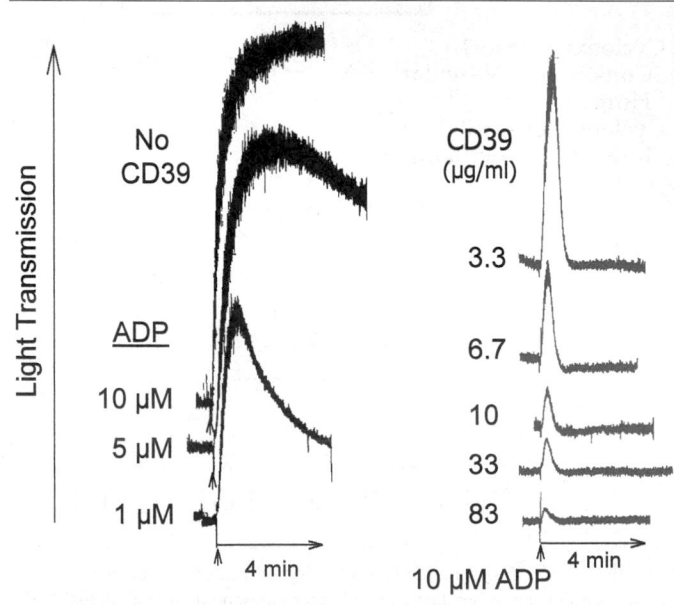

FIGURE 108-3   Purified soluble CD39 induces complete blockade of ADP-induced platelet aggregation. The response to increasing concentrations of ADP is shown on the *left*. The response to ADP is inhibited by increasing quantities of soluble CD39 shown on the *right*. The experiment demonstrates that blockade of platelet reactivity by purified soluble CD39 is far greater than the reduction in platelet activation when ADP as an agonist is diluted 10-fold. In the presence of only 3.3 μg/ml soluble CD39, platelet aggregation as induced by 10 μM ADP was abruptly terminated, with the curve rapidly returning to baseline.[2,3,11]

arrhythmia *in vivo*.[46,47] Thus, CD39 has been suggested to represent the next generation of cardioprotective and cerebroprotective molecules.[6-8,48-50]

PROTEIN C PATHWAY

The protein C pathway plays a critical role in thrombosis prevention and is an integral part of the host inflammatory response (described in detail in Chap. 107). This pathway is initiated on the endothelial cell surface when thrombin combines with the endothelial receptor protein thrombomodulin (TM). Although thrombin is capable of slowly activating protein C, the reaction is markedly inhibited in the presence of physiologic concentrations of calcium ions. Once thrombin is bound to TM, the rate of protein C activation is dramatically enhanced[51] and is dependent on the presence of calcium. The detailed biochemistry of this activation reaction has been reviewed elsewhere.[52,53] Another protein found predominantly in large vessels, the endothelial cell protein C receptor EPCR, can bind protein C and further augment its activation by the thrombin–TM complex.[54] Presumably the activated protein C (APC) can dissociate from EPCR and interact with protein S on either the endothelial cell or other membrane surface to exert its anticoagulant function. The function of APC is discussed in detail elsewhere in this book (see Chap. 107) and in other reviews[55-58] and per se is not discussed in this chapter.

THROMBOMODULIN

FUNCTIONS OF TM

The most well known function of TM is its role in protein C activation. However, TM has many other functions. When TM or its expression is altered, the extent to which observed effects result from compromise of protein C activation versus compromise of another function of TM is not obvious. Some of these functions include additional effects on thrombin. Any change in TM that alters the affinity for thrombin has multiple effects. When thrombin is bound to TM, thrombin can no longer convert fibrinogen to fibrin, activate factors V and VIII,[59] or activate platelets by interacting with the protease-activated receptors (PAR)s.[60,61] Thus, TM acts as a direct anticoagulant. The rates of thrombin inactivation by its inhibitors AT and protein C inhibitor (PCI) are enhanced when thrombin is complexed with TM.[62] This process leads to an estimated half-life of the thrombin–TM complex of 2 to 3 seconds.

TM promotes activation of plasma procarboxypeptidase B, also referred to as thrombin activatable fibrinolysis inhibitor (TAFI), by thrombin. This carboxypeptidase,[63] or carboxypeptidase R, causes partial inhibition of fibrin degradation by plasmin, presumably by removing carboxy-terminal lysine residues from fibrin, thereby decreasing fibrin binding to certain forms of plasminogen and plasmin (see Chap. 127). However, TAFI has functions other than its antifibrinolytic role. TAFI is the major enzyme responsible for removal of a C-terminal arginine from C5a,[64-66] leading to its inactivation. C5a is a potent anaphylotoxin generated during complement activation, and other vasoactive substances most likely are inactivated by this enzyme by a similar mechanism. TM accelerates the proteolytic inactivation of prourokinase (also called single-chain urokinase-type plasminogen activator [scu-PA]) by thrombin,[67,68] which may affect fibrinolysis and tissue remodeling.[69] Despite the antifibrinolytic affects of TM, many *in vivo* experiments have demonstrated that soluble TM infusion results in a net antithrombotic and/or antiinflammatory effect[62] (and references therein).

TM has direct effects on cell interactions independent of thrombin or APC production. The N-terminal "lectin-like" domain of TM can down-regulate expression of adhesion molecules on the endothelium

when injured.[70] This process in turn diminishes the adhesion of neutrophils and the resultant tissue damage. The effect is mediated by suppression of cytokine-induced activation of the mitogen-activated protein (MAP) kinase and nuclear factor (NF)-κB pathways. Mice engineered with this domain deleted have decreased survival after endotoxin exposure, more neutrophil accumulation in their lungs, and increased production of cytokines. These animals also develop larger infarcts after myocardial ischemia/reperfusion, most likely as a result of greater neutrophil infiltration. Interestingly, the isolated domain is capable of down-regulating these proinflammatory pathways both *in vivo* and *in vitro*.

TM can modulate cell proliferation in tumor cells, and this function is dependent on both the amino-terminal and cytoplasmic domains.[71] Isolates of lymphatic endothelial cells from lymphangiosarcomas and neonatal myocardia lacking the lectin-like domain of TM showed more rapid growth than wild-type cells (EM Conway, personal communication with permission). Conceivably, the effect on proliferation may result from direct involvement of TM in adhesion, leading to cell interactions involved in limiting cell growth.[72] Keratinocytes express high TM levels.[73] Cell lines treated with antibody to the N-terminal domain no longer maintain cell–cell contact. In addition, TM-negative melanoma cells transfected with full-length TM, but not TM missing the N-terminal domain, acquired the ability to grow in clusters. Growth of these tumors *in vivo* was affected by the form of TM expressed by the cells. Adhesion results from the lectin properties of the domain, as mannose and chondroitin sulfates A and C but not other sugars tested disperse TM-expressing cell clusters. The physiologic significance of this adhesion is not known.

TM plays a crucial role in fetal development independent of TM's effect on hemostasis. When the TM gene is deleted by homologous recombination in mice, embryos die on day 8.5, prior to development of a functional cardiovascular system,[74] implying that TM has functions in addition to its anticoagulant and fibrinolytic properties. TM[75] and EPCR[76] are highly expressed on the giant trophoblast cells of the placenta. If TM expression is maintained on these cells, TM null embryos survive.[77,78] TM (and/or APC?) also appears to counteract thrombin-dependent growth arrest of these cells, which is independent of clot formation.[79,80] Strong TM expression also has been observed on neural crest cells of the developing mouse embryo,[81,82] although the role of TM is unknown.

TM STRUCTURE AND RELATION TO FUNCTION

The domain structure of TM (Fig. 108-4)[58,62,83] was deduced from the cloned cDNA for the protein. The gene for TM lacks introns and is located on chromosome 20. The amino-terminal 226 residues of the mature protein show weak homology to lectin-like domains, as in the asialoglycoprotein receptor, and are involved in the constitutive internalization of the receptor.[84] As discussed above, this domain has been implicated in the down-regulation of adhesion proteins in response to endothelial injury[70] and cell adhesion.[72] Although the antiinflammatory activity of soluble TM in a model of glomerular injury was interpreted to result from TAFI activation,[66] the direct antiadhesion activity of this domain of soluble TM also may have contributed to the decreased leukocyte infiltration observed. This region is followed by six epidermal growth factor (EGF)-b type repeats. EGF domain 5 (EGF5) and EGF domain 6 (EGF6), particularly EGF5, contribute most of the binding affinity for thrombin, can block fibrinogen cleavage by thrombin, and accelerate scu-PA inactivation by thrombin.[85] However, this region cannot support protein C activation. EGF5 has been suggested to not exhibit the canonical disulfide bonding pattern.[86] This unusual disulfide pairing (1–2, 3–4, 5–6 rather than the usual 1–3, 2–4, 5–6) has been confirmed by x-ray crystal analysis.[87] A tight

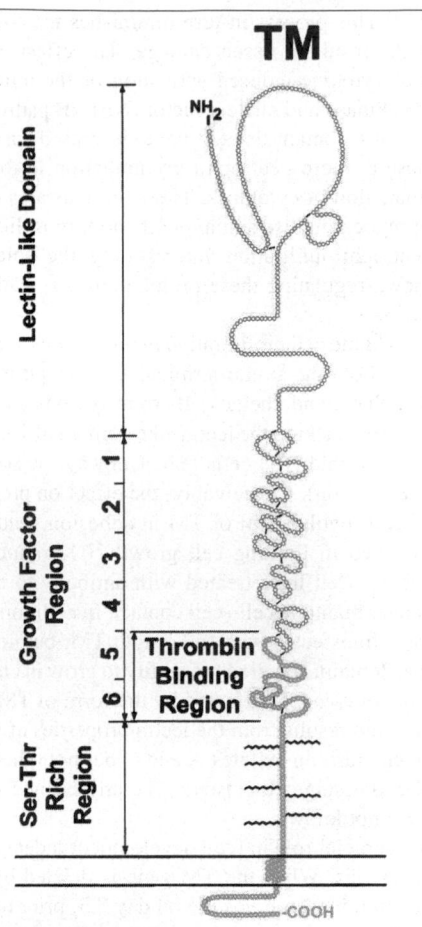

FIGURE 108-4 Domain structure of thrombomodulin (TM) as deduced from the amino acid sequence. Structures shown on the Ser-Thr–rich region of TM represent chondroitin sulfate attachment. See text for detailed descriptions. (Modified figure reprinted with permission from *J Biol Chem* 264:4743, 1989; copyright the American Society of Biochemistry and Molecular Biology, Inc., 1989.)

calcium binding site, important for protein C activation, is also present in EGF6.[87,88]

Although EGF4,5 can promote activation of protein C by thrombin,[89] rates approaching those of the intact TM molecule require the linkage region between EGF3 and EGF4 and the entire fourth, fifth, and sixth EGF modules.[90,91] A methionine in position 388 (between the fourth and fifth EGF domains), at least in the human molecule, is highly sensitive to oxidation. This oxidation leads to inactivation of the molecule.[92,93] Many studies involving x-ray crystallography and nuclear magnetic resonance analysis of mutations in TM, thrombin, and protein C have been performed to determine how these three proteins interact for efficient protein C activation. TM appears to supply at least part of the binding site for protein C through EGF domain 4. This scenario is supported by mutational studies and the crystal structure of EGF4,5,6 in complex with thrombin (see Chap. 107).[53,94,95] However, additional mutational and spectral data indicate TM binding also affects the conformation of thrombin (for details, see Chap. 107 and references).[53,94,95] EGF3 is required for catalysis of TAFI activation.[96] No specific function has been observed for EGF domain 2.

A 34-residue region rich in serine and threonine follows the EGF domains. The region contains several *O*-linked glycosylation sites and two potential chondroitin sulfate attachment sites. The region

apparently is elongated and serves as a spacer, positioning the TM binding sites above the cell surface.[97] The presence of chondroitin sulfate in this region has several functional consequences. It enhances the affinity of TM for thrombin, facilitates inhibition of thrombin by antithrombin (AT) and protein C inhibitor (PCI), modulates the calcium dependence of protein C activation,[58] and is directly involved in platelet factor 4 modulation of protein C activation.[98] Biochemical[99] and electron microscopic[100] experiments indicate the glycosaminoglycan chain can bind a second molecule of thrombin. Chondroitin sulfate also is required for the optimal acceleration of thrombin-mediated inactivation of scu-PA[85] and may be involved in the pathogenesis of malaria caused by *Plasmodium falciparum*.[101] Addition of chondroitin sulfate can be variable[102,103] and has been suggested to lead to functionally different TMs in different vascular beds.[103,104]

The 23-residue hydrophobic region corresponding to the transmembrane domain is the most highly conserved domain of TM among species.[105] This finding suggests the region may have an important, specific function, although none has yet been detected. The cytoplasmic domain of 38 residues contains several potential phosphorylation sites, one of which is phosphorylated following cell stimulation with phorbol myristate acetate.[106] Its presence also is required for the antiproliferative activity of TM.[71] Whether this requirement is because of a direct affect or because protein lacking this domain is shed and the soluble protein itself is mitogenic is not known.

CONTROL OF TM EXPRESSION

The TM gene contains a cAMP-responsive element in its 3′ untranslated region[107] and a retinoic acid response element in its 5′ untranslated region.[108,109] Agents that increase cAMP levels intracellularly increase TM expression,[107,110,111] as do retinoids. In addition, these same effectors, interleukin (IL)-4,[112] and vascular endothelial growth factor (VEGF)[113] blunt, if not totally block, the effect of suppressors of TM expression.[109,114] Whether protein kinase C–controlled pathways are involved in TM regulation is not known.[111,115,116] The effects of active phorbol esters are biphasic.[111] Heat shock also leads to a biphasic response.[117] The TM gene contains several tandem heat shock elements in its 5′ untranslated region. Although TM antigen does not respond early to heat in human umbilical vein endothelial culture, the message decreases significantly for 6 hours before rising dramatically and then continuing for at least 48 hours. Increased surface activity can be observed after 18 hours of treatment. This finding is in marked contrast to the normal response of heat-responsive genes, in which the response occurs within 1 hour of stress. In addition, the TM response does not attenuate as does classic heat shock protein expression. This finding suggests multiple regulatory mechanisms are operative. Augmentation of TM synthesis may protect the vasculature from further thrombotic damage during an inflammatory response. In line with this concept, histamine,[118] an additional inflammatory mediator, reportedly enhances TM synthesis.

In general, inflammatory mediators tend to decrease TM function, thereby sensitizing at least the involved areas of injury to thrombosis. Mediators include endotoxin, IL-1, tumor necrosis factor (TNF)-α,[111] transforming growth factor (TGF)-β,[119] and viral infection.[120] At least one case of dramatic TM loss in severe meningococcemia has been reported.[121] However, the successful use of protein C in this disease argues that complete loss of TM most likely is the exception.[122] Hypoxia also leads to decreased TM expression,[123] apparently through the cAMP-responsive element.[124] Because hypoxia also increases VEGF production, which reportedly induces TM expression,[123] predicting which pathway would dominate in any specific microenvironment *in vivo* is difficult.

TM expression is dramatically reduced over the surface of coronary atherosclerotic plaque,[125] which is expected to increase the thrombotic and proinflammatory balance in the area. Atherogenic stimuli, such as oxidized low-density lipoprotein (LDL),[126,127] transcriptionally down-regulate TM in endothelial cells. Homocysteine, another atherogenic stimulus, has multiple effects on endothelial TM expression at the nucleic acid and protein levels (reviewed by Lentz[128]) that overall appear to down-regulate TM function.

Although TM expression usually is limited to vascular endothelial cells, TM has been observed histochemically on vascular smooth muscle cells and monocytes within the vessel wall of atherosclerotic lesions.[129] Expression on smooth muscle cells may contribute to vessel passivation after injury. In injuries in which the endothelial layer is removed, as in rupture of an atheroma, the underlying smooth muscle cells can act as a site for focal clot formation. However, within a relatively short period, the cells undergo passivation, that is, they no longer support platelet adhesion or fibrin formation.[130] Induction of TM expression on the smooth muscle cells may contribute to this phenomenon[130-132] until the wound is reendothelialized.

TM is mitogenic for fibroblast and smooth muscle cells in culture.[129,133] However, cellular TM likely does not normally serve this function *in vivo*. In a rabbit model of injury, local overexpression of TM resulted in *reduced* neointima proliferation, leukocyte infiltration, and thrombosis.[134,135] How much of this protection results from thrombin binding and the concomitant local generation of APC and decreased signaling by thrombin through receptors[60] or from the direct antiproliferation and antiadhesion properties of the TM so expressed is not known.[70-72] Statins, at least in tissue culture, can up-regulate TM expression,[136,137] which may contribute to the beneficial effect of these drugs beyond their lipid-lowering properties.

TM is dramatically down-regulated in a rabbit model of a vein to artery graft, which mimics the common clinical situation.[138] Suppression of TM expression, and the resulting decrease in protein C activation, is prolonged and stays incomplete for more than 1 month, significantly impairing vein graft thromboresistance. Although an inflammatory reaction occurs in such grafts, the primary stimulus for TM loss is exposure of the vein segments to changes in wall tension as a result of arterial pressure.[139] TM on endothelial cells in culture is known to be down-regulated by sheer stress in the range of 15 dynes/cm^2.[140] Thromboresistance could be restored by overexpressing TM using an adenovirus system.[134,135] Unlike the arterial model, overexpression did not affect neointimal development in the vein graft model, possibly indicating different control pathways in arterial versus venous endothelium.

Another mechanism by which TM expression can be attenuated is through endothelial cell interaction with activated leukocytes, such as those present during inflammation. TM is sensitive to proteolytic release products,[141,142] and neutrophil elastase is the enzyme most commonly implicated in this process. In Wegener granulomatosis, wherein leukocyte infiltration occurs extensively, soluble TM levels increase significantly. In at least one patient who died of the disease, TM was essentially absent from the lung lesions.[143] TNF treatment increases TM release from endothelial cells by neutrophil elastase.[144-146] Because of TM proteolysis in response to inflammation or endothelial injury, TM measurements in plasma are believed to reflect endothelial injury in various disease states.[147,148] Leukocytes also may modulate TM activity by oxidation of the critical methionine.[92,141]

The major basic protein from the granules of eosinophils can interact with TM to inhibit its protein C activation potential.[149] The cationic protein released from platelet granules, platelet factor 4, seems to have opposite effects on TM. Platelet factor 4 can both inhibit the direct anticoagulant functions of TM[150] and enhance protein C activation *in vitro* and *in vivo*.[98,151]

ENDOTHELIAL PROTEIN C RECEPTOR

STRUCTURE OF EPCR

EPCR is a 220-amino-acid, type 1 transmembrane protein.[152-154] EPCR has two extracellular domains that show structural homology with the α- and β-domains of major histocompatibility complex (MHC) class 1 molecules, most notably the CD1d family. These proteins contain two α-helices that sit upon an eight-stranded β-sheet platform. Because three Cys residues are present in the extracellular domain, the possibility of cross-linking with another protein exists. An x-ray crystal structure of a soluble form of EPCR (sEPCR) in complex with the Gla domain of protein C has been described, confirming the structure deduced from the amino acid sequence (Fig. 108-5).[152,155] What could not be predicted from the DNA sequence is the presence of a phospholipid molecule in the groove that would be the "antigen-presenting" groove in the MHC proteins. The major phospholipid found in the crystal was phosphatidylcholine. The crystal was made from a form released from the cell upon synthesis. In the case of the CD1 family, apparently the groove can be "reloaded" with lipids during internalization/recycling.[156] Whether a similar process occurs with natural EPCR is not known. Earlier protein C and antibody binding experiments[157] confirmed that rather than binding to the "groove," the calcium-stabilized conformer of the Gla domain of protein C/APC[58,152] interacts with the distal end of the α-helices and does not interact with the phospholipid. The transmembrane domain contains two Gly-Gly sequences that are not commonly found in this region of membrane proteins. The cytoplasmic domain of human EPCR is only three amino acids long (Arg-Arg-Cys). The terminal Cys can be acylated with palmitate and may have functional consequences.[158]

Protein C and APC bind to EPCR with similar affinity, approximately 30 nM.[152] Binding requires the presence of calcium and is strengthened by the presence of magnesium ions. In addition, sEPCR normally found in plasma[159] is capable of binding both protein C and APC with equivalent affinity (see next section).

FUNCTION OF EPCR

EPCR augments protein C activation via the thrombin–TM complex, primarily by decreasing the K_m for protein C.[54,160] This finding has been confirmed *in vivo*.[161] The enhanced activation observed on cells can be recapitulated by incorporation of the two receptors (TM and EPCR) into phosphatidylcholine vesicles, indicating additional cellular proteins or architecture is not required.[102] Because sEPCR binds the ligands with the same affinity as the cellular form, sEPCR can compete with the cellular protein, thereby inhibiting protein C activation.[58] The APC–EPCR complex can still be inhibited by its protein inhibitors PCI and α1-antitrypsin.[162]

APC bound to EPCR undergoes a switch in function from an anticoagulant to an antiinflammatory molecule that is protective against septic shock.[55,163-165] EPCR may make a significant contribution by enhancing protein C activation.[161] APC can alter the gene expression profile of endothelial cells in culture.[166] APC bound to EPCR can activate the PARs, particularly PAR-1, resulting in altered gene function.[167] The expression profile observed is compatible with APC's antiapoptotic activity[166] and similar activity observed in stroke models.[168,169] However, reconciling how APC induces an antiinflammatory response through this receptor is difficult because thrombin induces proinflammatory responses via the same receptor.[170] Whether interactions with other molecules or specific temporal/spatial elements can explain the apparent discrepancy remains to be determined. EPCR also can constitutively translocate into the nucleus[171] and mediate APC but not protein C translocation to the nucleus, which is another possible method by which APC exerts its antiinflammatory activity.

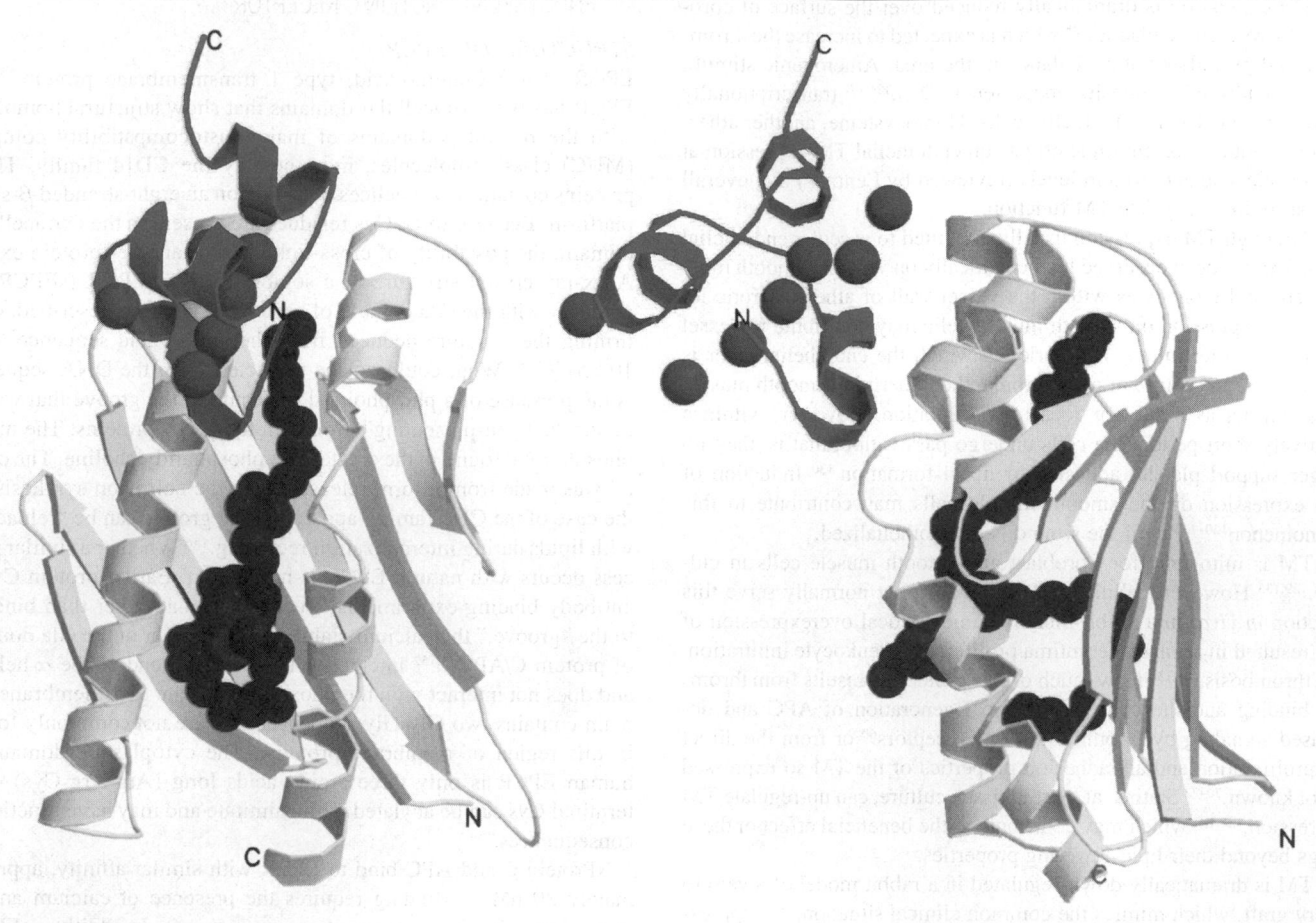

FIGURE 108-5   Ribbon models of two views of the x-ray crystal structure of the (EPCR)–protein C Gla domain complex. EPCR *(in gray)* is shown complexed to the Gla domain of protein C *(blue ribbon)*. A phospholipid molecule *(black spheres)* is bound in the central groove. *Dark blue spheres* represent Ca^{2+} ions bound to the Gla domain of protein C visible in the crystal structure. (Modified figure reprinted with permission from *J Biol Chem* 277:24851 2002; copyright the American Society of Biochemistry and Molecular Biology, Inc., 2002.)

sEPCR can bind to activated neutrophils[172] through PR3, a proteinase that is also the autoantigen of Wegener granulomatosis. Presumably, APC bound to EPCR can exert an effect on neutrophils. Preliminary studies suggest sEPCR binding to these cells blocks tight binding to endothelial cells.

Deletion of the EPCR gene by homologous recombination leads to early embryonic lethality at approximately day 9.5.[173] At this time, EPCR is highly expressed in the giant trophoblasts of the placenta but is not yet apparent by immunologic staining of the developing embryo in normal animals.[76] In contrast to TM knockout animals,[79] the placentas of EPCR knockout embryos show significant fibrin deposition at the fetal–maternal interface. Anticoagulation extends the viability of a subset of knockout embryos significantly to at least day 15, although no live births occur. Expression of less than 10 percent normal EPCR leads to the birth of viable animals.[174]

CONTROL OF EPCR EXPRESSION

Control of EPCR expression is complex. The gene structures for human and murine EPCR have been reported.[175,176] A thrombin response element and Sp1 site are conserved between the two species, although the human gene has multiple Sp1 sites. EPCR is expressed mainly on the large vessels, with decreasing immunostaining as smaller and smaller vessels are traversed,[177] except for the liver sinusoids and focal regions of the spleen. EPCR reportedly is expressed on microvascular

endothelium.[178] Some expression on the smaller vessels may be consistent with the observation of the major effect of blocking protein C binding to EPCR upon activation *in vivo*,[161] presumed to occur mainly within the microcirculation.

Inflammatory mediators have an interesting effect on EPCR expression. When endotoxin is administered to rats, EPCR mRNA increases rapidly.[179] The increase can be blocked by coinfusion of hirudin, indicating the rise most likely results from stimulation through the thrombin response element. Paradoxically, in both tissue culture and the rat model, although EPCR message was increased in response to thrombin, cellular EPCR protein was not. Instead, sEPCR produced by the action of a metalloproteinase[180] could be recovered from the cell supernatants or animal plasma. Significant sEPCR levels have been found in humans, and the concentration appears to be increased in certain disease states.[159] High sEPCR levels in some individuals may reflect a hypercoagulable state,[181] possibly resulting from the ability of sEPCR to inhibit cell surface activation of protein C. A haplotype associated with elevated sEPCR levels and an increased risk of thrombosis has been reported.[182]

EPCR and TM sometimes, but not always, are coordinately controlled in disease states. In the report of TM down-regulation in meningococcemia, EPCR also was missing on these vessels.[121] Loss of EPCR over atherosclerotic plaques also was seen.[125] Changes in EPCR expression were not observed in the rabbit vein graft model.[138] Similarly, although TM was down-regulated in a rat model of diabetes,

EPCR was not.[183] Induction of metalloprotease release of sEPCR was not reported in these studies.

ENDOTHELIAL CELL FIBRINOLYTIC SYSTEM

Plasmin, the major clot-dissolving protease, is formed upon cleavage of a single peptide bond within the zymogen plasminogen. Impairment of fibrinolytic assembly systems may play a central role in the etiology of occlusive vascular disease (see Chap. 127). The tightly regulated reaction is strongly influenced by cells of the blood vessel wall, including endothelial cells, smooth muscles cells, and macrophages, which express plasminogen activators, plasminogen activator inhibitors (PAIs), and fibrinolytic receptors. This section describes the interplay between the cells of the vascular wall and the fibrinolytic system in the maintenance of blood vessel patency and how vascular cells use the fibrinolytic system to execute the remodeling response to blood vessel injury.

ENDOTHELIAL CELL PRODUCTION OF FIBRINOLYTIC PROTEINS

Plasmin generation is a property of blood vessels. In 1958, Todd[184] demonstrated that fibrinolytic activity in human tissues is focally distributed, related consistently to blood vessels, especially veins, venous sinusoids, and, to a lesser extent, arteries. The activity was localized primarily to the wall of the blood vessel,[185] although plasminogen activator activity may be associated with certain individual extravascular cells.[186]

TISSUE PLASMINOGEN ACTIVATOR
Although endothelial cells cultured from multiple sources (umbilical vein, umbilical artery, pulmonary artery, vena cava) synthesize tissue plasminogen activator (t-PA) and the endothelium appears to be the principal source of t-PA in blood,[187] t-PA expression *in vivo* appears to be highly restricted to smaller vessels in specific anatomic locations. This pattern of expression likely reflects the heterogeneity of endothelial cells as they respond to a myriad of cues specific to a given tissue.[188] In the baboon, for example, neither t-PA antigen nor t-PA mRNA was detected in femoral artery or vein, carotid artery, or aorta, whereas both mRNA and protein were readily apparent in precapillary arterioles, postcapillary venules, and the vasa vasora ranging in diameter from 7 to 30 μm.[189] Similarly in the mouse lung, bronchial blood vessels displayed endothelial cell-associated t-PA antigen, whereas pulmonary blood vessels were uniformly negative.[190] t-PA expression at branch points of pulmonary blood vessels may reflect stimulation by laminar shear stress.[191]

Although *in vitro* studies suggest t-PA expression in cultured endothelial cells is regulated by a wide array of factors, only a few of these factors have been confirmed *in vivo*. Thrombin,[192] histamine,[193,194] oxygen radicals,[195] phorbol myristate acetate,[196] (1-deamino, 8-D-arginine) vasopressin (DDAVP),[197] and butyric acid liberated from dibutyryl cAMP[198] all increase t-PA mRNA in cultured endothelial cells. Thrombin and histamine appear to act via receptor-mediated activation of the protein kinase C pathway.[187] Laminar shear stress stimulates t-PA secretion[199] and steady-state mRNA levels.[200] Hyperosmotic stress and repetitive stretch also enhance t-PA expression.[201,202] In addition, differentiating agents, such as retinoids[203,204] and butyrate,[198] stimulate transcription of t-PA in endothelial cells *in vitro*.

In vivo, the circulating half-life of t-PA is approximately 5 minutes. Infusion of DDAVP, bradykinin, platelet-activating factor (PAF), ET, or thrombin is associated with acute release of t-PA, and a burst of fibrinolytic activity can be detected within minutes.[187] In the mouse lung, exposure to hyperoxia leads to 4.5-fold up-regulation of t-PA

mRNA in small-vessel endothelial cells.[190] TNF infusion into patients with malignancy is associated with increased t-PA,[205] whereas treatment of cultured endothelial cells with TNF either has no effect or decreases t-PA production.[206] Deficient release of t-PA in response to venous occlusion in humans has been associated with deep venous thrombotic vascular disease,[207] *atrophie blanche*, and other cutaneous vasculitides.[208]

UROKINASE PLASMINOGEN ACTIVATOR
In vivo, urokinase plasminogen activator (u-PA) is not a product of resting endothelium[209] but is produced primarily by renal tubular epithelium.[210] However, expression of u-PA mRNA in endothelium is strongly stimulated during wound repair and physiologic angiogenesis within ovarian follicles, corpus luteum, and maternal decidua.[211] Endothelial cells passaged in culture synthesize u-PA,[212] and expression of u-PA mRNA is stimulated by TNF by 5- to 30-fold.[213] Small increases in u-PA have been observed *in vitro* in response to IL-1 and lipopolysaccharide.[214–216]

The association of u-PA with the blood vessel wall appears to reflect its association with the u-PA receptor u-PAR. In the adult mouse, u-PAR mRNA is not normally detected by *in situ* hybridization in the endothelium of either large or small blood vessels.[217] However, upon stimulation with endotoxin, expression is detected in endothelium lining aorta, arteries, veins, and capillaries of a variety of organs, including heart, kidney, brain, and liver,[217] whereas the same stimulus leads to a dramatic decrease in expression in the renal tubules.[210] u-PAR may fulfill a variety of nonproteolytic functions ranging from directed cell migration to cellular adhesion, differentiation, and proliferation.[218]

PLASMINOGEN ACTIVATOR INHIBITOR-1

PAI-1 likely functions as a major regulator of plasmin generation in the vicinity of the endothelial cell. *In vitro*, PAI-1 appears to be associated mainly with the substratum of cultured human umbilical vein endothelial cells rather than the external face of the plasma membrane.[219,220] Thrombin, IL-1, TGF-β, TNF-α, and endotoxin all induce dramatic increases in steady-state PAI-1 message levels.[192,214,215,221] In addition, the LDL-like particle lipoprotein(a) [Lp(a)], which contains an apoprotein homologous to plasminogen, induces a two- to four-fold increase in PAI-1 mRNA without affecting mRNA for t-PA.[222] Heparin-binding growth factor-1 (endothelial cell growth factor) is a down-regulator of PAI-1 mRNA production by cultured endothelial cells. This agent has no effect on t-PA.[223] These studies suggest that *in vitro* synthesis and secretion of PAI-1 by endothelial cells are regulated independently of t-PA.

Elevated levels of circulating PAI-1 have been linked epidemiologically to risk for myocardial infarction.[207] Although quiescent endothelial cells express little or no PAI-1 *in vivo*, with the liver as the major source of plasma PAI-1, endothelial expression of PAI-1 is detected near neovascular sprouts that also express u-PA during decidual neovascularization in the ovary.[211] In addition, inflammatory cytokines are powerful stimuli for PAI-1 induction in a variety of tissues including liver. In rats and humans with active malignancy, TNF injection results in strikingly increased plasma PAI-1 concentrations.[187,205]

ANNEXIN 2

In contrast to the endothelial cell coreceptor for t-PA and plasminogen, annexin 2 appears to be expressed constitutively *in vivo* in association with blood vessels in a wide variety of tissues. In the adult chicken, endothelial cells of vessels in the dermis, lung, renal glomeruli, pancreas, liver, and meninges stain intensely positive by immunohistology.[224] Blood vessels of the developing mouse brain are strongly cross-

TABLE 108-3   FIBRINOLYTIC SYSTEM IN CARDIOVASCULAR DISEASE:
TRANSGENIC MOUSE MODELS

GENOTYPE	RESULT	REFERENCE
Atherogenesis		
PLG-/-ApoE-/-	Increased atherogenesis	252
t-PA-/-ApoE-/-	Unchanged atherogenesis	253
u-PA-/-ApoE-/-	Unchanged atherogenesis	253
PAI-1-/-ApoE-/-	Decrease in early plaque size; increase in advanced plaque size	254,255–256
Transplant Arteriosclerosis		
PLG-/-	Reduced leukocyte invasion in transplant model;	258
	Reduced extent of disease	
Coronary Ligation		
u-PA-/-	Protection from ventricular rupture, but poor revascularization and late death from heart failure	259
t-PA-/-	No protection	259
u-PAR -/-	No protection	259
Aortic Aneurysm		
u-PA-/-ApoE-/-	Protected	253
t-PA-/-ApoE-/-	Not protected	253
Early Oxidative Injury		
PAI-1 -/-	Attenuated thrombotic occlusion (rose bengal)	267
PAI-1 -/-	Attenuated thrombotic occlusion (FeCl₃)	268
u-PA -/-	Increased thrombosis (FeCl₃)	269
t-PA -/-	Increased thrombosis (FeCl₃)	269
Restenosis with Prominent Thrombosis		
PAI-1 -/-	No neointima (Cu cuff)	272
PAI-1 -/-	Reduced neointima (ligation)	371
	Reduced neointima (FeCl₃)	371
PAI-1 -/- ApoE-/-	Reduced neointima (FeCl₃)	271
Restenosis without Prominent Thrombosis		
PLG-/-	Reduced neointima (electrical)	260,261
t-PA-/-	No change (electrical or mechanical)	260,262
u-PA-/-	Reduced neointima (electrical or mechanical)	260,262
u-PA-/- t-PA-/-	Reduced neointima (electrical or mechanical)	260,262
u-PAR-/-	No change (electrical)	263
PAI-1-/-	Increased neointima (ligation)	372
PAI-1-/-	Increased neointima (electrical or mechanical)	264

PLG, plasminogen.

reactive.[225] In rats[226] and humans,[227] vascular endothelial cells are positive for annexin 2 in most tissues studied to date. The evidence that annexin 2 plays a role in maintaining vascular patency includes the following findings: (1) Individuals with acute promyelocytic leukemia that overexpress annexin 2 usually present with a hemorrhagic disorder.[228] (2) Systemic injection of annexin 2 can diminish thrombotic vascular occlusion following vascular injury.[229] (3) Annexin 2–deficient mice display fibrin deposition on microvessels and impaired clearance of arterial thrombi following vascular injury.[230] Expression of annexin 2 in neuronal-like PC12 cells is transcriptionally up-regulated upon stimulation with nerve growth factor, suggesting the potential for regulation by receptor tyrosine kinases.[231] In addition, the in vitro transition of human monocyte to macrophage is associated with a several-fold increase in annexin 2 protein and steady-state mRNA expression and an even more dramatic (8- to 10-fold) increase in cell surface expression.[232] These data suggest that annexin 2 is sub-ject to regulation in a variety of cell types found within and outside of the vasculature.

NONFIBRINOLYTIC FUNCTIONS OF PLASMIN

PLASMIN AND ANTICOAGULANT FUNCTION

Plasmin inactivates bovine factor Va in vitro by cleaving the heavy and light chains of this M_r 168,000 protein.[233] This lipid-dependent inactivation results in a series of plasmin-specific cleavages that are distinct from those produced by APC.[234] Inactivation of human factor V by plasmin may be preceded by transient generation of procoagulant fragments that subsequently are degraded to an inactive form.[235] Plasmin also can inactivate factor VIIIa, another coagulant cofactor that is structurally homologous to factor Va.[236] Finally, factor X is subject to a well-defined pattern of cleavage events, some of the products of which may stimulate t-PA–dependent plasminogen activation.[237]

PLASMIN AND PLATELET FUNCTION

The effects of plasmin on in vitro platelet function are complex. Platelet glycoprotein IIb/IIIa complex (GPIIb-IIIa) and glycoprotein Ib (GPIb), the cell surface receptors for fibrinogen and vWF, respectively, are plasmin substrates.[238,239] Thus, plasmin formation in the vicinity of a hemostatic plug could lead to impaired adhesion and poor aggregation in response to agonists. Plasmin generation is associated with platelet activation[240,241] and platelet inhibition[242] or disaggregation.[243] The ultimate effect of plasmin appears to depend upon the incubation conditions, particularly the dose and duration of plasmin treatment. These findings are of potential significance given reports that plasminogen can interact with platelets in a manner that is enhanced upon thrombin-mediated conversion of platelet fibrinogen to fibrin.[244] In vivo, prolonged bleeding times were found in patients 90 minutes after t-PA infusion for thrombolysis, suggesting early impairment of platelet function upon plasmin generation.[245] However, evidence also suggests platelets play a role in thrombotic reocclusion following successful thrombolytic therapy.[246]

FIBRINOLYTIC FUNCTION IN VASCULAR INJURY

A number of transgenic mouse models of vascular disease have begun to elucidate the complex role of the fibrinolytic system in atherosclerotic vascular disease (Table 108-3). In mice, the general effects of plasminogen deficiency include runting, fibrin deposition in intravascular and extravascular locations, and premature death.[247,248] In addition, the mice display impaired healing of cutaneous wounds,[249] a response that appears to depend largely on the fibrinolytic action of plasmin given that loss of fibrinogen eliminates the defects.[250] Migration of monocytes to sites of inflammation is also reduced.[251] Based on these results, impaired plaque formation might be expected in atherosclerosis-prone mice with plasminogen deficiency (Fig. 108-6). However, mice doubly deficient in plasminogen and apolipoprotein E (ApoE) showed an increased predisposition to atherosclerosis compared to animals deficient in ApoE alone.[252] Mice with ApoE deficiency combined with deficiency of either u-PA or t-PA showed the same predilection for early fatty streak and advanced plaque formation as was observed in mice with isolated ApoE deficiency, suggesting that complete elimination of plasmin-generating activity is required to exacerbate the proatherogenic state.[253] Finally, mice doubly deficient in Apo E and PAI-1 exhibited no change in early plaque size at the aortic root[254,255] and decreased early plaque size at the carotid bifurcation,[254,255] but increased advanced plaque size with accelerated deposition of matrix.[256] Thus, rather than promoting cellular invasion during initial plaque formation, plasmin may fulfill the more important role of degrading fibrin and other matrix-deposited constituents once

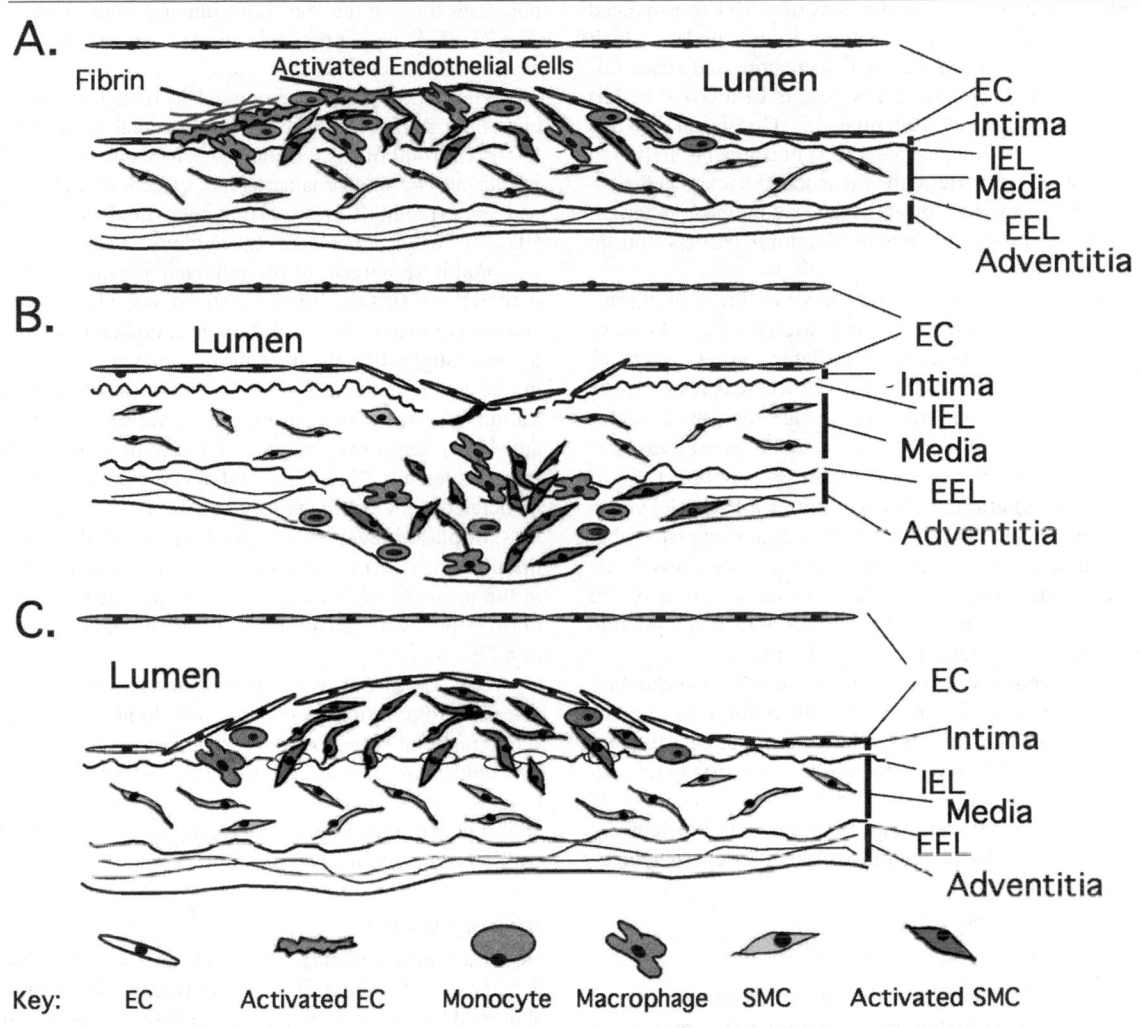

FIGURE 108-6   Schematic representation of the suggested role of the fibrinolytic system in vascular disease. *(A)* Plaque formation. Atheromatous plaque is thought to form in response to endothelial cell injury or perturbation. Following the initial injury,
perturbed endothelial cells may fail to clear fibrin on the blood vessel surface and may promote adhesion and invasion of leukocytes.
In addition, smooth muscle cells arising in the tunica media invade the developing plaque within the intima. Endothelial cells may
utilize cell surface receptors for focal activation of plasmin to maintain a thromboresistant vascular surface. Leukocytes, macrophages, and smooth muscle cells may use plasmin to migrate into the evolving plaque. *(B)* Aneurysm. Fragmentation and dissolution
of the elastic laminae of the arterial wall may occur upon matrix metalloproteinase activation via plasmin-dependent pathways,
possibly mediated by smooth muscle cells. Cells migrating outward toward the adventitial surface of the vessel induce further
matrix degradation and the potential for rupture. *(C)* Restenosis. In response to vascular injury, smooth muscle cells proliferate
and, with leukocytes, invade the subendothelial space establishing a thickened neointima that compromises vascular patency. In
all three scenarios, cell migration is thought to require plasmin activity, possibly in association with cell surfaces. EC, endothelial
cells; EEL, external elastic lamina, IEL, internal elastic lamina.

the lesion is initiated. Clearly, more studies are needed to clarify these
issues.

Plasmin may affect progression of the atherosclerotic plaque by
mediating invasion of leukocytes.[257] In the peritoneal cavity, recruitment of inflammatory cells is profoundly influenced by the presence
or absence of plasminogen.[251] In transplant-associated arteriosclerosis,
the extent of disease is significantly reduced in plasminogen-deficient
mice, reflecting, at least in part, reduced influx of macrophages, with
diminished medial necrosis, fragmentation of elastic laminae, and remodeling of the adventitia.[258]

During aneurysm formation, the fibrinolytic system assumes a central role (see Fig. 108-6). In a model of aortic aneurysm, u-PA but not
t-PA deficiency was associated with reduced medial destruction and
reduced activation of downstream plasmin-dependent matrix metal-

loproteinases.[253] Similarly, u-PA− but not t-PA−deficient mice were
protected from cardiac rupture secondary to ventricular aneurysm. In
this study, temporary administration of PAI-1 or tissue inhibitor of
metalloproteinase (TIMP)-1, the general matrix metalloproteinase inhibitor, completely protected wild-type mice from aortic rupture.[259]

Vascular remodeling may occur following acute arterial injury induced by interventions for vascular compromise and can lead to a
secondary phase of vascular compromise known as restenosis (see Fig.
108-6). Restenosis reflects leukocyte invasion, proliferation and migration of smooth muscle cells, deposition of extracellular matrix, and
reendothelialization, and it may require plasmin activity at several
stages. Electrical or mechanical injury studies in gene-targeted mice
indicate neointima formation requires intact expression of plasminogen and u-PA, but not t-PA.[260–262] Interestingly, loss of u-PAR has no

effect on neointima formation,[263] whereas loss of PAI-1 is associated with increased neointimal stenosis.[264] In these injury models, which do not induce severe thrombosis, vascular occlusion, and hence migration of smooth muscle cells and leukocytes, is believed to be impaired when fibrinolytic potential is attenuated.[265] Consistent with this hypothesis is the observation that stenosis in vein segments grafted to the arterial circulation did not require the presence of background plasminogen, suggesting that plasmin proteolysis may be most important in neointima formation in settings where structural barriers impede cellular invasion.[266]

In the ferric chloride, rose bengal, and copper cuff models, thrombosis is observed within minutes following arterial injury. In these systems, PAI-1 deficiency is associated with later and less extensive thrombotic occlusion of the injured artery,[267,268] whereas loss of u-PA is associated with more rapid and more significant thrombotic occlusion.[269] At the same time, the absence of PAI-1 led to reduced vascular stenosis, regardless of whether ApoE was absent[270,271] or present.[272] In balloon-injured rat carotid arteries, transduction of a PAI-1–expressing gene led to increased restenosis of the vessel, again suggesting that clearance of the initial thrombus has long-term effects on vessel patency and neointima formation.[273] In these models, the effect of the fibrinolytic system in clearing the initial thrombus, which may provide an initial scaffolding for later restenosis, predominates.

The fibrinolytic system may play an important role in modulating growth factor activity. Circulating levels of TGF-β are reduced in individuals with atherosclerosis, possibly reflecting impaired activation by plasmin.[274] In vitro, u-PA–mediated plasmin activity appears to generate active TGF-β, which is antiapoptotic for smooth muscle cells.[275] The in vitro mitogenic and chemotactic effects of basic fibroblast growth factor and platelet-derived growth factor depend upon u-PA and t-PA, respectively.[276]

FIBRINOLYTIC ASSEMBLY AND VASCULAR DISEASE

Both plasminogen and plasminogen activators can assemble on cell surface receptors in a manner that enhances the potential for plasmin activation (see Chap. 127). The major endothelial cell fibrinolytic receptors are u-PAR and annexin 2 (Fig. 108-7). Both receptors have significant roles in vascular homeostasis in gene-targeted mice.

LIPOPROTEIN(A)

Lp(a) is an LDL-like particle that is an independent risk factor for atherosclerosis.[277–280] Lp(a) contains apolipoprotein B-100 and a disulfide-linked moiety called apolipoprotein(a) [apo(a)]. Apo(a) shares a remarkable degree of homology with plasminogen,[281] including multiple tandem repeats of domains similar to kringle 4, a single region resembling kringle 5, and a pseudoprotease segment.[282] Plasminogen and apo(a) are genetically linked on chromosome 6 and may have arisen from a common ancestral gene.[283]

Whereas Lp(a) levels are only transiently responsive to diet,[284,285] plasma levels appear to be subject to mendelian inheritance.[286–288] Plasma Lp(a) concentrations seem to correlate inversely with the ratio of kringle 4 to kringle 5 encoding domains within the apo(a) gene,[289,290] such that larger apo(a) gene products are associated with lower plasma concentrations of apo(a). In addition, Lp(a) appears to represent an acute phase reactant in the postsurgical and postmyocardial infarction setting[287] and in patients with cancer,[288] suggesting a role for soluble inflammatory mediators in regulating Lp(a) synthesis or assembly. Apo(a) possesses a high-affinity lysine binding site within kringle 4 that closely resembles kringle 1 of plasminogen with its lysine-binding amino acid tetrad consisting of anionic Asp55 and Asp57 plus cationic Arg34 and Arg71.[291] Kringle 37 of the originally cloned apo(a) resembles plasminogen kringle 4 of plasminogen, which

possesses three of the four lysine binding amino acids (Asp55, Asp57, Arg-71).[292] In vivo, Lp(a) colocalizes histologically with fibrin in atheromatous tissue.[293]

When apo(a) is overexpressed in transgenic mice,[294] cell-associated plasmin activity is reduced such that the animals are resistant to t-PA thrombolysis.[295] Three mechanisms potentially explain the prothrombotic and proatherogenic effects of Lp(a). (1) Both Lp(a) and apo(a) inhibit Lys–plasminogen binding to endothelial cells (ID_{50} = 36-fold excess).[296] Lp(a) binds to annexin 2 in vitro[297] and can inhibit 95 percent of plasminogen activation by t-PA at the endothelial cell surface. The estimated dissociation constants for apo(a) and plasminogen with respect to the endothelial cell surface are comparable, suggesting that receptor occupancy in vivo is largely determined by the ambient level of Lp(a), because plasminogen concentrations do not appear to change significantly.[298–300] Furthermore, anti-Lp(a) cross-reactive material can be detected within atherosclerotic lesions.[297] (2) Endothelial cell exposure to Lp(a) in vitro is associated with enhanced levels of PAI-1 that were not found with LDL or plasminogen[222] but have been reported for very-low-density lipoprotein.[301] (3) Lp(a) may act as a competitive inhibitor of t-PA in the presence of fibrinogen[302] or as an uncompetitive inhibitor of fibrin-dependent enhancement of t-PA–induced plasmin generation.[303]

When Lp(a) was overexpressed in mice receiving a high-fat diet, atherosclerotic lesions containing both lipid and anti-apo(a) cross-reactive material were observed.[304] Deposition of both lipid and apo(a) was reduced in mice expressing apo(a) in which lysine binding sites had been mutated.[305] These data indicate that lysine binding sites of apo(a) play a role in its atherogenicity in vivo, possibly by competing with plasminogen for cell surface receptors.

HOMOCYSTEINE

HC is a thiol-containing amino acid that accumulates in nutritional deficiencies of vitamin B_6, vitamin B_{12}, or folic acid, or in inherited abnormalities of cystathionine β-synthase, methylene tetrahydrofolate reductase, or methionine synthase.[306] A meta-analysis of 27 studies including approximately 4000 patients showed HC was an independent risk factor for atherosclerosis of coronary, cerebral, and peripheral arteries.[307] Of ten subsequent prospective studies, eight demonstrate an increased risk of coronary heart disease, venous thromboembolism, cardiovascular complications, and death.[308] In vitro, HC-treated endothelial cells bind approximately 50 percent less t-PA than untreated cells and activated approximately 50 percent less plasminogen.[309] Mass spectrometry studies indicate that HC directly disables the t-PA binding domain of annexin 2 by forming a covalent adduction product with cysteine 9 within the tail domain of purified annexin 2.[310] HC further inhibits the ability of annexin 2 to bind t-PA with half-maximal effect observed at approximately 11 μM, a value close to the upper limit of normal for HC in plasma (14 μM). Thus, inhibition of t-PA–annexin 2 assembly on the endothelial cell may contribute to the prothrombotic, proatherogenic effect of HC.

ROLE OF ADHESION MOLECULES

A proinflammatory environment also is prothrombotic. Endothelial cells express molecules that regulate binding of leukocytes to their surface during inflammation. These interactions have both direct and indirect roles in hemostasis and thrombosis, as many of the cytokines and bioactive molecules that promote the inflammatory response also trigger the former. Moreover, the inflammatory response itself results in expression of adhesion molecules and mediators that secondarily promote hemostasis.

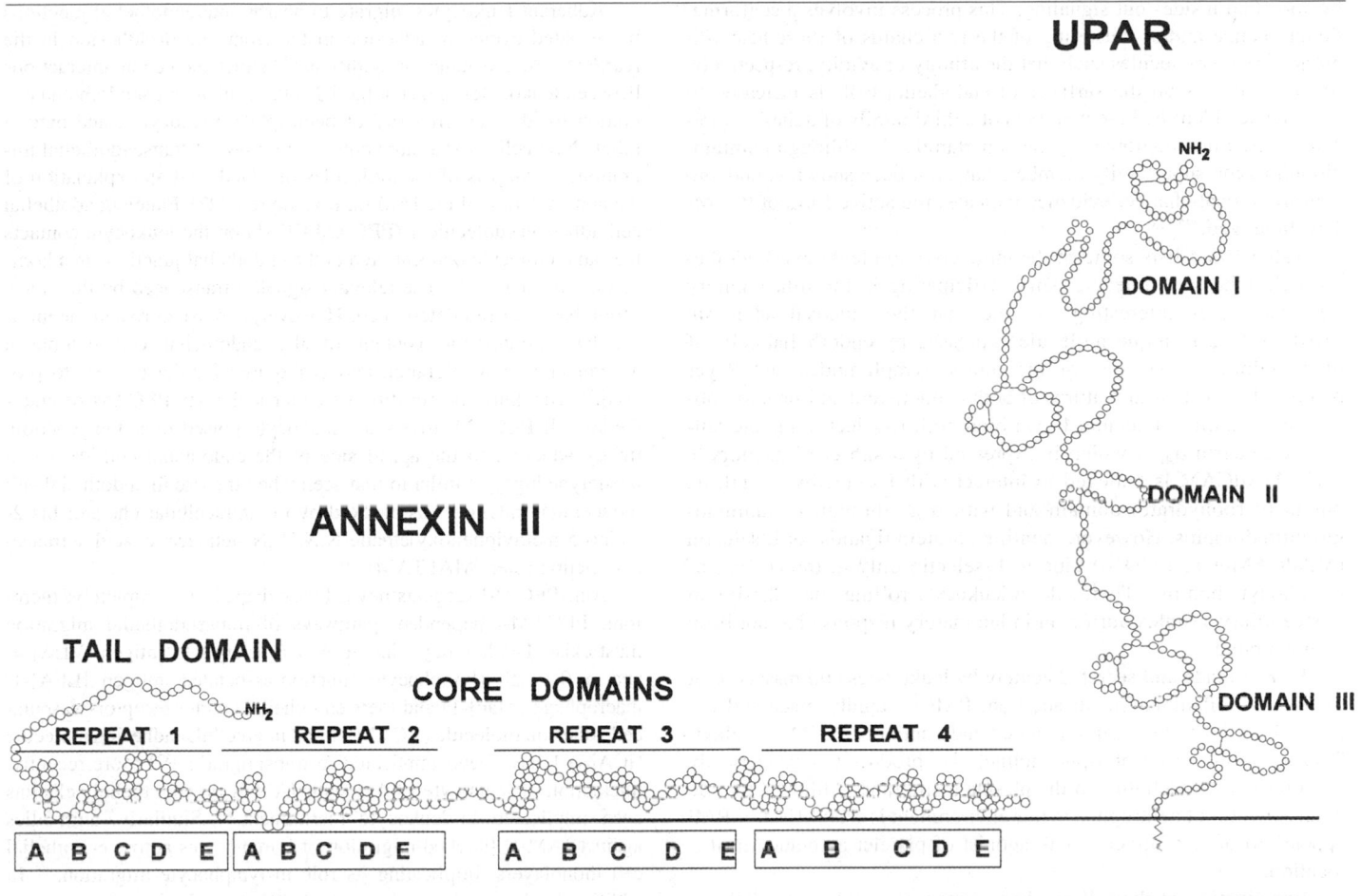

FIGURE 108-7   Two-dimensional representation of the structure of endothelial cell fibrinolytic receptors. Annexin 2 consists of a hydrophilic amino terminal tail domain (approximately 3 kDa) and a membrane-oriented carboxyl terminal core domain (approximately 33 kDa).[376,377] The tail domain contains residues required for t-PA binding. The core domain is composed of four homologous annexin repeats, each consisting of five α-helical regions (A through E) that contribute to calcium-dependent phospholipid binding sites. Repeat 2 appears to be most important for interaction of annexin 2 with the endothelial cell surface. Plasminogen binding requires lysine residue 307 within helix C of repeat 4. u-PAR is a 55- to 60-kDa, glycosylphosphatidylinositol-linked protein that consists of three disulfide-linked domains.[378] Domain I contains sequences required for u-PA binding. Domains II and III appear to mediate the receptor's interaction with matrix proteins such as vitronectin.

MOLECULAR CHANGES IN AN INFLAMMATORY MILIEU

IMMEDIATE CHANGES

Histamine produced locally at the site of inflammation by degranulation of resident tissue mast cells stimulates the overlying endothelial cells to express P-selectin on their surfaces. This change occurs within minutes and results from rapid fusion of Weibel-Palade bodies, with the plasma membrane bringing P-selectin to the surface. Along with P-selectin expression, fusion of the Weibel-Palade bodies results in release of vWF into the local environment. In addition to thrombin's ability to induce release of platelet α-granules and expression of P-selectin on the surface of platelets, thrombin can trigger the release of P-selectin that is expressed on the endothelial cell surface at sites of inflammation.

P-selectin serves as a receptor for P-selectin glycoprotein ligand (PSGL)-1 and probably other unidentified ligands on leukocytes. PSGL-1 is a specific sialomucin containing sialylated, fucosylated O-linked oligosaccharides and an unusual sulfated tyrosine residue motif.[311] Dimerization of PSGL-1 may be required for optimal recognition of P-selectin.[312] Adhesive interactions between P-selectin and its ligands result in tethering of passing leukocytes to, and rolling on, the surface of the endothelial cell—the first step in leukocyte emigration. L-selectin, another member of the selectin family of adhesion molecules, is constitutively expressed on the surfaces of most leukocytes. It binds to sialylated, fucosylated GP ligands expressed by endothelial cells in response to inflammation and to CD34 constitutively expressed by cells of endothelial venules.

The low-affinity reversible adhesions of leukocytes to the endothelium at the site of inflammation result in leukocyte rolling along the luminal surface. This stage slows down the movement of leukocytes and brings them into contact with a variety of chemical mediators that trigger the next stage of leukocyte emigration—tight adhesion to the endothelial surface. These mediators include surface-bound chemokines,[313] additional adhesion molecules expressed by the endothelium in response to inflammatory cytokines,[314] platelet-activating factor (PAF),[315] soluble chemokines,[316] and ligands that cross-link leukocyte CD31.[317–319] The variety of chemical signals that can trigger tight adhesion is large (reviewed in ref. 320) and may vary according to the nature of the inflammatory stimulus, the tissue involved, and the chronology of the response. However, all the factors seem to work by stimulating the activation of leukocyte integrin adhesion molecules by so-called inside–out signaling. This process involves a conformational change and/or clustering of the two chains of these heterodimeric surface molecules such that the affinity or avidity, respectively, for their ligands on the surfaces of endothelial cells is increased.[321] Any ligands identified are members of a third family of adhesion molecules, the immunoglobulin gene superfamily.[320] Although immunoglobulin gene superfamily members have not been shown to undergo conformational change, evidence indicates the active form of ICAM-1 is dimerized.[322,323]

Table 108-4 lists some of the more common leukocyte/endothelial cell adhesion molecule pairs participating in the inflammatory response. It is interesting to note that the mucosal addressin MAdCAM-1, a unique molecule expressed by endothelial cells of high endothelial venules of mesenteric lymph nodes and Peyer patches, has structural features of both a mucin and an immunoglobulin superfamily molecule. It can bind both L-selectin and the leukocyte integrin $\alpha_4\beta_7$, which is expressed by a subset of memory T cells. MAdCAM is believed to interact with L-selectin through its mucin (carbohydrate) domain and with $\alpha_4\beta_7$ through its immunoglobulin domains. However, identified protein ligands for L-selectin (MAdCAM-1 and CD34) bind to L-selectin only in the context of lymphocyte homing. Their role in leukocyte rolling and adhesion in postcapillary venules during an inflammatory response has not been demonstrated.

PAF is made and secreted acutely by leukocytes and mast cells at the site of inflammation. In addition, PAF is rapidly made and expressed on the surfaces of stimulated endothelial cells. PAF (1-alkyl-2-acetyl-sn-glycero-3-phosphocholine) is produced enzymatically from phosphatidylcholine in the plasma membrane. Although its role as an activator of neutrophils in this environment is established,[315] PAF appears to be a relatively weak agonist of platelet activation in this location.

Examination of the rolling phenomenon *in vivo* by intravital microscopy shows that leukocytes may roll on other leukocytes that already are tightly adherent. These interactions, which are promoted through L-selectin and PSGL-1 on the leukocytes, amplify the inflammatory process.[324,325]

Adherent leukocytes migrate to nearby interendothelial junctions by repeated cycles of adhesion in the front and disadhesion in the rear.[320,326] At the junction, additional distinct molecular interactions between leukocytes and endothelial cells regulate transendothelial migration for the vast majority of neutrophils, monocytes, and natural killer (NK) cells (for a more complete review of transendothelial migration, a synopsis of the molecules involved, and an explanation of the nomenclature of the JAM family, see ref. 327). Platelet/endothelial cell adhesion molecule-1 (PECAM/CD31) on the leukocyte contacts the same molecule concentrated at the endothelial junctions in a homophilic manner.[328–330] The relevant signal(s) transduced by this interaction has not been determined. However, a transient rise in the intracellular calcium ion content of the endothelial cell cytoplasm accompanies transmigration and is required for the process to proceed.[331] Blocking the function of either leukocyte PECAM or endothelial cell PECAM arrests the leukocyte poised over the junction, tightly adherent to the apical side of the endothelial cell,[330,332,333] a phenotype highly similar to that seen when the rise in endothelial cell intracellular calcium was blocked by the intracellular chelator bis(2-amino-5-methylphenoxy)ethane-N,N,N′,N′-tetraacetic acid tetraacetoxymethyl ester (MAPTAM).[331]

Anti-PECAM reagents never block diapedesis completely; therefore, PECAM-independent pathways of transendothelial migration must exist. The leukocyte integrins $\alpha_4\beta_1$ (very late antigen [VLA]-4) and $\alpha_L\beta_2/\alpha_M\beta_2$ (lymphocyte function-associated antigen [LFA]-1/macrophage [Mac]-1) and their endothelial counterreceptors vascular cell adhesion molecule (VCAM)-1 and intercellular adhesion molecule (ICAM)-1 have been implicated in transmigration.[320] More recently, interaction of leukocyte LFA-1 with JAM-A on endothelial cells has been implicated in leukocyte recruitment.[334] Similarly, antibodies against JAM-C blocked migration of lymphocytes across endothelial cell monolayers, implicating its role in lymphocyte migration.[335] In addition, under certain specialized conditions, pathways across the endothelial cell appear to bypass the intercellular junction.[336]

CD99, a GP expressed on the surfaces of leukocytes, platelets, and erythrocytes and concentrated at the endothelial cell borders, controls a step in diapedesis distal to the step controlled by PECAM,[337] inter-

TABLE 108-4 COMMON LEUKOCYTE-ENDOTHELIAL CELL ADHESION MOLECULE PAIRS IN INFLAMMATION

LEUKOCYTE MOLECULE	CD AND INTEGRIN NOMENCLATURE	LEUKOCYTES EXPRESSING[a]	ACTION	ENDOTHELIAL COUNTER LIGAND	CD NUMBER
L-selectin	CD62L	PMN, Mo, T, B, NK	Tethering, rolling	MAdCAM-1[b]	Pending
				Gp105-120	CD34
PSGL-1	CD162	PMN, Mo, T, B, NK	Tethering, rolling	P-selectin	CD62P
Sialyl Lewis X, ESL-1, CLA[c]	CD15s	PMN, Mo, T, B, NK	Tethering, rolling	E-selectin	CD62E
LFA-1	CD11a/CD18 ($\alpha_L\beta_2$)	PMN, Mo, T, B, NK	Tight adhesion	ICAM-1	CD54
				ICAM-2	CD102
				ICAM-3	CD50
			Adhesion, diapedesis	JAM-A	Pending
MAC-1	CD11b/CD18	PMN, Mo, NK	Tight adhesion	ICAM-1	CD54
VLA-4	CD49d/CD29	Mo, B, Eo[d] > NK, T	Tight adhesion,[e] rolling	VCAM-1	CD106
PECAM-1	CD31	PMN, Mo, NK, subsets of T	Diapedesis	PECAM-1	CD31
CD99	CD99	All leukocytes to varying degrees	Diapedesis	CD99	CD99
JAM-C?	Pending	T	Diapedesis	JAM-C?	Pending

[a] B, B lymphocytes; Eo, eosinophils; Mo, monocytes; NK, natural killer cells; PMN, neutrophils; T, T lymphocytes.

[b] MAdCAM-1 (mucosal addressin cell adhesion molecule) and CD34 are important for homing of T cells to lymph nodes via high endothelial venules. The protein structures bearing the L-selectin ligands, including CD15s, at sites of inflammation have not been identified.

[c] ESL-1 (E-selectin ligand), a protein with homology to fibroblast growth factor receptor, has been identified in mice. CLA (cutaneous lymphocyte antigen), a molecule on the surface of skin-homing T cells related to PSGL-1, directs them to skin via E-selectin expressed on dermal venules.

[d] Expression of VLA-4 on granulocytes is limited to eosinophils and basophils. Adult human neutrophils do not express VLA-4 under normal circumstances.

[e] Although VLA-4/VCAM-1 interactions are generally thought to be important for tight adhesion of leukocytes to endothelium, there are reports[373,374] that indicate leukocytes can use VLA-4 to roll on endothelial VCAM-1.

fering with homophilic interaction between leukocyte CD99 and endothelial cell CD99-arrested monocytes midway through diapedesis. Their leading edges were below the endothelial cell monolayer, whereas their trailing uropods remained on the apical surface of the endothelial cell.

At the onset of most acute inflammatory responses, vascular permeability transiently increases as a result of histamine release. The endothelial junctions are soon reestablished, and the junctions are closed to the leukocytes that arrive at the scene over the next hour. During diapedesis—the passage of leukocytes across the endothelium—leukocytes migrate in ameboid fashion across the junction between tightly apposed endothelial cells. Studies performed *in vivo* and *in vitro* indicate that, during diapedesis, leukocytes penetrate the vessel wall without breaching the vascular permeability barrier.[331,338] This process prevents exposure of subendothelial collagen and vWF deposits to circulating platelets. Although PECAM-1 has no known role in binding platelets to endothelial cells, PECAM-1 has been hypothesized to maintain the tight apposition of endothelial cells and leukocytes during diapedesis.[330]

ACUTE CHANGES

In addition to stimulation of immediate responses by endothelial cells, cytokines and inflammatory mediators released at the site of inflammation activate the surrounding endothelial cells to initiate new genetic programs. *De novo* synthesis of mRNA and protein leads to establishment of an inflammatory phenotype within several hours of exposure to adequate levels of the mediator. The changes induce a procoagulant and proadhesive phenotype in the endothelial cell.

Stimulated by inflammatory cytokines such as TNF-α or IL-1, vascular endothelial cells express several important cell adhesion molecules on their surface. E-selectin expression is induced within hours of cytokine stimulation. Expression peaks 4 to 6 hours *in vitro*. However, *in vivo* in the presence of interferon (IFN)-γ, expression is maintained over several days.[339,340] E-selectin mediates rolling of leukocytes bearing sialylated, fucosylated carbohydrate receptors similar to sialylated Lewis X antigen. This molecule is important for the slow rolling seen in some vascular beds.[341] P-selectin expression on the endothelial cell surface stimulated by thrombin or histamine is transient, but expression can be prolonged by IL-3,[342] IL-4, or oncostatin M stimulation[343] of human endothelium and by TNF-α stimulation of murine but not human endothelium.[344,345] Expression often lasts for hours to days. The prolonged expression requires *de novo* message and protein synthesis.

In general, expression of the immunoglobulin superfamily members ICAM-1 and VCAM-1 is induced by the same stimuli that induce E-selectin. Some specializations exist, at least *in vitro*. For example, IL-4 induces VCAM-1 but not E-selectin or ICAM-1 in microvascular endothelial cells.[346,347] These molecules serve as counter-receptors for the leukocyte integrins in the tight adhesion step, as discussed in the previous section.

CHRONIC CHANGES

Prolonged stimulation of endothelial cells with IFN-γ leads to expression of MHC class II molecules (HLA-DR and HLA-DQ) on their surfaces. This process requires several days *in vitro*. In human tissues such as skin and gut, class II expression is commonly seen even in the absence of overt inflammation and is thought to result from chronic exposure of these sites to subclinical inflammation and antigenic stimulation. Cytokines also can induce expression of CD40 ligand on endothelial cells. The significance of class II expression on endothelial cells is as follows. When costimulatory molecules such as CD40, ICAM-1, or LFA-3 are induced by inflammatory stimuli, the endothelial cell becomes capable (at least *in vitro*) of acting as an antigen-presenting cell that can stimulate CD4+ memory T cells. Although this process may not be a major threat in the normal host, the mechanism may stimulate graft rejection by the host when the endothelium belongs to an organ graft with foreign MHC class II.[348-350]

In contrast to these changes, expression of the adhesion molecule ICAM-2 does not change in response to inflammatory mediators. PECAM-1 shows a unique expression pattern in response to IFN-γ *in vitro*[351] and *in vivo*.[352] The distribution but not the absolute amount of PECAM on the surface changes as the molecule is no longer concentrated at intercellular borders but becomes expressed diffusely over the surface of the cell. *In vitro* chronic exposure of human umbilical vein endothelial cells to a combination of IFN-γ and TNF-α at relatively high doses leads to a decrease in total PECAM-1 expression.[353] Such a cytokine milieu could exist *in vivo*, but a similar phenotype has not been described.

ADHESION MOLECULES IN A THROMBOTIC MILIEU

In addition to the adhesive interactions germane to thrombosis and hemostasis, such an environment exposes leukocytes to ligands that promote their adhesion and recruitment to the vessel wall. For example, *in vitro* thrombin induces E-selectin expression and IL-8 secretion by human umbilical vein endothelial cells.[354] These changes are classically induced by inflammatory cytokines such as IL-1 and TNF-α. Table 108-5 lists some mediators that could have dual roles in inflammation and hemostasis/thrombosis.

TABLE 108-5   DUAL ROLES OF INFLAMMATORY MEDIATORS IN THROMBOSIS/HEMOSTASIS

MEDIATOR	ROLE IN INFLAMMATION	ROLE IN THROMBOSIS OR HEMOSTASIS
Histamine, thrombin	P-selectin expression induced on vascular endothelium	Degranulation of Weibel-Palade bodies; extrusion of vWF
Platelet-activating factor	Activation of leukocyte integrins	Activation of platelets
Expression of P-selectin glycoprotein ligand (PSGL-1)	Adhesion of leukocytes to endothelial P-selectin	Adhesion of platelets to adherent leukocytes via P-selectin bidirectionally
Adherent platelets	Leukocyte rolling on platelet P-selectin; tight adhesion to platelet membrane component	Thrombosis
Fibrinogen	Adhesion of leukocytes to fibrinogen via CD11b/CD18	Bridging of platelets to vWF and matrix via $\alpha_{IIb}\beta_{III}$
Thrombin	Induction of E-selectin expression and IL-8 secretion by endothelial cells	Activation of fibrinogen
Leukocyte integrin CD11b/CD18	Adhesion of leukocytes to endothelium; phagocytosis	Binding and activation of factor X; adhesion of platelets via GPIbα; adhesion of platelets via JAM-C

LEUKOCYTE–PLATELET AND ENDOTHELIAL CELL–PLATELET INTERACTIONS

Activated platelets bind to circulating lymphocytes in a P-selectin–dependent manner. The interaction can facilitate rolling on the endothelium[355] and allow homing of lymphocytes to peripheral lymph nodes in the absence of L-selectin, because P-selectin on the adherent platelets interacts with peripheral lymph node addressin.[356] In vitro, neutrophils are capable of rolling on immobilized platelets via PSGL-1 on the leukocyte interacting with degranulated P-selectin on platelet membranes.[357] Moreover, $\alpha_M\beta_2$(CD11b/CD18)-dependent arrest and tight adhesion of neutrophils to bound platelets following P-selectin–dependent rolling has been described.[357,358] The endothelial ligand for this process is not known. ICAM-2 has been found on the surface of activated platelets, but it is not a ligand for $\alpha_M\beta_2$. In fact, antibodies against neither ICAM-2 nor its neutrophil receptor α_L (CD11) blocked this adhesion.[358,359] On the other hand, neutrophil $\alpha_M\beta_2$ reportedly binds to fibrinogen, which may be present on the surfaces of activated platelets bound to $\alpha_{IIb}\beta_3$ (GPIIb-IIIa). Two additional platelet surface molecules, GPIbα and JAM-C, have been demonstrated as ligands for leukocyte CD11b/CD18.[360,361] GPIbα is part of the GP1b-IX-V complex, and JAM-C originally was described as a component of epithelial and endothelial cell tight junctions.

Platelets can interact with activated endothelial cells. Platelets express PSGL-1 and can use this expression to interact with P-selectin on the surfaces of activated endothelial cells.[362] Activated platelets also bind to endothelial cells via fibrinogen, fibrin, or vWF, forming a molecular bridge between platelet $\alpha_{IIb}\beta_3$ (GPIIb-IIIa) and endothelial cell $\alpha_v\beta_3$ and ICAM-1.

LEUKOCYTE–ENDOTHELIAL CELL MATRIX INTERACTIONS THAT PROMOTE COAGULATION

The same proinflammatory stimuli that stimulate de novo expression of E-selectin and VCAM-1 and augment expression of ICAM-1 for recruitment of leukocytes may stimulate synthesis and expression of TF by endothelial cells.[363] Furthermore, interaction of monocytes with endothelium stimulates TF production on monocytes. Adhesion of monocytic cell lines to cytokine-activated endothelial cells in culture leads to rapidly increased procoagulant activity as a result of TF induction. This effect is partially blocked by a monoclonal antibody directed against E-selectin on endothelium and is mimicked by cross-linking Lewis X on the monocyte cell lines.[364] A similar increase in TF gene expression can be induced by cross-linking α_4 or β_1 integrin chains, the components of VLA-4 on monocytic cell lines.[365]

A study of prolonged interaction of peripheral blood monocytes with human endothelial cells showed that within a few hours of transendothelial migration, monocytes in the collagen matrix expressed functional TF on their surfaces.[366] Over the next several days, approximately half of these monocytes had differentiated into immature dendritic cells and, bearing even higher levels of TF, migrated back across the intact endothelial cell monolayer in the abluminal-to-luminal direction. TF on the surface of monocytes was involved in this migration because it could be blocked by soluble fragments of TF. The same TF fragments blocked adhesion of endothelial cells to TF in vitro. Therefore, TF expressed by the emigrating dendritic cells was hypothesized to be directly involved in an adhesive step of this process and in any procoagulant role it may play.[366]

Leukocytes bound to P-selectin exposed on the surfaces of platelets on adherent thrombi promote conversion of fibrinogen to fibrin.[367] The leukocyte integrin CD11b/CD18 binds fibrinogen.[368] The same integrin has a conformational form that binds coagulation factor X.[369] Monocytic cells are capable of activating the bound factor X to Xa when activated,[370] defining a pathway for activation of factor X that is independent of TF.

REFERENCES

1. Marcus AJ, Safier LB: Thromboregulation: Multicellular modulation of platelet reactivity in hemostasis and thrombosis. *FASEB J* 7:516, 1993

2. Marcus AJ, Broekman MJ, Drosopoulos JHF, et al: Heterologous cell-cell interactions: Thromboregulation, cerebroprotection and cardioprotection by CD39 (NTPDase-1). *J Thromb Haemost* 1:2497, 2003.

3. Marcus AJ, Broekman MJ, Pinsky DJ: COX inhibitors and thromboregulation. *N Engl J Med* 347:1025, 2002.

4. Marcus AJ, Broekman MJ, Safier LB, et al: Formation of leukotrienes and other hydroxy acids during platelet-neutrophil interactions in vitro. *Biochem Biophys Res Commun* 109:130, 1982.

5. Weksler BB, Marcus AJ, Jaffe EA: Synthesis of prostaglandin I2 (prostacyclin) by cultured human and bovine endothelial cells. *Proc Natl Acad Sci U S A* 74:3922, 1999.

6. Marcus AJ, Safier LB, Hajjar KA, et al: Inhibition of platelet function by an aspirin-insensitive endothelial cell ADPase. Thromboregulation by endothelial cells. *J Clin Invest* 88:1690, 1991.

7. Marcus AJ, Broekman MJ, Drosopoulos JHF, et al: The endothelial cell ecto-ADPase responsible for inhibition of platelet function is CD39. *J Clin Invest* 99:1351, 1997.

8. Gayle RB, Maliszewski CR, Gimpel SD, et al: Inhibition of platelet function by recombinant soluble ecto-ADPase/CD39. *J Clin Invest* 101:1851, 1998.

9. Cines DB, Pollak ES, Buck CA, et al: Endothelial cells in physiology and in the pathophysiology of vascular disorders. *Blood* 91:3527, 1998.

10. Marcus AJ, Weksler BB, Jaffe EA, Broekman MJ: Synthesis of prostacyclin from platelet-derived endoperoxides by cultured human endothelial cells. *J Clin Invest* 66:979, 1980.

11. Pinsky DJ, Broekman MJ, Peschon JJ, et al: Elucidation of the thromboregulatory role of CD39/ectoapyrase in the ischemic brain. *J Clin Invest* 109:1031, 2002.

12. Ross R: Atherosclerosis: An inflammatory disease. *N Engl J Med* 340:115, 1999.

13. Widlansky ME, Gokce N, Keaney JF Jr, Vita JA: The clinical implications of endothelial dysfunction. *J Am Coll Cardiol* 42:1149, 2003.

14. Taubman MB, Fallon JT, Schecter AD, et al: Tissue factor in the pathogenesis of atherosclerosis. *Thromb Haemost* 78:200, 1997.

15. Virchow RLK: Gesammelte abhandlungen zur wissenschaftlichen medicin. Meidinger Sohn & Co., Frankfurt, 1856.

16. Hamberg M, Svensson J, Samuelsson B: Thromboxanes: A new group of biologically active compounds derived from prostaglandin endoperoxides. *Proc Natl Acad Sci U S A* 72:2994, 1975.

17. Piper PJ, Vane JR: Release of additional factors in anaphylaxis and its antagonism by anti-inflammatory drugs. *Nature* 223:29, 1969.

18. Moncada S, Gryglewski R, Bunting S, Vane JR: An enzyme isolated from arteries transforms prostaglandin endoperoxides to an unstable substance that inhibits platelet aggregation. *Nature* 263:663, 1976.

19. Whittaker N, Bunting S, Salmon J, et al: The chemical structure of prostaglandin X (prostacyclin). *Prostaglandins* 12:915, 1976.

20. Maclouf J, Folco G, Patrono C: Eicosanoids and iso-eicosanoids: Constitutive, inducible and transcellular biosynthesis in vascular disease. *Thromb Haemost* 79:691, 1998.

21. Herschman HR: Prostaglandin synthase 2. *Biochim Biophys Acta* 1299:125, 1996.

22. McAdam BF, Catella-Lawson F, Mardini IA, et al: Systemic biosynthesis of prostacyclin by cyclooxygenase (COX)-2: The human pharmacology of a selective inhibitor of COX-2. *Proc Natl Acad Sci U S A* 96:272, 1999.

23. Yaksh TL, Dirig DM, Malmberg AB: Mechanism of action of nonsteroidal anti-inflammatory drugs. *Cancer Invest* 16:509, 1998.

24. DeWitt DL, Smith WL: Cloning of sheep and mouse prostaglandin endoperoxide synthases. *Methods Enzymol* 187:469, 1990.

25. Xie WL, Chipman JG, Robertson DL, et al: Expression of a mitogen-responsive gene encoding prostaglandin synthase is regulated by mRNA splicing. *Proc Natl Acad Sci U S A* 88:2692, 1991.

26. Kurumbail RG, Stevens AM, Gierse JK, et al: Structural basis for selective inhibition of cyclooxygenase-2 by anti-inflammatory agents [published erratum appears in *Nature* 385:555, 1997]. *Nature* 384:644, 1996.

27. Smith WL, DeWitt DL: Prostaglandin endoperoxide H synthases-1 and -2. *Adv Immunol* 62:167, 1996.

28. Loll PJ, Picot D, Garavito RM: The structural basis of aspirin activity inferred from the crystal structure of inactivated prostaglandin H2 synthase. *Nat Struct Biol* 2:1, 1995.

29. Pouliot M, Gilbert C, Borgeat P, et al: Expression and activity of prostaglandin endoperoxide synthase-2 in agonist-activated human neutrophils. *FASEB J* 12:1109, 1998.

30. Dubois RN, Abramson SB, Crofford L, et al: Cyclooxygenase in biology and disease. *FASEB J* 12:1063, 1998.

31. Lipsky LPE, Abramson SB, Crofford L, et al: The classification of cyclooxygenase inhibitors. *J Rheumatol* 25:2298, 1998.

32. Furchgott RF, Zawadzki JV: The obligatory role of endothelial cells in the relaxation of arterial smooth muscle by acetylcholine. *Nature* 288:373, 1980.

33. Vichinsky EP: Pulmonary hypertension in sickle cell disease. *N Engl J Med* 350:373, 2004.

34. Marletta MA: Nitric oxide synthase structure and mechanism. *J Biol Chem* 268:1223, 1993.

35. Moncada S, Higgs EA: Molecular mechanisms and therapeutic strategies related to nitric oxide. *FASEB J* 9:1319, 1995.

36. Moncada S, Palmer RMJ, Higgs EA: Nitric oxide: Physiology, pathophysiology, and pharmacology. *Pharmacol Rev* 43:109, 1991.

37. Matsumoto A, Momomura S, Sugiura S, et al: Effect of inhaled nitric oxide on gas exchange in patients with congestive heart failure. *Ann Intern Med* 130:40, 1999.

38. Lentz SR, Sobey CG, Piegers DJ, et al: Vascular dysfunction in monkeys with diet-induced hyperhomocyst(e)inemia. *J Clin Invest* 98:24, 1996.

39. Stamler JS, Osborne JA, Jaraki O, et al: Adverse vascular effects of homocysteine are modulated by endothelium-derived relaxing factor and related oxides of nitrogen. *J Clin Invest* 91:308, 1993.

40. Upchurch GR Jr, Welch GN, Fabian AJ, et al: Homocyst(e)ine decrease bioavailable nitric oxide by a mechanism involving glutathione peroxidase. *J Biol Chem* 272:17012, 1997.

41. Voetsch B, Loscalzo J: Genetic determinants of arterial thrombosis. *Arterioscler Thromb Vasc Biol* 24:216, 2004.

42. Broekman MJ, Eiroa AM, Marcus AJ: Inhibition of human platelet reactivity by endothelium-derived relaxing factor from human umbilical vein endothelial cells in suspension. Blockade of aggregation and secretion by an aspirin-insensitive mechanism. *Blood* 78:1033, 1991.

43. Moore K, Wendon J, Frazer M, et al: Plasma endothelin immunoreactivity in liver disease and the hepatorenal syndrome. *N Engl J Med* 327:1774, 1992.

44. Rubanyi GM, Polokoff MA: Endothelins: Molecular biology, biochemistry, pharmacology, physiology, and pathophysiology. *Pharmacol Rev* 46:325, 1994.

45. Maliszewski CR, Delespesse GJ, Schoenborn MA, et al: The CD39 lymphoid cell activation antigen. Molecular cloning and structural characterization. *J Immunol* 153:3574, 1994.

46. Sesti C, Broekman MJ, Drosopoulos JHF, et al: Ectonucleotidase in cardiac sympathetic nerve endings modulates ATP-mediated feedback of norepinephrine release. *J Pharmacol Exp Ther* 300:605, 2002.

47. Sesti C, Koyama M, Broekman MJ, et al: Ectonucleotidase in sympathetic nerve endings modulates ATP and norepinephrine exocytosis in myocardial ischemia. *J Pharmacol Exp Ther* 306:238, 2003.

48. Kaczmarek E, Koziak K, Sevigny J, et al: Identification and characterization of CD39 vascular ATP diphosphohydrolase. *J Biol Chem* 271:33116, 1996.

49. Guckelberger O, Sun XF, Sevigny J, et al: Beneficial effects of CD39/ecto-nucleoside triphosphate diphosphohydrolase-1 in murine intestinal ischemia reperfusion injury. *Thromb Haemost* 91:576, 2004.

50. Marcus AJ, Broekman MJ, Drosopoulos JHF, et al: Metabolic control of excessive extracellular nucleotide accumulation by CD39/ectonucleotidase-1: Implications for ischemic vascular diseases. *J Pharmacol Exp Ther* 305:9, 2003.

51. Esmon CT, Owen WG: Identification of an endothelial cell cofactor for thrombin-catalyzed activation of protein C. *Proc Natl Acad Sci U S A* 78:2249, 1981.

52. Esmon CT: Anticoagulant properties of vascular cells: Thrombomodulin and protein C activation pathway, in *Vascular Control of Hemostasis*, edited by VWM Van Hinsbergh, pp 9–37. Harwood Academic, The Netherlands, 1996.

53. Esmon CT: Regulation of blood coagulation. *Biochim Biophys Acta* 1477:349, 2000.

54. Stearns-Kurosawa DJ, Kurosawa S, Mollica JS, et al: The endothelial cell protein C receptor augments protein C activation by the thrombin-thrombomodulin complex. *Proc Natl Acad Sci U S A* 93:10212, 1996.

55. Esmon CT: Protein C pathway in sepsis. *Ann Med* 34:598, 2002.

56. Esmon CT: Inflammation and thrombosis. *J Thromb Haemost* 1:1343, 2003.

57. Esmon CT: The protein C pathway. *Chest* 124:26S, 2003.

58. Esmon CT: Protein C, protein S, and thrombomodulin, in *Hemostasis and Thrombosis: Basic Principles and Clinical Practice*, 5th ed, edited by RW Colman, J Hirsh, VJ Marder, AW Clowes, JN George, SZ Goldhaber, pp 1–1822. Lippincott Williams & Wilkins, Philadelphia, 2005 (in press).

59. Esmon CT: The roles of protein C and thrombomodulin in the regulation of blood coagulation. *J Biol Chem* 264:4743, 1989.

60. Grinnell BW, Berg DT: Surface thrombomodulin modulates thrombin receptor responses on vascular smooth muscle cells. *Am J Physiol* 270:H603, 1996.

61. Lafay M, Laguna R, Le Bonniec BF, et al: Thrombomodulin modulates the mitogenic response to thrombin of human umbilical vein endothelial cells. *Thromb Haemost* 79:848, 1998.

62. Esmon CT: Anticoagulant protein C/thrombomodulin pathway, in *The Metabolic and Molecular Bases of Inherited Disease*, 8th ed., edited by CR Scriver, AL Beaudet, WS Sly, D Valle,Childs, B, Kinzler KW, Vogelstein B, pp 4327–4343. McGraw-Hill, New York, 2001.

63. Bajzar L, Manuel R, Nesheim M: Purification and characterization of TAFI, a thrombin activatable fibrinolysis inhibitor. *J Biol Chem* 270:14477, 1995.

64. Campbell WD, Okada N, Okada H: Carboxypeptidase R is an inactivator of complement-derived inflammatory peptides and an inhibitor of fibrinolysis. *Immunol Rev* 180:162, 2001.

65. Campbell WD, Lazoura E, Okada N, Okada H: Inactivation of C3a and C5a octapeptides by carboxypeptidase R and carboxypeptidase N. *Microbiol Immunol* 46:131, 2002.

66. Ikeguchi H, Fujita Y, Kato T, et al: Effects of human soluble thrombomodulin on experimental glomerulonephritis. *Kidney Int* 61:490, 2002.

67. de Munk GAW, Groeneveld E, Rijken DC: Acceleration of the thrombin inactivation of single chain urokinase-type plasminogen activator (pro-urokinase) by thrombomodulin. *J Clin Invest* 88:1680, 1991.

68. Molinari A, Giogetti C, Lansen J, et al: Thrombomodulin is a cofactor for thrombin degradation of recombinant single-chain urokinase plasminogen activator in vitro and in a perfused rabbit heart model. *Thromb Haemost* 67:226, 1992.

69. Preissner KT, May AE, Wohn KD, et al: Molecular crosstalk between adhesion receptors and proteolytic cascades in vascular remodeling. *Thromb Haemost* 78:88, 1997.

70. Conway EM, Van de WM, Pollefeyt S, et al: The lectin-like domain of thrombomodulin confers protection from neutrophil-mediated tissue damage by suppressing adhesion molecule expression via nuclear factor kappaB and mitogen-activated protein kinase pathways. *J Exp Med* 196: 565, 2002.

71. Zhang Y, Stern DM, Rosenberg RD, Nawroth P: Thrombomodulin modulates growth of tumor cells independent of its anticoagulant activity. *J Clin Invest* 101:1301, 1998.

72. Huang HC, Shi GY, Jiang SJ, et al: Thrombomodulin-mediated cell adhesion: Involvement of its lectin-like domain. *J Biol Chem* 278:46750, 2003.

73. Raife TJ, Lager DJ, Madison KC, et al: Thrombomodulin expression by human keratinocytes. Induction of cofactor activity during epidermal differentiation. *J Clin Invest* 93:1846, 1994.

74. Healy AM, Rayburn HB, Rosenberg RD, Weiler H: Absence of the blood-clotting regulator thrombomodulin causes embryonic lethality in mice before development of a functional cardiovascular system. *Proc Natl Acad Sci U S A* 92:850, 1995.

75. Weiler-Guettler H, Aird WC, Rayburn H, et al: Developmentally regulated gene expression of thrombomodulin in postimplantation mouse embryos. *Development* 122:2271, 1996.

76. Crawley JTB, Gu AM, Ferrell G, Esmon CT: Distribution of endothelial cell protein C/activated protein C receptor (EPCR) during mouse embryo development. *Thromb Haemost* 88:259, 2002.

77. Isermann B, Hendrickson SB, Hutley K, et al: Tissue-restricted expression of thrombomodulin in the placenta rescues thrombomodulin-deficient mice from early lethality and reveals a secondary developmental block. *Development* 128:827, 2001.

78. Isermann B, Hendrickson SB, Zogg M, et al: Endothelium-specific loss of murine thrombomodulin disrupts the protein C anticoagulant pathway and causes juvenile-onset thrombosis. *J Clin Invest* 108:537, 2001.

79. Weiler H, Isermann B: Thrombomodulin. *J Thromb Haemost* 1:1515, 2003.

80. Isermann B, Sood R, Pawlinski R, et al: The thrombomodulin-protein C system is essential for the maintenance of pregnancy. *Nat Med* 9:331, 2003.

81. Imada S, Yamaguchi H, Nagumo M, et al: Identification of fetomodulin, a surface marker protein of fetal development, as thrombomodulin by gene cloning and functional assays. *Dev Biol* 140:113, 1990.

82. Imada M, Imada S, Iwasaki H, et al: Fetomodulin: Marker surface protein of fetal development which is modulatable by cyclic AMP. *Dev Biol* 122:483, 1987.

83. Sadler JE: Thrombomodulin structure and function. *Thromb Haemost* 78:392, 1997.

84. Conway EM, Pollefeyt S, Collen D, Steiner-Mosonyi M: The amino terminal lectin-like domain of thrombomodulin is required for constitutive endocytosis. *Blood* 89:652, 1997.

85. Schenk-Braat EAM, Morser J, Rijken DC: Identification of the epidermal growth factor-like domains of thrombomodulin essential for the acceleration of thrombin-mediated inactivation of single-chain urokinase-type plasminogen activator. *Eur J Biochem* 268:5562, 2001.

86. White CE, Hunter MJ, Meininger DP, et al: The fifth epidermal growth factor-like domain of thrombomodulin does not have an epidermal growth factor-like disulfide bonding pattern. *Proc Natl Acad Sci U S A* 93:10177, 1996.

87. Fuentes-Prior P, Iwanaga Y, Huber R, et al: Structural basis for the anticoagulant activity of the thrombin-thrombomodulin complex. *Nature* 404:518, 2000.

88. Light DR, Glaser CB, Betts M, et al: The interaction of thrombomodulin with Ca2+. *Eur J Biochem* 262:522, 1999.

89. White CE, Hunter MJ, Meininger DP, et al: Large-scale expression, purification and characterization of small fragments of thrombomodulin:

90. The roles of the sixth domain and of methionine 388. *Protein Eng* 8: 1177, 1995.

90. Stearns DJ, Kurasawa S, Esmon CT: Micro-thrombomodulin: Residues 310-486 from the epidermal growth factor precursor homology domain of thrombomodulin will accelerate protein C activation. *J Biol Chem* 264:3352, 1989.

91. Suzuki K, Hayashi T, Nishioka J, et al: A domain composed of epidermal growth factor-like structures of human thrombomodulin is essential for thrombin binding and for protein C activation. *J Biol Chem* 264: 4872, 1989.

92. Glaser CB, Morser J, Clarke JH, et al: Oxidation of a specific methionine in thrombomodulin by activated neutrophil products blocks cofactor activity. *J Clin Invest* 90:2565, 1992.

93. Wood MJ, Becvar LA, Prieto JH, et al: NMR Structures reveal how oxidation inactivates thrombomodulin. *Biochemistry* 42:11932, 2003.

94. Dahlback B, Villoutreix BO: Molecular recognition in the protein C anticoagulant pathway. *J Thromb Haemost* 1:1525, 2003.

95. Rezaie AR, Yang L: Thrombomodulin allosterically modulates the activity of the anticoagulant thrombin. *Proc Natl Acad Sci U S A* 100: 12051, 2003.

96. Kokami K, Zheng X, Sadler JE: Activation of thrombin-activatable fibrinolysis inhibitor requires epidermal growth factor-like domain 3 of thrombomodulin and is inhibited competitively by protein C. *J Biol Chem* 273:12135, 1998.

97. Tsiang M, Lentz SR, Sadler JE: Functional domains of membrane-bound human thrombomodulin. EGF-like domains four to six and the serine/threonine-rich domain are required for cofactor activity. *J Biol Chem* 267:6164, 1992.

98. Dudek AZ, Pennell CA, Decker TD, et al: Platelet factor 4 binds to glycanated forms of thrombomodulin and to protein C. A potential mechanism for enhancing generation of activated protein C. *J Biol Chem* 272:31785, 1997.

99. Ye J, Esmon CT, Johnson AE: The chondroitin sulfate moiety of thrombomodulin binds a second molecule of thrombin. *J Biol Chem* 268:2373, 1993.

100. Weisel JW, Nagaswami C, Young TA, Light DR: The shape of thrombomodulin and interactions with thrombin as determined by electron microscopy. *J Biol Chem* 271:31485, 1996.

101. Gysin J, Pouvelle B, Le Tonqueze M, et al: Chondroitin sulfate of thrombomodulin is an adhesion receptor for plasmodium falciparum-infected erythrocytes. *Mol Biochem Parasitol* 88:267, 1997.

102. Xu J, Esmon NL, Esmon CT: Reconstitution of the human endothelial cell protein C receptor with thrombomodulin in phosphatidylcholine vesicles enhances protein C activation. *J Biol Chem* 274:6704, 1999.

103. Lin JH, McLean K, Morser J, et al: Modulation of glycosaminoglycan addition in naturally expresses and recombinant human thrombomodulin. *J Biol Chem* 269:25021, 1994.

104. Parkinson JF, Garcia JGN, Bang NU: Decreased thrombin activity of cell-surface thrombomodulin following treatment of cultured endothelial cells with b-D-xylose. *Biochem Biophys Res Commun* 169:177, 1990.

105. Dittman WA, Majerus PW: Structure and function of thrombomodulin: A natural anticoagulant. *Blood* 75:329, 1990.

106. Dittman WA, Kumada T, Sadler JE, Majerus PW: The structure and function of mouse thrombomodulin. Phorbol myristate acetate stimulates degradation and synthesis of thrombomodulin without affecting mRNA levels in hemangioma cells. *J Biol Chem* 263:15815, 1988.

107. Tazawa R, Yamamoto K, Suzuki K, et al: Presence of functional cyclic AMP responsive element in the 3'-untranslated region of the human thrombomodulin gene. *Biochim Biophys Res Commun* 200:1391, 1994.

108. Dittman WA, Nelson SC, Greer PK, et al: Characterization of thrombomodulin expression in response to retinoic acid and identification of a retinoic acid response element in the human thrombomodulin gene. *J Biol Chem* 269:16925, 1994.

109. Ishii H, Horie S, Kizaki K, Kazama M: Retinoic acid counteracts both the downregulation of thrombomodulin and the induction of tissue factor in cultured human endothelial cells exposed to tumor necrosis factor. *Blood* 80:2556, 1992.

110. Ohdama S, Takano S, Ohashi K, et al: Pentoxifylline prevents tumor necrosis factor-induced suppression of endothelial cell surface thrombodulin. *Thromb Res* 62:745, 1991.

111. Hirokawa K, Aoki N: Regulatory mechanisms for thrombomodulin expression in human umbilical vein endothelial cells in vitro. *J Cell Physiol* 147:157, 1999.

112. Kapiotis S, Besemer J, Bevec D, et al: Interleukin-4 counteracts pyrogen-induced downregulation of thrombomodulin in cultured human vascular endothelial cells. *Blood* 78:410, 1991.

113. Calnek DS, Grinnell BW: Thrombomodulin-dependent anticoagulant activity is regulated by vascular endothelial growth factor. *Exp Cell Res* 238:294, 1998.

114. Miyake S, Ohdama S, Tazawa R, Aoki N: Retinoic acid prevents cytokine-induced suppression of thrombomodulin expression on surface of human umbilical vascular endothelial cells. *Thromb Res* 68:483, 1999.

115. Herbert JM, Savi P, Laplace MC, et al: Chelerythrine, a selective protein kinase C inhibitor, counteracts pyrogen-induced expression of tissue factor without effect on thrombomodulin down-regulation in endothelial cells. *Thromb Res* 71:487, 1993.

116. Yang HL, Hseu YC, Lu FJ, Tsai HD: Humic acid reduces protein C-activating cofactor activity of thrombomodulin of human umbilical vein endothelial cells. *Br J Haem* 101:16, 1998.

117. Conway EM, Liu L, Nowakowski B, et al: Heat shock of vascular endothelial cells induces an up-regulatory transcriptional response of the thrombomodulin gene that is delayed in onset and does not attenuate. *J Biol Chem* 269:22804, 1994.

118. Hirokawa K, Aoki N: Up-regulation of thrombomodulin by activation of histamine H1 receptors in human umbilical-vein endothelial cells in vitro. *Biochem J* 276:739, 1991.

119. Ohji T, Urano H, Shirahata A, et al: Transforming growth factor beta1 and beta2 induce down-modulation of thrombomodulin in human umbilical vein endothelial cells. *Thromb Haemost* 73:812, 1995.

120. Key NS, Vercellotti GM, Winkelmann JC, et al: Infection of vascular endothelial cells with herpes simplex virus enhances tissue factor activity and reduces thrombomodulin expression. *Proc Natl Acad Sci U S A* 87:7095,1990.

121. Faust SN, Levin M, Harrison OB, et al: Dysfunction of endothelial protein C activation in severe meningococcal sepsis. *N Engl J Med* 345:408, 2001.

122. Rintala E, Kauppila M, Seppälä OP, et al: Protein C substitution in sepsis-associated purpura fulminans. *Crit Care Med* 28:2373, 2000.

123. Dufourcq P, Seigneur M, Pruvost A, et al: Membrane thrombomodulin levels are decreased during hypoxia and restored by cAMP and IBMX. *Thromb Res* 77:305, 1994.

124. Seigneur M, Dufourcq P, Belloc F, et al: Influence of pentoxifylline on membrane thrombomodulin levels in endothelial cells submitted to hypoxic conditions. *J Cardiovasc Pharmacol* 25(suppl 2):S85, 1995.

125. Laszik ZG, Zhou XJ, Ferrell GL, et al: Down-regulation of endothelial cell protein C receptor and thrombomodulin in coronary atherosclerosis. *Am J Pathol* 159:797, 2001.

126. Ishii H, Kizaki K, Horie S, Kazama M: Oxidized low density lipoprotein reduces thrombomodulin transcription in cultured human endothelial cells through degradation of the lipoprotein in lysosomes. *J Biol Chem* 271:8458, 1996.

127. Ishii H, Tezuka T, Ishikawa H, et al: Oxidized phospholipids in oxidized low-density lipoprotein downregulate thrombomodulin transcription in vascular endothelial cells through a decrease in the binding of RARb-

128. Lentz SR: Homocysteine and vascular dysfunction. *Life Sci* 61:1205, 1997.

129. Tohda G, Oida K, Okada Y, et al: Expression of thrombomodulin in atherosclerotic lesions and mitogenic activity of recombinant thrombomodulin in vascular smooth muscle cells. *Arterioscler Thromb Vasc Biol* 18:1861, 1998.

130. Ma SF, Garcia JGN, Reuning U, et al: Thrombin induces thrombomodulin mRNA expression via the proteolytically activated thrombin receptor in cultured bovine smooth muscle cells. *J Lab Clin Med* 129:611, 1997.

131. Fink LM, Eidt JF, Johnson K, et al: TM activity and localization. *Int J Dev Biol* 37:221, 1993.

132. Soff GA, Jackman RW, Rosenberg RD: Expression of thrombomodulin by smooth muscle cells in culture: Different effects of tumor necrosis factor and cyclic adenosine monophosphate on thrombomodulin expression by endothelial cells and smooth muscle cells in culture. *Blood* 77:515, 1991.

133. Hamada H, Ishii H, Sakyo K, et al: The epidermal growth factor-like domain of recombinant human thrombomodulin exhibits mitogenic activity for Swiss 3T3 cells. *Blood* 86:225, 1995.

134. Waugh JM, Yuksel E, Li J, et al: Local overexpression of thrombomodulin for in vivo prevention of arterial thrombosis in a rabbit model. *Circ Res* 84:84, 1999.

135. Waugh JM, Li-Hawkins J, Yuksel E, et al: Thrombomodulin overexpression to limit neointima formation. *Circulation* 102:332, 2000.

136. Masamura K, Oida K, Kanehara H, et al: Pitavastatin-induced thrombomodulin expression by endothelial cells acts via inhibition of small G proteins of the Rho family. *Arterioscler Thromb Vasc Biol* 23:512, 2003.

137. Shi JM, Wang JR, Zheng H, et al: Statins increase thrombomodulin expression and function in human endothelial cells by a nitric oxide-dependent mechanism and counteract tumor necrosis factor alpha-induced thrombomodulin downregulation. *Blood Coagul Fibrinolysis* 14:575, 2003.

138. Kim AY, Walinsky PL, Kolodgie FD, et al: Early loss of thrombomodulin expression impairs vein graft thromboresistance: Implications for vein graft failure. *Circ Res* 90:205, 2002.

139. Sperry JL, Deming CB, Bian C, et al: Wall tension is a potent negative regulator of in vivo thrombomodulin expression. *Circ Res* 92:41, 2003.

140. Malek AM, Jackman R, Rosenberg RD, Izumo S: Endothelial cell expression of TM is reversibly regulated by fluid shear stress. *Circ Res* 74:852, 1994.

141. MacGregor IA, Perrie AM, Donnelly SC, Haslett C: Modulation of human endothelial thrombomodulin by neutrophils and their release products. *Am J Respir Crit Care Med* 155:4, 1997.

142. Boehme MWJ, Galle P, Stremmel W: Kinetics of thrombomodulin release and endothelial cell injury by neutrophil-derived proteases and oxygen radicals. *Immunology* 107:340, 2002.

143. Ohdama S, Matsubara O, Aoki N: Plasma thrombomodulin in Wegener's granulomatosis as an indicator of vascular injuries. *Chest* 106:666, 1994.

144. Boehme MWJ, Deng Y, Raeth U, et al: Release of thrombomodulin from endothelial cells by concerted action of TNF-α and neutrophils: In vivo and in vitro studies. *Immunology* 87:134, 1996.

145. Key NS, Vercellotti GM, Esmon NL, et al: Neutrophils enhance procoagulant effects of tumor necrosis factor on endothelium by accelerating thrombomodulin loss: Role in endotoxin shock. *Clin Res* 37:601, 1989.

146. Abe H, Okajima K, Okabe H, et al: Granulocyte proteases and hydrogen peroxide synergistically inactivate thrombomodulin of endothelial cells in vitro. *J Lab Clin Med* 123:874, 1994.

147. Boffa MC: Considering cellular thrombomodulin distribution and its modulating factors can facilitate the use of plasma thrombomodulin as a reliable endothelial marker? *Haemostasis* 26:233, 1996.

148. Blann A, Seigneur M: Soluble markers of endothelial cell function: *Clin Hemorheol Microcirc* 17:3, 1997.

149. Slungaard A, Vercellotti GM, Tran T, et al: Eosinophil cationic granule proteins impair thrombomodulin function. A potential mechanism for thromboembolism in hypereosinophilic heart disease. *J Clin Invest* 91:1721, 1993.

150. Bourin MC, Ohlin AK, Lane DA, et al: Relationship between anticoagulant activities and polyanionic properties of rabbit thrombomodulin. *J Biol Chem* 263:8044, 1988.

151. Slungaard A, Fernandez JA, Griffin JH, et al: Platelet factor 4 enhances generation of activated protein C in vitro and in vivo. *Blood* 102:146, 2003.

152. Fukodome K, Esmon CT: Identification, cloning, and regulation of a novel endothelial cell protein C/activated protein C receptor. *J Biol Chem* 269:26486, 1994.

153. Esmon CT, Gu J, Xu J, et al: Regulation and functions of the protein C anticoagulant pathway. *Haematologica* 84:363, 1999.

154. Esmon CT, Xu J, Gu J, et al: Endothelial protein C receptor. *Thromb Haemost* 82:251, 1999.

155. Oganesyan V, Oganesyan N, Terzyan S, et al: The crystal structure of the endothelial protein C receptor and a bound phospholipid. *J Biol Chem* 277:24851, 2002.

156. Prigozy TI, Naidenko O, Qasba P, et al: Glycolipid antigen processing for presentation by CD1d molecules. *Science* 291:664, 2004.

157. Liaw PCY, Mather T, Oganesyan N, et al: Identification of the protein C/activated protein C binding sites on the endothelial cell protein C receptor: Implications for a novel mode of ligand recognition by a major histocompatibility complex class 1-type receptor. *J Biol Chem* 276:8364, 2001.

158. Xu J, Liaw PCY, Esmon CT: A novel transmembrane domain of the endothelial cell protein C receptor (EPCR) dictates receptor localization of sphingolipid-cholesterol rich regions on plasma membrane while EPCR palmitoylation modulates intracellular trafficking patterns. *Thromb Haemost* (suppl):695A, 1999.

159. Kurosawa S, Stearns-Kurosawa DJ, Hidari N, Esmon CT: Identification of functional endothelial protein C receptor in human plasma. *J Clin Invest* 100:411, 1997.

160. Fukodome K, Ye X, Tsuneyoshi N, et al: Activation mechanism of anticoagulant protein C in large blood vessels involving the endothelial cell protein C receptor. *J Exp Med* 187:1029, 1998.

161. Taylor FB Jr, Peer GT, Lockhart MS, et al: Endothelial cell protein C receptor plays an important role in protein C activation in vivo. *Blood* 97:1685, 2001.

162. Regan LM, Stearns-Kurosawa DJ, Kurosawa S, et al: The endothelial cell protein C receptor: Inhibition of activated protein C anticoagulant function without modulation of reaction with proteinase inhibitors. *J Biol Chem* 271:17499, 1996.

163. Esmon CT, Taylor FB, Snow TR: Inflammation and coagulation: Linked processes potentially regulated through a common pathway mediated by protein C. *Thromb Haemost* 66:160, 1991.

164. Esmon CT, Schwarz HP: An update on clinical and basic aspects of the protein C anticoagulant pathway. *Trends Cardiovasc Med* 5:141, 1995.

165. Taylor FB, Stearns-Kurosawa DJ, Kurasawa S, et al: The endothelial cell protein C receptor aids in host defense against *Escherichia coli* sepsis. *Blood* 95:1680, 2000.

166. Joyce DE, Gelbert L, Ciaccia A, et al: Gene expression profile of antithrombic protein C defines new mechanisms modulating inflammation and apoptosis. *J Biol Chem* 276:11199, 2001.

167. Riewald M, Petrovan RJ, Donner A, et al: Activation of endothelial cell protease activated receptor1 by the protein C pathway. *Science* 296:1880, 2002.

168. Cheng T, Liu D, Griffin JH, et al: Activated protein C blocks p53-mediated apoptosis in ischemic human brain endothelium and is neuroprotective. *Nat Med* 9:338, 2003.

169. Guo H, Liu D, Gelbard H, et al: Activated protein C prevents neuronal apoptosis via protease activated receptors 1 and 3. *Neuron* 41:563, 2004.

170. Coughlin SR: Thrombin signaling and protease-activated receptors. *Nature* 407:258, 2000.

171. Xu J, Esmon CT: Endothelial cell protein C receptor (EPCR) constitutively translocates into the nucleus and also mediates activated protein C, but not protein C, nuclear translocation. *Thromb Haemost* (suppl):206A, 1999.

172. Kurosawa S, Esmon CT, Stearns-Kurosawa DJ: The soluble endothelial protein C receptor binds to a proteinase-3/MAC-1 heterocomplex on neutrophils. *J Immunol* 165:4697, 2000.

173. Gu JM, Crawley JTB, Ferrell G, et al: Disruption of the endothelial cell protein C receptor gene in mice causes placental thrombosis and early embryonic lethality. *J Biol Chem* 277:43335, 2002.

174. Castellino FJ, Liang Z, Volkir SP, et al: Mice with severe deficiency of the endothelial protein C receptor gene develop, survive, and reproduce normally, and do not present with enhanced arterial thrombosis after challenge. *Thromb Haemost* 88:462, 2002.

175. Simmonds RE, Lane DA: Structural and functional implications of the intron/exon organization of the human endothelial cell protein C/activated protein C receptor (EPCR) gene: Comparison with the structure of CD1/major histocompatibility complex alpha1 and alpha2 domains. *Blood* 94:632, 1999.

176. Gu JM, Fukudome K, Esmon CT: Characterization and regulation of the 5′ flanking region of the murine endothelial protein C receptor gene. *J Biol Chem* 275:12481, 2000.

177. Laszik Z, Mitro A, Taylor FB, et al: Human protein C receptor is present primarily on endothelium of large vessels: Implications for the control of the protein C pathway. *Circulation* 96:3633, 1997.

178. Ye X, Fukudome K, Tsuneyoshi, et al: The endothelial cell protein C receptor (EPCR) functions as a primary receptor for protein C activation on endothelial cell in arteries, veins, and capillaries. *Biochem Biophys Res Commun* 259:671, 1999.

179. Gu JM, Katsuura Y, Ferrell GL, et al: Endotoxin and thrombin elevate rodent endothelial cell protein C receptor mRNA and increase receptor shedding in vivo. *Blood* 95:1687, 2000.

180. Xu J, Qu D, Esmon NL, Esmon CT: Metalloproteolytic release of endothelial cell protein C receptor. *J Biol Chem* 275:6038, 1999.

181. Stearns-Kurosawa DJ, Burgin C, Parker D, et al: Bimodal distribution of soluble endothelial protein C receptor levels in healthy populations. *J Thromb Haemost* 1:855, 2003.

182. Saposnik B, Reny HL, Gaussem P, et al: A haplotype of the EPCR gene is associated with increased plasma levels of sEPCR and is a candidate risk factor for thrombosis. *Blood* 103:1311, 2003.

183. Laszik ZG, Zho XJ, Silva FG, et al: Thrombomodulin (TM) but not endothelial cell protein C receptor (EPCR) mRNA is downregulated in streptozotocin-induced diabetic rat kidneys. *Mod Pathol* 16:267a, 2003.

184. Todd AS: Fibrinolysis autographs. *Nature* 181:495, 1958.

185. Todd AS: Localization of fibrinolytic activity in tissues. *Br Med Bull* 20:210, 1964.

186. Pandolfi M: Histochemistry of tissue plasminogen activator. *Thromb Diath Haemorrh* 34:661, 1975.

187. Van Hinsbergh VWM, Kooistra T, Emeis JJ, Koolwijk P: Regulation of plasminogen activator production by endothelial cells: Role in fibrinolysis and local proteolysis. *Int J Radiat Biol* 60:261, 1991.

188. Augustin HG, Kozian DH, Johnson RC: Differentiation of endothelial cells: Analysis of the constitutive and activated endothelial cell phenotypes. *Bioessays* 16:901, 1994.

189. Levin EG, del Zoppo GJ: Localization of tissue plasminogen activator in the endothelium of a limited number of vessels. *Am J Pathol* 144: 855, 1994.

190. Levin EG, Santell L, Osborn KG: The expression of endothelial tissue plasminogen activator in vivo: A function defined by vessel size and anatomic location. *J Cell Sci* 110:139, 1997.

191. Levin EG, Osborn KG, Schleuning WD: Vessel-specific gene expression in the lung: Tissue plasminogen activator is limited to bronchial arteries and pulmonary vessels of discrete size. *Chest* 114:68S, 1998.

192. Dichek D, Quertermous T: Thrombin regulation of mRNA levels of tissue plasminogen activator inhibitor-1 in cultured human umbilical vein endothelial cells. *Blood* 74:222, 1989.

193. Hanss M, Collen D: Secretion of tissue-type plasminogen activator and plasminogen activator inhibitor by cultured human endothelial cells: Modulation by thrombin, endotoxin, and histamine. *J Lab Clin Med* 109: 97, 1987.

194. Levin EG, Santell L: Stimulation and desensitization of tissue plasminogen activator release from human endothelial cells. *J Biol Chem* 263: 9360, 1988.

195. Shatos MA, Doherty JM, Orfeo T, et al: Modulation of the fibrinolytic response of cultured human vascular endothelium by extracellularly generated oxygen radicals. *J Biol Chem* 267:597, 1992.

196. Levin EG, Marotti KR, Santell L: Protein kinase C and the stimulation of tissue plasminogen activator release from human endothelial cells. *J Biol Chem* 264:16030, 1989.

197. Cugno M, Uziel L, Fabrizi I, et al: Fibrinolytic response in normal subjects to venous occlusion and DDAVP infusion. *Thromb Res* 56:625, 1989.

198. Kooistra T, Van den Berg J, Tons A, et al: Butyrate stimulates tissue type plasminogen activator synthesis in cultured human endothelial cells. *Biochem J* 247:605, 1987.

199. Diamond SL, Eskin SG, McIntire LV: Fluid flow stimulates tissue plasminogen activator secretion by cultured endothelial cells. *Science* 243:1483, 1989.

200. Diamond SL, Sharefkin JB, Dieffenbach C, et al: Tissue plasminogen activator messenger RNA levels increase in cultured human endothelial cells exposed to laminar shear stress. *J Cell Physiol* 143:364, 1990.

201. Levin EG, Santell L, Saljooque F: Hyperosmotic stress stimulates tissue plasminogen activator expression by a PKC-dependent pathway. *Am J Physiol* 265:C387, 1993.

202. Iba T, Shin T, Sonoda T, et al: Stimulation of endothelial secretion of tissue-type plasminogen activator by repetitive stretch. *J Surg Res* 50: 457, 1991.

203. Thompson EA, Nelles L, Collen D: Effect of retinoic acid on the synthesis of tissue-type plasminogen activator and plasminogen activator inhibitor 1 in human endothelial cells. *Eur J Biochem* 201:627, 1991.

204. Bulens F, Ibanez-Tallon I, Van Acker P, et al: Retinoic acid induction of human tissue-type plasminogen activator gene expression via a direct repeat element (DR5) located at -7 kilobases. *J Biol Chem* 270:7167, 1995.

205. Van Hinsbergh VWM, Bauer KA, Kooistra T, et al: Progress of fibrinolysis during tumor necrosis factor infusions in humans. Concomitant increase in tissue-type plasminogen activator, plasminogen activator inhibitor type-1, and fibrin(ogen) degradation products. *Blood* 76:2284, 1990.

206. Schleef RR, Bevilaqua MP, Sawdey M, et al: Cytokine activation of vascular endothelium: Effects on tissue-type plasminogen activator and type 1 plasminogen activator inhibitor. *J Biol Chem* 263:5797, 1988.

207. Hamsten A, Wiman B, De Faire U, Blomback M: Increased plasma levels of a rapid inhibitor of tissue plasminogen activator in young survivors of myocardial infarction. *N Engl J Med* 313:1557, 1985.

208. Pizzo SV, Murray JC, Gonias SL: Atrophie blanche: A disorder associated with defective release of tissue plasminogen activator. *Arch Pathol Lab Med* 110:517, 1986.

209. Kristensen P, Larson LI, Nielsen LS, et al: Human endothelial cells contain one type of plasminogen activator. *FEBS Lett* 168:33, 1984.

210. Yamamoto K, Loskutoff DJ: Fibrin deposition in tissues from endotoxin-treated mice correlates with decreases in the expression of urokinase-type but not tissue-type plasminogen activator. *J Clin Invest* 97: 2440, 1996.

211. Bacharach E, Itin A, Keshet E: In vivo patterns of expression of urokinase and its inhibitor PAI-1 suggest a concerted role in regulating physiological angiogenesis. *Proc Natl Acad Sci U S A* 89:10686, 1992.

212. Booyse FM, Scheinbuks J, Radek J, et al: Immunological identification and comparison of plasminogen activator forms in cultured normal human endothelial cells and smooth muscle cells. *Thromb Res* 24:495, 1981.

213. Van Hinsbergh VWM, Van den Berg EA, Fiers W, Dooijewaard G: Tumor necrosis factor induces the production of urokinase-type plasminogen activator by human endothelial cells. *Blood* 75:1991, 1990.

214. Sawdey M, Podor TJ, Loskutoff DJ: Regulation of type-1 plasminogen activator inhibitor gene expression in cultured bovine aortic endothelial cells. *J Biol Chem* 264:10396, 1989.

215. Van den Berg EA, Sprengers ED, Jaye M, et al: Regulation of plasminogen activator inhibitor-1 mRNA in human endothelial cells. *Thromb Haemost* 60:63, 1988.

216. Ellis V, Scully MF, Kakkar V: Plasminogen activation by single-chain urokinase in functional isolation. *J Biol Chem* 262:14998, 1987.

217. Almus-Jacobs F, Varki N, Sawdey MS, Loskutoff DJ: Endotoxin stimulates expression of the murine urokinase receptor gene in vivo. *Am J Pathol* 147:688, 1995.

218. Blasi F, Carmeliet P: UPAR: A versatile signaling orchestrator. *Nat Rev Mol Cell Biol* 3:932, 2002.

219. Schleef RR, Podor TJ, Dunne E, et al: The majority of type 1 plasminogen activator inhibitor associated with cultured human endothelial cells is located under the cells and is accessible to solution-phase tissue-type plasminogen activator. *J Cell Biol* 110:155, 1990.

220. Levin EG, Santell L: Association of a plasminogen activator inhibitor (PAI-1) with the growth substratum and membrane of human endothelial cells. *J Cell Biol* 105:2543, 1987.

221. Medina R, Socher SH, Han JH, Friedman PA: Interleukin-1, endotoxin, or tumor necrosis factor/cachectin enhance the level of plasminogen activator inhibitor messenger RNA in bovine aortic endothelial cells. *Thromb Res* 54:41, 1989.

222. Etingin OR, Hajjar DP, Hajjar KA, et al: Lipoprotein(a) regulates plasminogen activator inhibitor-1 expression in endothelial cells. *J Biol Chem* 266:2459, 1990.

223. Konkle B, Ginsburg D: The addition of endothelial cell growth factor and heparin to human endothelial cell cultures decrease plasminogen activator. *J Clin Invest* 82:579, 1988.

224. Greenberg ME, Brackenbury R, Edelman GM: Changes in the distribution of the 34-kdalton tyrosine kinase substrate during differentiation and maturation of chicken tissues. *J Cell Biol* 98:473, 1984.

225. Hamre KM, Chepenik KP, Goldowitz D: The annexins: Specific markers of midline structures and sensory neurons in the developing murine central nervous system. *J Comp Neurol* 352:421, 1995.

226. Gould KL, Cooper JA, Hunter T: The 46,000-dalton tyrosine kinase substrate is widespread, whereas the 36,000-dalton substrate is only expressed at high levels in certain rodent tissues. *J Cell Biol* 98:487, 1984.

227. Dreier R, Schmid KW, Gerke V, Riehemann K: Differential expression of annexins I, II, and IV in human tissues: An immunohistochemical study. *Histochem Cell Biol* 110:137, 1998.

228. Menell JS, Cesarman GM, Jacovina AT, et al: Annexin II and bleeding in acute promyelocytic leukemia. *N Engl J Med* 340:994, 1999.

229. Ishii H, Yoshida M, Hiraoka M, et al: Recombinant annexin II modulates impaired fibrinolytic activity in vitro and in rat carotid artery. *Circ Res* 89:1240, 2001.

230. Ling Q, Febbraio M, Deora B, et al: Annexin II is a key regulator of fibrin homeostasis and neoangiogenesis. *J Clin Invest* 113:38, 2004.

231. Jacovina AT, Zhong F, Khazanova E, et al: Neuritogenesis and the nerve growth factor-induced differentiation of PC-12 cells requires annexin II-mediated plasmin generation. *J Biol Chem* 276:49350, 2001.

232. Brownstein C, Deora AB, Jacovina AT, et al: Annexin II mediates plasminogen-dependent matrix invasion by human monocytes: Enhanced expression by macrophages. *Blood* 103:317, 2004.

233. Omar MN, Mann KG: Inactivation of Factor Va by plasmin. *J Biol Chem* 262:9750, 1987.

234. Esmon CT: The regulation of natural anticoagulant pathways. *Science* 235:1348, 1987.

235. Lee CD, Mann KG: Activation/inactivation of human factor V by plasmin. *Blood* 73:185, 1989.

236. McKee PA, Anderson JC, Switzer ME: Molecular structural studies of human factor VIII. *Ann N Y Acad Sci* 240:8, 1975.

237. Moser TL, Stack MS, Asplin I, et al: Angiostatin binds ATP synthase on the surface of human endothelial cells. *Proc Natl Acad Sci U S A* 96: 2811, 1999.

238. Stricker RB, Wong D, Shiu DT, et al: Activation of plasminogen by tissue plasminogen activator on normal and thrombasthenic platelets: Effects on surface proteins and platelet aggregation. *Blood* 68:275, 1986.

239. Adelman B, Michelson AD, Greenberg J, Handin RI: Proteolysis of platelet glycoprotein by plasmin is facilitated by plasmin lysine-binding regions. *Blood* 68:1280, 1986.

240. Schafer AI, Adelman B: Plasmin inhibition of platelet function and of arachidonate metabolism. *J Clin Invest* 75:456, 1985.

241. Puri RN, Zhou FX, Colman RF, Colman RW: Plasmin-induced platelet aggregation is accompanied by cleavage of aggregin and indirectly mediated by calpain. *Am J Physiol* 259:C862, 1990.

242. Schafer AI, Maas AK, Ware JA, et al: Platelet protein phosphorylation, elevation of cytosolic calcium, and inositol phospholipid breakdown in platelet activation induced by plasmin. *J Clin Invest* 78:73, 1986.

243. Loscalzo J, Vaughan DE: Tissue plasminogen activator promotes platelet disaggregation. *J Clin Invest* 79:1749, 1986.

244. Miles LA, Ginsberg MA, White JG, Plow EF: Plasminogen interacts with platelets through two distinct mechanisms. *J Clin Invest* 77:2001, 1986.

245. Gimple LW, Gold HK, Leinbach RC, et al: Correlation between template bleeding times and spontaneous bleeding during treatment of acute myocardial infarction with recombinant issue type plasminogen activator. *Blood* 80:581, 1989.

246. Coller BS: Platelets and thrombolytic therapy. *N Engl J Med* 322:33, 1990.

247. Ploplis VA, Carmeliet P, Vazirzadeh S, et al: Effects of disruption of the plasminogen gene on thrombosis, growth, and health in mice. *Circulation* 92:2585, 1995.

248. Bugge TH, Flick MJ, Daugherty CC, Degen JL: Plasminogen deficiency causes severe thrombosis but is compatible with development and reproduction. *Genes Dev* 9:794, 1995.

249. Romer J, Bugge TH, Pyke C, et al: Impaired wound healing in mice with a disrupted plasminogen gene. *Nat Med* 2:287, 1996.

250. Bugge TH, Kombrinck KW, Flick MJ, et al: Loss of fibrinogen rescues mice from the pleiotropic effects of plasminogen deficiency. *Cell* 87: 709, 1996.

251. Ploplis VA, French EL, Carmeliet P, et al: Plasminogen deficiency differentially affects recruitment of inflammatory cell populations in mice. *Blood* 91:2005, 1998.

252. Xiao Q, Danton MJS, Witte DP, et al: Plasminogen deficiency accel-

erates vessel wall disease in mice predisposed to atherosclerosis. *Proc Natl Acad Sci U S A* 94:10335, 1997.

253. Carmeliet P, Moons L, Lijnen R, et al: Urokinase-generated plasmin activates matrix metalloproteinases during aneurysm formation. *Nat Genet* 17:439, 1997.

254. Eitzman DT, Westrick RJ, Xu Z, et al: Plasminogen activator inhibitor-1 deficiency protects against atherosclerosis progression in the mouse carotid artery. *Blood* 96:4212, 2000.

255. Sjoland H, Eitzman DT, Gordon D, et al: Atherosclerosis progression in LDL receptor-deficient and apolipoprotein E-deficient mice is independent of genetic alterations in plasminogen activator inhibitor-1. *Arterioscler Thromb Vasc Biol* 20:846, 1999.

256. Luttun A, Lupu F, Storkebaum E, et al: Lack of plasminogen activator inhibitor-1 promotes growth and abnormal remodeling of advanced atherosclerotic plaque in apolipoprotein E-deficient mice. *Arterioscler Thromb Vasc Biol* 22:499, 2002.

257. Plow EF, Ploplis VA, Busuttil S, et al: A role of plasminogen in atherosclerosis and restenosis models in mice. *Thromb Haemost* 82(suppl 1):4, 1999.

258. Moons L, Wi C, Ploplis V, et al: Reduced transplant arteriosclerosis in plasminogen-deficient mice. *J Clin Invest* 102:1788, 1998.

259. Heymans S, Luttun A, Nuyens D, et al: Inhibition of plasminogen activators or matrix metalloproteinases prevents cardiac rupture but impairs therapeutic angiogenesis and causes cardiac failure. *Nat Med* 5: 1135, 2003.

260. Lijnen HR, Van Hoef B, Lupu F, et al: Function of the plasminogen/plasmin and matrix metalloproteinase systems after vascular injury in mice with targeted inactivation of fibrinolytic system genes. *Arterioscler Thromb Vasc Biol* 18:1035, 1998.

261. Carmeliet P, Moons L, Ploplis VA, et al: Impaired arterial neointima formation in mice with disruption of the plasminogen gene. *J Clin Invest* 99:200, 1997.

262. Carmeliet P, Moons L, Herbert JM, et al: Urokinase but not tissue plasminogen activator mediates arterial neointima formation in mice. *Circ Res* 81:829, 1997.

263. Carmeliet P, Moons L, Dewerchin M, et al: Receptor-independent role of urokinase-type plasminogen activator in pericellular plasmin and matrix metalloproteinase proteolysis during vascular wound healing in mice. *J Cell Biol* 140:233, 1998.

264. Carmeliet P, Moons L, Lijnen R, et al: Inhibitory role of plasminogen activator inhibitor-1 in arterial wound healing and neointima formation. *Circulation* 96:3180, 1997.

265. Konstantinides S, Schafer K, Loskutoff DJ: Do PAI-1 and vitronectin promote or inhibit neointima formation? *Arterioscler Thromb Vasc Biol* 22:1943, 2002.

266. Shi C, Patel A, Zhang D, et al: Plasminogen is not required for neointima formation in a mouse model of vein graft stenosis. *Circ Res* 84:883, 1999.

267. Eitzman DT, Westrick RJ, Nabel EG, Ginsburg D: Plasminogen activator inhibitor-1 and vitronectin promote vascular thrombosis in mice. *Blood* 95:577, 2000.

268. Konstantinides S, Schafer K, Thinnes T, Loskutoff DJ: Plasminogen activator inhibitor-1 and its cofactor vitronectin stabilize arterial thrombi following vascular injury in mice. *Circulation* 103:576, 2001.

269. Schafer K, Konstantinides S, Riedel C, et al: Different mechanisms of increased luminal stenosis after arterial injury in mice deficient for urokinase- or tissue-type plasminogen activator. *Circulation* 106:1847, 2002.

270. Schafer K, Muller K, Hecker A, et al: Enhanced thrombosis in atherosclerosis-prone mice is associated with increased arterial expression of plasminogen activator. *Arterioscler Thromb Vasc Biol* 23:2097, 2003.

271. Zhu Y, Farrehi PM, Fay WP: Plasminogen activator inhibitor type 1

enhances neointima formation after oxidative vascular injury in ather-osclerosis-prone mice. *Circulation* 103:3105, 2001.

272. Ploplis VA, Cornelissen I, Sandoval-Cooper MJ, et al: Remodeling of the vessel wall after copper-induced injury is highly attenuated in mice with a total deficiency of plasminogen activator inhibitor-1. *Am J Pathol* 158:107, 2001.

273. DeYoung MB, Tom C, Dichek DA: Plasminogen activator inhibitor type 1 increases neointima formation in balloon-injured rat carotid arteries. *Circulation* 104:1972, 2001.

274. Grainger DJ, Kemp PR, Metcalfe JC, et al: The serum concentration of active transforming growth factor-β is severely depressed in advanced atherosclerosis. *Nat Med* 1995;1:74, 1995.

275. Herbert JM, Carmeliet P: Involvement of u-PA in the anti-apoptotic activity of TGFbeta for vascular smooth muscle cells. *FEBS Lett* 413:401, 1997.

276. Herbert JM, Lamarche I, Carmeliet P: Urokinase and tissue-type plasminogen activator are required for the mitogenic and chemotactic effects of bovine fibroblast growth factor and platelet-derived growth factor-BB for vascular smooth muscle cells. *J Biol Chem* 272:23585, 1997.

277. Scanu AM, Fless GM: Lipoprotein(a) heterogeneity and biologic relevance. *J Clin Invest* 85:1709, 1990.

278. Utermann G: The mysteries of lipoprotein(a). *Science* 246:904, 1989.

279. Loscalzo J: Lipoprotein(a), a unique risk factor for atherothrombotic disease. *Arteriosclerosis* 10:672, 1990.

280. Hajjar KA, Nachman RL: The role of lipoprotein(a) in atherogenesis and thrombosis. *Ann Rev Med* 47:423, 1996.

281. Bauer PI, Machovich R, Buki KG, et al: Interaction of plasmin with endothelial cells. *Biochem J* 218:119, 1984.

282. McLean JW, Tomlinson JE, Kuang WJ, et al: CDNA sequence of human apolipoprotein(a) is homologous to plasminogen. *Nature* 330:132, 1987.

283. Weitkamp LR, Guttormsen SA, Schultz JS: Linkage between the loci for the Lp(a) lipoprotein (Lp) and plasminogen (PLG). *Hum Genet* 79:80, 1988.

284. Neven L, Khalil A, Pfaffinger D, et al: Rhesus monkey model of familial hypercholesterolemia: Relation between plasma Lp(a) levels, apo(a) isoforms and LDL-receptor function. *J Lipid Res* 31:633, 1990.

285. Pfaffinger D, Schuelke J, Kim C, et al: Relationship between apo(a) isoforms and Lp(a) density in subjects with different apo(a) phenotype: A study before and after a fatty meal. *J Lipid Res* 32:679, 1991.

286. Utermann G, Menzel HJ, Kraft HG, et al: Lp(a) glycoprotein phenotypes. *J Clin Invest* 80:458, 1987.

287. Maeda S, Abe A, Seishima M, et al: Transient changes of serum lipoprotein(a) as an acute phase protein. *Atherosclerosis* 78:145, 1989.

288. Wright LC, Sullivan DR, Muller M, et al: Elevated apolipoprotein(a) levels in cancer patients. *Int J Cancer* 43:241, 1989.

289. Gavish D, Azrolan N, Breslow JL: Fish oil reduces plasma Lp(a) levels and affects post-prandial association of apo(a) with triglyceride rich lipoproteins. *J Clin Invest* 84:2021, 1989.

290. Koschinsky ML, Beisiegel U, Henne-Bruns D, et al: Apolipoprotein(a) size heterogeneity is related to variable number of repeat sequences in its mRNA. *Biochemistry* 29:640, 1990.

291. Lerch PG, Rickli EE, Lergier W, Gillessen D: Localization of individual lysine-binding regions in human plasminogen and investigations on their complex-forming properties. *Eur J Biochem* 107:7, 1980.

292. Armstrong VW, Harrach B, Robenek H, et al: Heterogeneity of human lipoprotein Lp(a): Cytochemical and biochemical studies on the interaction of two Lp(a) species with the LDL receptor. *J Lipid Res* 31:429, 1990.

293. Wolf K, Rith M, Niendorf A, et al: Thrombosis: Cellular elements of the vasculature. *Circulation* 80, 1989.

294. Grainger DJ, Kemp PR, Liu AC, et al: Activation of transforming growth factor-beta is inhibited in transgenic apolipoprotein(a) mice. *Nature* 370:460, 1994.

295. Palabrica TM, Liu AC, Aronovitz MJ, et al: Antifibrinolytic activity of apolipoprotein(a) in vivo: Human apolipoprotein(a) transgenic mice are resistant to tissue plasminogen activator-mediated thrombolysis. *Nat Med* 1:256, 1995.

296. Petros AM, Ramesh V, Llinas M: NMR studies of aliphatic ligand binding to human plasminogen kringle 4. *Biochemistry* 28:1368, 1989.

297. Hajjar KA: The endothelial cell tissue plasminogen activator receptor: Specific interaction with plasminogen. *J Biol Chem* 266:21962, 1991.

298. Hajjar KA, Gavish D, Breslow J, Nachman RL: Lipoprotein(a) modulation of endothelial cell surface fibrinolysis and its potential role in atherosclerosis. *Nature* 339:303, 1989.

299. Gonzales-Gronow M, Edelberg JM, Pizzo SV: Further characterization of the cellular plasminogen binding site: Evidence that plasminogen 2 and lipoprotein a compete for the same site. *Biochemistry* 28:2374, 1989.

300. Miles LA, Fless GM, Levin EG, et al: A potential basis for the thrombotic risks associated with lipoprotein(a). *Nature* 339:301, 1989.

301. Stiko Rahm A, Wiman B, Hamsten A, Nilsson J: Secretion of plasminogen activator inhibitor-1 from cultured human umbilical vein endothelial cells is induced by very low density lipoprotein. *Arteriosclerosis* 10:1067, 1990.

302. Edelberg JM, Gonzalez-Gronow M, Pizzo SV: Lipoprotein(a) inhibition of plasminogen activation by tissue-type plasminogen activator. *Thromb Res* 57:155, 1990.

303. Loscalzo J, Weinfeld M, Fless G, Scanu AM: Lipoprotein(a), fibrin binding, and plasminogen activation. *Arteriosclerosis* 10:240, 1990.

304. Lawn RM, Wade DP, Hammer RE, et al: Atherogenesis in transgenic mice expressing human apolipoprotein(a). *Nature* 360:670, 1992.

305. Boonmark NW, Lou XJ, Schwartz K, et al: Modification of apolipoprotein(a) lysine binding site reduces atherosclerosis in transgenic mice. *J Clin Invest* 100:558, 1997.

306. Kraus JP: Molecular basis of phenotype expression in homocystinuria. *J Inherit Metab Dis* 17:383, 1994.

307. Boushey CJ, Beresford SAA, Omenn GS, Motulsky AG: A quantitative assessment of plasma homocysteine as a risk factor for vascular disease. *JAMA* 274:1049, 1995.

308. Refsum H, Ueland PM, Nygard O, Vollset SE: Homocysteine and cardiovascular disease. *Annu Rev Med* 49:31, 1998.

309. Hajjar KA: Homocysteine-induced modulation of tissue plasminogen activator binding to its endothelial cell membrane receptor. *J Clin Invest* 91:2873, 1993.

310. Hajjar KA, Mauri L, Jacovina AT, et al: Tissue plasminogen activator binding to the annexin II tail domain: Direct modulation by homocysteine. *J Biol Chem* 273:9987, 1998.

311. Wilkins PP, Moore KL, McEver RP, Cummings RD: Tyrosine sulfation of P-selectin glycoprotein ligand-1 is required for high affinity binding to P-selectin. *J Biol Chem* 270:22677, 1995.

312. Snapp KR, Craig R, Herron M, et al: Dimerization of P-selectin glycoprotein ligand-1 (PSGL-1) required for optimal recognition of P-selectin. *J Cell Biol* 142:263, 1998.

313. Tanaka Y, Adams Dh, Hubscher S, et al: T-cell adhesion induced by proteoglycan-immobilized cytokine MIP-1 beta. *Nature* 361:79, 1993.

314. Lo SK, Lee S, Ramos RA, et al: Endothelial-leukocyte adhesion molecule 1 stimulates the adhesive activity of leukocyte integrin CD3 [CD11B/CD18, Mac-1, alpha m beta 2] on human neutrophils. *J Exp Med* 173:1493, 1991.

315. Lorant DE, Patel KD, McIntyre TM, et al: Coexpression of GMP-140 and PAF by endothelium stimulated by histamine or thrombin: A juxtacrine system for adhesion and activation of neutrophils. *J Cell Biol* 115:223, 1991.

316. Huber AR, Kunkel SL, Todd RF, Weiss SL: Regulation of transendothelial neutrophil migration by endogenous interleukin-8. *Science* 254:99, 1991.

317. Tanaka Y, Albelda SM, Horgan KJ, et al: CD31 expressed on distinctive T cell subsets is a preferential amplifier of beta 1 integrin-mediated adhesion. *J Exp Med* 176:245, 1992.

318. Piali L, Albelda SM, Baldwin HS, et al: Murine platelet endothelial cell adhesion molecule (PECAM-1/CD31) modulates beta2 integrins on lymphokine-activated killer cells. *Eur J Immunol* 23:2464, 1993.

319. Berman ME, Muller WA: Ligation of platelet/endothelial cell adhesion molecule 1 (PECAM-1/CD31) on monocytes and neutrophils increases binding capacity of leukocyte CR3 (CD11b/CD18). *J Immunol* 154:299, 1995.

320. Carlos TM, Harlan JM: Leukocyte-endothelial cell adhesion molecules. *Blood* 84:2068, 1994.

321. Hynes RO: Integrins: Versatility, modulation, and signaling in cell adhesion. *Cell* 69:11, 1992.

322. Miller J, Knorr R, Ferrone M, et al: Intercellular adhesion molecule-1 dimerization and its consequences for adhesion mediated by lymphocyte function associated molecule-1. *J Exp Med* 182:1231, 1995.

323. Reilly PL, Woska RJR, Jeanfavre DD, et al: The native structure of intercellular adhesion molecule-1(ICAM-1) is a dimer. Correlation with binding to LFA-1. *J Immunol* 155:529, 1995.

324. Bargatze RF, Kurk S, Butcher EC, Jutila MA: Neutrophils roll on adherent neutrophils bound to cytokine-induced endothelial cells via L-selectin on the rolling cells. *J Exp Med* 180:1785, 1994.

325. Walcheck B, Moore KL, McEver RP, Kishimoto TK: Neutrophil-neutrophil interactions under hydrodynamic shear stress involve L-selectin and PSGL-1. *J Clin Invest* 98:1081, 1996.

326. Muller WA: Migration of leukocytes across the vascular intima. Molecules and mechanisms. *Trends Cardiovasc Med* 5:15, 1995.

327. Muller WA: Leukocyte-endothelial cell interactions in leukocyte transmigration and the inflammatory response. *Trends Immunol* 24:326, 2003.

328. Muller WA, Ratti CM, McDonnell SL, Cohn ZA: A human endothelial cell-restricted, externally disposed plasmalemmal protein enriched in intercellular junctions. *J Exp Med* 170:399, 1989.

329. Newman PJ, Berndt MC, Gorski J, et al: PECAM-1 [CD31] cloning and relation to adhesion molecules of the immunoglobulin gene superfamily. *Science* 247:1219, 1990.

330. Muller WA, Weigl SA, Deng X, Phillips DM: PECAM-1 is required for transendothelial migration of leukocytes. *J Exp Med* 178:449, 1993.

331. Huang AJ, Manning JE, Bandak TM, et al: Endothelial cell cytosolic free calcium regulates neutrophil migration across monolayers of endothelial cells. *J Cell Biol* 120:1371, 1993.

332. Liao F, Huynh HK, Eiroa A, et al: Migration of monocytes across endothelium and passage through extracellular matrix involve separate molecular domains of PECAM-1. *J Exp Med* 182:1337, 1995.

333. Liao F, Ali J, Greene T, Muller WA: Soluble domain 1 of platelet-endothelial cell adhesion molecule (PECAM) is sufficient to block transendothelial migration in vitro and in vivo. *J Exp Med* 185:1349, 1997.

334. Ostermann G, Weber KSC, Zernecke A, et al: JAM-1 is a ligand for the b2 integrin LFA-1 involved in transendothelial migration of leukocytes. *Nat Immunol* 3:151, 2002.

335. Johnson-Leger C, Aurrand-Lions M, Beltraminelli N, et al: Junctional adhesion molecule-2 (JAM-2) promotes lymphocyte transendothelial migration. *Blood* 100:2479, 2002.

336. Feng D, Nagy JA, Pyne K, et al: Neutrophils emigrate from venules by a transendothelial cell pathway in response to fMLP. *J Exp Med* 187:903, 1999.

337. Schenkel AR, Mamdouh Z, Chen X, et al: CD99 plays a major role in the migration of monocytes through endothelial junctions. *Nat Immunol* 3:2479, 2002.

338. Marchesi VT, Florey HW: Electron micrographic observations on the emigration of leukocytes. *J Exp Physiol* 45:343, 1960.

339. Leeuwenberg JFM, Von Asmuth EJ, Jeunhomme TM, Buurman WA: IFN-gamma regulates the expression of the adhesion molecule ELAM-1 and IL-6 production by human endothelial cells in vitro. *J Immunol* 145:2110, 1990.

340. Strindall J, Lundblad A, Pahlsson P: Interferon-gamma enhancement of E-selectin expression on endothelial cells is inhibited by monensin. *Scand J Immunol* 46:338, 1997.

341. Ley K, Arbones ML, Bosse R, et al: Sequential contribution of L- and P-selectin to leukocyte rolling in vivo. *J Exp Med* 181:669, 1995.

342. Khew-Goodall Y, Butcher E, Litwin MS, et al: Chronic expression of P-selectin on endothelial cells stimulated by the T-cell cytokine, interleukin-3. *Blood* 87:1432, 1999.

343. Yao L, Pan J, Setiadi H, et al: Interleukin-4 or oncostatin M induces a prolonged increase in P-selectin mRNA and protein in human endothelial cells. *J Exp Med* 184:81, 1996.

344. Jung U, Ley K: Regulation of E-selectin, P-selectin, and intercellular adhesion molecule-1 expression in mouse cremaster vasculature. *Microcirculation* 4:311, 1997.

345. Pan J, Xia L, Yao L, McEver RP: Tumor necrosis factor-alpha- or lipopolysaccharide-induced expression of the murine P-selectin gene in endothelial cells involves novel kappaB sites and a variant activating transcription factor/cAMP response element. *J Biol Chem* 273:10067, 1998.

346. Masinovsky B, Urdal D, Gallatin WM: IL-4 acts synergistically with IL-1 beta to promote lymphocyte adhesion to microvascular endothelium by induction of vascular cell adhesion molecule-1. *J Immunol* 145:2886, 1990.

347. Blease K, Seybold J, Adcock IM, et al: Interleukin-4 and lipopolysaccharide synergize to induce vascular adhesion molecule-1 expression in human lung microvascular endothelial cells. *Am J Respir Cell Mol Biol* 18:620, 1998.

348. Pober JS, Collins T, Gimbrone M, et al: Inducible expression of class II major histocompatibility complex antigens and the immunogenicity of vascular endothelium. *Transplantation* 41:141, 1986.

349. Savage COS, Hughes CCW, McIntyre BW, et al: CD4+ cells proliferate to HLA-DR+ allogeneic vascular endothelium. Identification of accessory interactions. *Transplantation* 56:128, 1993.

350. Pober JS, Orosz CG, Rose ML, Savage COS: Can graft endothelial cells initiate a host anti-graft immune response? *Transplantation* 61:343, 1996.

351. Romer LH, McLean NV, Horng-Chin Yet al: IFN-gamma and TNF-alpha induce redistribution of PECAM-1 [CD31] on human endothelial cells. *J Immunol* 154:6582, 1995.

352. Tang Q, Hendricks RL: Interferon gamma regulates platelet endothelial cell adhesion molecule-1 expression and neutrophil infiltration into herpes simplex virus-infected mouse corneas. *J Exp Med* 184:1435, 1996.

353. Rival Y, Del Maschio A, Rabiet MJ, et al: Inhibition of platelet endothelial cell adhesion molecule-1 synthesis and leukocyte transmigration in endothelial cells by the combined action of TNFα and IFNα. *J Immunol* 157:1233, 1996.

354. Kaplanski G, Fabrigoule M, Boulay V, et al: Thrombin induces endothelial type II activation in vitro: IL-1- and TNF-alpha-independent IL-8 secretion and E-selectin expression. *J Immunol* 158:5435, 1997.

355. Diacovo TG, Puri KD, Warnock RA, et al: Platelet-mediated lymphocyte delivery to high endothelial venules. *Science* 273:252, 1996.

356. Diacovo TG, Catalina MD, Siegelman MH, Von Adrian UH: Circulating activated platelets reconstitute lymphocyte homing and immunity in L-selectin-deficient mice. *J Exp Med* 187:197, 1998.

357. Buttrum SM, Hatton R, Nash GB: Selectin-mediated rolling of neutrophils on immobilized platelets. *Blood* 82:1165, 1993.

358. Diacovo TG, Roth SJ, Buccola JM, et al: Neutrophil rolling, arrest, and transmigration across activated, surface-adherent platelets via sequential action of P-selectin and the beta 2-integrin CD11b/CD18. *Blood* 88:146, 1996.

359. Diacovo TG, De Fougerolles AR, Bainton DF, Springer TA: A functional integrin ligand on the surface of platelets: Intercellular adhesion molecule-2. *J Clin Invest* 94:1243, 1994.

360. Simon DI, Chen Z, Xu H, et al: Platelet glycoprotein Ibα is a counter-receptor for the leukocyte integrin Mac-1 (CD11b/CD18). *J Exp Med* 192:193, 2000.

361. Santoso S, Sachs UJ, Kroll H, et al: The junctional adhesion molecule 3 (JAM-3) on human platelets is a counterreceptor for the leukocyte integrin Mac-1. *J Exp Med* 196:679, 2002.

362. Frenette PS, Denis CV, Weiss L, et al: P-selectin glycoprotein ligand 1 (PSGL-) is expressed on platelets and can mediate platelet-endothelial interactions in vivo. *J Exp Med* 191:1413, 2000.

363. Altieri DC: Coagulation assembly on leukocytes in transmembrane signaling and cell adhesion. *Blood* 81:569, 1993.

364. Lo SK, Cheung A, Zheng Q, Silverstein RL: Induction of tissue factor in monocytes by adhesion to endothelial cells. *J Immunol* 154:4768, 1995.

365. Fan ST, Mackman N, Cui MZ, Edgington TS: Integrin regulation of an inflammatory effector gene: Direct induction of the tissue factor promoter by engagement of b1 or a4 integrin chains. *J Immunol* 154:3266, 1995.

366. Randolph GJ, Luther T, Albrecht S, et al: Role of tissue factor adhesion of mononuclear phagocytes to and trafficking through endothelium. *Blood* 92:4167, 1998.

367. Palabrica T, Lobb R, Furie BC, et al: Leukocyte accumulation promoting fibrin deposition is mediated in vivo by P-selectin on adherent platelets. *Nature* 359:848, 1992.

368. Wright SD, Weitz JI, Huang AJ, et al: Complement receptor type [CR3, CD11b/CD18] of human polymorphonuclear leukocytes recognizes fibrinogen. *Proc Natl Acad Sci U S A* 85:7734, 1988.

369. Altieri DC, Morrisey JH, Edgington TS: Adhesive receptor Mac-1 co-ordinates the activation of factor X on stimulated cells of monocytic and myeloid differentiation: An alternative initiation of the coagulation protease cascade. *Proc Natl Acad Sci U S A* 85:7462, 1988.

370. Altieri DC, Edgington TS: The saturable high affinity association of factor X to ADP-stimulated monocytes defines a novel function of the Mac-1 receptor. *J Biol Chem* 263:7007, 1988.

371. Peng L, Bhatia N, Parker AC, et al: Endogenous vitronectin and plasminogen activator inhibitor-1 promote neointima formation in murine carotid arteries. *Arterioscler Thromb Vasc Biol* 22:934, 2002.

372. de Waard V, Armitage RJ, Carmeliet P, et al: Plasminogen activator inhibitor-1 and vitronectin protect against stenosis in a murine carotid ligation model. *Arterioscler Thromb Vasc Biol* 22:1978, 2002.

373. Alon R, Fassner PD, Carr MW, et al: The integrin VLA-4 supports tethering and rolling on VCAM-1. *J Cell Biol* 128:1243, 1995.

374. Berlin CBRF, Campbell JJ, Von Andrian UH, et al: Alpha 4 integrins mediate lymphocyte attachment and rolling under physiologic flow. *Cell* 80:413, 1995.

375. Serhan CN: Eicosanoids and related compounds, in *Arthritis and Allied Conditions: A Textbook of Rheumatology*, edited by WJ Koopman, LW Moreland, p 517. Lippincott Williams & Wilkins, Philadelphia, 2004.

376. Huber R, Berendes R, Burger A, et al: Crystal and molecular structure of human annexin V after refinement: Implications for structure, membrane binding and ion channel formation of the annexin family of proteins. *J Mol Biol* 223:683, 1992.

377. Huang K-S, Wallner BP, Mattaliano RJ, et al: Two human 35 kd inhibitors of phospholipase A2 are related to substrates of pp60 v-src and of the epidermal growth factor receptor/kinase. *Cell* 46:191, 1986.

378. Blasi F, Conese M, Moller LB, et al: The urokinase receptor: Structure, regulation and inhibitor-mediated internalization. *Fibrinolysis* 8:182, 1994.

CLASSIFICATION, CLINICAL MANIFESTATIONS, AND EVALUATION OF DISORDERS OF HEMOSTASIS

URI SELIGSOHN
KENNETH KAUSHANSKY

Evaluation of a hemostatic disorder is commonly initiated when (1) a patient or referring physician suspects a bleeding tendency, (2) a bleeding tendency is discovered in one or more family members, (3) an abnormal coagulation assay result is obtained from an individual as part of a routine examination, (4) an abnormal assay result is obtained from a patient during preparation for surgery, or (5) a patient has unexplained diffuse bleeding during or after surgery or following trauma. Evaluation of a possible hemostatic disorder in each of these scenarios is a stepwise process that requires knowledge of the various classes of hemostatic disorders commonly found under the particular circumstances. The patient's history, the results of physical examination, and an initial set of hemostatic tests usually enable a tentative diagnosis. However, more specific tests are commonly necessary to make a definitive diagnosis. This chapter reviews the necessary steps.

CLASSIFICATION OF HEMOSTATIC DISORDERS

Hemostatic disorders can conveniently be classified as either hereditary or acquired (Table 109-1). Alternatively, hemostatic disorders can be classified according to the mechanism of the defect. Of the acquired disorders, the thrombocytopenias are the most frequently encountered entities. Thrombocytopenias can result from reduced production of platelets, excessive destruction caused by antibodies or other consumptive processes, or pooling of platelets in the spleen, as in hypersplenism (see Chap. 110).

BLEEDING HISTORY

The bleeding history is a crucial element in the evaluation of a patient with a hemorrhagic disorder. The bleeding history helps define the subsequent diagnostic approach and the likelihood of future bleeding. Eliciting and interpreting all of the relevant information requires a systematic and methodical approach. The following points are worth considering.

1. Patients vary in their responses to hemorrhagic symptoms. Some patients ignore significant symptoms, whereas other patients are highly sensitive to even minor symptoms. When asked in standardized questionnaires, many normal, healthy people indicate they have excessive bleeding or bruising.[1,2] Therefore, some experts believe the question "Do you bruise easily?" is virtually worthless. Women more likely respond that they have excessive bleeding or bruising than do men.

2. Patients with severe hemorrhagic disorders invariably have very abnormal bleeding histories.

3. The diagnostic value of any specific symptom varies in the different disorders. Therefore, recognizing typical patterns of bleeding is important (Table 109-2). Unprovoked hemarthroses and muscle hemorrhages suggest one of the hemophilias, whereas mucocutaneous bleeding (epistaxis, gingival bleeding, menorrhagia) are more characteristic of patients with qualitative platelet disorders, thrombocytopenia, or von Willebrand disease.

4. Assessing the extent of hemorrhage against the background of any trauma or provocation that may have elicited the hemorrhage is important. If a patient has never had a significant hemostatic challenge, such as tooth extraction, surgery, trauma, or childbirth, the lack of a significant bleeding history is much less valuable in excluding a mild hemorrhagic disorder. For example, a significant percentage of patients with mild von Willebrand disease or mild forms of hemophilia may have negative bleeding histories,[1] even though they may be at considerable risk for excessive bleeding after surgery or other interventions. Thus, these diagnoses must be considered even in elderly patients if their first severe hemostatic challenge occurs at that age.

5. Obtaining objective confirmation of the subjective information conveyed in the bleeding history is valuable. Objective data include (1) previous hospital or physician visits for bleeding symptoms and the results of previous laboratory evaluations, (2) previous transfusions of blood products, and (3) a history of anemia and/or previous treatment with iron.

6. Although self-administered questionnaires may provide useful background information, they are not a substitute for a dialogue between physician and patient. Thus, history taking in general, but especially in the often subtle histories related to hemostatic disorders, is an intellectually active process involving data collection, hypothesis development, new question formulation, additional data gathering, and new hypothesis development. However, this procedure has its limitations even when it is carefully persued.[3,4]

7. A medication history is a crucial component of the bleeding history, with particular attention to nonprescription drugs, such as aspirin and nonsteroidal antiinflammatory agents, which may affect bleeding symptoms. A medication history is especially important in patients with thrombocytopenia, because drug-induced thrombocytopenia is common (see Chap. 110 and Table 109-1). Medication also may affect hemostasis through effects on the liver or kidney (see Chap. 120). The increased use of herbal and alternative medicines poses particular problems, because patients may not readily share information about what they are taking, and the dose they are taking of any particular active ingredient may be difficult to determine. Ginkgo and ginseng are the most commonly used herbals that can affect coagulation. Resources for assessing the effects and side effects of such therapies are limited, but books (e.g., *PDR for Herbal Medicines*), articles,[5] and Internet-based databases[6] are now available.

8. A nutrition history should be obtained to assess the likelihood of (1) vitamin K deficiency, especially if the patient also is taking broad-spectrum antibiotics, (2) vitamin C deficiency, especially if the patient has skin bleeding consistent with scurvy, and (3) general malnutrition and/or malabsorption. In patients taking oral anticoagulants, the patient should be counseled to try to maintain

TABLE 109-1   CLASSIFICATION OF DISORDERS OF HEMOSTASIS

Major Types	Disorders	Examples
Acquired	Thrombocytopenias	Autoimmune and alloimmune, drug-induced, hypersplenism, hypoplastic (primary, suppressive, myelophthisic), DIC, thrombotic thrombocytopenic purpura (see Chaps. 110 and 121)
	Liver diseases	Cirrhosis, acute hepatic failure, liver transplantation (see Chap. 120), thrombopoietin deficiency
	Renal failure	
	Vitamin K deficiency	Malabsorption syndrome, hemorrhagic disease of the newborn, prolonged antibiotic therapy, malnutrition, prolonged biliary obstruction
	Hematologic disorders	Acute leukemias (particularly promyelocytic), myelodysplasias, monoclonal gammopathies, essential thrombocythemia (see Chaps. 86, 87, and 111)
	Acquired antibodies against coagulation factors	Neutralizing antibodies against factors V, VIII, and XIII, accelerated clearance of antibody-factor complexes, e.g., acquired von Willebrand disease, hypoprothrombinemia associated with antiphospholipid antibodies (see Chaps. 118, 119, and 123)
	Disseminated intravascular coagulation	Acute (sepsis, malignancies, trauma, obstetric complications) and chronic (malignancies, giant hemangiomas, missed abortion) (see Chap. 121)
	Drugs	Antiplatelet agents, anticoagulants, antithrombins, and thrombolytic, myelosuppressive, hepatotoxic, and nephrotoxic agents (see Chaps. 21, 125–127)
	Vascular	Nonpalpable purpura ("senile," solar, and factitious purpura), use of corticosteroids, vitamin C deficiency, child abuse, thromboembolic, purpura fulminans; palpable-purpura (Henoch-Schönlein, vasculitis, dysproteinemias) (see Chap. 114), amyloidosis
Inherited	Deficiencies of coagulation factors	Hemophilia A (factor VIII deficiency), hemophilia B (factor IX deficiency), deficiencies of fibrinogen factors II, V, VII, X, XI, and XIII and von Willebrand disease (see Chaps. 115 116 117 118)
	Platelet disorders	Glanzmann thrombasthenia, Bernard-Soulier syndrome, platelet granule disorders. (see Chap. 112)
	Fibrinolytic disorders	α_2-Antiplasmin deficiency, plasminogen activator inhibitor-1 deficiency (see Chap. 127)
	Vascular	Hemorrhagic telangiectasias (see Chap. 114)
	Connective tissue disorders	Ehlers-Danlos syndrome (see Chap. 114)

Therefore, hereditary hemorrhagic telangiectasias, Cushing disease, scurvy, Ehlers-Danlos syndrome, and vasculitis must be considered in the differential diagnosis. Many primary dermatologic disorders also have a purpuric or hemorrhagic component and must also be considered in the differential diagnosis (see Chap. 114).

12. A family history is particularly important when hereditary disorders are considered. Patients usually will not spontaneously offer a history of consanguinity, so specific inquiry should be made about this possibility. A diagram of the patient's genealogic tree, extending back at least two generations, should be included to document consideration of genetic disorders. A sex-linked pattern of inheritance is consistent with hemophilia A or B (see Chap. 115). An autosomal dominant pattern is characteristic of most forms of von Willebrand disease (see Chap. 118). An autosomal recessive pattern is typical for all other coagulation factor deficiencies (see Chap. 116), inherited platelet disorders (see Chap. 112), and the rare severe, type 3 von Willebrand disease. Population genetic information may be helpful, for example, the higher prevalence of factor XI deficiency in Ashkenazi Jews (see Chap. 116).

13. The history should include information on diseases and organs that may affect hemostasis, such as cirrhosis, renal insufficiency, essential thrombocythemia, acute leukemia, systemic lupus erythematosus, and Gaucher disease (see Table 109-1).

Individual hemorrhagic symptoms often require detailed analysis before the significance of the symptoms with regard to the patient's diagnosis or proper therapy can be determined. Some of the more common symptoms are discussed below.

A. Epistaxis is one of the most common symptoms of platelet disorders and von Willebrand disease. It also is the most common symptom of hereditary hemorrhagic telangiectasias. In the latter condition, epistaxis almost always becomes more severe with advancing age. Epistaxis is not uncommon in normal children, but it usually resolves before puberty. Dry air heating systems can provoke epistaxis even in otherwise normal individuals. Bleeding confined to a single nostril more likely results from a local vascular problem than a systemic coagulopathy.

B. Gingival hemorrhage is very common in patients with both qualitative and quantitative platelet abnormalities and von Willebrand disease. Occasional gum bleeding occurs in normal individuals, especially with tooth brushing using a hard bristle tooth brush and dental hygiene procedures. Thus, establishing whether the bleeding is excessive may be difficult. Frequent gingival hemorrhage can occur in individuals with normal hemostasis if they have gingivitis.

C. Oral mucous membrane bleeding in the form of blood blisters is a common manifestation of severe thrombocytopenia. Such

a consistent level of vitamin K intake. Major alterations in diet should be discouraged unless accompanied by more frequent monitoring of the prothrombin time (PT). Similarly, new vitamins and food supplements should be checked for their vitamin K content.

9. Several tissues have high local levels of fibrinolytic activity. Such tissues include the urinary tract, endometrium, and mucous membranes of the nose and oral cavity. These sites are particularly likely to have prolonged oozing of blood after trauma in patients with hemostatic abnormalities. Excessive bleeding following tooth extraction is one of the most common manifestations.

10. Bleeding isolated to a single organ or system (e.g., hematuria, hematemesis, hemoptysis) less likely results from a hemostatic abnormality than a local cause such as a neoplasm, an ulcer, or angiodysplasia. Thus, careful anatomic evaluation of the involved organ or system should be performed.

11. Bleeding or excessive hemorrhage may result from blood vessel disorders and disorders of platelets or coagulation proteins.

TABLE 109-2 CLINICAL MANIFESTATIONS TYPICALLY ASSOCIATED WITH SPECIFIC HEMOSTATIC DISORDERS

CLINICAL MANIFESTATIONS	HEMOSTATIC DISORDERS
Mucocutaneous bleeding	Thrombocytopenias, platelet dysfunction, von Willebrand disease
Cephalhematomas in newborns, hemarthroses, hematuria, and intramuscular, intracerebral and retroperitoneal hemorrhages	Severe hemophilias A and B, severe deficiencies of factor VII, X, or XIII, severe type 3 von Willebrand disease, afibrinogenemia
Injury-related bleeding and mild spontaneous bleeding	Mild and moderate hemophilias A and B, severe factor XI deficiency, moderate deficiencies of fibrinogen and factors II, V, VII, or X, combined factors V and VIII deficiency, α_2-antiplasmin deficiency
Bleeding from stump of umbilical cord and habitual abortions	Afibrinogenemia, hypofibrinogenemia, dysfibrinogenemia, or factor XIII deficiency
Impaired wound healing	Factor XIII deficiency
Facial purpura in newborns	Glanzmann thrombasthenia, severe thrombocytopenia
Recurrent severe epistaxis and chronic iron deficiency anemia	Hereditary hemorrhagic telangiectasias

bleeding usually has a predilection for sites where teeth can traumatize the inner surface of the cheek.

D. Skin hemorrhage in the form of petechiae and ecchymoses are common manifestations of hemostatic disorders. However, skin hemorrhage also is common among individuals without hemostatic disorders. Excessive bruising is more common in women than men. Moreover, women frequently note that the severity of their bruising varies with the phase of their menstrual cycle, although the most severe phase of the cycle may differ in different women. Features that help establish the severity of skin hemorrhage include the size of the bruises, the frequency of bruising, whether the bruises occur spontaneously or only with trauma, and the appearance of bruises on regions of the body that usually are not traumatized, such as the trunk and back. The color of the bruise may yield information. Red bruises on the extensor surfaces of the arms and hands indicate loss of supporting tissues, as occurs in Cushing syndrome, glucocorticoid therapy, senile purpura, and damage from chronic sun exposure. Jet-black bruises may be caused by warfarin-induced skin necrosis and similar disorders.

E. Tooth extractions are common hemostatic challenges and may be helpful in defining the risk of bleeding. Molar extractions are greater hemostatic challenges than extractions of other teeth. Objective data regarding excessive bleeding based on the need for blood products or the need to pack or suture the extraction site are valuable.

F. Excessive bleeding in response to razor nicks is common in patients with platelet disorders or von Willebrand disease. If patients indicate they use an electric razor or a depilatory, ask if they ever used a blade razor and, if so, why they switched.

G. Hemoptysis almost never is the presenting symptom of a bleeding disorder and is rare even in patients with serious bleeding disorders. However, blood-tinged sputum in association with upper respiratory tract infections may be more common in patients with hemostatic disorders.

H. Hematemesis, like hemoptysis, almost never is the presenting symptom of a hemostatic disorder. However, a hemostatic disorder may exacerbate hematemesis because of an anatomic abnormality. Some hemostatic disorders more likely result in hematemesis because of a combination of effects, such as liver disease with esophageal varices and aspirin ingestion with gastritis.

I. Hematuria is rarely the presenting symptom of a hemostatic disorder except for the hemophilias. However, hemostatic disorders can exacerbate hematuria caused by other disorders, including simple urinary tract infections.

J. Hematochezia in individuals with normal hemostasis most often results from hemorrhoids, but von Willebrand disease and platelet disorders may contribute to repeated episodes of hematochezia when associated with a number of different underlying causes, including diverticuli, hemorrhoids, and angiodysplasia. Not infrequently, identifying the precise site of bleeding is difficult. Melena is also only rarely the presenting symptom of a hemorrhagic disorder. However, repeated episodes of melena may occur in patients with hemorrhagic disorders. Objective data about gastrointestinal bleeding include the number of previous endoscopic evaluations and any previous need for blood products.

K. The amount and duration of menstrual bleeding typically are excessive in women with platelet disorders and von Willebrand disease but may be difficult to establish by history. In general, menstrual bleeding is considered excessive if the patient indicates she has heavy flow for more than 3 days or total flow for more than 6 or 7 days. Objective data regarding menstrual bleeding includes whether a previous physician prescribed birth control pills to suppress menses, treated the patient with blood products, told the patient she was anemic, prescribed iron, performed a dilatation and curettage, performed an emergency hysterectomy to secure hemostasis, or performed an elective hysterectomy or other procedure to prevent excessive bleeding.

L. Childbirth poses a considerable hemostatic challenge; therefore, obtaining a detailed history of each pregnancy, including data on excessive bleeding and the need for transfusion, dilatation and curettage, hysterectomy, or iron therapy, is important. Repeated spontaneous abortions raise the possibility that the patient has a quantitative or qualitative abnormality of fibrinogen (see Chap. 117), factor XIII deficiency (see Chap. 116), or the antiphospholipid syndrome (see Chap. 123).

M. Hemarthroses are the hallmark abnormality in the hemophilias. They are rare except in severe factor VII deficiency and type 3 von Willebrand disease (see Chaps. 116 and 118). Because discoloration of the skin overlying the joint is unusual with hemarthroses, patients may not recognize that their symptoms are caused by bleeding into their joints. Therefore, inquiring about recurrent pain, swelling, and limitation of motion is important.

N. Excessive hemorrhage in response to surgical procedures provides vital prognostic information. Specific inquiry about tonsillectomy, which is a significant hemostatic challenge, is important, because patients often forget having undergone the procedure. If possible, the hospital records should be obtained because they commonly contain information the patient does not have. Especially important facts to inquire about are delays in hospital discharge and the need for blood products.

O. Excessive bleeding in response to circumcision is common in males with severe hemostatic disorders such as hemophilia A, hemophilia B, or Glanzmann thrombasthenia and often is the patient's first symptom. Delayed bleeding after circumcision or from the umbilical stump may be observed in patients with hemophilia A or B but is particularly characteristic of bleeding as the result of factor XIII deficiency.

P. Patients with vascular disorders secondary to connective tissue abnormalities such as Ehlers-Danlos syndrome may give a history of easily distensible skin or extraordinary ligament laxness ("double-jointed"). Manifestations of Cushing syndrome include rounded facies, purple striae, truncal obesity, and fat deposition at the back of the neck. Old photographs may be helpful in establishing a change in the patient's appearance.

PHYSICAL EXAMINATION

On physical examination, look for signs of bleeding or their sequelae and for signs of a possible underlying disorder that can cause the hemostatic derangement (see Table 109-1). Careful examination of the skin is essential for detecting petechiae and ecchymoses. These signs may be prominent on the legs, where the hydrostatic pressure is greatest, or around the hair follicles in vitamin C deficiency.

Telangiectasias may range from pinpoint erythematous dots that blanch with pressure to classic cherry angiomata ranging in size up to several centimeters. Many normal individuals develop increasing numbers of telangiectasias with aging. Patients with hereditary hemorrhagic telangiectasias have more florid lesions that characteristically affect the vermilion border of the lips and the tongue (including the underside of the tongue), but not all patients have these classic features. Thus, a systematic search of the integument is necessary. Spider telangiectasias found in patients with liver disease have a more splotchy and serpiginous appearance than the telangiectasias associated with hereditary hemorrhagic telangiectasias. In addition, the telangiectasias tend to be concentrated on the shoulders, chest, and face.

Chapter 114 details the differential diagnosis of nonpalpable purpuras and palpable purpuras. Hematomas, ecchymoses, and protracted oozing should be sought at venipuncture sites, injection sites, and arterial and venous catheter insertion sites. Joint deformities and limited joint mobility are suggestive of severe hemophilia A or B, severe deficiency of factor VII, or type 3 von Willebrand disease (see Chaps. 115, 116, and 118). Hyperelasticity of the skin and hyperextensibility of joints are typical of Ehlers-Danlos syndrome, and hyperextensibility of only the thumb probably is a variant.[7]

EVALUATION BASED ON BLEEDING HISTORY AND INITIAL HEMOSTATIC TESTS

The patient's history and results of physical examination provide important information on the likelihood of the patient having a hemostatic defect and the possible cause of the defect, if one is present. However, performing an initial set of tests, including (PT), activated partial thromboplastin time (aPTT), and platelet count, to broadly assess the major components of the hemostatic system is important for the following reasons. (1) The patient's history sometimes is unreliable. (2) The patient may have a mild hemostatic abnormality that has not manifested itself for lack of hemostatic challenge. (3) The patient may have developed an acquired hemostatic defect that has remained asymptomatic. (4) The tests may reveal more than one abnormality.[8]

Figure 109-1 shows a series of algorithms that integrate the patient's bleeding history and the results of the initial hemostatic tests. A prolonged aPTT as a sole abnormality can be caused by a deficiency of factor VIII, IX, XI, or XII or by an inhibitor, which can be either factor specific, such as an antibody against factor VIII, or factor nonspecific, such as heparin or a lupus anticoagulant (Fig. 109-1A). A prolonged PT as the sole finding can indicate a factor VII deficiency

or the presence of an inhibitor (Fig. 109-1B). Abnormalities of both PT and aPTT may indicate a deficiency of fibrinogen, prothrombin, factor V or X, an inhibitor to one of these factors, or a combined deficiency of coagulation factors (Fig. 109-1C).

To distinguish between a deficiency state and the presence of an inhibitor, repeating the PT and aPTT using a 1:1 mixture of the patient's plasma and normal plasma is useful. If the mixture normalizes the prolonged PT or aPTT, a deficiency state is likely. If the mixture still yields a significantly prolonged PT or aPTT, an inhibitor probably is present. Some inhibitors, such as antibodies to factor VIII, require time to inhibit the assay, whereas other inhibitors, such as lupus anticoagulant and heparin, do not. Therefore, incubating the mixture for 1 or 2 hours at 37°C (98.6°F) before performing the coagulation assay is desirable.

When the results of none of the initial tests (PT, aPTT, and platelet count) are abnormal and the patient exhibits bleeding manifestations, the bleeding time (BT), ristocetin cofactor (RCF) activity, and examination of the blood film can be helpful for distinguishing among various candidate hemostatic abnormalities. Although the BT can be useful in diagnosis, an experienced technician is a requisite for proper interpretation because the test is highly operator dependent. Figure 109-2 shows an algorithm that includes these secondary tests. Not infrequently, patients with type 1 and type 2 von Willebrand disease have normal findings on initial laboratory tests because factor VIII levels are sufficiently high (>30 U/dl) for a normal aPTT result (see Chap. 118). Examination of the blood film is helpful for distinguishing between Bernard-Soulier syndrome and von Willebrand disease because giant platelets are characteristic of the former (see Chap. 112). Distinguishing mild type von Willebrand disease from normal is difficult because of the broad distribution of von Willebrand factor level partly related to ABO blood types. In fact, some investigators have questioned whether patients with von Willebrand factor levels as low as 35 percent should be labeled as having von Willebrand disease.[9] The ristocetin-induced platelet aggregation test is useful for distinguishing type 2B and platelet-type von Willebrand disease from the other types of von Willebrand disease. In type 2B and platelet-type von Willebrand disease, an enhanced response to low concentrations of ristocetin is observed, whereas in the other types of von Willebrand disease, a decreased response is found. Total absence of platelet aggregates in a blood film prepared from nonanticoagulated blood and absent clot retraction are characteristic of Glanzmann thrombasthenia (see Chap. 112).

Another simple test that may be useful for distinguishing among hemostatic disorders is the thrombin time (i.e., time for plasma to clot after adding thrombin). The thrombin time is prolonged in (1) afibrinogenemia, hypofibrinogenemia, and dysfibrinogenemias (see Chap. 117), (2) the presence of heparin, (3) disseminated intravascular coagulation (DIC) that results because increased levels of fibrin(ogen) degradation products inhibit fibrin monomer polymerization (see Fig. 109-1D) (see Chap. 121), and (4) patients with amyloidosis and an immunoglobulin inhibitor of thrombin.[10]

PREOPERATIVE ASSESSMENT OF HEMOSTASIS

Surgical procedures are a great challenge to the hemostatic system; therefore, carefully assessing the risk of bleeding in every patient is important. The assessment is based on the bleeding history, the underlying disorder if any, the results of initial hemostatic tests (PT, aPTT, platelet count), and the type of surgery that is planned. Table 109-3 lists low-risk and high-risk conditions. A critical analysis of each potential cause of bleeding should be undertaken for the high-risk conditions.

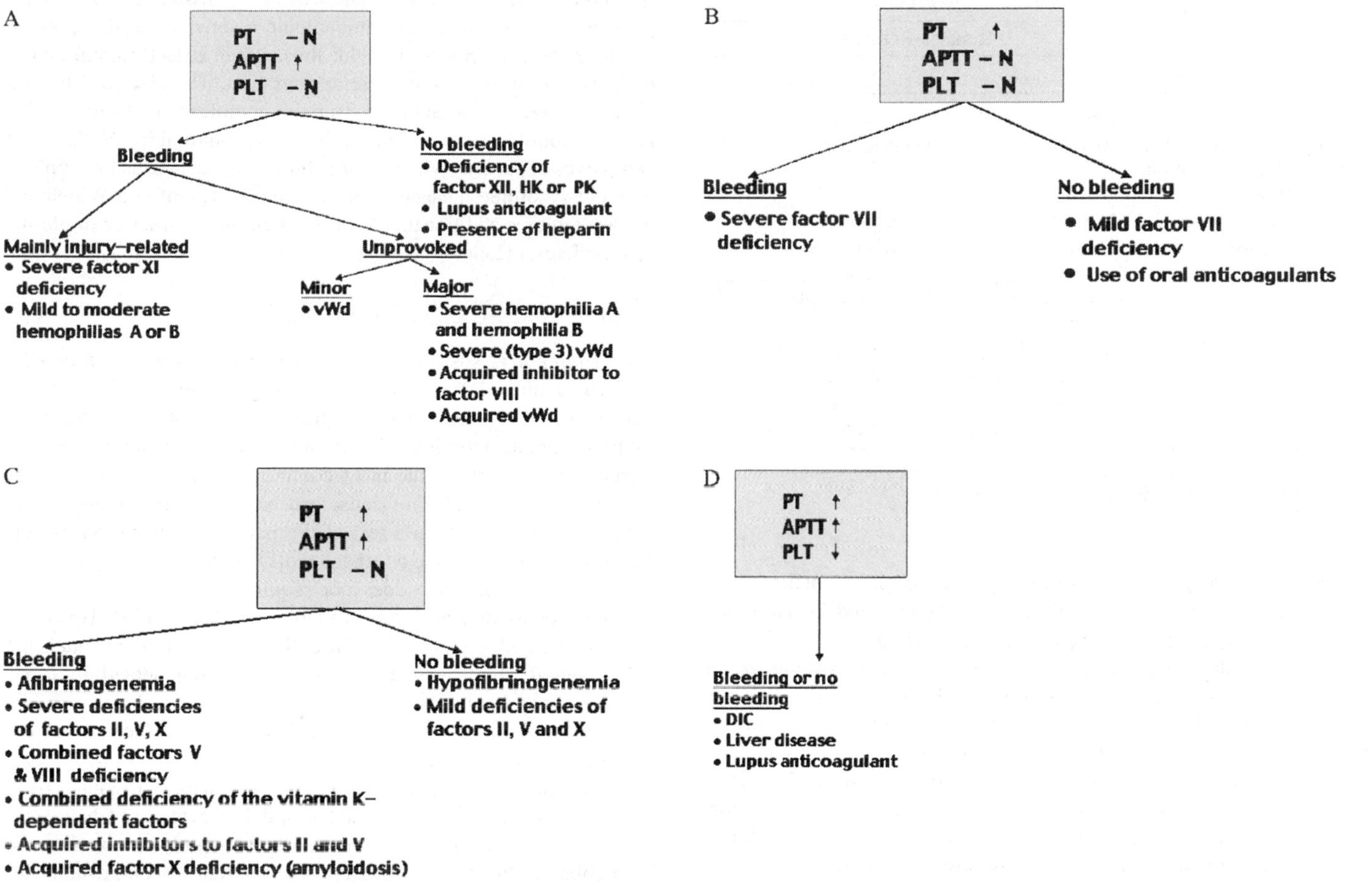

A

```
        PT  – N
        APTT ↑
        PLT – N
```

Bleeding ←   → No bleeding
                                        • Deficiency of
                                          factor XII, HK or PK
                                        • Lupus anticoagulant
                                        • Presence of heparin

Mainly injury–related   Unprovoked
• Severe factor XI
  deficiency   Minor   Major
• Mild to moderate   • vWd   • Severe hemophilia A
  hemophilias A or B   and hemophilia B
                                         • Severe (type 3) vWd
                                         • Acquired inhibitor to
                                           factor VIII
                                         • Acquired vWd

B

```
        PT   ↑
        APTT – N
        PLT  – N
```

Bleeding ←   → No bleeding
• Severe factor VII   • Mild factor VII
  deficiency   deficiency
                                        • Use of oral anticoagulants

C

```
        PT   ↑
        APTT ↑
        PLT  – N
```

Bleeding ←   → No bleeding
• Afibrinogenemia   • Hypofibrinogenemia
• Severe deficiencies   • Mild deficiencies of
  of factors II, V, X   factors II, V and X
• Combined factors V
  & VIII deficiency
• Combined deficiency of the vitamin K–
  dependent factors
• Acquired inhibitors to factors II and V
• Acquired factor X deficiency (amyloidosis)

D

```
        PT   ↑
        APTT ↑
        PLT  ↓
```

Bleeding or no
bleeding
• DIC
• Liver disease
• Lupus anticoagulant

FIGURE 109-1   Measures for establishing a tentative diagnosis of a hemostatic disorder using initial tests of hemostasis and the patient's history of bleeding. APTT, activated partial thromboplastin time; BT, bleeding time; DIC, disseminated intravascular coagulation; HK, high molecular weight kininogen; N, normal; PK, prekallikrein; PLT, platelets; PT, prothrombin time; vWd, von Willebrand disease.

In addition to the extent of the surgical trauma, the magnitude of the fibrinolytic activity at the surgical site must be considered. For example, prostatectomy carries considerable risk of prolonged bleeding because of the presence of high fibrinolytic activity in the urine. Some surgical procedures can be anticipated to cause hemostatic abnormalities, such as operations in which extracorporeal circulation is used (because the extracorporeal circuits and/or the anticoagulation cause platelet dysfunction) and operations on patients with extensive malignancies or brain injury, which can give rise to DIC. Finally, the ability to institute local hemostatic measures should be considered. Thus, liver, lung, and kidney biopsies, although considered minor procedures, have a significant risk of bleeding because local measures, such as direct pressure, cannot be used to control bleeding.

The initial hemostatic tests may provide other important information for managing patients undergoing surgery, such as (1) baseline values for future comparison if bleeding occurs, and (2) information about deficiencies of factor XII, prekallikrein, or high molecular weight kininogen, for which no treatment is necessary, or the lupus anticoagulant, for which anticoagulant prophylaxis may be indicated.

SPECIFIC ASSAYS FOR ESTABLISHING THE DIAGNOSIS

A tentative diagnosis can be made by following the stepwise process of evaluation outlined in Figs. 109-1 and 109-2. However, further testing usually is required to establish a definitive diagnosis.

THROMBOCYTOPENIAS

When the laboratory reports an abnormally low platelet count, looking at the blood film to exclude pseudothrombocytopenia as a result of anticoagulant-induced platelet clumping is essential.[11] Examination of

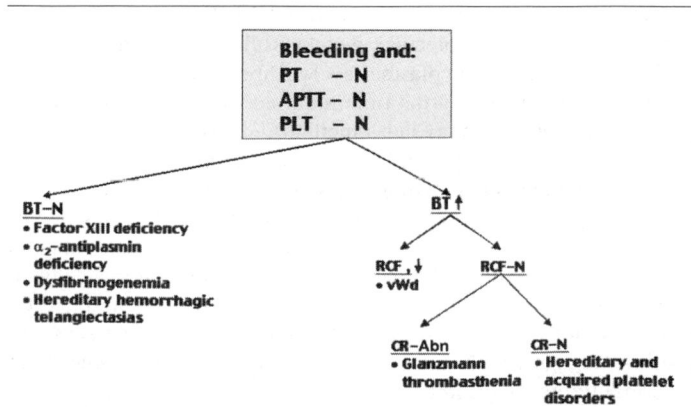

FIGURE 109-2   Tentative diagnoses in patients with bleeding manifestations and normal primary hemostatic tests using secondary tests. Abn, abnormal; APTT, activated partial thromboplastin time; BT, bleeding time; CR, clot retraction; N, normal; PK, prekallikrein; PLT, platelets; PT, prothrombin time; RCF, ristocetin cofactor activity; vWd, von Willebrand disease.

TABLE 109-3 EVALUATION OF BLEEDING RISK DURING SURGERY

ASSESSED FACTOR	RISK OF BLEEDING	
	LOW	HIGH
Bleeding history	Negative	Positive
Underlying conditions that compromise hemostasis (see Table 109-1)	Absent	Present
Initial hemostatic tests	Normal	Abnormal
Type of surgery	Minor	Major
	Not expected to induce a hemostatic defect	Expected to induce a hemostatic defect[a]
	At a site without local fibrinolysis	At a site with local fibrinolysis[b]
	Local hemostatic measures effective	Local hemostatic measures ineffective[c]

[a] Open heart surgery or brain surgery.
[b] Prostatectomy, tonsillectomy, oral or nasal surgery.
[c] Liver, lung, or kidney biopsy.

the blood film also can reveal the presence of: giant platelets, as in some inherited thrombocytopenias; giant platelets and Döhle bodies in leukocytes, as in May-Hegglin/Fechtner/Sebastian syndromes; moderately enlarged platelets, as in immune thrombocytopenia or other conditions associated with shortened platelet survival; small platelets, as in Wiskott-Aldrich syndrome; schistocytes and burr cells, as in the hemolytic uremic syndrome and thrombotic thrombocytopenic purpura, and occasionally in DIC; rouleaux formation, as in monoclonal gammopathies; macrocytosis and/or hypersegmentation, as in vitamin B_{12} or folic acid deficiency; and abnormal white blood cells, as in leukemias and myeloproliferative disorders. Chapter 110 further discusses the evaluation and differential diagnosis of the thrombocytopenias.

FACTOR DEFICIENCIES

Coagulation factors usually are assayed by measuring their clotting activity. The most common assays analyze the ability of dilutions of the patient's plasma to correct the clotting time of a plasma known to be deficient in the factor being measured (substrate plasma). The results are compared to the ability of dilutions of a normal reference plasma to correct the abnormality in the substrate plasma. The activities of factors II, V, VII, and X usually are determined in PT-based assays, whereas the activities of factors VIII, IX, XI, and XII, prekallikrein, and high molecular weight kininogen are measured in aPTT-based assays. The plasma level of fibrinogen most commonly is measured by assessing the time required for thrombin to clot the patient's diluted plasma (Clauss method).[12] Several assays of transglutaminase activity are available for measuring factor XIII activity,[13] but a simple qualitative test based on dissolving a fibrin clot in 5 M urea usually is sufficient (see Chap. 116). The RCF function of von Willebrand factor can be measured by the ability of the patient's plasma to support the agglutination of a suspension of formaldehyde-fixed normal platelets by ristocetin.[14] This activity is defined as *ristocetin cofactor activity*. As with the coagulation factor assays, the results using patient plasma are compared to the results obtained with a normal reference plasma.

To determine whether a coagulation factor activity deficiency results from a quantitative decrease in protein or a qualitative abnormality in the protein, immunologic assays can be performed using specific polyclonal or monoclonal antibodies to assess the presence of the protein, independent of its function. Electroimmunoassays, enzyme-linked immunosorbent assays (ELISAs), and immunoradiometric assays all have been used successfully. Crossed immunoelectrophoresis measures both the immunologic reactivity and the mobility of the protein in an electric field; thus, it can detect protein abnormalities that affect electrophoretic migration. The abnormalities include the presence of antibody–antigen complexes that migrate differently from the protein itself, such as antiprothrombin–prothrombin complexes in patients with systemic lupus erythematosus or antiphospholipid syndrome. Diagnosis of the specific type of von Willebrand disease requires additional tests of the multimeric structure of plasma and, perhaps, platelet von Willebrand factor.

INHIBITORS TO COAGULATION FACTORS

If an inhibitor is suspected as a result of a prolonged PT or PTT performed on a 1:1 mixture of the patient's plasma and normal plasma, further studies can help define the nature of the inhibitor and its titer. Among inhibitors that do not require incubation (i.e., immediate-type), perhaps the most common cause is the presence of heparin in the sample. This cause can be verified by finding a prolonged thrombin time on a test of the patient's plasma that is corrected with toluidine blue or other agents that neutralize heparin. The lupus anticoagulant also does not require incubation, and several methods for its detection are available (see Chap. 123). However, with lupus anticoagulant, the PT usually is less prolonged than is the aPTT, and aPTT reagents have markedly different sensitivity to lupus-type anticoagulant.

Immunoglobin inhibitors to specific coagulation factors may develop either after factor replacement therapy in patients with inherited deficiencies of coagulation factors (see Chaps. 115 and 116) or spontaneously in patients without factor deficiencies (see Chap. 119). Antibodies that neutralize factor activity frequently can be detected by incubating the patient's plasma with normal plasma, usually for 2 hours at 37°C (98.6°F), and then assaying the specific factor. The Bethesda assay originally was designed to quantify factor VIII inhibitors but can be modified to detect other inhibitors of coagulation factors[15] (see Chap. 115). Some inhibitors do not directly neutralize clotting activity; rather, they reduce factor levels by forming complexes with coagulation factors, which then are rapidly cleared from the circulation. Such plasmas do not produce prolonged clotting times when mixed 1:1 with normal plasma and thus may be confused with inherited deficiency states. More elaborate assays are required to identify this type of inhibitor, which may, for example, produce severe deficiencies of prothrombin in some patients with the antiphospholipid syndrome (see Chap. 123) and of von Willebrand factor in some acquired forms of von Willebrand disease (see Chap. 118).[16]

PLATELET FUNCTION DISORDERS

A prolonged BT suggests a platelet function disorder (inherited or acquired) or von Willebrand disease. Use of the RCF activity assay, platelet aggregation, and/or clot retraction are useful for initially assessing whether the patient has von Willebrand disease or a platelet function disorder (see Fig. 109-2). Chapter 112 contains a flow diagram of the steps required to diagnose the different qualitative disorders of platelet function. Additional platelet function assays and glycoprotein analysis may be required to establish the diagnosis.

REFERENCES

1. Miller CH, Graham JB, Goldin LR, Elston RC: Genetics of classic von Willebrand's disease: II. Optimal assignment of the heterozygous genotype (diagnosis) by discriminant analysis. *Blood* 54:137, 1979.

2. Wahlberg T, Blomback M, Hall P, Axelsson G: Application of indicators, predictors and diagnostic indices in coagulation disorders: I. Evaluation of a self-administered questionnaire with binary questions. *Methods Inf Med* 19:194, 1980.

3. Eikenboom JCJ, Rosendaal FR, Briet E: Value of the patient interview: All but consensus among haemostasis experts. *Haemostasis* 22:221, 1992.

4. Sramek A, Eikenboom JC, Briet E, et al: Usefulness of patient interview in bleeding disorders. *Arch Intern Med* 155:1409, 1995.

5. Miller LG: Herbal medicinals: Selected clinical considerations focusing on known or potential drug-herb interactions. *Arch Intern Med* 158:2200, 1998.

6. Horton RM: Alternative medicine resources on the internet. *Curr Pract Med* 1:71, 1998.

7. Kaplinsky C, Kenet G, Seligsohn U, Rechavi G: Association between hyperflexibility of the thumb and an unexplained bleeding tendency: Is it a rule of thumb? *Br J Haematol* 101:260, 1998.

8. Rapaport SI: Preoperative hemostatic evaluation: Which tests, if any? *Blood* 61:229, 1983.

9. Sadler JE: Von Willebrand disease type 1: A diagnosis in search of a disease. *Blood* 101:2089, 2003.

10. Gastineau DA, Gertz MA, Daniels TM, et al: Inhibitor of the thrombin time in systemic amyloidosis: A common coagulation abnormality. *Blood* 77:2637, 1991.

11. Payne BA, Pierre RV: Pseudothrombocytopenia: A laboratory artifact with potentially serious consequences. *Mayo Clin Proc* 59:123, 1984.

12. Clauss A: Gerinnungsphysiologische schnell methodes zur des fibrinogens. *Acta Haematol* 17:327, 1957.

13. Fickenscher K, Aab A, Stuber W: A photometric assay for blood coagulation factor XIII. *Thromb Haemost* 65:535, 1991.

14. McFarlane DE, Stibbe J, Kirby EP, et al: A method for assaying von Willebrand factor (ristocetin cofactor). *Thromb Diath Haemorrh* 34:306, 1975.

15. Kasper CK, Aledort L, Aronson D, et al: Proceedings: A more uniform measurement of factor VIII inhibitors. *Thromb Diath Haemorrh* 34:612, 1975.

16. Inbal A, Bank I, Zivelin A, et al: Acquired von Willebrand disease in a patient with angiodysplasia resulting from immune-mediated clearance of von Willebrand factor. *Br J Haematol* 96:179, 1997.

THROMBOCYTOPENIA

REYHAN DIZ-KÜÇÜKKAYA
FRANCISCA C. GUSHIKEN
JOSÉ A. LÓPEZ

This chapter describes the pathogenesis, clinical features, and management of patients with thrombocytopenia, defined as a platelet count less than 150 × 10⁹/liter. The causes of thrombocytopenia are many, but they can be grouped according to the distribution of platelets. Thus, a low platelet count could result from peripheral destruction by an immune or nonimmune mechanism, decreased production resulting from an inherited or acquired marrow disease, or splenic pooling. Pseudothrombocytopenia also should be considered in the differential diagnosis, particularly in asymptomatic patients, and results from *in vitro* clumping of platelets following blood collection.

The age at onset of thrombocytopenia reflects the prevailing diseases for each age range. The most likely causes of thrombocytopenia in newborns are neonatal alloimmune thrombocytopenia, infection, and passive transfer of antibodies from a mother with immune thrombocytopenic purpura (ITP). In children, ITP and acute viral infection are most common. The differential diagnosis of thrombocytopenia in adults is broad but is acquired in the vast majority of patients, usually associated with an underlying disease or because of an autoimmune process. Nevertheless, inherited thrombocytopenia should always be considered when evaluating a patient with mild to moderate thrombocytopenia that may not have a clinically significant history of bleeding. A large number of adult patients are diagnosed incidentally on routine examination. Careful examination of the blood film is the best means for narrowing the differential diagnosis. Platelet clumping supports the diagnosis

of pseudothrombocytopenia and obviates the need for further exhaustive workup and possible harmful interventions. Many of the congenital thrombocytopenias have recognizable changes in platelet morphology, such as giant or small platelets, abnormal platelet granules, or associated erythrocyte or leukocyte morphologic changes. Table 110-1 summarizes the most common causes of thrombocytopenia.

PLATELET KINETICS

Platelet kinetic studies have been performed *in vivo* to determine the pathophysiologic mechanisms in various thrombocytopenic states, particularly in complicated clinical situations. For instance, the thrombocytopenia seen in patients with human immunodeficiency virus (HIV) infection can result from many factors, including platelet destruction (because of an autoimmune mechanism or drug toxicity) or decreased platelet production because of malignancy or infection of the marrow.

Platelet kinetic studies are performed using autologous platelets, which are labeled *ex vivo* with radioactive isotopes and then infused back into the patient. The radioisotope indium-111 (¹¹¹In) oxine is most commonly used because it binds platelets very efficiently, which allows kinetic studies even in subjects with very low platelet counts.[1-3] Platelet recovery, platelet survival, and platelet turnover are calculated based on the radioactivity of blood samples drawn from the patient during the several days following injection of the radiolabeled platelets. Platelet recovery is determined by the percentage of radiolabeled platelets detected in blood 1 hour after the injection. It takes approximately 10 to 12 minutes for the platelets to pass through a normal spleen; nearly one third of reinfused platelets are sequestered during the first hour before reaching equilibrium with the circulating platelets.[4] The normal value of initial platelet recovery is between 50 and 70 percent. The initial platelet recovery is high in patients who have undergone splenectomy and low in patients with immune thrombocytopenia or hypersplenism.[4-6]

The mean life span of platelets is generally calculated in reference to a standard curve generated using radioactivity measurements taken over time in normal controls.[2] Under normal conditions, human platelets have a mean life span in the circulation of between 7 and 10 days.[7,8] Patients with thrombocytopenia because of platelet destruction have a markedly decreased platelet survival.[9,10] Patients with thrombocytopenia because of marrow failure have mildly decreased platelet survival because of the body's fixed daily consumption of platelets, which more closely approximates the number produced as the disease progresses.[11] Platelet turnover is a measure of the net effect of platelet production and platelet destruction under steady-state conditions.[10] Several studies using ¹¹¹In oxine have established that, under normal conditions, platelet turnover in humans ranges from 40 to 50 × 10⁹/liter per day.[10] Although a high platelet turnover is expected in patients with idiopathic thrombocytopenic purpura (ITP), platelet production measured as turnover is not always increased.[10] Low production may result from binding of the antibodies to megakaryocytes that inhibit their development or lead to their destruction, causing an inappropriate marrow response to the degree of thrombocytopenia.[12]

The number of platelets entering the circulation to maintain the platelet count defines platelet production rate. This rate is calculated from mean platelet life span (MPLS), platelet count, blood volume, and the initial platelet recovery. The normal rate of platelet production varies from 160 × 10⁹ to 280 × 10⁹ per day.

Platelet kinetic studies also usually measure hepatic and splenic platelet uptake, estimated by the radioactivity from these organs detected by a gamma camera connected to a computerized data collection system. Images are taken during the first hour after injection and fol-

Acronyms and abbreviations that appear in this chapter include: ACLA, anticardiolipin antibody; AIDS, acquired immunodeficiency syndrome; AML, acute myelogenous leukemia; APLA, antiphospholipid antibody; APS, antiphospholipid syndrome; ASH, American Society of Hematology; AZT, azidothymidine; BSS, Bernard-Soulier syndrome; CAMT, congenital amegakaryocytic thrombocytopenia; DIC, disseminated intravascular coagulation; EDTA, ethylenediaminetetraacetic acid; FPS, familial platelet syndrome; Gp, glycoprotein; HAART, highly active antiretroviral therapy; HELLP, microangiopathic hemolysis (H), elevated liver enzymes (EL), and low platelet (LP) counts; HIT, heparin-induced thrombocytopenia; HIV, human immunodeficiency virus; HSC, hematopoietic stem cell; Ig, immunoglobulin; IL, interleukin; ITP, idiopathic thrombocytopenic purpura; IVIg, intravenous immunoglobulin; KMS, Kasabach-Merritt syndrome; LDH, lactate dehydrogenase; MACA, modified antigen-capture enzyme-linked immunoadsorbent assay; MAIPA, monoclonal antibody-specific immobilization of platelet antigens assay; MDS, myelodysplastic syndrome; MPLS, mean platelet life span; NADPH, reduced nicotinamide adenine dinucleotide phosphate; NAIT, neonatal alloimmune thrombocytopenia; NMMHC, nonmuscle myosin heavy chain; PAICA, platelet-associated IgG characterization assay; PAIgG, platelet-associated immunoglobulin G; PlGF, placental growth factor; PNH, paroxysmal nocturnal hemoglobinuria; RAEB, refractory anemia with excess blasts; SLE, systemic lupus erythematosus; TAR, thrombocytopenia and absent radii; TPO, thrombopoietin; TTP, thrombotic thrombocytopenic purpura; TTP-HUS, thrombotic thrombocytopenic purpura and hemolytic uremic syndrome; VEGF, vascular endothelial growth factor; vWF, von Willebrand factor; WAS, Wiskott-Aldrich syndrome; WASP, Wiskott-Aldrich syndrome protein.

TABLE 110-1 CLASSIFICATION OF THROMBOCYTOPENIA

Pseudo-thrombocytopenia
  Platelet agglutination
  Platelet satellitism
  Antiphospholipid antibodies
  GpIIa-IIIa antagonists
  Giant platelets
  Miscellaneous associations
Impaired platelet production
  Congenital
    Autosomal dominant
      MYH9-related
        May-Hegglin anomaly
        Fechtner syndrome
        Epstein syndrome
        Sebastian syndrome
      Mediterranean macrothrombocytopenia
      Familial platelet syndrome with predisposition to acute myelogenous
        leukemia
      Thrombocytopenia with linkage to chromosome 10
      Paris-Trousseau syndrome
      Thrombocytopenia with radial synostosis
    Autosomal recessive
      Congenital amegakaryocytic thrombocytopenia
      Thrombocytopenia with absent radius (TAR) syndrome
      Bernard-Soulier syndrome (see Chap. 112)
      Gray platelet syndrome (see Chap. 112)
    X-linked thrombocytopenias
      Wiskott-Aldrich syndrome
      X-linked thrombocytopenia
      X-linked thrombocytopenia with dyserythrocytosis
  Acquired
    Marrow infiltration (see Chap. 42)
    Infectious disease
      HIV (see Chap. 83)
      Parvovirus (see Chap. 34)
      Cytomegalovirus (see Chap. 34)
      Others
    Radiotherapy and chemotherapy (see Chap. 19)
    Folic acid and vitamin B_{12} deficiency (see Chap. 39)
    Paroxysmal nocturnal hemoglobinuria (see Chap. 38)
    Acquired aplastic anemia (see Chap. 33)
    Myelodysplastic syndromes (see Chap. 86)
    Acquired pure megakaryocytic thrombocytopenia
Accelerated platelet destruction
  Immune-mediated thrombocytopenia
    Autoimmune thrombocytopenic purpura
      Idiopathic
      Secondary (infections, pregnancy-related, lymphoproliferative disorders,
        collagen vascular diseases)
    Alloimmune thrombocytopenia
      Neonatal thrombocytopenia
      Posttransfusion purpura
  Nonimmune thrombocytopenia
    Thrombotic microangiopathies
      Thrombotic thrombocytopenic purpura and hemolytic uremic syndrome
      Disseminated intravascular coagulopathy
      Kasabach-Merritt syndrome
    Platelet destruction by artificial surfaces
    Hemophagocytosis
Abnormal platelet distribution or pooling
  Splenomegaly (see Chap. 55)
  Hypersplenism (see Chap. 55)
  Hypothermia
  Massive transfusion
Drug-induced thrombocytopenia
  Heparin-induced thrombocytopenia (HIT) (see Chap. 124)
  Other drug-induced thrombocytopenias

lowed for 5 to 7 days. In normal subjects, platelet uptake by the liver and spleen usually is constant for 5 days. Thus, increased sequestration beyond this time is suggestive of increased platelet destruction. Patients with ITP and increased splenic sequestration respond better to splenectomy than do patients with liver sequestration only or with combined liver and splenic uptake.[13] The scan is useful for determining spleen size and other sites of platelet sequestration, such as an accessory spleen or congenital hemangiomas, which also are associated with thrombocytopenia.

SPURIOUS THROMBOCYTOPENIA (PSEUDOTHROMBOCYTOPENIA)

Spurious thrombocytopenia, also called *pseudothrombocytopenia*, is a relatively uncommon phenomenon caused by *ex vivo* agglutination of platelets. As a result of platelet clumping, platelet counts reported by automated counters may be much lower than the actual count in the blood because these devices cannot differentiate platelet clumps from individual cells. The incidences of pseudothrombocytopenia reported in different studies range from 0.09 to 0.21 percent, which would account for 15 to 30 percent of all cases of isolated thrombocytopenia.[14–21] An example of *ex vivo* platelet clumping is shown in Color Plate XII-1, accompanied by platelet–neutrophil satellitism (see below in section entitled "Platelet Satellitism").

ANTIBODY-INDUCED PLATELET AGGLUTINATION

Platelet agglutination *ex vivo* can be induced by antiplatelet antibodies or by activation of the platelets during collection. The responsible antibodies do not appear to be associated with a pathologic process, as they are found in normal individuals. One hypothesis put forth to explain their presence is that the antibodies are responsible for clearing aged and damaged platelets. Most antibodies implicated in pseudothrombocytopenia recognize platelet membrane glycoproteins that are modified or exposed when calcium is chelated. Typically, the artifact is most prominent in the presence of ethylenediaminetetraacetic acid (EDTA), but other anticoagulants, such as sodium citrate, sodium oxalate, acid citrate dextrose, and heparin, also can cause platelet clumping. The antibodies usually are of the immunoglobulin (Ig)G type; IgM and IgA antibodies also have been described.[22–24] Most antibodies react at room temperature; thus, the reaction can be prevented when the blood sample is kept at 37°C. In 20 percent of cases, the antibodies, usually of the IgM type, are reactive at both 22°C and 37°C.[23] Clumping usually is evident within 60 minutes after the blood is drawn but may require incubations of 2 to 3 hours. Agglutination can be reproduced by incubating plasma from patients with pseudothrombocytopenia with blood from normal individuals in the presence of EDTA.

In most cases, the antibodies are directed against glycoprotein IIb/IIIa (GpIIb-IIIa), a conclusion supported by the observation that platelets from patients with Glanzmann thrombasthenia, who lack the GpIIb-IIIa complex, fail to agglutinate in the presence of patient sera.[25–28] Moreover, pretreatment of fresh blood with anti–GpIIb-IIIa dramatically reduces EDTA-induced platelet agglutination.[29] The responsible epitope normally is cryptic and located in the GpIIb subunit. Low temperature and calcium chelation combine to change the conformation of GpIIb-IIIa and expose the epitope.[26]

PLATELET SATELLITISM

Antibodies directed against GpIIb-IIIa may react simultaneously with the leukocyte Fcγ receptor III (FcγRIII) and attach the platelets to neutrophils and monocytes, inducing a phenomenon known as platelet leukocyte satellitism,[25] another form of pseudothrombocytopenia. These antibodies fail to produce satellitism in the presence of platelets from patients with type I Glanzmann thrombasthenia or in the presence of neutrophils from patients with congenital absence of FcγRIII.[25] Typically, the platelets form a rosette around the periphery of leukocytes (see Color Plate XII-1). Neutrophils are most frequently involved, but the phenomenon also is occasionally observed with monocytes.[30,31] These antibodies also are naturally occurring, and their presence does not clearly correlate with any specific clinical situation, disease, or drug. As with the antibodies that induce only platelet clumping, exposure of a cryptic antigen on EDTA-treated platelets and leukocytes may trigger this phenomenon.

ANTIPHOSPHOLIPID ANTIBODIES

Some antiplatelet antibodies from patients with pseudothrombocytopenia cross-react with negatively charged phospholipids and may exhibit anticardiolipin activity.[32] The sera of these patients lose their ability to clump platelets when adsorbed onto either cardiolipin or activated normal platelets, supporting the hypothesis that antibody subpopulations directed against negatively charged phospholipids can bind to antigens modified by EDTA on the platelet membrane. Another possibility is that the antigens in this case are negatively charged phospholipids on the surface of platelets.

GLYCOPROTEIN IIB/IIIA ANTAGONISTS

Thrombocytopenia has been described in patients suffering from acute coronary syndromes treated with the GpIIb-IIIa antagonist abciximab.[33–35] Abciximab has been associated with both pseudothrombocytopenia and true thrombocytopenia. The mechanism for platelet clumping with abciximab is unknown, and the drug itself likely is not cross-linking the platelets because it is monovalent. More likely, other agglutinins bind GpIIb-IIIa at new epitopes induced by the combination of abciximab binding and calcium chelation. True abciximab-induced thrombocytopenia occurs in approximately 0.3 to 1 percent of patients treated with the drug.[36] The mechanism is unknown but may include formation of antibodies to a neoepitope expressed after binding of abciximab to GpIIb-IIIa or abciximab-induced platelet activation with subsequent platelet sequestration from the circulation. In some abciximab-treated patients, high antibody titers are detected in the plasma.

The incidence of pseudothrombocytopenia and thrombocytopenia related to abciximab was determined in four large placebo-controlled trials[34]: c7E3 Fab Antiplatelet Therapy in Unstable Refractory Angina (CAPTURE), Evaluation of 7E3 for the Prevention of Ischemic Complications (EPIC), Evaluation of Percutaneous Transluminal Coronary Angioplasty to Improve Long-term Outcome of c7E3 GpIIb-IIIa Receptor Blockade (EPILOG), and Evaluation of Platelet IIb-IIIa Inhibitor for Stenting (EPISTENT). In these studies, pseudothrombocytopenia accounted for more than one third of low platelet counts in patients undergoing coronary interventions and treated with abciximab. These studies demonstrated that pseudothrombocytopenia is a benign laboratory condition not associated with increased bleeding, stroke, transfusion requirements, or the need for repeat revascularization.

MISCELLANEOUS ASSOCIATIONS

Some studies have suggested that platelet agglutinins occur more frequently in hospitalized patients and in association with medical conditions such as autoimmune diseases, malignancy, liver disease, and sepsis.[21,37–40] However, others have found no association with any particular pathology or with use of specific drugs.[23]

One study showed that antibodies from patients with pseudothrombocytopenia can induce agglutination of donor platelets in the presence of EDTA. This agglutination was prevented by warming the donor platelets to 37°C or by pretreating the platelets with aspirin, prostaglandin F_1, apyrase, and monoclonal antibodies against GpIIb-IIIa that block the binding site for fibrinogen and the von Willebrand factor (vWF) or RGD peptide, which binds the site on GpIIb-IIIa that recognizes cytoadhesive proteins.[26] Whether the same reaction occurs *in vivo* is not known, but in that case the antibodies should have a slow reactivity or else a bleeding diathesis should be expected.

DIAGNOSIS

An automated platelet count must be confirmed by microscopic examination of the blood film. Automated cell counters identify platelets merely based on their small volumes, generally defined as volumes between 2 and 20 fl. Because the platelet clumps tend to exceed 20 fl, the clumps may be counted as leukocytes.[14] Thus, pseudothrombocytopenia may be accompanied by pseudoleukocytosis.[17,18,20] The greater the delay in processing of anticoagulated blood, the greater is the degree of platelet clumping and the greater the potential for artifact.[17]

Platelet clumping can be prevented by collecting the sample in EDTA and maintaining its temperature at 37°C. Even with these measures, however, clumping still will be present in approximately 20 percent of cases.[23] Another alternative is use of sodium citrate, which chelates calcium more weakly than does EDTA but still causes platelet clumping in approximately 10 to 20 percent of cases with EDTA-induced clumping. In some patients, an accurate platelet count can be obtained only by sampling blood directly into ammonium oxalate and manually counting the platelets using a Burker chamber.[23]

IMPLICATIONS

Platelet agglutinins are not associated with bleeding or thrombosis, so they appear to have no clinical implications. Transplacental transmission has been documented, but the pseudothrombocytopenia induced by these antibodies in the neonate resolves spontaneously.[41] No complications have been reported when platelet agglutinins are discovered during pregnancy.[41,42] Transfusion of blood products from patients with pseudothrombocytopenia produces an acceptable corrected count increment in the recipient, again supporting its benign nature.[19] Thus, the clinical importance of pseudothrombocytopenia concerns conditions with which it is confused rather than any pathology associated with the condition. It is important that this syndrome be recognized promptly to avoid unnecessary diagnostic tests and treatment.

THROMBOCYTOPENIA RESULTING FROM IMPAIRED PLATELET PRODUCTION

CONGENITAL THROMBOCYTOPENIA RESULTING FROM IMPAIRED PLATELET PRODUCTION

MYH9-RELATED THROMBOCYTOPENIA SYNDROMES

Genetics May-Hegglin anomaly, Fechtner syndrome, Sebastian syndrome, and Epstein syndrome are autosomal dominant macrothrombocytopenias with mutations in the *MYH9* gene,[43–47] located on chromosome 22q12-13. This gene encodes nonmuscle myosin heavy chain (NMMHC)-IIA, which is expressed in platelets, kidney, leukocytes and the cochlea.[48–52] Although these syndromes result from mutations in the *MYH9* gene, a clear phenotype-genotype relationship within each has not been determined. A suggestion is that they represent a class of allelic disorders with variable phenotypic expression leading to diversity among the group.[53]

Pathogenesis The NMMHC-IIA protein appears to be an important cytoskeletal contractile protein in hematopoietic cells.[50] One mutation in the *MYH9* gene rendered a highly unstable protein with abnormal organization of the megakaryocyte cytoskeleton.[54] It is attractive to postulate that defective MYH9 leads to defective megakaryocyte platelet shedding, thereby accounting for the reduced numbers and giant platelets seen in these disorders.

Clinical Findings Affected patients have the triad of thrombocytopenia, macrothrombocytes, and Döhle body-like inclusions in the leukocytes, except for those with Epstein syndrome, which lacks the latter, and various degrees of high-tone sensorineural deafness, nephritis, and cataracts.[44] Hematuria and proteinuria are manifestations of the glomerulonephritic lesions present in a proportion of patients. Selective high-tone hearing loss and cataracts also develop in varying proportions of patients. Patients may have a history of mild bleeding, but they may be completely asymptomatic and discovered incidentally. Conversely, patients may have a bleeding tendency despite a seemingly adequate platelet count and normal standard platelet function test results. Expression of GpIb-IX-V on the surface of platelets from May-Hegglin anomaly is reduced and could account for this finding.[48]

One hallmark feature of MYH9-related disorders is revealed on the blood film, where neutrophilic inclusions that appear blue with Wright-Giemsa stain are noted. The inclusions correspond to cytoplasmic aggregates of NMMHC-IIA, which are readily detected by immunocytochemistry.[55–58]

Treatment Patients with MYH9-related disorders may be misdiagnosed with ITP and subjected to inappropriate treatment with glucocorticoids, intravenous immunoglobulin (IVIg), or splenectomy. Thus, the patient and his/her relatives should be educated to avoid potentially dangerous treatments for presumed ITP. Treatment of MYH9-related disorders generally is supportive, with platelet transfusions given only in specific instances, such as uncontrolled bleeding, prior to major surgery, and with a complicated delivery. No prevention or treatment for the nonhematopoietic consequences of these disorders is known.

MEDITERRANEAN MACROTHROMBOCYTOPENIA

Mediterranean macrothrombocytopenia is a mild congenital thrombocytopenia with an autosomal dominant pattern of inheritance.[59] The condition initially was described in a group of 145 apparently healthy subjects from Italy and the Balkan Peninsula.[59] Because the undefined macrothrombocytopenia was not present in controls from northern Europe, it was named *Mediterranean macrothrombocytopenia*. Many of the patients shared clinical and molecular features with the heterozygous Bernard-Soulier syndrome phenotype.[60] Linkage analyses revealed a heterozygous Ala156Val missense substitution in the *GpIbα* gene (also known as *Bolzano mutation*), which is also present in patients with Bernard-Soulier syndrome (BSS). Patients with true autosomal hereditary thrombocytopenia without the mutation have a normal content of platelet glycoproteins, whereas the content is abnormal in those with the mutation, similar to that found in BSS heterozygotes.[60] The genetic abnormality responsible for Mediterranean thrombocytopenia in patients not bearing a BSS allele is not known and is considered a diagnosis of exclusion. No mutations of GpIbα, GpIbβ, GpV, or GpIX have been found.[61] The clinical manifestations of Mediterranean macrothrombocytopenia are variable, with the severity of bleeding related to both platelet number and function.

FAMILIAL PLATELET SYNDROME WITH PREDISPOSITION TO ACUTE MYELOGENOUS LEUKEMIA

Pathogenesis Familial platelet syndrome (FPS) with predisposition to acute myelogenous leukemia (AML) is a rare autosomal dominant condition characterized by qualitative and quantitative platelet defects resulting in pathologic bleeding and predisposition to the development of AML.[62] Genetic analysis of several pedigrees linked the causative defect to a mutation in the transcription factor Runx-1 (also known as AML1 and CBFA2).[63] Runx-1 binds to transcriptional complexes and regulates many genes important in hematopoiesis. Mutations of *Runx*-1 are commonly involved in the pathogenesis of sporadic leukemia and myelodysplastic syndromes (MDSs), stressing the importance of this transcriptional factor in normal hematopoiesis.[64] Genetic studies performed in animals engineered to have altered expression of *Runx*-1 and in humans affected with FPS/AML suggest that a deficiency of the full-length Runx-1 leads to an expanded population of undifferentiated hematopoietic stem cells (HSC).[65] In animal models, at least one functional copy of Runx-1 is required to affect definitive embryonic hematopoiesis. In contrast, patients with point mutations in one allele are predisposed to develop acute myeloid leukemia in adult life.[63,65]

Clinical Features The degree of thrombocytopenia in FPS/AML is mild to moderate. Platelets are of normal size and morphology but may have functional defects that lead to a prolonged bleeding time and clinical bleeding. The marrow may show decreased levels of megakaryocytic progenitors. The reason for the thrombocytopenia seen in this disorder is unknown, but the explanation may lie in the interaction of Runx-1 with the megakaryocytic transcription factors GATA-1 and Fli-1 (see Chap. 104).[66,67]

AUTOSOMAL DOMINANT THROMBOCYTOPENIA WITH LINKAGE TO HUMAN CHROMOSOME 10

This autosomal dominant thrombocytopenia has a genetic defect localized to 10p11-12 on the short arm of chromosome 10.[68,69] In one large kindred with the disorder, a missense mutation was identified within the gene *FLJ14813*a,[70] which encodes a putative tyrosine kinase of unknown function. Pedigree studies show that the thrombocytopenia segregates with incomplete differentiation of megakaryocytes. Megakaryocyte precursors from affected individuals produce low numbers of polyploid cells *in vitro*, with delayed nuclear and cytoplasmic differentiation when analyzed by electron microscopy.[68] Thus, the newly identified kinase (possibly a tyrosine kinase) seems to be involved in megakaryocyte endomitosis and terminal maturation. Affected family members have lifelong moderate thrombocytopenia, with a risk of bleeding proportionate to the degree of thrombocytopenia, but without any association with hematopoietic malignancy or progression to aplastic anemia.[68]

PARIS-TROUSSEAU SYNDROME

Paris-Trousseau syndrome and its variant Jacobsen syndrome are congenital dysmorphology syndromes in which affected individuals manifest trigonocephaly, facial dysmorphism, heart defects, and mental retardation.[71] Both disorders result from deletion of the long arm of chromosome 11 at 11q23, a region that includes the *FLI1* gene,[72] the product of which is a transcription factor involved in megakaryopoiesis.[73,74] The dominant inheritance pattern of Paris-Trousseau syndrome despite the presence of one normal allele seems to result from monoallelic expression of *FLI1* only during a brief window in megakaryocyte differentiation.[73,75] All affected patients have mild to moderate thrombocytopenia and dysfunctional platelets.[71] The blood film shows a subpopulation of platelets containing giant α-granules.[72] Marrow examination reveals two distinct subpopulations of megakaryocytes with expansion of immature megakaryocytic progenitors, dysmegakaryopoiesis, and many micromegakaryocytes.[73] Pathologic bleeding usually is mild.

THROMBOCYTOPENIA WITH RADIAL SYNOSTOSIS

Clinical Features Patients with amegakaryocytic thrombocytopenia with radioulnar synostosis present at birth with severe normocytic thrombocytopenia with absent marrow megakaryocytes, proximal radioulnar synostosis, and other skeletal anomalies such as clinodactyly and shallow acetabulae.[76] Bleeding complications are proportional to the degree of thrombocytopenia. Subsequent development of hypoplastic anemia and pancytopenia occurred in several individuals, suggesting that the defect is not limited to megakaryocytic progenitors.

Pathogenesis Genetic analysis of patients with thrombocytopenia and radioulnar synostosis revealed a mutation in *HoxA11*.[77] The Hox family of genes is characterized by a conserved DNA-binding domain termed the *homeobox*, a region that helps direct their transcriptional activity. These genes are known primarily for their role in embryonic development and cell fate determination. Studies have shown that members of Hox clusters A and B are expressed in HSCs. By manipulating the levels of HoxB4 and HoxA9 in mice, several investigators have shown that these genes are important in maintaining adequate numbers of HSC.[78] Although defects in *HoxA10* and *HoxA11* result in forearm defects and expression of each gene has been detected in HSC, only *HoxA10* has been shown to be expressed in megakaryocytes.[79] Mice that are genetically null for *HoxA11* have forearm defects and impaired fertility, but no description of hematopoiesis in these mice has been reported. Thus, how elimination of HoxA11 function alters thrombopoiesis is not clear, but the associated development of aplastic anemia suggests that the defect is at the level of the HSC.

CONGENITAL AMEGAKARYOCYTIC THROMBOCYTOPENIA

Congenital amegakaryocytic thrombocytopenia (CAMT) is a rare disease that in most cases presents with severe thrombocytopenia without physical abnormalities at birth. Bleeding complications usually are substantial because of the severe thrombocytopenia present in these children. The disorder progresses to aplastic anemia before age 3 to 5 years in most patients. CAMT results from mutations in the thrombopoietin receptor c-Mpl, rendering it deficient (type I CAMT) or of reduced function (type II CAMT).[80,81] The first patient in whom the pathogenesis of the disorder was identified displayed compound heterozygosity for two mutations in the *c-mpl* gene, both of which encoded truncated c-Mpl receptor polypeptides lacking all domains essential for intracellular signals.[82] Sequence analysis in eight patients with CAMT uncovered non-sense or missense mutations in all of them.[83]

Mutations of the thrombopoietin (TPO) receptor are associated with greatly reduced megakaryopoiesis, which correlates with the decreased number of megakaryocyte precursors seen in the marrow at birth. TPO affects megakaryocytes but also multipotent hematopoietic progenitors.[84–86] The gradual loss of CD34+ cells and hematopoietic progenitor cells in the blood and marrow of CAMT patients with increasing age, eventuating in marrow failure, establishes the critical role for TPO and c-Mpl in humans.[87] Marrow transplantation is the only curative therapy for CAMT.[88]

THROMBOCYTOPENIA WITH ABSENT RADIUS SYNDROME

The thrombocytopenia and absent radii (TAR) syndrome is a rare disease, first identified[89] in 1959, that occurs with an approximate frequency of one in 500,000 to 1,000,000 births. The inheritance pattern of TAR is unknown. The disease is characterized by the absence of both radii in the presence of both thumbs and thrombocytopenia.[90] The disorder can be associated with a broad range of congenital anomalies.[90] In a study of 34 patients with TAR syndrome, all cases had documented thrombocytopenia and bilateral radial aplasia, 47 percent had lower limb anomalies, 47 percent had intolerance to cow's milk, 23 percent had renal anomalies, and 15 percent had cardiac anomalies,[91] results consistent with previous reports.[92]

The thrombocytopenia in TAR syndrome usually is moderate, approximately 50×10^9 platelets/liter. It may be severe early in life but tends to improve with age. Thus, given a strong clinical suspicion, the diagnosis should not be excluded based on one isolated normal count. The etiology of the thrombocytopenia is unknown, but most authors agree the defect directly involves the megakaryocytes and causes an early arrest in megakaryopoiesis.[93] Serum TPO levels are normal,[94] and marrow cellularity is normal or increased. Megakaryocytes are low in number, or absent, or appear immature.

Affected patients can be managed with platelet transfusions and supportive treatment. Treatment usually is required only at early ages when the thrombocytopenia is more severe. Death is most commonly caused by bleeding in very young patients. In a review of 77 patients, only one death related to thrombocytopenia occurred after age 14 months.[92]

WISKOTT-ALDRICH SYNDROME

Definition, Genetics, and Pathogenesis Wiskott-Aldrich syndrome (WAS) is a rare X-linked immunodeficiency disorder characterized by microthrombocytopenia, eczema, recurrent infections, T cell deficiency, and increased risk for autoimmune and lymphoproliferative disorders.[95,96] The syndrome is caused by mutations of the *WASP* gene located on the short arm of the X chromosome (Xp11.22).[97–99] The product of this gene, the WAS protein (WASP), is expressed in hematopoietic cells. WASP regulates actin polymerization and coordinates reorganization of the actin cytoskeleton and signal transduction pathways that occur during cell movement and cell–cell interaction.[100] Microthrombocytopenia is the most consistent feature of WASP-associated disease, but the mechanism of reduced production and abnormal size remains incompletely understood. Mutant WASP is uniformly absent in platelets, even in the mildest patient phenotypes, suggesting a direct role of WASP deficiency in producing thrombocytopenia.[101] In some patients, destruction of platelets is increased as they may experience a significant rise in platelet count after splenectomy.[102] Because of a compromise in the cytoskeleton, a selective physical restriction to transmigration of larger platelets through the splenic vasculature leads to destruction of larger platelets in the spleen with resulting microthrombocytopenia.[103] Some studies have suggested a defect of platelet production, but the mechanism remains unclear.

Clinical Findings Clinically, the genetic defect produces cellular and humoral immunodeficiency, high susceptibility to autoimmune diseases, and increased risk for developing hematologic malignancies. This is the classic presentation, but the disease has a broad clinical spectrum that tends to correlate with the location and nature of the causative mutation.[100,103] More than 300 mutations have been described, and the clinical picture varies from mild microthrombocytopenia alone (also called *X-linked thrombocytopenia*) to the full-blown syndrome.[104,105]

Treatment HSC transplantation is the treatment of choice for patients with severe WAS. It corrects both thrombocytopenia and immunodeficiency and should always be considered, even in patients with milder phenotypes, because of the risk of developing hematologic malignancies.[106,107] Supportive treatment during acute bleeding and disease complications consists of platelet transfusions, antibiotics, and systemic glucocorticoids when eczema is severe. Patients with mild phenotypes and severe thrombocytopenia may respond to splenectomy, but the risk of infection in these already immunocompromised patients may outweigh the benefit. Some patients may have a rise in platelet count in response to prednisolone or methylprednisolone pulse therapy, but the response is only transient. The thrombocytopenia is not immune mediated. No platelet autoantibodies are present, and patients do not respond to IVIg therapy. Gene therapy, with retrovirus-mediated transfer of the *WASP* gene, is under active investigation and has shown promise in experimental animals.[108–110]

X-LINKED THROMBOCYTOPENIA WITH DYSERYTHROPOIESIS

A family of X-linked disorders of thrombocytopenia associated with dyserythropoiesis and thalassemia has been described.[111] GATA-1 is a transcription factor containing two zinc fingers: the C-terminal finger supports DNA binding and the N-finger stabilizes its binding to DNA and interacts with the cofactor Friend of GATA-1 (FOG-1). In several families, mutations in the N-finger are associated with macrothrombocytopenia and variable abnormalities in the erythroid lineage, whereas in other families mutations in the N-finger that disrupt the interaction of GATA-1 with FOG-1 lead to macrothrombocytopenia with dyserythropoietic anemia or β-thalassemia.[112] Although GATA-1 was first recognized for its vital role in erythropoiesis, GATA-1 and FOG-1 subsequently were shown to be critical for megakaryopoiesis,[113,114] as the GATA-1 consensus motif is found in the 5′ flanking regions of almost all characterized erythroid and megakaryocyte specific genes.[115] Although GATA-1 null mice die in embryogenesis of severe anemia, a megakaryocyte-specific deletion of the transcription factor allows sufficient erythropoiesis for survival, revealing the role of the transcription factor in megakaryopoiesis. These mice demonstrate hyperproliferation of immature low ploidy megakaryocyte progenitors associated with abnormal maturation and reduced expression of platelet specific genes.[116] Chapter 104 discusses the role of GATA-1 and FOG in megakaryopoiesis.

FANCONI ANEMIA

Patients with Fanconi anemia occasionally present with predominant thrombocytopenia, but the coexistent anemia and dysmorphogenesis usually make the diagnosis obvious. Chapter 33 discusses the disorder in greater detail.

THROMBOCYTOPENIA RESULTING FROM PLATELET TRAPPING

KASABACH-MERRITT SYNDROME

Definition Kasabach-Merritt syndrome (KMS) is defined as profound thrombocytopenia related to platelet trapping within a vascular tumor, either a Kaposi-like hemangioendothelioma or a tufted angioma.[117–120] The syndrome presents predominantly during infancy, but several adult cases have been reported.[121] These vascular tumors should be differentiated from vascular malformations such as classic benign hemangiomas. Benign hemangiomas usually are superficial, multiple, not associated with severe thrombocytopenia or disseminated intravascular coagulopathy (DIC), and usually disappear during childhood. On the other hand, Kaposi-like hemangioendothelioma and tufted angioma are low-grade malignant vascular tumors associated with high morbidity and mortality.

Histopathology Vascular tumors usually are solitary, may reach 20 cm in diameter, and may be superficial or invade internal organs and the retroperitoneum.[122–124] Superficial tumors can be recognized by the local red to purple discoloration of the skin.

The histologic types more frequently associated with KMS are Kaposi-like hemangioendothelioma and tufted angiomas or angioblastomas.[117,118,125,126] Kaposi-like hemangioendothelioma is a locally aggressive, low-grade malignant tumor characterized by infiltrating sheets or lobules of poorly formed vascular channels and aberrant lymphatic vessels. These tumors are composed predominantly of plump, round, oval, and/or spindled endothelial cells with hemosiderin deposits.[117] A tufted angioma is a lesion characterized by the presence of vascular tufts and aggregates of round dilated capillaries, lymphangiomatosis, microthrombi, and hemosiderin deposits.[117,118,127,128] Electron microscopic examination shows abnormal endothelial cells with prominent cytoplasmic projections and wide intercellular gaps, fibrin deposition, and platelet aggregates within the vessels.[118] The histology

of the tumor is useful for differentiating the vascular tumors associated with KMS from benign capillary hemangiomas.[129]

Clinical Findings Thrombocytopenia in KMS usually is severe and associated with DIC.[130] Contributing factors include "platelet trapping" by abnormally proliferating endothelium within the hemangioma[131,132] and platelet consumption associated with DIC. Platelet trapping has been demonstrated by immunohistochemical staining of the tumors with anti-CD61 antibodies (a marker of platelets and megakaryocytes)[133] and by nuclear studies using ^{51}Cr-labeled platelets[134] and ^{111}In platelet scintigraphy used to monitor response to therapy.[135,136] How platelets become trapped is not clear. Initial physical entrapment of the platelets within twisted abnormal vessels may favor their adhesion to abnormal endothelium, which may lead to platelet activation and aggregation followed by activation of the coagulation cascade, fibrin deposition, and formation of microthrombi. Excessive flow and shear rates generated by arteriovenous shunting within the tumor further increase the level of platelet activation. Continuous thrombus formation leads to platelet consumption and activation of the fibrinolytic cascade. Severe thrombocytopenia and DIC result.

Treatment and Course The mainstay of treatment is eradication of the tumor. Several specific therapeutic modalities have been proposed, but none has been established as consistently effective.[137] Among the therapies are high-dose glucocorticoids,[137] interferon-α,[137,138] vincristine,[139] cyclophosphamide,[140] combination chemotherapy,[141] and radiation.[142–144] For severe cases, interventions such as arterial embolization[145,146] surgical resection,[147,148] and pneumatic compression can be attempted.

The mortality rate for advanced KMS is approximately 12 percent and a higher rate when associated with retroperitoneal or intraabdominal tumors. Patients die of complications resulting from DIC, low platelet count, and infections secondary to immunosuppression.

ACQUIRED THROMBOCYTOPENIA RESULTING FROM IMPAIRED PLATELET PRODUCTION

THROMBOCYTOPENIA ASSOCIATED WITH HUMAN IMMUNODEFICIENCY VIRUS INFECTION

PREVALENCE

Thrombocytopenia is common in patients infected with HIV, with the prevalence of thrombocytopenia depending on the subpopulation of patients studied[149] (see Chap. 83). Among HIV-infected drug users, the prevalence is approximately 36.9 percent compared to 8.7 percent in drug users without HIV infection.[150] In homosexual men, the prevalence is approximately 16 percent in the HIV-infected group and 3 percent in the HIV-negative group.[150] The high prevalence of thrombocytopenia in homosexuals and intravenous drug users without HIV probably results from the high frequency of hepatitis in these populations. Thrombocytopenia occurs in approximately 19 percent of HIV-infected hemophiliacs and in 3 percent in the noninfected group.[151] One study showed that 50 percent of hemophiliacs manifested thrombocytopenia within 1 year of being diagnosed with an acquired immunodeficiency syndrome (AIDS)-defining illness.[151]

ETIOLOGY AND PHYSIOPATHOLOGY

Thrombocytopenia associated with HIV infection has numerous causes, many of which can be present simultaneously. These causes include accelerated platelet destruction primarily related to immune complexes, decreased platelet production, especially in advanced disease, splenic sequestration, and, rarely, platelet consumption associated with thrombotic thrombocytopenic purpura (TTP). Medications, concurrent infections such as hepatitis C, and hematologic malignancies may contribute to the development of thrombocytopenia[152–155] (see Chap. 83).

Accelerated Platelet Destruction Platelet kinetic studies performed in HIV-positive patients with thrombocytopenia demonstrate that the MPLS usually is very short, an indication of accelerated platelet destruction.[10,156] As opposed to the situation with ITP, in which the platelets are destroyed by antiplatelet antibodies directed against specific platelet antigens, in HIV platelet destruction results mainly from the nonspecific deposition of complement and immune complexes.[157,158] The levels of platelet-bound immunoglobulin and complement components are four times higher in these patients than in patients with ITP.[159–162]

HIV appears capable of triggering a large repertoire of immune complexes that participate in the destruction of platelets. Immune complexes containing anti-F(ab')2 antibodies are found in homosexual individuals with HIV and thrombocytopenia.[163] These immune complexes are composed of IgG anti-F(ab')2 antibodies that have a broad reactivity and react against F(ab')2 antibodies from control and from HIV-infected patients. Part of the immune complex bound to platelets has been proposed to correspond to IgG anti-F(ab')2 antibodies.[163]

Antibodies against CD4 and the CD4 receptor gp120 have been found in HIV-positive patients with and without thrombocytopenia.[164] Studies with affinity-purified anti-CD4 and anti-gp120 have shown that the antibodies are capable of forming complexes through their specificity-determining regions.[164–166] These immune complexes can bind platelets and have been postulated to play a role in the thrombocytopenia associated with HIV.

High-affinity antibodies against platelet GpIIIa have been eluted from the platelets of thrombocytopenic patients infected with HIV.[167] These antibodies react against a specific region on the molecule located between amino acids 49 and 66. That these antibodies are relevant pathophysiologically is supported by *in vivo* studies showing that administration of the antibodies systemically produces significant thrombocytopenia, an effect that can be prevented by coadministration of an albumin conjugate of GpIIIa49-66.[167] The presence of this immunodominant epitope appears unique to thrombocytopenia associated with HIV infection and may reflect cross-reactivity with antibodies directed against particular HIV antigens. Cross-reactivity of antibodies directed against viral antigens gp120 and p24 with platelet glycoproteins has been suggested in several studies.[168–173]

Antiidiotype antibodies directed against anti–GpIIIa49-66 can be detected in HIV patients, whether or not they are thrombocytopenic.[174] In the plasma, these antibodies (which usually are of the IgM type) are found as part of immune complexes. They are capable of blocking the destruction of platelets induced by anti–GpIIIa49-66. The levels of the antiidiotype antibodies appear to be inversely related to the degree of platelet destruction. Thus, the levels are higher in HIV patients without thrombocytopenia than in patients with thrombocytopenia.

One study has proposed that the mechanism of platelet destruction by anti–GpIIIa49-66 is independent of complement.[175] Anti–GpIIIa49-66 antibodies were shown to induce platelet fragmentation through the generation of reactive oxygen species such as H_2O_2 through the reduced nicotinamide adenine dinucleotide phosphate (NADPH) oxidase pathway. These findings where observed *in vitro* using inhibitors of reactive oxygen species and *in vivo* using p47phox-deficient mice lacking NADPH oxidase.[175,176]

Circulating immune complexes containing the head domain of talin (talin-H) have been described associated with thrombocytopenia in HIV.[177] Talin-H is a cleavage product of talin that can be generated by calpain when platelets become activated or by HIV-1 protease. Anti-talin antibodies have been detected in the serum of HIV patients with thrombocytopenia but not in controls subjects with ITP. These antibodies are highly mutated, suggesting an antigen-driven, affinity-matured response that may result from exposure of immunodominant epitopes on talin-H. The role of these antibodies in producing thrombocytopenia is unknown. The fact that they are directed against a cytoskeletal antigen argues against a causative role.

Decreased Platelet Production In addition to increased platelet destruction, reduced platelet production appears to play a role in the thrombocytopenia observed in HIV patients.[156,178,179] A direct effect of viral infection on platelet production is suggested by the observation that platelet production increases when patients are treated with zidovudine, an antiretroviral drug.[180] Infected patients with thrombocytopenia also have increased levels of TPO, again supporting the notion of ineffective platelet production in the origin of HIV-associated thrombocytopenia.[181,182] The defect appears to lie at the level of megakaryopoiesis, as decreased levels of megakaryocyte progenitors in marrow have been observed.[178,183]

How HIV decreases megakaryopoiesis is not known. The response to antiretroviral therapy suggests that the virus infects megakaryocytes or their precursors in the marrow. HIV-1 entry into cells requires sequential interaction of the viral envelope glycoprotein gp120 with CD4 and a coreceptor on the host cell plasma membrane, either C-C chemokine receptor-5 (CCR5) or CXC chemokine receptor-4 (CXCR4).[184] All of these receptors are expressed by megakaryocytes.[185,186] CD4, the receptor for HIV-1 on T cells, has been detected by flow cytometry in approximately 25 percent of human megakaryocytes at a density comparable to that of CD4+ T cells.[187] Anti-CD4 antibodies inhibit HIV infection of megakaryocytic cell lines *in vitro*.[188]

One study determined the biologic characteristics of HIV-1 in the marrow of HIV-1–infected patients and identified distinct amino acids in the third hypervariable loop (V3) of HIV-1 envelope glycoprotein gp120 that distinguish patients with thrombocytopenia from those without thrombocytopenia.[189] This study suggests that a particular strain of HIV-1 may be causally related to the development of thrombocytopenia, either by infection of megakaryocytes or their precursors or by infection of cells of the marrow microenvironment.[189,190]

Defective modulation of hematopoiesis by HIV-infected T lymphocytes can explain impairment of megakaryopoiesis. T cells from infected patients reduce the growth *in vitro* of colony-forming units for granulocytes, erythrocytes, monocytes/macrophages, and megakaryocytes.[191] A significant increase in the growth of these colonies in marrow from HIV-infected patients was observed when the cultures were depleted of T cells. Growth inhibition recurred upon readministration of the T cells. This effect was dependent on the ratio of T4 to T8 cells.[191]

Increased Platelet Consumption Patients with HIV are at higher risk for developing thrombotic microangiopathies.[192,193] A cohort study from New York found that one third of patients diagnosed with TTP also were infected with HIV. The incidence of TTP was much greater in the HIV-infected patients than in the general patient population, suggesting a causal association. In addition, several cases of recurrent thrombocytopenia in HIV patients refractory to conventional treatment who responded to plasma exchange have been reported. The mechanism may be akin to an autoimmune mechanism, as the levels of ADAMTS-13, a vWF-cleaving protease, reportedly are low.[194] One report shows absence of ADAMTS-13 in association with antibodies against the protease.

CLINICAL COURSE

Thrombocytopenic patients with HIV rarely experience clinically important bleeding (except, of course, those with hemophilia). The platelet counts rarely dip below 50×10^9/liter, and the thrombocytopenia often spontaneously resolves.[151,195-198] Thrombocytopenia in the early stages often is discovered through routine blood testing.[197] In the late stages of the disease, decreased platelet production may become more apparent, and marrow aspiration may be required to rule out infiltrative processes, although such processes are not routinely seen. One study examining the marrow in 42 patients with HIV infection found trilineage dysplasia, increased plasma cells and eosinophils, increased megakaryocytes, increased iron, and reticulin fibrosis.[199] Granulomata were found in two cases. Another study that reviewed marrow biopsies from 85 patients with HIV infection, at different stages, found increased cellularity in 72.9 percent, dysmyelopoiesis in 78.8 percent, plasma cell hyperplasia in 97.7 percent, lymphoid infiltration in 27 percent, and histiocytosis with or without granulomata in 11.7 percent.[200] In patients with end-stage AIDS, 28.2 percent had marrow hypoplasia. Opportunistic infections were seen occasionally, with agents such as *Mycobacterium avium*, *Cryptococcus neoformans*, *Toxoplasma gondii*, and *Leishmania donovani*. Malignancies were found in seven cases, including three cases of lymphoma.[200]

TREATMENT

Antiretroviral therapy is generally the first-line and most effective therapy for the thrombocytopenia associated with HIV infection.[197,201] Although improvements in platelet counts were previously achieved with zidovudine,[202-204] current combination antiretroviral regimens likely are more effective in increasing platelet counts as they are for enhancing CD4 cell counts and reducing HIV viral loads.[205] One retrospective study compared patients with severe thrombocytopenia treated with zidovudine to those treated with highly active antiretroviral therapy (HAART). After 6 months, HAART therapy more frequently resulted in complete and sustained recovery of platelet counts.[206] Responses were achieved even in those with azidothymidine (AZT)-resistant thrombocytopenia.

Management of patients with severe and symptomatic thrombocytopenia is similar to the management of patients with severe ITP. A retrospective study analyzed the response to prednisone, splenectomy, and other therapeutic modalities in 208 cases.[207] As in ITP, patients initially were treated with prednisone for 1 month; refractory or relapsed patients underwent splenectomy and/or other therapeutic modalities. An initial complete response with prednisone was seen in 38.8 percent of patients, a sustained remission that lasted for more than 6 months was observed in 18.7 percent, but only a few patients remained in remission. Splenectomy was performed in 63 patients, of whom 47 had an initial response, 41 had sustained remission, and 12 experienced sustained partial remission. Spontaneous remissions were observed in eight of 87 untreated cases. The patients who underwent splenectomy were more likely to experience a sustained complete remission. Similarly, another study of 185 HIV-infected patients showed an increase in the mean platelet count from 18×10^9/liter to 223×10^9/liter in those patients who underwent splenectomy, with a sustained response in 82 percent.[208] Neither AIDS progression rate nor AIDS-free survival was influenced by splenectomy. Thus, as in ITP, splenectomy is an effective therapy and appears to have no adverse effect on the progression of HIV disease.[209,210]

Other treatment modalities, such as IVIg[211,212] anti-D,[213] megakaryocyte growth factor,[214] and interferon-α,[215] have been used and reportedly were successful in particular cases.

CHEMOTHERAPY AND RADIATION THERAPY

The hematopoietic system appears to promptly recover after doses of chemotherapy and radiotherapy. However, heavily treated patients have a reduced tolerance to additional therapy, showing lower nadirs of blood counts, particularly platelets.[216] Depressed marrow function has been demonstrated up to 5 years following treatment. Hypoplastic syndromes or MDSs have been observed at late intervals. During the recovery phase, severe thrombocytopenia requires prompt attention. The current American Society of Clinical Oncology recommendations for platelet transfusions include prophylactic platelet transfusions when the platelet concentration is less than 10×10^9/liter (grade 4 toxicity), when the platelet concentration is less than 20×10^9/liter in patients with necrotic tumors (e.g., colorectal or bladder tumors), or when performance status is decreased.[217] Patients given multiple platelet transfusions may become refractory and show inadequate increments in the posttransfusion platelet counts. A platelet count increment less than 7×10^9/liter 1 hour posttransfusion or less than 20×10^9/liter 20 hours posttransfusion should raise the possibility of platelet refractoriness.[218] A true refractory state is encountered in less than half of patients treated for hematologic malignancies and results from alloimmunization against human leukocyte antigen (HLA) antigen on leukocytes in the transfused platelets. Other potential causes of poor platelet count increments following transfusion include fever, infections, bleeding, autoantibodies, and splenomegaly. Several strategies have been proposed in an effort to minimize the risks of allogeneic platelet transfusions, including routine transfusion of leukocyte-poor platelets[219] and transfusion of autologous cryopreserved platelets obtained with recombinant human TPO or with TPO mimetics.[220] A patient with thrombocytopenia refractory to platelet transfusion can be treated with HLA-compatible platelets or large quantities of platelet concentrates.[219]

Administration of growth factors, such as interleukin (IL)-1, IL-4, IL-6, IL-3,[221-223] or IL-11,[224-230] have been used to manage thrombocytopenia by stimulating uncommitted progenitors. Several studies have shown that administration of recombinant human (rh)TPO after chemotherapy reduces the degree and duration of thrombocytopenia[231-238]; however, additional studies are needed to validate the benefit of this drug in the treatment of myelosuppressive forms of thrombocytopenia.

NUTRITIONAL DEFICIENCIES AND ALCOHOL-INDUCED THROMBOCYTOPENIA

Mild thrombocytopenia occurs in approximately 20 percent of patients with megaloblastic anemia resulting from vitamin B_{12} deficiency in the United States.[239] The frequency may be higher in patients with folic acid deficiency because of the high frequency of concomitant alcohol abuse (see Chap. 39). One large study of 139 patients examined the rates of cytopenias associated with megaloblastic anemia in India.[240] In this study, 76 percent had isolated vitamin B_{12} deficiency, 7 percent had isolated folate deficiency, 9 percent had a combined deficiency, and 8 percent had normal vitamin levels. All by definition were anemic, and 80 percent had thrombocytopenia with mild to moderate depression of the platelet count. In more than half of those with thrombocytopenia, neutropenia was also present. The authors suggested that the cytopenias tended to progress from isolated anemia, to anemia plus thrombocytopenia, to pancytopenia, with the degree of cytopenia related to the severity of vitamin deficiency. Occasionally, thrombocytopenia is severe in the megaloblastic anemias and, when accompanied by fever, hepatomegaly, and splenomegaly, the presenting features may suggest acute leukemia. In these syndromes the primary mechanism of thrombocytopenia is ineffective platelet production[241]; marrow megakaryocyte number usually is normal or increased. Abnormalities of megakaryocyte morphology are much less distinctive than the characteristic erythroid and myeloid defects, but larger size and dispersed nuclear segments, rather than polyploid single nuclei, may be seen.[242]

Thrombocytopenia may be seen in association with vitamin B_{12} deficiency when the latter results from autoantibodies against parietal cells or intrinsic factor and is associated with immune thrombocytopenia.[243,244] Various other autoimmune disorders can coexist with pernicious anemia, including autoimmune vitiligo and autoimmune thyroiditis.[245]

Abnormalities of platelet function are sometimes seen associated with vitamin B_{12} deficiency.[246,247] Diminished platelet aggregation and reduced release of adenosine diphosphate and adenosine triphosphate from granular stores in response to different agonists have been reported, and vitamin deficiency has been suggested to induce an acquired storage pool disease[247] (see Chap. 39).

Thrombocytopenia has been reported in association with iron deficiency, although thrombocytosis is a much more common association (see Chap. 40). One study described thrombocytopenia in six iron-deficient children ranging in age from 14 months to 17 years, with the platelet counts ranging from 11 to 102×10^9/liter. In all patients, platelet counts returned to normal with iron repletion. Another study reported the case of a multiparous woman who presented with a platelet count of 9×10^9/liter, menorrhagia, and severe anemia because of iron deficiency. The marrow revealed no evidence of an underlying hematologic abnormality, and all findings resolved with repletion of iron stores.[248] These reports illustrate the extent to which severe iron deficiency can diminish the platelet count.

Thrombocytopenia in alcoholic patients almost always results from liver cirrhosis with congestive splenomegaly or from folic acid deficiency, but in some patients thrombocytopenia appears to result primarily from direct marrow suppression by alcohol of platelet production.[249,250] Suppression of platelet production sufficient to produce thrombocytopenia requires consumption of large quantities of ethanol over several days.[249] However, one study of guinea pigs allowed to ingest ethanol *ad libitum* showed that, although blood ethanol never reached measurable levels, the average platelet count declined 16 percent in the 4 weeks of study.[251] The platelets of the ethanol-imbibing guinea pigs were smaller than those of the control animals.

Thrombocytopenia induced by alcohol ingestion is accompanied by a decreased number of marrow megakaryocytes. Vacuolated proerythroblasts and granulocyte precursors are sometimes seen, as are multinuclear erythroblasts and megaloblasts.[252] Vacuolization of the periphery of mature megakaryocytes has been reported.[250] Thrombocytopenia usually resolves in 5 to 21 days with cessation of ethanol ingestion, sometimes with a transient rebound thrombocytosis. Thrombopoietin deficiency may contribute to thrombocytopenia in alcoholics with liver cirrhosis given that the liver is a major site of TPO synthesis.[253]

PAROXYSMAL NOCTURNAL HEMOGLOBINURIA

Thrombocytopenia in patients with paroxysmal nocturnal hemoglobinuria (PNH) primarily results from marrow failure (see Chap. 38). Decreased platelet production has been shown by kinetic studies using autologous radiolabeled platelets[254] and by *in vitro* studies using CD34+ cells from PNH patients.[255,256] These cells demonstrate decreased proliferation and differentiation of megakaryocyte progenitors, as is seen in aplastic anemia, suggesting a defect at the stem cell level.[256] Thrombocytopenia also may be explained by platelet consumption associated with ongoing thrombosis. The molecular bases of thrombophilia in these patients are unknown. Several mechanisms have been proposed, including excessive generation of platelet microvesicles released from complement injured and activated plate-

lets,[257,258] increased prothrombinase activity on C5b-C9 injured platelets,[259] increased tissue factor expression by complement injured CD55- and CD59-deficient monocytes and macrophages,[260] resistance to fibrinolytic stimuli because of detachment of the glycosylphosphatidylinositol-anchored urokinase plasminogen activator receptor from monocytes and neutrophils,[261,262] and elevated microparticles from damaged endothelium.[263]

MYELODYSPLASTIC SYNDROMES

MDSs are clonal myeloid disorders characterized by blood cytopenias in combination with a hypercellular marrow that often exhibit dysplastic changes in any of the three hematopoietic lineages[264–266] (see Chap. 86). Thrombocytopenia is present in approximately 50 percent of patients and usually occurs in conjunction with other cytopenias. Isolated thrombocytopenia at initial presentation occurs in less than 5 percent of cases.[267] Thrombocytopenia is seen more frequently in patients with oligoblastic myelogenous leukemia (refractory anemia with excess blasts [RAEB]) than in those with clonal cytopenias (refractory anemia and refractory anemia with ringed sideroblasts) (see Chap. 86).[268] Moreover, platelets from patients with MDS often display functional abnormalities (see Chaps. 86 and 113) and, when present, usually augment the thrombocytopenia-related bleeding disorder.

The presence of micromegakaryocytes or micromononuclear megakaryocytes in marrow from MDS patients indicates altered megakaryopoiesis. Normal megakaryocytes have a diameter of 25 to 35 μm and a peak ploidy of 16N, whereas micromegakaryocytes have a diameter less than 20 μm and a peak ploidy of 4N or 8N.[269–274] The relationship between these morphologic changes and the pathophysiology of abnormal megakaryopoiesis in MDS is unknown.

Maturation of megakaryocytes is arrested in MDS, as suggested by immunohistochemistry studies showing an increased number of megakaryocytic precursors in the marrow of affected patients.[272] Besides the maturational arrest, as measured by enumeration of denuded megakaryocytic nuclei, an increased rate of apoptosis has been detected in all subtypes of MDS.[275] Immunohistochemistry studies of the marrow biopsies from patients with MDS suggest that the mechanism of programmed cell death of megakaryocytes is independent of activated caspase 3 or cathepsin D.[276] Abnormal megakaryopoiesis seems to be worse and clinically more significant in the high-risk group of patients with MDS, such as those with RAEB.[268,277] Abnormal proliferation and differentiation of megakaryocytes have been observed *in vitro*, during evaluation of the number and growth of megakaryocyte colony-forming units of mononuclear cells in marrow from patients with MDS.[278,279] Although the TPO receptor is present on megakaryocytes of patients with MDS, *in vitro* administration of TPO overcomes the underlying maturation defect in only a subset of patient cells.[280] These findings suggest that the defective response may result from either a dysfunctional receptor or an abnormality in the downstream signaling pathway rather than from diminished expression of the receptor itself.[281] In accordance with this hypothesis, some studies have shown TPO induction of blast cell proliferation in marrow from patients with RAEB and the condition previously termed RAEB-T.[282–284] Many ongoing studies aim to identify the molecular bases of the hematopoietic insufficiency and the leukemic progression in patients with the MDSs.[267] Until this goal is achieved, supportive therapy in addition to chemotherapy and marrow transplantation remain the mainstays of therapy.

APLASTIC ANEMIA

Aplastic anemia is a pancytopenia that results from failure of marrow hematopoiesis (see Chap. 33). However, some patients with MDS or amegakaryocytic thrombocytopenia present with low platelet counts and then progress to pancytopenia and aplastic anemia.[285-287] In aplastic anemia, blood testing reveals markedly decreased cell counts, reticulocytopenia, and lack of circulating blasts.

A considerable amount of data support the hypothesis that aplastic anemia results from an autoimmune attack directed against HSC.[288-290] Activated Th1-type T cells that produce interferon-α, tumor necrosis factor, and IL-2 are responsible for suppression of the hematopoietic cell compartment. This cytotoxic activation leads to a Fas-mediated cell cycle arrest and death of CD34+ cells. The majority of cases are idiopathic; however, idiosyncratic reactions to some drugs, chemicals, and viruses have been implicated in the etiology (see Chap. 33).

The development of alloantibodies to platelets is a major problem in the supportive management of thrombocytopenia in patients with severe aplastic anemia. Leukocyte-reduced platelets are helpful in preventing alloimmunization. Cyclosporin A has been used to modulate alloimmunization in these patients. Platelet counts greater than 10×10^9/liter should be adequate to prevent catastrophic bleeding, except in the case of breeches in vascular integrity or surgical challenge. Experimental treatment with rhIL-11 (Neumega) and with recombinant TPO reportedly has been effective for treatment of thrombocytopenia in some patients with aplastic anemia.[291-293]

ACQUIRED PURE AMEGAKARYOCYTIC THROMBOCYTOPENIA

Thrombocytopenia because of pure aplasia or hypoplasia of megakaryocytes is rare.[294] More common are instances in which amegakaryocytic thrombocytopenia is seen preceding the development of full-blown myelodysplastic syndromes or aplastic anemia and is associated with subtle abnormalities of other lineages, such as macrocytosis and dyserythropoiesis.[295-299] Most commonly the disorder is caused by autoimmune suppression of megakaryocyte development, either idiopathic,[300] associated with autoimmune disorders such as systemic lupus erythematosus (SLE)[301] and eosinophilic fasciitis,[302] or associated with infections such as hepatitis C.[287] Antibodies against TPO[303] have been described to cause the disorder, as have antibodies against the TPO receptor.[304] Patients may achieve durable remission with therapies designed to blunt the autoimmune response, such as cyclosporine or anti-thymocyte globulin (ATG).[305]

THROMBOCYTOPENIA RESULTING FROM ACCELERATED PLATELET DESTRUCTION

AUTOIMMUNE (IDIOPATHIC) THROMBOCYTOPENIC PURPURA IN ADULTS

DEFINITION AND CLASSIFICATION

Immune (autoimmune, idiopathic) thrombocytopenic purpura is a common acquired autoimmune disorder defined by a low platelet count secondary to accelerated platelet destruction by antiplatelet antibodies. The diagnosis of ITP requires decreased platelets on the blood film and the exclusion of other causes of thrombocytopenia. Normal or increased numbers of marrow megakaryocytes are found in the majority of patients.[306] ITP can be classified based on the absence or presence of other diseases (primary or secondary), patient age (adult or childhood ITP), and duration of thrombocytopenia (acute or chronic). Antibody-mediated platelet destruction may develop in several infectious diseases, lymphoproliferative diseases, and autoimmune diseases, and in association with drug therapy (Table 110-2).

The presentation and management of ITP are different in adults and children. Childhood ITP typically is acute in onset. Boys and girls are equally affected, and the condition often develops after a viral

TABLE 110-2   CAUSES OF IMMUNE-MEDIATED THROMBOCYTOPENIA

1. Primary

   Idiopathic autoimmune thrombocytopenic purpura

2. Secondary

  A. Autoimmune diseases: systemic lupus erythematosus, antiphospholipid syndrome, autoimmune hepatitis, autoimmune thyroiditis

  B. Lymphoproliferative disorders: chronic lymphocytic leukemia, Hodgkin lymphoma, large granular lymphocytic leukemia

  C. Infections: human immunodeficiency virus, hepatitis C, *Helicobacter pylori*

  D. Myelodysplastic syndrome

  E. Agammaglobulinemia, hypogammaglobulinemia, immunoglobulin A deficiency

  F. Drugs: quinidine, gold, heparin, penicillin, procainamide, α-methyldopa, sulfamethoxazole

infection or vaccination. Although thrombocytopenia may be severe, it usually resolves spontaneously, within a few weeks up to 6 months.[307] In contrast to childhood ITP, adult ITP generally is a chronic disease of insidious onset, is predominant in women, and rarely resolves spontaneously (Table 110-3).

INCIDENCE

ITP is relatively common, but demographic studies have yielded a wide range of incidence rates largely because of differences in the age and gender distribution of the populations studied and differences in cutoff platelet counts used to define the syndrome. In one detailed study, the reported annual incidence of ITP was 5.5 per 100,000 persons when defined by a platelet count of less than 100×10^9/liter and 3.2 per 100,000 using a cutoff platelet count less than 50×10^9/liter.[308] The estimated female-to-male ratio was 1.7. The incidence of ITP increases with age, being twofold higher in populations older than 60 years than in those younger than 60 years.[308,309]

TABLE 110-3   CLINICAL FEATURES OF IDIOPATHIC THROMBOCYTOPENIC PURPURA IN CHILDREN AND ADULTS

	CHILDREN	ADULTS
Occurrence		
Peak age (years)	2–4	15–40
Sex (F:M)	Equal	1.2–1.7
Presentation		
Onset	Acute (most with symptoms <1 week)	Insidious (most with symptoms >2 months)
Symptoms	Purpura (<10% with severe bleeding)	Purpura (typically bleeding not severe)
Platelet count	Most <20,000/μl	Most <20,000/μl
Course		
Spontaneous remission	83%	2%
Chronic disease	24%	43%
Response to splenectomy	71%	66%
Eventual complete recovery	89%	64%
Morbidity and mortality		
Cerebral hemorrhage	<1%	3%
Hemorrhagic death	<1%	4%
Mortality of chronic refractory disease	2%	5%

PATHOPHYSIOLOGY

More than 50 years ago Harrington and colleagues provided the first evidence that ITP was caused by antiplatelet antibodies. In this pioneering work, normal volunteers were infused with the plasma from patients with ITP, resulting in severe thrombocytopenia in the recipients.[310,311] Subsequently, Shulman and coworkers[312] showed that the thrombocytopenic effect of ITP plasma was dose dependent and associated with globulin fraction. Additional findings suggested that splenic clearance was the major mechanism of thrombocytopenia.[312]

In the early 1970s, two groups showed that platelets from chronic ITP patients had elevated levels of platelet-associated immunoglobulin G (PAIgG).[313,314] Elevated levels of PAIgG later were seen often in nonimmune thrombocytopenic patients.[315,316] In 1982, the first platelet target was identified. Autoantibodies from patients with ITP were shown not to bind to platelets deficient in the GpIIb-IIIa complex (i.e., from patients with Glanzmann thrombasthenia).[317] In the late 1980s, two specific assays for the target antigens were described: the immunobead assay[318] and the monoclonal antibody-specific immobilization of platelet antigens assay (MAIPA) assay.[319] These assays showed that the majority of antiplatelet antibodies in patients with ITP are directed against GpIIb-IIIa (approximately 80%), and the remainder against the GpIb-IX complex and other platelet glycoproteins such as GpIV and GpIa-IIa.[320,321] Antibodies in some sera recognize several antigens. Most antiplatelet autoantibodies are IgG; the remainder are IgM and IgA. Antibody-coated platelets bind antigen-presenting cells through Fcγ receptors, primarily in the spleen but also in other organs of the mononuclear phagocyte system.[322,323] It has been postulated that platelet destruction also amplifies the immune response. The mechanism involves presentation of platelet antigens by activated antigen-presenting cells, which thereby activate both CD4+ T cell clones and antigen-specific T cell clones. These T cell clones, having different antigen specificities, induce different B cell clones to produce antibodies against distinct platelet antigens.[321-323]

In the initial studies with PAIgG, antibodies in ITP reportedly were polyclonal.[324] However, later studies showed that at least some ITP patients had clonal B cell proliferation, as determined by DNA analysis for immunoglobulin heavy- and light-chain rearrangements and by flow cytometry of B cells from blood and spleen for surface Ig light chains.[325,326]

Although ITP is antibody mediated, the autoantibodies are under the control of T helper cells and their cytokines. Abnormal T cell responses drive the differentiation of autoreactive B cell clones and autoantibody secretion. GpIIb-IIIa–reactive CD4+ T cells from patients with ITP promote the production of anti–GpIIb-IIIa antibodies capable of binding normal platelets,[327] and the clones respond to chemically modified GpIIb-IIIa and recombinant GpIIb-IIIa fragments but not to native GpIIb-IIIa. Thus, autoreactive CD4+ T helper cells in patients with ITP may recognize a modified GpIIb-IIIa molecule (the cryptic epitope theory[24]). Although specific GpIIb-IIIa peptide fragments have been identified that are recognized by autoreactive CD4+ T cells,[322,328,329] the initial event that induces these abnormalities is not clear.

Complement activation plays a role in thrombocytopenia in some patients with ITP. Increased platelet-associated C3, C4, and C9 have been demonstrated on the platelets from patients with ITP.[330,331] In vitro studies have shown that, in the presence of antiplatelet antibodies, C3 and C4 can bind platelets and cause their lysis.[332]

PLATELET PRODUCTION AND DESTRUCTION

Early studies of platelet survival demonstrated that platelet life span is shortened in ITP patients and returns to normal after splenectomy-induced remission.[333] Platelet transfusion only transiently increases a patient's platelet count, and the transfused platelets have shortened survival, reflecting the fact that the major problem in ITP is platelet destruction. The antibody-coated platelets are destroyed by tissue macrophages located primarily in the spleen and, to a lesser extent, in the liver and marrow.

The marrow responds to thrombocytopenia by increasing platelet production. The severity of thrombocytopenia in ITP patients reflects the balance between platelet destruction and platelet production. In most cases of ITP, the marrow has a normal or increased number of megakaryocytes. Because the target antigens of platelet autoantibodies may be present on the megakaryocytes and their progenitors, megakaryopoiesis is impaired in some patients with ITP, manifested by decreased numbers of megakaryocytes in marrow.[334] Autoantibodies against platelet glycoproteins may interfere with the maturation of megakaryocytes, resulting in reduced platelet production, contributing to the severity of thrombocytopenia in some ITP patients.[335] Antibodies that target the GpIb-IX-V complex may induce thrombocytopenia by decreasing platelet production, as GpIb autoantibodies have been shown to inhibit megakaryopoiesis in vitro,[335] and GpIb monoclonal antibodies inhibit proplatelet formation in vitro.[336]

The compensatory increase in platelet production in ITP is generally associated with large platelets on the blood film and an elevated mean platelet volume on automated cell counters. Large, young platelets have increased granular contents and enhanced function both in vitro and in vivo,[337-339] likely explaining the observation that the bleeding time is generally less severely affected in patients with ITP, even when severe, than in patients with thrombocytopenia from other causes with equivalent platelet levels. Although the mean platelet volume is increased, the ultrastructure of ITP platelets viewed by electron microscopy is similar to that of normal platelets.[340]

The large size and increased function of the platelets in ITP can be largely attributed to the actions of TPO, the major regulator of megakaryopoiesis and thrombopoiesis. TPO is synthesized in greatest quantity in the liver but is found in other organs (kidney, muscle), including the marrow in patients with ITP.[341] This protein hormone enhances megakaryocyte colony formation and increases the size, number, and ploidy of megakaryocytes and platelet production.[341-343] TPO levels are markedly elevated in patients with thrombocytopenia associated with megakaryocytic hypoplasia, disorders such as aplastic anemia or acute leukemia. The association of TPO levels with ITP is not clear. In most reports, ITP patients have normal or slightly elevated TPO levels whether measured in plasma or serum, but the levels are always lower than the concentrations found in thrombocytopenias resulting from megakaryocytic hypoplasia.[341-345] Most authorities believe this finding results from active TPO uptake and destruction by the expanded megakaryocyte mass in ITP.

GENETICS

ITP has been documented in monozygotic twins[346] and in some families.[347] As with other autoimmune disorders, heredity may contribute to the development of ITP and may affect the response to therapy. HLA class I and II allele frequencies in patients with ITP have been studied by several investigators, with inconsistent results. Some investigators reported an increased frequency of HLA Aw32, DRw2, DRB1*0410.[323,348-350] Investigation has focused on genetic differences associated with dysregulation of immune tolerance and humoral immunity, but results have been inconclusive. For example, genetic polymorphisms of CTLA-4, tumor necrosis factor, and Fcγ receptors IIA and IIIA have been suggested to influence the development of ITP and the response to therapy,[149,351,352] but as yet no strong association has been found.

CLINICAL FEATURES

ITP usually is a chronic disease in adults. Chronic ITP is traditionally defined as ITP with a platelet count less than 150×10^9/liter for more than 6 months. A significant portion of patients are diagnosed incidentally in routine complete blood counts. Symptoms and signs of ITP depend on the platelet count. Approximately one third of patients have platelet counts greater than 30×10^9/liter at diagnosis and no significant bleeding,[353] although bleeding symptoms are generally seen in patients with counts below this level. Purpura (ecchymoses and petechiae), epistaxis, menorrhagia, and gingival bleeding are common. Hematuria, hemoptysis, and gastrointestinal bleeding are less common. Intracerebral hemorrhage is rare and generally occurs in patients with platelet counts less than 10×10^9/liter and usually is associated with trauma or vascular lesions. The incidence of life-threatening complications is highest in patients older than 60 years; however, mortality rates are low in patients with ITP, even in those with severe thrombocytopenia.[353-356]

The purpuric lesions seen in ITP are not palpable, do not blanch with pressure, and often develop on distal regions of the extremities and on skin areas exposed to pressure (e.g., around tight belts and stockings and at tourniquet sites). Hemorrhagic bullae, which may develop in the buccal mucosa, generally reflect acute, severe thrombocytopenia. Bleeding after surgery, trauma, or tooth extraction is common.

Besides the physical findings associated with platelet-type bleeding, the history and physical examination usually are normal. Family history is especially important to discriminate familial thrombocytopenic syndromes from ITP. The spleen usually is not enlarged but may be palpable in some patients, a finding considered to occur with the same incidence as in normal adults.[357] Constitutional symptoms, such as fever, significant weight loss, marked splenomegaly, hepatomegaly, and lymphadenopathy, provide evidence against the possibility that the thrombocytopenia results from ITP and strongly suggest an alternative diagnosis.

LABORATORY FEATURES

Platelet Counts and Size Thrombocytopenia is defined as a blood platelet count less than 150×10^9/liter. The blood film usually demonstrates isolated thrombocytopenia without evidence of pseudothrombocytopenia. Platelet anisocytosis is a common finding in ITP. Mean platelet volume and platelet distribution width are increased. Platelets may be abnormally large or abnormally small. The former reflect accelerated platelet production,[358] and the latter platelet microparticles reflect platelet destruction.[359] The observation of giant platelets should trigger consideration of inherited platelet disorders, which often are misdiagnosed as ITP.[360] Bleeding time correlates inversely with platelet count if the count is less than 100×10^9/liter but may be normal in patients with mild or moderate thrombocytopenia.[361] The ultrastructure of ITP platelets viewed by electron microscopy is similar to that of normal platelets.[340]

Other Blood Findings Hemoglobin concentration and hematocrit are generally normal in patients with ITP. The presence of anemia that is not easily explained (e.g., resulting from iron deficiency in bleeding patients or associated with thalassemia minor in endemic areas) requires further investigation. Autoimmune hemolytic anemia with a positive Coombs test and reticulocytosis may accompany ITP; the association is termed *Evans syndrome*.[362] The latter syndrome can include immune neutropenia.[362] Neither erythrocyte poikilocytosis nor schistocytes should be present. Total leukocyte counts and differential are generally normal. Although atypical lymphocytes and eosinophilia may occur in children with ITP, leukocytosis and leukopenia with immature cells are not consistent with the diagnosis.[363]

Marrow examination, which is not always required to make a di-

agnosis of ITP, generally reveals normal or increased numbers of megakaryocytes of normal morphology, although a decreased number of megakaryocytes does not rule out ITP.[364] Erythropoiesis and myelopoiesis are normal. The American Society of Hematology (ASH) guidelines for ITP state that marrow aspiration is unnecessary in the initial evaluation of ITP if the patient is younger than 60 years, has a typical presentation, has a good response to first-line therapy, and if splenectomy is not being considered.[306] Nevertheless, some hematologists recommend that the marrow be evaluated to rule out leukemia and myelodysplasia, especially in children and those older than 40 years.[323,363]

Measuring Platelet Antibodies Because ITP is caused by autoantibodies, specific measurement of such antibodies is expected to provide useful diagnostic clues, much as the Coombs test is used to diagnose autoimmune hemolytic anemia. Various antiplatelet antibody tests have been described, but none is sufficiently sensitive or specific to be of widespread clinical use. Three types of antiplatelet antibody tests have been developed.

Phase 1 assays were developed after the demonstration that infusion of ITP plasma to healthy subjects resulted in platelet destruction.[310] In these, the patient's serum is incubated with control platelets, and platelet-dependent endpoints are measured, such as platelet aggregation or agglutination, granule release, or platelet lysis. Phase 1 tests are neither sensitive nor specific and are of no diagnostic value for ITP.[364,365]

Phase 2 assays measure PAIgG and other antibodies that can bind the platelet plasma membrane. Antibodies found in platelet granules and in the open canalicular system also are detected with these assays. In these assays, total and surface PAIgG can be measured with different methods.[366] PAIgG is increased in patients with ITP but is also found in healthy subjects and in patients with nonimmune thrombocytopenia. Normal platelets contain immunoglobulins in their α-granules, and plasma immunoglobulin levels affect the amount of immunoglobulins in platelets.[367-369] Although the sensitivity of phase 2 assays has been reported to be as high as 91 percent, the specificity is very low. PAIgG assays cannot discriminate immune from nonimmune thrombocytopenia.[316,366,367]

Phase 3 assays measure platelet glycoprotein-specific autoantibodies. Three techniques are most widely used: immunoblotting, immunoprecipitation, and glycoprotein immobilization assays. In the *immunoblot assay*, platelet membrane proteins are separated by electrophoresis, transferred to membranes, and the membranes incubated with the patient's serum. Serum autoantibodies bound to platelet proteins then are detected by radiolabeled or enzyme-conjugated antihuman IgG. Platelet autoantigens are identified based on their electrophoretic migration.[365,370] The sensitivity of the immunoblot assay is low, and nonspecific binding may occur with normal sera.[371] In the *immunoprecipitation assay*, platelet glycoprotein–autoantibody complexes are captured from the serum using Sepharose beads coated with staphylococcal protein A. This technique may be useful for identifying novel platelet antigens, but its sensitivity is low.[365] *Glycoprotein immobilization assays* include five different assays: microtiter well assay, immunobead assay, modified antigen-capture enzyme-linked immunoadsorbent assay (MACA), MAIPA, and platelet-associated IgG characterization assay (PAICA). The microtiter well assay is an indirect test, and both sensitivity and specificity are low.[365,372] The immunobead assay, MACA, MAIPA, and PAICA all appear to be more sensitive and specific than the microtiter well assay.[319] PAICA has several advantages because it can detect both surface and intracellular autoantibodies. These tests may be useful for discriminating immune from nonimmune thrombocytopenia and for monitoring response to treatment. Although phase 3 tests are specific, they are not sensitive enough for ITP screening.

DIFFERENTIAL DIAGNOSIS

The diagnosis of ITP is based on its clinical manifestations because no laboratory parameters can accurately diagnose the condition. The diagnosis is based on history, physical examination, blood count, and blood film. The ASH guidelines recommend no further diagnostic studies for the typical patient.

Additional tests, such as lupus anticoagulant, antiplatelet antibody testing, direct antiglobulin test, reticulocyte count, mean platelet volume, urinalysis, and thyroid function tests, are generally unnecessary but may be appropriate when other patient characteristics call attention to underlying disorders. Bleeding time, platelet survival study, serum complement, abdominal ultrasound, computed tomography, and PAIgG assays are unnecessary and inappropriate.[364] Antiphospholipid antibodies (lupus anticoagulant and anticardiolipin antibodies) are seen frequently in patients with ITP.[373] Although some researchers have reported these autoantibodies have no clinical significance,[207,374] others have found an increased risk for thrombosis in ITP patients with antiphospholipid antibodies[375,376] (see "Thrombocytopenia in Patients with Systemic Lupus Erythematosus" and "Thrombocytopenia in Patients with Antiphospholipid Syndrome" below).

THERAPY, COURSE, AND PROGNOSIS

The natural course of ITP is unknown, as most patients are treated with glucocorticoids. Studies conducted before the glucocorticoid era showed that ITP in adults typically is a chronic disease, with infrequent spontaneous remissions, in contrast to ITP in children. Even with glucocorticoid therapy, complete remission usually is not seen. An analysis of 12 series of 1761 adults with ITP reported a complete remission rate of only 25 percent with glucocorticoids and a mortality rate of 5 percent, predominantly because of intracerebral hemorrhage.[354] The risk of hemorrhagic complications is greater in patients older than 60 years.[308]

ITP may respond to various agents or manipulations, including glucocorticoids, splenectomy, IVIg, infused anti-D, danazol, and antineoplastic drugs such as vincristine and azathioprine. Thus, the patient's symptoms and initial response to therapy should dictate ongoing therapy.

INITIAL MANAGEMENT

Observation Because most ITP patients are diagnosed incidentally in routine evaluation, signs and symptoms of bleeding are important in determining whether any treatment is required. Patients with no bleeding and consistent platelet counts in excess of 50×10^9/liter do not require treatment and can be observed periodically. These patients are at low risk for clinically important bleeding and may safely undergo invasive procedures.[354,355,377] Patients with platelet counts between 30 and 50×10^9/liter generally do not experience clinically important bleeding but may manifest easy bruising. They usually do not require treatment. Careful followup is necessary for these patients because the clinical course is difficult to predict. Simple observation is not recommended for patients with platelet counts less than 20×10^9/liter, in those with platelet counts between 20 and 50×10^9/liter and significant mucosal bleeding, or in those with risk factors for bleeding, such as uncontrolled hypertension, peptic ulcer, or a vigorous lifestyle.[364]

Emergency Treatment of Acute Bleeding Resulting from Severe Thrombocytopenia Fortunately, bleeding symptoms generally are not severe in adult patients with ITP, even with very low platelet counts. However, life-threatening bleeding may occur in patients with platelet counts less than 10×10^9/liter. Emergent treatment should be instituted in patients with intracranial or gastrointestinal bleeding, massive hematuria, internal hematoma, or in need of emergent surgical intervention. The presence of extensive purpura or hemorrhagic bullae in mucosal tissues is a harbinger of life-threatening bleeding and war-

rants therapy. Patients with any of these findings should be hospitalized and monitored closely. High-dose parenteral glucocorticoid therapy (methyl prednisolone 1 g/day in divided doses for 3 days), IVIg (1 g/kg/day for 2 days), or IVIg and parenteral glucocorticoids in combination are generally recommended for those patients.[306] In most patients, IVIg increases the platelet count within 2 to 3 days.[306,323,354] Although platelet transfusions may not increase the platelet counts because the transfused platelets are destroyed rapidly, they nevertheless may contribute to the formation of platelet plugs at sites of bleeding and improve hemostasis. Platelet transfusions after IVIg infusion may increase the platelet count because IVIg may improve platelet survival.[378] Aminocaproic acid, which inhibits fibrinolysis, can be used to reduce bleeding[378] and is safe except in the presence of hematuria, in which it can cause thrombi of the glomeruli, renal pelves, and ureters. This agent does not affect platelet count or function. Aminocaproic acid usually is administered intravenously (initial dose 0.1 g/kg over 30 minutes, then given either by continuous infusion at 0.5–1 g/h or as an equivalent intermittent dose every 2–4 hours). Aminocaproic acid also can be administered orally in a similar dose in emergency situations because it is absorbed very rapidly from the gastrointestinal tract. Vincristine can be used in combination with glucocorticoid and IVIg treatment.[323]

Glucocorticoid Therapy Glucocorticoids are recommended as initial treatment for patients with platelet counts less than 20×10^9/liter and in patients with platelet counts between 20 and 50×10^9/liter and significant bleeding. Oral prednisone 1 to 2 mg/kg/day is generally accepted for initial treatment in patients with ITP. Glucocorticoids increase the platelet count through several mechanisms, including inhibition of phagocytosis of antibody-coated platelets by macrophages, decreasing autoantibody production, and improving marrow platelet production.[379,380] They also appear to reduce capillary leakage. Although no consensus exists regarding the duration of initial therapy, treatment should continue until platelet counts reach a safe range. Patients generally respond to initial glucocorticoid therapy within the first 3 weeks of treatment. In approximately two thirds of patients, platelet counts increase to greater than 50×10^9/liter within 1 week but decrease again when the prednisone dose is tapered.[306,354] Thus, in patients who respond, the recommendation is to continue glucocorticoid therapy 1 mg/kg/day for a total of 3 weeks before initiating the taper.

The glucocorticoid-dosing regimen that achieves the best response of the platelet count in patients with ITP is still under investigation. In addition to the standard 1 to 2 mg/kg/day dose of prednisone, lower doses[381,382] and high doses[383–386] have been investigated, with good results. Methylprednisolone or dexamethasone can be used for high-dose initial therapy by either oral or intravenous route.

The major drawback of glucocorticoid therapy is that the adverse effects may be worse than the disease itself. Facial swelling, weight gain, folliculitis, hyperglycemia, hypertension, cataracts, osteoporosis, opportunistic infections, and behavioral disturbances are common side effects and can be severe.[306,387] A study showed that a short course of treatment with high-dose glucocorticoids (dexamethasone 40 mg/day for 4 consecutive days) as initial therapy for ITP was well tolerated and effective[386] compared to standard-dose therapy. Despite this success, the use of this regimen as first-line therapy has not been validated.

Sustained remissions with glucocorticoids are infrequent, with reported rates ranging from 5 to 30 percent.[306,323] If the patient does not respond to 3 weeks of prednisone therapy, other therapeutic options should be considered.

Splenectomy Splenectomy was first demonstrated by Kaznelson in 1916 to be effective in patients with ITP.[388] Splenectomy is indicated in adult ITP patients whose platelet counts remain less than 10×10^9/liter and in patients whose platelet counts remain less than 30×10^9/liter and who continue to experience excessive bleeding after

4 to 6 weeks of appropriate medical treatment. Splenectomy also should be considered in patients who have experienced a transient response to primary treatment and have platelet counts less than 30 × 10⁹/liter after 3 months or who require continuous glucocorticoid therapy to maintain safe platelet counts.[306,388] At least 2 weeks before splenectomy, patients should be immunized with polyvalent pneumococcal vaccine, *Haemophilus influenzae* type B vaccine, and quadrivalent meningococcal polysaccharide vaccine,[389] because they are susceptible to overwhelming sepsis, especially from these bacterial infections, and immunization following splenectomy does not result in adequate protection rates (see Chap. 55). Patients with platelet counts less than 50 × 10⁹/liter, and especially less than 30 × 10⁹/liter, may require glucocorticoid and/or IVIg therapy before the procedure to reach platelet levels that minimize the risk of surgical bleeding. Platelet transfusions may be required during the perioperative period in severely thrombocytopenic patients.

Two thirds of patients who undergo splenectomy achieve normal platelet counts.[306,388] In the remaining third of patients, platelet counts recover only partially or transiently, and most of these patients relapse within 6 months of splenectomy. The duration of the disease prior to splenectomy does not affect the results of the procedure. Splenectomy can be performed even years after ITP is diagnosed.[390,391] Both the time required to reach a normal platelet count and the magnitude of platelet recovery are useful predictors of the long-term efficacy of splenectomy. In most cases, platelet counts recover within 10 days. Patients who attain a normal platelet count within 3 days of splenectomy or platelet counts greater than 500 × 10⁹/liter by day 10 generally have a good long-term response to splenectomy. Younger patients respond better to splenectomy.

The mortality rate associated with splenectomy is very low (<1%), even in patients with severe thrombocytopenia. The rate increases in older patients and in the presence of coexisting illnesses.[306,392] Splenectomized patients should be informed to be alert for the symptoms and signs of infection and be prepared for an emergency situation. Whether adults should be revaccinated at 10-year intervals is still debated.[306,392]

Laparoscopic splenectomy, first introduced in 1991, is an alternative to open splenectomy because the spleen is of normal size and vascularity in ITP patients. In experienced hands, laparoscopic splenectomy is cost effective and safe. Long-term and short-term benefits and complications are similar to those seen with open splenectomy. This procedure is limited by a high frequency of retained splenic tissue, especially in those with an accessory spleen, and increased risk of splenosis.[323,393] Splenic irradiation or splenic artery embolization can be used in glucocorticoid-resistant ITP patients in whom surgical splenectomy is contraindicated.[306,394] In patients refractory to splenectomy, the presence of accessory splenic tissue should be suspected, particularly if the blood film shows no evidence of splenectomy (i.e., pitting and Howell-Jolly bodies are absent in the erythrocytes; see Chap. 55). Such patients should be screened with sensitive radionuclide or magnetic resonance scans to identify residual splenic tissue.

Intravenous Immunoglobulin IVIg was first shown to be effective in childhood ITP in 1981.[395] IVIg increases the platelet count in more than 75 percent of patients with chronic ITP and normalizes the platelet count in approximately 50 percent of the patients.[306,387] The effect of IVIg is similar whether or not the patient is splenectomized and is transient, generally lasting only 3 to 4 weeks. The patient may become refractory with repeated infusions of IVIg.[396]

Postulated mechanisms for the action of IVIg include blockade of macrophage Fc receptors, which slows clearance of antibody-coated platelets, and antiidiotype neutralization of antiplatelet autoantibodies.[387,397] The recommended total dose of IVIg is 2 g/kg administered either as 0.4 g/kg/day on 5 consecutive days or as 1 g/kg/day on

2 consecutive days. For maintenance therapy, 0.5 to 1 g/kg as a single dose may be used. Adverse effects of IVIg therapy include headache, backache, nausea, fever, aseptic meningitis, alloimmune hemolysis, hepatitis, renal failure, pulmonary insufficiency, and thrombosis. Anaphylactic reactions may occur in patients with congenital IgA deficiency; therefore, IgA levels should be evaluated before IVIg infusions. The cost of IVIg is considerable, and it is not recommended as initial therapy in adult patients with ITP, except in the setting of life-threatening bleeding.[306]

Anti-(Rh) D Anti-(Rh) D is a γ-globulin containing high titers of antibodies against the Rhₒ (D) antigen of erythrocytes. It is administered intravenously for treatment of ITP. Anti-(Rh) D binds Rh-positive erythrocytes and leads to their destruction in the spleen. Because splenic Fc receptors are blocked, more antibody-coated platelets survive in the circulation.[398,399] A positive direct antiglobulin test, a decrease in serum haptoglobin levels, and mild and transient hemolysis occur in all Rh-positive patients after anti-(Rh) D infusion, generally without requiring a blood transfusion,[399] although serious hemolysis can occur. Anti-(Rh) D therapy is not effective in Rh-negative patients, and response rates are very low in splenectomized patients.

A single dose of 50 to 100 μg/kg is recommended, given by intravenous infusion over 3 to 5 minutes.[213,398–401] Adverse effects of anti-(Rh) D therapy are those seen with both γ-globulin infusion and autoimmune hemolytic anemia; symptoms include headache, asthenia, chills, fever, abdominal pain, diarrhea, vomiting, dizziness, and myalgia. Immediate anaphylactic reactions and both type I (IgE-mediated) and type III (immune complex-mediated) hypersensitivity reactions can occur.[213,306,398–400] Although anti-(Rh) D reportedly increases platelet counts in more than 70 percent of patients who are Rh-positive and not splenectomized[213] and may preclude the need for splenectomy,[400] a randomized, controlled trial comparing anti-D with conventional therapy showed no differences in the rates of spontaneous remission or the need for splenectomy.[401]

Treatments for Patients Refractory to Initial Therapies Approximately one third of patients with ITP do not respond to splenectomy or relapse after a short remission. The therapeutic options for those with moderate to severe thrombocytopenia after splenectomy are many; therapy should be tailored to the individual patient. Bleeding symptoms rather than platelet count should determine whether treatment is required. Patients with platelet counts greater than 30 × 10⁹/liter can be followed without therapy because their bleeding risk is very low. The treatment strategy is uncertain for patients with platelet counts less than 30 × 10⁹/liter. Observation without therapy may be appropriate if the patient has no signs of bleeding and has no risk factors for bleeding, such as uncontrolled hypertension or peptic ulcer disease. It is generally accepted that if splenectomy fails to produce a remission, other modalities likely will not produce a complete and long-lasting remission.[323,354,402] The main goal of therapy in these patients is prevention of bleeding.

Vinca alkaloids. Both vincristine and vinblastine transiently increase the platelet count in approximately 70 percent of ITP patients within 5 to 21 days but produce sustained remissions in only 10 percent of treated patients.[306,323,355,402] The recommended dose of vincristine is 1 to 2 mg and of vinblastine is 0.1 mg/kg (maximum 10 mg), both given by bolus injection at 1-week intervals for a minimum of three courses. It has been proposed that vinca alkaloids bind to platelet microtubules and thereby are transported to the spleen, where they subsequently inhibit the phagocytic functions of splenic macrophages. They may also stimulate megakaryopoiesis. Peripheral neuropathy, neutropenia, jaw pain, alopecia, and constipation are complications of treatment with vinca alkaloids.[402–405]

Cyclophosphamide. Cyclophosphamide, an alkylating drug, can be used orally (50–200 mg/day) or parenterally (1–1.5 g/m² IV every

4 weeks) in refractory ITP patients.[406,407] It increases platelet counts in 60 to 80 percent of ITP cases, and 20 to 40 percent of those patients will remain in remission for 2 to 3 years[306] after 2 to 3 months of therapy. Its action in increasing the platelet count involves immunosuppression. The major complications of cyclophosphamide therapy are marrow suppression, hemorrhagic cystitis, infertility, alopecia, and secondary malignancy.

Azathioprine. Azathioprine is a purine analogue that is converted to 6-mercaptopurine following gastrointestinal absorption. It also works through immunosuppression. An azathioprine dose ranging from 50 to 250 mg/day for at least 4 months seems to be necessary before its effectiveness can be evaluated. Azathioprine reportedly produced a sustained normalization of the platelet counts in up to 45 percent of refractory ITP patients.[408] As with other immunosuppressive drugs, major adverse effects are marrow suppression, possible increased risk of secondary malignancy, and teratogenesis.[306,402]

Danazol. Danazol is a synthetic androgen with reduced virilizing effects compared to other androgens and has been used for treatment of refractory ITP patients. Given at doses of 400 to 800 mg/day for at least 6 months, reported response rates range from 10 to 80 percent.[306,402] Danazol is postulated to decrease Fc receptor numbers on phagocytic cells by antagonizing the effects of estrogens.[355] Danazol should not be given to pregnant women or patients with liver disease. Common side effects of danazol therapy are weight gain, fluid retention, seborrhea, hirsutism, secondary amenorrhea, vocal changes, acne, hepatic toxicity, headache, lethargy, myalgia, and thrombocytopenia. Because liver dysfunction is common with danazol therapy, liver function should be evaluated monthly.[306,355,402]

Other therapies. Many other therapies, including interferon-α,[409] dapsone,[410] immunoadsorption with staphylococcal protein A,[411] cyclosporine,[412] ascorbic acid,[413] colchicine,[414] and plasmapheresis[415] have been studied for refractory ITP cases, but none has been clearly demonstrated to be effective. Several investigators have reported that rituximab, a monoclonal antibody against CD20, presumably by depleting the autoreactive B cell clone, is effective in the treatment of refractory ITP.[416–418]

Accessory Therapies Adjunctive therapies include agents designed to reduce bleeding without necessarily affecting the platelet count. For example, aminocaproic acid can be used for excessive menstrual bleeding in young women and may prevent blood loss.

THROMBOCYTOPENIA IN PATIENTS WITH ANTIPHOSPHOLIPID SYNDROME

Antiphospholipid syndrome (APS) is characterized by recurrent arterial and venous thrombosis and well-defined morbidity during pregnancy in the presence of antiphospholipid antibodies (APLA)[419] (see Chap. 123). APS may affect any system or organ in the body, including the heart, brain, kidney, skin, lung, and placenta. This syndrome is predominant in females (female-to-male ratio 5:1), especially during the childbearing years.[420] APLA (lupus anticoagulant: LA; anticardiolipin antibodies: ACLA) represent a heterogeneous family of antibodies that react with anionic phospholipids and phospholipid–protein complexes. Despite overwhelming evidence that APLA are associated with thrombosis, the mechanisms remain uncertain. Many have been proposed, including endothelial cell damage and apoptosis, inhibition of prostacyclin release from endothelial cells, inhibition of the protein C–protein S anticoagulant system, induction of tissue factor, activation of platelets, interference with antithrombin, impairment of fibrinolytic activity, and the effect of APL antibodies in inhibiting annexin V binding to membrane phospholipids, eliminating the antithrombotic effect of annexin V.[421–424]

APS is considered one of the most common causes of acquired thrombophilia. The syndrome is defined as "primary" in the absence of an underlying disease and "secondary" when associated with other diseases, especially SLE.[425,426]

Thrombocytopenia is reported in approximately 20 to 40 percent of patients with APS, usually is mild (70–120 $\times$ 10^9/liter), and does not require clinical intervention. Severe thrombocytopenia (platelet counts <50 $\times$ 10^9/liter) may be seen in 5 to 10 percent of patients.[427–429] Although thrombocytopenia was a clinical criterion used to define the syndrome in the initial classification of APS,[430] it was not included in the most recently proposed classification.[419] In this classification, patients with APLA and thrombocytopenia as the only associated clinical manifestation were defined as having "probable" or "possible" APS. ITP patients who present with APLA are at increased risk for thrombosis[375]; thus, measurement of APLA, especially lupus anticoagulant, in patients diagnosed with ITP may identify a subgroup at high risk for developing APS.

The pathogenesis of thrombocytopenia in APS is not clear. Evidence indicates APLA bind platelet membranes and cause platelet destruction, but the link is not definitive. Some investigators suggest that antibodies against platelet glycoproteins, rather than APLA, are responsible for thrombocytopenia in patients with APS. Antiglycoprotein antibodies are rare in patients with APS with normal platelet counts.[431,432] Antibodies against the GpIIb-IIIa or GpIb-IX-V complexes are found in approximately 40 percent of thrombocytopenic patients with APS.[433] Such antibodies do not cross-react with antibodies against phospholipids or β_2-glycoprotein I.[434] Immunosuppressive treatment in these patients increases the platelet count and reduces the titers of anti-Gp antibodies but not the titers of APLA.[374] These data suggest that thrombocytopenia is a secondary immune phenomenon that develops concomitantly with APS. Against this conclusion, platelet antigens in thrombocytopenic patients with APS were found to be different from those in ITP and display virtually no reactivity of the antibodies with membrane glycoproteins.[435]

Another issue of clinical importance in evaluating thrombocytopenia associated with APS is the risk for future development of thrombosis. In one study in which APS patients were divided into three groups according to platelet counts as nonthrombocytopenic, moderately thrombocytopenic (50–100 $\times$ 10^9/liter), or severely thrombocytopenic (<50 $\times$ 10^9/liter), the rates of future thrombosis were 40 percent, 32 percent, and 9 percent, respectively.[428] These data show that moderate thrombocytopenia does not prevent thrombosis in patients with APS. Antithrombotic prophylaxis should be considered in these patients.[427,428]

Although thrombocytopenia is a common finding in patients with APS, bleeding complications are rare, even with severe thrombocytopenia. Bleeding in an APS patient with moderate thrombocytopenia should trigger evaluation for the presence of antiprothrombin antibodies[436] and other disorders that may affect hemostasis, such as DIC and uremia. Severe thrombocytopenia may require therapy, with treatment strategies similar to those used for patients with ITP. Glucocorticoids are effective in only 15 percent of patients.[427] IVIg and immunosuppressive drugs such as cyclophosphamide can be used in patients with severe bleeding and "catastrophic" APS. Splenectomy is another option, producing sustained remission in approximately two thirds of patients.[207,437,438] Preoperative vaccinations should be administered to patients with ITP. Because of their increased risk of thrombosis, patients should be prophylactically anticoagulated in the immediate postoperative period.

Cases of thrombocytopenia correction using aspirin,[439,440] warfarin,[441,442] and antimalarial drugs have been reported.[443] Inhibition of platelet activation, aggregation, and platelet consumption have been suggested as helpful in increasing platelet counts in APS patients.

THROMBOCYTOPENIA IN PATIENTS WITH SYSTEMIC LUPUS ERYTHEMATOSUS

SLE is a complex autoimmune disease that primarily afflicts women of childbearing age. The autoimmune attack in SLE is not organ specific; it may affect any tissue in the body. The diagnostic criteria for SLE are based on a classification system proposed by the American College of Rheumatology. Patients with SLE should fulfill any four of 11 criteria.[444,445]

FREQUENCY OF THROMBOCYTOPENIA

Thrombocytopenia is common in patients with SLE, occurring in 20 to 40 percent of patients.[446] The causes are many and include platelet destruction (ITP, DIC, TTP with hemolytic uremic syndrome [TTP-HUS], sepsis), ineffective hematopoiesis (megaloblastic anemia), abnormal platelet pooling (hypersplenism), marrow hypoplasia (from drugs and infections), and dilutional thrombocytopenia related to therapy. Severe thrombocytopenia is relatively rare, seen in 5 percent of patients.[446] Although clinically significant bleeding is uncommon even in patients with severe thrombocytopenia, fatal gastrointestinal, cerebral, and pulmonary bleeding have been reported.

PATHOGENESIS OF THROMBOCYTOPENIA

Among the many potential contributors to thrombocytopenia in SLE patients, destruction of the platelets by autoantibodies is the major mechanism. Antiplatelet antibodies are present in up to 60 percent of SLE patients.[447,448] Although the presence of antiplatelet antibodies is correlated with low platelet counts and increased disease severity,[448] the mechanism of platelet destruction is not clear. Besides the antiplatelet antibodies, antiphospholipid antibodies (see "Thrombocytopenia in Patients with Antiphospholipid Syndrome" above) and circulating immune complexes that bind platelets nonspecifically may accelerate platelet destruction.[449] Specific antiplatelet antibodies, especially those against GpIIb-IIIa, have an important role in the pathogenesis of thrombocytopenia in SLE patients.[432,447,448]

In general, marrow megakaryocytes are normal or increased, and platelet production is not affected in SLE patients with thrombocytopenia. However, decreased numbers of megakaryocytes and even amegakaryocytic thrombocytopenia have been reported.[301,450] High levels of TPO in the serum, and both anti-TPO and anti-TPO receptor antibodies have been found in SLE patients,[451,452] the latter associated with a decrease in marrow megakaryocytes and thrombocytopenia.[452]

Thrombocytopenia in SLE has been associated with serious organ pathology, leading to neuropsychiatric disease,[453] renal disease,[454,455] and APS,[456] and is an independent indicator of poor prognosis.[455,457,458] A study of selected SLE families in which at least one affected member was thrombocytopenic reported genetic linkage to loci at chromosomes 11p13 and 1q22-23.[459] Severe lupus phenotype was much more common among patients with thrombocytopenia and their affected family members than in patients from families with no thrombocytopenic patients. Therefore, thrombocytopenia in a family member may herald severe lupus in familial SLE.

TREATMENT OF THROMBOCYTOPENIA

Although thrombocytopenia is a common finding in SLE, treatment strategies for severe thrombocytopenia are not well established. Because SLE ranges in severity from milder forms with easily controlled symptoms and signs to severe forms that may be fatal, the treatment of severe thrombocytopenia should be tailored to the individual patient. Patients with severe thrombocytopenia are generally treated with glucocorticoids as first-line therapy, but sustained remission is infrequent. Because most patients with severe thrombocytopenia also have nephritis and neurologic symptoms for which they receive immuno-

suppressive therapy either alone or combination with glucocorticoids, immunosuppressive drugs can be used as components of first-line therapy.[460–463] Because of its high cost and transient effect, IVIg is reserved for use in patients with emergent bleeding symptoms.[464,465] If initial therapy fails, splenectomy should be considered. Although case reports suggest that—in contrast to other autoimmune disorders—splenectomy increases complications in SLE patients and does not improve thrombocytopenia,[466–468] more comprehensive series indicate that splenectomy yields sustained remission in 61 percent of SLE patients with severe thrombocytopenia.[461] Danazol and hydroxychloroquine, when used with glucocorticoids, resulted in sustained remission rates of 50 percent and 64 percent of cases, respectively.

THROMBOCYTOPENIA DURING PREGNANCY

Evaluation of blood counts of pregnant women has shown that thrombocytopenia is the second most common hematologic problem in pregnancy, after anemia. Table 110-4 lists the major causes of thrombocytopenia in pregnancy (see Chap. 7).

Platelet counts tend to decrease during normal pregnancy. Mild thrombocytopenia, with platelet counts ranging from 120 to 150 × 10^9/liter, may be present, especially during the third trimester.[469,470] It is important to investigate the cause of thrombocytopenia and exclude the disorders associated with significant morbidity (see Table 110-4). A thorough history, blood pressure measurement, repeated blood count with a fresh sample, and examination of the blood film are the main steps in the diagnosis of pseudothrombocytopenia, leukemia, and microangiopathic disorders such as TTP; microangiopathic hemolysis (H), elevated liver enzymes (EL), and low platelet (LP) counts (HELLP) syndrome; and DIC in pregnant women with thrombocytopenia. Physical examination may be difficult in the third trimester, so an abdominal ultrasound may be required to detect organomegaly.

GESTATIONAL THROMBOCYTOPENIA

Gestational thrombocytopenia is detected in 5 to 7 percent of otherwise healthy pregnant women, accounting for approximately 74 percent of thrombocytopenia cases at term.[471–473] Gestational thrombocytopenia is a benign disorder and is not associated with an increased risk of bleeding. It is not associated with decreased platelet counts in the fetus. Platelet counts are generally greater than 70 × 10^9/liter[469–472] and usually return to normal after delivery. The pathogenesis of gestational thrombocytopenia is unknown. Several mechanisms have been pro-

TABLE 110-4   CAUSES OF THROMBOCYTOPENIA DURING PREGNANCY

Pseudothrombocytopenia
Gestational thrombocytopenia
Autoimmune thrombocytopenia
Antiphospholipid syndrome and systemic lupus erythematosus
Folate deficiency
Preeclampsia, eclampsia
HELLP (hemolysis, elevated liver function tests, low platelets) syndrome
Thrombotic thrombocytopenic purpura
Disseminated intravascular coagulation
Hypersplenism
Viral infections (human immunodeficiency virus, cytomegalovirus, Epstein-Barr virus)
Drug-induced thrombocytopenia
Marrow dysfunction (aplastic anemia, leukemia)
Acute fatty liver
Hereditary disorders (type IIb von Willebrand disease, May-Hegglin anomaly, hereditary macrothrombocytopenia)

posed, including hemodilution, a compensated state of subclinical co-agulopathy, endothelial cell injury, and immune destruction. Some authors have suggested platelet consumption by the placenta and hormonal depression of megakaryopoiesis as causes of gestational thrombocytopenia, as suggested by the rapid return of platelet count to normal after delivery and by the transient return to normal of platelet count during pregnancy in some cases of essential thrombocythemia.[473–476]

Discriminating gestational thrombocytopenia from immune thrombocytopenia can be difficult because ITP is also common in young women. Neither condition can be diagnosed by currently available tests. The diagnosis of ITP is favored if the patient had a previous episode of ITP unassociated with pregnancy or if the thrombocytopenia is severe and associated with bleeding that occurs in the first trimester. In healthy pregnant women, a platelet count greater than 75×10^9/liter late in pregnancy does not require intensive investigation at that time because bleeding is not likely in the woman or her newborn child.[477]

IMMUNE THROMBOCYTOPENIC PURPURA

ITP is responsible for 4 to 5 percent of all cases of pregnancy-associated thrombocytopenia.[471,473] It generally causes moderate to severe thrombocytopenia in the first trimester. No test for discriminating ITP from gestational thrombocytopenia is available. PAIgG is elevated in patients with ITP and in gestational thrombocytopenia.[478] Diagnosis of ITP in a pregnant woman requires the exclusion of other causes of thrombocytopenia. Given no suspicious clinical or laboratory features, marrow aspiration is considered unnecessary.[470] Diagnosis of ITP is important for the fetus because antiplatelet antibodies decrease the fetal platelet count and may cause bleeding.[472]

According to the ASH ITP guidelines, an ITP patient who has platelet counts greater than 50×10^9/liter should not be discouraged from becoming pregnant, but the patient who has platelet counts less than 10×10^9/liter after splenectomy should be advised of the high risk to the fetus.[471] ITP may exacerbate during pregnancy, but generally the platelet count returns to the prepregnancy level after delivery.

The approach to treatment of ITP during pregnancy is different from that in nonpregnant women because the potential side effects of the drugs may complicate both fetal development and the course of the pregnancy. Mother and fetus should be managed by close collaboration between a hematologist, an obstetrician, and a neonatologist. Although glucocorticoids are not teratogenic, they may induce gestational diabetes, osteoporosis, hypertension, or psychosis. Fetal side effects are minimal because approximately 90 percent of the glucocorticoid dose is metabolized in the placenta.[470] Cytotoxic drugs, such as vinca alkaloids, azathioprine, and cyclophosphamide, are potentially teratogenic. The rigors of splenectomy may induce preterm labor. IVIg is safe for the fetus but often is associated with maternal side effects. Experience with anti (Rh)-D therapy in pregnant women is limited. Platelet counts and bleeding symptoms are important for management of these patients. If the platelet count is greater than 30×10^9/liter and the patient has no bleeding symptoms, observation without therapy is appropriate. A pregnant women who has a platelet count less than 10×10^9/liter in any trimester, a platelet count of 10 to 30×10^9/liter in the third trimester, or signs of bleeding requires therapy. If the pregnant woman has no life-threatening bleeding symptoms, glucocorticoids are considered for initial therapy. A starting dosage of 1 mg/kg/day and then the minimal dose that will keep platelet counts greater than 50×10^9/liter are appropriate. If the platelet count is greater than 50×10^9/liter, vaginal delivery can be performed. If cesarean section or epidural anesthesia is required, the platelet count should be maintained over 80×10^9/liter.[470] IVIg is indicated in pa-

tients who have no response to glucocorticoid treatment, have life-threatening bleeding symptoms, and have platelet count less than 10×10^9/liter at term. A dosage of 400 mg/kg/day for 5 days or 1 g/kg/day for 2 days can be used. The transient effect and the cost of IVIg therapy should be considered. In patients who have no response to standard glucocorticoid and IVIg therapy and have bleeding symptoms, a combined therapy with high-dose glucocorticoids (1 g/day) and IVIg (1–2 g/kg/day) may increase platelet counts. Splenectomy can be performed in the second trimester if the patient has not responded to glucocorticoids and IVIg therapy and has a platelet count less than 10×10^9/liter or has bleeding symptoms. Platelet transfusions may be required in patients who have platelet counts less than 30×10^9/liter to prevent maternal bleeding during labor.[470,471]

Severe neonatal thrombocytopenia (platelet counts $<20 \times 10^9$/liter) occurs in 4 percent of ITP pregnancies and moderate neonatal thrombocytopenia (platelet counts $<50 \times 10^9$/liter) in 9 percent.[479] Severe bleeding occurs in less than 1 percent of the babies. Because earlier studies reported that thrombocytopenic neonates have an increased risk for intracranial hemorrhage, some physicians have recommended performing cesarean delivery for all women with ITP to avoid injuries to the fetus during passage through the pelvis.[480] However, no data have proved that cesarean delivery is an effective approach for reducing the occurrence of intracerebral hemorrhage in the thrombocytopenic fetus because of the rarity of intracerebral hemorrhage.[476] Measurement of platelet counts in infants before delivery, such as by percutaneous umbilical cord blood sampling or fetal scalp vein sampling after cervical dilatation, is not recommended routinely because the morbidity and mortality rates of these procedures are high (2%).[479,481,482] Maternal platelet count at delivery does not correlate with the infant's platelet count. In ITP patients who gave birth more than once, however, the first infant's platelet count at birth is an important predictor of severe thrombocytopenia in subsequent pregnancies and may justify further obstetric management.[476,481,483] On the other hand, discordances in degree of thrombocytopenia between dichorionic twins in ITP indicate that fetal factors also are important.[484] Although the risk of neonatal thrombocytopenia is higher in newborns of mothers with ITP, only a small percentage of newborns have severe thrombocytopenia, with the infrequent case of intracranial hemorrhage often associated with other risk factors such as prematurity and alloimmune thrombocytopenia. In a study in which platelet counts were obtained from 6770 pregnant women late in pregnancy and in 6103 of their newborns, severe neonatal thrombocytopenia was found in only one newborn of a thrombocytopenic mother.[477] There are no controlled studies describing the effects of antepartum treatment of the pregnant woman on the fetal platelet count. Treatment with glucocorticoids and IVIg has failed to improve the neonatal platelet count compared to counts obtained prepartum by serial fetal blood sampling.[485] IgG antibodies, especially IgG4, are transmitted in breast milk. Although ITP reportedly is not a contraindication to breast-feeding,[323] if the neonatal platelet count does not return to normal in the weeks after birth, a trial cessation of breast-feeding should be instituted.[476]

PREECLAMPSIA, ECLAMPSIA, AND HELLP SYNDROME

Preeclampsia, defined by hypertension and proteinuria, complicates 5 to 8 percent of all pregnancies. It usually becomes evident during the second trimester and is a major contributor to maternal and fetal morbidity and mortality[486,487] (see Chap. 7). *Eclampsia* is defined by the occurrence of acute neurologic abnormalities in a preeclamptic woman during the peripartum period.[487–489] Thrombocytopenia is seen in approximately 50 percent of women with preeclampsia, with the severity of thrombocytopenia correlating with the severity of the preeclampsia.[490]

PATHOGENESIS

Attempts to define the pathogenesis of preeclampsia have engendered numerous theories, to the point that the disorder has been termed *a disease of theories*.[491] One clear aspect of the pathogenesis is the requirement for a placenta, given that the condition can be produced in abdominal pregnancies and molar pregnancies.[492] The disease appears to be initiated by defective invasion of the uterine spiral arteries by placental cytotrophoblasts. During normal implantation, these cells convert from epithelial to endothelial morphology, a process called *pseudovasculogenesis*.[493,494] In preeclampsia, this process is defective, resulting in diminished maternal blood flow to the placenta and placental hypoxia. Through unknown mechanisms, the production of membrane and soluble forms of the vascular endothelial growth factor (VEGF) receptor fms-like tyrosine kinase-1 (Flt1) is increased,[495] with resultant increases of soluble Flt1 (sFlt1) in the amniotic fluid[496] and maternal circulation.[497] sFlt1 is the product of an alternately spliced form of the Flt1 mRNA, which lacks the transmembrane and cytoplasmic domains present in the full-length receptor. A large amount of evidence implicates sFlt1 as playing a key role in the pathogenesis of preeclampsia. By binding to VEGF and the related placental growth factor (PlGF), sFlt1 prevents their favorable effects on vascular endothelium. Its expression in rats produces a syndrome akin to preeclampsia: hypertension and proteinuria associated with glomerular endotheliosis (occlusion of glomerular capillaries by swollen endothelial cells). These findings strongly suggest that a tonic level of VEGF-like angiogenic factors is required to maintain the normal function of vascular endothelial cells. During pregnancy, PlGF appears to have a prominent role in this process, as expression in rats of soluble Flt-1, a VEGF receptor that does not bind PlGF, fails to produce a preeclampsia-like syndrome.[493,498,499]

The connection between preeclampsia and thrombocytopenia is not clear, although many cases have evidence of activation of blood coagulation detected by elevated levels of fibrin-degradation products and thrombin–antithrombin complexes[473] (see Chap. 121). Low levels of the vWF-cleaving metalloprotease ADAMTS-13 have also been described.[500]

A disorder related to preeclampsia/eclampsia is the HELLP syndrome, seen in the peripartum period and defined by the presence of microangiopathic hemolytic anemia, elevated liver enzymes, and low platelets. This disorder occurs more commonly in Caucasian women older than 25 years and is the most common cause of severe liver disease in pregnancy.[501] Microangiopathic hemolysis results from shearing of the erythrocytes as they pass through arterioles occluded by platelet–fibrin deposits. Adhesion and aggregation of platelets on damaged and activated endothelium presumably accounts for the low platelet count (see Chap. 49). HELLP shares a number of features with TTP, including the presence of microangiopathic hemolysis and thrombocytopenia. Involvement of the central nervous system is a more prominent feature of TTP, whereas HELLP more commonly displays severe liver function abnormalities[502] (see Chaps. 7, 49, and 124). Because the two syndromes can be confused with one other, one study attempted to distinguish the two by measuring the activity of ADAMTS-13, which usually is absent or severely deficient in TTP.[500] The study found that essentially all 17 patients in a cohort with the HELLP syndrome had mild to moderate reductions in the activity of ADAMTS-13 in the plasma, and none was severely deficient.

Delivery of the fetus is the most effective treatment for preeclampsia, eclampsia, and the HELLP syndrome. The nadir of the platelet count and the peak of serum lactate dehydrogenase (LDH) may occur postpartum, during the first postpartum day in most patients, but as late as 5 to 7 days in some. For patients with severe thrombocytopenia and microangiopathic hemolytic anemia, plasma exchange may be indicated if the fetus cannot be delivered or if improvement does not follow delivery. This treatment is empirically based on the similarity of the clinical picture to that of TTP. Postpartum day 3 often is considered the limit for supportive therapy in anticipation of a spontaneous recovery.[500] If thrombocytopenia and hemolysis (as assessed by serum LDH levels) continue to worsen beyond this time, intervention with plasma exchange is appropriate for the presumed diagnosis of TTP-HUS (see Chap. 124). At this point, TTP-HUS cannot be distinguished from atypical preeclampsia/eclampsia/HELLP syndrome, for which plasma exchange treatment may be beneficial.[503] Earlier intervention with plasma exchange is indicated for more severe clinical problems, such as neurologic abnormalities or acute, anuric renal failure.

As with TTP-HUS, recurrence of HELLP syndrome in subsequent pregnancies is a concern. In the absence of persistent hypertension between pregnancies, HELLP syndrome is uncommon in subsequent pregnancies (3%), but less severe complications are more common in subsequent pregnancies (preeclampsia 19% and preterm delivery 21%).[504]

NEONATAL ALLOIMMUNE THROMBOCYTOPENIA

Fetal–neonatal alloimmune thrombocytopenia (NAIT) is caused by the placental transfer of maternal alloantibodies against fetal platelet antigens inherited from the father. NAIT resembles neonatal alloimmune hemolytic anemia (Rh hemolytic disease of the newborn) in many aspects. In both diseases, maternal alloantibodies against fetal blood cell antigens cross the placenta and destroy antigen-positive cells, resulting in significant fetal/neonatal morbidity and mortality. However, unlike neonatal alloimmune hemolytic anemia, which tends to spare the first-born child, the first child is affected in 40 to 60 percent of NAIT cases.[470] Transplacental transfer of antiplatelet antibodies can occur in babies born from mothers with ITP. Maternal ITP rarely may cause serious thrombocytopenia or bleeding problems in the fetus, including intracranial hemorrhage. In cases of NAIT, thrombocytopenia tends to be more severe and the intracranial hemorrhage rate is higher (10–20%) compared with maternal ITP.[218] In contrast to maternal ITP, in NAIT the maternal platelet count is normal, a key differential diagnostic finding.

PREVALENCE AND PATHOGENESIS

The estimated frequency of NAIT varies from one in 500 to one in 2000 live births.[218,470,505] Maternal alloantibodies against human platelet antigens (HPAs) are responsible for platelet destruction in NAIT. In Caucasians, the most frequently implicated antigens are HPA-1a or Pl^{A1} (78% of cases) and HPA-5b or Br^a (19% of cases).[506] These antigens are rare in Asian populations. HPA-4a (80%) and HPA-3a (15%) are responsible for platelet destruction in most Asian NAIT cases.[507] Besides targeting the HPA system, anti–HLA-2 antibodies have been reported, but whether they are responsible for NAIT is not clear.[505,508,509]

The frequency of NAIT in Caucasians is lower than would be expected given that the incidence of HPA-1a negativity is 2.5 percent. Only 10 percent of HPA-1a–negative mothers exposed to HPA-1a–positive platelets during pregnancy become immunized. HPA alloimmunization is strongly correlated with the presence of specific class II HLA antigens, with increased risk demonstrated in HPA-1a–negative mothers expressing HLA-B8, HLA-DR3, and HLA-DR52a antigens.[470,510,511] The presence of HLA-DRB3*0101 allele in HPA-1a–negative women increases the NAIT risk as much as 140-fold.[511]

NAIT tends to be clinically more severe in cases with alloantibodies against HPA-1a.[218] HPA-1 (Pl^A) antigens are expressed on platelet GpIIIa. Anti–HPA-1a antibodies have been proposed to impair platelet aggregation, which may explain the severity of bleeding symptoms.[512]

CLINICAL FEATURES

IgG alloantibodies can cross the placenta as early as week 14 of pregnancy, and passage increases with gestational age.[505] These antibodies bind to fetal platelets and lead to their destruction. In severe cases, intracranial hemorrhage and hydrocephalus may develop and lead to fetal death. The diagnosis is difficult to make in the first fetus affected. An ultrasound scan may not help unless it detects bleeding or hydrocephalus. Unexplained fetal deaths in the maternal history or fetal hydrocephalus or bleeding in previous pregnancies may alert the physician to the possibility of NAIT. The diagnosis is made by fetal blood sampling.

Usually the diagnosis of NAIT is possible after birth. NAIT should be suspected in a thrombocytopenic neonate with extensive purpura or visceral hemorrhage but no evidence of sepsis, skeletal anomalies, or other systemic diseases that may cause thrombocytopenia, including maternal ITP. Affected babies may have no symptoms (13–59% of cases), or they may have bleeding symptoms (18–65% of cases) and evidence of intracranial hemorrhage (22–23%).[513] In a case series of 88 infants with NAIT resulting from anti–HPA-1a antibodies, 90 percent had purpura, 66 percent had hematomas, 30 percent had gastrointestinal bleeding, and 14 percent had intracerebral hemorrhage. Bleeding may be delayed, as the platelet count usually falls further during the first several days of life. Death or neurologic impairment occurs in up to 25 percent of infants. Platelet counts recover to normal in 1 to 2 weeks.[514]

The diagnosis of NAIT usually can be confirmed by tests for circulating maternal alloantibodies against fetal antigens (usually by MAIPA) or by platelet typing of the parents and neonate by either genotyping or enzyme-linked immunosorbent assay. These tests may fail to yield the diagnosis because private HPA antigens may be responsible for NAIT.[218,470,505]

MANAGEMENT

Postnatal The alternatives in the management of affected neonates are IVIg, glucocorticoids (alone or combined with IVIg), and platelet transfusions. IVIg and/or steroid therapy may increase platelet counts rapidly, although a substantial increase of platelet counts usually occurs after 24 to 72 hours.[506] In cases with severe bleeding, platelets should be transfused. Transfused platelets should be ABO and RhD compatible and HPA-1a–negative in the majority of cases.[515] Transfusion of washed and irradiated maternal platelets to the affected fetus is an alternative but may not be appropriate for several reasons. Washing of maternal platelets to eliminate maternal alloantibodies and irradiation to prevent graft-versus-host disease may damage the platelets.[218] Repeated platelet transfusions may be required.[470] One alternative in these cases is transfusion of platelets from HPA-1a–negative donors. Platelet counts usually increase rapidly after transfusion.[218,505]

Prenatal The treatment options in high-risk NAIT are maternal weekly IVIg administration with or without glucocorticoids, serial *in utero* platelet transfusions, *in utero* IVIg administration, and early delivery (after 32 weeks of gestation). Maternal IVIg administration at a dosage of 1 g/kg/week with or without glucocorticoids may increase fetal platelet counts,[516] although not all studies support this conclusion.[505,512] Direct administration of IVIg to the fetus also may not consistently raise fetal platelet counts.[517] In patients who do not respond to IVIg and glucocorticoid administration, serial matched platelet transfusions may be used. Matched platelet transfusions will only transiently increase the fetal platelet count because the transfused platelets also are targeted.[470] Serial platelet transfusions may increase the cumulative risk of hemorrhage and procedure-related hemorrhage and

fetal loss.[512] In severely thrombocytopenic fetuses, early delivery with cesarean section may help reduce the risk of intracranial hemorrhage.[512]

Current therapeutic alternatives for antenatal management of NAIT are unsatisfactory. Novel therapeutic strategies are under investigation, including vaccines and competitive molecules that competitively bind anti–HPA-1a antibodies.[515]

ABNORMAL PLATELET DISTRIBUTION OR POOLING

SPLENOMEGALY

Splenomegaly may lead to thrombocytopenia by inducing a reversible pooling of up to 90 percent of total body platelets.[518,519] This process can be thought of as an exaggeration of normal splenic pooling, in which approximately one third of the platelet mass is contained within the spleen at any one time (see Chap. 55). The survival of platelets within the spleen often is normal or may be moderately reduced. Thus, the total blood platelet pool in a patient with splenomegaly could be normal even when the counts measured in venous blood are only 20 percent of normal. In splenomegaly, platelet production usually is normal, as estimated by dividing the total body platelet mass by the platelet life span.[518]

Several lines of evidence support the concept that pooling is the major factor responsible for thrombocytopenia in uncomplicated splenomegaly. First, the fraction of radiolabeled platelets that can be recovered from the circulation after infusion into patients with hypersplenism is small, from 10 to 30 percent, in contrast to 60 to 80 percent in normal subjects and 90 to 100 percent in asplenic patients.[518,520] Second, epinephrine injected intravenously causes an immediate increase in the platelet count in both normal individuals and patients with splenomegaly. The increase in patients with splenomegaly is proportionally greater than the 30 to 40 percent seen in normal individuals.[518,521,522] Epinephrine causes constriction of the splenic artery, with a fivefold decrease in splenic blood flow and passive emptying of the spleen. Third, large quantities of platelets, three to seven times the number present in the circulation, can be flushed from enlarged spleens after surgical removal. Fourth, removal of large numbers of platelets from the circulation through apheresis is followed rapidly by replenishment from the splenic pool, without resulting thrombocytopenia.[519,523]

The fact that thrombocytopenia associated with increased splenic pooling does not result in increased platelet production indicates that the total blood platelet pool, not the blood platelet concentration in the systemic circulation, is responsible for feedback regulation of platelet production.

The most common disorder causing thrombocytopenia resulting from splenic pooling is chronic liver disease with portal hypertension and congestive splenomegaly. In patients with cirrhosis and portal hypertension, moderate thrombocytopenia is the rule. However, in such cases the thrombocytopenia often results from both splenic pooling and reduced production of TPO.

Thrombocytopenia associated with splenomegaly often is of no clinical importance. Signs and symptoms are related to the primary disorder, and bleeding manifestations result primarily from coagulation abnormalities caused by the underlying liver disease. This finding is consistent with the relatively moderate degree of thrombocytopenia, the near-normal total body content of platelets,[518] and the ability to mobilize platelets from the spleen to replenish losses.[523]

Because thrombocytopenia resulting from splenic pooling rarely is of clinical importance, no treatment is indicated. When splenectomy is performed for another reason, however, the platelet count predictably returns to normal and thrombocytosis may even occur.[518] Platelet counts may return to normal in patients following surgical correction of portal hypertension by portosystemic shunting.[524] Platelet transfusions usually are not needed for splenomegaly-associated thrombocytopenia and rarely produce significant increases in platelet count because as much as 90 percent of the transfused platelets will be sequestered in the spleen.

HYPERSPLENISM

Hypersplenism is distinguished from uncomplicated splenomegaly in that pooling is accompanied by increased destruction of platelets, leukocytes, and erythrocytes in association with increased marrow precursors of the deficient lines and correction of the cytopenia by splenectomy.[525–528] The clinical manifestations, laboratory findings, and specific treatment are aimed at the underlying disease[529] (see Chap. 55).

Imaging studies, such as computed tomographic scans, can be useful for defining the size of the spleen and identifying intrasplenic and extrasplenic disease. Magnetic resonance imaging defines blood flow patterns, which is especially useful for detecting portal or splenic vein thromboses. Cell survival studies using radiolabeled platelets or red blood cells may be helpful for identifying hypersequestration when weighing the need for splenectomy. Most patients with splenomegaly require therapy for the underlying disease rather than for thrombocytopenia.

THROMBOCYTOPENIA ASSOCIATED WITH MASSIVE TRANSFUSION

In the era before platelet transfusion, thrombocytopenia often accompanied severe hemorrhage with transfusion of stored blood. In the massively transfused patient, the severity of thrombocytopenia is related to the number of red cell transfusions but does not solely result from dilution of the platelets (see Chap. 54). Platelet counts may be higher than predicted, possibly by release of platelets from the spleen, or they may be lower than predicted because of consumption in microvascular lesions.[530] Fibrinogen deficiency develops earlier than thrombocytopenia when blood is replaced by red cell concentrates and plasma substitutes.[531] A study of patients requiring massive transfusion, defined as transfusion of 10 or more red cell units within 24 hours, demonstrated that mild thrombocytopenia ($47-100 \times 10^9$/liter) occurred in all patients after transfusion of 15 red cell units, and more severe thrombocytopenia ($25-61 \times 10^9$/liter) developed after 20 red cell units.[531,532] DIC, triggered by the disease responsible for the blood loss or the hypotension that commonly occurs with massive blood loss, may contribute to the thrombocytopenia. Management of the thrombocytopenia depends on its severity and the underlying condition. Routinely transfusing platelets in a fixed ratio to packed red blood cells is not necessary, although in general platelet concentrates are needed for every 10 U of red cells necessary to maintain an adequate erythrocyte mass.

THROMBOCYTOPENIA RESULTING FROM HYPOTHERMIA

Transient thrombocytopenia occurs during hypothermia when the body temperature falls below 25°C, in both animals and humans.[533] The degree of thrombocytopenia correlates with the severity of body temperature drop. Thus, thrombocytopenia is less severe in cardiac surgery patients supported by normothermic systemic perfusion (35–37°C) than in those supported by moderately hypothermic systemic perfusion (25–29°C).[534] In this case, the drop in platelet count likely results from splenic and hepatic pooling[535] and from cold activation and clearance of platelets. Cold induces clustering of the GpIb complex and rearrangement of its carbohydrate chains, which then serve as ligands for the macrophage integrin $\alpha_M\beta_2$, which mediates their clearance in hepatic macrophages.[536,537] In hypothermic dogs, radiolabeled platelets are sequestered in the spleen, liver, and other organs; the platelets return to the circulation when normal body temperature is restored.[533,538] The clinical relevance of these observations is illustrated by reports of patients, often elderly, who are hypothermic after periods of unconsciousness in inadequately heated rooms. In one report, a 69-year-old woman had 13 admissions over an 8-year period with repeated hypothermia, 31° to 34°C. On each admission she was thrombocytopenic (platelet count $7-39 \times 10^9$/liter). With no therapy other than rewarming, platelet counts returned to normal in 4 to 10 days.[539] However, a review of 75 patients admitted with hypothermia (body temperatures 26°–35°C) demonstrated that only three patients were thrombocytopenic.[539]

DRUG-INDUCED THROMBOCYTOPENIA

A number of drugs cause thrombocytopenia by inducing antibody formation that ultimately targets the megakaryocyte and/or platelet. The most severe and life-threatening is heparin-induced thrombocytopenia (HIT), an immune-mediated disorder caused by antibodies that recognize a neoepitope in platelet factor 4 exposed when it binds heparin. The result is activation of platelets and the coagulation cascade and, ultimately, thrombosis. HIT affects up to 5 percent of patients exposed to heparin (discussed in detail in Chap. 124).

Assessment of isolated thrombocytopenia in a patient taking several medications must be systematic, with drug-induced thrombocytopenia considered before the diagnosis of ITP is established.[471] This section discusses drugs, other than heparin and its analogues, that cause isolated thrombocytopenia by immune platelet destruction. Heparin is discussed in the section immediately below and more extensively in Chapter 124. Chapter 33 discusses drug-induced aplastic anemia with thrombocytopenia.

ETIOLOGY
Reviews of drug-induced thrombocytopenia often contain such extensive lists of implicated drugs, many of which are commonly used, that they are not helpful for decisions regarding which therapy to interrupt first. To address the issue of which drugs most likely cause thrombocytopenia, a systematic review of all published case reports defined levels of evidence to document the causal relation between the drug and thrombocytopenia.[540] This review distinguished drugs with definite or probable causal relationships from those for which the evidence was weaker.[540] Table 110-5 lists the drugs for which there is definite evidence of a causal role in producing thrombocytopenia (which includes recurrent thrombocytopenia with rechallenge in the same patient) and drugs for which the causal relation to thrombocytopenia has been validated by at least two reports with probable evidence (thus meeting all of the criteria for definite evidence except for the lack of rechallenge). Quinidine is by far the most commonly cited drug. Other commonly cited drugs are similar to drugs documented in a case control study.[541] A remarkable observation from the systematic review was how many case reports did not provide sufficient clinical information to allow a determination of even a probable causal relation.[471]

PATHOGENESIS
Thrombocytopenia is assumed to result from immune platelet destruction by drug-dependent antiplatelet antibodies. Initial experimental observations suggested that drug–antibody complexes bound to platelets via the platelet Fcγ receptor. This mechanism has been confirmed for HIT (see below in this section), but for other drugs, the drug-dependent antibodies appear to bind to platelets via their Fab regions.[542] The antigen on the platelet surface is formed by drug binding to a mem-

brane glycoprotein receptor, creating a structural change that initiates antibody formation in susceptible subjects. The new antigen may be a newly revealed sequence of a surface glycoprotein or a complex composed of the drug and a platelet surface protein. Most experimental studies have used drug-dependent antibodies isolated from patients with quinidine- or quinine-induced thrombocytopenia. The antigen targets are the major platelet surface glycoproteins (GpIb-IX and GpIIb-IIIa). Different drugs may provoke drug-dependent antibodies that preferentially react with one of these glycoproteins, or drug-dependent antibodies from a single patient may react with multiple epitopes on both glycoproteins. For example, a study of sera from 15 patients with quinine-induced thrombocytopenia demonstrated that, in the presence of quinine, the antibodies bound to two distinct domains on GpIb-IX, one on GpIbα and one on GpIX. Some patients had only one of the antibodies; some had both.[544] The same domains on GpIb-IX also appear to be the antigenic targets for quinidine-[543,544] and ranitidine-dependent[545] antiplatelet antibodies. Definition of the specific epitope involved in patient reactions with drug-dependent antibodies may not only elucidate the mechanism of drug-induced thrombocytopenia but also identify polymorphisms in GpIb-IX that cause sensitivity in producing drug-dependent antiplatelet antibodies. Sulfonamides, quinidine, and quinine are frequent causes of drug-induced thrombocytopenia. Studies of sera from 15 patients with thrombocytopenia caused by sulfamethoxazole or sulfisoxazole demonstrated that the antigenic epitope was part of GpIIb-IIIa.[546] Some antibodies from patients with quinidine- and quinine-dependent antiplatelet antibodies also react with GpIIb-IIIa.[547]

In addition to specificity for discrete epitopes on platelet surface glycoproteins, drug-dependent antibodies are highly specific for the structure of the drug. For example, no cross-reactivity occurs between quinidine and quinine-dependent antibodies or between sulfamethoxazole and sulfisoxazole-dependent antibodies, even though both pairs of drugs have similar structures. Therefore, the neoantigens produced by drug binding to platelets create discrete epitopes that are sensitive to minor changes in drug structure.

The implications of this mechanism for platelet destruction are apparent. A patient with prior sensitivity to the drug has preformed antibodies that immediately react with the altered platelets upon repeat drug exposure, as demonstrated. An exception to this situation is the immediate acute thrombocytopenia that may occur with initial administration of the new class of antithrombotic agents that block the platelet fibrinogen receptor GpIIb-IIIa.[36,548]

TABLE 110-5 DRUGS CAUSING THROMBOCYTOPENIA SUPPORTED BY ONE OR MORE PATIENT CASE REPORTS WITH LEVEL I (DEFINITE) EVIDENCE OR LEVEL II (PROBABLE) CLINICAL EVIDENCE*

DRUG	NO. OF PATIENT CASE REPORTS		SEVERITY OF BLEEDING	
	LEVEL I	LEVEL II	MAJOR	MINOR
Quinidine (Quinaglute, Cardioquin)	15	23	3	11
Quinine (Quinamm, Quindan)	4	3	2	4
Rifampin (Rifadin, Rimactane)	4	3	1	3
Trimethoprim/sulfamethoxazole (Bactrim, Septra)	3	7	4	2
Methyldopa (Aldomet)	3	3	0	1
Acetaminophen (Tylenol, Panadol)	3	2	2	1
Digoxin (Lanoxin)	3	0	0	2
Danazol (Danocrine)	2	4	0	4
Diclofenac (Cataflam, Voltaren)	2	2	0	2
Aminoglutethimide (Cytadren)	2	1	1	1
Amphotericin B (Amphocin, Fungizone)	2	1	0	0
Aminosalicylic acid (Paser)	2	1	1	1
Oxprenolol (Trasicor)	2	1	0	1
Vancomycin (Vancoled)	2	1	1	0
Levamisole (Ergamisol)	2	0	0	0
Meclofenamate (Meclodium)	2	0	0	0
Diatrizoate meglumine/diatrizoate sodium (Hypaque Meglumine)	2	0	0	0
Amiodarone (Cordarone)	2	0	0	0
Nalidixic acid (NegGram)	1	5	0	1
Cimetidine (Tagamet)	1	5	0	0
Chlorothiazide (Diuril)	1	2	0	1
Diatrizoate meglumine (Urografin)	1	2	0	2
Interferon-α (Roferon A, Intron A)	1	2	0	1
Sulfasalazine (Azulfidine)	1	2	0	0
Ethambutol (Myambutol)	1	1	1	0
Iopanoic acid (Telepaque)	1	1	0	1
Sulfisoxazole (Gantrisin)	1	1	0	1
Tamoxifen (Nolvadex)	1	0	0	0
Thiothixene (Navane)	1	0	0	0
Naphazoline (Privine, Vasocon-A)	1	0	0	0
Amrinone (Inocor)	1	0	0	0
Lithium (Lithonate, Eskalith)	1	0	0	0
Diazepam (Valium)	1	0	0	0
Haloperidol (Haldol)	1	0	0	0
Alprenolol (Aptin)	1	0	0	1
Tolmetin (Tolectin)	1	0	0	1
Nitroglycerin (Nitrogard, Nitroglyn)	1	0	0	0
Minoxidil (Loniten)	1	0	0	1
Diazoxide (Proglycem, Hyperstat)	1	0	0	0
Chlorpromazine (Thorazine)	1	0	0	0
Isoniazid (Nydrazid)	1	0	0	0
Cephalothin (Keflin)	1	0	0	0
Difluoromethylornithine (Eflornithine, Ornidyl)	1	0	0	0
Piperacillin (Pipracil)	1	0	0	1
Diethylstilbestrol (Stilphostrol)	1	0	0	0
Methicillin (Staphcillin)	1	0	0	1
Deferoxamine (Desferal)	1	0	0	0
Novobiocin (Albamycin)	1	0	0	0
Gold (Ridaura, Solganal)	0	11	3	3
Procainamide (Pronestyl)	0	7	0	0
Carbamazepine (Tegretol)	0	5	0	0
Hydrochlorothiazide (Aquazide-H, Esidrix)	0	4	0	2
Ranitidine (Zantac)	0	4	0	0
Chlorpropamide (Diabinese)	0	3	0	1
Oxyphenbutazone (Tandearil, Oxalid)	0	2	0	2
Sulindac (Clinoril)	0	2	0	1
Ibuprofen (Motrin)	0	2	0	2
Phenytoin (Dilantin)	0	2	0	1
Oxytetracycline (Terramycin)	0	2	0	0
Glibenclamide (Diabeta, Micronase)	0	2	0	1
Fluconazole (Diflucan)	0	2	0	0
Captopril (Capoten)	0	2	0	0
Ampicillin (Omnipen, Totacillin)	0	2	1	1

* The full list of articles reviewed, the database established by this review, and the methodology for establishing levels of evidence are available at http://moon.ouhsc.edu/jgeorge, which can be accessed through the *Williams Hematology*, 6th edition web page.
SOURCE: George and colleagues,[561] with permission.

These patients have been postulated to have preformed antibodies to epitopes exposed on GpIIb-IIIa by drug binding. These could be the same antibodies that cause *in vitro* EDTA-dependent platelet agglutination and pseudothrombocytopenia.[26,549,550]

Diagnosis The diagnosis can be made only by recovery from thrombocytopenia upon discontinuation of the drug and can be confirmed if thrombocytopenia recurs with rechallenge by the drug. Prompt recovery within 5 to 7 days is predictable.[540] Gold-induced thrombocytopenia is an exception because gold salts are retained for a long time within the body and thrombocytopenia can persist for months, becoming indistinguishable from ITP.[551] Rechallenge with a suspected drug is dangerous, because severe thrombocytopenia can develop rapidly with even very small doses. However, when any one of multiple drugs is involved and all are important for management, it may be appropriate to reintroduce them individually, followed by several days of close observation. In general, the smallest possible dose of the drug should be administered. The administration should be performed under direct supervision, with platelets available for bleeding should it occur. If rechallenge leads to thrombocytopenia, the patient should be advised to wear a Medic Alert bracelet. For common drugs, especially those that can be purchased without a prescription, it may be safer to supervise a rechallenge and unequivocally document risk rather than risk future unintentional use.

Laboratory assays can detect drug-dependent antibodies, and positive results can support a clinical diagnosis. However, the laboratory role remains largely investigational because results are not promptly available when a clinical decision must be made about discontinuing a drug. Furthermore, no laboratory test has been validated by continuing a suspected drug with no adverse effects following a negative laboratory test.

Drug-dependent antibodies can be detected by flow cytometric techniques,[546] MAIPA,[552] and solid-phase red cell adherence assays.[553] Strongly positive tests are apparent, but distinction of positive from negative tests is arbitrary and not yet clinically validated. Positive tests for heparin-dependent antibodies have been reported in patients without thrombocytopenia,[554–557] and patients with clinical evidence for drug-induced thrombocytopenia may have negative tests using multiple techniques.[545,546]

CLINICAL AND LABORATORY FEATURES

In patients with newly discovered thrombocytopenia, all medications should be identified. Not only prescription medications but also nonprescription drugs, such as products with acetaminophen,[540] and drinks that may include quinine ("tonic water") must be documented.[558,559]

Drug-induced thrombocytopenia typically produces profoundly low platelet counts. Among the 247 patient case reports with evidence for a definite or probable causal relation of the drug to thrombocytopenia, 23 patients (9%) had major bleeding, including two patients who died of bleeding,[540] and 68 patients (28%) had overt but minor bleeding; 96 patients (39%) had only purpura or trivial bleeding, and the remainder had no bleeding.[540] The time from beginning the drug to the initial occurrence of thrombocytopenia varies from 1 day to 3 years, but the median time is only 14 days. With rechallenge, acute thrombocytopenia may occur within minutes but almost always within 3 days.[540] Patients may have other signs and symptoms of drug sensitivity, such as nausea and vomiting, rash, fever, and abnormal liver function tests.[560] Laboratory data may demonstrate leukopenia, indicating multiple cell targets of the drug-dependent antibodies.[560] Patients who have systemic adverse reactions manifesting TTP-HUS are described in Chapter 124.

TREATMENT

Withdrawal of the offending drug is the most important therapeutic measure. Prednisone is commonly given because the distinction from ITP almost never is initially clear; however, it does not appear to influence recovery.[560] In patients with major bleeding, emergent treatment should be the same as for ITP: platelet transfusions, high doses of parenteral methylprednisolone, and possibly IVIg.[471]

REFERENCES

1. International Committee for Standardization in Hematology, Panel on Diagnostic Application of Radioisotopes in Hematology: Recommended methods for radioisotope platelet survival studies. *Blood* 50:1137, 1977.
2. International Committee for Standardization in Hematology, Panel on Diagnostic Applications of Radionuclides: Recommended method for indium-111 platelet survival studies. *J Nucl Med* 29:564, 1988.
3. Heyns AP, Badenhorst PN, Wessels P, et al: Indium-111-labelled human platelets: A method for use in severe thrombocytopenia. *Thromb Haemost* 52:226, 1984.
4. Brubaker DB, Marcus C, Holmes E: Intravascular and total body platelet equilibrium in healthy volunteers and in thrombocytopenic patients transfused with single donor platelets. *Am J Hematol* 58:165, 1998.
5. Heyns AD, Lotter MG, Badenhorst PN, Van Reenen O, Pieters H, Minnaar PC: Kinetics and fate of (111)Indium-oxine labeled blood platelets in asplenic subjects. *Thromb Haemost* 44:100, 1980.
6. Aster RH: Pooling of platelets in the spleen: Role in the pathogenesis of "hypersplenic" thrombocytopenia. *J Clin Invest* 45:645, 1966.
7. Hill-Zobel RL, McCandless B, Kang SA, et al: Organ distribution and fate of human platelets: Studies of asplenic and splenomegalic patients. *Am J Hematol* 23:231, 1986.
8. Heyns AD, Lotter MG, Badenhorst PN, et al: Kinetics, distribution and sites of destruction of 111indium-labeled human platelets. *Br J Haematol* 44:269, 1980.
9. Heyns AD, Lotter MG, Badenhorst PN, et al: Kinetics and sites of destruction of 111Indium-oxine-labeled platelets in idiopathic thrombocytopenic purpura: A quantitative study. *Am J Hematol* 12:167, 1982.
10. Leissinger CA: Platelet kinetics in immune thrombocytopenic purpura and human immunodeficiency virus thrombocytopenia. *Curr Opin Hematol* 8:299, 2001.
11. Hanson SR, Slichter SJ: Platelet kinetics in patients with bone marrow hypoplasia: Evidence for a fixed platelet requirement. *Blood* 66:1105, 1985.
12. Ballem PJ, Segal GM, Stratton JR, et al: Mechanisms of thrombocytopenia in chronic autoimmune thrombocytopenic purpura. Evidence of both impaired platelet production and increased platelet clearance. *J Clin Invest* 80:33, 1987.
13. Lamy T, Moisan A, Dauriac C, et al: Splenectomy in idiopathic thrombocytopenic purpura: Its correlation with the sequestration of autologous indium-111-labeled platelets. *J Nucl Med* 34:182, 1993.
14. Yoneyama A, Nakahara K: EDTA-dependent pseudothrombocytopenia—Differentiation from true thrombocytopenia. *Nippon Rinsho* 61:569, 2003.
15. Garcia SJ, Merino JL, Rodriguez M, et al: Pseudothrombocytopenia: Incidence, causes and methods of detection. *Sangre (Barc)* 36:197, 1991.
16. Payne BA, Pierre RV: Pseudothrombocytopenia: A laboratory artifact with potentially serious consequences. *Mayo Clin Proc* 59:123, 1984.
17. Savage RA: Pseudoleukocytosis due to EDTA-induced platelet clumping. *Am J Clin Pathol* 81:317, 1984.
18. Vicari A, Banfi G, Bonini PA: EDTA-dependent pseudothrombocytopaenia: A 12-month epidemiological study. *Scand J Clin Lab Invest* 48:537, 1988.
19. Sweeney JD, Holme S, Heaton WA, et al: Pseudothrombocytopenia in plateletpheresis donors. *Transfusion* 35:46, 1995.
20. Bartels PC, Schoorl M, Lombarts AJ: Screening for EDTA-dependent deviations in platelet counts and abnormalities in platelet distribution

histograms in pseudothrombocytopenia. *Scand J Clin Lab Invest* 57:629, 1997.

21. Bragnani G, Bianconcini G, Brogna R, Zoli G: Pseudothrombocytopenia: Clinical comment on 37 cases. *Minerva Med* 92:13, 2001.

22. Onder O, Weinstein A, Hoyer LW: Pseudothrombocytopenia caused by platelet agglutinins that are reactive in blood anticoagulated with chelating agents. *Blood* 56:177, 1980.

23. Bizzaro N: EDTA-dependent pseudothrombocytopenia: A clinical and epidemiological study of 112 cases, with 10-year follow-up. *Am J Hematol* 50:103, 1995.

24. Hoyt RH, Durie BG: Pseudothrombocytopenia induced by a monoclonal IgM kappa platelet agglutinin. *Am J Hematol* 31:50, 1989.

25. Bizzaro N, Goldschmeding R, Dem Borne AE: Platelet satellitism is Fc gamma RIII (CD16) receptor-mediated. *Am J Clin Pathol* 103:740, 1995.

26. Casonato A, Bertomoro A, Pontara E, et al: EDTA dependent pseudothrombocytopenia caused by antibodies against the cytoadhesive receptor of platelet gpIIB-IIIA. *J Clin Pathol* 47:625, 1994.

27. Nomura S, Nagata H, Oda K, et al: Effects of EDTA on the membrane glycoproteins IIb-IIIa complex—Analysis using flow cytometry. *Thromb Res* 47:47, 1987.

28. Schrezenmeier H, Muller H, Gunsilius E, et al: Anticoagulant-induced pseudothrombocytopenia and pseudoleucocytosis. *Thromb Haemost* 73:506, 1995.

29. Ryo R, Sugano W, Goto M, et al: Platelet release reaction during EDTA-induced platelet agglutinations and inhibition of EDTA-induced platelet agglutination by anti-glycoprotein II b/III a complex monoclonal antibody. *Thromb Res* 74:265, 1994.

30. Cohen AM, Lewinski UH, Klein B, Djaldetti M: Satellitism of platelets to monocytes. *Acta Haematol* 64:61, 1980.

31. Djaldetti M, Fishman P: Satellitism of platelets to monocytes in a patient with hypogammaglobulinaemia. *Scand J Haematol* 21:305, 1978.

32. Bizzaro N, Brandalise M: EDTA-dependent pseudothrombocytopenia. Association with antiplatelet and antiphospholipid antibodies. *Am J Clin Pathol* 103:103, 1995.

33. Schell DA, Ganti AK, Levitt R, Potti A: Thrombocytopenia associated with c7E3 Fab (abciximab). *Ann Hematol* 81:76, 2002.

34. Sane DC, Damaraju LV, Topol EJ, Cabot CF, et al: Occurrence and clinical significance of pseudothrombocytopenia during abciximab therapy. *J Am Coll Cardiol* 36:75, 2000.

35. Pinton P: Abciximab-induced thrombopenia during treatment of acute coronary syndromes by angioplasty. *Ann Cardiol Angeiol (Paris)* 47:351, 1998.

36. Berkowitz SD, Sane DC, Sigmon KN, et al: Occurrence and clinical significance of thrombocytopenia in a population undergoing high-risk percutaneous coronary revascularization. Evaluation of c7E3 for the Prevention of Ischemic Complications (EPIC) Study Group. *J Am Coll Cardiol* 32:311, 1998.

37. Berkman N, Michaeli Y, Or R, Eldor A: EDTA-dependent pseudothrombocytopenia: A clinical study of 18 patients and a review of the literature. *Am J Hematol* 36:195, 1991.

38. Mori M, Kudo H, Yoshitake S, et al: Transient EDTA-dependent pseudothrombocytopenia in a patient with sepsis. *Intensive Care Med* 26:218, 2000.

39. Bizzaro N, Fiorin F: Coexistence of erythrocyte agglutination and EDTA-dependent platelet clumping in a patient with thymoma and plasmocytoma. *Arch Pathol Lab Med* 123:159, 1999.

40. Matarazzo M, Conturso V, Di Martino M, et al: EDTA-dependent pseudothrombocytopenia in a case of liver cirrhosis. *Panminerva Med* 42:155, 2000.

41. Chiurazzi F, Villa MR, Rotoli B: Transplacental transmission of EDTA-dependent pseudothrombocytopenia. *Haematologica* 84:664, 1999.

42. Solanki DL, Blackburn BC: Spurious thrombocytopenia during pregnancy. *Obstet Gynecol* 65:14S, 1985.

43. Kelley MJ, Jawien W, Ortel TL, Korczak JF: Mutation of MYH9, encoding non-muscle myosin heavy chain A, in May-Hegglin anomaly. *Nat Genet* 26:106, 2000.

44. Seri M, Pecci A, Di Bari F, et al: MYH9-related disease: May-Hegglin anomaly, Sebastian syndrome, Fechtner syndrome, and Epstein syndrome are not distinct entities but represent a variable expression of a single illness. *Medicine (Baltimore)* 82:203, 2003.

45. Heath KE, Campos-Barros A, Toren A, et al: Nonmuscle myosin heavy chain IIA mutations define a spectrum of autosomal dominant macrothrombocytopenias: May-Hegglin anomaly and Fechtner, Sebastian, Epstein, and Alport-like syndromes. *Am J Hum Genet* 69:1033, 2001.

46. Balduini CL, Iolascon A, Savoia A: Inherited thrombocytopenias: From genes to therapy. *Haematologica* 87:860, 2002.

47. Shao XR, Li JZ, Ma J, et al: Clinical and molecular-biological study of a May-Hegglin anomaly family. *Zhonghua Xue Ye Xue Za Zhi* 25:548, 2004.

48. Di Pumpo M, Noris P, Pecci A, et al: Defective expression of GPIb/IX/V complex in platelets from patients with May-Hegglin anomaly and Sebastian syndromes. *Haematologica* 87:943, 2002.

49. Ghiggeri GM, Caridi G, Magrini U, et al: Genetics, clinical and pathological features of glomerulonephritis associated with mutations of nonmuscle myosin IIA (Fechtner syndrome). *Am J Kidney Dis* 41:95, 2003.

50. Toothaker LE, Gonzalez DA, Tung N, et al: Cellular myosin heavy chain in human leukocytes: Isolation of 5′ cDNA clones, characterization of the protein, chromosomal localization, and upregulation during myeloid differentiation. *Blood* 78:1826, 1991.

51. D'Apolito M, Guarnieri V, Boncristiano M, et al: Cloning of the murine non-muscle myosin heavy chain IIA gene ortholog of human MYH9 responsible for May-Hegglin, Sebastian, Fechtner, and Epstein syndromes. *Gene* 286:215, 2002.

52. Arrondel C, Vodovar N, Knebelmann B, et al: Expression of the non-muscle myosin heavy chain IIA in the human kidney and screening for MYH9 mutations in Epstein and Fechtner syndromes. *J Am Soc Nephrol* 13:65, 2002.

53. Kunishima S, Matsushita T, Kojima T, et al: Identification of six novel MYH9 mutations and genotype-phenotype relationships in autosomal dominant macrothrombocytopenia with leukocyte inclusions. *J Hum Genet* 46:722, 2001.

54. Deutsch S, Rideau A, Bochaton-Piallat ML, et al: Asp1424Asn MYH9 mutation results in an unstable protein responsible for the phenotypes in May-Hegglin anomaly/Fechtner syndrome. *Blood* 102:529, 2003.

55. Pujol-Moix N, Kelley MJ, Hernandez A, et al: Ultrastructural analysis of granulocyte inclusions in genetically confirmed MYH9-related disorders. *Haematologica* 89:330, 2004.

56. Kunishima S: May-Hegglin anomaly—From genome research to clinical laboratory. *Rinsho Byori* 51:898, 2003.

57. Kunishima S, Matsushita T, Kojima T, et al: Immunofluorescence analysis of neutrophil nonmuscle myosin heavy chain-A in MYH9 disorders: Association of subcellular localization with MYH9 mutations. *Lab Invest* 83:115, 2003.

58. Pecci A, Noris P, Invernizzi R, et al: Immunocytochemistry for the heavy chain of the non-muscle myosin IIA as a diagnostic tool for MYH9-related disorders. *Br J Haematol* 117:164, 2002.

59. Behrens WE: Mediterranean macrothrombocytopenia. *Blood* 46:199, 1975.

60. Savoia A, Balduini CL, Savino M, et al: Autosomal dominant macrothrombocytopenia in Italy is most frequently a type of heterozygous Bernard-Soulier syndrome. *Blood* 97:1330, 2001.

61. Noris P, Pecci A, Di Bari F, et al: Application of a diagnostic algorithm for inherited thrombocytopenias to 46 consecutive patients. *Haematologica* 89:1219, 2004.

62. Minelli A, Maserati E, Rossi G, et al: Familial platelet disorder with propensity to acute myelogenous leukemia: Genetic heterogeneity and

progression to leukemia via acquisition of clonal chromosome anomalies. *Genes Chromosomes Cancer* 40:165, 2004.

63. Song WJ, Sullivan MG, Legare RD, et al: Haploinsufficiency of CBFA2 causes familial thrombocytopenia with propensity to develop acute myelogenous leukaemia. *Nat Genet* 23:166, 1999.

64. Okuda T, van Deursen J, Hiebert SW, et al: AML1, the target of multiple chromosomal translocations in human leukemia, is essential for normal fetal liver hematopoiesis. *Cell* 84:321, 1996.

65. Michaud J, Wu F, Osato M, et al: In vitro analyses of known and novel RUNX1/AML1 mutations in dominant familial platelet disorder with predisposition to acute myelogenous leukemia: Implications for mechanisms of pathogenesis. *Blood* 99:1364, 2002.

66. Elagib KE, Racke FK, Mogass M, et al: RUNX1 and GATA-1 coexpression and cooperation in megakaryocytic differentiation. *Blood* 101:4333, 2003.

67. Geddis AE, Kaushansky K: Inherited thrombocytopenias: Toward a molecular understanding of disorders of platelet production. *Curr Opin Pediatr* 16:15, 2004.

68. Drachman JG, Jarvik GP, Mehaffey MG: Autosomal dominant thrombocytopenia: Incomplete megakaryocyte differentiation and linkage to human chromosome 10. *Blood* 96:118, 2000.

69. Savoia A, Del Vecchio M, Totaro A, et al: An autosomal dominant thrombocytopenia gene maps to chromosomal region 10p. *Am J Hum Genet* 65:1401, 1999.

70. Gandhi MJ, Cummings CL, Drachman JG: FLJ14813 missense mutation: A candidate for autosomal dominant thrombocytopenia on human chromosome 10. *Hum Hered* 55:66, 2003.

71. Grossfeld PD, Mattina T, Lai Z, et al: The 11q terminal deletion disorder: A prospective study of 110 cases. *Am J Med Genet* 129A:51, 2004.

72. Favier R, Jondeau K, Boutard P, et al: Paris-Trousseau syndrome: Clinical, hematological, molecular data of ten new cases. *Thromb Haemost* 90:893, 2003.

73. Raslova H, Komura E, Le Couedic JP, et al: FLI1 monoallelic expression combined with its hemizygous loss underlies Paris-Trousseau/Jacobsen thrombopenia. *J Clin Invest* 114:77, 2004.

74. Hart A, Melet F, Grossfeld P, et al: Fli-1 is required for murine vascular and megakaryocytic development and is hemizygously deleted in patients with thrombocytopenia. *Immunity* 13:167, 2000.

75. Shivdasani RA: Lonely in Paris: When one gene copy isn't enough. *J Clin Invest* 114:17, 2004.

76. Thompson AA, Woodruff K, Feig SA, et al: Congenital thrombocytopenia and radio-ulnar synostosis: A new familial syndrome. *Br J Haematol* 113:866, 2001.

77. Thompson AA, Nguyen LT: Amegakaryocytic thrombocytopenia and radio-ulnar synostosis are associated with HOXA11 mutation. *Nat Genet* 26:397, 2000.

78. Sauvageau G, Iscove NN, Humphries RK: In vitro and in vivo expansion of hematopoietic stem cells. *Oncogene* 23:7223, 2004.

79. Thorsteinsdottir U, Sauvageau G, Hough MR, et al: Overexpression of HOXA10 in murine hematopoietic cells perturbs both myeloid and lymphoid differentiation and leads to acute myeloid leukemia. *Mol Cell Biol* 17:495, 1997.

80. van den OS, de Haas M, dem Borne AE: Screening for c-mpl mutations in patients with congenital amegakaryocytic thrombocytopenia identifies a polymorphism. *Blood* 97:3675, 2001.

81. Tonelli R, Scardovi AL, Pession A, et al: Compound heterozygosity for two different amino-acid substitution mutations in the thrombopoietin receptor (c-mpl gene) in congenital amegakaryocytic thrombocytopenia (CAMT). *Hum Genet* 107:225, 2000.

82. Ihara K, Ishii E, Eguchi M, et al: Identification of mutations in the c-mpl gene in congenital amegakaryocytic thrombocytopenia. *Proc Natl Acad Sci U S A* 96:3132, 1999.

83. Ballmaier M, Germeshausen M, Schulze H, et al: C-mpl mutations are the cause of congenital amegakaryocytic thrombocytopenia. *Blood* 97:139, 2001.

84. Germeshausen M, Schulze H, Gaudig A, et al: Congenital amegakaryocytic thrombocytopenia (CAMT)—A defect of the thrombopoietin receptor c-Mpl. *Klin Padiatr* 213:155, 2001.

85. Germeshausen M, Ballmaier M, Welte K: Implications of mutations in hematopoietic growth factor receptor genes in congenital cytopenias. *Ann N Y Acad Sci* 938:305, 2001.

86. van den OS, Bruin M, Folman CC, et al: Mutations in the thrombopoietin receptor, Mpl, in children with congenital amegakaryocytic thrombocytopenia. *Br J Haematol* 110:441, 2000.

87. Ballmaier M, Germeshausen M, Krukemeier S, Welte K: Thrombopoietin is essential for the maintenance of normal hematopoiesis in humans: Development of aplastic anemia in patients with congenital amegakaryocytic thrombocytopenia. *Ann N Y Acad Sci* 996:17, 2003.

88. Al Ahmari A, Ayas M, Al Jefri A, et al: Allogeneic stem cell transplantation for patients with congenital amegakaryocytic thrombocytopenia (CAT). *Bone Marrow Transplant* 33:829, 2004.

89. Shaw S: Congenital hypoplastic thrombocytopenia with skeletal deformities in siblings. *Blood* 14:374, 1959.

90. Hall JG: Thrombocytopenia and absent radius (TAR) syndrome. *J Med Genet* 24:79, 1987.

91. Greenhalgh KL, Howell RT, Bottani A, et al: Thrombocytopenia-absent radius syndrome: A clinical genetic study. *J Med Genet* 39:876, 2002.

92. Hedberg VA, Lipton JM: Thrombocytopenia with absent radii. A review of 100 cases. *Am J Pediatr Hematol Oncol* 10:51, 1988.

93. Letestu R, Vitrat N, Masse A, et al: Existence of a differentiation blockage at the stage of a megakaryocyte precursor in the thrombocytopenia and absent radii (TAR) syndrome. *Blood* 95:1633, 2000.

94. Ballmaier M, Schulze H, Strauss G, et al: Thrombopoietin in patients with congenital thrombocytopenia and absent radii: Elevated serum levels, normal receptor expression, but defective reactivity to thrombopoietin. *Blood* 90:612, 1997.

95. Ochs HD: The Wiskott-Aldrich syndrome. *Clin Rev Allergy Immunol* 20:61, 2001.

96. Rengan R, Ochs HD: Molecular biology of the Wiskott-Aldrich syndrome. *Rev Immunogenet* 2:243, 2000.

97. Derry JM, Kerns JA, Weinberg KI, et al: WASP gene mutations in Wiskott-Aldrich syndrome and X-linked thrombocytopenia. *Hum Mol Genet* 4:1127, 1995.

98. Derry JM, Ochs HD, Francke U: Isolation of a novel gene mutated in Wiskott-Aldrich syndrome. *Cell* 78:635, 1994.

99. Villa A, Notarangelo L, Macchi P, et al: X-linked thrombocytopenia and Wiskott-Aldrich syndrome are allelic diseases with mutations in the WASP gene. *Nat Genet* 9:414, 1995.

100. Imai K, Nonoyama S, Ochs HD: WASP (Wiskott-Aldrich syndrome protein) gene mutations and phenotype. *Curr Opin Allergy Clin Immunol* 3:427, 2003.

101. Burns S, Cory GO, Vainchenker W, Thrasher AJ: Mechanisms of WASp-mediated hematologic and immunologic disease. *Blood*, 104:3454, 2004.

102. Notarangelo LD, Mazza C, Giliani S, et al: Missense mutations of the WASP gene cause intermittent X-linked thrombocytopenia. *Blood* 99:2268, 2002.

103. Zhu Q, Watanabe C, Liu T, et al: Wiskott-Aldrich syndrome/X-linked thrombocytopenia: WASP gene mutations, protein expression, and phenotype. *Blood* 90:2680, 1997.

104. Shcherbina A, Rosen FS, Remold-O'Donnell E: WASP levels in platelets and lymphocytes of Wiskott-Aldrich syndrome patients correlate with cell dysfunction. *J Immunol* 163:6314, 1999.

105. Lum LG, Tubergen DG, Corash L, Blaese RM: Splenectomy in the

management of the thrombocytopenia of the Wiskott-Aldrich syndrome. *N Engl J Med* 302:892, 1980.

106. Filipovich AH, Stone JV, Tomany SC, et al: Impact of donor type on outcome of bone marrow transplantation for Wiskott-Aldrich syndrome: Collaborative study of the International Bone Marrow Transplant Registry and the National Marrow Donor Program. *Blood* 97:1598, 2001.

107. Drachman JG: Inherited thrombocytopenia: When a low platelet count does not mean ITP. *Blood* 103:390, 2004.

108. Strom TS, Gabbard W, Kelly PF, et al: Functional correction of T cells derived from patients with the Wiskott-Aldrich syndrome (WAS) by transduction with an oncoretroviral vector encoding the WAS protein. *Gene Ther* 10:803, 2003.

109. Wada T, Jagadeesh GJ, Nelson DL, Candotti F: Retrovirus-mediated WASP gene transfer corrects Wiskott-Aldrich syndrome T-cell dysfunction. *Hum Gene Ther* 13:1039, 2002.

110. Klein C, Nguyen D, Liu CH, et al: Gene therapy for Wiskott-Aldrich syndrome: Rescue of T-cell signaling and amelioration of colitis upon transplantation of retrovirally transduced hematopoietic stem cells in mice. *Blood* 101:2159, 2003.

111. Freson K, Devriendt K, Matthijs G, et al: Platelet characteristics in patients with X-linked macrothrombocytopenia because of a novel GATA-1 mutation. *Blood* 98:85, 2001.

112. Mehaffey MG, Newton AL, Gandhi MJ, et al: X-linked thrombocytopenia caused by a novel mutation of GATA-1. *Blood* 98:2681, 2001.

113. Shivdasani RA, Fujiwara Y, McDevitt MA, Orkin SH: A lineage-selective knockout establishes the critical role of transcription factor GATA-1 in megakaryocyte growth and platelet development. *EMBO J* 16:3965, 1997.

114. Tsang AP, Fujiwara Y, Hom DB, Orkin SH: Failure of megakaryopoiesis and arrested erythropoiesis in mice lacking the GATA-1 transcriptional cofactor FOG. *Genes Dev* 12:1176, 1998.

115. Orkin SH: GATA-binding transcription factors in hematopoietic cells. *Blood* 80:575, 1992.

116. Vyas P, Ault K, Jackson CW, et al: Consequences of GATA-1 deficiency in megakaryocytes and platelets. *Blood* 93:2867, 1999.

117. Enjolras O, Wassef M, Mazoyer EA, et al: Infants with Kasabach-Merritt syndrome do not have "true" hemangiomas. *J Pediatr* 130:631, 1997.

118. Sarkar M, Mulliken JB, Kozakewich HP, et al: Thrombocytopenic coagulopathy (Kasabach-Merritt phenomenon) is associated with Kaposiform hemangioendothelioma and not with common infantile hemangioma. *Plast Reconstr Surg* 100:1377, 1997.

119. Vin-Christian K, McCalmont TH, Frieden IJ: Kaposiform hemangioendothelioma. An aggressive, locally invasive vascular tumor that can mimic hemangioma of infancy. *Arch Dermatol* 133:1573, 1997.

120. Hall GW: Kasabach-Merritt syndrome: Pathogenesis and management. *Br J Haematol* 112:851, 2001.

121. Cooper JG, Edwards SL, Holmes JD: Kaposiform haemangioendothelioma: Case report and review of the literature. *Br J Plast Surg* 55:163, 2002.

122. Hoeger PH, Helmke K, Winkler K: Chronic consumption coagulopathy due to an occult splenic haemangioma: Kasabach-Merritt syndrome. *Eur J Pediatr* 154:365, 1995.

123. Brasanac D, Janic D, Boricic I, et al: Retroperitoneal kaposiform hemangioendothelioma with tufted angioma-like features in an infant with Kasabach-Merritt syndrome. *Pathol Int* 53:627, 2003.

124. Mukhtar IA, Letts M: Hemangioma of the radius associated with Kasabach-Merritt syndrome: Case report and literature review. *J Pediatr Orthop* 24:87, 2004.

125. Fukunaga M, Ushigome S, Ishikawa E: Kaposiform haemangioendothelioma associated with Kasabach-Merritt syndrome. *Histopathology* 28:281, 1996.

126. Alvarez-Mendoza A, Lourdes TS, Ridaura-Sanz C, Ruiz-Maldonado R: Histopathology of vascular lesions found in Kasabach-Merritt syndrome: Review based on 13 cases. *Pediatr Dev Pathol* 3:556, 2000.

127. Jones EW, Orkin M: Tufted angioma (angioblastoma). A benign progressive angioma, not to be confused with Kaposi's sarcoma or low-grade angiosarcoma. *J Am Acad Dermatol* 20:214, 1989.

128. Wong SN, Tay YK: Tufted angioma: A report of five cases. *Pediatr Dermatol* 19:388, 2002.

129. Mueller BU, Mulliken JB: The infant with a vascular tumor. *Semin Perinatol* 23:332, 1999.

130. Mazoyer E, Enjolras O, Laurian C, et al: Coagulation abnormalities associated with extensive venous malformations of the limbs: Differentiation from Kasabach-Merritt syndrome. *Clin Lab Haematol* 24:243, 2002.

131. Lyons LL, North PE, Mac-Moune LF, et al: Kaposiform hemangioendothelioma: A study of 33 cases emphasizing its pathologic, immunophenotypic, and biologic uniqueness from juvenile hemangioma. *Am J Surg Pathol* 28:559, 2004.

132. Gilon E, Ramot B, Sheba C: Multiple hemangiomata associated with thrombocytopenia: Remarks on the pathogenesis of the thrombocytopenia in this syndrome. *Blood* 14:74, 1959.

133. Seo SK, Suh JC, Na GY, et al: Kasabach-Merritt syndrome: Identification of platelet trapping in a tufted angioma by immunohistochemistry technique using monoclonal antibody to CD61. *Pediatr Dermatol* 16: 392, 1999.

134. Brizel HE, Raccuglia G: Giant hemangioma with thrombocytopenia. Radioisotopic demonstration of platelet sequestration. *Blood* 26:751, 1965.

135. Shulkin BL, Argenta LC, Cho KJ, Castle VP: Kasabach-Merritt syndrome: Treatment with epsilon-aminocaproic acid and assessment by indium 111 platelet scintigraphy. *J Pediatr* 117:746, 1990.

136. Warrell RP Jr, Kempin SJ, Benua RS, et al: Intratumoral consumption of indium-111 labeled platelets in a patient with hemangiomatosis and intravascular coagulation (Kasabach-Merritt syndrome). *Cancer* 52: 2256, 1983.

137. Wananukul S, Nuchprayoon I, Seksarn P: Treatment of Kasabach-Merritt syndrome: A stepwise regimen of prednisolone, dipyridamole, and interferon. *Int J Dermatol* 42:741, 2003.

138. MacArthur CJ, Senders CW, Katz J: The use of interferon alfa-2a for life-threatening hemangiomas. *Arch Otolaryngol Head Neck Surg* 121: 690, 1995.

139. Haisley-Royster C, Enjolras O, Frieden IJ, et al: Kasabach-Merritt phenomenon: A retrospective study of treatment with vincristine. *J Pediatr Hematol Oncol* 24:459, 2002.

140. Blei F, Karp N, Rofsky N, et al: Successful multimodal therapy for kaposiform hemangioendothelioma complicated by Kasabach-Merritt phenomenon: Case report and review of the literature. *Pediatr Hematol Oncol* 15:295, 1998.

141. Hu B, Lachman R, Phillips J, et al: Kasabach-Merritt syndrome-associated kaposiform hemangioendothelioma successfully treated with cyclophosphamide, vincristine, and actinomycin D. *J Pediatr Hematol Oncol* 20:567, 1998.

142. Frevel T, Rabe H, Uckert F, Harms E: Giant cavernous haemangioma with Kasabach-Merritt syndrome: A case report and review. *Eur J Pediatr* 161:243, 2002.

143. Atahan IL, Cengiz M, Ozyar E, Gurkaynak M: Radiotherapy in the management of Kasabach-Merritt syndrome: A case report. *Pediatr Hematol Oncol* 18:471, 2001.

144. Ogino I, Torikai K, Kobayasi S, et al: Radiation therapy for life- or function-threatening infant hemangioma. *Radiology* 218:834, 2001.

145. Billio A, Pescosta N, Rosanelli C, et al: Treatment of Kasabach-Merritt syndrome by embolisation of a giant liver hemangioma. *Am J Hematol* 66:140, 2001.

146. Hosono S, Ohno T, Kimoto H, et al: Successful transcutaneous arterial embolization of a giant hemangioma associated with high-output cardiac failure and Kasabach-Merritt syndrome in a neonate: A case report. *J Perinat Med* 27:399, 1999.

147. Zukerberg LR, Nickoloff BJ, Weiss SW: Kaposiform hemangioendothelioma of infancy and childhood. An aggressive neoplasm associated with Kasabach-Merritt syndrome and lymphangiomatosis. *Am J Surg Pathol* 17:321, 1993.

148. George M, Singhal V, Sharma V, Nopper AJ: Successful surgical excision of a complex vascular lesion in an infant with Kasabach-Merritt syndrome. *Pediatr Dermatol* 19:340, 2002.

149. Pavkovic M, Georgievski B, Cevreska L, et al: CTLA-4 exon 1 polymorphism in patients with autoimmune blood disorders. *Am J Hematol* 72:147, 2003.

150. Mientjes GH, van Ameijden EJ, Mulder JW, et al: Prevalence of thrombocytopenia in HIV-infected and non-HIV infected drug users and homosexual men. *Br J Haematol* 82:615, 1992.

151. Ehmann WC, Rabkin CS, Eyster ME, Goedert JJ: Thrombocytopenia in HIV-infected and uninfected hemophiliacs. Multicenter Hemophilia Cohort study. *Am J Hematol* 54:296, 1997.

152. Ciernik IF, Cone RW, Fehr J, Weber R: Impaired liver function and retroviral activity are risk factors contributing to HIV-associated thrombocytopenia. Swiss HIV Cohort Study. *AIDS* 13:1913, 1999.

153. Dominguez A, Gamallo G, Garcia R, et al: Pathophysiology of HIV related thrombocytopenia: An analysis of 41 patients. *J Clin Pathol* 47:999, 1994.

154. Louache F, Vainchenker W: Thrombocytopenia in HIV infection. *Curr Opin Hematol* 1:369, 1994.

155. Brook MG, Ayles H, Harrison C, et al: Diagnostic utility of bone marrow sampling in HIV positive patients. *Genitourin Med* 73:117, 1997.

156. Van WV, Kotze HF, Heyns AP: Kinetics of indium-111-labelled platelets in HIV-infected patients with and without associated thrombocytopaenia. *Eur J Haematol* 62:332, 1999.

157. Kamiyama M, Arkel YS, Chen K, Shido K: Inhibition of platelet GPIIb/IIIa binding to fibrinogen by serum factors: Studies of circulating immune complexes and platelet antibodies in patients with hemophilia, immune thrombocytopenic purpura, human immunodeficiency virus-related immune thrombocytopenic purpura, and systemic lupus erythematosus. *J Lab Clin Med* 117:209, 1991.

158. Karpatkin S, Nardi MA, Hymes KB: Sequestration of anti-platelet GPIIIa antibody in rheumatoid factor immune complexes of human immunodeficiency virus 1 thrombocytopenic patients. *Proc Natl Acad Sci U S A* 92:2263, 1995.

159. Karpatkin S, Nardi M, Lennette ET, et al: Anti-human immunodeficiency virus type 1 antibody complexes on platelets of seropositive thrombocytopenic homosexuals and narcotic addicts. *Proc Natl Acad Sci U S A* 85:9763, 1988.

160. Fabris F, Cordiano I, Casonato A, et al: "Anti-platelet antibodies" in HIV infected haemophiliacs. *Folia Haematol Int Mag Klin Morphol Blutforsch* 117:709, 1990.

161. Bettaieb A, Oksenhendler E, Fromont P, et al: Immunochemical analysis of platelet autoantibodies in HIV-related thrombocytopenic purpura: A study of 68 patients. *Br J Haematol* 73:241, 1989.

162. Quadri MI, Lee CA, Goodall AH, et al: Antibodies to platelet glycoproteins in haemophiliacs infected with HIV. *Clin Lab Haematol* 14:109, 1992.

163. Yu JR, Lennette ET, Karpatkin S: Anti-F(ab')2 antibodies in thrombocytopenic patients at risk for acquired immunodeficiency syndrome. *J Clin Invest* 77:1756, 1986.

164. Karpatkin S, Nardi MA, Kouri YH: Internal-image anti-idiotype HIV-1gp120 antibody in human immunodeficiency virus 1 (HIV-1)-seropositive individuals with thrombocytopenia. *Proc Natl Acad Sci U S A* 89:1487, 1992.

165. Karpatkin S, Nardi M: Autoimmune anti-HIV-1gp120 antibody with antiidiotype-like activity in sera and immune complexes of HIV-1-related immunologic thrombocytopenia. *J Clin Invest* 89:356, 1992.

166. Karpatkin S, Nardi MA, Liu LX, et al: Production of a human anti-CD4 monoclonal antibody with antiidiotype to anti-HIV type 1 glycoprotein 120. *AIDS Res Hum Retroviruses* 11:509, 1995.

167. Nardi MA, Liu LX, Karpatkin S: GPIIIa-(49-66) is a major pathophysiologically relevant antigenic determinant for anti-platelet GPIIIa of HIV-1-related immunologic thrombocytopenia. *Proc Natl Acad Sci U S A* 94:7589, 1997.

168. Chia WK, Blanchette V, Mody M, et al: Characterization of HIV-1-specific antibodies and HIV-1-crossreactive antibodies to platelets in HIV-1-infected haemophiliac patients. *Br J Haematol* 103:1014, 1998.

169. Gonzalez-Conejero R, Rivera J, Rosillo MC, et al: Association of autoantibodies against platelet glycoproteins Ib/IX and IIb/IIIa, and platelet-reactive anti-HIV antibodies in thrombocytopenic narcotic addicts. *Br J Haematol* 93:464, 1996.

170. Samuel H, Nardi M, Karpatkin M, et al: Differentiation of autoimmune thrombocytopenia from thrombocytopenia associated with immune complex disease: Systemic lupus erythematosus, hepatitis-cirrhosis, and HIV-1 infection by platelet and serum immunological measurements. *Br J Haematol* 105:1086, 1999.

171. Bettaieb A, Oksenhendler E, Duedari N, Bierling P: Cross-reactive antibodies between HIV-gp120 and platelet gpIIIa (CD61) in HIV-related immune thrombocytopenic purpura. *Clin Exp Immunol* 103:19, 1996.

172. Bettaieb A, Fromont P, Louache F, et al: Presence of cross-reactive antibody between human immunodeficiency virus (HIV) and platelet glycoproteins in HIV-related immune thrombocytopenic purpura. *Blood* 80:162, 1992.

173. Hohmann AW, Booth K, Peters V, et al: Common epitope on HIV p24 and human platelets. *Lancet* 342:1274, 1993.

174. Nardi M, Karpatkin S: Antiidiotype antibody against platelet anti-GPIIIa contributes to the regulation of thrombocytopenia in HIV-1-ITP patients. *J Exp Med* 191:2093, 2000.

175. Nardi M, Feinmark SJ, Hu L, et al: Complement-independent Ab-induced peroxide lysis of platelets requires 12-lipoxygenase and a platelet NADPH oxidase pathway. *J Clin Invest* 113:973, 2004.

176. Nardi M, Tomlinson S, Greco MA, Karpatkin S: Complement-independent, peroxide-induced antibody lysis of platelets in HIV-1-related immune thrombocytopenia. *Cell* 106:551, 2001.

177. Koefoed K, Ditzel HJ: Identification of talin head domain as an immunodominant epitope of the anti-platelet antibody response in patients with HIV-1-associated thrombocytopenia. *Blood* 104:4054, 2004.

178. Cole JL, Marzec UM, Gunthel CJ, et al: Ineffective platelet production in thrombocytopenic human immunodeficiency virus-infected patients. *Blood* 91:3239, 1998.

179. Chelucci C, Federico M, Guerriero R, et al: Productive human immunodeficiency virus-1 infection of purified megakaryocytic progenitors/precursors and maturing megakaryocytes. *Blood* 91:1225, 1998.

180. Ballem PJ, Belzberg A, Devine DV, et al: Kinetic studies of the mechanism of thrombocytopenia in patients with human immunodeficiency virus infection. *N Engl J Med* 327:1779, 1992.

181. Espanol I, Muniz-Diaz E, Margall N, et al: Serum thrombopoietin levels in thrombocytopenic and non-thrombocytopenic patients with human immunodeficiency virus (HIV-1) infection. *Eur J Haematol* 63:245, 1999.

182. Young G, Loechelt BJ, Rakusan TA, et al: Thrombopoietin levels in HIV-associated thrombocytopenia in children. *J Pediatr* 133:765, 1998.

183. Zauli G, Catani L, Gibellini D, et al: Impaired survival of bone marrow GPIIb/IIIa+ megakaryocytic cells as an additional pathogenetic mechanism of HIV-1-related thrombocytopenia. *Br J Haematol* 92:711, 1996.

184. Sato T, Sekine H, Kakuda H, et al: HIV infection of megakaryocytic cell lines. *Leuk Lymphoma* 36:397, 2000.

185. Kowalska MA, Ratajczak J, Hoxie J, et al: Megakaryocyte precursors, megakaryocytes and platelets express the HIV co-receptor CXCR4 on their surface: Determination of response to stromal-derived factor-1 by megakaryocytes and platelets. *Br J Haematol* 104:220, 1999.

186. Riviere C, Subra F, Cohen-Solal K, et al: Phenotypic and functional evidence for the expression of CXCR4 receptor during megakaryocytopoiesis. *Blood* 93:1511, 1999.

187. Basch RS, Kouri YH, Karpatkin S: Expression of CD4 by human megakaryocytes. *Proc Natl Acad Sci U S A* 87:8085, 1990.

188. Kouri YH, Borkowsky W, Nardi M, et al: Human megakaryocytes have a CD4 molecule capable of binding human immunodeficiency virus-1. *Blood* 81:2664, 1993.

189. Voulgaropoulou F, Tan B, Soares M, et al: Distinct human immunodeficiency virus strains in the bone marrow are associated with the development of thrombocytopenia. *J Virol* 73:3497, 1999.

190. Voulgaropoulou F, Pontow SE, Ratner L: Productive infection of CD34+-cell-derived megakaryocytes by X4 and R5 HIV-1 isolates. *Virology* 269:78, 2000.

191. Stella CC, Ganser A, Hoelzer D: Defective in vitro growth of the hemopoietic progenitor cells in the acquired immunodeficiency syndrome. *J Clin Invest* 80:286, 1987.

192. Ahmed S, Sadiq A, Siddiqui AK, et al: Thrombotic thrombocytopenic purpura: A rare cause of thrombocytopenia in HIV-infected hemophiliacs. *Ann Hematol* 83:253, 2004.

193. Sutor GC, Schmidt RE, Albrecht H: Thrombotic microangiopathies and HIV infection: Report of two typical cases, features of HUS and TTP, and review of the literature. *Infection* 27:12, 1999.

194. Sahud MA, Claster S, Liu L, et al: Von Willebrand factor-cleaving protease inhibitor in a patient with human immunodeficiency syndrome-associated thrombotic thrombocytopenic purpura. *Br J Haematol* 116:909, 2002.

195. Peltier JY, Lambin P, Doinel C, et al: Frequency and prognostic importance of thrombocytopenia in symptom-free HIV-infected individuals: A 5-year prospective study. *AIDS* 5:381, 1991.

196. Glatt AE, Anand A: Thrombocytopenia in patients infected with human immunodeficiency virus: Treatment update. *Clin Infect Dis* 21:415, 1995.

197. Scaradavou A. HIV-related thrombocytopenia. *Blood Rev* 16:73, 2002.

198. Mannucci PM, Gringeri A: HIV-related thrombocytopenias. *Ann Ital Med Int* 15:20, 2000.

199. Sitalakshmi S, Srikrishna A, Damodar P: Haematological changes in HIV infection. *Indian J Pathol Microbiol* 46:180, 2003.

200. Diebold J, Tabbara W, Marche C, et al: Bone marrow changes at several stages of HIV infection, studied on bone marrow biopsies in 85 patients. *Arch Anat Cytol Pathol* 39:137, 1991.

201. Ananworanich J, Phanuphak N, Nuesch R, et al: Recurring thrombocytopenia associated with structured treatment interruption in patients with human immunodeficiency virus infection. *Clin Infect Dis* 37:723, 2003.

202. Ballem PJ, Belzberg A, Devine D, et al: Pathophysiology of thrombocytopenia associated with HIV infection in homosexual men. A preliminary report. *Blut* 59:111, 1989.

203. Panzer S, Stain C, Benda H, Mannhalter C: Effects of 3-azidothymidine on platelet counts, indium-111-labelled platelet kinetics, and antiplatelet antibodies. *Vox Sang* 57:120, 1989.

204. Swiss Group for Clinical Studies on the Acquired Immunodeficiency Syndrome (AIDS): Zidovudine for the treatment of thrombocytopenia associated with human immunodeficiency virus (HIV). A prospective study. *Ann Intern Med* 109:718, 1988.

205. Aboulafia DM, Bundow D, Waide S, et al: Initial observations on the efficacy of highly active antiretroviral therapy in the treatment of HIV-associated autoimmune thrombocytopenia. *Am J Med Sci* 320:117, 2000.

206. Carbonara S, Fiorentino G, Serio G, et al: Response of severe HIV-associated thrombocytopenia to highly active antiretroviral therapy including protease inhibitors. *J Infect* 42:251, 2001.

207. Stasi R, Stipa E, Masi M, et al: Long-term observation of 208 adults with chronic idiopathic thrombocytopenic purpura. *Am J Med* 98:436, 1995.

208. Oksenhendler E, Bierling P, Chevret S, et al: Splenectomy is safe and effective in human immunodeficiency virus-related immune thrombocytopenia. *Blood* 82:29, 1993.

209. Marroni M, Gresele P: Detrimental effects of high-dose dexamethasone in severe, refractory, HIV-related thrombocytopenia. *Ann Pharmacother* 34:1139, 2000.

210. Brown SA, Majumdar G, Harrington C, et al: Effect of splenectomy on HIV-related thrombocytopenia and progression of HIV infection in patients with severe haemophilia. *Blood Coagul Fibrinolysis* 5:393, 1994.

211. Majluf-Cruz A, Luna-Castanos G, Huitron S, Nieto-Cisneros L: Usefulness of a low-dose intravenous immunoglobulin regimen for the treatment of thrombocytopenia associated with AIDS. *Am J Hematol* 59:127, 1998.

212. Jahnke L, Applebaum S, Sherman LA, et al: An evaluation of intravenous immunoglobulin in the treatment of human immunodeficiency virus-associated thrombocytopenia. *Transfusion* 34:759, 1994.

213. Scaradavou A, Woo B, Woloski BM, et al: Intravenous anti-D treatment of immune thrombocytopenic purpura: Experience in 272 patients. *Blood* 89:2689, 1997.

214. Harker LA, Marzec UM, Novembre F, et al: Treatment of thrombocytopenia in chimpanzees infected with human immunodeficiency virus by pegylated recombinant human megakaryocyte growth and development factor. *Blood* 91:4427, 1998.

215. Marroni M, Gresele P, Landonio G, et al: Interferon-alpha is effective in the treatment of HIV-1-related, severe, zidovudine-resistant thrombocytopenia. A prospective, placebo-controlled, double-blind trial. *Ann Intern Med* 121:423, 1994.

216. Neben S, Hellman S, Montgomery M, et al: Hematopoietic stem cell deficit of transplanted bone marrow previously exposed to cytotoxic agents. *Exp Hematol* 21:156, 1993.

217. Schiffer CA, Anderson KC, Bennett CL, et al: Platelet transfusion for patients with cancer: Clinical practice guidelines of the American Society of Clinical Oncology. *J Clin Oncol* 19:1519, 2001.

218. Bishop JF, Matthews JP, Yuen K, et al: The definition of refractoriness to platelet transfusions. *Transfus Med* 2:35, 1992.

219. Helleberg C, Taaning EB, Johnsen HE: Transfusion-refractory thrombocytopenia during chemotherapy: Pathogenesis, frequency, and treatment. *Ugeskr Laeger* 157:5082, 1995.

220. Vadhan-Raj S, Kavanagh JJ, Freedman RS, et al: Safety and efficacy of transfusions of autologous cryopreserved platelets derived from recombinant human thrombopoietin to support chemotherapy-associated severe thrombocytopenia: A randomised cross-over study. *Lancet* 359:2145, 2002.

221. Leonardi V, Danova M, Fincato G, Palmeri S: Interleukin 3 in the treatment of chemotherapy induced thrombocytopenia. *Oncol Rep* 5:1459, 1998.

222. Farber L, Haus U, Fuchsel G, et al: Treatment of prolonged chemotherapy induced severe thrombocytopenia with recombinant human interleukin-3—A report on four cases. *Anticancer Drugs* 8:288, 1997.

223. Meden H, Fock M, Kuhn W: Effect of recombinant human interleukin-3 (rhIL-3) on persisting chemotherapy-induced thrombocytopenia. *Anticancer Drugs* 5:483, 1994.

224. Chu DT, Xu BH, Song ST, et al: Recombinant human interleukin-11 in the prevention of chemotherapy-induced thrombocytopenia. *Zhonghua Zhong Liu Za Zhi* 25:272, 2003.

225. Sun XF, Guan ZZ, Huang H, et al: Clinical study of rhIL-11 for prevention and treatment of chemotherapy-induced thrombocytopenia. *Ai Zheng* 21:892, 2002.

226. Chu DT, Xu BH, Song ST, et al: Recombinant human interleukin 11 (mega) promotes thrombopoiesis in cancer patients with chemotherapy-induced myelosuppression. *Zhongguo Shi Yan Xue Ye Xue Za Zhi* 9:314, 2001.

227. Smith JW: Tolerability and side-effect profile of rhIL-11. *Oncology (Huntingt)* 14:41, 2000.

228. Kaye JA: FDA licensure of NEUMEGA to prevent severe chemotherapy-induced thrombocytopenia. *Stem Cells* 16(suppl 2):207, 1998.

229. Tepler I, Elias L, Smith JW, et al: A randomized placebo-controlled trial of recombinant human interleukin-11 in cancer patients with severe thrombocytopenia due to chemotherapy. *Blood* 87:3607, 1996.

230. Kaye JA: Clinical development of recombinant human interleukin-11 to treat chemotherapy-induced thrombocytopenia. *Curr Opin Hematol* 3: 209, 1996.

231. Nichol JL, Hokom MM, Hornkohl A, et al: Megakaryocyte growth and development factor. Analyses of in vitro effects on human megakaryopoiesis and endogenous serum levels during chemotherapy-induced thrombocytopenia. *J Clin Invest* 95:2973, 1995.

232. Bai CM, Xu GX, Zhao YQ, et al: A multi-center clinical trial of recombinant human thrombopoietin in the treatment of chemotherapy-induced thrombocytopenia in patients with solid tumor. *Zhongguo Yi Xue Ke Xue Yuan Xue Bao* 26:437, 2004.

233. Bai CM, Zou XY, Zhao YQ, et al: The clinical study of recombinant human thrombopoietin in the treatment of chemotherapy-induced severe thrombocytopenia. *Zhonghua Yi Xue Za Zhi* 84:397, 2004.

234. Vadhan-Raj S, Patel S, Bueso-Ramos C, et al: Importance of predosing of recombinant human thrombopoietin to reduce chemotherapy-induced early thrombocytopenia. *J Clin Oncol* 21:3158, 2003.

235. Vadhan-Raj S: Clinical experience with recombinant human thrombopoietin in chemotherapy-induced thrombocytopenia. *Semin Hematol* 37: 28, 2000.

236. Nash RA, Kurzrock R, DiPersio J, et al: A phase I trial of recombinant human thrombopoietin in patients with delayed platelet recovery after hematopoietic stem cell transplantation. *Biol Blood Marrow Transplant* 6:25, 2000.

237. Shinjo K, Takeshita A, Nakamura S, et al: Serum thrombopoietin levels in patients correlate inversely with platelet counts during chemotherapy-induced thrombocytopenia. *Leukemia* 12:295, 1998.

238. Heits F, Katschinski DM, Wilmsen U, et al: Serum thrombopoietin and interleukin 6 concentrations in tumour patients and response to chemotherapy-induced thrombocytopenia. *Eur J Haematol* 59:53, 1997.

239. Stabler SP, Allen RH, Savage DG, Lindenbaum J: Clinical spectrum and diagnosis of cobalamin deficiency. *Blood* 76:871, 1990.

240. Sarode R, Garewal G, Marwaha N, et al: Pancytopenia in nutritional megaloblastic anaemia. A study from north-west India. *Trop Geogr Med* 41:331, 1989.

241. Slichter SJ, Harker LA: Thrombocytopenia: Mechanisms and management of defects in platelet production. *Clin Haematol* 7:523, 1978.

242. Epstein RD: Cells of the megakaryocytic series in pernicious anemia: In particular, the effect of specific therapy. *Am J Pathol* 25:239, 1949.

243. Rabinowitz AP, Sacks Y, Carmel R: Autoimmune cytopenias in pernicious anemia: A report of four cases and review of the literature. *Eur J Haematol* 44:18, 1990.

244. Junca J, Flores A, Granada ML, et al: The relationship between idiopathic thrombocytopenic purpura and pernicious anaemia. *Br J Haematol* 111:513, 2000.

245. Dittmar M, Kahaly GJ: Polyglandular autoimmune syndromes: Immunogenetics and long-term follow-up. *J Clin Endocrinol Metab* 88:2983, 2003.

246. Ingeberg S, Stoffersen E: Platelet dysfunction in patients with vitamin B12 deficiency. *Acta Haematol* 61:75, 1979.

247. Terade H, Niikura H, Mori H, et al: Megaloblastic anemia and platelet function—A qualitative platelet defect in pernicious anemia. *Rinsho Ketsueki* 31:254, 1990.

248. Berger M, Brass LF: Severe thrombocytopenia in iron deficiency anemia. *Am J Hematol* 24:425, 1987.

249. Sullivan LW, Adams WH, Liu YK: Induction of thrombocytopenia by thrombopheresis in man: Patterns of recovery in normal subjects during ethanol ingestion and abstinence. *Blood* 49:197, 1977.

250. Latvala J, Parkkila S, Niemela O: Excess alcohol consumption is common in patients with cytopenia: Studies in blood and bone marrow cells. *Alcohol Clin Exp Res* 28:619, 2004.

251. Smith CM, Tobin JD Jr, Burris SM, White JG: Alcohol consumption in the guinea pig is associated with reduced megakaryocyte deformability and platelet size. *J Lab Clin Med* 120:699, 1992.

252. Michot F, Gut J: Alcohol-induced bone marrow damage. A bone marrow study in alcohol-dependent individuals. *Acta Haematol* 78:252, 1987.

253. Wolber EM, Jelkmann W: Thrombopoietin: The novel hepatic hormone. *News Physiol Sci* 17:6, 2002.

254. Louwes H, Vellenga E, de Wolf JT: Abnormal platelet adhesion on abdominal vessels in asymptomatic patients with paroxysmal nocturnal hemoglobinuria. *Ann Hematol* 80:573, 2001.

255. Elebute MO, Rizzo S, Tooze JA, et al: Evaluation of the haemopoietic reservoir in de novo haemolytic paroxysmal nocturnal haemoglobinuria. *Br J Haematol* 123:552, 2003.

256. Nishimura J, Ware RE, Burnette A, et al: The hematopoietic defect in PNH is not due to defective stroma, but is due to defective progenitor cells. *Blood Cells Mol Dis* 29:159, 2002.

257. Hugel B, Socie G, Vu T, et al: Elevated levels of circulating procoagulant microparticles in patients with paroxysmal nocturnal hemoglobinuria and aplastic anemia. *Blood* 93:3451, 1999.

258. Gralnick HR, Vail M, McKeown LP, et al: Activated platelets in paroxysmal nocturnal haemoglobinuria. *Br J Haematol* 91:697, 1995.

259. Wiedmer T, Hall SE, Ortel TL, et al: Complement-induced vesiculation and exposure of membrane prothrombinase sites in platelets of paroxysmal nocturnal hemoglobinuria. *Blood* 82:1192, 1993.

260. Liebman HA, Feinstein DI: Thrombosis in patients with paroxysmal nocturnal hemoglobinuria is associated with markedly elevated plasma levels of leukocyte-derived tissue factor. *Thromb Res* 111:235, 2003.

261. Ninomiya H, Hasegawa Y, Nagasawa T, Abe T: Excess soluble urokinase-type plasminogen activator receptor in the plasma of patients with paroxysmal nocturnal hemoglobinuria inhibits cell-associated fibrinolytic activity. *Int J Hematol* 65:285, 1997.

262. Grunewald M, Siegemund A, Grunewald A, et al: Plasmatic coagulation and fibrinolytic system alterations in PNH: Relation to clone size. *Blood Coagul Fibrinolysis* 14:685, 2003.

263. Simak J, Holada K, Risitano AM, et al: Elevated circulating endothelial membrane microparticles in paroxysmal nocturnal haemoglobinuria. *Br J Haematol* 125:804, 2004.

264. Williams JL: The myelodysplastic syndromes and myeloproliferative disorders. *Clin Lab Sci* 17:223, 2004.

265. Lawrence LW: Refractory anemia and the myelodysplastic syndromes. *Clin Lab Sci* 17:178, 2004.

266. Bain B: The WHO classification of the myelodysplastic syndromes. *Exp Oncol* 26:166, 2004.

267. Hofmann WK, Kalina U, Koschmieder S, et al: Defective megakaryocytic development in myelodysplastic syndromes. *Leuk Lymphoma* 38: 13, 2000.

268. Hofmann WK, Ottmann OG, Ganser A, Hoelzer D: Myelodysplastic syndromes: Clinical features. *Semin Hematol* 33:177, 1996.

269. Kobayashi Y, Takahashi Y, Chikayama S, et al: Comparison of the DNA content of megakaryocytes identified immunologically with that identified morphologically. *Histochem Cell Biol* 108:115, 1997.

270. Kobayashi Y, Uoshima N, Kimura S, et al: Relationship between morphological classification of the degree of maturation and the ploidy of micromegakaryocytes in myelodysplastic syndrome patients. *Int J Hematol* 61:117, 1995.

271. Ohshima K, Kikuchi M, Takeshita M: A megakaryocyte analysis of the bone marrow in patients with myelodysplastic syndrome, myeloproliferative disorder and allied disorders. *J Pathol* 177:181, 1995.

272. Thiele J, Quitmann H, Wagner S, Fischer R: Dysmegakaryopoiesis in myelodysplastic syndromes (MDS): An immunomorphometric study of bone marrow trephine biopsy specimens. *J Clin Pathol* 44:300, 1991.

273. Mori H, Niikura H, Terada H, Fujita K: Morphological analysis of the megakaryocytes in myelodysplastic syndrome. *Rinsho Byori* 38:1347, 1990.

274. Thiele J, Titius BR, Kopsidis C, Fischer R: Atypical micromegakaryocytes, promegakaryoblasts and megakaryoblasts: A critical evaluation by immunohistochemistry, cytochemistry and morphometry of bone marrow trephines in chronic myeloid leukemia and myelodysplastic syndromes. *Virchows Arch* 62:275, 1992.

275. Hatfill SJ, Fester ED, Steytler JG: Apoptotic megakaryocyte dysplasia in the myelodysplastic syndromes. *Hematol Pathol* 6:87, 1992.

276. Houwerzijl EJ, Blom NR, van der Want JJ, et al: Increased peripheral platelet destruction and caspase-3-independent programmed cell death of bone marrow megakaryoctes in myelodysplastic patients. *Blood* 105:3472, 2005.

277. Hofmann WK, Kalina U, Wagner S, et al: Characterization of defective megakaryocytic development in patients with myelodysplastic syndromes. *Exp Hematol* 27:395, 1999.

278. Wang W, Matsuo T, Yoshida S, et al: Colony-forming unit-megakaryocyte (CFR-meg) numbers and serum thrombopoietin concentrations in thrombocytopenic disorders: An inverse correlation in myelodysplastic syndromes. *Leukemia* 14:1751, 2000.

279. Dan K, An E, Futaki M, et al: Megakaryocyte, erythroid, and granulocyte-macrophage colony formation in myelodysplastic syndromes. *Acta Haematol* 89:113, 1993.

280. Adams JA, Liu Yin JA, Brereton ML, et al: The in vitro effect of pegylated recombinant human megakaryocyte growth and development factor (PEG rHuMGDF) on megakaryopoiesis in normal subjects and patients with myelodysplasia and acute myeloid leukaemia. *Br J Haematol* 99:139, 1997.

281. Kalina U, Hofmann WK, Koschmieder S, et al: Alteration of c-mpl-mediated signal transduction in CD34(+) cells from patients with myelodysplastic syndromes. *Exp Hematol* 28:1158, 2000.

282. Luo SS, Ogata K, Yokose N, et al: Effect of thrombopoietin on proliferation of blasts from patients with myelodysplastic syndromes. *Stem Cells* 18:112, 2000.

283. Fontenay-Roupie M, Dupont JM, Picard F, et al: Analysis of megakaryocyte growth and development factor (thrombopoietin) effects on blast cell and megakaryocyte growth in myelodysplasia. *Leuk Res* 22:527, 1998.

284. Hashimoto S, Toba K, Fuse I, et al: Thrombopoietin activates the growth of megakaryoblasts in patients with chronic myeloproliferative disorders and myelodysplastic syndrome. *Eur J Haematol* 64:225, 2000.

285. Nishikawa M: Thrombocytopenia due to deficient platelet production. *Nippon Rinsho* 61:575, 2003.

286. King JA, Elkhalifa MY, Latour LF: Rapid progression of acquired amegakaryocytic thrombocytopenia to aplastic anemia. *South Med J* 90:91, 1997.

287. Slater LM, Katz J, Walter B, Armentrout SA: Aplastic anemia occurring as amegakaryocytic thrombocytopenia with and without an inhibitor of granulopoiesis. *Am J Hematol* 18:251, 1985.

288. Kondo Y, Molldrem JJ: Immune-induced cytopenia: Bone marrow failure syndrome. *Curr Hematol Rep* 3:178, 2004.

289. Maciejewski JP, Risitano A, Kook H, et al: Immune pathophysiology of aplastic anemia. *Int J Hematol* 76(suppl 1):207, 2002.

290. Nakao S: Immune mechanism of aplastic anemia. *Int J Hematol* 66:127, 1997.

291. Kurzrock R, Cortes J, Thomas DA, et al: Pilot study of low-dose interleukin-11 in patients with bone marrow failure. *J Clin Oncol* 19:4165, 2001.

292. Wang WX, Gong CL: Clinical report on treatment of thrombocytopenia with rhIL-11 (Mega) in 10 chronic aplastic anemia patients. *Zhongguo Shi Yan Xue Ye Xue Za Zhi* 10:375, 2002.

293. Brereton ML, Adams JA, Briggs M, Liu Yin JA: The in vitro effect of pegylated recombinant human megakaryocyte growth and development factor (PEGrHuMGDF) on megakaryopoiesis in patients with aplastic anaemia. *Br J Haematol* 104:119, 1999.

294. Hoffman R: Acquired pure amegakaryocytic thrombocytopenic purpura. *Semin Hematol* 28:303, 1991.

295. Antonijevic N, Terzic T, Jovanovic V, et al: Acquired amegakaryocytic thrombocytopenia: Three case reports and a literature review. *Med Pregl* 57:292, 2004.

296. Dewulf G, Gouin I, Pautas E, et al: Myelodisplasic syndromes diagnosed in a geriatric hospital: Morphological profile in 100 patients. *Ann Biol Clin (Paris)* 62:197, 2004.

297. Rochant H: Myelodysplastic syndromes: Unusual and mild forms. *Pathol Biol (Paris)* 45:579, 1997.

298. Kini J, Khadilkar UN, Dayal JP: A study of the haematologic spectrum of myelodysplastic syndrome. *Indian J Pathol Microbiol* 44:9, 2001.

299. Nand S, Godwin JE: Hypoplastic myelodysplastic syndrome. *Cancer* 62:958, 1988.

300. Zafar T, Yasin F, Anwar M, Saleem M: Acquired amegakaryocytic thrombocytopenic purpura (AATP): A hospital based study. *J Pak Med Assoc* 49:114, 1999.

301. Nagasawa T, Sakurai T, Kashiwagi H, Abe T: Cell-mediated amegakaryocytic thrombocytopenia associated with systemic lupus erythematosus. *Blood* 67:479, 1986.

302. Chaudhary UB, Eberwine SF, Hege KM: Acquired amegakaryocytic thrombocytopenia purpura and eosinophilic fasciitis: A long relapsing and remitting course. *Am J Hematol* 75:146, 2004.

303. Shiozaki H, Miyawaki S, Kuwaki T, et al: Autoantibodies neutralizing thrombopoietin in a patient with amegakaryocytic thrombocytopenic purpura. *Blood* 95:2187, 2000.

304. Katsumata Y, Suzuki T, Kuwana M, et al: Anti-c-Mpl (thrombopoietin receptor) autoantibody-induced amegakaryocytic thrombocytopenia in a patient with systemic sclerosis. *Arthritis Rheum* 48:1647, 2003.

305. Leach JW, Hussein KK, George JN: Acquired pure megakaryocytic aplasia report of two cases with long-term responses to antithymocyte globulin and cyclosporine. *Am J Hematol* 62:115, 1999.

306. George JN, Woolf SH, Raskob GE: Idiopathic thrombocytopenic purpura: A guideline for diagnosis and management of children and adults. American Society of Hematology. *Ann Med* 30:38, 1998.

307. Lusher JM, Iyer R: Idiopathic thrombocytopenic purpura in children. *Semin Thromb Hemost* 3:175, 1977.

308. Frederiksen H, Schmidt K: The incidence of idiopathic thrombocytopenic purpura in adults increases with age. *Blood* 94:909, 1999.

309. Neylon AJ, Saunders PW, Howard MR, et al: Clinically significant newly presenting autoimmune thrombocytopenic purpura in adults: A prospective study of a population-based cohort of 245 patients. *Br J Haematol* 122:966, 2003.

310. Harrington WJ, Minnich V, Hollingsworth JW, Moore CV: Demonstration of a thrombocytopenic factor in the blood of patients with thrombocytopenic purpura. *J Lab Clin Med* 38:1, 1951.

311. Altman L: Black and blue at the flick of a feather, in Anonymous: *Who Goes First?* p 273. Random House, New York, 1987.

312. Shulman NR, Weinrach RS, Libre EP, Andrews HL: The role of the reticuloendothelial system in the pathogenesis of idiopathic thrombocytopenic purpura. *Trans Assoc Am Physicians* 78:374, 1965.

313. McMillan R, Smith RS, Longmire RL, et al: Immunoglobulins associated with human platelets. *Blood* 37:316, 1971.

314. Dixon R, Rosse W, Ebbert L: Quantitative determination of antibody in idiopathic thrombocytopenic purpura. Correlation of serum and platelet-bound antibody with clinical response. *N Engl J Med* 292:230, 1975.

315. Mueller-Eckhardt C, Mueller-Eckhardt G, Kayser W, et al: Platelet as-

sociated IgG, platelet survival, and platelet sequestration in thrombocytopenic states. *Br J Haematol* 52:49, 1982.

316. Kelton JG, Powers PJ, Carter CJ: A prospective study of the usefulness of the measurement of platelet-associated IgG for the diagnosis of idiopathic thrombocytopenic purpura. *Blood* 60:1050, 1982.

317. van Leeuwen EF, van der Ven JT, Engelfriet CP, van dem Borne AE: Specificity of autoantibodies in autoimmune thrombocytopenia. *Blood* 59:23, 1982.

318. McMillan R, Tani P, Millard F, et al: Platelet-associated and plasma anti-glycoprotein autoantibodies in chronic ITP. *Blood* 70:1040, 1987.

319. Kiefel V, Santoso S, Weisheit M, Mueller-Eckhardt C: Monoclonal antibody-specific immobilization of platelet antigens (MAIPA): A new tool for the identification of platelet-reactive antibodies. *Blood* 70:1722, 1987.

320. Kiefel V, Santoso S, Kaufmann E, Mueller-Eckhardt C: Autoantibodies against platelet glycoprotein Ib/IX: A frequent finding in autoimmune thrombocytopenic purpura. *Br J Haematol* 79:256, 1991.

321. He R, Reid DM, Jones CE, Shulman NR: Spectrum of Ig classes, specificities, and titers of serum antiglycoproteins in chronic idiopathic thrombocytopenic purpura. *Blood* 83:1024, 1994.

322. McMillan R: Autoantibodies and autoantigens in chronic immune thrombocytopenic purpura. *Semin Hematol* 37:239, 2000.

323. Cines DB, Blanchette VS: Immune thrombocytopenic purpura. *N Engl J Med* 346:995, 2002.

324. Hymes K, Schur PH, Karpatkin S: Heavy-chain subclass of round antiplatelet IgG in autoimmune thrombocytopenic purpura. *Blood* 56:84, 1980.

325. van der HD, de Jong D, Limpens J, et al: Clonal B-cell populations in patients with idiopathic thrombocytopenic purpura. *Blood* 76:2321, 1990.

326. McMillan R, Lopez-Dee J, Bowditch R: Clonal restriction of platelet-associated anti-GPIIb/IIIa autoantibodies in patients with chronic ITP. *Thromb Haemost* 85:821, 2001.

327. Kuwana M, Kaburaki J, Ikeda Y: Autoreactive T cells to platelet GPIIb-IIIa in immune thrombocytopenic purpura. Role in production of antiplatelet autoantibody. *J Clin Invest* 102:1393, 1998.

328. Kuwana M, Kaburaki J, Kitasato H, et al: Immunodominant epitopes on glycoprotein IIb-IIIa recognized by autoreactive T cells in patients with immune thrombocytopenic purpura. *Blood* 98:130, 2001.

329. Semple JW: Pathogenic T-cell responses in patients with autoimmune thrombocytopenic purpura. *J Pediatr Hematol Oncol* 25(suppl 1):S11, 2003.

330. Hauch TW, Rosse WF: Platelet-bound complement (C3) in immune thrombocytopenia. *Blood* 50:1129, 1977.

331. Kurata Y, Curd JG, Tamerius JD, McMillan R: Platelet-associated complement in chronic ITP. *Br J Haematol* 60:723, 1985.

332. Tsubakio T, Tani P, Curd JG, McMillan R: Complement activation in vitro by antiplatelet antibodies in chronic immune thrombocytopenic purpura. *Br J Haematol* 63:293, 1986.

333. Aster RH, Keene WR: Sites of platelet destruction in idiopathic thrombocytopenic purpura. *Br J Haematol* 16:61, 1969.

334. Hoffman R, Zaknoen S, Yang HH, et al: An antibody cytotoxic to megakaryocyte progenitor cells in a patient with immune thrombocytopenic purpura. *N Engl J Med* 312:1170, 1985.

335. Chang M, Nakagawa PA, Williams SA, et al: Immune thrombocytopenic purpura (ITP) plasma and purified ITP monoclonal autoantibodies inhibit megakaryocytopoiesis in vitro. *Blood* 102:887, 2003.

336. Takahashi R, Sekine N, Nakatake T: Influence of monoclonal antiplatelet glycoprotein antibodies on in vitro human megakaryocyte colony formation and proplatelet formation. *Blood* 93:1951, 1999.

337. Bessman JD: The relation of megakaryocyte ploidy to platelet volume. *Am J Hematol* 16:161, 1984.

338. Thompson CB, Jakubowski JA: The pathophysiology and clinical relevance of platelet heterogeneity. *Blood* 72:1, 1988.

339. Saxon BR, Mody M, Blanchette VS, Freedman J: Reticulated platelet counts in the assessment of thrombocytopenic disorders. *Acta Paediatr Suppl* 424:65, 1998.

340. Hughes M, Webert K, Kelton JG: The use of electron microscopy in the investigation of the ultrastructural morphology of immune thrombocytopenic purpura platelets. *Semin Hematol* 37:222, 2000.

341. Kaushansky K: Thrombopoietin: The primary regulator of megakaryocyte and platelet production. *Thromb Haemost* 74:521, 1995.

342. Chang M, Qian JX, Lee SM, et al: Tissue uptake of circulating thrombopoietin is increased in immune-mediated compared with irradiated thrombocytopenic mice. *Blood* 93:2515, 1999.

343. Kosugi S, Kurata Y, Tomiyama Y, et al: Circulating thrombopoietin level in chronic immune thrombocytopenic purpura. *Br J Haematol* 93:704, 1996.

344. Porcelijn L, Folman CC, Bossers B, et al: The diagnostic value of thrombopoietin level measurements in thrombocytopenia. *Thromb Haemost* 79:1101, 1998.

345. Gouin-Thibault I, Cassinat B, Chomienne C, et al: Is the thrombopoietin assay useful for differential diagnosis of thrombocytopenia? Analysis of a cohort of 160 patients with thrombocytopenia and defined platelet life span. *Clin Chem* 47:1660, 2001.

346. Laster AJ, Conley CL, Kickler TS, et al: Chronic immune thrombocytopenic purpura in monozygotic twins: Genetic factors predisposing to ITP. *N Engl J Med* 307:1495, 1982.

347. Bizzaro N: Familial association of autoimmune thrombocytopenia and hyperthyroidism. *Am J Hematol* 39:294, 1992.

348. Karpatkin S, Fotino M, Winchester R: Hereditary autoimmune thrombocytopenic purpura: An immunologic and genetic study. *Ann Intern Med* 94:781, 1981.

349. Stanworth SJ, Turner DM, Brown J, et al: Major histocompatibility complex susceptibility genes and immune thrombocytopenic purpura in Caucasian adults. *Hematology* 7:119, 2002.

350. Evers KG, Thouet R, Haase W, Kruger J: HLA frequencies and haplotypes in children with idiopathic thrombocytopenic purpura (ITP). *Eur J Pediatr* 129:267, 1978.

351. Foster CB, Zhu S, Erichsen HC, et al: Polymorphisms in inflammatory cytokines and Fcgamma receptors in childhood chronic immune thrombocytopenic purpura: A pilot study. *Br J Haematol* 113:596, 2001.

352. Carcao MD, Blanchette VS, Wakefield CD, et al: Fcgamma receptor IIa and IIIa polymorphisms in childhood immune thrombocytopenic purpura. *Br J Haematol* 120:135, 2003.

353. Cortelazzo S, Finazzi G, Buelli M, et al: High risk of severe bleeding in aged patients with chronic idiopathic thrombocytopenic purpura. *Blood* 77:31, 1991.

354. George JN, el Harake MA, Raskob GE: Chronic idiopathic thrombocytopenic purpura. *N Engl J Med* 331:1207, 1994.

355. McMillan R: Therapy for adults with refractory chronic immune thrombocytopenic purpura. *Ann Intern Med* 126:307, 1997.

356. Schattner E, Bussel J: Mortality in immune thrombocytopenic purpura: Report of seven cases and consideration of prognostic indicators. *Am J Hematol* 46:120, 1994.

357. McIntyre OR, Ebaugh FG Jr: Palpable spleens in college freshmen. *Ann Intern Med* 66:301, 1967.

358. Burstein SA, Downs T, Friese P, et al: Thrombocytopoiesis in normal and sublethally irradiated dogs: Response to human interleukin-6. *Blood* 80:420, 1992.

359. Khan I, Zucker-Franklin D, Karpatkin S: Microthrombocytosis and platelet fragmentation associated with idiopathic/autoimmune thrombocytopenic purpura. *Br J Haematol* 31:449, 1975.

360. Lopez JA, Andrews RK, Afshar-Kharghan V, Berndt MC: Bernard-Soulier syndrome. *Blood* 91:4397, 1998.

361. Rodgers RP, Levin J: A critical reappraisal of the bleeding time. *Semin Thromb Hemost* 16:1, 1990.

362. Evans RS, Takahashi K, Duane RT, et al: Primary thrombocytopenic purpura and acquired hemolytic anemia; evidence for a common etiology. *Arch Intern Med* 87:48, 1951.

363. Vesely S, Buchanan GR, Cohen A, et al: Self-reported diagnostic and management strategies in childhood idiopathic thrombocytopenic purpura: Results of a survey of practicing pediatric hematology/oncology specialists. *J Pediatr Hematol Oncol* 22:55, 2000.

364. George JN, Raskob GE: Idiopathic thrombocytopenic purpura: Diagnosis and management. *Am J Med Sci* 316:87, 1998.

365. Chong BH, Keng TB: Advances in the diagnosis of idiopathic thrombocytopenic purpura. *Semin Hematol* 37:249, 2000.

366. Kelton JG, Murphy WG, Lucarelli A, et al: A prospective comparison of four techniques for measuring platelet-associated IgG. *Br J Haematol* 71:97, 1989.

367. George JN, Saucerman S, Levine SP, et al: Immunoglobulin G is a platelet alpha granule-secreted protein. *J Clin Invest* 76:2020, 1985.

368. George JN, Saucerman S: Platelet IgG, IgA, IgM, and albumin: Correlation of platelet and plasma concentrations in normal subjects and in patients with ITP or dysproteinemia. *Blood* 72:362, 1988.

369. Kelton JG, Denomme G: The quantitation of platelet-associated IgG on cohorts of platelets separated from healthy individuals by buoyant density centrifugation. *Blood* 60:136, 1982.

370. Beardsley DS, Spiegel JE, Jacobs MM, et al: Platelet membrane glycoprotein IIIa contains target antigens that bind anti-platelet antibodies in immune thrombocytopenias. *J Clin Invest* 74:1701, 1984.

371. Reid DM, Jones CE, Vostal JG, Shulman NR: Western blot identification of platelet proteins that bind normal serum immunoglobulins. Characteristics of a 95-Kd reactive protein. *Blood* 75:2194, 1990.

372. Nomura S, Yanabu M, Soga T, et al: Analysis of idiopathic thrombocytopenic purpura patients with antiglycoprotein IIb/IIIa or Ib autoantibodies. *Acta Haematol* 86:25, 1991.

373. Harris EN, Gharavi AE, Hegde U, et al: Anticardiolipin antibodies in autoimmune thrombocytopenic purpura. *Br J Haematol* 59:231, 1985.

374. Stasi R, Stipa E, Masi M, et al: Prevalence and clinical significance of elevated antiphospholipid antibodies in patients with idiopathic thrombocytopenic purpura. *Blood* 84:4203, 1994.

375. Diz-Kucukkaya R, Hacihanefioglu A, Yenerel M, et al: Antiphospholipid antibodies and antiphospholipid syndrome in patients presenting with immune thrombocytopenic purpura: A prospective cohort study. *Blood* 98:1760, 2001.

376. Funauchi M, Hamada K, Enomoto H, et al: Characteristics of the clinical findings in patients with idiopathic thrombocytopenic purpura who are positive for anti-phospholipid antibodies. *Intern Med* 36:882, 1997.

377. Lacey JV, Penner JA: Management of idiopathic thrombocytopenic purpura in the adult. *Semin Thromb Hemost* 3:160, 1977.

378. Baumann MA, Menitove JE, Aster RH, Anderson T: Urgent treatment of idiopathic thrombocytopenic purpura with single-dose gammaglobulin infusion followed by platelet transfusion. *Ann Intern Med* 104:808, 1986.

379. Gernsheimer T, Stratton J, Ballem PJ, Slichter SJ: Mechanisms of response to treatment in autoimmune thrombocytopenic purpura. *N Engl J Med* 320:974, 1989.

380. Bussel JB: Fc receptor blockade and immune thrombocytopenic purpura. *Semin Hematol* 37:261, 2000.

381. Mazzucconi MG, Francesconi M, Fidani P, et al: Treatment of idiopathic thrombocytopenic purpura (ITP): Results of a multicentric protocol. *Haematologica* 70:329, 1985.

382. Bellucci S, Charpak Y, Chastang C, Tobelem G: Low doses versus conventional doses of corticoids in immune thrombocytopenic purpura (ITP): Results of a randomized clinical trial in 160 children, 223 adults. *Blood* 71:1165, 1988.

383. Ozsoylu S, Irken G, Karabent A: High-dose intravenous methylprednisolone for acute childhood idiopathic thrombocytopenic purpura. *Eur J Haematol* 42:431, 1989.

384. Ozsoylu S, Sayli TR, Ozturk G: Oral megadose methylprednisolone versus intravenous immunoglobulin for acute childhood idiopathic thrombocytopenic purpura. *Pediatr Hematol Oncol* 10:317, 1993.

385. Albayrak D, Islek I, Kalayci AG, Gurses N: Acute immune thrombocytopenic purpura: A comparative study of very high oral doses of methylprednisolone and intravenously administered immune globulin. *J Pediatr* 125:1004, 1994.

386. Cheng Y, Wong RS, Soo YO, et al: Initial treatment of immune thrombocytopenic purpura with high-dose dexamethasone. *N Engl J Med* 349:831, 2003.

387. George JN, Vesely SK: Immune thrombocytopenic purpura—Let the treatment fit the patient. *N Engl J Med* 349:903, 2003.

388. Bell WR Jr: Long-term outcome of splenectomy for idiopathic thrombocytopenic purpura. *Semin Hematol* 37:22, 2000.

389. Atkinson WL, Pickering LK, Schwartz B, et al: General recommendations on immunization. Recommendations of the Advisory Committee on Immunization Practices (ACIP) and the American Academy of Family Physicians (AAFP). *MMWR Recomm Rep* 51:1, 2002.

390. Najean Y, Rain JD, Billotey C: The site of destruction of autologous 111In-labelled platelets and the efficiency of splenectomy in children and adults with idiopathic thrombocytopenic purpura: A study of 578 patients with 268 splenectomies. *Br J Haematol* 97:547, 1997.

391. Pizzuto J, Ambriz R: Therapeutic experience on 934 adults with idiopathic thrombocytopenic purpura: Multicentric Trial of the Cooperative Latin American group on Hemostasis and Thrombosis. *Blood* 64:1179, 1984.

392. Lortan JE: Management of asplenic patients. *Br J Haematol* 84:566, 1993.

393. Marcaccio MJ: Laparoscopic splenectomy in chronic idiopathic thrombocytopenic purpura. *Semin Hematol* 37:267, 2000.

394. Callis M, Palacios C, Lopez A, et al: Splenic irradiation as management of ITP. *Br J Haematol* 105:843, 1999.

395. Imbach P, Barandun S, d'Apuzzo V, et al: High-dose intravenous gammaglobulin for idiopathic thrombocytopenic purpura in childhood. *Lancet* 1:1228, 1981.

396. Bussel JB, Pham LC, Aledort L, Nachman R: Maintenance treatment of adults with chronic refractory immune thrombocytopenic purpura using repeated intravenous infusions of gammaglobulin. *Blood* 72:121, 1988.

397. Berchtold P, Dale GL, Tani P, McMillan R: Inhibition of autoantibody binding to platelet glycoprotein IIb/IIIa by anti-idiotypic antibodies in intravenous gammaglobulin. *Blood* 74:2414, 1989.

398. Hong F, Ruiz R, Price H, et al: Safety profile of WinRho anti-D. *Semin Hematol* 35:9, 1998.

399. Ware RE, Zimmerman SA: Anti-D: Mechanisms of action. *Semin Hematol* 35:14, 1998.

400. Waintraub SE, Brody JI: Use of anti-D in immune thrombocytopenic purpura as a means to prevent splenectomy: Case reports from two University Hospital Medical Centers. *Semin Hematol* 37:45, 2000.

401. George JN, Raskob GE, Vesely SK, et al: Initial management of immune thrombocytopenic purpura in adults: A randomized controlled trial comparing intermittent anti-D with routine care. *Am J Hematol* 74:161, 2003.

402. Blanchette V, Freedman J, Garvey B: Management of chronic immune thrombocytopenic purpura in children and adults. *Semin Hematol* 35:36, 1998.

403. Ahn YS, Byrnes JJ, Harrington WJ, et al: The treatment of idiopathic thrombocytopenia with vinblastine-loaded platelets. *N Engl J Med* 298:1101, 1978.

404. Jackson CW, Edwards CC: Evidence that stimulation of megakaryocytopoiesis by low dose vincristine results from an effect on platelets. *Br J Haematol* 36:97, 1977.

405. Tangun Y, Atamer T: More on vincristine in treatment of ITP. *N Engl J Med* 297:894, 1977.

406. Verlin M, Laros RK Jr, Penner JA: Treatment of refractory thrombocytopenic purpura with cyclophosphamine. *Am J Hematol* 1:97, 1976.

407. Reiner A, Gernsheimer T, Slichter SJ: Pulse cyclophosphamide therapy for refractory autoimmune thrombocytopenic purpura. *Blood* 85:351, 1995.

408. Quiquandon I, Fenaux P, Caulier MT, et al: Reevaluation of the role of azathioprine in the treatment of adult chronic idiopathic thrombocytopenic purpura: A report on 53 cases. *Br J Haematol* 74:223, 1990.

409. Sekreta CM, Baker DE: Interferon alfa therapy in adults with chronic idiopathic thrombocytopenic purpura. *Ann Pharmacother* 30:1176, 1996.

410. Godeau B, Durand JM, Roudot-Thoraval F, et al: Dapsone for chronic autoimmune thrombocytopenic purpura: A report of 66 cases. *Br J Haematol* 97:336, 1997.

411. Snyder HW Jr, Cochran SK, Balint JP Jr, et al: Experience with protein A-immunoadsorption in treatment-resistant adult immune thrombocytopenic purpura. *Blood* 79:2237, 1992.

412. Emilia G, Messora C, Longo G, Bertesi M: Long-term salvage treatment by cyclosporin in refractory autoimmune haematological disorders. *Br J Haematol* 93:341, 1996.

413. Godeau B, Bierling P: Treatment of chronic autoimmune thrombocytopenic purpura with ascorbate. *Br J Haematol* 75:289, 1990.

414. Strother SV, Zuckerman KS, LoBuglio AF: Colchicine therapy for refractory idiopathic thrombocytopenic purpura. *Arch Intern Med* 144:2198, 1984.

415. Bussel JB, Saal S, Gordon B: Combined plasma exchange and intravenous gammaglobulin in the treatment of patients with refractory immune thrombocytopenic purpura. *Transfusion* 28:38, 1988.

416. Stasi R, Pagano A, Stipa E, Amadori S: Rituximab chimeric anti-CD20 monoclonal antibody treatment for adults with chronic idiopathic thrombocytopenic purpura. *Blood* 98:952, 2001.

417. Narang M, Penner JA, Williams D: Refractory autoimmune thrombocytopenic purpura: Responses to treatment with a recombinant antibody to lymphocyte membrane antigen CD20 (rituximab). *Am J Hematol* 74:263, 2003.

418. Cooper N, Stasi R, Cunningham-Rundles S, et al: The efficacy and safety of B-cell depletion with anti-CD20 monoclonal antibody in adults with chronic immune thrombocytopenic purpura. *Br J Haematol* 125:232, 2004.

419. Wilson WA, Gharavi AE, Koike T, et al: International consensus statement on preliminary classification criteria for definite antiphospholipid syndrome: Report of an international workshop. *Arthritis Rheum* 42:1309, 1999.

420. Cervera R, Piette JC, Font J, et al: Antiphospholipid syndrome: Clinical and immunologic manifestations and patterns of disease expression in a cohort of 1,000 patients. *Arthritis Rheum* 46:1019, 2002.

421. Oosting JD, Derksen RH, Bobbink IW, et al: Antiphospholipid antibodies directed against a combination of phospholipids with prothrombin, protein C, or protein S: An explanation for their pathogenic mechanism? *Blood* 81:2618, 1993.

422. D'Cruz D, Hughes G: Antibodies, thrombosis and the endothelium. *Br J Rheumatol* 33:2, 1994.

423. Santoro SA: Antiphospholipid antibodies and thrombotic predisposition: Underlying pathogenetic mechanisms. *Blood* 83:2389, 1994.

424. Rand JH, Wu XX: Antibody-mediated interference with annexins in the antiphospholipid syndrome. *Thromb Res* 114:383, 2004.

425. Asherson RA, Khamashta MA, Ordi-Ros J, et al: The "primary" antiphospholipid syndrome: Major clinical and serological features. *Medicine (Baltimore)* 68:366, 1989.

426. Alarcon-Segovia D, Deleze M, Oria CV, et al: Antiphospholipid antibodies and the antiphospholipid syndrome in systemic lupus erythematosus. A prospective analysis of 500 consecutive patients. *Medicine (Baltimore)* 68:353, 1989.

427. Galli M, Finazzi G, Barbui T: Thrombocytopenia in the antiphospholipid syndrome. *Br J Haematol* 93:1, 1996.

428. Thrombosis and thrombocytopenia in antiphospholipid syndrome (idiopathic and secondary to SLE): First report from the Italian Registry. Italian Registry of Antiphospholipid Antibodies (IR-APA). *Haematologica* 78:313, 1993.

429. Cuadrado MJ, Mujic F, Munoz E, et al: Thrombocytopenia in the antiphospholipid syndrome. *Ann Rheum Dis* 56:194, 1997.

430. Harris EN: Antiphospholipid antibodies. *Br J Haematol* 74:1, 1990.

431. Godeau B, Piette JC, Fromont P, et al: Specific antiplatelet glycoprotein autoantibodies are associated with the thrombocytopenia of primary antiphospholipid syndrome. *Br J Haematol* 98:873, 1997.

432. Macchi L, Rispal P, Clofent-Sanchez G, et al: Anti-platelet antibodies in patients with systemic lupus erythematosus and the primary antiphospholipid antibody syndrome: Their relationship with the observed thrombocytopenia. *Br J Haematol* 98:336, 1997.

433. Galli M, Daldossi M, Barbui T: Anti-glycoprotein Ib/IX and IIb/IIIa antibodies in patients with antiphospholipid antibodies. *Thromb Haemost* 71:571, 1994.

434. Lipp E, von Felten A, Sax H, et al: Antibodies against platelet glycoproteins and antiphospholipid antibodies in autoimmune thrombocytopenia. *Eur J Haematol* 60:283, 1998.

435. Fabris F, Steffan A, Cordiano I, et al: Specific antiplatelet autoantibodies in patients with antiphospholipid antibodies and thrombocytopenia. *Eur J Haematol* 53:232, 1994.

436. Bernini JC, Buchanan GR, Ashcraft J: Hypoprothrombinemia and severe hemorrhage associated with a lupus anticoagulant. *J Pediatr* 123:937, 1993.

437. Font J, Jimenez S, Cervera R, et al: Splenectomy for refractory Evans' syndrome associated with antiphospholipid antibodies: Report of two cases. *Ann Rheum Dis* 59:920, 2000.

438. Hakim AJ, Machin SJ, Isenberg DA: Autoimmune thrombocytopenia in primary antiphospholipid syndrome and systemic lupus erythematosus: The response to splenectomy. *Semin Arthritis Rheum* 28:20, 1998.

439. Alarcon-Segovia D, Sanchez-Guerrero J: Correction of thrombocytopenia with small dose aspirin in the primary antiphospholipid syndrome. *J Rheumatol* 16:1359, 1989.

440. Alliot C, Messouak D, Albert F, Barrios M: Correction of thrombocytopenia with aspirin in the primary antiphospholipid syndrome. *Am J Hematol* 68:215, 2001.

441. Wisbey HL, Klestov AC: Thrombocytopenia corrected by warfarin in antiphospholipid syndrome. *J Rheumatol* 23:769, 1996.

442. Ames PR, Orefice G, Brancaccio V: Reversal of thrombocytopenia following oral anticoagulation in two patients with primary antiphospholipid syndrome. *Lupus* 4:491, 1995.

443. Suarez IM, Diaz RA, Aguayo CD, Pujol de la Llave E: Correction of severe thrombocytopenia with chloroquine in the primary antiphospholipid syndrome. *Lupus* 5:81, 1996.

444. Tan EM, Cohen AS, Fries JF, et al: The 1982 revised criteria for the classification of systemic lupus erythematosus. *Arthritis Rheum* 25:1271, 1982.

445. Hochberg MC: Updating the American College of Rheumatology revised criteria for the classification of systemic lupus erythematosus. *Arthritis Rheum* 40:1725, 1997.

446. Rabinowitz Y, Dameshek W: Systemic lupus erythematosus after "idiopathic" thrombocytopenic purpura: A review. *Ann Intern Med* 52:1, 1960.

447. Michel M, Lee K, Piette JC, et al: Platelet autoantibodies and lupus-associated thrombocytopenia. *Br J Haematol* 119:354, 2002.

448. Pujol M, Ribera A, Vilardell M, et al: High prevalence of platelet au-

toantibodies in patients with systemic lupus erythematosus. *Br J Haematol* 89:137, 1995.

449. McMillan R: Immune thrombocytopenia. *Clin Haematol* 12:69, 1983.

450. Griner PF, Hoyer LW: Amegakaryocytic thrombocytopenia in systemic lupus erythematosus. *Arch Intern Med* 125:328, 1970.

451. Fureder W, Firbas U, Nichol JL, et al: Serum thrombopoietin levels and anti-thrombopoietin antibodies in systemic lupus erythematosus. *Lupus* 11:221, 2002.

452. Kuwana M, Okazaki Y, Kajihara M, et al: Autoantibody to c-Mpl (thrombopoietin receptor) in systemic lupus erythematosus: Relationship to thrombocytopenia with megakaryocytic hypoplasia. *Arthritis Rheum* 46:2148, 2002.

453. Feinglass EJ, Arnett FC, Dorsch CA, et al: Neuropsychiatric manifestations of systemic lupus erythematosus: Diagnosis, clinical spectrum, and relationship to other features of the disease. *Medicine (Baltimore)* 55:323, 1976.

454. Miller MH, Urowitz MB, Gladman DD: The significance of thrombocytopenia in systemic lupus erythematosus. *Arthritis Rheum* 26:1181, 1983.

455. Mok CC, Lee KW, Ho CT, et al: A prospective study of survival and prognostic indicators of systemic lupus erythematosus in a southern Chinese population. *Rheumatology (Oxford)* 39:399, 2000.

456. Drenkard C, Villa AR, Alarcon-Segovia D, Perez-Vazquez ME: Influence of the antiphospholipid syndrome in the survival of patients with systemic lupus erythematosus. *J Rheumatol* 21:1067, 1994.

457. Reveille JD, Bartolucci A, Alarcon GS: Prognosis in systemic lupus erythematosus. Negative impact of increasing age at onset, black race, and thrombocytopenia, as well as causes of death. *Arthritis Rheum* 33:37, 1990.

458. Abu-Shakra M, Urowitz MB, Gladman DD, Gough J: Mortality studies in systemic lupus erythematosus. Results from a single center: II. Predictor variables for mortality. *J Rheumatol* 22:1265, 1995.

459. Scofield RH, Bruner GR, Kelly JA, et al: Thrombocytopenia identifies a severe familial phenotype of systemic lupus erythematosus and reveals genetic linkages at 1q22 and 11p13. *Blood* 101:992, 2003.

460. Boumpas DT, Austin HA III, Fessler BJ, et al: Systemic lupus erythematosus: Emerging concepts. Part 1: Renal, neuropsychiatric, cardiovascular, pulmonary, and hematologic disease. *Ann Intern Med* 122:940, 1995.

461. Arnal C, Piette JC, Leone J, et al: Treatment of severe immune thrombocytopenia associated with systemic lupus erythematosus: 59 cases. *J Rheumatol* 29:75, 2002.

462. Boumpas DT, Barez S, Klippel JH, Balow JE: Intermittent cyclophosphamide for the treatment of autoimmune thrombocytopenia in systemic lupus erythematosus. *Ann Intern Med* 112:674, 1990.

463. Roach BA, Hutchinson GJ: Treatment of refractory, systemic lupus erythematosus-associated thrombocytopenia with intermittent low-dose intravenous cyclophosphamide. *Arthritis Rheum* 36:682, 1993.

464. Maier WP, Gordon DS, Howard RF, et al: Intravenous immunoglobulin therapy in systemic lupus erythematosus-associated thrombocytopenia. *Arthritis Rheum* 33:1233, 1990.

465. Cohen MG, Li EK: Limited effects of intravenous IgG in treating systemic lupus erythematosus-associated thrombocytopenia. *Arthritis Rheum* 34:787, 1991.

466. Hall S, McCormick JL Jr, Greipp PR, et al: Splenectomy does not cure the thrombocytopenia of systemic lupus erythematosus. *Ann Intern Med* 102:325, 1985.

467. Rivero SJ, Alger M, Alarcon-Segovia D: Splenectomy for hemocytopenia in systemic lupus erythematosus. A controlled appraisal. *Arch Intern Med* 139:773, 1979.

468. Alarcon-Segovia D: Splenectomy has a limited role in the management of lupus with thrombocytopenia. *J Rheumatol* 29:1, 2002.

469. Burrows RF, Kelton JG: Incidentally detected thrombocytopenia in healthy mothers and their infants. *N Engl J Med* 319:142, 1988.

470. Letsky EA, Greaves M: Guidelines on the investigation and management of thrombocytopenia in pregnancy and neonatal alloimmune thrombocytopenia. Maternal and Neonatal Haemostasis Working Party of the Haemostasis and Thrombosis Task Force of the British Society for Haematology. *Br J Haematol* 95:21, 1996.

471. George JN, Woolf SH, Raskob GE, et al: Idiopathic thrombocytopenic purpura: A practice guideline developed by explicit methods for the American Society of Hematology. *Blood* 88:3, 1996.

472. Burrows RF, Kelton JG: Fetal thrombocytopenia and its relation to maternal thrombocytopenia. *N Engl J Med* 329:1463, 1993.

473. McCrae KR, Samuels P, Schreiber AD: Pregnancy-associated thrombocytopenia: Pathogenesis and management. *Blood* 80:2697, 1992.

474. Shehata N, Burrows R, Kelton JG: Gestational thrombocytopenia. *Clin Obstet Gynecol* 42:327, 1999.

475. Kaplan C, Forestier F, Dreyfus M, et al: Maternal thrombocytopenia during pregnancy: Diagnosis and etiology. *Semin Thromb Hemost* 21:85, 1995.

476. Dussel JB: Immune thrombocytopenia in pregnancy: Autoimmune and alloimmune. *J Reprod Immunol* 37:35, 1997.

477. Boehlen F, Hohlfeld P, Extermann P, et al: Platelet count at term pregnancy: A reappraisal of the threshold. *Obstet Gynecol* 95:29, 2000.

478. Lescale KB, Eddleman KA, Cines DB, et al: Antiplatelet antibody testing in thrombocytopenic pregnant women. *Am J Obstet Gynecol* 174:1014, 1996.

479. Gill KK, Kelton JG: Management of idiopathic thrombocytopenic purpura in pregnancy. *Semin Hematol* 37:275, 2000.

480. al Mofada SM, Osman ME, Kides E, et al: Risk of thrombocytopenia in the infants of mothers with idiopathic thrombocytopenia. *Am J Perinatol* 11:423, 1994.

481. Webert KE, Mittal R, Sigouin C, et al: A retrospective 11-year analysis of obstetric patients with idiopathic thrombocytopenic purpura. *Blood* 102:4306, 2003.

482. Stamilio DM, Macones GA: Selection of delivery method in pregnancies complicated by autoimmune thrombocytopenia: A decision analysis. *Obstet Gynecol* 94:41, 1999.

483. Christiaens GC, Nieuwenhuis HK, Bussel JB: Comparison of platelet counts in first and second newborns of mothers with immune thrombocytopenic purpura. *Obstet Gynecol* 90:546, 1997.

484. Moise KJ Jr, Cotton DB: Discordant fetal platelet counts in a twin gestation complicated by idiopathic thrombocytopenic purpura. *Am J Obstet Gynecol* 156:1141, 1987.

485. Kaplan C, Daffos F, Forestier F, et al: Fetal platelet counts in thrombocytopenic pregnancy. *Lancet* 336:979, 1990.

486. Silver RM, Branch DW, Scott JR: Maternal thrombocytopenia in pregnancy: Time for a reassessment. *Am J Obstet Gynecol* 173:479, 1995.

487. Mushambi MC, Halligan AW, Williamson K: Recent developments in the pathophysiology and management of pre-eclampsia. *Br J Anaesth* 76:133, 1996.

488. Leitch CR, Cameron AD, Walker JJ: The changing pattern of eclampsia over a 60-year period. *Br J Obstet Gynaecol* 104:917, 1997.

489. Thomas SV: Neurological aspects of eclampsia. *J Neurol Sci* 155:37, 1998.

490. McCrae KR: Thrombocytopenia in pregnancy: Differential diagnosis, pathogenesis, and management. *Blood Rev* 17:7, 2003.

491. Schlembach D: Pre-eclampsia—Still a disease of theories. *Fukushima J Med Sci* 49:69, 2003.

492. Brittain PC, Bayliss P: Partial hydatidiform molar pregnancy presenting with severe preeclampsia prior to twenty weeks gestation: A case report and review of the literature. *Milit Med* 160:42, 1995.

493. Luttun A, Carmeliet P: Soluble VEGF receptor Flt1: The elusive preeclampsia factor discovered? *J Clin Invest* 111:600, 2003.

494. Torry DS, Hinrichs M, Torry RJ: Determinants of placental vascularity. *Am J Reprod Immunol* 51:257, 2004.

495. Maynard SE, Min JY, Merchan J, et al: Excess placental soluble fms-like tyrosine kinase 1 (sFlt1) may contribute to endothelial dysfunction, hypertension, and proteinuria in preeclampsia. *J Clin Invest* 111:649, 2003.

496. Vuorela P, Helske S, Hornig C, et al: Amniotic fluid-soluble vascular endothelial growth factor receptor-1 in preeclampsia. *Obstet Gynecol* 95:353, 2000.

497. Zhou Y, McMaster M, Woo K, et al: Vascular endothelial growth factor ligands and receptors that regulate human cytotrophoblast survival are dysregulated in severe preeclampsia and hemolysis, elevated liver enzymes, and low platelets syndrome. *Am J Pathol* 160:1405, 2002.

498. Livingston JC, Chin R, Haddad B, et al: Reductions of vascular endothelial growth factor and placental growth factor concentrations in severe preeclampsia. *Am J Obstet Gynecol* 183:1554, 2000.

499. Torry DS, Wang HS, Wang TH, et al: Preeclampsia is associated with reduced serum levels of placenta growth factor. *Am J Obstet Gynecol* 179:1539, 1998.

500. Lattuada A, Rossi E, Calzarossa C, et al: Mild to moderate reduction of a von Willebrand factor cleaving protease (ADAMTS-13) in pregnant women with HELLP microangiopathic syndrome. *Haematologica* 88:1029, 2003.

501. Tank PD, Nadanwar YS, Mayadeo NM: Outcome of pregnancy with severe liver disease. *Int J Gynaecol Obstet* 76:27, 2002.

502. Egerman RS, Sibai BM: HELLP syndrome. *Clin Obstet Gynecol* 42:381, 1999.

503. Martin JN Jr, Files JC, Blake PG, et al: Postpartum plasma exchange for atypical preeclampsia-eclampsia as HELLP (hemolysis, elevated liver enzymes, and low platelets) syndrome. *Am J Obstet Gynecol* 172:1107, 1995.

504. Sibai BM, Ramadan MK, Chari RS, Friedman SA: Pregnancies complicated by HELLP syndrome (hemolysis, elevated liver enzymes, and low platelets): Subsequent pregnancy outcome and long-term prognosis. *Am J Obstet Gynecol* 172:125, 1995.

505. Kaplan C: Alloimmune thrombocytopenia of the fetus and the newborn. *Blood Rev* 16:69, 2002.

506. Mueller-Eckhardt C, Kiefel V, Grubert A, et al: 348 cases of suspected neonatal alloimmune thrombocytopenia. *Lancet* 1:363, 1989.

507. Ohto H: Neonatal alloimmune thrombocytopenia. *Nippon Rinsho* 55:2310, 1997.

508. Grainger JD, Morrell G, Yates J, Deleacy D: Neonatal alloimmune thrombocytopenia with significant HLA antibodies. *Arch Dis Child Fetal Neonatal Ed* 86:F200, 2002.

509. Chow MP, Sun KJ, Yung CH, et al: Neonatal alloimmune thrombocytopenia due to HLA-A2 antibody. *Acta Haematol* 87:153, 1992.

510. Davoren A, McParland P, Crowley J, et al: Antenatal screening for human platelet antigen-1a: Results of a prospective study at a large maternity hospital in Ireland. *BJOG* 110:492, 2003.

511. Williamson LM, Hackett G, Rennie J, et al: The natural history of fetomaternal alloimmunization to the platelet-specific antigen HPA-1a (PlA1, Zwa) as determined by antenatal screening. *Blood* 92:2280, 1998.

512. Jolly MC, Letsky EA, Fisk NM: The management of fetal alloimmune thrombocytopenia. *Prenat Diagn* 22:96, 2002.

513. Murphy MF, Hambley H, Nicolaides K, Waters AH: Severe fetomaternal alloimmune thrombocytopenia presenting with fetal hydrocephalus. *Prenat Diagn* 16:1152, 1996.

514. Kaplan C, Murphy MF, Kroll H, Waters AH: Feto-maternal alloimmune thrombocytopenia: Antenatal therapy with IvIgG and steroids—More questions than answers. European Working Group on FMAIT. *Br J Haematol* 100:62, 1998.

515. Ouwehand WH, Smith G, Ranasinghe E: Management of severe alloimmune thrombocytopenia in the newborn. *Arch Dis Child Fetal Neonatal Ed* 82:F173, 2000.

516. Porcelijn L, Kanhai HH: Fetal thrombocytopenia. *Curr Opin Obstet Gynecol* 10:117, 1998.

517. Weiner E, Zosmer N, Bajoria R, et al: Direct fetal administration of immunoglobulins: Another disappointing therapy in alloimmune thrombocytopenia. *Fetal Diagn Ther* 9:159, 1994.

518. Aster RH: Platelet sequestration studies in man. *Br J Haematol* 22:259, 1972.

519. Wadenvik H, Denfors I, Kutti J: Splenic blood flow and intrasplenic platelet kinetics in relation to spleen volume. *Br J Haematol* 67:181, 1987.

520. Savage B, McFadden PR, Hanson SR, Harker LA: The relation of platelet density to platelet age: Survival of low- and high-density 111indium-labeled platelets in baboons. *Blood* 68:386, 1986.

521. Wadenvik H, Kutti J: The effect of an adrenaline infusion on the splenic blood flow and intrasplenic platelet kinetics. *Br J Haematol* 67:187, 1987.

522. Vilen L, Freden K, Kutti J: Presence of a non-splenic platelet pool in man. *Scand J Haematol* 24:137, 1980.

523. Heyns AD, Badenhorst PN, Lotter MG, et al: Kinetics and mobilization from the spleen of indium-111-labeled platelets during platelet apheresis. *Transfusion* 25:215, 1985.

524. Lawrence SP, Lezotte DC, Durham JD, et al: Course of thrombocytopenia of chronic liver disease after transjugular intrahepatic portosystemic shunts (TIPSs). A retrospective analysis. *Dig Dis Sci* 40:1575, 1995.

525. Peck-Radosavljevic M: Hypersplenism. *Eur J Gastroenterol Hepatol* 13:317, 2001.

526. Eichner ER: Splenic function: Normal, too much, and too little. *Am J Med* 66:311, 1979.

527. Jacob HS: Hypersplenism: Mechanisms and management. *Br J Haematol* 27:1, 1974.

528. Cooney DP, Smith BA: The pathophysiology of hypersplenic thrombocytopenia. *Arch Intern Med* 121:332, 1968.

529. McCormick PA, Murphy KM: Splenomegaly, hypersplenism, and coagulation abnormalities in liver disease. *Baillieres Best Pract Res Clin Gastroenterol* 14:1009, 2000.

530. Reed RL, Ciavarella D, Heimbach DM, et al: Prophylactic platelet administration during massive transfusion. A prospective, randomized, double-blind clinical study. *Ann Surg* 203:40, 1986.

531. Hiippala ST, Myllyla GJ, Vahtera EM: Hemostatic factors and replacement of major blood loss with plasma-poor red cell concentrates. *Anesth Analg* 81:360, 1995.

532. Leslie SD, Toy PT: Laboratory hemostatic abnormalities in massively transfused patients given red blood cells and crystalloid. *Am J Clin Pathol* 96:770, 1991.

533. Villalobos TJ, Adelson E, Riley PA Jr, Crosby WH: A cause of the thrombocytopenia and leukopenia that occur in dogs during deep hypothermia. *J Clin Invest* 37:1, 1958.

534. Yau TM, Carson S, Weisel RD, et al: The effect of warm heart surgery on postoperative bleeding. *J Thorac Cardiovasc Surg* 103:1155, 1992.

535. Pina-Cabral JM, Ribeiro-da-Silva A, Almeida-Dias A: Platelet sequestration during hypothermia in dogs treated with sulphinpyrazone and ticlopidine—Reversibility accelerated after intra-abdominal rewarming. *Thromb Haemost* 54:838, 1985.

536. Hoffmeister KM, Felbinger TW, Falet H, et al: The clearance mechanism of chilled blood platelets. *Cell* 112:87, 2003.

537. Hoffmeister KM, Josefsson EC, Isaac NA, et al: Glycosylation restores survival of chilled blood platelets. *Science* 301:1531, 2003.

538. Reddick RL, Poole BL, Penick GD: Thrombocytopenia of hibernation. Mechanism of induction and recovery. *Lab Invest* 28:270, 1973.

539. Chan KM, Beard K: A patient with recurrent hypothermia associated with thrombocytopenia. *Postgrad Med J* 69:227, 1993.

540. George JN, Raskob GE, Shah SR, et al: Drug-induced thrombocytopenia: A systematic review of published case reports. *Ann Intern Med* 129: 886, 1998.

541. Kaufman DW, Kelly JP, Johannes CB, et al: Acute thrombocytopenic purpura in relation to the use of drugs. *Blood* 82:2714, 1993.

542. Christie DJ, Mullen PC, Aster RH: Fab-mediated binding of drug-dependent antibodies to platelets in quinidine- and quinine-induced thrombocytopenia. *J Clin Invest* 75:310, 1985.

543. Chong BH, Du XP, Berndt MC, et al: Characterization of the binding domains on platelet glycoproteins Ib-IX and IIb/IIIa complexes for the quinine/quinidine-dependent antibodies. *Blood* 77:2190, 1991.

544. Lopez JA, Li CQ, Weisman S, Chambers M: The glycoprotein Ib-IX complex-specific monoclonal antibody SZ1 binds to a conformation-sensitive epitope on glycoprotein IX: Implications for the target antigen of quinine/quinidine-dependent autoantibodies. *Blood* 85:1254, 1995.

545. Gentilini G, Curtis BR, Aster RH: An antibody from a patient with ranitidine-induced thrombocytopenia recognizes a site on glycoprotein IX that is a favored target for drug-induced antibodies. *Blood* 92:2359, 1998.

546. Curtis BR, McFarland JG, Wu GG, et al: Antibodies in sulfonamide-induced immune thrombocytopenia recognize calcium-dependent epitopes on the glycoprotein IIb/IIIa complex. *Blood* 84:176, 1994.

547. Visentin GP, Newman PJ, Aster RH: Characteristics of quinine- and quinidine-induced antibodies specific for platelet glycoproteins IIb and IIIa. *Blood* 77:2668, 1991.

548. Berkowitz SD, Harrington RA, Rund MM, Tcheng JE: Acute profound thrombocytopenia after C7E3 Fab (abciximab) therapy. *Circulation* 95: 809, 1997.

549. Fiorin F, Steffan A, Pradella P, et al: IgG platelet antibodies in EDTA-dependent pseudothrombocytopenia bind to platelet membrane glycoprotein IIb. *Am J Clin Pathol* 110:178, 1998.

550. Cancio LC, Cohen DJ: Heparin-induced thrombocytopenia and thrombosis. *J Am Coll Surg* 186:76, 1998.

551. Coblyn JS, Weinblatt M, Holdsworth D, Glass D: Gold-induced thrombocytopenia. A clinical and immunogenetic study of twenty-three patients. *Ann Intern Med* 95:178, 1981.

552. Nieminen U, Kekomaki R: Quinidine-induced thrombocytopenic purpura: Clinical presentation in relation to drug-dependent and drug-independent platelet antibodies. *Br J Haematol* 80:77, 1992.

553. Leach MF, Cooper LK, AuBuchon JP: Detection of drug-dependent, platelet-reactive antibodies by solid-phase red cell adherence assays. *Br J Haematol* 97:755, 1997.

554. Visentin GP, Malik M, Cyganiak KA, Aster RH: Patients treated with unfractionated heparin during open heart surgery are at high risk to form antibodies reactive with heparin:platelet factor 4 complexes. *J Lab Clin Med* 128:376, 1996.

555. Boon DM, van Vliet HH, Zietse R, Kappers-Klunne MC: The presence of antibodies against a PF4-heparin complex in patients on haemodialysis. *Thromb Haemost* 76:480, 1996.

556. Kappers-Klunne MC, Boon DM, Hop WC, et al: Heparin-induced thrombocytopenia and thrombosis: A prospective analysis of the incidence in patients with heart and cerebrovascular diseases. *Br J Haematol* 96:442, 1997.

557. Bauer TL, Arepally G, Konkle BA, et al: Prevalence of heparin-associated antibodies without thrombosis in patients undergoing cardiopulmonary bypass surgery. *Circulation* 95:1242, 1997.

558. Belkin GA: Cocktail purpura. An unusual case of quinine sensitivity. *Ann Intern Med* 66:583, 1967.

559. Siroty RR: Purpura on the rocks—With a twist. *JAMA* 235:2521, 1976.

560. Pedersen-Bjergaard U, Andersen M, Hansen PB: Drug-induced thrombocytopenia: Clinical data on 309 cases and the effect of corticosteroid therapy. *Eur J Clin Pharmacol* 52:183, 1997.

561. George JN, Raskob GE, Shah SR, Rizvi MA, Hamilton SA, Osborne S, Vondracek T: Drug-induced thrombocytopenia: A systematic review of published case reports. *Ann Intern Med* 138:239, 2003.

ESSENTIAL THROMBOCYTHEMIA AND THROMBOCYTOSIS

ANDREW I. SCHAFER

The three major pathophysiologic causes of thrombocytosis are (1) clonal, including essential (or primary) thrombocythemia and other myeloproliferative disorders; (2) familial, including rare cases of nonclonal myeloproliferation resulting from thrombopoietin mutations; and (3) reactive, in which thrombocytosis occurs secondary to a variety of acute and chronic clinical conditions. Essential thrombocythemia often is discovered incidentally from blood counts in asymptomatic individuals and is largely a diagnosis of exclusion. Major causes of morbidity and mortality are bleeding and thrombotic complications, the latter most commonly involving the arterial circulation. Reactive thrombocytosis usually does not cause these complications and does not require treatment. The indications for therapeutic intervention in essential thrombocythemia remain unsettled. Therapy to reduce the platelet count in essential thrombocythemia is generally indicated in patients with previous bleeding or thrombotic episodes or in those at high risk for such complications. The most commonly used drugs for cytoreduction of the platelet count are hydroxyurea, anagrelide, and recombinant interferon alpha. Use of antiplatelet agents is indicated in patients with essential thrombocythemia who had or now have a risk of arterial thrombotic or ischemic problems.

DEFINITION AND HISTORY

The upper limit of the normal platelet count generally is between 350,000/μl (350 $\times$ 10^9/liter) and 450,000/μl (450 $\times$ 10^9/liter). The value varies among different laboratories. In a sample of 10,000 healthy individuals aged 18 to 65 years, 99 (1%) had platelet counts greater than 400,000/μl. Among these individuals, thrombocytosis was confirmed in only eight at repeat examination 6 months to 1 year later.[1] The causes of thrombocytosis in which the platelet count exceeds the upper limit can be broadly categorized as (1) clonal, including essential thrombocythemia and other myeloproliferative disorders; (2) familial; and (3) reactive, or secondary (Table 111-1).

Essential (primary) thrombocythemia is one of a group of related chronic myeloproliferative disorders that includes polycythemia vera, chronic myelogenous leukemia (CML), and myeloid metaplasia with or without myelofibrosis. In retrospect, the earliest descriptions of essential thrombocythemia by Di Guglielmo[2] in 1920 and by Epstein and Goedel[3] in 1934 represented thrombocytosis in association with other disorders. This historical misclassification underscores the diagnostic uncertainty that may occur in patients with thrombocytosis.[4]

In 1960, essential thrombocythemia was established as a separate disease entity on a clinicopathologic basis.[5,6]

ETIOLOGY AND PATHOGENESIS

ESSENTIAL THROMBOCYTHEMIA (CLONAL THROMBOCYTOSIS)

As one of the myeloproliferative syndromes, essential thrombocythemia is a clonal disorder that arises in a primitive multipotential hematopoietic cell. The clonal nature of essential thrombocythemia was established by the discovery of a single glucose-6-phosphate dehydrogenase (G-6-PD) isoenzyme expressed in all blood cell lines of women with essential thrombocythemia who coincidentally were heterozygous for two types of G-6-PD: enzymes "A" and "B."[7] Subsequently, clonality in essential thrombocythemia and other myeloproliferative disorders was confirmed by several approaches using X-linked polymorphic markers in female patients.[8] However, essential thrombocythemia may not always be a clonal disease.[9,10] Although these findings suggest essential thrombocythemia is a more heterogeneous disorder than originally thought, the findings also highlight the potential pitfalls and technical limitations of X chromosome inactivation pattern analysis of clonality.[11] Other possible explanations for the findings of polyclonality in some essential thrombocythemia patients include failure to detect a small population of clonal cells against a polyclonal background,[11] progression of nonclonal essential thrombocythemia to clonal disease, or restriction of clonality in some patients to the megakaryocytic lineage.[4,12]

Despite the origin of essential thrombocythemia in a multipotential hematopoietic cell, the dominant phenotypic change involves the megakaryocyte lineage. The lesion affects erythropoiesis and granulopoiesis, but these changes usually are nominal at the time of diagnosis.[13] Alternatively, the mutation(s) may occur in a single multipotential hemopoietic stem cell, the lineage potential of which has become restricted to differentiation primarily into platelets.[14]

Thrombopoietin,[15] the ligand for the megakaryocytic growth factor receptor c-*mpl*, is the major humoral regulator of megakaryocytopoiesis and platelet production. Although thrombopoietin supports the entire continuum of megakaryocyte development from stem cell to platelet production, other cytokines (e.g., interleukin [IL]-6, IL-11) also exert actions at different stages, probably in synergy with thrombopoietin (see Chap. 105). Platelets themselves have an important role in regulating plasma thrombopoietin levels, as their receptors for thrombopoietin (c-*mpl*) remove it from plasma. Thus, as the platelet

TABLE 111-1   MAJOR CAUSES OF THROMBOCYTOSIS

I. Clonal thrombocytosis
   A. Essential (primary) thrombocythemia
   B. Other myeloproliferative disorders (polycythemia vera, chronic myelogenous leukemia, myeloid metaplasia, myelofibrosis)
II. Familial thrombocytosis
III. Reactive (secondary) thrombocytosis
   A. Transient reactive processes
      1. Acute blood loss
      2. Recovery ("rebound") from thrombocytopenia
      3. Acute infection, inflammation
      4. Response to exercise
   B. Sustained processes
      1. Iron deficiency
      2. Postsplenectomy, asplenic states
      3. Malignancies
      4. Chronic inflammatory and infectious diseases (inflammatory bowel disease, temporal arteritis, tuberculosis, chronic pneumonitis)
      5. Response to drugs (vincristine, epinephrine, all-*trans*-retinoic acid, some antibiotics, cytokines and growth factors)
      6. Hemolytic anemia

count drops, increased free plasma thrombopoietin levels stimulate megakaryocytopoiesis. Conversely, as the platelet count rises, depletion of free plasma thrombopoietin decreases megakaryocytopoiesis. This modulatory mechanism results in the steady-state level of platelet production. However, unlike the relationship between polycythemia vera and erythropoietin (EPO) levels, thrombopoietin levels are normal or even elevated in essential thrombocythemia[11,16] despite the increased platelet and megakaryocyte mass. The increased circulating levels of plasma thrombopoietin in essential thrombocythemia may result from abnormal thrombopoietin binding and consumption by the defective platelets and megakaryocytes of essential thrombocythemia.[17] In support of the latter, the expression of platelet c-mpl is strikingly reduced in essential thrombocythemia.[18,19]

Increased numbers of colony forming unit–megakaryocytes (CFU-Meg) have been cultured from the blood or marrow of patients with essential thrombocythemia compared with control subjects or patients with secondary thrombocytosis.[20–23] This finding has been attributed to increased sensitivity and responsiveness of essential thrombocythemia megakaryocytes to thrombopoietin.[24–26] CFU-Meg of patients with essential thrombocythemia are less sensitive to transforming growth factor β1, an endogenous inhibitor of megakaryocytopoiesis.[27] Thus, despite the decreased number and function of thrombopoietin receptors (c-mpl) on megakaryocytes of patients with essential thrombocythemia, increased megakaryocyte proliferation and platelet production result from hypersensitivity to stimulators and/or decreased sensitivity to negative regulators of megakaryocytopoiesis.

Several groups have recently found an identical acquired point mutation in the Janus kinase 2 (JAK2) gene in the blood cells of about 25 to 55 percent of patients with essential thrombocythemia (and the majority of patients with polycythemia vera).[134–137] JAK2 is a tyrosine kinase which functions as an intermediate between cell membrane receptors for hematopoietic growth factors and their downstream signaling molecules. The mutation encodes a valine-to-phenylalanine substitution at position 617 (V617F) in the autoinhibitory (JH2) domain of JAK2, thereby interrupting the normal regulation of JAK2 and rendering the enzyme constitutively active. The constitutively activated JAK2 can then initiate cell signaling and activation even in the absence of the normally required binding of growth factors to hematopoietic cells. This is consistent with earlier observations of endogenous or spontaneous in vitro growth of erythroid colonies cultured from the marrows of patients with polycythemia vera and essential thrombocythemia, as well as the above noted findings of increased responsiveness of essential thrombocythemia megakaryocytes to thrombopoietin. One study found that patients with the JAK2 V617F mutation had a significantly higher rate of complications (fibrosis, bleeding, and thrombosis) than those with mild-type JAK2.[137]

FAMILIAL THROMBOCYTOSIS

Rare cases of familial occurrence of thrombocytosis have been reported, generally inherited by autosomal dominant transmission. Specific mutations in the thrombopoietin gene, including exon skipping and single-nucleotide deletions in the 5′-untranslated region of the gene, have been described in these families. These mutations represent loss of translational repression and increased efficiency of mRNA translation,[28] leading to markedly elevated plasma thrombopoietin levels.[29,30] Other modes of inheritance with normal thrombopoietin levels now are recognized, so familial thrombocytosis is a genetically heterogeneous disorder. In one family, a unique, dominant-activating point mutation identified in the transmembrane domain of the c-mpl gene causes autonomous, thrombopoietin-independent, and IL-3–independent activation of intracellular signaling and cell survival.[31]

REACTIVE (SECONDARY) THROMBOCYTOSIS

By far the most common cause of thrombocytosis in general medical practice is a reactive or secondary process.[4] The degree of thrombocytosis cannot differentiate clonal from reactive causes (see "Differential Diagnosis" below). In one series of 732 medical and surgical patients with platelet counts 500,000/μl or higher, 88 percent had reactive thrombocytosis, most frequently secondary to surgery, infection, malignancy, and chronic inflammation.[32] Similarly, in another series of 280 hospitalized patients with platelets greater than 1,000,000/μl, 82 percent had reactive thrombocytosis.[33] In most cases, the underlying cause of secondary thrombocytosis is clinically overt. However, patients with subclinical causes of thrombocytosis (e.g., occult malignancy) pose the most vexing diagnostic problems for the clinician. Before attributing thrombocytosis to a clonal myeloproliferative disorder, which is largely a diagnosis of exclusion, the clinician must be confident that the elevated platelet count is not the result of an inapparent but potentially treatable underlying disease.

Secondary thrombocytosis may be a transient reactive process or a sustained condition (see Table 111-1), usually driven by elevated endogenous levels of thrombopoietin, other cytokines, or hormones produced by the underlying disorder.[34] The mechanisms are not well defined and likely are as complex and diverse as the underlying disorders causing it. For example, thrombocytosis may result from elevated levels of IL-6 and other cytokines that accompany many inflammatory disorders.[35] Thrombocytosis during all-trans-retinoic acid (ATRA) therapy for acute promyelocytic leukemia results from ATRA-induced transcriptional up-regulation of thrombopoietin, with resultant increased serum thrombopoietin levels.[36] Catecholamine-mediated thrombocytosis may result from platelet release from the spleen.

"Rebound" thrombocytosis following recovery from marrow suppression generally peaks 10 to 14 days after withdrawal of the offending drug (e.g., alcohol[37]) or replacement therapy for the cause of thrombocytopenia (e.g., for cobalamin deficiency[38]). The platelet count may transiently rise above normal limits with effective treatment for immune thrombocytopenic purpura.[39] Following splenectomy for any condition, the platelet count typically rises within the first week to 1,000,000/μl or higher and then gradually returns to normal within approximately 2 months. Reasons for persistent or extreme postsplenectomy thrombocytosis include unresolved hemolytic anemia or unmasking of a previously unrecognized myeloproliferative disorder.

CLINICAL FEATURES

CLINICAL PRESENTATION

In the past, essential thrombocythemia was considered the least common of the myeloproliferative disorders, typically affecting patients between the ages of 50 and 70 years, with an equal sex distribution. However, with frequent inclusion of platelet counts in most automated blood analysis, more asymptomatic patients are being uncovered with the incidental finding of thrombocytosis. The incidence of essential thrombocythemia in Olmsted County, Minnesota, was reported to be approximately 2.5 cases per 100,000 population annually.[40] The prevalence of the disease in Vicenza, Italy, was 40 cases per 100,000 persons, although this value may be an underestimate because the study excluded individuals older than 65 years.[1] The diagnosis of essential thrombocythemia is being made increasingly in younger individuals. The disease occasionally is found in children, and, as noted above in "Familial Thrombocytosis," rare familial cases have been reported.[29,30]

In contrast to some of the other myeloproliferative disorders, constitutional or hypermetabolic symptoms such as fever, sweats, and weight loss are highly uncommon in essential thrombocythemia. Physical findings usually are limited to mild splenomegaly, which is present in approximately 40 percent of patients. Echocardiography may reveal aortic and mitral valvular lesions, including leaflet thickening and vegetations, similar to the lesions described in nonbacterial thrombotic endocarditis.[41] The relationship of cardiac valve lesions to thromboembolic complications in essential thrombocythemia is unclear.

BLEEDING AND THROMBOTIC COMPLICATIONS

Bleeding and thrombotic complications are major causes of morbidity and mortality in essential thrombocythemia, as in the other myeloproliferative disorders.[42–46] The incidence of these hemostatic complications is unknown, varying markedly in different series. Some symptomatic patients exhibit an exclusive pattern of either bleeding or thrombotic problems, whereas others are paradoxically predisposed to both types of complications during the disease course. Some studies have suggested older patients are at markedly increased risk of hemostatic complications,[47] whereas younger patients are relatively protected from these problems.[48] However, other reports have documented no age-related differences[49,50] and have noted serious bleeding and thrombotic episodes even in younger patients.[51]

Therapeutic intervention in essential thrombocythemia (see "Therapy, Course, and Prognosis" below) should be guided by the underlying risk of thrombotic or bleeding complications in any individual patient. Table 111-2 summarizes the emerging consensus of clinical risks of either thrombosis or bleeding, as previously reviewed.[52–55] Risks of thrombosis in essential thrombocythemia include a previous history of thrombosis, associated cardiovascular risk factors (e.g., smoking), and advanced age. Patients with extreme thrombocytosis (platelet count >1,500,000/μl) have an increased risk of bleeding. Although some investigators have suggested use of aspirin and possibly other nonsteroidal antiinflammatory drugs is associated with a higher risk of bleeding in patients with essential thrombocythemia than in normal individuals, the degree of risk is uncertain. Other reported risk factors for hemostatic complications require specialized testing and must be confirmed in larger series. Essential thrombocythemia patients with monoclonal myelopoiesis appear to have a higher risk of thrombosis than those with polyclonal myelopoiesis.[9,56] The polycythemia rubra vera-1 (PRV-1) gene is overexpressed in the granulocytes of most patients with polycythemia vera but also in some patients with essential thrombocythemia.[57,58] The latter group appears to have a more aggressive clinical course, with increased risk of vascular complications, compared with PRV-1 negative essential thrombocythemia patients.[59] Reduced megakaryocyte expression of the thrombopoietin receptor c-*mpl* has likewise been associated with increased risk of thrombosis.[19] Increased risk of thromboembolism also has been reported in essential thrombocythemia patients with low serum EPO levels.[60] How these molecular markers of adverse clinical course in essential thrombocythemia (monoclonality, PRV-1 overexpression, reduced megakaryocyte c-*mpl*, and low EPO levels) relate to each other or to the clinical findings is unclear.

BLEEDING COMPLICATIONS

Bleeding complications of essential thrombocythemia are similar in nature to the bleeding complications seen in platelet or vascular disorders, occurring in superficial locations either spontaneously or after minimal trauma. The most common sites of hemorrhage are mucosal and gastrointestinal, although cutaneous, genitourinary tract, and postoperative bleeding also are seen.[45] Use of aspirin, which causes exaggerated prolongations of the bleeding time in patients with myeloproliferative disorders,[61] may lead to serious bleeding complications in occasional cases.[62]

THROMBOTIC COMPLICATIONS

In a series of 187 consecutive patients with essential thrombocythemia followed at a single institution, 50 percent had at least one thrombotic episode within 9 years after diagnosis.[63] Arterial thrombotic complications occur more frequently than venous thrombosis in essential thrombocythemia, although approximately 25 percent of all thrombotic events in these patients are deep vein thrombosis of the lower extremities.[45] The most common sites of arterial thrombosis in essential thrombocythemia involve the cerebrovascular, peripheral vascular, and coronary arterial circulations. Patients are particularly predisposed to certain specific types of thrombotic events, including both arterial and venous events.

Erythromelalgia and Digital Microvascular Ischemia Erythromelalgia is characterized by intense burning or throbbing pain in a patchy distribution in the extremities, most prominently involving the feet.[64,65] The pain tends to be exacerbated by heat, exercise, and dependency and to be relieved by cold exposure and elevation of the extremity. The pain often is accompanied by warmth, duskiness, and mottled erythema of the involved areas, sometimes resembling livedo reticularis. Erythromelalgia may be confused with Raynaud syndrome, reflex sympathetic dystrophy, shoulder–hand syndrome, or causalgia.[65] Histopathologic examination of biopsies of the affected areas typically shows arterial endothelial swelling, fibromuscular intimal proliferation, and vascular occlusion caused predominantly by platelet thrombi.[66]

Signs of digital microvascular ischemia, primarily involving the toes, may develop in essential thrombocythemia independently of erythromelalgia. Painful vascular insufficiency may progress to frank gangrene and necrosis of the digits unless treatment is promptly instituted. Because thrombosis involves the small vessels, physical examination usually reveals normal peripheral pulses, and arteriography shows patent major vessels.[67] Erythromelalgia and digital ischemia often respond promptly and dramatically to aspirin and reduction of the elevated platelet count.[67]

Cerebrovascular Ischemia A wide spectrum of neurologic complications occur in approximately 25 percent of patients with essential thrombocythemia.[68] The complications may be caused by cerebrovascular ischemia.[45,69,70] Central nervous system involvement may take the form of nonspecific symptoms, such as headache and dizziness; a vague sense of decreased mental acuity; or focal neurologic signs, such as anterior or posterior cerebral artery transient ischemic attacks, sei-

TABLE 111-2   CLINICAL RISKS OF THROMBOHEMORRHAGIC COMPLICATIONS IN ESSENTIAL THROMBOCYTHEMIA

	THROMBOSIS	BLEEDING
Increased risk	Previous history of thrombosis	Use of aspirin and other nonsteroidal antiinflammatory drugs
	Associated cardiovascular risk factors (especially smoking)	Extreme thrombocytosis (platelet count >1,500,000/μl)
	Advanced age (>60 years)	
	Inadequate control of thrombocytosis (in high-risk patients)	
No associated risk	Degree of thrombocytosis	Prolonged bleeding time
	In vitro platelet function	*In vitro* platelet function

SOURCE: Modified from Schafer.[52]

zures, or retinal artery occlusion. Ischemic stroke may be the presenting manifestation of essential thrombocythemia.[71] As in the digital ischemia syndromes, cerebrovascular ischemia usually responds promptly to aspirin and platelet reduction.

Recurrent Abortions and Fetal Growth Retardation Multiple placental infarctions, presumably caused by platelet thrombi, may result in placental insufficiency in some pregnant women with essential thrombocythemia.[72,73] This situation may lead to recurrent spontaneous abortions, fetal growth retardation, premature deliveries, or abruptio placentae.[72–74] These serious complications occur in approximately 50 percent of pregnancies in women with essential thrombocythemia[75] and have led to the use of aspirin during pregnancy in women with essential thrombocythemia.[74] However, the successful outcome of pregnancy in the absence of any specific therapy[76,77] and the lack of clinical trials evaluating treatment modalities make specific recommendations difficult. No correlation has been found between pregnancy outcome and the degree of maternal thrombocytosis, presence of disease complications, or specific therapy for thrombocythemia. To reduce the risk of maternal or neonatal bleeding complications, aspirin should be avoided for at least 1 week prior to delivery. A number of case reports have claimed successful pregnancies in women with essential thrombocythemia who were treated with interferon alpha, but no controlled trials have been undertaken to prove interferon alpha's efficacy.[78] Pregnancy does not adversely affect the natural history of essential thrombocythemia.[77]

Hepatic and Portal Vein Thromboses The myeloproliferative disorders are the most frequently identifiable underlying etiologies in patients presenting with hepatic vein thrombosis (Budd-Chiari syndrome).[79,80] The incidence of myeloproliferative disorders associated with either hepatic or portal vein thrombosis may be underestimated. Such patients have EPO-independent erythroid colony growth in marrow cultures, a diagnostic marker of a stem cell abnormality, even in the absence of overt clinical or hematologic manifestations of a myeloproliferative disorder.[80,81] Hepatic and portal vein thromboses are most commonly associated with polycythemia vera, but a number of cases associated with essential thrombocythemia have been described.[44]

LABORATORY FEATURES

BLOOD AND MARROW FINDINGS

Untreated patients with essential thrombocythemia have platelet counts that range from only slightly above the normal limits to several million per microliter. Some patients have mild leukocytosis and mild anemia. Platelet morphology on blood films typically shows large, pale blue staining, hypogranular platelets, and occasional nucleated megakaryocyte fragments that may have a lymphoblastoid appearance. Increased platelet turnover in essential thrombocythemia is indicated by the finding of increased reticulated platelets (young platelets) in the circulation, which can be detected by flow cytometric analysis of platelet RNA. Although both the percentage and the absolute number of reticulated platelets in blood are elevated in patients with essential thrombocythemia compared with healthy individuals, whether this finding can distinguish essential thrombocythemia from secondary (reactive) thrombocytosis is unclear.[82,83]

Serum thrombopoietin levels generally are normal or mildly elevated in clonal thrombocytosis (Chapter 105), and do not correlate with platelet count in these patients. Serum thrombopoietin levels are also usually elevated in reactive thrombocytosis, so this test cannot discriminate these patients from those with essential thrombocythemia. Plasma levels of IL-6 and C-reactive protein are low or undetectable

in clonal thrombocytosis, whereas levels may be elevated in secondary thrombocytosis, which often accompanies acute and chronic inflammatory states.[35]

Pseudohyperkalemia may be found in patients with extreme thrombocytosis or leukocytosis. It is diagnosed in thrombocytosis states when the serum potassium concentration exceeds the plasma potassium concentration. Pseudohyperkalemia is caused by release of intracellular potassium during blood clotting *in vitro*.[84]

Marrow pathology in essential thrombocythemia characteristically reveals increased cellularity with megakaryocytic hyperplasia. There cells are frequently giant megakaryocytes with increased ploidy that occur in clusters.[85] Significant dysplasia of the megakaryocytes is unusual, but large masses of platelet debris ("platelet drifts") typically are seen in marrow samples.[86]

Most patients with essential thrombocythemia have no cytogenetic abnormalities demonstrated using conventional techniques.[87] However, some patients who otherwise meet the diagnostic criteria of essential thrombocythemia have the Philadelphia chromosome based on cytogenetic analysis of the marrow.[88] Such patients generally do not have pronounced leukocytosis or other characteristic clinical features of CML. However, the natural history of their disease is more like that of CML than of essential thrombocythemia. Some patients with essential thrombocythemia have the *BCR-ABL* gene rearrangement in the absence of the Philadelphia chromosome, although the clinical implications of this are not clear.[89] Deletion of the long arm of chromosome 5 (5q-) has been reported in association with marked thrombocytosis.[90]

CLINICAL TESTS OF HEMOSTASIS

The bleeding time is prolonged in fewer than 20 percent of patients with essential thrombocythemia.[42,70] This test generally does not correlate with the degree of thrombocytosis or specific platelet function abnormalities. It does not reliably predict either a bleeding or a thrombotic tendency in patients with essential thrombocythemia.[91,92]

Platelet aggregation abnormalities in patients are variable. Reduced platelet responses to collagen, adenosine diphosphate, and arachidonic acid occur in less than one third of cases.[44] A characteristic aggregation abnormality is complete loss of platelet responsiveness to epinephrine. In contrast to platelet release defects (e.g., storage pool deficiency or aspirin-like defect) in which only the second wave of platelet aggregation is absent, even the primary wave of epinephrine-stimulated aggregation often is lost in essential thrombocythemia. An abnormal epinephrine-induced platelet response is the most frequent and sometimes only abnormality noted on aggregometry. This unusual abnormality also is observed in other myeloproliferative disorders.[42,44,70] Some patients have platelet hyperaggregability or spontaneous aggregation *in vitro*.[70,93]

ADDITIONAL PLATELET DEFECTS

A wide array of specific morphologic, biochemical, and metabolic platelet defects has been described in patients with essential thrombocythemia.[43] These abnormalities include acquired von Willebrand disease,[94] reduced α-adrenergic receptors associated with absent aggregation to epinephrine,[95] acquired storage pool disease,[92] impaired membrane procoagulant activity,[91] selective deficiency of 12-lipoxygenase,[96] abnormal membrane glycoproteins,[97] increased Fc receptors,[98] and reduced prostaglandin D_2 receptors.[99] Only some of these abnormalities are specific for the myeloproliferative disorders, and none of them has been directly demonstrated to be pathogenetically linked to clinical hemostatic complications.

DIFFERENTIAL DIAGNOSIS

DIAGNOSTIC CRITERIA FOR ESSENTIAL THROMBOCYTHEMIA

No tests are available that can establish with certainty the diagnosis of essential thrombocythemia; the disease remains largely a diagnosis of exclusion. For these reasons, a set of diagnostic criteria for essential thrombocythemia (Table 111-3) has been proposed.[100] The World Health Organization extended these criteria in 2001 to include characteristic marrow findings of increased number of enlarged, mature megakaryocytes.[85] The minimum platelet count of 600,000/μl used to establish the diagnosis of essential thrombocythemia has been challenged.[101] Thrombocythemia-related complications may occur in individual patients with only slight thrombocytosis or even with platelet counts in the upper normal range, and the natural history of these patients with early-stage essential thrombocythemia is comparable to that of patients meeting the original diagnostic criteria.[101]

DISTINCTION FROM OTHER MYELOPROLIFERATIVE DISORDERS

Most of the diagnostic criteria listed in Table 111-3 were designed to differentiate essential thrombocythemia from other myeloproliferative disorders associated with thrombocytosis. Polycythemia vera with thrombocytosis usually can be readily distinguished from essential thrombocythemia by the finding of erythrocytosis and an elevated red cell mass. This disease may be masked by concomitant iron deficiency, which can further increase the platelet count. However, a trial of iron therapy in such cases, which should be done cautiously, typically raises the hematocrit to polycythemic levels. CML with associated thrombocytosis sometimes is misdiagnosed as essential thrombocythemia until the diagnostic cytogenetic or DNA abnormalities characteristic of CML are revealed. Myeloid metaplasia and myelofibrosis are characterized by more marked, frequently massive, splenomegaly. Furthermore, in contrast to essential thrombocythemia, the blood film in myelofibrosis typically shows myelophthisic or leukoerythroblastic changes, and the marrow biopsy shows fibrosis. Some cases of apparent essential thrombocythemia actually represent the recently recognized entity of "prefibrotic myelofibrosis," which evolves into overt myelofibrosis.[102] Despite characteristic distinctions in clinical presentation in most cases, some myeloproliferative disorders represent "overlap" syndromes that cannot be clearly categorized. Most importantly, essential thrombocythemia cannot be diagnosed without excluding possible causes of reactive (or secondary) thrombocytosis.

DISTINCTION FROM SECONDARY THROMBOCYTOSIS

As is illustrated in the section on secondary thrombocytosis and Table 111-1, in the majority of patients with thrombocytosis the elevated platelet count is secondary to an underlying inflammatory disease, iron deficiency, or other disorders. A number of clinical and laboratory findings help distinguish between primary and secondary causes. The findings include the presence of an underlying disorder associated with thrombocytosis, persistence of high counts following correction of the suspected underlying cause, bleeding or thrombotic tendency without other explanation, abnormal platelet aggregation, presence of splenomegaly, and clustering of megakaryocytes and fibrosis on marrow examination.

The finding of the *JAK2* V617F mutation in patients with essential thrombocythemia and the other classical myeloproliferative disorders[134–137] should allow for a rapid, reliable and unambiguous molecular diagnosis to be made in a large number of patients in the future.[138]

REACTIVE (SECONDARY) THROMBOCYTOSIS

A large number of diverse processes are associated with reactive thrombocytosis (see Table 111-1). Although many are active systemic diseases that dominate the clinical picture in these patients, in some individuals subclinical disorders (e.g., occult cancer) may be responsible for the secondary thrombocytosis. In the latter cases, reactive thrombocytosis is particularly difficult to distinguish from essential thrombocythemia. Search for occult malignancy should involve thorough physical examination, including stools for occult blood, chest x-ray film, and further testing directed by systemic and localizing symptoms and signs.[4]

Table 111-4 summarizes clinical findings that may distinguish between clonal and reactive (secondary) thrombocytosis. Patients with reactive thrombocytosis generally do not have splenomegaly, unless enlargement of the spleen results from the underlying disease. Extreme thrombocytosis (platelet count >1,000,000/μl) by no means excludes a reactive or secondary process as its etiology. In a review of 280 consecutive hospitalized patients with reported platelet counts greater than 1,000,000/μl, 82 percent had reactive thrombocytosis and only 14 percent had myeloproliferative disorders.[33] Platelet morphology and platelet function typically are normal in reactive thrombocytosis, in contrast to essential thrombocythemia. Although marrow megakaryocytes are increased in number in both clonal and reactive thrombocytosis, their morphology is normal in the latter. In general, reactive

---

TABLE 111-3 DIAGNOSTIC CRITERIA FOR ESSENTIAL THROMBOCYTHEMIA

1. Platelet count >600,000/μl
2. Hemoglobin (13 g/dl) or normal red cell mass (males <36 ml/kg, females <32 ml/kg)
3. Stainable iron in marrow or failure of iron trial (<1 g/dl rise in hemoglobin after 1 month of iron therapy)
4. No Philadelphia chromosome
5. Collagen fibrosis of marrow
   A. Absent or
   B. <1/3 biopsy area without both splenomegaly and leukoerythroblastic reaction
6. No known cause for reactive thrombocytosis
7. Megakaryocytes in clumps

SOURCE: From Murphy et al.[100]

TABLE 111-4 CLINICAL FEATURES OF CLONAL AND REACTIVE (SECONDARY) THROMBOCYTOSIS

	CLONAL THROMBOCYTOSIS	REACTIVE THROMBOCYTOSIS
Splenomegaly	Yes, in ~40% of cases	No
Platelet morphology	Giant platelets	Normal platelets
Platelet function	Often abnormal	Normal
Bone marrow	Increased megakaryocytes; giant dysplastic forms with increased ploidy, associated with masses of platelet debris	Increased megakaryocytes; normal morphology
Thrombotic complications	Digital or cerebrovascular ischemia; large-vessel arterial or venous thrombosis	No
Bleeding complications	Increased risk	No
Underlying systemic disease	No	Often clinically apparent

SOURCE: Modified from Schafer.[4]

thrombocytosis, even when extreme, does not cause thrombotic or bleeding complications and hence does not require treatment (see "Therapy, Course, and Prognosis" below).

THERAPY, COURSE, AND PROGNOSIS

The therapeutic options described in the following are designed specifically for patients with clonal thrombocytosis (essential thrombocythemia and thrombocytosis associated with other myeloproliferative disorders) and not for patients with secondary or reactive thrombocytosis. Some reports have attempted to link reactive thrombocytosis with thrombotic complications; however, the thrombotic events in these cases usually can be attributed to the underlying systemic disease (e.g., cancer, postoperative state) rather than the secondary thrombocytosis per se. One exception might be the increased risk of thrombosis in patients who develop thrombocytosis following splenectomy for hemolytic anemias, most notably thalassemia, that are incompletely resolved by the surgical procedure.[103,104] Although identifying and attempting to treat the underlying systemic disease are important, no convincing evidence indicates therapy to reduce the platelet count or antiplatelet therapy is beneficial in patients with reactive thrombocytosis.

CYTOREDUCTION

INDICATIONS

The pivotal therapeutic decision in essential thrombocythemia is whether or not treatment is required to reduce the elevated platelet count. This issue is controversial because of the paucity of prospective, controlled trials determining the impact of platelet cytoreduction on morbidity and mortality in clonal thrombocythemia.

Although an association between the platelet count in thrombocythemia and the occurrence of thrombotic complications has been suggested, most retrospective studies have not supported such a correlation.[44,45,47,49,70] The prophylactic efficacy of platelet-lowering therapy in asymptomatic, low-risk essential thrombocythemia patients, irrespective of degree of thrombocytosis, remains untested. One prospective study of "high-risk" patients with essential thrombocythemia (age over 60 years and/or previous episodes of thrombosis) found that control of platelet count to levels less than $600,000/\mu l$ using hydroxyurea significantly reduced the incidence of thrombotic episodes over a median followup of 73 months.[54,105] The general consensus is that lowering the platelet count in patients with active or recurrent bleeding or thrombosis may result in symptomatic improvement. The indication for prompt cytoreduction is particularly strong in patients with microvascular digital[67] or cerebrovascular[69] ischemia syndromes.

THERAPEUTIC MODALITIES

When reduction of the platelet count is indicated for treatment of thrombocytosis, plateletpheresis[106–108] is generally reserved for selected cases of acute and threatening thrombotic and hemostatic problems. Reduction of the platelet count by this method is transient and may be followed by a rebound increase in thrombocytosis. Use of radiophosphorus and alkylating agents (e.g., melphalan, busulfan) has largely been abandoned because of their leukemogenic potential, except in selected older patients who cannot tolerate other drugs.[109]

Hydroxyurea, a nonalkylating myelosuppressive agent, is highly effective as initial therapy for essential thrombocythemia. Doses required for thrombocytosis control are generally 10 to 30 mg/kg/day. Blood counts should be checked within 7 days of initiating therapy and monitored frequently thereafter, because hydroxyurea can cause rapid myelosuppression. Maintenance doses should be individually adjusted according to blood counts. Continuous, orally administered daily treatment with hydroxyurea reduces the platelet count to less than $500,000/\mu l$ within 8 weeks in 80 percent of patients and provides long-term control without severe marrow toxicity or serious side effects.[110] Painful but reversible leg ulceration may occur with long-term hydroxyurea treatment.[111] Hydroxyurea initially was not considered leukemogenic, although the Polycythemia Vera Study Group noted a statistically insignificant trend to an increased incidence of acute leukemia with hydroxyurea use.[112] Studies[113,114] have suggested the leukemogenic potential of hydroxyurea, although its potential is not as great as that of radiophosphorus or alkylating agents. The subject is highly controversial.[115] The risk of leukemia with hydroxyurea is particularly increased after prolonged hydroxyurea use, when hydroxyurea is combined with other drugs, or in essential thrombocythemia patients with 17p chromosomal deletions.[114] These considerations are important when deciding on long-term hydroxyurea use in younger patients with essential thrombocythemia.

Anagrelide is effective for platelet cytoreduction in essential thrombocythemia and is now an alternative first-line therapy. This quinazoline derivative can be given orally and reduces platelet counts by inhibiting marrow megakaryocyte maturation.[116,117] The recommended starting dose is 0.5 mg qid or 1 mg bid, with dosage adjustments made at weekly intervals when needed, up to a maximum dose of 10 mg/day. The dose required to control the platelet count in average-size adults is approximately 2.0 to 3.0 mg/day.[118] The time to 50 percent reduction in the platelet count after the start of anagrelide therapy is approximately 11 days. Anagrelide reduces the platelet count without affecting the white blood cell count. Progressive anemia occurs in many patients.[119] Up to 30 percent of patients cannot tolerate anagrelide because of side effects, many of which result from its vasodilatory and positive inotropic actions, such as fluid retention, palpitations and arrhythmias, heart failure, and headaches. The side effects of anagrelide diminish over time, but use of the drug requires particular caution in elderly patients or those with heart disease. Platelet counts are well controlled while patients are taking the drug, but discontinuation of the drug leads to a rapid rise in the platelet count in most patients. Important adverse reactions include neurologic and gastrointestinal symptoms, palpitations, and fluid retention.[118,120]

A multi-center, randomized controlled trial compared hydroxyurea with anagrelide in patients with essential thrombocythemia at high risk of vascular events.[139] The two agents produced equivalent long-term control of the platelet count. Anagrelide was associated with an increased rate of arterial thrombosis, major bleeding, and myelofibrotic transformation, but decreased venous thrombosis. The authors concluded that hydroxyurea should remain first-line cytoreductive therapy in patients with essential thrombocythemia at high risk for vascular events.

Recombinant interferon alpha also is effective therapy for essential thrombocythemia.[121] This drug suppresses proliferation of the abnormal megakaryocyte clone and results in decreased megakaryocyte size and ploidy during therapy. Platelet counts are reduced to the normal or near-normal range in most patients within 1 month of starting interferon therapy. An effective regimen is to initially administer interferon subcutaneously at a dose of 3,000,000 units/day, with doses subsequently adjusted according to individual tolerance and response.[122,123] Suppression of the platelet count can be maintained for several years using lower doses of interferon administered by subcutaneous injection three times per week.[122] Thrombocytosis relapse occurs after interferon is discontinued.[122] Severe flu-like side effects are not infrequent but generally can be ameliorated by reducing the interferon dose and using acetaminophen. Side effects make interferon intolerable for approximately 20 percent of patients. Interferon therapy often is accompanied by some reduction in the white blood and platelet counts, but generally no effect on the hematocrit is noted. Although interferon alpha is nonleukemogenic, the toxicity and cost associated with long-term treatment with this drug make unlikely its use as first-line therapy in "low-risk" patients with essential thrombocythemia.[124] Because hydroxyurea is teratogenic and anagrelide crosses the placenta (with unknown safety implications), interferon alpha is the treatment of choice for high-risk women with essential thrombocythemia who are contemplating pregnancy.

Hemopoietic stem cell transplantation can be considered for highly selected, younger patients with essential thrombocythemia who have complicated, advanced disease.[125,126] The finding of the *JAK2* V617F mutation in a large number of patients with essential thrombocythemia should stimulate the development of targeted therapy against the mutant form of the kinase.[138]

ANTIPLATELET AGENTS

Aspirin can be highly effective adjunctive therapy in patients with essential thrombocythemia who have recurrent thrombotic complications, particularly digital or cerebrovascular ischemia. Aspirin (but not warfarin) improves the increased platelet turnover and the clinical symptoms of erythromelalgia.[127] However, aspirin may cause marked prolongation of the bleeding time and unpredictable serious bleeding in some patients with thrombocythemia.[61,62] Low-dose aspirin (100 mg/day) effectively prevented thrombotic complications without increasing risk of bleeding in a double-blind, placebo-controlled, randomized trial in patients with polycythemia vera who did not have contraindications to aspirin.[128] Whether these observations can be extended to patients with essential thrombocythemia is uncertain. Aspirin use in patients with essential thrombocythemia remains controversial. Some experts recommend caution, but others recommend routine use to prevent thrombosis unless patients have a specific contraindication, such as a history of bleeding.

COURSE AND PROGNOSIS

The major causes of morbidity and mortality in essential thrombocythemia are thrombosis and hemorrhage. In occasional patients, even in the absence of leukemogenic treatment, the disease terminates by converting to acute leukemia or myelodysplasia, or the disease evolves into myelofibrosis.[4,129-131] Although the other myeloproliferative disorders have the potential, to a greater or lesser degree, to spontaneously convert to acute leukemia, the association is less clear in essential thrombocythemia. Use of radiophosphorus or alkylating agents, and probably hydroxyurea, to treat essential thrombocythemia likely enhances the leukemic potential of the disease. A high proportion of patients with essential thrombocythemia who develop acute myeloid leukemia and myelodysplastic syndromes with hydroxyurea treatment had chromosome 17p deletions and other characteristics of the 17p-syndrome.[114,132] An earlier analysis of actuarial survival in essential thrombocythemia indicated no significant decrease in life expectancy.[133] However, the later, population-based Olmsted County Study suggested survival of patients with essential thrombocythemia was significantly worse than that of age- and sex-matched healthy controls.[40]

REFERENCES

1. Ruggeri M, Tosetto A, Frezzato M, Rodeghiero F: The rate of progression to polycythemia vera or essential thrombocythemia in patients with erythrocytosis or thrombocytosis. *Ann Intern Med* 139:470, 2003.

2. Di Guglielmo G: Erithroleucemia e piastrinemia. *Folia Med* 1:36, 1920.

3. Epstein E, Goedel A: Hämorrhagische thrombozythämie bei vaskulärer Schrumpfmilz. *Virchows Arch Pathol Anat Physiol Klin Med* 292:233, 1934.

4. Schafer AI: Thrombocytosis. *N Engl J Med* 350:1211, 2004.

5. Gunz FW: Hemorrhagic thrombocythemia: A critical review. *Blood* 15:706, 1960.

6. Ozer FL, Truax WE, Miesch DC, Levin WC: Primary hemorrhagic thrombocythemia. *Am J Med* 28:807, 1960.

7. Fialkow PJ, Faguet GB, Jacobsen RJ, et al: Evidence that essential thrombocythemia is a clonal disorder with origin in a multipotent cell. *Blood* 58:916, 1981.

8. Liu E, Jelinek J, Pastore YD, et al: Discrimination of polycythemias and thrombocytoses by novel, simple, accurate clonality assays and comparison with PRV-1 expression and BFU-E response to erythropoietin. *Blood* 101:3294, 2003.

9. Harrison CN, Gale RE, Machin SJ, Linch DC: A large proportion of patients with a diagnosis of essential thrombocythemia do not have a clonal disorder and may be at lower risk of thrombotic complications. *Blood* 93:417, 1999.

10. Shih LY, Lin TL, Lai CL, et al: Predictive values of X-chromosome inactivation pattern and clinicohematologic parameters for vascular complications in female patients with essential thrombocythemia. *Blood* 100:1596, 2002.

11. Harrison CN, Green AR: Essential thrombocythemia. *Hematol Oncol Clin North Am* 17:1175, 2003.

12. Nimer SD: Essential thrombocythemia: Another "heterogeneous disease" better understood? *Blood* 93:415, 1999.

13. Adamson JW, Fialkow PJ: The pathogenesis of myeloproliferative syndromes. *Br J Haematol* 38:299, 1978.

14. Ogawa M: Cellular mechanisms of myeloproliferative disorders. *Br J Haematol* 58:563, 1984.

15. Kaushansky K: Regulation of megakaryopoiesis, in *Thrombosis and Hemorrhage*, 3rd ed, edited by J Loscalzo, AI Schafer, p 120. Lippincott Williams & Wilkins, Philadelphia, 2003.

16. Kaushansky K: Etiology of the myeloproliferative disorders: The role of thrombopoietin. *Semin Hematol* 40(suppl 1):6, 2003.

17. Griesshammer M, Bangerter M, Schrezenmeier H: A possible role for thrombopoietin and its receptor c-Mpl in the pathobiology of essential thrombocythemia. *Semin Thromb Hemost* 23:419, 1997.

18. Horikawa Y, Matsumura I, Hashimoto K, et al: Markedly reduced expression of platelet c-Mpl receptor in essential thrombocythemia. *Blood* 90:4031, 1997.

19. Teofili L, Pierconti F, Di Febo A, et al: The expression pattern of c-Mpl in megakaryocytes correlates with thrombotic risk in essential thrombocythemia. *Blood* 100:714, 2002.

20. Mazur EM, Cohen JL, Bogart L: Growth characteristics of circulating hematopoietic progenitor cells from patients with essential thrombocythemia. *Blood* 71:1544, 1988.

21. Han ZC, Abgrall JF, et al: Spontaneous formation of megakaryocyte progenitors (CFU-MK) in primary thrombocythaemia. *Acta Haematol* 78:51, 1987.

22. Juvonen E, Partanen S, Ruutu T: Colony formation by megakaryocytic progenitors in essential thrombocythaemia. *Br J Haematol* 66:161, 1987.

23. Kimura H, Ishibashi T, Sato T, et al: Megakaryocytic colony formation (CFU-Meg) in essential thrombocythemia: Quantitative and qualitative abnormalities of bone marrow CFU-Meg. *Am J Hematol* 24:23, 1987.

24. Axelrad AA, Eskinazi D, Correa PN, Amato D: Hypersensitivity of circulating progenitor cells to megakaryocyte growth and development factor (PEG-rHu MDGF) in essential thrombocythemia. *Blood* 96:3310, 2000.

25. Kawasaki H, Nakano T, Kohdera U, Kobayashi Y: Hypersensitivity of megakaryocyte progenitors to thrombopoietin in essential thrombocythemia. *Am J Hematol* 68:194, 2001.

26. Mi JQ, Blanc-Jouvan F, Wang J, et al: Endogenous megakaryocytic colony formation and thrombopoietin sensitivity of megakaryocytic progen-

itor cells are useful to distinguish between essential thrombocythemia and reactive thrombocytosis. *J Hematother Stem Cell Res* 10:405, 2001.

27. Kuroda H, Matsunaga T, Terui T, et al: Decrease of Smad4 gene expression in patients with essential thrombocythaemia may cause an escape from suppression of megakaryopoiesis by transforming growth factor-β1. *Br J Haematol* 124:221, 2004.

28. Cazzola M, Skoda RC: Translational pathophysiology: A novel mechanism of human disease. *Blood* 95:3280, 2000.

29. Wiestner A, Schlemper RJ, Van der Maas APC, Skoda RC: An activating splice donor mutation in the thrombopoietin gene causing hereditary thrombocythemia. *Nat Genet* 18:49, 1998.

30. Kondo T, Okabe M, Sanada M, et al: Familial essential thrombocythemia associated with one-base deletion in the 5'-untranslated region of the thrombopoietin gene. *Blood* 92:1091, 1998.

31. Ding J, Komatsu H, Wakita A, et al: Familial essential thrombocythemia associated with a dominant-positive activating mutation of the c-MPL gene, which encodes for the receptor for thrombopoietin. *Blood* 103:4198, 2004

32. Griesshammer M, Bangertner M, Sauer T, et al: Aetiology and clinical significance of thrombocytosis: Analysis of 732 patients with an elevated platelet count. *J Intern Med* 245:295, 1999.

33. Buss DH, Cashell AW, O'Connor ML, et al: Occurrence, etiology, and clinical significance of extreme thrombocytosis: A study case of 280 cases. *Am J Med* 96:247, 1994.

34. Schafer AI: Thrombocytosis and thrombocythemia. *Blood Rev* 15:159, 2001.

35. Tefferi A, Ho TC, Ahmann GJ, et al: Plasma interleukin-6 and C-reactive protein levels in reactive versus clonal thrombocytosis. *Am J Med* 97:374, 1994.

36. Kinjo K, Miyakawa Y, Uchida H, et al: All-*trans* retinoic acid directly up-regulates thrombopoietin transcription in human bone marrow stromal cells. *Exp Hematol* 32:45, 2004.

37. Numminen H, Hillbom M, Juvela S: Platelets, alcohol consumption, and onset of brain infarction. *J Neurol Neurosurg Psychiatry* 61:376, 1996.

38. Ogston D, Dawson AA: Thrombocytosis following thrombocytopenia in man. *Postgrad Med J* 45:754, 1969.

39. Bierling P, Divine M, Farcet JP, et al: Persistent remission of adult chronic autoimmune thrombocytopenic purpura after treatment with high-dose intravenous immunoglobulin. *Am J Haematol* 25:271, 1987.

40. Mesa RA, Silverstein MN, Jacobsen SJ, et al: Population-based incidence and survival figures in essential thrombocythemia and agnogenic myeloid metaplasia: An Olmsted County Study 1976-1995. *Am J Hematol* 61:10, 1999.

41. Reisner SA, Rinkevich D, Markiewicz W, et al: Cardiac involvement in patients with myeloproliferative disorders. *Am J Med* 93:498, 1992.

42. Schafer AI: Bleeding and thrombosis in the myeloproliferative disorders. *Blood* 64:1, 1984.

43. Schafer AI: The primary and secondary hypercoagulable states, in *Molecular Mechanisms of Hypercoagulable States*, edited by AI Schafer, p 1. Landes, Austin, 1997.

44. Schafer AI: Essential thrombocythemia. *Prog Hemost Thromb* 10:69, 1991.

45. Randi ML, Stocco F, Rossi C, et al: Thrombosis and hemorrhage in thrombocytosis: Evaluation of a large cohort of patients (357 cases). *J Med* 22:213, 1991.

46. Ravandi-Kashani F, Schafer AI: Microvascular disturbances, thrombosis, and bleeding in thrombocythemia: Current concepts and perspectives. *Semin Thromb Hemost* 23:479, 1997.

47. Kessler CM, Klein HG, Havlik RJ: Uncontrolled thrombocytosis in chronic myeloproliferative disorders. *Br J Haematol* 50:157, 1982.

48. Hoagland HC, Silverstein MN: Primary thrombocythemia in the young patient. *Mayo Clin Proc* 53:578, 1978.

49. Grossi A, Rosseti S, Vannucchi AM, et al: Occurrence of haemorrhagic and thrombotic events in myeloproliferative disorders: A retrospective study of 108 patients. *Clin Lab Haematol* 10:167, 1988.

50. Randi ML, Casonato A, Fabris F, et al: The significance of thrombocytosis in old age. *Acta Hematol* 78:41, 1987.

51. Mitus AJ, Barbui T, Shulman LN, et al: Hemostatic complications in young patients with essential thrombocythemia. *Am J Med* 88:371, 1990.

52. Schafer AI: Management of thrombocythemia. *Curr Opin Hematol* 3:341, 1996.

53. Tefferi A, Silverstein MN, Hoagland HC: Primary thrombocythemia. *Semin Oncol* 22:334, 1995.

54. Cortelazzo S, Finazzi G, Ruggeri M, et al: Hydroxyurea for patients with essential thrombocythemia and a high risk of thrombosis. *N Engl J Med* 332:1132, 1995.

55. Barbui T, Finazzi G: Risk factors and prevention of vascular complications in polycythemia vera. *Semin Thromb Hemost* 23:455, 1997.

56. Chiusolo P, La Barbera EO, Laurenti L, et al: Clonal hemopoiesis and risk of thrombosis in young female patients with essential thrombocythemia. *Exp Hematol* 29:670, 2001.

57. Temerinac S, Klippel S, Strunck E, et al: Cloning of PRV-1, a novel member of the uPAR receptor superfamily, which is overexpressed in polycythemia rubra vera. *Blood* 95:2569, 2000.

58. Klippel S, Strunck E, Temerinac S, et al: Quantification of PRV-1 mRNA distinguishes polycythemia vera from secondary erythrocytosis. *Blood* 102:3569, 2003.

59. Johansson P, Rickstein A, Wennstrom L, et al: Increased risk for vascular complications in PRV-1 positive patients with essential thrombocythaemia. *Br J Haematol* 123:513, 2003.

60. Messinezy M, Westwood NB, El-Hemaidi I, et al: Serum erythropoietin values in erythrocytoses and in primary thrombocythaemia. *Br J Haematol* 117:47, 2002.

61. Barbui T, Buelli M, Cortelazzo S, et al: Aspirin and risk of bleeding in patients with thrombocythemia. *Am J Med* 83:265, 1987.

62. Tartaglia AP, Goldberg JD, Berk PD, Wasserman LR: Adverse effects of antiaggregating platelet therapy in the treatment of polycythemia vera. *Semin Hematol* 23:172, 1986.

63. Bazzan M, Tamponi G, Schinco P, et al: Thrombosis-free survival and life expectancy in 187 consecutive patients with essential thrombocythemia. *Ann Hematol* 78:539, 1999.

64. Mitchell SW: On a rare vaso-motor neurosis of the extremities, and on the maladies with which it may be confounded. *Am J Med Sci* 76:2, 1878.

65. Michiels JJ: Erythromelalgia and vascular complications in polycythemia vera. *Semin Thromb Hemost* 23:441, 1997.

66. Michiels JJ, ten Kate FWJ, Vuzevski VD, Abels J: Histopathology of erythromelalgia in thrombocythaemia. *Histopathology* 8:669, 1984.

67. Singh AK, Wetherley-Mein G: Microvascular occlusive lesions in primary thrombocythaemia. *Br J Haematol* 36:553, 1977.

68. Kesler A, Ellis MH, Manor Y, et al: Neurological complications of essential thrombocythemia (ET). *Acta Neurol Scand* 105:299, 2000.

69. Jabaily J, Iland JF, Laszlo J, et al: Neurologic manifestations of essential thrombocythemia. *Ann Intern Med* 99:513, 1983.

70. Hehlmann R, Jahn M, Baumann B, Köpcke W: Essential thrombocythemia. Clinical characteristics and course of 61 cases. *Cancer* 61:2487, 1988.

71. Arboix A, Besses C, Acin P, et al: Ischemic stroke as first manifestation of essential thrombocythemia. Report of six cases. *Stroke* 26:1463, 1995.

72. Falconer J, Pineo G, Blahey W, et al: Essential thrombocythemia associated with recurrent abortions and fetal growth retardation. *Am J Hematol* 25:345, 1987.

73. Mercer B, Drouin J, Jolly E, D'Anjou G: Primary thrombocythemia in pregnancy: A report of two cases. *Am J Obstet Gynecol* 159:127, 1988.

74. Snethlage W, ten Cate JW: Thrombocythaemia and recurrent late abortions: Normal outcome of pregnancies after antiaggregating treatment. Case report. *Br J Obstet Gynaecol* 93:386, 1986.

75. Wright CA, Tefferi A: A single institutional experience with 43 pregnancies in essential thrombocythemia. *Eur J Haematol* 66:152, 2001.

76. Sanada M: Three successful pregnancies in a woman with essential thrombocythemia. *Eur J Haematol* 42:215, 1989.

77. Beressi AH, Tefferi A, Silverstein MN, et al: Outcome analysis of 34 pregnancies in women with essential thrombocythemia. *Arch Intern Med* 155:1217, 1995.

78. Vantroyen B, Vanstraelen D: Management of essential thrombocythemia during pregnancy with aspirin, interferon alpha-2a and no treatment. A comparative analysis of the literature. *Acta Haematol* 107:158, 2002.

79. Mahmoud AE, Mendoza A, Meshikhes AN, et al: Clinical spectrum, investigations and treatment of Budd-Chiari syndrome. *Q J Med* 89:37, 1996.

80. De Stefano V, Teofili L, Leone G, Michiels JJ: Spontaneous erythroid colony formation as the clue to an underlying myeloproliferative disorder in patients with Budd-Chiari syndrome or portal vein thrombosis. *Semin Thromb Hemost* 23:411, 1997.

81. Valla D, Casadevall N, Huisse MG, et al: Etiology of portal vein thrombosis in adults. A prospective evaluation of primary myeloproliferative disorders. *Gastroenterology* 94:1063, 1988.

82. Rinder HM, Schuster JE, Rinder CS, et al: Correlation of thrombosis with increased platelet turnover in thrombocytosis. *Blood* 91:1288, 1998.

83. Robinson MSC, Harrison C, Mackie IJ, et al: Reticulated platelets in primary and reactive thrombocytosis. *Br J Haematol* 101:338, 1998.

84. Graber M, Subramani K, Corish D, Schwab A: Thrombocytosis elevates serum potassium. *Am J Kidney Dis* 12:116, 1988.

85. George TI, Arber DA: Pathology of the myeloproliferative diseases. *Hematol Oncol Clin North Am* 17:1101, 2003.

86. Wolf BC, Neiman RS: The bone marrow in myeloproliferative and dysmyelopoietic syndromes. *Hematol Oncol Clin North Am* 2:669, 1988.

87. Adeyinka A, Dewald GW: Cytogenetics of chronic myeloproliferative disorders and related myelodysplastic syndromes. *Hematol Oncol Clin North Am* 17:1129, 2003.

88. Emilia G, Luppi M, Ferrari MG, et al: Chronic myeloid leukemia with thrombocythemic onset may be associated with different BCR/ABL variant transcripts. *Cancer Genet Cytogenet* 101:75, 1998.

89. Blickstein D, Aviram A, Luboshitz J, et al: BCR-ABL transcripts in bone marrow aspirates of Philadelphia-negative essential thrombocythemia patients: Clinical presentation. *Blood* 90:2768, 1997.

90. Takahashi H, Furukawa T, Hashimoto S, et al: 5q- syndrome presenting chronic myeloproliferative disorders-like manifestation: A case report. *Am J Hematol* 64:120, 2000.

91. Walsh PN, Murphy S, Barry WE: The role of platelets in the pathogenesis of thrombosis and hemorrhage in patients with thrombocytosis. *Thromb Haemost* 38:1085, 1977.

92. Pareti FI, Gugliotta L, Mannucci L, et al: Biochemical and metabolic aspects of platelet dysfunction in chronic myeloproliferative disorders. *Thromb Haemost* 47:84, 1982.

93. Wu KK: Platelet hyperaggregability and thrombosis in patients with thrombocythemia. *Ann Intern Med* 88:7, 1978.

94. Budde U, van Genderen PJJ: Acquired von Willebrand disease in patients with high platelet counts. *Semin Thromb Hemost* 23:425, 1997.

95. Kaywin P, McDonough M, Insel P, Shattil SJ: Platelet function in essential thrombocythemia: Decreased epinephrine responsiveness associated with a deficiency of platelet α-adrenergic receptors. *N Engl J Med* 299:505, 1978.

96. Schafer AI: Deficiency of platelet lipoxygenase activity in myeloproliferative disorders. *N Engl J Med* 306:381, 1982.

97. Thibert V, Bellucci S, Cristofari M, et al: Increased platelet CD36 constitutes a common marker in myeloproliferative disorders. *Br J Haematol* 91:618, 1995.

98. Moore A, Nachman RL: Platelet Fc receptor: Increased expression in myeloproliferative disease. *J Clin Invest* 67:1064, 1981.

99. Cooper B, Schafer AI, Puchalsky D, Handin RI: Platelet resistance to prostaglandin D_2 in patients with myeloproliferative disorders. *Blood* 52:618, 1978.

100. Murphy S, Iland H, Rosenthal D, Laszlo J: Essential thrombocythemia: An interim report from the Polycythemia Vera Study Group. *Semin Hematol* 23:177, 1986.

101. Lengfelder E, Hochhaus A, Kronawitter U, et al: Should a platelet limit of $600 \times 10^9/l$ be used as a diagnostic criterion in essential thrombocythaemia? An analysis of the natural course including early stages. *Br J Haematol* 100:15, 1998.

102. Thiele J, Kvasnicka HM, Schmitt-Graeff A, et al: Follow-up examinations including sequential bone marrow biopsies in essential thrombocythemia (ET): A retrospective clinicopathological study of 120 patients. *Am J Hematol* 70:283, 2002.

103. Hirsh J, Dacie JV: Persistent post-splenectomy thrombocytosis and thromboembolism: A consequence of continuing anaemia. *Br J Haematol* 12:44, 1966.

104. Borgna Pignatti C, Carnelli V, Caruso V, et al: Thromboembolic events in beta thalassemia major: An Italian multicenter study. *Acta Hematol* 99:76, 1998.

105. Finazzi G, Ruggeri M, Rodeghiero F, Barbui T: Second malignancies in patients with essential thrombocythaemia treated with busulphan and hydroxyurea: Long-term follow-up of a randomized clinical trial. *Br J Haematol* 110:577, 2000.

106. Taft EG, Babcock RB, Scharman WB, Tartaglia AP: Plateletpheresis in the management of thrombocytosis. *Blood* 50:927, 1977.

107. Younger J, Umlas J: Rapid reduction of platelet count in essential hemorrhagic thrombocythemia by discontinuous flow plateletpheresis. *Am J Med* 64:659, 1978.

108. Orlin JB, Berkman EM: Improvement of platelet function following plateletpheresis in patients with myeloproliferative diseases. *Transfusion* 20:540, 1980.

109. Sedlacek SM, Curtis JL, Weintraub J, Levin J: Essential thrombocythemia and leukemic transformation. *Medicine* 65:353, 1986.

110. Löfvenberg E, Wahlin A: Management of polycythaemia vera, essential thrombocythaemia and myelofibrosis with hydroxyurea. *Eur J Haematol* 41:375, 1988.

111. Best PJ, Daoud MS, Pittelkow MR, Pettit RM: Hydroxyurea-induced leg ulceration in 14 patients. *Ann Intern Med* 128:29, 1998.

112. Kaplan ME, Mack K, Goldberg JD, et al: Long-term management of polycythemia vera with hydroxyurea: A progress report. *Semin Hematol* 23:167, 1986.

113. Weinfeld A, Swolin B, Westin J: Acute leukemia after hydroxyurea therapy in polycythaemia vera and allied disorders: Prospective study of efficacy and leukaemogenicity with therapeutic implications. *Eur J Haematol* 52:134, 1994.

114. Sterkers Y, Preudhomme C, Lai J-L, et al: Acute myeloid leukemia and myelodysplastic syndromes following essential thrombocythemia treated with hydroxyurea: High proportion of cases with 17p deletion. *Blood* 91:616, 1998.

115. Finazzi G, Ruggeri M, Rodeghiero F, Barbui T: Efficacy and safety of long-term use of hydroxyurea in young patients with essential thrombocythemia and a high risk of thrombosis. *Blood* 101:3749, 2003.

116. Thiele J, Kvasnicka HM, Fuchs N, et al: Anagrelide-induced bone marrow changes during therapy of chronic myeloproliferative disorders with thrombocytosis. An immunohistochemical and morphometric study of sequential trephine biopsies. *Haematologica* 88:1130, 2003.

117. Solberg LA, Tefferi A, Oles KJ, et al: The effects of anagrelide on human megakaryocytopoiesis. *Br J Haematol* 99:174, 1997.

118. Anagrelide Study Group: Anagrelide, a therapy for thrombocythemic states: Experience in 577 patients. *Am J Med* 92:69, 1992.

119. Storen EC, Tefferi A: Long-term use of anagrelide in young patients with essential thrombocythemia. *Blood* 97:863, 2001.

120. Petitt RM, Silverstein MN, Petrone ME: Anagrelide for control of thrombocythemia in polycythemia and other myeloproliferative disorders. *Semin Hematol* 34:51, 1997.

121. Ludwig H, Linkesch W, Gisslinger H, et al: Interferon alfa corrects thrombocytosis in patients with myeloproliferative disorders. *Cancer Immunol Immunother* 25:266, 1987.

122. Gisslinger H, Chott A, Scheithauer W, et al: Interferon in essential thrombocythaemia. *Br J Haematol* 79(suppl 1):42, 1991.

123. Gilles FJ: Maintenance therapy in the myeloproliferative disorders: The current options. *Br J Haematol* 79(suppl 1):92, 1991.

124. Elliott MA, Tefferi A: Interferon-α therapy in polycythemia vera and essential thrombocythemia. *Semin Thromb Hemost* 23:463, 1997.

125. Jurado M, Deeg H, Gooley T, et al: Haemopoietic stem cell transplantation for advanced polycythaemia vera or essential thrombocythaemia. *Br J Haematol* 112:392, 2001.

126. Wayne AS, Barrett AJ: Allogeneic hematopoietic stem cell transplantation for myeloproliferative disorders and myelodysplastic syndromes. *Hematol Oncol Clin North Am* 17:1243, 2003.

127. van Genderen PJJ, Michiels JJ, Van Strik R, et al: Platelet consumption in thrombocythemia complicated by erythromelalgia: Reversal by aspirin. *Thromb Haemost* 73:210, 1995.

128. Landolfi R, Marchioli R, the European Collaboration on Low-dose Aspirin in Polycythemia Vera (ECLAP) Investigators, et al: Efficacy and safety of low-dose aspirin in polycythemia vera. *N Engl J Med* 350:114, 2004.

129. Harrison CN: Current trends in essential thrombocythaemia. *Br J Haematol* 117:796, 2002.

130. Hoffman R: Quality of life issues in patients with essential thrombocythemia and polycythemia vera. *Semin Oncol* 29(suppl 10):3, 2002.

131. Cervantes F, Alvarez-Larran A, Talarn C, et al: Myelofibrosis with myeloid metaplasia following essential thrombocythaemia: Actuarial probability, presenting characteristics and evolution in a series of 195 patients. *Br J Haematol* 118:786, 2002.

132. Bernasconi P, Boni M, Cavigliano PM, et al: Acute myeloid leukemia (AML) having evolved from essential thrombocythemia (ET): Distinctive chromosome abnormalities in patients treated with pipobroman or hydroxyurea. *Leukemia* 16:2078, 2002.

133. Rozman C, Giralt M, Feliu E, et al: Life expectancy of patients with chronic nonleukaemic myeloproliferative disorders. *Cancer* 67:2658, 1991.

134. Baxter EJ, Scott LM, Campbell PJ, et al: Acquired mutation of the tyrosine kinase JAK2 in human myeloproliferative disorders. *Lancet* 365:1054, 2005.

135. Levine RL, Wadleigh M, Cools J, et al: Activating mutation in the tyrosine kinase *JAK2* in polycythemia vera, essential thrombocythemia, and myeloid metaplasia with myelofibrosis. *Cancer Cell* 7:387, 2005.

136. James C, Ugo V, Le Couedic J-P, et al: A unique clonal *JAK2* mutation leading to constitutive signaling causes polycythaemia vera. *Nature* 434:1144, 2005.

137. Kralovics R, Passamonti F, Buser AS, et al: A gain-of-function mutation of *JAK2* in myeloproliferative disorders. *N Engl J Med* 352:1179, 2005.

138. Kaushansky K: On the molecular origins of the chronic myeloproliferative disorders: it all makes sense. *Blood* 105:4187, 2005.

139. Green A, Campbell P, Buck G, et al: The Medical Research Council PT1 Trial in essential thrombocythemia. *Blood* 104:5a, 2004.

HEREDITARY QUALITATIVE PLATELET DISORDERS

BARRY S. COLLER
W. BEAU MITCHELL
DEBORAH L. FRENCH

Abnormalities of platelet function manifest themselves primarily as excessive hemorrhage at mucocutaneous sites, with ecchymoses, petechiae, epistaxis, gingival hemorrhage, and menorrhagia most common. Both quantitative and qualitative platelet abnormalities can produce these symptoms, so thrombocytopenia must be excluded (see Chap. 110) by performing a platelet count. A prolonged bleeding time in a patient with a normal platelet count is indicative of a qualitative platelet abnormality, von Willebrand disease (see Chap. 118), or afibrinogenemia (see Chap. 117). Chapter 113 discusses acquired qualitative platelet abnormalities. This chapter discusses the hereditary qualitative platelet abnormalities.

The hereditary qualitative platelet disorders can be classified according to the major locus of the defect (Table 112-1, Fig. 112-1). Thus, abnormalities of platelet glycoproteins, platelet granules, and signal transduction and secretion all can result in hemorrhagic diatheses and prolonged bleeding times. Glanzmann thrombasthenia results from abnormalities in either αIIb (GPIIb) or β3 (GPIIIa), resulting in loss or dysfunction of the αIIbβ3 (GPIIb-IIIa) receptor. This situation results in a profound defect in platelet aggregation and secondary defects in platelet adhesion and platelet coagulant activity. Loss of the platelet GPIb-IX-V complex because of abnormalities in GPIbα, GPIbβ, or GPIX results in the Bernard-Soulier syndrome, which is characterized by giant platelets and thrombocytopenia. The major defect is in platelet adhesion and results from a decrease in platelet interactions with von Willebrand factor, but abnormalities in αIIbβ3 activation and thrombin-induced aggregation also are present. Other defects in platelet α2β1 (GPIa-IIa) and GPVI and isolated defects in agonist receptors or proteins involved in signal transduction also may produce hemorrhagic symptoms, but these disorders are less well characterized. Abnormalities of platelet coagulant activity, that is, the ability of platelets to facilitate thrombin generation (see Chap. 106), also can lead to a hemorrhagic diathesis, but this platelet defect is unique in that it usually does not produce mucocutaneous hemorrhage or a prolonged bleeding time.

Acronyms and abbreviations that appear in this chapter include: ADP, adenosine diphosphate; ATP, adenosine triphosphate; BLOC, biogenesis of lysosome-related organelles complex; cAMP, cyclic adenosine monophosphate; cDNA, complementary deoxyribonucleic acid; CMV, cytomegalovirus; EDTA, ethylenediaminetetraacetic acid; HLA, human leukocyte antigen; Ig, immunoglobulin; MIDAS, metal ion-dependent adhesion site; rFVIIa, recombinant factor VIIa; VLDL, very-low-density lipoprotein.

GLYCOPROTEIN ABNORMALITIES

αIIbβ3 (GLYCOPROTEIN IIB/IIIA; CD41/CD61): GLANZMANN THROMBASTHENIA

DEFINITION AND HISTORY

Glanzmann thrombasthenia is an inherited hemorrhagic disorder characterized by severely reduced or absent platelet aggregation in response to multiple physiologic agonists because of qualitative or quantitative abnormalities of platelet glycoprotein αIIb (GPIIb; CD 41) and/or β3 (GPIIIa; CD61).

In 1918, Eduard Glanzmann,[1] a Swiss pediatrician, described a group of patients with hemorrhagic symptoms and "weak" platelets (i.e., thrombasthenia). Subsequent studies demonstrated that platelets from thrombasthenic patients failed to aggregate in response to physiologic agonists such as adenosine diphosphate (ADP), epinephrine, collagen, and thrombin[2–5]; had markedly reduced levels of platelet fibrinogen[2,4–6]; and had reduced or absent clot retraction.[7] In the mid-1970s, Nurden and Caen[8] and Phillips and colleagues[9] discovered that thrombasthenic platelets were deficient in both αIIb and β3. Later studies demonstrated that αIIb and β3 form a calcium-dependent complex in the platelet membrane that functions as a receptor for fibrinogen and other adhesive glycoproteins.[10–13] Cloning and sequencing of the complementary deoxyribonucleic acids (cDNAs) for αIIb[14] and β3[15] identified them as separate protein subunits that are members of the integrin receptor superfamily[16] and permitted the molecular biologic characterization of patients with the disorder. Identification of the DNA defects in selected patients has provided information on the structure-function relationships of the αIIbβ3 receptor and permitted DNA-based carrier detection and prenatal diagnosis.[17–82]

ETIOLOGY AND PATHOGENESIS

Glanzmann thrombasthenia is a rare disorder characterized by autosomal recessive inheritance with a worldwide distribution. In regions where consanguineous matings are common, groups of patients with the disorder have been identified. In several populations, founder mutations were identified by analyzing polymorphisms in the DNA surrounding the affected mutation. These populations include 42 patients from South India; 39 patients from the Iraqi-Jewish population in Israel; 46 Arab patients from Israel, Jordan, and Saudi Arabia; 30 patients from Italy; and a smaller number of patients from three Gypsy

TABLE 112-1   INHERITED DISORDERS OF PLATELET FUNCTION

I. Glycoprotein adhesion receptor abnormalities
    A. αIIbβ3 (glycoprotein IIb-IIIa; CD41/CD61): Glanzmann thrombasthenia
    B. Glycoproteins Ib (CD42b,c), IX (CD42a), and V: Bernard-Soulier syndrome
    C. Glycoprotein Ib (CD42b,c): Platelet-type (pseudo-) von Willebrand disease
    D. α2β1 (glycoprotein Ia-IIa; VLA-2; CD49b/CD29)
    E. Glycoprotein IV (CD36)
    F. Glycoprotein VI
    G. CD43: Wiskott-Aldrich syndrome (secondary abnormality)
II. Abnormalities of Platelet Granules
    A. δ-Storage pool deficiency
    B. Gray platelet syndrome: α-storage pool deficiency
    C. Paris-Trousseau/Jacobsen syndrome (giant α-granule)
    D. α,δ-Storage pool deficiency
    E. Quebec platelet disorder
III. Abnormalities of platelet coagulant activity
IV. Abnormalities of signal transduction and secretion
    A. Defects in platelet agonist receptors (ADP, epinephrine, thromboxane A$_2$) or agonist-specific signal transduction
    B. Defects in arachidonic acid metabolism
    C. Defects in phospholipase C, Gαq, calcium mobilization, and calcium responsiveness

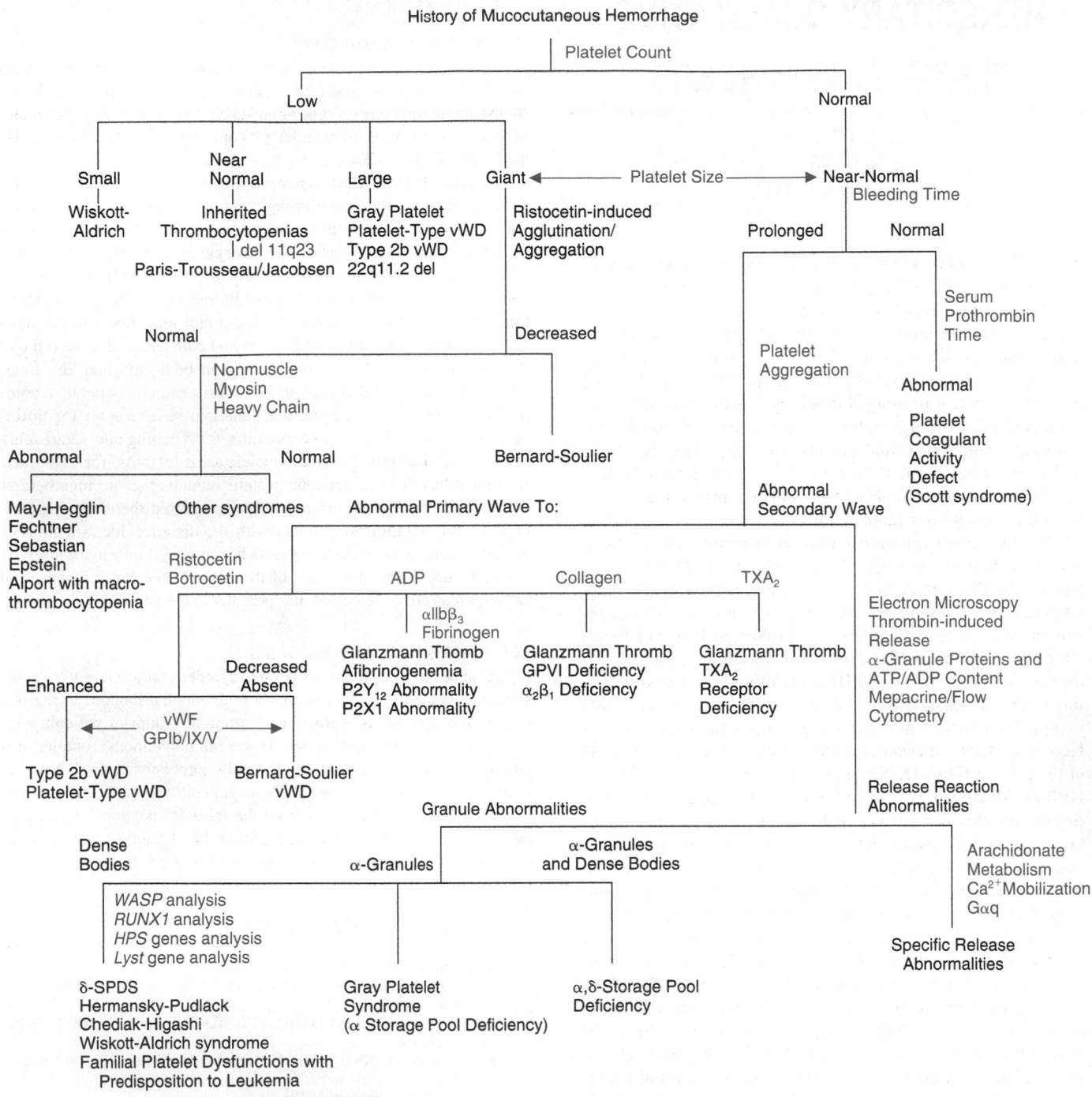

FIGURE 112-1　Evaluation of patients for abnormalities in platelet number or function. A reduced platelet count occurs in patients with purely quantitative platelet disorders (inherited or acquired) and in patients with inherited qualitative platelet disorders associated with thrombocytopenia. Platelet size (determined from the blood film and/or mean platelet volume) helps to separate the inherited quantitative platelet syndromes from the acquired thrombocytopenias and the inherited combined quantitative and qualitative thrombocytopenias (see Chap. 110). The Paris-Trousseau/Jacobsen syndrome is a rare inherited thrombocytopenia with giant α-granules in only a fraction of circulating platelets and deletion of chromosome 11q23.3-24. Very small platelets are characteristic of the Wiskott-Aldrich syndrome. Large platelets that lack purple granules are observed in the gray platelet syndrome (α-storage pool deficiency), but one must be certain that the stain is working properly and that no plasma factor is producing platelet degranulation. The diagnosis of gray platelet syndrome is confirmed by biochemical analysis of α-granule contents. Patients with platelet-type (pseudo-) von Willebrand disease (vWD) and type 2b vWD have moderate thrombocytopenia and large platelets. Studies of GPIb function and biochemistry described below establish the diagnosis. Patients who are hemizygous for GPIbβ because of deletion of 22q11.2 have variable thrombocytopenia and large platelets. The platelets in Bernard-Soulier syndrome are truly giant; the diagnosis is confirmed with biochemical and functional analyses of the GPIb-IX-V complex.

The bleeding time is prolonged in almost all patients with qualitative platelet disorders (although to various extents) except in platelet coagulant disorders, where the serum prothrombin time is the preferred screening assay. Other tests of platelet coagulant activity are used to establish the diagnosis. Platelet aggregation can separate patients into those with defects in the primary wave of platelet aggregation (dependent on fibrinogen, von Willebrand factor [vWF], their respective receptors, or other agonist receptors for collagen and ADP) and those with defects in the secondary wave of aggregation. Enhanced ristocetin-induced platelet families.[6,24,41,68,83–87] Perhaps the highest frequency of a Glanzmann thrombasthenia mutation is found in the Iraqi-Jewish population where the most common mutation causing Glanzmann thrombasthenia was found in six of 700 individuals.[41]

The platelet $\alpha IIb\beta 3$ receptor is required for platelet aggregation induced by all of the agonists thought to operate *in vivo* (ADP, epinephrine, thrombin, collagen, thromboxane A_2) (see Chap. 105).[10–12] Consequently, abnormalities in the receptor result in a failure of platelet plug formation at sites of vascular injury, leading to excessive bleeding and bruising.

The $\alpha IIb\beta 3$ receptor is responsible for uptake of fibrinogen from plasma into platelet α-granules,[88–91] so patients with Glanzmann thrombasthenia have markedly reduced levels of platelet fibrinogen.[2,4,5,92,93] Clot retraction requires platelets with intact $\alpha IIb\beta 3$ receptors,[94–96] presumably to make contact with fibrin, so patients with Glanzmann thrombasthenia usually have abnormal clot retraction.[2,7]

Defects in either αIIb or $\beta 3$ result in the same functional defect because both subunits are required for receptor function (see Chap. 105). Biosynthetic studies indicate that αIIb and $\beta 3$ form a complex in the rough endoplasmic reticulum soon after protein synthesis.[97–99] Subsequent posttranslational processing[100] and transport to the platelet membrane require that the complex be intact (Fig. 112-2).[101,102] Complex formation is required for transport from the endoplasmic reticulum to the Golgi,[97–100] so if either αIIb or $\beta 3$ is absent or unable to form a normal complex, the other subunit is degraded. Thus, a deficiency in either glycoprotein produces a deficiency in both. Because complex formation and transport to the Golgi also are required for proteolytic processing of pro-αIIb into its constituent $\alpha IIb\alpha$ and $\alpha IIb\beta$ subunits,[100] if complex formation and/or transport does not occur normally, the very small amount of residual αIIb will be pro-αIIb and not mature αIIb.[103]

$\beta 3$ (GPIIIa) can combine with the αV-integrin (CD51) subunit to form the $\alpha V\beta 3$ "vitronectin" receptor (see Fig. 112-2 and Chap. 105).[15,104,105] Despite its common name, this receptor can bind many of the same adhesive glycoproteins as $\alpha IIb\beta 3$, although some differences in ligand preference and binding sequences exist.[105–109] A small number of $\alpha V\beta 3$ receptors are present on platelets (50–100 per platelet).[108,110,111] Osteoclasts, endothelial cells, macrophages, and uterine cells, among others, also have $\alpha V\beta 3$ receptors.[112–114] In general,

Glanzmann thrombasthenia patients with defects in $\beta 3$ also are deficient in $\alpha V\beta 3$, whereas patients with defects in αIIb have either normal or increased numbers of platelet $\alpha V\beta 3$ receptors.[19,20,35,108,111,113] The one exception is a patient with a defect in $\beta 3$ (H280P) that interferes with $\alpha IIb\beta 3$ biogenesis to a much greater extent than $\alpha V\beta 3$ biogenesis.[65] At present, no evidence indicates that patients who lack $\alpha V\beta 3$ receptors in addition to $\alpha IIb\beta 3$ receptors have a more severe hemorrhagic diathesis or suffer from any other abnormalities, perhaps because alternative receptors containing αV associated with other β-subunits can substitute for $\alpha V\beta 3$.[111] Up-regulation of $\alpha 2\beta 1$ on osteoclasts of Iraqi-Jewish patients with Glanzmann thrombasthenia has been reported as a potential compensatory mechanism explaining the lack of bone changes despite the deficiency in osteoclast $\alpha V\beta 3$.

The molecular biologic abnormalities in more than 50 patients with Glanzmann thrombasthenia have been identified. They are listed in an Internet database that is updated continuously[40] (available at *http://med.mssm.edu/glanzmanndb*) and can be reached through the Williams Hematology web site (available at *http://www.williamshematology.com*). Figure 112-3 contains information on mutations of particular interest. Of note, many of the patients with identified mutations are compound heterozygotes rather than homozygotes, indicating that a sizable number of silent carriers are present in the population. Where consanguinity is common, the disorder more likely results from a homozygous mutation arising in a founder, but even under these circumstances more than one mutation may be present. Thus, in the Iraqi-Jewish population, in which consanguinity has been present from 586 BCE to the present, two separate mutations have been identified.[41] Most of the missense mutations result in decreased expression of $\alpha IIb\beta 3$ on the surface of platelets. This finding probably reflects the stringent structural requirements for proper folding and complex formation.

Mutations Within the Metal Ion-Dependent Adhesion Site of $\beta 3$ (GPIIIa) and the Interface with the αIIb (GPIIb) β-Propeller A metal coordination site or metal ion-dependent adhesion site (MIDAS) domain,[115] which is highly conserved in six integrin receptor α-chain subunits and required for ligand binding,[116] is also present in the βA (or I-like) domain of the $\beta 3$-subunit.[117] Mutagenesis and molecular modeling experiments suggested that a highly conserved DxSxS amino acid sequence[118] motif plus additional coordinating residues are

---

FIGURE 112-1 (CONTINUED) aggregation at low doses of ristocetin has been identified in patients with platelet-type vWD (who have a defect in the GPIb receptor that facilitates vWF binding) and in patients with type 2b vWD (who have an intrinsic defect in vWF) (see Chap. 118). These two diseases can be separated by analyzing the binding of the patient's vWF to normal platelets or the ability of cryoprecipitate or asialo-vWF to aggregate patient platelets. Confirmation of the diagnosis of platelet-type vWD requires analysis of GPIb.

Neither ristocetin nor the snake venom botrocetin induces platelet aggregation if the plasma lacks functional vWF, as in most cases of vWD (see Chap. 118), or if the platelets lack functional GPIb-IX complexes, as in Bernard-Soulier syndrome. The defect in vWD, but not Bernard-Soulier syndrome, can be corrected by adding normal plasma. Direct analysis of vWF and the platelet GPIb-IX complex confirms the diagnosis.

Patients whose plasma lacks fibrinogen (afibrinogenemia) (see Chap. 117) or whose platelets cannot bind fibrinogen because of abnormal $\alpha IIb\beta 3$ receptors (Glanzmann thrombasthenia) have no primary wave of platelet aggregation in response to ADP or epinephrine. Analysis of plasma fibrinogen and platelet $\alpha IIb\beta 3$ receptors can differentiate between the two groups. Isolated defects in the primary response to collagen have been observed in patients with abnormalities in platelet $\alpha 2\beta 1$ (GPIa-IIa) or GPVI. Platelet glycoprotein analysis can separate the two. Because antibodies to GPVI can result in receptor depletion from circulating platelets, a search for an antibody to GPVI should be undertaken. Other isolated defects in one or more of the ADP receptors or the thromboxane A_2 receptor result in decreased ADP-induced platelet aggregation, whereas isolated defects in the receptors for epinephrine or platelet activating factor lead to defects in primary aggregation in response to these agonists.

A heterogeneous group of platelet defects can result in an abnormal secondary wave of platelet aggregation in response to ADP and epinephrine and diminished responses to low doses of collagen and thrombin, but they can be broadly separated into granule defects and defects in the platelet release reaction. These two groups can be separated based on their release of granule contents in response to high doses of thrombin. Thrombin activation can overcome most or all of the release reaction abnormalities, so platelets from patients with these disorders will release normal amounts of granule contents. Patients with reduced granule contents have abnormal release responses even when activated with high doses of thrombin. α-Granule contents and dense body contents can be measured immunologically and biochemically. Electron microscopy can confirm the diagnosis of granule defects. Analysis of the genes or proteins implicated in the different granule defect abnormalities (Wiskott-Aldrich syndrome [WASP], Hermansky-Pudlak syndrome, Chédiak-Higashi syndrome [Lyst], inherited platelet disorder with predisposition to leukemia [RUNX1]) can establish the diagnosis. Release reaction abnormalities can be subcategorized by analyzing the response to arachidonic acid or a thromboxane A_2 analogue and by measuring release of arachidonic acid, calcium fluxes, $G\alpha q$, and phosphoinositide metabolism.

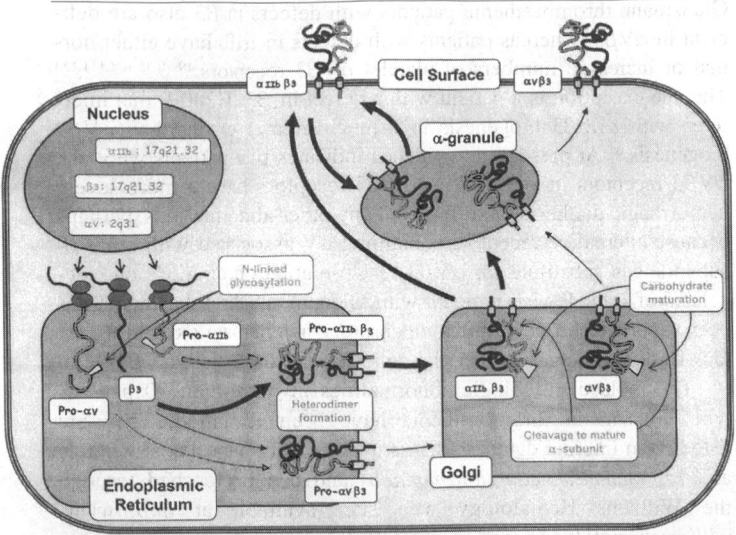

FIGURE 112-2 Biogenesis of integrin Receptors αIIbβ3 and αVβ3. The nuclear genes for αIIb (chromosome localization 17q21.32; gene designation ITGA2B; 30 exons), αV (2q31; ITGAV; 30 exons), and β3 (17q21.32; ITGB3; 14 exons) are transcribed into messenger RNA and translated by ribosomes attached to the membranes of the endoplasmic reticulum (ER). The proteins undergo initial glycosylation and form the αIIbβ3 and αVβ3 heterodimers in the ER. It is presumed that many more αIIbβ3 complexes form than αVβ3 complexes because the final copy number of platelet αIIbβ3 receptors is approximately 100,000 whereas the number is only 50 to 100 for αVβ3. This situation is shown schematically by the differences in the width of the arrows depicting αIIbβ3 versus αVβ3 complex formation. The heteroduplexes are transported to the Golgi, where the carbohydrate chains undergo modification to their mature structures and both αIIb and αV undergo proteolytic cleavage within a disulfide-bonded loop, resulting in two-chain forms of the receptor subunits. Mature αIIbβ3 receptors are transported to α-granule membranes, where they undergo cycling to and from the plasma membrane. This process results in the internalization of fibrinogen and perhaps other plasma proteins. αIIbβ3 may also be directly transported to the plasma membrane. Of the total of approximately 100,000 αIIbβ3 receptors, approximately two thirds are on the surface at any given time; the remaining one third can be brought to the surface by platelet activation. The distribution of αVβ3 between the plasma membrane and α-granules and the potential cycling of αVβ3 receptors between α granules and the plasma membrane have not been defined.

brought together in the three-dimensional structure of the β3-subunit to form a cation-binding sphere of the MIDAS domain.[115] This hypothesis was confirmed by the crystal structures of αVβ3 and later αIIbβ3 (see Figs. 105-13 and 112-3).[119,120] Thus, the β3 MIDAS is composed of Asp119, Ser121, Ser123, Glu220 and Asp251, but the region from R214 to A218, which is at the interface with the αIIb β-propeller, also contributes to the ligand-binding pocket. Adjacent to the MIDAS domain is a metal ion site termed ADMIDAS, in which calcium is coordinated by Ser123, Asp126, Asp127, and Met335 in unliganded αVβ3, but Asp251 substitutes for Met335 in the ligand-bound structures of both αVβ3 and αIIbβ3. The crystal structures also demonstrated that peptide ligands containing the RGD cell adhesion sequence interact with αVβ3 in part by coordination of the metal ion in the MIDAS by the aspartic acid in the RGD peptide.[121] The low molecular weight drugs eptifibatide and tirofiban, which block ligand binding to αIIb, have negatively charged regions that also interact with the MIDAS cation. The fibrinogen γ-chain C-terminal dodecapeptide mediates binding to αIIbβ3, but the precise manner in which it binds to the receptor has not been reported. A number of mutations in patients with Glanzmann thrombasthenia have been identified within the cation-binding sphere of the MIDAS domain (see Fig. 112-3). Two

mutations D119Y (Cam variant)[18] and D119N (patient NR)[122] are located within the conserved DxSxS amino acid motif and produce severe abnormalities of ligand binding to αIIbβ3 but do not affect α-IIbβ3 surface expression. Mutations at residues R214 and R216 result in abnormal αIIbβ3 receptors that are highly sensitive to dissociation by calcium chelation. A R217V mutation also produces a functionally defective receptor.[25,68,123,124] Further support for the importance of the MIDAS domain comes from studies in which the mutations D119N, R214W, D217N, E220Q, and E220K were introduced into CHO cells in vitro and shown to result in functional abnormalities.[125]

The interface between the αIIb β-propeller and the β3 βA (I-like) domain involves, in part, the interaction between β3 R261, contained in a four-amino-acid 3₁₀ helix, and a number of hydrophobic residues in the αIIb β-propeller arranged as inner and outer rings, making up a cage.[126] A β3 L262Y mutation adjacent to R261 results in disruption of the helix and an unstable αIIbβ3 complex that is expressed on the

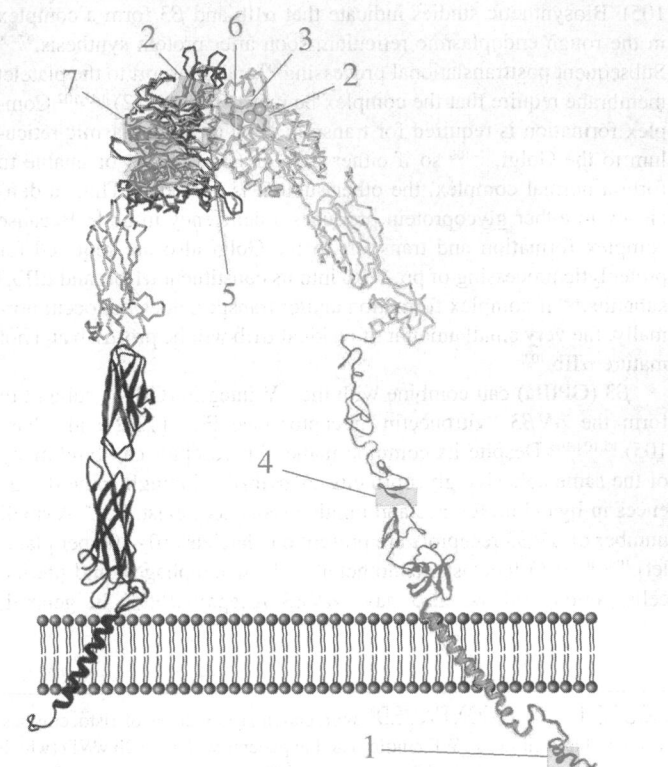

FIGURE 112-3 Diagram of αIIbβ3 structure and identification of select mutations causing Glanzmann thrombasthenia. A full listing of reported Glanzmann thrombasthenia mutations is available at the web site http://sinaicentral.mssm.edu/glanzmanndb. Details of the structure of αIIbβ3 are given in Figures 105-3 and 105-13. The αIIbβ3 structure depicted is a composite of data obtained from the headpiece of αIIbβ3,[120] the extracellular domains of αVβ3,[119] and the transmembrane and intracellular domains.[675] Among the missense mutations identified are those that (1) interfere with inside-out and outside-in signaling (β3 S752P),[22,135] (2) interfere with ligand binding to either the metal ion-dependent adhesion site (MIDAS) in β3 (β3 D119Y and D119N) or the αIIb component of the ligand binding site (Y143H, P145L/A, insert R160/T161),[18,51,76,122,131] (3) result in receptors that are sensitive to dissociation by divalent cation chelation (R214W, R214Q, R216Q),[23,25,33,123,124] (4) result in a constitutively active receptor (β3 C560R),[61] (5) alter the interface between αIIb and β3 and disrupt ligand binding (β3 L262P),[127] (6) result in a β3-protein that can complex more effectively with αV than αIIb (S162L, R216Q, H280P),[65] and (7) alter αIIb-propeller structure and prevent normal αIIbβ3 complex formation, processing, and/or transport.[34–39,74,75] (Adapted from Qin et al.,[674] Xiong et al.,[119] and Xiao et al.[120])

surface of platelets but is unable to bind fibrinogen.[127] Remarkably, the platelets of the patient with this mutation were able to bind fibrin and support clot retraction, suggesting different requirements for fibrinogen and fibrin binding.

Mutations Within the GPIIb (α-chain) β-Propeller Sequence
Based on their homology to another integrin α-subunit, the amino-terminal 450 amino acids of αIIb and the homologous region in αV, which contain the minimal ligand-binding sequence,[128] were predicted to fold into seven repeat (blade) β-propellers containing four cation-binding sites.[129] This prediction was confirmed by the crystal structures of both αV and αIIb.[120,130] The upper surface of the propeller interacts with the β3-subunit βA (or I-like) domain to form the head of the αIIbβ3 complex, which is the site of ligand binding. Each repeat (blade) contains four β-strands, with loops connecting the β-strands. The four calcium binding sites in αIIb, which are in β hairpin structures, are located in loops on the undersurface of the propeller. Ligand binding in αIIb has been localized to a hydrophobic (F160, Y190, F231) and negatively charged (D224) pocket that lies adjacent to the MIDAS domain in β3. It is composed of contributions from the loops that link blade 2 to blade 3 (residues 144–171), β-strand 2 to β-strand 3 in blade 3 (residues 186–193), and blade 3 to blade 4 (residues 223–236). αIIb contains a unique "cap" subdomain made up of four insertions in β-propeller loops (residues 72–88, 111–126, 147–166, 200–217) that plays a ligand-binding role similar to that of I domains in integrin receptors that contain I domains.[120]

Glanzmann thrombasthenia missense mutations located within the αIIb β-propeller (see Fig. 112-3) primarily affect transport of the αIIbβ3 complex to the cell surface,[34,35,37,39,55] but several missense mutations and an insertion result in functionally defective receptors. Thus, Y143H affects soluble ligand binding but not adhesion or clot retraction,[76] and P145A, which has been identified in several kindreds,[68,131] and P145L prevent ligand binding. A two-amino-acid insertion at residues 161 and 162, and a T176I missense mutation, also affect ligand binding.[43,51,132] An L183P mutation, which is near to but not in the loop containing Y190, affected both receptor expression and function.[53]

Mutations that Affect Receptor Activation Several β3 missense mutations (C560R, V193M) result in the receptor adopting a high-affinity ligand-binding state, which is paradoxical because the mutations result in a bleeding diathesis.[61,62] The cytoplasmic domain of β3 plays a functional role in integrin activation and the regulation of ligand binding.[22,133,134] Two Glanzmann thrombasthenia mutations have been identified in this region. One is an R724X nonsense mutation (patient R.M.)[45] that results in the deletion of the carboxy-terminal 39 residues of β3; the other is a β3 S752P missense mutation (patient P or Paris 1).[22,134,135] This latter patient is unusual because he had a generally mild history of excessive hemorrhage, but he had a prolonged bleeding time and his platelets did not aggregate in response to ADP. These mutations do not severely affect surface expression of platelet αIIbβ3 complexes, but both mutant receptors are unresponsive to agonist stimulation. Mammalian cell expression studies of these mutations show normal adhesion to immobilized fibrinogen but abnormal cell spreading. Cells expressing the S752P mutant receptors have reduced focal adhesion plaque formation, and cells expressing the R724X mutant receptors have undetectable tyrosine phosphorylation of the focal adhesion kinase pp125[FAK]. These mutations provide evidence for the role of the β3-cytoplasmic tail in inside-out signaling (i.e., platelet signals that lead to αIIbβ3 adopting a high-affinity ligand-binding conformation) and outside-in signaling (i.e., signaling to the interior of the platelet as a result of αIIbβ3 binding ligand).

CLINICAL FEATURES
The clinical manifestations of a total of 232 patients with Glanzmann thrombasthenia were the subject of two reviews. Table 112-2 sum-

TABLE 112-2 BLEEDING IN PATIENTS WITH GLANZMANN THROMBASTHENIA

	NO. OF AFFECTED PATIENTS	FREQUENCY (%)
Symptoms		
Menorrhagia	54/55	98
Easy bruising, purpura	152/177	86
Epistaxis	129/177	73
Gingival bleeding	97/177	55
Gastrointestinal hemorrhage	22/177	12
Hematuria	10/177	6
Hemarthrosis	5/177	3
Intracranial hemorrhage	3/177	2
Visceral hematoma	1/177	1
Severity		
Requirement for red cell transfusions		
Patients from literature*	32/48	67
Paris patients	54/64	84

* Data from 177 patients reviewed by George et al.,[6] of whom 113 were from the literature and 64 were studied in Paris.
SOURCE: From Coller BS: Inherited disorders of platelet function, in *Haemostasis and Thrombosis*, 3d ed, edited by AL Bloom, CD Forbes, DP Thomas, EGD Taddenham, pp 721–766. Churchill Livingstone, Edinburgh, 1994, with permission.

marizes data from 177 of these patients.[6,24] Menorrhagia occurs in nearly all patients, especially at the time of menarche. Purpura can be present immediately after birth but often is not dramatic. Petechiae of the face and subconjunctival hemorrhage associated with crying may be the first symptoms in neonates and babies. Epistaxis is a common symptom and can be life threatening.[6,24,136] It usually abates in adulthood. Gingival bleeding can be a chronic source of blood (and iron) loss, especially if the teeth are not kept in good repair. Gastrointestinal bleeding was only present in 12 percent of patients in one review[6] but was present in 49 percent of patients in another.[24] Gastrointestinal bleeding usually is intermittent, but identifying the bleeding site often is difficult. Patients with Glanzmann thrombasthenia and vascular abnormalities of the gastrointestinal tract, such as hereditary hemorrhagic telangiectasias or angiodysplasia can present severe challenges because bleeding may be recurrent and difficult to control.

Hemarthroses are rare and spontaneous cases even rarer, thus distinguishing Glanzmann thrombasthenia from the hemophilias and related illnesses. Having Glanzmann thrombasthenia undoubtedly increases the risk of excessive bleeding when the central nervous system has suffered trauma, but the rareness of spontaneous central nervous system bleeding is remarkable.[6,24]

Patients with Glanzmann thrombasthenia do not appear to bleed excessively during pregnancy, but immediate postpartum hemorrhage is common unless platelet transfusions are administered.[6] Delayed postpartum hemorrhage can be severe but may be less likely to occur in patients delivered by cesarean section.[6] Surgical procedures, including oral surgery, usually are complicated by excessive bleeding unless prophylactic platelet transfusions are administered.[6,24,137]

The hemorrhagic diathesis in Glanzmann thrombasthenia is notable for its variability and the lack of correlation between the biochemical platelet abnormalities and clinical severity.[6] Even within groups of patients such as Iraqi Jews, most of whom share the same genetic abnormality and have similar platelet function and biochemical profiles, a wide spectrum of clinical severity is observed.[24,41] Moreover, the severity of bleeding symptoms can vary significantly during the lifetime of individual patients. Thus, factors other than the platelet defect itself play important roles in determining the risk of bleeding.

Carriers of Glanzmann thrombasthenia usually are asymptomatic and generally have normal results on platelet function tests,[6,24] although a prolonged bleeding time has been reported in at least one heterozygote.[56]

LABORATORY FEATURES

Table 112-3 lists the characteristic laboratory data of patients with Glanzmann thrombasthenia. Patients have normal platelet counts and morphology, prolonged bleeding times, decreased or absent clot retraction, and abnormal platelet aggregation responses to physiologic stimuli. Platelets of patients with Glanzmann thrombasthenia have a normal (or near-normal) initial slope of high-dose ristocetin-induced aggregation, reflecting the normal levels of plasma von Willebrand factor and the normal platelet GPIb-IX content. At lower doses of ristocetin, however, when GPIb-IX–mediated activation of $\alpha IIb\beta3$ normally contributes to the aggregation response, patients have decreased second wave aggregation.[138] The interesting cyclical aggregation observed at high doses of ristocetin[139] probably reflects a complex interaction between ristocetin-induced binding of von Willebrand factor to GPIb-IX and inhibition of this interaction by released ADP.[140] Glanzmann thrombasthenia platelets undergo normal shape change in response to ADP and thrombin, demonstrating their ability to undergo metabolic and cytoskeletal changes in response to these agents. Similarly, high doses of thrombin and collagen produce normal release of dense body and α-granule contents.[2,4,141] The release reaction abnormalities observed with lower doses of these agents reflect the lack of augmentation of the release reaction normally produced by platelet aggregation.[2,138,142–144]

Platelets in whole blood or platelet-rich plasma adhere to glass because fibrinogen first becomes deposited on the glass and the platelets then adhere to the immobilized fibrinogen.[145,146] Platelets from patients with Glanzmann thrombasthenia fail to adhere to glass,[2,4,145]

TABLE 112-3   LABORATORY FEATURES OF GLANZMANN THROMBASTHENIA

I.   Platelet count: Normal
II. Bleeding time: Markedly prolonged
III. Tests of platelet function
    A. Platelet aggregation
       1. Epinephrine: No observable response
       2. ADP and thrombin: Shape change, but no aggregation
       3. Collagen: Shape change followed by variable increase in light transmission most likely resulting from progressive adhesion to collagen fibers (pseudoaggregation)
       4. Ristocetin: Normal initial slope of aggregation; at low doses, inhibition of second wave; at high doses, cyclical aggregation–disaggregation
    B. Aperture closure time (PFA-100): Prolonged
    C. Clot retraction: Absent or reduced
    D. Platelet release reaction: Decreased with epinephrine and low-dose ADP, thrombin, and collagen; normal with high-dose thrombin and collagen
    E. Interaction with glass (platelet retention test): Absent or reduced
    F. Platelet coagulant activity: Variably abnormal
    G. Microparticle formation: Variably abnormal
    H. *Ex vivo* interaction with deendothelialized blood vessels in flow chambers: Marked abnormality in platelet thrombus formation and defective platelet spreading; decreased platelet adhesion at high shear rates
IV. Tests of $\alpha IIb\beta3$ and $\alpha V\beta3$ receptors: Number and functional integrity
    A. $\alpha IIb\beta3$ content: Reduced or absent, except in variants
    B. $\alpha V\beta3$ content: Reduced or absent in patients with $\beta3$ defects; normal or increased in patients with αIIb defects
    C. Platelet binding of fibrinogen and other adhesive glycoproteins to $\alpha IIb\beta3$: Reduced or absent
    D. Platelet fibrinogen content: Markedly reduced, except in some variants

thus forming the basis of their abnormality in the glass bead retention assay.[147] Platelet coagulant activity has been variably reported as normal or abnormal,[2–5,148–150] probably as a result of variations in the assays used to assess this activity or individual patient differences. A defect in platelet microparticle formation and support of thrombin generation has been identified in some patients,[149–152] but not all patients appear to share this abnormality.[153] $\alpha IIb\beta3$ and $\alpha V\beta3$ have been shown to bind prothrombin, probably accounting for some of the abnormalities identified.[154,155]

In flow chamber studies, thrombasthenic platelets adhere normally to deendothelialized blood vessels at low and intermediate shear rates but do not spread normally or form platelet thrombi.[156–158] A defect in adhesion occurs at higher shear rates. A paradoxical increase in fibrin formation on these surfaces has been observed with thrombasthenic platelets, but the explanation for this phenomenon remains unknown.[159] In contrast to normal blood, blood from nearly all patients with Glanzmann thrombasthenia fails to occlude a 150-μm aperture in collagen-coated membranes under high sheer, in the presence of either ADP or epinephrine (PFA-100).[160,161]

Platelet $\alpha IIb\beta3$ and $\alpha V\beta3$ can be quantitated by several techniques, including monoclonal antibody binding (using flow cytometry or radiolabeled binding), immunoblotting, and surface labeling followed by sodium dodecyl sulfate-polyacrylamide gel electrophoresis. Based on the results of such studies, patients with Glanzmann thrombasthenia have been subcategorized by $\alpha IIb\beta3$ content into those with less than 5 percent of normal $\alpha IIb\beta3$ (type I), 5 to 20 percent (type II), or 50 percent or more (variants).[6,162] In one review of 64 patients, 78 percent were type I, 14 percent were type II, and 8 percent were variants.[6] The subtyping of Glanzmann thrombasthenia into type I, type II, and variants predated the identification of $\alpha IIb\beta3$ abnormalities as the cause of Glanzmann thrombasthenia and was based on functional data. With current methods of more precise laboratory analysis and recognition of the diverse clinical and functional abnormalities present in Glanzmann thrombasthenia, this categorization provides only limited information.

Measuring $\alpha V\beta3$ content is technically more demanding than measuring $\alpha IIb\beta3$ because so few $\alpha V\beta3$ receptors are present per platelet.[111] The $\alpha V\beta3$ level is useful, however, for making a preliminary assessment of whether the patient has a defect in αIIb or $\beta3$, because generally patients who lack $\beta3$ also lack $\alpha V\beta3$ receptors.[163] However, a $\beta3$ missense mutation (H280P) that differentially affected $\alpha IIb\beta3$ more than $\alpha V\beta3$ has been described.[65]

Fibrinogen binding studies assess the function of the $\alpha IIb\beta3$ complex.[10,11] One method consists of adding radiolabeled fibrinogen to platelets suspended in buffer (prepared by washing or gel filtration) and then measuring the binding of radioactivity when the platelets are stimulated with ADP[10,11] or a similar agonist. Fibrinogen also can be labeled with a fluorescent molecule and then flow cytometry used to measure fibrinogen binding. These techniques are most useful for detecting qualitative abnormalities of $\alpha IIb\beta3$ in patients with variant Glanzmann thrombasthenia. Binding of a monoclonal antibody (PAC1) to platelets gives similar information because the antibody only binds to the activated form of $\alpha IIb\beta3$.[164]

Carriers of Glanzmann thrombasthenia have essentially normal platelet function.[83] However, their platelets contain only approximately 60 percent of the normal number of $\alpha IIb\beta3$ receptors. The overlap in values between normals and carriers does not, however, permit unequivocal diagnosis of carriers by this technique.[165] Carrier detection is most accurately performed by DNA analysis when the defect is known, and advances in polymerase chain reaction technology allows such analysis even when using DNA obtained from cells in random urine samples.[21]

Platelet fibrinogen is reduced to approximately 10 percent of normal in patients with marked reductions in $\alpha IIb\beta 3^{2,5,92,93}$ but is variably reduced in patients with significant amounts of $\alpha IIb\beta 3$.[162,166,167] Its presence may provide insights into the nature of the functional defect.

DIFFERENTIAL DIAGNOSIS
A history of mucocutaneous hemorrhage, as opposed to hemarthroses and muscle hemorrhage, helps to differentiate disorders of platelet function (including von Willebrand disease and afibrinogenemia) from the hemophilias and related disorders. The symptoms of qualitative platelet function disorders and thrombocytopenia are essentially identical, so their differentiation depends on laboratory studies, most importantly the platelet count. Similarly, the symptoms of von Willebrand disease, afibrinogenemia, and the different qualitative platelet disorders often are indistinguishable, and again laboratory tests are required to make the definitive diagnosis. Hereditary disorders, such as Glanzmann thrombasthenia, usually are present at birth or have onset in early childhood. Thus, the history can be helpful in distinguishing inherited from acquired abnormalities. Figure 112-1 is a flow diagram depicting a logical series of steps that can be taken to evaluate patients with mucocutaneous hemorrhage.

Autoantibodies to $\alpha IIb\beta 3$ may produce the phenotype of Glanzmann disease and many of the characteristic laboratory abnormalities.[168–176] Mixing studies using patient plasma and normal platelets should identify these acquired autoimmune disorders.

THERAPY, COURSE, AND PROGNOSIS
Therapy involves both preventive measures and treatment of specific bleeding episodes. Dental hygiene is especially important for minimizing gingival hemorrhage. Antiplatelet agents should be avoided. Iron and folate may be needed in patients with ongoing hemorrhage sufficient to cause anemia and iron depletion. Hepatitis B vaccine should be administered early in life, using a small-gauge needle and with prolonged direct pressure to the injection site to prevent excessive bleeding.

Antifibrinolytic agents are useful in patients with gingival bleeding or who are undergoing tooth extractions. Either ε-aminocaproic acid (40 mg/kg given orally four times daily)[6] or tranexamic acid (0.5–1.0 g given orally three or four times daily)[177,178] has been recommended based on studies in patients with hemophilia A or B. Tranexamic acid usually produces fewer gastrointestinal side effects than ε-aminocaproic acid. These agents are contraindicated if disseminated intravascular coagulation is present. A tranexamic acid mouthwash (10 ml of a 5% solution used four times daily) is effective in controlling gum bleeding in patients treated with oral anticoagulants and in patients with hemophilia,[179] and this agent may be helpful in patients with Glanzmann thrombasthenia.

Antifibrinolytic agents may be effective in controlling menstrual bleeding in patients with relatively mild hemorrhagic symptoms. In those with more severe menorrhagia, hormonal therapy to suppress menses should be considered, although the long-term consequences of such therapy must be considered. Menorrhagia often is most severe at the time of menarche and can result in the need for emergency hysterectomy.[180] Thus, patients should be counseled to seek medical attention immediately at the time of menarche. Desmopressin (DDAVP) (see Chap. 118) usually does not normalize the bleeding time in patients with Glanzmann thrombasthenia,[6,181] but exceptions have been reported.[182] Anecdotal reports suggest desmopressin may improve hemostasis, even without normalizing the bleeding time.[182,183]

Topical agents can help arrest bleeding in Glanzmann thrombasthenia patients. Gelfoam (a form of resolvable, oxidized, regenerated cellulose) soaked in either tranexamic acid[184] or topical thrombin may be effective. Fibrin sealants prepared from a source of fibrinogen and

a source of thrombin, with or without antifibrinolytic agents or other components, have been used successfully in patients with Glanzmann thrombasthenia and in one study eliminated the need for platelet transfusion at the time of tooth extractions.[185,186] Bovine thrombin, however, has induced antibody formation to itself and contaminating factors V and XI. At least some antibodies to factor V have cross-reacted with human factor V and caused serious hemorrhage.[187–189] Immunoglobulin (Ig)E-mediated anaphylaxis has been reported with bovine topical thrombin.[190,191] A microfibrillar collagen hemostatic agent of bovine origin has been used to secure hemostasis in bleeding normal individuals. However, antibodies to bovine (and rabbit) tissue factor have been identified in some patients treated with this hemostatic agent, but the antibodies did not cross-react with human tissue factor or induce a hemorrhagic diathesis.[192] For dental procedures, custom splints of soft acrylic or celluloid help prevent excessive hemorrhage.[186,193]

Control of epistaxis can be particularly difficult. A stepwise approach has been described that involves the following: elevation of the head and local pressure; topical vasoconstriction with cottonoid pledgets and oxymetazoline; cauterization with silver nitrate or trichloroacetic acid; anterior packing; posterior packing; and, finally, arterial ligation or embolic occlusion of the internal maxillary artery.[136] When simple topical measures fail to control bleeding, platelet transfusions are administered.

Postpartum hemorrhage may benefit from administration of prostaglandin E_2 in Ringer lactate solution via continuous intrauterine irrigation.[194] This experimental technique has been effective in normal patients with severe postpartum hemorrhage, but additional data about its effectiveness in patients with platelet disorders are required.

Erythropoietin reportedly improved the bleeding time and glass bead column platelet retention in one patient with Glanzmann thrombasthenia, without producing a significant increase in hemoglobin concentration.[182] A positive effect of erythropoietin on platelet function, independent of an effect on hemoglobin, has also been reported in patients with uremia.[195–197]

Transfusion of platelets (see Chap. 132) is the mainstay of therapy for serious bleeding in Glanzmann thrombasthenia and as prophylaxis prior to surgery or other major hemostatic stresses. Judging the effect of transfusion on hemostasis prior to a procedure may be difficult because a platelet count increment may be difficult to establish above a normal baseline level, and the bleeding time has major limitations with regard to reproducibility and requires considerable operator skill. Shortening the closure time of the aperture of a collagen-coated membrane in the presence of ADP or epinephrine (PFA-100) has been recommended to monitor therapy.[198] One of the authors (B.S.C.) has used a prototype version of the Rapid Platelet Function Assay,[199] which assesses the ability of platelets activated with a thrombin receptor activating peptide to agglutinate fibrinogen-coated beads (unpublished data).

Because patients may require transfusions throughout their lifetimes, hepatitis B vaccine should be administered at an early age. All transfusions of platelets and packed red blood cells should be given with leukocyte-depletion filters to decrease the risk of alloimmunization[200] and cytomegalovirus (CMV) transmission.[201] Febrile transfusion reactions can be diminished by leukocyte depletion at the time of blood collection.[202,203] Even in patients who are refractory to platelets, leukocyte-depletion filters may improve the recovery of transfused platelets in the circulation.[204] Whenever possible, females of childbearing potential who are Rh negative should be given Rh-negative platelets. Platelets prepared by apheresis may have less erythrocyte contamination, but whether this reduction translates into decreased immunization is not clear.[205] If no alternative to Rh-positive platelets is available, patients should also receive anti-D therapy to neutralize the Rh antigen.[206] Use of only human leukocyte antigen (HLA)-matched platelets, even early in the course of the disease, to minimize the risk of alloimmunization may be justified.[207] Matching A, B, O blood group status in platelet transfusions is preferable because it may improve platelet response and will decrease the risk of a hemolytic transfusion reaction, which has been reported on rare occasions when transfusing type O platelets into type A individuals.[205] Use of platelets prepared by apheresis of a single individual compared with pooling of platelets concentrates obtained from whole blood donations will decrease the number of donor exposures but may increase the possibility of a severe reaction because more plasma ($\sim$200 ml) is transfused from a single individual with this product than with pooled donor platelets ($\sim$40–60 ml/U). Use of family members' platelets may be convenient, but if consideration is given to marrow transplantation from a family member, avoiding donations from family members may be advisable. Blood from family members should be irradiated to prevent transfusion-related graft-versus-host disease. Similarly, if bone marrow transplantation is considered and the patient has not already developed CMV infection, selecting blood from donors who do not have evidence of CMV infection may be desirable.

Platelet alloimmunization poses several different problems in patients with Glanzmann thrombasthenia, depending upon the antigen involved. In addition to antibodies directed at platelet proteins other than $\alpha IIb\beta 3$, such as HLA determinants, patients can make several different types of antibodies to αIIb and/or $\beta 3$, including antibodies to (1) the well-recognized polymorphic alloantigens on αIIb and $\beta 3$ (see Chap. 129)[208,209]; (2) other regions of $\alpha IIb\beta 3$ that are not involved in ligand binding; and (3) the ligand-binding regions of $\alpha IIb\beta 3$. Because the platelets from most patients with Glanzmann thrombasthenia lack $\alpha IIb\beta 3$ and thus the $\alpha IIb\beta 3$ alloantigens, antibodies against these determinants and against other nonligand-binding domains of $\alpha IIb\beta 3$ theoretically could be produced as a result of either transfusions or pregnancy. Such antibodies could result in refractoriness to platelet transfusions, a predisposition to developing posttransfusion purpura, or a predisposition to having children with neonatal isoimmune thrombocytopenia (see Chap. 110).[208] In one report, platelets from Pl[A2] (HPA1b/b) donors were less reactive with serum from a multiply transfused patient than platelets containing the Pl[A1] alloantigen, and platelets from Pl[A2] donors produced good platelet increments when transfused into the patient.[209] One possible case of neonatal thrombocytopenia in a Glanzmann patient has been reported, but an autoantibody could not be excluded.[210]

Development of antibodies that inhibit $\alpha IIb\beta 3$ function has the potential to make further platelet transfusions ineffectual, even if the platelets circulate. Several such cases have been reported.[6,210–214] The antibodies produced by the patients induce a thrombasthenic defect in the transfused normal platelets. If patients with antibodies to $\alpha IIb\beta 3$ (which block ligand binding) have severe hemorrhage, attempting to mechanically remove the offending plasma antibodies is reasonable, but the efficacy of such treatment is not defined and at best provides only short-term benefit.[214–216] Of note, at least one patient who had an inhibiting antibody for more than 15 years without significant hemorrhage has been reported.[6,217]

Allogeneic marrow transplantation has been reported in several patients with Glanzmann thrombasthenia. The first was a 5-year-old boy who had several severe gastrointestinal hemorrhages.[218] His bleeding diathesis was cured, and the patient was alive and well. However, he developed mild graft-versus-host disease 16 years after transplant.[219] The second patient, who required multiple hospital admissions to control bleeding but who had received a platelet transfusion only once, was transplanted at age 2.5 years from an HLA-identical sibling who was heterozygous for Glanzmann thrombasthenia.[220] She was well 19 months after the transplant. The third patient was trans-

planted at age 5 years with marrow from a sibling and did well.[221] The fourth patient, the sister of the first patient, was 16 years of age at the time of transplantation, and she also had an uneventful course.[219] Nonmyeloablative bone marrow transplantation has been performed successfully in a dog model of Glanzmann thrombasthenia.[222] *In utero* transplantation at 16 weeks' gestation of fetal liver cells from a 16-week fetus led to platelet alloantigen chimerism 3 weeks later (at the time of pregnancy termination), supporting the potential of such therapy for treating fetuses with Glanzmann thrombasthenia.[223]

Recombinant factor VIIa (rFVIIa) has been used to treat patients with Glanzmann thrombasthenia with considerable but not universal success. Rare thromboembolic complications have been reported in association with rFVIIa therapy.[198,224–227] The optimal dose and duration of therapy remain uncertain, as does the relative role of this treatment compared to platelet transfusion. Thus, the justification for rFVIIa is strongest for patients who have not responded to platelet transfusions, who are known to have antibodies that are associated with refractoriness to platelet transfusions, or who have antibodies to $\alpha IIb\beta 3$ that may inhibit platelet function. The mechanism(s) by which rFVIIa improves hemostasis in patients with Glanzmann thrombasthenia is still under study, but available data support several possibilities, including facilitated platelet–fibrin interactions,[228] enhanced thrombin generation and fibrin production on the platelet surface,[198,226,229] and enhanced adhesion of platelets to endothelial cell matrix and collagen.[230] Several of these phenomena can occur even in the absence of tissue factor.[228,230]

Progress in gene therapy approaches to correcting the genetic defect in Glanzmann thrombasthenia in megakaryocytes has been made.[231,232] Several animal models are available, including a β_3-null mouse model[233] and two dog models involving mutations in α_{IIb}.[234] Thus, as methods of marrow transplantation and gene transfer therapy improve, reassessing the risk-to-benefit ratios of these therapies for individual patients with Glanzmann thrombasthenia will become important.

Although Glanzmann thrombasthenia is a severe disease, the prognosis for survival is generally good. In one series, two of 64 patients died of hemorrhage; in another study, three of 43 patients died of hemorrhage.[6,24] A nationwide survey in Japan identified 98 Glanzmann thrombasthenia patients in 1976 and 192 patients in 1991.[235] The mortality rate decreased substantially during this time interval.

GLYCOPROTEIN Ib (CD42B,C), GLYCOPROTEIN IX (CD42A), AND GLYCOPROTEIN V: BERNARD-SOULIER SYNDROME

DEFINITION AND HISTORY

Bernard-Soulier syndrome is an inherited disorder of the platelet GPIb-IX-V complex characterized by thrombocytopenia, giant platelets, and a failure of platelets to bind GPIb ligands, most importantly, von Willebrand factor and thrombin.[236,237]

In 1948, Bernard and Soulier[238,239] described two children from a consanguineous family who had a severe bleeding disorder characterized by mucocutaneous hemorrhage. Evaluation of the patients' blood revealed variable thrombocytopenia and giant platelets. Beginning in the early 1970s, Bernard-Soulier syndrome platelets were shown to have a functional defect in von Willebrand factor-dependent platelet adhesion and agglutination.[240–242] In 1975, Nurden and Caen[243] identified an abnormality in platelet GPIb as the cause of the functional defect. Subsequent studies confirmed the defect in von Willebrand factor–GPIb interactions[244–246] and identified additional defects in platelet GPV and GPIX.[247,248] Later studies identified additional ligands for the GPIb-IX complex, including thrombin,[249] P-selectin,[250] leukocyte integrin $\alpha M\beta 2$,[251] high molecular weight kininogen,[252] and coagulation factors XI[253] and XII,[254] but the precise contributions of these interactions to the disorder are not well defined. A mouse model of Bernard-Soulier syndrome has been produced by gene targeting of GPIbα,[255] but mice deficient in GPV do not demonstrate the typical features of human Bernard-Soulier syndrome and paradoxically have an increased platelet response to thrombin.[256]

ETIOLOGY AND PATHOGENESIS

Epidemiology This rare disease, with a prevalence estimated as less than one in 1,000,000, has been reported from countries around the world.[68,236,239,247,257–326] Consanguinity is common in families with affected children[239] because the disorder usually is inherited as an autosomal recessive trait and because spontaneous mutations appear infrequently. However, an autosomal dominant form of the disease has been reported.[280]

Causes of Hemorrhage Six different features of Bernard-Soulier syndrome may contribute to the hemorrhagic diathesis: thrombocytopenia, abnormal platelet interactions with von Willebrand factor, abnormal platelet interactions with thrombin, abnormal platelet coagulant activity, abnormal platelet interactions with P-selectin, and abnormal platelet interactions with leukocyte integrin αMβ2.

The pathophysiology of thrombocytopenia is uncertain. Early studies suggested a marked shortening of platelet survival, presumably because of the decrease in platelet surface charge resulting from the GPIb defect.[327,328] Later studies using [111]Indium-oxine to label platelets reported more modest or no shortening of platelet survival, suggesting that ineffective thrombopoiesis and/or decreased thrombopoiesis contribute to thrombocytopenia.[329,330] Morphologic abnormalities have been identified in Bernard-Soulier syndrome megakaryocytes and may contribute to abnormal platelet production.[331] Based upon observations in other giant platelet syndromes (see Chap. 110), the large size of Bernard-Soulier platelets would tend to diminish the adverse hemostatic effects of the thrombocytopenia because the platelet mass is better preserved. However, in fact, the bleeding diathesis with Bernard-Soulier syndrome is more severe than expected from the thrombocytopenia, reinforcing the conclusion that a qualitative platelet defect is also present.[217,239]

The platelet GPIb-IX complex functions as a receptor for von Willebrand factor (see Chaps. 105 and 118).[236,332,333] This interaction is crucial for the adhesion of platelets to subendothelial surfaces, especially under high shear conditions, where von Willebrand factor acts as a bridge between the subendothelial matrix and the platelet.[157,158] The relative roles of subendothelial von Willebrand factor, plasma von Willebrand factor, and platelet von Willebrand factor are not completely defined, but they probably all contribute.[333] The interaction of von Willebrand factor with GPIb-IX initiates activation of αIIbβ3,[334] which can also bind to von Willebrand factor but at a different site on the molecule. The interaction of GPIb-IX with von Willebrand factor also directly contributes to platelet–platelet interactions.[335,336]

GPIb-IX–von Willebrand factor interactions can occur in platelet suspensions at high shear rates, which can lead to platelet activation with subsequent aggregation mediated by αIIbβ3.[333,337–339] Whether sustained shear rates *in vivo* ever reach the levels required to initiate von Willebrand factor binding is not established.

The platelets of patients with Bernard-Soulier syndrome have a decreased response to platelet activation by thrombin, especially at limiting concentrations of thrombin.[340–343] Bernard-Soulier platelets are deficient in two different proteins that interact with thrombin, namely, GPIbα, which binds thrombin,[249] and GPV, which is a thrombin substrate (see Chap. 105). The precise nature of the interactions of thrombin with GPIbα and its biologic consequences are unclear, but binding of thrombin to GPIbα can initiate signaling within the platelet, perhaps directly through GPIbα cross-linking or indirectly by augmenting other thrombin-dependent events at the platelet surface.[249]

Paradoxically, mice deficient in GPV actually have increased sensitivity to thrombin activation and increased thrombus formation, perhaps because GPV limits access of thrombin to GPIb.[344,345] Because thrombin is one of the major physiologic activators of platelets, this abnormality may also contribute to the hemorrhagic diathesis.

Bernard-Soulier platelets appear to be defective in supporting thrombin generation as judged by the serum prothrombin time,[346] a test performed with whole blood. However, in other tests of platelet coagulant activity, Bernard-Soulier platelets support coagulation as well as or better than normal platelets.[148,347] Defects in collagen-induced coagulant activity and the association of factors V, VIII, and XI with Bernard-Soulier platelets have been described,[347] but their significance is unclear. Similarly, GPIb-IX has been identified as a binding site for other proteins involved in coagulation, including high molecular weight kininogen and factors XI and XII, but the contributions of these interactions to the coagulant abnormality are uncertain.[252–254] Abnormal membrane lipids have also been reported.[348] Binding of von Willebrand factor to GPIb-IX has been implicated in fibrin-dependent, but not fibrin-independent, augmentation of platelet coagulant activity. Thus, fibrin-dependent coagulant activity likely is abnormal in Bernard-Soulier syndrome.[150] This finding may explain, at least in part, the variability in findings between the serum prothrombin time and some of the other assays, as the serum prothrombin time is one of the few assays used to assess platelet coagulant activity in which fibrin forms.

The mechanism(s) producing the giant platelets in Bernard-Soulier syndrome has not been identified, but because giant platelets are found in Bernard-Soulier syndrome variants in which GPIb-IX is present but is unable to bind ligand, the abnormality has been proposed to result from the inability of GPIb-IX to bind a postulated novel bone marrow ligand.[236] It cannot result from an inability to bind von Willebrand factor given that patients lacking von Willebrand factor do not have large platelets. Moreover, in a mouse model of Bernard-Soulier syndrome, restoring a receptor with the GPIb transmembrane and cytoplasmic domains, but not the ligand-binding domain, partially corrected both the thrombocytopenia and large platelet size.[349] A defect in GPIb-IX–mediated signaling also has been proposed to cause the large platelets, as a deficiency of phospholipase C has been described in Bernard-Soulier syndrome.[236,350] A mechanical alteration in the plasma membrane of Bernard-Soulier platelets has been identified by micropipette experiments showing the plasma membrane was more deformable than normal.[351] Megakaryocytes in Bernard-Soulier syndrome have increased ploidy and volume and alterations in the membrane demarcation system, granules, and microtubules.[330,331] Both the increased size and deformability may reflect the loss of normal interaction of GPIb-IX with the cytoskeleton via actin-binding protein (filamin-1) (see Chap. 105).

Bernard-Soulier platelets are deficient not only in GPIbα, GPIbβ, and GPIX, which are known to be associated as a complex, but also in GPV (see Chap. 105).[236,248,352] Of considerable interest is that all of these proteins share highly conserved leucine-rich regions.[236,332,333] One possible explanation for the loss of surface expression of all the proteins is that they must form a complex during biosynthesis in order to be transported to the surface.[333] Evidence supports the need for the presence of GPIbα, GPIbβ, and GPIX for optimal surface expression,[353] but data from mice deficient in GPV indicate this glycoprotein is not required for surface expression of the GPIb-IX complex.[344] Moreover, data from the Bernard-Soulier mouse expressing a chimeric GPIbα molecule in which the leucine-rich repeat domain was replaced with the external domain of another receptor indicate that complex formation does not require the GPIbα leucine-rich domain.[349]

At the molecular level, the platelets from different patients with Bernard-Soulier syndrome are heterogeneous. Many have no detectable GPIb, whereas others have variable amounts, up to 50 percent of normal.[236,267,269,274,276,350,354,355] Variability in the degree of concordance in the reduction of GPIb and the other deficient proteins also is observed.[282,356]

Molecular Biologic Defects The molecular biologic basis of Bernard-Soulier syndrome has been determined in a number of patients (Table 112-4). Defects have been identified in GPIbα, GPIbβ, and GPIX but not in GPV. Nearly half of the defects affect the leucine-rich repeats or the conserved flanking sequences, supporting the importance of these structural elements in the biogenesis and surface expression of the GPIb-IX-V complex (Fig. 112-4). Three patients homozygous for a deletion in the last two bases of codon 492 of GPIbα (nucleotides 1523 and 1524) resulting in a frameshift that alters the membrane-spanning region and leads to premature termination have been described, and another patient heterozygous for this deletion and a missense mutation of GPIbα has been described.[295,297,298,305] These defects appear to result in a poorly anchored GPIbα with GPIbα antigen present in plasma. Haplotype analysis indicated that the three identical mutations in Caucasians may have derived from a common founder. A homozygous Y88C defect in GPIbβ has been reported to cause Bernard-Soulier syndrome in two Japanese families, and heterozygotes with this mutation have a giant platelet syndrome.[298,312] Similarly, a patient heterozygous for a GPIbβ R17C mutation also had a giant platelet syndrome.[315] An N45S mutation in GPIX affecting leu-

cine-rich repeat 1 has been reported in at least eight different Caucasian patients.[304,316]

Bernard-Soulier syndrome in association with hemizygous deletion of GPIbβ and several neighboring genes on chromosome 22q11.2, the DiGeorge/velocardiofacial syndrome, has been reported in several patients.[290,323–326] Hemizygous mutations in the remaining GPIbβ allele include P96S and P29L.[324,325] In other studies of patients with the 22q11.2 deletion syndrome, modest reductions in platelet count and increases in platelet volume, as well as reduced platelet agglutination to ristocetin and decreased platelet GPIb-IX expression, have been variably reported, consistent with hemizygosity for GPIbβ.[301,357–360]

Several variants of Bernard-Soulier syndrome have been described. An autosomal dominant form has been ascribed to a heterozygous mutation in the second leucine-rich repeat (L57F).[280] Presumably, the abnormal GPIbα interferes with the function of the normal GPIbα. The affected patients have moderate bleeding symptoms, moderate thrombocytopenia, and giant platelets. The GPIb is unusually susceptible to proteolysis and functions ineffectively with regard to its interactions with von Willebrand factor. The Bolzano defect, which has been described in two patients, involves the sixth leucine-rich repeat of GPIbα (A156V). This mutation results in a GPIbα molecule that cannot bind von Willebrand factor but can bind thrombin. In one patient, the Bolzano defect was homozygous, and the patient had nearly normal levels of GPIb-IX-V complex.[275] In the other patient, it

TABLE 112-4　SELECT MOLECULAR BIOLOGIC ABNORMALITIES IN BERNARD-SOULIER SYNDROME

GPIbα MUTATIONS

PATIENT DESIGNATION	GENOTYPE	MUTATION	PHENOTYPE	AMINO ACID SUBSTITUTION	AFFECTED LEUCINE REPEATS	REFERENCE
Caucasian male	Heterozygous autosomal dominant	217C→T	Missense	L57F*	II	280
Bolzano variant male	Homozygous	515C→T	Missense	A156V	VI	283
Female	Compound heterozygous	515C→T	Missense	A156V	VI	306
		554-589del	Del: In frame	N169-Q180del→E181K	VII	
TP1, TP2	Heterozygous	515C→T	Missense	A156V	VII	684
Finnish female	Homozygous	1523ATdel	Del: Out of frame	Premature termination		305
Caucasian female	Homozygous	1523ATdel	Del: Out of frame	Premature termination		295
Caucasian female	Homozygous	1523ATdel	Del: Out of frame	Premature termination		296

GPIbβ MUTATIONS

PATIENT DESIGNATION	GENOTYPE	MUTATION	PHENOTYPE	AMINO ACID SUBSTITUTION	REFERENCE
SF	Heterozygous	124C→T	Missense	R17C	315
Japanese family I	Homozygous	338A→G	Missense	Y88C	312
Japanese family II	Compound	338*A→G	Missense	Y88C	298
	Heterozygous	457G→C	Missense	A108P	
NIH patient	Hemizgyous/22q11.2 del	C→T	Missense	P96S	324
Irish patient	Hemizgyous/22q11.2 del		Missense	P29L	325

GPIX MUTATIONS

PATIENT DESIGNATION	GENOTYPE	MUTATION	PHENOTYPE	AMINO ACID SUBSTITUTION	AFFECTED LEUCINE REPEATS	REFERENCE
Female	Compound heterozygous	110*A→G	Missense	D21G	N-Flank	282
		182A→G	Missense	N45S	I	
Caucasian male	Homozygous	182A→G	Missense	N45S	I	685
Finnish 5 families, 3 female, 2 male	Homozygous	182A→G	Missense	N45S	I	686
Patients 1–4	Homozygous	182A→G	Missense	N45S	I	307

* Amino acid numbering begins with the first amino acid of the mature protein (excluding the leader sequence) as +1. Amino acid numbers including the leader sequence are determined by adding 16 residues for GPIbα, 25 residues for GPIbβ, and 16 residues for GPIX.

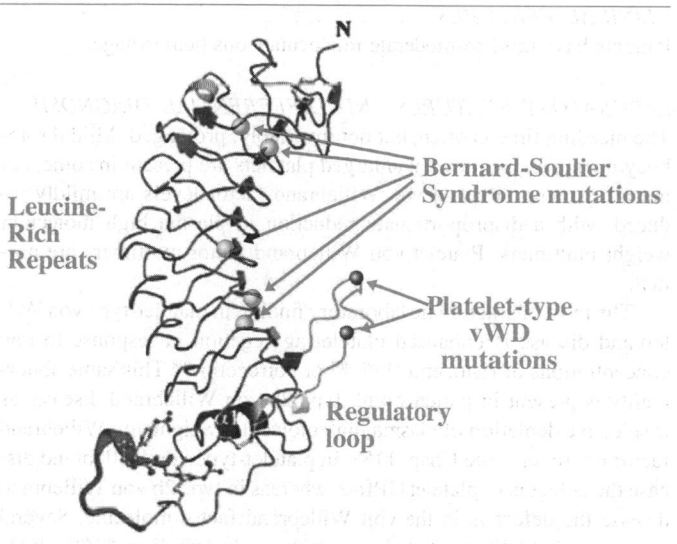

FIGURE 112-4 Localization of select missense mutations causing platelet-type von Willebrand disease (vWD) and Bernard-Soulier syndrome in the GPIbα N-terminal domain. Ribbon diagram of the topology of GPIbα N-terminal domain viewed from the side. The regulatory loop is colored *blue* with activating platelet-type vWD mutations G233V and M239V indicated as *open black balls*. Five Bernard-Soulier syndrome mutations, which cause loss of von Willebrand factor binding, are shown as *blue balls*. L57F and C65R localize to leucine-rich repeat (LRR) 2, with L129P, A156V, and L179del localized to the LRR5, LRR6, and LRR7 β-strands, respectively. The molecular structure of the sulfated tyrosine residues 276, 278, and 279 are shown. (Adapted from Uff et al.,[402] with permission.)

coexisted with a 12-amino-acid deletion and an amino acid substitution (Q181K); GPIbα platelet expression was markedly reduced in this patient.[306] A Japanese patient heterozygous for two mutations in GPIbβ, one of which produced an additional Cys at amino acid 88, had a mild bleeding disorder, significant amounts of functional platelet GPIb-IX-V complex, and very large platelets. Of note, the patient did not have thrombocytopenia. A defect in GPIbβ cross-linking to GPIbα was proposed as the cause of the abnormality.[298]

CLINICAL FEATURES

Epistaxis is the most common symptom of Bernard-Soulier syndrome (70%), with ecchymoses (58%), menometrorrhagia (44%), gingival hemorrhage (42%), and gastrointestinal bleeding (22%) also common.[239] Hemorrhagic symptoms that occur with lower frequency include posttraumatic bleeding (13%), hematuria (7%), cerebral hemorrhage (4%), and retinal hemorrhage (2%). Considerable variability in symptoms exists among patients,[217] even among patients within a single family.[236,361] A review that includes brief descriptions of the clinical features of 55 patients reported through 1998 has been published.[236]

LABORATORY FEATURES

Platelet Number and Morphology Thrombocytopenia is present in nearly all patients but varies in severity, ranging from approximately 20,000 platelets/μl to near-normal levels. Platelets are large on blood film. More than one third usually have diameters greater than 3.5 μm, and some are as large or larger than lymphocytes. By electron microscopy, platelets display only minor variations in vesicular structures and the open canalicular system,[239] but megakaryocytes have more notable abnormalities in their demarcation membranes.[331] The membrane of Bernard-Soulier platelets appears to be more deformable than

normal,[351] perhaps because GPIb ordinarily interacts with the platelet cytoskeleton (see Chap. 105).[362]

Bleeding Time The bleeding time almost always is prolonged, but the degree of prolongation varies. Closure times of the apertures of collagen-coated membranes are markedly prolonged in the presence of ADP or epinephrine (PFA-100).[160]

Platelet Aggregation The hallmark finding in the Bernard-Soulier syndrome is the failure of platelets to aggregate in response to ristocetin[241] or botrocetin,[244,363] agents that require von Willebrand factor–GPIb interactions, in von Willebrand disease, but not Bernard-Soulier syndrome, this defect can be corrected by adding normal plasma (or von Willebrand factor).

Although the large size of the platelets in Bernard-Soulier syndrome and the thrombocytopenia make performing platelet aggregation studies technically difficult, aggregation induced by ADP, epinephrine, or collagen generally is either normal or enhanced.[242,278,364] The response to thrombin usually is dose dependent, with essentially a normal response at high doses of thrombin[341] but with a prolonged lag phase and a diminished response at low doses of thrombin.[340,365]

Platelet Coagulant Activity The coagulant activity of Bernard-Soulier platelets has been variably reported as reduced, normal, or increased.[148,346,347] The variable presence of fibrin in the different assays used to assess platelet coagulant activity may account for these inconsistent results, because GPIb–von Willebrand factor interactions enhance platelet coagulant activity when fibrin is present but not when it is absent.[150]

Platelet–Thrombin Interactions Both GPIb and the seven transmembrane domain receptors are required for maximal response to thrombin.[249,365] Two somewhat different crystal structures of the interactions between thrombin and GPIbα have been reported. Since two molecules of thrombin may be able to bind to each GPIbα molecule and multiple sites on thrombin can interact with GPIbα, it is possible that free thrombin or thrombin adherent to fibrin clusters GPIb-IX-V complexes.[249,366,367] GPV, which is missing from the platelet surface in Bernard-Soulier syndrome, is cleaved by thrombin, but the cleavage is neither necessary nor sufficient for thrombin-induced platelet activation.[368,369] In fact, platelets of mice lacking GPV have increased responsiveness to thrombin, perhaps because GPV ordinarily limits access of thrombin to GPIbα or inhibits GPIbα cross-linking.[344,345]

***Ex Vivo* Interaction with Subendothelial Surfaces** Bernard-Soulier platelets demonstrate defective adhesion to subendothelial surfaces, especially at shear rates greater than 650 s⁻¹.[157,158,240,370] The results are similar to those in patients with von Willebrand disease.

Shear-Induced Platelet Aggregation Unlike normal platelets, Bernard-Soulier platelets are not aggregated by high shear rates.[337,338] The initial interaction in this process appears to be binding of von Willebrand factor to GPIb,[333] with subsequent activation of αIIbβ3, perhaps through signaling via the protein 14-3-3ζ associated with the cytoplasmic domain of GPIbα[339,371] or either Fcγ receptor IIA or the Fc receptor γ-chain, both of which have been identified as linked to the GPIb-IX complex and both of which are capable of initiating signal transduction (see Chap. 105).[372,373] Pathologic shear stress reportedly increased binding of α-actin to GPIb-IX as part of the signaling process.[374]

DIFFERENTIAL DIAGNOSIS

The differential diagnosis of Bernard-Soulier syndrome is discussed in the "Differential Diagnosis" of Glanzmann thrombasthenia above. Acquired Bernard-Soulier syndrome caused by autoantibodies,[375–379] as part of a juvenile myelodysplastic syndrome,[380,381] and in association with acute myelogenous leukemia has been reported.[381]

THERAPY, COURSE, AND PROGNOSIS

The therapy of Bernard-Soulier syndrome is essentially identical to that for Glanzmann thrombasthenia (see section on "Glanzman Thrombasthemia, Therapy, Course, and Prognosis"). Splenectomy has been performed when the diagnosis of immune thrombocytopenia was mistakenly made, but this procedure usually does not normalize the platelet count or improve the bleeding diathesis.[306] Oral contraceptives can control menorrhagia.[382] Desmopressin (DDAVP) has been variably effective in decreasing the bleeding time.[183,266,268,278,293,300,383–386] Platelet transfusions are effective when needed but carry a risk of alloimmunization, including the production of antibodies to the functional region of GPIb.[387,388] Factor VIIa infusion has been reported in several patients and may be beneficial, but the proper indications, dose, and duration are uncertain.[226,389] Patients have achieved successful pregnancies and deliveries, but serious delayed bleeding can occur, and emergency hysterectomy has been required to control the hemorrhage.[258,261,271,281,302,388] Neonatal thrombocytopenia presumed to result from maternal alloimmunization has been reported.[388] Two sisters with serious bleeding episodes who developed antibodies to the GPIb-IX-V complex and refractoriness to platelet transfusions underwent successful hematopoietic stem cell transplantation from an HLA-identical sibling.[390]

As with Glanzmann thrombasthenia, the prognosis of patients with Bernard-Soulier syndrome has improved as platelet transfusion support has become more readily available and other supportive measures have become more effective.

GLYCOPROTEIN Ib (CD42B,C): PLATELET-TYPE (PSEUDO-) VON WILLEBRAND DISEASE

DEFINITION AND HISTORY

A heterogeneous group of patients with mild-to-moderate bleeding symptoms, variably enlarged platelets, variable thrombocytopenia, and diminished plasma high molecular weight von Willebrand factor multimers has been described. The fundamental defect in these patients is thought to be an enhanced interaction between an abnormal platelet GPIb-IX receptor and normal plasma von Willebrand factor.[391–396] Because these patients have some of the hallmarks of von Willebrand disease but the defect is in platelet GPIb-IX, it has been termed both *pseudo-von Willebrand disease* and *platelet-type von Willebrand disease*.

ETIOLOGY AND PATHOGENESIS

A qualitative abnormality in GPIb is thought to be responsible for this disorder, with ongoing *in vivo* binding of high molecular weight von Willebrand multimers to platelets causing depletion of the plasma high molecular weight multimers. In addition, binding of von Willebrand factor to platelets may shorten platelet survival, perhaps accounting for the variable thrombocytopenia. Inheritance appears to be autosomal dominant.

Abnormalities in the M_r of GPIb identified in two families[396] may have resulted from a now-recognized polymorphism in GPIb (see Chap. 105) rather than being related to the functional disorder. Heterozygous point mutations in the GPIbα DNA (G233V, G233S, M239V) have been found in several different families.[397–401] All of these mutations are in the carboxy-terminal flanking sequence of the leucine-rich repeats, a region implicated in ligand binding (see Fig. 112-4).[236,332,333,402,403] Molecular modeling suggests that the M239V substitution produces a significant conformational change in the molecule,[404] and this was confirmed by crystallographic analysis.[405] Recombinant GPIbα fragments containing the G233V and M239V mutations demonstrated enhanced interactions with von Willebrand factor in several different systems, including those under shear stress.[406,407]

CLINICAL FEATURES

Patients have mild-to-moderate mucocutaneous hemorrhage.

LABORATORY FEATURES AND DIFFERENTIAL DIAGNOSIS

The bleeding time is often, but not invariably, prolonged. Mild thrombocytopenia and somewhat enlarged platelets are present in some, but not all, patients. Plasma von Willebrand factor levels are mildly reduced, with a disproportionate reduction in plasma high molecular weight multimers. Platelet von Willebrand factor multimers are normal.

The most characteristic laboratory finding in platelet-type von Willebrand disease is enhanced platelet aggregation in response to low concentrations of ristocetin[391–395,401] or botrocetin.[408] This same abnormality is present in patients with type 2b von Willebrand disease, as is selective depletion of plasma high molecular weight von Willebrand factor multimers (see Chap. 118). In platelet-type von Willebrand disease the defect is in platelet GPIbα, whereas in type 2b von Willebrand disease the defect is in the von Willebrand factor molecule. Several assays can help differentiate between these abnormalities[393,409–411]: (1) normal von Willebrand factor (in cryoprecipitate or purified) aggregates platelets from patients with platelet-type von Willebrand disease but not platelets from patients with type 2b von Willebrand disease; (2) isolated platelets from patients with platelet-type von Willebrand disease bind normal von Willebrand factor at lower concentrations of ristocetin than normal platelets or platelets from patients with type 2b von Willebrand disease; (3) plasma von Willebrand factor from patients with type 2b von Willebrand disease binds to normal platelets at lower than normal concentrations of ristocetin, whereas higher than normal concentrations of ristocetin are required for the plasma von Willebrand factor from patients with platelet-type von Willebrand factor to bind to normal platelets[410]; and (4) von Willebrand factor lacking sialic acid residues (asialo-von Willebrand factor) agglutinates platelets from patients with platelet-type von Willebrand disease in the presence of ethylenediaminetetraacetic acid (EDTA).[412]

THERAPY, COURSE, AND PROGNOSIS

Because normal von Willebrand factor (especially the high molecular weight forms) can bind excessively to the platelets of patients with platelet-type von Willebrand disease and potentially lead to rapid platelet clearance from the circulation, increasing the von Willebrand factor level by any means (desmopressin infusion or von Willebrand replacement with cryoprecipitate or von Willebrand factor concentrates) poses a potential risk for inducing thrombocytopenia.[409,413] It may be possible to estimate this risk by assessing whether the patient's platelets aggregate *ex vivo* in response to von Willebrand factor (as in cryoprecipitate).[392] Low-dose cryoprecipitate has successfully supported hemostasis, without inducing thrombocytopenia in patients at risk for having thrombocytopenia.[394,413,414] Currently, cryoprecipitate is generally less favored for von Willebrand factor replacement therapy than plasma-derived concentrates such as Humate-P, which is approved in the United States for the therapy of von Willebrand disease, because the latter are treated to reduce the risk of viral infection. Consideration also should be given to platelet transfusion in appropriate circumstances. Factor VIIa infusion may be beneficial but is experimental; it has the theoretical advantage of preventing excessive interactions between von Willebrand factor and the abnormal GPIbα receptor.[226,415]

α2β1 (GLYCOPROTEIN IA/IIA; VLA-2; CD49B/CD29)

α2β1 (GPIa-IIa) can mediate platelet adhesion to collagen and platelet activation under certain conditions (see Chap. 105). Nieuwenhuis and coworkers[416,417] reported a female patient with excessive posttraumatic bruising and menorrhagia but no epistaxis, gum bleeding, or excessive bleeding after tonsillectomy or appendectomy, whose platelets selectively failed to aggregate or undergo shape change in response to collagen. The bleeding time was markedly prolonged, and the patient's platelets failed to adhere and spread normally on subendothelial surfaces. The patient's platelets contained only approximately 15 to 25 percent of the normal amount of GPIa.[416,418] A reduction in GPIIa also was apparent.[416] Drawing conclusions about the physiologic role of GPIa-IIa in platelet function from this patient is difficult because her GPIa-IIa deficiency was incomplete, her bleeding symptoms were mild and variable, and some of the platelet function abnormalities (e.g., abnormal platelet–collagen interactions in the presence of the divalent chelating agent EDTA) are difficult to ascribe to the deficiency in GPIa-IIa.[416,419]

Another patient with GPIa deficiency has been described.[420] She had a history of mucocutaneous and postoperative bleeding. Her bleeding time was prolonged, and platelet aggregation in response to collagen was selectively reduced but not absent. In addition to her GPIa defect, the patient had little or no intact thrombospondin, and exogenous thrombospondin corrected the defect in platelet aggregation. The patient's hemorrhagic symptoms and platelet defects disappeared when she entered menopause.

GLYCOPROTEIN IV (CD36)

Approximately 3 percent of Japanese individuals, 2 percent of African-Americans, and 0.3 percent of Caucasians in the United States have platelets that lack GPIV (CD36).[421,422] Although GPIV (CD36) has been implicated in platelet interactions with collagen and thrombospondin[423,424] and in platelet–monocyte interactions,[425] individuals lacking GPIV (CD36) do not have a hemorrhagic diathesis. Platelets from these patients can bind thrombospondin via alternative receptors,[426] and controversy exists as to whether they have even a mild defect in adhesion to collagen.[427,428] GPIV (CD36) has been implicated as a receptor for very-low-density lipoprotein (VLDL), and binding of VLDL to GPIV (CD36) reportedly enhances collagen-induced platelet aggregation and thromboxane production.[429] Two forms of GPIV (CD36) deficiency have been described in Japan: type I in which both platelets and monocytes are deficient, and type II in which only platelets are deficient.[430] A C478T substitution leading to a Pro90Ser substitution and abnormal posttranslational modification is a common abnormality contributing to both type I and type II deficiencies. In the type I form, patients are homozygous for the abnormality, whereas in type II form, patients are doubly heterozygous for the Pro90Ser abnormality and an unidentified platelet-specific expression defect.[430,431] Other abnormalities that have been associated with type I deficiency include a dinucleotide deletion (539–540) in exon 5, a 161-bp deletion (331–491) corresponding to loss of exon 4, a nucleotide insertion at position 1159 in codon 317 leading to a frameshift and premature stop, and splice site mutations.[432–434] Other mutations have been identified in other populations.

GPIV (CD36) deficiency can result in refractoriness to platelet transfusions because of isoimmunization (see Chap. 132) and has been implicated in posttransfusion purpura (see Chap. 110).[435] GPIV (CD36) also has been implicated in monocyte binding of oxidized low-density lipoprotein and atherosclerosis, especially in diabetes, and myocardial uptake of long-chain fatty acids.[436–438] The abnormality in myocardial long-chain fatty acid uptake in individuals with type I GPIV (CD36) deficiency can be documented by nuclear medicine studies, and an association with hypertrophic cardiomyopathy may exist.[436,439] GPIV (CD36) has been implicated in the adherence of *Plasmodium falciparum* to erythrocytes, and different GPIV (CD36) mutations in African and Asian populations reportedly either predispose

to, or protect from, cerebral falciparum malaria.[440–443] GPIV (CD36)-mediated platelet clumping of *P. falciparum*-infected erythrocytes has been associated with malaria severity.[444]

GLYCOPROTEIN VI

GPVI can mediate platelet adhesion to collagen and is important in collagen-induced signal transduction (see Chap. 105). Four patients with mild-to-moderate bleeding disorders and variable deficiencies of platelet GPVI have been described; one had concomitant gray platelet syndrome (α-granule deficiency) and is discussed in the section on that disorder.[445–448] The other three patients had selective abnormalities in platelet–collagen interactions. Platelet GPVI deficiency associated with an autoantibody to GPVI has been described in three patients, one of whom also had systemic lupus erythematosis.[449–451] Studies in mice demonstrated that antibodies to GPVI can result in loss of GPVI from the platelet surface, even though the platelets continue to circulate.[452] Therefore, the deficiency of GPVI in these patients likely results from the autoantibody, especially in the one patient who had a normal GPVI nucleotide sequence and normal expression of platelet GPVI mRNA.[451] Whether the patients earlier reported as having GPVI deficiency also had an immune basis for their GPVI deficiency is unclear.

CD43: WISKOTT-ALDRICH SYNDROME

DEFINITION AND HISTORY

The Wiskott-Aldrich syndrome, which affects four of every million males worldwide, is an X chromosome-linked inherited disorder characterized by small platelets, thrombocytopenia, recurrent infections, and eczema, although only a minority of patients have all of the classic manifestations.[453–455] In addition, a variety of immunologic abnormalities affecting T lymphocyte function, immunoglobulin levels, cellular immunity, and responsiveness to polysaccharide antigens are commonly present.[453,455] The immune deficiency probably is responsible for an increase in lymphoreticular malignancies associated with the disorder. Death from infection, hemorrhage, or malignancy is common before adulthood.

ETIOLOGY AND PATHOGENESIS

The Wiskott-Aldrich syndrome protein (WASP) has been cloned and its amino acid sequence deduced from the cDNA. The protein contains a unique Wiskott homology domain, which also is present in a number of other genes that convey signals from the surface of cells to the actin cytoskeleton. Figure 112-5 depicts the other domains and their interactions with other proteins.[453] WASP is found in all hematopoietic stem cell-derived lineages. Signals from G-protein coupled receptors likely can initiate actin bundling via WASP. Most but not all patients with Wiskott-Aldrich syndrome have mutations in the WASP protein,[453] so other genes may be involved in the syndrome. Moreover, some patients with X-linked thrombocytopenia without the other associated features of Wiskott-Aldrich syndrome have mutations in WASP.[456] Of note, an apparently X-linked severe congenital neutropenia was found in a family with a constitutively activating mutation in WASP.[457] An international database of WASP mutations is available and can be accessed via the Williams Hematology 6th edition web page.[458]

A defect in the surface glycoprotein sialophorin (CD43, gp115, leukosialin) has been described in Wiskott-Aldrich syndrome.[459] CD43 is a carbohydrate-rich protein found in one form on T lymphocytes, B cells, and monocytes and in another form on neutrophils and platelets. The CD43 abnormalities most likely reflect aberrant O-linked oligosaccharide biosynthesis,[460] but the connection between the WASP defect and aberrant O-linked glycosidation is unknown. CD43 can bind

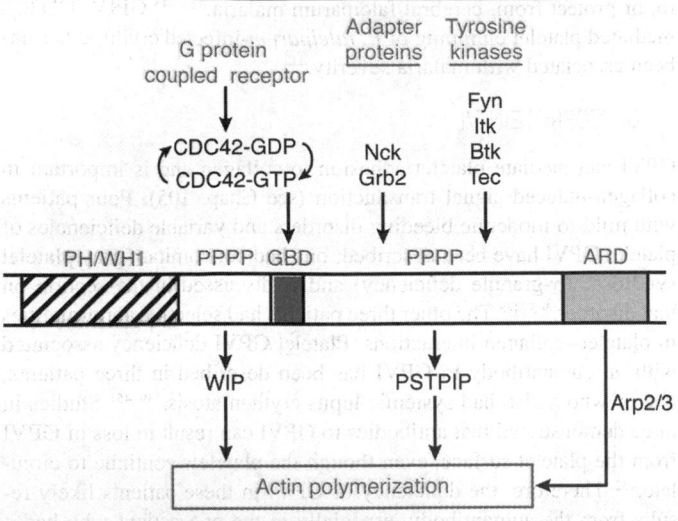

FIGURE 112-5   Domain structure of the Wiskott-Aldrich syndrome protein (WASP) and identification of molecules that interact with the protein.[675–678] The actin regulatory domain (ARD), also designated a VDA region, contains a WASP homology 2 domain (also called *verprolin homology domain*; V) followed by a "connecting" or "central" (C) region and an acidic (A) region. The intramolecular binding of the ARD region to the GTPase binding domain ([GBD] GBL or CRIB) produces autoinhibition of WASP. Binding of the small GTPase CDC42-GTP to the GBD releases the autoinhibition by interfering with binding of ARD to GBD. Phosphatidylinositol-4,5-bisphosphate also contributes to the activation. Binding of the actin-related protein (Arp) 2/3 complex, which is made up of seven proteins, to the ARD region promotes the nucleation of actin filaments. The WASP homology 1 (WH1) domain structurally resembles pleckstrin homology (PH) domains and is also termed EVH1 (Ena, vasodilatior-stimulated phosphoprotein or VASP homology 1). The WASP-interacting protein (WIP) binds to the polyproline (PPPP) region of the PH/WH1 domain and facilitates actin polymerization. The other polyproline region contains several consensus binding sites for proteins with SH3-binding domains. Adaptor proteins bind to this region and produce subcellular redistribution of WASP to sites where actin nucleation is required. The tyrosine kinases that bind to this region phosphorylate WASP itself and other substrate proteins. (Adapted from Sullivan,[453] with permission.)

intercellular adhesion molecule-1, a protein implicated in immune function,[461] so the CD43 abnormality may contribute to the immunodeficiency. Moreover, transgenic animals with overexpression of *O*-linked Core 2 GlcNAc transferase (an enzyme that modifies CD43 and is increased in Wiskott-Aldrich platelets and resting T lymphocytes) have defects in T cell function.[462] Deficiencies in platelet GPIb, perhaps also resulting from aberrant *O*-linked oligosaccharide synthesis, have been described in some patients with Wiskott-Aldrich syndrome,[459,463] but this finding is not invariant.[462,464] Deficiencies in integrin $\alpha 2$ have been recorded in some, but not all, patients.[459] Similarly, decreases in platelet $\alpha IIb\beta 3$ and GPIV have been reported based on flow cytometric studies even after normalizing for platelet size.[462]

The thrombocytopenia in Wiskott-Aldrich syndrome initially was ascribed to shortened platelet survival resulting from an intrinsic platelet defect because autologous platelet survival was found to be short and transfused normal platelets reportedly had normal survival.[465–467] However, a later study found normal autologous platelet recovery and only a modest decrease in platelet survival.[468] Because bone marrow megakaryocytes were not decreased, this finding indicated that ineffective thrombopoiesis also was contributing to the thrombocytopenia.[469] The normal level of reticulated platelets found in Wiskott-Aldrich syndrome despite the thrombocytopenia also indicates that ineffective thrombopoiesis may contribute to the thrombocytopenia.[462]

The alterations in platelet glycoproteins may contribute to these phenomena, but so might the elevated platelet-associated IgG levels founds on the platelets of patients with Wiskott-Aldrich syndrome.[462] Splenectomy consistently improves the platelet count,[470,471] which supports shortened survival as a major mechanism of thrombocytopenia. Postsplenectomy, immune thrombocytopenia as a common cause of recurrent severe thrombocytopenia and hemorrhage has been reported.[453,469,472]

The cause of the small size of the platelets is unknown but can reasonably be presumed to be related in part to an abnormality in the connection between the membrane and the cytoskeleton caused by the defect in the WASP because cytoskeletal elements have been demonstrated to be important in proplatelet production from megakaryocytes.[473] However, the spleen also appears to play a complex role in the platelet size defect because platelet size increases soon after splenectomy to near-normal values but then decreases to below normal again over a period of months.[466,470,474] Thrombocytopenia and small platelet size have been used to determine whether a fetus is affected with the syndrome, but a false-negative result has been reported, raising the possibility that platelet abnormalities develop late in gestation.[475]

Variant forms of Wiskott-Aldrich syndrome characterized by thrombocytopenia and X chromosome-linked inheritance have been reported,[456,476] some of which are associated with mutations of WASP.[456,477]

Platelets from most patients with Wiskott-Aldrich syndrome have qualitative and quantitative abnormalities. Most common is a deficiency in the storage pool of adenine nucleotides, producing a reduced positive feedback mechanism during platelet activation and aggregation.[465,467,476] Abnormalities in platelet energy metabolism also have been described.[467,478]

CLINICAL FEATURES
Hemorrhage, recurrent infections, eczema, and lymphoreticular malignancies dominate the clinical picture. Autoimmune diseases, including arthritis, vasculitis, autoimmune hemolytic anemia, and immune thrombocytopenia, may complicate the disorders.[472] Enormous variability exists in disease severity and even within individual kindreds.[453] Correlations between WASP gene mutations and clinical manifestations are inexact, but patients whose cells express full-length protein may have better immunologic function.[453,458]

LABORATORY FEATURES
The platelet count is variably reduced. Forty-four percent of patients in a large study had platelet counts $20,000/\mu l$ or less at the time of diagnosis, and the platelet volume is significantly reduced in nearly all patients.[454,469] Lymphopenia and eosinophilia are present in a minority of patients. The bleeding time usually is prolonged to a greater extent than would be expected from the platelet count. However, when the reduced platelet mass is considered, the bleeding time prolongation may not be inappropriate. Platelet aggregation and release of dense body contents are variably abnormal. Platelet ultrastructural abnormalities have been reported, but on balance platelet morphology appears to be essentially normal.[479]

Results of immunologic evaluations vary significantly, but some patients have decreased numbers of CD8+ T cells.[454] Serum IgG levels usually are normal, whereas serum IgM levels usually are depressed and serum IgA and IgE levels usually are elevated.[469] Variable deficiencies in immune response to antigenic challenge, especially polysaccharide antigens, are common.[469]

Flow cytometry can be used to assess quantitative abnormalities of WASP in peripheral blood mononuclear cells and may be useful for carrier detection under certain circumstances.[480,481] X-inactivation in some carriers of Wiskott-Aldrich syndrome is nonrandom, however, so caution is required in interpreting the results of such studies.[482]

THERAPY, COURSE, AND PROGNOSIS

Splenectomy usually, but not invariably, improves the thrombocytopenia and usually partially corrects the defect in platelet size, at least temporarily.[454,470,471] It also may improve platelet function. Thus, splenectomy should be considered in patients with excessive hemorrhage. Opportunistic infections present serious problems.[453,469,470] The risk of overwhelming bacterial sepsis after splenectomy is increased but can be reduced by use of pneumococcal, meningococcal, and *Haemophilus influenza* vaccines, prophylactic antibiotics, and intravenous immunoglobulin. Patients with Wiskott-Aldrich syndrome tend to have hypercatabolism of IgG and thus may require a higher dose and more frequent dosing of IgG.[469] If platelet transfusion is required to stop hemorrhage, the platelets should be irradiated to prevent transfusion-related graft-versus-host disease. Obtaining platelets from donors who are free of CMV is preferable.

Marrow transplantation can cure the disorder.[453,471] Because the prognosis is otherwise poor, transplantation before the onset of significant immunodeficiency has been recommended when a histocompatible donor is available.[453,471] Transplantation from matched unrelated donors can be successful in young patients, but the success rate declines after age 5 to 6 years.[469] Umbilical cord blood cells may be a useful alternative source of stem cells for transplantation (see Chap. 22).

GRANULE ABNORMALITIES

A heterogeneous group of disorders involving platelet granules has been described. They are broadly categorized into defects affecting dense granules (δ-storage pool deficiency), α-granules (α-storage pool deficiency, or gray platelet syndrome), or both dense bodies and α-granules (α,δ-storage pool deficiency). The familial platelet disorder with predisposition to leukemia syndrome is discussed under δ-storage pool deficiency because most patients have been described as having abnormalities of dense granules, but at least several patients have been found to have α-granule abnormalities.

δ-STORAGE POOL DEFICIENCY

DEFINITION AND HISTORY

Based on the original description by Weiss and colleagues[483] in 1969 and subsequent studies by other investigators,[484,485] δ-storage pool deficiency is a heterogeneous disorder characterized by a mild bleeding tendency, abnormalities in the second wave of platelet aggregation, and variable deficiencies of the contents of platelet dense granules.

ETIOLOGY AND PATHOGENESIS

δ-Storage pool deficiency can be a primary, inherited platelet disorder or a component of a multisystem disorder, such as Hermansky-Pudlak syndrome[486,487] (variable oculocutaneous albinism, excessive accumulation of ceroid-like material in lysosomes in monocyte-macrophage cells in bone marrow and other tissues, variable pulmonary fibrosis, inflammatory bowel disease, and hemorrhagic diathesis), Chediak-Higashi syndrome[488–491] (partial oculocutaneous albinism, giant lysosomal granules, and frequent pyogenic infections), and Wiskott-Aldrich syndrome (see Chap. 66). Other diseases have been associated with δ-storage pool deficiency (Ehlers-Danlos syndrome, osteogenesis imperfecta, thrombocytopenia with absent radii), but the relationship is less well established.[485] The mode of inheritance is not well defined,[485] but an autosomal dominant pattern for the primary form has been identified in some patients. Inheritance of the forms

associated with multisystem disorders follows the autosomal recessive and X-linked patterns characteristic of those disorders

Defects in platelet function and platelet granules in leukemia and myeloproliferative disorders were reported many years ago,[492] but they were originally presumed to be secondary to abnormalities of the leukemic clone or *in vivo* activation of platelets. An association between platelet granule defects (and other inherited platelet abnormalities) and a predisposition to acute myeloid leukemia subsequently was reported in several different families in which the platelet abnormalities antedated the leukemia and were linked, with one exception, to inherited mutations or a deletion in the gene *RUNX1 (AML1, CBFA2)*.[493–503] This gene is involved in the sporadic mutations and the t(8;21), t(3;21), and t(12;21) translocations found in more than 10 percent of patients with acute myelogenous leukemia.[494,504,505] Of note, all but one of the mutations of *RUNX1* affected the Runt domain.[500] The one exception, involving the transactivating domain (Y260X), was identified in a family with only mild thrombocytopenia and defects in platelet α-granules and α2-adrenergic receptors in addition to defects in dense bodies.[500] Another patient with a splice site mutation leading to a frameshift with premature termination in the Runt domain was found to have abnormal αIIbβ3 activation, decreased platelet pleckstrin phosphorylation, and a selective decrease in platelet protein kinase C-θ. The patient also had diminished platelet albumin and IgG, suggesting an α-granule abnormality, but normal levels of the α-granule proteins fibrinogen and β-thromboglobulin.[502] A partial α-granule abnormality was identified in another patient with this syndrome.[493] Whether α-granules were specifically studied in some of the other families is not clear, so this disorder possibly more generally affects both dense bodies and α-granules. The disorder is inherited as an autosomal dominant trait, and individuals generally have mild thrombocytopenia from birth and a bleeding disorder that is disproportionate to the thrombocytopenia. Prior to developing the leukemia, the bone marrow may be normal or demonstrate mild morphologic abnormalities in megakaryocytes or changes consistent with myelodysplasia. The overall frequency of leukemia is 35 percent, with a median age of onset of 33 years.

The etiology of primary human δ-storage pool deficiency is unknown, but based on data from animal models the deficiency most likely results from a defect intrinsic to hematopoietic precursors. In δ-storage pool deficiency associated with Hermansky-Pudlak syndrome, a total failure of δ-granule formation occurs as judged by electron microscopy of platelets and megakaryocytes[479] and by the absence of CD63 (ME491, LIMP-1, LAMP-3, granulophysin), a lysosomal and dense granule membrane protein of M_r 40,000 that is also found in melanosomes.[487,506,507] The defect in melanosomes accounts for the oculocutaneous albinism, and the defect in lysosomes results in accumulation of ceroid lipofuscin, a lipid–protein complex. Granulomatous colitis and pulmonary fibrosis are variably manifest. Abnormalities of seven separate genes have been implicated as the cause of this disorder (Figure 112-6). Hermansky-Pudlak syndrome is unusually common in patients from northwest Puerto Rico, and linkage analysis of patients from this area led to the identification of the abnormal gene in these patients *(HPS1)*. The gene codes for a 700-amino-acid protein that participates in complexes of proteins involved in the biogenesis of lysosome-related organelles complex (BLOC-3, BLOC-4, BLOC-5).[487] The mutation in the Puerto Rican kindreds is a 16-bp duplication in exon 15. Other mutations of the same gene have been identified in patients from other ethnic groups.[487,508] Mutations in the β3A subunit of the heterotetrameric AP3-complex (HPS2), a protein that facilitates the formation of vesicles of lysosomal lineage from membranes of the trans-Golgi network or late endosomes, have been identified in patients with Hermansky-Pudlak syndrome, and patients

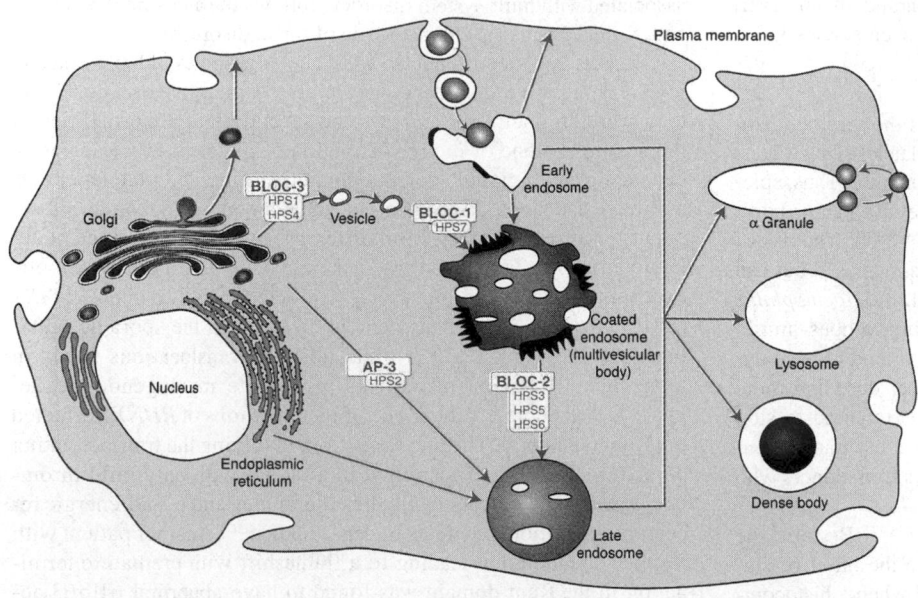

FIGURE 112-6   Hypothetical model of platelet granule formation and location of defects resulting in Hermansky-Pudlak syndrome (HPS). Early endosomes derive from invaginations from the plasma membrane, whereas membrane-bound structures from the Golgi and endoplasmic reticulum contribute to production of coated endosomes and late endosomes. Three multiprotein complexes termed *biogenesis of lysosome related organelles complex* (BLOC) are involved in the transport and interconversion of the different endosomal species. The gene products of HPS1 and HPS4 are involved in BLOC-3, whereas those of HPS3, HPS5, and HPS6 are involved in BLOC-2, and that of HPS7 contributes to BLOC-1. HPS2 results from mutations in adaptor complex-3 (AP-3). The endosomal species that contribute to α granules, lysosomes, and dense bodies have not been determined, but all three organelles are affected in HPS. α-Granules are in dynamic exchange with the plasma membrane, selectively taking up fibrinogen via αIIbβ3 receptors. (Adapted from M. Huizing and W. Gahl, National Human Genome Research Institute, National Institutes of Health, with permission.)

with mutations in this protein tend to also have neutropenia and childhood infections.[509]

Defects in the *HPS3* gene cause a relatively mild form of Hermansky-Pudlak syndrome, and pulmonary involvement is usually minimal.[510] *HPS4* encodes a protein that interacts with the *HPS1* protein in BLOC-3.[511–514] Patients with mutations in this gene tend to have severe disease and, like patients with defects in *HPS1*, pulmonary involvement is common. The gene products of *HPS5* and *HPS6* interact with the *HPS3* gene product to form BLOC-2,[515,516] whereas the protein implicated in HPS7 (*DTNBP1*) is a component of BLOC-1.[517]

In other forms of δ-storage pool disease, data obtained with uranaffin, a dye that specifically stains amine-containing granules, indicate that dense granule membranes are formed but not properly filled.[485,518,519] The defects in the different substances contained in dense granules are heterogeneous; some patients can secrete significant amounts of calcium and pyrophosphate even when adenine nucleotide secretion is nearly completely absent.[485]

Mutation of the *Lyst* gene have been found in 13 patients with Chediak-Higashi syndrome. The gene encodes a protein of estimated molecular mass of 429 kDa, predicted from domain analysis to participate in vesicle transport and interact with microtubules. An *HPS1*-like region also is present.[520]

The heterogeneity of human δ-storage pool deficiency is matched by a similar heterogeneity among animals with disorders associated with abnormal platelet dense granules. Thus, at least 16 separate inherited mouse defects have been reported to include dense granule deficiencies.[507,521–525] Of these defects, pale ear (*ep*) is linked to the mouse equivalent of the *HPS1* gene, pearl (*pe*) to the mouse equivalent of *HSP2* (β$_3$A subunit of AP-3 complex), cocoa to *HPS3*, light ear (*le*)

to *HPS4*, ruby-eye-2 (*ru2*) to *HPS5*, ruby-eye (*ru*) to *HPS6*, and sandy (*sdy*) to *HPS7*.[516,522,526,527] Another mouse mutation (the pallid mutation) has been genetically linked to protein 4.2.[521] The beige mouse and rat serve as models for Chediak-Higashi syndrome.[520,528] Several of these animal disorders are also characterized by abnormalities in lysosomes, pigment, and inner ear function.[521,522]

CLINICAL FEATURES

Patients with δ-storage pool deficiency as part of Hermansky-Pudlak syndrome may have severe, or even lethal, hemorrhage.[487,529,530] For all other forms of the disorder, the bleeding tendency is usually mild to moderate in severity.[485]

Mucocutaneous hemorrhage is most common, with excessive bruising and epistaxis and increased bleeding after delivery, tooth extractions, and surgical procedures. The bleeding symptoms can be considerably more severe, however, if patients are taking aspirin or other antiplatelet agents.[484,485]

LABORATORY FEATURES

The results of platelet function tests are variable among patients and even in the same patient over time, so providing precise diagnostic criteria is difficult.[479,483–485,531–534] The bleeding time usually is prolonged, and some correlation may exist between the severity of dense granule deficiency and bleeding time prolongation.[535] However, patients with δ-storage pool deficiency may have normal bleeding times. In one report, patients with δ-storage pool deficiency had normal aperture closure times using collagen/ADP, and only a minority had prolonged closure times with collagen/epinephrine (PFA-100). The sensitivity was similar to that of the bleeding time.[536] In another report, 13 of 19 patients had abnormal closure times, but the closure times did not correlate with bleeding symptoms.[530]

Platelet aggregation abnormalities are characteristic. ADP and epinephrine induce normal primary waves of aggregation, but the secondary waves are variably abnormal, and the defects range from minor to major. The dose of collagen used affects the results obtained in patients with δ-storage pool deficiency. Low doses accentuate the abnormality and high doses obscure it. Therefore, using the lowest dose that gives a strong response with normal platelets is important.[485] If aspirin treatment of normal platelets results in a diminished aggregation response, the dose of collagen probably is low enough to detect the abnormality in δ-storage pool-deficient platelets. Thrombin at high doses causes maximal release of platelet dense body contents, even when platelets have been treated with aspirin or have an intrinsic release reaction abnormality. Therefore, this reagent can distinguish between δ-storage pool deficiency (diminished release) and abnormalities of the platelet release reaction (normal release). Release of ATP from platelets can be measured by luminescence simultaneously with platelet aggregation using specially designed aggregometers.

More sophisticated tests can define further the extent of the platelet abnormality. The total platelet content of adenine nucleotides is reduced, and the ratio of total platelet ATP to ADP is increased because it more closely reflects the ratio in the cytoplasmic "metabolic" pool of adenine nucleotides (~8:1) rather than that of the "storage" pool in dense granules (~2:3) (see Chap. 105).[485,531,535] Platelet serotonin is variably reduced, with the lowest levels found in patients with Hermansky-Pudlak syndrome.[537] Serotonin can be taken up by platelets of patients with δ-storage pool deficiency, but serotonin is rapidly catabolized because it cannot be stored in dense granules.[537] Abnormalities in platelet secretion and arachidonic acid metabolism have been identified but are quite variable, and whether they result from the aggregation abnormalities is unclear.[485,538–540] Reduced levels of plasma and platelet von Willebrand factor activity in association with a decrease in plasma high molecular weight multimers and an increase in low molecular weight multimers have been reported in Hermansky-Pudlak syndrome.[541,542] Combined δ-storage pool disease in Hermansky-Pudlak syndrome and reduced von Willebrand factor activity may result in more severe bleeding,[541] but in one study no association between bleeding and von Willebrand factor levels could be identified.[542]

The decrease or absence of platelet dense bodies can be confirmed by electron microscopy, using either whole mounts[543,544] or thin sections of platelets fixed in the presence of calcium.[479] Some patients have abnormal granules.[519,533,545] Uranaffin and osmium may help to identify dense granules.[518,546] The fluorescent amine mepacrine can be used to quantify dense bodies by fluorescence microscopy or flow cytometry.[547,548]

Platelet thrombus formation on subendothelial surfaces is decreased in δ-storage pool deficiency, and a hematocrit-related defect in platelet adhesion has been noted.[158]

DIFFERENTIAL DIAGNOSIS
See "Differential Diagnosis" for Glanzmann thrombasthenia above.

THERAPY, COURSE, AND PROGNOSIS
The general principles of patient management are similar to those described for Glanzmann thrombasthenia. Patients should be specifically instructed to avoid aspirin or other antiplatelet agents. Short courses of glucocorticoids before surgery may reduce the operative risk,[485,549] but the effectiveness of this therapy is not clear. Although desmopressin did not shorten the bleeding time in three patients with δ-storage pool deficiency in the only reported double-blind, placebo-controlled trial,[550] it has been reported to shorten or normalize the bleeding time in some patients.[181,551–555] Possibly it improves hemostasis even though it does not normalize the bleeding time. In one patient with Hermansky-Pudlak syndrome, desmopressin did not prevent excessive hemorrhage after one cesarian section but did prevent excessive hemorrhage after another.[556] Cryoprecipitate reportedly corrects the bleeding time in patients with δ-storage pool deficiency,[557] but whether the response is the result of an increase in plasma von Willebrand factor or the infusion of platelet fragments and microparticles found in cryoprecipitate is unclear.[558,559] Platelet transfusions have been used to prevent and treat surgical and postpartum hemorrhage in patients with Hermansky-Pudlak syndrome, but most patients have mild symptoms and may not require platelet transfusion before delivery.[556,560] One patient with Hermansky-Pudlak underwent thyroidectomy uneventfully with prophylactic desmopressin, platelet transfusion, tranexamic acid, and recombinant factor VIIa; the latter two agents were given after the former two failed to correct the bleeding time.[561] Whether all of these measures were required to achieve hemostasis is not clear.

Patients with Hermansky-Pudlak syndrome suffer from a number of additional problems related to their albinism, colitis, and pulmonary fibrosis. In particular, they should avoid sun exposure. The antifibrotic agent pirfenidone may slow the progression of pulmonary fibrosis.[562]

GRAY PLATELET SYNDROME (α-GRANULE DEFICIENCY)

DEFINITION AND HISTORY
Although Fonio reported on a family with mucosal bleeding and hypogranular platelets in 1947,[681] and Kurstjens et al. in 1968[682] and

others subsequently reported similar patients with a deficiency of α-granules, the term gray platelet syndrome was coined by Raccuglia in 1971[563] when he reported on an 11-year-old girl with a lifelong bleeding tendency. Since then, a number of additional patients with isolated abnormalities in platelet α-granules have been reported,[447,564–583] including one patient with Goldenhar syndrome,[564] one patient with Marfan syndrome,[576] and one patient with concomitant GPVI deficiency.[447] The inheritance is not certain, but because many parents are normal and more than one sibling may be affected, at least some cases probably result from recessive inheritance.[578,581–583] A Japanese family with 24 affected members has been reported,[584] but these patients were atypical. They had only an approximate 50 percent reduction in platelet factor 4 and only a partial loss of platelet granularity. They also had apparently coincidental reductions in von Willebrand factor.

ETIOLOGY AND PATHOGENESIS
Studies using antibodies to the α-granule membrane protein P-selectin (CD62P) and other α-granule membrane proteins indicate that gray platelets contain α-granule membranes, but the membranes form abnormal vesicular structures rather than α-granules.[585,586] The P-selectin (CD62P) molecules join the plasma membrane when platelets are stimulated with thrombin, indicating the membranes can fuse with the plasma membrane. Antibodies specific for proteins contained in α-granules, such as fibrinogen and von Willebrand factor, identify small and misshapen α-granules in gray platelets, further supporting a defect in packaging, as does the observation that the von Willebrand factor lacks high molecular weight multimers.[581,587] Plasma levels of the α-granule proteins β-thromboglobulin and platelet factor 4 are normal or increased, indicating the defect is not in the synthesis of α-granule proteins.[564] One study of the megakaryocytes in patients with the gray platelet syndrome identified von Willebrand factor, platelet-derived growth factor, and platelet factor 4 in early megakaryocytes but also a failure of the proteins to be retained in α-granules as the megakaryocytes matured.[352] In another study, megakaryocytes were observed to have increased P-selectin staining, decreased von Willebrand staining, and extensive neutrophil emperipolesis (passage of blood cells through megakaryocytes), perhaps as a result of neutrophil interactions with P-selectin.[581] Emperipolesis of neutrophils has been postulated to result in megakaryocyte leakage of platelet-derived growth factor from platelet α-granules, which may be responsible for the mild reticulin fibrosis observed in some patients.[567,569,577,588,589] Bone marrow fibrosis has been associated with splenomegaly and evidence of extramedullary hematopoiesis.[577,581] The fibrosis does not, however, appear to be progressive. An association with pulmonary fibrosis has been reported,[574] raising the possibility of leakage of growth factors from megakaryocytes in the lung, but this remains speculative. In one family with three affected siblings, neutrophils were gray on blood film, and electron microscopy confirmed deceased numbers of secondary granules.[580]

The primary defect responsible for abnormal granule formation has not been identified, but it could involve membrane production, protein targeting, granule formation, or protein retention. The evidence for constant recycling of α-granules to and from the plasma membrane adds additional loci where defects may result in abnormalities in α-granules.[590]

The pathophysiology of the thrombocytopenia is uncertain, but reports of increased bone marrow megakaryocytes, shortened platelet survival, and elevated levels of plasma glycocalicin (a fragment of GPIbα) relative to the platelet count suggest that decreased platelet survival and/or ineffective thrombopoiesis contribute.[568,581,591]

CLINICAL FEATURES
Hemorrhagic manifestations usually are mild in the gray platelet syndrome, but severe bleeding has been noted in a patient with head trauma.[570]

LABORATORY FEATURES

Platelets appear as larger-than-normal, pale, ghost-like, oval forms on blood films. Often they can be extremely difficult to identify. Thrombocytopenia is common and can be moderately severe, with the count dropping below 50,000/μl. Platelet aggregation abnormalities are present, but the reported abnormalities vary considerably. ADP- and epinephrine-induced aggregation is normal or nearly normal. Collagen- and thrombin-induced aggregation tend to be more abnormal, but this finding is not consistent. Concomitant GPVI deficiency has been reported in one patient and, if the association is more widespread, may explain the variable abnormalities in collagen-induced aggregation.[447,571,575,592] The abnormal thrombin-induced aggregation was studied further in one patient. Abnormal platelet aggregation in response to thrombin receptor-activating peptide and normal numbers of thrombin PAR-1 receptors were found.[575] Additional abnormalities in phosphoinositide metabolism, protein phosphorylation, calcium mobilization, platelet factor Va, and platelet secretion have been described.[593–595] Thus, whether the α-granule protein deficiency, the defects in signal transduction, or both are responsible for the platelet aggregation abnormalities is unclear. The failure of α-granule proteins to fully correct the aggregation defects suggests that the signal transduction defects may be significant.[571]

Gray platelets are deficient in α-granule contents, including fibrinogen, von Willebrand factor, thrombospondin, platelet factor 4, β-thromboglobulin, and platelet-derived growth factor, proteins that can be analyzed by immunologic assays or polyacrylamide gel electrophoresis. Platelet IgG and albumin are less severely affected. Electron microscopy confirms a selective absence of α-granules, with normal numbers of dense granules.[479,569,587]

DIFFERENTIAL DIAGNOSIS

See "Differential Diagnosis" for Glanzmann thrombasthenia above. Degranulated platelets are sometimes observed in myelodysplastic and myeloproliferative disorders, but the clinical setting should provide enough information to establish the diagnosis. The platelets of some normal individuals degranulate *in vitro* when anticoagulated with EDTA and thus appear gray on blood film.[596]

THERAPY, COURSE, AND PROGNOSIS

The general measures for treating this disorder are similar to those for Glanzmann thrombasthenia. Desmopressin produces inconsistent correction of the bleeding time,[568,597] but hemostasis after a tooth extraction was acceptable after desmopressin treatment in one patient, even without correction of the bleeding time.[568] Antifibrinolytic therapy also may be beneficial.[570] Platelet transfusions are rarely needed but should be given for serious hemorrhage.

Thrombocytopenia can contribute to the hemostatic defect. Glucocorticoid therapy may increase the platelet count but usually does not result in a normal count.[563,568] The mechanism for this effect is unknown, but it raises the possibility that an immune mechanism contributes to the thrombocytopenia in some patients. Splenectomy resulted in normalization of the platelet count in two patients soon after the surgery,[563,577] but in one patient the count slowly decreased thereafter.[564]

DIMORPHIC DYSMORPHIC PLATELETS WITH GIANT α-GRANULES AND THROMBOCYTOPENIA (PARIS-TROUSSEAU/ JACOBSEN SYNDROME)

The Paris-Trousseau syndrome, a variant of Jacobsen syndrome, is a rare disorder that has been described in only 10 patients.[598–601] It is characterized by mental retardation, congenital thrombocytopenia, giant α-granules in only a fraction of circulating platelets, bone marrow

dysmegakaryopoiesis, and deletion of the distal part of either the maternally or paternally derived chromosome 11 (11q23.3-24). Thus, the inheritance is autosomal dominant. Although platelet survival is normal, bone marrow megakaryocytes expand dramatically as a result of an arrest in megakaryocyte development. Among the genes deleted is the transcription factor *FLI1*, which plays an important role in megakaryocyte development. Remarkably, during a period in early megakaryocyte development, only one of the two *FLI1* alleles appears to be expressed in any single megakaryocyte precursor, thus accounting for the inheritance pattern and the dimorphic platelet population containing both normal platelets and platelets with dysmorphic giant α-granules.[600,601] It also can explain the expansion of dysmorphic megakaryocytes in the bone marrow. Whether this gene defect also is responsible for the abnormalities in α-granules and mental function is unclear.

α,δ-STORAGE POOL DEFICIENCY

This rare disorder is characterized by moderate-to-severe defects in both α- and δ-granules, with heterogeneous expression in the few patients in whom it has been reported.[485,602] One severely affected patient also had decreased platelet P-selectin (CD62P), a point of distinction from other patients with the disorder and patients with gray platelet syndrome.[603] Clinical and laboratory features are similar to those of δ-storage pool deficiency. In general, the defect in dense granules is more severe than the defect in α-granules. Decreased α_2-adrenergic receptors[604] and increased platelet GPIV (CD36)[605] have been reported in isolated cases, as has an association with hematologic malignancy.[606]

QUEBEC PLATELET DISORDER

Originally termed *factor V Quebec*, the early description of this autosomal dominant disorder included severe bleeding after trauma, mild thrombocytopenia, decreased functional platelet factor V, and normal plasma factor V.[607,608] The bleeding time and epinephrine-induced platelet aggregation are abnormal. Subsequent studies demonstrated that the platelets of these patients had markedly reduced levels of multimerin and thrombospondin (see Chap. 105), and both reduced levels and proteolysis of a number of α-granule proteins, including factor V, fibrinogen, von Willebrand factor, and osteonectin.[609] Platelet factor 4 and β-thromboglobulin, which also are α-granule proteins, did not show evidence of proteolysis. The defect in the platelets of these patients appears to be excessive plasmin generation as a result of increased expression of urokinase-type plasminogen activator. The amount of plasminogen available for conversion to plasmin may affect the severity of the disorder.[610,611] Treatment with fibrinolytic inhibitors appears to be effective in controlling bleeding.[612] Because the platelet factor V abnormality is prominent, this defect also can be classified as a defect in platelet coagulant activity (see "Abnormalities of Platelet Coagulant Activity" below).

ABNORMALITIES OF PLATELET COAGULANT ACTIVITY

DEFINITION AND HISTORY

Patients whose platelets fail to facilitate thrombin generation are defined as having defects in platelet coagulant activity (see Chap. 105). Only a few patients with isolated defects in platelet coagulant activity have been described,[613–620] but minor defects secondary to abnormalities in platelet aggregation are more common. The patient Scott, described by Weiss and colleagues[613,614] in 1979, has been studied in detail, so patients with isolated abnormalities in platelet coagulant activity are commonly referred to as having Scott syndrome.[615–617]

ETIOLOGY AND PATHOGENESIS

The primary abnormality in the patient Scott appears to be a failure of platelets to undergo normal microvesiculation in response to several different stimuli.[614,621] This condition is thought to be responsible for the decreased translocation of phosphatidylserine to the platelet's outer membrane leaflet, which in turn is presumed to be responsible for decreased binding of factors Va–Xa and VIIIa–IXa.[621–624] Without platelet binding of these intermediates in blood coagulation, the reactions do not proceed at their normal rate. The patient Scott's defect and the defect in patient V.W. were not confined to platelets; their erythrocytes and lymphocytes demonstrated similar defects in microvesicle formation and/or coagulant activity.[618,619,625] Complementation studies using the patient's lymphocytes and a myeloma cell line suggested that the patient's cells lack a functional gene product.[626] Two other patients with sporadic defects in platelet coagulant activity have been described. In both cases, the most significant abnormality was in collagen plus thrombin-induced prothrombinase activity in the absence of added factor Va. In one of these patients, the abnormality may have resulted from a defect in α-granule factor V distinct from the abnormality found in Quebec platelet disorder (see "Quebec Platelet Disorder" above).[616] A French family with Scott syndrome in which the pattern of inheritance suggested autosomal recessive inheritance has been reported.[615] The platelets of the propositus were found to have a defect in protein tyrosine phosphorylation in response to thrombin and collagen plus thrombin, especially of an M_r 40,000 protein, suggesting a defect in signal transduction is responsible for the abnormality in coagulant activity.[617]

CLINICAL FEATURES

Platelet coagulant defects differ from other platelet function disorders in that the hemorrhagic manifestations are not primarily mucocutaneous. For example, the patient Scott did not have easy bruising or excessive bleeding after superficial cuts.[613,614] She did, however, have variably severe bleeding after tooth extractions, menorrhagia, severe postpartum hemorrhage requiring transfusions and hysterectomy, and a spontaneous pelvic hematoma. Bleeding after surgery was present in the two sporadic cases, but epistaxis and easy bruising were present in only one of the two patients.[616] In the French family, the 71-year-old female propositus had epistaxis, trauma-related hematomas, bleeding after tooth extractions, and severe postpartum hemorrhage.[615] Her two older sisters died from hemorrhage during childbirth.

LABORATORY FEATURES

The bleeding time usually is normal, which distinguishes platelet coagulant defects from other qualitative platelet abnormalities.[614–616] The serum prothrombin time, which reflects the completeness of clotting of whole blood as reflected in consumption of prothrombin, is consistently abnormal and serves as a convenient screening assay.[613,615,616] More specific assays of "platelet factor 3," the phenomenologic designation of all of the platelet's contributions to accelerating clot formation, are abnormal. A number of different techniques are used to measure platelet factor 3, however, so the results vary considerably.[627]

The patient Scott had normal platelet aggregation, normal platelet phospholipid content, normal to enhanced platelet adhesion to subendothelium with diminished thrombus formation, severely impaired fibrin formation on subendothelium, diminished factor Va binding to platelets and platelet microparticles, diminished platelet acceleration of both factor X activation and prothrombin activation, decreased microparticle formation, and decreased activation-dependent exposure of negatively charged phospholipids.[621,623,624,628,629] Platelet calpain, amino-phospholipid translocase, and phospholipid scramblase, en-

zymes that might contribute to the functional abnormalities, were normal. Abnormalities in exposure of negatively charged phospholipids and shedding of microparticles, measured by any one of several techniques, including the binding of annexin V to the surface of platelets and microparticles, have been consistent findings in all of the patients described.[615–619]

DIFFERENTIAL DIAGNOSIS

The normal bleeding time, abnormal serum prothrombin time, and, in several of the reported cases, the lack of the characteristic mucocutaneous pattern of bleeding distinguish platelet coagulant defects from the other qualitative platelet disorders. See "Differential Diagnosis" for Glanzmann thrombasthenia above.

THERAPY, COURSE, AND PROGNOSIS

Platelet or whole-blood transfusions have been effective as prophylaxis and as therapy for bleeding episodes.[613–616] Prothrombin complex concentrates, which may contain activated coagulation species that can bypass some of the activation steps, reportedly were effective in the patient Scott.[485] These preparations may induce thrombosis, so they should be reserved for serious hemorrhagic episodes.

ABNORMALITIES OF PLATELET AGONIST RECEPTORS, SIGNAL TRANSDUCTION, AND SECRETION

Platelet activation is a complex phenomenon involving agonist binding to receptors; signal transduction through G -protein coupled receptors and other types of receptors; phosphoinositol metabolism resulting in calcium mobilization and phosphorylation of target proteins; arachidonic acid metabolism leading to thromboxane A_2 production; activation of the $\alpha IIb\beta 3$ receptor, and release of granule contents (see Chap. 105). Defects involving any of these phenomena can result in impaired platelet function.[485,630]

Abnormalities in signal transduction usually produce only a minor hemorrhagic tendency, comparable to that caused by aspirin ingestion. Therapy is not always necessary, although desmopressin may be helpful for patients with more severe bleeding. Many patients with these defects likely do not come to medical attention. In addition, the abnormalities of only a small percentage of patients with defects in signal transduction have been defined at the molecular level.

DEFECTS IN PLATELET AGONIST RECEPTORS OR AGONIST-SPECIFIC SIGNAL TRANSDUCTION

THROMBOXANE A_2

A mutation in the thromboxane A_2 receptor (Arg60Leu) as the cause of an inherited bleeding disorder in several unrelated families from Japan has been described.[631,632] The mutation is in the first cytoplasmic loop of the receptor, and studies with recombinant mutated receptor indicate a defect in signal initiation rather than ligand binding. Both dominant and recessive inheritance patterns have been reported. The homozygotes had more severe abnormalities in phospholipase C activation. Nonetheless, the dominant inheritance in some patients suggests the possibility that the abnormal receptor acts in a dominant negative fashion.

ADENOSINE DIPHOSPHATE

Abnormalities in the response to ADP as a result of abnormalities in either P2Y12 or P2X1 ADP receptors in several kindreds with bleeding disorders have been described.[633–637] In one family with several affected members, the bleeding diathesis was moderately severe, with episodes of serious hemorrhage in association with surgery and trauma.[635] ADP induced only a small wave of platelet aggregation followed by a disaggregation wave and, consistent with the known role of P2Y12, failed to decrease cyclic adenosine monophosphate (cAMP) in platelets treated with prostaglandin E₁. The genetic abnormality was identified as a 2-bp deletion at codon 240 of P2Y12 resulting in a frameshift and premature termination.[638] Only the mutant allele was expressed, although no mutations were present in the coding region of the other allele. Similar results were found in two other kindreds with homozygous small deletions (one or two bp) that resulted in frameshifts and premature termination of protein synthesis.[633,636,637] Heterozygosity for one of these defects produced a pattern of platelet function similar to that described for primary secretion defects, suggesting that abnormalities in the ADP receptors may be mistaken for secretion defects.[637] In another kindred, the affected person had a lifelong history of excessive bruising and postsurgical and posttraumatic bleeding.[639] His bleeding time was prolonged, and his platelets demonstrated marked and selective abnormalities in binding and responding to ADP, but ADP-induced shape change was normal. Unlike the other patients, this patient's platelets were able to bind an ADP analogue.[639] He was found to have compound heterozygosity for missense mutations in P2Y12 (R256Q/R265W) that affected function but not surface expression.[639]

The 6-year-old patient with a heterozygous deletion of one amino acid in P2X1 had a history of petechiae, ecchymoses, and severe epistaxis requiring tranexamic acid and platelet transfusion.[640] She had isolated impairment of ADP-induced platelet aggregation. The patient was heterozygous for a deletion of a single leucine at position 351–354 in the second transmembrane domain. The exact site of the deletion could not be established because all of the residues are leucines. The mutant protein apparently caused a dominant negative effect on ATP- and ADP-induced P2X1 calcium channel activity.

EPINEPHRINE
Abnormalities of α-adrenergic receptors or α-adrenergic-specific signal transduction have been described in several patients.[641–644]

PLATELET-ACTIVATING FACTOR
A defect in the platelet-activating factor receptor or platelet-activating factor-specific signal transduction has been reported.[645]

DEFECTS IN SIGNAL TRANSDUCTION

DEFECTS IN ARACHIDONIC ACID METABOLISM
Arachidonic Acid Release from Phospholipids   Several patients whose platelets aggregated normally in response to arachidonic acid but not to ADP, epinephrine, and/or collagen have been described. The platelets of these patients did not release arachidonic acid normally in response to thrombin but appeared to have normal phospholipase A₂ activity, suggesting a defect in mobilizing sufficient calcium to activate the phospholipase.[646,647] A patient with Hermansky-Pudlak syndrome whose platelets had δ-storage pool deficiency and abnormal phospholipase A₂ activity has been reported.[648] Another patient whose platelets failed to release arachidonic acid normally has been identified.[649]

Cyclooxygenase (Prostaglandin H₂ Synthase-1) Deficiency   Deficient platelet cyclooxygenase (prostaglandin H₂ synthase-1) activity leading to impaired platelet function has been identified in a number of patients.[650–655] Platelets from such patients cannot make thromboxane from arachidonic acid but can make thromboxane from cyclic endoperoxides. If cyclooxygenase activity is deficient in endothelial cells, prostacyclin production also will be impaired, as demonstrated in one patient.[652] The clinical manifestations of patients with cyclooxygenase deficiency are of considerable interest because they presumably reflect the competing influences of thromboxane A2 and prosta-

cyclin. One patient had a mild bleeding disorder,[652] whereas another patient had evidence of a thrombotic vascular disease, including a transient ischemic attack.[653]

Thromboxane Synthase Deficiency   Presumed platelet thromboxane synthase deficiencies have been identified in two families based on the failed conversion of cyclic endoperoxides to thromboxane A₂.[656,657] An otherwise mild bleeding disorder associated with one life-threatening hemorrhage and a variably prolonged bleeding time was found in one patient.[657]

DEFECTS IN PHOSPHOLIPASE C, GαQ, CALCIUM MOBILIZATION, AND CALCIUM RESPONSIVENESS

Defects in platelet secretion and the second wave of platelet aggregation with weak agonists, such as epinephrine and ADP, but not strong agonists, such as high-dose collagen or thrombin, are commonly encountered. When aspirin ingestion is excluded and the platelets are capable of making at least some thromboxane A₂ in response to the weak agonists, the platelets' diminished response is inferred to result from one or more abnormalities of the thromboxane A₂ receptor (discussed in the section "Defects in Platelet Agonist Receptors or Agonist-Specific Signal Transduction, Thromboxane A₂," the signal transduction pathway involved in calcium mobilization, or the calcium-responsive mechanisms involved in platelet activation.[630,641,642,658–665] Because ADP acts synergistically with thromboxane A₂, some of these abnormalities may reflect a contribution from diminished ADP secretion or responsiveness.[637,646,666]

A platelet lineage-specific deficiency in phospholipase C-β₂ expression has been described in association with a mild hemorrhage disorder. No abnormality in the coding sequence of the protein was identified.[667–669] In addition, a selective deficiency of Gαq, a G protein implicated in signal transduction, has been described in association with a mild bleeding disorder and abnormal platelet aggregation and secretion.[670] This last defect is of particular interest because mice lacking Gαq reportedly have abnormal platelet function.[671] Two families with polymorphisms of the Gsα gene resulting in overexpression of the paternally imprinted large form of the protein have been reported.[672] This condition resulted in increased production of cAMP, an inhibitor of platelet activation in response to physiologic stimuli. Patients had prolonged bleeding times, excessive posttraumatic bleeding, mental retardation, and skeletal malformations.

REFERENCES

1. Glanzmann E: Hereditäre hämmorhagische thrombasthenie. *Beitr Pathol Bluplätchen J Kinderkt* 88:113, 1918.
2. Caen JP, Castaldi PA, Leclerc JC, et al: Congenital bleeding disorders with long bleeding time and normal platelet count: I. Glanzmann's thrombasthenia. *Am J Med* 41:4, 1966.
3. Hardisty RM, Dormandy KM, Hutton RA: Thrombasthenia: Studies on three cases. *Br J Haematol* 10:371, 1964.
4. Zucker MB, Pert JH, Hilgartner MW: Platelet function in a patient with thrombasthenia. *Blood* 28:524, 1966.
5. Weiss HJ, Kochwa S: Studies of platelet function and proteins in 3 patients with Glanzmann's thrombasthenia. *J Lab Clin Med* 71:153, 1968.
6. George JN, Caen JP, Nurden AT: Glanzmann's thrombasthenia: The spectrum of clinical disease. *Blood* 75:1383, 1990.
7. Caen JP: Glanzmann's thrombasthenia. *Clin Haematol* 1:383, 1972.
8. Nurden AT, Caen JP: An abnormal platelet glycoprotein pattern in three cases of Glanzmann's thrombasthenia. *Br J Haematol* 28:253, 1974.
9. Phillips DR, Jenkins CS, Luscher EF, Larrieu M: Molecular differences of exposed surface proteins on thrombasthenic platelet plasma membranes. *Nature* 257:599, 1975.

10. Peerschke EI: The platelet fibrinogen receptor. *Semin Hematol* 22:241, 1985.

11. Bennett JS: The platelet-fibrinogen interaction, in *Platelet Membrane Glycoproteins*, edited by JN George, AT Nurden, DR Phillips, p 193. Plenum, New York, 1985.

12. Phillips DR, Charo IF, Parise LV, Fitzgerald LA: The platelet membrane glycoprotein IIb-IIIa complex. *Blood* 71:831, 1988.

13. Plow EF, Ginsberg MH: Cellular adhesion: GPIIb-IIIa as a prototypic adhesion receptor. *Prog Hemost Thromb* 9:117, 1989.

14. Poncz M, Eisman R, Heidenreich R, et al: Structure of the platelet membrane glycoprotein IIb. Homology to the alpha subunits of the vitronectin and fibronectin membrane receptors. *J Biol Chem* 262:8476, 1987.

15. Fitzgerald LA, Steiner B, Rall SC Jr, et al: Protein sequence of endothelial glycoprotein IIIa derived from a cDNA clone. Identity with platelet glycoprotein IIIa and similarity to "integrin." *J Biol Chem* 262:3936, 1987.

16. Hynes RO: Integrins. Bidirectional, allosteric signaling machines. *Cell* 110:673, 2002.

17. Bray PF, Shuman MA: Identification of an abnormal gene for the GPIIIa subunit of the platelet fibrinogen receptor resulting in Glanzmann's thrombasthenia. *Blood* 75:881, 1990.

18. Loftus JC, O'Toole TE, Plow EF, et al: A β3 integrin mutation abolishes ligand binding and alters divalent cation-dependent conformation. *Science* 249:915, 1990.

19. Newman PJ, Seligsohn U, Lyman S, Coller BS: The molecular genetic basis of Glanzmann thrombasthenia in the Iraqi-Jewish and Arab populations in Israel. *Proc Natl Acad Sci U S A* 88:3160, 1991.

20. Burk CD, Newman PJ, Lyman S, et al: A deletion in the gene for glycoprotein IIb associated with Glanzmann's thrombasthenia. *J Clin Invest* 87:270, 1991.

21. Peretz H, Seligsohn U, Zwang E, et al: Detection of the Glanzmann's thrombasthenia mutations in Arab and Iraqi-Jewish patients by polymerase chain reaction and restriction analysis of blood or urine samples. *Thromb Haemost* 66:500, 1991.

22. Chen Y-P, Djaffar I, Pidard E: Ser752Pro mutation in the cytoplasmic domain of integrin β3 subunit and defective activation of platelet integrin αIIbβ3 (glycoprotein IIb-IIIa) in a variant of Glanzmann thrombasthenia. *Proc Natl Acad Sci U S A* 89:10169, 1992.

23. Bajt ML, Ginsberg MH, Frelinger AL III, et al: A spontaneous mutation of integrin αIIbβ3 (platelet glycoprotein IIb-IIIa) helps define a ligand binding site. *J Biol Chem* 267:3789, 1992.

24. Seligsohn U, Peretz H, Newman PJ, et al: Glanzmann thrombasthenia in Israel: Clinical, biochemical and molecular genetic characterization, in *Genetic Diversity Among Jews*, edited by B Bonne-Tamir, A Adam, p 275. Oxford University, New York, 1992.

25. Lanza F, Stierle A, Fournier D, et al: A new variant of Glanzmann's thrombasthenia (Strasbourg I). Platelets with functionally defective glycoprotein IIb-IIIa complexes and a glycoprotein IIIa Arg214Trp mutation. *J Clin Invest* 89:1995, 1992.

26. Kato A, Yamamoto K, Miyazaki S, et al: Molecular basis for Glanzmann's thrombasthenia (GT) in a compound heterozygote with glycoprotein IIb gene: A proposal for the classification of GT based on the biosynthetic pathway of glycoprotein IIb-IIIa complex. *Blood* 79:3212, 1992.

27. Gu J-M, Xu W-F, Wang X-D, et al: Identification of a nonsense mutation at amino acid 584-arginine of platelet glycoprotein IIb in patients with type I Glanzmann thrombasthenia. *Br J Haematol* 83:442, 1993.

28. Simsek S, Heyboer H, De Bruijne-Admiraal LG, et al: Glanzmann's thrombasthenia caused by homozygosity for a splice defect that leads to deletion of the first coding exon of the glycoprotein IIIa mRNA. *Blood* 81:2044, 1993.

29. Djaffar I, Caen JP, Rosa JP: A large alteration in the human platelet glycoprotein IIIa (integrin beta 3) gene associated with Glanzmann's thrombasthenia. *Hum Mol Genet* 2:2183, 1993.

30. Babu R, Nibu K, Jablonski L, Poncz M: Rapid diagnosis of Glanzmann thrombasthenia using a single-stranded conformational polymorphism analysis. *Thromb Haemost* 69:1018, 1993.

31. Li L, Bray PF: Homologous recombination among three intragene Alu sequences causes an inversion-deletion resulting in the hereditary bleeding disorder Glanzmann thrombasthenia. *Am J Hum Genet* 53:140, 1993.

32. Jin Y, Dietz HC, Nurden A, Bray PF: Single-strand conformation polymorphism analysis is a rapid and effective method for the identification of mutations and polymorphisms in the gene for glycoprotein IIIa. *Blood* 82:2281, 1993.

33. Djaffar I, Rosa JP: A second case of variant of Glanzmann's thrombasthenia due to substitution of platelet GPIIIa (integrin beta 3) Arg214 by Trp. *Hum Mol Genet* 2:2179, 1993.

34. Wilcox DA, Wautier JL, Pidard D, Newman PJ: A single amino acid substitution flanking the fourth calcium binding domain of alpha IIb prevents maturation of the alpha IIb beta 3 integrin complex. *J Biol Chem* 269:4450, 1994.

35. Poncz M, Rifat S, Coller BS, et al: Glanzmann thrombasthenia secondary to a Gly273Asp mutation adjacent to the first calcium-binding domain of platelet glycoprotein IIb. *J Clin Invest* 93:172, 1994.

36. Bourre R, Peyruchaud O, Bray PF, et al: A point mutation in the gene for platelet GPIIb leads to a substitution in a highly conserved amino acid located between the second and the third Ca++-binding domain [abstract]. *Blood* 86, 452a 1995.

37. Wilcox DA, Paddock CM, Lyman S, et al: Glanzmann thrombasthenia resulting from a single amino acid substitution between the second and third calcium-binding domains of GPIIb. Role of the GPIIb amino terminus in integrin subunit association. *J Clin Invest* 95:1553, 1995.

38. Ferrer M, Fernandez-Pinel M, Gonzalez-Manchon C, et al: A mutant (Arg327→His) GPIIb associated to thrombasthenia exerts a dominant negative effect in stably transfected CHO cells. *Thromb Haemost* 76:292, 1996.

39. Basani RB, Vilaire G, Shattil SJ, et al: Glanzmann thrombasthenia due to a two amino acid deletion in the fourth calcium-binding domain of alpha IIb: Demonstration of the importance of calcium-binding domains in the conformation of alpha IIb beta 3. *Blood* 88:167, 1996.

40. French DL, Coller BS: Hematologically important mutations: Glanzmann thrombasthenia. *Blood Cells Mol Dis* 23:39, 1997.

41. Rosenberg N, Yatuv R, Orion Y, et al: Glanzmann thrombasthenia caused by an 11.2-kb deletion in the glycoprotein IIIa (beta3) is a second mutation in Iraqi Jews that stemmed from a distinct founder. *Blood* 89:3654, 1997.

42. Milet S, Bourre F, Peyruchaud O, et al: Amino acid substitution Cys457 to Tyr in the β3 subunit of αIIbβ3 is involved in an atypical case of Glanzmann thrombasthenia [abstract]. *Thromb Haemost* 77:360, 1997.

43. Westrup D, Santoso S, Becker-Hagendorff K, et al: Transfection of GPIIbIIe176/IIIa (Frankfurt I) in mammalian cells [abstract]. *Thromb Haemost* 77:671, 1997.

44. Basani R, Bennett JS, Poncz M: A Glanzmann thrombasthenia variant due to an αIIb mutation suggests that an additional N-terminal loop is involved in ligand binding [abstract]. *Blood* 90(suppl 1):26a, 1997.

45. Wang R, Shattil SJ, Ambruso DR, Newman PJ: Truncation of the cytoplasmic domain of β3 in a variant form of Glanzmann thrombasthenia abrogates signaling through the integrin αIIbβ3 complex. *J Clin Invest* 100:2393, 1997.

46. Ward CM, Newman PJ: A Leu262Pro mutation in the integrin β3 subunit results in an αIIbβ3 complex which binds fibrin but not fibrinogen [abstract]. *Blood* 90:25a, 1997.

47. Ambo H, Kamata T, Handa M, et al: Three novel integrin beta3 subunit missense mutations (H280P, C560F, and G579S) in thrombasthenia, in-

cluding one (H280P) prevalent in Japanese patients. *Biochem Biophys Res Commun* 251:763, 1998.

48. Ambo H, Kamata T, Handa M, et al: Novel point mutations in the alphaIIb subunit (Phe289→Ser, Glu324→Lys and Gln747→Pro) causing thrombasthenic phenotypes in four Japanese patients. *Br J Haematol* 102:829, 1998.

49. Peyruchaud O, Nurden AT, Milet S, et al: R to Q amino acid substitution in the GFFKR sequence of the cytoplasmic domain of the integrin IIb subunit in a patient with a Glanzmann's thrombasthenia-like syndrome. *Blood* 92:4178, 1998.

50. Tadokoro S, Tomiyama Y, Honda S, et al: A Gln747→Pro substitution in the IIb subunit is responsible for a moderate IIbbeta3 deficiency in Glanzmann thrombasthenia. *Blood* 92:2750, 1998.

51. Honda S, Tomiyama Y, Shiraga M, et al: A two-amino acid insertion in the Cys146-Cys167 loop of the αIIb subunit is associated with a variant of Glanzmann thrombasthenia. *J Clin Invest* 102:1183, 1998.

52. Scott JP, III, Scott JP II, Chao YL, et al: A frameshift mutation at Gly975 in the transmembrane domain of GPIIb prevents GPIIb-IIIa expression: Analysis of two novel mutations in a kindred with type I glanzmann thrombasthenia. *Thromb Haemost* 80:546, 1998.

53. Grimaldi CM, Chen F, Wu C, et al: Glycoprotein IIb Leu214Pro mutation produces Glanzmann thrombasthenia with both quantitative and qualitative abnormalities in GPIIb/IIIa. *Blood* 91:1562, 1998.

54. Jackson DE, White MM, Jennings LK, Newman PJ: A Ser162→Leu mutation within glycoprotein (GP) IIIa (integrin beta3) results in an unstable alphaIIbbeta3 complex that retains partial function in a novel form of type II Glanzmann thrombasthenia. *Thromb Haemost* 80:42, 1998.

55. Ruan J, Peyruchaud O, Alberio L, et al: Double heterozygosity of the GPIIb gene in a Swiss patient with Glanzmann's thrombasthenia. *Br J Haematol* 102:918, 1998.

56. Ruan J, Schmugge M, Clemetson KJ, et al: Homozygous Cys542→Arg substitution in GPIIIa in a Swiss patient with type I Glanzmann's thrombasthenia. *Br J Haematol* 105:523, 1999.

57. Gonzalez-Manchon C, Fernandez-Pinel M, Arias-Salgado EG, et al: Molecular genetic analysis of a compound heterozygote for the glycoprotein (GP) IIb gene associated with Glanzmann's thrombasthenia: Disruption of the 674-687 disulfide bridge in GPIIb prevents surface exposure of GPIIb-IIIa complexes. *Blood* 93:866, 1999.

58. Tao J, Arias-Salgado EG, Gonzalez-Manchon C, et al: A novel (288delC) mutation in exon 2 of GPIIb associated with type I Glanzmann's thrombasthenia. *Br J Haematol* 111:96, 2000.

59. Tao J, Arias-Salgado EG, Gonzalez-Manchon C, et al: A 1063G→A mutation in exon 12 of glycoprotein (GP)IIb associated with a thrombasthenic phenotype: Mutation analysis of [324E]GPIIb. *Br J Haematol* 111:965, 2000.

60. Yatuv R, Rosenberg N, Zivelin A, et al: Identification of a region in glycoprotein IIIa involved in subunit association with glycoprotein IIb: Further lessons from Iraqi-Jewish Glanzmann thrombasthenia. *Blood* 98:1063, 2001.

61. Ruiz C, Liu CY, Sun QH, et al: A point mutation in the cysteine-rich domain of glycoprotein (GP) IIIa results in the expression of a GPIIb-IIIa (alphaIIbbeta3) integrin receptor locked in a high-affinity state and a Glanzmann thrombasthenia-like phenotype. *Blood* 98:2432, 2001.

62. Fullard J, Murphy R, O'Neill S, et al: A Val193Met mutation in GPIIIa results in a GPIIb/IIIa receptor with a constitutively high affinity for a small ligand. *Br J Haematol* 115:131, 2001.

63. Morel-Kopp MC, Melchior C, Chen P, et al: A naturally occurring point mutation in the beta3 integrin MIDAS-like domain affects differently alphavbeta3 and alphaIIIbbeta3 receptor function. *Thromb Haemost* 86:1425, 2001.

64. Vinciguerra C, Bordet JC, Beaune G, et al: Description of 10 new mutations in platelet glycoprotein IIb (alphaIIb) and glycoprotein IIIa (beta3) genes. *Platelets* 12:486, 2001.

65. Tadokoro S, Tomiyama Y, Honda S, et al: Missense mutations in the beta(3) subunit have a different impact on the expression and function between alpha(IIb)beta(3) and alpha(v)beta(3). *Blood* 99:931, 2002.

66. Nurden AT, Ruan J, Pasquet JM, et al: A novel 196Leu to Pro substitution in the beta3 subunit of the alphaIIbbeta3 integrin in a patient with a variant form of Glanzmann thrombasthenia. *Platelets* 13:101, 2002.

67. Arias-Salgado EG, Tao J, Gonzalez-Manchon C, et al: Nonsense mutation in exon-19 of GPIIb associated with thrombasthenic phenotype. Failure of GPIIb(delta597-1008) to form stable complexes with GPIIIa. *Thromb Haemost* 87:684, 2002.

68. D'Andrea G, Colaizzo D, Vecchione G, et al: Glanzmann's thrombasthenia: Identification of 19 new mutations in 30 patients. *Thromb Haemost* 87:1034, 2002.

69. Milet-Marsal S, Breillat C, Peyruchaud O, et al: Two different beta3 cysteine substitutions alter alphaIIb beta3 maturation and result in Glanzmann thrombasthenia. *Thromb Haemost* 88:104, 2002.

70. Bellucci S, Caen J: Molecular basis of Glanzmann's thrombasthenia and current strategies in treatment. *Blood Rev* 16:193, 2002.

71. Tanaka S, Hayashi T, Hori Y, et al: A Leu55 to Pro substitution in the integrin alphaIIb is responsible for a case of Glanzmann's thrombasthenia. *Br J Haematol* 118:833, 2002.

72. Nurden P, Poujol C, Winckler J, et al: A Ser752→Pro substitution in the cytoplasmic domain of beta3 in a Glanzmann thrombasthenia variant fails to prevent interactions between the alphaIIbbeta3 integrin and the platelet granule pool of fibrinogen. *Br J Haematol* 118:1143, 2002.

73. Nair S, Li J, Mitchell WB, et al: Two new beta3 integrin mutations in Indian patients with Glanzmann thrombasthenia: Localization of mutations affecting cysteine residues in integrin beta3. *Thromb Haemost* 88:503, 2002.

74. Milet-Marsal S, Breillat C, Peyruchaud O, et al: Analysis of the amino acid requirement for a normal alphaIIbbeta3 maturation at alpha-IIbGlu324 commonly mutated in Glanzmann thrombasthenia. *Thromb Haemost* 88:655, 2002.

75. Mitchell WB, Li JH, Singh F, et al: Two novel mutations in the alpha IIb calcium-binding domains identify hydrophobic regions essential for alpha IIbbeta 3 biogenesis. *Blood* 101:2268, 2003.

76. Kiyoi T, Tomiyama Y, Honda S, et al: A naturally occurring Tyr143His alpha IIb mutation abolishes alpha IIb beta 3 function for soluble ligands but retains its ability for mediating cell adhesion and clot retraction: Comparison with other mutations causing ligand-binding defects. *Blood* 101:3485, 2003.

77. Rosenberg N, Yatuv R, Sobolev V, et al: Major mutations in calf-1 and calf-2 domains of glycoprotein IIb in patients with Glanzmann thrombasthenia enable GPIIb/IIIa complex formation, but impair its transport from the endoplasmic reticulum to the Golgi apparatus. *Blood* 101:4808, 2003.

78. Yarali N, Fisgin T, Duru F, Kara A: Osteopetrosis and Glanzmann's thrombasthenia in a child. *Ann Hematol* 82:254, 2003.

79. Gonzalez-Manchon C, Arias-Salgado EG, Butta N, et al: A novel homozygous splice junction mutation in GPIIb associated with alternative splicing, nonsense-mediated decay of GPIIb-mRNA, and type II Glanzmann's thrombasthenia. *J Thromb Haemost* 1:1071, 2003.

80. Kannan M, Ahmed RP, Jain P, et al: Type I Glanzmann thrombasthenia: Most common subtypes in North Indians. *Am J Hematol* 74:139, 2003.

81. Srivastava A, Usher S, Nelson EJ, et al: Prenatal diagnosis of Glanzmann thrombasthenia. *Natl Med J India* 16:207, 2003.

82. Garcia LC, Breillat C, Lima M, et al: Mutations in the beta3 gene giving rise to type I Glanzmann thrombasthenia in two families in Portugal. *Platelets* 15:15, 2004.

83. Reichert N, Seligsohn U, Ramot B: Clinical and genetic studies of Glanzmann's thrombasthenia in Israel. *Thromb Diath Haemorrh* 34:806, 1975.

84. Awidi AS: Increased incidence of Glanzmann's thrombasthenia in Jordan as compared with Scandinavia. *Scand J Haematol* 30:218, 1983.

85. Khanduri U, Pullmood R, Sudarsanam A, et al: Glanzmann's thrombasthenia. A review and report of 42 cases from South India. *Thromb Haemost* 46:717, 1981.

86. Ahmed MA, Al Sohaibani MO, Al Mohaya SA, et al: Inherited bleeding disorders in the Eastern Province of Saudi Arabia. *Acta Haematol* 79: 202, 1988.

87. Awidi AS: Rare inherited bleeding disorders secondary to coagulation factors in Jordan: A nine-year study. *Acta Haematol* 88:11, 1992.

88. Handagama PJ, Shuman MA, Bainton DF: Incorporation of intravenously injected albumin, immunoglobulin G, and fibrinogen in guinea pig megakaryocyte granules. *J Clin Invest* 84:73, 1989.

89. Harrison P, Wilbourn BR, Debili N, et al: Uptake of plasma fibrinogen into the alpha granules of human megakaryocytes and platelets. *J Clin Invest* 84:1320, 1989.

90. Handagama P, Rappolee DA, Werb Z, et al: Platelet alpha-granule fibrinogen, albumin, and immunoglobulin G are not synthesized by rat and mouse megakaryocytes. *J Clin Invest* 86:1364, 1990.

91. Harrison P: Platelet α-granular fibrinogen. *Platelets* 3:1, 1992.

92. Coller BS, Seligsohn U, West SM, et al: Platelet fibrinogen and vitronectin in Glanzmann thrombasthenia: Evidence consistent with specific roles for glycoprotein IIb/IIIa and αVβ3 integrins in platelet protein trafficking. *Blood* 78:2603, 1991.

93. Disdier M, Legrand C, Bouillot C, et al: Quantitation of platelet fibrinogen and thrombospondin in Glanzmann's thrombasthenia by electroimmunoassay. *Thromb Res* 53:521, 1989.

94. Degos L, Dautigny A, Brouet JC, et al: A molecular defect in thrombasthenic platelets. *J Clin Invest* 56:236, 1975.

95. Cohen I, Gerrard JM, White JG: Ultrastructure of clots during isometric contraction. *J Cell Biol* 91:775, 1982.

96. Gartner TK, Ogilvie ML: Peptides and monoclonal antibodies which bind to platelet glycoproteins IIb and/or IIIa inhibit clot retraction. *Thromb Res* 49:43, 1988.

97. Duperray A, Troesch A, Berthier R, et al: Biosynthesis and assembly of platelet GPIIb-IIIa in human megakaryocytes: Evidence that assembly between pro-GPIIb and GPIIIa is a prerequisite for expression of the complex on the cell surface. *Blood* 74:1603, 1989.

98. Bodary SC, Napier MA, McLean JW: Expression of recombinant platelet glycoprotein IIbIIIa results in a functional fibrinogen-binding complex. *J Biol Chem* 264:18859, 1989.

99. O'Toole TE, Loftus JC, Plow EF, et al: Efficient surface expression of platelet GPIIb-IIIa requires both subunits. *Blood* 74:14, 1989.

100. Kolodziej MA, Vilaire G, Gonder D, et al: Study of the endoproteolytic cleavage of platelet glycoprotein IIb using oligonucleotide-mediated mutagenesis. *J Biol Chem* 266:23499, 1991.

101. Bennett JS: The molecular biology of platelet membrane proteins. *Semin Hematol* 27:186, 1990.

102. Kieffer N, Phillips DR: Platelet membrane glycoproteins: Functions in cellular interactions. *Annu Rev Cell Biol* 6:329, 1990.

103. Seligsohn U, Coller BS, Zivelin A, et al: Immunoblot analysis of platelet GPIIb in patients with Glanzmann thrombasthenia in Israel. *Br J Haematol* 72:415, 1989.

104. Zimrin AB, Eisman R, Vilaire G, et al: Structure of platelet glycoprotein IIIa. A common subunit for two different membrane receptors. *J Clin Invest* 81:1470, 1988.

105. Cheresh DA: Human endothelial cells synthesize and express an Arg-Gly-Asp-directed adhesion receptor involved in attachment to fibrinogen and von Willebrand factor. *Proc Natl Acad Sci U S A* 84:6471, 1987.

106. Smith JW, Cheresh DA: The Arg-Gly-Asp binding domain of the vitronectin receptor. *J Biol Chem* 263:18726, 1988.

107. Cheresh DA, Berliner SA, Vicente V, Ruggeri ZM: Recognition of distinct adhesive sites on fibrinogen by related integrins on platelets and endothelial cells. *Cell* 58:945, 1989.

108. Lawler J, Hynes RO: An integrin receptor on normal and thrombasthenic platelets which binds thrombospondin. *Blood* 74:2022, 1989.

109. Yokoyama K, Zhang XP, Medved L, Takada Y: Specific binding of integrin alpha v beta 3 to the fibrinogen gamma and alpha E chain C-terminal domains. *Biochemistry* 38:5872, 1999.

110. Lam SC, Plow EF, D'Souza SE, et al: Isolation and characterization of a platelet membrane protein related to the vitronectin receptor. *J Biol Chem* 264:3742, 1989.

111. Coller BS, Cheresh DA, Asch E, Seligsohn U: Platelet vitronectin receptor expression differentiates Iraqi-Jewish from Arab Patients with Glanzmann thrombasthenia in Israel. *Blood* 77:75, 1991.

112. Beckstead JH, Stenberg PE, McEver RP, et al: Immunohistochemical localization of membrane and alpha-granule proteins in human megakaryocytes: Application to plastic-embedded bone marrow biopsy specimens. *Blood* 67:285, 1986.

113. Krissansen GW, Elliott MJ, Lucas CM, et al: Identification of a novel integrin beta subunit expressed on cultured monocytes (macrophages). *J Biol Chem* 265:823, 1990.

114. Byzova TV, Rabbani R, D'Souza SE, Plow EF: Role of integrin alpha(v)beta3 in vascular biology. *Thromb Haemost* 80:726, 1998.

115. Lee JO, Rieu P, Arnaout MA, Liddington R: Crystal structure of the A domain from the alpha subunit of integrin CR3 (CD11b/CD18). *Cell* 80: 631, 1995.

116. Michishita M, Videm V, Arnaout MA: A novel divalent cation-binding site in the A domain of the beta 2 integrin CR3 (CD11b/CD18) is essential for ligand binding. *Cell* 72:857, 1993.

117. Tozer EC, Liddington RC, Sutcliffe MJ, et al: Ligand binding to integrin αIIbβ3 is dependent on a MIDAS-like domain in the beta3 subunit. *J Biol Chem* 271:21978, 1996.

118. Bajt ML, Loftus JC: Mutation of a ligand binding domain of beta 3 integrin. Integral role of oxygenated residues in alpha IIb beta 3 (GPIIb-IIIa) receptor function. *J Biol Chem* 269:20913, 1994.

119. Xiong JP, Stehle T, Diefenbach B, et al: Crystal structure of the extracellular segment of integrin alpha Vbeta3. *Science* 294:339, 2001.

120. Xiao T, Takagi J, Coller BS, et al: Structural basis for allostery in integrins and binding of ligand-mimetic therapeutics to the platelet receptor for fibrinogen. *Nature* 432:59, 2004.

121. Xiong JP, Stehle T, Zhang R, et al: Crystal structure of the extracellular segment of integrin alpha Vbeta3 in complex with an Arg-Gly-Asp ligand. *Science* 296:151, 2002.

122. Ward CM, Chao YL, Kato GJ, et al: Substitution of Asn, but not Tyr, for ASP119 of the β3 integrin subunit preserves fibrin binding and clot retraction [abstract]. *Blood* 90:26a, 1997.

123. Fournier DJ, Kabral A, Castaldi PA, Berndt MC: A variant of Glanzmann's thrombasthenia characterized by abnormal glycoprotein IIb/IIIa complex formation. *Thromb Haemost* 62:977, 1989.

124. Newman PJ, Weyerbusch-Bottum S, Visentin GP, et al: Type II Glanzmann thrombasthenia due to a destablizing amino acid substitution in platelet membrane glycoprotein IIIa [abstract]. *Thromb Haemost* 69: 1017, 1993.

125. Baker EK, Tozer EC, Pfaff M, et al: A genetic analysis of integrin function: Glanzmann thrombasthenia in vitro. *Proc Natl Acad Sci U S A* 94:1973, 1997.

126. Xiong JP, Stehle T, Diefenbach B, et al: Crystal structure of the extracellular segment of integrin alphaVbeta3. *Science* 294:339, 2001.

127. Ward CM, Kestin AS, Newman PJ: A Leu262Pro mutation in the integrin beta(3) subunit results in an alpha(IIb)-beta(3) complex that binds fibrin but not fibrinogen. *Blood* 96:161, 2000.

128. Loftus JC, Halloran CE, Ginsberg MH, et al: The amino-terminal one-third of alpha IIb defines the ligand recognition specificity of integrin alpha IIb beta 3. *J Biol Chem* 271:2033, 1996.

129. Springer TA: Folding of the N-terminal, ligand-binding region of integrin α-subunits into a β-propeller domain. *Proc Natl Acad Sci U S A* 94:65, 1997.

130. Xiong JP, Stehle T, Diefenbach B, et al: Crystal structure of the extracellular segment of integrin alpha Vbeta3. *Science* 294:339, 2001.

131. Basani RB, French DL, Vilaire G, et al: A naturally-occurring mutation near the amino terminus of αIIb defines a new region involved in ligand binding to αIIbβ3. *Blood* 95:180, 2000.

132. Kirchmaier CM, Westrup D, Becker-Hagendorff K, et al: A new variant of Glanzmann thrombasthenia (Frankfurt I) [abstract]. *Thromb Haemost* 73:1058, 1995.

133. Ylanne J, Chen Y, O'Toole TE, et al: Distinct functions of integrin alpha and beta subunit cytoplasmic domains in cell spreading and formation of focal adhesions. *J Cell Biol* 122:223, 1993.

134. Ylanne J, Huuskonen J, O'Toole TE, et al: Mutation of the cytoplasmic domain of the integrin beta 3 subunit. Differential effects on cell spreading, recruitment to adhesion plaques, endocytosis, and phagocytosis. *J Biol Chem* 270:9550, 1995.

135. Chen YP, O'Toole TE, Ylanne J, et al: A point mutation in the integrin beta 3 cytoplasmic domain (S752→P) impairs bidirectional signaling through alpha IIb beta 3 (platelet glycoprotein IIb-IIIa). *Blood* 84:1857, 1994.

136. Guarisco JL, Cheney ML, Ohene-Frempong K, et al: Limited septoplasty as treatment for recurrent epistaxis in a child with Glanzmann's thrombasthenia. *Laryngoscope* 97:336, 1987.

137. Seligsohn U, Rososhansky S: A Glanzmann's thrombasthenia cluster among Iraqi Jews in Israel. *Thromb Haemost* 52:230, 1984.

138. Coller BS, Peerschke EI, Scudder LE, Sullivan CA: A murine monoclonal antibody that completely blocks the binding of fibrinogen to platelets produces a thrombasthenic-like state in normal platelets and binds to glycoproteins IIb and/or IIIa. *J Clin Invest* 72:325, 1983.

139. Chediak J, Telfer MC, Vander LB, et al: Cycles of agglutination-disagglutination induced by ristocetin in thrombasthenic platelets. *Br J Haematol* 43:113, 1979.

140. Grant RA, Zucker MB, McPherson J: ADP-induced inhibition of von Willebrand factor-mediated platelet agglutination. *Am J Physiol* 230:1406, 1976.

141. Malmsten C, Kindahl H, Samuelsson B, et al: Thromboxane synthesis and the platelet release reaction in Bernard-Soulier syndrome, thrombasthenia Glanzmann and Hermansky-Pudlak syndrome. *Br J Haematol* 35:511, 1977.

142. Charo IF, Feinman RD, Detwiler TC: Interrelations of platelet aggregation and secretion. *J Clin Invest* 60:866, 1977.

143. Heptinstall S, Taylor PM: The effects of citrate and extracellular calcium ions on the platelet release reaction induced by adenosine diphosphate and collagen. *Thromb Haemost* 42:778, 1979.

144. Caen JP, Cronberg S, Levy-Toledano S, et al: New data on Glanzmann's thrombasthenia. *Proc Soc Exp Biol Med* 136:1082, 1971.

145. Zucker MB, Vroman L: Platelet adhesion induced by fibrinogen adsorbed onto glass. *Proc Soc Exp Biol Med* 131:318, 1969.

146. Stanford MF, Munoz PC, Vroman L: Platelets adhere where flow has left fibrinogen on glass. *Ann N Y Acad Sci* 416:504, 1983.

147. Zucker MB, McPherson J: Reactions of platelets near surfaces in vitro: Lessons from the platelet retention test. *Ann N Y Acad Sci* 283:128, 1977.

148. Bevers EM, Comfurius P, Nieuwenhuis HK, et al: Platelet prothrombin converting activity in hereditary disorders of platelet function. *Br J Haematol* 63:335, 1986.

149. Reverter JC, Beguin S, Kessels H, et al: Inhibition of platelet-mediated, tissue factor-induced thrombin generation by the mouse/human chimeric 7E3 antibody. Potential implications for the effect of c7E3 Fab treatment on acute thrombosis and "clinical restenosis." *J Clin Invest* 98:863, 1996.

150. Beguin S, Kumar R, Keularts I, et al: Fibrin-dependent platelet procoagulant activity requires GPIb receptors and von Willebrand factor. *Blood* 93:564, 1999.

151. Gemmell CH, Sefton MV, Yeo EL: Platelet-derived microparticle formation involves glycoprotein IIb-IIIa. Inhibition by RGDS and a Glanzmann's thrombasthenia defect. *J Biol Chem* 268:14586, 1993.

152. Nomura S, Komiyama Y, Matsuura E, et al: Participation of $\alpha_{IIb}\beta_3$ in platelet microparticle generation by collagen plus thrombin. *Haemostasis* 26:31, 1996.

153. Nomura S, Komiyama Y, Murakami T, et al: Flow cytometric analysis of surface membrane proteins on activated platelets and platelet-derived microparticles from healthy and thrombasthenic individuals. *Int J Hematol* 58:203, 1993.

154. Byzova TV, Plow EF: Networking in the hemostatic system. Integrin alphaiibbeta3 binds prothrombin and influences its activation. *J Biol Chem* 272:27183, 1997.

155. Byzova TV, Plow EF: Activation of alphaVbeta3 on vascular cells controls recognition of prothrombin. *J Cell Biol* 143:2081, 1998.

156. Tschopp TB, Weiss HJ, Baumgartner HR: Interaction of thrombasthenic platelets with subendothelium: Normal adhesion, absent aggregation. *Experientia* 31:113, 1975.

157. Sakariassen KS, Nievelstein PFEM, Coller BS, Sixma JJ: The role of platelet membrane glycoproteins Ib and IIb-IIIa in platelet adherence to human artery subendothelium. *Br J Haematol* 63:681, 1986.

158. Weiss HJ, Turitto VT, Baumgartner HR: Platelet adhesion and thrombus formation on subendothelium in platelets deficient in glycoproteins IIb-IIIa, Ib, and storage granules. *Blood* 67:322, 1986.

159. Weiss HJ, Turitto VT, Baumgartner HR: The role of shear rate and platelets in promoting fibrin formation on rabbit subendothelium: Studies utilizing patients with quantitative and qualitative platelet defects. *J Clin Invest* 78:1072, 1986.

160. Harrison P, Robinson M, Liesner R, et al: The PFA-100: A potential rapid screening tool for the assessment of platelet dysfunction. *Clin Lab Haematol* 24:225, 2002.

161. Buyukasik Y, Karakus S, Goker H, et al: Rational use of the PFA-100 device for screening of platelet function disorders and von Willebrand disease. *Blood Coagul Fibrinolysis* 13:349, 2002.

162. Lee H, Nurden AT, Thomaidis A, Caen JP: Relationship between fibrinogen binding and platelet glycoprotein deficiencies in Glanzmann's thrombasthenia type I and type II. *Br J Haematol* 48:47, 1981.

163. Coller BS, Seligsohn U, Peretz H, Newman PJ: Glanzmann thrombasthenia: New insights from an historical perspective. *Semin Hematol* 31:301, 1994.

164. Shattil SJ, Hoxie JA, Cunningham M, Brass LF: Changes in the platelet membrane glycoprotein IIb.IIIa complex during platelet activation. *J Biol Chem* 260:11107, 1985.

165. Coller BS, Seligsohn U, Zivelin A, et al: Immunologic and biochemical characterization of homozygous and heterozygous Glanzmann's thrombasthenia in Iraqi-Jewish and Arab populations of Israel: Comparison of techniques for carrier detection. *Br J Haematol* 62:723, 1986.

166. Karpatkin M, Howard L, Karpatkin S: Studies of the origin of platelet-associated fibrinogen. *J Lab Clin Med* 104:223, 1984.

167. Grimaldi CM, Chen F, Scudder LE, et al: A Cys374Tyr homozygous mutation of platelet glycoprotein IIIa (beta 3) in a Chinese patient with Glanzmann's thrombasthenia. *Blood* 88:1666, 1996.

168. Diminno G, Coraggio F, Cerbone AM, et al: A myeloma paraprotein with specificity for platelet glycoprotein IIIa in a patient with a fatal bleeding disorder. *J Clin Invest* 77:157, 1986.

169. Niessner H, Clemetson KJ, Panzer S, et al: Acquired thrombasthenia due to GPIIb/IIIa-specific platelet autoantibodies. *Blood* 68:571, 1986.

170. Kubota T, Tanoue K, Murohashi I, et al: Autoantibody against platelet glycoprotein IIb/IIIa in a patient with non-hodgkin's lymphoma. *Thromb Res* 53:379, 1989.

171. Malik U, Dutcher JP, Oleksowicz L: Acquired Glanzmann's thrombasthenia associated with Hodgkin's lymphoma: A case report and review of the literature. *Cancer* 82:1764, 1998.

172. Macchi L, Nurden P, Marit G, et al: Autoimmune thrombocytopenic purpura (AITP) and acquired thrombasthenia due to autoantibodies to GP IIb-IIIa in a patient with an unusual platelet membrane glycoprotein composition. *Am J Hematol* 57:164, 1998.

173. Thomas RV, Bessos H, Turner ML, et al: The successful use of plasma exchange and immunosuppression in the management of acquired Glanzmann's thrombasthenia. *Br J Haematol* 119:878, 2002.

174. Dinakaran S, Edwards MP, Hampton KK: Acquired Glanzmann's thrombasthenia causing prolonged bleeding following phacoemulsification. *Br J Ophthalmol* 87:1189, 2003.

175. Rawal A, Sarode R, Curtis BR, et al: Acquired Glanzmann's thrombasthenia as part of multiple-autoantibody syndrome in a pediatric heart transplant patient. *J Pediatr* 144:672, 2004.

176. Granel B, Swiader L, Veit V, et al: Pseudo-Glanzmann thrombasthenia in the course of autoimmune thrombocytopenic purpura. *Rev Med Interne* 19:823, 1998.

177. Ratnoff OD: Some therapeutic agents influencing hemostasis, in *Hemostasis and Thrombosis: Basic Principles and Clinical Practice*, edited by RW Colman, J Hirsh, VJ Marder, EW Salzman, p 1026. Lippincott, Philadelphia, 1987.

178. Berliner S, Horowitz I, Martinowitz U, et al: Dental surgery in patients with severe factor XI deficiency without plasma replacement. *Blood Coagul Fibrinolysis* 3:465, 1992.

179. Sindet-Pedersen S, Ramstrom G, Bernvil S, Blomback M: Hemostatic effect of tranexamic acid mouthwash in anticoagulant-treated patients undergoing oral surgery. *N Engl J Med* 320:840, 1989.

180. Markovitch O, Ellis M, Holzinger M, et al: Severe juvenile vaginal bleeding due to Glanzmann's thrombasthenia: Case report and review of the literature. *Am J Hematol* 57:225, 1998.

181. Mannucci PM: Desmopressin (DDAVP) for treatment of disorders of hemostasis. *Prog Hemost Thromb* 8:19, 1986.

182. Lethagen S, Karlsson MK: Erythropoietin and desmopressin obviated transfusion in a thromboasthenic Jehovah's witness undergoing scoliosis surgery. *Thromb Haemost* 2:11, 1996.

183. DiMichele DM, Hathaway WE: Use of DDAVP in inherited and acquired platelet dysfunction. *Am J Hematol* 33:39, 1990.

184. Tengborn L, Petruson B: A patient with Glanzmann thrombasthenia and epistaxis successfully teated with recombinant factor VIIa. *Thromb Haemost* 75:981, 1996.

185. Rakocz M, Lavie G, Martinowitz U: Glanzmann's thrombasthenia: The use of autologous fibrin glue in tooth extractions. *J Dent Child (Chic)* 62:129, 1995.

186. Chuansumrit A, Suwannuraks M, Sri-Udomporn N, et al: Recombinant activated factor VII combined with local measures in preventing bleeding from invasive dental procedures in patients with Glanzmann thrombasthenia. *Blood Coagul Fibrinolysis* 14:187, 2003.

187. Cmolik BL, Spero JA, Magovern GJ, Clark RE: Redo cardiac surgery: Late bleeding complications from topical thrombin-induced factor V deficiency. *J Thorac Cardiovasc Surg* 105:222, 1993.

188. Banninger H, Hardegger T, Tobler A, et al: Fibrin glue in surgery: Frequent development of inhibitors of bovine thrombin and human factor V. *Br J Haematol* 85:528, 1993.

189. Streiff MB, Ness PM: Acquired FV inhibitors: A needless iatrogenic complication of bovine thrombin exposure. *Transfusion* 42:18, 2002.

190. Tadokoro K, Ohtoshi T, Takafuji S, et al: Topical thrombin-induced IgE-mediated anaphylaxis: RAST analysis and skin test studies. *J Allergy Clin Immunol* 88:620, 1991.

191. Wai Y, Tsui V, Peng Z, et al: Anaphylaxis from topical bovine thrombin (Thrombostat) during haemodialysis and evaluation of sensitization among a dialysis population. *Clin Exp Allergy* 33:1730, 2003.

192. Tsuda H, Higashi S, Iwanaga S, et al: Development of antitissue factor antibodies in patients after liver surgery. *Blood* 82:96, 1993.

193. Jasmin JR, Dupont D, Velin P: Multiple dental extractions in a child with Glanzmann's thrombasthenia: Report of case. *J Dent Child (Chic)* 54:208, 1987.

194. Peyser MR, Kupferminc MJ: Management of severe postpartum hemorrhage by intrauterine irrigation with prostaglandin E2. *Am J Obstet Gynecol* 162:694, 1990.

195. Cases A, Escolar G, Reverter JC, et al: Recombinant human erythropoietin treatment improves platelet function in uremic patients. *Kidney Int* 42:668, 1992.

196. Tsao CJ, Kao RH, Cheng TY, et al: The effect of recombinant human erythropoietin on hemostatic status in chronic uremic patients. *Int J Hematol* 55:197, 1992.

197. Borawski J, Rydzewski A, Pawlak K, et al: Long-term effects of erythropoietin on platelet serotonin storage and platelet aggregation in hemodialysis patients with reference to ketanserin treatment. *Thromb Res* 90:171, 1998.

198. Bell JA, Savidge GF: Glanzmann's thrombasthenia proposed optimal management during surgery and delivery. *Clin Appl Thromb Hemost* 9: 167, 2003.

199. Smith JW, Steinhubl SR, Lincoff AM, et al: Rapid platelet-function assay (RPFA): An automated and quantitative cartridge-based method. *Circulation* 99:620, 1999.

200. The Trial to Reduce Alloimmunization to Platelets Study Group. Leukocyte reduction and ultraviolet B irradiation of platelets to prevent alloimmunization and refractoriness to platelet transfusions. *N Engl J Med* 337:1861, 1997.

201. Bowden RA, Slichter SJ, Sayers M, et al: A comparison of filtered leukocyte-reduced and cytomegalovirus (CMV) seronegative blood products for the prevention of transfusion-associated CMV infection after marrow transplant. *Blood* 86:3598, 1995.

202. Heddle NM, Klama L, Meyer R, et al: A randomized controlled trial comparing plasma removal with white cell reduction to prevent reactions to platelets. *Transfusion* 39:231, 1999.

203. Heddle NM, Klama L, Singer J, et al: The role of the plasma from platelet concentrates in transfusion reactions. *N Engl J Med* 331:625, 1994.

204. Saarinen UM, Kekomaki R, Siimes MA, Myllyla G: Effective prophylaxis against platelet refractoriness in multitransfused patients by use of leukocyte-free blood components. *Blood* 75:512, 1990.

205. Lozano M, Cid J: The clinical implications of platelet transfusions associated with ABO or Rh(D) incompatibility. *Transfus Med Rev* 17:57, 2003.

206. Anderson B, Shad AT, Gootenberg JE, Sandler SG: Successful prevention of post-transfusion Rh alloimmunization by intravenous Rho (D) immune globulin (WinRho SD). *Am J Hematol* 60:245, 1999.

207. Slichter SJ: Platelet transfusions a constantly evolving therapy. *Thromb Haemost* 66:178, 1991.

208. Newman PJ, McFarland JG, Aster RH: The alloimmune thrombocytopenias, in *Thrombosis and Hemorrhage*, edited by J Loscalzo, AI Schafer, p 531. Blackwell Scientific, Boston, 1994.

209. Conte R, Cirillo D, Ricci F, et al: Platelet transfusion in a patient affected by Glanzmann's thrombasthenia with antibodies against GPIIb-IIIa. *Haematologica* 82:73, 1997.

210. Jallu V, Pico M, Chevaleyre J, et al: Characterization of an antibody to the integrin beta 3 subunit (GP IIIa) from a patient with neonatal thrombocytopenia and an inherited deficiency of GP IIb-IIIa complexes in platelets (Glanzmann's thrombasthenia). *Hum Antibodies Hybridomas* 3:93, 1992.

211. Levy-Toledano S, Tobelem G, Legrand C, et al: Acquired IgG antibody occurring in a thrombasthenic patient: Its effect on human platelet function. *Blood* 51:1065, 1978.

212. Rosa JP, Kieffer N, Didry D, et al: The human platelet membrane glycoprotein complex GP IIb-IIIa expresses antigenic sites not exposed on the dissociated glycoproteins. *Blood* 64:1246, 1984.

213. Coller BS, Peerschke EI, Seligsohn U, et al: Studies on the binding of an alloimmune and two murine monoclonal antibodies to the platelet glycoprotein IIb-IIIa complex receptor. *J Lab Clin Med* 107:384, 1986.

214. Martin I, Kriaa F, Proulle V, et al: Protein A Sepharose immunoadsorption can restore the efficacy of platelet concentrates in patients with Glanzmann's thrombasthenia and anti-glycoprotein IIb-IIIa antibodies. *Br J Haematol* 119:991, 2002.

215. Ito K, Yoshida H, Hatoyama H, et al: Antibody removal therapy used successfully at delivery of a pregnant patient with Glanzmann's thrombasthenia and multiple anti-platelet antibodies. *Vox Sang* 61:40, 1991.

216. Kriaa F, Laurian Y, Hiesse C, et al: Five years' experience at one centre with protein A immunoadsorption in patients with deleterious allo/autoantibodies (anti-HLA antibodies, autoimmune bleeding disorders) and post-transplant patients relapsing with focal glomerular sclerosis. *Nephrol Dial Transplant* 10(suppl 6):108, 1995.

217. George JN, Nurden AT: Inherited disorders of the platelet membrane: Glanzmann's thrombasthenia and Bernard-Soulier syndrome, in *Hemostasis and Thrombosis: Basic Principles and Clinical Practice*, edited by RW Colman, J Hirsh, VJ Marder, EW Salzman, p 726. Lippincott, Philadelphia, 1987.

218. Bellucci S, Devergie A, Gluckman E, et al: Complete correction of Glanzmann's thrombasthenia by allogeneic bone marrow transplantation. *Br J Haematol* 59:635, 1985.

219. Bellucci S, Damaj G, Boval B, et al: Bone marrow transplantation in severe Glanzmann's thrombasthenia with antiplatelet alloimmunization. *Bone Marrow Transplant* 25:327, 2000.

220. Johnson A, Goodall AH, Downie CJ, et al: Bone marrow transplantation for Glanzmann's thrombasthenia. *Bone Marrow Transplant* 14:147, 1994.

221. McColl MD, Gibson BE: Sibling allogeneic bone marrow transplantation in a patient with type I Glanzmann's thrombasthenia. *Br J Haematol* 99:58, 1997.

222. Niemeyer GP, Boudreaux MK, Goodman-Martin SA, et al: Correction of a large animal model of type I Glanzmann's thrombasthenia by non-myeloablative bone marrow transplantation. *Exp Hematol* 31:1357, 2003.

223. Chen F, Xie Q, Jian Z, et al: Chimera formation of platelet GP II b Bak a/b by intrauterine transplantation of fetal liver stem cells. *Chin Med J (Engl)* 114:676, 2001.

224. Poon MC, d'Oiron R, Hann I, et al: Use of recombinant factor VIIa (NovoSeven) in patients with Glanzmann thrombasthenia. *Semin Hematol* 38:21, 2001.

225. d'Oiron R, Menart C, Trzeciak MC, et al: Use of recombinant factor VIIa in 3 patients with inherited type I Glanzmann's thrombasthenia undergoing invasive procedures. *Thromb Haemost* 83:644, 2000.

226. Poon M-C: Factor VIIa, in *Platelets*, edited by AD Michelson, p 867. Academic, San Diego, 2002.

227. Poon MC, d'Oiron R, von Depka M, et al: Prophylactic and therapeutic recombinant factor VIIa administration to patients with Glanzmann's thrombasthenia: Results of an international survey. *J Thromb Haemost* 2:1096, 2004.

228. Lisman T, Adelmeijer J, Heijnen HF, de Groot PG: Recombinant factor VIIa restores aggregation of alphaIIbbeta3-deficient platelets via tissue factor-independent fibrin generation. *Blood* 103:1720, 2004.

229. Galan AM, Tonda R, Pino M, et al: Increased local procoagulant action: A mechanism contributing to the favorable hemostatic effect of recombinant FVIIa in PLT disorders. *Transfusion* 43:885, 2003.

230. Lisman T, Moschatsis S, Adelmeijer J, et al: Recombinant factor VIIa enhances deposition of platelets with congenital or acquired alpha IIb beta 3 deficiency to endothelial cell matrix and collagen under conditions of flow via tissue factor-independent thrombin generation. *Blood* 101:1864, 2003.

231. Wilcox DA, Olsen JC, Ishizawa L, et al: Integrin alphaIIb promoter-targeted expression of gene products in megakaryocytes derived from retrovirus-transduced human hematopoietic cells. *Proc Natl Acad Sci U S A* 96:9654, 1999.

232. Wilcox DA, White GC: Gene therapy for platelet disorders, in *Platelets*, edited by AD Michelson, p 927. Academic, San Diego, 2000.

233. Hodivala-Dilke KM, Tsakiris DA, Rayburn H, et al: Beta3-integrin-deficient mice are a model for Glanzmann thrombasthenia showing placental defects and reduced survival. *J Clin Invest* 103:229, 1999.

234. Boudreaux MK, Lipscomb DL: Clinical, biochemical, and molecular aspects of Glanzmann's thrombasthenia in humans and dogs. *Vet Pathol* 38:249, 2001.

235. Yasunaga K, Nomura S: Statistical analysis of Glanzmann's thrombasthenia in Japan. *Acta Haematol* 89:165, 1993.

236. Lopez JA, Andrews RK, Afshar-Kharghan V, Berndt MC: Bernard-Soulier syndrome. *Blood* 91:4397, 1998.

237. Lopez JA, Berndt MC: The GPIb-IX-V complex, in *Platelets*, edited by AD Michelson, p 85. Academic, San Diego, 2002.

238. Bernard J, Soulier J-P: Sur une nouvelle variete de dystrophie thrombocytaire-hemorragipare congenitale. *Semin Hop Paris* 24:3217, 1948.

239. Bernard J: History of congenital hemorrhagic thrombocytopathic dystrophy. *Blood Cells* 9:179, 1983.

240. Weiss HJ, Tschopp TB, Baumgartner HR, et al: Decreased adhesion of giant (Bernard-Soulier) platelets to subendothelium. Further implications on the role of the von Willebrand factor in hemostasis. *Am J Med* 57:920, 1974.

241. Howard MA, Hutton RA, Hardisty RM: Hereditary giant platelet syndrome: A disorder of a new aspect of platelet function. *Br Med J* 2:586, 1973.

242. Bithell TC, Parekh SJ, Strong RR: Platelet-function studies in the Bernard-Soulier syndrome. *Ann N Y Acad Sci* 201:145, 1972.

243. Nurden AT, Caen JP: Specific roles for platelet surface glycoproteins in platelet function. *Nature* 255:720, 1975.

244. Howard MA, Perkin J, Salem HH, Firkin BG: The agglutination of human platelets by botrocetin: Evidence that botrocetin and ristocetin act at different sites on the factor VIII molecule and platelet membrane. *Br J Haematol* 57:25, 1984.

245. Moake JL, Olson JD, Troll JH, et al: Binding of radioiodinated human von Willebrand factor to Bernard-Soulier, thrombasthenic, and von Willebrand's disease platelets. *Thromb Res* 19:21, 1980.

246. Zucker MB, Kim SJ, McPherson J, Grant RA: Binding of factor VIII to platelets in the presence of ristocetin. *Br J Haematol* 35:535, 1977.

247. Berndt MC, Gregory C, Chong BH, et al: Additional glycoprotein defects in Bernard-Soulier's syndrome: Confirmation of genetic basis by parental analysis. *Blood* 62:800, 1983.

248. Clemetson KJ, McGregor JL, James E, et al: Characterization of the platelet membrane glycoprotein abnormalities in Bernard-Soulier syndrome and comparison with normal by surface-labeling techniques and high-resolution two-dimensional gel electrophoresis. *J Clin Invest* 70:304, 1982.

249. Vanhoorelbeke K, Ulrichts H, Romijn RA, et al: The GPIbalpha-thrombin interaction: Far from crystal clear. *Trends Mol Med* 10:33, 2004.

250. Romo GM, Dong JF, Schade AJ, et al: The glycoprotein Ib-IX-V complex is a platelet counterreceptor for P-selectin. *J Exp Med* 190:803, 1999.

251. Simon DI, Chen Z, Xu H, et al: Platelet glycoprotein Iba is a counterreceptor for the leukocyte integrin Mac-1 (CD11b/CD18). *J Exp Med* 192:193, 2000.

252. Bradford HN, Dela Cadena RA, Kunapuli SP, et al: Human kininogens regulate thrombin binding to platelets through the glycoprotein Ib-IX-V complex. *Blood* 90:1508, 1997.

253. Baglia FA, Badellino KO, Li CQ, et al: Factor XI binding to the platelet glycoprotein Ib-IX-V complex promotes factor XI activation by thrombin. *J Biol Chem* 277:1662, 2002.

254. Bradford HN, Pixley RA, Colman RW: Human factor XII binding to the glycoprotein Ib-IX-V complex inhibits thrombin-induced platelet aggregation. *J Biol Chem* 275:22756, 2000.

255. Ware J, Russell S, Ruggeri ZM: Generation and rescue of a murine model of platelet dysfunction: The Bernard-Soulier syndrome. *Proc Natl Acad Sci U S A* 97:2803, 2000.

256. Ramakrishnan V, Reeves PS, DeGuzman F, et al: Increased thrombin responsiveness in platelets from mice lacking glycoprotein V. *Proc Natl Acad Sci U S A* 96:13336, 1999.

257. McGill M, Jamieson GA, Drouin J, et al: Morphometric analysis of platelets in Bernard-Soulier syndrome: Size and configuration in patients and carriers. *Thromb Haemost* 52:37, 1984.

258. Michalas S, Malamitsi-Puchner A, Tsevrenis H: Pregnancy and delivery in Bernard-Soulier syndrome. *Acta Obstet Gynecol Scand* 63:185, 1984.

259. Suhasini G, Nanivadekar SA, Sawant PD, et al: Bernard-Soulier syndrome presenting as recurrent exsanguinating haematemesis. *Indian J Gastroenterol* 5:137, 1986.

260. Heslop HE, Hickton CM, Laird E, et al: Twin pregnancy and parturition in a patient with the Bernard Soulier syndrome. *Scand J Haematol* 37:71, 1986.

261. De Marco L, Fabris F, Casonato A, et al: Bernard-Soulier syndrome: Diagnosis by an ELISA method using monoclonal antibodies in 2 new unrelated patients. *Acta Haematol* 75:203, 1986.

262. Sheffer R, Ilan Y, Eldor A: Bernard-Soulier syndrome. *Harefuah* 111:119, 1986.

263. Ingerslev J, Stenbjerg S, Taaning E: A case of Bernard-Soulier syndrome: Study of platelet glycoprotein Ib in a kindred. *Eur J Haematol* 39:182, 1987.

264. Oki Y, Yoshioka K, Konishi M, et al: A case of Bernard-Soulier syndrome. *Nippon Naika Gakkai Zasshi* 76:1414, 1987.

265. de Moerloose P, Vogel JJ, Clemetson KJ, et al: Bernard-Soulier syndrome in a Swiss family. *Schweiz Med Wochenschr* 117:1817, 1987.

266. Cuthbert RJ, Watson HH, Handa SI, et al: DDAVP shortens the bleeding time in Bernard-Soulier syndrome. *Thromb Res* 49:649, 1988.

267. Drouin J, McGregor JL, Parmentier S, et al: Residual amounts of glycoprotein Ib concomitant with near-absence of glycoprotein IX in platelets of Bernard-Soulier patients. *Blood* 72:1086, 1988.

268. Mant MJ: DDAVP in Bernard-Soulier syndrome. *Thromb Res* 52:77, 1988.

269. Stevens MC, Blanchette VS, Freedman MH, et al: A variant form of Bernard-Soulier syndrome: Mild haemostatic defect associated with partial platelet GPIb deficiency. *Clin Lab Haematol* 10:443, 1988.

270. Shimamoto Y, Kaneoka H, Matsuzaki M, et al: Genetic markers and thrombin reaction in a family of Bernard-Soulier syndrome. *Nippon Ketsueki Gakkai Zasshi* 52:1155, 1989.

271. Peaceman AM, Katz AR, Laville M: Bernard-Soulier syndrome complicating pregnancy: A case report. *Obstet Gynecol* 73:457, 1989.

272. Nichols WL, Kaese SE, Gastineau DA, et al: Bernard-Soulier syndrome: Whole blood diagnostic assays of platelets. *Mayo Clin Proc* 64:522, 1989.

273. Ware J, Russell SR, Vicente V, et al: Nonsense mutation in the glycoprotein Ib alpha coding sequence associated with Bernard-Soulier syndrome. *Proc Natl Acad Sci U S A* 87:2026, 1990.

274. Finch CN, Miller JL, Lyle VA, Handin RI: Evidence that an abnormality in the glycoprotein Ib alpha gene is not the cause of abnormal platelet function in a family with classic Bernard-Soulier disease. *Blood* 75:2357, 1990.

275. De Marco L, Mazzucato M, Fabris F, et al: Variant Bernard-Soulier syndrome type Bolzano. A congenital bleeding disorder due to a structural and functional abnormality of the platelet glycoprotein Ib-IX complex. *J Clin Invest* 86:25, 1990.

276. Poulsen LO, Taaning E: Variation in surface platelet glycoprotein Ib expression in Bernard-Soulier syndrome. *Haemostasis* 20:155, 1990.

277. Ware J, Russell SR, Vicente V, et al: Nonsense mutation in the glycoprotein Ibalpha coding sequence associated with Bernard-Soulier syndrome. *Proc Natl Acad Sci U S A* 87:2026, 1990.

278. Waldenstrom E, Holmberg L, Axelsson U, et al: Bernard-Soulier syndrome in two Swedish families: Effect of DDAVP on bleeding time. *Eur J Haematol* 46:182, 1991.

279. Humphries JE, Yirinec BA, Hess CE: Atherosclerosis and unstable angina in Bernard-Soulier syndrome. *Am J Clin Pathol* 97:652, 1992.

280. Miller JL, Lyle VA, Cunningham D: Mutation of leucine-57 to phenylalanine in a platelet glycoprotein Ib alpha leucine tandem repeat occurring in patients with an autosomal dominant variant of Bernard-Soulier disease. *Blood* 79:439, 1992.

281. Avila MA, Jacyntho C, Santos ML, et al: Bernard-Soulier syndrome and pregnancy: A case report. *J Gynecol Obstet Biol Reprod (Paris)* 21:73, 1992.

282. Wright SD, Michaelides K, Johnson DJ, et al: Double heterozygosity for mutations in the platelet glycoprotein IX gene in three siblings with Bernard-Soulier syndrome. *Blood* 81:2339, 1993.

283. Ware J, Russell SR, Marchese P, et al: Point mutation in a leucine-rich repeat of platelet glycoprotein Ibalpha in the Bernard-Soulier syndrome. *J Clin Invest* 92:1213, 1993.

284. Simsek S, Admiraal LG, Modderman PW, et al: Identification of a homozygous single base pair deletion in the gene coding for the human platelet glycoprotein Ibalpha causing Bernard-Soulier syndrome. *Thromb Haemost* 72:444, 1994.

285. Simsek S, Noris P, Lozano M, et al: Cys209Ser mutation in the platelet membrane glycoprotein Ibalpha gene is associated with Bernard Soulier syndrome. *Br J Haematol* 88:839, 1994.

286. Kunishima S, Miura G, Fukutani H, et al: Bernard-Soulier syndrome Kagoshima: Ser 444-Stop mutation of glycoprotein (GP) Ibalpha resulting in circulating truncated GPIbalpha and surface expression of GPIbbeta and GPIX. *Blood* 84:3356, 1994.

287. Li C, Martin SE, Roth GJ: The genetic defect in two well-studied cases of Bernard-Soulier syndrome: A point mutation in the fifth leucine-rich repeat of platelet glycoprotein Iba. *Blood* 86:3805, 1995.

288. De La Salle C, Baas M-J, Lanza F, et al: A three-base deletion removing a leucine residue in a leucine-rich repeat of platelet glycoprotein Ibalpha associated with a variant of Bernard-Soulier syndrome (Nancy I). *Br J Haematol* 89:386, 1995.

289. Noda M, Fujimura K, Takafuta T, et al: Heterogenous expression of glycoprotein Ib, IX and V in platelets from two patients with Bernard-Soulier syndrome caused by different genetic abnormalities. *Thromb Haemost* 74:1411, 1995.

290. Budarf ML, Konkle BA, Ludlow LB, et al: Identification of a patient with Bernard-Soulier syndrome and a deletion in the DiGeorge/Velocardio-facial chromosomal region in 22q11.2. *Hum Mol Genet* 4:763, 1995.

291. Ludlow LB, Schick BP, Budarf ML, et al: Identification of a mutation in a GATA binding site of the platelet glycoprotein Ibbeta promoter resulting in the Bernard-Soulier syndrome. *J Biol Chem* 271:22076, 1996.

292. Li C, Pasquale DN, Roth GJ: Bernard-Soulier syndrome with severe bleeding: Absent platelet glycoprotein Ib alpha due to a homozygous one-base deletion. *Thromb Haemost* 76:670, 1996.

293. Martinez-Murillo C, Quintana-Gonzalez S, Ambriz-Fernandez R, et al: Utility of desmopressin in 4 cases of thrombocytopathies associated with giant platelets. *Rev Invest Clin* 49:281, 1997.

294. Kanaji T, Okamura T, Kuroiwa M, et al: Molecular and genetic analysis of two patients with Bernard-Soulier syndrome: Identification of new mutations in glycoprotein Ibalpha gene. *Thromb Haemost* 77:1055, 1997.

295. Kenny D, Newman PJ, Morateck PA, Montgomery RR: A dinucleotide deletion results in defective membrane anchoring and circulating soluble glycoprotein Ibalpha in a novel form of Bernard-Soulier syndrome. *Blood* 90:2626, 1997.

296. Afshar-Kharghan V, Lopez JA: Bernard-Soulier syndrome caused by a dinucleotide deletion and reading frameshift in the region encoding the glycoprotein Ibalpha transmembrane domain. *Blood* 90:2634, 1997.

297. Holmberg L, Karpman D, Nilsson I, Olofsson T: Bernard-Soulier syndrome Karlstad: Trp 498-Stop mutation resulting in a truncated glycoprotein Ibalpha that contains part of the transmembrane domain. *Br J Haematol* 98:57, 1997.

298. Kunishima S, Lopez JA, Kobayashi S, et al: Missense mutations of the glycoprotein (GP) Ib beta gene impairing the GPIb alpha/beta disulfide linkage in a family with giant platelet disorder. *Blood* 89:2404, 1997.

299. Noris P, Simsek S, Stibbe J, von dem Borne AEGK: A phenylalanine-55 to serine amino-acid substitution in the human glycoprotein IX leucine-rich repeat is associated with Bernard-Soulier syndrome. *Br J Haematol* 97:312, 1997.

300. Noris P, Arbustini E, Spedini P, et al: A new variant of Bernard-Soulier syndrome characterized by dysfunctional glycoprotein (GP) Ib and severely reduced amounts of GPIX and GPV. *Br J Haematol* 103:1004, 1998.

301. Van Geet C, Devriendt K, Eyskens B, et al: Velocardiofacial syndrome patients with a heterozygous chromosome 22q11 deletion have giant platelets. *Pediatr Res* 44:607, 1998.

302. Khalil A, Seoud M, Tannous R, et al: Bernard-Soulier syndrome in pregnancy: Case report and review of the literature. *Clin Lab Haematol* 20:125, 1998.

303. Kenny D, Morateck PA, Gill JC, Montgomery RR: The critical interaction of glycoprotein (GP) Ibb with GPIX-a genetic cause of Bernard-Soulier syndrome. *Blood* 93:2968, 1999.

304. Koskela S, Javela K, Jouppila J, et al: Variant Bernard-Soulier syndrome due to homozygous Asn45Ser mutation in the platelet glycoprotein (GP) IX in seven patients of five unrelated Finnish families. *Eur J Haematol* 62:256, 1999.

305. Koskela S, Partanen J, Salmi TT, Kekomaki R: Molecular characterization of two mutations in platelet glycoprotein (GP) Ibalpha in two Finnish Bernard-Soulier syndrome families. *Eur J Haematol* 62:160, 1999.

306. Margaglione M, D'Andrea G, Grandone E, et al: Compound heterozygosity (554-589 del, C515-T transition) in the platelet glycoprotein Ib alpha gene in a patient with a severe bleeding tendency. *Thromb Haemost* 81:486, 1999.

307. Sachs UJ, Kroll H, Matzdorff AC, et al: Bernard-Soulier syndrome due to the homozygous Asn-45Ser mutation in GPIX: An unexpected, frequent finding in Germany. *Br J Haematol* 123:127, 2003.

308. Watanabe R, Ishibashi T, Saitoh Y, et al: Bernard-soulier syndrome with a homozygous 13 base pair deletion in the signal peptide-coding region of the platelet glycoprotein Ib(beta) gene. *Blood Coagul Fibrinolysis* 14:387, 2003.

309. Strassel C, Pasquet JM, Alessi MC, et al: A novel missense mutation shows that GPIbbeta has a dual role in controlling the processing and stability of the platelet GPIb-IX adhesion receptor. *Biochemistry* 42:4452, 2003.

310. Kunishima S, Matsushita T, Ito T, et al: Novel nonsense mutation in the platelet glycoprotein Ibbeta gene associated with Bernard-Soulier syndrome. *Am J Hematol* 71:279, 2002.

311. Lanza F, De La SC, Baas MJ, et al: A Leu7Pro mutation in the signal peptide of platelet glycoprotein (GP)IX in a case of Bernard-Soulier syndrome abolishes surface expression of the GPIb-V-IX complex. *Br J Haematol* 118:260, 2002.

312. Kurokawa Y, Ishida F, Kamijo T, et al: A missense mutation (Tyr88 to Cys) in the platelet membrane glycoprotein Ibbeta gene affects GPIb/IX complex expression: Bernard-Soulier syndrome in the homozygous form and giant platelets in the heterozygous form. *Thromb Haemost* 86:1249, 2001.

313. Gonzalez-Manchon C, Larrucea S, Pastor AL, et al: Compound heterozygosity of the GPIbalpha gene associated with Bernard-Soulier syndrome. *Thromb Haemost* 86:1385, 2001.

314. Wang Z, Shi J, Han Y: A novel point mutation in the transmembrane domain of platelet glycoprotein IX gene identified in a Bernard-Soulier syndrome patient. *Zhonghua Xue Ye Xue Za Zhi* 22:464, 2001.

315. Kunishima S, Naoe T, Kamiya T, Saito H: Novel heterozygous missense mutation in the platelet glycoprotein Ib beta gene associated with isolated giant platelet disorder. *Am J Hematol* 68:249, 2001.

316. Vanhoorelbeke K, Schlammadinger A, Delville JP, et al: Occurrence of the Asn45Ser mutation in the GPIX gene in a Belgian patient with Bernard-Soulier syndrome. *Platelets* 12:114, 2001.

317. Rivera CE, Villagra J, Riordan M, et al: Identification of a new mutation in platelet glycoprotein IX (GPIX) in a patient with Bernard-Soulier syndrome. *Br J Haematol* 112:105, 2001.

318. Afshar-Kharghan V, Craig FE, Lopez JA: Bernard-Soulier syndrome in a patient doubly heterozygous for two frameshift mutations in the glycoprotein ib alpha gene. *Br J Haematol* 110:919, 2000.

319. Antonucci JV, Martin ES, Hulick PJ, et al: Bernard-Soulier syndrome: Common ancestry in two African American families with the GP Ib alpha Leu129Pro mutation. *Am J Hematol* 65:141, 2000.

320. Kunishima S, Tomiyama Y, Honda S, et al: Homozygous Pro74→Arg mutation in the platelet glycoprotein Ibbeta gene associated with Bernard-Soulier syndrome. *Thromb Haemost* 84:112, 2000.

321. Moran N, Morateck PA, Deering A, et al: Surface expression of glycoprotein ib alpha is dependent on glycoprotein ib beta: Evidence from a novel mutation causing Bernard-Soulier syndrome. *Blood* 96:532, 2000.

322. Kunishima S, Tomiyama Y, Honda S, et al: Cys97→Tyr mutation in the glycoprotein IX gene associated with Bernard-Soulier syndrome. *Br J Haematol* 107:539, 1999.

323. Lascone MR, Sacchelli M, Vittorini S, Giusti S: Complex conotruncal heart defect, severe bleeding disorder and 22q11 deletion: A new case of Bernard-Soulier syndrome and of 22q11 deletion syndrome? *Ital Heart J* 2:475, 2001.

324. Tang J, Stern-Nezer S, Liu PC, et al: Mutation in the leucine-rich repeat C-flanking region of platelet glycoprotein Ibbeta impairs assembly of von Willebrand factor receptor. *Thromb Haemost* 92:75, 2004.

325. Hillmann A, Nurden A, Nurden P, et al: A novel hemizygous Bernard-Soulier Syndrome (BSS) mutation in the amino terminal domain of glycoprotein (GP)Ibbeta: Platelet characterization and transfection studies. *Thromb Haemost* 88:1026, 2002.

326. Nakagawa M, Okuno M, Okamoto N, et al: Bernard-Soulier syndrome associated with 22q11.2 microdeletion. *Am J Med Genet* 99:286, 2001.

327. Grottum KA, Solum NO: Congenital thrombocytopenia with giant platelets: A defect in the platelet membrane. *Br J Haematol* 16:277, 1969.

328. Greenberg JP, Packham MA, Guccione MA, et al: Survival of rabbit-platelets treated in vitro with chymotrypsin, plasmin, trypsin, and neuraminidase. *Blood* 53:916, 1979.

329. Heyns Ad, Badenhorst PN, Wessels P, et al: Kinetics, in vivo redistribution and sites of sequestration of indium-111-labelled platelets in giant platelet syndromes. *Br J Haematol* 60:323, 1985.

330. Tomer A, Scharf RE, McMillan R, et al: Bernard-Soulier syndrome: Quantitative characterization of megakaryocytes and platelets by flow cytometric and platelet kinetic measurements. *Eur J Haematol* 52:193, 1994.

331. Nurden P, Nurden A: Giant platelets, megakaryocytes and the expression of glycoprotein Ib-IX complexes. *C R Acad Sci III* 319:717, 1996.
332. Ruggeri Z: The platelet glycoprotein Ib-IX complex. *Prog Hemost Thromb* 10:35, 1991.
333. Roth GJ: Developing relationships: Arterial platelet adhesion, glycoprotein Ib, and leucine-rich glycoproteins. *Blood* 77:5, 1991.
334. Yap CL, Hughan SC, Cranmer SL, et al: Synergistic adhesive interactions and signaling mechanisms operating between platelet glycoprotein Ib/IX and integrin alpha IIbbeta 3. Studies in human platelets ans transfected Chinese hamster ovary cells. *J Biol Chem* 275:41377, 2000.
335. Wu YP, Vink T, Schiphorst M, et al: Platelet thrombus formation on collagen at high shear rates is mediated by von Willebrand factor-glycoprotein Ib interaction and inhibited by von Willebrand factor-glycoprotein IIb/IIIa interaction. *Arterioscler Thromb Vasc Biol* 20:1661, 2000.
336. Kulkarni S, Dopheide SM, Yap CL, et al: A revised model of platelet aggregation. *J Clin Invest* 105:783, 2000.
337. Ikeda Y, Handa M, Kawano K, et al: The role of von Willebrand factor and fibrinogen in platelet aggregation under varying shear stress. *J Clin Invest* 87:1234, 1991.
338. Peterson DM, Stathopoulos NA, Giorgio TD, et al: Shear-induced platelet aggregation requires von Willebrand factor and platelet membrane glycoproteins Ib and IIb-IIIa. *Blood* 69:625, 1987.
339. Ruggeri ZM: Mechanisms of shear-induced platelet adhesion and aggregation. *Thromb Haemost* 70:119, 1993.
340. Jamieson GA, Okumura T: Reduced thrombin binding and aggregation in Bernard-Soulier platelets. *J Clin Invest* 61:861, 1978.
341. Nurden AT, George JN, Phillips DR: Human platelet membrane glycoproteins, in *Biochemistry of the Platelet*, edited by M Shuman, DR Phillips, p 159. Academic, New York, 1986.
342. Jandrot-Perrus M, Rendu F, Caen JP, et al: The common pathway for alpha- and gamma-thrombin-induced platelet activation is independent of GPIb: A study of Bernard-Soulier platelets. *Br J Haematol* 75:385, 1990.
343. De Marco L, Mazzucato M, Masotti A, et al: Function of glycoprotein Ib alpha in platelet activation induced by alpha-thrombin. *J Biol Chem* 266:23776, 1991.
344. Ramakrishnan V, Reeves PS, DeGuzman F, et al: Increased thrombin responsiveness in platelets from mice lacking glycoprotein V. *Proc Natl Acad Sci U S A* 96:13336, 1999.
345. Ni H, Ramakrishnan V, Ruggeri ZM, et al: Increased thrombogenesis and embolus formation in mice lacking glycoprotein V. *Blood* 98:368, 2001.
346. Caen J, Bellucci S: The defective prothrombin consumption in Bernard-Soulier syndrome. Hypotheses from 1948 to 1982. *Blood Cells* 9:389, 1983.
347. Walsh PN, Mills DC, Pareti FI, et al: Hereditary giant platelet syndrome. Absence of collagen-induced coagulant activity and deficiency of factor-XI binding to platelets. *Br J Haematol* 29:639, 1975.
348. Perret B, Levy-Toledano S, Plataviv M: Abnormal phospholipid organization in Bernard-Soulier platelets. *Thromb Res* 31:529, 1983.
349. Kanaji T, Russell S, Ware J: Amelioration of the macrothrombocytopenia associated with the murine Bernard-Soulier syndrome. *Blood* 100:2102, 2002.
350. McNicol A, Drouin J, Clemetson KJ, Gerrard JM: Phospholipase C activity in platelets from Bernard-Soulier syndrome patients. *Arterioscler Thromb* 13:1567, 1993.
351. White JG, Burris SM, Hasegawa D, Johnson M: Micropipette aspiration of human blood platelets: A defect in Bernard-Soulier's syndrome. *Blood* 63:1249, 1984.
352. Nurden AT: Congenital abnormalities of platelet membrane glycoproteins, in *Platelet Immunobiology, Molecular and Clinical Aspects*, edited by TJ Kunicki, JN George, p 95. Lippincott, Philadelphia, 1989.

353. Lopez JA, Leung B, Reynolds CC, et al: Efficient plasma membrane expression of a functional platelet glycoprotein Ib-IX complex requires the presence of its three subunits. *J Biol Chem* 267:12851, 1992.
354. Nurden AT, Didry-Dupies V, Rosa JP: Molecular defects of platelets in Bernard Soulier Syndrome. *Blood Cells* 9:333, 1983.
355. Nurden AT: Inherited abnormalities of platelets. *Thromb Haemost* 82:468, 1999.
356. Nurden AT, Jallu V, Hourdille P: GP Ib and Bernard-Soulier platelets. *Blood* 73:2225, 1989.
357. Lawrence S, McDonald-McGinn DM, Zackai E, Sullivan KE: Thrombocytopenia in patients with chromosome 22q11.2 deletion syndrome. *J Pediatr* 143:277, 2003.
358. Kato T, Kosaka K, Kimura M, et al: Thrombocytopenia in patients with 22q11.2 deletion syndrome and its association with glycoprotein Ib-beta. *Genet Med* 5:113, 2003.
359. Latger-Cannard V, Bensoussan D, Gregoire MJ, et al: Frequency of thrombocytopenia and large platelets correlates neither with conotruncal cardiac anomalies nor immunological features in the chromosome 22q11.2 deletion syndrome. *Eur J Pediatr* 163:327 2004.
360. Ryan AK, Goodship JA, Wilson DI, et al: Spectrum of clinical features associated with interstitial chromosome 22q11 deletions: A European collaborative study. *J Med Genet* 34:798, 1997.
361. George JN, Reimann TA, Moake JL, et al: Bernard-Soulier disease: A study of four patients and their parents. *Br J Haematol* 48:459, 1981.
362. Fox JEB: Linkage of a membrane skeleton to integral membrane glycoproteins in human platelets. Identification of one of the glycoproteins as glycoprotein Ib. *J Clin Invest* 76:1673, 1985.
363. Eaton LA Jr, Read MS, Brinkhous KM: Glycoprotein Ib bioassays. Activity levels in Bernard-Soulier syndrome and in stored blood bank platelets. *Arch Pathol Lab Med* 115:488, 1991.
364. Evensen SA, Solum NO, Grottum KA, Hovig T: Familial bleeding disorder with a moderate thrombocytopenia and giant blood platelets. *Scand J Haematol* 13:203, 1974.
365. Greco NJ, Tandon NN, Jones GD, et al: Contributions of glycoprotein Ib and the seven transmembrane domain receptor to increases in platelet cytoplasmic [Ca^{2+}] induced by a-thrombin. *Biochemistry* 35:906, 1996.
366. Celikel R, McClintock RA, Roberts JR, et al: Modulation of alpha-thrombin function by distinct interactions with platelet glycoprotein Ibalpha. *Science* 301:218, 2003.
367. Dumas JJ, Kumar R, Seehra J, et al: Crystal structure of the GpIbalpha-thrombin complex essential for platelet aggregation. *Science* 301:222, 2003.
368. McGowan EB, Ding A, Detwiler TC: Correlation of thrombin-induced glycoprotein V hydrolysis and platelet activation. *J Biol Chem* 258:11243, 1983.
369. Bienz D, Schnippering W, Clemetson KJ: Glycoprotein V is not the thrombin activation receptor on human blood platelets. *Blood* 68:720, 1986.
370. Caen JP, Nurden AT, Jeanneau C, et al: Bernard-Soulier syndrome: A new platelet glycoprotein abnormality. Its relationship with platelet adhesion to subendothelium and with the factor VIII von Willebrand protein. *J Lab Clin Med* 87:586, 1976.
371. Andrews RK, Harris SJ, McNally T, Berndt MC: Binding of purified 14-3-3 zeta signaling protein to discrete amino acid sequences within the cytoplasmic domain of the platelet membrane glycoprotein Ib-IX-V complex. *Biochemistry* 37:638, 1998.
372. Sullam PM, Hyun WC, Szollosi J, et al: Physical proximity and functional interplay of the glycoprotein Ib-IX-V complex and the Fc receptor FcgammaRIIA on the platelet plasma membrane. *J Biol Chem* 273:5331, 1998.
373. Falati S, Edmead CE, Poole AW: Glycoprotein Ib-V-IX, a receptor for von Willebrand factor, couples physically and functionally to the Fc

receptor γ-chain, Fyn, and Lyn to activate human platelets. *Blood* 94: 1648, 1999.

374. Feng S, Resendiz JC, Christodoulides N, et al: Pathological shear stress stimulates the tyrosine phosphorylation of alpha-actinin associated with the glycoprotein Ib-IX complex. *Biochemistry* 41:1100, 2002.

375. Stricker RB, Wong D, Saks SR, et al: Acquired Bernard-Soulier syndrome. Evidence for the role of a 210,000-molecular weight protein in the interaction of platelets with von Willebrand factor. *J Clin Invest* 76: 1274, 1985.

376. Deckmyn H, Vanhoorelbeke K, Peerlinck K: Inhibitory and activating human antiplatelet antibodies. *Baillieres Clin Haematol* 11:343, 1998.

377. Devine DV, Currie MS, Rosse WF, Greenberg CS: Pseudo-Bernard-Soulier syndrome: Thrombocytopenia caused by autoantibody to platelet glycoprotein Ib. *Blood* 70:428, 1987.

378. Varon D, Gitel SN, Varon N, et al: Immune Bernard Soulier-like syndrome associated with anti-glycoprotein-IX antibody. *Am J Hematol* 41: 67, 1992.

379. Beales IL: An acquired-pseudo Bernard-Soulier syndrome occurring with autoimmune chronic active hepatitis and anti-cardiolipin antibody. *Postgrad Med J* 70:305, 1994.

380. Berndt MC, Kabral A, Grimsley P, et al: An acquired Bernard-Soulier-like platelet defect associated with juvenile myelodysplastic syndrome. *Br J Haematol* 68:97, 1988.

381. Hicsonmez G, Gumruk F, Cetin M, et al: Bernard-Soulier-like functional platelet defect in myelodysplastic syndrome and in acute myeloblastic leukemia associated with trilineage myelodysplasia. *Turk J Pediatr* 37: 425, 1995.

382. Sharma JB, Buckshee K, Sharma S: Puberty menorrhagia due to Bernard Soulier syndrome and its successful treatment by "Ovral" hormonal tablets. *Aust N Z J Obstet Gynaecol* 31:369, 1991.

383. Greinacher A, Potzsch B, Kiefel V, et al: Evidence that DDAVP transiently improves hemostasis in Bernard-Soulier syndrome independent of von Willebrand-factor. *Ann Hematol* 67:149, 1993.

384. Kemahli S, Canatan D, Uysal Z, et al: DDAVP shortens bleeding time in Bernard-Soulier syndrome. *Thromb Haemost* 71:675, 1994.

385. Greinacher A, Potzsch B, Kiefel V, et al: Evidence that DDAVP transiently improves hemostasis in Bernard-Soulier syndrome independent of von Willebrand-factor. *Ann Hematol* 67:149, 1993.

386. Saade G, Homsi R, Seoud M: Bernard-Soulier syndrome in pregnancy; a report of four pregnancies in one patient, and review of the literature. *Eur J Obstet Gynecol Reprod Biol* 40:149, 1991.

387. Degos L, Tobelem G, Lethielleux P, et al: Molecular defect in platelets from patients with bernard-soulier syndrome. *Blood* 50:899, 1977.

388. Peng TC, Kickler TS, Bell WR, Haller E: Obstetric complications in a patient with Bernard-Soulier syndrome. *Am J Obstet Gynecol* 165:425, 1991.

389. Peters M, Heijboer H: Treatment of a patient with Bernard-Soulier syndrome and recurrent nosebleeds with recombinant factor VIIa. *Thromb Haemost* 80:352, 1998.

390. Locatelli F, Rossi G, Balduini C: Hematopoietic stem-cell transplantation for the Bernard-Soulier syndrome. *Ann Intern Med* 138:79, 2003.

391. Takahashi H: Studies on the pathophysiology and treatment of von Willebrand's disease: IV. Mechanism of increased ristocetin-induced platelet aggregation in von Willebrand's disease. *Thromb Res* 19:857, 1980.

392. Krizek DM, Rick ME, Williams SB, Gralnick HR: Cryoprecipitate transfusion in variant von Willebrand's disease and thrombocytopenia. *Ann Intern Med* 98:484, 1983.

393. Weiss HJ, Meyer D, Rabinowitz R, et al: Pseudo-von Willebrand's disease. An intrinsic platelet defect with aggregation by unmodified human factor VIII/von Willebrand factor and enhanced adsorption of its high-molecular-weight multimers. *N Engl J Med* 306:326, 1982.

394. Miller JL, Castella A: Platelet-type von Willebrand's disease: Characterization of a new bleeding disorder. *Blood* 60:790, 1982.

395. Gralnick HR, Williams SB, Shafer BC, Corash L: Factor VIII/von Willebrand factor binding to von Willebrand's disease platelets. *Blood* 60: 328, 1982.

396. Takahashi H, Handa M, Watanabe K, et al: Further characterization of platelet-type von Willebrand's disease in Japan. *Blood* 64:1254, 1984.

397. Miller JL, Cunningham D, Lyle VA, Finch CN: Mutation in the gene encoding the alpha chain of platelet glycoprotein Ib in platelet-type von Willebrand disease. *Proc Natl Acad Sci U S A* 88:4761, 1991.

398. Russell SD, Roth GJ: Pseudo-von Willebrand disease: A mutation in the platelet glycoprotein Ib alpha gene associated with a hyperactive surface receptor. *Blood* 81:1787, 1993.

399. Takahashi H, Murata M, Moriki T, et al: Substitution of Val for Met at residue 239 of platelet glycoprotein Ib alpha in Japanese patients with platelet-type von Willebrand disease. *Blood* 85:727, 1995.

400. Kunishima S, Heaton DC, Naoe T, et al: De novo mutation of the platelet glycoprotein Ib alpha gene in a patient with pseudo-von Willebrand disease. *Blood Coagul Fibrinolysis* 8:311, 1997.

401. Matsubara Y, Murata M, Sugita K, Ikeda Y: Identification of a novel point mutation in platelet glycoprotein Ibalpha, Gly to Ser at residue 233, in a Japanese family with platelet-type von Willebrand disease. *J Thromb Haemost* 1:2198, 2003.

402. Uff S, Clemetson JM, Harrison T, et al: Crystal structure of the platelet glycoprotein Ib(alpha) N-terminal domain reveals an unmasking mechanism for receptor activation. *J Biol Chem* 277:35657, 2002.

403. Huizinga EG, Tsuji S, Romijn RA, et al: Structures of glycoprotein Ibalpha and its complex with von Willebrand factor A1 domain. *Science* 297:1176, 2002.

404. Pincus MR, Carty RP, Miller JL: Structural implications of the substitution of Val for Met at residue 239 in the alpha chain of human platelet glycoprotein Ib. *J Protein Chem* 13:629, 1994.

405. Dumas JJ, Kumar R, McDonagh T, et al: Crystal structure of the wild-type von Willebrand factor A1-glycoprotein Ibalpha complex reveals conformation differences with a complex bearing von Willebrand disease mutations. *J Biol Chem* 279:23327, 2004.

406. Doggett TA, Girdhar G, Lawshe A, et al: Alterations in the intrinsic properties of the GPIbalpha-VWF tether bond define the kinetics of the platelet-type von Willebrand disease mutation, Gly233Val. *Blood* 102: 152, 2003.

407. Tait AS, Cranmer SL, Jackson SP, et al: Phenotype changes resulting in high-affinity binding of von Willebrand factor to recombinant glycoprotein Ib-IX: Analysis of the platelet-type von Willebrand disease mutations. *Blood* 98:1812, 2001.

408. Takahashi H, Nagayama R, Hattori A, Shibata A: Botrocetin- and polybrene-induced platelet aggregation in platelet-type von Willebrand disease. *Am J Hematol* 18:179, 1985.

409. Miller JL, Kupinski JM, Castella A, Ruggeri ZM: Von Willebrand factor binds to platelets and induces aggregation in platelet-type but not type IIB von Willebrand disease. *J Clin Invest* 72:1532, 1983.

410. Scott JP, Montgomery RR: The rapid differentiation of type IIb von Willebrand's disease from platelet-type (pseudo-) von Willebrand's disease by the "neutral" monoclonal antibody binding assay. *Am J Clin Pathol* 96:723, 1991.

411. Miller JL: Sorting out heightened interactions between platelets and von Willebrand factor. "IIB or not IIB?" is becoming an increasingly answerable question in the molecular era. *Am J Clin Pathol* 96: 681, 1991.

412. Miller JL, Ruggeri ZM, Lyle VA: Unique interactions of asialo von Willebrand factor with platelets in platelet-type von Willebrand disease. *Blood* 70:1804, 1987.

413. Takahashi H: Replacement therapy in platelet-type von Willebrand disease. *Am J Hematol* 18:351, 1985.

414. Miller JL: Platelet-type von Willebrand's disease. *Clin Lab Med* 4:319, 1984.

415. Fressinaud E, Signaud-Fiks M, Le Boterff C, Piot B: Use of recombinant factor VIIa (NovoSeven®) for dental extraction in a patient affected by platelet-type (pseudo-) von Willebrand disease [abstract]. *Haemophilia* 4:299, 1998.

416. Nieuwenhuis HK, Akkerman JWN, Houdijk WPM, Sixma JJ: Human blood platelets showing no response to collagen fail to express surface glycoprotein Ia. *Nature* 318:470, 1985.

417. Nieuwenhuis HK, Sakariassen KS, Houdijk WPM, et al: Deficiency of platelet membrane glycoprotein Ia associated with a decreased platelet adhesion to subendothelium: A defect in platelet spreading. *Blood* 68:692, 1986.

418. Beer JH, Nieuwenhuis HK, Sixma JJ, Coller BS: Deficiency of antibody 6F1 binding to the platelets of a patient with an isolated defect in platelet-collagen interaction [abstract]. *Circulation* 78(suppl):II, 1988.

419. Coller BS, Beer JH, Scudder LE, Steinberg MH: Collagen-platelet interactions: Evidence for a direct interaction of collagen with platelet GPIa/IIa and an indirect interaction with platelet GPIIb/IIa mediated by adhesive proteins. *Blood* 74:182, 1989.

420. Kehrel B, Balleisen L, Kokott R, et al: Deficiency of intact thrombospondin and membrane glycoprotein Ia in platelets with defective collagen-induced aggregation and spontaneous loss of disorder. *Blood* 71:1074, 1988.

421. Yamamoto N, Ikeda H, Tandon NN, et al: A platelet membrane glycoprotein (GP) deficiency in healthy blood donors: Nakᵃ-platelets lack detectable GPIV (CD36). *Blood* 76:1698, 1990.

422. Curtis BR, Aster RH: Incidence of the Nak(a)-negative platelet phenotype in African Americans is similar to that of Asians. *Transfusion* 36:331, 1996.

423. Asch AS, Barnwell J, Silverstein RL, Nachman RL: Isolation of the thrombospondin membrane receptor. *J Clin Invest* 79:1054, 1987.

424. Tandon NN, Kralisz U, Jamieson GA: Identification of glycoprotein IV (CD36) as a primary receptor for platelet-collagen adhesion. *J Biol Chem* 264:7576, 1989.

425. Silverstein RL, Asch AS, Nachman RL: Glycoprotein IV mediates thrombospondin-dependent platelet-monocyte and platelet-U937 cell adhesion. *J Clin Invest* 84:546, 1989.

426. Kehrel B, Kronenberg A, Schwippert B, et al: Thrombospondin binds normally to glycoprotein IIIb deficient platelets. *Biochem Biophys Res Commun* 179:985, 1991.

427. Tandon NN, Ockenhouse CF, Greco NJ, Jamieson GA: Adhesive functions of platelets lacking glycoprotein IV (CD36). *Blood* 78:2809, 1991.

428. Saelman EU, Kehrel B, Hese KM, et al: Platelet adhesion to collagen and endothelial cell matrix under flow conditions is not dependent on platelet glycoprotein IV. *Blood* 83:3240, 1994.

429. Englyst NA, Taube JM, Aitman TJ, et al: A novel role for CD36 in VLDL-enhanced platelet activation. *Diabetes* 52:1248, 2003.

430. Kashiwagi H, Tomiyama Y, Honda S, et al: Molecular basis of CD36 deficiency. Evidence that a 478C→T substitution (proline90→serine) in CD36 cDNA accounts for CD36 deficiency. *J Clin Invest* 95:1040, 1995.

431. Kashiwagi H, Tomiyama Y, Kosugi S, et al: Family studies of type II CD36 deficient subjects: Linkage of a CD36 allele to a platelet-specific mRNA expression defect(s) causing type II CD36 deficiency. *Thromb Haemost* 74:758, 1995.

432. Kashiwagi H, Tomiyama Y, Kosugi S, et al: Identification of molecular defects in a subject with type I CD36 deficiency. *Blood* 83:3545, 1994.

433. Kashiwagi H, Tomiyama Y, Nozaki S, et al: A single nucleotide insertion in codon 317 of the CD36 gene leads to CD36 deficiency. *Arterioscler Thromb Vasc Biol* 16:1026, 1996.

434. Hanawa H, Watanabe K, Nakamura T, et al: Identification of cryptic splice site, exon skipping, and novel point mutations in type I CD36 deficiency. *J Med Genet* 39:286, 2002.

435. Bierling P, Godeau B, Fromont P, et al: Posttransfusion purpura-like syndrome associated with CD36 (Naka) isoimmunization. *Transfusion* 35:777, 1995.

436. Nozaki S, Tanaka T, Yamashita S, et al: CD36 mediates long-chain fatty acid transport in human myocardium: Complete myocardial accumulation defect of radiolabeled long-chain fatty acid analog in subjects with CD36 deficiency. *Mol Cell Biochem* 192:129, 1999.

437. Griffin E, Re A, Hamel N, et al: A link between diabetes and atherosclerosis: Glucose regulates expression of CD36 at the level of translation. *Nat Med* 7:840, 2001.

438. Coburn CT, Knapp FF Jr, Febbraio M, et al: Defective uptake and utilization of long chain fatty acids in muscle and adipose tissues of CD36 knockout mice. *J Biol Chem* 275:32523, 2000.

439. Okamoto F, Tanaka T, Sohmiya K, Kawamura K: CD36 abnormality and impaired myocardial long-chain fatty acid uptake in patients with hypertrophic cardiomyopathy. *Jpn Circ J* 62:499, 1998.

440. Aitman TJ, Cooper LD, Norsworthy PJ, et al: Malaria susceptibility and CD36 mutation. *Nature* 405:1015, 2000.

441. Omi K, Ohashi J, Patarapotikul J, et al: CD36 polymorphism is associated with protection from cerebral malaria. *Am J Hum Genet* 72:364, 2003.

442. Pain A, Urban BC, Kai O, et al: A non-sense mutation in Cd36 gene is associated with protection from severe malaria. *Lancet* 357:1502, 2001.

443. Oquendo P, Hundt E, Lawler J, Seed B: CD36 directly mediates cytoadherence of Plasmodium falciparum parasitized erythrocytes. *Cell* 58:95, 1989.

444. Pain A, Ferguson DJ, Kai O, et al: Platelet-mediated clumping of Plasmodium falciparum-infected erythrocytes is a common adhesive phenotype and is associated with severe malaria. *Proc Natl Acad Sci U S A* 98:1805, 2001.

445. Moroi M, Jung SM, Okuma M, Shinmyozu K: A patient with platelets deficient in glycoprotein VI that lack both collagen-induced aggregation and adhesion. *J Clin Invest* 84:1440, 1989.

446. Ryo R, Yoshida A, Sugano W, et al: Deficiency of P62, a putative collagen receptor, in platelets from a patient with defective collagen-induced platelet aggregation. *Am J Hematol* 39:25, 1992.

447. Nurden P, Jandrot-Perrus M, Combrie R, et al: Severe deficiency of glycoprotein VI in a patient with gray platelet syndrome. *Blood* 104:107, 2004.

448. Arai M, Yamamoto N, Moroi M, et al: Platelets with 10% of the normal amount of glycoprotein VI have an impaired response to collagen that results in a mild bleeding tendency. *Br J Haematol* 89:124, 1995.

449. Sugiyama T, Okuma M, Ushikubi F, et al: A novel platelet aggregating factor found in a patient with defective collagen-induced platelet aggregation and autoimmune thrombocytopenia. *Blood* 69:1712, 1987.

450. Takahashi H, Moroi M: Antibody against platelet membrane glycoprotein VI in a patient with systemic lupus erythematosus. *Am J Hematol* 67:262, 2001.

451. Boylan B, Chen H, Rathore V, et al: Anti-GPVI-associated ITP: An acquired platelet disorder caused by autoantibody-mediated clearance of the GPVI/FcR{gamma}-chain complex from the human platelet surface. *Blood* 104:1350, 2004.

452. Nieswandt B, Schulte V, Bergmeier W, et al: Long-term antithrombotic protection by in vivo depletion of platelet glycoprotein VI in mice. *J Exp Med* 193:459, 2001.

453. Sullivan KE: Recent advances in our understanding of Wiskott-Aldrich syndrome. *Curr Opin Hematol* 6:8, 1999.

454. Sullivan KE, Mullen CA, Blaese RM, Winkelstein JA: A multiinstitutional survey of the Wiskott-Aldrich syndrome. *J Pediatr* 125:876, 1994.

455. Ochs HD: The Wiskott-Aldrich syndrome. *Semin Hematol* 35:332, 1998.

456. Thompson LJ, Lalloz MR, Layton DM: Unique and recurrent WAS gene mutations in Wiskott-Aldrich syndrome and X-linked thrombocytopenia. *Blood Cells Mol Dis* 25:218, 1999.

457. Devriendt K, Kim AS, Mathijs G, et al: Constitutively activating mutation in WASP causes X-linked severe congenital neutropenia. *Nat Genet* 27:313, 2001.

458. Zhu Q, Watanabe C, Liu T, et al: Wiskott-Aldrich syndrome/X-linked thrombocytopenia: WASP gene mutations, protein expression, and phenotype. *Blood* 90:2680, 1997.

459. Parkman R, Remold-O'Donnell E, Kenney DM, et al: Surface protein abnormalities in lymphocytes and platelets from patients with Wiskott-Aldrich syndrome. *Lancet* 2:1387, 1981.

460. Higgins EA, Siminovitch KA, Zhuang DL, et al: Aberrant O-linked oligosaccharide biosynthesis in lymphocytes and platelets from patients with the Wiskott-Aldrich syndrome. *J Biol Chem* 266:6280, 1991.

461. Rosenstein Y, Park JK, Hahn WC, et al: CD43, a molecule defective in Wiskott-Aldrich syndrome, binds ICAM-1. *Nature* 354:233, 1991.

462. Semple JW, Siminovitch KA, Mody M, et al: Flow cytometric analysis of platelets from children with the Wiskott-Aldrich syndrome reveals defects in platelet development, activation, and structure. *Br J Haematol* 97:747, 1997.

463. Higgins EA, Siminovitch KA, Zhuang DL, et al: Aberrant O-linked oligosaccharide biosynthesis in lymphocytes and platelets from patients with the Wiskott-Aldrich syndrome. *J Biol Chem* 266:6280, 1991.

464. Pidard D, Didry D, Le Deist F, et al: Analysis of the membrane glycoproteins of platelets in the Wiskott-Aldrich syndrome. *Br J Haematol* 69:529, 1988.

465. Grottum KA, Hovig T, Holmsen H, et al: Wiskott-Aldrich syndrome: Qualitative platelet defects and short platelet survival. *Br J Haematol* 17:373, 1969.

466. Murphy S, Oski FA, Naiman JL, et al: Platelet size and kinetics in hereditary and acquired thrombocytopenia. *N Engl J Med* 286:499, 1972.

467. Baldini MG: Nature of the platelet defect in the Wiskott-Aldrich syndrome. *Ann N Y Acad Sci* 201:437, 1972.

468. Ochs HD, Slichter SJ, Harker LA, et al: The Wiskott-Aldrich syndrome: Studies of lymphocytes, granulocytes, and platelets. *Blood* 55:243, 1980.

469. Ochs HD: The Wiskott-Aldrich syndrome. *Springer Semin Immunopathol* 19:435, 1998.

470. Litzman J, Jones A, Hann I, et al: Intravenous immunoglobulin, splenectomy, and antibiotic prophylaxis in Wiskott-Aldrich syndrome. *Arch Dis Child* 75:436, 1996.

471. Mullen CA, Anderson KD, Blaese RM: Splenectomy and/or bone marrow transplantation in the management of the Wiskott-Aldrich syndrome: Long-term follow-up of 62 cases. *Blood* 82:2961, 1993.

472. Akman IO, Ostrov BE, Neudorf S: Autoimmune manifestations of the Wiskott-Aldrich syndrome. *Semin Arthritis Rheum* 27:218, 1998.

473. Italiano JE, Hartwig JH: Megakaryocyte development and platelet formation, in *Platelets*, edited by AD Michelson, p 21. Academic, San Diego, 2002.

474. Lum LG, Tubergen DG, Corash L, Blaese RM: Splenectomy in the management of the thrombocytopenia of the Wiskott-Aldrich syndrome. *N Engl J Med* 302:892, 1980.

475. Lorenz P, Bollmann R, Hinkel GK, et al: False-negative prenatal exclusion of Wiskott-Aldrich syndrome by measurement of fetal platelet count and size. *Prenat Diagn* 11:819, 1991.

476. Stormorken H, Hellum B, Egeland T, et al: X-linked thrombocytopenia and thrombocytopathia: Attenuated Wiskott-Aldrich syndrome. Functional and morphological studies of platelets and lymphocytes. *Thromb Haemost* 65:300, 1991.

477. Villa A, Notarangelo L, Macchi P, et al: X-linked thrombocytopenia and Wiskott-Aldrich syndrome are allelic diseases with mutations in the WASP gene. *Nat Genet* 9:414, 1995.

478. Verhoeven AJ, van Oostrum IE, van Haarlem H, Akkerman JW: Impaired energy metabolism in platelets from patients with Wiskott-Aldrich syndrome. *Thromb Haemost* 61:10, 1989.

479. White JG: Inherited abnormalities of the platelet membrane and secretory granules. *Hum Pathol* 18:123, 1987.

480. Yamada M, Ariga T, Kawamura N, et al: Determination of carrier status for the Wiskott-Aldrich syndrome by flow cytometric analysis of Wiskott-Aldrich syndrome protein expression in peripheral blood mononuclear cells. *J Immunol* 165:1119, 2000.

481. Yamada M, Ohtsu M, Kobayashi I, et al: Flow cytometric analysis of Wiskott-Aldrich syndrome (WAS) protein in lymphocytes from WAS patients and their familial carriers. *Blood* 93:756, 1999.

482. Wengler G, Gorlin JB, Williamson JM, et al: Nonrandom inactivation of the X chromosome in early lineage hematopoietic cells in carriers of Wiskott-Aldrich syndrome. *Blood* 85:2471, 1995.

483. Weiss HJ, Chervenick PA, Zalusky R, Factor A: A familial defect in platelet function associated with impaired release of adenosine diphosphate. *N Engl J Med* 281:1264, 1969.

484. Nieuwenhuis HK, Akkerman JW, Sixma JJ: Patients with a prolonged bleeding time and normal aggregation tests may have storage pool deficiency: Studies on one hundred six patients. *Blood* 70:620, 1987.

485. Weiss HJ: Inherited disorders of platelet granules and signal transduction, in *Hemostasis and Thrombosis: Basic Principles and Clinical Practice*, edited by RW Colman, J Hirsh, VJ Marder, M Samama, p 673. Lippincott, Philadelphia, 1993.

486. Hermansky F, Pudlak P: Albinism associated with hemorrhagic diathesis and unusual pigmented reticular cells in the bone marrow: Report of two cases with histochemical studies. *Blood* 14:162, 1959.

487. Gahl WA, Brantly M, Kaiser-Kupfer MI, et al: Genetic defects and clinical characteristics of patients with a form of oculocutaneous albinism (Hermansky-Pudlak syndrome). *N Engl J Med* 338:1258, 1998.

488. Buchanan GR, Handin RI: Platelet function in the Chediak-Higashi syndrome. *Blood* 47:941, 1976.

489. Costa JL, Fauci AS, Wolff SM: A platelet abnormality in the Chediak-Higashi syndrome of man. *Blood* 48:517, 1976.

490. Boxer GJ, Holmsen H, Robkin L, et al: Abnormal platelet function in Chediak-Higashi syndrome. *Br J Haematol* 35:521, 1977.

491. Apitz-Castro R, Cruz MR, Ledezma E, et al: The storage pool deficiency in platelets from humans with the Chediak-Higashi syndrome: Study of six patients. *Br J Haematol* 59:471, 1985.

492. Cowan DH, Graham RC Jr, Baunach D: The platelet defect in leukemia. Platelet ultrastructure, adenine nucleotide metabolism, and the release reaction. *J Clin Invest* 56:188, 1975.

493. Gerrard JM, Israels ED, Biship AJ, et al: Inherited platelet-storage pool deficiency associated with a high incidence of acute myeloid leukaemia. *Br J Haematol* 79:246, 1991.

494. Ganly P, Walker LC, Morris CM: Familial mutations of the transcription factor RUNX1 (AML1, CBFA2) predispose to acute myeloid leukemia. *Leuk Lymphoma* 45:1, 2004.

495. Dowton SB, Beardsley D, Jamison D, et al: Studies of a familial platelet disorder. *Blood* 65:557, 1985.

496. Ho CY, Otterud B, Legare RD, et al: Linkage of a familial platelet disorder with a propensity to develop myeloid malignancies to human chromosome 21q22.1-22.2. *Blood* 87:5218, 1996.

497. Arepally G, Rebbeck TR, Song W, et al: Evidence for genetic homogeneity in a familial platelet disorder with predisposition to acute myelogenous leukemia (FPD/AML). *Blood* 92:2600, 1998.

498. Song WJ, Sullivan MG, Legare RD, et al: Haploinsufficiency of CBFA2 causes familial thrombocytopenia with propensity to develop acute myelogenous leukaemia. *Nat Genet* 23:166, 1999.

499. Buijs A, Poddighe P, van Wijk R, et al: A novel CBFA2 single-nucleotide mutation in familial platelet disorder with propensity to develop myeloid malignancies. *Blood* 98:2856, 2001.

500. Michaud J, Wu F, Osato M, et al: In vitro analyses of known and novel RUNX1/AML1 mutations in dominant familial platelet disorder with predisposition to acute myelogenous leukemia: Implications for mechanisms of pathogenesis. *Blood* 99:1364, 2002.

501. Walker LC, Stevens J, Campbell H, et al: A novel inherited mutation of the transcription factor RUNX1 causes thrombocytopenia and may predispose to acute myeloid leukaemia. *Br J Haematol* 117:878, 2002.

502. Sun L, Mao G, Rao AK: Association of CBFA2 mutation with decreased platelet PKC-theta and impaired receptor-mediated activation of GPIIb-IIIa and pleckstrin phosphorylation: Proteins regulated by CBFA2 play a role in GPIIb-IIIa activation. *Blood* 103:948, 2004.

503. Minelli A, Maserati E, Rossi G, et al: Familial platelet disorder with propensity to acute myelogenous leukemia: Genetic heterogeneity and progression to leukemia via acquisition of clonal chromosome anomalies. *Genes Chromosomes Cancer* 40:165, 2004.

504. Taketani T, Taki T, Takita J, et al: AML1/RUNX1 mutations are infrequent, but related to AML-M0, acquired trisomy 21, and leukemic transformation in pediatric hematologic malignancies. *Genes Chromosomes Cancer* 38:1, 2003.

505. Asou N: The role of a Runt domain transcription factor AML1/RUNX1 in leukemogenesis and its clinical implications. *Crit Rev Oncol Hematol* 45:129, 2003.

506. Nishibori M, Cham B, McNicol A, et al: The protein CD63 is in platelet dense granules, is deficient in a patient with Hermansky-Pudlak syndrome, and appears identical to granulophysin. *J Clin Invest* 91:1775, 1993.

507. Huizing M, Boissy RE, Gahl WA: Hermansky-Pudlak syndrome: Vesicle formation from yeast to man. *Pigment Cell Res* 15:405, 2002.

508. Hermos CR, Huizing M, Kaiser-Kupfer MI, Gahl WA: Hermansky-Pudlak syndrome type 1: Gene organization, novel mutations, and clinical-molecular review of non-Puerto Rican cases. *Hum Mutat* 20:482, 2002.

509. Dell'Angelica EC, Shotelersuk V, Aguilar RC, et al: Altered trafficking of lysosomal proteins in Hermansky-Pudlak syndrome due to mutations in the beta 3A subunit of the AP-3 adaptor. *Mol Cell* 3:11, 1999.

510. Huizing M, Anikster Y, Fitzpatrick DL, et al: Hermansky-Pudlak syndrome type 3 in Ashkenazi Jews and other non-Puerto Rican patients with hypopigmentation and platelet storage-pool deficiency. *Am J Hum Genet* 69:1022, 2001.

511. Nazarian R, Falcon-Perez JM, Dell'Angelica EC: Biogenesis of lysosome-related organelles complex 3 (BLOC-3): A complex containing the Hermansky-Pudlak syndrome (HPS) proteins HPS1 and HPS4. *Proc Natl Acad Sci U S A* 100:8770, 2003.

512. Martina JA, Moriyama K, Bonifacino JS: BLOC-3, a protein complex containing the Hermansky-Pudlak syndrome gene products HPS1 and HPS4. *J Biol Chem* 278:29376, 2003.

513. Suzuki T, Li W, Zhang Q, et al: Hermansky-Pudlak syndrome is caused by mutations in HPS4, the human homolog of the mouse light-ear gene. *Nat Genet* 30:321, 2002.

514. Anderson PD, Huizing M, Claassen DA, et al: Hermansky-Pudlak syndrome type 4 (HPS-4): Clinical and molecular characteristics. *Hum Genet* 113:10, 2003.

515. Huizing M, Helip-Wooley A, Dorward H, et al: IL-25 Hermansky-Pudlak syndrome: A model for abnormal vesicle formation and trafficking. *Pigment Cell Res* 16:584, 2003.

516. Zhang Q, Zhao B, Li W, et al: Ru2 and Ru encode mouse orthologs of the genes mutated in human Hermansky-Pudlak syndrome types 5 and 6. *Nat Genet* 33:145, 2003.

517. Li W, Zhang Q, Oiso N, et al: Hermansky-Pudlak syndrome type 7 (HPS-7) results from mutant dysbindin, a member of the biogenesis of lysosome-related organelles complex 1 (BLOC-1). *Nat Genet* 35:84, 2003.

518. Payne CM: A qualitative ultrastructural evaluation of the cell organelle specificity of the uranaffin reaction to normal human platelets. *Am J Clin Pathol* 31:62, 1984.

519. Weiss HJ, Lages B, Vicic W, et al: Heterogeneous abnormalities of platelet dense granule ultrastructure in 20 patients with congenital storage pool deficiency. *Br J Haematol* 83:282, 1993.

520. Huizing M, Anikster Y, Gahl WA: Hermansky-Pudlak syndrome and Chediak-Higashi syndrome: Disorders of vesicle formation and trafficking. *Thromb Haemost* 86:233, 2001.

521. White RA, Peters LL, Adkison LR, et al: The murine pallid mutation is a platelet storage pool disease associated with the protein 4.2 (pallidin) gene. *Nat Genet* 2:80, 1992.

522. Swank RT, Novak EK, McGarry MP, et al: Mouse models of Hermansky Pudlak syndrome: A review. *Pigment Cell Res* 11:60, 1998.

523. Shotelersuk V, Gahl WA: Hermansky-Pudlak syndrome: Models for intracellular vesicle formation. *Mol Genet Metab* 65:85, 1998.

524. Novak EK, Gautam R, Reddington M, et al: The regulation of platelet-dense granules by Rab27a in the ashen mouse, a model of Hermansky-Pudlak and Griscelli syndromes, is granule-specific and dependent on genetic background. *Blood* 100:128, 2002.

525. Suzuki T, Oiso N, Gautam R, et al: The mouse organellar biogenesis mutant buff results from a mutation in Vps33a, a homologue of yeast vps33 and Drosophila carnation. *Proc Natl Acad Sci U S A* 100:1146, 2003.

526. Zhen L, Jiang S, Feng L, et al: Abnormal expression and subcellular distribution of subunit proteins of the AP-3 adaptor complex lead to platelet storage pool deficiency in the pearl mouse. *Blood* 94:146, 1999.

527. Gautam R, Chintala S, Li W, et al: The Hermansky-Pudlak syndrome 3 (cocoa) protein is a component of the biogenesis of lysosome-related organelles complex-2 (BLOC-2). *J Biol Chem* 279:12935, 2004.

528. Spritz RA: Genetic defects in Chediak-Higashi syndrome and the beige mouse. *J Clin Immunol* 18:97, 1998.

529. Hardisty RM, Mills DC, Ketsa-Ard K: The platelet defect associated with albinism. *Br J Haematol* 23:679, 1972.

530. Harrison C, Khair K, Baxter B, et al: Hermansky-Pudlak syndrome: Infrequent bleeding and first report of Turkish and Pakistani kindreds. *Arch Dis Child* 86:297, 2002.

531. Pareti FI, Day HJ, Mills DC: Nucleotide and serotonin metabolism in platelets with defective secondary aggregation. *Blood* 44:789, 1974.

532. Holmsen H, Weiss HJ: Hereditary defect in the platelet release reaction caused by a deficiency in the storage pool of platelet adenine nucleotides. *Br J Haematol* 19:643, 1970.

533. White JG, Witkop CJ: Studies of platelets in a variant of the Hermansky-Pudlak syndrome. *Am J Pathol* 63:319, 1971.

534. Holmsen H, Weiss HJ: Further evidence for a deficient storage pool of adenine nucleotides in platelets from some patients with thrombocytopathia—"storage pool disease." *Blood* 39:197, 1972.

535. Akkerman JW, Nieuwenhuis HK, Mommersteeg-Leautaud ME, et al: ATP-ADP compartmentation in storage pool deficient platelets: Correlation between granule-bound ADP and the bleeding time. *Br J Haematol* 55:135, 1983.

536. Cattaneo M, Lecchi A, Agati B, et al: Evaluation of platelet function with the PFA-100 system in patients with congenital defects of platelet secretion. *Thromb Res* 96:213, 1999.

537. Weiss HJ, Tschopp TB, Rogers J, Brand H: Studies of platelet 5-hydroxytryptamine (serotonin) in storage pool disease and albinism. *J Clin Invest* 54:421, 1974.

538. Willis AL, Weiss HJ: A congenital defect in platelet prostaglandin production associated with impaired hemostasis in storage pool disease. *Prostaglandins* 4:783, 1973.

539. Holmsen H, Setkowsky CA, Lages B, et al: Content and thrombin-induced release of acid hydrolases in gel-filtered platelets from patients with storage pool disease. *Blood* 46:131, 1975.

540. Weiss HJ, Lages B: Platelet malondialdehyde production and aggregation responses induced by arachidonate, prostaglandin-G2, collagen, and epinephrine in 12 patients with storage pool deficiency. *Blood* 58:27, 1981.

541. Witkop CJ Jr, Bowie EJ, Krumwiede MD, et al: Synergistic effect of storage pool deficient platelets and low plasma von Willebrand factor on the severity of the hemorrhagic diathesis in Hermansky-Pudlak syndrome. *Am J Hematol* 44:256, 1993.

542. McKeown LP, Hansmann KE, Wilson O, et al: Platelet von Willebrand factor in Hermansky-Pudlak syndrome. *Am J Hematol* 59:115, 1998.

543. Israels SJ, McNicol A, Robertson C, Gerrard JM: Platelet storage pool deficiency: Diagnosis in patients with prolonged bleeding times and normal platelet aggregation. *Br J Haematol* 75:118, 1990.

544. Witkop CJ, Krumwiede M, Sedano H, White JG: Reliability of absent platelet dense bodies as a diagnostic criterion for Hermansky-Pudlak syndrome. *Am J Hematol* 26:305, 1987.

545. Weiss HJ, Ames RP: Ultrastructural findings in storage-pool disease and aspirin-like defects in platelets. *Am J Pathol* 71:447, 1973.

546. Richards JG, DaPrada M: Uranaffin reaction: A new cytochemical technique for the localization of adenine nucleotides in organelles storing biogenic amines. *J Histochem Cytochem* 25:1322, 1977.

547. Lorez HP, Richards JG, Da Prada M, et al: Storage pool disease: Comparative fluorescence microscopical, cytochemical and biochemical studies on amine-storing organelles of human blood platelets. *Br J Haematol* 43:297, 1979.

548. Gordon N, Thom J, Cole C, Baker R: Rapid detection of hereditary and acquired platelet storage pool deficiency by flow cytometry. *Br J Haematol* 89:117, 1995.

549. Mielke CH Jr, Levine PH, Zucker S: Preoperative prednisone therapy in platelet function disorders. *Thromb Res* 21:655, 1981.

550. Rao AK, Ghosh S, Sun L, et al: Mechanisms of platelet dysfunction and response to DDAVP in patients with congenital platelet function defects. A double-blind placebo-controlled trial. *Thromb Haemost* 74:1071, 1995.

551. Kobrinsky NL, Israels ED, Gerrard JM, et al: Shortening of bleeding time by 1-deamino-8-D-arginine vasopressin in various bleeding disorders. *Lancet* 1:1145, 1984.

552. Nieuwenhuis HK, Sixma JJ: 1-Desamino-8-D-arginine vasopressin (desmopressin) shortens the bleeding time in storage pool deficiency. *Ann Intern Med* 108:65, 1988.

553. Wijermans PW, van Dorp DB: Hermansky-Pudlak syndrome: Correction of bleeding time by 1-desamino-8D-arginine vasopressin. *Am J Hematol* 30:154, 1989.

554. van Dorp DB, Wijermans PW, Meire F, Vrensen G: The Hermansky-Pudlak syndrome. Variable reaction to 1-desamino-8D-arginine vasopressin for correction of the bleeding time. *Ophthalmic Paediatr Genet* 11:237, 1990.

555. Castaman G, Rodeghiero F: Consistency of responses to separate desmopressin infusion in patients with storage pool disease and isolated prolonged bleeding time. *Thromb Res* 69:407, 1993.

556. Zatik J, Poka R, Borsos A, Pfliegler G: Variable response of Hermansky-Pudlak syndrome to prophylactic administration of 1-desamino 8D-arginine in subsequent pregnancies. *Eur J Obstet Gynecol Reprod Biol* 104:165, 2002.

557. Gerritsen SW, Akkerman JW, Sixma JJ: Correction of the bleeding time in patients with storage pool deficiency by infusion of cryoprecipitate. *Br J Haematol* 40:153, 1978.

558. Coller BS, Hirschman RJ, Gralnick HR: Studies of the factor VIII/von Willebrand factor antigen on human platelets. *Thromb Res* 6:469, 1975.

559. George JN, Pickett EB, Heinz R: Platelet membrane microparticles in blood bank fresh frozen plasma and cryoprecipitate. *Blood* 68:307, 1986.

560. Wax JR, Rosengren S, Spector E, et al: DNA diagnosis and management of Hermansky-Pudlak syndrome in pregnancy. *Am J Perinatol* 18:159, 2001.

561. Pozo Pozo AI, Jimenez-Yuste V, Villar A, et al: Successful thyroidectomy in a patient with Hermansky-Pudlak syndrome treated with recombinant activated factor VII and platelet concentrates. *Blood Coagul Fibrinolysis* 13:551, 2002.

562. Gahl WA, Brantly M, Troendle J, et al: Effect of pirfenidone on the pulmonary fibrosis of Hermansky-Pudlak syndrome. *Mol Genet Metab* 76:234, 2002.

563. Raccuglia G: Gray platelet syndrome. A variety of qualitative platelet disorder. *Am J Med* 51:818, 1971.

564. Gerrard JM, Phillips DR, Rao GH, et al: Biochemical studies of two patients with the gray platelet syndrome. Selective deficiency of platelet alpha granules. *J Clin Invest* 66:102, 1980.

565. Levy-Toledano S, Caen JP, Breton-Gorius J, et al: Gray platelet syndrome: Alpha-granule deficiency. Its influence on platelet function. *J Lab Clin Med* 98:831, 1981.

566. Nurden AT, Kunicki TJ, Dupuis D, et al: Specific protein and glycoprotein deficiencies in platelets isolated from two patients with the gray platelet syndrome. *Blood* 59:709, 1982.

567. Coller BS, Hultin MB, Nurden AT: Isolated alpha-granule deficiency (gray platelet syndrome) with slight increase in bone marrow reticulin and possible glycoprotein and/or protease defect [abstract]. *Thromb Haemost* 50:211, 1983.

568. Kohler M, Hellstern P, Morgenstern E, et al: Gray platelet syndrome: Selective alpha-granule deficiency and thrombocytopenia due to increased platelet turnover. *Blut* 50:331, 1985.

569. Berndt MC, Castaldi PA, Gordon S, et al: Morphological and biochemical confirmation of gray platelet syndrome in two siblings. *Aust N Z J Med* 13:387, 1983.

570. Gootenberg JE, Buchanan GR, Holtkamp CA, Casey CS: Severe hemorrhage in a patient with gray platelet syndrome. *J Pediatr* 109:1017, 1986.

571. Srivastava PC, Powling MJ, Nokes TJ, et al: Grey platelet syndrome: Studies on platelet alpha-granules, lysosomes and defective response to thrombin. *Br J Haematol* 65:441, 1987.

572. Berrebi A, Klepfish A, Varon D, et al: Gray platelet syndrome in the elderly. *Am J Hematol* 28:270, 1988.

573. Wills EJ: Gray platelet syndrome. *Ultrastruct Pathol* 13:451, 1989.

574. Facon T, Goudemand J, Caron C, et al: Simultaneous occurrence of grey platelet syndrome and idiopathic pulmonary fibrosis: A role for abnormal megakaryocytes in the pathogenesis of pulmonary fibrosis? *Br J Haematol* 74:542, 1990.

575. Lages B, Sussman II, Levine SP, et al: Platelet alpha granule deficiency associated with decreased P-selectin and selective impairment of thrombin-induced activation in a new patient with gray platelet syndrome (alpha-storage pool deficiency). *J Lab Clin Med* 129:364, 1997.

576. Martinez-Murillo C, Payns Borrego E, Arzate Hernandez G, et al: Gray-platelet syndrome associated with Marfan disease in a Mexican family. *Sangre (Barc)* 39:287, 1994.

577. Jantunen E, Hanninen A, Naukkarinen A, et al: Gray platelet syndrome with splenomegaly and signs of extramedullary hematopoiesis: A case report with review of the literature. *Am J Hematol* 46:218, 1994.

578. Alkhairy KS: The gray platelet syndrome of four members of a Palestinian Arab family. *Emirates Medical Journal* 13:137, 1995.

579. Lutz P, Roth-Pougheon A, Wiesel ML, et al: Gray platelet syndrome. *Arch Fr Pediatr* 49:637, 1992.

580. Drouin A, Favier R, Masse JM, et al: Newly recognized cellular abnormalities in the gray platelet syndrome. *Blood* 98:1382, 2001.

581. Falik-Zaccai TC, Anikster Y, Rivera CE, et al: A new genetic isolate of gray platelet syndrome (GPS): Clinical, cellular, and hematologic characteristics. *Mol Genet Metab* 74:303, 2001.

582. Elliott MA, White JG, Charlesworth JE, et al: Gray platelet syndrome (GPS) in a native American female [abstract]. *Thromb Haemost* abstr 508:1163, 1999.

583. Laskey AL, Tobias JD: Anesthetic complications of the gray platelet syndrome. *Can J Anaesth* 47:1224, 2000.

584. Mori K, Suzuki S, Sugai K: Electron microscopic and functional studies on platelets in gray platelet syndrome. *Tohoku J Exp Med* 143:261, 1984.

585. Berger G, Masse JM, Cramer EM: Alpha-granule membrane mirrors the platelet plasma membrane and contains the glycoproteins Ib, IX, and V. *Blood* 87:1385, 1996.

586. Rosa JP, George JN, Bainton DF, et al: Gray platelet syndrome. Demonstration of alpha granule membranes that can fuse with the cell surface. *J Clin Invest* 80:1138, 1987.

587. Cramer EM, Vainchenker W, Vinci G, et al: Gray platelet syndrome: Immunoelectron microscopic localization of fibrinogen and von Willebrand factor in platelets and megakaryocytes. *Blood* 66:1309, 1985.

588. Caen JP, Deschamps JF, Bodevin E, et al: Megakaryocytes and myelofibrosis in gray platelet syndrome. *Nouv Rev Fr Hematol* 29:109, 1987.

589. Schmitt A, Jouault H, Guichard J, et al: Pathologic interaction between megakaryocytes and polymorphonuclear leukocytes in myelofibrosis. *Blood* 96:1342, 2000.

590. Wencel-Drake JD: Plasma membrane GPIIb/IIIa. Evidence for a cycling receptor pool. *Am J Clin Pathol* 136:61, 1990.

591. Steinberg MH, Kelton JG, Coller BS: Plasma glycocalicin: An aid in the classification of thrombocytopenic disorders. *N Engl J Med* 317:1037, 1987.

592. Greenberg-Sepersky SM, Simons ER, White JG: Studies of platelets from patients with the grey platelet syndrome. *Br J Haematol* 59:603, 1985.

593. Rendu F, Marche P, Hovig T, et al: Abnormal phosphoinositide metabolism and protein phosphorylation in platelets from a patient with the grey platelet syndrome. *Br J Haematol* 67:199, 1987.

594. Baruch D, Lindhout T, Dupuy E, Caen JP: Thrombin-induced platelet factor Va formation in patients with a gray platelet syndrome. *Thromb Haemost* 58:768, 1987.

595. Enouf J, Lebret M, Bredoux R, et al: Abnormal calcium transport into microsomes of grey platelet syndrome. *Br J Haematol* 65:437, 1987.

596. Cockbill SR, Burmester HB, Heptinstall S: Pseudo grey platelet syndrome: Grey platelets due to degranulation in blood collected into EDTA. *Eur J Haematol* 41:326, 1988.

597. Pfueller SL, Howard MA, White JG, et al: Shortening of bleeding time by 1-deamino-8-arginine vasopressin (DDAVP) in the absence of platelet von Willebrand factor in Gray platelet syndrome. *Thromb Haemost* 58:1060, 1987.

598. Breton-Gorius J, Favier R, Guichard J, et al: A new congenital dysmegakaryopoietic thrombocytopenia (Paris-Trousseau) associated with giant platelet alpha-granules and chromosome 11 deletion at 11q23. *Blood* 85:1805, 1995.

599. Favier R, Jondeau K, Boutard P, et al: Paris-Trousseau syndrome: Clinical, hematological, molecular data of ten new cases. *Thromb Haemost* 90:893, 2003.

600. Raslova H, Komura E, Le Couedic JP, et al: FLI1 monoallelic expression combined with its hemizygous loss underlies Paris-Trousseau/Jacobsen thrombopenia. *J Clin Invest* 114:77, 2004.

601. Shivdasani RA: Lonely in Paris: When one gene copy isn't enough. *J Clin Invest* 114:17, 2004.

602. Weiss HJ, Witte LD, Kaplan KL, et al: Heterogeneity in storage pool deficiency: Studies on granule-bound substances in 18 patients including variants deficient in alpha-granules, platelet factor 4, beta-thromboglobulin, and platelet-derived growth factor. *Blood* 54:1296, 1979.

603. Lages B, Shattil SJ, Bainton DF, Weiss HJ: Decreased content and surface expression of alpha-granule membrane protein GMP-140 in one of two types of platelet alpha delta storage pool deficiency. *J Clin Invest* 87:919, 1991.

604. Weiss HJ, Lages B: The response of platelets to epinephrine in storage pool deficiency: Evidence pertaining to the role of adenosine diphosphate in mediating primary and secondary aggregation. *Blood* 72:1717, 1988.

605. Jamieson GA, Okumara T, Fishback B, et al: Platelet membrane glycoproteins in thrombasthenia, Bernard-Soulier syndrome, and storage pool disease. *J Lab Clin Med* 93:652, 1979.

606. Gerrard JM, McNicol A: Platelet storage pool deficiency, leukemia, and myelodysplastic syndromes. *Leuk Lymphoma* 8:277, 1992.

607. Tracy PB, Giles AR, Mann KG, et al: Factor V (Quebec): A bleeding diathesis associated with a qualitative platelet Factor V deficiency. *J Clin Invest* 74:1221, 1984.

608. Janeway CM, Rivard GE, Tracy PB, Mann KG: Factor V Quebec revisited. *Blood* 87:3571, 1996.

609. Hayward CP, Rivard GE, Kane WH, et al: An autosomal dominant, qualitative platelet disorder associated with multimerin deficiency, abnormalities in platelet factor V, thrombospondin, von Willebrand factor, and fibrinogen and an epinephrine aggregation defect. *Blood* 87:4967, 1996.

610. Kahr WH, Zheng S, Sheth PM, et al: Platelets from patients with the Quebec platelet disorder contain and secrete abnormal amounts of urokinase-type plasminogen activator. *Blood* 98:257, 2001.

611. Sheth PM, Kahr WH, Haq MA, et al: Intracellular activation of the fibrinolytic cascade in the Quebec Platelet Disorder. *Thromb Haemost* 90:293, 2003.

612. McKay H, Derome F, Haq MA, et al: Bleeding risks associated with inheritance of the Quebec platelet disorder. *Blood* 104:159, 2004.

613. Weiss HJ, Vicic WJ, Lages BA, Rogers J: Isolated deficiency of platelet procoagulant activity. *Am J Med* 67:206, 1979.

614. Weiss HJ: Scott syndrome: A disorder of platelet coagulant activity. *Semin Hematol* 31:312, 1994.

615. Toti F, Satta N, Fressinaud E, et al: Scott syndrome, characterized by impaired transmembrane migration of procoagulant phosphatidylserine and hemorrhagic complications, is an inherited disorder. *Blood* 87:1409, 1996.

616. Weiss HJ, Lages B: Platelet prothrombinase activity and intracellular calcium responses in patients with storage pool deficiency, glycoprotein IIb-IIIa deficiency, or impaired platelet coagulant activity: A comparison with Scott syndrome. *Blood* 89:1599, 1997.

617. Dachary-Prigent J, Pasquet JM, Fressinaud E, et al: Aminophospholipid exposure, microvesiculation and abnormal protein tyrosine phosphorylation in the platelets of a patient with Scott syndrome: A study using physiologic agonists and local anaesthetics. *Br J Haematol* 99:959, 1997.

618. Zwaal RF, Comfurius P, Bevers EM: Scott syndrome, a bleeding disorder caused by defective scrambling of membrane phospholipids. *Biochim Biophys Acta* 1636:119, 2004.

619. Munnix IC, Harmsma M, Giddings JC, et al: Store-mediated calcium entry in the regulation of phosphatidylserine exposure in blood cells from Scott patients. *Thromb Haemost* 89:687, 2003.

620. Solum NO: Procoagulant expression in platelets and defects leading to clinical disorders. *Arterioscler Thromb Vasc Biol* 19:2841, 1999.

621. Sims PJ, Wiedmer T, Esmon CT, et al: Assembly of the platelet prothrombinase complex is linked to vesiculation on the platelet plasma membrane. Studies in Scott syndrome: An isolated defect in platelet procoagulant activity. *J Biol Chem* 264:137, 1989.

622. Miletich JP, Kane WH, Hofmann SL, et al: Deficiency of factor Xa-factor Va binding sites on the platelets of a patient with a bleeding disorder. *Blood* 54:1015, 1979.

623. Rosing J, Bevers EM, Comfurius P, et al: Impaired factor X and prothrombin activation associated with decreased phospholipid exposure in platelets from a patient with a bleeding disorder. *Blood* 65:1557, 1985.

624. Ahmad SS, Rawala-Sheikh R, Ashby B, Walsh PN: Platelet receptor-mediated factor X activation by factor IXa. High-affinity factor IXa receptors induced by factor VIII are deficient on platelets in Scott syndrome. *J Clin Invest* 84:824, 1989.

625. Bevers EM, Wiedmer T, Comfurius P, et al: Defective Ca(2+)-induced microvesiculation and deficient expression of procoagulant activity in erythrocytes from a patient with a bleeding disorder: A study of the red blood cells of Scott syndrome. *Blood* 79:380, 1992.

626. Kojima H, Newton-Nash D, Weiss HJ, et al: Production and characterization of transformed B-lymphocytes expressing the membrane defect of Scott syndrome. *J Clin Invest* 94:2237, 1994.

627. Weiss HJ: Platelet aggregation, adhesion and adenosine diphosphate release in thrombopathia (platelet factor 3 deficiency). A comparison with Glanzmann's thrombasthenia and von Willebrand's disease. *Am J Med* 43:570, 1967.

628. Zhou Q, Sims PJ, Wiedmer T: Expression of proteins controlling transbilayer movement of plasma membrane phospholipids in the B lymphocytes from a patient with Scott syndrome. *Blood* 92:1707, 1998.

629. Stout JG, Basse F, Luhm RA, et al: Scott syndrome erythrocytes contain a membrane protein capable of mediating Ca2+-dependent transbilayer migration of membrane phospholipids. *J Clin Invest* 99:2232, 1997.

630. Rao AK: Inherited defects in platelet signaling mechanisms. *J Thromb Haemost* 1:671, 2003.

631. Hirata T, Kakizuka A, Ushikubi F, et al: Arg60 to Leu mutation of the human thromboxane A2 receptor in a dominantly inherited bleeding disorder. *J Clin Invest* 94:1662, 1994.

632. Higuchi W, Fuse I, Hattori A, Aizawa Y: Mutations of the platelet thromboxane A2 (TXA2) receptor in patients characterized by the absence of TXA2-induced platelet aggregation despite normal TXA2 binding activity. *Thromb Haemost* 82:1528, 1999.

633. Cattaneo M, Lecchi A, Randi AM, et al: Identification of a new congenital defect of platelet function characterized by severe impairment of platelet responses to adenosine diphosphate. *Blood* 80:2787, 1992.

634. Cattaneo M, Lombardi R, Zighetti ML, et al: Deficiency of (33P)2MeS-ADP binding sites on platelets with secretion defect, normal granule stores and normal thromboxane A2 production. Evidence that ADP potentiates platelet secretion independently of the formation of large platelet aggregates and thromboxane A2 production. *Thromb Haemost* 77:986, 1997.

635. Nurden P, Savi P, Heilmann E, et al: An inherited bleeding disorder linked to a defective interaction between ADP and its receptor on platelets. Its influence on glycoprotein IIb-IIIa complex function. *J Clin Invest* 95:1612, 1995.

636. Conley PB, Delaney SM: Scientific and therapeutic insights into the role of the platelet P2Y12 receptor in thrombosis. *Curr Opin Hematol* 10:333, 2003.

637. Cattaneo M, Lecchi A, Lombardi R, et al: Platelets from a patient heterozygous for the defect of P2CYC receptors for ADP have a secretion defect despite normal thromboxane A2 production and normal granule stores: Further evidence that some cases of platelet "primary secretion defect" are heterozygous for a defect of P2CYC receptors. *Arterioscler Thromb Vasc Biol* 20:E101, 2000.

638. Hollopeter G, Jantzen HM, Vincent D, et al: Identification of the platelet ADP receptor targeted by antithrombotic drugs. *Nature* 409:202, 2001.

639. Cattaneo M, Zighetti ML, Lombardi R, et al: Molecular bases of defective signal transduction in the platelet P2Y12 receptor of a patient with congenital bleeding. *Proc Natl Acad Sci U S A* 100:1978, 2003.

640. Oury C, Toth-Zsamboki E, Van Geet C, et al: A natural dominant negative P2X1 receptor due to deletion of a single amino acid residue. *J Biol Chem* 275:22611, 2000.

641. Rao AK: Congenital disorders of platelet function: Disorders of signal transduction and secretion. *Am J Med Sci* 316:69, 1998.

642. Scrutton MC, Clare KA, Hutton RA, Bruckdorfer KR: Depressed responsiveness to adrenaline in platelets from apparently normal human donors: A familial trait. *Br J Haematol* 49:303, 1981.

643. Tamponi G, Pannocchia A, Arduino C, et al: Congenital deficiency of alpha-2-adrenoceptors on human platelets: Description of two cases. *Thromb Haemost* 58:1012, 1987.

644. Rao AK, Willis J, Kowalska MA, et al: Differential requirements for platelet aggregation and inhibition of adenylate cyclase by epinephrine. Studies of a familial platelet alpha 2-adrenergic receptor defect. *Blood* 71:494, 1988.

645. Pelczar-Wissner CJ, McDonald EG, Sussman II: Absence of platelet activating factor (PAF) mediated platelet aggregation: A new platelet defect. *Am J Hematol* 16:419, 1984.

646. Rao AK: Congenital disorders of platelet function. *Hematol Oncol Clin North Am* 4:65, 1990.

647. Fuse I: Disorders of platelet function. *Crit Rev Oncol Hematol* 22:1, 1996.

648. Rendu F, Breton-Gorius J, Trugnan G, et al: Studies on a new variant of the Hermansky-Pudlak syndrome: Qualitative, ultrastructural, and functional abnormalities of the platelet-dense bodies associated with a phospholipase A defect. *Am J Hematol* 4:387, 1978.

649. Holmsen H, Walsh PN, Koike K, et al: Familial bleeding disorder associated with deficiencies in platelet signal processing and glycoproteins. *Br J Haematol* 67:335, 1987.

650. Malmsten C, Hamberg M, Svensson J, Samuelsson B: Physiological role of an endoperoxide in human platelets: Hemostatic defect due to platelet cyclo-oxygenase deficiency. *Proc Natl Acad Sci U S A* 72:1446, 1975.

651. Lagarde M, Byron PA, Vargaftig BB, Dechavanne M: Impairment of platelet thromboxane A2 generation and of the platelet release reaction in two patients with congenital deficiency of platelet cyclo-oxygenase. *Br J Haematol* 38:251, 1978.

652. Pareti FI, Mannucci PM, D'Angelo A, et al: Congenital deficiency of thromboxane and prostacyclin. *Lancet* 1:898, 1980.

653. Rak K, Boda Z: Haemostatic balance in congenital deficiency of platelet cyclo-oxygenase. *Lancet* 2:44, 1980.

654. Horellou MH, Lecompte T, Lecrubier C, et al: Familial and constitutional bleeding disorder due to platelet cyclo-oxygenase deficiency. *Am J Hematol* 14:1, 1983.

655. Rao AK, Koike K, Day HJ, et al: Bleeding disorder associated with albumin-dependent partial deficiency in platelet thromboxane production. Effect of albumin on arachidonate metabolism in platelets. *Am J Clin Pathol* 83:687, 1985.

656. Defreyn G, Machin SJ, Carreras LO, et al: Familial bleeding tendency with partial platelet thromboxane synthetase deficiency: Reorientation of cyclic endoperoxide metabolism. *Br J Haematol* 49:29, 1981.

657. Mestel F, Oetliker O, Beck E, et al: Severe bleeding associated with defective thromboxane synthetase. *Lancet* 1:157, 1980.

658. Wu KK, Minkoff IM, Rossi EC, Chen YC: Hereditary bleeding disorder due to a primary defect in platelet release reaction. *Br J Haematol* 47:241, 1981.

659. Wu KK, Le Breton GC, Tai HH, Chen YC: Abnormal platelet response to thromboxane A2. *J Clin Invest* 67:1801, 1981.

660. Lages B, Malmsten C, Weiss HJ, Samuelsson B: Impaired platelet response to thromboxane-A2 and defective calcium mobilization in a patient with a bleeding disorder. *Blood* 57:545, 1981.

661. White JG: Structural defects in inherited and giant platelet disorders. *Adv Hum Genet* 19:133, 1990.

662. Samama M, Lecrubier C, Conard J, et al: Constitutional thrombocytopathy with subnormal response to thromboxane A2. *Br J Haematol* 48:293, 1981.

663. Lages B, Weiss HJ: Heterogeneous defects of platelet secretion and responses to weak agonists in patients with bleeding disorders. *Br J Haematol* 68:53, 1988.

664. Lages B, Weiss HJ: Impairment of phosphatidylinositol metabolism in a patient with a bleeding disorder associated with defects of initial platelet responses. *Thromb Haemost* 59:175, 1988.

665. Rao AK, Kowalska MA, Disa J: Impaired cytoplasmic ionized calcium mobilization in inherited platelet secretion defects. *Blood* 74:664, 1989.

666. Ramasamy I: Inherited bleeding disorders: Disorders of platelet adhesion and aggregation. *Crit Rev Oncol Hematol* 49:1, 2004.

667. Lee SB, Rao AK, Lee KH, et al: Decreased expression of phospholipase C-beta 2 isozyme in human platelets with impaired function. *Blood* 88:1684, 1996.

668. Mao GF, Vaidyula VR, Kunapuli SP, Rao AK: Lineage-specific defect in gene expression in human platelet phospholipase C-beta2 deficiency. *Blood* 99:905, 2002.

669. Yang X, Sun L, Ghosh S, Rao AK: Human platelet signaling defect characterized by impaired production of inositol-1,4,5-triphosphate and phosphatidic acid and diminished Pleckstrin phosphorylation: Evidence for defective phospholipase C activation. *Blood* 88:1676, 1996.

670. Gabbeta J, Yang X, Kowalska MA, et al: Platelet signal transduction defect with Galpha subunit dysfunction and diminished Galphaq in a patient with abnormal platelet responses. *Proc Natl Acad Sci U S A* 94:8750, 1997.

671. Offermanns S, Toombs CF, Hu YH, Simon MI: Defective platelet activation in G alpha(q)-deficient mice. *Nature* 389:183, 1997.

672. Freson K, Hoylaerts MF, Jaeken J, et al: Genetic variation of the extra-large stimulatory G protein alpha-subunit leads to Gs hyperfunc-

tion in platelets and is a risk factor for bleeding. *Thromb Haemost* 86:733, 2001.

673. Xiao T, Takagi J, Coller BS, et al.: Structural basis for allostery in integrins and binding of ligand-mimetic therapeutics. *Nature* 432:59, 2004.

674. Qin J, Vinogradova O, Plow EF: Integrin bidirectional signaling: A molecular view. *PLoS Biol* 2:726, 2004.

675. Badour K, Zhang J, Siminovitch KA: The Wiskott-Aldrich syndrome protein: Forging the link between actin and cell activation. *Immunol Rev* 192:98, 2003.

676. Millard TH, Sharp SJ, Machesky LM: Signaling to actin assembly via the WASP (Wiskott-Aldrich syndrome protein)-family proteins and the Arp2/3 complex. *Biochem J* 380:1, 2004.

677. Miki H, Takenawa T: Regulation of actin dynamics by WASP family proteins. *J Biochem (Tokyo)* 134:309, 2003.

678. Notarangelo LD, Ochs HD: Wiskott-Aldrich Syndrome: A model for defective actin reorganization, cell trafficking and synapse formation. *Curr Opin Immunol* 15:585, 2003.

679. Savoia A, Balduini CL, Savino M, et al: Autosomal dominant macrothrombocytopenia in Italy is most frequently a type of heterozygous Bernard-Soulier syndrome. *Blood* 97:1330, 2001.

680. Clemetson JM, Kyrle PA, Brenner B, Clemetson KJ: Variant Bernard-Soulier syndrome associated with a homozygous mutation in the leucine-rich domain of glycoprotein IX. *Blood* 84:1124, 1994.

681. Fonio A. La thrombocyotopathie granulopénique. *Rev d'Hémat* 2:149, 1947.

682. Kurstjens R, Bolt C, Vossen M, Haanen C. Familial thrombopathic thrombocytopenia. *Br J Haematol* 15:305, 1968.

ACQUIRED QUALITATIVE PLATELET DISORDERS

CHARLES S. ABRAMS
SANFORD J. SHATTIL
JOEL S. BENNETT

Acquired qualitative platelet disorders are frequent causes of abnormal platelet function *in vitro*, prolonged bleeding times, and occasionally mild bleeding diatheses. However, their clinical importance increases in the presence of thrombocytopenia or additional disorders of hemostasis. Acquired disorders of platelet function can be conveniently classified into those that result from drugs, hematologic diseases, and systemic disorders. Drugs are the most frequent cause of acquired qualitative platelet dysfunction. Aspirin is the most notable drug in this regard because of its frequent use, its irreversible effect on platelet prostaglandin synthesis, and its documented effect on hemostatic competency, although this effect is minimal in normal individuals. Other nonsteroidal antiinflammatory drugs reversibly inhibit platelet prostaglandin synthesis and usually have little effect on hemostasis. The antiplatelet effect of a number of drugs has proved useful in preventing arterial thrombosis but, as anticipated, excessive bleeding can be a complication of their use. In addition to aspirin, these drugs include the thienopyridines ticlopidine and clopidogrel, which primarily antagonize adenosine diphosphate-stimulated platelet aggregation, and drugs that specifically inhibit the platelet glycoprotein IIb/IIIa receptor. Other drugs used to treat thrombosis, such as heparin and fibrinolytic agents, also can impair platelet function *in vitro* and *ex vivo*, but the clinical significance of these observations are uncertain. High doses of the β-lactam antibiotics can impair platelet function *in vitro* and prolong the bleeding time, whereas clinically significant bleeding is unusual in the absence of a coexisting hemostatic defect. Similarly, a number of other drugs (including a variety of psychotropic, chemotherapeutic, and anesthetic agents) and a number of foods and food additives reportedly affect platelet function *in vitro*, but these effects do not appear to be clinically significant. Hematologic diseases associated with abnormal platelet function include marrow processes in which platelets may be intrinsically abnormal, such as the clonal myeloid diseases, dysproteinemias in which abnormal plasma proteins can impair platelet function, and acquired forms of von Willebrand disease. Of the systemic diseases, renal failure is most prominently associated with abnormal platelet function because of

retention of platelet inhibitory compounds. Platelet function may be abnormal in the presence of antiplatelet antibodies, following cardiopulmonary bypass, in association with liver disease, or in disseminated intravascular coagulation.

INTRODUCTION

Platelet function may be adversely affected by drugs and by hematologic and nonhematologic disorders. Because the use of aspirin and other nonsteroidal antiinflammatory drugs is pervasive in current medical practice, acquired platelet dysfunction is much more frequent than inherited platelet dysfunction. Acquired disorders of platelet function can be classified according to the underlying clinical condition with which they are associated (Table 113-1).

Although acquired disorders of platelet function usually produce mild effects, important exceptions to this rule exist, particularly when platelet dysfunction is associated with other hemostatic defects. If the patient does not present with a history of bleeding, predicting the risk of future bleeding may be difficult. This situation is not surprising because even patients with thrombocytopenia may experience little or no spontaneous bleeding until their platelet count is less than 10,000/μl. Furthermore, clinical assessment of these disorders is made problematic by difficulties in standardization and interpretation of the two most frequently used laboratory tests of platelet function: bleeding time and platelet aggregometry. These tests appear more useful in diagnosing platelet dysfunction than in predicting the risk of bleeding.[1-3]

DRUGS THAT AFFECT PLATELET FUNCTION

Drugs represent the most common cause of platelet dysfunction (Table 113-2).[4] For example, in an analysis of 72 hospitalized patients with a prolonged bleeding time, 54 percent were receiving large doses of antibiotics known to prolong the bleeding time and 10 percent were taking aspirin or other nonsteroidal antiinflammatory drugs.[5] Some drugs can prolong the bleeding time and either cause or exacerbate a

TABLE 113-1   ACQUIRED QUALITATIVE PLATELET DISORDERS

DRUGS THAT AFFECT PLATELET FUNCTION
Nonsteroidal antiinflammatory drugs
Thienopyridines (ticlopidine and clopidogrel)
GpIIb-IIIa receptor antagonists
Drugs that increase platelet cAMP
Antibiotics
Anticoagulants and fibrinolytic agents
Cardiovascular drugs
Volume expanders
Psychotropic agents and anesthetics
Oncologic drugs
Foods and food additives
Hematologic disorders associated with abnormal platelet function
Chronic myeloproliferative disorders
Leukemias and myelodysplastic syndromes
Dysproteinemias
Acquired von Willebrand disease
Systemic disorders associated with abnormal platelet function
Uremia
Antiplatelet antibodies
Cardiopulmonary bypass
Liver disease
Disseminated intravascular coagulation

Acronyms and abbreviations that appear in this chapter include: ADP, adenosine diphosphate; BCNU, bischloroethylnitrosourea; cAMP, cyclic adenosine monophosphate; cGMP, cyclic guanosine monophosphate; COX, cyclooxygenase; coxib, COX inhibitor; DDAVP, desmopressin (1-desamino-8-D-arginine vasopressin); DIC, disseminated intravascular coagulation; Epo, erythropoietin; Gp, glycoprotein; HIV, human immunodeficiency virus; Ig, immunoglobulin; ITP, idiopathic thrombocytopenic purpura; NO, nitric oxide; PG, prostaglandin; PGHS, prostaglandin endoperoxide H synthase; SLE, systemic lupus erythematosus; t-PA, tissue plasminogen activator; vWF, von Willebrand factor.

TABLE 113-2 DRUGS THAT INHIBIT PLATELET FUNCTION

Nonsteroidal antiinflammatory drugs

Aspirin, sulfinpyrazone, indomethacin, ibuprofen, sulindac, naproxen, phenylbutazone, meclofenamic acid, mefenamic acid, diflunisal, piroxicam, tolmetin, zomepirac

Thienopyridines

Ticlopidine, clopidogrel

GpIIb-IIIa antagonists

Abciximab, tirofiban, eptifibatide

Drugs that affect platelet cAMP levels or function

Prostacyclin, iloprost, dipyridamole, cilostazol

Antibiotics

Penicillins

Penicillin G, carbenicillin, ticarcillin, methicillin, ampicillin, piperacillin, azlocillin, mezlocillin, apalcillin, sulbenicillin, temocillin

Cephalosporins

Cephalothin, moxalactam, cefoxitin, cefotaxime, cefazolin

Nitrofurantoin

Miconazole

Anticoagulants, fibrinolytic agents, and antifibrinolytic agents

Heparin

Streptokinase, tissue plasminogen activator, urokinase

ε-Aminocaproic acid

Cardiovascular drugs

Nitroglycerin, isosorbide dinitrate, propranolol, nitroprusside, nifedipine, verapamil, diltiazem, quinidine

Volume expanders

Dextran, hydroxyethyl starch

Psychotropic drugs and anesthetics

Psychotropic drugs

Imipramine, amitriptyline, nortriptyline, chlorpromazine, promethazine, fluphenazine, trifluoperazine, haloperidol

Anesthetics

Local

Dibucaine, tetracaine, hexylcaine hydrochloride (Cyclaine), butacaine, dibucaine hydrochloride (Nupercaine), procaine, cocaine

General

Halothane

Oncologic drugs

Mithramycin, daunorubicin, BCNU

Miscellaneous drugs

Antihistamines

Diphenhydramine, chlorpheniramine, mepyramine

Radiographic contrast agent

Iopamidol, iothalamate, ioxaglate, meglumine diatrizoate, sodium diatrizoate

Other

Ketanserin

Foods and food additives

ω-3 Fatty acids, ethanol, chinese black tree fungus, onion extract ajoene, cumin, turmeric

bleeding diathesis. Other drugs may prolong the bleeding time but not cause bleeding, whereas many drugs only affect platelet function *ex vivo* or when they are added to platelets *in vitro*. The hematologist must understand the clinical significance of these distinctions.

ASPIRIN AND OTHER NONSTEROIDAL ANTIINFLAMMATORY DRUGS

ASPIRIN

Aspirin acetylates a serine residue at position 529 of the enzyme cyclooxygenase (COX), also known as prostaglandin endoperoxide H

synthase (PGHS). Acetylation of COX irreversibly inactivates the enzyme. Three isoforms of COX have been cloned (COX-1, COX-2, COX-3), but platelets have only COX-1, and endothelial cells have predominantly COX-2 (see Chap. 126 for the use of aspirin as an antithrombotic agent).[6,7] Inactivation of COX-1 prevents platelet synthesis of prostaglandin endoperoxides and the subsequent synthesis of thromboxane A_2 by thromboxane synthase, thereby inhibiting platelet responses that require these substances. Thus, platelet responses to adenosine diphosphate (ADP), epinephrine, arachidonic acid, and low doses of collagen and thrombin are affected, but almost no effect on the responses to higher doses of collagen or thrombin is observed.[8,9]

Platelet prostaglandin synthesis in an adult is nearly completely inhibited by a single 100-mg dose of aspirin or by 30 mg taken daily for 7 to 10 days.[10] Although small doses of aspirin irreversibly inhibit both platelet and endothelial cell COX,[11] they have no lasting effect on prostacyclin production by endothelial cells.[12] This situation results from the ability of endothelial cells to synthesize additional COX unaffected by aspirin (see "Cyclooxygenase Inhibitors" below).[13] *In vitro* studies also suggest that the presence of erythrocytes contributes to agonist-stimulated platelet reactivity,[14] an effect that can be inhibited by aspirin at doses greater than those required to inhibit platelet COX-1.[15] The optimal dose of aspirin required to minimize vascular events has been disputed. A meta-analysis suggests that doses varying between 50 and 1500 mg/day are equally efficacious.[16] This finding led many to suggest that lower doses should be prescribed to minimize gastrointestinal toxicity. However, even low doses of aspirin are associated with significant gastrointestinal hemorrhage.[17,18] Notably, concomitant administration of other nonsteroidal antiinflammatory drugs (see section on "Other Nonsteroidal Antiinflammatory Drugs") antagonizes the irreversible platelet inhibition induced by aspirin.[19]

Aspirin is one of the few drugs that prolongs the bleeding time in humans. It appears to do so by blocking aggregation rather than adhesion. In normal individuals, the effect on the bleeding time is slight (generally no more than 1.2–2.0 times the preaspirin bleeding time),[20,21] is observed in both males and females, and requires that almost all the COX in the circulating platelets be inhibited.[20] The sensitivity of the bleeding time to aspirin is dependent on such technical variables as the direction of the incision on the forearm and the degree of hydrostatic pressure applied to the arm.[22] The bleeding time may remain prolonged for 1 to 4 days after the aspirin has been discontinued, and platelet aggregation test results may remain abnormal for up to 1 week until affected platelets are replaced.[23]

The significance of aspirin ingestion on the hemostatic competency of normal individuals appears to be minimal. Nevertheless, patients chronically taking aspirin report a significant increase in bruising, epistaxis, and gastrointestinal blood loss.[24] The latter appears to be caused by a direct effect of the drug on the gastric mucosa.[25,26] Moreover, a slight, but not statistically significant, increase in hemorrhagic strokes was seen in a group of otherwise healthy physicians who took aspirin chronically as primary prophylaxis against myocardial infarction.[24] Aspirin also may increase bleeding in the mother and the neonate during parturition.[27] In addition, some, but not all, studies have shown that aspirin taken preoperatively increases the amount of blood loss following cardiothoracic surgery.[28,29] On the other hand, a retrospective analysis documented the safety of performing epidural and spinal anesthesia in patients who had ingested aspirin.[30] Although aspirin may increase the amount of blood loss following general surgery,[31] the significance of aspirin ingestion in this setting has never been tested in a prospective, randomized, double-blind study with objective end points. Many surgeons ask their patients to avoid aspirin, particularly prior to cardiothoracic, plastic, or neurosurgical procedures, in which the limits of tolerable bleeding are narrow.[32] Aspirin causes a marked prolongation of the bleeding time and precipitates hemorrhage in individuals with preexistent hemostatic defects, such as von Willebrand disease, hemophilia A, warfarin ingestion, uremia, and disorders of platelet function.[33–35] Whereas ingestion of ethanol has no direct effect on the bleeding time, it can potentiate the effect of aspirin.[36,37] Infusion of desmopressin (1-desamino-8-D-arginine vasopressin [DDAVP]) has been effective in correcting a prolonged bleeding time caused by aspirin.[38,39]

OTHER NONSTEROIDAL ANTIINFLAMMATORY DRUGS

Nonsteroidal antiinflammatory drugs such as indomethacin, ibuprofen, naproxen, phenylbutazone, and sulfinpyrazone inhibit platelet COX.[40] In contrast to aspirin, their effect is reversible and generally short lasting (<4 hours).[19] An exception is piroxicam, whose effect may last for days because of its prolonged half-life.[41] These drugs may cause transient prolongation of the bleeding time when given in therapeutic doses; however, this effect usually is not clinically significant.[42–44] Ibuprofen and probably other nonsteroidal antiinflammatory drugs bind to COX and block its acetylation by aspirin.[19] Thus, coadministration of nonsteroidal antiinflammatory drugs impairs the irreversible effects of aspirin on platelets. For this reason, patients who require both medications should ingest aspirin at least 2 hours prior to the other nonsteroidal antiinflammatory drug.

As evidence of the modest effect of these other nonsteroidal antiinflammatory drugs on platelet function, ibuprofen has been given safely to patients with hemophilia A.[45,46] However, when ibuprofen is given to patients with hemophilia and human immunodeficiency virus (HIV) receiving zidovudine, increased bleeding can occur.[47] Analgesics such as acetaminophen, sodium or choline salicylate, and narcotics neither inhibit COX nor prolong the bleeding time.[19,45,48,49]

CYCLOOXYGENASE INHIBITORS

COX inhibitors (coxibs) do not directly affect platelet function because they are relatively specific for COX-2, a COX isoform absent in platelets.[19] Through a COX-2 dependent pathway, endothelial cells synthesize prostacyclin, which inhibits platelet aggregation and smooth muscle proliferation.[50] Thus, coxibs could be prothrombotic by inhibiting the vascular protective effect of prostacyclin production by endothelial cells without impairing platelet activation. In the Vioxx Gastrointestinal Outcomes Research (VIGOR) trial, which was designed to compare the gastrointestinal toxicity of a coxib (rofecoxib) with a traditional nonsteroidal antiinflammatory drug (naproxen), a fivefold increase in the rate of myocardial infarction was observed in the group treated with the coxib.[51,52] This observation, along with a 3.9-fold excess of thromboembolic events in patients taking rofecoxib in the Adenomatous Polyp Prevention on Vioxx (APPROVe) trial, led to the withdrawal of rofecoxib from the world market.[53] Whether other coxibs that are less specific for COX-2 also are associated with vascular complications remains to be established.

THIENOPYRIDINES

The thienopyridines ticlopidine and clopidogrel are used as antithrombotic agents in arterial diseases (see Chap. 126). They may be more effective than aspirin in the secondary prevention of cerebrovascular and cardiovascular events.[54–60] The antithrombotic effects of thienopyridines and aspirin may be additive and beneficial in preventing thrombotic complications associated with unstable angina or after coronary artery stent placement.[56,58,59,61,62] In other clinical situations, such as treatment of ischemic stroke or transient ischemic attacks, the benefit of adding a thienopyridine to aspirin therapy does not appear to outweigh the added hemorrhagic risk.[63,64]

Ticlopidine and clopidogrel differ from aspirin in the mechanism of their antiplatelet activity and their toxicity profile. Both thienopyridines are prodrugs that depend on metabolites to competitively inhibit the platelet ADP receptor P2Y12.[65–73] Ticlopidine 250 mg by mouth twice per day or clopidogrel 75 mg once per day inhibits platelet aggregation ex vivo and prolongs the bleeding time in humans. The degree of prolongation of the bleeding time is equivalent to or greater than that of aspirin, and the effect of thienopyridines and aspirin appears additive.[59,74] Effects of ticlopidine and clopidogrel on platelet aggregation and the bleeding time may be seen within 24 to 48 hours of the first dose but are not maximal for 4 to 6 days. A loading dose of clopidogrel 300 mg followed by a daily dose of 75 mg/day shortens the time required for the maximal antiplatelet effect.[75] The effects of these drugs may persist for 4 to 10 days after they have been discontinued, as a result of their extended half-life after multiple doses or an irreversible effect on platelets.[65]

Ticlopidine administration has been associated with potentially serious hematologic complications, including neutropenia (<1200/μl in 2.4% of individuals)[65,76,77] and, less commonly, aplastic anemia, and thrombocytopenia.[78,79] In addition, at least one of 5000 patients treated with ticlopidine develops thrombotic thrombocytopenic purpura.[80–82] Results from a large clinical trial suggest that hematologic complications may be less common with clopidogrel.[54] One study suggested that clopidogrel is rarely associated with thrombotic thrombocytopenic purpura (1/270,000 patients treated),[83] although this rate is close to the incidence of this disease in the general population. Because of its toxicity profile, clopidogrel essentially has replaced ticlopidine in the United States.

GLYCOPROTEIN IIB/IIIA RECEPTOR ANTAGONISTS

Drugs that specifically impair the function of platelet glycoprotein IIb/IIIa (GpIIb-IIIa; $\alpha_{IIb}\beta_3$) have been developed for short-term use as antithrombotic agents in the setting of ischemic coronary artery disease.[84–86] Abciximab, eptifibatide, and tirofiban are three US Food and Drug Administration-approved GpIIb-IIIa inhibitors that are structurally dissimilar, but all rapidly impair platelet aggregation. Abciximab is a human-murine chimeric Fab fragment, eptifibatide is a cyclic heptapeptide, and tirofiban is a nonpeptide mimetic. Because inherited GpIIb-IIIa abnormalities result in the bleeding disorder Glanzmann thrombasthenia,[87,88] the finding that these drugs can predispose to bleeding is not surprising. In the Evaluation of c7E3 for the Prevention of Ischemic Complications (EPIC), a clinical trial of the efficacy of abciximab in patients undergoing percutaneous coronary angioplasty, 14 percent of patients given abciximab experienced major bleeding compared to 7 percent of patients given placebo.[89] However, the patients were also given aspirin and heparin. When the heparin dose was decreased in the subsequent Evaluation in PTCA to Improve Long-term Outcome with Abciximab GP IIb/IIIa Blockade (EPILOG) trial, the incidence of major bleeding in patients receiving abciximab decreased to 2.0 percent compared to 3.1 percent in the control group, which received heparin and aspirin alone.[90] Nonetheless, in both EPIC and EPILOG, minor bleeding was significantly more frequent in patients given abciximab and standard-dose heparin compared to patients given standard-dose heparin alone, attesting to the ability of a GpIIb-IIIa antagonist to impair normal hemostasis. In the Platelet Receptor Inhibition in Ischemic Syndrome Management in Patients Limited by Unstable Signs and Symptoms (PRISM-PLUS) trial of tirofiban and the Platelet Glycoprotein IIb/IIIa in Unstable Angina: Receptor Suppression Using Integrilin Therapy (PURSUIT) trial of eptifibatide, major and minor bleeding were slightly more frequent in patients receiving the study drug compared to controls.[91,92] Similarly, patients receiving the oral GpIIb-IIIa inhibitors xemilofiban and sibrafiban for 30 and 28 days, respectively, frequently experienced mucocutaneous bleeding similar to that experienced by patients with thrombasthenia.[93,94]

The risk of bleeding in patients undergoing percutaneous coronary intervention given GpIIb-IIIa antagonists can be minimized by using low-dose heparin (such as 70 U/kg as in EPILOG),[90] by avoiding treatment of patients who are receiving warfarin at therapeutic doses, by early vascular sheath removal, and by meticulous care of vascular puncture sites.[95] Platelet transfusions appear to rapidly reverse the defect in platelet function in patients receiving abciximab, primarily by decreasing the extent of GpIIb-IIIa blockade. The ability of platelet transfusion to reverse the effects of the other GpIIb-IIIa antagonists is less clear, but these drugs have short half-lives if renal and hepatic function are normal. When bleeding requiring intervention occurs, platelet transfusion in an attempt to decrease the concentration of platelet-bound drug should be considered.

Thrombocytopenia occurring within 24 hours of initiating therapy has been observed in small numbers of patients following the administration of all types of GpIIb-IIIa antagonists.[91,92,94-96] In the EPIC trial, the incidence of platelet counts less than 100,000/μl and less than 50,000/μl in patients receiving abciximab for the first time was 3.9 and 0.9 percent, respectively.[96] The incidence of profound thrombocytopenia after administration of abciximab was confirmed in subsequent publications.[89,90,97,98] Thrombocytopenia has been reported in patients receiving eptifibatide, tirofiban, and a variety of small molecule RDG- and non-RGD based GpIIb-IIIa inhibitors. The incidence of thrombocytopenia has varied from 0 to 13 percent in several studies, depending on the specific inhibitor studied.[91,92,94,96,99-102] The mechanism responsible for the decrease in platelet count is uncertain but may be related to the presence of preexisting anti-GpIIb-IIIa antibodies that recognize epitopes on GpIIb-IIIa exposed by binding of the GpIIb-IIIa antagonist (ligand-induced binding sites).[103] Whether prescreening patients for preexisting antibodies will reduce the incidence of severe thrombocytopenia is unknown.[104] The thrombocytopenia usually reverses readily when the drug is stopped, but it also may be reversed by platelet transfusion if clinically indicated.[95] Thrombocytopenia in patients receiving GpIIb-IIIa antagonists must be differentiated from pseudothrombopenia resulting from drug-induced platelet clumping, from heparin-induced thrombocytopenia in patients receiving heparin concurrently, and from other causes of thrombocytopenia depending on the clinical circumstances.[105,106] Identifying thrombocytopenia early is particularly important because GpIIb-IIIa antagonists are administered as long infusions, and the drug should be stopped as soon as true thrombocytopenia has been confirmed. In most cases of profound thrombocytopenia, a platelet count obtained 2 to 4 hours after initiating therapy provides evidence of a significantly decreased platelet count.

DRUGS THAT AFFECT PLATELET CYCLIC NUCLEOTIDE LEVELS OR FUNCTION

The pyrimidopyrimidine derivative dipyridamole inhibits cyclic nucleotide phosphodiesterase, resulting in the intracellular accumulation of cyclic adenosine monophosphate (cAMP). Dipyridamole also may inhibit the breakdown of cyclic guanosine monophosphate (cGMP), resulting in the potentiation of a nitric oxide (NO) effect.[107] Although dipyridamole inhibits platelet function in vitro, its clinical utility is controversial.[108,109] A meta-analysis failed to demonstrate a benefit for the addition of dipyridamole to aspirin therapy.[110] However, many of the older dipyridamole trials used formulations with limited bioavailability.[111] The European Stroke Prevention Study 2 (ESPS 2) reported benefit to patients receiving dipyridamole for prevention of stroke and transient ischemic attack, although no difference in mortality between patients taking dipyridamole and placebo or among patients taking dipyridamole plus aspirin compared to either dipyridamole or aspirin alone was observed.[112] The basis for the benefit of dipyridamole in the ESPS 2 trial is unclear but could result from the higher dipyridamole

dosage or the sustained release dipyridamole preparation used in the trial.

Intravenous infusions of prostaglandin PG (E$_1$), prostacyclin, or stable analogues of prostacyclin stimulate platelet adenylyl cyclase, causing an increase in platelet cAMP levels and a decrease in platelet responsiveness.[113-115] These agents cause a transient prolongation of the bleeding time and inhibit platelet shape change, aggregation, and secretion. However, their clinical utility is limited by their short half-life and side effects, which include peripheral vasodilatation.[113,116] Cilostazol, a phosphodiesterase III inhibitor, has been approved in the United States for treatment of peripheral vascular disease[117] and may be useful in the prevention of cardiac stent occlusion.[118] NO and organic nitrates such as nitroglycerin inhibit platelet function in vitro, probably by activating guanylyl cyclase, thereby increasing cGMP.[119] Their effect on in vivo platelet function is uncertain. High concentrations of caffeine and theophylline also inhibit platelet phosphodiesterases in vitro.

ANTIBIOTICS

The various penicillins contain a β-lactam ring and a unique side chain. Most penicillins cause a dose-dependent prolongation of the bleeding time in normal volunteers.[120] Because they reduce platelet aggregation and secretion and ristocetin-induced platelet agglutination, they may affect both platelet adhesion and platelet activation. Tests of platelet aggregation are abnormal in at least 50 to 75 percent of individuals receiving large doses (at least several grams per day) of carbenicillin, penicillin G, ticarcillin, ampicillin, nafcillin, and azlocillin and in 25 to 50 percent of patients taking piperacillin, azlocillin, apalcillin, or mezlocillin.[120-122] Differences in the antiplatelet effects of these antibiotics probably relate to differences in blood levels and drug potency. Their effect on platelets is maximal 1 to 3 days after administration and may remain for several days after the antibiotic has been stopped, suggesting that the effect of these antibiotics on platelets in vivo is irreversible.

Penicillins may impair the interaction of agonists and von Willebrand factor (vWF) with the platelet membrane.[123] When many penicillins are incubated with washed platelets, albeit at concentrations higher than those attained in vivo, they inhibit the interaction of vWF and agonists, such as ADP and epinephrine, with their platelet receptors.[124] The relative in vitro antiplatelet potency of the penicillins correlates well with their lipid solubility and with the inhibitory potency of the isolated side chains.[125] Moreover, the inhibitory effect of penicillin G on platelet function in vitro is potentiated by the presence of probenecid.[126] When platelet function was tested after intravenous administration of penicillin, oxacillin or mezlocillin for 3 to 17 days to patients or normal volunteers, irreversible inhibition of agonist-induced aggregation was noted, along with a 40% reduction in low-affinity thromboxane A$_2$ receptors.[127] Thus, penicillins probably inhibit platelet function by binding to one or more membrane components necessary for adhesive interactions with the vessel wall or for stimulus-response coupling.

Clinically significant bleeding has been associated with use of carbenicillin, penicillin G, ticarcillin, and nafcillin but is far less common than prolongation of the bleeding time.[120,128] Patients with coexisting hemostatic defects (e.g., thrombocytopenia, vitamin K deficiency, uremia) may be particularly prone to this complication. On the other hand, high doses of penicillin G did not increase gastrointestinal blood loss in a thrombocytopenic rabbit model.[129] In our experience, bleeding resulting from antibiotic-induced platelet dysfunction is uncommon and unpredictable. Because β-lactam-induced platelet dysfunction resolves with time following drug cessation, this class of drugs should be considered as a cause of bleeding only in the appropriate clinical setting. A similar pattern of platelet dysfunction has been reported with some cephalosporins or related antibiotics but not with others.[120,130,131] Broad-spectrum antibiotics can cause a bleeding diathesis attributable to vitamin K deficiency. Nitrofurantoin, a structurally unrelated antibiotic, may cause mild prolongation of the bleeding time and impair platelet aggregation when blood levels of the drug are higher than 20 μM.[132] Miconazole, an antifungal agent, has been shown to inhibit human and rabbit platelet COX in vitro and rabbit platelet cyclooxygenase after intravenous infusion.[133]

ANTICOAGULANTS, FIBRINOLYTIC AGENTS, AND ANTIFIBRINOLYTIC AGENTS

Heparin predisposes to bleeding primarily through its anticoagulant effect, but it also may affect platelet function. For example, a bolus injection of heparin 100 U/kg can cause a significant prolongation of the bleeding time in normal subjects and in patients prior to cardiopulmonary bypass, suggesting that therapeutic doses of heparin impair platelet function.[134] Heparin likely impairs platelet function by inhibiting the generation and action of thrombin, a potent platelet agonist. In vitro studies also suggest that heparin enhances platelet aggregation induced by other platelet agonists.[135] Heparin binds to a single class of high-affinity binding sites on resting platelets and to an additional class of lower-affinity binding sites on fully activated platelets.[136] High heparin doses have been found to impair vWF-dependent platelet function, possibly by binding to the heparin-binding domain of vWF.[137] The contributions of these effects on platelet function to the bleeding complications of heparin therapy are uncertain.

Bleeding during fibrinolytic therapy results predominantly from the combined effects of structural lesions in blood vessels and the fibrin(ogen)olytic activity of the agent used. However, pharmacologic doses of streptokinase, urokinase, and tissue plasminogen activator (t-PA) can affect platelet function.[138] High concentrations of plasmin ex vivo cause platelet aggregation.[139] Moreover, marked increases in the urinary excretion of the thromboxane A_2 metabolite 2,3-dinor-TxB$_2$ have been detected in patients receiving streptokinase or t-PA for coronary thrombolysis, suggesting that in vivo platelet activation had occurred during infusion of the drug.[140,141] Nevertheless, several in vitro studies indicate that plasmin generation has an inhibitory effect on platelet function. First, very high levels of fibrin(ogen) degradation products, coupled with very low levels of fibrinogen, may impair platelet aggregation.[142] Second, plasminogen can bind to platelets[143] and, after its conversion to plasmin, enzymatically degrade platelet GpIb, impairing the interaction of platelets with vWF.[144,145] Third, plasmin can inhibit platelet arachidonic acid metabolism.[146] Fourth, t-PA promotes the disaggregation of platelet aggregates, presumably by inducing lysis of the fibrinogen that mediates aggregate formation.[147] Finally, after initial activation, platelets incubated with plasmin and recombinant t-PA in vitro become refractory to activation by other agonists.[148] Whether any of the in vitro and ex vivo observations apply to the in vivo situation and are clinically significant remains to be determined.[149] The antifibrinolytic drug ε-aminocaproic acid can increase the bleeding time when administered for several days at doses of at least 24 g/day.[150]

CARDIOVASCULAR DRUGS

Administration of nitroprusside (which increases platelet cGMP),[151–155] nitroglycerine,[156] and propranolol[157,158] can decrease platelet aggregation and secretion ex vivo. Nitroprusside can increase the bleeding time twofold when administered at infusion rates of 6 to 8 μg/kg/min, whereas trimethaphan, another effective parenteral antihypertensive agent, does not.[151,159] As mentioned previously in the section entitled "Drugs that Affect Platelet Cyclic Nucleotide Levels or Function,"

inhalation of NO, which is advocated for treatment of pulmonary hypertension and adult respiratory distress syndrome, can impair agonist-induced platelet aggregation ex vivo, although effects on the bleeding time have been variable.[160–162] The clinical significance of these observations is unclear. "Calcium channel blockers," such as verapamil, nifedipine, and diltiazem, inhibit platelet aggregation when added at very high concentrations to washed platelets.[163] This effect is seen primarily with epinephrine-induced aggregation and does not appear to be related to calcium channel blockade. For example, verapamil can act as an α_2-adrenergic receptor antagonist at concentrations that inhibit platelet function.[164] At therapeutic doses, calcium channel blockers do not prolong the bleeding time, although one agent, nisoldipine, reportedly inhibited agonist-induced calcium transients and platelet aggregation after 10 days of oral administration.[165] At high concentrations, the antiarrhythmic drug quinidine reportedly caused mild prolongation of the bleeding time and potentiated the effect of aspirin.[166]

VOLUME EXPANDERS

Dextran is a neutral polysaccharide that is heterogeneous in molecular size. Two preparations with average molecular weights of 40,000 and 70,000 are in clinical use. Dextran infusions may prolong the bleeding time in normal subjects and in patients with von Willebrand disease, but this effect has not been observed in most normal subjects.[167–169] Infused dextran adsorbs to the platelet surface and can impair platelet aggregation, secretion, and procoagulant activity. The maximal effect of dextran may require several hours, suggesting that larger molecules with a slower clearance rate are responsible.[167] Curiously, the drug has no effect when added to platelet-rich plasma.[167] Dextran infusion produces a modest reduction in plasma vWF antigen and ristocetin cofactor activity.[168] Despite these effects on primary hemostasis and the use of dextran in the operative setting as a volume expander or for antithrombotic prophylaxis, prospective studies indicate that dextran is not associated with significant postoperative bleeding unless it is administered together with low-dose heparin.[170,171] Hydroxyethyl starch, another volume expander, although generally safe, may prolong the bleeding time and predispose to hemorrhage, particularly if it is administered in doses exceeding 20 ml/kg of a 6 percent solution. A lower dose of hydroxyethyl starch may contribute to bleeding if it is administered simultaneously with low-dose heparin, is given to patients with a preexistent hemostatic defect, or is given to patients after major cardiothoracic surgery.[172–175] Different hydroxyethyl starch preparations vary with regard to the average number of hydroxymethyl groups per glucose unit, which may affect intravascular survival and effects on hemostasis.[176,177]

PSYCHOTROPIC DRUGS, ANESTHETICS, AND COCAINE

Platelets from patients taking antidepressants or phenothiazines may exhibit impaired aggregation responses, but this effect is not associated with bleeding.[178,179] The effect on aggregation has been attributed to inhibition of intracellular signaling molecules such as protein kinase C.[180] Selective serotonin reuptake inhibitors, such as paroxetine, have been shown to decrease serotonin storage within platelets.[181] Fluoxetine does not appear to impair in vitro platelet aggregation and only rarely has been associated with clinical bleeding.[182,183] General anesthesia with halothane or propofol may cause a slight prolongation of the bleeding time, most likely because of an effect on calcium signaling, but with adverse effect on surgical hemostasis.[184,185] In addition to an association with thrombocytopenia, cocaine has been reported to either inhibit platelet function[186,187] or induce platelet activation.[188] Heroin decreases platelet NO production.[189] The clinical relevance of these observations is unknown.

ONCOLOGIC DRUGS

Administration of mithramycin to a total dose of 6 to 21 mg has been associated with mucocutaneous bleeding, an increase in the bleeding time, and decreased platelet aggregation.[190] An *ex vivo* defect in platelet secretion and secondary aggregation has been reported in patients with solid tumors within 48 hours of receiving infusions of autologous bone marrow and high-dose chemotherapy consisting of cisplatin, cyclophosphamide, and either bischloroethylnitrosourea (BCNU) or melphelan.[191] Both daunorubicin and BCNU can inhibit platelet aggregation and secretion when added to platelet-rich plasma, but as single agents they have not been shown to cause clinically significant platelet dysfunction.[192-194] Administration of recombinant forms of thrombopoietin to thrombocytopenic patients with cancer results in production of normally functioning platelets.[195,196]

MISCELLANEOUS AGENTS

The immunosuppressive drug cyclosporine A reportedly enhanced ADP-stimulated platelet aggregation *in vitro*.[197-199] Whether this effect contributes to the thrombotic thrombocytopenic purpura syndrome associated with this drug is unclear. Antihistamines,[200] the serotonin antagonist ketanserin,[201] and some radiographic contrast agents[202,203] can impair platelet aggregation responses *ex vivo* by unknown mechanisms.

FOODS AND FOOD ADDITIVES

The effect of certain foods and food additives on platelet function must be considered. For example, a diet rich in fish oils containing ϖ-3 fatty acids (eicosapentaenoic acid; docosahexaenoic acid) causes a slight prolongation of the bleeding time.[204] These fatty acids act by reducing the platelet content of arachidonic acid and by competing with arachidonic acid for COX.[205,206] Easy bruising noted after eating Chinese food has been attributed to an antiplatelet effect of the black tree fungus.[207] A component of extract of onion can inhibit platelet arachidonic acid metabolism.[208] Ajoene, a component of garlic, is an inhibitor of fibrinogen binding and platelet aggregation.[209,210] Extracts of two commonly used spices, cumin and turmeric, inhibit platelet aggregation and eicosanoid biosynthesis.[211]

HEMATOLOGIC DISORDERS ASSOCIATED WITH ABNORMAL PLATELET FUNCTION

CHRONIC MYELOPROLIFERATIVE DISORDERS

DEFINITION AND HISTORY
Bleeding and thrombosis are significant causes of morbidity and mortality in the chronic myeloproliferative disorders: essential thrombocythemia, polycythemia rubra vera, myelofibrosis with myeloid metaplasia, and chronic myelogenous leukemia.[212-215] Thrombocytosis is a constant finding in essential thrombocythemia, but the differential diagnosis includes these other myeloproliferative disorders as well as other diseases (see Chap. 85).[216]

ETIOLOGY AND PATHOGENESIS
Several factors contribute to the hemostatic abnormalities in the myeloproliferative disorders:

1. Increased whole-blood viscosity in polycythemia vera: The engorgement of blood vessels associated with polycythemia is a risk factor for thrombosis and bleeding, particularly in postoperative situations.[217,218]
2. Intrinsic defects in platelet function: A number of intrinsic platelet defects in the myeloproliferative disorders have been reported.

However, the bleeding time is prolonged in only a minority of patients, and bleeding can occur in individuals with normal bleeding times.[213,219]

3. Elevated platelet counts: The contribution of an elevated platelet count, by itself, to the risk of hemorrhage and thrombosis is controversial.[220-224] A number of retrospective studies indicate the risk of abnormal hemostasis cannot be confidently predicted from the degree of thrombocytosis.[213]
4. Leukocyte and/or endothelial dysfunction might contribute to the thrombotic phenotype in some individuals, perhaps through leukocyte–platelet and leukocyte–endothelial cell interactions.[213,225]

Under the light or electron microscope, platelets in these disorders may be larger or smaller than normal, may be abnormally shaped, and may exhibit a reduction in the number of storage granules.[226] In essential thrombocythemia, platelet survival may be modestly reduced.[227] A number of functional and biochemical abnormalities have been described in platelets from patients with myeloproliferative disorders. The most frequently encountered functional abnormality is a decrease in platelet aggregation and secretion in response to epinephrine, ADP, or collagen.[213,228] The defect in epinephrine-induced aggregation often includes absence of the primary wave of aggregation, which is unusual in other conditions. This effect does not result simply from an elevated platelet count, as it is not encountered in reactive thrombocytosis.[216,229] Thus, loss of platelet responsiveness to epinephrine may be useful in confirming the presence of a myeloproliferative disorder.

Reduced platelet aggregation and secretion in the myeloproliferative disorders have been associated with one or more of the following: decreased agonist-induced release of arachidonic acid from membrane phospholipids[230,231]; reduced conversion of arachidonic acid to prostaglandin endoperoxides or lipoxygenase products[232]; reduced platelet responsiveness to thromboxane A_2[233,234]; deficiency of dense or α-granules[235,236]; deficiency of integrin $\alpha_2\beta_1$, resulting in variable changes in platelet responsiveness to collagen[237]; and decreased numbers of α2-adrenergic receptors associated with reduced or absent platelet responses to epinephrine.[238,239] On the other hand, spontaneous platelet aggregation in a patient with essential thrombocythemia and thrombosis has been reported,[240] as has increased thromboxane biosynthesis by platelets from patients with essential thrombocythemia[241] or polycythemia vera.[242]

Reduction in platelet procoagulant activity has been reported in some patients with myeloproliferative disorders and thrombocytosis.[243] Also reported are specific platelet membrane abnormalities, including decreased expression and activation of integrin GpIIb-IIIa,[244] decreased amounts of the GpIb-V-IX complex, resulting in an acquired form of Bernard-Soulier syndrome,[245] decreased numbers of receptors for prostaglandin PGD$_2$,[246] increased numbers of FcγRIIa receptors,[247] an increase in GpIV (CD36) with[248,249] or without[250] a corresponding decrease in GpIb, and impaired expression of thrombopoietin receptors in polycythemia vera[251] and essential thrombocythemia.[252] An acquired form of von Willebrand disease has been observed in several individuals with chronic myelogenous leukemia and other myeloproliferative syndromes; see "Acquired von Willebrand Disease" below.[253] In these cases, a reduction in the plasma level of the high molecular weight vWF multimers was observed;[254] in some patients, the vWF abnormality was corrected transiently by DDAVP infusion.[249,255] In other patients, the abnormalities were partially or completely corrected by cytoreductive therapy.[253,256]

Several features of the platelet functional defects noted *in vitro* require emphasis relative to the clinical setting. First, none is unique to a particular myeloproliferative disorder. Second, the relative frequency of these features has varied widely in reported series. Third, none has been predictive of bleeding or thrombosis. Fourth, although the myeloproliferative disorders comprise several distinct clinicopathologic entities, they represent clonal abnormalities of hematopoiesis. Therefore, platelets may acquire structural and biochemical abnormalities as they develop from a clone of abnormal megakaryocytes.

CLINICAL AND LABORATORY FEATURES

Bleeding occurs in approximately one third of patients with myeloproliferative disorders and contributes to mortality in 10 percent. Thrombosis also occurs in one third of cases, contributing to mortality in 15 to 40 percent.[213,219] Most symptomatic patients experience either bleeding or thrombosis; however, some develop both complications during the course of their disease. Bleeding usually involves the skin or mucous membranes but also may occur after surgery or trauma. Thrombosis can involve arteries or veins and may occur in unusual locations, such as the hepatic, portal, and mesenteric circulations.[257–259] Full-blown or latent myeloproliferative disorders account for a substantial proportion of patients with Budd-Chiari syndrome or portal vein thrombosis.[257,260] Individuals with essential thrombocythemia may experience ischemia and necrosis of the fingers and toes resulting from digital artery thrombosis, microvascular occlusion in the coronary circulation, and transient neurologic symptoms resulting from cerebrovascular occlusion.[261] A syndrome of redness and burning pain in the extremities, termed *erythromelalgia*, is strongly associated with essential thrombocythemia and polycythemia vera and is thought to result, in part, from arteriolar platelet thrombi, although it also may have vasculopathic and neuropathic components.[261,263] Predicting the risk of bleeding or thrombosis in an asymptomatic patient has been difficult,[220] but an increased number of reticulated platelets in patients with thrombocytosis, thought to reflect an increase in platelet turnover, has been associated with an increased risk for thrombosis.[264] Vascular complications are more likely to occur in patients older than 60 years and in patients with other risk factors for vascular disease.[265,266]

THERAPY

Therapy should be considered for symptomatic patients, for patients older than 60 years, and for individuals about to undergo surgery. The treatment of polycythemia vera is discussed in Chapter 56 and has been reviewed.[266] Treatment includes correction of polycythemia, maintenance of normal red cell mass,[267] and treatment of the underlying disorder.[213,219,259,268,269] Platelet count reduction to less than 400,000/μl in patients with thrombocytosis, either by plateletpheresis or cytoreductive agents, has generally been associated with clinical improvement.[219,259,270]

Effective agents used to decrease the platelet count include the ribonuclease reductase inhibitor hydroxyurea,[271] interferon alpha, and anagrelide[266,270,272,273] (see Chap. 111). In a prospective, randomized trial of 114 "high-risk" individuals with essential thrombocythemia who either were older than 60 years or had a history of thrombosis, hydroxyurea significantly reduced the incidence of new thrombosis from 24 to 3.6 percent.[271] Anagrelide, an imidazoquinazolin derivative, is thought to decrease platelet counts by specifically impairing megakaryocyte maturation. Anagrelide has essentially no effect on red and white cells counts and is not known to be leukemogenic. Nevertheless, 10 to 20 percent of patients experience neurologic, gastrointestinal, and cardiac side effects, particularly fluid retention, necessitating discontinuation of the drug. Recently, the Medical Research Council of Great Britain conducted a randomized clinical trial of 809 patients with essential thrombocythemia, testing the efficacy and side effects of aspirin combined with either anagrelide or hydroxyurea. The authors found that after a mean follow up of 39 months, patients on the aspirin and anagrelide arm had developed statistically significant increased numbers of arterial thrombosis, bleeding complications, myelofibrotic

transformation, and side effects leading to cessation of the anagrelide than did patients treated with aspirin and hydroxyurea. The authors concluded that hydroxyurea should remain first-line therapy in patients with ET at high risk for vascular events. In addition to this form of preventive therapy, during an episode of acute bleeding, DDAVP infusion may temporarily improve hemostasis if the patient has an acquired storage pool defect or acquired von Willebrand disease.[235,255]

Low-dose aspirin (100–300 mg/day) may be useful in patients with essential thrombocythemia and thrombosis, particularly those with erythromelalgia or with digital or cerebrovascular ischemia.[263,274] However, the evidence to date is largely anecdotal, and aspirin can exacerbate a bleeding tendency in patients with myeloproliferative disorders.[266,275] In a double-blind, placebo-controlled study of 518 patients with polycythemia vera who were judged to have no contraindications to daily low-dose (100 mg) aspirin, subjects in the aspirin arm exhibited a reduced risk of nonfatal arterial/venous cardiovascular end points. Although aspirin was well tolerated, no effect of aspirin on overall and cardiovascular mortality was observed.[276] As previously noted,[267] this study population was heavily pretreated to normalize the platelet count, although some individuals possibly had residual elevations in red cell mass. Consequently, the safety and efficacy of aspirin documented in this study may not be relevant to all patients with polycythemia vera.

Essential thrombocythemia in pregnancy poses special challenges because of an apparent increased risk for unsuccessful pregnancy, thrombotic or bleeding complications, and potential teratogenicity of hydroxyurea. Interferon has been recommended if platelet cytoreduction is warranted and aspirin if microvascular symptoms are present. Low-dose heparin at conventional doses is recommended for prophylaxis or treatment of venous thrombosis, followed by oral anticoagulant therapy for 6 weeks in the puerperium.[266]

LEUKEMIAS AND MYELODYSPLASTIC SYNDROMES

CLINICAL AND LABORATORY FEATURES

The most frequent cause of bleeding in these disorders is thrombocytopenia. However, abnormal platelet function *in vitro* has been described in acute myelogenous leukemia and may be clinically significant in some patients. In acute myelogenous leukemia and its variants, platelets may be larger than normal, abnormally shaped, and exhibit a marked variation in the number of granules (see Chap. 87). Decreased aggregation, serotonin release, and platelet procoagulant activity may occur in response to ADP, epinephrine, or collagen. The functional abnormalities may result from either acquired storage pool deficiency or a defect in the process of platelet activation.[277–279] These defects are intrinsic to the platelet and probably relate to the fact that the megakaryocytes from which platelets are derived have originated from a leukemic stem cell. Bleeding in the acute leukemias usually responds to platelet transfusions and to treatment of the underlying disease. Similar platelet abnormalities may be seen in the myelodysplastic syndromes.[277,280,281] In these syndromes, platelets appear to be less uniformly affected, perhaps because of a residual population of normal platelets admixed with those from the malignant clone.

Reduced platelet aggregation has been reported in children with acute lymphocytic leukemia.[278] Unless the leukemia is biphenotypic, ascribing the platelet defect to the leukemic process itself is difficult. Platelets are normal in children with lymphoblastic leukemia in complete remission[282] (see Chap. 91). Hairy cell leukemia is a lymphoproliferative disease in which platelet dysfunction in rare cases complicates the clinical picture (see Chap. 93). Bleeding is responsible for death in 8 percent of patients. It usually results from thrombocytopenia rather than platelet dysfunction.[283] Some patients exhibit storage pool deficiency or a defect in the process of platelet activation, and these abnormalities reportedly disappear following splenectomy.[284] However, this finding should be interpreted with caution because splenectomy usually corrects the thrombocytopenia as well. Acquired von Willebrand disease in association with hairy cell leukemia has been reported.[285]

DYSPROTEINEMIAS

DEFINITION AND HISTORY

Platelet dysfunction is observed in approximately one third of patients with IgA myeloma or Waldenström macroglobulinemia, 15 percent of patients with IgG myeloma, and occasionally in patients with monoclonal gammopathy of undetermined significance.[286] In addition to platelet dysfunction, other causes of bleeding should be considered in these patients, including hyperviscosity syndrome,[287] thrombocytopenia, complications of amyloidosis (such as amyloid angiopathy)[288] or acquired factor X deficiency,[289,290] and, rarely, a circulating heparin-like anticoagulant[291,292] or systemic fibrino(gen)lysis.[293,294] The myeloma protein may affect *in vitro* coagulation tests by interfering with fibrin polymerization and with the function of other coagulation proteins (see Chaps. 99, 100, 101, and 102)

ETIOLOGY AND PATHOGENESIS

The bleeding time may be prolonged in patients with dysproteinemias, even in the absence of clinical bleeding. The platelet defect is caused by the monoclonal protein. Some monoclonal immunoglobulins have been suggested to interact with the platelet surface to interfere nonspecifically with platelet adhesion or stimulus–response coupling. This concept is supported by the observations that platelet dysfunction is more common when the concentration of the paraprotein in plasma or on the platelet membrane is very high[295] such that platelet aggregation, secretion, clot retraction, and platelet procoagulant activity may all be affected and that normal platelets acquire these defects when incubated with the purified monoclonal immunoglobulin.[296]

In some cases, specific interactions of the monoclonal protein with platelets have been described. One IgA myeloma protein inhibited the ability of a suspension of aortic connective tissue to aggregate normal platelets.[297] The bleeding time and bleeding diathesis of the patient from whom this myeloma protein was obtained were corrected by removing the protein by plasmapheresis. In another patient, an IgG myeloma protein bound specifically to the platelet integrin β_3 subunit. Both the intact immunoglobulin and its F(ab')$_2$ fragment inhibited the binding of fibrinogen to activated platelets, thus inducing a thrombasthenic-like state.[298] Several patients with myeloma, benign monoclonal gammopathy, or chronic lymphocytic leukemia reportedly have an acquired form of von Willebrand disease in which the plasma level of vWF is reduced or the high molecular weight multimers of vWF are lacking.[299–301]

THERAPY

When clinically significant platelet dysfunction occurs in a patient with a dysproteinemia, cytoreductive therapy should be considered as a means to reduce the production and plasma level of the monoclonal immunoglobulin.[286] Plasmapheresis can control bleeding by reducing the level of abnormal protein and can be life-saving during acute bleeds.[302,303] Cryoprecipitate, DDAVP, intravenous γ-globulin, and/or plasmapheresis may be transiently effective in patients with acquired von Willebrand disease.[300,301,304,305]

ACQUIRED VON WILLEBRAND DISEASE

Acquired von Willebrand disease is a relatively rare disorder that typically occurs in the setting of an autoimmune or clonal hematologic disease.[306,307] The latter disorders include myeloma,[301,304] Waldenstrom macroglobulinemia,[308] low-grade non-Hodgkin lymphoma,[309,310] chronic lymphocytic leukemia,[311] and myeloproliferative disorders.[253] In many hematologic disorders, a specific anti-vWF antibody is present,[301,304,312] whereas in autoimmune disorders, anti-vWF antibodies are part of a generalized autoimmune response.[313] When acquired von Willebrand disease occurs in other clinical situations such as cancer or hypothyroidism, it may result from nonspecific direct absorption of vWF onto tumor cells[285,314–316] or decreased vWF production.[317,318]

Mucocutaneous bleeding and a prolonged bleeding time should raise the suspicion of acquired von Willebrand disease in patients without a prior personal or family history of bleeding. This is especially important in patients with known autoimmune disease or lymphoproliferative or myeloproliferative disorders.[319] Diagnostic evaluation includes measurements of factor VIII coagulant activity, vWF antigen, and ristocetin cofactor activity. The presence of an *in vitro* inhibitor may or may not be detected, depending on whether the antibody binds to vWF and neutralizes its function or merely leads to accelerated vWF clearance by the reticuloendothelial system.[319] Patient management includes infusions of desmopressin,[301,311,313] vWF-containing factor VIII concentrates,[320] or high-dose intravenous immunoglobulin.[262,307,321,322] The latter has been efficacious in patients when acquired von Willebrand disease is associated with a lymphoproliferative disorder or monoclonal paraprotein and most likely acts by delaying vWF clearance via mononuclear phagocyte system blockade, although other mechanisms have been postulated.[262,323,324] Treatment of the underlying associated disease is helpful only sometimes.[319]

SYSTEMIC DISORDERS ASSOCIATED WITH ABNORMAL PLATELET FUNCTION

UREMIA

DEFINITION AND HISTORY

In the predialysis era, hemorrhage occurred in approximately 50 percent of uremic patients and was a cause of death in approximately 30 percent.[325,326] With the advent of dialysis, the frequency of spontaneous hemorrhage in patients with renal failure has decreased.[326] Experience with percutaneous renal biopsy in several thousand patients with renal disease supports the notion that the hemostatic defect in patients with renal disease usually is mild. Although the incidence of small perirenal hematomas following biopsy may be as high as 85 percent when patients are examined by computerized tomography, gross hematuria is observed in only 5 to 10 percent of cases and usually is transient.[327,328] Severe bleeding following biopsy requiring surgical intervention is even less common and usually can be attributed to factors other than a uremic hemostatic defect, such as needle lacerations of the kidney or spleen, anomalous vessels, heparin anticoagulation, or the presence of amyloid in the kidney.

ETIOLOGY AND PATHOGENESIS

The hemostatic defect in uremia has been attributed to abnormal platelet function,[329] and defects in every phase of platelet function have been reported.[326] The basis for the defective platelet adhesion observed in uremic patients appears to be multifactorial.[330–332] One prominent factor is renal failure-associated anemia.[333] In an *ex vivo* perfusion system, a lowered hematocrit causes a platelet adhesion defect that can be corrected by increasing the hematocrit to 30 percent or higher.[330] In uremic patients, successful treatment of anemia with red blood cell transfusion or recombinant human erythropoietin (Epo) results in partial or complete correction of prolonged bleeding times when the hematocrit is increased to 27 to 32 percent.[329,334–338] The influence of anemia on primary hemostasis is not unique to uremia. In normal individuals, the bleeding time correlates with the hematocrit, even though both sets of values are in the normal range and bleeding times can be prolonged in patients with severe anemia of any etiology.[333] Red cells may have a beneficial effect on hemostasis because they displace platelets to the periphery of the column of circulating blood.[339] In addition, they may enhance platelet reactivity.[14]

Correction of anemia does not return the bleeding time to normal in all uremic individuals. Thus other factors likely impair platelet adhesion.[330] Ristocetin-induced platelet aggregation, an *in vitro* surrogate for vWF binding to the platelet GpIb-IX-V complex, may be decreased in uremia. However, vWF levels in plasma, measured either immunologically or functionally by ristocetin cofactor activity, are normal or elevated in renal failure,[340] and qualitative vWF abnormalities have not been uniformly observed.[331,341] Moreover, mixing studies using uremic platelets and normal plasma, and vice versa, did not demonstrate consistent quantitative or qualitative abnormalities in GpIb-IX-V.[331,341,342] Nonetheless, uremic plasma can inhibit platelet adhesion to everted, deendothelialized human umbilical artery segments, whereas uremic platelets adhere normally in the presence of normal plasma.[331] Because the defective adhesion was independent of the vWF present in uremic plasma, an unidentified component of uremic plasma appeared to be responsible for adhesion defect.[331] In another perfusion system using rabbit vessels, uremic platelets exhibited markedly reduced spreading on the subendothelium, a defect attributed to impaired vWF binding to platelet $\alpha_{IIb}\beta_3$.[343] Because vWF binding to $\alpha_{IIb}\beta_3$ requires platelet stimulation, these results suggest a uremia-induced defect in platelet activation.

In addition to defective vWF binding to $\alpha_{IIb}\beta_3$,[343] a number of other reports have described defective platelet activation in uremia. Uremic platelets reportedly exhibit reduced fibrinogen binding, aggregation, and secretion in response to a variety of agonists.[344] This abnormality may be retained by platelets after their separation from uremic plasma; in some cases, uremic plasma imparted the defect to normal platelets.[344] The ability of activated platelets to provide a procoagulant surface for generation of activated factor X and thrombin is consistently reduced in uremia.[345] The biochemical reactions required for platelet aggregation, secretion, and procoagulant activity can be impaired in uremic platelets. These reactions include agonist-induced increases in cytoplasmic free calcium,[346] release of arachidonic acid from platelet phospholipids,[325] and conversion of released arachidonic acid to prostaglandin endoperoxides and thromboxane A$_2$.[347–350] Decreased platelet-dense granule ADP and serotonin have been observed in uremia,[351] as has an increased level of cAMP.[352] Because ADP and serotonin are platelet agonists and cAMP is an inhibitor of platelet function, these abnormalities could contribute to an activation defect.

A number of dialyzable and nondialyzable substances have been reported to be responsible for the platelet function defects in uremia. *Ex vivo* platelet aggregation can be inhibited by small dialyzable substances, such as guanidinosuccinic acid and phenolic acids, and by poorly characterized "middle molecules" at concentrations found in uremic plasma.[353] Moreover, platelet function improves after patients are placed on dialysis.[354] Venous and arterial tissue segments from uremic patients produce more prostacyclin than segments from normal individuals, an abnormality that is not corrected by dialysis.[355] Altered NO metabolism has been observed in uremia. In a rat model of uremia, prolonged bleeding times and defective platelet adhesion were normalized by an inhibitor of NO formation,[356] suggesting that increased NO synthesis by endothelial cells and/or platelets is at least partially responsible for the defective platelet function seen in uremia.[357] However, why renal failure increases NO synthesis is not entirely clear, although exposing endothelial cells to guanidinosuccinic acid can mimic the effects of NO, suggesting that retained guanidinosuccinic acid is the relevant substrate.[358] Uremia has been reported to up-reg-

ulate the y$^+$ amino acid transport system for L-arginine transport into platelets, enabling platelets to maintain or enhance NO synthesis, even in the face of uremia-induced low circulating L-arginine concentrations.[359,360] On the other hand, some substances found in high concentrations in uremic plasma, such as urea and parathyroid hormone, play no role in platelet dysfunction.

Two additional factors must be considered when a patient with renal failure exhibits a bleeding tendency: concurrent medications and thrombocytopenia. Aspirin can prolong the bleeding time inordinately in uremia. Unlike aspirin's effect on COX, this effect is transient and correlates with blood levels of aspirin.[33,34] Bleeding may be potentiated by the administration of heparin during hemodialysis. In this situation, use of an ethylene-vinyl alcohol copolymer hollow-fiber dialyzer or intermittent saline infusion and high blood flow rates may eliminate the need for heparin.[361] β-Lactam antibiotics that prolong the bleeding time may have a greater effect in uremic patients and increase the occurrence of bleeding, particularly if renal clearance of the antibiotic is reduced.[362]

Mild thrombocytopenia has been reported in patients with chronic renal failure, particularly in those on dialysis,[363] because of diminished marrow production and decreased platelet survival.[364] In one study, thrombocytopenia was more prevalent after many years of hemodialysis and with concomitant hepatitis C infection. Serum thrombopoietin levels in hemodialysis patients are increased,[363,365] perhaps reflecting a decrease in megakaryocyte mass. Nonetheless, when the platelet count is less than 100,000/μl, consideration must be given to whether a systemic disease or medication that can also cause thrombocytopenia, such as multiple myeloma, systemic vasculitis, hemolytic uremic syndrome, eclampsia, renal allograft rejection, or heparin, is responsible.

CLINICAL AND LABORATORY FEATURES

Despite the advent of dialysis, abnormal platelet function in uremia remains a clinical issue because it may contribute to serious bleeding in some patients with renal failure, particularly following surgical procedures or trauma or in conjunction with anatomic lesions of the gastrointestinal tract and because it often is associated with a prolonged bleeding time.[347,361] Although the bleeding time has often been used as an indication of hemorrhagic risk in uremia, critical reviews of the published literature indicate the data are not sufficient to use the bleeding time for this purpose.[2,366] Moreover, in specific circumstances where therapy for a uremic bleeding diathesis is necessary, the uremic platelet defect usually can be successfully treated.

THERAPY

Abnormal platelet aggregation and a prolonged bleeding time are common in uremic patients but by themselves are not indications for therapeutic intervention. The frequency of excessive bleeding after biopsies or other surgical procedures in uremic patients who have not received specific treatment is not known, but it may be uncommon. Thus, if bleeding complicates a procedure, a thorough search for causes of bleeding other than uremia should be initiated without assuming that uremia is the cause. Several therapeutic maneuvers can either partially or completely correct an abnormal bleeding time in uremic patients, and anecdotal observations indicate they also may improve hemostasis. Because prospective studies comparing various treatment regimens have not been performed, the choice of therapy should be based on the severity of the bleeding, anticipated severity of the hemostatic stress imposed by surgery or trauma, predicted duration of the therapeutic effect, and risks of therapy.

Dialysis Intensive dialysis can correct the bleeding time and bleeding diathesis in many patients but is only partially effective in other patients.[367] Peritoneal dialysis and hemodialysis are equally effective.[367,368] If a patient who is undergoing dialysis bleeds, increasing the intensity of the dialysis may be worthwhile.

Red Cell Transfusion Increasing the hematocrit, via red blood cell transfusion or treatment with recombinant human Epo, is associated with correction of the bleeding time and a suggestion of diminished clinical bleeding in uremic individuals. Improvement or normalization of the bleeding time is observed at hematocrits of 27 to 32 percent,[329,334–337] and the beneficial effects of transfusion and DDAVP may be additive.[369] Moreover, a number of reports suggest that Epo has an effect on platelets that is independent of an increase in hematocrit,[338] perhaps the result of an increased number of young platelets in the circulation.[370]

Desmopressin (1-Desamino-8-D-Arginine Vasopressin) DDAVP is a vasopressin analogue whose pressor effects (V_1 vasopressin receptors) are substantially less than its antidiuretic effects (V_2 vasopressin receptors). DDAVP causes release of vWF from tissue stores, predominantly endothelial cells, and reportedly shortens the bleeding time in 50 to 75 percent of patients with uremia. In many cases, surgery has been performed safely after administration of this drug, although no controlled trial has been performed.[371] DDAVP usually is administered intravenously at a dose of 0.3 μg/kg over 15 to 30 minutes (maximum dose 20 μg), but it also is effective at this dose when given subcutaneously.[371] Alternatively, the drug can be given intranasally.[372] Improvement in the bleeding time is seen within 30 to 60 minutes of administration, lasts for approximately 4 hours, and roughly correlates with the rise in plasma vWF levels and the appearance in the circulation of high molecular weight vWF multimers.[371] However, DDAVP is efficacious in patients whose plasma contains normal or increased amounts of vWF, suggesting that mechanisms in addition to changes in the quantity or quality of circulating vWF are involved.[371] In some patients, the drug has been given repeatedly at 12- to 24-hour intervals, although tachyphylaxis can occur.[373]

Side effects of DDAVP are mild and uncommon, They include a 10 to 15 percent decrease in mean arterial pressure, a 20 to 30 percent increase in pulse rate, facial flushing, water retention, and hyponatremia leading to seizures. The latter is more common after repeated administration and when fluids are given freely.[371] Water retention and hyponatremia have not been observed in patients whose kidneys cannot respond to the hormone. Several uremic and nonuremic individuals with atherosclerosis reportedly developed stroke or myocardial infarction after DDAVP administration, although such complications appear to be rare.[374,375] If dialysis is not effective, DDAVP is the treatment of choice for uremic bleeding, particularly if only a short-term effect is required.[371]

Conjugated Estrogens Conjugated estrogens reportedly shorten the bleeding time in most, but not all, uremic individuals, both in uncontrolled studies and in randomized, double-blind studies.[376–379] They also may be useful in some patients with uremia who bleed from gastrointestinal telangiectasia.[380] Conjugated estrogens usually are administered at a dose of 0.6 mg/kg intravenously for 5 days. Shortening of the bleeding time may be seen within 72 hours of the first dose; the maximal effect occurs within 5 to 7 days and can persist for up to 14 days. Lower doses have not been effective.[378] One report suggests oral conjugated estrogens are effective at a dose of 50 mg/day, but this regimen has not been compared to the parenteral regimen in a controlled study.[381] Because no changes in the plasma levels or multimer distribution of vWF have been noted with this treatment, the active component in conjugated estrogens, 17β-estradiol, has been postulated to act through an estrogen receptor mechanism.[382] Endothelial cells contain such receptors, but platelets do not.

Cryoprecipitate In uncontrolled studies, cryoprecipitate infusions reportedly shortened the bleeding time in uremic patients and ameliorated bleeding.[383] However, other studies reported inconsistent results.[384] Conceivably, hemostasis is promoted by either the vWF or the platelet microparticles found within cryoprecipitate preparations.[385] However, the uncertain efficacy of cryoprecipitate argues against its routine use for uremic bleeding.

ANTIPLATELET ANTIBODIES

DEFINITION AND HISTORY

Antibody binding to the platelets occurs in several pathologic conditions, including idiopathic thrombocytopenic purpura (ITP), systemic lupus erythematosus (SLE), and platelet alloimmunization, and can produce thrombocytopenia because of decreased platelet survival. In most instances, the surviving platelets function normally. Less commonly, bleeding times are shorter than expected for the degree of thrombocytopenia, suggesting enhanced platelet function.[386] Occasionally platelet function is impaired. Thus, a platelet count greater than 30,000 to 40,000/μl is generally regarded as "safe"[387] but cannot always be assumed to be in patients with immune thrombocytopenia.

ETIOLOGY AND PATHOGENESIS

The mechanism by which autoantibodies or alloantibodies impair platelet function usually is not apparent. In several cases, however, antibody binding to specific platelet glycoproteins has been responsible. Most antiplatelet antibodies are directed against the GpIIb-IIIa ($\alpha_{IIb}\beta_3$) complex, but antibodies directed against GpIb-IX-V, GpIa-IIa (integrin $\alpha_2\beta_1$), and GpIV also have been detected.[388,389] In most instances, the functional consequences of antibody binding are obscured by the presence of thrombocytopenia. In a few cases, antibody had no effect on platelet function *in vitro*.[390] Nonetheless, several patients with normal platelet counts and autoantibodies against GpIIb-IIIa had absent platelet aggregation and a bleeding diathesis reminiscent of Glanzmann thrombasthenia.[391–394] Similarly, two IgG autoantibodies against GpIb that selectively inhibit ristocetin-induced platelet aggregation have been reported. In one patient, lymphadenopathy and polyclonal hypergammaglobulinemia were associated with a prolonged bleeding time and clinical bleeding.[395] In the second patient, the clinical significance of the antibody's selective effect on GpIb function was obscured by severe thrombocytopenia.[396] In two other patients, impaired collagen-induced platelet aggregation was associated with autoantibodies against $\alpha_2\beta_1$.[397,398] Finally, a human monoclonal antibody derived from a patient with SLE was shown to react with a 32-kDa antigen on the surface of activated platelets and inhibit the second wave of platelet aggregation induced by ADP or a thromboxane A_2 analogue.[399]

In addition to interfering with the function of membrane components, some antibodies can activate platelets and induce aggregation and secretion. *In vitro*, antibodies can activate platelets through immune complex binding to platelet Fc receptors, by depositing sublytic quantities of the membrane attack complex of complement (C5b-9) on the cell surface,[400] or by binding to a specific membrane antigen.[401] The prototypic example of this phenomenon is heparin-induced thrombocytopenia in which antibodies bound to neoepitopes exposed on the platelet factor 4 molecule by heparin binding activate platelets by binding to platelet Fc receptors.[402]

CLINICAL AND LABORATORY FEATURES

Platelet dysfunction should be suspected in any patient with ITP or SLE who has mucocutaneous bleeding with a platelet count that is not ordinarily associated with this complication [e.g., $\geq$40,000/μl]. In such cases, the bleeding time may be longer than expected for the platelet count. The clinical spectrum of autoimmune platelet dysfunction may include some individuals, usually women, with "easy bruising" and a normal platelet count. These patients may have ITP with "compensated thrombocytolysis" because a substantial proportion of them have circulating antiplatelet antibodies and megathrombocytes.[403]

Patients with antiplatelet antibodies may exhibit defective platelet function *in vitro*, even if they do not manifest a prolonged bleeding time or excessive bleeding. In two series, 13 of 19 patients with ITP demonstrated impaired platelet aggregation to ADP, epinephrine, or collagen.[404,405] Similarly, 22 of 35 patients with SLE had reduced platelet aggregation in response to these agonists.[406,407] The functional abnormalities appeared to be antibody mediated because IgG purified from the plasma or eluted from the platelets of some of the patients inhibited the aggregation of normal platelets.

Several aspects of platelet function may be impaired by antiplatelet antibodies. Some antiplatelet antibodies may inhibit the adhesion of platelets to the subendothelial matrix[408] The most frequently reported abnormality is absence of platelet aggregation in response to low concentrations of collagen and absence of the second wave of aggregation in response to ADP or epinephrine. This pattern is identical to that seen in individuals with congenital storage pool disease. In fact, both ITP and SLE may be associated with an acquired form of storage pool disease manifested by a reduced platelet content of dense and α-granule components.[409,410] In one report, platelets in ITP also exhibited an activation defect manifested by impaired conversion of arachidonic acid to thromboxane A_2.[411]

THERAPY
Antibody-mediated platelet dysfunction and bleeding almost always occur in the setting of immune thrombocytopenia. Therapeutic efforts should be directed to the treatment of these disorders.

CARDIOPULMONARY BYPASS

DEFINITION AND HISTORY
Circulating blood through an extracorporeal bypass circuit during cardiac surgery induces a variety of hemostatic defects. The most significant of these defects are thrombocytopenia, platelet dysfunction, and hyperfibrinolysis.[412-414] At their extreme, these defects can result in substantial postoperative bleeding that may last hours to days after bypass. Approximately 5 percent of patients experience excessive postoperative bleeding after extracorporeal bypass. About half of the bleeding results from surgical causes; much of the remainder results from qualitative platelet defects and hyperfibrinolysis.

ETIOLOGY AND PATHOGENESIS
Thrombocytopenia is a consistent feature of bypass surgery.[134,413] Typically, platelet counts decrease to 50 percent of presurgical levels by 25 minutes after initiation of bypass, but thrombocytopenia can occur within 5 minutes and may persist for as long as several days.[412,414,415] The major factor responsible for thrombocytopenia is hemodilution from priming the pump with colloid or crystalloid solutions, but it often is more profound than can be accounted for by hemodilution alone.[414-416] Platelet adhesion to artificial surfaces in the circuit has been demonstrated by scanning electron micrography.[417] The mechanism of this interaction is uncertain, but it may result from deposition of fibrinogen onto the bypass circuit and platelet adhesion mediated by GpIIb-IIIa.[418] Less common causes of thrombocytopenia during bypass are disseminated intravascular coagulation (DIC), sequestration of damaged platelets in the liver, and heparin-induced thrombocytopenia.[419]

Qualitative platelet defects are the primary nonstructural hemostatic defects induced by the bypass circuit[413,420] and are manifest as prolonged bleeding times, abnormal *ex vivo* platelet aggregation, decreased ristocetin-induced platelet agglutination, deficiency of platelet α- and δ-granules, release of soluble CD40 ligand, and generation of platelet microparticles.[412,414,415,421-424] The severity of these abnormalities correlates with the duration of extracorporeal bypass,[425] and the defects generally resolve within 2 to 24 hours.[413]

Bypass-induced defects in platelet function likely result from platelet activation and fragmentation[423,426] from hypothermia, contact with fibrinogen-coated synthetic surfaces, contact with the blood–air interface, cardiotomy suction, and exposure to traces of thrombin, plasmin, ADP, or complement.[418,427-429] Exposure to thrombin during bypass reportedly reduced subsequent platelet response to the thrombin receptor-activating peptide and was associated with increased postoperative blood loss.[430] Drugs such as heparin, protamine, GpIIb-IIIa antagonists, and aspirin and production of fibrin degradation products also can impair platelet function.[134,431-433] Controversy exists about the significance of these defects *in vivo*. Some investigators have suggested that the entire qualitative platelet defect results from use of heparin during bypass surgery and its inhibitory effect on thrombin activity.[431] However, such heparin use would not account for the bleeding diathesis that can exist hours after reversal of heparin.

Hyperfibrinolysis may contribute to the bleeding diathesis associated with cardiopulmonary bypass.[434,435] This effect likely results from thrombus formation in the pericardial cavity, followed by local and subsequently systemic fibrinolysis.[434] The relevance of hyperfibrinolysis to postbypass bleeding is bolstered by the efficacy of antifibrinolytic therapy in minimizing cardiopulmonary bypass surgery blood loss.

THERAPY
Preoperative evaluation of cardiac surgical candidates should include a history of bleeding in either the patient or family members. Some authors recommend a screening prothrombin time, partial prothrombin time, and bleeding time even in individuals with no history of bleeding,[436] but the validity of this approach is controversial.[437] Regardless, prophylactic transfusion of allogeneic blood components is not indicated.[413,438,439] Studies of the preoperative use of recombinant human Epo in anemic patients or Epo plus autologous blood donation in nonanemic patients suggest that these approaches are reasonable.[440-442] Cells savers now are often used during bypass surgery, and the collected washed autologous red blood cells are reinfused after completion of cardiopulmonary bypass. In addition, blood collected from chest tube drainage has been reinfused to minimize allogeneic transfusions.[443] The safety of transfusing large quantities of blood by this technique is not fully been established.[444]

A number of maneuvers have been attempted to reduce the hemostatic abnormalities associated with cardiac surgery. These techniques include coating the artificial surfaces of cardiopulmonary bypass devices with heparin,[445-449] using centrifugal rather than roller pumps,[450] performing coronary artery surgery without bypass,[451,452] and using a number of pharmacologic agents.[453] Several pharmacologic maneuvers have been attempted to assist in the management of postoperative bleeding. Postoperative patients with a prolonged bleeding time and excessive blood loss may respond to DDAVP, as evidenced by shortening of the bleeding time. However, results of trials with this agent have been contradictory, with some studies showing a reduced blood loss and others showing no benefit.[454,455] Based on the assumption that platelet activation during bypass could be a major cause of postoperative platelet dysfunction, infusion of platelet activation inhibitors such as PGE_1, prostacyclin, or stable prostacyclin analogues has been carried out in animal models and in humans. By increasing platelet cAMP and reducing platelet responsiveness, these agents prevent bypass-induced thrombocytopenia and platelet dysfunction. However, randomized trials using prostacyclin and its analogue iloprost did not show a clear overall benefit, in part because of significant toxicity, including hypotension.[113,116] Recombinant factor

VIIa has been used successfully for treatment of uncontrolled postoperative bleeding.[456,457]

Evidence exists that inhibition of fibrinolysis using aprotinin, ε-aminocaproic acid, and tranexamic acid reduces mediastinal blood loss and transfusion requirements.[453] The effects of aprotinin, a broad-spectrum protease inhibitor, have been well studied. Aprotinin may exert a protective effect on platelets,[458–461] but it does inhibit hyperfibrinolysis, and this may be its sole beneficial activity at low dosages.[460,462] Treatment with aprotinin usually is started preoperatively and continued for the duration of surgery, with reported reductions of blood loss of 50 percent.[15,459] It has been applied topically to the pericardium to inhibit local fibrinolytic activity.[463] Little evidence supports the concern that aprotinin causes a postoperative hypercoagulable state leading to coronary graft occlusion.[464] Its major toxicities include allergic reactions, particularly in patients who received the drug within the past 6 months, and pancreatitis.[465]

The most important determinant of blood loss following cardiopulmonary surgery is the surgical procedure itself. If excessive nonsurgical postoperative bleeding occurs, verify that the patient is no longer hypothermic and that heparin has been fully reversed. At this point, administration of pharmacologic agents and judicious transfusions of platelets, cryoprecipitate, fresh-frozen plasma, and red blood cells are appropriate.

MISCELLANEOUS DISORDERS

Chronic liver disease of various causes reportedly results in a prolonged bleeding time and reduced platelet aggregation and procoagulant activity.[466–468] The prolonged bleeding time in such patients may respond to DDAVP infusion.[469] However, the existence of a platelet function defect specific to liver disease was placed in doubt by a study of 60 patients with cirrhosis in whom aggregation studies and bleeding times were compatible with the degree of thrombocytopenia.[470] The cause of the bleeding diathesis associated with fulminant or end-stage liver disease is multifactorial and includes decreased coagulation factor production, fibrinolysis, dysfibrinogenemia, thrombocytopenia resulting from hypersplenism and thrombopoietin deficiency,[471,472] and occasionally DIC.[468] Thus, the prolonged bleeding time reported in some patients with severe liver disease may result from multiple factors, including thrombocytopenia, hypofibrinogenemia, and anemia, none of which implies an intrinsic defect in platelet function.[473]

Patients with DIC may exhibit reduced platelet aggregation and acquired storage pool deficiency.[474,475] These disorders result from platelet activation in vivo by thrombin or other agonists. Alternatively, elevated levels of fibrin(ogen) degradation products and low fibrinogen levels that accompany DIC may contribute to the platelet defect. Although purified low molecular weight fibrinogen degradation products can impair platelet aggregation, this effect requires concentrations of degradation products unlikely to occur in vivo.[476] Furthermore, hypofibrinogenemia would contribute to a defect in aggregation only in extreme cases because the fibrinogen concentration in normal plasma is at least 15-fold greater than that required to saturate platelet fibrinogen receptors.[477] Finally, assessing the significance of platelet dysfunction in most patients with DIC is difficult because of the simultaneous presence of thrombocytopenia and other hemostatic defects.

A prolonged bleeding time and decreased platelet aggregation and secretion in response to epinephrine or ADP have been reported in patients with Bartter syndrome. The platelet abnormalities have been suggested to result from an inhibitory plasma factor, possibly a prostaglandin.[478] The paradoxical ability of aspirin to correct the prolonged bleeding time supports this contention.

Isolated cases of a slight prolongation of the bleeding time and/or ex vivo platelet function defects in a number of other clinical conditions have been reported. These situations include nonthrombocytopenic purpura with eosinophilia,[479–481] atopic asthma and hay fever,[482] acute respiratory failure,[483] and Wilms tumor elaborating hyaluronic acid.[484] The clinical significance of these associations is not clear.

REFERENCES

1. Rodgers RP, Levin J: A critical reappraisal of the bleeding time. *Semin Thromb Hemost* 16:1, 1990.
2. Lind SE: The bleeding time does not predict surgical bleeding. *Blood* 77:2547, 1991.
3. Carr ME Jr: In vitro assessment of platelet function. *Transfus Med Rev* 11:106, 1997.
4. George J, Shattil S: The clinical importance of acquired abnormalities of platelet function. *N Engl J Med* 324:27, 1991.
5. Wisloff F, Godal H: Prolonged bleeding time with adequate platelet count in hospital patients. *Scand J Haematol* 27:45, 1981.
6. Smith W, Garavito R, DeWitt D: Prostaglandin endoperoxide H synthases (cyclooxygenases)-1 and -2. *J Biol Chem* 271:33157, 1996.
7. Chandrasekharan NV, Dai H, Roos KL, et al: COX-3, a cyclooxygenase-1 variant inhibited by acetaminophen and other analgesic/antipyretic drugs: Cloning, structure, and expression. *Proc Natl Acad Sci U S A* 99: 13926, 2002.
8. Weiss H, Aledort L: Impaired platelet/connective tissue reaction in man after aspirin ingestion. *Lancet* 2:495, 1967.
9. O'Brien JR: Effect of salicylates on human platelets. *Lancet* 1:1431, 1968.
10. Patrono C: Aspirin as an antiplatelet drug. *N Engl J Med* 330:1287, 1994.
11. Kyrle PA, Eichler HG, Jager U, Lechner K: Inhibition of prostacyclin and thromboxane A2 generation by low-dose aspirin at the site of plug formation in man in vivo. *Circulation* 75:1025, 1987.
12. Clarke RJ, Mayo G, Price P, FitzGerald GA: Suppression of thromboxane A2 but not of systemic prostacyclin by controlled-release aspirin. *N Engl J Med* 325:1137, 1991.
13. Jaffe EA, Weksler BB: Recovery of endothelial cell prostacyclin production after inhibition by low doses of aspirin. *J Clin Invest* 63:532, 1979.
14. Marcus AJ, Safier LB: Thromboregulation: Multicellular modulation of platelet reactivity in hemostasis and thrombosis. *FASEB J* 7:516, 1993.
15. Rich JB: The efficacy and safety of aprotinin use in cardiac surgery. *Ann Thorac Surg* 66:S6, 1998.
16. Johnson ES, Lanes SF, Wentworth CE 3rd, et al: A metaregression analysis of the dose-response effect of aspirin on stroke. *Arch Intern Med* 159:1248, 1999.
17. A comparison of two doses of aspirin (30 mg vs 283 mg a day) in patients after a transient ischemic attack or minor ischemic stroke. The Dutch TIA Trial Study Group. *N Engl J Med* 325:1261, 1991.
18. Derry S, Loke YK: Risk of gastrointestinal haemorrhage with long term use of aspirin: Meta-analysis. *BMJ* 321:1183, 2000.
19. Catella-Lawson F, Reilly MP, Kapoor SC, et al: Cyclooxygenase inhibitors and the antiplatelet effects of aspirin. *N Engl J Med* 345:1809, 2001.
20. Kallmann R, Nieuwenhuis HK, Groot PG, et al: Effects of low doses of aspirin 10 mg and 30 mg daily, on bleeding time, thromboxane production and 6-keto-PGF1a excretion in healthy subjects. *Thromb Res* 45: 355, 1987.
21. Nakajima H, Takami H, Yamagata K, et al: Aspirin effects on colonic mucosal bleeding. *Dis Colon Rectum* 40:1484, 1997.
22. Mielke CHJr: Aspirin prolongation of the template bleeding time: Influence of venostasis and direction of incision. *Blood* 60:1139, 1982.
23. Hirsh J, Salzman EW, Harker L, et al: Aspirin and other platelet active drugs. Relationship among dose, effectiveness, and side effects. *Chest* 95:12S, 1989.

24. Final report on the aspirin component of the ongoing physicians' health study. Steering Committee of the Physicians' Health Study Research Group. *N Engl J Med* 321:129, 1989.

25. Page IH: Salicylate damage to the gastric mucosal barrier. *N Engl J Med* 276:1307, 1967.

26. Leonards JR, Levy G: The role of dosage form in aspirin-induced gastrointestinal bleeding. *Clin Pharmacol* 8:400, 1969.

27. Stuart MJ, Gross SJ, Elrad H, Graeber JE: Effects of acetylsalicylic-acid ingestion on maternal and neonatal hemostasis. *N Engl J Med* 307:909, 1982.

28. Ferraris VA, Ferraris SP, Lough FC, Berry WR: Preoperative aspirin ingestion increases operative blood loss after coronary artery bypass grafting. *Ann Thorac Surg* 45:71, 1988.

29. Sethi GK, Copeland JG, Goldman S, et al: Implications of preoperative administration of aspirin in patients undergoing coronary artery bypass grafting. Department of Veterans Affairs Cooperative Study on Antiplatelet Therapy. *J Am Coll Cardiol* 15:15, 1990.

30. Horlocker TT, Wedel DJ, Offord KP: Does preoperative antiplatelet therapy increase the risk of hemorrhagic complications associated with regional anesthesia? *Anesth Analg* 70:631, 1990.

31. Kitchen L, Erichson RB, Sideropoulos H: Effect of drug-induced platelet dysfunction on surgical bleeding. *Am J Surg* 143:215, 1982.

32. Kennedy BM: Aspirin and surgery: A review. *Ir Med J* 77:363, 1984.

33. Livio M, Benigni A, Vigano G, et al: Moderate doses of aspirin and risk of bleeding in renal failure. *Lancet* 1:414, 1986.

34. Gaspari F, Vigano G, Orisio S, et al: Aspirin prolongs bleeding time in uremia by a mechanism distinct from platelet cyclooxygenase inhibition. *J Clin Invest* 79:1788, 1987.

35. Chesebro JH, Fuster V, Elveback LR, et al: Trial of combined warfarin plus dipyridamole or aspirin therapy in prosthetic heart valve replacement: Danger of aspirin compared with dipyridamole. *Am J Cardiol* 51:1537, 1983.

36. Deykin D, Janson P, McMahon L: Ethanol potentiation of aspirin-induced prolongation of the bleeding time. *N Engl J Med* 306:852, 1982.

37. Rosove MH, Hocking WG, Harwig SS, Perloff JK: Studies of beta-thromboglobulin, platelet factor 4, and fibrinopeptide A in erythrocytosis due to cyanotic congenital heart disease. *Thromb Res* 29:225, 1983.

38. Kobrinsky NL, Israels ED, Gerrard JM, et al: Shortening of bleeding time by 1-deamino-8-D-arginine vasopressin in various bleeding disorders. *Lancet* 1:1145, 1984.

39. Lethagen S, Rugarn P: The effect of DDAVP and placebo on platelet function and prolonged bleeding time induced by oral acetyl salicylic acid intake in healthy volunteers. *Thromb Haemost* 67:185, 1992.

40. Simon LS, Mills JA: Drug therapy: Nonsteroidal antiinflammatory drugs (first of two parts). *N Engl J Med* 302:1179, 1980.

41. McQueen EG, Facoory B, Faed JM: Non-steroidal anti-inflammatory drugs and platelet function. *N Z Med J* 99:358, 1986.

42. Buchanan GR, Martin V, Levine PH, et al: The effects of "anti-platelet" drugs on bleeding time and platelet aggregation in normal human subjects. *Am J Clin Pathol* 68:355, 1977.

43. Nadell J, Bruno J, Varady J, Segre EJ: Effect of naproxen and of aspirin on bleeding time and platelet aggregation. *J Clin Pharmacol* 14:176, 1974.

44. Mielke CH Jr, Kahn SB, Muschek LD, et al: Effects of zomepirac on hemostasis in healthy adults and on platelet function in vitro. *J Clin Pharmacol* 20:409, 1980.

45. Thomas P, Hepburn B, Kim HC, Saidi P: Nonsteroidal anti-inflammatory drugs in the treatment of hemophilic arthropathy. *Am J Hematol* 12:131, 1982.

46. McIntyre BA, Philp RB, Inwood MJ: Effect of ibuprofen on platelet function in normal subjects and hemophiliac patients. *Clin Pharmacol Ther* 24:616, 1978.

47. Ragni MV, Miller BJ, Whalen R, Ptachcinski R: Bleeding tendency,

48. Kasper CK, Rapaport SI: Bleeding times and platelet aggregation after analgesics in hemophilia. *Ann Intern Med* 77:189, 1972.

49. Mielke CH Jr: Comparative effects of aspirin and acetaminophen on hemostasis. *Arch Intern Med* 141:305, 1981.

50. FitzGerald GA: Cardiovascular pharmacology of nonselective nonsteroidal anti-inflammatory drugs and coxibs: Clinical considerations. *Am J Cardiol* 89:26D 2002.

51. Bombardier C, Laine L, Reicin A, et al: Comparison of upper gastrointestinal toxicity of rofecoxib and naproxen in patients with rheumatoid arthritis. VIGOR Study Group. *N Engl J Med* 343:1520, 2000.

52. Ray WA, Stein CM, Daugherty JR, et al: COX-2 selective non-steroidal anti-inflammatory drugs and risk of serious coronary heart disease. *Lancet* 360:1071, 2002.

53. Fitzgerald GA: Coxibs and cardiovascular disease. *N Engl J Med* 351:1709, 2004.

54. A randomized, blinded, trial of clopidogrel versus aspirin in patients at risk of ischaemic events (CAPRIE). CAPRIE Steering Committee. *Lancet* 348:1329, 1996.

55. Rupprecht HJ, Darius H, Borkowski U, et al: Comparison of antiplatelet effects of aspirin, ticlopidine, or their combination after stent implantation. *Circulation* 97:1046, 1998.

56. Leon MB, Baim DS, Popma JJ, et al: A clinical trial comparing three antithrombotic-drug regimens after coronary-artery stenting. Stent Anticoagulation Restenosis Study Investigators. *N Engl J Med* 339:1665, 1998.

57. Sharis PJ, Cannon CP, Loscalzo J: The antiplatelet effects of ticlopidine and clopidogrel. *Ann Intern Med* 129:394, 1998.

58. Schomig A, Neumann FJ, Kastrati A, et al: A randomized comparison of antiplatelet and anticoagulant therapy after the placement of coronary-artery stents. *N Engl J Med* 334:1084, 1996.

59. Yusuf S, Zhao F, Mehta SR, et al: Effects of clopidogrel in addition to aspirin in patients with acute coronary syndromes without ST-segment elevation. *N Engl J Med* 345:494, 2001.

60. Bhatt DL, Chew DP, Hirsch AT, et al: Superiority of clopidogrel versus aspirin in patients with prior cardiac surgery. *Circulation* 103:363, 2001.

61. Bossavy JP, Thalamas C, Sagnard L, et al: A double-blind randomized comparison of combined aspirin and ticlopidine therapy versus aspirin or ticlopidine alone on experimental arterial thrombogenesis in humans. *Blood* 92:1518, 1998.

62. Steinhubl SR, Berger PB, Mann JT 3rd, et al: Early and sustained dual oral antiplatelet therapy following percutaneous coronary intervention: A randomized controlled trial. *JAMA* 288:2411, 2002.

63. Diener HC, Bogousslavsky J, Brass LM, et al: Aspirin and clopidogrel compared with clopidogrel alone after recent ischaemic stroke or transient ischaemic attack in high-risk patients (MATCH): Randomized, double-blind, placebo-controlled trial. *Lancet* 364:331, 2004.

64. Rothwell PM: Lessons from MATCH for future randomized trials in secondary prevention of stroke. *Lancet* 364:305, 2004.

65. McTavish D, Faulds D, Goa KL: Ticlopidine. An updated review of its pharmacology and therapeutic use in platelet-dependent disorders. *Drugs* 40:238, 1990.

66. Hardisty RM, Powling MJ, Nokes TJ: The action of ticlopidine on human platelets. Studies on aggregation, secretion, calcium mobilization and membrane glycoproteins. *Thromb Haemost* 64:150, 1990.

67. Humbert M, Nurden P, Bihour C, et al: Ultrastructural studies of platelet aggregates from human subjects receiving clopidogrel and from a patient with an inherited defect of an ADP-dependent pathway of platelet activation. *Arterioscler Thromb Vasc Biol* 16:1532, 1996.

68. Hechler B, Eckly A, Ohlmann P, et al: The P2Y1 receptor, necessary but not sufficient to support full ADP-induced platelet aggregation, is not the target of the drug clopidogrel. *Br J Haematol* 103:858, 1998.

platelet function, and pharmacokinetics of ibuprofen and zidovudine in HIV(+) hemophilic men. *Am J Hematol* 40:176, 1992.

69. Geiger J, Honig-Liedl P, Schanzenbacher P, Walter U: Ligand specificity and ticlopidine effects distinguish three human platelet ADP receptors. *Eur J Pharmacol* 351:235, 1998.

70. Geiger J, Brich J, Honig-Liedl P, et al: Specific impairment of human platelet P2Y(AC) ADP receptor-mediated signaling by the antiplatelet drug clopidogrel. *Arterioscler Thromb Vasc Biol* 19:2007, 1999.

71. Savi P, Laplace MC, Maffrand JP, Herbert JM: Binding of [3H]-2-methylthio ADP to rat platelets: Effect of clopidogrel and ticlopidine. *J Pharmacol Exp Ther* 269:772, 1994.

72. Daniel JL, Dangelmaier C, Jin J, et al: Molecular basis for ADP-induced platelet activation: I. Evidence for three distinct ADP receptors on human platelets. *J Biol Chem* 273:2024, 1998.

73. Jantzen HM, Gousset L, Bhaskar V, et al: Evidence for two distinct G-protein-coupled ADP receptors mediating platelet activation. *Thromb Haemost* 81:111, 1999.

74. De Caterina R, Sicari R, Bernini W, et al: Benefit/risk profile of combined antiplatelet therapy with ticlopidine and aspirin. *Thromb Haemost* 65:504, 1991.

75. Helft G, Osende JI, Worthley SG, et al: Acute antithrombotic effect of a front-loaded regimen of clopidogrel in patients with atherosclerosis on aspirin. *Arterioscler Thromb Vasc Biol* 20:2316, 2000.

76. Hass WK, Easton JD, Adams HP Jr, et al: A randomized trial comparing ticlopidine hydrochloride with aspirin for the prevention of stroke in high-risk patients. Ticlopidine Aspirin Stroke Study Group. *N Engl J Med* 321:501, 1989.

77. Gent M, Blakely JA, Easton JD, et al: The Canadian American Ticlopidine Study (CATS) in thromboembolic stroke. *Lancet* 1:1215, 1989.

78. Mataix R, Ojeda E, Perez MC, Jimenez S: Ticlopidine and severe aplastic anaemia. *Br J Haematol* 80:125, 1992.

79. Garnier G, Taillan B, Pesce A, et al: Ticlopidine and severe aplastic anaemia. *Br J Haematol* 81:459, 1992.

80. Bennett CL, Weinberg PD, Rozenberg-Ben-Dror K, et al: Thrombotic thrombocytopenic purpura associated with ticlopidine. A review of 60 cases. *Ann Intern Med* 128:541, 1998.

81. Steinhubl SR, Tan WA, Foody JM, Topol EJ: Incidence and clinical course of thrombotic thrombocytopenic purpura due to ticlopidine following coronary stenting. EPISTENT Investigators. Evaluation of Platelet IIb/IIIa Inhibitor for Stenting. *JAMA* 281:806, 1999.

82. Chen DK, Kim JS, Sutton DM: Thrombotic thrombocytopenic purpura associated with ticlopidine use: A report of 3 cases and review of the literature. *Arch Intern Med* 159:311, 1999.

83. Bennett CL, Connors JM, Carwile JM, et al: Thrombotic thrombocytopenic purpura associated with clopidogrel. *N Engl J Med* 342:1773, 2000.

84. Lefkovits J, Plow EF, Topol EJ: Platelet glycoprotein IIb/IIIa receptors in cardiovascular medicine. *N Engl J Med* 332:1553, 1995.

85. Nurden AT, Poujol C, Durrieu-Jais C, Nurden P: Platelet glycoprotein IIb/IIIa inhibitors: Basic and clinical aspects. *Arterioscler Thromb Vasc Biol* 19:2835, 1999.

86. Bennett JS, Mousa S: Platelet function inhibitors in the Year 2000. *Thromb Haemost* 85:395, 2001.

87. French DL, Seligsohn U: Platelet glycoprotein IIb/IIIa receptors and Glanzmann's thrombasthenia. *Arterioscler Thromb Vasc Biol* 20:607, 2000.

88. Nurden AT: Inherited abnormalities of platelets. *Thromb Haemost* 82:468, 1999.

89. Use of a monoclonal antibody directed against the platelet glycoprotein IIb/IIIa receptor in high-risk coronary angioplasty. The EPIC Investigation. *N Engl J Med* 330:956, 1994.

90. Platelet glycoprotein IIb/IIIa receptor blockade and low-dose heparin during percutaneous coronary revascularization. The EPILOG Investigators. *N Engl J Med* 336:1689, 1997.

91. Inhibition of the platelet glycoprotein IIb/IIIa receptor with tirofiban in

unstable angina and non-Q-wave myocardial infarction. Platelet Receptor Inhibition in Ischemic Syndrome Management in Patients Limited by Unstable Signs and Symptoms (PRISM-PLUS) Study Investigators. *N Engl J Med* 338:1488, 1998.

92. Inhibition of platelet glycoprotein IIb/IIIa with eptifibatide in patients with acute coronary syndromes. The PURSUIT Trial Investigators. Platelet Glycoprotein IIb/IIIa in Unstable Angina: Receptor Suppression Using Integrilin Therapy. *N Engl J Med* 339:436, 1998.

93. Simpfendorfer C, Kottke-Marchant K, Lowrie M, et al: First chronic platelet glycoprotein IIb/IIIa integrin blockade. A randomized, placebo-controlled pilot study of xemilofiban in unstable angina with percutaneous coronary interventions. *Circulation* 96:76, 1997.

94. Cannon CP, McCabe CH, Borzak S, et al: Randomized trial of an oral platelet glycoprotein IIb/IIIa antagonist, sibrafiban, in patients after an acute coronary syndrome: Results of the TIMI 12 trial. Thrombolysis in Myocardial Infarction. *Circulation* 97:340, 1998.

95. Ferguson JJ, Kereiakes DJ, Adgey AA, et al: Safe use of platelet GP IIb/IIIa inhibitors. *Eur Heart J* 19(suppl D):D40, 1998.

96. Berkowitz SD, Sane DC, Sigmon KN, et al: Occurrence and clinical significance of thrombocytopenia in a population undergoing high-risk percutaneous coronary revascularization. Evaluation of c7E3 for the Prevention of Ischemic Complications (EPIC) Study Group. *J Am Coll Cardiol* 32:311, 1998.

97. Randomized placebo-controlled trial of abciximab before and during coronary intervention in refractory unstable angina: The CAPTURE Study. *Lancet* 349:1429, 1997.

98. Jubelirer SJ, Koenig BA, Bates MC: Acute profound thrombocytopenia following C7E3 Fab (Abciximab) therapy: Case reports, review of the literature and implications for therapy. *Am J Hematol* 61:205, 1999.

99. Giugliano RP, McCabe CH, Sequeira RF, et al: First report of an intravenous and oral glycoprotein IIb/IIIa inhibitor (RPR 109891) in patients with recent acute coronary syndromes: Results of the TIMI 15A and 15B trials. *Am Heart J* 140:81, 2000.

100. Comparison of sibrafiban with aspirin for prevention of cardiovascular events after acute coronary syndromes: A randomized trial. The SYMPHONY Investigators. Sibrafiban versus Aspirin to Yield Maximum Protection from Ischemic Heart Events Post-acute Coronary Syndromes. *Lancet* 355:337, 2000.

101. Hongo RH, Brent BN: Association of eptifibatide and acute profound thrombocytopenia. *Am J Cardiol* 88:428, 2001.

102. McClure MW, Berkowitz SD, Sparapani R, et al: Clinical significance of thrombocytopenia during a non-ST-elevation acute coronary syndrome. The platelet glycoprotein IIb/IIIa in unstable angina: Receptor suppression using Integrilin therapy (PURSUIT) trial experience. *Circulation* 99:2892, 1999.

103. Abrams CS, Cines DB: Platelet glycoprotein IIb/IIIa inhibitors and thrombocytopenia: Possible link between platelet activation, autoimmunity and thrombosis. *Thromb Haemost* 88:888, 2002.

104. Brassard JA, Curtis BR, Cooper RA, et al: Acute thrombocytopenia in patients treated with the oral glycoprotein IIb/IIIa inhibitors xemilofiban and orbofiban: Evidence for an immune etiology. *Thromb Haemost* 88:892, 2002.

105. Christopoulos CG, Machin SJ: A new type of pseudothrombocytopenia: EDTA-mediated agglutination of platelets bearing Fab fragments of a chimaeric antibody. *Br J Haematol* 87:650, 1994.

106. Sane DC, Damaraju LV, Topol EJ, et al: Occurrence and clinical significance of pseudothrombocytopenia during abciximab therapy. *J Am Coll Cardiol* 36:75, 2000.

107. Ivy DD, Kinsella JP, Ziegler JW, Abman SH: Dipyridamole attenuates rebound pulmonary hypertension after inhaled nitric oxide withdrawal in postoperative congenital heart disease. *J Thorac Cardiovasc Surg* 115:875, 1998.

108. Gresele P, Arnout J, Deckmyn H, Vermylen J: Mechanism of the anti-

platelet action of dipyridamole in whole blood: Modulation of adenosine concentration and activity. *Thromb Haemost* 55:12, 1986.

109. FitzGerald GA: Dipyridamole. *N Engl J Med* 316:1247, 1987.

110. Collaborative meta-analysis of randomized trials of antiplatelet therapy for prevention of death, myocardial infarction, and stroke in high risk patients. *Br J Med* 324:71, 2002.

111. Reilly M, FitzGerald GA: Gathering intelligence on antiplatelet drugs: The view from 30,000 feet. When combined with other information overviews lead to conviction. *BMJ* 324:59, 2002.

112. Diener HC, Cunha L, Forbes C, et al: European Stroke Prevention Study 2. Dipyridamole and acetylsalicylic acid in the secondary prevention of stroke. *J Neurol Sci* 143:1, 1996.

113. Walker ID, Davidson JF, Faichney A, et al: A double-blind study of prostacyclin in cardiopulmonary bypass surgery. *Br J Haematol* 49:415, 1981.

114. Huddleston CB, Wareing TH, Clanton JA, Bender HW Jr: Amelioration of the deleterious effects of platelets activated during cardiopulmonary bypass: Comparison of a thromboxane synthetase inhibitor and a prostacyclin analogue. *J Thorac Cardiovasc Surg* 89:190, 1985.

115. Fisher CA, Kappa JR, Sinha AK, et al: Comparison of equimolar concentrations of iloprost, prostacyclin, and prostaglandin E1 on human platelet function. *J Lab Clin Med* 109:184, 1987.

116. Fish KJ, Sarnquist FH, van Steennis C, et al: A prospective, randomized study of the effects of prostacyclin on platelets and blood loss during coronary bypass operations. *J Thorac Cardiovasc Surg* 91:436, 1986.

117. Sorkin EM, Markham A: Cilostazol. *Drugs Aging* 14:63, 1999.

118. Yoshitomi Y, Kojima S, Sugi T, et al: Antiplatelet treatment with cilostazol after stent implantation. *Heart* 80:393, 1998.

119. Loscalzo J, Welch G: Nitric oxide and its role in the cardiovascular system. *Prog Cardiovasc Dis* 38:87, 1995.

120. Sattler FR, Weitekamp MR, Ballard JO: Potential for bleeding with the new beta-lactam antibiotics. *Ann Intern Med* 105:924, 1986.

121. Pillgram-Larsen J, Wisloff F, Jorgensen JJ, et al: Effect of high-dose ampicillin and cloxacillin on bleeding time and bleeding in open-heart surgery. *Scand J Thorac Cardiovasc Surg* 19:45, 1985.

122. Fass RJ, Copelan EA, Brandt JT, et al: Platelet-mediated bleeding caused by broad-spectrum penicillins. *J Infect Dis* 155:1242, 1987.

123. Cazenave JP, Packham MA, Guccione MA, Mustard JF: Effects of penicillin G on platelet aggregation, release, and adherence to collagen. *Proc Soc Exp Biol Med* 142:159, 1973.

124. Shattil SJ, Bennett JS, McDonough M, Turnbull J: Carbenicillin and penicillin G inhibit platelet function in vitro by impairing the interaction of agonists with the platelet surface. *J Clin Invest* 65:329, 1980.

125. Fletcher C, Pearson C, Choi SC, et al: In vitro comparison of antiplatelet effects of beta-lactam penicillins. *J Lab Clin Med* 108:217, 1986.

126. Packham MA, Rand ML, Perry DW, et al: Probenecid inhibits platelet responses to aggregating agents in vitro and has a synergistic inhibitory effect with penicillin G. *Thromb Haemost* 76:239, 1996.

127. Burroughs SF, Johnson GJ: Beta-lactam antibiotic-induced platelet dysfunction: Evidence for irreversible inhibition of platelet activation in vitro and in vivo after prolonged exposure to penicillin. *Blood* 75:1473, 1990.

128. Sattler FR, Weitekamp MR, Sayegh A, Ballard JO: Impaired hemostasis caused by beta-lactam antibiotics. *Am J Surg* 155:30, 1988.

129. Giles AR, Greenwood P, Tinlin S: A platelet release defect induced by aspirin or penicillin G does not increase gastrointestinal blood loss in thrombocytopenic rabbits. *Br J Haematol* 57:17, 1984.

130. Andrassy K, Koderisch J, Trenk D, et al: Hemostasis in patients with normal and impaired renal function under treatment with cefodizime. *Infection* 15:348, 1987.

131. Brown RB, Klar J, Lemeshow S, et al: Enhanced bleeding with cefoxitin or moxalactam. Statistical analysis within a defined population of 1,493 patients. *Arch Intern Med* 146:2159, 1986.

132. Rossi EC, Levin NW: Inhibition of primary ADP-induced platelet aggregation in normal subjects after administration of nitrofurantoin (Furadantin). *J Clin Invest* 52:2457, 1973.

133. Ishikawa S, Manabe S, Wada O: Miconazole inhibition of platelet aggregation by inhibiting cyclooxygenase. *Biochem Pharmacol* 35:1787, 1986.

134. Khuri SF, Valeri CR, Loscalzo J, et al: Heparin causes platelet dysfunction and induces fibrinolysis before cardiopulmonary bypass. *Ann Thorac Surg* 60:1008, 1995.

135. Salzman EW, Rosenberg RD, Smith MH, et al: Effect of heparin and heparin fractions on platelet aggregation. *J Clin Invest* 65:64, 1980.

136. Horne MK 3rd, Chao ES: Heparin binding to resting and activated platelets. *Blood* 74:238, 1989.

137. Sobel M, McNeill PM, Carlson PL, et al: Heparin inhibition of von Willebrand factor-dependent platelet function in vitro and in vivo. *J Clin Invest* 87:1787, 1991.

138. Coller BS: Platelets and thrombolytic therapy. *N Engl J Med* 322:33, 1990.

139. Niewiarowski S, Senyi AF, Gillies P: Plasmin-induced platelet aggregation and platelet release reaction. Effects on hemostasis. *J Clin Invest* 52:1647, 1973.

140. Fitzgerald DJ, Catella F, Roy L, FitzGerald GA: Marked platelet activation in vivo after intravenous streptokinase in patients with acute myocardial infarction. *Circulation* 77:142, 1988.

141. Kerins DM, Roy L, FitzGerald GA, Fitzgerald DJ: Platelet and vascular function during coronary thrombolysis with tissue-type plasminogen activator. *Circulation* 80:1718, 1989.

142. Thorsen LI, Brosstad F, Gogstad G, et al: Competitions between fibrinogen with its degradation products for interactions with the platelet-fibrinogen receptor. *Thromb Res* 44:611, 1986.

143. Miles LA, Ginsberg MH, White JG, Plow EF: Plasminogen interacts with human platelets through two distinct mechanisms. *J Clin Invest* 77:2001, 1986.

144. Adelman B, Michelson AD, Loscalzo J, et al: Plasmin effect on platelet glycoprotein Ib-von Willebrand factor interactions. *Blood* 65:32, 1985.

145. Stricker RB, Wong D, Shiu DT, et al: Activation of plasminogen by tissue plasminogen activator on normal and thrombasthenic platelets: Effects on surface proteins and platelet aggregation. *Blood* 68:275, 1986.

146. Schafer AI, Adelman B: Plasmin inhibition of platelet function and of arachidonic acid metabolism. *J Clin Invest* 75:456, 1985.

147. Loscalzo J, Vaughan DE: Tissue plasminogen activator promotes platelet disaggregation in plasma. *J Clin Invest* 79:1749, 1987.

148. Penny WF, Ware JA: Platelet activation and subsequent inhibition by plasmin and recombinant tissue-type plasminogen activator. *Blood* 79:91, 1992.

149. Winters KJ, Eisenberg PR, Jaffe AS, Santoro SA: Dependence of plasmin-mediated degradation of platelet adhesive receptors on temperature and Ca2+. *Blood* 76:1546, 1990.

150. Green D, Ts'ao CH, Cerullo L, et al: Clinical and laboratory investigation of the effects of epsilon-aminocaproic acid on hemostasis. *J Lab Clin Med* 105:321, 1985.

151. Hines R, Barash PG: Infusion of sodium nitroprusside induces platelet dysfunction in vitro. *Anesthesiology* 70:611, 1989.

152. Kroll MH, Schafer AI: Biochemical mechanisms of platelet activation. *Blood* 74:1181, 1989.

153. Anfossi G, Russo I, Massucco P, et al: Studies on inhibition of human platelet function by sodium nitroprusside. Kinetic evaluation of the effect on aggregation and cyclic nucleotide content. *Thromb Res* 102:319, 2001.

154. Bozzo J, Hernandez MR, Galan AM, et al: Antiplatelet effects of sodium nitroprusside in flowing human blood: Studies under normoxic and hypoxic conditions. *Thromb Res* 97:217, 2000.

155. Jang EK, Azzam JE, Dickinson NT, et al: Roles for both cyclic GMP

and cyclic AMP in the inhibition of collagen-induced platelet aggregation by nitroprusside. *Br J Haematol* 117:664, 2002.

156. Schafer AI, Alexander RW, Handin RI: Inhibition of platelet function by organic nitrate vasodilators. *Blood* 55:649, 1980.

157. Weksler BB, Gillick M, Pink J: Effect of propranolol on platelet function. *Blood* 49:185, 1977.

158. Leon R, Tiarks CY, Pechet L: Some observations on the in vivo effect of propranolol on platelet aggregation and release. *Am J Hematol* 5:117, 1978.

159. Hines R: Preservation of platelet function during trimethaphan infusion. *Anesthesiology* 72:834, 1990.

160. Hogman M, Frostell C, Arnberg H, Hedenstierna G: Bleeding time prolongation and NO inhalation. *Lancet* 341:1664, 1993.

161. Samama CM, Diaby M, Fellahi JL, et al: Inhibition of platelet aggregation by inhaled nitric oxide in patients with acute respiratory distress syndrome. *Anesthesiology* 83:56, 1995.

162. Gries A, Bode C, Peter K, et al: Inhaled nitric oxide inhibits human platelet aggregation, P-selectin expression, and fibrinogen binding in vitro and in vivo. *Circulation* 97:1481, 1998.

163. Ring ME, Corrigan JJ Jr, Fenster PE: Effects of oral diltiazem on platelet function: Alone and in combination with "low dose" aspirin. *Thromb Res* 44:391, 1986.

164. Barnathan ES, Addonizio VP, Shattil SJ: Interaction of verapamil with human platelet alpha-adrenergic receptors. *Am J Physiol* 242:H19, 1982.

165. Fujinishi A, Takahara K, Ohba C, et al: Effects of nisoldipine on cytosolic calcium, platelet aggregation, and coagulation/fibrinolysis in patients with coronary artery disease. *Angiology* 48:515, 1997.

166. Lawson D, Mehta J, Mehta P, et al: Cumulative effects of quinidine and aspirin on bleeding time and platelet α_2-adrenoceptors: Potential mechanism of bleeding diathesis in patients receiving this combination. *J Lab Clin Med* 108:581, 1986.

167. Weiss HJ: The effect of clinical dextran on platelet aggregation, adhesion, and ADP release in man: In vivo and in vitro studies. *J Lab Clin Med* 69:37, 1967.

168. Aberg M, Hedner U, Bergentz SE: Effect of dextran 70 on factor VIII and platelet function in von Willebrand's disease. *Thromb Res* 12:629, 1978.

169. Mishler JMT: Synthetic plasma volume expanders: Their pharmacology, safety, and clinical efficacy. *Clin Haematol* 13:75, 1984.

170. Kelton JG, Hirsh J: Bleeding associated with antithrombotic therapy. *Semin Hematol* 17:259, 1980.

171. Korttila K, Lauritsalo K, Sarmo A, et al: Suitability of plasma expanders in patients receiving low-dose heparin for prevention of venous thrombosis after surgery. *Acta Anaesthesiol Scand* 27:104, 1983.

172. Cope JT, Banks D, Mauney MC, et al: Intraoperative hetastarch infusion impairs hemostasis after cardiac operations. *Ann Thorac Surg* 63:78, 1997.

173. Ruttmann TG, James MF, Aronson I: In vivo investigation into the effects of haemodilution with hydroxyethyl starch (200/0.5) and normal saline on coagulation. *Br J Anaesth* 80:612, 1998.

174. Roberts JS, Bratton SL: Colloid volume expanders. Problems, pitfalls, and possibilities. *Drugs* 55:621, 1998.

175. Avorn J, Patel M, Levin R, Winkelmayer WC: Hetastarch and bleeding complications after coronary artery surgery. *Chest* 124:1437, 2003.

176. Treib J, Haass A, Pindur G: Coagulation disorders caused by hydroxyethyl starch. *Thromb Haemost* 78:974, 1997.

177. Scharbert G, Deusch E, Kress HG, et al: Inhibition of platelet function by hydroxyethyl starch solutions in chronic pain patients undergoing peridural anesthesia. *Anesth Analg* 99:823, 2004.

178. Svehla C, Spankova H, Mlejnkova M: The effect of tricyclic antidepressive drugs on adrenaline and adenosine diphosphate induced platelet aggregation. *J Pharm Pharmacol* 18:616, 1966.

179. Warlow C, Ogston D, Douglas AS: Platelet function after the administration of chlorpromazine to human subjects. *Haemostasis* 5:21, 1976.

180. Morishita S, Aoki S, Watanabe S: Different effect of desipramine on protein kinase C in platelets between bipolar and major depressive disorders. *Psychiatry Clin Neurosci* 53:11, 1999.

181. Hergovich N, Aigner M, Eichler HG, et al: Paroxetine decreases platelet serotonin storage and platelet function in human beings. *Clin Pharmacol Ther* 68:435, 2000.

182. Alderman CP, Seshadri P, Ben-Tovim DI: Effects of serotonin reuptake inhibitors on hemostasis. *Ann Pharmacother* 30:1232, 1996.

183. Pai VB, Kelly MW: Bruising associated with the use of fluoxetine. *Ann Pharmacother* 30:786, 1996.

184. Corbin F, Blaise G, Sauve R: Differential effect of halothane and forskolin on platelet cytosolic Ca2+ mobilization and aggregation. *Anesthesiology* 89:401, 1998.

185. Aoki H, Mizobe T, Nozuchi S, Hiramatsu N: In vivo and in vitro studies of the inhibitory effect of propofol on human platelet aggregation. *Anesthesiology* 88:362, 1998.

186. Heesch CM, Negus BH, Steiner M, et al: Effects of in vivo cocaine administration on human platelet aggregation. *Am J Cardiol* 78:237, 1996.

187. Jennings LK, White MM, Sauer CM, et al: Cocaine-induced platelet defects. *Stroke* 24:1352, 1993.

188. Togna G, Graziani M, Sorrentino C, Caprino L: Prostanoid production in the presence of platelet activation in hypoxic cocaine-treated rats. *Haemostasis* 26:311, 1996.

189. Batista A, Macedo T, Tavares P, et al: Nitric oxide production and nitric oxide synthase expression in platelets from heroin abusers before and after ultrarapid detoxification. *Ann N Y Acad Sci* 965:479, 2002.

190. Ahr DJ, Scialla SJ, Kimbali DB Jr: Acquired platelet dysfunction following mithramycin therapy. *Cancer* 41:448, 1978.

191. Panella TJ, Peters W, White JG, et al: Platelets acquire a secretion defect after high-dose chemotherapy. *Cancer* 65:1711, 1990.

192. Pogliani EM, Fantasia R, Lambertenghi-Deliliers G, Cofrancesco E: Daunorubicin and platelet function. *Thromb Haemost* 45:38, 1981.

193. McKenna R, Ahmad T, Ts'ao CH, Frischer H: Glutathione reductase deficiency and platelet dysfunction induced by 1,3-bis(2-chloroethyl)-1-nitrosourea. *J Lab Clin Med* 102:102, 1983.

194. Karolak L, Chandra A, Khan W, et al: High-dose chemotherapy-induced platelet defect: Inhibition of platelet signal transduction pathways. *Mol Pharmacol* 43:37, 1993.

195. O'Malley CJ, Rasko JE, Basser RL, et al: Administration of pegylated recombinant human megakaryocyte growth and development factor to humans stimulates the production of functional platelets that show no evidence of in vivo activation. *Blood* 88:3288, 1996.

196. Vadhan-Raj S, Murray LJ, Bueso-Ramos C, et al: Stimulation of megakaryocyte and platelet production by a single dose of recombinant human thrombopoietin in patients with cancer. *Ann Intern Med* 126:673, 1997.

197. Vanrenterghem Y, Roels L, Lerut T, et al: Thromboembolic complications and haemostatic changes in cyclosporin-treated cadaveric kidney allograft recipients. *Lancet* 1:999, 1985.

198. Cohen H, Neild GH, Patel R, et al: Evidence for chronic platelet hyperaggregability and in vivo activation in cyclosporin-treated renal allograft recipients. *Thromb Res* 49:91, 1988.

199. Grace AA, Barradas MA, Mikhailidis DP, et al: Cyclosporine A enhances platelet aggregation. *Kidney Int* 32:889, 1987.

200. Thomson C, Forbes CD, Prentice CR: A comparison of the effects of antihistamines on platelet function. *Thromb Diath Haemorrh* 30:547, 1973.

201. Platelet function during long-term treatment with ketanserin of claudicating patients with peripheral atherosclerosis. A multi-center, double-blind, placebo-controlled trial. The PACK Trial Group. *Thromb Res* 55:13, 1989.

202. Parvez Z, Moncada R, Fareed J, Messmore HL: Antiplatelet action of intravascular contrast media. Implications in diagnostic procedures. *Invest Radiol* 19:208, 1984.

203. Rao AK, Rao VM, Willis J, et al: Inhibition of platelet function by contrast media: Iopamidol and ioxaglate versus iothalamate. Work in progress. *Radiology* 156:311, 1985.

204. Goodnight SH Jr, Harris WS, Connor WE: The effects of dietary omega 3 fatty acids on platelet composition and function in man: A prospective, controlled study. *Blood* 58:880, 1981.

205. Moncada S, Higgs EA: Arachidonate metabolism in blood cells and the vessel wall. *Clin Haematol* 15:273, 1986.

206. Leaf A, Weber PC: Cardiovascular effects of n-3 fatty acids. *N Engl J Med* 318:549, 1988.

207. Hammerschmidt DE: Szechwan purpura. *N Engl J Med* 302:1191, 1980.

208. Srivastava KC: Onion exerts antiaggregatory effects by altering arachidonic acid metabolism in platelets. *Prostaglandins Leukot Med* 24:43, 1986.

209. Apitz-Castro R, Ledezma E, Escalante J, Jain MK: The molecular basis of the antiplatelet action of ajoene: Direct interaction with the fibrinogen receptor. *Biochem Biophys Res Commun* 141:145, 1986.

210. Apitz-Castro R, Escalante J, Vargas R, Jain MK: Ajoene, the antiplatelet principle of garlic, synergistically potentiates the antiaggregatory action of prostacyclin, forskolin, indomethacin and dipyridamole on human platelets. *Thromb Res* 42:303, 1986.

211. Srivastava KC: Extracts from two frequently consumed spices—cumin (Cuminum cymium) and turmeric (Curcuma longa)—inhibit platelet aggregation and alter eicosanoid biosynthesis in human blood platelets. *Prostaglandins Leukot Essent Fatty Acids* 37:57, 1989.

212. Landolfi R: Bleeding and thrombosis in myeloproliferative disorders. *Curr Opin Hematol* 5:327, 1998.

213. Schafer AI: Thrombocytosis and thrombocythemia. *Blood Rev* 15:159, 2001.

214. Pearson TC: The risk of thrombosis in essential thrombocythemia and polycythemia vera. *Semin Oncol* 29:16, 2002.

215. Kessler CM: Propensity for hemorrhage and thrombosis in chronic myeloproliferative disorders. *Semin Hematol* 41:10, 2004.

216. Schafer AI: Thrombocytosis. *N Engl J Med* 350:1211, 2004.

217. Wasserman LR, Gilbert HS: The treatment of polycythemia vera. *Med Clin North Am* 50:1501, 1966.

218. Murphy S: Polycythemia vera. *Dis Mon* 38:153, 1992.

219. Elliott MA, Tefferi A: Pathogenesis and management of bleeding in essential thrombocythemia and polycythemia vera. *Curr Hematol Rep* 3:344, 2004.

220. Kessler CM, Klein HG, Havlik RJ: Uncontrolled thrombocytosis in chronic myeloproliferative disorders. *Br J Haematol* 50:157, 1982.

221. Bellucci S, Janvier M, Tobelem G, et al: Essential thrombocythemias. Clinical evolutionary and biological data. *Cancer* 58:2440, 1986.

222. Lahuerta-Palacios JJ, Bornstein R, Fernandez-Debora FJ, et al: Controlled and uncontrolled thrombocytosis. Its clinical role in essential thrombocythemia. *Cancer* 61:1207, 1988.

223. Mitus AJ, Barbui T, Shulman LN, et al: Hemostatic complications in young patients with essential thrombocythemia. *Am J Med* 88:371, 1990.

224. McIntyre KJ, Hoagland HC, Silverstein MN, Petitt RM: Essential thrombocythemia in young adults. *Mayo Clin Proc* 66:149, 1991.

225. Villmow T, Kemkes-Matthes B, Matzdorff AC: Markers of platelet activation and platelet-leukocyte interaction in patients with myeloproliferative syndromes. *Thromb Res* 108:139, 2002.

226. Maldonado JE, Pintado T, Pierre RV: Dysplastic platelets and circulating megakaryocytes in chronic myeloproliferative diseases: I. The platelets: Ultrastructure and peroxidase reaction. *Blood* 43:797, 1974.

227. Bautista AP, Buckler PW, Towler HM, et al: Measurement of platelet life-span in normal subjects and patients with myeloproliferative disease with indium oxine labeled platelets. *Br J Haematol* 58:679, 1984.

228. Schafer AI: Essential thrombocythemia. *Prog Hemost Thromb* 10:69, 1990.

229. Ginsberg AD: Platelet function in patients with high platelet counts. *Ann Intern Med* 82, 1975.

230. Jubelirer SJ, Russel F, Vaillancourt R, Deykin D: Platelet arachidonic acid metabolism and platelet function in ten patients with chronic myelogenous leukemia. *Blood* 56:728, 1980.

231. Pareti FI, Gugliotta L, Mannucci L, et al: Biochemical and metabolic aspects of platelet dysfunction in chronic myeloproliferative disorders. *Thromb Haemost* 47:84, 1982.

232. Schafer AI: Deficiency of platelet lipoxygenase activity in myeloproliferative disorders. *N Engl J Med* 306:381, 1982.

233. Ushikubi F, Okuma M, Kanaji K, et al: Hemorrhagic thrombocytopathy with platelet thromboxane A2 receptor abnormality: Defective signal transduction with normal binding activity. *Thromb Haemost* 57:158, 1987.

234. Okuma M, Takayama H, Uchino H: Subnormal platelet response to thromboxane A_2 in a patient with chronic myeloid leukaemia. *Br J Haematol* 51:469, 1982.

235. Mohri H: Acquired von Willebrand disease and storage pool disease in chronic myelocytic leukemia. *Am J Hematol* 22:391, 1986.

236. Malpass TW, Savage B, Hanson SR, et al: Correlation between prolonged bleeding time and depletion of platelet dense granule ADP in patients with myelodysplastic and myeloproliferative disorders. *J Lab Clin Med* 103:894, 1984.

237. Handa M, Watanabe K, Kawai Y, et al: Platelet unresponsiveness to collagen: Involvement of glycoprotein Ia-IIa (alpha 2 beta 1 integrin) deficiency associated with a myeloproliferative disorder. *Thromb Haemost* 73:521, 1995.

238. Kaywin P, McDonough M, Insel PA, Shattil SJ: Platelet function in essential thrombocythemia: Decreased epinephrine responsiveness associated with a deficiency of platelet alpha-adrenergic receptors. *N Engl J Med* 299:505, 1978.

239. Swart SS, Pearson D, Wood JK, Barnett DB: Functional significance of the platelet alpha2-adrenoceptor: Studies in patients with myeloproliferative disorders. *Thromb Res* 33:531, 1984.

240. Nurden P, Bihour C, Smith M, et al: Platelet activation and thrombosis: Studies in a patient with essential thrombocythemia. *Am J Hematol* 51:79, 1996.

241. Rocca B, Ciabattoni G, Tartaglione R, et al: Increased thromboxane biosynthesis in essential thrombocythemia. *Thromb Haemost* 74:1225, 1995.

242. Landolfi R, Ciabattoni G, Patrignani P, et al: Increased thromboxane biosynthesis in patients with polycythemia vera: Evidence for aspirin-suppressible platelet activation in vivo. *Blood* 80:1965, 1992.

243. Walsh PN, Murphy S, Barry WE: The role of platelets in the pathogenesis of thrombosis and hemorrhage in patients with thrombocytosis. *Thromb Haemost* 38:1085, 1977.

244. Kaplan R, Gabbeta J, Sun L, et al: Combined defect in membrane expression and activation of platelet GPIIb-IIIa complex without primary sequence abnormalities in myeloproliferative disease. *Br J Haematol* 111:954, 2000.

245. Berndt MC, Kabral A, Grimsley P, et al: An acquired Bernard-Soulier-like platelet defect associated with juvenile myelodysplastic syndrome. *Br J Haematol* 68:97, 1988.

246. Cooper B, Schafer AI, Puchalsky D, Handin RI: Platelet resistance to prostaglandin D2 in patients with myeloproliferative disorders. *Blood* 52:618, 1978.

247. Moore A, Nachman RL: Platelet Fc receptor. Increased expression in myeloproliferative disease. *J Clin Invest* 67:1064, 1981.

248. Bolin RB, Okumura T, Jamieson GA: Changes in distribution of platelet membrane glycoproteins in patients with myeloproliferative disorders. *Am J Hematol* 3:63, 1977.

249. Eche N, Sie P, Caranobe C, et al: Platelets in myeloproliferative disorders: III. Glycoprotein profile in relation to platelet function and platelet density. *Scand J Haematol* 26:123, 1981.

250. Thibert V, Bellucci S, Cristofari M, et al: Increased platelet CD36 constitutes a common marker in myeloproliferative disorders. *Br J Haematol* 91:618, 1995.

251. Moliterno AR, Hankins WD, Spivak JL: Impaired expression of the thrombopoietin receptor by platelets from patients with polycythemia vera. *N Engl J Med* 338:572, 1998.

252. Li J, Xia Y, Kuter DJ: The platelet thrombopoietin receptor number and function are markedly decreased in patients with essential thrombocythaemia. *Br J Haematol* 111:943, 2000.

253. Budde U, Schaefer G, Mueller N, et al: Acquired von Willebrand's disease in the myeloproliferative syndrome. *Blood* 64:981, 1984.

254. van Genderen PJ, Budde U, Michiels JJ, et al: The reduction of large von Willebrand factor multimers in plasma in essential thrombocythaemia is related to the platelet count. *Br J Haematol* 93:962, 1996.

255. Mohri H, Ohkubo T: Acquired von Willebrand's syndrome due to an inhibitor of IgG specific for von Willebrand's factor in polycythemia rubra vera. *Acta Haematol* 78:258, 1987.

256. van Genderen PJ, Prins FJ, Lucas IS, et al: Decreased half-life time of plasma von Willebrand factor collagen binding activity in essential thrombocythaemia: Normalization after cytoreduction of the increased platelet count. *Br J Haematol* 99:832, 1997.

257. Mitchell MC, Boitnott JK, Kaufman S, et al: Budd-Chiari syndrome: Etiology, diagnosis, and management. *Medicine (Baltimore)* 61:199, 1982.

258. Murphy S: Thrombocytosis and thrombocythaemia. *Clin Haematol* 12:89, 1983.

259. Schafer AI: Bleeding and thrombosis in the myeloproliferative disorders. *Blood* 64:1, 1984.

260. Valla D, Casadevall N, Huisse MG, et al: Etiology of portal vein thrombosis in adults. A prospective evaluation of primary myeloproliferative disorders. *Gastroenterology* 94:1063, 1988.

261. Singh AK, Wetherley-Mein G: Microvascular occlusive lesions in primary thrombocythaemia. *Br J Haematol* 36:553, 1977.

262. van Genderen PJ, Terpstra W, Michiels JJ, et al: High-dose intravenous immunoglobulin delays clearance of von Willebrand factor in acquired von Willebrand disease. *Thromb Haemost* 73:891, 1995.

263. Michiels JJ, Berneman ZN, Schroyens W, Van Vliet HH: Pathophysiology and treatment of platelet-mediated microvascular disturbances, major thrombosis and bleeding complications in essential thrombocythaemia and polycythaemia vera. *Platelets* 15:67, 2004.

264. Rinder HM, Schuster JE, Rinder CS, et al: Correlation of thrombosis with increased platelet turnover in thrombocytosis. *Blood* 91:1288, 1998.

265. Besses C, Cervantes F, Pereira A, et al: Major vascular complications in essential thrombocythemia: A study of the predictive factors in a series of 148 patients. *Leukemia* 13:150, 1999.

266. Barbui T, Barosi G, Grossi A, et al: Practice guidelines for the therapy of essential thrombocythemia. A statement from the Italian Society of Hematology, the Italian Society of Experimental Hematology and the Italian Group for Bone Marrow Transplantation. *Haematologica* 89:215, 2004.

267. Spivak J: Daily aspirin: Only half the answer. *N Engl J Med* 350:99, 2004.

268. Kaplan ME, Mack K, Goldberg JD, et al: Long-term management of polycythemia vera with hydroxyurea: A progress report. *Semin Hematol* 23:167, 1986.

269. Gilbert HS: Modern treatment strategies in polycythemia vera. *Semin Hematol* 40:26, 2003.

270. Barbui T, Finazzi G: Treatment indications and choice of a platelet-lowering agent in essential thrombocythemia. *Curr Hematol Rep* 2:248, 2003.

271. Cortelazzo S, Finazzi G, Ruggeri M, et al: Hydroxyurea for patients with essential thrombocythemia and a high risk of thrombosis. *N Engl J Med* 332:1132, 1995.

272. Pescatore SL, Lindley C: Anagrelide: A novel agent for the treatment of myeloproliferative disorders. *Expert Opin Pharmacother* 1:537, 2000.

273. Fruchtman SM, Petitt RM, Gilbert HS, et al, and the Anagrelide Study Group: Anagrelide: analysis of long-term efficacy, safety and leukemogenic potential in myeloproliferative disorders. *Leuk Res* 29:481, 2005.

274. Michiels JJ, Abels J, Steketee J, et al: Erythromelalgia caused by platelet-mediated arteriolar inflammation and thrombosis in thrombocythemia. *Ann Intern Med* 102:466, 1985.

275. Van Genderen PJJ, Mulder PGH, Waleboer M, et al: Prevention and treatment of thrombotic complications in essential thrombocythaemia: Efficacy and safety of aspirin. *Br J Haematol* 97:179, 1997.

276. Landolfi R, Marchioli R, Kutti J, et al: Efficacy and safety of low-dose aspirin in polycythemia vera. *N Engl J Med* 350:114, 2004.

277. Sultan Y, Caen JP: Platelet dysfunction in preleukemic states and in various types of leukemia. *Ann N Y Acad Sci* 201:300, 1972.

278. Cowan DH, Haut MJ: Platelet function in acute leukemia. *J Lab Clin Med* 79:893, 1972.

279. Cowan DH, Graham RC Jr, Baunach D: The platelet defect in leukemia. Platelet ultrastructure, adenine nucleotide metabolism, and the release reaction. *J Clin Invest* 56:188, 1975.

280. Meschengieser S, Blanco A, Maugeri N, et al: Platelet function and intraplatelet von Willebrand factor antigen and fibrinogen in myelodysplastic syndromes. *Thromb Res* 46:601, 1987.

281. Zeidman A, Sokolover N, Fradin Z, et al: Platelet function and its clinical significance in the myelodysplastic syndromes. *Hematol J* 5:234, 2004.

282. Pui CH, Jackson CW, Chesney C: Normal platelet function after therapy for acute lymphocytic leukemia. *Arch Intern Med* 143:73, 1983.

283. Westbrook CA, Golde DW: Clinical problems in hairy cell leukemia: Diagnosis and management. *Semin Oncol* 11:514, 1984.

284. Rosove MH, Naeim F, Harwig S, Zighelboim J: Severe platelet dysfunction in hairy cell leukemia with improvement after splenectomy. *Blood* 55:903, 1980.

285. Roussi JH, Houbouyan LL, Alterescu R, et al: Acquired von Willebrand's syndrome associated with hairy cell leukaemia. *Br J Haematol* 46:503, 1980.

286. Lackner H: Hemostatic abnormalities associated with dysproteinemias. *Semin Hematol* 10:125, 1973.

287. Perkins HA, MacKenzie MR, Fudenberg HH: Hemostatic defects in dysproteinemias. *Blood* 35:695, 1970.

288. Rapoport M, Yona R, Kaufman S, et al: Unusual bleeding manifestations of amyloidosis in patients with multiple myeloma. *Clin Lab Haematol* 16:349, 1994.

289. Furie B, Greene E, Furie BC: Syndrome of acquired factor X deficiency and systemic amyloidosis in vivo studies of the metabolic fate of factor X. *N Engl J Med* 297:81, 1977.

290. McPherson RA, Onstad JW, Ugoretz RJ, Wolf PL: Coagulopathy in amyloidosis: Combined deficiency of factors IX and X. *Am J Hematol* 3:225, 1977.

291. Palmer RN, Rick ME, Rick PD, et al: Circulating heparan sulfate anticoagulant in a patient with a fatal bleeding disorder. *N Engl J Med* 310:1696, 1984.

292. Chapman GS, George CB, Danley DL: Heparin-like anticoagulant associated with plasma cell myeloma. *Am J Clin Pathol* 83:764, 1985.

293. Liebman H, Chinowsky M, Valdin J, et al: Increased fibrinolysis and amyloidosis. *Arch Intern Med* 143:678, 1983.

294. Meyer K, Williams EC: Fibrinolysis and acquired alpha-2 plasmin inhibitor deficiency in amyloidosis. *Am J Med* 79:394, 1985.

295. McGrath KM, Stuart JJ, Richards F 2nd: Correlation between serum IgG, platelet membrane IgG, and platelet function in hypergammaglobulinaemic states. *Br J Haematol* 42:585, 1979.

296. Kasturi J, Saraya AK: Platelet functions in dysproteinaemia. *Acta Haematol* 59:104, 1978.

297. Vigliano EM, Horowitz HI: Bleeding syndrome in a patient with IgA myeloma: Interaction of protein and connective tissue. *Blood* 29:823, 1967.

298. DiMinno G, Coraggio F, Cerbone AM, et al: A myeloma paraprotein with specificity for platelet glycoprotein IIIa in a patient with a fatal bleeding disorder. *J Clin Invest* 77:157, 1986.

299. Mannucci PM, Lombardi R, Bader R, et al: Studies of the pathophysiology of acquired von Willebrand's disease in seven patients with lymphoproliferative disorders or benign monoclonal gammopathies. *Blood* 64:614, 1984.

300. Takahashi H, Nagayama R, Tanabe Y, et al: DDAVP in acquired von Willebrand syndrome associated with multiple myeloma. *Am J Hematol* 22:421, 1986.

301. Mohri H, Noguchi T, Kodama F, et al: Acquired von Willebrand disease due to inhibitor of human myeloma protein specific for von Willebrand factor. *Am J Clin Pathol* 87:663, 1987.

302. Wallace MR, Simon SR, Ershler WB, Burns SL: Hemorrhagic diathesis in multiple myeloma. *Acta Haematol* 72:340, 1984.

303. Hyman BT, Westrick MA: Multiple myeloma with polyneuropathy and coagulopathy. A case report of the polyneuropathy, organomegaly, endocrinopathy, M-protein, and skin change (POEMS) syndrome. *Arch Intern Med* 146:993, 1986.

304. Bovill EG, Ershler WB, Golden EA, et al: A human myeloma-produced monoclonal protein directed against the active subpopulation of von Willebrand factor. *Am J Clin Pathol* 85:115, 1986.

305. Silberstein LE, Abrahm J, Shattil SJ: The efficacy of intensive plasma exchange in acquired von Willebrand's disease. *Transfusion* 27:234, 1987.

306. Michiels JJ, Budde U, van der Planken M, et al: Acquired von Willebrand syndromes: Clinical features, aetiology, pathophysiology, classification, and management. *Best Pract Res Clin Haematol* 14:401, 2001.

307. Kumar S, Pruthi RK, Nichols WL: Acquired von Willebrand disease. *Mayo Clin Proc* 77:181, 2002.

308. Mazurier C, Parquet-Gernez A, Descamps J, et al: Acquired von Willebrand's syndrome in the course of Waldenstrom's disease. *Thromb Haemost* 44:115, 1980.

309. Handin RI, Martin V, Moloney WC: Antibody-induced von Willebrand's disease: A newly defined inhibitor syndrome. *Blood* 48:393, 1976.

310. Van Genderen PJJ, Vink T, Michiels JJ, et al: Acquired von Willebrand disease caused by an autoantibody selectively inhibiting the binding of von Willebrand factor to collagen. *Blood* 84:3378, 1994.

311. Goudemand J, Samor B, Caron C, et al: Acquired type II von Willebrand's disease: Demonstration of a complexed inhibitor of the von Willebrand factor-platelet interaction and response to treatment. *Br J Haematol* 68:227, 1988.

312. Mohri H, Hisanaga S, Mishima A, et al: Autoantibody inhibits binding of von Willebrand factor to glycoprotein Ib and collagen in multiple myeloma: Recognition sites present on the A1 loop and A3 domains of von Willebrand factor. *Blood Coagul Fibrinolysis* 9:91, 1998.

313. Igarashi N, Miura M, Kato E, et al: Acquired von Willebrand's syndrome with lupus-like serology. *Am J Pediatr Hematol Oncol* 11:32, 1989.

314. Scott JP, Montgomery RR, Tubergen DG, Hays T: Acquired von Willebrand's disease in association with Wilm's tumor: Regression following treatment. *Blood* 58:665, 1981.

315. Rao KP, Kizer J, Jones TJ, et al: Acquired von Willebrand's syndrome associated with an extranodal pulmonary lymphoma. *Arch Pathol Lab Med* 112:47, 1988.

316. Tefferi A, Hanson CA, Kurtin PJ, et al: Acquired von Willebrand's disease due to aberrant expression of platelet glycoprotein Ib by marginal zone lymphoma cells. *Br J Haematol* 96:850, 1997.

317. Levesque H, Borg JY, Cailleux N, et al: Acquired von Willebrand's syndrome associated with decrease of plasminogen activator and its inhibitor during hypothyroidism. *Eur J Med* 2:287, 1993.

318. Aylesworth CA, Smallridge RC, Rick ME, Alving BM: Acquired von Willebrand's disease: A rare manifestation of postpartum thyroiditis. *Am J Hematol* 50:217, 1995.

319. Tefferi A, Nichols WL: Acquired von Willebrand disease: Concise review of occurrence, diagnosis, pathogenesis, and treatment. *Am J Med* 103:536, 1997.

320. Joist JH, Cowan JF, Zimmerman TS: Acquired von Willebrand's disease. Evidence for a quantitative and qualitative factor VIII disorder. *N Engl J Med* 298:988, 1978.

321. Macik BG, Gabriel DA, White GC 2nd, et al: The use of high-dose intravenous gamma-globulin in acquired von Willebrand syndrome. *Arch Pathol Lab Med* 112:143, 1988.

322. White LA, Chisholm M: Gastrointestinal bleeding in acquired von Willebrand's disease: Efficacy of high-dose immunoglobulin where substitution treatments failed. *Br J Haematol* 84:332, 1993.

323. Rinder MR, Richard RE, Rinder HM: Acquired von Willebrand's disease: A concise review. *Am J Hematol* 54:139, 1997.

324. Van Genderen PJ, Papatsonis DN, Michiels JJ, et al: High-dose intravenous gammaglobulin therapy for acquired von Willebrand disease. *Postgrad Med J* 70:916, 1994.

325. Rao AK: Uraemic platelets. *Lancet* 1:913, 1986.

326. Boccardo P, Remuzzi G, Galbusera M: Platelet dysfunction in renal failure. *Semin Thromb Hemost* 30:579, 2004.

327. Rosenbaum R, Hoffstein PE, Stanley RJ, Klahr S: Use of computerized tomography to diagnose complications of percutaneous renal biopsy. *Kidney Int* 14:87, 1978.

328. Diaz-Buxo JA, Donadio JVJ: Complications of percutaneous renal biopsy: An analysis of 1,000 consecutive biopsies. *Clin Nephrol* 4:223, 1975.

329. Weigert AL, Schafer AI: Uremic bleeding: Pathogenesis and therapy. *Am J Med Sci* 316:94, 1998.

330. Castillo R, Lozano T, Escolar G, et al: Defective platelet adhesion on vessel subendothelium in uremic patients. *Blood* 68:337, 1986.

331. Zwaginga JJ, Ijsseldijk MJW, Beeser-Visser N, et al: High von Willebrand factor concentration compensates a relative adhesion defect in uremic blood. *Blood* 75:1498, 1990.

332. Zwaginga JJ, Ijsseldijk I, De Groot PG, et al: Defects in platelet adhesion and aggregate formation in uremic bleeding disorder can be attributed to factors in plasma. *Arterioscler Thromb* 11:733, 1991.

333. Valeri CR, Cassidy G, Pivacek LE, et al: Anemia-induced increase in the bleeding time: Implications for treatment of nonsurgical blood loss. *Transfusion* 41:977, 2001.

334. Livio M EG, Marchesi D, et al: Uraemic bleeding: Role of anaemia and beneficial effect of red cell transfusions. *Lancet* 2:1013, 1982.

335. Fernandez F, Goudable C, Sie P, et al: Low haematocrit and prolonged bleeding time in uraemic patients: Effect of red cell transfusions. *Br J Haematol* 59:139, 1985.

336. Moia M, Mannucci PM, Vizzotto L, et al: Improvement in the haemostatic defect of uraemia after treatment with recombinant human erythropoietin. *Lancet* 2:1227, 1987.

337. Vigano G, Benigni A, Mendogni D, et al: Recombinant human erythropoietin to correct uremic bleeding. *Am J Kidney Dis* 18:44, 1991.

338. Tang WW, Stead RA, Goodkin DA: Effects of epoetin alfa on hemostasis in chronic renal failure. *Am J Nephrol* 18:263, 1998.

339. Turrito VT, Weiss HJ: Red blood cells: Their dual role in thrombus formation. *Science* 207:541, 1980.

340. Casonato A, Pontara E, Vertolli UP, et al: Plasma and platelet von Willebrand factor abnormalities in patients with uremia: Lack of correlation with uremic bleeding. *Clin Appl Thromb Hemost* 7:81, 2001.

341. Sloand EM, Sloand JA, Prodouz K, et al: Reduction of platelet glycoprotein Ib in uremia. *Br J Haematol* 77:375, 1991.

342. Gralnick HR, McKeown LP, Williams SB, et al: Plasma and platelet von Willebrand factor defects in uremia. *Am J Med* 85:806, 1988.

343. Escolar G, Cases A, Bastida E, et al: Uremic platelets have a functional defect affecting the interaction of von Willebrand factor with glycoprotein IIb-IIIa. *Blood* 76:1336, 1990.

344. Di Minno G, Cerbone A, Usberti M, et al: Platelet dysfunction in uremia: II. Correction by arachidonic acid of the impaired exposure of fibrinogen receptors by adenosine diphosphate or collagen. *J Lab Clin Med* 108: 246, 1986.

345. Rabiner SF, Hrodek O: Platelet factor 3 in normal subjects and patients with renal failure. *J Clin Invest* 47:901, 1968.

346. Ware JA, Clark BA, Smith M, Salzman EW: Abnormalities of cytoplasmic Ca^{2+} in platelets from patients with uremia. *Blood* 73:172, 1989.

347. Mannucci PM, Remuzzi G, Pusineri F, et al: Deamino-8-arginine vasopressin shortens the bleeding time in uremia. *N Engl J Med* 308:8, 1983.

348. Winter M, Frampton G, Bennett A, et al: Synthesis of thromboxane B_2 in uraemia and the effects of dialysis. *Thromb Res* 30:265, 1983.

349. Bloom A, Greaves M, Preston FE, Brown CB: Evidence against a platelet cyclooxygenase defect in uraemic subjects on chronic haemodialysis. *Br J Haematol* 62:143, 1986.

350. Remuzzi G, Benigni A, Dodesini P, et al: Reduced platelet thromboxane formation in uremia: Evidence for a functional cyclooxygenase defect. *J Clin Invest* 71:762, 1983.

351. Eknoyan G, Brown CH: Biochemical abnormalities of platelets in renal failure. Evidence for decreased platelet serotonin, adenosine diphosphate and Mg-dependent adenosine triphosphatase. *Am J Nephrol* 1:17, 1981.

352. Vlachoyannis J, Schoeppe W: Adenylate cyclase activity and cAMP content of human platelets in uraemia. *Eur J Clin Invest* 12:379, 1982.

353. Bazilinski N, Shaykh M, Dunea G, et al: Inhibition of platelet function by uremic middle molecules. *Nephron* 40:423, 1985.

354. Remuzzi G, Livio M, Marchiaro G, et al: Bleeding in renal failure: Altered platelet function in chronic uraemia only partially corrected by haemodialysis. *Nephron* 22:347, 1978.

355. Livio M, Benigni A, Remuzzi G: Coagulation abnormalities in uremia. *Semin Nephrol* 5:82, 1985.

356. Remuzzi G, Perico N, Zoja C, et al: Role of endothelium-derived nitric oxide in the bleeding tendency of uremia. *J Clin Invest* 86:1768, 1990.

357. Aiello S, Noris M, Todeschini M, et al: Renal and systemic nitric oxide synthesis in rats with renal mass reduction. *Kidney Int* 52:171, 1997.

358. Noris M, Remuzzi G: Uremic bleeding: Closing the circle after 30 years of controversies? *Blood* 94:2569, 1999.

359. Mendes Ribeiro AC, Brunini TM, Ellory JC, Mann GE: Abnormalities in L-arginine transport and nitric oxide biosynthesis in chronic renal and heart failure. *Cardiovasc Res* 49:697, 2001.

360. Brunini TM, Yaqoob MM, Novaes Malagris LE, et al: Increased nitric oxide synthesis in uraemic platelets is dependent on L-arginine transport via system y(+)L. *Pflugers Arch* 445:547, 2003.

361. Remuzzi G: Bleeding disorders in uremia: Pathophysiology and treatment. *Adv Nephrol* 18:171, 1989.

362. Andrassy K, Ritz E: Uremia as a cause of bleeding. *Am J Nephrol* 5: 313, 1985.

363. Ando M, Iwamoto Y, Suda A, et al: New insights into the thrombopoietic status of patients on dialysis through the evaluation of megakaryocytopoiesis in bone marrow and of endogenous thrombopoietin levels. *Blood* 97:915, 2001.

364. George CRP, Slichter SJ, Quadracci LJ: A kinetic evaluation of hemostasis in renal disease. *N Engl J Med* 291:1111, 1974.

365. Linthorst GE, Folman CC, van Olden RW, von dem Borne AE: Plasma thrombopoietin levels in patients with chronic renal failure. *Hematol J* 3:38, 2002.

366. Peterson P, Hayes TE, Arkin CF, et al: The preoperative bleeding time test lacks clinical benefit. *Arch Surg* 133:134, 1998.

367. Stewart JH, Castaldi PA: Uraemic bleeding: A reversible platelet defect corrected by dialysis. *Q J Med, New Series XXXVI* 143:409, 1967.

368. Lindsay RM, Friesen M, Koens F, et al: Platelet function in patients on long-term peritoneal dialysis. *Clin Nephrol* 6:335, 1976.

369. Gotti E, Mecca G, Valentino C, et al: Renal biopsy in patients with acute renal failure and prolonged bleeding time. *Lancet* 2:978, 1984.

370. Tassies D, Reventer JC, Cases A, et al: Effect of recombinant human erythropoietin treatment on circulating reticulated platelets in uremic patients: Association with early improvement in platelet function. *Am J Hematol* 59:105, 1998.

371. Mannucci PM: Desmopressin: A non-transfusional form of treatment for congenital and acquired bleeding disorders. *Blood* 72:1449, 1988.

372. Rose EH, Aledort LM: Nasal spray desmopressin (DDAVP) for mild hemophilia A and von Willebrand disease. *Ann Intern Med* 114:563, 1991.

373. Canavese C, Salomone M, Pacitti A, et al: Reduced response of uraemic bleeding time to repeated doses of desmopressin. *Lancet* 1:867, 1985.

374. Byrnes JJ, Larcada A, Moake JL: Thrombosis following desmopressin for uremic bleeding. *Am J Hematol* 28:63, 1988.

375. Mannucci PM: Desmopressin and thrombosis. *Lancet* 2:675, 1989.

376. Liu YK, Kosfeld RE, Marcum SG: Treatment of uremic bleeding with conjugated estrogen. *Lancet* 2:887, 1984.

377. Livio M, Mannucci PM, Vigano G, et al: Conjugated estrogens for the management of bleeding associated with renal failure. *N Engl J Med* 315:731, 1986.

378. Vigano G, Gaspari F, Locatelli M, et al: Dose-effect and pharmacokinetics of estrogens given to correct bleeding time in uremia. *Kidney Int* 34:853, 1988.

379. Heistinger M, Stockenhuber F, Schneider B, et al: Effect of conjugated estrogens on platelet function and prostacyclin generation in CRF. *Kidney Int* 38:1181, 1990.

380. Bronner MH, Pate MD, Cunningham JT: Estrogen-progesterone therapy for bleeding of gastrointestinal telangiectasias in chronic renal failure. *Ann Intern Med* 105:371, 1986.

381. Shemin D, Elnour M, Amarantes B, Abuelo JG: Oral estrogens decrease bleeding time and improve clinical bleeding in patients with renal failure. *Am J Med* 89:436, 1990.

382. Vigano G, Zoja C, Corna D, et al: 17 β-estradiol is the most active component of the conjugated estrogen mixture active on uremic bleeding by a receptor mechanism. *Mol Pharmacol* 252:344, 1990.

383. Janson PA, Jubelirer SJ, Weinstein MS, Deykin D: Treatment of bleeding tendency in uremia with cryoprecipitate. *N Engl J Med* 303:1318, 1980.

384. Triulzi DJ, Blumber N: Variability in response to cryoprecipitate treatment for hemostatic defects in uremia. *Yale J Biol Med* 63:1, 1990.

385. George JN: Platelet membrane microparticles in blood bank fresh frozen plasma and cryoprecipitate. *Blood* 68:307, 1986.

386. Thompson AR, Harker LA: Approach to bleeding disorders, in *Manual of Hemostasis and Thrombosis*, 3rd ed, p 57. FA Davis, Philadelphia, 1983.

387. George JN, Woolf SH, Raskob GE, et al: Idiopathic thrombocytopenic purpura: A practice guideline developed by explicit methods for the American Society of Hematology. *Blood* 88:3, 1996.

388. George JN, El-Harake MA, Raskob GE: Chronic idiopathic thrombocytopenic purpura. *N Engl J Med* 331:1207, 1994.

389. McMillan R: Antiplatelet antibodies in chronic adult immune thrombocytopenic purpura: Assays and epitopes. *J Pediatr Hematol Oncol* 25(suppl 1):S57, 2003.

390. Uesugi Y, Fuse I, Toba K, et al: Acquired immune thrombocytopenia caused by IgG antiglycoprotein Ib antibody in a patient with Hodgkin's disease. *Acta Haematol* 98:217, 1997.

391. Meyer M, Kirchmaier CM, Schirmer A, et al: Acquired disorder of platelet function associated with autoantibodies against membrane glycoprotein IIb-IIIa complex-1. Glycoprotein analysis. *Thromb Haemost* 65: 491, 1991.

392. Balduini CL, Grignani G, Sinigaglia F, et al: Severe platelet dysfunction in a patient with autoantibodies against membrane glycoproteins IIb-IIIa. *Haemostasis* 7:98, 1987.

393. Balduini CL, Bertolino G, Noris P, et al: Defect of platelet aggregation and adhesion induced by autoantibodies against platelet glycoprotein IIIa. *Thromb Haemost* 68:208, 1992.

394. Fuse I, Higuchi W, Narita M, et al: Overproduction of antiplatelet antibody against glycoprotein IIb after splenectomy in a patient with Evans syndrome resulting in acquired thrombasthenia. *Acta Haematol* 99:83, 1998.

395. Stricker RB, Wong D, Saks SR, et al: Acquired Bernard-Soulier syndrome: Evidence for the role of a 210,000-molecular weight protein in the interaction of platelets with von Willebrand factor. *J Clin Invest* 76: 1274, 1985.

396. Devine DV, Currie MS, Rosse WF, Greenberg CS: Pseudo-Bernard-Soulier syndrome: Thrombocytopenia caused by autoantibody to platelet glycoprotein Ib. *Blood* 70:428, 1987.

397. Deckmyn H, Zhang J, Van Houtte E, Vermylen J: Production and nucleotide sequence of an inhibitory human IgM autoantibody directed against platelet glycoprotein Ia/IIa. *Blood* 84:1968, 1994.

398. Dromigny A, Triadou P, Lesavre P, et al: Lack of platelet response to collagen associated with autoantibodies against glycoprotein (GP) Ia/IIa and Ib/IX leading to the discovery of SLE. *Hematol Cell Ther* 38:355, 1996.

399. Xu H, Frojmovic MM, Wong T, Rauch J: P32, a platelet autoantigen recognized by an SLE-derived autoantibody that inhibits platelet aggregation. *J Autoimmun* 8:97, 1995.

400. Wiedmer T, Ando B, Sims PJ: Complement C5b-9-stimulated platelet secretion is associated with a calcium-initiated activation of cellular protein kinases. *J Biol Chem* 262:13674, 1987.

401. Sugiyama T, Okuma M, Ushikubi F, et al: A novel platelet aggregating factor found in a patient with defective collagen-induced platelet aggregation and autoimmune thrombocytopenia. *Blood* 69:1712, 1987.

402. Warkentin TE: Heparin-induced thrombocytopenia: Pathogenesis and management. *Br J Haematol* 121:535, 2003.

403. Lackner H, Karpatkin S: On the "easy bruising" syndrome with normal platelet count: A study of 75 patients. *Ann Intern Med* 83:190, 1975.

404. Clancy R, Jenkins E, Firkin B: Qualitative platelet abnormalities in idopathic thrombocytopenic purpura. *N Engl J Med* 286:622, 1972.

405. Heyns DA, Fraser J, Retief FP: Platelet aggregation in chronic idiopathic thrombocytopenic purpura. *J Clin Pathol* 31:1239, 1978.

406. Regan MG, Lackner H, Karpatkin S: Platelet function and coagulation profile in lupus erythematosus. *Am J Med* 81:462, 1974.

407. Dorsch CA, Meyerhoff J: Mechanisms of abnormal platelet aggregation in systemic lupus erythematosus. *Arthritis Rheum* 25:966, 1982.

408. Nieuwenhuis HK, Zwaginga JJ, Sixma JJ: Analysis of patients with a prolonged bleeding time. *Thromb Haemost* 58:527, 1987.

409. Weiss HJ, Rosove MH, Lages BA, Kaplan KL: Acquired storage pool deficiency with increased platelet-associated IgG. *Am J Med* 69:711, 1980.

410. Meyerhoff J, Dorsch CA: Decreased platelet serotonin levels in systemic lupus erythematosus. *Arthritis Rheum* 24:1495, 1981.

411. Stuart MJ, Kelton JG, Allen JB: Abnormal platelet function and arachidonate metabolism in chronic idiopathic thrombocytopenic purpura. *Blood* 58:326, 1981.

412. Harker LA, Malpass TW, Branson HE, et al: Mechanism of abnormal bleeding in patients undergoing cardiopulmonary bypass: Acquired transient platelet dysfunction associated with selective alpha-granule release. *Blood* 56:824, 1980.

413. Woodman RC, Harker LA: Bleeding complications associated with cardiopulmonary bypass. *Blood* 76:1680, 1990.

414. Mammen EF, Koets MH, Washington BC, et al: Hemostasis changes during cardiopulmonary bypass surgery. *Semin Thromb Hemost* 11:281, 1985.

415. Khuri SF, Wolfe JA, Josa M, et al: Hematologic changes during and after cardiopulmonary bypass and their relationship to the bleeding time and nonsurgical blood loss. *J Thorac Cardiovasc Surg* 104:94, 1992.

416. Martin JF, Daniel TD, Trowbridge EA: Acute and chronic changes in platelet volume and count after cardiopulmonary bypass induced thrombocytopenia in man. *Thromb Haemost* 57:55, 1987.

417. Chandler AB, Hutson MS: Platelet plug formation in an extracorporeal unit. *Am J Clin Pathol* 64:101, 1975.

418. Lindon JN, McManama, Kushner L: Does the conformation of adsorbed fibrinogen dictate platelet interactions with artificial surfaces? *Blood* 68: 355, 1986.

419. Singer RL, Mannion JD, Bauer TL, et al: Complications from heparin-induced thrombocytopenia in patients undergoing cardiopulmonary bypass. *Chest* 104:1436, 1993.

420. Bick RL: Hemostasis defects associated with cardiac surgery, prosthetic devices, and other extracorporeal circuits. *N Engl J Med* 22:1446, 1986.

421. McKenna R, Bachmann F, Whittaker B, et al: The hemostatic mechanism after open heart surgery: II. Frequency of abnormal platelet functions during and after extracorporeal circulation. *J Thorac Cardiovasc Surg* 70:298, 1975.

422. Beurling-Harbury C, Galvan CA: Acquired decrease in platelet secretory ADP associated with increased post-operative bleeding in post-cardiopulmonary bypass patients and in patients with severe valvular heart disease. *Blood* 52:13, 1978.

423. Abrams CS, Ellison N, Budzynski AZ, Shattil S: Direct detection of activated platelets and platelet-derived microparticles in humans. *Blood* 75:128, 1990.

424. Nannizzi-Alaimo L, Rubenstein MH, Alves VL, et al: Cardiopulmonary bypass induces release of soluble CD40 ligand. *Circulation* 105:2849, 2002.

425. Wahba A, Rothe G, Lodes H, et al: The influence of the duration of cardiopulmonary bypass on coagulation, fibrinolysis and platelet function. *Thorac Cardiovasc Surg* 49:153, 2001.

426. George JN, Pickett EB, Saucerman S, et al: Platelet surface glycoproteins. Studies on resting and activated platelets and platelet membrane microparticles in normal subjects, and observations in patients during adult respiratory distress syndrome and cardiac surgery. *J Clin Invest* 78:340, 1986.

427. Bachmann F, McKenna R, Cole ER, Najafi H: The hemostatic mechanism after open heart surgery. I. Studies on plasma coagulation factors and fibrinolysis in 512 patients after extracorporeal circulation. *J Thorac Cardiovasc Surg* 70:76, 1975.

428. Gluszko P, Ricinski B, Musial J, et al: Fibrinogen receptors in platelet adhesion to surfaces of extracorporeal circuit. *Am J Physiol* 252:H615, 1987.

429. van den Dengen JJAM, Karliczek GF, Brenken W, et al: Clinical study of blood trauma during perfusion with membrane and bubble oxygenators. *Thorac Cardiovasc Surg* 83:108, 1982.

430. Ferraris VA, Ferraris SP, Singh A, et al: The platelet thrombin receptor and postoperative bleeding. *Ann Thorac Surg* 65:352, 1998.

431. Kestin AS, Valeri CR, Khuri SF, et al: The platelet function defect of cardiopulmonary bypass. *Blood* 82:107, 1993.

432. Weksler BB, Pett SB, Alonso D, et al: Differential inhibition of aspirin of vascular prostaglandin synthesis in atherosclerotic patients. *N Engl J Med* 308:800, 1983.

433. Levy JH: Pharmacologic preservation of the hemostatic system during cardiac surgery. *Ann Thorac Surg* 72:S1814, 2001.

434. Tabuchi N, De Haan J, Boonstra PW, Van Oeveren W: Activation of fibrinolysis in the pericardial cavity during cardiopulmonary bypass. *J Thorac Cardiovasc Surg* 106:828, 1993.

435. Hunt BJ, Parratt RN, Segal HC, et al: Activation of coagulation and fibrinolysis during cardiothoracic operations. *Ann Thorac Surg* 65:712, 1998.

436. Rapaport SI: Preoperative hemostatic evaluation: Which tests, if any? *Blood* 61:229, 1983.

437. Magovern JA, Sakert T, Benckart DH, et al: A model for predicting transfusion after coronary artery bypass grafting. *Ann Thorac Surg* 61: 27, 1996.

438. Simon TA, Akl BF, Murphy W: Controlled trial of routine administration of platelet concentrates in cardiopulmonary bypass surgery. *Ann Thorac Surg* 37:359, 1987.

439. Wasser MNJM, Houbiers JGA, D'Amaro J, et al: The effect of fresh versus stored blood on post-operative bleeding after coronary bypass surgery: A prospective randomized study. *Br J Haematol* 72:81, 1989.

440. Sowade O, Warnke H, Scigalla P, et al: Avoidance of allogeneic blood transfusions by treatment with epoetin beta (recombinant human erythropoietin) in patients undergoing open-heart surgery. *Blood* 89:411, 1997.

441. Shimpo H, Mizumoto T, Onoda K, et al: Erythropoietin in pediatric cardiac surgery: Clinical efficacy and effective dose. *Chest* 111:1565, 1997.

442. Schmoeckel M, Nollert G, Mempel M, et al: Effects of recombinant human erythropoietin on autologous blood donation before open heart surgery. *Thorac Cardiovasc Surg* 41:364, 1993.

443. Axford TC, Dearani JA, Ragno G, et al: Safety and therapeutic effectiveness of reinfused shed blood after open heart surgery. *Ann Thorac Surg* 57:615, 1994.

444. Griffith LD, Billman GF, Daily PO, Lane TA: Apparent coagulopathy caused by infusion of shed mediastinal blood and its prevention by washing of the infusate. *Ann Thorac Surg* 47:400, 1989.

445. Hsu LC: Heparin-coated cardiopulmonary bypass circuits: Current status. *Perfusion* 16:417, 2001.

446. Spijker HT, Graaff R, Boonstra PW, et al: On the influence of flow conditions and wetability on blood material interactions. *Biomaterials* 24:4717, 2003.

447. Lappegard KT, Fung M, Bergseth G, et al: Effect of complement inhibition and heparin coating on artificial surface-induced leukocyte and platelet activation. *Ann Thorac Surg* 77:932, 2004.

448. Weerwind PW, Caberg NE, Reutelingsperger CP, et al: Exposure of procoagulant phospholipids on the surface of platelets in patients undergoing cardiopulmonary bypass using non-coated and heparin-coated extracorporeal circuits. *Int J Artif Organs* 25:770, 2002.

449. Johnell M, Elgue G, Larsson R, et al: Coagulation, fibrinolysis, and cell activation in patients and shed mediastinal blood during coronary artery bypass grafting with a new heparin-coated surface. *J Thorac Cardiovasc Surg* 124:321, 2002.

450. Linneweber J, Chow TW, Kawamura M, et al: In vitro comparison of blood pump induced platelet microaggregates between a centrifugal and roller pump during cardiopulmonary bypass. *Int J Artif Organs* 25:549, 2002.

451. Nuttall GA, Erchul DT, Haight TJ, et al: A comparison of bleeding and transfusion in patients who undergo coronary artery bypass grafting via sternotomy with and without cardiopulmonary bypass. *J Cardiothorac Vasc Anesth* 17:447, 2003.

452. Lo B, Fijnheer R, Castigliego D, et al: Activation of hemostasis after coronary artery bypass grafting with or without cardiopulmonary bypass. *Anesth Analg* 99:634, 2004.

453. Despotis GJ, Avidan MS, Hogue CW Jr: Mechanisms and attenuation of hemostatic activation during extracorporeal circulation. *Ann Thorac Surg* 72:S1821, 2001.

454. Hackmann T, Gascoyne R, Naiman SC, et al: A trial of desmopressin to reduce blood loss in uncomplicated cardiac surgery. *N Engl J Med* 321:1437, 1989.

455. Seear MD, Wadsworth LD, Rogers PC, et al: The effect of desmopressin acetate (DDAVP) on postoperative blood loss after cardiac operations in children. *J Thorac Cardiovasc Surg* 98:217, 1989.

456. Pychynska-Pokorska M, Moll JJ, Krajewski W, Jarosik P: The use of recombinant coagulation factor VIIa in uncontrolled postoperative bleeding in children undergoing cardiac surgery with cardiopulmonary bypass. *Pediatr Crit Care Med* 5:246, 2004.

457. Herbertson M: Recombinant activated factor VII in cardiac surgery. *Blood Coagul Fibrinolysis* 15(suppl 1):S31, 2004.

458. van Oeveren W, Harder MP, Roozendaal KJ, et al: Aprotinin protects platelets against the initial effect of cardiopulmonary bypass. *J Thorac Cardiovasc Surg* 99:788, 1990.

459. Speekenbrink RG, Wildevuur CR, Sturk A, Eijsman L: Low-dose and high-dose aprotinin improve hemostasis in coronary operations. *J Thorac Cardiovasc Surg* 112:523, 1996.

460. Orchard MA, Goodchild CS, Prentice CR, et al: Aprotinin reduces cardiopulmonary bypass-induced blood loss and inhibits fibrinolysis without influencing platelets. *Br J Haematol* 85:533, 1993.

461. Wahba A, Black G, Koksch M, et al: Aprotinin has no effect on platelet activation and adhesion during cardiopulmonary bypass. *Thromb Haemost* 75:844, 1996.

462. Mastroroberto P, Chello M, Zofrea S, Marchese AR: Suppressed fibrinolysis after administration of low-dose aprotinin: Reduced level of plasmin-alpha2-plasmin inhibitor complexes and postoperative blood loss. *Eur J Cardiothorac Surg* 9:143, 1995.

463. Khalil PN, Ismail M, Kalmar P, et al: Activation of fibrinolysis in the pericardial cavity after cardiopulmonary bypass. *Thromb Haemost* 92: 568, 2004.

464. Bidstrup BP, Underwood SR, Sapsford RN, Streets EM: Effect of aprotinin (Trasylol) on aorta-coronary bypass graft patency. *J Thorac Cardiovasc Surg* 105:147, 1993.

465. Dietrich W, Spath P, Ebell A, Richter JA: Prevalence of anaphylactic reactions to aprotinin: Analysis of two hundred forty-eight reexposures to aprotinin in heart operations. *J Thorac Cardiovasc Surg* 113:194, 1997.

466. Krauss JS, Jonah MH: Platelet dysfunction (thrombocytopathy) in extrahepatic biliary obstruction. *South Med J* 75:506, 1982.

467. Hillbom M, Muuronen A, Neiman J: Liver disease and platelet function in alcoholics. *Br Med J* 295:581, 1987.

468. Amitrano L, Guardascione MA, Brancaccio V, Balzano A: Coagulation disorders in liver disease. *Semin Liver Dis* 22:83, 2002.

469. Mannucci PM, Vicente V, Vianello L, et al: Controlled trial of desmopressin in liver cirrhosis and other conditions associated with a prolonged bleeding time. *Blood* 67:1148, 1986.

470. Stein SF, Harker LA: Kinetic and functional studies of platelets, fibrinogen, and plasminogen in patients with hepatic cirrhosis. *J Lab Clin Med* 99:217, 1982.

471. Peck-Radosavljevic M, Wichlas M, Zacherl J, et al: Thrombopoietin induces rapid resolution of thrombocytopenia after orthotopic liver transplantation through increased platelet production. *Blood* 95:795, 2000.

472. Giannini E, Botta F, Borro P, et al: Relationship between thrombopoietin serum levels and liver function in patients with chronic liver disease related to hepatitis C virus infection. *Am J Gastroenterol* 98:2516, 2003.

473. Violi F, Leo R, Vezza E, et al: Bleeding time in patients with cirrhosis: Relation with degree of liver failure and clotting abnormalities. C.A.L.C. Group. Coagulation Abnormalities in Cirrhosis Study Group. *J Hepatol* 20:531, 1994.

474. Pareti FI, Capitanio A, Mannucci L: Acquired storage pool disease in

platelets during disseminated intravascular coagulation. *Blood* 48:511, 1976.

475. Pareti FI, Capitanio A, Mannucci L, et al: Acquired dysfunction due to the circulation of "exhausted" platelets. *Am J Med* 69:235, 1980.

476. Solum NO, Rigollot C, Budzynski A, Marder VJ: A quantitative evaluation of the inhibition of platelet aggregation by low molecular weight degradation products of fibrinogen. *Br J Haematol* 24:619, 1973.

477. Bennett JS, Vilaire G: Exposure of platelet fibrinogen receptors by ADP and epinephrine. *J Clin Invest* 64:1393, 1979.

478. Stoff JS, Stemerman M, Steer M, et al: A defect in platelet aggregation in Bartter's syndrome. *Am J Med* 68:171, 1980.

479. Lim SH, Tan CE, Agasthian T, Chew LS: Acquired platelet dysfunction with eosinophilia: Review of seven adult cases. *J Clin Pathol* 42:950, 1989.

480. Poon MC, Ng SC, Coppes MJ: Acquired platelet dysfunction with eosinophilia in white children. *J Pediatr* 126:959, 1995.

481. Laosombat V, Wongchanchailert M, Sattayasevana B, et al: Acquired platelet dysfunction with eosinophilia in children in the south of Thailand. *Platelets* 12:5, 2001.

482. Szczeklik A, Milner PC, Birch J, et al: Prolonged bleeding time, reduced platelet aggregation, altered PAF-acether sensitivity and increased platelet mass are a trait of asthma and hay fever. *Thromb Haemost* 56:283, 1986.

483. Carvalho AC, Quinn DA, DeMarinis SM, et al: Platelet function in acute respiratory failure. *Am J Hematol* 25:377, 1987.

484. Bracey AW, Wu AH, Aceves J, et al: Platelet dysfunction associated with Wilms tumor and hyaluronic acid. *Am J Hematol* 24:247, 1987.

THE VASCULAR PURPURAS

PHILLIP H.A. LEE
RICHARD L. GALLO

Purpura, the clinical manifestation of red blood cell extravasation into mucosa or skin, results from various conditions, including rheumatologic, infectious, dermatologic, traumatic, and hematologic disorders. This chapter does not consider purpura resulting from quantitative or functional deficiencies of platelets or coagulation factors as causes of purpura; these causes are discussed in other chapters of this book. The differential diagnosis of the disparate causes of nonthrombocytopenic purpura is best approached by stratifying purpura into three types of lesions: (1) palpable or retiform and noninflammatory, such as hyperglobulinemic purpura of Waldenström, (2) palpable or nonpalpable but inflammatory, such as Henoch-Schönlein purpura, or (3) nonpalpable and noninflammatory, such as senile purpura. By accounting for palpability, presence or absence of inflammation, size, and shape, the number of possible diagnoses for a particular lesion can be significantly reduced. Tables 114-1, 2, and 3 list the numerous and diverse types of vascular purpura in one of these three categories.

DEFINITION AND DIAGNOSTIC APPROACH

Purpura, from the Latin for purple, is a visible hemorrhage into mucous membranes or skin. Purpuric lesions do not blanch completely upon compression compared to erythema, which blanches completely. Blanching is commonly tested by compressing skin lesions with a glass slide, referred to as diascopy (see Color Plates XXV-1 and XXV-2). Certain conditions give rise to lesions that mimic purpura with incomplete blanching upon diascopy but are not purpura because hemorrhage has not occurred. These disorders include conditions in which red cells are obstructed or move slowly, as in tortuous veins.

Determining if a lesion is palpable is the first step in evaluating purpuric lesions, and can narrow the differential diagnosis (Fig. 114-1). The causes of palpability are varied and include fibrin deposition, localized edema, significant cellular infiltration, and extravasation of red cells under subcutaneous fat.

Inspecting the lesion for inflammatory changes is the next step in evaluating purpuric lesions. The presence, localization, and degree of pain, the presence of erythema, and palpation for warmth and localized swelling are signs of inflammation and suggest a vasculitis or immune complex disorder.

The shape of a purpuric lesion, either round or retiform (branching), is important in assessing the lesion. In the absence of accompanying inflammation, retiform purpuric lesions suggest small vessel occlusion. A retiform, inflammatory purpuric lesion supports the diagnosis of vasculitis as a result of immunoglobulin (Ig) complex formation.[1] Small, focal areas of hemorrhage are referred to as *pete-*

chiae (≤4 mm). Larger lesions are referred to as *intermediate* or *mid-size purpura* (>4 mm but <1 cm) or *ecchymoses* (≥1 cm).[2]

Purpuric lesions commonly are purple, but they can take on a variety of colors depending on the age of the lesion and the hemoglobin saturation of the extravasated red blood cells. Ecchymosis usually starts as blue or purple, evolves to a greenish brown, and finally changes to yellow as hemoglobin slowly degrades to bilirubin.[2] Although the color of an ecchymosis has been used to establish the age of the trauma site, this usage is unreliable.[3,4]

Purpuric lesions also can be caused by hemostatic disorders, such as abnormalities in platelets or coagulation factors. However, this chapter does not address etiologies of purpura resulting from hemostatic defects. Tables 114-1 through 114-3 classify etiologies discussed in this chapter.

PALPABLE OR RETIFORM, NONINFLAMMATORY PURPURIC LESIONS (TABLE 114-1)

DYSPROTEINEMIAS

CRYOGLOBULINEMIA

Cryoglobulinemia refers to the presence in plasma of cold-insoluble Igs[5] and is a secondary finding associated with several disease states. Symptoms occur when the abnormal protein precipitates at the temperatures present in superficial venules in the skin and acral parts of the body. Cryoglobulinemia syndromes are divided into three main types based on the Ig composition of the precipitate. Type I cryoglobulinemia results from the accumulation of monoclonal IgG, IgM, or IgA. It is most commonly seen in association with lymphoproliferative disorders, such as myeloma, Waldenström macroglobulinemia, or lymphoma.[6] Type II, or mixed, cryoglobulinemia involves formation of complexes composed of polyclonal IgG with monoclonal Igs, typically IgM with anti-IgG specificity. Exposure to exogenous antigens appears to cause polyclonal Ig production, as these complexes have antibody activity against bacteria, viruses, and fungi. Mixed cryoglobulinemia is commonly seen secondary to hepatitis C virus (HCV) infection.[7] First-line treatment of HCV-associated mixed cryoglobulinemia includes use of interferon alpha, often with adjunct glucocorticoids or plasmapheresis.[8] In addition, direct treatment of the HCV infection with ribavirin and interferon therapy ameliorates associated lymphoproliferative disorders.[9,10] Deposition of these complexes on vessel walls leads to vascular damage and subsequent increased vessel permeability. Tissue deposition in nerves, joints, and skin gives rise to

TABLE 114-1   PALPABLE OR RETIFORM, NONINFLAMMATORY PURPURIC LESIONS

A. Dysproteinemias
  1. Cryoglobulinemia
  2. Waldenström hyperglobulinemic purpura
  3. Light-chain vasculopathy
  4. Cryofibrinogenemia
B. Thrombotic
  1. Heparin necrosis
  2. Warfarin necrosis
  3. Protein C and S deficiency
  4. Paroxysmal nocturnal hemoglobinuria
  5. Antiphospholipid syndrome
  6. Livedoid vasculitis
C. Embolic
  1. Cholesterol emboli
  2. Cutaneous calciphylaxis
  3. Emboli from atrial myxoma
D. Arthropod bites

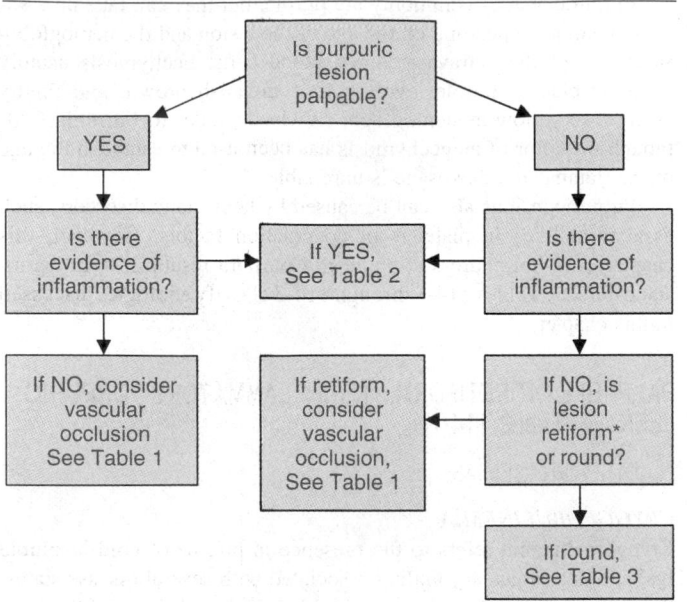

* Retiform refers to a branching, stellate pattern

FIGURE 114-1   Bedside approach to purpuric lesion diagnosis.

the hallmark findings of mixed cryoglobulinemia: weakness, arthralgias, and purpura. This purpura often is palpable and is accompanied by areas of hemorrhagic necrosis (see Color Plate XXV-3) and occasionally follicular pustular purpura. Other cutaneous manifestations include lower extremity ulcerations, urticaria, Raynaud phenomena, and subungual purpura (see Color Plate XXV-4).[11,12]

Type III cryoglobulinemia is characterized by complexes of polyclonal Igs. It is associated with a variety of infections, systemic lupus erythematous, and post-streptococcal glomerulonephritis. The association with immune complex disorders makes difficult the evaluation of tissue injury directly resulting from type III cryoglobulin formation.[6] Thus, little is known about the pathophysiology of this cryoglobulinemic syndrome.

WALDENSTRÖM HYPERGLOBULINEMIC PURPURA

A polyclonal increase of Igs, most commonly IgG, appears to be responsible for the varied cutaneous findings seen in this benign hypergammaglobulinemic purpura. Waldenström[13] first described a hyperproteinemic syndrome characterized by hypergammaglobulinemia, recurrent purpura, elevated erythrocyte sedimentation rate, and anemia. The syndrome is most commonly seen in young women. It has been associated with a large number of autoimmune disorders, including systemic lupus erythematosus, rheumatoid arthritis, Sjögren syndrome, polymyositis, and multiple sclerosis.[14] Discrete to confluent collections of lower limb petechiae are the most common skin findings (see Color Plate XXV-5).[15] Reticulate purpura with accompanying hemorrhagic blisters has also been described in a 75-year-old man with this disorder.[16] These purpuric lesions usually are self-limited but they commonly recur. They are associated with exposure to cold temperatures or increases in hydrostatic pressures, as with use of tight stockings or upon prolonged standing.[17] Development of edema and arthralgias in involved extremities has been described.[18]

Common histologic findings include perivascular infiltrates, hemorrhage, vascular necrosis, and leukocytoclastic vasculitis. In addition to the polyclonal increase in IgA, IgM, or IgG, serum may include cryoglobulinemia, rheumatoid factor, or antinuclear antibodies.[19] Imbalances in IgG subclass expressions, usually resulting from a decrease

in IgG2, have been described and appear to be associated with recurrent infections in these patients.[18] Development of antibodies directed against lymphocytes may result in lymphopenia. Antibodies against Ro/SSA were discovered in up to 78 percent of patients in one series, suggesting that screening for anti-Ro/SSA should be considered in patients suspected of having hyperglobulinemia.[20]

LIGHT-CHAIN VASCULOPATHY

Precipitates of Ig light chains that form crystalline deposits in the skin can cause palpable purpura with hemorrhagic vesicles. For instance, an 82-year-old man and a 34-year-old-woman were found by direct immunofluorescence to have crystalline deposits containing monoclonal λ light-chain serum components in their skin.[21] Both patients developed ischemic necrosis and rapidly progressive renal failure consistent with the findings of extensive deposition of light-chain crystals in multiple tissues. Although clinical presentation suggested a systemic vasculitis, no histologic signs of inflammation were seen. Light-chain vasculopathy with cutaneous findings has been described in a 37-year-old man with multiple myeloma. Intravascular deposition of crystals containing IgG and λ light chains was found by immunohistochemical analysis. This obstructive vasculopathy manifested as gangrene of the feet and intestinal perforation.[22]

CRYOFIBRINOGENEMIA

Cryofibrinogenemia was first described by Korst and Kratochvil in 1955. Cryofibrinogenemia is a form of dysproteinemia characterized by formation of an abnormal cold-precipitable fibrinogen in the blood that may lead to cutaneous manifestations such as cyanosis, erythema, Raynaud phenomenon, and palpable purpura, most often distributed on the nose, ears, and distal extremities.[23] Cryofibrinogen is a complex of multiple cold-insoluble proteins, including fibrin, fibrinogen, fibrin split products, and albumin. The pathogenesis of cryofibrinogenemia is unclear but may be an inhibition of normal fibrinolysis. Cryofibrinogenemia is most commonly seen as a secondary form associated with thromboembolic disorders, metastatic malignancies, and collagen vascular disease, but a familial form has been described.[24] Treatment options include plasmapheresis, fibrinolytics, and stanozolol, an anabolic steroid with fibrinolytic capacity.[25]

THROMBOTIC PURPURA

HEPARIN NECROSIS

Cutaneous reactions to heparin administration vary greatly, ranging from an urticarial rash, likely resulting from histamine release, to purpuric plaques with cutaneous ulceration or necrosis.[26] Cases have been described after both subcutaneous and intravenous administration secondary to a delayed-type hypersensitivity reaction to the medication, with skin lesions appearing within 1 to 2 weeks after treatment initiation.[27,28] Development of cutaneous lesions secondary to heparin therapy is closely associated with heparin-induced thrombocytopenia (HIT), which also can manifest as necrotic purpuric lesions after heparin therapy. Because HIT results from generation of heparin-dependent platelet-activating antibodies,[29] the platelet count should be measured in any patient developing a skin reaction following heparin initiation.

WARFARIN NECROSIS

The development of painful erythematous plaques and nodules is a potential complication of warfarin (Coumadin) therapy. These plaques and nodules can rapidly become hemorrhagic and necrotic, leading to large areas of infarction with subsequent skin sloughing.[30] Presence of a black eschar in the central area of necrosis is common. Warfarin-induced necrosis is more common in women. It has a prevalence between 0.01 and 0.1 percent and typically presents 3 to 10 days after treatment initiation.[31,32] Late-onset warfarin necrosis has been reported in a patient who developed palpable purpura with rapid progression to hemorrhagic bullae on her abdomen and thighs 56 days after initiation of warfarin treatment for heart valve replacement.[33] Although warfarin necrosis tends to develop in areas of greatest fat deposition, such as the breasts, thighs, and buttocks, acral areas including the penis, fingers, and toes also can be involved (see Color Plate XXV-6).[34] Warfarin necrosis results from the rapidly decreased level of the vitamin K-dependent natural anticoagulation factor protein C. Microvascular occlusion of dermal and subcutaneous vessels is seen on histologic analysis. The mechanism of thrombi formation is unclear. However, immunohistochemical evaluation of these lesions revealed the presence of tissue necrosis factor and induction of endothelial cell adhesion molecules.[28] Treatment involves prompt cessation of warfarin therapy and occasionally surgical intervention if gangrenous tissue develops.[35] Methicillin-resistant *Staphylococcus aureus* infection of widely involved areas of warfarin necrosis can lead to fatal septic shock.[33] Because patients with protein C deficiency have increased susceptibility to warfarin necrosis, heparin should be administered prior to initiation of warfarin therapy in this patient population.[36]

PROTEIN C AND S DEFICIENCY

Congenital and acquired deficiencies of either protein C or S can lead to palpable necrotic purpura and ecchymosis.[37–41] Erythematous purpuric lesions associated with homozygous protein C deficiency can develop within hours of birth and can rapidly progress to hemorrhagic necrotic lesions (see Chap. 122). Acquired deficiencies of protein C have been associated with autoantibodies to protein C, antibiotics administration, and liver disease.[42] Acquired protein S deficiency occurring after varicella infection is associated with generation of anti-protein S Igs.[43,44] Protein repletion with fresh-frozen plasma is effective as initial treatment for protein C or S deficiency to help clear cutaneous lesions and venous occlusion, whereas lifelong warfarin treatment is used for recurrence prevention.[36,45,46] Liver transplantation also has been successful.[47,48]

PAROXYSMAL NOCTURNAL HEMOGLOBINURIA

Paroxysmal nocturnal hemoglobinuria is a clonal hematopoietic disorder resulting in defective production of glycosylphosphatidylinositol-anchored cell surface proteins, including at least two responsible for regulating complement binding to the erythrocyte membrane (see Chap. 38).[49] Cutaneous manifestations of the disorder are secondary to its associated hypercoagulable state and include palpable purpura, ecchymosis, necrosis, and hemorrhagic bullae.[50,51] A rare association with pyoderma gangrenosum has been described.[52] Histologic analysis may show evidence of microvascular fibrin thrombi.[51]

ANTIPHOSPHOLIPID SYNDROME

Antiphospholipid syndrome is a disease characterized by a hypercoagulable state associated with the presence of antibodies against phospholipids, such as anticardiolipin and lupus anticoagulant (see Chap. 123).[53] Approximately 40 percent of patients with antiphospholipid syndrome present with cutaneous lesions secondary to both large-vessel and microvascular thrombosis.[54] Skin manifestations include ecchymosis, livedo reticularis, ulcerations, bullae, and extensive cutaneous necrosis (see Color Plates XXV-7 and XXV-8).[54,55] Acute bullous purpura rarely occurs concurrently.[56]

LIVEDOID VASCULITIS

Livedoid vasculitis was first described by Bard and Winkelmann in 1967. Livedoid vasculitis, also known as segmental hyalinizing vasculitis, is a chronic disorder characterized by the development of lower

extremity ulceration with subsequent healing to atrophie blanche, ivory-white stellate scars commonly surrounded by hyperpigmented areas, and telangiectasia (see Color Plate XXV-9).[57] These lesions result from small-vessel thrombi, as early histologic analysis shows fibrin deposition. The condition evolves into hyalinization of lower dermal vessels accompanied by epidermal atrophy.[58] Although livedoid vasculitis most commonly is idiopathic, it has been associated with polyarteritis nodosum, antiphospholipid syndrome, and systemic lupus erythematous.[59,60] No treatment modality has been consistently beneficial, but common therapies include antiplatelet medications, glucocorticoids, and dapsone. Ketanserin, an S2 serotoninergic receptor blocker, psoralen plus ultraviolet-A therapy, and intravenous Igs have each been successful.[58]

EMBOLIC PURPURA

CHOLESTEROL CRYSTAL EMBOLI

Cholesterol crystal emboli, also known as atheroemboli, are responsible for a syndrome characterized by lower extremity pain and a mottled or net-like red to blue discoloration termed *livedo reticularis*, but with preservation of peripheral pulses. Livedo reticularis is the most common cutaneous finding, but other common findings include purpura, ulcerations, cyanosis, and gangrene (see Color Plates XXV-10 and XXV-11).[61] Clinical signs and symptoms include fever, myalgias, altered mental state, acutely elevated blood pressure, elevated erythrocyte sedimentation rate, eosinophilia, and acute renal failure. Cholesterol crystal emboli usually dislodge from atherosclerotic lesions in the descending aorta, which explains the propensity for lower extremity findings. Peripheral pulses are not decreased because cholesterol crystal emboli occlude only smaller vessels. The syndrome is more prevalent in older men and has been associated with vascular procedures and anticoagulant use. A definitive diagnosis can be made if birefringent cholesterol crystals are found within blood vessel lumen in the absence of vasculitis.[62] No effective treatment exists for cholesterol crystal emboli. Antithrombotics should be avoided because they may exacerbate the condition. Supportive care includes hydration, control of elevated blood pressure, and renal dialysis to lessen the potential for end-organ damage.

CUTANEOUS CALCIPHYLAXIS

Calciphylaxis is characterized by the formation of cutaneous, subcutaneous, and vascular calcifications most commonly seen in patients with end-stage renal disease. Calcification of small- and medium-size blood vessels results from the development of secondary hyperparathyroidism, a common occurrence in these patients. Approximately 4 percent of hemodialysis-dependent patients suffer from calciphylaxis, and less than half of these patients survive 5 years after diagnosis.[63] Risk factors associated with calciphylaxis include smoking, female gender, chronic alkalosis as a result of renal dialysis, diabetes mellitus, and hyperlipidemia. Prolonged glucocorticoid use in rheumatoid arthritis patients may contribute to cutaneous calciphylaxis without associated renal disease.[64] The skin lesions initially present as reddish-purple plaques but soon evolve to tender, gangrenous ulcers or reticular hemorrhagic necrosis. Treatment often involves a combination of medical and surgical intervention. Diphosphonates, a low-phosphate diet, and antibiotics for secondary infection have been successful.[63]

EMBOLI FROM ATRIAL MYXOMA

Acral purpuric lesions can occur secondary to emboli arising from left atrial myxomas.[65] The lesions may develop cutaneous necrosis, splinter hemorrhages, and palpable purpura. Cyanosis, livedo reticularis, and lower extremity ulcerations can occur.

ARTHROPOD BITES

Bites from bed bugs *Cimex lectularius* can give rise to localized purpuric macules or papules, whereas bites from kissing bugs *Reduviidae* often manifest as urticaria with hemorrhagic bulla.[66] Cutaneous findings after envenomation from the brown recluse spider *Loxosceles reclusa* include purpuric necrosis with surrounding erythema evolving to ulcer formation. Lesions from brown recluse spider bites tend to spread in a gravitationally dependent fashion.

PALPABLE AND NONPALPABLE, INFLAMMATORY PURPURIC LESIONS (TABLE 114-2)

PYODERMA GANGRENOSUM

Pyoderma gangrenosum is an idiopathic skin eruption characterized by tender, fluctuant nodules with surrounding erythema that spread peripherally and ulcerate. A raised, violaceous rim surrounds the ulcers with necrotic pustules at their center (see Color Plate XXV-12).[67] Once considered pathognomonic for ulcerative colitis, an increasing number of systemic disorders have been found to be associated with pyoderma gangrenosum, including several rheumatologic conditions, hematologic disorders, and solid tumors.[68] Although pyoderma gangrenosum is classified into four main clinical variants (ulcerative, pustular, bullous, vegetative), all share the histopathologic finding of a central necrotizing, neutrophilic infiltration, surrounded by a perivascular and intramural lymphocytic infiltration. Treatment of pyoderma gangrenosum involves wound care and systemic immunosuppressants, such as glucocorticoids and/or cyclosporine.[69]

SWEET SYNDROME

Acute, febrile neutrophilic dermatosis, also known as Sweet syndrome, is characterized by the acute manifestation of painful erythematous and violaceous papules, nodules, and plaques accompanied by fever and elevated neutrophil count.[70] These papules, which most commonly appear on the face, neck, and upper extremities, tend to coalesce, forming well-circumscribed, irregularly bordered plaques (see Color Plate XXV-13). In addition to the skin, a number of organ systems can be involved, including the central nervous system, kidneys, lungs, and bones.[71] Although classically more prominent in women 30 to 50 years old, the syndrome also is seen in young adults and children. The development of Sweet syndrome is associated with respiratory and urinary infections, pregnancy, malignancy, medications, and inflamma-

TABLE 114-2   PALPABLE AND NONPALPABLE, INFLAMMATORY PURPURIC LESIONS

A. Pyoderma gangrenosum
B. Sweet syndrome
C. Behçet disease
D. Serum sickness
E. Henoch-Schönlein purpura
F. Infections
G. Waldenström hypergammaglobulinemia (see Table 114-1)
H. Erythema multiforme
I. Cutaneous polyarteritis nodosum
J. Paraneoplastic vasculitis
K. Drug-induced vasculitis
L. Antineutrophil cytoplasmic antibody-associated vasculitidis
   1. Wegener granulomatosis
   2. Churg-Strauss syndrome
   3. Microscopic angiitis

tory bowel disease. Histologic analysis shows a distinct neutrophilic infiltrate in the superficial dermis with dermal edema. Although systemic glucocorticoids are the preferred treatment, clofazimine, dapsone, indomethacin, and cyclosporine also have been successful.[72]

BEHÇET DISEASE

Behçet disease is classified as a neutrophilic dermatosis, but Behçet disease is an inflammatory disorder that affects multiple organ systems. Clinical features include cutaneous manifestations, such as palpable purpura, infiltrative erythema, and papular/pustular lesions; oral mucosal and genital ulcers; arthralgias; and gastrointestinal and central nervous system involvement.[73] Genetic studies have shown an association between Behçet disease and the human leukocyte antigen (HLA) B51.[74] Interestingly, histologic analysis commonly shows leukocytoclastic or lymphocytic vasculitis, which has prompted some investigators to suggest Behçet disease should be categorized as a vasculitis rather than a neutrophilic dermatosis.

SERUM SICKNESS

Serum sickness refers to the systemic manifestation of immune complex formation and deposition. Cutaneous lesions such as urticarial and morbilliform eruptions predominate, but palpable purpura and erythema multiforme (EM) also are often seen. Serum sickness associated with infection or medical therapy can result in specific characteristic lesions. For example, use of antithymocyte globulin for marrow failure causes 75 percent of patients to develop serpiginous bands of erythema and purpura on the sides of their hands and feet (see Color Plate XXV-14).[75] These characteristic lesions consistently appear 1 to 2 days prior to the onset of systemic symptoms of serum sickness, which include fever and malaise. Analysis of biopsies by direct immunofluorescence reveals deposition of IgM, IgE, IgA, and C3.[76] The deposits appear to activate neutrophils, leading to release of lysozymal enzymes and, in turn, provoking dermal vasculitis.[77]

HENOCH-SCHÖNLEIN PURPURA

Henoch-Schönlein purpura was first described by Dr. William Heberden in 1801.[78] Henoch-Schönlein purpura is a predominantly pediatric vasculitic syndrome characterized by the acute onset of abdominal pain and lower extremity eruption of diffuse urticarial plaques and palpable purpura. Schönlein later recognized in 1837 the association of the syndrome with arthritis. Henoch reported the association of the syndrome with gastrointestinal manifestations in 1874 and renal involvement in 1899. Henoch-Schönlein purpura is the most common vasculitis occurring in children. It predominantly affects patients 2 to 20 years old; 90 percent of patients are younger than 10 years.[79] In pediatric cases, boys are more commonly affected than girls (2:1); however, adult males and females are affected equally. The etiology of the syndrome remains unclear, but many environmental triggers have been associated with its onset. Reported triggers include viral (hepatitis B virus, HCV, parvovirus B19, HIV) and bacterial (*Streptococcus* species, *S. aureus*, *Salmonella* species) infections in children, and medications (nonsteroidal antiinflammatory drugs [NSAIDs], angiotensin-converting enzyme inhibitors, antibiotics), food allergies, and insect bites in adults.[80] A specific genetic risk factor for the disorder is complement factor 4 (C4) deficiency.[81] Leukocytoclastic vasculitis as a feature of Henoch-Schönlein purpura is the result of immune complex and complement deposition on vessel walls. Immunohistochemical detection of IgA immune complexes and increased serum IgA levels are common laboratory findings in these patients.[82] Furthermore, complement activation in these patients leads to formation of the cytolytic complex C5b-9, the membrane attack complex.[83] Elevated levels of thrombomodulin, tissue plasminogen activator, and plasminogen activator inhibitor-1 correlate with endothelial injury and fibrinolytic activity in the acute phase of the disease.[84] Increased tumor necrosis factor, interleukin (IL)-1, and IL-6 serum levels and biopsies of lesions suggest a role for these cytokines in disease pathogenesis.[85]

Henoch-Schönlein purpura is a multiorgan system syndrome, but its most characteristic features are its cutaneous manifestations. Skin eruptions often begin acutely as urticarial papules and plaques evolving to palpable and nonpalpable purpura over the lower extremities and buttocks (see Color Plate XXV-15). Other common clinical features include nephritis, arthritis, and abdominal pain.[86] Renal involvement is more common in adults than in children, but the long-term prognosis is similar; approximately 90 percent of children and adults recover renal function.[87,88] Testicular pain and scrotal swelling can occur.[89] The white cell count, platelet count, and C-reactive protein levels usually are elevated in pediatric patients.[90]

Henoch-Schönlein purpura usually is self-limited, and treatment is supportive. Use of immunosuppressive drugs, such as glucocorticoids, are reserved for patients with renal involvement.[78] Persistent purpura, severe abdominal symptoms, and diminished plasma coagulation factor XIII activity are predictive of renal involvement and should prompt initiation of glucocorticoid therapy at the onset of disease in appropriate patients.[91] The self-limited course of the disorder may result from enhanced apoptosis of offending immune cells that reduces the severity of the acute inflammatory response.[92]

INFECTIONS

Analysis of skin lesions associated with an infection can provide important hints that help identify the responsible pathogen. Purpura associated with infection may result from (1) direct invasion of vessels with subsequent vascular occlusion, (2) septic emboli, (3) vascular effects of toxins, and (4) immune complex formation.[93] The morphology of these purpuric lesions may be nonspecific; however, several pathogens lead to characteristic findings.

BACTERIAL INFECTIONS

Gram-positive and gram-negative bacterial infections give rise to a large array of purpuric patterns, depending on the bacterial virulence and the patient's immune status. Purpuric patterns range from simple macules and papules to ulcers and necrosis. Purpura fulminans, a syndrome consisting of fever, disseminated intravascular coagulation, acral purpura, and hypotension, occurs as a result of bacterial sepsis (see Chap. 121). Although purpura fulminans most commonly is seen in immunocompromised hosts, an association between purpura fulminans and bacterial pathogens in immunocompetent hosts has been described.[94] Similarly characteristic in immunocompromised patients, ecthyma gangrenosum is seen with gram-negative sepsis resulting from *Pseudomonas aeruginosa, Klebsiella* species, *or Escherichia coli* infection (see Color Plate XXV-16). These cutaneous lesions begin as erythematous or purpuric macules that evolve into erythematous plaques with surrounding purpura and progress rapidly to hemorrhagic vesicles or bullae surrounded by a halo of normal skin with an erythematous rim.[95] The vesicle or bullae can rupture, leaving an ulcer with a necrotic center. Facial purpura and livedo reticularis may be seen arising during fulminant pneumococcal infection in asplenic patients.[96]

Twenty percent of febrile hospitalized children with petechiae had invasive bacterial infections secondary to pathogens, including *Neisseria meningitidis, Haemophilus influenzae* type B, and *Streptococcus pneumoniae*.[97] Sepsis secondary to *N. meningitidis* can produce a characteristic pattern of purpuric lesions. Erythematous papules can quickly progress to numerous petechiae combined with violaceous reticular purpuric lesions (see Color Plate XXV-17).[47] Although whether these lesions are a direct effect of endotoxin on the vasculature or invasion of blood vessels by the pathogen is unclear, the finding of petechiae in a patient with symptoms and signs of bacterial meningitis is predictive of meningococcal meningitis.[98] Approximately 7 percent of children with fever and petechiae seen in emergency rooms are diagnosed with meningococcemia.[99] Cutaneous ischemic lesions, such as symmetric peripheral gangrene, may emerge secondary to fibrin deposition. Adult patients with purpura fulminans as a result of meningococcemia have significantly depressed antithrombin III and protein C and S levels, which may explain the tendency toward fibrin deposition. Rapid clinical improvement has been seen in meningococcemia patients treated with antithrombin III or protein C concentrates.[100-102]

Borrelia burgdorferi infection gives rise to erythema migrans, the characteristic lesion of Lyme disease. Although this lesion classically is a nonpurpuric erythematous expanding plaque, it can include a central hemorrhagic bulla (see Color Plate XXV-18). Other cutaneous findings associated with *B. burgdorferi* infection include papular urticaria, Henoch-Schönlein-like purpura, and morphea.[103]

VIRAL INFECTIONS

Purpuric lesions can be a manifestation of a viral infection. The adenovirus and enterovirus families of viruses have been associated with development of fever and petechiae in children.[104] Parvovirus B19 can produce a syndrome of petechiae or purpuric papules progressing to confluent purpuric papules or plaques in a glove and sock distribution. In addition to the cutaneous findings, the "gloves and socks syndrome" is characterized by fever and occasionally leukopenia.[105] Purpura in the axilla and chest has also been described during parvovirus B19 infection (see Color Plate XXV-19).[106] Histopathologic analysis of these purpuric lesions show an evolution from superficial perivascular lymphocytic infiltrate to a dermatitis accompanied by necrotic keratinocytes and hemorrhage.[107] Another virus that causes purpuric lesions is the Hantaan virus. The Hantaan virus causes a syndrome of hemorrhagic fever and renal failure accompanied by headache, vomiting, and cutaneous and mucosal petechiae and ecchymosis.[108]

FUNGAL INFECTIONS

Use of immunosuppressive agents for minimizing organ transplantation rejection or treating malignancy is increasing.[109] In these settings, disseminated or locally invasive fungal infections can give rise to petechiae and hemorrhagic necrosis. Common pathogens in disseminated disease include *Candida* (see Color Plate XXV-20), *Aspergillus* (see Color Plate XXV-21), *Histoplasma*, and *Fusarium*.[110] Disseminated candidiasis can cause ecthyma gangrenosum in immunocompromised patients. A skin biopsy obtained in these cases can be diagnostic.[111]

PARASITIC INFECTIONS

Immunocompromised patients are at risk for developing purpuric lesions secondary to parasitic infections, such as strongyloidiasis. Disseminated strongyloidiasis, characterized by larva currens, a serpiginous urticarial eruption caused by the migration of filariform larvae through the dermis, in immunocompromised patients can be fatal.[112] Cutaneous involvement includes widespread reticular purpura involving the arms, legs, and abdomen (see Color Plate XXV-22).[113]

RICKETTSIAL INFECTIONS

Infections caused by *Rickettsia* species can lead to purpuric lesions because of their direct invasion of endothelial cell cytoplasm and nuclei. This situation is followed by vascular medial and intimal necrosis and subsequent thrombosis and hemorrhage.[93] For example, cutaneous lesions in Rocky Mountain spotted fever range from petechiae (see Color Plate XXV-23) to hemorrhagic necrosis (see Color Plate XXV-24).

ERYTHEMA MULTIFORME

EM is a cutaneous disorder characterized by the development of crops of well-demarcated, erythematous target lesions with central clearing most commonly triggered by infection or drug exposure (see Color Plate XXV-25). The severity of this disorder ranges from mild, referred to as *EM minor*, to severe, referred to as *EM major*, or Stevens-Johnson syndrome.[114] EM can be triggered by a number of viruses (herpes simplex, mycoplasma, adenovirus, cytomegalovirus) and medications (sulfonamides, penicillins, phenylbutazone, phenytoin, NSAIDS).[115,116] A cellular allergic reaction coupled with impaired histamine metabolism resulting from decreased histamine-N-methyltransferase activity may be responsible for target lesion formation.[117] Treatment for mild cases is supportive, whereas glucocorticoid use often is warranted in severe cases.

CUTANEOUS POLYARTERITIS NODOSUM

Classic polyarteritis nodosum is a systemic small-size and medium-size vessel vasculitis that most commonly involves the skin, heart, liver, and kidneys. A relatively benign cutaneous form lacks significant systemic involvement.[118] Tender erythematous nodules with occasional retiform purpura localized on both upper and lower extremities and the face are characteristic (see Color Plate XXV-26). Findings in the benign cutaneous form include arthralgias, arthritis, myalgias, and fever. Histologic analysis of involved skin shows deep dermal arterial necrosis with infiltration of neutrophils and eosinophils and fibrin deposition. NSAIDs and prednisone, alone or in combination, are effective treatment. Cases of cutaneous polyarteritis nodosum can progress to systemic disease.[119] Thus, long-term followup of patients diagnosed with the benign cutaneous form is important.[120]

PARANEOPLASTIC VASCULITIS

Cutaneous paraneoplastic vasculitis is associated with hematologic neoplasia[121] and less commonly with carcinomas of the lung, colon, breast, and cervix.[122–124] Cutaneous manifestations include petechiae, urticaria, and palpable purpura and often are intensely pruritic. In lymphoproliferative and myeloproliferative disorders, the lesions often precede the development of the malignancy by an average of 10 months (see Color Plate XXV-27).[125] Histologic analysis of these lesions shows necrotizing leukocytoclastic vasculitis with neutrophilic infiltration.

DRUG-INDUCED VASCULITIS

A long list of drugs reportedly cause a vasculitis resulting in erythematous purpuric lesions, including allopurinol, cefaclor, hematopoietic colony-stimulating factors, D-penicillamine, furosemide (see Color Plate XXV-28), hydralazine, isotretinoin, methotrexate, phenytoin, minocycline, and propylthiouracil.[126]

ANTINEUTROPHIL CYTOPLASMIC ANTIGEN-ASSOCIATED VASCULITIDES

WEGENER GRANULOMATOSIS

Wegener granulomatosis, a small- to medium-vessel vasculitis most commonly affecting the upper and lower respiratory tracts and kidneys, is strongly associated with the development of antineutrophil cytoplasmic antibodies (ANCAs). Skin involvement has been reported in 35 to 50 percent of cases.[127] Cutaneous eruptions include a com-

bination of palpable purpura, oral ulcers, and erythematous cutaneous and subcutaneous nodules (see Color Plate XXV-29). Necrotizing vasculitis, palisading granulomas, and granulomatous vasculitis are characteristic findings on histologic analysis of involved skin.[128]

CHURG-STRAUSS SYNDROME

Churg-Strauss syndrome is characterized by granulomatous inflammation in the lungs associated with asthma and eosinophilia. Cutaneous findings such as ulcers, palpable purpura, cutaneous nodules, and infarcts of fingers and toes may develop.[129] Laboratory features include eosinophilia, elevated IgE levels, and a positive ANCA. Histologic analysis commonly reveals granulomatous inflammation and necrotizing vasculitis of small- to medium-size blood vessels.[128]

MICROSCOPIC ANGIITIS

As opposed to Wegener granulomatosis and Churg-Strauss syndrome, microscopic angiitis is a predominantly small-vessel vasculitis that is associated with ANCA. It differs from other small-vessel vasculitidis, such as cryoglobulinemic vasculitis and Henoch-Schönlein purpura, in its absence or paucity of immune complex deposition.[130] Clinical features include necrotizing glomerulonephritis, pulmonary capillaritis, and cutaneous eruptions such as palpable purpura and nodules.[128] Histologic assessment shows necrotizing vasculitis of small vessels and minimal, if any, immune complex deposition.

NONPALPABLE, NONINFLAMMATORY, ROUND PURPURIC LESIONS (TABLE 114-3)

INCREASED TRANSMURAL PRESSURE GRADIENT

Acute increases in vascular transmural pressure gradients lead to extravasation of red blood cells resulting in nonpalpable, noninflammatory petechiae and larger purpuric lesions. One cause is dramatically increased intravascular pressure, as seen in postictal purpura,[131] weightlifting,[132] postemesis facial purpura,[133] prolonged Valsalva maneuver, and childbirth. Acute decreases in extravascular negative pressure, referred to as *suction purpura*, resulting from gas mask, kissing, or cupping can increase this gradient, resulting in well-circumscribed lesions shaped like the causative device.[134] Development of petechiae in mountain climbers has been described, presumably as a result of significantly reduced atmospheric pressures at high elevations.[135] In

TABLE 114-3   NONPALPABLE, NONINFLAMMATORY, ROUND PURPURIC LESIONS[a]

A. Increased transmural pressure gradient
B. Drug reactions
C. Coagulation disorders
D. Decreased vessel integrity without trauma
   1. Senile purpura
   2. Excess glucocorticoid (Cushing syndrome, glucocorticoid treatment)
   3. Scurvy—vitamin C deficiency
   4. Systemic amyloidosis
   5. Connective tissue disorders (Ehlers-Danlos syndrome, pseudoxanthoma elasticum)
   6. Mitochondrial encephalomyopathy with lactic acidosis and stroke-like syndrome (MELAS)
E. Trauma
F. Waldenström hypergammaglobulinemic purpura (see Table 114-1)
G. Schamberg disease (progressive pigmentary dermatosis)

[a] This category includes the purpura resulting from quantitative and qualitative abnormalities of platelets and of coagulation proteins, which are discussed in this text in "Hemostasis and Thrombosis."

addition, lower extremity venous incompetence, predominantly at the medial ankle, can result in macules or patches of yellowish-brown purpura. Poor clearing of hemosiderin, a red blood cell breakdown product, leading to unsightly persistent lesions occurs for unclear reasons.[136]

THROMBOCYTOPENIAS

Idiopathic thrombocytopenic purpura,[137] thrombotic thrombocytopenic purpura,[138] and other thrombocytopenias (see Chaps. 110, 112, 113, and 124) lead to petechiae and purpura, which are generally gravity dependent or seen at sites of minimal trauma.

DRUG REACTIONS

A large list of medications reportedly result in vasculitic and nonvasculitic purpuric eruptions.[139] Nevertheless, any drug being used by a patient with a purpuric lesion should be regarded with suspicion. These lesions most often appear to result from a hypersensitivity reaction to a drug.

COAGULATION DISORDERS

A large number of disorders manifest with increased bruising, including but not limited to anticoagulant use, vitamin K deficiency, and poor hepatic function (see Chap. 109).

DECREASED VESSEL INTEGRITY WITHOUT TRAUMA

SENILE PURPURA
Synonymous with actinic purpura, senile purpura refers to the easy bruising seen in the aged, commonly appearing on the dorsal aspect of the hands and forearms (see Color Plates XXV-30 and XXV-31). Degeneration of skin extracellular matrix components that leaves dermal capillaries unsupported and vulnerable to shearing injuries is a major cause.[140] A correlation between senile purpura and zinc deficiency has been reported.[141]

EXCESS GLUCOCORTICOID
The presence of excess endogenous (Cushing syndrome) or exogenous (therapeutic use) glucocorticoids can result in dermal thinning and vessel fragility.[142] Consequently, nonpalpable purpuric lesions tend to arise after slight or even undetected trauma.

SCURVY–VITAMIN C DEFICIENCY
Vitamin C (ascorbic acid) deficiency is rare but can occur in cases of severe malnutrition. The deficiency disrupts normal collagen production, resulting in blood vessel fragility leading to parafollicular petechiae and larger purpuric plaques, most commonly on the lower extremities (see Color Plate XXV-32).[143] Cutaneous features include follicular hyperkeratosis, poor wound healing, and bent or corkscrew-shaped body hairs.[144] Although the deficiency usually is diagnosed clinically, plasma vitamin C levels can confirm the diagnosis in atypical cases. The treatment is vitamin C administration.

SYSTEMIC AMYLOIDOSIS
Systemic amyloidosis results from clonal proliferation of plasma cells leading to subsequent deposition of modified Ig light chain in vital organs (see Chaps. 100 and 101).[145] It can present as a primary disorder or as a consequence of myeloma. Waxy, purpuric cutaneous and mucocutaneous lesions result when light-chain aggregates deposit in dermal blood vessels (see Color Plates XXV-33 and XXV-34). Palmo-digital purpura has been reported as the sole cutaneous finding in myeloma-associated systemic amyloidosis.[146] A localized form, called *primary cutaneous amyloidosis*, caused by local dermal infiltration of plasma cells can occur in which skin lesions are largely indistinguishable from those seen in the systemic form of the disease.[145] Such skin infiltrates reduce vascular integrity, increasing the likelihood of purpura development after increased intramural vascular pressure. Classically, this condition has been described as *postproctoscopic periorbital purpura*.

CONNECTIVE TISSUE DISORDERS
Ehlers-Danlos Syndrome This disorder is a rare autosomal dominant syndrome that results from a mutation of a gene in collagen synthesis, leading to loss of skin elasticity, joint hypermobility, and systemic organ tissue fragility. Cutaneous findings include thin skin and a tendency to develop nonpalpable purpuric lesions as a result of dermal blood vessel fragility (see Color Plate XXV-35).[147] A correlation has been reported between increased thumb flexibility and unexplained bleeding tendencies, suggesting that many of these patients have a modified form of Ehlers-Danlos syndrome.[148]

Pseudoxanthoma Elasticum Pseudoxanthoma elasticum is a genetic disorder characterized by mineralization and fragmentation of elastin in the skin, retina, and blood vessels. This autosomally inherited disease is associated with a mutation in the ABCC6 gene, an ATP-binding cassette transporter, which may play an important role in connective tissue turnover.[149] Cutaneous lesions include small white or yellow papules or larger confluent areas of purpura or necrosis.

Mitochondrial Encephalomyopathy with Lactic Acidosis and Stroke-like Episodes Syndrome Nonpalpable purpuric lesions on the palms and soles can occur in mitochondrial encephalomyopathy with lactic acidosis and stroke-like episodes (MELAS) syndrome.[150] This disorder, one of a family of mitochondrial encephalomyopathies, is associated with a mutation in the gene for a mitochondrial transfer RNA.[151] Skin manifestations include hypertrichosis and ichthyosis. Transmission electron microscopy of involved skin reveals evidence of endothelial degeneration and morphologically irregular mitochondria.

TRAUMA

Focal ecchymosis and other purpuric lesions can result from trauma. Characteristic patterns of purpuric lesions are clues used in forensic examinations. For example, traumatic asphyxia is characterized by cervicofacial cyanosis and swelling, petechiae, and subconjunctival hemorrhage, usually resulting from strangulation or crush injury to the upper aspect of the thorax.[152,153] Factitious purpura, often related to deliberate suction purpura, should be considered in the differential diagnosis of purpura in situations where no organic disorder is found.[154] Furthermore, care should be taken in distinguishing a subungal hematoma from a subungal melanoma or nevi (see Color Plate XXV-36). These entities can be distinguished by inspection of the proximal nail fold which should be clear of pigmentation in the case of subungual hematoma.

SCHAMBERG DISEASE

Schamberg disease, also referred to as progressive pigmentary purpura, is the most common of a family of benign pigmented dermatoses. It is characterized by the development of "cayenne pepper" petechiae on a background of hyperpigmented oval patches often seen in tibial regions bilaterally (see Color Plate XXV-37).[155] Although the etiology remains unclear, histologic analysis reveals capillaritis with a perivascular infiltrate of dendritic cells, suggesting this disease involves a cell-mediated immune response. Extravasated red blood cells and hemosiderin-laden macrophage are commonly seen. Although Schamberg disease usually follows a chronic benign course, progression to cutaneous T cell lymphoma has been reported in young males.

REFERENCES

1. Piette WW: The differential diagnosis of purpura from a morphologic perspective. *Adv Dermatol* 9:3, discussion 24, 1994.
2. Piette WW: Hematologic diseases, in *Fitzpatrick's Dermatology in General Medicine*, 6th ed, edited by IM Freedburg, AZ Eisen, K Wolff, KF Austen, LA Goldsmith, SI Katz, p 1523. McGraw-Hill, New York, 2003.
3. Langlois NE, Gresham GA: The ageing of bruises: A review and study of the colour changes with time. *Forensic Sci Int* 50:227, 1991.
4. Stephenson T: Ageing of bruising in children. *J R Soc Med* 90:312, 1997.
5. Winfield JB: Cryoglobulinemia. *Hum Pathol* 14:350, 1983.
6. Feiner HD: Pathology of dysproteinemia: Light chain amyloidosis, non-amyloid immunoglobulin deposition disease, cryoglobulinemia syndromes, and macroglobulinemia of Waldenstrom. *Hum Pathol* 19:1255, 1988.
7. Agnello V, Romain PL: Mixed cryoglobulinemia secondary to hepatitis C virus infection. *Rheum Dis Clin North Am* 22:1, 1996.
8. Dispenzieri A: Symptomatic cryoglobulinemia. *Curr Treat Options Oncol* 1:105, 2000.
9. Agnello V, Mecucci C, Casato M: Regression of splenic lymphoma after treatment of hepatitis C virus infection. *N Engl J Med* 347:2168, 2002.
10. Casato M, Mecucci C, Agnello V, et al: Regression of lymphoproliferative disorder after treatment for hepatitis C virus infection in a patient with partial trisomy 3, Bcl-2 overexpression, and type II cryoglobulinemia. *Blood* 99:2259, 2002.
11. Gorevic PD, Kassab HJ, Levo Y, et al: Mixed cryoglobulinemia: Clinical aspects and long-term follow-up of 40 patients. *Am J Med* 69:287, 1980.
12. Cohen SJ, Pittelkow MR, Su WP: Cutaneous manifestations of cryoglobulinemia: Clinical and histopathologic study of seventy-two patients. *J Am Acad Dermatol* 25:21, 1991.
13. Waldenström J: Clinical methods for determination of hyperproteinemia and their practical value for diagnosis. *Nord Med* 20:2288, 1943.
14. Ferreiro JE, Pasarin G, Quesada R, Gould E: Benign hypergammaglobulinemic purpura of Waldenstrom associated with Sjogren's syndrome. Case report and review of immunologic aspects. *Am J Med* 81:734, 1986.
15. Finder KA, McCollough ML, Dixon SL, et al: Hypergammaglobulinemic purpura of Waldenstrom. *J Am Acad Dermatol* 23:669, 1990.
16. Tan E, Ng SK, Tan SH, Wong GC: Hypergammaglobulinaemic purpura presenting as reticulate purpura. *Clin Exp Dermatol* 24:469, 1999.
17. Malaviya AN, Kaushik P, Budhiraja S, et al: Hypergammaglobulinemic purpura of Waldenstrom: Report of 3 cases with a short review. *Clin Exp Rheumatol* 18:518, 2000.
18. Al-Mayouf SM, Ghonaium A, Bahabri S: Hypergammaglobulinaemic purpura associated with IgG subclass imbalance and recurrent infection. *Clin Rheumatol* 19:499, 2000.
19. Oosterkamp HM, van der Pijl H, Derksen J, et al: Arthritis and hypergammaglobulinemic purpura in hypersensitivity pneumonitis. *Am J Med* 100:478, 1996.
20. Miyagawa S, Fukumoto T, Kanauchi M, et al: Hypergammaglobulinaemic purpura of Waldenstrom and Ro/SSA autoantibodies. *Br J Dermatol* 134:919, 1996.
21. Stone GC, Wall BA, Oppliger IR, et al: A vasculopathy with deposition of lambda light chain crystals. *Ann Intern Med* 110:275, 1989.
22. Usuda H, Emura I, Naito M: Crystal globulin-induced vasculopathy accompanying ischemic intestinal lesions of a patient with myeloma. *Pathol Int* 46:165, 1996.
23. Sankarasubbaiyan S, Scott G, Holley JL: Cryofibrinogenemia: An addition to the differential diagnosis of calciphylaxis in end-stage renal disease. *Am J Kidney Dis* 32:494, 1998.
24. van Geest AJ, van Dooren-Greebe RJ, Andriessen MP, et al: Familial primary cryofibrinogenemia. *J Eur Acad Dermatol Venereol* 12:47, 1999.
25. Helfman T, Falanga V: Stanozolol as a novel therapeutic agent in dermatology. *J Am Acad Dermatol* 33:254, 1995.
26. Wutschert R, Piletta P, Bounameaux H: Adverse skin reactions to low molecular weight heparins: Frequency, management and prevention. *Drug Saf* 20:515, 1999.
27. Arnold J, Cohen H: Heparin-induced skin necrosis. *Br J Haematol* 111:992, 2000.
28. Hermes B, Haas N, Henz BM: Immunopathological events of adverse cutaneous reactions to coumarin and heparin. *Acta Derm Venereol* 77:35, 1997.
29. Chong BH: Heparin-induced thrombocytopenia. *J Thromb Haemost* 1:1471, 2003.
30. Horn JR, Danziger LH, Davis RJ: Warfarin-induced skin necrosis: Report of four cases. *Am J Hosp Pharm* 38:1763, 1981.
31. Chan YC, Valenti D, Mansfield AO, Stansby G: Warfarin induced skin necrosis. *Br J Surg* 87:266, 2000.
32. Harenberg J, Hoffmann U, Huhle G, et al: Cutaneous reactions to anticoagulants. Recognition and management. *Am J Clin Dermatol* 2:69, 2001.
33. Scarff CE, Baker C, Hill P, Foley P: Late-onset warfarin necrosis. *Australas J Dermatol* 43:202, 2002.
34. Stone MS, Rosen T: Acral purpura: An unusual sign of coumarin necrosis. *J Am Acad Dermatol* 14:797, 1986.
35. Cole MS, Minifee PK, Wolma FJ: Coumarin necrosis—A review of the literature. *Surgery* 103:271, 1988.
36. Segel GB, Francis CA: Anticoagulant proteins in childhood venous and arterial thrombosis: A review. *Blood Cells Mol Dis* 26:540, 2000.
37. Auletta MJ, Headington JT: Purpura fulminans. A cutaneous manifestation of severe protein C deficiency. *Arch Dermatol* 124:1387, 1988.
38. Marlar RA, Neumann A: Neonatal purpura fulminans due to homozygous protein C or protein S deficiencies. *Semin Thromb Hemost* 16:299, 1990.
39. Kemahli S, Alhenc-Gelas M, Gandrille S, et al: Homozygous protein C deficiency with a double variant His 202 to Tyr and Ala 346 to Thr. *Blood Coagul Fibrinolysis* 9:351, 1998.
40. Gladson CL, Groncy P, Griffin JH: Coumarin necrosis, neonatal purpura fulminans, and protein C deficiency. *Arch Dermatol* 123:1701a, 1987.
41. Mahasandana C, Suvatte V, Chuansumrit A, et al: Homozygous protein S deficiency in an infant with purpura fulminans. *J Pediatr* 117:750, 1990.
42. Gruber A, Blasko G, Sas G: Functional deficiency of protein C and skin necrosis in multiple myeloma. *Thromb Res* 42:579, 1986.
43. Levin M, Eley BS, Louis J, et al: Postinfectious purpura fulminans caused by an autoantibody directed against protein S. *J Pediatr* 127:355, 1995.
44. van Ommen CH, van Wijnen M, de Groot FG, et al: Postvaricella purpura fulminans caused by acquired protein s deficiency resulting from antiprotein s antibodies: Search for the epitopes. *J Pediatr Hematol Oncol* 24:413, 2002.
45. Branson HE, Katz J, Marble R, Griffin JH: Inherited protein C deficiency and coumarin-responsive chronic relapsing purpura fulminans in a newborn infant. *Lancet* 2:1165, 1983.
46. Sills RH, Marlar RA, Montgomery RR, et al: Severe homozygous protein C deficiency. *J Pediatr* 105:409, 1984.
47. Baselga E, Drolet BA, Esterly NB: Purpura in infants and children. *J Am Acad Dermatol* 37:673, quiz 706, 1997.
48. Pescatore SL: Clinical management of protein C deficiency. *Expert Opin Pharmacother* 2:431, 2001.
49. Hillman RS, Ault, KA: The dysplastic and sideroblastic anemias, in *Hematology in Clinical Practice*, 2nd ed, edited by J Morgan, P Hanley, p 151. McGraw-Hill, New York, 1998.
50. Berlin JM, Queen JR: Lower extremity purpura. *Arch Dermatol* 138:831, 2002.
51. White JM, Watson K, Arya R, Du Vivier AW: Haemorrhagic bullae in a case of paroxysmal nocturnal haemoglobinuria. *Clin Exp Dermatol* 28:504, 2003.

52. Goulden V, Bond L, Highet AS: Pyoderma gangrenosum associated with paroxysmal nocturnal haemoglobinuria. *Clin Exp Dermatol* 19:271, 1994.

53. Cuadrado MJ, Lopez-Pedrera C: Antiphospholipid syndrome. *Clin Exp Med* 3:129, 2003.

54. DiFrancesco LM, Burkart P, Hoehn JG: A cutaneous manifestation of antiphospholipid antibody syndrome. *Ann Plast Surg* 51:517, 2003.

55. Sammaritano LR, Gharavi AE, Lockshin MD: Antiphospholipid antibody syndrome: Immunologic and clinical aspects. *Semin Arthritis Rheum* 20:81, 1990.

56. Martin L, Armingaud P, Georgescu V, et al: Acute bullous purpura associated with hyperhomocysteinemia and antiphospholipid antibodies. *J Am Acad Dermatol* 49:S161, 2003.

57. Bard JW, Winkelmann RK: Livedo vasculitis. Segmental hyalinizing vasculitis of the dermis. *Arch Dermatol* 96:489, 1967.

58. Ravat FE, Evans AV, Russell-Jones R: Response of livedoid vasculitis to intravenous immunoglobulin. *Br J Dermatol* 147:166, 2002.

59. Mimouni D, Ng PP, Rencic A, et al: Cutaneous polyarteritis nodosa in patients presenting with atrophie blanche. *Br J Dermatol* 148:789, 2003.

60. Acland KM, Darvay A, Wakelin SH, Russell-Jones R: Livedoid vasculitis: A manifestation of the antiphospholipid syndrome? *Br J Dermatol* 140:131, 1999.

61. Falanga V, Fine MJ, Kapoor WN: The cutaneous manifestations of cholesterol crystal embolization. *Arch Dermatol* 122:1194, 1986.

62. Pennington M, Yeager J, Skelton H, Smith KJ: Cholesterol embolization syndrome: Cutaneous histopathological features and the variable onset of symptoms in patients with different risk factors. *Br J Dermatol* 146:511, 2002.

63. Trent JT, Kirsner RS: Calciphylaxis: Diagnosis and treatment. *Adv Skin Wound Care* 14:309, 2001.

64. Korkmaz C, Dundar E, Zubaroglu I: Calciphylaxis in a patient with rheumatoid arthritis without renal failure and hyperparathyroidism: The possible role of long-term steroid use and protein S deficiency. *Clin Rheumatol* 21:66, 2002.

65. McAllister SM, Bornstein AM, Callen JP: Painful acral purpura. *Arch Dermatol* 134:789, 1998.

66. Zhu YI, Stiller MJ: Arthropods and skin diseases. *Int J Dermatol* 41:533, 2002.

67. Shankar S, Sterling JC, Rytina E: Pustular pyoderma gangrenosum. *Clin Exp Dermatol* 28:600, 2003.

68. Crowson AN, Mihm MC Jr, Magro C: Pyoderma gangrenosum: A review. *J Cutan Pathol* 30:97, 2003.

69. Gettler S, Rothe M, Grin C, Grant-Kels J: Optimal treatment of pyoderma gangrenosum. *Am J Clin Dermatol* 4:597, 2003.

70. Cohen PR, Kurzrock R: Sweet's syndrome: A neutrophilic dermatosis classically associated with acute onset and fever. *Clin Dermatol* 18:265, 2000.

71. Nobeyama Y, Kamide R: Sweet's syndrome with neurologic manifestation: Case report and literature review. *Int J Dermatol* 42:438, 2003.

72. Cohen PR, Kurzrock R: Sweet's syndrome: A review of current treatment options. *Am J Clin Dermatol* 3:117, 2002.

73. Chen KR, Kawahara Y, Miyakawa S, Nishikawa T: Cutaneous vasculitis in Behcet disease: A clinical and histopathologic study of 20 patients. *J Am Acad Dermatol* 36:689, 1997.

74. Yurdakul S, Hamuryudan V, Yazici H: Behcet syndrome. *Curr Opin Rheumatol* 16:38, 2004.

75. Bielory L, Gascon P, Lawley TJ, et al: Human serum sickness: A prospective analysis of 35 patients treated with equine anti-thymocyte globulin for bone marrow failure. *Medicine (Baltimore)* 67:40, 1988.

76. Bielory L, Yancey KB, Young NS, et al: Cutaneous manifestations of serum sickness in patients receiving antithymocyte globulin. *J Am Acad Dermatol* 13:411, 1985.

77. Jegasothy BV: Immune complexes in the reactive inflammatory vascular dermatoses. *Dermatol Clin* 3:185, 1985.

78. Ballinger S: Henoch-Schonlein purpura. *Curr Opin Rheumatol* 15:591, 2003.

79. Saulsbury FT: Henoch-Schonlein purpura. *Curr Opin Rheumatol* 13:35, 2001.

80. Fervenza FC: Henoch-Schonlein purpura nephritis. *Int J Dermatol* 42:170, 2003.

81. Jin DK, Kohsaka T, Koo JW, et al: Complement 4 locus II gene deletion and DQA1*0301 gene: Genetic risk factors for IgA nephropathy and Henoch-Schonlein nephritis. *Nephron* 73:390, 1996.

82. Levinsky RJ, Barratt TM: IgA immune complexes in Henoch-Schonlein purpura. *Lancet* 2:1100, 1979.

83. Kawana S, Shen GH, Kobayashi Y, Nishiyama S: Membrane attack complex of complement in Henoch-Schonlein purpura skin and nephritis. *Arch Dermatol Res* 282:183, 1990.

84. Besbas N, Erbay A, Saatci U, et al: Thrombomodulin, tissue plasminogen activator and plasminogen activator inhibitor-1 in Henoch-Schonlein purpura. *Clin Exp Rheumatol* 16:95, 1998.

85. Besbas N, Saatci U, Ruacan S, et al: The role of cytokines in Henoch-Schonlein purpura. *Scand J Rheumatol* 26:456, 1997.

86. Sharieff GQ, Francis K, Kuppermann N: Atypical presentation of Henoch-Schonlein purpura in two children. *Am J Emerg Med* 15:375, 1997.

87. Coppo R, Mazzucco G, Cagnoli L, et al: Long-term prognosis of Henoch-Schonlein nephritis in adults and children. Italian Group of Renal Immunopathology Collaborative Study on Henoch-Schonlein purpura. *Nephrol Dial Transplant* 12:2277, 1997.

88. Blanco R, Martinez-Taboada VM, Rodriguez-Valverde V, et al: Henoch-Schonlein purpura in adulthood and childhood: Two different expressions of the same syndrome. *Arthritis Rheum* 40:859, 1997.

89. Mintzer CO, Nussinovitch M, Danziger Y, et al: Scrotal involvement in Henoch-Schonlein purpura in children. *Scand J Urol Nephrol* 32:138, 1998.

90. Lin SJ, Huang JL, Hsieh KH: Clinical and laboratory correlation of acute Henoch-Schonlein purpura in children. *Zhonghua Min Guo Xiao Er Ke Yi Xue Hui Za Zhi* 39:94, 1998.

91. Kaku Y, Nohara K, Honda S: Renal involvement in Henoch-Schonlein purpura: A multivariate analysis of prognostic factors. *Kidney Int* 53:1755, 1998.

92. Ozaltin F, Besbas N, Uckan D, et al: The role of apoptosis in childhood Henoch-Schonlein purpura. *Clin Rheumatol* 22:265, 2003.

93. Kingston ME, Mackey D: Skin clues in the diagnosis of life-threatening infections. *Rev Infect Dis* 8:1, 1986.

94. Cnota JF, Barton LL, Rhee KH: Purpura fulminans associated with Streptococcus pneumoniae infection in a child. *Pediatr Emerg Care* 15:187, 1999.

95. El Baze P, Thyss A, Caldani C, et al: Pseudomonas aeruginosa O-11 folliculitis. Development into ecthyma gangrenosum in immunosuppressed patients. *Arch Dermatol* 121:873, 1985.

96. Rusonis PA, Robinson HN, Lamberg SI: Livedo reticularis and purpura: Presenting features in fulminant pneumococcal septicemia in an asplenic patient. *J Am Acad Dermatol* 15:1120, 1986.

97. Van Nguyen Q, Nguyen EA, Weiner LB: Incidence of invasive bacterial disease in children with fever and petechiae. *Pediatrics* 74:77, 1984.

98. Mancebo J, Domingo P, Blanch L, et al: The predictive value of petechiae in adults with bacterial meningitis. *JAMA* 256:2820, 1986.

99. Baker RC, Seguin JH, Leslie N, et al: Fever and petechiae in children. *Pediatrics* 84:1051, 1989.

100. Fourrier F, Lestavel P, Chopin C, et al: Meningococcemia and purpura fulminans in adults: Acute deficiencies of proteins C and S and early treatment with antithrombin III concentrates. *Intensive Care Med* 16:121, 1990.

101. Rintala E, Seppala OP, Kotilainen P, et al: Protein C in the treatment of coagulopathy in meningococcal disease. *Crit Care Med* 26:965, 1998.

102. Rintala E, Kauppila M, Seppala OP, et al: Protein C substitution in sepsis-associated purpura fulminans. *Crit Care Med* 28:2373, 2000.

103. Berger BW: Dermatologic manifestations of Lyme disease. *Rev Infect Dis* 11(suppl 6):S1475, 1989.

104. Nielsen HE, Andersen EA, Andersen J, et al: Diagnostic assessment of haemorrhagic rash and fever. *Arch Dis Child* 85:160, 2001.

105. Perez-Ferriols A, Martinez-Aparicio A, Aliaga-Boniche A: Papular-purpuric "gloves and socks" syndrome caused by measles virus. *J Am Acad Dermatol* 30:291, 1994.

106. Shiraishi H, Umetsu K, Yamamoto H, et al: Human parvovirus (HPV/B19) infection with purpura. *Microbiol Immunol* 33:369, 1989.

107. Smith SB, Libow LF, Elston DM, et al: Gloves and socks syndrome: Early and late histopathologic features. *J Am Acad Dermatol* 47:749, 2002.

108. Bruno P, Hassell LH, Brown J, et al: The protean manifestations of hemorrhagic fever with renal syndrome. A retrospective review of 26 cases from Korea. *Ann Intern Med* 113:385, 1990.

109. Radentz WH: Opportunistic fungal infections in immunocompromised hosts. *J Am Acad Dermatol* 20:989, 1989.

110. Helm TN, Longworth DL, Hall GS, et al: Case report and review of resolved fusariosis. *J Am Acad Dermatol* 23:393, 1990.

111. Fine JD, Miller JA, Harrist TJ, Haynes HA: Cutaneous lesions in disseminated candidiasis mimicking ecthyma gangrenosum. *Am J Med* 70:1133, 1981.

112. von Kuster LC, Genta RM: Cutaneous manifestations of strongyloidiasis. *Arch Dermatol* 124:1826, 1988.

113. Ronan SG, Reddy RL, Manaligod JR, et al: Disseminated strongyloidiasis presenting as purpura. *J Am Acad Dermatol* 21:1123, 1989.

114. Stampien TM, Schwartz RA: Erythema multiforme. *Am Fam Physician* 46:1171, 1992.

115. Yang YH, Tsai MJ, Tsau YK, et al: Clinical observations of erythema multiforme in children. *Acta Paediatr Taiwan* 40:107, 1999.

116. Roujeau JC: Clinical aspects of skin reactions to NSAIDs. *Scand J Rheumatol Suppl* 65:131, 1987.

117. Imamura S, Horio T, Yanase K, et al: Erythema multiforme: Pathomechanism of papular erythema and target lesion. *J Dermatol* 19:524, 1992.

118. Siberry GK, Cohen BA, Johnson B: Cutaneous polyarteritis nodosa. Reports of two cases in children and review of the literature. *Arch Dermatol* 130:884, 1994.

119. Minkowitz G, Smoller BR, McNutt NS: Benign cutaneous polyarteritis nodosa. Relationship to systemic polyarteritis nodosa and to hepatitis B infection. *Arch Dermatol* 127:1520, 1991.

120. Chen KR: Cutaneous polyarteritis nodosa: A clinical and histopathological study of 20 cases. *J Dermatol* 16:429, 1989.

121. Farrell AM, Stern SC, El-Ghariani K, et al: Splenic lymphoma with villous lymphocytes presenting as leucocytoclastic vasculitis. *Clin Exp Dermatol* 24:19, 1999.

122. Ponge T, Boutoille D, Moreau A, et al: Systemic vasculitis in a patient with small-cell neuroendocrine bronchial cancer. *Eur Respir J* 12:1228, 1998.

123. Callen JP: Cutaneous leukocytoclastic vasculitis in a patient with an adenocarcinoma of the colon. *J Rheumatol* 14:386, 1987.

124. Nakajima H, Ikeda M, Yamamoto Y, Kodama H: Large annular purpura and paraneoplastic purpura in a patient with Sjogren's syndrome and cervical cancer. *J Dermatol* 27:40, 2000.

125. Greer JM, Longley S, Edwards NL, et al: Vasculitis associated with malignancy. Experience with 13 patients and literature review. *Medicine (Baltimore)* 67:220, 1988.

126. ten Holder SM, Joy MS, Falk RJ: Cutaneous and systemic manifestations of drug-induced vasculitis. *Ann Pharmacother* 36:130, 2002.

127. Daoud MS, Gibson LE, DeRemee RA, et al: Cutaneous Wegener's granulomatosis: Clinical, histopathologic, and immunopathologic features of thirty patients. *J Am Acad Dermatol* 31:605, 1994.

128. Csernok E, Gross WL: Primary vasculitides and vasculitis confined to skin: Clinical features and new pathogenic aspects. *Arch Dermatol Res* 292:427, 2000.

129. Otani Y, Anzai S, Shibuya H, et al: Churg-Strauss syndrome (CSS) manifested as necrosis of fingers and toes and liver infarction. *J Dermatol* 30:810, 2003.

130. Jennette JC, Thomas DB, Falk RJ: Microscopic polyangiitis (microscopic polyarteritis). *Semin Diagn Pathol* 18:3, 2001.

131. Reis JJ, Kaplan PW: Postictal hemifacial purpura. *Seizure* 7:337, 1998.

132. Pierson JC, Suh PS: Powerlifter's purpura: A valsalva-associated phenomenon. *Cutis* 70:93, 2002.

133. Alcalay J, Ingber A, Sandbank M: Mask phenomenon: Postemesis facial purpura. *Cutis* 38:28, 1986.

134. Metzker A, Merlob P: Suction purpura. *Arch Dermatol* 128:822, 1992.

135. Forster PJ: Microvascular fragility at high altitude. *Br Med J (Clin Res Ed)* 296:1004, 1988.

136. Danielsson G, Eklof B, Grandinetti A, et al: Deep axial reflux, an important contributor to skin changes or ulcer in chronic venous disease. *J Vasc Surg* 38:1336, 2003.

137. Beardsley DS: Pathophysiology of immune thrombocytopenic purpura. *Blood Rev* 16:13, 2002.

138. Tsai HM: Advances in the pathogenesis, diagnosis, and treatment of thrombotic thrombocytopenic purpura. *J Am Soc Nephrol* 14:1072, 2003.

139. Bruinsma W: The file of side effects to the skin: A guide to drug eruptions. *Semin Dermatol* 8:141, 1989.

140. Feinstein RJ, Halprin KM, Penneys NS, et al: Senile purpura. *Arch Dermatol* 108:229, 1973.

141. Haboubi NY, Haboubi NA, Gyde OH, et al: Zinc deficiency in senile purpura. *J Clin Pathol* 38:1189, 1985.

142. Capewell S, Reynolds S, Shuttleworth D, et al: Purpura and dermal thinning associated with high dose inhaled corticosteroids. *BMJ* 300:1548, 1990.

143. Nguyen RT, Cowley DM, Muir JB: Scurvy: A cutaneous clinical diagnosis. *Australas J Dermatol* 44:48, 2003.

144. Hirschmann JV, Raugi GJ: Adult scurvy. *J Am Acad Dermatol* 41:895, quiz 907, 1999.

145. Breathnach SM: Amyloid and amyloidosis. *J Am Acad Dermatol* 18:1, 1988.

146. Vella FS, Simone B, Antonaci S: Palmodigital purpura as the only skin abnormality in myeloma-associated systemic amyloidosis. *Br J Haematol* 120:917, 2003.

147. Germain DP: Clinical and genetic features of vascular Ehlers-Danlos syndrome. *Ann Vasc Surg* 16:391, 2002.

148. Kaplinsky C, Kenet G, Seligsohn U, Rechavi G: Association between hyperflexibility of the thumb and an unexplained bleeding tendency: Is it a rule of thumb? *Br J Haematol* 101:260, 1998.

149. Hu X, Plomp AS, Van Soest S, et al: Pseudoxanthoma elasticum: A clinical, histopathological, and molecular update. *Surv Ophthalmol* 48:424, 2003.

150. Horiguchi Y, Fujii T, Imamura S: Purpuric cutaneous manifestations in mitochondrial encephalomyopathy. *J Dermatol* 18:295, 1991.

151. Kubota Y, Ishii T, Sugihara H, et al: Skin manifestations of a patient with mitochondrial encephalomyopathy with lactic acidosis and stroke-like episodes (MELAS syndrome). *J Am Acad Dermatol* 41:469, 1999.

152. Kondo T, Betz P, Eisenmenger W: Retrospective study on skin reddenings and petechiae in the eyelids and the conjunctivae in forensic physical examinations. *Int J Legal Med* 110:204, 1997.

153. Lowe L, Rapini RP, Johnson TM: Traumatic asphyxia. *J Am Acad Dermatol* 23:972, 1990.

154. Yates VM: Factitious purpura. *Clin Exp Dermatol* 17:238, 1992.

155. Tristani-Firouzi P, Meadows KP, Vanderhooft S: Pigmented purpuric eruptions of childhood: A series of cases and review of literature. *Pediatr Dermatol* 18:299, 2001.

HEMOPHILIA A AND HEMOPHILIA B

HAROLD R. ROBERTS

MIGUEL ESCOBAR

GILBERT C WHITE II

The clinical manifestations of hemophilia A and hemophilia B result from deficiency of factors VIII and IX, respectively, are clinically indistinguishable, and occur in mild, moderate, and severe forms. They are the only blood clotting disorders inherited in a sex-linked pattern. The severe forms of hemophilia A and hemophilia B are characterized mainly by frequent hemarthroses leading to chronic crippling hemarthropathy when not treated very early or prophylactically. Highly purified concentrates, prepared from human plasma or manufactured by recombinant technology, are available for treatment and are considered safe and effective. In addition, prophylactic treatment is recommended, when feasible, for all severely affected patients. The main complication of treatment is the development of antibody inhibitors against either factor VIII or factor IX, which are more common in patients with hemophilia A than in patients with hemophilia B.

HEMOPHILIA A (CLASSIC HEMOPHILIA, FACTOR VIII DEFICIENCY)

DEFINITION AND HISTORY

Hemophilia A is an X chromosome-linked hereditary disorder caused by defective synthesis or by synthesis of dysfunctional factor VIII molecules. Hemophilia A is less common than von Willebrand disease (vWD), but it is more common than other inherited clotting factor abnormalities. The estimated incidence of hemophilia A is only one in every 5000 to 7000 live male births. It occurs in all ethnic groups in all parts of the world.[1]

Sex-linked hemophilia was recognized in the second century, when a rabbi correctly deduced that sons of hemophilic carriers were at risk for bleeding following circumcision.[2] In the 19th century, several authors noted the sex-linked inheritance pattern of the disease and ascribed the hemorrhagic episodes to delayed blood coagulation. Morawitz[3] developed the classic theory of blood coagulation, which recognized two major reactions: (1) conversion of prothrombin to thrombin by a tissue substance that Morawitz termed *thrombokinase*, and (2) conversion of fibrinogen to fibrin by thrombin. In 1911, Addis[4]

Acronyms and abbreviations that appear in this chapter include: AAV, adeno-associated virus; AIDS, acquired immune deficiency syndrome; aPTT, activated partial thromboplastin time; BT, bleeding time; BU, Bethesda unit; CJD, Creutzfeldt-Jakob disease; CRM, cross-reacting material; CT, computed tomography; DDAVP, 1-desamino-8-D-arginine vasopressin (desmopressin); EACA, ε-amino caproic acid; FEIBA, factor VIII inhibitor bypassing activity; HIV, human immunodeficiency virus; Ig, immunoglobulin; MRI, magnetic resonance imaging; PT, prothrombin time; PTT, partial thromboplastin time; RFLP, restriction fragment length polymorphism; vWD, von Willebrand disease; vWF, von Willebrand factor; VNTR, variable number of tandem repeats.

demonstrated that thrombin formed more slowly in hemophilic blood than in normal blood and that the defect could be corrected by small amounts of normal plasma. However, he incorrectly theorized that hemophilia resulted from prothrombin deficiency. As protein purification techniques improved throughout the 1930s and 1940s, thrombokinase was resolved into several distinct components. Brinkhous[5] demonstrated that the prothrombin content of hemophilic plasma was normal and that the basic defect in hemophilia was the delayed conversion of prothrombin to thrombin. The defect could be corrected by a fraction of normal plasma containing the antihemophilic factor, later named *factor VIII*. In 1947, Pavlovsky[6] observed that when blood from one patient with hemophilia whom he was studying was transfused into another patient, the prolonged clotting time in the recipient was corrected. At the time, Pavlovsky did not recognize that he was dealing with two different types of hemophilia. This fact was recognized by Aggeler and coworkers[7] in 1952, when they described a patient deficient in "plasma thromboplastin component," a blood clotting factor different from factor VIII. A deficiency of "plasma thromboplastin component," later termed *factor IX*, is expressed clinically as hemophilia B.[8]

In 1964, a proposal to organize the growing number of coagulation factors into a cascade, or waterfall, mechanism was put forth.[9,10] In this scheme, each zymogen clotting factor was activated to a protease that subsequently acted on the next zymogen until thrombin ultimately was produced. In this scheme, factors VIII and IX were considered proenzymes. Later, however, factor VIII was shown not to be a proenzyme but rather a cofactor that, when activated by thrombin, acted as an essential cofactor for factor IXa. The cascade hypothesis has been modified so that the primary role of the tissue factor–factor VII complex in the initiation of coagulation is emphasized (see Chap. 106).[11]

ETIOLOGY AND PATHOGENESIS

Hemophilia A is a heterogeneous disorder resulting from defects in the factor VIII gene that leads to reduced circulating levels of functional factor VIII. The reduced activity can result from a decreased amount of factor VIII protein, the presence of a functionally abnormal protein, or a combination of both. For factor VIII to be an effective cofactor for factor IXa, it must first be activated by thrombin, a reaction that results in the formation of a heterotrimer composed of the A_1, A_2, and A_3, C_1, and C_2 domains of factor VIII in a complex with calcium (see Chap. 106).[12] Activated factor VIII (factor VIIIa) and activated factor IX (factor IXa) associate on the surface of activated platelets, forming a functional factor X-activating complex ("tenase" or "Xase").[13] In the presence of factor VIIIa, the rate of factor X activation by factor IXa is dramatically enhanced. That hemophilia A and hemophilia B have similar clinical manifestations is not surprising, because both factor VIIIa and factor IXa are required to form the Xase complex. The lack of either activated factor leads to a similar lack of platelet surface Xase activity. In patients with hemophilia, clot formation is delayed because thrombin generation is markedly decreased. The clot that is formed is friable, easily dislodged, and highly susceptible to fibrinolysis, all of which lead to excessive bleeding.

GENETICS

Hemophilia A is an X chromosome-linked recessive disorder that occurs almost exclusively in males. Approximately 30 percent of the mutations arise *de novo*. Figure 115-1 shows the inheritance pattern of hemophilia A and hemophilia B. All the sons of affected hemophilic males are normal, whereas all the daughters are obligatory carriers of the factor VIII defect. Sons of carriers have a 50 percent chance of being affected, whereas daughters of carriers have a 50 percent chance of being carriers themselves.

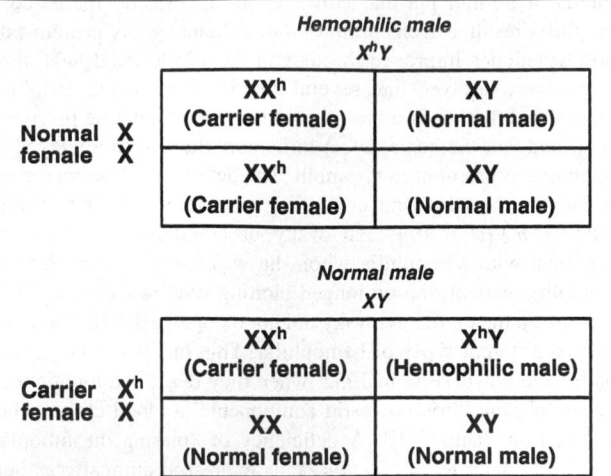

FIGURE 115-1   Inheritance pattern of hemophilia A. X, normal; X^h, abnormal X chromosome with the hemophilic gene; X^hY, hemophilic male; XX, normal female; XX^h, carrier female; XY, normal male; Y, normal.

The factor VIII gene is very large, approximately 186 kb, with approximately 9 kb of exons. The gene contains 26 exons and 25 intervening sequences or introns. The size and complexity of the gene have made difficult the pinpointing, on a routine basis, of specific mutations resulting in hemophilia. Nevertheless, the factor VIII gene

has been cloned and sequenced, and numerous specific mutations have been described.[14,15]

Hemophilia A can result from multiple alterations in the factor VIII gene, including gene rearrangements; missense mutations, in which a single base substitution leads to an amino acid change in the molecule; nonsense mutations, which result in a stop codon; abnormal splicing of the gene; deletions of all or portions of the gene; or insertions of genetic elements.[14] The genetic defects leading to hemophilia have been reviewed.[15] Table 115-1 presents a summary of the different 142 mutations as of 2003.[16]

One of the most common mutations, accounting for 40 to 50 percent of patients, is a unique combined gene inversion and crossing over that disrupts the factor VIII gene.[17,18] Figures 115-2 and 115-3 show schematically the factor VIII gene. Within intron 22 are two other genes: (1) F8A, which is transcribed in the 5' direction, and (2) F8B, which is transcribed in the 3' direction of the factor VIII gene. The hatched boxes in Fig. 115-3 show two other homologous sequences (a_2, a_3) 5' to the F8A gene that lies within intron 22 (a_1). The presence of an extragenic F8A sequence 5' to the F8A gene within intron 22 is central to the inversion and translocation of the factor VIII gene from exon 1 to exon 22. The mechanism is homologous recombination between the F8A gene sequence that lies within intron 22 and one of the homologous sequences of the F8A gene 5' to the factor VIII gene. During meiosis, crossing over of homologous sequences occurs between the F8A gene nested in intron 22 and the extragenic F8A sequence 5' to intron 22 so that transcription of the complete factor VIII sequence is interrupted (Fig. 115-3). Many patients with an inversion are susceptible to development of antifactor VIII inhibitor antibodies.

Of the different insertions in the factor VIII gene that have been reported, a few are LINE (L_1) elements that are transposon sequences, that is, sequences that have been inserted frequently throughout the genome.[19] Most insertions result in severe hemophilia.

Like many mutations causing disease states, mutations in the factor VIII gene occur frequently at CpG dinucleotides.[19] Because the restriction fragment enzyme TaqI recognizes the sequence TCGA, CpG mutations at this site can be directly detected by loss of a TaqI cleavage site. Codons for the amino acid arginine (CGA) are frequently affected by mutations at CG doublets. A C→T transition often results in a stop codon (Fig. 115-4). A stop codon results in synthesis of a truncated factor VIII molecule and usually is associated with severe hemophilia.

A G→A transition results in a missense mutation, which often leads to a dysfunctional factor VIII molecule and may be associated with mild, moderate, or severe hemophilia. Some missense mutations result in the production of normal or near-normal amounts of factor VIII antigen, while the coagulant activity may be dramatically or only slightly reduced. Many other single-base substitutions have been described, resulting in hemophilia of varying degrees of severity.

Large deletions in the factor VIII gene almost always are associated with severe hemophilia. However, cases in which a small deletion that does not change the reading frame of

TABLE 115-1   SUMMARY OF DIFFERENT MUTATIONS REPORTED FOR HEMOPHILIA A AS OF 2003

	POINT MUTATIONS			DELETIONS		
EXON	MISSENSE[a]	NONSENSE (STOP)	SPLICING[b]	SMALL	LARGE	INSERTIONS
1	14	1	4	2	—	0
2	5	1	5	6	—	2
3	24	0	3	4	—	0
4	24	5	2	1		1
5	11	1	7	3		1
6	6	0	3	4		2
7	32	4	0	6		0
8	21	4	1	8		1
9	22	3	1	5		1
10	10	1	0	4		0
11	27	1	3	1		1
12	20	5	2	0		1
13	23	3	2	4		1
14	37	39	3	63	—	31
15	13	1	4	2	—	0
16	18	4	2	5	—	0
17	24	3	1	5	—	4
18	26	4	1	3	—	3
19	14	4	5	3	—	1
20	5	1	0	0	—	1
21	5	4	0	0	—	1
22	16	5	5	3	—	1
23	25	1	4	6	—	0
24	10	3	3	3	—	2
25	11	2	1	4	—	2
26	19	3	0	7	—	0
Total	462	100	62	152	120	57

[a] Includes 9 missense mutations that are predicted to affect splice junctions.
[b] In the case of intronic substitutions, splice mutations are referred to the preceding exon.
SOURCE: HAMPSTeRS web site, with permission. Available at: www.europium.csc.mrc.ac.uk.

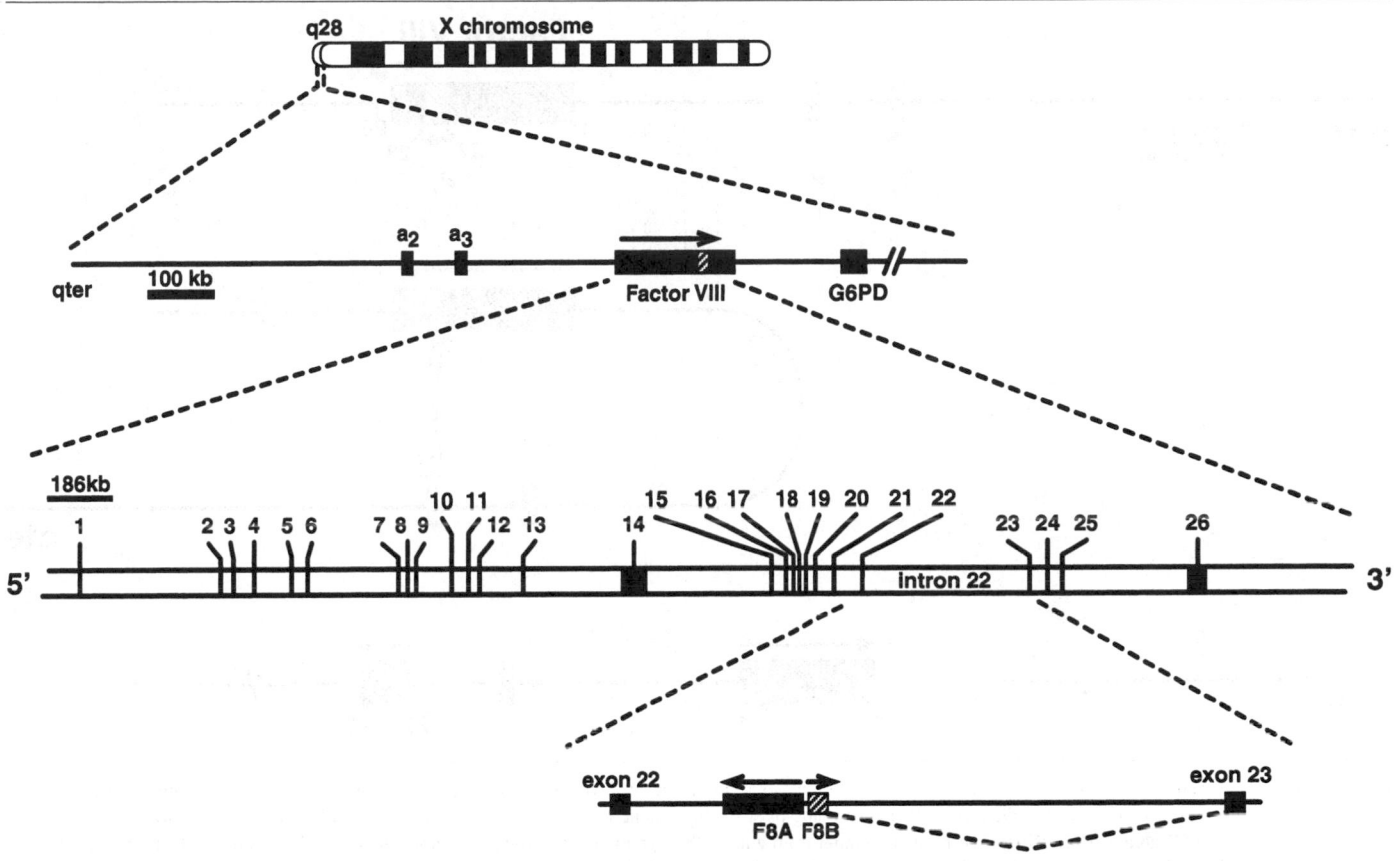

FIGURE 115-2   Schematic representation of the factor VIII gene. The factor VIII gene is located at q28 on the X chromosome. The region of the factor VIII gene is enlarged on the *second line*. Two genes are designated a₂ and a₃ 5′ to the factor VIII gene. The *hatched area* indicated on the factor VIII gene corresponds to intron 22 shown on the *third line*. Within intron 22 *(fourth line)* are two nested genes, one designated *F8A*, which is transcribed in a direction opposite to that of the whole factor VIII gene and is homologous to the a₂ and a₃ genes shown on *line 2*. (From Kazazian HK, Tuddenham EGD, Antonorakis SE: Hemophilia A: Deficiency of coagulation factor VIII, in *Metabolic and Molecular Basis of Inherited Diseases*, 8th ed, vol 4, edited by CR Scriver, AL Beaudet, WS Sly, D Valle, B Childs, KW Kinzler, B Vogelstein, p 4367. McGraw-Hill, New York, 1995, with permission.)

the gene results in milder disease have been described. Patients with large deletions who have no detectable factor VIII antigen are thought to also be more susceptible to the development of anti-factor VIII antibodies, although antibodies clearly also occur in patients without deletions.[14,19]

Hemophilia A in females is extremely rare, although affected female offspring from a hemophilic father and carrier mother have been reported. Hemophilia A may occur in females with X chromosome abnormalities such as Turner syndrome, X chromosome mosaicism, and other X chromosome defects.[20,21] If the normal X chromosome is inactivated disproportionately ("imbalanced X inactivation") in a carrier female, factor VIII levels may be sufficiently low to cause bleeding manifestations. Usually, these manifestations are mild but may be serious during surgical procedures or in instances of significant trauma.

PRENATAL DIAGNOSIS AND CARRIER DETECTION

A careful and complete family history is important for carrier detection.[22] All daughters of a hemophilic father are obligatory carriers of the hemophilic defect. If a known carrier has a daughter, the daughter has a 50 percent chance of being a carrier.

Carrier detection is important when a daughter of a known carrier or a female offspring of a hemophilic patient wishes to become pregnant. If resources for advanced carrier detection are not available, a careful family history can be taken and factor VIII coagulant activity and the von Willebrand factor (vWF) antigen level measured. The ratio

of vWF to factor VIII is higher in carrier females than in noncarriers; thus, determining the ratio adds to test sensitivity. Carriers generally have 50 percent or less of the normal factor VIII level. When these data are added to the family history, the probability of whether a woman is a carrier can be calculated.[23,24] However, the physician or genetic counselor must carefully explain to the subjects being tested that the test results carry a significant error rate, and accurate determination of the carrier state using the ratio of factor VIII to vWF cannot be guaranteed.

Carriers who harbor the intron 22 inversion can be identified using the Southern blot technique. Where the capability exists, analysis of the complete coding region can be performed using gradient gel electrophoresis and single-stranded conformation polymorphism technology or by restriction fragment length polymorphism (RFLP) analysis.[22]

Use of markers for RFLP is simpler than direct sequencing of the coding region of the factor VIII gene, but use of the RFLP technique requires that the pedigree analyses include at least one hemophilic male whose mother is heterozygous for one or more RFLP markers. Figure 115-5 shows an example of RFLP analysis.[25,26] The polymorphic markers include the variable number of tandem repeats (VNTR) in introns 13 and 22 and *Bcl*I and *Xba*I restriction sites. The female III-2 has the same polymorphic marker in intron 13 and the same *Xba*I restriction site as her hemophilic brother, carrier mother, and hemophilic grandfather. In contrast, the female III-1 inherits markers that are not linked with hemophilia.

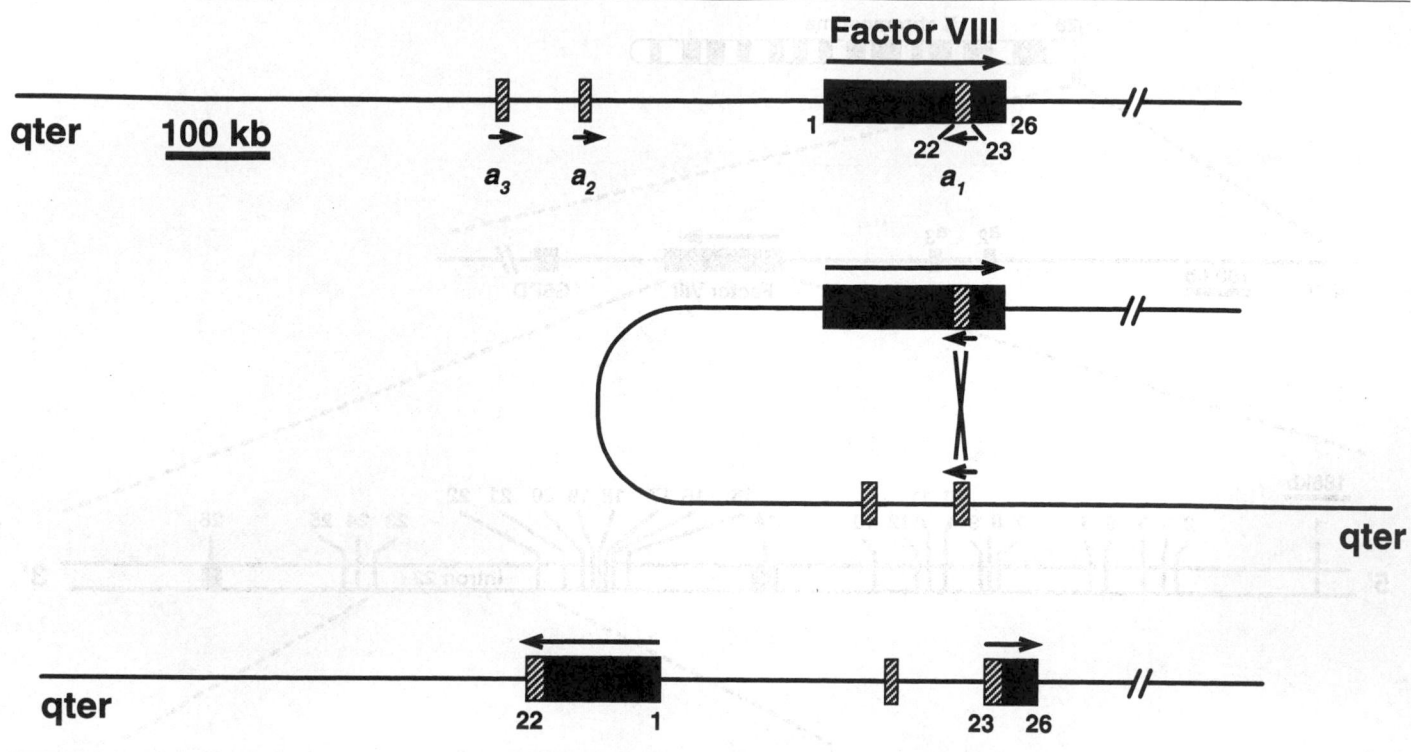

FIGURE 115-3   Schematic representation of inversion and crossing-over at intron 22. Inversion and crossing-over of the a_3 gene with its homologous sequence a_1 nested within intron 22 are shown. *(Middle panel)* When crossing-over of the a_1 gene nested within intron 22 and the a_3 gene extragenic to factor VIII occurs, a portion of the factor VIII gene is transcribed in a reverse manner from exon 1 through exon 22. (From SE Antonarakis, HH Kazazian, EG Tuddenham: Molecular etiology of factor VIII deficiency in hemophilia A. *Hum Mutat* 5:1, 1995, with permission.)

Prenatal diagnosis of hemophilia now can be performed almost routinely. If a carrier female has a fetus that can be identified as a female by chromosomal analysis of cells obtained by amniocentesis (approximately week 16) or by chorionic villus sampling at week 10 of gestation, little concerns exists regarding whether the female fetus is a carrier because carriers usually have no bleeding tendency. If the fetus is male, sufficient cells can be obtained to perform DNA analysis using the methods described above. The decision on whether to carry an affected fetus to term should be decided by the parents after they are appropriately counseled and provided with all the necessary information. Because the severity of hemophilia usually is consistent within a given family, the parents' decision is facilitated by their prior experience.

CLINICAL FEATURES

Hemophilia A is characterized by excessive bleeding into various organs of the body. Soft tissue hematomas and hemarthroses leading to severe, crippling hemarthropathy are highly characteristic of the disease. The disease has been broadly classified as *mild, moderate,* and *severe,* although overlap exists between categories. Table 115-2 shows a classification based on the severity of clinical manifestations. A range of plasma factor VIII concentrations in percentages of normal and in units per milliliter is given for each severity category. Occasionally, patients with very low factor VIII clotting activity are mildly affected clinically. Some patients with factor VIII levels compatible with severe hemophilia may exhibit mild symptoms because of the coinheritance of the factor V Leiden mutation (R506Q) with the hemophilic gene.[27] However, in some patients with "severe" hemophilia with a "milder" bleeding diathesis, neither the factor V Leiden mutation nor other known "prothrombotic" markers have been found.[28] Severely affected patients (<1 percent factor VIII) frequently experience bleeding without known trauma other than that associated with

the usual day-to-day activities. Without effective treatment, recurrent hemarthroses, resulting in chronic hemophilic arthropathy, occur by young adulthood and are highly characteristic of the severe form of the disorder. Severely affected patients are subject to serious hemor-

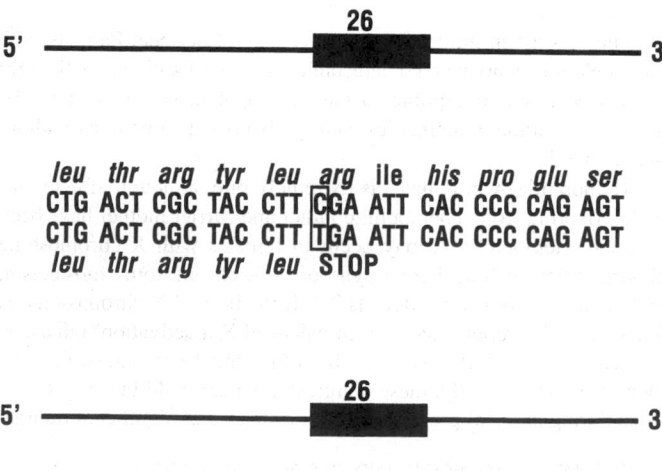

FIGURE 115-4   Examples of mutations and CG doublets. *Black box* denotes exon 26. A C→T transition results in a stop codon (TGA), whereas a G→A transition results in substitution of a glutamine for an arginine residue.

rhages that may dissect through tissue planes, ultimately leading to compromise of vital organs. However, bleeding episodes are intermittent, and some patients do not hemorrhage for weeks or months. Except for intracranial bleeding, sudden death because of hemorrhage is rare.

Moderately affected patients with hemophilia have occasional hematomas and hemarthroses usually, but not always, associated with known trauma. These patients have greater than 1 to 5 percent factor VIII activity. Although hemarthroses occur in moderately affected patients, hemarthropathy is less disabling than that occurring in severely affected patients.

Mildly affected patients with hemophilia (6–30% factor VIII) have infrequent bleeding episodes. The disease may go undiagnosed and be discovered only because of excessive hemorrhage postoperatively, following trauma, or after the toss and tumble of contact sports.

Most carriers have approximately 50 percent factor VIII activity and experience no bleeding difficulty, even with surgical procedures. Carriers with factor VIII levels less than 50 percent, usually because of extremely imbalanced X chromosome inactivation, may experience excessive bleeding after trauma (e.g., childbirth or surgery); therefore, a factor VIII level should be obtained for all carriers.

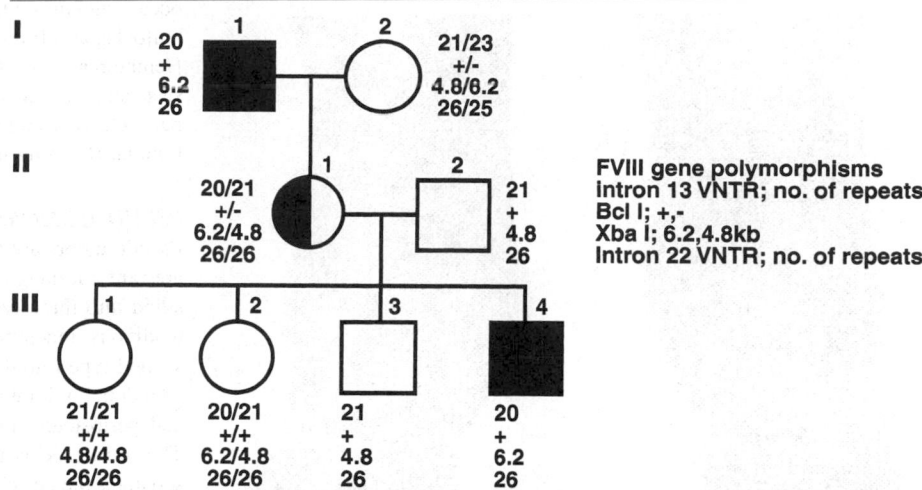

FVIII gene polymorphisms
Intron 13 VNTR; no. of repeats
Bcl I; +,-
Xba I; 6.2,4.8kb
Intron 22 VNTR; no. of repeats

FIGURE 115-5   Use of RFLP and VNTR for carrier diagnosis of hemophilia. The carrier female (II-1) is informative for polymorphisms at intron 13 and the XbaI site but not informative for markers on BclI or intron 22. III-2 is a carrier of the hemophilic trait with markers similar to the hemophilic grandfather (I-1) and hemophilic brother (III-4). VNTR is a variable number of tandem repeats; BclI and XbaI are sites cleaved by these restriction endonucleases. (From AC Goodeve, IR Peake: Diagnosis of hemophilia A and B carriers and prenatal diagnosis, in Haemophilia, edited by CD Forbes, L Aledort, R Madhok, p 63. Chapman & Hall, London, 1997, with permission.)

HEMARTHROSES

Bleeding into joints accounts for approximately 75 percent of bleeding episodes in severely affected patients with hemophilia A.[29] The normal synovium has few cells, but numerous capillaries beneath the synovial layer can be damaged by the mechanical trauma associated with daily use of joints. The joints most frequently involved, in decreasing order of frequency, are knees, elbows, ankles, shoulders, wrists, and hips. Hinge joints much more likely are involved than are ball and socket joints. Hemarthroses usually occur when an affected child begins to walk.

Hemarthroses sometimes are heralded by an aura of mild discomfort that, over a period of minutes to hours, becomes progressively painful. The joint usually swells, becomes warm, and exhibits limited motion. Occasionally the patient experiences a mild fever. Significant and sustained fever, however, suggests an infected joint. Bleeding into the knee joint is more easily detected by physical findings than is bleeding into either the elbow or shoulder. When bleeding stops, the blood resorbs, and the symptoms subside over a period of several days. If hemarthroses are treated early and the joint is not chronically involved, pain usually subsides in 6 to 8 hours and disappears in 12 to 24 hours. However, repeated hemorrhage into the joints eventually results in extensive destruction of articular cartilage, synovial hyperplasia, and other reactive changes in the adjacent bone and tissues. Acute bleeding into a chronically affected joint may be difficult to distinguish from the pain of degenerative arthritis.

One of the major complications of repeated hemarthroses is joint deformity complicated by muscle atrophy and soft tissue contractures (Fig. 115-6). Figure 115-7 shows the various radiologic stages of progressive destruction of joint cartilage and adjacent bone. Osteoporosis and cystic areas in the subchondral bone may develop, and progressive loss of joint space occurs.

Repeated bleeding into a joint results in synovial hypertrophy and inflammation. The synovium is thickened and folded, leading to lim-

ited joint motion. The result is a tendency for repeated hemorrhages leading to a so-called target joint. The joints most often involved are the knees, ankles, and elbows, which become chronically swollen. Bleeding into such a joint with significant synovial hypertrophy usually is less painful than is bleeding into a normal joint, but pain nevertheless may occur. Chronic synovitis may persist for months or years unless the condition is adequately treated.

Infection of hemophilic joints is not common but must be suspected in all patients with fever, leukocytosis, or other systemic manifestations. Rapid diagnosis is mandatory, because infection of such joints leads to rapid loss of joint architecture and function. A painful swollen joint may require aspiration, which should be performed by experienced personnel using meticulous aseptic techniques and appropriate factor replacement therapy.

HEMATOMAS

Hematomas are characteristic of blood clotting factor deficiencies. They usually are not seen, for example, in uncomplicated thrombocytopenia. Hemorrhage into subcutaneous connective tissues or into muscles may occur with or without known trauma. Hematomas, once formed, may stabilize and slowly resorb without treatment. However,

TABLE 115-2   CLINICAL CLASSIFICATION OF HEMOPHILIA

CLASSIFICATION	FACTOR VIII LEVEL	CLINICAL FEATURES
Severe	≤1% of normal (≤0.01 U/ml)	1. Spontaneous hemorrhage from early infancy
		2. Frequent spontaneous hemarthroses and other hemorrhages, requiring clotting factor replacement
Moderate	1–5% of normal (0.01–0.05 U/ml)	1. Hemorrhage secondary to trauma or surgery
		2. Occasional spontaneous hemarthroses
Mild	6–30% of normal (0.06–0.30 U/ml)	1. Hemorrhage secondary to trauma or surgery
		2. Rare spontaneous hemorrhage

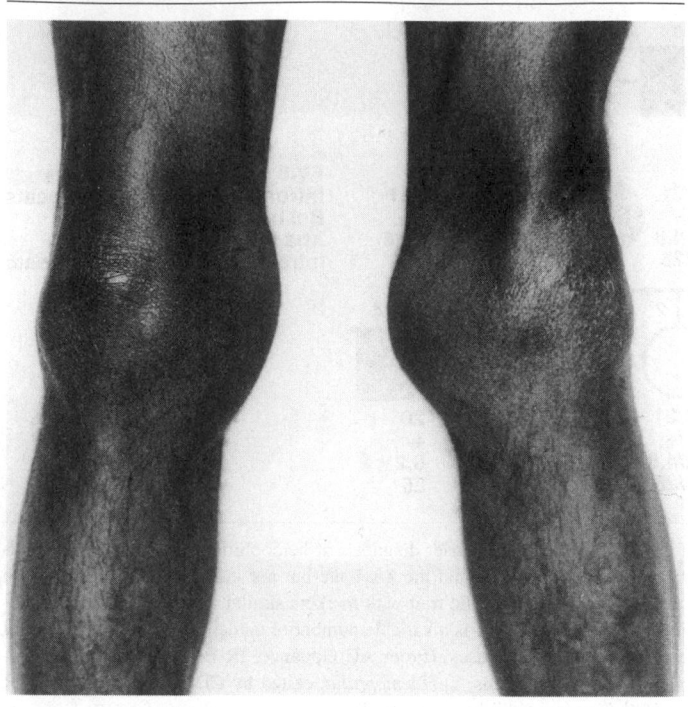

FIGURE 115-6　Hemophilic arthropathy. The chronic effects of repeated hemorrhage into the knee of a severely affected hemophilic are seen.

in moderately and severely affected patients, hematomas have a tendency to enlarge progressively and to dissect in all directions. Retroperitoneal hematomas can dissect through the diaphragm, into the chest, and into the soft tissues of the neck, compromising the airway. They also may compromise renal function by causing ureteral obstruction. Figure 115-8 shows the computed tomographic (CT) scan of a retroperitoneal hemorrhage. Other hematomas expand locally and compress adjacent organs, blood vessels, and nerves. A rare, and often fatal, complication of an abdominal hematoma is perforation and drainage into the colon. Subcutaneous hematomas are known to dissect into muscle. Pharyngeal and retropharyngeal hematomas, sometimes complicating simple colds, may enlarge and obstruct the airway. Hemorrhage in or around the airway is a potentially life-threatening situation that requires prompt administration of factor VIII. Hemorrhages

occur into muscle in the following order of frequency: calf, thigh, buttocks, and forearm. Bleeding into the iliopsoas muscle is frequent. Hematomas in these areas may lead to muscle contractures, nerve palsies, and muscle atrophy. Bleeding into the tongue or frenulum is particularly frequent in young children and usually is caused by trauma. Bleeding into the myocardium is extremely unusual.

PSEUDOTUMORS (BLOOD CYSTS)

Pseudotumors are blood cysts that occur in soft tissues or bone. They are rare but dangerous complications of hemophilia.[30] They are classified into three types. One type is a simple cyst that is confined by tendinous attachments within the fascial envelope of a muscle. The second type initially develops as a simple cyst in soft tissues such as a tendon, but it interferes with the vascular supply to the adjacent bone and periosteum, resulting in cyst formation and resorption of bone. The third type is thought to result from subperiosteal bleeding that separates the periosteum from the bony cortex (Fig. 115-9). The extent of periosteal stripping is limited by the aponeurotic or tendinous attachments. Most pseudotumors are not associated with pain unless rapid growth or nerve compression occurs. As the volume of the cyst increases, the cyst compresses and destroys the adjacent muscle, nerve, and/or bone. Pseudotumors usually contain either serosanguineous fluid or a viscous brownish material surrounded by a fibrous membrane. The pseudotumors have a tendency to expand over several years and eventually become multiloculated. Some reach enormous size and involve so many structures that the pseudotumors are inoperable. Erosion through surrounding tissues and penetration into viscera or through the skin can occur, usually as a late event. Sinus tracts from the pseudotumor predispose to infection and septicemia. Pseudotumors develop primarily in the lower half of the body, usually in the thigh, buttock, or pelvis, but they can occur anywhere, including the temporal bone. The small bones of the hands or feet are most frequently affected in younger patients. CT or magnetic resonance imaging (MRI) are useful for diagnosis. Needle biopsies of pseudotumors should be avoided because of the risk of infection and hemorrhage. The only reliable treatment is operative removal of the entire mass. The pseudotumor likely will re-form if it is not completely removed.

HEMATURIA

Almost all severely affected patients with hemophilia experience episodes of hematuria. The urine may be brown or red, depending upon the rate of bleeding. Most bleeding arises from the renal pelvis, usually

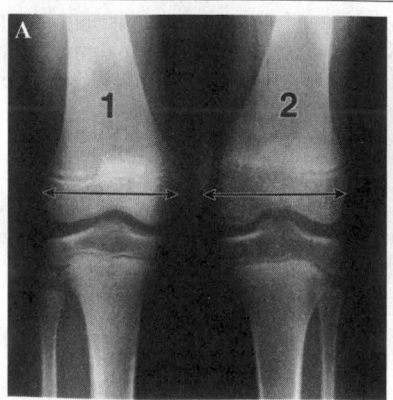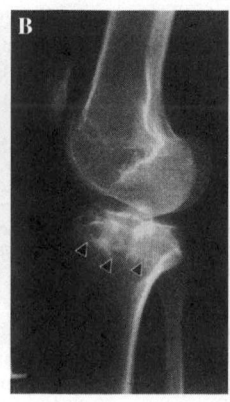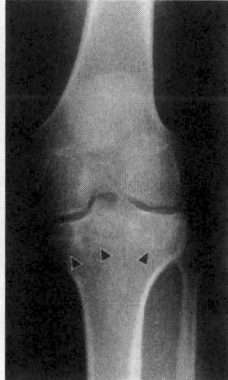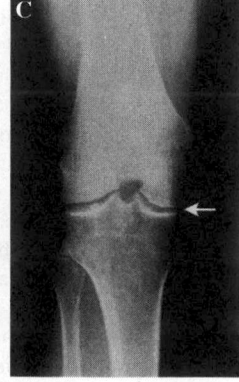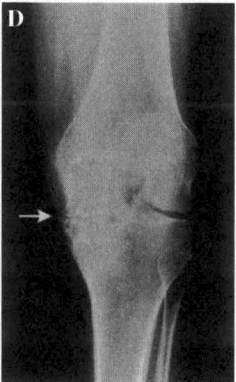

FIGURE 115-7　Various radiologic stages of hemophilic arthropathy. Stages 0 (normal joint) and 1 (fluid in the joint) are not shown. (A) Stage 2. Some osteoporosis and epiphyseal overgrowth are present in knee 2. Epiphysis is wider in knee 2 than in knee 1 (arrows). (B) Stage 3. Subchondral bone cysts (arrowheads). Joint spaces exhibit irregularities. (C) Stage 4. Prominent bone cysts with marked narrowing of joint space (arrow). (D) Stage 5. Obliteration of joint space with epiphyseal overgrowth (arrow).

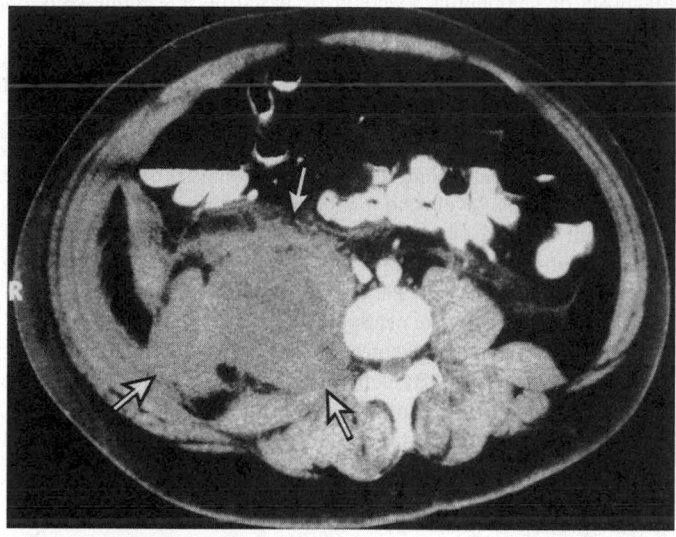

FIGURE 115-8 CT scan of a retroperitoneal hematoma in a patient with severe hemophilia A. Extent of the hematoma is indicated by the *arrows*.

from one kidney but occasionally from both kidneys. A structural lesion should be considered as a cause of hematuria. Initially, when necessary, intravenous pyelography, ultrasound, or other appropriate studies of the genitourinary tract should be used for diagnosis, although frequently no lesions are detected except for filling defects caused by clots. If the hematuria clears upon urination, bleeding from the lower genitourinary tract should be suspected. Severe renal colic may occur when clots obstruct the ureters. If the hematuria is minimal and painless and the patient's history suggests no genitourinary pathology, the physician is justified in waiting a few days for bleeding to cease. If bleeding continues, treatment with factor VIII may be necessary.

NEUROLOGIC COMPLICATIONS

Intracranial bleeding is the most dangerous hemorrhagic event in hemophilic patients.[31] Hemorrhage into the central nervous system may be "spontaneous" but usually follows trauma, which may be trivial. Symptoms often occur soon after trauma, but sometimes bleeding is delayed. For example, symptoms of a subdural hematoma may be delayed for several weeks. Hemorrhage into the brain parenchyma or a subdural or epidural hematoma should always be suspected in hemophilic patients with unusual headaches (Fig. 115-10). When intracranial bleeding is suspected, the patient should be treated immediately with factor VIII. Diagnostic procedures, such as CT scans or MRI studies, should be delayed until after treatment is initiated. Although lumbar puncture has been performed safely in severe hemophilic patients without replacement therapy, replacing factor VIII to a level of approximately 50 percent of normal prior to the procedure is safer.

Hemorrhage into the spinal canal is a highly uncommon neurologic complication in hemophilia but can result in paraplegia. Bleeding may occur within the spinal cord itself, but epidural bleeding compressing the cord is more common.[31]

Peripheral nerve compression is a frequent complication of muscle hematomas, particularly in the extremities. Compression of the femoral nerve by an iliopsoas muscle hematoma can result in sensory loss over the lateral and anterior thigh, weakness and atrophy of the quadriceps, and loss of the patellar reflex. The ulnar nerve is the next most frequently involved peripheral nerve. Bleeding may occur in any muscle and may compress local neural blood supply. This situation can be followed by permanent neuromuscular defects and multiple contractures.

MUCOUS MEMBRANE HEMORRHAGE

Mucous membrane bleeding is common in hemophilia. Epistaxis and hemoptysis, often resulting from allergic reactions or trauma, can be associated with local structural lesions involving the upper and/or lower respiratory tract. Treatment of epistaxis by cautery or nasal packing sometimes is followed by recurrent bleeding because of sloughing of the cauterized area or dislodging of a poorly formed clot when the packing is removed. Peptic ulcer disease occurs approximately five times more frequently in the adult hemophilia A population than in the general male population.[32] Ingestion of antiinflammatory drugs for relief of pain of hemophilic arthropathy is a frequent cause of upper gastrointestinal hemorrhage, and a history of ingestion of aspirin and other antiinflammatory drugs should be specifically addressed when assessing the etiology of such bleeding.[33]

DENTAL AND SURGICAL BLEEDING

Severe hemophilia usually is diagnosed in childhood, so patients are treated preoperatively and postoperatively to prevent bleeding. Mildly or sometimes moderately affected patients may go unrecognized until surgery results in excessive bleeding at the surgical site. Bleeding may be delayed for several hours or, occasionally, for several days. Surgery in such patients is characterized by poor wound healing because of

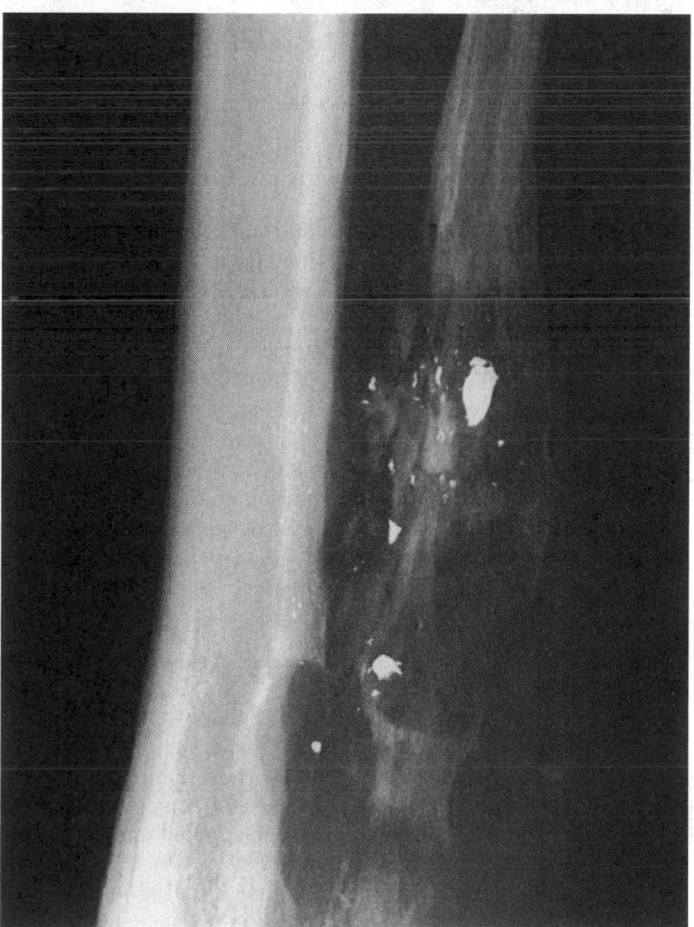

FIGURE 115-9 Pseudotumor of the fibula in a severely affected hemophilic. Note the virtual destruction with cysts and calcifications. The tibia also is involved.

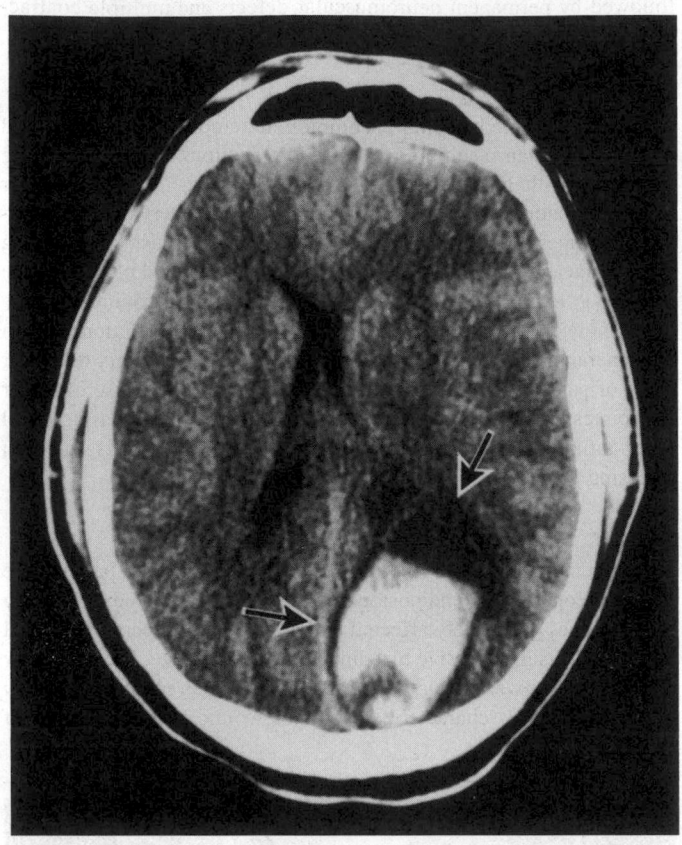

FIGURE 115-10 CT scan of an intracerebral hematoma in a severely affected hemophilic. The lesion is indicated by the *arrows*. Note compression of the ventricles.

poor clot formation. Prolonged bleeding and subsequent infection of the wound hematoma may further complicate healing. Appropriate factor VIII replacement therapy can prevent intraoperative and postoperative hemorrhages.

Dental extraction is the most frequent surgical procedure performed on hemophilic patients. Loss of deciduous teeth seldom causes excessive bleeding, but extraction of permanent teeth may result in excessive hemorrhage that can persist intermittently for several days to weeks unless appropriate treatment is administered. In the untreated patient with severe hemophilia, life-threatening, dissecting pharyngeal and/or sublingual hematomas may result from dental procedures or from administration of regional block anesthesia.

LABORATORY FEATURES

Patients with severe hemophilia A characteristically have a prolonged activated partial thromboplastin time (aPTT). The prothrombin time (PT), thrombin clotting time, and bleeding time (BT) are normal, although some investigators have reported minor increases in BT. Different combinations of aPTT reagents and instrumentation exhibit varying sensitivities to factor VIII levels. In mild hemophilia, the aPTT may be only slightly prolonged or at the upper limit of normal, especially if factor VIII activity is 20 percent or greater of normal. The aPTT is corrected when hemophilic plasma is mixed with an equal volume of normal plasma and not corrected when mixed with plasma of a known patient with hemophilia A. If the hemophilic plasma contains an inhibitor antibody against factor VIII, the aPTT on a similar mixture is prolonged, although incubation of the mixture for 1 or 2 hours at 37°C may be required to detect a prolongation. A definitive

diagnosis of hemophilia A should be based on a specific assay for factor VIII activity.

Functional factor VIII coagulant activity is measured by one-stage clotting assays based on aPTT.[34] Chromogenic assays for factor VIII activity also are used widely but do not always agree with one-stage assays.[34] Factor VIII antigen is measured by immunologic assays, which detect normal and most abnormal factor VIII molecules. If the factor VIII antigen level is normal but the clotting activity is reduced, the patient has a dysfunctional factor VIII molecule. Such patients have antigen-positive hemophilia, also referred to as *cross-reacting material* (CRM) *positive*.[35] Patients in whom both the factor VIII antigen level and activity are nearly undetectable are *CRM negative*.

Factor VIII activity is expressed as percent of normal or as units per milliliter of plasma. By definition, 1 U of factor VIII equals the amount of factor VIII in 1 ml of pooled fresh normal human plasma. Also by definition, 1 U of factor VIII per milliliter is 100 percent of normal.

DIFFERENTIAL DIAGNOSIS

Von Willebrand disease sometimes is confused with hemophilia A. The basic defect in vWD is reduced activity of vWF, which acts as a carrier of factor VIII *in vivo* (see Chap. 118). Thus, in vWD, factor VIII levels are reduced, although considerable variability exists. Although factor VIII is synthesized normally in patients with vWD, the half-life of factor VIII is shortened because the vWF "carrier" molecule is decreased or absent. Other abnormalities in vWD that distinguish vWD from hemophilia A are prolonged BT, decreased vWF antigen level, and decreased ristocetin-induced platelet agglutination. One variant of vWD that is particularly difficult to distinguish from hemophilia A is vWD–Normandy, in which vWF activities are normal but factor VIII levels are low. Several mutations causing vWD–Normandy have been described, but all of them result in decreased binding of factor VIII to vWF. The results is shortening of the intravascular survival of factor VIII and thus reduced factor VIII activity. The Normandy variant should be suspected in patients with mild hemophilia who do not exhibit a sex-linked recessive inheritance pattern.[36]

Hemophilia A must be distinguished from other hereditary blood clotting factor deficiencies that exhibit a prolonged aPTT, including deficiencies of factors IX, XI, and XII, prekallikrein, and high molecular weight kininogen. Only deficiencies of factors VIII and IX cause chronic crippling hemarthroses with a family history suggestive of an X-linked bleeding disorder. Only specific assays can distinguish hemophilia A from factor IX deficiency (hemophilia B). Factor XI deficiency occurs in males and females and is a milder hemorrhagic disorder compared to severe hemophilia A or B. Factor XI deficiency can be confused with mild hemophilia A or B, but specific assays distinguish them. Deficiencies of factor XII, prekallikrein, and high molecular weight kininogen can be distinguished from hemophilia because they are not associated with bleeding. Mild hemophilia A, with factor VIII levels of approximately 15 percent of normal, must be distinguished from combined deficiency of factors V and VIII.[37] Both PT and aPTT are moderately prolonged in the combined disorder.

THERAPY

GENERAL

General principles applicable to therapy for hemophilia A include avoidance of aspirin, nonsteroidal antiinflammatory drugs, and other agents that interfere with platelet aggregation. Acetaminophen or cyclooxygenase (COX)-2 inhibitors such as celecoxib or rofecoxib have been recommended, but these drugs can be harmful when taken in excessive doses. Patients should be advised of the numerous over-the-counter analgesics that contain aspirin or other antiplatelet agents. Addictive narcotic agents should be used with great caution and only when clearly indicated, because drug dependency can be a major problem in this disease. In general, intramuscular injections should be avoided unless the patient receives adequate replacement therapy. In the absence of prophylactic therapy, patients with hemophilia A must be treated as early as possible to avoid bleeding complications. Surgical procedures in hemophilic patients should be scheduled early in the week to avoid "weekend crises." Ample supplies of factor VIII should be available in the blood bank or pharmacy to ensure rapid access to treatment when needed. All hemophilic patients should have access to home treatment and periodic examinations at a comprehensive hemophilia diagnostic and treatment center. Prophylactic therapy should be considered in all severely affected patients.

FACTOR VIII REPLACEMENT THERAPY

Hemorrhagic episodes in patients with hemophilia A can be managed by replacing factor VIII. Several plasma products are available for use in raising factor VIII to hemostatic levels. Fresh-frozen plasma and cryoprecipitate both contain factor VIII and once were the only products available for treatment. A disadvantage of plasma is that large volumes must be infused to achieve and maintain even minimal factor VIII levels. The highest factor VIII level that can be achieved with plasma is approximately 20 percent of normal, which is not always attainable or sufficient for hemostasis. Cryoprecipitate, containing approximately 80 U of factor VIII in 10 ml of solution, can be used to attain normal factor VIII levels, but individual bags of cryoprecipitate must be pooled, the factor VIII dose can only be estimated, and the product must be stored frozen. Several commercial lyophilized factor VIII concentrates, using cryoprecipitate of pooled normal human plasmas as starting material (2000–20,000 donors), are available and do not have the disadvantages of plasma and cryoprecipitate (Table 115-3). Factor VIII concentrates have been sterilized by heating in solution, by superheating to 80°C after lyophilization, or by exposure to organic solvent–detergents that inactivate enveloped viruses, including human immunodeficiency virus (HIV) and hepatitis B and C viruses, but do not inactivate parvovirus or hepatitis A.[38,39] Parvovirus

infection does not occur frequently in hemophilia A patients because parvovirus is transmitted by cellular elements of the blood. Nevertheless, seroconversion to B19 parvovirus has been observed in patients receiving plasma-derived concentrates undergoing solvent–detergent extraction or pasteurization. Hepatitis A has occurred in patients receiving plasma-derived concentrates inactivated by solvent–detergent techniques.[40]

Some of these products contain significant amounts of vWF (see Table 115-3). Plasma-derived factor VIII concentrates prepared by monoclonal antibody techniques, and subjected to one of the procedures mentioned above, are highly purified and, barring breakdown in manufacturing techniques, are generally safe in terms of transmission of viral diseases.

Factor VIII produced by recombinant DNA techniques is available, safe, and effective (see Table 115-3). One of the newer factor VIII products, Advate, is manufactured without exposure to animal or human protein. This product was developed because of fear of transmission of new-variant Creutzfeldt-Jakob disease (CJD) disease by blood products. This concern was accelerated by a single report of possible transmission of CJD to a patient who received a blood transfusion from a donor who later developed new-variant CJD.[41] In addition to human factor VIII, porcine factor VIII can be of great benefit in hemophilic patients with factor VIII antibodies because the human anti-factor VIII antibody may not cross-react with porcine factor VIII. A comprehensive list of factor VIII concentrates is available.[42,43]

The dose of factor VIII can be determined as follows. If 1 U of factor VIII per milliliter of plasma is considered 100 percent of normal, the dose required to raise the level to a given value depends upon the patient's plasma volume (approximately 5% of body weight in kilograms) and the level to which factor VIII is to be raised. Thus, the plasma volume of a 70-kg adult is approximately equivalent to 3500 ml (5% × 70 kg = 3.5 kg = 3500g, approximately equivalent to 3500 ml). To achieve normal factor VIII levels of 1 U/ml (100%), 3500 U of factor VIII should be given. This scenario assumes a 100 percent recovery of the administered dose. Recovery has approached 100 percent in studies but depends upon the method of assay and the factor VIII standard used for comparison.[44] After the initial dose of factor VIII, further doses of factor VIII are based on a half-life of 8 to 12 hours. Thus, after a loading dose of 3500 U of factor VIII, a dose of 1750 U could be given in 12 hours. However, for practical purposes, the dose of factor VIII is based on the knowledge that 1 U of factor VIII per kilogram of body weight raises the circulating factor VIII level approximately 0.02 U/ml. Thus, to raise the factor VIII level to 100 percent, that is, 1 U/ml, the dose of factor VIII required is approximately 50 U per kilogram of body weight, assuming the patient's baseline factor VIII level is less than 1 percent of normal. The site and severity of hemorrhage determine the frequency and dose of factor VIII to be infused. Table 115-4 summarizes the recommended doses of factor VIII for various types of hemorrhage.[44] These doses are not based on rigorous randomized studies, and recommendations vary among hemophilia centers. Given the high cost of factor VIII, some physicians prefer the lower doses.

Factor VIII can be given as a constant infusion. Following a loading dose to raise factor VIII to the desired level, 150 to 200 U of factor VIII per hour can be infused. Factor VIII levels can be conveniently monitored in blood obtained from veins other than the vein into which factor VIII was infused. In selected patients, factor VIII can be given outside the hospital in a continuous infusion using pump devices.[45]

TABLE 115-3 CURRENTLY AVAILABLE FACTOR VIII PRODUCTS[a]

	ORIGIN	VIRAL INACTIVATION
Intermediate purity		
Humate P[b]	Plasma	Pasteurization[c]
Profilate SD[b]	Plasma	Solvent–detergent[d]
High purity		
Koate HP[b]	Plasma	Solvent–detergent[d]
Alphanate	Plasma	Pasteurization[c]
Monarc M	Plasma	Solvent–detergent
Hyate C	Porcine plasma	
Ultrapure[e]		
Hemofil M	Plasma	Solvent–detergent[d]
Monoclate P	Plasma	Pasteurization[c]
Recombinant		
Advate[h]	CHO cells	Solvent–detergent
Recombinate[e]	CHO cells[f]	Solvent–detergent
Kogenate[e]	BHK cells[g]	Solvent–detergent
Refacto (B-domain deleted)	CHO cells[f]	Solvent–detergent

[a] Additional concentrates are available in Europe.
[b] Contains vWF.
[c] Pasteurization at 60°C for 10 h.
[d] Solvent–detergent: TNBP + polysorbate 88.
[e] Human albumin added; insignificant vWF.
[f] Chinese hamster ovarian cells.
[g] Baby hamster kidney cells.
[h] Not exposed to human protein during manufacture.

DDAVP (DESMOPRESSIN)

During the 1970s, 1-desamino-8-D-arginine vasopressin (DDAVP; desmopressin) was found to cause a transient increase in factor VIII in normal subjects and in patients with mild to moderate hemophilia.

TABLE 115-4   DOSES OF FACTOR VIII FOR TREATMENT OF HEMORRHAGE[a]

SITE OF HEMORRHAGE	DESIRED FACTOR VIII LEVEL (% OF NORMAL)	FACTOR VIII DOSE[b] (U/KG BODY WEIGHT)	FREQUENCY OF DOSE[c] (EVERY NO. OF HOURS)	DURATION (DAYS)
Hemarthroses	30–50	~25	12–24	1–2
Superficial intramuscular hematoma	30–50	~25	12–24	1–2
Gastrointestinal tract	~50	~25	12	7–10
Epistaxis	30–50	~25	12	Until resolved
Oral mucosa	30–50	~25	12	Until resolved
Hematuria	30–100	~25–50	12	Until resolved
Central nervous system	50–100	50	12	At least 7–10 days
Retropharyngeal	50–100	50	12	At least 7–10 days
Retroperitoneal	50–100	50	12	At least 7–10 days

[a] Mild or moderately affected patients may respond to DDAVP, which should be used in lieu of blood or blood products whenever possible.

[b] Factor VIII may be administered in a continuous infusion if the patient is hospitalized. After initial bolus, approximately 150 U of factor VIII per hour usually are sufficient in an average-size adult. Doses are given every 12–24 hours.

[c] The frequency of dosing and duration of therapy can be adjusted, depending on the severity and duration of the patient's bleeding episode.

Patients with severe hemophilia A do not respond.[46] After a dose of DDAVP, 0.3 μg per kilogram body weight, factor VIII levels increase twofold to threefold above baseline in most, but not all, mildly or moderately affected hemophilia A patients. A concentrated intranasal spray of DDAVP also can be used (150 μg in each nostril).[47] The degree of response to the drug should always be determined in patients before a bleeding episode, because occasionally mildly or moderately affected patients do not respond. The peak response to DDAVP usually occurs 30 to 60 minutes after infusion. In patients with mild or moderate hemophilia A and in carriers whose baseline factor VIII levels are less than 0.5 U/ml, DDAVP may be used in lieu of blood products. The mechanism by which DDAVP increases factor VIII is unknown.

Repeated administration of DDAVP results in a diminished response to the agent (tachyphylaxis). In many patients, the response to the second DDAVP dose averages 30 percent less than the response to the first dose, and the response rate may be even less after additional doses.[48] DDAVP is a potent antidiuretic. As a result, hyponatremia in some patients whose water intake exceeds approximately 1 liter per 24 hours has been reported. No convincing evidence indicates DDAVP administration is associated with thrombosis in hemophilic patients.

ANTIFIBRINOLYTIC AGENTS

Antifibrinolytic agents, such as ε-aminocaproic acid (EACA) and tranexamic acid, have been used to enhance hemostasis in patients with hemophilia A.[49,50] Fibrinolytic inhibitors may be given as adjunctive therapy for bleeding from mucous membranes and are particularly valuable as adjunctive therapy for dental procedures. The usual oral dose of tranexamic acid for adults is 1 g four times per day. EACA can be given as a loading dose of 4 to 5 g followed by 1 g/hour in adults. Another regimen is 4 g every 4 to 6 hours orally for 2 to 8 days, depending upon the severity of the bleeding episode. Antifibrinolytic agents are particularly useful as adjunctive therapy. However, antifibrinolytic therapy is contraindicated in the presence of hematuria.

FIBRIN GLUE

Fibrin glue, otherwise known as *fibrin tissue adhesives*, has been used as adjunctive therapy to factor VIII in hemophilic patients.[51] Briefly, fibrin glue contains fibrinogen, thrombin, and factor XIII. Fibrinolytic inhibitors are added to some commercial products. The fibrinogen–factor XIII mixture is placed on the injury site and clotted with a human thrombin solution containing calcium. As a result, the fibrin clot is cross-linked and anchored to tissue. It is especially useful for hemostasis in patients undergoing dental surgery, who receive a preextraction bolus of factor VIII followed by application of fibrin glue to the tooth socket. Fibrin glue also has been used as adjunctive therapy

to factor VIII following orthopedic procedures and circumcision. It has been particularly valuable for controlling bleeding when applied to the bed of a surgical wound following removal of large pseudotumors. Some hemophilia centers prepare their own "homemade" fibrin glue using cryoprecipitate as a source of fibrinogen and factor XIII. In some cases, bovine thrombin preparations are used for clotting the fibrinogen solution. Bovine thrombin can result in complications because bovine thrombin is contaminated with small amounts of bovine factor V. As a result, human antibodies to bovine factor V and thrombin may develop in patients receiving such products. These antibodies may cross-react with human factor V and/or human thrombin, resulting in a transient hemorrhagic disorder.[52]

TREATMENT OF MINOR OR MODERATE HEMORRHAGE

On occasion, superficial cuts and abrasions are managed with local measures, that is, application of pressure sometimes suffices to control bleeding, although oozing may continue intermittently for several hours. Topical thrombin is of no value in this type of bleeding. In general, cautery should be avoided because bleeding may restart when the cauterized area sloughs.

When replacement therapy for epistaxis is needed, the factor VIII level should be raised to approximately 30 to 50 percent of normal. For treatment of hematuria, patients should be instructed to drink large quantities of fluids. If hematuria is mild, uncomplicated, and painless, factor VIII replacement is not necessary unless the hematuria persists. Gross or protracted hematuria may require replacement therapy. In these patients, factor VIII levels of at least 50 percent of normal are needed, and therapy should be continued until bleeding stops.

Hemophilic patients requiring endoscopic procedures first should be treated with factor VIII to raise levels to at least 0.5 U/ml. Only one dose may be necessary if endoscopy is uncomplicated. In cases of severe abrasions or perforations following endoscopy, factor VIII replacement should be continued until lesion healing is complete. For expanding soft tissue hematomas, factor VIII therapy should be started immediately and maintained until the hematoma begins to resolve. With effective therapy, the patient usually experiences rapid relief from pain. For treatment of acute hemarthroses, prompt administration of factor VIII decreases the occurrence of extensive degenerative joint changes, deformity, and muscle wasting. For chronic synovitis and for bleeding into "target" joints, daily administration of factor VIII to raise levels to 100 percent of normal for 6 to 8 weeks may be indicated.

TREATMENT OF MAJOR NONSURGICAL HEMORRHAGES

Any hemorrhage in a patient with hemophilia A may become major, but the following hemorrhages are common and frequently life-threatening: retropharyngeal, retroperitoneal, and central nervous system bleeding, whether subdural, subarachnoid, or into the brain parenchyma.[53]

For treatment of retropharyngeal bleeding, particularly that associated with a sensation of tightness in the throat, pain in the neck, dysphagia, or difficulty breathing, patients should receive factor VIII immediately in doses sufficient to raise factor VIII levels to normal (1.0 U/ml). Near-normal levels should be maintained until bleeding ceases and the hematoma begins to resolve. For retroperitoneal hemorrhage, early treatment is required, and therapy should be continued for 7 to 10 days; otherwise, bleeding may recur upon resumption of activity. Immediate administration of factor VIII, sufficient to raise the level to normal, should be started upon the first sign of an intracranial hemorrhage or following a history of head trauma. Even asymptomatic patients with a history of head trauma should receive at least one dose of factor VIII as a prophylactic measure, and this dose should be given before diagnostic procedures such as CT scan. Treatment of a known intracranial hemorrhage should be maintained for a minimum of 7 to 10 days, and the circulating factor VIII level should be kept normal throughout this period. Evacuation of subdural hematomas and surgical removal of hematomas involving the brain parenchyma can be performed, depending upon location. Despite aggressive replacement therapy, however, mortality from central nervous system bleeding is high.

REPLACEMENT OF FACTOR VIII FOR SURGICAL PROCEDURES

For major surgical procedures, factor VIII should be raised to normal levels before operation and maintained for 7 to 10 days or until healing is well underway. Treatment can be started a few hours before surgery and continued intraoperatively. Postoperatively, factor VIII levels should be monitored at least one or two times per day to ensure adequate levels are maintained. Because factor VIII may be "consumed" during surgery, doses of factor VIII higher than normal may be required. Thus, factor VIII levels should be measured during surgery and in the postoperative period. Bone and joint surgery may require longer periods of factor VIII coverage. Replacement of knee, hip, and elbow joints now is possible, and several weeks of replacement therapy may be needed.[54]

HOME THERAPY

Home therapy using available factor VIII concentrates was introduced in the United States in 1977 and was a major advance in the treatment of all forms of hemophilia.[55] Children as young as 3 years can be treated at home by parents or other reliable adults. Patients 6 years and older can be taught to treat themselves with factor VIII in the correct dose for an appropriate length of time. The training of patients and their families for home therapy is best accomplished in a regional comprehensive hemophilia diagnostic and treatment center or an affiliate of one of these centers. Patients are given an adequate supply of factor concentrates and the paraphernalia required for intravenous administration. Prompt treatment of hemarthroses and hematomas made possible by home therapy markedly improved the morbidity and mortality associated with hemophilia. In addition, the quality of life of hemophilia A patients improved dramatically.[56,57]

PROPHYLACTIC THERAPY

The advent of stable and safe factor VIII concentrates has made prophylactic therapy for hemophilia A in severely affected patients feasible. Administration of 40–50 U of factor VIII per kilogram of body weight three times per week markedly decreases the frequency of hemophilic arthropathy and other long-term effects of hemorrhagic episodes.[58,59] Institution of prophylactic therapy for severely affected patients has been recommended when such therapy is available. For prophylactic therapy to be successful, patients should be selected for their reliability in managing central venous catheter devices.[60,61] Analysis of the economic impact of prophylactic therapy, weighing the benefits against the high costs of factor VIII concentrates, suggests the clinical benefit of prophylaxis is warranted, as evidenced by significant improvement in the clinical condition of patients and improvement in quality of life.[62]

LIVER TRANSPLANTATION AND GENE THERAPY

Normal livers have been transplanted successfully into patients with hemophilia, with resulting cure of the hemophilic condition.[63,64] The procedure is performed not only to cure hemophilia but also for therapy for chronic hepatitis that afflicts many of the older hemophilic patients. As advances in modulation of graft-versus-host disease continue, the use of liver transplantation for cure of hemophilia may increase.

Gene replacement therapy for classic hemophilia offers an ideal approach for prophylactic therapy or even for a final cure of the disorder. Gene therapy trials in human hemophilic patients have included *ex vivo* transduction of human fibroblasts with a plasmid containing the factor VIII gene and subsequent implantation of the transduced cells into patients,[65] and infusion of a retroviral vector containing the cDNA for B domainless factor VIII.[66] Although no serious side effects were observed in either trial, in both trials the expression level of factor VIII was low (approximately 1% of normal) and persisted for only a few months to 1 year. Despite these disappointing early results, however, gene therapy still may hold promise for cure of hemophilia. Factor VIII is a difficult protein to express not only because of its large size but also because it must transit the endoplasmic reticulum–Golgi apparatus, which requires chaperone proteins for proper protein folding and other posttranslational modifications.[67,68] Molecular manipulations of factor VIII such that the protein is easier to express should make gene therapy with factor VIII more feasible in the future. Large and small animal models of hemophilia A exist and can be used to test new approaches to gene therapy.[69,70] Development of better viral and nonviral vectors is possible and promises to improve chances for future successful gene transfer in hemophilic patients.

COURSE AND PROGNOSIS

After the advent of factor VIII concentrates in the 1960s, the morbidity and mortality from bleeding in hemophilia were significantly reduced, and by the late 1970s the life span of hemophilia A patients began to approach that of normal individuals. However, use of replacement therapy has not been without significant complications. Prior to 1985, common and serious adverse side effects of treatment included the following: chronic liver disease resulting from hepatitis B and C and, from about 1978, infection with HIV.[71] Factor VIII concentrates were prepared from many thousands of donors, making contamination of lots of factor VIII concentrates highly likely. With the introduction of heat- or solvent–detergent-treated concentrates in 1985, contamination of blood products with these viruses has been eliminated for all practical purposes. However, acquired immune deficiency syndrome (AIDS) became a leading cause of death in older patients with hemophilia.[71] Chronic liver disease in hemophilia A patients resulting from transfusion-related hepatitis B and C may be accelerated by HIV infection and by the associated hepatotoxicity of antiviral drug therapy.[72] Fortunately, patients treated after 1985 can expect almost normal life spans free of the complications of hepatitis, AIDS, and other currently recognized bloodborne viral diseases. However, the development of antibodies (inhibitors, circulating anticoagulants) against factor VIII has been, and continues to be, one of the more serious complications of replacement therapy.

FACTOR VIII INHIBITORS

Other than the transmission of viral diseases by factor VIII infusions, the main complication of hemophilia A is the development of specific inhibitor antibodies that neutralize factor VIII.[73] Current debate centers around the true frequency of antifactor VIII inhibitors in severe hemophilia A patients. However, analysis reveals the frequency of inhibitors in a large group of patients was approximately 40 percent in patients with large deletions and approximately 35 percent in patients with nonsense mutations.[74] When the whole population of hemophilia A patients is included, the overall incidence of inhibitor formation appears to be approximately 20 percent over a long followup. Frequent testing for inhibitors in previously untreated patients receiving newer highly purified factor VIII products from plasma or by recombinant technology revealed the frequent occurrence of transient inhibitors to factor VIII, many of which were of low titer and did not necessitate cessation of treatment with the same product. Although still a matter of uncertainty, the risk of inhibitors does not appear to be higher with use of highly purified plasma or recombinant products than the risk reported in earlier studies using products of lower purity.[75,76] However, this observation is not an indication that development of factor VIII inhibitors may not be related to the nature of factor VIII product.[76] At least one outbreak of inhibitors appeared to be related to treatment with a specific plasma-derived factor VIII product of intermediate purity. Fortunately, inhibitors disappeared from the affected patients when use of the product was stopped.[77]

Table 115-5 lists the factors related to development of inhibitors. They arise most frequently in severely affected patients, many of whom have gross gene rearrangements or inversion of the factor VIII gene. Inhibitors usually appear early in life, after approximately 100 exposure days to factor VIII replacement.

Factor VIII inhibitors are antibodies (almost always alloantibodies, although some mild hemophilic patients develop autoantibodies against the factor), most often of the immunoglobulin (Ig)G class and frequently restricted to the IgG4 subclass.[73] Antibodies against the A_2 and C domains of factor VIII are most common. These antibodies interfere with the interactions of factor VIII with other hemostatic components (for review see ref. 78).

Early diagnosis of factor VIII inhibitors is essential. Although the presence of an inhibitor can be suspected on clinical grounds, as when a patient does not respond to conventional doses of factor VIII, laboratory diagnosis is required for confirmation. Factor VIII inhibitors are time and temperature dependent. The prolonged aPTT of the plasma of a patient without an inhibitor is corrected when mixed 1:1 with normal plasma even after incubation at 37°C for 1 to 2 hours. In contrast, the partial thromboplastin time (PTT) of a 1:1 mixture of plasma from a patient with an inhibitor and normal plasma is prolonged after incubation at 37°C for 1 to 2 hours. Specific diagnosis rests upon demonstrating that an appropriate dilution of the patient's plasma, when added to normal plasma, specifically neutralizes factor VIII and not other blood clotting factors that influence PTT (i.e., factors IX, XI, XII, prekallikrein, high molecular weight kininogen). The demonstration that the inhibitor is specific for factor VIII distinguishes it from inhibitors of other clotting factors, the lupus anticoagulant, and nonspecific inhibitors. A common assay for an inhibitor is the Bethesda assay. In the Bethesda assay, the patient's plasma is diluted such that, when the plasma is mixed with an equal volume of normal pooled human plasma and incubated for 2 hours, the factor VIII activity in the mixture is decreased by 50 percent.[79] A modification of the Bethesda assay is the Nijmegen assay, in which the pH of the sample over the 2-hour incubation period is controlled.[80]

Several approaches to treatment of factor VIII inhibitors are available (Table 115-6). Use of these treatments requires knowledge of

TABLE 115-5 RISK FACTORS FOR DEVELOPMENT OF ANTI-FACTOR VIII ANTIBODIES IN HEMOPHILIA A PATIENTS

- Disease severity: 80% of hemophilia A patients with inhibitors have <1% factor VIII activity
- Exposure to factor VIII concentrates: majority of high-titer inhibitors develop after <90 days of exposure to factor VIII
- Genetic factors
  1. Family history of inhibitor development
  2. Negative correlation with HLA Cw5 antigen
  3. Molecular defects: inversion and crossing-over defect in intron 22, gene deletions, and nonsense point mutations resulting in patients without factor VIII antigen
- Method of purification of factor VIII concentrate

SOURCE: Roberts HR: Inhibitors and their management, in *Haemophilia & Other Bleeding Disorders*, edited by C Rizza, G Lowe, p. 371. WB Saunders, New York, 1997, with permission.

whether the patient with an inhibitor is a "high" or "low" responder and whether the bleeding episode requiring treatment is minor or major.[81]

High-Responder Patients Approximately 60 percent of patients who have inhibitors are high responders. *High responders* are defined as patients whose inhibitor titer is higher than 10 Bethesda units (BU) at baseline or whose initial inhibitor titer is less than 10 BU but rises to greater than 10 BU after administration of factor VIII. Thus, high responders who are not treated with factor VIII for long periods may have a sustained high level of inhibitor, or they may have a very low to undetectable level of inhibitor until they are challenged with factor VIII.

Major bleeding episodes in a high-responder patient whose initial inhibitor titer is less than 10 BU should be treated with either human or porcine factor VIII (if the porcine product is available) (Table 115-6). With this rationale, when the initial titer is low, sufficient factor VIII can be administered to neutralize the inhibitor and attain adequate factor VIII levels for hemostasis. Although factor VIII inhibitor bypassing agents can be used (see below), they are not as reliable as factor VIII in achieving hemostasis, and their effect cannot be adequately monitored with specific laboratory tests. If human factor VIII is used, a loading dose of 10,000 to 15,000 U may be required, followed by up to 1000 U of factor VIII per hour depending upon the factor VIII level. All patients with inhibitors should be tested to determine whether their inhibitor cross-reacts with porcine factor VIII, as measured in the Bethesda assay, in which porcine factor VIII replaces human factor VIII. If the inhibitor does not cross-react with porcine factor VIII, the inhibitor can be administered in doses of 50 to 100 U per kilogram of body weight every 8 to 12 hours.

In high-responder patients whose initial inhibitor titer is less than 10 BU and who experience a minor bleeding episode, the agent of choice is a factor VIII inhibitor bypassing agent. Recombinant factor VIIa in doses of 90 to 120 μg per kilogram of body weight or higher every 2 to 3 hours is safe and effective in most hemorrhagic episodes.[81] The dosing frequency is based on a factor VIIa plasma half-life of approximately 2 to 3 hours. The mechanisms of action of factor VIIa have been investigated using *in vitro* techniques. After coagulation is initiated by the tissue factor/factor VII pathway, factor VIIa at recommended doses is hypothesized to activate factor X on the surface of activated platelets, even in the absence of additional tissue factor activity.[82] Factor Xa then can associate with factor Va and convert prothrombin to thrombin. Because activated platelets are localized to the site of vessel injury, thrombin generation by factor VIIa is localized to the site of bleeding. This process may account for the reported safety of factor VIIa.[82] If this agent is not available, activated or unactivated prothrombin complex concentrates may be used. Factor VIII can also be used but should be avoided in most instances in view of an anamnestic response of the inhibitor to factor VIII.

High-responder patients whose initial inhibitor titer is greater than 10 BU usually do not respond to even high doses of human factor VIII. If the inhibitor cross-reacts with porcine factor, this product too may be ineffective. Thus, in high-responder patients whose initial inhibitor titer is greater than 10 BU and who experience a major or minor bleeding episode, recombinant factor VIIa or an activated prothrombin complex concentrate containing factor VIII inhibitor bypassing activity (FEIBA) can be used.[83] If these agents are not available, unactivated prothrombin complex concentrates or exchange transfusion can be considered (see Table 115-6).

Low-Responder Patients Low-responder patients are arbitrarily defined as patients whose inhibitor titer is less than 10 BU even after challenge with factor VIII. For major bleeding episodes, high doses of human or porcine factor VIII can be used as recommended above. For minor bleeds, recombinant factor VIIa, or prothrombin complex concentrates (activated or unactivated), are recommended because some "low" responders convert to high responders when they are challenged repeatedly with factor VIII.

Nonactivated or activated prothrombin complex concentrates contain variable amounts of activated factors, including factors VIIa, IXa, and Xa. The activated products have higher concentrations of activated factors than do unactivated products. How these agents "bypass" the inhibitors is not known, but one postulated mechanism is enhancement of the tissue factor–factor VIIa pathway of coagulation. FEIBA reportedly contains a complex of prothrombin and factor Xa that can bind to membrane surfaces and enhance thrombin generation.

Other approaches to treatment of inhibitors include immunosuppression, removal of the antibody by plasmapheresis, adsorption of the antibody on an affinity column during plasma exchange, and administration of intravenous γ-globulin. The Malmö protocol uses nearly all of these approaches in combination, including extracorporeal adsorption of antibody to a Sepharose A column, administration of cyclophosphamide, daily administration of factor VIII, and intravenous γ-globulin.[84]

The most promising approach to eradication of an inhibitor is use of immune tolerance regimens. The basis of this approach is administration of daily doses of factor VIII until the inhibitor titer is undetectable.[85] Low-dose and high-dose regimens have been described (Table 115-7). Factor VIII inhibitor bypassing agents are used for acute bleeds that occur during immune tolerance induction. Various approaches to treatment of factor VIII inhibitors have been compiled.[86]

Other immunosuppressive drugs, including cyclosporine and rituximab, have been used in attempts to eradicate alloantibody inhibitors in hemophilic patients. However, these agents, although occasionally successful, seem to be more effective in acquired hemophilia resulting from autoantibodies against factor VIII.

INFECTIOUS COMPLICATIONS

Hepatitis Almost all multitransfused patients with hemophilia treated before 1985 were infected with one or more agents of viral hepatitis. Although many infected patients did not suffer acute symptoms, at least 50 percent developed chronic persistent or chronic active hepatitis that led to cirrhosis.[87] Hepatitis C and B viruses are commonly associated with chronic liver disease. Many adult hemophilic patients treated with concentrates before 1985 have antibodies to hepatitis B surface antigen, and some of them have circulating hepatitis B surface antigen. The antigen-positive adult patients frequently have a superimposed infection with the delta agent, leading to severe active hepatitis and cirrhosis and an increased risk of hepatocellular carcinoma.[88,90] Therapy with recombinant interferon alpha and ribavirin can reduce viral load and improve survival of affected patients.[91] All patients with hemophilia should be vaccinated against hepatitis A and hepatitis B.

Human Immunodeficiency Virus Many of the older, severely affected hemophilia A patients who were treated before 1985 have antibodies to HIV, indicating infection with the virus. The incidence of HIV antibodies in mildly affected patients is much lower and correlates with treatment with factor VIII concentrates before viral inactivation procedures were used. In one study, 14 percent of patients treated only with cryoprecipitate from 1979 to 1985 were infected with HIV, whereas 88 percent of patients treated with factor VIII concentrates became infected.[92] Screening of donor populations and new techniques for preparing factor VIII concentrates since 1985 have eliminated the risk of HIV transmission.

TABLE 115-6   TREATMENT OF INHIBITORS IN HEMOPHILIA A PATIENTS

TYPE OF PATIENT	INITIAL TITER	MINOR HEMORRHAGE[a]	MAJOR HEMORRHAGE[a]
High responder	<10 BU	Recombinant factor VIIa; prothrombin complex concentrates; activated prothrombin complex concentrates	Human factor VIII; recombinant factor VIIa; porcine factor VIII; prothrombin complex concentrates; activated prothrombin complex concentrates
High responder	>10 BU	Recombinant factor VIIa; prothrombin complex concentrates; activated prothrombin complex concentrates	Porcine factor VIII; recombinant factor VIIa; prothrombin complex concentrates; plasma exchange + high-dose factor VIII
Low responder	<10 BU	Recombinant factor VIIa; prothrombin complex concentrates; activated prothrombin complex concentrates	High-dose human factor VIII; recombinant factor VIIa; porcine factor VIII; activated prothrombin complex concentrates

[a] Choice of agents for treatment of major and minor hemorrhage are listed. Some physicians will choose the first product listed as the agent of choice, but the choice varies among physicians.
SOURCE: Roberts HR: Inhibitors and their management, in *Haemophilia & Other Bleeding Disorders*, edited by C Rizza, G Lowe, p 376, WB Saunders, New York, 1997, with permission.

TABLE 115-7   EXAMPLES OF TOLERANCE PROTOCOLS FOR HEMOPHILIA A INHIBITOR PATIENTS

IMMUNE TOLERANCE PROTOCOLS	DOSE	INITIAL RESPONSE
High-dose regimen	100 U/kg factor VIII two times per day until antibody reaches 1 BU/ml, then 150 U/kg factor VIII per day until factor VIII half-life is normal	In 16 of 21 patients, titer fell to <1 BU/ml
Low-dose regimen	50 U/kg factor VIII per day	9 of 12 patients responded
Netherlands protocol	25 U/kg factor VIII per day	11 of 18 patients responded

SOURCE: Roberts HR: Inhibitors and their management, in *Haemophilia & Other Bleeding Disorders*, edited by C Rizza, G Lowe, p 379, WB Saunders, New York, 1997, with permission.

Risk of Viral Disease Transmission by New Factor VIII Products
Available factor VIII concentrates are considered safe and effective, and almost no risk of transmitting currently known viral diseases is associated with these products. However, occasional exceptions have been observed. For example, solvent–detergent extraction does not inactivate viruses without lipid envelopes, including hepatitis A virus and parvovirus. As a result, outbreaks of hepatitis A have been reported in patients receiving some solvent–detergent-treated products. These outbreaks of viral diseases usually are related to breakdowns during the manufacturing process.

Prions Prions are infectious particles consisting of proteinaceous material devoid of a nucleic acid genome.[93] They are thought to be variant forms of a normal protein with an altered conformation. The "infectious" nature of prions may result from their ability to bind to other proteins and induce similar conformational changes in them such that new "infectious" particles can be generated. Prions are responsible for several neurodegenerative disorders, including CJD in humans, scrapie in sheep, and spongiform encephalopathy in cows. Prions are resistant to all currently available viral inactivation techniques. Although prion diseases generally are transmitted by ingestion of infected neural tissues, a new variant of CJD appears to occur in people who have eaten beef from cows infected with a form of prion causing bovine spongiform encephalopathy.[94] This form of CJD has been reported mainly in the United Kingdom and in certain other European countries and has been related to the bovine disease. For example, prions have been found in tonsillar tissue of patients with new-variant CJD, heightening concern about whether prions of this type might be transmitted by blood products.[95] One case of a patient suspected of contracting new-variant CJD following transfusion of a blood product from a donor later found to be infected has been reported.[41] Conclusive data are lacking, so continued vigilance is necessary. For this reason, certain plasma products prepared from blood of donors in the United Kingdom have been withdrawn until more data are available. As yet, no evidence of hemophilic patients being infected with CJD from blood products has been reported.

HEMOPHILIA B (FACTOR IX DEFICIENCY, CHRISTMAS FACTOR DEFICIENCY)

DEFINITION AND HISTORY

Hemophilia B is clinically indistinguishable from hemophilia A. It is a sex-linked, recessive hemorrhagic disease characterized by decreased factor IX clotting activity. In 1952, Aggeler and colleagues[7] and Biggs and colleagues[9] observed the existence of another X chromosome-linked bleeding disorder that was clinically similar to classic hemophilia. The deficient factor has been designated *factor IX*, and the disease is called *hemophilia B*. Other synonyms for factor IX include *plasma thromboplastin component* and *Christmas factor*, named after the family in which the factor was described.

ETIOLOGY AND PATHOGENESIS

Hemophilia B occurs in one of every 25,000 to 30,000 male births. As with hemophilia A, hemophilia B is found in all ethnic groups and has no geographic predilection.

Factor IX is a vitamin K-dependent, single-chain glycoprotein consisting of 415 amino acids. It is activated by the factor VIIa–tissue factor complex, or factor XIa, forming the active enzyme factor IXa (see Chap. 106). Once activated, factor IXa activates factor X in the presence of factor VIIIa, phospholipid (activated platelets), and calcium. Factor VIIIa is a necessary cofactor for activity of factor IXa. Therefore, deficiency of either factor IX or VIII leads to a similar lack

of factor X-activating activity. Factor Xa converts prothrombin to thrombin in the presence of factor Va, activated platelets, and calcium. Thus, deficiency of factor IX results in delayed conversion of prothrombin to thrombin, which is the cause of the bleeding tendency. Hemophilia B can result from either the absence or the dysfunction of factor IX molecules. Clinical severity of hemophilia B is roughly correlated with factor IX functional activity.

GENETICS AND MOLECULAR BIOLOGY

The factor IX gene is located on the long arm of the X chromosome. It is approximately 33 kb long, which is much smaller than the gene for factor VIII.[97] Because it is less complex, the factor IX gene has been studied in greater detail than the factor VIII gene. Figure 115-11 shows a schematic diagram of the gene and the protein product. The protein consists of a signal peptide that targets the protein for secretion from the hepatocyte to the circulation. The propeptide is necessary for posttranslational modification of 12 amino-terminal glutamic acid residues by an intracellular vitamin K-dependent carboxylase. The propeptide is cleaved from the mature protein before it enters the circulation. The next domain contains the 12 γ-carboxyglutamic acid (Gla) residues necessary for calcium-dependent lipid binding. The activation peptide is cleaved from the zymogen form of factor IX by either factor VIIa/TF or factor XIa, resulting in the two-chain active enzyme factor IXaβ. The catalytic triad (histidine 221, aspartic acid 229, serine 365) resides on the heavy chain (see Chap. 106).

Eight hundred ninety-six distinct mutations in the factor IX gene have been reported in the factor IX database, including more than 500 distinct amino acid substitutions and 41 complete gene deletions.[98,99] More than 30 percent of factor IX mutations occur at CpG dinucleotides. These mutations often involve critical arginine residues that result in a dysfunctional molecule.[99–102] Many mutations have been reported in more than one kindred, and some of these mutations derive from the same "founder."[103] As predicted by genetic theory of X chromosome-linked recessive disorders, approximately one third of mutations resulting in hemophilia B arise *de novo*.

Mutations in regulatory regions of the factor IX gene have been identified. Particularly interesting examples are mutations in the 5' promoter region that lead to the hemophilia B Leiden phenotype (Table 115-8). This disorder is characterized by very low levels of factor IX antigen and of activity at birth and during early childhood. The levels gradually rise to 60 percent of normal or greater following puberty, apparently in response to endogenous androgen synthesis. Several different mutations in the promoter region of the factor IX gene disrupt binding of transcription factors, resulting in reduced transcription of the factor IX gene.[103–106] The hormonal changes occurring at puberty apparently can overcome the transcription defect and maintain hemostatically adequate levels of factor IX.

Hemophilia Bm, a unique form of hemophilia B, is characterized by a deficiency of factor IX clotting activity and a prolonged ox brain PT. The original hemophilia B patient with a prolonged ox brain PT had the surname Martin, which led to the term *hemophilia Bm*.[107] A number of missense mutations affecting amino acid residues at positions 180, 181, and 182 of the protein and several residues close to the active site region have been identified in patients with the characteristic findings of hemophilia Bm. These mutations result in a factor IX molecule that exhibits abnormal interaction with ox brain tissue factor.[107]

Hemophilia B inheritance is similar to that of hemophilia A. All daughters of affected males are obligatory carriers, whereas all sons are normal. Female carriers may have factor IX levels ranging from less than 10 to 100 percent of normal, but the mean level is approximately 50 percent of normal. Carriers of hemophilia B usually are

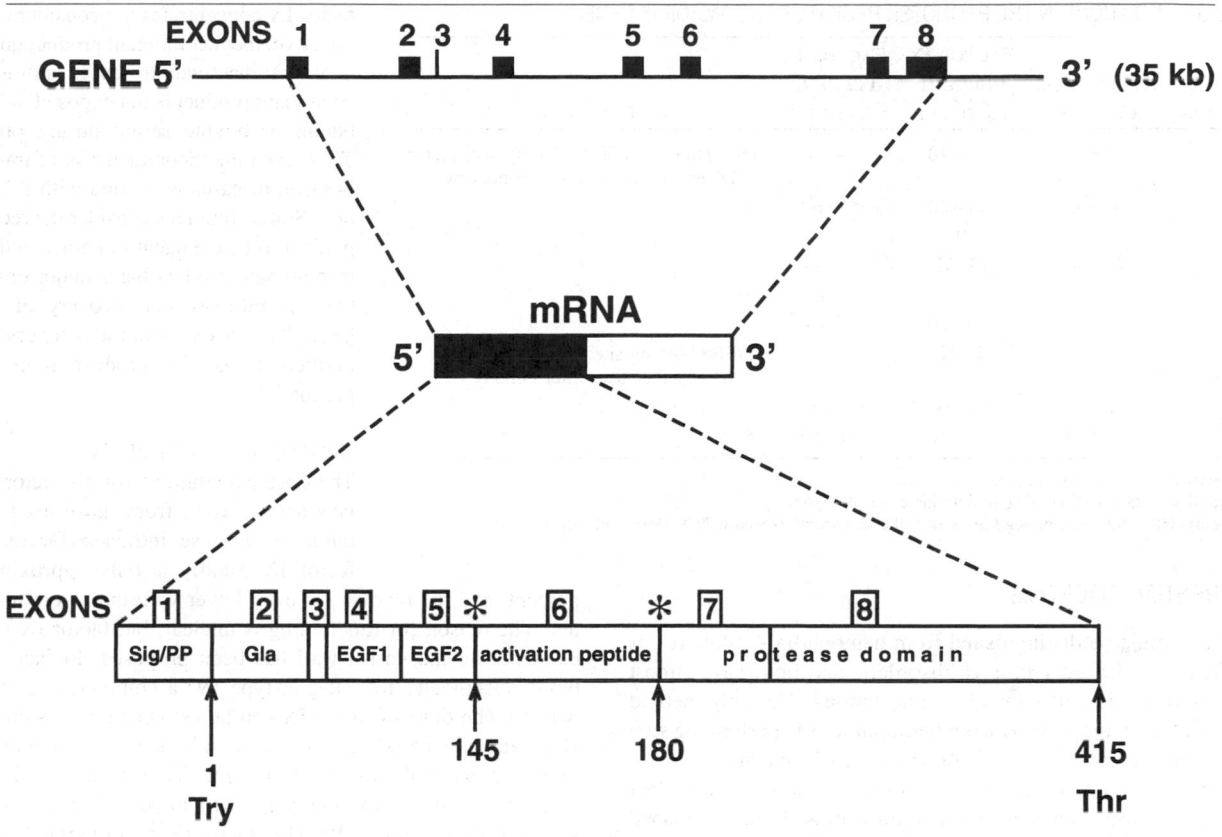

FIGURE 115-11   Schematic diagram of the factor IX gene, the messenger RNA, and the protein. Exons are depicted by the *black boxes*. The *white* 3' portion of the RNA is untranslated. The diagram of the protein shows the domains and the exons that encode each portion of the protein. The cleavage sites of factor XIa or factor VIIa–tissue factor complex are indicated by *asterisks*.

asymptomatic, except in cases of extreme X chromosome inactivation, X mosaicism, Turner syndrome, or testicular feminization.[108] When the level of factor IX activity is less than 25 percent of normal, abnormal bleeding may occur, especially after trauma.

CARRIER DETECTION AND PRENATAL DIAGNOSIS

Carrier detection and genetic screening sometimes are possible through use of DNA probes to directly identify mutations. As with factor VIII, mutations at CpG nucleotide pairs disrupt *Taq*I cleavage sites and therefore can be directly detected by restriction endonuclease mapping. More commonly, RFLP analysis is used. Prenatal diagnosis has been reliably accomplished by RFLP analysis of DNA obtained by chorionic villus sampling as early as 8 to 10 weeks after conception.[109] This procedure also can be performed on fetal cells obtained by amniocentesis and is more accurate than fetal blood sampling for factor IX activity and factor IX antigenic material. Direct sequencing of the factor IX gene can be used for carrier detection but is not available in most laboratories.

CLINICAL FEATURES

Bleeding episodes in patients with hemophilia B are clinically identical to episodes in patients with hemophilia A. (See "Clinical Features" under "Hemophilia A.") When patients are inadequately treated, repeated hemarthroses leading to chronic, crippling hemarthropathy occur. Hematoma formation with dissection into surrounding tissues is common. Hematuria, bleeding from mucous membranes, and other bleeding manifestations are as described in the section on hemophilia A. The physical, psychological, vocational, and social aspects of the disease are similar to those encountered with hemophilia A. Classification of hemophilia B is based on clinical severity and roughly correlates with the level of factor IX coagulant activity. Severe disease usually is associated with factor IX levels of less than 1 percent of normal, moderate disease is associated with factor IX levels of 1 to 5 percent, and mild disease is associated with factor IX levels ranging from 5 to 40 percent of normal.

The occurrence of factor IX inhibitor antibodies is much less common in hemophilia B patients than in hemophilia A patients. Only approximately 3 percent of severely affected patients develop inhibitors.

LABORATORY FEATURES

The screening tests used in the diagnosis of hemophilia A also are used in the diagnosis of hemophilia B. In most cases of hemophilia B, PT is normal and PTT is prolonged. However, specific assay of factor IX coagulant activity is required for definitive diagnosis. The most commonly used test is a one-stage clotting assay based on PTT. Determination of factor IX antigen levels is valuable in further classifying the disorder. PTs usually are normal in hemophilia B, but occasionally they are prolonged, especially when ox brain thromboplastin is the source of tissue factor (hemophilia Bm). Factor IX in patients with hemophilia Bm competes with factor X for activation by the factor VIIa–tissue factor complex, resulting in a prolonged PT. Because most PT reagents contain rabbit brain or human tissue factor, the PTs recorded for patients with hemophilia Bm usually are normal, and the hemophilia Bm subtype is not identified. In all forms of hemophilia B, the bleeding time usually is normal.

TABLE 115-8 MUTATIONS IN THE PROMOTER REGION OF THE FACTOR IX GENE

NUCLEOTIDE SUBSTITUTION	NUCLEOTIDE CHANGE	FACTOR IX PERCENT ACTIVITY	FACTOR IX PERCENT ANTIGEN	COMMENTS
−21	T→G	<1–70	—	Disruption of HNF-4 binding site; factor IX activity increases after puberty
−20	T→A	<1–60	<1–60	a
−20	T→C	9	—	a
−6	G→A	13–70	—	a
−5	A→T	3	—	a
6	T→A	<2–20	—	a
8	T→C	1–32	—	C/EBP binding site: factor IX clotting activity increases after puberty
13	A→G	<1–60	<1–60	b
13	delete 1	<1–60	<1–60	b

a Factor IX activity increases after puberty.
b C/EBP binding site: factor IX clotting activity increases after puberty.
SOURCE: Roberts HR: Molecular biology of hemophilia B. *Thromb Haemost* 70:3, 1993, with permission.

DIFFERENTIAL DIAGNOSIS

Hemophilia B must be distinguished from hemophilia A. Both forms are inherited as X-linked recessive disorders, and both have almost identical hemorrhagic and clinical manifestations. The only method for differentiating hemophilia B from hemophilia A is performing specific assays for factors VIII and IX on the patient's plasma.

Inherited and acquired deficiencies of other vitamin K-dependent factors, liver disease, and warfarin overdose must be distinguished from hemophilia B. In these cases, not only factor IX but all other vitamin K-dependent clotting factors, including prothrombin, factor VII, and factor X, are decreased. Acquired antibodies specific for factor IX occur in nonhemophilic patients but are very rare.

THERAPY

FACTOR IX REPLACEMENT

The basic treatment of hemophilia B is replacement of factor IX. Several products are available for use (Table 115-9). The older factor IX-containing products often are referred to as *prothrombin complex concentrates*. These products, which are prepared from large pools of human plasma (several thousand donors), contain not only factor IX but also prothrombin, factors VII and X, and proteins C and S. In addition, the products may contain small amounts of activated factors, such as factors VIIa, IXa, and Xa. Some of these products have been associated with thromboembolic events, presumably resulting from contamination with the activated components. Deep venous thrombosis and disseminated intravascular coagulation have been reported in some patients receiving large doses of prothrombin complex concentrates, but these complications seem to occur less frequently with currently available products than with earlier preparations. Nevertheless, prothrombin complex concentrates are not the best choice for replacement therapy in hemophilia B, even though the prothrombin complex concentrates are much less expensive than the highly purified factor IX concentrates. When prothrombin complex concentrates are used for replacement therapy, factor IX levels greater than 50 percent of normal should not be exceeded in order to minimize the risk of thrombosis. Use of these products in factor IX-deficient patients with liver dysfunction may be hazardous because the activated factors contaminating these preparations may not be cleared efficiently by a diseased liver, and thrombosis might be induced (see Chap. 121).

Table 115-9 lists the highly purified factor IX products. Some products are prepared from human plasma; one product (BeneFix) is produced by recombinant DNA technology. Although all available factor IX concentrates are considered safe and effective, the recombinant product undergoes a final viral inactivation step. In addition, the recombinant product is not exposed to human albumin or bovine serum during preparation. Thus, even the theoretical risk of transmission of prion diseases is averted with this preparation. Some clinicians consider the recombinant product to be the agent of choice, although the recombinant product has a major drawback in that the intravascular recovery of factor IX generally is lower than the recovery of highly purified factor IX product prepared from plasma.[110]

DOSING OF FACTOR IX

The dose calculations for all factor IX products are different from those used in hemophilia A because intravascular recovery of factor IX usually is only approximately 50 percent, and the recovery is even lower with the recombinant product. The reason for this finding is unclear, but factor IX binding to elements on the vessel wall has been proposed. In fact, factor IX binds specifically to collagen type IV, a component of the vessel wall.[111] The dose of factor IX can be estimated by assuming that 1 U of factor IX per kilogram body weight increases circulating factor IX by 1 percent of normal or 0.01 U/ml. Thus, to achieve 100 percent of normal (using only highly purified factor IX products) in a severely affected patient, 100 U of factor IX per kilogram body weight should be given as a bolus, followed by half this amount every 12 to 18 hours. Dosing should be monitored by assays of factor IX before and after bolus administration. Factor IX also can be administered as a constant infusion after the bolus administration. The dose of factor IX to be infused per hour can be estimated based on a factor IX half-life of 18 to 24 hours. Thus, in a 60-kg adult who receives highly purified factor IX, 6000 U of the factor should raise the factor IX level to approximately 100 percent of normal. Over the next 12 to 18 hours, the level decreases by approximately 50 percent. Thus, the patient needs approximately 3000 U of factor IX during that period or 250 U of factor IX per hour as an infusion. These calculations are only estimates of average responses, so factor IX dosing should be monitored by factor IX assays and the dose adjusted appropriately. Prophylactic therapy for hemophilia B also can be attempted in individuals selected in the same manner as that described for hemophilia A patients. The prophylactic dose of factor IX is 25 to 40 U/kg of body weight two times per week.

TABLE 115-9 CURRENTLY AVAILABLE FACTOR IX PRODUCTS[a]

	ORIGIN	VIRAL INACTIVATION
Intermediate purity (prothrombin complex concentrates)		
Konyne 80	Plasma	Dry heat 80°C
Proplex T	Plasma	Dry heat 60°C
Profilnine SD	Plasma	Solvent–detergent
Bebulin VH	Plasma	Vapor heating
High purity		
Mononine	Plasma	Ultra filtration; chemical
Alphanine	Plasma	Solvent–detergent
Recombinant		
BeneFix	CHO cells	Pasteurization

a Additional factor IX concentrates are available in Europe.
SOURCE: *Hematology 1997*, p 36, American Society of Hematology, Washington, DC, 1997, with permission.

Although currently available factor IX concentrates are safe in terms of transmission of HIV and hepatitis B and C viruses, patients treated prior to 1985 may have been infected with these agents.

COURSE AND PROGNOSIS

Unless treated properly, severe hemophilia B is fraught with the same complications of recurrent hemorrhages as hemophilia A. Thus, hemarthroses and chronic hemophilic arthropathy are common in inadequately treated patients. In addition to joint deformities, chronic active hepatitis and chronic persistent hepatitis are common in patients treated before 1985. Approximately 50 percent of older and severely affected patients now are HIV positive. Patients treated after 1985 are not likely to have contracted HIV and can expect to have a relatively normal life span.

Patients with severe hemophilia B may develop inhibitory antibodies against factor IX, making treatment very difficult.[112,113] Approximately 3 percent of patients with severe hemophilia B develop specific inhibitor antibodies, frequently restricted in immunoglobulin composition to the IgG4 subclass and κ light chains.[114] Most inhibitors can be detected when the aPTT of a mixture of normal plasma and the patient's plasma is prolonged. In contrast to the inhibitors in hemophilia A patients, inhibitor antibodies against factor IX are not time and temperature dependent; thus, incubating the mixtures for 2 hours at 37°C usually is not necessary. Inhibitors to factor IX can be quantitated by modifying the Bethesda method for detecting factor VIII inhibitors. Many patients with inhibitors have mutations that result in the absence of circulating factor IX antigen, most commonly deletions and nonsense mutations.

TREATMENT OF FACTOR IX INHIBITORS

When the inhibitor titer is less than 10 BU/ml, the factor IX inhibitor possibly can be neutralized using large doses of highly purified factor IX concentrates. However, when the inhibitor titer is greater than 5 to 10 BU/ml, acute bleeding in patients should be treated with the same agents used to bypass factor VIII inhibitors (see Table 115-6). Recombinant factor VIIa in doses of 90 to 120 μg per kilogram body weight administered intravenously every 2 to 3 hours can be used. Alternatively, activated or nonactivated prothrombin complex concentrates can be used (see Table 115-6).

Induction of immune tolerance can be attempted in hemophilia B patients using daily infusions of highly purified factor IX preparations. However, significant adverse reactions, including anaphylaxis and nephrotic syndrome, have been reported in severely affected patients.[115] Of the reported cases, many patients were younger than 12 years and suffered from severe hemophilia B as a result of large deletions of the factor IX gene. The nephrotic syndrome may be transient and remit upon cessation of factor IX replacement. The etiology of the nephrotic syndrome is not known. Patients with hemophilia B and factor IX antibodies who experience anaphylaxis with factor IX infusions should be treated with factor VIIa concentrates because both unactivated and activated prothrombin complex concentrates contain factor IX.

GENE THERAPY FOR HEMOPHILIA B

Long-term correction of hemophilia B has been achieved in animal models.[116] Transduction of muscle cells by an adeno-associated virus (AAV) vector containing a factor IX construct resulted in phenotypic correction of the clotting defect in hemophilia B dogs for more than 17 months.[116] Likewise, transduction of hepatocytes with an AAV vector containing factor IX DNA reportedly corrected the hemophilia defect in hemophilia B mice and dogs for approximately 7 and 8 months, respectively. Sustained factor IX levels up to 25 percent of normal

were obtained in one study in mice,[117] whereas levels exceeding 100 percent were achieved in another study.[117,119] The results in animals are encouraging and suggest that permanent corrections of the hemophilic defect using gene transfer technology in humans are possible. Clinical trials of gene transfer therapy for hemophilia B using AAV vectors containing factor IX cDNA were started in humans but have been stopped because of mild increases in liver enzyme levels.[120] These setbacks are considered temporary, and further trials hopefully will resume.[121] One of the interesting approaches to gene therapy for hemophilia B has been the introduction of an AAV vector containing the cDNA of factor VII, which, when secreted, becomes activated.[122] When factor VIIa is expressed in hemophilia B mice, even at low levels, the animals experience fewer bleeding episodes. No thromboembolic side effects were noted. Although gene transfer trials for hemophilic patients currently are suspended, ongoing studies of new vectors and in animal models of hemophilia are encouraging.

REFERENCES

1. Brinkhous KM: A short history of hemophilia, with some comments on the word "hemophilia," in *Handbook of Hemophilia*, edited by KM Brinkhous, HC Hemker, p 3. Elsevier, New York, 1975.
2. Katznelson JL: Hemophilia, with special reference to the Talmud. *Heb Med J* 1:165, 1956.
3. Morawitz P: Die Chemie der Blutgerinnung. *Ergeb Physiol* 4:307, 1905.
4. Addis T: The pathogenesis of hereditary haemophilia. *J Pathol Bacteriol* 15:427, 1911.
5. Brinkhous KM: A study of the clotting defect in hemophilia. The delayed formation of thrombin. *Am J Med Sci* 198:509, 1939.
6. Pavlovsky A: Contribution to the pathogenesis of hemophilia. *Blood* 2:185, 1947.
7. Aggeler PM, White SG, Glendenning MB: Plasma thromboplastin component (PTC) deficiency: A new disease resembling hemophilia. *Proc Soc Exp Biol Med* 79:692, 1952.
8. Wright IS: The nomenclature of blood clotting factors. *Thromb Diath Haemorrh* 7:381, 1962.
9. Macfarlane RG: An enzyme cascade in the blood clotting mechanism, and its function as a biological amplifier. *Nature* 202:498, 1964.
10. Davie EW, Ratnoff OD: Waterfall sequence for intrinsic blood clotting. *Science* 145:1310, 1964.
11. Broze GR Jr: Tissue factor pathway inhibitor and the revised theory of coagulation. *Annu Rev Med* 46:103, 1995.
12. Fay PJ: Reconstitution of human factor VIII from isolated subunits. *Arch Biochem Biophys* 262:525, 1988.
13. Roberts HR, Monroe DM, Oliver JA, et al: Newer concepts of blood coagulation. *Haemophilia* 4:331, 1998.
14. Tuddenham EGD: Factor VIII, in *Molecular Basis of Thrombosis and Hemostasis*, edited by KA High, HR Roberts, p 167. Marcel Dekker, New York, 1995.
15. Hemophilia A mutation, structure, test and resource site (HAMSTeRS). Available at: http://europium.csc.mrc.ac.uk. Accessed January 2005.
16. Tuddenham EGD, Cooper DN, Gitschier J, et al: Haemophilia A: Database of nucleotide substitutions, deletions, insertions and rearrangements of the factor VIII gene. *Nucleic Acids Res* 22:4851, 1996.
17. Lakich D, Kazazian HH, Antonarakis SE, Gitschier J: Inversions disrupting the factor VIII gene are a common cause of severe hemophilia A. *Nat Genet* 5:236, 1993.
18. Higuchi M, Kazazian HH Jr, Kasch L, et al: Molecular characterization of severe hemophilia A suggests that about half the mutations are not within the coding regions and splice junctions of the factor VIII gene. *Proc Natl Acad Sci U S A* 88:7405, 1991.
19. Antonarakis SE, Youssoufian H, Kazazian H: Molecular genetics of hemophilia in man (factor VIII deficiency). *Mol Biol Med* 4:81, 1987.

20. Mori PG, Pasino M, Vadala CR, et al: Haemophilia "A" in a 46Xi(Xq) female. *Br J Haematol* 43:143, 1979.

21. Gitschier J, Kogan S, Diamond C, Levinson B: Genetic basis of hemophilia A. *Thromb Haemost* 66:37, 1991.

22. Liu Q, Feng J, Buzin C, et al: Detection of virtually all mutations-SSCP (DOVAM-S): A rapid method for mutation scanning with virtually 100% sensitivity. *Biotechniques* 26:936, 1999.

23. Peake IR, Lillicrap DP, Boulyjenkov V, et al: Report of a joint WHO/WFH meeting on control of haemophilia: Carrier detection and prenatal diagnosis. *Blood Coagul Fibrinolysis* 4:313, 1993.

24. Ljung RC: Prenatal diagnosis of haemophilia. *Haemophilia* 5:84, 1999.

25. Goodeve AC, Peake IR: Diagnosis of hemophilia A and B carriers and prenatal diagnosis, in *Haemophilia*, edited by CD Forbes, L Aledort, R Madhok, p 63. Chapman & Hall, London, 1997.

26. Poon MC, Hoar DI, Low S, et al: Hemophilia A carrier detection by restriction fragment length polymorphism analysis and discriminant analysis based on ELISA of factor VIII and vWf. *J Lab Clin Med* 119:751, 1992.

27. Nichols WC, Amano K, Cacheris PM, et al: Moderation of hemophilia A phenotype by the factor V R506Q mutation. *Blood* 88:1183, 1996.

28. Arbini AA, Mannucci PM, Bauer K: Low prevalence of the factor V Leiden mutation among "severe" hemophiliacs with a "milder" bleeding diathesis. *Thromb Haemost* 74:1255, 1995.

29. Gilbert MS: Musculoskeletal complications of haemophilia: The joint. *Haemophilia* 6:34, 2000.

30. Gilbert MS: The hemophilic pseudotumor. *Prog Clin Biol Res* 324:257, 1990.

31. Hanley JP, Ludlam CA: Central and peripheral nervous system bleeding, in *Hemophilia*, edited by CD Forbes, L Aledort, R Madhok, p 87. Chapman & Hall, London, 1997.

32. Schulman S, Rehnberg AS, Hein M, et al: Helicobacter pylori causes gastrointestinal hemorrhage in patients with congenital disorders. *Thromb Haemost* 89:741, 2003.

33. Griffin PH, Chopra S: Spontaneous intramural gastric hematoma: A unique presentation for hemophilia. *Am J Gastroenterol* 80:430, 1985.

34. Cinotti S, Longo G, Messori A, et al: Reproducibility of one-stage, two-stage and chromogenic assays of factor VIII activity: A multi-center study. *Thromb Res* 61:385, 1991.

35. Hoyer LW, Breckenridge RT: Immunologic studies of antihemophilic factor (AHF, factor VIII): Cross-reacting material in a genetic variant of hemophilia A. *Blood* 32:962, 1968.

36. Tully EA, Gaucher C, Jorieux S, et al: Expression of von Willebrand factor "Normandy." An autosomal mutation that mimics hemophilia A. *Proc Natl Acad Sci U S A* 88:6377, 1991.

37. Seligsohn U, Zwang E, Zivelin A: Combined factor V and factor VIII deficiency among non-Ashkenazi Jews. *N Engl J Med* 307:1191, 1982.

38. Santagostino E, Mannucci PM, Gringeri A, et al: Transmission of parvovirus B_{19} by coagulation factor concentrates exposed to 100 degrees C of heat after lyophilization. *Transfusion* 37:517, 1997.

39. Robertson BH, Alter MJ, Bell BP, et al: Hepatitis A virus sequence detected in clotting factor concentrates associated with disease transmission. *Biologicals* 26:95, 1998.

40. Souci JM, Robertson BH, Bell BP, et al: Hepatitis A virus infections associated with clotting factor concentrate in the United States. *Transfusion* 38:573, 1998.

41. Llewelyn CA, Hewitt PE, Knight RS, et al: Possible transmission of variant Creutzfeldt-Jakob disease by blood transfusion. *Lancet* 363:411, 2004.

42. World Federation of Hemophilia web site. Available at: http://www.wfh.org. Accessed January 2005.

43. International Society on Thrombosis and Haemostasis web site. Available at: http://www.med.unc.edu/isth/welcome. Accessed January 2005.

44. Escobar MA: Treatment on demand—In vivo dose finding studies. *Haemophilia* 9:360, 2003.

45. Schulman S: Continuous infusion. *Haemophilia* 9:368, 2003.

46. Rodeghiero F, Castaman G, Di Bona E, Ruggeri M: Consistency of responses to repeated DDAVP infusions in patients with von Willebrand's disease and hemophilia A. *Blood* 74:1997, 1989.

47. Lusher JM: Response to l-deamino-8-D-arginine vasopressin in von Willebrand disease. *Haemostasis* 24:276, 1994.

48. Mannucci PM, Bettega D, Cattaneo M: Patterns of development of tachyphylaxis in patients with haemophilia and von Willebrand disease after repeated doses of desmopressin (DDAVP). *Br J Haematol* 82:87, 1992.

49. Porte RJ, Leebeek FW: Pharmacological strategies to decrease transfusion requirements in patients undergoing surgery. *Drugs* 62:2193, 2002.

50. Ghosh K, Shetty S, Jijina F, Mohanty D: Role of epsilon amino caproic acid in the management of haemophilic patients with inhibitors. *Haemophilia* 10:58, 2004.

51. Martinowitz U, Saltz R: Fibrin sealant. *Curr Opin Haematol* 3:395, 1996.

52. Ortel TL, Charles LA, Keller FG, et al: Topical thrombin and acquired coagulation factor inhibitors: Clinical spectrum and laboratory diagnosis. *Am J Hematol* 45:128, 1994.

53. Revel-Vilk S, Golomb MR, Achonu C, et al: Effect of intracranial bleeds on the health and quality of life of boys with hemophilia. *J Pediatr* 144:490, 2004.

54. Rodriguez-Merchan EC: Orthopaedic surgery in persons with haemophilia. *Thromb Haemost* 89:34, 2003.

55. Rabiner SF, Telfer MC: Home transfusion for patients with hemophilia A. *N Engl J Med* 283:1011, 1977.

56. Teitel JM, Barnard D, Israels S, et al: Home management of haemophilia. *Haemophilia* 10:118, 2004.

57. Manco-Johnson MJ, Riske B, Kasper CK: Advances in care of children with hemophilia. *Semin Thromb Hemost* 29:585, 2003.

58. Nilsson IM, Berntorp E, Lofqvist T, Pettersson H: Twenty-five years' experience of prophylactic treatment in severe haemophilia A and B. *J Intern Med* 232:25, 1992.

59. Carcao MD, Aledort L: Prophylactic factor replacement in hemophilia. *Blood Rev* 18:101, 2004.

60. Price VE, Carcao M, Connolly B, et al: A prospective, longitudinal study of central venous catheter-related deep venous thrombosis in boys with hemophilia. *J Thromb Haemost* 2:737, 2004.

61. Lofqvist T, Nilsson IM, Berntorp E, Pettersson H: Haemophilia prophylaxis in young patients—A long-term follow-up. *J Intern Med* 241:395, 1997.

62. Globe DR, Curtis RG, Koerper MA: Utilization of care in haemophilia: A resource-based method for cost analysis from the Haemophilia Utilization Group Study (HUGS). *Haemophilia* 10(suppl 1):63, 2004.

63. Bontempo FA, Lewis JH, Gorenc TJ, et al: Liver transplantation in hemophilia A. *Blood* 69:1721, 1987.

64. Wilde J, Teixeira P, Bramhall SR, et al: Liver transplantation in haemophilia. *Br J Haematol* 117:952, 2002.

65. Roth DA, Tawa NE Jr, O'Brien JM, et al: Nonviral transfer of the gene encoding coagulation factor VIII in patients with severe hemophilia A. *N Engl J Med* 344:1735, 2001.

66. Powell JS, Ragni MV, White GC 2nd, et al: Phase 1 trial of FVIII gene transfer for severe hemophilia A using a retroviral construct administered by peripheral intravenous infusion. *Blood* 102:2038, 2003.

67. Pipe SW: Coagulation factors with improved properties for hemophilia gene therapy. *Semin Thromb Hemost* 30:227, 2004.

68. Kaufman RJ: Good things come in small packages for hemophilia. *J Thromb Haemost* 1:2472, 2003.

69. Wilcox DA, Shi Q, Nurden P, et al: Induction of megakaryocytes to synthesize and store a releasable pool of human factor VIII. *J Thromb Haemost* 1:274, 2003.

70. Miao HZ, Sirachainan N, Palmer L, et al: Bioengineering of coagulation factor VIII for improved secretion. *Blood* 103:3412, 2004.

71. Levetow LB, Sox HCJ, Stoto MA: *HIV and the Blood Supply: An Analysis of Crisis Decision Making, Institute of Medicine*, p 1. National Academy Press, Washington, DC, 1994.

72. Santagostino E, De Filippi F, Rumi MG, et al: Sustained suppression of hepatitis C virus by high doses of interferon and ribavirin in adult hemophilic patients. *Transfusion* 44:790, 2004.

73. Lollar P: Pathogenic antibodies to coagulation factors: I. Factor VIII and factor IX. *J Thromb Haemost* 2:1082, 2004.

74. Goodeve A: The incidence of inhibitor development according to specific mutations—and treatment. *Blood Coagul Fibrinolysis* 14(suppl 1): 17, 2003.

75. Lusher JM: Is the incidence and prevalence of inhibitors greater with recombinant products? No. *J Thromb Haemost* 2:863, 2004.

76. Hoots WK, Lusher J: High-titer inhibitor development in hemophilia A: Lack of product specificity. *J Thromb Haemost* 2:358, 2004.

77. Peerlinck K, Arnout J, Gilles JH, et al: A higher than expected incidence of factor VIII inhibitors in multitransfused haemophilia A patients treated with an intermittent purity pasteurized factor VIII concentrate. *Thromb Haemost* 69:115, 1993.

78. Parker ET, Healey JF, Barrow RT, et al: Reduction of the inhibitory antibody response to human factor VIII in hemophilia A mice by mutagenesis of the A2 domain B cell epitope. *Blood* 104:704, 2004.

79. Kasper CK: Laboratory tests for factor VIII inhibitors, their variation, significance and interpretation. *Blood Coagul Fibrinolysis* 2:S7, 1991.

80. Verbruggen B, Novakova I, Wessels H, et al: The Nijmegen modification of the Bethesda assay for factor VIII:C inhibitors: Improved specificity and reliability and specificity. *Thromb Haemost* 73:247, 1995.

81. Roberts HR: The use of agents that by-pass factor VIII inhibitors in patients with hemophilia. *Vox Sang.* 77 (supp 1):38, 1999.

82. Monroe DM, Roberts HR: Mechanism of action of high-dose factor VIIa: Points of agreement and disagreement. *Arterioscler Thromb Vasc Biol* 23:8, 2003.

83. Varadi K, Negrier C, Berntorp E, et al: Monitoring the bioavailability of FEIBA with a thrombin generation assay. *J Thromb Haemost* 1:2374, 2003.

84. Makris M: Systematic review of the management of patients with haemophilia A and inhibitors. *Blood Coagul Fibrinolysis* 15(suppl 1):S25, 2004.

85. Brackmann HH, Effenberger W, Heiss L, et al: Immune tolerance induction: A role for recombinant activated factor VII (rVIIa)? *Eur J Haematol* 63:18, 1998.

86. http://www.hemostasis-forum.org. Accessed January 2005.

87. Triger DR, Preston FE: Chronic liver disease in haemophiliacs. *Br J Haematol* 74:241, 1990.

88. Lemon SM, Becherer PR, Wang JG, et al: Hepatitis delta infection among multiply-transfused hemophiliacs. *Prog Clin Biol Res* 364:351, 1991.

89. Rosina F, Saracco G, Rizzetto M: Risk of post-transfusion infection with the hepatitis delta virus. A multicenter study. *N Engl J Med* 312:1488, 1985.

90. Gerritzen A, Brackmann H, Van Loo B, et al: Chronic delta hepatitis in haemophiliacs. *J Med Virol* 34:188, 1991.

91. Gotto J, Dusheiko GM: Hepatitis C and treatment with pegylated interferon and ribavirin. *Int J Biochem Cell Biol* 36:1874, 2004.

92. Gjerset GF, Clements MJ, Counts RB, et al: Treatment type and amount influenced human immunodeficiency virus seroprevalence of patients with congenital bleeding disorders. *Blood* 78:1623, 1991.

93. Prusiner SB: Molecular biology of prion diseases. *Science* 252:1515, 1991.

94. Lee CA, Ironside JW, Bell JE, et al: Retrospective neuropathological review of prion disease in U.K. haemophilic patients. *Thromb Haemost* 80:909, 1998.

95. Farrugia A: Risk of variant Creutzfeldt-Jakob disease from factor concentrates: Current perspectives. *Haemophilia* 8:350, 2002.

96. Biggs R, Douglas AS, Macfarlane RG: Christmas disease: A condition previously mistaken for hemophilia. *Br Med J* 12:1373, 1952.

97. Kurachi K, Davie EW: Isolation and characterization of a cDNA coding for factor IX. *Proc Natl Acad Sci U S A* 79:6461, 1982.

98. Noyes CM, Griffith MJ, Roberts HR, Lundblad RL: Identification of the molecular defect in factor IX Chapel Hill: Substitution of a histidine for an arginine at position 145. *Proc Natl Acad Sci U S A* 80: 4200, 1983.

99. http://www.kcl.ac.uk/ip/petergreen/intro.html Accessed January 2005.

100. Monroe DM, McCord DM, Huang MN, et al: Functional consequences of an arginine 180 to glutamine mutation in factor IX Hilo. *Blood* 73: 1540, 1989.

101. Bertina RM, van der Linden IK, Mannucci PM, et al: Mutations in hemophilia Bm occur at the Arg 180-Val activation site or in the catalytic domain of factor IX. *J Biol Chem* 265:10876, 1990.

102. Bottema CD, Ketterling RP, Ii S, et al: Missense mutations and evolutionary conservation of amino acids: Evidence that many of the amino acids in factor IX function as "spacer" elements. *Am J Hum Genet* 49: 820, 1991.

103. Ketterling RP, Bottema CD, Phillips JA III, Sommer SS: Evidence that descendants of three founders constitute about 25% of hemophilia B in the United States. *Genomics* 10:1093, 1991.

104. Briet E, Bertina RM, van Tilburg NH, Veltkamp JJ: Hemophilia B Leyden: A sex-linked hereditary disorder that improves after puberty. *N Engl J Med* 306:788, 1982.

105. Crossley M, Ludwig M, Stowell KM, et al: Recovery from hemophilia B Leyden: An androgen-responsive element in the factor IX promoter. *Science* 257:377, 1992.

106. Reijnen MJ, Sladek FM, Bertina RM, Reitsma PH: Disruption of a binding site for hepatocyte nuclear factor 4 results in hemophilia B Leyden. *Proc Natl Acad Sci U S A* 89:6300, 1992.

107. Hamaguchi N, Roberts HR, Stafford DW: Mutations in the catalytic region of factor IX that are related to the subclass hemophilia Bm. *Biochem* 32:6324, 1993.

108. Lusher JM, McMillan CW: Severe factor VIII and factor IX deficiency in females. *Am J Med* 65:637, 1978.

109. McGraw RA, Davis LM, Lundblad RL, et al: Structure and function of factor IX: Defects in haemophilia B. *Clin Haematol* 14:359, 1985.

110. White GC, Bebe A, Nielsen B: Recombinant factor IX. *Thromb Haemost* 78:261, 1997.

111. Wolberg AS, Stafford DW, Erie DA: Human factor IX binds to specific sites on the collagenous domain of collagen IV. *J Biol Chem* 272:16717, 1997.

112. Kim HC, McMillan CW, White GC, et al: Purified factor IX using monoclonal immunoaffinity technique: Clinical trials in hemophilia B and comparison to prothrombin complex concentrates. *Blood* 79:568, 1992.

113. Briet E, Reisner HM, Roberts HR: Inhibitors in Christmas disease, in *Factor VIII Inhibitors*, edited by LW Hoyer, p 408. Alan R. Liss, New York, 1984.

114. High KA: Factor IX: Molecular structure, epitopes, and mutations associated with inhibitor formation, in *Inhibitors to Coagulation Factors*, edited by LM Aledort, LW Hoyer, JM Lusher, HM Reisner, CG White, p 79. Plenum, New York, 1995.

115. Warrier I, Ewenstein BM, Koerper MA, et al: Factor IX inhibitors and anaphylaxis in hemophilia B. *J Pediatr Hematol Oncol* 19:23, 1997.

116. Herzog RW, Yang EY, Couto LB, et al: Long term correction of hemophilia B by gene transfer of blood coagulation factor IX mediated by adeno-associated viral vector. *Nat Med* 5:56, 1999.

117. Arruda VR, Schuettrumpf J, Herzog RW, et al: Safety and efficacy of factor IX gene transfer to skeletal muscle in murine and canine hemophilia B models by adeno-associated viral vector serotype 1. *Blood* 103: 85, 2004.

118. Wang L, Takabe K, Bidlingmaier SM, et al: Sustained correction of bleeding disorder in hemophilia B mice by gene therapy. *Proc Natl Acad Sci U S A* 96:3906, 1999.

119. Kay MA, Manno CS, Ragni PJ, et al: Evidence for gene transfer and expression of factor IX in haemophilia B patients treated with AAV vector. *Nat Genet* 24:257, 2000.

120. Kaiser J: Gene therapy: Side effects sideline hemophilia trial. *Science* 304:1423, 2004.

121. High KA: Clinical gene transfer studies for hemophilia B. *Semin Thromb Hemost* 30:257, 2004.

122. Margaritis P, Arruda VR, Aljamali M, et al: Novel therapeutic approach for hemophilia using gene delivery of an engineered secreted activated Factor VII. *J Clin Invest* 113:1025, 2004.

INHERITED DEFICIENCIES OF COAGULATION FACTORS II, V, VII, X, XI, AND XIII AND COMBINED DEFICIENCIES OF FACTORS V AND VIII AND OF THE VITAMIN K-DEPENDENT FACTORS

URI SELIGSOHN

ARIELLA ZIVELIN

AIDA INBAL

Bleeding tendencies caused by inherited deficiencies of one or more coagulation factors are rare disorders distributed worldwide. Homozygotes or compound heterozygotes for the mutant genes responsible for these defects exhibit bleeding manifestations that are of variable severity and usually related to the extent of the decreased activity of the particular coagulation factor. Heterozygotes for the various deficiencies rarely display a bleeding tendency. Numerous mutations have been identified in genes encoding coagulation factors II, VII, X, V, XI, and XIII. For some factors, such as factors II, VII, and X, mutations giving rise to dysfunctional proteins predominate, whereas for other factors, such as factors V, XI, and XIII, true protein deficiencies usually are found. Combined deficiency of factors V and VIII, inherited as an autosomal recessive trait, results from mutations in genes encoding two proteins that transport factors V and VIII out of the endoplasmic reticulum to the Golgi compartment. The very rare combined deficiency of the vitamin K-dependent coagulation factors can be caused by mutations in the gene encoding for a carboxylase that γ-carboxylates glutamic acid residues in these proteins or in the gene encoding vitamin K epoxide reductase. Treatment of patients with the various coagulation factor deficiencies may be necessary during spontaneous bleeding episodes, during and after surgical procedures, and for prevention of intracranial hemorrhage. In most deficiency states, plasma replacement has been used, but

specific concentrates of all the vitamin K-dependent factors and of factors VII, XI, and XIII are available.

Inherited deficiencies of the coagulation factors other than factor VIII (hemophilia A) and factor IX (hemophilia B) are rare bleeding disorders that have been described in most populations. The severity of bleeding manifestations in affected patients, who usually are homozygotes or compound heterozygotes for a mutant gene, is variable and usually related to the extent of the deficiency. Some patients have only mild bruising or display excessive bleeding only following trauma. Other patients with less than 1 percent of normal factor VII, XIII, or X activity exhibit intracranial hemorrhages and hemarthroses similar to those of patients with severe hemophilias A and B.

The study of these disorders has significantly advanced the understanding of the pathophysiology of blood coagulation mechanisms (see Chap. 106). Following characterization of the genes encoding for the coagulation factors, a host of mutations causing the various deficiencies have been identified (Table 116-1). Use of molecular genetic techniques has established the molecular basis for two disorders that have been enigmas for several decades. The inherited combined deficiency of factors V and VIII was shown to be caused by mutations in two genes encoding for transporter proteins carrying factors V and VIII from the endoplasmic reticulum to the Golgi apparatus, and the combined deficiency of all vitamin K-dependent factors was shown to result from mutations in two genes encoding for the carboxylase that introduces γ-carboxyl groups into these coagulation factors and for the vitamin K epoxide reductase (VKOR) that replenishes the resources of active vitamin K, respectively.

This chapter reviews the clinical, biochemical, and genetic aspects of the inherited deficiencies of coagulation factors that cause bleeding tendencies other than the hemophilias (see Chap. 115) and von Willebrand disease (see Chap. 118). Published mutations causing the coagulation factor deficiencies reviewed in this chapter and their characteristics have been compiled and placed on the International Society of Thrombosis and Hemostasis web site (http://www.med.unc.edu/isth/) under databases. This list will be periodically updated.

FACTOR II DEFICIENCY

DEFINITION

Inherited factor II (prothrombin) deficiency presents in two forms: type I, true deficiency (hypoprothrombinemia), or type II, in which dysfunctional prothrombin is produced (dysprothrombinemia). These autosomal recessive disorders are rare, genetically heterogeneous, and characterized by a mild to moderate bleeding tendency. Both types of prothrombin deficiency impair the generation or function of thrombin, the central enzyme of the blood coagulation system.

MOLECULAR FEATURES AND BIOCHEMISTRY

Prothrombin is an M_r approximately 72,000 protein that is structurally homologous with other members of the vitamin K-dependent proteins, factors VII, IX, and X, protein C, protein S, and bone γ-carboxyglutamic acid (Gla) protein. Prothrombin is synthesized in the liver as a prepropeptide of 622 amino acids. Prothrombin is composed of the following domains: a prepropeptide domain (residues −43 to −1), a Gla domain (residues 1–37), kringle 1 domain (F1; residues 38–155), kringle 2 domain (F2; residues 156–271), and catalytic domain (residues 272–579).[1–3] The prepropeptide domain is responsible for protein processing, targeting, and carboxylation, and it is removed prior to secretion from the cell. The Gla domain constitutes the amino-terminus of the mature prothrombin molecule and contains the 10 glutamic acid residues that are posttranslationally modified through action

TABLE 116-1   MUTATIONS CAUSING RARE BLEEDING DISORDERS

				NUMBER OF MUTATIONS BY TYPE					
DEFICIENCY	GENE	GENE SIZE[a]	PROMOTER	MISSENSE	NONSENSE	SPLICING	INSERTION/ DELETION	GROSS DELETION	TOTAL NUMBER
Prothrombin	Prothrombin	20.3		33	2	2	5		42
Factor V	Factor V	72.3		11	8	5	14		38
Factor VII	Factor VII	14.2	7	85+2[b]	8	17	14		133
Factor X	Factor X	26.7		47+1[b]		5	5	2	60
Factor XI	Factor XI	22.7		27	11	7	8		53
Factor XIII	Factor XIII A	176.6		29	4	10	14	1	58
Factor XIII	Factor XIII B	28.0		1		1	2		4
Combined factors V and VIII	LMAN1 (ERGIC-53)	29.4		1[b]	3	4	10		18
Combined factors V and VIII	MCFD2	13.9		2		2	3		7
Vitamin K dependent factors	γ-glutamyl carboxylase	12.4		2					2
Vitamin K dependent factors	Vitamin K epoxide reductase			1					1

[a] Gene size is based on the human genome working draft available at http://genome.ucsc.edu. It varies somewhat from the original gene size reports.
[b] Initiation codon.
For detailed information on the mutations included in this table see http://www.med.unc.edu/isth/.

of vitamin K-dependent carboxylase to Gla. As a result of this modification, prothrombin acquires the capacity to bind calcium and membranes containing acidic phospholipids. The kringle domain contains two extensively folded, disulfide-bonded "kringle" motifs, the functions of which are not fully understood.[4] They are present in diverse proteins and are thought to mediate protein–protein interactions. For example, the second kringle mediates interaction of prothrombin with activated factor V (factor Va).[5] The catalytic domain contains the enzyme's active site, which is responsible for fibrinogen cleavage. The residues characteristic for the serine protease family, His363, Asp419, and Ser525, constitute a charge relay system responsible for bond cleavage. The crystal structure of prothrombin has not been determined, but the crystal structure of human α-thrombin complexed with *D-Phe-Pro-Arg chloromethylketone* (an inhibitor that is a transition state analogue covalently bound to the enzyme) has been determined.[6]

The prothrombin gene is located on chromosome 11 near the centromere.[7] It is 20 kb long and consists of 14 exons separated by 13 introns. Comparison of the organization of the prothrombin gene shows homology with the organization of other vitamin K-dependent serine protease genes, with the highest degree of homology in the part encoding the Gla domain. An unusual feature of the prothrombin gene is the presence of 41 copies of Alu-repetitive sequences in the upstream and intervening sequences.[8,9] The function, if any, of these sequences is unknown.

Prothrombin plays a central role in coagulation, functioning in both tissue factor and surface activation pathways. Prothrombin is converted to its proteolytically active form thrombin by the prothrombinase complex consisting of activated factor X (factor Xa), factor Va, and phospholipid surface of platelets and other cells (see Chap. 106). Two forms of thrombin are generated: meizothrombin if prothrombin is cleaved at residue 320, and α-thrombin if cleavage occurs first at residue 271, yielding prothrombin fragment 1.2, and subsequently at residue 320. The α-thrombin A-chain (residues 272–320) formed by factor Xa cleavage is encoded by exons 8 and 9. The B-chain (residues 321–579) containing the catalytic site and regulatory elements is encoded by exons 9 to 14.

Thrombin is a multifunctional serine protease. In addition to converting fibrinogen to fibrin (see Chap. 117) thrombin also activates (1) platelets by cleavage of the protease-activated receptor (PAR)-1 and

PAR-4, initiating signals leading to adhesion and aggregation; (2) factors V, VIII, and XI, promoting generation of additional thrombin; (3) factor XIII, which leads to cross-linking of fibrin; (4) plasminogen, converting it to plasmin and thereby activating the fibrinolytic system; (5) thrombin-activatable fibrinolysis inhibitor (TAFI), which leads to fibrinolysis inhibition; and (6) protein C after binding to thrombomodulin in the presence of endothelial protein C receptor (see Chap. 107). Thrombin also stimulates wound healing through its action as a growth factor and its proangiogenic activity.[10]

GENETICS

Abnormalities of prothrombin are inherited in an autosomal recessive manner. Among individuals with type I deficiency, heterozygotes exhibit prothrombin levels that are approximately 50 percent of normal, whereas homozygotes display levels that typically are less than 10 percent of normal. Prothrombin activity and antigen levels are reduced concordantly in these patients, who are designated as cross-reacting material (CRM) negative (CRM−). Heterozygotes for type II deficiency exhibit a prothrombin activity level approximately 50 percent of normal, with antigen levels that are normal or nearly normal. Homozygotes display a prothrombin activity level 1 to 20 percent of normal, with antigen levels that are either normal (CRM+) or partially reduced (CRMred). Compound heterozygotes with one type I deficiency allele and one type II deficiency allele have been reported. They typically have a prothrombin activity level between 1 and 20 percent, with antigen levels between 13 and 50 percent of normal. Undetectable plasma prothrombin probably is incompatible with life, as inferred from the embryonic and neonatal lethality of prothrombin knockout mice.[11]

Forty-two mutations that cause prothrombin deficiency have been identified, of which 33 are missense, two nonsense, five small deletions/insertions, and two splicing mutations (see Table 116-1). Type II deficiency (dysprothrombinemias) results from missense mutations that are located throughout the gene. However, many mutations are in the catalytic domain, imparting dysfunction of thrombin [Arg418Trp (Tokushima, Molise), Met337Thr (Himi I), Arg388His (Himi II), Arg382His, Arg382Cys (Quick I, Corpus Christi), Gly558Val (Quick II), Glu466Ala (Salakta, Frankfurt), Arg517Gln (Greenville), Gly548Ala

(Perija), Lys556Thr (Scranton)].[12–21] Other mutations give rise to abnormally slow activation of prothrombin [Arg271Cys (Barcelona, Madrid, Obihirio), Arg271His (Padua, Dhahran), Arg320His (San Antonio), Arg457Gln (Puerto Rico I)].[15–25] Nine mutations were identified in patients with type I deficiency, of which four were present in homozygotes. Two mutations clustered in distinct populations suggest common ancestry: prothrombin Puerto Rico I reported in five unrelated families from Puerto Rico, and prothrombin Perija, which is found in 35 percent of Yukba Indians living in a small village in Venezuela.[25–27]

A number of polymorphisms have been identified in the prothrombin gene. One of these polymorphisms, a G→A change at nucleotide 20210 in the 3' untranslated region of the prothrombin gene, is associated with increased plasma levels of prothrombin and an increased tendency to venous thrombosis.[28] The 20210A variant increases the efficiency of prothrombin mRNA processing and stability (see. Chap 122).[29]

CLINICAL MANIFESTATIONS

Inherited type I and II deficiencies are characterized by mild to moderate mucocutaneous and soft tissue bleeding that usually correlates with the degree of functional prothrombin deficiency. With prothrombin levels less than 1 percent of normal, bleeding may occur spontaneously or following trauma. Surgical bleeding may be significant. Menorrhagia, epistaxis, gingival bleeding, easy bruising, and subcutaneous hematomas may occur. Hemarthrosis has been observed but is less frequent than in the hemophilias. In patients with prothrombin activities 2 to 5 percent of normal, bleeding is variable. Some individuals bleed following minimal trauma, whereas others are asymptomatic. Patients with prothrombin activity 5 to 50 percent of normal usually bleed only following major trauma and surgery, or they do not bleed at all.

DIFFERENTIAL DIAGNOSIS

The activated partial thromboplastin time (aPTT) and prothrombin time (PT) are variably prolonged in inherited hypoprothrombinemia and dysprothrombinemia, but thrombin time is normal. The diagnosis of a prothrombin abnormality is established by demonstrating decreased functional levels of prothrombin. Both functional and antigenic levels of prothrombin should be determined in cases of possible prothrombin deficiency in order to establish the presence of dysprothrombinemia. Although acquired prothrombin deficiency is infrequent (e.g., in patients with antiphospholipid antibodies who have a bleeding tendency), family studies are helpful in establishing the diagnosis of an inherited deficiency.

Prothrombin can be activated by enzymes of several snake venoms, and the pattern of activation can provide clues to the nature of the prothrombin abnormality. Activation of prothrombin by Taipan viper venom and by *Pseudonaja textilis* venom is independent of factor V. Thus, normal Taipan viper venom or *Pseudonaja textilis* venom times with an abnormal classic one-stage assay for prothrombin implies a defect in the region of prothrombin that binds factor V. *Echis carinatus* venom activates prothrombin in the absence of factor V, phospholipid, and calcium and therefore can be used with other prothrombin activators to test the requirement for each of these components. Plasma prothrombin immunoelectrophoresis is useful for the diagnosis of dysprothrombinemias.

Prolonged aPTT and PT with a normal thrombin time are seen in inherited factor V and factor X deficiency, acquired conditions such as vitamin K deficiency, therapeutic or surreptitious use of warfarin, liver disease, and lupus anticoagulants. These various disorders are readily distinguished by taking the patient's history and performing additional factor assays (see Chap. 109).

THERAPY

Replacement therapy in patients with inherited prothrombin deficiencies consists of administration of prothrombin complex concentrates containing coagulation factors II, VII, IX, and X. These concentrates are heated or treated with solvent–detergent, processes that remove HIV, hepatitis B, hepatitis C, and other viruses but do not remove parvovirus, hepatitis A virus,[30–33] and other possible bloodborne agents such as prions causing Creutzfeldt-Jacob disease and its new variant. Thus, these concentrates are not without risk. In addition to the zymogen forms of factors II, VII, IX, and X, prothrombin complex concentrates contain small amounts of activated forms of some of these factors. As a result, their administration may cause venous thromboembolism, myocardial infarction, or stroke.[34] The risk of thrombosis appears to increase with the dose; thus, repeated administration of small doses probably is safer.

Fresh-frozen plasma is effective but confers a very low but measurable risk of HIV and hepatitis B and C virus transmission. Solvent–detergent-treated fresh-frozen plasma has been developed, providing increased safety. However, because solvent–detergent-treated fresh-frozen plasma is prepared from large pools of plasma, it may increase the risk of transmitting agents that are not destroyed by solvent–detergent treatment.

In many cases, the decision is not what to use for treatment but whether treatment is needed. Bruises and mild superficial bleeding generally do not require replacement therapy. The biologic half-life of prothrombin is approximately 3 days, so in many cases a single treatment is sufficient for prevention of surgical bleeding or arrest of significant bleeding.

FACTOR VII DEFICIENCY

DEFINITION AND HISTORY

Hereditary deficiency of factor VII, first described by Alexander and colleagues[35] in 1951, is a rare autosomal recessive disorder that has been observed in most populations. Among the rare clotting factor deficiencies described in this chapter and recorded in the United Kingdom, Italy, Iran, and the United States, the relative frequency of factor VII deficiency is by far the highest.[36,37] The disorder is symptomatic mainly in homozygotes or compound heterozygotes, and the symptoms vary greatly from mild to severe. A presumptive diagnosis can be easily made, because factor VII deficiency is the only coagulation disorder that produces a prolonged PT and a normal aPTT (see Chap. 109).

BIOCHEMISTRY AND MOLECULAR FEATURES

Human factor VII is a single-chain glycoprotein (Mr ~50,000) that is secreted from the liver parenchymal cells as a zymogen. The mature protein consists of 406 amino acids organized in three main domains: a Gla domain at the N-terminus containing 10 Gla residues, a growth factor domain in the center, and a serine protease domain at the C-terminus.[38] Vitamin K is required for formation of the Gla residues that bind calcium ions and permit interactions with phospholipid membranes. The factor VII gene spans approximately 12.8 kb[39] and is located on chromosome 13q34,[40,41] 2.8 kb upstream from the factor X gene.[42] The gene contains a pre-pro leader sequence and seven exons that encode the mature protein. Promoter and silencer elements of the 5' flanking region have been characterized.[43,44] Factor VII zymogen circulates in blood at an extremely low concentration (~500 ng/ml)[45] and has the shortest half-life of all coagulation factors (5 hours).[46]

Factor VII is converted to activated factor VII (factor VIIa) by cleavage of an Arg152-Ile153 bond, resulting in a two-chain molecule held together by a disulfide bond. The cleavage can be caused by factor

Xa,[47] activated factor IX (factor IXa),[48] activated factor XII (factor XIIa),[48,49] thrombin,[47] and factor VIIa in the presence of tissue factor in an autoactivation process.[50] Binding of factor VII to tissue factor strikingly enhances these reactions.[51–55]

Factor VIIa can be detected in plasma by a sensitive assay using a recombinant soluble form of tissue factor.[56] The mean concentration of plasma factor VIIa is 3.6 ng/ml in normal individuals, which is 0.76 percent of the total factor VII mass in plasma. The half-life of factor VIIa is relatively long (~2.5 hours)[57] compared to other activated coagulation factors. Factor IXa, which activates factor VII,[48] probably is responsible for the basal levels of plasma factor VIIa in normal individuals, but its origin is unknown. This supposition is supported by the observation that patients with severe hemophilia B, unlike patients with severe hemophilia A, have a very low concentration of circulating factor VIIa.[58,59] Moreover, hemophilia B patients acquire normal levels of factor VIIa within a few hours of purified factor IX infusion.[60]

The initial generation of thrombin that heralds blood coagulation occurs when blood is exposed to tissue factor present in the subendothelium, in tissues, or on the surface of stimulated monocytes (see Chap. 106). The exposed tissue factor forms a complex with circulating factor VIIa, which activates factor X, and factor Xa converts prothrombin to thrombin in the presence of factor Va (of an unidentified source), negatively charged phospholipids, and calcium ions. The factor VIIa–tissue factor complex also activates factor IX.[61] Once factor VIII is activated by the initial amounts of generated thrombin, factor IXa in the presence of factor VIIIa, negatively charged phospholipids, and calcium ions activates factor X at a rate 50-fold higher than the rate of factor X activation by factor VIIa–tissue factor complex.[62]

When factor VII is completely lacking, as in knockout mice, fatal hemorrhage occurs perinatally.[63] Mice lacking tissue factor die during the embryonal phase because of abnormalities in the vascular wall,[64] whereas transgenic mice, rescued by incorporation of approximately 1 percent human tissue factor activity, develop normally and exhibit normal hemostasis.[65]

GENETICS

Factor VII deficiency is inherited as an autosomal recessive trait. The disorder manifests in homozygotes or compound heterozygotes, some of whom are also homozygotes for polymorphisms associated with reduced factor VII levels.[53,66,67]

The heterogeneity of factor VII deficiency was apparent in 1971, when two of four patients studied were found to have dysfunctional factor VII demonstrable by the presence of antibody-neutralizing material.[68] Later studies confirmed these observations and classified subjects with factor VII deficiency into CRM−, CRM+ (having normal levels of factor VII antigen), and CRM-reduced.[69,70] The latter two categories predominated.[70] Further complexity emanated from observations of variable reactivities of plasma from individuals with factor VII deficiency to bovine, rabbit, and human tissue factor.[70] Following the characterization of the factor VII gene, the heterogeneity of factor VII deficiency was confirmed. At the time of this writing, more than 130 mutations have been reported (see Table 116-1). The mutations are distributed throughout the gene, and most are missense mutations. Seven single-base substitutions are in the promoter region; four disrupt binding to transcriptional factors such as the hepatocyte nuclear factor-4 and SP1.[71–74] Two homozygotes bearing such mutations exhibited a very severe bleeding tendency.[71,72] Four mutations (Phe24del, Asn57Asp, Arg79Gln, Gln100Arg) affect binding to tissue factor.[75–79] The Arg152Gln mutation located at the cleavage site prevents activation of the factor VII zymogen,[77] and other mutations at the catalytic domain impair factor VIIa activity on its substrates.

Most mutations causing factor VII deficiency have been observed in individual patients. However, one missense mutation (Ala244Val) was detected in 102 (84%) of 121 independent mutant alleles discerned in 88 unrelated patients in Israel.[75] Most subjects were of Iranian and Moroccan-Jewish origin and shared an identical haplotype, consistent with a founder effect. In the general Iranian-Jewish and Moroccan-Jewish populations, the prevalences of the Ala244Val allele are 0.023 and 0.025, respectively.[67]

The Dubin-Johnson syndrome caused by mutations in the multidrug resistance protein-2 is associated with factor VII deficiency in Iranian and Moroccan Jews.[80] This association probably reflects the high consanguinity rates, the relatively high prevalence of the Ala244Val mutation in both populations, a high prevalence of an MRP2 Ile1173Phe mutation in Iranian Jews, and a high prevalence of the MRP2 Arg1150His mutation in Moroccan Jews.[81]

Several additional clusters of mutations were reported. (1) Ala294Val, with or without a deletion of nt C at position 11128, prevails in patients from Poland and Germany but also was identified in other Europeans.[66,82,83] All subjects bearing Ala294Val have an identical haplotype, suggesting common ancestry.[82] (2) Twelve unrelated families from Norway carry Gln100Arg.[77] (3) IVS7+5 was detected in six unrelated patients from the Lazio region in Italy. All bear the same haplotype, suggesting a founder effect.[84] (4) Gly331Ser was identified in 10 Italian and four German patients on one haplotype.[85] The widely distributed and common Arg304Gln mutation probably is a recurrent mutation.[86]

Three polymorphisms in the factor VII gene are associated with reduced plasma levels of factor VII. The first polymorphism, an Arg353Gln substitution, results in impaired secretion of factor VII from cells[87] and gives rise to a 20 to 25 percent decrease in plasma factor VII level in heterozygotes and a 40 to 50 percent decrease in homozygotes.[88,89] The allele frequency of the Arg353Gln polymorphism varies significantly in different populations. For example, the observed frequency is only 3.5 percent in Japanese subjects,[90] whereas the frequency is 8 percent in Afro-Caribbeans,[91] 9 percent in North Europeans,[91] and 21 percent in Italians.[92] The highest allele frequencies are in Gujaratis (25%) and Dravidian Indians (29%).[93] The second polymorphism associated with a diminished factor VII level is a decanucleotide insertion upstream from the 5′ end of the gene at −323, which confers a 33 percent decrease in the promoter activity.[44] The relative effects of this polymorphism and the Arg353Gln polymorphism on factor VII level are difficult to assess because linkage disequilibrium exists between these markers.[89] A third polymorphism associated with factor VII level is a hypervariable region 4 polymorphism (HVR4) in intron 7.[94] The variable number of tandem repeats (five to eight copies of 37 bp) apparently influences the splicing efficiency. The effect of the variable repeats on factor VII level are less conspicuous than the decanucleotide insertion at the promoter region and the Arg353Gln polymorphism.

All homozygotes for the Ala244Val mutation also are homozygotes for the Arg353Gln polymorphism.[67,75] In coexpression studies performed in COS-1 and BHK cells, the two gene alterations have an additive effect in reducing secretion of factor VII.[75,95]

CLINICAL FEATURES

Bleeding manifestations occur in homozygotes and in compound heterozygotes for factor VII deficiency. Heterozygotes who have partial factor VII deficiency usually do not bleed excessively even following trauma,[46,96] but a registry in North America recorded bleeding manifestations, mostly mild, in 36 percent of apparent heterozygotes.[37] Patients who have factor VII activity less than 1 percent of normal frequently present with a disease that is indistinguishable from severe hemophilia A or hemophilia B. Such patients are afflicted by hemarthroses leading to severe arthropathy[46,97] and can present with life-threatening intracerebral hemorrhage.[46,98] Patients with slightly higher levels of factor VII can also manifest such severe bleeding episodes, but this finding seems to be exceptional because most patients with factor VII activity of 5 percent of normal or more have a much milder disease, characterized by epistaxis, gingival bleeding, menorrhagia, and easy bruising. Dental extractions, tonsillectomy, and surgical procedures involving the urogenital tracts frequently are accompanied by bleeding when no prior therapy is instituted.[46] In contrast, surgical procedures such as laparotomy, herniorrhaphy, appendectomy, and hysterectomy have been uneventful.[46] This apparent discrepancy can be explained by different extents of local fibrinolysis exhibited by the respective traumatized tissues. Factor VII levels rise during pregnancy in healthy females[99] but do not change in homozygous patients with the deficiency.[100] Nevertheless, postpartum hemorrhage has not been observed in patients with factor VII deficiency, except for a few instances.[46,101] Inhibitors to factor VII have not been described in patients with inherited factor VII deficiency.

Venous and arterial thromboses have been described in several patients. A survey of 514 cases with severe or partial factor VII deficiency recorded seven patients with venous thrombosis and one patient with arterial thrombosis.[102] In six of the eight patients, the thrombotic event occurred after surgery or labor. These data suggest factor VII deficiency confers no protection against thrombosis.

LABORATORY FEATURES

A normal aPTT and a prolonged PT in a patient with a lifelong history of a mild or severe bleeding tendency is consistent with the diagnosis of factor VII deficiency (see Chap. 109). The prolonged PT can be corrected by normal serum (containing factor VII) but not by barium sulfate-absorbed plasma (devoid of factor VII). Determining the diagnosis depends on a specific assay of factor VII activity using known factor VII-deficient plasma. Factor VII antigen can be measured by a commercial enzyme-linked immunosorbent assay (ELISA). Factor VIIa can be measured by a clotting assay using soluble tissue factor, which is insensitive to native factor VII,[56] or by an ELISA using an antibody that exhibits 3000-fold greater reactivity with factor VIIa than with factor VII.[103] Heterozygous carriers have reduced mean levels of factor VII activity, but the range of activity overlaps with normal values. Factor VII activity also can be decreased when the subject being studied has vitamin K deficiency, which occurs frequently. Detection of heterozygotes can be facilitated by concomitant measurements of factor VII activity and antigen levels following administration of vitamin K. Because many factor VII deficiency states are CRM+ or CRM-reduced,[69,70] findings of reduced factor VII activity and significantly higher factor VII antigen level are consistent with heterozygosity.[104] A more definitive approach is identifying the mutant gene in the involved family and tracking it among family members.

DIFFERENTIAL DIAGNOSIS

The common causes of acquired factor VII deficiency must be excluded before diagnosing inherited factor VII deficiency. These causes include liver disease, vitamin K deficiency, and use of warfarin and related anticoagulants. Very rare hereditary defects that must be distinguished from factor VII deficiency are the combined deficiency of all vitamin K-dependent factors (see "Combined Deficiency of the Vitamin K-Dependent Factors," below), combined deficiency of factors VII and X,[105] and combined deficiency of factors VII and IX.[106]

THERAPY

Replacement therapy is unnecessary for minor bleeding episodes. Local hemostasis for skin lacerations and administration of an antifibrinolytic agent for menorrhagia, epistaxis, and gingival hemorrhage usually are sufficient to arrest bleeding. Replacement therapy is essential in patients who present with severe hemorrhage, such as hemarthrosis or intracerebral bleeding. When surgery is required, the following factors should be considered: (1) the site of surgery, as dental extractions, tonsillectomy, nose surgery, and urologic interventions likely are associated with bleeding because of local fibrinolysis; (2) history of bleeding, as patients who have experienced hemarthroses, intracerebral hemorrhage, or other severe bleeding episodes have a much higher risk of bleeding than those who have not had such symptoms; (3) basic level of factor VII, as patients with very low activities (<3% of normal) more likely will bleed; (4) trough factor VII level 20 to 25 percent of normal probably is sufficient even when extensive trauma is present[46,107]; (5) volume overload should be expected if plasma is used as the replacement material; (6) short half-life of factor VII (~5 hours)[46]; and (7) safety of the blood component to be used.

When plasma is used for major surgery, a loading dose of 15 ml/kg should be administered, followed by 4 ml/kg every 6 hours for 7 to 10 days. Diuretics or even plasmapheresis may be necessary because of volume overload.[107] Prothrombin complex concentrates containing activated clotting factors[57] can be used, but they confer a risk of thrombosis.[108] Specific factor VII concentrates have been used successfully in series of patients.[109] The dose during surgery usually ranges between 8 and 40U/kg given at 4- to 6-hour intervals. Another option is use of recombinant factor VIIa, which has been successful in managing patients with hemarthroses and during surgery.[110,111] During surgery, recombinant factor VIIa doses of 20 to 25 μg/kg were used at intervals of 2 to 3 hours. In children and in females during pregnancy, the half-life of factor VIIa is even shorter than the usual 2.5 hours, so treating such patients is a challenge.

FACTOR X DEFICIENCY

Factor X deficiency, a moderate to severe bleeding tendency, is an autosomal recessive disorder first reported by Telfer and colleagues[112] and Hougie and colleagues.[113]

BIOCHEMISTRY AND MOLECULAR FEATURES

The gene encoding factor X is located on chromosome 13q34-qter, adjacent to the gene encoding factor VII.[114,115] The gene spans approximately 25 kb and is composed of eight exons.[116] The factor X gene shows significant homology with the genes of other vitamin K-dependent serine proteases, which suggests all of these multidomain genes evolved from a common ancestral gene.[117]

The protein encoded by the factor X gene is 488 amino acids long. A 23-amino-acid signal peptide that targets factor X as a secretory protein and is removed by a signal peptidase is located at the N-terminus. The Gla domain forms the N-terminus of the mature protein and contains 11 Gla residues that are responsible for calcium and phospholipid binding.[118] Adjacent to the Gla domain is a short aromatic amino acid stack of predominantly hydrophobic amino acids, followed by the epidermal growth factor domain, which contains two epidermal growth factor motifs that are believed to mediate protein–protein interactions. The heavily glycosylated 52-amino-acid activation peptide of factor X separates the epidermal growth factor domain from the C-terminal catalytic domain.

Factor X undergoes proteolytic processing in the endoplasmic reticulum so that circulating factor X is a two-chain, disulfide-linked protein consisting of a 17-kDa light chain composed of the Gla and epidermal growth factor domains and a 40-kDa heavy chain composed of the activation and catalytic domains.[119] Factor X can be activated by a complex of negatively charged phospholipids, factor IXa, and factor VIIIa or by membrane-bound factor VIIa–tissue factor.[120] Factor X also can be activated by a component of Russell's Viper venom,[121] by trypsin, and, in an autocatalytic reaction, by factor Xa. In each case, activation of factor X is accomplished by proteolytic cleavage and subsequent removal of the activation peptide. Factor Xa, in turn, activates prothrombin to thrombin in a reaction that requires negatively charged phospholipids, calcium ions, and factor Va.

GENETICS

Factor X deficiency is inherited in an autosomal recessive manner. Heterozygotes have factor X levels that are approximately 50 percent of normal and are generally asymptomatic. The genetic defects causing a deficiency of factor X are classified according to functional and immunologic analysis as CRM+, CRM−, and CRM-reduced.

The 60 mutations that cause factor X deficiency consist of large deletions, small frameshift deletions, nonsense mutations, and missense mutations. The deletion mutations result in impaired protein synthesis or in synthesis of unstable or dysfunctional proteins. CRM+ variants may affect factor X function in several ways. Activation through the tissue factor pathway may be affected when the mutations are located in the Gla domain, as in Glu7Gly (St. Louis II), Glu14Lys (Vorarlberg), and Glu19Ala.[122–124] Activation through factor IXa is affected by Thr318Met (Roma).[125] Activation of factor X through Russell's viper venom is almost intact by the Pro343Ser (Friuli)[126] mutation, whereas its activation through the intrinsic and tissue factor pathways is only 5 to 9 percent of normal. Missense mutations also may affect synthesis or secretion, thus producing CRM− phenotypes, as with factor X Santo Domingo (Gly-20Arg) and the Stuart mutation (Val298Met).[127,128]

CLINICAL MANIFESTATIONS

The clinical manifestations of factor X deficiency are related to the functional levels of factor X. Individuals with severe factor X deficiency and functional factor X levels less than 1 percent of normal bleed spontaneously and following trauma. Bleeding occurs primarily into joints and soft tissues, from the umbilical cord and mucous membranes.[129] Menorrhagia may be especially problematic in women. More unusual bleedings are intracerebral hemorrhage, intramural intestinal bleeding (which can produce symptoms like those of an acute abdomen), urinary tract bleeding, and soft tissue bleeding with development of hemorrhagic pseudocysts or pseudotumors. In individuals homozygous for moderate or mild deficiencies of factor X and in heterozygotes, bleeding is less common, usually occurring only after trauma or during or after surgery. Such patients may experience easy bruising as the only clinical manifestation.

DIFFERENTIAL DIAGNOSIS

The diagnosis of factor X deficiency is suggested by assays demonstrating prolonged PT and aPTT. The Russell's viper venom time, which is based on the activation of factor X by the venom, is prolonged in most cases. The thrombin time is normal. The diagnosis of factor X deficiency depends on demonstrating an isolated deficiency of factor X by a specific factor X assay.

Prolonged PT and aPTT and a normal thrombin time can be observed in patients with prothrombin deficiency, factor V deficiency, multiple factor deficiencies, vitamin K deficiency, liver disease, and lupus anticoagulants. These disorders are distinguished from factor X deficiency by measuring the levels of factor X and other specific factors, including factors II, V, VII, and IX (see Chap. 109).

Inherited factor X deficiency must be differentiated from various acquired causes of isolated factor X deficiency, such as systemic amyloidosis.[130–133] Factor X deficiency that sometimes occurs in this disorder can result from (1) selective binding of factor X to the amyloid fibrils, which can be erroneously attributed to the presence of an inhibitor when exogenously infused factor X is rapidly removed from the circulation[131,132]; and (2) presence of abnormal factor X molecules with reduced activity versus antigen level.[133] Amyloidosis associated with factor X deficiency resulting from both causes is generally of the primary type. Acquired isolated factor X deficiency has been reported in association with respiratory infections, spindle cell thymoma, fungicide exposure, renal and adrenal adenocarcinoma, acute myelogenous leukemia, and methylbromide use.

THERAPY

Therapy for inherited factor X deficiency usually is administration of heated and solvent–detergent-treated prothrombin complex concentrates containing factor X, in addition to factors II, VII, and IX. Use of these concentrates carries a low risk of transmission of bloodborne viruses. However, a risk of thrombosis, including venous thromboembolism, diffuse intravascular coagulation, and myocardial infarction,[34,134] which is thought to be dose dependent, exists. As a result, administration of doses greater than 2000 U is not recommended. If a larger dose is needed, divided doses are recommended.

For soft tissue, mucous membrane, and joint hemorrhages, the aim of treatment should be maintaining a factor X level at least 30 percent of normal. For more serious hemorrhages, a factor X level 50 to 100 percent of normal should be the goal. The biologic half-life of factor X is 24 to 40 hours.[135,136] Based on this value, if continued treatment is needed, prothrombin complex concentrates should be administrated every 24 hours until hemostasis is achieved. Fresh-frozen plasma containing factor X at a concentration of 1 U/ml also can be used to treat patients with factor X deficiency. The issue of volume overload with plasma and the relative merits of using solvent–detergent-treated plasma are discussed above for therapy of prothrombin deficiency.

COMBINED DEFICIENCY OF THE VITAMIN K-DEPENDENT FACTORS

In 1966, McMillan and Roberts[137] reported the first case of severe hereditary deficiency of coagulation factors II, VII, IX, and X. The combined deficiency of these vitamin K-dependent factors is a very rare autosomal recessive disorder described in only 14 families to date.[138] It can be manifested by a mild or severe bleeding tendency. Protein C and protein S levels were reduced in patients in whom these proteins were assayed.[139,140]

For full function, vitamin K-dependent proteins must undergo γ-carboxylation of glutamic acid residues. This reaction is driven by a carboxylase that uses oxygen and reduced vitamin K to introduce carbon dioxide to glutamic acid residues, yielding vitamin K 2,3-epoxide. This change enables vitamin K-dependent proteins to bind calcium ions and become associated with membranes containing negatively charged phospholipids. VKOR, the target of inhibition by warfarin, then reduces vitamin K 2,3-epoxide, thereby replenishing reduced vitamin K. Mutations in the genes encoding for γ-glutamyl carboxylase and VKOR cause the combined deficiency of the vitamin K-dependent factors by impairing production of fully functional γ-carboxylated vitamin K-dependent factors. Two described missense mutations in the carboxylase gene (Arg394Leu, Trp501Ser) inflict direct impairment of γ-carboxylation,[141,142] whereas a mutation in VKOR (Arg98Trp), observed in two unrelated families, abrogates recycling of vitamin K 2,3-epoxide to reduced vitamin K.[143]

Administration of large doses of vitamin K has improved hemostasis and partially corrected the levels of factors in several cases.[138,140] Fresh-frozen plasma or prothrombin complex concentrate can be used for replacement therapy in patients who do not respond to vitamin K administration.[144]

FACTOR V DEFICIENCY

DEFINITION AND HISTORY

Hereditary factor V deficiency, initially described as parahemophilia,[145] is a rare autosomal recessive disorder manifested in homozygotes as a moderate bleeding tendency. The prevalence of the disorder is unknown, and no specific ethnic or population clusters have been reported.

BIOCHEMISTRY AND MOLECULAR FEATURES

Human plasma factor V is a high molecular weight (Mr ~330,000) single-chain glycoprotein that consists of 2196 amino acids.[146,147] Analysis of the approximately 7-kb factor V cDNA showed that the protein is organized according to the following domain structure: A_1-A_2-B-A_3-C_1-C_2.[148] The A- and C-domains have approximately 40 percent homology with analogous domains in factor VIII. The large B-domain shows no homology with the corresponding B-domain of factor VIII. The gene contains 25 exons[148] and was mapped to chromosome 1q21-25.[149] Factor V is converted to its activated form following several proteolytic cleavages by thrombin[150] or factor Xa.[151] These cleavages remove the B-domain and yield factor Va, which consists of a heavy chain (A_1-A_2 domains) associated by Ca^{2+} with a light chain (A_3-C_1-C_2 domains).[146,147] The light chain contains the binding sites for membrane phospholipids, prothrombin, and activated protein C; both light and heavy chains probably are necessary for factor Xa binding.[147]

Assembly of factors Va and Xa on the phospholipid membrane of platelets in the presence of calcium ions forms the prothrombinase complex, which catalyzes the conversion of prothrombin to thrombin.[146] Exclusion of factor Va from the prothrombinase complex reduces the rate of thrombin generation by four orders of magnitude.[146] Factor V is synthesized by the liver[152] and by megakaryocytes.[153,154] Its plasma concentration is approximately 7 μg/ml,[155] and its half-life is 12 to 15 hours.[156] Approximately 20 percent of factor V in whole blood is localized in the α-granules of platelets,[157] where it is complexed with an extremely large protein multimerin.[158] Factor V can be absorbed from plasma.[159] Although it undergoes partial proteolysis, its cofactor activity is preserved.[157,160] Its release from platelets upon their activation exerts an important hemostatic effect, because patients with an inherited defect of α-granule proteins, including platelet factor V, have a severe bleeding tendency.[161,162]

Factor Va is inactivated by activated protein C through limited proteolysis at Arg506, Arg306, and Arg679 in the presence of protein S, calcium ions, and either platelet or endothelial cell membrane phospholipids.[163] Partial protection from this cleavage is provided by factor Xa when bound to factor Va.[164] Partial resistance to inactivation by activated protein C occurs when the cleavage sites Arg306 and Arg506 are mutated (see Chaps. 107 and 122).

GENETICS

Factor V deficiency is inherited as an autosomal recessive trait. Heterozygotes, whose plasma factor V activity ranges between 26 and 60 percent of normal, usually are asymptomatic.[165] Assays of factor V antigen indicate most homozygotes and compound heterozygotes have a true deficiency rather than a dysfunctional protein. A total of 38 distinct mutations are identified, of which 11 are missense, 14 are small insertions/deletions, eight are nonsense, and five are splice site mutations (see Table 116-1). Most mutations cause truncations and are localized throughout the gene. Several mutations have interesting features. One, a Tyr1702Cys transition, was identified in eight unrelated families, of whom six were Italian. The frequency of this mutant allele in Italy is 0.002.[166,167] Another mutation, a Ala221Val (New Brunswick) alteration, characterized in the homozygous state by activity and antigen levels of 29 and 39 percent of normal, displays decreased stability of the expressed protein.[168] Three additional mutations exhibit decreased secretion of the protein from producing cells.[169,170] Remarkably, the Gln773ter and Arg1133ter mutations and a 4-bp deletion mutation, all present in exon 13 and predicted to result in partial truncation of the B-domain and complete truncation of the A3-, C1-, and C2-domains, cause no bleeding or only a mild bleeding tendency in affected patients having factor V antigen and activity levels 1 percent of normal.[171–173] This finding contrasts with the phenotype of factor V knockout mice, which have defective embryonic development and early hemorrhagic death.[174]

Subjects who are compound heterozygotes for factor V Arg506Gln (factor V Leiden) and for a factor V null allele have normal hemostasis (despite reduced factor V clotting activity). However, because they are phenotypically homozygous for activated protein C resistance, these patients may present with thrombosis (see Chap. 122).[175–179]

Among several polymorphisms detected in the factor V gene, the His1299Arg in exon 13 is particularly interesting because it is associated with a reduced plasma factor V level.[180] Moreover, in two heterozygotes for factor V R506Q (factor V Leiden) who presented with thrombosis, reduced factor V activity resulting from the His1299Arg polymorphism conferred a pseudohomozygous phenotype for activated protein C resistance.[180]

Factor V Quebec initially was described as an autosomal dominant disorder with severe bleeding manifestations.[181] Affected patients had platelet factor V activity 2 to 4 percent of normal, slightly reduced platelet factor V antigen, moderately decreased plasma factor V activity, and mild thrombocytopenia. The inactive platelet factor V in these patients is caused by abnormal proteolysis of several platelet α-granule proteins,[161,162,182] including fibrinogen, von Willebrand factor, thrombospondin, and factor V complexed with multimerin.[158] Thus, factor V Quebec, described in two unrelated families,[181,182] is a deficiency of platelet factor V activity secondary to a generalized platelet defect.

CLINICAL MANIFESTATIONS

Homozygous patients whose factor V level ranges from less than 1 to 10 percent of normal exhibit a lifelong bleeding tendency. Manifestations include, in decreasing order of frequency, ecchymoses, epistaxis, gingival bleeding, hemorrhage following minor lacerations, and menorrhagia.[156] Bleeding from other sites is less common, but instances of hemarthroses unrelated to trauma and intracerebral hemorrhage have been reported.[36] Trauma, dental extractions, and surgery confer a high risk of excessive bleeding.

Venous and arterial thromboses have been described in patients with factor V levels ranging between 2 and 14 percent of normal.[183–185] These observations indicate that factor V deficiency, like deficiencies of other coagulation factors, does not provide protection against thrombosis.[186] Factor V deficiency deprives activated protein C of one of its essential substrates, thereby down-regulating the inhibitory function of the protein C system. As previously discussed in "Genetics," this situation is highlighted in patients with thrombosis who are compound heterozygotes for a factor V deficiency allele and an allele bearing the factor V Leiden mutation.[175–179]

Only two patients with hereditary factor V deficiency developed an inhibitor after receiving plasma transfusions.[187,188] The inhibitor disappeared in one patient, but a low titer of the inhibitor persisted in the other patient.[188]

DIFFERENTIAL DIAGNOSIS

Hereditary factor V deficiency must be distinguished from hereditary combined deficiency of factors V and VIII, acquired factor V deficiency associated with severe liver dysfunction or disseminated intravascular coagulation (DIC), and from a deficiency related to an acquired inhibitor to factor V. In both factor V deficiency and combined deficiency of factors V and VIII, PT and aPTT are prolonged, inheritance is autosomal recessive, and bleeding manifestations are similar. Therefore, an assay of factor VIII is essential for distinguishing between these entities (see Chap. 109). The clinical manifestations of severe liver disease or DIC are sufficient to allow easy distinction between acquired and inherited factor V deficiency.

THERAPY

Patients with epistaxis and gingival bleeding may respond to tranexamic acid (1g qid), and local hemostatic measures may suffice for minor lacerations. If these measures fail, severe spontaneous bleeding occurs, or surgery is performed, fresh-frozen plasma replacement should be given. The following factors should be considered when planning plasma replacement therapy: (1) half-life of factor V is approximately 12 to 14 hours; (2) a factor V level of 25 percent of normal usually is adequate even for major surgery[189,190]; (3) surgical procedures at sites such as the urogenital tract, oral cavity, and nose having high local fibrinolytic activity likely will result in excessive bleeding, and late bleeding may occur. Infusion of a loading dose of 20 ml/kg of fresh-frozen plasma followed by 5 to 10 ml/kg every 12 hours for 7 to 10 days usually is adequate to ensure hemostasis during and after surgery.

COMBINED DEFICIENCY OF FACTORS V AND VIII

DEFINITION AND HISTORY

Combined deficiency of factors V and VIII, first described in 1954,[191] is a rare moderate bleeding disorder that is transmitted as an autosomal recessive trait.[192] Affected homozygotes have plasma levels of factors V and VIII ranging from 5 to 30 percent of normal.[193] The disorder results from a deficiency of either mannose-binding lectin LMAN1, also called endoplasmic reticulum–Golgi intermediate compartment protein ERGIC-53, or multiple combined factor deficiency protein MCFD2, which form a specific calcium-dependent cargo receptor complex for the endoplasmic reticulum to Golgi transport of factors V and VIII.[194,195] The disorder has been detected in many populations, but a relatively high frequency occurs among Tunisian and Middle-Eastern Jews residing in Israel[192] and among Iranians.[196]

BIOCHEMISTRY AND MOLECULAR GENETIC FEATURES

Factors V and VIII are essential coagulation factors that circulate in plasma as precursors. Upon limited proteolysis by thrombin or factor Xa and in concert with negatively charged phospholipid surfaces, factors V and VIII exhibit profound cofactor activities for activation of factor X by factor IXa and for activation of prothrombin by factor Xa, respectively. Inactivation of factors Va and VIIIa is accomplished by activated protein C in the presence of protein S and phospholipids through several proteolytic cleavages at distinct sites. Factors V and VIII have similar domain organizations with partial homology (see "Factor V Deficiency" above and Chap. 106).

The pathogenesis of combined deficiency of factors V and VIII puzzled investigators for more than 40 years. The enigma was resolved by the finding that the disease stems from a deficiency of either one of two interacting proteins, LMAN1 and MCFD2, which play a role in the specific transport of factors V and VIII from the endoplasmic reticulum to the Golgi en route to their secretion from cells that produce them.[194,195] Homozygosity mapping in nine unrelated Jewish families demonstrated that the LMAN1 gene was localized on the long arm of chromosome 18.[197,198] Genetic linkage studies and recombination analysis localized the gene to an approximately 2.5-centimorgan (cM) region,[197] and the involved protein was identified as a 53-kDa transmembrane protein hexamer of ERGIC.[199,200] All 18 mutations identified in the LMAN1 gene predicted either a truncated protein product or no protein at all.[194,201,202] The MCFD2 gene was localized to the short arm of chromosome 2. Of the seven mutations identified, five seem to result in loss of MCFD2 protein expression and two in defective binding to LMAN1.[195] Formation of a calcium-dependent LMAN1–MCFD2 protein complex is essential for transport of factors V and VIII from the endoplasmic reticulum to the Golgi. Hence, deficiency in either subunit gives rise to a phenotypically indistinguishable combined deficiency of factors V and VIII.

Because all patients with the combined deficiency have residual plasma levels of factor V and VIII ranging from 5 to 30 percent of normal, alternative mechanisms of intracellular transport of factor V and VIII probably exist.

The defect is inherited as an autosomal recessive trait, and consanguinity in affected families is common.[192,193,195,196]

A distinct founder haplotype was found in patients belonging to five unrelated families of Tunisian-Jewish origin bearing a T→C transition in intron 9 at a donor splice site of the LMAN1 gene.[197] All five families originated from an ancient Jewish community that has resided on the island of Djerba for more than two millennia. A survey of this community, which presently is living in Israel, disclosed that the mutation is prevalent at an allele frequency of 0.0107.[203] Another founder effect for a G insertion in exon 1 of the LMAN1 gene was observed in five unrelated Jewish families of Middle-Eastern origin.[197]

CLINICAL MANIFESTATIONS

Homozygous patients exhibit spontaneous and posttraumatic bleeding. Menorrhagia, epistaxis, easy bruising, and gingival hemorrhage are common observations.[193,196] Hemarthrosis, unrelated to trauma, was described in approximately 20 percent of cases.[193,196] Hematuria, gastrointestinal hemorrhage, and spontaneous intracranial hemorrhage are less common.[196] Dental extractions and surgical procedures almost always are accompanied by excessive bleeding when the missing factors are not replaced. Interestingly, bleeding was noted in only one of six Jewish infant patients who underwent circumcision on day 8 of life.[192] In contrast, Muslim patients bled excessively following circumcision performed at age 5 to 7 years.[196] Postpartum hemorrhage was noted in 13 of 17 women.[193,196]

Heterozygotes exhibit slight but significantly reduced mean levels of factors V and VIII.[192] In a literature survey of 161 heterozygotes, 22 reported having significant bleeding manifestations.[204] However, no correlation between the factor V or VIII level and bleeding tendency was noted.[193,204]

DIFFERENTIAL DIAGNOSIS

Coincidental association between hemophilia A and factor V deficiency is estimated to be extremely rare.[205] The association has been reported in only five families.[206–210] Features that help distinguish between this association and the combined deficiency are the following: (1) Consanguinity frequently is present in parents of patients with combined deficiency of factors V and VIII. (2) Independent segregation of factor V and factor VIII deficiency can be observed among immediate relatives of patients with the coincidental association. (3) Concordant reductions in levels of factors V and VIII more likely occur in patients afflicted by the combined deficiency. Hereditary factor V deficiency can be confused with combined deficiency of factors V and VIII because the two entities are inherited as autosomal recessive traits, have similar manifestations, and are characterized by prolonged PT and aPTT. Therefore, assays of factors V and VIII are essential for making the distinction (see Chap. 109).

THERAPY

An antifibrinolytic agent such as tranexamic acid or ε-aminocaproic acid can be helpful in patients exhibiting menorrhagia, epistaxis, or gingival bleeding. Patients with severe bleeding episodes or patients undergoing surgical procedures, including dental extractions, should receive fresh-frozen plasma as replacement for factor V and cryoprecipitate or factor VIII concentrate as a source of factor VIII. Desmopressin can be used to increase factor VIII level,[193] but this treatment sometimes fails.[211] As with other clotting factor deficiencies, replacement therapy in patients undergoing major surgery should be maintained for 7 to 10 days after the operation. Hemostatically safe levels of factor V and VIII have not been established, but given the significant bleeding experienced by patients with factor V and VIII levels up to 30 percent of normal, a reasonable aim is trough factor levels greater than 50 percent of normal during and after surgery. Volume overload can be a serious problem but can be circumvented by plasma exchange and concomitant use of a factor VIII concentrate.[211]

FACTOR XI DEFICIENCY

DEFINITION AND HISTORY

Factor XI deficiency initially was described as a "new hemophilia" in two sisters and their maternal uncle by Rosenthal and colleagues[212] in 1953. The deficiency was erroneously thought to be transmitted as an autosomal dominant disorder with variable expressivity. Later studies clearly established that, in most cases, the mode of transmission of factor XI deficiency is autosomal recessive.[213,214] The disorder is exhibited in homozygotes or compound heterozygotes as a mild to moderate bleeding tendency that is mainly injury related. Affected subjects are rarely encountered in most populations except for Jewish persons, particularly of Ashkenazi origin, among whom the deficiency is common.[214]

Until 1991, factor XI was regarded as one of the "contact" coagulation factors, functioning in the initiation of the intrinsic coagulation system. Numerous studies showed that when blood or plasma is exposed to negatively charged surfaces in vitro, a series of reactions involving factor XII, high molecular weight kininogen (HK), and prekallikrein (PK) yields α-factor XIIa. α-Factor XIIa then activates factor XI, and factor XIa in turn activates factor IX in the presence of calcium ions, thereby propagating the intrinsic coagulation system. All attempts to ascribe to the contact activation pathway an essential function in vivo have been futile because, unlike factor XI deficiency, severe deficiencies of factor XII, HK, and PK have not been associated with a bleeding tendency. Studies in 1991 showed that factor XI can be activated by thrombin,[215,216] thereby bypassing the contact reactions. This finding and new observations on the involvement of factor XI in the intrinsic coagulation system (see Chap. 106) and in the fibrinolytic system (see "Biochemistry and Molecular Features," below) explain why factor XI is important for hemostasis, whereas factor XII, HK and PK probably are not.

BIOCHEMISTRY AND MOLECULAR FEATURES

Factor XI is a glycoprotein that consists of two identical 80-kDa polypeptide chains linked by a disulfide bond.[217] Each subunit contains 607 amino acids with a serine protease domain at the C-terminus and four tandem repeats of 90 or 91 amino acids, designated "apple domains," at the N-terminus. A disulfide bond is formed between Cys321 residues in the fourth apple domain of each monomer.[218] In blood, factor XI is complexed noncovalently with HK through binding primarily to the apple 2 domain and secondarily to other apple domains.[219] The normal plasma concentration of factor XI is 4 μg/ml. The 23-kb gene encoding for factor XI consists of 15 exons and 14 introns[220] and is located on chromosome 4q34-35.[221]

Activation of factor XI involves cleavage of an Arg369-Ile370 bond, yielding a heavy chain containing the four apple domains linked by a disulfide bond to a light chain that contains the catalytic domain.[217] Each activated molecule thus contains two catalytic sites. Factor XI adhered to negatively charged surfaces by HK can be activated by α-factor XIIa or through autoactivation by factor XIa,[222] but whether these reactions occur in vivo is doubtful. The major activator of factor XI in vivo is thrombin,[215,216] and the reaction occurs mainly on the surface of activated platelets. Factor XI binds through its apple 3 domain to lipid rafts on activated platelets containing glycoprotein Ib–IX–V complex. This glycoprotein complex also binds thrombin; thus, both substrate and enzyme are colocalized at the same site.[223] Optimal binding of factor XI to these membrane rafts requires HK (and Zn^{2+}) or prothrombin (and Ca^{2+}) (see Chap. 106). Factor XI activation also can occur on the fibrin surface after a clot forms.[224] Conceivably, one subunit of the factor XI dimer binds to the platelets and the other subunit binds to factor IX.[225] Factor XIa, once generated, activates factor IX by limited proteolysis of two peptide bonds in the presence of calcium ions.[226] Factor IXa then activates factor X in the presence of factor VIIIa, negatively charged phospholipids, and calcium ions. Thus, additional thrombin is generated through thrombin-mediated activation of factor XI.

The presence of factor XI is essential for activation of procarboxypeptidase B by thrombin. When this procarboxypeptidase B, also termed thrombin-activatable fibrinolysis inhibitor (TAFI), is activated, it removes terminal lysine residues from fibrin, which impairs binding of certain forms of plasminogen to fibrin and disrupts tissue plasminogen activator-induced plasmin generation in the blood clot.[227] Thus, activated TAFI is a strong inhibitor of fibrinolysis. Large amounts of thrombin are necessary for TAFI activation, but the reaction is substantially augmented when thrombin is bound to thrombomodulin.[228] It follows that impaired generation of thrombin, for example, in inherited deficiency of factor VIII, IX, or XI, not only delays clot formation but also enhances premature lysis of clots.[229] Activation of factor XI by thrombin, particularly within the blood clot, is essential for adequate TAFI activation and protection of the clot from lysis in vitro[230,231] and in vivo.[232] These data fit well with clinical observations in factor XI-deficient patients of bleeding that commonly occurs at sites exhibiting local fibrinolytic activity[233] and with the effective prevention of such episodes by antifibrinolytic agents[234] (see "Therapy" below).

Factor XI is synthesized by the liver. The case of acquired factor XI deficiency as a result of liver transplantation from a donor who, in retrospect, had the deficiency has been reported.[235]

GENETICS

INHERITANCE

In most cases, factor XI deficiency is inherited as an autosomal recessive trait characterized by plasma factor XI levels less than 15 percent of normal in homozygotes and compound heterozygotes.[213,214,233] In heterozygotes, factor XI levels frequently range between 25 and 70 percent of normal but can be higher.[214,236] Exceptional cases of patients in whom dominantly transmitted heterozygosity is associated with a significant bleeding tendency and factor XI levels of approximately 10 to 20 percent of normal (see "Mutations," below) have been described. Factor XI deficiency as a result of a dysfunctional protein is exceedingly rare. In a study of 125 patients of various ethnic origins, none had discordant levels of factor XI activity and antigen.[237] Only several cases of patients with deficiency of factor XI activity and seemingly normal antigen levels have been described.[238–241]

MUTATIONS

Three mutations, designated type I, II, and III, were first described in six Ashkenazi-Jewish patients with severe factor XI deficiency.[242] The type I mutation is a G→A change at the splice site of the last intron of the gene. The type II mutation is a G→T change in exon 5 at Glu117 leading to a stop codon −TAA. The type III mutation is a T→ C change in exon 9 that results in a substitution of Phe283 by Leu in the fourth apple domain of the protein. A fourth mutation designated type IV, later identified in another Ashkenazi-Jewish patient, consists of a 14-bp deletion at the intron N−exon 14 junction.[243] Of the four mutations, the predominant mutations in Jewish persons are types II and III. Forty-nine additional mutations have been reported in non-Jewish and Jewish patients of various origins (see Table 116-1). Twenty-six are missense mutations, 10 nonsense mutations, seven deletions and/or insertions, and six splice site mutations. Expression of 12 missense mutations, five located in the apple 4 domains in the catalytic domain and two in the apple 1 domain, revealed impaired factor XI secretion from transfected cells.[244–246] For one of these mutations (Phe283Leu) in the apple 4 domain, impaired secretion was related to defective dimerization.[218,244]

The homodimeric structure of factor XI implies that for certain mutations in heterozygotes, the mutant allele imparts a dominant negative effect by impairing secretion of wild-type mutant heterodimers. Cotransfection experiments with Gly400Val or Trp569Ser yielded decreased secretion of wild-type factor XI by 50 percent.[247] The heterozygotes for these mutations manifest a significant bleeding tendency and a factor XI level as low as 10 percent of normal.

The Gly555Glu mutation located two amino acids before the active serine yields a dysfunctional protein that is normally activated by factor XIIa or thrombin, but its activated form fails to activate factor IX and is resistant to inhibition by antithrombin.[239]

ETHNIC DISTRIBUTION AND PREVALENCE

Most patients with factor XI deficiency are Jewish.[213,214,233,236] Several instances of vertical transmission of severe factor XI deficiency in Ashkenazi-Jewish families (consistent with pseudodominance) suggested the gene frequency in this segment of Jewish individuals is very high. The high frequency was found in two surveys of this population performed in Israel.[214,248]

Types II and III are the predominant mutations causing factor XI deficiency in Jewish persons.[233,249] Of 590 mutant alleles in 295 unrelated patients with severe deficiency we analyzed, 577 (97.8%) were either type II (306 alleles) or type III (271 alleles). Screening of the general Ashkenazi-Jewish population for these mutations disclosed allele frequencies of 0.0217 for type II mutation and 0.0254 for type III mutation.[250] Hence, the estimated frequency of subjects with severe factor XI deficiency in Ashkenazi Jews is 1:450 and of heterozygotes for both types of mutation is 1:11. These data indicate factor XI deficiency is the most frequent hereditary disorder in this population. Interestingly, the type II mutation was observed in Iraqi Jews with a similar allele frequency of −0.0167[250] but in Palestinian Arabs and in Sephardic and other Middle-Eastern Jews at frequencies of 0.0065 and

0.0027, respectively.[251] In sharp contrast, the type III mutation was not detected among 1343 Jewish persons of non-Ashkenazi origin or in 313 Palestinian Arabs.[251]

A second cluster of patients with factor XI deficiency was observed in Basques living in southwestern France in whom the predominant mutation is a Cys38Arg substitution.[246] The frequency of this mutant allele in the general Basque population is 0.005. A third cluster of factor XI-deficient patients was reported in Caucasians residing in or originating from the United Kingdom.[252] The mutation, a Cys128stop nonsense alteration, is predicted to produce a truncated protein and has an estimated allele frequency of 0.01 in the general British Caucasian population.

FOUNDER EFFECTS

Haplotype analysis based on examination of factor XI gene polymorphisms disclosed distinct founder effects for type II and type III mutations.[251] In view of the similar prevalences of the type II mutation in Iraqi Jews and Ashkenazi Jews, the presence of the type II mutation in Palestinian Arabs and Sephardic Jews, and the historical information about the divergence of these populations 2000 to 2500 years ago, the type II mutation seems to have occurred in ancient times. Type III mutation, which is confined to Ashkenazi Jews, probably stemmed from a founder who lived in more recent times. Evidence supporting these hypotheses has been reported.[253] Haplotype analyses have suggested founder effects for the Cys38Arg mutation in Basques and for the Cys128stop mutation in British Caucasians.[246,252]

CLINICAL FEATURES

BLEEDING MANIFESTATIONS IN HOMOZYGOTES AND COMPOUND HETEROZYGOTES

Most bleeding manifestations in homozygotes and compound heterozygotes are injury related. Excessive bleeding can occur at the time of injury or begin several hours or days following trauma. Some patients with severe factor XI deficiency may not bleed at all following trauma.[213] In other patients, the bleeding tendency varies depending upon the hemostatic challenge.[233,236] The apparent inconsistencies now can be partially explained by the patient's genotype, which affects the extent of the deficiency, and by the variable sites of injury.[233,236,254,255] Homozygotes for the type III missense mutation, whose mean factor XI level was 9.7 percent of normal, had significantly fewer injury-related bleeding events than homozygotes for the type II mutation with a mean factor XI level of 1.2 percent of normal. Surgical procedures involving tissues with high fibrinolytic activity (urinary tract, tonsils, nose, tooth sockets) frequently are associated with excessive bleeding in patients with severe factor XI deficiency, irrespective of the genotype.[233] A significantly lower frequency of bleeding complications follows surgical interventions at sites without excessive local fibrinolysis, such as appendicectomy, cholecystectomy, circumcision, and orthopedic surgery.[233,255] Site-related bleeding tendency now can be understood in light of the demonstrated function of factor XI in preventing clot lysis (see "Biochemistry and Molecular Features," above).

Spontaneous bleeding manifestations such as menorrhagia, gingival bleeding, ecchymoses, and epistaxis occur in patients with severe factor XI deficiency but are uncommon.[254,255] Postpartum hemorrhage occurs in only 24 percent of affected women.[256]

BLEEDING MANIFESTATIONS IN HETEROZYGOTES

Whether heterozygotes exhibit a bleeding tendency (except for those bearing mutations causing a dominant negative effect) has been a matter of debate. In one extensive study, heterozygotes had almost no bleeding complications following a variety of surgical procedures, including operations at sites with enhanced local fibrinolysis.[213] In another study, all heterozygotes who underwent urologic surgery did well except for one patient whose factor XI level was 25 percent of normal.[248] In contrast with these observations, other studies identified a bleeding tendency, particularly following injury in 33 percent,[236] 48 percent,[254] and 20 percent[255] of heterozygotes. Variable definitions of what constitutes a bleeding tendency[257] can only partially explain this discrepancy. A more likely explanation for the variable manifestations in heterozygotes is the coexistence of additional hemostatic abnormalities in patients who do bleed. Thus, heterozygotes who were defined as bleeders tended to have lower levels of factor VIII and von Willebrand factor and to have blood group O, which is associated with reduced von Willebrand factor levels. Moreover, in another study, most heterozygotes who presented with a bleeding tendency also had a platelet function abnormality.[258] A study that assessed the risk of bleeding in patients from 45 families showed that the odds ratio for bleeding was 13.0 in homozygotes and compound heterozygotes but was only 2.6 in heterozygotes.[255]

A conclusion can be made that heterozygotes for factor XI deficiency may display a small risk of bleeding but that this risk is significantly lower than the risk of bleeding exhibited by homozygotes and compound heterozygotes.

THROMBOSIS

Although factor XI plays an essential role in blood coagulation and fibrinolysis, severe factor XI deficiency, unlike the hemophilias, does not confer protection against myocardial infarction. Of 96 unrelated patients older than 35 years with severe factor XI deficiency, 16 had a myocardial infarction.[259] Venous thromboembolism was described in two other reports,[252,260] but whether this finding suggests no protection against venous thrombosis requires many more observations. Thrombotic events have been described in patients with severe factor XI deficiency following infusion of factor XI concentrates (see "Therapy" below).

ASSOCIATION OF FACTOR XI DEFICIENCY WITH OTHER DISORDERS

Factor XI deficiency has been described in patients with Gaucher disease.[261–263] In view of the independent segregation of the two disorders,[261] the coincidental occurrence of Gaucher disease and hereditary factor XI deficiency appears to stem from the high frequency of the respective mutant genes in the Ashkenazi-Jewish population. Patients with Noonan syndrome reportedly exhibited factor XI deficiency and a bleeding tendency.[264] However, later studies showed that in addition to factor XI deficiency, patients with Noonan syndrome display several other abnormalities in coagulation factors and platelet function for which no explanation has been provided.[265,266] A variety of other inherited disorders of hemostasis have been described in association with factor XI deficiency, including von Willebrand disease,[267,268] factor VIII deficiency,[236,269,270] and factor VII deficiency.[271] Because of the high prevalence of factor XI deficiency in Jewish persons, these associations are expected to occur in this population.

ACQUIRED INHIBITORS

Inhibitors that neutralize factor XI activity have been described in patients with severe hereditary factor XI deficiency who received plasma replacement therapy. Of 118 Israeli patients examined, seven had an inhibitor to factor XI.[272] All the patients belonged to a subgroup of 21 patients who were homozygotes for the Glu117stop mutation and had received plasma prior to development of the inhibitor. Of six additional patients who received plasma and had an inhibitor, five had the same genotype and one was homozygous for another null mutation, Gln88stop.[240] Thus, approximately one third of patients who are homozygous for a null mutation can be expected to develop an inhibitor.

Inhibitors that were characterized are of the IgG type recognizing different epitopes of factor XI and giving rise to impaired binding to HK, abrogation of activation by thrombin and factor XIIa, and diminished activation of factor IX. Spontaneous bleeding manifestations do not seem to be aggravated by the development of the inhibitors. However, in one patient whose antibody titer was extremely high, spontaneous bleeding occurred.[273] Securing hemostasis during and after surgery in such cases is a great challenge (see "Therapy" below).

LABORATORY FEATURES

Patients with factor XI deficiency have a prolonged aPTT and normal PT (see Chap. 109). All homozygotes and compound heterozygotes have aPTTs that are longer than two standard deviations above the normal mean.[274] However, aPTT values in heterozygotes substantially overlap the normal range.[233,274] Consequently, screening of patients for a hemostatic abnormality prior to surgery (which is recommended for Jewish patients because of the high prevalence of factor XI deficiency) identifies all patients with a severe factor XI deficiency. The diagnosis is established by an aPTT-based assay using factor XI-deficient plasma.[213] Factor XI antigen can be measured by ELISA.[239] Analysis of DNA polymerase chain reaction and restriction enzyme digestion can identify the patient's genotype.[233,242,249] Mean factor XI levels and aPTT values in type II homozygotes are 1.2 percent of normal and 108 seconds, respectively; in compound heterozygotes for the type II and type III mutations are 3.3 percent of normal and 85 seconds, respectively; and in type III homozygotes are 9.7 percent of normal and 67 seconds, respectively.[233,249] Although one study reported heterozygotes for the type II mutation have a significantly lower mean factor XI level than heterozygotes for the type III mutation,[233] another study found similar values in patients bearing the two genotypes.[249]

THERAPY

PATIENTS WITH A SEVERE DEFICIENCY

Patients with severe factor XI deficiency who must undergo a surgical procedure should be carefully evaluated and meticulously prepared for the operation. A negative history of excessive bleeding following previous procedures does not preclude an increased bleeding tendency. Other hemostatic abnormalities and the presence of an inhibitor to factor XI should be excluded. Aspirin or other antiplatelet agents should not be given during the week prior to surgery.

When choosing the treatment modality and the intensity of treatment, the following factors should be considered: (1) patient's age and history of cardiovascular disease, as use of plasma may create volume overload and use of a factor XI concentrate can induce thrombosis (see "Thrombosis," below); (2) baseline plasma level of factor XI, as homozygotes with levels approximately 10 percent of normal have a lower risk of bleeding compared to homozygotes or compound heterozygotes with lower levels (except when procedures are performed at sites with high local fibrinolytic activity[233]; (3) presence of an inhibitor to factor XI, as plasma or factor XI concentrate cannot be used in such patients; (4) use of an antifibrinolytic agent should be considered in patients undergoing operation at a site with high local fibrinolytic activity, as in dental or urologic surgery; (5) PT and platelet count should be tested; (6) safety, as transmission of infectious agents and allergic reactions are more common following plasma transfusions compared to factor XI concentrate; however, concentrates can induce thrombosis; (7) half-life of factor XI, as a mean half life of 52 hours was recorded following infusions of a factor XI concentrate[275] and 45 hours following plasma transfusion.[276]

Patients undergoing dental extractions do not require replacement therapy. Tranexamic acid administration (1 g qid) starting 12 hours before surgery until 7 days after surgery effectively prevents bleeding.[234] ε-Aminocaproic acid (5–6 g qid) given similarly is expected to achieve the same results. For major surgery or surgery at sites with high levels of local fibrinolysis, fresh-frozen plasma should be transfused for 10 to 14 days, targeting trough factor XI levels 45 percent of normal.[277] For surgery at tissues not displaying high levels of local fibrinolysis, fresh-frozen plasma can be transfused for 5 to 7 days, targeting trough factor XI levels 30 percent of normal. Following prostatectomy and bladder operations, continuous flushing of the bladder with saline containing tranexamic acid 0.5 to 1 g/liter can be helpful for hemostasis. For nose surgery or tonsillectomy, apart from replacement therapy, tranexamic acid or ε-aminocaproic acid given as for dental extraction should be considered. No plasma replacement therapy is necessary during or after labor unless excessive bleeding occurs.[256]

Two viral-inactivated factor XI concentrates have been used for treatment of patients with factor XI deficiency.[275,278,279] However, infusions of the two concentrates result in laboratory signs of DIC.[280,281] Pulmonary embolism and arterial thrombosis, including fatal cases, have been reported in patients receiving the concentrates,[282,283] albeit mostly in elderly patients who had preexisting cardiovascular disease and were given a dose greater than 30 U/kg. Consequently, these concentrates must be used with great caution.

PATIENTS WITH PARTIAL FACTOR XI DEFICIENCY

Heterozygotes with a negative history of a bleeding tendency who do not exhibit any other hemostatic abnormality and whose plasma factor XI level is more than 40 percent of normal probably do not require treatment while undergoing surgery.[248] However, if a positive bleeding history is elicited in such patients, a detailed investigation of the hemostatic system should be performed. If another abnormality is found, adequate measures should be taken to correct that abnormality, in addition to replacement therapy for 5 days targeting trough factor XI levels 45 percent of normal.

PATIENTS WITH INHIBITOR TO FACTOR XI

Most reported patients have not exhibited aggravation of bleeding tendency following development of an inhibitor. Consequently, when such patients undergo dental extraction, use of tranexamic acid and fibrin glue may be sufficient,[284] but limited evidence supporting this contention is available. Activated prothrombin complex[273,285] and recombinant factor VIIa[286] have been used successfully for major surgical procedures, and an in vitro study revealed that abnormal thrombin generation in the plasma of patients with an inhibitor was corrected by adding moderate amounts of factor VIIa.[272]

FACTOR XIII DEFICIENCY

DEFINITION AND HISTORY

Factor XIII (fibrin-stabilizing factor) is a plasma transglutaminase that cross-links γ-glutamyl-ε-lysine residues of fibrinogen chains, thereby stabilizing the fibrin clot. Severe deficiency of factor XIII, first described by Duckert and colleagues[287] in 1960, causes a moderate to severe hemorrhagic disorder, recurrent abortions, and impaired wound healing in some patients.

BIOCHEMISTRY AND MOLECULAR FEATURES

Plasma factor XIII is an Mr approximately 340,000 heterotetramer composed of two catalytic A-subunits and two carrier B-subunits linked by noncovalent bonds. The average concentration of the A_2B_2 tetramer in plasma is approximately 22 μg/ml, and its half-life is 9 to 14 days.[288] The A-subunit (Mr ~82,000) contains an activation peptide, the catalytic site of factor XIII, and a calcium binding site.[289] It is structurally homologous with the a chain of tissue transglutaminase,[290] the a chain of keratinocyte transglutaminase,[291] and band 4.2 of erythrocytes,[292] although the latter lacks transglutaminase activity. The first 37 amino acids of the N-terminus of the factor XIII A-subunit constitute an activation peptide that is removed by thrombin cleavage of an Arg37-Gly38 bond in the presence of calcium ions.[293] An active site sulfhydryl residue, which is characteristic for this class of enzymes, is located at Cys314. Two calcium-binding domains, which have weak homology with the canonical EF calcium-binding hands of calmodulin, flank the active site cysteine.

The three-dimensional structure of factor XIII A-subunit determined by x-ray crystallography disclosed the A-subunit is divided into four sequential domains: β-sandwich (Glu43-Phe184), catalytic core (Asn185-Arg515), and two barrel domains (Ser516-Thr628, Ile629-Arg727).[294] The catalytic triad Cys314-His373-Asp396 is very similar to the Cys-His-Asp triad of papain-like cysteine proteases.

The two B-subunits of factor XIII function as carrier proteins for the A-subunits,[295,296] stabilizing them in the circulation and regulating the calcium-dependent activation of factor XIII. The B-subunit of Mr, approximately 76,500, is composed of 10 homologous consensus or "sushi" repeats.[297] Each repeat is approximately 60 amino acids long and contains four disulfide bonds, with Cys1 linked to Cys3 and Cys2 linked to Cys4. The function of these repeats is unknown.

The gene for the factor XIII A-subunit is located on chromosome 6p24-p25.[298,299] It spans more than 170 kb and is composed of 15 exons, ranging in size from 63 to 1688 bp.[300] Exon 1 consists of the 5′ noncoding region, and exon 2 encodes for the activation peptide (amino acid 1-37). In general, conservation among genes of the transglutaminase family is observed.[293] For example, the sequences encompassing the active site thiol are encoded by exon 7; the calcium-binding sequences are encoded by exons 6 and 11; and the fibrin binding sequences are encoded by exons 3 and 5.

The B-subunit gene is located on chromosome 1q31-q32.1.[301] Interestingly, a number of other genes encoding for proteins with "sushi" repeats also are located on chromosome 1. The gene for the B-subunit spans 28 kb and is composed of 12 exons.[297] The first exon encodes the leader sequence, whereas exons 2 through 11 each encodes a single "sushi" repeat. Exon 12 encodes the C-terminus.

Factor XIII A-subunit is synthesized in megakaryocytes and is packed into newly formed platelets.[302] Monocytes and tissue macrophages/histiocytes in the placenta, uterus, and liver also produce A-subunits.[288,303] Because factor XIII-A subunit lacks the signal sequence, it cannot be released by the classic secretory pathway through the Golgi. Conceivably, factor XIII A-subunit is released into the circulation from cells as a consequence of cell injury.[300]

The B-subunit is synthesized in the liver.[304,305] Assembly of the A- and B-subunits probably occurs in the circulation.

Factor XIII circulates in plasma as an inactive tetramer (A_2B_2). Cleavage of the Arg37-Gly38 peptide bond of the A-subunit by thrombin releases a 4500-kDa activation peptide that is required for activation of the tetramer.[306] Thereafter, calcium ions induce dissociation of the A- and B-subunits. In the absence of inhibitory B-subunits, the active site sulfhydryl residue of the A-subunit is exposed and proteolytically activated (activated factor XIII [factor XIIIa]).[288] Fibrin polymer is an important cofactor for generation of factor XIIIa.[307]

Factor XIIIa catalyzes the formation of peptide bonds between adjacent molecules of fibrin monomer, thus imparting chemical and mechanical stability to a clot. The peptide bond that is formed consists of an amide bond between the γ-carbonyl group of glutamine and the ε-amino group of lysine. In fibrin, this amide bond is located between Aα-chain sequences and between γ-chain sequences. The γ-chain links occur between Gln398 or Gln399 on the γ-chain of one fibrin molecule and Lys406 on the γ-chain of another fibrin molecule.[308] Cross-linking sites in the Aα-chain have been identified as Gln221, Gln237, Gln328, and Gln366. Lysine residues that function as acceptor sites for the transglutaminase reaction include Lys208, Lys224, Lys418, Lys508, Lys556, and Lys562.[307] Factor XIIIa also cross-links α2-antiplasmin to the α-chain of fibrin,[309] thereby increasing the resistance of fibrin to plasmin degradation, and cross-links fibronectin to the α-chain of fibrin,[310] thereby affecting the mechanical properties of the clot and increasing cell adhesion. A number of other proteins also are substrates for factor XIIIa, including factor V, plasminogen activator inhibitor-2, collagen, thrombospondin, von Willebrand factor, vinculin, vitronectin, actin, myosin, and lipoprotein(a), but the physiologic significance of these reactions is less clear.[288]

GENETICS

Inherited factor XIII deficiency is transmitted in an autosomal recessive fashion. Parents of affected individuals typically are asymptomatic, and consanguinity is common. Deficiency of the factor XIII A-subunit is the predominant abnormality and occurs at a frequency of approximately one in two million.[36] At the time of this writing, 58 mutations causing factor XIII A-subunit deficiency have been reported, of which 29 are missense mutations, four are nonsense mutations, 10 are splice site mutations, 14 are small deletions/insertions, and one is a gross deletion in the A-subunit gene (see Table 116-1). In four mutations (Arg77His, Arg661Ter, Leu660Pro, and nt2045 G→A, the last nucleotide of exon 14),[311–314] a founder effect has been suggested, but definitive proof has been provided only for Leu660Pro, which is prevalent in Palestinian Arabs, and nt2045 G→A alteration, which was observed in five families from Pakistan.[313,314]

Six common nonsynonymous polymorphisms have been identified in the A-subunit gene.[315] One is a common G→T alteration resulting in Val34Leu substitution that affects factor XIII function.[307] Some but not all studies found the Leu34 allele was protective against myocardial infarction and venous thrombosis.[307]

Four mutations causing deficiency of B-subunits have been described. One is a missense mutation (Cys430Phe); the remaining are small deletions/insertions.[316]

CLINICAL MANIFESTATIONS

Factor XIII deficiency causes formation of blood clots that are unstable and susceptible to fibrinolytic degradation by plasmin. As a result, affected individuals have an increased tendency to bleed. Factor XIII A-subunit knockout mice manifest bleeding into the thoracic cavity, peritoneum, and subcutis.[317] In humans, bleeding from the umbilical stump during the first few days of life is common, and intracranial hemorrhage is observed more frequently than in other inherited bleeding disorders. This finding forms the basis for recommending prophylaxis against intracranial hemorrhage by regular replacement therapy. Ecchymoses, hematomas, and prolonged bleeding following trauma also are characteristic. Hemarthroses and bleeding into the muscles are less common than in the hemophilias. Bleeding following trauma may be delayed for 12 to 36 hours in some patients, whereas immediate bleeding occurs in other patients.

Delayed wound healing occurs in approximately 15 percent of patients deficient in factor XIII A-subunit. The exact mechanism by which factor XIII, or its activated form, exerts its beneficial effect on wound healing is unknown. However, the demonstrated proangiogenic effect of factor XIIIa suggests that, in the absence of factor XIII, decreased vascularization of the wound results in improper repair.[318]

Habitual abortions are commonly observed in affected patients and in mice deficient in factor XIII A-subunit.[319] In affected women, for-

mation of the cytotrophoblastic shell is impaired.[320] Conceivably, factor XIII A-subunit deficiency at the implantation site abrogates fibrin/fibronectin cross-linking, which is essential for attachment of the placenta to the uterus.[321]

DIFFERENTIAL DIAGNOSIS

PT and aPTT are normal in factor XIII deficiency (see Chap. 109). Because of increased fibrin breakdown, levels of fibrin degradation products may be increased and result in a minimally prolonged thrombin time. This finding may be the only clue to the diagnosis based on simple coagulation screening tests. Diagnosis of factor XIII deficiency is established by demonstrating increased clot solubility in 5 M urea, dilute monochloroacetic acid, or acetic acid. Factor XIII activity also can be determined quantitatively by measuring its ability to catalyze the incorporation of fluorescent or radioactive amines into proteins such as casein and by using commercial kits.[322] Factor XIII A-subunit antigen can be measured by electroimmunoassay[323] or ELISA.[324]

The disorder is easily differentiated from other deficiencies of plasma coagulation factors by demonstrating normal results of screening coagulation tests and increased fibrin solubility. Deficiency of α2-antiplasmin may cause an increased tendency to bleed, also with normal screening tests and increased clot solubility. A specific assay for α2-antiplasmin is required to distinguish between the two disorders. However, patients with α2-antiplasmin deficiency appear to have a milder bleeding disorder and do not manifest umbilical cord or intracranial hemorrhages. A family history and a lifelong history of bleeding help distinguish inherited factor XIII deficiency from an acquired inhibitor or other causes of the deficiency.

THERAPY

Replacement therapy for factor XIII deficiency is highly satisfactory because of the small quantities of factor XIII needed for effective hemostasis and the long half-life of factor XIII (10–14 days). Plasma-derived, virus-inactivated concentrates of factor XIII are available[325] and are the treatment of choice. Fresh frozen plasma and solvent detergent-treated plasma can be used when the concentrates are unavailable. The low plasma levels of factor XIII required to control bleeding (5% of normal) and the long half-life of factor XIII make prophylactic therapy feasible. Thus, prophylactic therapy with factor XIII concentrate at a regimen of 10 to 20 U/kg every 5 to 6 weeks is sufficient to secure normal hemostasis. During pregnancy, more frequent replacement therapy is needed to prevent fetal loss.[326] A one-time infusion of 10 to 20 U/kg is sufficient when impaired wound healing occurs.

In patients with hereditary factor XIII deficiency, development of an inhibitor is very rare and to date has been reported in only three cases.[37,326]

REFERENCES

1. Walz DA, Hewett-Emmett D, Seegers WH: Amino acid sequence of human prothrombin fragments 1 and 2. *Proc Natl Acad Sci U S A* 74: 1969, 1977.
2. Butkowski RJ, Elion J, Downing MR, Mann KG: Primary structure of human prethrombin 2 and alpha-thrombin. *J Biol Chem* 252:4942, 1977.
3. Degen SJ, MacGillivray RT, Davie EW: Characterization of the complementary deoxyribonucleic acid and gene coding for human prothrombin. *Biochemistry* 22:2087, 1983.
4. Degen SJ, Sun WY: The biology of prothrombin. *Crit Rev Eukaryot Gene Expr* 8:203, 1998.

5. Kotkow KJ, Deitcher SR, Furie B, Furie BC: The second kringle domain of prothrombin promotes factor Va-mediated prothrombin activation by prothrombinase. *J Biol Chem* 270:4551, 1995.

6. Bode W, Mayr I, Baumann U, et al: The refined 1.9 A crystal structure of human α-thrombin interaction with D-Phe-Pro-Arg chloromethylketone and significance of the Tyr-Pro-Pro-Trp insertion segment. *EMBO J* 8:3467, 1989.

7. Royle NJ, Irwin DM, Koschnsky ML, et al: Human genes encoding prothrombin and ceruloplasmin map to 11p11-q12 and 3q21-24, respectively. *Somat Cell Mol Genet* 13:285, 1987.

8. Degen SJ, Davie EW: Nucleotide sequence of the gene for human prothrombin. *Biochemistry* 26:6165, 1987.

9. Bancroft JD, Schaefer LA, Degen SJ: Characterization of the Alu-rich 5'-flanking region of the human prothrombin-encoding gene: Identification of a positive *cis*-acting element that regulates liver-specific expression. *Gene* 95:253, 1990.

10. Moser M, Patterson C: Thrombin and vascular development: A sticky subject. *Arterioscler Thromb Vasc Biol* 23:922, 2003.

11. Sun WY, Witte DP, Degen JL, Colbert MC, et al: Prothrombin deficiency results in embryonic and neonatal lethality in mice. *Proc Natl Acad Sci U S A* 95:7597, 1998.

12. Miyata T, Moita T, Inomoto T, et al: Prothrombin Tokushima, a replacement of arginine-418 by tryptophan that impairs the fibrinogen clotting activity of derived thrombin Tokushima. *Biochemistry* 26:1117, 1987.

13. Morishita E, Saito M, Asakura H, et al: Prothrombin Himi: An abnormal prothrombin characterized by a defective thrombin activity. *Thromb Res* 62:697, 1991.

14. Akhavan S, De Cristofaro R, Peyvandi F, et al: Molecular and functional characterization of a natural homozygous Arg67His mutation in the prothrombin gene of a patient with a severe procoagulant defect contrasting with a mild hemorrhagic phenotype. *Blood* 100:1347, 2002.

15. O'Marcaigh AS, Nichols WL, Hassinger NL, et al: Genetic analysis and functional characterization of prothrombins Corpus Christi (Arg382-Cys), Dhahran (Arg271-His), and hypoprothrombinemia. *Blood* 88:2611, 1996.

16. Henriksen RA, Mann KG: Identification of the primary structural defect in the dysthrombin thrombin Quick I: Substitution of cysteine for arginine-382. *Biochemistry* 27:9160, 1988.

17. Henriksen RA, Mann KG: Substitution of valine for glycine-558 in the congenital dysthrombin thrombin Quick II alters primary substrate specificity. *Biochemistry* 28:2078, 1989.

18. Miyata T, Aruga R, Umeyama H, et al: Prothrombin Salakta: Substitution of glutamic acid-466 by alanine reduces the fibrinogen clotting activity and the esterase activity. *Biochemistry* 31:7457, 1992.

19. Henriksen RA, Dunham CK, Miller LD, et al: Prothrombin Greenville, Arg517→Gln, identified in an individual heterozygous for dysprothrombinemia. *Blood* 91:2026, 1998.

20. Sekine O, Sugo T, Ebisawa K, et al: Substitution of Gly-548 to Ala in the substrate binding pocket of prothrombin Perija leads to the loss of thrombin proteolytic activity. *Thromb Haemost* 87:282, 2002.

21. Sun WY, Smirnow D, Jenkins ML, Degen SJ: Prothrombin Scranton: Substitution of an amino acid residue involved in the binding of Na⁺ (Lys-556 to Thr) leads to dysprothrombinemia. *Thromb Haemost* 85:651, 2001.

22. Diuguid DL, Rabiet MJ, Furie BC, Furie B: Molecular defects of factor IX Chicago-2 (Arg 145→His) and prothrombin Madrid (Arg 271→Cys): Arginine mutations that preclude zymogen activation. *Blood* 74:193, 1989.

23. James HL, Kim DJ, Zheng DQ, Girolami A: Prothrombin Padua I: Incomplete activation due to an amino acid substitution at a factor Xa cleavage site. *Blood Coagul Fibrinolysis* 5:841, 1994.

24. Sun WY, Burkart MC, Holahan JR, Degen SJ: Prothrombin San Antonio: A single amino acid substitution at a factor Xa activation site (Arg320 to His) results in dysprothrombinemia. *Blood* 95:711, 2000.

25. Lefkowitz JB, Weller A, Nuss R, et al: A common mutation, Arg457→Gln, links prothrombin deficiencies in the Puerto Rican population. *J Thromb Haemost* 1:2381, 2003.

26. Ruiz-Saez A, Luengo J, Rodriguez A, et al: Prothrombin Perija: A new congenital dysprothrombinemia in an Indian family. *Thromb Res* 44:587, 1986.

27. Ruiz-Saez A, Bosch N, Echenagucia M, et al: High prevalence of an abnormal prothrombin in an Indian population of Venezuela [abstract]. *Thrombosis Haemost* 73:1438, 1995.

28. Poort SR, Rosendaal FR, Reitsma PH, Bertina RM: A common genetic variation in the 3'-untranslated region of the prothrombin gene is associated with elevated plasma prothrombin levels and an increase in venous thrombosis. *Blood* 88:3698, 1996.

29. Gehring NH, Frede U, Neu-Yilik G, et al: Increased efficiency of mRNA 3' end formation: A new genetic mechanism contributing to hereditary thrombophilia. *Nat Genet* 28:389, 2001.

30. Mannucci PM: Outbreak of hepatitis A among Italian patients with haemophilia. *Lancet* 339:819, 1992.

31. Gerritzen A, Schneweis KE, Brackmann HH, et al: Acute hepatitis A in haemophilias. *Lancet* 340:1231, 1992.

32. Ragni MV, Koch WC, Jorda JA: Parvovirus B19 infection in patients with hemophilia. *Transfusion* 36:238, 1996.

33. Yee TT, Cohen BJ, Pasi KJ, Lee CA: Transmission of symptomatic parvovirus B19 infection by clotting factor concentrate. *Br J Haematol* 93:457, 1996.

34. Lusher JM: Thrombogenicity associated with factor IX complex concentrates. *Semin Hematol* 28:3, 1991.

35. Alexander B, Goldstein R, Landwehr G, Cook CD: Congenital SPCA deficiency: A hitherto unrecognized coagulation defect with hemorrhage rectified by serum and serum fractions. *J Clin Invest* 30:596, 1951.

36. Peyvandi F, Duga S, Akhavan S, Mannucci PM: Rare coagulation deficiencies. *Haemophilia* 8:308, 2002.

37. Acharya SS, Coughlin A, Dimichele DM: Rare Bleeding Disorder Registry: Deficiencies of factors II V, VII X, XIII, fibrinogen and dysfibrinogenemias. *J Thromb Haemost* 2:248, 2004.

38. Hagen FS, Gray CL, O'Hara P, et al: Characterization of a cDNA coding for human factor VII. *Proc Natl Acad Sci U S A* 83:2412, 1986.

39. O'Hara PJ, Grant FJ, Haldeman BA, et al: Nucleotide sequence of the gene coding for human factor VII, a vitamin K-dependent protein participating in blood coagulation. *Proc Natl Acad Sci U S A* 84:5158, 1987.

40. Ott R, Pfeiffer RA: Evidence that activities of coagulation factors VII and X are linked to chromosome 13 (q34). *Hum Hered* 34:123, 1984.

41. Gilgenkrantz S, Briquel ME, Andre E, et al: Structural genes of coagulation factors VII and X located on 13q34. *Ann Genet* 29:32, 1986.

42. Miao CH, Leytus SP, Chung DW, Davie EW: Liver-specific expression of the gene coding for human factor X, a blood coagulation factor. *J Biol Chem* 267:7395, 1992.

43. Greenberg D, Miao CH, Ho WT, et al: Liver-specific expression of the human factor VII gene. *Proc Natl Acad Sci U S A* 92:12347, 1995.

44. Pollak ES, Hung HL, Godin W, et al: Functional characterization of the human factor VII 5'-flanking region. *J Biol Chem* 271:1738, 1996.

45. Fair DS: Quantitation of factor VII in the plasma of normal and warfarin-treated individuals by radioimmunoassay. *Blood* 62:784, 1983.

46. Marder VJ, Shulman NR: Clinical aspects of congenital factor VII deficiency. *Am J Med* 37:182, 1964.

47. Radcliffe R, Nemerson Y: Activation and control of factor VII by activated factor X and thrombin: Isolation and characterization of a single chain form of factor VII. *J Biol Chem* 250:388, 1975.

48. Seligsohn U, Osterud B, Brown SF, et al: Activation of human factor VII in plasma and in purified systems: Roles of activated factor IX, kallikrein, and activated factor XII. *J Clin Invest* 64:1056, 1979.

49. Radcliffe R, Bagdasarian A, Colman R, Nemerson Y: Activation of bovine factor VII by Hageman factor fragments. *Blood* 50:611, 1977.

50. Nakagaki T, Foster DC, Berkner KL, Kisiel W: Initiation of the extrinsic pathway of blood coagulation: Evidence for the tissue factor dependent autoactivation of human coagulation factor VII. *Biochemistry* 30:10819, 1991.

51. Rapaport SI, Rao LV: The tissue factor pathway: How it has become a "prima ballerina." *Thromb Haemost* 74:7, 1995.

52. Banner DW, D'Arcy A, Chene C, et al: The crystal structure of the complex of blood coagulation factor VIIa with soluble tissue factor. *Nature* 380:41, 1996.

53. Cooper DN, Millar DS, Wacey A, et al: Inherited factor VII deficiency: Molecular genetics and pathophysiology. *Thromb Haemost* 78:151, 1997.

54. Edgington TS, Dickinson CD, Ruf W: The structural basis of function of the TF-VIIa complex in the cellular initiation of coagulation. *Thromb Haemost* 78:401, 1997.

55. Morrissey JH, Neuenschwander PF, Huang Q, et al: Factor VIIa–tissue factor: Functional importance of protein-membrane interactions. *Thromb Haemost* 78:112, 1997.

56. Morrissey JH, Macik BG, Neuenschwander PF, Comp PC: Quantitation of activated factor VII levels in plasma using a tissue factor mutant selectively deficient in promoting factor VII activation. *Blood* 81:734, 1993.

57. Seligsohn U, Kasper CK, Osterud B, Rapaport SI: Activated factor VII: Presence in factor IX concentrates and persistence in the circulation after infusion. *Blood* 53:828, 1979.

58. Miller BC, Hultin MB, Jesty J: Altered factor VII activity in hemophilia. *Blood* 65:845, 1985.

59. Wildgoose P, Nemerson Y, Hansen LL, et al: Measurement of basal levels of factor VIIa in hemophilia A and B patients. *Blood* 80:25, 1992.

60. Eichinger S, Mannucci PM, Tradati F, et al: Determinants of plasma factor VIIa levels in humans. *Blood* 86:3021, 1995.

61. Osterud B, Rapaport SI: Activation of factor IX by the reaction product of tissue factor and factor VII: Additional pathway for initiating blood coagulation. *Proc Natl Acad Sci U S A* 74:5260, 1977.

62. Butenas S, Van't Veer C, Mann KG: Evaluation of the initiation phase of blood coagulation using ultrasensitive assays for serine proteases. *J Biol Chem* 272:21527, 1997.

63. Rosen ED, Chan JC, Idusogie E, et al: Mice lacking factor VII develop normally but suffer fatal perinatal bleeding. *Nature* 390:290, 1997.

64. Carmeliet P, Mackman N, Moons L, et al: Role of tissue factor in embryonic blood vessel development. *Nature* 383:73, 1996.

65. Parry GC, Erlich JH, Carmeliet P, et al: Low levels of tissue factor are compatible with development and hemostasis in mice. *J Clin Invest* 101:560, 1998.

66. Arbini AA, Bodkin D, Lopaciuk S, Bauer KA: Molecular analysis of Polish patients with factor VII deficiency. *Blood* 84:2214, 1994.

67. Tamary H, Fromovich Y, Shalmon L, et al: Ala244Val is a common, probably ancient mutation causing factor VII deficiency in Moroccan and Iranian Jews. *Thromb Haemost* 76:283, 1996.

68. Goodnight SH Jr, Feinstein DI, Osterud B, Rapaport SI: Factor VII antibody-neutralizing material in hereditary and acquired factor VII deficiency. *Blood* 38:1, 1971.

69. Mariani G, Mazzucconi MG, Hermans J, et al: Factor VII deficiency: Immunological characterization of genetic variants and detection of carriers. *Br J Haematol* 48:7, 1981.

70. Triplett DA, Brandt JT, Batard MA, et al: Hereditary factor VII deficiency: Heterogeneity defined by combined functional and immunochemical analysis. *Blood* 66:1284, 1985.

71. Arbini AA, Pollak ES, Bayleran JK, et al: Severe factor VII deficiency due to a mutation disrupting a hepatocyte nuclear factor 4 binding site in the factor VII promoter. *Blood* 89:176, 1997.

72. Carew JA, Pollak ES, High KA, Bauer KA: Severe factor VII deficiency due to a mutation disrupting an Sp1 binding site in the factor VII promoter. *Blood* 92:1639, 1998.

73. Nagaizumi K, Inaba H, Suzuki T, et al: Two double heterozygous mutations in the F7 gene show different manifestations. *Br J Haematol* 119:1052, 2002.

74. Carew JA, Pollak ES, Lopaciuk S, Bauer KA: A new mutation in the HNF4 binding region of the factor VII promoter in a patient with severe factor VII deficiency. *Blood* 96:4370, 2000.

75. Fromovich-Amit Y, Zivelin A, Rosenberg N, et al: Characterization of mutations causing factor VII deficiency in 61 unrelated Israeli patients. *J Thromb Haemost* 2:1774, 2004.

76. Leonard BJN, Chen Q, Blajchman MA, et al: Factor VII deficiency caused by a structural variant N57D of the first epidermal growth factor domain. *Blood* 91:142, 1998.

77. Chaing S, Clarke B, Sridhara S, et al: Severe factor VII deficiency caused by mutations abolishing the cleavage site for activation and altering binding to tissue factor. *Blood* 83:3524, 1994.

78. Kavlie A, Orning L, Grindflek A, et al: Characterization of a factor VII molecule carrying a mutation in the second epidermal growth factor-like domain. *Thromb Haemost* 79:1136, 1998.

79. Kemball-Cook G, Johnson DJD, Takamiya O, et al: Coagulation factor VII Gln^{100}→Arg. Amino acid substitution at the epidermal growth factor 2-protease domain interface results in severely reduced tissue factor binding and procoagulant function. *J Biol Chem* 273:8516, 1998.

80. Seligsohn U, Shani M, Ramot B, et al: Dubin-Johnson syndrome in Israel: II. Association with factor VII deficiency. *Q J Med* 39:569, 1970.

81. Mor-Cohen R, Zivelin A, Rosenberg N, et al: Identification and functional analysis of two novel mutations in the multidrug resistance protein 2 gene in Israeli patients with Dubin-Johnson syndrome. *J Biol Chem* 276:36923, 2001.

82. Wulff K, Herrmann FH: Twenty two novel mutations of the factor VII gene in factor VII deficiency. *Hum Mutat* 15:489, 2000.

83. Giansily-Blaizot M, Aguilar-Martinez P, Biron-Andreani C, et al: Analysis of the genotypes and phenotypes of 37 unrelated patients with inherited factor VII deficiency. *Eur J Hum Genet* 9:105, 2001.

84. Bernardi F, Patracchini P, Gemmati D, et al: Molecular analysis of factor VII deficiency in Italy: A frequent mutation (FVII Lazio) in a repeated intronic region. *Hum Genet* 92:446, 1993.

85. Etro D, Pinotti M, Wulff K, et al: The Gly331Ser mutation in factor VII in Europe and the Middle East. *Haematologica* 88:1434, 2003.

86. Bernardi F, Liney DL, Patracchini P, et al: Molecular defects in CRM+ factor VII deficiencies: Modeling of missense mutations in the catalytic domain of FVII. *Br J Haematol* 86:610, 1994.

87. Hunault M, Arbini AA, Lopaciuk S, et al: The Arg^{353} Gln polymorphism reduces the level of coagulation factor VII: In vivo and in vitro studies. *Arterioscler Thromb Vasc Biol* 17:2825, 1997.

88. Green F, Kelleher C, Wilkes H, et al: A common genetic polymorphism associated with lower coagulation factor VII levels in healthy individuals. *Arterioscler Thromb* 11:540, 1991.

89. Bernardi F, Marchetti G, Pinotti M, et al: Factor VII gene polymorphisms contribute about one-third of the factor VII level variation in plasma. *Arterioscler Thromb Vasc Biol* 16:72, 1996.

90. Kario K, Narita N, Matsuo T, et al: Genetic determinants of plasma factor VII activity in the Japanese. *Thromb Haemost* 73:617, 1995.

91. Lane A, Cruickshank JK, Mitchell J, et al: Genetic and environmental determinants of factor VII coagulant activity in ethnic groups at differing risk of coronary heart disease. *Atherosclerosis* 94:43, 1992.

92. La Coviello L, Di Castelnuovo A, DeKnijff P, et al: Polymorphisms in the coagulation factor VII gene and the risk of myocardial infarction. *N Engl J Med* 338:79, 1998.

93. Saha N, Liu Y, Hong CK, et al: Association of factor VII genotype with

plasma factor VII activity and antigen levels in healthy Indian adults and interaction with triglycerides. *Arterioscler Thromb* 14:1923, 1994.

94. Marchetti G, Gemmati D, Patracchini P, et al: PCR detection of a repeat polymorphism within the F7 gene. *Nucleic Acids Res* 19:4570, 1991.

95. Hunault M, Arbini AA, Carew JA, Bauer KA: Mechanism underlying factor VII deficiency in Jewish populations with the Ala244Val mutation. *Br J Haematol* 105:1101, 1999.

96. Hall CA, Rapaport SI, Ames SB, et al: A clinical and family study of hereditary proconvertin (factor VII) deficiency. *Am J Med* 37:172, 1964.

97. Mariani G, Mazzucconi MG: Factor VII congenital deficiency: Clinical picture and classification of the variants. *Haemostasis* 13:169, 1983.

98. Ragni MV, Lewis JH, Spero JA, Hasiba U: Factor VII deficiency. *Am J Hematol* 10:79, 1981.

99. de Moerloose P, Amiral J, Vissac AM, Reber G: Longitudinal study on activated factors XII and VII levels during normal pregnancy. *Br J Haematol* 100:40, 1998.

100. Seligsohn U, Peyser MR, Toaff R, et al: Severe hereditary deficiency of factor VII during pregnancy: Evidence for the absence of transplacental diffusion of factor VII. *Thromb Diath Haemorrh* 24:146, 1970.

101. Robertson LE, Wasserstrum N, Banez E, et al: Hereditary factor VII deficiency in pregnancy: Peripartum treatment with factor VII concentrate. *Am J Hematol* 40:38, 1992.

102. Mariani G, Herrmann FH, Schulman S, et al: Thrombosis in inherited factor VII deficiency. *J Thromb Haemost* 1:2153, 2003.

103. Philippou H, Adami A, Amersey RA, et al: A novel specific immunoassay for plasma two-chain factor VIIa: Investigation of FVIIa levels in normal individuals and in patients with acute coronary syndromes. *Blood* 89:767, 1997.

104. Mariani G, Hermans J, Orlando M, et al: Carrier detection in factor VII congenital deficiency. *Br J Haematol* 60:687, 1985.

105. Boxus G, Slacmeulder M, Ninane J: Combined hereditary deficiency in factors VII and X revealed by a prolonged partial thromboplastin time. *Arch Pediatr* 4:44, 1997.

106. Hall C, London AR, Moynihan AC, Dodds WJ: Hereditary factor VII and IX deficiencies in a large kindred. *Br J Haematol* 29:319, 1975.

107. Briet E, Onvlee G: Hip surgery in a patient with severe factor VII deficiency. *Haemostasis* 17:273, 1987.

108. Cederbaum AI, Blatt PM, Roberts HR: Intravascular coagulation with use of human prothrombin complex concentrates. *Ann Intern Med* 84:683, 1976.

109. Perry DJ: Factor VII deficiency. *Blood Coag Fibrinolysis Suppl* 14:S47, 2003.

110. Mariani G, Testa MG, Di Paolantonio T, et al: Use of recombinant, activated factor VII in the treatment of congenital factor VII deficiencies. *Vox Sang* 77:131,1999.

111. Tcheng WY, Donkin J, Konzal S, Wong WY: Recombinant factor VIIa in a patient with severe congenital factor VII deficiency. *Haemophilia* 10:295, 2004.

112. Telfer TP, Denson KW, Wright DW: A "new" coagulation defect. *Br J Haematol* 2:308, 1956.

113. Hougie C, Barrow EM, Graham JB: Stuart clotting defect: I. Segregation of an hereditary hemorrhagic state from the heterogeneous group heretofore called "stable factor" (SPCA, proconvertin, factor VII) deficiency. *J Clin Invest* 36:485, 1957.

114. Scambler PJ, Williamson R: The structural gene for human coagulation factor X is located on chromosome 13q34. *Cytogenet Cell Genet* 39:231, 1985.

115. Royle NJ, Fung MR, McGillivray RT, Hamerton JL: The gene for clotting factor 10 is mapped to 13q32-qter. *Cytogenet Cell Genet* 41:185, 1986.

116. Leytus SP, Foster DC, Kurachi K, Davie EW: Gene for human factor

117. Neurath H: Evolution of proteolytic enzymes. *Science* 224:350, 1984.

118. McMullen BA, Fujikawa K, Kisiel W, et al: Complete amino acid sequence of the light chain of human blood coagulation factor X: Evidence for identification of residue 63 as beta-hydroxyaspartic acid. *Biochemistry* 22:2875, 1983.

119. Jackson CM: Characterization of two glycoprotein variants of bovine factor X and demonstration that the factor X zymogen contains two polypeptide chains. *Biochemistry* 11:4873, 1972.

120. Fujikawa K, Coan MH, Legaz ME, Davie EW: The mechanism of activation of bovine factor X (Stuart factor) by intrinsic and extrinsic pathways. *Biochemistry* 13:5290, 1974.

121. Fujikawa K, Legaz ME, Davie EW: Bovine factor X (Stuart factor): Mechanism of activation by protein from Russell's viper venom. *Biochemistry* 11:4892, 1972.

122. Rudolph AE, Mullane MP, Porche-Sorbet R, et al: Factor X St. Louis II. Identification of a glycine substitution at residue 7 and characterization of the recombinant protein. *J Biol Chem* 271:28601, 1996.

123. Watzke HH, Lechner K, Roberts HR, et al: Molecular defect (Gla+14-Lys) and its functional consequences in a hereditary factor X deficiency (factor X "Vorarlberg"). *J Biol Chem* 265:11982, 1990.

124. Pinotti M, Marchetti G, Baroni M, et al: Reduced activation of the Gla19Ala FX variant via the extrinsic coagulation pathway results in symptomatic CRM^{red} FX deficiency. *Thromb Haemost* 88:236, 2002.

125. De Stefano V, Leone G, Ferrelli R, et al: Factor X Roma: A congenital factor X variant defective at different degrees in the intrinsic and the extrinsic activation. *Br J Haematol* 69:387, 1988.

126. James HL, Girolami A, Fair DS: Molecular defect in coagulation factor X$_{Friuli}$ results from a substitution of serine for proline at position 343. *Blood* 77:317, 1991.

127. Watzke HH, Wallmark A, Hamaguchi N, et al: Factor X Santo Domingo: Evidence that the severe clinical phenotype arises from a mutation blocking secretion. *J Clin Invest* 88:1685, 1991.

128. Cooper DN, Millar DS, Wacey A, et al: Inherited factor X deficiency: Molecular genetics and pathophysiology. *Thromb Haemost* 78:161, 1997.

129. Peyvandi F, Mannucci PM, Lak M, et al: Congenital factor X deficiency: Spectrum of bleeding symptoms in 32 Iranian patients. *Br J Haematol* 102:626, 1998.

130. Howell M: Acquired factor X deficiency associated with systemic amyloidosis: A report of a case. *Blood* 21:739, 1963.

131. Furie B, Greene E, Furie BC: Syndrome of acquired factor X deficiency and systemic amyloidosis: In vivo studies of the metabolic fate of factor X. *N Engl J Med* 297:81, 1977.

132. Furie B, Voo L, McAdam KP, Furie BC: Mechanism of factor X deficiency in systemic amyloidosis. *N Engl J Med* 304:827, 1981.

133. Fair DS, Edgington TS: Heterogeneity of hereditary and acquired factor X deficiencies by combined immunochemical and functional analyses. *Br J Haematol* 59:235, 1985.

134. Blatt PM, Lundblad RL, Kingdon HS, et al: Thrombogenic materials in prothrombin complex concentrates. *Ann Intern Med* 81:766, 1974.

135. Biggs R, Denson KWE: The fate of prothrombin and factors VII, IX, and X transfused to patients deficient in these factors. *Br J Haematol* 9:532, 1963.

136. Roberts HR, Lechler E, Webster WP, Penick GD: Survival of transfused factor X in patients with Stuart disease. *Thromb Diath Haemorrh* 18:305, 1965.

137. McMillan CW, Roberts HR: Congenital combined deficiency of coagulation factors II, VII, IX and X: Report of a case. *N Engl J Med* 274:1313, 1966.

138. Fregin A, Rost S, Wolz W, et al: Homozygosity mapping of a second

X: A blood coagulation factor whose gene organization is essentially identical with that of factor IX and protein C. *Biochemistry* 25:5098, 1986.

gene locus for hereditary combined deficiency of vitamin K-dependent clotting factors to the centromeric region of chromosome 16. *Blood* 100: 3229, 2002.

139. Samama M, Bertina RM, Conard J, Horellou MH: Combined congenital deficiency in protein C and in factors II, VII, IX, and X. *Thromb Haemost* 50:359, 1983.

140. Brenner B, Tavori S, Zivelin A, et al: Hereditary deficiency of all vitamin K–dependent procoagulants and anticoagulants. *Br J Haematol* 75:537, 1990.

141. Spronk HM, Farah RA, Buchanan GR, et al: Novel mutation in the gamma-glutamyl carboxylase gene resulting in congenital combined deficiency of all vitamin K-dependent blood coagulation factors. *Blood* 96: 3650, 2000.

142. Soute BA, Jin DY, Spronk HM, et al: Characteristics of recombinant W501S mutated human gamma-glutamyl carboxylase. *J Thromb Haemost* 2:597, 2004.

143. Rost S, Fregin A, Ivaskevicius V, et al: Mutations in VKORC1 cause warfarin resistance and multiple coagulation factor deficiency type 2. *Nature* 427:537, 2004.

144. Goldsmith GH, Pence RE, Ratnoff OD, et al: Studies on a family with combined deficiencies of vitamin K–dependent coagulation factors. *J Clin Invest* 69:1253, 1982.

145. Owren PA: Parahemophilia: Hemorrhagic diathesis due to absence of a previously unknown factor. *Lancet* 1:446, 1947.

146. Tracy PB, Mann KG: Abnormal formation of the prothrombinase complex: Factor V deficiency and related disorders. *Hum Pathol* 18:162, 1987.

147. Kane WH, Davie EW: Blood coagulation factors V and VIII: Structural and functional similarities and their relationship to hemorrhagic and thrombotic disorders. *Blood* 71:539, 1988.

148. Cripe LD, Moore KD, Kane WH: Structure of the gene for human coagulation factor V. *Biochemistry* 31:3777, 1992.

149. Wang H, Riddell DC, Guinto ER, et al: Localization of the gene encoding human factor V to chromosome 1q21-25. *Genomics* 2:324, 1988.

150. Suzuki K, Dahlback B, Stenflo J: Thrombin-catalyzed activation of human coagulation factor V. *J Biol Chem* 257:6556, 1982.

151. Foster WB, Nesheim ME, Mann KG: The factor Xa-catalyzed activation of factor V. *J Biol Chem* 258:13970, 1983.

152. Wilson DB, Salem HH, Mruk JS, et al: Biosynthesis of coagulation factor V by human hepatocellular carcinoma cell line. *J Clin Invest* 73: 654, 1983.

153. Gewirtz AM, Keefer M, Doshi K, et al: Biology of human megakaryocyte factor V. *Blood* 67:1639, 1986.

154. Yang TL, Pipe SW, Yang A, Ginsburg D: Biosynthetic origin and functional significance of murine platelet factor V. *Blood* 102:2851, 2003.

155. Tracy PB, Eide LL, Bowie EJ, Mann KG: Radioimmunoassay of factor V in human plasma and platelets. *Blood* 60:59, 1982.

156. Seeler RA: Parahemophilia: Factor V deficiency. *Med Clin North Am* 56:119, 1972.

157. Viskup RW, Tracy PB, Mann KG: The isolation of human platelet factor V. *Blood* 69:1188, 1987.

158. Hayward CP, Furmaniak-Kazmierczak E, Cieutat AM, et al: Factor V is complexed with multimerin in resting platelet lysates and colocalizes with multimerin in platelet alpha-granules. *J Biol Chem* 270:19217, 1995.

159. Camire RM, Pollak ES, Kaushansky K, Tracy PB: Secretable human platelet-derived factor V originates from the plasma pool. *Blood* 92: 3035, 1998.

160. Gould WR, Silveira JR, Tracy PB: Unique in vivo modifications of coagulation factor V produce a physically and functionally distinct platelet-derived cofactor: Characterization of purified platelet-derived factor V/Va. *J Biol Chem* 279:2383, 2004.

161. Hayward CP, Rivard GE, Kane WH, et al: An autosomal dominant, qualitative platelet disorder associated with multimerin deficiency, abnormalities in platelet factor V, thrombospondin, von Willebrand factor, and fibrinogen and an epinephrine aggregation defect. *Blood* 87:4967, 1996.

162. Janeway CM, Rivard GE, Tracy PB, Mann KG: Factor V Quebec revisited. *Blood* 87:3571, 1996.

163. Suzuki K, Stenflo J, Dahlback B, Teodorsson B: Inactivation of human coagulation factor V by activated protein C. *J Biol Chem* 258:1914, 1983.

164. Nesheim ME, Canfield WM, Kisiel W, Mann KG: Studies of the capacity of factor Xa to protect factor Va from inactivation by activated protein C. *J Biol Chem* 257:1443, 1982.

165. Mitterstieler G, Muller W, Geir W: Congenital factor V deficiency: A family study. *Scand J Haematol* 21:9, 1978.

166. Castoldi E, Simioni P, Kalafatis M, et al: Combinations of 4 mutations (FV R506Q, FV H1299R, FV Y1702C, PT 20210G/A) affecting the prothrombinase complex in a thrombophilic family. *Blood* 96:1443, 2000.

167. Castoldi E, Lunghi B, Mingozzi F, et al: A missense mutation (Y1702C) in the coagulation factor V gene is a frequent cause of factor V deficiency in the Italian population. *Haematologica* 86:629, 2001.

168. Steen M, Miteva M, Villoutreix BO, et al: Factor V New Brunswick: Ala221Val associated with FV deficiency reproduced in vitro and functionally characterized. *Blood* 102, 1316, 2003.

169. Duga S, Montefusco MC, Asselta R, et al: Arg2074Cys missense mutation in the C2 domain of factor V causing moderately severe factor V deficiency: Molecular characterization by expression of the recombinant protein. *Blood* 101:173, 2003.

170. Montefusco MC, Duga S, Asselta R, et al: Clinical and molecular characterization of 6 patients affected by severe deficiency of coagulation factor V: Broadening of the mutational spectrum of factor V gene and in vitro analysis of the newly identified missense mutations. *Blood* 102: 3210, 2003.

171. Van Wijk R, Nieuwenhuis K, van den Berg M, et al: Five novel mutations in the gene for human blood coagulation factor V associated with type I factor V deficiency. *Blood* 98:358, 2001.

172. Van Wijk R, Montefusco MC, Duga S, et al: Coexistence of a novel homozygous nonsense mutation in exon 13 of the factor V gene with the homozygous Leiden mutation in two unrelated patients with severe factor V deficiency. *Br J Haematol* 114:871, 2001.

173. Guasch JF, Cannegieter S, Reitsma PH, et al: Severe coagulation factor V deficiency caused by a 4 bp deletion in the factor V gene. *Br J Haematol* 101:32, 1998.

174. Cui J, O'Shea KS, Purkayastha A, et al: Fatal haemorrhage and incomplete block to embryogenesis in mice lacking coagulation factor V. *Nature* 384:66, 1996.

175. Guasch JF, Lensen RP, Bertina RM: Molecular characterization of a type I quantitative factor V deficiency in a thrombosis patient that is "pseudohomozygous" for activated protein C resistance. *Thromb Haemost* 77:252, 1997.

176. Simioni P, Scudeller A, Radossi P, et al: "Pseudohomozygous" activated protein C resistance due to double heterozygous factor V defects (factor V Leiden mutation and type I quantitative factor V defect) associated with thrombosis: Report of two cases belonging to two unrelated kindreds. *Thromb Haemost* 75:422, 1996.

177. Zehnder JL, Jain M: Recurrent thrombosis due to compound heterozygosity for factor V Leiden and factor V deficiency. *Blood Coagul Fibrinolysis* 7:361, 1996.

178. Girolami A, Simioni P, Venturelli U, et al: Factor V antigen levels in APC resistance, in factor V deficiency and in combined APC resistance and factor V deficiency (pseudohomozygous for APC resistance). *Blood Coagul Fibrinolysis* 8:245, 1997.

179. Delahousse B, Iochmann S, Pouplard C, et al: Pseudo-homozygous activated protein C resistance due to coinheritance of heterozygous factor V Leiden mutation and type I factor V deficiency: Variable expression when analyzed by different activated protein C resistance functional assays. *Blood Coagul Fibrinolysis* 8:503, 1997.

180. Lunghi B, Iacoviello L, Gemmati D, et al: Detection of new polymorphic markers in the factor V gene: Association with factor V levels in plasma. *Thromb Haemost* 75:45, 1996.

181. Tracy PB, Giles AR, Mann KG, et al: Factor V (Quebec): A bleeding diathesis associated with a qualitative platelet factor V deficiency. *J Clin Invest* 74:1221, 1984.

182. Hayward CP, Cramer EM, Kane WH, et al: Studies of a second family with the Quebec platelet disorder: Evidence that the degradation of the alpha-granule membrane and its soluble contents are not secondary to a defect in targeting proteins to alpha-granules. *Blood* 89:1243, 1997.

183. Miller SP: Coagulation dynamic in factor V deficiency: A family study with a note on the occurrence of thrombophlebitis. *Thromb Diath Haemorrh* 13:500, 1965.

184. Reich NE, Hoffman GC, de Wolfe VG, Van Ordstrand HS: Recurrent thrombophlebitis and pulmonary emboli in congenital factor 5 deficiency. *Chest* 69:113, 1976.

185. Manotti C, Quintavalla R, Pini M, et al: Thromboembolic manifestations and congenital factor V deficiency: A family study. *Haemostasis* 19:331, 1989.

186. Goodnough LT, Saito H, Ratnoff OD: Thrombosis or myocardial infarction in congenital clotting factor abnormalities and chronic thormbocytopenias: A report of 21 patients and a review of 50 previously reported cases. *Medicine (Baltimore)* 62:248, 1983.

187. Fratantoni JC, Hilgartner M, Nachman RL: Nature of the defect in congenital factor V deficiency: Study in a patient with an acquired circulating anticoagulant. *Blood* 39:751, 1972.

188. Mazzucconi MG, Solinas S, Chistolini A, et al: Inhibitor to factor V in severe factor V congenital deficiency: A case report. *Nouv Rev Fr Hematol* 27:303, 1985.

189. Webster WP, Roberts HR, Penick GD: Hemostasis in factor V deficiency. *Am J Med Sci* 248:194, 1964.

190. Tanis BC, van der Meer FJ, Bloem RM, Vlasveld LT: Successful excision of a pseudotumour in a congenitally factor V deficient patient. *Br J Haematol* 100:380, 1998.

191. Oeri J, Matter M, Isenschmid H, et al: Angeborener Mangel an Faktor V (Parahaemophilie) verbunden mit echter Haemophilie A bein zwei Brudern. *Med Probl Paediatr* 1:575, 1954.

192. Seligsohn U, Zivelin A, Zwang E: Combined factor V and factor VIII deficiency among non-Ashkenazi Jews. *N Engl J Med* 307:1191, 1982.

193. Seligsohn U: Combined factor V and factor VIII deficiency, in *Factor VIII: Von Willebrand Factor*, vol 2, edited by J Seghatchian, GT Savidge, p 89. CRC Press, Boca Raton, 1989.

194. Nichols WC, Seligsohn U, Zivelin A, et al: Mutations in the ER-Golgi intermediate compartment protein ERGIC-53 cause combined deficiency of coagulation factors V and VIII. *Cell* 93:61, 1998.

195. Zhang B, Cunningham MA, Nichols WC, et al: Bleeding due to disruption of a cargo-specific ER-to-Golgi transport complex. *Nat Genet* 34:220, 2003.

196. Peyvandi F, Tuddenham EG, Akhtari AM, et al: Bleeding symptoms in 27 Iranian patients with the combined deficiency of factor V and factor VIII. *Br J Haematol* 100:773, 1998.

197. Nichols WC, Seligsohn U, Zivelin A, et al: Linkage of combined factors V and VIII deficiency to chromosome 18q by homozygosity mapping. *J Clin Invest* 99:596, 1997.

198. Neerman-Arbez M, Antonarakis SE, Blouin JL, et al: The locus for combined factor V-factor VIII deficiency (F5F8D) maps to 18q21, between D18S849 and D18S1103. *Am J Hum Genet* 61:143, 1997.

199. Schindler R, Itin C, Zerial M, et al: ERGIC-53, a membrane protein of the ER-Golgi intermediate compartment, carries an ER retention motif. *Eur J Cell Biol* 61:1, 1993.

200. Schweizer A, Fransen JA, Bachi T, et al: Identification, by a monoclonal antibody, of a 53-kD protein associated with a tubulo-vesicular compartment at the *cis*-side of the Golgi apparatus. *J Cell Biol* 107:1643, 1988.

201. Nichols WC, Terry VH, Matthew MA, et al: ERGIC-53 gene structure and mutation analysis in 19 combined factors V and VIII deficiency families. *Blood* 93:2261, 1999.

202. Neerman-Arbez M, Johnson KM, Morris MA, et al: Molecular analysis of the ERGIC-53 gene in 35 families with combined factor V-factor VIII deficiency (F5F8D). *Blood* 93:2253, 1999.

203. Segal A, Zivelin A, Rosenberg N, et al: A mutation in LMAN 1 (ERGIC-53) causing combined factor V and factor VIII deficiency is prevalent in Jews originating from the island of Djerba in Tunisia. *Blood Coagul Fibrinolysis* 15:99, 2004.

204. Fischer RR, Giddings JC, Roisenberg I: Hereditary combined deficiency of clotting factors V and VIII with involvement of von Willebrand factor. *Clin Lab Haematol* 10:53, 1988.

205. Soff GA, Levin J, Bell WR: Familial multiple coagulation factor deficiencies: I. Review of the literature: Differentiation of single hereditary disorders associated with multiple factor deficiencies from coincidental concurrence of single factor deficiency state. *Semin Thromb Hemost* 7:112, 1981.

206. Gobbi F: Heredity of combined deficiency of AHG and proaccelerin. *Scand J Haematol* 3:222, 1966.

207. Girolami A, Gastaldi G, Patrassi G, Galletti A: Combined congenital deficiency of factor V and factor VIII: Report of a further case with some considerations on the hereditary transmission of this disorder. *Acta Haematol* 55:234, 1976.

208. Mazzone D, Fichera A, Pratico G, Sciacca F: Combined congenital deficiency of factor V and factor VIII. *Acta Haematol* 68:337, 1982.

209. Bartlett JA, Sweeney JD, Sadowsky D: Exodontia in combined factor V and factor VIII deficiency. *Br J Oral Maxillofac Surg* 43:537, 1985.

210. Tsurumi H, Takahashi T, Moriwaki H, Muto Y: Congenital combined deficiency of factor V and factor VIII with acquired ichthyosis, epidermodysplasia verruciformis, and immunological abnormalities. *Am J Hematol* 40:320, 1992.

211. Sallah AS, Angchaisuksiri P, Roberts HR: Use of plasma exchange in hereditary deficiency of factor V and factor VIII. *Am J Hematol* 52:229, 1996.

212. Rosenthal RL, Dreskin OH, Rosenthal N: A new hemophilia like disease caused by deficiency of a third plasma thromboplastin factor. *Proc Soc Exp Biol Med* 82:171, 1953.

213. Rapaport SI, Proctor RR, Patch NJ, Yettra M: The mode of inheritance of PTA deficiency: Evidence for the existence of major PTA deficiency and minor PTA deficiency. *Blood* 18:149, 1961.

214. Seligsohn U: High gene frequency of factor XI (PTA) deficiency in Ashkenazi-Jews. *Blood* 51:1223, 1978.

215. Gailani D, Broze GJ Jr: Factor XI activation in a revised model of blood coagulation. *Science* 253:909, 1991.

216. Naito K, Fujikawa K: Activation of human blood coagulation factor XI independent of factor XII: Factor XI is activated by thrombin and factor XIa in the presence of negatively charged surfaces. *J Biol Chem* 266:7353, 1991.

217. McMullen BA, Fujikawa K, Davie EW: Location of the disulfide bonds in human coagulation factor XI: The presence of tandem apple domains. *Biochemistry* 30:2056, 1991.

218. Meijers JCM, Mulvihill ER, Davie EW, Chung DW: Apple four in human blood coagulation factor XI mediates dimer formation. *Biochemistry* 31:4680, 1992.

219. Renne T, Gailani D, Meijers JC, Muller-Esterl W: Characterization of

the H-kininogen-binding site on factor XI: A comparison of factor XI and plasma prekallikrein. *J Biol Chem* 277:4892, 2002.

220. Asakai R, Davie EW, Chung DW: Organization of the gene for human factor XI. *Biochemistry* 26:7221, 1987.

221. Kato A, Asakai R, Davie EW, Aoki N: Factor XI gene (F11) is located on the distal end of the long arm of human chromosome 4. *Cytogenet Cell Genet* 52:77, 1989.

222. Bouma BN, Griffin JH: Human blood coagulation factor XI: Purification, properties, and mechanism of activation by activated factor XII. *J Biol Chem* 252:6432, 1977.

223. Baglia FA, Shrimpton CN, Lopez JA, Walsh PN: The glycoprotein Ib-IX-V complex mediates localization of factor XI to lipid rafts on the platelet membrane. *J Biol Chem* 278:21744, 2003.

224. Von dem Borne PA, Meijers JC, Bouma BN: Effect of heparin on the activation of factor XI by fibrin-bound thrombin. *Thromb Haemost* 76: 347, 1996.

225. Gailani D, Ho D, Sun MF, et al: Model for a factor IX activation complex on blood platelets: Dimeric conformation of factor XIa is essential. *Blood* 97:3117, 2001.

226. Osterud B, Bouma BN, Griffin JH: Human blood coagulation factor IX: Purification, properties, and mechanism of activation by activated factor XI. *J Biol Chem* 253:5946, 1978.

227. Bouma BN, Meijers JC: Thrombin-activatable fibrinolysis inhibitor (TAFI, plasma procarboxypeptidase B, procarboxypeptidase R, procarboxypeptidase U). *J Thromb Haemost* 1:1566, 2003.

228. Bajzar L, Morser J, Nesheim M: TAFI, or plasma procarboxypeptidase B, couples the coagulation and fibrinolytic cascades through the thrombin-thrombomodulin complex. *J Biol Chem* 271:16603, 1996.

229. Broze GJ Jr, Higuchi DA: Coagulation-dependent inhibition of fibrinolysis: Role of carboxypeptidase-U and the premature lysis of clots from hemophilic plasma. *Blood* 88:3815, 1996.

230. Von dem Borne PA, Meijers JC, Bouma BN: Feedback activation of factor XI by thrombin in plasma results in additional formation of thrombin that protects fibrin clots from fibrinolysis. *Blood* 86:3035, 1995.

231. Von dem Borne PA, Bajzar L, Meijers JC, et al: Thrombin-mediated activation of factor XI results in a thrombin-activatable fibrinolysis inhibitor-dependent inhibition of fibrinolysis. *J Clin Invest* 99:2323, 1997.

232. Minnema MC, Friederich PW, Levi M, et al: Enhancement of rabbit jugular vein thrombolysis by neutralization of factor XI: In vivo evidence for a role of factor XI as an anti-fibrinolytic factor. *J Clin Invest* 101:10, 1998.

233. Asakai R, Chung DW, Davie EW, Seligsohn U: Factor XI deficiency in Ashkenazi Jews in Israel. *N Engl J Med* 325:153, 1991.

234. Berliner S, Horowitz I, Martinowitz U, et al: Dental surgery in patients with severe factor XI deficiency without plasma replacement. *Blood Coagul Fibrinolysis* 3:465, 1992.

235. Clarkson K, Rosenfeld B, Fair J, et al: Factor XI deficiency acquired by liver transplantation. *Ann Intern Med* 115:877, 1991.

236. Bolton-Maggs PH, Young Wan-Yin B, McCraw AH, et al: Inheritance and bleeding in factor XI deficiency. *Br J Haematol* 69:521, 1988.

237. Saito H, Ratnoff OD, Bouma BN, Seligsohn U: Failure to detect variant (CRM+) plasma thromboplastin antecedent (factor XI) molecules in hereditary plasma thromboplastin antecedent deficiency: A study of 125 patients of several ethnic backgrounds. *J Lab Clin Med* 106:718, 1985.

238. Mannhalter C, Hellstern P, Deutsch E: Identification of a defective factor XI cross-reacting material in a factor XI-deficient patient. *Blood* 70:31, 1987.

239. Zivelin A, Ogawa T, Bulvik S, et al: Severe Factor XI deficiency caused by a Gly^{555} to Glu mutation (factor XI-Glu^{555}): A cross-reactive material positive variant defective in factor IX activation. *J Thromb Haemost* 2: 1782, 2004.

240. Quelin F, Trossaert M, Sigaud M, et al: Molecular basis of severe factor XI deficiency in seven families from the west of France. Seven novel mutations, including an ancient Q88X mutation. *J Thromb Haemost* 2: 71, 2004.

241. Martincic D, Zimmerman SA, Ware RE, et al: Identification of mutations and polymorphisms in the factor XI genes of an African-American family by dideoxy fingerprinting. *Blood* 92:3309, 1998.

242. Asakai R, Chung DW, Ratnoff OD, Davie EW: Factor XI (plasma thromboplastin antecedent) deficiency in Ashkenazi Jews is a bleeding disorder that can result from three types of point mutations. *Proc Natl Acad Sci U S A* 86:7667, 1989.

243. Peretz H, Zivelin A, Usher S, Seligsohn U: A 14-bp deletion (codon 554 del AAGgtaacagagtg) at exon 14/intron N junction of the coagulation factor XI gene disrupts splicing and causes severe factor XI deficiency. *Hum Mutat* 8:77, 1996.

244. Meijers JC, Davie EW, Chung DW: Expression of human blood coagulation factor XI: Characterization of the defect in factor XI type III deficiency. *Blood* 79:1435, 1992.

245. Pugh RE, McVey JH, Tuddenham EGD, Hancock JF: Six point mutations that cause factor XI deficiency. *Blood* 85:1509, 1995.

246. Zivelin A, Bauduer F, Ducout L, et al: Factor XI deficiency in French Basques is caused predominantly by an ancestral Cys38Arg mutation in the factor XI gene. *Blood* 99:2448, 2002.

247. Kravtsov DV, Wu W, Meijers JC, et al: Dominant factor XI deficiency caused by mutations in the factor XI catalytic domain. *Blood* 104:128, 2004.

248. Sidi A, Seligsohn U, Jonas P, Many M: Factor XI deficiency: Detection and management during urological surgery. *J Urol* 119:528, 1978.

249. Hancock JF, Wieland K, Pugh RE, et al: A molecular genetic study of factor XI deficiency. *Blood* 77:1942, 1991.

250. Shpilberg O, Peretz H, Zivelin A, et al: One of the two common mutations causing factor XI deficiency in Ashkenazi Jews (type II) is also prevalent in Iraqi Jews, who represent the ancient gene pool of Jews. *Blood* 85:429, 1995.

251. Peretz H, Mulai A, Usher S, et al: The two common mutations causing factor XI deficiency in Jews stem from distinct founders: One of ancient Middle Eastern origin and another of more recent European origin. *Blood* 90:2654, 1997.

252. Bolton-Maggs PHB, Peretz H, Butler R, et al: A common ancestral mutation (C128X) occurring in 11 non-Jewish families from the U.K. with factor XI deficiency. *J Thromb Haemost* 2:918, 2004.

253. Goldstein DB, Reich DE, Bradman N, et al: Age estimates of two common mutations causing factor XI deficiency: Recent genetic drift is not necessary for elevated disease incidence among Ashkenazi Jews. *Am J Hum Genet* 64:1071, 1999.

254. Bolton-Maggs PH, Patterson DA, Wensley RT, Tuddenham EG: Definition of the bleeding tendency in factor XI-deficient kindreds: A clinical and laboratory study. *Thromb Haemost* 73:194, 1995.

255. Brenner B, Laor A, Lupo H, et al: Bleeding predictors in factor-XI-deficient patients. *Blood Coagul Fibrinolysis* 8:511, 1997.

256. Salomon O, Steinberg DM, Tamarin I, et al: Plasma replacement therapy during labor is not mandatory for women with severe factor XI deficiency. *Blood Coagul Fibrinolysis* 16:37, 2005.

257. Eikenboom JC, Rosendaal FR, Briet E: Value of the patient interview: All but consensus among haemostasis experts. *Haemostasis* 22:221, 1992.

258. Peter MK, Meili EO, Von Felten A: Factor XI deficiency: Do patients with hemorrhagic diathesis also have hemostasis defects? *Schweiz Med Wochenschr* 126:999, 1996.

259. Salomon O, Steinberg DM, Dardik R, et al: Inherited factor XI deficiency confers no protection against acute myocardial infarction. *J Thromb Haemost* 1:658, 2003.

260. Brodsky JB, Burgess GE: Pulmonary embolism with factor XI deficiency. *JAMA* 534:1156, 1975.

261. Seligsohn U, Zitman D, Many A, Klibansky C: Coexistence of factor XI (plasma thromboplastin antecedent) deficiency and Gaucher's disease. *Isr J Med Sci* 12:1448, 1976.

262. Berrebi A, Malnick SD, Vorst EJ, Stein D: High incidence of factor XI deficiency in Gaucher's disease. *Am J Hematol* 40:153, 1992.

263. Billett HH, Rizvi S, Sawitsky A: Coagulation abnormalities in patients with Gaucher's disease: Effect of therapy. *Am J Hematol* 51:234, 1996.

264. Kitchens CS, Alexander JA: Partial deficiency of coagulation factor XI as a newly recognized feature of Noonan syndrome. *J Pediatr* 102:224, 1983.

265. Sharland M, Patton MA, Talbot S, et al: Coagulation-factor deficiencies and abnormal bleeding in Noonan's syndrome. *Lancet* 339:19, 1992.

266. Singer ST, Hurst D, Addiego JE Jr: Bleeding disorders in Noonan syndrome: Three case reports and review of the literature. *J Pediatr Hematol Oncol* 19:130, 1997.

267. Chediak J, Lambert E, Johnson EI, Telfer MC: Combined severe factor XI deficiency and von Willebrand's disease. *Am J Clin Pathol* 74:108, 1980.

268. Tavori S, Brenner B, Tatarsky I: The effect of combined factor XI deficiency with von Willebrand factor abnormalities on haemorrhagic diathesis. *Thromb Haemost* 63:36, 1990.

269. Lian EC, Deykin D, Harkness DR: Combined deficiencies of factor VIII (AHF) and factor XI (PTA). *Am J Hematol* 1:319, 1976.

270. Berg LP, Varon D, Martinowitz U, et al: Combined factor VII/factor VIII/factor XI deficiency may cause intra-familial clinical variability in haemophilia A among Ashkenazi Jews. *Blood Coagul Fibrinolysis* 5:59, 1994.

271. Berube C, Ofosu FA, Kelton JG, Blajchman MA: A novel congenital haemostatic defect: Combined factor VII and factor XI deficiency. *Blood Coagul Fibrinolysis* 3:357, 1992.

272. Salomon O, Zivelin A, Livnat T, et al: Prevalence, causes, and characterization of factor XI inhibitors in patients with inherited factor XI deficiency. *Blood* 101:4783, 2003.

273. Stern DM, Nossel HL, Owen J: Acquired antibody to factor XI in a patient with congenital factor XI deficiency. *J Clin Invest* 69:1270, 1982.

274. Seligsohn U, Modan M: Definition of the population at risk of bleeding due to factor XI deficiency in Ashkenazic Jews and the value of activated partial thromboplastin time in its detection. *Isr J Med Sci* 17:413, 1981.

275. Bolton-Maggs PHB, Wensley RT, Kernoff PBA, et al: Production and therapeutic use of a factor XI concentrate from human plasma. *Thromb Haemost* 67:314, 1992.

276. Inbal A, Epstein O, Blickstein D, et al: Evaluation of solvent/detergent treated plasma in the management of patients with hereditary and acquired coagulation disorders. *Blood Coagul Fibrinolysis* 4:599, 1993.

277. Seligsohn U: Factor XI deficiency. *Thromb Haemost* 70:68, 1993.

278. De Raucourt MH, Aurousseau MH, Denninger MH, et al: Use of a factor XI concentrate in three severe factor XI-deficient patients. *Blood Coagul Fibrinolysis* 6:486, 1995.

279. Aledort LM, Forster A, Maksoud J, Isola L: BPL factor XI concentrate: Clinical experience in the U.S.A. *Haemophilia* 3:59, 1997.

280. Mannucci PM, Bauer KA, Santagostino E, et al: Activation of the coagulation cascade after infusion of a factor XI concentrate in congenitally deficient patients. *Blood* 84:1314, 1994.

281. Richards EM, Makris MM, Cooper P, Preston FE: In vivo coagulation activation following infusion of highly purified factor XI concentrate. *Br J Haematol* 96:293, 1997.

282. Bolton-Maggs PHB, Colvin BT, Satchi G, et al: Thrombogenic potential of factor XI concentrate. *Lancet* 344:748, 1994.

283. Briggs N, Harman C, Dash CH: A decade of experience with factor XI concentrate. *Haemophilia* 2:14, 1996.

284. Rakocz M, Mazar A, Varon D, et al: Dental extractions in patients with bleeding disorders. *Oral Surg Oral Med Oral Pathol* 75:280, 1993.

285. Connelly NR, Brull SJ: Anesthetic management of a patient with factor XI deficiency and factor XI inhibitor undergoing a cesarean section. *Anesth Analg* 76:1365, 1993.

286. Hedner U: Factor VIIa in the treatment of haemophilia. *Blood Coagul Fibrinolysis* 1:307, 1990.

287. Duckert F, Jung E, Sherling DH: An undescribed congenital haemorrhagic diathesis probably due to fibrin stabilizing factor deficiency. *Thromb Diath Haemorrh* 5:179, 1960.

288. Muszbek L, Adany R, Mikkola H: Novel aspects of blood coagulation factor XIII: I. Structure, distribution, activation, and function. *Crit Rev Clin Lab Sci* 33:357, 1996.

289. Chung SI, Lewis MS, Folk JE: Relationships of the catalytic properties of human plasma and platelet transglutaminases (activated blood coagulation factor XIII) to their subunit structures. *J Biol Chem* 249:940, 1974.

290. Gentile V, Saydak M, Chiocca EA, et al: Isolation and characterization of cDNA clones to mouse macrophage and human endothelial cell tissue transglutaminases. *J Biol Chem* 266:478, 1991.

291. Phillips MA, Stewart BE, Qin Q, et al: Primary structure of keratinocyte transglutaminase. *Proc Natl Acad Sci U S A* 87:9333, 1990.

292. Sung LA, Chien S, Chang LS, et al: Molecular cloning of human protein 4.2: A major component of the erythrocyte membrane. *Proc Natl Acad Sci U S A* 87:955, 1990.

293. Lorand L, Graham RM: Transglutaminases: Crosslinking enzymes with pleiotropic functions. *Nat Rev Mol Cell Biol* 4:140, 2003.

294. Yee VC, Pedersen LC, Le Trong I, et al: Three-dimensional structure of a transglutaminase: Human blood coagulation factor XIII. *Proc Natl Acad Sci U S A* 91:7296, 1994.

295. Lorand L, Gray AJ, Brown K, Credo RB, et al: Dissociation of the subunit structure of fibrin stabilizing factor during activation of the zymogen. *Biochem Biophys Commun* 56:914, 1974.

296. Mary A, Achyuthan KE, Greenberg CS: B-Chains prevent the proteolytic inactivation of the a-chains of plasma factor XIII. *Biochem Biophys Acta* 966:328, 1988.

297. Bottenus RE, Ichinose A, Davie EW: Nucleotide sequence of the gene for the b subunit of human factor XIII. *Biochemistry* 29:11195, 1990.

298. Board PG, Webb GC, McKee J, Ichinose A: Localization of the coagulation factor XIII A subunit gene (F13A) to chromosome bands 6p24-p25. *Cytogenet Cell Genet* 48:25, 1988.

299. Weisberg LJ, Shiu DT, Greenberg CS, et al: Localization of the gene for coagulation factor XIII a-chain to chromosome 6 and identification of sites of synthesis. *J Clin Invest* 79:649, 1987.

300. Ichinose A, Davie EW: Characterization of the gene for the a subunit of human factor XIII (plasma transglutaminase), a blood coagulation factor. *Proc Natl Acad Sci U S A* 85:5829, 1988.

301. Webb GC, Coggan M, Ichinose A, Board PG: Localization of the coagulation factor XIII B subunit gene (F13B) to chromosome bands 1q31-32.1 and restriction fragment length polymorphism at the locus. *Hum Genet* 81:157, 1989.

302. Adany R, Kiss A, Muszbek L: Factor XIII: A marker of mono- and megakaryocytopoiesis. *Br J Haematol* 67:167, 1987.

303. Inbal A, Muszbek L, Lubetsky A et al: Platelets but not monocytes contribute to the plasma levels of factor XIII subunit A in patients undergoing autologous peripheral blood stem cell transplantation. *Blood Coagul Fibrinolysis* 15:249, 2004.

304. Wolpl A, Lattke H, Board PG, et al: Coagulation factor XIII A and B subunits in bone marrow and liver transplantation. *Transplantation* 43:151, 1987.

305. Nagy JA, Kradin RL, McDonagh J: Biosynthesis of factor XIII A and B subunits. *Adv Exp Med Biol* 231:29, 1988.

306. Takagi T, Doolittle RF: Amino acid sequence studies on factor XIII and the peptide released during its activation by thrombin. *Biochemistry* 13:750, 1974.

307. Ariens RA, Lai TS, Weisel JW, et al: Role of factor XIII in fibrin clot formation and effects of genetic polymorphisms. *Blood* 100:743, 2002.

308. Varadi A, Scheraga HA: Localization of segments essential for polymerization and for calcium binding in the gamma-chain of human fibrinogen. *Biochemistry* 25:519, 1986.

309. Sakata Y, Aoki N: Cross-linking of alpha 2-plasmin inhibitor to fibrin by fibrin-stabilizing factor. *J Clin Invest* 65:290, 1980.

310. Mosher DF, Schad PE, Vann JM: Cross-linking of collagen and fibronectin by factor XIIIa: Localization of participating glutaminyl residues to a tryptic fragment of fibronectin. *J Biol Chem* 255:1181, 1980.

311. Peyvandi F, Tagliabue L, Menegatti M, et al: Phenotype-genotype characterization of 10 families with severe A subunit factor XIII deficiency. *Hum Mutat* 23:98, 2004.

312. Mikkola H, Syrjala M, Rasi V, et al: Deficiency in the A-subunit of coagulation factor XIII: Two novel point mutations demonstrate different effects on transcript level. *Blood* 84:517, 1994.

313. Inbal A, Yee VC, Kornbrot N, et al: Factor XIII deficiency due to a Leu660Pro mutation in the factor XIII subunit-a gene in three unrelated Palestinian Arab families. *Thromb Haemost* 77:1062, 1997.

314. Aslam S, Standen GR, Khurshid M, Bilwani F: Molecular analysis of six factor XIII-A-deficient families in Southern Pakistan. *Br J Haematol* 109:463, 2000.

315. Cargill M, Altshuler D, Ireland J, et al: Characterization of single-nucleotide polymorphisms in coding regions of human genes. *Nat Genet* 22:231, 1999.

316. Ichinose A: Physiopathology and regulation of factor XIII. *Thromb Haemost* 86:57, 2001.

317. Lauer P, Metzner HJ, Zettlmeissl G, et al: Targeted inactivation of the mouse locus encoding coagulation factor XIII-A: Hemostatic abnormalities in mutant mice and characterization of the coagulation deficit. *Thromb Haemost* 88:967, 2002.

318. Dardik R, Solomon A, Loscalzo J, et al: Novel proangiogenic effect of factor XIII associated with suppression of thrombospondin 1 expression. *Arterioscler Thromb Vasc Biol* 23:1472, 2003.

319. Koseki-Kuno S, Yamakawa M, Dickneite G, Ichinose A: Factor XIII A subunit-deficient mice developed severe uterine bleeding events and subsequent spontaneous miscarriages. *Blood* 102:4410, 2003.

320. Asahina T, Kobayashi T, Okada Y, et al: Maternal blood coagulation factor XIII is associated with the development of cytotrophoblastic shell. *Placenta* 21:388, 2000.

321. Inbal A, Muszbek L: Coagulation factor deficiencies and pregnancy loss. *Semin Thromb Hemost* 29:171, 2003.

322. Fickenscher K, Aab A, Stuber W: A photometric assay for blood coagulation factor XIII. *Thromb Haemost* 65:535, 1991.

323. Berliner S, Lusky A, Zivelinet al: Hereditary factor XIII deficiency: Report of four families and definition of the carrier state. *Br J Haematol* 56:495, 1984.

324. Katona E, Haramura G, Karpati L, et al: A simple, quick one-step ELISA assay for the determination of complex plasma factor XIII (A2B2). *Thromb Haemost* 83:268, 2000.

325. Gootenberg JE: Factor concentrates for the treatment of factor XIII deficiency. *Curr Opin Hematol* 5:372, 1998.

326. Anwar R, Miloszewski KJ: Factor XIII deficiency. *Br J Haematol* 107:468, 1999.

HEREDITARY FIBRINOGEN ABNORMALITIES

MICHAEL W. MOSESSON

Hereditary fibrinogen abnormalities comprise two classes of plasma fibrinogen defects: (1) type I, afibrinogenemia or hypofibrinogenemia (antithrombin I deficiency), which has absent or low plasma fibrinogen antigen levels, and (2) type II, dysfibrinogenemia or hypodysfibrinogenemia, which shows normal or reduced antigen levels associated with disproportionately low functional activity. In afibrinogenemia, most mutations of the FGA, FGB, or FGG fibrinogen genes involve null or missense mutations, usually causing truncations of the affected chain and failure of intracellular fibrinogen assembly and/or secretion. In certain hypofibrinogenemic kindreds, assembled fibrinogen molecules are produced and retained in the rough endoplasmic reticulum of hepatocytes, causing endoplasmic reticulum storage disease. Type I deficiencies are associated with mild to severe bleeding. Thromboembolism also occurs, sometimes spontaneously, but more often in association with infusions of fibrinogen-rich fractions. These thrombophilic manifestations result from the absence or severe reduction of plasma fibrinogen levels, eliminating or reducing nonsubstrate thrombin binding to fibrin (antithrombin I).

Hereditary dysfibrinogenemias are characterized by biosynthesis of a structurally abnormal fibrinogen molecule that exhibits reduced functional properties in relation to the level of fibrinogen antigen. Type II disorders are commonly associated with bleeding, thrombophilia, or both bleeding and thrombophilia, or they do not manifest any symptoms. Hypodysfibrinogenemia is a subcategory of this disorder. Occasional patients develop avascular osteonecrosis, a thrombophilic disorder. Certain mutations involving fibrinogen αC domain are associated with renal amyloidosis, in which an abnormal fragment from the fibrinogen αC domain is deposited in the kidneys. The basis for thrombophilia in type II fibrinogen abnormalities often is uncertain but may involve defective calcium binding, other thrombophilic risk factors, impaired tissue-type plasminogen activator-mediated fibrinolysis, resistance to fibrinolysis, defective fibrin polymerization, defective thrombin binding, or antithrombin I deficiency (hypodysfibrinogenemia).

INTRODUCTION

This chapter provides information on the molecular basis for abnormal fibrinogen and fibrin function in most of the hereditary conditions described. More detailed and thoroughly annotated reviews have been published.[1-5] A compilation of the published literature on inherited fibrinogen abnormalities up to 1994 is available.[6] A registry for new hereditary fibrinogen abnormalities[7] can be accessed at *http://www.geht.org/databaseang/fibrinogen/*.

In addition to being the precursor molecule for the insoluble fibrin clot, fibrinogen in circulation participates in numerous other biologic processes. Fibrinogen binds plasminogen, α_2-antiplasmin, fibronectin, and factor XIII. It binds to platelets and supports platelet aggregation. After fibrinogen is converted to fibrin by thrombin, it provides nonsubstrate binding sites for thrombin ("antithrombin I") and binds to vascular endothelial and other cells, plasma or tissue matrix components such as fibronectin and glycosaminoglycans, and peptide growth factors. Fibrin provides a template for assembly and activation of the fibrinolytic system and is the major substrate for the enzyme plasmin (see Chap. 127). Both fibrinogen and fibrin also serve as substrates for plasma factor XIII and other cellular transglutaminases that catalyze covalent cross-linking.

STRUCTURE AND SYNTHESIS

Fibrinogen is a 340-kDa plasma protein that circulates at a concentration of 1.5 to 3.5 mg/ml ($\sim$4–10 μM). Each fibrinogen molecule is approximately 45 nm in length. The core structure consists of two outer D domains and a central E domain connected through coiled-coil regions (Figure 117-1).[1,8] The molecule exhibits a twofold axis of symmetry perpendicular to the long axis,[9-11] consisting of two sets of three polypeptide chains (Aα, Bβ, γ) that are joined in their amino-terminal regions by disulfide bridges to form the E domain.[8,12-14] Most Aα chains are composed of 610 residues, Bβ chains 461 residues, and γA, the predominant form of the γ chain, 411 residues.[8] A minor γ-chain variant termed γ', which amounts to approximately 8 percent of the γ-chain population,[15] is composed of 427 residues having a unique C-terminal amino acid sequence.[16] A subclass of human fibrinogen molecules termed *fibrinogen-420* contains homodimeric Aα isoforms termed α_E that contain a unique globular 236-residue C-terminal extension beyond Aα 610 termed α_EC, which is coded for by exon VI of the FGA gene.[17,18] The α_EC structure contains a recognition site for leukocyte β_2-integrins[19] that is functionally similar to the $\alpha_M\beta_2$ (Mac-1) receptor site in the γ subdomain of the fibrinogen D domain.[20]

Fibrinogen is synthesized by hepatocytes.[21,22] Three separate fibrinogen genes code for γ (FGG), Aα (FGA), and Bβ (FGB) chains. These genes are clustered in a region of 50 kb on human chromosome 4q28-31.[23-26] Synthesis of fibrinogen at the transcriptional level is controlled by regulatory sequences in the immediate proximity of each gene, thus assuring coordinated synthesis of the chains in response to stimuli such as acute or chronic inflammation and injury, or pregnancy.[27-29] Subsequent to hepatic assembly of the constituent polypeptide chains and the addition of carbohydrate side chains, the mature molecule is secreted into the circulation, where it exhibits a half-life of approximately 4 days and a fractional catabolic rate of 25 percent per day.[30,31] In addition to plasma fibrinogen, blood contains an internalized intracellular fibrinogen pool that is stored within platelet α-granules. Both megakaryocytes and platelets are capable of internalizing plasma fibrinogen via the fibrinogen glycoprotein IIb/IIIa (GpIIb-IIIa; $\alpha_{IIb}\beta_3$) receptor.[32-34] This process is specifically dependent upon GpIIb-IIIa binding to the C-terminal platelet recognition sequence that is present on γA chains but is conspicuously absent from γ' chains. Thus, internalized platelet fibrinogen molecules contain only γ_A chains.[33-37] Interestingly, although the mutant γA chains of fibrinogen Paris I contain a normal C-terminal platelet recognition sequence, Paris I γA chains are not taken up by platelets.[38]

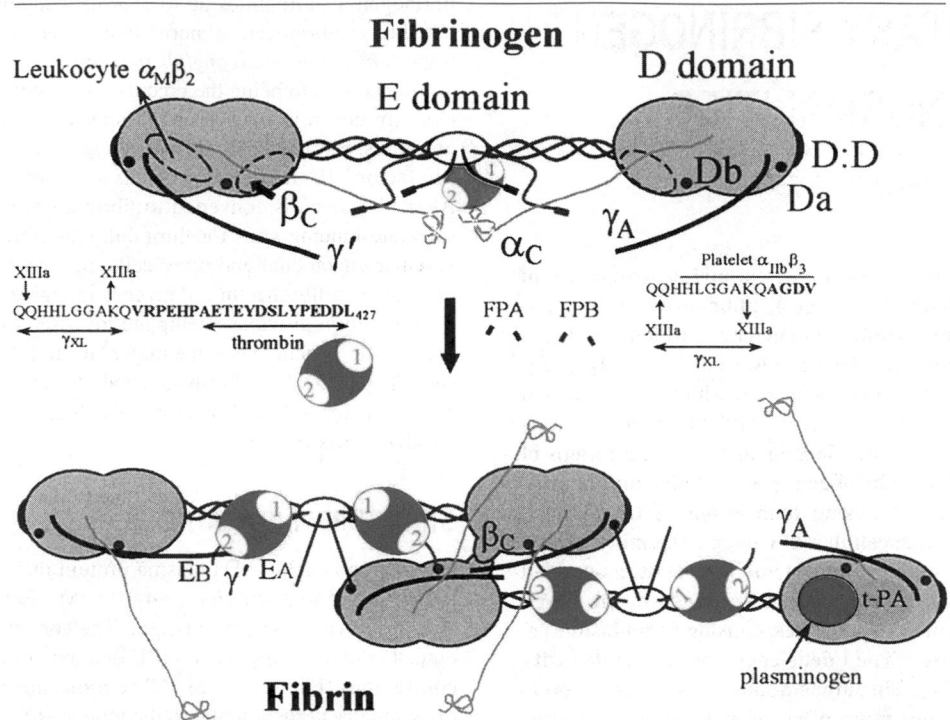

FIGURE 117-1   Structures of fibrinogen and fibrin, their major association sites, and their interactions with thrombin. (Thrombin exosites are numbered in the *white ovals.*) The C-terminal sequences of the γ' and γ_A chains are shown, including the factor XIII cross-linking sites. Following E_B:Db interactions, rearrangements in the β_C region of the D domain permit lateral β_C:β_C contacts.[68] The locations of the tissue-type plasminogen activator and plasminogen binding sites in the fibrin D domain are indicated. The cryptic binding site in fibrinogen for $\alpha_M\beta_2$ is indicated. (Adapted from MW Mosesson.[3])

FIBRINOGEN CONVERSION TO FIBRIN AND NETWORK ASSEMBLY

Conversion of fibrinogen to a fibrin clot occurs in three distinct phases: (1) enzymatic cleavage by thrombin to produce fibrin monomeric units; (2) self-assembly of fibrin units to form an organized polymeric structure; and (3) covalent cross-linking of fibrin by factor XIII or XIIIa. In the first phase of conversion to fibrin, cleavage of fibrinogen at Aα16R/17G* and later Bβ14R/15G cleavage results in release of fibrinopeptides A (FPA) and B (FPB), respectively,[39–41] concomitant with exposure of E_A and E_B polymerization sites. One portion of the E_A site is located at the amino-terminal end of the fibrin α chain composing the amino-terminal Aα17-20 GPRV sequence.[42,43] Another portion of this site is in the amino-terminal region of the fibrinogen Bβ chain, specifically in the β15-42 sequence.[44–48] The E_A site in fibrin interacts with the constitutive complementary association site Da in the D domain of another molecule (the so-called *D:E interaction*) to initiate the fibrin assembly process.[41,49–51] The Da site is encompassed by γ337-379 of the D-domain γ-chain module.[52,53]

Da:E_A associations (D:E) result in formation of double-stranded fibrils in which fibrin molecules become aligned in an end-to-middle, staggered overlapping arrangement (Figure 117-2).[54–57] Fibrils subsequently undergo branching by lateral fibril associations ("bilateral branch junctions") in which two fibrils converge to form a four-stranded "bilateral" fibril junction. Progressive lateral associations among fibrils result in larger fibril bundles, now called *fibers*. A second

type of junction called *equilateral branching* is formed by three fibrils converging to form a three-member junction.[58] Together these two types of branch junctions provide scaffolding for the clot network, the ultimate structure of which is governed by several variables, including salt concentration, pH, and thrombin concentration.[59–61]

FPB (Bβ1-14) release occurs more slowly than FPA release[39–41] and exposes an independent polymerization site, E_B,[62] beginning with β15-18.[42,43] GHRP interacts with a Db site in the β-chain module of the D domain encompassed by β397-432.[63,64] FPB cleavage is accelerated by fibrin polymerization, whereas FPA cleavage is independent of fibrin polymerization.[65–67] E_B:Db interaction is not required for lateral fibril associations, but it contributes to lateral association by inducing rearrangements in the β_C region that permit β_C:β_C contacts to occur.[68]

Another domain termed αC originates at Aα_{220} near where the Aα chain emerges from the D domain and terminates at Aα_{610}.[69] Fibrin clots from plasma fibrinogen molecules lacking more than 100 C-terminal αC domain residues (e.g., plasma fraction I-9)[70,71] display prolonged thrombin times, develop reduced turbidity, and produce thinner fibers,[72–74] indicating αC participates in lateral fibril associations.[75] In addition, αC domains, which tend to be noncovalently tethered in the vicinity of the E domain,[10] become dissociated as a result of FPB cleavage.[76,77] This process evidently makes αC domains available for noncovalent interaction with other such domains, thereby promoting lateral fibril associations and fibrin network assembly. A considerable number of dysfibrinogenemias are associated with irregularities in this region of the molecule.

In addition to the interactive sites between D and E domains, other self-association sites in D domains contribute to fibrin assembly. These sites are termed *D:D* and γ_{XL}, respectively.[78–80] Intermolecular inter-

---

*A one-letter abbreviation for amino acids is used in this chapter. A, alanine; C, cysteine; D, aspartic acid; E, glutamic acid; F, phenylalanine; G, glycine; H, histidine; I, isoleucine; K, lysine; L, leucine; M, methionine; N, asparagine; P, proline; Q, glutamine; R, arginine; S, serine; T, threonine; V, valine; W, tryptophan; Y, tryosine.

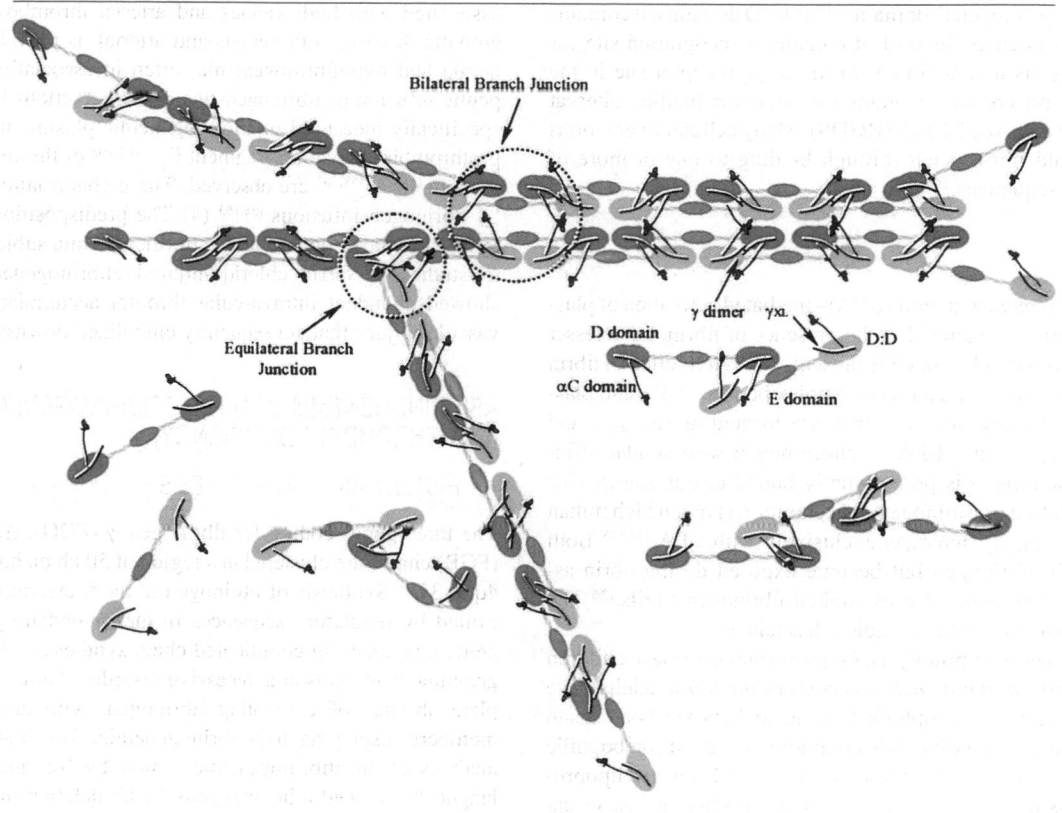

FIGURE 117-2   Schematic diagram of fibrin assembly and γ chain cross-linking. Fibrin molecules are represented in different color schemes for ease of recognition. The two types of branch junctions are indicated, and the preferred positioning of cross-linked γ chains "transversely" between fibril strands is shown. The αC domains are depicted extending between fibrils and sometimes interacting with other αC domains. (Adapted from MW Mosesson.[2])

actions between D:D sites, which are situated at the distal ends of D domains in fibrin, promote end-to-end alignment of assembling fibrin units.[78,79] X-ray crystal structures show that the interface for the D:D sites lies between γ275R and γ300S,[53] but other nearby γ chain residues contribute to or perturb this site, as evidenced by impaired D:D interactions in dysfibrinogenemic molecules such as fibrinogen Kurashiki I (γ268G$\rightarrow$E).[81]

The γ_{XL} site is situated in the C-terminal region of each γ chain. It contains a factor XIIIa cross-linking site that lies between γ398/399Q and γ406K. In the major γ-chain subtype γ_A, the γ_{XL} site overlaps the platelet fibrinogen receptor $\alpha_{IIb}\beta_3$ binding site between γ_A400 and 411.[82,83] In the γ'-chain variant, the platelet binding site is absent. These chains instead contain an acidic C-terminal sequence beginning at γ'408 and ending at γ'427.[16] Because the cross-linking site is retained, γ' chains undergo cross-linking at the same rate as γ_A chains,[84] therefore implying that the γ398 to γ406 sequence comprises the cross-linking site and plays a significant but incompletely defined role in promoting self-association at the γ_{XL} site. Although γ' chains do not bind to platelets, their unique sequence binds plasma factor XIII through the B subunits, thereby serving as a carrier protein for factor XIII in plasma[85] and acting to sharply down-regulate XIII-mediated cross-linking activity in blood.[86] The γ' chains also bind to thrombin with relatively high affinity.[87]

CROSS-LINKING BY FACTOR XIII

In the presence of factor XIIIa, fibrin undergoes intermolecular covalent cross-linking by forming ε-(γ-glutamyl) lysine isopeptide bonds.[88,89] Cross-linking of γ chains occurs first with formation of γ dimers,[90] which occur as reciprocal bridges between lysine at position

406 of one γ chain and glutamine at position 398 or 399 of another chain (see Figure 117-2).[91–93] The resulting γ-chain cross-linked clot becomes more rigid and resistant to deformation and exhibits almost perfect elasticity up to a maximum stretch of 1.8-fold.[94-96] Cross-linked γ chains are situated "transversely" between the strands of each fibril, and in this position they account for the mechanical properties of cross-linked fibrin.[4,5] Slower cross-linking among α chains creates α-chain oligomers and α-polymers.[97] Cross-linking between α chains and γ chains also occurs.[59,98] Other plasma proteins, notably α_2-plasmin inhibitor and fibronectin, become cross-linked to α chains,[99–103] and this process may be mediated by nonthrombin-activated factor XIII (plasma protransglutaminase).[86]

CELLULAR AND OTHER BINDING SITES ON FIBRIN(OGEN)

In addition to the role played by GHRP in mediating fibrin assembly, the β15-42 sequence binds heparin[104,105] and through this sequence promotes endothelial cell binding[105,106] via the endothelial cell receptor VE-cadherin.[107] Exposure of the β15-42 sequence also promotes platelet spreading,[108] fibroblast proliferation,[109] endothelial cell spreading, proliferation and capillary tube formation,[107,109,110] and release of von Willebrand factor.[111,112]

A high-affinity monocyte and neutrophil integrin binding site ($\alpha_M\beta_2$, Mac-1) is located in the fibrinogen D domain at a site corresponding to the confluence of γ190-202 and γ377-395, which form two antiparallel β strands.[20,113] In addition, a minor subclass of human fibrinogen molecules ("fibrinogen-420"), amounting to 1 to 3 percent of the fibrinogen in plasma, contain a globular structure termed α_E, which is appended to Aα chains immediately following the C-terminal αC domains.[17] Its structure is largely superimposable on the γ_C and

β_C constituents in fibrinogen D domains. Unlike D domains, it contains no polymerization pockets; instead, it contains a recognition site for leucocyte β_2 integrins that is similar to the $\alpha_M\beta_2$ receptor site in the D domain.[19] Fibrinogen also contains two integrin binding sites at Aα95-98 (RGDF) and Aα572-575 (RGDS). Many cellular interactions with fibrinogen and fibrin occur through binding to one or more of these recognition sequences.[1]

FIBRINOLYSIS

Tissue-type plasminogen activator (t-PA)–mediated activation of plasminogen is markedly accelerated in the presence of fibrin, but a lesser effect is seen when only fibrinogen is present.[114,115] Activation in fibrin occurs through formation of a ternary complex between t-PA and plasminogen.[114] Two binding sites in fibrin are located at A$\alpha_{148-160}$ and $\gamma_{312-324}$.[116–118] A$\alpha_{148-160}$ binds t-PA or plasminogen with similar affinity,[119–121] but plasminogen is preferentially bound at this site *in vivo* because the circulating plasminogen concentration is much higher than that of t-PA.[122,123] $\gamma_{312-324}$ interacts exclusively with t-PA.[124,125] Both sites are cryptic in fibrinogen but become exposed during fibrin assembly or during formation of cross-linked fibrinogen fibrils.[126] The exposure is reversible after the complex dissociates.[122]

As a related aspect of fibrinolysis, *Legg-Perthes disease* in children and the counterpart *idiopathic osteonecrosis of the hip* in adults have been associated with thrombophilia leading to hypoxic bone death *inter alia*.[127–135] Affected individuals commonly have a thrombophilic clinical profile, often exhibiting hypofibrinolysis and elevated lipoprotein Lp(a) or plasminogen-activator inhibitor (PAI)-1 levels. Occasionally these subjects are homozygotic for the factor V Leiden defect, but more commonly they are heterozygotic for the factor V Leiden defect, protein C deficiency, or protein S deficiency. Avascular osteonecrosis has been reported in adults with hypodysfibrinogenemia (fibrinogen Keokuk[136]) and dysfibrinogenemia (fibrinogen Cedar Rapids[103]).

THROMBIN BINDING TO FIBRINOGEN AND FIBRIN (ANTITHROMBIN I)

Thrombin binding to its substrate fibrinogen is mediated through a fibrinogen recognition site in thrombin, termed *exosite 1*.[137–139] The binding site for FPA cleavage is contained within residues 1 to 51 of the N-terminal Aα chain, whereas the binding site for FPB cleavage is at least partly in the N-terminal Bβ chain.[65,87,140,141]

The nonsubstrate binding potential of fibrin for thrombin is referred to as *antithrombin I*[3] and was first identified by Seegers and colleagues[142] more than 60 years ago. Two classes of nonsubstrate thrombin binding sites are present in fibrin. "Low-affinity" binding represents a residual aspect of fibrinogen substrate recognition in the fibrin E domain, whereas "high-affinity" binding is associated with the presence of a variant γ chain termed γ'.[87] Two thrombin "exosite 1" binding sites are present in each fibrin E domain, and the site includes Aα27-50,[143,144] Bβ 68A, Bβ69D, and other residues, as detailed in the x-ray structure of cocrystallized thrombin and fibrin fragment E.[141] In contrast, γ' chains bind mainly to thrombin exosite 2[145,146] and mainly account for the high-affinity thrombin binding component in fibrin. Simultaneous low-affinity site binding to thrombin "exosite 1" plus γ' chain binding to "exosite 2" contribute to the net activity of the high-affinity component.[146,147]

The concept that antithrombin I (fibrin) is a physiologically important regulator of thrombin generation in clotting blood is based upon a considerable number of observations and reports. (1) Fibrin from certain dysfibrinogens, notably fibrinogen New York I[148] and Naples I,[147,149,150] exhibit reduced thrombin binding capacity and are

associated with both venous and arterial thrombosis. (2) Thromboembolic disease, both venous and arterial, is prevalent in afibrinogenemia and hypofibrinogenemia, often in association with the therapeutic infusion of fibrinogen-rich plasma fractions.[136,151–161] (3) When specifically measured in afibrinogenemic plasma, increased levels of prothrombin activation fragment F_{1+2}[162,163] or thrombin–antithrombin III complexes[158,162] are observed. These abnormalities are normalized by fibrinogen infusions.[158,163] (4) The predisposition to occlusive arterial thromboembolism in an afibrinogenemia subject[158] is analogous to studies of ferric chloride-injured afibrinogenemic mice, which showed abundant intravascular thrombi accumulating at the site of vascular injury that subsequently embolized downstream.[164]

AFIBRINOGENEMIA AND HYPOFIBRINOGENEMIA (ANTITHROMBIN I DEFICIENCY)

HISTORY AND PATHOGENESIS

The three genes coding for fibrinogen γ (FGG), Aα (FGA), and Bβ (FGB) chains are clustered in a region of 50 kb on human chromosome 4q28-31.[26] Synthesis of fibrinogen at the transcriptional level is controlled by regulatory sequences in the immediate proximity of each gene, thus assuring coordinated chain synthesis.[27–29] Classic afibrinogenemia is an autosomal recessive disorder characterized by the complete absence of circulating fibrinogen, with heterozygotic family members displaying hypofibrinogenemia. The first reported genetic analysis of an afibrinogenemic family by Neerman-Arbez and colleagues[165] showed a homozygous 11-kb deletion in FGA that caused the condition. Since then, numerous other fibrinogen gene mutations have been described in FGA, FGB, and FGG that result in afibrinogenemia, and these were summarized up to 2001 by Neerman-Arbez.[166] Most are null mutations (frameshift, nonsense, or splice site)[166–171] or missense mutations,[172,173] each predicted to cause a total lack of the corresponding fibrinogen chain in the homozygous state. However, afibrinogenemia also occurs in subjects displaying compound heterozygosity of FGB[174] in which a previously described nonsense mutation in the FBG coding region[168] was combined with a missense mutation in the FGB coding region (Bβ444G→S), resulting in afibrinogenemia, thus emphasizing the importance of an intact C-terminal Bβ chain for successful fibrinogen assembly and secretion.

HYPOFIBRINOGENEMIA

Hypofibrinogenemias are featured by low antigenic concentrations (<1.5 mg/ml or <4.4 μM) of structurally normal fibrinogen or at least plasma fibrinogen containing molecules that show a normal thrombin time reactivity and polymerization potential (Table 117-1). Hypofibrinogenemia occurs in heterozygotic members of afibrinogenemic families or in certain kindreds consisting only of heterozygotic individuals. This disorder overlaps with "*hypodysfibrinogenemia*," in which structurally altered or dysfunctional fibrinogen molecules are found at reduced levels along with the normal fibrinogen that is coded for on one of the alleles.[175]

MUTATIONS CAUSING HEPATIC ENDOPLASMIC RETENTION AND HYPOFIBRINOGENEMIA

The hypofibrinogenemia caused by the fibrinogen Brescia mutation (γ284G→R) involves defective intracellular transport.[176] This γ-chain substitution causes fibrinogen retention within the rough endoplasmic reticulum and leads to chronic liver cirrhosis. Fibrinogen molecules in circulation are normal but are hypersialated. The fibrinogen Hamilton mutation (Bβ316D→Y) also may result in defective intracellular transport, although biopsy material was not available for examination.[177] Fibrinogen Aguadilla[178] is a heterozygotic γ375R→W point

TABLE 117-1 MUTATIONS CAUSING HYPOFIBRINOGENEMIA

MUTATION	NAME	INHERITANCE PATTERN	ETIOLOGY/PATHOLOGY	CLINICAL MANIFESTATIONS	REFERENCES
Bβ41Y→tag	Tottori II	Heterozygotic	Nonsense mutation/Bβ chain truncation	Mild bleeding	281
Bβ316D→Y	Hamilton	Heterozygotic	Retention within the RER?	Menorrhagia	177
Bβ255R→H + noncontributory Bβ148K→N	Merivale	Compound heterozygotic	Loss of essential contact with β414 in the D domain/protein instability	None	183
Bβ172L→Q Bβ17R→stop	None	Compound heterozygotic	Missense→activation of a cryptic acceptor splice site, plus a nonsense mutation	Moderate bleeding	184
Bβ intron 6 splice site	Avon	Heterozygotic	Bβ chain truncation	None	282
Bβ440W→stop	Mt. Eden	Heterozygotic	Bβ chain truncation	Mild epistaxis	169
γ82A→G Bβ235P→L + noncoding Aα/Bβ mutations	Dunedin	Compound heterozygotic	Aberrant helical packing in the coiled-coil region	None	181
γ82A→G γIVS-2 gt→at	Waikato	Compound heterozygotic	Aberrant helical packing in the coiled-coil region	Pregnancy-associated bleeding and miscarriage	175, 182
γ153C→R	Matsumoto IV	Heterozygotic	Missense mutation/defective assembly and secretion	None	283
γ284G→R	Brescia	Heterozygotic	Retention within the RER	Chronic liver cirrhosis	176
γ345N→D	Stuttgart	Heterozygotic	—	None	258
γ371T→I	Muncie	Heterozygotic	Retention within the RER?	Bleeding	284
γ375R→W	Aguadilla	Heterozygotic	Retention within the RER	Abnormal liver function tests	178

RER = rough endoplasmic reticulum.

mutation that causes endoplasmic reticulum storage disease (ERSD) and hypofibrinogenemia. Other types of fibrinogen mutations may cause ERSD, as four morphologically distinguishable types of fibrinogen inclusion bodies have been described in liver biopsies.[179,180]

COMPOUND HETEROZYGOSITY AND HYPOFIBRINOGENEMIA

A novel γ82A→G mutation was the cause of hypofibrinogenemia in a normal male subject who also had Bβ235P→L and two other noncoding mutations of the FGA and FGB genes.[181] Residue γ82 is located in the triple helix region that separates the E and D domains, and aberrant packing of these helices may explain the decreased concentration of fibrinogen molecules with this phenotype. Another female hypofibrinogenemic subject with the γ82A→G mutation had a history of recurrent, pregnancy-associated bleeding and miscarriage.[182] In addition, she had a gt splice sequence mutation in intron 2 of FGG (γIVS-2 gt→at). This second mutation would have resulted in premature γ-chain truncation and explains the phenotypic homogeneity of the γ82A→G mutation. In a compound heterozygous FGB point mutation (Fibrinogen Merivale), the Bβ255R→H mutation resulted in hypofibrinogenemia,[183] but a concomitant Bβ148K→N mutation (Fibrinogen Merivale II) was expressed in plasma fibrinogen without functional or clinical consequences. A female with severe hypofibrinogenemia and moderate bleeding was a compound heterozygote for two FBG mutations.[184] The first was a novel Bβ missense mutation (Bβ172L→Q) that activated a cryptic splice site in FGB exon 4, resulting in a truncated Bβ chain. Second, the subject had a previously described nonsense mutation at Bβ17 that would have led to afibrinogenemia in the homozygous condition.

CLINICAL FEATURES

It is logical to refer to congenital afibrinogenemia or hypofibrinogenemia as *congenital antithrombin I deficiency*[3] in the same context that

factor VIII deficiency is referred to as *hemophilia A*. Fibrin formation is an important regulator of thrombin generation in clotting blood; see "Thrombin Binding to Fibrinogen and Fibrin (Antithrombin I)." Thromboembolic disease, both venous and arterial, is prevalent in afibrinogenemia and in hypofibrinogenemia, often in association with therapeutic infusion of fibrinogen-rich plasma fractions.[136,151–161]

A moderate level of hypofibrinogenemia on any basis generally is not expected to be accompanied by bleeding as clinically significant as occurs in afibrinogenemia. In the γ82A→G mutation, the Bβ172L→Q mutation, and several other hypofibrinogenemias, bleeding was the predominant clinical finding, whereas the Fibrinogen Merivale subject and several other hypofibrinogenemics were without clinical symptoms. It is important to emphasize, however, that low fibrinogen levels, per se, are commonly associated with thrombophilia, both venous and arterial, often in association with therapeutic infusions containing fibrinogen.[151–154,159] Thus, the finding that hypofibrinogenemic subjects are bleeders, or even that they are asymptomatic, does not preclude superimposition of thromboembolic complications at some time based on *de facto* antithrombin I deficiency.

LABORATORY FEATURES

All measurements of plasma fibrinogen that are based upon the appearance of a fibrin clot yield abnormal results in afibrinogenemic and in most profoundly hypofibrinogenemic patients. Routine tests, such as prothrombin time, partial thromboplastin time, and thrombin time, are prolonged. These abnormalities can be corrected by the addition of normal plasma or purified fibrinogen. The clinical diagnosis is established by immunologic measurements of fibrinogen concentration, backed by genomic sequencing analyses. The platelet fibrinogen content in most cases of afibrinogenemia is negligible.[185] Related coagulation abnormalities include a prolonged bleeding time and abnormal platelet aggregation. These abnormalities can be corrected by infusion of plasma or fibrinogen concentrates.[185–187]

THERAPY, COURSE, AND PROGNOSIS

Patients with afibrinogenemia or hypofibrinogenemia may require replacement therapy with fibrinogen-rich fractions to control bleeding episodes or in preparation for surgery. Fibrinogen-rich cryoprecipitate has been used during pregnancy to prevent spontaneous abortion and to assist in carrying pregnancies to term.[188] Development of antifibrinogen antibodies has been reported.[189] More importantly, both venous and arterial thromboembolic disease are prevalent in afibrinogenemia and hypofibrinogenemia, particularly in association with therapeutic infusion of fibrinogen-rich plasma fractions.[136,151-161] Thus, infusion of fibrinogen-enriched fractions must be undertaken with an outlook for incipient thromboembolic complications. Based upon the reported experience of Schuepbach and colleagues,[161] when fibrinogen infusion is performed on an elective basis or when the indication for fibrinogen infusion is not life threatening, the recommendation is to infuse small doses of fibrinogen on a frequent basis, such as the doses reported by Cattaneo and colleagues,[187] until fibrinogen levels reach approximately 0.5 mg/ml, after which the amount of fibrinogen infused can be increased to reach the desired fibrinogen level. Although little experience in this matter has been reported, low molecular weight heparin (LMWH) can be included with the initial infusions of fibrinogen. However, treating an overt or life-threatening bleeding episode with this drug combination is a challenging situation. Schuepbach and colleagues[161] reported successfully managing a spontaneous and recurring episode of arterial thrombosis in an afibrinogenemic patient using various combinations of LMWH, unfractionated heparin, low-dose aspirin, and hirudin plus continuous fibrinogen infusions. Lepirudin (Refludan, Schering), which reportedly binds both free and clot-bound thrombin, appeared to be particularly effective in managing the problem. After a prolonged course, their patient was successfully discharged and maintained on LMWH, low-dose aspirin, and fibrinogen replacement therapy.

DYSFIBRINOGENEMIA

DEFINITION AND HISTORY

Most "dysfibrinogenemias" are caused by point mutations in the coding region of one of the three fibrinogen genes. With some exceptions, they result in impairment of some aspect of fibrinogen conversion and the fibrin assembly process (Table 117-2). Most of these dysfibrinogens are expressed in plasma at normal antigenic levels; therefore, they are recognized by the combination of a prolonged thrombin time, normal levels of fibrinogen antigen, and low functional levels of fibrinogen. More than 260 cases of congenital dysfibrinogenemia had been reported by 1994,[6] and at the time of this writing that number has grown to well over 400. Approximately 25 percent of the reported families with dysfibrinogenemia have a history of bleeding, and in approximately 20 percent a tendency toward thrombosis was observed.[6] Sometimes both bleeding and thrombophilia prevail.

The abnormality in blood most commonly but not always (e.g., Hanss and colleagues[190]) is revealed by a prolonged thrombin-mediated clotting time. With some exceptions, the described mutants carry the name of the city of origin of the family. In some dysfibrinogenemic families, an associated fibrinogen-related organ pathology, including *renal amyloidosis* or *avascular osteonecrosis*, is present (Tables 117-2 and 117-3).

ETIOLOGY, PATHOGENESIS, AND CLINICAL AND LABORATORY FEATURES

Dysfibrinogenemic abnormalities usually are reflected in one or more phases of the fibrinogen-fibrin conversion and fibrin assembly process,

including (1) impaired release of fibrinopeptides, (2) defects in fibrin polymerization, and (3) defective factor XIIIa-mediated cross-linking. Other significant abnormalities involve related aspects of fibrin(ogen) function or metabolism, such as catabolism, abnormal tissue deposition, defective assembly of the fibrinolytic system, abnormal interactions with platelets, endothelial cells, or calcium binding.

ABNORMAL FIBRINOPEPTIDE RELEASE OR A DEFECTIVE E_A OR E_B SITE

Fibrinogen Detroit was the first abnormal fibrinogen in which the specific mutation was identified ($A\alpha 19R{\rightarrow}S$).[191] This mutation is located at the fibrin E_A polymerization site (i.e., GPRV) and results in impaired fibrin polymerization and a bleeding tendency. Amino acid substitutions at this site in other kindreds are associated with bleeding in some cohorts (Munich I, $A\alpha 19R{\rightarrow}N$; Mannheim I, $A\alpha 19R{\rightarrow}G$) and with thrombosis in other cohorts (Aarhus, $R19R{\rightarrow}G$; Kumamoto, $A\alpha 19R{\rightarrow}G$[192]). In many cases the mechanism for thrombophilia remains unclear, but coexisting risk factors may contribute to the clinical manifestations. Furthermore, the inability of a mutant fibrin to effectively bind and sequester thrombin (antithrombin I deficiency) may play a role in such a clinical presentation, an aspect that has not been evaluated in most situations. $A\alpha 18P{\rightarrow}L$ (Kyoto II)[193] is associated with a bleeding tendency because of a defective E_A polymerization site. Fibrinogen Nijmegen ($B\beta 44R{\rightarrow}C$)[194] exhibits abnormal polymerization (consistent with an abnormal E_A polymerization site) plus abnormal t-PA–induced plasminogen activation and binding[195] but does not exhibit impaired fibrinopeptide release like fibrinogen Naples I ($B\beta 68A{\rightarrow}T$).[147,149,150,196] Bleeding that occurs under conditions involving defective fibrinopeptide release or production of a defective E_A polymerization site likely is related to the reduced polymerization potential of the mutant fibrins that are produced, with resulting defective clot formation.

Dysfibrinogenemias with a structural alteration in the $A\alpha 7$ to 12 segment of the FPA sequence (Lille, Mitaka II, Rouen I) exhibit defective thrombin–substrate binding and impaired FPA release. Fibrinogen Milano XII, a compound heterozygotic defect, shows delayed release of FPA and FPB that is related to the $A\alpha 16R{\rightarrow}C$ mutation and is asymptomatic. Only Mitaka II displayed a bleeding tendency. Delayed FPA release also is associated with dysfibrinogens manifesting a structural defect in the N-terminal region of the $B\beta$ chain, including fibrinogen New York I ($B\beta 9$-72 deletion),[44] fibrinogen Naples I ($B\beta 68A{\rightarrow}T$),[147,149,150,196] and dysfibrinogenemias involving substitutions at the FPB cleavage site $B\beta 14R{\rightarrow}C$ or $B\beta G15C$ (Ise,[6] Fukuoka II[197]).

Thrombin cleaves each $A\alpha$ chain at 16R/17G to release FPA. The most common mutation is located at $A\alpha 16$, with Arg replacement leading to delayed ($R{\rightarrow}H$) or absent ($R{\rightarrow}C$) FPA release. Most subjects, especially those who are heterozygous, have no bleeding tendencies. Some patients with a bleeding tendency are homozygous for the defect (Metz,[198] Giessen I,[199] Bicêtre I[6]) or have other demonstrable abnormalities, such as an abnormal von Willebrand factor[200] or impaired cross-linking.[201] $A\alpha 17G{\rightarrow}V$ in Bremen I[202] results in delayed FPA release and a modest impairment of fibrin monomer polymerization, indicating a defect also is present at the E_A polymerization site resulting from change of GPRV to VPRV. This defect is associated with a bleeding tendency and delayed wound healing.

FPB release results in exposure of the E_B polymerization site,[62,203] but this does not occur in mutant $B\beta$ chains with Cys substitutions at the FPB cleavage site $B\beta 14R{\rightarrow}C$ (see Table 117-2) and in fibrinogen New York I, which exhibits deletion of $B\beta 9$-72, corresponding to exon 2 of the $B\beta$ chain gene.[44] Impaired FPB release also occurs in dysfibrinogenemias having a mutation involving FPB cleavage, including $B\beta 15G{\rightarrow}C$ (fibrinogens Ise,[6] Fukuoka II,[197] Kosai, and Ogasa[204]), and

TABLE 117-2 MUTATIONS RESULTING IN DYSFIBRINOGENEMIA

MUTATION	NAME	INHERITANCE PATTERN	ETIOLOGY/PATHOLOGY	CLINICAL MANIFESTATIONS	REFERENCES
Aα9L→P	Magdeburg I	Heterozygotic	Delayed FPA release	None	285
Aα11E→G	Mitaka II	Heterozygotic	Delayed FPA release	Bleeding	6
Aα16R→H	Bicêtre I, Giessen I, etc. (>30)	Heterozygotic	Delayed FPA release	Bleeding (variable)	6, 199, 200, 201
Aα16R→C	Metz I, Zurich I, etc. (>15)	Heterozygotic	Delayed FPA release	Bleeding (variable)	6, 198
Aα16R→C-albumin γ165G→R	Milano XII	Compound heterozygotic	Delayed FPA and FPB release/modified plasmin digestion of fragment D because of γ165G→R	None	286
AαG 17→V	Bremen I	Heterozygotic	Delayed FPA release	Bleeding	202
Aα18P→L	Kyoto II	Heterozygotic	Abnormal polymerization	Bleeding	193
Aα19R→S	Detroit	Heterozygotic	Abnormal polymerization	Bleeding	6, 191
Aα19R→N	Munich I	Heterozygotic	Abnormal polymerization	Bleeding	6
Aα19R→G	Mannheim I	Heterozygotic	Abnormal polymerization	Bleeding	6
Aα19R→G	Aarhus I, Kumamoto	Heterozygotic	?	Thrombophilia	6, 192
Aα141R→S N-glycosylation Aα139	Lima	Heterozygotic	Abnormal polymerization normalized by desialation	None	247
Aα272 in frame insert	Champagne au Mont d'Or	Heterozygotic	39-residue duplication and insert/normal thrombin time and fibrinogen level	Thrombophilia	190
Aα434S→N-glycosylated	Caracas II	Heterozygotic	Impaired fibrin gelation with thinner fibers	None	245, 246
Aα451I+t(frameshift) →WSstop	Milano III	Homozygotic	Disulfide-linked albumin/severe fibrin polymerization defect	Thrombophilia	235, 236
Aα494del/ frameshift→ Aα517stop	Perth	Heterozygotic	23 new residues/thinner clot fibers	Menorrhagia, easy bruising	244
A499del/frameshift→ Aα518Cstop-albumin	San Giovanni Rotundo	Heterozygotic	Defective polymerization	None	287
Aα522del/ frameshift →548stop	None	Heterozygotic	Renal deposit of a 49-residue peptide beginning Aα499-421	Renal amyloidosis	255
Aα524del/frameshift/ 547 stop	None	Heterozygotic	Renal deposit of an Aα-chain fragment	Renal amyloidosis	254
Aα526E→V	None	Heterozygotic	Renal deposit of an Aα-chain fragment	Renal amyloidosis	252, 253
Aα554R→L	None	Heterozygotic	Renal deposition of Aα 499 through 580	Renal amyloidosis	250, 251
Aα554R→C-albumin	Dusart	Heterozygotic	Abnormal clot structure and fibrinolysis, accelerated fibrinogen cross-linking, defective plasminogen binding	Thrombophilia	237–242
Bβ14R→C-albumin	Ijmuiden	Heterozygotic	Large fibrinogen complexes; disulfide-linked albumin	Thrombophilia	194
Bβ15G→C	Ise, Fukuoka II	Heterozygotic	Defective lateral association	None	6, 197
Bβ15G→C-albumin	Kosai	Heterozygotic	Defective FPB release	Arteriosclerosis obliterans	204
Bβ15G→C-albumin	Ogasa	Heterozygotic	Defective FPB release	None	204
Bβ9-72del (Exon II)	New York I	Heterozygotic	Defective thrombin binding to fibrin	Thrombophilia	6, 44, 205
Bβ44R→C	Nijmegen	Heterozygotic	Impaired tissue-type plasminogen activator-mediated fibrinolysis	Thrombophilia	194, 195
Bβ68A→T	Naples I	Homozygotic	Defective thrombin binding	Thrombophilia	147, 149, 150
Bβ236Y→stop	Lozanne	Heterozygotic	Truncated Bβ chain participates in chain assembly/ thrombin time normal	Thrombophilia	190
Bβ335A→T	Pontoise	Heterozygotic	Defective polymerization	None	217
γ268G→E	Kurashiki	Heterozygotic	Impaired D:D interactions	None	81, 218
γ275R→C	Baltimore IV, Milano IV, Morioka I, Osaka II, Tochigi I, Tokyo II, Villajoyosa I, etc.	Heterozygotic	Impaired D:D interactions	None	6,79, 219, 260, 261, 288
γ275R→C	Bologna I, Cedar Rapids	Heterozygotic	Impaired D:D interactions	Thrombophilia	103, 259
γ275R→H	Barcelona IV, Claro I, Essen I, Osaka III, Perugia I, Saga I	Heterozygotic	Impaired D:D interactions	None	6, 261, 262, 289

(Continued)

TABLE 117-2   MUTATIONS RESULTING IN DYSFIBRINOGENEMIA (*Continued*)

MUTATION	NAME	INHERITANCE PATTERN	ETIOLOGY/PATHOLOGY	CLINICAL MANIFESTATIONS	REFERENCES
γ275R→H	Haifa I, Barcelona III, Bergamo II	Heterozygotic	Impaired D:D interactions	Thrombophilia	6, 220, 261, 262
γ275R→S	Kamogawa	Heterozygotic	Impaired D:D interactions	None	290
γ280Y→C	Banks Peninsula	Heterozygotic	Impaired D:D interactions	Bleeding	291
γ292G→V	Baltimore I	Heterozygotic	Impaired D:D site function?	Bleeding, thrombophilia	6, 222, 292
γ308N→I	Baltimore III	Heterozygotic	—	None	6, 223
γ308N→K	Kyoto I	Heterozygotic	—	None	6, 224
γ308N→K	Bicêtre II	Heterozygotic	?	Thrombophilia	6, 225
γ308N→K	Matsumoto II	Heterozygotic	—	Bleeding	226, 293
γ310M→T, 308N-glycosylation	Asahi I, Frankfurt VII	Heterozygotic	—	Bleeding	6, 227, 229
γ318D→G	Giessen IV	Heterozygotic	Defective calcium binding	Bleeding, thrombophilia	6, 259
γdel319N,320D	Vlissingen	Heterozygotic	Defective calcium binding	Thrombophilia	229, 230
γdel319N,320D	Otsu I	Heterozygotic	Defective calcium binding	None	273
γ329Q→R	Nagoya I	Heterozygotic	Defective polymerization	None	212
γ330D→Y	Kyoto III	Heterozygotic	Defective polymerization	None	224
γ330D→V	Milano I	Heterozygotic	Defective polymerization	None	211
γ337N→K	Bern I	Heterozygotic	Defective polymerization	None	214
γ350/insert/γ351G→S	Paris I	Heterozygotic	Absent XIIIa-mediated γ-chain cross-linking, defective ADP-induced platelet aggregation	Wound dehiscence	38, 228, 231–233
γ357A→T	Frankfurt I	Heterozygotic	Defective platelet aggregation	Bleeding	294
γ358S→C-albumin	Milano VII	Heterozygotic	Defective fibrin polymerization	None	215
γ361N→K	Poissy II	Heterozygotic	Impaired release of FPB, defective fibrin polymerization	Abruptio placenta in propositus	216
γ364D→H	Matsumoto I	Heterozygotic	Defective fibrin polymerization	None	208
γ364D→V	Melun I	Heterozygotic	Defective fibrin polymerization	Thrombophilia	209
γ375R→G	Osaka V	Heterozygotic	Defective high-affinity calcium binding and lack of protective effect of calcium on fibrinolysis	None	213
γ380K→N-glycosylated	Kaiserslautern	Heterozygotic	Defect normalized with calcium or by removing sialic acid residues	Thrombophilia	269, 270

TABLE 117-3   MUTATIONS CAUSING HYPODYSFIBRINOGENEMIA

MUTATION	NAME	INHERITANCE PATTERN	ETIOLOGY/PATHOLOGY	CLINICAL MANIFESTATIONS	REFERENCES
Aα20V→D	Canterbury	Heterozygotic	Intracellular cleavage of Aα1→19R by furin	Mild bleeding	256
Aα268R→Q/frameshift/QEP stop	Otago	Heterozygotic/homozygotic	Diminished assembly or secretion	Bleeding	243
Aα328Q→stop Aα IVS4 gt→tt	Keokuk	Compound heterozygotic	Aα splice site mutation and premature stop codon	Bleeding, miscarriage (♀), aseptic hip necrosis; thrombosis after fibrinogen infusion	136
Aα452G→WSstop	Milano III	Homozygotic/heterozygotic	Premature Aα-chain termination after 453	Thrombophilia	235, 236
Aα461K→stop	Marburg	Homozygotic	Premature Aα-chain termination	Bleeding, thrombophilia	234, 274
Aα476M→H/frameshift/CLAstop	Lincoln	Heterozygotic	Frameshift and premature Aα-chain termination after 479	Bleeding	295
γ326C→Y-albumin	Suhl	Heterozygotic	Defective polymerization	Thrombophilia	258
γ327A→T	Tokyo V	Heterozygotic	Defective fibrin assembly, cross-linking, fibrinolysis, altered Ca²⁺ binding function	Thrombophilia	257
γ336M→I	Hannover VI	Heterozygotic	Defective polymerization	Thrombophilia	258
γ354Y→C-albumin	Homburg VII	Heterozygotic	Defective polymerization	Thrombophilia	258
γ378S→P	Philadelphia	Heterozygotic	Hypercatabolism	Moderate to severe bleeding	31, 296

fibrinogen Naples I (Bβ68A→T)[147,149,150,196] and New York I.[44,205] Fibrinogen Nijmegen (BβR44R→C)[149] does not exhibit impaired fibrinopeptide release but rather abnormal polymerization.

THERAPY, COURSE, AND PROGNOSIS

When bleeding occurs under conditions involving defective fibrinopeptide release or production of a defective E_A polymerization site, the bleeding condition likely is related to the reduced polymerization potential of the mutant fibrins, with resulting defective clot formation. In general, if bleeding is severe, replacement therapy with fibrinogen-rich components such as cryoprecipitate or other fibrinogen concentrate is warranted. The mechanism for thrombophilia remains unclear in many cases. However, the inability of a mutant fibrin to bind thrombin effectively (antithrombin I defect or deficiency) may play a role in such clinical presentations, and special therapeutic precautions may be required (see "Afibrinogenemia and Hypofibrinogenemia [Antithrombin I Deficiency]" above).

POLYMERIZATION DEFECTS IN THE D DOMAIN

Fibrin assembly initially involves Da:E_A site interactions that drive the formation of staggered overlapping end-to-middle molecular associations resulting in double-stranded fibrils. In addition, two other distinct association sites are present in each D domain, termed γ_{XL} and D:D. In the following sections, these sites are considered in terms of known congenital abnormalities of fibrinogen. Some of these changes have been considered in terms of x-ray crystal structures.[206,207]

Da SITE

D domain mutations are associated with defective fibrin polymerization, and many are located in the region of the Da site. These mutations include fibrinogen Matsumoto I (γ364D→H)[208] and fibrinogen Melun I (γ364D→V).[209] The latter is associated with thrombophilia. Other dysfibrinogenemias that induce functional changes at the Da site include Kyoto III (γ330D→Y),[210] Milano I (γ330D→V),[211] Nagoya I (γQ329R),[212] Osaka V (γ375R→G),[213] and Bern I (γ337N→K).[214] Fibrinogen Milano VII (γ358S→C-albumin) molecules, which are disulfide linked to albumin,[215] displayed a marked polymerization defect. How this abnormality relates to abnormal polymerization is not clear, because the location itself does not appear to contribute to Da site function, and removal of albumin did not normalize the defect. None of these last-mentioned dysfibrinogens have thrombotic or bleeding manifestations. The Poissy II propositus experienced abruptio placenta and disseminated intravascular coagulation, but all other family members were asymptomatic.[216]

Db SITE

To date, no dysfibrinogenemias that specifically involve this site in the D domain have been described. Most mutations involving this region of the Bβ chain present as afibrinogenemias or hypofibrinogenemias and thus usually are not manifested in gene products.[166,174,177] The substitution in fibrinogen Pontoise (Bβ335A→T)[217] results in a new N-linked glycosylation site, and the molecule exhibits defective polymerization. The polymerization defect may be related to steric modifications or a charge effect on the polymerization process, but it likely is not directly related to an abnormality in the GHRP binding pocket, per se.[68]

D:D SITE

The interface for the end-to-end D:D site lies between γ275R and γ300S, with γ280T contacting γ275R at the D:D interface.[53] The nearby γ-chain residues also contribute to the site, as evidenced by

functional impairment of D:D interactions in molecules such as fibrinogen Kurashiki I (γ268G→E).[81,218] Fibrinogen Tokyo II[79,219] is one of many reported γ275R→C-substituted dysfibrinogens and was the first to be characterized in terms of its defective D:D site interactions. Several other γ275-substituted mutants have R substituted by H or S (see Table 117-2). Tokyo II fibrin displayed normal D:E associations and normal γ chain cross-linking. Factor XIIIa-cross-linked fibrinogen polymers were defective in that otherwise linear double-stranded fibrils were disorganized due to failure of normal end-to-end molecular associations. For the same reason, Tokyo II fibrin showed increased fiber branching.[79] The same type of abnormal fibrin branching has been shown for fibrinogen Haifa I (γ275R→H),[220] a case in which thrombophilia was prominent. Fibrinogen Banks Peninsula (γ280Y→C),[221] which is associated with mild bleeding, shows the same type of polymerization defect as described for Tokyo II fibrinogen, because the Cys substitution at γ280 disrupts the normal D:D contact with γ275R.

Fibrinogen Baltimore I (γ292G→V)[6] may represent another example of defective D:D site function, although its characteristics are not the same as those of fibrinogen Tokyo II. The Baltimore I patient had a history of recurrent thrombosis, pulmonary embolism, and mild bleeding.[222] Electron microscopy of fibrin networks showed thinner, relatively more branched fibers. Cross-linking of γ chains was normal, as seems to be characteristic of purely D:D defective molecules, but α-polymer formation was delayed although correctable. Other γ-chain mutations also may cause abnormal D:D site function. These include mutations at γ308N→I (Baltimore III)[223] or 308N→K (Kyoto I)[224]; Bicêtre II[225]; Matsumoto II[226]; and glycosylation at γ308N because of a γ310M→T mutation (Asahi I).[227]

γ_XL SITE

The γ_{XL} self-association site contains the factor XIIIa cross-linking sequence and overlaps the platelet fibrinogen receptor $\alpha_{IIb}\beta_3$ binding site. No mutations specifically involving this region of the molecule have been reported, although markedly impaired to absent γ-chain cross-linking at this site has been documented in fibrinogen Asahi I[227] and fibrinogen Paris I.[228] Fibrinogen Asahi I has a carbohydrate group incorporated at γ308N that may sterically interfere with cross-linking at the γ_{XL} site, although it does not interfere with factor XIIIa–mediated incorporation of amine donors at γ398Q. A dysfibrinogen with the same γ310M→T substitution as Asahi I (Frankfurt VII)[229] reportedly displays abnormal adenosine diphosphate (ADP)-induced platelet aggregation, probably by sterically hindering the C-terminal platelet binding sequence at the γ_{XL} site. Fibrinogen Vlissingen[230] (γdel 319N,320D) also displayed abnormal platelet aggregation,[229] probably resulting from disruption of its calcium binding site. These dysfibrinogens are also discussed in "Thrombophilia Related to Dysfibrinogenemia and Hypodysfibrinogenemia" below.

The fibrinogen Paris I abnormality is characterized by markedly impaired fibrin polymerization and clot retraction[231] but is not associated with clinical bleeding or thrombophilia, although the propositus displayed surgical wound dehiscence. The defect (γ350/insert/γ351G→S) involves a point mutation in intron 8 that results in insertion of a 15-amino-acid sequence after γ350 and substitution of S for G at γ351.[232] The $\gamma_{Paris I}$ chains have a normal C-terminal sequence beyond γ351,[232,233] yet despite this finding, the γ_{XL} site does not participate in factor-XIIIa–mediated γ-chain cross-linking nor can amine donors such as dansyl cadaverine be incorporated into these chains.[228] Furthermore, $\gamma_{Paris I}$ chains manifest defective ADP-induced platelet aggregation,[233] and $\gamma_{Paris I}$-containing molecules are not incorporated into platelets.[38] These findings suggest that marked conformational changes have occurred in the Paris I γ chain that makes the C-terminal sequence unavailable for any functions attributable to the γ_{XL} site.

αC DOMAIN

Fibrinogen Marburg[234] is a homozygous hypodysfibrinogenemia lacking amino acid residues Aα461-610. This abnormality is discussed in "Thrombophilia Related to Dysfibrinogenemia and Hypodysfibrinogenemia" below, as is fibrinogen Milano III, another Aα-chain truncation dysfibrinogenemic mutant.[235,236] Fibrinogen Dusart (Aα554R→C-albumin)[237–242] also is discussed in "Thrombophilia Related to Dysfibrinogenemia and Hypodysfibrinogenemia" below. Fibrinogen Otago,[243] an Aα-chain truncation mutant, displays hypodysfibrinogenemia (see Table 117-3) and is associated with a bleeding tendency. Fibrinogen Perth, a heterozygous dysfibrinogenemic Aα truncation mutant is associated with menorrhagia and easy bruising.[244]

Fibrinogen Caracas II (Aα434S→N-glycosylated)[245] is characterized by impaired fibrin gelation that is related to N-glycosylation. The fibrin ultrastructure shows thinner, less well-ordered fibers.[246] The carbohydrate group may interfere with fibrin polymerization in the same way as the bulky albumin group does in the case of fibrinogen Dusart, or possibly the problem is related to repulsive forces generated by its negative charge. In contrast to several other thrombophilic dysfibrinogenemias located in this region of the molecule, this dysfibrinogenemia is clinically silent. Fibrinogen Lima (Aα141R→S + Aα139N-glycosylation)[247] is a homozygous dysfibrinogenemia discovered in a family without a history of bleeding or thrombosis. The glycosylation site is located in the proximal portion of the D domain and evidently does not interfere with D:E or D:D interactions nor with fibrin-dependent plasminogen activation by t-PA. It most likely interferes with lateral fibril associations resulting from the repulsive negative charge on the carbohydrate group, since desialation normalizes the defect.

Renal Amyloidosis Renal amyloidosis can result from deposition of an abnormal fragment of fibrinogen mutated in the αC domain. Hereditary amyloidosis is characterized by progressive extracellular deposition of an amyloid protein in various organs. The disorder is associated with autosomal mutations of several plasma proteins: transerythretin, gelsolin, apolipoprotein A1, lysozyme, and fibrinogen.[248,249] Patients with transerythretin-associated amyloidoses, the most common form, have peripheral neuropathy and cardiomyopathy as major clinical manifestations, but they also develop gastrointestinal dysfunction, nephropathy, sexual impotence, vitreous opacification, and cerebral hemorrhage. In amyloidosis related to apolipoprotein A1, lysozyme, and fibrinogen, renal amyloid deposition has been the major finding. In the first such description for fibrinogen, amyloid fibrils from the kidney of a patient with hereditary renal amyloidosis (HRA) contained a fibrinogen Aα-chain fragment covering residues 499 through 580 and included an Aα554R→L mutation.[250] The propositus developed nephrotic syndrome and azotemia at age 36 years and required renal transplantation at the age of 40. A second renal transplantation for the same condition was performed when the patient was 50 years of age. After the patient died of septicemia, an autopsy revealed the same amyloid deposition in the transplanted kidney as had been found in the original and first transplanted kidneys. Another kindred with the same Aα554R→L abnormality developed HRA much later in life, between the sixth and eighth decades.[251] It is important to note that substitution of C for R at the same position Aα554, such as occurred in fibrinogens Dusart and Chapel Hill III, did not result in amyloidosis but instead caused a different functional impairment and a thrombophilic profile.

An Aα526E→V mutation has been described in four families with HRA manifested in the fifth to seventh decades of life.[252,253] In one kindred,[252] plasma fibrinogen levels and thrombin times were in the normal range, and the distributions of normal and mutant Aα chains

were equal, indicating a heterozygous defect. In another kindred, HRA was recognized in the fourth to fifth decades of life,[254] and genomic sequencing showed a nucleotide deletion that caused a frameshift after position Aα524 that produced an abnormal sequence and chain termination after position 547. A similar frameshift mutation was observed after Aα521 in another kindred with the onset of HRA as early as the second decade and resulted in renal deposition of a 49-residue hybrid peptide whose N-terminal 23 amino acids were identical to Aα499 to 521.[255] The remaining 26 amino acids in the peptide resulting from a frameshift at codon 522 had a unique sequence that terminated at position 547.

Therapy and Course Renal transplantation is not a curative solution for HRA-related renal failure, because continuing fibrinogen-related amyloid deposition ultimately results in allograft destruction.[250,255] Chronic renal dialysis could be a medium-term temporizing approach for managing renal failure, but liver transplantation should be considered a curative alternative to chronic dialysis.

HYPODYSFIBRINOGENEMIA

CLINICAL FEATURES

The clinical presentation in patients in this category ranges from bleeding to thrombophilia, or both. In fibrinogen Canterbury (Aα20V→D), the E_A polymerization site and the entire FPA sequence (i.e., Aα1 to 19) are missing.[256] This situation occurs because the AαV20D mutation created a cleavage site at R19 (RGPRD) for the intracellular enzyme furin, and the mutant Aα chain was cleaved intracellularly at that site prior to secretion, creating a sequence beginning with Aα20D. A mild bleeding tendency exists in this situation.

Thrombophilic hypodysfibrinogen Tokyo V was identified in a 43-year-old man with recurrent arterial and venous thromboembolism and a heterozygous γ-chain mutation (γ327A→T) that also created a new N-linked glycosylation site at γN325.[257] The γ-chain mutation is in the vicinity of the calcium binding site, the Da polymerization site, and the t-PA binding site. Although it amounts to only 22 percent of the total γ-chain population in the plasma fibrinogen, its presence nevertheless resulted in several functional abnormalities, including marked impairment of fibrin polymerization, reduced to absent XIIIa-mediated cross-linking of the mutant γ chain, globally defective α-polymerization, and a large proportion of soluble cross-linked fibrin. In addition, Tokyo V-derived fibrin was resistant to t-PA–mediated fibrinolysis and displayed altered function of the high-affinity calcium binding site in the γ chain. Although not yet proved, the hypodysfibrinogenemia might be related to hypercatabolism. Taken together, these data suggest that fibrinolysis-resistant thrombin-bound Tokyo V fibrin polymers may be released to the circulation and partly account for the severe thromboembolic episodes in the patient.

Two siblings with severe hypodysfibrinogenemia (fibrinogen Keokuk) have experienced lifelong trauma-related bleeding, repeated miscarriages in the female member of the kindred, and recurrent thromboembolism on two separate occasions in the male sibling after cryoprecipitate infusions following surgery.[136] Each sibling was a compound heterozygote for an Aα328Q→stop mutation causing a truncated Aα chain of 35 kDa and an Aα chain splice site mutation (Aα IVS4 gt→tt) that has previously been described in afibrinogenemia.[166,175] Compound heterozygosity was required for expression of severe hypodysfibrinogenemia and for clinical symptoms, since simple heterozygotic family members were entirely asymptomatic. It is noteworthy that the sibling who twice experienced thromboembolic complications following infusions of cryoprecipitate had been treated with long-term "anticoagulants" or LMWH and aspirin. Also noteworthy is that the first surgery was replacement of the left hip because of *aseptic necrosis*, and in that context the laboratory findings included a prolonged clot lysis time and elevated PAI-1.

ETIOLOGIC AND THERAPEUTIC CONSIDERATIONS

Thrombophilia in the Tokyo V patient may be related to several factors, including reduced fibrinolysis, increased levels of soluble cross-linked fibrin in the circulation, and deficient antithrombin I activity. In fibrinogen Keokuk, the bleeding and repeated miscarriages may be related to the very low levels of functional fibrinogen in the circulation. On the other hand, recurrent thromboembolism was associated with infusion of fibrinogen-rich cryoprecipitate, and this situation falls into the category of antithrombin I deficiency; see "Thrombin Binding to Fibrinogen and Fibrin (Antithrombin I)." Other severe hypodysfibrinogenemias associated with thrombophilia include fibrinogens Suhl (γ326C$\rightarrow$Y-albumin), Hannover VI (γ336M$\rightarrow$I), and Homburg VII (γ354Y$\rightarrow$C-albumin).[258] The pathophysiology in these cases also may be related to antithrombin I deficiency.

DYSFIBRINOGENEMIA AND AVASCULAR OSTEONECROSIS

CLINICAL FEATURES

Avascular osteonecrosis of the hip in adults and Legg-Perthes disease in children has been associated with thrombophilia leading to hypoxic bone death[127–135] *inter alia*. Affected individuals often have a thrombophilic profile, often exhibiting hypofibrinolysis and an elevated Lp(a) or PAI-1 level. One affected member of this family had undergone hip replacement surgery for aseptic necrosis of the femoral head and exhibited defective fibrinolysis and elevated PAI-1. Hypodysfibrinogenemia likely was causally related to the osteonecrosis that had occurred. Treatment with LMWH (Enoxaparin) reportedly has been effective in slowing the progression of osteonecrosis[133,135] and would have been recommended if osteonecrosis had not progressed to an irreversible extent.

THERAPEUTIC CONSIDERATIONS

One thrombophilic member of the Cedar Rapids kindred exhibited defective fibrinolysis and was heterozygotic for factor V Leiden. She had undergone bilateral hip arthroplasty for avascular necrosis of the femoral heads. She also had developed bilateral necrosis of the femoral condyles. It seems likely that the dysfibrinogenemia and associated conditions were causally related to the osteonecrosis that had occurred. Because treatment with LMWH (Enoxaparin) reportedly has been effective in slowing the progression of osteonecrosis,[133,135] had the relationship been recognized, this treatment would have been recommended in the Cedar Rapids patient. A male sibling in the hypodysfibrinogenemic Keokuk kindred displayed thromboembolism following cryoprecipitate infusion in preparation for hip replacement for aseptic necrosis.[136] Antithrombin I deficiency is the likely incipient cause for the thromboembolism that occurred, and LMWH might have been considered earlier in the course of the patient's hip disease.

THROMBOPHILIA RELATED TO DYSFIBRINOGENEMIA AND HYPODYSFIBRINOGENEMIA

Dysfibrinogenemia or hypodysfibrinogenemia associated with thromboembolic disorders occurs in approximately 20 percent of dysfibrinogenemic families,[6,259] and thrombophilia as an aspect of afibrinogenemia or hypofibrinogenemia has already been discussed (see "Dysfibrinogenemia"). Among dysfibrinogenemic families, thrombotic problems related to pregnancy are common, particularly spontaneous abortion and postpartum thromboembolism. Most of the thrombophilic kindreds identified to date are listed in Tables 117-2 and 117-3, and some of the potential mechanisms for the thrombophilic condition are considered below.

Fibrinogen Nijmegen is associated with abnormal t-PA–induced plasminogen activation but normal fibrinopeptide release.[194,195] Abnormal high molecular weight fibrinogen complexes and albumin-linked fibrinogen molecules were also found. Fibrinogen Ijmuiden was similar to Nijmegen in these respects and also showed abnormal FPB release.[194] The polymerization abnormality shown by both fibrinogens may cause abnormal t-PA–mediated plasminogen activation, which in turn may contribute to thrombophilia.

Of the numerous dysfibrinogenemic families found to have an amino acid substitution at position 275R of the γ chain (see Table 117-2), all but five were asymptomatic at the time of the Cedar Rapids report. Of the families reporting thrombophilia, two had γ275R$\rightarrow$C, Bologna I[259] and Cedar Rapids,[103] and three had γ275R$\rightarrow$H substitutions. The γ275R$\rightarrow$H Haifa I patient[260] presented at the age of 30 with arterial occlusions, Barcelona III with venous thrombosis,[261] and Bergamo II with pulmonary embolism associated with pregnancy.[262] Clearly there is no simple direct linkage between this type of structural abnormality and thromboembolism, and other contributory conditions must be considered. Several genetic risk factors have been implicated in the pathogenesis of venous thromboembolism, including abnormalities of protein C, protein S, antithrombin III, plasminogen, prothrombin, fibrinogen, plasma homocysteine levels, and factor V.[263,264] The factor V defect is manifested as resistance to degradation by activated protein C resulting from a mutation in the factor V gene leading to substitution of Q for R at position 506, commonly referred to as factor V Leiden (see Chap. 122).[265–268]

Fibrinogen Cedar Rapids is a heterozygous dysfibrinogenemia in which thromboembolic disease was associated with pregnancy in three second-generation family members.[103] Each affected family member was heterozygous for the factor V Leiden defect, whereas the parents and their siblings manifested either the factor V Leiden defect (paternal) or fibrinogen Cedar Rapids (maternal) and were asymptomatic. These observations suggest that coexpression of factor V Leiden and fibrinogen Cedar Rapids is associated with thrombophilia, but the mechanism by which they contribute to the thrombophilic state is not clear. Another possible example of such concurrent conditions is found in fibrinogen Giessen IV (γ318D$\rightarrow$G).[259]

The defect in fibrinogen Melun I (γ364D$\rightarrow$V)[209] is situated in a position that interferes with Da site function. This family has a pervasive history of venous thromboembolic disease in the heterozygous state. Presumably, defective Da:E$_A$ site interactions contributed to the thrombophilia that has been observed. However, an anomaly (D364H) at the same site (fibrinogen Matsumoto I)[208] is not associated with thrombophilia. As in other situations of this kind, more information is needed to resolve this paradoxical situation.

Fibrinogen Kaiserslautern (γ380K$\rightarrow$N-glycosylated)[269,270] was described in a 34-year-old woman who developed a cerebral sinus thrombosis after cesarean section even though other members of her family with the functional defect were asymptomatic. The site of the abnormality is far removed from either the Da polymerization pocket or the D:D association site. The polymerization defect is normalized with calcium or by removing sialic acid residues and thus appears to result from electrostatic repulsion between condensing fibrils. The mechanism for the thrombophilia is unclear.

DEFECTS IN THE CALCIUM BINDING SITE OF THE γ CHAIN

A high-affinity calcium binding site in the γ chain is located between residues 311 and 336 and involves residues at γ318D, γ320D, γ322F, γ324G, and γ328E.[53,230,271] The calcium site is important for the structural integrity of the D domain and provides a protective effect against plasmin cleavage of the γ chain.[272] Fibrinogen Vlissingen (γdel319N,320D)[230] was identified in a woman who had been hospitalized because of pulmonary embolism. Fibrin polymerization was delayed in both the presence and the absence of calcium. Deletion of γ-chain residues 319 and 320 resulted in defective calcium binding and probable allosterically mediated dysfunction of the Da polymerization site and possibly the D:D site. Abnormal ADP-induced platelet aggregation also has been reported for this abnormal fibrinogen,[229] implying impaired function at the γ_{XL} site. Similarly, the fibrinogen Giessen IV (γ318D→G)[259] defect results in defective calcium binding and polymerization and was reported in an 18-year-old woman with recurrent venous thrombosis and mild bleeding, who also was heterozygous for the factor V Leiden defect. However, the relationship between the calcium binding defect and thrombophilia, as in many situations, is not clear, since the identical deletion in fibrinogen Otsu I (γdel319N,320D)[273] was asymptomatic. Furthermore, fibrinogen Osaka V (γ375R→G)[213] showed defective calcium binding and lack of the protective effect of calcium on fibrinolysis, yet it is asymptomatic.

MUTATIONS INVOLVING C-TERMINAL REGIONS OF Aα OR Bβ CHAIN

Fibrinogen Marburg[234] is a homozygous hypodysfibrinogenemia lacking amino acid residues Aα461-610 because of a stop codon at position 461 of the Aα chain. Its unpaired cysteine residue at position 442 forms a disulfide bridge with albumin and other substances.[274] The Marburg patient suffered from severe uterine bleeding after cesarian section, pelvic vein thrombosis, and recurrent thromboembolic disease. The effect of antithrombin I deficiency as a causative element in this syndrome should be considered. Another homozygous truncation mutant (Aα451I+t[frameshift]→WSstop), fibrinogen Milano III,[235,236] also is associated with recurrent venous thrombosis. Unlike fibrinogen Marburg, this mutant fibrinogen circulates at normal levels. The abnormality is associated with defective lateral fibril association and comes about by a single base insertion after Aα451, resulting in a frameshift and a premature stop codon at 453S. Because of premature Aα-chain termination, an unpaired Cys residue is present at position 442, and, like Marburg, Milano III is associated with covalent linkage of albumin to the Aα chain. The thrombophilia may be causally related to formation of fine fibrin clots, which are resistant to fibrinolysis.[240,275,276]

Hanss and colleagues[190] used gel electrophoresis to screen for fibrinogen mutations in patients with a thrombophilic profile and normal thrombin times and plasma fibrinogen levels. They found two novel dysfibrinogenemias in a cohort of 217 consecutive patients with familial or early onset thrombosis. The first patient (fibrinogen Champagne au Mont d'Or) showed a 39-residue duplication and in-frame insertion at Aα 272. The second patient (fibrinogen Lozanne) had a heterozygous mutation at Bβ236 resulting in a stop codon, but the truncated Bβ chain nevertheless could participate in molecular assembly. The basis for thrombophilia in these patients is obscure.

DUSART SYNDROME

Fibrinogen Dusart (Aα554R→C-albumin) has been studied extensively.[237–242] The defect is the same as that in fibrinogen Chapel Hill III,[6,277] which also presented with thrombophilia. Dusart fibrinogen displays reduced plasminogen binding,[238,242] impaired fibrin-dependent t-PA activation,[238] and abnormal fibrin polymerization and clot structure[237,239–241] that is normalized by removing the affected region of the molecule.[241] In addition to these abnormalities, fibrinogen Dusart molecules show an enhanced self-association tendency that is di-

rectly related to the Aα-chain defect, and the fibrinogen cross-linking rate is accelerated.[242] These several events, including the hypofibrinolysis caused by the abnormal clot structure itself, may collectively contribute to the thrombophilia.

The fibrinogen Caracas V abnormality (Aα532S→C) is located in about the same region of the Aα chain as the Dusart and Chapel Hill III anomalies. This dysfibrinogenemia has been associated with both venous and arterial thrombotic diseases in several members of the kindred.[259,278] Electron microscopy of Caracas V fibrin revealed no differences from normal,[279] suggesting that expression of the defect is different from Dusart.

THROMBIN BINDING DEFECTS (DEFECTIVE ANTITHROMBIN I)

Low-affinity nonsubstrate thrombin binding sites are found in fibrin E domains and represent a residual aspect of fibrinogen substrate recognition of thrombin exosite 1.[87,141] As outlined in the "Introduction" above, there is also a higher-affinity thrombin binding component present in fibrin that is found in variant γ' chains. This site binds to thrombin exosite 2.[145,146] Cooperative binding of thrombin exosite I at the low-affinity sites in the E domain of fibrin plus thrombin exosite 2 binding to the γ' chains account for the measured high-affinity thrombin binding component. Homozygous members of the fibrinogen Naples I kindred (Bβ68A→T)[147,149,150] showed markedly impaired thrombin binding, which was the proximate cause for the thrombophilia presented by the patients, including juvenile arterial stroke, thrombotic abdominal aortic occlusions, and postoperative deep venous thrombosis. In contrast, heterozygous members of the kindred were asymptomatic. Careful analyses in two homozygotes showed that low-affinity thrombin binding to fibrin was absent and resulted from the absence of thrombin binding in the E domain. However, residual thrombin binding was present at the high-affinity site in the γ' chain of these subjects, albeit reduced in relation to the measured affinity in normal γ' chain-containing fibrin. Cooperative binding to thrombin exosite 1 plus γ' chain binding to thrombin exosite 2 contribute to formation of the high-affinity thrombin binding component.[146,147] In heterozygotic Naples I subjects, sufficient low-affinity binding activity is present to yield normal high-affinity binding association constants, but this situation does not hold for the homozygotic subjects.[147] This combination of events undoubtedly contributes to the profound antithrombin I defect. The fibrinogen New York I (Bβ9-72del) subject exhibited defective nonsubstrate thrombin binding, concomitant with recurrent venous thrombosis and fatal pulmonary embolism.[205] Fibrinogens Kumamoto and Aarhus I (both Aα19R→G) are each associated with thrombosis, and reduced thrombin binding to fibrin has been reported for Kumamoto.[192]

THERAPEUTIC CONSIDERATIONS

Patients with thrombophilic dysfibrinogenemias and hypodysfibrinogenemias are heterogeneous with respect to their molecular abnormalities and the causes of their thromboembolic problems. Bleeding, especially when associated with hypodysfibrinogenemia (e.g., fibrinogen Marburg), can be managed by fibrinogen infusion, but the same precautions should be taken as outlined for infusing fibrinogen-rich concentrates in afibrinogenemic patients. Patients with potentially life-threatening thrombophilic manifestations, as occurs with fibrinogen Cedar Rapids, have been successfully managed with plasma exchange prior to major surgery.[280] However, insufficient data exist to suggest that this type of treatment is more effective than more general measures for managing potential thromboembolism. Long-term management strategies for thrombophilic dysfibrinogenemia are the same as the strategies for patients with recurrent thromboembolism and include long-term anticoagulation.

REFERENCES

1. Mosesson MW, Siebenlist KR, Meh DA: The structure and biological features of fibrinogen and fibrin. *Ann N Y Acad Sci* 936:11, 2001.
2. Mosesson MW: Fibrinogen gamma chain functions. *J Thromb Haemost* 1:2318, 2003.
3. Mosesson MW: Antithrombin I. Inhibition of thrombin generation in plasma by fibrin formation. *Thromb Haemost* 89:9, 2003.
4. Mosesson MW: The fibrin cross-linking debate: Cross-linked gamma-chains in fibrin fibrils bridge "transversely" between strands: Yes. *J Thromb Haemost* 2:388, 2004
5. Mosesson MW: Cross-linked γ chains in fibrin fibrils are situated "transversely" between its strands. *J Thromb Haemost* 2:1469, 2004.
6. Ebert RF: *Index of Variant Human Fibrinogens.* CRC Press, Boca Raton, 1994.
7. Hanss M, Biot F: A database for human fibrinogen variants. *Ann N Y Acad Sci* 936:89, 2001.
8. Henschen A, Lottspeich F, Kehl M, Southan C: Covalent structure of fibrinogen. *Ann N Y Acad Sci* 408:28, 1983.
9. Slayter HS: Electron microscopic studies of fibrinogen structure: Historical perspectives and recent experiments. *Ann N Y Acad Sci* 408:131, 1983.
10. Mosesson MW, Hainfeld JF, Haschemeyer RH, Wall JS: Identification and mass analysis of human fibrinogen molecules and their domains by scanning transmission electron microscopy. *J Mol Biol* 153:695, 1981.
11. Williams RC: Morphology of fibrinogen monomers and fibrin polymers. *Ann N Y Acad Sci* 408:180, 1983.
12. Blombäck B, Hessel B, Hogg D: Disulfide bridges in NH₂-terminal part of human fibrinogen. *Thromb Res* 8:639, 1976.
13. Huang S, Cao Z, Davie EW: The role of amino-terminal disulfide bonds in the structure and assembly of human fibrinogen. *Biochem Biophys Res Commun* 190:488, 1993.
14. Zhang JZ, Redman CM: Role of interchain disulfide bonds on the assembly and secretion of human fibrinogen. *J Biol Chem* 269:652, 1994.
15. Finlayson JS, Mosesson MW: Heterogeneity of human fibrinogen. *Biochemistry* 2:42, 1963.
16. Wolfenstein-Todel C, Mosesson MW: Carboxy-terminal amino acid sequence of a human fibrinogen γ chain variant (γ'). *Biochemistry* 20:6146, 1981.
17. Grieninger G: Contribution of the αEC domain to the structure and function of fibrinogen-420. *Ann N Y Acad Sci* 936:44, 2001.
18. Mosesson MW, DiOrio JP, Hernandez I, et al: The ultrastructure of fibrin-420 and the fibrin-420 polymer. *Biophys Chem* 112:209, 2004.
19. Lishko VK, Yakubenko VP, Hertzberg KM, et al: The alternatively spliced alpha(E)C domain of human fibrinogen-420 is a novel ligand for leukocyte integrins alpha(M)beta(2) and alpha(X)beta(2). *Blood* 98:2448, 2001.
20. Ugarova TP, Solovjov DA, Zhang L, et al: Identification of a novel recognition sequence for integrin αMβ2 within the γ-chain of fibrinogen. *J Biol Chem* 273:22519, 1998.
21. Barnhart MI, Cress DC, Noonan SM, Walsh RT: Influence of fibrinolytic products on hepatic release and synthesis of fibrinogen. *Thromb Haemost* 39(suppl):143, 1970.
22. Fuller GM, Nickerson JM, Adams MA: Translation and cotranslational events in fibrinogen synthesis. *Ann N Y Acad Sci* 408:440, 1983.
23. Olaisen B, Teissberg P, Gedde-Dahl T Jr: Fibrinogen γ chain locus is on chromosome 4 in man. *Hum Genet* 61:24, 1982.
24. Chung DW, Rixon MW, Que BG, Davie EW: Cloning of fibrinogen genes and their cDNA. *Ann N Y Acad Sci* 408:449, 1983.
25. Crabtree GR, Kant JA, Fornace AJ Jr, et al: Regulation and characterization of the mRNA for the Aα, Bβ and γ chains of fibrinogen. *Ann N Y Acad Sci* 408:457, 1983.
26. Kant J, Fornace AJ Jr, Saxe D, et al: Organization and evolution of the human fibrinogen locus on chromosome four. *Proc Natl Acad Sci U S A* 82:2344, 1985.
27. Fowlkes DM, Mullis NT, Comeau CM, Crabtree GR: Potential basis for regulation of the coordinately expressed fibrinogen genes: Homology in the 5' flanking regions. *Proc Natl Acad Sci U S A* 81:2313, 1984.
28. Huber P, Laurent M, Dalmon J: Human beta-fibrinogen gene expression. Upstream sequences involved in its tissue specific expression and its dexamethasone and interleukin 6 stimulation. *J Biol Chem* 265:5695, 1990.
29. Liu Z, Fuller GM: Detection of a novel transcription factor for the Aα fibrinogen gene in response to interleukin-6. *J Biol Chem* 270:7580, 1995.
30. Collen D, Tytgat GN, Claeys H, Piessens R: Metabolism and distribution of fibrinogen I. *Br J Haematol* 22:681, 1972.
31. Martinez J, Holburn RR, Shapiro SS, Erslev AJ: Fibrinogen Philadelphia. A hereditary hypodysfibrinogenemia characterized by fibrinogen hypercatabolism. *J Clin Invest* 53:600, 1974.
32. Harrison P, Wilbourn B, Debili N, et al: Uptake of plasma fibrinogen into the alpha granules of human megakaryocytes and platelets. *J Clin Invest* 84:320, 1989.
33. Handagama P, Scarborough RM, Shuman MA, Bainton DF: Endocytosis of fibrinogen into megakaryocytes and platelet α-granules is mediated by αIIbb₃ (glycoprotein IIb-IIIa). *Blood* 82:135, 1993.
34. Handagama P, Amrani DL, Shuman MA: Endocytosis of fibrinogen into hamster megakaryocyte α granules is dependent on a dimeric γA configuration. *Blood* 85:1790, 1995.
35. Mosesson MW, Homandberg GA, Amrani DL: Human platelet fibrinogen gamma chain structure. *Blood* 63:990, 1984.
36. Francis CW, Nachman RL, Marder VJ: Plasma and platelet fibrinogen differ in gamma chain content. *Thromb Haemost* 51:84, 1984.
37. Kunicki TJ, Newman PJ, Amrani DL, Mosesson MW: Human platelet fibrinogen: Purification and hemostatic properties. *Blood* 66:808, 1985.
38. Jandrot-Perrus M, Mosesson MW, Denninger M-H, Ménaché D: Studies of platelet fibrinogen from a subject with a congenital plasma fibrinogen abnormality (fibrinogen Paris I). *Blood* 54:1109, 1979.
39. Scheraga HA, Laskowski M Jr: The fibrinogen-fibrin conversion. *Adv Protein Chem* 12:1, 1957.
40. Blombäck B: Studies on the action of thrombotic enzymes on bovine fibrinogen as measured by N-terminal analysis. *Arkiv Kemi* 12:321, 1958.
41. Blombäck B, Hessel B, Hogg D, Therkildsen L: A two-step fibrinogen-fibrin transition in blood coagulation. *Nature* 275:501, 1978.
42. Laudano AP, Doolittle RF: Studies on synthetic peptides that bind to fibrinogen and prevent fibrin polymerization. *Proc Natl Acad Sci U S A* 75:3085, 1978.
43. Laudano AP, Doolittle RF: Studies on synthetic peptides that bind to fibrinogen and prevent fibrin polymerization: Structural requirements and species differences. *Biochemistry* 19:1013, 1980.
44. Liu CY, Koehn JA, Morgan FJ: Characterization of fibrinogen New York 1. *J Biol Chem* 260:4390, 1985.
45. Pandya BV, Cierniewski CS, Budzynski AZ: Conservation of human fibrinogen conformation after cleavage of the Bβ chain NH₂-terminus. *J Biol Chem* 260:2994, 1985.
46. Shimizu A, Saito Y, Inada Y: Distinctive role of histidine-16 of the Bβ chain of fibrinogen in the end-to-end association of fibrin. *Proc Natl Acad Sci U S A* 83:591, 1986.
47. Siebenlist KR, DiOrio JP, Budzynski AZ, Mosesson MW: The polymerization and thrombin-binding properties of des-(B beta 1-42)-fibrin. *J Biol Chem* 265:18650, 1990.
48. Pandya BV, Gabriel JL, O'Brien J, Budzynski AZ: Polymerization site in the β chain of fibrin: Mapping of the Bβ1-55 sequence. *Biochemistry* 30:162, 1991.

49. Kudryk B, Reuterby J, Blombäck B: Adsorption of plasmic fragment D to thrombin modified fibrinogen-sepharose. *Thromb Res* 2:297, 1973.

50. Kudryk B, Collen D, Woods KR, Blombäck B: Evidence for localization of polymerization sites in fibrinogen. *J Biol Chem* 249:3322, 1974.

51. Olexa SA, Budzynski AZ: 1980. Evidence for four different polymerization sites involved in human fibrin formation. *Proc Natl Acad Sci U S A* 77:1374, 1980.

52. Shimizu A, Nagel GM, Doolittle RF: Photoaffinity labeling of the primary fibrin polymerization site: Isolation of a CNBr fragment corresponding to γ 337-379. *Proc Natl Acad Sci U S A* 89:2888, 1992.

53. Spraggon G, Everse SJ, Doolittle RF: Crystal structures of fragment D from human fibrinogen and its crosslinked counterpart from fibrin. *Nature* 389:455, 1997.

54. Ferry JD: The mechanism of polymerization of fibrinogen. *Proc Natl Acad Sci U S A* 38:566, 1952.

55. Krakow W, Endres GF, Siegel BM, Scheraga HA: An electron microscopic investigation of the polymerization of bovine fibrin monomer. *J Mol Biol* 71:95, 1972.

56. Fowler WE, Hantgan RR, Hermans J, et al: Structure of the fibrin protofibril. *Proc Natl Acad Sci U S A* 78:4872, 1981.

57. Hantgan R, McDonagh J, Hermans J: Fibrin assembly. *Ann N Y Acad Sci* 408:344, 1983.

58. Mosesson MW, DiOrio JP, Siebenlist KR, et al: Evidence for a second type of fibril branch point in fibrin polymer networks, the trimolecular junction. *Blood* 82:1517, 1993.

59. Mosesson MW, Siebenlist KR, Amrani DL, DiOrio JP: Identification of covalently linked trimeric and tetrameric D domains in crosslinked fibrin. *Proc Natl Acad Sci U S A* 86:1113, 1989.

60. Hewat EA, Tranqui L, Wade RH: Electron microscope structural study of modified fibrin and a related modified fibrinogen aggregate. *J Mol Biol* 170:203, 1983.

61. Blombäck B, Carlsson K, Fatah K, et al: Fibrin in human plasma: Gel architectures governed by rate and nature of fibrinogen activation. *Thromb Res* 75:521, 1994.

62. Shainoff JR, Dardik BN: Fibrinopeptide B in fibrin assembly and metabolism: Physiologic significance in delayed release of the peptide. *Ann N Y Acad Sci* 408:254, 1983.

63. Everse SJ, Spraggon G, Veerapandian L, et al: Crystal structure of fragment double-D from human fibrin with two different bound ligands. *Biochemistry* 37:8637, 1998.

64. Medved LV, Litvinovich SV, Ugarova TP, et al: Localization of a fibrin polymerization site complimentary to Gly-His-Arg sequence. *FEBS Lett* 320:239, 1993.

65. Martinelli RA, Scheraga HA: Steady-state kinetic study of the bovine thrombin-fibrinogen interaction. *Biochemistry* 19:2343, 1980.

66. Hurlet-Jensen A, Cummins HZ, Nossel HL, Liu CY: Fibrin polymerization and release of fibrinopeptide B by thrombin. *Thromb Res* 27:419, 1982.

67. Ruf W, Bender A, Lane DA, et al: Thrombin-induced fibropeptide B release from normal and variant fibrinogens: Influence of inhibitors of fibrin polymerization. *Biochim Biophys Acta* 965:169, 1988.

68. Yang Z, Mochalkin I, Doolittle RF: A model of fibrin formation based on crystal structures of fibrinogen and fibrin fragments complexed with synthetic peptides. *Proc Natl Acad Sci U S A* 97:14156, 2000.

69. Weisel JW, Medved LV: The structure and function of the αC domains of fibrinogen. *Ann N Y Acad Sci* 936:312, 2001.

70. Mosesson MW, Finlayson JS, Umfleet RA, Galanakis DK: Human fibrinogen heterogeneities: I. Structural and related studies of plasma fibrinogens which are high solubility catabolic intermediates. *J Biol Chem* 247:5210, 1972.

71. Mosesson MW, Galanakis DK, Finlayson JS: Comparison of human plasma fibrinogen subfractions and early plasmic fibrinogen derivatives. *J Biol Chem* 249:4656, 1974.

72. Mosesson MW, Sherry S: The preparation and properties of human fibrinogen of relatively high solubility. *Biochemistry* 5:2829, 1966.

73. Mosesson MW: Fibrinogen heterogeneity. *Ann N Y Acad Sci* 408:97, 1983.

74. Hasegawa N, Sasaki S: Location of the binding site "b" for lateral polymerization of fibrin. *Thromb Res* 57:183, 1990.

75. Medved' LV, Gorkun OV, Manyakov VF, Belitser VA: The role of fibrinogen αC-domains in the fibrin assembly process. *FEBS Lett* 181:109, 1985.

76. Veklich YI, Gorkun OV, Medved LV, et al: Carboxyl-terminal portions of the a chains of fibrinogen and fibrin. *J Biol Chem* 268:13577, 1993.

77. Gorkun OV, Veklich YI, Medved LV, et al: Role of the αC domains of fibrin in clot formation. *Biochemistry* 33:6986, 1994.

78. Mosesson MW, Siebenlist KR, Hainfeld JF, Wall JS: The covalent structure of factor XIIIa crosslinked fibrinogen fibrils. *J Struct Biol* 115:88, 1995.

79. Mosesson MW, Siebenlist KR, DiOrio JP, et al: The role of fibrinogen D domain intermolecular association sites in the polymerization of fibrin and fibrinogen Tokyo II (γ275 Arg→Cys). *J Clin Invest* 96:1053, 1995.

80. Siebenlist KR, Meh DA, Wall JS, et al: Orientation of the carboxy-terminal regions of fibrin γ chain dimers determined from the crosslinked products formed in mixtures of fibrin, fragment D, and factor XIIIa. *Thromb Haemost* 74:1113, 1995.

81. Niwa K, Takebe M, Sugo T, et al: A γ Gly-268 to Glu substitution is responsible for impaired fibrin assembly in a homozygous dysfibrinogen Kurashiki. *Blood* 87:4686, 1996.

82. Kloczewiak M, Timmons S, Hawiger J: Recognition site for the platelet receptor is present on the 15-residue carboxy-terminal fragment of the γ-chain of human fibrinogen and is not involved in the fibrin polymerization reaction. *Thromb Res* 29:249, 1983.

83. Kloczewiak M, Timmons S, Lukas TJ, Hawiger J: Platelet receptor recognition site on human fibrinogen. Synthesis and structure-function relationship of peptides corresponding to the C-terminal segment of the γ chain. *Biochemistry* 23:1767, 1984.

84. Wolfenstein-Todel C, Mosesson MW: Human plasma fibrinogen heterogeneity: Evidence for an extended carboxyl-terminal sequence in a normal gamma chain variant (γ'). *Proc Natl Acad Sci U S A* 77:5069, 1980.

85. Siebenlist KR, Meh DA, Mosesson MW: Plasma factor XIII binds specifically to fibrinogen molecules containing γ' chains. *Biochemistry* 35:10448, 1996.

86. Siebenlist KR, Meh D, Mosesson MW: Protransglutaminase (factor XIII) mediated crosslinking of fibrinogen and fibrin. *Thromb Haemost* 86:1221, 2001.

87. Meh DA, Siebenlist KR, Mosesson MW: Identification and characterization of the thrombin binding sites on fibrin. *J Biol Chem* 271:23121, 1996.

88. Matacic S, Loewy AG: The identification of isopeptide crosslinks in insoluble fibrin. *Biochem Biophys Res Commun* 30:356, 1968.

89. Pisano JJ, Finlayson JS, Peyton MP: Crosslink in fibrin polymerized by factor XIII: ε-(γ-glutamyl)lysine. *Science* 160:892, 1968.

90. Chen R, Doolittle RF: Identification of the polypeptide chains involved in the cross-linking of fibrin. *Proc Natl Acad Sci U S A* 63:420, 1969.

91. Chen R, Doolittle RF: γ-γ Cross-linking sites in human and bovine fibrin. *Biochemistry* 10:4486, 1971.

92. Doolittle RF, Chen R, Lau F: Hybrid fibrin: Proof of the intermolecular nature of γ-γ cross-linking units. *Biochem Biophys Res Commun* 44:94, 1971.

93. Purves LR, Purves M, Brandt W: Cleavage of fibrin-derived D-dimer into monomers by endopeptidase from puff adder venom (bitis arietans) acting at cross-linked sites of the γ chain. Sequence of carboxy-terminal cyanogen bromide γ-chain fragments. *Biochemistry* 26:4640, 1987.

94. Shimizu A, Ferry JD: Ligation of fibrinogen by factor XIIIa with di-thiothreitol: Mechanical properties of ligated fibrinogen gels. *Biopolymers* 27:703, 1988.

95. Roska FJ, Ferry JD, Lin JS, Anderegg JW: Studies of fibrin film: II. Small-angle x-ray scattering. *Biopolymers* 21:1833, 1982.

96. Roska FJ, Ferry JD: Studies of fibrin film: I. Stress relaxation and bi-refringence. *Biopolymers* 21:1811, 1982.

97. McKee PA, Mattock P, Hill RL: Subunit structure of human fibrinogen, soluble fibrin, and cross-linked insoluble fibrin. *Proc Natl Acad Sci U S A* 66:738, 1970.

98. Shainoff JR, Urbanic DA, DiBello PM: Immunoelectrophoretic characterizations of the cross-linking of fibrinogen and fibrin by factor XIIIa and tissue transglutaminase. *J Biol Chem* 266:6429, 1991.

99. Stathakis NE, Mosesson MW, Chen AB, Galanakis DK: Cryoprecipitation of fibrin-fibrinogen complexes induced by the cold-insoluble globulin of plasma. *Blood* 51:1211, 1978.

100. Tamaki T, Aoki H: Cross-linking of α_2-plasmin inhibitor and fibronectin to fibrin by fibrin-stabilizing factor. *Biochim Biophys Acta* 661:280, 1981.

101. Sobel JH, Ehrlich PH, Birken S, et al: Monoclonal antibody to the region of fibronectin involved in cross-linking to human fibrin. *Biochemistry* 22:4175, 1983.

102. Kimura S, Aoki N: Cross-linking site in fibrinogen for alpha 2-plasmin inhibitor. *J Biol Chem* 261:15591, 1986.

103. Siebenlist KR, Mosesson MW, Meh DA, et al: Coexisting dysfibrinogenemia (γR275C) and factor V Leiden deficiency associated with thromboembolic disease (fibrinogen Cedar Rapids). *Blood Coagul Fibrinolysis* 11:293, 2000.

104. Odrljin TM, Shainoff JR, Lawrence SO, Simpson-Haidaris PJ: Thrombin cleavage enhances exposure of a heparin binding domain in the N-terminus of the fibrin β chain. *Blood* 88:2050, 1996.

105. Odrljin TM, Francis CW, Sporn LA, et al: Heparin binding domain of fibrin mediates its binding to endothelial cells. *Arterioscler Thromb Vasc Biol* 16:1544, 1996.

106. Erban JK, Wagner DD: A 130-kDa protein on endothelial cells binds to amino acids 15-42 of the B beta chain of fibrinogen. *J Biol Chem* 267:2451, 1992.

107. Bach TL, Barsigian C, Yaen CH, Martinez J: Endothelial cell VE-cadherin functions as a receptor for the β15-42 sequence of fibrin. *J Biol Chem* 273:30719, 1998.

108. Hamaguchi M, Bunce LA, Sporn LA, Francis CW: Spreading of platelets on fibrin is mediated by the amino terminus of the β chain including peptide β 15-42. *Blood* 81:2348, 1993.

109. Sporn LA, Bunce LA, Francis CW: Cell proliferation on fibrin: Modulation by fibrinopeptide cleavage. *Blood* 86:1801, 1995.

110. Chalupowicz DG, Chowdhury ZA, Bach TL, et al: Fibrin II induces endothelial cell capillary tube formation. *J Cell Biol* 130:207, 1995.

111. Ribes JA, Bunce LA, Francis CW: Mediation of fibrin-induced release of von Willebrand factor from cultured endothelial cells by the fibrin β chain. *J Clin Invest* 84:435, 1989.

112. Francis CW, Bunce LA, Sporn LA: Endothelial cell responses to fibrin mediated by FPB cleavage and the amino terminus of the β chain. *Blood Cells* 19:291, 1993.

113. Altieri DC, Plescia J, Plow EF: The structural motif glycine 190-valine 202 of the fibrinogen γ chain interacts with CD11b/CD18 integrin ($\alpha_M\beta_2$, Mac-1) and promotes leukocyte adhesion. *J Biol Chem* 268:1847, 1993.

114. Hoylaerts M, Rijken DC, Lijnen HR, Collen D: Kinetics of the activation of plasminogen by human tissue plasminogen. *J Biol Chem* 257:2912, 1982.

115. Ranby M: Studies on the kinetics of plasminogen activation by tissue plasminogen activator. *Biochim Biophys Acta* 704:461, 1982.

116. Schielen WJ, Voskuilen M, Tesser GI, Nieuwenhuizen W: The sequence A alpha-(148-160) in fibrin, but not in fibrinogen, is accessible to monoclonal antibodies. *Proc Natl Acad Sci U S A* 86:8951, 1989.

117. Schielen WJ, Adams HP, van Leuven K, et al: The sequence gamma-(312-324) is a fibrin-specific epitope. *Blood* 77:2169, 1991.

118. Schielen WJG, Adams HPHM, Voskuilen M, et al: The sequence Aα-(154-159) of fibrinogen is capable of accelerating the tPA catalyzed activation of plasminogen. *Blood Coagul Fibrinolysis* 2:465, 1991.

119. Lezhen TI, Kudinov SA, Medved' LV: Plasminogen-binding site of the thermostable region of fibrinogen fragment D. *FEBS Lett* 197:59, 1986.

120. Bosma PJ, Rijken DC, Nieuwenhuizen W: Binding of tissue-type plasminogen activator to fibrinogen fragments. *Eur J Biochem* 172:399, 1988.

121. de Munk GA, Caspers MP, Chang GT, et al: Binding of tissue-type plasminogen activator to lysine, lysine analogues, and fibrin fragments. *Biochemistry* 28:7318, 1989.

122. Yakovlev S, Makogonenko E, Kurochkina N, et al: Conversion of fibrinogen to fibrin: Mechanism of exposure of tPA- and plasminogen-binding sites. *Biochemistry* 39:15730, 2000.

123. Nieuwenhuizen W: Fibrin-mediated plasminogen activation. *Ann N Y Acad Sci* 936:237, 2001.

124. Yonekawa O, Voskuilen M, Nieuwenhuizen W: Localization in the fibrinogen gamma-chain of a new site that is involved in the acceleration of the tissue-type plasminogen activator-catalysed activation of plasminogen. *Biochem J* 283(Pt 1):187, 1992.

125. Grailhe P, Nieuwenhuizen W, Angles-Cano E: Study of tissue-type plasminogen activator binding sites on fibrin using distinct fragments of fibrinogen. *Eur J Biochem* 219:961, 1994.

126. Mosesson MW, Siebenlist KR, Voskuilen M, Nieuwenhuizen W: Evaluation of the factors contributing to fibrin-dependent plasminogen activation. *Thromb Haemost* 79:796, 1998.

127. Glueck CJ, Glueck HI, Greenfield D, et al: Protein C and S deficiency, thrombophilia, and hypofibrinolysis: Pathophysiologic causes of Legg Perthes disease. *Pediatr Res* 35:383, 1994.

128. Glueck CJ, Glueck HI, Welch M, et al: Familial idiopathic osteonecrosis mediated by familial hypofibrinolysis with high levels of plasminogen activator inhibitor. *Thromb Haemost* 71:195, 1994.

129. Glueck CJ, Freiberg R, Glueck HI, et al: Hypofibrinolysis: A common, major cause of osteonecrosis. *Am J Hematol* 45:156, 1994.

130. Glueck CJ, Freiberg R, Glueck HI, et al: Idiopathic osteonecrosis, hypofibrinolysis, high plasminogen activator inhibitor, high lipoprotein(a), and therapy with Stanozolol. *Am J Hematol* 48:213, 1995.

131. Glueck CJ, Freiberg R, Tracy T, et al: Thrombophilia and hypofibrinolysis: Pathophysiologies of osteonecrosis. *Clin Orthop* 334:43, 1997.

132. Gruppo R, Glueck CJ, Wall E, et al: Legg-Perthes disease in three siblings, two heterozygous and one homozygous for the factor V Leiden mutation. *J Pediatr* 132:885, 1998.

133. Glueck CJ, Freiberg RA, Fontaine RNP, et al: Hypofibrinolysis, thrombophilia, osteonecrosis. *Clin Orthop* 386:19, 2001.

134. Posan E, Szepesi K, Gaspar L, et al: Thrombotic and fibrinolytic alterations in the aseptic necrosis of femoral head. *Blood Coagul Fibrinolysis* 14:243, 2003.

135. Glueck CJ, Freiberg RA, Wang P: Role of thrombosis in osteonecrosis. *Curr Hematol Rep* 2:417, 2003.

136. Lefebvre P, Velasco PT, Dear A, et al: Severe hypodysfibrinogenemia in compound heterozygotes of the fibrinogen AalphaIVS4 + 1G→T mutation and an AalphaGln328 truncation (fibrinogen Keokuk). *Blood* 103:2571, 2004.

137. Fenton JW II, Olson TA, Zabinski MP, Wilner GD: Anion-binding exosite of human α-thrombin and fibrin(ogen) recognition. *Biochemistry* 27:7106, 1988.

138. Stubbs MT, Bode W: A player of many parts: The spotlight falls on thrombin's structure. *Thromb Res* 69:1, 1993.

139. Mosesson MW, Hernandez I, Siebenlist KR: Evidence that catalytically-inactivated thrombin forms non-covalently linked dimers that bridge between fibrin/fibrinogen fibers and enhance fibrin polymerization. *Biophys Chem* 110:93, 2004.

140. Scheraga HA: Interaction of thrombin and fibrinogen and the polymerization of fibrin monomer. *Ann N Y Acad Sci* 408:330, 1983.

141. Pechik I, Madrazo J, Mosesson MW, et al: Crystal structure of the complex between thrombin and the central "E" region of fibrin. *Proc Natl Acad Sci U S A* 101:2718, 2004.

142. Seegers WH, Nieft M, Loomis EC: Note on the adsorption of thrombin on fibrin. *Science* 101:520, 1945.

143. Vali Z, Scheraga HA: Localization of the binding site on fibrin for the secondary binding site of thrombin. *Biochemistry* 27:1956, 1988.

144. Binnie CG, Lord ST: A synthetic analog of fibrinogen α27-50 is an inhibitor of thrombin. *Thromb Haemost* 65:165, 1991.

145. Lovely RS, Moaddel M, Farrell DH: Fibrinogen γ′ chain binds thrombin exosite II. *J Thromb Haemost* 1:124, 2003.

146. Pospisil CH, Stafford AR, Fredenburgh JC, Weitz JI: Evidence that both exosites on thrombin participate in its high affinity interaction with fibrin. *J Biol Chem* 278:21584, 2003.

147. Meh DA, Mosesson MW, Siebenlist KR, et al: Fibrinogen Naples I (Bβ A68T) non-substrate thrombin binding capacities. *Thromb Res* 103:63, 2001.

148. Liu CY, Nossel HL, Kaplan KL: Defective thrombin binding by abnormal fibrin associated with recurrent thrombosis [abstract]. *Thromb Haemost* 42:79, 1979.

149. Koopman J, Haverkate F, Lord ST, et al: Molecular basis of fibrinogen Naples associated with defective thrombin binding and thrombophilia. Homozygous substitution of B beta 68 Ala—Thr. *J Clin Invest* 90:238, 1992.

150. Di Minno G, Martinez J, Cirillo F, et al: A role for platelets and thrombin in the juvenile stroke of two siblings with defective thrombin-absorbing capacity of fibrin(ogen). *Arterioscler Thromb* 11:785, 1991.

151. Caen J, Faur Y, Inceman S, et al: Nécrose ischémique bilatérale dans un cas de grande hypofibrinogénémie congénitale. *Nouv Rev Fr Hematol* 4:321, 1964.

152. Marchal G, Duhamel G, Samama M, Flandrin G: Thrombose massive des vaisseaux d'un membre au cours d'une hypofibrinémie congénitale. *Hémostase* 4:81, 1964.

153. Nilsson IM, Niléhn J-E, Cronberg S, Nordén G: Hypofibrinogenemia and massive thrombosis. *Acta Med Scand* 180:65, 1966.

154. Ingram GI, McBrien DJ, Spencer H: Fatal pulmonary embolism in congenital fibrinopenia. *Acta Haematol* 35:56, 1966.

155. Mackinnon HH, Fekete JF: Congenital afibrinogenemia: Vascular changes and multiple thrombosis induced by fibrinogen infusions and contraceptive medication. *Can Med Assoc J* 140:597, 1971.

156. Cronin C, Fitzpatrick D, Temperly I: Multiple pulmonary emboli in a patient with afibrinogenaemia. *Acta Haematol* 7:53, 1988.

157. Drai E, Taillan B, Schneider S, et al: Thrombose portale révélatrice d'une afibrinogénémie congénitale. *Presse Med* 21:1820, 1992.

158. Dupuy E, Soria C, Molho P, et al: Embolized ischemic lesions of toes in an afibrinogenemic patient: Possible relevance to in vivo circulating thrombin. *Thromb Res* 102:211, 2001.

159. Chafa O, Chellali T, Sternberg C, et al: Severe hypofibrinogenemia associated with bilateral ischemic necrosis of toes and fingers. *Blood Coagul Fibrinolysis* 6:549, 1995.

160. Lak M, Keihani M, Elahi F, et al: Bleeding and thrombosis in 55 patients with inherited afibrinogenaemia. *Br J Haematol* 107:204, 1999.

161. Schuepbach RA, Meili EO, Schneider E, et al: Lepirudin therapy for thrombotic complications in congential afibrinogenemia. *Thromb Haemost* 91:1044, 2004.

162. de Bosch N, Sáez A, Soria C, et al: Coagulation profile in afibrinogenemia [abstract]. *Thromb Haemost* 78(suppl):625, 1997.

163. Korte W, Feldges A: Increased prothrombin activation in a patient with congenital afibrinogenemia is reversible by fibrinogen substitution. *Clin Invest* 72:396, 1994.

164. Ni H, Denis CV, Subbarao S, et al: Persistence of platelet thrombus formation in arterioles of mice lacking both von Willebrand factor and fibrinogen. *J Clin Invest* 106:385, 2000.

165. Neerman-Arbez M, Honsberger A, Antonarakis SE, Morris MA: Deletion of the fibrinogen [correction of fibrogen] alpha-chain gene (FGA) causes congenital afibrogenemia. *J Clin Invest* 103:215, 1999.

166. Neerman-Arbez M: The molecular basis of inherited afibrinogenaemia. *Thromb Haemost* 86:154, 2001.

167. Spena S, Duga S, Asselta R, et al: Congenital afibrinogenemia: First identification of splicing mutations in the fibrinogen Bbeta-chain gene causing activation of cryptic splice sites. *Blood* 100:4478, 2002.

168. Asselta R, Spena S, Duga S, et al: Analysis of Iranian patients allowed the identification of the first truncating mutation in the fibrinogen Bbeta-chain gene causing afibrinogenemia. *Haematologica* 87:855, 2002.

169. Homer VM, Brennan SO, Ockelford P, George PM: Novel fibrinogen truncation with deletion of Bbeta chain residues 440-461 causes hypofibrinogenaemia. *Thromb Haemost* 88:427, 2002.

170. Remijn JA, van Wijk R, Nieuwenhuis HK, et al: Molecular basis of congenital afibrinogenaemia in a Dutch family. *Blood Coagul Fibrinolysis* 14:299, 2003.

171. Neerman-Arbez M, Vu D, Abu-Libdeh B, et al: Prenatal diagnosis for congenital afibrinogenemia caused by a novel nonsense mutation in the FGB gene in a Palestinian family. *Blood* 101:3492, 2003.

172. Duga S, Asselta R, Santagostino E, et al: Missense mutations in the human beta fibrinogen gene cause congenital afibrinogenemia by impairing fibrinogen secretion. *Blood* 95:1336, 2000.

173. Duga S, Asselta R, Santagostino E, et al: Involvement of fibrinogen Bbeta-chain gene in the pathogenesis of congenital afibrinogenemia [abstract]. *Thromb Haemost* 86(suppl):P1108, 2001.

174. Vu D, Bolton-Maggs PH, Parr JR, et al: Congenital afibrinogenemia: Identification and expression of a missense mutation in FGB impairing fibrinogen secretion. *Blood* 102:4413, 2003.

175. Brennan SO, Fellowes AP, George PM: Molecular mechanisms of hypo- and afibrinogenemia. *Ann N Y Acad Sci* 936:91, 2001.

176. Brennan SO, Wyatt J, Medicina D, et al: Fibrinogen Brescia: Hepatic endoplasmic reticulum storage and hypofibrinogenemia because of a gamma284 Gly→Arg mutation. *Am J Pathol* 157:189, 2000.

177. Brennan SO, Wyatt JM, May S, et al: Hypofibrinogenemia due to novel 316 Asp→Tyr substitution in the fibrinogen Bbeta chain. *Thromb Haemost* 85:450, 2001.

178. Brennan SO, Maghzal G, Shneider BL, et al: Novel fibrinogen gamma375 Arg→Trp mutation (fibrinogen Aguadilla) causes hepatic endoplasmic reticulum storage and hypofibrinogenemia. *Hepatology* 36:652, 2002.

179. Callea F, Brisigotti M, Fabbretti G, et al: Hepatic endoplasmic reticulum storage diseases. *Liver* 12:357, 1992.

180. Medicina D, Fabbretti G, Brennan SO, et al: Genetic and immunological characterization of fibrinogen inclusion bodies in patients with hepatic fibrinogen storage and liver disease. *Ann N Y Acad Sci* 936:522, 2001.

181. Brennan SO, Fellowes AP, Faed JM, George PM: Hypofibrinogenemia in an individual with 2 coding (gamma82 A→G and Bbeta235 P→L) and 2 noncoding mutations. *Blood* 95:1709, 2000.

182. Wyatt J, Brennan SO, May S, George PM: Hypofibrinogenaemia with compound heterozygosity for two gamma chain mutations: gamma 82 Ala→Gly and an intron two GT→AT splice site mutation. *Thromb Haemost* 84:449, 2000.

183. Maghzal GJ, Brennan SO, Fellowes AP, et al: Familial hypofibrinogenaemia associated with heterozygous substitution of a conserved arginine residue; Bbeta255 Arg→His (Fibrinogen Merivale). *Biochim Biophys Acta* 1645:146, 2003.

184. Asselta R, Duga S, Spena S, et al: Missense or splicing mutation? The case of a fibrinogen Bbeta-chain mutation causing severe hypofibrinogenemia. *Blood* 103:3051, 2004.

185. Weiss HJ, Rogers J: Fibrinogen and platelets in the primary arrest of bleeding. Studies in two patients with congenital afibrinogenemia. *N Engl J Med* 285:369, 1971.

186. Girolami A, De Marco L, Virgolini L, et al: Platelet adhesiveness and aggregation in congenital afibrinogenemia. An investigation of three patients with post-transfusion, cross-correction studies between two of them. *Blut* 30:87, 1975.

187. Cattaneo M, Bettega D, Lombardi R, et al: Sustained correction of the bleeding time in an afibrinogenaemic patient after infusion of fresh frozen plasma. *Br J Haematol* 82:388, 1992.

188. Inamoto Y, Terao T: First report of case of congenital afibrinogenemia with successful delivery. *Am J Obstet Gynecol* 153:803, 1985.

189. De Vries A, Rosenberg T, Kochwa S, Boss JH: Precipitating antifibrinogen antibody appearing after fibrinogen infusions in a patient with congenital afibrinogenemia. *Am J Med* 30:486, 1961.

190. Hanss MM, Ffrench PO, Mornex JF, et al: Two novel fibrinogen variants found in patients with pulmonary embolism and their families. *J Thromb Haemost* 1:1251, 2003.

191. Blomback M, Blomback B, Mammen EF, Prasad AS: Fibrinogen Detroit: A molecular defect in the N-terminal disulphide knot of human fibrinogen? *Nature* 218:134, 1968.

192. Yamaguchi FI, Sugo T, Hashimoto Y, et al: Fibrinogen Kumamoto with an Aα Arg19→Gly substitution associated clinically with thrombosis. *Fibrinolysis* 10(suppl 4):23, 1996.

193. Yoshida N, Okuma M, Hirata H, et al: Fibrinogen Kyoto II, a new congenitally abnormal molecule, characterized by the replacement of A alpha proline-18 by leucine. *Blood* 78:149, 1991.

194. Koopman J, Haverkate F, Grimbergen J, et al: Abnormal fibrinogens IJmuiden (B beta Arg14—Cys) and Nijmegen (B beta Arg44—Cys) form disulfide-linked fibrinogen-albumin complexes. *Proc Natl Acad Sci U S A* 89:3478, 1992.

195. Engesser L, Koopman J, de Munk G, et al: Fibrinogen Nijmegen: Congenital dysfibrinogenemia associated with impaired t-PA mediated plasminogen activation and decreased binding of t-PA. *Thromb Haemost* 60:113, 1988.

196. Lord ST, Strickland E, Jayjock E: Strategy for recombinant multichain protein synthesis: Fibrinogen Bβ-chain variants as thrombin substrates. *Biochemistry* 35:2342, 1996.

197. Kamura T, Tsuda H, Yae Y, et al: An abnormal fibrinogen Fukuoka II (Gly-B beta 15→Cys) characterized by defective fibrin lateral association and mixed disulfide formation. *J Biol Chem* 270:29392, 1995.

198. Soria J, Soria C, Samama M, et al: Detection of fibrinogen abnormality in dysfibrinogenemia: Special report of fibrinogen Metz characterized by an amino acid substitution located at the peptide bond cleaved by thrombin, in *Fibrinogen—Recent Biochemical and Medical Aspects*, edited by A Henschen, H Graeff, F Lottspeich, p 129. W de Gruyter, Berlin, 1982.

199. Alving BM, Henschen AH: Fibrinogen Giessen I: A congenital homozygously expressed dysfibrinogenemia with A alpha 16 Arg—His substitution. *Am J Hematol* 25:479, 1987.

200. Siebenlist KR, Prchal JT, Mosesson MW: Fibrinogen Birmingham: A heterozygous dysfibrinogenemia (Aα 16 Arg→His) containing heterodimeric molecules. *Blood* 71:613, 1988.

201. Carrell N, McDonagh J: Fibrinogen Chapel Hill II: Defective in reactions with thrombin, factor XIIIa and plasmin. *Br J Haematol* 52:35, 1982.

202. Wada Y, Niwa K, Maekawa H, et al: A new type of congenital dysfibrinogen, fibrinogen Bremen, with an A alpha Gly-17 to Val substitution associated with hemorrhagic diathesis and delayed wound healing. *Thromb Haemost* 70:397, 1993.

203. Shainoff JR, Dardik BN: Fibrinopeptide B and aggregation of fibrinogen. *Science* 204:200, 1979.

204. Hirota-Kawadobora M, Terasawa F, Yonekawa O, et al: Fibrinogens

205. Kosai and Ogasa: Bbeta15Gly→Cys (GGT→TGT) substitution associated with impairment of fibrinopeptide B release and lateral aggregation. *J Thromb Haemost* 1:275, 2003.

205. Liu CY, Wallen P, Handley DA: Fibrinogen New York I: The structural, functional, and genetic defects and an hypothesis of the role of fibrin in the regulation of coagulation and fibrinolysis, in *Fibrinogen, Fibrin Formation and Fibrinolysis*, edited by DA Lane, A Henschen, MK Jasani, p 79. W de Gruyter, Berlin, 1986.

206. Côté HCF, Lord ST, Pratt KP: γ-chain dysfibrinogenemias: Molecular structure-function relationships of naturally occurring mutations in the γ chain of human fibrinogen. *Blood* 92:2195, 1998.

207. Everse SJ, Spraggon G, Doolittle RF: A three-dimensional consideration of variant human fibrinogens. *Thromb Haemost* 80:1, 1998.

208. Okumura N, Furihata K, Terasawa F, et al: Fibrinogen Matsumoto I: A gamma 364 Asp→His (GAT→CAT) substitution associated with defective fibrin polymerization. *Thromb Haemost* 75:887, 1996.

209. Bentolila S, Samama MM, Conard J, et al: Association of dysfibrinogenemia and thrombosis. Apropos of a family (Fibrinogen Melun) and review of the literature. *Ann Med Interne (Paris)* 146:575, 1995.

210. Terukina S, Yamazumi K, Okamoto K, et al: Fibrinogen Kyoto III: A congenital dysfibrinogen with a gamma aspartic acid-330 to tyrosine substitution manifesting impaired fibrin monomer polymerization. *Blood* 74:2681, 1989.

211. Reber P, Furlan M, Rupp C, et al: Characterization of fibrinogen Milano I: Amino acid exchange gamma 330 Asp→Val impairs fibrin polymerization. *Blood* 67:1751, 1986.

212. Miyata T, Furukawa K, Iwanaga S, et al: Fibrinogen Nagoya, a replacement of glutamine-329 by arginine in the gamma chain that impairs the polymerization of fibrin monomer. *J Biochem (Tokyo)* 105:10, 1989.

213. Yoshida N, Hirata H, Morigami Y, et al: Characterization of an abnormal fibrinogen Osaka V with the replacement of gamma-arginine 375 by glycine. The lack of high affinity calcium binding to D-domains and the lack of protective effect of calcium on fibrinolysis. *J Biol Chem* 267: 2753, 1992.

214. Steinmann C, Reber P, Jungo M, et al: Fibrinogen Bern I: Substitution gamma 337 Asn→Lys is responsible for defective fibrin monomer polymerization. *Blood* 82:2104, 1993.

215. Steinmann C, Bogli C, Jungo M, et al: A new substitution, gamma 358 Ser→Cys, in fibrinogen Milano VII causes defective fibrin polymerization. *Blood* 84:1874, 1994.

216. Mathonnet F, Guillon L, Detruit H, et al: Fibrinogen Poissy II (gammaN361K): A novel dysfibrinogenemia associated with defective polymerization and peptide B release. *Blood Coagul Fibrinolysis* 14: 293, 2003.

217. Kaudewitz H, Henschen A, Soria J, Soria C: Fibrinogen Pontoise—A genetically abnormal fibrinogen with defective fibrin polymerization but normal fibrinopeptide release, in *Fibrinogen, Fibrin Formation and Fibrinolysis*, edited by DA Lane, A Henschen, MK Jasani, p 91. W de Gruyter, Berlin, 1986.

218. DiOrio JP, Mosesson MW, Matsuda M: Fibrinogen Kurashiki (γG268E) fibrin network structure. *Microsc Microanal* 4(suppl 2):1160, 1998.

219. Matsuda M, Baba M, Morimoto K, Nakamikawa C: "Fibrinogen Tokyo II." An abnormal fibrinogen with an impaired polymerization site on the aligned DD domain of fibrin molecules. *J Clin Invest* 72:1034, 1983.

220. Siebenlist KR, Mosesson MW, Di Orio JP, et al: The polymerization of fibrin prepared from fibrinogen Haifa (gamma 275Arg→His). *Thromb Haemost* 62:875, 1989.

221. Fellowes AP, Brennan SO, Ridgway HJ, et al: Electrospray ionization mass spectrometry identification of fibrinogen Banks Peninsula (gamma280Tyr→Cys): A new variant with defective polymerization. *Br J Haematol* 101:24, 1998.

222. Beck EA, Charache P, Jackson DP: A new inherited coagulation disorder caused by an abnormal fibrinogen ("Fibrinogen Baltimore"). *Nature* 208:143, 1965.

223. Bantia S, Bell WR, Dang CV: Polymerization defect of fibrinogen Baltimore III due to a gamma Asn308→Ile mutation. *Blood* 75:1659, 1990.

224. Yoshida N, Terukina S, Okuma M, et al: Characterization of an apparently lower molecular weight gamma-chain variant in fibrinogen Kyoto I. The replacement of gamma-asparagine 308 by lysine which causes accelerated cleavage of fragment D1 by plasmin and the generation of a new plasmin cleavage site. *J Biol Chem* 263:13848, 1988.

225. Grailhe P, Boyer-Neumann C, Haverkate F, et al: The mutation in fibrinogen Bicetre II (gamma Asn308→Lys) does not affect the binding of t-PA and plasminogen to fibrin. *Blood Coagul Fibrinolysis* 4:679, 1993.

226. Okumura N, Furihata K, Terasawa F, et al: Fibrinogen Matsumoto II: Gamma 308 Asn→Lys (AAT→AAG) mutation associated with bleeding tendency. *Br J Haematol* 94:526, 1996.

227. Yamazumi K, Shimura K, Terukina S, et al: A gamma methionine-310 to threonine substitution and consequent N-glycosylation at gamma asparagine-308 identified in a congenital dysfibrinogenemia associated with posttraumatic bleeding, fibrinogen Asahi. *J Clin Invest* 83:1590, 1989.

228. Mosesson MW, Amrani DL, Ménaché D: Studies on the structural abnormality of fibrinogen Paris I. *J Clin Invest* 57:782, 1976.

229. Galanakis DK, Spitzer SG, Scharrer I, Peerschke EIB: Impaired platelet aggregation support by two dysfibrinogens: A γ319-320 deletion and a γ310 Met→Thr substitution [abstract]. *Thromb Haemost* 69:2564, 1993.

230. Koopman J, Haverkate F, Briet E, Lord ST: A congenitally abnormal fibrinogen (Vlissingen) with a 6-base deletion in the gamma-chain gene, causing defective calcium binding and impaired fibrin polymerization. *J Biol Chem* 266:13456, 1991.

231. Menache D: Constitutional and familial abnormal fibrinogen. *Thromb Diath Haemorrh* (suppl 13):173, 1964.

232. Rosenberg JB, Newman PJ, Mosesson MW, et al: Paris I dysfibrinogenemia: A point mutation in intron 8 results in insertion of a 15 amino acid sequence in the fibrinogen γ-chain. *Thromb Haemost* 69:217, 1993.

233. Denninger MH, Jandrot-Perrus M, Elion J, et al: ADP-induced platelet aggregation depends on the conformation or availability of the terminal gamma chain sequence of fibrinogen. Study of the reactivity of fibrinogen Paris 1. *Blood* 70:558, 1987.

234. Koopman J, Haverkate F, Grimbergen J, et al: Fibrinogen Marburg: A homozygous case of dysfibrinogenemia, lacking amino acids A alpha 461-610 (Lys 461 AAA→stop TAA). *Blood* 80:1972, 1992.

235. Furlan M, Steinmann C, Jungo M, et al: A frameshift mutation in Exon V of the A alpha-chain gene leading to truncated A alpha-chains in the homozygous dysfibrinogen Milano III. *J Biol Chem* 269:33129, 1994.

236. Furlan M, Steinmann C, Jungo M, Lammle B: Binding of calcium ions and their effect on clotting of fibrinogen Milano III, a variant with truncated A alpha-chains. *Blood Coagul Fibrinolysis* 7:331, 1996.

237. Soria J, Soria C, Caen P: A new type of congenital dysfibrinogenaemia with defective fibrin lysis—Dusard syndrome: Possible relation to thrombosis. *Br J Haematol* 53:575, 1983.

238. Lijnen HR, Soria J, Soria C, et al: Dysfibrinogenemia (fibrinogen Dusard) associated with impaired fibrin-enhanced plasminogen activation. *Thromb Haemost* 51:108, 1984.

239. Koopman J, Haverkate F, Grimbergen J, et al: Molecular basis for fibrinogen Dusart (A alpha 554 Arg→Cys) and its association with abnormal fibrin polymerization and thrombophilia. *J Clin Invest* 91:1637, 1993.

240. Collet JP, Soria J, Mirshahi M, et al: Dusart syndrome: A new concept of the relationship between fibrin clot architecture and fibrin clot degradability: Hypofibrinolysis related to an abnormal clot structure. *Blood* 82:2462, 1993.

241. Siebenlist KR, Mosesson MW, DiOrio JP, et al: The polymerization of fibrinogen Dusart (A alpha 554 Arg→Cys) after removal of carboxy terminal regions of the A alpha-chains. *Blood Coagul Fibrinolysis* 4:61, 1993.

242. Mosesson MW, Siebenlist KR, Hainfeld JF, et al: The relationship between the fibrinogen D domain self-association/crosslinking site (γXL) and the fibrinogen Dusart abnormality (Aα R554C-albumin). *J Clin Invest* 97:2342, 1996.

243. Ridgway HJ, Brennan SO, Faed JM, George PM: Fibrinogen Otago: A major alpha chain truncation associated with severe hypofibrinogenaemia and recurrent miscarriage. *Br J Haematol* 98:632, 1997.

244. Homer VM, Mullin JL, Brennan SO, et al: Novel Aalpha chain truncation (fibrinogen Perth) resulting in low expression and impaired fibrinogen polymerization. *J Thromb Haemost* 1:1245, 2003.

245. Maekawa H, Yamazumi K, Muramatsu S, et al: An Aα Ser 434 to N-glycosylated Asn substitution in a dysfibrinogen, fibrinogen Caracas II, characterized by impaired fibrin gel formation. *J Biol Chem* 266:11575, 1991.

246. Woodhead JL, Nagaswami C, Matsuda M, et al: The ultrastructure of fibrinogen Caracas II molecules, fibers, and clots. *J Biol Chem* 271:4946, 1996.

247. Maekawa H, Yamazumi K, Muramatsu S, et al: Fibrinogen Lima: A homozygous dysfibrinogen with an A alpha-arginine-141 to serine substitution associated with extra N-glycosylation at A alpha-asparagine-139. Impaired fibrin gel formation but normal fibrin-facilitated plasminogen activation catalyzed by tissue-type plasminogen activator. *J Clin Invest* 90:67, 1992.

248. Benson MD: Amyloidosis, in *The Metabolic Basis of Inherited Disease*, edited by CR Scriver, AL Beaudet, WS Sly, DV Valle, p 4159. McGraw-Hill, New York, 1995.

249. Lachmann HJ, Booth DR, Booth SE, et al: Misdiagnosis of hereditary amyloidosis as AL (primary) amyloidosis. *N Engl J Med* 346:1786, 2002.

250. Benson MD, Liepnieks J, Uemichi T, et al: Hereditary renal amyloidosis associated with a mutant fibrinogen alpha-chain. *Nat Genet* 3:252, 1993.

251. Uemichi T, Liepnieks JJ, Gertz MA, Benson MD: Fibrinogen A alpha chain Leu 554: An African-American kindred with late onset renal amyloidosis. *Amyloid* 5:188, 1998.

252. Uemichi T, Liepnieks JJ, Benson MD: Hereditary renal amyloidosis with a novel variant fibrinogen. *J Clin Invest* 93:731, 1994.

253. Uemichi T, Liepnieks JJ, Alexander F, Benson MD: The molecular basis of renal amyloidosis in Irish-American and Polish-Canadian kindreds. *QJM* 89:745, 1996.

254. Uemichi T, Liepnieks JJ, Yamada T, et al: A frame shift mutation in the fibrinogen A alpha chain gene in a kindred with renal amyloidosis. *Blood* 87:4197, 1996.

255. Hamidi AL, Liepnieks JJ, Uemichi T, et al: Renal amyloidosis with a frame shift mutation in fibrinogen alpha-chain gene producing a novel amyloid protein. *Blood* 90:4799, 1997.

256. Brennan SO, Hammonds B, George PM: Aberrant hepatic processing causes removal of activation peptide and primary polymerisation site from fibrinogen Canterbury (A alpha 20 Val→Asp). *J Clin Invest* 96:2854, 1995.

257. Hamano A, Mimuro J, Aoshima M, et al: Thrombophilic dysfibrinogen Tokyo V with the amino acid substitution of gammaAla327Thr: Formation of fragile but fibrinolysis-resistant fibrin clots and its relevance to arterial thromboembolism. *Blood* 103:3045, 2004.

258. Meyer M, Franke K, Richter W, et al: New molecular defects in the gamma subdomain of fibrinogen D-domain in four cases of (hypo)dysfibrinogenemia: Fibrinogen variants Hannover VI, Homburg VII, Stuttgart and Suhl. *Thromb Haemost* 89:637, 2003.

259. Haverkate F, Samama M: Familial dysfibrinogenemia and thrombophil-

ia. Report on a study of the SSC Subcommittee on Fibrinogen. *Thromb Haemost* 73:151, 1995.

260. Brook JG, Tabori S, Tatarsky I, et al: Fibrinogen "Haifa"; A new fibrinogen variant. A case report. *Haemostasis* 13:277, 1983.

261. Borrell M, Gari M, Coll I, et al: Abnormal polymerization and normal binding of plasminogen and t-PA in three new dysfibrinogenaemias: Barcelona III and IV (gamma Arg 275→His) and Villajoyosa (gamma Arg 275→Cys). *Blood Coagul Fibrinolysis* 6:198, 1995.

262. Reber P, Furlan M, Henschen A, et al: Three abnormal fibrinogen variants with the same amino acid substitution (gamma 275 Arg→His): Fibrinogens Bergamo II, Essen and Perugia. *Thromb Haemost* 56:401, 1986.

263. Bick RL, Kaplan H: Syndromes of thrombosis and hypercoagulability. Congenital and acquired causes of thrombosis. *Med Clin North Am* 82:409, 1998.

264. Dahlback B: Inherited thrombophilia: Resistance to activated protein C as a pathogenic factor of venous thromboembolism. *Blood* 85:607, 1995.

265. Bertina RM, Koeleman BP, Koster T, et al: Mutation in blood coagulation factor V associated with resistance to activated protein C. *Nature* 369:64, 1994.

266. Zoller B, Dahlback B: Linkage between inherited resistance to activated protein C and factor V gene mutation in venous thrombosis. *Lancet* 343:1536, 1994.

267. Greengard JS, Sun X, Xu X, et al: Activated protein C resistance caused by Arg506Gln mutation in factor Va. *Lancet* 343:1361, 1994.

268. Voorberg J, Roelse J, Koopman R, et al: Association of idiopathic venous thromboembolism with single point-mutation at Arg506 of factor V. *Lancet* 343:1535, 1994.

269. Ridgway HJ, Brennan SO, Loreth RM, George PM: Fibrinogen Kaiserslautern (gamma 380 Lys to Asn): A new glycosylated fibrinogen variant with delayed polymerization. *Br J Haematol* 99:562, 1997.

270. Brennan SO, Loreth RM, George PM: Oligosaccharide configuration of fibrinogen Kaiserslautern: Electrospray ionisation analysis of intact gamma chains. *Thromb Haemost* 80:263, 1998.

271. Dang CV, Ebert RF, Bell WR: Localization of a fibrinogen calcium binding site between gamma-subunit positions 311 and 336 by terbium fluorescence. *J Biol Chem* 260:9713, 1985.

272. Haverkate F, Timan G: Protective effect of calcium in the plasmin degradation of fibrinogen and fibrin fragments D. *Thromb Res* 10:803, 1977.

273. Terasawa F, Hogan KA, Kani S, et al: Fibrinogen Otsu I: A gamma Asn319,Asp320 deletion dysfibrinogen identified in an asymptomatic pregnant woman. *Thromb Haemost* 90:757, 2003.

274. Sugo T, Nakamikawa C, Takebe M, et al: Factor XIIIa cross-linking of the Marburg fibrin: Formation of alpha and gamma-heteromultimers and the alpha-chain-linked albumin gamma complex, and disturbed protofibril assembly resulting in acquisition of plasmin resistance relevant to thrombophilia. *Blood* 91:3282, 1998.

275. Gabriel DA, Muga K, Boothroyd EM: The effect of fibrin structure on fibrinolysis. *J Biol Chem* 267:24259, 1992.

276. Carr ME Jr, Alving BM: Effect of fibrin structure on plasmin-mediated dissolution of plasma clots. *Blood Coagul Fibrinolysis* 6:567, 1995.

277. Wada Y, Lord ST: A correlation between thrombotic disease and a specific fibrinogen abnormality (Aα 554 Arg→Cys) in two unrelated kindred, Dusart and Chapel Hill III. *Blood* 84:3709, 1994.

278. Marchi R, Lundberg U, Grimbergen J, et al: Fibrinogen Caracas V, an abnormal fibrinogen with an Aalpha 532 Ser→Cys substitution associated with thrombosis. *Thromb Haemost* 84:263, 2000.

279. Marchi R, Arocha-Pinango CL, Gil F: Electron microscopy studies of 7 patients with dysfibrinogenemia and some of their relatives. *Rev Iberoamer Thromb Hemostasia* 3:185, 1990.

280. Mosesson MW, Siebenlist KR, Olson JD: Thrombophilia associated with dysfibrinogenemia [fibrinogen Cedar Rapids (γR275C)] and a heterozygous factor V Leiden defect [abstract]. *Thromb Haemost* 78(suppl):382, 1997.

281. Mimuro J, Hamano A, Tanaka T, et al: Hypofibrinogenemia caused by a nonsense mutation in the fibrinogen Bbeta chain gene. *J Thromb Haemost* 1:2356, 2003.

282. Homer VM, Brennan SO, George PM: Novel fibrinogen Bbeta gene mutation causing hypofibrinogenaemia. *Thromb Haemost* 88:1066, 2002.

283. Terasawa F, Okumura N, Kitano K, et al: Hypofibrinogenemia associated with a heterozygous missense mutation gamma153Cys to Arg (Matsumoto IV): In vitro expression demonstrates defective secretion of the variant fibrinogen. *Blood* 94:4122, 1999.

284. Brennan SO, Wyatt JM, Fellowes AP, et al: Gamma371 Thr→Ile substitution in the fibrinogen gammaD domain causes hypofibrinogenaemia. *Biochim Biophys Acta* 1550:183, 2001.

285. Meyer M, Kutscher G, Sturzebecher J, et al: Fibrinogen Magdeburg I: A novel variant of human fibrinogen with an amino acid exchange in the fibrinopeptide A (Aalpha 9, Leu→Pro). *Thromb Res* 109:145, 2003.

286. Bolliger-Stucki B, Lord ST, Furlan M: Fibrinogen Milano XII: A dysfunctional variant containing 2 amino acid substitutions, Aalpha R16C and gamma G165R. *Blood* 98:351, 2001.

287. Margaglione M, Vecchione G, Santacroce R, et al: A frameshift mutation in the human fibrinogen Aalpha-chain gene (Aalpha(499)Ala frameshift stop) leading to dysfibrinogen San Giovanni Rotondo. *Thromb Haemost* 86:1483, 2001.

288. Steinmann C, Bogli C, Jungo M, et al: Fibrinogen Milano V: A congenital dysfibrinogenaemia with a gamma 275 Arg→Cys substitution. *Blood Coagul Fibrinolysis* 5:463, 1994.

289. Steinmann C, Jungo M, Beck EA, et al: Fibrinogen Claro: Another dysfunctional fibrinogen variant with gamma 275 arginine→histidine substitution. *Thromb Res* 81:145, 1996.

290. Niwa K, Kawata Y, Madoiwa S, et al: Fibrinogen Kamogawa: A new type of gamma Arg-275 to Ser substitution characterized by delayed fibrin gel formation [abstract]. *Thromb Haemost* 73:1229, 1995.

291. Fellowes AP, Brennan SO, Ridgway HJ, et al: Electrospray ionization mass spectrometry identification of fibrinogen Banks Peninsula (gamma280Tyr→Cys): A new variant with defective polymerization. *Br J Haematol* 101:24, 1998.

292. Bantia S, Mane SM, Bell WR, Dang CV: Fibrinogen Baltimore I: Polymerization defect associated with a gamma 292Gly—Val (GGC—GTC) mutation. *Blood* 76:2279, 1990.

293. Okumura N, Terasawa F, Fujita K, et al: Evidence that heterodimers exist in the fibrinogen Matsumoto II (gamma308N→K) proband and participate in fibrin fiber formation. *Thromb Res* 107:157, 2002.

294. Galanakis DK, Peerschke EIB, Spitzer S, Scharrer I: Fibrinogen Frankfurt I, a γ357 Ala→Thr substitution associated with impaired fibrin polymerization and decreased platelet aggregation support. *Blood* 86(suppl 1):76a, 1995.

295. Ridgway HJ, Brennan SO, Gibbons S, George PM: Fibrinogen Lincoln: A new truncated alpha chain variant with delayed clotting. *Br J Haematol* 93:177, 1996.

296. Keller MA, Martinez J, Baradet TC, et al: Fibrinogen Philadelphia, a hypodysfibrinogenemia characterized by abnormal polymerization and fibrinogen hypercatabolism due to γ S378P mutation. *Blood* 105:3162, 2005.

CHAPTER 118

VON WILLEBRAND DISEASE

JILL JOHNSEN
DAVID GINSBURG

von Willebrand factor (vWF) is a central component of hemostasis that serves as a carrier for factor VIII and an adhesive link between platelets and the injured blood vessel wall. Abnormalities in vWF function result in von Willebrand disease (vWD), the most common inherited bleeding disorder in humans. The overall prevalence of vWD has been estimated to be as high as 1 percent of the general population, although the prevalence of clinically significant disease probably is closer to 1:1000. vWD is associated with either quantitative deficiency (types 1 and 3) or qualitative abnormalities of vWF (type 2). The uncommon type 3 variant is the most severe form of vWD and is characterized by very low or undetectable levels of vWF, a severe bleeding diathesis, and a generally autosomal recessive pattern of inheritance. Type 1 vWD, the most common variant, is characterized by vWF that is normal in structure and function but decreased in quantity (ranging from 20 to 50 percent of normal). In type 2 vWD, the vWF is abnormal in structure and/or function. Type 2A vWD is associated with selective loss of the largest and most functionally active vWF multimers. Type 2A is further subdivided into group 1, resulting from mutations that interfere with biosynthesis and secretion, and group 2, in which the mutant vWF exhibits an increased sensitivity to proteolysis in plasma. Type 2N vWD is characterized by mutations within the factor VIII binding domain of vWF, leading to disproportionately decreased factor VIII and a disorder resembling mild hemophilia A but with autosomal recessive inheritance. Type 2B vWD results from mutations clustered within the vWF A1 domain, in a segment critical for binding to the platelet glycoprotein Ib receptor. These mutations produce a "gain of function" resulting in spontaneous vWF binding to platelets and clearance of the resulting platelet complexes, leading to thrombocytopenia and loss of the most active (large) vWF multimers. Type 1 vWD often can be effectively managed by treatment with 1-desamino-8-D-arginine vasopressin (DDAVP [desmopressin]), which produces a twofold to threefold increase in plasma vWF level. Response to DDAVP is generally poor in type 3 and most of the type 2 vWD variants. These disorders often require treatment with factor replacement in the form of plasma or selected factor VIII concentrates containing large quantities of intact vWF multimers.

Acronyms and abbreviations that appear in this chapter include: ADAMTS13, *a* *d*isintegrin *a*nd *m*etalloprotease with *t*hrombo*s*pondin type 1 motifs; Ag, antigen; aPTT, activated partial thromboplastin time; cDNA, complementary DNA; DDAVP, 1-desamino-8-D-arginine vasopressin (desmopressin); ELISA, enzyme-linked immunosorbent assay; ER, endoplasmic reticulum; FVIII, factor VIII; Gp, glycoprotein; HHT, hereditary hemorrhagic telangiectasia; mRNA, messenger RNA; RIPA, ristocetin-induced platelet aggregation; vWD, von Willebrand disease; vWF, von Willebrand factor.

DEFINITION AND HISTORY

In 1926, Eric von Willebrand[1] described a bleeding disorder in 24 of 66 members of a family from the Åland Islands. Both sexes were afflicted, and the bleeding time was prolonged despite normal platelet counts and normal clot retraction. von Willebrand distinguished this condition from the other hemostatic diseases known at the time and recognized its genetic basis, calling the disorder "hereditary pseudohemophilia" but incorrectly characterizing the inheritance as X-linked dominant. von Willebrand's confusion about the inheritance pattern probably resulted, at least in part, from the greater recognition of bleeding symptoms in women because of the hemostatic stresses of menstruation and parturition. The proband in the original family, Hjördis, was 5 years old at the time of von Willebrand's initial evaluation and ultimately died at age 13 years during her fourth menstrual cycle. Four of Hjördis' sisters died between the ages of 2 and 4 years, and deaths among family members during childbirth were noted.

An apparently similar disorder was independently reported in the United States by Minot and others in 1928. The original family in the Åland Islands was reexamined by von Willebrand and Jürgens in 1933, leading to the conclusion that the defect in this disorder resulted from an impairment of platelet function. It was not until 1953 that Alexander and Goldstein demonstrated reduced levels of coagulation factor VIII (FVIII) in von Willebrand disease (vWD) patients, along with prolonged bleeding time. This observation was confirmed by others, including studies of the original von Willebrand pedigree by Nilsson and coworkers. In the late 1950s, the latter group demonstrated that a fraction of plasma referred to as "I-O" could correct the FVIII deficiency and normalize the bleeding time, indicating that the defect in vWD resulted from deficiency of a plasma factor rather than an intrinsic platelet abnormality. Infusion of fraction I-O promptly increased the FVIII level in a hemophilic patient, whereas in vWD the FVIII level rose gradually, peaking at 5 to 8 hours. Fraction I-O prepared from a hemophilia A patient corrected the defect in vWD, demonstrating that these disorders resulted from deficiencies of distinct plasma factors (reviewed in refs. 2 and 3).

It was not until 1971 that Zimmerman, Ratnoff, and Powell[4] prepared the first antibodies against what was thought to be a highly purified form of FVIII. This FVIII-related antigen was found to be normal in hemophilia A patients but decreased in vWD. This puzzle finally was resolved with the demonstration that von Willebrand factor (vWF) and FVIII are closely associated, with greater than 98 percent of the mass of the complex composed of vWF (see "The Interaction of vWF with Factor VIII"). Thus, antibodies raised against this complex predominantly recognize vWF. The first direct assay of vWF function was based on the observation that the antibiotic ristocetin induced thrombocytopenia and the demonstration by Howard and Firkin[5] that ristocetin-induced platelet aggregation (RIPA) was absent in some vWD patients. Weiss and coworkers[6] used this observation to develop a quantitative assay for vWF function that remains a mainstay of laboratory evaluation for vWD to this day. In 1973, several groups succeeded in dissociating vWF from FVIII procoagulant activity.[7,8]

Final proof that vWF and FVIII are independent proteins encoded by distinct genes came with the complementary DNA (cDNA) cloning of the two molecules in 1984 and 1985.[9–14] These discoveries also marked the beginning of the molecular genetic era for the study of vWF and FVIII, leading to the identification of gene mutations in many patients with hemophilia and vWD and considerable insight into the structure and function of these related proteins.

Table 118-1 summarizes the current nomenclature and terminology for FVIII and vWF. vWD is a heterogenous disorder with more than 20 variants described. The previous complex and confusing classification has been consolidated and simplified into six distinct

TABLE 118-1 VON WILLEBRAND FACTOR AND FACTOR VIII TERMINOLOGY

Factor VIII

Antihemophilic factor, the protein that is reduced in plasma of patients with classic hemophilia A and vWD and is measured in standard coagulation assays

Factor VIII activity (factor VIII:C)

Coagulant property of the factor VIII protein (this term is sometimes used interchangeably with factor VIII)

Factor VIII antigen (VIII:Ag)

Antigenic determinant(s) on factor VIII measured by immunoassays, which may use polyclonal or monoclonal antibodies

von Willebrand factor (vWF)

Large multimeric glycoprotein that is necessary for normal platelet adhesion, a normal bleeding time, and stabilizing factor VIII

von Willebrand factor antigen (vWF:Ag)

Antigenic determinant(s) on vWF measured by immunoassays, which may use polyclonal or monoclonal antibodies; *inaccurate designations of historical interest only* include factor VIII-related antigen (VIIIR:Ag), factor VIII antigen, AHF antigen, and AHF-like antigen

Ristocetin cofactor activity (vWF:RCo)

Property of vWF that supports ristocetin-induced agglutination of washed or fixed normal platelets

types,[15,16] as summarized in Table 118-2. Type 3 vWD is associated with very low or undetectable levels of vWF and severe bleeding. Type 1 vWD is characterized by concordant reductions in FVIII activity, vWF antigen, and ristocetin cofactor activity, generally ranging from 20 to 50 percent of normal, in association with normal vWF multimer structure. Type 2 vWD is heterogeneous and further divided into four

subtypes (2A, 2B, 2M, 2N). Type 2A vWD is characterized by a disproportionately low level of ristocetin cofactor activity relative to vWF antigen and absence of large- and intermediate-size multimers. Type 2B vWD also is associated with reduced high molecular weight vWF multimers but as a result of an abnormal vWF molecule with increased affinity for platelet glycoprotein (Gp) Ib. Functional abnormalities in vWF also can result in defective interactions with platelets, as in type 2M vWD, or decreased FVIII binding to vWF, designated type 2N vWD and characterized by mild to moderate FVIII deficiency. Many other subtypes have been reported, including platelet-type (pseudo-) vWD, which is an intrinsic platelet disorder resulting from mutations in GpIb (see Chap. 112). Finally, acquired forms of vWD occur, resulting in accelerated loss of circulating vWF because of antibody formation.

ETIOLOGY AND PATHOGENESIS

vWF is synthesized exclusively in endothelial cells and megakaryocytes and has two major functions in hemostasis. First, vWF serves as the initial critical bridge between circulating platelets and the injured blood vessel wall, accounting for the apparent defect in platelet function and prolonged bleeding time observed in vWD patients. The vWF monomer is assembled into higher-order multimers, a structure required for optimal adhesive function. Second, vWF serves as the carrier in plasma for FVIII, ensuring its stability and localizing it to the initial platelet plug for participation in thrombin generation and fibrin clot formation (see Chap. 106). This tight, noncovalent interaction between vWF and FVIII accounts for the copurification of these two molecules and the resulting initial confusion as to the origin of

TABLE 118-2 CLASSIFICATION OF VON WILLEBRAND DISEASE

TYPE	MOLECULAR CHARACTERISTICS	INHERITANCE	FREQUENCY	FACTOR VIII ACTIVITY	vWF ANTIGEN	RISTOCETIN COFACTOR ACTIVITY	RIPA	PLASMA vWF MULTIMER STRUCTURE
1	Partial quantitative vWF deficiency	Autosomal dominant, incomplete penetrance	1–30:1000; most common vWD variant (>70% of vWD)	Decreased	Decreased	Decreased	Decreased or normal	Normal
3	Severe quantitative reduction or absence of vWF	Autosomal recessive (or codominant)	$1–5:10^6$	Markedly decreased	Very low or absent	Very low or absent	Absent	Usually absent
2A	Qualitative vWF defect; loss of large vWF multimers	Usually autosomal dominant	≈10–15% of clinically significant vWD	Decreased to normal	Usually low	Markedly decreased	Decreased	Largest and intermediate multimers absent
2B	Qualitative vWF defect; increased vWF–platelet interaction (GpIb)	Autosomal dominant	Uncommon variant (<5% of clinical vWD)	Decreased to normal	Usually low	Decreased to normal	Increased to low concentrations of ristocetin	Largest multimers reduced/absent
2M	Qualitative vWF defect; decreased vWF-platelet interaction	Usually autosomal dominant	Rare (case reports)	Variably decreased	Variably decreased	Decreased	Variably decreased	Normal and occasionally ultralarge forms
2N	Qualitative vWF defect; decreased vWF–FVIII binding capacity	Autosomal recessive	Uncommon; heterozygotes may be prevalent in some populations	Decreased	Normal	Normal	Normal	Normal
Platelet-type (pseudo-)	Platelet defect; decreased platelet–vWF interactions	Autosomal dominant	Rare	Decreased to normal	Decreased to normal	Decreased	Increased to low concentrations of ristocetin	Largest multimers absent

hemophilia and vWD. FVIII is encoded by the FVIII gene on the X chromosome (see Chaps. 106 and 115), whereas vWF is encoded by a distinct gene on human chromosome 12.

vWF GENE AND COMPLEMENTARY DEOXYRIBONUCLEIC ACID

The vWF cDNA initially was cloned from endothelial cells[11–14] and the corresponding gene mapped to the short arm of chromosome 12 (12p13.3).[11] The vWF messenger RNA (mRNA) is approximately 9 kb in length, encoding a primary translation product of 2813 amino acid residues with an estimated M_r of 310,000. Comparison of the primary peptide sequence obtained from plasma vWF[17] with the vWF cDNA sequence established the pre-propolypeptide nature of vWF.[18] Pre-propolypeptide vWF is composed of a 22-amino-acid signal peptide, a 741-amino-acid precursor polypeptide (propeptide) termed vWF antigen II, and the mature subunit.[11,18–21] Cleavage of the 741-amino-acid propeptide from the amino-terminus produces the mature vWF subunit of 2050 amino acids (Fig. 118-1).

Analysis of the vWF sequence identifies four distinct types of repeated domains: three A domains, three B domains, two C domains, and four D domains.[19,22] The first pair of D domains is tandemly arranged in the vWF propeptide, followed by a partial and full D domain at the N-terminus of the mature subunit. The final complete D domain is separated by a segment of more than 600 amino acids containing the triplicated A domains. The repeated domain structure of vWF suggests that the gene evolved via a complex series of partial duplications, although exon structure is not highly conserved between homologous domains.

Comparison of the vWF amino acid sequence to other proteins identifies a superfamily of related proteins that all share sequence similarity with the vWF A domains.[23] The common theme among these potentially evolutionarily related genes is a role in extracellular matrix or adhesive function. Consistent with this notion, vWF functional domains for binding to the platelet receptor GpIb and specific ligands within the extracellular matrix have been localized to the vWF A repeats. A potential relationship between the vWF C domains and portions of thrombospondin and procollagen has been proposed.[24]

The vWF gene spans 178 kb and is divided into 52 exons.[25] Exons range in size from 40 bases to 1.4 kb (exon 28). The latter exon is unusually large, encoding the entire A1 and A2 domains and containing most of the known type 2A and all of the type 2B vWD mutations. The concentration of these defects within one exon has facilitated the identification of human mutations responsible for these vWD variants (see "Molecular Genetics of von Willebrand Disease" below). A partial, nonfunctional duplication of the vWF gene, termed a pseudogene, is located on human chromosome 22.[26] The pseudogene duplicates the middle portion of the vWF gene, from exons 23 to 34, and includes the intervening sequences. The pseudogene is approximately 97 percent identical in sequence to the authentic vWF gene, indicating it is of fairly recent evolutionary origin.[27] Gene conversion involving the pseudogene, possibly through recombination with the large homologous exon 28 sequence, has been proposed as a mechanism for introducing mutations into the vWF gene.[28–30]

vWF is synthesized exclusively in megakaryocytes and endothelial cells and, as a result, has frequently been used as a specific histochemical marker to identify cells of endothelial cell origin. Although generally assumed to mark all endothelial cells, vWF is expressed at widely varying levels among endothelial cells, depending on the size and location of the associated blood vessel.[31,32] A careful survey in the

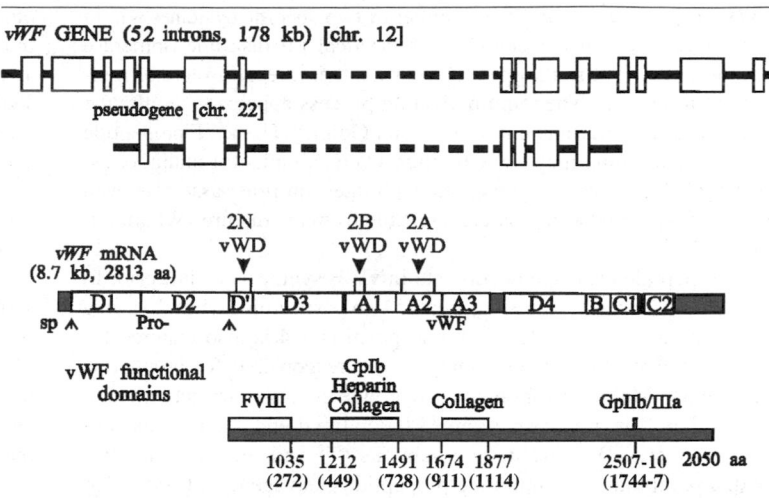

FIGURE 118-1   Schematic diagram of the human von Willebrand factor (vWF) gene, mRNA, and protein. The vWF gene and pseudogene are depicted at the top, with boxes representing exons and the solid black line representing introns. The vWF mRNA encoding the full prepro-vWF subunit is depicted in the middle as the bar and lettered boxes. The locations of signal peptide (sp) and propeptide (Pro) cleavage sites are indicated by arrowheads, and the lettered boxes denote regions of internally repeated sequence. The approximate localizations for known vWF functional domains within the mature vWF subunit are indicated at the bottom. Numbers underneath the domains refer to amino acid residues numbered from the ATG start site; numbers in parentheses indicate the amino acid residue position in the mature vWF subunit. aa = amino acid; chr = chromosome. (Adapted from D Ginsburg and EJW Bowie,[248] with permission.)

mouse identified wide differences in the level of vWF mRNA, with five to 50 times higher concentrations in the lung and brain, particularly in small vessels, than in comparable vessels in the liver and kidney. In general, the higher levels of vWF mRNA and antigen were found in the endothelial cells of large vessels rather than in microvasculature, and in venous rather than arterial endothelial cells.[32]

Specific DNA sequences within or near the proximal promoter of the vWF gene appear to be required for endothelial-specific gene expression,[33–35] although additional important regulatory elements likely exist outside of this region, perhaps at a great distance. A portion of the human vWF promoter from −487 to +246 targets vWF expression to blood vessels of the yolk sac and a subset of endothelial cells in the adult brain of the mouse.[36]

VON WILLEBRAND FACTOR BIOSYNTHESIS

The processing steps involved in the biosynthesis of vWF are similar in megakaryocytes and endothelial cells (reviewed in refs. 37 and 38). vWF is first synthesized as a large precursor monomer polypeptide (see Fig. 118-1). vWF is unusually rich in cysteine, which accounts for 8.3 percent of its amino acid content. All cysteines in the mature vWF molecule are involved in disulfide bonds.[39] Pro-vWF monomers are assembled into dimers through disulfide bonds at both C-termini, and only dimers are exported from the endoplasmic reticulum (ER).[39–41]

Glycosylation begins in the ER, with 12 potential N-linked glycosylation sites present on the mature subunit and three on the propeptide. Extensive additional posttranslational modification of vWF occurs in the Golgi apparatus, including the addition of multiple O-linked carbohydrate structures, sulfation, and multimerization through the formation of disulfide bonds at the N-termini of adjacent dimers. vWF is the only protein known to undergo extensive disulfide bond formation at this late stage, and this unique process appears to be catalyzed by a novel disulfide isomerase activity present within the vWF propeptide.[42] Mutations at either of two specific cysteines within the propeptide that are thought to be critical for disulfide isomerase activity, or a shift in the spacing between them, result in loss of multimer formation.[42] The multimerization process appears to require the slightly acidic environment of the distal Golgi.[43] The vWF propeptide self-associates and may serve to align vWF subunits for multimer assembly.[44] However, the propeptide facilitates multimer assembly even when coexpressed as a separate molecule from the mature vWF monomer.[45,46]

Propeptide cleavage occurs late in vWF synthesis or just prior to secretion. Cleavage occurs adjacent to two basic amino acids, Lys-Arg at positions −2 and −1. An Arg at position −4 is also required for recognition by the intracellular protease responsible for propeptide cleavage.[47] Multimerization and propeptide cleavage are not linked to each other. The multimers secreted by cultured endothelial cells contain both pro-vWF and mature subunits,[48,49] and recombinant vWF with a point mutation inhibiting propeptide cleavage is still assembled into normal multimer structures.[50] Although propeptide cleavage appears to occur primarily intracellularly, cleavage also may occur after secretion.

vWF is secreted from endothelial cells via both constitutive and regulated pathways.[37] vWF is stored in tubular structures within the α-granules of platelets and within the Weibel-Palade bodies in endothelial cells[51,52] (reviewed in ref. 53). Weibel-Palade bodies are derived from the Golgi apparatus and are found in most endothelial cells, although the number varies considerably. Although a number of other hemostatic proteins are also stored in the platelet α-granule, the Weibel-Palade body appears to be relatively specific for vWF and its propeptide.[54,55] vWF and FVIII colocalize in storage granules, and vWF appears to play a key role in trafficking FVIII to Weibel-Palade bodies.[56] The transmembrane glycoprotein P-selectin is found in the membranes of both the α-granule and the Weibel-Palade body.[57] The only other known components of the Weibel-Palade body are tissue plasminogen activator, a thrombolytic secreted protein, and CD63, a lysosomal protein also found on activated platelets.[58–60]

Regulated secretion of vWF from its storage site in the Weibel-Palade body is triggered by a number of secretagogues, including thrombin,[61] fibrin,[62] histamine,[63] and the C5b-9 complement complex.[64] The secretagogue desmopressin acetate (1-desamino-8-D-arginine vasopressin [DDAVP]), a vasopressin analogue, is used clinically for its capacity to cause a marked release of vWF and FVIII *in vivo* by acting through type 2 vasopressin receptors to induce secretion from the Weibel-Palade bodies in endothelial cells.[65] Constitutive secretion of vWF occurs evenly at the apical and basolateral surfaces, whereas regulated secretion from the Weibel-Palade body is highly polarized in the basolateral direction.[66] Constitutively secreted multimers are of relatively small size, whereas the multimers stored within the Weibel-Palade body are the largest, most biologically potent form.[55,67] The vWF stored in platelet α-granules is enriched for large multimers.[68] The N-terminal D domains appear to be required for vWF storage, with deletion of any of the individual domains resulting in constitutive secretion.[69,70] Cleavage of the vWF propeptide appears to be required for efficient formation of storage granules.[71]

The concentration of vWF in plasma is approximately 10 μg/ml, with approximately 15 percent of circulating vWF localized to the platelet compartment.[72] Bone marrow transplants between normal and vWD pigs demonstrate that platelet vWF is derived entirely from synthesis within the marrow and does not contribute to the normal plasma vWF pool.[73–75] These studies also demonstrate that both the plasma and the platelet vWF pools are required for full hemostasis, although the plasma pool appears to be more critical.

Plasma vWF is further processed in the circulation through cleavage by a specific protease, identified as ADAMTS13 (*a d*isintegrin *and m*etalloprotease with *t*hrombo*s*pondin type 1 motifs), resulting in reduction in the size of the largest multimers (reviewed in ref. 76). The major proteolytic cleavage site maps to the peptide bond between Tyr842 and Met843 in the vWF A2 domain,[77] and recombinant vWF missing the A2 domain is resistant to proteolysis.[78] vWF carrying a subgroup of type 2A vWD mutations exhibits increased susceptibility to cleavage by this protease[79] and is the proposed mechanism for the selective loss of large vWF multimers in this group of patients (see "Molecular Genetics of von Willebrand Disease" below). Increased vWF susceptibility to proteolysis by ADAMTS13 has also been described in a subset of type 1 vWD patients, but the clinical significance of this finding is unclear as increased proteolysis appears to occur only under certain conditions.[80,81] Decreased ADAMTS13 activity, resulting from either congenital deficiency or acquired inhibitors, plays a central role in the pathophysiology of thrombotic thrombocytopenic purpura (see Chap. 124).

FUNCTION OF VON WILLEBRAND FACTOR

vWF is a large multivalent adhesive protein that plays an important role in platelet attachment to subendothelial surfaces, platelet aggregation at sites of vessel injury, and stabilization of coagulation FVIII in the circulation. Not only is the interaction of vWF and FVIII important for the protection of FVIII from inactivation or degradation, FVIII bound to vWF may localize to cells and/or sites, where it can more readily participate in the promotion of blood coagulation and/or thrombus formation.

vWF is required for adhesion of platelets to subendothelium, particularly at moderate to high shear force. vWF performs this bridging function by binding to two platelet receptors, GpIb and GpIIb-IIIa, and to specific ligands such as collagen within the exposed subendothelium at sites of vascular injury (reviewed in refs. 82 and 83). Binding of vWF to its platelet receptors generally does not occur in the circulation under normal conditions. However, the interaction of vWF with exposed ligands in the vessel wall, combined with high shear stress conditions, facilitates vWF binding to platelet GpIb and subsequent platelet adhesion and activation. Activation of platelets leads to the exposure of the GpIIb-IIIa complex, an integrin receptor that can bind to fibrinogen, vWF, and other ligands, to form the platelet–platelet bridges required for thrombus propagation. Platelet adhesion to vWF immobilized at a site of injury appears to be a two-step process, with the initial tethering of the rapidly moving platelet dependent on vWF–GpIb interaction and subsequent firm adhesion occurring through GpIIb-IIIa after platelet activation[84,85] (see Chap. 105).

VON WILLEBRAND FACTOR BINDING
TO THE VESSEL WALL

vWF binds to the vessel wall at sites of vascular endothelial injury (reviewed in ref. 82). vWF binds to several different types of collagens, including types I through VI. Two distinct binding domains for the fibrillar collagen types I and III have been localized to specific segments within the vWF A1 and A3 repeats (see Fig. 118-1),[86,87] and a potential third domain has been identified in the propeptide.[88] Studies of recombinant vWF suggest that the A3 collagen-binding domain is the most important.[89,90] The physiologic relevance of vWF interactions with fibrillar collagens has been questioned, because vWF still binds to extracellular matrix depleted of these molecules by treatment with collagenase.[91] vWF binds to the nonfibrillar collagen type VI, which is resistant to collagenase[92] and colocalizes with vWF in the subendothelium.[93] Type VI collagen supports the binding of vWF under high shear through cooperative interactions between binding domains within the vWF A1 and A3 repeat.[94] Although vWF binding has been demonstrated in a number of other potential components of the subendothelium, including glycosaminoglycans[95,96] and sulfatides,[97] the biologic significance of these interactions remains to be demonstrated.

VON WILLEBRAND FACTOR BINDING TO PLATELETS

vWF interacts with platelets to mediate platelet aggregation and platelet localization to sites of vascular injury (reviewed in ref. 82 and Chap. 105). vWF interacts with a receptor complex on the surface of platelets composed of the disulfide-linked GpIbα and GpIbβ chains noncovalently associated with GpIX and GpV. The binding site for vWF is within a 293-amino-acid segment at the N-terminus of GpIbα and requires sulfation of several key tyrosine residues for optimal binding.[98] The GpIbα binding domain within vWF lies within the A1 segment, within the disulfide loop formed between the cysteine residues at 509 and 695 (see Fig. 118-1).[99,100] Scanning mutagenesis studies of recombinant vWF characterized a number of amino acid residues within the vWF A1 domain that are critical for binding to GpIb and for interaction with botrocetin.[101] Several mutations were identified that increase platelet binding, an effect similar to that of mutations associated with type 2B vWD (see "Molecular Genetics of von Willebrand Disease" below). These natural and synthetic mutations cluster in a small area on the surface of the vWF A1 domain structure, as revealed by x-ray crystallographic studies.[102] The structure of the A1 domain closely resembles that of other previously studied A domains, including the vWF A3 domain.[103–105] The structure of GpIb in complex with the vWF A1 domain has been solved, providing new insight into the structural basis for the gain of function mutations associated with type 2B vWD.[106]

Ristocetin binds to both vWF and platelets, but the mechanism by which it enhances vWF–GpIb interaction is poorly understood.[107,108] The snake venom botrocetin appears to induce GpIb binding through a different alteration in the vWF A1 domain and is used to study this interaction.[105]

The Arg-Gly-Asp-Ser (RGDS) sequence at amino acids 1744 to 1747 of the mature vWF subunit serves as the binding site within vWF for GpIIb-IIIa. The latter complex, also known as $\alpha_{IIb}\beta_3$, is a member of the integrin family of cell surface receptors. GpIIb-IIIa undergoes a conformational change to a high-affinity ligand binding state following platelet activation and, in addition to vWF, can bind a number of other adhesive proteins, including fibrinogen. Although vWF is present in blood at much lower concentrations than is fibrinogen, evidence suggests vWF is a critical ligand under flow conditions.[84,85] An RGD sequence is present in the vWF propeptide (vWF antigen II), although its functional significance is unknown.

INTERACTION OF VON WILLEBRAND FACTOR WITH FACTOR VIII

The noncovalent interaction between FVIII and vWF is required for the stability of FVIII in the circulation, as evident from FVIII levels less than 10 percent observed in most severe vWD patients. Although each vWF subunit appears to carry a binding site for FVIII, the stoichiometry for the vWF–FVIII complex found in normal plasma is approximately 1 to 2 FVIII molecules per 100 vWF monomers.[109] FVIII bound to vWF is protected from proteolytic degradation by activated protein C (reviewed in refs. 110 and 111).

The FVIII binding domain within vWF has been localized to the first 272 N-terminal amino acids of the mature subunit,[112] with antibody studies suggesting a particularly critical role for amino acids 78 to 96.[113,114] The mutations identified in patients with type 2N vWD, in which vWF binding to FVIII is specifically affected (see "Molecular Genetics of von Willebrand Disease" below) are clustered in this region, including the most common type 2N mutation at Arg91.[115] Of note, the same amino acid substitution at Arg89 is a common poly-

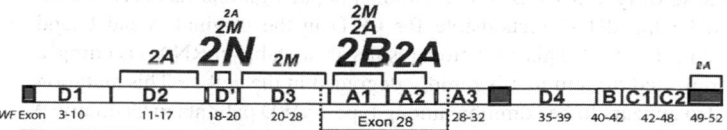

FIGURE 118-2 von Willebrand disease (vWD) mutations. The von Willebrand factor (vWF) domain locations of all reported mutations associated with type 2A, 2B, 2M, and 2N vWD are shown. *Lettering size* represents the proportion of total mutations reported within the designated vWF domain of that subtype, with *larger letters* indicating more mutations. Type 1 and Type 3 vWD associated mutations have been reported throughout the *vWF* gene. The relative positions of the vWF gene exons are shown at the *bottom*. (Mutation data from WC Nichols and D Ginsburg,[119] and the vWD mutation database available at *http://www.shef.ac.uk/vwf/.*)

morphism that does not affect FVIII binding.[116] The corresponding binding site for vWF on FVIII includes an acidic region at the N-terminus of the light chain (residues 1669–1689)[117] and requires sulfation of Tyr1680 for optimal binding.[118] Thrombin cleavage after Arg1689 activates and releases FVIII from vWF. Thus, vWF may serve to efficiently deliver FVIII to the sites of clot formation, where it can complex with factor IXa on the platelet surface.

MOLECULAR GENETICS OF VON WILLEBRAND DISEASE

vWD is an extremely heterogenous and complex disorder, with more than 20 distinct subtypes reported (reviewed in refs. 119 and 120). Many mutations within the vWF gene have been identified (Fig. 118-2). A list is maintained by a consortium of vWD investigators and can be accessed through the Internet at http://www.shef.ac.uk/vwf/. These findings form the basis for the simplified classification of vWD outlined in Table 118-2[15,16] and used throughout this chapter. Types 1 and 3 vWD are defined as pure quantitative deficiencies of vWF that are either partial (type 1) or complete (type 3). Type 2 vWD is characterized by qualitative abnormalities of vWF structure and/or function. The quantity of vWF found in type 2 vWD may be normal, but usually it is mildly to moderately decreased (see Table 118-2).

TYPE 3 VON WILLEBRAND DISEASE

Patients with type 3 vWD account for 1 to 5 percent of clinically significant vWD, have very low or undetectable levels of plasma and platelet vWF antigen and ristocetin cofactor activity, and generally present early in life with severe bleeding.[121] FVIII coagulant activity is markedly reduced but usually detectable at levels of 3 to 10 percent of normal. Type 3 vWD appears to be inherited as an autosomal recessive trait in most families, but parents of affected individuals may have mildly reduced vWF levels and occasionally are diagnosed as having mild type 1 vWD.

Mutations associated with type 3 vWD have been reported throughout the *vWF* gene (available at *http://www.shef.ac.uk/vwf/*). Southern blot analysis has identified gross gene deletion as the molecular mechanism for type 3 vWD in only a small subset of families.[26,122–124] However, large deletions may confer an increased risk for the development of alloantibodies against vWF.[26,124] A similar correlation has been reported for hemophilia B (see Chap. 115). Comparative analysis of vWF genomic DNA and platelet vWF mRNA has identified nondeletion defects resulting in complete loss of vWF mRNA expression as a molecular mechanism in some patients with type 3 vWD.[125,126] A number of nonsense and frameshift mutations that would be predicted to result in loss of vWF protein expression or in expression of a markedly truncated or disrupted protein have been identified in some type 3 vWD families (see Fig. 118-2).[119,127–129] A frameshift mutation in exon 18 appears to be a particularly common cause of type 3 vWD in the Swedish population and has been shown to be the defect responsible for vWD in the original Åland Island pedigree.[130,131] This mutation results in a stable mRNA encoding a truncated protein that is rapidly degraded in the cell.[132] This mutation also appears to be common among type 3 vWD patients in Germany[133] but not in the United States.[132]

TYPE 1 VON WILLEBRAND DISEASE

Type 1 is the most common form, accounting for approximately 70 percent of vWD patients. Type 1 vWD is generally autosomal dominant in inheritance and is associated with coordinate reductions in FVIII, ristocetin cofactor activity, and vWF antigen with maintenance of the full complement of multimers (Fig. 118-3). Subgroups within type 1 vWD have been proposed based on the relative levels of vWF present in the plasma and platelet pools,[134–137] but this distinction is not generally used in clinical practice.

Type 1 vWF often is assumed to simply represent the heterozygous form of type 3 vWD. However, the majority of heterozygous carriers of vWF gene deletions and carriers of vWF mRNA expression defects[26,123,125,126] are asymptomatic and have normal vWF laboratory values, consistent with an autosomal recessive pattern of inheritance for type 3 vWD. Nonetheless, in some families with nonsense or frameshift mutations, heterozygotes with apparent type 1 vWD have been identified, indicating that some, but probably not all (see below), type 1 vWD result from such defects within the vWF gene (see Fig. 118-2). Mutations that give rise to defective vWF subunits that interfere in a dominant negative way with the normal allele may be particularly likely to cause symptomatic vWD in the heterozygote.[129] Mutations have been identified at several cysteine residues in the vWF D3 domain and in the vWF propeptide of patients with moderately severe type 1 vWD. vWF carrying one of these mutations is retained in the ER, where it is proposed to exert a dominant negative effect on vWF derived from the normal allele via heterodimerization and degradation.[138,139]

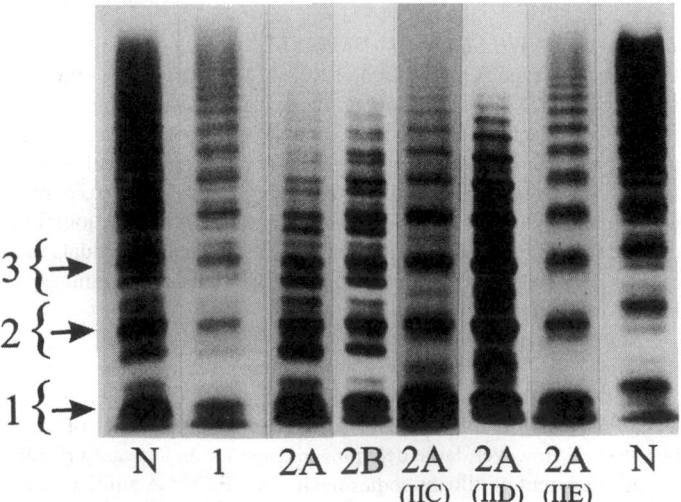

FIGURE 118-3   Agarose gel electrophoresis of plasma von Willebrand factor (vWF). vWF multimers from plasma of patients with various subtypes of von Willebrand disease (vWD) are shown. The *brackets to the left* encompass three individual multimer subunits, including the main band and its associate satellite bands. N indicates normal control lanes. Lanes 5 through 7 are rare variants of type 2A vWD. The former designations for these variants are indicated in *parentheses below the lanes* (IIC, IID, IIE). (Adapted from SD Berkowitz, ZM Ruggeri, TS Zimmerman TS,[249] with permission.)

To date, most mutation studies and genetic linkage analysis of type 1 vWD have been consistent with defects within the vWF gene. Although no single mutation can explain the majority of type 1 vWD, a report identified a common *vWF* founder mutation, Tyr1584Cys, in 14 percent of Canadian type 1 vWD patients and possibly a similar proportion of patients in the United Kingdom.[140] Given the complex biosynthesis and processing of vWF, defects at a number of other loci could be expected to result in quantitative vWF abnormalities (reviewed in ref. 129). This concept is supported by a study of families with type 1 vWD in which bleeding histories and low ristocetin cofactor activities did not always cosegregate with genetic markers at the vWF locus.[141] Of interest, a mouse model for type 1 vWD associated with an up to 20-fold reduction in plasma vWF results from an unusual mutation in a glycosyltransferase gene, leading to aberrant posttranslation processing of vWF and accelerated clearance from plasma.[142] A similar mechanism may explain the modifying effect of the ABO blood group glycosyltransferases on plasma vWF level.[143]

The diagnosis of type 1 vWD can be confounded by the incomplete penetrance of the disease, the wide range of vWF levels in "normals," the inherent difficulties in obtaining reliable bleeding histories, and borderline laboratory results. An alternative strategy has been proposed to classify some patients for whom the diagnosis of vWD is ambiguous as "low vWF," recognizing that these patients may have an increased risk for bleeding without labeling them as type 1 vWD.[144] This proposal has not yet been tested in clinical practice.

TYPE 2A VON WILLEBRAND DISEASE

Type 2A is the most common qualitative variant of vWD and is generally associated with autosomal dominant inheritance and selective loss of the large and intermediate vWF multimers from plasma (see Fig. 118-3). A 176-kDa proteolytic fragment present in normal individuals is markedly increased in quantity in many type 2A vWD patients. This fragment results from proteolytic cleavage of the peptide bond between Tyr842 and Met843.[77,145] Based on this observation, initial DNA sequence analysis in patients centered on vWF exon 28, in the region encoding this segment of the vWF protein, leading to the identification of the first point mutations responsible for vWD.[146] Since then, a large number of mutations have been identified, accounting for the majority of type 2A vWD patients.[119] Most of these mutations are clustered within a 134-amino-acid segment of the vWF A2 domain (between Gly742 and Glu875; see Fig. 118-3). The most common mutation, Arg834Trp, appears to account for approximately one third of type 2A vWD patients.[119,127]

Expression of recombinant vWF containing type 2A vWD mutations has identified two distinct molecular mechanisms for the loss of large vWF multimers characteristic of this disorder.[147] In the first subset, classified as group 1, the type 2A vWD mutation results in a defect in intracellular transport, with retention of mutant vWF in the ER. In the second subset, classified as group 2, mutant vWF is normally processed and secreted *in vitro*; thus loss of multimers *in vivo* presumably occurs because of increased susceptibility to proteolysis in plasma[77,147–150] at the same Tyr842-Met843 site cleaved by ADAMTS13.[76,81]

The multimer structure of platelet vWF correlates well with this subclassification. Group 1 patients show loss of large vWF multimers within platelets because of defective synthesis, whereas group 2 patients have normal vWF multimers within the protected environment of the α-granule.[147] These observations confirm the earlier subclassification of type 2A vWD based on platelet multimers.[134] Subclassification into group 1 or 2 might be expected to predict response to desmopressin therapy but remains to be demonstrated.

In addition to the major class of type 2A vWD described above, a number of rare variants previously classified as types IIC to IIH, type

IB, and "platelet discordant" now are included in the new, more general type 2A category. Most of these rare variants were distinguished based on subtle differences in the multimer pattern (see Fig. 118-3; reviewed in ref. 120). The IIC variant usually is inherited as an autosomal recessive trait and is associated with loss of large multimers and a prominent dimer band. Several mutations have been identified in the vWF propeptide of these patients,[151,152] presumably interfering with multimer assembly. A mutation at the C-terminus of vWF, interfering with dimer formation, was described in a patient with the IID variant.[153] Most of the other reported variants of type 2A vWD are rare, often limited to single case reports.

TYPE 2B VON WILLEBRAND DISEASE

Type 2B vWD usually is inherited as an autosomal dominant disorder and is characterized by thrombocytopenia and loss of large vWF multimers. The plasma vWF in type 2B vWD binds to normal platelets in the presence of lower concentrations of ristocetin than does normal vWF and often binds spontaneously. Accelerated clearance of the resulting complexes between platelets and the large, most adhesive forms of vWF accounts for the thrombocytopenia and the characteristic multimer pattern (see Fig. 118-3).

The peculiar functional abnormality characteristic of type 2B vWD suggested a molecular defect within the GpIb binding domain of vWF. For this reason, initial DNA sequence analysis focused on the corresponding portion of vWF exon 28.[154,155] All of these mutations are located within the vWF A1 domain, at one surface of the described crystallographic structure.[102,106] The four most common mutations are clustered within a 35-amino-acid stretch between Arg543 and Arg578 (see Fig. 118-2). Together these mutations account for more than 80 percent of type 2B vWD patients.[127] Functional analysis of mutant recombinant vWF[156-160] confirms that these single amino acid substitutions are sufficient to account for increased GpIb binding and the resulting characteristic type 2B vWD phenotype.

Three families that exhibit enhanced vWF binding to GpIb but a normal distribution of vWF multimers have been described. These variants, previously referred to as type I New York, type I Malmö, and type I Sydney, now all are designated as type 2B vWD. Type I New York and type I Malmö have now been shown to be caused by the same mutation, Pro503Leu. This mutation is located within the cluster of type 2B mutations in the vWF A1 domain and results in a similar increase in platelet GpIb binding.[161]

TYPE 2N VON WILLEBRAND DISEASE

Hemophilia A results from defects in the *FVIII* gene and is inherited in an X-linked recessive manner (see Chap. 115). Rare families in which the inheritance of hemophilia appears to be autosomal, based on the occurrence of affected females or direct transmission from an affected father, have been reported.[162,163] Several cases of an apparent autosomal recessive decrease in FVIII have resulted from decreased binding of FVIII by vWF.[164-166] This disorder has also been referred to as vWD Normandy, after the province of origin of the first patient. DNA sequence analysis has identified a total of 37 mutations associated with this disorder, which are summarized in the ISTH SSC vWF Database (available at *http://www.shef.ac.uk/vwf/*), all located at the vWF N terminus (see Fig. 118-2). One of these mutations, Arg91Gln, appears to be particularly common and may contribute to variability in the severity of type 1 vWD in some cases.[167]

TYPE 2M VON WILLEBRAND DISEASE

This category is reserved for rare vWD variants in which a defect in vWF platelet-dependent function leads to significant bleeding but vWF multimer structure is not affected (although some have subtle multimer abnormalities). Most of these variants previously were classified as

type I. The variant previously referred to as type B is associated with absent ristocetin cofactor activity but normal platelet binding with other agonists. This variant results from a mutation in the A1 domain (Gly561Ser).[168] Mutations have been identified in a number of other families with normal vWF multimers and disproportionately decreased ristocetin cofactor activity.[120,169] Several families with a vWD variant (vWD Vicenza) characterized by larger than normal vWF multimers have been described.[170] Genetic linkage analysis indicates the defect lies within the vWF gene.[171] Although mutations within the vWF gene reportedly are associated with vWD Vicenza,[172] the underlying molecular mechanism responsible for the vWD Vicenza phenotype remains controversial.[173]

CLINICAL FEATURES

INHERITANCE

Type 1 vWD is the most common form of vWD, with a prevalence estimated to be as high as 1 percent.[174,175] Type 1 vWD generally is transmitted as an autosomal dominant disorder and accounts for approximately 70 percent of clinically significant vWD. However, disease expressivity is variable, and penetrance is incomplete.[129] Laboratory values and clinical symptoms can vary considerably, even within the same individual, and establishing a definite diagnosis of vWD often is difficult. In two large families with type 1 vWD, only 65 percent of individuals with both an affected parent and an affected descendent had significant clinical symptoms.[176] For comparison, 23 percent of the unrelated spouses of the patients, who presumably did not have a bleeding disorder, were judged to have a positive bleeding history.

A number of factors modify vWF levels, including ABO blood group, secretor blood group, estrogens, thyroid hormone, age, and stress.[177-179] ABO blood group is the best characterized of these factors. A genome-wide linkage screen has confirmed strong linkage between the ABO locus and vWF levels.[180] Mean vWF antigen levels are approximately 75 percent for type O individuals and 123 percent for type AB individuals compared to a pool of normal donor plasmas. Thus, differentiating between a low–normal value and mild type 1 vWD in blood group O individuals may be difficult. The variable expressivity and incomplete penetrance of type 1 vWD have complicated the determination of accurate incidence figures for vWD, with estimates ranging from as high as 1 percent[174,175] to as low as two to 10 per 100,000.[181]

In general, the type 2 variants are more uniformly penetrant. Type 2A and type 2B vWD account for the vast majority of patients with qualitative vWF abnormalities. No accurate incidence figures are available for these subtypes, but the type 2 variants are generally believed to compose 20 to 30 percent of all vWD diagnoses. The type 2 variants generally are autosomal dominant in inheritance, although type 2N and other rare cases of apparent recessive inheritance have been reported.

Estimates of prevalence for severe (type 3) vWD range from 0.5 to 5.3 per 1,000,000.[182-184] This variant frequently is defined as autosomal recessive in inheritance, but this finding is not consistent. As described in "Type 3 von Willebrand Disease" above, one or both parents of a severe vWD patient frequently are clinically asymptomatic and often have entirely normal laboratory test results, but many families have been reported in which one or both parents appear to be affected with classic type 1 vWD. Thus, in some families, severe vWD may represent the homozygous form of type 1 vWD. In this model, the apparent recessive inheritance in a subset of families could simply be the result of the incomplete penetrance of type 1 vWD. Alternatively, a fundamental difference in the molecular mechanisms responsible for type 1 and type 3 vWD may exist.[129]

CLINICAL SYMPTOMS

Mucocutaneous bleeding is the most common symptom in patients with type 1 vWD.[176] Importantly, more than 20 percent of normal individuals may have a positive bleeding history.[185] This observation, together with the limited sensitivity and specificity of the currently available laboratory tests (see "Laboratory Features" below), makes the diagnosis of mild vWD difficult and probably contributes to the wide range of prevalence figures for type 1 vWD reported in the literature.

Approximately 60 percent of type 1 vWD patients have epistaxis, 40 percent have easy bruising and hematomas, 35 percent have menorrhagia, and 35 percent have gingival bleeding. Gastrointestinal bleeding occurs in approximately 10 percent of patients.[186] An apparent association between hereditary hemorrhagic telangiectasia (HHT) and vWD had been reported in several families. The causative genes in HHT have been identified and are located on chromosomes 9q33-34, and 12q13[187] (see Chap. 115), distinct from the *vWF* gene on chromosome 12p13. However, because inheriting vWD likely increases the severity of bleeding from HHT, the diagnosis more likely will be made in patients inheriting both defects.[188] Mucocutaneous bleeding is common after trauma, with approximately 50 percent of patients reporting bleeding after dental extraction, approximately 35 percent after trauma or wounds, 25 percent postpartum, and 20 percent postoperatively. Hemarthroses in patients with moderate disease are rare and generally are encountered only after major trauma. The bleeding symptoms can be variable among patients within the same family and even in the same patient over time. An individual may experience postpartum bleeding with one pregnancy but not with others. Clinical symptoms in mildly to moderately affected type 1 individuals often ameliorate by the second or third decade of life. Aside from an infrequent type 3 patient, death from bleeding rarely occurs in vWD.

Patients with type 3 vWD can suffer from severe clinical bleeding and experience hemarthroses and muscle hematomas, as in severe hemophilia A (see Chap. 115). The bleeding time is very prolonged. After infusion of vWF-containing plasma fractions, some patients develop anti-vWF antibodies that neutralize vWF. Development of antibodies has been correlated with the presence of gene deletions.[26,124]

Thrombocytopenia is a common feature of type 2B vWD and is not seen in any other form of vWD. Most patients experience thrombocytopenia only at times of increased vWF production or secretion, such as during physical effort, during pregnancy, in newborn infants, postoperatively, or if an infection develops. The platelet count rarely drops sufficiently to contribute to clinical bleeding.[189,190] Infants with type 2B vWD may present with neonatal thrombocytopenia, which can be confused with neonatal sepsis or congenital thrombocytopenia.

Patients who are homozygous or compound heterozygous for type 2N vWD generally have normal levels of vWF antigen and ristocetin cofactor activity and normal vWF platelet adhesive function. However, FVIII levels are moderately decreased, resulting in a mild to moderate hemophilia-like phenotype.[115] In contrast to patients with classic hemophilia A (FVIII deficiency), these patients do not respond to infusion of purified FVIII and should be treated with vWF-containing concentrates. Heterozygotes for this disorder may have mildly decreased FVIII levels but are generally asymptomatic. Although type 2N vWD appears to be considerably less common than classic hemophilia A, it should be considered in the differential diagnosis of FVIII deficiency, particularly if any features suggest an autosomal pattern of inheritance. Although the FVIII level rarely drops below 5 percent, at least one type 2N vWD mutation has been associated with FVIII levels as low as 1 percent when coinherited with a type 3 vWD allele.[191] The latter observation suggests that a diagnosis of type 2N vWD should also be considered in patients with marked reductions of FVIII.

LABORATORY FEATURES

In the initial laboratory evaluation of patients suspected by history of having vWD, the following tests are routinely performed: assay of FVIII activity, vWF antigen (vWF:Ag), and ristocetin cofactor activity. In a large epidemiologic study, the ristocetin cofactor assay was more sensitive than the vWF:Ag for the diagnosis of type 1 vWD.[192] Other tests that are commonly used include the bleeding time, RIPA, and vWF multimer analysis. Routine coagulation studies, such as prothrombin time or activated partial thromboplastin time (aPTT), are generally not useful in the evaluation of vWD. As noted above in "Molecular Genetics of von Willebrand Disease; Type 1 von Willebrand Disease," results of these tests can be normal in some patients with type 1 vWD. In addition, the wide range of normal and the considerable overlap with the levels observed in type 1 vWD make borderline levels difficult to interpret. A variety of concurrent diseases and drugs can modify the results of individual tests, including aspirin or other nonsteroidal antiinflammatory drugs, which often prolong the bleeding time. Many conditions, such as pregnancy, age, time of menstrual cycle, hypothyroidism or hyperthyroidism, uremia, recent exercise, liver disease, infection, diabetes, estrogen therapy, or myeloproliferative syndromes, affect FVIII activity, vWF:Ag, and ristocetin cofactor activity levels. These values can be regarded as acute-phase reactants, and many minor illnesses can increase their levels to normal. Even controlling for many of these factors, the coefficients of variation of repeated vWF:Ag and ristocetin cofactor assays in a single person are large.[193] For this reason, repeated measurements usually are necessary, and the diagnosis of vWD or its exclusion should not be based on a single set of laboratory values unless the results are well below or well above the limits of normal.

BLEEDING TIME

The bleeding time has long been used as a standard screening test for vWD and other abnormalities of platelet function.[194] However, results can vary considerably with the experience of the operator and a variety of other factors, and its value as a screening test has been questioned. Furthermore, although bleeding time does not prolong with FVIII deficiency, low FVIII levels have been shown to correlate with operative bleeding.[83] The general consensus is that the bleeding time should not be used for routine patient screening in the preoperative setting.[195-197] Although the bleeding time also probably should not be used as a routine screening test for vWD, it may still be of value in selected patients when taken together with the clinical history and the results of other laboratory tests. It also may be useful as a means of monitoring therapy in some settings.

FACTOR VIII

FVIII levels in vWD patients generally are coordinately decreased along with plasma vWF. Levels in type 3 vWD generally range from 3 to 10 percent. In contrast, the levels in type 1 and the type 2 vWD variants (other than 2N) are variable and usually only mildly or moderately decreased. The FVIII level in type 2N vWD is more severely decreased but rarely to less than 5 percent. aPTT can be prolonged in vWD, although only as a reflection of the reduced FVIII level.

VON WILLEBRAND FACTOR ANTIGEN

Plasma vWF:Ag usually is quantitated by electroimmunoassay, radioimmunoassay, or an enzyme-linked immunosorbent assay (ELISA) technique. In type 1 vWD, the vWF:Ag assay usually parallels the ristocetin cofactor activity, but it has lower specificity and sensitivity than the ristocetin cofactor assay. In patients with type 2A vWD, the vWF:Ag usually is low but can be normal.[193]

RISTOCETIN COFACTOR ACTIVITY

The standard measure of vWF activity quantitates the ability of plasma vWF to agglutinate platelets via platelet membrane GpIbα in the presence of ristocetin,[198] also referred to as the *ristocetin cofactor assay*. Normal platelets washed free of plasma vWF are used either as fresh platelets or after formalin fixation. This assay reportedly is the most sensitive and specific single test for detection of vWD.[192] An ELISA alternative to the standard platelet-based ristocetin cofactor activity assay has been developed.[199] However, the assay has high interassay and interlaboratory variability,[200,201] leading the UK Haemophilia Centre Doctors' Organization vWD working party to recommend use of only platelet-based ristocetin cofactor activity assays.[202] Ristocetin cofactor activity is generally decreased coordinately with vWF: Ag and FVIII in type 1 vWD patients. In type 2 vWD variants, ristocetin cofactor activity can be disproportionately decreased, as is usually the case in type 2A variants (and sometimes type 2B) because of the greater dependence of ristocetin-mediated platelet–vWF interaction on the presence of larger vWF multimers and in type 2M because of decreased vWF–platelet interactions (see Table 118-2).

RISTOCETIN-INDUCED PLATELET AGGLUTINATION

Similar to the ristocetin cofactor assay, the RIPA assay also measures platelet agglutination caused by ristocetin-mediated vWF binding to platelet membrane glycoprotein Ibα. In the case of RIPA, ristocetin is added directly to patient platelet-rich plasma. This activity is generally reduced in most vWD patients. Hyperresponsiveness to RIPA results either from a type 2B vWD mutation or an intrinsic defect in the platelet (platelet-type or pseudo-vWD). In these disorders, patient platelet-rich plasma agglutinates spontaneously or at ristocetin concentrations of only 0.2 to 0.7 mg/ml. At these concentrations, normal platelet-rich plasma does not agglutinate. Type 2B and platelet-type vWD can be distinguished by RIPA experiments performed with separated patient platelets or plasma mixed with the corresponding component from a normal individual.

MULTIMER ANALYSIS

Analysis of plasma vWF multimers is critical for the proper diagnosis and subclassification of vWD (see Fig. 118-3). This is generally accomplished by agarose gel electrophoresis of plasma vWF to separate vWF multimers based on molecular size, with the largest multimers migrating more slowly than the intermediate or smaller multimers. The multimers can be visualized by autoradiography after incubation with ^{125}I-monospecific antihuman vWF antibody or by nonradioactive immunologic techniques. The normal multimeric distribution is an orderly ladder of major protein bands of increasing molecular weight, going from the smallest to the largest vWF multimers (see Fig. 118-3). Each normal multimer has a fine structure consisting of one major component and two to four satellite bands.[203] Type 2B and most of the type 2A variants initially were distinguished from each other based on subtle variations in the satellite band pattern.

ADDITIONAL LABORATORY TESTS

Because of the variable sensitivity and specificity of laboratory testing for vWD, additional select diagnostic studies may be useful in the classification of vWD patients. When type 2N vWD is suspected, vWF:FVIII binding capacity can be measured.[166] A specific assay of FVIII binding to vWF has been developed and is used to confirm the diagnosis of type 2N vWD.[204] Although this assay is widely used in European hemostasis laboratories, its availability in the United States currently is limited to a few specialized reference laboratories.

A number of other assays for vWF activity have been developed. Assays based upon vWF collagen binding activity reportedly complement vWF ristocetin cofactor activity in detecting type 2 vWD variants.[205,206] A new functional assay, the PFA-100 system, measures platelet binding under high shear,[207,208] but application of the PFA-100 in the diagnosis or monitoring of vWD is controversial.[83,202] Additional assays can measure platelet agglutination induced by botrocetin and other snake venom proteins.[209] None of these assays currently is available in the routine clinical laboratory.

With advances in understanding the molecular genetics of vWD, it now is possible to precisely diagnose and subclassify many variants of vWD based on specific DNA mutations identified in the research laboratory. DNA testing for type 2N vWD now is clinically available using a panel of mutations that accounts for the majority, but not all, of reported type 2N patients. Unfortunately, DNA testing for other subtypes of vWD currently is not available in the clinical setting. As molecular testing is gradually introduced into the clinical laboratory, DNA diagnosis should be particularly straightforward for type 2B vWD, where a panel of four mutations detects more than 80 percent of patients. Similar panels of mutations should be able to correctly identify the defect in the majority of type 2A vWD. Analysis of type 3 and type 1 vWD will be more complex, because the currently known mutations account only for a small subset of these patients, except in selected populations.[130]

PRENATAL TESTING

Given the mild clinical phenotype of most patients with the common variants of vWD, prenatal diagnosis for the purpose of deciding on terminating the pregnancy is rarely performed. However, type 3 vWD patients often have a profound bleeding disorder, similar to or more severe than classic hemophilia, so some families may request prenatal diagnosis. In cases of vWD in which the precise mutation is known, DNA diagnosis can be performed rapidly and accurately by polymerase chain reaction from amniotic fluid or chorionic villus biopsies.[210] In cases where the mutation is unknown, diagnosis still can be attempted by genetic linkage analysis using the large panel of known polymorphisms within the vWF gene.[211] One of these polymorphisms, a TCTA tetranucleotide repeat of variable length in intron 40, is particularly useful, with more than 100 known polymorphic alleles. Several cases of successful prenatal diagnosis have been reported.[210,212,213] Although all cases of vWD analyzed to date appear to be linked to the vWF gene, the possibility of locus heterogeneity (i.e., a similar phenotype resulting from a mutation in a gene other than vWF) should be considered.[129]

DIFFERENTIAL DIAGNOSIS

PLATELET-TYPE (PSEUDO-) VON WILLEBRAND DISEASE

Platelet-type (pseudo-) vWD is a platelet defect that phenotypically mimics vWD (see Chap. 112).[214] The plasma vWD lacks the largest multimers, RIPA is enhanced at low concentrations of ristocetin, and thrombocytopenia of variable degree is often present. Clinically, these patients have primarily mucocutaneous bleeding. Molecular analysis has identified mutations within the GpIbα chain as the molecular basis for pseudo-vWD. These mutations are located within the segment of GpIb that encodes the vWF binding domain and appear to induce the conformational change complementary to that produced in the corresponding fragment of vWF by type 2B vWD mutations.[106,214]

The specialized RIPA test should be performed at low ristocetin concentrations to distinguish type 2B and platelet-type vWD from type 2A vWD. Purified plasma vWF or cryoprecipitate causes platelet aggregation when added to platelet-rich plasma from patients with platelet-type vWD, distinguishing this disorder from type 2B vWD. In addition, type 2B vWD plasma transfers the enhanced RIPA to normal platelets, whereas plasma from patients with platelet-type vWD interacts normally with control platelets.

ACQUIRED VON WILLEBRAND DISEASE

Acquired vWD is a relatively rare acquired bleeding disorder that usually presents as a late-onset bleeding diathesis in a patient with no prior bleeding history and a negative family history of bleeding (reviewed in ref. 215). Decreased levels of FVIII, vWF:Ag, and ristocetin cofactor activity are common, and the bleeding time usually is prolonged. Acquired vWD usually is associated with another underlying disorder and reportedly occurs in patients with myeloproliferative disorders,[216] benign or malignant B cell disorders,[217] hypothyroidism,[218] autoimmune disorders,[219] several solid tumors (particularly Wilms tumor),[220] cardiac or vascular defects (notably aortic stenosis),[221] or in association with several drugs, including ciprofloxacin and valproic acid.[222,223]

A variety of B cell disorders have been associated with the development of anti-vWF autoantibodies. In most cases the acquired vWD appears to result from rapid clearance of vWF induced by the circulating inhibitor, although these antibodies also may interfere with vWF function. Hypothyroidism results in decreased vWF synthesis,[218] and, in some cases of malignancy, the acquired vWD is thought to result from selective adsorption of vWF to the tumor cells. In acquired vWD associated with valvular heart disease or certain drugs, vWF may be lost by accelerated destruction or proteolysis.[222,223]

Although the vWF multimers in acquired vWD usually exhibit a type 2A pattern with relative depletion of the large multimer forms, acquired vWD can manifest as a wide range of vWD phenotypes.[219,215] Distinguishing acquired vWD from genetic vWD can be difficult, because testing for the associated autoantibodies is generally not available in the clinical setting. The diagnosis often rests on the late onset of the disease, the absence of a family history, and the identification of an associated underlying disorder.

Management of acquired vWD is generally aimed at treating the underlying disorder. vWF levels and bleeding symptoms often improve with successful treatment of hypothyroidism or an associated malignancy. Refractory patients have been treated with corticosteroids, plasma exchange, intravenous γ-globulin, DDAVP, and vWF-containing FVIII concentrates.[215,223]

THERAPY, COURSE, AND PROGNOSIS

The mainstays of therapy for vWD are DDAVP, which induces secretion of both vWF and FVIII, and replacement therapy with vWF-containing plasma concentrates. The choice of treatment in any given patient depends upon the type and severity of vWD, the clinical setting, and the type of hemostatic challenge that must be met. Type 1 patients are most often treated with DDAVP alone, types 2A and 2B with a combination of DDAVP and a vWF-containing FVIII product, and type 2N and type 3 patients with vWF-containing concentrates.[224] A previous history of trauma or surgery and the success of previous treatment are important parameters to include in the assessment of risk of bleeding. Prophylaxis generally is not used except in anticipation of hemostatic challenges, such as dental extractions, and in the most severe type 3 vWD patients[225] who exhibit recurrent hemarthroses or gastrointestinal bleeding. In general a correlation exists between normal hemostasis and correction of the bleeding time and FVIII activity but does not occur in all cases. FVIII has been found to be the most important determinant of soft tissue and postoperative hemorrhage, but no laboratory test clearly correlates with mucosal bleeding or response to therapy.[83]

DESMOPRESSIN (DDAVP)

DDAVP is an analogue of antidiuretic hormone that acts through type 2 vasopressin receptors to induce secretion of FVIII and vWF, likely via cyclic adenosine monophosphate-mediated secretion from the Weibel-Palade bodies in endothelial cells.[65] DDAVP administered to healthy subjects causes sustained increases of FVIII and ristocetin cofactor activity for approximately 4 hours.[226] DDAVP also releases tissue plasminogen activator, presumably from endothelial cells. Patients with type 1 vWD treated with DDAVP release unusually high molecular weight vWF multimers into the circulation for 1 to 3 hours after the infusion.[226,227] Therapy with DDAVP increases FVIII activity, vWF:Ag, and ristocetin cofactor activity to two to five times the basal level and, in many instances, corrects the bleeding time of type 1 vWD patients.

DDAVP has become a mainstay for treatment of mild hemophilia and vWD[228] because it is relatively inexpensive, widely available, and avoids the risks of plasma-derived products. Approximately 80 percent of type 1 vWD patients have excellent responses to DDAVP. It is regularly used in the setting of mild to moderate bleeding and for prophylaxis of patients undergoing surgical procedures. DDAVP is administered at a dose of $0.3\mu g/kg$ continuous intravenous infusion over 30 minutes. DDAVP also is available for subcutaneous injection (at the same $0.3\mu g/kg$ dose) and in intranasal form (at a fixed dose of $300\mu g$ for adults and $150\mu g$ for children), which appears to be similar in efficacy to intravenous administration,[229,230] although the response may be more variable.

The response to DDAVP in any given individual with vWD is generally reproducible and predicts response to future doses. In one study, 22 type 1 vWD patients showed a departure of less than 20 percent from the mean FVIII peak level calculated from two separate infusions. In addition, the consistency of response in one patient reliably predicted the future response of that patient and other affected family members.[231] For patients requiring repeated infusions of DDAVP, FVIII activity and vWF responses may not be of the same magnitude as after the first infusion. Although this decay in response has considerable individual variability, after one infusion of DDAVP per day for 4 days, the responses on days 2 to 4 were reduced approximately 30 percent compared to day 1.[229–232]

Therefore, in patients for whom DDAVP is potentially the treatment of choice, a test dose should be given at the planned therapeutic dose and route in advance of the first required course of treatment with measurements of before and after vWF and FVIII:C (coagulant property) levels to ensure an adequate therapeutic response. For patients with type 1 vWD who are undergoing surgical procedures, DDAVP can be administered 1 hour before surgery and approximately every 12 hours thereafter for up to two to four doses before loss of clinically significant response. The response of FVIII and ristocetin cofactor activity should be monitored when DDAVP is administered at frequent intervals. vWF-containing FVIII concentrates and/or cryoprecipitate should be available for transfusion as backup.

Approximately 20 to 25 percent of patients with vWD do not respond adequately to DDAVP. Type 2 vWD patients are less likely to have a response than type 1 patients,[233] and nearly all patients with type 3 vWD cannot respond. The response to DDAVP of patients with type 2A vWD is variable. Although most patients respond only transiently, some patients exhibit complete hemostatic correction after DDAVP infusion.[234,235] The differences in DDAVP efficacy among type 2A patients have been hypothesized to correspond to the type of mutation, with better responses predicted in patients with group 2 mutations. A prospective study of the biologic response to DDAVP in well-characterized vWD patients included type 2A vWD patients with both group 1 and group 2 defects. Although patients with group 2 mutations had greater improvements in vWF ristocetin cofactor activity and bleeding time than patients with group 1 defects, neither groups could be classified as responders.[233]

Common side effects of DDAVP administration are mild cutaneous vasodilatation resulting in a feeling of heat, facial flushing, tachycardia, tingling, and headaches. The potential for dilutional hyponatremia, especially in elderly and very young patients, requires appropriate attention to fluid restriction because it may result in seizures. Isolated reports of acute arterial thrombosis associated with administration of DDAVP have been reported, but the risk appears to be low when judged against the total number of patients treated. However, DDAVP is contraindicated in patients with unstable coronary artery disease because of increased risk for thrombotic events, such as myocardial infarction.[83] As above, patients receiving DDAVP at closely spaced intervals of less than 24 to 48 hours can develop tachyphylaxis.[232]

Many experts consider DDAVP to be contraindicated in the treatment of type 2B vWD, as the high molecular weight vWF released from storage sites has an increased affinity for binding to GpIb and might be expected to induce spontaneous platelet aggregation and worsening thrombocytopenia.[236] However, two reports indicated successful use of DDAVP in type 2B vWD patients, with an associated shortening or correction of the bleeding time and variable thrombocytopenia.[237,238] Although type 2N patients can exhibit increased FVIII:C levels after DDAVP, in some cases the FVIII:C levels rapidly decline in the absence of stabilizing normal vWF, attenuating clinical efficacy. Type 2M patients generally do not have a satisfactory response to DDAVP.[233,239]

VON WILLEBRAND FACTOR REPLACEMENT THERAPY

It is important to determine the response to DDAVP for each individual in order to avoid the unnecessary use of plasma products. For type 3 vWD patients and other patients unresponsive to DDAVP, the use of selected virus-inactivated, vWF-containing FVIII concentrates is generally safe and effective.[240] Cryoprecipitate has been successfully used in the past, but because it is not currently treated to inactivate viruses, it is less desirable. Solvent detergent-treated plasma is available, and cryoprecipitate prepared from such plasma may be an appropriate choice. It is important to note that most standard FVIII concentrates and all recombinant FVIII products are not effective in vWD because they lack clinically significant quantities of vWF. Although such products can substantially increase circulating FVIII:C, the infused factor is short-lived in the circulation in the absence of stabilizing vWF.[241] Only preparations that contain large quantities of vWF with well-preserved multimer structure are suitable for use in vWD patients. Humate-P and Alphanate both are acceptable commercial vWF-containing plasma concentrates that have been evaluated in vWD replacement therapy in clinical studies, although other vWF-containing FVIII concentrates also may be effective (reviewed in ref. 83).

In practice, vWD replacement therapy dosing and timing has been largely empiric. Recommendations for therapy have been outlined based upon the degree and nature of hemorrhage.[83,242] The recommended treatment goals are similar to the posttreatment FVIII:C and vWF activity level goals currently used in clinical practice.[224] The objective is to elevate FVIII:C and vWF activity until bleeding stops and healing is complete. In general, replacement goals of FVIII:C and vWF activity should be greater than 50 to 80 percent for major trauma, surgery, or central nervous system hemorrhage, greater than 50 percent FVIII:C and vWF activity for delivery and in the postpartum period,

greater than 30 to 50 percent FVIII:C and vWF activity for dental extractions and minor surgery, and 20 to 80 percent FVIII:C and vWF activity for mucous membrane bleeding or menorrhagia. Laboratory monitoring of posttreatment FVIII:C and vWF levels is important in guiding therapy and avoiding supratherapeutic replacement doses (>200%), which have been associated with increased risk for thrombosis.[243,244]

In patients who have concomitant thrombocytopenia associated with or in addition to vWD, it may be necessary to transfuse platelets in addition to FVIII concentrates. If clinical bleeding continues, additional replacement therapy must be given and searches undertaken for other hemostatic defects. Type 3 vWD patients receiving multiple transfusions can develop antibodies directed against vWF, and continued replacement with vWF-containing concentrates is contraindicated because of the risk of anaphylaxis.[245,246] A variety of approaches to the management of vWD inhibitors, similar to the treatment of FVIII inhibitors in hemophilia A (see Chap. 115), have been tried. Immunosuppression, recombinant FVIII, and recombinant factor VIIa reportedly have been useful in patients with type 3 vWD who developed anti-vWF antibodies.

OTHER NONREPLACEMENT THERAPIES

Estrogens or oral contraceptives have been used empirically for treatment of menorrhagia. In addition to their effects on the ovaries and uterus, estrogens tend to increase plasma vWF levels. Patients with vWD frequently normalize their levels of FVIII, vWF:Ag, and ristocetin cofactor activity during pregnancy. The mechanism of action of estrogens may be partly related to the increased production of vWF through a direct effect on endothelial cells.[247] In pregnant patients with type 1 vWD, the FVIII and ristocetin cofactor activities usually rise above 50 percent. These patients usually do not require any specific therapy at the time of parturition. In contrast, individuals who have 30 percent or less FVIII or variant forms of vWD are more likely to require prophylactic therapy with DDAVP or plasma products before delivery. Postpartum hemorrhage within the first few days after parturition may be related to the relatively rapid return to prepregnancy levels of FVIII and vWF activities, and postpartum hemorrhage in all forms of vWD may occur as long as 1 month postpartum. Therefore, laboratory monitoring is recommended at term and for 2 weeks postpartum to identify patients at risk for immediate and/or delayed bleeding complications.

Fibrinolytic inhibitors, such as ε-aminocaproic acid or tranexamic acid, have been used effectively in some vWD patients. Antifibrinolytics are commonly used alone or in conjunction with DDAVP or a plasma-derived vWF replacement product in patients with mucous membrane bleeding or undergoing dental extraction.[224] Fibrinolytic inhibitors are generally well tolerated but rarely can cause nausea or diarrhea and are contraindicated in patients with gross hematuria.

REFERENCES

1. von Willebrand EA: Hereditär Pseudohemofili. *Finska Läkarsällskapetes Handl* 67:7, 1926.
2. Hoyer LW: Von Willebrand's disease. *Prog Hemost Thromb* 3:231, 1976.
3. Nilsson IM: Von Willebrand's disease—Fifty years old. *Acta Med Scand* 201:497, 1977.
4. Zimmerman TS, Ratnoff OD, Powell AE: Immunologic differentiation of classic hemophilia (Factor VIII deficiency) and von Willebrand disease. *J Clin Invest* 50:244, 1971.
5. Howard MA, Firkin BG: Ristocetin: A new tool in the investigation of platelet aggregation. *Thromb Diath Haemorrh* 76:362, 1971.

6. Weiss HJ, Rogers J, Brand H: Defective ristocetin-induced platelet aggregation in von Willebrand's disease and its correction by Factor VIII. *J Clin Invest* 52:2697, 1973.

7. Weiss HJ, Hoyer LW: Von Willebrand factor: Dissociation from antihemophilic factor procoagulant activity. *Science* 182:1149, 1973.

8. Zimmerman TS, Edgington TS: Factor VIII Coagulant activity and Factor VIII-like antigen: Independent molecular entities. *J Exp Med* 138:1015, 1973.

9. Gitschier J, Wood WI, Goralka TM, et al: Characterization of the human factor VIII gene. *Nature* 312:326, 1984.

10. Toole JJ, Knopf JL, Wozney JM, et al: Molecular cloning of a cDNA encoding human antihaemophilic factor. *Nature* 312:342, 1984.

11. Ginsburg D, Handin RI, Bonthron DT, et al: Human von Willebrand factor (vWF): Isolation of complementary DNA (cDNA) clones and chromosomal localization. *Science* 228:1401, 1985.

12. Lynch DC, Zimmerman TS, Collins CJ, et al: Molecular cloning of cDNA for human von Willebrand factor: Authentication by a new method. *Cell* 41:49, 1985.

13. 13. Sadler JE, Shelton-Inloes BB, Sorace JM, et al: Cloning and characterization of two cDNAs coding for human von Willebrand factor. *Proc Natl Acad Sci U S A* 82:6394, 1985.

14. Verweij CL, de Vries CJM, Distel B, et al: Construction of cDNA coding for human von Willebrand factor using antibody probes for colony-screening and mapping of the chromosomal gene. *Nucleic Acids Res* 13:4699, 1985.

15. Sadler JE: A revised classification of von Willebrand disease. *Thromb Haemost* 71:520, 1994.

16. Sadler JE, Gralnick HR: Commentary: A new classification for von Willebrand disease. *Blood* 84:676, 1994.

17. Titani K, Kumar S, Takio K, et al: Amino acid sequence of human von Willebrand Factor. *Biochem* 25:3171, 1986.

18. Fay PJ, Kawai Y, Wagner DD, et al: Propolypeptide of von Willebrand factor circulates in blood and is identical to von Willebrand antigen II. *Science* 232:995, 1986.

19. Bonthron DT, Handin RI, Kaufman RJ, et al: Structure of pre-pro-von Willebrand factor and its expression in heterologous cells. *Nature* 324:270, 1986.

20. Bonthron DT, Orr EC, Mitsock LM, et al: Nucleotide sequence of pre-pro-von Willebrand factor cDNA. *Nucleic Acids Res* 14:7125, 1986.

21. Shelton-Inloes BB, Broze GJ Jr, Miletich JP, Sadler JE: Evolution of human von Willebrand Factor: cDNA sequence polymorphisms, repeated domains, and relationship to von Willebrand antigen II. *Biochem Biophys Res Commun* 144:657, 1987.

22. Shelton-Inloes BB, Titani K, Sadler JE: cDNA sequences for human von Willebrand Factor reveal five types of repeated domains and five possible protein sequence polymorphisms. *Biochem* 25:3164, 1986.

23. Colombatti A, Bonaldo P: The superfamily of proteins with von Willebrand factor Type A-like domains: One theme common to components of extracellular matrix, hemostasis, cellular adhesion, and defense mechanisms. *Blood* 77:2305, 1991.

24. Hunt LT, Barker WC: von Willebrand factor shares a distinctive cysteine-rich domain with thrombospondin and procollagen. *Biochem Biophys Res Commun* 144:876, 1987.

25. Mancuso DJ, Tuley EA, Westfield LA, et al: Structure of the gene for human von Willebrand factor. *J Biol Chem* 264:19514, 1989.

26. Shelton-Inloes BB, Chehab FF, Mannucci PM, et al: Gene deletions correlate with the development of alloantibodies in von Willebrand Disease. *J Clin Invest* 79:1459, 1987.

27. Mancuso DJ, Tuley EA, Westfield LA, et al: Human von Willebrand factor gene and pseudogene: Structural analysis and differentiation by polymerase chain reaction. *Biochemistry* 30:253, 1991.

28. Zhang ZP, Blomback M, Nyman D, Anvret M: Mutations of von Willebrand factor gene in families with von Willebrand disease in the Aland Islands. *Proc Natl Acad Sci U S A* 90:7937, 1993.

29. Eikenboom JC, Vink T, Briet E, et al: Multiple substitutions in the von Willebrand factor gene that mimic the pseudogene sequence. *Proc Natl Acad Sci U S A* 91:2221, 1994.

30. Eikenboom JC, Castaman G, Vos HL, et al: Characterization of the genetic defects in recessive type 1 and type 3 von Willebrand disease patients of Italian origin. *Thromb Haemost* 79:709, 1998.

31. Rand JH, Badimon L, Gordon RE, et al: Distribution of von Willebrand factor in porcine intima varies with blood vessel type and location. *Arteriosclerosis* 7:287, 1987.

32. Yamamoto K, de Waard V, Fearns C, Loskutoff DJ: Tissue distribution and regulation of murine von Willebrand factor gene expression in vivo. *Blood* 92:2791, 1998.

33. Jahroudi N, Lynch DC: Endothelial-cell-specific regulation of von Willebrand factor gene expression. *Mol Cell Biol* 14:999, 1994.

34. Harvey PJ, Keightley AM, Lam YM, et al: A single nucleotide polymorphism at nucleotide-1793 in the von Willebrand factor (VWF) regulatory region is associated with plasma VWF:Ag levels. *Br J Haematol* 109:349, 2000.

35. Guan J, Guillot PV, Aird WC: Characterization of the mouse von Willebrand factor promoter. *Blood* 94:3405, 1999.

36. Aird WC, Jahroudi N, Weiler-Guettler H, et al: Human von Willebrand factor gene sequences target expression to a subpopulation of endothelial cells in transgenic mice. *Proc Natl Acad Sci U S A* 92:4567, 1995.

37. Wagner DD: Cell biology of von Willebrand factor. *Annu Rev Cell Biol* 6:217, 1990.

38. de Wit TR, van Mourik JA: Biosynthesis, processing and secretion of von Willebrand factor: Biological implications. *Best Pract Res Clin Haematol* 14:241, 2001.

39. Marti T, Rosselet SJ, Titani K, Walsh KA: Identification of disulfide-bridged substructures within human von Willebrand factor. *Biochem* 26:8099, 1987.

40. Wagner DD, Lawrence SO, Ohlsson-Wilhelm BM, et al: Topology and order of formation of interchain disulfide bonds in von Willebrand factor. *Blood* 69:27, 1987.

41. Voorberg J, Fontijn R, Calafat J, et al: Assembly and routing of von Willebrand factor variants: The requirements for disulfide-linked dimerization reside within the carboxy-terminal 151 amino acids. *J Cell Biol* 113:195, 1991.

42. Mayadas TN, Wagner DD: Vicinal cysteines in the prosequence play a role in von Willebrand factor multimer assembly. *Proc Natl Acad Sci U S A* 89:3531, 1992.

43. Mayadas TN, Wagner DD: In vitro multimerization of von Willebrand factor is triggered by low pH: Importance of the propolypeptide and free sulfhydryls. *J Biol Chem* 264:13497, 1989.

44. Wagner DD, Fay PJ, Sporn LA, et al: Divergent fates of von Willebrand factor and its propolypeptide (von Willebrand antigen II) after secretion from endothelial cells. *Proc Natl Acad Sci U S A* 84:1955, 1987.

45. Verweij CL, Hart M, Pannekoek H: Expression of variant von Willebrand factor (vWF) cDNA in heterologous cells: Requirement of the pro-polypeptide in vWF multimer formation. *EMBO J* 6:2885, 1987.

46. Wise RJ, Pittman DD, Handin RI, et al: The propeptide of von Willebrand factor independently mediates the assembly of von Willebrand multimers. *Cell* 52:229, 1988.

47. Rehemtulla A, Kaufman RJ: Preferred sequence requirements for cleavage of pro-von Willebrand propeptide-processing enzymes. *Blood* 79:2349, 1992.

48. Wagner DD, Marder VJ: Biosynthesis of von Willebrand protein by human endothelial cells: Processing steps and their intracellular localization. *J Cell Biol* 99:2123, 1984.

49. Lynch DC, Zimmerman TS, Ling EH, Browning PJ: An explanation for minor multimer species in endothelial cell-synthesized von Willebrand factor. *J Clin Invest* 77:2048, 1986.

50. Verweij CL, Hart M, Pannekoek H: Proteolytic cleavage of the precursor of von Willebrand Factor is not essential for multimer formation. *J Biol Chem* 263:7921, 1988.

51. Weibel ER, Palade GE: New cytoplasmic components in arterial endothelia. *J Biol Chem* 23:101, 1964.

52. Wagner DD, Olmsted JB, Marder VJ: Immunolocalization of von Willebrand protein in Weibel-Palade bodies of human endothelial cells. *J Cell Biol* 95:355, 1982.

53. Hannah MJ, Williams R, Kaur J, et al: Biogenesis of Weibel-Palade bodies. *Semin Cell Dev Biol* 13:313, 2002.

54. McCarroll DR, Levin EG, Montgomery RR: Endothelial cell synthesis of von Willebrand antigen II, von Willebrand factor, and von Willebrand factor/von Willebrand antigen II complex. *J Clin Invest* 75:1089, 1985.

55. Ewenstein BM, Warhol MJ, Handin RI, Pober JS: Composition of the von Willebrand factor storage organelle (Weibel-Palade body) isolated from cultured human umbilical vein endothelial cells. *J Cell Biol* 104:1423, 1987.

56. Rosenberg JB, Foster PA, Kaufman RJ, et al: Intracellular trafficking of factor VIII to von Willebrand factor storage granules. *J Clin Invest* 101:613, 1998.

57. Bonfanti R, Furie BC, Furie B, Wagner DD: PADGEM (GMP140) is a component of Weibel-Palade bodies of human endothelial cells. *Blood* 73:1109, 1989.

58. Metzelaar MJ, Wijngaard PLJ, Peters PJ, et al: CD63 Antigen: A novel lysosomal membrane glycoprotein, cloned by a screening procedure for intracellular antigens in eukaryotic cells. *J Biol Chem* 266:3239, 1991.

59. Vischer UM, Wagner DD: CD63 is a component of Weibel-Palade bodies of human endothelial cells. *Blood* 82:1184, 1993.

60. Huber D, Cramer EM, Kaufmann JE, et al: Tissue-type plasminogen activator (t-PA) is stored in Weibel-Palade bodies in human endothelial cells both in vitro and in vivo. *Blood* 99:3637, 2002.

61. Levine JD, Harlan JM, Harker LA, et al: Thrombin-mediated release of factor VIII antigen from human umbilical vein endothelial cells in culture. *Blood* 60:531, 1982.

62. Ribes JA, Francis CW, Wagner DD: Fibrin induces release of von Willebrand factor from endothelial cells. *J Clin Invest* 79:117, 1987.

63. Hamilton KK, Sims PJ: Changes in cytosolic Ca2+ associated with von Willebrand factor release in human endothelial cells exposed to histamine. Study of microcarrier cell monolayers using the fluorescent probe indo-1. *J Clin Invest* 79:600, 1987.

64. Hattori R, Hamilton KK, McEver RP, Sims PJ: Complement proteins C5b-9 induce secretion of high molecular weight multimers of endothelial von Willebrand factor and translocation of granule membrane protein GMP-140 to the cell surface. *J Biol Chem* 264:9053, 1989.

65. Kaufmann JE, Oksche A, Wollheim CB et al: Vasopressin-induced von Willebrand factor secretion from endothelial cells involves V2 receptors and cAMP. *J Clin Invest* 106:107, 2000.

66. Sporn LA, Marder VJ, Wagner DD: Differing polarity of the constitutive and regulated secretory pathways for von Willebrand factor in endothelial cells. *J Cell Biol* 108:1283, 1989.

67. Sporn LA, Marder VJ, Wagner DD: Inducible secretion of large, biologically potent von Willebrand factor multimers. *Cell* 46:185, 1986.

68. Fernandez MF, Ginsberg MH, Ruggeri ZM, et al: Multimeric structure of platelet factor VIII/von Willebrand factor: The presence of larger multimers and their reassociation with thrombin-stimulated platelets. *Blood* 60:1132, 1982.

69. Wagner DD, Saffaripour S, Bonfanti R, et al: Induction of specific storage organelles by von Willebrand factor propolypeptide. *Cell* 64:403, 1991.

70. Voorberg J, Fontijn R, Calafat J, et al: Biogenesis of Von Willebrand factor-containing organelles in heterologous transfected CV-1 cells. *EMBO J* 12:749, 1993.

71. Journet AM, Saffaripour S, Cramer EM, et al: Von Willebrand factor storage requires intact prosequence cleavage site. *Eur J Cell Biol* 60:31, 1993.

72. Nachman RL, Jaffe EA: Subcellular platelet factor VIII antigen and von Willebrand factor. *J Exp Med* 141:1101, 1975.

73. Bowie EJW, Solberg LA Jr, Fass DN, et al: Transplantation of normal bone marrow into a pig with severe von Willebrand's disease. *J Clin Invest* 78:26, 1986.

74. Nichols TC, Samama CM, Bellinger DA, et al: Function of von Willebrand factor after crossed bone marrow transplantation between normal and von Willebrand disease pigs: Effect on arterial thrombosis in chimeras. *Proc Natl Acad Sci U S A* 92:2455, 1995.

75. André P, Brouland JP, Roussi J, et al: Role of plasma and platelet von Willebrand factor in arterial thrombogenesis and hemostasis in the pig. *Exp Hematol* 26:620, 1998.

76. Chung DW, Fujikawa K: Processing of von Willebrand Factor by ADAMTS-13. *Biochem* 41:11065, 2003.

77. Dent JA, Berkowitz SD, Ware J, et al: Identification of a cleavage site directing the immunochemical detection of molecular abnormalities in type IIA von Willebrand factor. *Proc Natl Acad Sci U S A* 87:6306, 1990.

78. Lankhof H, Damas C, Schiphorst ME, et al: von Willebrand factor without the A2 domain is resistant to proteolysis. *Thromb Haemost* 77:1008, 1997.

79. Tsai H-M, Sussman II, Ginsburg D, et al: Proteolytic cleavage of recombinant type 2A von Willebrand factor mutants R834W and R834Q: Inhibition by doxycycline and by monoclonal antibody VP-1. *Blood* 89:1954, 1997.

80. Bowen DJ, Collins PW: An amino acid polymorphism in von Willebrand factor correlates with increased susceptibility to proteolysis by ADAMTS13. *Blood* 103:941, 2004.

81. Bowen DJ: Increased susceptibility of von Willebrand factor to proteolysis by ADAMTS13: Should the multimer profile be normal or type 2A? *Blood* 103:3246, 2004.

82. Ruggeri ZM, Ware J, Ginsburg D: von Willebrand factor, in *Thrombosis and Hemorrhage*, edited by J Loscalzo, AI Schafer, p 246. Lippincott Williams & Wilkins, Philadelphia, 2003.

83. Mannucci PM: Treatment of von Willebrand's Disease. *N Engl J Med* 351:683, 2004.

84. Savage B, Saldívar E, Ruggeri ZM: Initiation of platelet adhesion by arrest onto fibrinogen or translocation on von Willebrand factor. *Cell* 84:289, 1996.

85. Savage B, Almus-Jacobs F, Ruggeri ZM: Specific synergy of multiple substrate-receptor interactions in platelet thrombus formation under flow. *Cell* 94:657, 1998.

86. Kalafatis M, Takahashi Y, Girma J-P, Meyer D: Localization of a collagen-interactive domain of human von Willebrand factor between amino acid residues Gly 911 and Glu 1365. *Blood* 70:1577, 1987.

87. Pareti FI, Niiya K, McPherson JM, Ruggeri ZM: Isolation and characterization of two domains of human von Willebrand Factor that interact with fibrillar collagen types I and III. *J Biol Chem* 262:13835, 1987.

88. Takagi J, Sekiya F, Kasahara K, et al: Inhibition of platelet-collagen interaction by propolypeptide of von Willebrand factor. *J Biol Chem* 264:6017, 1989.

89. Cruz MA, Yuan H, Lee JR, et al: Interaction of the von Willebrand factor (vWF) with collagen. Localization of the primary collagen-binding site by analysis of recombinant vWF A domain polypeptides. *J Biol Chem* 270:10822, 1995.

90. Lankhof H, Van Hoeij M, Schiphorst ME, et al: A3 domain is essential for interaction of von Willebrand factor with collagen type III. *Thromb Haemost* 75:950, 1996.

91. Wagner DD, Urban-Pickering M, Marder VJ: von Willebrand protein binds to extracellular matrices independently of collagen. *Proc Natl Acad Sci U S A* 81:471, 1984.

92. Rand JH, Patel ND, Schwartz E, et al: 150-kD von Willebrand factor binding protein extracted from human vascular subendothelium is Type VI collagen. *J Clin Invest* 88:253, 1991.

93. Rand JH, Wu X-X, Potter BJ, et al: Co-localization of von Willebrand factor and type VI collagen in human vascular subendothelium. *Am J Pathol* 142:843, 1993.

94. Mazzucato M, Spessotto P, Masotti A, et al: Identification of domains responsible for von Willebrand factor type VI collagen interaction mediating platelet adhesion under high flow. *J Biol Chem* 274:3033, 1999.

95. Fretto LJ, Fowler WE, McCaslin DR, et al: Substructure of human von Willebrand factor: Proteolysis by V8 and characterization of two functional domains. *J Biol Chem* 261:15679, 1986.

96. Fujimura Y, Titani K, Holland LZ, et al: A heparin-binding domain of human von Willebrand factor. Characterization and localization to a tryptic fragment extending from amino acid residue Val[449] to Lys[728]. *J Biol Chem* 262:1734, 1987.

97. Christophe O, Obert B, Meyer D, Girma J-P: The binding domain of von Willebrand factor to sulfatides is distinct from those interacting with glycoprotein Ib, heparin, collagen and residues between amino acid residues Leu 512 and Lys 673. *Blood* 78:2310, 1991.

98. Marchese P, Murata M, Mazzucato M, et al: Identification of three tyrosine residues of glycoprotein IBα with distinct roles in von Willebrand factor and α-thrombin binding. *J Biol Chem* 270:9571, 1995.

99. Fujimura Y, Titani K, Holland LZ, et al: von Willebrand Factor: A reduced and alkylated 52/48-kDa fragment beginning at amino acid residue 449 contains the domain interacting with platelet glycoprotein Ib. *J Biol Chem* 261:381, 1986.

100. Mohri H, Fujimura Y, Shima M, et al: Structure of the von Willebrand Factor domain interacting with glycoprotein Ib. *J Biol Chem* 263:17901, 1988.

101. Matsushita T, Sadler JE: Identification of amino acid residues essential for von Willebrand factor binding to platelet glycoprotein Ib. Charged-to-alanine scanning mutagenesis of the A1 domain of human von Willebrand factor. *J Biol Chem* 270:13406, 1995.

102. Emsley J, Cruz M, Handin RI, Liddington R: Crystal structure of the von Willebrand factor A1 domain and implications for the binding of platelet glycoprotein Ib. *J Biol Chem* 273:10396, 1998.

103. Bienkowska J, Cruz M, Atiemo A, et al: The von Willebrand factor A3 domain does not contain a metal ion-dependent adhesion site motif. *J Biol Chem* 272:25162, 1997.

104. Huizinga EG, Van der Plas RM, Kroon J, et al: Crystal structure of the A3 domain of human von Willebrand factor: Implications for collagen binding. *Structure* 5:1147, 1997.

105. Fukuda K, Doggett TA, Bankston LA, et al: Structural basis of von Willebrand factor activation by the snake toxin botrocetin. *Structure (Camb)* 10:943, 2002.

106. Huizinga EG, Tsuji S, Romijn RA, et al: Structures of glycoprotein Ibalpha and its complex with von Willebrand factor A1 domain. *Science* 297:1176, 2002.

107. Scott JP, Montgomery RR, Retzinger GS: Dimeric ristocetin flocculates proteins, binds to platelets, and mediates von Willebrand factor-dependent agglutination of platelets. *J Biol Chem* 266:8149, 1991.

108. Berndt MC, Du XP, Booth WJ: Ristocetin-dependent reconstitution of binding of von Willebrand factor to purified human platelet membrane glycoprotein Ib-IX complex. *Biochem* 27:633, 1988.

109. Vlot AJ, Koppelman SJ, Van den Berg MH, et al: The affinity and stoichiometry of binding of human factor VIII to von Willebrand factor. *Blood* 85:3150, 1995.

110. Sadler JE: Biochemistry and genetics of von Willebrand factor. *Annu Rev Biochem* 67:395, 1998.

111. Vlot AJ, Koppelman SJ, Bouma BN, Sixma JJ: Factor VIII and von Willebrand factor. *Thromb Haemost* 79:456, 1998.

112. Foster PA, Fulcher CA, Marti T, et al: A major factor VIII binding domain resides within the amino-terminal 272 amino acid residues of von Willebrand factor. *J Biol Chem* 262:8443, 1987.

113. Bahou WF, Ginsburg D, Sikkink R, et al: A monoclonal antibody to von Willebrand factor (vWF) inhibits factor VIII binding. Localization of its antigenic determinant to a nonadecapeptide at the amino terminus of the mature vWF polypeptide. *J Clin Invest* 84:56, 1989.

114. Ginsburg D, Bockenstedt PL, Allen EA, et al: Fine mapping of monoclonal antibody epitopes on human von Willebrand factor using a recombinant peptide library. *Thromb Haemost* 67:166, 1992.

115. Mazurier C: von Willebrand disease masquerading as haemophilia A. *Thromb Haemost* 67:391, 1992.

116. Cacheris PM, Nichols WC, Ginsburg D: Molecular characterization of a unique von Willebrand disease variant. A novel mutation affecting von Willebrand factor/factor VIII interaction. *J Biol Chem* 266:13499, 1991.

117. Lollar P, Hill-Eubanks DC, Parker CG: Association of the Factor VIII light chain with von Willebrand Factor. *J Biol Chem* 263:10451, 1988.

118. Leyte A, van Schijndel HB, Niehrs C, et al: Sulfation of Tyr[1680] of human blood coagulation factor VIII is essential for the interaction of Factor VIII with von Willebrand factor. *J Biol Chem* 266:740, 1991.

119. Nichols WC, Ginsburg D: von Willebrand disease. *Medicine* 76:1, 1997.

120. Nichols WC, Cooney KA, Ginsburg D, Ruggeri ZM: von Willebrand disease, in *Thrombosis and Hemorrhage*, edited by J Loscalzo, AI Schafer, p 539. Lippincott Williams & Wilkins, Philadelphia, 2003.

121. Zimmerman TS, Abildgaard CF, Meyer D: The factor VIII abnormality in severe von Willebrand's disease. *N Engl J Med* 301:1307, 1979.

122. Ngo KY, Glotz VT, Koziol JA, et al: Homozygous and heterozygous deletions of the von Willebrand factor gene in patients and carriers of severe von Willebrand Disease. *Proc Natl Acad Sci U S A* 85:2753, 1988.

123. Peake IR, Liddell MB, Moodie P, et al: Severe Type III von Willebrand's disease caused by deletion of Exon 42 of the von Willebrand factor gene: Family studies that identify carriers of the condition and a compound heterozygous individual. *Blood* 75:654, 1990.

124. Mancuso DJ, Tuley EA, Castillo R, et al: Characterization of partial gene deletions in type III von Willebrand disease with alloantibody inhibitors. *Thromb Haemost* 72:180, 1994.

125. Nichols WC, Lyons SE, Harrison JS, et al: Severe von Willebrand disease due to a defect at the level of von Willebrand factor mRNA expression: Detection by exonic PCR-restriction fragment length polymorphism analysis. *Proc Natl Acad Sci U S A* 88:3857, 1991.

126. Eikenboom JCJ, Ploos van Amstel HK, Reitsma PH, Briët E: Mutations in severe, type III von Willebrand's disease in the Dutch population: Candidate missense and nonsense mutations associated with reduced levels of von Willebrand factor messenger RNA. *Thromb Haemost* 68:448, 1992.

127. Ginsburg D, Sadler JE: von Willebrand Disease: A database of point mutations, insertions, and deletions. *Thromb Haemost* 69:177, 1993.

128. Eikenboom JCJ, Castaman G, Vos HL, et al: Characterization of the genetic defects in recessive type 1 and type 3 von Willebrand disease patients of Italian origin. *Thromb Haemost* 79:709, 1998.

129. Mohlke KL, Ginsburg D: von Willebrand disease and quantitative deficiency of von Willebrand factor. *J Lab Clin Med* 130:252, 1997.

130. Zhang ZP, Falk G, Blombäck M, et al: A single cytosine deletion in exon 18 of the von Willebrand factor gene is the most common mutation in Swedish vWD type III patients. *Hum Mol Genet* 1:767, 1992.

131. Zhang ZP, Blombäck M, Nyman D, Anvret M: Mutations of von Willebrand factor gene in families with von Willebrand disease in the Åland Islands. *Proc Natl Acad Sci U S A* 90:7937, 1993.

132. Mohlke KL, Nichols WC, Rehemtulla A, et al: A common frameshift mutation in von Willebrand factor does not alter mRNA stability but interferes with normal propeptide processing. *Br J Haematol* 95:184, 1996.

133. Schneppenheim R, Krey S, Bergmann F, et al: Genetic heterogeneity of severe von Willebrand disease type III in the German population. *Hum Genet* 94:640, 1994.

134. Weiss HJ, Piétu G, Rabinowitz R, et al: Heterogeneous abnormalities in the multimeric structure, antigenic properties, and plasma-platelet content of factor VIII/von Willebrand factor in subtypes of classic (type I) and variant (type IIA) von Willebrand's disease. *J Lab Clin Med* 101: 411, 1983.

135. Hoyer LW, Rizza CR, Tuddenham EGD, et al: Von Willebrand factor multimer patterns in von Willebrand's disease. *Br J Haematol* 55:493, 1983.

136. Mannucci PM, Lombardi R, Bader R, et al: Heterogeneity of Type I von Willebrand disease: Evidence for a subgroup with an abnormal von Willebrand factor. *Blood* 66:796, 1985.

137. Mannucci PM: Platelet von Willebrand factor in inherited and acquired bleeding disorders. *Proc Natl Acad Sci U S A* 92:2428, 1995.

138. Eikenboom JCJ, Matsushita T, Reitsma PH, et al: Dominant type 1 von Willebrand disease caused by mutated cysteine residues in the D3 domain of von Willebrand factor. *Blood* 88:2433, 1996.

139. Bodo I, Katsumi A, Tuley EA, et al: Type 1 von Willebrand disease mutation Cys1149Arg causes intracellular retention and degradation of heterodimers: A possible general mechanism for dominant mutations of oligomeric proteins. *Blood* 98:2973, 2001.

140. O'Brien LA, James PD, Othman M, et al: Founder von Willebrand factor haplotype associated with type 1 von Willebrand disease. *Blood* 102: 549, 2003.

141. Castaman G, Eikenboom JC, Bertina RM, Rodeghiero F: Inconsistency of association between type 1 von Willebrand disease phenotype and genotype in families identified in an epidemiological investigation. *Thromb Haemost* 82:1065, 1999.

142. Mohlke KL, Purkayastha AA, Westrick RJ, et al: *MvWf*, a dominant modifier of murine von Willebrand factor, results from altered lineage-specific expression of a glycosyltransferase. *Cell* 96:111, 1999.

143. Ginsburg D: Molecular genetics of von Willebrand disease. *Thromb Haemost* 82:585, 1999.

144. Sadler JE: Von Willebrand disease type 1: A diagnosis in search of a disease. *Blood* 101:2089, 2003.

145. Berkowitz SD, Dent JA, Roberts J, et al: Epitope mapping of the von Willebrand factor subunit distinguishes fragments present in normal and type IIA von Willebrand Disease from those generated by plasmin. *J Clin Invest* 79:524, 1987.

146. Ginsburg D, Konkle BA, Gill JC, et al: Molecular basis of human von Willebrand disease: Analysis of platelet von Willebrand factor mRNA. *Proc Natl Acad Sci U S A* 86:3723, 1989.

147. Lyons SE, Bruck ME, Bowie EJW, Ginsburg D: Impaired intracellular transport produced by a subset of type IIA von Willebrand disease mutations. *J Biol Chem* 267:4424, 1992.

148. Dent JA, Galbusera M, Ruggeri ZM: Heterogeneity of plasma von Willebrand factor multimers resulting from proteolysis of the constituent subunit. *J Clin Invest* 88:774, 1991.

149. Gralnick HR, Williams SB, McKeown LP, et al: In vitro correction of the abnormal multimeric structure of von Willebrand factor in Type IIA von Willebrand's disease. *Proc Natl Acad Sci U S A* 82:5968, 1985.

150. Kunicki TJ, Montgomery RR, Schullek J: Cleavage of human von Willebrand factor by platelet calcium-activated protease. *Blood* 65:352, 1985.

151. Schneppenheim R, Thomas KB, Krey S, et al: Identification of a candidate missense mutation in a family with von Willebrand disease type IIC. *HumGenet* 95:681, 1995.

152. Gaucher C, Diéval J, Mazurier C: Characterization of von Willebrand factor gene defects in two unrelated patients with type IIC von Willebrand disease. *Blood* 84:1024, 1994.

153. Schneppenheim R, Brassard J, Krey S, et al: Defective dimerization of von Willebrand factor subunits due to a Cys→Arg mutation in type IID von Willebrand disease. *Proc Natl Acad Sci U S A* 93:3581, 1996.

154. Cooney KA, Nichols WC, Bruck ME, et al: The molecular defect in type IIB von Willebrand disease. Identification of four potential missense mutations within the putative GpIb binding domain. *J Clin Invest* 87:1227, 1991.

155. Ribba AS, Lavergne JM, Bahnak BR, et al: Duplication of a methionine within the glycoprotein Ib binding domain of von Willebrand factor detected by denaturing gradient gel electrophoresis in a patient with Type IIB von Willebrand disease. *Blood* 78:1738, 1991.

156. Cooney KA, Ginsburg D: Comparative analysis of type 2B von Willebrand disease mutations: Implications for the mechanism of von Willebrand factor to binding platelets. *Blood* 87:2322, 1996.

157. Cooney KA, Lyons SE, Ginsburg D: Functional analysis of a type IIB von Willebrand disease missense mutation: Increased binding of large von Willebrand factor multimers to platelets. *Proc Natl Acad Sci U S A* 89:2869, 1992.

158. Ware J, Dent JA, Azuma H, et al: Identification of a point mutation in type IIB von Willebrand disease illustrating the regulation of von Willebrand factor affinity for the platelet membrane glycoprotein Ib-IX receptor. *Proc Natl Acad Sci U S A* 88:2946, 1991.

159. Kroner PA, Kluessendorf ML, Scott JP, Montgomery RR: Expressed full-length von Willebrand factor containing missense mutations linked to type IIB von Willebrand disease shows enhanced binding to platelets. *Blood* 79:2048, 1992.

160. Randi AM, Jorieux S, Tuley EA, et al: Recombinant von Willebrand factor Arg[578]→Gln: A type IIB von Willebrand disease mutation affects binding to glycoprotein Ib but not to collagen or heparin. *J Biol Chem* 267:21187, 1992.

161. Holmberg L, Dent JA, Schneppenheim R, et al: von Willebrand factor mutation enhancing interaction with platelets in patients with normal multimeric structure. *J Clin Invest* 91:2169, 1993.

162. Veltkamp JJ, van Tilburg NH: Autosomal Haemophilia: A variant of von Willebrand's disease. *Br J Haematol* 26:141, 1974.

163. Graham JB, Barrow ES, Roberts HR, et al: Dominant inheritance of hemophilia A in three generations of women. *Blood* 46:175, 1975.

164. Mazurier C, Gaucher C, Jorieux S, et al: Evidence for a von Willebrand factor defect in factor VIII binding in three members of a family previously misdiagnosed mild haemophilia A and haemophilia A carriers: Consequences for therapy and genetic counseling. *Br J Haematol* 76: 372, 1990.

165. Mazurier C, Diéval J, Jorieux S, et al: A new von Willebrand Factor (vWF) defect in a patient with factor VIII (FVIII) deficiency but with normal levels and multimeric patterns of both plasma and platelet vWF. Characterization of abnormal vWF/FVIII interaction. *Blood* 75:20, 1990.

166. Nishino M, Girma J-P, Rothschild C, et al: New variant of von Willebrand disease with defective binding to factor VIII. *Blood* 74:1591, 1989.

167. Eikenboom JCJ, Reitsma PH, Peerlinck KMJ, Briët E: Recessive inheritance of von Willebrand's disease type I. *Lancet* 341:982, 1993.

168. Rabinowitz I, Tuley EA, Mancuso DJ, et al: von Willebrand disease type B: A missense mutation selectively abolishes ristocetin-induced von Willebrand factor binding to platelet glycoprotein Ib. *Proc Natl Acad Sci U S A* 89:9846, 1992.

169. Meyer D, Fressinaud E, Gaucher C, et al: Gene defects in 150 unrelated French cases with type 2 von Willebrand disease: From the patient to the gene. *Thromb Haemost* 78:451, 1997.

170. Mannucci PM, Lombardi R, Castaman G, et al: von Willebrand disease "Vicenza" with larger-than-normal (supranormal) von Willebrand factor multimers. *Blood* 71:65, 1988.

171. Randi AM, Sacchi E, Castaman GC, et al: The genetic defect of type I von Willebrand disease "Vicenza" is linked to the von Willebrand factor gene. *Thromb Haemost* 69:173, 1993.

172. Casonato A, Pontara E, Sartorello F, et al: Reduced von Willebrand factor survival in type Vicenza von Willebrand disease. *Blood* 99:180, 2002.

173. Castaman G, Rodeghiero F, Mannucci PM: The elusive pathogenesis of von Willebrand disease Vicenza. *Blood* 99:4243, 2002.

174. Rodeghiero F, Castaman G, Dini E: Epidemiological investigation of the prevalence of von Willebrand's disease. *Blood* 69:454, 1987.

175. Werner EJ, Broxson EH, Tucker EL, et al: Prevalence of von Willebrand disease in children: A multiethnic study. *J Pediatr* 123:893, 1993.

176. Miller CH, Graham JB, Goldin LR, Elston RC: Genetics of classic von Willebrand's disease: I. phenotypic variation within families. *Blood* 54:117, 1979.

177. Gill JC, Endres-Brooks J, Bauer PJ, et al: The effect of ABO blood group on the diagnosis of von Willebrand Disease. *Blood* 69:1691, 1987.

178. Orstavik KH, Kornstad L, Reisner H, Berg K: Possible effect of secretor locus on plasma concentration of Factor VIII and von Willebrand factor. *Blood* 73:990, 1989.

179. O'Donnell J, Boulton FE, Manning RA, Laffan MA: Genotype at the secretor blood group locus is a determinant of plasma von Willebrand factor level. *Br J Haematol* 116:350, 2002.

180. Souto JC, Almasy L, Soria JM, et al: Genome-wide linkage analysis of von Willebrand factor plasma levels: Results from the GAIT project. *Thromb Haemost* 89:468, 2003.

181. Sadler JE: Von Willebrand disease type 1: A diagnosis in search of a disease. *Blood* 101:2089, 2003.

182. Weiss HJ, Ball AP, Mannucci PM: Incidence of severe von Willebrand's disease. *N Engl J Med* 307:127, 1982.

183. Berliner SA, Seligsohn U, Zivelin A, et al: A relatively high frequency of severe (type III) von Willebrand's disease in Israel. *Br J Haematol* 62:535, 1986.

184. Mannucci PM, Bloom AL, Larrieu MJ, et al: Atherosclerosis and von Willebrand factor: I. Prevalence of severe von Willebrand's disease in western Europe and Israel. *Br J Haematol* 57:163, 1984.

185. Nosek-Cenkowska B, Cheang MS, Pizzi NJ, et al: Bleeding/bruising symptomatology in children with and without bleeding disorders. *Thromb Haemost* 65:237, 1991.

186. Silwer J: von Willebrand's disease in Sweden. *Acta Paediatr Scand* 238(suppl):1, 1973.

187. van den DS, Mummery CL, Westermann CJ: Hereditary hemorrhagic telangiectasia: An update on transforming growth factor beta signaling in vasculogenesis and angiogenesis. *Cardiovasc Res* 58:20, 2003.

188. Iannuzzi MC, Hidaka N, Boehnke ML, et al: Analysis of the relationship of von Willebrand disease (vWD) and hereditary hemorrhagic telangiectasia and identification of a potential type IIA vWD mutation (IIe865 to Thr). *Am J Hum Genet* 48:757, 1991.

189. Rick ME, Williams SB, Sacher RA, McKeown LP: Thrombocytopenia associated with pregnancy in a patient with Type IIB von Willebrand's disease. *Blood* 69:786, 1987.

190. Mazurier C, Parquet-Gernez A, Goudemand J, et al: Investigation of a large kindred with type IIB von Willebrand's disease, dominant inheritance and age-dependent thrombocytopenia. *Br J Haematol* 69:499, 1988.

191. Schneppenheim R, Budde U, Krey S, et al: Results of a screening for von Willebrand disease type 2N in patients with suspected haemophilia A or von Willebrand disease type 1. *Thromb Haemost* 76:598, 1996.

192. Rodeghiero F, Castaman G, Tosetto A: von Willebrand factor antigen is less sensitive than ristocetin cofactor for the diagnosis of Type I von Willebrand disease: results based on a epidemiological investigation. *Thromb Haemost* 64:349, 1990.

193. Abildgaard CF, Suzuki Z, Harrison J, et al: Serial studies in von Willebrand's disease: Variability versus "variants." *Blood* 56:712, 1980.

194. Harker LA, Slichter SJ: The bleeding time as a screening test for evaluation of platelet function. *N Engl J Med* 287:155, 1972.

195. Lind SE: The bleeding time does not predict surgical bleeding. *Blood* 77:2547, 1991.

196. De Caterina R, Lanza M, Manca G, et al: Bleeding time and bleeding: An analysis of the relationship of the bleeding time test with parameters of surgical bleeding. *Blood* 84:3363, 1994.

197. Peterson P, Hayes TE, Arkin CF, et al: The preoperative bleeding time test lacks clinical benefit: College of American Pathologists' and American Society of Clinical Pathologists' position article. *Arch Surg* 133:134, 1998.

198. Weiss HJ, Hoyer LW, Rickles FR, et al: Quantitative assay of a plasma factor deficient in von Willebrand's disease that is necessary for platelet aggregation. *J Clin Invest* 52:2708, 1973.

199. Murdock PJ, Woodhams BJ, Matthews KB, et al: von Willebrand factor activity detected in a monoclonal antibody-based ELISA: An alternative to the ristocetin cofactor platelet agglutination assay for diagnostic use. *Thromb Haemost* 78:1272, 1997.

200. Preston FE: Assays for von Willebrand factor functional activity: A U.K. NEQAS survey. National External Quality Assessment Scheme. *Thromb Haemost* 80:863, 1998.

201. Favaloro EJ, Henniker A, Facey D, Hertzberg M: Discrimination of von Willebrand's disease (VWD) subtypes: Direct comparison of von Willebrand factor:collagen binding assay (VWF:CBA) with monoclonal antibody (MAB) based VWF-capture systems. *Thromb Haemost* 84:541, 2000.

202. Laffan M, Brown SA, Collins PW, et al: The diagnosis of von Willebrand disease: A guideline from the U.K. Haemophilia Centre Doctors' Organization. *Haemophilia* 10:199, 2004.

203. Ruggeri ZM, Zimmerman TS: The complex multimeric composition of Factor VIII/von Willebrand Factor. *Blood* 57:1140, 1981.

204. Mazurier C, Meyer D: Factor VIII binding assay of von Willebrand factor and the diagnosis of type 2N von Willebrand disease - results of an international survey. On behalf of the Subcommittee on von Willebrand Factor of the Scientific and Standardization Committee of the ISTH. *Thromb Haemost* 76:270, 1996.

205. Favaloro EJ, Dean M, Grispo L, et al: von Willebrand's disease: Use of collagen binding assay provides potential improvement to laboratory monitoring of desmopressin (DDAVP) therapy. *Am J Hematol* 45:205, 1994.

206. Riddell AF, Jenkins PV, Nitu-Whalley IC, et al: Use of the collagen-binding assay for von Willebrand factor in the analysis of type 2M von Willebrand disease: A comparison with the ristocetin cofactor assay. *Br J Haematol* 116:187, 2002.

207. Fressinaud E, Veyradier A, Truchaud F, et al: Screening for von Willebrand disease with a new analyzer using high shear stress: A study of 60 cases. *Blood* 91:1325, 1998.

208. Cattaneo M, Federici AB, Lecchi A, et al: Evaluation of the PFA-100 system in the diagnosis and therapeutic monitoring of patients with von Willebrand disease. *Thromb Haemost* 82:35, 1999.

209. Fujimura Y, Kawasaki T, Titani K: Snake venom proteins modulating the interaction between von Willebrand factor and platelet glycoprotein Ib. *Thromb Haemost* 76:633, 1996.

210. Bignell P, Standen GR, Bowen DJ, et al: Rapid neonatal diagnosis of von Willebrand's disease by use of the polymerase chain reaction. *Lancet* 336:638, 1990.

211. Sadler JE, Ginsburg D: A database of polymorphisms in the von Willebrand factor gene and pseudogene. *Thromb Haemost* 69:185, 1993.

212. Peake IR, Bowen D, Bignell P, et al: Family studies and prenatal diagnosis in severe von Willebrand Disease by polymerase chain reaction

amplification of a variable number tandem repeat region of the von Willebrand factor gene. *Blood* 76:555, 1990.

213. Mannhalter C, Kyrle PA, Brenner B, Lechner K: Rapid neonatal diagnosis of Type IIB von Willebrand disease using the polymerase chain reaction. *Blood* 77:2538, 1991.

214. Miller JL: Platelet-type von Willebrand disease. *Thromb Haemost* 75:865, 1996.

215. Kumar S, Pruthi RK, Nichols WL: Acquired von Willebrand disease. *Mayo Clin Proc* 77:181, 2002.

216. Budde U, Schaefer G, Mueller N, et al: Acquired von Willebrand's disease in the myeloproliferative syndrome. *Blood* 64:981, 1984.

217. Mannucci PM, Lombardi R, Bader R, et al: Studies of the pathophysiology of acquired von Willebrand's disease in seven patients with lymphoproliferative disorders or benign monoclonal gammopathies. *Blood* 64:614, 1984.

218. Rogers JS, Shane SR, Jencks FS: Factor VIII activity and thyroid function. *Ann Intern Med* 97:713, 1982.

219. Viallard JF, Pellegrin JL, Vergnes C, et al: Three cases of acquired von Willebrand disease associated with systemic lupus erythematosus. *Br J Haematol* 105:532, 1999.

220. Scott JP, Montgomery RR, Tubergen DG, Hays T: Acquired von Willebrand's disease in association with Wilm's tumor: Regression following treatment. *Blood* 58:665, 1981.

221. Warkentin TE, Moore JC, Morgan DG: Aortic stenosis and bleeding gastrointestinal angiodysplasia: Is acquired von Willebrand's disease the link? *Lancet* 340:35, 1992.

222. Castaman G, Lattuada A, Mannucci PM, Rodeghiero F: Characterization of two cases of acquired transitory von Willebrand syndrome with ciprofloxacin: Evidence for heightened proteolysis of von Willebrand factor. *Am J Hematol* 49:83, 1995.

223. Tefferi A, Nichols WL: Acquired von Willebrand disease: Concise review of occurrence, diagnosis, pathogenesis, and treatment. *Am J Med* 103:536, 1997.

224. Cohen AJ, Kessler CM, Ewenstein BM: Management of von Willebrand disease: A survey on current clinical practice from the haemophilia centres of North America. *Haemophilia* 7:235, 2001.

225. Sumner M, Williams J: Type 3 von Willebrand disease: Assessment of complications and approaches to treatment: Results of a patient and Hemophilia Treatment Center Survey in the United States. *Haemophilia* 10:360, 2004.

226. Mannucci PM, Ruggeri ZM, Pareti FI, Capitanio A: 1-Deamino-8-D-arginine vasopressin: A new pharmacological approach to the management of haemophilia and von Willebrand's diseases. *Lancet* 1:869, 1977.

227. Ruggeri ZM, Mannucci PM, Lombardi R, et al: Multimeric composition of factor VIII/von Willebrand Factor following administration of DDAVP: Implications for pathophysiology and therapy of von Willebrand's disease subtypes. *Blood* 59:1272, 1982.

228. Mannucci PM: Desmopressin (DDAVP) in the treatment of bleeding disorders: The first 20 years. *Blood* 90:2515, 1997.

229. Lethagen S, Harris AS, Nilsson IM: Intranasal desmopressin (DDAVP) by spray in mild hemophilia A and von Willebrand's disease type I. *Blut* 60:187, 1990.

230. Rose EH, Aledort LM: Nasal spray desmopressin (DDAVP) for mild hemophilia A and von Willebrand disease. *Ann Intern Med* 114:563, 1991.

231. Rodeghiero F, Castaman G, Di Bona E, Ruggeri M: Consistency of responses to repeated DDAVP infusions in patients with von Willebrand's disease and hemophilia A. *Blood* 74:1997, 1989.

232. Mannucci PM, Bettega D, Cattaneo M: Patterns of development of tachyphylaxis in patients with haemophilia and von Willebrand disease after repeated doses of desmopressin (DDAVP). *Br J Haematol* 82:87, 1992.

233. Federici AB, Mazurier C, Berntorp E, et al: Biologic response to desmopressin in patients with severe type 1 and type 2 von Willebrand disease: Results of a multicenter European study. *Blood* 103:2032, 2004.

234. de la Fuente B, Kasper CK, Rickles FR, Hoyer LW: Response of patients with mild and moderate hemophilia A and von Willebrand's disease to treatment with desmopressin. *Ann Intern Med* 103:6, 1985.

235. Gralnick HR, Williams SB, McKeown LP, et al: DDAVP in type IIa von Willebrand's disease. *Blood* 67:465, 1986.

236. Holmberg L, Nilsson IM, Borge L, et al: Platelet aggregation induced by 1-desamino-8-D-arginine vasopressin (DDAVP) in Type IIB von Willebrand's disease. *N Engl J Med* 309:816, 1983.

237. Casonato A, Sartori MT, De Marco L, Girolami A: 1-Desamino-8-D-arginine vasopressin (DDAVP) infusion in Type IIB von Willebrand's disease: Shortening of bleeding time and induction of a variable pseudothrombocytopenia. *Thromb Haemost* 64:117, 1990.

238. McKeown LP, Connaghan G, Wilson O, et al: 1-desamino-8-arginine-vasopressin corrects the hemostatic defects in type 2B von Willebrand's disease. *Am J Hematol* 51:158, 1996.

239. Mazurier C, Gaucher C, Jorieux S, Goudemand M, et al: Biological effect of desmopressin in eight patients with type 2N ("Normandy") von Willebrand disease. *Br J Haematol* 88:849, 1994.

240. Foster PA: A perspective on the use of FVIII concentrates and cryoprecipitate prophylactically in surgery or therapeutically in severe bleeds in patients with von Willebrand disease unresponsive to DDAVP: Results of an international survey. *Thromb Haemost* 74:1370, 1995.

241. Morfini M, Mannucci PM, Tenconi PM, et al: Pharmacokinetics of monoclonally-purified and recombinant factor VIII in patients with severe von Willebrand disease. *Thromb Haemost* 70:270, 1993.

242. Pasi KJ, Collins PW, Keeling DM, et al: Management of von Willebrand disease: A guideline from the U.K. Haemophilia Centre Doctors' Organization. *Haemophilia* 10:218, 2004.

243. Makris M, Colvin B, Gupta V, et al: Venous thrombosis following the use of intermediate purity FVIII concentrate to treat patients with von Willebrand's disease. *Thromb Haemost* 88:387, 2002.

244. Mannucci PM, Chediak J, Hanna W, et al: Treatment of von Willebrand disease with a high-purity factor VIII/von Willebrand factor concentrate: A prospective, multicenter study. *Blood* 99:450, 2002.

245. Mannucci PM, Tamaro G, Narchi G, et al: Life-threatening reaction to factor VIII concentrate in a patient with severe von Willebrand disease and alloantibodies to von Willebrand factor. *Eur J Haematol* 39:467, 1987.

246. Bergamaschini L, Mannucci PM, Federici AB, et al: Posttransfusion anaphylactic reactions in a patient with severe von Willebrand disease: Role of complement and alloantibodies to von Willebrand factor. *J Lab Clin Med* 125:348, 1995.

247. Harrison RL, McKee PA: Estrogen stimulates von Willebrand Factor production by cultured endothelial cells. *Blood* 63:657, 1984.

248. Ginsburg D, Bowie EJW: Molecular genetics of von Willebrand disease. *Blood* 79:2507, 1992.

249. Berkowitz SD, Ruggeri ZM, Zimmerman TS: von Willebrand Disease, in *Coagulation and Bleeding Disorders. The Role of Factor VIII and von Willebrand Factor*, edited by TS Zimmerman, ZM Ruggeri, p 215. Marcel Dekker, New York, 1989.

ANTIBODY-MEDIATED COAGULATION FACTOR DEFICIENCIES

JOZEF VERMYLEN

JEF ARNOUT

Antibody-mediated coagulation factor deficiencies are uncommon acquired conditions that can lead to uncontrollable hemorrhage. The most frequently observed example is acquired hemophilia A, which is associated with older age, autoimmune and malignant disorders, the postpartum period, and use of drugs such as penicillin and sulfonamides. Unlike isoantibodies that develop in hemophilia A patients, autoantibodies that develop in patients with acquired hemophilia A are amenable to immunosuppressive therapy. Prothrombin deficiency can occur in patients with lupus anticoagulant and is associated with bleeding. Autoantibodies against factor V or factor XIII can cause bleeding. Acquired factor X deficiency is rare; but when it occurs, acquired factor X deficiency usually is associated with amyloidosis (AL) as a result of adsorption of factor X to the amyloid fibrils.

INTRODUCTION

Coagulation factor deficiencies are inherited or acquired. The causes of acquired coagulation factor deficiency include (1) impaired synthesis, for example, vitamin K deficiency or liver disease (see Chap. 120); (2) accelerated catabolism, as in disseminated intravascular coagulation (DIC) (see Chap. 121), and thrombolytic therapy (see Chap. 127); (3) antibody-mediated neutralization of activity; and (4) accelerated clearance from the circulation. The main entities caused by autoantibodies to coagulation factors are acquired hemophilia A, prothrombin deficiency complicating the antiphospholipid syndrome (see Chap. 123), acquired factor V deficiency, and acquired factor XIII deficiency. Accelerated removal of factor X occurs in light chain amyloidosis (AL) and results in factor X deficiency.

ACQUIRED HEMOPHILIA A

DEFINITION AND HISTORY

Acquired hemophilia A is a sudden deficiency of factor VIII caused by the development of factor VIII autoantibodies, usually of the IgG class, which occurs in subjects with no previous history of a bleeding disorder. The concept of circulating anticoagulants as a cause of bleeding was first introduced in the 1950s, as reviewed in 1961.[1]

EPIDEMIOLOGY

Autoimmune factor VIII deficiency is uncommon. A population-based study of consecutive patients with acquired hemophilia A in South Wales, United Kingdom, yielded an annual incidence rate of 1.34 cases per million. The median age at presentation was 70 years.[2] The disorder is evenly distributed between males and females. In a large multicenter survey, approximately 50 percent of patients had associated or concomitant disorders that were recognized at the time of autoantibody detection.[3] Rheumatoid arthritis, systemic lupus erythematosus, and other immunologic disorders, such as drug reactions, accounted for almost half of the associated conditions. Among the drugs that have been implicated are penicillin, sulfonamides, isoniazid, hydralazine, procainamide, methyldopa, interferon alpha, and phenytoin. Malignant disorders also have been implicated; however, because most patients with acquired hemophilia A are older, whether the association is coincidental or reflects a paraneoplastic phenomenon is not clear. Eight percent of the cases occur during the postpartum period.[3] In such women, the acquired factor VIII antibodies usually are identified 2 to 5 months after delivery but sometimes after 12 months.

ETIOLOGY AND PATHOGENESIS

Acquired hemophilia is an autoimmune disorder. The pathogenesis of autoimmunity is incompletely understood. For many years, prevailing thought maintained that, in the normal state of the immune system, autoimmunity did not occur because of clonal deletion of autoreactive cells, while the major repertoire of T and B cells was directed toward recognizing foreign antigens. The current view maintains that a low level of autoreactivity is physiologic and even essential for normal immune function, and that survival of naive T and B cells in the peripheral tissues requires continuous exposure to autoantigens.[4] Because autoreactivity is physiologic, the challenge is understanding why and how it becomes pathogenic. Autoreactivity at the B cell level involves autoantibody production. Normal serum contains antibodies that are called "natural" because they are generated in the absence of deliberate immunization or exposure to foreign antigens.[5] Most natural antibodies in healthy people are autoantibodies produced by autoreactive B cells in response to autoantigens.[6] Autoantibodies against factor VIII can be detected in the serum of most healthy people,[7] but their activity normally is neutralized by the simultaneous presence of a second autoantibody against the idiotype of the first antibody. Therefore, the lack of autoimmunity does not result from the absence of autoreactive lymphocytes but from maintenance of a state of active tolerance in these lymphocytes. Tolerance signaling occurs in lymphocytes when antigen is chronically encountered, which ensures lymphocyte survival. Autoimmunity occurs when tolerance signaling fails and causes formation of larger amounts of natural autoantibodies, such as the natural autoantibody to factor VIII. Therefore, autoimmunity is considered a loss of active self-control.[8] Such reduced self-control, which occurs at old age, during the postpartum period, and with exposure to specific drugs, predisposes patients to development of acquired hemophilia A.

CLINICAL FEATURES

Autoimmune factor VIII deficiency is one of the major causes of spontaneous life-threatening bleeding in the elderly. The cardinal clinical feature is unexplained bleeding of sudden onset. The condition may consist of extensive subcutaneous bruising, spontaneous bleeding in closed compartments such as joints, or bleeding into large muscles, the retroperitoneal space, gastrointestinal tract, and urinary tract. Joint bleeding is not life-threatening. However, joint bleeding is extremely painful because of the very high pressure that develops within the joint, and it can give rise to joint deformity. Bleeding in poorly defined compartments can be life- or limb-threatening because the bleeding does not cease spontaneously, possibly leading to exsanguination, displacement, and compression of organs, nerves, and blood vessels by massive hematomas. Occasionally, uncontrollable hemorrhage follow-

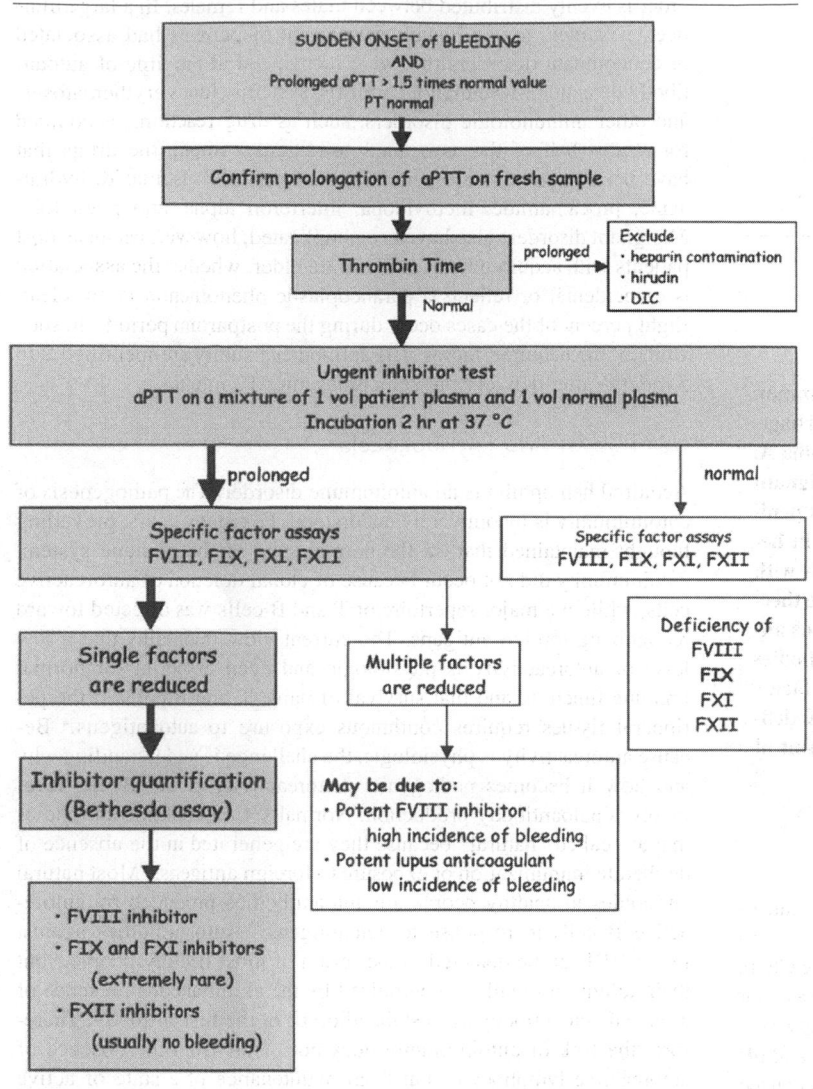

FIGURE 119-1   Flow chart for laboratory diagnosis of acquired hemophilia. When no inhibitor is found, an assay for factor XIII should be performed. FIX, factor IX; FVIII, factor VIII; FXI, factor XI; FXII, factor XII.

ing a minor invasive procedure, such as insertion of a central venous line, is the initial manifestation of the disorder.

LABORATORY FEATURES

Acquired hemophilia A is characterized by a prolonged activated partial thromboplastin time (aPTT) that is not normalized when plasma from the patient is mixed with normal plasma (in a deficiency state, a limited amount of normal plasma corrects the coagulation disturbance). A thrombin time assay should be performed to exclude heparin contamination of the sample. Prothrombin time (PT) and platelet count are characteristically normal. Specific factor VIII assays usually reveal a level less than 5 percent of normal. The neutralizing autoantibody can be quantified using the Bethesda assay,[9] which also is used for quantification of isoantibodies to factor VIII that may develop in hemophiliacs following therapeutic exposure to factor VIII (see Chap. 115). One Bethesda unit corresponds to the amount of antibody that halves factor VIII activity of normal plasma following incubation of 2 hours at 37°C. In some patients, slight residual factor VIII activity is detected despite the presence of relatively high antibody titers. Presumably such antibodies only partially interfere with expression of

clotting activity.[10] When high titers of factor VIII inhibitors are present, activity of factors XII, XI, and IX may be artificially depressed. However, if the assays are repeated in increasing dilutions of patient plasma in factor-deficient plasma, then the true levels of factors XII, XI, and IX emerge while factor VIII activity remains at the lower levels. Figure 119-1 outlines the diagnostic procedure for identifying acquired hemophilia A and its differentiation from other diagnoses.

DIFFERENTIAL DIAGNOSIS

Distinction of acquired hemophilia A from hemophilia A or von Willebrand disease is evidenced by bleeding that is of recent onset and not lifelong. Acquired von Willebrand disease may be more difficult to distinguish from acquired hemophilia A, but typically patients with acquired von Willebrand disease have a prolonged bleeding time and low levels of von Willebrand factor (see Chaps. 109 and 118). A strong lupus anticoagulant may interfere with the one-stage clotting assay of factor VIII (see Chap. 123) but also can prolong the one-stage clotting assays of factors IX, XI, and XII. Dilution of a sample containing such a lupus anticoagulant restores a normal level of factor VIII (and of the other factors), whereas dilution of a sample containing an antibody against factor VIII fails to correct the low level of factor VIII (see Chap. 109). A lupus anticoagulant only rarely is associated with a sudden onset of bleeding symptoms.

THERAPY

As soon as the diagnosis of acquired hemophilia is suspected, a number of preventive measures must be taken. All invasive procedures, including intramuscular injections, arterial punctures, and placement of central venous lines should be avoided because the procedures may cause catastrophic bleeding. When such procedures cannot be avoided, they should only be performed after hemostatic therapy (see next section). Intake of aspirin or other drugs that may affect hemostasis should be prohibited. Sites of venous puncture require prolonged application of local pressure. Therapy consists of immediate measures for an acute bleeding episode and long-term elimination of the autoantibody.

IMMEDIATE HEMOSTATIC MEASURES

Instances of bleeding from tooth sockets sometimes can be controlled by local application of a fibrin glue and use of an oral antifibrinolytic drug (ε-aminocaproic acid or tranexamic acid) to delay resorption of the fibrin plug. Desmopressin, which induces release of endogenous stores of factor VIII, can be effective but only in patients with very low inhibitor titers. In patients with a low-titer inhibitor (less than 5 Bethesda units per ml), intravenous administration of very high doses of factor VIII (500 units per kilogram body weight) may temporarily normalize the factor VIII level and arrest the bleeding. Administration of factor VIII in patients with acquired hemophilia A usually does not provoke an anamnestic response, that is, a further rise in natural antibody level. This finding contrasts with the frequent (sometimes profound) increase of isoantibodies that occurs in patients with hemophilia A following administration of factor VIII concentrates. In patients with a higher titer of autoantibodies against factor VIII, correcting hemostasis simply by administering factor VIII is not possible.

Activated Concentrates An alternative strategy for achieving hemostasis is use of activated clotting factor concentrates that "bypass" the inhibitor. Activated prothrombin concentrates containing prothrombin and factors VII and X (the latter two partially activated) may render thrombin generation less dependent on factor VIII. Their efficacy has been shown in both hemophiliacs and nonhemophiliacs with antibodies to factor VIII.[11,12] One disadvantage of these plasma derivatives is that the active principle is not precisely defined and quantified. Recombinant activated factor VII, on the other hand, is a clearly defined and quantified active agent. It binds to negatively charged phospholipids on activated platelets and locally generates sufficient amounts of thrombin that is hemostatically effective. The recommended dose of recombinant factor VIIa is 90 to 120 μg/kg body weight in intravenous boluses repeated every 2 hours until the hemorrhagic condition improves.[13] The disadvantages of activated prothrombin concentrates and recombinant factor VIIa are unpredicted hemostatic efficacy, rare thrombotic complications, and the extremely high cost of the products.

Use of Porcine Factor VIII The autoantibodies to human factor VIII usually show lower cross-reactivity to porcine factor VIII. In some countries, porcine factor VIII is available for treatment of bleeding in patients with factor VIII inhibitors and yields satisfactory results.[14,15] This animal protein usually gives rise to an anamnestic anti-factor VIII response. Although the porcine concentrate is not subjected to viral inactivation processes during production, no evidence indicates porcine virus transmission with this concentrate.[16]

IMMUNODEPLETION AND SUPPRESSION

Extracorporeal immunoadsorption of antibody on protein A Sepharose columns[17,18] in combination with administration of high doses of factor VIII and immunosuppressive therapy (or intravenous immunoglobulin) also has been advocated but requires highly specialized equipment and entails very high cost. Exchange plasmapheresis to reduce the level of circulating antibody usually is not sufficiently effective or feasible in hemodynamically unstable bleeding patients.

Occasional cases of high-dose intravenous immunoglobulin by itself dramatically reducing the antibody titer, presumably because the immunoglobulin contains neutralizing antiidiotypic antibodies, have been reported.[19] However, the outcome of this mode of treatment is unpredictable.

In contrast to the hemophilia A patient with an inhibitor, the patient with acquired hemophilia may respond well to immunosuppressive therapy. Initial treatment consists of prednisone. If no response is seen within a few weeks, cyclophosphamide should be added. The value of this combination was documented in a prospective randomized trial.[20] Other treatments with cyclosporin,[21] rituximab,[22] and 2-chlorodeoxyadenosine[23] have been used, but the experience is limited.

COURSE AND PROGNOSIS

Mortality in patients with acquired hemophilia A is high. Mortality in a large series was 22 percent,[3] with similar rates observed in other reports.[2,24] A meta-analysis revealed that malignancy, older age at diagnosis, and poor response to therapy were associated with poor prognosis. Patients with an underlying autoimmune disorder had a better prognosis, and women at the postpartum period had the best outcome. Autoantibodies occurring during pregnancy or after drug reactions may disappear spontaneously in the postpartum period or when the drug reaction subsides. Spontaneous disappearance of idiopathic autoantibodies has been recorded.[3,25]

Completely eradicating the inhibitor may not always be feasible. Some patients manage well with a low-titer inhibitor, and a balance must be sought between the residual risk posed by the inhibitor and the side effects of immunosuppressive therapy.

ANTIBODY-MEDIATED PROTHROMBIN DEFICIENCY

Although antibodies to prothrombin are frequently found in the antiphospholipid syndrome,[26] prothrombin deficiency is rare because the antiprothrombin antibodies in this syndrome usually are of moderate affinity and do not significantly affect circulating prothrombin levels. The lupus anticoagulant-hypoprothrombinemia syndrome was first described by Rapaport and colleagues[27] in an 11-year-old girl with systemic lupus erythematosus and severe bleeding. Since the initial report, this syndrome has been documented in 29 pediatric patients, often following viral infection, and less frequently in adult patients.[28] Such patients have prolonged prothrombin and partial thromboplastin times. The diagnosis is established based on a selective deficiency of prothrombin in an adequately diluted sample and normal levels of the other vitamin K-dependent clotting factors. If the bleeding problems are considerable, immunosuppressive therapy may be an option.

ACQUIRED FACTOR X DEFICIENCY IN AMYLOIDOSIS

Isolated factor X deficiency can be one feature of AL amyloidosis. In a study of 368 consecutive patients with systemic AL amyloidosis, 32 (8.7%) had factor X levels less than 50 percent of normal.[29] Eighteen of the 32 patients had bleeding manifestations that were more frequent and severe in the 12 patients with factor X less than 25 percent of normal; bleeding was fatal in two patients. Radiolabeled factor X is cleared at an extremely fast rate from blood in these patients because of specific binding of factor X to amyloid fibrils.[30] The extent of factor X deficiency in a given patient depends on the affinity of the amyloid immunoglobulin light-chain fibrils for factor X and the mass of amyloid that is exposed to the circulating blood.

Factor X deficiency is characterized by prolonged prothrombin and partial thromboplastin times. Factor X activity is markedly reduced, whereas the other vitamin K-dependent clotting factors usually are within the normal range. The bleeding tendency in patients sometimes is aggravated by perivascular deposits of amyloid causing vascular fragility. When an invasive procedure is planned, treatment with a prothrombin complex concentrate may be considered, taking into account the very rapid disappearance of the infused factor X.

Ten factor X-deficient patients received high-dose melphalan chemotherapy followed by autologous stem cell transplantation.[29] Of seven patients who were alive 1 year after transplantation, four had a complete hematologic response and an increased factor X level. Removal of a large spleen infiltrated with amyloid can correct the factor X deficiency.[31]

ACQUIRED FACTOR V DEFICIENCY

Between 1955 and 2002, 126 cases of antibodies against factor V were documented in the medical literature, 87 in the last decade of the survey. Of these 87 cases, two thirds were associated with exposure to bovine thrombin.[32] Bovine thrombin has been used frequently for surgical hemostasis. Until 1999, bovine thrombin-derived fibrin sealant was the only product available in the United States. Presumably, antibodies developing in patients exposed to bovine thrombin are against bovine factor V that contaminates the bovine thrombin preparation. These antibodies cross-react with human factor V, leading to the acquired factor V deficiency. The cross-reacting antibodies tend to disappear spontaneously. Bovine thrombin now has largely been replaced by human thrombin in hemostatic preparations. The overall prognosis of factor V inhibitors is good, with the best prognosis observed in patients exposed to bovine thrombin and the worst prognosis in patients with "idiopathic" inhibitors.[33] The patients have a moderate bleeding tendency. Both prothrombin and partial thromboplastin times are prolonged. Assay of factor V reveals a markedly decreased level. The presence of neutralizing antibody is confirmed by the disappearance of factor V activity when dilutions of patient plasma are added to normal plasma. Immunoadsorption and plasmapheresis seem to be the most effective modes of therapy in acute severe bleeding.[33] Hypothetically, activated prothrombin complex concentrates or recombinant factor VIIa acting in concert with activated platelets could be useful. Platelets contain an activated form of factor V in the α-granules that may be protected from the circulating antibody. Rapid interaction of secreted factor V, surface-bound factor VIIa, factor Xa, and prothrombin, all assembled on activated platelets, may prevent neutralization by the factor V antibody and induce local thrombin formation, resulting in hemostasis. Long-term eradication of the inhibitor may require immunosuppressive therapy. Successful use of high-dose intravenous immunoglobulin has been reported.[34]

ACQUIRED FACTOR XIII DEFICIENCY

Fewer than 30 patients with neutralizing antibodies against factor XIII have been described. Provoking factors are autoimmune disorders such as systemic lupus erythematosus, drugs such as isoniazid, procainamide, practolol, or phenytoin, and old age.[35,36] The clinical picture consists of bruising, gastrointestinal hemorrhage, and cerebral bleeding. Unless suspected, the diagnosis may not be simple because results of all screening coagulation tests, such as PT or aPTT, are normal. The lack of fibrin stabilization because of factor XIII deficiency can be demonstrated by enhanced solubilization of clots in 5 M urea. Specific factor XIII assays are available and demonstrate markedly reduced factor XIII activity. The presence of a neutralizing antibody is confirmed by mixing experiments. Treatment of severe bleeding can be attempted with antifibrinolytic agents or infusion of factor XIII concentrate.[35] Immunosuppressive therapy can eliminate the autoantibody.

REFERENCES

1. Margolius A Jr, Jackson DP, Ratnoff OD: Circulating anticoagulants: A study of 40 cases and a review of the literature. *Medicine (Baltimore)* 40:145, 1961.

2. Collins P, Macartney N, Davies R, et al: A population based, unselected, consecutive cohort of patients with acquired haemophilia A. *Br J Haematol* 124:86, 2004.

3. Green D, Lechner K: A survey of 215 non-hemophilic patients with inhibitors to factor VIII. *Thromb Haemost* 45:200, 1981.

4. Dighiero G, Rose NR: Critical self-epitopes are key to the understanding of self-tolerance and autoimmunity. *Immunol Today* 20:423, 1999.

5. Coutinho A, Kazatchkine MD, Avremeas S: Natural autoantibodies. *Curr Opin Immunol* 7:812, 1995.

6. Hayakawa K, Asano M, Shinton SA, et al: Positive selection of natural autoreactive B cells. *Science* 285:112, 1999.

7. Gilles JG, Saint-Remy JMR: Healthy subjects produce both anti-factor VIII and specific antiidiotypic antibodies. *J Clin Invest* 94:1496, 1994.

8. Bach JF: Autoimmune diseases as the loss of active "self-control." *Ann N Y Acad Sci* 998:11, 2003.

9. Kasper CK, Aledort LM, Counts RB, et al: A more uniform measurement of factor VIII inhibitors. *Thromb Diath Haemorrh* 34:869, 1975.

10. Jacquemin M, Benhida A, Peerlinck K, et al: A human antibody directed to the factor VIII C1 domain inhibits factor VIII cofactor activity and binding to von Willebrand factor. *Blood* 95:156, 2000.

11. Lusher JM, Shapiro SS, the Hemophilia Study Group, et al: Efficacy of prothrombin complex concentrates in hemophiliacs with antibodies to factor VIII: A multicenter therapeutic trial. *N Engl J Med* 303:421, 1980.

12. Lusher JM: Factor VIII inhibitors: Etiology, characterization, natural history and management. *Ann N Y Acad Sci* 509:89, 1987.

13. Hay CR, Négrier C, Ludlam CA: The treatment of bleeding in acquired haemophilia with recombinant factor VIIa: A multicenter study. *Thromb Haemost* 78:1463, 1997.

14. Brettler DB, Forsberg AD, Levine PH, et al: The use of porcine factor VIII concentrate (Hyate C) in the treatment of patients with inhibitor antibodies to factor VIII:C: A multicenter U.S. trial. *Arch Intern Med* 149:1381, 1989.

15. Morrison AE, Ludlam CA, Kessler CM: Use of porcine factor VIII in the treatment of patients with acquired hemophilia. *Blood* 81:1513, 1993.

16. Giangrande PLF, Kessler CM, Jenkins CE, et al: Viral pharmacovigilance study of haemophiliacs receiving porcine factor VIII. *Haemophilia* 8:798, 2002.

17. Nilsson IM, Jonsson S, Sundqvist SB: A procedure for removing high titer antibodies by extracorporeal protein-A Sepharose in hemophilia: Substitution therapy and surgery in a patient with hemophilia B and antibodies. *Blood* 58:38, 1981.

18. Rivard GE, St Louis J, Lacroix S, et al: Immunoadsorption for coagulation factor inhibitors: A retrospective critical appraisal of 10 consecutive cases from a single institution. *Haemophilia* 9:711, 2003.

19. Sultan Y, Maisonneuve P, Kazatchkine MD, Nydegger UE. Anti-idiotypic suppression of autoantibodies to factor VIII (antihaemophilic factor) by high-dose intravenous gammaglobin. *Lancet* ii:765, 1984.

20. Green D, Rademaker AW, Briët E: A prospective, randomized trial of prednisone and cyclophosphamide in the treatment of patients with factor VIII autoantibodies. *Thromb Haemost* 70:753, 1993.

21. Schulman S, Langevitz P, Livnek A, et al: Cyclosporine therapy for acquired factor VIII inhibitor in a patient with systemic lupus erythematosus. *Thromb Haemost* 76:344, 1996.

22. Wiestner A, Cho HJ, Asch AS, et al: Rituximab in the treatment of acquired factor VIII inhibitors. *Blood* 100:3426, 2002.

23. Sallah S, Wan JS: Efficacy of 2-chlorodeoxyadenosine in refractory factor VIII inhibitors in persons without hemophilia. *Blood* 101:943, 2003.

24. Delgado J, Jimenez-Yuste V, Hernandez-Navarro F, Villar A: Acquired haemophilia: Review and meta-analysis focused on therapy and prognostic factors. *Br J Haematol* 121:26, 2003.

25. Lottenberg R, Kentro TB, Kitchens CS: Acquired hemophilia: A natural history study of 16 patients with factor VIII inhibitors receiving little or no therapy. *Arch Intern Med* 147:1077, 1987.

26. Arnout J, Vermylen J: Current status and implications of autoimmune antiphospholipid antibodies in relation to thrombotic disease. *J Thromb Haemost* 1:931, 2003.

27. Rapaport SI, Ames SB, Duvall BJ: A plasma coagulation defect in systemic lupus erythematous arising from hypoprothrombinemia combined with anti-prothrombinase activity. *Blood* 15:212, 1960.

28. Baca V, Montiel G, Meillon L, et al: Diagnosis of lupus anticoagulant in the lupus anticoagulant-hypoprothrombinemia syndrome: Report of two cases and review of the literature. *Am J Hematol* 71:200, 2002.

29. Choufani EB, Sanchorawala V, Ernst T, et al: Acquired factor X deficiency in patients with amyloid light-chain amyloidosis: Incidence, bleeding manifestations, and response to high-dose chemotherapy. *Blood* 97:1885, 2001.

30. Furie B, Voo L, McAdam KPWJ, Furie BC: Mechanism of factor X deficiency in amyloidosis. *N Engl J Med* 304:827, 1981.

31. Greipp PR, Kyle RA, Bowie EJW: Factor X deficiency in primary amyloidosis: Resolution after splenectomy. *N Engl J Med* 301:1050, 1979.

32. Streiff MB, Ness PM: Acquired factor V inhibitors: A needless iatrogenic complication of bovine thrombin exposure. *Transfusion* 42:18, 2002.

33. Knöbl P, Lechner K: Acquired factor V inhibitors. *Baillieres Clin Haematol* 11:305, 1998.

34. de Raucourt E, Barbier C, Sinda P, et al: High-dose intravenous immunoglobulin treatment in two patients with acquired factor V inhibitors. *Am J Hematol* 74:187, 2003.

35. Tosetto A, Rodeghiero F, Gatti E, et al: An acquired hemorrhagic disorder of fibrin crosslinking due to IgG antibodies to FXIII, successfully treated with F XIII replacement and cyclophosphamide. *Am J Hematol* 48:34, 1995.

36. Ahmad F, Solymoss S, Poon M-C, et al: Characterization of an acquired IgG inhibitor of coagulation factor XIII in a patient with systemic lupus erythematosus. *Br J Haematol* 93:700, 1996.

HEMOSTATIC DYSFUNCTION RELATED TO LIVER DISEASES AND LIVER TRANSPLANTATION

TON LISMAN
PHILIP G. DE GROOT

Liver disease is associated with substantial changes in the hemostatic system, which include thrombocytopenia and platelet dysfunction, defects in thrombin generation, defective fibrin formation resulting from dysfibrinogenemia, and augmented fibrinolysis. The net effect of these hemostatic derangements is a bleeding tendency that is manifested particularly during invasive procedures. The greatest challenge to hemostasis in a patient with liver disease occurs during liver transplantation when the hemostatic system is further compromised. The impaired clearance of activated clotting factors during the anhepatic phase and the release of activators of coagulation and fibrinolysis from the donor liver following reperfusion are the main causes for the severe derangement in hemostatic balance. Thus, liver transplantation is accompanied by massive blood loss and requires multiple perioperative transfusions.

INTRODUCTION

Chronic or acute liver failure initiated by, for example, viral hepatitis, alcohol abuse, or acetaminophen intoxication results in substantial changes in the hemostatic system.[1] Because the liver is involved in the synthesis of many hemostatic proteins, reduced amounts of these proteins are found if the synthetic function of the liver is compromised. Furthermore, a diseased liver has a reduced ability to clear activated hemostatic proteins, activators of fibrinolysis, or protein–inhibitor complexes from the circulation. A reduced platelet count and impaired platelet function also are commonly observed in patients with liver disease. Taken together, these alterations lead to a bleeding tendency that is particularly evident during major invasive procedures, such as liver transplantation. On the other hand, thrombosis of the portal vein and the hepatic artery may occur in patients with liver disease or following liver transplantation. This chapter considers the hemostatic changes in patients with liver disease and during liver transplantation and reviews the currently available therapeutic modalities.

PATHOGENESIS

PLATELETS

THROMBOCYTOPENIA

A mild to moderate thrombocytopenia (platelet counts between 50,000 and 100,000/μl) is frequently present in patients with liver disease.

Acronyms and abbreviations that appear in this chapter include: ADAMTS-13, a disintegrin-like and metalloprotease with thrombospondin type 1 repeats; DIC, disseminated intravascular coagulation; PAI, plasminogen-activator inhibitor; TAFI, thrombin-activatable fibrinolysis inhibitor; TFPI, tissue factor pathway inhibitor; t-PA, tissue plasminogen activator; vWF, von Willebrand factor.

The main causes for thrombocytopenia are increased platelet sequestration in the spleen because of congestive splenomegaly related to portal hypertension[2,3] and reduced thrombopoietin production by the liver.[4] Alternative mechanisms of thrombocytopenia include a reduced platelet half-life possibly related to autoantibodies[5] and, in patients with alcohol-induced liver disease, folic acid deficiency and defective platelet production as consequences of toxic effects of alcohol on megakaryocytopoiesis.[6] Low-grade disseminated intravascular coagulation (DIC) may result in further platelet consumption,[7] but its presence in patients with liver disease is controversial.[8]

PLATELET FUNCTION DEFECTS

Platelet aggregation in response to various agonists frequently is diminished in patients with liver disease.[9] Also, the interaction of platelets with extracellular matrix components under flow conditions is impaired.[10] Defective platelet function results from impaired signal transduction,[11] decreased levels of proaggregatory components in the platelet granules,[12] proteolysis of platelet membrane proteins presumably as a result of excessive plasmin formation,[13] and increased production of the endothelial-derived platelet inhibitors nitric oxide and prostacyclin.[14] The presence of abnormal high-density lipoprotein also may impair platelet function,[15] and the presence of a reduced hematocrit may contribute to defective platelet–vessel wall interaction.[16]

VON WILLEBRAND FACTOR

Profoundly elevated levels of von Willebrand factor (vWF) frequently are observed in patients with liver disease and were suggested to result from endothelial damage possibly mediated by bacterial infection.[17] vWF mRNA and protein expression in the liver itself are substantially enhanced in cirrhosis.[18] Increased as well as normal vWF activity measured by ristocetin or botrocetin-induced agglutination has been reported; thus, the net effect of increased vWF level on hemostasis in these patients is not clear.[9,17,19] A further confounding effect is related to the finding of reduced levels of the vWF-cleaving protease, a disintegrin-like and metalloprotease with thrombospondin type 1 repeats (ADAMTS-13), in patients with liver disease,[20] suggesting that in addition to elevated vWF levels, increased amounts of the more hemostatically active high molecular weight vWF multimers may circulate. On the other hand, other proteases, such as plasmin and elastase, can contribute to vWF proteolysis in patients with liver disease.[21]

COAGULATION AND ANTICOAGULATION

PROCOAGULANT FACTORS

The liver is the site of synthesis of most procoagulant proteins; therefore, decreased levels of coagulation factors V, VII, IX, X, and XI and prothrombin are commonly observed in patients with liver failure.[22] In contrast, factor VIII level is increased and may be related to the elevated level of its carrier protein vWF and to decreased hepatic expression of low-density lipoprotein-related receptor, which is involved in clearance of factor VIII from the circulation.[18] Furthermore, unlike other coagulation factors, factor VIII is synthesized primarily by hepatic sinusoidal endothelial cells, which may maintain the capacity to synthesize factor VIII when liver function is severely compromised.[23]

Qualitative defects in clotting factors can arise as a consequence of hepatic failure. Because of vitamin K deficiency or decreased production of the vitamin K-dependent carboxylase, a proportion of circulating vitamin K-dependent factors II, VII, IX, and X may be deficient in γ-carboxylated glutamic acid residues, which impairs their function.[24] The markedly increased levels of des-γ-carboxyprothrombin in patients with hepatocellular carcinoma can be used to distinguish between malignant and nonmalignant liver disease.[25]

ANTICOAGULANT FACTORS

Levels of anticoagulant protein C, protein S, antithrombin, heparin cofactor II, and α_2-macroglobulin are decreased in patients with liver disease, a consequence of reduced synthesis.[1,26] As tissue factor pathway inhibitor (TFPI) is mainly synthesized by endothelial cells, normal levels of this protein are present in patients with hepatic failure,[27] although one study found decreased levels.[28]

DYSFIBRINOGENEMIA

Fibrinogen levels are in the normal range in patients with chronic liver disease but may be decreased in patients with decompensated cirrhosis or acute liver failure.[29] A qualitative defect in fibrinogen is common in all types of liver disease. The dysfibrinogen is characterized by an increased content of sialic acid,[30] possibly caused by enhanced tissue levels of glycosyltransferases.[31] Hypersialisation of fibrinogen impairs polymerization but does not affect the interaction of fibrinogen with platelets.[32]

FIBRINOLYTIC SYSTEM

SYNTHESIS OF PROTEINS INVOLVED IN FIBRINOLYSIS

Except for tissue plasminogen activator (t-PA) and plasminogen-activator inhibitor (PAI)-1, all proteins involved in fibrinolysis are synthesized by the liver. Consequently, liver disease leads to decreased plasma levels of plasminogen, α_2-antiplasmin, thrombin-activatable fibrinolysis inhibitor (TAFI), and factor XIII.[33–35] Plasma levels of t-PA are elevated as a consequence of enhanced secretion from endothelial cells and/or reduced clearance by the diseased liver.[36] PAI-1 plasma levels also are increased but not to the same extent as t-PA,[37] except in patients with acute hepatic failure in whom PAI-1 levels are substantially increased.[38]

HYPERFIBRINOLYSIS

Accelerated lysis of fibrin clots prepared in plasma of patients with chronic liver disease was described in 1914.[39] Since then, *in vitro* hyperfibrinolysis has been demonstrated by using various clot lysis assays and by measurement of plasma levels of indicators of fibrinolysis such as D-dimer, fibrin(ogen) degradation products, and plasmin–antiplasmin complexes.[8,26,40–42]

Hyperfibrinolysis in cirrhosis has been associated with low-grade DIC induced by endotoxemia.[43,44] This relationship was deduced from the presence of elevated markers of coagulation and fibrinolysis in plasma of patients with liver disease, such as prothrombin fragment 1+2, fibrinopeptide A, D-dimers, thrombin–antithrombin complexes, and plasmin–antiplasmin complexes. However, the increased levels of these markers may result from their decreased clearance by the liver rather than from DIC. More importantly, postmortem studies showed little evidence of fibrin deposition in organs of patients with liver disease, which is the hallmark of "classic" DIC (see Chap. 121).[45] Thus, whether or not low-grade DIC plays a role in uncomplicated liver disease is unknown.

In patients with acute liver failure, the elevated PAI-1 levels lead to a hypofibrinolytic state.[34,38] However, despite the apparent hypofibrinolysis, plasma levels of D-dimer, indicative of augmented fibrinolysis, were increased in such patients.[38]

PATIENT VARIABILITY

Variable hemostatic profiles are observed in patients with different liver diseases. Thus, patients with cholestatic liver disease, such as primary biliary cirrhosis, have a milder hemostatic defect compared to patients with other types of cirrhosis.[46] In alcoholic cirrhosis, the platelet dysfunction is further aggravated by direct toxic effects of ethanol. In acute liver disease caused by paracetamol overdose, factor II, V, VII, and X levels are significantly lower and factor VIII level significantly higher than in stable cirrhosis.[22] Moreover, the hemostatic disorder in all types of liver disease hypothetically can be ameliorated by the presence of factor V Leiden or the prothrombin G20210A mutation.

CLINICAL FEATURES

LIVER DISEASE

HEMOSTATIC BALANCE

Alterations in the hemostatic system in patients with liver disease include both prohemostatic and antihemostatic changes (Table 120-1). However, the net result of these hemostatic changes leans more toward a bleeding tendency than toward a thrombotic tendency. Among the major causes of bleeding are the combined effects of thrombocytopenia and platelet dysfunction and the reduced levels of clotting factors. The contribution of hyperfibrinolysis is less certain.[34,40,47]

BLEEDING COMPLICATIONS

Bleeding in patients with liver disease may not be related only to impaired hemostasis. Local causes, such as esophageal varices[48] are common. Hemostasis-related bleeding consists of bruising, purpura, epistaxis, gingival bleeding, menorrhagia, gastrointestinal bleeding, and bleeding associated with invasive procedures. Bleeding following liver biopsy is uncommon but usually is immediate when it occurs,[49] which argues against a role for hyperfibrinolysis in causing bleeding because typical hyperfibrinolytic bleeding occurs hours or days after trauma or surgery.[50]

A larger and more pronounced bleeding risk is encountered when patients undergo major surgery, such as liver transplantation (see "Liver Transplantation").

THROMBOSIS

Patients with liver disease may develop thrombosis in the portal and mesenteric veins. These complications presumably are caused by (1) decreased levels of the inhibitors of coagulation, antithrombin, protein C, and protein S, (2) the common inherited thrombophilias such as factor V Leiden, prothrombin G20210A, and homozygous methylenetetrahydrofolate reductase C677T,[51] and (3) alterations in blood flow in the splanchnic venous bed as a consequence of portal hypertension. The prevalence of portal vein thrombosis in patients with cirrhosis without hepatocellular carcinoma was thought to have an incidence of

TABLE 120-1   ALTERATIONS IN THE HEMOSTATIC SYSTEM IN PATIENTS WITH LIVER DISEASE THAT CONTRIBUTE TO BLEEDING (LEFT) OR COUNTERACT BLEEDING (RIGHT)

CHANGES THAT IMPAIR HEMOSTASIS	CHANGES THAT PROMOTE HEMOSTASIS
Thrombocytopenia	Elevated levels of vWF
Platelet function defects	Decreased levels of ADAMTS-13
Enhanced production of nitric oxide and prostacyclin	Elevated levels of factor VIII
Low levels of factors II, V, VII, IX, X, and XI	Decreased levels of protein C, protein S, antithrombin, α_2-macroglobulin, and heparin cofactor II
Vitamin K deficiency	Low levels of plasminogen
Dysfibrinogenemia	
Low levels of α_2-antiplasmin, factor XIII, and TAFI	
Elevated t-PA levels	

SOURCE: Modified from the European Association for the Study of the Liver from Lisman et al.[1] with permission.

six per 1000 (0.6%).[52] However, later studies found a much higher incidence of eight per 100 (8%), which may be related to improved imaging techniques.[51]

LIVER TRANSPLANTATION

PREANHEPATIC PHASE

In the first stage of liver transplantation—removal of the diseased liver—no significant worsening of the preoperative hemostatic impairment is usually observed.[53] Blood loss during this phase can result from extensive surgical damage, such as transsection of collaterals and abnormality of hemostasis. The major factors determining bleeding in this phase are the extent of preoperative hemostatic failure, the experience and skill of the surgeon, and the presence of portal hypertension.

ANHEPATIC PHASE

Following removal of the diseased liver, more significant hemostatic changes that occur contribute to the bleeding tendency. Because activated clotting factors are not removed from the circulation during this phase, DIC can develop, and consumption of platelets and clotting factors further compromises hemostasis. Laboratory signs of DIC have been observed in most studies.[54] Moreover, both primary and secondary hyperfibrinolysis may contribute to bleeding during the anhepatic phase. Primary hyperfibrinolysis is a consequence of the defective clearance of t-PA,[55] and secondary hyperfibrinolysis results from DIC. The role of defective clearance of activators of fibrinolysis in inducing hyperfibrinolysis was demonstrated in a study that compared orthotopic with heterotopic liver transplantation. In heterotopic liver transplantation, in which there is no anhepatic phase, no hyperfibrinolysis was observed.[56]

REPERFUSION PHASE

Probably the most severe hemostatic changes during liver transplantation occur after reperfusion of the donor liver. The donor liver contributes to bleeding observed during this phase by multiple mechanisms. Platelets are trapped in the graft, giving rise to an aggravation of thrombocytopenia and causing damage to the graft as the sequestered platelets induce endothelial cell apoptosis.[57] Activators of coagulation (tissue factor) and fibrinolysis (t-PA) are released by the graft as a result of endothelial damage.[55,58] This results in primary fibrinolysis and DIC with secondary fibrinolysis. The graft releases heparinlike material that inhibits coagulation. In addition, other factors such as hypothermia, metabolic acidosis, and hemodilution adversely affect hemostasis during this phase. The levels of platelets and hemostatic proteins are at their nadir after reperfusion and rise gradually during the early postoperative period. However, the levels of procoagulant factors rise more rapidly than do the levels of anticoagulant factors,[58] which results in a temporary hypercoagulable state that can induce hepatic artery thrombosis exhibited in approximately 5 percent of patients soon after transplantation.[59] A transiently increased level of PAI-1 immediately after surgery may contribute to the development of hepatic artery thrombosis.[60]

THERAPY

LIVER DISEASE

Spontaneous bleeding is uncommon in patients with stable liver disease. Bleeding occurs if gastroesophageal varices rupture, but treatment for this type of bleeding is not primarily aimed at correction of hemostasis. In patients who bleed severely as a consequence of impaired hemostasis, particularly following invasive procedures, therapy is aimed at correcting hemostasis by means of platelet and plasma

transfusion, administration of vitamin K, and/or use of antifibrinolytic agents, such as tranexamic acid or aprotinin.

PREPARATION FOR LIVER BIOPSY

Bleeding following liver biopsy is uncommon[49] but is often a serious problem when it occurs. Therefore, stringent contraindications for liver biopsy have been formulated that include a prothrombin time more than 3 to 5 seconds of control, a platelet count less than $50,000/\mu l$, a bleeding time longer than 10 minutes, and use of nonsteroidal anti-inflammatory drugs in the preceding 7 to 10 days.[61] However, these cutoff values differ among treatment centers.[62,63] It has been argued that, in general, the bleeding time is not a predictor of bleeding associated with invasive procedures,[64] but some evidence suggests that in patients undergoing liver biopsy, a prolonged bleeding time is associated with an increased bleeding risk.[65] When a biopsy is required despite these contraindications, the risk of bleeding should be decreased by prior transfusion of platelets and plasma.

HEMOSTATIC MANAGEMENT DURING LIVER TRANSPLANTATION

BLOOD PRODUCTS

Transfusion of a combination of blood products usually is required to correct the hemostatic derangements associated with liver transplantation.[66] The guidelines for transfusion differ among transplantation centers and are based on empirical data rather than on controlled trials. Red cells usually are transfused to maintain a hematocrit of 25 to 30 percent. As red cells promote localization of platelets at the vessel wall and possibly thrombin generation, transfusion of red cells can improve hemostasis. Fresh-frozen plasma is transfused to maintain the prothrombin time less than 3 seconds above control, but volume overload can create a problem. Prothrombin complex concentrates also can be used, but they carry a risk of thrombotic complications and correct only the deficiency of vitamin K-dependent factors. Fibrinogen concentrate or cryoprecipitate is also used when transfusion of plasma fails to raise the fibrinogen levels greater than 0.7 to 1 g/liter. Platelets are transfused to maintain the platelet count greater than $50,000/\mu l$.

In a multicenter study, the total blood loss during liver transplantation was between 2100 and 9000 ml[67] when only blood products and not prohemostatic agents such as aprotinin or recombinant factor VIIa (see below) were used. In these patients, between 1500 and 6250 ml of red cells (autologous and allogeneic) and between 1725 and 2400 ml of fresh-frozen plasma were transfused. Forty-four percent of the patients required platelet transfusions and 13 percent needed transfusion of cryoprecipitate. In another single-center study, the severity of liver disease, increased preoperative serum urea concentration, operative cold ischemia time, and use of autologous red cell transfusion were independent predictors of transfusion requirements.[68] Furthermore, a decline in transfusion requirements was noted during the years in which the study was performed.

ANTIFIBRINOLYTIC DRUGS

Hyperfibrinolysis is thought to contribute significantly to impaired hemostasis during the anhepatic and reperfusion phases. Synthetic antifibrinolytics, such as tranexamic acid (a lysine analogue) and aprotinin (a serine protease inhibitor) are frequently used and reduce red cell and plasma transfusion.[67,69] These agents also improve hemostasis by modulating vascular tone, preserving platelet function, and inhibiting inflammation.[70,71]

NOVEL STRATEGIES

Novel strategies aimed at correcting multiple hemostatic defects simultaneously are needed. A new agent, recombinant factor VIIa, which originally was developed for treatment of hemophilia A patients with an inhibitor to factor VIII (see Chap. 115), reduces transfusion requirements in patients undergoing liver transplantation.[72] Although the mechanism of action of recombinant factor VIIa is not completely understood, improved platelet function, enhanced fibrin formation, and augmented stabilization of the fibrin clot have been demonstrated.[73,74] Large clinical trials are needed to verify the benefit and safety of recombinant factor VIIa in liver transplantation.

REFERENCES

1. Lisman T, Leebeek FWG, de Groot PG: Haemostatic abnormalities in patients with liver disease. *J Hepatol* 37:280, 2002.

2. Aster RH: Pooling of platelets in the spleen: Role in the pathogenesis of "hypersplenic" thrombocytopenia. *J Clin Invest* 45:645, 1966.

3. Schmidt KG, Rasmussen JW, Bekker C, Madsen PE: Kinetics and in vivo distribution of 111-In-labelled autologous platelets in chronic hepatic disease: Mechanisms of thrombocytopenia. *Scand J Haematol* 34:39, 1985.

4. Goulis J, Chau TN, Jordan S, et al: Thrombopoietin concentrations are low in patients with cirrhosis and thrombocytopenia and are restored after orthotopic liver transplantation. *Gut* 44:754, 1999.

5. Kajihara M, Kato S, Okazaki Y, et al: A role of autoantibody-mediated platelet destruction in thrombocytopenia in patients with cirrhosis. *Hepatology* 37:1267, 2003.

6. Levine RF, Spivak JL, Meagher RC, Sieber F: Effect of ethanol on thrombopoiesis. *Br J Haematol* 62:345, 1986.

7. Carr JM: Disseminated intravascular coagulation in cirrhosis. *Hepatology* 10:103, 1989.

8. Ben Ari Z, Osman E, Hutton RA, Burroughs AK: Disseminated intravascular coagulation in liver cirrhosis: Fact or fiction? *Am J Gastroenterol* 94:2977, 1999.

9. Escolar G, Cases A, Vinas M, et al: Evaluation of acquired platelet dysfunctions in uremic and cirrhotic patients using the platelet function analyzer (PFA-100): Influence of hematocrit elevation. *Haematologica* 84:614, 1999.

10. Ordinas A, Escolar G, Cirera I, et al: Existence of a platelet-adhesion defect in patients with cirrhosis independent of hematocrit: Studies under flow conditions. *Hepatology* 24:1137, 1996.

11. Laffi G, Marra F, Failli P, et al: Defective signal transduction in platelets from cirrhotics is associated with increased cyclic nucleotides. *Gastroenterology* 105:148, 1993.

12. Laffi G, Marra F, Gresele P, et al: Evidence for a storage pool defect in platelets from cirrhotic patients with defective aggregation. *Gastroenterology* 103:641, 1992.

13. Michelson AD, Barnard MR: Plasmin-induced redistribution of platelet glycoprotein Ib. *Blood* 76:2005, 1990.

14. Cahill PA, Redmond EM, Sitzmann JV: Endothelial dysfunction in cirrhosis and portal hypertension. *Pharmacol Ther* 89:273, 2001.

15. Desai K, Mistry P, Bagget C, et al: Inhibition of platelet aggregation by abnormal high density lipoprotein particles in plasma from patients with hepatic cirrhosis. *Lancet* 1:693, 1989.

16. Turitto VT, Baumgartner HR: Platelet interaction with subendothelium in a perfusion system: Physical role of red blood cells. *Microvasc Res* 9:335, 1975.

17. Ferro D, Quintarelli C, Lattuada A, et al: High plasma levels of von Willebrand factor as a marker of endothelial perturbation in cirrhosis: Relationship to endotoxemia. *Hepatology* 23:1377, 1996.

18. Hollestelle MJ, Geertzen HG, Straatsburg IH, et al: Factor VIII expression in liver disease. *Thromb Haemost* 91:267, 2004.

19. Beer JH, Clerici N, Baillod P, et al: Quantitative and qualitative analysis of platelet GPIb and von Willebrand factor in liver cirrhosis. *Thromb Haemost* 73:601, 1995.

20. Mannucci PM, Canciani MT, Forza I, et al: Changes in health and disease of the metalloprotease that cleaves von Willebrand factor. *Blood* 98:2730, 2001.

21. Federici AB, Berkowitz SD, Lattuada A, Mannucci PM: Degradation of von Willebrand factor in patients with acquired clinical conditions in which there is heightened proteolysis. *Blood* 81:720, 1993.

22. Kerr R, Newsome P, Germain L, et al: Effects of acute liver injury on blood coagulation. *J Thromb Haemost* 1:754, 2003.

23. Hollestelle MJ, Thinnes T, Crain K, et al: Tissue distribution of factor VIII gene expression in vivo—A closer look. *Thromb Haemost* 86:855, 2001.

24. Blanchard RA, Furie BC, Jorgensen M, et al: Acquired vitamin K-dependent carboxylation deficiency in liver disease. *N Engl J Med* 305:242, 1981.

25. Marrero JA, Su GL, Wei W, et al: Des-gamma carboxyprothrombin can differentiate hepatocellular carcinoma from nonmalignant chronic liver disease in American patients. *Hepatology* 37:1114, 2003.

26. Vukovich T, Teufelsbauer H, Fritzer M, et al: Hemostasis activation in patients with liver cirrhosis. *Thromb Res* 77:271, 1995.

27. Bajaj MS, Kuppuswamy MN, Saito H, et al: Cultured normal human hepatocytes do not synthesize lipoprotein-associated coagulation inhibitor: Evidence that endothelium is the principal site of its synthesis. *Proc Natl Acad Sci U S A* 87:8869, 1990.

28. Oksuzoglu G, Simsek H, Haznedaroglu IC, Kirazli S: Tissue factor pathway inhibitor concentrations in cirrhotic patients with and without portal vein thrombosis. *Am J Gastroenterol* 92:303, 1997.

29. de Maat MP, Nieuwenhuizen W, Knot EA, et al: Measuring plasma fibrinogen levels in patients with liver cirrhosis. The occurrence of proteolytic fibrin(ogen) degradation products and their influence on several fibrinogen assays. *Thromb Res* 78:353, 1995.

30. Francis JL, Armstrong DJ: Acquired dysfibrinogenaemia in liver disease. *J Clin Pathol* 35:667, 1982.

31. Martinez J, MacDonald KA, Palascak JE: The role of sialic acid in the dysfibrinogenemia associated with liver disease: Distribution of sialic acid on the constituent chains. *Blood* 61:1196, 1983.

32. Harfenist EJ, Packham MA, Mustard JF: Effects of variant gamma chains and sialic acid content of fibrinogen upon its interactions with ADP-stimulated human and rabbit platelets. *Blood* 64:1163, 1984.

33. Stein SF, Harker LA: Kinetic and functional studies of platelets, fibrinogen, and plasminogen in patients with hepatic cirrhosis. *J Lab Clin Med* 99:217, 1982.

34. Lisman T, Leebeek FW, Mosnier LO, et al: Thrombin-activatable fibrinolysis inhibitor deficiency in cirrhosis is not associated with increased plasma fibrinolysis. *Gastroenterology* 121:131, 2001.

35. Biland L, Duckert F, Prisender S, Nyman D: Quantitative estimation of coagulation factors in liver disease. The diagnostic and prognostic value of factor XIII, factor V and plasminogen. *Thromb Haemost* 39:646, 1978.

36. Leiper K, Croll A, Booth NA, et al: Tissue plasminogen activator, plasminogen activator inhibitors, and activator-inhibitor complex in liver disease. *J Clin Pathol* 47:214, 1994.

37. Leebeek FWG, Kluft C, Knot EAR, et al: A shift in balance between profibrinolytic and antifibrinolytic factors causes enhanced fibrinolysis in cirrhosis. *Gastroenterology* 101:1382, 1991.

38. Pernambuco JR, Langley PG, Hughes RD, et al: Activation of the fibrinolytic system in patients with fulminant liver failure. *Hepatology* 18:1350, 1993.

39. Goodpasture EW: Fibrinolysis in chronic hepatic insufficiency. *Johns Hopkins Hosp Bull* 25:330, 1914.

40. Francis RB Jr, Feinstein DI: Clinical significance of accelerated fibrinolysis in liver disease. *Haemostasis* 14:460, 1984.

41. Colucci M, Binetti BM, Branca MG, et al: Deficiency of thrombin activatable fibrinolysis inhibitor in cirrhosis is associated with increased plasma fibrinolysis. *Hepatology* 38:230, 2003.

42. Wilde JT, Kitchen S, Kinsey S, et al: Plasma D-dimer levels and their relationship to serum fibrinogen/fibrin degradation products in hypercoagulable states. *Br J Haematol* 71:65, 1989.

43. Violi F, Ferro D, Basili S, et al: Hyperfibrinolysis resulting from clotting activation in patients with different degrees of cirrhosis. *Hepatology* 17:78, 1993.

44. Violi F, Ferro D, Basili S, et al: Association between low-grade disseminated intravascular coagulation and endotoxemia in patients with liver cirrhosis. *Gastroenterology* 109:531, 1995.

45. Oka K, Tanaka K: Intravascular coagulation in autopsy cases with liver diseases. *Thromb Haemost* 42:564, 1979.

46. Segal H, Cottam S, Potter D, Hunt BJ: Coagulation and fibrinolysis in primary biliary cirrhosis compared with other liver disease and during orthotopic liver transplantation. *Hepatology* 25:683, 1997.

47. Violi F, Ferro D, Basili S, et al: Hyperfibrinolysis increases the risk of gastrointestinal hemorrhage in patients with advanced cirrhosis. *Hepatology* 15:672, 1992.

48. Sharara AI, Rockey DC: Gastroesophageal variceal hemorrhage. *N Engl J Med* 345:669, 2001.

49. Piccinino F, Sagnelli E, Pasquale G, Giusti G: Complications following percutaneous liver biopsy. A multicentre retrospective study on 68,276 biopsies. *J Hepatol* 2:165, 1986.

50. Lee MH, Vosburgh E, Anderson K, McDonagh J: Deficiency of plasma plasminogen activator inhibitor 1 results in hyperfibrinolytic bleeding. *Blood* 81:2357, 1993.

51. Amitrano L, Brancaccio V, Guardascione MA, et al: Inherited coagulation disorders in cirrhotic patients with portal vein thrombosis. *Hepatology* 31:345, 2000.

52. Okuda K, Ohnishi K, Kimura K, et al: Incidence of portal vein thrombosis in liver cirrhosis. An angiographic study in 708 patients. *Gastroenterology* 89:279, 1985.

53. Kang YG, Martin DJ, Marquez J, et al: Intraoperative changes in blood coagulation and thrombelastographic monitoring in liver transplantation. *Anesth Analg* 64:888, 1985.

54. Porte RJ, Knot EAR, Bontempo FA: Hemostasis in liver transplantation. *Gastroenterology* 97:488, 1989.

55. Porte RJ, Bontempo FA, Knot EA, et al: Systemic effects of tissue plasminogen activator-associated fibrinolysis and its relation to thrombin generation in orthotopic liver transplantation. *Transplantation* 47:978, 1989.

56. Bakker CM, Metselaar HJ, Groenland TN, et al: Increased fibrinolysis in orthotopic but not in heterotopic liver transplantation: the role of the anhepatic phase. *Transplant Int* 5(suppl 1):S173, 1992.

57. Sindram D, Porte RJ, Hoffman MR, et al: Platelets induce sinusoidal endothelial cell apoptosis upon reperfusion of the cold ischemic rat liver. *Gastroenterology* 118:183, 2000.

58. Suzumura N, Monden M, Gotoh M, et al: Coagulation disorders during orthotopic liver transplantation: Inhibition of tissue thromboplastin activity by its antibody. *Transplant Proc* 21:2367, 1989.

59. Kok T, Slooff MJ, Thijn CJ, et al: Routine Doppler ultrasound for the detection of clinically unsuspected vascular complications in the early postoperative phase after orthotopic liver transplantation. *Transplant Int* 11:272, 1998.

60. Lisman T, Leebeek FWG, Meijer K, et al: Recombinant factor VIIa improves clot formation but not fibrinolytic potential in patients with cirrhosis and during liver transplantation. *Hepatology* 35:616, 2002.

61. Bravo AA, Sheth SG, Chopra S: Liver biopsy. *N Engl J Med* 344:495, 2001.

62. Sue M, Caldwell SH, Dickson RC, et al: Variation between centers in technique and guidelines for liver biopsy. *Liver* 16:267, 1996.

63. Mayoral W, Lewis JH: Percutaneous liver biopsy: What is the current approach? Results of a questionnaire survey. *Dig Dis Sci* 46:118, 2001.

64. Rodgers RP, Levin J: A critical reappraisal of the bleeding time. *Semin Thromb Hemost* 16:1, 1990.

65. Boberg KM, Brosstad F, Egeland T, et al: Is a prolonged bleeding time associated with an increased risk of hemorrhage after liver biopsy? *Thromb Haemost* 81:378, 1999.

66. Ozier Y, Steib A, Ickx B, et al: Haemostatic disorders during liver transplantation. *Eur J Anaesthesiol* 18:208, 2001.

67. Porte RJ, Molenaar IQ, Begliomini B, et al: Aprotinin and transfusion requirements in orthotopic liver transplantation: A multicentre randomised double-blind study. EMSALT Study Group. *Lancet* 355:1303, 2000.

68. Hendriks HG, Van der MJ, Klompmaker IJ, et al: Blood loss in orthotopic liver transplantation: A retrospective analysis of transfusion requirements and the effects of autotransfusion of cell saver blood in 164 consecutive patients. *Blood Coagul Fibrinolysis* 11(suppl 1):S87, 2000.

69. Boylan JF, Klinck JR, Sandler AN, et al: Tranexamic acid reduces blood loss, transfusion requirements, and coagulation factor use in primary orthotopic liver transplantation. *Anesthesiology* 85:1043, 1996.

70. Cumming AD, Nimmo GR, Craig KJ, et al: Vasoactive effects of aprotinin. *Agents Actions Suppl* 38:211, 1992.

71. Peters DC, Noble S: Aprotinin: An update of its pharmacology and therapeutic use in open heart surgery and coronary artery bypass surgery. *Drugs* 57:233, 1999.

72. Hendriks HG, Meijer K, de Wolf JT, et al: Reduced transfusion requirements by recombinant factor VIIa in orthotopic liver transplantation: A pilot study. *Transplantation* 71:402, 2001.

73. Lisman T, de Groot PG: Mechanism of action of recombinant activated factor VII. *TATM* 5:5, 2003.

74. Tonda R, Galan AM, Pino M, et al: Hemostatic effect of activated recombinant factor VII (rFVIIa) in liver disease: studies in an in vitro model. *J Hepatol* 39:954, 2003.

DISSEMINATED INTRAVASCULAR COAGULATION

URI SELIGSOHN
W. KEITH HOOTS

When procoagulants are produced or introduced into the blood and overcome the anticoagulant mechanisms of coagulation, thrombin is generated, which can lead to disseminated intravascular coagulation. The clinical manifestations of intravascular coagulation include (1) multiorgan dysfunction caused by microthrombi, (2) bleeding caused by consumption of platelets, fibrinogen, factor V, and factor VIII, and (3) secondary fibrinolysis. Exposure of blood to tissue factor is the most common trigger. This event can occur when mononuclear phagocytes and endothelial cells are induced to generate and express tissue factor during the systemic inflammatory response syndrome (e.g., gram-negative and gram-positive infections, fungemia, burns, severe trauma) or when contact is established between blood and tissue factor constitutively present on membranes of cells foreign to blood (e.g., malignant, placental, brain, adventitial cells, or traumatized tissues). Laboratory features include thrombocytopenia, reduced fibrinogen level, elevated levels of D-dimer and fibrin(ogen) degradation products, and prolonged partial thromboplastin, prothrombin, and thrombin times. Several underlying disorders affect these hemostatic parameters and can lead to a false-positive diagnosis of disseminated intravascular coagulation (e.g., liver disease-related coagulation abnormalities and thrombocytopenia) or to a false-negative diagnosis (e.g., pregnancy-related high fibrinogen levels). Reexamining these variables every 6 to 8 hours may permit a specific diagnosis. Early detection, vigorous treatment of the underlying disorder, and support of vital functions are essential for survival of affected patients. Blood component therapy is pertinent in patients who bleed excessively, whereas heparin administration is indicated in a limited number of circumstances. Infusion of recombinant activated protein C, which exerts antiinflammatory and anticoagulant effects, reduces mortality caused by sepsis-related intravascular coagulation. Intravascular coagulation and the underlying disorders causing it contribute to a high rate of mortality. The severity of organ dysfunction, extent of hemostatic failure, and increasing patient age have been associated with a grave prognosis.

Acronyms and abbreviations that appear in this chapter include: APACHE, Acute Physiology and Chronic Health Evaluation; APL, acute promyelocytic leukemia; aPTT, activated partial thromboplastin time; ARDS, adult respiratory distress syndrome; AT, antithrombin; DIC, disseminated intravascular coagulation; FDP, fibrinogen degradation product; HELLP, hemolysis, elevated liver enzymes, low platelet count; IL, interleukin; LCAD, long-chain acyl-CoA dehydrogenase; LPS, lipopolysaccharide; MP, microparticle; NF-κB, nuclear factor-κB; NO, nitric oxide; PAI, plasminogen-activator inhibitor; PAR, protease-activated receptor; TAFI, thrombin activatable fibrinolysis inhibitor; TAT, thrombin–antithrombin; TF, tissue factor; TFPI, tissue factor pathway inhibitor; TNF, tumor necrosis factor; t-PA, tissue plasminogen activator; vWF, von Willebrand factor.

DEFINITION AND HISTORY

Disseminated intravascular coagulation (DIC) is a clinicopathologic syndrome in which widespread intravascular coagulation is induced by procoagulants that are introduced or produced in the blood and overcome the natural anticoagulant mechanisms. Perturbation of the endothelium in the microcirculation along with stimulated inflammatory cells play a key role in this mechanism. DIC may cause tissue ischemia from occlusive microthrombi and bleeding from the consumption of platelets and coagulation factors and the anticoagulant effect of products of secondary fibrinolysis. DIC complicates a variety of disorders, and the complexity of its pathophysiology has made it the subject of a voluminous literature.[1-7]

In 1834, Dupuy[8] reported that injection of brain material into animals caused widespread clots in blood vessels, thus providing the first description of DIC. In 1865, Trousseau[9] described the tendency to thrombosis, sometimes disseminated, in cachectic patients with malignancies. In 1873, Naunyn[10] showed that disseminated thrombosis could be evoked by intravenous injection of dissolved red cells, and Wooldridge[11,12] demonstrated that the procoagulant involved was a substance contained in the stroma of the red cells.

The mechanism by which DIC can lead to bleeding was clarified only in 1961, when Lasch and coworkers[13] introduced the concept of consumption coagulopathy, and McKay[1] established that DIC is a pathogenetic feature of a variety of diseases. Sizable series of cases were first described in the late 1960s, following the introduction of defined laboratory criteria for DIC.[14] Yet despite the vast experience that has been accumulated, DIC still constitutes a major clinicopathologic and therapeutic challenge.

PATHOLOGY

Diffuse multiorgan bleeding, hemorrhagic necrosis, microthrombi in small blood vessels, and thrombi in medium and large blood vessels are common findings at autopsy, although patients who had unequivocal clinical and laboratory signs of DIC may not have confirming postmortem findings.[15,16] Conversely, some patients in whom clinical and laboratory signs were not consistent with DIC had typical autopsy findings.[17,18] This occasional lack of correlation among clinical, laboratory, and pathologic findings remains unexplained.

Organs most frequently involved by diffuse microthrombi are the lungs and kidneys, followed by the brain, heart, liver, spleen, adrenal glands, pancreas, and gut. Acute tubular necrosis is more frequent than is renal cortical necrosis.[15] A significant proportion of patients with chronic DIC have nonbacterial thrombotic endocarditis involving mainly the mitral and aortic valves.[19] Moreover, in a retrospective pathologic study, approximately 50 percent of patients with nonbacterial thrombotic endocarditis had DIC.[20] These heart lesions can be a source of arterial embolization, leading to infarction of the brain, kidneys, and myocardium.

PATHOGENESIS

MICROVASCULAR ENDOTHELIUM, MONONUCLEAR PHAGOCYTE SYSTEM, AND DISSEMINATED INTRAVASCULAR COAGULOPATHY

In addition to being the biologic highway, blood and blood vessels are quintessential components of the host immunity against foreign pathogens and defense against organ and tissue injury. The endothelium of the capillary bed in conjunction with fixed, circulating, and migratory mononuclear inflammatory cells are mainstays of this host defense. Together, they operate as an interacting microvascular-mononuclear phagocyte system, which is maintained in a state of normalcy by complex and tightly regulated cellular and chemical processes.[21] It is the extreme perturbation of these integrated systems that constitutes the *sine qua non* for most patients with DIC. Following injury or infection, the integrity of the endothelium is compromised, cells of the mononuclear phagocyte system are activated by cytokine and hormonal signals, additional cytokines and surface receptors are up-regulated, procoagulant proteins and platelets are activated, the endothelium changes from an anticoagulant to procoagulant surface, and fibrinolysis is impeded. This sequence of events is typical for the so-called *systemic inflammatory response syndrome* and can lead to microvascular thrombosis with ensuing multiorgan dysfunction and eventually to multiorgan failure. When bacteria are the cause of a systemic inflammatory response, the severity of the syndrome can be graded as sepsis, severe sepsis, and septic shock,[22] with stepwise increases in the rates of DIC, multiorgan dysfunction, and mortality.[23–26]

This sequence can be aborted by natural inhibitors of coagulation and by quenching the inflammatory signals (e.g., activated protein C) that lead to restoration of homeostasis and elimination of the risk for progressive microangiopathy (see "Role of Protein C Pathway and Serine Protease Inhibitors" below). These salutary events restore the equilibrium when disease processes known to predispose to DIC are not overwhelming in their presentation and/or when the injury to the host is partially localized, thereby forestalling dissemination. However, in instances of extreme injury/infection, the unregulated microvascular-mononuclear phagocyte system interactions amplify their own dysfunction in response to tissue ischemia and necrosis. When all regulation is lost, DIC is the outcome. When the precarious situation hangs in the balance, a partial or nonovert state of DIC occurs. Figure 121-1 displays the conditions causing DIC, the initiating pathways, and the clinical and laboratory consequences.

ROLE OF CYTOKINES AND TISSUE FACTOR

Cytokines with molecular weights less than 80 kDa and circulating at picomolar concentrations exert inflammatory effects. Their biologic activities are proinflammatory (e.g., tumor necrosis factor [TNF]-α, interleukin [IL]-1, IL-12, IL-6), antiinflammatory (e.g., IL-4, IL-10, IL-13), and inhibitory of other cytokines (e.g., soluble TNF receptors, IL-1 receptors, and IL-1 receptor antagonist).[27] Plasma concentrations of these mediators underestimate local concentrations, which are higher and induce an intense inflammatory and procoagulant response. IL-1 and TNF-α work synergistically to up-regulate tissue factor (TF) on both monocytes[28] and endothelial cells. IL-12 helps to sustain activation of the coagulation system in primates.[29] In contrast, IL-10 attenuates this response.[29–31] Cytokine expression normally is tightly regulated. For example, activated protein C inhibits endotoxin-induced up-regulation of TNF-α, IL-1, IL-6, and IL-8 by monocytes and macrophages. Once TF is expressed on the membrane of monocytes and endothelial cells, it initiates coagulation by forming a complex with factor VII or VIIa, leading to thrombin generation and fibrin and platelet deposition[32,33] (see Chap. 106). Coagulation triggered by TF also can occur when blood is exposed to cells that constitutively express TF on their membrane, for example, to adventitial and extravascular tissue cells following injury, to circulating malignant cells, or to placental or amniotic cells[34] (see Figure 121-1).

DAMAGE TO ENDOTHELIAL CELLS

Absence of the endothelial surfaces at sites of injury exposes platelets to collagen, initiating platelet adhesion and activation, and potentially exposes blood to TF constitutively present on adventitial cells. TF present on circulating monocyte-derived microparticles (MPs) also accumulates on activated platelets by binding of P-selectin glycoprotein ligand 1 of the MP to platelet P-selectin.[35] These processes initiate thrombin generation, which is amplified by the assembly of procoa-

gulants on the surface of activated platelets (see "Amplifying Role of Thrombin" below). Damage to the endothelium also causes release of plasminogen-activator inhibitor (PAI)-1 inhibiting fibrinolysis, and because tissue plasminogen activator (t-PA) is released from the endothelium in response to stimulation by thrombin, its depletion from endothelial cells can further compromise fibrinolysis.[21,36] Loss of large expanses of endothelial surfaces also attenuates thrombin clearance by thrombomodulin and glycosaminoglycan receptors expressed primarily on microvascular endothelial cells.[37] In primates, endothelial damage that is not extreme, such as moderate endotoxemia, results in an initial endothelial damage that can be controlled by natural regulators such as thrombomodulin, activated protein C, and glycosaminoglycans. Blood samples taken hours later indicate a secondary increase in inflammatory markers consistent with an ischemia–reperfusion injury. This model system is a paradigm for the concept of nonovert DIC.[38]

Injury or hyperstimulation of endothelium elicits release of ultra-large molecular weight forms of von Willebrand factor (vWF) from Weibel-Palade bodies that may accentuate microvascular thrombosis. Conceivably, these ultra-large vWF forms have a longer half-life in DIC because of a decreased level of the vWF-cleaving protease,[39] giving rise to platelet deposition and aggregation, a scenario analogous to thrombotic thrombocytopenic purpura (see Chap. 124).

AMPLIFYING ROLE OF THROMBIN

Thrombin generated by the TF pathway amplifies both clotting and inflammation through its various activities: (1) it activates platelets, giving rise to platelet aggregation and augmenting platelet functions in coagulation; (2) it activates factors VIII, V, and XI, yielding further thrombin generation; (3) it activates proinflammatory factors via protease-activated receptors (PARs); (4) it activates factor XIII to factor XIIIa, which covalently cross-links fibrin clots, thereby making them insoluble; (5) it activates thrombin-activatable fibrinolysis inhibitor (TAFI), making clots resistant to fibrinolysis; and (6) it increases expression of adhesion molecules, such as L-selectin, thereby promoting the inflammatory effects of leukocytes.[40] Paradoxically, at low concentrations, thrombin exhibits both antiinflammatory and anticoagulant effects because it binds to thrombomodulin and activates protein C to the activated form, which, in turn, down-regulates inflammation and serves as an "off switch" for further thrombin generation (see Chap. 107).

There is a hierarchy of sensitivity to thrombin: vascular endothelium and its associated anticoagulant and fibrinolytic functions are most responsive to thrombin stimulation, platelets are intermediate, and fibrinogen is least sensitive, requiring the highest concentration of thrombin for cleavage.[21]

ROLE OF THE COMPLEMENT SYSTEM

Activation of complement by inflammation or injury (particularly C5 and C5-9) induces intracellular calcium fluxes, with a resultant increase in the exposure of negatively charged phospholipids on the surfaces of inflammatory cells and platelets, thereby accelerating the rate of coagulation reactions. In addition, these calcium fluxes result in shedding of MPs from the activated cells contributing to the procoagulant effect. Coagulation and inflammation also interface through complement in that the C4b binding protein can become a procoagulant and proinflammatory by binding protein S, thereby diminishing free protein S levels and yielding a slower rate of activated protein C activity in cleaving factors Va and VIIIa. This process permits factors Va and VIIIa to enhance thrombin generation and slows quenching of inflammation via the endothelial protein C receptor pathway.

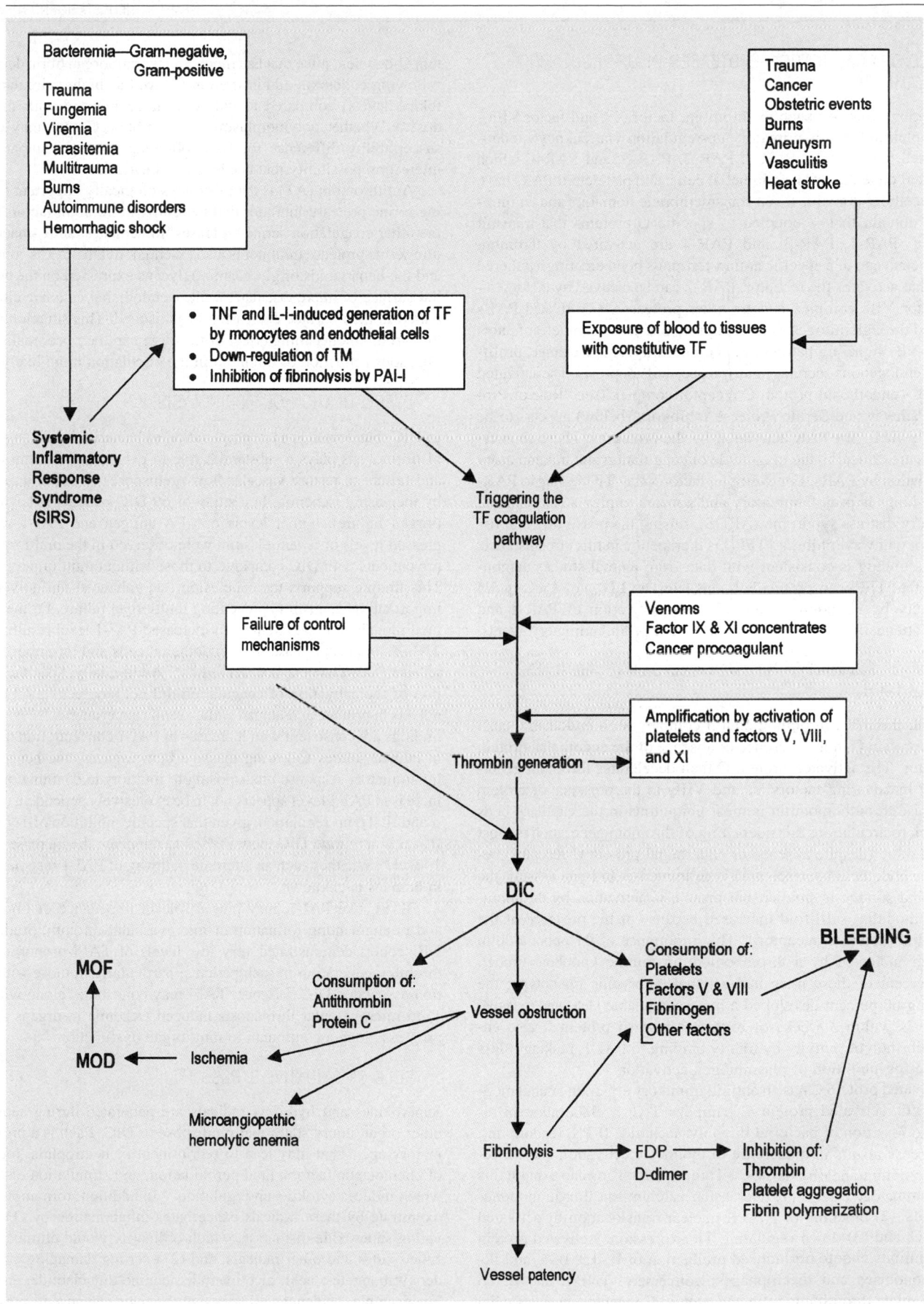

FIGURE 121-1   Major initiation mechanisms and consequences of disseminated intravascular coagulation (DIC). FDP, fibrinogen degradation product; IL, interleukin; MOD, multiorgan dysfunction; MOF, multiorgan failure; PAI, plasminogen-activator inhibitor; TF, tissue factor; TNF, tumor necrosis factor.

ROLE OF COAGULATION PROTEASES IN UP-REGULATING INFLAMMATION

Coagulation proteases such as thrombin, factor Xa, and factor VIIa–TF complex induce inflammatory up-regulation via leukocyte, endothelial cell, and platelet PAR-1, PAR-2, PAR-3, and PAR-4, which are located on leukocytes, endothelial cells, and platelets.[41] PARs have an extracellular domain, seven transmembrane domains, and an intracellular domain that is coupled to specific G-proteins that transmit signaling. PAR-1, PAR-3, and PAR-4 are activated by thrombin through cleavage of a specific amino-terminus bond creating a tethered ligand that activates the receptor. PAR-2 can be cleaved by factor Xa–TF–factor VIIa complex and by other proteases.[42] Activated PARs then lead through mitogen-activated protein kinase and nuclear factor-κB (NF-κB) signaling pathways to cell motility, shape change, proliferation, endogenous secretagogue release, and apoptosis. The activated protein C–endothelial protein C receptor complex (see "Role of Protein C Pathway and Serine Protease Inhibitors" below) appears to be the "off switch" for PAR activation by the proteases. These counterbalances are critical to the magnitude of coagulation and inflammatory up-regulation by PARs. For example, factor VIIa–TF binding to PAR-2 in the lungs is proinflammatory and appears to play a role in acute respiratory distress syndrome (ARDS), raising the possibility that tissue factor pathway inhibitor (TFPI) is therapeutic in this circumstance.[38,43] This finding is consistent with data from animal studies demonstrating that TFPI can protect baboons from an LD_{100} of *Escherichia coli*, likely by impeding factor VIIa–TF activation of PAR-2 and thereby attenuating release of IL-6 and other proinflammatory agents.

ROLE OF PROTEIN C PATHWAY AND SERINE PROTEASE INHIBITORS

As noted, thrombin-thrombomodulin complexes on endothelial cells activate protein C in the presence or absence of the endothelial protein C receptor. The activated protein C then decelerates thrombin generation by inactivating factors Va and VIIIa in the presence of protein S. Because thrombomodulin is most ubiquitous in the capillary beds of the microcirculation, this quenching of thrombin generation is most efficient there (despite absence of endothelial protein C receptor) because the endothelial surface area is so immense. In large vessels, the endothelial surface is smaller, but protein C activation by thrombin-thrombomodulin is 10-fold increased because of the presence of the endothelial protein C receptor.[40] The importance of thrombomodulin is further indicated by a thrombomodulin murine knockout model. Forty percent of these mice had a lethal embryonic phenotype; the remaining 60 percent developed a hypercoagulable state and massive thrombosis within 3 weeks of birth.[40] Activated protein C also enhances fibrinolytic activity by tightly binding to PAI-1, making it less available for inhibition of plasminogen activation.

Activated protein C has an antiinflammatory effect. In animal models of DIC, activated protein C dampens TNF-α elaboration in response to injection of bacterial lipopolysaccharide (LPS) (endotoxin). This process results in a decrease in monocyte activation and the resultant toxicity to nearby tissues.[44] Three mechanisms can explain this antiinflammatory effect: (1) decreasing calcium ion flux in mononuclear cells, (2) blocking of NF-κB nuclear translocation by activated protein C, and (3) down-regulating TF expression. Activated protein C also inhibits endotoxin-induced production of IL-1β, IL-6, and IL-8 by monocytes and macrophages; conversely, TNF-α and IL-1β down-regulate thrombomodulin and protein C receptor on endothelial cell surfaces, making them unavailable for thrombin binding and neutralization.[45]

That activated protein C levels may be rate limiting in broad physiologic ranges is suggested by studies of transgenic heterozygous protein C-deficient mice that had much greater intraorgan fibrin deposition following endotoxin administration (as well as higher circulating cytokine levels) compared to wild-type mice injected with the same dose.[46] Whether polymorphisms in the protein C gene may cause a susceptibility difference for DIC following sepsis in humans is an interesting possibility that needs to be elucidated.

Antithrombin (AT) is the most physiologically important circulating serine protease inhibitor that neutralizes thrombin, factor Xa, and the other coagulation serine proteases. In neonates, an α_2-macroglobulin serine protease inhibitor is also essential. In DIC, AT is consumed, and the heparinoids or glycosaminoglycans expressed on the endothelial surface of microvascular/capillary endothelial cells are either impaired in their surface expression or jettisoned. This situation negates the thrombin quenching effect of the large capillary bed, making promiscuous activation of thrombin in the circulation more likely.[47,48]

DYSREGULATION OF FIBRINOLYSIS

In DIC that develops as a complication of bacterial sepsis, impedance of fibrinolysis plays a substantial role in persistent microthrombosis, and failure to restore vascular flow predisposes to organ impairment by increasing ischemia. In a study of 69 DIC patients (31 with multiorgan failure), higher levels of t-PA antigen and PAI-1 with depressed levels of α_2-antiplasmin were observed in the multiorgan failure patients with DIC compared to those without multiorgan failure.[49] This finding supports the conclusion that enhanced fibrinolysis is an important mechanism in preventing multiorgan failure. Further, in animal models of endotoxemia, an increased PAI-1 level resulting from TNF-α–induced release from endothelial cells and thrombin-induced release from platelets is observed.[50–53] Additionally, specific prevention of the activation of coagulation did not stop activation of fibrinolysis in primate and human endotoxemia experiments.[38,50,51,54] These findings are consistent with increases in PAI-1 concentration observed in human studies following massive burn injuries, another systemic inflammatory response predisposing to multiorgan dysfunction.[55] The increased PAI-1 level appears not to be exclusively dependent on TNF-α and IL-1β up-regulation, given that specific inhibition of TNF-α and IL-1β in a murine DIC model failed to attenuate the increase in PAI-1 level.[56] Whether such an alternate pathway of PAI-1 response exists in humans is unknown.

TAFI, like PAI-1, may play a role in impedance of fibrinolysis and in augmenting formation of microvascular thrombi. Studies in a DIC cohort demonstrated very low levels of TAFI proportionate to thrombin generation in such patients, particularly in those with infection-associated DIC.[57] Hence, TAFI may contribute (along with PAI-1) to microvascular thrombosis-induced ischemia in organs that can progress along a continuum to multiorgan dysfunction.

ROLE OF OXIDATIVE STRESS

Superoxides and hydroxyl radicals are generated during sepsis and other organ injury states that predispose to DIC. Each is a proinflammatory agent that may lead to recruitment of neutrophils, formation of chemotactic factors, lipid peroxidation, and stimulation of NF-κB, which induces cytokine up-regulation.[58] In addition, formation of peroxynitrate by these radicals exacerbates inflammation by (1) deactivating superoxide dismutase, which ordinarily would eliminate these superoxides and other radicals, and (2) exerting damaging effects on deoxyribonucleic acid, nicotinamide adenine dinucleotide, and ATP. For example, evidence indicates that the poor response to pressors in shock-like states associated with DIC may be directly related to their deactivation by superoxides.

Adding further insult, high levels of superoxide impair vascular response to nitrous oxide, thereby creating an imbalance in the signaling to vascular cells. Because of the strategic importance of an intact endothelium for attenuating any microangiopathic process, the most devastating effect of excessive generation of superoxides and associated free radicals may be their role in inducing endothelial apoptosis, which would exacerbate capillary leak.[58]

ROLE OF VASOACTIVE MOLECULES

Vasoactive substances play a critical role in the evolution of DIC. The vasodilatory agent nitric oxide (NO) and the vasoconstrictor endothelin have been measured in experimental rat models of DIC induced by both TF infusion and LPS infusion.[59] LPS infusion increased both NO and endothelin remarkably, whereas TF infusion increased NO more than did LPS but did not stimulate endothelin significantly. The differential stimuli/response mechanisms may help explain the previously discussed phenomenon that LPS-induced DIC so prominently displays tissue infarction leading to multiorgan dysfunction (e.g., sepsis) compared to DIC, which is predominately induced by TF release (e.g., head trauma).

ROLE OF NEUTROPHILS AND CELL–CELL INTERACTION

The endothelium not only is critical for homeostasis and its damage a *sine qua non* for DIC, but its interaction with the other cells of the microvasculature and mononuclear phagocyte system is critical for the evolution of microangiopathies. Activated neutrophils that adhere to the injured endothelium release clastase, which augments DIC by (1) inhibiting thrombomodulin function, (2) causing detachment of endothelial cells, and (3) inhibiting fibrinolysis,[60] probably by degrading fibrinolytic proteases. Endothelial–neutrophil interaction in blood of trauma patients with DIC and/or multiorgan dysfunction results in increased circulating levels of cell adhesion molecules (L-, P-, and E-selectins, intercellular adhesion molecule-1, vascular cell adhesion molecule-1), thrombomodulin, and elastase. These changes are indicative of neutrophil activation and endothelial injury and correlate with DIC and multiorgan dysfunction scores.[61] Thus, a relationship exists between inflammation and thrombosis in posttrauma DIC. Depletion of these cell adhesive molecules and the associated tight junctions they maintain induces one of the hallmarks of DIC, the capillary leak syndrome.

INFLAMMATORY VERSUS PROCOAGULANT INITIATORS OF DISSEMINATED INTRAVASCULAR COAGULOPATHY

In experimental models, a marked difference exists in the pathophysiology of TF-induced DIC (comparable in many respects to the DIC following head trauma) and endotoxin-induced DIC (modeled to replicate sepsis-associated DIC), even when the amount of thrombin generated is identical. Circulating endotoxin associated with sepsis in rats is much more likely to be characterized by fibrinolytic blockade by PAI-1 with ensuing ischemia and multiorgan dysfunction because of failure to clear microthrombi.[62]

Primates in which only thrombin generation was induced survived, whereas animals injected with an LD_{100} dose of *E. coli*, which induced both thrombin generation and inflammation, died despite comparable thrombin levels as indicated by measurements of thrombin–antithrombin (TAT) complexes.[21] These findings may explain why sepsis-induced DIC in patients is much more likely to result in multiorgan failure than is DIC caused only by thrombin generation (e.g., snake bites).[27]

OTHER INITIATORS OF DISSEMINATED INTRAVASCULAR COAGULOPATHY

Less common initiators of DIC are a cancer procoagulant that directly activates factor X, snake venoms that activate factor X or prothrombin, and activated coagulation factors that are variably contained in prothrombin complex and factor XI concentrates (see "Specific Underlying Disorders" below).

CONSUMPTION OF HEMOSTATIC FACTORS

The widespread generation of thrombin in DIC induces deposition of fibrin, which leads to the consumption of substantial amounts of platelets, fibrinogen, factors V and VIII, protein C, AT, and components of the fibrinolytic system. This situation results in massive depletion of these components that is further aggravated because of their decreased synthesis by the liver, which frequently is affected in DIC. Depending on the magnitude and nature of component depletion, bleeding, enhanced thrombosis, or both can result. Bleeding can be promoted by fibrinolysis-derived fibrin degradation products (FDPs) that exhibit anticoagulant and antiplatelet aggregation effects (see Figure 121-1). Microangiopathic hemolytic anemia also occurs as a result of blood cells passing through vessels that are partially occluded by thrombi.

CLINICAL FEATURES

Numerous disorders can provoke DIC (see Fig. 121-1), but only a few constitute major causes, as can be inferred from retrospective clinical studies.[4,7,63–66] Infectious diseases and malignant disorders together account for approximately two thirds of DIC cases in the major series, except for one study[7] that included a disproportionately large number of obstetric cases (Table 121-1). Trauma was a major cause of DIC in two series,[63,64] probably reflecting the specialized nature of the clinical material in the two centers.

Clinical manifestations are attributable to DIC, the underlying disease, or both. Bleeding manifestations were common in all series of DIC cases, but considerable variation existed in the relative frequency of shock and of dysfunction of the liver, kidney, lungs, and central nervous system (Table 121-2). These variations probably reflect the different nature of the underlying disorders in the respective series.

TABLE 121-1   RELATIVE FREQUENCY (%) OF MAJOR UNDERLYING DISEASES IN SERIES OF CASES WITH DISSEMINATED INTRAVASCULAR COAGULOPATHY

REFERENCE NO.	N	INFECTIOUS DISEASES	MALIGNANT DISEASE	SURGERY AND TRAUMA	LIVER DISEASES	OBSTETRIC DISORDERS	MISCELLANEOUS DISEASES
4	60	41	30	2	5	2	20
63	118	40	7	24	4	4	21
64	346	26	24	19	8	—	23
65	503	15	61	2	6	4	12
66	345	16	55	—	4	5	20
7	361	15	6	14	3	38	24

TABLE 121-2   FREQUENCY (%) OF CLINICAL MANIFESTATIONS IN SERIES OF CASES WITH DISSEMINATED INTRAVASCULAR COAGULOPATHY

REFERENCE NO.	N	BLEEDING	THROMBOEMBOLISM	RENAL DYSFUNCTION	LIVER DYSFUNCTION	RESPIRATORY DYSFUNCTION	CENTRAL NERVOUS SYSTEM MANIFESTATIONS	SHOCK	ACRAL CYANOSIS
4	60	87	22	67	*	78	65	*	14
67	89	76	23	39	*	*	11	*	0
63	118	64	8	25	22	16	2	14	0
124	47	87	47	40	†	38	†	†	†
64	346	77	†	†	†	†	†	†	†
7	361	73	11	61	57	37	13	55	13‡

* Difficulties in defining relationship to disseminated intravascular coagulopathy.
† Not mentioned.
‡ Including necrotizing purpura and acral gangrene.

BLEEDING

Acute DIC frequently is heralded by hemorrhage into the skin at multiple sites.[4,63] Petechiae, ecchymoses, and oozing from venipunctures, arterial lines, catheters, and injured tissues are common. Bleeding also may occur on mucosal surfaces. Hemorrhage may be life threatening, with massive bleeding into the gastrointestinal tract,[63] lungs,[4] central nervous system, or orbit.[7] Patients with chronic DIC usually exhibit only minor skin and mucosal bleeding.

THROMBOSIS AND THROMBOEMBOLISM

Extensive organ dysfunction can result from microvascular thrombi or from venous and/or arterial thromboembolism. For example, involvement of the skin can cause hemorrhagic bullae, acral necrosis, and gangrene.[4,7] Thrombosis of major veins and arteries and pulmonary embolism occur but are rare.[4,63] Cerebral embolism can complicate nonbacterial thrombotic endocarditis in patients with chronic DIC.[20]

SHOCK

Both the diseases underlying DIC and the DIC itself can cause shock. For example, septicemia and excessive blood loss because of trauma or obstetric complications by themselves can cause shock. Whatever the cause of shock, its advent in cases with DIC is a serious adverse event.

RENAL DYSFUNCTION

Renal cortical ischemia induced by microthrombosis of afferent glomerular arterioles and acute tubular necrosis related to hypotension are the major causes of renal dysfunction in DIC. Oliguria, anuria, azotemia, and hematuria were observed in 25 to 67 percent of the cases in all series (see Table 121-2).

LIVER DYSFUNCTION

Hepatocellular dysfunction sufficient to cause jaundice has been reported in 22 percent[63] and 57 percent[7] of patients with DIC. Infectious diseases and prolonged hypotension contribute to hepatic dysfunction.

CENTRAL NERVOUS SYSTEM DYSFUNCTION

Microthrombi, macrothrombi, emboli, and hemorrhage in the cerebral vasculature all have been held responsible for the nonspecific neurologic symptoms and signs displayed by patients with DIC.[4,67] These manifestations include coma, delirium, transient focal neurologic symptoms, and signs of meningeal irritation. Careful exclusion of causes other than DIC is essential.

PULMONARY DYSFUNCTION

Symptoms and signs of respiratory dysfunction in DIC range from transient hypoxemia in mild cases to pulmonary hemorrhage and ARDS in severe cases. Whereas pulmonary hemorrhage is specific for DIC,[4,68] ARDS is not.[69–71] Pulmonary hemorrhage is heralded by hemoptysis, dyspnea, and chest pain. Physical examination reveals rales, wheezing, and occasionally a pleural friction rub. Chest imaging shows diffuse infiltration resulting from excessive intraalveolar hemorrhage. ARDS is characterized by tachypnea, auscultatory silence, hypoxemia, low lung compliance, normal wedge pressure, and "white lungs" on chest images.[70] It stems from severe damage to the pulmonary vascular endothelium, which permits egress of blood components into the pulmonary interstitium and alveoli. This situation leads to intraalveolar hyaline membrane formation and severe respiratory insufficiency. ARDS can be caused by septic shock, severe trauma, fat embolism, amniotic fluid embolism, and heat stroke, all of which can also incite DIC. Yet only a fraction of patients with ARDS exhibit signs of DIC.[69] When DIC and ARDS are simultaneously triggered, each aggravates the other. Regardless of the mechanism, ARDS is a serious complication in patients with DIC.

MORTALITY

Both DIC and its underlying disorders contribute to the high mortality rate. Mortality correlates independently with the extent of organ dysfunction,[63] the degree of hemostatic failure,[17,62,63] and increasing age.[63] Mortality rates in major series of patients with DIC ranged from 31 to 86 percent,[63,64,72] whether or not heparin was administered.

LABORATORY FEATURES AND DIAGNOSIS

Simple laboratory tests in conjunction with clinical considerations are used for establishing the diagnosis of DIC. Algorithms designed by the Scientific and Standardization Committee of the International Society of Thrombosis and Haemostasis for overt DIC and nonovert DIC (impending DIC or a microvascular injury state that has not yet progressed to DIC) are available.[73,74] The simple tests include platelet count, prothrombin time (PT), fibrinogen level, and fibrin-related markers, such as fibrin degradation products or D-dimer. Caution should be exercised when using these laboratory parameters in the algorithms described below because an underlying disease by itself can cause an abnormality. For example, impairment of hemostasis and/or thrombocytopenia unrelated to DIC can arise from hepatic disease and from marrow involvement by leukemia. Impaired hemostasis also may occur normally in the neonatal period. Conversely, the elevated levels of some hemostatic components that are normally observed during pregnancy may obscure the presence of DIC. These limitations in laboratory diagnosis of DIC can be overcome by repeated testing following the dynamics of the process.

Figure 121-2 presents an algorithm and scoring system by which the diagnosis of overt DIC is made. It is imperative that one of the underlying disorders known to be associated with DIC be present.

Pending validation by prospective studies, a score of 5 or more is consistent with overt DIC. A score less than 5 may indicate nonovert DIC. Overt DIC scoring may be useful for daily monitoring therapy but has not been validated.

Criteria for nonovert DIC have been more difficult to establish.[73,75] In the algorithm for nonovert DIC,[73] the global coagulation tests are scored as with the overt DIC algorithm; however, when scoring by the algorithm is being serially repeated, improvement in any laboratory test confers a negative score (rather than a zero or neutral score). This "trend" scoring allows longitudinal assessment of the patient's microangiopathy and, when therapy has been instituted, inference on whether the therapy has improved the course of the disease. Measurements of several markers for assessing the risk of progression from nonovert to overt DIC and prediction of multiorgan dysfunction are potentially valuable and in the future can be accommodated in the nonovert DIC score. For example, and as discussed, impaired fibrinolysis may play a particularly important role in multiorgan dysfunction resulting from DIC of sepsis. Therefore, assaying PAI-1, plasmin–antiplasmin complexes, or TAFI in septic patients may be important. Another highly sensitive early marker of impending DIC is a monoclonal antibody against activated protein C that identifies a calcium ion-dependent epitope involved in factor Va inactivation.[54] Whether serial measurement of vWF cleaving protease also will identify individuals at risk early in their disease course or will help differentiate individuals with microangiopathy who are not prone to progress needs further data.[39,76]

One new method that has proved highly sensitive and specific for nonovert (impending) DIC is the partial thromboplastin test biphasic waveform analysis.[77,78] This test, which requires specific instrumentation, detects the presence of precipitates of a complex of very-low-density lipoprotein and C-reactive protein that appears very early in DIC. When such complexes first appear in the plasma of individuals with diseases known to predispose to DIC, they confer a greater than 90 percent sensitivity and specificity for that individual subsequently developing DIC and having a higher mortality rate.[79]

Linking prognostic determinants from critical care measurement scores such as Acute Physiology and Chronic Health Evaluation (APACHE-II) to DIC scores is an important goal. In addition, certain biochemical indicators of organ dysfunction may imply a DIC risk. For example, serial assessment of arterial lactate has proved to be a reliable prognostic indicator of DIC development among patients with the systemic inflammatory response syndrome.[80]

SPECIFIC UNDERLYING DISORDERS

INFECTIOUS DISEASES

Bacterial infections are among the most common causes of DIC. Certain patients are particularly vulnerable to infection-induced DIC: (1) immune-compromised hosts, (2) pregnant women with reduced plasma protein S levels and diminished fibrinolytic activity, (3) asplenic patients whose ability to clear bacteria, particularly pneumococci, is impaired,[81] and (4) newborns whose coagulation inhibitory

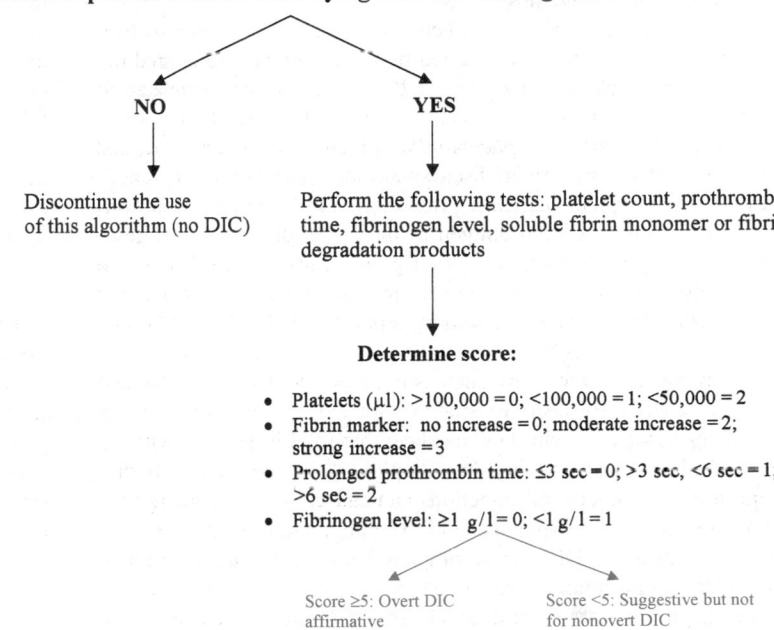

Does the patient have an underlying disorder causing DIC?

NO — Discontinue the use of this algorithm (no DIC)

YES — Perform the following tests: platelet count, prothrombin time, fibrinogen level, soluble fibrin monomer or fibrin degradation products

Determine score:

- Platelets (μl): >100,000 = 0; <100,000 = 1; <50,000 = 2
- Fibrin marker: no increase = 0; moderate increase = 2; strong increase = 3
- Prolonged prothrombin time: ≤3 sec = 0; >3 sec, <6 sec = 1; >6 sec = 2
- Fibrinogen level: ≥1 g/l = 0; <1 g/l = 1

Score ≥5: Overt DIC affirmative

Score <5: Suggestive but not for nonovert DIC

FIGURE 121-2   Algorithm for establishing the diagnosis of overt disseminated intravascular coagulation (DIC). (Adapted from the recommendations of the Scientific Standardization Committee of the International Society of Thrombosis and Haemostasis.[73])

systems are immature. Infections are frequently superimposed on trauma and malignancies, which themselves are potential triggers of DIC. In addition, infections can aggravate bleeding and thrombosis by directly inducing thrombocytopenia, hepatic dysfunction, and shock associated with diminished blood flow in the microcirculation.

Infections (gram-negative, gram-positive, and fungal) elicit the systemic inflammatory response syndrome, the severity of which is graded as sepsis, severe sepsis, or septic shock.[82] DIC under these circumstances is an intermediary mechanism of microvascular dysfunction and organ failure[83] that is triggered by the following processes: (1) TF expression by monocytes and endothelial cells stimulated by IL-1β and TNF-α, (2) IL-6–induced suppression of AT synthesis, destruction of AT by neutrophil elastase, and decreased availability of its cofactor glycosaminoglycan at the perturbed endothelium,[84] (3) impaired function of the protein C system because of decreased synthesis of proteins C and S and down-regulation of endothelial thrombomodulin and endothelial protein C receptor,[85] and (4) deranged fibrinolysis caused by increased production of PAI-1, the main inhibitor of fibrinolysis.[60] An extensive study of markers of DIC in patients with severe sepsis disclosed remarkable similarities among gram-negative, gram-positive, and fungal infections and greater derangements in nonsurvivors.[86]

Extreme examples of sepsis-related DIC are (1) streptococcus A toxic shock syndrome, characterized by deep tissue infection, vascular collapse, vascular leakage, and multiorgan failure; a streptococcal M protein forms complexes with fibrinogen, and these complexes bind to β_2 integrins of neutrophils leading to their activation[87]; and (2) meningococcemia, a fulminant gram-negative infection characterized by extensive hemorrhagic necrosis, DIC, and shock. The extent of hemostatic derangement in patients with meningococcemia correlates with prognosis.[88,89] More frequent gram-negative infections associated with DIC are caused by *Pseudomonas aeruginosa*, *E. coli*, and *Proteus vulgaris*. Patients affected by such bacteremias may have only laboratory signs of DIC (nonovert DIC) or may have severe DIC, especially when shock develops.[62,73,90]

Among the gram-positive infections, *Staphylococcus aureus* bacteremia can cause DIC accompanied by renal cortical and dermal necrosis.[91] The mechanism by which DIC is elicited may be related to an α-toxin that activates platelets and induces IL-1 secretion by macrophages.[92] *Streptococcus pneumoniae* infection has been associated with the Waterhouse-Friderichsen syndrome[93] and acral gangrene,[94] particularly in asplenic patients.[81] Initiation of DIC in these conditions is ascribed to the capsular antigen of the bacterium and to antigen–antibody complex formation.[95] Other gram-positive bacteria that can cause DIC are the anaerobic clostridia. Clostridial bacteremia is a highly lethal disease characterized by septic shock, DIC, renal failure, and hemolytic anemia.[96]

Common viral infections, such as influenza, varicella, rubella, and rubeola, have rarely been associated with DIC.[97] However, purpura fulminans associated with DIC has been reported in patients with infections and either hereditary thrombophilias[98] or acquired antibodies to protein S.[99] Other viral infections can cause "hemorrhagic fevers" characterized by fever, hypotension, bleeding, and renal failure. Laboratory evidence of DIC can accompany Korean, rift valley, and dengue-related hemorrhagic fevers,[100–102] but apparently not the Argentine hemorrhagic fever.[103] Release of TF from cells in which viruses replicate[104] and increased levels of TNF-α have been suggested as mechanisms for initiation of the TF pathway in these conditions.[105]

PURPURA FULMINANS

Purpura fulminans is a severe, often lethal form of DIC in which extensive areas of the skin over the extremities and buttocks undergo hemorrhagic necrosis.[106,107] The disease affects infants and children predominantly[106,108] and occasionally adults.[109] Diffuse microthrombi in small blood vessels, necrosis, and occasionally vasculitis are present in biopsies of skin lesions. Onset can be within 2 to 4 weeks of a mild infection such as scarlet fever, varicella, or rubella or can occur during an acute viral or bacterial infection in patients with acquired[108] or hereditary thrombophilias[98] affecting the protein C inhibitory pathway. Homozygous protein C deficiency presents in neonates soon after birth as purpura fulminans,[110] with or without extensive thrombosis.[111] Patients affected by purpura fulminans are acutely ill with fever, hypotension, and hemorrhage from multiple sites; they frequently have typical laboratory signs of DIC.[106,108] Excision of necrotic skin areas and grafting are indispensable at a later stage.

SOLID TUMORS

Trousseau[9] was the first to describe the propensity to thrombosis of patients with cancer and cachexia, and evidence for malignancy-related primary fibrino(geno)lysis and/or DIC was provided 75 years ago.[112–114]

In 182 patients with malignant disorders, excessive bleeding was recorded in 75 cases, venous thrombosis in 123, migratory thrombophlebitis in 96, arterial thrombosis in 45, and arterial embolism resulting from nonbacterial thrombotic endocarditis in 31.[115] Multifocal hemorrhagic infarctions of the brain, caused by fibrin microemboli and manifested as disorders of consciousness, have been described.[116] Patients with solid tumors and DIC are more prone to thrombosis than to bleeding, whereas patients with leukemia and DIC are more prone to hemorrhage.

Bleeding and thromboembolism stem from the DIC that is initiated by exposure of blood to TF present in carcinomas.[117] Another mechanism for triggering the coagulation system is via activation of factor X by a cysteine proteinase termed *cancer procoagulant*.[118] Interactions of P- and L-selectins with mucin from mucinous adenocarcinoma can

induce formation of platelet microthrombi and probably constitute a third mechanism.[119] Depending on the rate and quantity of exposure or influx of shed vesicles from tumors containing TF,[120] a nonovert or overt DIC develops.[121] For instance, a patient may be asymptomatic or present with venous thromboembolism if the tumor cells expose or release TF slowly or intermittently and the ensuing utilization of fibrinogen and platelets is compensated by increased production of these components. Conversely, massive thrombosis[122] or severe bleeding[123,124] may supervene in a patient whose circulation is deluged by TF.

Patients with solid tumors are vulnerable to risk factors and additional triggers of DIC that can aggravate thromboembolism and bleeding. Risk factors include advanced age, stage of the disease, and use of chemotherapy or antiestrogen therapy.[125,126] Triggers include septicemia, immobilization, and involvement of the liver by metastases that impede the function of the liver in controlling DIC. Microangiopathic hemolytic anemia frequently is induced by DIC in patients with malignancies and is particularly severe in patients with widespread intravascular metastases of mucin-secreting adenocarcinomas.[127]

LEUKEMIAS

In 1935, bleeding and a low fibrinogen level were observed in a patient with acute myelocytic leukemia.[128] Since then, numerous reports on DIC and fibrinolysis complicating the course of acute leukemias have been published. Although relatively uncommon among the acute leukemias, acute promyelocytic leukemia (APL) is the entity most frequently associated with life-threatening hemorrhage (see Chap. 87). The pathogenesis of hemostatic disturbance in APL is related to properties of the malignant cells and their interaction with the host's endothelial cells.[129] APL cells express TF and the cancer procoagulant that can initiate coagulation, and they release IL-1β and TNF-α, which down-regulate endothelial thrombomodulin thereby compromising the protein C anticoagulant pathway. APL cells also express increased amounts of annexin II, which mediates augmented conversion of plasminogen to plasmin (see Chap. 127).[130] The overall results of these processes are DIC and hyperfibrinolysis. All-*trans*-retinoic acid, currently used for induction and maintenance therapy of APL, inhibits *in vitro* and *in vivo* the deleterious effect of APL cells and has led to a reduced frequency of early hemorrhagic death.[129]

In adult patients with acute lymphoblastic leukemia, a high incidence of DIC, particularly during induction therapy without L-asparaginase, has been described.[131] The pathogenesis of DIC in these patients is not clear.

TRAUMA

When DIC complicates trauma, it usually occurs in severely injured patients. Extensive exposure of TF to the blood circulation and hemorrhagic shock probably are the most immediate triggers of DIC in such instances. Later, however, DIC can be induced within the framework of the systemic inflammatory response syndrome that commonly follows multiorgan trauma. The levels of TNF-α, IL-1β, PAI-1, circulating TF, plasma elastase derived from neutrophils, and soluble thrombomodulin all can be elevated in patients with signs of DIC,[132] predicting multiorgan dysfunction (ARDS included) and death.[133] Careful monitoring of laboratory signs of DIC, reduced fibrinolytic activity, and perhaps low AT levels[134] also are useful for predicting the outcome of such patients.

DIC can be aggravated in patients with severe trauma who require massive blood replacement because stored blood components are diluted and do not contain sufficient amounts of viable platelets and factors V and VIII. Acidosis and hypotension further aggravate bleeding.[135] Infection commonly occurs in such patients and may contribute to the DIC.

The time interval between trauma and medical intervention correlates with the development and magnitude of DIC. Experience during the Vietnam War proved that fast evacuation and prompt medical care reduce the risk of DIC.[136]

BRAIN INJURY

Brain injury can be associated with DIC, most likely because the injury exposes the abundant TF of brain tissue to blood. DIC can cause serious bleeding,[137] but transfusion of platelets and plasma components can arrest bleeding.[138] Specimens of contused brain obtained during surgery in patients with head injury and of liver, lungs, kidneys, and pancreas obtained during autopsy revealed microthrombi in arterioles and venules.[139,140] In adults and children with head injuries, a high rate of mortality occurred when DIC was present.[141] A laboratory DIC score has predictive value for prognosis in patients with head injuries, thereby supplementing the Glasgow coma score.[141,142] Hence, bleeding in patients with DIC related to brain injury can be managed by replacement therapy but carries a grave prognosis.

BURNS

TF exposed to blood at sites of burned tissue, the systemic inflammatory response syndrome induced by the burn, and the commonly present superimposed infections all can trigger DIC. Bleeding, laboratory tests indicative of DIC, and vascular microthrombi in biopsies of undamaged skin have been described in patients with extensive burns.[143] Kinetic studies with labeled fibrinogen and labeled platelets disclosed that, in addition to systemic consumption of hemostatic factors, significant local consumption occurs in burned areas.[144] Laboratory signs of DIC are associated with organ failure, and the extent of protein C and AT deficiencies correlates with a poor outcome.[145] A clinicopathologic study of 139 patients who died during treatment for a severe burn disclosed that 18 percent had cerebral infarctions caused by septic arterial occlusions or DIC and approximately 4 percent had intracranial hemorrhage.[146]

LIVER DISEASES

Very complicated derangements of hemostasis occur in patients with severe liver disease and during liver transplantation (see Chap. 120). Synthesis of most coagulation factors and natural anticoagulants (protein C, protein S, and AT) and of the main components of the fibrinolytic system (plasminogen, TAFI, and α_2-antiplasmin) is reduced. In addition, the capacity of the liver to clear the circulation of activated factors IX, X, and XI and of t-PA is decreased. Moreover, thrombocytopenia is common as a result of hypersplenism and decreased production of thrombopoietin by the liver. The similarities between the hemostatic defects observed in patients with liver disease and in patients with DIC are striking and have evoked an ongoing controversy as to whether or not DIC contributes to hemostatic derangements associated with liver disease.[147,148]

Several laboratory and clinical observations support the hypothesis that DIC accompanies hepatic disorders. They include a shortened half-life of radiolabeled fibrinogen and prolongation of fibrinogen half-life by administration of heparin[149,150]; failure of replacement therapy to significantly increase the levels of hemostatic factors (suggesting continuous consumption)[151]; and increased blood levels of D-dimer,[152] TAT complexes,[153,154] and fibrinopeptide A,[155] all consistent with ongoing thrombin generation.

Other observations and considerations argue against the hypothesis that DIC accompanies liver diseases. They include (1) an extremely low incidence (2.2%) of microthrombosis in the tissues of patients who die of liver disease[156] and (2) causes other than, or inconsistent with, DIC for the deranged findings in liver disease. Examples of alternative explanations include the following: (A) a prolonged thrombin time may result from acquired dysfibrinogenemia[157]; (B) low levels of coagulation factors and inhibitors may result from reduced synthesis[158]; (C) increased FDP levels may be a consequence of primary fibrinogenolysis induced by reduced synthesis of α_2-antiplasmin and PAI-1 by decreased clearance of t-PA; (D) factor VIII levels are commonly increased rather than decreased[159]; (E) the kinetic data show that the apparently excessive consumption of fibrinogen can be explained by loss of fibrinogen into extravascular spaces[160]; and (F) fibrinogen and plasminogen do not appear to be removed rapidly when labeled endogenously by ^{75}Se-selenomethionine.[161]

A third hypothesis maintains that patients with liver disease usually do not present with DIC but are extremely sensitive to the various triggers of DIC in view of their impeded capacity to clear procoagulants and to synthesize essential components of the coagulation, inhibitory, and fibrinolytic systems. Patients with primary or metastatic liver disease who undergo a peritoneovenous shunt operation for severe ascites are more likely to develop DIC than are patients with ascites who undergo the same procedure because of other causes.[162]

What, then, should be the approach to patients with liver disease and bleeding without an apparent local cause? First, possible underlying causes of DIC should be considered and identified, and then a hemostatic profile should be examined at frequent intervals in order to detect any dynamic changes that may be helpful in recognizing DIC. The sensitive assays that reflect thrombin generation (TAT complex and prothrombin fragments 1.2) or concomitant thrombin and plasmin generation (D-dimer) may help establish the diagnosis of DIC in a patient with liver disease.[163]

HEAT STROKE

Heat stroke is a syndrome characterized by a rise in body temperature to over 42°C that follows collapse of the thermoregulatory mechanism. The following predisposing factors have been identified: high environmental temperature, strenuous physical activity, infection, dehydration, and lack of acclimatization.[164,165] Extensive hemorrhage, unclottable blood, and venous engorgement were found as early as 1838 in postmortem examination of patients who died of heat stroke.[166] Investigations have confirmed that a severe hemorrhagic diathesis and multiple organ failure often accompany heat stroke.[164,167,168] Diffuse fibrin deposition and hemorrhagic infarctions are found in fatal human cases.[167] DIC associated with profound fibrin(ogen)olysis is evident in patients with heat stroke.[168–170] The possible triggers of DIC in patients with heat stroke include endothelial cell damage[171] and TF released from heat-damaged tissues.

The severity of the syndrome and the stage of its development affect the type and magnitude of hemostatic alterations.[168–170] Thus, in a study of 56 patients, three groups were discernible: nonbleeders, bleeders without DIC but with slight consumption of hemostatic factors, and bleeders with typical signs of DIC.[168] Prompt cooling and support of vital functions have substantially reduced the high mortality that was commonly observed in early studies.[164]

SNAKE BITES

Several species of snakes belonging to the Viperidae family produce venoms that have a wide range of activities affecting hemostasis. Prominent among these species are the *Vipera, Echis (E. carinatus* or *E. coloratus), Aspis, Crotalus, Bothrops,* and *Agkistrodon.* Venoms of these snakes contain enzymes or peptides that exert the following activities: (1) thrombin-like activity, cleaving fibrinopeptide A from the

Aα chain of fibrinogen *(Agkistrodon rhodostoma)*; (2) activation of prothrombin even in the absence of calcium ions *(E. carinatus)*; (3) activation of factors X and V (Russell viper venom); (4) fibrinogenolytic activity *(Agkistrodon acutus)*[172]; (5) induction of thrombocytopenia by platelet aggregation[172]; (6) inhibition of platelet aggregation by the low molecular weight arginine-glycine-aspartic acid–containing peptides from a variety of snake species[173]; (7) activation of protein C[174]; and (8) activities causing damage to endothelial cells, leading to bleeding, tissue ischemia, and edema. Interestingly, victims of snake bites rarely experience excessive bleeding or thromboembolism, in spite of the serious derangements in hemostatic tests and findings that are sometimes consistent with DIC.[175–177]

The major symptoms and signs related to envenomation are vomiting, diarrhea, apprehension, hypotension, local swelling, ischemia, and necrosis. Consequently, treatment for victims of snake bites consists of immediate immobilization, administration of antivenom and fluids, and other general measures to preserve vital functions. Local incisions, cooling, and application of tourniquet should be avoided.[172,178]

INFUSION OF FACTOR IX AND FACTOR XI CONCENTRATES

Concentrates of the vitamin K-dependent clotting factors are used to treat patients with hemophilia B and patients with other hereditary or acquired coagulation factor deficiencies (see Chaps. 115 and 116). Instances of severe DIC were reported in patients after infusion of these concentrates and were related to the presence of factors IXa and Xa in the concentrates and to liver dysfunction that impaired the capacity to clear these activated factors.[179,180] Newly prepared factor IX concentrates appear to be less thrombogenic because they are almost completely free of activated clotting factors. Nevertheless, prothrombin complex concentrates should not be given as replacement therapy to patients with DIC, and patients with hepatic dysfunction should receive prothrombin complex concentrates only as a last resort, preferably only after their nonthrombogenicity has been established.

Two factor XI concentrates, produced in England and France, have been shown to induce activation of the coagulation and fibrinolytic systems.[181,182] Infusions of these concentrates have been associated with severe thrombotic events in several patients,[183] but no instances of severe DIC have been observed. Contributing factors in the development of DIC are cardiovascular diseases, cancer, and surgery.

HEMANGIOMAS

In 1940, Kasabach and Merritt described the association between giant hemangioma and a bleeding tendency occurring mainly in infants. The pathogenesis and management of this syndrome have been reviewed.[184] Studies using radiolabeled fibrinogen[185] and platelets[186] provided evidence that within the hemangioma, consumption of platelets and fibrinogen occurs because of localized intravascular clotting and excessive fibrinogenolysis. Conceivably, concomitant local activation of the coagulation pathway and release of large amounts of t-PA by the abnormal endothelium lining the tumor vessels occur. Microangiopathic hemolytic anemia and laboratory signs of DIC and fibrinolysis have been demonstrated in patients with giant hemangiomas.[187] Accelerated growth of these hemangiomas in infants is associated with augmented consumption of hemostatic factors, which can be effectively treated with irradiation, glucocorticoids, and interferon.[188] Spontaneous mild to moderate bleeding manifestations have been observed, but severe bleeding generally occurs only after surgery or trauma.

Extensive vascular malformation may persist and cause pain, probably resulting from thrombosis, and bleeding following trauma, which is related to the localized or generalized consumption of clotting factors and platelets and hyperfibrinolysis.[189] Graded permanent elastic

compression, when possible, and low molecular weight heparin constitute the only effective treatment in such cases.

AORTIC ANEURYSM

An association between aortic aneurysm and DIC is well documented.[190–192] In a series of patients with aortic aneurysm, 40 percent had elevated levels of fibrin(ogen) split products, but only 4 percent had significant bleeding and laboratory evidence of DIC.[191] Several factors predispose patients with aortic aneurysms to the development of DIC: a large surface area,[191] dissection,[190] and expansion of the aneurysm.[192] Clinical and laboratory signs of DIC should be carefully sought in patients with an aortic aneurysm because bleeding may seriously complicate surgical repair of the aneurysm.[193,194] The initiation of localized and generalized intravascular coagulation can be ascribed to activation of the TF pathway by the abundant amounts of TF present in atherosclerotic plaques.[195] When patients present with significant bleeding or when surgery is planned, hemostatic defects should be sought and corrected by low molecular weight heparin.[196] Stent-grafting, which is a common procedure for repair of aortic aneurysms, was complicated by DIC and death in two patients, of whom one had cirrhosis and the other underwent a lengthy procedure.[197,198] However, a study of 31 such patients failed to detect DIC following stent-grafting of thoracic aneurysms.[199]

TRANSFUSION REACTION

DIC accompanies incompatible blood transfusion, in which massive hemolysis is commonly associated with excessive bleeding with widespread thrombosis in fatal cases.[200] The trigger of DIC in these cases cannot be simply ascribed to the release of red cell stroma, as patients with massive oxidative hemolysis because of glucose-6-phosphate dehydrogenase deficiency do not develop DIC.[201] Rather, extensive antigen–antibody reaction appears to cause DIC as a result of release of elastase and TNF-α from neutrophils,[202] and activation of monocytes that release TNF-α express TF and complement, with assembly of the membrane attack complex inflicting damage to endothelial cells.[203]

DISSEMINATED INTRAVASCULAR COAGULOPATHY DURING PREGNANCY

Pregnancy predisposes patients to DIC for at least three reasons: (1) pregnancy itself produces a hypercoagulable state, manifested by evidence of low-grade thrombin generation, with elevated levels of fibrin monomer complexes and fibrinopeptide A; (2) pregnancy is associated with reduced fibrinolytic activity because of increased plasma levels of PAI-1; and (3) pregnancy is associated with a decline in the plasma level of protein S. DIC may be difficult to diagnose during pregnancy because of the high initial levels of coagulation factors such as fibrinogen, factor VIII, and factor VII. Progressive reductions in these factors, however, can confirm or exclude the diagnosis of DIC in suspected cases.[204] Thrombocytopenia may be particularly helpful in determining whether DIC is present, provided other causes of thrombocytopenia are excluded.[205]

ABRUPTIO PLACENTAE

The dramatic clinical presentation of abruptio placentae was first reported by DeLee[206] in 1901, but the immediate cause of sudden rupture of uterine spiral arteries and detachment of the placenta is still unknown. Placental abruption is a leading cause of perinatal death.[207] Older multiparous women or patients with one of the hypertensive disorders of pregnancy are thought to be at highest risk.[207] The severe hemostatic failure accompanying abruptio placentae is the result of acute DIC emanating from the introduction of large amounts of TF into the blood circulation from the damaged placenta and uterus.[207,208] Abruptio placentae occurs in 0.2 to 0.4 percent of pregnancies,[209,210] but only 10 percent of these cases are associated with DIC.[205] Different grades of severity are found among those who develop DIC, with only the more severe forms resulting in shock and fetal death. Rapid volume replenishment and evacuation of the uterus is the treatment of choice.[207] Transfusion of cryoprecipitate, fresh-frozen plasma, and platelets should be given when profuse bleeding occurs.[205] However, in the absence of severe bleeding, administration of blood components may not be necessary because depleted coagulation factors increase rapidly following delivery. Heparin or antifibrinolytic agents are not indicated.

AMNIOTIC FLUID EMBOLISM

This rare catastrophic disorder described by Steiner and Lushbaugh[211] in 1941 occurs only in one in 8000 to one in 80,000 deliveries. A maternal mortality rate of 86 percent was reported in a 1979 review of 272 cases,[212] but in a later population-based study the maternal mortality (26.4 percent) was significantly lower.[213] Patients predisposed to amniotic fluid embolism are multiparous women whose pregnancies are postmature with large fetuses and women undergoing a tumultuous labor after pharmacologic or surgical induction. Apparently, amniotic fluid is introduced into the maternal circulation through tears in the chorioamniotic membranes, rupture of the uterus, and injury of uterine veins.[212] The trigger of DIC probably is TF present in amniotic fluid.[214] The mechanical obstruction of pulmonary blood vessels by fetal debris, meconium, and other particulate matter in the amniotic fluid enhances local fibrin–platelet thrombus formation and fibrinolysis. The extensive occlusion of the pulmonary arteries and an acute anaphylactoid response reminiscent of severe systemic inflammatory response syndrome provoke sudden dyspnea, cyanosis, acute cor pulmonale, left ventricular dysfunction, shock, and convulsions. These symptoms are followed within minutes to several hours by severe bleeding in 37 percent of patients.[212] Hemorrhage is particularly severe from the atonic uterus, puncture sites, gastrointestinal tract, and other organs. The best prospect for decreasing mortality lies in early termination of parturition in patients at high risk and prevention of hypertonic and tetanic uterine contractions during labor. When the syndrome is recognized, immediate termination of pregnancy under pulmonary and cardiovascular support is essential.

PREECLAMPSIA AND ECLAMPSIA

Thrombocytopenia described in early reports of eclampsia[215] and widespread deposition of fibrin in blood vessels observed in fatal cases[216] were interpreted as evidence of DIC triggered by placental TF exposure to the circulation.[217] A critical analysis of the literature concluded that the thrombocytopenia in these patients stems from endothelial injury rather than DIC.[218] However, other investigators provided evidence for significant DIC in preeclampsia and eclampsia.[215] Moreover, in a large series of patients, a good correlation was noted between the clinical severity and abnormalities in platelet counts and fibrin(ogen) degradation products.[219] Also consistent with DIC were results of assays of sensitive parameters of thrombin generation and activation of fibrinolysis, such as TAT complexes, D-dimer, and fibrinopeptide Bβ1–42.[205,220] Despite these observations, administration of heparin to patients with preeclampsia and eclampsia has not resulted in convincing benefits.[221,222]

HELLP SYNDROME

The syndrome of hemolysis (H), elevated liver enzymes (EL), low platelet count (LP), and severe epigastric pain is a complication of pregnancy-induced hypertension.[223] Seventy percent of the cases occur during the third trimester of pregnancy and 30 percent occur during

the postpartum period.[224] HELLP syndrome occurs more often in whites, multipara, and women older than 35 years.[222] Liver biopsy findings of fibrin deposition in hepatic blood vessels[225] and laboratory tests consistent with DIC in a significant proportion of patients[224,226] imply that DIC plays a role in the pathogenesis of the syndrome. Hepatic imaging in 33 patients revealed subcapsular hematomas in 13 and intraparenchymal hemorrhage in 6.[227] What actually triggers DIC in these cases is not known but has been related to endothelial dysfunction.[222] Multiple organ dysfunctions manifested by acute renal failure, ascites, pulmonary edema, and severe hemorrhage resulting from DIC may develop, leading to significant maternal and perinatal mortality rates.[222] Management of patients with HELLP syndrome consists of supportive care, careful monitoring, and blood component replacement therapy. With few exceptions, immediate delivery, not necessarily by cesarian section, is indicated.[222] HELLP syndrome tends to recur in subsequent gestations.[228]

SEPSIS DURING PREGNANCY

Gram-negative bacteria, group A streptococci, and *Clostridium perfringens* are among the more common causes of sepsis during pregnancy. These infections are frequently associated with fulminant DIC. The pathogens gain entry into the circulation during abortion, via amnionitis that may follow invasive procedures or rupture of membranes, by endometritis developing during labor, and by way of the urinary tract. Approximately 40 percent of bacteremic patients experience shock, which is associated with significant mortality.[229] In addition, a high rate of bleeding and organ dysfunction affects the kidneys, lungs, and central nervous system. In recent years this complication of pregnancy is rarely seen.[205]

Treatment of all cases of sepsis-related DIC should include antibiotics, support of vital functions, and surgical intervention to remove any local nidus of infection. Abortion or even hysterectomy may require consideration.

DEAD FETUS SYNDROME

Several weeks after intrauterine fetal death, approximately one third of patients may exhibit laboratory signs of DIC, occasionally accompanied by bleeding.[205,230] Apparently, TF from the retained dead fetus or placenta slowly enters the maternal circulation and initiates DIC, which sometimes is accompanied by significant fibrinolysis. This complication currently is rarely observed because labor is induced promptly after the diagnosis of fetal death is made. However, if labor induction is unavoidably delayed, serial blood coagulation tests should be performed.

The entity of fetal death and DIC can occur following the demise of one of multiple gestations. If it occurs at term, therapy is started as discussed. If it occurs prior to fetal maturity, prolonged administration of heparin can be useful.[230] Interestingly, when selective termination of the life of an anomalous fetus is performed in women with multiple pregnancies, hemostatic abnormalities develop in only approximately 3 percent of cases.[231]

ACUTE FATTY LIVER

Acute fatty liver of pregnancy is a rare disorder that occurs during the third trimester of pregnancy. It can lead to hepatic failure, encephalopathy, and death of the mother and fetus.[232–235] In 15 to 20 percent of cases, acute fatty liver of pregnancy is associated with fetal homozygosity or compound heterozygosity for long-chain acyl-CoA dehydrogenase (LCAD) deficiency.[236] Infants born with LCAD deficiency fail to thrive and are prone to liver failure and death. LCAD is one of four enzymes taking part in β-oxidation of fatty acids in mitochondria. When it is deficient, accumulation of medium- and long-chain fatty acid occurs. One predominant mutation (G1528C) accounts for 65 to 90 percent of cases with the deficiency. The precise mechanism by which LCAD deficiency in the fetus causes the severe liver disease in the heterozygous mother is unclear. The acute fatty liver disease of pregnancy is characterized by severe liver dysfunction, renal failure, hypertension, and signs of DIC.[233,237] The typical histologic feature is microvesicular fatty infiltration of the liver. Exceedingly low levels of AT and other laboratory signs of DIC were observed in a series of 28 patients, but no definite clinical benefit from AT concentrate infusion was achieved.[237] The primary therapy for these patients is early delivery and supportive care, which yield a maternal survival of 90 percent and perinatal survival of more than 85 percent.[233,238] Pancreatitis is a potentially lethal complication of acute fatty liver of pregnancy.[239]

NEWBORNS

Newborns have a limited capacity to cope with triggers of DIC for several reasons: (1) their ability to clear soluble fibrin and activated factors is reduced; (2) their fibrinolytic potential is decreased because of a low plasminogen level; and (3) their capacity to synthesize coagulation factors and inhibitors is limited.[240,241] Criteria for diagnosis of DIC in newborns are different from those for diagnosis in adults.[242] Important to consider are the physiologic hemostatic findings common at this age, which include low levels of the vitamin K-dependent factors, reduced AT and protein C levels, and prolonged thrombin time. The laboratory evidence of DIC in the newborn is based on the progressive decline of hemostatic parameters, thrombocytopenia, and reduced levels of fibrinogen, factor V, and factor VIII.[240,243]

DIC occurs in sick neonates and particularly in those who are premature. More than one underlying cause usually can be identified in newborns with DIC. The most frequent underlying conditions are sepsis, hyaline membrane disease (respiratory distress syndrome), asphyxia, necrotizing enterocolitis, intravascular hemolysis, abruptio placentae, and eclampsia.[240,241,243,244]

Bleeding from multiple sites is the most common manifestation of DIC in newborns, with intracranial hemorrhage being the most life-threatening condition. No clinical manifestations of DIC are apparent in approximately 20 percent of neonates,[244] so a high index of suspicion in patients at risk is essential.

THERAPY

Controlled studies of patients with DIC are difficult to perform in view of the variabilities in DIC triggers, clinical presentations, and grades of severity. Figure 121-3 shows general guidelines for management of patients with DIC, but decisions regarding treatment must be individualized after careful consideration of all clinically important aspects.

TREATMENT OF UNDERLYING DISORDERS AND VITAL SUPPORT

The survival of patients with DIC depends on vigorous treatment of the underlying disorder to alleviate or remove the inciting injurious cause. For sepsis-induced DIC, treatment includes aggressive use of intravenous organism-directed antibiotics. In the case of head trauma following a fall or sudden impact, treatment is initiated after the inciting event has set into motion microvascular–mononuclear phagocyte interactive events that provide diagnostic evidence of DIC. Efforts to control increasing intracranial pressure and to stop central nervous system bleeding surgically constitute treatment of the underlying disease. Other examples of vigorous treatment of underlying conditions are hysterectomy in patients with abruptio placentae, resection of aortic aneurysm, and debridement of crushed tissues.

Intensive support of vital functions is required.[245] Volume replacement and correction of hypotension, acidosis, and oxygenation improve blood flow through the microcirculation to restore toward equilibrium the functions of the microvascular–mononuclear phagocyte system. Careful monitoring of pulmonary, cardiac, and renal function enables prompt institution of supportive measures, such as use of a respirator for better oxygenation, inotropic drugs for improvement of cardiac output, and maintenance of electrolyte balance.[246]

BLOOD COMPONENT THERAPY

Treatment of the underlying disease and vital support are necessary but usually insufficient to treat DIC or forestall progression of nonovert DIC to overt DIC. Equally aggressive intervention to treat the specific injuries occurring to the microvasculature–mononuclear phagocyte system is required. These interventions include replacing the coagulation factors, natural anticoagulant, fibrinolytic proteins, and platelets that are actively consumed during DIC (see Fig. 121-1). This process requires judicious use of blood components, particularly fresh-frozen plasma, in an effort to replete the plasma proteins that are deficient because of the consumption process and the often-seen reduction in their production by a liver that itself is impaired by the microangiopathic process.[247]

One of the major challenges of infusion of fresh-frozen plasma in these dire circumstances is the propensity of the added volume to exacerbate capillary leak. This situation can increase the risk of inducing or worsening pulmonary edema and, by extension, predispose to ARDS and induce ascites or anasarca. One clinical strategy that may be helpful in the critical care setting in which fresh-frozen plasma is needed to treat DIC is to concentrate all infusion medications to the minimum volume of crystalloid that is feasible and to replace insensible and other losses required for fluid replenishment and maintenance with fresh-frozen plasma by infusion. Despite efforts to maximize the amount of fresh-frozen plasma that can be infused safely, replacement of deficient blood components rarely suffices to treat DIC, even when all the adjunctive therapies for systemic inflammatory response syndrome and multiorgan dysfunction are applied.[248]

Platelet transfusion is often required in DIC to prevent bleeding into already ischemic or damaged organs (particularly the central nervous system). Fortunately, the transfusion is required only when platelet consumption or decreased production by impaired megakaryopoiesis results in a precariously low platelet count. The threshold platelet count that should prompt transfusion is patient- and disease-specific because in many instances DIC microangiopathy can induce multiorgan failure long before the bleeding risk from DIC ever comes into play.

Cryoprecipitate can be used to rapidly raise the fibrinogen and factor VIII levels, particularly when bleeding is part of the DIC and fibrinogen level is less than 1g/liter. Cryoprecipitate has at least four to five times the mass of fibrinogen per milliliter of infusate compared to fresh-frozen plasma. Otherwise, usually sufficient fibrinogen is present in the fresh-frozen plasma being infused to treat mild to moderate hypofibrinogemia in DIC states.

Replacement therapy for thrombocytopenia should consist of 6 to 10 U platelet concentrate to raise the platelet count to between 50,000 and 100,000/μl; for hypofibrinogenemia (<1 g/liter) should consist of 8 to 10 units of cryoprecipitate; and for depletion or maintenance of other hemostatic components should consist of 1 to 2 U fresh-frozen plasma, depending on the severity of the depletion and the patient's body weight. Replacement therapy may need to be repeated every 8 hours, with adjustment of doses according to platelet count, PT, activated partial thromboplastin time (aPTT), fibrinogen level, and volume status. Fibrin(ogen) degradation products and D-dimer are not useful for monitoring therapy because their clearance can be delayed, espe-

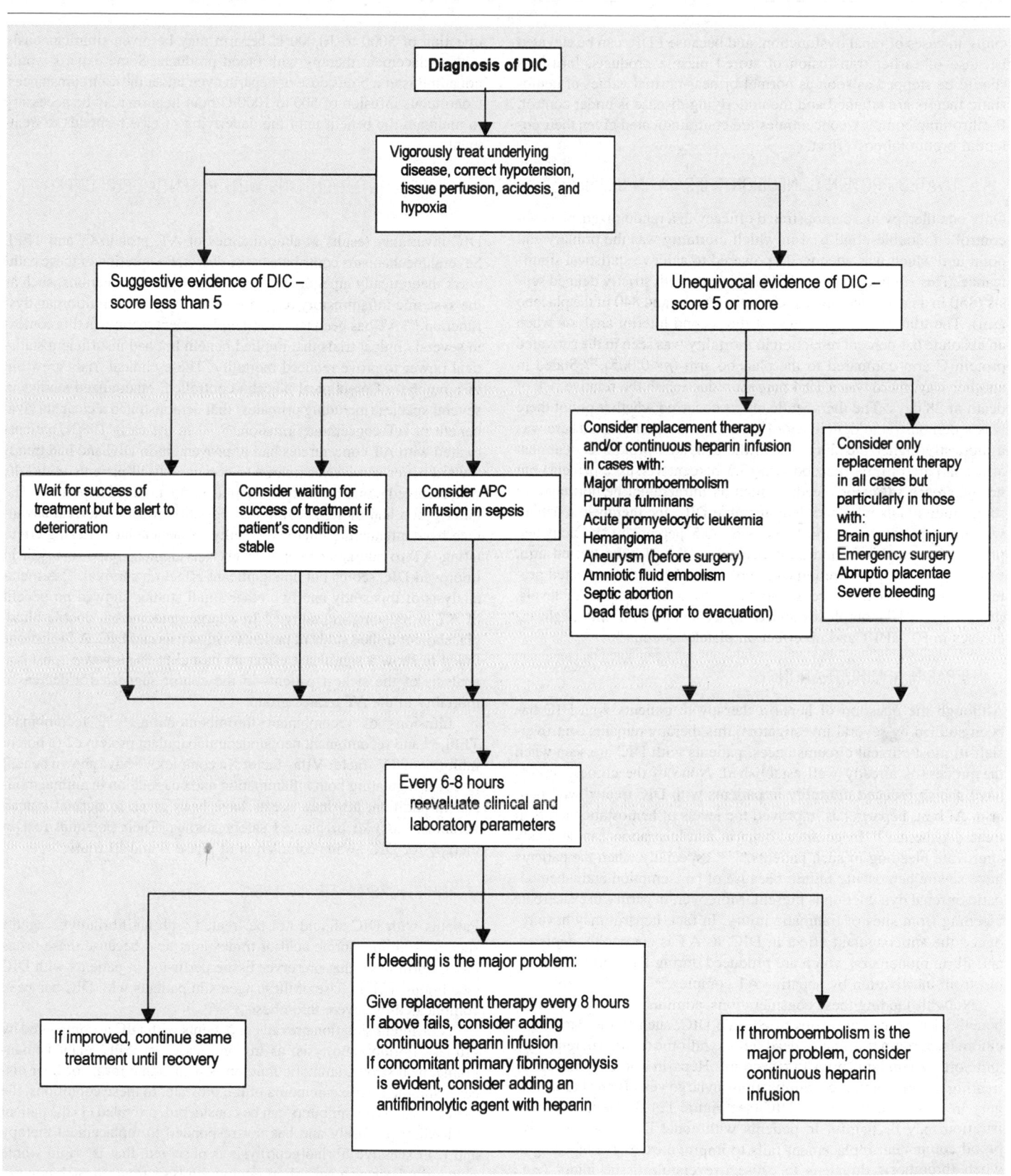

FIGURE 121-3   General guidelines for initial treatment and follow-up of patients with disseminated intravascular coagulation (DIC). The success of management is related to taking rapid, vigorous measures against the underlying disease, support of vital functions, close clinical observation, thoughtful consideration in each individual patient, availability of 24-hour coagulation laboratory services, and an adequate supply of platelet concentrate, cryoprecipitate, fresh-frozen plasma, and packed red cells for replacement therapy. Heparin, when indicated, should be administered by continuous infusion. The basis and limitations of each of the outlined recommendations are detailed throughout the text. APC, activated protein C.

cially in cases of renal dysfunction, and because FDPs can be elevated because of earlier transfusion of stored plasma products. Infusions should be stopped as soon as normal or near-normal values of hemostatic factors are attained and the underlying disease is under control. Prothrombin complex concentrates are contraindicated given their potential prothrombotic effect.

ACTIVATED PROTEIN C INFUSION THERAPY IN SEPSIS

Only one therapy has demonstrated efficacy in a randomized, placebo-controlled, double-blind trial in which mortality was the primary end point and which was adequately powered to achieve statistical significance. This study randomized 1690 patients with strictly defined sepsis (850 in an activated protein C treatment arm and 840 in the placebo arm). The trial was discontinued at the second interim analysis when an absolute 6.1 percent reduction in mortality was seen in the activated protein C arm compared to the placebo arm ($p<0.005$).[249] Stated in another way, there was a 19.4 percent reduction in the relative risk of death at 28 days. The therapeutic effect occurred whether or not there was a demonstrable deficiency of protein C at enrollment. There was a modestly higher bleeding risk in the activated protein C treatment arm compared to the placebo arm (3.5 percent versus 2 percent) but no difference in major bleeding such as intracranial hemorrhage. In septic individuals who had demonstrable DIC, the therapeutic benefit was more pronounced; mortality was 30.5 percent in the activated protein C-treated arm and 52.4 percent in the placebo-treated arm. Coagulation studies were indicative of direct benefit of activated protein C on the associated coagulopathy with an increase in AT levels, decrease in TAT complexes and D-dimer levels, with only slight increases in PT, aPTT and no effect on platelet count.[250]

HEPARIN ADMINISTRATION

Although the question of heparin therapy in patients with DIC has been studied by several investigators, this therapy remains controversial. In most clinical circumstances, patients with DIC are seen when the process is already well established. None of the clinical reports have shown reduced mortality in patients with DIC treated with heparin. At best, heparin has improved the levels of hemostatic factors in treated patients.[251] In contrast, heparin administration can seriously aggravate bleeding in such patients,[67,124] especially when the patients have severe hemostatic failure because of consumption and when hepatic or renal dysfunction is present. Moreover, heparin can exacerbate bleeding from sites of traumatic injury. In fact, heparin may have reduced the anticoagulant effect in DIC, as AT is commonly depleted, and fibrin monomers, which are produced during DIC, protect thrombin from inactivation by heparin–AT complex.[252]

Notwithstanding these considerations, administration of heparin is beneficial in some categories of chronic DIC, such as metastatic carcinomas, purpura fulminans, dead fetus syndrome (at time of removal), and aortic aneurysm (prior to resection). Heparin also is indicated for treating thromboembolic complications in large vessels and before surgery in patients with chronic DIC (see Figure 121-3). Heparin administration may be helpful in patients with acute DIC when intensive blood component replacement fails to improve excessive bleeding or when thrombosis threatens to cause irreversible tissue injury (e.g., acute cortical necrosis of the kidney or digital gangrene).

Heparin should be used cautiously in all these conditions. In patients with chronic DIC because of metastatic carcinoma, dead fetus syndrome, and aortic aneurysm, continuous infusion of heparin 500 to 750 U/hour without a bolus injection may be sufficient. If no response is obtained within 24 hours, escalating dosages can be used. In hyperacute DIC cases, such as mismatched transfusion, amniotic fluid embolism, septic abortion, and purpura fulminans, intravenous bolus injection of 5000 to 10,000 U heparin may be given simultaneously with replacement therapy with blood products. Some experts would not administer a bolus dose of heparin even under these circumstances. Continuous infusion of 500 to 1000 U/hour heparin may be necessary to maintain the benefit until the underlying disease responds to treatment.

CLINICAL INTERVENTIONS WITH POTENTIAL BUT UNPROVEN EFFICACY

DIC invariably results in abnormalities of AT, protein C, and TFPI. Several mechanisms contribute to the defect. Restoration of these pathways theoretically ameliorates the DIC and its complications, such as the systemic inflammatory response syndrome and/or multiorgan dysfunction.[249] AT has been tested as a replacement therapy in this context in several clinical trials that implied benefit but had insufficient statistical power to prove reduced mortality. These clinical trials grew out of a number of preclinical placebo-controlled, randomized studies in several species (including primates) that demonstrated a clear survival benefit of AT concentrate infusion.[253–255] In the early 1980s, patients treated with AT concentrates had improvement in DIC and had trends toward better survival compared to comparably ill patients with DIC who received either placebo or AT plus unfractionated heparin.[256] The latter group had more bleeding that possibly offset a survival advantage from attenuating microangiopathy. A decade later, raising circulating AT to supraphysiologic levels was demonstrated to result in improved DIC scores but no significant effect on survival.[257] A meta-analysis of this study and two other small studies showed no benefit of AT in reducing mortality.[258] In a large randomized, double-blind, placebo-controlled study of patients with sepsis and DIC, AT infusions failed to show a significant effect on mortality.[259] However, post hoc analysis of the sickest patients in the cohort suggested a decreased mortality in the AT treated group.

Infusions of recombinant thrombomodulin,[260–262] recombinant TFPI,[263] and recombinant nematode anticoagulant protein c2 (a potent inhibitor of TF–factor VIIa–factor Xa complex)[264] have shown benefit in down-regulating both inflammation and coagulation in animal models. In addition, all three agents have been given to normal human volunteers as part of phase I safety studies. Their potential role in therapy for DIC awaits completion of phase II and III trials.

INHIBITORS OF FIBRINOLYSIS

Patients with DIC should not be treated with antifibrinolytic agents such as ε-aminocaproic acid or tranexamic acid because these drugs block fibrinolysis that preserves tissue perfusion in patients with DIC (see Figure 121-1). Use of these agents in patients with DIC has been complicated by severe thrombosis.[265,266]

A different situation prevails in patients with DIC accompanied by primary fibrino(geno)lysis, as in some cases of APL, giant hemangioma, heat stroke, amniotic fluid embolism, some forms of liver disease, and metastatic carcinoma of the prostate. In these conditions, the use of fibrinolytic inhibitors can be considered, provided (1) the patient is bleeding profusely and has not responded to replacement therapy and (2) excessive fibrino(geno)lysis is observed, that is, rapid whole blood clot lysis or a very short euglobulin lysis time. In such circumstances, use of antifibrinolytic agents should be preceded by replacement of depleted blood components and continuous heparin infusion.

EXPERIMENTAL THERAPEUTIC APPROACHES

Several different strategies are undergoing preclinical evaluation in animal models of DIC. One strategy focuses on the role cell adhesive molecules play in murine DIC. Mice are primed with anti–Ly-6 (a glycosylphosphoinositol protein in neutrophils), which causes these circulating granulocytes to adhere and aggregate on the endothelial surface with concomitant recruitment of monocytes and platelets to an injured endothelial site.[267] Infusion of antibodies to both P- and E-selectin plus heparin dramatically attenuated the microangiopathy in these mice. A similar mitigation of inflammation and procoagulant activation can be demonstrated when P- and E-selectin knockout mice are infused with heparin alone.[268]

In addition to recombinant analogues of natural antiproteases, specially engineered inhibitors of serine protease activation (e.g., factor Xa) are being tested.[268] In another approach, selective blockade of covalent cross-linking of fibrin monomer by inhibition of factor XIIIa has been demonstrated to prevent LPS-induced DIC in a rabbit model.[269] Further, weak antithrombin inhibitors in the thioglycoside class have a beneficial effect in animal models of LPS-induced DIC.[270]

In weighing all potential DIC treatments, the wide variations in both the primary disease and its secondary effects giving rise to DIC should be considered. This is particularly true when agents developed for other coagulopathic conditions are applied to the discrete symptoms of the DIC syndrome. For example, applications of recombinant factor VIIa for treatment of massive hemorrhage in obstetric patients must be viewed with caution because of the potential of this preparation to potentiate thrombin generation.[271,272]

REFERENCES

1. McKay DG: *Disseminated Intravascular Coagulation: An Intermediary Mechanism of Disease.* Harper and Row, New York, 1965.

2. Hardaway RM: *Syndromes of Disseminated Intravascular Coagulation with Special Reference to Shock and Hemorrhage.* Charles C. Thomas, Springfield, 1966.

3. Mammen EF, Anderson GF, Barnhard MI (eds): Disseminated intravascular coagulation. *Thromb Diath Haemorrh Suppl* 36, 1969.

4. Minna JD, Robboy SJ, Colman RW: *Disseminated Intravascular Coagulation in Man.* Charles C. Thomas, Springfield, 1974.

5. Bick RL: *Disseminated Intravascular Coagulation and Related Syndromes.* CRC Press, Boca Raton, 1983.

6. Abe T, Yamanaka M (eds): *Disseminated Intravascular Coagulation. Bibliotheca Haematologica,* no 49. Karger, Basel, 1983.

7. Larcan A, Lambert H, Gerard A: *Consumption Coagulopathies.* Masson, New York, 1987.

8. Dupuy M: Injections de matière cérébrale dans les veines. *Gas Med Paris* 2:524, 1834.

9. Trousseau A: Phlegmasia alba dolens. *Clin Med (Hotel Dieu Paris)* 695, 1865.

10. Naunyn C: Untersuchungen uber Blutgerinnung im lebeden tiere und ihre Folgen. *Arch Exp Pathol Pharmacol* 1, 1873.

11. Wooldridge LC: Note on the relation of the red blood corpuscles to coagulation. *Practitioner* 38:187, 1886.

12. Wooldridge LC: Ueber intravasculare gerinnungen. *Arch Ant Physiol Abt (Leipzig)* 397, 1886.

13. Lasch HG, Krecke HJ, Rodriguez-Erdman F, et al: Verbrauchskoagu-lopathien (Patogenese und Therapie). *Folia Haematol (Frankf)* 6:325, 1961.

14. Merskey C, Johnson AJ, Kleiner GJ, et al: The defibrination syndrome: Clinical features and laboratory diagnosis. *Br J Haematol* 13:528, 1967.

15. Robboy SJ, Major MC, Colman RW, Minna JD: Pathology of disseminated intravascular coagulation (DIC). Analysis of 26 cases. *Hum Pathol* 3:327, 1972.

16. Wilde JT, Roberts KM, Greaves M, Preston FE: Association between necropsy evidence of disseminated intravascular coagulation and coagulation variables before death in patients in intensive care units. *J Clin Pathol* 41:138, 1988.

17. Kim HS, Suzuki M, Lie JT, Titus JL: Clinically unsuspected disseminated intravascular coagulation (DIC). An autopsy survey. *Am J Clin Pathol* 66:31, 1976.

18. Watanabe T, Imamura T, Nakagaki K, Tanaka K: Disseminated intravascular coagulation in autopsy cases. Its incidence and clinicopathologic significance. *Pathol Res Pract* 165:311, 1979.

19. Sugiura M, Hiraoka K, Ohkawa S, et al: A clinico-pathological study on cardiac lesions in 64 cases of disseminated intravascular coagulation. *Jpn Heart J* 18:57, 1977.

20. Kim HS, Suzuki M, Lie JT, Titus JL: Nonbacterial thrombotic endocarditis (NBTE) and disseminated intravascular coagulation (DIC). *Arch Pathol Lab Med* 101:65, 1977.

21. Taylor FB Jr: Response of anticoagulant pathways in disseminated intravascular coagulation. *Semin Thromb Hemost* 27:619, 2001.

22. American College of Chest Physicians/Society of Critical Care Medicine Consensus Conference: Definitions for sepsis and organ failure and guidelines for the use of innovative therapies in sepsis. *Crit Care Med* 20:864, 1992.

23. Fourrier F, Chopin C, Goudemand J, et al: Septic shock, multiple organ failure, and disseminated intravascular coagulation. Compared patterns of antithrombin III, protein C, and protein S deficiencies. *Chest* 101:816,1992.

24. Rangel-Frausto MS, Pittet D, Costigan M, et al: The natural history of the systemic inflammatory response syndrome (SIRS). A prospective study. *JAMA* 273:117, 1995.

25. Gando S, Kameue T, Nanzaki S, Nakanishi Y: Disseminated intravascular coagulation is a frequent complication of systemic inflammatory response syndrome. *Thromb Haemost* 75:224, 1996.

26. Gando S, Nanzaki S, Morimoto Y, et al: Tissue factor pathway inhibitor response does not correlate with tissue factor-induced disseminated intravascular coagulation and multiple organ dysfunction syndrome in trauma patients. *Crit Care Med* 29:262, 2001.

27. Hotchkiss RS, Karl IE: The pathophysiology and treatment of sepsis. *N Engl J Med* 348:138, 2003.

28. Edwards RL, Rickles FR: The role of human T cells (and T cell products) for monocyte tissue factor generation. *J Immunol* 125:606, 1980.

29. Lauw FN, Dekkers PE, te Velde AA, et al: Interleukin-12 induces sustained activation of multiple host inflammatory mediator systems in chimpanzees. *J Infect Dis* 179:646,1999.

30. Schwager I, Jungi TW: Effect of human recombinant cytokines on the induction of macrophage procoagulant activity. *Blood* 83:152, 1994.

31. Ramani M, Ollivier V, Khechai F, et al: Interleukin-10 inhibits endotoxin-induced tissue factor mRNA production by human monocytes. *FEBS Lett* 334:114, 1993.

32. Gando S, Kameue T, Morimoto Y, et al: Tissue factor production not balanced by tissue factor pathway inhibitor in sepsis promotes poor prognosis. *Crit Care Med* 30:1729, 2002.

33. Gando S, Kameue T, Matsuda N, et al: Combined activation of coagulation and inflammation has an important role in multiple organ dysfunction and poor outcome after severe trauma. *Thromb Haemost* 88:943, 2002.

34. Edgington TS, Mackman N, Brand K, Ruf W: The structural biology of expression and function of tissue factor. *Thromb Haemost* 66:67, 1991.

35. Falatis S, Liu Q, Gross P, et al: Accumulation of tissue factor into developing thrombi in vivo is dependent upon microparticle P-selectin glycoprotein ligand 1 and platelet P-selectin. *J Exp Med* 197:1585, 2003.

36. Gelehrter TD, Sznycer-Laszuk R: Thrombin induction of plasminogen activator-inhibitor in cultured human endothelial cells. *J Clin Invest* 77:165, 1986.

37. Isermann B, Hendrickson SB, Zogg M, et al: Endothelium-specific loss of murine thrombomodulin disrupts the protein C anticoagulant pathway and causes juvenile-onset thrombosis. *J Clin Invest* 108:537, 2001.

38. ten Cate H, Schoenmakers SH, Franco R, et al: Microvascular coagulopathy and disseminated intravascular coagulation. *Crit Care Med* 29(suppl):S95, discussion S97, 2001.

39. Loof AH, van Vliet HH, Kappers-Klunne MC: Low activity of von Willebrand factor-cleaving protease is not restricted to patients suffering from thrombotic thrombocytopenic purpura. *Br J Haematol* 112:1087, 2001.

40. Esmon CT: Protein C anticoagulant pathway and its role in controlling microvascular thrombosis and inflammation. *Crit Care Med* 29(suppl 7):S48, discussion S51, 2001.

41. Coughlin SR: Thrombin signaling and protease-activated receptors. *Nature* 407:258, 2000.

42. Versteeg HH, Peppelenbosch MP, Spek CA: The pleiotropic effects of tissue factor: A possible role for factor VIIa-induced intracellular signaling? *Thromb Haemost* 86:1353, 2001.

43. Ruf W, Riewald M: Tissue factor-dependent coagulation protease signaling in acute lung injury. *Crit Care Med* 31(suppl 4):S231, 2003.

44. White B, Schmidt M, Murphy C, et al: Activated protein C inhibits lipopolysaccharide-induced nuclear translocation of nuclear factor kappaB (NF-kappaB) and tumour necrosis factor alpha (TNF-alpha) production in the THP-1 monocytic cell line. *Br J Haematol* 110:130, 2000.

45. van der Poll T, de Jonge E, Levi M: Regulatory role of cytokines in disseminated intravascular coagulation. *Semin Thromb Hemost* 27:639, 2001.

46. Levi M, Dorffler-Melly J, Reitsma P, et al: Aggravation of endotoxin-induced disseminated intravascular coagulation and cytokine activation in heterozygous protein-C-deficient mice. *Blood* 101:4823, 2003.

47. Hoots WK: Coagulation disorders in the head-injured patient, in *Neurotrauma*, edited by RK Narayan, JE Wilberger, JT Pevlishock. McGraw-Hill, New York, 1996.

48. Faulk WP, Labarre CA: Antithrombin III in normal and transplanted hearts: Indications of vascular disease. *Semin Hematol* 31 (suppl):26, 1994.

49. Asakura H, Ontachi Y, Mizutani T, et al: An enhanced fibrinolysis prevents the development of multiple organ failure in disseminated intravascular coagulation in spite of much activation of blood coagulation. *Crit Care Med* 29:1164, 2001.

50. Levi M, de Jonge E, van der Poll T: New strategies for disseminated intravascular coagulation based on current understanding of pathophysiology. *Ann Med* 36:41, 2004.

51. Hack CE: Fibrinolysis in disseminated intravascular coagulation. *Semin Thromb Hemost* 27:633, 2001.

52. Taylor FB Jr: Response of anticoagulant pathways in disseminated intravascular coagulation. *Semin Thromb Hemost* 27:619, 2001.

53. Montes R, Rodriguez-Whilhelmi P, Hurtado V, et al: The endotoxin-induced plasminogen activator inhibitor-1 increase in rabbits is not tumor necrosis factor-alpha dependent and can occur in the absence of interleukin-1beta. *Thromb Haemost* 88:639, 2002

54. Liaw PC, Ferrell G, Esmon CT: A monoclonal antibody against activated protein C allows rapid detection of activated protein C in plasma and reveals a calcium ion dependent epitope involved in factor Va inactivation. *J Thromb Haemost* 1:662, 2003.

55. Aoki K, Aikawa N, Sekine M, et al: Elevation of plasma free PAI-1 levels as an integrated endothelial response to severe burns. *Burns* 27:569, 2001.

56. Norman KE, Cotter MJ, Stewart JB, et al: Combined anticoagulant and antiselectin treatments prevent lethal intravascular coagulation. *Blood* 101:921, 2003.

57. Watanabe R, Wada H, Watanabe Y, et al: Activity and antigen levels of thrombin-activatable fibrinolysis inhibitor in plasma of patients with disseminated intravascular coagulation. *Thromb Res* 104:1, 2001.

58. Salvemini D, Cuzzocrea S: Oxidative stress in septic shock and disseminated intravascular coagulation. *Free Radic Biol Med* 33:1173, 2002.

59. Asakura H, Okudaira M, Yoshida T, et al: Induction of vasoactive substances differs in LPS-induced and TF-induced DIC models in rats. *Thromb Haemost* 88:663, 2002.

60. Slofstra SH, Spek CA, ten Cate H: Disseminated intravascular coagulation. *Hematol J* 4:295, 2003.

61. Gando S, Kameue T, Matsuda N, et al: Combined activation of coagulation and inflammation has an important role in multiple organ dysfunction and poor outcome after severe trauma. *Thromb Haemost* 88:943, 2002.

62. Asakura HY, Suga K, Aoshima Y, et al: Marked difference in pathophysiology between tissue factor- and lipopolysaccharide-induced disseminated intravascular coagulation models in rats. *Crit Care Med* 30:161, 2002.

63. Siegal T, Seligsohn U, Aghai E, Modan M: Clinical and laboratory aspects of disseminated intravascular coagulation (DIC): A study of 118 cases. *Thromb Haemost* 39:122, 1978.

64. Spero JA, Lewis JH, Hasiba U: Disseminated intravascular coagulation. Findings in 346 patients. *Thromb Haemost* 43:28, 1980.

65. Matsuda M, Aoki N: Statistics on underlying and causative diseases of DIC in Japan. A cooperative study, in *Disseminated Intravascular Coagulation*, edited by T Abe, M Yamanaka, p 15. Karger, Basel, 1983.

66. Kobayashi N, Maekawa T, Takada M, Tanaka H: Criteria for diagnosis of DIC on the analysis of clinical and laboratory findings in 345 patients collected by the research committee on DIC in Japan, in *Disseminated Intravascular Coagulation*, edited by T Abe, M Yamanaka, p 265. Karger, Basel, 1983.

67. Al-Mondhiry H: Disseminated intravascular coagulation. Experience in a major cancer center. *Thromb Diath Haemorrh* 34:181, 1975.

68. Katsumura Y, Ohtsubo K: Incidence of pulmonary thromboembolism, infarction and hemorrhage in disseminated intravascular coagulation: A necroscopic analysis. *Thorax* 50:160, 1995.

69. Bone RC, Francis PB, Pierce AK: Disseminated intravascular coagulation with the adult respiratory distress syndrome. *Am J Med* 61:585, 1976.

70. Rinaldo JE, Christman JW: Mechanisms and mediators of the adult respiratory distress syndrome. *Clin Chest Med* 11:621, 1990.

71. Kollef MH, Schuster DP: The acute respiratory distress syndrome. *N Engl J Med* 332:27, 1995.

72. Colman RW, Robboy SJ, Minna JD: Disseminated intravascular coagulation. A reappraisal. *Annu Rev Med* 30:359, 1979.

73. Taylor FB Jr, Toh CH, Hoots WK, et al: Towards definition, clinical and laboratory criteria, and a scoring system for disseminated intravascular coagulation. *Thromb Haemost* 86:1327, 2001.

74. Wada H, Gabazza EC, Asakura H, Koike KK, et al: Comparison of diagnostic criteria for disseminated intravascular coagulation (DIC): Diagnostic criteria of the International Society of Thrombosis and Hemostasis and of the Japanese Ministry of Health and Welfare for overt DIC. *Am J Hematol* 74:17, 2003.

75. Wada H, Yamamuro M, Inoue A, et al: Comparison of the responses of global tests of coagulation with molecular markers of neutrophil, endothelial, and hemostatic system perturbation in the baboon model of E. colisepsis—Toward a distinction between uncompensated overt DIC and compensated non-overt DIC. *Thromb Haemost* 86:1489, 2001.

76. Moore JC, Hayward CP, Warkentin TE, Kelton JG: Decreased von Willebrand factor protease activity associated with thrombocytopenic disorders. *Blood* 98:1842, 2001.

77. Toh CH, Samis J, Downey C, et al: Biphasic transmittance waveform in the APTT coagulation assay is due to the formation of a Ca(++)-dependent complex of C-reactive protein with very-low-density lipoprotein and is a novel marker of impending disseminated intravascular coagulation. *Blood* 100:2522, 2002.

78. Toh CH, Giles AR: Waveform analysis of clotting test optical profiles in the diagnosis and management of disseminated intravascular coagulation (DIC). *Clin Lab Haematol* 24:321, 2002.

79. Toh CH: Laboratory testing in disseminated intravascular coagulation. *Semin Thromb Hemost* 27:653, 2001.

80. Kobayashi S, Gando S, Morimoto Y, et al: Serial measurement of arterial lactate concentrations as a prognostic indicator in relation to the incidence of disseminated intravascular coagulation in patients with systemic inflammatory response syndrome. *Surg Today* 31:853, 2001.

81. Bisno AL, Freeman JC: The syndrome of asplenia, pneumococcal sepsis, and disseminated intravascular coagulation. *Ann Intern Med* 72:389, 1970.

82. Levy MM, Fink MP, Marshall JC, et al: 2001 SCCM/ESICM/ACCP/ATS/SIS International Sepsis Definitions Conference. *Crit Care Med* 31:1250, 2003.

83. Levi M, De Jong E, Vander Poll T: Sepsis and disseminated intravascular coagulation. *J Thromb Thrombolysis* 16:43, 2003.

84. Okajma K: Regulation of inflammatory responses by natural anticoagulants. *Immunol Rev* 184:258, 2001.

85. Faust SN, Levin M, Harrison OB, et al: Dysfunction of endothelial protein C activation in severe meningococcal sepsis. *N Engl J Med* 345:408, 2001.

86. Kinasewitz GT, Yan SB, Basson B, et al: Universal changes in biomarkers of coagulation and inflammation occur in patients with severe sepsis, regardless of causative micro-organism [ISRCTN74215569]. *Crit Care* 8:R82, 2004.

87. Herwald H, Cramer H, Morgelin M, et al: M protein, a classical bacterial virulence determinant, forms complexes with fibrinogen that induce vascular leakage. *Cell* 116:367, 2004.

88. Vik-Mo H, Lote K, Nordoy A: Disseminated intravascular coagulation in patients with meningococcal infection: Laboratory diagnosis and prognostic factors. *Scand J Infect Dis* 10:187, 1978.

89. Kornelisse RF, Hazelzet JA, Hop WC, et al: Meningococcal septic shock in children: Clinical and laboratory features, outcome, and development of a prognostic score. *Clin Infect Dis* 25:640, 1997.

90. Dempfle CA: Coagulopathy of sepsis. *Thromb Haemost* 91:213, 2004.

91. Murray HW, Tuazon CU, Sheagren JN: Staphylococcal septicemia and disseminated intravascular coagulation. *Arch Intern Med* 137:844, 1977.

92. Bhakdi S, Muhly M, Mannhardt U, et al: Staphylococcal alpha toxin promotes blood coagulation via attack on human platelets. *J Exp Med* 168:527, 1988.

93. Ratnoff OD, Nebehay WG: Multiple coagulative defects in a patient with Waterhouse-Friderichsen syndrome. *Ann Intern Med* 56:627, 1962.

94. Stossel TP, Levy R: Intravascular coagulation associated with pneumococcal bacteremia and symmetrical peripheral gangrene. *Arch Intern Med* 125:876, 1970.

95. Rytel MW, Dee TH, Ferstenfeld JE, Hensley GT: Possible pathogenetic role of capsular antigens in fulminant pneumococcal disease with disseminated intravascular coagulation (DIC). *Am J Med* 57:889, 1974.

96. De Virgilio C, Klein S, Chang L, et al: Clostridial bacteremia: Implications for the surgeon. *Am Surg* 57:388, 1991.

97. Cosgriff TM: Viruses and hemostasis. *Rev Infect Dis* 11(suppl 4):S672, 1989.

98. Inbal A, Kenet G, Zivelin A, et al: Purpura fulminans induced by disseminated intravascular coagulation following infection in two unrelated children with double heterozygosity for factor V Leiden and protein S deficiency. *Thromb Haemost* 77:1086, 1997.

99. Levin M, Eley BS, Louis J, et al: Postinfectious purpura fulminans caused by an autoantibody directed against protein S. *J Pediatr* 127:355, 1995.

100. Lee M, Lee JS, Kim BK: Disseminated intravascular coagulation in Korean hemorrhagic fever. *Bibl Haematol* 49:181, 1983.

101. Peters CJ, Liu CT, Anderson GW Jr, et al: Pathogenesis of viral hemorrhagic fevers: Rift Valley fever and Lassa fever contrasted. *Rev Infect Dis* 11(suppl 4):S743, 1989.

102. Srichaikul T, Nimmannitya S: Haematology in dengue and dengue haemorrhagic fever. *Baillieres Best Pract Res Clin Haematol* 13:261, 2000.

103. Molinas FC, de Bracco MM, Maiztegui JI: Hemostasis and the complement system in Argentine hemorrhagic fever. *Rev Infect Dis* 11(suppl 4):S762, 1989.

104. Grob C: Tissue factor initiation of disseminated intravascular coagulation in filovirus infection. *Med Hypotheses* 45:380, 1995.

105. Vitarana T, de Silva H, Withana N, Gunasekera C: Elevated tumour necrosis factor in dengue fever and dengue haemorrhagic fever. *Ceylon Med J* 36:63, 1991.

106. Hjort PF, Rapaport SI, Jorgensen L: Purpura fulminans. Report of a case successfully treated with heparin and hydrocortisone. Review of 50 cases from the literature. *Scand J Haematol* 1:69, 1964.

107. Carpenter CT, Kaiser AB: Purpura fulminans in pneumococcal sepsis: Case report and review. *Scand J Infect Dis* 29:479, 1997.

108. Gerson WT, Dickerman JD, Bovill EG, Golden E: Severe acquired protein C deficiency in purpura fulminans associated with disseminated intravascular coagulation: Treatment with protein C concentrate. *Pediatrics* 91:418, 1993.

109. Tishler M, Abramov AL, Seligsohn U, Kahn Y: Purpura fulminans in an adult. *Isr J Med Sci* 22:820, 1986.

110. Branson HE, Katz J, Marble R, Griffin JH: Inherited protein C deficiency and a coumarin-responsive chronic relapsing purpura fulminans syndrome in a newborn infant. *Lancet* 2:1156, 1983.

111. Seligsohn U, Berger A, Abend M, et al: Homozygous protein C deficiency manifested by massive venous thrombosis in the newborn. *N Engl J Med* 310, 1984.

112. Jurgens R, Trautwein H: über Fibrinopenic (Fibrinogenopenie) beim Erwaschsenen, nebst Bemerkungen über die herkunft des Fibrinogens. *Dtsch Arch Klin Med* 169:28, 1930.

113. Goad KE, Gralnick HR: Coagulation disorders in cancer. *Hematol Oncol Clin North Am* 10:457, 1996.

114. Desancho MT, Rand JH: Bleeding and thrombotic complications in critically ill patients with cancer. *Crit Care Clin* 17:599, 2001.

115. Sack GH Jr, Levin J, Bell WR: Trousseau's syndrome and other manifestations of chronic disseminated coagulopathy in patients with neoplasms: Clinical, pathophysiologic, and therapeutic features. *Medicine (Baltimore)* 56:1, 1977.

116. Collins RC, Al-Mondhiry H, Chernik NL, et al: Neurologic manifestations of intravascular coagulation in cancer: A clinicopathologic analysis of 12 cases. *Neurology* 25:795, 1975.

117. Szczepanski M, Bardadin K, Zawadzki J, Pypno W: Procoagulant activity of gastric, colorectal and renal cancer is factor VII-dependent. *J Cancer Res Clin Oncol* 114:519, 1988.

118. Falanga A, Gordon SG: Isolation and characterization of cancer procoagulant: A cysteine proteinase from malignant tissue. *Biochemistry* 24:5558, 1985.

119. Wahrenbrock M, Borsig L, Le D, et al: Selectin-mucin interactions as a probable molecular explanation for the association of Trousseau syndrome with mucinous adenocarcinomas. *J Clin Invest* 112:853, 2003.

120. Dvorak HF, Quay SC, Orenstein NS, et al: Tumor shedding and coagulation. *Science* 212:923, 1981.

121. Pineo GF, Regoeczi E, Hatton MWC, Brain MC: The activation of coagulation by extracts of mucus: A possible pathway of intravascular coagulation accompanying adenocarcinomas. *J Lab Clin Med* 82:255, 1973.

122. Bell WR, Starksen NF, Tong S, Proterfield JK: Trousseau's syndrome. Devastating coagulopathy in the absence of heparin. *Am J Med* 79:423, 1985.

123. Sallah S, Wan JY, Nguyen NP, Hanrahan LR, Sigounas G: Disseminated intravascular coagulation in solid tumors: Clinical and pathologic study. *Thromb Haemostasis* 86:828, 2001.

124. Mant MJ, King EG: Severe, acute disseminated intravascular coagulation. A reappraisal of its pathophysiology, clinical significance and therapy based on 47 patients. *Am J Med* 67:557, 1979.

125. Sutherland DE, Weitz IC, Liebman HA: Thromboembolic complications of cancer: Epidemiology, pathogenesis, diagnosis, and treatment. *Am J Hematol* 72:43, 2003.

126. Agnes Y, Lee Y: Epidemiology and management of venous thromboembolism in patients with cancer. *Thromb Res* 110:167, 2003.

127. Seligsohn U, Weber H, Yoran C, et al: Microangiopathic hemolytic anemia and defibrination syndrome in metastatic carcinoma of the stomach. *Isr J Med Sci* 4:69, 1968.

128. Risak E: Die Fibrinopenie. *Z Klin Med* 128:606, 1935.

129. Falanga A, Rickles FR: Pathogenesis and management of the bleeding diathesis in acute promyelocytic leukaemia. *Best Pract Res Clin Haematol* 16:463, 2003.

130. Menell JS, Cesarman GM, Jacovina AT, et al: Annexin II and bleeding in acute promyelocytic leukemia. *N Engl J Med* 340:994, 1999.

131. Sarris A, Cortes J, Kantarjian H, et al: Disseminated intravascular coagulation in adult acute lymphoblastic leukemia: Frequent complications with fibrinogen levels less than 100 mg/dl. *Leuk Lymphoma* 21:85, 1996.

132. Gando S: Disseminated intravascular coagulation in trauma patients. *Semin Thromb Hemost* 27:585, 2001.

133. Gando S, Kameue T, Matsuda N, et al: Combined activation of coagulation and inflammation has an important role in multiple organ dysfunction and poor outcome after severe trauma. *Thromb Haemost* 88:943, 2002.

134. Owings JT, Bagley M, Gosselin R, et al: Effect of critical injury on plasma antithrombin activity: Low antithrombin levels are associated with thromboembolic complications. *J Trauma* 41:396, 1996.

135. Armand R, Hess JR: Treating coagulopathy in trauma patients. *Transfus Med Rev* 17:223, 2003.

136. Simmons RL, Collins JA, Heisterkamp CA, et al: Coagulation disorders in combat casualties: I. Acute changes after wounding: II. Effect of massive transfusion: III. Post-resuscitative changes. *Ann Surg* 169:455, 1969.

137. Goodnight SH, Kenover G, Rapaport SI, et al: Defibrination after brain-tissue destruction. A serious complication of head injury. *N Engl J Med* 290:1043, 1974.

138. Scherer RU, Spangenberg P: Procoagulant activity in patients with isolated severe head trauma. *Crit Care Med* 26:149, 1998.

139. Kaufman HH, Hui KS, Mattson JC, et al: Clinicopathological correlations of disseminated intravascular coagulation in patients with head injury. *Neurosurgery* 15:34, 1984.

140. Stein SC, Chen XH, Sinson GP, Smith DH: Intravascular coagulation: A major secondary insult in nonfatal traumatic brain injury. *J Neurosurg* 97:1373, 2002.

141. Olson JD, Kaufman HH, Moake J, et al: The incidence and significance of hemostatic abnormalities in patients with head injuries. *Neurosurgery* 24:825, 1989.

142. Selladurai BM, Vickneswaran M, Duraisamy S, Atan M: Coagulopathy in acute head injury—a study of its role as a prognostic indicator. *Br J Neurosurg* 11:398, 1997.

143. McManus WF, Eurenius K, Pruitt BA: Disseminated intravascular coagulation in burned patients. *J Trauma* 13:416, 1973.

144. Simon TL, Current PW, Harker LA: Kinetic characterization of hemostasis in thermal injury. *J Lab Clin Med* 82:702, 1977.

145. Garcia-Avello A, Lorente JA, Cesar-Perez J, et al: Degree of hypercoagulability and hyperfibrinolysis is related to organ failure and prognosis after burn trauma. *Thromb Res* 89:59, 1998.

146. Winkelman MD, Galloway PG: Central nervous system complications of thermal burns. A postmortem study of 139 patients. *Medicine (Baltimore)* 71:271, 1992.

147. Carr JM: Disseminated intravascular coagulation in cirrhosis. *Hepatology* 10:103, 1989.

148. Joist JH: AICF and DIC in liver cirrhosis: Expressions of a hypercoagulable state. *Am J Gastroenterol* 94:2801, 1999.

149. Tytgat GN, Collen D, Verstraete M: Metabolism of fibrinogen in cirrhosis of the liver. *J Clin Invest* 50:1960, 1971.

150. Coleman M, Finlayson N, Bettigole RE, et al: Fibrinogen survival in cirrhosis: Improvement by "low dose" heparin. *Ann Intern Med* 83:79, 1975.

151. Tytgat GN, Piesens J, Collen D, De Groote J: Experience with exchange transfusion in the treatment of hepatic coma. *Digestion* 1:257, 1968.

152. Carr JM, McKinney M, McDonagh J: Diagnosis of DIC: Role of D-dimer. *Am J Clin Pathol* 91:280, 1989.

153. Paramo JA, Rifon J, Fernandez J, et al: Thrombin activation and increased fibrinolysis in patients with chronic liver disease. *Blood Coagul Fibrinolysis* 2:227, 1991.

154. Van Wersch JWJ, Russel MG, Lustermans FA: The extent of diffuse intravascular coagulation and fibrinolysis in patients with liver cirrhosis. *Eur J Clin Chem Clin Biochem* 30:275, 1992.

155. Coccheri S, Mannucci PM, Palaret G, et al: Significance of plasma fibrinopeptide A and high molecular weight fibrinogen in patients with liver cirrhosis. *Br J Haematol* 52:503, 1982.

156. Oka K, Tanaka K: Intravascular coagulation in autopsy cases with liver diseases. *Thromb Haemost* 42:564, 1979.

157. Palascak JE, Martinez J: Dysfibrinogenemia associated with liver disease. *J Clin Invest* 60:89, 1977.

158. Ben Ari Z, Osman E, Hutton RA, Burroughs AK: Disseminated intravascular coagulation in liver cirrhosis: Fact or fiction? *Am J Gastornterol* 94:2977, 1999.

159. Corrigan JJ, Bennett BB, Bueffel B: The value of factor VIII levels in acquired hypofibrinogenemia. *Am J Clin Pathol* 60:897, 1973.

160. Straub PW: Diffuse intravascular coagulation in liver disease? *Semin Thromb Haemost* 4:29, 1977.

161. Canoso RT, Hutton RA, Deykin D: The hemostatic defect of chronic liver disease. Kinetic studies using ^{75}Se-Selenomethionine. *Gastroenterology* 76:540, 1979.

162. Tempero MA, Davis RB, Reed E, Edney J: Thrombocytopenia and laboratory evidence of disseminated intravascular coagulation after shunts for ascites in malignant disease. *Cancer* 55:2718, 1985.

163. Bakker CM, Knot EA, Stibbe J, Wilson JH: Disseminated intravascular coagulation in liver cirrhosis. *J Hepatol* 15:330, 1992.

164. Shibolet S, Coll R, Gilat T, et al: Heatstroke: Its clinical picture and mechanism in 36 cases. *Q J Med* 36:525, 1967.

165. Shibolet S, Lancaster MC, Danon Y: Heat stroke: A review. *Aviat Space Environ Med* 47:280, 1976.

166. Wakefield EG, Hall WW: Heat injuries: A preparatory study for experimental heat stroke. *JAMA* 89:92, 1927.

167. Malamud N, Naymaker W, Custer RP: Heat stroke. A clinicopathology study of 125 fatal cases. *Milit Surg* 99:397, 1946.

168. Mustafa KY, Omer O, Khogali M, et al: Blood coagulation and fibrinolysis in heat stroke. *Br J Haematol* 61:517, 1985.

169. Al-Mashhadani SA, Gader AG, al-Harthi SS, et al: The coagulopathy of heat stroke: Alterations in coagulation and fibrinolysis in heat stroke patients during the pilgrimage (Haj) to Makkah. *Blood Coagul Fibrinolysis* 5:731, 1994.

170. Bouchama A, Bridey F, Hammami MM, et al: Activation of coagulation and fibrinolysis in heatstroke. *Thromb Haemost* 76:909, 1996.

171. Sohal RS, Sun SC, Colcolough HL, et al: Heat stroke. An electron microscopy study of endothelial cell damage and disseminated intravascular coagulation. *Arch Intern Med* 122:43, 1968.

172. Seegers WH, Ouyang C: Snake venoms and blood coagulation, in *Snake Venoms*, edited by C-Y Lee, p 684. Springer-Verlag, Berlin, 1979.

173. Huang TF, Holt JC, Lukasiwic H, Niewiarowski S: Trigamin: A low molecular weight peptide inhibiting fibrinogen interaction with platelet receptors expressed on glycoprotein IIb-IIIa complex. *J Biol Chem* 262: 16157, 1987.

174. Klein JD, Walker FJ: Purification of a protein C activator from the venom of the southern copperhead snake (Agkistrodon contortrix). *Biochemistry* 25:4175, 1986.

175. Schulchynska-Castel H, Dvilansky A, Keynan A: Echis colorata bites: Clinical evaluation of 42 patients. A retrospective study. *Isr J Med Sci* 22:880, 1986.

176. Weiss HJ, Phillips LL, Hopewell WS, et al: Heparin therapy in a patient bitten by a saw-scaled viper (Echis carinatus), a snake whose venom activated prothrombin. *Am J Med* 54:653, 1973.

177. Fainaru M, Eisenberg S, Manny N, Hershko C: The natural course of defibrination syndrome caused by Echis colorata venom in man. *Thromb Diath Haemorrh* 31:420, 1974.

178. Efrati P: Symptomatology, pathology and treatment of the bites of viperid snakes, in *Snake Venoms*, edited by C-Y Lee, p 956, Springer-Verlag, Berlin, 1979.

179. Cederbaum AI, Blatt PM, Roberts HR: Intravascular coagulation with use of human prothrombin complex concentrates. *Ann Intern Med* 84: 683, 1976.

180. Hultin MB: Activated clotting factors in factor IX concentrates. *Blood* 54:1028, 1979.

181. Mannucci PM, Bauer KA, Santagostino E, et al: Activation of the coagulation cascade after infusion of a factor XI concentrate in congenitally deficient patients. *Blood* 84:1314, 1994.

182. Richards EM, Makris MM, Cooper P, Preston FE: In vivo coagulation activation following infusion of highly purified factor XI concentrate. *Br J Haematol* 96:293, 1997.

183. Bolton-Maggs PH, Colvin BT, Satchi BT, et al: Thrombogenic potential of factor XI concentrate. *Lancet* 344:748, 1994.

184. Hall GW: Kasabach-Merritt syndrome: Pathogenesis and management. *Br J Haematol* 112:851, 2001.

185. Straub PW, Kessler S, Schreiber A, Frick PG: Chronic intravascular coagulation in Kasabach-Merritt syndrome. Preferential accumulation of fibrinogen ^{131}I in a giant hemangioma. *Arch Intern Med* 129:475, 1972.

186. Warrell RP, Kempin SJ, Benua RS, et al: Intra-tumoral consumption of indium-111 labeled platelets in a patient with hemangiomatosis and intravascular coagulation (Kasabach-Merritt syndrome). *Cancer* 52:2256, 1983.

187. Propp RP, Scharfman WB: Hemangioma-thrombocytopenia syndrome associated with microangiopathic hemolytic anemia. *Blood* 28:623, 1966.

188. Hesselmann S, Micke O, Marquardt T, et al: Case report: Kasabach-Merritt syndrome: A review of the therapeutic options and a case report of successful treatment with radiotherapy and interferon alpha. *Br J Radiol* 75:180, 2002.

189. Mazoyer E, Enjolras O, Laurian C, et al: Coagulation abnormalities associated with extensive venous malformations of the limbs: Differentiation from Kasabach-Merritt syndrome. *Clin Lab Haematol* 24:243, 2002.

190. Fine NL, Applebaum J, Elguezabal A, Castleman L: Multiple coagulation defects in association with dissecting aneurysm. *Arch Intern Med* 119:522, 1967.

191. Fisher DI, Yawn DH, Crawford S: Preoperative disseminated intravascular coagulation associated with aortic aneurysm. *Arch Surg* 118:1252, 1983.

192. Bieger R, Vreeken J, Stibbe J, Loeliger EA: Arterial aneurysm as a cause of consumption coagulopathy. *N Engl J Med* 285:152, 1971.

193. ten Cate JW, Timmers H, Becker AE: Coagulopathy in ruptured or dissecting aortic aneurysm. *Am J Med* 59:171, 1975.

194. Mulcare RJ, Royster TS, Phillips LL: Intravascular coagulation in surgical procedures on the abdominal aorta. *Surg Gynecol Obstet* 143:730, 1976.

195. Wilcox JN, Smith KM, Schwartz SM, Gordon D: Localization of tissue factor in the normal vessel wall and in the atherosclerotic plaque. *Proc Natl Acad Sci U S A* 86:2839, 1989.

196. Cummins D, Segal H, Hunt BJ, et al: Chronic disseminated intravascular coagulation after surgery for abdominal aortic aneurysm: Clinical and haemostatic response to dalteparin. *Br J Haematol* 113:658, 2001.

197. Ohara N, Miyata T, Oshiro H, et al: Adverse outcome following transfemoral stent-graft repair of an abdominal aortic aneurysm in a patient with severe liver dysfunction: Report of a case. *Surg Today* 30:764, 2000.

198. Cross KS, Bouchier-Hayes D, Leahy AL: Consumptive coagulopathy following endovascular stent repair of abdominal aortic aneurysm. *Eur J Vasc Endovasc Surg* 19:94, 2000.

199. Shimazaki T, Ishimaru S, Kawaguchi S, et al: Blood coagulation and fibrinolytic response after endovascular stent grafting of thoracic aorta. *J Vasc Surg* 37:1213, 2003.

200. Krevans JR, Jackson DP, Conley CL, Hartmann RC: The nature of the hemorrhagic disorder accompanying hemolytic transfusion reactions in man. *Blood* 12:834, 1957.

201. Mannucci PM, Lobina GF, Caocci L, Dioguardi N: Effect on blood coagulation of massive intravascular haemolysis. *Blood* 33:207, 1969.

202. Butler J, Parker D, Pillai R, et al: Systemic release of neutrophil elastase and tumour necrosis factor alpha following ABO incompatible blood transfusion. *Br J Haematol* 79:525, 1991.

203. Hamilton K, Hattori R, Esmon C, Sims P: Complement proteins C5b-9 induce vesiculation of the endothelial plasma membrane and expose catalytic surface for assembly of the prothrombinase enzyme complex. *J Biol Chem* 265:3809, 1990.

204. Weiner CP: The obstetric patient and disseminated intravascular coagulation. *Clin Perinatol* 13:705, 1986.

205. Letsky EA: Disseminated intravascular coagulation. *Best Pract Res Clin Obstet Gynecol* 15:623, 2001.

206. DeLee JB: A case of fatal hemorrhagic diathesis with premature detachment of the placenta. *Am J Obstet Gynecol* 44:785, 1901.

207. Eskes TK: Abruptio placentae. A "classic" dedicated to Elizabeth Ramsey. *Eur J Obstet Gynecol Reprod Biol* 75:63, 1997.

208. Kuczynski J, Uszynski W, Zekanowska E, et al: Tissue factor (TF) and tissue factor pathway inhibitor (TFPI) in the placenta and myometrium. *Europ J Obstet Gynecol Reprod Biol* 105:15, 2002.

209. Pritchard JA, Brekken AL: Clinical and laboratory studies on severe abruptio placentae. *Am J Obstet Gynecol* 97:681, 1967.

210. Diekmann WJ: Blood chemistry and renal function in abruptio placentae. *Am J Obstet Gynecol* 31:734, 1936.

211. Steiner PE, Lushbaugh CC: Maternal pulmonary embolism by amniotic fluid as a cause of obstetric shock and unexpected deaths in obstetrics. *JAMA* 117:1245, 1941.

212. Morgan M: Amniotic fluid embolism. *Anaesthesia* 34:20, 1979.

213. Gilbert WM, Danielsen B: Amniotic fluid embolism: Decreased mortality in a population-based study. *Obstet Gynecol* 93:973, 1999.

214. Uszynski M, Zekanowska E, Uszynski W, Kuczynski J: Tissue factor (TF) and tissue factor pathway inhibitor (TFPI) in amniotic fluid and blood plasma: Implications for the mechanism of amniotic fluid embolism. *Europ J Obstet Gynecol Rep Biol* 95:163, 2001.

215. Stahnke E: Über das Verhalten der blutplattchen bei Eklampsie. *Zentralbl Gynak* 46:391, 1922.

216. McKay DG, Marrill SJ, Weiner AE, et al: The pathologic anatomy of eclampsia, bilateral renal cortical necrosis, pituitary necrosis, and other acute fatal complications of pregnancy, and its possible relationship to the generalized Shwartzman phenomenon. *Am J Obstet Gynecol* 55:507, 1953.

217. Page EW: On the pathogenesis of pre-eclampsia and eclampsia. *J Obstet Gynecol Br Commonwealth* 79:883, 1972.

218. Gibson B, Hunter D, Neame PB, Kelton JG: Thrombocytopenia in pre-eclampsia and eclampsia. *Semin Thromb Haemost* 8:234, 1982.

219. Giles C: Intravascular coagulation in gestational hypertension and pre-eclampsia: The value of haematological screening tests. *Clin Lab Haematol* 4:351, 1982.

220. Borok Z, Weitz J, Owen J, et al: Fibrinogen proteolysis and platelet alpha granule release in pre-eclampsia/eclampsia. *Blood* 63:525, 1984.

221. Broughton Pipkin F, Rubin PC: Pre-eclampsia—The "disease of theories." *Br Med Bull* 50:381, 1994.

222. Norwitz ER, Hsu CD, Repke JT: Acute complications of preeclampsia. *Clin Obstet Gynecol* 45:308, 2002.

223. Weinstein L: Syndrome of hemolysis, elevated liver enzymes, and low platelet count: a severe consequence of hypertension in pregnancy. *Am J Obstet Gynecol* 142:159, 1982.

224. Sibai BM, Ramadan MK, Usta I, et al: Maternal morbidity and mortality in 442 pregnancies with hemolysis, elevated liver enzymes, and low platelets. *Am J Obstet Gynecol* 169:1000, 1993.

225. Aarnoudse JG, Houthoff JH, Weits K, et al: A syndrome of liver damage and intravascular coagulation in the last trimester of normotensive pregnancy. A clinical and histopathological study. *Br J Obstet Gynaecol* 93:145, 1986.

226. Audibert F, Friedman SA, Frangieh AY, Sibai BM: Clinical utility of strict diagnostic criteria for the HELLP (hemolysis, elevated liver enzymes, and low platelets) syndrome. *Am J Obstet Gynecol* 175:460, 1996.

227. Barton JR, Sibai BM: Hepatic imaging in HELLP syndrome (hemolysis, elevated liver enzymes, and low platelet count). *Am J Obstet Gynecol* 174:1820, 1996.

228. Sullivan CA, Magann EF, Perry KG Jr, et al: The recurrence risk of the syndrome of hemolysis, elevated liver enzymes, and low platelets (HELLP) in subsequent gestations. *Am J Obstet Gynecol* 171:940, 1994.

229. Lee W, Clark SL, Cotton DB, et al: Septic shock during pregnancy. *Am J Obstet Gynecol* 159:410, 1988.

230. Romero R, Copel JA, Hobbins JC: Intrauterine fetal demise and hemostatic failure: The fetal death syndrome. *Clin Obstet Gynecol* 28:24, 1985.

231. Berkowitz RL, Stone JL, Eddleman KA: One hundred consecutive cases of selective termination of an abnormal fetus in a multifetal gestation. *Obstet Gynecol* 90:606, 1997.

232. Bacq Y, Riely CA: Acute fatty liver of pregnancy: The hepatologist's view. *Gastroenterologist* 1:257, 1993.

233. Usta IM, Barton JR, Amon EA, et al: Acute fatty liver of pregnancy: An experience in the diagnosis and management of fourteen cases. *Am J Obstet Gynecol* 171:1342, 1994.

234. Pereira SP, O'Donohue J, Wendon J, Williams R: Maternal and perinatal outcome in severe pregnancy-related liver disease. *Hepatology* 26:1258, 1997.

235. Rahman TM, Wendon J: Severe hepatic dysfunction in pregnancy. *Q J Med* 95:343, 2002.

236. Ibdah JA, Yang Z, Bennett MJ: Liver disease in pregnancy and fetal fatty acid oxidation defects. *Mol Genet Metab* 71:182, 2000.

237. Castro MA, Goodwin TM, Shaw KJ, et al: Disseminated intravascular coagulation and antithrombin III depression in acute fatty liver of pregnancy. *Am J Obstet Gynecol* 174:211, 1996.

238. Watson WJ, Seeds JW: Acute fatty liver of pregnancy. *Obstet Gynecol Surv* 45:585, 1990.

239. Moldenhauer JS, O'Brien JM, Barton JR, Sibai B: Acute fatty liver of pregnancy associated with pancreatitis: A life-threatening complication. *Am J Obstet Gynecol* 190:502, 2004.

240. Hathaway WE, Mull MM, Peschet GS: Disseminated intravascular coagulation in the newborn. *Pediatrics* 43:233, 1969.

241. Corrigan JJ: Activation of coagulation and disseminated intravascular coagulation in the newborn. *Am J Pediatr Hematol Oncol* 1:245, 1979.

242. Williams MD, Chalmers EA, Gibson BE: The investigation and management of neonatal haemostasis and thrombosis. *Br J Haematol* 119:295, 2002.

243. Woods WG, Luban NL, Hilgartner MW, Miller DR: Disseminated intravascular coagulation in the newborn. *Am J Dis Child* 133:44, 1979.

244. Corrigan JJ: Disseminated intravascular coagulopathy. *Pediatr Rev* 1:37, 1979.

245. Gentilello LM, Pierson DJ: Trauma critical care. *Am J Respir Crit Care Med* 163:604, 2001.

246. Schupp M, Swanevelder JL, Peek GJ, et al: Postoperative extracorporeal membrane oxygenation for severe intraoperative SIRS 10 h after multiple trauma. *Br J Anaesth* 90:91, 2003.

247. Mueller MM, Bomke B, Seifried E: Fresh frozen plasma in patients with disseminated intravascular coagulation or in patients with liver diseases. *Thromb Res* 107(suppl 1):S9, 2002.

248. Stegmayr BG, Banga R, Berggren L, et al: Plasma exchange as rescue therapy in multiple organ failure including acute renal failure. *Crit Care Med* 31:1730, 2003.

249. Bernard GR, Vincent JL, Laterre PF, et al: Efficacy and safety of recombinant human activated protein C for severe sepsis. *N Engl J Med* 344:699, 2001.

250. Bernard GR, Ely EW, Wright TJ, et al: Safety and dose relationship of recombinant human activated protein C for coagulopathy in severe sepsis. *Crit Care Med* 29:2051, 2001.

251. Corrigan JJ, Jordan CM: Heparin therapy in septicemia with disseminated intravascular coagulation. *N Engl J Med* 283:778, 1970.

252. Hogg PJ, Jackson CM: Fibrin monomer protects thrombin from inactivation by heparin-antithrombin III: Implications for heparin efficacy. *Proc Natl Acad Sci U S A* 86:3619, 1989.

253. Cowan PJ, Aminian A, Barlow H, et al: Protective effects of recombinant human antithrombin III in pig-to-primate renal xenotransplantation. *Am J Transplant* 2:520, 2002.

254. Dickneite G, Kroez M: Treatment of porcine sepsis with high-dose antithrombin III reduces tissue edema and effusion but does not increase risk for bleeding. *Blood Coagul Fibrinolysis* 12:459, 2001.

255. Dickneite G, Paques EP: Reduction of mortality with antithrombin III in septicemic rats: A study of Klebsiella pneumoniae induced sepsis. *Thromb Haemost* 69:98, 1993.

256. Blauhut B, Necek S, Vinazzer H, Bergmann H: Substitution therapy with an antithrombin III concentrate in shock and DIC. *Thromb Res* 27:271, 1982.

257. Fourrier F, Chopin C, Goudemand J, et al: Septic shock, multiple organ failure, and disseminated intravascular coagulation. Compared patterns of antithrombin III, protein C, and protein S deficiencies. *Chest* 101:816, 1992.

258. Messori A, Vacca F, Vaiani M, Trippoli S: Antithrombin III in patients admitted to intensive care units: A multicenter observational study. *Crit Care* 6:447, 2002.

259. Warren BL, Eid A, Singer P, et al: Caring for the critically ill patient. High-dose antithrombin III in severe sepsis: A randomized controlled trial. *JAMA* 286:1869, 2001.

260. Faust SN, Heyderman RS, Levin M: Coagulation in severe sepsis: A central role for thrombomodulin and activated protein C. *Crit Care Med* 29(suppl 7):S62, discussion S67, 2001.

261. Maruyama I: Recombinant thrombomodulin and activated protein C in the treatment of disseminated intravascular coagulation. *Thromb Haemost* 82:718, 1999.

262. Nakashima M, Kanamaru M, Umemura K, Tsuruta K: Pharmacokinetics and safety of a novel recombinant soluble human thrombomodulin, ART-123, in healthy male volunteers. *J Clin Pharmacol* 38:40, 1998.

263. Creasey AA, Chang AC, Feigen L, et al: Tissue factor pathway inhibitor reduces mortality from Escherichia coli septic shock. *J Clin Invest* 91: 2850, 1993.

264. de Pont AC, Moons AH, de Jonge E, et al: Recombinant nematode anticoagulant protein c2, an inhibitor of tissue factor/factor VIIa, attenuates coagulation and the interleukin-10 response in human endotoxemia. *J Thromb Haemost* 2:65, 2004.

265. Naeye RL: Thrombotic state after a hemorrhagic diathesis, a possible complication of therapy with epsilon-aminocaproic acid. *Blood* 19:694, 1962.

266. Gralnick HR, Greipp P: Thrombosis with epsilon aminocaproic acid therapy. *Am J Clin Pathol* 56:151, 1971.

267. Norman KE, Cotter MJ, Stewart JB, et al: Combined anticoagulant and antiselectin treatments prevent lethal intravascular coagulation. *Blood* 101:921, 2003.

268. Asakura H, Ichino T, Yoshida T, et al: Beneficial effect of JTV-803, a new synthetic inhibitor of activated factor X, against both lipopolysaccharide-induced and tissue factor-induced disseminated intravascular coagulation in rat models. *Blood Coagul Fibrinolysis* 13:233, 2002.

269. Lee SY, Chang SK, Lee IH, et al: Depletion of plasma factor XIII prevents disseminated intravascular coagulation-induced organ damage. *Thromb Haemost* 85:464, 2001.

270. Szabo G, Barabas E, Kedves R, et al: Effect of some new thioglycosides on endotoxin-induced disseminated intravascular coagulation in rabbits. *Thromb Res* 107:357, 2002.

271. Moscardo F, Perez F, de la Rubia J, et al: Successful treatment of severe intra-abdominal bleeding associated with disseminated intravascular coagulation using recombinant activated factor VII. *Br J Haematol* 114: 174, 2001.

272. Zupancic Salek S, Sokolic V, Viskovic T, et al: Successful use of recombinant factor VIIa for massive bleeding after caesarean section due to HELLP syndrome. *Acta Haematol* 108:162, 2002.

HEREDITARY THROMBOPHILIA

URI SELIGSOHN
JOHN H. GRIFFIN

Thrombophilia **is defined as a genetically determined increased likelihood of thrombosis.** *Thromboembolism* **is a multicausal disease involving one or more genetic defects in conjunction with acquired risk factors such as trauma, immobility, malignancy, inflammation, pregnancy, oral contraceptive use, or autoimmune disease. The two most common hereditary defects in Caucasians (found in a substantial proportion of patients presenting with venous thrombosis) include activated protein C resistance caused by replacement of Arg506 by Gln in the factor V gene (factor V Leiden) and a prothrombin single nucleotide polymorphism (G20210A) that causes elevated plasma prothrombin levels. Also common are hyperhomocysteinemia and increased plasma levels of factor VIII that can result from identified and unidentified genetic defects or from acquired conditions. Less common genetic abnormalities include deficiencies of the anticoagulant proteins, protein C, protein S, or antithrombin. The majority of these thrombophilic defects either enhance procoagulant reactions or hamper anticoagulant mechanisms, thus causing a prothrombotic state resulting from hypercoagulability of the blood. Venous thrombosis is the most common manifestation of thrombophilia, although a minority of patients, particularly those with other vascular risk factors, also develop arterial thrombosis. Less usual presentations include visceral or cerebral vein thrombosis, second- or third-trimester pregnancy loss, placental abruption, or severe preeclampsia. Laboratory assays are widely available to identify the majority of patients with thrombophilia. Knowledge of these disorders affects patient management, including the duration of anticoagulant treatment, the need for prophylactic antithrombotic agents, and counseling involving the relative risks of pregnancy and use of oral contraceptives or hormone replacement.**

DEFINITION AND HISTORY

Hereditary thrombophilia hereinafter termed *thrombophilia* is defined as a genetically determined increased risk of thrombosis. Table 122-1 lists the major genetic defects associated with venous thrombosis and the predisposing risk factors. Interaction among the genetic defects and the acquired predisposing factors is the common cause of venous thrombosis (Figure 122-1).

The first description of thrombophilia caused by a hereditary deficiency of an anticoagulant protein was by Egeberg[1] in 1965. Mem-

bers of the family described in the report suffered from recurrent venous thrombosis, and the disorder was inherited in an autosomal dominant pattern. The plasma of affected family members had reduced amounts of antithrombin III, an inhibitor to thrombin, which at present is termed *antithrombin*. Another thrombophilia, hereditary dysfibrinogenemia, was described by Beck and coworkers[2] in the same year. In 1976, Stenflo and coworkers[3] purified and characterized an anticoagulant factor from bovine plasma that was designated *protein C* because it was in the third peak on a chromatogram. Subsequently, the first patients with heterozygous protein C deficiency (approximately 50% of normal plasma level) and venous thrombosis in young adults were described by Griffin and colleagues.[4] Three years later, protein S deficiency was reported in several families with thrombosis by Schwarz and coworkers[5] and Comp and coworkers.[6,7] Initial searches for deficiencies of antithrombin, protein C, and protein S in patients with idiopathic venous thrombosis were disappointing because only 5 to 20 percent of such patients had one of these inherited disorders.[8] This situation changed dramatically in 1993 when Dahlback and coworkers reported that venous thrombosis often is associated with hereditary resistance to activated protein C (APC).[9,10] In 1994, three laboratories reported that the underlying genetic defect for most patients with APC resistance (APCR) involved the factor V mutation of Arg506 to Gln, a defect now referred to as *factor V Leiden*.[11–13] At about the same time, mild to moderate hyperhomocysteinemia was recognized as a risk factor for venous thrombosis,[14] although a predisposition to arterial vascular disease because of elevated homocysteine levels had been known since 1969.[15] In 1996, a single nucleotide polymorphism in the 3′-untranslated region of prothrombin (G20210A) was identified and linked to familial venous thromboembolism by Poort and colleagues.[16] Subsequently, elevated levels of factor VIII were defined as another risk factor for venous thrombosis that is clustered in families, but to date no causal genetic factor has been discerned.[17–19]

Specific thrombophilic risk factors can be identified in approximately 70 percent of patients presenting with an unprovoked first or recurrent episode of venous thromboembolism.[20–22] Patients with venous thrombosis may have more than one hereditary thrombophilia[22]

TABLE 122-1   THROMBOPHILIAS AND PREDISPOSING RISK FACTORS FOR VENOUS THROMBOEMBOLISM

THROMBOPHILIAS	PREDISPOSING RISK FACTORS FOR VENOUS THROMBOSIS
Common	
Factor V Leiden	Surgery or trauma
Prothrombin G20210A	Prolonged immobilization
Increased factor VIII level*	Increasing age
Homozygous C677T polymorphism in methylene tetrahydrofolate reductase†	Malignant neoplasms
Rare	Myeloproliferative diseases
Protein C deficiency	Superficial vein thrombosis
Protein S deficiency	Previous venous thrombosis
Antithrombin deficiency	Pregnancy and puerperium
Very rare	Use of female hormones
Dysfibrinogenemia	Antiphospholipid antibodies
Homozygous homocystinuria	Hyperhomocysteinemia
	Activated protein C resistance unrelated to a factor V mutation
	Varicose veins

* Heritability is inferred. No gene alteration has been discerned.
† Weak thrombophilia associated with hyperhomocysteinemia in patients with deficiencies of folic acid or vitamin B$_{12}$.

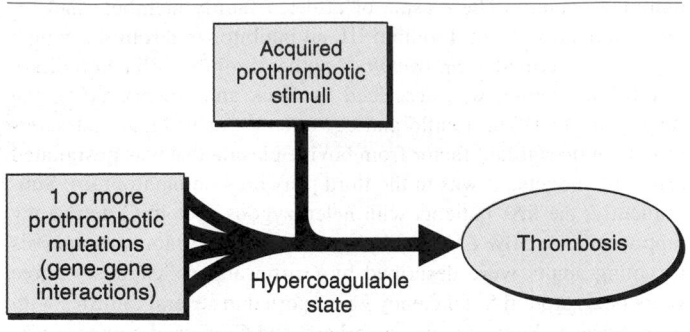

FIGURE 122-1   Paradigm for genetic contribution to venous thrombosis. Clinically significant venous thrombosis most often follows from the simultaneous presence of an acquired risk factor for thrombosis and one or more genetic factors that convey thrombotic risk. The presence of two genetic factors (i.e., gene–gene interaction) greatly increases the likelihood of thrombosis. Mild genetic risk factors include activated protein C resistance with or without factor V Leiden; the prothrombin G20210A polymorphism causing elevated plasma prothrombin levels; and heterozygous deficiency of protein C, protein S, or antithrombin. Hyperhomocysteinemia is a mild risk factor. Elevated levels (>150% of normal) of various coagulation factors, including factors VIII, XI, and IX and fibrinogen, also appear to be mild risk factors for venous thrombosis. Venous thrombosis patients frequently have two or more genetic risk factors. (From AI Schafer,[454] with permission.)

associated with acquired abnormalities, such as antiphospholipid antibodies, malignancy, myeloproliferative diseases, or inflammatory disorders (see Table 122-1). Currently known thrombophilias usually are not associated with arterial thrombosis. However, in association with other risk factors such as smoking or diabetes, up to 10 percent of arterial thromboses are associated with thrombophilia.[23–25]

PATHOGENESIS

Thrombosis often is associated with defects in normal, physiologic hemostatic mechanisms that are essential to avoid bleeding. Pathogenesis of thrombosis, according to Virchow's classic triad, involves abnormalities in the vessel wall, blood flow (i.e., stasis) and/or changes in the blood components. Risk of venous thrombosis is amplified by both the number and the nature of risk factors present in a given subject, whether genetic or acquired (see Figure 122-1). Identification of defects in specific blood components, especially plasma factors, thus far has provided most of the molecular insights into the pathogenesis of thrombophilia, whereas abnormalities in the vessel wall or in blood flow appear to constitute acquired risk factors for venous thrombosis.[26] Figure 122-2 presents the major mechanisms of the normal control of coagulation and inherited thrombophilias. Control of coagulation is achieved by the protein C pathway and antithrombin. In the protein C pathway, thrombin bound to thrombomodulin activates protein C, which in turn inactivates activated factor V and factor VIII in the presence of protein S, thereby down-regulating the generation of thrombin. The neutralization of thrombin is achieved by antithrombin bound to heparan sulfate. In the inherited thrombophilias, a deficiency of antithrombin, protein C, or protein S, aberrant activity of factor V, or increased activity of prothrombin results in decreased neutralization of thrombin or increased generation of thrombin. The two most commonly identifiable genetic defects contributing to thrombophilia involve plasma factors, namely, APC-resistant factor V Leiden and elevated prothrombin levels caused by the prothrombin G20210A polymorphism. Elevated factor VIII levels are associated with increased risk of venous thrombosis and of its recurrence. Although the genetic causes are unknown for elevated levels of other clotting factors (XI and IX), such elevations mildly amplify the risk. Overall, these coagulation factor abnormalities cause an imbalance between the procoagulant and anticoagulant forces in blood with potential mechanistic

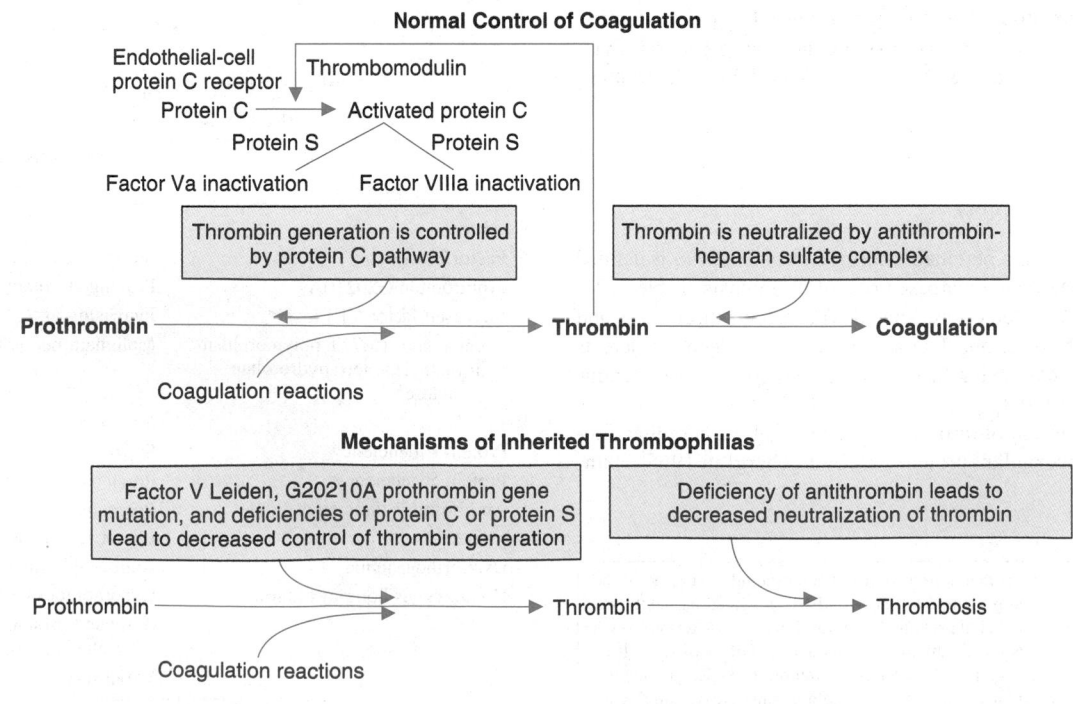

FIGURE 122-2   Major mechanisms involved in the normal control of coagulation and inherited thrombophilias. (From U Seligsohn and A Lubetsky,[39] with permission.)

contributions to thrombosis. Other plasma protein defects contribute to decreased fibrinolytic potential that is caused by either defective molecules (e.g., dysfibrinogenemia, dysplasminogenemia) or abnormal levels of normal molecules (e.g., thrombin-activatable fibrinolysis inhibitor [TAFI]) (see Chap. 127).

Venous thrombosis and markers of hypercoagulability each is estimated to manifest approximately 30 to 60 percent heritability,[27–29] where the term *heritability* indicates the relative contributions of heredity versus contributions of environment. Although thrombophilic risk factors are discernible in the majority of patients with unprovoked thrombosis, these risk factors are relatively mild and probably are enhanced by additional risk factors. For example, venous function exhibits from 30 to 60 percent heritability,[30] suggesting that thrombophilic risk factors can be identified that directly affect endothelium or vessel wall defects that contribute to the pathogenesis of venous thrombosis.

Males are at greater risk for venous thrombosis than are females. For example, male gender is associated with a higher risk of recurrent venous thromboembolism[31] for reasons that presently are unclear. Male gender is well known as a risk factor for arterial atherothrombosis, and, intriguingly, atherosclerosis is associated with venous thrombosis.[32] An association between dyslipoproteinemia and venous thrombosis has been described in males (see below "Other Potential Thrombophilic Disorders").

Tissue factor-bearing microparticles in blood play essential roles in experimental thrombogenesis in animal models,[33,34] and cellular microparticles appear to provide novel mechanisms for cell–cell signaling and communications. This finding suggests that genetically determined cellular processes that regulate the life cycle of prothrombotic (or antithrombotic) microparticles derived from cells of the endothelium and/or bloodborne cells, such as leukocytes or platelets, eventually can be identified as significant thrombophilic factors.

Inflammation contributes to thrombogenesis through various mechanisms, some of which may prove to be genetic and eventually identified as significant thrombophilic factors.[35–38] For example, elevated levels of C reactive protein and of certain cytokines, such as interleukin-1 or interleukin-6, are associated with venous thrombosis, and these proinflammatory agents likely are influenced by genetic factors.

EPIDEMIOLOGY

The prevalences of factor V Leiden and prothrombin G20210A vary substantially in human populations. Factor V Leiden and prothrombin G20210A are exceedingly rare in Africans and Orientals, whereas the mean prevalence of heterozygotes in healthy Caucasians is 4.8 and 2.7 percent, respectively (Table 122-2).[39] A particularly high prevalence of heterozygous factor V Leiden (11%–14%) was reported in Southern Sweden and in Arabs.[22,40] Founder effects were demonstrated for both factor V Leiden and prothrombin G20210A, suggesting that they occurred after the evolutionary separation of non-Africans from Africans and after the divergence of Caucasians and Orientals.[41,42] The relatively high prevalence of factor V Leiden in Caucasians has been attributed to potential evolutionary advantages, such as decreased bleeding during labor[43] and menstruation,[44] amelioration of acquired and inherited bleeding tendencies,[45,46] and better survival in sepsis.[47]

TABLE 122-2 FREQUENCY OF THROMBOPHILIAS IN HEALTHY SUBJECTS AND UNSELECTED AND SELECTED PATIENTS WITH VENOUS THROMBOSIS*

THROMBOPHILIA	HEALTHY SUBJECTS		UNSELECTED PATIENTS		SELECTED PATIENTS	
	N	PERCENT AFFECTED	N	PERCENT AFFECTED	N	PERCENT AFFECTED
Factor V Leiden	16,150†	4.8	1,142	18.8	162	40
	2,192‡	0.05				
Prothrombin G20210A	11,932†	2.7	2,884	7.1	551	16
	1,811‡	0.06				
Protein C deficiency	15,070	0.2–0.4	2,008	3.7	767	4.8
Protein S deficiency	3,788	0.16–0.21	2,008	2.3	649	4.3
Antithrombin deficiency	9,669	0.02	2,008	1.9	649	4.3

* Adapted from ref. 39 and 48.
† Caucasians.
‡ Africans and Asians.

The frequency of thrombophilias is significantly higher in unselected patients with unprovoked venous thrombosis than in healthy subjects (see Table 122-2).[39,48] A further twofold increase in the frequency of thrombophilia is demonstrable in selected patients with venous thrombosis who are likely, on clinical grounds, to have thrombophilia.

Because factor V Leiden and prothrombin G20210A are relatively common, their coinheritance[49] or inheritance with deficiencies of protein C, protein S, or antithrombin[50–53] is not rare. Studies of family members affected by two thrombophilic factors have shown an accentuated risk of venous thrombosis.[49–53] Thrombophilia also interacts with common acquired causes of venous thrombosis, such as hyperhomocysteinemia, use of female hormones, and antiphospholipid antibodies to increase the risk.

MAJOR HEREDITARY DEFECTS

HEREDITARY RESISTANCE TO ACTIVATED PROTEIN C

BIOCHEMISTRY AND MOLECULAR FEATURES

The term *APCR* is defined as an abnormally reduced anticoagulant response of a subject's plasma to APC based on *in vitro* testing. A "normal" range for response to APC is established for the various coagulation or other related assay conditions used to assess response to APC.[9,54,55]

Theoretically, any genetic abnormality of a protein C pathway component that interferes with the expression of APC activity can cause APCR, as could acquired abnormalities such as antibodies against protein C pathway components.[56,57] Although the causes of many cases of acquired APCR are unknown, the majority (>90%) of hereditary APCR subjects have the same genetic abnormality, factor V Leiden with a G1691A alteration causing Arg506Gln substitution. This gene alteration arose in a single Caucasian founder approximately 21,000 to 34,000 years ago.[41] The molecular mechanism for APCR in such probands involves resistance of Gln506-factor Va to proteolytic inactivation by APC,[11,58,59] with kinetic studies showing that the Gln506-variant is inactivated 10 times slower than normal Arg506-factor Va.[59,60] Gln506-factor Va, whether activated by thrombin or factor Xa, is partially but not entirely resistant to APC, implying that inactivation of Gln506-factor Va by APC can occur *in vivo*, albeit at a reduced rate. Explanation for only a partial resistance to APC derives from the fact that cleavage of factor Va by APC at Arg306 also occurs, causing complete loss of factor Va activity, although this cleavage is slower than that at the Arg506 site.[59,61] This finding helps explain why APCR resulting from Gln506-factor V is a rather mild risk factor for venous thrombosis and why a combination of genetic risk factors or a combination of a genetic risk factor and acquired risk factors for venous thrombosis is found in a significant fraction of symptomatic patients (see Figure 122-1).

Additional molecular defects contribute to thrombosis in hereditary APCR. In purified clotting factor reaction mixtures, factor V enhances inactivation of factor VIIIa by APC in the presence of protein S,[62] and APC-resistant subjects carrying factor V Leiden reportedly are defective in this APC cofactor activity.[63,64] This cofactor activity also is impaired in patients with venous thrombosis who are pseudo-homozygous for an Ile359Thr mutation in factor V with a null allele factor V-Glu119Stop.[65] APCR caused by rare factor V mutations that replace Arg306 by Thr[66] or Gly[67] has been reported, although the relationship to relative risks of thrombosis has not been established.[68] The reason why these mutated proteins may not confer a risk of thrombosis probably is related to their preserved APC cofactor activity toward factor VIIIa.[69] A factor V haplotype, designated R2, has been associated with mild APCR.[70] The molecular mechanisms and thrombotic risks associated with the R2 factor V haplotype that contains normal Arg506 remain to be defined, although the R2 haplotype appears to be only a risk factor when present with the Gln506-factor V allele.[71]

APC is a normal component of blood that contributes to antithrombotic surveillance mechanisms and prevents thrombosis (see Chap. 107).[72] Normal subjects have a mean APC concentration of 2.3 ng/ml (38 pM) in the circulation,[73] and the in vivo half-life of APC in normal adult human subjects and in freshly drawn whole blood is approximately 22 minutes.[74,75] Thus, the protein C pathway undergoes continuous activation in vivo. In normal subjects, an inverse relationship exists between levels of circulating APC and thrombin.[76] One report suggests circulating APC deficiency is associated with venous thrombosis.[77] APC levels are increased when thrombin is acutely generated, as occurs during disseminated intravascular coagulation, ischemia, or surgical procedures.

Because circulating APC has such a long half-life, it provides systemic anticoagulation to down-regulate thrombin generation and to limit extension of hemostatic plugs. Hence, genetic or acquired defects that impair the response to APC are understandably prothrombotic. Elevated plasma levels of prothrombin fragment F1+2 and thrombin–antithrombin complexes are found in many subjects heterozygous or homozygous for Gln506-factor V,[78–81] presumably reflecting impairment of the expression of APC's anticoagulant activity.

CLINICAL FEATURES

Deep and superficial venous thromboses are the most common manifestations of this disorder, whereas primary pulmonary embolism appears to be relatively less frequent than in subjects with deficiencies in antithrombin, protein C, or protein S.[82–84] In patients with post-thrombotic and nonpostthrombotic venous leg ulcers, 38 and 16 percent, respectively, had factor V Leiden.[85,86] Cerebral, hepatic, portal, and upper extremity venous thromboses have been reported in patients with factor V Leiden.[87,88] About half of venous thrombosis patients with factor V Leiden will have unprovoked venous thromboembolism, with 20 percent occurring after surgery and 30 percent in women who are pregnant or taking birth control pills.[89] Pregnancy loss and other obstetric complications occur at an increased rate in women with factor V Leiden (see "Hereditary Thrombophilias During Pregnancy And Puerperium").

The risk of venous thrombosis in subjects with factor V Leiden is somewhat lower than in patients from families with deficiencies of antithrombin or protein C.[90,91] Nonetheless, because factor V Leiden

is so common among known thrombophilic factors, it accounts for the largest proportion of patients presenting with a first thromboembolic event (20%– 25%).[92] The relative risk of deep and superficial vein thrombosis in patients heterozygous for factor V Leiden is increased by fourfold to eightfold[93–95] and fourfold, respectively,[96] although lower risks have been reported.[97] The risk of idiopathic venous thromboembolism for men increases with age, from a relative risk of 1.2 at age 40 to 50 years to 6 for those 70 years and older.[93] First-degree relatives of symptomatic carriers of the factor V mutation develop thromboses at a mean rate of 0.45 percent per year (0.25% per year in the 15- to 30-year age group, and 1.1% per year in those older than 60 years).[89,91]

Homozygotes for factor V Leiden have an odds ratio (OR) for venous thrombosis of 50 to 100, and it is estimated that approximately half of such individuals will experience a clinically significant episode during their lives.[98] Although thrombosis in homozygotes is substantially more common than in heterozygotes, the disorder is far less severe than in subjects with homozygous deficiency of protein C, or protein S, consistent with the emerging paradigm for a physiologic cellular protein C pathway (see Chap. 107). Despite the increased thrombotic risk, the presence of factor V Leiden does not increase overall mortality.[99–102]

Coronary artery thrombosis has been notably associated with the factor V Leiden mutation in young women[23] and men[25] also displaying other vascular risk factors. The relative risk of myocardial infarction in carriers of V Leiden from the Netherlands was 1.4, which increased to threefold to sixfold if other risk factors, such as obesity, smoking, hypertension, or diabetes, were present.[103] However, another large study of men who survived a first myocardial infarction that occurred when they were younger than 45 years failed to find an association with factor V Leiden.[104] Although prothrombin G20210A is associated with peripheral arterial disease, this is not the case for factor V Leiden.[105] In children, factor V Leiden is associated with cerebral infarction or venous thrombosis[106–108] and confers a relative risk of 2.6 for central venous catheter-related thrombosis.[109]

PREDISPOSING FACTORS FOR THROMBOSIS

Although isolated factor V Leiden is associated with a relatively mild hypercoagulable state, the risk of thrombosis is greatly magnified when other prothrombotic disorders also are present. These additional risk factors may be hereditary or acquired, for example, protein C deficiency, protein S deficiency, the prothrombin G20210A polymorphism, elevated levels of factor VIII (see "Elevated Factor VIII Levels"), acquired antiphospholipid antibodies, hyperhomocysteinemia, prolonged immobility, surgery, malignancy, or use of contraceptives or pregnancy[92] (see Table 122-2). In a study of 129 homozygotes for factor V Leiden, environmental risk factors were present in 81 percent of women and 29 percent of men during their first thrombotic episode.[110]

LABORATORY ASSAYS

Coagulation assays and DNA-based assays are available for the identification of patients with APCR. Plasma-based coagulation tests depend on the relative prolongation of the activated partial thromboplastin time (aPTT) or other coagulation screening tests caused by the addition of purified APC. Individuals with resistance to APC have less prolongation of the aPTT than normal. Although an aPTT assay using patient's plasma originally was used, many current assays use factor V-deficient plasma,[58] which makes the test informative for most patients with lupus anticoagulant, pregnant patients, patients with inflammatory states, and patients on oral anticoagulants. The test is sensitive and specific compared with the genetic test for factor V Leiden.[111] An abnormally low APCR is associated with venous thrombosis, in both the presence and absence of the factor V Leiden mutation[112,113] and with ischemic stroke.[114,115] Thus, there is clinically relevant information obtained from the classic aPTT-based APCR test using patient's plasma that is not obtained using factor V-deficient substrate plasma. Tissue factor-based APCR assays can provide additional information about plasma components that differentially modulate the protein C pathway,[116–118] such as "anticoagulant" high-density lipoprotein or glucosylceramide and possibly as yet unidentified factors that are altered by oral contraceptive usage. The presence of platelets or platelet microparticles in plasma tested for APCR using aPTT assays,[119–121] and autoantibodies against APC,[57] can reduce the anticoagulant response to APC, indicating the need to carefully prepare plasma prior to testing.

Many DNA-based assays for the factor V Leiden polymorphism are available. Genomic DNA is isolated, amplified by polymerase chain reaction (PCR), subjected to restriction fragment length polymorphism analysis, and analyzed for G or A at nucleotide 1691.[11] Plasma coagulation tests are often used for screening patients, followed by confirmation of positive results with the DNA assay. Only DNA tests clearly distinguish factor V Leiden heterozygosity from homozygosity. "Pseudohomozygotes" who are heterozygous for factor V Leiden and for a dysfunctional factor V allele have very low APC resistance ratios in the plasma test but are heterozygous by the DNA assay for factor V Leiden.[122]

PROTHROMBIN G20210A GENE ALTERATION

BIOCHEMISTRY AND MOLECULAR FEATURES

Replacement of G by A at nt 20210 in the 3'-untranslated region of the prothrombin gene augments translation and stability of prothrombin mRNA.[123] This process results in elevated synthesis and secretion of prothrombin by the liver. The elevated level of plasma prothrombin with a mean of 132 percent of normal in heterozygotes[16] may contribute directly to increased thrombotic risk by causing increased thrombin generation[124] or decreased fibrinolytic activity because of enhanced activation of TAFI.[125] Another basis for prothrombotic action might derive from the ability of prothrombin to inhibit APC's inactivation of factor Va.[126]

CLINICAL FEATURES

The prothrombin gene mutation is found largely in Caucasian populations.[42] In contrast to factor V Leiden, the frequency of the mutation seems to increase from northern Europe to southern Europe, that is, only 1.7 percent of the population in northern Europe has the abnormality compared with 3 to 5 percent in southern Europe and the Middle East.[127,128] The prothrombin gene mutation is associated with venous thrombosis in all age groups.[129] When sequential patients presenting with a first venous thromboembolism are analyzed, 4 to 8 percent have the mutation, and the relative risk of thrombosis in subjects with prothrombin 20210A is increased approximately twofold to 5.5-fold.[16,20,130–135] For patients with superficial vein thrombosis, an OR of 4.3 (95% confidence interval 1.5–12.6) was reported.[96]

As in other forms of hereditary thrombophilia, the prothrombin gene mutation has been found in patients with thrombosis in unusual sites, particularly hepatic, portal, and cerebral sinus vein thrombosis.[88,136–141] For example, in a study of 40 patients with cerebral vein thrombosis, 20 percent had the gene defect (OR 10.2). Many of these thromboses were in young women taking oral contraceptives, which raises the likelihood of thrombosis even higher (i.e., OR 150).[138]

Individuals who are homozygous for the prothrombin gene mutation appear more likely than heterozygotes to develop thrombosis.[142–144]

The prothrombin gene mutation appears generally not to be overrepresented in unselected patients with cerebral vascular or coronary artery disease.[145–149] However, certain selected groups of patients with arterial thrombosis have an increased likelihood of carrying the mutation.[103,105,131,143,150–152] A meta-analysis of studies of patients with documented arterial events disclosed only a modest association with prothrombin G20210A, but when the analysis was limited to patients younger than 55 years, the association was more robust (OR 1.66; 95% confidence interval 1.13–2.46).[153]

Notably, a large proportion of a group of young women with acute unexplained spinal cord infarction had the mutation.[154] All were taking oral contraceptives, and most were smokers.

LABORATORY FEATURES

Identification of the mutation in the 3'-untranslated region of the prothrombin gene requires DNA analysis following PCR amplification of the pertinent region.[16] Although prothrombin levels are elevated, assay of prothrombin activity or prothrombin antigen usually is not sufficiently sensitive or specific for the presence of the mutation or as a more effective predictor of thrombosis.[155–157] Interestingly, when an A19911G polymorphism in the prothrombin gene is coinherited with G20210A, it increases the risk of venous thrombosis.[158]

HYPERHOMOCYSTEINEMIA

BIOCHEMISTRY AND MOLECULAR FEATURES

Homocysteine is an intermediate in the metabolism of the sulfur-containing amino acids methionine and cysteine and participates in several metabolic pathways. Remethylation of homocysteine to generate methionine requires the vitamin B_{12}-dependent enzyme methionine synthase and 5-methyltetrahydrofolate, which are part of a metabolic pathway that recycles tetrahydrofolate and 5-methyltetrahydrofolate and involves the enzyme methylenetetrahydrofolate reductase (MTHFR). For synthesis of cysteine from homocysteine, a transsulfuration pathway first involves condensation of homocysteine with serine to generate cystathionine by the vitamin B_6-dependent enzyme cystathionine β-synthase, then deamination and cleavage of cystathionine to yield cysteine and α-ketobutyrate are accomplished by the vitamin B_6-dependent enzyme cystathioninase.

A plasma homocysteine level above the normal range defines hyperhomocysteinemia.[159] Severe hyperhomocysteinemia (plasma levels >100 μmol/L), also identifiable as homocystinuria, occurs in approximately one in 200,000 to 300,000 individuals in the general population and is transmitted as an autosomal recessive trait. The most common causes for homocysteinuria are mutations in cystathionine β-synthase. Rarely, other mutations in 5,10-MTHFR, or methionine synthase give rise to homocystinuria. Such severe abnormalities are associated with neurologic abnormalities, mental retardation, ectopia lentis, premature cardiovascular disease, stroke, venous thrombosis, and arterial thrombosis.[159] The most common genetic cause of mild hyperhomocysteinemia involves an MTHFR gene polymorphism, nt C677T, which causes a conservative replacement of Ala222 by Val that results in a variant enzyme with reduced specific activity and increased thermolability. Homozygosity for TT at nt 677 occurs in 10 to 20 percent of healthy Caucasians and 10 percent of Orientals but is rare in Africans.[160] The MTHFR C677T polymorphism can be associated with mild hyperhomocysteinemia, particularly when plasma folate level is low.[161] A second polymorphism, ntA1298C, also can be associated with mild hyperhomocysteinemia. Suboptimal levels of folate or vitamin B_6 or B_{12} can contribute to acquired mild to moderate hyperhomocysteinemia by providing inadequate cofactor levels to support the enzymes that regulate homocysteine metabolism. Other causes for hyperhomocysteinemia are renal failure, hypothyroidism, smoking, excessive coffee consumption, inflammatory bowel disease, psoriasis, and rheumatoid arthritis.[162]

The exact mechanisms by which hyperhomocysteinemia causes increased risk of thrombosis have not been defined. Deleterious effects on the endothelium, enhanced smooth muscle proliferation, induction of tissue factor by monocytes, reduced cleavage of factor Va by APC, suppression of heparan sulfate synthesis, and down-regulation of thrombomodulin all have been described, but these effects were mainly based on *in vitro* studies that used homocysteine concentrations that exceeded the highest pathologic levels observed in homocystinuria.[162]

CLINICAL FEATURES

Retrospective case control studies have shown an association between hyperhomocysteinemia and venous thromboembolism. Two meta-analyses of these studies estimated similar pooled ORs of 2.5 (95% CI 1.8–3.5) and 3.0 (95% CI 2.1–4.2), respectively.[163,164] In a non-population-based prospective study of men, a significant association between increased homocysteine level (>95th percentile) and idiopathic venous thrombosis was found.[165] In contrast, a prospective nested case control study (longitudinal investigation of thromboembolism etiology) that included 303 cases and 635 controls demonstrated that the highest quintile of serum homocysteine level carried a nonstatistically significant adjusted OR of 1.55 (95% CI 0.91–2.6) compared to the lowest quintile.[166] Nevertheless, a significant association was observed when the analysis was limited to subjects 45 to 64 years old, with OR 2.05 (95% CI 1.1–3.8). Thus, whether or not hyperhomocysteinemia causes venous thrombosis requires further exploration. Cerebral vein thrombosis has been associated with hyperhomocysteinemia. In a large case control study involving 121 patients and 242 controls, the estimated risk conferred by hyperhomocysteinemia was represented by an OR of 19.5 (95% CI 5.7–67.3).[167]

Conflicting results have been reported regarding a possible association between homozygous MTHFR C677T and venous thrombosis. A meta-analysis of 31 studies comprising 4901 cases with venous thrombosis and 7886 controls revealed a borderline degree of risk with pooled OR 1.2 (95% CI 1.1–1.4), but after exclusion of cases with thrombophilias the estimated pooled OR was 1.5 (95% CI 1.2–1.9).[168]

Regarding cardiovascular disease, numerous retrospective case control studies have found a significant association with hyperhomocysteinemia after adjustment for confounding factors. For an increment of 5 μmol/L homocysteine in plasma, the ORs for coronary heart disease, cerebrovascular disease, and peripheral vascular disease were 1.5, 1.6, and 6.8, respectively.[169] Meta-analysis of 30 prospective or retrospective studies involving more than 5000 cases with ischemic heart disease and more than 1100 cases with stroke showed that a decrease of approximately 3 μmol/L in homocysteine level was associated with an 11 percent lower risk of ischemic heart disease and a 19 percent lower risk of stroke.[170] Also, an association, albeit modest, is observed between homozygosity for MTHFR C677T and cardiovascular disease. Meta-analysis of 40 case control studies involving more than 11,000 patients with coronary heart disease and more than 12,000 controls yielded an OR of 1.16 (95% CI 1.05–1.28) and, in the presence of a low folate status, an OR of 1.44 (95% CI 1.12–1.83).[171] Similar results were obtained in another meta-analysis that included patients with cerebrovascular and peripheral vascular diseases.[153] No increased risk was demonstrated in pooled data from North American study groups compared to European study groups. This difference was attributed to the lower intake of vitamin supplements and higher homocysteine levels for Europeans.[171]

LABORATORY FEATURES

Plasma homocysteine concentrations can be measured by high-pressure liquid chromatography or immunoassay. Both fasting levels and levels after methionine loading have been used to assess hyperhomocysteinemia.[172,173] Although the methionine loading test may detect

additional subjects with hyperhomocysteinemia,[174] relatively few centers have used the test because of practical difficulties involved.[162] Blood samples for homocysteine levels should be obtained in the fasting state, kept cold, and centrifuged immediately. Individual measurements reflect average homocysteine concentrations over time (e.g., 4 weeks) reasonably well.[175] Serum homocysteine levels are higher than plasma levels, and male values are higher than female values.[176]

The MTHFR C677T substitution creates a cleavage site for HinfI; thus, its detection is possible by PCR to amplify a flanking sequence and digestion by the restriction enzyme.[177] Mutations causing homozygous homocystinuria have mainly been identified in the cystathionine β-synthase gene with more than 130 mutations described.[178] Of these mutations, the T833C and G919A polymorphisms are prevalent and can be detected by relatively simple methods.[178,179] However, detection of these mutations is rarely needed because heterozygotes do not manifest hyperhomocysteinemia.

PROTEIN C DEFICIENCY

BIOCHEMISTRY AND MOLECULAR FEATURES

Protein C is one of the vitamin K-dependent proteins that is synthesized in the liver and circulates in plasma as a serine protease zymogen. Protein C is activated by limited proteolysis by thrombin bound to thrombomodulin, with additional acceleration by an endothelial protein C receptor (EPCR) (see Chap. 107).[180,181] APC is a potent anticoagulant enzyme that down-regulates the blood coagulation pathways by proteolytic and irreversible inactivation of factors Va and VIIIa with protein S serving as a cofactor in these reactions (see Figure 122-2). Thus, decreased levels of protein C zymogen may impair the natural inhibition of thrombin generation and contribute to hypercoagulability. Acting directly on cells, APC alters gene expression profiles, down-regulates inflammatory reactions, and inhibits p53-mediated apoptosis of ischemic human brain endothelium.[182] These protective direct effects of APC on endothelial cells require EPCR and protease activated receptor 1 (see Chap. 107).[182–184] This APC cellular pathway likely helps explain the success of APC in reducing mortality in patients with severe sepsis,[185] whereas antithrombin and tissue factor pathway inhibitor (TFPI), two other natural plasma anticoagulants, failed to do so.[186,187] Moreover, discovery of the cellular pathway and APC's pharmacologic success in severe sepsis imply that thrombosis in protein C deficiency arises, in part, because of a deficiency in APC cellular pathway activity.

More than 150 mutations in the protein C gene have been identified (see http://www.xs4all.nl/%7Ereitsma/Prot_C_home.htm). Type I protein C deficiency is defined as a disorder with parallel reductions in plasma antigen and anticoagulant activity levels, whereas type II deficiency, associated with circulating dysfunctional molecules, involves normal plasma levels of antigen but low levels of anticoagulant activity.

CLINICAL FEATURES

Heterozygous protein C deficiency occurs in 0.2 to 0.4 percent of normal individuals[188,189] and is found in approximately 4 to 5 percent of consecutive outpatients with objectively confirmed deep venous thrombosis.[190] Deficiency of protein C is linked to thrombosis (OR 6.5–8).[90,190,191] The mean age of first thrombotic event has been reported to be similar (approximately 45 years) in patients with factor V Leiden and protein C deficiency.[192] Heterozygotes for protein C deficiency have a normal survival.[193]

Variability in clinical expression is a hallmark of the disorder. Subjects identified by screening large numbers of normal individuals (e.g., blood donors) in most instances have neither a personal nor a family history of thromboembolism.[188,189] The discrepancy in thrombosis rates between these surveys and studies of families who have striking thrombotic symptoms can be explained in part by the coinheritance of factor V Leiden or other thrombophilic loci.[194,195] Polymorphisms in the promotor region of the protein C gene resulting in lower levels of protein C in some of the families can be involved.[196]

Deep and superficial venous thromboses are the most common clinical presentations of protein C deficiency.[197–200] By age 45 years, up to 50 percent of heterozygous subjects in clinically affected families will have venous thromboembolism, and half of the episodes will be spontaneous.[201] Protein C deficiency has been linked to unusual sites of venous thrombosis, including the cerebral and mesenteric veins.[197,202] Arterial thrombosis seems to be uncommon, although ischemic stroke and other arterial occlusive events have been reported.[90,203]

Homozygous protein C deficiency with protein C levels of less than 1 percent of normal causes neonatal purpura fulminans and massive thrombosis in affected infants.[204,205] In a similar scenario, "warfarin skin necrosis" (large areas of thrombotic skin necrosis) appears over central areas of the body (breast, abdomen, genitalia) in subjects with heterozygous protein C deficiency given warfarin (see Color Plate XXV).[206] In such patients, the vitamin K antagonist rapidly induces a fall in protein C activity from approximately 50 percent of normal to very low levels because of the short half-life of protein C (approximately 8 hours).[207,208] Because the half-lives of prothrombin, factor IX, and factor X are much longer, a transient hypercoagulable state may arise at the onset of vitamin K antagonist therapy.[208]

LABORATORY FEATURES

Most laboratories screen for protein C deficiency with a protein C activity assay that uses a highly specific snake venom protease to activate protein C.[209,210] Protein C activity is best assessed with an assay that uses a coagulation rather than a chromogenic end point to identify the greatest number of patients with protein C deficiency.[211] Immunoassays are used to distinguish type I defects (reduced antigen and activity) from type II disorders (normal antigen, reduced activity).[212] Normal ranges for protein C increase with age (4% per decade), so results must be interpreted against these age-specific norms.[209] Protein C gene promotor polymorphisms influence plasma concentrations of the protein, which can vary from 94 to 106 percent,[196,213] and liver disease or use of oral contraceptives can lower or raise protein C levels, respectively (Table 122-3).[214] Consequently, protein C levels of less than 55 percent of normal (in the absence of oral anticoagulant therapy, vitamin K deficiency, or overt liver disease) suggest protein C deficiency, but levels from 55 to 70 percent must be considered borderline, and repeated testing or family studies should be undertaken.[211] Use of DNA-based assays to identify patients with hereditary protein C deficiency is impractical because of the numerous mutations that have been described.

The diagnosis of hereditary protein C deficiency in patients receiving warfarin is particularly difficult. Protein C antigen levels can be compared with antigen levels for other vitamin K-dependent clotting factors, but only if careful control ranges are established for the ratios of protein C to two other vitamin K-dependent factors.[4,215] In most situations, a waiting period of at least 2 weeks after discontinuation of anticoagulant therapy is necessary for a reliable diagnosis. Warfarin should not be restarted before laboratory results are available in order to reduce the possibility of warfarin-induced skin necrosis in patients who are later found to have protein C deficiency. In cases of neonatal purpura fulminans, testing of parents can be useful.

PROTEIN S DEFICIENCY

BIOCHEMISTRY AND MOLECULAR FEATURES

Protein S is one of the vitamin K-dependent coagulation proteins but differs from them by not containing a serine protease domain. It enhances the anticoagulant activity of APC; hence, currently available functional assays of protein S measure APC cofactor activity using protein S-depleted plasma as substrate. Protein S is principally synthesized in the liver, but other organs may be important sites for its synthesis, including the endothelium, kidney, testes, and brain (see Chap. 107). Protein S reversibly associates with the plasma complement factor C4b-binding protein (C4BP), previously known as proline-rich lipoprotein. In normal plasma, approximately 60 percent of protein S is bound to C4BP and 40 percent is free. Importantly, only the free form of protein S functions as a cofactor for APC. Because protein S is a cofactor for APC, decreased levels of free protein S may impair the down-regulation of thrombin generation and contribute to hyper-

TABLE 122-3 ACQUIRED CONDITIONS THAT CAN YIELD ABNORMAL TEST RESULTS OF THROMBOPHILIA

TESTS*	ACQUIRED CONDITIONS THAT CAN CAUSE ABNORMAL TEST RESULTS
APCR (decreased ratio)	Pregnancy, use of oral contraceptives, stroke, presence of lupus anticoagulant,† increased factor VIII levels,† autoantibodies against activated protein C, use of oral anticoagulants†
Factor V Leiden	—
Prothrombin G20210A	—
Hyperhomocysteinemia	Deficiencies of folate, vitamin B$_{12}$, or vitamin B$_6$, old age, renal failure, excessive consumption of coffee, smoking
Increased factor VIII levels	Pregnancy, use of oral contraceptives, exercise, stress, older age, acute phase response, liver disease, hyperthyroidism
Presence of lupus anticoagulant	Systemic lupus erythematosus, antiphospholipid syndrome, autoimmune disease, liver disease, hyperthyroidism, healthy subjects
Increased titer of anticardiolipin antibody	Same as lupus anticoagulant, infectious diseases
Decreased level of protein C	Liver disease, use of oral anticoagulants, vitamin K deficiency, childhood, disseminated intravascular coagulation, presence of autoantibodies against protein C
Decreased level of free protein S	Liver disease, use of oral anticoagulants, vitamin K deficiency, pregnancy, use of oral contraceptives, nephrotic syndrome, childhood, presence of autoantibodies against protein S, disseminated intravascular coagulation
Decreased level of antithrombin	Use of heparin, thrombosis, disseminated intravascular coagulation, liver disease, nephrotic syndrome
Increased level of fibrinogen	Acute phase reaction, pregnancy, old age, atherosclerosis, smoking
Increased level of factor IX	—
Increased level of factor XI	—
Homozygous MTHFR C677T	—
Dysfibrinogenemia	Neonates, liver disease

* Tests are listed in a decreasing order of priority.
† Normal ratios are expected when activated protein C resistance (APCR) is measured in samples diluted with factor V–depleted plasma.

coagulability (see Figure 122-2). Protein S also exhibits anticoagulant activity that is independent of APC by directly binding to and inhibiting factors Va, VIIIa, and Xa, suggesting that deficiency of protein S also contributes to hypercoagulability by failing to inhibit these factors (see Chap. 107). Protein S also has cytoprotective, antiapoptotic activity *in vitro* and *in vivo* in murine ischemic stroke models (see Chap. 107).

Three types of protein S deficiency have been characterized. Type I protein S deficiency is defined as parallel reductions in both antigen and anticoagulant activity levels in plasma. Type II deficiency, which is associated with circulating dysfunctional molecules, involves normal plasma levels of free protein S antigen but low levels of anticoagulant activity. Type III deficiency involves low free protein S level while total protein S antigen usually is in the low to normal range. More than 150 mutations causing protein S deficiency have been described (http://archive.uwcm.ac.uk/uwcm/mg/hgmd/search.html).[216]

CLINICAL FEATURES

In several studies, approximately 2 to 3 percent of unselected outpatients presenting with venous thromboembolism had low levels of protein S (see Table 122-2).[190,217,218] A higher prevalence is seen in patients younger than 50 years and in patients with a personal or family history of venous thrombosis. The OR for thrombosis in patients with free protein S deficiency has been variably reported as 1.6,[190] 2.4,[217] 8.5,[90] and 11.5[219] Deep venous thrombosis and pulmonary embolism are the most common forms of thrombosis associated with protein S deficiency, although superficial vein thrombophlebitis and thrombosis in unusual sites also occur.[197–199] As in other forms of thrombophilia, approximately 50 percent of thromboses are unprovoked.[198] Arterial thrombosis has been reported in a significant number of protein S-deficient patients, particularly in those who smoke or have other thrombotic risk factors.[24,220,221] Neonatal purpura fulminans has been reported in two rare patients with homozygous or compound heterozygous protein S deficiency having very low levels of protein S.[222–224] Warfarin-induced skin necrosis has been reported in association with protein S deficiency.[225]

Analysis of four prospective studies showed that the incidence of venous thromboembolism in asymptomatic protein S-deficient relatives of symptomatic probands was 0.7 to 2.2 percent per year. About half of these events occurred during well-known risk periods, but incidence rates were decreased by prophylactic use of oral anticoagulants.[226]

LABORATORY FEATURES

Laboratory assays of plasma protein S must be chosen and interpreted with care because the protein circulates both free and bound to C4BP. Moreover, normal ranges differ for males compared with females, depend on age, and can be reduced in a variety of conditions (see below). Free protein S antigen and APC cofactor anticoagulant activity are better parameters than total protein S antigen in screening for hereditary protein S deficiency.[190,227] Free protein S antigen can be assayed using monoclonal antibodies specific for free protein S.[228,229] Protein S activity assays may be affected by coexisting APCR, although the second-generation assays in which factor V-deficient plasma is used as substrate have improved specificity.[230–232] Assessment of total and free protein S plus protein S activity should allow classification of patients with protein S defects into types I, II, or III. Type I and type III deficiencies may be phenotypic variants of the same disease given the finding that, within families, different individuals carrying the same DNA mutation in the protein S gene can present with laboratory findings indicating either type I or type III deficiency.[227] Type II deficiency, that is, normal free protein S antigen with reduced protein S activity, is uncommon,[211] so screening patients with free protein S

antigen levels is clinically reasonable. In normal subjects, an excellent correlation is seen between free protein S antigen and anticoagulant activity. The lower limit of the normal range for free protein S is lower in females than in males (55% vs. 65%).[233] Protein S is remarkably sensitive to hormonal status in females.

The high frequency of acquired protein S deficiency makes identification of hereditary defects more difficult. Oral contraceptives and hormone replacement therapy decrease plasma protein S levels. Reduced levels of free protein S are regularly found during pregnancy (e.g., as low as 20%–30% of normal),[234,235] in patients who are taking oral anticoagulants, and in patients with disseminated intravascular coagulation, liver disease, nephrotic syndrome, inflammatory conditions, and acute thromboembolism (see Table 122-3).[236–239] Protein S deficiency can occur in concert with the lupus anticoagulant[240,241] and as a result of autoantibodies to protein S following varicella or other infections in children.[242,243] Thus, these acquired conditions leading to low protein S levels should be excluded and tests repeated before making a diagnosis of hereditary thrombophilia. Family studies may be useful. Diagnosis of hereditary protein S deficiency using DNA techniques is not favored unless the defect has previously been established in the family because numerous different mutations in the protein S gene cause protein S deficiency.

ANTITHROMBIN DEFICIENCY

BIOCHEMISTRY AND MOLECULAR FEATURES

Antithrombin is a plasma protease inhibitor that neutralizes thrombin and factors Xa, IXa, and XIa by irreversibly forming 1:1 complexes in reactions accelerated by heparin or by heparan sulfate on endothelial surfaces (see Chap. 107). Therefore, defects in antithrombin compromise the normal inhibition of the coagulation pathways and cause a hypercoagulable state (see Figure 122-2). Antithrombin deficiency is classified into two major categories. Type I antithrombin deficiency is defined by low levels of both antigen and activity assayed in the absence or presence of heparin. Approximately 100 mutations causing type I deficiency have been described and include major deletion frameshifts and point mutations. Type II deficiency is defined by the presence of normal levels of antigen with defects that affect either the inhibitor's active center, which complexes with the target enzyme's active site, or the inhibitor's heparin binding site, which mediates heparin-dependent acceleration of antithrombin activity. Type II antithrombin deficiency is further subdivided into type IIa with mutations affecting the reactive site, type IIb involving mutations in the heparin binding site, and type IIc that includes a pleiotropic group of mutations. A database of more than 125 mutations in the antithrombin gene is available[244] (http://archive.uwcm.ac.uk/uwcm/mg/hgmd/search.html). Severe deficiency of antithrombin (<5% of normal) is rare, involves defects in heparin-dependent enhancement of antithrombin (type IIb), and is associated with severe venous and arterial thrombosis.[245–248] Type I antithrombin deficiency is found in 0.023 percent of normal individuals in Scotland, whereas type II defects, mostly observed in asymptomatic individuals, are more common and are found in 0.16 percent of people screened.[249]

CLINICAL FEATURES

Antithrombin deficiency is found in approximately 1 to 2 percent of consecutive unselected patients younger than 70 years with a first objectively documented venous thrombosis.[90–92] The frequency is higher in selected patients with venous thrombosis (see Table 122-2). The OR for thrombosis in patients with antithrombin deficiency is approximately 10 to 20, which is notably greater than in subjects heterozygous for factor V Leiden.[90,92,190,250] No evidence indicates differences in clinical severity between patients with heterozygous type I defects and those with type II mutations involving the thrombin binding site. Mortality rates are not increased in these patients.[251,252] Patients with type II mutations of the heparin binding site have few, if any, thrombotic episodes, although homozygous mutations affecting the heparin binding site are associated with thromboembolism.[253,254]

Venous thrombosis of the lower extremities, which occurs at an early age and peaks in the second decade of life, is the most common symptom in antithrombin deficiency.[253] Superficial venous thrombosis appears to be somewhat less common than in protein C or protein S deficiency or in APCR.[90,197,198] Thromboses in unusual sites, such as the mesenteric, hepatic, or cerebral veins, have been reported.[197,198,255] Arterial thrombosis occurs infrequently (approximately 1% of affected patients).[256,257] Almost 70 percent of patients present with the first thrombotic event before age 35 years and 85 percent before age 50 years.[253] Patients with severe antithrombin deficiency, that is, activity levels less than 5 percent, are rare, most likely because the profound deficiency state causes fetal loss *in utero*. A few infants with homozygous defects involving the heparin binding region of the molecule have survived, but most have suffered severe venous and arterial thrombosis.[245–248,254] No patients homozygous for reactive center defects have been identified, leading to the speculation that complete deficiency of antithrombin in humans is incompatible with life. Complete antithrombin deficiency in knockout mice results in death of the embryo.[258]

Resistance to the anticoagulant effects of heparin has been observed in some patients with antithrombin deficiency. Both acute thrombosis and several days of heparin therapy can decrease antithrombin levels, occasionally to as low as 50 percent of normal, which may lead to an erroneous diagnosis of hereditary antithrombin deficiency.[259,260] Other acquired conditions leading to low levels of antithrombin are common and include liver disease, disseminated intravascular coagulation, nephrotic syndrome, chemotherapy with asparaginase, and preeclampsia (see Table 122-3).[261–265]

Prospective studies of asymptomatic thrombophilic relatives of symptomatic probands with antithrombin deficiency demonstrated that the incidence of venous thrombosis (unprovoked or provoked by acquired risk factors) was 4 percent per year.[266] Collectively, the observations in patients with antithrombin deficiency indicate that, among the thrombophilias, this entity imparts the most severe clinical manifestations.

LABORATORY FEATURES

Antithrombin deficiency screening assays should first be performed in the presence of heparin because defects may involve either the reactive center of the inhibitor or the heparin binding site. If initial results are abnormal, then assays that measure the ability of the inhibitor to neutralize thrombin in the absence of heparin (progressive antithrombin activity) should be performed to characterize the abnormality. Antithrombin activity assays that use a chromogenic substrate are widely available.[266] Most laboratories now use factor Xa or bovine thrombin in their antithrombin assays to avoid the inhibitory effects of heparin cofactor II on human thrombin. The normal range for plasma antithrombin levels in healthy subjects is narrow (i.e., 84–116%).[267] Antithrombin antigen measurements are used to help distinguish type I from type II defects. Crossed immunoelectrophoresis using an antithrombin antibody in the presence and absence of heparin can help identify defects in the heparin binding portion of the molecule.

In general, patients with type I deficiency and many of those with type II disorders involving the thrombin binding site have antithrombin activity levels of 40 to 60 percent. Levels of 60 to 80 percent can be caused by other type II defects but frequently result from acquired antithrombin deficiency (see Table 122-3). If these confounding conditions are present, measurement of antithrombin level should be repeated and family studies performed if possible.

ELEVATED FACTOR VIII LEVELS

BIOCHEMISTRY AND MOLECULAR FEATURES

Increased factor VIII levels are commonly observed in association with increasing age and body mass index, pregnancy, surgery, chronic inflammation, liver disease, hyperthyroidism, diabetes mellitus, and exercise (see Table 122-3).[268] The ABO blood group system exerts a substantial effect on factor VIII level and von Willebrand factor level, with non-O subjects having significantly higher levels than subjects with blood group O. The mechanisms by which these conditions cause elevated factor VIII levels have not been elucidated, but augmented synthesis of factor VIII or down-regulation of low-density lipoprotein-related receptor protein, the liver protein that clears factor VIII from the circulation,[269] is possible. In the Leiden population-based case control study on venous thrombosis, increased factor VIII activity and antigen levels were defined as risk factors independent of all other causes of elevated factor VIII levels and other thrombophilias.[17,268] This observation was confirmed by other studies,[270,271] and the elevated factor VIII levels in patients with venous thrombosis were found to persist over time.[271] Clustering of increased factor VIII levels in families of patients with venous thrombosis suggests heritability,[18,19] but no gene alteration has been described. How elevated factor VIII levels increase the risk of thrombosis is unknown. The suggestion that increased factor VIII levels enhance thrombin generation[268] has been disputed.[272] It is possible that elevated levels of factor VIII increase the risk of venous thrombosis by diminishing the anticoagulant effect of APC, thereby causing acquired APC resistance.[268]

CLINICAL FEATURES

The clinical presentation of patients with venous thrombosis and elevated factor VIII levels does not differ from that of patients with other thrombophilias. The relative risk of venous thrombosis is correlated with the extent of increase in factor VIII level. Thus, subjects with factor VIII levels of 100 to 125 percent of normal have an OR of 2.3 (95% CI 1.3–3.8) and those with factor VIII levels of 150 percent of normal or higher have an OR of 4.8 (95% CI 2.3–10).[17] Interestingly, the prevalence of increased factor VIII levels (>150% of normal) in healthy controls of the Leiden study was 10 percent versus 25 percent in patients with a first event of venous thrombosis. This finding suggests that increased factor VIII level is one of the most frequent risk factors of venous thrombosis. Moreover, elevated factor VIII is significantly associated with recurrent venous thrombosis (see Recurrent Venous Thrombosis in Thrombophilias).

In a study of families of patients who had venous thrombosis and harbored factor V Leiden, the frequency of elevated factor VIII level among relatives was 33 percent.[273] Among relatives who did not carry factor V Leiden, those whose factor VIII levels were 150 percent or more of normal had an annual risk of venous thrombosis of 0.38 percent, whereas those who had levels less than 150 percent of normal had an incidence of only 0.13 percent per year.

LABORATORY FEATURES

Factor VIII activity is measured by a one-stage assay using factor VIII-depleted plasma and normal reference plasma. Assaying factor VIII antigen is not necessary because factor VIII antigen level correlates well with factor VIII activity, provided plasma is carefully separated and stored at −70°C. Factor VIII should not be assayed close to the time of the thrombotic event or when an acute phase reaction is predicted. An assay in more than one blood sample is advisable.

HIGH LEVELS OF OTHER COAGULATION FACTORS

Increased levels of other factors have been associated with an increased risk for venous thrombosis.[274] The Leiden population-based case control study revealed that in patients with factor IX levels greater than 129 percent of normal (90th percentile in controls), the OR for venous thrombosis was 2.3 (95% CI 1.6–3.5).[275] Adjustments for confounding factors and other hereditary thrombophilias showed that increased factor IX level was an independent risk factor. A "dose–response" relationship also was demonstrated, such that the higher the level, the higher the risk. The thrombotic risk was more pronounced in women than in men and was particularly high in premenopausal women not using oral contraceptives (OR 12.4; 95% CI 3.3–47.2) and in postmenopausal women (OR 6.2; 95% CI 2.4–15.9).

Similar observations were made regarding elevated levels of factor XI in the Leiden study.[276] The adjusted OR for venous thrombosis in patients with factor XI levels above the 90th percentile (121% of normal) compared to those who had factor XI levels at or below the 90th percentile was 2.2 (95% CI 1.5–3.2). Stratification of subjects according to factor XI levels disclosed an increase in the relative risk of thrombosis concordant with increasing factor XI levels.

Elevated levels of fibrinogen have been demonstrated to confer a risk of venous thrombosis in the Leiden study.[277] However, reanalysis of the data and adjustments for all possible confounding factors disclosed that the estimated risk was small and confined to subjects older than 45 years.[278]

Regarding possible effects of elevated levels of other coagulation factors (e.g., factors II, V, X, XII), no convincing evidence has been provided.[274]

HEREDITARY THROMBOTIC DYSFIBRINOGENEMIA

Dysfibrinogenemias are defined as qualitative defects in the fibrinogen molecule resulting from mutations in one of the genes encoding for one of the three polypeptide chains (see Chap. 117). The hereditary dysfibrinogenemias represent a heterogeneous group of abnormalities that are asymptomatic in 55 percent of cases. They cause thrombosis with or without bleeding in 20 percent of patients or a bleeding tendency in 25 percent of patients.[279]

BIOCHEMISTRY AND MOLECULAR FEATURES

For normal hemostasis, fibrin is formed after release of fibrinopeptides Aα and Bβ from fibrinogen because of proteolysis by thrombin and subsequent polymerization of fibrin monomers. Fibrin then is stabilized by covalent cross-links introduced by factor XIIIa. Plasmin-dependent proteolysis of fibrin, either to limit formation or growth of a thrombus or to clear fibrin in a timely and normal fashion during healing, is essential. Defects in fibrinogen that cause abnormal fibrinolysis can cause thrombosis, either because fibrin is not cleared in a normal fashion or because the growth of a normal hemostatic plug is not limited. Specific defects causing hypofibrinolysis can involve alterations of plasmin cleavage sites in fibrin or of sites that promote assembly of components of the fibrinolytic system, for example, binding sites for plasminogen or plasminogen activators (see Chap. 117). Numerous mutations causing structural defects in fibrinogen have been reported, most of which are point mutations that give rise to single amino acid substitutions. The mode of transmission of dysfibrinogenemias is autosomal dominant.

CLINICAL FEATURES

Venous thrombosis exhibited in approximately 20 percent of patients with hereditary dysfibrinogenemias usually occurs at a young age (27–32 years).[280] When a large number of patients presenting with venous thromboembolism were screened, dysfibrinogenemia was found in only 0.8 percent.[280] An occasional patient has both thrombosis and bleeding (usually postpartum hemorrhage). An increased rate of pregnancy-associated thrombosis, spontaneous abortion, and stillbirth have been described.

LABORATORY FEATURES

Prolongation of a dilute thrombin time and/or reptilase time because of delayed fibrin polymerization is common in patients with dysfibrinogenemia, as is a disparity between measurement of immunoreactive and clottable fibrinogen. More sophisticated testing often demonstrates abnormal fibrinogen structure or resistance of fibrin to fibrinolysis. Unfortunately, no assays are readily available that measure the key properties of fibrinogen likely to cause thrombosis in patients with dysfibrinogenemia, so this defect may be underdiagnosed.

HEREDITARY DEFECTS IN THE FIBRINOLYTIC SYSTEM

Associations between mutations or polymorphisms in the genes encoding for plasminogen and plasminogen-activator inhibitor (PAI)-1 and venous thrombosis are not firmly established.[281–284] Both types of plasminogen deficiency, hypoplasminogenemia (type I) and dysplasminogenemia (type II), have been described in patients with venous thrombosis (particularly in Japan), but other studies failed to determine that isolated plasminogen deficiency is a risk factor for venous thrombosis.[283] Severe plasminogen deficiency with levels of 5 to 6 percent of normal is a rare entity that is manifested by a pseudomembranous disease affecting mucous membranes, for example, the eyes (ligneous conjunctivitis), but surprisingly not by venous thrombosis.[285] Mild to moderate plasminogen deficiency was observed in 28 of 9611 blood donors (0.26 percent) in Scotland.[286] Further analysis of 19 of these subjects and family members (20 with hypoplasminogenemia and four with dysplasminogenemia) disclosed that only one subject who had venous thrombosis also was heterozygous for prothrombin G20210A.[283]

Increased levels of PAI-1, assumed to cause hypofibrinolysis, have been related to a 4G/5G insertion/deletion at nucleotide −675 of the gene promoter. Homozygotes for the 4G allele have 25 percent higher levels of PAI-1 than homozygotes for the 5G allele.[282] Several studies suggested that the 4G genotype was associated with an increased risk of venous thrombosis, but a prospective population-based study of 308 subjects with venous thrombosis and 640 controls failed to demonstrate a significant association.[284] Another study that focused on potential factors affecting recurrence of venous thrombosis failed to show an association between levels of PAI-1, tissue plasminogen activator, or euglobulin clot lysis time with recurrence.[287]

Increased levels of TAFI (above the 90th percentile in controls, i.e., >122 U/dl) have been associated with an increased risk of venous thrombosis (OR 1.7; 95% CI 1.1–2.5) in the Leiden study,[288] which indicates this parameter is a mild risk factor. Recurrent venous thrombosis has been associated with increased TAFI level (see "Recurrent Venous Thrombosis in Thrombophilias"). TAFI is activated by thrombin mostly after blood clots are formed and activated TAFI suppresses fibrinolysis by removing carboxy-terminal lysine residues from fibrin polymers that otherwise promote the binding of tissue plasminogen activator and plasminogen to fibrin. Several polymorphisms in the TAFI gene, many of which are in linkage disequilibrium, were shown to affect plasma TAFI level.[289] However, no association between TAFI polymorphisms and venous thrombosis has been reported.

Protein C inhibitor (PCI) is another protein that exhibits an antifibrinolytic effect by inhibiting tissue plasminogen activator and urokinase, albeit exerting (1) a profibrinolytic effect (inhibition of TAFI activation by thrombin–thrombomodulin complex); (2) an anticoagulant effect (inhibition of thrombin, factor Xa, and factor XIa); and (3) a procoagulant effect (inhibition of APC).[290]

In the Leiden study, PCI levels above the 95th percentile of controls (136% of normal) were associated with an increased relative risk of venous thrombosis with an OR of 1.6 (95% CI 0.9–2.8) compared to PCI levels below the 95th percentile.[291] No other studies on the role of PCI have been reported.

Taken together, of all components of the fibrinolytic system, only increased levels of TAFI and PCI constitute mild risk factors for venous thrombosis. At the present time, their measurement is performed only in specialized laboratories.

OTHER POTENTIAL THROMBOPHILIC DISORDERS

Thrombomodulin is an endothelial receptor that binds thrombin with very high affinity and promotes protein C activation.[180,292] Several mutations in the thrombomodulin gene have been discovered in families with thrombosis.[293–295] The gene alterations are scattered throughout the thrombomodulin gene, and some are associated with variable levels of soluble thrombomodulin in plasma,[294] reduced expression, and impaired function.[296] None of the mutations has been shown to be firmly associated with venous thrombosis. A population-based study demonstrated no difference in plasma levels of soluble thrombomodulin in patients with venous thrombosis and controls.[297]

EPCR is an endothelial transmembrane protein that promotes interaction between protein C and the thrombin–thrombomodulin complex (see Chap. 107). Changes in the endothelial EPCR have been suggested to be associated with an increased risk of venous thrombosis. A soluble form of EPCR lacking the transmembrane and intracellular domains is present in plasma of normal individuals over a broad range of concentrations (70–200 ng/ml), and the plasma level is strongly influenced by EPCR haplotype.[298–301] Soluble EPCR inhibits APC activity and fails to augment activation of protein C by thrombin–thrombomodulin complex. Hence, high levels of soluble EPCR have been suggested to promote thrombosis. Elevated concentrations of soluble EPCR have been observed in approximately 18 percent of healthy individuals bearing a relatively common haplotype.[299,301] In a study of 338 patients with venous thrombosis compared to controls, an A_3 haplotype constituted a risk factor with ORs of 2.5 (95% CI 1.4–4.5) in men but only 1.3 (95% CI 0.8–2.2) in women.[299] However, another study of a similar size did not confirm these findings.[300] Another gene alteration, a 23-bp insertion into exon 3 of the EPCR gene, has been suggested to confer a risk of venous thrombosis,[302,303] but another study failed to confirm this finding.[304]

A polymorphism in protease activated receptor 1, a receptor that mediates APC's cytoprotective effects on endothelial cells (see Chap. 107), is associated with thrombosis in males.[305]

Low levels of TFPI have also been implicated in the Leiden and other studies to constitute a weak risk factor of venous thrombosis.[306,307] Measuring plasma levels of TFPI poses several challenges. Circulating TFPI represents only 10 to 15 percent of the total TFPI in the intravascular space because most is bound to the endothelium. In plasma, some TFPI is lipoprotein associated, and this association can reduce TFPI functional activity.[308,309] Several polymorphisms in the TFPI gene have been described, but no firm association with venous thrombosis has been discerned. "TFPI resistance," presumably resulting from impaired inhibition of factors VIIa and Xa, reportedly was more prevalent in patients with venous thrombosis who had no other defects than in controls.[310,311] Tests of "TFPI resistance," such as APCR, measure the anticoagulant response of a test plasma to exogenously added TFPI in a prothrombin time performed with diluted tissue factor. Further studies are needed to confirm this finding and clarify the mechanism involved.

Other potential thrombophilias include various forms of dyslipidemia. Dyslipidemia and dyslipoproteinemia are well-recognized risk factors for arterial atherothrombosis. Accumulating evidence supports the concept that dyslipidemia is associated with venous thrombosis,[118,312–323] and the incidence of venous thrombosis is reduced by lipid-lowering drugs, such as statins.[321,322] In approximately 25 percent of venous thrombosis patients younger than 55 years, low levels of plasma glucosylceramide, a glycosphingolipid anticoagulant cofactor for APC, are found,[118] and young adult patients with venous thrombosis have low levels of high-density protein particles.[323] No clear genetic cause for the observed associations between venous thrombosis and dyslipidemia has been firmly established. Interestingly, spontaneous venous thrombosis is associated with clinically silent atherosclerotic vascular disease; thus, "atherosclerosis may induce venous thrombosis, or the two conditions may share common risk factors."[312] Because multiple genes control lipid and lipoprotein metabolism and determine the plasma levels of the various lipoprotein subclasses, these genes should be studied to identify genetic contributions to dyslipoproteinemia in venous thrombosis patients.

NEW METHODS FOR THROMBOPHILIA DISCOVERY

Discovery of thrombophilia risk factors is an important challenge for future genetic studies. Because of the strong evidence for a high degree of heredity in venous thrombosis and in causative hypercoagulability factors,[324–328] one would posit the existence of a significant number of common, mild genetic risk factors for venous thrombosis yet to be discovered. Most humans who are heterozygous for factor V Leiden will not experience a clinically significant episode of venous thrombosis in their lifetime. Moreover, even the combination of factor V Leiden with a single acquired risk factor, such as pregnancy, generally does not result in venous thrombosis. Consequently, in factor V Leiden subjects, other risk factors, whether genetic, acquired, or both, are prerequisite to increasing the sum of the contributions of multiple risk factors in a person's life at any given age and situation (e.g., trauma, malignancy, pregnancy, surgery) that result in a clinical episode of venous thrombosis (see Figure 122-1).[92] Hence, venous thrombosis is not just a multifactorial disease; it likely is a multigenic disease in many or even most patients. The goal of much future effort will be identifying common genetic risk factors for venous thrombosis and quantitating the amount of risk that such factors carry with the related goal of assessing gene–gene and gene–environment interactions (see "Interactions Between the Different Thrombophilias And Between Thrombophilia And Environmental Factors").

Methods for future discovery of thrombophilias will draw heavily on the human genome, which will initially provide the necessary platform from which to proceed to discover genotypes underlying venous thrombosis.[329] Studies will use both the candidate gene approach in which suspected genes are studied in great detail[330] and the quantitative trait loci (QTL) approach[331,332] in which traits or phenotypes are linked to sites within the genome without an a priori prejudice for genetic locus. In the Genetic Analysis of Idiopathic Thrombosis project and in other studies using QTL methodology, investigators have started to provide remarkable information about potential genetic influences on various plasma risk factors (e.g., protein C and protein S levels, APCR ratios, levels of various clotting factors) that affect venous thrombosis.[194,324,331–336]

Both the feasibility and expense of future thrombophilia human genome linkage studies will benefit from the latest screening methodologies and the extensive data for single nucleotide polymorphisms. At least 2.8 million of the estimated 10 million single nucleotide polymorphisms in the human genome are known and publicly available (http://snp.cshl.org). Moreover, the human genome contains relatively large haplotype blocks such that not all polymorphisms must be studied for rigorous linkage studies.[337,338] An international research consortium is engaged to provide a human haplotype map, the "HapMap," to facilitate disease association studies. In spite of the availability of these new databases, some fundamental challenges remain and have been reviewed.[329,339,340] For example, false-positive results in genetic association studies have notoriously appeared. This situation had a number of potential explanations, among them the confounding effects of population stratification, which refers to differences in allele frequencies between cases and controls because of systematic differences in ancestry rather than a disease association. This factor can be potentially overcome by careful study design and use of large numbers of subjects and genetic loci. Another complication can arise from fundamental assumptions about the extent to which common gene variants (found in >2% of study subjects) versus rare variants (<1% of study subjects) contribute to an observed phenotype. At present, insufficient data have accrued to be definitive about this potential problem. However, of note, studies of genetic variation in subjects with very low levels of serum high-density lipoprotein cholesterol showed that rare variants in two genes, apolipoprotein AI and the ABC transporter A1, are found in 10 to 15 percent of the subjects.[341–343] This finding raises the concern that perhaps rare variants in a number of key genes contribute to the studied phenotype such that these important risk factors elude detection. These and other difficulties notwithstanding, a genome-scale, sequence-based approach to venous thrombosis association studies holds great promise for future discovery of thrombophilias.[330,331]

INTERACTIONS BETWEEN DIFFERENT THROMBOPHILIAS AND BETWEEN THROMBOPHILIA AND ENVIRONMENTAL FACTORS

Gene–gene interactions or gene–environmental interactions play a profound role in the pathogenesis of venous thromboembolism (see Figure 122-1). Multiple hereditary thrombophilic defects, or gene–gene interactions, are found in up to 15 percent of patients presenting with venous thormboembolism.[20] Factor V Leiden has been reported in combination with protein C deficiency,[50,344,345] protein S deficiency,[51,52] antithrombin deficiency,[53] prothrombin 20210A mutation,[346–350] hyperhomocysteinemia[165,351,352] and increased factor VIII and TAFI levels.[353,354] All studies demonstrated that these combined defects were associated with an increased risk for venous thrombosis and/or its recurrence. Increased risks of thrombosis have been described in subjects with prothrombin G20210A and protein S deficiency[355] or hyperhomocysteinemia.[356] A pooled analysis of eight case control studies that included 2310 patients with venous thrombosis and 3204 controls showed that the OR for venous thrombosis in heterozygotes for both factor V Leiden and prothrombin G20210A was 20 (95% CI 11.1–36.1).[357] In another study based on retrospective analysis of 400 relatives of 226 probands with factor V Leiden and venous thrombosis, the estimated annual incidence rate of venous thrombosis was 4.8 percent in subjects heterozygous for both factor V Leiden and inherited deficiency of protein C or protein S.[358] In families with combined defects, thromboses occurred not only more frequently in carriers of two thrombophilias but also at an early age.[50–53,355]

Apart from the strong gene–gene interactions, gene–environment interactions are frequent and impart an augmented increased risk for thrombosis. Oral contraceptives and hormone replacement therapy substantially enhance the risk of venous thrombosis in women with factor V Leiden and other thrombophilias. Of women who develop venous thromboembolism during pregnancy, 28 to 46 percent will carry the factor V mutation.[20,359–361] During pregnancy and puerperium, heterozygotes for factor V Leiden have a threefold increase in the

relative risk of venous thromboembolism and a 3.9-fold increased risk of its recurrence compared to women who are not carriers.[361] Several studies have examined the risks of thromboembolism in women with factor V Leiden using third-generation oral contraceptives. A highly significant increase of 30- to 80-fold in the OR for thrombosis was noted, with an absolute increase in risk from 0.8 to 28.5 per 10,000 women per year.[362,363] Even higher risks are seen in women homozygous for factor V Leiden mutation.[364] Among users of oral contraceptives, a 16-fold increased risk was observed in carriers of prothrombin G20210A compared to a sixfold increased risk in noncarriers.[365] Carriers of prothrombin G20210A also have an excessive risk for cerebral vein thrombosis while using oral contraceptives (OR 149; 95% CI 31–711).[366] Deficiencies of antithrombin, protein C, and protein S also interact with the use of oral contraceptives and synergistically increase the risk of venous thrombosis[367] that occurs in many women within 6 months of starting the pills.[368] The joint effect of increased factor VIII levels ($\geq$150% of normal) and use of oral contraceptives gave an OR of 10.3 (95% CI 3.7–28.9), which was indicative of an additive effect.[369]

Similar synergistic effects have been observed in women receiving hormone replacement therapy who are carriers of factor V Leiden or prothrombin G20210A.[370] Possible interactions between other thrombophilias and hormone replacement therapy have not been sufficiently explored.

RECURRENT VENOUS THROMBOSIS IN THROMBOPHILIAS

All patients with venous thrombosis, whether or not they have a thrombophilia, are prone to recurrent thromboses for many years after the first incident. Recurrence is fatal in approximately 5 percent of patients[371] and in one third of patients is associated with the postthrombotic syndrome.[372] Recurrent venous thrombosis requires prolonged therapy with anticoagulants, which itself carries a significant risk of major hemorrhage. Recurrence is more common in men, the elderly, patients who are immobilized, patients with cancer, patients who have had an unprovoked thrombotic event, patients with persistent residual venous thrombi, pulmonary embolism, or increased D-dimer levels, and patients who previously had recurrent thrombosis.[372–376]

The effect of inherited thrombophilias on recurrent venous thrombosis has been assessed mainly in retrospective studies. Recurrent venous thrombosis is more common in patients with a deficiency of antithrombin, protein C, or protein S.[377] Whether or not heterozygosity for factor V Leiden confers a risk of recurrent venous thrombosis has been controversial because of conflicting data. In the prospective Physicians Health Study, factor V Leiden was associated with a fourfold to fivefold increased risk of recurrent venous thrombosis.[378] In a different 10-year followup study after a first episode of venous thrombosis, the prevalence of recurrence was 55 percent among carriers of factor V Leiden compared to 23 percent in noncarriers,[379] yielding a significant hazard ratio of 2.4 (95% CI 1.4–4.1). In contrast, three large followup studies performed in Sweden, Austria, and the United Kingdom failed to demonstrate an increased risk of recurrent venous thrombosis among factor V Leiden heterozygotes.[380–382] Homozygotes for factor V Leiden probably have increased relative risk for recurrent venous thrombosis.[383]

The risk of recurrence conferred by prothrombin G20210A has been uncertain. Two studies showed an increased risk,[379,384] but other studies demonstrated no difference in recurrence rate between heterozygous carriers and noncarriers.[381,382,385,386] In patients who are double heterozygotes for factor V Leiden and prothrombin G20210A, the risk of recurrent venous thrombosis is substantial, with an adjusted OR of 9.1 (95% CI 1.3–63).[387] A similar observation was made in children with venous thrombosis.[388]

Hyperhomocysteinemia exerts an increased risk for recurrent venous thrombosis. In one study of 185 patients with a history of recurrent venous thrombosis, 46 (25%) had homocysteine concentrations above the 90th percentile. The adjusted OR (taking into account age, gender, and menopausal status) was 2.0 (95% CI 1.5–2.7).[389] In another study, the relative risk for recurrent venous thrombosis in patients with homocysteine levels above the 95th percentile was 2.7 (95% CI 1.3–5.8) compared to patients with homocysteine concentration below the 95th percentile. At 24-month followup, 19.2 percent of patients with hyperhomocysteinemia had developed a recurrent episode compared to 6.3 percent of patients with the lower levels of homocysteine.[390] A third study confirmed these observations and revealed that the risk for combined factor V Leiden and MTHFR C677T homozygosity was significantly increased (OR 18.7; 95% CI 3.3–108).[352] A less strong association between hyperhomocysteinemia and recurrence was observed in a population-based prospective study.[166]

Increased levels of factor VIII have been associated with an increased risk for recurrent venous thrombosis.[391] The likelihood of recurrence at 24-month followup was 37 percent in patients with factor VIII levels above the 90th percentile compared to 5 percent in patients with lower levels. A similar observation was made by the same authors regarding increased factor IX levels. When both factor VIII and factor IX levels were elevated, the relative risk of recurrence was 6.6-fold.[392] Various combinations of elevated levels of factors VIII, IX, and XI and TAFI have been implicated in increasing the recurrence rate.[392,393]

HEREDITARY THROMBOPHILIAS DURING PREGNANCY AND PUERPERIUM

Hereditary thrombophilias have been associated with major complications of pregnancy, such as placental abruption, preeclampsia, early and late fetal loss, and intrauterine growth restriction (IUGR), all probably related to compromised blood flow and thrombosis in the maternal–placental–fetal blood circulation[394,395] and maternal venous thromboembolism. For some of these complications, the evidence for an association with thrombophilias is robust (venous thromboembolism and stillbirth), but for others the evidence is suggestive (placental abruption, severe preeclampsia), controversial (early fetal loss), and probably negative (preeclampsia and IUGR).

VENOUS THROMBOEMBOLISM

Although venous thromboembolism occurs in only 1:1000 pregnancies, pulmonary embolism is the major cause of maternal death. Pregnancy can be regarded as an acquired thrombophilia because, during gestation factor VIII and fibrinogen levels increase, protein S levels decrease, fibrinolysis diminishes (because of increased PAI-1 and PAI-2 levels), and acquired APCR occurs. Moreover, venous flow in the lower limbs declines, particularly in the left iliac vein because of compression by the right iliac and ovarian arteries. The ensuing stasis and hypercoagulability explain why venous thrombosis mainly affects the left iliofemoral vein in approximately 80 percent of pregnancy-related venous thromboses. Approximately 50 percent of women with venous thromboembolism detected during pregnancy or puerperium have an underlying hereditary thrombophilia in addition to the acquired risks.[396] The risk of venous thrombosis during pregnancy also depends on the type of thrombophilia. A review of uncontrolled retrospective studies found that venous thrombosis occurred in 30 to 60 percent of patients with antithrombin deficiency compared to 10 to 20 percent of patients with protein C or protein S deficiency.[397] In one of the studies, among 129 asymptomatic women who were relatives of patients with protein C or protein S deficiency, the relative risk of

venous thrombosis during pregnancy and puerperium was eight times more in those who had a deficiency than in unaffected women.[398]

The relative risks for thrombosis in heterozygotes and homozygotes for factor V Leiden were estimated to be 5.3 (95% CI 3.7–7.6) and 25.4 (95% CI 8.8–66), respectively; for prothrombin G20210A heterozygotes was 6.1 (95% CI 3.4–11.2), and for double heterozygotes for factor V and prothrombin G20210A was 84 (95% CI 19–369).[399] A less profound relative risk for double heterozygotes (9.2) was observed in another study.[400] The estimated probabilities of developing venous thrombosis in women with these thrombophilias were 0.26 percent for heterozygous factor V Leiden, 0.37 percent for heterozygous prothrombin G20210A, 1.5 percent for homozygous factor V Leiden, 4.7 percent for double heterozygotes (factor V Leiden and prothrombin G20210A), 7.2 percent for antithrombin deficiency, and 0.8 percent for protein C deficiency.[399] When additional risks were present, such as previous thrombotic events or a familial history of venous thrombosis, these probabilities were further increased. Other, less well-studied acquired risk factors that can enhance the risk in women with a thrombophilia are obesity, age over 35 years, cesarean section, gross varicose vein, and prolonged immobility.[396] In 57 percent of women with pregnancy-related venous thrombosis, the event occurs during the puerperium irrespective of the presence or absence of an hereditary thrombophilia.[401]

FETAL LOSS

RECURRENT FETAL LOSS

Recurrent habitual abortions (three or more consecutive fetal losses) occur in 1 to 2 percent of women.[402] An early study showed that in patients with deficiencies of antithrombin, protein C, or protein S, the relative risk of habitual abortions was increased (OR 2.0; 95% CI 1.2–3.3).[403] A meta-analysis of 31 studies showed that for women with factor V Leiden heterozygosity, the risk of early and late recurrent fetal loss was significantly increased (OR 2.01; 95% CI 1.1–3.6; and OR 7.8; 95% CI 2.8–21.7, respectively).[404] Analysis of the exact time during gestation of recurrent abortions in a large cohort of 491 patients with adverse outcomes of pregnancy revealed an increased risk in patients with factor V Leiden or prothrombin G20210A only when fetal losses occurred after week 14 of gestation.[405] A meta-analysis also concluded that factor V Leiden is primarily associated with second- and third-trimester recurrent fetal losses.[406] Conceivably, late recurrent pregnancy loss reflects thrombosis of placental vessels, whereas other causes prevail at early stages of gestation. In another meta-analysis, factor V Leiden (16 studies) and prothrombin G20210A (seven studies) were shown to confer a similar increase in the relative risk for recurrent fetal losses with OR 2.0 (95% CI 1.5–2.7) and 2.0 (95% CI 1.0–4.0), respectively.[407]

STILLBIRTH

Third-trimester fetal death is rare in developed countries and has been associated with pregnancy-induced hypertension, diabetes mellitus, hydrops fetalis, uterine infections, and congenital anomalies. In many cases, the cause of stillbirth remains unexplained. Several case control studies have shown that in such unexplained cases, the prevalence of thrombophilias is significantly increased[408–412] and that thrombosis and infarcts in the placenta are commonly observed.[409,410] The prevalence of thrombophilias in cases compared to controls was 21 percent versus 4 percent in one study,[409] 16 percent versus 6 percent in a second study,[410] and 43 percent versus 15 percent in a third study.[411] Analysis of the data disclosed that protein S deficiency and factor V Leiden predominated in the studies of unexplained stillbirth, with pooled ORs of 16.2 (95% CI 5.0–52) and 6.1 (95% CI 2.8–13.2), respectively.[412]

Prothrombin G20210A is significantly associated with stillbirth, yielding ORs of 2.3 (95% CI 1.3–4) and 3.3 (95% CI 1.1–10.3) in two studies.[409,411] Recurrent late fetal death also occurs more frequently in thrombophilic women.[413]

PLACENTAL ABRUPTION

The cause of placental abruption, a life-threatening condition for both mother and fetus, has not been determined. Predisposing factors include pregnancy-induced hypertension, advanced age, great parity, chorioamnionitis, smoking, and previous abruption. High prevalences of thrombophilias, particularly factor V Leiden, have been found in such patients.[394,414,415] In an analysis of controlled studies published through 2002, the pooled ORs for heterozygous and homozygous factor V Leiden were 6.7 (95% CI 2–21.6) and 16.9 (95% CI 2–142), respectively.[412] Two studies showed that heterozygous prothrombin G20210A constitutes a significant risk factor for placental abruption,[394,415] estimated in one of these studies to have an OR of 12.2 (95% CI 2.4–30).[415] Hyperhomocysteinemia also is a significant risk factor, with a pooled OR of 3.5 (95% CI 1.5–8.1).[412]

INTRAUTERINE GROWTH RESTRICTION

IUGR is a significant cause of neonatal and maternal morbidity. It is defined as birth weight lower than the 10th percentile. Several studies suggested that IUGR is associated with factor V Leiden, prothrombin G20210A, and homozygous MTHFR C677T.[394,416–419] In contrast, a large case control study of the mothers of 493 neonates with IUGR and the mothers of 472 neonates with normal birth weights (at or above the 10th percentile) demonstrated no significant difference in the frequency of factor V Leiden and prothrombin G20210A between cases and controls.[420] Multiple infarcts, thromboses of blood vessels, and perivillous fibrin deposition that were found in the placentas of thrombophilic women who had IUGR, preeclampsia, and abruption were suggested to constitute the link between thrombophilia and these adverse complications of pregnancy.[421] However, two studies of placentas in cohorts of women with these complications found similar frequencies of pathologic findings in those who had or did not have thrombophilia.[422,423] Also, measurements of blood flow parameters in the maternal–placental–fetal unit that were determined by ultrasound Doppler revealed no significant differences between women with and without thrombophilia.[424] Collectively, these data cast doubt upon a significant association between IUGR and thrombophilias.

PREECLAMPSIA

Preeclampsia complicates 2 to 8 percent of pregnancies and is a major cause of maternal morbidity, prematurity, and neonatal death.[425] In preeclampsia, impaired trophoblastic implantation and diminished placental perfusion occur, leading to production by the placenta of components that are released into the maternal circulation and cause widespread endothelial dysfunction. This process results in secretion of vasopressors with ensuing hypertension, activation of the coagulation system, reduced organ perfusion, increased vascular permeability, proteinuria, and edema.[426] One such component, a soluble fms-like tyrosine kinase 1 (sFlt1), was shown to be produced in excessive amounts by preeclamptic placentas.[427] This factor is a splice variant of the vascular endothelial growth factor (VEGF) receptor that acts as a potent antagonist of VEGF. Increased plasma concentrations of sFlt1 and decreased concentrations of VEGF were found in women with preeclampsia, and administration of sFlt1 to pregnant rats induced hypertension, proteinuria, and glomerular endotheliosis, the hallmarks of preeclampsia.[427] What causes the increased synthesis of sFlt1 and whether other factors play a role in the pathogenesis of preeclampsia are unknown.

Thrombophilias have been implicated as possible causes or enhancers of preeclampsia. A systematic review of case control studies that included from 21 to 284 patients disclosed significant associations between preeclampsia and deficiencies of antithrombin, protein C, and protein S, with pooled ORs of 7.1 to 21.5.[412] For heterozygous factor V Leiden, heterozygous prothrombin G20210A, homozygous MTHFR C677T, and hyperhomocysteinemia, the pooled OR ratios were 1.6 to 2.2 and for homozygous factor V Leiden the OR was 3.7 (95% CI 0.9–15.6). The data on factor V Leiden, prothrombin G20210A and MTHFR C677T contrast with the findings of a large population-based study that included 404 patients with preeclampsia, 303 patients with gestational hypertension, and 164 controls.[428] The study failed to demonstrate a significant difference between cases and controls regarding the prevalence of heterozygosities for factor V Leiden, prothrombin G20210A, and homozygosity for MTHFR C677T. This study also included a meta-analysis of studies that involved only appropriate inclusion criteria. The meta-analysis showed no overall association between preeclampsia and factor V Leiden, prothrombin G20210A, or homozygous MTHFR C677T. Further analysis restricted to patients with severe preeclampsia revealed a significant association with factor V Leiden (pooled OR 2.84; 95% CI 1.95–4.14) and with homozygous MTHFR C677T (OR 1.5; 95% CI 1.0–2.2) but no significant association with prothrombin G20210A (OR 1.76; 95% CI 0.79–3.91).[428] The differences in the described studies and analyses were attributed to the relatively small size of many studies, different inclusion criteria, and bias caused by the variable prevalences of the prothrombotic polymorphisms in controls.[429] Taken together, preeclampsia does not appear to be associated with thrombophilia, but certain thrombophilias may act in concert with other more prominent factors in causing severe preeclampsia.

DIAGNOSIS

In unselected patients with venous thrombosis, testing for the more frequent thrombophilias (APCR, factor V Leiden, prothrombin G20210A, hyperhomocysteinemia, deficiency of protein C, protein S, or antithrombin, increased factor VIII levels) is expected to yield at least one thrombophilia in 30 percent (or more) of cases.[39] In selected patients, this proportion is 70 percent or even higher.[20] Table 122-3 lists in a decreasing order of priority the abnormal parameters that can be searched for. Tests for lupus anticoagulant, anticardiolipin antibody titer, and homocysteine concentration should be performed because of their relatively high frequency and known interaction with thrombophilias. Acquired conditions can produce abnormal test results that may lead to an erroneous diagnosis of a thrombophilia (Table 122-3).

Who should be tested, which tests should be performed, and when is the right time after venous thrombosis to test patients with a suspected thrombophilia are debatable issues. Some of the considerations have been discussed by experts for several organizations such as the American College of Medical Genetics[430] and the College of the American Pathologists,[407,431] and recommendations have been made. Addressing these issues can be facilitated by evaluating the following: (1) what is the likelihood a given patient will be affected; (2) which are the tests that are predicted to yield abnormal results more frequently; (3) will the testing for thrombophilia change the approach to therapy and prophylaxis; (4) what is the likelihood of recurrence if a given thrombophilia is found; (5) what is the cost; (6) will abnormal results induce anxiety in a given patient and family; and (7) will abnormal results have an effect on health insurance.

Based in part on published recommendations (levels 1 and 2),[407,431] reviews of other experts,[432,433] and the experience of the authors of this chapter as reviewed elsewhere,[39] the patients who meet one of the following criteria should be tested for thrombophilia: (1) unprovoked venous thrombosis in subjects younger than 50 years; (2) the presence of a family history of venous thrombosis; (3) cerebral or visceral vein thrombosis; (4) three or more unexplained abortions or one or more stillbirths; (5) recurrent thrombotic events; (6) heparin-induced thrombocytopenia (see below); and (7) venous thromboembolism provoked by pregnancy, oral contraceptives, or hormone replacement therapy.

The high-priority tests to be performed are APCR, factor V Leiden, prothrombin G20210A, levels of homocysteine, factor VIII, protein C, protein S, and antithrombin, and lupus anticoagulant and anticardiolipin antibody titer. If all results are normal, a search for dysfibrinogenemia, measurements of fibrinogen, factor IX and factor XI levels, and testing for MTHFR C677T can be considered. Testing asymptomatic females who are first-degree relatives for the particular thrombophilia found in the proband should be considered prior to pregnancy or use of oral contraceptives. When deficiencies of protein C, protein S, or antithrombin are found in the proband, testing of all immediate relatives is recommended. Whether or not immediate relatives should be tested for factor V Leiden and prothrombin G20210A is controversial. Proponents of testing for these parameters argue there is a 50 percent chance of finding the same genotype in immediate relatives and a 2.5 percent chance of finding homozygosity for the same defect or double heterozygosity for factor V Leiden and prothrombin G20210A in siblings because one of the parents is an obligatory carrier and the other has an approximately 1:10 chance of carrying either gene alteration if they are Caucasians. Although incidence rates of thrombosis are less than 0.7 percent per year for heterozygotes, over a span of 30 to 40 years the cumulative incidence becomes significant and prophylaxis can decrease it. For homozygotes and double heterozygotes, the risk is much higher. Opponents to testing argue that anxiety because of stigmatization, health insurance issues, and cost are too great. These are difficult issues. Patients should participate in the decision on whether or not testing is performed.

Testing for thrombophilia is not necessary for patients who had distal vein thrombosis following trauma or surgery because such patients have a very low recurrence rate (1.5% per year).[434] Similarly, patients whose event was associated with active cancer or an intravascular device should not be tested. Testing patients older than 50 years who had unprovoked venous thromboembolism or patients whose event was related to use of estrogen receptor modulators is controversial.[431]

The optimal time for performing tests in most patients is 6 months after the thrombotic event, when the decision as to whether or not treatment should be continued must be made. The results of examinations performed earlier can be misleading, because thrombosis itself can cause low antithrombin levels and elevated levels of factor VIII. At 6 months, while the patient is still undergoing oral anticoagulant therapy, all high-priority tests (see above) can be performed except for proteins C and protein S, which are decreased because of oral anticoagulant therapy. The patients then can be switched to treatment with low molecular weight heparin for 2 weeks and subsequently tested for protein C activity and the level of free protein S antigen. Upon completion of the evaluation and assessment of the risks of thrombosis recurrence and bleeding, a decision can be made regarding discontinuation of treatment or its extension (see "Therapy").

In patients who are younger than 50 years and who had arterial thrombosis with no atherosclerotic risk factors or evidence for atherosclerosis, the high-priority tests should be performed as outlined for patients with venous thrombosis (see Table 122-3). All patients who had heparin-induced thrombocytopenia and thrombosis, such as arterial thrombosis while taking heparin or within 30 days of its discontinuation, should be tested.

THERAPY

Patients with a known thrombophilia who present with venous thromboembolism should be treated with a standard regimen of heparin overlapped with warfarin until an international normalized ratio of 2.0 to 3.0 is obtained on 2 consecutive days (see Chap. 125). This regimen is sufficient for the prevention of skin necrosis, which may occur during the initiation of warfarin therapy in patients with a protein C deficiency. The chief goals of therapy are to prevent recurrent venous thromboembolism, which is fatal in 5 percent of cases.[371] Recurrent thromboses also increase the risk of venous insufficiency[372] and impose a consideration for indefinite anticoagulant therapy, which carries a significant risk of bleeding. Warfarin therapy reduces the risk of recurrence by 90 to 95 percent, but the annual risk of fatal hemorrhage is 0.25 percent.[435] Consequently, the benefits and hazards associated with increasing the duration of therapy should be carefully evaluated and discussed with each patient, with consideration of the patient's preference and clinical and laboratory risk factors that increase susceptibility to recurrent venous thrombosis or hemorrhage. Comprehensive, evidence-based guidelines for therapy cannot yet be formulated, but several reviews have provided reasonable approaches to treatment that are based partly on evidence and partly on expert views.[39,436-440]

During the initiation of therapy, patients are classified according to their likelihood of having thrombophilia. Patients with the lowest likelihood are those who present with distal vein thrombosis after surgery or trauma. Such patients are treated for 3 months by anticoagulants, and no tests for thrombophilia are performed because of a very low recurrence rate (see above). All other patients are treated with warfarin for 6 months,[39,438-441] after which they are examined for the presence of thrombophilia (as outlined in "Diagnosis" above) and assessed for risks of recurrence and hemorrhage. Based on this assessment, treatment is discontinued, continued for 6 to 18 more months, or continued indefinitely. Table 122-4 summarizes possible indications for therapy extension.

In patients with hyperhomocysteinemia, we recommend indefinite treatment with folic acid, supplemented by vitamins B_6 and B_{12} if

TABLE 122-4   POSSIBLE INDICATIONS FOR EXTENSION OF ANTICOAGULANT THERAPY BEYOND 6 MONTHS IN PATIENTS WITH THROMBOPHILIA

LENGTH OF EXTENSION	INDICATION
6–18 months*	Deficiency of protein C or protein S
	Elevated factor VIII level
	Active cancer
	Severe venous insufficiency
	Iliofemoral venous thrombosis
	Persistence of inciting causes†
Indefinite	Life-threatening event
	Cerebral or visceral vein thrombosis
	Recurrent event
	Antithrombin deficiency
	Combined thrombophilias
	Presence of antiphospholipid antibodies

* An extension should be carefully evaluated and probably not applied in patients with a great risk of bleeding, e.g. age >70 years, history of stroke or gastrointestinal bleeding, renal failure, or poorly controlled anticoagulant therapy.
† Examples include immobilization, absolute necessity for female hormone, estrogen modulation therapy.

normal levels of homocysteine are not achieved with folic acid alone. Annual testing of serum vitamin B_{12} levels is advisable to prevent potential deleterious effects of folic acid in patients with vitamin B_{12} deficiency.

All patients with venous thrombosis of the legs should wear fitted compression stockings for at least 2 years. This measure reduces the incidence of the postthrombotic syndrome by 50 percent.[442] Pregnant patients with thrombophilia who develop venous thromboembolism should be treated similarly to pregnant women without a thrombophilia who have such a complication. Detailed guidelines are available.[443,444] The preferable anticoagulant is low molecular weight heparin, which carries a much smaller risk than heparin for heparin-induced thrombocytopenia, osteoporosis, or bleeding. Warfarin should be avoided because of embryopathy that can occur between 6 of 12 weeks of gestation or central nervous system abnormalities that have been observed during all trimesters.[443,444] The dose of low molecular weight heparin used throughout pregnancy should be targeted at anti–factor Xa levels of 0.5 to 1.2 U/ml 4 to 6 hours after administering low molecular weight heparin given twice per day. Heparin treatment should be continued for 6 weeks following delivery or replaced by oral anticoagulants (see Chap. 125).

Specific therapies are available for some thrombophilic disorders. Antithrombin concentrates, including a recombinant preparation, can be administered for surgery, major trauma, and at the time of delivery in patients with antithrombin deficiency.[445–448] Protein C and APC concentrates are available and can be useful in infants or children with homozygous protein C deficiency or in heterozygous subjects during surgery or other major stresses.[449–451]

PROPHYLAXIS

For thrombophilic patients who had venous thromboembolism, prophylactic measures should be part of their therapy from its initiation. Measures include weight loss (if necessary), avoiding immobility, and discontinuation of female hormone therapy and smoking (if relevant). Following diagnosis of a thrombophilia, the patient must be educated on thrombophilias, future risks of thrombosis (during surgery, air travel, pregnancy, trauma), risk of bleeding during anticoagulant therapy, familial implications, and need for prophylactic therapy during high-risk situations. Followup is advisable for reiteration of prophylactic measures, updating the patient about new tests and therapy, and maintenance of normal homocysteine levels. If gross varicose veins are present, surgery should be considered under appropriate prophylaxis with heparin.

Low molecular weight heparin should be given at prophylactic doses prior to surgery, during pregnancy and for 6 weeks following delivery, during periods of immobilization, and prior to air travel for more than 4 hours. Use of an antithrombin concentrate should be considered during surgery and delivery in patients with antithrombin deficiency.

Prophylactic oral anticoagulant therapy usually is not warranted in subjects who have not suffered a thrombotic event but who are found to have thrombophilia because of family testing or some other reason. In this instance, the risk of hemorrhage because of warfarin clearly outweighs the risk of thrombosis. However, during exposure to risk periods, use of prophylactic anticoagulant therapy has been suggested to decrease the occurrence of venous thrombosis.[452] Use of low molecular weight heparin for 6 weeks postpartum has been advocated.[39,453]

Patients with thrombophilia who had adverse outcomes of pregnancy, such as fetal loss, preeclampsia, and placental abruption, have been treated with low molecular weight heparin resulting in uncontrolled small-scale studies with good outcomes. A review of these studies is available.[395] Until results of controlled studies become available, it seems reasonable to use low molecular weight heparin prophylaxis throughout pregnancy and 6 weeks postpartum in women with thrombophilia who had three or more abortions, stillbirth, placental abruption, or severe preeclampsia but not in women who had IUGR or preeclampsia.

REFERENCES

1. Egeberg O: Inherited antithrombin deficiency causing thrombophilia. *Thromb Diath Haemorrh* 13:516, 1963.
2. Beck EA, Charache P, Jackson DP: A new inherited coagulation disorder caused by an abnormal fibrinogen ("fibrinogen Baltimore"). *Nature* 208:143, 1965.
3. Stenflo J, Fernlund P, Egan W, Roepstorff P: Vitamin K-dependent modifications of glutamic acid residues in prothrombin. *Proc Natl Acad Sci U S A* 71:2730, 1974.
4. Griffin JH, Evatt B, Zimmerman TS, Kleiss AJ: Deficiency of protein C in congenital thrombotic disease. *J Clin Invest* 68:1370, 1981.
5. Schwarz HP, Fischer M, Hopmeier P, et al: Plasma protein S deficiency in familial thrombotic disease. *Blood* 64:1297, 1984.
6. Comp PC, Nixon RR, Cooper MR, Esmon CT: Familial protein S deficiency is associated with recurrent thrombosis. *J Clin Invest* 74:2082, 1984.
7. Comp PC, Esmon CT: Recurrent venous thromboembolism in patients with a partial deficiency of protein S. *N Engl J Med* 311:1525, 1984.
8. Koeleman BP, Reitsma PH, Bertina RM: Familial thrombophilia: A complex genetic disorder. *Semin Hematol* 34:256, 1997.
9. Dahlback B, Carlsson M, Svensson PJ: Familial thrombophilia due to a previously unrecognized mechanism characterized by poor anticoagulant response to activated protein C: Prediction of a cofactor to activated protein C. *Proc Natl Acad Sci U S A* 90:1004, 1993.
10. Svensson PJ, Dahlbäck B: Resistance to activated protein C as a basis for venous thrombosis. *N Engl J Med* 330:517, 1994.
11. Bertina RM, Koeleman BPC, Koster T, et al: Mutation in blood coagulation factor V associated with resistance to activated protein C. *Nature* 369:64, 1994.
12. Greengard JS, Sun X, Xu X, et al: Activated protein C resistance caused by Arg506Gln mutation in factor Va. *Lancet* 343:1361, 1994.
13. Voorberg J, Roelse J, Koopman R, et al: Association of idiopathic venous thromboembolism with single point-mutation at Arg506 of factor V. *Lancet* 343:1535, 1994.
14. Bienvenu T, Ankri A, Chadefaux B, et al: Elevated total plasma homocysteine, a risk factor for thrombosis. Relation to coagulation and fibrinolytic parameters. *Thromb Res* 70:123, 1993.
15. McCully KS: Vascular pathology of homocystinemia: Implications for the pathogenesis of arteriosclerosis. *Am J Pathol* 56:111, 1969.
16. Poort SR, Rosendaal FR, Reitsma PH, Bertina RM: A common genetic variation in the 3′-untranslated region of the prothrombin gene is associated with elevated plasma prothrombin levels and an increase in venous thrombosis. *Blood* 88:3698, 1996.
17. Koster T, Blann AD, Briët E, et al: Role of clotting factor VIII in effect of von Willebrand factor on occurrence of deep-vein thrombosis. *Lancet* 345:152, 1995.
18. Kamphuisen PW, Lensen R, Houwing-Duistermatt JJ, et al: Heritability of elevated factor VIII antigen levels in factor V Leiden families with thrombophilia. *Br J Haematol* 109:519, 2000.
19. Schambeck CM, Hinney K, Haubitz I, et al: Familial clustering of high factor VIII levels in patients with venous thromboembolism. *Arterioscler Thromb Vasc Biol* 21:289, 2001.
20. Salomon O, Steinberg DM, Zivelin A, et al: Single and combined prothrombotic factors in patients with idiopathic venous thromboembo-

lism—Prevalence and risk assessment. *Arterioscler Thromb Vasc Biol* 19:511, 1999.

21. Bertina RM: Genetic approach to thrombophilia. *Thromb Haemost* 86: 92, 2001.

22. Seligsohn U, Zivelin A: Thrombophilia as a multigenic disorder. *Thromb Haemost* 78:297, 1997.

23. Rosendaal FR, Siscovick DS, Schwartz SM, et al: Factor V Leiden (resistance to activated protein C) increases the risk of myocardial infarction in young women. *Blood* 89:2817, 1997.

24. Zoller B, Garcia de Frutos P, Dahlback B: A common 4G allele in the promoter of the plasminogen activator inhibitor-1 (PAI-1) gene as a risk factor for pulmonary embolism and arterial thrombosis in hereditary protein S deficiency. *Thromb Haemost* 79:802, 1998.

25. Inbal A, Freimark D, Modan B, et al: Synergistic effects of prothrombotic polymorphisms and atherogenic factors on the risk of myocardial infarction in young males. *Blood* 93:2186, 1999.

26. Anderson FA Jr, Spencer FA: Risk factors for venous thromboembolism. *Circulation* 107(23 suppl 1):I9, 2003.

27. Souto JC, Almasy L, Borrell M, et al: Genetic susceptibility to thrombosis and its relationship to physiological risk factors: The GAIT study. Genetic Analysis of Idiopathic Thrombophilia. *Am J Hum Genet* 67: 1452, 2000.

28. Ariens RA, De Lange M, Snieder H, et al: Activation markers of coagulation and fibrinolysis in twins: Heritability of the prethrombotic state. *Lancet* 359:667, 2002.

29. Heit JA, Phelps MA, Ward SA, et al: Familial segregation of venous thromboembolism. *J Thromb Haemost* 2:731, 2004.

30. Brinsuk M, Tank J, Luft FC: Heritability of venous function in humans. *Arterioscler Thromb Vasc Biol* 24:207, 2004.

31. Kyrle PA, Minar L, Bialonczyk C, et al: The risk of recurrent venous thromboembolism in men and women. *N Engl J Med* 350:2558, 2004.

32. Prandoni P, Bilora F, Marchen A, et al: An association between atherosclerosis and venous thrombosis. *N Engl J Med* 348:1435, 2003.

33. Bogdanov VY, Balasubramanian V, Hathcock J, et al: Alternatively spliced human tissue factor: A circulating, soluble, thrombogenic protein. *Nat Med* 9:458, 2003.

34. Chou J, Mackman N, Merrill-Skoloff G, et al: Hematopoietic cell-derived microparticle tissue factor contributes to fibrin formation during thrombus propagation. *Blood* 104:3190, 2004.

35. Esmon CT: Coagulation and inflammation. *J Endotoxin Res* 9:192, 2003.

36. Levi M, Van der Poll T, Buller HR: Bidirectional relation between inflammation and coagulation. *Circulation* 109:2698, 2004.

37. Krieger E, Van Der Loo B, Amann-Vesti BR, et al: C-reactive protein and red cell aggregation correlate with late venous function after deep venous thrombosis. *J Vasc Surg* 40:644, 2004.

38. Reitsma PH, Rosendaal FR: Activation of innate immunity in patients with venous thrombosis: The Leiden thrombophilia study. *J Thromb Haemost* 2:619, 2004.

39. Seligsohn U, Lubetsky A: Genetic susceptibility to venous thrombosis. *N Engl J Med* 344:1222, 2001.

40. Prochazka M, Happach C, Marsal K, et al: Factor V Leiden in pregnancies complicated by placental abruption. *Br J Obstet Gynaecol* 110:462, 2003.

41. Zivelin A, Griffin JH, Xu X, et al: A single genetic origin for a common caucasian risk factor for venous thrombosis. *Blood* 89:397, 1997.

42. Zivelin A, Rosenberg N, Faier S, et al: A single genetic origin for the common prothrombotic G20210A polymorphism in the prothrombin gene. *Blood* 92:1119, 1998.

43. Lindqvist PG, Svensson PJ, Dahlback B, Marsal K: Factor V Q^{506} mutation (activated protein C resistance) associated with reduced intrapartum blood loss: A possible evolutionary selection mechanism. *Thromb Haemost* 79:69, 1998.

44. Lindqvist PG, Zoller B, Dahlback B: Improved hemoglobin status and reduced menstrual blood loss among female carriers of factor V Leiden: An evolutionary advantage? *Thromb Haemost* 86:1122, 2001.

45. Corral J, Iniesta JA, Gonzalez-Conejero R, et al: Polymorphisms of clotting factors modify the risk for primary intracranial hemorrhage. *Blood* 97:2979, 2001.

46. Nichols WC, Amano K, Cacheris PM, et al: Moderation of hemophilia A phenotype by the factor V R506Q mutation. *Blood* 88:1183, 1996.

47. Kerlin BA, Yan SB, Isermann BH, et al: Survival advantage associated with heterozygous factor V Leiden mutation in patients with severe sepsis and in mouse endotoxemia. *Blood* 102:3085, 2003.

48. Beauchamp NJ, Dykes AC, Parikh N, et al: The prevalence of, and molecular defects underlying, inherited protein S deficiency in the general population. *Br J Haematol* 125:647, 2004.

49. De Stefano V, Martinelli I, Mannucci PM, et al: The risk of recurrent deep venous thrombosis among heterozygous carriers of both factor V Leiden and the G20210A prothrombin mutation. *N Engl J Med* 341:801, 1999.

50. Koeleman BPC, Reitsma PH, Allaart CF, Bertina RM: Activated protein C resistance as an additional risk factor for thrombosis in protein C deficient families. *Blood* 84:1031, 1994.

51. Zoller B, Berntsdotter A, Garcia de Frutos P, Dahlback B: Resistance to activated protein C as an additional genetic risk factor in hereditary deficiency of protein S. *Blood* 85:3518, 1995.

52. Koeleman PBC, Van Rumpt D, Hamulyak K, et al: Factor V Leiden: An additional risk factor for thrombosis in protein S deficient families? *Thromb Haemost* 74:580, 1995.

53. van Boven HH, Vandenbroucke JP, Briet E, Rosendaal FR: Gene-gene and gene-environment interactions determine risk of thrombosis in families with inherited antithrombin deficiency. *Blood* 94:2590, 1999.

54. Koster T, Rosendaal FR, Deronde H, et al: Venous thrombosis due to poor anticoagulant response to activated protein-C. Leiden Thrombophilia Study. *Lancet* 342:1503, 1993

55. Griffin JH, Evatt B, Wideman C, Fernandez JA: Anticoagulant protein C pathway defective in majority of thrombophilic patients. *Blood* 82: 1989, 1993.

56. Oosting JD, Derksen RHWM, Bobbink IWG, et al: Antiphospholipid antibodies directed against a combination of phospholipids with prothrombin, protein C, or protein S: An explanation for their pathogenic mechanism? *Blood* 81:2618, 1993.

57. Zivelin A, Gitel S, Griffin JH, et al: Extensive venous and arterial thrombosis associated with an inhibitor to activated protein C. *Blood* 94:895, 1999.

58. Sun X, Evatt B, Griffin JH: Blood coagulation factor Va abnormality associated with resistance to activated protein C in venous thrombophilia. *Blood* 83:3120, 1994.

59. Heeb MJ, Kojima Y, Greengard JS, Griffin JH: Activated protein C resistance: Molecular mechanisms based on studies using purified Gln506-factor V. *Blood* 85:3405, 1995.

60. Rosing J, Hoekema L, Nicolaes GA, et al: Effects of protein S and factor Xa on peptide bond cleavages during inactivation of factor Va and factor VaR506Q by activated protein C. *J Biol Chem* 270:27852, 1995.

61. Gale, AJ, Xu, X, Pellequer, JL, et al: Interdomain engineered disulfide bond permitting elucidation of mechanisms of inactivation of coagulation factor Va by activated protein C. *Prot Sci* 11:2091, 2002.

62. Shen L, Dahlback B: Factor V and protein S as synergistic cofactors to activated protein C in degradation of factor VIIIa. *J Biol Chem* 269: 18735, 1994.

63. Dahlback B, Hildebrand B: Inherited resistance to activated protein C is corrected by anticoagulant cofactor activity found to be a property of factor V. *Proc Natl Acad Sci U S A* 91:1396, 1994.

64. Nicolaes, GA, Dahlback, B: Factor V and thrombotic disease: Description of a Janus-faced protein. *Arterioscler Thromb Vasc Biol* 22:530, 2002.

65. Steen M, Norstrom EA, Tholander A-L, et al: Functional characterization of factor V-Ile359Thr: A novel mutation associated with thrombosis. *Blood* 103:3381, 2004.

66. Williamson D, Brown K, Luddington R, et al: Factor V Cambridge: A new mutation (Arg[306]→Thr) associated with resistance to activated protein C. *Blood* 91:1140, 1998.

67. Chan WP, Lee CK, Kwong YL, et al: A novel mutation of Arg[306] of factor V gene in Hong Kong Chinese. *Blood* 91:1135, 1998.

68. Franco RF, Maffei FH, Lourenco D, et al: Factor VArg[306]→Thr (factor V Cambridge) and factor V Arg[306]→Gly mutations in venous thrombotic disease. *Br J Haematol* 103:888, 1998.

69. Norstrom E, Thorelli E, Dahlback B: Functional characterization of recombinant FV Hong Kong and FV Cambridge. *Blood* 100:524, 2002.

70. Bernardi F, Faioni EM, Castoldi E, et al: A factor V genetic component differing from factor V R506Q contributes to the activated protein C resistance phenotype. *Blood* 90:1552, 1997.

71. Alhenc-Gelas M, Nicaud V, Gandrille S, et al: The factor V gene A4070G mutation and the risk of venous thrombosis. *Thromb Haemost* 81:193, 1999.

72. Griffin JH: Blood coagulation. The thrombin paradox [see news; comment]. *Nature* 378:337, 1995.

73. Gruber A, Griffin JH: Direct detection of activated protein C in blood from human subjects. *Blood* 79:2340, 1992.

74. Okajima K, Koga S, Kaji M, et al: Effect of protein C and activated protein C on coagulation and fibrinolysis in normal human subjects. *Thromb Haemost* 63:48, 1990.

75. Heeb MJ, Gruber A, Griffin JH: Identification of divalent metal ion-dependent inhibition of activated protein C by alpha 2-macroglobulin and alpha 2-antiplasmin in blood and comparisons to inhibition of factor Xa, thrombin, and plasmin. *J Biol Chem* 266:17606, 1991.

76. Fernandez JA, Petaja J, Gruber A, Griffin JH: Activated protein C correlates inversely with thrombin levels in resting healthy individuals. *Am J Hematol* 56:29, 1997.

77. Espana F, Vaya A, Mira Y, et al: Low level of circulating activated protein C is a risk factor for venous thromboembolism. *Thromb Haemost* 86:1368, 2001.

78. Greengard JS, Eichinger S, Griffin JH, Bauer KA: Variability of thrombosis among homozygous siblings with resistance to activated protein C due to an Arg→Gln mutation in the gene for factor V. *N Engl J Med* 331:1559, 1994.

79. Martinelli I, Bottasso B, Duca F, et al: Heightened thrombin generation in individuals with resistance to activated protein C. *Thromb Haemost* 75:703, 1996.

80. Simioni P, Scarano L, Gavasso S, et al: Prothrombin fragment 1+2 and thrombin-antithrombin complex levels in patients with inherited APC resistance due to factor V Leiden mutation. *Br J Haematol* 92:435, 1996.

81. Zoller B, Holm J, Svensson P, Dahlback B: Elevated levels of prothrombin activation fragment 1+2 in plasma from patients with heterozygous Arg[506] to Gln mutation in the factor V gene (APC-resistance) and/or inherited protein S deficiency. *Thromb Haemost* 75:270, 1996.

82. Desmarais S, De Moerloose P, Reber G, et al: Resistance to activated protein C in an unselected population of patients with pulmonary embolism. *Lancet* 347:1374, 1996.

83. Turkstra F, Karemaker R, Kuijer PMM, et al: Is the prevalence of the factor V Leiden mutation in patients with pulmonary embolism and deep vein thrombosis really different? *Thromb Haemost* 81:345, 1999.

84. de Moerloose P, Reber G, Perrier A, et al: Prevalence of factor V Leiden and prothrombin G20210A mutations in unselected patients with venous thromboembolism. *Br J Haematol* 110:125, 2000.

85. Munkvad S, Jorgensen M: Resistance to activated protein C: A common anticoagulant deficiency in patients with venous leg ulceration. *Br J Dermatol* 134:296, 1996.

86. Hafner J, Kuhne A, Schar B, et al: Factor V Leiden mutation in postthrombotic and non-postthrombotic venous ulcers. *Arch Dermatol* 137:599, 2001.

87. Janssen HL, Meinardi JR, Vleggaar FP, et al: Factor V Leiden mutation, prothrombin gene mutation, and deficiencies in coagulation inhibitors associated with Budd-Chiari syndrome and portal vein thrombosis: Results of a case control study. *Blood* 96:2364, 2000.

88. Bombeli T, Basic A, Fehr J: Prevalence of hereditary thrombophilia in patients with thrombosis in different venous systems. *Am J Hematol* 70:126, 2002.

89. Middeldorp S, Henkens CMA, Koopman MMW, et al: The incidence of venous thromboembolism in family members of patients with factor V Leiden mutation and venous thrombosis. *Ann Intern Med* 128:15, 1998.

90. Martinelli I, Mannucci PM, De Stefano V, et al: Different risks of thrombosis in four coagulation defects associated with inherited thrombophilia: A study of 150 families. *Blood* 92:2353, 1998.

91. Bucciarelli P, Rosendaal FR, Tripodi A, et al: Risk of venous thromboembolism and clinical manifestations in carriers of antithrombin, protein C, protein S deficiency, or activated protein C resistance—A multicenter collaborative family study. *Arterioscler Thromb Vasc Biol* 19:1026, 1999.

92. Rosendaal FR: Venous thrombosis: A multicausal disease. *Lancet* 353:1167, 1999.

93. Ridker PM, Glynn RJ, Miletich JP, et al: Age-specific incidence rates of venous thromboembolism among heterozygous carriers of factor V Leiden mutation. *Ann Intern Med* 126:528, 1997.

94. Ridker PM, Hennekens CH, Lindpaintner K, et al: Mutation in the gene coding for coagulation factor V and the risk of myocardial infarction, stroke, and venous thrombosis in apparently healthy men. *N Engl J Med* 332:912, 1995.

95. Price DT, Ridker PM: Factor V Leiden mutation and the risks for thromboembolic disease: A clinical perspective. *Ann Intern Med* 127:895, 1997.

96. Martinelli I, Cattaneo M, Taioli E, et al: Genetic risk factors for superficial vein thrombosis. *Thromb Haemost* 82:1215, 1999.

97. Juul K, Tybjaerg-Hansen A, Schnohr P, et al: Factor V Leiden and the risk for venous thromboembolism in the adult Danish population. *Ann Intern Med* 140:330, 2004.

98. Rosendaal FR, Koster T, Vandenbroucke JP, Reitsma PH: High risk of thrombosis in patients homozygous for factor V Leiden (activated protein C resistance). *Blood* 85:1504, 1995.

99. Mari D, Mannucci PM, Duca F, et al: Mutant factor V (Arg506Gln) in healthy centenarians. *Lancet* 347:1044, 1996.

100. Heijmans BT, Westendorp RGJ, Knook DL, et al: The risk of mortality and the factor V Leiden mutation in a population-based cohort. *Thromb Haemost* 80:607, 1998.

101. Hille ETM, Westendorp RGJ, Vandenbroucke JP, Rosendaal FR: Mortality and causes of death in families with the factor V Leiden mutation (resistance to activated protein C). *Blood* 89:1963, 1997.

102. Rees DC, Liu YT, Cox MJ, et al: Factor V Leiden and thermolabile methylenetetrahydrofolate reductase in extreme old age. *Thromb Haemost* 78:1357, 1997.

103. Doggen CJM, Cats VM, Bertina RM, Rosendaal FR: Interaction of coagulation defects and cardiovascular risk factors—Increased risk of myocardial infarction associated with factor V Leiden or prothrombin 20210A. *Circulation* 97:1037, 1998.

104. Atherosclerosis, Thrombosis, and Vascular Biology Italian Study Group: No evidence of association between prothrombotic gene polymorphisms and the development of acute myocardial infarction at a young age. *Circulation* 107:1117, 2003.

105. Reny JL, Alhenc-Gelas M, Fontana P, et al: The factor II G20210A gene polymorphism, but not factor V Arg506Gln, is associated with peripheral arterial disease: Results of a case-control study. *J Thromb Haemost* 2:1334, 2004.

106. Becker S, Heller CH, Gropp F, et al: Thrombophilic disorders in children with cerebral infarction. *Lancet* 352:1756, 1998.

107. Nowak-Gottl U, Koch HG, Aschka I, et al: Resistance to activated protein C (APCR) in children with venous or arterial thromboembolism. *Br J Haematol* 92:992, 1996.

108. Sifontes MT, Nuss R, Hunger SP, et al: Activated protein C resistance and the factor V Leiden mutation in children with thrombosis. *Am J Hematol* 57:29, 1998.

109. Van Rooden CJ, Rosendaal FR, Meinders AE, et al: The contribution of factor V Leiden and prothrombin G20210A mutation to the risk of central venous catheter-related thrombosis. *Haematologica* 89:201, 2004.

110. Ehrenforth S, Nemes L, Mannhalter C, et al: Impact of environmental and hereditary risk factors on the clinical manifestation of thrombophilia in homozygous carriers of factor V:G1691A. *J Thromb Haemost* 2:430, 2004.

111. Tripodi A, Negri B, Bertina RM, Mannucci PM: Screening for the FV: Q506 mutation: Evaluation of thirteen plasma-based methods for their diagnostic efficacy in comparison with DNA analysis. *Thromb Haemost* 77:436, 1997.

112. De Visser MCH, Rosendaal FR, Bertina RM: A reduced sensitivity for activated protein C in the absence of factor V Leiden increases the risk of venous thrombosis. *Blood* 93:1271, 1999.

113. Rodeghiero F, Tosetto A: Activated protein C resistance and factor V Leiden mutation are independent risk factors for venous thromboembolism. *Ann Intern Med* 130:643, 1999.

114. Fisher M, Fernandez JA, Ameriso SF, et al: Activated protein C resistance in ischemic stroke not due to factor V arginine506→glutamine mutation. *Stroke* 27:1163, 1996.

115. Van der Bom JG, Bots ML, Haverkate F, et al: Reduced response to activated protein C is associated with increased risk for cerebrovascular disease. *Ann Intern Med* 125:265, 1996.

116. Le DT, Griffin JH, Greengard JS, et al: Use of a generally applicable tissue factor-dependent factor V assay to detect activated protein C-resistant factor Va in patients receiving warfarin and in patients with a lupus anticoagulant. *Blood* 85:1704, 1995.

117. Griffin JH, Kojima K, Banka CL, et al: High-density lipoprotein enhancement of anticoagulant activities of plasma protein S and activated protein C. *J Clin Invest* 103:219, 1999.

118. Deguchi H, Fernandez JA, Pabinger I, et al: Plasma glucosylceramide deficiency as potential risk factor for venous thrombosis and modulator of anticoagulant protein C pathway. *Blood* 97:1907, 2001.

119. Stearns-Kurosawa DJ, Kurosawa S, Mollica JS, et al: The endothelial cell protein C receptor augments protein C activation by the thrombin-thrombomodulin complex. *Proc Natl Acad Sci U S A* 93: 10212, 1996.

120. Cooper PC, Abuzenadah A, Preston FE: APC resistance test, a new phenomenon—The role of platelets. *Br J Haematol* 86(suppl):33, 1999.

121. Shizuka R, Kanda T, Amagai H, Kobayashi I: False-positive activated protein C (APC) sensitivity ratio caused by freezing and by contamination of plasma with platelets. *Thromb Res* 78:189, 1995.

122. Simioni P, Scudeller A, Radossi P, et al: "Pseudo homozygous" activated protein C resistance due to double heterozygous factor V defects (factor V Leiden mutation and type I quantitative factor V defect) associated with thrombosis: Report of two cases belonging to two unrelated kindreds. *Thromb Haemost* 75:422, 1996.

123. Carter AM, Sachchithananthan M, Stasinopoulos S, et al: Prothrombin G20210A is a bifunctional gene polymorphism. *Thromb Haemost* 87: 846, 2002.

124. Kyrle PA, Mannhalter C, Beguin S, et al: Clinical studies and thrombin generation in patients homozygous or heterozygous for the G20210A mutation in the prothrombin gene. *Arterioscler Thromb Vasc Biol* 18: 1287, 1998.

125. Colucci M, Binetti BM, Tripodi A, et al: Hyperprothrombinemia associated with prothrombin G20210A mutation inhibits plasma fibrinolysis through a TAFI-mediated mechanism. *Blood* 103:2157, 2003.

126. Smirnov MD, Safa O, Esmon NL, Esmon CT: Inhibition of activated protein C anticoagulant activity by prothrombin. *Blood* 94:3839, 1999.

127. Rosendaal FR, Doggen CJM, Zivelin A, et al: Geographic distribution of the 20210 G to A prothrombin variant. *Thromb Haemost* 79:706, 1998.

128. Souto JC, Coll I, Llobet D, et al: The prothrombin 20210A allele is the most prevalent genetic risk factor for venous thromboembolism in the Spanish population. *Thromb Haemost* 80:366, 1998.

129. Rosendaal FR, Vos HL, Poort SL, Bertina RM: Prothrombin 20210A variant and age at thrombosis. *Thromb Haemost* 79:444, 1998.

130. Leroyer C, Mercier B, Oger E, et al: Prevalence of 20210 A allele of the prothrombin gene in venous thromboembolism patients. *Thromb Haemost* 80:49, 1998.

131. Arruda VR, Annichino-Bizzacchi JM, Gonçalves MS, Costa FF: Prevalence of the prothrombin gene variant (nt20210A) in venous thrombosis and arterial disease. *Thromb Haemost* 78:1430, 1997.

132. Margaglione M, Brancaccio V, Giuliani N, et al: Increased risk for venous thrombosis in carriers of the prothrombin G→A^{20210} gene variant. *Ann Intern Med* 129:89, 1998.

133. Hillarp A, Zoller B, Svensson PJ, Dahlback B: The 20210 A allele of the prothrombin gene is a common risk factor among Swedish outpatients with verified deep venous thrombosis. *Thromb Haemost* 78:990, 1997.

134. Cumming AM, Keeney S, Salden A, et al: The prothrombin gene G 20210A variant: Prevalence in a U.K. anticoagulant clinic population. *Br J Haematol* 98:353, 1997.

135. Brown K, Luddington R, Williamson D, et al: The risk of venous thromboembolism associated with a G to A transition at position 20210 in the 3′-untranslated region of the prothrombin gene. *Br J Haematol* 98:907, 1997.

136. De Stefano V, Chiusolo P, Paciaroni K, et al: Hepatic vein thrombosis in a patient with mutant prothrombin 20210A allele. *Thromb Haemost* 80:519, 1998.

137. Darnige L, Jezequel P, Amoura Z, et al: Mesenteric venous thrombosis in two patients heterozygous for the 20210 A allele of the prothrombin gene. *Thromb Haemost* 80:703, 1998.

138. Martinelli I, Sacchi E, Landi G, et al: High risk of cerebral-vein thrombosis in carriers of a prothrombin-gene mutation and in users of oral contraceptives. *N Engl J Med* 338:1793, 1998.

139. Biousse V, Conard J, Brouzes C, et al: Frequency of the 20210 G→A mutation in the 3′-untranslated region of the prothrombin gene in 35 cases of cerebral venous thrombosis. *Stroke* 29:1398, 1998.

140. Chamouard P, Pencreach E, Maloisel F, et al: Frequent factor II G20210A mutation in idiopathic portal vein thrombosis. *Gastroenterology* 116:144, 1999.

141. Reuner KH, Ruf A, Grau A, et al: Prothrombin gene G20210→A transition is a risk factor for cerebral venous thrombosis. *Stroke* 29:1765, 1998.

142. Zawadzki C, Gaveriaux V, Trillot N, et al: Homozygous G20210A transition in the prothrombin gene associated with severe venous thrombotic disease: Two cases in a French family. *Thromb Haemost* 80:1027, 1998.

143. De Stefano V, Chiusolo P, Paciaroni K, et al: Prothrombin G20210A mutant genotype is a risk factor for cerebrovascular ischemic disease in young patients. *Blood* 91:3562, 1998.

144. Howard TE, Marusa M, Channell C, Duncan A: A patient homozygous for a mutation in the prothrombin gene 3'-untranslated region associated with massive thrombosis. *Blood Coagul Fibrinolysis* 8:316, 1997.

145. Ferraresi P, Marchetti G, Legnani C, et al: The heterozygous 20210 G/A prothrombin genotype is associated with early venous thrombosis in inherited thrombophilias and is not increased in frequency in artery disease. *Arterioscler Thromb Vasc Biol* 17:2418, 1997.

146. Corral J, Gonzalez-Conejero R, Lozano ML, et al: The venous thrombosis risk factor 20210 A allele of the prothrombin gene is not a major risk factor for arterial thrombotic disease. *Br J Haematol* 99:304, 1997.

147. Eikelboom JW, Baker RI, Parsons R, et al: No association between the 20210 G/A prothrombin gene mutation and premature coronary artery disease. *Thromb Haemost* 80:878, 1998.

148. Redondo M, Watzke HH, Stucki B, et al: Coagulation factors II, V, VII, and X, prothrombin gene 20210G→A transition, and factor V Leiden in coronary artery disease—High factor V clotting activity is an independent risk factor for myocardial infarction. *Arterioscler Thromb Vasc Biol* 19:1020, 1999.

149. Ridker PM, Hennekens CH, Miletich JP: G20210A mutation in prothrombin gene and risk of myocardial infarction, stroke, and venous thrombosis in a large cohort of U.S. men. *Circulation* 99:999, 1999.

150. Rosendaal FR, Siscovick DS, Schwartz SM, et al: A common prothrombin variant (20210 G to A) increases the risk of myocardial infarction in young women. *Blood* 90:1747, 1997.

151. Franco RF, Trip MD, Ten Cate H, et al: The 20210 G→A mutation in the 3'-untranslated region of the prothrombin gene and the risk for arterial thrombotic disease. *Br J Haematol* 104:50, 1999.

152. Gardemann A, Arsic T, Katz N, et al: The factor II G20210A and factor V G1691A gene transitions and coronary heart disease. *Thromb Haemost* 81:208, 1999.

153. Kim RJ, Becker RC: Association between factor V Leiden, prothrombin G20210A, and methylenetetrahydrofolate reductase C677T mutations and events of the arterial circulatory system: A meta-analysis of published studies. *Am Heart J* 146:948, 2003.

154. Mercier E, Quere I, Campello C, et al: The 20210A allele of the prothrombin gene is frequent in young women with unexplained spinal cord infarction. *Blood* 92:1840, 1998.

155. Simioni P, Tormene D, Manfrin D, et al: Prothrombin antigen levels in symptomatic and asymptomatic carriers of the 20210A prothrombin variant. *Br J Haematol* 103:1045, 1998.

156. Makris M, Preston FE, Beauchamp NJ, et al: Co-inheritance of the 20210A allele of the prothrombin gene increases the risk of thrombosis in subjects with familial thrombophilia. *Thromb Haemost* 78:1426, 1997.

157. Ceelie H, Bertina RM, van Hylckama Vlieg A, et al: Polymorphisms in the prothrombin gene and their association with plasma prothrombin levels. *Thromb Haemost* 85:1066, 2001.

158. Perez-Ceballos E, Corral J, Alberca I, et al: Prothrombin A19911G and G20210A polymorphisms' role in thrombosis. *Br J Haematol* 118:610, 2002.

159. Mudd SH, Levy Hl, Skovby F: Disorders of transsulfuration, in *The Metabolic and Molecular Bases of Inherited Disease*, edited by CR Scriver, AL Beaudet, WS Sly, D Valle, p 1279. McGraw-Hill, New York, 1995.

160. Rosenberg N, Murata M, Ikeda Y, et al: The frequent 5,10-methylenetetrahydrofolate reductase C677T polymorphism is associated with a common haplotype in whites, Japanese, and Africans. *Am J Hum Genet* 70:758, 2002.

161. Jacques PF, Bostom AG, Williams RR, et al: Relation between folate status, a common mutation in methyltetrahydrofolate reductase, and plasma homocysteine concentrations. *Circulation* 93:7,1996.

162. Key NS, McGlennen RC: Hyperhomocyst(e)inemia and thrombophilia. *Arch Pathol Lab Med* 126:1367, 2002.

163. den Heijer M, Rosendaal FR, Blom HJ, et al: Hyperhomocysteinemia and venous thrombosis: A meta-analysis. *Thromb Haemost* 80:874, 1998.

164. Ray JG: Meta-analysis of hyperhomocysteinemia as a risk factor for venous thromboembolic disease. *Arch Intern Med* 158:2101, 1998.

165. Ridker PM, Hennekens CH, Selhub J, et al: Interrelation of hyperhomocyst(e)inemia, factor V Leiden, and risk of future venous thromboembolism. *Circulation* 95:1777, 1997.

166. Tsai AW, Cushman M, Tsai MY, et al: Serum Homocysteine, thermolabile variant of methylenetetrahydrofolate reductase (MTHFR), and venous thromboembolism: Longitudinal investigation of thromboembolism etiology (LITE). *Am J Hematol* 72:192, 2003.

167. Martinelli I, Battaglioli T, Pedotti P, et al: Hyperhomocysteinemia in cerebral vein thrombosis. *Blood* 102:1363, 2003.

168. Ray JG, Shmorgun D, Chan WS: Common C677T polymorphism of the methylenetetrahydrofolate reductase gene and the risk of venous thromboembolism: Meta-analysis of 31 studies. *Pathophysiol Haemost Thromb* 32:51, 2002.

169. Boushey CJ, Beresford SA, Omenn GS, Motulsky AG: A quantitative assessment of plasma homocysteine as a risk factor for vascular disease. Probable benefits of increasing folic acid intakes. *JAMA* 274:1049, 1995.

170. Homocysteine Studies Collaboration: Homocysteine and risk of ischemic heart disease and stroke. *JAMA* 288:2015, 2002.

171. Klerk M, Verhoef P, Clarke R, et al: MTHFR 677C→T polymorphism and risk of coronary heart disease: A meta-analysis. *JAMA* 288:2023, 2002.

172. Pfeiffer CM, Huff DL, Smith SJ, et al: Comparison of plasma total Homocysteine measurements in 14 laboratories: An international study. *Clin Chem* 45:1261, 1999.

173. Tripodi A, Chantarangkul V, Lombardi R, et al: Multicenter study of homocysteine measurement—Performance characteristics of different methods, influence of standards on interlaboratory agreement of results. *Thromb Haemost* 85:291, 2001.

174. Bostom AG, Jacques PF, Nadeau MR, et al: Post-methionine load hyperhomocysteinemia in persons with normal fasting total plasma homocysteine: Initial results from the NHLBI Family Heart Study. *Atherosclerosis* 116:147, 1995.

175. Garg UC, Zheng ZJ, Folsom AR, et al: Short-term and long-term variability of plasma homocysteine measurement. *Clin Chem* 43:141, 1997.

176. Jacobsen DW, Gatautis VJ, Green R, et al: Rapid HPLC determination of total homocysteine and other thiols in serum and plasma: Sex differences and correlation with cobalamin and folate concentrations in healthy subjects [see comments]. *Clin Chem* 40:873, 1994.

177. Frosst P, Blom HJ, Milos R, et al: A candidate genetic risk factor for vascular disease: A common mutation in methylenetetrahydrofolate reductase. *Nat Genet* 10:111,1995.

178. Moat SJ, Bao L, Fowler B, et al: The molecular basis of cystathionine beta-synthase (CBS) deficiency in U.K. and U.S. patients with homocystinuria. *Hum Mutat* 23:206,2004.

179. Tsai MY, Hanson NQ, Bignell MK, Schwichtenberg KA: Simultaneous detection and screening of T833C and G919A mutations of the cystathionine beta-synthase gene by single-strand conformational polymorphism. *Clin Biochem* 29:473, 1996.

180. Esmon CT: Role of coagulation inhibitors in inflammation. *Thromb Haemost* 86:51, 2001.

181. Esmon CT: Structure and functions of the endothelial cell protein C receptor. *Crit Care Med* 32:S298, 2004.

182. Cheng T, Liu D, Griffin JH, et al: Activated protein C blocks p53-mediated apoptosis in ischemic human brain endothelium and is neuroprotective. *Nat Med* 9:338, 2003.

183. Riewald M, Petrovan RJ, Donner A, et al: Activation of endothelial cell protease activated receptor 1 by the protein C pathway. *Science* 296: 1880, 2002.

184. Mosnier LO, Griffin JH: Inhibition of staurosporine-induced apoptosis of endothelial cells by activated protein C requires protease activated receptor-1 and endothelial cell protein C receptor. *Biochem J* 373:65, 2003.

185. Bernard GR, Vincent JL, Laterre PF, et al: Efficacy and safety of re-combinant human activated protein C for severe sepsis. *N Engl J Med* 344:699, 2001.

186. Warren BL, Eid A, Singer P, et al: For the KyberSept trail study group. High-dose antithrombin III in severe sepsis: A randomized controlled trial. *JAMA* 286:1869, 2001.

187. Abraham E, Reinhart K, Opal S, et al: For the OPTIMIST trial study group. Efficacy and safety of tifacogin (recombinant tissue factor path-way inhibitor) in severe sepsis: A randomized controlled trail. *JAMA* 290:238, 2003.

188. Miletich J, Sherman L, Broze G: Absence of thrombosis in subjects with heterozygous protein C deficiency. *N Engl J Med* 317:991, 1987.

189. Tait RC, Walker ID, Reitsma PH, et al: Prevalence of protein C defi-ciency in the healthy population. *Thromb Haemost* 73:87, 1995.

190. Koster T, Rosendaal FR, Briët E, et al: Protein C deficiency in a con-trolled series of unselected outpatients: An infrequent but clear risk fac-tor for venous thrombosis (Leiden thrombophilia study). *Blood* 85:2756, 1995.

191. Folsom AR, Aleksic N, Wang L, et al: Protein C, antithrombin, and venous thromboembolism incidence a prospective population-based study. *Arterioscler Thromb Vasc Biol* 22:1018, 2002.

192. Lensen RPM, Rosendaal FR, Koster T, et al: Apparent different throm-botic tendency in patients with factor V Leiden and protein C deficiency due to selection of patients. *Blood* 88:4205, 1996.

193. Allaart CF, Rosendaal FR, Noteboom WMP, et al: Survival in families with hereditary protein C deficiency 1820 to 1993. *BMJ* 311:910, 1995.

194. Hasstedt SJ, Scott BT, Callas PW, et al: Genome scan of venous throm-bosis in a pedigree with protein C deficiency. *J Thromb Haemost* 2:868, 2004.

195. Brenner B, Zivelin A, Lanir N, et al: Venous thromboembolism asso-ciated with double heterozygosity for R506Q mutation of factor V and for T298M mutation of protein C in a large family of a previously de-scribed homozygous protein C-deficient newborn with massive throm-bosis. *Blood* 88:877, 1996.

196. Spek CA, Koster T, Rosendaal FR, et al: Genotypic variation in the promoter region of the protein C gene is associated with plasma protein C levels and thrombotic risk. *Arterioscler Thromb Vasc Biol* 15:214, 1995.

197. Pabinger I, Schneider B: Thrombotic risk in hereditary antithrombin III, protein C, or protein S deficiency—A cooperative, retrospective study. *Arterioscler Thromb Vasc Biol* 16:742, 1996.

198. De Stefano V, Leone G, Mastrangelo S, et al: Clinical manifestations and management of inherited thrombophilia: Retrospective analysis and follow-up after diagnosis of 238 patients with congenital deficiency of antithrombin III, protein C, protein S. *Thromb Haemost* 72:352, 1994.

199. Pabinger I, Kyrle PA, Heistinger M, et al: The risk of thromboembolism in asymptomatic patients with protein C and protein S deficiency: A prospective cohort study. *Thromb Haemost* 71:441, 1994.

200. Van den Belt AGM, Sanson BJ, Simioni P, et al: Recurrence of venous thromboembolism in patients with familial thrombophilia. *Arch Intern Med* 157:2227, 1997.

201. Allaart CF, Poort SR, Rosendaal FR, et al: Increased risk of venous thrombosis in carriers of hereditary protein C deficiency defect. *Lancet* 341:134, 1993.

202. De Bruijn SFTM, Stam J, Koopman MMW, Vandenbroucke JP: Cere-bral venous sinus thrombosis study: Case-control study of risk of cere-bral sinus thrombosis in oral contraceptive users who are carriers of hereditary prothrombotic conditions. *BMJ* 316:589, 1998.

203. Camerlingo M, Finazzi G, Casto L, et al: Inherited protein C deficiency and nonhemorrhagic arterial stroke in young adults. *Neurology* 41:1371, 1991.

204. Branson HE, Katz J, Marble R, Griffin JH: Inherited protein C deficiency and coumarin-responsive chronic relapsing purpura fulminans in a new-born infant. *Lancet* 2:1165, 1983.

205. Seligsohn U, Berger A, Abend M, et al: Homozygous protein C defi-ciency manifested by massive venous thrombosis in the newborn. *N Engl J Med* 310:559, 1984.

206. McGehee WG, Klotz TA, Epstein DJ, Rapaport SI: Coumarin necrosis associated with hereditary protein C deficiency. *Ann Intern Med* 101: 59, 1984.

207. Vigano D'A, Comp PC, Esmon CT, D'Angelo A: Relationship between protein C antigen and anticoagulant activity during oral anticoagulation and in selected disease states. *J Clin Invest* 77:416, 1986.

208. Weiss P, Soff GA, Halkin H, Seligsohn U: Decline of proteins C and S and factors II, VII, IX, and X during the initiation of warfarin therapy. *Thromb Res* 45:783, 1987.

209. Miletich JP: Laboratory diagnosis of protein C deficiency. *Semin Thromb Hemost* 16:169, 1990.

210. Francis RBJ, Seyfert U: Rapid amidolytic assay of protein C in whole plasma using an activator from the venom of Agkistrodon contortrix. *Am J Clin Pathol* 87:619, 1987.

211. Aiach M, Borgel D, Gaussem P, et al: Protein C and protein S deficien-cies. *Semin Hematol* 34:205, 1997.

212. Berdeaux DH, Abshire TC, Marlar RA: Dysfunctional protein C defi-ciency (Type II). A report of 11 cases in 3 American families and review of the literature. *Am J Clin Pathol* 99:677, 1993.

213. Aiach M, Nicaud V, Alhenc-Gelas M, et al: Complex association of protein C gene promoter polymorphism with circulating protein C levels and thrombotic risk. *Arterioscler Thromb Vasc Biol* 19:1573, 1999.

214. Tait RC, Walker ID, Islam SI, et al: Protein C activity in healthy vol-unteers—Influence of age, sex, smoking, and oral contraceptives. *Thromb Haemost* 70:281, 1993.

215. Bertina RM, Broekmans AW, Van der Linden IK, Mertens K: Protein C deficiency in a Dutch family with thrombotic disease. *Thromb Hae-most* 48:1, 1982.

216. Gandrille S, Borgel D, Sala N, et al: Protein S deficiency: A database of mutations—Summary of the first update. *Thromb Haemost* 84:918, 2000.

217. Faioni EM, Valsecchi C, Palla A, et al: Free protein S deficiency is a risk factor for venous thrombosis. *Thromb Haemost* 78:1343, 1997.

218. Heijboer H, Brandjes DPM, Büller HR, et al: Deficiencies of coagula-tion-inhibiting and fibrinolytic proteins in outpatients with deep-vein thrombosis. *N Engl J Med* 323:1512, 1990.

219. Simmonds RE, Ireland H, Lane DA, et al: Clarification of the risk for venous thrombosis associated with hereditary protein S deficiency by investigation of a large kindred with a characterized gene defect. *Ann Intern Med* 128:8, 1998.

220. Coller BS, Owen J, Jesty J, et al: Deficiency of plasma protein S, protein C, or antithrombin III and arterial thrombosis. *Arteriosclerosis* 7:456, 1987.

221. Allaart CF, Aronson DC, Ruys T, et al: Hereditary protein S deficiency in young adults with arterial occlusive disease. *Thromb Haemost* 64: 206, 1990.

222. Mahasandana C, Suvatte V, Chuansumrit A, et al: Homozygous protein S deficiency in an infant with purpura fulminans. *J Pediatr* 117:750, 1990.

223. Pegelow CH, Ledford M, Young JN, Zilleruelo G: Severe protein S deficiency in a newborn. *Pediatrics* 89:674, 1992.

224. Pung-Amritt P, Poort SR, Vos HL, et al: Compound heterozygosity for one novel and one recurrent mutation in a Thai patient with severe pro-tein S deficiency. *Thromb Haemost* 81:189, 1999.

225. Grimaudo V, Gueissaz F, Hauert J, et al: Necrosis of skin induced by coumarin in a patient deficient in protein S. *BMJ* 298:233, 1989.

226. Langlois NJ, Wells PS: Risk of venous thromboembolism in relatives of symptomatic probands with thrombophilia: A systematic review. *Thromb Haemost* 90:17, 2003.

227. Zoller B, Garcia de Frutos P, Dahlback B: Evaluation of the relationship between protein S and C4b-binding protein isoforms in hereditary protein S deficiency demonstrating type I and type III deficiencies to be phenotypic variants of the same genetic disease. *Blood* 85:3524, 1995.

228. Wolf M, Boyer-Neumann C, Peynaud-Debayle E, et al: Clinical applications of a direct assay of free protein S antigen using monoclonal antibodies. A study of 59 cases. *Blood Coagul Fibrinolysis* 5:187, 1994.

229. Amiral J, Grosley B, Boyer-Neumann C, et al: New direct assay of free protein S antigen using two distinct monoclonal antibodies specific for the free form. *Blood Coagul Fibrinolysis* 5:179, 1994.

230. Faioni EM, Boyer-Neumann C, Franchi F, et al: Another protein S functional assay is sensitive to resistance to activated protein C. *Thromb Haemost* 72:648, 1994.

231. Brunet D, Barthet MC, Morange PE, et al: Protein S deficiency: Different biological phenotypes according to the assays used. *Thromb Haemost* 79:446, 1998.

232. Wolf M, Boyer-Neumann C, Leroy-Matheron C, et al: Functional assay of protein S in 70 patients with congenital and acquired disorders. *Blood Coagul Fibrinolysis* 2:705, 1991.

233. Gari M, Falkon L, Urrutia T, et al: The influence of low protein S plasma levels in young women, on the definition of normal range. *Thromb Res* 73:149, 1994.

234. Comp PC, Thurnau GR, Welsh J, Esmon CT: Functional and immunologic protein S levels are decreased during pregnancy. *Blood* 68:881, 1986.

235. Malm J, Laurell M, Dahlback B: Changes in the plasma levels of vitamin K-dependent proteins C and S and of C4b-binding protein during pregnancy and oral contraception. *Br J Haematol* 68:437, 1988.

236. Comp PC, Doray D, Patton D, Esmon CT: An abnormal plasma distribution of protein S occurs in functional protein S deficiency. *Blood* 67:504, 1986.

237. D'Angelo A, Vigano-D'Angelo S, Esmon CT, Comp PC: Acquired deficiencies of protein S. Protein S activity during oral anticoagulation, in liver disease, and in disseminated intravascular coagulation. *J Clin Invest* 81:1445, 1988.

238. Vigano-D'Angelo S, D'Angelo A, Kaufman CE, et al: Protein S deficiency occurs in the nephrotic syndrome. *Ann Intern Med* 107:42, 1987.

239. Aadland E, Odegaard OR, Roseth A, Try K: Free protein S deficiency in patients with chronic inflammatory bowel disease. *Scand J Gastroenterol* 27:957, 1992.

240. Parke AL, Weinstein RE, Bona RD, et al: The thrombotic diathesis associated with the presence of phospholipid antibodies may be due to low levels of free protein S. *Am J Med* 93:49, 1992.

241. Song KS, Park YS, Kim HK: Prevalence of anti-protein S antibodies in patients with systemic lupus erythematosus. *Arthritis Rheum* 43:557, 2000.

242. Levin M, Eley BS, Louis J, et al: Postinfectious purpura fulminans caused by an autoantibody directed against protein S. *J Pediatr* 127:355, 1995.

243. D'Angelo A, Della Valle P, Crippa L, et al: Brief report: Autoimmune protein S deficiency in a boy with severe thromboembolic disease. *N Engl J Med* 328:1753, 1993.

244. Lane DA, Bayston T, Olds RJ, et al: Antithrombin mutation database: 2nd (1997) update. For the Plasma Coagulation Inhibitors Subcommittee of the Scientific and Standardization Committee of the International Society on Thrombosis and Haemostasis. *Thromb Haemost* 77:197, 1997.

245. Sakuragawa N, Takahashi K, Kondo S, Koide T: Antithrombin III Toyama: A hereditary abnormal antithrombin III of a patient with recurrent thrombophlebitis. *Thromb Res* 31:305, 1983.

246. Fischer AM, Cornu P, Sternberg C, et al: Antithrombin III Alger: A new homozygous AT III variant. *Thromb Haemost* 55:218, 1986.

247. Okajima K, Ueyama H, Hashimoto Y, et al: Homozygous variant of antithrombin III that lacks affinity for heparin, AT III Kumamoto. *Thromb Haemost* 61:20, 1989.

248. Boyer C, Wolf M, Vedrenne J, et al: Homozygous variant of antithrombin III: AT III Fontainebleau. *Thromb Haemost* 56:18, 1986.

249. Tait RC, Walker ID, Perry DJ, et al: Prevalence of antithrombin deficiency in the healthy population. *Br J Haematol* 87:106, 1994.

250. Van Boven HH, Vandenbroucke JP, Briët E, Rosendaal FR: Gene-gene and gene-environment interactions determine risk of thrombosis in families with inherited antithrombin deficiency. *Blood* 94:2590, 1999.

251. Rosendaal FR, Heijboer H, Briet E, et al: Mortality in hereditary antithrombin III deficiency—1830 to 1989. *Lancet* 337:260, 1991.

252. Van Boven HH, Olds RJ, Thein S-L, et al: Hereditary antithrombin deficiency: Heterogeneity of the molecular basis and mortality in Dutch families. *Blood* 84:4209, 1994.

253. Hirsh J, Piovella F, Pini M: Congenital antithrombin III deficiency. Incidence and clinical features. *Am J Med* 87(suppl 3B):34S, 1989.

254. Kuhle S, Lane DA, Jochmanns K, et al: Homozygous antithrombin deficiency type II (99 Leu to Phe mutation) and childhood thromboembolism. *Thromb Haemost* 86:1007, 2001.

255. Nakase H, Kawasaki T, Itani T, et al: Budd-Chiari syndrome and extrahepatic portal obstruction associated with congenital antithrombin III deficiency. *J Gastroenterol* 36:341, 2001.

256. Coller BS, Owen J, Jesty J, et al: Deficiency of plasma protein S, protein C, or antithrombin III and arterial thrombosis. *Arteriosclerosis* 7:456, 1987.

257. Nishimura M, Shimada J, Ito K, et al: Acute arterial thrombosis with antithrombin III deficiency in nephritic syndrome: Report of a case. *Surg Today* 30:663, 2000.

258. Ishiguro K, Kojima T, Kadomatsu K, et al: Complete antithrombin deficiency in mice results in embryonic lethality. *J Clin Invest* 106:873, 2000.

259. De Boer AC, van Riel LA, den Ottolander GJ: Measurement of antithrombin III, alpha 2-macroglobulin and alpha 1-antitrypsin in patients with deep venous thrombosis and pulmonary embolism. *Thromb Res* 15:17, 1979.

260. Marciniak E, Gockerman JP: Heparin-induced decrease in circulating antithrombin-III. *Lancet* 2:581, 1977.

261. Von Kaulla E, Von Kaulla KN: Antithrombin 3 and diseases. *Am J Clin Pathol* 48:69, 1967.

262. Damus PS, Wallace GA: Immunologic measurement of antithrombin III-heparin cofactor and alpha2 macroglobulin in disseminated intravascular coagulation and hepatic failure coagulopathy. *Thromb Res* 6:27, 1975.

263. Kauffmann RH, Veltkamp JJ, van Tilburg NH, Van Es LA: Acquired antithrombin III deficiency and thrombosis in the nephrotic syndrome. *Am J Med* 65:607, 1978.

264. Buchanan GR, Holtkamp CA: Reduced antithrombin III levels during L-asparaginase therapy. *Med Pediatr Oncol* 8:7, 1980.

265. Weenink GH, Treffers PE, Vijn P, et al: Antithrombin III levels in preeclampsia correlate with maternal and fetal morbidity. *Am J Obstet Gynecol* 148:1092, 1984.

266. Kottke-Marchant K, Duncan A: Antithrombin deficiency: Issues in laboratory diagnosis. *Arch Pathol Lab Med* 126:1326, 2002.

267. Demers C, Henderson P, Blajchman MA, et al: An antithrombin III assay based on factor Xa inhibition provides a more reliable test to identify congenital antithrombin III deficiency than an assay based on thrombin inhibition. *Thromb Haemost* 69:231, 1993.

268. Kamphuisen PW, Eikenboom JC, Bertina RM: Elevated factor VIII levels and the risk of thrombosis. *Arterioscler Thromb Vasc Biol* 21:731, 2001.

269. Saenko EL, Yakhyaev AV, Mikhailenko I, et al: Role of the low density lipoprotein-related protein receptor in mediation of factor VIII catabolism. *J Biol Chem* 274:37685, 1999.

270. O'Donnell J, Tuddenham EG, Manning R, et al: High prevalence of elevated factor VIII levels in patients referred for thrombophilia screening: Role of increased synthesis and relationship to the acute phase reaction. *Thromb Haemost* 77:825, 1997.

271. Kraaijenhagen RA, In't Anker PS, Koopman MM, et al: High plasma concentration of factor VIIIc is a major risk factor for venous thromboembolism. *Thromb Haemost* 83:5, 2000.

272. Siegemund A, Petros S, Siegemund T, et al: The endogenous thrombin potential and high levels of coagulation factor VIII, factor IX and factor XI. *Blood Coagul Fibrinolysis* 15:241, 2004.

273. Lensen R, Bertina RM, Vandenbroucke JP, Rosendaal FR: High factor VIII levels contribute to the thrombotic risk in families with factor V Leiden. *Br J Haematol* 114:380, 2001.

274. Tripodi A: Levels of coagulation factors and venous thromboembolism. *Haematologica* 88:705, 2003.

275. Van Hyleckama Vlieg A, van der Linden IK, Bertina RM, Rosendaal FR: High levels of factor IX increase the risk of venous thrombosis. *Blood* 95:3678, 2000.

276. Meijers JC, Tekelenburg WL, Bouma BN, et al: High levels of coagulation factor XI as a risk factor for venous thrombosis. *N Engl J Med* 342:696, 2000.

277. Kamphuisen PW, Eikenboom JC, Vos HL, et al: Increased levels of factor VIII and fibrinogen in patients with venous thrombosis are not caused by acute phase reactions. *Thromb Haemost* 81:680, 1999.

278. Van Hylckama Vlieg A, Rosendaal FR: High levels of fibrinogen are associated with the risk of deep venous thrombosis mainly in the elderly. *J Thromb Haemost* 1:2677, 2003.

279. Hayes T: Dysfibrinogenemia and thrombosis. *Arch Pathol Lab Med* 126:1387, 2002.

280. Haverkate F, Samama M: Familial dysfibrinogenemia and thrombophilia. Report on a study of the SSC Subcommittee on Fibrinogen. *Thromb Haemost* 73:151, 1995.

281. Prins MH, Hirsh J: A critical review of the evidence supporting a relationship between impaired fibrinolytic activity and venous thromboembolism. *Arch Intern Med* 151:1721, 1991.

282. Francis CW: Plasminogen activator inhibitor-1 levels and polymorphisms. *Arch Pathol Lab Med* 126:1401, 2002.

283. Tefts K, Tait CR, Walker ID, et al: A K19E missense mutation in the plasminogen gene is a common cause of familial hypoplasminogenaemia. *Blood Coagul Fibrinolysis* 14:411, 2003.

284. Folsom AR, Cushman M, Heckbert SR, et al: Prospective study of fibrinolytic markers and venous thromboembolism. *J Clin Epidemiol* 56:598, 2003.

285. Schuster V, Mingers AM, Seidenspinner S, et al: Homozygous mutations in the plasminogen gene of two unrelated girls with ligneous conjunctivitis. *Blood* 90:958, 1997.

286. Tait RC, Walker ID, Conkie JA, et al: Isolated familial plasminogen deficiency may not be a risk factor for thrombosis. *Thromb Haemost* 76:1004, 1996.

287. Crowther MA, Roberts J, Roberts R, et al: Fibrinolytic variables in patients with recurrent venous thrombosis: A prospective cohort study. *Thromb Haemost* 85:390, 2001.

288. Van Tilburg NH, Rosendaal FR, Bertina RM: Thrombin activatable fibrinolysis inhibitor and the risk for deep vein thrombosis. *Blood* 95:2855, 2000.

289. Henry M, Aubert H, Morange PE, et al: Identification of polymorphisms in the promoter and the 3' region of the TAFI gene: Evidence that plasma TAFI antigen levels are strongly genetically controlled. *Blood* 97:2053, 2001.

290. Mosnier LO, Elisen MG, Bouma BN, Meijers JC: Protein C inhibitor regulates the thrombin-thrombomodulin complex in the up- and down-regulation of TAFI activation. *Thromb Haemost* 86:1057, 2001.

291. Meijers JC, Marquart JA, Bertina RM, et al: Protein C inhibitor (plasminogen activator inhibitor-3) and the risk of venous thrombosis. *Br J Haematol* 118:604, 2002.

292. Van de Wouwer M, Collen D, Conway EM: Thrombomodulin-protein C-EPCR system integrated to regulate coagulation and inflammation. *Arterioscler Thromb Vasc Biol* 24:1, 2004.

293. Ohlin AK, Marlar RA: The first mutation identified in the thrombomodulin gene in a 45-year-old man presenting with thromboembolic disease. *Blood* 85:330, 1995.

294. Ohlin AK, Marlar RA: Thrombomodulin gene defects in families with thromboembolic disease—A report on four families. *Thromb Haemost* 81:338, 1999.

295. Ohlin AK, Norlund L, Marlar RA: Thrombomodulin gene variations and thromboembolic disease. *Thromb Haemost* 78:396, 1997.

296. Kunz G, Ohlin AK, Adami A, et al: Naturally occurring mutations in the thrombomodulin gene leading to impaired expression and function. *Blood* 99:3646, 2002.

297. Aleksic N, Folsom AR, Cushman M, et al: Prospective study of the A455V polymorphism in the thrombomodulin gene, plasma thrombomodulin, and incidence of venous thromboembolism: The LITE study. *J Thromb Haemost* 1:88, 2003.

298. Stearns-Kurosawa DJ, Burgin C, Parker D, et al: Bimodal distribution of soluble endothelial protein C receptor levels in healthy populations. *J Thromb Haemost* 1:855, 2003.

299. Saposnik B, Reny JL, Gaussem P, et al: A haplotype of the EPCR gene is associated with increased plasma levels of sEPCR and is a candidate risk factor for thrombosis. *Blood* 103:1311, 2004.

300. Medina P, Navarro S, Estelles A, et al: Contribution of polymorphisms in the endothelial protein C receptor gene to soluble endothelial protein C receptor and circulating activated protein C levels, and thrombotic risk. *Thromb Haemost* 91:905, 2004.

301. Uitte de Willige S, Van Marion V, Rosendaal FR, et al: Haplotypes of the EPCR gene, plasma sEPCR levels and the risk of deep venous thrombosis. *J Thromb Haemost* 2:1305, 2004.

302. von Depka M, Czwalinna A, Eisert R, et al: Prevalence of a 23 bp insertion in exon 3 of the endothelial cell protein C receptor gene in venous thrombophilia. *Thromb Haemost* 86:1360, 2001.

303. Biguzzi E, Merati G, Liaw PC, et al: A 23bp insertion in the endothelial protein C receptor (EPCR) gene impairs EPCR function. *Thromb Haemost* 86:945, 2001.

304. Poort SR, Vos HL, Rosendaal FR, Bertina RM: The endothelial protein C receptor (EPCR) 23 bp insert mutation and the risk of venous thrombosis. *Thromb Haemost* 88:160, 2002.

305. Arnaud E, Nicaud V, Poirier O, et al: Protective effect of a thrombin receptor (protease-activated receptor 1) gene polymorphism toward venous thromboembolism. *Arterioscl Thromb Vasc Biol* 20:585, 2000.

306. Dahm A, Van Hylckama Vlieg A, Bendz B, et al: Low levels of tissue factor pathway inhibitor (TFPI) increase the risk of venous thrombosis. *Blood* 101:4387, 2003.

307. Amini-Nekoo A, Futers TS, Moia M, et al: Analysis of the tissue factor pathway inhibitor gene and antigen levels in relation to venous thrombosis. *Br J Haematol* 113:537, 2001.

308. Kato H: Regulation of the function of vascular wall cells by tissue factor pathway inhibitor. Basic and Clinical Aspects. *Arterioscl Thromb Vasc Biol* 22:539, 2002.

309. Caplice NM, Panetta C, Peterson TE, et al: Lipoprotein (a) binds and inactivates tissue factor pathway inhibitor: A novel link between lipoproteins and thrombosis. *Blood* 98:2980, 2001.

310. Tardy-Poncet B, Tardy B, Laporte S, et al: Poor anticoagulant response to tissue factor pathway inhibitor in patients with venous thrombosis. *J Thromb Haemost* 1:507, 2003.

311. Bombeli T, Piccapietra B, Boersma J, Fehr J: Decreased anticoagulant response to tissue factor pathway inhibitor in patients with venous thromboembolism and otherwise no evidence of hereditary or acquired thrombophilia. *Thromb Haemost* 91:80, 2004.

312. Prandoni P, Bilora F, Marchen A, et al: An association between atherosclerosis and venous thrombosis. *N Engl J Med* 348:1435, 2003.

313. Griffin JH, Fernandez JA, Deguchi H: Plasma lipoproteins, hemostasis, and thrombosis. *Thromb Haemost* 86:386, 2001.

314. Kawasaki T, Kambayashi J, Ariyoshi H, et al: Hypercholesterolemia as a risk factor for deep-vein thrombosis. *Thromb Res* 88:67, 1997.

315. Gonzalez-Ordonez AJ, Venta R, Venados N, et al: Association between sensitivity for activated protein C (APC) and lipid or lipoprotein levels. *Thromb Haemost* 88:1069, 2002.

316. Vaya A, Mira Y, Ferrando F, et al: Hyperlipidaemia and venous thromboembolism in patients lacking thrombophilic risk factors. *Br J Haematol* 118:255, 2002.

317. Gonzalez-Ordonez AJ, Fernandez-Carreira JM, Fernandez-Alvarez CR, et al: The concentrations of soluble vascular cell adhesion molecule-1 and lipids are independently associated with venous thromboembolism. *Haematologica* 88:1035, 2003.

318. Doggen CJ, Smith NL, Lemaitre RN, et al: Serum lipid levels and the risk of venous thrombosis. *Arterioscler Thromb Vasc Biol* 24:1970, 2004.

319. Cushman M, Tsai AW, White RH, et al: Deep vein thrombosis and pulmonary embolism in two cohorts: The longitudinal investigation of thromboembolism etiology. *Am J Med* 117:19, 2004.

320. Kaba NK, Francis CW, Moss AJ, et al: Effects of lipids and lipid-lowering therapy on hemostatic factors in patients with myocardial infarction. *J Thromb Haemost* 2:718, 2004.

321. Grady D, Wenger NK, Herrington D, et al: Postmenopausal hormone therapy increases risk for venous thromboembolic disease. The Heart and Estrogen/Progestin Replacement Study. *Ann Intern Med* 132:689, 2000.

322. Ray JG, Mamdani M, Tsuyuki RT, et al: Use of statins and the subsequent development of deep vein thrombosis. *Arch Intern Med* 161:1405, 2001.

323. Deguchi H, Pecheniuk NM, Elias DJ, et al: High density lipoprotein deficiency and dyslipoproteinemia associated with venous thrombosis. (in press), 2005.

324. Souto JC, Almasy L, Borrell M, et al: Genetic susceptibility to thrombosis and its relationship to physiological risk factors: The GAIT study. Genetic Analysis of Idiopathic Thrombophilia. *Am J Hum Genet* 67:1452, 2000.

325. Ariens RA, De Lange M, Snieder H, et al: Activation markers of coagulation and fibrinolysis in twins: Heritability of the prethrombotic state. *Lancet* 359:667, 2002.

326. Heit JA, Phelps MA, Ward SA, et al: Familial segregation of venous thromboembolism. *J Thromb Haemost* 2:731, 2004.

327. Vossen CY, Hasstedt SJ, Rosendaal FR, et al: Heritability of plasma concentrations of clotting factors and measures of a prethrombotic state in a protein C-deficient family. *J Thromb Haemost* 2:242, 2004.

328. Dunn EJ, Ariens RA, De Lange M, et al: Genetics of fibrin clot structure: A twin study. *Blood* 103:1735, 2004.

329. Botstein D, Risch N: Discovering genotypes underlying human phenotypes: Past successes for Mendelian disease, future approaches for complex disease. *Nat Genet* 33(suppl):228, 2003.

330. Rosendaal PR: Genetic studies in complex disease: The case proassociation studies. *J Thromb Haemost* 1:1679, 2003.

331. Souto JC: Genetic studies in complex disease: The case prolinkage studies. *J Thromb Haemost* 1:1676, 2003.

332. Blangero J, Williams JT, Almasy L: Novel family-based approaches to genetic risk in thrombosis. *J Thromb Haemost* 1:1391, 2003.

333. Soria JM, Almasy L, Souto JC, et al: A new locus on chromosome 18 that influences normal variation in activated protein C resistance phenotype and factor VIII activity and its relation to thrombosis susceptibility. *Blood* 101:163, 2003.

334. Almasy L, Soria JM, Souto JC, et al: A quantitative trait locus influencing free plasma protein S levels on human chromosome 1q results from the genetic analysis of idiopathic thrombophilia (GAIT) project. *Arterioscler Thromb Vasc Biol* 23:508, 2003.

335. Buil A, Soria JM, Souto JC, et al: Protein C levels are regulated by a quantitative trait locus on chromosome 16. Results from the genetic analysis of idiopathic thrombophilia (GAIT) project. *Arterioscier Thromb Vasc Biol* 24:1321, 2004.

336. Berger M, Mattheisen M, Kulle B, et al: High factor VIII levels in venous thromboembolism show linkage to imprinted loci on chromosomes 5 and 11. *Blood* 105:638, 2004.

337. Gabriel SB, Schaffner SF, Nguyen H, et al: The structure of haplotype blocks in the human genome. *Science* 296:2225, 2002.

338. Sabeti PC, Reich DE, Higgins JM, et al: Detecting recent positive selection in the human genome from haplotype structure. *Curr Biol* 13: R86, 2003.

339. Freedman ML, Reich D, Penney KL, et al: Assessing the impact of population stratification on genetic association studies. *Nae Genet* 36: 388, 2004.

340. Marchini J, Cardon LR, Phillips MS, Donnelly P: The effects of human population structure on large genetic association studies. *Nat Genet* 36: 512, 2004.

341. Cohen JC, Kiss RS, Pertsemlidis A, et al: Multiple rare alleles contribute to low plasma levels of HDL cholesterol. *Science* 305:869, 2004.

342. Frikke-Schmidt R, Nordestgaard BG, Jensen GB, Tybjaerg-Hansen A: Genetic variation in ABC transporter A1 contributes to HDL cholesterol in the general population. *J Clin Invest* 114:1343, 2004.

343. Pajukanta P: Do DNA sequence variants in ABCA1 contribute to HDL cholesterol levels in the general population? *J Clin Invest* 114:1244, 2004.

344. Gandrille S, Greengard JS, Alhenc-Gelas M, et al: Incidence of activated protein C resistance caused by the ARG 506 GLN mutation in factor V in 113 unrelated symptomatic protein C-deficient patients. The French Network on the behalf of INSERM. *Blood* 86:219, 1995.

345. Brenner B, Zivelin A, Lanir N, et al: Venous thromboembolism associated with double heterozygosity for R506Q mutation of factor V and for T298M mutation of protein C in a large family of a previously described homozygous protein C deficient newborn with massive thrombosis. *Blood* 88:877, 1996.

346. Tosetto A, Rodeghiero F, Martinelli I, et al: Additional genetic risk factors for venous thromboembolism in carriers of the factor V Leiden mutation. *Br J Haematol* 103:871, 1998.

347. Ehrenforth S, Prondsinski MV, Aygören-Pürsün E, et al: Study of the prothrombin gene 20210 GA variant in FV:Q^{506} carriers in relationship to the presence or absence of juvenile venous thromboembolism. *Arterioscler Thromb Vasc Biol* 19:276, 1999.

348. De Stefano V, Martinelli I, Mannucci PM, et al: The risk of recurrent deep venous thrombosis among heterozygous carriers of both factor V Leiden and the G20210A prothrombin mutation. *N Engl J Med* 341:801, 1999.

349. Howard TE, Marusa M, Boisza J, et al: The prothrombin gene 3'-untranslated region mutation is frequently associated with factor V Leiden in thrombophilic patients and shows ethnic-specific variation in allele frequency. *Blood* 91:1092, 1998.

350. Zoller B, Svensson PJ, Dahlback B, Hillarp A: The A20210 allele of the prothrombin gene is frequently associated with the factor V Arg 506 to Gln mutation but not with protein S deficiency in thrombophilic families. *Blood* 91:2210, 1998.

351. Mandel H, Brenner B, Berant M, et al: Coexistence of hereditary homocystinuria and Factor V Leiden—Effect on thrombosis. *N Engl J Med* 334:763, 1996.

352. Keijzer MB, den Heijer M, Blom HJ, et al: Interaction between hyperhomocysteinemia, mutated methylenetetrahydrofolate reductase (MTHFR) and inherited thrombophilic factors in recurrent venous thrombosis. *Thromb Haemost* 88:723, 2002.

353. Lensen R, Bertina RM, Vandenbroucke JP, Rosendaal FR: High factor VIII levels contribute to the thrombotic risk in families with factor V Leiden. *Br J Haematol* 114:380, 2001.

354. Libourel EJ, Bank I, Meinardi JR, et al: Co-segregation of thrombophilic disorders in factor V Leiden carriers: The contributions of factor VIII, factor XI, thrombin activatable fibrinolysis inhibitor and lipoprotein(a) to the absolute risk of venous thromboembolism. *Haematologica* 87:1068, 2002.

355. Castaman G, Tosetto A, Cappellari A, et al: The A20210 allele in the prothrombin gene enhances the risk of venous thrombosis in carriers of inherited protein S deficiency. *Blood Coagul Fibrinolysis* 11:321, 2000.

356. De Stefano V, Zappacosta B, Persichilli S, et al: Prevalence of mild hyperhomocysteinaemia and association with thrombophilic genotypes (factor V Leiden and prothrombin G20210A) in Italian patients with venous thromboembolic disease. *Br J Haematol* 106:564, 1999.

357. Emmerich J, Rosendaal FR, Cattaneo M, et al: Combined effect of factor V Leiden and prothrombin 20210A on the risk of venous thromboembolism-pooled analysis of 8 case-control studies including 2,310 cases and 3,204 controls. Study Group for Pooled-Analysis in Venous Thromboembolism. *Thromb Haemost* 86:809, 2001.

358. Meinardi JR, Middeldorp S, de Kam PJ, et al: Risk of venous thromboembolism in carriers of factor V Leiden with a concomitant inherited thrombophilic defect: A retrospective analysis. *Blood Coagul Fibrinolysis* 12:713, 2001.

359. Dizon-Townson DS, Nelson LM, Jang H, et al: The incidence of the factor V Leiden mutation in an obstetric population and its relationship to deep vein thrombosis. *Am J Obstet Gynecol* 176:883, 1997.

360. Hallak M, Senderowicz J, Cassel A, et al: Activated protein C resistance (factor V Leiden) associated with thrombosis in pregnancy. *Am J Obstet Gynecol* 176:889, 1997.

361. Bokarewa MI, Bremme K, Blomback M: Arg^{506}-Gln mutation in factor V and risk of thrombosis during pregnancy. *Br J Haematol* 92:473, 1996.

362. Bloemenkamp KWM, Rosendaal FR, Helmerhorst FM, et al: Enhancement by factor V Leiden mutation of risk of deep-vein thrombosis associated with oral contraceptives containing third-generation progestagen. *Lancet* 346:1593, 1995.

363. Vandenbroucke JP, Koster T, Brit E, et al: Increased risk of venous thrombosis in oral-contraceptive users who are carriers of factor V Leiden mutation. *Lancet* 344:1453, 1994.

364. Rintelen C, Mannhalter C, Ireland H, et al: Oral contraceptives enhance the risk of clinical manifestation of venous thrombosis at a young age in females homozygous for factor V Leiden. *Br J Haematol* 93:487, 1996.

365. Martinelli I, Taioli E, Bucciarelli P, et al: Interaction between the G20210A mutation of the prothrombin gene and oral contraceptive use in deep vein thrombosis. *Arterioscler Thromb Vasc Biol* 19:700, 1999.

366. Martinelli I, Sacchi E, Landi G, et al: High risk of cerebral-vein thrombosis in carriers of a prothrombin-gene mutation and in users of oral contraceptives. *N Engl J Med* 338:1793, 1998.

367. Bloemenkamp KW, Helmerhorst FM, Rosendaal FR, Vandenbroucke JP: Thrombophilias and gynaecology. *Best Pract Res Clin Obstet Gynaecol* 17:509, 2003.

368. Bloemenkamp KW, Rosendaal FR, Helmerhorst FM, Vandenbroucke JP: Higher risk of venous thrombosis during early use of oral contraceptives in women with inherited clotting defects. *Arch Intern Med* 160:49, 2000.

369. Bloemenkamp KW, Helmerhorst FM, Rosendaal FR, Vandenbroucke JP: Venous thrombosis, oral contraceptives and high factor VIII levels. *Thromb Haemost* 82:1024, 1999.

370. Rosendaal FR, Vessey M, Rumley A, et al: Hormonal replacement therapy, prothrombotic mutations and the risk of venous thrombosis. *Br J Haematol* 116:851, 2002.

371. Douketis JD, Kearon C, Bates S, et al: Risk of fatal pulmonary embolism in patients with treated venous thromboembolism. *JAMA* 279:458, 1998.

372. Prandoni P, Lensing AW, Cogo A, et al: The long-term clinical course of acute deep venous thrombosis. *Ann Intern Med* 125:1, 1996.

373. Prandoni P, Lensing AW, Piccioli A, et al: Recurrent venous thromboembolism and bleeding complications during anticoagulant treatment in patients with cancer and venous thrombosis. *Blood* 100:3484, 2002.

374. Prandoni P, Lensing AW, Prins MH, et al: Residual venous thrombosis as a predictive factor of recurrent venous thromboembolism. *Ann Intern Med* 137:955, 2002.

375. Eichinger S, Weltermann A, Minar E, et al: Symptomatic pulmonary embolism and the risk of recurrent venous thromboembolism. *Arch Intern Med* 164:92, 2004.

376. Palareti G, Legnani C, Cosmi B, et al: Risk of venous thromboembolism recurrence: High negative predictive value of D-dimer performed after oral anticoagulation is stopped. *Thromb Haemost* 87:7, 2002.

377. Van den Belt AG, Sanson BJ, Simioni P, et al: Recurrence of venous thromboembolism in patients with familial thrombophilia. *Arch Intern Med* 157:2227, 1997.

378. Ridker PM, Miletich JP, Stampfer MJ, et al: Factor V Leiden and risks of recurrent idiopathic venous thromboembolism. *Circulation* 92:2800, 1995.

379. Simioni P, Prandoni P, Lensing AW, et al: Risk for subsequent venous thromboembolic complications in carriers of the prothrombin or the factor V gene mutation with a first episode of deep-vein thrombosis. *Blood* 96:3329, 2000.

380. Eichinger S, Weltermann A, Mannhalter C, et al: The risk of recurrent venous thromboembolism in heterozygous carriers of factor V Leiden and a first spontaneous venous thromboembolism. *Arch Intern Med* 162:2357, 2002.

381. Baglin T, Luddington R, Brown K, Baglin C: Incidence of recurrent venous thromboembolism in relation to clinical and thrombophilic risk factors: Prospective cohort study. *Lancet* 362:523, 2003.

382. Lindmarker P, Schulman S, Sten-Linder M, et al: The risk of recurrent venous thromboembolism in carriers and non-carriers of the G1691A allele in the coagulation factor V gene and the G20210A allele in the prothrombin gene. DURAC Trial Study Group. Duration of anticoagulation. *Thromb Haemost* 81:684, 1999.

383. Procare Group: Is recurrent venous thromboembolism more frequent in homozygous patients for the factor V Leiden mutation than in heterozygous patients? *Blood Coagul Fibrinolysis* 14:523, 2003.

384. Miles JS, Miletich JP, Goldhaber SZ, et al: G20210A mutation in the prothrombin gene and the risk of recurrent venous thromboembolism. *J Am Coll Cardiol* 37:215, 2001.

385. Eichinger S, Minar E, Hirschl M, et al: The risk of early recurrent venous thromboembolism after oral anticoagulant therapy in patients with the G20210A transition in the prothrombin gene. *Thromb Haemost* 81:14, 1999.

386. De Stefano V, Martinelli I, Mannucci PM, et al: The risk of recurrent venous thromboembolism among heterozygous carriers of the G20210A prothrombin gene mutation. *Br J Haematol* 113:630, 2001.

387. Meinardi JR, Middeldorp S, De Kam PJ, et al: The incidence of recurrent venous thromboembolism in carriers of factor V Leiden is related to concomitant thrombophilic disorders. *Br J Haematol* 116:625, 2002.

388. Nowak-Gottl U, Junker R, Kreuz W, et al: Risk of recurrent venous thrombosis in children with combined prothrombotic risk factors. *Blood* 97:858, 2001.

389. Den Heijer M, Blom HJ, Gerrits WB, et al: Is hyperhomocysteinaemia a risk factor for recurrent venous thrombosis? *Lancet* 345:882, 1995.

390. Eichinger S, Stumpflen A, Hirschl M, et al: Hyperhomocysteinemia is a risk factor of recurrent venous thromboembolism. *Thromb Haemost* 80:566, 1998.

391. Kyrle PA, Minar E, Hirschl M, et al: High plasma levels of factor VIII and the risk of recurrent venous thromboembolism. *N Engl J Med* 343:457, 2000.

392. Weltermann A, Eichinger S, Bialonczyk C, et al: The risk of recurrent venous thromboembolism among patients with high factor IX levels. *J Thromb Haemost* 1:28, 2003.

393. Eichinger S, Schonauer V, Weltermann A, et al: Thrombin-activatable fibrinolysis inhibitor and the risk for recurrent venous thromboembolism. *Blood* 103:3773, 2004.

394. Kupferminc MJ, Eldor A, Steinman N, et al: Increased frequency of genetic thrombophilia in women with complications of pregnancy. *N Engl J Med* 340:9, 1999.

395. Brenner B: Clinical management of thrombophilia-related placental vascular complications. *Blood* 103:4003, 2004.

396. Greer IA: Inherited thrombophilia and venous thromboembolism. *Best Pract Res Clin Obstet Gynaecol* 17:413, 2003.

397. Girling J, de Swiet M: Inherited thrombophilia and pregnancy. *Curr Opin Obstet Gynecol* 10:135, 1998.

398. Friederich PW, Sanson BJ, Simioni P, et al: Frequency of pregnancy-related venous thromboembolism in anticoagulant factor-deficient women: Implications for prophylaxis. *Ann Intern Med* 125:955, 1996.

399. Zotz RB, Gerhardt A, Scharf RE: Inherited thrombophilia and gestational venous thromboembolism. *Best Pract Res Clin Haematol* 16:243, 2003.

400. Martinelli I, Legnani C, Bucciarelli P, et al: Risk of pregnancy-related venous thrombosis in carriers of severe inherited thrombophilia. *Thromb Haemost* 86:800, 2001.

401. Martinelli I, De Stefano V, Taioli E, et al: Inherited thrombophilia and first venous thromboembolism during pregnancy and puerperium. *Thromb Haemost* 87:791, 2002.

402. Hatasaka HH: Recurrent miscarriage: Epidemiologic factors, definitions, and incidence. *Clin Obstet Gynecol* 37:625, 1994.

403. Sanson BJ, Friederich PW, Simioni P, et al: The risk of abortion and stillbirth in antithrombin-, protein C-, and protein S-deficient women. *Thromb Haemost* 75:387, 1996.

404. Rey E, Kahn SR, David M, Shrier I: Thrombophilic disorders and fetal loss: A meta-analysis. *Lancet* 361:901, 2003.

405. Roque H, Paidas MJ, Funai EF, et al: Maternal thrombophilias are not associated with early pregnancy loss. *Thromb Haemost* 91:290, 2004.

406. Kovalevsky G, Gracia CR, Berlin JA, et al: Evaluation of the association between hereditary thrombophilia and recurrent pregnancy loss: A meta-analysis. *Arch Intern Med* 164:558, 2004.

407. Press RD, Bauer KA, Kujovich JL, Heit JA: Clinical utility of factor V Leiden (R506Q) testing for the diagnosis and management of thromboembolic disorders. *Arch Pathol Lab Med* 126:1304, 2002.

408. Preston FE, Rosendaal FR, Walker ID, et al: Increased fetal loss in women with heritable thrombophilia. *Lancet* 348:913, 1996.

409. Gris JC, Quere I, Monpeyroux F, et al: Case-control study of the frequency of thrombophilic disorders in couples with late fetal loss and no thrombotic antecedent the Nimes Obstetricians and Haematologists Study5 (NOHA5). *Thromb Haemost* 81:891, 1999.

410. Martinelli I, Taioli E, Cetin I, et al: Mutations in coagulation factors in women with unexplained late fetal loss. *N Engl J Med* 343:1015, 2000.

411. Many A, Elad R, Yaron Y, et al: Third-trimester unexplained intrauterine fetal death is associated with inherited thrombophilia. *Obstet Gynecol* 99:684, 2002.

412. Alfirevic Z, Roberts D, Matlew V: How strong is the association between maternal thrombophilia and adverse pregnancy outcome? A systematic review. *Eur J Obstet Gynecol Reprod Biol* 101:6, 2002.

413. Martinelli I, Taioli E, Cetin I, Mannucci PM: Recurrent late fetal death in women with and without thrombophilia. *Thromb Haemost* 87:358, 2002.

414. Wiener-Megnagi Z, Ben-Shlomo I, Goldberg Y, Shalev E: Resistance to activated protein C and the Leiden mutation: High prevalence in patients with abruption placentae. *Am J Obstet Gynecol* 179:1565, 1998.

415. Facchinetti F, Marozio L, Grandone E, et al: Thrombophilic mutations are a main risk factor for placental abruption. *Haematologica* 88:785, 2003.

416. Kupferminc MJ, Many A, Bar-Am A, et al: Mid-trimester severe intrauterine growth restriction is associated with a high prevalence of thrombophilia. *Br J Obst Gynaecol* 109:1373, 2002.

417. Martinelli P, Grandone E, Colaizzo D, et al: Familial thrombophilia and the occurrence of fetal growth restriction. *Haematologica* 86:428, 2001.

418. Grandone E, Margaglione M, Colaizzo D, et al: Lower birth-weight in neonates of mothers carrying factor V G1691A and factor II A(20210) mutations. *Haematologica* 87:177, 2002.

419. Kupferminc MJ, Peri H, Zwang E, et al: High prevalence of the prothrombin gene mutation in women with intrauterine growth retardation, abruption placentae, and second trimester loss. *Acta Obstet Gynecol Scand* 79:963, 2000.

420. Infante-Rivard C, Rivard GE, Yotov WV, et al: Absence of association of thrombophilia polymorphisms with intrauterine growth restriction. *N Engl J Med* 347:19, 2002.

421. Kupferminc MJ, Eldor A: Inherited thrombophilia and gestational vascular complications. *Semin Thromb Hemost* 29:185, 2003.

422. Mousa HA, Alfirevicl Z: Do Placental lesions reflect thrombophilia state in women with adverse pregnancy outcome? *Hum Reprod* 15:1830, 2000.

423. Sikkema JM, Franx A, Bruinse HW, et al: Placental pathology in early onset pre-eclampsia and intra-uterine growth restriction in women with and without thrombophilia. *Placenta* 23:337, 2002.

424. Salomon O, Seligsohn U, Steinberg DM et al: The common prothrombotic factors in nulliparous women do not compromise blood flow in the feto-maternal circulation and are not associated with preeclampsia or intrauterine growth restriction. *Am J Obstet Gynecol* 191:2002, 2004.

425. Duley L: Pre-eclampsia and the hypertensive disorders of pregnancy. *Br Med Bull* 67:161, 2003.

426. Roberts JM, Lain KY: Recent insights into the pathogenesis of pre-eclampsia. *Placenta* 23:359, 2002.

427. Maynard SE, Min JY, Merchan J, et al: Excess placental soluble fms-like tyrosine kinase 1 (sFlt1) may contribute to endothelial dysfunction, hypertension, and proteinuria in preeclampsia. *J Clin Invest* 111:649, 2003.

428. Morrison ER, Miedzybrodzka ZH, Campbell DM, et al: Prothrombotic genotypes are not associated with pre-eclampsia and gestational hypertension: Results from a large population-based study and systematic review. *Thromb Haemost* 87:779, 2002.

429. Greer IA: Thrombophilia: Implications for pregnancy outcome. *Thromb Res* 109:73, 2003.

430. Grody WW, Griffin JH, Taylor AK, et al: American College of Medical Genetics consensus statement on factor V Leiden mutation testing. *Genet Med* 3:139, 2001.

431. Van Cott EM, Laposata M, Prins MH: Laboratory evaluation of hypercoagulability with venous or arterial thrombosis. *Arch Pathol Lab Med* 126:1281, 2002.

432. Tripodi A, Mannucci PM: Laboratory investigation of thrombophilia. *Clin Chem* 47:1597, 2001.

433. Bauer KA: The thrombophilias: Well-defined risk factors with uncertain therapeutic implications. *Ann Intern Med* 135:367, 2001.

434. Schulman S: Duration of anticoagulants in acute or recurrent venous thromboembolism. *Curr Opin Pulm Med* 6:321, 2000.

435. Hirsh J, Kearon C, Ginsberg J: Duration of anticoagulant therapy after first episode of venous thrombosis in patients with inherited thrombophilia. *Arch Intern Med* 157:2174, 1997.

436. Kearon C, Crowther M, Hirsh J: Management of patients with hereditary hypercoagulable disorders. *Annu Rev Med* 51:169, 2000.

437. Bauer KA: Management of thrombophilia. *J Thromb Haemost* 1:1429, 2003.

438. Geerts WH, Pineo GF, Heit JA, et al: Prevention of venous thromboembolism: The seventh ACCP conference on antithrombotic and thrombolytic therapy. *Chest* 126:338S, 2004.

439. Kearon C: Long-term management of patients after venous thromboembolism. *Circulation* 110(9 suppl 1):110, 2004.

440. Bates SM, Ginsberg JS: Clinical practice. Treatment of deep-vein thrombosis. *N Engl J Med* 351:268, 2004.

441. Schulman S, Rhedin AS, Lindmarker P, et al: A comparison of six weeks with six months of oral anticoagulant therapy after a first episode of venous thromboembolism. Duration of Anticoagulation Trial Study Group. *N Engl J Med* 332:1661, 1995.

442. Brandjes DP, Buller HR, Heijboer H: Randomized trial of effect of compression stockings in patients with symptomatic proximal-vein thrombosis. *Lancet* 349:759, 1997.

443. Ginsberg JS, Bates SM: Management of venous thromboembolism during pregnancy. *J Thromb Haemost* 1:1435, 2003.

444. Bowles L, Cohen H: Inherited thrombophilias and anticoagulation in pregnancy. *Best Pract Res Clin Obstet Gynaecol* 17:471, 2003.

445. Lechner K, Kyrle PA: Antithrombin III concentrates—Are they clinically useful? *Thromb Haemost* 73:340, 1995.

446. Bucur SZ, Levy JH, Despotis GJ, et al: Uses of antithrombin III concentrate in congenital and acquired deficiency states. *Transfusion* 38:481, 1998.

447. Menache D, O'Malley JP, Schorr JB, et al: Evaluation of the safety, recovery, half-life, and clinical efficacy of antithrombin III (human) in patients with hereditary antithrombin III deficiency. *Blood* 75:33, 1990.

448. Konkle BA, Bauer KA, Weinstein R: Use of recombinant human antithrombin in patients with congenital antithrombin deficiency undergoing surgical procedures. *Transfusion* 43:390, 2003.

449. Vukovich T, Auberger K, Weil J, et al: Replacement therapy for a homozygous protein C deficiency-state using a concentrate of human protein C and S. *Br J Haematol* 70:435, 1988.

450. Manco-Johnson M, Nuss R: Protein C concentrate prevents peripartum thrombosis. *Am J Hematol* 40:69, 1992.

451. Gerson WT, Dickerman JD, Bovill EG, Golden E: Severe acquired protein C deficiency in purpura fulminans associated with disseminated intravascular coagulation: Treatment with protein C concentrate. *Pediatrics* 91:418, 1993.

452. Sanson BJ, Simioni P, Tormene D, et al: The incidence of venous thromboembolism in asymptomatic carriers of a deficiency of antithrombin, protein C, or protein S: A prospective cohort study. *Blood* 94:3702, 1999.

453. Martinelli I: Pros and cons of thrombophilia testing: Pros. *J Thromb Haemost* 1:410, 2003.

454. Schafer AI: Hypercoagulable states: Molecular genetics to clinical practice. *Lancet* 344:1739, 1994.

THE ANTIPHOSPHOLIPID SYNDROME

JACOB H. RAND
LISA SENZEL

The antiphospholipid (aPL) syndrome is an acquired disorder in which patients have thrombotic manifestations and/or recurrent spontaneous pregnancy loss, with laboratory evidence of autoantibodies that recognize anionic phospholipid–protein complexes. The disorder is considered secondary when it occurs in the presence of systemic lupus erythematosus or other major autoimmune conditions and primary when it occurs in their absence. The deep veins of the lower extremities are the most frequent sites of thrombosis, but thromboembolism can involve almost any portion of the arterial or venous circulations. Additional reported manifestations of aPL syndrome include immune thrombocytopenia, livedo reticularis, stroke, atherosclerosis, pulmonary hypertension, and sensorineural hearing loss. Rare patients have a catastrophic form of aPL syndrome in which disseminated large- and small-vessel thrombi occur with accompanying multiorgan ischemia and infarction. This form of the disorder may mimic the presentation of thrombotic thrombocytopenic purpura or disseminated intravascular coagulation.

The antigenic targets for the antibodies generated in this condition appear to be epitopes on phospholipid-binding proteins such as β_2 glycoprotein I (β_2GPI) rather than phospholipid itself. The syndrome is recognized by laboratory evidence for the presence of antibodies against these phospholipid–protein cofactor complexes that are detected by enzyme-linked immunosorbent assays (anticardiolipin, antiphosphatidyl serine, or anti-β_2GPI assays) or by coagulation assays ("lupus anticoagulants") that paradoxically report the inhibition of phospholipid-dependent coagulation reactions. Several conditions, including syphilis, Lyme disease, hepatitis C, alcoholic liver injury, human immunodeficiency virus infection, and multiple sclerosis, are associated with increased levels of antibodies directed against anionic phospholipids themselves but not against protein cofactors. These conditions are not associated with an increased risk of thrombosis.

Patients with spontaneous vascular thrombosis and aPL syndrome should be treated with anticoagulant therapy. Catastrophic aPL syndrome may require additional therapy with high-dose anticoagulants, plasmapheresis, and immunosuppressive agents. Patients with recurrent spontaneous pregnancy losses and aPL syndrome generally require treatment with aspirin and heparin for the major portion of their pregnancies and may need additional prophylaxis against deep vein thrombosis during the postpartum period. Because aPL test results may be abnormal in conditions other than aPL syndrome, patients should not be committed to antithrombotic therapy based on the results of laboratory tests alone. The clinician should have documented evidence—or at least a very high suspicion—for thromboembolism or pregnancy losses before administering treatment. In patients treated with warfarin, care should be taken to confirm that coagulation tests for monitoring oral anticoagulant therapy reflect true reductions in the levels of the vitamin K-dependent coagulation proteins and not acquired hypoprothrombinemia or lupus anticoagulants.

DEFINITION AND HISTORY

The antiphospholipid (aPL) antibody syndrome is a disorder in which vascular thrombosis or recurrent pregnancy losses occur in patients with laboratory evidence for antibodies against phospholipids or phospholipid-binding protein cofactors. The presence of these antibodies is detectable with immunoassays using solid-phase phospholipids and protein cofactors as antigenic targets or with coagulation assays that demonstrate the inhibition of phospholipid-dependent coagulation reactions known as the lupus anticoagulant (LA) phenomenon. The syndrome was first proposed to be a distinct entity, "the anticardiolipin (aCL) syndrome," in 1985[1] and soon was renamed the "aPL syndrome."[2] The disorder is classified as primary if no other autoimmune condition such as systemic lupus erythematosus (SLE) is concurrent and secondary in the presence of such disorders (Figure 123-1). The clinical presentations and the courses of thrombosis of patients with the primary and secondary disorders do not appear to be different.[3] In view of the apparent multiplicity of antigens recognized by the antibodies (see "Antigenic Specificities" below) and the ambiguous pathophysiology, other names for the condition, such as the "aPL/cofactor syndrome,"[4] the "antibody-mediated thrombosis syndrome,"[5,6] and the eponym "Hughes syndrome"[7] have been proposed.

The first laboratory evidence for the disorder was the observation of the "biologic false-positive" serologic test for syphilis (BFP syphilis test), described by Moore and Mohr[8] in 1952. This laboratory anomaly was found to often be associated with SLE[9] and with an "anticoagulant" phenomenon,[10] but its clinical significance was not known. In the early 1950s, the development of coagulation tests that used a phospholipid extract of animal brain (cephalin) to accelerate coagulation reactions[11] led to the recognition of abnormalities that were attributed to the presence of an anticoagulant in patients with SLE, frequently with BFP syphilis tests. This phenomenon was named the "lupus anticoagulant."[12] Although the first report of patients with these anticoagulants described bleeding manifestations,[13] these in vitro anticoagulants were associated with bleeding problems in vivo only if other hemostatic defects were present, such as hypoprothrombinemia, thrombocytopenia, platelet function abnormalities, or specific inhibitors of blood coagulation factors.[10] The subsequent finding that these anticoagulants were associated with thrombotic and embolic manifestations[14] and with recurrent pregnancy loss was surprising.[15,16] A major step leading to the identification of aPL syndrome occurred in 1983 when a quantitative test was developed to assay antibodies against the anionic phospholipid known as cardiolipin (diphosphatidylglycerol), which is the primary antigen in the syphilis test reagent.[17]

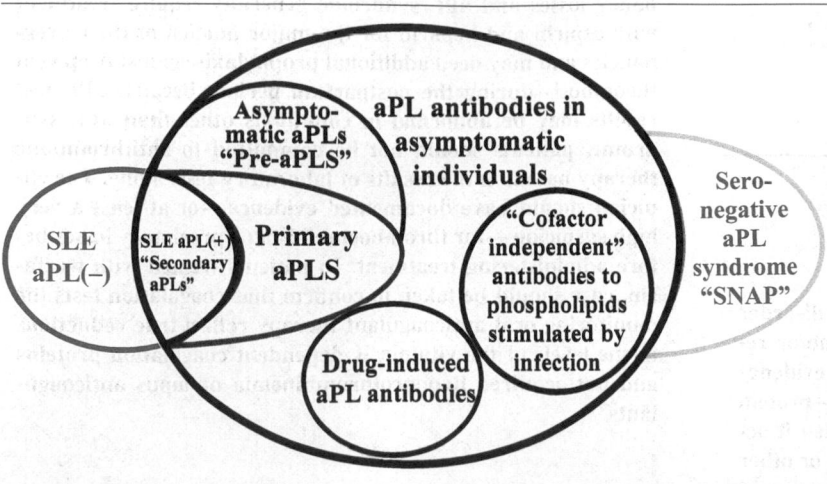

FIGURE 123-1 Conceptual framework for classifying patients having antibodies against phospholipid and phospholipid-binding proteins. *Large thick-walled circle* includes all patients having antibodies against phospholipid. The group includes patients with antiphospholipid (aPL) syndrome (aPLS; primary, secondary, and asymptomatic) and patients having antibodies but without the autoimmune thrombotic syndrome. Outside the large circle are patients with sero-negative aPL syndrome ("SNAP") and patients with systemic lupus erythematosus (SLE) lacking aPL antibodies.

It is important for the clinician to distinguish the class of patients who have the autoimmune thrombotic disorder referred to as aPL syndrome (whether primary or secondary) from patients having aPL antibodies but without the clinical syndrome (see Figure 123-1). The latter include completely asymptomatic and otherwise apparently normal healthy people, patients with infections that induce antibodies recognizing anionic phospholipids directly, and patients taking medications such as chlorpromazine or procainamide. Among the asymptomatic normal healthy population are some individuals who are at high risk for thrombosis but have not yet manifested the clinical disorder ("pre-aPL syndrome"). Also considered are patients suspected of having a seronegative form of the disorder (seronegative aPL syndrome [SNAP]).

ETIOLOGY AND PATHOGENESIS

ETIOLOGY

The genesis of the antibodies in this disorder and even their antigenic specificities are not well established. The disorder is generally considered to fall into the category of "autoimmune" conditions. Although antibodies against anionic phospholipid moieties arise during the course of infections such as syphilis and Lyme disease, those antibodies are generally distinct from antibodies generated by patients with the syndrome because they recognize phospholipid epitopes directly (i.e., they are not "cofactor dependent") and are not associated with the clinical manifestations of the syndrome. In contrast (as described in "Antigenic Specificities" below), the antibodies generated in patients with the syndrome recognize epitopes that include protein cofactors, primarily β_2GPI, and thus often are referred to as "cofactor dependent."

GENETIC PREDISPOSITION

Familial clustering of raised aPL antibody levels[18] and human leukocyte antigen (HLA) linkages[19–22] indicate that the antibodies probably occur in response to some antigenic challenge in a genetically susceptible host. In one study, the strongest association with aPL was the HLA-DR53 haplotypes, some of which include DQ7, whereas the

HLA-B8, DR17, DQ2 haplotypes closely associated with SLE were significantly decreased in patients with primary and secondary aPL syndrome.[20]

POSSIBLE ETIOLOGIC AGENTS

There are intriguing reports of aPL syndrome arising in patients with infections (in contrast to patients having antibodies against phospholipid alone without the syndrome, whose relationship to infection has been well established). aPL antibodies have been reported in patients with postvaricella purpura fulminans[23] or venous thrombosis,[24] in patients with varicella pneumonia and spontaneous tibial artery thrombosis,[25] and in patients with hepatitis C.[26] An association of aPL and mesenteric and femoropopliteal thrombosis in a patient with cytomegalovirus (CMV) infection has been reported.[27] Also, β_2GPI cofactor-dependent antibodies against cardiolipin, phosphatidyl serine, and phosphatidyl ethanolamine have been identified in sera from patients with parvovirus B19.[28] aCL antibodies having β_2GPI dependence and LA activity have been generated in rabbits immunized with lipid A and lipoteichoic acid, suggesting that some bacteria contribute to the production of pathogenic aPL antibodies.[29]

It has been proposed that cellular apoptosis, with the resulting exposure of anionic phospholipids on the cell surface, triggers the generation of aPL antibodies.[30–32] aPL antibodies induced in mice by immunization with a CMV-derived peptide cause thrombosis and activation of endothelial cells.[33] Molecular mimicry between β_2GPI-related synthetic peptides and structures within bacteria, viruses, tetanus toxoid, and CMV is a cause for experimental aPL syndrome.[34]

PATHOGENESIS

The pathophysiologic mechanism(s) of this syndrome has remained obscure, in part because of the apparent multiplicity of antigenic determinants recognized by the antibodies. Also, a large number of effects have been described for the antibodies *in vitro* and in cell culture systems (Table 123-1). Many of these effects, including the paradoxical LA phenomenon, are a consequence of the multiple roles involving phospholipids in the hemostatic system and in biologic processes in general and simply may reflect antibody-mediated effects on phospholipid-dependent processes that may not be relevant *in vivo*.

RELATIONSHIP OF ANTIBODIES TO CLINICAL MANIFESTATIONS: EVIDENCE FROM ANIMAL STUDIES

Although the relationship of aPL antibodies to the disease process—that is, whether cause, effect, or epiphenomenon—has been much debated, convincing evidence from experimental animal models of aPL syndrome indicates that aPL antibodies can play a causal role in the development of thrombosis and pregnancy loss. Mice immunized against β_2GPI develop aPL antibodies and pregnancy wastage.[35] Exposure to aPL antibodies causes fetal wastage in rats[36]and mice, in a manner requiring complement C3 activation.[37] Mice infused with aPL antibodies develop significantly larger thrombi after experimental vascular injury than mice infused with control antibodies, but this enhancement is abrogated in E-selectin–deficient mice.[38] Monoclonal human aCL antibodies derived from patients with aPL syndrome promote thrombosis in mice.[39] Atherosclerosis in a susceptible mouse model (low-density lipoprotein [LDL] receptor knockout mouse) was accelerated by immunization with human aCL antibodies from an aPL syndrome patient, suggesting that these antibodies play a role in the

TABLE 123-1   MECHANISMS PROPOSED FOR THE ANTIPHOSPHOLIPID
SYNDROME

Disruption of annexin A5 shield
Altered eicosanoid synthesis
Injury to endothelium
Induction of endothelial receptors for cell adhesion molecules
Increase of endothelin-1
Induction of tissue factor expression on monocytes and endothelial cells
Induction of apoptosis
Interference with protein C pathway
    Antiphospholipid binding to proteins C and S
    Inhibition of activation of protein C
    Acquired activated protein C resistance
Inhibition of heparan sulfate–antithrombin complex formation
Cross-reactivity with oxidized low-density lipoprotein
Increase of plasminogen activator inhibitor-1
Reduced fibrinolysis by impairment of autoactivation of factor XII and by
    antibodies to tissue-type plasminogen activator
Platelet activation
Activation of complement
Antibodies against tissue factor pathway inhibitor
Concentration of prothrombin locally

development of atherosclerosis in patients with aPL syndrome.[40] Remarkably, in contrast, passive administration of aCL antibodies to atherosclerosis-prone, LDL receptor-deficient mice reduced plaque formation.[41] A monoclonal anti-β_2GPI antibody and its Fab$_2$ fragments, but not the Fab$_1$ fragments, promoted thrombosis in an animal model of photochemically induced vessel damage.[42] In mice injected with immunoglobulin (Ig)G-aPL syndrome, fluvastatin blunted the resulting thrombogenic and inflammatory responses (adhesion of leukocytes to endothelial cells).[43]

A direct causal relationship between aPL antibodies and thrombotic manifestations or pregnancy losses in humans has not yet been proved. Some patients with aPL antibodies may manifest thrombosis and pregnancy loss by coincidence. The fact that elevated levels of antibodies are detectable in a significant proportion of asymptomatic individuals has raised questions about their predictive value.[44–46]

ANTIGENIC SPECIFICITIES

Some aPL antibodies recognize phospholipids directly without protein cofactors.[47] Purified aPL antibodies from patients with the syndrome generally do not bind directly to purified phospholipid in the absence of a source of serum proteins.[48,49] These usually are "dependent" upon a serum phospholipid-binding protein, known as β_2GPI or apolipoprotein H, for recognition of the phospholipid in enzyme-linked immunosorbent assays (ELISAs). In contrast, antibodies against phospholipid that arise during the immunologic response to syphilis infection are not "cofactor dependent" and recognize the anionic phospholipid epitopes directly.[50]

β_2GPI is a highly glycosylated single-chain plasma protein composed of 326 amino acids with a molecular weight of 50 kDa (Figure 123-2) that appears to be the major, but not the only, cofactor for recognition of anionic phospholipid by aPL antibodies.[51] The protein is a member of the "complement control protein" or "short consensus repeat" superfamily.[52] The protein, which contains five repeating short consensus repeat (SCR) stretches of approximately 60 amino acid residues,[53] is thought to insert into phospholipid bilayers through a cationic segment near the carboxy-terminus of SCR domain V (Figure 123-2). The dimerization of the protein, via aPL IgG recognition of epitopes in the other domains, increases the affinity of the antibody–

protein complex for membrane phospholipids.[53,54] Evidence indicates that β_2GPI itself may be one of the major epitopes for aPL antibodies[55,56] or may, in complex with phospholipids, form an antigenic site.

The physiologic function of β_2GPI has not been established. Homozygous β_2GPI-null mice appear to be free of disease, anatomically and histologically.[57] Thrombin generation was found to be defective, but the reason for the defect is unknown. The protein may play a role early in the reproductive process, as fewer than expected numbers of homozygous β_2GPI-null offspring are born from heterozygous parents.[57] β_2GPI has been shown to bind to endothelial cells via annexin II, a protein that also serves as a receptor for plasminogen and tissue plasminogen activator.[58] Antibody binding to β_2GPI on the endothelial surface can increase the expression of adhesion molecules on the membrane (see "Effects of aPL Antibodies on Vascular Endothelial Cells," below).

Additional candidate cofactors and antigenic targets have been identified,[59] including prothrombin (factor II), coagulation factor V, protein C, protein S, annexin A5, high and low molecular weight kininogens, and factor VII/VIIa.[60] In the presence of cardiolipin and β_2GPI, protein C can be a target of aCL, leading to protein C dysfunction.[61] Also, antibodies of some aPL patients cross-react with heparin and inhibit the formation of antithrombin–thrombin complexes.[62]

Oxidation of phospholipids may be necessary for aPL antibody recognition.[63,64] The epitopes for some aPL antibodies appear to be adducts of oxidized phospholipid and protein such as β_2GPI.[65] Thus, some affinity-purified cardiolipin-binding antibodies in sera from patients with SLE appear to cross-react with oxidized LDL.[66] Elevated levels of the latter antibodies have been proposed to be markers for arterial thrombosis[67] but the point is controversial.[68]

Antimitochondrial M5 type antibodies reportedly are a serologic

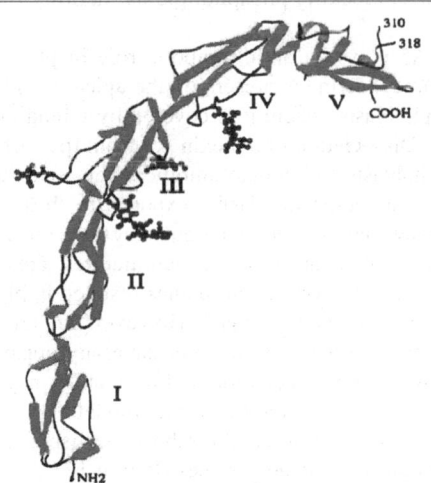

FIGURE 123-2   Structure of human blood plasma β_2 glycoprotein I (β_2GPI). Ribbon model of β_2GPI based upon crystal structure. The protein is composed of an extended chain of five short consensus repeat (SCR) domains having a "fishhook" appearance. The structure of SCR domain V deviates from the standard fold of the four other domains and forms the putative phospholipid-binding site. The structural data suggest a simple membrane-binding mechanism in which the cationic patch of domain V has an affinity for anionic phospholipid. The stretch of Ser311 to Lys317 forms a hydrophobic loop that inserts into the lipid bilayer and positions Trp316 at the interface region between the acyl chains and the phosphate head groups of the lipids, thereby anchoring the β_2GPI in the membrane. Current data support the hypothesis that antiphospholipid (aPL) antibodies reactive against β_2GPI mainly recognize epitopes on domains I and II and that antibody-mediated dimerization of β_2GPI markedly increases the affinity of β_2GPI for phospholipid. (From B Bouma, PG de Groot, JM van den Elsen, et al.,[53] with permission.)

marker for aPL syndrome distinct from anticardiolipin and anti-β_2GPI antibodies. These antibodies, unlike aCL and anti-β_2GPI IgG antibodies, are not significantly associated with thrombosis, but they are associated with thrombocytopenia and recurrent fetal loss.[69]

PROPOSED PATHOGENIC MECHANISMS

Because almost any of the biologic processes that involve or require phospholipids may be affected by the presence of antibodies that bind to the phospholipids (either directly or via cofactors), any proposed aPL-mediated effects that are based on *in vitro* studies must be evaluated for *in vivo* relevance. Also, any plausible explanation for aPL syndrome needs to account for the paradox of the LA phenomenon. Table 123-1 summarizes the current hypotheses for pathogenic mechanisms in aPL syndrome. Several of these effects could act in concert and cause the clinical manifestations.

Antiphospholipid Antibody-Mediated Disruption of the Annexin A5 Anticoagulant Shield   Annexin A5 (placental anticoagulant protein-I, vascular anticoagulant-α) has potent anticoagulant properties *in vitro* that are based on its high affinity for anionic phospholipids and its capacity to displace coagulation factors from phospholipid surfaces.[70] To date, more than 160 annexin proteins have been identified in both animal and plant cells.[71] These proteins are very similar in structure. Most of the members consist of four highly homologous cassette domains of approximately 70 amino acids each. The uniqueness of each protein is believed to reside largely in the structure of its amino-terminal sequences.

Annexin A5 significantly prolongs phospholipid-dependent coagulation reactions by forming two-dimensional clusters that displace coagulation proteins from phospholipid surfaces.[70] This clustering property likely is of functional importance because it permits the formation of a protective shield of annexin A5 over the phospholipid surface, blocking phospholipid availability for coagulation reactions.

Annexin A5 plays an antithrombotic role in physiologic conditions. Phosphatidyl serine is present on the apical membranes of syncytialized trophoblasts, where it is covered by a binding layer of annexin A5.[72–74] Dissociation of annexin A5 from the surface of human placental trophoblasts and human umbilical vein endothelial cells accelerates the coagulation of plasma exposed to those cells.[75] Thus, annexin A5 may play a thrombomodulatory role on the surfaces of cells lining the placental and systemic vasculatures. Treatment of pregnant mice with antiannexin A5 antibodies resulted in placental necrosis, fibrosis, and pregnancy loss.[76] However, an annexin A5-null mouse has been reported and does not have any apparent disease.[77] This discrepancy is not understood and ultimately may be explained by compensating factors in the transgenic model.

aPL antibodies may promote thrombosis by displacing annexin A5 from phospholipid membrane surfaces (Figure 123-3).[78] Annexin A5 is markedly reduced on the apical membranes of human placentas of women with aPL antibodies compared to placentas of women with uncomplicated term deliveries, non–aPL-related pregnancy losses, and elective pregnancy terminations.[75,79] Moreover, IgG fractions from aPL syndrome patients reduce the quantity of annexin A5 on cultured trophoblasts and endothelial cells and accelerate the coagulation of plasma exposed to these cells.[75] Monoclonal aPL antibodies disrupt the crystal structure of the annexin A5 anticoagulant shield (Figure 123-4), allowing exposure of phospholipids and acceleration of coagulation reactions.

Whereas the displacement of annexin A5 occurs via aPL antibodies, some investigators have identified aPL patients with antibodies that recognize annexin A5 directly.[80,81] Antiannexin A5 antibodies from patients with aPL syndrome can induce apoptosis in cultured human umbilical vein endothelial cells.[82]

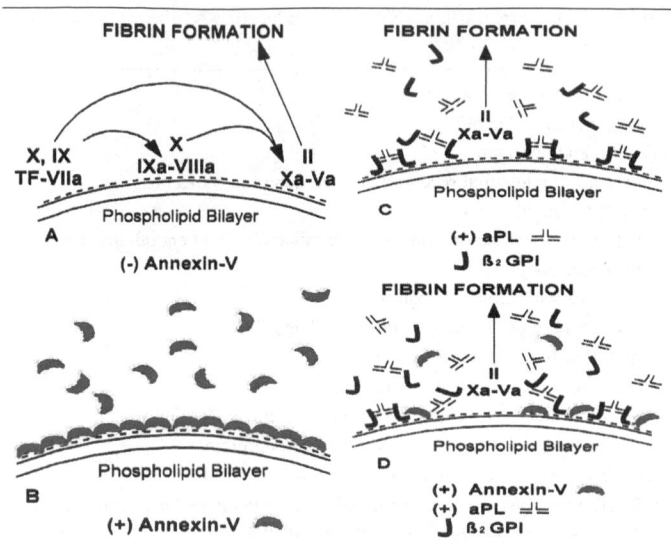

FIGURE 123-3   Model for the mechanism of the "lupus anticoagulant effect" and for a "lupus procoagulant effect." *(A)* Anionic phospholipids (negative charges), when exposed on the apical surface of the cell membrane bilayer, serve as potent cofactors for the assembly of four different coagulation complexes—two tissue factor (TF)–VIIa complexes, IXa–VIIIa complex, and Xa–Va complex—and thereby accelerate blood coagulation. TF complexes yield factors IXa and Xa; IXa complex yields factor Xa; and factor Xa formed from both of these reactions is the active enzyme in the prothrombinase complex, which yields factor IIa (thrombin) that in turn cleaves fibrinogen to form fibrin. *(B)* Annexin A5, in the absence of antiphospholipid (aPL) antibodies, serves as a potent anticoagulant by forming clusters that bind with high affinity to the anionic phospholipid surface and shield the surface from the assembly of the phospholipid-dependent coagulation complexes. *(C)* In the absence of annexin A5, aPL antibodies can prolong the coagulation times by reducing the access of coagulation factors to anionic phospholipids. This process may result in a "lupus anticoagulant" effect. *(D)* In the presence of annexin A5, antiphospholipid antibodies, either directly or via interaction with protein-phospholipid cofactors, disrupt the ability of annexin A5 to cluster on the phospholipid surface. This process results in a net increase of the amount of anionic phospholipid available for promoting coagulation reactions. The aPL–cofactor complexes expose significantly more phospholipids by disrupting the annexin A5 shield than they block by direct binding. This situation manifests in the net acceleration of coagulation *in vitro* and in thrombophilia *in vivo*. (From JH Rand, XX Wu, HAM Andree, et al.,[78] with permission.)

Effects of Antiphospholipid Antibodies on Vascular Endothelial Cells   aPL antibodies have been found to recognize, injure, and/or activate cultured vascular endothelial cells.[83–86] Cultured endothelial cells incubated with aPL express increased levels of cell adhesion molecules,[87] an effect that may be mediated by β_2GPI,[88] increase the adhesion of leukocytes to the vascular wall, and promote inflammation and thrombosis. However, not all studies have been able to demonstrate such an effect.[89] Incubation of cultured endothelial cells with aPL results in increased expression of tissue factor.[90,91] Activation of endothelial cells by anti-β_2GPI antibodies is followed by redistribution of nuclear factor-κB from the cytoplasm to the nucleus, a process that is accompanied by increased expression of tissue factor and of the leukocyte adhesion molecules intercellular adhesion molecule (ICAM)-1, vascular cell adhesion molecule (VCAM)-1, and E-selectin. Inhibition of the nuclear translocation of nuclear factor-κB abolished the response to these antibodies. In an immortalized human microvascular endothelial cell model, the signaling cascade has been shown to involve TRAF6 and MyD88 but not TRAF2 and to show the same kinetics as interleukin (IL)-1 receptor-activated kinase phosphorylation, suggesting involvement of the Toll-like receptor family.[92] The pattern of effects of the anti-β_2GPI anti-

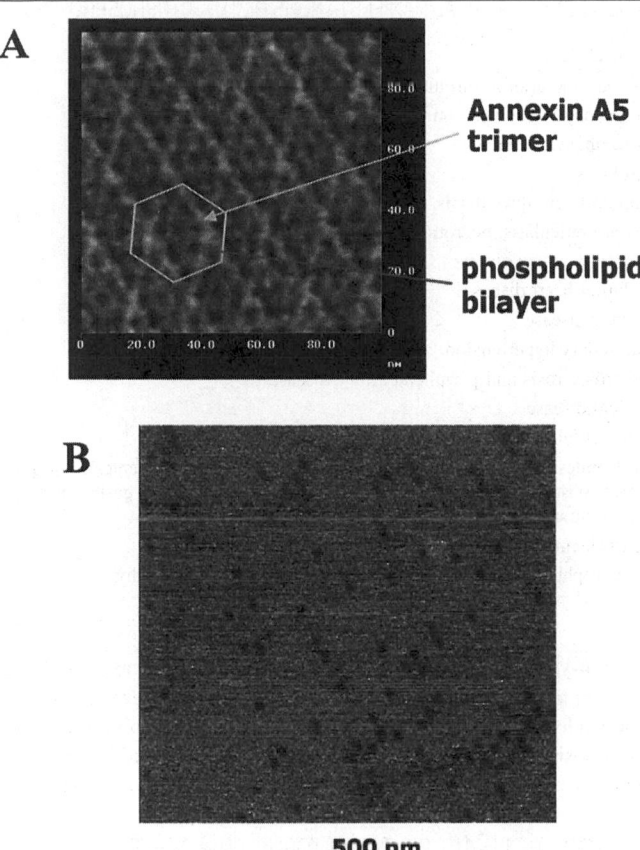

Annexin A5 trimer

phospholipid bilayer

500 nm

FIGURE 123-4 Morphologic evidence for disruption of the annexin A5 anticoagulant shield by antiphospholipid (aPL) antibodies. *(A)* Atomic force image of the two-dimensional crystallization of annexin A5 over a phospholipid bilayer. Each of the circular structures that composes each row is a trimer of annexin A5. The crystal covers nearly 100 percent of the phospholipid bilayer. *(B)* Effects of a monoclonal aPL antibody together with β_2 glycoprotein I (β_2GPI) on the crystal structure of annexin A5. aPL β_2GPI results in marked disruption of the annexin A5 crystal. (From JH Rand, XX Wu, AS Quinn, et al.,[301] with permission.)

bodies is comparable to activation by lipopolysaccharide or IL-1 but different from activation by tumor necrosis factor. aPL antibody-induced adhesion of leukocytes to endothelium with concurrent thrombosis was confirmed *in vivo* in a murine model of vascular injury, where it was shown to be mediated by ICAM-1, VCAM-1, and P-selectin.[93] As mentioned above, aPL antibodies that recognize annexin A5 induce apoptosis in endothelial cells.[82] Endothelial-derived microparticles are detectable in normal human blood and are increased in patients with LA.[94] Significantly increased plasma levels of endothelin-1, which is thought to play a role in arterial tone, vasospasm, and thrombotic arterial occlusion, were found in aPL syndrome patients with arterial thrombosis.[95] Human monoclonal aCL antibodies induced an increase in preproendothelin-1 mRNA.

Immune Complexes The IgG$_2$ subtype of aPL is most closely associated with thrombosis[87]; thus, complement fixation may play an important role in aPL-mediated thrombosis. High-titer aCL IgG antibodies have been shown to bind complement C5b-9, as demonstrated by a monoclonal antibody.[96] Also, the concentration and avidity of aPL antibodies were higher in fractions that were enriched for circulating immune complexes.[97] Blockade of complement activation using a C3 convertase inhibitor or genetic deletion of C3 protected mice from pregnancy complications induced by aPL antibodies.[98,99]

Induction of Tissue Factor Activity by Leukocytes aPL antibodies can promote tissue factor synthesis by leukocytes.[100,101] In one study, the ability of IgG to stimulate monocyte tissue factor expression was associated with decreased free protein S and increased prethrombotic markers in the plasma.[102]

Interference with Components of the Protein C Pathway The protein C pathway, one of the important endogenous antithrombotic mechanisms (see Chap. 107), is initiated when thrombin binds to thrombomodulin on endothelial cells. This binding modifies the substrate specificity of thrombin. The enzyme loses its procoagulant specificities and cleaves protein C to activated protein C (APC). In the presence of the free form of protein S, APC proteolyzes coagulation factors Va and VIIIa. aPL antibodies can interfere with the protein C system by (1) decreasing the activation of protein C by the thrombomodulin–thrombin complex; (2) inhibiting the assembly of the protein C complex; (3) inhibiting the activity of protein C, directly or via its cofactor protein S; and (4) binding to factors Va and VIIIa in a manner that protects them from proteolysis by APC.[59] In addition, some patients with aPL syndrome have protein S deficiency.[103,104]

Inhibition of the Antithrombin Pathway Antithrombin is a member of the serine protease inhibitor family. Individuals with inherited deficiencies of antithrombin are at increased risk for deep vein thrombosis (see Chap. 122). The antithrombotic activity of this protein is markedly accelerated by the presence of heparin or *in vivo* by heparan sulfate proteoglycans. At least some aPL antibodies cross-react with heparin and heparinoid molecules (which are highly polyanionic) and inhibit their effect on acceleration of antithrombin activity.[62]

Effects of Antiphospholipid Antibodies on Platelets and Eicosanoid Metabolism aPL antibodies can stimulate platelet aggregation.[105] Circulating activated (CD62-positive) platelets were detected by flow cytometry in the majority of a group of primary aPL syndrome patients with neurologic disease, suggesting the existence of a relationship among activated platelets, aCL, and the neurologic disorders.[106] Some studies have shown that aPL antibodies may alter the balance of eicosanoid synthesis toward prothrombotic moieties, as indicated by the presence of an increased quantity of thromboxane metabolites in the urine of aPL patients compared to controls.[107,108] However, other studies have not found aPL antibodies to affect eicosanoid metabolism.[109,110] Dimers of β_2GPI, which mimic effects of β_2GPI–antiβ_2GPI antibody complexes, increase platelet adhesion to collagen and thrombus formation in a flow system. These effects can be abrogated by inhibition of thromboxane synthesis.[111]

Additional Effects aPL antibodies may show cross-reactivity against oxidized LDL[63,64,66] and thereby may be associated with an increased risk of atherosclerosis.[112] Fibrinolysis has been suggested to be impaired in aPL syndrome, as females with the disorder have been described as having elevated plasminogen activator inhibitor-1 levels.[103] Fibrinolysis also may be impaired via anti-β_2GPI-mediated inhibition of the autoactivation of factor XII[113] and the ensuing reductions of kallikrein and urokinase. Autoantibodies against tissue factor pathway inhibitor[114] and tissue-type plasminogen activator[115] have been reported in patients with aPL syndrome. In a flow system, LA IgGs enhanced binding of prothrombin to phospholipid and augmented thrombin production, suggesting antibody-mediated increase in the local concentration of prothrombin as a mechanism for enhanced coagulation.[116]

Although aPL antibodies are unquestionably associated with thrombosis, a significant number of individuals with positive aPL screening tests are asymptomatic. At present, distinguishing asymptomatic individuals who are at increased risk for future thromboembolic events and pregnancy losses ("pre-aPL syndrome") from patients having antibodies that are not associated with the thrombotic disorder is not possible (see Figure 123-1). The current available data from animal models support a causal role for the antibodies in the development of thrombosis. However, the primary pathogenic process might be the exposure of thrombogenic anionic phospholipids through some other process, and the development of aPL could be the effect of autoimmune reactivity to anionic phospholipids in susceptible individuals. For example, the surfaces of apoptotic cells promote procoagulant activity,[117] and aPL antibodies have been shown to bind to phospholipid exposed by apoptotic thymocytes.[31] Thus, aPL antibodies may be both an effect and a cause of thrombosis. Anionic phospholipids, exposed during blood clotting, could trigger immunologic recognition and formation of aPL antibodies, which then could promote a vicious cycle through their thrombogenic properties. Finally, aPL could be an epiphenomenon or a surrogate marker and not directly involved in the cause and effect relationships of this disease process.

CLINICAL FEATURES

Patients generally present with thrombotic manifestations, that is, evidence for vasoocclusion or end-organ ischemia or infarction, and/or pregnancy losses and complications. The usual age of patients at the time of presentation with thrombosis is approximately 35 to 45 years,[118] with the disease rarely presenting after age 60 years.[119] Men and women are equally susceptible.[118] The thrombotic manifestations may occur in the setting of a concurrent autoimmune condition such as SLE ("secondary aPL syndrome") or as an independent autoimmune disorder ("primary aPL syndrome"). No differences have been observed between the arterial and venous distributions of thromboses of primary and secondary aPL patients.[120]

SYSTEMIC VASCULAR THROMBOSIS

Patients may present with spontaneous venous and/or arterial thrombosis or embolism, which may involve any site in the vasculature. The syndrome should be especially suspected when unusual sites are involved or when a patient experiences recurrent thromboses with no other cause.[121] Nevertheless, most patients present with deep vein thrombosis of the lower extremities, similar to most patients with venous thromboembolism and to patients with other thrombophilias.[122] In one study of patients with radiologic evidence of thrombosis, 59 percent had thrombi limited to the venous circulation, 28 percent had solely arterial thromboses, and 13 percent had both types of events.[121] Deep vein thrombosis of the legs was the most common finding, occurring in approximately half of the patients. Other sites of venous thrombotic events included pulmonary embolism, thoracic veins (superior vena cava, subclavian vein, or jugular vein), and abdominal or pelvic veins.[121] Patients may present with stroke, cerebral venous thrombosis, upper extremity venous thrombosis,[122] myocardial infarction, adrenal infarction, acalculous gallbladder infarction, aortic thrombosis with renal infarction,[123] and mesenteric artery thrombosis[124] (Table 123-2).

Thrombosis may occur spontaneously or in the presence of a predisposing factor such as estrogen hormone replacement therapy, oral contraceptives,[120,125] vascular stasis, surgery, or trauma. Women are at particularly high risk for venous thrombosis during pregnancy and in the postpartum period.[120] Some patients with venous thrombosis, but generally not with arterial thrombosis,[126] have concurrent genetic thrombophilic conditions such as heterozygosity for the factor V Leiden polymorphism.[126–129] Having a history of a thromboembolic event is a major risk factor for future thromboembolism. The risk of recurrence increases to approximately 30 percent in patients with a first episode of venous thromboembolism who also have aCL antibodies.[130] The risk of recurrence correlates with the titer of antibodies.[130]

TABLE 123-2   CLINICAL MANIFESTATIONS OF THE ANTIPHOSPHOLIPID SYNDROME

Venous and arterial thromboembolism
Pregnancy losses and complications
Thrombocytopenia
Stroke
Cerebral vein thrombosis
Livedo reticularis, necrotizing skin vasculitis
Coronary artery disease
Valvular heart disease
Kidney disease
Pulmonary hypertension, acute respiratory distress syndrome
Atherosclerosis and peripheral artery disease
Retinal disease
Adrenal failure, hemorrhagic adrenal infarction
Gastrointestinal manifestations: Budd-Chiari syndrome, mesenteric and portal vein obstructions, hepatic infarction, esophageal necrosis, gastric and colonic ulceration, gallbladder necrosis
Sensorineural hearing loss
Catastrophic antiphospholipid syndrome with microangiopathy

A 4-year prospective study of 360 patients with aPL antibodies reported that previous thrombosis and aCL titer greater than 40 U are independent predictors of thrombosis.[131] Remarkably, other than thrombosis, hematologic malignancies including non-Hodgkin lymphoma were the major causes of death in this group of patients.

SYSTEMIC LUPUS ERYTHEMATOSUS AND OTHER AUTOIMMUNE CONDITIONS

aPL syndrome is classified within the category of autoimmune disorders. Patients may have concurrent features of other autoimmune conditions such as SLE. From 0 to 40 percent of SLE patients have elevated levels of aPL antibodies. In one study of 47 patients with SLE and aPL antibodies who were diagnosed with aPL syndrome, approximately 50 percent had thrombosis, approximately 50 percent had thrombocytopenia, and approximately 40 percent had neuropsychiatric manifestations, consisting mainly of cerebrovascular ischemic disease.[132] Immune thrombocytopenia probably is the most common concurrent condition in patients with aPL syndrome. aPL syndrome has been associated with myasthenia gravis,[133] Budd-Chiari syndrome in the setting of SLE,[134] Graves disease,[135] autoimmune hemolytic anemia, progressive systemic sclerosis,[136] Evan syndrome,[137] and secondary Sjögren syndrome in the presence of SLE.[138] A direct association between relapsing polychondritis and aPL syndrome is not evident.[139] The elevated levels of aPL antibodies in patients with that disorder appear to occur in the individuals who also have SLE. aCL antibodies are present early in the course of giant cell arteritis and disappear within a few weeks of initiating corticosteroid therapy.[140] Takayasu arteritis[141] and polyarteritis nodosa[142] have been associated with aPL syndrome.

STROKE AND OTHER NEUROLOGIC CONDITIONS

Prospective analysis for the presence of aPL antibodies in stroke patients in the Antiphospholipid Antibody Stroke Study (APASS) demonstrated that elevated levels of aCL antibodies are associated with increased risk for developing stroke but not with subsequent thromboembolic events.[143] However, patients who tested positive for both aCL and LA tended to have more subsequent thromboocclusive events than patients who tested negative for both (31.7% vs. 24.0%, $p = 0.07$).[144] aPL syndrome should be suspected in young patients with transient ischemic attacks or stroke, particularly when the usual risk factors for cerebrovascular disease are absent.[145] aPL-associated stroke has been reported with other medical conditions, such as Crohn disease[146] and liver transplantation.[147] Although most aPL patients presenting with stroke have arterial thromboembolic strokes that are clinically indistinguishable from arteriosclerotic strokes in general patients, some aPL patients actually have cerebral venous thrombosis.[148] aPL patients with cerebral venous thrombosis tend to be younger and have more extensive involvement of the venous system than do aPL-negative patients with the disorder.[148] In one series of 40 cases of cerebral venous thrombosis, three patients (8%) had elevated aPL antibody levels, and two of these three patients were heterozygous for the factor V Leiden polymorphism.[149] Superior sagittal sinus thrombosis is associated with primary aPL syndrome.[150]

Additional neurologic abnormalities associated with aPL antibodies include seizures, chorea, migraines, Guillain-Barré syndrome, transient global amnesia, dementia, diabetic peripheral neuropathy, and orthostatic hypotension.[151] Recurrent acute transverse myelopathy has been described with aPL syndrome.[152–156] However, in one study of 315 SLE patients, including 10 with a history of transverse myelopathy, the disorder was not associated with aPL antibodies.[157] A high incidence of elevated aCL antibody levels occurs in patients with multiple sclerosis (in one series, 9% had IgG antibodies and 44% had IgM antibodies).[158] However, no clinical distinction has been observed between aPL-positive and aPL-negative multiple sclerosis patients. The significance of the antibodies in this disease is not known. An increased prevalence of LA and aCL antibodies in psychotic patients, even in the absence of chlorpromazine or other antipsychotic drugs, has been reported.[159] In this study, 32 percent (11/34) of the unmedicated psychotic patients had laboratory evidence for aPL antibodies.[159]

CATASTROPHIC ANTIPHOSPHOLIPID SYNDROME

The catastrophic aPL syndrome (CAPS), a rare form of the syndrome, is characterized by severe widespread vascular occlusions, sometimes leading to death. Patients present with evidence for severe multiorgan ischemia/infarction, usually with concurrent microvascular thrombosis. Patients with CAPS can present with massive venous thromboembolism, respiratory failure, stroke, abnormal liver enzymes, renal impairment, adrenal insufficiency, and areas of cutaneous infarction. Respiratory failure usually results from acute respiratory distress syndrome (ARDS) and diffuse alveolar hemorrhage. Laboratory evidence for disseminated intravascular coagulation is frequently present. Reviews of 130 patients with CAPS showed that a majority were female, with a mean age in the late thirties but ranging from childhood to old age.[160,161] Most had either primary aPL syndrome or SLE. A minority had other autoimmune conditions including Sjögren syndrome, scleroderma, and rheumatoid arthritis. Precipitating factors believed to contribute to the development of CAPS in some patients included infections, drugs (sulfur-containing diuretics, captopril, oral contraceptives), surgical procedures, and cessation of prior anticoagulant therapy. Patients usually presented with multiple organ failure that develop over a very short period of time. Most patients manifested evidence of microangiopathy affecting predominantly small vessels of the kidneys, lungs, brain, heart, and liver. Only a minority of patients experienced large-vessel occlusions. Death occurred in approximately half of patients, but relapse was rare in survivors. Preliminary CAPS classification criteria and treatment guidelines were accepted during the 10th International Congress on aPL.[162,163] Diagnostic criteria include evidence of involvement of at least three organs, systems, and/or tissues, development of manifestations simultaneously or in less than 1 week, histopathologic confirmation of small-vessel occlusion, and laboratory confirmation of the presence of aPL.[163]

PREGNANCY LOSSES, OBSTETRIC COMPLICATIONS, AND INFERTILITY

For a comprehensive review of the topic, see Galli and Barbui.[164] Most studies have estimated the prevalence of aPL antibodies among general obstetric populations to be approximately 5 percent or less. Most patients are not clinically affected.[165] Among obstetric patients with recurrent fetal losses, approximately 16 to 38 percent of patients have aPL antibodies.

Women with aPL syndrome often present with a history of recurrent (usually defined as three or more) pregnancy losses. Pregnancies occurring in women with aPL antibodies are at significantly increased risk for miscarriage, prematurity, intrauterine growth retardation, and preeclampsia.[166] Pregnancy losses including stillbirth occur in the second trimester or later, but in approximately half of patients they also occur in the first trimester. Pregnant patients with aPL syndrome are more prone to developing deep vein thrombosis during pregnancy or the puerperium. Rarely, pregnant patients develop CAPS.[167,168] The best predictor for pregnancy loss in a patient who tests positive for aPL antibodies is not the degree of laboratory abnormality but whether the patient has a history of previous pregnancy loss or thrombosis.[131,169]

Coagulation mechanisms are activated in pregnant women with aPL syndrome. Prothrombin activation fragment F1.2, a marker for thrombin generation, is increased in pregnant patients with aPL antibodies and a previous history of pregnancy losses compared to control healthy non-aPL pregnant women.[170] Histologic abnormalities were found in many, but not all, placentas of aPL patients.[171] One study did not define a morphologic lesion specific for aPL syndrome but did describe a higher frequency of decreased vasculosyncytial membranes, the presence of villous fibrosis, hypovascular villi, increased syncytial knots, and evidence of thrombosis or infarction.[172] Studies of placental pathology in patients with aPL antibodies but without a prior history of fetal loss showed that approximately half had uteroplacental vascular pathology, approximately half had evidence of thrombotic occlusion, and approximately one third had chronic villitis and/or decidual plasma cell infiltrates.[173,174]

Thrombotic occlusions and vascular pathology may be consequences of the marked decrease of the placental anticoagulant protein annexin A5, which has been described on the apical membranes of aPL placental syncytiotrophoblasts.[79] Reduction of this protein, which normally coats the interface between the maternal and fetal circulations, may disrupt a constitutive antithrombotic mechanism within the intervillous blood circulation.[73,76] This process accelerates coagulation within the maternal side of the maternal–fetal interface.

Controversy exists about whether aPL syndrome is a cause of reproductive failure (i.e., infertility) in patients undergoing *in vitro* fertilization. Although most studies have reported an increased prevalence of elevated aPL antibody levels among women undergoing *in vitro* fertilization, prospective studies demonstrate that the presence of aPL antibodies does not significantly affect either the implantation or ongoing pregnancy rates.[175] A randomized trial of heparin and aspirin for women with *in vitro* fertilization failure and aPL antibodies did not show any improvement in pregnancy or implantation rates.[176]

BLEEDING

Occasional patients with aPL syndrome exhibit a bleeding tendency. The presence of a concurrent coagulopathy needs to be excluded in these patients (Table 123-3). Severe bleeding because of acquired hypoprothrombinemia has been reported.[177,178] The diagnosis may be missed when coagulation abnormalities are attributed only to the LA effect, so a specific assay for prothrombin should be performed when the prothrombin time is prolonged. Other associated bleeding causes

TABLE 123-3 CAUSES OF BLEEDING IN THE ANTIPHOSPHOLIPID
SYNDROME

Hypoprothrombinemia
Thrombocytopenia
Acquired platelet function abnormality
Acquired inhibitor to specific coagulation factor, e.g., factor VIII

in aPL syndrome include acquired thrombocytopathies, associated thrombocytopenia (usually immune mediated), and acquired inhibitors against specific coagulation factors, such as factor VIII.

CUTANEOUS MANIFESTATIONS

Cutaneous manifestations may occur as the first sign of aPL syndrome.[179] Noninflammatory vascular thrombosis is the most frequent histopathologic feature observed. Livedo reticularis is relatively common, occurring in 24 percent of a series of 1000 aPL patients,[180] and occasionally presents in a necrosing form.[181] Necrotizing vasculitis, livedoid vasculitis, thrombophlebitis, cutaneous ulceration and necrosis, erythematous macules, purpura, ecchymoses, painful skin nodules, and subungual splinter hemorrhages can occur. Rarely, aPL syndrome is associated with anetoderma (macular atrophy), discoid lupus erythematosus, cutaneous T cell lymphoma, or disorders that closely resemble Sneddon or Degos syndromes. Patients with systemic sclerosis who are aCL positive have more widespread skin and visceral involvement than those who are aCL negative with the disorder.[182]

CORONARY ARTERY DISEASE

aPL antibodies have been associated with increased susceptibility to coronary artery disease, particularly premature atherosclerosis.[183] Antiprothrombin antibodies reportedly were a predictor of myocardial infarction in middle-aged men, and one study found that the joint effect of antiprothrombin antibodies with other known risk factors was multiplicative.[184] Coronary artery disease appears to be associated with antibodies against oxidized LDL. aPL syndrome should be considered in patients who lack the usual risk factors for coronary artery disease or who have evidence for thrombotic or embolic coronary occlusion without angiographic evidence of atherosclerotic disease. aPL antibodies appear to be a risk factor for restenosis after percutaneous transluminal coronary angioplasty, where restenosis with recurrent ischaemia appears to occur earlier and more frequently.[185,186]

VALVULAR HEART DISEASE

Approximately 35 percent of patients with primary aPL syndrome have cardiac valvular abnormalities detected by echocardiography.[187] Approximately 20 percent of cardiac patients with valvular heart disease have evidence for aPL antibodies compared with approximately 10 percent of matched control subjects.[188] Valvular abnormalities occur in approximately half of patients with SLE and aPL antibodies (Figure 123-5). Valvulopathy includes leaflet thickening, vegetations, regurgitation, and stenosis.[189] The mitral valve is mainly affected, followed by the aortic valve.[190] aPL syndrome valvular lesions consist mainly of superficial or intravalvular fibrin deposits in association with variable degrees of vascular proliferation, fibroblast influx, fibrosis, and calcification. These conditions result in valve thickening, fusion, and rigidity, sometimes leading to functional abnormalities. Inflammation is not a prominent feature of this lesion.[191] Deposits of immunoglobulins, including aCL antibodies, and of complement components are common in the affected valves of patients with primary and secondary aPL syndrome.[192] In a prospective followup of 89 patients with severe, nonspecific valvular heart disease, thromboembolic

events were significantly more frequent in the aPL-positive group than in the aPL-negative group. However, presence of aPLs was not an independent risk factor for thromboembolic events in the multivariate analysis.[193] One study of patients with SLE, progressive systemic sclerosis, rheumatoid arthritis, and primary aPL syndrome did not find a relationship between increased aCL antibodies and valvular abnormalities.[194]

PERIPHERAL VASCULAR DISEASE

One prospective study found that approximately one third of patients with peripheral arterial disease undergoing bypass grafting procedures had elevated aPL antibody levels (mostly aCL antibodies).[195] Although these patients did not appear to be at increased risk for reocclusion, this finding may have been the result of the higher frequency of anticoagulant therapy given to these patients. An unusual pattern of premature aortoiliac atherosclerosis in women younger than 50 years appears to be associated with the presence of aPL antibodies in approximately 40 percent of patients.[196] Intraarterial thromboembolic events are common at presentation and complicate surgical management.

PULMONARY MANIFESTATIONS

In addition to pulmonary thromboembolism, patients with aPL syndrome may present with *in situ* thrombosis in pulmonary vessels. aPL antibodies have been described in patients with pulmonary hypertension.[197–199] In one prospective trial of 38 consecutive patients with precapillary pulmonary hypertension, approximately 30 percent had aPL antibodies with various phospholipid specificities.[198] aPL syndrome has been diagnosed in patients presenting with refractory noninflammatory pulmonary vasculopathy.[200,201] The majority of patients with CAPS, described above in "Catastrophic aPL Syndrome," have dyspnea, and most of these individuals have ARDS.[160]

GASTROINTESTINAL MANIFESTATIONS

Gastrointestinal manifestations of aPL syndrome include Budd-Chiari syndrome, hepatic infarction, esophageal necrosis with perforation, intestinal ischemia and infarction, pancreatitis, and colonic ulceration. Primary biliary cirrhosis,[202] acute acalculous cholecystitis with gallbladder necrosis,[203,204] and giant gastric ulceration have been associated with aPL antibody syndrome.[205] Cases of primary aPL syndrome associated with mesenteric inflammatory venoocclusive disease[206] and with mesenteric and portal venous obstruction[207] have been reported.

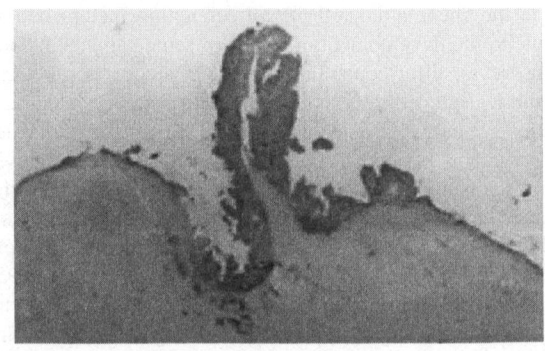

FIGURE 123-5 Verrucose lesion of the mitral valve from a patient with antiphospholipid syndrome secondary to systemic lupus erythematosus. (From M Hojnik, J George, L Ziporen, Y Shoenfeld,[190] with permission.)

THROMBOCYTOPENIA

Approximately 20 to 40 percent of patients with aPL syndrome have varying degrees of thrombocytopenia. The thrombocytopenia usually is mild or moderate and rarely is significant enough to cause bleeding complications or affect anticoagulant therapy.[208,209] Most cases appear to be immune mediated. Whether aPL antibodies themselves can directly reduce platelet counts or whether the thrombocytopenia reflects a common autoimmune background mediated by different antibody populations is not clear. Antibodies directed against major platelet membrane glycoproteins may play a role in the thrombocytopenia. According to one study, the majority of patients with aPL syndrome and thrombocytopenia had antibodies against glycoprotein IIb/IIIa (GPIIa-IIIa) complex and/or GPIb-IX complex.[210] However, in another study, no correlation was found between the presence of antibodies against platelet GPIIb-IIIa, GPIb-IX, and thrombocytopenia, and the eluted platelet antibodies did not have any LA activity.[211] Conversely, aPL antibodies and antibodies against platelet membrane glycoprotein were present simultaneously in approximately 70 percent of patients with immune-mediated thrombocytopenia.[212] In a prospective cohort study, 5-year thrombosis-free survival of aPL-positive and aPL-negative ITP patients was 39 percent and 98 percent, respectively,[213] indicating that thrombocytopenia itself is not protective against thrombosis in these patients.

RETINAL ABNORMALITIES

The diagnosis of aPL antibody retinopathy should be suspected in patients with diffuse retinal vasoocclusion, particularly when characterized by involvement of arteries and veins, neovascularization at presentation, and symptoms of systemic rheumatologic disease.[214] aPL antibodies were present in 5 to 33 percent of patients with retinal vein occlusion.[215,216] Cilioretinal artery occlusion,[217] optic neuropathy,[218] and severe vasoocclusive retinopathy[219] have been described with aPL syndrome.

LIVER DISEASES

aPL antibody levels frequently are elevated in patients with chronic liver disease of various causes. In one prospective study of patients with liver disease, approximately half of patients with alcoholic liver disease and one third of patients with chronic hepatitis C virus had elevated aPL antibody levels. The frequency was even higher in patients with more severe cirrhosis.[220] In another study, 22 percent of patients with chronic hepatitis C had aCL antibodies.[26] Because hepatitis C infection has been associated with other autoimmune disorders, such as rheumatoid arthritis, SLE, polymyositis, and thyroid disease,[221] aPL antibodies in this condition also may be autoimmune in origin. In hepatitis C virus-infected patients with manifestations of aPL syndrome, the most common features were intraabdominal thrombosis and myocardial infarction.[222]

KIDNEY DISEASES

aPL syndrome may affect the renal system. Patients may present with renal artery stenosis and/or thrombosis, renal infarction, renal vein thrombosis, and glomerulonephritis that is distinct from vasoocclusive disease.[180,223] An entity named "aPL syndrome nephropathy" has been described, which consists of a vasoocclusive disease of small-size intrarenal vessels.[224] This nephropathy features fibrous intimal hyperplasia, focal cortical atrophy, and thrombotic microangiopathy. A review of 29 consecutive renal biopsies from patients with primary aPL syndrome, performed at two institutions over 22 years, described 20 cases of aPL syndrome nephropathy and nine cases with other distinct pathologic features.[223] These features included membranous nephropathy, minimal change disease/focal segmental glomerulonephritis, mesangial C3 nephropathy, and pauci-immune crescentic glomerulonephritis.

"SERONEGATIVE" ANTIPHOSPHOLIPID SYNDROME

Some patients present with the clinical picture of aPL syndrome, but they have no laboratory evidence of aPL in their serum at the time of initial presentation and develop laboratory evidence for the antibodies several months later (see Figure 123-1).[225]

ANTIPHOSPHOLIPID SYNDROME AND ACQUIRED IMMUNODEFICIENCY SYNDROME

Although patients with HIV-1 infection frequently have elevated aPL antibody levels, they rarely have thrombotic manifestations. In one series, 64 percent of HIV-1 patients had elevated aCL antibody levels.[226] However, most of these positive patients also had antibodies against phosphatidyl choline and very few had antibodies to β_2GPI, antiprothrombin antibodies, LA, BFP syphilis, or thrombosis.[226] In HIV-infected patients with manifestations of aPL syndrome, the most common features were avascular bone and cutaneous necrosis.[222]

ANTIPHOSPHOLIPID SYNDROME IN CHILDREN

aPL syndrome has been reported among pediatric patients in whom diverse clinical features are common as in adults.[197] aPL-related thrombosis seems to constitute a significant proportion of childhood thromboses. Approximately one third of children suffering a thrombotic event have circulating aPL antibodies, and more than two thirds of children with idiopathic cerebral ischemia have evidence of elevated aPL antibody levels.[227] One study reported a high prevalence of aCL antibody levels in children (7/10) who suffered acute cerebral infarction.[228] A variety of neurologic disorders, including migraine, benign intracranial hypertension, and unilateral movement disorders, such as hemichorea and hemidystonia other than stroke, have been associated with aPL antibodies in children.[229] The catastrophic form of the syndrome is rare in children.[230]

OTHER MANIFESTATIONS

Acute adrenal failure secondary to bilateral infarction of the adrenal glands has been reported as the first manifestation of primary aPL syndrome.[231] Adrenal hemorrhage has been reported.[232] aPL antibodies have been associated with bone marrow necrosis.[233] Sudden acute sensorineural hearing loss in patients with SLE or lupus-like syndromes has been described as a manifestation of aPL syndrome.[234]

LABORATORY FEATURES

Diagnosis of aPL syndrome requires the demonstration of antibodies against phospholipids and/or relevant protein cofactors. This determination is most commonly obtained through immunoassays that detect aCL, antiphosphatidyl serine, anti-β_2GPI, or antiprothrombin antibodies or through evidence for interference with phospholipid-dependent coagulation assays known as the "lupus anticoagulant" phenomenon (Table 123-4). The laboratory diagnosis of aPL syndrome frequently is problematic. Research criteria have been developed to identify patients with the "definite" autoimmune aPL syndrome[235] (Table 123-5). These criteria are not for clinical diagnostic use but are designed for clinical research studies. At present, no single test is sufficient for diagnosing the disorder. Therefore, when the disorder is suspected, a panel of tests, including syphilis testing, antibodies against cardiolipin, phosphatidyl serine, and β_2GPI, and coagulation tests for LA should be performed.

TABLE 123-4 DIAGNOSTIC TESTS FOR THE ANTIPHOSPHOLIPID SYNDROME

Immunoassays
  Serologic test for syphilis ("biologic false positive")
  Anticardiolipin antibodies
  Antiphosphatidyl serine antibodies
  Anti–β_2GPI antibodies
  Antiprothrombin antibodies
Coagulation Tests
  aPTT with mixing incubation studies, aPL-sensitive and insensitive reagents and platelet neutralization procedure
  Dilute Russell viper venom time
  Kaolin clotting time
  Tissue thromboplastin inhibition test
  Hexagonal phase array test
  Textarin/Ecarin test

APL = antiphospholipid; aPTT = activated partial thromboplastin time; β_2GPI = β_2 glycoprotein I.

IMMUNOASSAYS

ANTICARDIOLIPIN ANTIBODY ASSAYS

Most patients with the condition are identified by elevated levels of aCL antibodies. The precursor of this assay, the "biologic false-positive" VDRL test for syphilis, in which cardiolipin is the primary antigen, is itself a qualitative aPL test. High levels of aCL antibodies are predictive for an increased risk of thrombosis. During a 10-year followup of patients with elevated levels of aCL antibodies, approximately 50 percent of patients who presented with the antibodies but without clinical manifestations of the syndrome subsequently developed the syndrome.[236] The presence of elevated titers of aCL antibodies 6 months after an episode of venous thromboembolism is a predictor for increased risk of recurrence and of death.[130] Women with IgM antibodies, IgG aCL antibody titer less than 20 IgG binding units, and no LA do not appear to be at risk for aPL syndrome.[237] In contrast, women with an IgG aCL titer greater than 20 binding units or a positive LA were more likely to develop complications.[237] With respect to stroke, elevated levels of aCL antibodies of IgG or IgM isotype are a significant risk factor.[238] aPL antibodies also are an independent risk factor for stroke in young women.[239] In APASS, 41 percent of patients who met study criteria, including those who experienced an ischemic stroke within 30 days, tested aPL positive.[144]

As mentioned previously, most patients found to have elevated aCL antibodies during the course of general screening studies do not have aPL syndrome. The prevalence of positive tests in the asymptomatic "normal" population has generally ranged from approximately 3 to 10 percent. In a prospective study of 2132 consecutive Spanish patients with venous thromboembolism, 4.1 percent had elevated levels of aCL antibodies (i.e., about the same prevalence as in the asymptomatic healthy population).[240] In a group of healthy young women, 18.2 percent had elevated levels of aCL antibodies and 12.8 percent tested LA positive.[241] Many individuals have antibody levels that are elevated in response to microbial infections and are not associated with thrombotic complications. Patients with syphilis, Lyme disease, and other infections may be misdiagnosed with aPL syndrome based on elevated aCL antibody levels when concurrent stroke or arterial thrombosis is present, so these conditions must always be ruled out in susceptible patients.

aPL syndrome has been described primarily with elevated levels of aCL IgG antibodies, but it also occurs with elevated levels of IgM antibodies. aCL antibody isotype distributions may vary in different ethnic groups.[242] Although all four IgG subclasses are found in auto-

immune aCL, the presence of IgG2 is significantly associated with thrombotic complications.[243] A polymorphism in the Fcγ receptor IIA expressed on platelets, monocytes, and endothelial cells efficiently recognizing IgG2 may be a genetic marker for aPL syndrome.[244,245] This polymorphism affects predisposition to aPL syndrome under a recessive model, whereas it confers risk for SLE in an additive manner.[246]

In a systematic literature review, 15 of 28 studies showed significant associations between aCL antibodies and thrombosis.[247] In all cases, a correlation existed between higher antibody titers and high odds ratios for thrombosis. Elevated levels of aCL antibodies, whether high or low titer, were significantly associated with both myocardial infarction and cerebral stroke. Only high-titer aCL antibodies significantly increased the risk of deep vein thrombosis.

Some patients with elevated IgA aCL antibodies with aPL syndrome have been reported. However, determination of IgA aCL antibodies does not appear to be helpful in diagnosing aPL syndrome or in explaining thrombotic events or fetal loss because the prevalence of true positivity to IgA aCL antibodies is extremely low. For example, in one study of 795 patients, IgA aPL was found in only two patients, both of whom were also positive to IgG aPL.[248] This finding is in contrast to IgA anti-β_2GPI antibodies, which appear to be significantly associated with thrombosis.[247]

Approximately 20 percent of patients taking procainamide have moderate to high levels of aCL antibodies.[249] In these patients, the antibodies are associated with anti-β_2GPI specificity. However, the predictive significance of procainamide-induced aPL for thrombosis is not known. Treatment with chlorpromazine is frequently associated with the development of aCL antibodies. These antibodies are rarely associated with thrombosis,[250] and whether they are cofactor dependent is not clear.

ANTIPHOSPHATIDYL SERINE ANTIBODY ASSAY

Because cardiolipin is present in intracellular membranes and is not exposed to coagulation proteins *in vivo*, tests for antibodies against phosphatidyl serine, which is normally present in the inner leaflet of the plasma membrane, have been hypothesized to be more relevant pathophysiologically. Phosphatidyl serine is also exposed on syncytialized cells, on apoptotic cells, and on activated platelets. Antibodies to phosphatidyl serine (aPS) correlate more specifically with aPL syndrome than aCL antibodies, particularly in arterial thrombosis.[251,252]

ASSAYS FOR ANTIBODIES AGAINST OTHER PHOSPHOLIPIDS

Antibodies against the zwitterionic phospholipid phosphatidyl ethanolamine have been associated with thrombosis and APC resistance.[253]

TABLE 123-5 SAPPORO INVESTIGATIONAL CRITERIA FOR DIAGNOSIS OF ANTIPHOSPHOLIPID SYNDROME.[235]

Clinical
  Vascular thromboses (one or more episodes of arterial, venous, or small-vessel thrombosis)
  Pregnancy morbidity
Laboratory
  aCL IgG and/or IgM antibody present in medium or high titer on two or more occasions, at least 6 weeks apart, measured by standard ELISA for β_2GPI-dependent aCL antibodies
  Lupus anticoagulant in plasma, on two or more occasions, at least 6 weeks apart
Definite aPL syndrome is considered to be present if at least one of the clinical criteria and one of the laboratory criteria are met.

aCL = anticardiolipin; aPL = antiphospholipid; β_2GPI = β_2 glycoprotein I; ELISA = enzyme-linked immunosorbent assay; Ig = immunoglobulin.

Some studies have suggested that antiphosphatidyl ethanolamine antibodies occur in aPL syndrome in the absence of antibodies against cardiolipin or other anionic phospholipids.[254] Some investigators have advocated testing for antibodies against a panel of phospholipids other than cardiolipin,[254-257] others have disagreed,[258] and one group recommends using a mixture of anionic and zwitterionic phospholipids to test for antibodies.[259] Antiphosphatidylinositol antibodies are prevalent in young patients with cerebral ischemia.[260,261]

ANTI-β_2 GLYCOPROTEIN I ANTIBODY ASSAY

β_2GPI is believed to be the major protein cofactor for aPL antibodies. ELISAs for anti-β_2GPI antibodies are considered to be more specific but less sensitive for aPL syndrome than aCL assays.[262] Although these antibodies usually are present in conjunction with abnormal aCL and aPS antibodies, some patients with aPL syndrome present with antibodies to β_2GPI but without antibodies detectable in standard aPL assays.[263,264] Despite their higher specificity for aPL syndrome (98%), β_2GPI antibodies alone cannot be relied upon for the diagnosis because of their low sensitivity (40–50%).[265,266] Concurrent testing for aCL and aPS antibodies and LA is advised.

In a systematic literature review, 34 of 60 studies showed significant associations between anti-β_2GPI antibodies and thrombosis.[247] None of the studies were prospective. Of the 10 studies that included multivariate analysis, only two confirmed that IgG anti-β_2GPI antibodies were independent risk factors for venous thrombosis. Anti-β_2GPI antibodies were more often associated with venous than arterial events. IgA anti-β_2GPI antibodies were always significantly associated with thrombosis. Interlaboratory variation is a problem with anti-β_2GPI antibody assays.[267]

ANTIPROTHROMBIN ANTIBODY ASSAY

Prothrombin is considered the second major cofactor for aPL antibodies. In a systematic literature review, 17 of 46 studies showed significant associations between antiprothrombin antibodies and thrombosis.[247] Of the eight studies that included multivariate analysis, two confirmed that antiprothrombin antibodies were independent risk factors for thrombosis, and three other studies showed that antiprothrombin antibodies added to the risk borne by LA or aCL antibodies.

ANTIFACTOR VII/VIIA ANTIBODY ASSAY

Antibody to factor VII/VIIa was seen in 22 of 33 patients with aPL syndrome.[268] The IgM class correlated with arterial thrombosis and the IgG class with venous thrombosis.

COAGULATION TESTS

LUPUS ANTICOAGULANTS

One of the most enigmatic features of aPL syndrome is the frequent presence of the LA phenomenon *in vitro*.[269,270] Although commonly used, the term *lupus anticoagulant* is a misnomer because it is not restricted to patients with SLE. LAs act by limiting the quantity of phospholipid available to support coagulation reactions (listed in Table 123-6), thus prolonging the coagulation times. The common denominator for the various LA tests is that they detect inhibition of phospholipid-dependent blood coagulation reactions.[10] A number of different methods have been devised to detect the LA phenomenon,

TABLE 123-6 PHOSPHOLIPID-DEPENDENT COAGULATION REACTIONS

Tissue factor–factor VII (VIIa)-mediated activations of factors X and IX
Factor IXa and factor VIIIa activation of factor X to factor Xa
Factor Xa and factor Va activation of prothrombin to thrombin

including modifications of the activated partial thromboplastin time (aPTT) test with LA-sensitive and LA-insensitive reagents, kaolin clotting time, dilute Russell viper venom time (dRVVT), tissue thromboplastin inhibition time, hexagonal phase array test, and platelet neutralization procedure.

The results of LA tests can be so variable that even specialized laboratories may frequently disagree as to the results of LA tests. For example, three surveys in the United Kingdom have shown that although most laboratories can agree with regard to their identification of plasmas containing strong positive LA activity, they frequently disagree about plasmas that are known to have weak LA activity (these are missed in approximately half the cases) and frequently misdiagnose factor IX-deficient LA-negative plasmas as being LA positive.[271]

The presence of LA activity is more predictive and more specific for the occurrence of thrombosis or pregnancy loss than aCL ELISA assays in lupus patients[272] and others. In a meta-analysis of the risk for aPL-associated venous thromboembolism in individuals with aPL antibodies without underlying autoimmune disease or previous thrombosis for a 15-year period, the mean odds ratios were 1.6 for aCL antibodies, 3.2 for high titers of aCL, and 11.0 for LA.[273] In a systematic literature review, 12 of 12 studies showed significant associations between LA and thrombosis, with odds ratios from 5.7 to 9.4.[247] LA increased the risks of arterial and venous events to the same extent. Only 15 of 28 studies showed significant associations between aCL and thrombosis. In APASS,[144] positivity for both LA and aCL, but not for aCL alone, predicted a higher risk of recurrent thromboocclusive events in patients with first ischemic stroke.

In addition to their role in immunoassays for aPL antibodies, the protein cofactors play a role in LA activity.[7] In the case of β_2GPI, the LA activity of anti-β_2GPI antibodies appears to depend on their epitope specificity. Anti-β_2GPI monoclonal antibodies s directed against the third and fourth domains of β_2GPI have a LA effect, whereas anti-β_2GPI monoclonal antibodies directed against the fifth domain and the carboxy-terminal region of the fourth sushi domain show no LA-like activity.[274] Although LA can result from antiprothrombin antibodies, removal of antiprothrombin antibodies does not eliminate LA activity in the majority of plasmas.[7]

Why the LA test, a test for *in vitro* anticoagulant activity, is the marker that correlates best with *in vivo* thrombosis in aPL syndrome is not clear. Possibly the LA effect "reports" aPL antibody–phospholipid/cofactor complexes having the highest affinities and avidities for the antigens and the most potent ability to displace endogenous phospholipid-binding anticoagulant proteins that shield anionic phospholipids from participating in coagulation reactions.[78] This explanation for the LA phenomenon and a "lupus procoagulant" mechanism have been described in detail.[78]Figure 123-3 presents a model.

DILUTE RUSSELL VIPER VENOM TIME

dRVVT is considered to be one of the most sensitive of the LA tests. The test is performed by using Russell viper venom (RVV) in a system containing limiting quantities of diluted rabbit brain phospholipid. RVV directly activates coagulation factor X, leading to formation of fibrin clot. LA prolongs dRVVT by interfering with assembly of the prothrombinase complex. To ensure that prolongation of the clotting time is not a result of a factor deficiency, the procedure includes mixture of patient and control plasmas. The presence of heparin may interfere with coagulation and can yield a falsely abnormal test result unless a neutralizing agent is present.

ACTIVATED PARTIAL THROMBOPLASTIN TIME TESTS

Prolongation of the aPTT detects some LAs, and, in the general population, LAs reportedly were the most frequent cause of prolonged aPTT tests.[275] The various reagents available for performing aPTTs vary widely with regard to sensitivity to LA, so knowing which reagents are used is important. When the aPTT of a particular plasma sample is prolonged and not "correctable" by mixture with normal plasma, the presence of an "anticoagulant" or "inhibitor" should be suspected. The LA needs to be differentiated from inhibitors of specific coagulation factors and from anticoagulants such as heparin. Besides specific assays to exclude the latter two possibilities, the clinician should check whether the aPTT normalizes when an LA-insensitive aPTT reagent is used or when the assay is performed using frozen washed platelets as the source of phospholipid, a procedure referred to as the *platelet neutralization procedure*. The effects of incubation with normal plasma may be helpful in differentiating LAs from coagulation factor inhibitors. aPTTs performed on mixtures of normal plasma and plasma containing a factor VIII inhibitor usually show no prolongation immediately after mixing but marked prolongation with incubation for 1 to 2 hours at 37°C, whereas LA-containing plasmas usually prolong the aPTT immediately after mixing with normal plasma and show no further prolongation with incubation. However, in rare patients, both types of anticoagulants—LA and specific coagulation factor inhibitors—coexist. Specific coagulation factor inhibitor assays should clarify this issue. Of note, LAs may result in artifactual decreases in coagulation factor levels using the standard assays because they are based on aPTT. Patients can be misdiagnosed as having multiple coagulation factor deficiencies. This problem usually can be avoided by using an aPTT reagent that is insensitive to LA for the specific factor assays or by repeating the coagulation factor assays following dilution of the plasma samples. The latter results in complete or partial normalization of coagulation factor levels with progressive dilution.

KAOLIN CLOTTING TIME

This assay depends upon the ability of aPL antibodies to block the availability of trace quantities of phospholipid present in centrifuged plasma from participation in coagulation reactions. Some authors maintain that the kaolin clotting time–LA test reflects dependence on prothrombin as a cofactor and is less likely to be associated with thrombosis than the dRVVT, which appears to be more dependent on β_2GPI.[276,277]

TISSUE THROMBOPLASTIN INHIBITION TEST

This test is a prothrombin time assay done with diluted tissue factor–phospholipid complex. It can be performed with standard and recombinant tissue factor.[278,279] The results are expressed as a ratio of the patient to control clotting times.

HEXAGONAL PHASE ARRAY TEST

aPL antibodies can recognize phosphatidyl ethanolamine in the hexagonal phase array configuration but not in the lamellar phase. The principle of this test is that incubation of plasma with the hexagonal phase phosphatidyl ethanolamine should absorb the LA antibodies, if present, and therefore normalize a prolonged aPTT because of LA.

TEXTARIN/ECARIN TEST

This test depends on the different coagulation mechanisms initiated by two snake venoms: textarin activates prothrombin via a phospholipid-dependent pathway, and ecarin activates prothrombin even in the absence of phospholipid.[279]

DIFFERENTIAL DIAGNOSIS

Patients with aPL syndrome usually present with vascular occlusion, recurrent pregnancy losses, or abnormal coagulation screening test results. When vascular occlusion occurs in the setting of a known au-toimmune disorder such as SLE, then the possibility of vasculitis must be considered. Patients with CAPS may appear to have other multi-system vasooclusive disorders, such as thrombotic thrombocytopenic purpura or disseminated vasculitis, and may present with laboratory findings of disseminated intravascular coagulation.

The differential diagnosis of a prolonged aPTT includes hereditary and acquired coagulation factor deficiencies, inhibitors to coagulation proteins (e.g. acquired hemophilia A, see Chap. 119), and the presence, or use, of anticoagulants. The diagnosis of an LA is clarified through plasma mixing studies and specific factor assays. A positive aPL ELISA helps confirm the diagnosis.

When an elevated level aPL antibody level is detected, the clinician must consider the possibility that the patient has an infectious etiology for the antibodies. These antibodies occur frequently in syphilis, Lyme disease, HIV-1, and hepatitis C. Also, elevated antibodies may be artifactual and result from increased immunoglobulin levels.[280] In such cases, diagnosis is aided by specific tests for suspected infection, quantitative measurement of serum immunoglobulins, and subtraction of background controls using uncoated microtiter wells. Antipsychotic or other medications should be excluded as causative agents.

THERAPY, COURSE, AND PROGNOSIS

Physician opinions differ concerning treatment of patients with aPL syndrome. Prospective studies are in progress to examine the utility of specific anticoagulant regimens in the prophylaxis treatment of recurrent thromboembolism in patients with aPL antibodies. Overall, there is general agreement that patients with recurrent spontaneous thrombosis require long-term, and perhaps lifelong, anticoagulant therapy and patients with recurrent spontaneous pregnancy losses require antithrombotic therapy for most of the gestational period. Differences arise in the approach to treatment of patients with single thrombotic events, significant thrombotic events in the distant past, and thrombotic events that were not spontaneous. Opinions also vary widely on the treatment of asymptomatic pregnant women with aPL antibodies, especially if they are older or have fertility difficulties.

THROMBOSIS

No evidence indicates that acute treatment of patients presenting with thrombosis in aPL syndrome should be any different from that of patients with other thrombotic etiologies. For patients treated with intravenous unfractionated heparin, care must be taken to determine whether the patient has a preexisting LA that can interfere with aPTT monitoring of heparin levels. If so, then the heparin concentration can be estimated with one of the LA-insensitive aPTT reagents, with a specific heparin assay, or with the activated coagulation time test, which usually is insensitive to LAs. The issue of aPTT monitoring also can be handled by treatment with a low molecular weight heparin (LMWH).

Patients who experienced spontaneous thromboembolism and have evidence for aPL syndrome should be treated with long-term oral anticoagulant therapy. Studies have yielded varying results regarding the recommended intensity of anticoagulant therapy. For example, a prospective study on the treatment of venous thromboembolism concluded that an INR in the range from 2.0 to 3.0 will prevent recurrences.[130] A retrospective study of a variety of patients with aPL syndrome showed that a higher intensity (INR > 3.0) was necessary for preventing recurrences.[281] In one retrospective study, 6 of 16 patients (37%) followed over 6 to 42 months developed deep venous thrombosis despite oral anticoagulation (INR 1.5–3.0).[282] Another study of secondary aPL syndrome concluded that conventional management of thromboembolic manifestations with heparin and/or oral anticoagulants did not prevent either recurrent thromboses or fatal outcomes.[132]

A prospective randomized trial of 114 patients showed no benefit of high-intensity warfarin (INR 3.1–4.0) compared to moderate-intensity warfarin (INR 2.0–3.0) thromboprophylaxis in patients with aPL antibodies and previous thrombosis.[283] Recurrent thromboses were rare in both groups. Most patients were not treated with aspirin. Furthermore, APASS showed no benefit of warfarin (median INR 1.9) over aspirin for prevention of recurrent thromboocclusive events in aPL-positive patients with first ischemic stroke.[144] However, most patients in this study had low-positive or moderate aCL IgG titers, and the high prevalence of aPL immunoreactivity (41%) suggested that nonspecific immune activation may have caused some of the aPL antibodies.

A high titer of aCL (>30 U/ml) is not sufficient to justify prophylactic anticoagulation therapy in otherwise healthy asymptomatic patients.[282] The same conclusion can be applied to patients with LAs who have not experienced thrombotic or embolic events. Anticoagulant therapy can be considered for occasional asymptomatic patients, such as those with convincing family histories for thromboembolic complications of aPL syndrome who themselves manifest significant laboratory abnormalities, patients with SLE who have significant aPL laboratory abnormalities, and patients who have other reasons for being at increased risk for thrombosis (e.g., severe valvular heart disease).[193]

An important practical consequence of the LA effect is that prothrombin time and INR results have been reported to be falsely elevated in some patients with aPL syndrome and LAs treated with warfarin anticoagulant therapy.[284] As with aPTT, the prothrombin time reagents differ with regard to their sensitivity to LAs, and different LAs vary significantly with regard to their effects on prothrombin time.[285] Alternative tests, such as specific chromogenic coagulation factor assays for vitamin K-dependent proteins or the "prothrombin and proconvertin time," have been suggested as useful for confirming the appropriate warfarin effect in these patients.[284] However, a multicenter study found that all but one of the commercial thromboplastins in use at nine centers provided acceptable INR values for aPL syndrome patients with LA.[286] Thus, new thromboplastins should be checked for their responsiveness to LA prior to their use in monitoring oral anticoagulant treatment in patients with aPL syndrome.

Cases of fibrinolytic treatment of patients with primary aPL syndrome for extensive thrombosis of the common femoral and iliac veins extending to the lower vena cava,[287] acute ischemic stroke,[288] and acute myocardial infarction[289] have been reported. Treatment with the antimalarial drug hydroxychloroquine may have an antithrombotic effect in patients with aPL syndrome and SLE.[290,291] The potential effectiveness of this treatment has been supported by animal studies.[292]

Patients with CAPS require aggressive immunosuppressive therapy in the form of high-dose glucocorticoids in addition to anticoagulation. Second-line therapies, including intravenous immunoglobulin and/or plasma exchange, are necessary in the absence of a clinical response or in the presence of ongoing thrombosis despite treatment. Third-line treatments include fibrinolytics, cyclophosphamide, and prostacyclin.[163]

Experimental therapies for aPL syndrome include specific antiidiotypic or anti-CD4 antibodies, IL-3, ciprofloxacin or bromocriptine, and bone marrow transplantation.[293] Other new pharmacologic strategies under consideration but still unproved include statins, angiotensin-converting enzyme inhibitors to inhibit monocyte tissue factor expression, a β_2GPI-specific B cell tolerogen known as LJP 1082, and oral direct thrombin inhibitors.[101]

PREGNANCY LOSS

A systematic review of randomized trials on aPL antibody-positive women with recurrent pregnancy loss evaluated 10 trials on 627 women. Three trials on aspirin alone showed no significant reduction in pregnancy loss, whereas heparin plus aspirin (two trials) significantly reduced pregnancy loss compared to aspirin alone. Prednisone plus aspirin (two trials) resulted in a significant increase in prematurity but no significant reduction in pregnancy loss. Intravenous immunoglobulin did not add significant benefit to heparin plus aspirin (one trial), and heparin plus aspirin was superior to prednisone plus aspirin (one trial). High-dose and low-dose heparin did not show significantly different results (one trial).[294]

Women with a history of three or more spontaneous pregnancy losses and evidence of aPL antibodies should be treated with a combination of low-dose aspirin (75–81 mg/day) and prophylactic doses of unfractionated heparin. Treatment should be started as soon as pregnancy is documented and continued until delivery in order to reduce the rate of late complications.[164,295] In especially high-risk situations, induction of early delivery may be necessary. Prophylactic doses of heparin (i.e., 5000 U q 12 h subcutaneous) should be started approximately 4 to 6 hours after delivery, if significant bleeding has ceased, and continued until the patient is fully ambulatory. For patients who experienced systemic thromboembolism, oral anticoagulant therapy is warranted for at least 6 weeks after delivery. The duration of postpartum treatment for patients who did not experience vascular thrombosis or embolism is not known, although many physicians recommend prophylactic treatment for the puerperium. Treatment with LMWHs produces results similar to treatment with unfractionated heparin[296]; however, at the time of writing these drugs have not been approved in the United States for use during pregnancy. The potential benefits of LMWH include once-daily injections, decreased rate of allergic reactions, including heparin-induced thrombocytopenia, and the possibility of decreased bone loss compared to unfractionated heparins.

The presence of aPL antibodies during pregnancy, without any history of spontaneous pregnancy losses, other attributable pregnancy complications, thrombosis, or embolism, does not require treatment. A prospective study of an untreated general obstetric population found that 2 to 3 percent of nonpregnant patients had low-titer increases of aCL antibodies, with a live birth rate of approximately 60 percent among these patients. The Organizing Group of the Antiphospholipid Antibody Treatment Trial randomly assigned 19 women with one or no prior spontaneous abortions and no history of thrombosis or thrombocytopenia to low-dose aspirin or no treatment and found that both groups were at such a low risk for pregnancy losses that prophylactic therapy seemed unwarranted.[297]

Although prednisone may improve the outcomes of pregnant patients with aPL syndrome, the benefit is associated with significant toxicity.[297] Thus, both corticosteroids and intravenous IgG should be considered only for patients who are refractory to anticoagulant therapy, who have a severe immune thrombocytopenia or other significant bleeding problem, or who have a contraindication to heparin therapy. Treatment with the combination of prednisone and heparin should be avoided, when possible, because this combination markedly increases the risk of osteopenia and vertebral fractures.[298] A randomized placebo-controlled pilot study evaluated treatment of aPL-positive pregnant women with intravenous immunoglobulin.[299] All the women were treated with heparin and low-dose aspirin. No differences were observed in live birth rates or placental insufficiency, and differences in fetal growth restriction were not statistically significant. A meta-analysis failed to demonstrate a benefit of intravenous immunoglobulin in women with unexplained recurrent miscarriages; however, this finding remains controversial.[300] Hopefully the Antiphospholipid Syndrome

Collaborative Registry (APSCORE), a clinical trial that is recruiting patients at the time of writing, will contribute toward resolving questions regarding the nature, dosage, and duration of treatment.

REFERENCES

1. Hughes GR: The anticardiolipin syndrome. *Clin Exp Rheumatol* 3:285, 1985.
2. Harris EN, Hughes GRV, Gharavi AE: The antiphospholipid antibody syndrome. *J Rheumatol Suppl* 13:210, 1987.
3. Vianna JL, Khamashta MA, Ordi Ros J, et al: Comparison of the primary and secondary antiphospholipid syndrome: A European Multicenter Study of 114 patients. *Am J Med* 96:3, 1994.
4. Alarcon-Segovia D, Cabral AR: The concept and classification of antiphospholipid/cofactor syndromes. *Lupus* 5:364, 1996.
5. Roubey RA, Hoffman M: From antiphospholipid syndrome to antibody-mediated thrombosis. *Lancet* 350:1491, 1997.
6. Vermylen J, Hoylaerts MF, Arnout J: Antibody-mediated thrombosis. *Thromb Haemost* 78:420, 1997.
7. Hughes GR, Khamashta MA, Gharavi AE, Wilson WA: *Lupus* (Special Issue 8th International Symposium on Antiphospholipid Antibodies) 7(suppl 2), 1998.
8. Moore JE, Mohr CF: Biologically false positive serological tests for syphilis: Type, incidence, and cause. *J Am Med Assoc* 150:467, 1952.
9. Moore JE, Lutz WB: Natural history of systemic lupus erythematosus: Approach to its study through chronic biologic false positive reactors. *J Chronic Dis* 1:297, 1955.
10. Shapiro SS, Thiagarajan P: Lupus anticoagulants. *Prog Hemost Thromb* 6:263, 1982.
11. Bell WN, Alton HG: A brain extract as a substitute for platelet suspensions in the thromboplastin generation test. *Nature* 174:880, 1955.
12. Feinstein DI, Rapaport SI: Acquired inhibitors of blood coagulation. *Prog Hemost Thromb* 1:75, 1972.
13. Conley CL, Hartmann RC: A hemorrhagic disorder caused by circulating anticoagulant in patients with disseminated lupus erythematosus. *J Clin Invest* 31:621, 1952.
14. Bowie WEJ, Thompson JH, Pascuzzi CA, Owen GA: Thrombosis in systemic erythematosus despite circulating anticoagulants. *J Clin Invest* 62:416, 1963.
15. Beaumont JL: Acquired hemorrhagic syndrome caused by a circulating anticoagulant; inhibition of the thromboplastic function of the blood platelets; description of a specific test. *Vox Sang* 25:1, 1954.
16. Nilsson IM, Astedt B, Hedner U, Berezin D: Intrauterine death and circulating anticoagulant ("antithromboplastin"). *Acta Med Scand* 197:153, 1975.
17. Harris EN, Gharavi AE, Boey ML, et al: Anticardiolipin antibodies: Detection by radioimmunoassay and association with thrombosis in systemic lupus erythematosus. *Lancet* 2:1211, 1983.
18. Hellan M, Kuhnel E, Speiser W, et al: Familial lupus anticoagulant: A case report and review of the literature. *Blood Coagul Fibrinolysis* 9:195, 1998.
19. Sebastiani GD, Galeazzi M, Morozzi G, Marcolongo R: The immunogenetics of the antiphospholipid syndrome, anticardiolipin antibodies, and lupus anticoagulant. *Semin Arthritis Rheum* 25:414, 1996.
20. Goldstein R, Moulds JM, Smith CD, Sengar DP: MHC studies of the primary antiphospholipid antibody syndrome and of antiphospholipid antibodies in systemic lupus erythematosus. *J Rheumatol* 23:1173, 1996.
21. Granados J, Vargas AG, Drenkard C, et al: Relationship of anticardiolipin antibodies and antiphospholipid syndrome to HLA-DR7 in Mexican patients with systemic lupus erythematosus (SLE). *Lupus* 6:57, 1997.
22. Wilson WA, Gharavi AE: Genetic risk factors for aPL syndrome. *Lupus* 5:398, 1996.
23. Manco Johnson MJ, Nuss R, Key N, et al: Lupus anticoagulant and protein S deficiency in children with postvaricella purpura fulminans or thrombosis. *J Pediatr* 128:319, 1996.
24. Barcat D, Constans J, Seigneur M, et al: Deep venous thrombosis in an adult with varicella. *Rev Med Interne* 19:509, 1998.
25. Peyton BD, Cutler BS, Stewart FM: Spontaneous tibial artery thrombosis associated with varicella pneumonia and free protein S deficiency. *J Vasc Surg* 27:563, 1998.
26. Prieto J, Yuste JR, Beloqui O, et al: Anticardiolipin antibodies in chronic hepatitis C: Implication of hepatitis C virus as the cause of the antiphospholipid syndrome [see comments]. *Hepatology* 23:199, 1996.
27. Labarca JA, Rabaggliati RM, Radrigan FJ, et al: Antiphospholipid syndrome associated with cytomegalovirus infection: Case report and review. *Clin Infect Dis* 24:197, 1997.
28. Loizou S, Cazabon JK, Walport MJ, et al: Similarities of specificity and cofactor dependence in serum antiphospholipid antibodies from patients with human parvovirus B19 infection and from those with systemic lupus erythematosus. *Arthritis Rheum* 40:103, 1997.
29. Gotoh M, Matsuda J: Induction of anticardiolipin antibody and/or lupus anticoagulant in rabbits by immunization with lipoteichoic acid, lipopolysaccharide, and lipid A. *Lupus* 5:593, 1996.
30. Eschwege V, Freyssinet JM: The possible contribution of cell apoptosis and necrosis to the generation of phospholipid-binding antibodies. *Ann Med Interne Paris* 147(suppl 1):33, 1996.
31. Price BE, Rauch J, Shia MA, et al: Anti-phospholipid autoantibodies bind to apoptotic, but not viable, thymocytes in a beta 2-glycoprotein I-dependent manner. *J Immunol* 157:2201, 1996.
32. Pittoni V, Isenberg D: Apoptosis and antiphospholipid antibodies. *Semin Arthritis Rheum* 28:163, 1998.
33. Gharavi AE, Pierangeli SS, Espinola RG, et al: Antiphospholipid antibodies induced in mice by immunization with a cytomegalovirus-derived peptide cause thrombosis and activation of endothelial cells in vivo. *Arthritis Rheum* 46:545, 2002.
34. Blank M, Asherson RA, Cervera R, Shoenfeld Y: Antiphospholipid syndrome infectious origin. *J Clin Immunol* 24:12, 2004.
35. Garcia CO, Kanbour-Shakir A, Tang H, et al: Induction of experimental antiphospholipid antibody syndrome in PL/J mice following immunization with beta 2 GPI. *Am J Reprod Immunol* 37:118, 1997.
36. Matalon ST, Shoenfeld Y, Blank M, et al: Antiphosphatidylserine antibodies affect rat yolk sacs in culture: A mechanism for fetal loss in antiphospholipid syndrome. *Am J Reprod Immunol* 51:144, 2004.
37. Holers VM, Girardi G, Mo L, et al: Complement C3 activation is required for antiphospholipid antibody-induced fetal loss. *J Exp Med* 195:211, 2002.
38. Espinola RG, Liu X, Colden-Stanfield M, et al: E-Selectin mediates pathogenic effects of antiphospholipid antibodies. *J Thromb Haemost* 1:843, 2003.
39. Pierangeli SS, Liu X, Espinola R, et al: Functional analyses of patient-derived IgG monoclonal anticardiolipin antibodies using in vivo thrombosis and in vivo microcirculation models. *Thromb Haemost* 84:388, 2000.
40. George J, Afek A, Gilburd B, et al: Atherosclerosis in LDL-receptor knockout mice is accelerated by immunization with anticardiolipin antibodies. *Lupus* 6:723, 1997.
41. Nicolo D, Goldman BI, Monestier M: Reduction of atherosclerosis in low-density lipoprotein receptor-deficient mice by passive administration of antiphospholipid antibody. *Arthritis Rheum* 48:2974, 2003.
42. Jankowski M, Vreys I, Wittevrongel C, et al: Thrombogenicity of beta 2-glycoprotein I-dependent antiphospholipid antibodies in a photochemically induced thrombosis model in the hamster. *Blood* 101:157, 2003.
43. Ferrara DE, Liu X, Espinola RG, et al: Inhibition of the thrombogenic and inflammatory properties of antiphospholipid antibodies by fluvastatin in an in vivo animal model. *Arthritis Rheum* 48:3272, 2003.

44. Vila P, Hernandez MC, Lopez Fernandez MF, Batlle J: Prevalence, follow-up, and clinical significance of the anticardiolipin antibodies in normal subjects. *Thromb Haemost* 72:209, 1994.

45. Jones JV, Eastwood BJ, Jones E, et al: Antiphospholipid antibodies in a healthy population: Methods for estimating the distribution. *J Rheumatol* 22:55, 1995.

46. Ginsberg JS, Wells PS, Brill Edwards P, et al: Antiphospholipid antibodies and venous thromboembolism. *Blood* 86:3685, 1995.

47. Sorice M, Circella A, Griggi T, et al: Anticardiolipin and anti-beta 2-GPI are two distinct populations of autoantibodies. *Thromb Haemost* 75:303, 1996.

48. Galli M, Comfurius P, Maassen C, et al: Anticardiolipin antibodies (ACA) directed not to cardiolipin but to a plasma protein cofactor. *Lancet* 335:1544, 1990.

49. McNeil HP, Simpson RJ, Chesterman CN, Krilis SA: Anti-phospholipid antibodies are directed against a complex antigen that includes a lipid-binding inhibitor of coagulation: Beta 2-glycoprotein I (apolipoprotein H). *Proc Natl Acad Sci U S A* 87:4120, 1990.

50. Roubey RA, Pratt CW, Buyon JP, Winfield JB: Lupus anticoagulant activity of autoimmune antiphospholipid antibodies is dependent upon beta 2-glycoprotein I. *J Clin Invest* 90:1100, 1992.

51. Schultz DR: Antiphospholipid antibodies: Basic immunology and assays. *Semin Arthritis Rheum* 26:724, 1997.

52. Goldsmith GH, Pierangeli SS, Branch DW, et al: Inhibition of prothrombin activation by antiphospholipid antibodies and beta 2-glycoprotein 1. *Br J Haematol* 87:548, 1994.

53. Bouma B, de Groot PG, van den Elsen JM, et al: Adhesion mechanism of human beta(2)-glycoprotein I to phospholipids based on its crystal structure. *EMBO J* 18:5166, 1999.

54. Willems GM, Janssen MP, Pelsers MM, et al: Role of divalency in the high-affinity binding of anticardiolipin antibody-beta 2 glycoprotein I complexes to lipid membranes. *Biochemistry* 35:13833, 1996.

55. Pengo V, Biasiolo A, Brocco T, et al: Autoantibodies to phospholipid-binding plasma proteins in patients with thrombosis and phospholipid-reactive antibodies. *Thromb Haemost* 75:721, 1996.

56. Roubey RA, Eisenberg RA, Harper MF, Winfield JB: "Anticardiolipin" autoantibodies recognize beta 2-glycoprotein I in the absence of phospholipid. Importance of Ag density and bivalent binding. *J Immunol* 154:954, 1995.

57. Sheng Y, Reddel SW, Herzog H, et al: Impaired thrombin generation in beta 2-glycoprotein I null mice. *J Biol Chem* 276:13817, 2001.

58. Ma K, Simantov R, Zhang JC, et al: High affinity binding of beta 2-glycoprotein I to human endothelial cells is mediated by annexin II. *J Biol Chem* 275:15541, 2000.

59. de Groot PG, Horbach DA, Derksen RH: Protein C and other cofactors involved in the binding of antiphospholipid antibodies: Relation to the pathogenesis of thrombosis. *Lupus* 5:488, 1996.

60. Bidot CJ, Jy W, Horstman LL, et al: Factor VII/VIIa: A new antigen in the anti-phospholipid antibody syndrome. *Br J Haematol* 120:618, 2003.

61. Atsumi T, Khamashta MA, Amengual O, et al: Binding of anticardiolipin antibodies to protein C via beta2-glycoprotein I (beta2-GPI): A possible mechanism in the inhibitory effect of antiphospholipid antibodies on the protein C system. *Clin Exp Immunol* 112:325, 1998.

62. Shibata S, Harpel PC, Gharavi A, et al: Autoantibodies to heparin from patients with antiphospholipid antibody syndrome inhibit formation of antithrombin III-thrombin complexes. *Blood* 83:2532, 1994.

63. Witztum JL, Horkko S: The role of oxidized LDL in atherogenesis: Immunological response and anti-phospholipid antibodies. *Ann N Y Acad Sci* 811:88, 1997.

64. Horkko S, Miller E, Dudl E, et al: Antiphospholipid antibodies are directed against epitopes of oxidized phospholipids. Recognition of cardiolipin by monoclonal antibodies to epitopes of oxidized low density lipoprotein. *J Clin Invest* 98:815, 1996.

65. Horkko S, Miller E, Branch DW, et al: The epitopes for some antiphospholipid antibodies are adducts of oxidized phospholipid and beta2 glycoprotein 1 (and other proteins). *Proc Natl Acad Sci U S A* 94:10356, 1997.

66. Vaarala O, Puurunen M, Lukka M, et al: Affinity-purified cardiolipin-binding antibodies show heterogeneity in their binding to oxidized low-density lipoprotein. *Clin Exp Immunol* 104:269, 1996.

67. Amengual O, Atsumi T, Khamashta MA, et al: Autoantibodies against oxidized low-density lipoprotein in antiphospholipid syndrome. *Br J Rheumatol* 36:964, 1997.

68. Romero FI, Amengual O, Atsumi T, et al: Arterial disease in lupus and secondary antiphospholipid syndrome: Association with anti-beta2-glycoprotein I antibodies but not with antibodies against oxidized low-density lipoprotein. *Br J Rheumatol* 37:883, 1998.

69. La Rosa L, Covini G, Galperin C, et al: Anti-mitochondrial M5 type antibody represents one of the serological markers for anti-phospholipid syndrome distinct from anti-cardiolipin and anti-beta2-glycoprotein I antibodies. *Clin Exp Immunol* 112:144, 1998.

70. Andree HAM, Hermens WT, Hemker HC, Willems GM: Displacement of factor Va by annexin V, in *Phospholipid Binding and Anticoagulant Action of Annexin V*, p 73. Universitaire Pers Maastricht, The Netherlands, 1992.

71. Gerke V, Moss SE: Annexins: From structure to function. *Physiol Rev* 82:331, 2002.

72. Lyden TW, Vogt E, Ng AK, et al: Monoclonal antiphospholipid antibody reactivity against human placental trophoblast. *J Reprod Immunol* 22:1, 1992.

73. Krikun G, Lockwood CJ, Wu XX, et al: The expression of the placental anticoagulant protein, annexin V, by villous trophoblasts: Immunolocalization and in vitro regulation. *Placenta* 15:601, 1994.

74. Vogt E, Ng AK, Rote NS: Antiphosphatidylserine antibody removes annexin-V and facilitates the binding of prothrombin at the surface of a choriocarcinoma model of trophoblast differentiation. *Am J Obstet Gynecol* 177:964, 1997.

75. Rand JH, Wu XX, Andree HA, et al: Pregnancy loss in the antiphospholipid-antibody syndrome—A possible thrombogenic mechanism. *N Engl J Med* 337:154, 1997.

76. Wang X, Campos B, Kaetzel MA, Dedman JR: Annexin V is critical in the maintenance of murine placental integrity. *Am J Obstet Gynecol* 180:1008, 1999.

77. Brachvogel B, Dikschas J, Moch H, et al: Annexin A5 is not essential for skeletal development. *Mol Cell Biol* 23:2907, 2003.

78. Rand JH, Wu XX, Andree HAM, et al: Antiphospholipid antibodies accelerate plasma coagulation by inhibiting annexin-V binding to phospholipids: A "lupus procoagulant" phenomenon. *Blood* 92:1652, 1998.

79. Rand JH, Wu XX, Guller S, et al: Reduction of annexin-V (placental anticoagulant protein-I) on placental villi of women with antiphospholipid antibodies and recurrent spontaneous abortion. *Am J Obstet Gynecol* 171:1566, 1994.

80. Matsuda J, Saitoh N, Gohchi K, et al: Anti-annexin V antibody in systemic lupus erythematosus patients with lupus anticoagulant and/or anticardiolipin antibody. *Am J Hematol* 47:56, 1994.

81. Matsuda J, Gotoh M, Saitoh N, et al: Anti-annexin antibody in the sera of patients with habitual fetal loss or preeclampsia [letter]. *Thromb Res* 75:105, 1994.

82. Nakamura N, Ban T, Yamaji K, et al: Localization of the apoptosis-inducing activity of lupus anticoagulant in an annexin V-binding antibody subset. *J Clin Invest* 101:1951, 1998.

83. Dueymes M, Levy Y, Ziporen L, et al: Do some antiphospholipid antibodies target endothelial cells? *Ann Med Interne(Paris)* 147(suppl 1):22, 1996.

84. Del-Papa N, Raschi E, Catelli L, et al: Endothelial cells as a target for

antiphospholipid antibodies: Role of anti-beta 2 glycoprotein I antibodies. *Am J Reprod Immunol* 38:212, 1997.

85. Matsuda J, Gotoh M, Gohchi K, et al: Anti-endothelial cell antibodies to the endothelial hybridoma cell line (EAhy926) in systemic lupus erythematosus patients with antiphospholipid antibodies. *Br J Haematol* 97:227, 1997.

86. Navarro M, Cervera R, Teixido M, et al: Antibodies to endothelial cells and to beta 2-glycoprotein I in the antiphospholipid syndrome: Prevalence and isotype distribution. *Br J Rheumatol* 35:523, 1996.

87. Simantov R, Lo SK, Gharavi A, et al: Antiphospholipid antibodies activate vascular endothelial cells. *Lupus* 5:440, 1996.

88. Meroni PL, Papa ND, Beltrami B, et al: Modulation of endothelial cell function by antiphospholipid antibodies. *Lupus* 5:448, 1996.

89. Hanly JG, Hong C, Issekutz A: Beta 2-glycoprotein I and anticardiolipin antibody binding to resting and activated cultured human endothelial cells. *J Rheumatol* 23:1543, 1996.

90. Branch DW, Rodgers GM: Induction of endothelial cell tissue factor activity by sera from patients with antiphospholipid syndrome: A possible mechanism of thrombosis. *Am J Obstet Gynecol* 168:206, 1993.

91. Oosting JD, Derksen RH, Blokzijl L, et al: Antiphospholipid antibody positive sera enhance endothelial cell procoagulant activity—Studies in a thrombosis model. *Thromb Haemost* 68:278, 1992.

92. Raschi E, Testoni C, Bosisio D, et al: Role of the MyD88 transduction signaling pathway in endothelial activation by antiphospholipid antibodies. *Blood* 101:3495, 2003.

93. Pierangeli SS, Espinola RG, Liu X, Harris EN: Thrombogenic effects of antiphospholipid antibodies are mediated by intercellular cell adhesion molecule-1, vascular cell adhesion molecule-1, and P-selectin. *Circ Res* 88:245, 2001.

94. Combes V, Simon AC, Grau GE, et al: In vitro generation of endothelial microparticles and possible prothrombotic activity in patients with lupus anticoagulant. *J Clin Invest* 104:93, 1999.

95. Atsumi T, Khamashta MA, Haworth RS, et al: Arterial disease and thrombosis in the antiphospholipid syndrome: A pathogenic role for endothelin 1. *Arthritis Rheum* 41:800, 1998.

96. Stewart MW, Etches WS, Gordon PA: Antiphospholipid antibody-dependent C5b-9 formation. *Br J Haematol* 96:451, 1997.

97. Arfors L, Lefvert AK: Enrichment of antibodies against phospholipids in circulating immune complexes (CIC) in the anti-phospholipid syndrome (APLS). *Clin Exp Immunol* 108:47, 1997.

98. Salmon JE, Girardi G, Holers VM: Complement activation as a mediator of antiphospholipid antibody induced pregnancy loss and thrombosis. *Ann Rheum Dis* 61(suppl 2):ii46, 2002.

99. Salmon JE, Girardi G: The role of complement in the antiphospholipid syndrome. *Curr Dir Autoimmun* 7:133, 2004.

100. Martini F, Farsi A, Gori AM, et al: Antiphospholipid antibodies (aPL) increase the potential monocyte procoagulant activity in patients with systemic lupus erythematosus. *Lupus* 5:206, 1996.

101. Roubey RA: New approaches to prevention of thrombosis in the antiphospholipid syndrome: Hopes, trials, and tribulations. *Arthritis Rheum* 48:3004, 2003.

102. Reverter JC, Tassies D, Font J, et al: Hypercoagulable state in patients with antiphospholipid syndrome is related to high induced tissue factor expression on monocytes and to low free protein S. *Arterioscler Thromb Vasc Biol* 16:1319, 1996.

103. Ames PR, Tommasino C, Iannaccone L, et al: Coagulation activation and fibrinolytic imbalance in subjects with idiopathic antiphospholipid antibodies—A crucial role for acquired free protein S deficiency. *Thromb Haemost* 76:190, 1996.

104. Crowther MA, Johnston M, Weitz J, Ginsberg JS: Free protein S deficiency may be found in patients with antiphospholipid antibodies who do not have systemic lupus erythematosus. *Thromb Haemost* 76:689, 1996.

105. Lin YL, Wang CT: Activation of human platelets by the rabbit anticardiolipin antibodies. *Blood* 80:3135, 1992.

106. Emmi L, Bergamini C, Spinelli A, et al: Possible pathogenetic role of activated platelets in the primary antiphospholipid syndrome involving the central nervous system. *Ann N Y Acad Sci* 823:188, 1997.

107. Lellouche F, Martinuzzo M, Said P, et al: Imbalance of thromboxane/prostacyclin biosynthesis in patients with lupus anticoagulant. *Blood* 78:2894, 1991.

108. Kaaja R, Julkunen H, Viinikka L, Ylikorkala O: Production of prostacyclin and thromboxane in lupus pregnancies: Effect of small dose of aspirin. *Obstet Gynecol* 81:327, 1993.

109. Hasselaar P, Derksen RH, Blokzijl L, De Groot PG: Thrombosis associated with antiphospholipid antibodies cannot be explained by effects on endothelial and platelet prostanoid synthesis. *Thromb Haemost* 59:80, 1988.

110. Schinco PC, Marranca D, Bazzan M, et al: Lupus anticoagulant: Interference with in vivo prostaglandin production and with platelet sensitivity to prostacyclin. *Scand J Rheumatol* 21:124, 1992.

111. Lutters BC, Derksen RH, Tekelenburg WL, et al: Dimers of beta 2-glycoprotein I increase platelet deposition to collagen via interaction with phospholipids and the apolipoprotein E receptor 2'. *J Biol Chem* 278:33831, 2003.

112. Vaarala O: Antiphospholipid antibodies and atherosclerosis. *Lupus* 5:442, 1996.

113. Schousboe I, Rasmussen MS: Synchronized inhibition of the phospholipid mediated autoactivation of factor XII in plasma by beta 2-glycoprotein I and anti-beta 2-glycoprotein I. *Thromb Haemost* 73:798, 1995.

114. Forastiero RR, Martinuzzo ME, Broze GJ: High titers of autoantibodies to tissue factor pathway inhibitor are associated with the antiphospholipid syndrome. *J Thromb Haemost* 1:718, 2003.

115. Cugno M, Cabibbe M, Galli M, et al: Antibodies to tissue-type plasminogen activator (tPA) in patients with antiphospholipid syndrome: Evidence of interaction between the antibodies and the catalytic domain of tPA in 2 patients. *Blood* 103:2121, 2004.

116. Field SL, Hogg PJ, Daly EB, et al: Lupus anticoagulants form immune complexes with prothrombin and phospholipid that can augment thrombin production in flow. *Blood* 94:3421, 1999.

117. Casciola Rosen L, Rosen A, Petri M, Schlissel M: Surface blebs on apoptotic cells are sites of enhanced procoagulant activity: Implications for coagulation events and antigenic spread in systemic lupus erythematosus. *Proc Natl Acad Sci U S A* 93:1624, 1996.

118. Stone JH, Amend WJ, Criswell LA: Outcome of renal transplantation in systemic lupus erythematosus. *Semin Arthritis Rheum* 27:17, 1997.

119. Piette JC, Cacoub P: Antiphospholipid syndrome in the elderly: Caution. *Circulation* 97:2195, 1998.

120. Krnic BS, O'Connor CR, Looney SW, et al: A retrospective review of 61 patients with antiphospholipid syndrome. Analysis of factors influencing recurrent thrombosis. *Arch Intern Med* 157:2101, 1997.

121. Provenzale JM, Ortel TL, Allen NB: Systemic thrombosis in patients with antiphospholipid antibodies: Lesion distribution and imaging findings. *AJR Am J Roentgenol* 170:285, 1998.

122. Martinelli I, Cattaneo M, Panzeri D, et al: Risk factors for deep venous thrombosis of the upper extremities. *Ann Intern Med* 126:707, 1997.

123. Poux JM, Boudet R, Lacroix P, et al: Renal infarction and thrombosis of the infrarenal aorta in a 35-year-old man with primary antiphospholipid syndrome. *Am J Kidney Dis* 27:721, 1996.

124. Kojima E, Naito K, Iwai M, et al: Antiphospholipid syndrome complicated by thrombosis of the superior mesenteric artery, co-existence of smooth muscle hyperplasia. *Intern Med* 36:528, 1997.

125. Girolami A, Zanon E, Zanardi S, et al: Thromboembolic disease developing during oral contraceptive therapy in young females with antiphospholipid antibodies. *Blood Coagul Fibrinolysis* 7:497, 1996.

126. Montaruli B, Borchiellini A, Tamponi G, et al: Factor V Arg506→Gln mutation in patients with antiphospholipid antibodies. *Lupus* 5:303, 1996.

127. Simantov R, Lo SK, Salmon JE, et al: Factor V Leiden increases the risk of thrombosis in patients with antiphospholipid antibodies. *Thromb Res* 84:361, 1996.

128. Schutt M, Kluter H, Hagedorn GM, et al: Familial coexistence of primary antiphospholipid syndrome and factor V Leiden. *Lupus* 7:176, 1998.

129. Brenner B, Vulfsons SL, Lanir N, Nahir M: Coexistence of familial antiphospholipid syndrome and factor V Leiden: Impact on thrombotic diathesis. *Br J Haematol* 94:166, 1996.

130. Schulman S, Svenungsson E, Granqvist S: Anticardiolipin antibodies predict early recurrence of thromboembolism and death among patients with venous thromboembolism following anticoagulant therapy. Duration of Anticoagulation Study Group. *Am J Med* 104:332, 1998.

131. Finazzi G, Brancaccio V, Moia M, et al: Natural history and risk factors for thrombosis in 360 patients with antiphospholipid antibodies: A four-year prospective study from the Italian Registry. *Am J Med* 100:530, 1996.

132. Petrovic R, Petrovic M, Novicic SD, et al: Anticardiolipin antibodies and clinical spectrum of antiphospholipid syndrome in patients with systemic lupus erythematosus. *Vojnosanit Pregl* 55:23, 1998.

133. Shoenfeld Y, Lorber M, Yucel T, Yazici H: Primary antiphospholipid syndrome emerging following thymectomy for myasthenia gravis: Additional evidence for the kaleidoscope of autoimmunity [see comments]. *Lupus* 6:474, 1997.

134. Yun YY, Yoh KA, Yang HI, et al: A case of Budd-Chiari syndrome with high antiphospholipid antibody in a patient with systemic lupus erythematosus. *Korean J Intern Med* 11:82, 1996.

135. Hofbauer LC, Spitzweg C, Heufelder AE: Graves' disease associated with the primary antiphospholipid syndrome. *J Rheumatol* 23:1435, 1996.

136. Chun WH, Bang D, Lee SK: Antiphospholipid syndrome associated with progressive systemic sclerosis. *J Dermatol* 23:347, 1996.

137. Frolow M, Jankowski M, Swadzba J, Musial J: Evans' syndrome with antiphospholipid-protein antibodies. *Pol Merkuriusz Lek* 1:344, 1996.

138. Cervera R, Garcia Carrasco M, Font J, et al: Antiphospholipid antibodies in primary Sjogren's syndrome: Prevalence and clinical significance in a series of 80 patients. *Clin Exp Rheumatol* 15:361, 1997.

139. Zeuner M, Straub RH, Schlosser U, et al: Anti-phospholipid-antibodies in patients with relapsing polychondritis. *Lupus* 7:12, 1998.

140. Meyer O, Nicaise P, Moreau S, et al: Antibodies to cardiolipin and beta 2 glycoprotein I in patients with polymyalgia rheumatica and giant cell arteritis. *Rev Rhum Engl Ed* 63:241, 1996.

141. Yokoi K, Hosoi E, Akaike M, et al: Takayasu's arteritis associated with antiphospholipid antibodies. Report of two cases. *Angiology* 47:315, 1996.

142. Dasgupta B, Almond MK, Tanqueray A: Polyarteritis nodosa and the antiphospholipid syndrome. *Br J Rheumatol* 36:1210, 1997.

143. Antiphospholipid Antibodies and Stroke Study Group (APASS): Anticardiolipin antibodies and the risk of recurrent thrombo-occlusive events and death. *Neurology* 48:91, 1997.

144. Levine SR, Brey RL, Tilley BC, et al: Antiphospholipid antibodies and subsequent thrombo-occlusive events in patients with ischemic stroke. *JAMA* 291:576, 2004.

145. Weingarten K, Filippi C, Barbut D, Zimmerman RD: The neuro-imaging features of the cardiolipin antibody syndrome. *Clin Imaging* 21:6, 1997.

146. Mevorach D, Goldberg Y, Gomori JM, Rachmilewitz D: Antiphospholipid syndrome manifested by ischemic stroke in a patient with Crohn's disease. *J Clin Gastroenterol* 22:141, 1996.

147. Bronster DJ, Gousse R, Fassas A, Rand JH: Anticardiolipin antibody-associated stroke after liver transplantation. *Transplantation* 63:908, 1997.

148. Carhuapoma JR, Mitsias P, Levine SR: Cerebral venous thrombosis and anticardiolipin antibodies. *Stroke* 28:2363, 1997.

149. Deschiens MA, Conard J, Horellou MH, et al: Coagulation studies, factor V Leiden, and anticardiolipin antibodies in 40 cases of cerebral venous thrombosis. *Stroke* 27:1724, 1996.

150. Nagai S, Horie Y, Akai T, et al: Superior sagittal sinus thrombosis associated with primary antiphospholipid syndrome—Case report. *Neurol Med Chir (Tokyo)* 38:34, 1998.

151. Brey RL, Escalante A: Neurological manifestations of antiphospholipid antibody syndrome. *Lupus* 7(suppl 2):S67, 1998.

152. Matsushita T, Kanda F, Yamada H, Chihara K: Recurrent acute transverse myelopathy: An 83-year-old man with antiphospholipid syndrome. *Rinsho Shinkeigaku* 37:987, 1997.

153. Ruiz AG, Guzman RJ, Flores FJ, Garay MJ: Refractory hiccough heralding transverse myelitis in the primary antiphospholipid syndrome. *Lupus* 7:49, 1998.

154. Takamura Y, Morimoto S, Tanooka A, Yoshikawa J: Transverse myelitis in a patient with primary antiphospholipid syndrome—A case report. *No To Shinkei* 48:851, 1996.

155. Campi A, Filippi M, Comi G, Scotti G: Recurrent acute transverse myelopathy associated with anticardiolipin antibodies. *AJNR Am J Neuroradiol* 19:781, 1998.

156. Smyth AE, Bruce IN, McMillan SA, Bell AL: Transverse myelitis: A complication of systemic lupus erythematosus that is associated with the antiphospholipid syndrome. *Ulster Med J* 65:91, 1996.

157. Mok CC, Lau CS, Chan EY, Wong RW: Acute transverse myelopathy in systemic lupus erythematosus: Clinical presentation, treatment, and outcome. *J Rheumatol* 25:467, 1998.

158. Sugiyama Y, Yamamoto T: Characterization of serum anti-phospholipid antibodies in patients with multiple sclerosis. *Tohoku J Exp Med* 178:203, 1996.

159. Schwartz M, Rochas M, Weller B, et al: High association of anticardiolipin antibodies with psychosis. *J Clin Psychiatry* 59:20, 1998.

160. Asherson RA: The catastrophic antiphospholipid syndrome 1998. A review of the clinical features, possible pathogenesis, and treatment. *Lupus* 7(suppl 2):S55, 1998.

161. Asherson RA, Cervera R, Piette JC, et al: Catastrophic antiphospholipid syndrome: Clues to the pathogenesis from a series of 80 patients. *Medicine (Baltimore)* 80:355, 2001.

162. Asherson RA, Cervera R, de Groot PG, et al: Catastrophic antiphospholipid syndrome: International consensus statement on classification criteria and treatment guidelines. *Lupus* 12:530, 2003.

163. Erkan D, Cervera R, Asherson RA: Catastrophic antiphospholipid syndrome: Where do we stand? *Arthritis Rheum* 48:3320, 2003.

164. Galli M, Barbui T: Antiphospholipid antibodies and pregnancy. *Best Pract Res Clin Haematol* 16:211, 2003.

165. Lockshin MD: Pregnancy loss and antiphospholipid antibodies. *Lupus* 7(suppl 2):S86, 1998.

166. Rai R, Regan L: Obstetric complications of antiphospholipid antibodies. *Curr Opin Obstet Gynecol* 9:387, 1997.

167. Ornstein MH, Rand JH: An association between refractory HELLP syndrome and antiphospholipid antibodies during pregnancy; a report of 2 cases. *J Rheumatol* 21:1360, 1994.

168. Neuwelt CM, Daikh DI, Linfoot JA, et al: Catastrophic antiphospholipid syndrome: Response to repeated plasmapheresis over three years. *Arthritis Rheum* 40:1534, 1997.

169. Ramsey-Goldman R, Kutzer JE, Kuller LH, et al: Pregnancy outcome and anti-cardiolipin antibody in women with systemic lupus erythematosus. *Am J Epidemiol* 138:1057, 1993.

170. Zangari M, Lockwood CJ, Scher J, Rand JH: Prothrombin activation fragment (F1.2) is increased in pregnant patients with antiphospholipid antibodies. *Thromb Res* 85:177, 1997.

171. Locatelli A, Patane L, Ghidini A, et al: Pathology findings in preterm

placentas of women with autoantibodies: A case-control study. *J Matern Fetal Neonatal Med* 11:339, 2002.

172. Out HJ, Bruinse HW, Christiaens GC, et al: Prevalence of antiphospholipid antibodies in patients with fetal loss. *Ann Rheum Dis* 50:553, 1991.

173. Salafia CM, Cowchock FS: Placental pathology and antiphospholipid antibodies: A descriptive study. *Am J Perinatol* 14:435, 1997.

174. Salafia CM, Parke AL: Placental pathology in systemic lupus erythematosus and phospholipid antibody syndrome. *Rheum Dis Clin North Am* 23:85, 1997.

175. Backos M, Rai R, Regan L: Antiphospholipid antibodies and infertility. *Hum Fertil (Camb)* 5:30, 2002.

176. Stern C, Chamley L, Norris H, et al: A randomized, double-blind, placebo-controlled trial of heparin and aspirin for women with in vitro fertilization implantation failure and antiphospholipid or antinuclear antibodies. *Fertil Steril* 80:376, 2003.

177. Vivaldi P, Rossetti G, Galli M, Finazzi G: Severe bleeding due to acquired hypoprothrombinemia-lupus anticoagulant syndrome. Case report and review of literature. *Haematologica* 82:345, 1997.

178. Hudson N, Duffy CM, Rauch J, et al: Catastrophic haemorrhage in a case of paediatric primary antiphospholipid syndrome and factor II deficiency. *Lupus* 6:68, 1997.

179. Gibson GE, Su WP, Pittelkow MR: Antiphospholipid syndrome and the skin. *J Am Acad Dermatol* 36:970, 1997.

180. Asherson RA, Cervera R: The antiphospholipid syndrome: Multiple faces beyond the classical presentation. *Autoimmun Rev* 2:140, 2003.

181. Aronoff DM, Callen JP: Necrosing livedo reticularis in a patient with recurrent pulmonary hemorrhage. *J Am Acad Dermatol* 37:300, 1997.

182. Picillo U, Migliaresi S, Marcialis MR, et al: Clinical setting of patients with systemic sclerosis by serum autoantibodies. *Clin Rheumatol* 16: 378, 1997.

183. Vaarala O: Antiphospholipid antibodies and myocardial infarction. *Lupus* 7(suppl 2):S132, 1998.

184. Vaarala O, Puurunen M, Manttari M, et al: Antibodies to prothrombin imply a risk of myocardial infarction in middle-aged men. *Thromb Haemost* 75:456, 1996.

185. Ludia C, Domenico P, Monia C, et al: Antiphospholipid antibodies: A new risk factor for restenosis after percutaneous transluminal coronary angioplasty? *Autoimmunity* 27:141, 1998.

186. Chambers-JD J, Haire HD, Deligonul U: Multiple early percutaneous transluminal coronary angioplasty failures related to lupus anticoagulant. *Am Heart J* 132:189, 1996.

187. Niaz A, Butany J: Antiphospholipid antibody syndrome with involvement of a bioprosthetic heart valve. *Can J Cardiol* 14:951, 1998.

188. Bouillanne O, Millaire A, de Groote P, et al: Prevalence and clinical significance of antiphospholipid antibodies in heart valve disease: A case-control study. *Am Heart J* 132:790, 1996.

189. Nesher G, Ilany J, Rosenmann D, Abraham AS: Valvular dysfunction in antiphospholipid syndrome: Prevalence, clinical features, and treatment. *Semin Arthritis Rheum* 27:27, 1997.

190. Hojnik M, George J, Ziporen L, Shoenfeld Y: Heart valve involvement (Libman-Sacks endocarditis) in the antiphospholipid syndrome. *Circulation* 93:1579, 1996.

191. Garcia TR, Amigo MC, De-la-Rosa A, et al: Valvular heart disease in primary antiphospholipid syndrome (PAPS): Clinical and morphological findings. *Lupus* 5:56, 1996.

192. Ziporen L, Goldberg I, Arad M, et al: Libman-Sacks endocarditis in the antiphospholipid syndrome: Immunopathologic findings in deformed heart valves. *Lupus* 5:196, 1996.

193. Bulckaen HG, Puisieux FL, Bulckaen ED, et al: Antiphospholipid an-

tibodies and the risk of thromboembolic events in valvular heart disease. *Mayo Clin Proc* 78:294, 2003.

194. Gabrielli F, Alcini E, Prima MA, et al: Cardiac involvement in connective tissue diseases and primary antiphospholipid syndrome: Echocardiographic assessment and correlation with antiphospholipid antibodies. *Acta Cardiol* 51:425, 1996.

195. Lee RW, Taylor-LM J, Landry GJ, et al: Prospective comparison of infrainguinal bypass grafting in patients with and without antiphospholipid antibodies. *J Vasc Surg* 24:524, 1996.

196. Gagne PJ, Vitti MJ, Fink LM, et al: Young women with advanced aortoiliac occlusive disease: New insights. *Ann Vasc Surg* 10:546, 1996.

197. von-Scheven E, Athreya BH, Rose CD, et al: Clinical characteristics of antiphospholipid antibody syndrome in children. *J Pediatr* 129:339, 1996.

198. Karmochkine M, Cacoub P, Dorent R, et al: High prevalence of antiphospholipid antibodies in precapillary pulmonary hypertension. *J Rheumatol* 23:286, 1996.

199. Miyashita Y, Koike H, Misawa A, et al: Asymptomatic pulmonary hypertension complicated with antiphospholipid syndrome case [see comments]. *Intern Med* 35:912, 1996.

200. Kerr JE, Poe R, Kramer Z: Antiphospholipid antibody syndrome presenting as a refractory noninflammatory pulmonary vasculopathy [see comments]. *Chest* 112:1707, 1997.

201. Maggiorini M, Knoblauch A, Schneider J, Russi EW: Diffuse microvascular pulmonary thrombosis associated with primary antiphospholipid antibody syndrome [see comments]. *Eur Respir J* 10:727, 1997.

202. Hoffman M, Burke M, Fried M, et al: Primary biliary cirrhosis associated with antiphospholipid syndrome. *Isr J Med Sci* 33:681, 1997.

203. Date K, Shirai Y, Hatakeyama K: Antiphospholipid antibody syndrome presenting as acute acalculous cholecystitis. *Am J Gastroenterol* 92: 2127, 1997.

204. Dessailloud R, Papo T, Vaneecloo S, et al: Acalculous ischemic gallbladder necrosis in the catastrophic antiphospholipid syndrome. *Arthritis Rheum* 41:1318, 1998.

205. Kalman DR, Khan A, Romain PL, Nompleggi DJ: Giant gastric ulceration associated with antiphospholipid antibody syndrome [see comments]. *Am J Gastroenterol* 91:1244, 1996.

206. Gul A, Inanc M, Ocal L, et al: Primary antiphospholipid syndrome associated with mesenteric inflammatory veno-occlusive disease. *Clin Rheumatol* 15:207, 1996.

207. Lee HJ, Park JW, Chang JC: Mesenteric and portal venous obstruction associated with primary antiphospholipid antibody syndrome. *J Gastroenterol Hepatol* 12:822, 1997.

208. Galli M, Finazzi G, Barbui T: Thrombocytopenia in the antiphospholipid syndrome. *Br J Haematol* 93:1, 1996.

209. Cuadrado MJ, Mujic F, Munoz E, et al: Thrombocytopenia in the antiphospholipid syndrome. *Ann Rheum Dis* 56:194, 1997.

210. Macchi L, Rispal P, Clofent SG, et al: Anti-platelet antibodies in patients with systemic lupus erythematosus and the primary antiphospholipid antibody syndrome: Their relationship with the observed thrombocytopenia. *Br J Haematol* 98:336, 1997.

211. Panzer S, Gschwandtner ME, Hutter D, et al: Specificities of platelet autoantibodies in patients with lupus anticoagulants in primary antiphospholipid syndrome. *Ann Hematol* 74:239, 1997.

212. Lipp E, von-Felten A, Sax H, et al: Antibodies against platelet glycoproteins and antiphospholipid antibodies in autoimmune thrombocytopenia. *Eur J Haematol* 60:283, 1998.

213. Diz-Kucukkaya R, Hacihanefioglu A, Yenerel M, et al: Antiphospholipid antibodies and antiphospholipid syndrome in patients presenting

with immune thrombocytopenic purpura: A prospective cohort study. *Blood* 98:1760, 2001.

214. Dunn JP, Noorily SW, Petri M, et al: Antiphospholipid antibodies and retinal vascular disease. *Lupus* 5:313, 1996.

215. Coniglio M, Platania A, Di Nucci GD, et al: Antiphospholipid-protein antibodies are not an uncommon feature in retinal venous occlusions. *Thromb Res* 83:183, 1996.

216. Glacet BA, Bayani N, Chretien P, et al: Antiphospholipid antibodies in retinal vascular occlusions. A prospective study of 75 patients. *Arch Ophthalmol* 112:790, 1994.

217. Dori D, Gelfand YA, Brenner B, Miller B: Cilioretinal artery occlusion: An ocular complication of primary antiphospholipid syndrome. *Retina* 17:555, 1997.

218. Reino S, Munoz RF, Cervera R, et al: Optic neuropathy in the "primary" antiphospholipid syndrome: Report of a case and review of the literature. *Clin Rheumatol* 16:629, 1997.

219. Au A, O'Day J: Review of severe vaso-occlusive retinopathy in systemic lupus erythematosus and the antiphospholipid syndrome: Associations, visual outcomes, complications and treatment. *Clin Experiment Ophthalmol* 32:87, 2004.

220. Biron C, Andreani H, Blanc P, et al: Prevalence of antiphospholipid antibodies in patients with chronic liver disease related to alcohol or hepatitis C virus: Correlation with liver injury. *J Lab Clin Med* 131:243, 1998.

221. McMurray RW: Hepatitis C-associated autoimmune disorders. *Rheum Dis Clin North Am* 24:353, 1998.

222. Ramos-Casals M, Cervera R, Lagrutta M, et al: Clinical features related to antiphospholipid syndrome in patients with chronic viral infections (hepatitis C virus/HIV infection): Description of 82 cases. *Clin Infect Dis* 38:1009, 2004.

223. Fakhouri F, Noel LH, Zuber J, et al: The expanding spectrum of renal diseases associated with antiphospholipid syndrome. *Am J Kidney Dis* 41:1205, 2003.

224. Nochy D, Daugas E, Droz D, et al: The intrarenal vascular lesions associated with primary antiphospholipid syndrome. *J Am Soc Nephrol* 10:507, 1999.

225. Miret C, Cervera R, Reverter JC, et al: Antiphospholipid syndrome without antiphospholipid antibodies at the time of the thrombotic event: Transient "seronegative" antiphospholipid syndrome? *Clin Exp Rheumatol* 15:541, 1997.

226. Abuaf N, Laperche S, Rajoely B, et al: Autoantibodies to phospholipids and to the coagulation proteins in AIDS. *Thromb Haemost* 77:856, 1997.

227. Ravelli A, Martini A: Antiphospholipid antibody syndrome in pediatric patients. *Rheum Dis Clin North Am* 23:657, 1997.

228. Baca V, Garcia RR, Ramirez LM, et al: Cerebral infarction and antiphospholipid syndrome in children. *J Rheumatol* 23:1428, 1996.

229. Angelini L, Zibordi F, Zorzi G, et al: Neurological disorders, other than stroke, associated with antiphospholipid antibodies in childhood. *Neuropediatrics* 27:149, 1996.

230. Falcini F, Taccetti G, Ermini M, et al: Catastrophic antiphospholipid antibody syndrome in pediatric systemic lupus erythematosus. *J Rheumatol* 24:389, 1997.

231. Marie I, Levesque H, Heron F, et al: Acute adrenal failure secondary to bilateral infarction of the adrenal glands as the first manifestation of primary antiphospholipid antibody syndrome [letter]. *Ann Rheum Dis* 56:567, 1997.

232. Espinosa G, Santos E, Cervera R, et al: Adrenal involvement in the antiphospholipid syndrome: Clinical and immunologic characteristics of 86 patients. *Medicine (Baltimore)* 82:106, 2003.

233. Paydas S, Kocak R, Zorludemir S, Baslamisli F: Bone marrow necrosis in antiphospholipid syndrome. *J Clin Pathol* 50:261, 1997.

234. Naarendorp M, Spiera H: Sudden sensorineural hearing loss in patients with systemic lupus erythematosus or lupus-like syndromes and antiphospholipid antibodies. *J Rheumatol* 25:589, 1998.

235. Wilson WA, Gharavi AE, Koike T, et al: International consensus statement on preliminary classification criteria for definite antiphospholipid syndrome: Report of an international workshop. *Arthritis Rheum* 42:1309, 1999.

236. Shah NM, Khamashta MA, Atsumi T, Hughes GR: Outcome of patients with anticardiolipin antibodies: A 10 year follow-up of 52 patients. *Lupus* 7:3, 1998.

237. Silver RM, Porter TF, van Leeuwen I, et al: Anticardiolipin antibodies: Clinical consequences of "low titers". *Obstet Gynecol* 87:494, 1996.

238. Tuhrim S, Rand JH, Wu XX, et al: Elevated anticardiolipin antibody titer is a stroke risk factor in a multiethnic population independent of isotype or degree of positivity. *Stroke* 30:1561, 1999.

239. Brey RL, Stallworth CL, McGlasson DL, et al: Antiphospholipid antibodies and stroke in young women. *Stroke* 33:2396, 2002.

240. Mateo J, Oliver A, Borrell M, et al: Laboratory evaluation and clinical characteristics of 2,132 consecutive unselected patients with venous thromboembolism—Results of the Spanish Multicentric Study on Thrombophilia (EMET-Study). *Thromb Haemost* 77:444, 1997.

241. Brey RL, Stallworth CL, McGlasson DL, et al: Antiphospholipid antibodies and stroke in young women. *Stroke* 33:2396, 2002.

242. Molina JF, Gutierrez US, Molina J, et al: Variability of anticardiolipin antibody isotype distribution in 3 geographic populations of patients with systemic lupus erythematosus. *J Rheumatol* 24:291, 1997.

243. Sammaritano LR: Significance of aPL IgG subclasses. *Lupus* 5:436, 1996.

244. Sammaritano LR, Ng S, Sobel R, et al: Anticardiolipin IgG subclasses: Association of IgG2 with arterial and/or venous thrombosis. *Arthritis Rheum* 40:1998, 1997.

245. Atsumi T, Caliz R, Amengual O, et al: Fcgamma receptor IIA H/R131 polymorphism in patients with antiphospholipid antibodies. *Thromb Haemost* 79:924, 1998.

246. Karassa FB, Bijl M, Davies KA, et al: Role of the Fcgamma receptor IIA polymorphism in the antiphospholipid syndrome: An international meta-analysis. *Arthritis Rheum* 48:1930, 2003.

247. Galli M, Luciani D, Bertolini G, Barbui T: Anti-beta 2-glycoprotein I, antiprothrombin antibodies, and the risk of thrombosis in the antiphospholipid syndrome. *Blood* 102:2717, 2003.

248. Selva-O'Callaghan A, Ordi-Ros J, Monegal-Ferran F et al: IgA anticardiolipin antibodies—Relation with other antiphospholipid antibodies and clinical significance. *Thromb Haemost* 79:282, 1998.

249. Merrill JT, Shen C, Gugnani M, et al: High prevalence of antiphospholipid antibodies in patients taking procainamide. *J Rheumatol* 24:1083, 1997.

250. Karmochkine M, Piette JC, Mazoyer E, et al: Antiphospholipid antibodies: Cause of thrombosis or an epiphenomenon? *Presse Med* 24:267, 1995.

251. Lopez LR, Dier KJ, Lopez D, et al: Anti-beta 2-glycoprotein I and antiphosphatidylserine antibodies are predictors of arterial thrombosis in patients with antiphospholipid syndrome. *Am J Clin Pathol* 121:142, 2004.

252. Audrain MA, El Kouri D, Hamidou MA, et al: Value of autoantibodies to beta(2)-glycoprotein 1 in the diagnosis of antiphospholipid syndrome. *Rheumatology (Oxford)* 41:550, 2002.

253. Esmon NL, Smirnov MD, Esmon CT: Lupus anticoagulants and thrombosis: The role of phospholipids. *Haematologica* 82:474, 1997.

254. Berard M, Chantome R, Marcelli A, Boffa MC: Antiphosphatidylethanolamine antibodies as the only antiphospholipid antibodies. I. Association with thrombosis and vascular cutaneous diseases. *J Rheumatol* 23:1369, 1996.

255. Rauch J, Janoff AS: Antibodies against phospholipids other than cardiolipin: Potential roles for both phospholipid and protein. *Lupus* 5:498, 1996.

256. Yetman DL, Kutteh WH: Antiphospholipid antibody panels and recurrent pregnancy loss: Prevalence of anticardiolipin antibodies compared with other antiphospholipid antibodies. *Fertil Steril* 66:540, 1996.

257. de Maistre E, Gobert B, Bene MC, et al: Comparative assessment of phospholipid-binding antibodies indicates limited overlapping. *J Clin Lab Anal* 10:6, 1996.

258. Branch DW, Silver R, Pierangeli S, et al: Antiphospholipid antibodies other than lupus anticoagulant and anticardiolipin antibodies in women with recurrent pregnancy loss, fertile controls, and antiphospholipid syndrome. *Obstet Gynecol* 89:549, 1997.

259. Laroche P, Berard M, Rouquette AM, et al: Advantage of using both anionic and zwitterionic phospholipid antigens for the detection of antiphospholipid antibodies. *Am J Clin Pathol* 106:549, 1996.

260. Panarelli P, Viola-Magni MP, Albi E: Antiphosphatidylinositol antibody in deep venous thrombosis patients. *Int J Immunopathol Pharmacol* 16:61, 2003.

261. Toschi V, Motta A, Castelli C, et al: High prevalence of antiphosphatidylinositol antibodies in young patients with cerebral ischemia of undetermined cause. *Stroke* 29:1759, 1998.

262. Amengual O, Atsumi T, Khamashta MA, et al: Specificity of ELISA for antibody to beta 2-glycoprotein I in patients with antiphospholipid syndrome. *Br J Rheumatol* 35:1239, 1996.

263. Alarcon-Segovia D, Mestanza M, Cabiedes J, Cabral AR: The antiphospholipid/cofactor syndromes: II. A variant in patients with systemic lupus erythematosus with antibodies to beta 2-glycoprotein I but no antibodies detectable in standard antiphospholipid assays. *J Rheumatol* 24:1545, 1997.

264. Cabral AR, Amigo MC, Cabiedes J, Alarcon-Segovia D: The antiphospholipid/cofactor syndromes: A primary variant with antibodies to beta 2-glycoprotein-I but no antibodies detectable in standard antiphospholipid assays. *Am J Med* 101:472, 1996.

265. Sanmarco M, Soler C, Christides C, et al: Prevalence and clinical significance of IgG isotype anti-beta 2-glycoprotein I antibodies in antiphospholipid syndrome: A comparative study with anticardiolipin antibodies. *J Lab Clin Med* 129:499, 1997.

266. Day HM, Thiagarajan P, Ahn C, et al: Autoantibodies to beta2-glycoprotein I in systemic lupus erythematosus and primary antiphospholipid antibody syndrome: Clinical correlations in comparison with other antiphospholipid antibody tests. *J Rheumatol* 25:667, 1998.

267. Reber G, Schousboe I, Tincani A, et al: Inter-laboratory variability of anti-beta2-glycoprotein I measurement. A collaborative study in the frame of the European Forum on Antiphospholipid Antibodies Standardization Group. *Thromb Haemost* 88:66, 2002.

268. Bidot CJ, Jy W, Horstman LL, et al: Factor VII/VIIa: A new antigen in the anti-phospholipid antibody syndrome. *Br J Haemol* 120:618, 2003.

269. Shapiro SS: The lupus anticoagulant/antiphospholipid syndrome. *Annu Rev Med* 47:533, 1996.

270. Triplett DA: Lupus anticoagulants/antiphospholipid-protein antibodies: The great imposters. *Lupus* 5:431, 1996.

271. Jennings I, Kitchen S, Woods TA, et al: Potentially clinically important inaccuracies in testing for the lupus anticoagulant: An analysis of results from three surveys of the U.K. National External Quality Assessment Scheme (NEQAS) for Blood Coagulation. *Thromb Haemost* 77:934, 1997.

272. Somers E, Magder LS, Petri M: Antiphospholipid antibodies and incidence of venous thrombosis in a cohort of patients with systemic lupus erythematosus. *J Rheumatol* 29:2531, 2002.

273. Nojima J, Suehisa E, Akita N, et al: Risk of arterial thrombosis in patients with anticardiolipin antibodies and lupus anticoagulant. *Br J Haematol* 96:447, 1997.

274. Takeya H, Mori T, Gabazza EC, et al: Anti-beta2-glycoprotein I (beta2GPI) monoclonal antibodies with lupus anticoagulant-like activity enhance the beta2GPI binding to phospholipids. *J Clin Invest* 99:2260, 1997.

275. Kitchens CS: Prolonged activated partial thromboplastin time of unknown etiology: A prospective study of 100 consecutive cases referred for consultation. *Am J Hematol* 27:38, 1988.

276. Galli M, Barbui T: Prothrombin as cofactor for antiphospholipids. *Lupus* 7(suppl 2):S37, 1998.

277. Galli M, Finazzi G, Bevers EM, Barbui T: Kaolin clotting time and dilute Russell's viper venom time distinguish between prothrombin-dependent and beta 2-glycoprotein I-dependent antiphospholipid antibodies. *Blood* 86:617, 1995.

278. Liu HW, Wong KL, Lin CK, et al: The reappraisal of dilute tissue thromboplastin inhibition test in the diagnosis of lupus anticoagulant. *Br J Haematol* 72:229, 1989.

279. Forastiero RR, Cerrato GS, Carreras LO: Evaluation of recently described tests for detection of the lupus anticoagulant. *Thromb Haemost* 72:728, 1994.

280. Lenzi R, Rand JH, Spiera H: Anticardiolipin antibodies in pregnant patients with systemic lupus erythematosus. *N Engl J Med* 314:1392, 1986.

281. Khamashta MA, Cuadrado MJ, Mujic F, et al: The management of thrombosis in the antiphospholipid-antibody syndrome. *N Engl J Med* 332:993, 1995.

282. Urfer C, Pichler WJ, Helbling A: Antiphospholipid antibodies syndrome: Follow-up of patients with a high antiphospholipid antibodies titer. *Schweiz Med Wochenschr* 126:2136, 1996.

283. Crowther MA, Ginsberg JS, Julian J, et al: A comparison of two intensities of warfarin for the prevention of recurrent thrombosis in patients with the antiphospholipid antibody syndrome. *N Engl J Med* 349:1133, 2003.

284. Moll S, Ortel TL: Monitoring warfarin therapy in patients with lupus anticoagulants. *Ann Intern Med* 127:177, 1997.

285. Della VP, Crippa L, Safa O, et al: Potential failure of the International Normalized Ratio (INR) System in the monitoring of oral anticoagulation in patients with lupus anticoagulants. *Ann Med Interne (Paris)* 147(suppl 1):10, 1996.

286. Tripodi A, Chantarangkul V, Clerici M, et al: Laboratory control of oral anticoagulant treatment by the INR system in patients with the antiphospholipid syndrome and lupus anticoagulant. Results of a collaborative study involving nine commercial thromboplastins. *Br J Haematol* 115:672, 2001.

287. Camps GM, Guil M, Sanchez LJ, et al: Fibrinolytic treatment in primary antiphospholipid syndrome. *Lupus* 5:627, 1996.

288. Julkunen H, Hedman C, Kauppi M: Thrombolysis for acute ischemic stroke in the primary antiphospholipid syndrome. *J Rheumatol* 24:181, 1997.

289. Ho YL, Chen MF, Wu CC, et al: Successful treatment of acute myocardial infarction by thrombolytic therapy in a patient with primary antiphospholipid antibody syndrome. *Cardiology* 87:354, 1996.

290. Petri M: Thrombosis and systemic lupus erythematosus: The Hopkins Lupus Cohort perspective [editorial]. *Scand J Rheumatol* 25:191, 1996.

291. Wallace DJ: The use of chloroquine and hydroxychloroquine for noninfectious conditions other than rheumatoid arthritis or lupus: A critical review. *Lupus* 5(suppl 1):S59, 1996.

292. Edwards MH, Pierangeli S, Liu X, et al: Hydroxychloroquine reverses thrombogenic properties of antiphospholipid antibodies in mice. *Circulation* 96:4380, 1997.

293. Krause I, Blank M, Shoenfeld Y: Immunomodulation of experimental APS: Lessons from murine models. *Lupus* 5:458, 1996.

294. Empson M, Lassere M, Craig JC, Scott JR: Recurrent pregnancy loss with antiphospholipid antibody: A systematic review of therapeutic trials. *Obstet Gynecol* 99:135, 2002.

295. Rai R: Obstetric management of antiphospholipid syndrome. *J Autoimmun* 15:203, 2000.

296. Backos M, Rai R, Baxter N, et al: Pregnancy complications in women with recurrent miscarriage associated with antiphospholipid antibodies treated with low dose aspirin and heparin. *Br J Obstet Gynaecol* 106: 102, 1999.

297. Cowchock S, Reece EA: Do low-risk pregnant women with antiphospholipid antibodies need to be treated? Organizing Group of the Antiphospholipid Antibody Treatment Trial. *Am J Obstet Gynecol* 176:1099, 1997.

298. Cowchock S: Treatment of antiphospholipid syndrome in pregnancy. *Lupus* 7(suppl 2):S95, 1998.

299. Branch DW, Peaceman AM, Druzin M, et al: A multicenter, placebo-controlled pilot study of intravenous immune globulin treatment of antiphospholipid syndrome during pregnancy. The Pregnancy Loss Study Group. *Am J Obstet Gynecol* 182:122, 2000.

300. Daya S, Gunby J, Porter F, et al: Critical analysis of intravenous immunoglobulin therapy for recurrent miscarriage. *Hum Reprod Update* 5:475, 1999.

301. Rand JH, Wu XX, Quinn AS, et al: Human monoclonal antiphospholipid antibodies disrupt the annexin a5 anticoagulant crystal shield on phospholipid bilayers: Evidence from atomic force microscopy and functional assay. *Am J Pathol* 163:1193, 2003

ANTIBODY-MEDIATED THROMBOTIC DISORDERS: IDIOPATHIC THROMBOTIC THROMBOCYTOPENIC PURPURA AND HEPARIN-INDUCED THROMBOCYTOPENIA

J. EVAN SADLER
MORTIMER PONCZ

Idiopathic thrombotic thrombocytopenic purpura (TTP) is associated with microangiopathic hemolytic anemia, thrombocytopenia, and microvascular thrombosis that results in variable injury of the central nervous system, kidney, and other organs. Most cases of idiopathic TTP are caused by autoantibodies to ADAMTS13, a metalloprotease that normally cleaves von Willebrand factor (vWF) and thereby inhibits vWF-dependent platelet aggregation. Idiopathic TTP almost uniformly is fatal if untreated. Most patients respond to plasma exchange, although a large fraction of patients have relapsing disease. Clinically similar idiopathic thrombotic microangiopathy can occur with normal ADAMTS13 levels. Secondary thrombotic microangiopathy occurs in association with metastatic cancer, infections, organ and hematopoietic stem cell transplantation, and certain drugs. Secondary thrombotic microangiopathy has a much lower likelihood of responding to plasma exchange and a lower survival rate.

Heparin-induced thrombocytopenia (HIT) is a significant complication of treatment with heparin, especially unfractionated, high molecular weight heparin. It is associated with mild-to-moderate thrombocytopenia, although the main concern is the high frequency of both arterial and venous thrombotic complications. HIT is an immune complex-based disorder involving heparin/platelet factor 4 complexes. Immediate cessation of heparin is required, but the risk of subsequent thrombosis remains high. Direct thrombin inhibitors are the present-day treatment of choice for limiting thrombotic complications.

Acronyms and abbreviations that appear in this chapter include: ADAMTS, a disintegrin and metalloprotease with thrombospondin type 1 repeats; APLS, antiphospholipid syndrome; aPTT, activated partial thromboplastin time; DDAVP, desmopressin, 1-deamino-(8-D-arginine)-vasopressin; D+HUS, diarrhea-associated hemolytic uremic syndrome; D-HUS, diarrhea-negative hemolytic uremic syndrome; Gp, glycoprotein; HELLP, hemolysis, elevated liver enzymes, and low platelets; HIT, heparin-induced thrombocytopenia; HMW, high molecular weight; HUS, hemolytic uremic syndrome; Ig, immunoglobulin; LDH, lactate dehydrogenase; LMW, low molecular weight; MCP, membrane cofactor protein; MTHFR, methylenetetrahydrofolate reductase; PT, prothrombin time; SLE, systemic lupus erythematosus; TTP, thrombotic thrombocytopenic purpura; vWF, von Willebrand factor.

IDIOPATHIC THROMBOTIC THROMBOCYTOPENIC PURPURA

DEFINITION AND HISTORY

Thrombotic microangiopathy refers to a combination of microangiopathic hemolytic anemia, thrombocytopenia, and microvascular thrombosis, regardless of cause or specific tissue involvement. Various kinds of thrombotic microangiopathy differ with regard to pathogenesis and prognosis but can be difficult to distinguish because their clinical features overlap.

Idiopathic thrombotic thrombocytopenic purpura (TTP) is a form of thrombotic microangiopathy in which tissue injury can affect any organ but often results in neurologic damage and fever. Renal involvement is common, but oliguric renal failure is not. Idiopathic TTP usually is associated with acquired autoantibodies that inhibit a disintegrin and metalloprotease thrombospondin type 1 repeats (ADAMTS)13. Idiopathic TTP occurs in patients without other medical conditions that sometimes cause thrombotic microangiopathy, such as metastatic cancer, systemic infection, solid organ or hematopoietic stem cell transplantation, radiation exposure, chemotherapy, certain other drugs, or various other causes of disseminated intravascular coagulation.

Congenital TTP, or Upshaw-Schulman syndrome, refers to TTP that is caused by inherited deficiency of ADAMTS13.

Hemolytic uremic syndrome (HUS) refers to thrombotic microangiopathy that mainly affects the kidney and usually causes oliguric or anuric renal failure. *Diarrhea-associated* or *typical* HUS (D+HUS) is caused by enteric infection with Shiga toxin-producing gram-negative bacilli and usually is associated with a prodrome of diarrhea. *Diarrhea-negative* or *atypical* HUS (D-HUS) is not associated with diarrhea or Shiga toxin-producing organisms and occurs in patients without an obvious predisposing condition.

Most examples of thrombotic microangiopathy that can be attributed to a predisposing medical condition are considered *secondary thrombotic microangiopathy*, independent of the pattern of tissue involvement. For these heterogeneous disorders, the most important clinical intervention is correcting the underlying "primary" condition. With a few specific exceptions, ADAMTS13 levels are normal and plasma exchange is ineffective.

Eli Moschcowitz[1,2] reported the first detailed clinical description of idiopathic TTP in 1924. The patient was a 16-year-old girl with fever, severe anemia, leukocytosis, petechiae, and hemiparesis. Her renal function was not impaired, but the urine contained albumin, hyaline casts, and granular casts. She became comatose and died 2 weeks after her first symptoms. At autopsy, hyaline thrombi were found diffusely in terminal arterioles and capillaries, particularly of the heart and kidney. For many years, patients with similar findings were described as having Moschcowitz disease. The name *TTP* was proposed in 1947[3] and widely adopted thereafter.

In 1955, the term *hemolytic uremic syndrome* (HUS) was proposed for thrombotic microangiopathy occurring in children and associated with acute anuric renal failure, which is uncommon in TTP.[4] Childhood HUS often was preceded by a diarrheal illness and, unlike TTP in adults, the prognosis was favorable. The majority of patients survived and recovered normal renal function with only supportive care.[5]

In 1966, a review of 272 published cases defined the major clinical features of TTP.[6] Most patients were females between the ages of 10 and 39 years. The symptoms and physical findings included a classic pentad of severe thrombocytopenia, hemolytic anemia with numerous fragmented red cells or schistocytes, neurologic findings, renal damage, and fever. Mortality exceeded 90 percent: the average hospital stay was only 14 days before death, and 80 percent of patients lived fewer than 90 days after onset of symptoms. However, dramatic recoveries occurred in some cases following splenectomy.

This grim prognosis was recorded before the recognition that blood or plasma infusions improved the outcome of TTP. A few reports, including one from Moschowitz[2] in 1925, had suggested that blood transfusion sometimes induced dramatic responses.[7,8] However, interest in transfusion therapy increased after 1976, when whole blood exchange transfusions reportedly induced prompt remissions in eight of 14 patients.[9] Similar responses were described after plasmapheresis with plasma replacement.[10] One remarkable case report showed that plasmapheresis was effective if the replacement fluid was plasma or cryoprecipitate-depleted plasma but ineffective if the replacement fluid contained just albumin.[11] Furthermore, simple plasma infusions without plasmapheresis could induce sustained remissions, suggesting that replacement of a missing plasma factor sometimes was sufficient to ameliorate TTP.[11]

A similar congenital disorder first described by Schulman and colleagues[12] and Upshaw[13] is characterized by autosomal recessive inheritance and chronic relapsing thrombotic microangiopathy from infancy. Congenital TTP, or Upshaw-Schulman syndrome, shared many features with idiopathic TTP in adults, including the consistent response to plasma.[13]

These reports led to the widespread adoption of plasma therapy for TTP, and two studies published in 1991 provided compelling evidence for its efficacy. Plasma infusion was associated with 91 percent survival in 108 patients, an impressive improvement over historical experience.[14] In the same year, a prospective randomized comparison of plasma exchange and plasma infusion in 102 patients with TTP was reported.[15] Long-term survival was 78 percent for the plasma exchange group and 63 percent for the plasma infusion group, a significant difference in favor of plasma exchange.

A link between TTP and von Willebrand factor (vWF) was proposed in 1982, based on studies of four patients with chronic relapsing TTP.[16] Their plasma vWF multimers were much larger than those of healthy controls and similar in size to the vWF multimers secreted by endothelial cells. Patients with TTP were proposed to lack a depolymerase activity, perhaps a protease or a reductase, that shortens newly secreted vWF multimers *in vivo* and produces the multimer distribution of normal plasma. The absence of this depolymerase would cause the persistence of "unusually large" vWF, which promotes intravascular platelet aggregation, thrombocytopenia, and microvascular thrombosis. Plasma exchange therapy could provide the missing depolymerase activity, or it could remove other factors that provoke clinical relapses.

A candidate depolymerase was identified in 1996, when a metalloprotease in plasma was shown to cleave vWF multimers subjected to high fluid shear stress or mild protein denaturants.[17,18] Soon thereafter, children with congenital TTP were shown to have inherited deficiency of this metalloprotease,[19] and adults with acquired idiopathic TTP were shown to have autoantibody inhibitors of the enzyme.[20,21] The vWF-cleaving protease was purified,[22,23] cloned,[24,25] and named ADAMTS13, a new member of the ADAMTS family of metalloproteases.[26] Simultaneously, the *ADAMTS13* locus was identified by linkage analysis in families affected by congenital TTP, and causative *ADAMTS13* mutations were characterized.[27]

Clinical studies confirmed the association of severe ADAMTS13 deficiency with congenital TTP and acquired idiopathic TTP. In contrast, ADAMTS13 deficiency is almost unknown in HUS or secondary thrombotic microangiopathy. Consequently, ADAMTS13 levels correlate with differences in pathophysiology and prognosis.

ETIOLOGY AND PATHOGENESIS

Unregulated vWF-dependent platelet thrombosis appears to be the mechanism underlying congenital TTP and most instances of idiopathic TTP. Large vWF multimers mediate platelet adhesion at sites of vascular injury by binding to connective tissue and glycoprotein

(Gp)Ib on the platelet surface (see Chapter 118). The vWF subunit from which multimers are constructed has a modular structure consisting of five types of conserved structural motifs (Fig. 124-1). vWF multimers bind to collagen through domain A3 and to platelet GpIb through domain A1. When platelets bind to vWF under conditions of high fluid shear stress, the vWF multimer is stretched and the Tyr1605–Met1606 bond within domain A2 becomes accessible to the metalloprotease ADAMTS13 (Fig. 124-2), which cleaves it and thereby may release any adherent platelets. ADAMTS13 deficiency prevents this feedback inhibition and leads to microvascular platelet thrombosis.

Idiopathic TTP usually is caused by polyclonal immunoglobulin (Ig)G autoantibodies that inhibit ADAMTS13 (Fig. 124-3).[20,21] The antibodies usually bind the cysteine-rich or spacer domain and often bind to the CUB domains and first thrombospondin-1 repeat; they bind less frequently to other thrombospondin-1 repeats, the metalloprotease domain, or the propeptide.[28,29] Noninhibitory IgG and IgM antibodies have been identified, although their significance is unknown.[30]

The composition of the lesions in idiopathic TTP is consistent with a pathophysiologic role of vWF-dependent platelet thrombosis. Amorphous thrombi and subendothelial hyaline deposits may be found in the small arterioles and capillaries of any organ but are particularly common (in order of decreasing severity) in the myocardium, pancreas, kidney, adrenal gland, and brain. The liver and lung are relatively spared. The lesions consist mainly of platelets and vWF, with little fibrin and few inflammatory cells. They often include focal endothelial cell proliferation.[31–33] The histologic findings in congenital TTP are similar.[34] In contrast, D+HUS mainly affects the renal cortex, which often shows extensive necrosis. Lesions occur infrequently in the pancreas, brain, adrenal glands, and myocardium. The thrombi of HUS typically involve glomerular capillaries and arterioles and are composed mainly of fibrin with few platelets.[33,35]

Factors other than ADAMTS13 deficiency have been proposed to contribute to idiopathic TTP, although a causal relationship has not been established. These factors include platelet agglutinating proteins distinct from vWF,[36] antibodies that activate endothelial cells[37] or bind CD36 and activate platelets,[38] and circulating factors causing endothelial cell apoptosis.[39]

Secondary thrombotic microangiopathy is an infrequent complication in many different settings, and the pathophysiology is heterogeneous. Endothelial injury may be a common feature, although the mechanism of injury probably varies and in most cases is not understood. With the exception of some drug-induced TTP, severe ADAMTS13 deficiency is not observed.[40,41] Autopsy studies in a few patients with secondary thrombotic microangiopathy suggest that microvascular thrombosis tends to be limited to the kidney.[41–43]

EPIDEMIOLOGY

The incidence of idiopathic TTP in the United States has been estimated at 3.8 per million per year.[44,45] Seasonal or geographical trends have not been observed consistently. Idiopathic TTP is relatively uncommon before age 20 years, with a peak incidence between ages 30 and 50 years.[44,45] Across many reports the female-to-male ratio averages approximately 2:1, but female preponderance is more pronounced before age 50 years and the ratio approaches equality after age 60 years.[44,45] Other risk factors for idiopathic TTP include African ancestry[44,46,47] and obesity.[46,48] Women have a tendency to present during late pregnancy or peripartum (reviewed in references 31 and 49). Congenital TTP[50] and secondary thrombotic microangiopathy[46,47] affect the genders almost equally.

Heritable risk factors probably affect susceptibility to idiopathic TTP. For example, identical twin sisters developed idiopathic TTP at

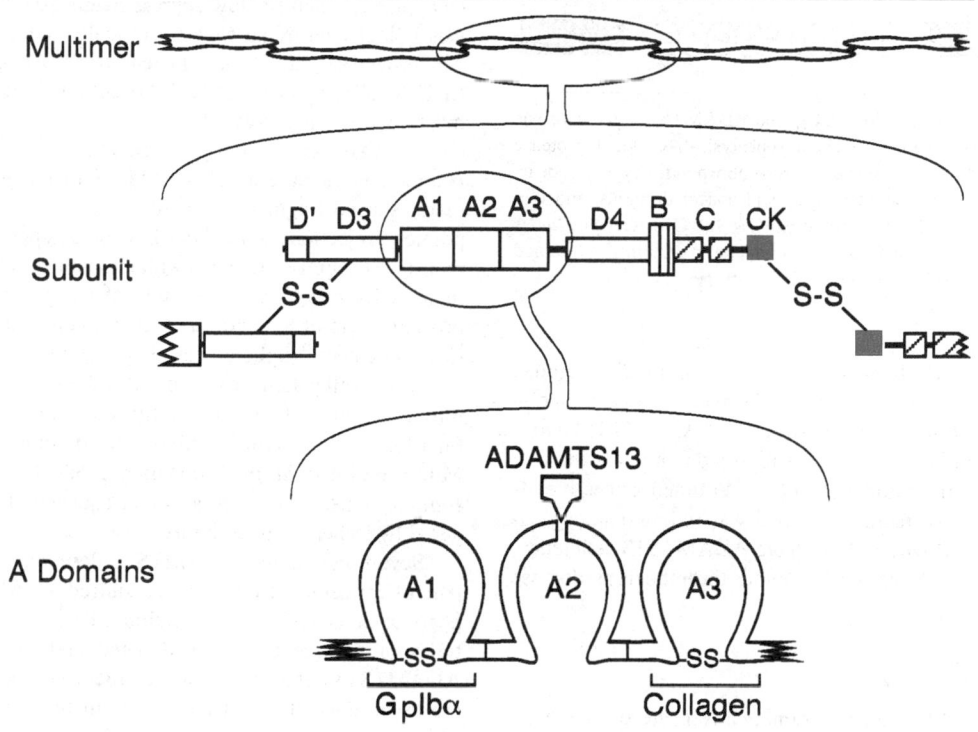

FIGURE 124-1   Structure of von Willebrand factor. Multimeric von Willebrand factor *(top)* is composed of identical subunits with five kinds of structural motifs, including three A domains, three B domains, two C domains, two complete and one partial D domains, and a cystine knot (CK) domain. Subunits *(middle)* are linked into multimers by disulfide bonds between C-terminal CK domains and N-terminal D3 domains. Domain A1 *(bottom)* binds platelet glycoprotein Ibα (GpIbα), domain A3 binds collagen in extracellular matrix, and domain A2 contains a Tyr-Met bond that is susceptible to cleavage by ADAMTS13.

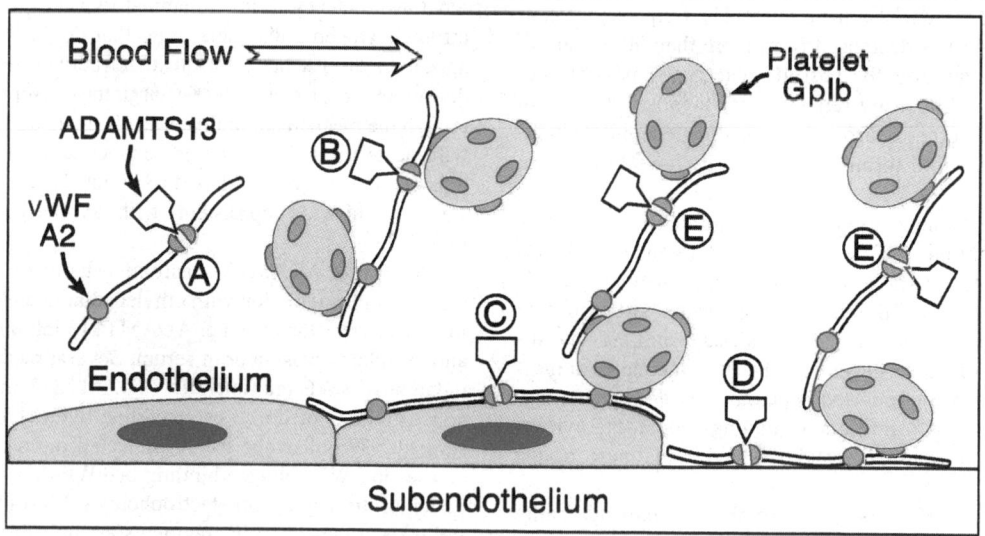

FIGURE 124-2   Regulation of von Willebrand factor (vWF)-dependent platelet thrombosis by ADAMTS13. Endothelial cells secrete vWF as "unusually large" multimers that enter the circulation (A, B) or adhere to the cell surface (C). vWF also binds to connective tissue at sites of vascular injury (D). Under conditions of high fluid shear stress, platelets may adhere to vWF in solution (B) or on surfaces (C, D) through platelet glycoprotein Ib (GpIb). vWF also can recruit platelets to other adherent platelets (E). ADAMTS13 cleaves the A2 domain of the vWF subunit, severing the multimer. This reaction is slow for vWF in solution (A) but occurs rapidly when platelets adhere to vWF under high fluid shear conditions in suspension (B) or on surfaces (C–E), presumably as a consequence of conformational changes induced by tensile force on vWF. Failure of this mechanism can cause TTP. (From JE Sadler,[272] with permission.).

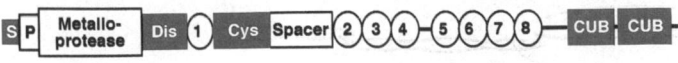

FIGURE 124-3   Structure of ADAMTS13. The ADAMTS13 precursor has a signal peptide (S), a short propeptide (P), a reprolysin-like metalloprotease domain, disintegrin-like domain (Dis), eight thrombospondin type 1 repeats (numbered), characteristic cysteine-rich (Cys) and spacer domains, and two CUB domains (named for motifs in complement C1r and C1s, *Xenopus laevis* urinary epidermal growth factor, and bone morphogenetic protein 1). (Adapted from X Zheng, D Chung, TK Takayama, et al.,[24] with permission.).

age 23 and 24 years. Both women had autoantibodies against ADAMTS13 and responded completely to plasma exchange, with disappearance of the inhibitors and normalization of ADAMTS13 activity.[51] A low frequency of HLA-DR53 was reported in adults with TTP or HUS, suggesting an immunogenetically determined protective effect.[52] A high prevalence of factor V Leiden was reported among patients with idiopathic TTP who did not have ADAMTS13 deficiency, suggesting that inherited risk factors for venous thrombosis predispose to thrombotic microangiopathy.[53]

CLINICAL FEATURES

The onset of idiopathic TTP can be dramatically acute or insidious, developing over weeks. Approximately one third of patients have symptoms of hemolytic anemia.[6,31] Thrombocytopenia typically causes petechiae or purpura. Oral, gastrointestinal, or genitourinary bleeding is less common but can be severe.

Systemic microvascular thrombosis can affect any organ, and the consequences are variable. Renal involvement is common, but acute renal failure occurs in fewer than 10 percent of cases.[31,46,47] Neurologic findings can be transient or persistent and may include headache, visual disturbances, vertigo, personality change, confusion, lethargy, syncope, coma, seizures, aphasia, hemiparesis, and other focal sensory or motor deficits.[6,31] Many patients have fever. The frequency of neurologic findings or fever has decreased from more than 90 percent to approximately 50 percent over the past 40 years,[46,47,54] possibly because these features no longer are required for diagnosis of TTP. In rare instances, stroke or other neurologic events precede microangiopathic hemolytic anemia and thrombocytopenia by days[55] to several weeks.[56,57]

Cardiac involvement may cause myocardial infarction, congestive heart failure, or arrhythmias.[31] Direct pulmonary involvement is uncommon, but severe acute respiratory distress syndrome may occur,[58] possibly secondary to cardiac failure.[31] Gastrointestinal symptoms are common and can include abdominal pain, nausea, vomiting, and diarrhea.[6,31] Physical examination may suggest acute pancreatitis or mesenteric ischemia. One review reported hepatomegaly and splenomegaly in one fifth of cases.[6] Infrequent findings include Raynaud phenomenon, chest pain, arthralgia, myalgia, and retinal hemorrhage or detachment.[6,31]

The clinical features of secondary thrombotic microangiopathy usually are dominated by the underlying condition.

LABORATORY FEATURES

The symptoms and signs of idiopathic TTP are nonspecific. The diagnosis depends on laboratory testing to document microangiopathic hemolytic anemia and thrombocytopenia, without another cause such as disseminated intravascular coagulation. Almost all patients have, anemia and one third have hemoglobin values below approximately 6 g/dl.[6,31] Thrombocytopenia typically is severe, and half of patients

have platelet counts below approximately 20,000/μl.[6,31,46,47,54] Hemolysis is indicated by an elevated reticulocyte count and serum lactate dehydrogenase (LDH) and a decreased serum haptoglobin. The median LDH level is approximately 1200 U/liter.[14,15,46,47,54] Coombs test almost always is negative.[14,15,31]

The characteristic morphologic feature of TTP on the blood film is a marked increase in schistocytes. Schistocytes are jagged or irregularly shaped fragments of split red cells with two or more sharply pointed projections, sometimes having the appearance of military helmets (see Chap. 28). Patients with idiopathic TTP often have markedly increased schistocytes; in a study of six patients, schistocytes comprised a mean of 8.3 percent of all red cells with a range of 1 percent to 18.4 percent.[59] Spherocytes also may be seen.

Almost all patients have normal values for plasma fibrinogen, prothrombin time (PT), and activated partial thromboplastin time (aPTT),[14,15,31] reflecting a minor role of blood coagulation in TTP. Mildly elevated fibrin degradation products have been reported in some patients,[31,60] perhaps as a consequence of fibrin generation triggered by ischemic tissue injury.

Severe congenital ADAMTS13 deficiency (<5%) is characteristic of congenital TTP. Severe acquired ADAMTS13 deficiency appears to be specific for idiopathic TTP,[20,21,61,62] although the sensitivity of the association is debated and the frequency of severe ADAMTS13 deficiency in idiopathic TTP depends on how patients are ascertained. If adult patients with thrombotic microangiopathy are selected with no plausible secondary cause, no diarrheal prodrome, and no features suggestive of HUS (e.g., oliguria, severe hypertension, dialysis, serum creatinine >3.5 mg/dl), then at least 80 percent may have undetectable ADAMTS13 activity and the majority will have easily detectable autoantibody inhibitors.[20,21,47,63] Among less highly selected patients, severe ADAMTS13 deficiency and inhibitors are less prevalent.[46]

ADAMTS13 levels tend to vary inversely with vWF level.[64] ADAMTS13 levels are normal to moderately decreased in newborns, during pregnancy, after surgery, and in chronic liver cirrhosis, chronic renal insufficiency, acute inflammatory states, sepsis, and a variety of thrombocytopenic disorders other than TTP.[62,64] ADAMTS13 levels appear to drop acutely by up to 50 percent after administration of desmopressin [1-deamino-(8-D-arginine)-vasopressin (DDAVP)], although the mechanism of this effect is unclear.[65] In rare cases, patients with acute viral hepatitis[66] or venoocclusive disease after stem cell transplantation[67] have ADAMTS13 levels less than 5 percent transiently, which is consistent with synthesis of ADAMTS13 in liver.[24,25,27]

Assays for ADAMTS13 activity usually are performed on citrated plasma; anticoagulation with ethylenediaminetetraacetic acid irreversibly inactivates the enzyme. ADAMTS13 inhibitors can be assayed in anticoagulated plasma or in serum. Several methods that rely on degradation of vWF multimers by ADAMTS13 in the presence of low concentrations of urea[17] or guanidine hydrochloride[18] have been described. vWF cleavage then is detected indirectly by measuring decreases in vWF-collagen binding or vWF-dependent platelet agglutination or directly by gel electrophoresis.[68] Rapid assay methods using small recombinant vWF fragments as the substrate are under development.[69]

Other laboratory tests should be considered to detect conditions that may cause thrombotic microangiopathy by mechanisms other than ADAMTS13 deficiency. The tests include microbiologic and serologic tests for Shiga toxin-producing organisms, tests for antiphospholipid antibody syndrome or factor V Leiden, serologies for systemic lupus erythematosus and other autoimmune diseases, and testing suitable for potential causes of secondary thrombotic microangiopathy.

DIFFERENTIAL DIAGNOSIS

The diagnosis of TTP should be considered for any patient with microangiopathic hemolytic anemia and thrombocytopenia, without evidence of disseminated intravascular coagulation and without features associated with D⁺HUS, such as a prodromal diarrheal illness and acute oliguric or anuric renal failure. These criteria can only be approximate, however, because many diseases associated with secondary thrombotic microangiopathy can produce overlapping clinical and laboratory findings. As a consequence, making a diagnosis of TTP can be a challenge, and a wide differential diagnosis often must be considered (Table 124-1).

Schistocytes occur in a variety of conditions other than TTP, although the level seldom enters the 1 to 18 percent range typical of idiopathic TTP.[59] For example, schistocytes were seen in the blood film of 58 percent of healthy controls, with a mean of 0.05 percent and a range of 0 to 0.27 percent of all red cells.[59] Up to 0.6 percent schistocytes were observed in patients with chronic renal failure, pre-

TABLE 124-1 CLASSIFICATION AND DIFFERENTIAL DIAGNOSIS OF THROMBOTIC MICROANGIOPATHY

Congenital TTP (Upshaw-Schulman syndrome)
  Inherited ADAMTS13 deficiency
Idiopathic TTP
  With acquired ADAMTS13 deficiency
  Without acquired ADAMTS13 deficiency
Secondary thrombotic microangiopathy
  Infections and disseminated intravascular coagulation
  Tissue transplant-associated with
    Chemotherapy or radiation injury
    Tissue rejection
    Graft-versus-host disease
  Cancer
    Trousseau syndrome
    Metastatic carcinoma
    Erythroleukemia
  Pregnancy associated (preeclampsia, eclampsia, HELLP syndrome)
  Autoimmune disorders
    Evans syndrome
    Systemic lupus erythematosus and other vasculitides
    Antiphospholipid syndrome
  Drugs (commonly implicated)
    Autoimmune with anti-ADAMTS13 antibodies:
      Ticlopidine
      Clopidogrel (mechanism may be variable)
    Autoimmune without anti-ADAMTS13 antibodies
      Quinine
    Dose-related toxicity
      Mitomycin C
      Gemcitabine
      Cyclosporine
      Tacrolimus
  Postoperative
  Malignant hypertension
Hemolytic uremic syndrome
  Diarrhea positive (Infectious, Shiga toxin-associated)
    Sporadic
    Epidemic
  Diarrhea negative
    Inherited complement regulatory protein deficiencies (factor H, membrane cofactor protein, factor I)

eclampsia, or properly functioning prosthetic heart valves.[59] Severe hemolysis and marked schistocytosis occur in patients with defective mechanical heart valves. Patients receiving marrow allografts or autografts for a variety of indications had a mean of 0.7 percent schistocytes 6 weeks after transplantation, with a range of 0 to approximately 4 percent schistocytes.[70,71] Approximately 10 percent of patients had at least 1.3 percent schistocytes, placing them at risk for diagnosis of thrombotic microangiopathy.[71]

CONGENITAL THROMBOTIC THROMBOCYTOPENIC PURPURA

Congenital TTP is caused by homozygosity or compound heterozygosity for inactivating mutations in the *ADAMTS13* gene[27] on chromosome 9q34 (reviewed in reference [72]). The mutations usually impair the synthesis or secretion of ADAMTS13. The mutation R475S in the cysteine-rich domain permits the circulation in plasma of significant amounts of inactive ADAMTS13. Approximately 10 percent of Japanese individuals are heterozygous for this variant.[73] As yet no evidence convincingly indicates locus heterogeneity in congenital TTP.

The clinical findings in congenital TTP are similar to the findings in idiopathic TTP, except for age of onset. Most children with congenital ADAMTS13 deficiency have neonatal jaundice and hemolysis but no evidence of ABO blood group or Rh incompatibility. Approximately half of the children continue to have a chronic relapsing course from infancy. The remaining children usually develop symptoms in their late teens or early twenties. Females may present during their first pregnancy, possibly because vWF levels are increased late in pregnancy. In either case, acute exacerbations often are triggered by infections, otitis media, surgery, or other inflammatory stress.[50] One patient suffered an acute attack after receiving desmopressin (DDAVP), which stimulates the release of vWF from endothelial cell stores.[74] As in acquired idiopathic TTP, most patients with congenital TTP have some renal involvement with proteinuria, hematuria, or a mildly elevated serum creatinine, although anuria and chronic renal failure are uncommon.[75]

Congenital TTP can be treated with periodic infusions of fresh-frozen plasma or an equivalent virucidally treated product, if available. The half-life of ADAMTS13 is 2 to 3 days,[76] and the level of ADAMTS13 required to avoid symptoms is approximately 5 percent of normal. From 5 to 10 ml/kg of plasma every 2 to 3 weeks usually is sufficient to prevent symptoms.[77–80] The frequency of relapses varies considerably among patients, and continuous prophylaxis with plasma may not be necessary in all cases.

SECONDARY THROMBOTIC MICROANGIOPATHY

Infections and Disseminated Intravascular Coagulation Conditions resulting in disseminated intravascular coagulation sometimes cause microangiopathic changes and thrombocytopenia with little alteration in blood coagulation tests, which can suggest a diagnosis of TTP. Infections may trigger disease in patients with severe ADAMTS13 deficiency, but more commonly infections cause secondary thrombotic microangiopathy by other mechanisms (Table 124-2). Secondary thrombotic microangiopathy resulting from infections may respond to antimicrobial or antiviral therapy but generally not to plasma exchange.

Thrombotic microangiopathy, often with acute renal failure, is a rare complication of invasive infections with *Streptococcus pneumoniae*. A surveillance study in Atlanta, Georgia, identified HUS in 0.6 percent of pneumococcal infections in children younger than 2 years.[81] Patients usually have pneumococcal pneumonia or meningitis, with normal plasma fibrinogen and normal or minimally prolonged PT and aPTT.[81,82] The pathophysiology is thought to involve bacterial neuraminidase, made by *S. pneumoniae* and some other organisms, which removes sialic acid residues from cell surface glycoproteins and ex-

TABLE 124-2 INFECTIOUS AGENTS ASSOCIATED WITH SECONDARY THROMBOTIC MICROANGIOPATHY

BACTERIA	REFERENCE
Actinomyces turicensis	273
Campylobacter jejuni	274–276
Enterobacter	277
Escherichia coli (without Shiga toxin)	278
Escherichia coli (with Shiga toxin)	279–281
Group A streptococci	277
Legionella pneumophila	282, 283
Pseudomonas aeruginosa	277
Salmonella typhi	284
Staphylococcus aureus	277
Shigella dysenteriae	285
Streptococcus pneumoniae	277, 286, 287
Yersinia pseudotuberculosis	288
Fungi	
Aspergillus fumigatus	277, 289
Blastomyces species	277
Candida albicans	277
Candida glabrata	290
Candida krausei	290
Viruses	
Coxsackie B	291–293
Cytomegalovirus	277
Echovirus	294
Epstein-Barr	295
HIV (usually with a bacterial infectious complication)	277, 296
Herpes simplex	297
HSV-6	298
HTLV-1	299
Influenza	300, 301
Parvovirus B19	302
Rickettsia	
Rickettsia rickettsii	277, 303
Mycoplasma	
Mycoplasma pneumoniae	304, 305

poses Thomsen-Friedenreich antigen (T antigen) that normally is cryptic. T antigen is recognized by naturally occurring antibodies that fix complement, causing hemolysis and damaging the renal microvasculature.[82] Exchange transfusion has been proposed to stop hemolysis by replacing T antigen-bearing red blood cells and removing circulating neuraminidase, but the efficacy of this treatment is controversial.[83]

Tissue Transplants Recipients of solid organ transplants can develop thrombotic microangiopathy, often dominated by renal involvement associated with immunosuppression by cyclosporine or tacrolimus.[84,85] These drugs appear to damage renal endothelial cells directly and can cause neurotoxicity, adding another feature suggestive of TTP.[86] Similarly, hematopoietic stem cell transplant recipients may develop thrombotic microangiopathy associated with high-dose chemotherapy or radiation, immunosuppressive drugs, graft-versus-host disease, or infections.[43] ADAMTS13 levels are normal,[40,41] and plasma therapy is generally ineffective.[43,87]

Cancer Thrombotic microangiopathy occurs in a small fraction of patients with almost any cancer but most commonly with adenocarcinoma of the pancreas, lung, prostate, stomach, colon, ovary, breast, or unknown primary site.[88] In most cases, the cancer is widely metastatic. These cancers also are associated with Trousseau syndrome or paraneoplastic hypercoagulability and thrombosis. Manifestations include arterial thromboembolism, nonbacterial thrombotic endocar-

ditis, venous thrombosis, and hemorrhage.[88] Most patients have variable prolongation of PT and aPTT and increased fibrin degradation products. These signs of disseminated intravascular coagulation often are intermittent, however,[88] which can suggest a diagnosis of TTP. The thrombosis of Trousseau syndrome may respond to anticoagulation with heparin but not warfarin.[88] Abundant schistocytes have been described in acute erythroleukemia.[89,90] Severe ADAMTS13 deficiency almost never occurs in cancer-associated thrombotic microangiopathy, and plasma exchange usually is ineffective.[46,47,91]

Pregnancy-Associated Thrombotic Microangiopathy The differential diagnosis of thrombotic microangiopathy in pregnancy includes preeclampsia, eclampsia, HELLP syndrome (hemolysis, elevated liver enzymes, and low platelets), acute fatty liver of pregnancy, abruptio placenta, amniotic fluid embolism, and retained products of conception (see Chap. 121). In addition, pregnancy can trigger disease in patients with congenital or acquired ADAMTS13 deficiency. In most case series of TTP, between 12 and 31 percent of patients are women who are pregnant, usually in the third trimester, or immediately postpartum.[49] Distinguishing among these various conditions may be possible only by following the course of disease after delivery.

Severe ADAMTS13 deficiency has not been observed in HELLP syndrome, and ADAMTS13 assays may help differentiate it from idiopathic TTP.[92] Women with congenital ADAMTS13 deficiency or idiopathic TTP have been carried through pregnancy successfully with plasma therapy.[93,94]

Autoimmune Disorders Autoimmune thrombocytopenia may be confused with idiopathic TTP if other causes of microangiopathic hemolytic anemia are present. Asymptomatic thrombocytopenia may be the only finding in idiopathic TTP, as demonstrated by a previous or subsequent episode of disease. Patients in whom idiopathic TTP and autoimmune thrombocytopenia appeared to occur simultaneously or sequentially have been described.[95] Evans syndrome (autoimmune hemolytic anemia with autoimmune thrombocytopenia) usually can be distinguished from TTP by a positive Coombs test and by the prominence of spherocytes relative to schistocytes in the blood film. Heparin-induced thrombocytopenia (HIT) may resemble idiopathic TTP, with thrombocytopenia and disseminated arterial and venous thrombosis. In the former condition, the patient has heparin exposure.

Systemic lupus erythematosus (SLE) can cause autoimmune hemolysis and thrombocytopenia, and lupus vasculitis can cause microangiopathic changes, renal insufficiency, and neurologic defects consistent with TTP. Vasculitis associated with other autoimmune disorders can pose a similar diagnostic problem. Although ADAMTS13 deficiency is uncommon among patients with SLE,[96] in rare cases they develop autoimmune ADAMTS13 deficiency and idiopathic TTP that responds to plasma exchange.[97] Conversely, patients with idiopathic TTP and autoantibodies against ADAMTS13 may have other markers of autoimmune disease, including antinuclear or anti-DNA antibodies, polyarthritis, discoid lupus, or ulcerative colitis.[98,99] High-titer antinuclear and anti-DNA antibodies, a positive Coombs test, decreased serum complement, and histologic or clinical evidence of active vasculitis suggest a diagnosis of thrombotic microangiopathy secondary to SLE, whereas the absence of these signs plus severe ADAMTS13 deficiency favors a diagnosis of idiopathic TTP.

Thrombotic microangiopathy can develop in patients with antiphospholipid syndrome (APLS), with or without concurrent SLE (see Chap. 123). Among 46 reported cases, the clinical features resembled HUS, catastrophic APLS, malignant hypertension, idiopathic TTP, or HELLP syndrome. One third of patients presented during pregnancy or in the postpartum period.[100] Mortality was 22 percent; recovery occurred in 34 percent of patients treated with glucocorticoids and 73 percent of patients treated with plasma exchange.[100]

Thrombotic microangiopathy occurs in patients with progressive systemic sclerosis, particularly in association with acute scleroderma renal crisis and malignant hypertension. Treatment with angiotensin-converting enzyme inhibitors is effective. The value of plasma exchange therapy is uncertain.[101]

Drug-Induced Thrombotic Microangiopathy Among the drugs associated with thrombotic microangiopathy (Table 124-3), the antiplatelet drugs ticlopidine and clopidogrel are unusual because they appear to induce autoantibody inhibitors of ADAMTS13, effectively causing idiopathic TTP. Thrombotic microangiopathy occurs in 200 to 625 per million users of ticlopidine, usually between 2 and 12 weeks after starting therapy.[102] ADAMTS13 levels typically are undetectable, and IgG inhibitors of ADAMTS13 are present.[103] Plasma exchange appears to be effective. The disease usually resolves within 2 weeks of discontinuing the drug, and relapses have not been reported.[102] The incidence of TTP with clopidogrel is lower and is estimated to be four per million users. TTP usually develops within the first 2 weeks of clopidogrel treatment and may be less responsive to plasma exchange therapy compared to ticlopidine-associated TTP.[104] ADAMTS13 deficiency and IgG inhibitors were found in two patients with clopidogrel-associated TTP after coronary artery stenting.[105]

Other drugs associated with thrombotic microangiopathy do not cause severe ADAMTS13 deficiency. Comprehensive lists including single case reports can be found in Table 124-3 and in several reviews.[106–108] Drugs commonly implicated include selected antineoplastic agents, cyclosporine A, tacrolimus, and quinine.

Mitomycin C is an alkylating agent that is used in a variety of chemotherapy regimens for anal carcinoma and many adenocarcinomas. It appears to cause dose-dependent nephrotoxicity, with renal failure occurring in approximately 16 percent of patients who receive a cumulative dose of at least 50 mg.[109] About half of the patients with renal toxicity also develop thrombotic microangiopathy, usually 4 to 8 weeks after the latest dose. Mitomycin C-induced thrombotic microangiopathy does not respond to plasma exchange and has a high mortality rate of approximately 70 percent within 4 months of onset.[110]

Gemcitabine is a nucleoside analogue often used for carcinoma of the pancreas, bladder, or lung. Thrombotic microangiopathy with renal failure reportedly occurs with an incidence of 0.015 percent,[111] although the incidence at one institution was 0.3 percent.[112] The time to develop thrombotic microangiopathy was 6 to 8 months, with a cumulative dose of 9 to 56 g/m^2.[111,112] Death or disability usually results from cancer progression or renal failure, not from extrarenal manifestations of thrombotic microangiopathy.

Cyclosporine and tacrolimus are structurally distinct immunosuppressive drugs that indirectly inhibit calcineurin and suppress T cell activation. Both agents cause dose-dependent nephrotoxicity, neurotoxicity, and thrombotic microangiopathy.[113–115] Renal damage is thought to involve toxic effects on endothelium.[113] Thrombotic microangiopathy can develop during the first few weeks of treatment, and its etiology may be difficult to determine because graft rejection, graft-versus-host disease, and systemic infections can cause similar microangiopathic changes.[113,116] Thrombotic microangiopathy often remits with dose reduction or substitution of other immunosuppressive drugs and may not recur if therapy with cyclosporine or tacrolimus is reinstituted. Plasma exchange has been used as additional therapy but has not been shown to modify the course of disease.[116–118]

Quinine accounts for up to 11 percent of all cases of thrombotic microangiopathy in some series. It has a high risk of chronic renal failure and a high mortality.[106] Most patients are women. Severe thrombotic microangiopathy occurs suddenly within several hours after drug ingestion, with fever, abdominal pain, nausea, vomiting, diarrhea, and oliguric renal failure. Many patients have low fibrinogen, abnormal coagulation test results, abnormal liver function, and leu-

TABLE 124-3   DRUGS AND TOXINS ASSOCIATED WITH SECONDARY THROMBOTIC MICROANGIOPATHY

	REFERENCE
Immune-mediated	
Quinine	306
Ticlopidine	307, 308
Clopidogrel	309, 310
Antineoplastic agents	
All-*trans*-retinoic acid	311
Bleomycin plus cisplatinum	312, 313
Carmustine	306
Chlorozotocin	314
Cytosine arabinoside	315
Daunorubicin	315
Deoxycoformycin	316
Estramustine	317
Gemcitabine	318, 319
Lomustine (CCNU)	320
Mitomycin C	321, 322
Tamoxifen (when combined with mitomycin C)	323
Immunosuppressive and antiinflammatory agents	
Cyclosporine	324, 325
Tacrolimus	326, 327
Penicillamine	328, 329
Muromonab-CD3 (OKT3)	330
Interferon-α	331, 332
Interferon-β	333
Antibiotics	
Ciprofloxacin	334
Clarithromycin	335
Cephalosporin	336
Piperacillin	337
Rifampicin	338
Metronidazole	339
Pentostatin	306
Sulfonamides	340
Penicillin	341
Ampicillin	341
Oxophenarsine	342
Valacyclovir	343, 344
Hormones	
Estrogen/progestogen oral contraceptives	345
Mestranol, norethindrone	346
17 β-estradiol transdermal patch	347
Conjugated estrogens	348
Illicit drugs	
Cocaine	349–351
Heroin	352
Ecstasy	353
Lipid lowering agents	
Atorvastatin	354
Simvastatin	355
H$_2$-receptor antagonists	
Cimetidine	356
Famotidine	356
Vaccinations	
Polio vaccination	357
Measles/mumps/rubella vaccination	358
Bacillus Calmette-Guerin (intravesicular)	359
Influenza vaccination	360
Miscellaneous	
Bee sting	361,362
Bupropion	363
Chlorpropamide	364
Procainamide	364
Iodine	364
Carbon monoxide	365
Chloronaphthalene (in varnish)	366

kopenia. Neurologic changes are common and include altered mental status, coma, and seizures.[119–121] ADAMTS13 levels are normal.[108] In a series of 17 patients, 14 required dialysis, eight developed chronic renal failure, and four died. Three of the deaths occurred during the initial illness and one occurred during chronic hemodialysis 5 years after a second episode.[120] The mechanism appears to involve a broad range of quinine-dependent antibodies against platelets, endothelium, and other cells.[106] Removal of the antibodies by plasma exchange may be beneficial,[119,120] although recovery without plasma exchange also is common.[121]

Postoperative Thrombotic Microangiopathy Thrombotic microangiopathy after major surgery appears to be a distinct syndrome, occurring 5 to 9 days postoperatively and lacking features of disseminated intravascular coagulation.[122] Most cases have followed cardiovascular procedures, with a few reported after gastrointestinal or orthopedic surgery. Patients can have many causes of thrombocytopenia, anemia, altered mental status, renal insufficiency, and fever, so thrombotic microangiopathy may be overlooked. The pathogenesis of postoperative thrombotic microangiopathy is unclear, although rapid responses to plasma exchange have been described.

Malignant Hypertension Malignant hypertension is associated with microangiopathic hemolytic anemia, thrombocytopenia, neurologic symptoms, and renal insufficiency[123] and therefore may resemble idiopathic TTP.

DIARRHEA-ASSOCIATED HEMOLYTIC UREMIC SYNDROME

The clinical features of idiopathic TTP and HUS can overlap. D+HUS can occur at any age but affects mainly children younger than 10 years. Symptoms develop within a few days to 2 weeks after a diarrheal illness, which sometimes includes hemorrhagic colitis. The disease occurs sporadically or in epidemics. In either case the disease is associated with ingestion of foods or other materials contaminated with Shiga toxin-producing bacteria. *Escherichia coli* O157:H7 accounts for at least 80 percent of cases in many series, but D+HUS can be caused by other toxin-bearing *E. coli* serotypes[124] or by *Shigella dysenteriae* type 1.[125] From 1 to 20 percent of patients with diarrhea caused by Shiga toxin-producing *E. coli* are thought to develop D+HUS, with the acute onset of microangiopathic hemolytic anemia, thrombocytopenia, and renal injury.[126–128] Renal signs may include proteinuria, hematuria, hypertension, and oliguria or anuria. Usually the PT and aPTT are normal or minimally prolonged, plasma fibrinogen is normal or elevated, and fibrin degradation products may be moderately elevated.[129] ADAMTS13 levels are normal in D+HUS.[130,131]

Among 3476 patients with HUS, 9 percent died and 3 percent developed end-stage renal failure; these values vary considerably among studies.[132] Central nervous system involvement (seizures, coma, or stroke) occurs in 20 to 40 percent of patients and correlates with a higher risk of death or end-stage renal failure.[124,132] Recurrences after kidney transplantation for D+HUS are uncommon.

In a study of 268 patients with HUS, 59 percent had prodromal diarrhea plus bacteriologic or serologic evidence of infection by Shiga toxin-producing *E. coli*; 21 percent had only diarrhea, and 10 percent had only positive bacteriologic or serologic studies. All three groups had a similar prognosis: approximately 1 percent died and 73 percent recovered normal renal function. These results emphasize the variability in symptoms and signs among patients with HUS caused by Shiga toxin. In contrast, the 11 percent of patients with neither diarrhea nor documented *E. coli* infection had a significantly worse outcome; 10 percent died and only 34 percent recovered normal renal function.[124]

No beneficial effect of plasma therapy has been proven for Shiga toxin-associated HUS.[133–135] The role of antibacterial therapy for enteritis caused by toxin-producing *E. coli* is controversial. Some reports suggest antibiotics increase the risk of HUS, although one meta-analysis of available studies did not support this conclusion.[136]

DIARRHEA-NEGATIVE HEMOLYTIC UREMIC SYNDROME AND INHERITED COMPLEMENT REGULATORY DEFECTS

Atypical HUS or D−HUS is much less common than D+HUS, and its causes are heterogeneous. A sizable minority results from inherited defects in complement factor H,[137–142] membrane cofactor protein (MCP, CD46),[143,144] or factor I.[145] Factor H is a plasma cofactor that promotes inactivation of complement C3b by the plasma serine protease factor I and accelerates the dissociation of factor Bb from the alternative complement convertase C3bBb complex. Factor H and MCP are structurally and functionally similar, but MCP is a transmembrane protein found on the surface of almost all cells. Mutations in these genes impair the regulation of the alternative complement pathway, causing increased endothelial deposition of C3b that attracts phagocytes, promotes membrane attack complex formation, and induces microvascular thrombosis. Some patients have mutations in both factor H alleles or both MCP alleles, but most are heterozygous, suggesting that partial deficiency predisposes to disease. The clinical presentation may be sporadic, recessive, or dominant. Many patients develop HUS in childhood, but some experience their first episode in adulthood or remain asymptomatic. Occasional patients have long intervals between exacerbations, which may appear to be precipitated by infections, other illness, or pregnancy.

The clinical course correlates with the locus that is mutated. HUS associated with factor H deficiency has responded at least transiently to intensive plasma therapy (20–40 ml/kg once or twice per week by infusion or plasma exchange).[142,146,147] The disease often recurs in transplanted kidneys,[137,138,141,142] probably because kidney transplantation does not alter the underlying complement defect. Factor H is synthesized in the liver, and a combined liver and kidney transplant was curative in one case.[148] In contrast, MCP is membrane associated, and the value of plasma therapy has not been established for HUS associated with MCP deficiency. Disease has not recurred after kidney transplantation in three instances,[143] presumably because MCP in the transplanted kidney protects it from complement attack.

THERAPY

PLASMA EXCHANGE

The mainstay of therapy for idiopathic TTP is plasma exchange (Table 124-4), which removes antibody inhibitors of ADAMTS13 and replenishes the enzyme. With the potential exception of factor H deficiency,[142,146,147] APLS,[100] and quinine-induced disease,[119,120] no compelling evidence indicates that plasma therapy is effective for thrombotic microangiopathy caused by any mechanism other than ADAMTS13 deficiency. Regardless of mechanism, however, the clinical features are variable and overlapping. Consequently, plasma exchange sometimes can be used to treat apparent HUS or secondary thrombotic microangiopathy, particularly in adults, based on the possibility that such patients have an atypical presentation of idiopathic TTP that will respond.

After diagnosing idiopathic TTP or determining that the diagnosis is sufficiently likely to justify treatment, plasma exchange therapy should be started immediately. Studies establishing the value of plasma therapy have excluded most forms of secondary thrombotic microangiopathy,[14,15] so the efficacy of plasma exchange has been demonstrated directly only for idiopathic TTP. The optimal plasma dose is not known, but a common practice is to perform plasma exchange once daily at a volume of 40 or 60 ml/kg, equivalent to 1 or 1.5 plasma volumes. For refractory disease, the intensity of plasma

TABLE 124-4   APPROACH TO TREATMENT AND MONITORING OF IDIOPATHIC THROMBOTIC THROMBOCYTOPENIC PURPURA

Treatment

  Glucocorticoids (e.g., prednisone 2 mg/kg/day or equivalent)

  Plasma exchange 1.5 volume per day

  Plasma infusion 15–30 ml/kg if plasma exchange will be delayed >12 hours

  Continue until complete response for 3 days (platelets >150,000/μl, LDH normal), then decrease plasma exchange to every other day for two more treatments and stop

  If response is durable, taper glucocorticoids

Monitoring

  Neurologic status

  Hemoglobin and platelet count

  Blood film for schistocytes

  LDH

  Serum electrolytes, calcium, blood urea nitrogen, creatinine

Common complications

  Cardiac arrhythmias

  Catheter-associated bleeding or thrombosis

  Citrate toxicity (hypocalcemia, alkalosis)

  Minor allergic reactions to plasma

LDH=lactate dehydrogenase.

exchange can be increased to 1 plasma volume twice daily.[149] Prompt treatment is essential. If plasma exchange must be delayed more than a few hours, plasma should be given by simple infusion at 20 to 40 ml/kg total dose per day, consistent with the patient's ability to tolerate the fluid load.

The replacement fluid should contain ADAMTS13. Satisfactory results have been obtained with fresh-frozen plasma,[14,15] solvent/detergent-treated plasma,[150] or plasma cryosupernatant.[151] The incidence of allergic reactions may be lower with solvent/detergent-treated plasma than with fresh-frozen plasma,[152] but the incidence of thrombosis is increased.[153] Cryosupernatant is depleted in the largest vWF multimers but has normal ADAMTS13 levels,[77] which could make cryosupernatant particularly suitable for treatment of TTP. Nevertheless, a randomized trial suggests that cryosupernatant is equivalent but not superior to fresh-frozen plasma for the initial treatment of TTP.[151] Based on a retrospective analysis, methylene blue-treated plasma may be less effective than fresh-frozen plasma,[154] despite having a similar concentration of ADAMTS13.[155]

Serious catheter-related complications of plasma exchange therapy occur in approximately 30 percent of patients and include pneumothorax and hemorrhage, cardiac perforation, venous thrombosis, and bacterial or fungal infections.[156,157] Regardless of the platelet count, catheter insertion generally can be performed safely without platelet transfusion.[156,158] Hives or pruritic reactions to fresh-frozen plasma occur in one to two thirds of patients but usually can be managed by premedication with antihistamines. High-volume plasma exchange causes metabolic alkalosis and hypocalcemia and may cause unintentional platelet removal.[159,160] Serious complications attributable to plasma are much less common, occurring in approximately 4 percent of patients, and include bronchospasm, anaphylaxis, and serum sickness.[156,157,161]

Plasma exchange should be continued daily until the patient has a complete response, as shown by a platelet count greater than 150,000/μl, LDH within the normal range, and resolution of nonfocal neurologic symptoms.[135,149] The optimal schedule for tapering or discontinuing therapy has not been determined. A typical strategy is to continue plasma exchange until the patient sustains a complete response for 3 days and then reduce the frequency of plasma exchange to every other day (or twice per week) for several days. If the disease remains quiescent, then treatment can be stopped and the patient monitored closely for recurrence.

GLUCOCORTICOIDS

Idiopathic TTP often is an autoimmune disease, and use of glucocorticoids is logical, although a beneficial effect has not been demonstrated conclusively. Similar results have been reported with[14] and without[15] glucocorticoids. Common practice is to give prednisone or equivalent at a total daily dose of 1 or 2 mg/kg, in one or two doses, for the duration of plasma exchange, followed by tapering. An alternative regimen is methylprednisolone 1 g intravenously daily for 3 days.[135]

ANTIPLATELET AGENTS

Use of antiplatelet agents in TTP is controversial. Aspirin and dipyridamole often are combined with plasma exchange but have not been shown conclusively to modify the course of idiopathic TTP.[15,162] To reduce the rate of relapse, ticlopidine was given for 1 year following successful treatment with plasma exchange,[162] but this study was not controlled adequately and ticlopidine can cause TTP.[102] Low-dose aspirin (e.g., 80 mg/day) has been suggested for thromboprophylaxis, once the platelet count exceeds 50,000/μl.[135]

PLATELET TRANSFUSION

Transfusion of platelets may correlate with acute deterioration and death in TTP.[14,31,163] Therefore, platelet transfusions are relatively contraindicated and should be reserved for treatment of life-threatening hemorrhage, preferably after plasma exchange treatment has been initiated. Platelets generally need not be given prophylactically before establishing venous access.[156,158] Platelets have been transfused before emergency surgery, immediately after preparation by intensive plasma exchange.[163]

IMMUNOSUPPRESSIVE THERAPY

Idiopathic TTP that is refractory to plasma exchange may respond to immunosuppression. Anecdotal experience suggests that vincristine may be beneficial, although its efficacy is difficult to assess. Dosing schedules have included 2 mg intravenously on day 1 followed by 1 mg on days 4 and 7,[164] or 2 mg intravenously per week for 2 to 14 weeks.[165] Although it can cause secondary thrombotic microangiopathy, cyclosporine has been used for treatment of refractory idiopathic TTP with some apparent responses.[166,167]

Other cytotoxic immunosuppressive regimens have included oral or intravenous cyclophosphamide, oral azathioprine (reviewed in reference 168), cyclophosphamide, doxorubicin, vincristine, and prednisone (CHOP) combination chemotherapy,[169] autologous stem cell transplantation,[170] and rituximab.[28,171–173]

Rituximab is a monoclonal antibody against CD20, which is expressed on B lymphocytes. It may be preferable to alkylating agents for treatment of women of childbearing age. Case reports describe 18 patients with refractory idiopathic TTP treated with rituximab 375 mg/m² weekly for two to eight doses. Glucocorticoids and vincristine were given simultaneously in four cases and cyclophosphamide in two cases.[28,57,171–177] Fifteen patients had durable complete responses within 2 to 5 weeks of the first dose of rituximab, two patients had partial responses, and one had no response. One patient with lung cancer and thrombotic microangiopathy was treated similarly but did not respond.[172] Rituximab can be removed by plasma exchange, although the efficiency of removal is unknown. Consequently, rituximab should be administered shortly after a session of plasma exchange, and the next plasma exchange should be delayed from 1 to several days if the patient's condition allows.[171]

SPLENECTOMY

Many reports suggest that splenectomy can result in lasting remissions or reduce the frequency of relapses for some patients with idiopathic TTP refractory to plasma exchange or immunosuppressive therapy.[178] Laparoscopic splenectomy can be performed safely in most patients.[179] The mechanism by which splenectomy acts is unknown but may involve the removal of a major site of anti-ADAMTS13 antibody production.[180]

OTHER TREATMENTS

Extracorporeal protein A immunoadsorption can remove anti-ADAMTS13 IgG, which could increase the intravascular survival of endogenous or transfused ADAMTS13. In practice, the results have been disappointing. The single-use devices available in the United States can remove 550 mg IgG per treatment compared to a normal plasma IgG concentration of 8 to 15 g/liter. The few reported responses may reflect a coincidental decline of disease activity or the proposed but undocumented changes in antiidiotype antibodies.[181] Higher-capacity immunoadsorption methods could be more effective. Prostacyclin analogues[182,183] or high-dose intravenous Igs[184,185] have been used, without convincing evidence of efficacy.

SUPPORTIVE THERAPY

Daily laboratory monitoring should include complete blood count with platelet count and levels of LDH, electrolytes, blood urea nitrogen, and creatinine. Because of the high incidence of cardiac damage,[31] continuous electrocardiographic monitoring and periodic assessment of cardiac enzymes should be considered. Patients should receive supplemental folic acid and vaccination for hepatitis B.[135] Minor allergic reactions, metabolic alkalosis, and hypocalcemia associated with plasma exchange should be prevented by appropriate adjustments in therapy.

After the platelet count increases to above 50,000/μl, prophylaxis for venous thromboembolism can be instituted with compression stockings, low molecular weight heparin,[153] and low-dose aspirin.[135]

COURSE AND PROGNOSIS

The long-term mortality of idiopathic TTP treated with plasma exchange ranges from 10 to 20 percent. Most deaths occur within a few days after presentation, and almost all occur within the first month.[14,15,43,47,186–188] The duration of illness is highly variable. Complete response occurs after an average of 9 to 16 days of plasma exchange, and almost all responders are encompassed by a range from 2 to 40 days.[14,15,43,47,186–188] Renal function abnormalities usually resolve over a similar time course.[54] Within the 2 weeks following a complete response, 25 to 50 percent of patients have an acute exacerbation that requires further treatment with plasma exchange. Some patients have repeated exacerbations over several months.[43,186,187]

Relapses, defined as recurrences of disease more than 30 days after a complete response, occur in up to one third of patients. Most relapses occur during the first year, but they have been documented up to 13 years after diagnosis.[43,47,186–189] Relapsing patients typically respond to plasma exchange. Relapses in idiopathic TTP are associated with severe ADAMTS13 deficiency and detectable ADAMTS13 autoantibody inhibitors.[47]

The signs of relapsing TTP can be atypical. Isolated thrombocytopenia may herald a relapse, and stroke or other thrombosis may precede overt thrombotic microangiopathy by days to months.[57,190] Evaluation for relapsing TTP should be considered for any symptom compatible with thrombotic microangiopathy, especially in association with a common trigger of relapse such as infection, surgery, or pregnancy.[50,191]

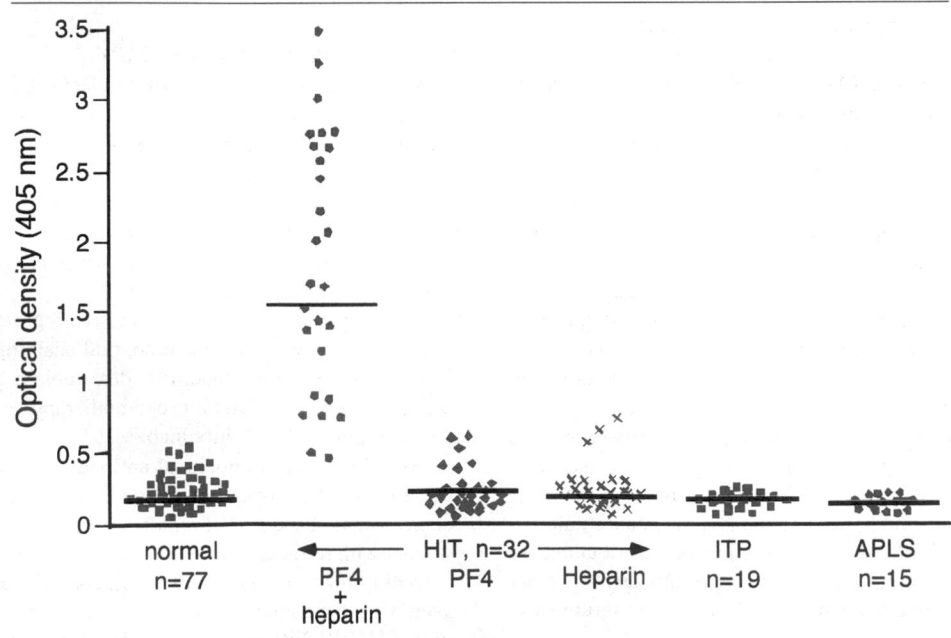

FIGURE 124-4 Heparin/platelet factor 4 (PF4)-based enzyme-linked immunosorbent assay showing heparin-induced thrombocytopenia (HIT) specificity among the thrombocytopenias. Studies were performed using sera from patients with each of the clinical conditions depicted using the indicated number of samples. All platelets were coated with equimolar amounts of PF4 and unfractionated heparin except as indicated. APLS = antiphospholipid syndrome; ITP, immune thrombocytopenic purpura. (Adapted from G Arepally, C Reynolds, A Tomaski, et al.,[220] with permission.).

Data on late sequelae of idiopathic TTP are scanty. Late sequelae may include severe persistent neurologic deficits in 5 to 13 percent,[189,192,193] chronic renal insufficiency in up to 25 percent,[149,193] and dialysis-dependent renal failure in 6 to 8 percent.[99,193]

HEPARIN-INDUCED THROMBOCYTOPENIA

DEFINITION AND HISTORY

HIT is a complication of heparin therapy in which the platelet count falls by more than 50 percent or falls to below 150,000/mm³ in association with heparin therapy. A substantial incidence of arterial and/or venous thromboembolic complications is noted in this disorder.

Although clinical use of heparin as an anticoagulant began in the late 1950s, it was not until the early 1970s that a small percentage of treated patients were noted to develop a complication consisting of thrombocytopenia with paradoxical, life-threatening thromboemboli (for a historical review see reference 194). In the 1980s, it became clear that HIT was caused by IgG antibodies that activated platelets. It also was recognized that HIT could be divided into two types: classic type I disease, which is the focus of this chapter, and type II, which is a benign condition associated with a mild, immediate, and transient decrease in platelet number with no immune basis and no increased risk of thrombosis.[195] In the late 1980s and early 1990s, it became clear that HIT antibodies activated both platelets and endothelial cells.[196,197] Further analysis showed that platelet activation involved an immune complex as blocking platelet FcγRIIA inhibited platelet activation by HIT sera *in vitro*.[198] The antigenic immune complex involved heparin bound to the platelet-specific chemokine platelet factor 4 (PF4).[199] Currently, the greatest challenge of this disorder is development of strategies for its prevention or treatment.

EPIDEMIOLOGY

The frequency of HIT in a hospitalized population depends on the nature of the heparin used, duration of heparin exposure, and clinical setting. Heparin is a negatively charged polysaccharide, enzymatically derived from either bovine or porcine intestines.[200] These products are not homogeneous for either polymer length or sequence. The frequency of HIT in nonsurgical settings is clearly higher in patients treated with unfractionated, high molecular weight (HMW) heparin (1–5%) than in patients treated with low molecular weight (LMW) heparin (0.2–1%).[201–205] Bovine-derived heparin may be associated with a higher incidence of HIT than porcine heparin.[201,206] Newer, synthetic pentasaccharide anticoagulants probably have a much lower or no risk of inducing HIT.[207]

No route of unfractionated, HMW heparin delivery protects against development of HIT.[203,208] The only recourse to preventing HIT development is limiting the exposure time[209] and avoiding heparin flushes thereafter.[210] Heparin-bonded catheters can underlie the development of HIT.[211,212]

The greatest clinical risk factors for developing HIT are the patient's age and the nature of the patient's medical condition. HIT may occur in pediatric patients, but its incidence and severity are much lower than in adults.[213] Patients treated for medical conditions have a lower risk of developing HIT than patients undergoing surgical procedures. Whether certain subgroups of medical patients, such as hemodialysis patients or pregnant women, have a particularly low incidence of HIT is not clear.[214,215] Among surgical patients, those undergoing coronary artery bypass grafting, orthopedic procedures, or isolated limb perfusion are particularly vulnerable to developing HIT.[204,216,217]

Determination of the incidence of thrombosis in various settings has been hampered by the infrequency of HIT, the need to carefully document both the diagnosis and the thrombotic complications. Nevertheless, some prospective studies suggest that the incidence of thrombosis is between 35 and 58 percent in patients with documented HIT.[204,218,219] The risk of thromboembolic complications is not altered by discontinuing heparin therapy.[219] The ratio of arterial to venous thrombi is high (0.7:1).[219]

ETIOLOGY AND PATHOGENESIS

HIT is an immune complex disorder of heparin therapy involving heparin–PF4 complexes. Such antibodies are not demonstrable in other forms of thrombocytopenia (Fig. 124-4).[220] A murine model involving mice that are transgenic for both human FcγRIIA and human PF4 supports the importance of heparin–PF4 immune complexes in the development of both thrombocytopenia and thrombosis in HIT.[221] Normally, mice lack platelet FcγRIIA. HIT antibodies do not recognize mice PF4 complexed to heparin. In a murine HIT model, mice were infused with an HIT-like monoclonal antibody termed *KKO*[222] and then given a course of heparin injections (Fig. 124-5, *A*). Only mice with platelets expressing both FcγRIIA and human PF4 developed thrombocytopenia (Fig. 124-5, *B*) and thrombosis. These studies demonstrate that four components are necessary to induce HIT in a

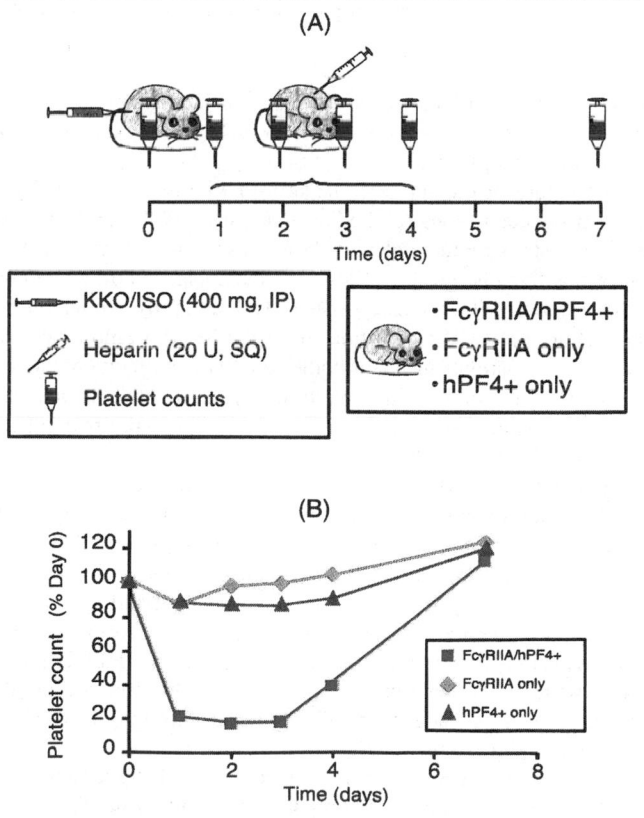

FIGURE 124-5   Murine model of heparin-induced thrombocytopenia (HIT). *(A)* Schema of the protocol for HIT mice model. The types of animals studied are shown in the *right lower-hand corner*. FcγRIIA, mice transgenic for the FcγRIIA receptor; hPF4+, mice transgenic for human platelet factor 4 (hPF4) expressed in megakaryocytes. On day 0, mice received the HIT-like monoclonal antibody KKO intraperitoneally (IP). On days 1–4, they were injected with heparin. On days 0, 1–4 and 7, blood was drawn. *(B)* Platelet counts in each set of transgenic mice at various times in relation to heparin exposure. (Adapted from MP Reilly, SM Taylor, NK Hartman, et al.,[221] with permission.)

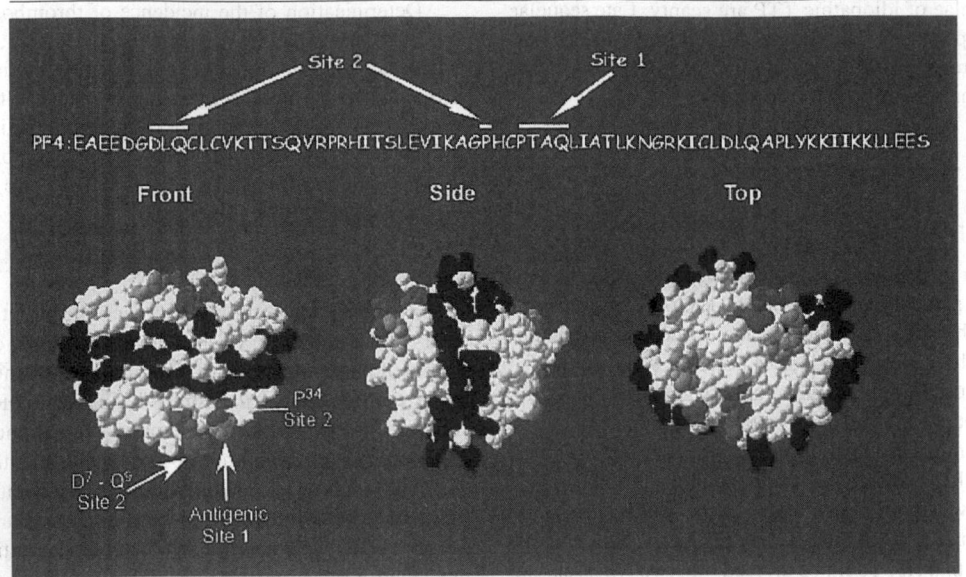

FIGURE 124-6 Platelet factor 4 (PF4) tetramer structure. *(Top)* Linear sequence of PF4 and the regions known to contribute to heparin-induced thrombocytopenia (HIT) antigenicity when PF4 is complexed to heparin *(boxed)*. *(Bottom)* Three views of the PF4 tetramer with the positively charged residues shown in *dark gray*. The sites at which HIT neoepitopes are exposed on the PF4 tetramer are indicated in shades of *light and medium gray*. (Adapted from ZQ Li, W Liu, KS Park, et al.,[225] with permission.)

mouse: (1) human PF4 released by platelets, (2) platelet FcγRIIA, (3) heparin infusion, and (4) presence of an IgG antibody that recognizes heparin-PF4 complexes.

The nature of the antigenic heparin-PF4 complex is partially defined. At concentrations reached at injury sites, PF4 exists as a tetramer.[223] Crystal structure analysis shows this tetramer is encircled by a ring of positive charge (Fig. 124-6),[223] and heparin is thought to bind to this region.[224] Two closely spaced HIT antibody recognition domains (Fig. 124-6)[225] are distinct from the heparin-binding domain. About half of patients have antibodies that react with one or the other heparin-binding domain, and one third of patients have no antibodies that react to either domain, suggesting the presence of other potential HIT antigenic sites on PF4.

Studies have shown that tetrameric PF4 and unfractionated heparin must be at an approximately 1:1 molar ratio to display optimal HIT antigenicity.[226,227] At this ratio, an ultra-large complex (>670 kDa) of PF4 and heparin forms and likely is the antigen functioning in HIT.[228] At higher or lower ratios, PF4 usually forms small and less antigenic heparin-PF4 complexes. LMW heparin inefficiently forms ultra-large complexes that may explain the lower incidence of HIT in patients treated with LMW heparin. The pentasaccharide fondaparinux does not bind PF4 at all, suggesting that fondaparinux may be useful for prevention and treatment of HIT.

Other studies in mice provide insights into why thrombosis is so prevalent in patients with HIT compared to patients with other immune complex disorders. Studies of transgenic mice overexpressing platelet PF4 demonstrated impaired thrombus formation. Infusion of heparin into these mice at a dose that fully anticoagulates normal mice paradoxically enhanced thrombus formation at a site of vascular injury[229] (Fig. 124-7). This model simulates the clinical setting of HIT. Many of the patients are elderly with atherosclerotic vascular changes and/ or have underlying sites of vascular injury. Release of excess PF4 at these vascular sites interferes with thrombosis until heparin is infused, after which a paradoxical increase in the capacity to form thrombi

occurs (Fig. 124-8). More platelets are incorporated into the growing thrombus, which contributes to thrombocytopenia, development of immune complexes that activate platelets, and formation of procoagulant platelet microparticles.[230]

As part of this cycle of increased activation, HIT antibodies bind to endothelial cells likely via a PF4–surface glycosaminoglycan complex[197,231] that appears to be heparin independent. This binding may

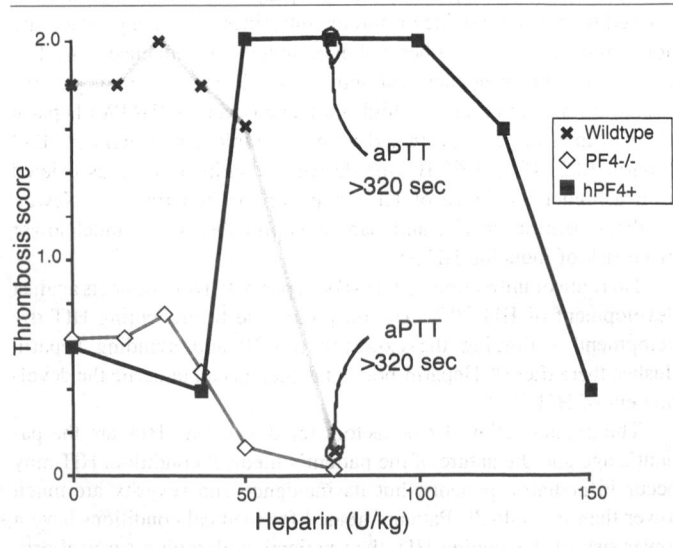

FIGURE 124-7 Role of platelet factor 4 (PF4) in thrombosis. An FeCl₃ injury of the carotid artery was induced, and vessel occlusion was monitored. A score of 2 indicates stable total occlusion, a score of 1 indicates unstable total occlusion, and a score 0 indicates that no stable total occlusion occurred. aPTT, activated partial thromboplastin time; hPF4+, transgenic mice overexpressing human PF4; PF4−/−, PF4 knockout mice.

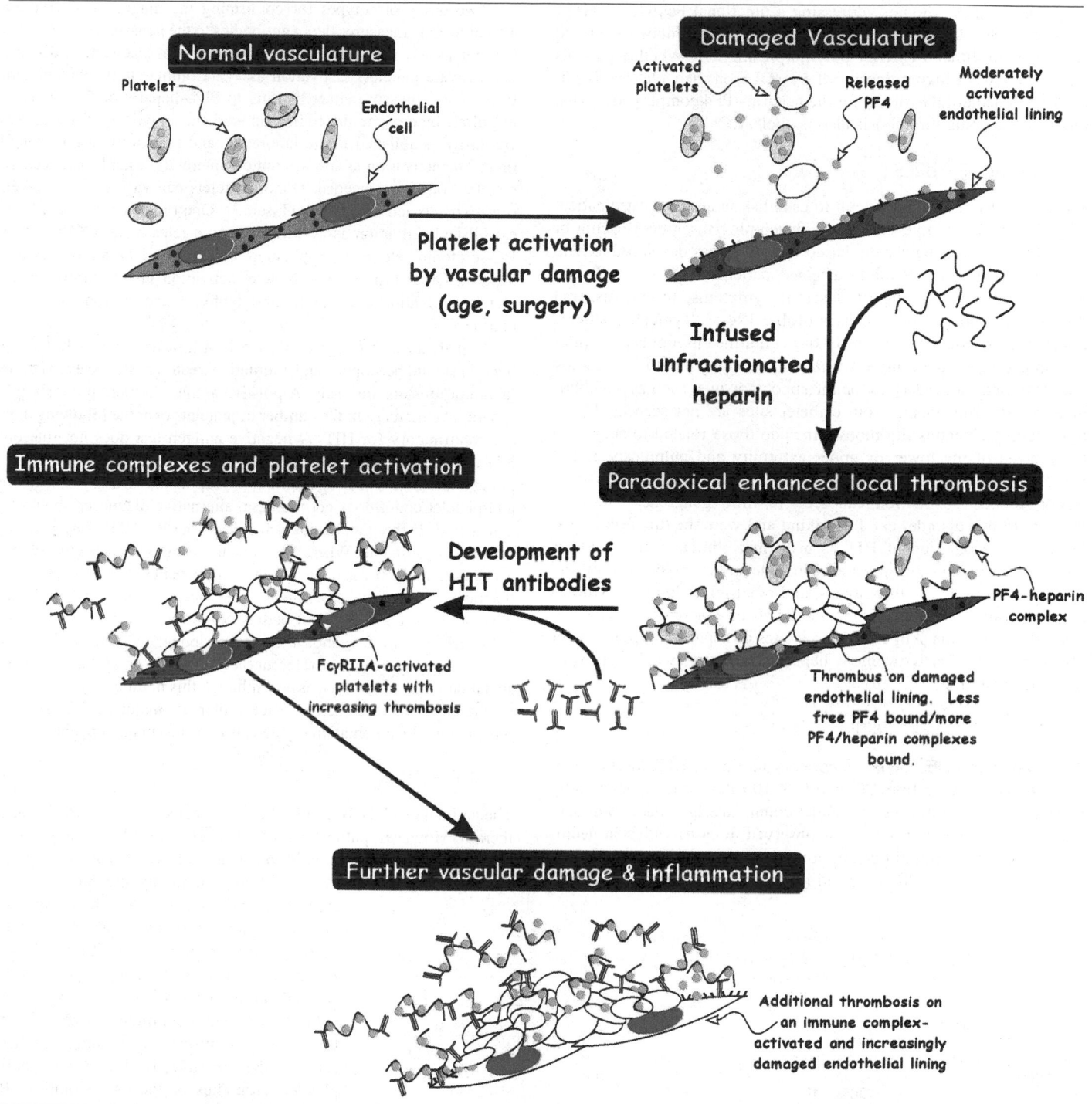

FIGURE 124-8   Model of early events in the etiology of heparin-induced thrombocytopenia (HIT). Patients develop a clinical condition associated with chronic release of platelet factor 4 (PF4) from platelets *(top right)*. Administration of heparin leads to paradoxically increased local thrombosis as a consequence of more PF4 release *(middle right)*. Neoepitopes exposed on the circulating large, stoichiometric PF4–heparin complexes induce an immune response *(middle left)*. Immune complexes composed of heparin–PF4 and the HIT antibody form, enhancing local thrombosis through additional platelet activation *(middle left)* and probably promote clearance of platelets in the spleen (not shown), both of which lead to thrombocytopenia. Additionally, the immune complexes contribute to local activation of endothelial cells *(bottom)* and macrophages, causing an inflammatory process that contributes to development of thrombosis.

further increase vascular activation, augmenting local thrombosis. Additionally, HIT antibodies activate monocytes in a PF4–surface glycosaminoglycan-dependent fashion[232,233] that requires activation through surface FcγRIIA[234] and leads to increased tissue factor expression within hours.

A number of polymorphisms have been examined, but none has shown a clear association with an increased risk for developing HIT or thrombosis. Thus, no clear association was shown with the known thrombophilic polymorphisms of factor V Leiden, prothrombin G20210A, methylenetetrahydrofolate reductase (MTHFR) C677T, or

$\alpha_{IIb}\beta_3$ and $\alpha_1\beta_2$.[235] Studies addressing a functional FcγRIIA R/H131 polymorphism showed that HIT, with or without thrombosis, occurred equally with either FcγRIIA polymorphism.[236,237] Whether patients with HIT have a higher density of FcγRIIA on their platelets is unclear.[238] Whether IgG affinity for the heparin–PF4 complex affects the risk of developing thrombosis also is unclear.[236,239]

CLINICAL FEATURES

The diagnosis of HIT is difficult to establish in a complicated patient who can have multiple causes for developing thrombocytopenia or thrombosis. A scoring system based on "4Ts" was developed to help maintain focus on potentially affected patients.[240] The four Ts are thrombocytopenia, timing of onset of symptoms, thrombosis, and thrombocytopenia of other causes (Table 124-5). Typically, patients develop thrombocytopenia 5 to 10 days after the onset of heparin therapy unless exposure occurred within the preceding month.[240] Bleeding manifestations secondary to the thrombocytopenia, such as petechiae, nose bleeds, and oozing from catheter sites are not seen in HIT.[204] Symptoms of venous thrombosis include those related to deep vein thrombosis of the lower or upper extremity and pulmonary embolism,[204,241] adrenal infarctions,[242] and cerebral venous thrombosis.[243] Major venous obstruction can lead to limb gangrene.[244] Arterial thrombi in this disorder can be striking and were the first feature that led to the recognition of HIT as a distinct clinical entity.[194] Other common thrombotic complications include stroke, myocardial infarction, mesenteric artery thrombosis, and renal infarction.[245,246] Thrombosis of grafts and prosthetic devices has been reported.[244,247] Gangrenous changes in the skin can occur at sites of heparin injections[248] but also can occur after intravenous heparin[249] or after switching to warfarin (Coumadin).[250]

LABORATORY FEATURES

Thrombocytopenia is the key laboratory finding in HIT. Most often it is moderate, ranging from 20 to 100×10^9/liter, or is represented by a 50 to 70 percent decline in platelet count. Rarely is the thrombocytopenia more severe or absent, as observed in cases with skin necrosis.[251] Although thrombin generation increases in HIT, patients rarely have decompensated disseminated intravascular coagulation.[252]

Two assay prototypes for confirming the diagnosis of HIT are available. One measures the Ig antibodies to the heparin–PF4 complex (antigen assay), and the other measures heparin-dependent antibodies that activate platelets (activation assay). Commercially available antigen assays measure either binding to PF4–heparin or PF4–polyvinylsulfate by enzyme-linked immunosorbent assay.[199,253] These assays are easily established in the laboratory and have a rapid turnaround time. The activation assays are not commercially established because platelet donors are needed. Donor platelets can vary greatly in their sensitivity to activation by HIT sera.[230] One of the earliest and best-established activation assays, the serotonin release assay,[254] involves ^{14}C-serotonin release from platelets induced by HIT antibodies and heparin. Other tests include platelet activation in a heparin-induced platelet activation assay,[255] luminography,[256] and microparticle generation.[230]

In patients with a high clinical risk of having HIT (Table 124-5), heparin should be stopped and alternative treatment started even before laboratory results are ready. A positive antigen test and particularly a progressive increase in the number of platelets over the following days are confirmatory for HIT. A negative antigen test does not rule out HIT and should be repeated after 24 hours while the patient is undergoing alternative anti-coagulant therapy. If the repeat assay is negative and platelet count does not increase, alternative diagnoses should be considered. If the platelet count increases but the HIT assay is negative, HIT is probable. Where the clinical setting is not straightforward, a negative antigen assay encourages the consideration of alternative diagnoses. A positive test can be false because many patients who develop anti-PF4/heparin antibodies do not necessarily go on to develop HIT.[209] An activation assay takes longer to perform and may require sending sera to a reference center. This assay has a greater specificity than the antigen assay, although this finding may vary based on the experience of the reference center. Its major usefulness is in *post factum* documentation of the cause of thrombocytopenia.

DIFFERENTIAL DIAGNOSIS

The hallmark of HIT is the onset of thrombocytopenia during heparin therapy. However, patients who develop HIT often have complicated medical and surgical conditions, many of which can also cause thrombocytopenia. These conditions commonly include disorders associated with increased peripheral destruction of platelets but rarely are associated with decreased platelet production (Table 124-6). A common cause of thrombocytopenia is dilutional thrombocytopenia following cardiopulmonary bypass operations, but this condition slowly improves over time. Another cause is the formation of drug-related, antiplatelet antibodies or the use of anti-$\alpha_{IIb}\beta_3$ drugs such as abciximab.[257] Posttransfusion purpura can begin approximately 1 week after blood transfusion,[258] and often the patient has a history of pregnancies and/or prior transfusion exposures. Sepsis and disseminated intravascular coagulation can present initially with thrombocytopenia as the most prominent manifestation, although often these processes rapidly progress, distinguishing themselves from HIT. TTP and HUS can present with thrombocytopenia as one of the first manifestations. Often, the ensuing clinical course and examination of the blood films distinguish these diseases from HIT. SLE and APLS can

TABLE 124-5 THE FOUR Ts SCORE OF 6–8 IS HIGH RISK FOR HEPARIN-INDUCED THROMBOCYTOPENIA, 4–5 IS INTERMEDIATE RISK, AND 0–3 IS LOW RISK

CLINICAL SIGN	POINTS PER CATEGORY		
	0	1	2
Thrombocytopenia (acute)	Very low nadir ($<10\times10^3$/mm³) or $<30\%$ fall	Low nadir ($10-20\times10^3$/mm³) or 30–50% fall	Moderate nadir (20–100×10^3/mm³) or $>50\%$ fall
Timing of first event (thrombocytopenia or thrombosis)	≤4 days (unless prior heparin exposure in last 3 months)	Within 5–10 days (but not well documented) or ≤1 day (with exposure in last 31–100 days)	Documented occurrence in 5–10 days or ≤1 day (with exposure in last 30 days)
Thrombotic-related event	None	Common thrombi (deep vein thrombosis or line thrombus) or recurrent thrombus; erythematous skin lesion or not suspected thrombus	Major vessel thrombus or skin necrosis or skin lesion at site of heparin infusion
Thrombocytopenia (other causes)	Definite other cause is present	Possible other cause is present	No other strong explanation for thrombocytopenia

SOURCE: Adapted from Warkentin.[240]

TABLE 124-6   ALTERNATIVE CAUSES OF CLINICAL CONDITIONS
SIMULATING HEPARIN-INDUCED THROMBOCYTOPENIA

Thrombocytopenia
  Increased destruction
    Acute immune thrombocytopenic purpura
    Dilutional thrombocytopenia
    Posttransfusion purpura
    Drug-induced thrombocytopenia
      Quinidine, quinine, trimethoprim-sulfamethoxazole, rifampicin, carbamazepine, diclofenac, ibuprofen
      Integrin $\alpha_{IIb}\beta_3$ inhibitors: abciximab, tirofiban, eptifibatide
  Decreased production
    Postsepsis
    Chemotherapy
    Malignancy
    Drug related
Thrombocytopenia and thrombosis
  Consumptive thrombohemorrhagic disorders
    Sepsis and disseminated intravascular coagulation
    Malignancies
    Disseminated intravascular coagulation in pregnancy or after snake bite
    Thrombotic thrombocytopenic purpura
    Hemolytic uremic syndrome
    Systemic lupus erythematosus
    Antiphospholipid syndrome
Thrombosis alone
  Venous stasis
  Central catheters
  Vasculitis

be confused with HIT because these conditions cause both thrombocytopenia and thrombosis.

THERAPY

Despite greater understanding of the molecular basis of HIT and the availability of a number of new therapeutic agents, management is problematic. Prospective studies of patients with HIT indicate that without treatment, more than 50 percent can develop thrombosis over the ensuing days to weeks.[204,218,219] Current therapies can reduce, but not eliminate, the risk of this life-threatening complication. For prevention of HIT, many authorities prefer using LMW heparin because it confers a lower risk of HIT than HMW heparin.[203–205] Heparin exposure should be limited to the period of high thrombotic risk. Institution of a hospital-wide policy of daily platelet counts in patients receiving heparin therapy may allow early detection of thrombocytopenia and earlier intervention. In addition, elimination of heparin usage in flushes for maintaining patent catheter lines and in impregnation of catheters with heparin decreases the incidence of HIT. Finally, the development of alternative agents to replace heparin therapy, such as synthetic pentasaccharides that do not bind to PF4, may decrease the incidence of HIT. Coumadin should not be used as the sole initial treatment of HIT because of the increased risk of untoward thrombosis.[250] LMW heparin should not replace HMW heparin because of cross-reactivity.[258]

Three accepted drugs are used for treatment of patients with HIT: danaparoid sodium (no longer available in the United States), recombinant hirudin (lepirudin), and argatroban. Danaparoid is a mixture of LMW heparinoids consisting of heparan sulfate, dermatan sulfate, and chondroitin sulfate. It has much greater anti-factor Xa activity than antithrombin activity.[259] Danaparoid is an effective anticoagulant[260] that inhibits HIT antibody-induced platelet aggregation *in vitro*.[261]

PF4–danaparoid complexes have little cross-reactivity with HIT antibodies.[262] Studies suggest danaparoid use improves platelet count recovery and decreases the incidence of serious thrombosis and death in patients with HIT.[263]

The other two drugs, lepirudin and argatroban, directly inhibit thrombin.[264] Both drugs are given intravenously and have rapid onset of action. Lepirudin binds to two sites on thrombin, the catalytic site and a fibrinogen-binding site, whereas argatroban binds only to the active site. Lepirudin prolongs the aPTT, so this test can be used to monitor effective dosing. Lepirudin is excreted in the urine, and its dosage must be adjusted in patients with renal failure.[265] Lepirudin induces antilepirudin antibodies in approximately half of patients who receive the drug. These antibodies rarely alter biologic activity but tend to prolong the drug's half-life, necessitating careful monitoring by aPTT.[266] Argatroban is synthesized from arginine and is rapidly metabolized in the liver.[267] It affects both aPTT and PT.[268] Use of lepirudin and argatroban is efficacious; the incidence of thrombotic complications is reduced, perhaps by half, and the time to platelet count recovery is shortened.[218,269–271] However, bleeding complications can occur. As with danaparoid, lepirudin or argatroban should be given until patients recover from the thrombocytopenia before adding and then switching to a prolonged course of an oral anticoagulant. With argatroban treatment, this switch is slightly more complicated because both argatroban and coumadin prolong the international normalized ratio.[268]

COURSE AND PROGNOSIS

Unrecognized HIT can lead to life-threatening thrombosis in approximately 50 percent of patients. The percentage of patients with an adverse outcome remains high even if heparin therapy is withdrawn immediately. Intervention with either of the direct thrombin inhibitors or danaparoid suggests that the length of time of thrombocytopenia, and more importantly, the percent of patients developing significant thrombosis can be reduced significantly with a generally acceptable increased incidence of significant bleeding. The prognosis likely will improve with increasing experience in the care of these patients. Whether alternative treatments based on increased insights into the pathophysiology of HIT will allow more rapid and more effective intervention remains to be seen.

REFERENCES

1. Moschcowitz E: Hyaline thrombosis of the terminal arterioles and capillaries: A hitherto undescribed disease. *Proc N Y Pathol Soc* 24:21, 1924.

2. Moschcowitz E: An acute febrile pleiochromic anemia with hyaline thrombosis of the terminal arterioles and capillaries. *Arch Intern Med* 36:89, 1925.

3. Singer K, Bornstein FP, Wile SA: Thrombotic thrombocytopenic purpura. Hemorrhagic diathesis with generalized platelet thromboses. *Blood* 2:542, 1946.

4. Gasser VC, Bautier D, Steck A, et al: Hämolytisch-ürämische Syndrome: Bilaterale Nierenrindennekrosen bei akuten erworbenen hämolytischen Anämien. *Schweiz Med Wochenschr* 85:905, 1955.

5. Kibel MA, Barnard PJ: The haemolytic-uraemic syndrome: A survey in Southern Africa. *S Afr Med J* 42:692, 1968.

6. Amorosi EL, Ultmann JE: Thrombotic thrombocytopenic purpura: Report of 16 cases and review of the literature. *Medicine* 45:139, 1966.

7. Rubinstein MA, Kagan BM, Macgillviray MH, et al: Unusual remission in a case of thrombotic thrombocytopenic purpura syndrome following fresh blood exchange transfusions. *Ann Intern Med* 51:1409, 1959.

8. Monnens LA, Retera RJ: Thrombotic thrombocytopenic purpura in a neonatal infant. *J Pediatr* 71:118, 1967.

9. Bukowski RM, Hewlett JS, Harris JW, et al: Exchange transfusions in the treatment of thrombotic thrombocytopenic purpura. *Semin Hematol* 13:219, 1976.

10. Bukowski RM, King JW, Hewlett JS: Plasmapheresis in the treatment of thrombotic thrombocytopenic purpura. *Blood* 50:413, 1977.

11. Byrnes JJ, Khurana M: Treatment of thrombotic thrombocytopenic purpura with plasma. *N Engl J Med* 297:1386, 1977.

12. Schulman I, Pierce M, Lukens A, Currimbhoy Z: Studies on thrombopoiesis: I. A factor in normal human plasma required for platelet production; chronic thrombocytopenia due to its deficiency. *Blood* 16:943, 1960.

13. Upshaw JD Jr: Congenital deficiency of a factor in normal plasma that reverses microangiopathic hemolysis and thrombocytopenia. *N Engl J Med* 298:1350, 1978.

14. Bell WR, Braine HG, Ness PM, Kickler TS: Improved survival in thrombotic thrombocytopenic purpura-hemolytic uremic syndrome. Clinical experience in 108 patients. *N Engl J Med* 325:398, 1991.

15. Rock GA, Shumak KH, Buskard NA, et al: Comparison of plasma exchange with plasma infusion in the treatment of thrombotic thrombocytopenic purpura. Canadian Apheresis Study Group. *N Engl J Med* 325: 393, 1991.

16. Moake JL, Rudy CK, Troll JH, et al: Unusually large plasma factor VIII: von Willebrand factor multimers in chronic relapsing thrombotic thrombocytopenic purpura. *N Engl J Med* 307:1432, 1982.

17. Furlan M, Robles R, Lämmle B: Partial purification and characterization of a protease from human plasma cleaving von Willebrand factor to fragments produced by in vivo proteolysis. *Blood* 87:4223, 1996.

18. Tsai H-M: Physiologic cleavage of von Willebrand factor by a plasma protease is dependent on its conformation and requires calcium ion. *Blood* 87:4235, 1996.

19. Furlan M, Robles R, Solenthaler M, et al: Deficient activity of von Willebrand factor-cleaving protease in chronic relapsing thrombotic thrombocytopenic purpura. *Blood* 89:3097, 1997.

20. Furlan M, Robles R, Galbusera M, et al: von Willebrand factor-cleaving protease in thrombotic thrombocytopenic purpura and the hemolytic-uremic syndrome. *N Engl J Med* 339:1578, 1998.

21. Tsai HM, Lian EC: Antibodies to von Willebrand factor-cleaving protease in acute thrombotic thrombocytopenic purpura. *N Engl J Med* 339: 1585, 1998.

22. Fujikawa K, Suzuki H, McMullen B, Chung D: Purification of human von Willebrand factor-cleaving protease and its identification as a new member of the metalloproteinase family. *Blood* 98:1662, 2001.

23. Gerritsen HE, Robles R, Lammle B, Furlan M: Partial amino acid sequence of purified von Willebrand factor-cleaving protease. *Blood* 98: 1654, 2001.

24. Zheng X, Chung D, Takayama TK, et al: Structure of von Willebrand factor-cleaving protease (ADAMTS13), a metalloprotease involved in thrombotic thrombocytopenic purpura. *J Biol Chem* 276: 41059, 2001.

25. Soejima K, Mimura N, Hirashima M, et al: A novel human metalloprotease synthesized in the liver and secreted into the blood: Possibly, the von Willebrand factor-cleaving protease? *J Biochem* 130:475, 2001.

26. Hurskainen TL, Hirohata S, Seldin MF, Apte SS: ADAM-TS5, ADAM-TS6, and ADAM-TS7, novel members of a new family of zinc metalloproteases. General features and genomic distribution of the ADAM-TS family. *J Biol Chem* 274:25555, 1999.

27. Levy GG, Nichols WC, Lian EC, et al: Mutations in a member of the ADAMTS gene family cause thrombotic thrombocytopenic purpura. *Nature* 413:488, 2001.

28. Zheng X, Pallera AM, Goodnough LT, et al: Remission of chronic thrombotic thrombocytopenic purpura after treatment with cyclophosphamide and rituximab. *Ann Intern Med* 138:105, 2003.

29. Klaus C, Plaimauer B, Studt JD, et al: Epitope mapping of ADAMTS13 autoantibodies in acquired thrombotic thrombocytopenic purpura. *Blood* 103:4514, 2004.

30. Scheiflinger F, Knobl P, Trattner B, et al: Nonneutralizing IgM and IgG antibodies to von Willebrand factor-cleaving protease (ADAMTS-13) in a patient with thrombotic thrombocytopenic purpura. *Blood* 102:3241, 2003.

31. Ridolfi RL, Bell WR: Thrombotic thrombocytopenic purpura. Report of 25 cases and review of the literature. *Medicine* 60:413, 1981.

32. Asada Y, Sumiyoshi A, Hayashi T, et al: Immunohistochemistry of vascular lesion in thrombotic thrombocytopenic purpura, with special reference to factor VIII related antigen. *Thromb Res* 38:469, 1985.

33. Hosler GA, Cusumano AM, Hutchins GM: Thrombotic thrombocytopenic purpura and hemolytic uremic syndrome are distinct pathologic entities. A review of 56 autopsy cases. *Arch Pathol Lab Med* 127:834, 2003.

34. Wallace DC, Lovric A, Clubb JS, Carseldine DB: Thrombotic thrombocytopenic purpura in four siblings. *Am J Med* 58:724, 1975.

35. Inward CD, Howie AJ, Fitzpatrick MM, et al: Renal histopathology in fatal cases of diarrhoea-associated haemolytic uraemic syndrome. British Association for Paediatric Nephrology. *Pediatr Nephrol* 11:556, 1997.

36. Siddiqui FA, Lian EC: Characterization of platelet agglutinating protein p37 purified from the plasma of a patient with thrombotic thrombocytopenic purpura. *Biochem Mol Biol Int* 30:385, 1993.

37. Praprotnik S, Blank M, Levy Y, et al: Anti-endothelial cell antibodies from patients with thrombotic thrombocytopenic purpura specifically activate small vessel endothelial cells. *Int Immunol* 13:203, 2001.

38. Schultz DR, Arnold PI, Jy W, et al: Anti-CD36 autoantibodies in thrombotic thrombocytopenic purpura and other thrombotic disorders: Identification of an 85 kD form of CD36 as a target antigen. *Br J Haematol* 103:849, 1998.

39. Mitra D, Jaffe EA, Weksler B, et al: Thrombotic thrombocytopenic purpura and sporadic hemolytic-uremic syndrome plasmas induce apoptosis in restricted lineages of human microvascular endothelial cells. *Blood* 89:1224, 1997.

40. van der Plas RM, Schiphorst ME, Huizinga EG, et al: von Willebrand factor proteolysis is deficient in classic, but not in bone marrow transplantation-associated, thrombotic thrombocytopenic purpura. *Blood* 93: 3798, 1999.

41. Arai S, Allan C, Streiff M, et al: Von Willebrand factor-cleaving protease activity and proteolysis of von Willebrand factor in bone marrow transplant-associated thrombotic microangiopathy. *Hematol J* 2:292, 2001.

42. Iwata H, Kami M, Hori A, et al: An autopsy-based retrospective study of secondary thrombotic thrombocytopenic purpura. *Haematologica* 86: 669, 2001.

43. George JN, Li X, McMinn JR, et al: Thrombotic thrombocytopenic purpura-hemolytic uremic syndrome following allogeneic HPC transplantation: A diagnostic dilemma. *Transfusion* 44:294, 2004.

44. Torok TJ, Holman RC, Chorba TL: Increasing mortality from thrombotic thrombocytopenic purpura in the United States—Analysis of national mortality data 1968-1991. *Am J Hematol* 50:84, 1995.

45. Miller DP, Kaye JA, Shea K, et al: Incidence of thrombotic thrombocytopenic purpura/hemolytic uremic syndrome. *Epidemiology* 15:208, 2004.

46. Vesely SK, George JN, Lammle B, et al: ADAMTS13 activity in thrombotic thrombocytopenic purpura-hemolytic uremic syndrome: Relation to presenting features and clinical outcomes in a prospective cohort of 142 patients. *Blood* 102:60, 2003.

47. Zheng XL, Kaufman RM, Goodnough LT, Sadler JE: Effect of plasma exchange on plasma ADAMTS13 metalloprotease activity, inhibitor level, and clinical outcome in patients with idiopathic and nonidiopathic thrombotic thrombocytopenic purpura. *Blood* 103:4043, 2004.

48. Nicol KK, Shelton BJ, Knovich MA, Owen J: Overweight individuals are at increased risk for thrombotic thrombocytopenic purpura. *Am J Hematol* 74:170, 2003.

49. McMinn JR, George JN: Evaluation of women with clinically suspected thrombotic thrombocytopenic purpura-hemolytic uremic syndrome during pregnancy. *J Clin Apheresis* 16:202, 2001.

50. Furlan M, Lämmle B: Aetiology and pathogenesis of thrombotic thrombocytopenic purpura and haemolytic uraemic syndrome: The role of von Willebrand factor-cleaving protease. *Best Pract Res Clin Haematol* 14:437, 2001.

51. Studt JD, Hovinga JA, Radonic R, et al: Familial acquired thrombotic thrombocytopenic purpura: ADAMTS13 inhibitory autoantibodies in identical twins. *Blood* 103:4195, 2004.

52. Joseph G, Smith KJ, Hadley TJ, et al: HLA-DR53 protects against thrombotic thrombocytopenic purpura/adult hemolytic uremic syndrome. *Am J Hematol* 47:189, 1994.

53. Raife TJ, Lentz SR, Atkinson BS, et al: Factor V Leiden: A genetic risk factor for thrombotic microangiopathy in patients with normal von Willebrand factor-cleaving protease activity. *Blood* 99:437, 2002.

54. Thompson CE, Damon LE, Ries CA, Linker CA: Thrombotic microangiopathies in the 1980s: Clinical features, response to treatment, and the impact of the human immunodeficiency virus epidemic. *Blood* 80:1890, 1992.

55. Piastra M, Curro V, Chiaretti A, et al: Intracranial hemorrhage at the onset of thrombotic thrombocytopenic purpura in an infant: Therapeutic approach and intensive care management. *Pediatr Emerg Care* 17:42, 2001.

56. O'Brien TE, Crum ED: Atypical presentations of thrombotic thrombocytopenic purpura. *Int J Hematol* 76:471, 2002.

57. Tsai H-M, Shulman K: Rituximab induces remission of cerebral ischemia caused by thrombotic thrombocytopenic purpura. *Eur J Haematol* 70:183, 2003.

58. Chang JC, Aly ES: Acute respiratory distress syndrome as a major clinical manifestation of thrombotic thrombocytopenic purpura. *Am J Med Sci* 321:124, 2001.

59. Burns ER, Lou Y, Pathak A: Morphologic diagnosis of thrombotic thrombocytopenic purpura. *Am J Hematol* 75:18, 2004.

60. Takahashi H, Tatewaki W, Nakamura T, et al: Coagulation studies in thrombotic thrombocytopenic purpura, with special reference to von Willebrand factor and protein S. *Am J Hematol* 30:14, 1989.

61. Veyradier A, Obert B, Houllier A, et al: Specific von Willebrand factor-cleaving protease in thrombotic microangiopathies: A study of 111 cases. *Blood* 98:1765, 2001.

62. Bianchi V, Robles R, Alberio L, et al: Von Willebrand factor-cleaving protease (ADAMTS13) in thrombocytopenic disorders: A severely deficient activity is specific for thrombotic thrombocytopenic purpura. *Blood* 100:710, 2002.

63. Tsai HM: Is severe deficiency of ADAMTS-13 specific for thrombotic thrombocytopenic purpura? Yes. *J Thromb Haemost* 1:625, 2003.

64. Mannucci PM, Canciani MT, Forza I, et al: Changes in health and disease of the metalloprotease that cleaves von Willebrand factor. *Blood* 98:2730, 2001.

65. Reiter RA, Knobl P, Varadi K, Turecek PL: Changes in von Willebrand factor-cleaving protease (ADAMTS13) activity after infusion of desmopressin. *Blood* 101:946, 2003.

66. Kavakli K, Canciani MT, Mannucci PM: Plasma levels of the von Willebrand factor-cleaving protease in physiological and pathological conditions in children. *Pediatr Hematol Oncol* 19:467, 2002.

67. Park YD, Yoshioka A, Kawa K, et al: Impaired activity of plasma von Willebrand factor-cleaving protease may predict the occurrence of hepatic veno-occlusive disease after stem cell transplantation. *Bone Marrow Transplant* 29:789, 2002.

68. Studt JD, Bohm M, Budde U, et al: Measurement of von Willebrand factor-cleaving protease (ADAMTS-13) activity in plasma: A multicenter comparison of different assay methods. *J Thromb Haemost* 1:1882, 2003.

69. Kokame K, Matsumoto M, Fujimura Y, Miyata T: VWF73, a region from D1596 to R1668 of von Willebrand factor, provides a minimal substrate for ADAMTS-13. *Blood* 103:607, 2004.

70. Zomas A, Saso R, Powles R, et al: Red cell fragmentation (schistocytosis) after bone marrow transplantation. *Bone Marrow Transplant* 22:777, 1998.

71. Kanamori H, Takaishi Y, Takabayashi M, et al: Clinical significance of fragmented red cells after allogeneic bone marrow transplantation. *Int J Hematol* 77:180, 2003.

72. Kokame K, Miyata T: Genetic defects leading to hereditary thrombotic thrombocytopenic purpura. *Semin Hematol* 41:34, 2004.

73. Kokame K, Matsumoto M, Soejima K, et al: Mutations and common polymorphisms in *ADAMTS13* gene responsible for von Willebrand factor-cleaving protease activity. *Proc Natl Acad Sci U S A* 99:11902, 2002.

74. Hara T, Kitano A, Kajiwara T, et al: Factor VIII concentrate-responsive thrombocytopenia, hemolytic anemia, and nephropathy. Evidence that factor VIII:von Willebrand factor is involved in its pathogenesis. *J Pediatr Hematol Oncol* 8:324, 1986.

75. Veyradier A, Obert B, Haddad E, et al: Severe deficiency of the specific von Willebrand factor-cleaving protease (ADAMTS 13) activity in a subgroup of children with atypical hemolytic uremic syndrome. *J Pediatr* 142:310, 2003.

76. Furlan M, Robles R, Morselli B, et al: Recovery and half-life of von Willebrand factor-cleaving protease after plasma therapy in patients with thrombotic thrombocytopenic purpura. *Thromb Haemost* 81:8, 1999.

77. Allford SL, Harrison P, Lawrie AS, et al: Von Willebrand factor-cleaving protease activity in congenital thrombotic thrombocytopenic purpura. *Br J Haematol* 111:1215, 2000.

78. Kinoshita S, Yoshioka A, Park YD, et al: Upshaw-Schulman syndrome revisited: A concept of congenital thrombotic thrombocytopenic purpura. *Int J Hematol* 74:101, 2001.

79. Barbot J, Costa E, Guerra M, et al: Ten years of prophylactic treatment with fresh-frozen plasma in a child with chronic relapsing thrombotic thrombocytopenic purpura as a result of a congenital deficiency of von Willebrand factor-cleaving protease. *Br J Haematol* 113:649, 2001.

80. Sasahara Y, Kumaki S, Ohashi Y, et al: Deficient activity of von Willebrand factor-cleaving protease in patients with Upshaw-Schulman syndrome. *Int J Hematol* 74:109, 2001.

81. Cabrera GR, Fortenberry JD, Warshaw BL, et al: Hemolytic uremic syndrome associated with invasive Streptococcus pneumoniae infection. *Pediatrics* 101:699, 1998.

82. Brandt J, Wong C, Mihm S, et al: Invasive pneumococcal disease and hemolytic uremic syndrome. *Pediatrics* 110:371, 2002.

83. Crookston KP, Reiner AP, Cooper LJ, et al: RBC T activation and hemolysis: Implications for pediatric transfusion management. *Transfusion* 40:801, 2000.

84. Singh N, Gayowski T, Marino IR: Hemolytic uremic syndrome in solid-organ transplant recipients. *Transplant Int* 9:68, 1996.

85. Pham PT, Peng A, Wilkinson AH, et al: Cyclosporine and tacrolimus-associated thrombotic microangiopathy. *Am J Kidney Dis* 36:844, 2000.

86. Chohan R, Vij R, Adkins D, et al: Long-term outcomes of allogeneic stem cell transplant recipients after calcineurin inhibitor-induced neurotoxicity. *Br J Haematol* 123:110, 2003.

87. Sarode R, McFarland JG, Flomenberg N, et al: Therapeutic plasma exchange does not appear to be effective in the management of thrombotic thrombocytopenic purpura/hemolytic uremic syndrome following bone marrow transplantation. *Bone Marrow Transplant* 16:271, 1995.

88. Sack GH Jr, Levin J, Bell WR: Trousseau's syndrome and other manifestations of chronic disseminated coagulopathy in patients with neoplasms: clinical, pathophysiologic, and therapeutic features. *Medicine* 56:1, 1977.

89. Atkins JN, Muss HB: Schistocytes in erythroleukemia. *Am J Med Sci* 289:110, 1985.

90. Domingo-Claros A, Larriba I, Rozman M, et al: Acute erythroid neoplastic proliferations. A biological study based on 62 patients. *Haematologica* 87:148, 2002.

91. Fontana S, Gerritsen HE, Kremer Hovinga J, et al: Microangiopathic haemolytic anaemia in metastasizing malignant tumours is not associated with a severe deficiency of the von Willebrand factor-cleaving protease. *Br J Haematol* 113:100, 2001.

92. Lattuada A, Rossi E, Calzarossa C, et al: Mild to moderate reduction of a von Willebrand factor cleaving protease (ADAMTS-13) in pregnant women with HELLP microangiopathic syndrome. *Haematologica* 88:1029, 2003.

93. Ezra Y, Rose M, Eldor A: Therapy and prevention of thrombotic thrombocytopenic purpura during pregnancy: A clinical study of 16 pregnancies. *Am J Hematol* 51:1, 1996.

94. George JN: The association of pregnancy with thrombotic thrombocytopenic purpura-hemolytic uremic syndrome. *Curr Opin Hematol* 10:339, 2003.

95. Baron BW, Martin MS, Sucharetza BS, et al: Four patients with both thrombotic thrombocytopenic purpura and autoimmune thrombocytopenic purpura: The concept of a mixed immune thrombocytopenia syndrome and indications for plasma exchange. *J Clin Apheresis* 16:179, 2001.

96. Mannucci PM, Vanoli M, Forza I, et al: Von Willebrand factor cleaving protease (ADAMTS-13) in 123 patients with connective tissue diseases (systemic lupus erythematosus and systemic sclerosis). *Haematologica* 88:914, 2003.

97. Güngör T, Furlan M, Lämmle B, et al: Acquired deficiency of von Willebrand factor-cleaving protease in a patient suffering from acute systemic lupus erythematosus. *Rheumatology (Oxford)* 40:940, 2001.

98. Ahmed S, Siddiqui AK, Chandrasekaran V: Correlation of thrombotic thrombocytopenic purpura disease activity with von Willebrand factor-cleaving protease level in ulcerative colitis. *Am J Med* 116:786, 2004.

99. Coppo P, Bengoufa D, Veyradier A, et al: Severe ADAMTS13 deficiency in adult idiopathic thrombotic microangiopathies defines a subset of patients characterized by various autoimmune manifestations, lower platelet count, and mild renal involvement. *Medicine* 83:233, 2004.

100. Espinosa G, Bucciarelli S, Cervera R, et al: Thrombotic microangiopathic haemolytic anaemia and antiphospholipid antibodies. *Ann Rheum Dis* 63:730, 2004.

101. Steen VD: Scleroderma renal crisis. *Rheum Dis Clin North Am* 29:315, 2003.

102. Bennett CL, Davidson CJ, Raisch DW, et al: Thrombotic thrombocytopenic purpura associated with ticlopidine in the setting of coronary artery stents and stroke prevention. *Arch Intern Med* 159:2524, 1999.

103. Tsai HM, Rice L, Sarode R, et al: Antibody inhibitors to von Willebrand factor metalloproteinase and increased binding of von Willebrand factor to platelets in ticlopidine-associated thrombotic thrombocytopenic purpura. *Ann Intern Med* 132:794, 2000.

104. Zakarija A, Bandarenko N, Pandey DK, et al: Clopidogrel-associated TTP: An update of pharmacovigilance efforts conducted by independent researchers, pharmaceutical suppliers, and the Food and Drug Administration. *Stroke* 35:533, 2004.

105. Bennett CL, Connors JM, Carwile JM, et al: Thrombotic thrombocytopenic purpura associated with clopidogrel. *N Engl J Med* 342:1773, 2000.

106. Medina PJ, Sipols JM, George JN: Drug-associated thrombotic thrombocytopenic purpura-hemolytic uremic syndrome. *Curr Opin Hematol* 8:286, 2001.

107. Pisoni R, Ruggenenti P, Remuzzi G: Drug-induced thrombotic microangiopathy: Incidence, prevention, and management. *Drug Saf* 24:491, 2001.

108. Dlott JS, Danielson CF, Blue-Hnidy DE, McCarthy LJ: Drug-induced thrombotic thrombocytopenic purpura/hemolytic uremic syndrome: A concise review. *Ther Apher Dial* 8:102, 2004.

109. Valavaara R, Nordman E: Renal complications of mitomycin C therapy with special reference to the total dose. *Cancer* 55:47, 1985.

110. Lesesne JB, Rothschild N, Erickson B, et al: Cancer-associated hemolytic-uremic syndrome: Analysis of 85 cases from a national registry. *J Clin Oncol* 7:781, 1989.

111. Fung MC, Storniolo AM, Nguyen B, et al: A review of hemolytic uremic syndrome in patients treated with gemcitabine therapy. *Cancer* 85:2023, 1999.

112. Humphreys BD, Sharman JP, Henderson JM, et al: Gemcitabine-associated thrombotic microangiopathy. *Cancer* 100:2664, 2004.

113. Remuzzi G, Bertani T: Renal vascular and thrombotic effects of cyclosporine. *Am J Kidney Dis* 13:261, 1989.

114. Bechstein WO: Neurotoxicity of calcineurin inhibitors: Impact and clinical management. *Transpl Int* 13:313, 2000.

115. Scott LJ, McKeage K, Keam SJ, Plosker GL: Tacrolimus: A further update of its use in the management of organ transplantation. *Drugs* 63:1247, 2003.

116. Roy V, Rizvi MA, Vesely SK, George JN: Thrombotic thrombocytopenic purpura-like syndromes following bone marrow transplantation: An analysis of associated conditions and clinical outcomes. *Bone Marrow Transplant* 27:641, 2001.

117. Dzik WH, Georgi BA, Khettry U, Jenkins RL: Cyclosporine-associated thrombotic thrombocytopenic purpura following liver transplantation—Successful treatment with plasma exchange. *Transplantation* 44:570, 1987.

118. Trimarchi HM, Truong LD, Brennan S, et al: FK506-associated thrombotic microangiopathy: Report of two cases and review of the literature. *Transplantation* 67:539, 1999.

119. Gottschall JL, Neahring B, McFarland JG, et al: Quinine-induced immune thrombocytopenia with hemolytic uremic syndrome: Clinical and serological findings in nine patients and review of literature. *Am J Hematol* 47:283, 1994.

120. Kojouri K, Vesely SK, George JN: Quinine-associated thrombotic thrombocytopenic purpura-hemolytic uremic syndrome: Frequency, clinical features, and long-term outcomes. *Ann Intern Med* 135:1047, 2001.

121. Knower MT, Bowton DL, Owen J, Dunagan DP: Quinine-induced disseminated intravascular coagulation: Case report and review of the literature. *Intensive Care Med* 29:1007, 2003.

122. Naqvi TA, Baumann MA, Chang JC: Post-operative thrombotic thrombocytopenic purpura: A review. *Int J Clin Pract* 58:169, 2004.

123. Capelli JP, Wesson GL Jr, Erslev AV: Malignant hypertension and red cell fragmentation syndrome. Report of a case. *Ann Intern Med* 64:128, 1966.

124. Gianviti A, Tozzi AE, De Petris L, et al: Risk factors for poor renal prognosis in children with hemolytic uremic syndrome. *Pediatr Nephrol* 18:1229, 2003.

125. Bhimma R, Rollins NC, Coovadia HM, Adhikari M: Post-dysenteric hemolytic uremic syndrome in children during an epidemic of Shigella dysentery in Kwazulu/Natal. *Pediatr Nephrol* 11:560, 1997.

126. Griffin PM, Ostroff SM, Tauxe RV, et al: Illnesses associated with Escherichia coli O157:H7 infections. A broad clinical spectrum. *Ann Intern Med* 109:705, 1988.

127. Bell BP, Griffin PM, Lozano P, et al: Predictors of hemolytic uremic

syndrome in children during a large outbreak of Escherichia coli O157: H7 infections. *Pediatrics* 100:E12, 1997.

128. Havelaar AH, Van Duynhoven YT, Nauta MJ, et al: Disease burden in The Netherlands due to infections with Shiga toxin-producing Escherichia coli O157. *Epidemiol Infect* 132:467, 2004.

129. Proesmans W: The role of coagulation and fibrinolysis in the pathogenesis of diarrhea-associated hemolytic uremic syndrome. *Semin Thromb Hemost* 27:201, 2001.

130. Tsai HM, Chandler WL, Sarode R, et al: von Willebrand factor and von Willebrand factor-cleaving metalloprotease activity in *Escherichia coli* O157:H7-associated hemolytic uremic syndrome. *Pediatr Res* 49:653, 2001.

131. Hunt BJ, Lämmle B, Nevard CH, et al: von Willebrand factor-cleaving protease in childhood diarrhoea-associated haemolytic uraemic syndrome. *Thromb Haemost* 85:975, 2001.

132. Garg AX, Suri RS, Barrowman N, et al: Long-term renal prognosis of diarrhea-associated hemolytic uremic syndrome: A systematic review, meta-analysis, and meta-regression. *JAMA* 290:1360, 2003.

133. Loirat C, Sonsino E, Hinglais N, et al: Treatment of the childhood haemolytic uraemic syndrome with plasma. A multicentre randomized controlled trial. The French Society of Paediatric Nephrology. *Pediatr Nephrol* 2:279, 1988.

134. Rizzoni G, Claris-Appiani A, Edefonti A, et al: Plasma infusion for hemolytic-uremic syndrome in children: results of a multicenter controlled trial. *J Pediatr* 112:284, 1988.

135. Allford SL, Hunt BJ, Rose P, Machin SJ: Guidelines on the diagnosis and management of the thrombotic microangiopathic haemolytic anaemias. *Br J Haematol* 120:556, 2003.

136. Safdar N, Said A, Gangnon RE, Maki DG: Risk of hemolytic uremic syndrome after antibiotic treatment of Escherichia coli O157:H7 enteritis: A meta-analysis. *JAMA* 288:996, 2002.

137. Landau D, Shalev H, Levy-Finer G, et al: Familial hemolytic uremic syndrome associated with complement factor H deficiency. *J Pediatr* 138:412, 2001.

138. Caprioli J, Bettinaglio P, Zipfel PF, et al: The molecular basis of familial hemolytic uremic syndrome: Mutation analysis of factor H gene reveals a hot spot in short consensus repeat 20. *J Am Soc Nephrol* 12: 297, 2001.

139. Richards A, Buddles MR, Donne RL, et al: Factor H mutations in hemolytic uremic syndrome cluster in exons 18-20, a domain important for host cell recognition. *Am J Hum Genet* 68:485, 2001.

140. Pérez-Caballero D, González-Rubio C, Gallardo ME, et al: Clustering of missense mutations in the C-terminal region of factor H in atypical hemolytic uremic syndrome. *Am J Hum Genet* 68:478, 2001.

141. Neumann HP, Salzmann M, Bohnert-Iwan B, et al: Haemolytic uraemic syndrome and mutations of the factor H gene: A registry-based study of German speaking countries. *J Med Genet* 40:676, 2003.

142. Dragon-Durey MA, Fremeaux-Bacchi V, Loirat C, et al: Heterozygous and homozygous factor H deficiencies associated with hemolytic uremic syndrome or membranoproliferative glomerulonephritis: Report and genetic analysis of 16 cases. *J Am Soc Nephrol* 15:787, 2004.

143. Richards A, Kemp EJ, Liszewski MK, et al: Mutations in human complement regulator, membrane cofactor protein (CD46), predispose to development of familial hemolytic uremic syndrome. *Proc Natl Acad Sci U S A* 100:12966, 2003.

144. Noris M, Brioschi S, Caprioli J, et al: Familial haemolytic uraemic syndrome and an MCP mutation. *Lancet* 362:1542, 2003.

145. Fremeaux-Bacchi V, Dragon-Durey MA, Blouin J, et al: Complement factor I: A susceptibility gene for atypical haemolytic uraemic syndrome. *J Med Genet* 41:e84, 2004.

146. Stratton JD, Warwicker P: Successful treatment of factor H-related haemolytic uraemic syndrome. *Nephrol Dial Transplant* 17:684, 2002.

147. Filler G, Radhakrishnan S, Strain L, et al: Challenges in the management of infantile factor H associated hemolytic uremic syndrome. *Pediatr Nephrol* 19:908, 2004.

148. Remuzzi G, Ruggenenti P, Codazzi D, et al: Combined kidney and liver transplantation for familial haemolytic uraemic syndrome. *Lancet* 359: 1671, 2002.

149. George JN: How I treat patients with thrombotic thrombocytopenic purpura-hemolytic uremic syndrome. *Blood* 96:1223, 2000.

150. Evans G, Llewelyn C, Luddington R, et al: Solvent/detergent fresh frozen plasma as primary treatment of acute thrombotic thrombocytopenic purpura. *Clin Lab Haematol* 21:119, 1999.

151. Zeigler ZR, Shadduck RK, Gryn JF, et al: Cryoprecipitate poor plasma does not improve early response in primary adult thrombotic thrombocytopenic purpura (TTP). *J Clin Apheresis* 16:19, 2001.

152. McCarthy LJ: Evidence-based medicine for apheresis: An ongoing challenge. *Ther Apher Dial* 8:112, 2004.

153. Yarranton H, Cohen H, Pavord SR, et al: Venous thromboembolism associated with the management of acute thrombotic thrombocytopenic purpura. *Br J Haematol* 121:778, 2003.

154. Alvarez-Larran A, Del Rio J, Ramirez C, et al: Methylene blue-photo-inactivated plasma vs. fresh-frozen plasma as replacement fluid for plasma exchange in thrombotic thrombocytopenic purpura. *Vox Sang* 86:246, 2004.

155. Cardigan R, Allford S, Williamson L: Levels of von Willebrand factor-cleaving protease are normal in methylene blue-treated fresh-frozen plasma. *Br J Haematol* 117:253, 2002.

156. Rizvi MA, Vesely SK, George JN, et al: Complications of plasma exchange in 71 consecutive patients treated for clinically suspected thrombotic thrombocytopenic purpura-hemolytic-uremic syndrome. *Transfusion* 40:896, 2000.

157. McMinn JR Jr, Thomas IA, Terrell DR, et al: Complications of plasma exchange in thrombotic thrombocytopenic purpura-hemolytic uremic syndrome: A study of 78 additional patients. *Transfusion* 43:415, 2003.

158. Doerfler ME, Kaufman B, Goldenberg AS: Central venous catheter placement in patients with disorders of hemostasis. *Chest* 110:185, 1996.

159. Marques MB, Huang ST: Patients with thrombotic thrombocytopenic purpura commonly develop metabolic alkalosis during therapeutic plasma exchange. *J Clin Apheresis* 16:120, 2001.

160. Perdue JJ, Chandler LK, Vesely SK, et al: Unintentional platelet removal by plasmapheresis. *J Clin Apheresis* 16:55, 2001.

161. Reutter JC, Sanders KF, Brecher ME, et al: Incidence of allergic reactions with fresh frozen plasma or cryo-supernatant plasma in the treatment of thrombotic thrombocytopenic purpura. *J Clin Apheresis* 16:134, 2001.

162. Bobbio-Pallavicini E, Gugliotta L, Centurioni R, et al: Antiplatelet agents in thrombotic thrombocytopenic purpura (TTP). Results of a randomized multicenter trial by the Italian Cooperative Group for TTP. *Haematologica* 82:429, 1997.

163. Coppo P, Lassoued K, Mariette X, et al: Effectiveness of platelet transfusions after plasma exchange in adult thrombotic thrombocytopenic purpura: A report of two cases. *Am J Hematol* 68:198, 2001.

164. Ferrara F, Annunziata M, Pollio F, et al: Vincristine as treatment for recurrent episodes of thrombotic thrombocytopenic purpura. *Ann Hematol* 81:7, 2002.

165. Bobbio-Pallavicini E, Porta C, Centurioni R, et al: Vincristine sulfate for the treatment of thrombotic thrombocytopenic purpura refractory to plasma-exchange. The Italian Cooperative Group for TTP. *Eur J Haematol* 52:222, 1994.

166. Pasquale D, Vidhya R, DaSilva K, et al: Chronic relapsing thrombotic thrombocytopenic purpura: Role of therapy with cyclosporine. *Am J Hematol* 57:57, 1998.

167. Itala M, Remes K: Excellent response of refractory life-threatening thrombotic thrombocytopenic purpura to cyclosporine treatment. *Clin Lab Haematol* 26:65, 2004.

168. Allan DS, Kovacs MJ, Clark WF: Frequently relapsing thrombotic thrombocytopenic purpura treated with cytotoxic immunosuppressive therapy. *Haematologica* 86:844, 2001.

169. Spiekermann K, Wormann B, Rumpf KW, Hiddemann W: Combination chemotherapy with CHOP for recurrent thrombotic thrombocytopenic purpura. *Br J Haematol* 97:544, 1997.

170. Passweg JR, Rabusin M, Musso M, et al: Haematopoetic stem cell transplantation for refractory autoimmune cytopenia. *Br J Haematol* 125:749, 2004.

171. Yomtovian R, Niklinski W, Silver B, et al: Rituximab for chronic recurring thrombotic thrombocytopenic purpura: A case report and review of the literature. *Br J Haematol* 124:787, 2004.

172. Sallah S, Husain A, Wan JY, Nguyen NP: Rituximab in patients with refractory thrombotic thrombocytopenic purpura. *J Thromb Haemost* 2:834, 2004.

173. Fakhouri F, Teixeira L, Delarue R, et al: Responsiveness of thrombotic thrombocytopenic purpura to rituximab and cyclophosphamide. *Ann Intern Med* 140:314, 2004.

174. Gutterman LA, Kloster B, Tsai H-M: Rituximab therapy for refractory thrombotic thrombocytopenic purpura. *Blood Cells Mol Dis* 28:385, 2002.

175. Chemnitz J, Draube A, Scheid C, et al: Successful treatment of severe thrombotic thrombocytopenic purpura with the monoclonal antibody rituximab. *Am J Hematol* 71:105, 2002.

176. Stein GY, Zeidman A, Fradin Z, et al: Treatment of resistant thrombotic thrombocytopenic purpura with rituximab and cyclophosphamide. *Int J Hematol* 80:94, 2004.

177. Ahmad A, Aggarwal A, Sharma D, et al: Rituximab for treatment of refractory/relapsing thrombotic thrombocytopenic purpura (TTP). *Am J Hematol* 77:171, 2004.

178. Aqui NA, Stein SH, Konkle BA, et al: Role of splenectomy in patients with refractory or relapsed thrombotic thrombocytopenic purpura. *J Clin Apheresis* 18:51, 2003.

179. Katkhouda N, Hurwitz MB, Rivera RT, et al: Laparoscopic splenectomy: Outcome and efficacy in 103 consecutive patients. *Ann Surg* 228:568, 1998.

180. Kremer Hovinga JA, Studt JD, Demarmels Biasiutti F, et al: Splenectomy in relapsing and plasma-refractory acquired thrombotic thrombocytopenic purpura. *Haematologica* 89:320, 2004.

181. Levy J, Degani N: Correcting immune imbalance: The use of Prosorba column treatment for immune disorders. *Ther Apher Dial* 7:197, 2003.

182. Bobbio-Pallavicini E, Porta C, Tacconi F, et al: Intravenous prostacyclin (as epoprostenol) infusion in thrombotic thrombocytopenic purpura. Four case reports and review of the literature. Italian Cooperative Group for Thrombotic Thrombocytopenic Purpura. *Haematologica* 79:429, 1994.

183. Sagripanti A, Carpi A, Rosaia B, et al: Iloprost in the treatment of thrombotic microangiopathy: Report of thirteen cases. *Biomed Pharmacother* 50:350, 1996.

184. Centurioni R, Bobbio-Pallavicini E, Porta C, et al: Treatment of thrombotic thrombocytopenic purpura with high-dose immunoglobulins. Results in 17 patients. Italian Cooperative Group for TTP. *Haematologica* 80:325, 1995.

185. Dervenoulas J, Tsirigotis P, Bollas G, et al: Efficacy of intravenous immunoglobulin in the treatment of thrombotic thrombocytopaenic purpura. A study of 44 cases. *Acta Haematol* 105:204, 2001.

186. Sarode R, Gottschall JL, Aster RH, McFarland JG: Thrombotic thrombocytopenic purpura: Early and late responders. *Am J Hematol* 54:102, 1997.

187. Bandarenko N, Brecher ME: United States Thrombotic Thrombocytopenic Purpura Apheresis Study Group (US TTP ASG): Multicenter survey and retrospective analysis of current efficacy of therapeutic plasma exchange. *J Clin Apheresis* 13:133, 1998.

188. Lara PN Jr, Coe TL, Zhou H, et al: Improved survival with plasma exchange in patients with thrombotic thrombocytopenic purpura-hemolytic uremic syndrome. *Am J Med* 107:573, 1999.

189. Shumak KH, Rock GA, Nair RC: Late relapses in patients successfully treated for thrombotic thrombocytopenic purpura. Canadian Apheresis Group. *Ann Intern Med* 122:569, 1995.

190. Downes KA, Yomtovian nR, Tsai HM, et al: Relapsed thrombotic thrombocytopenic purpura presenting as an acute cerebrovascular accident. *J Clin Apheresis* 19:86, 2004.

191. Anstadt MP, Carwile JM, Guill CK, et al: Relapse of thrombotic thrombocytopenic purpura associated with decreased VWF cleaving activity. *Am J Med Sci* 323:281, 2002.

192. Rose M, Eldor A: High incidence of relapses in thrombotic thrombocytopenic purpura. Clinical study of 38 patients. *Am J Med* 83:437, 1987.

193. Hayward CP, Sutton DM, Carter WH Jr, et al: Treatment outcomes in patients with adult thrombotic thrombocytopenic purpura-hemolytic uremic syndrome. *Arch Intern Med* 154:982, 1994.

194. Warkentin TE: History of heparin-induced thrombocytopenia, in *Heparin-Induced Thrombocytopenia*, edited by TE Warkentin, A Greinacher, p 1. Marcel Dekker, New York, 2004.

195. Chong BH, Berndt MC: Heparin-induced thrombocytopenia. *Blut* 58:53, 1989.

196. Fratantoni JC, Pollet R, Gralnick HR: Heparin-induced thrombocytopenia: Confirmation of diagnosis with in vitro methods. *Blood* 45:395, 1975.

197. Cines DB, Tomaski A, Tannenbaum S: Immune endothelial-cell injury in heparin-associated thrombocytopenia. *N Engl J Med* 316:581, 1987.

198. Kelton JG, Sheridan D, Santos A, et al: Heparin-induced thrombocytopenia: laboratory studies. *Blood* 72:925, 1988.

199. Amiral J, Bridey F, Dreyfus M, et al: Platelet factor 4 complexed to heparin is the target for antibodies generated in heparin-induced thrombocytopenia. *Thromb Haemost* 68:95, 1992.

200. Merton RE, Thomas DP, Havercroft SJ, et al: High and low affinity heparin compared with unfractionated heparin as antithrombotic drugs. *Thromb Haemost* 51:254, 1984.

201. Green D, Martin GJ, Shoichet SH, et al: Thrombocytopenia in a prospective, randomized, double-blind trial of bovine and porcine heparin. *Am J Med Sci* 288:60, 1984.

202. Verma AK, Levine M, Shalansky SJ, et al: Frequency of heparin-induced thrombocytopenia in critical care patients. *Pharmacotherapy* 23:745, 2003.

203. Pouplard C, May MA, Iochmann S, et al: Antibodies to platelet factor 4-heparin after cardiopulmonary bypass in patients anticoagulated with unfractionated heparin or a low-molecular-weight heparin: Clinical implications for heparin-induced thrombocytopenia. *Circulation* 99:2530, 1999.

204. Warkentin TE, Levine MN, Hirsh J, et al: Heparin-induced thrombocytopenia in patients treated with low-molecular-weight heparin or unfractionated heparin. *N Engl J Med* 332:1330, 1995.

205. Lindhoff-Last E, Nakov R, Misselwitz F, et al: Incidence and clinical relevance of heparin-induced antibodies in patients with deep vein thrombosis treated with unfractionated or low-molecular-weight heparin. *Br J Haematol* 118:1137, 2002.

206. Ansell J, Slepchuk N Jr, Kumar R, et al: Heparin induced thrombocytopenia: A prospective study. *Thromb Haemost* 43:61, 1980.

207. D'Amico EA, Villaca PR, Gualandro SF, et al: Successful use of Arixtra in a patient with paroxysmal nocturnal hemoglobinuria, Budd-Chiari syndrome and heparin-induced thrombocytopenia. *J Thromb Haemost* 1:2452, 2003.

208. Girolami B, Prandoni P, Stefani PM, et al: The incidence of heparin-induced thrombocytopenia in hospitalized medical patients treated with subcutaneous unfractionated heparin: A prospective cohort study. *Blood* 101:2955, 2003.

209. Bauer TL, Arepally G, Konkle BA, et al: Prevalence of heparin-associated antibodies without thrombosis in patients undergoing cardiopulmonary bypass surgery. *Circulation* 95:1242, 1997.

210. Doty JR, Alving BM, McDonnell DE, Ondra SL: Heparin-associated thrombocytopenia in the neurosurgical patient. *Neurosurgery* 19:69, 1986.

211. Almeida JI, Liem TK, Silver D: Heparin-bonded grafts induce platelet aggregation in the presence of heparin-associated antiplatelet antibodies. *J Vasc Surg* 27:896, 1998.

212. Laster J, Silver D: Heparin-coated catheters and heparin-induced thrombocytopenia. *J Vasc Surg* 7:667, 1988.

213. Ranze O, Ranze P, Magnani HN, Greinacher A: Heparin-induced thrombocytopenia in paediatric patients—A review of the literature and a new case treated with danaparoid sodium. *Eur J Pediatr* 158(suppl 3):S130, 1999.

214. O'Shea SI, Sands JJ, Nudo SA, Ortel TL: Frequency of anti-heparin-platelet factor 4 antibodies in hemodialysis patients and correlation with recurrent vascular access thrombosis. *Am J Hematol* 69:72, 2002.

215. Lindhoff-Last E, Bauersachs R: Heparin-induced thrombocytopenia-alternative anticoagulation in pregnancy and lactation. *Semin Thromb Hemost* 28:439, 2002.

216. Warkentin TE, Roberts RS, Hirsh J, Kelton JG: An improved definition of immune heparin-induced thrombocytopenia in postoperative orthopedic patients. *Arch Intern Med* 163:2518, 2003.

217. Masucci IP, Calis KA, Bartlett DL, et al: Thrombocytopenia after isolated limb or hepatic perfusions with melphalan: The risk of heparin-induced thrombocytopenia. *Ann Surg Oncol* 6:476, 1999.

218. Greinacher A, Eichler P, Lubenow N, et al: Heparin-induced thrombocytopenia with thromboembolic complications: Meta-analysis of 2 prospective trials to assess the value of parenteral treatment with lepirudin and its therapeutic aPTT range. *Blood* 96:846, 2000.

219. Wallis DE, Workman DL, Lewis BE, et al: Failure of early heparin cessation as treatment for heparin-induced thrombocytopenia. *Am J Med* 106:629, 1999.

220. Arepally G, Reynolds C, Tomaski A, et al: Comparison of PF4/heparin ELISA assay with the 14C-serotonin release assay in the diagnosis of heparin-induced thrombocytopenia. *Am J Clin Pathol* 104:648, 1995.

221. Reilly MP, Taylor SM, Hartman NK, et al: Heparin-induced thrombocytopenia/thrombosis in a transgenic mouse model requires human platelet factor 4 and platelet activation through FcgammaRIIA. *Blood* 98:2442, 2001.

222. Arepally GM, Kamei S, Park KS, et al: Characterization of a murine monoclonal antibody that mimics heparin-induced thrombocytopenia antibodies. *Blood* 95:1533, 2000.

223. Zhang X, Chen L, Bancroft DP, et al: Crystal structure of recombinant human platelet factor 4. *Biochemistry* 33:8361, 1994.

224. Stuckey JA, St Charles R, Edwards BF: A model of the platelet factor 4 complex with heparin. *Proteins* 14:277, 1992.

225. Li ZQ, Liu W, Park KS, et al: Defining a second epitope for heparin-induced thrombocytopenia/thrombosis antibodies using KKO, a murine HIT-like monoclonal antibody. *Blood* 99:1230, 2002.

226. Greinacher A, Potzsch B, Amiral J, et al: Heparin-associated thrombocytopenia: isolation of the antibody and characterization of a multimolecular PF4-heparin complex as the major antigen. *Thromb Haemost* 71:247, 1994.

227. Horne MK 3rd, Alkins BR: Platelet binding of IgG from patients with heparin-induced thrombocytopenia. *J Lab Clin Med* 127:435, 1996.

228. Rauova L, Poncz M, McKenzie SE, et al: High molecular weight complexes of heparin and PF4 are central to the pathogenesis of heparin-induced thrombocytopenia. *Blood* 102:126a, 2003.

229. Eslin DE, Zhang C, Samuels KJ, et al: Transgenic mice studies demonstrate a role for platelet factor 4 in thrombosis: Dissociation between anticoagulant and antithrombotic effect of heparin. *Blood* (in press), 104:3173, 2004.

230. Warkentin TE, Hayward CP, Boshkov LK, et al: Sera from patients with heparin-induced thrombocytopenia generate platelet-derived microparticles with procoagulant activity: An explanation for the thrombotic complications of heparin-induced thrombocytopenia. *Blood* 84:3691, 1994.

231. Visentin GP, Malik M, Cyganiak KA, Aster RH: Patients treated with unfractionated heparin during open heart surgery are at high risk to form antibodies reactive with heparin:platelet factor 4 complexes. *J Lab Clin Med* 128:376, 1996.

232. Pouplard C, Iochmann S, Renard B, et al: Induction of monocyte tissue factor expression by antibodies to heparin-platelet factor 4 complexes developed in heparin-induced thrombocytopenia. *Blood* 97:3300, 2001.

233. Arepally GM, Mayer IM: Antibodies from patients with heparin-induced thrombocytopenia stimulate monocytic cells to express tissue factor and secrete interleukin-8. *Blood* 98:1252, 2001.

234. Ma AD, Arepally G: HIT antibodies and monocyte signaling. *Blood* 100:16a, 2002.

235. Carlsson LE, Lubenow N, Blumentritt C, et al: Platelet receptor and clotting factor polymorphisms as genetic risk factors for thromboembolic complications in heparin-induced thrombocytopenia. *Pharmacogenetics* 13:253, 2003.

236. Arepally G, McKenzie SE, Jiang XM, et al: Fc gamma RIIA H/R 131 polymorphism, subclass-specific IgG anti-heparin/platelet factor 4 antibodies and clinical course in patients with heparin-induced thrombocytopenia and thrombosis. *Blood* 89:370, 1997.

237. Carlsson LE, Santoso S, Baurichter G, et al: Heparin-induced thrombocytopenia: new insights into the impact of the FcgammaRIIa-R-H131 polymorphism. *Blood* 92:1526, 1998.

238. Chong BH, Pilgrim RL, Cooley MA, Chesterman CN: Increased expression of platelet IgG Fc receptors in immune heparin-induced thrombocytopenia. *Blood* 81:988, 1993.

239. Suh JS, Malik MI, Aster RH, Visentin GP: Characterization of the humoral immune response in heparin-induced thrombocytopenia. *Am J Hematol* 54:196, 1997.

240. Warkentin TE: Heparin-induced thrombocytopenia: Pathogenesis and management. *Br J Haematol* 121:535, 2003.

241. Hong AP, Cook DJ, Sigouin CS, Warkentin TE: Central venous catheters and upper-extremity deep-vein thrombosis complicating immune heparin-induced thrombocytopenia. *Blood* 101:3049, 2003.

242. Rowland CH, Woodford PA, De Lisle-Hammond J, Nair B: Heparin-induced thrombocytopenia-thrombosis syndrome and bilateral adrenal haemorrhage after prophylactic heparin use. *Aust N Z J Med* 29:741, 1999.

243. Kyritsis AP, Williams EC, Schutta HS: Cerebral venous thrombosis due to heparin-induced thrombocytopenia. *Stroke* 21:1503, 1990.

244. Towne JB, Bernhard VM, Hussey C, Garancis JC: White clot syndrome. Peripheral vascular complications of heparin therapy. *Arch Surg* 114:372, 1979.

245. Warkentin TE, Kelton JG: A 14-year study of heparin-induced thrombocytopenia. *Am J Med* 101:502, 1996.

246. Nand S, Wong W, Yuen B, et al: Heparin-induced thrombocytopenia with thrombosis: Incidence, analysis of risk factors, and clinical outcomes in 108 consecutive patients treated at a single institution. *Am J Hematol* 56:12, 1997.

247. Lipton ME, Gould D: Case report: Heparin-induced thrombocytopenia—A complication presenting to the vascular radiologist. *Clin Radiol* 45:137, 1992.

248. Wutschert R, Piletta P, Bounameaux H: Adverse skin reactions to low molecular weight heparins: Frequency, management and prevention. *Drug Saf* 20:515, 1999.

249. Warkentin TE: Heparin-induced skin lesions. *Br J Haematol* 92:494, 1996.

250. Srinivasan AF, Rice L, Bartholomew JR, et al: Warfarin-induced skin necrosis and venous limb gangrene in the setting of heparin-induced thrombocytopenia. *Arch Intern Med* 164:66, 2004.

251. Warkentin TE: Heparin-induced thrombocytopenia: IgG-mediated platelet activation, platelet microparticle generation, and altered procoagulant/anticoagulant balance in the pathogenesis of thrombosis and venous limb gangrene complicating heparin-induced thrombocytopenia. *Transfus Med Rev* 10:249, 1996.

252. Betrosian AP, Theodossiades G, Lambroulis G, et al: Heparin-induced thrombocytopenia with pulmonary embolism and disseminated intravascular coagulation associated with low-molecular-weight heparin. *Am J Med Sci* 325:45, 2003.

253. Visentin GP, Ford SE, Scott JP, Aster RH: Antibodies from patients with heparin-induced thrombocytopenia/thrombosis are specific for platelet factor 4 complexed with heparin or bound to endothelial cells. *J Clin Invest* 93:81, 1994.

254. Cines DB, Kaywin P, Bina M, et al: Heparin-associated thrombocytopenia. *N Engl J Med* 303:788, 1980.

255. Greinacher A, Michels I, Kiefel V, Mueller-Eckhardt C: A rapid and sensitive test for diagnosing heparin-associated thrombocytopenia. *Thromb Haemost* 66:734, 1991.

256. Stewart MW, Etches WS, Boshkov LK, Gordon PA: Heparin-induced thrombocytopenia: An improved method of detection based on lumi-aggregometry. *Br J Haematol* 91:173, 1995.

257. Abrams CS, Cines DB: Thrombocytopenia after treatment with platelet glycoprotein IIb/IIIa inhibitors. *Curr Hematol Rep* 3:143, 2004.

258. Greinacher A, Michels I, Mueller-Eckhardt C: Heparin-associated thrombocytopenia: The antibody is not heparin specific. *Thromb Haemost* 67:545, 1992.

259. Meuleman DG: Orgaran (Org 10172): Its pharmacological profile in experimental models. *Haemostasis* 22:58, 1992.

260. Skoutakis VA: Danaparoid in the prevention of thromboembolic complications. *Ann Pharmacother* 31:876, 1997.

261. Chong BH, Ismail F, Cade J, et al: Heparin-induced thrombocytopenia: Studies with a new low molecular weight heparinoid, Org 10172. *Blood* 73:1592, 1989.

262. Newman PM, Swanson RL, Chong BH: Heparin-induced thrombocytopenia: IgG binding to PF4-heparin complexes in the fluid phase and cross-reactivity with low molecular weight heparin and heparinoid. *Thromb Haemost* 80:292, 1998.

263. Chong BH, Gallus AS, Cade JF, et al: Prospective randomized open-label comparison of danaparoid with dextran 70 in the treatment of heparin-induced thrombocytopaenia with thrombosis: A clinical outcome study. *Thromb Haemost* 86:1170, 2001.

264. Hermann JP, Kutryk MJ, Serruys PW: Clinical trials of direct thrombin inhibitors during invasive procedures. *Thromb Haemost* 78:367, 1997.

265. Vanholder R, Camez A, Veys N, et al: Pharmacokinetics of recombinant hirudin in hemodialyzed end-stage renal failure patients. *Thromb Haemost* 77:650, 1997.

266. Fischer KG, Liebe V, Hudek R, et al: Anti-hirudin antibodies alter pharmacokinetics and pharmacodynamics of recombinant hirudin. *Thromb Haemost* 89:973, 2003.

267. Okamoto S, Hijikata A, Kikumoto R, et al: Potent inhibition of thrombin by the newly synthesized arginine derivative No 805. The importance of stereo-structure of its hydrophobic carboxamide portion. *Biochem Biophys Res Commun* 101:440, 1981.

268. Hursting MJ, Zehnder JL, Joffrion JL, et al: The International Normalized Ratio during concurrent warfarin and argatroban anticoagulation: Differential contributions of each agent and effects of the choice of thromboplastin used. *Clin Chem* 45:409, 1999.

269. Lubenow N, Eichler P, Leitz T, Greinacher A: Meta-analysis of three prospective studies of lepirudin in the prevention of thrombosis in patients with heparin-induced thrombocytopenia. *Blood* 100:501a, 2002.

270. Lewis BE, Wallis DE, Berkowitz SD, et al: Argatroban anticoagulant therapy in patients with heparin-induced thrombocytopenia. *Circulation* 103:1838, 2001.

271. Matthai WH, Hursting MJ, Lewis BE: Argatroban use in patients with a history of heparin-induced thrombocytopenia who require acute anticoagulation. *Blood* 98:45a, 2001.

272. Sadler JE: A new name in thrombosis, ADAMTS13. *Proc Natl Acad Sci U S A* 99:11552, 2002.

273. Riegert-Johnson DL, Sandhu N, Rajkumar SV, Patel R: Thrombotic thrombocytopenic purpura associated with a hepatic abscess due to Actinomyces turicensis. *Clin Infect Dis* 35:636, 2002.

274. Denneberg T, Friedberg M, Holmberg L, et al: Combined plasmapheresis and hemodialysis treatment for severe hemolytic-uremic syndrome following Campylobacter colitis. *Acta Paediatr Scand* 71:243, 1982.

275. Chamovitz BN, Hartstein AI, Alexander SR, et al: Campylobacter jejuni-associated hemolytic-uremic syndrome in a mother and daughter. *Pediatrics* 71:253, 1983.

276. Morton AR, Yu R, Waldek S, et al: Campylobacter induced thrombotic thrombocytopenic purpura. *Lancet* 2:1133, 1985.

277. George JN, Vesely SK, Terrell DR: The Oklahoma Thrombotic Thrombocytopenic Purpura-Hemolytic Uremic Syndrome (TTP-HUS) Registry: A community perspective of patients with clinically diagnosed TTP-HUS. *Semin Hematol* 41:60, 2004.

278. Coppo P, Adrie C, Azoulay E, et al: Infectious diseases as a trigger in thrombotic microangiopathies in intensive care unit (ICU) patients? *Intensive Care Med* 29:564, 2003.

279. Griffin PM, Ostroff SM, Tauxe RV, et al: Illnesses associated with *Escherichia coli* O157:H7 infections. A broad clinical spectrum. *Ann Intern Med* 109:705, 1988.

280. Bell BP, Griffin PM, Lozano P, et al: Predictors of hemolytic uremic syndrome in children during a large outbreak of *Escherichia coli* O157:H7 infections. *Pediatrics* 100:E12, 1997.

281. Havelaar AH, Van Duynhoven YT, Nauta MJ, et al: Disease burden in The Netherlands due to infections with Shiga toxin-producing *Escherichia coli* O157. *Epidemiol Infect* 132:467, 2004.

282. Chang JC, Kathula SK: Various clinical manifestations in patients with thrombotic microangiopathy. *J Investig Med* 50:201, 2002.

283. Riggs SA, Wray NP, Waddell CC, et al: Thrombotic thrombocytopenic purpura complicating Legionnaires' disease. *Arch Intern Med* 142:2275, 1982.

284. Albaqali A, Ghuloom A, Al Arrayed A, et al: Hemolytic uremic syndrome in association with typhoid fever. *Am J Kidney Dis* 41:709, 2003.

285. Bhimma R, Rollins NC, Coovadia HM, Adhikari M: Post-dysenteric hemolytic uremic syndrome in children during an epidemic of Shigella dysentery in Kwazulu/Natal. *Pediatr Nephrol* 11:560, 1997.

286. Cabrera GR, Fortenberry JD, Warshaw BL, et al: Hemolytic uremic syndrome associated with invasive Streptococcus pneumoniae infection. *Pediatrics* 101:699, 1998.

287. Brandt J, Wong C, Mihm S, et al: Invasive pneumococcal disease and hemolytic uremic syndrome. *Pediatrics* 110:371, 2002.

288. Prober CG, Tune B, Hoder L: Yersinia pseudotuberculosis septicemia. *Am J Dis Child* 133:623, 1979.

289. Guidotti TL, Luetzeler J, di Sant' Agnese PA, Escaro DU: Fatal disseminated aspergillosis in a previously well young adult with cystic fibrosis. *Am J Med Sci* 283:157, 1982.

290. Safdar A, van Rhee F, Henslee-Downey JP, et al: Candida glabrata and Candida krausei fungemia after high-risk allogeneic marrow transplantation: No adverse effect of low-dose fluconazole prophylaxis on incidence and outcome. *Bone Marrow Transplant* 28:873, 2001.

291. Berberich FR, Cuene SA, Chard RL Jr, Hartmann JR: Thrombotic thrombocytopenic purpura. Three cases with platelet and fibrinogen survival studies. *J Pediatr* 84:503, 1974.

292. Glasgow LA, Balduzzi P: Isolation of Coxsackie virus group A, type 4, from a patient with hemolytic-uremic syndrome. *N Engl J Med* 273:754, 1965.

293. Ray CG, Tucker VL, Harris DJ, et al: Enteroviruses associated with the hemolytic-uremic syndrome. *Pediatrics* 46:378, 1970.

294. O'Regan S, Robitaille P, Mongeau JG, McLaughlin B: The hemolytic uremic syndrome associated with ECHO 22 infection. *Clin Pediatr (Phila)* 19:125, 1980.

295. Shashaty GG, Atamer MA: Hemolytic uremic syndrome associated with infectious mononucleosis. *Am J Dis Child* 127:720, 1974.

296. Thompson CE, Damon LE, Ries CA, Linker CA: Thrombotic microangiopathies in the 1980s: Clinical features, response to treatment, and the impact of the human immunodeficiency virus epidemic. *Blood* 80:1890, 1992.

297. Myers TJ, Wakem CJ, Ball ED, Tremont SJ: Thrombotic thrombocytopenic purpura: Combined treatment with plasmapheresis and antiplatelet agents. *Ann Intern Med* 92:149, 1980.

298. Matsuda Y, Hara J, Miyoshi H, et al: Thrombotic microangiopathy associated with reactivation of human herpesvirus-6 following high-dose chemotherapy with autologous bone marrow transplantation in young children. *Bone Marrow Transplant* 24:919, 1999.

299. Ucar A, Fernandez HF, Byrnes JJ, et al: Thrombotic microangiopathy and retroviral infections: A 13-year experience. *Am J Hematol* 45:304, 1994.

300. Chan JCM, Eleff MG, Campbell RAA: The hemolytic-uremic syndrome in nonrelated adopted siblings. *J Pediatr* 75:1050, 1969.

301. Wasserstein A, Hill G, Goldfarb S, Goldberg M: Recurrent thrombotic thrombocytopenic purpura after viral infection. Clinical and histologic simulation of chronic glomerulonephritis. *Arch Intern Med* 141:685, 1981.

302. Kok RHJ, Wolfhagen MJHM, Klosters G: A syndrome resembling thrombotic thrombocytopenic purpura associated with human parvovirus B19 infection. *Clin Infect Dis* 32:311, 2001.

303. Turner RC, Chaplinski TJ, Adams HG: Rocky Mountain spotted fever presenting as thrombotic thrombocytopenic purpura. *Am J Med* 81:153, 1986.

304. Reynolds PM, Jackson JM, Brine JA, Vivian AB: Thrombotic thrombocytopenic purpura—Remission following splenectomy. Report of a case and review of the literature. *Am J Med* 61:439, 1976.

305. Bar Meir E, Amital H, Levy Y, et al: Mycoplasma-pneumoniae-induced thrombotic thrombocytopenic purpura. *Acta Haematol* 103:112, 2000.

306. George JN, Vesely SK, Terrell DR: The Oklahoma Thrombotic Thrombocytopenic Purpura-Hemolytic Uremic Syndrome (TTP-HUS) Registry: A community perspective of patients with clinically diagnosed TTP-HUS. *Semin Hematol* 41:60, 2004.

307. Bennett CL, Davidson CJ, Raisch DW, et al: Thrombotic thrombocytopenic purpura associated with ticlopidine in the setting of coronary artery stents and stroke prevention. *Arch Intern Med* 159:2524, 1999.

308. Tsai HM, Rice L, Sarode R, et al: Antibody inhibitors to von Willebrand factor metalloproteinase and increased binding of von Willebrand factor to platelets in ticlopidine-associated thrombotic thrombocytopenic purpura. *Ann Intern Med* 132:794, 2000.

309. Zakarija A, Bandarenko N, Pandey DK, et al: Clopidogrel-associated TTP: An update of pharmacovigilance efforts conducted by independent researchers, pharmaceutical suppliers, and the Food and Drug Administration. *Stroke* 35:533, 2004.

310. Bennett CL, Connors JM, Carwile JM, et al: Thrombotic thrombocytopenic purpura associated with clopidogrel. *N Engl J Med* 342:1773, 2000.

311. Fujita H, Takemura S, Hyo R, et al: Pulmonary embolism and thrombotic thrombocytopenic purpura in acute promyelocytic leukemia treated with all-trans retinoic acid. *Leuk Lymphoma* 44:1627, 2003.

312. van der Heijden M, Ackland SP, Deveridge S: Haemolytic uraemic syndrome associated with bleomycin, epirubicin, and cisplatin chemotherapy—A case report and review of the literature. *Acta Oncol* 37:107, 1998.

313. Palmisano J, Agraharkar M, Kaplan AA: Successful treatment of cisplatin-induced hemolytic uremic syndrome with therapeutic plasma exchange. *Am J Kidney Dis* 32:314, 1998.

314. Kressel BR, Ryan KP, Duong AT, et al: Microangiopathic hemolytic anemia, thrombocytopenia, and renal failure in patients treated for adenocarcinoma. *Cancer* 48:1738, 1981.

315. Byrnes JJ, Baquerizo H, Gonzalez M, Hensely GT: Thrombotic thrombocytopenic purpura subsequent to acute myelogenous leukemia chemotherapy. *Am J Hematol* 21:299, 1986.

316. Sakai C, Takagi T, Wakatsuki S, Matsuzaki O: Hemolytic-uremic syndrome due to deoxycoformycin: A report of the second case. *Intern Med* 34:593, 1995.

317. Tassinari D, Sartori S, Panzini I, et al: Hemolytic-uremic syndrome during therapy with estramustine phosphate for advanced prostatic cancer. *Oncology* 56:112, 1999.

318. Fung MC, Storniolo AM, Nguyen B, et al: A review of hemolytic uremic syndrome in patients treated with gemcitabine therapy. *Cancer* 85:2023, 1999.

319. Humphreys BD, Sharman JP, Henderson JM, et al: Gemcitabine-associated thrombotic microangiopathy. *Cancer* 100:2664, 2004.

320. Laffay DL, Tubbs RR, Valenzuela R, et al: Chronic glomerular microangiopathy and metastatic carcinoma. *Hum Pathol* 10:433, 1979.

321. Valavaara R, Nordman E: Renal complications of mitomycin C therapy with special reference to the total dose. *Cancer* 55:47, 1985.

322. Lesesne JB, Rothschild N, Erickson B, et al: Cancer-associated hemolytic-uremic syndrome: Analysis of 85 cases from a national registry. *J Clin Oncol* 7:781, 1989.

323. Montes A, Powles TJ, O'Brien ME, et al: A toxic interaction between mitomycin C and tamoxifen causing the haemolytic uraemic syndrome. *Eur J Cancer* 29A:1854, 1993.

324. Dzik WH, Georgi BA, Khettry U, Jenkins RL: Cyclosporine-associated thrombotic thrombocytopenic purpura following liver transplantation—Successful treatment with plasma exchange. *Transplantation* 44:570, 1987.

325. Remuzzi G, Bertani T: Renal vascular and thrombotic effects of cyclosporine. *Am J Kidney Dis* 13:261, 1989.

326. Trimarchi HM, Truong LD, Brennan S, et al: FK506-associated thrombotic microangiopathy: Report of two cases and review of the literature. *Transplantation* 67:539, 1999.

327. Scott LJ, McKeage K, Keam SJ, Plosker GL: Tacrolimus: A further update of its use in the management of organ transplantation. *Drugs* 63:1247, 2003.

328. Ahmed F, Sumalnop V, Spain DM, Tobin MS: Thrombohemolytic thrombocytopenic purpura during penicillamine therapy. *Arch Intern Med* 138:1292, 1978.

329. Harrison EE, Hickman JW: Hemolytic anemia and thrombocytopenia associated with penicillamine ingestion. *South Med J* 68:113, 1975.

330. Abramowicz D, Pradier O, Marchant A, et al: Induction of thromboses within renal grafts by high-dose prophylactic OKT3. *Lancet* 339:777, 1992.

331. Ravandi-Kashani F, Cortes J, Talpaz M, Kantarjian HM: Thrombotic microangiopathy associated with interferon therapy for patients with chronic myelogenous leukemia: Coincidence or true side effect? *Cancer* 85:2583, 1999.

332. Al-Zahrani H, Gupta V, Minden MD, et al: Vascular events associated with alpha interferon therapy. *Leuk Lymphoma* 44:471, 2003.

333. Ubara Y, Hara S, Takedatu H, et al: Hemolytic uremic syndrome associated with beta-interferon therapy for chronic hepatitis C. *Nephron* 80:107, 1998.

334. Allan DS, Thompson CM, Barr RM, et al: Ciprofloxacin-associated hemolytic-uremic syndrome. *Ann Pharmacother* 36:1000, 2002.

335. Alexopoulou A, Dourakis SP, Kaloterakis A: Thrombotic thrombocytopenic purpura in a patient treated with clarithromycin. *Eur J Haematol* 69:191, 2002.

336. Baron BW, Van Besien K, Hoffman PC, et al: Thrombotic thrombocytopenic purpura after cephalosporin administration: A possible relationship. *Transfusion* 43:1317, 2003.

337. Yata Y, Miyagiwa M, Inatsuchi S, et al: Thrombotic thrombocytopenia purpura caused by piperacillin successfully treated with plasma infusion. *Ann Hematol* 79:593, 2000.

338. Fahal IH, Williams PS, Clark RE, Bell GM: Thrombotic thrombocytopenic purpura due to rifampicin. *BMJ* 304:882, 1992.

339. Powell HR, Davidson PM, McCredie DA, et al: Haemolytic-uraemic syndrome after treatment with metronidazole. *Med J Aust* 149:222, 1988.

340. Castelman B, McNeely BU: Case records of the Massachusetts General Hospital. Case 1-1968. *N Engl J Med* 278:36, 1968.

341. Parker JC, Barrett DA 2nd: Microangiopathic hemolysis and thrombocytopenia related to penicillin drugs. *Arch Intern Med* 127:474, 1971.

342. Symmers WS: Thrombotic microangiopathy (thrombotic thrombocytopenic purpura) associated with acute haemorrhagic leucoencephalitis and sensitivity to oxophenarsine. *Brain* 79:511, 1956.

343. Bell WR, Chulay JD, Feinberg JE: Manifestations resembling thrombotic microangiopathy in patients with advanced human immunodeficiency virus (HIV) disease in a cytomegalovirus prophylaxis trial (ACTG 204). *Medicine* 76:369, 1997.

344. Feinberg JE, Hurwitz S, Cooper D, et al: A randomized, double-blind trial of valaciclovir prophylaxis for cytomegalovirus disease in patients with advanced human immunodeficiency virus infection. AIDS Clinical Trials Group Protocol 204/Glaxo Wellcome 123-014 International CMV Prophylaxis Study Group. *J Infect Dis* 177:48, 1998.

345. Hauglustaine D, Van Damme B, Vanrenterghem Y, Michielsen P: Recurrent hemolytic uremic syndrome during oral contraception. *Clin Nephrol* 15:148, 1981.

346. McShane PM, Bern MM, Schiff I: Thrombotic thrombocytopenic purpura associated with oral contraceptives: A case report. *Am J Obstet Gynecol* 145:762, 1983.

347. Liang R, Wong RW, Cheng IK: Thrombotic thrombocytopenic purpura and 17 beta-estradiol transdermal skin patch. *Am J Hematol* 52:334, 1996.

348. Au WY, Chan KW, Lam CC, Young K: A post-menopausal woman with anuria and uterus bulk: The spectrum of estrogen-induced TTP/HUS. *Am J Hematol* 71:59, 2002.

349. Keung YK, Morgan D, Cobos E: Cocaine-induced microangiopathic hemolytic anemia and thrombocytopenia simulating thrombotic thrombocytopenia purpura. *Ann Hematol* 72:155, 1996.

350. Volcy J, Nzerue CM, Oderinde A, Hewan-Iowe K: Cocaine-induced acute renal failure, hemolysis, and thrombocytopenia mimicking thrombotic thrombocytopenic purpura. *Am J Kidney Dis* 35:E3, 2000.

351. Tumlin JA, Sands JM, Someren A: Hemolytic-uremic syndrome following "crack" cocaine inhalation. *Am J Med Sci* 299:366, 1990.

352. Peces R, Diaz-Corte C, Baltar J, et al: Haemolytic-uraemic syndrome in a heroin addict. *Nephrol Dial Transplant* 13:3197, 1998.

353. Schirren CA, Berghaus TM, Sackmann M: Thrombotic thrombocytopenic purpura after Ecstasy-induced acute liver failure. *Ann Intern Med* 130:163, 1999.

354. Dlott JS, Danielson CF, Blue-Hnidy DE, McCarthy LJ: Drug-induced thrombotic thrombocytopenic purpura/hemolytic uremic syndrome: A concise review. *Ther Apher Dial* 8:102, 2004.

355. McCarthy LJ, Porcu P, Fausel CA, et al: Thrombotic thrombocytopenic purpura and simvastatin. *Lancet* 352:1284, 1998.

356. Kallal SM, Lee M: Thrombotic thrombocytopenic purpura associated with histamine H2-receptor antagonist therapy. *West J Med* 164:446, 1996.

357. Blecher TE, Raper AB: Early diagnosis of thrombotic microangiopathy by paraffin sections of aspirated bone-marrow. *Arch Dis Child* 42:158, 1967.

358. Karim Y, Masood A: Haemolytic uraemic syndrome following mumps, measles, and rubella vaccination. *Nephrol Dial Transplant* 17:941, 2002.

359. Peyriere H, Klouche K, Beraud JJ, et al: Fatal systemic reaction after multiple doses of intravesical bacillus Calmette-Guerin for polyposis. *Ann Pharmacother* 34:1279, 2000.

360. Brown RC, Blecher TE, French EA, Toghill PJ: Thrombotic thrombocytopenic purpura after influenza vaccination. *BMJ* 2:303, 1973.

361. Jones MB, Armitage JO, Stone DB: Self-limited TTP-like syndrome after bee sting. *JAMA* 242:2212, 1979.

362. Ashley JR, Otero H, Aboulafia DM: Bee envenomation: A rare cause of thrombotic thrombocytopenic purpura. *South Med J* 96:588, 2003.

363. Mele L, Voso MT, Fianchi L, et al: Thrombotic thrombocytopenic purpura-hemolytic uremic syndrome after bupropion treatment for smoking cessation. *Blood Coagul Fibrinolysis* 14:77, 2003.

364. Amorosi EL, Ultmann JE: Thrombotic thrombocytopenic purpura: Report of 16 cases and review of the literature. *Medicine* 45:139, 1966.

365. Stonesifer LD, Bone RC, Hiller FC: Thrombotic thrombocytopenic purpura in carbon monoxide poisoning. Report of a case. *Arch Intern Med* 140:104, 1980.

366. Pilz P: Moschcowitz syndrome with involvement of the central nervous system. Light optical studies on the genesis of hemolytic anemia and vascular changes. *Virchows Arch* 366:59, 1975.

VENOUS THROMBOSIS

GARY E. RASKOB

RUSSELL D. HULL

GRAHAM F. PINEO

Venous thromboembolism (venous thrombosis and or pulmonary embolism) is a common disorder with an annual incidence of 117 per 100,000 persons. The incidence increases with age. Most clinically important pulmonary emboli arise from proximal deep vein thrombosis (thrombosis involving the popliteal, femoral, or iliac veins). Upper extremity deep vein thrombosis also may lead to clinically important pulmonary embolism. The clinical features of deep vein thrombosis and pulmonary embolism are nonspecific. Objective diagnostic testing is required to confirm or exclude the presence of venous thromboembolism. Strategies for diagnosis or exclusion of venous thromboembolism include tests for the detection of pulmonary embolism [lung scanning, computed tomography (CT), or pulmonary angiography], tests for deep vein thrombosis of the legs (ultrasound or venography), and measurement of plasma D-dimer. Spiral CT is a useful test for ruling in the diagnosis of pulmonary embolism if positive results are obtained, but it should not be used alone to exclude the diagnosis because the test is insensitive for subsegmental emboli, which may be clinically important in patients with impaired cardiopulmonary function. Anticoagulant therapy is the preferred treatment for most patients with acute venous thromboembolism. Initial treatment with continuous intravenous heparin, subcutaneous low molecular weight heparin, or subcutaneous fondaparinux (a synthetic pentasaccharide), followed by long-term treatment with an oral vitamin K antagonist such as warfarin sodium, is effective for preventing recurrent venous thromboembolism. Use of low molecular weight heparin or fondaparinux enables outpatient therapy and is the preferred initial therapy for most patients. Intravenous heparin is preferred for patients with severe renal impairment. Thrombolytic therapy is indicated for patients with pulmonary embolism who present with cardiovascular collapse and in selected patients who have clinical or echocardiographic findings of right ventricular impairment. The role of thrombolytic therapy for patients with deep vein thrombosis is limited because whether systemic or catheter-directed thrombolysis reduces the incidence of the postthrombotic syndrome is unknown. Insertion of a vena cava filter is effective for preventing major pulmonary embolism and is indicated for patients with acute venous thromboembolism who have an absolute contraindication to anticoagulant therapy or who have recurrent venous thromboembolism despite adequate anticoagulant treatment. Anticoagulant treatment should be continued for at least 3 months in patients with a first episode of venous thromboembolism secondary to a reversible risk factor. Indefinite anticoagulant therapy should be considered for patients with idiopathic venous thromboembolism, certain thrombophilias, or at least two episodes of venous thromboembolism.

DEFINITION AND HISTORY

Venous thrombosis commonly develops in the deep veins of the leg or the arm or in the superficial veins of these extremities. Superficial venous thrombosis is a relatively benign disorder unless extension into the deep venous system develops. Thrombosis involving the deep veins of the leg is divided into two prognostic categories: (1) calf vein thrombosis, in which thrombi remain confined to the deep calf veins; and (2) proximal vein thrombosis, in which thrombosis involves the popliteal, femoral, or iliac veins.[1]

Pulmonary emboli originate from thrombi in the deep veins of the leg in at least 90 percent of patients. Other less common sources of pulmonary embolism include the deep pelvic veins, renal veins, inferior vena cava, right side of the heart, and axillary veins. Most clinically important pulmonary emboli arise from proximal deep vein thrombosis of the leg. Upper extremity deep vein thrombosis also may lead to pulmonary embolism.[2] Deep vein thrombosis and/or pulmonary embolism are referred to collectively as *venous thromboembolism*.

Venous thromboembolism is a common disorder. The estimated annual incidence of symptomatic venous thromboembolism is 117 cases per 100,000 population.[3] This incidence translates to more than 250,000 patients each year in the United States. The incidence of venous thromboembolism increases with each decade over age 60 years. Given the large proportion of the United States population that soon will enter the older age group, venous thromboembolism will be an increasingly important national health problem.[3]

Effective prophylaxis against venous thromboembolism is available for most high-risk patients. Use of prophylaxis is more effective for preventing death and morbidity from venous thromboembolism than is treatment of the established disease. Evidence-based recommendations for prevention of venous thromboembolism are available.[4]

Historically, venous thromboembolism usually occurred in sick hospitalized patients. The burden of illness from venous thromboembolism has shifted to the community setting such that most patients now present as outpatients to their primary care physician or to the emergency room. Reasons for this shift are the greatly reduced lengths of hospital stay for most surgical procedures or medical conditions and the discharge of patients from the hospital either before the period of risk of venous thromboembolism has ended or who have subclinical venous thrombi that subsequently evolve and lead to symptomatic deep vein thrombosis or pulmonary embolism. The shift in burden of illness from the hospital to the community setting has led to an emphasis on effective and safe methods for outpatient diagnosis and management.

ETIOLOGY AND PATHOGENESIS

Venous thrombi are composed mainly of fibrin and red blood cells, with variable numbers of platelets and leukocytes. The formation, growth, and breakdown of venous thromboemboli reflect a balance between thrombogenic stimuli and protective mechanisms. The thrombogenic stimuli first identified by Virchow in the 19th century are (1) venous stasis, (2) activation of blood coagulation, and (3) vein damage. The protective mechanisms are (1) inactivation of activated coagulation factors by circulating inhibitors (e.g., antithrombin bound to heparan sulfate at blood vessel walls and activated protein C), (2) clearance of activated coagulation factors and soluble fibrin polymer

Acronyms and abbreviations that appear in this chapter include: aPTT, activated partial thromboplastin time; CT, computed tomography; ELISA, enzyme-linked immunosorbent assay; INR, international normalized ratio; LMW, low molecular weight; MRI, magnetic resonance imaging.

complexes by mononuclear phagocytes and the liver, and (3) lysis of fibrin by fibrinolytic enzymes derived from plasma and endothelial cells.

Acquired and inherited risk factors for venous thromboembolism have been identified and are shown in Table 125-1 (see also Chaps. 117, 122, and 123). The risk of thromboembolism increases when more than one predisposing factor is present.

Activated protein C resistance is the most common hereditary abnormality predisposing to venous thrombosis. The defect results from substitution of glutamine for arginine at residue 506 in the factor V molecule, making factor V resistant to proteolysis by activated protein C. The gene mutation is commonly designated *factor V Leiden* and follows autosomal dominant inheritance. Patients who are homozygous for the factor V Leiden mutation have a markedly increased risk of thromboembolism and present with clinical thromboembolism at a younger age (median 31 years) than those who are heterozygous (median age 46 years).[5] Factor V Leiden is present in approximately 5 percent of the normal Caucasian population, 16 percent of patients with a first episode of deep vein thrombosis, and up to 35 percent of patients with idiopathic deep vein thrombosis.[6] Prothrombin G20210A is another gene mutation that predisposes to venous thromboembolism. It is present in approximately 2 to 3 percent of apparently healthy individuals and in 7 percent of those with deep vein thrombosis.[7] An inherited abnormality cannot be detected in up to 40 to 60 percent of patients with idiopathic deep vein thrombosis, suggesting that other gene mutations are present and have an etiologic role (see Chap. 122).

Pulmonary embolism occurs in at least 50 percent of patients with objectively documented proximal vein thrombosis.[1] Many of these emboli are asymptomatic. The clinical importance of pulmonary embolism depends on the size of the embolus and the patient's cardiorespiratory reserve. Usually only part of the thrombus embolizes, and 30 to 70 percent of patients with pulmonary embolism detected by angiography also have identifiable deep vein thrombosis of the legs.[8] Deep vein thrombosis and pulmonary embolism are not separate disorders but a continuous syndrome of venous thromboembolism in which the initial clinical presentation may be symptoms of either deep vein thrombosis or pulmonary embolism. Therefore, strategies for diagnosis of venous thromboembolism include both tests for detection of pulmonary embolism (lung scanning, computed tomography [CT], or pulmonary angiography)[8–10] and tests for deep vein thrombosis of the legs (ultrasound or venography)[11–13] (see "Objective Testing for Pulmonary Embolism" and "Objective Testing for Deep Vein Thrombosis" below).

TABLE 125-1 RISK FACTORS FOR THROMBOEMBOLISM*

ACQUIRED	HEREDITARY THROMBOPHILIAS
Advancing age (as of age 40 years)	Activated protein C resistance
History of prior thromboembolic event	Prothrombin G20210A
Recent surgery	Antithrombin deficiency
Recent trauma	Protein C deficiency
Prolonged immobilization	Protein S deficiency
Certain forms of cancer	Dysfibrinogenemia
Congestive heart failure	
Recent myocardial infarction	
Paralysis of legs	
Estrogen use	
Pregnancy or postpartum period	
Varicose veins	
Obesity	
Antiphospholipid antibody syndrome	
Hyperhomocysteinemia	

* See also Chap. 122

CLINICAL FEATURES

VENOUS THROMBOSIS

The clinical features of venous thrombosis include leg pain, tenderness, and swelling, a palpable cord representing a thrombosed vessel, discoloration, venous distention, prominence of the superficial veins, and cyanosis. The clinical diagnosis of deep vein thrombosis is highly nonspecific because each of the symptoms or signs can be caused by nonthrombotic disorders. The rare exception is the patient with phlegmasia cerulea dolens (occlusion of the whole venous circulation, extreme swelling of the leg, and compromised arterial flow), in whom the diagnosis of massive iliofemoral thrombosis is obvious. This syndrome occurs in less than 1 percent of patients with symptomatic venous thrombosis. In most patients, the symptoms and signs are nonspecific. In 50 to 85 percent of patients, the clinical suspicion of deep vein thrombosis is not confirmed by objective testing.[10–12] Patients with minor symptoms and signs may have extensive deep venous thrombi. Conversely, patients with florid leg pain and swelling, suggesting extensive deep vein thrombosis, may have negative results by objective testing. Patients can be assigned pretest probabilities of deep vein thrombosis based on the their clinical features and history. However, these clinical pretest probabilities are neither sufficiently high to give anticoagulant treatment nor sufficiently low to withhold treatment without performing further diagnostic testing.

PULMONARY EMBOLISM

The clinical features of acute pulmonary embolism include the following symptoms and signs that may overlap: (1) transient dyspnea and tachypnea in the absence of other clinical features, (2) pleuritic chest pain, cough, hemoptysis, pleural effusion, and pulmonary infiltrates noted on chest radiogram caused by pulmonary infarction or congestive atelectasis (also known as *ischemic pneumonitis* or *incomplete infarction*), (3) severe dyspnea and tachypnea and right-sided heart failure, (4) cardiovascular collapse with hypotension, syncope, and coma (usually associated with massive pulmonary embolism), and (5) several less common and nonspecific clinical presentations, including unexplained tachycardia or arrhythmia, resistant cardiac failure, wheezing, cough, fever, anxiety/apprehension, and confusion. All of these clinical features are nonspecific and can be caused by a variety of cardiorespiratory disorders. Objective diagnostic testing is mandatory to confirm or exclude the presence of pulmonary embolism.

LABORATORY FEATURES

Venous thromboembolism is associated with nonspecific laboratory changes that constitute the acute phase response to tissue injury. This response includes elevated levels of fibrinogen and factor VIII, increases in leukocyte and platelet counts, and systemic activation of blood coagulation, fibrin formation, and fibrin breakdown, with increases in plasma concentrations of prothrombin fragment 1.2, fibrinopeptide A, complexes of thrombin–antithrombin, and fibrin degradation products. All of these changes are nonspecific and may occur as a result of surgery, trauma, infection, inflammation, or infarction. None of the reported laboratory changes can be used to predict the development of venous thromboembolism.

The fibrin breakdown fragment D-dimer can be measured by an enzyme-linked immunosorbent assay (ELISA) or by a latex agglutination assay. Some of these assays have a rapid turnaround time and some are quantitative. A negative D-dimer result is useful for excluding the diagnosis in patients with suspected deep vein thrombosis or suspected pulmonary embolism[10,14] (see "Objective Testing for Pulmonary Embolism" and "Objective Testing for Deep Vein Thrombosis" below). A positive result is highly nonspecific.

DIFFERENTIAL DIAGNOSIS OF DEEP VEIN THROMBOSIS

The differential diagnosis in patients with clinically suspected deep vein thrombosis includes muscle strain or tear, direct twisting injury to the leg, lymphangitis or lymphatic obstruction, venous reflux, popliteal cyst, cellulitis, leg swelling in a paralyzed limb, and abnormality of the knee joint. An alternate diagnosis frequently is not evident at presentation, so excluding deep vein thrombosis is not possible without objective testing. The cause of symptoms often can be determined by careful followup once deep vein thrombosis has been excluded by objective testing. In approximately 25 percent of patients, however, the cause of pain, tenderness, and swelling remains uncertain even after careful followup.[13]

OBJECTIVE TESTING FOR DEEP VEIN THROMBOSIS

The objective diagnostic imaging tests that have a role in patients with clinically suspected deep vein thrombosis are ultrasound imaging and venography. Both of these tests have been validated by properly designed clinical trials, including prospective studies with long-term followup that have established the safety of withholding anticoagulant treatment in patients with negative test results.[11–13] Impedance plethysmography historically was a useful noninvasive test for deep vein thrombosis, but the wide availability of ultrasound imaging supplanted impedance plethysmography as the first-line noninvasive test in most centers.

Ultrasound imaging using vein compression is effective for identifying patients with proximal vein thrombosis. Compression ultrasonography of the proximal veins performed at presentation (and, if normal, repeated once 5–7 days later) can safely replace venography in symptomatic patients.[11] In selected centers with experienced ultrasonography staff, a single comprehensive evaluation of the proximal and calf veins with duplex ultrasonography may be sufficient and, if negative, a repeat test is not required.[12] However, the positive predictive value of a positive ultrasound result isolated to the calf veins is uncertain and may vary among centers based on expertise and thrombosis prevalence. Therefore, the number of repeat ultrasound evaluations avoided by evaluating the calf veins is partially offset by an increased number of patients with positive ultrasound results confined to the calf, for whom additional diagnostic testing and/or anticoagulant treatment is required. Most patients with a negative ultrasound result at presentation require a followup visit to establish the alternate diagnosis and to guide further care, so the return visit for a repeat ultrasound at 5 to 7 days has added practical value and is complied with by most patients.[11] Venography continues to have an important role in selected patients, such as those in whom ultrasonography is unavailable or inconclusive or in whom repeat testing is impractical.

Measurement of plasma D-dimer has been extensively evaluated as an exclusion test in patients with clinically suspected deep vein thrombosis.[14] The different D-dimer assays (ELISA, quantitative rapid ELISA, latex agglutination, or whole blood agglutination) have different sensitivities, specificities, and likelihood ratios for deep vein thrombosis. ELISA and quantitative rapid ELISA have high sensitivity (96%) and negative likelihood ratios of approximately 0.10 for deep vein thrombosis in symptomatic patients. Thus, for excluding deep vein thrombosis in symptomatic patients, a negative D-dimer result by a quantitative rapid ELISA technique is as diagnostically useful as a negative result by duplex ultrasonography.[14] Measurement of D-dimer using an appropriate assay method can be combined with ultrasound imaging. If the two tests are negative at presentation, repeat ultrasound

imaging can be safely avoided.[15] Use of the D-dimer test for patient care decisions depends on the local availability of an appropriate assay that has high sensitivity and has been validated by clinical outcome studies. Figure 125-1 shows a practical approach for the diagnosis of suspected deep vein thrombosis.

Diagnosis of acute recurrent deep vein thrombosis is particularly challenging because recurrent symptoms such as pain and swelling are common in patients with deep vein thrombosis despite adequate anticoagulant therapy, and because both ultrasound imaging and venography have limitations for excluding the presence of acute recurrent deep vein thrombosis.[16] Compression ultrasound may remain abnormal for 1 year in 50 percent of patients and even longer in some patients[17] because of persistent noncompressibility of the vein caused by fibrous organization of the original thrombus. Venography is of limited value for excluding the diagnosis of recurrent deep vein thrombosis because of obliteration or recanalization of the previously affected venous segments or nonfilled venous segments. Thus, measurement of plasma D-dimer may be particularly useful as an exclusion test in patients with suspected acute recurrent deep vein thrombosis. However, use of D-dimer must be evaluated separately in this patient group because many patients with a past history of venous thromboembolism are receiving long-term oral anticoagulant therapy, which has the potential to cause a false negative D-dimer result. Promising initial results were obtained in one study,[18] but further studies in larger numbers of patients are needed before the use of a negative D-dimer to exclude acute recurrent deep vein thrombosis is routinely recommended.

DIFFERENTIAL DIAGNOSIS OF PULMONARY EMBOLISM

The differential diagnosis in patients with suspected pulmonary embolism includes cardiopulmonary disorders for each of the modes of presentation (see above in "Pulmonary Embolism"). For the presentation of dyspnea and tachypnea, they include atelectasis, pneumonia, pneumothorax, acute pulmonary edema, bronchitis, bronchiolitis, and acute bronchial obstruction. For pulmonary infarction exhibited by pleuritic chest pain or hemoptysis, they include pneumonia, pneumothorax, pericarditis, pulmonary or bronchial neoplasm, bronchiectasis, acute bronchitis, tuberculosis, diaphragmatic inflammation, myositis, muscle strain, and rib fracture. For the clinical presentation of right-sided heart failure, they include myocardial infarction, myocarditis, and cardiac tamponade. For cardiovascular collapse, they include myocardial infarction, acute massive hemorrhage, gram-negative septicemia, cardiac tamponade, and spontaneous pneumothorax.

OBJECTIVE TESTING FOR PULMONARY EMBOLISM

The objective diagnostic imaging tests include lung radionuclide scanning, spiral computed tomography (CT), pulmonary angiography, magnetic resonance imaging (MRI), and objective testing for proximal deep vein thrombosis. Measurement of plasma D-dimer is useful as an exclusion test.

SPIRAL COMPUTED TOMOGRAPHY IMAGING

Spiral CT imaging is highly sensitive for large emboli (segmental or larger arteries) but is much less sensitive for emboli in subsegmental pulmonary arteries.[10,19] Such emboli may be clinically important in patients with severely impaired cardiorespiratory reserve. Therefore, a negative result by spiral CT should not be used alone to exclude the diagnosis of pulmonary embolism. Spiral CT is a useful test for ruling in the diagnosis of pulmonary embolism if positive results are ob-

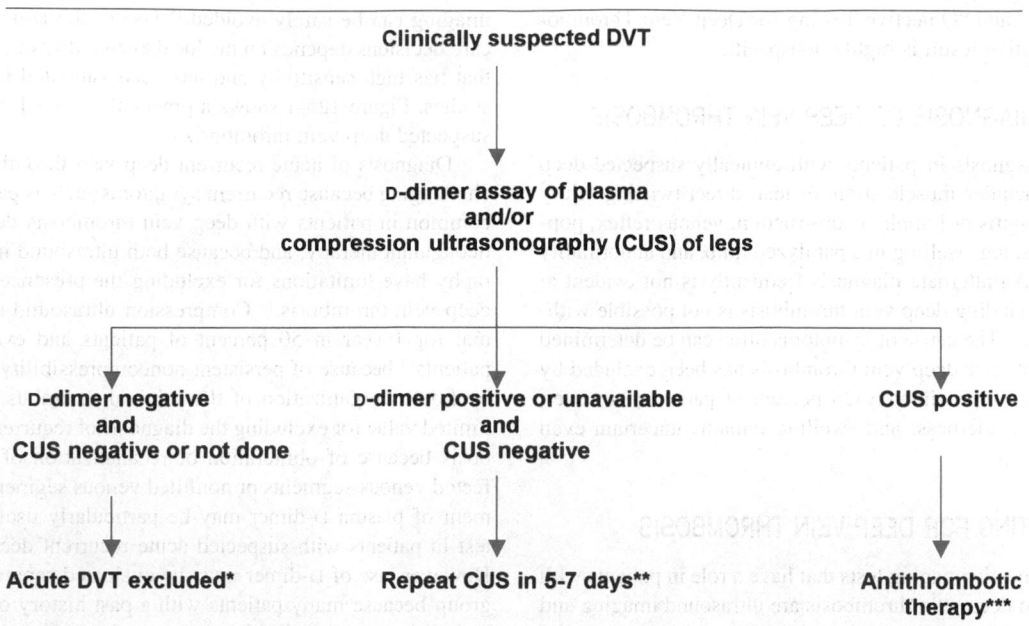

FIGURE 125-1   Diagnosis of patients with suspected first episode of deep vein thrombosis (DVT). *Negative D-dimer can be used to exclude acute DVT, without the need for further diagnostic testing with compression ultrasonography (CUS), provided the D-dimer is measured using an appropriately validated technique (see reference 14). Similarly, a negative D-dimer can be used with a negative CUS at presentation to exclude acute DVT without the need for a repeat CUS.[15] **CUS is performed with imaging of the common femoral vein in the groin and of the popliteal vein in the popliteal fossa extending distally 10 cm from mid-patella. A repeat CUS is required in 5 to 7 days to detect extending calf vein thrombi.[11] In selected centers with the expertise, a single negative result of full-leg duplex ultrasonography (CUS plus flow evaluation) may be sufficient to exclude acute DVT.[12] ***CUS that indicates noncompressibility of deep vein segments is highly predictive of DVT (>95%) and provides an indication for antithrombotic therapy in most patients. If CUS is positive at a single site isolated in the groin, additional testing with venography, computed tomography, or magnetic resonance imaging should be performed because of the potential for false-positive CUS results from disorders producing vein compression in the groin (e.g., tumor mass).

tained. A filling defect of a segmental or larger artery on spiral CT is associated with a high probability (>90%) of pulmonary embolism.

RADIONUCLIDE LUNG SCANNING

Radionuclide lung scanning continues to have an important role in the diagnosis of suspected pulmonary embolism. A normal perfusion lung scan excludes the diagnosis of clinically important pulmonary embolism.[9,20] A normal perfusion lung scan is found in approximately 10 percent of patients with suspected pulmonary embolism seen at academic health centers or tertiary referral centers. A high-probability lung scan result (i.e., large perfusion defects with ventilation mismatch) has a positive predictive value for pulmonary embolism of 85 percent and provides a diagnostic endpoint to give antithrombotic treatment in most patients.[9,20,21] A high-probability lung scan is found in approximately 10 to 15 percent of symptomatic patients. For patients with a history of pulmonary embolism, careful comparison of the lung scan results to the most recent lung scan is required to ensure the perfusion defects are new. Further diagnostic testing may be indicated for patients with a high-probability lung scan result who are at high risk for major bleeding, to reduce the likelihood of a false-positive diagnosis. The remaining lung scan patterns are nondiagnostic and are found in 70 percent of patients with suspected pulmonary embolism. These lung scan results have been called "low-probability" (matching ventilation-perfusion abnormalities or small perfusion defects), "intermediate probability," or indeterminate (because the perfusion defects correspond to an area of abnormality on chest x-ray film). Further diagnostic testing is required in these patients because,

regardless of the pretest clinical suspicion, the posttest probabilities of pulmonary embolism associated with these lung scan results are neither sufficiently high to give antithrombotic treatment nor sufficiently low to withhold therapy. The uncommon exception is the patient with a low clinical suspicion and a so-called "low-probability" lung scan result. However, even in these patients, objective testing for deep vein thrombosis with ultrasound and/or measurement of plasma D-dimer is without risk for the patient and may provide added diagnostic value (see "Objective Testing for Deep Vein Thrombosis" below).

OBJECTIVE TESTING FOR DEEP VEIN THROMBOSIS

Objective testing for deep vein thrombosis is useful in patients with suspected pulmonary embolism, particularly those with nondiagnostic lung scan results[22,23] or negative or inconclusive spiral CT results. [24] Detection of proximal vein thrombosis by objective testing provides an indication for anticoagulant treatment, regardless of the presence or absence of pulmonary embolism, and prevents the need for further testing. A negative result by objective testing for deep vein thrombosis does not exclude the presence of pulmonary embolism.[25] If the patient has adequate cardiorespiratory reserve, then serial noninvasive testing for proximal vein thrombosis can be used as an alternative to pulmonary angiography, and withholding anticoagulant therapy is safe if repeated ultrasound testing of the legs is negative.[23,24] The rationale is that the clinical objective in such patients is to prevent recurrent pulmonary embolism, which is unlikely in the absence of proximal vein thrombosis. For patients with inadequate cardiorespiratory reserve, the clinical objective is to prevent death and morbidity from an existing

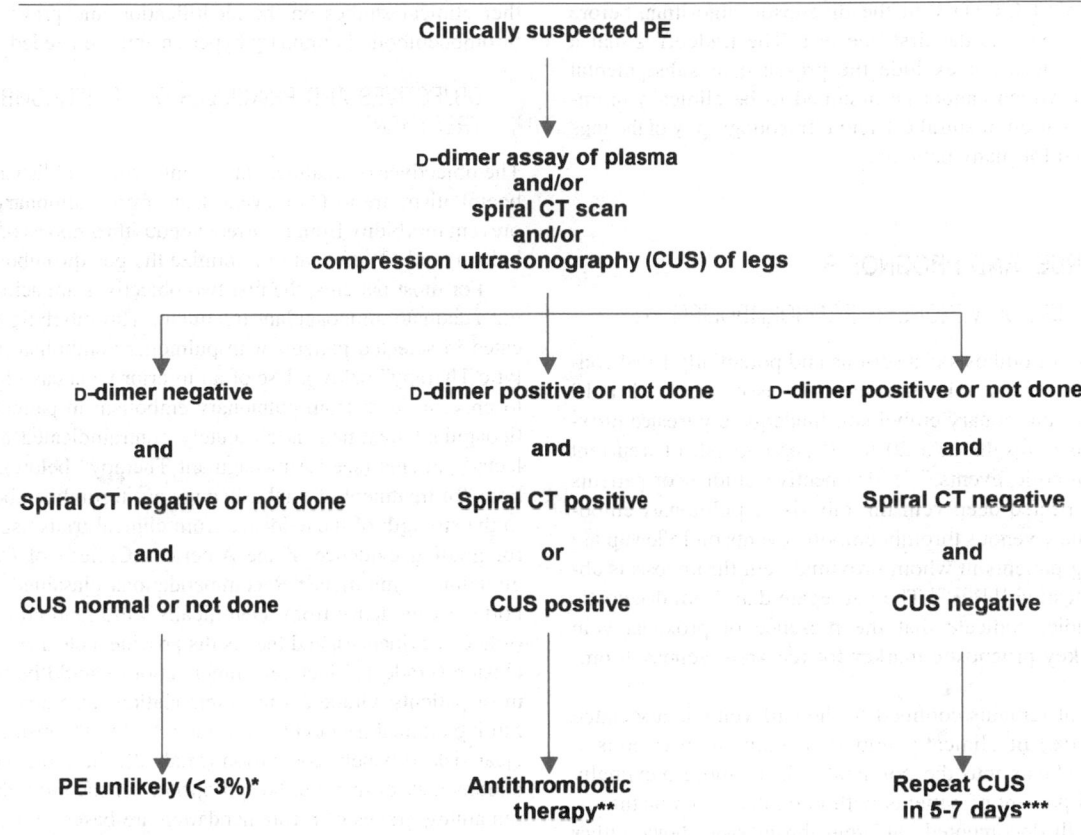

Clinically suspected PE

**D-dimer assay of plasma
and/or
spiral CT scan
and/or
compression ultrasonography (CUS) of legs**

D-dimer negative	D-dimer positive or not done	D-dimer positive or not done
and	and	and
Spiral CT negative or not done	Spiral CT positive	Spiral CT negative
and	or	and
CUS normal or not done	CUS positive	CUS negative
PE unlikely (< 3%)*	Antithrombotic therapy**	Repeat CUS in 5-7 days***

FIGURE 125-2   Diagnosis of patients with suspected pulmonary embolism (PE). *Negative D-dimer alone can be used as an exclusion test with high sensitivity (>96%) provided the D-dimer is measured using an appropriately validated technique.[10,14] Similarly, a negative D-dimer can be used with negative spiral computed tomography (CT) and/negative compression ultrasonography (CUS) as an exclusion approach. However, negative spiral CT should not be used alone to exclude the diagnosis of PE.[19] **Positive spiral CT in segmental or greater arteries, or a positive CUS of the legs, provides an indication for antithrombotic therapy. ***If a validated D-dimer technique is unavailable or if the result is positive, spiral CT can be used with CUS in patients with adequate cardiorespiratory reserve (see text for further details). If both tests are negative at presentation, CUS should be repeated in 5 to 7 days, and antithrombotic therapy can be withheld if CUS remains negative.[74] If lung scanning is used instead of or prior to spiral CT, a normal perfusion scan excludes clinically important PE, and a high-probability lung scan result is an indication for antithrombotic therapy in most patients. The remaining lung scan patterns are nondiagnostic. Because nondiagnostic patterns occur in 70 percent of patients, many centers have moved to spiral CT as the main imaging test for suspected PE.

embolus. In such patients, even a relatively small embolus may be an important contributing factor to their impaired cardiopulmonary function, and further testing for the presence or absence of pulmonary embolism is needed. Definitive testing for the presence or absence of embolism in the lung should be pursued among patients with features that may indicate an alternate source of embolism to proximal deep vein thrombosis of the leg (e.g., upper extremity thrombosis, renal vein thrombosis, pelvic vein thrombosis, or right-heart thrombus).

D-DIMER ASSAY

The assay for plasma D-dimer is useful as an exclusion test, provided an appropriately validated test is available. A negative result by the rapid quantitative ELISA for D-dimer has a negative likelihood ratio similar to that of a normal perfusion scan.[14] A positive D-dimer result is not useful diagnostically.

MAGNETIC RESONANCE IMAGING

MRI appears to be highly sensitive for pulmonary embolism and is a promising diagnostic approach. However, clinically important interobserver variation exists in the sensitivity for pulmonary embolism,

ranging from 70 to 100 percent.[26] Further studies are required to determine the clinical role of MRI in the diagnosis of patients with suspected pulmonary embolism.

PULMONARY ANGIOGRAPHY

Pulmonary angiography using selective catheterization of the pulmonary arteries is a relatively safe technique for patients who do not have pulmonary hypertension or cardiac failure.[9,20] If the expertise is available, pulmonary angiography should be used when other approaches are inconclusive and when definitive knowledge about the presence or absence of embolism in the lung is required.

Figure 125-2 summarizes the approach to diagnosis of suspected pulmonary embolism. The optimal combination and sequence of diagnostic testing is not completely resolved. Therefore, the specific approach used will depend on the local availability of technology and expertise with the different diagnostic techniques. An appropriately validated assay for plasma D-dimer, if available, provides a simple and rapid first-line exclusion test. Because the lung scan is nondiagnostic in 70 percent of patients and because a CT scan can often be obtained faster and easier than a radionuclide lung scan, many centers have moved to using spiral CT early in the diagnostic algorithm, before lung scanning and even as the first-line test. The tradeoff is that a negative spiral CT does not exclude the presence of subsegmental pulmonary emboli, which cannot be assumed to be clinically unimportant. The combination of spiral CT and ultrasonography of the legs is a useful approach for many patients.

THERAPY, COURSE, AND PROGNOSIS

CLINICAL COURSE OF VENOUS THROMBOEMBOLISM

Proximal deep vein thrombosis is a serious and potentially lethal condition. Untreated proximal vein thrombosis is associated with a 10 percent rate of fatal pulmonary embolism. Inadequately treated proximal vein thrombosis results in a 20 to 50 percent risk of recurrent venous thromboembolic events.[27–29] Prospective studies of patients with clinically suspected deep vein thrombosis or pulmonary embolism indicate that new venous thromboembolic events on followup are rare (≤2%) among patients in whom proximal vein thrombosis is absent by objective testing.[11,15,22–24] The aggregate data from diagnostic and treatment studies indicate that the presence of proximal vein thrombosis is the key prognostic marker for recurrent venous thromboembolism.

Thrombosis that remains confined to the calf veins is associated with low risk (≤1%) of clinically important pulmonary embolism. Extension of thrombosis into the popliteal vein or more proximally occurs in 15 to 25 percent of patients with untreated calf vein thrombosis.[1] Patients with documented calf vein thrombosis should either receive anticoagulant treatment to prevent extension or undergo monitoring for proximal extension using serial noninvasive tests.

The postthrombotic syndrome is a frequent complication of deep vein thrombosis.[30] Patients with the postthrombotic syndrome complain of pain, heaviness, swelling, cramps, and itching or tingling of the affected leg. Ulceration may occur. The symptoms usually are aggravated by standing or walking and improve with rest and elevation of the leg. A prospective study documented a 25 percent incidence of moderate-to-severe postthrombotic symptoms 2 years after the initial diagnosis of proximal vein thrombosis in patients who were treated with initial heparin and oral anticoagulants for 3 months.[31] The study also demonstrated that ipsilateral recurrent venous thrombosis is strongly associated with subsequent development of moderate or severe postthrombotic symptoms. Thus, prevention of ipsilateral recurrent deep vein thrombosis likely reduces the incidence of the postthrombotic syndrome. Application of a properly fitted graded compression stocking, as soon after diagnosis as the patient's symptoms will allow and continued for at least 2 years, is effective in reducing the incidence of postthrombotic symptoms, including moderate-to-severe symptoms.[32]

Chronic thromboembolic pulmonary hypertension is a serious complication of pulmonary embolism. Historically, thromboembolic pulmonary hypertension was believed to be relatively rare and to occur only several years after the diagnosis of pulmonary embolism. A prospective cohort study provides important new information on the incidence and timing of thromboembolic pulmonary hypertension.[33] The results indicate that thromboembolic pulmonary hypertension is more common and occurs earlier than previously thought. On prospective followup of 223 patients with documented pulmonary embolism, the cumulative incidence of chronic thromboembolic pulmonary hypertension was 3.8 percent at 2 years after diagnosis, despite state-of-the-art treatment for pulmonary embolism. The strongest independent risk factors were a history of pulmonary embolism (odds ratio 19) and idiopathic pulmonary embolism at presentation (odds ratio 5.7).[33] Fur-

ther clinical studies on the identification and prevention of chronic thromboembolic pulmonary hypertension are needed.

OBJECTIVES AND PRINCIPLES OF ANTITHROMBOTIC TREATMENT

The objectives of treatment in patients with established venous thromboembolism are to (1) prevent death from pulmonary embolism, (2) prevent morbidity from recurrent venous thrombosis or pulmonary embolism, and (3) prevent or minimize the postthrombotic syndrome.

For most patients, the first two objectives are achieved by providing adequate anticoagulant treatment. Thrombolytic therapy is indicated in selected patients with pulmonary embolism (see "Thrombolytic Therapy" below). Use of an inferior vena cava filter is indicated to prevent death from pulmonary embolism in patients in whom anticoagulant treatment is absolutely contraindicated and in other selected patients (see "Anticoagulant Therapy" below). Recommendations for treatment of established venous thromboembolism are linked to the strength of the evidence from clinical trials using the approach for grading evidence of the American College of Chest Physicians guideline committee.[34] Recommendations classified as 1A are supported by evidence from scientifically valid randomized clinical trials (grade A evidence), and the results provide a clear risk-to-benefit conclusion (grade 1). Such recommendations should be implemented for most patients. Grade 2A recommendations also are supported by definitive clinical trial evidence (grade A,) but the results indicate a less clear risk-to-benefit conclusion (grade 2); therefore, such recommendations may or may not be appropriate for the individual patient. The remaining grades of recommendation are based on nondefinitive evidence (grade B or C) and are less strong (see Chap. 21).

ANTICOAGULANT THERAPY

Anticoagulant therapy is the treatment of choice for most patients with proximal vein thrombosis or pulmonary embolism (grade 1A). The absolute contraindications to anticoagulant treatment include intracranial bleeding, severe active bleeding, recent brain, eye, or spinal cord surgery, and malignant hypertension. Relative contraindications include recent major surgery, recent cerebrovascular accident, active gastrointestinal tract bleeding, severe hypertension, severe renal or hepatic failure, and severe thrombocytopenia (platelets <50,000/μl).

HEPARIN AND LOW MOLECULAR WEIGHT HEPARIN

Patients with proximal deep vein thrombosis require both adequate initial anticoagulant treatment with heparin or low molecular weight (LMW) heparin and adequate long-term anticoagulant therapy to prevent recurrent venous thromboembolism.[27,28,34] Adequate anticoagulant treatment reduces the incidence of recurrent venous thromboembolism during the first 3 months after diagnosis from 25 percent to 5 percent or less.[27–29]

Initial therapy with continuous intravenous heparin has been the standard approach to treatment of deep vein thrombosis or pulmonary embolism for more than 20 years. During the 1990s, LMW heparin given by subcutaneous injection once or twice daily was evaluated by clinical trials and shown to be as effective and safe as continuous intravenous heparin for the initial treatment of patients with proximal deep vein thrombosis and submassive pulmonary embolism.[34,35] The advantage of LMW heparin is that it does not require anticoagulant monitoring (grade 1A). LMW heparin given subcutaneously once or twice daily is preferred over intravenous unfractionated heparin for the initial treatment of most patients with either deep vein thrombosis or submassive pulmonary embolism (grade 1A).[34] LMW heparin enables outpatient therapy for many patients with uncomplicated proximal vein thrombosis. Intravenous unfractionated heparin remains the preferred approach for initial anticoagulant therapy in patients with severe renal failure (grade 1A).[34] Initial treatment with LMW heparin or unfractionated heparin should be continued for at least 5 days (grade 1A). Table 125-2 lists the specific LMW drug regimens that have been effective in the initial treatment of venous thromboembolism.

If unfractionated heparin is used for initial therapy, it is important to achieve an adequate anticoagulant effect, defined as an activated partial thromboplastin time (aPTT) above the lower limit of therapeutic range within the first 24 hours.[36,37] Failure to achieve an adequate aPTT effect early during therapy is associated with a high incidence (25%) of recurrent venous thromboembolism.[36] Two thirds of the recurrent events occur between 2 and 12 weeks after the initial diagnosis, despite treatment with oral anticoagulants.[37] The clinical trial data indicate that initial management with either unfractionated heparin or LMW heparin is critical to the patient's long-term outcome.[37]

The synthetic pentasaccharide fondaparinux, which inhibits factor Xa, has been evaluated by large randomized clinical trials.[38,39] These studies indicate fondaparinux is as effective and safe as LMW heparin for treatment of established deep vein thrombosis and as effective and safe as intravenous heparin for treatment of symptomatic submassive pulmonary embolism. Fondaparinux has been approved by the US FDA for the initial treatment of established deep vein thrombosis or submassive pulmonary embolism. It is given subcutaneously once daily at a dose of 7.5 mg for patients weighing between 50 and 100 kg (85% of all patients evaluated in the clinical trials), 5 mg for patients weighing less than 50 kg, and 10 mg for patients weighing more than 100 kg.[38,39]

ORAL ANTICOAGULANTS

Long-term anticoagulant therapy is required to prevent a high frequency (15–25%) of symptomatic extension of thrombosis and/or recurrent venous thromboembolic events.[27,34,40] Oral anticoagulant treatment using a vitamin K antagonist (e.g., sodium warfarin) currently is the preferred approach for long-term treatment in most patients (grade 1A). Treatment with adjusted doses of unfractionated heparin or LMW heparin is indicated for selected patients in whom vitamin K antagonists are contraindicated (e.g., pregnant women) or impractical, or in patients with concurrent cancer for whom LMW heparin regimens have been shown to be more effective and safer.[34,41,42] Treatment with a vitamin K antagonist is started with initial heparin or LMW heparin therapy and then overlapped for 4 to 5 days (grade 1A).

The preferred intensity of the anticoagulant effect of treatment with a vitamin K antagonist has been established by clinical trials.[34,43–46]

TABLE 125-2   REGIMENS OF LOW MOLECULAR-WEIGHT HEPARIN AND FONDAPARINUX FOR TREATMENT OF VENOUS THROMBOEMBOLISM

Drug	Regimen
Enoxaparin	1.0 mg/kg bid*
Dalteparin	200 IU/kg once daily†
Tinzaparin	175 IU/kg once daily‡
Nadroparin	6150 IU bid for 50–70 kg¶
Reviparin	4200 IU bid for 46–60 kg§
Fondaparinux	7.5 mg once daily for 50–100 kg‖

* A once-daily regimen of 1.5 mg/kg can be used but probably is less effective in patients at high risk of recurrence, such as those with cancer.
† After 1 month, can be followed by 150 IU/kg once daily as an alternative to an oral vitamin K antagonist for long-term treatment.
‡ This regimen can also be used for long-term treatment as an alternative to an oral vitamin K antagonist.
¶ 4100 IU bid if patient weighs <50 kg or 9200 IU bid if patient weighs >70kg.
§ 3500 IU bid if patient weighs 35–45 kg or 6300 IU bid if patient weighs >60 kg.
‖ 5 mg once daily if patient weighs <50 kg or 10 mg once daily if patient weighs >100 kg.

The dose of vitamin K antagonist should be adjusted to maintain the international normalized ratio (INR) between 2.0 and 3.0 (grade 1A). High-intensity vitamin K antagonist treatment (INR 3.0–4.0) probably should not be used because it has not improved effectiveness in patients with the antiphospholipid syndrome and recurrent thrombosis[45] and has caused more bleeding.[46] Low-intensity therapy (INR 1.5–1.9) is not recommended because it is less effective than standard intensity treatment (INR 2.0–3.0) and does not reduce bleeding complications.[44]

DURATION OF ANTICOAGULANT THERAPY AND RECURRENT VENOUS THROMBOEMBOLISM

The appropriate duration of oral anticoagulant treatment for venous thromboembolism using a vitamin K antagonist has been evaluated by multiple randomized clinical trials.[34,43,47–52] Treatment should be continued for at least 3 months in patients with a first episode of proximal vein thrombosis or pulmonary embolism secondary to a transient (reversible) risk factor (grade 1A). Stopping treatment at 4 to 6 weeks resulted in an increased incidence of recurrent venous thromboembolism during the following 6 to 12 months (absolute risk increase 8%). In contrast, treatment for 3 to 6 months resulted in a low rate of recurrent venous thromboembolism during the following 1 to 2 years (annual incidence 3%).

Patients with a first episode of idiopathic venous thromboembolism should be treated for at least 6 to 12 months[34] (grade 1A). However, loss of benefit is seen upon withdrawal of anticoagulant treatment at 12 months, with similar rates of recurrent venous thromboembolism at 2 years among patients treated for 6 months or 1 year.[52] Therefore, patients with a first episode of idiopathic deep vein thrombosis should be considered for indefinite anticoagulant therapy (grade 2A). This decision should be individualized, taking into consideration the estimated risk of recurrent venous thromboembolism, risk of bleeding, and patient compliance and preference. If indefinite anticoagulant treatment is given, the risk-benefit of continuing such treatment should be reassessed at periodic intervals.

A variety of prothrombotic conditions or markers reportedly are associated with an increased risk of recurrent venous thromboembolism. These conditions include deficiencies of the naturally occurring inhibitors of coagulation such as antithrombin, protein C, and protein S, specific gene mutations including factor V Leiden and prothrombin 20210A, elevated levels of coagulation factor VIII, elevated levels of homocysteine, and the presence of antiphospholipid antibodies (see Chaps. 122 and 123). The presence of residual deep vein thrombosis assessed by compression ultrasonography,[53] elevated levels of plasma D-dimer after discontinuation of anticoagulant treatment,[54] and male gender[55] have been associated with an increased incidence of recurrent thromboembolism. However, the available data are limited to subgroup analyses of randomized trials and data from observational studies. No randomized trials have been performed, a priori, in these subgroups of patients with thrombophilic conditions to evaluate the risk-benefit of different durations of anticoagulant treatment, so no definitive recommendations can be made.[34]

For patients with a first episode of venous thromboembolism and documented antiphospholipid antibodies or two or more thrombophilic conditions (e.g., combined factor V Leiden and prothrombin 20210A gene mutations), the recommended duration of treatment is at least 12 months,[34] with consideration of indefinite anticoagulant treatment. For patients with a first episode of venous thromboembolism who have documented deficiency of antithrombin, protein C, or protein S, or the factor V Leiden or prothrombin 20210A gene mutation, hyperhomocysteinemia, or high factor VIII levels (>90th percentile), the duration of treatment should be individualized after the patients have completed at least 6 to 12 months of anticoagulant therapy.[34] Some of these patients also may be candidates for indefinite therapy.

Oral vitamin K antagonist treatment should be given indefinitely for most patients with a second episode of objectively documented venous thromboembolismm[34,50] (grade 2A), because stopping treatment at 3 to 6 months in these patients results in a high incidence (21%) of recurrent venous thromboembolism during the following 4 years. The risk of recurrent thromboembolism during 4-year followup was reduced by 87 percent (from 21% to 3%) by continuing anticoagulant treatment, but this benefit is partially offset by an increase in the cumulative incidence of major bleeding (from 3% to 9%).[50]

Use of LMW heparin for long-term treatment of venous thromboembolism has been evaluated in clinical trials.[41,42] The studies indicate that long-term treatment with subcutaneous LMW heparin for 3 to 6 months is at least as effective as, and in cancer patients is more effective than, an oral vitamin K antagonist adjusted to maintain the INR between 2.0 and 3.0. LMW heparin also was associated with less bleeding complications because of a reduction in minor bleeding. Therefore, patients with venous thromboembolism and concurrent cancer should be treated with LMW heparin for the first 3 to 6 months of long-term treatment (grade 1A). The patients then should receive anticoagulation indefinitely or until the cancer resolves. The regimens of LMW heparin that are established as effective for long-term treatment are dalteparin 200 U/kg once daily for 1 month, followed by 150 U/kg daily thereafter or tinzaparin 175 U/kg once daily.

ANTICOAGULANT THERAPY DURING PREGNANCY

Adjusted dose subcutaneous heparin is an appropriate long-term anticoagulant regimen for pregnant patients with venous thromboembolism. LMW heparin does not cross the placenta, and initial experience suggests these agents are safe for treatment of venous thromboembolism in pregnant patients.[56,57] With regard to safety advantages, LMW heparin causes less thrombocytopenia and potentially less osteoporosis than unfractionated heparin. An additional advantage is that LMW heparin is effective when given once daily, whereas unfractionated heparin requires twice-daily injection. Large randomized trials comparing the efficacy and safety of LMW heparin with unfractionated heparin in pregnant patients have not been completed. The key uncertainty about use of LMW heparin for treatment of venous thromboembolism during pregnancy is whether the regimens established as effective for initial and long-term therapy in nonpregnant patients, who do not require anticoagulant monitoring, can be generalized to pregnant patients. A study indicates no major change in the peak anti-Xa levels over the course of pregnancy in most patients treated with a once-daily therapeutic LMW heparin regimen (tinzaparin 175 U/kg).[57] Measurement of the anti-Xa level indicates if major pharmacokinetic changes are occurring in the individual patient, particularly during the third trimester. However, the appropriate therapeutic range for the anti-Xa level to be achieved by LMW heparin treatment has not been established by properly designed clinical outcome studies. Measurement of the anti-Xa level may provide reassurance that major drug accumulation is not occurring. However, the appropriate dose adjustments in response to a decreased anti-Xa level are uncertain. The choice between adjusted dose unfractionated heparin or LMW heparin therapy during pregnancy is a clinical judgment in the individual patient. The patient should be informed of the pros and cons discussed above and their preference factored into the decision. Evidence-based guidelines for antithrombotic therapy during pregnancy are available.[58]

DIRECT THROMBIN INHIBITOR

The oral direct thrombin inhibitor ximelagatran has been evaluated for the extended long-term treatment of venous thromboembolism.[59] The results indicate that ximelagatran at a dose of 24 mg twice daily is highly effective for extended anticoagulant treatment of venous thromboembolism after an initial 6 months of standard anticoagulant therapy and is associated with an incidence of major bleeding of approximately 1 percent per year. Ximelagatran has the advantage that it does not require anticoagulant monitoring and dose titration in the individual patient. However, it does require periodic monitoring of liver function to detect potential hepatotoxicity. Ximelagatran has been approved in Europe for extended treatment of venous thromboembolism, after an initial course of standard anticoagulant treatment, but at the time of this writing has not received approval by the FDA. Ximelagatran is undergoing evaluation in clinical trials for the initial treatment of venous thromboembolism.

SIDE EFFECTS OF ANTICOAGULANT THERAPY

Bleeding Bleeding is the most common side effect of anticoagulant therapy. Bleeding can be classified as major or minor according to standardized international criteria. *Major bleeding* is defined as clinically overt bleeding resulting in a decline of hemoglobin of at least 2g/dl, transfusion of at least 2 U of packed red cells, or bleeding that is retroperitoneal or intracranial. The rates of major bleeding in clinical trials of initial therapy with intravenous heparin, LMW heparin, or fondaparinux are 1 to 2 percent.[35,38,39] Patients at increased risk of major bleeding are those who underwent surgery or experienced trauma within the previous 14 days; those with a history of gastrointestinal bleeding, peptic ulcer disease, or genitourinary bleeding; and those with miscellaneous conditions predisposing to bleeding, such as thrombocytopenia, liver disease, and multiple invasive lines.

Major bleeding occurs in approximately 2 percent of patients during the first 3 months of oral anticoagulant treatment using a vitamin K antagonist and in 1 to 3 percent per year of treatment thereafter.[60] A meta-analysis suggests the clinical impact of major bleeding during long-term oral vitamin K antagonist treatment is greater than widely appreciated.[60] The estimated case fatality rate for major bleeding is 13 percent, and the rate of intracranial bleeding was 1.15 per 100 patient-years.[60] These risks are important considerations in the decision about extended or indefinite anticoagulant therapy in patients with venous thromboembolism. Further studies regarding the clinical impact of major bleeding associated with long-term therapy using the thrombin inhibitor ximelagatran in larger numbers of patients are needed.

Heparin-Induced Thrombocytopenia (See also Chap. 124.) Heparin or LMW heparin may cause thrombocytopenia. In large clinical studies of acute venous thromboembolism treatment, thrombocytopenia occurred in fewer than 1 percent of more than 2000 patients treated with unfractionated heparin or LMW heparin.[36,37] Nevertheless, heparin-induced thrombocytopenia can be a serious complication when accompanied by extension or recurrence of venous thromboembolism or the development of arterial thrombosis. Such complications may precede or coincide with the fall in platelet count and have been associated with a high rate of limb loss and a high mortality. Heparin in all forms should be discontinued when the diagnosis of heparin-induced thrombocytopenia is made on clinical grounds, and treatment with an alternative anticoagulant such as danaparoid, lepirudin, or argatroban should be initiated. Treatment with an oral vitamin K antagonist should be started or resumed once the thrombocytopenia resolves. It is given in low daily doses overlapping for at least 5 days with the alternative anticoagulant that is discontinued once a stable INR is achieved.

Heparin-Induced Osteoporosis   Osteoporosis may occur as a result of long-term treatment with heparin or LMW heparin (usually after more than 3 months). The earliest clinical manifestation of heparin-associated osteoporosis usually is nonspecific low back pain primarily involving the vertebrae or the ribs. Patients also may present with spontaneous fractures. Up to one third of patients treated with long-term heparin may have subclinical reduction in bone density. Whether these patients are predisposed to future fractures is not known. The incidence of symptomatic osteoporosis in clinical trials of LMW heparin treatment for 3 to 6 months was very low and are not increased compared to warfarin treatment. Patients with osteoporosis or fractures often had other risk factors such as bone metastases.

Other Side Effects of Heparin   Heparin or LMW heparin may cause elevated liver transaminase levels. These elevations are of unknown clinical significance and usually return to normal after the heparin or LMW heparin is discontinued. Awareness of this biochemical effect is important so as to avoid unnecessary interruption of heparin therapy and unnecessary liver biopsies in patients who may develop elevated transaminase levels during heparin or LMW heparin therapy. Additional rare side effects of heparin include hypersensitivity and skin reactions, such as necrosis, alopecia, and hyperkalemia occurring as a result of hypoaldosteronism.

Ximelagatran treatment may cause elevated liver transaminase enzyme levels. In the Thrombin Inhibitor in Venous Thromboembolism (THRIVE) III trial,[59] an elevated level of alanine aminotransferase more than threefold the upper limit of normal occurred in 6.4 percent of patients given ximelagatran compared with 1.2 percent of patients who received placebo. The transaminase elevations usually occurred after 4 weeks of treatment. The clinical consequences of this laboratory finding are not completely understood, and further details on the clinical importance of this finding will be important. Monitoring of liver transaminase enzymes will be required with oral direct thrombin-inhibitor treatment, which partially offsets the advantage of lack of anticoagulant monitoring.

THROMBOLYTIC THERAPY

Thrombolytic therapy is indicated for patients with pulmonary embolism who present with evidence of vascular collapse (hypotension and/or syncope) and for selected patients with pulmonary embolism who have clinical findings of right ventricular failure or echocardiographic evidence of right ventricular hypokinesia. Thrombolytic therapy provides more rapid lysis of pulmonary emboli and more rapid restoration of right ventricular function and pulmonary perfusion than does anticoagulant treatment.[61] An effective regimen is 100 mg of recombinant tissue plasminogen activator by intravenous infusion over 2 hours (50 mg/hour). Heparin then is given by continuous infusion once the thrombin time or aPTT is less than twice the control value.[61] The starting infusion dose is 1000 U/hour. Chapter 127 provides further details of thrombolytic therapy.

The role of thrombolytic therapy in patients with deep vein thrombosis is limited. Thrombolytic therapy may be indicated in patients with acute massive proximal vein thrombosis (phlegmasia cerulea dolens with impending venous gangrene) or in occasional patients with extensive iliofemoral vein thrombosis who have severe symptoms because of venous outflow obstruction. Thrombolytic therapy can be given by systemic infusion or catheter-directed infusion. Whether systemic or catheter-directed thrombolysis reduces the incidence of the postphlebitic syndrome is uncertain. The catheter-directed approach may be associated with a lower risk of major bleeding, particularly

intracranial bleeding, than systemic injection, but further clinical trials are required to determine the role of catheter-directed thrombolytic therapy in patients with deep vein thrombosis.

INFERIOR VENA CAVA FILTER

Insertion of an inferior vena cava filter is indicated for patients with acute venous thromboembolism and an absolute contraindication to anticoagulant therapy and the rare patients who have objectively documented recurrent venous thromboembolism during adequate anticoagulant therapy.

Insertion of a vena cava filter is effective for preventing important pulmonary embolism. However, use of a filter results in an increased incidence of recurrent deep vein thrombosis 1 to 2 years after insertion (increase in cumulative incidence at 2 years increases from 12% to 21%).[62] Long-term anticoagulant treatment should be started as soon as safely possible after placement of a vena cava filter to prevent morbidity from recurrent deep vein thrombosis.

REFERENCES

1. Moser KM, Lemoine JR: Is embolic risk conditioned by localization of deep venous thrombosis? *Ann Intern Med* 94:439, 1981.

2. Prandoni P, Polistena P, Bernardi E, et al: Upper-extremity deep vein thrombosis. Risk factors, diagnosis, and complications. *Arch Intern Med* 157:57, 1997.

3. Silverstein MD, Heit JA, Mohr DN, et al: Trends in the incidence of deep vein thrombosis and pulmonary embolism. A 25-year population-based study. *Arch Intern Med* 158:585, 1998.

4. Geerts W, Pineo G, Heit J, et al: Prevention of venous thromboembolism: The Seventh ACCP Conference on Antithrombotic and Thrombolytic Therapy. *Chest* 126(3 suppl):338S, 2004.

5. Rosendaal FR, Koster T, Vandenbroucke JP, Reitsma PH: High risk of thrombosis in patients homozygous for Factor V Leiden (activated Protein C resistance). *Blood* 85:1504, 1995.

6. Simioni P, Prandoni P, Lensing AWA, et al: The risk of recurrent venous thromboembolism in patients with an Arg[506]→Gln mutation in the gene for factor V (factor V Leiden). *N Engl J Med* 336:399, 1997.

7. Rosendaal FR, Doggen CJM, Zivelin A, et al: Geographic distribution of the 20210 G to A prothrombin variant. *Thromb Haemost* 79:706, 1998.

8. Hull R, Hirsh J, Carter C, et al: Diagnostic value of ventilation-perfusion lung scanning in patients with suspected pulmonary embolism. *Chest* 88:819, 1985.

9. PIOPED Investigators: Value of the ventilation/perfusion scan in acute pulmonary embolism: Results of the Prospective Investigation of Pulmonary Embolism Diagnosis (PIOPED). *JAMA* 263:2753, 1990.

10. Kruip M, Leclercq M, van der Heul C, et al: Diagnostic strategies for excluding pulmonary embolism in clinical outcome studies. A systematic review. *Ann Intern Med* 138;941, 2003.

11. Birdwell BG, Raskob GE, Whitsett TL, et al: The clinical validity of normal compression ultrasonography in outpatients suspected of having deep venous thrombosis. *Ann Intern Med* 128:1, 1998.

12. Stevens S, Elliott CG, Chan K, et al: Withholding anticoagulation after a negative result on Duplex ultrasonography for suspected symptomatic deep venous thrombosis. *Ann Intern Med* 140:985, 2004.

13. Hull R, Hirsh J, Sackett DL, et al: Clinical validity of a negative venogram in patients with clinically suspected venous thrombosis. *Circulation* 64:622, 1981.

14. Stein P, Hull RD, Patel K, et al: D-dimer for the exclusion of acute venous thrombosis and pulmonary embolism. A systematic review. *Ann Intern Med* 140:589, 2004.

15. Bernardi E, Prandoni P, Lensing AW, et al: D-dimer testing as an adjunct to ultrasonography in patients with clinically suspected deep-vein thrombosis: Prospective cohort study. *BMJ* 317:1037, 1998.

16. Hull RD, Carter CJ, Jay RM, et al: The diagnosis of acute, recurrent deep-vein thrombosis: A diagnostic challenge. *Circulation* 67:901, 1983.

17. Prandoni P, Cogo A, Bernardi, et al:A simple ultrasound approach for detection of recurrent proximal-vein thrombosis vein diameter. *Circulation* 88:1730, 1993.

18. Rathbun S, Whitsett T, Raskob G: Negative D-dimer to exclude recurrent deep-vein thrombosis in symptomatic patients. *Ann Intern Med* 141: 839, 2004.

19. Rathbun S, Whitsett T, Raskob G: Sensitivity and specificity of helical computed tomography in the diagnosis of pulmonary embolism: A systematic review. *Ann Intern Med* 132:227, 2000.

20. Hull R, Raskob G, Coates G, Panju A: Clinical validity of a normal perfusion lung scan in patients with suspected pulmonary embolism. *Chest* 97:23, 1990.

21. Miniati M, Prediletto A, Fornichi B, et al: Accuracy of clinical assessment in the diagnosis of pulmonary embolism. *Am J Respir Crt Care Med* 159:864, 1999

22. Hull RD, Raskob GE, Ginsberg JS, et al: A noninvasive strategy for the treatment of patients with suspected pulmonary embolism. *Arch Intern Med* 154:289, 1994.

23. Kearon C, Ginsberg J, Hirsh J: The role of venous ultrasonography in the diagnosis of suspected deep vein thrombosis and pulmonary embolism. *Ann Intern Med* 129:1044, 1998.

24. van Strijen M, de Monye W, Schiereck J, et al: Single–detector helical computed tomography as the primary diagnostic test in suspected pulmonary embolism: A multicenter clinical management study of 510 patients. *Ann Intern Med* 138:307, 2003.

25. Turkstra F, Kuijer P, van Beck EJ, et al: Diagnostic utility of ultrasonography of leg veins in patients suspected of having pulmonary embolism. *Ann Intern Med* 126:775, 1997.

26. Meaney JFM, Weg JG, Chenevert TL, et al: Diagnosis of pulmonary embolism with magnetic resonance angiography. *N Engl J Med* 336:1422, 1997.

27. Hull R, Delmore T, Genton E, et al: Warfarin sodium versus low-dose heparin in the long-term treatment of venous thrombosis. *N Engl J Med* 301:855, 1979.

28. Hull R, Raskob G, Hirsh J, et al: Continuous intravenous heparin compared with intermittent subcutaneous heparin in the initial treatment of proximal vein thrombosis. *N Engl J Med* 315:1109, 1986.

29. Brandjes D, Heijboer H, Buller H, et al: Acenocoumarol and heparin compared with acenocoumarol alone in the initial treatment of proximal-vein thrombosis. *N Engl J Med* 327:1485, 1992.

30. Kahn S, Ginsberg J: Relationship between deep venous thrombosis and the postthrombotic syndrome. *Arch Intern Med* 164:17, 2004.

31. Prandoni P, Lensing AWA, Cogo A, et al: The long-term clinical course of acute deep venous thrombosis. *Ann Intern Med* 125:1, 1996.

32. Brandjes D, Buller H, Heijboer H, et al: Randomized trial of the effect of compression stockings in patients with symptomatic proximal–vein thrombosis. *Lancet* 349:759, 1997.

33. Pengo V, Lensing A, Prins M, et al: Incidence of chronic thromboembolic pulmonary hypertension after pulmonary embolism. *N Engl J Med* 350:2257, 2004.

34. Buller H, Agnelli G, Hull R, et al: Antithrombotic therapy for venous thromboembolic disease: The Seventh ACCP Conference on Antithrombotic and Thrombolytic Therapy. *Chest* 126(3 suppl):401S, 2004; published erratum appear in *Chest* 127:416, 2005.

35. Quinlan D, McQuillan A, Eikelboom J: Low-molecular-weight heparin compared with intravenous unfractionated heparin for treatment of pulmonary embolism. *Ann Intern Med* 140:175, 2004.

36. Hull RD, Raskob GE, Brant RF, et al: Relation between the time to achieve the lower limit of the APTT therapeutic range and recurrent venous thromboembolism during heparin treatment for deep vein thrombosis. *Arch Intern Med* 157:2562, 1997.

37. Hull RD, Raskob GE, Brant RF, et al: The importance of initial heparin treatment on long-term clinical outcomes of antithrombotic therapy: The emerging theme of delayed recurrence. *Arch Intern Med* 157:2317, 1997.

38. Buller H, Davidson B, Decousus H, et al: Fondaparinux or enoxaparin for the initial treatment of symptomatic deep venous thrombosis. A randomized trial. *Ann Intern Med* 140:867, 2004.

39. Matisse Investigators: Subcutaneous fondaparinux versus intravenous unfractionated heparin in the initial treatment of pulmonary embolism. *N Engl J Med* 349:1695, 2003.

40. Lagerstedt C, Olsson C, Fagher B, et al: Need for long-term anticoagulant treatment in symptomatic calf-vein thrombosis. *Lancet* 2(8454): 515, 1986.

41. Lee A, Levine M, Baker R, et al: Low-molecular-weight heparin versus coumadin for the prevention of recurrent venous thromboembolism in patients with cancer. *N Engl J Med* 349:146, 2003.

42. Hull R, Pineo G, Mah A, et al: A randomized trial evaluating long-term low-molecular weight heparin therapy for three months versus intravenous heparin followed by warfarin sodium. *Blood* 100:148a, 2002.

43. Ridker P, Goldhaber S, Danielson E, et al: Long-term low-intensity warfarin therapy for the prevention of recurrent venous thromboembolism. *N Engl J Med* 348:1425, 2003.

44. Kearon C, Ginsberg J, Kovacs M, et al: Comparison of low-intensity warfarin therapy with conventional intensity warfarin therapy for long-term prevention of recurrent venous thromboembolism. *N Engl J Med* 349:631, 2003.

45. Crowther M, Ginsberg J, Julian J, et al: A comparison of two intensities of warfarin for the prevention of recurrent thrombosis in patients with the antiphospholipid antibody syndrome. *N Engl J Med* 349:1133, 2003.

46. Hull R, Hirsh J, Jay R, et al: Different intensities of oral anticoagulant therapy in the treatment of proximal-vein thrombosis. *N Engl J Med* 307:1676, 1982.

47. Optimum duration of anticoagulation for deep-vein thrombosis and pulmonary embolism. Research Committee of the British Thoracic Society. *Lancet* 340:873, 1992.

48. Schulman S, Rhedin A-S, Lindmarker P, et al: A comparison of six weeks with six months of oral anticoagulant therapy after a first episode of venous thromboembolism. *N Engl J Med* 332:1661, 1995.

49. Levine M, Hirsh J, Gent M, et al: Optimal duration of oral anticoagulant therapy: A randomized trial comparing four weeks with three months of warfarin in patients with proximal deep-vein thrombosis. *Thromb Haemost* 74:606, 1995.

50. Schulman S, Granqvist S, Holmström M, et al: The duration of oral anticoagulant therapy after a second episode of venous thromboembolism. *N Engl J Med* 336:393, 1997.

51. Kearon C, Gent M, Hirsh J, et al: A comparison of three months of anticoagulation with extended anticoagulation for a first–episode of idiopathic venous thromboembolism. *N Engl J Med* 340:901, 1999.

52. Agnelli G, Prandoni P, Santamaria M, et al: Three months versus one year of oral anticoagulant therapy for idiopathic deep-venous thrombosis. *N Engl J Med* 345:165, 2001.

53. Prandoni P, Lensing A, Prins M, et al: Residual venous thrombosis as a predictive factor of recurrent venous thromboembolism. *Ann Intern Med* 137:955, 2002.

54. Eichinger S, Minar E, Bialonczyk C, et al: D-dimer levels and risk of recurrent venous thromboembolism. *JAMA* 290:1071, 2003.

55. Kyrle P, Minar E, Bialonczyk, et al: The risk of recurrent venous thromboembolism in men and women. *N Engl J Med* 350:2558, 2004.

56. Pettila V, Kaaja R, Leinonen P, et al: Thromboprophylaxis with low molecular weight heparin (dalteparin) in pregnancy. *Thromb Res* 96: 275, 1999.

57. Smith M, Norris L, Steer P, et al: Tinzaparin sodium for thrombosis treatment and prevention during pregnancy. *Am J Obstet Gynecol* 190: 495, 2004.

58. Ginsberg J, Hirsh J: Antithrombotic therapy during pregnancy: The Seventh ACCP Conference on Antithrombotic and Thrombolytic Therapy. *Chest* 126(3 suppl):627S, 2004.

59. Schulman S, Wahlander K, Lundstrom T, et al: Secondary prevention of venous thromboembolism with the oral direct thrombin inhibitor ximelagatran. The THRIVE III Study. *N Engl J Med* 349:1713, 2003.

60. Linkins L, Choi P, Douketis J: Clinical impact of bleeding in patients taking oral anticoagulant therapy for venous thromboembolism. A meta-analysis. *Ann Intern Med* 139:893, 2003.

61. Goldhaber SZ, Haire WD, Feldstein ML, et al: Alteplase versus heparin in acute pulmonary embolism: Randomized trial assessing right-ventricular function and pulmonary perfusion. *Lancet* 341:507, 1993.

62. Decousus H, Leizorovicz A, Parent F, et al: A clinical trial of vena caval filters in the prevention of pulmonary embolism in patients with proximal deep-vein thrombosis. *N Engl J Med* 338:409, 1998.

ATHEROTHROMBOSIS: DISEASE INITIATION, PROGRESSION, AND TREATMENT

EMILE R. MOHLER III
ANDREW I. SCHAFER

The consequences of atherosclerotic vascular disease are the leading cause of morbidity and mortality in the developed countries of the world and are rapidly approaching that status in the developing world. This chapter reviews the pathologic mechanisms of atherosclerotic disease development and progression and details the interaction of these processes with the coagulation system. The earliest morphologically visible lesion of arterial atherosclerosis, the fatty streak, already is an advanced metabolic and immunologic locus that manifests as abnormalities of vascular tone, inflammation, cellular growth, and endothelial cell dysfunction. After years to decades, the lesions advance to form plaques that grow and eventually either impinge on the arterial lumen or rupture. Rupture of a vulnerable plaque is a catastrophic event that, through activation of both platelets and the coagulation cascade, triggers thrombosis, which leads to complete occlusion and tissue ischemia. Based on an increased understanding of the pathogenesis and consequences of atheromatous plaque development and progression, medical management of atherothrombotic syndromes has improved and is reviewed for the coronary, cerebrovascular and peripheral arteries.

ATHEROSCLEROSIS

Atherothrombosis describes a disease process that includes atherosclerosis and thrombosis in the artery. In the 1850s, Virchow[1] described atherosclerosis as an inflammatory process with insudation of plasma constituents into the vessel wall. Approximately 50 years later, Anitschkow in Russia noted atherosclerosis developing in rabbits fed a relatively high cholesterol diet. Although the involvement of inflammation in atherosclerosis has been known for more than 100 years,

the molecular mechanisms of atherosclerotic disease initiation and progression have only become clearer over the past decade.[2]

Lipid accumulation in the arterial intima, a fatty streak (Table 126-1), can occur in adolescents and may progress in paroxysmal fashion to a hemodynamically significant lesion causing arterial insufficiency. Autopsy studies of young soldiers and young trauma victims indicated that occult coronary atherosclerotic plaques are present in healthy individuals in their teens and 20s.[3,4] In addition, intracoronary ultrasound studies demonstrated the presence of coronary atherosclerosis in 37 percent of healthy heart donors aged 20 to 29 years, 60 percent of those aged 30 to 39 years, and 85 percent of those older than 50 years.[5] Several theories have been espoused for this propitious condition. One of these well-recognized theories is the *response to injury hypothesis* whereby the inciting event that predisposes to atherosclerosis is injury to the endothelial lining of the artery. This hypothesis was formulated in animal studies that showed vessel narrowing and intimal thickening after endothelial denudation with angioplasty.[6] However, human pathologic studies of early atherosclerotic plaques indicate that endothelium is structurally present but is dysfunctional. The dysfunctional state of endothelium includes abnormalities in vascular tone, inflammation, growth, and thrombosis. Atherosclerotic risk factors contribute to endothelial dysfunction and promote atherosclerosis. This section describes the mechanisms responsible for endothelial dysfunction and the impact of atherosclerotic risk factors.

ENDOTHELIAL DYSFUNCTION

Cardiovascular risk factors and abnormal blood rheology are thought to result in endothelial dysfunction that predisposes the aorta and arteries to atherosclerotic plaque development, sparing the arterioles and capillaries (Fig. 126-1). *Endothelial dysfunction* is a term that encompasses perturbations in the diverse physiologic functions of normal arteries, including regulation of vascular tone, inflammation, growth, and preservation of blood fluidity. Lipid accumulation[7] and endothelial dysfunction are intimately connected and seminal to the initiation and progression of atherosclerosis. Endothelial dysfunction occurs early in the development of plaque and is systemic in nature, afflicting vessels throughout the arterial circulation without gross evidence of atherosclerotic plaque formation. Emerging data indicate that proatherosclerotic genes are up-regulated and antiatherosclerotic genes are down-regulated in areas of turbulent blood flow, as seen at branch points of arteries,[8] resulting in vascular adhesion molecule expression and recruitment of monocytes but not granulocytes.[9] The atherosclerotic plaque initially may expand outward rather than inward into the vessel wall, making some significant lesions difficult to visualize by angiography. The components of the mature atherosclerotic lesion include smooth muscle cells, macrophages, T lymphocytes, and calcification, in addition to accumulation of lipoproteins.[10] Later in the process, increased activity of matrix metalloproteinases in the atherosclerotic cap predisposes to plaque rupture or ulceration, resulting in tissue factor (TF) exposure and platelet adhesion, culminating in thrombus formation.[11] The thrombus may undergo endogenous fibrinolysis with plaque healing or become occlusive and produce organ damage (e.g., myocardial infarction [MI]). In severe lesions, lamellar bone, presumably from endochondral calcification, may appear.[12] The following sections describe in detail the major manifestations of endothelial dysfunction that occur early in the atherosclerotic process.

ABNORMAL VASCULAR TONE

The importance of the endothelium in maintaining vascular tone was first recognized when endothelial cells of rabbit aorta were inadvertently removed and resulted in paradoxical vasoconstriction after administration of acetylcholine.[13] The major endothelium-dependent vasodilator normally produced was found to be nitric oxide (NO), a free radical gas with multiple physiologic properties,[14] including in-

TABLE 126-1   GLOSSARY OF TERMS

Fatty streak	Early accumulation of cholesterol in the intima of an artery
Atherosclerotic lesion	Accumulation of cholesterol, sclerotic tissue, inflammatory cells, smooth muscle cells, and calcium in a lesion that develops in the intima of the artery wall
Vulnerable plaque	Atherosclerotic plaque with high degree of inflammation, vulnerable to rupture or ulceration
Endothelial dysfunction	Abnormal function of endothelial cells lining the lumen of an artery
Foam cells	Lipid-laden macrophages
Scavenger receptors	Cell surface receptors on macrophages that bind and facilitate internalization into the cell of substances such as oxidized low-density lipoprotein and products of apoptotic cells

TABLE 126-2   CARDIOVASCULAR RISK FACTORS THAT CAUSE IMPAIRED ENDOTHELIUM-DEPENDENT VASODILATATION

Smoking
Dyslipidemia
Hypertension
Diabetes mellitus
Hyperhomocysteinemia

hibition of platelet aggregation and inflammation and stimulation of angiogenesis. Numerous studies indicate that the endothelium does not vasodilate appropriately in the setting of traditional and emerging cardiovascular risk factors. Cardiovascular risk factors (Table 126-2) are thought to reduce NO availability through a variety of mechanisms, including increased oxidative stress, and in so doing create an environment conducive to development of atherosclerosis.[15] A reduction in NO synthesis is thought to occur because of decreased availability of tetrahydrobiopterin, an essential cofactor for synthesis of NO.[16] Administration of sepiapterin, a substrate for tetrahydrobiopterin, improves endothelial dysfunction.[17]

High cholesterol levels are thought to produce oxygen free radicals that may inactivate NO. NO synthases are the enzymes responsible for converting L-arginine to NO (Fig. 126-2). The enzyme may be perturbed by modified low-density lipoprotein (LDL), resulting in decreased NO production.[18] Supplementation of the diet with L-arginine leads to improvement in endothelial-dependent vasodilatation.[19] Elevated levels of asymmetric dimethylarginine (ADMA), an endogenous competitive inhibitor of NO synthase, found in patients with hypercholesterolemia and diabetes, also may result in decreased NO availability.[20,21] Oxidized LDL is thought to increase the elaboration of ADMA by endothelial cells and decrease its degradation by the enzyme dimethylarginine dimethylaminohydrolase.[22] Administration of acetylcholine to patients with elevated serum LDL[23] and relatively low high-density lipoprotein (HDL)[24] may result in abnormal vasoconstriction, which can be reversed with nitroglycerin (an endothelium-independent vasodilator).[25] Intravenous infusion of HDL improves endothelial-mediated vasodilatation through improved NO availability.[26]

The decreased vasodilatory capacity because of dyslipidemia may facilitate the development of coronary ischemia.

Impaired endothelial vasodilatation is noted with advanced aging,[27] when the hands are exposed to cold, and during mental stress. The impairment may be mediated by increased production of endothelin, a potent vasoconstrictor.[28–30] Infection with concomitant inflammation is associated with impaired endothelial vasodilatation. For example, repeated infection with *Chlamydia pneumoniae* results in endothelial dysfunction via impaired NO availability.[31] The combination of coronary artery disease and elevated serum levels of high-sensitivity C-reactive protein (hsCRP) is an independent predictor of abnormal endothelial vasoreactivity.[32] External radiation therapy also results in endothelial dysfunction and may explain the increased risk of atherosclerosis in patients receiving mantle irradiation for Hodgkin lymphoma.[33]

ENDOTHELIAL INFLAMMATION

The endothelium does not routinely interact with inflammatory cells but is poised to express adhesion molecules after stimulation with inflammatory mediators. An inflammatory response is thought to begin in the vessel wall after "invasion" of pathogenic lipoproteins.[9,34] The presence of lipoproteins, especially oxidized LDL, results in expression of adhesion molecules such as vascular cell adhesion molecule (VCAM)-1 on the luminal surface of endothelial cells, leading to adherence of monocytes (Fig. 126-3).[35] Endothelial expression of adhesion molecules and recruitment of monocytes can be regarded as endothelial dysfunction because these events may occur in the absence of morphologic

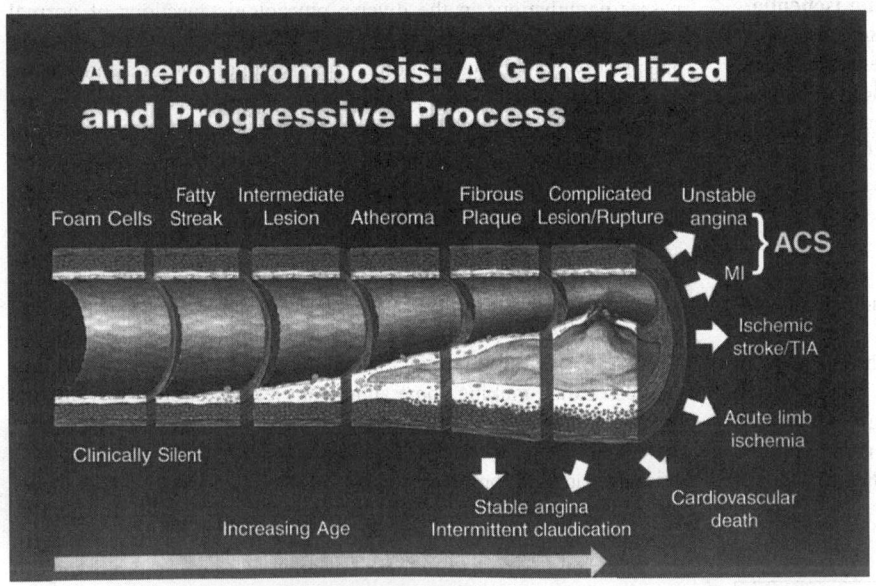

FIGURE 126-1   Schematic diagram showing the life span of the atherosclerotic plaque, beginning with the fatty streak and resulting in a thrombotic event. Cardiovascular risk factors and disturbed blood flow at branch points of vessels are thought to cause endothelial dysfunction that results in atherosclerotic plaque development in the aorta and conduit arteries. Early lipid accumulation in the intimal layer is called the *fatty streak*. A series of stimuli, including lipid peroxidation, are thought to signal adhesion molecule expression on the endothelium, which results in monocyte adhesion and diapedesis into the intimal space. The monocytes develop into macrophages and become sessile with accumulation of lipid (foam cells). Smooth muscle cells, primarily from the media, enter the plaque and participate in cap formation. The plaque accumulates hydroxyapatite mineral and forms calcific deposits. Matrix metalloproteinases also accumulate in the lesion and may predispose to plaque rupture or ulceration resulting in tissue factor exposure and thrombus formation. Risk factor modification favors a more stable plaque, which may have relatively less lipid accumulation and more sclerotic tissue than an unstable plaque. Severe lesions may even develop lamellar bone. ACS, acute coronary syndrome; TIA, transient ischemic attack. (Adapted from HC Stary et al. *Circulation* 92: 1335, 1995.)

changes in the vessel wall. Inflammation may develop without the demonstrable presence of an external microbial pathogen. The complex interactions of inflammation and oxidative stress on the initiation and progression of atherosclerosis are reviewed in more detail in "Inflammatory Response and Oxidative Stress" below.

ABNORMAL CONTROL OF VASCULAR GROWTH: SMOOTH MUSCLE CELLS AND EXTRACELLULAR MATRIX

Normal endothelium inhibits vascular smooth muscle cell proliferation.[36] The specific function of vascular smooth muscle cells in atherosclerosis is unclear. However, evidence indicates that, in early atherosclerosis, vascular smooth muscle cells contribute to the development of atheroma through production of proinflammatory mediators such as monocyte chemoattractant protein (MCP)-1 and VCAMs. Although smooth muscle cells primarily play a role in modulating vascular tone, they also are involved in the control of extracellular matrix formation and degradation through matrix modulators such as proteases, protease inhibitors, matrix proteins, and integrins (Fig. 126-4).

The importance of vascular smooth muscle cells in controlling the synthesis of matrix molecules is evident at the clinical level. They provide a thick, fibrous cap that promotes stability and inhibits plaque rupture and ulceration. Evidence indicates that vascular smooth muscle cells which undergo apoptosis, especially at the shoulder region of the plaque, may create a more unstable cap.[37] Both intact vascular smooth muscle cells and fibroblasts are thought to stabilize plaques through modulation of extracellular calcification and formation of a fibrocalcific plaque.

Vascular smooth muscle cells arise primarily from the medial layer and are considered monoclonal in origin.[38] Evidence also indicates that vascular smooth muscle cells may originate from the adventitia.[39] The rate and timing of smooth muscle cell replication is unclear. It may occur at a constant low rate throughout the development of the atherosclerotic lesion or episodically at a higher rate.[40,41] Evidence from animal studies indicates that new intimal cells may originate from outside the vessel wall from subpopulations of bone marrow- and non–bone marrow-derived circulating cells.[42–45] Smooth muscle progenitor cells circulating in blood may contribute to the arterial remodeling that occurs after angioplasty and after bypass graft surgery.[46]

Vascular proliferation and inflammation are linked processes. Impaired NO bioactivity because of inflammation contributes to vascular smooth muscle proliferation.[6] Overexpression of an NO synthase results in reduction of atherosclerotic or restenotic lesion formation in rabbits through both inhibition of vascular smooth muscle cell proliferation and inhibition of adhesion and chemoattractant molecule expression, with subsequent reduction of vascular mononuclear cell infiltration.[47,48] Thus, the vascular smooth muscle cell participates in the atherosclerotic process by affecting lipoprotein retention, modulating inflammation, and controlling plaque stability through formation of the fibrous cap. Several vascular disorders involve vascular smooth muscle proliferation as the primary pathophysiologic mechanism, including in-stent restenosis, transplant vasculopathy, and vein bypass graft failure.[49] Drug-eluting vascular stents that release agents such as sirolimus and paclitaxel interfere with the cell cycle and inhibit restenosis.[50]

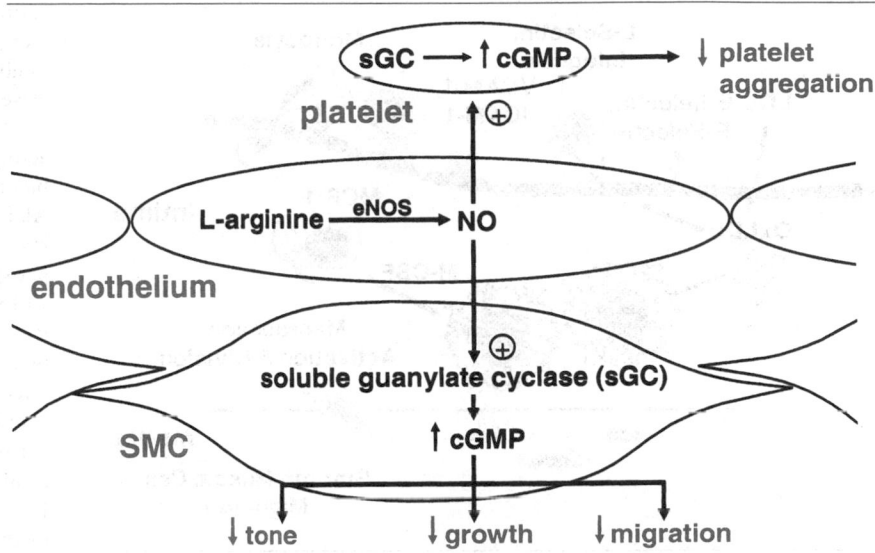

FIGURE 126-2   Vascular tone depends on endothelial production and release of various vasoconstricting and vasodilating substances. The endothelial-derived vasodilators include nitric oxide (NO) and prostacyclin. Nitric oxide is generated from the amino acid L-arginine by constitutive endothelial NO synthase (eNOS, or NOSIII). The enzyme is stimulated by blood flow across the endothelial surface (shear stress) or by chemical mediators, such as acetylcholine, which stimulate receptors on the endothelial surface. NO diffuses to the underlying smooth muscle cells (SMC), where it stimulates guanylate cyclase to generate cyclic guanosine V monophosphate (cGMP), which causes smooth muscle relaxation and vasodilatation. It also diffuses into blood, where it increases intraplatelet cGMP and thereby inhibits platelet adhesion and aggregation.

ABNORMAL ENDOTHELIAL CONTROL OF BLOOD FLUIDITY

Endothelial cells normally elaborate a number of antithrombotic substances. Some of these substances are released into blood whereas others are properties of the unactivated endothelial cell surface. These antiplatelet, anticoagulant, and profibrinolytic activities of endothelium, some of which also possess vasodilatory properties (e.g., prostacyclin, NO), act in concert to promote blood fluidity under normal circumstances.[51] Acute activation or chronic dysfunction of endothelial cells alters the hemostatic balance, transforming them from predominantly antithrombotic to prothrombotic cells.[52]

To this end, endothelial cells modulate the activities of thrombin in health and disease. In the presence of intact and normally functioning endothelium, the prothrombotic actions of thrombin are quenched and the antithrombotic actions of the enzyme predominate. Thrombin binds to thrombomodulin, an integral membrane protein expressed by endothelial cells, and activates protein C in the presence of endothelial protein C receptor, another endothelial cell protein (see Chap. 107). Activated protein C, in concert with its cofactor, protein S, has anticoagulant and profibrinolytic actions. It degrades by proteolytic digestion factors Va and VIIIa and inactivates plasminogen activator inhibitor (PAI)-1. Simultaneously, by binding to thrombomodulin, enzymatically active procoagulant thrombin is removed from the circulation, thereby limiting its availability to catalyze fibrin formation. Endothelial dysfunction causes loss of thrombomodulin activity from the vascular surface. In fact, increased circulating plasma levels of free thrombomodulin represent a marker of endothelial damage. In addition to the role of thrombomodulin in clearance of circulating thrombin, the procoagulant activity of thrombin is normally blocked by endothelial cells through the action of antithrombin, which binds to heparin-like glycosaminoglycans on their luminal surface, thereby catalyzing the inactivation of thrombin by antithrombin. Like thrombomodulin, this thrombin-neutralizing action of endothelial heparan sulfate glycosaminoglycans is lost with endothelial dysfunction.

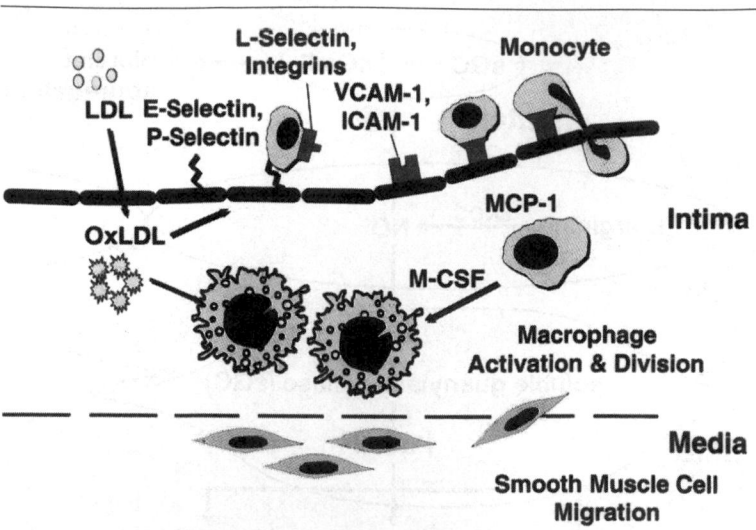

FIGURE 126-3   Atherosclerotic lesion initiation is stimulated by oxidized low-density lipoprotein (OxLDL). Induction of inflammatory gene products in vascular cells is activated by nuclear factor-κB transcription factor, which results in increased expression of cellular adhesion molecules. The adhesion molecules have specific functions for endothelial leukocyte interaction. The selectins tether and trap monocytes and other leukocytes. Vascular cell adhesion molecule-1 (VCAM-1) and intracellular adhesion molecule-1 (ICAM-1) mediate firm attachment of these leukocytes to the endothelial layer. Oxidized LDL also augments expression of monocyte chemoattractant protein-1 (MCP-1) and macrophage colony stimulating factor (M-CSF). MCP-1 mediates the attraction of monocytes and leukocytes and facilitates diapedesis through the endothelium into the intima. M-CSF is an important cytokine for the transformation of monocytes to macrophage foam cells. Macrophages express scavenger receptors and internalize oxidized LDL during their transformation into foam cells. Smooth muscle cells migrate from the media into the intima and participate in the formation of a fibrous atheroma. (Adapted from S Kinlay, AP Selwyn, P Libby: Inflammation, the endothelium, and the acute coronary syndromes. *J Cardiovasc Pharmacol* 32[suppl 3]:S62, 1998.)

Endothelial cells do not normally express TF, but they do so upon activation by inflammatory cytokines or exposure to endothelium-activating levels of homocysteine or free thrombin. The procoagulant effects of expression of TF by dysfunctional endothelial cells is potentially compounded by loss of TF pathway inhibitor, which normally is synthesized by endothelial cells.

Normal endothelium is profibrinolytic. It synthesizes and releases tissue-type plasminogen activator (t-PA); it possesses binding sites for t-PA and plasminogen to provide a surface for the concentrated assembly of the fibrinolytic complex and thereby enhance local plasmin generation; and it fails to produce significant amounts of PAI-1. This profibrinolytic state is converted to an antifibrinolytic state in the presence of endothelial dysfunction. In activated or dysfunctional endothelium, PAI-1 gene expression and PAI-1 secretion are induced; simultaneously, the profibrinolytic properties of normal endothelium are lost (see Chap. 108).

The antithrombotic profile of normal endothelium also manifests through the elaboration of several antiplatelet substances. NO is constitutively released into blood by normal endothelial cells and inhibits platelet adhesion and aggregation by stimulating platelet soluble guanylyl cyclase and raising intraplatelet levels of cyclic GMP (see Fig. 126-2).[53] Physiologic flow and shear forces maintain the activity of endothelial (endothelium-derived) nitric oxide synthase (eNOS)[54,55] under normal circumstances. Vascular cell-derived carbon monoxide, a product of heme catabolism by heme oxygenase, may have similar antiplatelet activity.[56] Prostacyclin (prostaglandin I$_2$ [PGI$_2$]) likewise is released basally by normal endothelial cells and inhibits platelet aggregation by inducing platelet adenylyl cyclase and raising intraplatelet levels of cyclic AMP.[57]

NO, carbon monoxide, and PGI$_2$ are labile autacoids, acting only in the immediate vicinity of their release into blood from endothelial cells. An endothelial surface ecto-ADPase (CD39) also blocks platelet activity by metabolizing and disposing of platelet aggregatory adenosine diphosphate (ADP).[58] In endothelial dysfunction, these various antiplatelet activities are lost, and endothelial release of von Willebrand factor is increased, which promotes platelet adhesion. In the case of NO, oxidative stress in the microenvironment of endothelial dysfunction actually "uncouples" eNOS activity[55,59] to preferentially generate superoxide over NO. Oxygen free radicals bind any remaining available NO to produce the toxic product peroxinitrite. Bioactive NO is further reduced in endothelial dysfunction by the presence of ADMA, which competes to block eNOS and limit NO production.[54,60]

INFLAMMATORY RESPONSE AND OXIDATIVE STRESS

INNATE IMMUNITY AND ATHEROSCLEROSIS
The endothelial response to injury manifests as a chronic inflammatory response that involves both innate and adaptive immunity.[61] Innate immunity provides the first line of defense for the host and involves several cell types, most importantly macrophages and dendritic cells, which express a limited number of highly conserved sensing molecules such as scavenger receptors and Toll-like receptors.[61,62] Ligation of a pathogen or other substances (such as lipopolysaccharides, aldehyde-derivatized proteins, mannans, teichoic acids) elicits endocytosis or activation of endothelial cells (e.g., through nuclear factor-κB) that results in an inflammatory response (see Chaps. 16 and 17).[62,63] Proinflammatory cytokines, such as tumor necrosis factor (TNF)-α and interleukin (IL)-1, magnify the innate inflammatory response.

Innate defense involves soluble factors, such as complement and hsCRP, which are involved in atherosclerotic lesion formation.[64] hsCRP has been found to be an important and independent predictor for cardiovascular events.[65] Accumulating evidence indicates the molecule also may be involved in the development of atherosclerosis because hsCRP is secreted by macrophages.[66] Natural antibodies that are generated in the absence of known antigen stimulation, mainly immunoglobulin (Ig)M, provide an immediate response against bacteria and viruses but also may be involved in atherosclerosis. For example, innate B lymphocytes, the so-called *B1 cells*, express a restricted set of germ-line–encoded antigen receptors that may bind oxidized LDL.

ADAPTIVE IMMUNITY AND ATHEROSCLEROSIS
Compared to innate immunity, adaptive immunity is slower but more precise (see Chap. 18).[61] T cells can be activated by dendritic cells and macrophages, whereas most antigens cannot stimulate B cells without assistance from CD4+ T cells, which recognize the peptide–major histocompatibility complex (MHC) complexes on B cells. By genetic recombination, the number of T cell and B cell receptors that can be formed is almost unlimited and far exceed the number of pattern recognition receptors used by the innate immune system. Most CD4+ cells are cytokine-secreting T helper (Th) cells and express αβ–T cell receptors, which interact with MHC class II molecules. A smaller number of Th cells express γδ–T cell receptors, which interact with the

nonpolymorphic, nonclassic MHC molecules, CD1, which present certain antigens (particularly lipids and glycolipids). Th cells are classified according to the cytokines they secrete. Th1 cells secrete interferon (IFN)-γ and IL-2 and promote cell-mediated immunity (see Chap. 78). Th2 cells secrete IL-4, IL-5, IL-10, and IL-13 and help B cells produce antibodies. CD8+ T cells are primarily cytotoxic killer cells, although they can secrete cytokines, such as TNF-α, IFN-γ, and lymphotoxin. Some thymus-independent antigens can activate these cells without the help of T cells. Oxidized LDL is considered such an antigen because it expresses multiple copies of oxidation-specific epitopes on a single LDL particle.

ADHESION MOLECULES AND ATHEROSCLEROSIS

Monocyte recruitment to inflammatory foci initially involves the expression of endothelial cell selectins, which mediate monocyte rolling on the endothelium (see Fig. 126-3). The rolling phenomenon is followed by a firmer attachment to endothelial cells mediated by integrins. Perhaps the most important of these is VCAM-1, which is up-regulated in cultured endothelial cells in the presence of oxidized LDL. The appearance of this molecule before the development of grossly visible atherosclerotic lesions supports oxidized LDL as an initial recruiter of macrophages. Granulocytes are conspicuously absent in any phase of atherosclerotic lesion development. The finding of reduced atherosclerosis in VCAM-1−deficient mice further supports the important role of macrophages and VCAM-1 in the pathogenesis of atherosclerosis.[67–69] Other adhesion molecules, such as P-selectin and intracellular cell adhesion molecule (ICAM)-1, also may be involved in monocyte adhesion at sites of lesion formation.[70]

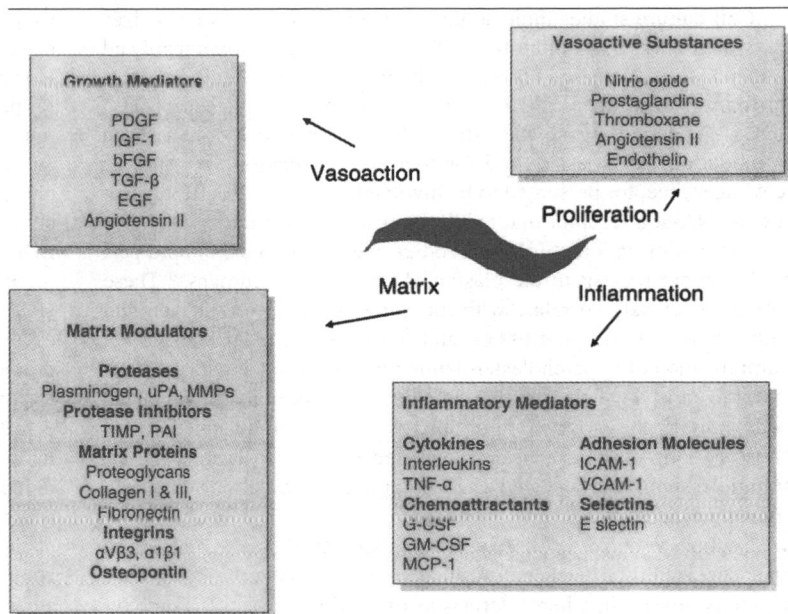

FIGURE 126-4 Vascular smooth muscle cells mediate vascular proliferation, inflammation, matrix composition, and contraction. Many of these mediators have multiple functions. For example, angiotensin is a vasoconstrictor, but it also stimulates proliferation and inflammation. This is only a partial list of mediators secreted by vascular smooth muscle cells. bFGF, basic fibroblast growth factor; EGF, epidermal growth factor; G-CSF, granulocyte colony stimulating factor; GM-CSF, granulocyte-monocyte colony stimulating factor; ICAM, intracellular adhesion molecule; IGF, insulin-like growth factor; MCP, monocyte chemoattractant protein; MMPs, matrix metalloproteinases; PAI, plasminogen activator inhibitor; PDGF, platelet-derived growth factor; TGF-β, transforming growth factor β; TIMP, tissue inhibitor of metalloproteinases; TNF, tumor necrosis factor alpha; uPA, urokinase-type plasminogen activator; VCAM, vascular cell adhesion molecule. (Adapted from VJ Dzau, RC Braun-Dullaeus, DG Sedding,[49] with permission.).

CHEMOKINES AND ATHEROSCLEROSIS

The chemoattractant MCP-1 facilitates recruitment of monocytes to atherosclerotic lesions, as noted in studies of mouse models of atherosclerosis, such as apolipoprotein E (ApoE-/-) or LDL receptor (LDLR-/-) deficient mice fed a western-style diet. When these mice are crossed to the model lacking MCP-1 or its receptor CCR-2, lesion development decreases significantly.[71–73]

MACROPHAGES AND ATHEROSCLEROSIS

Macrophages are essential for the clearance of modified lipoproteins and the efflux of lipoprotein-derived cholesterol to HDL receptors for reverse cholesterol transport, the process by which HDL removes cholesterol from cells. Multiple lines of evidence indicate that macrophages promote lesion initiation and progression. For example, hypercholesterolemic mice become markedly resistant to atherosclerosis if they are bred to macrophage-deficient animals.[74]

The earliest grossly visible sign of atherosclerosis is the fatty streak, which is composed mainly of macrophage foam cells containing relatively large amounts of cholesterol. Foam cells also can derive from smooth muscle cells, as these cells can express scavenger receptors when appropriately activated.[75,76] Formation of the fatty streak is thought to begin with adherence of circulating monocytes to activated endothelial cells at sites in the arterial system prone to atherosclerotic disease, such as at branch points in vessels. Multiple chemoattractant molecules have been identified in these nascent lesions, which recruit monocytes and induce their diapedesis into the subendothelial space where they further differentiate into macrophages.

LIPID PEROXIDATION AND ATHEROSCLEROSIS

Macrophages control the amount of cholesterol loading by down-regulating the native LDL receptor. Therefore, knowing how cholesterol is taken up into macrophages is important. Cell culture experiments revealed a "foam cell paradox," in which macrophages engulf only modified lipids. Treatment of native LDL with copper or acetic anhydride (causing acetylation) led to increased LDL uptake through use of the scavenger receptor, leading to the formation of lipid-laden macrophages. These experiments led to the peroxidation theory of atherosclerosis,[77–80] whereby LDL modification is an essential step in the development of foam cells. Although the precise mechanisms responsible for LDL oxidation remain unclear, enzymes including myeloperoxidase, inducible NO synthase, and reduced nicotinamide adenine dinucleotide phosphate (NADPH) oxidases are involved in the process.[81,82] Of note, macrophages express each of these enzymes, which normally are used as antimicrobial reactive oxygen species essential for native immunity.[83] Thus, accumulation of cholesterol in the macrophage occurs via scavenger (not LDL) receptors of oxidized (and not native) LDL.

SCAVENGER RECEPTORS AND ATHEROSCLEROSIS

Conserved pattern recognition receptors expressed by macrophages include scavenger receptors A and B1 and CD36, all of which internalize oxidized LDL.[84,85] Macrophages express various genes in response to oxidized LDL, including peroxisome proliferator-activated receptor-gamma and adenosine triphosphate binding cassette transporter A1, which profoundly influence macrophage-mediated inflammation and atherosclerotic activity.

Cell culture studies indicate that scavenger receptor A recognizes acetylated LDL but, unlike the LDL receptor, is not down-regulated in response to increased cholesterol content and thus likely accounts for foam cell formation.[86] However, no evidence indicates that acetyl LDL is generated *in vivo*, indicating other modifications of LDL, such as oxidation, may be required for foam cell formation.[87–89] Another scavenger receptor presumed to be involved in the atherosclerotic process is CD36, a receptor that avidly binds oxidized LDL.

Circulating IgG and IgM antibodies against products of lipid peroxidation are present in the plasma of animals and humans.[90] These antibodies closely correlate with measures of lipid peroxidation and with atherosclerotic progression and regression in murine models.[91] Immunization of hypercholesterolemic rabbits and mice with products of oxidized LDL, such as malonyldialdehyde LDL or copper-oxidized LDL, inhibits the progression of atherosclerotic lesion formation.[92–95] These experiments have been interpreted to indicate that an immunologic response to oxidized LDL components can alter the atherosclerotic process.

Leukocyte-derived 5-lipoxygenase also contributes to atherosclerosis susceptibility in mice.[96] Animal studies indicate the importance of lipoxygenases in atherosclerosis as disruption of the 12/15-lipoxygenase gene diminishes atherosclerosis in ApoE-deficient mice, and overexpression of 15-lipoxygenase in vascular endothelium accelerates early atherosclerosis in LDL receptor-deficient mice.[97,98]

ACCUMULATION OF LDL IN THE VASCULAR WALL

Three potential factors lead to accumulation of LDL in the vascular wall: increased permeability of the endothelium, prolonged retention of lipoproteins in the intima, and slow removal of lipoproteins from the vessel wall. Rabbits fed a high-cholesterol diet develop aortic wall lesions at specific lesion-susceptible sites; however, endothelial permeability is not increased at those sites, indicating that LDL is selectively retained in these regions.[99,100] Retention of LDL molecules likely results from their adherence to proteoglycans in the vessel wall.[101] LDL genetically engineered to not bind to proteoglycans is hypothesized to be less atherogenic than native LDL.[7]

Oxidized LDL and its products, oxidized phospholipids and oxysterols, have other properties that make them potentially proatherogenic.[80] These properties include proinflammatory characteristics, such as chemotactic signaling for monocytes, smooth muscle cells, and T lymphocytes (but not for B lymphocytes or neutrophils, neither of which is found in lesions) and increased expression of VCAM-1 on, and stimulation of MCP-1 release from, endothelial cells.[102] Oxidized LDL also may contribute to instability of the atherosclerotic plaque via induction of type 1 metalloproteinase expression and increase in TF activity.[35] For oxidized LDL to be a ligand for the scavenger receptor, extensive degradation of the polyunsaturated fatty acid in the sn-2 position of phospholipids by oxidation is essential.

To test the oxidized LDL hypothesis, several clinical studies have been conducted using antioxidant vitamins, most commonly vitamin E; however, most of the published reports provide negative results.[103,104] At the present time, treatment with vitamin E at doses of 400 to 800 IU daily does not seem adequate to prevent cardiovascular events. However, these studies have been inadequate to prove or disprove the hypothesis; other antioxidant combinations may prove more beneficial.

HIGH-DENSITY LIPOPROTEIN AND ATHEROSCLEROSIS

A low level of HDL cholesterol is a strong predictor of adverse cardiovascular events, presumably because the low level is associated with insufficient reverse cholesterol transport.[105,106] Animal studies using liver-directed gene transfer of human ApoA-I resulted in signifi-

cant promotion of reverse cholesterol transport and regression of preexisting atherosclerotic lesions in LDL receptor-deficient mice.[107,108] However, HDL has additional antiatherogenic properties that may confer protection against atherosclerosis.[109] For example, HDL is protective against oxidation of LDL, at least in part because of paraoxonase, an enzyme physically associated with HDL that degrades organophosphates.[110] Paraoxonase polymorphisms are associated with increased risk of cardiovascular disease, also indicating that oxidized LDL is an important factor in atherosclerotic development.[111]

Research studies currently are evaluating novel ways to increase HDL levels or to use ApoA-I variants and mimetics that hopefully will cause regression of atherosclerosis. Cholesteryl ester transfer protein promotes the transfer of cholesteryl esters from antiatherogenic HDLs to proatherogenic ApoB-containing lipoproteins, including very-low-density lipoproteins (VLDLs), VLDL remnants, intermediate density lipoproteins (IDLs), and LDLs. A deficiency of this molecule results in increased HDL levels and decreased LDL levels, a lipid profile that is antiatherogenic. A clinical study in humans showed that inhibition of the transfer protein increased HDL levels.[112] Clinical trials evaluating the effect of inhibition of cholesteryl ester transfer protein on atherosclerosis and cardiovascular events are underway. Along similar lines, delivery of a mutant form of ApoA1 (ApoA-1 Milano) resulted in regression of plaque size as measured by intravascular ultrasound in a small phase II clinical trial.[113] Studies evaluating the effect of ApoA1 mimetics on atherosclerosis also are underway.[114]

CD40, CD40 LIGAND, AND ATHEROSCLEROSIS

Studies indicate that human atherosclerotic lesions express the immune mediator CD40 and its soluble ligand sCD40L. Increasing evidence indicates the CD40–sCD40L signaling pathway plays a central role in several inflammatory processes, including atherosclerosis and graft rejection following transplantation. Interruption of CD40 signaling in hyperlipidemic mice reduces the size of aortic atherosclerotic lesions and their lipid, macrophage, and T lymphocyte content.[115] Atorvastatin, lovastatin, pravastatin, and simvastatin reduce IFN-γ–induced CD40 expression in a dose-dependent manner. Activation of atheroma-associated cells with human recombinant sCD40L is reduced when cells are treated with statins. In addition, retrospective ex vivo immunostaining of human carotid atherosclerotic lesions of patients treated with simvastatin for more than 3 months revealed less CD40 expression and atheroma-associated cells compared with patients who were not treated with the drug. A reduction in sCD40L has been associated with pravastatin or cerivastatin therapy.[116] These findings support the notion that statins have antiinflammatory and cholesterol-lowering effects.

TRANSFORMING GROWTH FACTOR-β AND ATHEROSCLEROSIS

Transforming growth factor (TGF)-β is a cytokine secreted by macrophages, smooth muscle cells, and the Th3 subset of Th cells that has multiple regulatory functions. TGF-β is speculated to contribute to plaque stabilization because it stimulates collagen synthesis and is fibrogenic. One study found that inhibition of TGF-β signaling by neutralizing antibodies led to a larger plaque size with an unstable phenotype.[117] Further studies are needed to clarify the role of TGF-β in atherosclerotic plaque initiation and growth.

INFECTION AND ATHEROSCLEROSIS

Several infectious agents have been implicated as pathogens in atherosclerosis.[118] A well-studied infectious pathogen is *Chlamydia pneumoniae*. Animals infected with this agent develop atherosclerosis, and patients with cardiovascular disease have higher titers of antibodies against this pathogen. Viruses, such as herpes simplex and cytomegalovirus, also have been implicated in human atherosclerotic lesion formation. Poor dental hygiene with associated gingivitis may invoke cellular immune activation and provoke atherosclerosis by cytokines or antibodies.[119] Endogenous proteins, such as heat shock proteins, have been implicated in atherosclerosis. One study showed that progression of carotid disease correlated with antibodies against heat shock proteins 65 and 60.[120]

SPLENECTOMY AND ATHEROSCLEROSIS

The relationship between the immune system and atherosclerosis is complex, as evident from an animal study that showed splenectomy of cholesterol-fed ApoE-/- mice led to significantly increased atherosclerosis.[121] This proatherogenic effect was rescued by transfer of either purified B cells or T cells from the spleens of atherosclerotic ApoE-/- donors. A long-term study of soldiers who underwent splenectomy after trauma found the soldiers had a twofold increased incidence of coronary artery disease, providing evidence that the spleen has antiatherogenic activity.[122] Further studies are needed to determine if splenectomy significantly impacts the atherosclerotic process.

ATHEROSCLEROTIC PLAQUE

PLAQUE CLASSIFICATION

The American Heart Association classification of atherosclerotic plaques into types I through VIII is based on lesion composition and structure (Fig. 126-5).[10,123] Type I through III atherosclerotic plaques have foam cells organized in a fatty streak, ranging from those not visible on close examination (type I) to those that are apparent on examination (type III). Type I through III lesions are small and clinically silent, whereas type IV through VI lesions may obstruct the lumen and produce a clinical event. Type IV lesions contain a confluent pool of lipid and in most patients do not cause anginal symptoms because of the ability of the artery to remodel outward. Type V lesions contain a fibromuscular cap resulting from replacement of tissue disrupted by accumulated lipid and hematoma or organized thrombotic deposits. Type VI lesions involve thrombosis that may be either mural or obstructive. Of note, a type IV lesion may develop type VI changes without ever passing through a type V change and accumulating significant fibrous tissue. Plaques that are complex and primarily composed of calcium are type VII lesions or, if fibrous tissue predominates, are type VIII lesions.

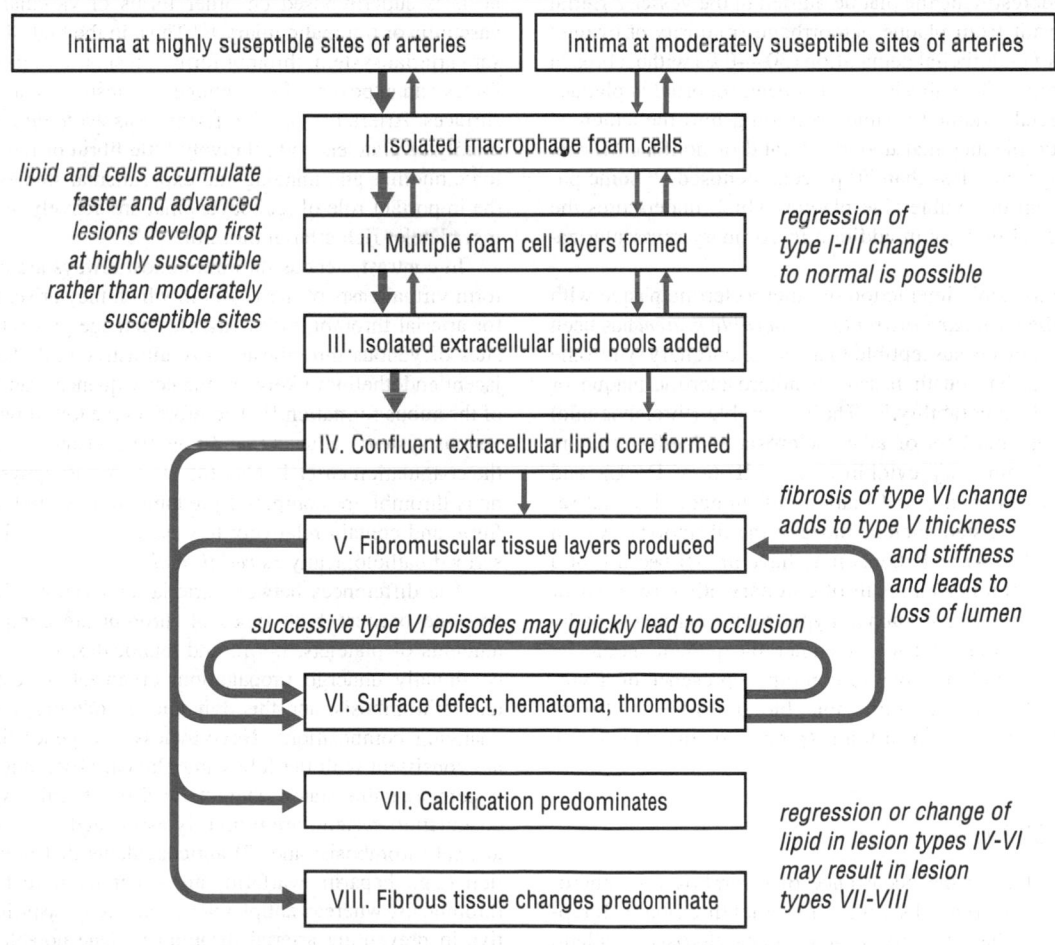

FIGURE 126-5   Flow diagram in *center column* indicates pathways in evolution and progression of human atherosclerotic lesions. *Roman numerals* indicate histologically characteristic types of lesions. The direction of *arrows* indicates sequence in which characteristic morphologies may change. From type I to type IV, changes in lesion morphology occur primarily because of increasing accumulation of lipid. The *loop* between types V and VI illustrates how lesions increase in surfaces. Thrombotic deposits may develop repeatedly over varied time spans in the same location and may be the principal mechanism for gradual occlusion of medium-sized arteries. (From HC Stary,[123] with permission.).

VULNERABLE PLAQUE AND THE VULNERABLE PATIENT

The pathologic mechanisms responsible for converting chronic coronary atherosclerosis to an acute coronary event result, in part, from *plaque disruption*, a term that was synonymously used with *plaque rupture*.[124,125] The term *vulnerable plaque* was used by Muller and colleagues[126,127] to describe rupture-prone plaques as the underlying cause of most clinical coronary events. The current definition for "vulnerable plaque" includes all thrombosis-prone plaques and those with a high probability of undergoing rapid progression, thus becoming culprit plaques (Fig. 126-6).[128] Criteria for development of the vulnerable plaque have been proposed based on histopathologic study of culprit plaques (Table 126-3).[128] The major criteria involve the presence of active inflammation, a thin cap with large lipid core, endothelial denudation with superficial platelet aggregation, a fissured plaque, and stenosis greater than 90 percent. The minor criteria for a vulnerable plaque include superficial calcified nodule, glistening yellow plaque, intraplaque hemorrhage, endothelial dysfunction, and outward (positive) remodeling. Some studies indicate plaques that are heavily calcified and without a significant lipid core are more stable.[12,129]

An important concept concerning plaque remodeling is that atherosclerotic plaques commonly grow outward (positive remodeling) before a luminal stenosis occurs.[130] Therefore, a contrast dye coronary angiogram may underestimate the plaque burden in the vessel. Arterial thrombosis may result from plaque hemorrhage (majority of events) or occur in an area of endothelial denudation (30–40%) without breach of the intimal space.[131] Thrombosis has also been reported in plaques that have a superficial calcified nodule protruding into the lumen.[131] Most atherosclerotic plaques that underlie a fatal or nonfatal MI are, as shown by angiography, less than 70 percent stenosed.[132] Some patients have more than one vulnerable plaque, which underscores the importance of medical therapy in addition to coronary revascularization.[133]

Because of the dynamic interaction of atherosclerotic plaque with circulating blood, the term *cardiovascular vulnerable patient* has been proposed to define subjects susceptible to an acute coronary syndrome (ACS) or sudden cardiac death based on atherosclerotic plaque or blood or myocardial vulnerability.[134] The vulnerable (thrombogenic) blood includes serum markers of atherosclerosis and inflammation, such as hsCRP, inflammatory cytokines (e.g., IL-6, sCD40L), and hypercoagulable factors. The blood markers of vulnerability that reflect the hypercoagulable state include those of the fibrinolytic system and platelets (Table 126-4).[134] Patients may have an MI because of a nonfatal or fatal arrhythmia as a result of coronary atherosclerosis or other nonatherosclerotic disease, such as hypertrophic cardiomyopathy or right ventricular dysplasia. Thus, a vulnerable patient should be considered from the standpoint of the combined presence of a vulnerable atherosclerotic plaque, vulnerable blood (prone to thrombosis), and/or vulnerable myocardium (prone to life-threatening arrhythmia).

ARTERIAL THROMBOSIS

Atherothrombosis refers to the occurrence of thrombosis on atherosclerotic lesions,[135,136] the typical setting for arterial thrombosis. It represents the acute event that converts chronic atherosclerosis—a silent, asymptomatic, progressive disease—into symptomatic, life-threatening clinical complications, including acute MI, stroke, and critical limb ischemia. The previous section described in detail the current concepts of the consecutive stages of atherosclerotic lesion development[137]: (1) endothelial cell dysfunction and activation, recruitment of inflammatory leukocytes, and accumulation of extracellular lipids in the intima; (2) smooth muscle cell migration and proliferation, synthesis of extra-

cellular matrix, and transformation of recruited macrophages to lipid-laden foam cells due to accumulation of oxidized LDLs; (3) matrix degradation by metalloproteinases and weakening of the fibrous cap. This section discusses the mechanisms of coagulation activation that culminates in arterial thrombus formation following plaque rupture. Importantly, however, arterial thrombosis does not always follow this sequence of events. In some cases, thrombus forms on atherosclerotic plaques as a result of superficial erosion of the luminal surface, without breakdown of an underlying plaque fibrous cap.

Thrombosis is not simply the final occlusive event. It also contributes to atherosclerosis lesion development. Intraplaque hemorrhage and *in situ* thrombosis localizes thrombin activity within plaques.[138] Thus, atheroma evolution is not only a proliferative process but also involves thrombosis.[136]

PATHOLOGY OF ARTERIAL THROMBI

Fundamental pathologic and pathophysiologic distinctions exist between arterial and venous thrombi (Table 126-5). Arterial thrombi usually are occlusive. However, nonocclusive mural thrombi often occur in the lumina of the heart chambers and large arteries, such as the aorta and the iliac and common carotid arteries. Arterial thrombi develop almost invariably upon preexisting abnormal intimal surfaces, which typically are atherosclerotic lesions. Less commonly, arterial thrombosis is superimposed on other forms of vascular disease, such as vasculitis or traumatic injury.[139] Thus, in the high-flow and high-pressure arterial system, thrombi form in response to increased local shear forces and exposure of thrombogenic substances on damaged vascular surfaces. Arterial thrombi, referred to as *white thrombi*, are composed mainly of platelets and relatively little fibrin or red cells. Histopathologic findings and imaging and experimental studies have highlighted the important role of leukocytes that are actively recruited into growing, platelet-rich arterial thrombi.[140,141]

In contrast, venous thrombi almost always are occlusive and may form virtual casts of the vessel in which they arise. Unlike the setting for arterial thrombi, gross vascular damage generally is not found at sites of venous thrombosis. Any ultrastructural abnormalities of adjacent endothelium likely are the consequences rather than the causes of thrombus formation.[142] Therefore, in the low-flow and low-pressure venous system, reduced blood flow (stasis) and systemic activation of the coagulation cascade play the primary pathophysiologic roles. Venous thrombi are composed predominantly of red cells enmeshed in fibrin and contain relatively few platelets; hence, they have been described pathologically as *red thrombi*.

The differences between arterial and venous thrombosis are not absolute because both types of thrombi are composed of different amounts of platelets, fibrin, and leukocytes. In addition, all thrombi continually undergo propagation, organization, embolization, lysis, and rethrombosis, and this dynamic remodeling results in constantly changing compositions. Nevertheless, the generalizations described are consistent with the following clinical observations: (1) hereditary hypercoagulable states, characterized by chronic hyperactivity of the coagulation system, are primarily associated with venous rather than arterial thrombosis; and (2) anticoagulants that prevent fibrin formation (e.g., heparin, warfarin) are generally used to prevent venous thrombosis, whereas antiplatelet agents (e.g., aspirin) are more effective in preventing arterial thrombosis. One notable exception, however, is that oral anticoagulants are the treatment of choice for patients with artificial (both prosthetic and biologic) heart valves.

SITE-SPECIFIC ARTERIAL THROMBOSIS

The model of atherothrombosis described has been best characterized in coronary arteries. This pathophysiology may not be entirely applicable to arterial thrombosis at other sites. It cannot be assumed that

Different Types of Vulnerable Plaque

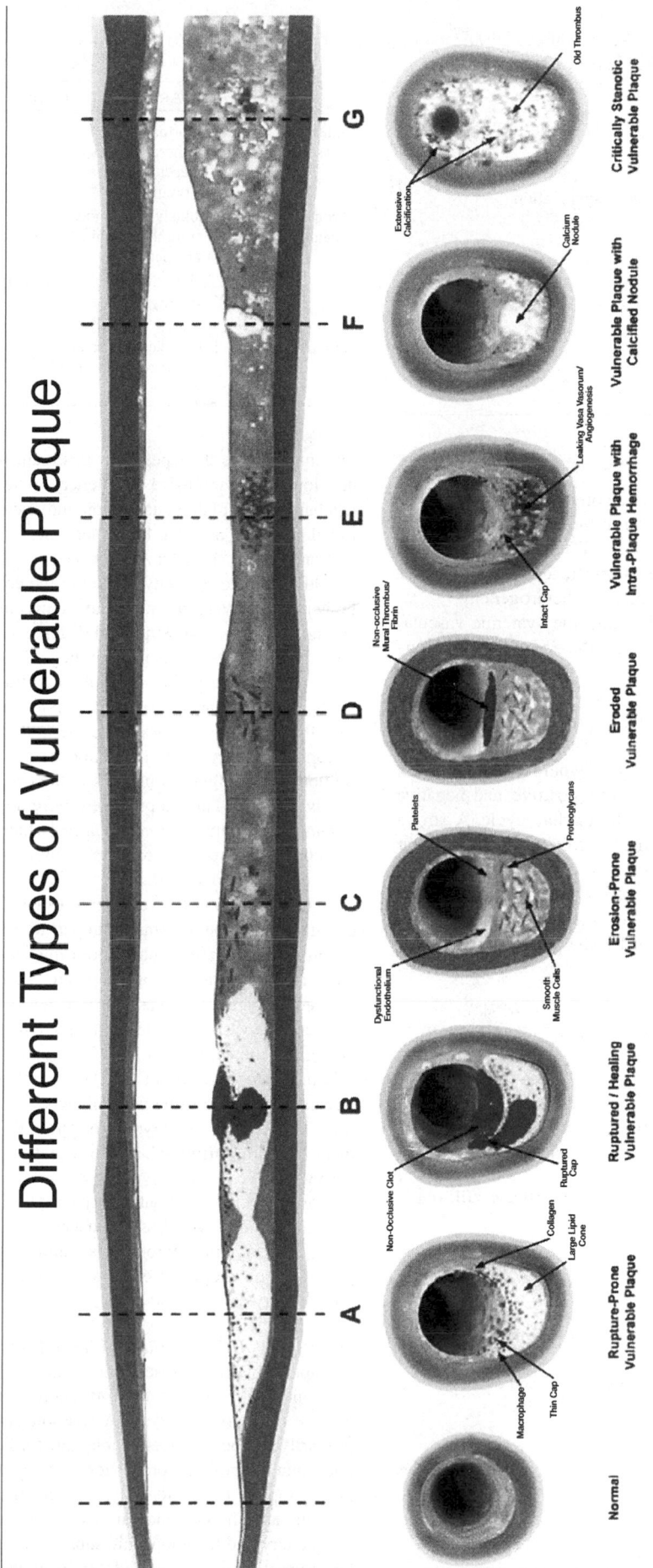

FIGURE 126-6   Different types of vulnerable plaque as underlying cause of acute coronary events and sudden cardiac death. (*A*) Rupture-prone plaque with large lipid core and thin fibrous cap infiltrated by macrophages. (*B*) Ruptured plaque with subocclusive thrombus and early organization. (*C*) Erosion-prone plaque with proteoglycan matrix in a smooth muscle cell-rich plaque. (*D*) Eroded plaque with subocclusive thrombus. (*E*) Intraplaque hemorrhage secondary to leaking vasa vasorum. (*F*) Calcific nodule protruding into the vessel lumen. (*G*) Chronically stenotic plaque with severe calcification, old thrombus, and eccentric lumen. (From M Naghavi, P Libby, E Falk, et al.,[128] with permission.).

TABLE 126-3 CRITERIA FOR DEFINING THE VULNERABLE PLAQUE, BASED ON THE STUDY OF CULPRIT PLAQUES

Major criteria
  Active inflammation (monocyte/macrophage and sometimes T cell infiltration)
  Thin cap with large lipid core
  Endothelial denudation with superficial platelet aggregation
  Fissured plaque
  Stenosis >90%
Minor criteria
  Superficial calcified nodule
  Glistening yellow
  Intraplaque hemorrhage
  Endothelial dysfunction
  Outward (positive) remodeling

SOURCE: From Naghavi et al.[128] with permission.

the local determinants of thrombosis that are operative in the coronary arteries are identical to those encountered in the cerebrovascular and peripheral arterial circulations. Basic regional differences may involve (1) distribution and composition of atherosclerotic lesions, (2) variable local rheology, and (3) underlying vascular cell heterogeneity.

Atherosclerosis is highly localized within the systemic vasculature.[143] Lesion formation particularly affects the carotid artery bifurcation, coronary arteries (especially the left coronary artery bifurcation), abdominal aorta (especially its posterior wall downstream of the renal arteries, but with little disease usually present in the upstream thoracic aorta), and profunda femoral arteries. These lesion-prone sites in the arterial circulation correspond to regions where wall shear stress is very low and may even oscillate between positive and negative directions (i.e., reversal of flow) during the cardiac cycle. A strong correlation exists between local hemodynamic conditions of low shear stress and the development of atherosclerotic plaque formation and intimal thickening.[143–145] However, as arteries become progressively diseased and stenoses develop at these sites, the local hemodynamics change. Stenotic flows are characterized by sharp increases in shear

TABLE 126-4 BLOOD HYPERCOAGULABILITY FACTORS THAT MAY CONTRIBUTE TO PATIENT VULNERABILITY TO CORONARY HEART DISEASE EVENTS

1. Markers of blood hypercoagulability
  Decreased anticoagulation factors (e.g., proteins C and S, antithrombin)
  Prothrombotic gene polymorphisms (e.g., factor V Leiden, G20210A prothrombin mutation)
  Increased coagulation factors (e.g., fibrinogen, factors VII and VIII, von Willebrand factor)
2. Increased platelet activation
  (e.g., gene polymorphisms of platelet integrin $\alpha_{IIb}\beta_3$, integrin $\alpha_2\beta_1$, GpIb-IX)
3. Decreased endogenous fibrinolysis activity
  (e.g., reduced t-PA, increased PAI-1, certain PAI-1 polymorphisms)
4. Other thrombogenic factors
  (e.g., anticardiolipin antibodies, thrombocytosis, sickle cell disease, polycythemia, diabetes mellitus, hyperhomocysteinemia, hypercholesterolemia)
5. Increased viscosity
6. Transient hypercoagulability
  (e.g., smoking, dehydration, infection, adrenergic surge, cocaine, estrogens, postprandial.)

SOURCE: Modified from Naghavi et al.[134]
PAI-1=type 1 plasminogen-activator inhibitor; t-PA=tissue plasminogen activator.

TABLE 126-5 PATHOPHYSIOLOGIC DIFFERENCES BETWEEN ARTERIAL AND VENOUS THROMBI

	ARTERIAL THROMBI	VENOUS THROMBI
Underlying vasculature	Abnormal Atherosclerosis Vasculitis Trauma	Normal
Thrombus pathology	Occlusive or nonocclusive (mural thrombi in large arteries)	Occlusive
	"White thrombus" composed mainly of platelets	"Red thrombus" composed mainly of fibrin, red cells
Pathophysiology	Local shear stress and thrombogenic vascular surface	Stasis and hypercoagulability

rate that achieve their peak just upstream of the stenosis throat, with development of intensive turbulence downstream of the stenosis. The mechanisms of platelet activation and accumulation that initiate arterial thrombosis at these high-shear sites are described below in the section entitled "Platelet Activation."

Striking heterogeneity is seen in the composition of atherothrombotic plaques, even within the same individual.[146] In addition to plaque composition, the basic structural differences between different arteries contribute to differences in thrombogenic substrates that are exposed upon arterial injury. For example, carotid and iliac arteries contain relatively more elastic fibers and proportionately fewer smooth muscle cells than coronary arteries.[147] Furthermore, ACSs typically result from disruption of only modestly stenotic, lipid-rich plaques, whereas disruption-prone, high-risk plaques in the carotid arteries usually are severely stenotic. Thus, a proposed more appropriate term is *high-risk plaque* rather than *vulnerable plaque* (which connotes its composition) to define a disruption-prone or thrombosis-prone plaque in different parts of the circulation.[146]

The pathophysiology of arterial thrombosis at different sites in the circulation may be determined in part by vascular bed-specific heterogeneity of endothelial and smooth muscle cells. Endothelial cell-derived anticoagulant and procoagulant activities are differentially expressed throughout the vascular tree. The heterogeneity of endothelial cells and the vascular bed-specific signaling pathways that control endothelial gene expression have been considered to play an important role in the localization of arterial thrombosis.[148,149] Heterogeneity of vascular smooth muscle cells likewise exists throughout the arterial tree. They vary in embryonic origin and, with subsequent development, acquire various phenotypes that can be traced to preferential sites within vessel walls.[150]

Less is known about the pathophysiology of cerebrovascular thrombosis, and even less about peripheral arterial thrombosis, than about coronary artery thrombosis. Future research in these areas should permit the development of more rational antithrombotic strategies in noncoronary artery thrombosis.

OVERVIEW OF ARTERIAL THROMBOTIC PROCESS

Disruption of an atherosclerotic plaque triggers an explosive cascade of events that results in the formation of a platelet-rich thrombus at the site of arterial injury.[151] Activation of coagulation is determined primarily by local factors (Table 126-6). Focal loss of the antithrombotic and vasodilator properties of endothelium is compounded by plaque rupture or erosion. These events trigger the local activation of platelets and the coagulation system by exposure of blood to previously encrypted thrombogenic substances. The local milieu for thrombus formation is aggravated by focal vasoconstriction, rapidly in-

TABLE 126-6 LOCAL AND SYSTEMIC DETERMINANTS OF ARTERIAL
THROMBOSIS

Local factors
  1. Loss of antithrombotic and vasodilator properties of endothelium
  2. Plaque rupture or erosion
  3. Exposure of platelet-activating and procoagulant substances
       Extracellular matrix
       Anionic phospholipids
       Tissue factor
  4. Vasoconstriction
  5. Increased shear stress
  6. Recruitment of leukocytes
Systemic factors
  1. Systemic state of activation of platelets and coagulation
       Acquired
       Genetic
  2. Adrenergic state
  3. Hyperlipidemia
  4. Diabetes mellitus

creased shear forces, and platelet-mediated recruitment of leukocytes. Platelet and coagulation activation are inseparable, reciprocally self-amplifying processes (Fig. 126-7). Activation of platelets generates procoagulant properties on their cell surfaces. Combined with nonplatelet-dependent local activators of the coagulation cascade, platelet activation culminates in the formation of thrombin, which itself is a potent stimulus for further platelet activation. Superimposed on these dominant local determinants of arterial thrombosis, the thrombotic process may be modulated by systemic, circulating factors (Table 126-6). The factors include the systemic state of activation of platelets and coagulation, which may be governed by acquired or genetic factors and by hormonal influences (e.g., adrenergic state).

Arterial thrombi generally are localized to the site of acute vascular injury. They are prevented from extending beyond this site by restoration of hemostatic balance that promotes blood fluidity along adjacent healthy endothelial surfaces. Thrombus propagation may occur, however, through a bloodborne pool of thrombogenic substances that originate at the site of vascular injury and thrombosis. These substances can be in the form of platelet and other cellular microparticles and circulating active TF derived from leukocytes activated within the thrombus.[151-153]

Thrombus persistence within an artery depends on the local balance among prothrombotic, antithrombotic, and fibrinolytic factors.[136] Ulcerated and thrombotic atherosclerotic plaques, particularly in the aorta, tend to persist or recur.[135,154,155] Atherosclerotic plaques of the aortic arch have been detected in almost one third of patients with cryptogenic stroke.[156] Aortic plaques more than 4 mm thick are significant independent predictors of recurrent cerebral infarction and other vascular events.[157]

PLATELET ACTIVATION

Disruption of an advanced atherosclerotic plaque results in abrupt exposure of highly thrombogenic material to flowing blood. This process leads locally to both thrombin generation and platelet activation, which operate simultaneously in a mutually self-amplifying process. Plaque rupture, and the development of new intimal surface irregularities, also suddenly alters local rheologic characteristics, increasing local shear rates. Increased shear stress resulting from sudden changes in degree

of stenosis following rupture is compounded by increased focal vasoconstriction induced by thrombin, thromboxane A_2, and other vasoactive substances released in the milieu of acute injury.

In addition to exposure of platelet-activating substances, the high levels of shear stress directly stimulate platelet-rich thrombus formation. Platelets adhere preferentially at the throat of the stenosis, where shear rates are highest. Shear rates in healthy arteries that are subject to thrombosis normally range from approximately 200 s^{-1} (internal carotid arteries) to 500 s^{-1} (left main coronary artery). With severe stenosis and plaque rupture, local peak shear rates can approximate 100,000 s^{-1}.[143] Increased shear rate promotes platelet transport, forcing the concentration of platelets outward toward the injured vessel wall to which they can adhere.

At high shear rates (>1000 s^{-1}), platelets must be initially tethered to the vascular surface through interaction between platelet membrane glycoprotein (Gp) Ib and von Willebrand factor bound to collagen.[158] Platelet adhesion also involves collagen binding to platelet collagen receptor ($\alpha_2\beta_1$ and GpVI). Other matrix constituents that become exposed to platelets and serve as adhesive ligands include fibronectin, laminin, fibrinogen, and fibrin. These initial adhesive interactions induce intracellular signaling pathways that activate platelets. High shear stress also activates platelets both directly[159] and by lowering the threshold of platelet activation by chemical agonists to which platelets are exposed in the microenvironment of the arterial thrombus.[160] Thus, following adhesion, platelets are explosively activated by several interacting pathways: (1) intracellular signaling initiated by the adhesion event itself, (2) direct action of locally increased shear stress, and (3) agonists released (e.g., ADP, thromboxane A_2) and generated (e.g., thrombin) at the site of vascular injury.

Finally, the occlusive arterial platelet thrombus is generated by the aggregation of platelets. This process is mediated by several alternative ligands (von Willebrand factor, fibrinogen, fibronectin) that bind to their activated receptors in the platelet $\alpha_{IIb}\beta_3$ complex. Stability of the platelet aggregate is induced by additional ligand–receptor interactions, including CD40L binding to $\alpha_{IIb}\beta_3$.[161] Platelet thrombus stabi-

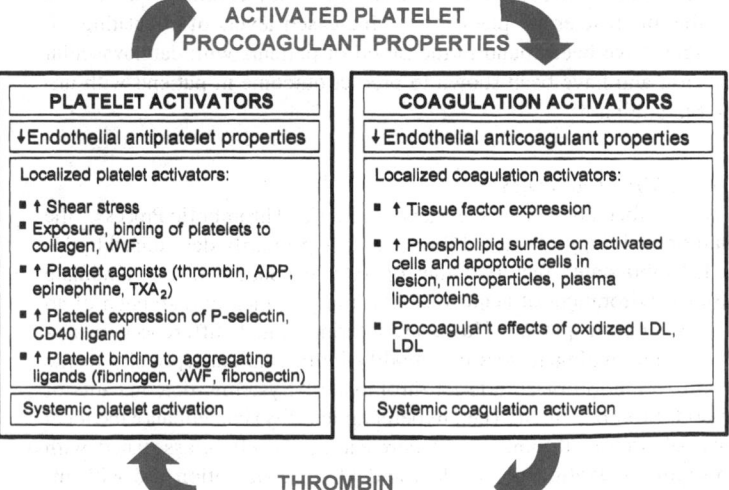

FIGURE 126-7 Atherothrombosis. Reciprocal, mutually amplifying activators of platelets and coagulation occurring on atherosclerotic lesions. ADP, adenosine diphosphate; LDL, low-density lipoprotein; TXA$_2$, thromboxane A$_2$; vWF, von Willebrand factor.

lization is designed to counteract shear forces that promote not only the formation of arterial thrombi but also their embolization.

The importance of the inflammatory component of arterial thrombosis,[141] which is characterized by complex interactions among leukocytes, endothelial cells, and platelets, is increasingly being recognized. Activated platelets recruit leukocytes to the site of vascular damage, promoting their adhesion to endothelium and their activation on endothelium-bound chemokines.

TISSUE FACTOR AND PHOSPHOLIPIDS

TF is a cell surface-bound transmembrane protein that normally is not exposed to circulating blood. When expressed, TF initiates coagulation by binding to factor VIIa and activates factors IX and X, thereby triggering the common pathway of coagulation and the formation of thrombin. Strong evidence indicates that TF, particularly the TF expressed on macrophages, is the principal thrombogenic factor in the lipid-rich core of atherosclerotic plaques.[136,162–164]

Upon rupture of the atherosclerotic plaque, exposure of vascular TF to flowing blood initiates the coagulation cascade. Coagulation reactions are accelerated on the surfaces of activated platelets and on other activated cells in the microenvironment of vascular injury. The surfaces of these activated cells express anionic phospholipids, particularly phosphatidylserine. Apoptotic cells, with which advanced lesions are enriched, likewise translocate phospholipids from the inner to the outer leaflet of the cell membrane.[165] Plasma lipoproteins can provide a phospholipid surface for the assembly of enzymatic complexes of the coagulation cascade; in particular, oxidized LDL, LDL, and VLDL have procoagulant effects.[137,166–168]

Arterial thrombosis is triggered by the acute exposure of circulating blood to TF and anionic phospholipids, leading to explosive thrombin formation. Thrombin, a potent platelet agonist, further fuels the platelet activation process described in the previous section. These reactions create a self-amplifying process that is tightly localized to the site of vascular injury. The arterial thrombus is further contained to this site by the dissipation of prothrombotic stimuli and restoration of normal, antithrombotic endothelium in adjacent areas of the vessel wall.

Some degree of thrombus propagation can be mediated by the thrombogenicity of bloodborne TF. Active TF most likely circulates in the form of microparticles shed from leukocytes and apoptotic cells in the atherosclerotic plaque.[146,152] Increased levels of circulating TF antigen have been found in the blood of patients with cardiovascular disease and have been shown to predict outcome in patients with unstable angina.[169]

SYSTEMIC FACTORS

As described above in "Overview of Arterial Thrombotic Process," the pathophysiology of arterial thrombosis is primarily determined by local, "solid-state" factors[136] that operate in concert in the immediate microenvironment of acute vascular injury, typically disruption of an atherosclerotic plaque. However, interindividual differences in systemic, circulating factors can modify individual susceptibility to the focal formation of an arterial thrombus.[170] Systemic determinants of blood thrombogenicity (i.e., hypercoagulability) can enhance the local risk of arterial thrombosis. Atherosclerosis itself is associated with systemic activation of platelets and blood coagulation and with increased fibrin turnover.[161,171,172]

Genetic determinants of the coagulation system may exert modifying effects on susceptibility to arterial thrombosis. The known hypercoagulable states that predispose to venous thrombosis (e.g., factor V Leiden, prothrombin gene mutation, antithrombin, protein C and pro-

tein S deficiency) generally are not associated with increased risk of arterial thrombosis. However, decreased mortality from ischemic heart disease has been noted in patients with hemophilia A or B and even in carriers of hemophilia.[173] This finding most likely results from reduced arterial thrombotic tendency in these individuals because early atherogenesis itself does not appear to be significantly affected by the coexistence of hemophilia.[174] Conversely, some epidemiologic studies have correlated elevated factor VIII levels with coronary and cerebrovascular disease. Increased fibrinogen levels are more strongly and consistently associated than are factor VIII levels with both subclinical atherosclerosis and clinical cardiovascular events.[175] Although increased fibrinogen and factor VIII levels represent risk factors for atherothrombosis, whether this situation is a cause or consequence of disease is not clear.

Several lines of evidence suggest that genetic determinants of increased platelet reactivity likewise enhance focal determinants of arterial thrombosis. Animal models of atherosclerosis in pigs and mice with von Willebrand disease suggest that an extremely low or absent von Willebrand factor level exerts a protective effect on the development and distribution of atherosclerotic lesions,[176,177] although these observations are inconclusive. Whether[178] or not[174] von Willebrand disease protects against development of human atherosclerosis remains in dispute. Nevertheless, increased plasma levels of von Willebrand factor are associated with risk of clinical cardiovascular events, albeit only moderately,[179] similar to the situation with hemophilia (see above).

Polymorphisms in platelet membrane Gp receptors have been considered to increase platelet reactivity, thereby potentially contributing to susceptibility to arterial thrombosis.[180,181] The first such genetic variation reported involves the PLA1/PLA2 polymorphism, which results in a Leu33Pro substitution in the β_3 subunit of the platelet integrin $\alpha_{IIb}\beta_3$ complex. The 33Pro allele was found to be associated with risk of MI in young individuals.[182] A number of subsequent studies provided conflicting data on a relationship between this polymorphism and arterial thrombosis.[180] Other platelet receptor polymorphisms that have been inconclusively linked to risk of cardiovascular disease include three different polymorphisms of the GpIb gene and a polymorphism of the collagen receptor integrin $\alpha_2\beta_1$. In some of these cases, the polymorphisms are associated with increased density of the corresponding platelet receptor. However, as is the case for the soluble hemostatic factors, lack of a clear relationship among genotype, phenotype, and clinical manifestations has failed to establish convincing cause-and-effect relationships for any of these genetic variations.

Although none of these individual hemostatic protein or platelet polymorphisms plays a clear, dominant role in the pathophysiology of arterial thrombosis, future application of microarray technologies may reveal combinations of polymorphisms that, in aggregate, influence disease.[180]

High blood levels of catecholamines likely contribute systemically to localized arterial thrombus formation. Catecholamines may be increased by physical or emotional stress or by cigarette smoking, thereby triggering acute cardiovascular events in these settings. In addition to their vasoactive actions, catecholamines are direct platelet agonists and enhance shear stress-induced platelet activation.[160,183,184]

Changes in lipid metabolism may exert systemic prothrombotic actions. The thrombogenicity of lipoprotein (a) has been attributed to its structural similarity to plasminogen, leading to reduced plasmin formation and impaired thrombolysis.[155] Elevated LDL cholesterol can contribute to blood hypercoagulability.[185] The prothrombotic state of diabetes involves multiple mechanisms, including platelet hyperreactivity and increased leukocyte procoagulant activity.[155]

ISCHEMIC VASCULAR DISEASE

MYOCARDIAL INFARCTION

Myocardial infarction is a term that reflects a loss of cardiac myocytes (necrosis) caused by prolonged ischemia. In the past, MI was defined by the combination of two of three characteristics: typical symptoms (i.e., chest discomfort), a rise in serum enzymatic markers derived from myocardial cells, and a typical electrocardiographic pattern involving the development of Q waves. The advent of sensitive and specific serologic biomarkers and precise imaging techniques have led to the development of revised criteria for MI.[185] For example, patients can be diagnosed with a "non-Q wave or non-ST segment elevation" MI (NSTEMI) if certain criteria are met. The criteria agreed upon by the American College of Cardiology and the European Society of Cardiology for acute, evolving, or recent MI [186] are as follows:

1. Typical rise and gradual fall (troponin) or more rapid rise and fall (creatinine kinase-MB isoform) or biochemical markers of myocardial necrosis with at least one of the following: (A) ischemic symptoms; (B) development of pathologic Q waves on the electrocardiogram (ECG); (C) electrocardiographic changes indicative of ischemia (ST segment elevation or depression); or (D) coronary artery intervention (e.g., coronary angioplasty)
2. Pathologic findings of an acute MI

The criteria for established MI [186] (i.e., event that occurred in the past) is any one of the following criteria:

1. Development of new pathologic Q waves on serial ECGs. The patient may or may not remember previous symptoms. Biochemical markers of myocardial necrosis may have normalized, depending on the length of time since the infarct developed.
2. Pathologic findings of a healed or healing MI

CLINICAL FEATURES OF ACUTE CORONARY SYNDROMES

Stable angina pectoris is chest discomfort caused by a narrowed coronary artery that does not allow sufficient oxygen delivery to meet the metabolic demands of the myocardium. *Unstable angina* is defined clinically as a change in the pattern of stable angina to more frequent or more severe symptoms or the development of angina at rest. The term *acute coronary syndrome* (ACS) has evolved as a useful description of the spectrum of patients presenting with angina pectoris caused by unstable angina through MI.[187] The underlying pathologic mechanism for the development of ACS is a vulnerable atherosclerotic plaque with either plaque rupture or plaque ulceration leading to thrombosis. Unstable angina and non-ST segment MI are differentiated by laboratory tests that confirm MI and by cardiac imaging that identifies a regional left ventricular wall-motion abnormality.

Angina pectoris can be associated with other symptoms, such as diaphoresis, dizziness, nausea, clamminess, and fatigue. Some patients with ACS present with atypical symptoms rather than chest pain. The presentation may be dyspnea alone, nausea and/or vomiting, palpitations/syncope, or cardiac arrest. Rarely, patients with diabetes mellitus and other patients have a "silent MI" diagnosed incidentally on ECG or cardiac imaging study.

The initial ECG may not be diagnostic in patients with ACS. In one clinical study, the ECG was not diagnostic in 45 percent and was normal in 20 percent of patients who subsequently were shown to have experienced an acute MI.[188,189] ST segment elevation and Q waves are consistent with acute MI, but other conditions, such as acute pericarditis with early repolarization variant and hypertrophic cardiomyopathy with Q waves, may mimic MI.

LABORATORY FEATURES OF ACUTE MYOCARDIAL INFARCTION

A variety of serum biomarkers are used to evaluate patients with suspected acute MI. The three most commonly used tests are (1) troponin I and troponin T, (2) creatine kinase (CK) and its isoform CK-MB, and 3) myoglobin. An elevated serum concentration of one or more of the three biomarkers is seen in almost all patients with acute MI. The preferred biomarkers are the troponins because the troponin assays are more specific than the other tests.

THERAPY FOR ACUTE CORONARY SYNDROMES

Therapy for Acute Myocardial Infarction The initial management of patients with ST elevation MI depends upon prompt recognition and therapy to reduce morbidity and mortality. A carefully coordinated plan of care is essential for optimal results in patients with ST elevation MI, given that multiple therapies usually are initiated simultaneously. The goals of therapy are to reduce ischemic pain, stabilize hemodynamic status, and treat coronary ischemia. The American College of Cardiology (ACC)/American Heart Association (AHA) guidelines for management of patients with acute MI are available on the ACC web site.[190]

Antiplatelet Agents. Unless contraindicated, all patients with acute MI should be given antiplatelet therapy. The Antiplatelet Trialists' Collaboration indicated a 30 percent reduction in vascular events with an absolute benefit of 38 vascular events prevented per 1000 patients at 1 month with antiplatelet therapy.[191] Aspirin 325 mg/day or an ADP receptor blocker such as clopidogrel is commonly used. Contraindications to antiplatelet therapy include active bleeding, coagulopathy, and severe, untreated hypertension (a relative contraindication). The combination of dipyridamole and aspirin has not been proven to provide incremental clinical benefit over aspirin alone.

β-Adrenergic Blockade. The control of heart rate with β-adrenergic blocker agents has been efficacious in the setting of acute MI or unstable angina.[190] An intravenous β-blocker such as metoprolol or atenolol in 3- to 5-mg bolus doses at 2-minute intervals should be administered with the goal of achieving a resting heart rate below 70 bpm. Patients with reduced left ventricular systolic function and signs of heart failure can be given a test dose of intravenous esmolol. After the patient receives adequate reperfusion therapy and is hemodynamically stable, an oral β-blocker is prescribed and continued on an outpatient basis.

Management of Chest Pain. A cornerstone of ischemic pain management has been intravenous nitroglycerin (beginning at 5–10 μg/min) in combination with morphine sulfate if necessary. Nitroglycerin also may improve hypertension and symptoms of heart failure, if present. Intravenous nitroglycerin therapy has not been proven to improve mortality and usually is discontinued within 24 to 48 hours of presentation.[190] Patients who have taken drugs (e.g., sildenafil) for erectile dysfunction within the preceding 24 hours are at increased risk for vasodilatation and hypotension, so caution is advised in these patients when intravenous nitroglycerin is given.

Reperfusion Therapy. The overriding goal of treatment of MI is restoration of myocardial blood flow and salvage of myocardial tissue. A decision should be made immediately whether the patient will undergo a primary (direct) percutaneous coronary intervention (PCI) or receive a thrombolytic agent. The currently preferred approach is PCI, but the relative advantages and limitations of each therapy should be considered. The most important factor to consider is whether PCI is immediately available. Several randomized trials indicate enhanced survival with PCI compared to thrombolysis, with a lower rate of intracranial hemorrhage and recurrent MI.[192–194] Transfer to a center that can provide PCI, if necessary, should be accomplished in less than 2 hours.[195]

Thrombolytic therapy should be given immediately if PCI cannot be performed promptly.[196] Prior to thrombolysis, the patient should be initially assessed for possible contraindications, which include active bleeding, history of cerebral vascular disease, intracranial neoplasm, drug allergy, and trauma.[190] A systolic blood pressure greater than 175 torr is a relative contraindication but should not prohibit therapy, especially if the pressure can be rapidly controlled. Many different thrombolytic regimens with different dosing schemes are available. Streptokinase was the first thrombolytic agent tested but has proved less effective than alteplase.[197] In addition, streptokinase is antigenic and can cause an allergic reaction, particularly with repeat administration. Other thrombolytic agents, such as tenecteplase and reteplase, have reportedly similar results compared to alteplase.[198] Tenecteplase is popular on hospital formularies because of its relatively easy single-bolus administration and reported lower rate of noncerebral bleeding.[199] A half-dose of thrombolytic agent in combination with platelet integrin $\alpha_{IIb}\beta_3$ inhibitors was successful in restoring coronary blood flow.[200,201] However, trials do not show a significant survival benefit compared to conventional thrombolytic therapy, and bleeding complications are increased, especially in the elderly.[202] Thus, this approach is not widely used for patients with acute MI.

Anticoagulation. Heparin, both unfractionated and low molecular weight, is commonly used in patients with acute MI. The exact role of heparin therapy with different thrombolytic agents is evolving. Patients who undergo primary PCI usually are given unfractionated heparin 7500 U subcutaneously twice daily or low molecular weight heparin, e.g., enoxaparin, 1 mg/kg twice daily unless contraindications are evident. For patients receiving intravenous unfractionated heparin, the recommended dose is an initial 60 to 70 units/kg bolus (maximum 5000 U) followed by 12 to 15 U/kg/hour (maximum 1000 U/hour) as continuous infusion with monitoring of the activated partial thromboplastin time (aPTT) measured at 6 hours. The heparin dose is adjusted to maintain an aPTT between 50 and 75 seconds.

The American College of Chest Physicians (ACCP) consensus conference recommends maintaining the aPTT at 50 to 75 seconds for short-term use. Heparin should be continued beyond this period only in the case of high risk of systemic or venous thrombolembolism.[203] Patients can be switched to a subcutaneously administered heparin or converted to oral warfarin during the high-risk period. The Coumadin-Aspirin Reinfarction Study (CARS) did not show a significant benefit with the combination of low-dose warfarin (1 or 3 mg) and aspirin 80 mg daily compared to aspirin 160 mg daily monotherapy on cardiovascular morbidity in patients who had an MI.[204]

Statins. All patients with MI should be started on a 3-hydroxy-3-methylglutaryl-coenzyme A reductase inhibitor (statin) unless the MI was caused by a nonatherosclerotic process such as coronary vasospasm, vasculitis, or embolus. Numerous studies indicate that statins reduce the risk of subsequent MI by approximately 30 to 50 percent.[104] Current evidence suggests that a serum LDL level less than 80 mg/dl with statin treatment is more efficacious in retarding atherosclerotic disease progression than a serum LDL level of 100 mg/dl or above.[205]

Therapy for Unstable Angina Pectoris and Non-ST Elevation Myocardial Infarction The distinction between unstable angina and NSTEMI initially may be difficult because levels of troponins and/or CK-MB may not be elevated until hours after presentation. Similar to acute MI, the initial treatment of unstable angina and NSTEMI includes supplemental oxygen, pain control, and bed rest.[187] Nitrates, given either intravenously or subcutaneously, are the treatment of choice for angina pectoris. β-Blockers also are routinely given to patients with unstable angina to relieve symptoms of angina and reduce the risk of progression to MI.

Treatment of unstable angina and NSTEMI involves administration of an antiplatelet agent and anticoagulation.[187] Thrombolytic therapy is not beneficial in patients with unstable angina, and its use is associated with a paradoxical increase in the incidence of MI. Antiplatelet treatment, most commonly aspirin at a dose of 325 mg daily, was shown in the Antithrombotic Trialists' Collaboration to reduce the combined end point of subsequent nonfatal MI, nonfatal stroke, or vascular death (8.0% vs. 13.3%) in patients with non-ST segment elevation ACS.[206] Clinical trials involving patients with non-ST segment elevation ACS have demonstrated significantly reduced cardiovascular events and mortality with aspirin administration.[207–209] Some patients do not benefit from aspirin, and this finding has generated an interest as to whether these patients are "aspirin resistant." Nonrandomized studies indicate that aspirin resistance may occur, but because of the limitations of these studies, the definition and prognostic significance of this phenomenon are uncertain.[210–213]

The thienopyridine clopidogrel (75 mg/day) is effective in reducing the risk of MI and mortality in patients with unstable angina.[190,214] The combination of aspirin and clopidogrel has been tested in patients with NSTEMI and unstable angina. The combination of these antiplatelet agents resulted in improved survival and decreased progression to MI.[215] The patients with non-ST segment elevation ACS who underwent PCI benefited the most from the combination of aspirin and clopidogrel.[216] However, the combination was associated with an increase in major bleeding and reoperation for bleeding in patients who underwent coronary artery bypass grafting (CABG). Therefore, a 5-day but preferably a 7-day period off clopidogrel is recommended before CABG.[187,217]

A meta-analysis of randomized clinical trials found that intravenous platelet integrin $\alpha_{IIb}\beta_3$ inhibitors substantially benefited patients with non-ST segment elevation ACS undergoing coronary intervention.[209] The integrin $\alpha_{IIb}\beta_3$ receptor antagonist abciximab (ReoPro) is a monoclonal antibody fragment that reduces short-term and long-term clinical events in patients with ACS undergoing angioplasty with or without stent placement.[218–220] Other platelet integrin $\alpha_{IIb}\beta_3$ antagonists, such as tirofiban[221–223] and integrilin,[224] also are effective and safe in treating unstable angina when combined with heparin anticoagulation.[225] Current guidelines from an ACC/AHA task force and the ACCP consensus conference recommend administration of an integrin $\alpha_{IIb}\beta_3$ inhibitor, in addition to aspirin and heparin, for patients with unstable angina/NSTEMI undergoing planned PCI.[187,203]

Either intravenous heparin or subcutaneous heparin reduces the rate of MI and death, and relieves anginal pain, when used in combination with an antiplatelet agent.[227] Intravenous heparin usually is given as a 5000-U bolus followed by continuous infusion. Low-molecular-weight heparins can be substituted for unfractionated heparin. Some studies have shown superior efficacy of low-molecular-weight heparins, but other studies have not indicated a significant difference.[187,228] Direct thrombin inhibitors, such as hirudin, have been shown to reduce the rate of death, non-fatal MI, and refractory angina compared to heparin.[229] Although efficacious in treating ACS, direct thrombin inhibitors are more expensive than heparin and have a higher risk of bleeding and need for transfusion; therefore, they are not used routinely at this time.[230] However, the ACCP recommends lepirudin (recombinant hirudin), argatroban, bivalirudin, or danaproid in patients with a history of heparin-associated thrombocytopenia.[226]

Therapy for Stable Angina Pectoris Patients with stable angina pectoris can be treated with either medical management or revascularization.[231] Limited clinical trial data comparing revascularization, either percutaneous or surgical, to medical therapy are available. The older trials evaluating percutaneous and surgical revascularization were limited by several factors: antiplatelet treatment, angiotensin-converting enzyme inhibitors and aggressive lipid lowering with statins were not given as background medical therapy of angina. Given these limitations, determining whether revascularization is better than medical management for long-term care of patients with stable angina in modern practice is difficult.

Both PCI and coronary bypass surgery significantly reduce angina. The Coronary Artery Surgery Study (CASS) showed more patients remained symptom-free after CABG compared to medical therapy 5 years after the procedure.[232] At 10 years, however, no significant difference in symptoms was observed. Clinical trials showed significant improvement in angina with PCI compared to medical therapy; however, patients who underwent the former had similar rates of death and MI as those undergoing medical therapy and were less likely to have angina and more likely to have undergone a coronary bypass graft.[231]

Restenosis is a complex process involving inflammation, cellular proliferation, thrombosis, and matrix deposition. Restenosis occurring after PCI may result in flow-limiting luminal narrowing in 20 to 30 percent of therapeutically dilated vessels.[233] Numerous pharmacologic agents, including heparin,[234] have been given in an attempt to reduce the restenosis rate but have met with limited or no success. Intraarterial radiation (brachytherapy) reduces the restenosis rate but is cumbersome to perform because of radiation safety issues. Drug-eluting arterial stents, including the immunosuppressive macrocyclic lactone rapamycin (Sirolimus)[235–238] and the chemotherapeutic agent paclitaxel (Taxol), have been shown to significantly reduce the rate of restenosis. Because drug-eluting stents were not available at the time of the previous clinical trials, extrapolating the benefits of PCI versus CABG or over medical therapy is difficult. The medical management of patients with stable angina pectoris should include antiplatelet therapy, statin drug treatment, a β-blocker, an angiotensin-converting enzyme inhibitor, and a long-acting nitrate.[231]

PERIPHERAL ARTERIAL DISEASE

Peripheral arterial disease (PAD) is a term that encompasses any arterial disease of the lower extremities, upper extremities, and iliac vessels. It most commonly results from atherosclerosis. Patients who have atherosclerotic disease that compromises blood flow to the extremities may present with exertional pain in a muscle group, called *claudication* (derived from the Latin *claudicare* meaning "to limp"). Claudication is an intermittent but reproducible discomfort of a defined group of muscles that is induced by exercise and relieved with rest.[239] Acute limb ischemia is a relatively rare problem in patients with PAD. In general it is caused by *in situ* thrombosis or an embolic event from arrhythmias, such as atrial fibrillation, or after manipulation of an artery or aorta with a catheter. Approximately 4 percent of patients with claudication progress to *critical limb ischemia*, which is defined as rest pain and/or foot ulceration that heralds impending tissue loss.

The 5-year mortality rate is estimated to be 30 percent in patients with PAD.[240] Approximately 75 percent of mortality results from a cardiovascular event, such as MI or stroke.[240] The ankle-brachial index is a noninvasive measure of limb vascular pressure in the lower extremities and has been noted in several studies to be predictive of cardiovascular events.[239] However, a decreased index is not just a predictor but is a physical finding that indicates significant atherosclerotic plaque burden is present. Other noninvasive imaging studies for PAD include the combination of segmental pressures and pulse volume recordings,[241,242] duplex Doppler ultrasound,[243,244] and magnetic resonance imaging.[245]

Medical therapy for patients with PAD includes risk factor modification, antiplatelet therapy, and treatment of claudication symptoms with exercise rehabilitation and possible pharmacologic agents. The risk factors for development of peripheral atherosclerosis include cigarette smoking, diabetes mellitus, hypertension, and dyslipidemia. Aggressive management of risk factors for PAD is recommended to prevent disease progression.[246] Some emerging risk factors for PAD

include hyperhomocysteinemia[247] and elevated fibrinogen levels.[239] Treatment with antiplatelet agents reduces the risk of cardiovascular events, such as MI and stroke, in patients with PAD.[239] The Antithrombotic Trialists' Collaboration evaluated 9214 patients with PAD enrolled in 42 trials and found that use of aspirin 75 to 325 mg/day resulted in a proportional reduction of 23 percent in serious vascular events.[206] Evaluation of patients with PAD in the Physicians' Health Study found that aspirin 325 mg every other day decreased the need for peripheral artery surgery.[248] However, no difference between the aspirin and placebo groups with regard to development of claudication was observed. Several studies have evaluated the ADP receptor blockers ticlopidine and clopidogrel. Meta-analysis of randomized studies found that ticlopidine treatment was associated with reduced mortality, especially from cardiovascular events.[249] Clopidogrel is considered a safer drug of the same class and was evaluated in 19,185 patients in the Clopidogrel versus Aspirin in Patients at Risk of Ischaemic Events (CAPRIE) study.[214] A dose of clopidogrel 75 mg/day had a modest but significant advantage over aspirin 325 mg/day in preventing stroke, MI, and peripheral vascular disease. Subgroup analysis revealed that the patients with PAD benefited the most with clopidogrel treatment. Antiplatelet therapy should be offered to all patients with PAD unless contraindicated by allergy or comorbidities.

The options for treating claudication symptoms include exercise rehabilitation, pharmacologic agents, and a revascularization procedure. Several studies indicate exercise rehabilitation improves the symptoms of claudication, and a supervised program is better than an unstructured program.[250] Two drugs are approved by the FDA for treatment of claudication symptoms: pentoxifylline, a methylxanthine derivative that may improve abnormal red cell deformability and reduce blood viscosity, and cilostazol, a type III phosphodiesterase inhibitor with antiplatelet and vasodilating properties. Cilostazol is generally considered more effective than pentoxifylline for improving walking distance in patients with claudication.[251] The addition of cilostazol to either aspirin or clopidogrel does not increase the bleeding time or bleeding risk.[252] A revascularization procedure in patients with stable, intermittent claudication generally is reserved for those with severe lifestyle-limiting symptoms or manifestation of critical limb ischemia.

CEREBROVASCULAR DISEASE

The etiology of ischemic stroke is multifactorial and can be categorized into embolic, small-vessel disease, large-vessel disease, and cryptogenic. Carotid artery disease accounts for approximately 30 percent of strokes. Major risk factors for developing carotid artery atherosclerosis are hypertension, diabetes, smoking, and dyslipidemia.[253,254] Emerging risk factors for stroke include hyperhomocysteinemia and an elevated plasma level of lipoprotein (a). An elevated hsCRP level is a risk factor associated with ischemic stroke in both men and women. However, at this time hsCRP is not routinely measured as an additional marker for increased risk of stroke. Similar to coronary and PAD, control of atherosclerotic risk factors is essential in the primary prevention of stroke in patients with evidence of carotid atherosclerosis and for those who have undergone carotid endarterectomy.[255,256]

Carotid endarterectomy is indicated for patients with symptoms and a greater than 50 percent stenosis or for patients who are asymptomatic with a greater than 60 to 70 percent stenosis of the common carotid or internal carotid arteries.[257,258] Carotid stents with embolic protection appear promising for treatment of carotid atherosclerosis.[259]

Two antiplatelet drug regimens are approved for prevention of stroke: clopidogrel and the combination of aspirin 25 mg and dipyridamole 200 mg daily. Approval of clopidogrel is based on the CAPRIE study, which showed a reduction in the combined endpoint of stroke,

MI, and death in patients treated with clopidogrel 75 mg/day compared to aspirin 325 mg/day.[214] The FDA indication for dipyridamole/aspirin is primarily based on the European Stroke Protection Study 2, which noted a reduction in stroke with the combination of dipyridamole 200 mg and aspirin 25 mg given together (Aggrenox) twice per day.[260] Fish oil (omega-3 fatty acids) lowers triglycerides and VLDLs and may reduce serum viscosity by lowering fibrinogen. Some studies suggest that fish oil consumption lowers the risk of ischemic stroke. The effect of fish oils on carotid atherosclerosis is unknown.[261,262]

ATHEROEMBOLISM

Atheromatous embolism refers to the dislodgment into the bloodstream of arterial plaque material, including cholesterol crystals ("cholesterol embolism") from ulcerated vascular plaques. The cholesterol embolization syndrome involves systemic microembolism to the end arteries of almost any circulatory bed. Atheroembolism most characteristically originates from lesions in the abdominal aorta and ileofemoral arteries. Cholesterol emboli that lodge in an arteriole incite an acute inflammatory response, followed by a foreign body reaction, intravascular thrombus formation, endothelial proliferation, and eventually fibrosis. These processes generally result in ischemia that sometimes leads to infarction and necrosis.[263] Mortality rate of clinically diagnosed atheroembolism can be as high as 80 percent, depending on the anatomic location and size of the vascular beds involved.[264]

Patients with atheroembolism, including the cholesterol embolization syndrome, generally have advanced atherosclerosis, often complicated by a history of hypertension, diabetes mellitus, renal failure, or aortic aneurysms. Atherosclerotic plaques can disrupt and embolize spontaneously; however, the clinical syndrome typically is triggered by vascular intervention, including vascular surgery, catheterization, angioplasty, endarterectomy, or angiography.[265,266] Anticoagulation or thrombolytic therapy may be risk factors with atheroembolism.[264] Clinical presentation depends on the sites of embolization. When these sites involve the distal extremity microcirculation, the "blue toe syndrome" may develop. The syndrome presents with the acute appearance of painful and tender discoloration or mottled blue and patchy appearance of one or more toes that may progress to ulceration and gangrene. Other common cutaneous manifestations are livedo reticularis involving the legs, buttocks or abdomen, painful nodules, and purpura.[263] Cerebrovascular embolism can cause transient neurologic abnormalities. Cholesterol emboli lodged in retinal arterial bifurcations can be visualized by ophthalmoscopy as bright, refractile, yellow rectangular crystals. Visceral organs most commonly affected by atheroembolism include the kidneys, sometimes causing renal failure, and the gastrointestinal tract, where abdominal pain, ischemic colitis, and bleeding may ensue.

Diagnosis is based on clinical presentation associated with imaging evidence of atherosclerosis of the arterial supply of affected organs.[264] Transient eosinophilia occurs in most cases.[265] Treatment of atheroembolism should include surgical removal or bypass of the source of emboli. No medical treatment modalities have been established to be effective. Anticoagulation or fibrinolytic therapy may increase the risk of further atheroembolism.[267]

REFERENCES

1. Virchow R: *Cellular Pathology: As Based upon Physiological and Pathological Histology.* Dover, New York, 1863.
2. Ross R: Atherosclerosis—An inflammatory disease. *N Engl J Med* 340: 115, 1999.
3. Enos WF, Holmes RH, Beyer J: Coronary disease among United States soldiers killed in action in Korea; preliminary report. *JAMA* 152:1090, 1953.
4. Joseph A, Ackerman D, Talley JD, et al: Manifestations of coronary atherosclerosis in young trauma victims—An autopsy study. *J Am Coll Cardiol* 22:459, 1993.
5. Tuzcu EM, Kapadia SR, Tutar E, et al: High prevalence of coronary atherosclerosis in asymptomatic teenagers and young adults: Evidence from intravascular ultrasound. *Circulation* 103:2705, 2001.
6. Ross R: Atherosclerosis-an inflammatory disease. *N Engl J Med* 340: 115, 1999.
7. Skalen K, Gustafsson M, Rydberg EK, et al: Subendothelial retention of atherogenic lipoproteins in early atherosclerosis. *Nature* 417:750, 2002.
8. Passerini AG, Polacek DC, Shi C, et al: Coexisting proinflammatory and antioxidative endothelial transcription profiles in a disturbed flow region of the adult porcine aorta. *Proc Natl Acad Sci U S A* 101:2482, 2004.
9. Libby P, Ridker PM, Maseri A: Inflammation and atherosclerosis. *Circulation* 105:1135, 2002.
10. Stary HC, Chandler AB, Dinsmore RE, et al: A definition of advanced types of atherosclerotic lesions and a histological classification of atherosclerosis. A report from the Committee on Vascular Lesions of the Council on Arteriosclerosis, American Heart Association. *Circulation* 92:1355, 1995.
11. Galis ZS, Khatri JJ: Matrix metalloproteinases in vascular remodeling and atherogenesis: The good, the bad, and the ugly. *Circ Res* 90:251, 2002.
12. Hunt JL, Fairman R, Mitchell ME, et al: Bone formation in carotid plaques: A clinicopathological study. *Stroke* 33:1214, 2002.
13. Furchgott RF, Zawadzki JV: The obligatory role of endothelial cells in the relaxation of arterial smooth muscle by acetylcholine. *Nature* 288: 373, 1980.
14. Furchgott RF: Endothelium-derived relaxing factor: Discovery, early studies, and identification as nitric oxide. *Biosci Rep* 19:235, 1999.
15. Harrison DG, Cai H: Endothelial control of vasomotion and nitric oxide production. *Cardiol Clin* 21:289, 2003.
16. Landmesser U, Dikalov S, Price SR, et al: Oxidation of tetrahydrobiopterin leads to uncoupling of endothelial cell nitric oxide synthase in hypertension. *J Clin Invest* 111:1201, 2003.
17. Tiefenbacher CP, Bleeke T, Vahl C, et al: Endothelial dysfunction of coronary resistance arteries is improved by tetrahydrobiopterin in atherosclerosis [in process citation]. *Circulation* 102:2172, 2000.
18. Kinlay S, Plutzky J: Effect of lipid-lowering therapy on vasomotion and endothelial function. *Curr Cardiol Rep* 1:238, 1999.
19. Creager MA, Gallagher SJ, Girerd XJ, et al: L-arginine improves endothelium-dependent vasodilation in hypercholesterolemic humans. *J Clin Invest* 90:1248, 1992.
20. Boger RH, Bode-Boger SM, Szuba A, et al: Asymmetric dimethylarginine (ADMA): A novel risk factor for endothelial dysfunction: Its role in hypercholesterolemia. *Circulation* 98:1842, 1998.
21. Cooke JP: Does ADMA cause endothelial dysfunction? *Arterioscler Thromb Vasc Biol* 20:2032, 2000.
22. Ito A, Tsao PS, Adimoolam S, et al: Novel mechanism for endothelial dysfunction: Dysregulation of dimethylarginine dimethylaminohydrolase. *Circulation* 99:3092, 1999.
23. Ludmer PL, Selwyn AP, Shook TL, et al: Paradoxical vasoconstriction induced by acetylcholine in atherosclerotic coronary arteries. *N Engl J Med* 315:1046, 1986.
24. Kuhn FE, Mohler ER, Satler LF, et al: Effects of high density lipoprotein on acetylcholine induced coronary vasoreactivity. *Am J Cardiol* 68: 1425, 1991.
25. Kuhn FE, Mohler ER, Rackley CE: Cholesterol and lipoproteins: Beyond atherosclerosis. *Clin Cardiol* 15:883, 1992.

26. Spieker LE, Sudano I, Hurlimann D, et al: High-density lipoprotein restores endothelial function in hypercholesterolemic men. *Circulation* 105:1399, 2002.

27. Celermajer DS, Sorensen KE, Spiegelhalter DJ, et al: Aging is associated with endothelial dysfunction in healthy men years before the age-related decline in women. *J Am Coll Cardiol* 24:471, 1994.

28. Ghiadoni L, Donald AE, Cropley M, et al: Mental stress induces transient endothelial dysfunction in humans. *Circulation* 102:2473, 2000.

29. Ghiadoni L, Virdis A, Magagna A, et al: Effect of the angiotensin II type 1 receptor blocker candesartan on endothelial function in patients with essential hypertension. *Hypertension* 35(1 Pt 2):501, 2000.

30. Boltwood MD, Taylor CB, Burke MB, et al: Anger report predicts coronary artery vasomotor response to mental stress in atherosclerotic segments. *Am J Cardiol* 72:1361, 1993.

31. Liuba P, Karnani P, Pesonen E, et al: Endothelial dysfunction after repeated Chlamydia pneumoniae infection in apolipoprotein E-knockout mice. *Circulation* 102:1039, 2000.

32. Fichtlscherer S, Rosenberger G, Walter DH, et al: Elevated C-reactive protein levels and impaired endothelial vasoreactivity in patients with coronary artery disease. *Circulation* 102:1000, 2000.

33. Beckman JA, Thakore A, Kalinowski BH, et al: Radiation therapy impairs endothelium-dependent vasodilation in humans. *J Am Coll Cardiol* 37:761, 2001.

34. Glass CK, Witztum JL: Atherosclerosis. The road ahead. *Cell* 104:503, 2001.

35. Steinberg D: Atherogenesis in perspective: Hypercholesterolemia and inflammation as partners in crime. *Nat Med* 8:1211, 2002.

36. Ross R, Glomset JA: Atherosclerosis and the arterial smooth muscle cell: Proliferation of smooth muscle is a key event in the genesis of the lesions of atherosclerosis. *Science* 180:1332, 1973.

37. Fuster V, Lewis A: Conner Memorial Lecture. Mechanisms leading to myocardial infarction: Insights from studies of vascular biology. *Circulation* 90:2126, 1994.

38. Schwartz SM, Murry CE: Proliferation and the monoclonal origins of atherosclerotic lesions. *Annu Rev Med* 49:437, 1998.

39. Scott NA, Cipolla GD, Ross CE, et al: Identification of a potential role for the adventitia in vascular lesion formation after balloon overstretch injury of porcine coronary arteries. *Circulation* 93:2178, 1996.

40. Gordon D, Reidy MA, Benditt EP, Schwartz SM: Cell proliferation in human coronary arteries. *Proc Natl Acad Sci U S A* 87:4600, 1990.

41. O'Brien ER, Alpers CE, Stewart DK, et al: Proliferation in primary and restenotic coronary atherectomy tissue. Implications for antiproliferative therapy. *Circ Res* 73:223, 1993.

42. Sata M, Saiura A, Kunisato A, et al: Hematopoietic stem cells differentiate into vascular cells that participate in the pathogenesis of atherosclerosis. *Nat Med* 8:403, 2002.

43. Hillebrands JL, Klatter FA, van den Hurk BM, et al: Origin of neointimal endothelium and alpha-actin-positive smooth muscle cells in transplant arteriosclerosis. *J Clin Invest* 107:1411, 2001.

44. Campbell JH, Han CL, Campbell GR: Neointimal formation by circulating bone marrow cells. *Ann N Y Acad Sci* 947:18, 2001.

45. Shimizu K, Sugiyama S, Aikawa M, et al: Host bone-marrow cells are a source of donor intimal smooth-muscle-like cells in murine aortic transplant arteriopathy. *Nat Med* 7:738, 2001.

46. Simper D, Stalboerger PG, Panetta CJ, et al: Smooth muscle progenitor cells in human blood. *Circulation* 106:1199, 2002.

47. Der Leyen HE, Gibbons GH, Morishita R, et al: Gene therapy inhibiting neointimal vascular lesion: In vivo transfer of endothelial cell nitric oxide synthase gene. *Proc Natl Acad Sci U S A* 92:1137, 1995.

48. Qian H, Neplioueva V, Shetty GA, et al: Nitric oxide synthase gene therapy rapidly reduces adhesion molecule expression and inflammatory cell infiltration in carotid arteries of cholesterol-fed rabbits. *Circulation* 99:2979, 1999.

49. Dzau VJ, Braun-Dullaeus RC, Sedding DG: Vascular proliferation and atherosclerosis: New perspectives and therapeutic strategies. *Nat Med* 8:1249, 2002.

50. Lemos PA, Lee CH, Degertekin M, et al: Early outcome after sirolimus-eluting stent implantation in patients with acute coronary syndromes: Insights from the Rapamycin-Eluting Stent Evaluated At Rotterdam Cardiology Hospital (RESEARCH) registry. *J Am Coll Cardiol* 41:2093, 2003.

51. Blann AD: Endothelial cell activation, injury, damage and dysfunction: Separate entities or mutual terms? *Blood Coagul Fibrinolysis* 11:623, 2000.

52. Sagripanti A, Carpi A: Antithrombotic and prothrombotic activities of the vascular endothelium. *Biomed Pharmacother* 54:107, 2000.

53. Feil R, Lohmann SM, De Jonge H, et al: Cyclic GMP-dependent protein kinases and the cardiovascular system: Insights from genetically modified mice. *Circ Res* 93:907, 2003.

54. Gonzalez MA, Selwyn AP: Endothelial function, inflammation, and prognosis in cardiovascular disease. *Am J Med* 115(suppl 8A):99S, 2003.

55. Anderson TJ: Nitric oxide, atherosclerosis and the clinical relevance of endothelial dysfunction. *Heart Fail Rev* 8:71, 2003.

56. Tulis DA, Durante W, Liu X, et al: Adenovirus-mediated heme oxygenase-1 gene delivery inhibits injury-induced vascular neointima formation. *Circulation* 104:2710, 2001.

57. Sachais BS: Platelet-endothelial interactions in atherosclerosis. *Curr Atheroscler Rep* 3:412, 2001.

58. Marcus AJ, Broekman MJ, Drosopoulos JH, et al: Metabolic control of excessive extracellular nucleotide accumulation by CD39/ecto-nucleotidase-1: Implications for ischemic vascular diseases. *J Pharmacol Exp Ther* 305:9, 2003.

59. Landmesser U, Merten R, Spiekermann S, et al: Vascular extracellular superoxide dismutase activity in patients with coronary artery disease: Relation to endothelium-dependent vasodilation. *Circulation* 101:2264, 2000.

60. Cooke JP: Does ADMA cause endothelial dysfunction? *Arterioscler Thromb Vasc Biol* 20:2032, 2000.

61. Binder CJ, Chang MK, Shaw PX, et al: Innate and acquired immunity in atherogenesis. *Nat Med* 8:1218, 2002.

62. Medzhitov R: Toll-like receptors and innate immunity. *Nat Rev Immunol* 1:135, 2001.

63. Medzhitov R, Janeway CAJr: Decoding the patterns of self and nonself by the innate immune system. *Science* 296:298, 2002.

64. Vlaicu R, Niculescu F, Rus HG, Cristea A: Immunohistochemical localization of the terminal C5b-9 complement complex in human aortic fibrous plaque. *Atherosclerosis* 57:163, 1985.

65. Ridker PM: Clinical application of C-reactive protein for cardiovascular disease detection and prevention. *Circulation* 107:363, 2003.

66. Yasojima K, Schwab C, McGeer EG, McGeer PL: Generation of C-reactive protein and complement components in atherosclerotic plaques. *Am J Pathol* 158:1039, 2001.

67. Dansky HM, Barlow CB, Lominska C, et al: Adhesion of monocytes to arterial endothelium and initiation of atherosclerosis are critically dependent on vascular cell adhesion molecule-1 gene dosage. *Arterioscler Thromb Vasc Biol* 21:1662, 2001.

68. Cybulsky MI, Gimbrone MA Jr: Endothelial expression of a mononuclear leukocyte adhesion molecule during atherogenesis. *Science* 251:788, 1991.

69. Cybulsky MI, Iiyama K, Li H, et al: A major role for VCAM-1, but not ICAM-1, in early atherosclerosis. *J Clin Invest* 107:1255, 2001.

70. Collins RG, Velji R, Guevara NV, et al: P-Selectin or intercellular adhesion molecule (ICAM)-1 deficiency substantially protects against atherosclerosis in apolipoprotein E-deficient mice. *J Exp Med* 191:189, 2000.

71. Boring L, Gosling J, Cleary M, Charo IF: Decreased lesion formation in CCR2-/- mice reveals a role for chemokines in the initiation of atherosclerosis. *Nature* 94:894, 1998.

72. Gu L, Okada Y, Clinton SK, et al: Absence of monocyte chemoattractant protein-1 reduces atherosclerosis in low density lipoprotein receptor-deficient mice. *Mol Cell* 2:275, 1998.

73. Gosling J, Slaymaker S, Gu L, et al: MCP-1 deficiency reduces susceptibility to atherosclerosis in mice that overexpress human apolipoprotein B. *J Clin Invest* 103:773, 1999.

74. Smith JD, Trogan E, Ginsberg M, et al: Decreased atherosclerosis in mice deficient in both macrophage colony-stimulating factor (op) and apolipoprotein E. *Proc Natl Acad Sci U S A* 92:8264, 1995.

75. Pitas RE: Expression of the acetyl low density lipoprotein receptor by rabbit fibroblasts and smooth muscle cells. Up-regulation by phorbol esters. *J Biol Chem* 265:12722, 1990.

76. Endemann G, Stanton LW, Madden KS, et al: CD36 is a receptor for oxidized low density lipoprotein. *J Biol Chem* 268:11811, 1993.

77. Steinberg D, Parthasarathy S, Carew TE, et al: Beyond cholesterol: Modifications of low-density lipoprotein that increase its atherogenicity. *N Engl J Med* 320:915, 1989.

78. Witztum JL, Steinberg D: Role of oxidized low density lipoprotein in atherogenesis. *J Clin Invest* 88:1785, 1991.

79. Goldstein JL, Ho YK, Basu SK, Brown MS: Binding site on macrophages that mediates uptake and degradation of acetylated low density lipoprotein, producing massive cholesterol deposition. *Proc Natl Acad Sci U S A* 76:333, 1979.

80. Navab M, Hama SY, Reddy ST, et al: Oxidized lipids as mediators of coronary heart disease. *Curr Opin Lipidol* 13:363, 2002.

81. Sugiyama S, Okada Y, Sukhova GK, et al: Macrophage myeloperoxidase regulation by granulocyte macrophage colony-stimulating factor in human atherosclerosis and implications in acute coronary syndromes. *Am J Pathol* 158:879, 2001.

82. Brennan ML, Penn MS, Van LF, et al: Prognostic value of myeloperoxidase in patients with chest pain. *Obstet Gynecol Surv* 59:267, 2004.

83. Babior BM: Phagocytes and oxidative stress. *Am J Med* 109:33, 2000.

84. Suzuki H, Kurihara Y, Takeya M, et al: A role for macrophage scavenger receptors in atherosclerosis and susceptibility to infection. *Nature* 386:292, 1997.

85. Febbraio M, Podrez EA, Smith JD, et al: Targeted disruption of the class B scavenger receptor CD36 protects against atherosclerotic lesion development in mice. *J Clin Invest* 105:1049, 2000.

86. Kodama T, Reddy P, Kishimoto C, Krieger M: Purification and characterization of a bovine acetyl low density lipoprotein receptor. *Proc Natl Acad Sci U S A* 85:9238, 1988.

87. Henriksen T, Mahoney EM, Steinberg D: Enhanced macrophage degradation of low density lipoprotein previously incubated with cultured endothelial cells: Recognition by receptors for acetylated low density lipoproteins. *Proc Natl Acad Sci U S A* 78:6499, 1981.

88. Steinbrecher UP, Parthasarathy S, Leake DS, et al: Modification of low density lipoprotein by endothelial cells involves lipid peroxidation and degradation of low density lipoprotein phospolipids. *Proc Natl Acad Sci U S A* 81:3883, 1984.

89. Steinberg D, Parthasarathy S, Carew TE, et al: Beyond cholesterol. Modifications of low-density lipoprotein that increase its atherogenicity. *N Engl J Med* 320:915, 1989.

90. Shaw PX, Horkko S, Chang MK, et al: Natural antibodies with the T15 idiotype may act in atherosclerosis, apoptotic clearance, and protective immunity. *J Clin Invest* 105:1731, 2000.

91. Tsimikas S, Palinski W, Witztum JL: Circulating autoantibodies to oxidized LDL correlate with arterial accumulation and depletion of oxidized LDL in LDL receptor-deficient mice. *Arterioscler Thromb Vasc Biol* 21:95, 2001.

92. Palinski W, Ord VA, Plump AS, et al: ApoE-deficient mice are a model of lipoprotein oxidation in atherogenesis. Demonstration of oxidation-specific epitopes in lesions and high titers of autoantibodies to malondialdehyde-lysine in serum. *Arterioscler Thromb* 14:605, 1994.

93. Ameli S, Hultgardh-Nilsson A, Regnstrom J, et al: Effect of immunization with homologous LDL and oxidized LDL on early atherosclerosis in hypercholesterolemic rabbits. *Arterioscler Thromb Vasc Biol* 16:1074, 1996.

94. Freigang S, Horkko S, Miller E, et al: Immunization of LDL receptor-deficient mice with homologous malondialdehyde-modified and native LDL reduces progression of atherosclerosis by mechanisms other than induction of high titers of antibodies to oxidative neoepitopes. *Arteriocler Thromb Vasc Biol* 18:1972, 1998.

95. Zhou X, Caligiuri G, Hamsten A, et al: LDL immunization induces T-cell-dependent antibody formation and protection against atherosclerosis. *Arterioscler Thromb Vasc Biol* 21:108, 2001.

96. Mehrabian M, Allayee H, Wong J, et al: Identification of 5-lipoxygenase as a major gene contributing to atherosclerosis susceptibility in mice. *Circ Res* 91:120, 2002.

97. Cyrus T, Witztum JL, Rader DJ, et al: Disruption of the 12/15-lipoxygenase gene diminishes atherosclerosis in apo E-deficient mice. *J Clin Invest* 103:1597, 1999.

98. Harats D, Shaish A, George J, et al: Overexpression of 15-lipoxygenase in vascular endothelium accelerates early atherosclerosis in LDL receptor-deficient mice. *Arterioscler Thromb Vasc Biol* 20:2100, 2000.

99. Schwenke DC: Comparison of aorta and pulmonary artery: I. Early cholesterol accumulation and relative susceptibility to atheromatous lesions. *Circ Res* 81:338, 1997.

100. Schwenke DC: Comparison of aorta and pulmonary artery: II. LDL transport and metabolism correlate with susceptibility to atherosclerosis. *Circ Res* 81:346, 1997.

101. Camejo G, Hurt-Camejo E, Wiklund O, Bondjers G: Association of apo B lipoproteins with arterial proteoglycans: Pathological significance and molecular basis. *Atherosclerosis* 139:205, 1998.

102. Rajavashisth TB, Andalibi A, Territo MC, et al: Induction of endothelial cell expression of granulocyte and macrophage colony-stimulating factors by modified low-density lipoproteins. *Nature* 344:254, 1990.

103. MRC/BHF Heart Protection Study of antioxidant vitamin supplementation in 20,536 high-risk individuals: A randomised placebo-controlled trial. *Lancet* 360:23, 2002.

104. Brown BG, Zhao XQ, Chait A, et al: Simvastatin and niacin, antioxidant vitamins, or the combination for the prevention of coronary disease. *N Engl J Med* 345:1583, 2001.

105. Gordon T, Kannel WB, Castelli WP, Dawber TR: Lipoproteins, cardiovascular disease, and death. The Framingham study. *Arch Intern Med* 141:1128, 1981.

106. Rader DJ: Regulation of reverse cholesterol transport and clinical implications. *Am J Cardiol* 92(4A):42J, 2003.

107. Tangirala RK, Tsukamoto K, Chun SH, et al: Regression of atherosclerosis induced by liver-directed gene transfer of apolipoprotein A-I in mice. *Circulation* 100:1816, 1999.

108. Zhang Y, Zanotti I, Reilly MP, et al: Overexpression of apolipoprotein A-I promotes reverse transport of cholesterol from macrophages to feces in vivo. *Circulation* 108:661, 2003.

109. Rader DJ: High-density lipoproteins and atherosclerosis. *Am J Cardiol* 90(8A):62i, 2002.

110. Shih DM, Gu L, Xia YR, et al: Mice lacking serum paraoxonase are susceptible to organophosphate toxicity and atherosclerosis. *Nature* 394:284, 1998.

111. Mackness MI, Mackness B, Durrington PN, et al: Paraoxonase and coronary heart disease. *Curr Opin Lipidol* 9:319, 1998.

112. Brousseau ME, Schaefer EJ, Wolfe ML, et al: Effects of an inhibitor of cholesteryl ester transfer protein on HDL cholesterol. *N Engl J Med* 350:1505, 2004.

113. Nissen SE, Tsunoda T, Tuzcu EM, et al: Effect of recombinant ApoA-I Milano on coronary atherosclerosis in patients with acute coronary syndromes: A randomized controlled trial. *JAMA* 290:2292, 2003.

114. Navab M, Anantharamaiah GM, Reddy ST, et al: Human apolipoprotein AI mimetic peptides for the treatment of atherosclerosis. *Curr Opin Investig Drugs* 4:1100, 2003.

115. Mach F, Schonbeck U, Sukhova GK, et al: Reduction of atherosclerosis in mice by inhibition of CD40 signaling. *Nature* 394:200, 1998.

116. Cipollone F, Mezzetti A, Porreca E, et al: Association between enhanced soluble CD40L and prothrombotic state in hypercholesterolemia effects of statin therapy. *Circulation* 106:399, 2002.

117. Mallat Z, Gojova A, Marchiol-Fournigault C, et al: Inhibition of transforming growth factor-beta signaling accelerates atherosclerosis and induces an unstable plaque phenotype in mice. *Circ Res* 89:930, 2001.

118. Libby P, Egan D, Skarlatos S: Roles of infectious agents in atherosclerosis and restenosis: An assessment of the evidence and need for future research. *Circulation* 96:4095, 1997.

119. Beck JD, Pankow J, Tyroler HA, Offenbacher S: Dental infections and atherosclerosis. *Am Heart J* 138(5 Pt 2):S528, 1999.

120. Mayr M, Kiechl S, Willeit J, et al: Infections, immunity, and atherosclerosis: Associations of antibodies to Chlamydia pneumoniae, Helicobacter pylori, and cytomegalovirus with immune reactions to heat-shock protein 60 and carotid or femoral atherosclerosis. *Circulation* 102:833, 2000.

121. Caligiuri G, Nicoletti A, Poirier B, Hansson GK: Protective immunity against atherosclerosis carried by B cells of hypercholesterolemic mice. *J Clin Invest* 109:745, 2002.

122. Robinette CD, Fraumeni JF Jr: Splenectomy and subsequent mortality in veterans of the 1939-1945 war. *Lancet* 2:127, 1977.

123. Stary HC: Natural history and histological classification of atherosclerotic lesions: An update. *Arterioscler Thromb Vasc Biol* 20:1177, 2000.

124. Falk E: Plaque rupture with severe pre-existing stenosis precipitating coronary thrombosis. Characteristics of coronary atherosclerotic plaques underlying fatal occlusive thrombi. *Br Heart J* 50:127, 1983.

125. Davies MJ, Thomas AC: Plaque fissuring—The cause of acute myocardial infarction, sudden ischaemic death, and crescendo angina. *Br Heart J* 53:363, 1985.

126. Muller JE, Tofler GH, Stone PH: Circadian variation and triggers of onset of acute cardiovascular disease. *Circulation* 79:733, 1989.

127. Muller JE, Abela GS, Nesto RW, Tofler GH: Triggers, acute risk factors, and vulnerable plaques: The lexicon of a new frontier. *J Am Coll Cardiol* 23:809, 1994.

128. Naghavi M, Libby P, Falk E, et al: From vulnerable plaque to vulnerable patient: A call for new definitions and risk assessment strategies: Part I. *Circulation* 108:1664, 2003.

129. Beckman JA, Ganz J, Creager MA, et al: Relationship of clinical presentation and calcification of culprit coronary artery stenoses. *Arterioscler Thromb Vasc Biol* 21:1618, 2001.

130. Glagov S, Weisenberg E, Zarins CK, et al: Compensatory enlargement of human atherosclerotic coronary arteries. *N Engl J Med* 316:1371, 1987.

131. Virmani R, Kolodgie FD, Burke AP, et al: Lessons from sudden coronary death: A comprehensive morphological classification scheme for atherosclerotic lesions. *Arterioscler Thromb Vasc Biol* 20:1262, 2000.

132. Casscells W, Naghavi M, Willerson JT: Vulnerable atherosclerotic plaque: A multifocal disease. *Circulation* 107:2072, 2003.

133. Uchida Y, Nakamura F, Tomaru T, et al: Prediction of acute coronary syndromes by percutaneous coronary angioscopy in patients with stable angina. *Am Heart J* 130:195, 1995.

134. Naghavi M, Libby P, Falk E, et al: From vulnerable plaque to vulnerable patient: A call for new definitions and risk assessment strategies: Part II. *Circulation* 108:1772, 2003.

135. Schoen FJ: Blood vessels, in *Pathologic Basis of Disease*, edited by V Kumar, AK Abbas, N Fausto, p 511. Elsevier Saunders, Philadelphia, 2005.

136. Karnicki K, Owen WG, Miller RS, McBane RD: Factors contributing to individual propensity for arterial thrombosis. *Arterioscler Thromb Vasc Biol* 22:1495, 2002.

137. Wagner DD, Burger PC: Platelets in inflammation and thrombosis. *Arterioscler Thromb Vasc Biol* 23:2131, 2003.

138. Schafer AI: The primary and secondary hypercoagulable states, in *Molecular Mechanisms of Hypercoagulable States*, edited by AI Schafer, p 1. Austin: Landes Bioscience, 1997.

139. Badimon L: Atherosclerosis and thrombosis: Lessons from animal models. *Thromb Haemost* 86:356, 2001.

140. Robbie L, Libby P: Inflammation and atherothrombosis. *Ann N Y Acad Sci* 947:167, 2001.

141. Khrenov AV, Ananyeva NM, Griffin JH, Saenko EL: Coagulation pathways in atherothrombosis. *Trends Cardiovasc Med* 12:317, 2002.

142. Smith EB: Fibrin deposition and fibrin degradation products in atherosclerotic plaques. *Thromb Res* 75:329, 1994.

143. Wootton DM, Ku DN: Fluid mechanics of vascular systems, diseases, and thrombosis. *Annu Rev Biomed Eng* 1:299, 1999.

144. He X, Ku DN: Pulsatile flow in the human left coronary artery bifurcation: Average conditions. *J Biomech Eng* 118:74, 1996.

145. Ku DN, Giddens DP, Zarins CK, Glagov S: Pulsatile flow and atherosclerosis in the human carotid bifurcation. Positive correlation between plaque location and low oscillating shear stress. *Arteriosclerosis* 5:293, 1985.

146. Corti R, Fuster V, Badimon JJ: Pathogenetic concepts of acute coronary syndromes. *J Am Coll Cardiol* 41(4 suppl S):7S, 2003.

147. Badimon JJ, Ortiz AF, Meyer B, et al: Different response to balloon angioplasty of carotid and coronary arteries: Effects on acute platelet deposition and intimal thickening. *Atherosclerosis* 140:307, 1998.

148. Rosenberg RD: Vascular-bed-specific hemostasis and hypercoagulable states: Clinical utility of activation peptide assays in predicting thrombotic events in different clinical populations. *Thromb Haemost* 86:41, 2001.

149. Aird WC: Endothelial cell heterogeneity. *Crit Care Med* 31(suppl 4):S221, 2003.

150. Gittenberger-De Groot AC, DeRuiter MC, Bergwerff M, Poelmann RE: Smooth muscle cell origin and its relation to heterogeneity in development and disease. *Arterioscler Thromb Vasc Biol* 19:1589, 1999.

151. Fitzgerald DJ: Vascular biology of thrombosis: The role of platelet-vessel wall adhesion. *Neurology* 57(5 suppl 2):S1, 2001.

152. Giesen PL, Rauch U, Bohrmann B, et al: Blood-borne tissue factor: Another view of thrombosis. *Proc Natl Acad Sci U S A* 96:2311, 1999.

153. Freyssinet JM: Cellular microparticles: What are they bad or good for? *J Thromb Haemost* 1:1655, 2003.

154. Tunick PA, Kronzon I: Embolism from the aorta: Atheroemboli and thromboemboli. *Curr Treat Options Cardiovasc Med* 3:181, 2001.

155. Rauch U, Osende JI, Fuster V, et al: Thrombus formation on atherosclerotic plaques: Pathogenesis and clinical consequences. *Ann Intern Med* 134:224, 2001.

156. Amarenco P, Cohen A, Tzourio C, et al: Atherosclerotic disease of the aortic arch and the risk of ischemic stroke. *N Engl J Med* 331:1474, 1994.

157. Cohen A, Tzourio C, Bertrand B, et al: Aortic plaque morphology and vascular events: A follow-up study in patients with ischemic stroke. FAPS Investigators. French Study of Aortic Plaques in Stroke. *Circulation* 96:3838, 1997.

158. Ruggeri ZM: Platelets in atherothrombosis. *Nat Med* 8:1227, 2002.

159. Kulkarni S, Dopheide SM, Yap CL, et al: A revised model of platelet aggregation. *J Clin Invest* 105:783, 2000.

160. Wagner CT, Kroll MH, Chow TW, et al: Epinephrine and shear stress synergistically induce platelet aggregation via a mechanism that partially bypasses VWF-GP IB interactions. *Biorheology* 33:209, 1996.

161. Andre P, Prasad KS, Denis CV, et al: CD40L stabilizes arterial thrombi by a beta3 integrin-dependent mechanism. *Nat Med* 8:247, 2002.

162. Moons AH, Levi M, Peters RJ: Tissue factor and coronary artery disease. *Cardiovasc Res* 53:313, 2002.

163. Toschi V, Gallo R, Lettino M, et al: Tissue factor modulates the thrombogenicity of human atherosclerotic plaques. *Circulation* 95:594, 1997.

164. Mach F, Schonbeck U, Bonnefoy JY, et al: Activation of monocyte/macrophage functions related to acute atheroma complication by ligation of CD40: Induction of collagenase, stromelysin, and tissue factor. *Circulation* 96:396, 1997.

165. Tedgui A, Mallat Z: Apoptosis as a determinant of atherothrombosis. *Thromb Haemost* 86:420, 2001.

166. Moyer MP, Tracy RP, Tracy PB, et al: Plasma lipoproteins support prothrombinase and other procoagulant enzymatic complexes. *Arterioscler Thromb Vasc Biol* 18:458, 1998.

167. Khrenov A, Sarafanov A, Ananyeva N, et al: Molecular basis for different ability of low-density and high-density lipoproteins to support activity of the intrinsic Xase complex. *Thromb Res* 105:87, 2002.

168. Ananyeva NM, Kouiavskaia DV, Shima M, Saenko EL: Intrinsic pathway of blood coagulation contributes to thrombogenicity of atherosclerotic plaque. *Blood* 99:4475, 2002.

169. Soejima H, Ogawa H, Yasue H, et al: Heightened tissue factor associated with tissue factor pathway inhibitor and prognosis in patients with unstable angina. *Circulation* 99:2908, 1999.

170. Endler G, Mannhalter C: Polymorphisms in coagulation factor genes and their impact on arterial and venous thrombosis. *Clin Chim Acta* 330:31, 2003.

171. Sueishi K, Ichikawa K, Kato K, et al: Atherosclerosis: Coagulation and fibrinolysis. *Semin Thromb Hemost* 24:255, 1998.

172. Koenig W, Rothenbacher D, Hoffmeister A, et al: Plasma fibrin D-dimer levels and risk of stable coronary artery disease: Results of a large case-control study. *Arterioscler Thromb Vasc Biol* 21:1701, 2001.

173. Sramek A, Kriek M, Rosendaal FR: Decreased mortality of ischaemic heart disease among carriers of haemophilia. *Lancet* 362:351, 2003.

174. Sramek A, Reiber JH, Gerrits WB, Rosendaal FR: Decreased coagulability has no clinically relevant effect on atherogenesis: Observations in individuals with a hereditary bleeding tendency. *Circulation* 104:762, 2001.

175. Haverkate F: Levels of haemostatic factors, arteriosclerosis, and cardiovascular disease. *Vasc Pharmacol* 39:109, 2002.

176. Badimon L, Badimon JJ, Chesebro JH, Fuster V: von Willebrand factor and cardiovascular disease. *Thromb Haemost* 70:111, 1993.

177. Methia N, Andre P, Denis CV, et al: Localized reduction of atherosclerosis in von Willebrand factor-deficient mice. *Blood* 98:1424, 2001.

178. Bilora F, Dei RC, Girolami B, et al: Do hemophilia A and von Willebrand disease protect against carotid atherosclerosis? A comparative study between coagulopathics and normal subjects by means of carotid echo-color Doppler scan. *Clin Appl Thromb Hemost* 5:232, 1999.

179. van der Meer IM, Brouwers GJ, Bulk S, et al: Genetic variability of von Willebrand factor and risk of coronary heart disease: The Rotterdam Study. *Br J Haematol* 124:343, 2004.

180. Simmonds RE, Hermida J, Rezende SM, Lane DA: Haemostatic genetic risk factors in arterial thrombosis. *Thromb Haemost* 86:374, 2001.

181. Williams MS, Bray PF: Genetics of arterial prothrombotic risk states. *Exp Biol Med (Maywood)* 226:409, 2001.

182. Weiss EJ, Bray PF, Tayback M, et al: A polymorphism of a platelet glycoprotein receptor as an inherited risk factor for coronary thrombosis. *N Engl J Med* 334:1090, 1996.

183. Birk AV, Leno E, Robertson HD, et al: Interaction between ATP and catecholamines in stimulation of platelet aggregation. *Am J Physiol Heart Circ Physiol* 284:H619, 2003.

184. Ikarugi H, Taka T, Nakajima S, et al: Norepinephrine, but not epinephrine, enhances platelet reactivity and coagulation after exercise in humans. *J Appl Physiol* 86:133, 1999.

185. Rauch U, Osende JI, Chesebro JH, et al: Statins and cardiovascular diseases: The multiple effects of lipid-lowering therapy by statins. *Atherosclerosis* 153:181, 2000.

186. Alpert JS, Thygesen K, Antman E, Bassand JP: Myocardial infarction redefined—A consensus document of The Joint European Society of Cardiology/American College of Cardiology Committee for the redefinition of myocardial infarction. *J Am Coll Cardiol* 36:959, 2000.

187. Braunwald E, Antman EM, Beasley JW, et al: ACC/AHA 2002 guideline update for the management of patients with unstable angina and non-ST-segment elevation myocardial infarction—Summary article: A report of the American College of Cardiology/American Heart Association task force on practice guidelines (Committee on the Management of Patients With Unstable Angina). *J Am Coll Cardiol* 40:1366, 2002.

188. Fesmire FM, Percy RF, Bardoner JB, et al: Usefulness of automated serial 12-lead ECG monitoring during the initial emergency department evaluation of patients with chest pain. *Ann Emerg Med* 31:3, 1998.

189. Pope JH, Ruthazer R, Beshansky JR, et al: Clinical features of emergency department patients presenting with symptoms suggestive of acute cardiac ischemia: A multicenter study. *J Thromb Thrombolysis* 6:63, 1998.

190. Ryan TJ, Antman EM, Brooks NH, et al: 1999 Update: ACC/AHA guidelines for the management of patients with acute myocardial infarction. A report of the American College of Cardiology/American Heart Association Task Force on Practice Guidelines (Committee on Management of Acute Myocardial Infarction). *J Am Coll Cardiol* 34:890, 1999.

191. Antiplatelet Trialists' Collaboration: Collaborative overview of randomised trials of antiplatelet therapy—I: Prevention of death, myocardial infarction, and stroke by prolonged antiplatelet therapy in various categories of patients. *BMJ* 308:81, 1994.

192. Grines CL, Browne KF, Marco J, et al: A comparison of immediate angioplasty with thrombolytic therapy for acute myocardial infarction. The Primary Angioplasty in Myocardial Infarction Study Group. *N Engl J Med* 328:673, 1993.

193. Le May MR, Labinaz M, Davies RF, et al: Stenting versus thrombolysis in acute myocardial infarction trial (STAT). *J Am Coll Cardiol* 37:985, 2001.

194. Keeley EC, Boura JA, Grines CL: Primary angioplasty versus intravenous thrombolytic therapy for acute myocardial infarction: A quantitative review of 23 randomised trials. *Lancet* 361:13, 2003.

195. Keeley EC, Grines CL: Primary coronary intervention for acute myocardial infarction. *JAMA* 291:736, 2004.

196. Boersma E, Mercado N, Poldermans D, et al: Acute myocardial infarction. *Lancet* 361:847, 2003.

197. Califf RM, White HD, Van de WF, et al: One-year results from the Global Utilization of Streptokinase and TPA for Occluded Coronary Arteries (GUSTO-I) trial. GUSTO-I Investigators. *Circulation* 94:1233, 1996.

198. Llevadot J, Giugliano RP, Antman EM: Bolus fibrinolytic therapy in acute myocardial infarction. *JAMA* 286:442, 2001.

199. Brieger DB, Mak KH, White HD, et al: Benefit of early sustained reperfusion in patients with prior myocardial infarction (the GUSTO-I trial). Global Utilization of Streptokinase and TPA for occluded arteries. *Am J Cardiol* 81:282, 1998.

200. Lincoff AM, Califf RM, Van de WF, et al: Mortality at 1 year with combination platelet glycoprotein IIb/IIIa inhibition and reduced-dose fibrinolytic therapy vs conventional fibrinolytic therapy for acute myocardial infarction: GUSTO V randomized trial. *JAMA* 288:2130, 2002.

201. Wallentin L, Bergstrand L, Dellborg M, et al: Low molecular weight heparin (dalteparin) compared to unfractionated heparin as an adjunct to rt-PA (alteplase) for improvement of coronary artery patency in acute myocardial infarction-the ASSENT Plus study. Eur Heart J 24:897, 2003.

202. Savonitto S, Armstrong PW, Lincoff AM, et al: Risk of intracranial haemorrhage with combined fibrinolytic and glycoprotein IIb/IIIa inhibitor therapy in acute myocardial infarction. Dichotomous response as a function of age in the GUSTO V trial. Eur Heart J 24:1807, 2003.

203. Harrington RA, Becker RC, Ezekowitz M, et al: Antithrombotic therapy for coronary artery disease. The Seventh ACCP Conference on Antithrombotic and Thrombolytic Therapy. Chest 126(suppl 3):513S, 2004.

204. Randomised double-blind trial of fixed low-dose warfarin with aspirin after myocardial infarction. Coumadin Aspirin Reinfarction Study (CARS) Investigators. Lancet 350:389, 1997.

205. Cannon CP, Braunwald E, McCabe CH, et al: Comparison of Intensive and Moderate Lipid Lowering with Statins after Acute Coronary Syndromes. N Engl J Med 350:1495, 2004.

206. Antithrombotic Trialists' Collaboration: Collaborative meta-analysis of randomised trials of antiplatelet therapy for prevention of death, myocardial infarction, and stroke in high risk patients. BMJ 324:71, 2002.

207. Lewis HD Jr, Davis JW, Archibald DG, et al: Protective effects of aspirin against acute myocardial infarction and death in men with unstable angina. Results of a Veterans Administration Cooperative Study. N Engl J Med 309:396, 1983.

208. Cairns JA, Gent M, Singer J, et al: Aspirin, sulfinpyrazone, or both in unstable angina. Results of a Canadian multicenter trial. N Engl J Med 313:1369, 1985.

209. Boersma E, Harrington RA, Moliterno DJ, et al: Platelet glycoprotein IIb/IIIa inhibitors in acute coronary syndromes: A meta-analysis of all major randomised clinical trials. Lancet 359:189, 2002.

210. McKee SA, Sane DC, Deliargyris EN: Aspirin resistance in cardiovascular disease: A review of prevalence, mechanisms, and clinical significance. Thromb Haemost 88:711, 2002.

211. Eikelboom JW, Hirsh J, Weitz JI, et al: Aspirin-resistant thromboxane biosynthesis and the risk of myocardial infarction, stroke, or cardiovascular death in patients at high risk for cardiovascular events. Circulation 105:1650, 2002.

212. Gum PA, Kottke-Marchant K, Welsh PA, et al: A prospective, blinded determination of the natural history of aspirin resistance among stable patients with cardiovascular disease. J Am Coll Cardiol 41:961, 2003.

213. Schafer AI: Genetic and acquired determinants of individual variability of response to antiplatelet drugs. Circulation 108:910, 2003.

214. CAPRIE Steering Committee: A randomised, blinded, trial of clopidogrel versus aspirin in patients at risk of ischaemic events (CAPRIE). Lancet 348:1329, 1996.

215. Yusuf S, Zhao F, Mehta SR, et al: Effects of clopidogrel in addition to aspirin in patients with acute coronary syndromes without ST-segment elevation. N Engl J Med 345:494, 2001.

216. Mehta SR: Aspirin and clopidogrel in patients with ACS undergoing PCI: CURE and PCI-CURE. J Invasive Cardiol 15(suppl B):17B, 2003.

217. Hongo RH, Ley J, Dick SE, Yee RR: The effect of clopidogrel in combination with aspirin when given before coronary artery bypass grafting. J Am Coll Cardiol 40:231, 2002.

218. Antoniucci D, Rodriguez A, Hempel A, et al: A randomized trial comparing primary infarct artery stenting with or without abciximab in acute myocardial infarction. J Am Coll Cardiol 42:1879, 2003.

219. Antoniucci D, Migliorini A, Parodi G, et al: Abciximab-Supported infarct artery stent implantation for acute myocardial infarction and long-term survival. A prospective, multicenter, randomized trial comparing infarct artery stenting plus abciximab with stenting alone. Circulation 109:1704, 2004.

220. Kandzari DE, Hasselblad V, Tcheng JE, et al: Improved clinical outcomes with abciximab therapy in acute myocardial infarction: A systematic overview of randomized clinical trials. Am Heart J 147:457, 2004.

221. Topol EJ, Moliterno DJ, Herrmann HC, et al: Comparison of two platelet glycoprotein IIb/IIIa inhibitors, tirofiban and abciximab, for the prevention of ischemic events with percutaneous coronary revascularization. N Engl J Med 344:1888, 2001.

222. Huynh T, Theroux P, Snapinn S, Wan Y: Effect of platelet glycoprotein IIb/IIIa receptor blockade with tirofiban on adverse cardiac events in women with unstable angina/non-ST-elevation myocardial infarction (PRISM-PLUS Study). Am Heart J 146:668, 2003.

223. Servoss SJ, Wan Y, Snapinn SM, et al: Tirofiban therapy for patients with acute coronary syndromes and prior coronary artery bypass grafting in the PRISM-PLUS trial. Am J Cardiol 93:843, 2004.

224. Blankenship JC, Sigmon KN, Pieper KS, et al: Effect of eptifibatide on angiographic complications during percutaneous coronary intervention in the IMPACT (Integrilin to Minimize Platelet Aggregation and Coronary Thrombosis) II Trial. Am J Cardiol 88:969, 2001.

225. Nguyen CM, Harrington RA: Glycoprotein IIb/IIIa receptor antagonists: A comparative review of their use in percutaneous coronary intervention. Am J Cardiovasc Drugs 3:423, 2003.

226. Warkentin TE, Greinacher A: Heparin-induced thrombocytopenia: recognition, treatment, and prevention. The Seventh ACCP Conference on Antithrombotic and Thrombolytic Therapy. Chest 126(suppl 3):311S, 2004.

227. Braunwald E: Application of current guidelines to the management of unstable angina and non-ST-elevation myocardial infarction. Circulation 108(16 suppl 1):III28, 2003.

228. Braunwald E, Antman EM, Beasley JW, et al: ACC/AHA guidelines for the management of patients with unstable angina and non-ST-segment elevation myocardial infarction. A report of the American College of Cardiology/American Heart Association Task Force on Practice Guidelines (Committee on the Management of Patients With Unstable Angina). J Am Coll Cardiol 36:970, 2000.

229. Direct Thrombin Inhibitor Trialists' Collaborative Group: Direct thrombin inhibitors in acute coronary syndromes: Principal results of a meta-analysis based on individual patients' data. Lancet 359:294, 2002.

230. Eikelboom JW, French J: Management of patients with acute coronary syndromes: What is the clinical role of direct thrombin inhibitors? Drugs 62:1839, 2002.

231. Gibbons RJ, Abrams J, Chatterjee K, et al: ACC/AHA 2002 guideline update for the management of patients with chronic stable angina—Summary article: A report of the American College of Cardiology/American Heart Association Task Force on practice guidelines (Committee on the Management of Patients With Chronic Stable Angina). J Am Coll Cardiol 41:159, 2003.

232. Kaiser GC, Davis KB, Fisher LD, et al: Survival following coronary artery bypass grafting in patients with severe angina pectoris (CASS). An observational study. J Thorac Cardiovasc Surg 89:513, 1985.

233. Mintz GS, Kimura T, Nobuyoshi M, Leon MB: Intravascular ultrasound assessment of the relation between early and late changes in arterial area and neointimal hyperplasia after percutaneous transluminal coronary angioplasty and directional coronary atherectomy. Am J Cardiol 83:1518, 1999.

234. Wilensky RL, Tanguay JF, Ito S, et al: Heparin infusion prior to stenting (HIPS) trial: Final results of a prospective, randomized, controlled trial evaluating the effects of local vascular delivery on intimal hyperplasia. Am Heart J 139:1061, 2000.

235. Morice MC, Serruys PW, Sousa JE, et al: A randomized comparison of a sirolimus-eluting stent with a standard stent for coronary revascularization. N Engl J Med 346:1773, 2002.

236. Moses JW, Leon MB, Popma JJ, et al: Sirolimus-eluting stents versus standard stents in patients with stenosis in a native coronary artery. N Engl J Med 349:1315, 2003.

237. Schofer J, Schluter M, Gershlick AH, et al: Sirolimus-eluting stents for treatment of patients with long atherosclerotic lesions in small coronary arteries: Double-blind, randomised controlled trial (E-SIRIUS). *Lancet* 362:1093, 2003.

238. Schampaert E, Cohen EA, Schluter M, et al: The Canadian study of the sirolimus-eluting stent in the treatment of patients with long de novo lesions in small native coronary arteries (C-SIRIUS). *J Am Coll Cardiol* 43:1110, 2004.

239. Mohler ER III: Peripheral arterial disease: Identification and implications. *Arch Intern Med* 163:2306, 2003.

240. Weitz JI, Byrne J, Clagett GP, et al: Diagnosis and treatment of chronic arterial insufficiency of the lower extremities: A critical review. *Circulation* 94:3026, 1996.

241. Carter SA: Clinical measurement of systolic pressures in limbs with arterial occlusive disease. *JAMA* 207:1869, 1969.

242. Darling RC, Raines JK, Brener BJ, Austen WG: Quantitative segmental pulse volume recorder: A clinical tool. *Surgery* 72:873, 1972.

243. Symes JF, Graham AM, Mousseau M: Doppler waveform analysis versus segmental pressure and pulse-volume recording: Assessment of occlusive disease in the lower extremity. *Can J Surg* 27:345, 1984.

244. Kohler TR, Nance DR, Cramer MM, et al: Duplex scanning for diagnosis of aortoiliac and femoropopliteal disease: A prospective study. *Circulation* 76:1074, 1987.

245. Perreault P, Edelman MA, Baum RA, et al: MR angiography with gadofosveset trisodium for peripheral vascular disease: Phase II trial. *Radiology* 229:811, 2003.

246. Mohler ER III: Treatment of risk factors and antiplatelet therapy, in *Peripheral Arterial Disease: Diagnosis and Treatment*, edited by JD Coffman, RT Eberhardt, p 159. Humana Press, Totowa, NJ, 2002.

247. Malinow MR, Kang SS, Taylor LM, et al: Prevalence of hyperhomocyst(e)inemia in patients with peripheral arterial occlusive disease. *Circulation* 79:1180, 1989.

248. Goldhaber SZ, Manson JE, Stampfer MJ, et al: Low-dose aspirin and subsequent peripheral arterial surgery in the Physicians' Health Study. *Lancet* 340:143, 1992.

249. Girolami B, Bernardi E, Prins MH, et al: Antithrombotic drugs in the primary medical management of intermittent claudication: A meta-analysis. *Thromb Haemost* 81:715, 1999.

250. Gardner AW, Poehlman ET: Exercise rehabilitation programs for the treatment of claudication pain. A meta-analysis. *JAMA* 274:975, 1995.

251. Reilly MP, Mohler ER III: Cilostazol: Treatment of intermittent claudication. *Ann Pharmacother* 35:48, 2001.

252. Wilhite DB, Comerota AJ, Schmieder FA, et al: Managing PAD with multiple platelet inhibitors: The effect of combination therapy on bleeding time. *J Vasc Surg* 38:710, 2003.

253. Bogousslavsky J, Regli F, van Melle G: Risk factors and concomitants of internal carotid artery occlusion or stenosis. A controlled study of 159 cases. *Arch Neurol* 42:864, 1985.

254. Whisnant JP: Modeling of risk factors for ischemic stroke. The Willis Lecture. *Stroke* 28:1840, 1997.

255. Heart Protection Study Collaborative Group: MRC/BHF Heart Protection Study of cholesterol lowering with simvastatin in 20,536 high-risk individuals: A randomised placebo-controlled trial. *Lancet* 360:7, 2002.

256. Mohler ER III, Delanty N, Rader DJ, Raps EC: Statins and cerebrovascular disease: Plaque attack to prevent brain attack. *Vasc Med* 4:269, 1999.

257. Moore WS, Barnett HJ, Beebe HG, et al: Guidelines for carotid endarterectomy. A multidisciplinary consensus statement from the Ad Hoc Committee, American Heart Association. *Circulation* 91:566, 1995.

258. Rothwell PM, Eliasziw M, Gutnikov SA, et al: Analysis of pooled data from the randomised controlled trials of endarterectomy for symptomatic carotid stenosis. *Lancet* 361:107, 2003.

259. Brown MM: Carotid artery stenting—Evolution of a technique to rival carotid endarterectomy. *Am J Med* 116:273, 2004.

260. Diener HC, Cunha L, Forbes C, et al: European Stroke Prevention Study 2. Dipyridamole and acetylsalicylic acid in the secondary prevention of stroke. *J Neurol Sci* 143:1, 1996.

261. Iso H, Sato S, Umemura U, et al: Linoleic acid, other fatty acids, and the risk of stroke. *Stroke* 33:2086, 2002.

262. He K, Rimm EB, Merchant A, et al: Fish consumption and risk of stroke in men. *JAMA* 288:3130, 2002.

263. Donohue KG, Saap L, Falanga V: Cholesterol crystal embolization: An atherosclerotic disease with frequent and varied cutaneous manifestations. *J Eur Acad Dermatol Venereol* 17:504, 2003.

264. Voetsch B, Afshar-Kharghan V, Loscalzo J, Schafer AI: Less common thrombotic and embolic disorders, in *Thrombosis and Hemorrhage*, edited by J Loscalzo, AI Schafer, p 707. Lippincott Williams & Wilkins, Philadelphia, 2003.

265. Bashore TM, Gehrig T: Cholesterol emboli after invasive cardiac procedures. *J Am Coll Cardiol* 42:217, 2003.

266. Funabiki K, Masuoka H, Shimizu H, et al: Cholesterol crystal embolization (CCE) after cardiac catheterization: A case report and a review of 36 cases in the Japanese literature. *Jpn Heart J* 44:767, 2003.

267. Applebaum RM, Kronzon I: Evaluation and management of cholesterol embolization and the blue toe syndrome. *Curr Opin Cardiol* 11:533, 1996.

FIBRINOLYSIS AND THROMBOLYSIS

KATHERINE A. HAJJAR

CHARLES W. FRANCIS

An understanding of the molecular mechanisms of fibrinolysis has led to major advances in fibrinolytic and antifibrinolytic therapy. Characterization of the genes for all the major fibrinolytic proteins has revealed the structure and function of the relevant serine proteases, their inhibitors, and their receptors. Analysis of the cell biology of plasmin generation has led to an appreciation for the fundamental role of cellular receptors and other cofactors. The development of genetically engineered animals deficient in one or more fibrinolytic protein(s) has demonstrated unexpected roles for these proteins in intravascular and extravascular settings. In addition, genetic analysis of human deficiency syndromes has revealed specific mutations that result in human disorders reflective of either fibrinolytic deficiency with thrombosis or fibrinolytic excess with hemorrhage. All of these advances have led to the development of more effective and safer protocols for fibrinolytic therapy and for the rational use of antifibrinolytic agents under certain specific circumstances.

BASIC CONCEPTS OF FIBRINOLYSIS

Fibrin, the insoluble end product of the action of thrombin on fibrinogen, is found in intravascular and extravascular settings. In response to injury, cross-linked fibrin, the final product of the coagulation cascade, is deposited in tissues and blood vessels. Once fibrin is no longer needed, the fibrinolytic system is activated, converting fibrin to its soluble degradation products through the action of the serine protease, plasmin (Fig. 127-1, A).

Under physiologic conditions, fibrinolysis is precisely regulated by the measured participation of activators, inhibitors, and cofactors.[1] In addition, cell surface receptors provide specialized, protected en-

Acronyms and abbreviations that appear in this chapter include: α_2-PI, α_2-plasmin inhibitor; aPTT, activated partial thromboplastin time; ASK, Australian Streptokinase; ATLANTIS, Alteplase Thrombolysis for Acute Noninterventional Therapy in Ischemic Stroke; bFGF, basic fibroblast growth factor; cAMP, cyclic adenosine monophosphate; CT, computed tomography; DIC, disseminated intravascular coagulation; DNA, deoxyribonucleic acid; EACA, ε-aminocaproic acid; ECASS, European Cooperative Acute Stroke Study; FDA, Food and Drug Administration; HC, homocysteine; IL, interleukin; KIU, kallikrein inhibitor unit; LDL, low-density lipoprotein; LRP, low-density lipoprotein receptor-related protein; MAST-E, Multicenter Acute Stroke Trial—Europe; MAST-I, Multicenter Acute Stroke Trial—Italy; MI, myocardial infarction; MMP, matrix metalloproteinase; MRI, magnetic resonance imaging; mRNA, messenger ribonucleic acid; MT1-MMP, membrane type 1 matrix metalloproteinase; PAI, plasminogen-activator inhibitor; PROACT, Prolyse in Acute Cerebral Thromboembolism; PT, prothrombin time; STILE, Surgery versus Thrombolysis for Ischemia of the Lower Extremity; TAFI, thrombin-activatable fibrinolysis inhibitor; TGF-β, transforming growth factor β; TOPAS, Thrombolysis or Peripheral Arterial Surgery; t-PA, tissue-plasminogen activator; u-PA, urokinase-plasminogen activator; u-PAR, urokinase-plasminogen activator receptor.

vironments where plasmin can be generated without compromise by circulating inhibitors[2] (Fig. 127-1, B). Endothelial cells, monocytes, macrophages, myeloid cells, and some tumor cells express protein receptor sites for plasminogen, tissue-plasminogen activator (t-PA), and/or urokinase. The broad in vitro substrate specificity of plasmin suggests it plays an important role in extravascular events such as modification of growth and differentiation factors, matrix proteins, and procoagulant molecules. This chapter reviews the fundamental features of plasmin generation, considers the major clinical syndromes resulting from abnormalities in fibrinolysis, and discusses approaches to fibrinolytic and antifibrinolytic therapy.

COMPONENTS OF THE FIBRINOLYTIC SYSTEM

PLASMINOGEN

Plasminogen is synthesized primarily in the liver.[3,4] It is an M_r approximately 92,000 single-chain proenzyme that circulates in plasma at a concentration of approximately 1.5 μM[5] (Table 127-1). The plasma half-life of plasminogen in adult males is approximately 2 days.[6] Its 791 amino acids are cross-linked by 24 disulfide bridges, 16 of which give rise to five homologous triple-loop structures called kringles[7] (Fig. 127-2). The first (K1) and fourth (K4) of these 80-amino-acid structures of M_r approximately 10,000 impart high-affinity and low-affinity lysine binding, respectively.[8] The lysine-binding domains of plasminogen appear to mediate its specific interactions with fibrin, cell surface receptors, and other proteins, including its circulating inhibitor α_2-antiplasmin (α_2-AP).[9–13]

Posttranslational modification of plasminogen results in two glycosylation variants (forms 1 and 2)[14–16] (see Table 127-1). O-linked oligosaccharide, which consists of sialic acid, galactose, and galactosamine resident on Thr345, is common to the two forms. Only form 2, which is composed of sialic acid, galactose, glucosamine, and mannose, contains N-linked oligosaccharide on Asn288. The carbohydrate portion of plasminogen appears to regulate its affinity for cellular receptors and may specify its physiologic degradation pathway.

Activation of plasminogen results from cleavage of a single Arg-Val peptide bond at position 560–561,[17] giving rise to the active protease plasmin (see Table 127-1). Plasmin contains a typical serine protease catalytic triad (His602, Asp645, Ser740)[5] but exhibits broad substrate specificity compared to other proteases of this class.[18] The circulating form of plasminogen, amino-terminal glutamic acid plasminogen (Glu-PLG), is readily converted by limited proteolysis to several modified forms known collectively as Lys-PLG.[19,20] Hydrolysis of the Lys77-Lys78 peptide bond gives rise to a conformationally modified form of the zymogen that more readily binds fibrin, displays twofold to threefold higher avidity for cellular receptors, and is activated 10 to 20 times more rapidly than is Glu-PLG.[10,17,21] Lys-PLG normally does not circulate in plasma[17] but has been identified on cell surfaces.[22]

Spanning 52.5 kb of deoxyribonucleic acid (DNA) on chromosome 6q26-27, the plasminogen gene consists of 19 exons[23,24] and directs expression of a 2.7-kb messenger ribonucleic acid (mRNA)[7] (see Fig. 127-2). The 5' upstream region of the plasminogen gene contains two regulatory elements common to genes for acute phase reactants (CTGGGA) and six interleukin (IL)-6–responsive elements.[24] Moreover, plasminogen gene activity is stimulated by the acute phase mediator IL-6 both in vitro and in vivo.[25] The gene is closely linked and structurally related to that of apolipoprotein(a), an apoprotein associated with the highly atherogenic low-density lipoprotein (LDL)-like particle lipoprotein(a)[26] and more distantly related to other kringle-containing proteins, such as t-PA, urokinase-plasminogen activator (u-PA), hepatocyte growth factor, and macrophage stimulating protein.[27–31] The significance of the latter two proteins to the fibrinolytic system remains to be determined.

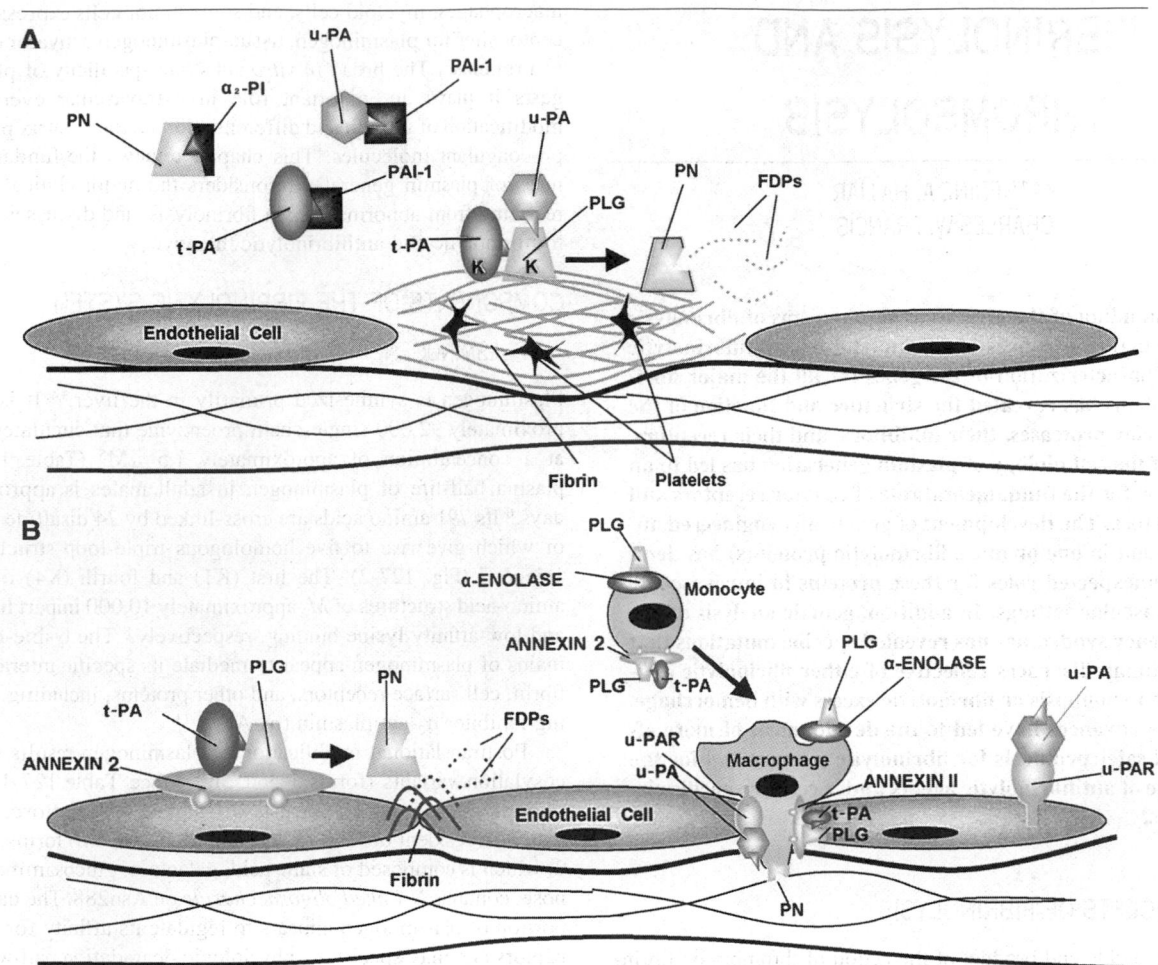

FIGURE 127-1   Overview of the fibrinolytic system. *(A)* Fibrin-based plasminogen (PLG) activation. The zymogen plasminogen is converted to the active serine protease plasmin (PN) through the action of tissue-plasminogen activator (t-PA) or urokinase-plasminogen activator (u-PA). The activity of t-PA is greatly enhanced by its assembly with plasminogen through lysine residues (K) on a fibrin-containing thrombus. u-PA acts independently of fibrin. Both t-PA and u-PA can be inhibited by plasminogen-activator inhibitor-1 (PAI-1), the main physiologic regulator of PA activity. By binding to fibrin, plasmin is protected from its major inhibitor α_2-plasmin inhibitor (α_2-PI). Bound plasmin degrades cross-linked fibrin, giving rise to soluble fibrin degradation products (FDPs). *(B)* Sites of cell surface plasminogen activation. On the blood vessel wall, endothelial cells, like monocytes and macrophages, express the u-PA receptor (u-PAR) and annexin 2, a coreceptor for t-PA and PLG that augments the efficiency of plasmin generation. Circulating monocytes and macrophages have cell surface α-enolase, a potential receptor for PLG.

PHYSIOLOGIC FUNCTIONS OF PLASMIN(OGEN)

Development of the plasminogen-deficient mouse has contributed significantly to our understanding of the physiologic function of the serine protease plasmin. Mice made completely plasminogen deficient through gene targeting undergo normal embryogenesis and development, are fertile, and survive to adulthood (Table 127-2).[32,33] In addition to runting and ligneous conjunctivitis,[34] these animals display a predisposition to thrombosis with spontaneous thrombi appearing in the liver, stomach, colon, rectum, lung, and pancreas; fibrin deposition in the liver; and ulcerative lesions in the gastrointestinal tract and rectum. These results suggest that plasminogen is not strictly required for normal development but does play a crucial role in postnatal intravascular and extravascular fibrinolysis.

PLASMINOGEN ACTIVATORS

TISSUE-PLASMINOGEN ACTIVATOR

t-PA is one of two major endogenous plasminogen activators. It consists of 527 amino acids composing an M_r approximately 72,000 gly-

coprotein[35] (see Table 127-1). t-PA contains five structural domains, including a fibronectin-like "finger," an epidermal growth factor-like domain, two "kringle" structures homologous to those of plasminogen, and a serine protease domain (see Fig. 127-2). Cleavage of the Arg275-Ile276 peptide bond by plasmin converts t-PA to a disulfide-linked, two-chain form.[35] Although single-chain t-PA is less active than two-chain t-PA in the fluid phase, both forms demonstrate equivalent activity when bound to fibrin.[36]

The two glycosylation forms of t-PA are distinguishable by the presence (type 1) or absence (type 2) of a complex *N-linked* oligosaccharide moiety on Asn184[37,38] (see Table 127-1). Both types contain high-mannose carbohydrate on Asn117, complex oligosaccharide on Asn448, and an *O-linked* α-fucose residue on Thr61.[39] The carbohydrate moieties of t-PA may modulate its functional activity, regulate its binding to cell surface receptors, and specify degradation pathways.

Located on chromosome 8p12-q11.2, the gene for human t-PA is encoded by 14 exons spanning a total of 36.6 kb[40–42] (see Fig. 127-2). Although exon one encodes a 58-nucleotide mRNA leader sequence,

TABLE 127-1 FIBRINOLYTIC PROTEINS

A. PROTEASES

PROPERTY	PLASMINOGEN	T-PA	U-PA
Molecular mass	92,000	72,000	54,000
Amino acids	791	527	411
Chromosome	6	8	10
Site of synthesis	Liver	Endothelium	Endothelium, kidney
Plasma concentration			
nM	1500	0.075	0.150
μg/ml	140	0.005	0.008
Plasma half-life	48 h	5 min	8 min
N-glycosylation (%)	2	13	7
Form 1	—	Asn117, Asn184, Asn448	Asn302
Form 2	Asn288	Asn117, —, Asn448	—
O-glycosylation			
α-Fucose	—	Thr61	Thr18
Complex	Thr345	—	—
Two-chain cleavage site	Arg560-Val561	Arg275-Ile276	Lys158-Ile159
Heavy-chain domains			
Finger	No	Yes	No
Growth factor	No	Yes	Yes
Kringles (no.)	5	2	1
Light-chain catalytic triad	His602, Asp645, Ser740	His322, Asp371, Ser478	His204, Asp255, Ser356

B. MAJOR SERPIN INHIBITORS

PROPERTY	α-PI	PAI-1	PAI-2
		Major Serpin Inhibitors	
Molecular mass	70,000	52,000	60,000 (glycosylated)
			47,000 (nonglycosylated)
Amino acids	452	402	393
Chromosome	18	7	18
Site of synthesis	Kidney, liver	Endothelium	Placenta
		Monocytes/macrophages	Monocytes/macrophages
		Hepatocytes	Tumor cells
		Adipocytes	
Plasma concentration			
nM	900	0.1–0.4	ND
μg/ml	50	0.02	ND
Serpin reactive site	Arg364-Met365	Arg346-Met347	Arg358-Thr359
Specificity	Plasmin	u-PA = t-PA	u-PA > t-PA

C. RECEPTORS

PROPERTY	U-PAR	ANNEXIN 2	LRP	MANNOSE RECEPTOR
		Receptors		
Molecular mass	55,000–60,000	36,000	600,000	175,000
Amino acids	313	339	4544	1456
Chromosome	19	15	12	10
Source	Endothelial cells	Endothelial cells	Hepatocytes	Macrophages
	Monocytes/macrophages	Monocytes/macrophages	Monocytes/macrophages	
	Fibroblasts	Myeloid cells	Fibroblasts	
	Tumor cells	Smooth muscle cells		
Ligand(s)	u-PA	t-PA, plasminogen	u-PA/PAI-1	t-PA
			u-PA/PAI-2	
			t-PA/PAI-1; PN/α_2-PI	

α_2-PI = α_2-plasmin inhibitor; LRP = low-density-lipoprotein receptor-like protein; ND = not determined; PAI-1 = plasminogen activator inhibitor type 1; PAI-2 = plasminogen activator inhibitor type 2; PN = plasmin; t-PA = tissue-plasminogen activator; u-PA = urokinase-plasminogen activator; u-PAR = urokinase-plasminogen activator receptor.

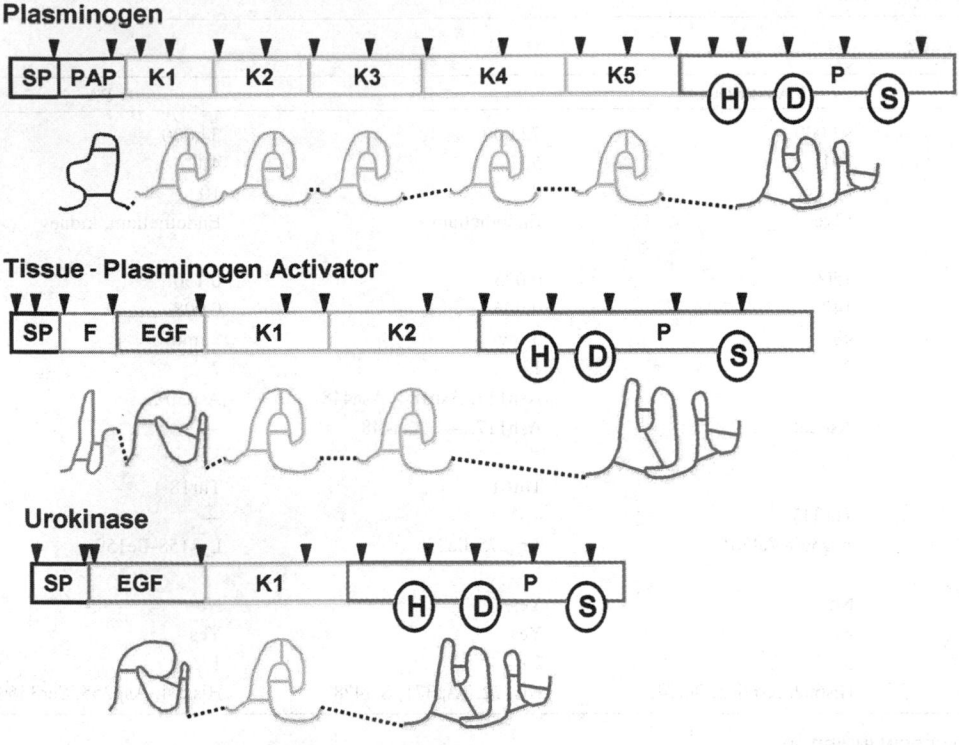

FIGURE 127-2   Structure–function relationships of plasminogen, tissue-plasminogen activator (t-PA), and urokinase-plasminogen activator (u-PA). Alignment of the intron-exon structure of plasminogen, t-PA, and u-PA genes with functional protein domains. Protein domains are labeled signal peptide (SP), preactivation peptide (PAP), "kringle" domains (K), fibronectin-like "finger" (F), epidermal growth factor-like domain (EGF), and protease. The position of catalytic triad amino acids histidine (H), aspartic acid (D), and serine (S) are shown within individual protease domains. The positions of individual introns relative to amino acid encoding exons are indicated with *inverted triangles*.

each of the structural domains of t-PA is encoded by one or two of the remaining 13 exons. This finding suggests the t-PA gene arose by an evolutionary process called *exon shuffling*, whereby functionally related genes evolved through rearrangement of exons encoding autonomous domains. Consistent with this hypothesis, deletion of exons encoding the fibronectin-like finger or kringle 2, but not kringle 1, domains of t-PA results in expression of mutants resistant to the cofactor activity of fibrin, while catalytic activity in the absence of fibrin remains intact.[43]

The proximal promoter of the human t-PA gene contains binding sequences for potentially important transcriptional factors, including AP1, NF1, SP1, and AP2,[44,45] as well as a possible cyclic adenosine monophosphate (cAMP)-responsive element.[46] *In vitro*, many agents exert small effects on the expression of t-PA mRNA, but relatively few enhance t-PA synthesis without also augmenting plasminogen-activator inhibitor (PAI)-1 synthesis. Agents that regulate t-PA gene expression independently of PAI-1 include histamine, butyrate, retinoids, arterial shear stress, and dexamethasone.[47–52] Forskolin, which increases intracellular cAMP levels, reportedly decreases synthesis of both t-PA and PAI-1.[45,53]

t-PA is synthesized and secreted primarily by endothelial cells. However, expression of t-PA appears to be restricted to 7- to 30-μm diameter precapillary arterioles, postcapillary venules, and vasa vasora. Much less expression is seen in endothelial cells of the femoral artery, femoral vein, carotid artery, and aorta.[54] In the mouse lung, bronchial artery endothelial cells express t-PA antigen, especially at branch points, whereas pulmonary blood vessels are uniformly negative.[48,55–57] Release of t-PA is governed by a variety of stimuli, such

as thrombin, histamine, bradykinin, epinephrine, acetylcholine, arginine vasopressin, gonadotropins, exercise, venous occlusion, and shear stress.[47,48,58,59] Its circulating half-life is exceedingly short ($\sim$5 minutes). Functionally, t-PA itself is a poor activator of plasminogen. However, the catalytic efficiency of t-PA–dependent plasmin generation (k_{cat}/K_m) increases by at least two orders of magnitude[21] because of a dramatic increase in affinity (decreased K_m) between t-PA and its substrate plasminogen in the presence of fibrin. Although it is expressed by extravascular cells, t-PA appears to be the major intravascular activator of plasminogen.[18]

UROKINASE

The second endogenous plasminogen activator, single-chain u-PA or prourokinase, is an M_r approximately 54,000 glycoprotein consisting of 411 amino acids (see Table 127-1). u-PA contains an epidermal growth factor-like domain and a single plasminogen-like "kringle." It possesses a classic catalytic triad (His204, Asp255, Ser356) within its serine protease domain[60] (see Fig. 127-2). Cleavage of the Lys158-Ile159 peptide bond by plasmin or kallikrein converts single-chain u-PA to a disulfide-linked two-chain derivative.[61] Located on chromosome 10, the human u-PA gene is encoded by 11 exons spanning 6.4 kb and is expressed by endothelial cells, macrophages, renal epithelial cells, and some tumor cells.[62,63] Its intron-exon structure is closely related to that of the t-PA gene.

Circumstantial evidence suggests u-PA synthesis is induced during neoplastic transformation, possibly through a mechanism involving transcription factors AP1 and AP2.[64] Other agents that appear to induce expression of u-PA *in vitro* include hormones, angiogenic growth fac-

TABLE 127-2   GENETIC MOUSE MODELS RELEVANT TO FIBRINOLYSIS

GENOTYPE	PHENOTYPE	REFERENCE
Gene Deletion Models		
Plasminogen		
PLG−/−	Spontaneous thrombosis, runting, premature death	32, 414
	Fibrin in liver, lungs, stomach; gastric ulcers	32, 414
	Impaired wound healing; ligneous conjunctivitis	34, 216
	Impaired monocyte recruitment	218
	Impaired neointima formation after electrical injury	219
	Impaired dissemination of *Borrelia burgdorferi*	220
	Reduced excitotoxic neuronal cell death in brain	221
Plasminogen Activators		
t-PA−/−	Reduced lysis of fibrin clot	80
	Increased endotoxin-induced thrombosis	80
u-PA−/−	Occasional fibrin in liver/intestine	80
	Rectal prolapse; ulcers of eyelids, face, ears	80
	Reduced macrophage degradation of fibrin	80
	Increased endotoxin-induced thrombosis	80
u-PA−/− t-PA−/−	Reduced growth, fertility, life span; cachexia	80
	Fibrin deposits in liver, gonads, lungs	80
	Ulcers in intestine, skin, ears; rectal prolapse	80
	Impaired clot lysis	80
Inhibitors		
PAI-1−/−	Mildly increased lysis of fibrin clot	114
	Resistance to endotoxin-induced thrombosis	415
LRP−/−	Embryonic lethal day 13.5 post-conception	171, 172
Receptors		
u-PAR−/−	Essentially normal	416
	Reduced macrophage PLG activation *in vitro*	416
	Normal matrix degradation	416
Annexin 2	Mild runting, fibrin deposition in microvasculature	165
	Impaired clearance of arterial thrombi	165
	Impaired postnatal neoangiogenesis	165
Overexpression Models		
Apo(a)+/+	Atherosclerotic lesions with high-fat diet	417
	Reduced cell-associated plasmin and activation of TGF-β	418
	Resistance to t-PA−mediated clot lysis	419
Apo(a)ΔLBS+/+	Reduced lipid deposition	420
PAI-1+++/+++	Venous thrombosis	113
	Tail necrosis, hind foot edema	
u-PA+++/+++	Fatal neonatal hemorrhage	421
	Impaired learning	422

tors, and cAMP.[52] Inflammatory cytokines, such as IL-1 and lipopolysaccharide, induce only small increments in u-PA expression, whereas tumor necrosis factor and transforming growth factor β (TGF-β) have a more dramatic (5- to 30-fold) effect.[65–67]

Two-chain u-PA occurs in a high molecular weight form (M_r 54,000) and a low molecular weight form (M_r 33,000) that differ by the presence and absence, respectively, of a 135-residue amino-terminal fragment released by plasmin cleavage between Lys135-Lys136.[68,69] Although the two forms are capable of activating plasminogen, only the high molecular weight form binds to the u-PA receptor (u-PAR). u-PA has much lower affinity for fibrin than does t-PA and is an effective plasminogen activator both in the presence and in the absence of fibrin.[70,71] The extent to which prourokinase possesses intrinsic plasminogen-activating capacity is controversial.[72,73]

ACCESSORY PLASMINOGEN ACTIVATORS AND FIBRINOLYSINS

Under certain conditions, proteases traditionally classified within the intrinsic arm of the coagulation cascade are capable of activating plasminogen directly. However, these proteases, which include kallikrein, factor XIa, and factor XIIa,[74–76] normally account for no more than 15 percent of total plasmin-generating activity in plasma.[77] In addition, the membrane type 1 matrix metalloproteinase (MT1-MMP) appears to exert fibrinolytic activity in the absence of plasminogen and may explain the unexpectedly mild phenotype observed in plasminogen-deficient mice.[78]

PHYSIOLOGIC FUNCTION OF PLASMINOGEN ACTIVATORS

Although abnormalities of the t-PA release mechanism have been reported,[79] no clinical examples of complete deficiency of t-PA or u-PA in humans are available. Thus, the most compelling studies of the physiologic functions of these proteins come from gene disruption analyses (see Table 127-2).[80] Both u-PA and t-PA null deletion mice exhibit normal fertility and embryonic development. However, u-PA-/- mice developed rectal prolapse, nonhealing ulcerations of the face and eyelids and occasional fibrin deposition in tissues. Although they show normal rates of pulmonary clot lysis, endotoxin-induced thrombus formation is significantly enhanced. t-PA−deficient mice display a normal spontaneous phenotype. However, these animals have a decreased rate of lysis of artificially induced pulmonary thrombi and enhanced thrombus formation in response to endotoxin injection. Doubly deficient (t-PA-/-; u-PA-/-) mice exhibit rectal prolapse, nonhealing ulceration, runting, and cachexia, with extensive fibrin deposition in the liver, intestine, gonads, and lung. Not surprisingly, clot lysis is markedly impaired. These findings demonstrate that t-PA and u-PA are not essential for normal embryologic development but do play crucial roles in lysis of artificially induced thrombi and in fibrinolytic surveillance in the adult.

INHIBITORS OF FIBRINOLYSIS

PLASMIN INHIBITORS

The action of plasmin is negatively modulated by a family of serine protease inhibitors called *serpins*[81] (see Table 127-1). All serpins share a mechanism of action, which consists of forming an irreversible complex with the active site serine of the target protease following proteolytic cleavage of the inhibitor by the target protease. Within such a complex, both protease and inhibitor lose their activity.

$α_2$-plasmin inhibitor ($α_2$-PI), a single-chain glycoprotein of M_r approximately 70,000, circulates in plasma at relatively high concentrations (~0.9 μM) and displays a plasma half-life of 2.4 days[82] (see Table 127-1). This serpin contains approximately 13 percent carbohydrate by mass and consists of 452 amino acids with two disulfide bridges.[83] In humans, the gene is located on chromosome 18 and contains 10 exons distributed over 16 kb of DNA.[84] The promoter region of the α_2-PI gene contains a hepatitis B-like enhancer element that directs tissue-specific expression in the liver.[83] α_2-PI is also a constituent of platelet α-granules.[85] Plasmin released into flowing blood or in the vicinity of a platelet-rich thrombus is immediately neutralized upon forming an irreversible 1:1 stoichiometric, lysine binding site-dependent complex with α_2-PI. Interaction with plasmin is accompanied by cleavage of the Arg364-Met365 peptide bond, and the resulting covalent complexes are cleared in the liver.

Several additional proteins can act as plasmin inhibitors (see Table 127-1). α_2-Macroglobulin is an M_r 725,000 dimeric protein synthesized by endothelial cells and macrophages and is found in platelet α-granules. This nonserpin inhibits plasmin, with approximately 10 percent of the efficiency exhibited as α_2-PI[86] forming noncovalent complexes with several distinct serine proteases. C_1-esterase inhibitor also can serve as an inhibitor of t-PA in plasma.[79] Protease nexin[87] may function as a noncirculating cell surface inhibitor of trypsin, thrombin, factor Xa, urokinase, or plasmin, resulting in protease-inhibitor complexes that are endocytosed via a specific nexin receptor.[88]

PLASMINOGEN-ACTIVATOR INHIBITORS

Plasminogen-Activator Inhibitor-1   Of the two major PAIs[89] (see Table 127-1), PAI-1 is the most ubiquitous. This M_r approximately 52,000 single-chain glycoprotein contains no cysteines. It is released by endothelial cells, monocytes, macrophages, hepatocytes, adipocytes, and platelets.[90–92] PAI-1 release is stimulated by many cytokines, growth factors, and lipoproteins common to the global inflammatory response.[66,93–95] The PAI-1 gene consists of nine exons that span 12.2 kb on chromosome 7q21.3-q22.[96] The serpin reactive site is located at Arg346-Met347, and activity of this labile serpin is stabilized upon complex formation with vitronectin, a component of plasma and pericellular matrix.[97,98]

The upstream regulatory region of the human PAI-1 gene contains a strong endothelial cell/fibroblast-specific element within the first 187 bp of the 5'-flanking region,[99,100] a glucocorticoid-responsive enhancer between positions −90 and +75,[100] and TGF-β–responsive elements between bases −791 and −546 and bases −328 and −186.[101] TGF-β stimulates fos and jun, the two components of the AP1 complex, and an AP1-binding site (GGAGTCA) is located at −672 to −666 upstream of the PAI-1 cap site.[102] Agents that enhance expression of PAI-1 at the message level, the protein level, or both without affecting t-PA synthesis include the inflammatory cytokines lipopolysaccharide, IL-1, tumor necrosis factor alpha,[65,66,93,94,103,104] TGF-β, and basic fibroblast growth factor (bFGF),[67,93,101,105] very-low-density lipoprotein and lipoprotein(a),[106,107] angiotensin II,[108] thrombin,[109,110] and phorbol esters.[111] In addition, endothelial cell PAI-1 is down-regulated by forskolin[44,53] and by endothelial cell growth factor in the presence of heparin.[112]

PAI-1 is the most important and rapidly acting physiologic inhibitor of both t-PA and u-PA. Transgenic mice that overexpress PAI-1 exhibit thrombotic occlusion of tail veins and swelling of hind limbs within 2 weeks of birth (see Table 127-2).[113] On the other hand, mice deficient in PAI-1 exhibit normal fertility, viability, tissue histology, and development but no evidence of hemorrhage.[114] These observations contrast with the moderately severe bleeding disorder observed in a patient with complete PAI-1 deficiency.[115]

Plasminogen-Activator Inhibitor-2   Originally purified from human placenta,[89,116] PAI-2 is a 393-amino-acid member of the serpin family whose reactive site is the Arg358-Thr359 peptide bond[116] (see Table 127-1). The gene encoding PAI-2 is located on chromosome 18q21-23, spans 16.5 kb, and contains eight exons.[117] PAI-2 exists as both an M_r 47,000 nonglycosylated intracellular form and an M_r 60,000 glycosylated form secreted by leukocytes and fibrosarcoma cells. Functionally, PAI-2 inhibits both two-chain t-PA and two-chain u-PA with comparable efficiency (second-order rate constants 10^5 $M^{-1}s^{-1}$). However, PAI-2 is less effective toward single-chain t-PA (second-order rate constant 10^3 $M^{-1}s^{-1}$) and does not inhibit prourokinase.

Significant PAI-2 levels are found in human plasma only during pregnancy. The gene's 5'-untranslated region is not yet characterized.[116] The 3'-downstream sequences include the TTATTTAT motif, which has been identified with inflammatory mediators.[118,119] In macrophages in vitro, PAI-2 secretion is enhanced by endotoxin and phorbol esters,[119,120] and dexamethasone decreases PAI-2 expression in HT-1080 cells.[52]

CELLULAR RECEPTORS

Although structurally diverse, cell surface fibrinolytic receptors can be classified into two groups whose integrated actions likely are essential for homeostatic control of plasmin activity[2] (see Table 127-1). "Activation" receptors localize and potentiate plasminogen activation, whereas "clearance" receptors eliminate plasmin and plasminogen activators from the blood or focal microenvironments.

ACTIVATION RECEPTORS

Plasminogen Receptors   Plasminogen receptors are a diverse group of proteins expressed on a wide array of cell types.[2] Reported receptors include α-enolase, glycoprotein IIb/IIIa complex, the Heymann nephritis antigen, amphoterin, and annexin 2, which are expressed primarily on monocytoid cells,[121] platelets,[122] renal epithelial cells,[123] neuroblastoma cells,[124] and endothelial cells,[125,126] respectively. These binding proteins commonly interact with the kringle structures of plasminogen through carboxyl-terminal lysine residues.[121]

Urokinase-Plasminogen Activator Receptor   u-PAR is expressed on monocytes, macrophages, fibroblasts, endothelial cells, and a variety of tumor cells[2] (see Table 127-1). u-PAR cDNA was cloned and sequenced from a human fibroblast cDNA library[127] and encodes a protein of 313 amino acids with a 21-residue signal peptide. The gene consists of seven exons distributed over 23 kb of genomic DNA, which places this glycoprotein within the Ly-1/elapid venom toxin superfamily of cysteine rich proteins.[128,129] u-PAR is anchored to the plasma membrane through glycosyl phosphatidylinositol linkages.[130] u-PA when bound to its receptor maintains its activity and susceptibility to the physiologic inhibitor PAI-1.[131] Formation of u-PA–PAI-1 complexes appears to hasten clearance of u-PA by hepatic or monocytoid cells.[131–134]

u-PAR appears to play a novel role in cellular signaling and adhesion events.[135] u-PAR binds the adhesive glycoprotein vitronectin at a site distinct from the u-PA binding domain,[136,137] and u-PA–transfected renal epithelial cells acquire enhanced adhesion to vitronectin while they lose their adhesion to fibronectin.[138] Furthermore, u-PAR colocalizes with integrins in focal contacts and at the leading edge of migrating cells.[139] It associates with caveolin, which is a major component of caveolae, structures that are abundant in endothelial cells and thought to participate in signaling events.[140–142] Thus, integrin function may be regulated by u-PAR, signifying an integrated relationship between cellular adhesion and proteolysis.

Annexin 2   Annexin 2 is a member of the annexin superfamily of calcium-dependent, phospholipid-binding proteins.[143] It is highly conserved and is abundantly expressed on endothelial cells,[144–147] monocyte/macrophages,[148] myeloid cells,[149] developing neuronal cells,[150] and some tumor cells.[151–153] All 50 annexin family members have in common a conserved C-terminal "core" region and a more variable N-terminal "tail."[154] The human annexin 2 gene consists of 13 exons distributed over 40 kb of genomic DNA on chromosome 15 (15q21).[155]

Annexin 2 is unique among fibrinolytic receptors in that it possesses binding affinity for both plasminogen (K_d 114 nM)[125] and t-PA (K_d 30 nM)[126] but not for u-PA.[126] In a fluid phase system of purified proteins, native human annexin 2 stimulates the catalytic efficiency of t-PA−dependent plasminogen activation by 60-fold.[156] This effect is completely inhibited in the presence of lysine analogues or upon treatment of annexin 2 with carboxypeptidase B, also termed *thrombin-activatable fibrinolysis inhibitor* (TAFI), an agent that removes basic carboxyl-terminal amino acids. Although it lacks a classic signal peptide, annexin 2 is constitutively translocated to the endothelial cell surface within 16 hours of its biosynthesis. It binds cell surface phospholipid via core repeat 2, which contains the linear amino acid sequence KGLGT and downstream aspartate residue (Asp161) that together constitute a classic "annexin" motif.[157] The annexin 2 heterotetramer, which consists of two annexin monomers and two p11 subunits, may have even greater stimulatory effects on t-PA−dependent plasmin generation.[146]

Plasminogen and t-PA appear to bind to distinct domains. Lys307 appears to be crucial for effective interaction of plasminogen with annexin 2.[156] The atherogenic LDL-like particle lipoprotein(a) competes with plasminogen for binding to annexin 2 *in vitro*,[158] thereby reducing cell surface plasmin generation. This mechanism may reduce fibrinolytic surveillance at the blood vessel wall. t-PA binding to annexin 2 requires a domain consisting of residues 8-13 (LCKLSL) within the receptor's amino-terminal "tail" domain.[159] This sequence is a target for homocysteine (HC), a thiol-containing amino acid that accumulates in association with nutritional deficiencies of vitamin B_6, vitamin B_{12}, or folic acid or in inherited abnormalities of cystathionine β-synthase, methylenetetrahydrofolate reductase, or methionine synthase,[160] and it is associated with atherothrombotic disease.[160–162] *In vitro*, HC impairs the intrinsic fibrinolytic system of the endothelial cell by approximately 50 percent[163] by forming a covalent derivative with Cys 9 of annexin 2, thus preventing its interaction with t-PA.[159] The half-maximal dose of HC for inhibition of t-PA binding to annexin 2 is approximately 11 μM HC, a value close to the upper limit of normal for HC in plasma (14 μM).

Several studies suggest a physiologic role for annexin 2 in fibrin homeostasis. First, blast cells from human patients with acute promyelocytic leukemia overexpress annexin 2 in proportion to their degree of hyperfibrinolytic coagulopathy.[149] Second, arterial thrombosis in rats can be significantly attenuated by pretreatment with intravenous annexin 2.[164] Finally, mice with total deficiency of annexin 2 display impaired clearance of artificial arterial thrombi, fibrin deposition in the microvasculature, and angiogenic defects in a variety of tissues.[165]

CLEARANCE RECEPTORS

Both u-PA and t-PA are cleared from the circulation via the liver.[166] *In vitro*, clearance of t-PA−PAI-1 complexes appears to be mediated by a large two-chain receptor called the *low-density lipoprotein receptor-related protein* (LRP).[167–169] This complex interaction requires both growth factor and finger domains of t-PA. An additional M_r 39,000 "receptor-associated protein" copurifies with LRP and may regulate the binding and uptake of LRP ligands.[170] LRP "knockout" embryos undergo developmental arrest by 13.5 days after conception, suggesting that regulation of serine protease activity is crucial for early embryogenesis.[171,172]

Although several PAI-1−independent clearance pathways for t-PA have been proposed[166] to involve the large LRP subunit,[173] the mannose receptor,[174] or an α-fucose−specific receptor,[175] *in vivo* studies in mice suggest that LRP and the mannose receptor play a dominant role in t-PA clearance[176]

FIBRINOLYTIC ACTIONS OF PLASMIN

DEGRADATION OF FIBRINOGEN

Fibrinogen possesses distinct proteolytic cleavage sites for plasmin and thrombin (Fig. 127-3). Plasmin cleaves carboxyl-terminal Aα and N-terminal fibrinopeptide B moieties, whereas thrombin primarily releases fibrinopeptide A, exposing the Gly-Pro-Arg tripeptide sequence and allowing fibrinogen to polymerize and form insoluble fibrin.[177] Plasmin cleavage of fibrinogen (M_r 340,000) initially produces carboxyl-terminal fragments from the α-chain within the D domain of fibrinogen (Aα fragment).[178–181] Simultaneously, but more slowly, the N-terminal segments of the β-chains are cleaved, releasing a peptide containing fibrinopeptide B. The resulting M_r approximately 250,000 molecule is termed *fragment X*, which is a clottable form of fibrinogen. Additional cleavage events may release the Bβ fragment from the β-chain's carboxyl-terminus. In a series of subsequent reactions, plasmin cleaves the three polypeptide chains that connect the D and E domains, giving rise to free D domain (M_r ~100,000) plus the binodular D-E fragment known as *fragment Y* (M_r ~150,000). Finally, domains D and E are separated from each other, and some of the N-terminal fibrinopeptide A sites on domain E are modified. Although fragment X can be converted to fibrin by thrombin, fragments Y, D, and E all are nonclottable and, in fact, may inhibit the spontaneous polymerization of fibrinogen.[182]

DEGRADATION OF FIBRIN

Plasmin degradation of fibrin leads to a distinct set of molecular products.[183] Species similar to fragments Y, D, and E but lacking fibrinopeptide sites are released from noncross-linked fibrin. If fibrin has been extensively cross-linked by factor XIII, however, the resulting D fragments are cross-linked to an E domain fragment. Assay of cross-linked D-dimer fragments is used clinically to identify disseminated intravascular coagulation (DIC) associated with excessive plasmin-mediated fibrinolysis. Several biologic activities, including inhibition of platelet function,[184] potentiation of the hypotensive effects of bradykinin,[185] chemotaxis,[186] and immune modulation, have been ascribed to fibrin breakdown products.[187]

TISSUE-PLASMINOGEN ACTIVATOR-MEDIATED PLASMINOGEN ACTIVATION

With or without fibrin, t-PA−mediated activation of plasminogen follows Michaelis-Menten kinetics.[21] In the absence of fibrin, t-PA is a weak activator of plasminogen. However, in the presence of fibrin, the catalytic efficiency (k_{cat}/K_m) of t-PA−dependent plasminogen activation is enhanced by at least two orders of magnitude. This process is the basis for its specificity as a lytic agent in the treatment of thrombosis. The affinity between t-PA and plasminogen in the absence of fibrin is low (K_m 65 μM) but increases significantly in its presence (K_m 0.16 μM), even though the catalytic rate constant remains essentially unchanged (k_{cat} ~0.05 s^{-1}). When plasmin forms on the fibrin surface, both its lysine binding sites and its active site are occupied. Thus, it is relatively protected from α_2-AP, its physiologic inhibitor.[188] Interaction of t-PA with fibrin probably is initiated by its "finger" domain. However, once fibrin is modified by plasmin, carboxy-terminal lysine residues are generated and become binding sites for kringle 2 of t-PA and kringles 1 and 4 of plasminogen.[189] Therefore, fibrin accelerates its own destruction by (1) enhancing the catalytic efficiency of plasmin formation by t-PA, (2) protecting plasmin from α_2-PI, its

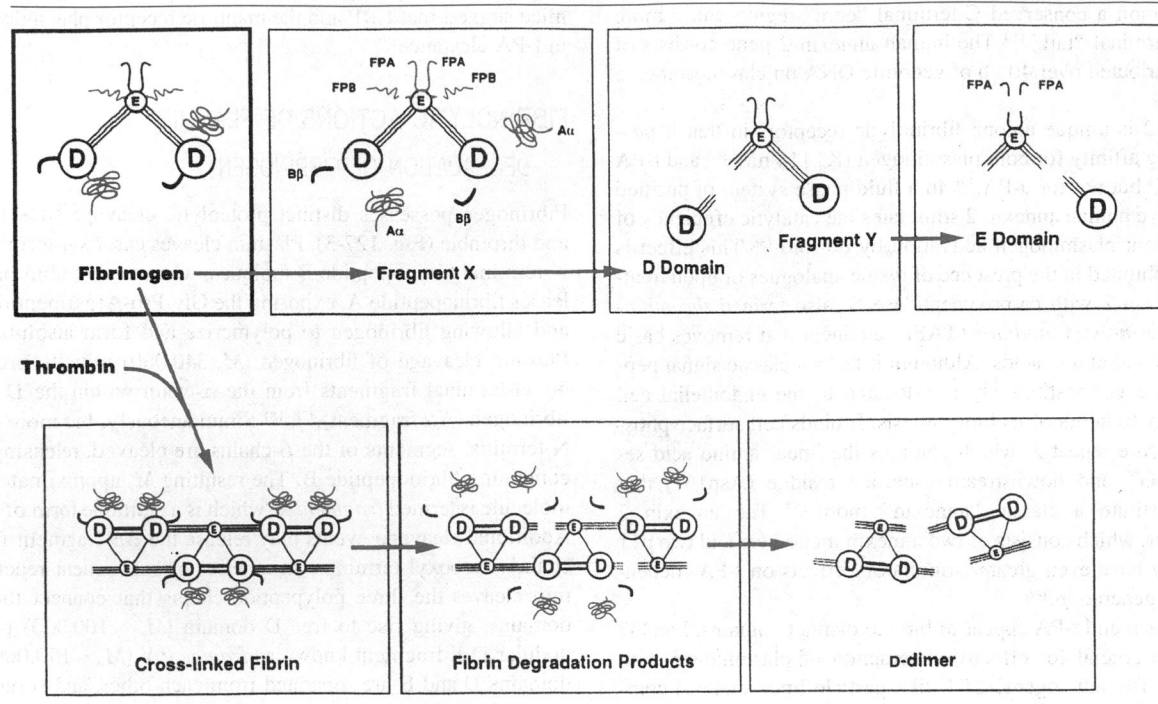

FIGURE 127-3   Degradation of fibrinogen and cross-linked fibrin by plasmin. *(Top)* Plasmin initially cleaves the C-terminal regions of the α- and β-chains within the D domain of fibrinogen, releasing the Aα and Bβ fragments. In addition, a fragment containing fibrinopeptide B (FPB) from the N-terminal region of the β-chain is released, giving rise to the intermediate fragment known as "fragment X." Subsequently, plasmin cleaves the three polypeptide chains connecting D and E domains, giving rise to fragments D, E, and Y. *(Bottom)* Fibrinogen can also be polymerized by thrombin to form fibrin. When degrading cross-linked fibrin, plasmin initially cleaves the C-terminal region of the α- and β-chains within the D domain. Subsequently, some of the connecting regions between the D and E domains are severed. Fibrin ultimately is solubilized upon hydrolysis of additional peptide bonds within the central portions of the coiled-coil connectors, giving rise to fibrin degradation products such as D-dimer. (From with KA Hajjar,[1] with permission.)

physiologic inhibitor, and (3) providing new binding sites for plasminogen and t-PA once its degradation has started.

UROKINASE-PLASMINOGEN ACTIVATOR-MEDIATED PLASMIN GENERATION

For activation of Glu-PLG by u-PA in a fibrin-free system, reported Michaelis constants (K_m) vary from 1.4 to 200 μM, whereas catalytic rate constants (k_{cat}) range from 0.26 to 1.48 s^{-1}.[1] Interestingly, activation of Glu-PLG by two-chain u-PA is increased in the presence of fibrin by approximately 10-fold even though u-PA does not bind to fibrin.[190] In contrast, single-chain u-PA has considerable fibrin specificity. This finding may reflect neutralization by fibrin of components in plasma that impair plasminogen activation.[191] It also may reflect a conformational change in plasminogen upon binding to fibrin.[192] Important to recognize, however, is that the intrinsic plasminogen activating potential of single-chain u-PA is less than 1 percent that of two-chain u-PA.[1] Two-chain u-PA has been used effectively as a thrombolytic agent for many years.[193]

THROMBIN-ACTIVATABLE FIBRINOLYSIS INHIBITOR

TAFI is a plasma carboxypeptidase with specificity for carboxy-terminal arginine and lysine residues that acts as a potent inhibitor of fibrinolysis.[194] Identical to the previously cloned carboxypeptidase B[195] and the previously isolated carboxypeptidase U,[196] this single-chain M_r 60,000 polypeptide circulates in plasma at concentrations of approximately 75 nM and undergoes limited proteolysis in the presence of thrombin, which leads to its activation.[197] The profibrinolytic effect of activated protein C in plasma results from its ability to in-

activate coagulation factors Va and VIIIa, thereby preventing activation of prothrombin and inhibiting activation of TAFI.[194] The profibrinolytic effect of activated protein C in an *in vitro* plasma-based system was TAFI dependent.[198] In a system of purified components, TAFI down-regulated t-PA−induced fibrinolysis half-maximally at a concentration of approximately 1 nM, which is 2 percent of its concentration in plasma.[199] Both inhibition of the intrinsic pathway of coagulation and inhibition of TAFI activity resulted in a doubling of endogenous clot lysis in an *in vivo* rabbit jugular vein model of thrombolysis.[200] Carboxypeptidases in plasma may regulate plasminogen binding to cell surface receptors and to fibrin.[201]

NONFIBRINOLYTIC ACTIONS OF PLASMIN

PLASMIN AS A TISSUE REMODELER

Many *in vitro* studies suggest a role for plasmin in tissue remodeling. Basement membrane proteins such as thrombospondin,[202] laminin,[203] fibronectin,[204] and fibrinogen[205] are readily degraded by plasmin *in vitro*, suggesting possible roles in inflammation,[206] tumor cell invasion,[207] embryogenesis,[208] ovulation,[209] neurodevelopment,[210,211] and prohormone activation.[212–214] Plasmin also activates matrix metalloproteinases (MMPs) 3 and 13, thereby facilitating the degradation of matrix proteins, such as the collagens, laminin, fibronectin, vitronectin, elastin, aggrecan, and tenascin C.[215] On the other hand, MMP activation apparently can proceed in the absence of plasminogen, possibly providing the basis for the mild phenotype observed in plasminogen null homozygote animals.[78]

A role for plasmin in tissue remodeling is further supported by *in vivo* observations in plasminogen-deficient mice (see Table 127-2). Impaired wound healing is observed in the plasminogen "knockout"[216] and is reversed upon simultaneous deletion of fibrinogen.[217] Plasminogen-deficient mice also display diminished recruitment of monocytes in response to intraperitoneal thioglycolate[218] and impaired neointima formation following electrical injury to blood vessels.[219] In studies of *Borrelia burgdorferi*, the agent of Lyme disease, dissemination of the spirochete within its arthropod vector *Ixodes dammini* is absolutely dependent upon host plasminogen even though the deer tick contains no fibrin.[220] Furthermore, kainate-induced excitotoxicity and attendant neuronal cell dropout in the hippocampus are not observed in plasminogen knockout mice but do occur in fibrinogen-deficient animals.[221] The latter two studies may define new roles for plasmin that appear to be unrelated to fibrin degradation.

Plasmin may play a role in the activation of growth factors and in the blood vessel's proliferative response to injury. TGF-β is an M_r 25,000 homodimeric polypeptide whose effects on vascular cell growth and differentiation are pleiomorphic.[222] In culture, cell-associated plasmin appears to convert latent TGF-β to its physiologically relevant active state. Inhibition of wound healing in this system was dependent upon active TGF-β, and activation of this agent could be blocked in the presence of plasmin inhibitors such as aprotinin or α_2-PI. Activation of TGF-β by plasmin may reflect alteration of its tertiary structure upon cleavage of an amino-terminal glycopeptide.[223] Once activated by plasmin, TGF-β can stimulate production of PAI-1, thus impairing further activation of plasminogen.

The role of the fibrinolytic system in vascular remodeling during atherosclerosis appears to be complex.[224] Atherogenesis appears to be a response to vascular insult.[225] In the evolution of an injury to the endothelial cell lining of blood vessels, deposition of intravascular fibrin and organization of a thrombus occur. As the injury heals, fibrin participates in plaque growth and luminal narrowing. Evidence of the importance of fibrinolytic balance in this process is the finding, in the absence of PAI-1, of less neointima formation and reduced luminal stenosis, possibly because of more rapid resolution of fibrin.[226] In areas of the vasculature where injury is not associated with fibrin deposition, however, absence of PAI-1 may lead to enhanced lesion formation, as cells that invade the developing plaque may require plasmin activity for their directed migration.[227]

ANGIOSTATIN AND RELATED PLASMINOGEN FRAGMENTS

Angiostatin is a circulating inhibitor of angiogenesis originally isolated from the urine of Lewis lung carcinoma-bearing mice.[228] This M_r approximately 38,000 fragment of plasminogen is identical to kringles 1 through 4. It inhibits bFGF-stimulated endothelial cell proliferation *in vitro*, possibly by inducing apoptosis,[229] and blocks new blood vessel formation in both the chick chorioallantoic membrane and mouse cornea assays. In several experimental animal models of metastasis, exogenous angiostatin induces dormancy of tumors critically dependent upon an intact blood supply.[230] Inhibition of primary and metastatic tumor growth is seen upon implantation of tumor cells stably transfected with an angiostatin gene in a murine fibrosarcoma model.[231] The cellular target or receptor for angiostatin is unknown, although an endothelial cell binding site distinct from annexin 2 has been proposed.[232] In other studies, kringle 5 of plasminogen was an even more potent inhibitor of growth factor-stimulated endothelial cell proliferation.[233] Angiostatin may be a promising new approach to antitumor therapy.[234]

The mechanism of angiostatin formation is a topic of intense investigation. Lewis lung carcinoma-associated macrophages stimulated with tumor-derived granulocyte-macrophage colony stimulating factor express high levels of metalloelastase, which can produce angiostatin from the parent molecule plasminogen.[235] Alternatively, angiostatin can form *in vitro* upon exposure of plasmin to a plasmin reductase followed by an unidentified serine protease secreted by cultured Chinese hamster ovary or HT1080 cells.[236] MMP7, MMP9,[237] an urokinase in the presence of free sulfhydryl donors[238] also have been proposed as angiostatin-generating agents. These studies suggest the possibility of multiple pathways for angiostatin generation.

DISORDERS OF PLASMIN GENERATION

FIBRINOLYTIC DEFICIENCY AND THROMBOSIS

Partial human plasminogen deficiency was first described in a 31-year-old man with a history of repeated episodes of thrombophlebitis, intracranial and mesenteric venous thrombosis, and pulmonary embolism.[239] Reduced plasminogen activity (50% of normal) in the patient's plasma was traced to an Ala601Thr point mutation, and several additional patients with this defect or related substitutions have since been described.[240] Acquired plasminogen deficiency, as may occur in liver disease, sepsis, and Argentine hemorrhagic fever resulting from decreased synthesis and/or increased catabolism, frequently has been associated with thrombotic vascular occlusion.[241]

Congenital plasminogen deficiency has been classified into two types.[242] In type I, the concentration of immunoreactive plasminogen is reduced in parallel with functional activity. Although no examples of complete aplasminogenemia have been reported in humans, type I mutations giving rise to reduced production of plasminogen (e.g., Ser572Pro) have been reported.[243] In a study of consecutive patients with thrombophilia, the prevalence of plasminogen deficiency was 1.9 percent.[244] Approximately half of these individuals had other risk factors, such as deficiency of antithrombin III, protein C, or protein S or resistance to activated protein C. Among 93 patients with type I plasminogen deficiency, the prevalence of thrombosis was 24 percent, or 9 percent when the propositi were excluded.[245] These data suggest that, compared with other thrombophilic conditions, the risk of thrombosis in inherited plasminogen deficiency is not as high[245] (see Chap. 122).

In one well-documented case of type I plasminogen deficiency, an infant with less than 1 percent of normal plasminogen antigen and activity presented with hydrocephalus, central nervous system malformations, poor wound healing, and recurrent respiratory infections, but no family history of thrombosis. His severe ligneous conjunctivitis, that is, development of fibrinous membrane over the eyes, resolved completely upon infusion of lys-plasminogen.[246] This case illustrates the importance of plasminogen in extravascular fibrinolysis and underscores the role of plasminogen deficiency as a relatively weak predisposing risk factor for thrombosis.[242]

In type II plasminogen deficiency, immunoreactive protein is normal but functional activity is reduced.[240] In a study of a Japanese cohort, 94 percent of 129 families with type II dysplasminogenemia had the Ala601Thr mutation, whereas 3 percent and 1 percent had the Val355Phe and Asp676Asn mutation, respectively.[247] In this study, approximately 27 percent of individuals with dysplasminogenemia had a clinical history of thrombosis. A number of additional plasminogen polymorphisms[248–250] and clinically significant dysplasminogenemias[251] have been reported.

Mutations in t-PA or urokinase have not been clinically linked to thrombophilia. However, defects in plasminogen activator release from the vessel wall and increased inhibition of t-PA by PAI-1 both have been associated with a thrombotic diathesis.[252–254] Increased circulating PAI-1 levels appear to be an independent risk factor for vascular reocclusion in young survivors of myocardial infarction (MI).[255] In addition, increased levels of PAI-1 have been associated with deep vein thrombosis in patients undergoing hip replacement surgery[256] and in individuals with insulin resistance.[257] With regard to the latter studies, however, bear in mind that PAI-1 itself is an acute phase reactant and thus may not be directly responsible for the observed prothrombotic tendency.[258]

ENHANCED FIBRINOLYSIS AND BLEEDING

Enhanced fibrinolysis resulting from congenital or acquired loss of fibrinolytic inhibitor activity is associated with a bleeding diathesis.[259] Patients with congenital deficiency of α_2-PI may present with a severe hemorrhagic disorder resulting from impaired inactivation of plasmin and premature lysis of the hemostatic plug.[260] Acquired α_2-PI deficiency may be seen in patients with severe liver disease resulting from decreased synthesis, DIC from consumption, nephrotic syndrome from urinary losses, or during thrombolytic therapy, which induces excessive utilization of the inhibitor.[260]

Patients with acute promyelocytic leukemia demonstrate excessive expression of annexin 2 on their developmentally arrested promyelocytes. Bleeding in this disorder is accompanied by evidence of high levels of plasmin generation and depletion of α_2-PI. Bleeding resolves upon initiation of all-*trans*-retinoic acid therapy, which eliminates expression of promyelocyte annexin 2, probably through a transcriptional mechanism.[149]

Complete loss of PAI-1 expression resulting in hemorrhage in a 9-year-old child was associated with severe hemorrhage in the setting of trauma or surgery.[115] This autosomal recessive trait reflected a frameshift mutation within exon 4 that induced a premature stop codon. This case demonstrates that the function of PAI-1 in humans apparently is limited to regulation of fibrinolysis.

DEVELOPMENTAL REGULATION OF THE FIBRINOLYTIC SYSTEM

In the resting, nonstressed state, the plasmin-generating potential in the newborn is significantly less than that of the adult.[261] Although the amino acid composition and apparent molecular mass of neonatal plasminogen are indistinguishable from those of the adult protein,[262,263] plasma concentrations of plasminogen in the neonate are approximately 50 percent of adult levels.[262,264,265] On the other hand, levels of histidine-rich glycoprotein, a carrier protein that may limit plasminogen's interaction with fibrin, are reduced by 50 to 80 percent in healthy term newborns.[266] Finally, plasminogen in the neonate is heavily glycosylated, less readily activated by t-PA, and only weakly bound to the endothelial cell surface.[263]

Although t-PA antigen and activity levels in the healthy newborn are reduced by 63 and 75 percent, respectively, compared with adult values,[265] stressed infants, such as those with severe congenital heart disease or respiratory distress syndrome, may have t-PA antigen levels that are increased by up to eightfold.[267,268] In contrast, the principal plasmin inhibitors undergo only minimal change from birth to adulthood.[264,269–271] Thus, reduced fibrinolytic activity may contribute to the thrombogenic state commonly observed in newborns,[272] but this predilection may be reversed under conditions of physiologic stress.

FIBRINOLYTIC ACTIVITY DURING PREGNANCY AND PUERPERIUM

Pregnancy is a hypofibrinolytic state.[273] Both plasminogen and fibrinogen levels in plasma increase by 50 to 60 percent during the third trimester. Overall fibrinolytic activity, as reflected in euglobulin lysis activity, is reduced, and increased fibrin deposition is suggested by increasing D-dimer levels throughout pregnancy.[274] Between week 20 of pregnancy and term, PAI-1 levels increase to three times their normal level whereas PAI-2 levels rise to 25 times their level during early pregnancy.[273] Less dramatic increases in both u-PA and t-PA levels also are observed. Within 1 hour of delivery, concentrations of both PAI-1 and PAI-2 begin to decrease and return to normal within 3 to 5 days.[273]

In preeclampsia, the hemostatic and fibrinolytic imbalances seen in pregnancy are further exaggerated.[275] Circulating PAI-1 levels exceed the levels in normal pregnancy, and fibrin deposition is seen in glomerular capillaries and spiral arteries of the placenta. Interestingly, levels of PAI-2, a marker of placental function, are reduced during preeclampsia compared with normal pregnancy, and the decrease correlates with intrauterine growth retardation of the fetus.

FIBRINOLYTIC THERAPY

The goal of thrombolytic therapy is rapid restoration of flow in an occluded vessel achieved by accelerating fibrinolytic proteolysis of the thrombus. The fibrinolytic system functions physiologically to remove fibrin deposits through the action of plasmin, but this process often is too slow to prevent tissue injury following acute vascular occlusion. Because arterial thrombosis immediately renders distal tissue ischemic with rapid onset of dysfunction and necrosis, a critical problem is minimizing time to restoration of flow. Thrombolytic therapy should be viewed as one part of an overall antithrombotic plan that frequently includes anticoagulants, antiplatelet agents, and mechanical approaches, all designed to rapidly restore flow, prevent reocclusion, and promote healing. Fibrinolytic therapy for acute MI was first attempted in 1958 by Fletcher and colleagues.[276] Since then, advances in biochemistry and pharmacology and the results of numerous clinical trials have led to approval of several therapeutic agents and to the routine use of thrombolysis in common clinical conditions, including acute MI, stroke, occlusive peripheral vascular disease, deep vein thrombosis, and pulmonary embolism. Thrombolytic therapy for MI is discussed in Chap. 126 and for deep vein thrombosis and pulmonary embolism in Chap. 125. The pharmacology of thrombolytic agents is discussed in Chap. 21.

PRINCIPLES OF THERAPY

All fibrinolytic drugs are enzymes that accelerate the conversion of plasminogen to plasmin, a serine protease that degrades the insoluble fibrin clot matrix into soluble derivatives. Plasminogen, normally found in plasma at micromolar concentrations, also binds specifically to fibrin. Physiologically, fibrinolysis is carefully regulated. Small amounts of plasminogen activator present in the blood or secreted locally by endothelial cells at the site of fibrin deposition convert fibrin-bound plasminogen to plasmin that acts locally to slowly dissolve the fibrin deposit, thereby liberating soluble degradation products of fibrin. The biochemical properties of fibrin, plasminogen activators, and inhibitors promote plasmin generation on the fibrin matrix but prevent its activation in the blood. The basic principle of all fibrinolytic therapy, therefore, is administration of pharmacologic amounts of plasminogen activator to achieve a high local concentration at the site of the thrombus and thereby accelerate conversion of plasminogen to plasmin and increase the rate of fibrin dissolution. If large amounts of plasminogen activator overwhelm the natural regulatory systems, plasmin may be formed in the blood, resulting in degradation of susceptible proteins, the "lytic state."[277] Additionally, because high concentrations of activator are not limited to the site of thrombosis, fibrin deposits at other sites, including physiologic hemostatic plugs needed at sites of injury, may dissolve and cause local bleeding, often exacerbated by the hypocoagulable state caused by plasmic proteolysis of proteins in the blood (Fig. 127-4).

Several therapeutic agents are available and approved for thrombolytic use (Table 127-3). Most are produced by recombinant methods, whereas others derive from natural sources and can be antigenic, causing allergic reactions. The degree of "fibrin specificity" also varies, so the intensity of action at the site of thrombosis must be compared to proteolysis of plasma proteins. The plasma half-life of most agents is short, ranging from 5 minutes for t-PA to as long as 70 minutes for anistreplase. The method of administration (bolus or continuous intravenous) and duration of therapy are determined by the half-life and by the specific condition being treated.

An important issue for treatment is use of systemic versus local or regional administration. Systemic therapy is delivered by peripheral vein, offers the advantage of simplicity, and does not require specialized facilities. However, this approach results in a greater risk of bleeding because large doses must be administered to achieve a sufficiently high concentration at the site of thrombosis. Regional delivery with a catheter placed close to the proximal end of the thrombus can deliver a high local concentration with a smaller total dose. This method increases the local effect and limits systemic exposure, although a portion of the drug delivered does reach the systemic circulation. For some indications, such as therapy for peripheral vascular disease, the catheter is positioned within the thrombus for direct drug administration and optimum effectiveness.

Fibrinolytic therapy should be viewed as one part of a combined antithrombotic strategy. For best results, thrombolytic therapy typically is given as soon as the patient presents with acute symptoms. This therapy accelerates thrombus dissolution by increasing fibrinolysis, but the overall process of thrombosis is dynamic, with concurrent fibrin formation and platelet deposition. Therefore, the change in thrombus size results from a balance of these processes, and fibrinolytic therapy often is administered in combination with an anticoagulant to block fibrin formation and with an antiplatelet agent to limit continued platelet deposition. Anticoagulant therapy is routinely continued after completion of fibrinolytic therapy to prevent thrombotic reocclusion stimulated by the procoagulant effects of the original lesion and by prothrombotic effects of fibrinolytic therapy itself. Finally, neither fibrinolytic therapy nor anticoagulant or antiplatelet drugs alters some local pathologic lesions, such as the atherosclerotic plaque, and mechanical approaches such as percutaneous coronary angioplasty play a vital role in successful therapy.

Fibrinolytic therapy typically results in proteolytic changes in the blood because plasminogen activation is not limited to the thrombus. These effects are complex and include reduced fibrinogen, increased fibrinogen degradation products, and decreased plasminogen and α_2-PI. Screening coagulation tests, including the activated partial thromboplastin time (aPTT), prothrombin time (PT), and thrombin clotting time, will be prolonged, depending on the intensity of the lytic state. Tests reflecting plasminogen activation, such as the euglobulin clot lysis time, will be abnormal. Platelet membrane proteins may be degraded, resulting in abnormal platelet function.[278–280] Overall, these effects contribute to a hypocoagulable state that may be beneficial in contributing to vessel patency but also may exacerbate a bleeding complication. The magnitude of the changes depends on the dose of plasminogen activator administered and its degree of fibrin specificity. Thus, high doses of a nonspecific activator, such as streptokinase,

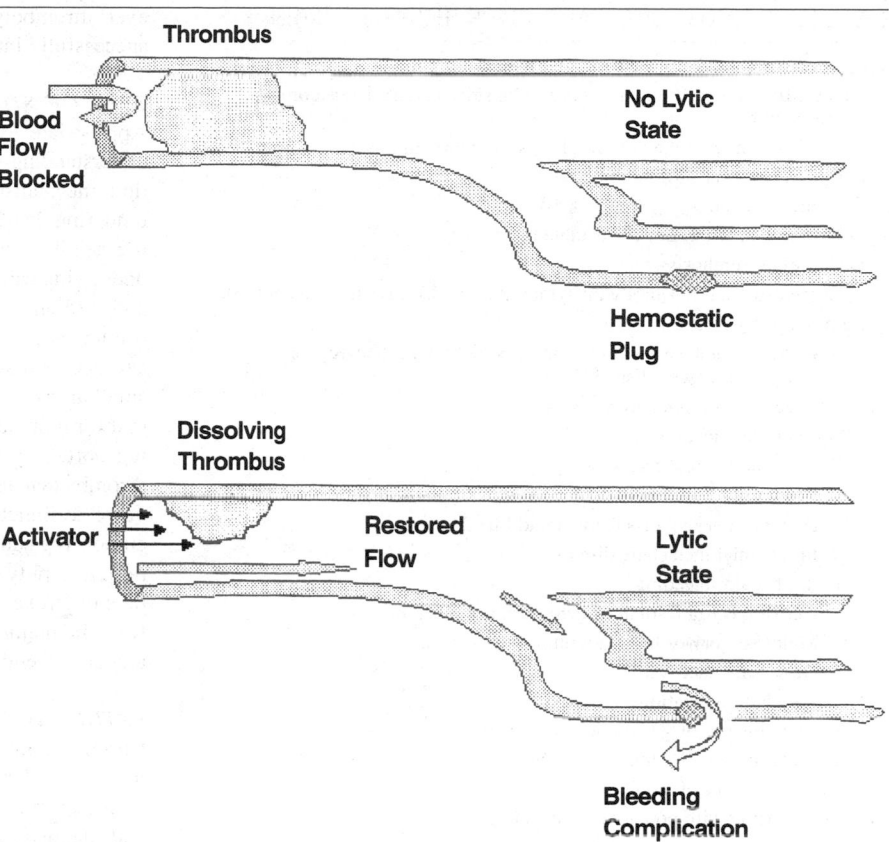

FIGURE 127-4 Multiple actions of fibrinolytic agents. Fibrinolytic therapy by pharmacologic doses of plasminogen activators causes a hypocoagulable "lytic state" that dissolves the clot, thereby resuming blood flow, but at the same time potentially accelerating lysis of physiologic hemostatic plugs at sites of vessel injury, giving rise to bleeding.

cause a marked lytic state, whereas a fibrin-specific agent such as reteplase administered as therapy for acute MI has a much lesser effect. Monitoring the hemostatic changes of the lytic state is of limited clinical value because the changes are not strongly predictive of either thrombolysis or bleeding complications.[281–284]

The decision to administer fibrinolytic therapy and the choice of agent and regimen depend on careful consideration of risks and ben-

TABLE 127-3 COMPARISON OF PLASMINOGEN ACTIVATORS

AGENT (REGIMEN)	SOURCE (APPROVED/ AVAILABLE)	ANTIGENIC	HALF-LIFE (MIN)
Streptokinase (infusion)	Streptococcus (Y/Y)	Yes	20
Urokinase (infusion)	Cell culture; recombinant (Y/N)	No	15
Alteplase (t-PA) (infusion)	Recombinant (Y/Y)	No	5
Anistreplase (bolus)	Streptococcus + plasma product (Y/N)	No	70
Reteplase (double bolus)	Recombinant (Y/Y)	No	15
Saruplase (scu-PA) (infusion)	Recombinant (N/N)	No	5
Staphylokinase (infusion)	Recombinant (N/N)	Yes	
Tenecteplase (bolus)	Recombinant (Y/Y)	No	15

TABLE 127-4 SELECTION OF PATIENTS FOR THROMBOLYTIC THERAPY

Treat those most likely to respond and benefit
  Acute MI: Within 12 hours of onset. Consider percutaneous coronary intervention
  Stroke: Ischemic stroke within 3 hours of symptom onset
  Peripheral arterial obstruction
    Acute occlusions
    Distal obstruction not correctable by surgery
  Deep vein thrombosis
    Large proximal thrombi with symptoms for <7 days (see Chap. 125)
  Pulmonary embolism
    Massive or submassive embolism, especially with hemodynamic compromise (see Chap. 125)
Prevent bleeding complications
  Major contraindications
    Risk of intracranial bleeding
      Recent head trauma or central nervous system surgery
      History of stroke or subarachnoid bleed
      Intracranial metastatic disease
    Risk of major bleeding
      Active gastrointestinal or genitourinary bleeding
      Major surgery or trauma within 7 days
      Dissecting aneurysm
  Relative contraindications
    Remote history of gastrointestinal bleeding
    Remote history of genitourinary bleeding
    Remote history of peptic ulcer
    Other lesion with potential for bleeding
    Recent minor surgery or trauma
    Severe, uncontrolled hypertension
    Coexisting hemostatic abnormalities
    Pregnancy

efits for an individual patient (Table 127-4). For patients with acute MI or stroke, a higher tolerance of bleeding complications is accepted because lytic therapy can be life-saving and can limit disability. Indeed, an overall improvement in outcome of stroke treatment is seen even though the rate of intracranial hemorrhage clearly is increased. Timing of treatment is critical, with greater benefit achieved with earlier administration. With venous disease, the potential benefits are less. However, fibrinolytic therapy for acute pulmonary embolism with hemodynamic compromise may be life-saving. Bleeding becomes more problematic for treatment of deep vein thrombosis because the benefit of rapid symptomatic relief and possible reduction in long-term complications is less dramatic. The risks of bleeding must be considered in all patients. Local bleeding complications at the site of vascular intervention are frequent, and catheterization sites must be closely monitored. Major bleeding complications involving the gastrointestinal tract, retroperitoneum, and especially intracranial hemorrhage may be life-threatening.

THROMBOLYTIC THERAPY FOR STROKE

Stroke is the third leading cause of death in the United States, with an annual incidence of 700,000, including 500,000 new episodes per year. Stroke also is the leading cause of serious disability. The incidence has been declining, most likely related to the control of risk factors. Total numbers are increasing, however, because of the increasing age of the population. Antithrombotic therapy plays an important role in management, primarily with use of aspirin in prevention (see Chap. 125) and anticoagulation for atrial fibrillation (see Chap. 126). However, thrombolytic therapy is the only approach currently available to successfully intervene during the acute stage.

TYPE OF STROKE

Appropriate use of thrombolytic therapy for stroke is based on an understanding of its pathogenesis. Ischemic stroke is caused by multiple mechanisms that suddenly block arterial flow in a brain vessel, rendering distal tissue ischemic with immediate dysfunction and leading rapidly to necrosis if blood flow is not restored. The most common underlying cause of ischemic stroke is atherosclerosis involving large- and medium-size arteries in the neck and cranium. Arterial thrombosis originates on disrupted atherosclerotic plaque and is the most common cause of stroke, but transient ischemic attack and stroke involving small arteries can result from embolization of platelet–fibrin thrombi that form on atherosclerotic vessels in the carotid arteries and ascending aorta. Up to 25 percent of strokes result from embolization of thrombi that form in the heart in association with atrial fibrillation, valve dysfunction, artificial valves, and endocardial thrombi. These emboli typically are relatively large and cause serious cortical infarction. A variety of uncommon vascular diseases account for small numbers of stroke, and up to 30 percent have no defined etiology. Therefore, the majority of strokes are caused by thrombi or thromboemboli and are potentially susceptible to thrombolytic therapy.

PATHOPHYSIOLOGY OF THE LESION

Current approaches to thrombolytic therapy for stroke are based on imaging to define the etiology, results of clinical trials, and experience with thrombolysis for acute MI. Modern computed tomography (CT) and magnetic resonance imaging (MRI) can identify ischemic areas quite early and localize areas of hemorrhage. Additionally, arteriography may be useful in some cases and can identify accurately obstructed vessels and follow the course of recanalization during thrombolytic therapy. Clinical studies have generally followed the successful designs used for MI that demonstrated the critical pathologic role of the occluded vessel, the importance of early recanalization in preserving myocardium, the impressive decrease in morbidity and mortality resulting from early reperfusion, and characterization of the bleeding risk. The experience with thrombolytic treatment of stroke also highlights important differences from MI. The arterial anatomy of the brain is more complex, the time from onset of ischemia to irreversible necrosis is shorter, the risk and consequences of bleeding are greater, and more variability exists in the thrombo(embolic) occluding lesion. Further, the occlusive platelet–fibrin thrombus that precipitates MI is quite small and has a consistent structure. In contrast, the occlusive lesion causing ischemic stroke may be a large *in situ* thrombus, small platelet–fibrin embolus, or large embolus of varying age and composition originating from the left atrium. Overall, results with thrombolysis for stroke have made a smaller impact than for treatment of MI, largely based on these differences.

EARLY THROMBOLYTIC STUDIES

The current therapeutic approach began with small studies in the 1980s, followed by large multicenter, randomized controlled trials throughout the 1990s and still ongoing. Early studies were small, open labeled, and used streptokinase, urokinase, and t-PA given intravenously or intraarterially to determine the dose, recanalization rate, hemorrhagic potential, and clinical predictors of response.[285–300] The principal findings were that recanalization of occluded vessels could be achieved, recanalization often resulted in clinical improvement, treatment was necessary very early after presentation, and the rate of intracranial hemorrhage and hemorrhagic transformation within the ischemic area was high. Phase II studies were performed to define the optimum dosage of intravenous t-PA and the time window from symptom onset to treatment as a basis for larger phase III trials. The current approach to thrombolytic therapy for stroke is based on the results of the large clinical trials primarily performed with recombinant t-PA (Table 127-5). Generally, these studies administered intravenous t-PA within 3 hours of symptom onset and demonstrated clinically significant improvements in outcomes.

TISSUE-PLASMINOGEN ACTIVATOR THERAPY

The National Institute of Neurological Disorders and Stroke (NINDS) study demonstrated the benefit of t-PA most clearly. This trial was a two-part randomized, double-blind, placebo-controlled study.[301] Part I involved 291 patients and tested whether t-PA had activity as indicated by clinical findings at 24 hours. Part II enrolled 333 patients, and the primary endpoint was clinical outcome at 3 months. All patients were treated with a total dose of 0.9 mg/kg t-PA within 3 hours of symptom onset. The combined results showed a 30 percent improvement in objectively characterized clinical outcomes at 3 months from a rate of 21 percent to 38 percent of patients with no or minimal disability. This benefit persisted at 12 months and was observed despite a 10-fold increase in early symptomatic intracranial hemorrhage from 0.6 percent to 6.4 percent. There was no difference between the groups in mortality at 3 months. This study formed the basis of the 1996 US Food and Drug Administration (FDA) approval of intravenous t-PA for treatment of stroke.

The European Cooperative Acute Stroke Study (ECASS) study had a similar design and included 622 subjects with moderate-to-severe symptoms who were randomized to placebo or t-PA at a higher dose of 1.1 mg/kg within 6 hours of symptom onset.[302] No significant differences were observed between the groups in the primary endpoint of functional status at 90 days and in 30-day mortality. The t-PA group showed some benefits in secondary endpoints, such as neurologic recovery at 90 days, shorter hospital stay, and more rapid recovery. The ECASS II study included 800 patients randomized to receive either rt-PA or placebo within 6 hours of symptom onset, with stratification for presentation up to 3 hours after symptom onset or between 3 and 6 hours.[303] No significant benefit of thrombolytic therapy was seen using the primary endpoint of functional capacity at 90 days. The Alteplase Thrombolysis for Acute Noninterventional Therapy in Ischemic Stroke (ATLANTIS) study evaluated the safety of rt-PA in a double-blind, placebo-controlled study with administration of drug between 3 to 5 hours after symptom onset.[304] rt-PA was administered at a dosage of 0.9 mg/kg over 1 hour. The primary endpoint of excellent neurologic recovery was observed in 32 percent of placebo and 34 percent of rt-PA–treated patients. No significant difference in secondary functional endpoints was observed. Early symptomatic intracranial hemorrhage occurred in 1.1 percent of control and 7 percent of rt-PA–treated patients. A nonsignificant trend toward increased mortality with rt-PA treatment at 90 days was observed (6.9% vs. 11.0%, $P = 0.09$).

STREPTOKINASE THERAPY

Streptokinase has been evaluated in three large stroke trials. The Australian Streptokinase (ASK) study was a double-blind, placebo-controlled trial of 340 patients randomized within 4 hours of symptom onset to receive placebo or 1.5 million U of streptokinase over 1 hour.[305] The early results showed an increase in unfavorable outcomes

TABLE 127-5 MAJOR FIBRINOLYTIC THERAPY TRIALS OF STROKE

STUDY	NO. OF PATIENTS	TIME (H)	DRUG	THROMBOLYTIC DOSE*†	MAIN EFFICACY RESULT
NINDS	624	≤3	t-PA, IV	0.9 mg/kg	Reduced disability at 3 months
ECASS I	620	≤6	t-PA, IV	1.1 mg/kg	No significant difference
ECASS II	800	≤6	t-PA, IV	0.9 mg/kg	No significant difference
ATLANTIS	613	≤6‡	t-PA, IV	0.9 mg/kg	No significant difference
ASK	340	≤4	SK, IV	1.5 million U	Increased morbidity and mortality
MAST-I	622	≤6	SK, IV¶	1.5 million U	Increased mortality
MAST-E	310	≤6	SK, IV§	1.5 million U	Increased mortality
PROACT II	180	≤6	Pro-UK,‖ IA	9 mg	Improved 3-month outcome

* All placebo-controlled
† All given over 1 hour except PROACT II, which was given over 2 hours.
‡ 547/613 within 3–5 hours
¶ 2 × 2 factorial design with aspirin (ASA) 300 mg/day.
§ ASA 100 mg/day.
‖ Pro-UK and placebo group also received heparin.

in streptokinase-treated patients, and the study was prematurely terminated. The death rate at 90 days was significantly higher in patients receiving streptokinase. Evidence of an improved outcome in the streptokinase group was seen in the small subgroup of 70 patients who entered the trial within 3 hours of symptom onset. The Multicenter Acute Stroke Trial—Italy (MAST-I) examined benefits and risks of streptokinase treatment with or without aspirin in 622 patients with acute ischemic stroke who presented within 6 hours of symptom onset using a 2 × 2 design.[306] Patients received 1.5 million U of streptokinase over 1 hour, and aspirin was given at a dose of 300 mg/day. Interim analysis resulted in early termination because streptokinase treatment was associated with a 2.7-fold increase in fatality at 10 days as a result of an increased death rate among patients receiving the combination of streptokinase and aspirin. The Multicenter Acute Stroke Trial—Europe (MAST-E) enrolled 310 patients with moderate-to-severe ischemia in the distribution of the middle cerebral artery who were randomized to receive placebo or 1.5 million U of streptokinase over 1 hour within 6 hours of symptom onset in a double-blind study.[307] The outcome endpoint of mortality or severe disability was not significantly different between the two groups. However, the mortality rate at 10 days was higher in patients who received streptokinase compared with placebo (34.0% vs. 18.2%, $P < 0.02$) primarily because of hemorrhagic transformation of infarcts.

INTRAARTERIAL THROMBOLYSIS

Potential advantages of intraarterial administration include delivery of a higher concentration of an activator proximally or directly into the thrombus using an appropriately placed catheter, more accurate anatomic diagnosis, ability to observe the course of recanalization, and lower total doses of drug that might reduce intracranial hemorrhage. Problems with this approach include the need for specialized facilities and experienced personnel available at all times to perform arteriography and selective catheterization. These requirements generally result in longer times before treatment can be delivered, which is a critical variable in treatment success. Several small open-label trials observed a high rate of recanalization and apparent clinical benefit with intraarterial therapy using urokinase, streptokinase, or t-PA, but hemorrhagic transformation was a frequent problem.[288,292,295,298,308–313] Intraarterial therapy may have particular value in acute basilar artery occlusion, which has a very high mortality but clinical recovery in up to 50 percent of patients receiving intraarterial thrombolysis.

The Prolyse in Acute Cerebral Thromboembolism (PROACT) and PROACT II trials evaluated recombinant human prourokinase by catheter-directed intraarterial administration. The PROACT trial included 26 patients with occlusion in the territory of the middle cerebral artery who received intraarterial prourokinase and heparin and 14 patients treated with heparin alone.[314] A significantly higher recanalization rate with prourokinase treatment but no increase in intracranial hemorrhage was observed. This finding led to the larger PROACT II trial, a randomized, placebo-controlled open-label trial that included 180 patients with acute occlusion of the middle cerebral artery who were treated within 6 hours of symptom onset with either heparin alone or 9 mg of intraarterial prourokinase plus heparin.[315] The recanalization rate was significantly higher with prourokinase (66% vs. 18%, $P < 0.001$). Functional improvement at 90 days also was superior. Symptomatic intracranial hemorrhage occurred in 10 percent of patients treated with prourokinase and 2 percent of controls. These results, although promising, did not lead to FDA approval of intraarterial prourokinase for treatment of stroke. Cochrane Reviews of these studies are available.[316,317]

Overall, these studies show that treatment of acute stroke with thrombolytic therapy can lead to recanalization of the occluded artery and improvement in clinical outcomes. A critical issue is the time from symptom onset to the start of therapy. Evidence is clear that earlier treatment results in better results. The need for very early treatment currently is the single largest limitation to greater application of thrombolytic therapy for stroke.[318-320] Fewer than 5 percent of stroke patients currently receive t-PA treatment because treatment is limited to patients who present within 3 hours of symptom onset and because of the additional contraindication to thrombolytic therapy. The greatest impediment is the delay from the time patients experience symptoms to the time they appear in the emergency room. Focused community educational efforts must be made if this treatment is to have a greater impact. The rate of intracranial hemorrhage is high, principally because of hemorrhagic transformation within ischemic tissue. Despite early deaths and increased morbidity in patients affected with intracranial hemorrhage, the overall functional results among stroke patients can be improved. The results are critically dependent on the dose and choice of thrombolytic agent. Clinical studies with intravenous t-PA showed better results, whereas streptokinase was associated with an unacceptably high rate of intracranial hemorrhage. Whether this difference results from intrinsic properties of these agents or dose and treatment intensity remains controversial.

Thrombolytic therapy for stroke is an area of intense investigation aimed at increasing the proportion of patients who can be successfully treated. This process will require motivating patients to seek medical attention earlier and extending the successful treatment period beyond 3 hours after symptom onset. An additional goal is to reduce intracranial hemorrhage by identifying patients at greatest risk using newer imaging modalities. Studies are evaluating newer agents, including reteplase and tenecteplase. The combination of potent antiplatelet therapy using a glycoprotein IIb/IIIa antagonist with a lower dose of a thrombolytic agent may improve results.[321-323] Other studies are examining the combination of intravenous and intraarterial therapy[324] and the adjunctive use of low-intensity ultrasound to accelerate fibrinolysis.[325,326]

Current recommendations limit thrombolytic therapy for stroke to patients who present within 3 hours of symptom onset.[327-329] The approved therapy consists of 0.9 mg/kg (maximum 90 mg) of t-PA administered intravenously, with 10 percent as an initial bolus and the remainder infused over 60 minutes. The best results are obtained in patients who meet strict eligibility requirements (Table 127-6). Treatment of patients who present beyond 3 hours is not recommended. Patients should be closely monitored for bleeding complications, es-

TABLE 127-6 GUIDELINES FOR t-PA IN STROKE

ELIGIBILITY
Diagnosis of ischemic stroke with significant neurologic deficit
Time from symptom onset to therapy ≤3 hours
Exclusions
Prior intracranial hemorrhage
Major surgery within 14 days
Gastrointestinal or urinary tract bleeding within 21 days
Arterial puncture in noncompressible site
Recent lumbar puncture
Intracranial surgery, serious head trauma, or prior stroke within 3 months
Minor neurologic deficit
Seizure at time of stroke onset
Clinical findings of subarachnoid hemorrhage
Active bleeding
Persistent systolic BP >185 and/or diastolic BP >110 or requiring aggressive treatment
Arteriovenous malformation or aneurysm
Evidence of hemorrhage on CT scan
Platelets <100,000/mm³
INR >1.5 on warfarin
Elevated PTT on heparin
Blood glucose <40 or >400 mg/dl

pecially intracranial hemorrhage. Facilities should be available for managing bleeding complications. Careful attention to management of blood pressure and other comorbidities is critical.

PERIPHERAL VASCULAR DISEASE

Most peripheral vascular disease results from atherosclerosis that progressively limits flow distally in the legs, resulting in clinical presentation with symptoms of claudication, rest pain, and tissue loss in severe cases. Typically, occlusive disease of the leg vessels is only one aspect of generalized atherosclerosis also involving the coronary and cerebral circulation. Treatment seeks to reduce disease progression through amelioration of risk factors and to decrease symptoms by improving flow through exercise, medication, and endovascular or surgical approaches to revascularization. Thrombolysis has very little role in treatment of chronic symptoms.

Acute peripheral arterial occlusion presents with the sudden onset of new, severe leg symptoms or critical acute worsening of chronic ischemia. It often involves embolic or acute thrombotic occlusion of leg arteries. The presentation usually is urgent, and the goals of treatment are to preserve limb function through restoration of flow. Anticoagulation typically is administered to prevent thrombus extension, whereas thrombolytic therapy or surgery can be used to restore perfusion.

The role of thrombolysis in acute peripheral arterial occlusion has evolved from the early application of systemic treatment to the current use of local arterial infusion. Large prospective studies have helped define the role of thrombolysis in relation to surgical intervention. The current approach uses thrombolysis in conjunction with both endovascular and surgical procedures for comprehensive treatment to maximize amputation-free survival. Unique challenges for thrombolytic therapy for peripheral arterial occlusion include the large size of arterial thrombi in comparison with coronary or cranial thrombi and the variable sites of occlusion extending from proximal aortoiliac disease to infrapopliteal small-vessel occlusion often seen in diabetics. Additionally, patients often have serious vascular comorbidities, including hypertension, diabetes, and coronary or cerebrovascular disease, which increase risk of bleeding and other operative complications.

Early approaches consisted of systemic thrombolytic therapy using streptokinase. The results of small studies demonstrated evidence of reperfusion in approximately 40 percent of patients, with greater success in treating occlusions of recent onset. Both embolic and thrombotic occlusions responded, and bleeding complications occurred in up to one third of patients.[330] Following the 1974 report by Dotter and colleagues[331] of successful thrombolysis in peripheral arterial occlusion using locally administered thrombolysis, practice moved progressively to the nearly exclusive use of local intraarterially administered treatment. Advantages include delivery of a high concentration of drug directly to the site of thrombosis, the ability to follow the course of treatment using the treatment catheter, and identification of local vascular lesions requiring endovascular or surgical treatment after recanalization.

Treatment involves obtaining arterial access from a remote site, followed by fluoroscopic guidance of the catheter to the site of obstruction. A guidewire is extended through the thrombus, and an infusion catheter is advanced to administer drug directly into the thrombus. This process is an important determinant of success, which is significantly less if the infusion is administered proximal to, but not within, the clot. Therapy is delivered by continuous infusion over a prolonged period of hours to days and requires close monitoring and a large dose of thrombolytic agent. Successful reperfusion occurs in approximately three fourths of patients overall. Intraarterial t-PA or urokinase is more effective than either intravenous t-PA or intravenous streptokinase.[332]

The relative roles of thrombolysis and surgery were explored in several prospective studies over the past 10 years. Ouriel and colleagues[333] reported the results of a prospective, randomized trial of 114 patients with limb-threatening ischemia of less than 7 days' duration who were assigned to receive either intraarterial urokinase or primary operative intervention. Thrombolytic therapy resulted in a 70 percent recanalization rate, and the frequency of limb salvage was the same in both groups at 1 year. However, a survival advantage was seen in patients who received primary thrombolytic therapy, resulting primarily from a decrease in the occurrence of in-hospital complications. The Surgery versus Thrombolysis for Ischemia of the Lower Extremity (STILE) trial enrolled 393 patients with nonembolic, native arterial or graft occlusion of less than 6 months' duration who were randomized to undergo the optimal surgical procedure or catheter-directed thrombolysis with either t-PA or urokinase.[334] The study was terminated prematurely because of lower ongoing or recurrent ischemia at 30 days in surgically treated patients. Some benefit to thrombolysis was observed, however, as patients with symptoms of fewer than 14 days' duration who were treated with thrombolysis had a lower amputation rate. More than half of patients who received thrombolysis had a decrease in the magnitude of the surgical procedure eventually required. No difference was seen in results with use of either t-PA or urokinase.

The Thrombolysis or Peripheral Arterial Surgery (TOPAS) I study compared recombinant urokinase or surgery for initial therapy for acute lower extremity ischemia of less than 14 days' duration in 213 patients who were randomized to one of three doses of urokinase or to surgery for initial therapy.[335] A dose of 4000 IU/min selected as the optimum urokinase dose resulted in complete clot lysis in 71 percent of patients, with hemorrhagic complications in 2 percent. One-year mortality and amputation-free survival were similar in the urokinase and surgery groups. A significant reduction in the frequency and magnitude of surgical interventions eventually required in patients randomized to initial thrombolysis was seen. The larger TOPAS II study included 544 patients with acute arterial obstruction of less than 14 days' duration.[336] Patients were randomized to either initial therapy with catheter-directed intraarterial recombinant urokinase or to sur-

gery. Recanalization occurred in 80 percent of patients who received urokinase. Amputation-free survival at 1 year was not significantly different between the two groups (65% with urokinase vs. 70% with surgery). Fewer patients in the thrombolysis group required surgical procedures by 6 months. Major hemorrhagic complications were significantly more frequent with urokinase (13%) compared to 6 percent with surgery ($P = 0.005$), with four episodes of intracranial hemorrhage occurring in the urokinase group.

Studies have investigated modified thrombolytic regimens. Reteplase appears to be equally effective as t-PA or urokinase with comparable recanalization rates, clinical outcomes, and bleeding complications.[337,338] Prourokinase also gave similar overall results to urokinase in a phase II study.[339] In an open-label trial, staphylokinase, a highly fibrin-specific plasminogen activator, given to 191 patients with peripheral arterial occlusion of less than 120 days' duration resulted in revascularization in 83 percent.[340] Occasional allergic reactions occurred, and severe bleeding complications were comparable to those with other agents. The addition of abciximab, a glycoprotein IIb/IIIa inhibitor, to urokinase resulted in more rapid clot-like lysis in a randomized study of 70 patients.[341] Good results also were reported with reteplase and abciximab.[342] Intraoperative thrombolysis during thromboembolectomy has been used to improve clearance of distal thromboemboli successfully.[343–346] Mechanical devices have been used with thrombolysis.[347]

Based on available studies, thrombolysis should be viewed as one part of a combined, comprehensive management approach to peripheral arterial occlusion. Early, accurate angiographic diagnosis is important. With appropriate intrathrombic catheter positioning, recanalization can be achieved in a high percentage of patients. The improved clinical condition and better angiographic studies available after reperfusion allow a more optimum choice of definitive endovascular or surgical procedures, and surgery can be avoided in some patients. Thrombolysis has particular appeal for patients with serious comorbidities that increase surgical risk and for lysis of thrombi in small distal vessels that are surgically inaccessible. Cochrane Reviews of studies are available,[348,349] and an excellent review has been provided from the Working Party on Thrombolysis in the Management of Limb Ischemia, which provides practical recommendations for management and an overview of dosing regimens for various thrombolytic agents.[350]

OTHER INDICATIONS

Small series and case reports have reported successful use of thrombolytic therapy for treatment of acute venous and arterial occlusions in a wide variety of sites. Judging the effectiveness based on the available reports is difficult, but thrombolytic therapy certainly is a reasonable choice for treatment of serious acute, symptomatic thrombosis based on a clinical appraisal of bleeding risks and potential benefit. Reports document successful treatment of intraabdominal thrombosis including Budd-Chiari syndrome,[351] portal vein thrombosis,[352–354] and mesenteric vein thrombosis.[354–356] Thrombolytic agents are used frequently to open thrombosed central venous catheters that are occluded with clot.[357–360] Thrombotic occlusion of access devices for hemodialysis is a major clinical problem, and thrombolysis, often in combination with mechanical approaches, often is successful in removing thrombus.[361–365]

MANAGEMENT OF BLEEDING COMPLICATIONS

Bleeding complications occur more frequently with fibrinolytic than with anticoagulant therapy and require rapid diagnosis and management. Two problems contribute to excess bleeding. First, the fibrinolytic effect is not limited to the site of thrombosis but usually is systemic. Therefore, any hemostatic plugs needed to prevent bleeding at sites of vascular injury caused either by catheters needed for treatment or within pathologic lesions in the brain, gastrointestinal tract, or elsewhere are susceptible to dissolution. Second, fibrinolytic therapy creates a systemic hypocoagulable state to a varying degree that is dependent on the dose and type of agent administered.

The most serious complication is intracranial hemorrhage, which occurs in approximately 1 percent of patients and is associated with high mortality and serious disability in survivors. Risk factors for intracranial hemorrhage include prior stroke, serious head trauma, intracranial surgery, tumor or vascular disease, such as aneurysms or arteriovenous malformations, and uncontrolled hypertension.[366] These conditions are strong contraindications to fibrinolytic therapy. The most common bleeding complications are related to invasive vascular procedures, such as placement of arterial and venous catheters. Some bleeding at these sites is frequent and is not a reason for interrupting therapy if the bleeding can be managed with local pressure or other simple measures. The problem can be minimized by limiting venous and arterial punctures and by early institution of local measures. Major bleeding may result from preexisting lesions, such as gastrointestinal ulcers or genitourinary lesions. Minor bleeding complications, such as ecchymoses and microscopic hematuria, are frequent and troublesome but of little clinical consequence.

Before administering thrombolytic therapy, the clinician should be familiar with these bleeding complications and prepared to manage any that develop (Table 127-7).[367] The first step is accurate diagnosis, recognizing that deep bleeding into tissues may appear only as pain and swelling. Intracranial hemorrhage often presents with headache, altered neurologic status, and vomiting. These symptoms represent an emergency, and management should include immediate imaging and neurosurgical consultation.

Treatment of bleeding complications involves measures directed at the local site and correction of the systemic hypocoagulable state resulting from proteolysis of plasma proteins and platelets. Initial management includes discontinuation of the fibrinolytic agent, which will be cleared rapidly because most such agents have a short half-life. For serious bleeding, an antifibrinolytic agent such as ε-aminocaproic acid (EACA) can be administered to block fibrinolysis. This step is of value only if the fibrinolytic agent remains in the blood, and its appropriate use depends on knowledge of the clearance rate of the agent administered. Replacement therapy to correct the hemostatic defect caused by systemic plasminemia is the next step. Fibrinogen replacement often is needed and can be accomplished by administration of 5 to 10 bags of cryoprecipitate. Fresh-frozen plasma can be used to replace

TABLE 127-7   TREATMENT OF FIBRINOLYTIC BLEEDING

If intracranial bleed is suspected, obtain imaging, consult neurosurgery, and correct hemostasis as follows.

For major bleeding:

Perform diagnostic test: aPTT, platelet count, fibrinogen.

Attend to local hemostatic problems. Apply pressure if bleeding is related to arterial puncture. Proceed with general supportive measures, including intravenous fluid hydration and transfusion of packed red cells if indicated. Proceed with diagnostic evaluation for gastrointestinal or genitourinary tract bleeding.

Correct abnormal hemostasis:

Prevent further fibrinolysis: stop fibrinolytic therapy; consider EACA or aprotinin.

Replacement therapy to repair hemostasis defect induced by fibrinolytic therapy: give cryoprecipitate 5–10 U and 2 U fresh-frozen plasma; consider platelet transfusion.

Correct other hemostatic defects: stop anticoagulant and antiplatelet agents; consider protamine to reverse heparin.

other hemostatic proteins. Replacement treatment should be monitored with repeated coagulation tests. Administration of platelet concentrates can also be useful because fibrinolytic therapy results in platelet dysfunction from proteolysis of surface proteins. Replacement of platelets, however, may not be of consistent value because the circulating fibrin(ogen) degradation products induced by fibrinolytic therapy can inhibit the function of infused platelets. Additionally, all other anticoagulant and antiplatelet agents should be discontinued. Heparin effect can be reversed by administration of protamine sulfate, and desmopressin may be of some value in reversing platelet dysfunction.

ANTIFIBRINOLYTIC THERAPY

PRINCIPLES OF THERAPY

The fibrinolytic system functions physiologically to remove fibrin deposits by converting plasminogen to plasmin, which proteolytically degrades and then solubilizes the fibrin matrix. This carefully regulated process is initiated as fibrin is formed but functions slowly, allowing for removal of fibrin after its physiologic need is passed. Pathologic processes that cause abnormal regulation can cause either bleeding or thrombosis, and pharmacologic agents have been developed to inhibit fibrinolysis for treatment of bleeding. They have been used in two different situations. First, excessive systemic fibrinolytic activation can cause a hemorrhagic diathesis associated with certain pathologic conditions and during fibrinolytic therapy. Second, the normal process of fibrinolysis may contribute to local bleeding by prematurely removing needed hemostatic plugs. Inhibition of fibrinolysis can improve hemostasis in both situations (Table 127-8). Care must be exercised using antifibrinolytic agents for treatment of bleeding in complicated clinical situations where thrombosis also may occur, because inhibiting fibrinolysis can worsen thrombosis. For example, in patients with DIC, excessive activation of both the coagulation and fibrinolytic systems can result in clinical manifestations of both bleeding and thrombosis. In this situation, inhibiting fibrinolysis to treat bleeding can precipitate or worsen thrombosis (see Chap. 121).

ANTIFIBRINOLYTIC AGENTS

ε-AMINOCAPROIC ACID AND TRANEXAMIC ACID

Two antifibrinolytic agents, EACA and tranexamic acid, are synthetic lysine analogues. Fibrinolysis is accelerated by binding of plasminogen to lysine residues on fibrin, and these agents inhibit fibrinolysis by competitively blocking this binding.[368–371] Both agents can be administered orally or intravenously, have rapid absorption after oral administration, and are excreted primarily through the kidneys. Only EACA is approved for use in the United States. Differences in the two agents are primarily in their pharmacology. Tranexamic acid is approximately 10-fold more potent than EACA because tranexamic acid has a higher binding affinity. Both drugs have a short half-life of 2 to 4 hours, so they must be administered frequently. EACA can be administered intravenously at a loading dose of approximately 100 mg/kg over 30 to 60 minutes followed by a continuous infusion of up to 1 g/hour, or the dose can be divided for intermittent administration. For oral treatment, the same loading dose can be administered, followed by a maximum 24 g/day in divided doses given every 1 to 6 hours as indicated. Use of tranexamic acid follows similar principles. The intravenous dose is 10 mg/kg followed by 10 mg/kg every 2 to 6 hours as needed. It also can be administered orally at a dosage of 25mg/kg given three or four times daily. Both EACA and tranexamic acid are generally well tolerated, but patients must be observed for possible thrombotic complications. Additionally, thrombotic ureteral obstruction can occur in patients with upper urinary tract bleeding, and such patients should be treated only after careful consideration. The

TABLE 127-8   PRINCIPAL USES OF ANTIFIBRINOLYTIC AGENTS

CONDITION	COMMENT
Systemic Fibrinolysis	
α_2–plasmin inhibitor or PAI-1 deficiency	Rare inherited disorders
Acute promyelocytic leukemia	Must distinguish fibrinolysis from disseminated intravascular coagulation
Cirrhosis and liver transplantation	Occasional cases of cirrhosis; common in anhepatic phase of liver transplantation
Malignancy	Occasional cases of prostate and other carcinomas
Disseminated intravascular coagulation	Must be used with caution; thrombosis can result
Cardiopulmonary bypass	Decreases blood loss and transfusion needs
Fibrinolytic therapy	Can be used to treat bleeding complications
Localized Fibrinolysis	
Hemophilia and von Willebrand disease	Decreases bleeding after dental extractions and possibly other procedures
Prostatectomy	Can decrease postoperative bleeding
Kasabach-Merritt syndrome	May shrink hemangioma
Menorrhagia	Often decreases bleeding

risks of ureteral obstruction can be decreased by ensuring high urine flow. Thrombotic complications can occur in patients with hypercoagulability, and thrombotic events can be precipitated or worsened in patients with DIC. Myonecrosis is a rare complication. Minor complications, including rash, abdominal discomfort, nausea, and vomiting, have been reported.

APROTININ

Aprotinin is a naturally occurring proteinase inhibitor obtained from bovine lung. It inhibits several proteinases, including trypsin, kallikrein, and plasmin, through interaction with the catalytic site.[372–374] It has both antiinflammatory and antifibrinolytic properties. Because it is a polypeptide, it must be administered intravenously. It distributes throughout the total extracellular space with an initial plasma half-life of approximately 150 minutes and a terminal elimination phase with a half-life of approximately 10 hours. Its most common and approved use in the United States is for reducing perioperative blood loss and blood transfusions in patients undergoing cardiopulmonary bypass. Because of the possibility of allergic reactions, a small test dose is recommended. After the test dose, a loading dose of 1 or 2 million kallikrein inhibitor units (KIU) is given, followed by a constant infusion of either 250,000 or 500,000 KIU/hour.

THERAPY FOR SYSTEMIC FIBRINOLYSIS

Excessive systemic fibrinolytic activation can lead to bleeding from premature lysis of hemostatic plugs and from the hypocoagulable state resulting from the lytic state. Inhibiting fibrinolysis can be useful in treating bleeding complications. Laboratory evaluation can aid in diagnosis and in followup of response to treatment. Excessive fibrinolysis is caused by increased plasminogen activator and may result in a shortened euglobulin clot lysis time, decreased plasminogen, decreased α_2-PI, increased plasmin–antiplasmin complexes, decreased fibrinogen, and increased fibrinogen degradation products. Screening tests, including PT and aPTT, may be prolonged. Distinguishing between abnormal hemostasis resulting from DIC or from systemic fibrinolysis can be difficult. Useful features include a more prominent decrease in fibrinogen and increase in fibrinogen degradation products and relatively less thrombocytopenia and elevation of D-dimer with primary fibrinolysis. Serial measurement of selected tests may be use-

ful in following the course of therapy, as the low fibrinogen and elevated fibrinogen degradation products may normalize.

Rare inherited deficiencies of either α_2-PI or PAI-1 can cause a lifelong bleeding disorder. Inherited deficiency of α_2-PI is an autosomal recessive condition, with a severe lifelong bleeding disorder occurring in patients with homozygous deficiency.[375,376] Individuals with heterozygous deficiency often are asymptomatic but may have a mild bleeding disorder that worsens with age. α_2-PI deficiency caused by synthesis of a dysfunctional molecule with a mutation near the reactive site has been reported and causes a bleeding disorder. Other reports describe an inherited bleeding disorder resulting from PAI-1 deficiency, in which affected patients bleed after surgery or trauma.[377–379] Treatment with antifibrinolytic agents has been effective in these bleeding conditions.

Antifibrinolytic therapy can be useful in the more common acquired systemic hyperfibrinolytic conditions. Acute promyelocytic leukemia often is associated with a severe bleeding disorder that may have elements of both DIC and systemic fibrinolysis in addition to thrombocytopenia. Administration of ϵACA to inhibit fibrinolysis can be useful.[380–382] However, antifibrinolytic therapy must be used with care in such patients to avoid thrombosis. Treatment can be given in combination with heparin. The hemostatic abnormality associated with severe liver disease is complex and includes elements of decreased synthesis of coagulation factors and inhibitors, abnormal clearance, thrombocytopenia, abnormal platelet function, and synthesis of abnormal proteins. In this setting, fibrinolysis can contribute to bleeding and occasionally is the primary abnormality.[383–385] During orthotopic liver transplantation, accelerated fibrinolysis often contributes to bleeding, particularly during the anhepatic phase of surgery. Treatment with antifibrinolytic agents can improve bleeding complications and decrease blood loss (see Chap. 120).[386–389]

Primary fibrinolysis with bleeding occurs rarely with some malignant tumors, including prostatic carcinoma,[386–395] and with heat stroke.[396] Fibrinolytic activation routinely occurs as a compensatory mechanism in consumption coagulopathy and occasionally is prominent, resulting in a short euglobulin lysis time, decreased plasminogen, and other manifestations of fibrinolysis. Distinguishing between the contribution of excessive fibrinolysis and the contribution of consumption coagulopathy to the development of bleeding complications is difficult. Management of DIC (see Chap. 121) involves treatment of the underlying condition, replacement of coagulation factors, and occasionally administration of heparin. If fibrinolytic activation is prominent and other measures do not control bleeding, then antifibrinolytic therapy can be helpful. It should be used with caution, however, because inhibiting physiologic fibrinolysis can exacerbate underlying thrombotic events.

The contact system is activated during cardiopulmonary bypass, resulting in alterations in the coagulation, fibrinolytic, and complement systems.[397,398] Both postoperative bleeding and the need for large transfusion volumes can be major problems. Several trials of antifibrinolytic therapy have established that total blood loss and transfusion requirements can be reduced, with Trasylol (aprotinin injection) often used for this purpose.[397–402] Antifibrinolytic therapy also can be useful for treating bleeding associated with some snakebites and following administration of fibrinolytic therapy (see "Antifibrinolytic Therapy").

Excessive bleeding associated with a local lesion in the absence of systemic fibrinolysis may respond to antifibrinolytic therapy. Bleeding following dental extractions in patients with hemophilia or von Willebrand disease can be reduced.[403–406] The oral mucosa is rich in fibrinolytic activity, and inhibition of normal fibrinolysis prevents premature dissolution of hemostatic thrombi and prevents local bleeding. Fibrinolytic activity is high in the urinary system and may contribute to excessive bleeding following prostatectomy. Because EACA and tranexamic acid are excreted through the kidneys, their concentration in the urine is high, and antifibrinolytic therapy can inhibit local fibrinolysis and decrease postprostatectomy bleeding.[407,408] Similarly, endometrial fibrinolysis contributes to menstrual bleeding, and antifibrinolytic therapy can be useful for treating menorrhagia in patients with hemostatic abnormalities or with normal hemostasis in whom other specific therapy is ineffective.[409,410] Antifibrinolytic therapy may be useful in rare cases of Kasabach-Merritt syndrome with symptomatic or expanding hemangioma and consumption coagulopathy. Inhibiting fibrinolysis can result in local thrombosis with shrinkage of the lesion.[411,412] Antifibrinolytic therapy has been used for treatment of gastrointestinal or genitourinary bleeding in patients with severe thrombocytopenia, ulcerative colitis, hereditary hemorrhagic telangiectasia, traumatic hyphema, following tonsillectomy, and subarachnoid hemorrhage. Caution is advised in the latter condition, because rebleeding may decrease with antifibrinolytic therapy but vasospasm and distal ischemia may worsen.[413]

REFERENCES

1. Hajjar KA: The molecular basis of fibrinolysis, in *Hematology of Infancy and Childhood*, edited by DG Nathan, SH Orkin, D Ginsburg, AT Look, p 1497. WB Saunders, Philadelphia, 2003.
2. Hajjar KA: Cellular receptors in the regulation of plasmin generation. *Thromb Haemost* 74:294, 1995.
3. Raum D, Marcus D, Alper CA, et al: Synthesis of human plasminogen by the liver. *Science* 208:1036, 1980.
4. Bohmfalk J, Fuller G: Plasminogen is synthesized by primary cultures of rat hepatocytes. *Science* 209:408, 1980.
5. Castellino FJ: Biochemistry of human plasminogen. *Semin Thromb Hemost* 10:18, 1984.
6. Collen D, Tytgat G, Claeys H, et al: Metabolism of plasminogen in healthy subjects. Effect of tranexamic acid. *J Clin Invest* 51:1310, 1972.
7. Forsgren M, Raden B, Israelsson M, et al: Molecular cloning and characterization of a full-length cDNA clone for human plasminogen. *FEBS Lett* 213:254, 1987.
8. Miles LA, Dahlberg CM, Plow EF: The cell-binding domains of plasminogen and their function in plasma. *J Biol Chem* 263:11656, 1988.
9. Markus G, DePasquale JL, Wissler FC: Quantitative determination of the binding of epsilon-aminocaproic acid to native plasminogen. *J Biol Chem* 253:727, 1978.
10. Markus G, Priore RL, Wissler FC: The binding of tranexamic acid to native (glu) and modified (lys) human plasminogen and its effect on conformation. *J Biol Chem* 254:1211, 1979.
11. Hajjar KA, Harpel PC, Jaffe EA, et al: Binding of plasminogen to cultured human endothelial cells. *J Biol Chem* 261:11656, 1986.
12. Miles LA, Plow EF: Cellular regulation of fibrinolysis. *Thromb Haemost* 66:32, 1991.
13. Rakoczi I, Wiman B, Collen D: On the biologic significance of the specific interaction between fibrin, plasminogen, and antiplasmin. *Biochim Biophys Acta* 540:295, 1978.
14. Hayes ML, Castellino FJ: Carbohydrate of the human plasminogen variants: I. Carbohydrate composition, glycopeptide isolation, and characterization. *J Biol Chem* 254:8768, 1979.
15. Hayes ML, Castelino FJ: Carbohydrate of the human plasminogen variants: II. Structure of the asparagine-linked oligosaccharide unit. *J Biol Chem* 254:8772, 1979.
16. Hayes ML, Castellino FJ: Carbohydrate of the human plasminogen variants: III. Structure of the O-glycosidically-linked oligosaccharide unit. *J Biol Chem* 254:8777, 1979.
17. Holvoet P, Lijnen HR, Collen D: A monoclonal antibody specific for lys-plasminogen. *J Biol Chem* 260:12106, 1985.
18. Saksela O: Plasminogen activation and regulation of proteolysis. *Biochim Biophys Acta* 823:35, 1985.
19. Wallen P, Wiman B: Characterization of human plasminogen: I. On the relationship between different molecular forms of plasminogen demonstrated in plasma and found in purified preparations. *Biochim Biophys Acta* 221:20, 1970.
20. Wallen P, Wiman B: Characterization of human plasminogen: II. Separation and partial characterization of different molecular forms of human plasminogen. *Biochim Biophys Acta* 157:122, 1972.
21. Hoylaerts M, Rijken DC, Lijnen HR, Collen D: Kinetics of the activation of plasminogen by human tissue plasminogen activator: Role of fibrin. *J Biol Chem* 257:2912, 1982.
22. Glenney JR: Purification of calpactins I and II and isolation of N-terminal tail of calpactin I. *Meth Enzymol* 196:65, 1991.
23. Murray JC, Buetow KH, Donovan M, et al: Linkage disequilibrium of plasminogen polymorphisms and assignment of the gene to human chromosome 6q26-6q27. *Am J Hum Genet* 40:338, 1987.
24. Petersen TE, Martzen MR, Ichinose A, Davie EW: Characterization of the gene for human plasminogen, a key proenzyme in the fibrinolytic system. *J Biol Chem* 265:6104, 1990.
25. Jenkins GR, Seiffert D, Parmer RJ, Miles LA: Regulation of plasminogen gene expression by interleukin-6. *Blood* 89:2394, 1997.
26. McLean JW, Tomlinson JE, Kuang WJ, et al: CDNA sequence of human apolipoprotein(a) is homologous to plasminogen. *Nature* 330:132, 1987.
27. Nakamura T, Nishizawa T, Hagiya M, et al: Molecular cloning and expression of human hepatocyte growth factor. *Nature* 342:440, 1989.
28. Weissbach L, Treadwell BV: A plasminogen-related gene is expressed in cancer cells. *Biochem Biophys Res Commun* 186:1108, 1992.
29. Yoshimura T, Yuhki N, Wang MH, et al: Cloning, sequencing, and expression of human macrophage stimulating protein (MSP, MST 1) confirms MSP as a member of the family of kringle proteins and locates the MSP gene on chromosome 3. *J Biol Chem* 268:15461, 1993.
30. Byrne CD, Schwartz K, Meer K, et al: The human apolipoprotein(a)/plasminogen gene cluster contains a novel homologue transcribed in liver. *Arterioscler Thromb* 14:534, 1994.
31. Ichinose A: Multiple members of the plasminogen-apolipoprotein(a) gene family associated with thrombosis. *Biochemistry* 31:3113, 1992.
32. Bugge TH, Flick MJ, Daugherty CC, Degen JL: Plasminogen deficiency causes severe thrombosis but is compatible with development and reproduction. *Genes Dev* 9:794, 1995.
33. Carmeliet P, Collen D: Gene targeting and gene transfer studies of the plasminogen/plasmin system: Implications in thrombosis, hemostasis, neointima formation, and atherosclerosis. *FASEB J* 9:934, 1995.
34. Drew AF, Kaufman AH, Kombrinck KW, et al: Ligneous conjunctivitis in plasminogen-deficient mice. *Blood* 91:1616, 1998.
35. Pennica D, Holmes WE, Kohr WJ, et al: Cloning and expression of human tissue-type plasminogen activator cDNA in E. coli. *Nature* 301:214, 1983.
36. Tate KM, Higgins DL, Holmes WE, et al: Functional role of proteolytic cleavage at arginine-275 of human tissue plasminogen activator as assessed by site-directed mutagenesis. *Biochemistry* 26:338, 1987.
37. Pohl G, Kenne L, Nilsson B, Einarsson M: Isolation and characterization of three different carbohydrate chains from melanoma tissue plasminogen activator. *Eur J Biochem* 170:69, 1987.
38. Spellman MW, Basa LJ, Leonard CK, Chakel JA: Carbohydrate structures of tissue plasminogen activator expressed in Chinese hamster ovary cells. *J Biol Chem* 264:14100, 1989.
39. Harris RJ, Leonard CK, Guzzetta AW: Tissue plasminogen activator has an O-linked fucose attached to threonine-61 in the epidermal growth factor domain. *Biochemistry* 30:2311, 1991.
40. Ny T, Elgh F, Lund B: Structure of the human tissue-type plasminogen activator gene: Correlation of intron and exon structures to functional and structural domains. *Proc Natl Acad Sci U S A* 81:5355, 1984.

41. Browne MJ, Tyrrell AWR, Chapman CG, et al: Isolation of a human tissue-type plasminogen activator genomic clone and its expression in mouse L cells. *Gene* 33:279, 1985.

42. Degen SJF, Rajput B, Reich E: The human tissue plasminogen activator gene. *J Biol Chem* 261:6872, 1986.

43. Van Zonnefeld A-J, Veerman H, Pannekoek H: Autonomous functions of structural domains on human tissue-type plasminogen activator. *Proc Natl Acad Sci U S A* 83:4670, 1986.

44. Feng P, Ohlsson M, Ny T: The structure of the TATA-less rat tissue-type plasminogen activator gene. *J Biol Chem* 265:2022, 1990.

45. Kooistra T, Bosma PJ, Toet K, et al: Role of protein kinase C and cyclic adenosine monophosphate in the regulation of tissue-type plasminogen activator, plasminogen activator inhibitor-1, and platelet-derived growth factor mRNA levels in human endothelial cells. Possible involvement of proto-oncogenes c-jun and c-fos. *Arterioscler Thromb* 11:1042, 1991.

46. Medcalf RL, Ruegg M, Schleuning WD: A DNA motif related to the cAMP-responsive element and an exon-located activator protein-2 binding site in the human tissue-type plasminogen activator gene promoter cooperate in basal expression and convey activation by phorbol ester and cAMP. *J Biol Chem* 265:14618, 1990.

47. Kooistra T, Van den Berg J, Tons A, et al: Butyrate stimulates tissue type plasminogen activator synthesis in cultured human endothelial cells. *Biochem J* 247:605, 1987.

48. Diamond SL, Eskin SG, McIntire LV: Fluid flow stimulates tissue plasminogen activator secretion by cultured human endothelial cells. *Science* 243:1483, 1989.

49. Hanss M, Collen D: Secretion of tissue-type plasminogen activator and plasminogen activator inhibitor by cultured human endothelial cells: Modulation by thrombin, endotoxin, and histamine. *J Lab Clin Med* 109:97, 1987.

50. Thompson EA, Nelles L, Collen D: Effect of retinoic acid on the synthesis of tissue-type plasminogen activator and plasminogen activator inhibitor 1 in human endothelial cells. *Eur J Biochem* 201:627, 1991.

51. Kooistra T, Opdenberg JP, Toet K, et al: Stimulation of tissue-type plasminogen activator synthesis by retinoids in cultured human endothelial cells and rat tissue *in vivo*. *Thromb Haemost* 65:565, 1991.

52. Medcaf RL, Van den Berg E, Schleuning WD: Glucocorticoid-modulated gene expression of tissue- and urinary-type plasminogen activator and plasminogen activator inhibitor-1 and 2. *J Cell Biol* 106:971, 1988.

53. Santell L, Levin EG: Cyclic AMP potentiates phorbol ester stimulation of tissue plasminogen activator release and inhibits secretion of plasminogen activator inhibitor-1 from human endothelial cells. *J Biol Chem* 263:16802, 1988.

54. Levin EG, del Zoppo GJ: Localization of tissue plasminogen activator in the endothelium of a limited number of vessels. *Am J Pathol* 144:855, 1994.

55. Levin EG, Santell L, Osborn KG: The expression of endothelial tissue plasminogen activator in vivo: A function defined by vessel size and anatomic location. *J Cell Sci* 110:139, 1997.

56. Levin EG, Osborn KG, Schleuning WD: Vessel-specific gene expression in the lung: Tissue plasminogen activator is limited to bronchial arteries and pulmonary vessels of discrete size. *Chest* 114:68S, 1998.

57. Diamond SL, Sharefkin JB, Dieffenbach C, et al: Tissue plasminogen activator messenger RNA levels increase in cultured human endothelial cells exposed to laminar shear stress. *J Cell Physiol* 143:364, 1990.

58. Dichek D, Quertermous T: Thrombin regulation of mRNA levels of tissue plasminogen activator inhibitor-1 in cultured human umbilical vein endothelial cells. *Blood* 74:222, 1989.

59. Levin EG, Marotti KR, Santell L: Protein kinase C and the stimulation of tissue plasminogen activator release from human endothelial cells. *J Biol Chem* 264:16030, 1989.

60. Kasai S, Arimura H, Nishida M, Suyama T: Primary structure of single-chain pro-urokinase. *J Biol Chem* 260:12382, 1985.

61. Gunzler WA, Steffens GJ, Otting F, et al: Structural relationship between high and low molecular mass urokinase. *Physiol Chem Phys Med NMR* 363:133, 1982.

62. Riccio A, Grimaldi G, Verde P, et al: The human urokinase-plasminogen activator gene and its promoter. *Nucleic Acids Res* 13:2759, 1985.

63. Holmes WE, Pennica D, Blaber M, et al: Cloning and expression of the gene for pro-urokinase in *Escherichia coli*. *Biotechnology* 3:923, 1985.

64. Schmitt M, Wilhelm O, Janicke F, et al: Urokinase-type plasminogen activator (uPA) and its receptor (CD87): A new target for tumor invasion and metastasis. *J Obstet Gynaecol* 21:151, 1995.

65. Van Hinsbergh VWM, Van den Berg EA, Fiers W, Dooijewaard G: Tumor necrosis factor induces the production of urokinase-type plasminogen activator by human endothelial cells. *Blood* 10:1991, 1990.

66. Medina R, Socher SH, Han JH, Friedman PA: Interleukin-1, endotoxin, or tumor necrosis factor/cachectin enhance the level of plasminogen activator inhibitor messenger RNA in bovine aortic endothelial cells. *Thromb Res* 54:41, 1989.

67. Gerwin BI, Keski-Oja J, Seddon M, et al: TGF beta 1 modulation of urokinase and PAI-1 expression in human bronchial epithelial cells. *Am J Pathol* 259:262, 1990.

68. Stump DC, Lijnen HR, Collen D: Purification and characterization of a novel low molecular weight form of single-chain urokinase-type plasminogen activator. *J Biol Chem* 261:17120, 1986.

69. Steffens GJ, Gunzler WA, Olting F, et al: The complete amino acid sequence of low molecular mass urokinase from human urine. *Physiol Chem Phys Med NMR* 363:1043, 1982.

70. Lijnen HR, Zamarron C, Blaber M, et al: Activation of plasminogen by pro-urokinase. *J Biol Chem* 261:1253, 1986.

71. Gurewich V, Pannell R, Louie S, et al: Effective and fibrin-specific clot lysis by a zymogen precursor from urokinase (pro-urokinase). A study *in vitro* and in two animal species. *J Clin Invest* 73:1731, 1984.

72. Lijnen HR, Van Hoef B, DeCock F, Collen D: The mechanism of plasminogen activation and fibrin dissolution by single chain urokinase-type plasminogen activator in a plasma milieu *in vitro*. *Blood* 73:1864, 1989.

73. Petersen LC, Lund LR, Nielsen LS, et al: One-chain urokinase-type plasminogen activator from human sarcoma cells is a precursor with little or no intrinsic activity. *J Biol Chem* 263:11189, 1988.

74. Colman RW: Activation of plasminogen by human plasma kallikrein. *Biochem Biophys Res Commun* 35:273, 1968.

75. Mandle RJ, Kaplan AP: Hageman factor-dependent fibrinolysis: Generation of fibrinolytic activity by the interaction of human activated factor XI and plasminogen. *Blood* 54:850, 1979.

76. Goldsmith GH, Saito H, Ratnoff OD: The activation of plasminogen by Hageman factor (factor XII) and Hageman factor fragments. *J Clin Invest* 62:54, 1978.

77. Ouimet H, Loscalzo J: Fibrinolysis, in *Thrombosis and Hemorrhage*, edited by J Loscalzo, AI Schafer, p 127. Blackwell Scientific, Boston, 1994.

78. Hiraoka N, Allen E, Apel IJ, et al: Matrix metalloproteinases regulate neovascularization by acting as pericellular fibrinolysins. *Cell* 95:365, 1998.

79. Huisman LG, Van Griensven JM, Kluft C: On the role of C1-inhibitor as inhibitor of tissue-type plasminogen activator in human plasma. *Thromb Haemost* 73:466, 1995.

80. Carmeliet P, Schoonjans L, Kieckens L, et al: Physiological consequences of loss of plasminogen activator gene function in mice. *Nature* 368:419, 1994.

81. Travis J, Salvesan GS: Human plasma proteinase inhibitors. *Annu Rev Biochem* 52:655, 1983.

82. Aoki N: Genetic abnormalities of the fibrinolytic system. *Semin Thromb Haemost* 10:42, 1984.

83. Holmes WE, Nelles L, Lijnen HR: Primary structure of human alpha2-antiplasmin, a serine protease inhibitor (serpin). *J Biol Chem* 262:1659, 1987.

84. Hirosawa S, Nakamura Y, Miura O, et al: Organization of the human alpha2-antiplasmin inhibitor gene. *Proc Natl Acad Sci U S A* 85:6836, 1988.

85. Plow EF, Collen D: The presence and release of alpha-2-antiplasmin from human platelets. *Blood* 58:1069, 1981.

86. Aoki N, Moroi M, Tachiya K: Effects of alpha-2-plasmin inhibitor on fibrin clot lysis. Its comparison with alpha-2-macroglobulin. *Thromb Haemost* 39:22, 1978.

87. Scott RW, Bergman BL, Bajpai A, et al: Protease nexin: Properties and a modified purification procedure. *J Biol Chem* 260:7029, 1985.

88. Cunningham DD, Van Nostrand WE, Farrell DH, Campbell CH: Interactions of serine proteases with cultured fibroblasts. *J Cell Biochem* 32: 281, 1986.

89. Sprengers ED, Kluft D: Plasminogen activator inhibitors. *Blood* 69:381, 1987.

90. Ny T, Sawdey M, Lawrence D, et al: Cloning and sequence of a cDNA coding for the human beta-migrating endothelial-cell-type plasminogen activator inhibitor. *Proc Natl Acad Sci U S A* 83:6776, 1986.

91. Kruithof EKO: Plasminogen activator inhibitor type 1: Biochemical, biological, and clinical aspects. *Blood Coagul Fibrinolysis* 2:59, 1988.

92. Samad F, Yamamoto K, Loskutoff DJ: Distribution and regulation of plasminogen activator inhibitor-1 in murine adipose tissue in vivo. *J Clin Invest* 97:37, 1996.

93. Sawdey M, Podor TJ, Loskutoff DJ: Regulation of type-1 plasminogen activator inhibitor gene expression in cultured bovine aortic endothelial cells. *J Biol Chem* 264:10396, 1989.

94. Van Hinsbergh VWM, Kooistra T, Van den Berg EA, et al: Tumor necrosis factor increases the production of plasminogen activator inhibitor in human endothelial cells in vitro and in rats in vivo. *Blood* 72: 1467, 1988.

95. Van den Berg EA, Sprengers ED, Jaye M, et al: Regulation of plasminogen activator inhibitor-1 mRNA in human endothelial cells. *Thromb Haemost* 60:63, 1988.

96. Loskutoff DJ, Linders M, Keijer J, et al: Structure of the human plasminogen activator inhibitor-1 gene: Non-random distribution of introns. *Biochemistry* 26:3763, 1987.

97. Mottonen J, Strand A, Symersky J, et al: Structural basis of latency in plasminogen activator inhibitor-1. *Nature* 355:270, 1992.

98. Declerck PJ, De Mol M, Alessi MC, et al: Purification and characterization of a plasminogen activator inhibitor-1 binding protein from human plasma. Identification as multimeric form of S protein (vitronectin). *J Biol Chem* 263:15454, 1988.

99. Bosma PJ, Van den Berg EA, Kooistra T, et al: Human plasminogen activator inhibitor-1 gene: Promoter and structural nucleotide sequences. *J Biol Chem* 263:9129, 1988.

100. Van Zonnefeld AJ, Curriden SA, Loskutoff DJ: Type 1 plasminogen activator inhibitor gene: Functional analysis and glucocorticoid regulation of its promoter. *Proc Natl Acad Sci U S A* 85:5525, 1988.

101. Westerhausen DR, Hopkins WE, Billadello JJ: Multiple transforming growth factor beta-inducible elements regulate expression of the plasminogen activator inhibitor type-1 gene in HepG2 cells. *J Biol Chem* 266:1092, 1991.

102. Keeton MR, Curriden SA, Van Zonneveld AJ, Loskutoff DJ: Identification of regulatory sequences in the type 1 plasminogen activator inhibitor gene responsive to transforming growth factor. *J Biol Chem* 266: 23048, 1991.

103. Emeis JJ, Kooistra T: Interleukin 1 and lipopolysaccharide induce an inhibitor of tissue-type plasminogen activator in vivo and in cultured endothelial cells. *J Exp Med* 163:1260, 1986.

104. Schleef RR, Bevilaqua MP, Sawdey M, et al: Cytokine activation of vascular endothelium: Effects on tissue-type plasminogen activator and type 1 plasminogen activator inhibitor. *J Biol Chem* 263:5797, 1988.

105. Craik CS, Rutter WJ, Fletternick R: Splice junctions: Association with variation in protein structure. *Science* 220:1125, 1983.

106. Stiko-Rahm A, Wiman B, Hamsten A, Nilsson J: Secretion of plasminogen activator inhibitor-1 from cultured human umbilical vein endothelial cells is induced by very low density lipoprotein. *Arterioscler Thromb Vasc Biol* 10:1067, 1990.

107. Etingin OR, Hajjar DP, Hajjar KA, et al: Lipoprotein(a) regulates plasminogen activator inhibitor-1 expression in endothelial cells. *J Biol Chem* 266:2459, 1990.

108. Vaughan DE, Shen C, Lazo S: Angiotensin II induces plasminogen activator inhibitor synthesis in vitro. *Circulation* 86:I, 1992.

109. Gelehrter TD, Scyncer-Laszuk R: Thrombin induction of plasminogen activator-inhibitor synthesis in vitro. *J Clin Invest* 77:165, 1986.

110. Van Hinsbergh VWM, Sprengers ED, Kooistra T: Effect of thrombin on the production of plasminogen activators and PA inhibitor-1 by human foreskin microvascular endothelial cells. *Thromb Haemost* 57:148, 1987.

111. Scarpati EM, Sadler JE: Regulation of endothelial cell coagulant properties. Modulation of tissue factor, plasminogen activator inhibitors, and thrombomodulin by phorbol 12-myristate 13-acetate and tumor necrosis factor. *J Biol Chem* 264:20705, 1989.

112. Konkle BA, Kollros PR, Kelly MD: Heparin-binding growth factor-1 modulation of plasminogen activator inhibitor-1 expression. *J Biol Chem* 265:21867, 1990.

113. Erickson LA, Fici GJ, Lund JE, et al: Development of venous occlusions in transgenic mice for the plasminogen activator inhibitor-1 gene. *Nature* 346:74, 1990.

114. Carmeliet P, Kieckens L, Schoonjans L, et al: Plasminogen activator inhibitor-1 gene-deficient mice: I. Generation by homologous recombination and characterization. *J Clin Invest* 92:2746, 1993.

115. Fay WP, Shapiro AD, Shih JL, et al: Complete deficiency of plasminogen activator inhibitor type 1 due to a frame-shift mutation. *N Engl J Med* 327:1729, 1992.

116. Ye RD, Wun T-C, Sadler JE: CDNA cloning and expression in Escherichia coli of a plasminogen activator inhibitor from human placenta. *J Biol Chem* 262:3718, 1987.

117. Ye RD, Aherns SM, Le Beau MM, et al: Structure of the gene for human plasminogen activator inhibitor-2. The nearest mammalian homologue of chicken ovalbumin. *J Biol Chem* 264:5495, 1989.

118. Antalis TM, Clok MA, Barnes T, et al: Cloning and expression of a cDNA coding for a human monocyte-derived plasminogen activator inhibitor. *Proc Natl Acad Sci U S A* 85:985, 1988.

119. Schleuning WD, Medcalf RL, Hession C, et al: Plasminogen activator inhibitor 2: Regulation of gene transcription during phorbol ester-mediated differentiation of U-937 human histiocytic lymphoma cells. *Mol Cell Biol* 7:4564, 1987.

120. Chapman HA, Stone OL: A fibrinolytic inhibitor of human alveolar macrophages. Induction with endotoxin. *Am Rev Respir Dis* 132:569, 1985.

121. Miles LA, Dahlberg CM, Plescia J, et al: Role of cell surface lysines in plasminogen binding to cells: Identification of alpha-enolase as a candidate plasminogen receptor. *Biochemistry* 30:1682, 1991.

122. Miles LA, Ginsberg MA, White JG, Plow EF: Plasminogen interacts with platelets through two distinct mechanisms. *J Clin Invest* 77:2001, 1986.

123. Kanalas JJ, Makker SP: Identification of the rat Heymann nephritis autoantigen (GP330) as a receptor site for plasminogen. *J Biol Chem* 266: 10825, 1991.

124. Barnathan ES, Kuo A, Van der Keyl H, et al: Tissue-type plasminogen activator binding to human endothelial cells: Evidence for two distinct binding sites. *J Biol Chem* 263:7792, 1988.

125. Hajjar KA: The endothelial cell tissue plasminogen activator receptor: Specific interaction with plasminogen. *J Biol Chem* 266:21962, 1991.

126. Hajjar KA, Hamel NM: Identification and characterization of human endothelial cell membrane binding sites for tissue plasminogen activator and urokinase. *J Biol Chem* 265:2908, 1990.

127. Roldan AL, Cubellis MV, Masucci MT, et al: Cloning and expression of the receptor for human urokinase plasminogen activator, a central molecule in cell surface, plasmin-dependent proteolysis. *EMBO J* 9:467, 1990.

128. Casey JR, Petranka JG, Kottra J, et al: The structure of the urokinase-type plasminogen activator receptor gene. *Blood* 84:1151, 1994.

129. Behrendt N, Ronne E, Ploug M, et al: The human receptor for urokinase plasminogen receptor. *J Biol Chem* 265:6453, 1990.

130. Ploug M, Ronne E, Behrendt N, et al: Cellular receptor for urokinase plasminogen activator. Carboxyl-terminal processing and membrane anchoring by glycosylphosphatidylinositol. *J Biol Chem* 266:1926, 1991.

131. Cubellis MV, Andreasson P, Ragno P, et al: Accessibility of receptor-bound urokinase to type-1 plasminogen activator inhibitor. *Proc Natl Acad Sci U S A* 86:4828, 1989.

132. Ellis V, Wun TC, Behrendt N, et al: Inhibition of receptor-bound urokinase by plasminogen activator inhibitor. *J Biol Chem* 265:9904, 1990.

133. Cubellis MV, Wun TC, Blasi F: Receptor-mediated internalization and degradation of urokinase is caused by its specific inhibitor PAI-1. *EMBO J* 9:1079, 1990.

134. Ellis V, Behrendt N, Dano K: Plasminogen activation by receptor-bound urokinase. *J Biol Chem* 266:12752, 1991.

135. Chapman HA: Plasminogen activators, integrins, and the coordinated regulation of cell adhesion and migration. *Curr Opin Cell Biol* 9:714, 1997.

136. Waltz DA, Chapman HA: Reversible cellular adhesion to vitronectin linked to urokinase receptor occupancy. *J Biol Chem* 269:14746, 1994.

137. Wei Y, Waltz DA, Rao N, et al: Identification of the urokinase receptor as an adhesion receptor for vitronectin. *J Biol Chem* 269:32380, 1994.

138. Wei Y, Lukashev M, Simon DI, et al: Regulation of integrin function by the urokinase receptor. *Science* 273:1551, 1996.

139. Xue W, Kindzelskii AL, Todd RF, Petty HR: Physical association of complement receptor type 3 and urokinase-type plasminogen activator in neutrophil membranes. *J Immunol* 152:4630, 1994.

140. Stahl A, Mueller BM: The urokinase-type plasminogen activator receptor, a GPI-linked protein, is localized in caveolae. *J Cell Biol* 129:335, 1995.

141. Anderson RG: Caveolae: Where incoming and outgoing messengers meet. *Proc Natl Acad Sci U S A* 90:10909, 1993.

142. Okamoto T, Schlegel A, Scherer PE, Lisanti MP: Caveolins, a family of scaffolding proteins for organizing "preassembled signaling complexes" at the plasma membrane. *J Biol Chem* 273:5419, 1998.

143. Raynal P, Pollard HB: Annexins: The problem of assessing the biologic role for a gene family of multifunctional calcium- and phospholipid-binding proteins. *Biochim Biophys Acta* 1197:63, 1994.

144. Chung CY, Erickson HP: Cell surface annexin II is a high affinity receptor for the alternatively spliced segment of tenascin-C. *J Cell Biol* 126:539, 1994.

145. Wright JF, Kurosky A, Wasi S: An endothelial cell-surface form of annexin II binds human cytomegalovirus. *Biochem Biophys Res Commun* 198:983, 1994.

146. Kassam G, Choi KS, Ghuman J, et al: The role of annexin II tetramer in the activation of plasminogen. *J Biol Chem* 273:4790, 1998.

147. Siever DA, Erickson HP: Extracellular annexin II. *Int J Biochem Cell Biol* 29:1219, 1997.

148. Falcone DJ, Borth W, Khan KM, Hajjar KA: Plasminogen-mediated matrix invasion and degradation by macrophages is dependent on surface expression of annexin II. *Blood* 97:777, 2001.

149. Menell JS, Cesarman GM, Jacovina AT, et al: Annexin II and bleeding in acute promyelocytic leukemia. *N Engl J Med* 340:994, 1999.

150. Lee TH, Rhim T, Kim SS: Prothrombin kringle 2 domain has a growth inhibitory activity against basic fibroblast growth factor-stimulated capillary endothelial cells. *J Biol Chem* 273:28805, 1998.

151. Tressler RJ, Updyke TV, Yeatman TJ, Nicolson GL: Extracellular annexin is associated with divalent cation-dependent tumor cell adhesion of metastatic RAW 117 large-cell lymphoma cells. *J Cell Biochem* 53:265, 1993.

152. Yeatman TJ, Updyke TV, Kaetzel MA, et al: Expression of annexins on the surfaces of non-metastatic human and rodent tumor cells. *Clin Exp Metastasis* 11:37, 1993.

153. Tressler RJ, Nicolson GL: Butanol-extractable and detergent-solubilized cell surface components from murine large cell lymphoma cells associated with adhesion to organ microvessel endothelial cells. *J Cell Biochem* 48:162, 1992.

154. Swairjo MA, Seaton BA: Annexin structure and membrane interactions: A molecular perspective. *Annu Rev Biophys Biomol Struct* 23:193, 1994.

155. Spano F, Raugei G, Palla E, et al: Characterization of the human lipocortin-2-encoding multigene family: Its structure suggests the existence of a short amino acid unit undergoing duplication. *Gene* 95:243, 1990.

156. Cesarman GM, Guevara CA, Hajjar KA: An endothelial cell receptor for plasminogen/tissue plasminogen activator: II. Annexin II-mediated enhancement of t-PA-dependent plasminogen activation. *J Biol Chem* 269:21198, 1994.

157. Hajjar KA, Guevara CA, Lev E, et al: Interaction of the fibrinolytic receptor, annexin II, with the endothelial cell surface: Essential role of endonexin repeat 2. *J Biol Chem* 271:21652, 1996.

158. Hajjar KA, Gavish D, Breslow J, Nachman RL: Lipoprotein(a) modulation of endothelial cell surface fibrinolysis and its potential role in atherosclerosis. *Nature* 339:303, 1989.

159. Hajjar KA, Mauri L, Jacovina AT, et al: Tissue plasminogen activator binding to the annexin II tail domain: Direct modulation by homocysteine. *J Biol Chem* 273:9987, 1998.

160. Kraus JP: Molecular basis of phenotype expression in homocystinuria. *J Inherit Metab Dis* 17:383, 1994.

161. Boushey CJ, Beresford SAA, Omenn GS, Motulsky AG: A quantitative assessment of plasma homocysteine as a risk factor for vascular disease. *JAMA* 274:1049, 1995.

162. Refsum H, Ueland PM, Nygard O, Vollset SE: Homocysteine and cardiovascular disease. *Ann Revu Med* 49:31, 1998.

163. Hajjar KA: Homocysteine-induced modulation of tissue plasminogen activator binding to its endothelial cell membrane receptor. *J Clin Invest* 91:2873, 1993

164. Ishii H, Yoshida M, Hiraoka M, et al: Recombinant annexin II modulates impaired fibrinolytic activity in vitro and in rat carotid artery. *Circ Res* 89:1240, 2001.

165. Ling Q, Febbraio M, Deora B, et al: Annexin II is a key regulator of fibrin homeostasis and neoangiogenesis. *J Clin Invest* 113:38, 2004.

166. Bu G, Warshawsky I, Schwartz AL: Cellular receptors for the plasminogen activators. *Blood* 83:3427, 1994.

167. Beiseigel U, Weber W, Ihrke G, et al: The LDL-receptor-related protein, LRP, is an apolipoprotein E-binding protein. *Nature* 341:162, 1989.

168. Brown MS, Herz J, Kowal RC: The low-density lipoprotein receptor-related protein: Double agent or decoy? *Curr Opin Lipidol* 2:65, 1991.

169. Orth K, Madison EL, Gething MJ, Sambrook JF: Complexes of tissue-type plasminogen activator and its serpin inhibitor plasminogen-activator inhibitor type 1 are internalized by means of the low density lipoprotein receptor-related protein/alpha-2-macroglobulin receptor. *Proc Natl Acad Sci U S A* 89:7422, 1992.

170. Herz J, Goldstein JL, Strickland DK, et al: 39 kDa protein modulates binding of ligands to low density lipoprotein receptor-related protein/alpha-2-macroglobulin receptor. *J Biol Chem* 266:21232, 1991.

171. Herz J, Clouthier DE, Hammer RE: LDL receptor-related protein internalizes and degrades uPA-PAI-1 complexes and is essential for embryo implantation. *Cell* 71:411, 1992.

172. Herz J, Clouthier DE, Hammer RE: Correction: LDL receptor-related protein internalizes and degrades uPA-PAI-1 complexes and is essential for embryo implantation. *Cell* 73:428, 1993.

173. Bu G, Morton PA, Schwartz AL: Identification and partial characterization by chemical cross-linking of a binding protein for tissue-type plasminogen activator (t-PA) on rat hepatoma cells. *J Biol Chem* 267:15595, 1992.

174. Otter M, Barrett-Bergshoeff MM, Rijken DC: Binding of tissue type plasminogen activator by the mannose receptor. *J Biol Chem* 266:13931, 1991.

175. Greenberg M, Ziff E: Stimulation of 3T3 cells induces transcription of the c-fos proto-oncogene. *Nature* 311:433, 1984.

176. Narita M, Bu G, Herz J, Schwartz AL: Two receptor systems are involved in the plasma clearance of tissue-type plasminogen activator (t-PA) in vivo. *J Clin Invest* 96:1164, 1995.

177. Bailey K, Bettelheim FR, Lorand L, Middlebrook WR: Action of thrombin in the clotting of fibrinogen. *Nature* 167:233, 1951.

178. Doolittle RF: The molecular biology of fibrin, in *The Molecular Basis of Blood Diseases*, edited by G Stamatoyannopoulos, AW Nienhuis, PW Majerus, H Varmus, p 701. WB Saunders, Philadelphia, 1994.

179. Marder VJ, Budzynski AZ: Data for defining fibrinogen and its plasmic degradation products. *Thromb Diath Haemorrh* 33:199, 1975.

180. Furlan M, Kemp G, Beck EA: Plasmic degradation of fibrinogen. *Biochim Biophys Acta* 400:95, 1975.

181. Gaffney PJ, Dobos P: A structural aspect of human fibrinogen suggested by its plasmin degradation. *FEBS Lett* 15:13, 1971.

182. Latallo ZS, Flether AP, Alkjaersig N, Sherry S: Inhibition of fibrin polymerization by fibrinogen proteolysis products. *Am J Physiol* 202:681, 1962.

183. Pizzo SV, Schwartz ML, Hill RL, McKee PA: The effect of plasmin on the subunit structure of human fibrin. *J Biol Chem* 248:4574, 1973.

184. Culasso DE, Donati MB, DeGaetano G, et al: Inhibition of human platelet aggregation by plasmin digests of human and bovine preparations: Role of contaminating factor VIII-related material. *Blood* 44:169, 1974.

185. Buluk K, Malofiegen M: The pharmacologic properties of fibrinogen degradation products. *Br J Pharmacol* 35:79, 1969.

186. Richardson DL, Pepper DS, Kay AB: Chemotaxis for human monocytes by fibrinogen degradation products. *Br J Haematol* 32:507, 1976.

187. Girmann G, Pees H, Schwarze G, Scheulen PG: Immunosuppression by micromolecular fibrin-fibrinogen degradation products in cancer. *Nature* 259:399, 1976.

188. Wiman B, Collen D: On the kinetics of the reaction between human antiplasmin and plasmin. *Eur J Biochem* 84:573, 1978.

189. Van Zonnefeld AJ, Veerman H, Pannekoek H: On the interaction of the finger and the kringle-2 domain of tissue-type plasminogen activator with fibrin: Inhibition of kringle-1 binding to fibrin by epsilon-aminocaproic acid. *J Biol Chem* 261:14214, 1986.

190. Camiolo SM, Thorsen S, Astrup T: Fibrinogenolysis and fibrinolysis with tissue plasminogen activator, urokinase, streptokinase-activated human globulin and plasmin. *Proc Soc Exp Biol Med* 138:277, 1971.

191. Lijnen HR, Zamarron C, Blaber M, et al: Activation of plasminogen by prourokinase: I. Mechanism. *J Biol Chem* 261:1253, 1986.

192. Pannell R, Black J, Gurewich V: Complementary modes of action of tissue-type plasminogen activator and pro-urokinase by which their synergistic effect on clot lysis may be explained. *J Clin Invest* 81:853, 1988.

193. Bell W: Fibrinolytic therapy: Indications and management, in: *Hematology: Basic Principles and Practice*, edited by R Hoffman, EJ Benz, SJ Shattil, B Furie, HJ Cohen, LE Silberstein, p 1814. Churchill Livingstone, New York, 1995.

194. Nesheim M, Wang W, Boffa M, et al: Thrombin, thrombomodulin and TAFI in the molecular link between coagulation and fibrinolysis. *Thromb Haemost* 78:386, 1997.

195. Eaton DL, Malloy BE, Tsai SP, et al: Isolation, molecular cloning, and partial characterization of a novel carboxypeptidase B from plasma. *J Biol Chem* 269:21833, 1991.

196. Wang W, Hendriks DF, Scharpe SS: Carboxypeptidase U, a plasma carboxypeptidase with high affinity for plasminogen. *J Biol Chem* 269:15937, 1994.

197. Bajzar L, Manuel R, Nesheim M: Purification and characterization of TAFI, a thrombin activatable fibrinolysis inhibitor. *J Biol Chem* 270:14477, 1995.

198. Bajzar L, Nesheim ME, Tracy PB: The profibrinolytic effect of activated protein C in clots formed from plasma is TAFI-dependent. *Blood* 88:2093, 1996.

199. Bajzar L, Morser J, Nesheim M: TAFI, or plasma procarboxypeptidase B, couples the coagulation and fibrinolytic cascades through the thrombin-thrombomodulin complex. *J Biol Chem* 271:16603, 1996.

200. Minnema MC, Friederich PW, Levi M, et al: Enhancement of rabbit jugular vein thrombolysis by neutralization of factor XI: In vivo evidence for a role of factor XI as an anti-fibrinolytic factor. *J Clin Invest* 101:10, 1998.

201. Redlitz A, Tan AK, Eaton D, Plow EF: Plasma carboxypeptidases as regulators of the plasminogen system. *J Clin Invest* 96:2534, 1995.

202. Coligan JE, Slayter HS: Structure of thrombospondin. *J Biol Chem* 259:3944, 1984.

203. Ott U, Odermatt E, Engel J, et al: Protease resistance and conformation of laminin. *Eur J Biochem* 123:63, 1982.

204. Aplin JD, Hughes RC: Complex carbohydrates of the extracellular matrix structures, interactions, and biologic roles. *Biochim Biophys Acta* 694:375, 1982.

205. Marder VJ, Sherry S: Thrombolytic therapy: Current status. *N Engl J Med* 318:1512, 1988.

206. Unkeless JC, Gordon S, Reich E: Secretion of plasminogen activator by stimulated macrophages. *J Exp Med* 139:834, 1974.

207. Ossowski L, Reich E: Antibodies to plasminogen activator inhibit human tumor metastasis. *Cell* 35:611, 1983.

208. Strickland SE, Reich E, Sherman MI: Plasminogen activator in early embryogenesis: Enzyme production by trophoblast and parietal endoderm. *Cell* 9:231, 1976.

209. Strickland SE, Beers WH: Studies on the role of plasminogen activator in ovulation. *J Biol Chem* 254:5694, 1976.

210. Moonen G, Grau-Wagemans MP, Selak I: Plasminogen activator-plasmin system and neuronal migration. *Nature* 298:753, 1982.

211. Pittman RN, Ivins JK, Buettner HM: Neuronal plasminogen activators: Cell surface binding sites and involvement in neurite outgrowth. *J Neurosci* 9:4269, 1989.

212. Virji MA, Vassalli JD, Estensen D, Reich E: Plasminogen activator of islets of Langerhans: Modulation by glucose and correlation with insulin production. *Proc Natl Acad Sci U S A* 77:875, 1980.

213. Geiger M, Binder BR: Plasminogen activation in diabetes mellitus. *J Biol Chem* 259:2976, 1984.

214. Russell J, Schneider AB, Katzhendler J, et al: Modification of human placental lactogen with plasmin. *J Biol Chem* 254:2296, 1979.

215. Loskutoff DJ, Quigley JP: PAI-1, fibrosis, and the elusive provisional fibrin matrix. *J Clin Invest* 106:1441, 2000.

216. Romer J, Bugge TH, Pyke C, et al: Impaired wound healing in mice with a disrupted plasminogen gene. *Nat Med* 2:287, 1996.

217. Bugge TH, Kombrinck KW, Flick MJ, et al: Loss of fibrinogen rescues mice from the pleiotropic effects of plasminogen deficiency. *Cell* 87:709, 1996.

218. Ploplis VA, French EL, Carmeliet P, et al: Plasminogen deficiency differentially affects recruitment of inflammatory cell populations in mice. *Blood* 91:2005, 1998.

219. Carmeliet P, Moons L, Ploplis VA, et al: Impaired arterial neointima formation in mice with disruption of the plasminogen gene. *J Clin Invest* 99:200, 1997.

220. Coleman JL, Gebbia JA, Piesman J, et al: Plasminogen is required for efficient dissemination of B. burfdorferi in ticks and for enhancement of spirochetemia in mice. *Cell* 89:1111, 1997.

221. Chen ZL, Strickland SE: Neuronal death in the hippocampus is promoted by plasmin-catalyzed degradation of laminin. *Cell* 91:917, 1997.

222. Sporn MB, Roberts AB, Wakefield LM, Assoian RK: Transforming growth factor-beta: Biological function and chemical structure. *Science* 233:532, 1986.

223. Lyons RM, Gentry LE, Purchio AF, Moses HL: Mechanism of activation of latent recombinant transforming growth factor beta1 by plasmin. *J Cell Biol* 110:1361, 1990.

224. Konstantinides S, Schafer K, Loskutoff DJ: Do PAI-1 and vitronectin promote or inhibit neointima formation? *Arterioscler Thromb Vasc Biol* 22:1943, 2002.

225. Ross R: Atherosclerosis: An inflammatory disease. *N Engl J Med* 340:115, 1999.

226. Konstantinides S, Schafer K, Thinnes T, Loskutoff DJ: Plasminogen activator inhibitor-1 and its cofactor vitronectin stabilize arterial thrombi following vascular injury in mice. *Circulation* 103:576, 2001.

227. Peng L, Bhatia N, Parker AC, et al: Endogenous vitronectin and plasminogen actvator inhibitor-1 promote neointima formation in murine carotid arteries. *Arterioscler Thromb Vasc Biol* 22:934, 2002.

228. O'Reilly MS, Holmgren L, Shing Y, et al: Angiostatin: A novel angiogenesis inhibitor that mediates the suppression of metastases by a Lewis lung carcinoma. *Cell* 79:315, 1995.

229. Lucas R, Holmgren L, Garcia I, et al: Multiple forms of angiostatin induce apoptosis in endothelial cells. *Blood* 92:4730, 1998.

230. O'Reilly MS, Holmgren L, Chen C, Folkman J: Angiostatin induces and sustains dormancy of human primary tumors in mice. *Nat Med* 2:689, 1996.

231. Cao Y, O'Reilly MS, Marshall B, et al: Expression of angiostatin cDNA in a murine fibrosarcoma suppresses primary tumor growth and produces long-term dormancy of metastases. *J Clin Invest* 101:1055, 1998.

232. Moser TL, Pizzo SV, Enghild JJ, et al: Isolation of an angiostatin receptor from the membranes of human umbilical vein endothelial cells. *Fibrinol Proteol* 11:39, 1997.

233. Cao Y, Chen A, Seong SSA, et al: Kringle 5 of plasminogen is a novel inhibitor of endothelial cell growth. *J Biol Chem* 272:22924, 1997.

234. Griscelli F, Li H, Bennaceur-Griscelli A, et al: Angiostatin gene transfer: Inhibition of tumor growth in vivo by blockage of endothelial cell proliferation associated with a mitosis arrest. *Proc Natl Acad Sci U S A* 95:6367, 1998.

235. Dong Z, Kumar R, Yang X, Fidler I: Macrophage-derived metallo-elastase is responsible for the generation of angiostatin in Lewis lung carcinoma. *Cell* 88:801, 1997.

236. Stathakis P, Fitzgerald M, Matthias LJ, et al: Generation of angiostatin by reduction and proteolysis of plasmin: Catalysis by a plasmin reductase secreted by cultured cells. *J Biol Chem* 272:20641, 1997.

237. Patterson BC, Sang QXA: Angiostatin-converting enzyme activities of human matrilysin (MMP-7) and gelatinase B/type IV collagenase (MMP-9). *J Biol Chem* 272:28823, 1997.

238. Gately S, Twardowski P, Stack MS, et al: The mechanism of cancer-mediated conversion of plasminogen to the angiogenesis inhibitor angiostatin. *Proc Natl Acad Sci U S A* 94:10868, 1998.

239. Aoki N, Moroi M, Sakata Y, et al: Abnormal plasminogen: A hereditary molecular abnormality found in a patient with recurrent thrombosis. *J Clin Invest* 61:1186, 1978.

240. Ichinose A, Espling ES, Takamatsu J, et al: Two types of abnormal genes for plasminogen in families with a predisposition for thrombosis. *Proc Natl Acad Sci U S A* 88:115, 1991.

241. Lijnen HR, Collen D: Congenital and acquired deficiencies of components of the fibrinolytic system and their relationship to bleeding or thrombosis. *Blood Coagul Fibrinolysis* 3:67, 1989.

242. Robbins KC: Dysplasminogenemia. *Prog Cardiovasc Dis* 34:295, 1992.

243. Azuma H, Mima N, Shirakawa M, et al: Molecular pathogenesis of type I congenital plasminogen deficiency: Expression of recombinant human mutant plasminogens in mammalian cells. *Blood* 89:183, 1997.

244. Demarmels Biasiutti F, Sulzer I, Stucki B, et al: Is plasminogen deficiency a thrombotic risk factor? A study on 23 thrombophilic patients and their family members. *Thromb Haemost* 80:167, 1998.

245. Sartori MT, Patrassi GM, Theodoridis P, et al: Heterozygous type I plasminogen deficiency is associated with an increased risk for thrombosis: A statistical analysis of 20 kindreds. *Blood Coagul Fibrinolysis* 5:889, 1994.

246. Schott D, Dempfle CE, Beck P, et al: Therapy with a purified plasminogen concentrate in an infant with ligneous conjunctivitis and homozygous plasminogen deficiency. *N Engl J Med* 339:1679, 1998.

247. Tsutsumi S, Saito T, Sakata T, et al: Genetic diagnosis of dysplasminogenemia: Detection of an Ala601-Thr mutation in 118 out of 125 families and identification of a new Asp676-Asn mutation. *Thromb Haemost* 76:135, 1996.

248. Summaria L, Arzadon L, Bernabe P, Robbins KC: Studies on the isolation of the multiple molecular forms of human plasminogen and plasmin by isoelectric focusing methods. *J Biochem Biophys* 247:4691, 1972.

249. Hobart MJ: Genetic polymorphism of human plasminogen. *Ann Hum Genet* 42:419, 1979.

250. Raum D, Marcus D, Alper CA: Genetic polymorphism of human plasminogen. *Am J Hum Genet* 32:681, 1980.

251. Robbins KC: Classification of abnormal plasminogens: Dysplasminogenemias. *Semin Thromb Haemost* 16:217, 1990.

252. Rakoczi I, Chamone D, Collen D, Verstraete M: Prediction of postoperative leg vein thrombosis in gynaecological patients. *Lancet* 1:509, 1978.

253. Nilsson IM, Ljungner H, Tengborn L: Two different mechanisms in patients with venous thrombosis and defective fibrinolysis: Low concentrations of plasminogen activator or increased concentration of plasminogen activator inhibitor. *Br Med J* 290:1453, 1985.

254. Juhan-Vague I, Valadier J, Alessi MC, et al: Deficient t-PA release and elevated PA inhibitor levels in patients with spontaneous or recurrent leg thrombosis. *Thromb Haemost* 57:67, 1987.

255. Hamsten A, Wiman B, De Faire U, Blomback M: Increased plasma levels of a rapid inhibitor of tissue plasminogen activator in young survivors of myocardial infarction. *N Engl J Med* 313:1557, 1985.

256. Paramo JA, Alfaro MJ, Rocha E: Postoperative changes in the plasmatic levels of tissue-type plasminogen activator and its fast-acting inhibitor: Relationship to deep vein thrombosis and influence of prophylaxis. *Thromb Haemost* 54:713, 1985.

257. Juhan-Vague I, Roul C, Alessi MC, et al: Increased plasminogen activator inhibitor activity in non-insulin dependent diabetic patients: Relationship with plasma insulin. *Thromb Haemost* 61:370, 1989.

258. Juhan-Vague I, Alessi MC, Joly P, et al: Plasma plasminogen activator inhibitor-1 in angina pectoris: Influence of plasma insulin and acute-phase response. *Arterioscler Thromb Vasc Biol* 9:362, 1989.

259. Stump DC, Taylor FB, Nesheim ME, et al: Pathologic fibrinolysis as a cause of clinical bleeding. *Semin Thromb Hemost* 16:260, 1990.

260. Saito H: Alpha-2-plasmin inhibitor and its deficiency states. *J Lab Clin Med* 112:671, 1988.

261. Suarez CR, Walenga J, Mangogna LC, Fareed J: Neonatal and maternal fibrinolysis: Activation at time of birth. *Am J Hematol* 19:365, 1985.

262. Summaria L: Comparison of human normal, full-term, fetal and adult plasminogen by physical and clinical analyses. *Haemostasis* 19:266, 1989.

263. Edelberg JM, Enghild JJ, Pizzo SV, Gonzales-Gronow M: Neonatal plasminogen displays altered cell surface binding and activation kinetics: Correlation with increased glycosylation of the protein. *J Clin Invest* 86:107, 1990.

264. Andrew M, Brooker L, Leaker M, et al: Fibrin clot lysis by thrombolytic agents is impaired in newborns due to a low plasminogen concentration. *Thromb Haemost* 68:325, 1992.

265. Corrigan JJ, Sleeth JJ, Jeter MA, Lox CD: Newborn's fibrinolytic mechanism: Components and plasmin generation. *Am J Hematol* 32:273, 1989.

266. Corrigan JJ, Jeter MA: Histidine-rich glycoprotein and plasminogen plasma levels in term and preterm newborns. *Am J Dis Child* 144:825, 1990.

267. Corrigan JJ, Jeter MA: Tissue-type plasminogen activator, plasminogen activator inhibitor, and histidine-rich glycoprotein in stressed human newborns. *Pediatrics* 89:43, 1992.

268. Brus F, Van Oeveren W, Okkern A, Oetomo SB: Activation of the plasma clotting, fibrinolytic, and kinin-kallikrein system in preterm infants with severe idiopathic respiratory distress syndrome. *Pediatric Res* 36:647, 1994.

269. Cederholm-Williams SA, Spencer JAD, Wilkerson AR: Plasma levels of selected haemostatic factors in newborn babies. *Thromb Res* 23:555, 1981.

270. Andrew M, Paes B, Milner R, et al: Development of the human coagulation system in the full-term infant. *Blood* 70:165, 1987.

271. Andrew M, Massicotte-Nolan PM, Karpatkin M: Plasma protease inhibitors in premature infants: Influence of gestational age, postnatal age, and health status. *Proc Soc Exp Biol Med* 173:495, 1983.

272. Corrigan JJ: Thrombosis and thromboembolism, in *Hemorrhagic and Thrombotic Disease in Childhood and Adolescence*, edited by JJ Corrigan, p 147. Churchill Livingstone, New York, 1985.

273. Bonnar J, Daly L, Sheppard BL: Changes in the fibrinolytic system during pregnancy. *Semin Thromb Hemost* 16:221, 1990.

274. Hellgren M: Hemostasis during pregnancy and puerperium. *Haemostasis* 26:244, 1996.

275. Schjetlein R, Haugen G, Wisloff F: Markers of intravascular coagulation and fibrinolysis in preeclampsia: Association with intrauterine growth retardation. *Acta Obstet Gynecol Scand* 76:541, 1997.

276. Fletcher AP, Alkjaersig N, Smyrniotis FE, Sherry S: The treatment of patients suffering from early myocardial infarction with massive and prolonged streptokinase therapy. *Trans Assoc Am Physicians* 71:287, 1958.

277. Sherry S, Fletcher AP, Alkjaersig N: Fibrinolysis and fibrinolytic activity in man. *Physiol Rev* 39:343, 1959.

278. Adelman B, Michelson AD, Loscalzo J, et al: Plasmin effect on platelet glycoprotein Ib-von Willebrand factor interactions. *Blood* 65:32, 1985.

279. Loscalzo J, Vaughan DE: Tissue plasminogen activator promotes platelet disaggregation in plasma. *J Clin Invest* 79:1749, 1987.

280. Rudd MA, George D, Amarante P, et al: Temporal effects of thrombolytic agents on platelet function in vivo and their modulation by prostaglandins. *Circ Res* 67:1175, 1990.

281. The urokinase pulmonary embolism trial. A national cooperative study. *Circulation* 47(2 suppl):II1, 1973.

282. Marder VJ: Relevance of changes in blood fibrinolytic and coagulation parameters during thrombolytic therapy. *Am J Med* 83:15, 1987.

283. Rao AK, Pratt C, Berke A, et al: Thrombolysis in Myocardial Infarction (TIMI) Trial—Phase I: Hemorrhagic manifestations and changes in plasma fibrinogen and the fibrinolytic system in patients treated with recombinant tissue plasminogen activator and streptokinase. *J Am Coll Cardiol* 11:1, 1988.

284. Timmis GC, Gangadharan V, Ramos RG, et al: Hemorrhage and the products of fibrinogen digestion after intracoronary administration of streptokinase. *Circulation* 69:1146, 1984.

285. Abe T, Kazama M, Naito I, et al: Clinical evaluation for efficacy of tissue culture urokinase (TCUK) on cerebral thrombosis by means of multicenter double blind study. *Blood Vessels* 12:321, 1981.

286. Abe T, Kazama M, Naito I, et al: Clinical effect of urokinase (60,000 units/day) on cerebral infarction comparative study by means of multiple center double blind test. *Blood Vessels* 12:342, 1981.

287. Atarashi J, Otomo E, Araki G, et al: Clinical utility of urokinase in the treatment of acute stage of cerebral thrombosis: Multi-center double-blind study in comparison with placebo. *Clin Eval* 13:659, 1985.

288. del Zoppo GJ, Ferbert A, Otis S, et al: Local intra-arterial fibrinolytic therapy in acute carotid territory stroke. A pilot study. *Stroke* 19:307, 1988.

289. Fletcher AP, Alkjaersig N, Lewis M, et al: A pilot study of urokinase therapy in cerebral infarction. *Stroke* 7:135, 1976.

290. Hacke W, Zeumer H, Ferbert A, et al: Intra-arterial thrombolytic therapy improves outcome in patients with acute vertebrobasilar occlusive disease. *Stroke* 19:1216, 1988.

291. Hanaway J, Torack R, Fletcher AP, Landau WM: Intracranial bleeding associated with urokinase therapy for acute ischemic hemispheral stroke. *Stroke* 7:143, 1976.

292. Matsumoto K, Satoh K: *Topical Intraarterial Urokinase Infusion for Acute Stroke*. Springer-Verlag, Heidelberg, 1991.

293. Meyer JS, Gilroy J, Barnhart MI, Johnson JF: Therapeutic thrombolysis in cerebral thromboembolism. Double-blind evaluation of intravenous plasmin therapy in carotid and middle cerebral arterial occlusion. *Neurology* 13:927, 1963.

294. Meyer JS, Gilroy J, Barnhart MI, Johnson JF: Anticoagulants plus streptokinase therapy in progressive stroke. *JAMA* 189:373, 1964.

295. Mori E, Tabuchi M, Yoshida T, Yamadori A: Intracarotid urokinase with thromboembolic occlusion of the middle cerebral artery. *Stroke* 19:802, 1988.

296. Mori E: *Fibrinolytic Recanalization Therapy in Acute Cerebrovascular Thromboembolism*. Springer-Verlag, Heidelberg, 1991.

297. Otomo E, Araki G, Itoh E, et al: Clinical efficacy of urokinase in the treatment of cerebral thrombosis. *Clin Eval* 13:711, 1985.

298. Theron J, Courtheoux P, Casasco A, et al: Local intraarterial fibrinolysis in the carotid territory. *AJNR Am J Neuroradiol* 10:753, 1989.

299. Zeumer H, Freitag HJ, Grzyska U, Neunzig HP: Local intra-arterial fibrinolysis in acute vertebrobasilar occlusion. Technical developments and recent results. *Neuroradiology* 31:336, 1989.

300. Zeumer H, Freitag HJ, Zanella F, et al: Local intra-arterial fibrinolytic therapy in patients with stroke: Urokinase versus recombinant tissue plasminogen activator (r-TPA). *Neuroradiology* 35:159, 1993.

301. Tissue plasminogen activator for acute ischemic stroke. The National Institute of Neurological Disorders and Stroke rt-PA Stroke Study Group. *N Engl J Med* 333:1581, 1995.

302. Hacke W, Kaste M, Fieschi C, et al: Intravenous thrombolysis with recombinant tissue plasminogen activator for acute hemispheric stroke. The European Cooperative Acute Stroke Study (ECASS). *JAMA* 274:1017, 1995.

303. Hacke W, Kaste M, Fieschi C, et al: Randomised double-blind placebo-controlled trial of thrombolytic therapy with intravenous alteplase in acute ischaemic stroke (ECASS II). Second European-Australasian Acute Stroke Study Investigators. *Lancet* 352:1245, 1998.

304. Clark WM, Wissman S, Albers GW, et al: Recombinant tissue-type plasminogen activator (Alteplase) for ischemic stroke 3 to 5 hours after symptom onset. The ATLANTIS Study: A randomized controlled trial. Alteplase Thrombolysis for Acute Noninterventional Therapy in Ischemic Stroke. *JAMA* 282:2019, 1999.

305. Donnan GA, Davis SM, Chambers BR, et al: Streptokinase for acute ischemic stroke with relationship to time of administration: Australian Streptokinase (ASK) Trial Study Group. *JAMA* 276:961, 1996.

306. Randomised controlled trial of streptokinase, aspirin, and combination of both in treatment of acute ischaemic stroke. Multicentre Acute Stroke Trial—Italy (MAST-I) Group. *Lancet* 346:1509, 1995.

307. Thrombolytic therapy with streptokinase in acute ischemic stroke. The Multicenter Acute Stroke Trial—Europe Study Group. *N Engl J Med* 335:145, 1996.

308. Barnwell SL, Clark WM, Nguyen TT, et al: Safety and efficacy of delayed intraarterial urokinase therapy with mechanical clot disruption for thromboembolic stroke. *AJNR Am J Neuroradiol* 15:1817, 1994.

309. Barr JD, Mathis JM, Wildenhain SL, et al: Acute stroke intervention with intraarterial urokinase infusion. *J Vasc Interv Radiol* 5:705, 1994.

310. Casto L, Caverni L, Camerlingo M, et al: Intra-arterial thrombolysis in acute ischaemic stroke: Experience with a superselective catheter embedded in the clot. *J Neurol Neurosurg Psychiatry* 60:667, 1996.

311. Jansen O, von Kummer R, Forsting M, et al: Thrombolytic therapy in acute occlusion of the intracranial internal carotid artery bifurcation. *AJNR Am J Neuroradiol* 16:1977, 1995.

312. Nesbit GM, Clark WM, O'Neill OR, Barnwell SL: Intracranial intraarterial thrombolysis facilitated by microcatheter navigation through an occluded cervical internal carotid artery. *J Neurosurg* 84:387, 1996.

313. Tarr R, Taylor CL, Selman WR, et al: Good clinical outcome in a patient with a large CT scan hypodensity treated with intra-arterial urokinase after an embolic stroke. *Neurology* 47:1076, 1996.

314. del Zoppo GJ, Higashida RT, Furlan AJ, et al: PROACT: A phase II randomized trial of recombinant pro-urokinase by direct arterial delivery in acute middle cerebral artery stroke. PROACT Investigators. Prolyse in Acute Cerebral Thromboembolism. *Stroke* 29:4, 1998.

315. Furlan A, Higashida R, Wechsler L, et al: Intra-arterial prourokinase for acute ischemic stroke. The PROACT II study: A randomized controlled trial. Prolyse in Acute Cerebral Thromboembolism. *JAMA* 282:2003, 1999.

316. Liu M, Wardlaw J: Thrombolysis (different doses, routes of administration and agents) for acute ischaemic stroke. *Cochrane Database Syst Rev* CD000514, 2000.

317. Wardlaw JM, Zoppo G, Yamaguchi T, Berge E: Thrombolysis for acute ischaemic stroke. *Cochrane Database Syst Rev* CD000213, 2003.

318. Broderick JP, William M: Feinberg Lecture: Stroke therapy in the year 2025: Burden, breakthroughs, and barriers to progress. *Stroke* 35:205, 2004.

319. Kleindorfer D, Khoury J, Alwell K, et al: Eligibility for rt-PA in acute ischemic stroke: A population-based study. *Stroke* 34:281, 2003.

320. Kothari RU, Pancioli A, Liu T, et al: Cincinnati Prehospital Stroke Scale: Reproducibility and validity. *Ann Emerg Med* 33:373, 1999.

321. Abciximab in acute ischemic stroke: A randomized, double-blind, placebo-controlled, dose-escalation study. The Abciximab in Ischemic Stroke Investigators. *Stroke* 31:601, 2000.

322. Qureshi AI, Suri MF, Khan J, et al: Abciximab as an adjunct to high-risk carotid or vertebrobasilar angioplasty: Preliminary experience. *Neurosurgery* 46:1316, 2000.

323. Qureshi AI, Ali Z, Suri MF, et al: Intra-arterial third-generation recombinant tissue plasminogen activator (reteplase) for acute ischemic stroke. *Neurosurgery* 49:41, 2001.

324. Ernst R, Pancioli A, Tomsick T, et al: Combined intravenous and intra-arterial recombinant tissue plasminogen activator in acute ischemic stroke. *Stroke* 31:2552, 2000.

325. Alexandrov AV, Demchuk AM, Felberg RA, et al: High rate of complete recanalization and dramatic clinical recovery during tPA infusion when continuously monitored with 2-MHz transcranial Doppler monitoring. *Stroke* 31:610, 2000.

326. Francis CW: Ultrasound-enhanced thrombolysis. *Echocardiography* 18:239, 2001.

327. Adams HP Jr, Adams RJ, Brott T, et al: Guidelines for the early management of patients with ischemic stroke: A scientific statement from the Stroke Council of the American Stroke Association. *Stroke* 34:1056, 2003.

328. Broderick JP, Hacke W: Treatment of acute ischemic stroke: Part I: Recanalization strategies. *Circulation* 106:1563, 2002.

329. Kaste M, Thomassen L, Grond M, et al: Thrombolysis for acute ischemic stroke: A consensus statement of the 3rd Karolinska Stroke Update, October 30-31, 2000. *Stroke* 32:2717, 2001.

330. Brogden RN, Speight TM, Avery GS: Streptokinase: A review of its clinical pharmacology, mechanism of action and therapeutic uses. *Drugs* 5:357, 1973.

331. Dotter CT, Rosch J, Seaman AJ: Selective clot lysis with low-dose streptokinase. *Radiology* 111:31, 1974.

332. Ouriel K: Current status of thrombolysis for peripheral arterial occlusive disease. *Ann Vasc Surg* 16:797, 2002.

333. Ouriel K, Shortell CK, DeWeese JA, et al: A comparison of thrombolytic therapy with operative revascularization in the initial treatment of acute peripheral arterial ischemia. *J Vasc Surg* 19:1021, 1994.

334. Results of a prospective randomized trial evaluating surgery versus thrombolysis for ischemia of the lower extremity. The STILE trial. *Ann Surg* 220:251, 1994.

335. Ouriel K, Veith FJ, Sasahara AA: Thrombolysis or peripheral arterial surgery: Phase I results. TOPAS Investigators. *J Vasc Surg* 23:64, 1996.

336. Ouriel K, Veith FJ, Sasahara AA: A comparison of recombinant urokinase with vascular surgery as initial treatment for acute arterial occlusion of the legs. Thrombolysis or Peripheral Arterial Surgery (TOPAS) Investigators. *N Engl J Med* 338:1105, 1998.

337. Castaneda F, Swischuk JL, Li R, et al: Declining-dose study of reteplase treatment for lower extremity arterial occlusions. *J Vasc Interv Radiol* 13:1093, 2002.

338. Ouriel K, Katzen B, Mewissen M, et al: Reteplase in the treatment of peripheral arterial and venous occlusions: A pilot study. *J Vasc Interv Radiol* 11:849, 2000.

339. Ouriel K, Kandarpa K, Schuerr DM, et al: Prourokinase versus urokinase for recanalization of peripheral occlusions, safety and efficacy: The PURPOSE trial. *J Vasc Interv Radiol* 10:1083, 1999.

340. Heymans S, Vanderschueren S, Verhaeghe R, et al: Outcome and one year follow-up of intra-arterial staphylokinase in 191 patients with peripheral arterial occlusion. *Thromb Haemost* 83:666, 2000.

341. Duda SH, Tepe G, Luz O, et al: Peripheral artery occlusion: Treatment with abciximab plus urokinase versus with urokinase alone—A randomized pilot trial (the PROMPT Study). Platelet Receptor Antibodies in Order to Manage Peripheral Artery Thrombosis. *Radiology* 221:689, 2001.

342. Drescher P, McGuckin J, Rilling WS, Crain MR: Catheter-directed thrombolytic therapy in peripheral artery occlusions: Combining reteplase and abciximab. *AJR Am J Roentgenol* 180:1385, 2003.

343. Cohen LH, Kaplan M, Bernhard VM: Intraoperative streptokinase. An adjunct to mechanical thrombectomy in the management of acute ischemia. *Arch Surg* 121:708, 1986.

344. Comerota AJ, White JV, Grosh JD: Intraoperative intra-arterial thrombolytic therapy for salvage of limbs in patients with distal arterial thrombosis. *Surg Gynecol Obstet* 169:283, 1989.

345. Parent FN, Bernhard VM, Pabst TS, et al: Fibrinolytic treatment of residual thrombus after catheter embolectomy for severe lower limb ischemia. *J Vasc Surg* 9:153, 1989.

346. Quinones-Baldrich WJ, Zierler RE, Hiatt JC: Intraoperative fibrinolytic therapy: An adjunct to catheter thromboembolectomy. *J Vasc Surg* 2:319, 1985.

347. Vedantham S, Vesely TM, Parti N, et al: Lower extremity venous thrombolysis with adjunctive mechanical thrombectomy. *J Vasc Interv Radiol* 13:1001, 2002.

348. Berridge DC, Kessel D, Robertson I: Surgery versus thrombolysis for acute limb ischaemia: Initial management. *Cochrane Database Syst Rev* CD002784, 2002.

349. Kessel D, Berridge D, Robertson I: Infusion techniques for peripheral arterial thrombolysis. *Cochrane Database Syst Rev* 1:CD000985, 2004.

350. Thrombolysis in the management of lower limb peripheral arterial occlusion—A consensus document. Working Party on Thrombolysis in the Management of Limb Ischemia. *Am J Cardiol* 81:207, 1998.

351. Menon KV, Shah V, Kamath PS: The Budd-Chiari syndrome. *N Engl J Med* 350:578, 2004.

352. Aytekin C, Boyvat F, Kurt A, et al: Catheter-directed thrombolysis with transjugular access in portal vein thrombosis secondary to pancreatitis. *Eur J Radiol* 39:80, 2001.

353. Ciccarelli O, Goffette P, Laterre PF, et al: Transjugular intrahepatic portosystemic shunt approach and local thrombolysis for treatment of early posttransplant portal vein thrombosis. *Transplantation* 72:159, 2001.

354. Tateishi A, Mitsui H, Oki T, et al: Extensive mesenteric vein and portal vein thrombosis successfully treated by thrombolysis and anticoagulation. *J Gastroenterol Hepatol* 16:1429, 2001.

355. Calin GA, Calin S, Ionescu R, et al: Successful local fibrinolytic treatment and balloon angioplasty in superior mesenteric arterial embolism: A case report and literature review. *Hepatogastroenterology* 50:732, 2003.

356. Savassi-Rocha PR, Veloso LF: Treatment of superior mesenteric artery embolism with a fibrinolytic agent: Case report and literature review. *Hepatogastroenterology* 49:1307, 2002.

357. Haire WD, Atkinson JB, Stephens LC, Kotulak GD: Urokinase versus recombinant tissue plasminogen activator in thrombosed central venous catheters: A double-blinded, randomized trial. *Thromb Haemost* 72:543, 1994.

358. Semba CP, Deitcher SR, Li X, et al: Treatment of occluded central venous catheters with alteplase: Results in 1,064 patients. *J Vasc Interv Radiol* 13:1199, 2002.

359. Shen V, Li X, Murdock M, et al: Recombinant tissue plasminogen activator (alteplase) for restoration of function to occluded central venous catheters in pediatric patients. *J Pediatr Hematol Oncol* 25:38, 2003.

360. Timoney JP, Malkin MG, Leone DM, et al: Safe and cost effective use of alteplase for the clearance of occluded central venous access devices. *J Clin Oncol* 20:1918, 2002.

361. Cooper SG: Original report. Pulse-spray thrombolysis of thrombosed hemodialysis grafts with tissue plasminogen activator. *AJR Am J Roentgenol* 180:1063, 2003.

362. Cynamon J, Pierpont CE: Thrombolysis for the treatment of thrombosed hemodialysis access grafts. *Rev Cardiovasc Med* 3(suppl 2):84, 2002.

363. Daeihagh P, Jordan J, Chen J, Rocco M: Efficacy of tissue plasminogen activator administration on patency of hemodialysis access catheters. *Am J Kidney Dis* 36:75, 2000.

364. Hilleman DE, Dunlay RW, Packard KA: Reteplase for dysfunctional hemodialysis catheter clearance. *Pharmacotherapy* 23:137, 2003.

365. Shrivastava D, Lundin AP, Dosunmu B, et al: Salvage of clotted jugular vein hemodialysis catheters. *Nephron* 68:77, 1994.

366. Sobel BE: Intracranial bleeding, fibrinolysis, and anticoagulation. Causal connections and clinical implications. *Circulation* 90:2147, 1994.

367. Sane DC, Califf RM, Topol EJ, et al: Bleeding during thrombolytic therapy for acute myocardial infarction: Mechanisms and management. *Ann Intern Med* 111:1010, 1989.

368. Alkjaersig N, Fletcher AP, Sherry S: Epsilon-Aminocaproic acid: An inhibitor of plasminogen activation. *J Biol Chem* 234:832, 1959.

369. Andersson L, Nilsson IM, Nilehn JE, et al: Experimental and clinical studies on AMCA, the antifibrinolytically active isomer of p-aminomethyl cyclohexane carboxylic acid. *Scand J Haematol* 2:230, 1965.

370. Brockway WJ, Castellino FJ: The mechanism of the inhibition of plasmin by xi-aminocaproic acid. *J Biol Chem* 14:4641, 1971.

371. McNicol GP, Fletcher AP, Alkjaersig N, et al: The absorption, distribution and excretion of xi-aminocaproic acid following oral or intravenous administration to man. *J Lab Clin Med* 59:15, 1962.

372. Huber R, Kukla D, Ruhlmann A, Steigemann W: Pancreatic trypsin inhibitor (Kunitz): I. Structure and function. *Cold Spring Harb Symp Quant Biol* 36:141, 1972.

373. Ruhlmann A, Kukla D, Schwager P, et al: Structure of the complex formed by bovine trypsin and bovine pancreatic trypsin inhibitor. Crystal structure determination and stereochemistry of the contact region. *J Mol Biol* 77:417, 1973.

374. Wiman B: On the reaction of plasmin or plasmin-streptokinase complex with aprotinin or alpha 2-antiplasmin. *Thromb Res* 17:143, 1980.

375. Aoki N, Moro M, Matsuda M, Tachiya K: The behavior of alpha-2 plasmin inhibitor in fibrinolytic states. *J Clin Invest* 60:361, 1977.

376. Aoki N, Sakata Y, Matsuda M, Tateno K: Fibrinolytic states in a patient with congenital deficiency of alpha 1-plasmin inhibitor. *Blood* 55:483, 1980.

377. Dieval J, Nguyen G, Gross S, et al: A lifelong bleeding disorder associated with a deficiency of plasminogen activator inhibitor type 1. *Blood* 77:528, 1991.

378. Fay WP, Shapiro AD, Shih JL, et al: Brief report: Complete deficiency of plasminogen-activator inhibitor type 1 due to a frame-shift mutation. *N Engl J Med* 327:1729, 1992.

379. Lee MH, Vosburgh E, Anderson K, McDonagh J: Deficiency of plasma plasminogen activator inhibitor 1 results in hyperfibrinolytic bleeding. *Blood* 81:2357, 1993.

380. Avvisati G, Ten Cate JW, Buller HR, Mandelli F: Tranexamic acid for control of haemorrhage in acute promyelocytic leukemia. *Lancet* ii:122, 1989.

381. Rodeghiero F, Avvisati G, Castaman G, et al: Early deaths and antihemorrhagic treatments in acute promyelocytic leukemia. A GIMEMA retrospective study in 268 consecutive patients. *Blood* 75:2112, 1990.

382. Schwartz BS, Williams EC, Conlan MG, Mosher DF: Epsilon-aminocaproic acid in the treatment of patients with acute promyelocytic leukemia and acquired alpha-2-plasmin inhibitor deficiency. *Ann Intern Med* 105:873, 1986.

383. Booth NA, Anderson JA, Bennett B: Plasminogen activators in alcoholic cirrhosis: Demonstration of increased tissue type and urokinase type activator. *J Clin Pathol* 37:772, 1984.

384. Hayashi T, Kamogawa A, Ro S, et al: Plasma from patients with cirrhosis increases tissue plasminogen activator release from vascular endothelial cells in vitro. *Liver* 18:186, 1998.

385. Violi F, Basili V, Ferro D, et al: Association between high values of D-dimer and tissue-plasminogen activator activity and first gastrointestinal bleeding in cirrhotic patients. *Thromb Haemost* 76:177, 1996.

386. Boylan JF, Klinck JR, Sandler AN, et al: Tranexamic acid reduces blood loss, transfusion requirements, and coagulation factor use in primary orthotopic liver transplantation. *Anesthesiology* 85:1043, 1996.

387. Kaspar M, Ramsay MA, Nguyen AT, et al: Continuous small-dose tranexamic acid reduces fibrinolysis but not transfusion requirements during orthotopic liver transplantation. *Anesth Analg* 85:281, 1997.

388. Segal HC, Hunt BJ, Cottam S, et al: Fibrinolytic activity during orthotopic liver transplantation with and without aprotinin. *Transplantation* 58:1356, 1994.

389. Soilleux H, Gillon MC, Mirand A, et al: Comparative effects of small and large aprotinin doses on bleeding during orthotopic liver transplantation. *Anesth Analg* 80:349, 1995.

390. Al-Mondhiry H, Manni A, Owen J, Gordon R: Hemostatic effects of hormonal stimulation in patients with metastatic prostate cancer. *Am J Hematol* 28:141, 1988.

391. Bennett B, Croll AM, Robbie LA, Herriot R: Tumour cell u-PA as a cause of fibrinolytic bleeding in metastatic disease. *Br J Haematol* 99:570, 1997.

392. Mannucci PM, Cugno M, Bottasso B, et al: Changes in fibrinolysis in patients with localized tumors. *Eur J Cancer* 26:83, 1990.

393. Meijer K, Smid WM, Geerards S, van der Meer J: Hyperfibrinogenolysis in disseminated adenocarcinoma. *Blood Coagul Fibrinolysis* 9:279, 1998.

394. Webber MM, Waghray A: Urokinase-mediated extracellular matrix degradation by human prostatic carcinoma cells and its inhibition by retinoic acid. *Clin Cancer Res* 1:755, 1995.

395. Zacharski LR, Memoli VA, Ornstein DL, et al: Tumor cell procoagulant and urokinase expression in carcinoma of the ovary. *J Natl Cancer Inst* 85:1225, 1993.

396. Bouchama A, Bridey F, Hammami MM, et al: Activation of coagulation and fibrinolysis in heatstroke. *Thromb Haemost* 76:909, 1996.

397. Harker LA: Bleeding after cardiopulmonary bypass. *N Engl J Med* 314:1446, 1986.

398. Williams GD, Bratton SL, Nielsen NJ, Ramamoorthy C: Fibrinolysis in pediatric patients undergoing cardiopulmonary bypass. *J Cardiothorac Vasc Anesth* 12:633, 1998.

399. Horrow JC, Hlavacek J, Strong MD, et al: Prophylactic tranexamic acid decreases bleeding after cardiac operations. *J Thorac Cardiovasc Surg* 99:70, 1990.

400. Horrow JC, Van Riper DF, Strong MD, et al: Hemostatic effects of tranexamic acid and desmopressin during cardiac surgery. *Circulation* 84:2063, 1991.

401. Munoz JJ, Birkmeyer NJ, Birkmeyer JD, et al: Is epsilon-aminocaproic acid as effective as aprotinin in reducing bleeding with cardiac surgery? A meta-analysis. *Circulation* 99:81, 1999.

402. Soslau G, Horrow J, Brodsky I: Effect of tranexamic acid on platelet ADP during extracorporeal circulation. *Am J Hematol* 38:113, 1991.

403. Havel M, Grabenwoger F, Schneider J, et al: Aprotinin does not decrease early graft patency after coronary artery bypass grafting despite reducing postoperative bleeding and use of donated blood. *J Thorac Cardiovasc Surg* 107:807, 1994.

404. Laub GW, Riebman JB, Chen C, et al: The impact of aprotinin on coronary artery bypass graft patency. *Chest* 106:1370, 1994.

405. Lemmer JH Jr, Stanford W, Bonney SL, et al: Aprotinin for coronary bypass operations: Efficacy, safety, and influence on early saphenous vein graft patency. A multicenter, randomized, double-blind, placebo-controlled study. *J Thorac Cardiovasc Surg* 107:543, 1994.

406. Sindet-Pedersen S, Stenbjerg S: Effect of local antifibrinolytic treatment with tranexamic acid in hemophiliacs undergoing oral surgery. *J Oral Maxillofac Surg* 44:703, 1986.

407. Blomback M, Johansson G, Johnsson H, et al: Surgery in patients with von Willebrand's disease. *Br J Surg* 76:398, 1989.

408. Hedlund PO: Antifibrinolytic therapy with Cyklokapron in connection with prostatectomy. A double blind study. *Scand J Urol Nephrol* 3:177, 1969.

409. Callender ST, Warner GT, Cope E: Treatment of menorrhagia with tranexamic acid. A double-blind trial. *Br Med J* 4:214, 1970.

410. Ong YL, Hull DR, Mayne EE: Menorrhagia in von Willebrand disease successfully treated with single daily dose tranexamic acid. *Haemophilia* 4:63, 1998.

411. Ortel TL, Onorato JJ, Bedrosian CL, Kaufman RE: Antifibrinolytic therapy in the management of the Kasabach Merritt syndrome. *Am J Hematol* 29:44, 1988.

412. Stahl RL, Henderson JM, Hooks MA, et al: Therapy of the Kasabach-Merritt syndrome with cryoprecipitate plus intra-arterial thrombin and aminocaproic acid. *Am J Hematol* 36:272, 1991.

413. Roos YB, Vermeulen M, Rinkel GJ, et al: Systematic review of antifibrinolytic treatment in aneurysmal subarachnoid haemorrhage. *J Neurol Neurosurg Psychiatry* 65:942, 1998.

414. Ploplis VA, Carmeliet P, Vazirzadeh S, et al: Effects of disruption of the plasminogen gene on thrombosis, growth, and health in mice. *Circulation* 92:2585, 1995.

415. Carmeliet P, Stassen JM, Schoonjans L, et al: Plasminogen activator inhibitor-1 gene-deficient mice: II. Effects on hemostasis, thrombosis, and thrombolysis. *J Clin Invest* 92:2756, 1993.

416. Dewerchin M, Van Nuffelen A, Wallays G, et al: Generation and characterization of urokinase receptor-deficient mice. *J Clin Invest* 97:870, 1996.

417. Lawn RM, Wade DP, Hammer RE, et al: Atherogenesis in transgenic mice expressing human apolipoprotein(a). *Nature* 360:670, 1992.

418. Grainger DJ, Kemp PR, Liu AC, et al: Activation of transforming growth factor-beta is inhibited in transgenic apolipoprotein(a) mice. *Nature* 370:460, 1994.

419. Palabrica TM, Liu AC, Aronovitz MJ, et al: Antifibrinolytic activity of apolipoprotein(a) *in vivo*: Human apolipoprotein(a) transgenic mice are resistant to tissue plasminogen activator-mediated thrombolysis. *Nat Med* 1:256, 1995.

420. Boonmark NW, Lou XJ, Schwartz K, et al: Modification of apolipoprotein(a) lysine binding site reduces atherosclerosis in transgenic mice. *J Clin Invest* 100:558, 1997.

421. Heckel JL, Sandgren EP, Degen JL, et al: Neonatal bleeding in transgenic mice expressing urokinase-type plasminogen activator. *Cell* 62:447, 1990.

422. Meiri N, Masos T, Rosenblum K, et al: Overexpression of urokinase-type plasminogen activator in transgenic mice is correlated with impaired learning. *Proc Natl Acad Sci U S A* 91:3196, 1994.

TRANSFUSION MEDICINE

ERYTHROCYTE ANTIGENS AND ANTIBODIES

MARION E. REID

LONI CALHOUN

LAWRENCE D. PETZ

Human red blood cells (RBCs) bear numerous cell surface structures that can be recognized as antigens by the immune system of individuals who lack that particular structure. Characterization of RBC antigens and antibodies has been the basis of pretransfusion compatibility testing, thereby minimizing the risk of hemolytic transfusion reactions. Such characterization has provided insights into understanding the etiology of hemolytic disease of the newborn. Biochemical and molecular studies have led to definition of the biologic functions of molecules expressing blood group antigens. These molecules play a critical role in susceptibility to infection by malarial parasites, some viruses, and bacteria. Diverse inherited and acquired diseases are associated with alteration of RBC antigen expression, and these alterations often play a role in the clinical manifestations of these diseases. Although erythrocytes traditionally have been considered relatively inert containers of hemoglobin, in fact they are active in a variety of physiologic processes.

DEFINITIONS AND HISTORY

A *blood group system* is a group of antigens encoded by alleles at a single gene locus or at gene loci so closely linked that crossing over does not occur or is very rare. An *antigen collection* is a group of antigens that are phenotypically, biochemically, or genetically related, but the genes encoding them have not been identified.[1]

Placement of a blood group antigen into a system or collection follows a natural progression. First, an antibody is discovered, usually in the serum of a multiparous woman or a multiply transfused recipient, and is found to have a unique pattern of reactivity. Using traditional serologic methods, the antibody can be used to study basic biochemical properties of the corresponding antigen, to enable recognition of the pattern of inheritance of the antigen in families and in populations, to identify red blood cells (RBCs) that lack the antigen, and to search for an antithetical antigen. A newly recognized antigen can be evaluated using biochemical and molecular genetic methods. Identified characteristics, such as prevalence of positive reactions or sensitivity or resistance to specific enzymes, are compared to known systems and collections.

The majority of genes encoding blood group antigens have been cloned and sequenced,[2] and the molecular basis of most blood group

antigens has been determined.[3–6] Details on the alleles associated with blood group antigens and phenotypes can be obtained from the following web site: *http://www.aecom.yu.edu*.

RBC blood group antigens are inherited carbohydrate or protein structures located on the outside surface of the RBC membrane. Most of the protein blood group antigens are carried on integral transmembrane proteins; however, a few are carried on glycosyl phosphatidylinositol (GPI)-linked proteins. Some antigens are carbohydrates attached to proteins or lipids, some require a combination of a specific portion of protein and carbohydrates, and a few antigens are carried on proteins that are adsorbed from the plasma. Some transmembrane proteins interact with other transmembrane proteins (e.g., band 3 and glycophorin A [GPA]; Kell and Kx; Rh and RhAG), with lipids (e.g., Rh), or with proteins in the membrane skeleton (e.g., band 3 and ankyrin, glycophorin C [GPC] and protein 4.1 and p55). Many of the proteins carrying blood group antigens reside in the erythrocyte membrane as complexes.[7–10] Many components carrying blood group antigens have been assigned cluster of differentiation (CD) numbers (Table 128-1; see Chap. 14). In human blood grouping, agglutination of RBCs usually serves as the detectable endpoint.[11] Our ability to detect and identify blood group antigens and antibodies has contributed significantly to current safe blood transfusion practice, reducing the deaths from hemolytic disease of the newborn (HDN) from 40 to 2 percent and supporting patients receiving chemotherapy or organ transplantation.

The naming of blood group antigens usually does not follow the classic convention wherein dominant traits are given capital letters and recessive traits are designated with lowercase letters. For example, in the ABO blood group system the recessive O phenotype is encoded by a gene designated *O*, whereas in the MNS system the genes *S* and *s* are codominant. To standardize terminology used to describe RBC blood groups, the International Society of Blood Transfusion (ISBT) Committee for Terminology for Red Cell Surface Antigens recommends using the traditional name for an antigen for verbal communication and a numerical system in computer databases. The committee has placed blood group antigens into four categories: (1) genetically discrete blood group systems; (2) serologically, biochemically, or genetically related antigens in blood group collections; (3) series of low-incidence antigens; and (4) series of high-incidence antigens. Each system and collection has been given a number and letter designation, and each antigen within the system is numbered sequentially in order of discovery. To date, 29 blood group systems and five antigen collections are defined (see Table 128-1).[1,5,6,12–14] Over time, notations devised to describe blood group antigens have changed. A single letter (e.g., A, D, K), a symbol with a superscript (e.g., Fy^a, Jk^b, Lu^a), a symbol with a number (e.g., Fy3, Lu4, K12), and three to four letters (e.g., VEL, LAN, FPPT) are all used, sometimes within the same blood group system.

BLOOD GROUP SYSTEMS

Tables 128-1 and 128-2 summarize the characteristics of common blood group antigens. The following sources provide more detail: Issitt and Anstee,[5] Reid and Lomas-Francis,[6] Mollison and colleagues,[15] Daniels,[4] Cartron and Rouger,[16] and Brecher and colleagues.[11] In the interest of space, reviews or books are referenced in place of original reports.

ABO BLOOD GROUP SYSTEM

The ABO blood group system was the first system described and remains the most significant used for transfusion medicine. A mismatch of ABO may be fatal, whereas a mismatch of other blood groups initially is harmless. This situation occurs because anti-A and anti-B usu-

TABLE 128-1 INTERNATIONAL SOCIETY OF BLOOD TRANSFUSION-DEFINED BLOOD GROUP SYSTEMS AND ANTIGEN COLLECTIONS WITH CHROMOSOME AND GENE

CONVENTIONAL NAME	ISBT SYMBOL (NO.)	CHROMO-SOME LOCATION	ISBT GENE NAME (ISGN IF DIFFERENT)	ASSOCIATED ANTIGENS [NULL PHENOTYPE]	FUNCTION OF RBC MEMBRANE COMPONENT (CD NO.)	DISEASE ASSOCIATION
Blood Group Systems						
ABO	ABO (001)	9q34.2	*ABO*	A, B, A,B, A1 [group O]	Glycocalyx (CD235)	Altered expression in some hematologic disorders
MNS	MNS (002)	4q31.21	*MNS (GYPA, GYPB)*	M, N, S, s, U, He, Mi^a, Vw, M^c, Mur, M^g, Vr, M^e, Mt^a, St^a, Ri^a, Cl^a, and 26 more [En(a–); U–; M^{k}M^k]	Binds microbe glycocalyx, complement regulation, chaperone for band 3	Decreased *P. falciparum* invasion, may be receptor for *E. coli*
P	P1 (003)	22q11.2-qter	*P1*	P1	Glycocalyx	
Rh	RH (004)	1p36.11	*RHD, RHCE (RH)*	D, C, E, c, e, f, C^w, C^x, V, G, hr^S, VS, D^w, Rh29, Go^a, hr^B, Rh32, Rh33, and 30 more [Rh$_{null}$]	Possibly transports CO$_2$ (CD240)	Hemolytic anemia, hereditary stomatocytosis, hematologic malignancies
Lutheran	LU (005)	19q13.2	*LU*	Lu^a, Lu^b, Lu3, Lu4, Lu5, Lu6, Lu7, Lu8, Lu9, Lu11, Lu12, Lu13, and 7 more [Recessive Lu(a–b–)]	Binds laminin (CD239)	Increased expressions possibly involved in vasoocclusion in sickle cell disease
Kell	KEL (006)	7q34	*KEL*	K, k, Kp^a, Kp^b, Ku, Js^a, Js^b, and 17 more [K$_0$ or K$_{null}$]	Cleaves big endothelin-3 to ET-3, a potent vasoconstrictor (CD238)	
Lewis	LE (007)	19p13.3	*LE (FUT3)*	Le^a, Le^b, Le^{ab}, Le^{bh}, ALe^b, BLe^b [Le(a–b–)]	Glycocalyx, Le^b is receptor for *H. pylori*	Increased expression in fucosidosis, Lewis antibodies may be important in graft rejection
Duffy	FY (008)	1q23.2	*FY (DARC)*	Fy^a, Fy^b, Fy3, Fy4, Fy5, Fy6 [Fy(a–b–)]	Chemokine, *Plasmodium vivax* receptor (CD234)	Resistance to *P. vivax* invasion
Kidd	JK (009)	18q12.3	*JK (HUT11, SE4AI)*	Jk^a, Jk^b, Jk3 [Jk(a–b–)]	Urea transporter	Impaired urea transport, urine concentrating defect
Diego	DI (010)	17q21.31	*DI (SLC4A1; AE1)*	Di^a, Di^b, Wr^a, Wr^b, Wd^a, Rb^a, and 14 more	Anion exchanger (CD233)	Southeast Asian ovalocytosis, hereditary spherocytosis, renal tubular acidosis
Yt	YT (011)	7q22	*Yt (ACHE)*	Yt^a, Yt^b	Acetylcholinesterase	Absent from PNH III RBCs
Xg	XG (012)	Xp22.33	*XG (XG, MIC2)*	Xg^a, CD99	Adhesion molecules (CD99)	
Scianna	SC (013)	1p34.2	*SC (ERMAP)*	Sc1, Sc2, Sc3, Rd [Sc:–1,–2,–3]	Possible adhesion	
Dombrock	DO (014)	12p12.3	*DO (ART4)*	Do^a, Do^b, Gy^a, Hy, Jo^a [Gy(a–)]	Enzymatic	Absent from PNH III RBCs
Colton	CO (015)	7p14	*CO (AQP1)*	Co^a, Co^b, Co3 [Co(a–b–)]	Water transport	Monosomy 7, inability to maximally concentrate urine, congenital dyserythropoietic anemia
Landsteiner-Wiener	LW (016)	19p13.2	*LW (ICAM)*	LW^a, LW^{ab}, LW^b [LW(a–b–)]	Binds CD11/CD18, ligand for integrins (CD242)	Depressed in pregnancy and some malignant diseases
Chido/Rogers	CH/RG (017)	6p21.32	*C4A,C4B*	CH1, CH2, Rg1, and 6 more	Complement components	Certain phenotypes have increased susceptibility to certain autoimmune conditions and infections
H	Hh (018)	19q13.33	*H (FUT1)*	H [Bombay, Oh]	Glycocalyx (CD173)	Decreased in some tumor cells, increased in hematopoietic stress
Kx	XK (019)	Xp21.1	*XK*	Kx [McLeod]	Possible neurotransmitter, function in RBCs not known	Acanthocytosis, muscular dystrophy, hemolytic anemia; McLeod syndrome sometimes associated with CGD
Gerbich	GE (020)	2q14.3	*GE (GYPC)*	Ge2, Ge3, Ge4, Wb, Ls^a, An^a, Dh^a [Leach phenotype]	Membrane attachment; interacts with 4.1R and p55 (CD236)	Hereditary elliptocytosis, hemolytic anemia, decreased 4.1R and p55
Cromer	CROMER (021)	1q32.2	*CROM (DAF)*	Cr^a, Tc^a, Tc^b, Tc^c, Dr^a, Es^a, IFC, WES^a, WES^b, UMC, GUTI, SERF [Inab phenotype]	Complement regulation, binds C3b, disassembles C3/C5 convertase (CD55)	Absent from PNH III RBCs, Dr^a is the receptor for uropathogenic *E. coli*

TABLE 128-1 INTERNATIONAL SOCIETY OF BLOOD TRANSFUSION-DEFINED BLOOD GROUP SYSTEMS AND ANTIGEN COLLECTIONS WITH CHROMOSOME AND GENE (*CONTINUED*)

CONVENTIONAL NAME	ISBT SYMBOL (NO.)	CHROMO-SOME LOCATION	ISBT GENE NAME (ISGN IF DIFFERENT)	ASSOCIATED ANTIGENS [NULL PHENOTYPE]	FUNCTION OF RBC MEMBRANE COMPONENT (CD NO.)	DISEASE ASSOCIATION
Knops	KN (022)	1q32.2	*KN (CR1)*	Kn^a, Kn^b, McC^a, Sl^a, Yk^a, McC^b, Vil, Sl3	Complement regulation, binds C3b and C4b, mediates phagocytosis (CD35)	Antigens depressed in certain autoimmune and malignant conditions
Indian	IN (023)	11p13	*IN (CD44)*	In^a, In^b	Binds hyaluronic acid, mediates adhesion of leukocytes (CD44)	Depressed in pregnancy, congenital dyserythropoietic anemia
	Ok (024)	19p13.3	*OK (BSB)*	Ok^a	Possible adhesion (CD147)	
	Raph (025)	11p15.5	*MER2 (CD151)*	MER2 [Raph−]	Adhesion molecule involved in kidney function (CD151)	Renal disease
	JMH (026)	15q24.1	*JMH (SEMA-L)*	JMH	Adhesion molecule, function in RBCs not known (CD108)	Absent from PNH III RBCs
	I (027)	6p24.2	*IGNT*	I [I−; i adult]	Glycocalyx	Congenital cataracts in Asians
	Globoside (028)	3q26.1	*P (β3GALT3, βGalNAcT1)*	P [P−]	Glycocalyx	Receptor *E. coli* and Parvovirus B19
	GIL (029)	9p13.3	*GIL (AQP3)*	GIL [GIL−]	Glycerol/water/urea transporter	
Antigen Collections						
Cost	COST (205)	—	—	Cs^a, Cs^b		
Ii	I (207)	—	—	i		
Er	ER (208)	—	—	Er^a, Er^b		
(P, P^k, LKE)	GLOB (209)	—	—	P^k, LKE		
(Lewis-like: Le^c, Le^d)	Unnamed: (210)	—	—	Le^c, Le^d		
Low incidence series	— (700)	—	—	19		
High incidence series	— (901)	—	—	11		

SOURCE: GL Daniels et al.,[13] PD Issitt and DJ Anstee,[5] and ME Reid and C Lomas-Francis.[6]
ISGN = International Society for Gene Nomenclature.

ally are present in the blood of adults lacking the corresponding antigen. These antibodies are stimulated by the ubiquitous distribution of the antigen that forms part of the membrane structure of many bacteria, plants, and animals. For this reason, all donor blood for transfusion is tested and labeled with the ABO group. The four main phenotypes are A, B, AB, and O, the latter indicating a lack of both A and B antigens. The sugars defining A and B antigens are added to carbohydrate chains carrying the H antigen (fucose), which is "hidden" by the A or B sugar. Thus group A or B erythrocytes appear to have less H antigen than group O cells. Nonetheless, H is found on all human erythrocytes except those in rare individuals of the O$_h$ (Bombay) phenotype.

Anti-A or anti-B can cause intravascular hemolysis when ABO-incompatible RBCs are transfused. Because A and B antigens also are expressed on most tissue cells, ABO compatibility is a significant consideration in solid organ transplantation. However, ABO incompatibility only rarely causes clinical HDN because antibodies directed against A and B antigens are predominantly immunoglobulin (Ig)M, which do not cross the placenta, and because A and B antigens are not fully developed on RBCs from a fetus.

Although the ABO blood group system has only four phenotypes, more than 90 alleles have been identified by DNA analyses. The *ABO* gene was cloned in 1990 following purification of A transferase.[17,18] A and B transferase have only four amino acid differences in the catalytic domain, two of which (Leu266Met and Gly268Ala) are primarily responsible for substrate specificity.[19] The group O phenotype results from mutations in A or B alleles that cause loss of glycosyltransferase activity. The most common group O (O$_1$) results from a single nucleotide deletion near the 5′ end of the gene that causes a frameshift and early termination with no active enzyme production.[20] The *ABO* gene has seven exons, and A or B subgroups (with only few exceptions) result from a variety of mutations in exon 7 that cause alterations in the catalytic domain of the glycosyltransferase (reviewed by Chester and Olsson[21]). The rare B(A), A(B), and *cis*-AB phenotypes expressing both A and B antigens result from variant glycosyltransferases that have a combination of A- and B-specific residues.[22,23] Numerous common and rare *ABO* alleles have been reported, and current information is available on the blood group antigen gene mutation database web site (*http://www.aecom.yu.edu*). In addition to single point mutations, recombinations and gene rearrangements can result in hybrids with unexpected activity of the transferase. This situation makes typing of ABO by DNA analysis difficult to interpret.[24] The function of the ABO system is not known, although several disease associations are well established.

TABLE 128-2 SUMMARY OF COMMON BLOOD GROUP SYSTEMS OR COLLECTIONS AND THEIR ANTIGENS

Blood Group (Year Recognized)	Common Phenotypes	Frequency White/Black (%)	No. Antigen Copies on Adult RBC × 10³	Dosage (See Text)	Cord Cell Expression	Biochemistry	Antigen Distribution in Blood, Fluids, and Tissues	Comments
ABO (1901)	A B AB O	40/27 11/10 4/4 45/29	AB: ~800–1000	A/B: not evident	Weak: ~1/3 adult expression	Carbohydrate on type 1, 2, 3 and 4 precursor chains	RBC, lymphs, plts	Most significant antigens in transfusion and transplantation
H (1948)	AB	4/4	H: ~1700	H expression depends on ABO: $O>A_2>$ $B>A_2B>A_1>$ A_1B	Main RBC carrier: bands 3 and 4.5	Attached to lipids in plasma and protein in secretions	Plasma, secretions; broad tissue distribution; most epithelial/endothelial cells	Weak subgroups result from variant transferases
Rh (1940)	Haplotype R_1 Dce r ce R_2 DcE R_0 Dce r' Ce r'' cE R_z DCE r'' CE	42/17 37/26 14/11 4/44 2/2 1/0 <1 <1	D on R_1R_2: 15–33 R_1R_1: 14–19 R_0r: 12–20 R_1r: 9–14 c on cc: 70–85 Cc: 37–53 e on ee: 18–24 Ee: 13–14	D: not evident C and c: yes E and e: yes	Normal adult	Multipass, nonglycosylated protein: 30–32 kDa; 417 aa C: serine 103/c: proline 103 E: proline 226/e: alanine 226 Forms "Rh complex" with LW, GPB, and Rh-related glycoprotein (chromosome 6)	Possible cation transport Possible role in RBC membrane integrity	D most significant antigen after A and B Three causes for weak D expression (see text) Nulls: amorphic type and regulator type
Lewis (1946)	Le(a+b−) Le(a+b+) Le(a−b−) Le(a+b+)	22/23 72/55 6/22 Rare	Le^a: ~3	Not evident	Weak: adult expression at age 2 years	Carbohydrate on type 1 precursor chains only Attached to lipids in plasma and protein in secretions	Plasma and secretion antigen; on RBC, lymphs, plts only by adsorption of plasma antigen	Le antigens depend on Le/Se interaction; Le/Se = Le(a−b+), ABH secretor; Le/sese = Le(a+b−), ABH nonsecretor; lele = Le(a−b−), Sese status not apparent Le(a−b+) express some Le^a, do not make anti-Le^a Women test Le(a−b−) during pregnancy
Ii (1956)	I adult (↑I↓i) I_{int} (↑I↑i) i cord (↓I↑i) i adult (↓I↑i)	Common Rare Common <1:10,000	I: ~500	Not evident	Strong i; weak I. Adult expressions at age 2 years	Carbohydrate on ABH active chains; lipid on RBC, protein in plasma	Broad tissue distribution; RBCs, plts, lymphs, granulos, monos; also in plasma, secretions (e.g., milk, saliva, urine)	I and i expression are inversely proportional but not products of alleles
P1 (1927) GLOB (1951)	P_1; P+P+P+ P_2; P+P+P+ p; P^k−P−P_1− P_1^k; P^k+P−P_1+ P_2^k; P^k+P−P_1−	79/94 21/6 Rare Rare Rarest	P_1: ~500 Globoside: ~15,000	Not evident, but inherited variations exist; e.g., P_1 may be normal, strong, or weak	Weak: adult expression by 7 years	Carbohydrate on RBC and plasma glycolipids; not in secretions	RBC, lymphs, plts, monos, fibroblasts, uroepithelial cells	P_1-like antigen is associated with pigeon and earthworm protein and parasitic infections
MNS (M: 1927) (S: 1947)	M+N− M+N+ M−N+ S+s− S+s+ S−s+ S−s−U−	28/26 50/44 22/30 11/3 44/28 45/69 0/<1	GPA: ~800 GPB: ~200	Yes	Normal adult	Single-pass sialoglycoprotein type 1 GPA: 43 kDa, 131 aa, carries MN GPB: 25 kDa, 72 aa, carries SsU; part of Rh complex	RBCs plus renal capillary epithelial/endothelium	GPA and GPB carry multiple antigens and many genetic variants exist: variant forms of MNSs, hybrids of GPA-GPB from crossover Can have absence of GPA, GPB, or both
Kell (1946) (Kp^a/Js^a: 1957)	K−k+ K+k+ K+k− Kp(a−b+) Kp(a+b+) Kp(a+b−) Js(a−b+) Js(a+b+) Js(a+b−)	91/98 8.8/2 0.2/rare 97.7/100 2.3/rare Rare/O 100/80 Rare/19 0/1	Kell: 2–6	Yes	Normal adult	Single-pass glycoprotein type II highly folded with S=S bonds: 93 kDa, 732 aa K/k: Met 193 Thr Kp^a/Kp^b: Trp 281Arg Js^a/Js^b: Pro 597Leu	Kell: RBC plus bone marrow and fetal liver tissue; not on brain, kidney, adult liver Kx: RBC plus skeletal/heart muscle, neurologic tissues	System of high- and low-frequency antigens Common phenotype: k, Kp^b, Js^b Kell antigen expression depends on both Kell and Xk genes K_{null} lacks Kell antigens, has Kx Kx_{null} has poor Kell antigen expression (McLeod phenotype) Other causes of poor Kell expression: cis Kp^a, Ge−, K_{mod}, autoantibody
Duffy (1950)	Fy(a+b−)Fy3+ Fy(a+b+)Fy3+ Fy(a−b+)Fy3+ Fy(a−b−)Fy3−	17/9 49/1 34/22 Rare/68	Fy^a: 6–13	Yes, but not always evident because of Fy gene (see text)	Normal: adult levels at 12 weeks	Multipass glycoprotein: 35–45 kDa, 338 aa Fy^a/Fy^b Gly 42Asp	RBC plus brain, colon, lung, spleen, thyroid, thymus, kidney, endothelium; not in liver or placenta tissue	Fy(a−b−) blacks do not express Fy^b on their RBC, but routinely express it on other tissues and seldom make anti-Fy^b
Kidd (1951)	Jk(a+b−)Jk3+ Jk(a+b+)Jk3+ Jk(a−b+)Jk3+ Jk(a−b−)Jk3−	28/57 49/34 23/9 <1%	Jk^a: ~14	Yes	Normal adult	Multipass protein: ~43 kDa, 391 aa 1 potential N-glycan Jk^a/Jk^b: Asp284 Asn	RBC specific	Important cause of DHTR Nulls are unable to fully concentrate urine; dominant inhibitor In(Jk) has weak Jk antigen
Lutheran (1951)	Lu(a+b−)Lu3+ Lu(a+b+)Lu3+ Lu(a−b+)Lu3+ Lu(a−b−)Lu3−	0.15/− 7.5/0 92.3/− Very rare — Polynesians	Lu^b: 1.5–4	Yes, but family variations exist	Weak: adult levels at 15 years	Single-pass glycoprotein type I: 85 kDa, 597 aa 78 kD B-CAM 5 Ig superfamily domains: two variable, three constant Lu^a/Lu^b: His77Arg	RBC plus brain, heart, kidney, lung, pancreas, placenta, skeletal muscle	System of high- and low-frequency antigens Dominant inhibitor In(Lu) and X-linked inhibitor (XS2) have weak Lu antigens First known autosomal linkage to Se

aa = amino acids; DHTR = delayed hemolytic transfusion reactions; GPA = glycophorin A; GPB = glycophorin B; granulos = granulocytes; Ig = immunoglobulin; ISBT = International Society of Blood Transfusion; lymphs = lymphocytes; monos = monocytes; plts = platelets; RBC = red blood cell; B-CAM = B cell adhesion molecule.

RH BLOOD GROUP SYSTEM

The Rh (not Rhesus) system is the second most important blood group system in transfusion medicine because antigen-positive RBCs frequently immunize antigen-negative individuals through transfusion and pregnancy.

Inheritance of Rh antigens is determined by a complex of two closely linked genes: one encodes the protein carrying D antigen (RhD); the other encodes the protein carrying C or c and E or e antigens (RhCE). RBCs from Rh-positive people have both RhD and RhCE, whereas Rh-negative RBCs have only RHCE. In the Rh system, eight common antigen combinations or haplotypes are possible: Dce (R_0, Rh_0), DCe (R_1, Rh_1), DcE (R_2, Rh_2), DCE (R_z, Rh_z), ce (r, rh), Ce (r′, hr′), cE (r″, hr″), and CE (ry, rh″). The letter "d" is commonly used to designate the lack of D, but there is no d antigen or anti-d.

Several nomenclatures can be used to describe Rh genes and antigens. The Fisher-Race nomenclature, which uses CDE terminology, is more commonly used for antigens; the Wiener nomenclature, which uses Rh designations, is favored for haplotypes and gene complexes; and the Rosenfield and Rubinstein nomenclature, which uses numerical designations, was introduced to allow analyses without bias.[25]

The Rh blood group system has 48 antigens (ABO has four). By far the most important and immunogenic antigen is D (Rh_0 in Weiner terminology, referring to Weiner's discovery that a Rhesus monkey injected with human RBCs would produce antibody that agglutinated 85% of white New Yorkers). For most clinical purposes, testing individuals for the D antigen and classifying them as D+ (or Rh-positive), or D− or (Rh-negative) is sufficient. Approximately 85 percent of the Caucasian population is Rh-positive, and 15 percent is Rh-negative. Most Rh-negative recipients produce anti-D if they receive Rh-positive blood. Anti-D can cause hemolysis in adults following an Rh-mismatched transfusion and in the newborn (HDN) if antibodies were raised in the mother from a prior transfusion or pregnancy. The risk of anti-D sensitization by transfusion is eliminated by matching. The risk of anti-D sensitization in pregnancy is minimized by passive immunization of mothers at risk against D. Thus donors and recipients are routinely typed and matched for D.

The antigens C, c, E, and e are less immunogenic and become important in patient care only after the corresponding antibody develops or when the basic Rh haplotype must be determined. The remaining 40+ antigens are other Rh protein epitopes whose corresponding antibodies are seldom encountered. Some are encoded by variant Rh alleles and appear as antithetical antigens to C, c, E, or e or as related "extra" antigens. Others are referred to as *compound* antigens or *cis* gene products. For example, the protein produced by the gene *ce* encodes c, e, and f (or ce) antigen. Other compound specificities include Ce (rh^i), cE, CE, V (ce^s), and Ce^s. Still other Rh antigens are related to the complex "mosaic" nature of D and e antigens. If immunized, individuals who lack a part of D or e and make antibody to the portion they lack can present with a challenging serologic picture. For example, the D+ person who lacks part of the D epitope and makes an antibody to the missing portion appears to make alloanti-D because normal D+ RBCs carry all D epitopes.[26]

Some, but not all, individuals who lack part of the D antigen (partial D) have weak expression of D on their red cells that is detected only by antiglobulin test. Having a *C* gene in transposition to a *D* gene (e.g., *Dce/Ce* or *DCe/Ce* genotypes) also can weaken expression of D in some individuals. A third type of weak D expression results from inheriting a *D* gene that encodes all epitopes of D, but in less than normal quantity.

DNA analyses have revealed the molecular basis underlying antigens and phenotypes in the Rh blood group system. A list of the alleles that have been described to date is available at *http://www.aecom.yu.edu*. Rh blood group orthologs are present in nonhuman primates and other species on the evolutionary tree.[27] Rh functions as a CO_2 or perhaps an ammonium transporter.

OTHER BLOOD GROUP SYSTEMS

In terms of transfusion and HDN, the other blood group systems and their antigens become important only when antibody develops. Transfusion service laboratories identify (antibody identification) the specificity and characterize the reactivity of antibodies detected in routine testing (antibody screening). Once this information is known, the blood bank assesses the clinical significance of the antibody and selects the most appropriate blood for transfusion. Tables 128-1 and 128-2 summarize the number of antigens in each blood group system and other relevant information. A detailed description of all the blood group antigens is beyond the scope of this chapter. Because the molecular bases of most blood group antigens and phenotypes are known,[6] DNA analysis can be used to type transfused patients and to identify the fetus at risk for HDN.[28]

GENERAL IMMUNOLOGY OF BLOOD GROUP ANTIGENS

An *antigen* is a substance that can evoke an immune response when introduced into an immunocompetent host and react with the antibody produced from that immune response. Its structure and stereochemical fit with its antibody determine its specificity. An antigen can have several *epitopes*, or *antigenic determinants*, each of which is capable of eliciting an antibody response.

The ability of an antigen to stimulate an immune response is called *immunogenicity*, and its ability to react with an antibody is called *antigenicity*. These primary characteristics are affected by antigen size, shape, rigidity, and the number and location of the determinants on the red cell membrane.

IMMUNOGENICITY

Immunogenicity depends on many antigen characteristics, not just the number of antigen sites. For example, a K+Fy(a+) RBC carries 7 to 17×10^3 Fy^a antigen sites but only 3 to 6×10^3 K antigen sites. Yet such cells are nine times more likely to stimulate the formation of anti-K than of anti-Fy^a.[15,29]

Relative immunogenicity is estimated by comparing the actual incidence with which an antibody is found to the calculated likelihood of a possible immunizing event. Although numbers vary, researchers agree that after A and B, the D antigen is most immunogenic (>80% of Rh-negative individuals produce anti-D after receiving a single Rh-positive unit), followed by K, which stimulates anti-K in 10 percent of cases.[15] The antigens c and E are 1/3 as immunogenic; K, Fy^a is 1/25 as potent; and Jk^a is 1/50 to 1/100 times as potent.[29]

ANTIGEN EXPRESSION

NUMBER OF ANTIGEN SITES

The number of antigen sites per RBC has been estimated by measuring the uptake of ^{125}I-labeled antibody or of ferritin-conjugated anti-IgG. Numbers vary widely among blood group systems (see Table 128-2).

ANTIGEN DEVELOPMENT ON FETAL ERYTHROCYTES

Most RBC antigens can be detected early in fetal development (A, B, and H antigens can be detected at 5–6 weeks' gestation), but not all are fully developed at birth. A, B, H, I, P1, Lu^a, Lu^b, Yt^a, Xg^a, Vel, Bg, Knops, and Dombrock antigen expression is considerably weaker

TABLE 128-3　BIOCHEMISTRY OF COMMON CARBOHYDRATE AND ANTIGENS ON GLYCOPHORIN A

SPECIFICITY	STRUCTURE	GENE FOR BOLDED DETERMINANT
i	—Gal(β1→4)GlcNAc(β1→3)Gal(β1→4)GLcNAc(β1→3)Gal—R—	
I	—Gal(β1→4)GlcNAc(β1→6) 　　　　　　　　　　　　　　　　 ⟩Gal(β1→4)GlcNAc(β1→3)Gal—R —Gal(β1→4)GlcNAc(β1→3)	IGNT
H	Gal(β1→4 or β1→3)GlcNAc(β1→3)Gal–R 　　　　　│ 　　Fuc(α1→2)	H (FUT1)
A	GalNAc(α1→3)Gal(β1→4 or β1→3)GlcNAc(β1→3)Gal–R 　　　　　　　　│ 　　　　Fuc(α1→2)	A
B	Gal(α1→3)Gal(β1→4 or β1→3)GlcNAc(β1→3)Gal–R 　　　　│ 　　Fuc(α1→2)	B
Le^a	Gal(β1→3)GlcNAc(β1→3)Gal–R 　　　　│ 　Fuc(α1→4)	LE (FUT3)
Le^b	Gal(β1→3)GlcNAc(β1→3)Gal–R 　　│　　│ Fuc(α1→2)Fuc(α1→4)	SE (FUT2)
P	Gal(α1→4)Gal(β1→4)Glc–Cer	Pk*
P	GalNAc(β1→3)Gal(α1→4)Gal(β1→4)Glc–Cer	β3GALT3
P$_1$	Gal(α1→4)Gal(β1→4)GlcNAc(β1→3)Gal(α1→4)Gal(β1→4)Glc–Cer	P1
M	▽　　▽　　▽ Ser—Ser—Thr—Thr—Gly—(GPA chain: 131 amino acids)	GYPA(M)
N	▽　　▽　　▽ Leu—Ser—Thr—Thr—GluA—(GPA chain: 131 amino acids)	GYPA(N)
S	▽　　▽　　▽ Leu—Ser—Thr—Thr—GluA—Met29—(GPB chain: 72 amino acids)	GPYB(S)
S	▽　　▽　　▽ Leu—Ser—Thr—Thr—GluA—Thr29—(GPB chain: 72 amino acids)	GPYB(s)

* Proposed gene.
Immunodominant sugars and amino acids are indicated in bold.
GPA = glycophorin A; GPB = glycophorin B; R = primary glycolipid attachment Glc-Ger, primary glycoprotein attachment GlcNAc-Asp;　　　—Gal—GalNAc—NeuNAc.
　　　　　　　　　　　　　　▽ =
　　　　　　　　　　　　　　　│
　　　　　　　　　　　　　NeuNac

on cord erythrocytes than on RBCs from adults. Le^a, sometimes Le^b, Ch/Rg, AnWj, and Sd^a, are not readily detectable, although 50 percent of cord samples type Le(a+) with more sensitive test methods. Full expression of A, B, H, I, and Lewis antigens usually is present by age 3 years, whereas full expression of P1 and Lutheran antigens may not occur until age 7 years.

VARIATION IN ANTIGEN EXPRESSION

RBCs from individuals who are homozygous for an allele typically have a greater number of antigen sites than do individuals who are heterozygous. Consequently, their RBCs can react more strongly with antibody. This difference in expression and antigen–antibody reactivity because of zygosity is known as *dosage*. For example, RBCs from a homozygous *MM* individual carry a double dose of M antigen and

react more strongly with anti-M than do RBCs from a *MN* heterozygous individual carrying only a single dose of M. Antithetical antigens C/c, E/e, M/N, S/s, and Jk^a/Jk^b commonly show dosage. Dosage is less obvious with D, K/k, and Lu^a/Lu^b antigens. It typically is more apparent within a family than between families. Dosage within the Duffy system also may not be serologically obvious because Fy(a+b−) or Fy(a−b+) phenotypes are seen in either homozygous (*Fy^{a}Fy^a* or *Fy^{b}Fy^b*) or heterozygous (*Fy^{a}Fy* or *Fy^{b}Fy*) individuals (see Table 128-2).

Some blood group antigens are inherited as closely linked genes or haplotypes. Haplotype pairings and gene interaction (either *cis* or *trans*) also can affect phenotypic expression. For example, the pairing of *C* in *trans* position to *D* can result in weak expression of D (see "Rh Blood Group System" above), whereas *E* in *cis* position with *D* is associated with strong expression of D. Among the common phenotypes, R$_2$R$_2$ RBCs carry the strongest expression of D. In the Kell system, *Kp^a* is associated with weakened expression of *cis* k and Js^b.

Still other antigens are affected by regulator genes.[30] *In(Lu)* is a dominant inhibitor gene that suppresses expression of Lutheran, P1, i, and many other antigens.[31] The dominant inhibitor *In(Jk)* suppresses expression of Jk^a and Jk^b antigens.[32] Rare variants of the *RHAG* gene depress or prevent expression of the Rh antigens (see "Rh$_{null}$ Syndrome" below).

BIOCHEMISTRY OF ERYTHROCYTE ANTIGENS

An antibody typically recognizes an epitope consisting of four to five amino acids on linear proteins or one to seven sugars. Alternatively, the antibody-binding site may encompass a more complex three-dimensional structure with branches or folds, and recognition may depend on both amino acids and sugars. Tables 128-2 and 128-3 and Figure 128-1 summarize blood group biochemistry and antigen structure.[4,6,15,16,33]

CARBOHYDRATE ANTIGENS

Polysaccharides with blood group activity are made by sequential addition of specific sugars (or sugar derivatives) to specific precursors by specific transferases. Sugars commonly involved are galactose (Gal), N-acetyl-galactosamine (GalNAc), N-acetyl-glucosamine (GlcNAc), fucose (Fuc), and N-acetyl-neuraminic acid (NeuNAc).

ABO, Lewis, and P blood group specificity depends on an immunodominant sugar, usually terminally located, the polysaccharide to which the sugar is attached, and the type of linkage involved. I/i specificity is defined by a series of sugars on the inner portion of ABH saccharide chains. The presence of at least two repeating Gal(β1→4)GlcNAc(β1→3)Gal units in a linear structure defines i activity. I activity involves these same sugars in branched form (see Table 128-3). The *I* gene encodes the transferase responsible for branching [β(1–6)glucosaminyltransferase]. During the first years of a child's life, linear chains are modified into branched chains, resulting in the appearance of I antigens.[34] The i antigen is reduced on RBCs from fetuses and infants. A rare i phenotype occurs in adults [see section on "I phenotype (i Adult)"].

Polysaccharide chains are attached to glycoproteins in secretions (on type 2 chains), to glycolipids (on type 1 chains) in plasma, and to both on the RBC membrane. Approximately 70 percent of A, B, H, and I antigens on the RBC membrane are carried on glycoproteins, primarily on the anion transporter, but also on the glucose transporter, the Rh glycoprotein, and others. Approximately 10 percent of these antigens are on NeuNAc-rich glycoproteins, 5 percent on simple glycolipids, and the remainder on polyglycosyl ceramide.[15] P, P^k, and P1 antigens are found on glycolipids both on the membrane and in plasma.[35]

Lewis antigens are unique because they occur only on type 1 polysaccharide chains, which are precursors found in plasma and secretions but not made by RBC. Hence, they are plasma and secretion antigens and exist on RBCs only by adsorption of Lewis substance from plasma. The *Le* (or *FUT3*) gene encodes an $\alpha(1-4)$fucosyltransferase. Whether the resulting antigen is Le^a or Le^b depends on the secretor gene *Se* (or *FUT2*), which encodes an $\alpha(1-2)$fucosyltransferase.

PROTEIN ANTIGENS

Protein structures that carry blood group antigens can be grouped into three categories: (1) those that make a single pass through the erythrocyte membrane, (2) those that make multiple passes through the membrane, and (3) those that are attached to the membrane through a covalent linkage to lipid (GPI-linked) (see Fig. 128-1).

Single-pass proteins include GPA with M and N antigens, glycophorin B (GPB) with S, s, and U antigens, glycophorins C and D with Gerbich antigens, and the proteins encoded by Kell, Lutheran, LW, Indian, Knops, Xg, Ok, and Scianna genes. Most of these proteins have an extracellular amino-terminus and an intracellular carboxyl-terminus (referred to as *type I*). An exception to this is Kell glycoprotein, in which the terminal positions are reversed: the carboxyl-terminus is extracellular and the amino-terminus is intracellular (*type II*).

Most proteins that make multiple passes through the erythrocyte membrane have both carboxyl- and amino-terminal ends that are intracellular, are hydrophobic, and have a transport function. Rh, Diego, Colton, Kidd, Kx, GIL, and Raph proteins are included in this category. The gene product of the Duffy gene also is a multipass protein, but it has an extracellular amino-terminus and has homology with a family of cytokine receptors.[36]

Lipid-linked proteins have their carboxyl-terminus attached to the lipid GPI and are said to be GPI linked or anchored. Cromer, Yt, Dombrock, and JMH proteins belong to this category. GPI-linked proteins are of special interest to hematologists because defective synthesis of the GPI anchor is responsible for paroxysmal nocturnal hemoglobinuria (PNH).[37,38] Thus PNH-III RBCs lack all proteins attached by a GPI anchor, including those carrying the blood groups mentioned.

EFFECT OF ENZYMES AND OTHER CHEMICALS ON ERYTHROCYTE ANTIGENS

Expression of an RBC antigen is determined by its exposure as a result of its position on the cell surface and its biochemical structure. It can

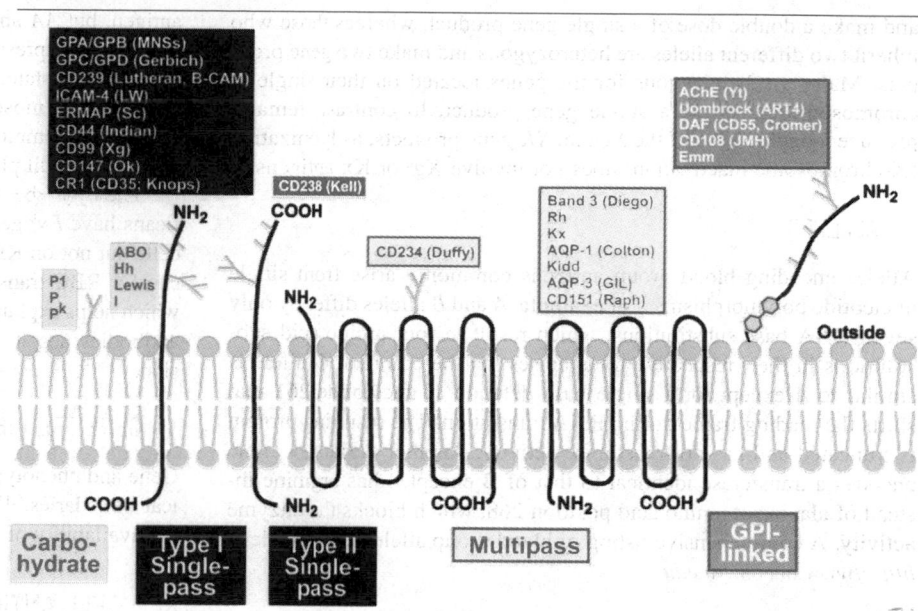

FIGURE 128-1 Erythrocyte membrane structures carrying blood group activity.

be modified with enzymes and other chemicals. These reagents are used in serologic testing to help identify complex mixtures of antibodies and to help characterize antibody specificity when identity is not apparent.

Proteolytic enzymes, such as ficin, papain, bromelin, trypsin, and α-chymotrypsin, cleave proteins from the erythrocyte membrane at specific amino acids. Enzyme treatment of RBCs cleaves certain protein antigens and allows carbohydrate and other protected protein antigens to react more strongly with their antibody. The reactivity of antibodies to A, B, H, I, P1, Lewis, Rh, and Kidd antigens is strongly enhanced after enzyme treatment of the RBCs, whereas reactivity of antibodies to M, N, Fy^a, Fy^b, and many minor antigens (Xg^a, Ch, Rg, JMH, Indian, Pr, Tn, Ge2, Ge4, and some examples of Yt^a) is reduced or eliminated. S and s are variably affected by enzyme treatment, and Kell and Lutheran antigens are relatively unaffected.[5,6]

Reagents that reduce disulfide bonds, such as 2-mercaptoethanol (2-ME), dithiothreitol (DTT), and 2-aminoethylisothiouronium bromide (AET), denature Kell blood group antigens but enhance Kx. Reducing reagents also denature the minor antigens LW, Scianna, Indian, JMH, and Yt^a and weaken Lutheran, Dombrock, Cromer, Knops, AnWj, and MER2 antigens.[5,6]

Acid treatment of RBCs, which is frequently used to remove IgG from RBCs, can weaken or completely denature antigens in the Kell blood group system. Chloroquine treatment of erythrocytes (also sometimes used to remove IgG from RBCs) at room temperature has little effect on most antigens. However, treatment for 30 minutes at 37°C can weaken expression of many antigens, including Fy^b, Lu^b, Yt^a, JMH, and those in the Rh, Dombrock, and Knops systems.

GENETICS OF ERYTHROCYTE ANTIGENS

Protein antigens are direct gene products: the gene encodes a protein that expresses one or more antigenic epitopes. Carbohydrate antigens, made by transferase action, are considered indirect gene products. Most blood group genes are located on autosomes; only two, *Xg* and *XK*, are located on the X chromosome (see Table 128-1 for gene and chromosome location).

Most genes that encode blood group antigens have two or more alleles. Individuals who inherit two identical alleles are homozygous and make a double dose of a single gene product, whereas those who inherit two different alleles are heterozygous and make two gene products. Males are hemizygous for the genes located on their single X chromosome and make a single gene product. In contrast, females produce a double dose of the *Xg* and *XK* gene products, as lyonization (X-chromosome inactivation) does not involve Xg^a or Kx antigens.[39]

ALLELES

Alleles encoding blood group antigens commonly arise from single nucleotide polymorphisms. For example, *A* and *B* alleles differ by only seven DNA base substitutions, which result in four amino acid substitutions in their respective transferases.[4–6] The common *O* allele is similar to *A* except for a single base deletion at nucleotide 261 that shifts the reading frame during RNA translation. The resulting protein is truncated and has no transferase activity. Another variant *O* allele encodes a transferase identical to that of B except it has arginine instead of alanine at amino acid position 268, which blocks the enzyme activity. A comprehensive listing of blood group alleles is available at *http://www.aecom.yu.edu*.

GENE COMPLEXES

Some blood group genes are complexes of several closely linked genes or loci that evolved through duplication of an ancestral gene. The antigens they encode are inherited within families as a "packet" or haplotype with no or few crossovers. Blood group examples include the Rh system with its genes *RHD* and *RHCE*, and the MNS system with its genes *GYPA* and *GYPB*.

Duplication of the RH gene appears to have occurred more than 500 million years ago. *RHD* and *RHCE* show remarkable homology between them and with the *RHAG* gene, which encodes the Rh glycoprotein RhAG. *GPYA* and *GPYB* probably arose by duplication of an ancestral *GPYA* gene encoding the N antigen.[40] The most common MNSs complex is Ns, followed by Ms, MS, and NS.

In both Rh and MNS systems, other antigens arose by further mutations, deletions, and rearrangements within the gene complex. Unequal pairing of *GYPA* and *GYPB* during meiosis, with subsequent recombination, resulted in several hybrids, such as *GYP(A-B)* (called Lepore type, by analogy with a similar hemoglobin hybrid), which encodes a protein with the amino-terminal end of GPA but the carboxyl-terminal end of glycophorin B. Anti–Lepore-type hybrids, *GYP(B-A)* (amino-terminal end of glycophorin B and carboxyl-terminal end of glycophorin A), and other rearrangements [*GYP(B-A-B)* and *GYP(A-B-A)*] are known. Within the Rh complex, hybrids of *RH(D-CE-D)* and *RH(CE-D-CE)* have been identified.[4–6] Such hybrids can result in altered antigen expression and new antigen epitopes.

Kell and Lutheran antigens were thought to arise from large gene complexes of four or more loci, each having two or more alleles: *K/k*, *Kp^a/Kp^b/Kp^c*, *Js^a/Js^b*, and *K^{11}/K^{17}* for Kell and *Lu^a/Lu^b*, *Lu^6/Lu^9*, *Lu^8/Lu^{14}*, and *Au^a/Au^b* for Lutheran. However, Kell and Lutheran proteins now are known to be single gene products that carry multiple antigens. The most common alleles in humans are *kKp^{b}Js^{b}K^{11}* and *Lu^{b}Lu^{6}Lu^{8}Au^a*. Antigens of lower prevalence (K, Kp^a/Kp^c, or Js^a, and Lu^a, Lu9, Lu14, or Au^b) arose from separate point mutations.

SILENT ALLELES

Some blood group alleles are amorphs, or silent, that is, they do not produce a recognizable antigen, although they may encode a product that is simply not detected with standard test methods. As discussed with regard to the ABO system, *A* and *B* genes produce transferases that add GalNAc or Gal, respectively, to the same precursor, but *O* produces no active enzyme. *AB* individuals express both A and B antigen, but *AA* and *AO* individuals express only A, and *BB* and *BO* individuals express only B. Amorphic alleles are recognized only in a homozygous state, and the result is a "null" phenotype. Null phenotypes exist in most blood group systems (see Table 128-1). Group O is the most common, followed by Fy(a−b−) and Le(a−b−) in Africans. Other null phenotypes are rare.

The Fy(a−b−) phenotype is especially interesting. Fy(a−b−) Africans have *Fy^b* genes that express normal Fy^b glycoprotein on tissue cells but not on RBCs. A mutation that disrupts the GATA-1 binding site for RBC transcription has been identified in these individuals,[41] which helps explain why many Fy(a−b−) Africans do not make Duffy antibodies despite exposure to antigen-positive RBCs from transfusion.

GENE FREQUENCIES

Gene and phenotype frequencies vary widely with race and geographical boundaries.[6,11,42,43] This information is needed when estimating the availability of compatible blood and the probability of HDN.

RED CELL ANTIGENS IN HEALTH AND DISEASE

EXPRESSION OF RED CELL ANTIGENS IN OTHER BODY TISSUES AND FLUIDS

Antigens in the Rh and Kidd blood group systems are present only on RBCs and have not been detected on platelets, lymphocytes, or granulocytes or in plasma, other body tissues, or secretions (saliva, milk, amniotic fluid).[5,6,15] MNSs, Lutheran, Kell, and Duffy antigens are found on RBCs and other body tissues (see Table 128-2).

ABH antigens have broad tissue distribution. In embryos, A, B, and H antigens are detectable on all endothelial cells and all epithelial cells except those of the central nervous system. ABH, Lewis, I, and P blood group antigens are in plasma and on platelets and lymphocytes. Granulocytes carry I antigen but no ABH. ABH on platelets and lymphocytes may be acquired at least in part by adsorption of plasma antigen. Lewis antigen is acquired only by adsorption. Secretions (saliva, milk, sweat, semen, and urine, but not cerebral spinal fluid) contain A, B, H, I, and Lewis antigens but no P or Globoside system antigens. Sd^a antigen is found in most body secretions, with the greatest concentration in urine.[5,15]

ASSOCIATIONS OF RED CELL ANTIGENS WITH DISEASE

ANTIGENS ASSOCIATED WITH POSSIBLE SUSCEPTIBILITY TO DISEASE

Some blood groups are statistically associated with medical conditions or disease (Table 128-4).[5,6,15,44–46] For example, blood group A is more common in persons with cancer of the salivary glands, stomach, colon, or ovary and with thrombosis (because of higher levels of factors VIII, V, and IX). Blood group O is more common in patients with duodenal and gastric ulcers, rheumatoid arthritis, and von Willebrand disease.

Associations with infection arise when microorganisms carry structures with blood group activity. *Yersinia pestis* carries H-like antigen, and the smallpox virus is associated with A-like antigen, making group O and A individuals, respectively, more susceptible. The presence of blood group antibody and/or soluble blood group antigen in secretions may help confer protection. Having anti-B may offer protection against *Salmonella*, *Shigella*, *Neisseria gonorrhoeae*, and some *Escherichia coli* infections. An association exists between nonsecretion of ABH antigen and susceptibility to *Candida albicans*, *Neisseria meningitidis*, *Streptococcus pneumoniae*, and *Haemophilus influenzae*.[45]

TABLE 128-4 BLOOD GROUP ANTIGENS AND ANTIBODIES ASSOCIATED WITH DISEASE

Phenotypes Associated with Disease Susceptibility

Group A	Carcinoma of the salivary glands, stomach, colon, rectum, ovary, uterus, cervix, bladder (T1 and T2 tumors); idiopathic thrombocytopenic purpura, coronary thrombosis, thrombosis (oral contraceptives), pernicious anemia, giardiasis, meningococcal meningitis infections
Group B	*Escherichia coli* urinary tract infection, gonorrhea
Group O	Duodenal and gastric ulcers, rheumatoid arthritis, von Willebrand disease, typhoid, paratyphoid, cholera
ABH nonsecretors	Duodenal ulcers, spondylarthropathies; increased susceptibility to *Candida albicans, Neisseria meningitidis, Streptococcus pneumoniae, Haemophilus influenzae*
Le(a−b−)	Sjögren syndrome
Group O, Le(a−b+)	*Helicobacter pylori*
Globoside	Parvovirus

Phenotypes Associated with Disease Resistance

p (PP$_1$P^k−)	Pyelonephritogenic infections of *E. coli*
Fy(a−b−)	*Plasmodium vivax, Plasmodium knowlesi*
Tn−, Cad−, En(a−), U−, Ge−	*Plasmodium falciparum*

Diseases Associated with Altered Antigen Expression

Weakened AB	Leukemia, preleukemia, Hodgkin disease, aplastic anemia, bacterial infections
Weakened MN	Bacterial infections, preleukemia, leukemia (Tn, T, Tk activation)
Enhanced i	Thalassemia, sickle cell disease, HEMPAS, Diamond-Blackfan anemia, myeloblastic or sideroblastic erythropoiesis, refractory anemia
Acquired A (Tn)	Preleukemia, acute myelogenous leukemia
Acquired B	Bacterial infections, gastrointestinal lesions or malignancies
Acquired T, Tk	Bacterial infections
Acquired K antigens	*Enterococcus faecium*
Acquired Jk^b antigen	*E. faecium* or *Micrococcus* infection
Absent Cromer, Yt, Dombrock, JMH antigens	Paroxysmal nocturnal hemoglobinuria
Weakened target antigens (Rh, Kell, Kidd, LW)	Autoimmune hemolytic anemia
Weakened I, Rh, S, s, U, Kp^b, Jk^a, Xg^a, or En^a	Stomatocytic hereditary elliptocytosis

Diseases Associated with Null Phenotypes

Rh$_{null}$ (D−C−E−c−e−)	Hereditary stomatocytosis, mild hemolytic anemia
McLeod phenotype (Kx−)	Hereditary acanthocytosis, mild hemolytic anemia
Ge− (Leach type)	Hereditary elliptocytosis, mild hemolytic anemia
Bombay (Oh)	Leukocyte adhesion deficiency II (some)
I− (i Adult)	Congenital cataracts in Asians (some)
Co(a−b−), Co:−3	Inability to maximally concentrate urine
MER2−	Kidney disease

Diseases Associated with Antibody Production

Anti-I, -IH, -i, -H, -Pr	Cold agglutinin disease
Anti-"Rh," -"Kell," -U, -Wr^b	Warm autoimmune hemolytic anemia
Anti-I	*Mycoplasma pneumoniae*, chronic lymphocytic leukemia, Hodgkin disease
Anti-i	Infectious mononucleosis, reticuloendothelial diseases
Anti-I^T	Hodgkin disease
Anti-K	Enterocolitis, bacterial infections (*E. coli* 0125:B15, *Campylobacter jejuni, E. coli*)
Anti-P1	Parasitic infections: hydatid cyst disease, liver flukes
Anti-PP$_1$P^k	Early spontaneous abortions
Anti-P	Paroxysmal cold hemoglobinuria, early spontaneous abortions, lymphoma
Anti-NF	Renal dialysis (formaldehyde exposure)
Anti-Forssman	Neoplastic disorders
Anti-Rx	Virally induced hemolysis
Decreased anti-A or −B	Agammaglobulinemia or hypogammaglobulinemia

"Null" Phenotypes Associated with Biologic Differences but No Disease

Group O	Lack GalNAc or Gal on terminal Gal
Bombay	Lack Fuc on terminal Gal
Le(a−b−)	Lack Fuc on terminal GlcNAc
M−N− or En(a−)	Lack or have altered GPA
S−s−U−	Lack or have altered GPB
Wr(a−b−)	Lack or have altered GPA
M^k phenotype	Lack GPA and GPB
K$_0$	Lack Kell glycoprotein
Jk(a−b−)	Lack or have altered Jk protein, reduced ability to concentrate urine
Lu(a−b−)	Lack or have reduced or altered Lu glycoprotein; RBC may show poikilocytosis, potassium loss, increased hemolysis during storage
LW(a−b−)	Lack or have altered LW glycoprotein
Do(a−b−), Gy(a−)	Lack a GPI-linked protein (Do glycoprotein)
Sc: −1, −2, −3	Lack or have altered Sc glycoprotein

SOURCE: Modified from PD Issitt and DJ Anstee,[5] G Daniels,[4] and ME Reid and C Lomas-Francis.[6]
HEMPAS = hereditary erythroblastic multinuclearity with positive acidified serum lysis test.

A number of disease associations with globoside have been identified. *Streptococcus suis*, which can cause meningitis and septicemia in humans, binds exclusively to P^k antigen. A class of toxins secreted by *Shigella dysenteriae*, *Vibrio cholerae*, and *Vibrio parahaemolyticus* have binding specificity for $Gal(\alpha1\rightarrow4)$-$Gal(\beta1\rightarrow4)$. In addition, globoside is the receptor of human parvovirus B19.[35] Some strains of *E. coli* use the disaccharide receptor $Gal(\alpha1\rightarrow4)$-$Gal\beta$ on uroepithelial cells to gain entry to the urinary tract receptors associated with P_1, P, and P^k antigens.[5,45,47,48] People with the rare p phenotype (P null) lack this disaccharide and are not susceptible to acute pyelonephritis from such *E. coli* strains.

PHENOTYPES ASSOCIATED WITH DISEASE RESISTANCE

Erythrocytes lacking Fy^a and Fy^b antigens are not infected by the malarial parasite *Plasmodium vivax* or by the simian malarial parasite *Plasmodium knowlesi*. These parasites attach to the Fy(a−b−) RBC membrane, but penetration does not take place. The Fy6 antigen is the critical receptor for *P. vivax* attachment.[5,49,50] *Plasmodium falciparum* attaches to RBC glycophorins and their O-linked oligosaccharides (carrying NeuNAc). RBCs with the following phenotypes have a decreased rate of infection: M−N− (GPA-deficient), S−s−U− (GPB-deficient), Ge− (Leach type or GPC-deficient), and Cad- and Tn-positive RBCs (which have abnormal O-linked sugars).[49]

DISEASES ASSOCIATED WITH ALTERED ANTIGEN EXPRESSION

Antigen expression can be altered with inherited and acquired disease. Inherited changes are fixed and consistent; acquired changes can disappear with remission or recovery. In some diseases, antigen expression weakens; in others, antigen expression increases or new antigens appear.

Weakened ABH expression on RBCs has been noted in acute myeloid leukemias and may result from reduced transferase activity.[5,15] Normal antigen expression returns with disease remission. Transient weakened expression of target antigen also occurs in some cases of autoimmune hemolytic anemia.[51] Weak Rh, Kell, and Kidd blood group activity has been reported with concurrent autoantibody.[5,15]

Increased expression of i on RBCs is associated with inherited disorders, such as thalassemia, sickle cell disease, Diamond-Blackfan syndrome, and hereditary erythroblastic multinuclearity with a positive acidified serum test (HEMPAS). Increased i expression also is noted with acquired conditions that decrease the red cell maturation time in the marrow, such as myeloblastic or sideroblastic erythropoiesis, refractory anemia, and excessive phlebotomy.[15,45,52] Expression of the *de novo* antigen Tn is caused by a galactosyltransferase deficiency acquired by somatic mutation in a population of stem cells. The antigen is present on RBCs, platelets, and granulocytes arising from these stem cells. This condition (seen as persistent mixed-field agglutination because of the presence of both normal and abnormal cell clones) causes other RBC changes, such as depressed MN expression, enhanced H, and reduced NeuNAc content. Tn antigen exposure is associated with preleukemia and acute myelomonocytic leukemia.[15,45] Other crypt antigens (T, Tk) occur as a result of infection when microbes produce enzymes that remove some sugars and expose new ones. Group A individuals can appear to acquire a B antigen when bacterial deacetylase removes the acetyl group on GalNAc.[53,54] This phenomenon is associated with severe infection, gastrointestinal lesions, and malignancies.

RBCs may acquire blood group activity when they adsorb material from certain microorganisms. Group B activity has been associated with *E. coli*86 and *Proteus vulgaris* infection, and K antigen with *Enterococcus faecium*. Acquired Jk^b-like activity has been associated with *E. faecium* and *Micrococcus* infections, although the mechanism is not clear.[55]

DISEASES ASSOCIATED WITH ABSENT ANTIGENS OR NULL PHENOTYPES

Rh_{null} SYNDROME

The Rh_{null} phenotype is associated with hereditary stomatocytosis, hemolytic anemia (usually mild and well compensated), and a lack of proteins carrying Rh antigen. The Rh protein resides in the RBC membrane, interacts with other membrane glycoproteins and possibly the membrane skeleton, and may help regulate or organize the lipids within the red cell membrane bilayer.[9,10,46] Hence, it is an important determinant of membrane shape and expression of other antigens. Rh_{null} cells have depressed expression or absence of S, s, U, LW, and Fy5 antigens.

Most Rh_{null} red cells are stomatocytes or occasionally spherocytes and demonstrate increased osmotic fragility, increased potassium permeability, and higher potassium pump activity. They have reduced cation and water content and a relative deficiency of membrane cholesterol.[46] Although these abnormalities are assumed to contribute to shortened *in vivo* survival, Rh_{null} RBCs survive normally in splenectomized patients, suggesting their removal is related more to splenic clearance because of shape rather than some other intrinsic factor.[46]

Two genetic mechanisms account for the Rh_{null} phenotype. Persons with the amorphic type are homozygous for the silent RhCE gene on a deleted *RHD* background. Individuals with the more common regulator type of Rh_{null} have normal Rh genes but an altered (silenced) *RHAG* gene. RhAG is required for expression of Rh antigens. Individuals with the Rh_{mod} phenotype have similar membrane and clinical anomalies associated with Rh_{null} syndrome but demonstrate some Rh antigen expression. The reduced expression of Rh antigens results from the presence of an altered form of RhAG.[25,27,56]

McLEOD PHENOTYPE

Numerous males (but no females) with the McLeod phenotype have been identified. These individuals have acanthocytosis, decreased RBC survival, very weak expression of Kell blood group antigens, lack of Kx antigen on RBCs, and a well-compensated hemolytic anemia.[57]

Kx, a 37-kDa protein encoded by the *XK* gene, interacts with the RBC membrane skeleton and helps stabilize the membrane. The absence of Kx is associated with a lipid deficiency in the membrane bilayer that may be critical to the Kell glycoprotein and general membrane shape. RBCs with the McLeod phenotype show a defect in water transport, increased mobility of phosphatidylcholine across the membrane, and increased phosphorylation of protein band 3 and β-spectrin.[57,58]

After age 40 years, patients with the McLeod phenotype develop a slowly progressive form of muscular dystrophy that is associated with areflexia, choreiform movements, and cardiomegaly, leading to cardiomyopathy. They have elevated levels of serum creatine kinase and carbonic anhydrase III. Some patients with the McLeod phenotype and X-linked chronic granulomatous disease (CGD) have a deletion of both the *XK* and *Phox-91* (see Chap. 66). The McLeod phenotype results from deletions or point mutations on the X chromosome near the *XK* gene at position Xp21[59] (for details, see *www.nefo.med.uni-muechen.de*).

GERBICH NEGATIVE PHENOTYPE

The *GYPC* gene on chromosome 2 encodes two proteins: GPC, with antigens Ge3 and Ge4 (the Ge2 portion is "hidden" by the Ge4-bearing terminal end), and its shorter partner glycophorin D (GPD), with antigens Ge2 (now exposed) and Ge3. GPC and GPD interact with membrane skeleton proteins 4.1 and p55, which are involved in cell deformability and membrane stability. Gerbich-negative RBCs of the Leach type (Ge:−2,−3,−4) lack both GPC and GPD, have reduced protein 4.1, and elliptocytosis but exhibit normal survival *in vivo*.[60]

BOMBAY (OH) PHENOTYPE

Rare people with the Le(a−b−) Bombay phenotype have a silenced gene that encodes the fucose transporter. As a consequence, all cells lack fucose. Without fucose, neutrophils lack sialyl Le^X and thus cannot roll and ingest bacteria. These patients have a high white blood cell count and severe recurrent infections. The condition is called *leukocyte adhesion deficiency II* (LADII) or congenital disorder of glycosylation II.[61,62]

I PHENOTYPE (i ADULT)

The gene encoding the I-branching ∝-1,6-N-acetylglucosaminyltransferase *(IGNT)* has three alternative forms of exon 1, with common exons 2 and 3. Mutations in exon 2 or 3 silence *IGNT* and give rise to the form of I-negative phenotype associated with congenital cataracts in Asians.[63,64] Mutations in exon 1C *(IGnTC or IGnT3)* silence the gene in RBCs but not in other tissues and lead to the I-negative phenotype (i adult) without cataracts.[65]

CO(a−b−), CO:−3 PHENOTYPE

Antigens of the Colton blood group system are carried on the water transporter (aquaporin). Although an absence of this protein from the RBC membrane was thought to be incompatible with life, in reality these rare individuals have been shown only to be unable to maximally concentrate urine.[66]

MER2−PHENOTYPE

The MER2 antigen in the Raph blood group system is carried on CD151.[67] Rare individuals who lack CD151 have chronic renal failure.[68]

OTHER NULL PHENOTYPES

The other rare null phenotypes are not associated with RBC shape changes or with hemolytic anemia.[45] However, patients with null phenotypes can develop RBC antibodies that make it difficult to find compatible blood to avoid the otherwise serious hemolytic transfusion reactions. For example, people with the Bombay phenotype (O$_h$ or H$_{null}$) demonstrate no red cell abnormality but make potent hemolytic anti-H as well as anti-A and anti-B. These antibodies are incompatible with all RBCs except those from other persons with the Bombay phenotype. Likewise, p individuals (PP$_1$P^k-negative) or P^k individuals (P-negative) can make hemolytic antibodies to the antigens they lack. Anti-PP$_1$P^k and anti-P also are associated with spontaneous abortions in the first trimester.[15] Women with such antibodies (notably IgG anti-P), even those with a history of spontaneous abortions, have delivered viable infants after plasmapheresis.[69]

Null phenotypes in the MNSs and Lutheran systems are interesting because several types of null phenotypes are known. Within the MNSs blood group system, people may lack GPA [En(a−) or MN-negative], GPB (SsU-negative), or both (M^{k}M^k phenotype).[44,45] The rare Lu(a−b−) phenotype is caused by a dominant inhibitor called *In(Lu)*, by homozygous pairing of the silent allele *Lu*, or by a recessive sex-linked inhibitor *XS2*.[5,15] Only the *LuLu*-type null [recessive Lu(a−b−)] is associated with high-prevalence antibody because the inhibitor type nulls produce small amounts of Lutheran antigen. *In(Lu)* type, Lu(a−b−) RBCs have low expression of CD44 and have varying degrees of poikilocytosis and acanthocytosis. RBCs of this type tend to

hemolyze more quickly during storage, even though they demonstrate normal osmotic fragility.[70]

The Jk(a−b−) phenotype is caused by the silent alleles *JkJk* or the dominant inhibitor *In(Jk)*. RBCs having the Jk(a−b−) phenotype resist lysis in 2M urea,[71] a solution commonly used in automated platelet counting systems. No significant clinical abnormalities have been identified to date, although Jk(a−b−) individuals have reduced ability to concentrate urine.[72]

The following diagnosis are made more easily from appropriate blood grouping: Rh syndrome, McLeod syndrome, and LADII.

ANTIERYTHROCYTE ANTIBODIES

IMMUNOLOGY OF RED CELL ANTIBODIES

Blood group antibodies are classified as autoantibodies if they are specific for *self-antigens* present on the patient's own RBC and as *alloantibodies* if they react with antigens present on the RBC of other people. Alloantibodies also can be classified according to their mode of sensitization as *naturally occurring* (no apparent sensitization) or *immune* (following sensitization). Table 128-5 summarizes the common antierythrocyte antibodies.[4–6,15]

IMMUNOGLOBULIN CLASSES ASSOCIATED WITH BLOOD GROUP ACTIVITY

IMMUNOGLOBULIN G

IgG is the predominant antibody made in an immune response and constitutes approximately 80 percent of total serum Ig (see Chap. 77). These antibodies, when specific for RBC antigens, can lyse transfused antigen-positive RBCs. Receptors on macrophages in the liver and spleen allow the macrophages to remove IgG-coated RBCs from the circulation. IgG blood group antibodies also are capable of fixing complement, although some subclasses do so less efficiently than others: IgG3 > IgG1 > IgG2 > IgG4. How well an IgG antierythrocyte antibody binds complement depends on the surface density and location of the recognized antigen. This situation occurs because C1q, the initiator of the classic complement cascade, requires binding of at least two IgG molecules to the RBC within a span of 20 to 30 nm to initiate the complement cascade.[15] For example, IgG anti-D rarely binds complement, presumably because most D sites are spaced too far apart.[15] Most IgG blood group antibodies do not agglutinate saline-suspended RBCs, presumably because the IgG molecule is too small to span the distance between RBCs, although some exceptions are known (i.e., potent IgG examples of anti-A, anti-B, anti-M, and anti-K. Some IgG anti-D can directly agglutinate RBCs with the D−− phenotype.) Instead, most IgG antibodies sensitize RBCs at 37°C and are detected with the help of an antiglobulin reagent.[11]

IMMUNOGLOBULIN M

IgM is a pentamer of five basic units (having μ heavy chains plus a short J, or joining, chain) and makes up only approximately 4 percent of total serum Ig (see Chap. 77). IgM is the first class of Ig produced by a fetus and is the predominant antibody in a primary immune response, but it does not cross the placenta. Because of their pentameric structure, even low-affinity IgM blood group antibodies can agglutinate RBCs and activate complement. Both hemolyzing and agglutinating abilities of IgM molecules are destroyed by reducing reagents, such as 2-ME and DTT. IgM antibodies of low affinity may agglutinate RBCs only at temperatures below 37°C. Such antibodies still may fix complement onto the RBC membrane *in vivo*, presumably by binding to red cells at the lower temperatures of the extremities and activating the complement cascade. Because such IgM antibodies dissociate from RBCs at higher temperatures, their reactivity may be detected in rou-

TABLE 128-5 SUMMARY OF ANTIERYTHROCYTE ANTIBODIES

Blood Group	Antibody	Ig Class		Serologic Activity			Activates Complement	Implicated in		Antigen Frequency (%)		Comments
		IgM	IgG	RT	37°C-AHG	ENZ/DTT		HTR	HDN	Whites	Blacks	
Antibodies More Commonly Encountered												
ABO	A	Most	Some	Most	Most	I/nc	Yes	Yes	Mild	40	27	A/B: very clinically significant, sometimes IgA
	B	Most	Some	Most	Most	I/nc	Yes	Yes	Mild	11	20	
	A_1	Most	Rare	Most	Rare	I/nc	Rare	Rare	No	30	—	A1: usually not clinically significant
	H	Most	Rare	Most	Rare	I/nc	Rare	Rare	—	>99.9	—	H: usually weak autoantibody, but strong alloantibody in O_h
Rh	D	Some	Most	Some	Most	I/nc	No	Yes	Sev	85	92	D: most common immune antibody
	C	Few	Most	—	Most	I/nc	No	Yes	Sev	70	33	C: often found with D
	E	Some	Most	S	Most	I/nc	No	Yes	Sev	30	21	Ec: often found together
	c	—	Most	—	Most	I/nc	No	Yes	Sev	80	97	Autoantibodies commonly directed against Rh protein
	E	—	Most	—	Most	I/nc	No	Yes	Mild–sev	98	99	All: clinically significant
	f(ce)	—	M	—	Most	I/nc	No	Yes	Sev	64	—	
	C^w	Some	Most	—	Most	I/nc	No	Yes	Sev	1	—	
	V	—	Most	—	Most	I/nc	No	Yes	Sev	<1	30	
Lewis	Le^a	Most	Rare	Most	Some	I/nc	Yes	Rare	No	22	23	Common in pregnancy
	Le^b	Most	Rare	Most	Some	I/nc	Yes	No	No	72	55	Not clinically significant Le(a−b−) individuals commonly make anti-Le^a
Ii	i	Most	—	Most	Some	I/nc	Yes	Rare	No	>99.9	>99.9	I: common autoantibody, rare significant alloantibody
	I	Most	—	Most	Some	I/nc	Yes	No	Mild	100	100	i: rare autoantibody
P	P_1	Most	Rare	Most	Some	I/nc	Few	Rare	No	79	94	P_1: usually not clinically significant
(GLOB)	P	Most	Few	Most	Some	I/nc	Yes	Yes	No–mild	>99.9	>99.9	P: Donath-Landsteiner antibody in PNH
	PP_1P^k	Most	Few	Most	Some	I/nc	Yes	Yes	Mild–sev	>99.9	>99.9	
MNSs	M	Some	Some	Most	Few	D/nc	No	Rare	(R)	78	70	M: common, usually not clinically significant
	N	Some	Some	Most	Rare	D/nc	No	Rare	(R)	72	74	
	S	Some	Some	Some	Most	V/nc	Some	Yes	Mild	55	31	N: rare, usually not clinically significant
	s̄	Few	Most	Few	Most	V/nc	Rare	Yes	Mild–sev	89	97	
	U	—	Most	—	Most	nc/nc	Rare	Yes	Mild–mod	100	99.7	SsU: clinically significant autoantibody specificities reported
Kell	K	Some	Most	Few	Most	nc/D	Rare	Yes	Mild–sev	9	2	K: very common immune antibody
	k	—	Most	Rare	Most	nc/D	No	Yes	Mild–sev	99.9	—	
	Kp^a	—	Most	Rare	Most	nc/D	No	Yes	Mild–mod	2.3	—	Autoantibodies reported
	Kp^b	—	Most	Rare	Most	nc/D	No	Yes	Mild–mod	>99.9	100	
	Js^a	—	Most	Rare	Rare	nc/D	No	Yes	Mild–sev	—	20	
	Js^b	—	Most	—	—	nc/D	No	Yes	Mild–sev	>99.9	99	
Duffy	Fy^a	—	Most	Rare	Most	D/nc	Rare	Yes	Mild–sev	66	10	Fy^a: common immune antibody
	Fy^b	—	Most	Rare	Most	D/nc	Rare	Yes	Mild	83	23	
Kidd	Jk^a	Few	Most	Rare	Most	I/nc	Yes	Yes	Mild–mod	77	92	Jk^a: associated with delayed HTR; hemolytic; disappears quickly from serum
	Jk^b	Few	Most	Rare	Most	I/nc	Yes	Yes	No–mild	72	41	
Lutheran	Lu^a	Some	Few	Most	Few	nc(V)/D	No	N	N–mild	7.7	—	Mild RBC destruction
	Lu^b	Some	Some	Few	Most	nc(V)/D	No	Yes	Mild	99.9	—	

TABLE 128-5 SUMMARY OF ANTIERYTHROCYTE ANTIBODIES (CONTINUED)

BLOOD GROUP	ANTIBODY	IG CLASS		SEROLOGIC ACTIVITY			ACTIVATES COMPLEMENT	IMPLICATED IN		ANTIGEN FREQUENCY (%)		COMMENTS
		IGM	IGG	RT	37°C-AHG	ENZ/DTT		HTR	HDN	WHITES	BLACKS	
Antibodies Less Commonly Encountered												
Xg	Xgᵃ	Some	Most	Rare	Most	D/nc	Some	No	No	64(m) 89(f)	— —	Xgᵃ: poor immunogen
Yt	Ytᵃ	—	Most	N	Most	D(V)/D(V)	No	No–mod	No	99.7	—	Yt: some antibody examples clinically significant, others not
	Ytᵇ	—	Most	N	M	D(V)/D	No	?	No	8	—	
Ch/Rg	Ch	Rare	Most	—	Most	D/nc	No	No	No	96	—	Ch/Rg: associated with C4 complement, clinically insignificant antibodies
	Rg		Most	—	Most	D/nc	No	No	No	98	—	
Colton	Coᵃ		Most	Some	Most	nc/nc	No	No	Mild–sev	99.9	—	
	Coᵇ		Most	Some	Most	nc/nc	Rare	No–mod	Mild	10	—	
Cost	Csᵃ		Most	—	Most	nc/nc	No	No	No	96	98	
Cromer	General group		Most	—	Most	nc/D	No	No–mild	No	>99.9	>99.9	
Diego	Diᵃ		Most	Some	Most	nc/nc	Rare	Yes	Mild–sev	R	—	Diᵃ: antigen found in South American Indians and Asians
	Diᵇ		Most	N	Most	nc/nc	No	Yes	Mild	100	—	
Dombrock	Doᵃ		Most	N	Most	nc/D(V)	No	Yes	Mild	67	—	Doᵃ Doᵇ: poor immunogens
	Doᵇ		Most	N	Most	nc/D(V)	No	Yes	No	83	—	Hy− and Jo(a−): found only in blacks
	Hy		Most	—	Most	nc(I)/D(V)	No	Yes	Mild	>99	—	Gy(a−) (Do$_{null}$) found in eastern Europeans and Japanese
	Gyᵃ		Most	—	Most	nc(I)/D(V)	No	Yes	Mild	>99	—	
	Joᵃ		Most	—	Most	nc(I)/D(V)	No	No	No	>99	—	
Gerbich	General group		Most	—	Most	D/nc	Yes	N–mod	(+DAT)	>99.9	>99.9	Ge: located on glycophorins C and D
Indian	Inᵃ		Most	—	Most	D/D	No	Yes	(+DAT)	<0.1	<0.1	In: located on CD44 adhesion protein
	Inᵇ		Most	—	Most	D/D	No	Yes	(+DAT)	99	96	
Knops	Knᵃ		Most	—	Most	D/D/nc	No	No	No	98	99	Knops antigens associated with CR1 (complement) receptor, clinically insignificant antibodies
	McCᵃ		Most	—	Most	D/D	No	No	No	98	94	
	Ykᵃ		Most	—	Most	D/D	No	No	No	92	98	
Scianna	Sc1		Most	—	Most	nc/D	Yes	No	Mild	>99.9	—	Sc1: some antibodies react in serum but not plasma
	Sc2		Most	—	Most	nc/D	No	No	Mild	1	—	
	Sc3		Most	—	Most	nc(I)/?	No	No–mild	No	>99.9	—	
High	JMH		Most	—	Most	D/D	No	No	No	>99.9	>99.9	JMH: carrier protein CDw108

AHG = antiglobulin phase; D = decreased; +DAT = positive direct antiglobulin test result; DTT = dithiothreitol-treated RBC; ENZ = enzyme-treated RBCs; f = female; GPI = glycosyl phosphatidylinositol; HDN = hemolytic disease of the newborn; HTR = hemolytic transfusion reactions; I = increased; M = most; m = male, mod = moderate; nc = no significant change using pretreated cells; RT = room temperature; S = some; sev = severe; V = variable.

tine antiglobulin tests by virtue of the complement components that remain bound to the red cell membrane.

IMMUNOGLOBULIN A

IgA is the primary Ig in body secretions, where it exists predominantly as a dimer with a secretory component (see Chap. 77). IgA does not cross the placenta or fix complement, but aggregated IgA can activate the alternative pathway of complement, and IgA can trigger cell-mediated events. Multimeric IgA antibodies in serum are seen as hemagglutinins in blood bank tests and most often are associated with anti-A or anti-B.

IMMUNOGLOBULIN IN THE FETUS AND NEWBORN

Young fetuses acquire low levels of maternal IgG, possibly by diffusion across the placenta. These levels rise significantly between 20 and 33 weeks' gestation as a selective transport system matures and maternal IgG is actively transported across the placenta. Thus almost all blood group antibodies detected in the fetus and newborn originate from the mother and disappear within the first few months of life.

Actual fetal antibody production begins shortly before birth with low levels of IgM, followed by IgG and IgA several weeks after birth. Antibody production continues to increase with age until adult levels are reached. Anti-A and anti-B usually are readily detected by age 2 to 6 months.

Because of this late immune response in the newborn and because maternal antibody is so predominant at birth, blood bank standards permit abbreviated testing on neonates younger than 4 months.[73] If available, the mother's serum is used (and preferred) for identifying antibodies in a newborn and for cross-matching units of blood.

NATURALLY OCCURRING ANTIBODIES

NATURALLY OCCURRING ANTIBODIES IN DEVELOPMENT
An antibody is said to be *naturally occurring* when it is found in the serum of an individual who has never been exposed to the antigen through transfusion or pregnancy. These antibodies most likely are heteroagglutinins produced in response to substances in the environment that are similar to RBC antigens.

Evidence supporting this concept has come from studies on the formation of anti-B in chickens.[74] Chicks raised in a normal environment made anti-B within the first 30 days of life, whereas chicks raised in a germ-free environment did not make anti-B by day 60. Naturally occurring alloanti-A and alloanti-B in humans, also called *isoagglutinins*, can increase in titer following ingestion or inhalation of suitable bacteria.[75]

However, a great many antigens that likely are not present in the environment have been associated with naturally occurring antibodies, so the stimulus for naturally occurring antibodies is not clearly known.

BLOOD GROUP ASSOCIATIONS AND OCCURRENCE OF NATURALLY OCCURRING ANTIBODIES
Naturally occurring alloantibodies are commonly associated with the carbohydrate antigens of the ABO, Lewis, and P blood group systems. Anti-A and anti-B are expected in people who lack the corresponding antigens, as are antibodies specific for H, PP_1P^k, or P antigens. Naturally occurring antibodies reactive with A1, Le^a, Le^b, or P1 determinants also are seen frequently. Carbohydrate antigens, especially those with repetitive epitopes, can stimulate B cells to make specific antibody without the aid of helper T cells. Such thymus-independent immune responses typically result in antigen-specific antibodies of the IgM class.[76]

Within other systems,[15] anti-Sd^a, anti-Vw, and anti-Wr^a are found in up to 2 percent of normal people. Other less common antibody specificities in approximate order of descending occurrence are M, S, N, Ge, K, Lu^a, Di^a, and Xg^a. Rh antigens are thought to reside only on RBCs, but apparent naturally occurring anti-D has been reported in 0.15 percent of Rh-negative donors and anti-E in more than 0.1 percent of Rh-positive donors when more sensitive enzyme detection methods are used. Examples of naturally occurring anti-C, anti-C^w, and anti-C^x also have been described.

Some naturally occurring antibodies exist as autoagglutinins (anti-H and anti-I). Patients with autoimmune hemolytic anemia can produce many antibodies to low-incidence antigens with no specific stimulus, in addition to autoantibody.[5,6,15,51]

CHARACTERISTICS OF NATURALLY OCCURRING ALLOANTIBODIES
Most naturally occurring antibodies are IgM, but some have an IgG component and a few are predominantly IgG. Some anti-A or anti-B may even be of the IgA class. Antibodies that cause direct agglutination of saline-suspended RBCs most commonly are of the IgM class. However, even IgG antibodies may cause agglutination of RBCs when they bind antigens that are present at high density on the RBC membrane, such as the ABO or MN antigens. With the exception of anti-A and anti-B, most common naturally occurring antibodies do not react

at body temperature and are considered clinically insignificant. However, if they are found to react at 37°C, providing cross-match compatible blood for transfusion is prudent.

ANTIBODIES GENERATED IN RESPONSE TO IMMUNIZATION: IMMUNE ANTIBODIES

IMMUNE ANTIBODIES IN DEVELOPMENT
Immune antibodies are produced following exposure to foreign RBC antigens through pregnancy or transfusion. The primary immune response is seen several weeks to several months after the first exposure to antigen. IgM usually is associated with early primary responses, but whether it is always the first antibody class made is unclear. In most individuals, IgG soon predominates. This process is characteristic of a thymus-dependent immune response, where T cells help induce B cells to undergo isotype switching from IgM to IgG.[76]

In a secondary or anamnestic response, antibody concentration starts to increase several days to several weeks following exposure, and IgG may rise to very high levels. Some IgG antibodies remain detectable 30 years after a stimulus. Others, especially Kidd antibodies, can disappear after several months and are more commonly associated with delayed hemolytic transfusion reactions.[5,6,15]

BLOOD GROUP ASSOCIATIONS AND OCCURRENCE OF IMMUNE ANTIBODIES
Immune antibodies are found more commonly in individuals who have been multiply transfused than in multiparous women. This situation occurs because in pregnancy the immunizing dose of red cells often is too small to elicit a primary response, and the foreign antigens are limited to those of the father.[15]

Anti-D used to be the most common immune antibody, but with the advent of Rh matching of donors and recipients in the late 1940s and use of Rh Ig prophylaxis since the 1970s, its incidence has sharply decreased. Anti-D is present in 0.27 to 0.56 percent of transfusion recipients, 0.10 to 0.20 percent of pregnant women, and 0.16 to 0.25 percent of healthy blood donors.[15]

In contrast, the occurrence of immune antibodies other than anti-D has increased. Specificities other than anti-D have been reported in approximately 0.6 percent of transfusion recipients, 0.14 percent of pregnant women, and 0.19 percent of healthy blood donors. Pooled data from three 5-year periods and approximately 300,000 patients suggest the absolute occurrence of Rh antibodies other than anti-D is 0.22 percent, anti-K 0.19 percent, anti-Fy^a 0.05 percent, and anti-Jk^a 0.035 percent.[15]

The rate of alloimmunization in sickle cell anemia was 18.6 percent in one survey, and 55 percent of the immunized patients made more than one antibody. The most common specificities were anti-C, anti-E, and anti-K.[15]

CHARACTERISTICS OF IMMUNE ANTIBODIES
Immune antibodies most often are IgG but may be IgM and sometimes are IgA. Most immune antibodies react at body temperature and are considered clinically significant, except those directed against Bg, Kn^a, McC^a, Sl^a, Yk^a, Cs^a, JMH, and sometimes Lutheran antigens.

CLINICAL SIGNIFICANCE OF ERYTHROCYTE ANTIBODIES

Information about the clinical significance of alloantibodies is available under Patient Services, Immunohematology at *www.nybloodcenter.org*.

HEMOLYTIC TRANSFUSION REACTIONS

Clinically significant antibodies are capable of destroying transfused RBCs. The severity of the reaction varies with antigen density and antibody characteristics.

Antibodies commonly associated with intravascular hemolysis include anti-A, anti-B, anti-Jk[a], and anti-Jk[b]. ABO incompatibility is the most potent cause of immediate hemolytic reactions because A and B antigens are so strongly expressed on RBCs and the antibodies so efficiently bind complement. Kidd antibodies are associated more often with delayed hemolytic reactions because they typically are difficult to detect and disappear quickly from the circulation. IgG anti-Jk[a] appears to bind complement only when traces of IgM anti-Jk[a] are present.[15] Anti-PP1Pk, anti-Vel, and anti-Le[a] have been associated with hemolysis, but such examples are rare.

Extravascular hemolysis occurs with IgG1 and IgG3 antibodies that react at body temperature, that is, immune antibodies reactive with Rh, Kidd, Kell, Duffy, or Ss antigens. These antibodies make up the bulk of clinically significant antibodies. Antibodies not expected to cause RBC destruction are those that react only at temperatures below 37°C and IgG antibodies of the IgG2 or IgG4 subclass.[15]

HEMOLYTIC DISEASE OF THE NEWBORN

HDN is caused by blood group incompatibility between a sensitized mother and her antigen-positive fetus (see Chap. 53). The antibodies most significant in HDN are those that cross the placenta (IgG1 and IgG3), react at body temperature to cause red cell destruction, and are directed against well-developed RBC antigens. ABO incompatibility most commonly is seen, but ABO HDN is clinically mild, presumably because the antigens are not fully expressed at birth. Antibodies directed against the D antigen can cause severe HDN, and fetal health should be carefully monitored when anti-D titers are greater than 1:16. The severity of HDN is less predictable with other blood group antibodies and can vary from mild to severe. For example, anti-K not only causes red cell hemolysis but also may suppress erythropoiesis.[77]

AUTOIMMUNE HEMOLYTIC ANEMIA

Autoimmune hemolytic anemia is caused by the production of "warm-" or "cold-" reactive autoantibodies directed against RBC antigens.[51] Production can be triggered by disease, viral infection, or drugs; from breakdown in immune system tolerance to self-antigens; or from exposure to foreign antigens that induce antibodies that cross-react with self-RBC antigens. Autologous specificity is not always obvious because antigen expression can be depressed when autoantibody is present.[51]

Warm autoantibodies react best at 37°C and are primarily IgG (rarely IgM or IgA). Most are directed against the Rh protein, but Wr[b], Kell, Kidd, and U blood group specificities have been reported.

Cold-reactive autoantibodies are primarily IgM. They react best at temperatures below 25°C but can agglutinate RBCs or activate complement at or near 37°C, causing hemolysis or vascular occlusion upon exposure to cold.[15] Patients with cold agglutinin disease often have C3d on their RBCs, which can provide some protection from hemolysis. Most cold-reactive autoantibodies have anti-I activity. Reactivity with i, H, Pr, P, or other antigenic specificities is much less common.

The biphasic cold-reactive IgG antibody associated with paroxysmal cold hemoglobinuria ("Donath-Landsteiner" antibody) typically reacts with the high-prevalence antigen P. It attaches to RBCs in the cold and very efficiently activates complement before it dissociates at warmer temperatures.

DISEASES ASSOCIATED WITH ANTIBODY PRODUCTION

Table 128-4 lists diseases associated with specific antibody production. These antibodies cause autoimmune hemolytic anemia only if the patient carries the corresponding antigen.

SEROLOGIC DETECTION OF ERYTHROCYTE ANTIGENS AND ANTIBODIES

ABO

ABO grouping is the single most important test performed in the blood bank because it is the fundamental basis for determining blood compatibility. ABO grouping is determined by testing RBCs with licensed antisera to identify the A or B antigens they carry (forward, or cell, grouping) and by reacting the corresponding serum or plasma with known A and B cells to identify the antibodies present (reverse, or serum, grouping). Positive reactions are seen as hemagglutination or hemolysis, and the results of one test should confirm the results of the other.

If results are discrepant or reactions are weaker than expected, the cause must be investigated before the ABO group can be interpreted with confidence. Discrepancies can be related to RBC anomalies, serum anomalies, or both, and they may be associated with disease.[5,11,15,45,78] Common causes, excluding clerical and technical error, are listed in Table 128-6. If the ABO group of a patient cannot be determined, group O blood can be used for transfusion.

RH

The D type is the next most important test performed for blood compatibility. Individuals who type D+ are called *Rh positive*, and those who type D− are called *Rh negative*, provided controls are acceptable. Blood donors and pregnant women who type D− using standard typing sera are tested further for weak D expression using more sensitive methods, such as an indirect antiglobulin test. Donors with weak D antigen are considered Rh positive. Testing for weak D is optional for transfusion recipients.[73]

EXTENDED ANTIGEN PHENOTYPING

Reagent antisera to detect other common antigens (e.g., CcEe, MNSs, Kk, Fy[a]Fy[b], Jk[a]Jk[b]) are available but are used only when identification of the red cell phenotype is essential to antibody identification, blood

TABLE 128-6   COMMON CAUSES OF ABO DISCREPANCIES

Red cells may appear to have	
Weak or missing antigens	Weak subgroup of A or B antigen
	Excess soluble A or B antigen in plasma
	Disease-associated loss (leukemia)
	ABO nonidentical marrow transplantation
	ABO nonidentical RBC transfusions
Extra antigens	Positive direct antiglobulin test
	Antibody to reagent additive or dye
	Rouleaux or cold agglutinin on cells
	Disease-associated acquisition (polyagglutination)
Serum may appear to have	
Weak or missing antibody	Age-related (newborns or the very elderly)
	Disease-associated immunosuppression
	Congenital hypogammaglobulinemia
	ABO nonidentical marrow transplantation
Extra antibody	Alloantibodies (A$_1$, Le[a], Le[b], P$_1$, M, N)
	Autoantibodies (I, i, H, Pr, P)
	Rouleaux
	Antibodies to additives in reagent RBCs
	Passive antibody acquisition from transfusion or from passenger lymphocytes in organ transplantation

compatibility, determination of zygosity, or paternity or forensic issues. Extended phenotyping is especially important to patients who are at high risk for alloimmunization from chronic blood transfusion, for example, those with sickle cell anemia or thalassemia. Ideally, an extended RBC phenotype of these patients should be determined prior to initiation of transfusion therapy.

ANTIBODY SCREEN

The antibody screen, or indirect antiglobulin test, detects "atypical" or "unexpected" antibodies in the serum (i.e., other than anti-A and anti-B) using group O reagent red cells that are known to carry most common antigens. The methods used must be able to detect clinically significant antibodies. Typically, serum or plasma and screening cells are incubated at 37°C with an additive to potentiate antibody–antigen reactions, then an indirect antiglobulin test is performed. Hemagglutination or hemolysis at any point is a positive reaction, indicating the presence of naturally occurring or immune alloantibody or autoantibody. The antibody screen will not detect all atypical antibodies in serum, such as antibodies to low-incidence antigens not present on screening cells and antibodies that are not apparent at 37°C and in the antiglobulin phase.

DIRECT ANTIGLOBULIN TEST

The direct antiglobulin test (direct Coombs test) detects antibody or complement bound to RBCs *in vivo*. Red cells are washed free of serum and then mixed with antiglobulin reagents that agglutinate RBCs coated with IgG or the C3 component of complement.

Positive direct antiglobulin test results are associated with the following: (1) transfusion reactions, in which recipient alloantibody coats transfused donor RBCs or transfused donor antibody coats recipient RBCs; (2) HDN, in which maternal antibody crosses the placenta and coats fetal RBCs; (3) autoimmune hemolytic anemias, in which autoantibody coats the patient's own RBCs; (4) drug or drug–antibody complex interactions with RBCs that sometimes lead to hemolysis; (5) passenger lymphocyte syndrome, in which transient antibody produced by passenger lymphocytes from a transplanted organ coats recipient RBCs; and (6) hypergammaglobulinemia, in which Igs nonspecifically adsorb onto circulating RBCs.

A positive direct antiglobulin test result does not always indicate decreased red cell survival. As many as 10 percent of hospital patients and 0.1 percent of blood donors have a positive direct antiglobulin test result with no clinical indication of hemolysis.[11]

COMPATIBILITY TESTING

Compatibility testing refers to a collection of donor and recipient tests that are performed prior to red cell transfusion. The collecting facility

tests donors for ABO, Rh, and unexpected antibody. However, transfusing hospitals retest the ABO (and D on Rh-negative units) to verify the accuracy of the blood label.[73] Routine recipient testing includes an ABO, Rh, and antibody screening on a blood sample collected within 3 days of the intended transfusion. Results are checked against historical records to verify ABO, Rh, and antibody status.[73]

If the recipient has a negative antibody screening test result and no history of clinically significant antibodies, a serologic immediate spin cross-match between recipient serum and donor red cells or a "computer cross-match" (wherein computer software compares the ABO test results of both donor and recipient) is required to confirm ABO compatibility.[11,73]

If clinically significant antibodies are detected in a recipient's serum or previously were identified, red cell components should test negative for the corresponding antigens and should be cross-match compatible at 37°C and by the antiglobulin test. The chance of finding compatible units usually reflects the antigen incidence in the general population, that is, 91 percent of units should be compatible with a patient making anti-K because 9 percent of the population is K+. This reasoning will not be valid if the local donor population varies significantly from the general population. When more than one antibody is present, the probability of finding compatible blood is the product of the prevalence (probability) of each independent antigen tested. For example, only 21 percent of units will be compatible for the recipient having both anti-K and anti-Jk^a: [0.91 for K−] × [0.23 for Jk(a−)] = 0.21.

When multiple clinically significant antibodies or antibodies directed against high-incidence antigens are present, finding compatible units may be extremely difficult. Antibody producers should be encouraged to give autologous units prior to their elective blood needs. If the patient is not a candidate for autologous donation, compatible units may be found by testing the patient's siblings or by asking regional blood suppliers to check their rare donor inventories and files. Such procurement requires additional time.

Repeat donor testing and cross-matching are not performed for plasma and platelet components, but the recipient's ABO and Rh phenotypes must be known for appropriate selection of components. Table 128-7 gives general ABO-Rh compatibility guidelines.

ANTIBODY IDENTIFICATION

All unexpected antibodies should be investigated. Those detected in serum or plasma as an ABO discrepancy, a positive antibody screening result, or an incompatible cross-match are identified using a panel of eight to 16 different group O cells that have been typed for antigens corresponding to clinically significant antibodies. Serum reactions with these RBCs are compared to their antigen typing to determine

TABLE 128-7   ABO-RH COMPATIBILITY GUIDELINES

	ANTIGEN ON RED CELLS	ANTIBODY IN SERUM	COMPATIBLE BLOOD GROUPS	
			RECIPIENT SERUM	RECIPIENT CELLS
If recipient blood group is				
A	A	Anti-B	A, O	A, AB
B	B	Anti-A	B, O	B, AB
O	O	Anti-A, anti-B	O	O, A, B, AB
AB	A, B	None	AB, A, B, O	AB
Rh-positive	D	None	Rh positive, Rh negative	Rh not considered
Rh-negative	—	Anti-D only if immunized	Rh-negative	Rh not considered

Whole blood must be identical to recipient's blood group. RBC products must be compatible with recipient's serum. Plasma products should be compatible with recipient's RBCs. Platelet and cryoprecipitate products should be compatible with recipient's RBCs, but any ABO group can be given if compatible units are not available.

specificity.[11] For example, an antibody that reacts with all K+ RBCs but not with K− cells most likely is anti-K.

A control of autologous RBCs and serum is tested concurrently with panel RBCs. Absence of reactivity with autologous cells implies the antibody is an alloantibody, whereas a positive result suggests autoantibody or a positive direct antiglobulin test result. Once antibody specificity is identified, the patient's RBCs are tested for the corresponding antigen. If the alloantibody is anti-K, the cells should type K−. Such antigen typing helps to confirm serum findings.

When antibody is detected both on red cells (a positive direct antiglobulin test result) and in serum, only the antibody in serum is identified unless a review of the medical or transfusion history offers evidence that the antibodies might be different. When antibody is detected only on RBCs and in vivo hemolysis is suspected, the antibody can be eluted from the patient's RBCs and tested against panel RBCs to identify the specificity.

REFERENCES

1. Lewis M, Anstee DJ, Bird GWG, et al: Blood group terminology 1990. ISBT working party on terminology for red cell surface antigens. Vox Sang 58:152, 1990.
2. Lögdberg L, Reid ME, Miller JL: Cloning and genetic characterization of blood group carrier molecules and antigens. Transfus Med Rev 16:1, 2002.
3. Cartron JP, Bailly P, Le Van Kim C, et al: Insights into the structure and function of membrane polypeptides carrying blood group antigens. Vox Sang 74(suppl 2):29, 1998.
4. Daniels G: Human Blood Groups, 2nd ed. Blackwell Science, Oxford, 2002.
5. Issitt PD, Anstee DJ: Applied Blood Group Serology, 4th ed. Montgomery Scientific, Durham, NC, 1998.
6. Reid ME, Lomas-Francis C: Blood Group Antigen Facts Book, 2nd ed. Academic, San Diego, 2003.
7. Telen MJ: Erythrocyte blood group antigens: Not so simple after all. Blood 85:299, 1995.
8. Cartron JP, Colin Y: Structural and functional diversity of blood group antigens. Transfus Clin Biol 8:163, 2001.
9. Bruce LJ, Ghosh S, King MJ, et al: Absence of CD47 in protein 4.2-deficient hereditary spherocytosis in man: An interaction between the Rh complex and the band 3 complex. Blood 100:1878, 2002.
10. Reid ME, Mohandas N: Red blood cell blood group antigens: Structure and function. Semin Hematol 41:93, 2004.
11. Brecher ME, Combs MR, Drew MJ, et al: Technical Manual, 14th ed. American Association of Blood Banks, Bethesda, 2002.
12. Daniels GL, Cartron JP, Fletcher A, et al: International Society of Blood Transfusion Committee on terminology for red cell surface antigens: Vancouver report. Vox Sang 84:244, 2003.
13. Daniels GL, Anstee DJ, Cartron J-P, et al: Blood group terminology 1995. ISBT working party on terminology for red cell surface antigens. Vox Sang 69:265, 1995.
14. Garratty G, Dzik WH, Issitt PD, et al: Terminology for blood group antigens and genes: Historical origins and guidelines in the new millennium. Transfusion 40:477, 2000.
15. Mollison PL, Engelfriet CP, Contreras M: Blood Transfusion in Clinical Medicine, 10th ed. Blackwell Science, Oxford, 1997.
16. Cartron J-P, Rouger P: Blood Cell Biochemistry, Vol 6. Molecular Basis of Human Blood Group Antigens. Plenum, New York, 1995.
17. Clausen H, White T, Takio K, et al: Isolation to homogeneity and partial characterization of a histo-blood group A defined Fucα1→2Galα1→3-N-acetylgalactosaminyltransferase from human lung tissue. J Biol Chem 265:1139, 1990.
18. Yamamoto F, Marken J, Tsuji T, et al: Cloning and characterization of DNA complementary to human UDP-GalNAc: Fucα1→2Galα1→3GalNAc transferase (histo-blood group A transferase) mRNA. J Biol Chem 265:1146, 1990.
19. Yamamoto F, Hakomori S: Sugar-nucleotide donor specificity of histo-blood group A and B transferases is based on amino acid substitutions. J Biol Chem 265:19257, 1990.
20. Yamamoto F, Clausen H, White T, et al: Molecular genetic basis of the histo-blood group ABO system. Nature 345:229, 1990.
21. Chester MA, Olsson ML: The ABO blood group gene: A locus of considerable genetic diversity. Transfus Med Rev 15:177, 2001.
22. Yamamoto F, McNeill PD, Kominato Y, et al: Molecular genetic analysis of the ABO blood group system: 2. cis-AB alleles. Vox Sang 64:120, 1993.
23. Yamamoto F, McNeill PD, Yamamoto M, et al: Molecular genetic analysis of the ABO blood group system: 3. A(X) and B(A) alleles. Vox Sang 64:171, 1993.
24. Olsson ML, Chester MA: Polymorphism and recombination events at the ABO locus: A major challenge for genomic ABO blood grouping strategies. Transfus Med 11:295, 2001.
25. Avent ND, Reid ME: The Rh blood group system: A review. Blood 95:375, 2000.
26. Tippett P, Lomas-Francis C, Wallace M: The Rh antigen D: Partial D antigens and associated low incidence antigens. Vox Sang 70:123, 1996.
27. Huang C-H, Liu PZ, Cheng JG: Molecular biology and genetics of the Rh blood group system. Semin Hematol 37:150, 2000.
28. Reid ME: Applications of DNA-based assays in blood group antigen and antibody identification. Transfusion 43:1748, 2003.
29. Giblett ER: A critique of the theoretical hazard of inter vs. intra-racial transfusion. Transfusion 1:233, 1961.
30. Tippett P: Regulator genes affecting red cell antigens. Transfus Med Rev 4:56, 1990.
31. Marsh WL, Johnson CL, Mueller KA: Proposed new notation for the In(Lu) modifying gene. Transfusion 24:371, 1984.
32. Okubo Y, Yamaguchi H, Nagao N, et al: Heterogeneity of the phenotype Jk(a-b-) found in Japanese. Transfusion 26:237, 1986.
33. Clausen H, Hakomori S: ABH and related histo-blood group antigens; immunochemical differences in carrier isotypes and their distribution. Vox Sang 56:1, 1989.
34. Hakomori S: Blood group ABH and Ii antigens of human erythrocytes: Chemistry, polymorphism, and their developmental change. Semin Hematol 18:39, 1981.
35. Spitalnik PF, Spitalnik SL: The P blood group system: Biochemical, serological, and clinical aspects. Transfus Med Rev 9:110, 1995.
36. Pogo AO, Chaudhuri A: The Duffy protein: A malarial and chemokine receptor. Semin Hematol 37:122, 2000.
37. Yomtovian R, Prince GM, Medof ME: The molecular basis for paroxysmal nocturnal hemoglobinuria. Transfusion 33:852, 1993.
38. Araten DJ, Swirsky D, Karadimitris A, et al: Cytogenetic and morphological abnormalities in paroxysmal nocturnal haemoglobinuria. Br J Haematol 115:360, 2001.
39. Tippett P, Ellis NA: The Xg blood group system: A review. Transfus Med Rev 12:233, 1998.
40. Cartron J-P, Rahuel C: Human erythrocyte glycophorins: Protein and gene structure analyses. Transfus Med Rev 6:63, 1992.
41. Tournamille C, Colin Y, Cartron JP, Le Van Kim C: Disruption of a GATA motif in the Duffy gene promoter abolishes erythroid gene expression in Duffy-negative individuals. Nat Genet 10:224, 1995.
42. Mourant AE, Kopec AC, Domaniewska-Sobczak K: Distribution of the Human Blood Groups and Other Polymorphisms, 2nd ed. Oxford University, London, 1976.
43. Mollison PL, Engelfriet CP, Contreras M: Blood Transfusion in Clinical Medicine, Blackwell Science, London, 1997.

44. Mourant AE, Kopec AC, Domaniewska-Sobczak K: *Blood Groups and Diseases: A Study of Associations of Disease as with Blood Groups and Other Polymorphisms.* Oxford University, Oxford, 1978.

45. Reid ME, Bird GW: Associations between human red cell blood group antigens and disease. *Transfus Med Rev* 4:47, 1990.

46. Issitt PD: Null red blood cell phenotypes: Associated biological changes. *Transfus Med Rev* 7:139, 1993.

47. Kallenius G, Mollby R, Svenson SB, et al: Occurrence of P-fimbriated *Escherichia coli* in urinary tract infections. *Lancet* 2:1369, 1981.

48. Kallenius G, Svenson S, Mollby R, et al: Structure of carbohydrate part of receptor on human uroepithelial cells for pyelonephritogenic *Escherichia coli. Lancet* 2:604, 1981.

49. Hadley TJ, Miller LH, Haynes JD: Recognition of red cells by malaria parasites: The role of erythrocyte-binding proteins. *Transfus Med Rev* 5:108, 1991.

50. Nichols ME, Rubinstein P, Barnwell J, et al: A new human Duffy blood group specificity defined by a murine monoclonal antibody. Immunogenetics and association with susceptibility to *Plasmodium vivax. J Exp Med* 166:776, 1987.

51. Petz LD, Garratty G: *Acquired Immune Hemolytic Anemias,* 2nd ed. Churchill Livingstone, New York, 2003.

52. Carratty G: *Blood Group Antigens and Disease.* American Association of Blood Banks, Arlington, 1983.

53. Gerbal A, Maslet C, Salmon C: Immunological aspects of the acquired B antigen. *Vox Sang* 28:398, 1975.

54. Gerbal A, Ropars C, Gerbal R, et al: Acquired B antigen disappearance by in vitro acetylation associated with A1 activity restoration. *Vox Sang* 31:64, 1976.

55. Moulds JM, Moulds JJ: Blood group associations with parasites, bacteria, and viruses. *Transfus Med Rev* 14:302, 2000.

56. Cartron JP: Molecular basis of red cell protein antigen deficiencies. *Vox Sang* 78:7, 2000.

57. Lee S, Russo D, Redman CM: The Kell blood group system: Kell and XK membrane proteins. *Semin Hematol* 37:113, 2000.

58. Marsh WL, Redman CM: The Kell blood group system: A review. *Transfusion* 30:158, 1990.

59. Danek A, Rubio JP, Rampoldi L, et al: McLeod neuroacanthocytosis: Genotype and phenotype. *Ann Neurol* 50:755, 2001.

60. Reid ME, Spring FA: Molecular basis of glycophorin C variants and their associated blood group antigens. *Transfus Med* 4:139, 1994.

61. Luhn K, Wild MK, Eckhardt M, et al: The gene defective in leukocyte adhesion deficiency II encodes a putative GDP-fucose transporter. *Nat Genet* 28:69, 2001.

62. Etzioni A, Tonetti M: Leukocyte adhesion deficiency II-from A to almost Z. *Immunol Rev* 178:138, 2000.

63. Yu L-C, Twu Y-C, Chang C-Y, Lin M: Molecular basis of the adult i phenotype and the gene responsible for the expression of the human blood group I antigen. *Blood* 98:3840, 2001.

64. Inaba N, Hiruma T, Togayachi A, et al: A novel I—branching b-1,6-*N*-acetylglucosaminyltransferase involved in human blood group I antigen expression. *Blood* 101:2870, 2003.

65. Yu LC, Twu YC, Chou ML, et al: The molecular genetics of the human I locus and molecular background explaining the partial association of the adult i phenotype with congenital cataracts. *Blood* 101:2081, 2003.

66. Agre P, King LS, Yasui M, et al: Aquaporin water channels: From atomic structure to clinical medicine. *J Physiol (Lond)* 542:3, 2002.

67. Daniels GL, Levene C, Berrebi A, et al: Human alloantibodies detecting a red cell antigen apparently identical to MER2. *Vox Sang* 55:161, 1988.

68. Crew VK, Green CA, Daniels G, Anstee DJ: Renal failure associated with an inactivating mutation in the human *CD151* gene of three individuals lacking the MER2 blood group [abstract]. *Blood* 102(11 Part 1): 4a, 2003.

69. Rock JA, Shirey RS, Braine HG, et al: Plasmapheresis for the treatment of repeated early pregnancy wastage associated with anti-P. *Obstet Gynecol* 66(suppl 3):57S, 1985.

70. Udden MM, Umeda M, Hirano Y, Marcus DM: New abnormalities in the morphology, cell surface receptors, and electrolyte metabolism of In(Lu) erythrocytes. *Blood* 69:52, 1987.

71. Heaton DC, McLoughlin K: Jk(a-b-) red blood cells resist urea lysis. *Transfusion* 22:70, 1982.

72. Sands JM: Molecular mechanisms of urea transport. *J Membr Biol* 191: 149, 2003.

73. Standards Committee of American Association of Blood Banks: *Standards for Blood Banks and Transfusion Services,* 22nd ed. American Associations of Blood Banks, Bethesda, 2003.

74. Springer GF, Horton RE, Forbes M: Origin of anti-human blood group B agglutinins in white leghorn chicks. *J Exp Med* 110:221, 1959.

75. Springer GF, Horton RE: Blood group isoantibody stimulation in man by feeding blood group-active bacteria. *J Clin Invest* 48:1280, 1969.

76. Roitt I, Brostoff J, Male DK: *Immunology,* 6th ed. Mosby, London, 2001.

77. Vaughan JI, Warwick R, Letsky E, et al: Erythropoietic suppression in fetal anemia because of Kell alloimmunization. *Am J Obstet Gynecol* 171:247, 1994.

78. Quinley ED: *Immunohematology: Principles and Practice,* 2nd ed. Lippincott, Philadelphia, 1998.

HUMAN LEUKOCYTE AND PLATELET ANTIGENS

KAREN A. SULLIVAN

THOMAS J. KIPPS

The human leukocyte antigens (HLAs) are polymorphic cell surface glycoproteins that present antigen peptide fragments to T cell receptors. The HLAs are encoded by multiple, closely linked genes, located in a 4-Mb region of DNA on chromosome 6, that compose the major histocompatibility complex (MHC) and play a central role in the regulation of immune responses. In general, the MHC genes are inherited as a single unit in simple mendelian fashion. The products of the MHC HLA-A, HLA-B, and HLA-C genes are called _class I antigens_. Class I antigens are expressed on essentially all tissues in the body and present small peptide fragments to CD8+ T cells. The HLA-DR, HLA-DQ, and HLA-DP genes of the MHC encode class II antigens. Class II antigens present antigen peptide fragments to CD4+ T cells and are limited in expression primarily to B cells, monocytes, and macrophages. The HLA antigens are the principal barriers to transplantation. The degree of similarity between donor and recipient HLA antigens determines the risk of allograft rejection and, in the case of stem cell transplantation, the risk of graft-versus-host disease. In addition to the HLAs, platelets express glycoproteins that can be recognized by autoantibodies or by antibodies made by recipients of platelet transfusions. The latter result from platelet alloantigens that reflect polymorphism in the genes encoding major platelet glycoproteins. Immune responses to platelet alloantigens are involved in the pathogenesis of several clinical syndromes, including neonatal alloimmune thrombocytopenia, posttransfusion purpura, and refractory responses to platelet transfusion. This chapter describes the major platelet autoantigens and outlines typing strategies used for effective platelet transfusion therapy or treatment of neonatal alloimmune thrombocytopenia.

Acronyms and abbreviations that appear in this chapter include: β_2M, β_2-microglobulin; CTL, cytotoxic T lymphocyte; ER, endoplasmic reticulum; F-SSCP, fluorescent-based single-stranded conformation polymorphism; GVHD, graft-versus-host disease; HLA, human leukocyte antigen; HPA, human platelet antigen; HTC, homozygous typing cells; ILT, immunoglobulin-like transcript; IMGT, ImMunoGeneTics; LMP, low molecular weight protein; MHC, major histocompatibility complex; MLC, mixed lymphocyte culture; MLR, mixed lymphocyte reaction; NK, natural killer; PCR, polymerase chain reaction; PLT, prime lymphocyte test; RFLP, restriction fragment length polymorphism; SSCP, single-stranded conformation polymorphism; SSOP, sequence-specific oligonucleotide probe hybridization; SSP, sequence-specific primer amplification; TAP, transporter-associated-with-antigen processing; TCR, T cell receptor; TNF, tumor necrosis factor; WMDA, World Marrow Donor Association.

HUMAN LEUKOCYTE ANTIGENS

DEFINITION

The human leukocyte antigens (HLAs) are highly polymorphic glycoproteins encoded by a cluster of genes on the short arm of chromosome 6.[1] The genes encoding the HLAs compose the major histocompatibility complex (MHC) because, next to the ABO system, the MHC is the principal barrier to transplantation. As products of the genes influencing the outcome of transplanted tissue or organs, the HLA molecules are called _histocompatibility antigens_. The biologic function of HLA molecules, however, is the presentation of antigenic peptides to T cells (see Chap. 78).

The HLA antigens are divided into six major groups: HLA-A, HLA-B, HLA-C, HLA-DR, HLA-DQ, and HLA-DP. These groups are subdivided into classes of antigens designated class I and class II, representing the two types of HLA molecules. The HLA-A, HLA-B, and HLA-C antigens are the classic class I antigens. A few "nonclassic" class I molecules are designated HLA-E, HLA-F, and HLA-G. The HLA-DR, HLA-DQ, and HLA-DP antigens are the class II antigens. The classic class I antigens were the first and most easily identified on leukocytes by antigen and antibody reactions, that is, by serologic techniques. The class II antigens originally were defined by lymphocyte proliferation assays such as the mixed lymphocyte reaction (MLR) or primed lymphocyte test (PLT) and only later were identified by serologic techniques. The antigens identified by such cellular assays were designated _HLA-Dw_. The HLA-Dw antigens (or specificities) now are known to be an _in vitro_ measure of T cell responses to the cumulative effects of the allotypic HLA-DR, HLA-DQ, and HLA-DP antigens. The class I antigens are ubiquitous in tissue distribution, found on most nucleated cells of the body. HLA class II antigens have a more restricted distribution than class I antigens. Class II antigens primarily are found on B lymphocytes, monocytes, macrophages, dendritic cells, and endothelial cells. However, class II antigens can be induced on other cell types through activation.[2]

Class I antigens are encoded by genes at the HLA-A, HLA-B, and HLA-C loci on chromosome 6. Class II antigens are encoded by genes at the HLA-DR, HLA-DQ, and HLA-DP loci on the chromosome. Class I and class II protein molecules are highly homologous to each other, that is, they share most of their amino acid sequences. However, the amino acid residues at small segments of the molecules vary from each other. These areas of variability (polymorphism) in amino acid sequences distinguish individual HLA molecules and confer antigen specificity. Each HLA locus can code for one of many HLA antigens. Thus, each HLA locus has multiple alleles (alternative or variant forms of genes). Although multiple possible alleles encode different antigens, each individual carries only one of the possible alleles at each HLA locus on each chromosome. Therefore, each person expresses only two of the many HLA-A antigens, two HLA-B antigens, and so on. Table 129-1 provides a complete list of recognized antigens.[3]

BIOCHEMISTRY

CLASS I ANTIGENS

Classic HLA Class I Antigens The HLA-A, HLA-B, and HLA-C molecules are transmembrane glycoproteins with an M_r of 56,000.[4] They are heterodimers consisting of noncovalently bound protein chains: an α heavy chain ($M_r = 45,000$) and a β light chain ($M_r = 11,000$). The α heavy chain is the polymorphic glycoprotein encoded by the HLA genes. It consists of an NH2-terminal extracellular hydrophilic region, a transmembrane hydrophobic region, and an intracellular hydrophilic region, the COOH-terminus. The extracellular region of the α heavy chain consists of three domains (α_1, α_2, α_3) based upon its folding and disulfide bonding. Each of these domains contains approximately 90 amino acids. Antigenic specificity resides in the α_1 and

TABLE 129-1 COMPLETE LISTING OF RECOGNIZED HLA SPECIFICITIES

A	B			C	D*	DR			DQ	DP
A1	B5	B47	B77(15)	Cw1	Dw1	DR1	DR13(6)	DR51	DQ1	DPw1
A2	B7	B48	B78	Cw2	Dw2	DR103	DR14(6)	DR52	DQ2	DPw2
A203	B703	B49(21)	B81	Cw3	Dw3	DR2	DR1403	DR53	DQ3	DPw3
A210	B8	B50(21)		Cw4	Dw4	DR3	DR1404		DQ4	DPw4
A3	B12	B51(5)		Cw5	Dw5	DR4	DR15(2)		DQ5(1)	DPw5
A9	B13	B5102		Cw6	Dw6	DR5	DR16(2)		DQ6(1)	DPw6
A10	B14	B5103	Bw4	Cw7	Dw7	DR6	DR17(3)		DQ7(3)	
A11	B15	B52(5)	Bw6	Cw8	Dw8	DR7	DR18(3)		DQ8(3)	
A19	B16	B53		Cw9(w3)	Dw9	DR8			DQ9(3)	
A23(9)	B17	B54(22)		Cw10(w3)	Dw10	DR9				
A24(9)	B18	B55(22)			Dw11(w7)	DR10				
A2403	B21	B56(22)			Dw12	DR11(5)				
A25(10)	B22	B57(17)			Dw13	DR12(5)				
A26(10)	B27	B58(17)			Dw14					
A28	B2708	B59			Dw15					
A29(19)	B35	B60(40)			Dw16					
A30(19)	B37	B61(40)			Dw17(w7)					
A31(19)	B38(16)	B62(15)			Dw18(w6)					
A32(19)	B39(16)	B63(15)			Dw19(w6)					
A33(19)	B3901	B64(14)			Dw20					
A34(10)	B3902	B65(14)			Dw21					
A36	B40	B67			Dw22					
A43	B4005	B70			Dw23					
A66(10)	B41	B71(70)			Dw24v					
A68(28)	B42	B72(70)			Dw25					
A69(28)	B44(12)	B73			Dw26					
A74(19)	B45(12)	B75(15)								
A80	B46	B76(15)								

Numbers in parentheses indicate the broad antigens for which the adjacent antigen is a split (variant).
*No single molecule is associated with HLA-D. Each HLA-D specificity is the cumulative effect of allogeneic differences of multiple class II molecules.

α_2 extracellular domains (Fig. 129-1, B). The β light chain is β_2-microglobulin (β_2M), a nonpolymorphic globular protein encoded by a gene on chromosome 15, which stabilizes the class I molecule on the cell surface.

Nonclassic HLA Class I Antigens In addition to the classic class I molecules are three types of nonclassic HLA class I molecules that each has a biochemical structure similar to that of classic HLA class I molecules.[5,6] These nonclassic HLA class I molecules include HLA-E, HLA-F, and HLA-G. These nonclassic HLA class I molecules are relatively nonpolymorphic in comparison to the classic HLA class I antigens and appear capable of binding a more limited array of different peptides. For example, the peptide-binding site of the relatively nonpolymorphic HLA-E molecules is highly hydrophobic. The binding grooves of the other nonclassic HLA class I antigens appear similarly restricted. Although tetramers of these molecules indicate that each can complex with β_2M,[7] whether HLA-F molecules physiologically complex with β_2M *in vivo* is uncertain.

CLASS II ANTIGENS

The class II antigens also are transmembrane glycoproteins formed by two noncovalently bound protein chains[8]: an α heavy chain (M_r = 34,000) and a β light chain (M_r = 29,000). Both chains are encoded by genes in the HLA region. Class II HLA molecules, like class I molecules, also consist of an extracellular hydrophilic NH_2-terminal region, a hydrophobic transmembrane region, and an intracellular COOH-terminus region. Unlike class I molecules, however, the extracellular region of each chain contains only two domains. The two domains of the α-chain are designated α_1 and α_2, and the two domains

of the β-chain are designated β_1 and β_2. The α-chain of HLA-DR is constant for all HLA-DR molecules, whereas the β-chain is polymorphic and determines the specificity of the molecule. Both the α- and β-chains of HLA-DQ and HLA-DP molecules are polymorphic, although the α-chain is less so than the β-chain. Polymorphism of class II molecules resides predominantly in the β_1 domain of the β-chain. The α_2 and β_2 domains show significant amino acid homology with β_2M, α_3 domains of HLA class I molecules, and immunoglobulin constant-region domains (see Chap. 78).

STRUCTURE

Crystallization of the HLA-A2 class I antigen and subsequently the HLA-DR1 class II antigen has greatly increased our knowledge of the structure and function of the HLA molecules.[9,10] The first and second α-chain domains of HLA-A2 form an interactive platform composed of a single β-pleated sheet "floor" topped by two α-helical structures with a cleft or groove between the α helices. This interactive structure is distal to the cell surface and is supported by the α_3 domain of the HLA α heavy chain and the β_2M molecule (see Fig. 129-1). The structure of HLA-DR1 is essentially similar to the structure of class I HLA molecules. In the case of class II, however, the α_1 domain of the α-chain and the β_1 domain of the β-chain form the interactive structure of two α helices and a β-pleated sheet floor. The tertiary structure of the α_2 and β_2 domains corresponds to β_2M and the class I α_3 domain, respectively. Polymorphic residues of the HLA class I and class II molecules are predominantly at positions within the α helices and the floor formed by the β-pleated sheet. Antigenic peptide fragments are

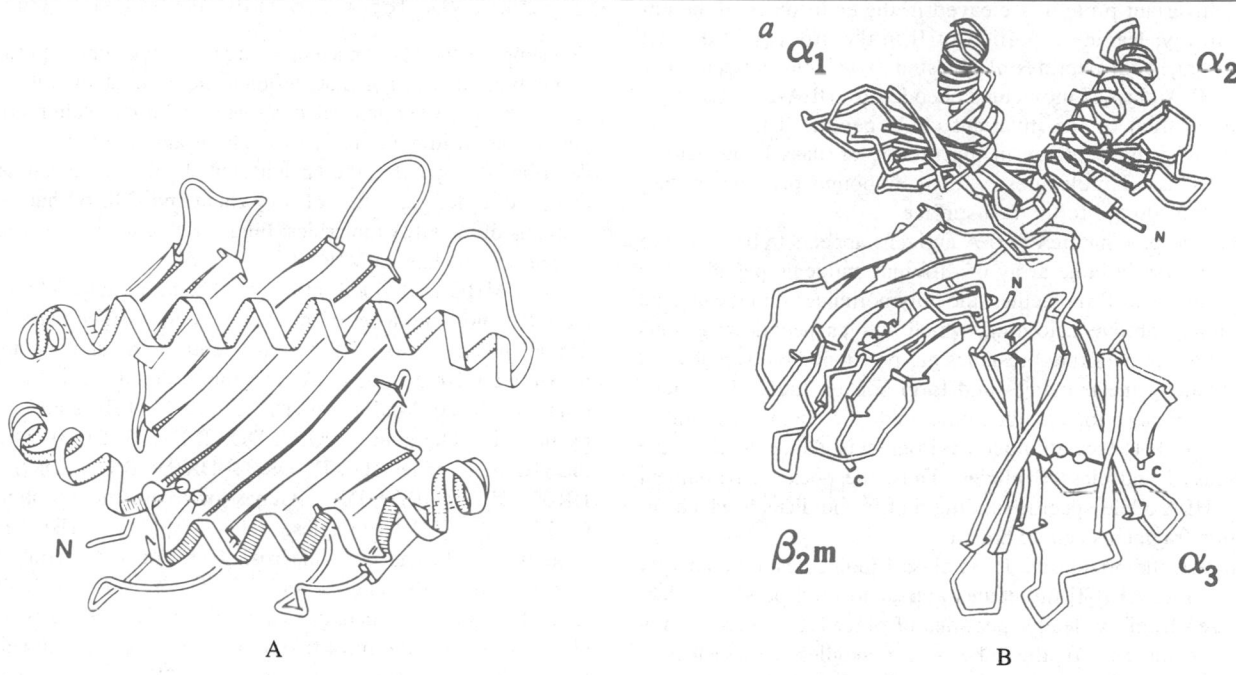

FIGURE 129-1   Schematic representation of the HLA-A2 molecule. *(A)* β strands are shown as *broad arrows* and the α helices as *helical ribbons*. A "pocket" or "groove" is formed by the α helices and a β-pleated sheet. The former form the rim of the pocket, and the latter forms the floor. The groove holds the processed piece of antigen for presentation to the T cell receptor in the orientation shown. N, amino-terminus of the chain. *(B)* Schematic representation of the entire molecule showing the four domains of the molecule. The α helices are present in the α₁ and α₂ domains. C and N represent the carboxy-terminus and amino-terminus of the two chains forming the molecule, respectively. (Both diagrams from PJ Bjorkman and colleagues.[9] From *Nature* 329:506, 1987, with permission. Copyright 1987 Macmillan Journals Limited.)

bound within the groove of the interactive structure for presentation to the T cell receptor (TCR) (see Chap. 78).[11,12]

TISSUE DISTRIBUTION

HLA antigen expression is especially high on leukocytes. Because of their easy availability, lymphocytes are used to identify HLA types. However, class I HLA-A, HLA-B, and HLA-C antigens are found on most normal tissues, including platelets.[13] Although platelets express class I antigens, they often lack expression of some HLA-B antigens and most HLA-C antigens.[14] Evidence indicates that some of the HLA antigens on platelets are absorbed from the plasma.[15] The class II antigens HLA-DR, HLA-DP, and HLA-DQ are more restricted in their distribution, being found primarily on B lymphocytes. Class II antigens may be found to a lesser degree on dendritic cells, endothelial cells, monocytes, macrophages, and activated, but not resting, T cells.[8] Expression or increased expression of class II antigens can be induced by treatment with interferon gamma.

Expression of the nonclassic HLA class I molecules HLA-G and HLA-F appears more restricted than that of other HLA antigens. Expression of HLA-G molecules is mostly confined to the placental trophoblast. Although the genes encoding HLA-F molecules are transcribed in a variety of cell types, whether the molecules are expressed on the cell surface plasma membrane is not known.

FUNCTION OF THE HUMAN LEUKOCYTE ANTIGENS

The function of the class I and class II molecules is to bind peptide fragments that have been derived by the intracellular degradation of protein antigens and to present them to T cells (see Chap. 78). TCR recognition of MHC peptide complexes is restricted by the class of HLA molecule.[16] CD4+ T cells recognize antigen peptides bound by

class II molecules, and CD8+ T cells recognize antigen peptides bound by class I molecules (see Chap. 78). Both classes of HLA molecules bind peptide fragments in the groove or cleft formed by the β-pleated sheet floor and the two α helices of the molecule, that is, the interactive platform (see Fig. 129-1).[11,12] The class I binding groove is closed at each end with conserved amino acid residues that bind amino-terminal and carbonyl-terminal peptide residues. Because the groove is closed at each end, binding peptides are restricted in length to eight to 11 amino acid residues. The middle portions of binding peptides can bulge out toward the TCR. The class II binding groove, on the other hand, is open at each end and binds peptides of between 15 and 24 residues in an extended conformation.

In addition to presenting antigen to different T cell subsets and binding peptides of different lengths, class I and class II molecules differ with regard to the source or type of peptide antigen they present.[17] Class I molecules present peptides derived from endogenous proteins synthesized within the cell (cytosol), such as virus-encoded proteins. Class II molecules present peptides derived from exogenous antigens that are ingested by the cell, such as bacterial pathogens. Class I molecules are assembled in the endoplasmic reticulum (ER), and peptides must be transported into the ER to bind empty class I molecules. Genes encoding the low molecular weight protein (LMP) and transporter-associated-with-antigen processing (TAP) complex map within the MHC complex. The products of these genes function in antigen peptide production (LMP), transport of peptides into the ER, and assembly of peptide–class I complexes (TAP). Class I molecules are unstable without bound peptide and are rapidly degraded. Class II molecules also are assembled in the ER as multimers of three class II molecules with invariant chain (Ii or CD74) proteins inserted in their grooves. The invariant chain is required for folding, transport, and peptide loading of class II molecules. The invariant protein is cleaved in the endosomes of the endocytic pathway, leaving a portion of Ii in the groove (CLIP) that then is exchanged for peptides of digested exogenous antigens. The nonclassic HLA class II molecules encoded by HLA-DM genes facilitate dissociation of the invariant chain peptide, CLIP, and the loading of antigenic peptides in the groove of class II molecules. Class I and class II molecules, with their bound peptides, subsequently are transported to the cell surface.

The polymorphic nature of HLA antigens appears to be related to the need to present a huge array of different antigenic peptides. For both class I and class II molecules, the polymorphic residues clustered in their binding groove determine which antigen peptide fragments can bind. These polymorphic residues are positioned outward toward the TCR or along the α helices and form pockets along the groove that have preferences for certain amino acid side chains of peptides. The binding pockets create unique environments characteristic of the different class I and class II alleles. Thus, the pocket environment determines HLA allele-specific binding motifs and dictates which antigen peptide fragments can be bound.

In contrast, the nonclassic HLA class I molecules are relatively nonpolymorphic. HLA-E molecules appear to bind peptides selectively derived from the leader peptides of other HLA class I heavy chains. The complexes of these HLA-E molecules with such peptides can serve as ligands for the natural killer (NK) cell receptors CD94:NKG2A and CD94:NKG2C (see Chap. 79).[6,18] HLA-E may be expressed by some tumors that have very low expression of the classic HLA class I molecules (e.g., HLA-A, HLA-B, HLA-C), raising the possibility that HLA-E contributes to the resistance of such tumors to recognition and clearance by NK cells.[19] Tetramers made of HLA-G molecules were found to interact with immunoglobulin-like transcript (ILT)-2 and ILT-4 receptors and may serve as receptors for NK cells.[7] In addition, studies suggest that HLA-G molecules play a role in regulating maternal–fetal immune interactions and in circumventing NK cell recognition of certain tumors.[20–22] The functional role of HLA-F molecules is not established.

GENETICS OF THE MAJOR HISTOCOMPATIBILITY COMPLEX

The genes of the MHC encompass a DNA segment of approximately 4000 kb on the short arm of chromosome 6. In addition to genes that encode the HLA antigens are other genes whose protein products also play a role in immune responses. The α and β terminology used to describe HLA genes is the same as, but should not be confused with, that used to designate the α heavy-chain and β light-chain structural domains of the HLA molecules. Figure 129-2 shows the arrangement of genes in the human MHC.[23]

The MHC is divided into several gene regions: class I genes, class II genes, and a set of intervening genes called class III genes. The HLA class II loci are the most centromeric and encompass approximately 1000 kb of DNA. They are ordered sequentially, beginning with the HLA-DP genes (DPβ2, DPα2, DPβ1, DPα1), followed by the HLA-DQ genes (DQβ2, DQα2, DQβ3, DQβ1, DQα1) and the HLA-DR genes (DRβ1, DRβ2, DRβ3, DRβ4, DRβ5, DRβ6, DRβ7, DRβ8, DRβ9, DRα). Genes for complement proteins (C4A, C4B, Bf, C2), 21-hydroxylase deficiency (21A, 21B), heat shock protein (hsp70), and tumor necrosis factor (TNF) separate the class II region from the class I region.[23] These genes are collectively termed *class III* and encompass approximately 1000 kb of DNA. The class I genes are the most telomeric, covering approximately 2000 kb of DNA, and include, in order, class III, HLA-B, HLA-C, and HLA-A genes. Interspersed within the class I and class II regions are other genes, some involved in antigen processing (LMP), some involved in peptide transport (TAP) and loading (HLA-DMA, HLA-DMB), some that are nonfunctional (i.e., pseudogenes), and some whose functions await elucidation. Table 129-2 lists the currently recognized HLA genes.

Class I antigens are encoded by a single α-chain gene at each locus, that is, HLA-A, HLA-B, and HLA-C. Class II antigens are encoded by one α-chain gene and one β-chain gene. Genetic polymorphism is found in both the α- and β-chains of HLA-DP and HLA-DQ, although to a lesser degree in the α-chain. All detected serologic specificities, however, appear to reside on the β-chain. The HLA-DR molecules are

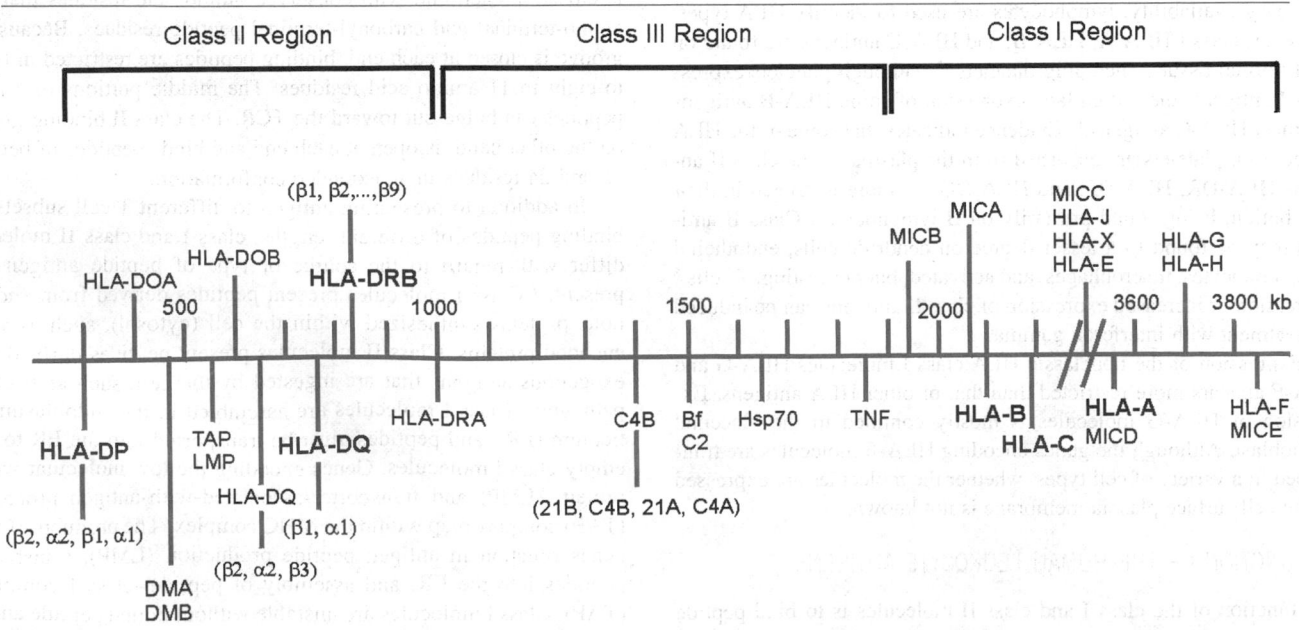

FIGURE 129-2   Representative diagram of the genes of the major histocompatibility complex on chromosome 6. The centromere is on the *left side*. For discussion, see "Genetics of the Major Histocompatibility Complex." (Adapted and simplified from R Campbell and J Trowsdale.[23])

TABLE 129-2 NAMES FOR GENES IN THE HLA REGION

NAME	PRODUCT
Class I genes	
HLA-A	Class I α-chain
HLA-B	Class I α-chain
HLA-C	Class I α-chain
HLA-E	Nonclassic class I α-chain
HLA-F	Nonclassic class I α-chain
HLA-G	Nonclassic class I α-chain
HLA-H	Class I pseudogene
HLA-J	Class I pseudogene
HLA-K	Class I pseudogene
HLA-L	Class I pseudogene
Class II genes	
HLA-DRA	DR α-chain
HLA-DRB1	DR β₁-chain determining specificities DR1, DR2, DR3, etc.
HLA-DRB2	Pseudogene with DR β-like sequences
HLA-DRB3	DR β₃-chain determining DR52 and Dw24, Dw25, Dw26 specificities
HLA-DRB4	DR β₄-chain determining DR53
HLA-DRB5	DR β₅-chain determining DR51
HLA-DRB6	DRB pseudogene found with DR1, DR2, DR10
HLA-DRB7	DRB pseudogene found with DR4, DR7, DR9
HLA-DRB8	DRB pseudogene found with DR4, DR7, DR9
HLA-DRB9	DRB pseudogene, isolated fragment
HLA-DQA1	DQ α-chain as expressed
HLA-DQB1	DQ β-chain as expressed
HLA-DQA2	DQ α-chain–related sequence, not expressed
HLA-DQB2	DQ β-chain–related sequence, not expressed
HLA-DQB3	DQ β-chain–related sequence, not expressed
HLA-DOA	DO α-chain
HLA-DOB	DO β-chain
HLA-DMA	DM α-chain
HLA-DMB	DM β-chain
HLA-DPA1	DP α-chain as expressed
HLA-DPB1	DP β-chain as expressed
HLA-DPA2	DP α-chain–related pseudogene
HLA-DPB2	DP β-chain–related pseudogene
Other	
TAP1	ABC (ATP binding cassette) transporter
TAP2	ABC (ATP binding cassette) transporter
LMP2	Protease-related sequence
LMP7	Protease-related sequence
MICA	Class I chain-related gene
MICB	Class I chain-related gene
MICC	Class I chain-related pseudogene
MICD	Class I chain-related pseudogene
MICE	Class I chain-related pseudogene

SOURCE: Adapted from JG Bodmer and coworkers.[24]

unique in that the product of one α-chain gene, which is not polymorphic, combines with any one of the products of the four functional β-chain genes (DRB1, DRB3, DRB4, DRB5) to generate class II molecules that have different serologic specificities. All HLA-DR antigens except DR51, DR52, and DR53 arise from polymorphism in the DRB1 gene. Most individuals express two β-chain gene products per chromosome or haplotype, one from DRB1 and another from DRB3, DRB4, or DRB5. Exceptions are individuals with the DR1, DR103, DR10, and DR8 antigens in whom only the DRB1 gene is expressed. The DR51, DR52, and DR53 serologic specificities are encoded by the DRB5, DRB3, and DRB4 genes, respectively. Different combinations of DRB1 alleles and DRB3, DRB4, or DRB5 are expressed, depending on the haplotype. DRB3 (DR52) is found on haplotypes with the DRB1 alleles encoding DR3, DR5, DR6, DR11, DR12, DR13, DR14, DR1403, DR1404, DR17, and DR18. DRB4 (DR53) is found with the DRB1 alleles encoding DR4, DR7, and DR9. DRB5 is found with DRB1 alleles encoding DR2, DR15, and DR16.

With the presence of genes that encode complement components or molecules involved in antigen processing (LMP1, LMP7) or peptide transport into the ER (TAP1, TAP2), the MHC is a complex of genes that encode molecules that are immunologically relevant.

NOMENCLATURE

Distinguishing polymorphic variations that are defined serologically or by cellular assay from those that are defined by molecular techniques is important. Serologically and cellularly defined entities are designated as *specificities* or *antigens*, whereas the terms *gene* and *allele* are reserved for loci defined by nucleic acid analyses.[3] As new loci, genes, alleles, and antigens within the MHC are recognized, the terminology used is standardized by the World Health Organization through an HLA Nomenclature Committee. The reports of this committee describe the naming of new HLA genes, alleles, and serologic specificities.[3,24] The latest report also contains complete lists of all the accepted genes and alleles and the serologically and cellularly defined specificities.[24]

The number of MHC class I and class II gene alleles is too numerous to include here (Table 129-3).[3,6,24] In 1998, the ImMunoGeneTics (IMGT)/HLA database became the official repository for HLA sequences.[25] The web site provides tools for sequence analysis and for submission of new data into the IMGT/HLA database. The

TABLE 129-3 NUMBER OF HLA ALLELES

REGION	LOCUS	NO. OF ALLELES
Class I		
HLA-A	A	324
HLA-B	B	591
HLA-C	Cw	174
HLA-E	E	5
HLA-F	F	2
HLA-G	G	14
Class II		
HLA-DR	DRA	3
	DRB1	380
	DRB2	1
	DRB3	41
	DRB4	13
	DRB5	18
	DRB6	3
	DRB7	2
	DRB8	1
	DRB9	1
HLA-DQ	DQA1	28
	DQB1	57
HLA-DP	DPA1	22
	DPB1	110
HLA-DM	DMA	4
	DMB	6
HLA-DO	DOA	8
	DOB	8

database is updated quarterly and is available at *http://www.ebi.ac.uk/imgt/hla/funding.html*. As of July 2004, the database contained more than 1500 HLA allele sequences (Table 129-3).

The HLA-A and HLA-B antigens were defined and many antigens named before the MHC was recognized as a multilocus system. Instead of changing the numbers already assigned to accepted antigens, subsequent HLA-A and HLA-B specificities and alleles continue to be numbered jointly as if they were products of a single locus (e.g., A34, B35, A36, B37). For all other HLA loci, alleles and specificities are numbered consecutively within that locus (e.g., Cw1, Cw2, etc., DR1, DR2, etc., DQ1, DQ2, etc.). The DNA-based, serologic-based, or cellular-based terminology is acceptable for use. Cellular terminology is used infrequently. Table 129-4 provides a comparison of serologic and DNA-based terminology.[26]

GENES ENCODING HUMAN LEUKOCYTE ANTIGENS

New class I region genes are designated as HLA followed by a letter in alphabetical order, omitting D (e.g., HLA-E, HLA-F, etc.). All class II genes are designated as D, followed by a letter that identifies a locus that is defined by location within the class II region of the chromosome and by the similarity of its genes (e.g., HLA-DQ, HLA-DP, etc.). The locus letter is followed by the letter A or B for α- or β-chain gene, and the A or B is followed by a number in cases of more than one α- or β-chain gene to a locus (DQA1, DQB1, DQA2, DQB2, etc.; see Table 129-2 and Fig. 129-2).

HUMAN LEUKOCYTE ANTIGEN ALLELES

New alleles of HLA genes are recognized through DNA sequencing of at least several clones. Alleles are designated using the gene name (e.g., DRB1) followed by an asterisk (*), followed by a four-digit number. The first two digits of the number identify any previously characterized antigen; the latter two digits identify the allele/variant. This method was chosen to maintain as much as possible the relationship between alleles and serologic specificities. For example, DRB1*1201 designates an allele of the protein formerly defined serologically as DR12, which itself was a serologically defined variant (split) of DR5. Currently, seven alleles have been identified as associated with DR12. As new alleles of a gene are sequenced and accepted, they are numbered consecutively.

In 1990, a five-digit number was introduced to distinguish alleles with synonymous nucleotide substitutions, that is, different DNA nucleotide sequences but unchanged amino acid sequences and thus unchanged expressed proteins. Examples are the DRB1*12021 and

TABLE 129-4   COMPARISON OF HLA TERMINOLOGY FOR TYPING RESOLUTION

Serologic typing/antigen level
   HLA-A1, B8, Cw1, DR17, DR52, DQ2
Molecular typing
   Low resolution: gene group
      HLA-A*01, B*08, Cw*01, DRB1*03, DRB3*02, DQB1*02
   High resolution: allele level
      HLA-A*0101, B*0801, Cw*0102, DRB1*0301, DRB3*0201, DQB1*0201
   Intermediate resolution: multiple but limited alleles*
      Class I HLA-A*0101/0102, B*0801/0802/0803, Cw*0101/0102
      Class II HLA-DRB1*0301/0304, DRB3*0201/0202, DQB1*0201/0203

* The National Marrow Donor Program (NMDP) has established codes to identify multiple allelic possibilities in an effort to facilitate selection of possible marrow donors. For example, HLA-A*0101/0102 = HLA-A*01AB and DRB1*0301/0304 = DRB1*03AD. (*www.marrow-donor.org*).

DRB1*12022 alleles. However, a fifth digit can accommodate only nine variants, and the number of variants for A*0201 already is six. Therefore, an extra digit has been introduced to allow for up to 99 synonymous variants of an allele.[27] Thus, these examples become DRB1*120201 and DRB1*120202.

The convention of using a five-digit code to describe a relationship between alleles and the serologic specificity has started to break down because the number of alleles for some genes already is approaching the maximum of 99. The B*15 group is one example for which 73 alleles already have been named. Therefore, a second number series will be used to extend the first one series. In the case of B*15, the second number series will be B*95.[27]

FREQUENCIES AND RACIAL DISTRIBUTION OF HUMAN LEUKOCYTE ANTIGENS

Different races and ethnic groups can vary greatly with regard to the frequency with which HLA antigens are found.[6,28,29] For example, HLA-A36 and HLA-B42 are infrequent in Caucasians compared to other ethnic groups. Similarly, although HLA-B46 is found in other populations, it occurs at a high frequency among Asians. Similar racial or ethnic differences continue to be noted using molecular techniques.[29]

HUMAN LEUKOCYTE ANTIGEN TYPING

Tissue typing for HLA antigens can be performed using a number of methods of varying degrees of sophistication and complexity, for example, mixed lymphocyte culture (MLC), PLT, cytotoxic T lymphocyte (CTL) clones, two-dimensional electrophoresis, isoelectric focusing, protein sequencing, and molecular assays. The most frequent procedures used in the clinical laboratory have been serologic and cellular assays. However, with the advent of the polymerase chain reaction (PCR) (see Chap. 9), DNA-based typing is becoming common for class I and class II and has essentially replaced cellular assays for the definition of HLA-DR, HLA-DQ, and HLA-DP (i.e., HLA-D) and, in some laboratories, has completely replaced serologic testing.

SEROLOGY

Serologic specificities (antigens) are recognized only if the serologic reagents identify products encoded by accepted allelic DNA sequences. For example, the newer serologic specificities of HLA-A2, corresponding to the allele sequences HLA-A*0203 and HLA-A*0210, are designated as HLA-A203 and HLA-A210. Similarly, the class II serologic specificity that is the product of the DRB1*0103 allele is designated DR103. Because new serologic specificities are based on a correlation with an identified DNA sequence, the designation *w* for *workshop* or provisional characterization has been dropped. Exceptions to this rule are HLA-C locus specificities, to avoid confusion with complement components; Dw and DP specificities, defined by MLR or PLT; and Bw4 and Bw6, to distinguish them from other B locus specificities. Bw4 and Bw6 are public antigens (i.e., epitopes or serologic specificities) defined by amino acid residues at positions 79, 80, and 83 on the class I α-chain.[30] Public antigens are epitopes shared by multiple HLA antigens. All HLA-B α-chains carry either Bw4 or Bw6; a few HLA-A α-chains carry Bw4.

The microcytotoxicity test has been the fundamental tissue typing procedure used for defining HLA antigens for more than 30 years.[31] In this assay, a suspension of lymphocytes is incubated with human alloantisera in a microtiter tray.[32] Rabbit serum is added as a source of complement. Cell death is evaluated microscopically and determined by the uptake of a vital dye or by immunofluorescence. Antibody panels generally consist of two to four sera that recognize the same specificity. This process requires that patients be tested with approximately 150 different reagents for class I and another 80 to 150 reagents for class II. Antisera usually are obtained from multiparous women and multiply transfused individuals, or they can be obtained from patients who have rejected allografts. Monoclonal HLA antibodies are used occasionally along with human alloantisera. Serology for HLA-DR and HLA-DQ requires enrichment for B lymphocytes. In addition, many antisera contain reactivity to class I antigens and HLA-DR and HLA-DQ. Before their use as anti–class II reagents, such sera must be absorbed with cells that express only class I antigens (e.g., platelets). HLA-DP antigens also may be characterized by monoclonal antibodies, although these antigens generally are not included in clinical serologic typing. Serologic definition of HLA antigens is important for patients destined to receive repeated platelet transfusions. It also is important in typing patients and donors for solid organ transplantation and in the initial investigation of families of patients requiring marrow or stem cell transplantation.

CELLULAR ASSAYS

The HLA-D region of the MHC (HLA-DR, HLA-DQ, HLA-DP) initially was identified by the capacity to stimulate allogeneic T cells in an MLR.[33] Initially HLA-D was thought to be a separate locus. Although no molecule could be associated with HLA-D, a large number of HLA-D specificities have been recognized (see Table 129-1). HLA-Dw specificity now clearly is the cumulative effect of allogeneic differences of multiple class II molecules.

Mixed Lymphocyte Reaction   MLR involves coculturing for several days the stimulator cells from one individual with the responder lymphocytes from another individual. Stimulator cells are prevented from proliferating by irradiation or exposure to mitomycin C. The responder cells that recognize alloantigens expressed by stimulator cells are induced to proliferate. Stimulator cells are B cells and monocytes (i.e., antigen-presenting cells). T lymphocytes are responding cells. A radioactive nucleotide, usually ^{3}H-thymidine, is added during the last 6 to 18 hours of culture to measure newly synthesized DNA. The amount of radioactive thymidine incorporated into the DNA of responder cells is generally proportional to the degree of HLA-D disparity between responder and stimulator cells. The average degree of stimulation between cells from family members that share one HLA-D haplotype is approximately half that found between cells from family members that differ for both HLA-D haplotypes. Cells from family members that share both HLA-D haplotypes (e.g., HLA-identical siblings) ordinarily do not stimulate each other. Similarly, cells from nonrelated individuals who share both HLA-D haplotypes generally stimulate each other minimally, if at all.

HLA-Dw specificities are identified using homozygous typing cells.[34] Homozygous typing cells (HTC) are obtained from progeny of consanguineous marriages who have inherited identical chromosomal HLA-D regions from each parent and are homozygous for all HLA-D region loci (DR, DQ, DP). HTC do not stimulate cells from individuals who have the same HLA-D haplotype. However, they stimulate and respond to cells from individuals who are HLA-D heterozygous or fully disparate from them (Table 129-5). Unfortunately, MLR testing for patients with hematologic malignancies often is not successful because leukemic cells generally are poor stimulators in the MLR with responder cells from almost any donor.

MLR response does not require prior sensitization of the responding individual and is an *in vitro* measure of an *in vivo* allograft response. Thus, MLR measures the biologic effect of multiple proteins that are intimately involved in immune response. Other biologic *in vitro* correlates of an allograft response include PLT and CTL assays. CTL are generated in an MLR and are the effectors of a cellular allograft response.

Table 129-5 gives the results of a typical MLR. Data can be expressed as (1) gross counts per minute; (2) a stimulation index (i.e., ratio of $A + B_x$ to $A + A_x$, where A is the responding cell and A_x and B_x are irradiated stimulating cells); or (3) a relative response, or the percentage of maximum stimulation observed when a cell is tested against cells from an unrelated panel. Controls include cultures of cell A, A_x, B, B_x, each responder cell population alone, and cells from two unrelated individuals to gauge the ability of cells A and B to respond to and stimulate allogeneic cells.

Primed Lymphocyte Test   HLA-DP antigens were classified originally using the PLT.[35] PLT is a secondary MLR. Lymphocytes primed to antigen during an initial MLR respond only to the priming antigen in a secondary MLR.

Although the CTL assay can be used to identify specificities and to help assess the degree of risk of allograft rejection or graft-versus-host disease (GVHD) in stem cell transplantation, it is a time-consuming, complex assay that mainly is used in research laboratories.

MOLECULAR TYPING

Development of PCR has radically changed the approach to HLA typing (see Chap. 9).[36,37] A number of DNA-based methods can be used for HLA typing, such as sequence-specific primer amplification (SSP), sequence-specific oligonucleotide probe hybridization (SSOP), restriction fragment length polymorphism (RFLP), single-stranded conformation polymorphism (SSCP), heteroduplex formation, and nucleotide sequencing. All of these methods involve amplification from genomic DNA of selected portions of HLA genes with appropriate oligonucleotide primer pairs. Generally, exons 3 and 4 of class I genes and exon 2 of class II genes are amplified. These exons are the gene fragments encoding most of the polymorphisms of the class I and class II molecules. The most common methods currently used for HLA typing are SSP and SSOP. In typing by SSOP, genomic DNA is isolated and amplified with oligonucleotide primer pairs specific for HLA gene fragments. The amplified DNA then is analyzed using a panel of oligonucleotide probes that hybridize with specific nucleotide sequences present in the amplified gene fragment. Oligonucleotide probes are labeled with either a radioactive isotope (usually ^{32}P) or a nonradioactive label such as biotin-avidin. Either amplified DNA is immobilized on a solid support (e.g., nylon membrane or plastic disk) and labeled probes are added (hybridization), or unlabeled probes are linked to the solid support and amplified DNA, which is labeled during PCR, is added (reverse hybridization). Successful hybridization results in a detectable "dot" or band (Fig. 129-3A). Typing by SSP requires multiple independent PCR reactions. Genomic DNA is isolated and added to a panel of oligonucleotide primer pairs. Each primer pair has specificity for certain nucleotide sequences within the selected exon(s) of the HLA genes. PCR is performed, and the resulting amplified products are analyzed by gel electrophoresis. Assignment of HLA type (i.e., genes and alleles) is based on the presence or absence of amplified product (as a band) from each reaction (Fig. 129-3B). As with serologic typing, the HLA type of the test sample is determined by the pattern with which the amplified gene fragments hybridize with the panel of different probes (SSOP) or by the pattern of products amplified in SSP.

DNA-based typing of HLA is generally performed at two levels, the first using reagents (probes or primer pairs) that detect all alleles of an HLA gene (low resolution) and the second using reagents with specificity for selected alleles (high resolution). Low-resolution typing identifies the HLA gene at the serologic or antigen level (e.g., HLA-

TABLE 129-5 IDENTIFICATION OF HLA-D ANTIGENS USING HOMOZYGOUS TYPING CELLS

RESPONDING CELL	FATHER$_M$*	MOTHER$_M$	CHILD 1$_M$	CHILD 2$_M$	CHILD 5$_M$	Dw3 HTC$_M$	Dw5 HTC$_M$	Dw2 HTC$_M$	Dw6 HTC$_M$
Father(ab)†	810‡	18,450	5,140	5,400	6,800	930	750	16,700	17,750
Mother(cd)	9,250	520	3,210	2,900	3,500	8,600	9,740	640	550
Child 1(ac)	3,400	4,600	440	640	9,980	650	9,345	375	10,650
Child 2(ac)	4,100	4,800	550	550	8,760	675	8,600	460	11,120
Child 5(bd)	2,350	2,300	8,260	7,550	345	8,840	320	11,550	575

* The subscript M indicates mitomycin-treated stimulating cell.
† Genotype code.
‡ Counts per minute.

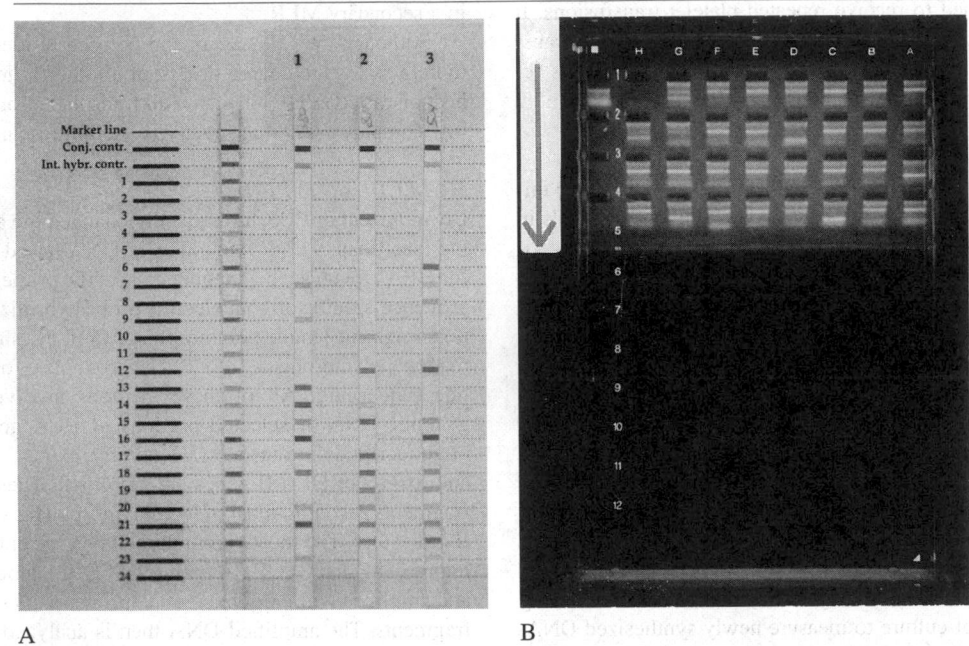

FIGURE 129-3 Examples of sequence-specific oligonucleotide probe hybridization (SSOP) and sequence-specific primer amplification (SSP) DNA-based typing. *(A)* SSOP. In this example, probes specific for HLA-DPB1 alleles are immobilized on nylon strips. Genomic DNA isolated from three individuals was added to oligonucleotide primer pairs that amplify all DPB1 alleles and incorporate a label into the DNA during polymerase chain reaction (PCR). Visible bands indicate specific hybridization of amplified DNA fragments with selected probes. The *left-most column* identifies controls and individual probe locations on the strip. The *second column from the left* is a graphical representation of the expected (typical) intensity of hybridization with each probe. Each numbered strip represents the hybridization of amplified DNA fragments from each individual with specific probes. The pattern of hybridization for the individual tested on strip 1 indicates the presence of the DPB1*0201 and DPB1*1001 alleles. The patterns of hybridization on strips 2 and 3 indicate the presence of the DPB1*2201 and DPB1*3101 alleles and the DPB1*0301 and DPB1*0401 alleles, respectively. *(B)* SSP. Example of low-resolution SSP typing of one individual for class II. Isolated genomic DNA was added to a panel of oligonucleotide primer pairs specific for DRB1, DRB3, DRB4, DRB5, or DQB1 alleles. Each mixture also contains a primer pair that amplifies a non-HLA DNA nucleotide sequence that is common to all individuals as a positive control for amplification. Following PCR, each reaction mixture was analyzed by gel electrophoresis. The various bands seen at each position and moving in the direction of electrophoresis are as follows:

- Unamplified genomic DNA (>1000 bp)
- Positive amplification control (~700 bp)—not always seen with a specific product
- Specific product (~75–350 bp)—seen only in wells that amplify the sample's alleles, that is, 1G, 2H, 2D, 3A, 4G, 4C
- Primer dimers (usually <75 bp)—result from primer excess, and the primers form a dimer with each other. Not always seen, but some may be very bright.

Position 1H contains a negative control consisting of appropriate primer pairs but no added genomic DNA. The band to the left of position 1H is a marker consisting of different-size DNA fragments to help determine base pair product size. Analysis of the pattern of amplified specific products identifies the class II type of this individual as HLA-DRB1*01, DRB1*04; DRB4*01; DQB1*03, DQB1*05 or, in serologic terms, HLA-DR1, DR4; DR53; DQ3, DQ5.

A*02, HLA-DRB1*01, etc.). High-resolution typing identifies specific alleles (e.g., HLA-A*0201, DRB1*0103, etc.). A third level is called *intermediate resolution*. In intermediate resolution, more than one allele of an HLA gene could be the correct one (e.g., DRB1*0302/0303/0304/0309; see Table 129-4). If primers or probes are unavailable, and if it is necessary to clarify the specific allele, then nucleotide sequencing of amplified product can be performed. Although nucleotide sequencing is thought by many to be the definitive method, it is costly, time consuming, and currently used more commonly in research laboratories.

Molecular typing has revealed greater polymorphism in the genes encoding HLA antigens than was previously detected.[24] For example, multiple alleles at HLA loci each encodes a molecule with the same serologic specificity (e.g., HLA-A2 serologic specificity is associated with >20 HLA-A2 alleles). Molecular typing has elucidated the origin of the class II public antigens HLA-DR51, HLA-DR52, and HLA-DR53. Unlike the Bw4 and Bw6 class I public antigens that result from amino acid substitutions on the class I α-chain, separate DRB genes encode the HLA-DR51, HLA-DR52, and HLA-DR53 antigens. Furthermore, DNA-based typing has helped to reveal the relationship of HLA-DR, HLA-DQ, and HLA-DP to HLA-Dw specificities. For example, HLA-DR4 appeared to be one antigen, even though it was associated with several different HLA-Dw specificities. To date, 32 alleles of DR4 have been identified by molecular analysis, and each of the Dw specificities identified for DR4 is associated with a specific DR4 allele.

Use of molecular testing has a number of advantages over serologic typing. First, DNA-based typing does not require isolation of viable lymphocyte populations but can be performed using any nucleated cell source. Second, DNA-based assays have increased accuracy and specificity. HLA antigens have a high degree of homogeneity, and alloantisera produced against them can be cross-reactive. This cross-reactivity can lead to inconsistent assignment of individual specificities.

INHERITANCE OF HUMAN LEUKOCYTE ANTIGENS

The genes of the MHC demonstrate more polymorphism than any other genetic system, that is, multiple alleles exist for each locus. Each individual, however, has one allele for each locus per chromosome and, therefore, encodes two HLA antigens per locus. Additionally, the antigens at each HLA locus are codominant, that is, each is expressed independently of the other. The identification of each HLA antigen of an individual is called a *phenotype*. Two unrelated individuals who express the same HLA antigens are *HLA-phenotype identical*.

Because HLA genes are closely linked on chromosome 6, recombination within the MHC is rare (≤1%), and a complete set of HLA genes usually is inherited from each parent as a unit. The genes inherited from one parent are referred to as a *haplotype*. Maternal and paternal haplotypes can be identified through family studies. Identification of both the paternal and the maternal haplotypes in an individual provides a *genotype*. Siblings who inherit the same haplotypes are termed *HLA identical*. Those who inherit the same haplotype from one parent but a different haplotype from the other parent are called *haplo-identical*. Finally, siblings who inherit different haplotypes from each parent are *HLA nonidentical*. In general, family studies consist of testing for the HLA-A, HLA-B, HLA-C, HLA-DR, and HLA-DQ antigens to identify haplotypes and to rule out genetic recombination within the MHC complex. Because HLA genes are inherited together on a single chromosome, four combinations of

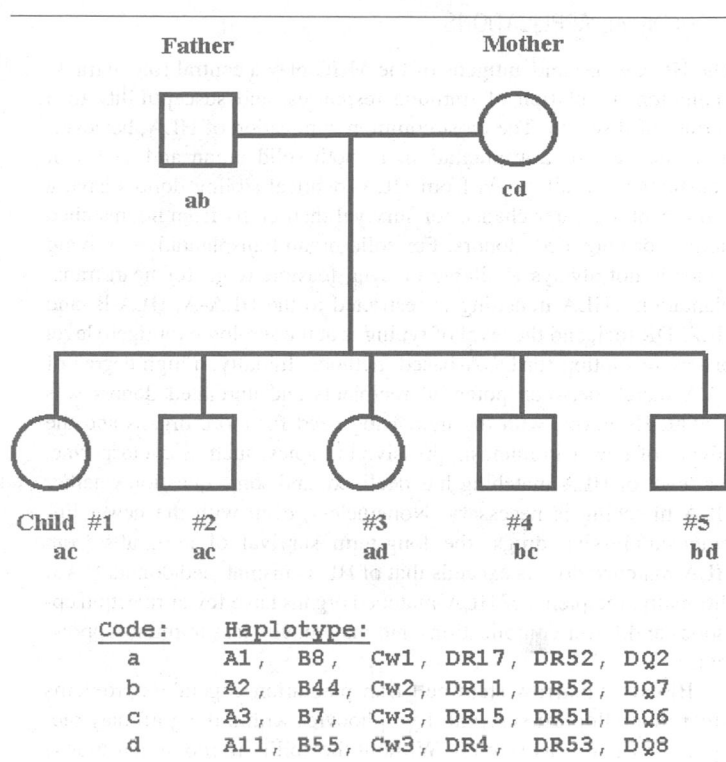

Code:	Haplotype:					
a	A1,	B8,	Cw1,	DR17,	DR52,	DQ2
b	A2,	B44,	Cw2,	DR11,	DR52,	DQ7
c	A3,	B7,	Cw3,	DR15,	DR51,	DQ6
d	A11,	B55,	Cw3,	DR4,	DR53,	DQ8

FIGURE 129-4   Representation of the inheritance of human leukocyte antigen. Each of the four parental chromosomes (haplotypes) is coded by a letter: *a* and *b* represent the paternal haplotypes; *c* and *d* represent the maternal haplotypes. Each child inherits one paternal haplotype (*a* or *b*) and one maternal haplotype (*c* or *d*).

maternal and paternal haplotypes are possible, provided no meiotic recombination between HLA genes occurs (Fig. 129-4). Thus, there is a 1 in 4 (25%) chance that two siblings will be HLA identical, a 2 in 4 (50%) chance that two siblings will be HLA haplo-identical, and a 1 in 4 (25%) chance that two siblings will be HLA nonidentical. All progeny are haplo-identical with their parents unless recombination has occurred.

LINKAGE DISEQUILIBRIUM

Because HLA is so highly polymorphic, the chance that two unrelated individuals are HLA identical could be astronomical. However, the situation is somewhat alleviated because the HLA system displays a phenomenon known as *linkage disequilibrium*, that is, certain HLA alleles are inherited together on the same chromosome more often than would be predicted if HLA loci were at equilibrium. At equilibrium, the frequency of an allele at one locus is independent of the frequencies of alleles at linked loci. For example, the gene frequency of HLA-A1 in North American Caucasians is 0.138 and that of HLA-B8 is 0.09. Given no preferential association between HLA-A1 and HLA-B8, then the frequency of the HLA-A1, B8 haplotype, predicted by equilibrium, should be 0.0124 (0.138 × 0.09 = 0.0124). However, population studies show that the actual frequency of the HLA-A1, B8 haplotype in this particular population is greater than that predicted by equilibrium, that is, 0.0609. The degree of linkage disequilibrium is defined as the observed frequency minus its expected frequency, 0.0485 in this example. Although the particular alleles found in linkage disequilibria differ for various racial groups, all racial groups display significant disequilibria.

CLINICAL APPLICATIONS

The HLA genes and antigens of the MHC play a central role in transplantation, regulation of immune responses, and susceptibility to a variety of diseases. The most common application of HLA, however, is in the field of transplantation. In both solid organ and stem cell transplantation, allografts from HLA-identical sibling donors have a significantly greater chance for survival than grafts from nonmatched family, or unrelated, donors. For solid organ transplantation, a living donor is not always available or even feasible (e.g., for heart transplantation). HLA matching is restricted to the HLA-A, HLA-B, and HLA-DR loci, and the level of typing is at the serologic (antigen) level or low resolution for DNA-based methods. Initially, a high degree of HLA match between potential recipients and unrelated donors was sought. However, with the increasing need for more organs and the advent of newer immunosuppressive therapies, such as cyclosporine, the level of HLA matching has declined, and some question whether HLA matching is necessary. Nonetheless, even with the newer immunosuppressive drugs, the long-term survival of allografts from HLA-matched donors exceeds that of HLA-mismatched donors.[30] Additionally, recipients of HLA-matched organs have fewer rejection episodes and fewer complications and may require less immunosuppression.

Blood or marrow stem cell transplantation engenders problems other than allograft survival. Lymphocytes within the graft may recognize host cells as foreign. Without the ability to mount a response to such host reactive cells, patients receiving stem cell allografts are prone to GVHD (see Chap. 22).[38,39] With HLA-identical sibling donors, disease-free survival of 80 to 90 percent can be achieved for some malignant and nonmalignant hematologic disorders.[39] However, less than 30 percent of individuals have an HLA-identical sibling. Thus, alternative donors, such as phenotypically matched unrelated volunteers and partially matched family members, must be considered. However, the risks and incidence of graft failure and GVHD are higher than seen with HLA-identical siblings and increase with increased HLA disparity. Fortunately, molecular typing has improved the accuracy of matching unrelated donors, allowing for improved outcomes.

The HLA criteria for selecting an appropriate stem cell donor vary among transplant centers and, within a center, depend on the transplant protocol. Within families, typing for HLA-A, HLA-B, HLA-DR, and HLA-DQ at the serologic or DNA-based low-resolution level is generally sufficient to identify all haplotypes, potential recombinants, and HLA-identical pairs. In those circumstances where the haplotypes are unclear, DNA-based, allele-level typing is recommended. For unrelated volunteer donors, allele-level molecular typing of HLA-A, HLA-B, HLA-C, HLA-DR, and HLA-DQ provides the best opportunity for a successful outcome and reduced GVHD. The World Marrow Donor Association (WMDA) published guidelines for the extent of HLA typing recommended for transplant centers and donor registries that participate in the exchange of stem cells for allogeneic transplantation.[40] Briefly, the WMDA recommends typing the HLA-A, HLA-B, and HLA-DR loci using DNA-based testing at the low-resolution level at a minimum.

PLATELET ANTIGENS

Platelets express antigens that can be recognized by autoantibodies or by antibodies made by recipients of platelet transfusions. HLA antigens are present on platelets, as judged by absorption, fluorescence, and complement fixation. In addition, platelets possess platelet-spe-cific antigens that are unrelated to erythrocyte or leukocyte isoantigens (see Chap. 14).

Platelet antigens can be targeted by autoantibodies, resulting in immune thrombocytopenia. A dominant platelet antigen recognized by the autoantibodies of many patients with autoimmune thrombocytopenia is platelet glycoprotein GPIIb/IIIa (otherwise called $\alpha_{IIb}\beta_3$ or CD41/CD61), although other platelet glycoproteins also may be targeted by autoantibodies.[41,42] Chapter 110 discusses this condition.

PLATELET ALLOANTIGENS

Platelet alloantigens, also referred to as *platelet isoantigens*, are substances that induce production of alloantibodies when platelets bearing such antigens are infused into patients who lack the specific alloantigen.[43] Immune responses to platelet alloantigens are involved in the pathogenesis of several clinical syndromes, including neonatal alloimmune thrombocytopenia, posttransfusion purpura, and refractory responses to platelet transfusion.[44] Immune thrombocytopenia can be an unusual complication of a type of GVHD in which donor lymphocytes make alloantibodies specific for the platelets produced by the recipient of an organ allograft.[45]

Patients can lack a particular platelet-associated antigen altogether because they have defective alleles of the gene encoding the antigen (see Chap. 112). Such patients can make antibodies against platelets of virtually all donors that bear the platelet-associated antigen. For example, patients with Bernard-Soulier syndrome, who lack platelet GPIb-V-IX, or patients with Glanzmann thrombasthenia, who lack expression of GPIIb (CD41) and GPIIIa (CD61), can be induced to make broadly reactive antiplatelet antibodies (see Chap. 112).[46,47] Several percent of Japanese individuals and approximately 0.3 percent of Caucasians are deficient in CD36, one of the major platelet glycoproteins, also known as *GPIV*.[48] Because these patients lack a platelet antigen, they can develop antiplatelet antibodies specific for the deficient platelet protein after they receive transfusions of platelets from normal donors or after pregnancy.

More commonly, platelet-specific alloantigens result from genetic polymorphism in genes encoding functional platelet proteins.[43,49] These alloantigens first were defined by antiplatelet antibodies discovered in the sera of multiparous females who gave birth to infants with neonatal thrombocytopenia. Many of these alloantigens subsequently were found to recognize allotypic determinants of platelet-associated membrane glycoproteins, such as GPIIb/IIIa (CD41/CD61). Each of these allotypic determinants may be generated by only a single amino acid substitution in a major platelet-associated glycoprotein (Table 129-6).[50] However, glycosylation may contribute to or influence the expression of certain human platelet antigen (HPA) epitopes, such as those associated with HPA-3.[51] In any case, these amino acid substitutions generally do not appear to affect the platelet function *in vitro*. However, conceivably the genetic polymorphism in platelet glycoproteins may be associated with more subtle differences in platelet physiology that can contribute to the relative risk for thrombosis and/or atherosclerosis.[52-54]

A nomenclature for human platelet alloantigens has been adopted to replace the old complex "classic" nomenclatures that previously were developed independently in laboratories throughout the world (see Table 129-6).[55] At least 10 HPAs have been defined at the molecular level. Each has two alleles, designated by the suffix *a* or *b*. These alleles are expressed by platelets codominantly (see Table 129-6). The *a* allele generally is the more prevalent allele; however, allelic frequencies vary among different racial groups (see Table 129-6).[56-60] For example, HPA-1b is expressed on the platelets of approximately

TABLE 129-6   HUMAN PLATELET ANTIGENS

ALLOANTIGEN	CLASSIC NAME	PLATELET GLYCOPROTEIN	POLYMORPHISM	GENE FREQUENCY		
				EUROPEAN	AFRICAN	ASIAN
GPIIb/GPIIIa ($\alpha_{IIb}\beta_3$) (CD41/CD61)						
HPA-1a	Pl^{AI}, Zw^a	GPIIIa (β_3)	CD61-Leu$_{33}$	0.85	0.89	>0.99
HPA-1b	Pl^{A2}, Zw^b	GPIIIa (β_3)	CD61-Pro$_{33}$	0.15	0.12	<0.01
HPA-3a	Bak^a, Lek^a	GPIIb (α_{IIb})	CD41-Ile$_{843}$	0.61		0.37
HPA-3b	Bak^b	GPIIb (α_{IIb})	CD41-Ser$_{843}$	0.39		0.63
HPA-4a	Pen^a, Yuk^b	GPIIIa (β_3)	CD61-Arg$_{185}$	>0.99		0.99
HPA-4b	Pen^b, Yuk^a	GPIIIa (β_3)	CD61-Gln$_{143}$	<0.01		0.01
HPA-6a		GPIIIa (β_3)	CD61-Arg$_{143}$	>0.99	>0.99	>0.99
HPA-6b	Ca, Tu	GPIIIa (β_3)	CD61-Gln$_{489}$	<0.01	<0.01	<0.01
HPA-7a		GPIIIa (β_3)	CD61-Pro$_{407}$	>0.99	>0.99	>0.99
HPA-7b	Mo	GPIIIa (β_3)	CD61-Ala$_{407}$	<0.01	<0.01	<0.01
HPA-8a		GPIIIa (β_3)	CD61-Arg$_{636}$	>0.99	>0.99	>0.99
HPA-8b	Sr^a	GPIIIa (β_3)	CD61-Cys$_{636}$	<0.01	<0.01	<0.01
HPA-9a	Max^a	GPIIb (α_{IIb})	CD41-Val$_{837}$	0.97		
HPA-9b	Max^b	GPIIb (α_{IIb})	CD41-Met$_{837}$	0.03		
HPA-10a	La^b	GPIIIa (β_3)	CD61-Arg$_{62}$	>0.99	>0.99	>0.99
HPA-10b	La^a	GPIIIa (β_3)	CD61-Gln$_{62}$	<0.01	<0.01	<0.01
GPIa/IIa ($\alpha_2\beta_1$) (CD49b/CD29)						
HPA-5a	Br^b Zav^b Hc^a	GPIa (α_2)	CD49b-Glu$_{505}$	0.89	0.79	0.97
HPA-5b	Br^a Zav^a Hc^b	GPIa (α_2)	CD49b-Lys$_{505}$	0.11	0.21	0.03
GPIb-IX-V (CD42/CD42d)						
HPA-2a	Ko^b Sib^b	GPIbα	CD42b-Thr$_{145}$	0.93	0.82	0.92
HPA-2b	Ko^a Sib^a	GPIbα	CD42b-Met$_{145}$	0.07	0.18	0.08

15 percent of persons of European ancestry but of less than 1 percent of persons of Asian ancestry.

The glycoproteins associated with the alloantigens and the HPA alloantigens are listed in the Alloantigens column (see Table 129-6). The terms used prior to the HPA system for designating the alloantigen are listed in the Classic Name column. The platelet glycoproteins corresponding to the respective alloantigen are listed in the Platelet Glycoprotein column. The Polymorphism column lists the protein using the CD designation (see Chap. 14) followed by the three-letter code for the amino acid residue found at the polymorphic position (indicated in subscript). The gene frequencies for the major ethnic groups in the United States are listed in the *European, African,* and *Asian* columns, with the approximate gene frequencies calculated from several different surveys).

In addition to the recognized HPAs, several other platelet alloantigens can be recognized by antiplatelet alloantibodies and account for neonatal alloimmune thrombocytopenia. Two alloantigens, designated *Gro^a* and *Oe^a*, are associated with GPIIIa (CD61).[61,62] Another potential alloantigen, designated *Va^a*, is associated with the GPIIb/IIIa complex (CD41/CD61).[63] Two others, designated *La^a* and *Ly^a*, are localized to the GPIb-IX-V complex.[64,65] Another alloantigen results from genetic polymorphism in the gene encoding CD109 (see Chap. 14), accounting for the Gov alloantigen system.[66,67] The less common allele encoding any one of these alloantigens may be present at very low gene frequencies.

HPA alleles HPA-4b, HPA-6b, HPA-7b, HPA-8b, HPA-9b, and HPA-10b present at gene frequencies less than 0.1 percent are designated *private* alleles (see Table 129-6). Some of these alleles, such as HPA-7b or HPA-8b,[61] are extremely rare. For this reason, the alloantigens encoded by such alleles likely do not account for most cases of posttransfusion purpura but can be found on isolated cases of neonatal alloimmune thrombocytopenia in selected families. On the other hand, alleles present at gene frequencies greater than 2 percent within the population are designated as *public* alleles. These alleles more likely encode the alloantigens that are targeted by antiplatelet alloantibodies.

The frequency of patients who express the more common HPA allele is greater than the gene frequency for that allele in the population. Using the classic Hardy-Weinberg equation [$a^2 + 2(ab) + b^2 = 1$], the proportion of individuals who are homozygous for the *a* allele (*a/a*) is the squared product of the gene frequency for *a* in the population (or a^2). Similarly, the proportion of cases that are homozygous for *b* is the squared product of the gene frequency for *b* (or b^2). The proportion of cases that are heterozygous (either *a/b* or *b/a*) is two times the product of the gene frequency for *a* times that for *b*. Because there are two alleles, the sum of all these products should equal 100 percent (or 1). Using such considerations for example, persons of European ancestry have a $(0.85)^2$ (72%) chance of being homozygous for HPA-1a and a 26 percent chance of being heterozygous for HPA-1a/ HPA-1b but only a $(0.15)^2$ (2%) chance of being homozygous for HPA-1b (see Table 129-6). As such, even though the gene frequency of HPA-1a is 85 percent, 98 percent of the population has at least one HPA-1a allele and will not make alloantibodies against the HPA-1a epitope. Similarly, a person being homozygous for HPA private antigens would be highly unusual. As such, alloantibodies against HPA-4a, HPA-6a, HPA-7a, HPA-8a, HPA-9a, and HPA-10a likely do not account for immune thrombocytopenia. Conversely, most persons lack the *b* allele of HPA private antigens and thus potentially can develop alloantibodies to HPA-4b, HPA-6b, HPA-7b, HPA-8b, HPA-9b, and HPA-10b alloantigens.

ANTIPLATELET ANTIBODIES AFTER TRANSFUSION

Patients who are homozygous for a given allele can develop antiplatelet alloantibodies after receiving transfusions of platelets or cells that express the other allele.[68] Generally, a few transfusions of unmatched platelets can be given to patients without adverse effects. However, the risk for developing antiplatelet antibodies increases with each successive platelet transfusion. Patients who receive multiple transfusions of red blood cells also may develop antiplatelet or anti-HLA antibodies against leukocytes contaminating the red blood cell preparation.

After repeated platelet transfusions, the patient may become sensitized, possibly developing antibodies that shorten the life span of the transfused cells. The number of unmatched transfusions required to elicit such antibodies is variable. Some patients never make antibodies, whereas others become refractory after receiving only a few platelet transfusions. Other patients, often multiparous women, may have clinically significant antiplatelet antibodies prior to receiving any platelet transfusions. Approximately half of all patients who receive repetitive platelet transfusions eventually produce antibodies against antigens on the transfused platelets. These antibodies may be directed against platelet-specific alloantigens, HLA antigens, or both.

Antibodies against some HPA-allelic determinants can inhibit platelet function. Anti–HPA-1 alloantibodies, for example, can inhibit clot retraction and platelet aggregation, presumably because they block the binding of GPIIb/IIIa ($\alpha_{IIb}\beta_3$) to fibrinogen. Moreover, anti–HPA-4 alloantibodies can completely inhibit aggregation of HPA-4 platelets that are homozygous for allele recognized by the alloantibodies because the epitope recognized by anti–HPA-4 alloantibodies is found on β_3 at amino acid position 143, which is in close proximity to the RGD-binding domain of the $\alpha_{IIb}\beta_3$ integrin. On the other hand, other anti–HPA-alloantibodies, such as alloantibodies specific for HPA-3, may not significantly interfere with platelet function but nonetheless can cause Fc-mediated platelet destruction and immune thrombocytopenia.[69]

If the patient develops anti-HLA antibodies that shorten the survival of unmatched transfused platelets, HLA-matched platelets may be more effective for subsequent transfusions. The patient and prospective platelet donors generally are matched for serologic identity at the HLA-A and HLA-B loci. Platelets derived from such HLA-matched donors generally survive longer in highly immunized patients than the platelets received from random donors.

In some cases, the platelet alloantigens of donors must be typed in order to provide effective platelet transfusion therapy.[70] Different techniques for phenotyping are well established and easy to perform, but they rely on the availability of antisera.[71] The molecular genetic basis for the clinically most relevant alloantigens has been elucidated, thus facilitating widespread platelet alloantigen typing.[62]

Typing for HPA status can be achieved using PCR (see Chap. 9), with subsequent analysis of the amplified gene fragment using restriction enzymes, sequence-specific primers, dot-blot hybridization, or a fluorescent-based single-stranded conformation polymorphism (F-SSCP) technique.[72–78] These techniques have proved to be highly useful in identifying the platelet genotype of fetuses at risk for neonatal alloimmune thrombocytopenia,[79] establishing the diagnosis of post-transfusion purpura, or identifying causes of refractory responses to platelet transfusions. Molecular methods for detecting HPA status also should facilitate clinical studies on the association of certain HPA alleles with relative risk for thrombosis[53] or response to therapy for immune thrombocytopenia.[80]

REFERENCES

1. Breuning MH, van den Berg-Loonen EM, Bernini LF, et al: Localization of HLA on the short arm of chromosome 6. *Hum Genet* 37:131, 1977.
2. Berrih S, Arenzana-Seisdedos F, Cohen S, et al: Interferon-gamma modulates HLA class II antigen expression on cultured human thymic epithelial cells. *J Immunol* 135:1165, 1985.
3. Bodmer JG, Marsh SG, Albert ED, et al: Nomenclature for factors of the HLA system 1991. WHO Nomenclature Committee for factors of the HLA system. *Tissue Antigens* 39:161, 1992.
4. Thorsby E: Structure and function of HLA molecules. *Transplant Proc* 19:29, 1987.
5. O'Callaghan CA, Bell JI: Structure and function of the human MHC class Ib molecules HLA-E, HLA-F, and HLA-G. *Immunol Rev* 163:129, 1998.
6. Marsh SG, Parham P, Barber LD: *The HLA Facts Book.* Facts Book Series. Academic, San Diego, 2000.
7. Allan DS, Lepin EJ, Braud VM, et al: Tetrameric complexes of HLA-E, HLA-F, and HLA-G. *J Immunol Methods* 268:43, 2002.
8. Trowsdale J: Genetics and polymorphism: Class II antigens. *Br Med Bull* 43:15, 1987.
9. Bjorkman PJ, Saper MA, Samraoui B, et al: Structure of the human class I histocompatibility antigen, HLA-A2. *Nature* 329:506, 1987.
10. Brown JH, Jardetzky TS, Gorga JC, et al: Three-dimensional structure of the human class II histocompatibility antigen HLA-DR1. *Nature* 364:33, 1993.
11. Bjorkman PJ, Saper MA, Samraoui B, et al: The foreign antigen binding site and T cell recognition regions of class I histocompatibility antigens. *Nature* 329:512, 1987.
12. Stern LJ, Brown JH, Jardetzky TS, et al: Crystal structure of the human class II MHC protein HLA-DR1 complexed with an influenza virus peptide. *Nature* 368:215, 1994.
13. Fugger L, Tisch R, Libau R, et al: The role of the major histocompatibility complex (HLA) genes in disease, in *The Metabolic Basis of Inherited Disease*, 7th ed, edited by CR Scriver, AL Beaudet, WS Sly, D Valle, p 555. McGraw-Hill, New York, 1995.
14. Mueller-Eckhardt G, Hauck M, Kayser W, Mueller-Eckhardt C: HLA-C antigens on platelets. *Tissue Antigens* 16:91, 1980.
15. Lalezari P, Driscoll AM: Ability of thrombocytes to acquire HLA specificity from plasma. *Blood* 59:167, 1982.
16. Zinkernagel RM, Doherty PC: Restriction of in vitro T cell-mediated cytotoxicity in lymphocytic choriomeningitis within a syngeneic or semiallogeneic system. *Nature* 248:701, 1974.
17. Mak T, Simard J: *Handbook of Immune Response Genes.* Plenum, New York, 1998.
18. Moretta L, Biassoni R, Bottino C, et al: Human NK cells and their receptors. *Microbes Infect* 4:1539, 2002.
19. Algarra I, Garcia-Lora A, Cabrera T, et al: The selection of tumor variants with altered expression of classical and nonclassical MHC class I molecules: Implications for tumor immune escape. *Cancer Immunol Immunother* 53:904, 2004.
20. Carosella ED, Moreau P, Le Maoult J, et al: HLA-G molecules: From maternal-fetal tolerance to tissue acceptance. *Adv Immunol* 81:199, 2003.
21. Seliger B, Abken H, Ferrone S: HLA-G and MIC expression in tumors and their role in anti-tumor immunity. *Trends Immunol* 24:82, 2003.
22. Hofmeister V, Weiss EH: HLA-G modulates immune responses by diverse receptor interactions. *Semin Cancer Biol* 13:317, 2003.
23. Campbell R, Trowsdale J: A map of the human major histocompatibility complex. *Immunol Today* 18:43, 1997.
24. Bodmer JG, Marsh SG, Albert ED, et al: Nomenclature for factors of the HLA system 1998. *Tissue Antigens* 53:407, 1999.

25. Marsh SG: HLA nomenclature and the IMGT/HLA sequence database. *Novartis Found Symp* 254:165, 2003.

26. Schreuder GM, Hurley CK, Marsh SG, et al: The HLA dictionary 1999: A summary of HLA-A, -B, -C, -DRB1/3/4/5, -DQB1 alleles and their association with serologically defined HLA-A, -B, -C, -DR and -DQ antigens. *Tissue Antigens* 54:409, 1999.

27. Marsh SG, Albert ED, Bodmer WF, et al: Nomenclature for factors of the HLA system. *Tissue Antigens* 60:407, 2002.

28. Baur M, Danilors J: Population analysis of HLA-A, B, C, DR and other genetic markers. in *Histocompatibility 1980*, edited by P Terasaki, pp. 955–993. UCLA Tissue Typing Laboratory, Los Angeles, 1980.

29. Gjertson D, Su-Hui L: HLA-A/B and -DRB1/DQB1 allele level haplotype frequencies, in *HLA*, edited by D Gjertson, P Teresaki, p X. American Society for Histocompatibility and Immunogenetics, Lenexa, 1998.

30. Parham P: Histocompatibility typing—Mac is back in town. *Immunol Today* 9:127, 1988.

31. Sullivan K, Amos D: The HLA system and its detection, in *Manual of Clinical Laboratory Immunology*, 3rd ed, edited by N Rose, H Friedman, J Fahey, p 835. American Society for Microbiology, Washington, DC, 1986.

32. Terasaki PI, McClelland JD: Microdroplet assay of human serum cytotoxins. *Nature* 204:998, 1964.

33. DuPont B, Hansen JA: Human mixed-lymphocyte culture reaction: Genetics, specificity, and biological implications. *Adv Immunol* 23:107, 1976.

34. Jorgensen F, Lamm LU, Kissmeyer-Nielsen F: Mixed lymphocyte cultures with inbred individuals: An approach to MLC typing. *Tissue Antigens* 3:323, 1973.

35. Shaw S, Johnson AH, Shearer GM: Evidence for a new segregant series of B cell antigens that are encoded in the HLA-D region and that stimulate secondary allogenic proliferative and cytotoxic responses. *J Exp Med* 152:565, 1980.

36. Saiki RK, Gelfand DH, Stoffel S, et al: Primer-directed enzymatic amplification of DNA with a thermostable DNA polymerase. *Science* 239:487, 1988.

37. Erlich H, Bugawan T: HLA class II gene polymorphism: DNA typing, evolution, and relationship to disease susceptibility, in *PCR Technology: Principles and Applications for DNA Amplification*, edited by H Erlich, pp. 193–208. Stockton, New York, 1989.

38. Martin PJ, Gooley T, Anasetti C, et al: HLAs and risk of acute graft-vs.-host disease after marrow transplantation from an HLA-identical sibling. *Biol Blood Marrow Transplant* 4:128, 1998.

39. Petersdorf EW, Gooley TA, Anasetti C, et al: Optimizing outcome after unrelated marrow transplantation by comprehensive matching of HLA class I and II alleles in the donor and recipient. *Blood* 92:3515, 1998.

40. Hurley CK, Wade JA, Oudshoorn M, et al: A special report: Histocompatibility testing guidelines for hematopoietic stem cell transplantation using volunteer donors. Quality Assurance and Donor Registries Working Groups of the World Marrow Donor Association. *Hum Immunol* 60:347, 1999.

41. Wadenvik H, Stockelberg D, Hou M: Platelet proteins as autoantibody targets in idiopathic thrombocytopenic purpura. *Acta Paediatr Suppl* 424:26, 1998.

42. Beardsley DS, Ertem M: Platelet autoantibodies in immune thrombocytopenic purpura. *Transfus Sci* 19:237, 1998.

43. Davis GL: Platelet specific alloantigens. *Clin Lab Sci* 11:356, 1998.

44. Warkentin TE, Smith JW: The alloimmune thrombocytopenic syndromes. *Transfus Med Rev* 11:296, 1997.

45. West KA, Anderson DR, McAlister VC, et al: Alloimmune thrombocytopenia after organ transplantation. *N Engl J Med* 341:1504, 1999.

46. Bierling P, Fromont P, Elbez A, et al: Early immunization against platelet glycoprotein IIIa in a newborn Glanzmann type I patient. *Vox Sang* 55:109, 1988.

47. Li C, Pasquale DN, Roth GJ: Bernard-Soulier syndrome with severe bleeding: Absent platelet glycoprotein Ib alpha due to a homozygous one-base deletion. *Thromb Haemost* 76:670, 1996.

48. Ikeda H: Platelet membrane protein CD36. *Hokkaido Igaku Zasshi* 74:99, 1999.

49. Newman PJ, Valentin N: Human platelet alloantigens: Recent findings, new perspectives. *Thromb Haemost* 74:234, 1995.

50. Santoso S, Kiefel V: Human platelet-specific alloantigens: Update. *Vox Sang* 74(suppl 2):249, 1998.

51. Lyman S, Aster RH, Visentin GP, Newman PJ: Polymorphism of human platelet membrane glycoprotein IIb associated with the Baka/Bakb alloantigen system. *Blood* 75:2343, 1990.

52. Nurden AT: Polymorphisms of human platelet membrane glycoproteins: Structure and clinical significance. *Thromb Haemost* 74:345, 1995.

53. Bray PF: Integrin polymorphisms as risk factors for thrombosis. *Thromb Haemost* 82:337, 1999.

54. Goldschmidt-Clermont PJ, Roos CM, Cooke GE: Platelet PlA2 polymorphism and thromboembolic events: From inherited risk to pharmacogenetics. *J Thromb Thrombolysis* 8:89, 1999.

55. Rozman P: Platelet antigens. The role of human platelet alloantigens (HPA) in blood transfusion and transplantation. *Transpl Immunol* 10:165, 2002.

56. Holensteiner A, Walchshofer S, Adler A, et al: Human platelet antigen gene frequencies in the Austrian population. *Haemostasis* 25:133, 1995.

57. Tanaka S, Taniue A, Nagao N, et al: Genotype frequencies of the human platelet antigen, Ca/Tu, in Japanese, determined by a PCR-RFLP method. *Vox Sang* 70:40, 1996.

58. Tanaka S, Ohnoki S, Shibata H, et al: Gene frequencies of human platelet antigens on glycoprotein IIIa in Japanese. *Transfusion* 36:813, 1996.

59. Kim HO, Jin Y, Kickler TS, et al: Gene frequencies of the five major human platelet antigens in African American, white, and Korean populations. *Transfusion* 35:863, 1995.

60. Kekomaki S, Partanen J, Kekomaki R: Platelet alloantigens HPA-1, -2, -3, -5, and -6b in Finns. *Transfus Med* 5:193, 1995.

61. Simsek S, Vlekke AB, Kuijpers RW, et al: A new private platelet antigen, Groa, localized on glycoprotein IIIa, involved in neonatal alloimmune thrombocytopenia. *Vox Sang* 67:302, 1994.

62. Kroll H, Kiefel V, Santoso S: Clinical aspects and typing of platelet alloantigens. *Vox Sang* 74(suppl 2):345, 1998.

63. Kekomaki R, Raivio P, Kero P: A new low-frequency platelet alloantigen, Vaa, on glycoprotein IIbIIIa associated with neonatal alloimmune thrombocytopenia. *Transfus Med* 2:27, 1992.

64. Peyruchaud O, Bourre F, Morel-Kopp MC, et al: HPA-10w(b) (La(a)): Genetic determination of a new platelet-specific alloantigen on glycoprotein IIIa and its expression in COS-7 cells. *Blood* 89:2422, 1997.

65. Kiefel V, Vicariot M, Giovangrandi Y, et al: Alloimmunization against Iy, a low-frequency antigen on platelet glycoprotein Ib/IX as a cause of severe neonatal alloimmune thrombocytopenic purpura. *Vox Sang* 69:250, 1995.

66. Kelton JG, Smith JW, Horsewood P, et al: Gova/b alloantigen system on human platelets. *Blood* 75:2172, 1990.

67. Bordin JO, Kelton JG, Warner MN, et al: Maternal immunization to Gov system alloantigens on human platelets. *Transfusion* 37:823, 1997.

68. McFarland JG: Alloimmunization and platelet transfusion. *Semin Hematol* 33:315, 1996.

69. Glade-Bender J, McFarland JG, Kaplan C, et al: Anti-HPA-3A induces

severe neonatal alloimmune thrombocytopenia. *J Pediatr* 138:862, 2001.

70. Kekomaki R: Use of HLA- and HPA–matched platelets in alloimmunized patients. *Vox Sang* 74(suppl 2):359, 1998.

71. Kaplan C: Evaluation of serological platelet antibody assays. *Vox Sang* 74(suppl 2):355, 1998.

72. Unkelbach K, Kalb R, Santoso S, et al: Genomic RFLP typing of human platelet alloantigens Zw(PlA), Ko, Bak, and Br (HPA-1, -2, -3, -5). *Br J Haematol* 89:169, 1995.

73. Panzer S, Kaplan C: Report on the 1997 International Society of Blood Transfusion Workshop for Genotyping of Platelet Alloantigens. Platelet and Granulocyte Workshop ISBT. *Transfus Med* 8:125, 1998.

74. McFarland JG: Platelet and neutrophil alloantigen genotyping in clinical practice. *Transfus Clin Biol* 5:13, 1998.

75. Quintanar A, Jallu V, Legros Y, Kaplan C: Human platelet antigen genotyping using a fluorescent SSCP technique with an automatic sequencer. *Br J Haematol* 103:437, 1998.

76. Metcalfe P, Cavanagh G, Hurd C, Ouwehand WH: HPA genotyping by PCR-SSP: Report of 4 exercises. *Vox Sang* 77:40, 1999.

77. Santoso S, Kiefel V: Human platelet alloantigens. *Wien Klin Wochenschr* 113:806, 2001.

78. Hurd CM, Cavanagh G, Schuh A, et al: Genotyping for platelet-specific antigens: Techniques for the detection of single nucleotide polymorphisms. *Vox Sang* 83:1, 2002.

79. Skupski DW, Bussel JB: Alloimmune thrombocytopenia. *Clin Obstet Gynecol* 42:335, 1999.

80. Nomura S, Matsuzaki T, Yamaoka M, et al: Genetic analysis of HLA- and HPA-typing in idiopathic (autoimmune) thrombocytopenic purpura patients treated with cepharanthine. *Autoimmunity* 30:99, 1999.

BLOOD PROCUREMENT AND SCREENING

JEFFREY McCULLOUGH

Blood procurement is a vital national priority that is met in the United States by volunteer donors and a pluralistic blood collection program that includes the American Red Cross, independent community blood centers, and hospitals. More than 13 million units of whole blood are collected from approximately 10 million donors annually. Recruitment of donors is preceded by a medical history and limited physical examination. The donated blood is subjected to as many as 15 tests, which include determination of blood type, examination for red cell antibodies, and a series of studies for infectious agents that may be transmitted by blood transfusion. The process usually starts with donations from random, unrelated donors but may include autologous, patient-specific, or patient-directed donors in special circumstances. In some cases, collection of red cells, platelets, leukocytes, or plasma is achieved by hemapheresis. Plasma for the subsequent manufacture of derivatives such as albumin and intravenous immunoglobulin is obtained from paid donors by for-profit organizations different from those that collect whole blood and prepare blood components.

The meticulous attention to donor risk characteristics and the use of sensitive assays to detect infectious agents that may be transmitted by blood have greatly improved the safety of blood as a therapeutic product in countries that apply these practices. Nevertheless, a risk of viral and bacterial infection, albeit small, remains. The introduction of nucleic acid amplification and bacterial detection techniques to detect microbial contaminants are the latest steps to further decrease the risk of acquiring an infection through transfusion.

OVERVIEW OF THE BLOOD BANKING SYSTEM

SYSTEM IN THE UNITED STATES

The United States has a pluralistic rather than a single national system of blood collection.[1,2] In the United States during 1997, approximately 12,602,000 units of blood donated by approximately 10,000,000 people were available for use (Table 130-1). Approximately 92 percent of the blood was collected in 150 regional blood centers, hospitals collected 8 percent, and approximately 1 percent was imported from Western Europe.[3] Approximately 5 percent of the units donated in the United States were autologous donations, and another 1.5 percent were directed donations, that is, blood given by family or friends for a specific patient. Of red cells collected, 93.8 percent of allogeneic, 65.3 percent of autologous, and 39.5 percent of directed donor red cells were transfused.[3] Blood collection increased during the 1970s and 1980s, but after the AIDS epidemic, collections have declined,[3] and the excess of supply over usage is decreasing. A single organization, the American Red Cross, collect approximately 45 percent of the blood through its network of approximately 40 regional blood centers. Community blood centers and hospitals collect the remainder. Community blood centers are individual, locally operated, nonprofit organizations, whereas the American Red Cross is a national corporation with a single Food and Drug Administration (FDA) license and set of operating procedures for all its regional centers.

All whole blood for transfusion in the United States is donated by volunteers; however, costs are incurred in the collection, testing, production, and distribution of blood components. Blood banks are nonprofit organizations that pass on these costs to hospitals. In the past, patients possibly could partially reduce the cost of blood by arranging for replacement of the blood they used. This practice has generally been discontinued because of the demand it places on the patient or family during the difficult time of the illness. Instead, blood banks assume the responsibility of ensuring that the community's blood needs are met by developing public education and donor recruitment programs.

Some areas of the United States are able to provide more blood than is needed locally, and other areas are unable to collect enough blood to meet their local needs. The misalignment of blood use and blood availability is a long-standing phenomenon. Several inventory-sharing systems are used to move blood around the United States in order to alleviate the shortages, but these systems are complex and fragile arrangements that are not always effective. As a result, blood shortages occasionally occur in some areas of the United States.

Blood is considered a drug, and all aspects of the selection of donors, collection, processing, testing, preservation, and dispensing are regulated by the FDA as specified in the Code of Federal Regulations. The requirements in the code define the procedures, records, staff proficiency, specific testing, and donor medical requirements that blood banks must follow. Additional standards are formulated by the American Association of Blood Banks (AABB), a voluntary organization that accredits blood banks. During the past decade, the FDA has required that blood banks implement good manufacturing practices similar to those used by pharmaceutical manufacturers. This requirement has had a major impact on the manner in which blood banks function.[1,2,4]

INTERNATIONAL PRACTICES

Considerable difference exists in the availability of blood and blood components throughout the world.[5-7] In general, this difference is related to the extent of development in the country and the country's health care system. For instance, in the developing world, "transfusion practice is fragmented and disorganized and it is difficult, if not impossible, to provide the five basic blood components . . . in an adequate supply."[8] These countries usually do not have an organized blood supply system, and no system for obtaining a blood supply for the general community may be in place. Patients may be required to arrange for the blood they need, so donors may be friends or family members of patients or even individuals who have been paid by the patient's family to donate the blood needed. Considerable evidence exists that blood from paid donors is more likely to transmit disease.[9] Donor screening may not be as extensive, transmissible disease testing may be lacking, equipment may be reused, and the blood collected into containers may be unsuitable for preparation of components. These difficulties may be compounded by the presence of endemic transfusion-transmissible diseases for which screening is difficult or expensive and thus not performed as extensively as in more developed countries.

The World Health Organization has estimated that approximately 75 to 90 million units of blood are collected annually worldwide.[10,11]

Acronyms and abbreviations that appear in this chapter include: AABB, American Association of Blood Banks; CPD, citrate, phosphate, dextrose; FDA, Food and Drug Administration; G-CSF, granulocyte colony stimulating factor; U, units.

TABLE 130-1   US BLOOD SUPPLY SYSTEM IN 1997*

	NUMBER	PERCENT
Total Units Whole Blood	12,602,000	100
Blood centers (190)	11,550,000	92
Hospitals (621)	1,052,000	8
Red Blood Cell Transfusions	11,517,000	100
Allogeneic	10,929,000	94.9
Autologous	420,000	3.6
Directed	81,000	0.7
Other	89,000	0.8
Discarded	666,000	5.4
Platelets		
SDP collected	981,000	54
Platelet concentrates	4,991,000	46
Total platelets transfused*	9,037,000	83
Fresh Frozen Plasma	3,320,000	—
Cryoprecipitate	816,000	—

* Data from MT Sullivan et al.[3]
SDP = single-donor platelet concentrate prepared by plateletpheresis.
One SDP is equivalent to six platelet concentrates.

The amount of blood collected in relation to the population ranges from 50 donations per 1000 population in industrialized countries to 5 to 15 per 1000 in developing countries and 1 to 5 per 1000 in the least developed countries. Thus, a concentration of blood transfusion is observed in industrialized countries. In developed countries, especially Western Europe and parts of Asia, a governmental agency usually oversees the blood collection activities, although the extent to which the government sets requirements and monitors or inspects the blood collection system varies.[12] Where national blood programs have been developed, usually a national blood policy is established that includes definition of the organization(s) responsible for the program, source of funding, type of blood donation, and regulations ensuring blood safety.[5,6] In these countries, the basic processes of donor medical screening, blood collection, laboratory testing, and preparation of blood components are similar to the US system. In virtually all developed countries, blood is donated by volunteers and not paid donors.[13] The blood may be collected by hospitals, community-based regional blood centers, or a combination of these facilities. The supply systems and sharing among hospitals and blood centers vary with the extent of development of the country's blood supply system. The basic blood components—red cells, platelets, plasma, and cryoprecipitate—usually are available, and apheresis instruments are used to collect platelets. Plasma derivatives such as albumin, coagulation factor VIII, and immune globulins are available. In many countries, these plasma derivatives are prepared from plasma collected from volunteer donors instead of the paid donor plasma used to prepare these derivatives in the United States. Thus, the availability of blood and its components around the world varies widely, from inadequate supplies and uncertain safety to sophisticated supply systems and component availability equal to or surpassing those of the United States.

PROCUREMENT OF PLASMA DERIVATIVES

The plasma industry is separate from the blood banking system described above in the section "Overview of the Blood Banking System." Plasma can be subjected to a fractionation process to produce several medically valuable products referred to as *plasma derivatives*. Examples are albumin, coagulation factor concentrates, immune serum globulins, and 19 others. Plasma fractionation is performed in a manufacturing plant setting, in batches of up to 10,000 liters involving the pooling of plasma from as many as 50,000 donors. Plasma for man-

ufacture or fractionation into derivatives can be obtained from units of whole blood, but this amount of plasma is not adequate to meet the needs for plasma derivatives. Therefore, large amounts of plasma are obtained by plasmapheresis, in which only the plasma and not red cells or platelets are removed. Individuals can donate plasma up to two times per week and usually are paid because of this more extensive time commitment. This plasma collection system usually is operated by for-profit organizations and functions separately from the system for whole-blood donation.

Approximately 11.5 million liters of plasma are collected annually in the United States,[14] although exact figures are not known because most plasma is collected by for-profit organizations. Twenty-two plasma derivatives are approved for licensure by the FDA (Table 130-2). Some derivatives are produced by only one manufacturer; other derivatives are produced by up to six different manufacturers. Thus, disruption in the sources of plasma or in one manufacturer's plant can have serious consequences and create shortages of certain derivatives.

The remainder of this chapter describes the blood collection system operated by voluntary community organizations to provide cellular and whole-blood–derived components.

RECRUITMENT OF BLOOD DONORS

Although most Americans will require a blood transfusion at some time in their lives, less than 5 percent of the total population, or less than 10 percent of those eligible to donate, have ever done so.[14] Most donors give once or infrequently; thus, much of the nation's blood supply comes from a small number of dedicated frequent donors.[14] Blood donors are more likely than the general population to be male, age 30 to 50 years, Caucasian, employed, and have more education and higher income.[14] Some studies of the social psychology and motivation of blood donors have been conducted,[15] but the process is not well understood. It is generally believed that the most effective way to get someone to donate blood is to ask him/her personally. Factors such as the convenience of donation, peer pressure, receipt of blood by a family member, and perceived community needs are important factors that are superimposed onto the individual's basic social commitments. Usually blood donors are asked to give to the general community supply. Some donors are asked to give for a specific patient, which is referred to as *directed donation*. Such donations may be easier to obtain and leave the donor with a stronger sense of satisfaction because of the personal nature of the donation.[14]

The heightened concerns about blood safety during the past decade have resulted in expanded requirements for the suitability for blood donation. Thus, a larger proportion of the population of potential donors is being excluded. The expanded requirements, along with the aging population, geographic and ethnic shifts in the population, and people's changing priorities, are causing a shrinking donor pool. Thus, understanding the motivation of blood donors and the psychosocial factors leading to blood donation will be increasingly important.

WHOLE-BLOOD DONOR SCREENING

The approach to the selection of blood donors is designed around two themes: (1) ensuring the safety of the donor and (2) obtaining a high-quality blood component that is as safe as possible for the recipient. Some specific steps that are taken to ensure that blood is as safe as possible are the use of only volunteer blood donors, questioning of donors about their general health before their donation is scheduled, obtaining a medical history including specific risk factors before donation, conducting a physical examination before donation, laboratory testing of donated blood, checking the donor's identity against a donor deferral registry,[16] and providing a method by which the donor can confidentially designate the unit as unsuitable for transfusion after the donation is completed.[14]

MEDICAL HISTORY

The questions designed to protect the safety of the donor include whether the donor is under the care of a physician and has a history of cardiovascular or lung disease, seizures, present or recent pregnancy, recent donation of blood or plasma, recent major illness or surgery, unexplained weight loss, or unusual bleeding. Use of medications and age also are documented. Questions designed to protect the safety of the recipient include those related to the donor's general health, presence of a bleeding disorder, history of receipt of growth hormone, and occurrence of or exposure to patients with hepatitis or other liver disease, AIDS (or symptoms of AIDS), Chagas disease, or babesiosis. A history also is obtained regarding the injection of drugs, receipt of coagulation factor concentrates, blood transfusion, tattoos, acupuncture, body piercing, organ or tissue transplant, travel to areas endemic for malaria, recent immunizations, contact with persons with hepatitis or other transmissible diseases, ingestion of medications (especially aspirin), presence of a major illness or surgery, or previous notice of a positive test for a transmissible disease. In addition, several questions are related to AIDS risk behavior, including whether the potential donor has had sex with anyone with AIDS, given or received money or drugs for sex, (for males) had sex with another male, or (for females) had sex with a male who has had sex with another male. This series of sex-related questions is highly specific and has changed the interaction and relationship between the donor and the blood bank.

Situations may arise in which the donor's physician believes donation would be safe but the blood bank does not accept the donor. For instance, donors with a history of cancer, other than minor skin cancer or carcinoma *in situ* of the cervix, usually are rejected because the genesis of malignant disease is not known. The donor is questioned about medications. Some medications may make the donor unsuitable because of the condition requiring the medication, whereas other medications may be potentially harmful to the recipient. Many other conditions must be evaluated individually by the blood bank physician, and that physician's assessment of conformance with FDA regulations, which view blood as a pharmaceutical, may not always coincide with the personal physician's view of the health of the patient who is the potential blood donor.

PHYSICAL AND LABORATORY EXAMINATION OF THE BLOOD DONOR

The examination includes determination of the temperature, pulse, blood pressure, weight, and blood hemoglobin concentration. The FDA has mandated limits for each of these factors. In addition, the donor's general appearance is assessed for any signs of illness or the influence of drugs or alcohol. The skin at the venipuncture site is examined for signs of intravenous drug abuse, lesions suggestive of

TABLE 130-2 PLASMA DERIVATIVE PRODUCTS AND THEIR USES

Albumin	Restoration of plasma volume subsequent to shock, trauma, surgery, and burns
α-1 Proteinase inhibitor	Treatment of emphysema caused by a genetic deficiency
Antihemophilic factor	Treatment or prevention of bleeding in patients with hemophilia A
Antiinhibitor coagulant	Treatment of bleeding episodes in the presence of factor VIII inhibitor complex
Antithrombin III	Treatment of bleeding episodes associated with liver disease, antithrombin III deficiency, and thromboembolism
Cytomegalovirus immune globulin	Passive immunization subsequent to exposure to cytomegalovirus
Factor IX complex	Prophylaxis and treatment of hemophilia B bleeding episodes and other bleeding disorders
Factor XIII	Treatment of bleeding and disorders of wound healing resulting from factor XIII deficiency
Fibrinogen	Treatment of hemorrhagic diathesis in hypofibrinogenemia, dysfibrinogenemia, and afibrinogenemia
Fibrinolysin	Dissolution of intravascular clots
Haptoglobin	Supportive therapy in viral hepatitis and pernicious anemia
Hepatitis B immune globulin	Passive immunization subsequent to exposure to hepatitis B
IgM-enriched immune globulin	Treatment and prevention of septicemia and septic shock resulting from toxin liberation in the course of antibiotic treatment
Immune globulin (intravenous and intramuscular)	Treatment of agammaglobulinemia and hypogammaglobulinemia; passive immunization for hepatitis A and measles
Plasma protein fraction	Restoration of plasma volume subsequent to shock, trauma, surgery, and burns
Rabies immune globulin	Passive immunization subsequent to exposure to rabies
Rh$_O$(D) immune globulin	Treatment and prevention of hemolytic disease of fetus and newborn resulting from Rh incompatibility and incompatible blood transfusions
Rubella immune globulin	Passive immunization subsequent to exposure to German measles
Serum cholinesterase	Treatment of prolonged apnea after administration of succinylcholine chloride
Tetanus immune globulin	Passive immunization subsequent to exposure to tetanus
Vaccinia immune globulin	Passive immunization subsequent to exposure to smallpox
Varicella-zoster immune globulin	Passive immunization subsequent to exposure to chicken pox

SOURCE: From information provided by the American Blood Resources Association.

Kaposi sarcoma, and local lesions that would make sterilizing the skin difficult and thus lead to contamination of the blood unit during venipuncture.

COLLECTION OF WHOLE BLOOD

BLOOD CONTAINERS

Blood must be collected into single-use, sterile, FDA-licensed containers. The containers are made of plasticized material that is biocompatible with blood cells and allows diffusion of gases in order to provide optimal cell preservation. These blood containers are combinations of bags that allow separation of the whole blood into its components in a closed system, thus minimizing the chance of bacterial contamination while making storage of the components for days or weeks possible. Plasticizers from the bags accumulate in red cell components during storage and can be found in tissues of multitransfused patients. However, no evidence indicates that transfusion of this material causes clinical problems.[17]

PREPARATION OF THE VENIPUNCTURE SITE

The blood should be drawn from an area free of skin lesions, and the phlebotomy site should be properly decontaminated. The site is scrubbed with a soap solution, followed by the application of tincture of iodine or iodophor complex solution. The selection of the venipuncture site and its decontamination are important steps because bacterial contamination of blood can be a serious or even fatal complication of transfusion.[18–21]

VENIPUNCTURE AND BLOOD COLLECTION

The venipuncture is done with a needle that should be used only once in order to prevent contamination. The blood must flow freely and be mixed with anticoagulant frequently as the blood fills the container to prevent the development of small clots. The actual time for collection of 450 ml usually is approximately 7 minutes and almost always is less than 10 minutes. During blood donation, cardiac output falls slightly, but heart rate changes little. A slight decrease in systolic pressure results, with a rise in peripheral resistance and diastolic blood pressure.[22]

Usually 450 ml ($\pm$10%) is collected, although some blood banks now collect 500 ml from larger donors. This amount is mixed with 63 to 70 ml of anticoagulant composed of citrate, phosphate, and dextrose (CPD). The amount of blood withdrawn must be within prescribed limits in order to maintain the proper ratio with the anticoagulant; otherwise, the blood cells may be damaged and/or anticoagulation may not be satisfactory. Although the red cells can be stored in the CPD-anticoagulant solution, customarily almost all the anticoagulated plasma is removed and the red cells resuspended in a solution that provides optimum red cell preservation. Some blood containers divert the first few milliliters so that no bacteria enter the container of transfusible blood.

POSTDONATION OBSERVATION AND ADVERSE REACTIONS TO BLOOD DONATION

An untoward reaction occurs after approximately 4 percent of blood donations, but fortunately most of the reactions are not serious.[23–25] Donors who have reactions are more likely to be younger, unmarried, have a higher predonation heart rate and lower diastolic blood pressure, and to be first-time or infrequent donors.[26] The most common reactions to blood donation are weakness, cool skin, and diaphoresis. More extensive but still moderate reactions are dizziness, pallor, hypertension, and bradycardia. Bradycardia usually is considered a sign of a vasovagal reaction rather than hypotensive or cardiovascular shock, where tachycardia would be expected. In a more severe form, this kind of reaction may progress to loss of consciousness, convulsions, and involuntary passage of urine or stool. These symptoms also are thought to result from vasovagal reactions rather than hypovolemia.[23,25] Other reactions include nausea and vomiting; hyperventilation, sometimes leading to twitching or muscle spasms; hematoma at the venipuncture site; convulsions; and serious cardiac difficulties. Such serious reactions are rare.[23,24,27] Injury of the brachial nerve and resulting pain and/or paresthesia may occur as a result of needle puncture of the nerve or compression from a hematoma.[28,29]

Donors are advised to drink extra fluids to replace lost blood volume and to avoid strenuous exercise for the remainder of the day of donation. The latter advice is given to prevent fainting and to minimize the possibility of hematoma development at the venipuncture site. Some donors are subject to lightheadedness or even fainting if they change position quickly. Therefore, donors are advised not to return to work for the remainder of the day if they have an occupation where fainting would be hazardous to themselves or others.

SPECIAL BLOOD DONATIONS

In several situations involving blood donation, the blood is not obtained from the community's general blood supply. Examples of such situations include autologous donation, directed donation, patient-specific donation, and therapeutic bleeding. In some of these situations, the FDA requirements for blood donation may not apply.

AUTOLOGOUS DONOR BLOOD

Autologous blood donation is an old concept but was little used until the AIDS epidemic raised fears of blood transfusion among both patients and physicians. Individuals can donate blood for their own use if the need for blood can be anticipated and a donation plan developed. Most commonly this situation occurs with elective surgery.

Autologous blood for transfusion can be obtained by preoperative donation, acute normovolemic hemodilution, intraoperative salvage, and postoperative salvage, but only preoperative donation is discussed here. If patient candidates for autologous blood donation meet the usual FDA criteria for blood donation, their blood can be "crossed over," that is, used for other patients if the original autologous donor has no need for the blood. This practice is no longer allowed by AABB standards. If the autologous donor does not meet the FDA criteria for blood donation, the blood must be specially labeled, segregated during storage, and discarded if it is not used by that specific patient. Thus, the autologous blood donation should be collected only for procedures with a substantial likelihood that the blood will be used.[30] Without this type of planning, a very high rate of wastage of autologous blood is observed, estimated at 65 percent in 1997.[3] Thus, the cost of autologous blood is high.[31]

No age or weight restrictions exist for autologous donation.[14] Pregnant women can donate, but this practice is not recommended routinely because these patients rarely require transfusion. The autologous donor's hemoglobin may be lower (11 g/dl) than that required for routine donors (12.5 g/dl), and autologous donors may donate as often as every 72 hours up to 72 hours prior to the planned surgery, although usually only 2 to 4 U of blood can be obtained before the hemoglobin falls below 11 g/dl. Autologous blood donors can be given erythropoietin and iron to increase the number of units of blood they can donate,[32] although the value of erythropoietin is dubious because this strategy has not been shown to reduce the need for allogeneic donor blood and only results in the ability to donate one additional unit of blood.[33] Contraindications for autologous blood donation include bacteremia, symptomatic angina, recent seizures, and symptomatic valvular heart lesions. However, the final decision on whether to withdraw blood from an autologous donor rests with the medical director of the blood bank. Often consultation between the donor's (patient's) physician and the blood bank physician is necessary to decide on a wise course of action.

Autologous blood must be typed for ABO and Rh antigens.[14] If the unit is to be shipped to another facility for transfusion, it must be tested for transmissible diseases similar to allogeneic blood.[14] If any of the transmissible disease tests are positive, the unit must be labeled with a biohazard label. This labeling sometimes is confusing or disconcerting to physicians but is required by the FDA to alert health care personnel to the hazard presented by the potentially infectious blood.

DIRECTED DONOR BLOOD

Directed donors are friends or relatives who wish to give blood for a specific patient because the patient hopes those donors will be safer than the regular blood supply. In general, the data do not indicate that directed donors have a lower incidence of transmissible disease markers[34,35] and thus do not support a realistic rationale for these donations. Moreover, when friends or relatives are asked to donate blood, they may be reluctant to disclose risk factors that would preclude them from voluntary donation, which actually increases risk. Some blood banks refuse directed donations, but most accept them as a service to the patients. However, because the blood becomes part of the community's general blood supply if it is not used for the originally intended patient, directed donors must meet all the usual FDA requirements for routine blood donation.

PATIENT-SPECIFIC DONATION

In a few situations, appropriate transfusion therapy involves collecting blood from a particular donor for a particular patient. Examples are donor-specific transfusions prior to kidney transplantation, maternal platelets for a fetus projected to have alloimmune neonatal thrombocytopenia, or family members of a patient with a rare blood type. In these situations, donors must meet all the usual FDA requirements, except that they may donate as often as every 3 days so long as the hemoglobin remains above the normal donor minimum of 12.5 g/dl.[14] These units must undergo all routine laboratory testing.[14]

THERAPEUTIC BLEEDING

Blood can be collected as part of the therapy of diseases such as polycythemia vera or hemochromatosis. Often the patient or physician asks that the blood be used for transfusion as a way of comforting the patient. However, usually such blood is not used for transfusion because the donors do not meet the FDA standards for donor health. As the genetic basis of hemochromatosis has become better understood, blood removed from these patients has been proposed for transfusion, although the subject remains controversial.[36,37]

COLLECTION AND PRODUCTION OF BLOOD COMPONENTS BY APHERESIS

Blood components can be obtained by apheresis rather than prepared from a standard unit of whole blood. In apheresis, the donor's anticoagulated whole blood is passed through an instrument in which the blood is separated into red cells, plasma, and a leukocyte/platelet fraction (see Chap. 25). Several semiautomated blood cell separator instruments are available for collection of platelets, granulocytes, peripheral blood stem cells, mononuclear cells, or plasma.[14] All of these instruments use centrifugation to separate the blood components.[38] Some apheresis procedures involve two venipunctures with continuous flow of blood from the donor through the blood cell separator; others can be accomplished with a single venipuncture and intermittent blood withdrawal and return. Apheresis has been used to collect 2 U of red cells[39–42] or various combinations of components.[43]

PLATELETPHERESIS

Platelet concentrates are produced from whole blood, but use of plateletpheresis has been increasing. By 1997, 54 percent of platelets produced in the United States were produced by plateletpheresis.[3] Plateletpheresis requires approximately 90 minutes, during which approximately 4000 to 5000 ml of the donor's blood is processed through the blood cell separator. The process results in a platelet concentrate with a volume of approximately 200 ml and containing approximately 4.0×10^{11} platelets and less than 0.5 ml red cells. Currently manufactured blood cell separators produce a platelet concentrate that contains less than 5×10^6 leukocytes and thus can be considered leukocyte depleted. Following plateletpheresis, the donor's platelet count declines by approximately 30 percent and does not return to preplateletpheresis levels for approximately 4 days (see Chap. 132).[44]

COLLECTION OF RED CELLS BY APHERESIS

Chronic shortages of group O red cells stimulated interest in the use of apheresis for collecting the equivalent of 2 U of red cells from some donors, especially group O.[39–42] The collection procedure is similar to other apheresis procedures, except that red cells are retained rather than returned to the donor. The red cells usually have a very high hematocrit as they are removed from the instrument, but an additive solution is incorporated and the red cells can be stored for the usual

42 days. The red cell products obtained by apheresis have a more standard volume than red cells prepared from whole blood, but otherwise red cells obtained by apheresis have the same characteristics as those produced from whole blood. Donors for 2-U red cell apheresis must meet weight and hemoglobin standards specified for each instrument. Because 2 U of red cells are removed, donors may donate only every 4 months. Double-unit red cell collection allows fewer donor visits, may increase red cell availability, and possibly reduces the patients' donor exposure if both donor units are given to the same patient. Apheresis for 2-U red cell collection is becoming popular and seems to be taking its place in the mixture of blood component production activities.

LEUKAPHERESIS

Leukapheresis has been used to produce a granulocyte concentrate for transfusion therapy of infections unresponsive to antibiotics.[14] In the past, leukapheresis provided only a marginally adequate dose of granulocytes for therapeutic benefit,[38] and its use had declined to very low levels (see Chap. 25). Leukapheresis usually is a more lengthy and complex procedure than plateletpheresis. Because the efficiency of granulocyte extraction from whole blood is less than for platelets, the leukapheresis procedure involves processing 6500 to 8000 ml of donor blood for approximately 3 hours.[38] To increase the separation of granulocytes from other blood components, hydroxyethyl starch is added to the blood cell separator flow system.[38] In addition, glucocorticoids have been administered to the donor to increase the peripheral blood granulocyte count and thus increase the yield. Granulocyte colony stimulating factor (G-CSF) has been administered to granulocyte donors to achieve much larger increases in granulocyte count and a much greater granulocyte yield.[45–49] Transfusion of these high-yield granulocyte concentrates results in substantially increased granulocyte count and has led to renewed interest in granulocyte transfusions (see Chap. 25).[50]

PLASMAPHERESIS

Plasmapheresis originally was developed using sets of multiple attached bags. This method is time consuming, cumbersome, and involves disconnecting the blood bags from the donor, resulting in the chance of returning the blood to the wrong donor; therefore, this method is no longer used. During the past few years, semiautomated instruments have become available that require less operator involvement than the bag systems while producing larger volumes of plasma more rapidly. The volume of plasma that can be collected depends on the size of the donor. Plasmapheresis usually can be performed in approximately 30 minutes to produce up to 750 ml of plasma. Few red cells are removed. The procedure can be repeated up to two times per week, so theoretically a donor could provide up to approximately 50 liters of plasma in 1 year.

SELECTION OF APHERESIS DONORS

The selection of donors for apheresis uses the same criteria as for whole-blood donation.[14] Because of the unique nature of apheresis, some additional donor requirements are necessary. Many apheresis procedures involve two venipunctures and continuous blood flow, so good venous access is important. No more than 15 percent of the donor's blood should be extracorporeal during apheresis; thus, the donor's size is considered when making decisions about specific apheresis procedures or instruments to be used. Following plateletpheresis, the donor's platelet count declines by approximately 30 percent and does not return to preplateletpheresis levels for approximately 4 days.[44] Donors may undergo plateletpheresis every 48 hours; however, if they are donating more often than every 8 weeks, a platelet count must be obtained to ensure that the count is at least 150,000/μl (1.5 × 10^{11}/liter).[31] Apheresis donors of 2-U red cells must wait 4 months before they may donate again. Following leukapheresis of G-CSF–stimulated donors, the granulocyte count decreases slightly, the platelet count decreases by 20 to 25 percent, and the hematocrit decreases by approximately 1 percent.[47,48] Thus, the platelet count must be monitored in donors undergoing frequent leukaphereses. Because a plateletpheresis concentrate would be the sole source of platelets for the transfusion, the donor must not have taken aspirin for at least 3 days. For donors undergoing plasmapheresis more often than once every 8 weeks, the serum protein must be at least 6 g/dl. In addition, a protein electrophoresis or a quantitative immunoglobulins assay should be obtained every 4 months, and the results must be normal to allow further donation.[14] The amount of blood components removed from apheresis donors must be monitored. Not more than 200 ml of red cells per 2 months or approximately 1500 ml of plasma per week can be removed.[14] The laboratory testing of donors and apheresis components for transmissible diseases is the same as for whole-blood donation. Thus, the likelihood of disease transmission from apheresis components is the same as from whole blood.

REACTIONS IN APHERESIS DONORS

Apheresis donors can experience the same kind of reactions as whole-blood donors. In addition, apheresis donors experience a higher incidence of paresthesias, probably because of the infusion of citrate used to anticoagulate the donor's blood while it is in the cell separator.[51,52] This type of reaction is managed by slowing the flow rate of the instrument, which slows the rate of citrate infusion. The additional donor selection and monitoring requirements for apheresis prevent the development of reactions or complications resulting from excess removal of blood cells or plasma. In leukapheresis, donors can be given glucocorticoid and/or G-CSF to elevate the granulocyte count, and the sedimenting agent hydroxyethyl starch is used in the cell separator to improve the granulocyte yield. When G-CSF is used, approximately 60 percent of donors experience side effects, usually myalgia, arthralgia, headache, or flu-like symptoms.[45–49] This rate of side effects may be higher if the donors also receive glucocorticoids.[48] The major side effect of hydroxyethyl starch is blood volume expansion manifested by headache and/or hypertension.[14] Donor selection techniques are intended to minimize the likelihood of hypertension resulting from hydroxyethyl starch.

LABORATORY TESTING OF DONATED BLOOD

Each unit of whole blood or each apheresis component undergoes a standard battery of tests (Table 130-3), including tests for blood type, red cell antibodies, and transmissible diseases. Additional tests, such as those for cytomegalovirus or HLA antibodies to aid in directed transfusions, may be done. Ten tests, eight of which have been introduced since 1985, are performed for transmissible diseases. The total number of test results for each unit of donated blood is approximately 15, depending on the specific methodology used. In addition, because each unit of whole blood is separated into several components and a donor history record and two or three tubes of blood for tests are available, each donation generates up to 30 different data elements. All data are amalgamated to ensure that they are satisfactory for release of the blood into the transfusion inventory. Because busy blood collection centers deal with hundreds of donors each day, this virtual explosion of data has made essential the need for blood banks to operate sophisticated computer systems and, where possible, automated laboratory testing equipment. Thus, the modern blood center uses

TABLE 130-3 LABORATORY TESTS OF DONATED BLOOD

AGENT	DISEASE
Treponema	Syphilis
Hepatitis B$_S$ antigen	Hepatitis B
Hepatitis B$_C$ antibody	Hepatitis B
	Hepatitis non-A, non-B
Hepatitis C antibody	Hepatitis C
Hepatitis C nucleic acids	Hepatitis C
HIV-1 and HIV-2 antibody	AIDS
HIV antigen	AIDS
HIV nucleic acids	AIDS
HTLV-I antibody	Leukemia
	Lymphoma
	Tropical paresis
HTLV-II antibody	Disease unknown
CMV*	CMV disease
Optional	
CMV antibody	
HLA antibody	
Other RBC antigens	

* Of use for immunodeficient recipients.
AIDS = acquired immunodeficiency syndrome; CMV = cytomegalovirus; HIV = human immunodeficiency virus; HLA = human leukocyte antigen; HTLV = human T lymphotropic virus.

pharmaceutical-type manufacturing processes to ensure accuracy and cost effectiveness.[2,4,14]

SAFETY OF THE BLOOD SUPPLY

Ironically, the improvements in blood safety have occurred at a time of the public's increased fear of transfusion and the more cautious use of blood components by physicians. The steps in donor selection and laboratory testing described have resulted in the nation's blood supply being safer than ever.[53–56] Each step in the overall process of donor evaluation and testing adds to blood safety in important ways. For instance, in San Francisco, California, changes in the medical history and donor selection criteria resulted in a 90 percent decrease in the HIV infectivity of the blood supply, even before the introduction of a test specific for HIV.[53] The introduction of new tests for transmissible diseases has further reduced the proportion of infectious donors. Screening of the donor's identity against donor deferral registries detects individuals who previously were deferred as blood donors but who for various reasons attempt to donate again. These and many other changes have resulted in improved blood safety. The risk of acquiring a transfusion-transmitted disease ranges from 1 per 150,000 U for hepatitis B to 1 per 2,135,000 U for HIV (Table 130-4). Thus, although

TABLE 130-4 TRANSFUSION-TRANSMITTED DISEASE*

	STRONG AND KATZ 2002	DODD ET AL. 2002	TABOR 2002	TOTAL US CASES*
Hepatitis C	1,200,000	1,935,000	625,000	6
Hepatitis B	150,000	—	150,000	80+
HTLV-I/HTLV-II	641,000	—	—	20+
HIV	1,400,000	2,135,000	769,230	5

* Calculated based on transfusion of 12,000,000 U of blood annually and Dodd incidence figures.
+ Calculations based on data from Strong and Katz.
HIV = human immunodeficiency virus; HTLV = human T lymphotropic virus.
SOURCE: Strong DM, Katz L: *Trends Mol Med* 8:355, 2002, and Dodd RY, Notari EP, Stramor SL: *Transfusion* 42:975, 2002.

the blood supply is safer than ever,[53–63] transfusion is not risk free and should be undertaken only after careful consideration of the patient's clinical situation and specific blood component needs (see Chap. 131).

REFERENCES

1. McCullough J: The nation's changing blood supply system. *JAMA* 269: 2239, 1993.

2. McCullough J: The continuing evolution of the nation's blood supply system. *Am J Clin Pathol* 105:689, 1996.

3. Sullivan MT, McCullough J, Schreiber GB, Wallace EL: Blood collection and transfusion in the United States in 1997. *Transfusion* 42:1253, 2002.

4. Zuck TF: Current good manufacturing practices. *Transfusion* 35:95, 1995.

5. Koistinen J: Organization of blood transfusion services in developing countries. *Vox Sang* 64:247, 1994.

6. Koistinen J, Westphal R: Blood transfusion worldwide, in *Transfusion Medicine, a European Course on Blood Transfusion*, coordinated by W van Aken, B Genetet. Centre Nationale d'Enseignement à Distance, Paris, 1994.

7. Emanuel JC: Blood transfusion systems in economically restricted countries. *Vox Sang* 64:267, 1994.

8. Beal R: Transfusion science and practice in developing countries: A high frequency of empty shelves. *Transfusion* 33:276, 1993.

9. Eastlund T: Monetary blood donation incentives and the risk of transfusion-transmitted infection. *Transfusion* 38:874, 1998.

10. World Health Day 2000: Some Facts. Available from WHO, Essential Health Technology, Geneva, Switzerland.

11. Leikola J: How much blood for the world? *Vox Sang* 54:1, 1988.

12. McCullough J: National blood programs in developed countries. *Transfusion* 36:1019, 1996.

13. Barker LF, Westphal RG: Voluntary, nonremunerated blood donation: Still a world health goal? *Transfusion* 38:803, 1998.

14. McCullough J: *Transfusion Medicine*, 2nd edition. Elsevier, Philadelphia, 2005:1–584.

15. Piliavin JA, Callero PL (eds): *Giving Blood. The Development of an Altruistic Identity*. Johns Hopkins University, Baltimore, 1991.

16. Grossman BJ, Springer KM, Zuck TF: Blood donor deferral registries: Highlights of a conference. *Transfusion* 32:868, 1992.

17. Rubin RJ, Ness PM: What price progress? An update on vinyl plastic blood banks. *Transfusion* 29:3358, 1989.

18. Morduchowicz G, Pitlik SD, Huminer D, et al: Transfusion reactions due to bacterial contamination of blood and blood products. *Rev Infect Dis* 13:307, 1991.

19. Sazama K: Reports of 355 transfusion-associated deaths: 1976 through 1985. *Transfusion* 30:583, 1990.

20. Klein HG, Dodd RY, Ness PM, et al: Current status of microbial contamination of blood components: Summary of a conference. *Transfusion* 37:95, 1997.

21. Kuehnert MJ, Roth VR, Haley NR, et al: Transfusion-transmitted bacterial infection in the United States, 1998 through 2000. *Transfusion* 41: 1492, 2001.

22. Logic JR, Johnson SA, Smith JJ: Cardiovascular and hematologic responses to phlebotomy in blood donors. *Transfusion* 3:83, 1963.

23. Ogata H, Iinuma N, Nagashima K, Akabane T: Vasovagal reactions in blood donors. *Transfusion* 20:679, 1980.

24. Kasprisin DO, Glynn SH, Taylor F, Miller KA: Moderate and severe reactions in blood donors. *Transfusion* 32:23, 1992.

25. Popovsky MA: Vasovagal donor reactions: An important issue with implications for the blood supply. *Transfusion* 42:1534, 2002.

26. Callahan R, Edelman EB, Smith MS, Smith JJ: Study of the incidence and characteristics of blood donor "reactors." *Transfusion* 3:76, 1963.

27. Popovsky MA, Whitaker B, Arnold NL: Severe outcomes of allogeneic and autologous blood donation: Frequency and characterization. *Transfusion* 35:734, 1995.

28. Newman BH, Waxman DA: Blood donation-related neurologic needle injury: Evaluation of 2 years' worth of data from a large blood center. *Transfusion* 36:213, 1996.

29. Berry PR, Wallis WE: Venipuncture nerve injuries. *Lancet* 1:1236, 1997.

30. Axelrod FB, Pepkowitz SH, Goldfinger D: Establishment of a schedule of optimal preoperative collection of autologous blood. *Transfusion* 29: 677, 1989.

31. Birkmeyer JD, Goodnough LT, AuBuchon JP, et al: The cost-effectiveness of preoperative autologous blood donation for total hip and knee replacement. *Transfusion* 33:544, 1993.

32. Goodnough LT, Rednick S, Price TH, et al: Increased preoperative collection of autologous blood with recombinant human erythropoietin therapy. *N Engl J Med* 321:1163, 1989.

33. Spivak JL: Recombinant human erythropoietin and its role in transfusion medicine. *Transfusion* 34:1, 1994.

34. Starkey NM, MacPherson JL, Bolgiano DC, et al: Markers for transfusion-transmitted disease in different groups of blood donors. *JAMA* 262: 3452, 1989.

35. Williams AE, Kleinman S, Gilcher RO, et al: The prevalence of infectious disease markers in directed versus homologous blood donations [abstract]. *Transfusion* 32:45S, 1992.

36. Jeffrey G, Adams PC: Blood from patients with hereditary hemochromatosis—A wasted resource? *Transfusion* 39:549, 1999.

37. Sacher RA: Hemochromatosis and blood donors: A perspective. *Transfusion* 39:551, 1999.

38. McLeod BC, Price TH, Drew MI (eds): *Apheresis: Principles and Practice*. AABB, Bethesda, MD, 1997.

39. Meyer D, Bolgiano DC, Sayers M, et al: Red cell collection by apheresis technology. *Transfusion* 33:819, 1993.

40. Shi PA, Ness PM: Two-unit red cell apheresis and its potential advantages over traditional whole-blood donation. *Transfusion* 39:219, 1999.

41. Gilcher RO: It's time to end RBC shortages. *Transfusion* 43:1658, 2003.

42. Snyder EL, Elfath MD, Taylor H, et al: Collection of two units of leukoreduced RBCs from a single donation with a portable multiple-component collection system. *Transfusion* 43:1695, 2003.

43. Smith JW, Gilcher RO: Red blood cells, plasma, and other new apheresis-derived blood products: Improving product quality and donor utilization. *Transfus Med Rev* 13:118, 1999.

44. Lasky L, Lin A, Kahn R, McCullough J: Donor platelet response and product quality assurance in plateletpheresis. *Transfusion* 21:247, 1981.

45. Bensinger WI, Price TH, Dale DC, et al: The effects of daily recombinant human granulocyte-colony-stimulating factor administration on normal granulocyte donors undergoing leukapheresis. *Blood* 81:1883, 1993.

46. Dale DC, Liles WC, Llewellyn C, et al: Neutrophil transfusions: Kinetics and functions of neutrophils mobilized with granulocyte colony-stimulating factor (G-CSF) and dexamethasone. *Transfusion* 38:713, 1998.

47. McCullough J, Clay M, Herr G, et al: Effects of granulocyte colony stimulating factor (G-CSF) on potential normal granulocyte donors. *Transfusion* 39:1136, 1999.

48. Hester J, Dignani MC, Anaissie EJ, et al: Collection and transfusion of granulocyte concentrates from donors primed with granulocyte stimulating factor and response of myelosuppressed patients with established infection. *J Clin Apheresis* 10:188, 1995.

49. Liles WC, Huang JE, Llewellyn C, et al: A comparative trial of granulocyte-colony-stimulating factor and dexamethasone, separately and in combination, for the mobilization of neutrophils in the peripheral blood of normal volunteers. *Transfusion* 37:182, 1997.

50. Strauss RG: Neutrophil (granulocyte) transfusions in the new millennium. *Transfusion* 38:710, 1998.

51. Olson PR, Cox C, McCullough J: Laboratory and clinical effects on the infusion of ACD solution during plateletpheresis. *Vox Sang* 33:79, 1977.

52. Bolan CD, Greer SE, Cecco SA, et al: Comprehensive analysis of citrate effects during plateletpheresis in normal donors. *Transfusion* 41:1165, 2001.

53. Busch MP, Young MJ, Transfusion Safety Study Group, et al: Risk of human immunodeficiency virus (HIV) transmission by blood transfusions before the implementation of HIV-1 antibody screening. *Transfusion* 31:4, 1991.

54. Cumming PD, Wallace EL, Schorr JB, Dodd RY: Exposure of patients to human immunodeficiency virus through the transfusion of blood components that test antibody-negative. *N Engl J Med* 321:941, 1989.

55. Busch MP, Bernard EE, Khayam-Bashi H, et al: Evaluation of screened blood donations from human immunodeficiency virus type 1 infection by culture and DNA amplification of pooled cells. *N Engl J Med* 325:1, 1991.

56. Donahue JG, Munoz A, Ness PM, et al: The declining risk of post-transfusion hepatitis C virus infection. *N Engl J Med* 327:369, 1992.

57. Dodd RY: The risk of transfusion-transmitted infection. *N Engl J Med* 327:419, 1992.

58. Nelson KE, Donahue JG, Munoz A, et al: Transmission of retroviruses from seronegative donors by transfusion during cardiac surgery. *Ann Intern Med* 117:554, 1992.

59. Kleinman S, Alter H, Busch M, et al: Increased detection of hepatitis C virus (HCV)-infected blood donors by a multiple-antigen HCV enzyme immunoassay. *Transfusion* 32:805, 1992.

60. Williams AE, Thomson RA, Schreiber GB, et al: Estimates of infectious disease risk factors in U.S. blood donors. *JAMA* 277:967, 1997.

61. Sloand EM, Pitt E, Klein HG: Safety of the blood supply. *JAMA* 274:1368, 1995.

62. Lackritz EM, Satten GA, Aberle-Grasse J, et al: Estimated risk of transmission of the human immunodeficiency virus by screened blood in the United States. *N Engl J Med* 333:1721, 1995.

63. Schreiber GB, Busch MP, Kleinman SH: The risk of transfusion-transmitted viral infections. *N Engl J Med* 334:1685, 1996.

PRESERVATION AND CLINICAL USE OF ERYTHROCYTES AND WHOLE BLOOD

ERNEST BEUTLER

Transfusion of whole blood or of red cell concentrates is important in the treatment of acute blood loss and of anemia. Red cells can be stored at 4°C for 5 weeks in media that are specially designed to preserve the physical and biochemical integrity of the erythrocytes and that maintain their viability after reinfusion. Citrate-phosphate-dextrose with adenine (CPDA) is commonly used for the collection of blood. The use of whole blood as a therapeutic agent has been almost entirely replaced by the use of blood fractions. Red cells can be stored in residual plasma or in additive solutions such as AS-1, a solution containing glucose, adenine, and mannitol. Erythrocytes can also be frozen after addition of a cryoprotective agent such as glycerol, and such cells can be stored for years. A variety of "blood substitutes" based either on hemoglobin or perfluorocarbons have been designed, but all have a short intravascular half-life and have not yet been found to be clinically useful.

Transfusion of red cells can cause febrile reactions, usually as a result of residual leukocytes, and the transmission of infectious diseases such as HIV and hepatitis. Other adverse effects include pulmonary hypersensitivity reactions, incompatible transfusions because of either unsuspected antigens or human error, and, in immunocompromised recipients, graft-versus-host disease.

Although the association of blood with life and vitality was recognized by primitive man, the transfusion of blood was not undertaken until after Harvey had described the circulation of the blood in 1628. During the following 40 years, animal blood was transfused directly into animals and humans, sometimes with unfortunate results.[1] Interest in blood transfusion waned, and it was not until 1828 that Blundell[2] successfully treated postpartum hemorrhage by direct transfusion of human blood. However, the mortality associated with transfusion was approximately 33 percent,[3] a figure surprisingly a little lower than the calculated frequency of ABO incompatibility.

Safe and effective transfusion therapy had to await the discovery of red cell blood group antigens by Landsteiner[4] and the development of nontoxic anticoagulants so that blood could be stored and used for indirect transfusions.[5–7] In 1937, Fantus[8] described the establishment at Cook County Hospital in Chicago of a blood bank for the collection, storage, and compatibility testing of blood for transfusion therapy.

Acronyms and abbreviations that appear in this chapter include: ADP, adenosine diphosphate; AIHA, autoimmune hemolytic anemia; AMP, adenosine monophosphate; ATP, adenosine triphosphate; BPG, bisphosphoglycerate; CPD, citrate-phosphate-dextrose; CPDA-1, citrate-phosphate-dextrose with adenine; DIC, disseminated intravascular coagulation; DPG, diphosphoglycerate; HLA, human leukocyte antigen; IMP, inosine monophosphate; PIP, phosphate, inosine, and pyruvate.

Extensive experience with transfusion therapy accumulated during World War II.[9,10] Subsequently, major technical developments included the introduction of closed plastic equipment consisting of tubing and bags that minimize the risk of bacterial contamination, the availability of a practical refrigerated centrifuge that facilitates separation of components, and the introduction of automated equipment for continuous-flow cell separations.[11,12]

PRINCIPLES OF STORAGE AND PRESERVATION OF BLOOD

Erythrocytes are preserved by either liquid storage at 4°C or frozen storage with various cryoprotective agents at either −80 or −150°C. During liquid storage, red blood cells undergo changes that lead to a loss in viability and a diminished capacity to offload oxygen. When stored red blood cells are reinfused into the circulation, some perish within a few hours, but the remainder appear to return to an entirely normal state. The survival of those cells not removed within the first 24 hours is normal.[13]

Many attempts have been made to devise a means of predicting the proportion of transfused erythrocytes that remain viable. The adenosine triphosphate (ATP) level of the erythrocytes enjoys a reputation as a predictor of viability of red blood cells after reinfusion that is poorly deserved.[14,15] The osmotic fragility and plasma hemoglobin levels are also of little value in predicting the viability of stored red blood cells. Indeed, the increase in osmotic fragility of stored erythrocytes results almost entirely from their becoming loaded with lactate. Not freely diffusible, this exerts an unbalanced osmotic effect when osmotic fragility is tested in saline solutions.[16]

Stored red blood cells develop multiple and complex changes in membrane structure.[17] Although it has been suggested that the exposure of phosphatidyl serine on the outer membrane, which has increasingly been implicated as a signal of red cell aging (see Chap. 31), may play a role in the loss of viability of stored erythrocytes,[18] this does not seem to be the case.[19–21] The critical changes associated with loss of viability have not been identified, so that of necessity preservative solutions are evaluated by red cell survival studies in volunteers. The standard that is generally applied is that 75 percent of the transfused red blood cells remains in the circulation 24 hours after administration.

After reinfusion, stored red blood cells need to function properly in delivering oxygen to the tissues. The loss of 2,3-bisphosphoglycerate (2,3-BPG, 2,3-diphosphoglycerate [2,3-DPG]) (see Chap. 45) during storage results in an increase in oxygen affinity that may compromise the ability of the stored erythrocytes to deliver oxygen to the tissues.[22,23] After reinfusion, the red cell 2,3-BPG level returns to half-normal in 4 hours and to normal in 24 hours.[24,25] Although the clinical significance of 2,3-BPG loss in stored blood is difficult to assess,[26] there is general agreement that blood with nearly normal oxygen affinity should be used for massive transfusions, particularly in infants, older patients, and patients with cardiovascular and pulmonary disease.

Ideally, preservative solutions for erythrocytes should ensure maximum viability for the longest possible storage time and should allow optimal oxygen delivery. Unfortunately, with commonly used preservative solutions, optimal storage conditions for either of the two critical components, ATP and 2,3-BPG, usually produce adverse effects on the other. The effect of various preservative solutions on maintenance of ATP and 2,3-BPG levels during liquid storage is summarized in Table 131-1.

LIQUID PRESERVATION OF ERYTHROCYTES

The preservative solutions used for the storage of whole blood or red blood cells contain glucose and a citrate buffer at an acid pH. The citrate ion chelates calcium and thus prevents coagulation of the blood, glucose sustains the metabolism of red blood cells during storage, and the acid pH counteracts the marked rise of pH that occurs when blood

TABLE 131-1   PRESERVATION OF ATP AND 2,3-BPG RED CELL CONCENTRATIONS DURING STORAGE IN DIFFERENT PRESERVATIVE SOLUTIONS

	STORAGE PERIOD (WEEKS)							
	1		2		3		4	
	ATP	2,3-BPG	ATP	2,3-BPG	ATP	2,3-BPG	ATP	2,3-BPG
ACD	90	60	80	10	60	5	40	5
CPD	75	120	70	85	65	40	40	10
ACD−0.5 mM adenine	85	110	85	70	80	30	65	10
CPD−0.5 mM adenine	95	100	90	40	85	10	70	5
CPD + PIP (10 mM phosphate, 5 mM inosine, 5 mM pyruvate)	70	150	60	150	55	105	45	35
Addition PIP at 14 days					80	120	70	100

NOTE: Whole blood stored at 4°C. Values are in percent of initial values and are approximate because there is considerable variation from donor to donor.
SOURCE: Modified from de Verdier, Åkerblom, Arturson, et al.[76,229]

is cooled to 4°C.[27] The two preservative solutions of this type in use until CPD-adenine was introduced in 1978 were acid-citrate-dextrose (ACD) and citrate-phosphate-dextrose (CPD) (see below).

When whole blood or packed red blood cells are stored in either ACD or CPD, a series of well-defined biochemical changes, designated collectively as the storage lesion, take place in the erythrocytes (Table 131-2). The concentration of red cell ATP falls gradually during storage.[25,27] As ATP is dephosphorylated, the levels of adenosine diphosphate (ADP) and adenosine monophosphate (AMP) rise at first but diminish with time, as AMP is irreversibly deaminated to inosine monophosphate (IMP), which is ultimately broken down to hypoxanthine.[28] When the ATP level declines to 0.4 mM or less, the capacity of red blood cells to phosphorylate glucose is impaired, and their viability is lost. The level of 2,3-BPG and consequently the hemoglobin oxygen affinity change rapidly in ACD blood. Some 40 percent of the 2,3-BPG is lost in the first week of storage, resulting in a significant increase in oxygen affinity. After 2 weeks' storage, nearly all of the 2,3-BPG has disappeared from blood stored in ACD solution. The loss of 2,3-BPG occurs more slowly in blood stored in CPD solution, because of its higher pH.[29] The oxygen affinity and 2,3-BPG levels remain nearly normal during the first week of storage and then fall rapidly. Potassium rapidly leaks from the stored blood cells, and sodium seeps in[30] because the sodium-potassium ATPase is exquisitely sensitive to changes in temperature. The osmotic fragility of the red blood cells gradually increases, but this change is largely an artifact produced by the intracellular accumulation of lactate.[16] Some erythrocytes undergo spontaneous lysis, causing a rise of plasma hemoglobin levels. Di-(2-ethylhexyl) phthalate plasticizer leached from the polyvinyl chloride plastic in which whole blood and red cell preparations are stored retards hemolysis and improves the viability of the cells when they are reinfused.[31] Microvesicles filled with hemoglobin begin to form.[32] Erythrocytes stored at 4°C also show a progressive increase in rigidity as measured by their rate of flow through filters. Their loss of deformability correlates to some extent with the loss of ATP.[33] Because some residual leukocytes are invariably present, various cytokines are also found in stored blood,[34] and these may play a role in some transfusion reactions. This seems to be the case when certain types of apparatus are used for intraoperative salvage of erythrocytes.[35] Blood collected in ACD or CPD will yield a 70 percent 24-hour survival of transfused red blood cells for up to 21 days of storage.

Major efforts have been directed toward development of preservative solutions that will maintain adequate erythrocyte levels of ATP and 2,3-BPG. Addition of adenine to give a final concentration of 0.25 to 0.75 mM at the beginning of storage helps to prevent the loss of ATP[36] because it can serve as a substrate for synthesis of adenine nucleotides (see Chap. 45). The addition of adenine does not prevent the loss of 2,3-BPG and may slightly hasten its depletion.

The addition of adenine alone at the end of storage is not helpful if red blood cells have lost a substantial portion of their ATP. Under these circumstances, they are unable to phosphorylate glucose and thus are unable to synthesize adenine nucleotides or to phosphorylate ADP and AMP to ATP. If inosine is supplied, ATP formation can occur even when red cell ATP levels are very low. The phosphorolysis of inosine yields ribose-1-phosphate, which can be metabolized to yield high-energy phosphates and maintain 2,3-BPG levels (see Chap. 45). The addition of inosine either at the beginning of storage or before infusion of ATP-depleted blood markedly improves the storage viability of red blood cells,[36] but a concentration of inosine of approximately 10 mM is required. Infusion of inosine or of the hypoxanthine formed by its catabolism may result in dangerous hyperuricemia.

The reported capacity of ascorbic acid to maintain 2,3-BPG levels[37,38] results from contaminating oxalate,[39–41] which seems to exert its function largely by inhibiting pyruvate kinase.[40] Certain xanthone derivatives exert a direct effect on the oxygen dissociation curve of hemoglobin and, in addition, elevate red cell 2,3-BPG levels[42] because of their inhibitory effect on 2,3-BPG phosphatase.[43] Dihydroxyacetone is metabolized by erythrocytes and helps to maintain 2,3-BPG levels during storage.[44–46] Periodic agitation of blood during storage improves the maintenance of 2,3-BPG levels in some preservatives, probably by preventing a localized decrease in pH in the gravity-sedimented red blood cells[47] but has little effect on red blood cells in blood collected in CPD solution.[48] Several other additives have been used experimentally to maintain or restore 2,3-BPG levels of stored red blood cells. The 2,3-BPG content of stored blood can be restored to normal or supranormal levels[49] by incubating the erythrocytes with phosphate, inosine, and pyruvate (PIP). Both 2,3-BPG and ATP levels in outdated blood can be restored by incubation with PIP and adenine. Phosphoenolpyruvate can enter red blood cells when they are suspended in a slightly acidic solution, and it has also been proposed that this source of metabolic energy may be useful in red cell preservation.[50] The rejuvenated erythrocytes can be recovered by centrifugation and washing and either used for transfusion or frozen for future use.[51]

TABLE 131-2   EFFECT OF STORAGE IN ACD ON ERYTHROCYTE PROPERTIES

ALTERATION	ATP	2,3-BPG	VIABILITY
Increased pH	Increase	Increase	Increase
Decreased pH	Decrease	Decrease	Decrease
Increased P_i	Increase		Unchanged
+Adenine	Increase	Decrease	Increase
+Inosine	Increase	Increase	Increase

P_i = inorganic phosphate.

Preservative solutions that contain high concentrations of inorganic phosphate, are hypotonic, and contain ammonium have been found to maintain 2,3 BPG and ATP levels for a prolonged time.[52,53] The effects of such solutions are primarily a function of the ammonium, which relieves phosphofructokinase inhibition by ATP, and of phosphate[54,55]; however, hypotonic additive media without ammonium also improve ATP and 2,3-BPG preservation in some[56] but not in other[57] circumstances.

ADDITIVE SOLUTIONS

The conversion of whole blood into components requires the removal of a significant fraction of both plasma and red cell preservative solution from the red blood cells. Red cell preservation, however, can be optimized if a nutrient solution is added to the isolated red blood cells.[58] The initial blood collection can be into CPD solution or half-strength CPD (0.5CPD).[59] The nutrient solutions that have been developed generally contain glucose as a source of energy, adenine to help support ATP levels, and mannitol to prevent hemolysis. The mechanism by which mannitol exerts this effect is unknown. Originally added to such solutions for osmotic support,[60] it has been shown that its osmotic effect is not the mechanism of action.[61] Several different additive solutions are now available in the United States (AS-3, Nutricell, Cutter Labs, Berkeley, CA; AS-1, Adsol, Fenwall Labs, Morton Grove, IL) and in Sweden.[62] ATP levels are well maintained and good survival is obtained after 42 days storage with the use of additive solutions, but the 2,3-BPG level is reduced by 90 percent at 42 days.[63,64] The loss of 2,3-BPG can be prevented by incorporating bicarbonate and a CO_2 trap into the system.[65]

FROZEN STORAGE OF ERYTHROCYTES

Uncontrolled freezing and thawing of erythrocytes results in hemolysis. Freeze-thaw injury is dependent on the rate of freezing, the physical structure of ice, and the properties of water, cell membranes, and solutions at various temperatures. One theory of freeze-thaw hemolysis suggests that slowly cooled red blood cells are damaged by osmotic dehydration as they are exposed to increasing extracellular electrolyte concentration and osmolality as water is removed by freezing.[66] Irreversible biochemical changes in the membrane may result from the prolonged exposure of the dehydrated, hypertonic red cell to temperatures insufficiently low to prevent biochemical alterations.[67] If such changes are prevented, then lysis of the red blood cells may occur on return to isotonicity because of the excess solute content acquired during the hypertonic phase of freezing.[68] Although the precise biochemical and biophysical changes leading to hemolysis are not fully understood, empirical methods have been developed for the practical freeze preservation of red blood cells. Preservation of erythrocytes by freezing retards or arrests the deleterious biochemical changes that occur during liquid storage.[69] Frozen cells are considered to have a storage time of at least 10 years but have maintained satisfactory viability for as long as 21 years.[70] Under some conditions, it is possible to preserve the metabolic activity and physical integrity of erythrocytes after lyophilization,[71,72] but the usefulness of such cells for transfusion purposes has not been documented.

Glycerol is the most commonly used cryoprotective agent for freeze preservation of erythrocytes. Hydroxyethyl starch[73] and dextran[74] also appear to have desirable cryoprotective properties. The most commonly utilized technique currently is a slow freezing method in which the red blood cells are equilibrated with 40 to 50 percent glycerol and cooled to -80 to $-120°C$.[75] All methods of freeze preservation of erythrocytes involving the use of cryoprotective agents re-

quire the technical capability for introducing and removing high concentrations of the cryoprotective agent (glycerol) under sterile conditions. Frozen red blood cells must be thawed and the glycerol removed gradually by washing in glycerol solutions of decreasing concentration to prevent osmotic hemolysis. Under optimum conditions of processing, storage, and cell washing, greater than 80 percent of the freeze-preserved red blood cells from 1 U of blood will survive and function normally after transfusion. Such thawed and washed red blood cells must be used within 24 hours because processing breaks the closed system and introduces the possibility of bacterial contamination.

WHOLE BLOOD PREPARATIONS

Most clinical situations require the use of specific blood components, and the use of whole blood is limited to correction or prevention of hypovolemia in patients with severe acute blood loss.

ACD, CPD, AND CPDA-1 WHOLE BLOOD

ACD and CPD are the two preservative-anticoagulant solutions used exclusively in the past in the United States. They have been largely superseded by adenine-containing solutions. Blood is currently collected and stored in bags manufactured from plastic films.

For each 100 ml of whole blood, there should be 15 ml of ACD solution or 14 ml of CPD or CPDA-1. The ACD solution (formula A) contains 8.0 g of citric acid ($C_6H_8O_7 \cdot H_2O$), 22 g of sodium citrate ($Na_3C_6H_5O_7 \cdot 2H_2O$), and 24.5 g of glucose ($C_6H_{12}O_6 \cdot H_2O$) per liter. CPD is a modified ACD solution that is slightly less acid and therefore improves the preservation of 2,3-BPG (see Table 131-1). It contains 3.27 g of citric acid, 23.6 g of sodium citrate, 25.5 g of glucose, and 2.22 g of $NaH_2PO_4 \cdot H_2O$ per liter.

Adenine is incorporated into CPD or ACD preservatives in amounts sufficient to provide a concentration of 0.25 to 0.75 mM to increase the shelf-life of the stored red blood cells.[76] CPDA-1 contains CPD modified to contain 125 percent of the usual concentration of glucose and adenine to provide a final concentration of 0.25 mM. Although still suboptimal, the higher glucose concentration provides an additional supply for cells packed immediately after collection so that the blood may be fractionated into components.[77,78]

One unit of whole blood may contain from 405 to 495 ml of blood.[75] The volume of each anticoagulant solution used for 450 ml of whole blood is 67.5 ml of ACD or 63 ml of CPD or CPDA-1 solution. The total fluid volume actually administered in transfusing 450 ml of whole blood is 517.5 ml of ACD and 513 ml of CPD collected blood. If the volume collected is between 300 and 405 ml, the red blood cells can be used for transfusion if they are labeled "Low Volume Unit __ ml. Red Blood Cells."[75]

With proper collection and storage at 2 to 6°C, ACD whole blood and CPD whole blood can be used within 21 days after its collection. The 21-day storage limit has been established based on survival of 70 percent of the transfused erythrocytes at 24 hours after transfusion. Blood collected in CPDA-1 is licensed for 35 days' storage. Whole blood is rarely administered in modern transfusion practice.

FRESH BLOOD

Requests for "fresh" blood are usually justified by the recognition that there is a relatively rapid loss of platelets, leukocytes, and some coagulation factors with liquid storage, as well as a progressive increase in the levels of undesirable products such as potassium, ammonium, and hydrogen ions.[79,80] Blood stored at 4°C over 48 hours using ACD, CPD, or their adenine-containing derivatives is depleted of viable platelets.[81] Factor V remains at adequate levels (>80%) for at least 5 days,[82] factor VIII remains above 80 percent of its original level for 1 to 2 days,[82] and factor XI activity rapidly falls to approximately 20 percent of its original level within the first week of storage.[83] All other clotting factors appear to be stable during liquid storage.[84–86]

Blood "freshness" cannot be precisely defined because it depends upon the storage stability of the particular component in blood that is needed. The loss of platelets and coagulation factors in stored whole blood may be a consideration in massive transfusions following trauma or surgery. Thrombocytopenia and decreased levels of labile coagulation factors with oozing of blood may occur when more than the patient's blood volume[12] (12–14 U) is replaced by banked blood within a 24-hour period.[87] In such cases, packed red blood cells, fresh-frozen plasma, and platelet concentrates are superior to "fresh" whole blood.

Whole blood less than 5 to 7 days old may be indicated when changes in stored blood, such as increased plasma potassium and ammonium and a decreased pH, must be avoided, as in patients with advanced renal or liver disease or newborn infants who are given exchange transfusions.

In a seriously ill patient massively transfused with 2- or 3-week-old banked blood, the low levels of 2,3-BPG may compromise tissue oxygenation. Although the 2,3-BPG levels are regenerated within a day or so,[24,25] it is probably prudent to administer a significant proportion of CPD blood less than 5 days old or ACD blood less than 2 days old.[22] It is also appropriate to provide patients with refractory anemias red blood cells that are less than 10 days old to avoid the infusion of nonviable cells that add unnecessarily to the patient's iron burden.

ERYTHROCYTE PREPARATIONS

Four types of erythrocyte preparations are in common use: packed red blood cells, washed red blood cells, leukocyte-reduced red blood cells, and frozen red blood cells. Washed red blood cells can be obtained from liquid stored blood by saline washing using a continuous-flow cell separator or from frozen erythrocytes that have been extensively washed to remove the cryoprotective agent.

PACKED RED BLOOD CELLS

At any time before the expiration date of the blood, erythrocytes can be separated and recovered from ACD, CPD, or CPDA-1 whole blood by centrifugation and removal of plasma to give a hematocrit of 60 to 90 percent. Red blood cells packed to a hematocrit of less than 80 percent or sedimented red blood cells stored at 1 to 6°C are suitable for transfusion for the full shelf life of the preservative-anticoagulant solution (21 or 35 days). Red blood cells packed to a higher hematocrit do not survive as well, chiefly because they exhaust available glucose.[77,78,88] If the blood is exposed to the external environment during preparation, the packed or sedimented red blood cells must be transfused within 24 hours.[89]

Red blood cells rather than whole blood should be used for the treatment of all patients who require transfusion because of a red cell mass deficit. Packed red blood cells and balanced salt solutions appear to be as effective as whole blood in correcting the blood loss that occurs at surgery.[90]

Red blood cells are administered in the same fashion as is whole blood. The rate of administration may be slower with packed red blood cells but approaches that of whole blood if a 17-gauge or larger needle is used, if a diluting solution such as saline is used,[91] or if the red blood cells have been stored in an additive solution.[92]

LEUKOCYTE-REDUCED RED BLOOD CELLS

There are three major reasons for the use of leukocyte-reduced red blood cells: (1) to prevent or avoid nonhemolytic febrile reactions resulting from antibodies to white cells and platelets in the recipient exposed to previous transfusions or pregnancies (see "Delayed Hemolytic Reaction" below); (2) to prevent sensitization of patients with aplastic anemia who may be candidates for marrow transplantation; and (3) to minimize transmission of viral disease such as HIV or cytomegalovirus. To prevent febrile reactions, 1 U of red blood cells should contain no more than 5×10^8 leukocytes; for the prevention of alloimmunization and to minimize transmission of viral diseases, it has been recommended that no more than 5×10^6 leukocytes remain.[75] It has also been suggested that leukocytes in transfused blood may have an undesirable immunomodulatory effect, and the effect of leukoreduction on outcomes has been appraised in several large studies.[93,94] The results of these studies do not reveal a convincing advantage for leukoreduction.

Three types of leukocyte-poor red cell preparations have been defined[75]: "Red Blood Cells, Leukocytes Removed by Centrifugation," "Red Blood Cells, Leukocytes Removed by Washing," and "Red Blood Cells, Leukocytes Removed by Filtration." The best preparations are those produced by filtration, passing the whole blood or packed cells through specially designed filters.[93,95,96] Universal leukoreduction of red cell preparations is being used increasingly in blood banks,[97] with a decrease in the number of febrile reactions observed.[98]

WASHED RED BLOOD CELLS

Washed red blood cells are usually obtained from whole blood. Packed red blood cells collected by centrifugation can be washed with saline using either manual batch centrifugation or continuous-flow cell separators.[99] Washed red blood cells must be used within 24 hours after processing because of the risk of bacterial contamination during preparation. Frozen red blood cells are an excellent, albeit expensive, source of washed red blood cells.

Washed red blood cells are indicated in the rare patient who is hypersensitive to plasma. Such patients develop an allergic or febrile reaction following whole blood transfusion that can be reproduced with the injection of even a small quantity of plasma. Some of these patients have a deficiency of immunoglobulin (Ig) A and have formed antibodies to IgA from a previous transfusion or pregnancy.[100] Saline-washed red blood cells may be indicated in neonatal transfusions[101] to reduce the quantity of anticoagulant, metabolic breakdown products, extracellular potassium, and risk of cytomegalovirus infection (see "Hazards of Transfusion Therapy" below).

FROZEN RED BLOOD CELLS

Frozen red blood cells have a shelf life measured in years[70] rather than weeks, which simplifies the efficient management of blood inventories. They are somewhat leukocyte poor and relatively free of plasma. Frozen red blood cells are admirably suited for autotransfusion (see "Autologous Transfusions" below). Other advantages include availability of an inventory of rare blood,[102,103] reduction in sensitization to histocompatibility antigens for potential transplant recipients as compared to unfiltered red blood cells, and more efficient inventory control. However, 1 U of frozen blood costs two to three times as much as 1 U stored in the liquid state.

It is possible to "rejuvenate" liquid stored erythrocytes at the end of the storage period by incubating with inosine, glucose, phosphate, and adenine.[104] Such rejuvenated erythrocytes can then be stored in a frozen state and transfused at a later time.[105] The economic soundness of such practices has not been established.

ARTIFICIAL BLOOD SUBSTITUTES

Some functions of blood, such as maintaining circulating volume and oncotic pressure, can be replaced with various crystalloid and colloid macromolecules such as dextran and hydroxyethyl starch (see Chap. 54). These blood substitutes, however, do not provide for oxygen transport.

Materials with the potential for supporting oxygen transport, such as stroma-free hemoglobin solutions, liposome-encapsulated hemoglobin, and perfluorocarbons, have been under active investigation.[106] Interest in such preparations has largely been driven by fear of transmitting microbial disease through blood transfusion and by the long shelf life such preparations might offer. The latter might be particularly important in stockpiling supplies for various types of unanticipated catastrophes.

Perfluorochemicals are large organic compounds in which all the hydrogen atoms are replaced by fluorine. Per unit volume solutions bind almost three times the oxygen carried by blood. They are chemically inert and are not metabolized but require emulsification with surfactants to be miscible with blood. Rats survived up to 8 hours following complete replacement of their blood with liquid fluorocarbon. A perfluorocarbon-hydroxyethyl starch preparation developed in Japan and marketed as Fluosol-DA (Green Corp., Osaka, Japan), that requires concurrent administration of 60 to 100 percent oxygen, has been used experimentally in human volunteers and in a few patients, but no evidence of therapeutic value has been found.[107] Moreover, the use of perfluorocarbons has been associated with pulmonary reactions, cytotoxicity, complement activation, retention of the fluorocarbon in the liver and spleen, and vulnerability to oxygen toxicity.[108]

Stroma-free hemoglobin solutions have been investigated as oxygen-carrying blood substitutes.[109] Their usefulness is limited because of toxicity,[110,111] high affinity for oxygen, and a very short intravascular half-life (2–4 hours). Hemoglobin complexes and recombinant mutant hemoglobin molecules have been prepared that will increase the intravascular life span to 10 to 12 hours, and some of these have a more favorable oxygen affinity.[112] Numerous clinical studies of hemoglobin solutions have been conducted.[113] With some preparations, significant hypertension occurs after infusion, and although this has been thought to result from the binding and depletion of nitric oxide, giving rise to vasospasm, the actual mechanism is not entirely clear.[114]

Hemoglobin has also been encapsulated in artificially prepared liposomes, enabling the addition of 2,3-BPG to achieve near-normal oxygen-hemoglobin dissociation properties.[115,116] The relatively short life span of liposomes, problems in scaling up the process, nonuniformity of liposome size, complement activation,[117] and difficulties in assuring sterility make it unlikely that such encapsulated hemoglobin preparations will ever have any clinical utility.

TRANSFUSION THERAPY

A patient should be transfused only when specific, well-established indications are present and, in practically all cases, with blood components rather than whole blood. Informed consent should be obtained from patients except in life-threatening emergencies. Patients who are candidates for transfusion should be provided with specific information regarding the risks and benefits of the proposed transfusion therapy, and the discussion should be documented by an entry in the patient's medical record.[118]

INDICATIONS FOR TRANSFUSION THERAPY

A major clinical indication for transfusion therapy is the need to restore and maintain the volume of circulating blood to prevent or treat shock, as in hemorrhage or trauma. Probably more than 50 percent of the blood transfused is in the support of surgery.[119] Another indication is the need for specific cellular or protein components such as erythrocytes, specific coagulation factors, or platelets. Exchange transfusions may be required to remove deleterious materials from the blood, in the past primarily in infants for hemolytic disease of the newborn. Blood is also used to maintain the circulation as in extracorporeal or cardiac bypass shunts.[120,121]

HEMORRHAGE AND SHOCK

A major indication for transfusion of blood or components is existing or anticipated hemorrhage (see Chap. 54). Treatment of acute blood loss should be devoted to volume support and only secondarily be concerned with loss of red cell mass. A loss of approximately 1 liter of blood in a patient without cardiovascular disease can be treated with electrolyte solutions. Colloids for volume support and possibly red blood cells may be needed with losses of 1 to 2 liters. Acute blood losses in excess of 2 to 3 liters require correction of both volume deficiency and red cell mass loss.[122]

If the history and the clinical picture suggest that the patient has sustained a significant loss of blood, replacement therapy with whole blood or red blood cells is indicated. Clinical[123] and experimental[90] observations in hypovolemic (hemorrhagic) shock suggest that the combination of packed red blood cells with crystalloids or albumin is as effective as whole blood in correcting a volume deficit. Blood of any age within the usual storage limits is suitable. Many patients who have sustained blood loss do not need a whole blood transfusion and should not be exposed to the associated risks (see "Hazards of Transfusion Therapy" below).

SURGERY

The loss of 500 ml of blood during a surgical procedure is well tolerated by the average patient. Maintaining normovolemia with crystalloid solutions appeared to be a significant factor in preventing morbidity and mortality. One hundred patients undergoing major surgery with blood losses greater than 1000 ml were treated with Hartmann solution (lactated Ringer solution: NaCl 102 mEq/liter, KCl 4 mEq/liter, CaCl$_2$ 3.5 mEq/liter, sodium lactate 27 mEq/liter), using two to three times the estimated volume of blood lost. Postoperative mortality and morbidity were not affected by the use of crystalloid rather than blood, and there were no unexpected complications.[124] Even patients undergoing open heart surgery have been managed successfully without transfusions[125] despite a severe, acute decrease in red blood cell mass.

BURNS

Initially, volume resuscitation is required in patients with severe burns because of the marked increase in permeability of the microcirculation in burned tissue.[126] Patients with a burn injury of more than 25 percent surface area require large volumes of balanced salt solutions during the initial 24 hours.[127,128] Plasma loss, which ensues during the next 5 days, can be corrected with plasma and colloids. The progressive development of anemia during the early post-burn period is best treated with packed red blood cells.

ANEMIA

Blood transfusion of patients with chronic stable anemia is probably unjustifiable if the hemoglobin level is above 7 g per 100 ml unless the patient is elderly or severe cardiac or pulmonary disease is present. There is probably significant misuse of blood transfusions in patients with chronic anemia. Data from 300 hospitals over a 1-year period (1974) revealed that 401 nonoperated patients with anemia were transfused, even though they had a hemoglobin concentration greater than

10 g per 100 ml.[129] Audit criteria for the evaluation of transfusion practice have been established.[130]

Multiple, repeated transfusions of whole blood or packed red blood cells have been used to suppress erythropoiesis in patients with thalassemia and sickle cell diseases (see Chaps. 46 and 47). However, transfusional hemochromatosis (see Chap. 40) may limit the usefulness of this therapy of managing the hemoglobinopathies. One approach to the control of iron accumulation in transfusion-dependent patients with thalassemia is the use of red blood cells enriched in their content of young red blood cells, "neocytes." Young red blood cells are obtained based on size and density using a continuous-flow cell separator.[131–133] The administration of neocytes has been associated with a decreased transfusion requirement.[131,134] However, in spite of the fact that with modern equipment "neocyte" preparations can be prepared without too much difficulty,[134] they are costly and their routine use has been limited. Furthermore, the effectiveness of transfused "neocytes" may be less than predicted by in vitro and in vivo studies.[135]

OTHER INDICATIONS

The clinical uses of other types of blood components are presented in Chapters 22 (leukocytes, dendritic cells, stem cells) and 132 (platelets).

MODE OF ADMINISTRATION

The most important action the physician or nurse can take before administering blood or a blood product is to read the label to verify that the unit to be used is the one selected by the laboratory for that particular patient (see "Hazards of Transfusion Therapy" below).

Blood need not be warmed before its use unless unusually large amounts must be given (>3 liters) at a rapid rate (>100 ml/min).[136] At the usual rate of administration (500 ml in 1–2 hours), the agglutinates that may occur in patients with high-titer cold agglutinins are usually dispersed as the transfused blood reaches body temperature.

Blood should be administered slowly during the first 30 minutes to minimize the amount given if an untoward reaction occurs. It is safe to transfuse 1000 ml of citrated blood within a period of 2 to 3 hours to the average patient without cardiovascular disease.[136]

Drugs or medications should not be added to blood or components. Several intravenous solutions are incompatible with banked blood and should not be administered through the blood lines. Aqueous dextrose solutions cause agglomeration (clumping) and hemolysis of red blood cells, and calcium-containing solutions such as Ringer lactate may exceed the calcium-binding capacity of the citrate in the anticoagulated blood with formation of clots.[137,138] Physiologic saline is compatible with all blood components.

Most transfusion therapy is administered intravenously. A vein in the forearm or antecubital fossa is ordinarily used, although any accessible vein or a central line may be employed. Infrequently used routes for the administration of blood and components are intraarterial and intraperitoneal. Because of the hazards, transfusion into an artery should be reserved for patients who have failed to respond to rapid, large-volume intravenous transfusion.

Intraperitoneal transfusions may be indicated for children in whom suitable veins are difficult to find and occasionally for the fetus in utero.[139,140] Intrauterine transfusion is hazardous to the fetus and is only used when the fetus is hydropic or at high risk of becoming so before 34 to 35 weeks of gestation. A high degree of skill is required, and the procedure is carried out only at tertiary prenatal centers. The blood can be given into an umbilical blood vessel under ultrasonic guidance. Intraperitoneal transfusion has also been given but is not useful for the nonbreathing, moribund hydropic fetus who might be salvaged with direct intravascular transfusion. When the umbilical vessels are inaccessible or too small, the use of intracardiac transfusion may be feasible.[141]

SPECIAL SITUATIONS

SINGLE-UNIT TRANSFUSIONS

Single-unit transfusions have sometimes been condemned as an unwarranted use of blood.[142] However, single-unit transfusions are often justifiable. Examples include elderly surgical patients with coronary disease, patients who have sustained an acute loss of 2 or 3 U who achieve circulatory stability with 1 U, and patients whose bleeding during surgery or from the gastrointestinal tract is controlled after transfusion of the first unit. Single-unit transfusion in such cases represents good judgment and therapeutic skill.[143,144]

AUTOLOGOUS TRANSFUSIONS

In autologous transfusions (autotransfusion), blood removed from a patient is returned to the patient's circulation after storage or blood lost at or immediately after surgery is reinfused. This now accounts for more than 5 percent of the transfusions administered in the United States.[145] Transfusion of autologous blood averts some problems associated with the use of homologous donor blood, such as febrile and allergic reactions, immunologic incompatibilities that may lead to hemolysis, alloimmunization, and transmission of disease.

Three variations of autotransfusion have been used: preoperative blood collection, with storage for a variable time and retransfusion during surgery; immediate preoperative phlebotomy and hemodilution, with postoperative return of the phlebotomized blood[146]; and intraoperative collection of shed blood with reinfusion during surgery.[147] Equipment designed for intraoperative autotransfusion is commercially available.[148–150]

In many elective surgical procedures, the recipient can predeposit autologous blood.[151] In some patients, the amount of predeposited autologous blood may be increased through the use of recombinant human erythropoietin therapy.[152] Predeposited autologous blood also may be frozen and represents the ideal product for patients with rare blood types (e.g., Rh-null) or for patients with antibodies in numbers and combinations that make it nearly impossible to find compatible units of blood.

DIRECTED OR DESIGNATED DONATIONS

Donors recruited from among family members or friends (donor-specific), contrary to expectation, are no safer than volunteer blood donors. Fatal graft-versus-host reactions have been reported involving unusual HLA similarities between close relatives (see "Graft-versus-Host Disease" below).

BLOOD FOR EXCHANGE TRANSFUSIONS

Exchange transfusions are used to treat the newborn who has severe hemolytic disease resulting from a fetomaternal blood group incompatibility, glucose-6-phosphate deficiency, or an unknown cause (see Chaps. 6, 45, and 53).

Exchange transfusions have been simplified by the introduction of equipment that automatically harvests blood components from an individual (see Chap. 25).

BLOOD FOR PATIENTS WITH AUTOIMMUNE HEMOLYTIC DISEASE

The provision of compatible red blood cells for patients with autoimmune hemolytic anemia (AIHA) is one of the most difficult and challenging problems in transfusion medicine.[153] Compatibility usually cannot be assured because of the effect of autoantibodies on routine serologic tests. Transfusion management of the patient with AIHA involves a risk-to-benefit judgment, namely: Does the need for increased oxygen-carrying capacity justify the risks of a possible hemolytic reaction? Transfusion should be avoided in these patients whenever possible.[154,155]

Ideally, donor blood should be selected so that it lacks those antigens corresponding to the antibodies in the recipient, whether autoimmune or alloimmune. Patients with red cell autoantibodies are serologically incompatible with their own red blood cells and with those of most, if not all, donors. Such patients, if previously transfused or pregnant, may also have clinically significant alloantibodies difficult to detect in the presence of the autoantibody.

Usually no autoantibody specificity can be established, and it may be impossible to find serologically compatible blood. However, it may be possible to find units that react more weakly than others. A variety of time-consuming serologic procedures are available to detect alloantibodies in the presence of autoantibodies, but it may require ^{51}Cr survival studies to establish compatibility. Many of these patients will tolerate hemoglobin levels of 5 to 7 g per 100 ml and should not be transfused. If life-threatening anemia is present, a transfusion may be required even in the face of serologic incompatibility. In such cases, blood should be selected that is at least as compatible as the patient's cells in their own serum. Packed red blood cells rather than whole blood should be used, and sometimes packed red blood cells less than 10 days old may be indicated to minimize the number and frequency of transfusions required.

BLOOD FOR EMERGENCIES

Emergencies in which no time is available to type, select, and crossmatch compatible blood should be a rare occurrence, except for trauma, unexpected intraoperative hemorrhage, massive gastrointestinal bleeding, or ruptured aneurysm.[156]

If the urgency of the patient's need justifies the administration of uncross-matched blood, type O, Rh-negative blood with low plasma anti-A and anti-B titers can be used. Unfortunately, tests for donor anti-A and anti-B levels are not done routinely. The use of packed red blood cells will reduce the quantity of anti-A or anti-B administered. It is preferable, however, to use ABO group and Rh type-specific blood, which is usually available within 15 minutes if the patient's blood is available for testing. Administration of uncross-matched group-specific blood will prevent hemolysis that may occur if a high-titered anti-A or anti-B group O blood is given to a non-O recipient. If 15 to 30 minutes are available, an abbreviated antibody screen can be carried out using low ionic strength conditions.[157] Group- and type-specific uncross-matched blood with a negative antibody screen provides compatibility for the recipient equivalent to that of cross-matched blood in essentially all cases.[158] The routine cross-match should be carried out retrospectively to identify any incompatibility when uncross-matched or partially cross-matched blood is administered.

BLOOD FOR TRANSPLANT RECIPIENTS

Kidney Grafts Random donor blood transfusions can result in allogeneic immunization,[159,160] and in the early days of transplantation they were avoided in order to prevent the possibility of inducing anti-HLA antibodies in potential transplant recipients. However, a series of reports from 1973 to 1978 surprisingly demonstrated that kidney transplant patients who had received multiple blood transfusions before transplantation actually had better graft survival.[161-163] This was particularly true of patients of African and Caribbean descent,[164] two groups that often demonstrate lower kidney graft survival rates than age- and gender-matched patients of European descent. Although the mechanism of this apparent paradox is still not clear, the purposeful administration of random donor blood transfusions became common practice. In kidney transplant patients with living related donors, the

blood transfusions were given from the related donor, a practice called "donor-specific transfusion."[165] The beneficial effect appears to be mediated by the HLA antigens expressed on donor leukocytes, probably monocytes but possibly also B cells.[166,167] In patients receiving donor-specific transfusions, the coadministration of low-dose azathioprine (Imuran) reduced the risk of sensitization to the donor HLA antigens from 30 percent to less than 10 percent.[168] That an immunosuppressive drug with antiproliferative effects on B cells could reduce the risk of antibody-mediated sensitization without altering the beneficial effect on graft survival supported the hypothesis that blood transfusions could generate some form of suppressor cell phenomenon, presumably mediated by memory T cells. An alternative theory is that blood transfusions represent a selection process for patients prone to be "responders" to certain donor HLA antigens. In other words, if a patient is sensitized by a specific HLA antigen after a transfusion, then that antigen is avoided when matching that patient for the kidney transplant and better graft survival results.

The current practice of blood transfusion in kidney transplantation has been changed dramatically by three developments: the introduction of cyclosporine and erythropoietin and the increasing concern over the danger of exposure to random donor transfusions. Cyclosporine is so potent an immunosuppressive drug that its use has challenged any additional beneficial effect of blood transfusions,[169,170] and the blood transfusion effect is no longer demonstrable in kidney transplantation,[164] even in patients of African and Caribbean descent. The only possible exception is that patients transplanted when younger than 15 years still demonstrate a small transfusion effect. The widespread use of erythropoietin has ended the routine practice of blood transfusions to treat the anemia of end-stage renal disease.

Marrow Grafts Previous blood transfusions, especially from the intended donor, are associated with a high rate of marrow graft rejection in patients with aplastic anemia but are not a serious problem in marrow transplantation of leukemic patients.[171] ABO incompatibility in otherwise histocompatible donors does not appear to affect the marrow transplant outcome.[172] There is a need to avoid an immediate transfusion reaction caused by the red blood cells in the marrow inoculum when an ABO-incompatible engraftment is carried out. Such a complication may be averted by removing anti-A or anti-B from the recipient by plasma exchange, by neutralization *in vivo*, or by removing mature red blood cells from the inoculum.[172] Indications for blood component therapy in marrow transplantation have been reviewed.[173] Because of the risk of infection with cytomegalovirus in immunosuppressed patients, marrow recipients who are seronegative are generally transfused only with blood products from donors who are seronegative for cytomegalovirus.[174]

Liver Grafts Unusually large volumes of blood and the ability to recognize and correct complex hemostatic deficiencies are required for liver transplantation.[175] The demand for blood is influenced by the underlying liver disease, the nature of the preoperative coagulation defect,[176] and the intraoperative blood loss associated with surgery on a large vascular organ. An additional problem is that the large number of donors increases the risk of disease transmission (see "Hazards of Transfusion Therapy" below). In a 1987 study, the mean number of donor exposures per patient receiving a liver transplant ranged from 170 to 200 U, [175] but more recently the use of blood products has declined drastically, with 32.0 percent of patients receiving no red cell transfusions, and 19.4 percent not receiving any blood products during the transplant.

HAZARDS OF TRANSFUSION THERAPY

Transfusion therapy, even under ideal conditions, carries a significant risk of an adverse reaction.[174] Such reactions are associated with significant morbidity and, in some cases, with a fatal outcome. Most of the reported fatalities involve human error. In one study of 70 fatalities, 56 percent resulted from acute hemolytic reactions. Half of these were preventable because they involved an ABO mismatch resulting from human error. Seventy-five percent of the fatalities resulted from administration of correctly cross-matched blood to the wrong patient.[177] Two subsequent reviews of FDA fatality reports from 1976 to 1983[178] and from 1976 to 1985[179] continue to confirm these findings, that is, a majority of transfusion fatalities are managerial/clerical and not technical failures. Based on a study in New York state, the risk of a matching error was estimated at one per 18,000 transfusions.[180]

Up to 20 percent of all transfusions may lead to some type of adverse reaction.[181] The precise risk is difficult to estimate because many reactions may be clinically occult, accuracy of reporting is poor, the risk is influenced by the nature of the recipient population, the source of donor blood, and the diligence and expertise of the blood bank laboratory staff.

An additional problem is that approximately half of transfusions are given to anesthetized patients.[119,182] If a reaction is suspected, the transfusion should be immediately discontinued and appropriate laboratory tests and clinical studies undertaken to establish the diagnosis and institute appropriate therapy (see below).

Transfusion reactions may be categorized as either immediate or delayed.

IMMEDIATE TRANSFUSION REACTIONS

Symptoms of an immediate reaction begin within minutes to hours and are nonspecific with respect to etiology. They may include chills, fever, urticaria, tachycardia, dyspnea, nausea and vomiting, tightness in the chest, chest and back pain, hypotension, bronchospasm, angioneurotic edema, anaphylaxis, shock, pulmonary edema, and congestive failure. In the anesthetized patient undergoing surgery, an immediate transfusion reaction may manifest itself as generalized oozing of blood from the operative site and by shock that is not corrected by the administration of blood.

Immediate transfusion reactions may be hemolytic, febrile, or may be caused by contaminated blood. The symptoms may not reflect the severity of the reaction. An etiologic diagnosis usually requires additional laboratory studies.

Acute Hemolytic Transfusion Reactions   Hemolytic transfusion reactions may be associated with a variety of signs and symptoms, such as fever, low-back pain, sensations of chest compression, hypotension, nausea, and vomiting. Two mechanisms may account for hemolysis of transfused red blood cells: (1) intravascular breakdown, most commonly resulting from an incompatibility in the ABO system, or (2) destruction occurring in the extravascular space, that is, the macrophage system of the spleen, liver, and bone marrow.

Important pathogenetic mechanisms in intravascular hemolysis are disseminated intravascular coagulation (DIC) and a series of hemodynamic alterations leading to ischemic necrosis of tissues, notably the kidneys (see Chap. 121).[183,184] Abnormal bleeding resulting from a consumptive coagulopathy may develop in one half to one third of patients who develop major intravascular hemolysis following an incompatible transfusion.[185,186]

Infrequently an asymptomatic hemolytic transfusion reaction occurs without demonstrable antibody.[187] Such patients do not show the expected hemoglobin increment following transfusion and have hemoglobinuria and hemoglobinemia. Such reactions are rare, and the absence of demonstrable antibody requires postulating a direct cell-mediated destruction of the incompatible red blood cells.

The clinical management of a hemolytic transfusion reaction should include immediate termination of the transfusion and institution of measures to correct shock, maintain renal circulation, and correct the bleeding diathesis. The risk of serious sequelae is proportional to the volume of incompatible blood transfused. Severe complications rarely follow the transfusion of less than 200 ml of red blood cells.[183] If a hemolytic reaction is suspected, therapy designed to correct bleeding and to protect the kidneys (see below) should be begun promptly without waiting for the laboratory studies to confirm its presence.

The laboratory diagnosis of an acute hemolytic reaction is based on evidence of hemolysis (hemoglobinemia and/or hemoglobinuria) and of a blood group incompatibility (antibodies in the recipient reacting with blood group antigens on transfused red blood cells). A sample of blood carefully drawn to avoid artifactual hemolysis is centrifuged for cell separation. The plasma is examined for hemoglobin (pink) or methemalbumin (brown) and is compared with the pretransfusion specimen. The urine should be examined for hemoglobin and urinary output monitored. The entire typing and cross-match procedure should be repeated to identify the blood group incompatibility. The patient and the blood transfused should be retyped, the cross-match reconfirmed, the patient's red blood cells examined for the presence of bound immunoglobulins and/or complement (antiglobulin or Coombs test), and the patient's serum tested for the presence of blood group alloantibodies. The donor's plasma should be examined for the presence of antibodies that may react with the patient's red blood cells.

The major effort in a hemolytic reaction should be directed toward control of bleeding, if it is present, and prevention of acute tubular necrosis. If bleeding is the result of DIC (see Chap. 121), heparin may be helpful, particularly in pregnant women.[186,188] Heparin therapy is not without potential risk, and its use should be restricted to cases in which a severe reaction has been confirmed. To be effective, heparin should be used early in the course of DIC.[186] When intravascular coagulation is controlled, the depleted coagulation factors can be restored by transfusing fibrinogen-rich cryoprecipitate, platelet concentrates, and fresh-frozen plasma.[189]

The prevention of renal complications relies on maintaining renal blood flow. Systolic blood pressure should be maintained above 100 mm Hg, if necessary by administration of intravenous fluids and transfusion. Mannitol has been used by some to protect against renal failure,[190,191] but others rely solely on diuretics.[136,192] If mannitol is used, it should be given in quantities sufficient to maintain a urine flow of 100 ml/hour. Initially, 100 ml of a 20 percent solution are infused intravenously in 5 minutes. This dose can be repeated if diuresis does not occur, but not more than 100 g of mannitol should be given in a 24-hour period. Diuretics such as furosemide (40–80 mg IV) or ethacrynic acid (50–100 mg IV) may be more effective in maintaining renal blood flow.

If anuria ensues, standard measures for management of the anuric patient should be instituted.

Febrile Reactions   A febrile response associated with the administration of blood may be the result of a hemolytic reaction, sensitivity to leukocytes or platelets, bacterial pyrogens, or unidentifiable causes. Febrile reactions resulting from bacterial pyrogens have become uncommon with the introduction of commercially manufactured disposable transfusion equipment.

The decision to stop the administration of blood in a febrile reaction is a difficult one. Many but not all febrile reactions can be tolerated by the patient with supportive care, such as antipyretics and antihistamines. A chill, however, may herald a more serious reaction, such as a hemolytic reaction, or may be the result of grossly contaminated blood. Unfortunately, reliable guidelines are not available to help with this decision. Clinicians should exercise their best judgment but should not hesitate to stop the transfusion if there is any doubt about the underlying cause of the reaction.

A frequent cause of a nonhemolytic febrile reaction is sensitization to white cell or platelet antigens.[174] Clinically there is a temperature rise during the administration of blood or shortly thereafter. The temperature continues to rise for 2 to 6 hours after cessation of transfusion, and the fever may persist for 12 hours. Occasionally there may be more severe manifestations, and, rarely, a drop in blood pressure with nausea and vomiting, accompanied by chest and back pains. Reactions as the result of leukocyte antigens have a good prognosis but may be confused with a hemolytic transfusion reaction. Nonhemolytic febrile reactions account for up to 30 percent of all recognized reactions. Usually at least seven transfusions are required to induce sensitization to leukocyte antigens in men, nonparous women, or children. In gravid or parous women, reactions may occur with the first or second transfusion. Diagnosis depends on laboratory demonstration of HLA or non-HLA antibodies to white cell antigens, usually leukoagglutinins or lymphocytotoxins. Most reactions of this type are associated with sensitivity to granulocytes, but sensitivity to lymphocytes or to platelets can also cause the reaction. Treatment is supportive. Most of these reactions can be prevented if the blood or red blood cells are passed through a leukocyte filter. If they persist, pretreatment with an antipyretic agent, such as acetaminophen, or with glucocorticoids may be helpful.

Transfusion-related Lung Injury (TRALI; Noncardiogenic Pulmonary Edema) Incompatibility to leukocyte antigens may also produce pulmonary edema of noncardiac origin, with acute respiratory distress, chills, fever, and tachycardia usually occurring within 4 hours of transfusion.[174,193] Once considered to be a rare complication, it is being recognized with increasing frequency.[194] Chest x-ray films show bilateral diffuse, patchy pulmonary densities without cardiac enlargement.[195] Leukocyte incompatibility can be demonstrated in most cases. Sometimes recipient antibodies react with donor leukocytes,[196] and passively transferred donor antibodies react with the recipient leukocytes[193,196] or with recently transfused (interdonor) leukocytes. It is unclear why only a relatively few individuals respond to leukocyte incompatibility by the pulmonary hypersensitivity reaction instead of the usual febrile response. The reaction can also occur with platelet concentrates, fresh-frozen plasma, whole blood, and packed red blood cells. Almost 25 percent of multiparous women donors have leukoagglutinins and lymphocytoxins that can cause these reactions. Therapy is supportive. In a healthy recipient, the symptoms subside in less than 24 hours, with pulmonary infiltrates clearing within 4 days. The reaction in a compromised recipient, however, can be fatal.[197] The frequency of this reaction has been estimated as one in 5000 transfusions.[198]

A catastrophic reaction to reinfusion of blood collected with the Cell-Saver apparatus has been documented.[35] Termed *disseminated intravascular inflammation*, this disorder is characterized by massive fluid accumulation, rapidly developing anemia, thrombocytopenia, and bleeding. The outcome is frequently fatal. This syndrome is believed to result from the release of cytokines by leukocytes directly contacting the polycarbonate surface of the separating bowl used in the apparatus, and it has been suggested that it can be avoided by exercising care in the aspiration of material from the operative field, avoiding aspiration of cellular debris, irrigating fluid, and blood that has been greatly diluted into the salvage apparatus.

Allergic Reactions Transfusions of blood or blood products in some patients may result in generalized pruritus and urticaria. Occasionally there may be bronchospasm, angioneurotic edema, or anaphylaxis. The cause of allergic reactions is poorly understood. It has been suggested that they are caused by sensitivity to plasma proteins or other agents passively transferred from the donor to the recipient. Subsequent exposure of the recipient to the antigen through medication or possibly allergens in food precipitates the reaction. Antibodies to leukocytes or platelets do not seem causally related to urticarial reactions.[199] These reactions are usually mild and respond readily to parenteral antihistamines. Serious reactions require the prompt parenteral administration of epinephrine.

Anti-IgA in IgA-Deficient Recipients Severe anaphylactoid transfusion reactions can occur in IgA-deficient patients who have formed anti-IgA.[200] Such patients either lack or have a marked deficiency of IgA and have developed an IgG or occasionally IgM anti-IgA that may be either class-specific (IgA) or allotype-specific (Am).[201] Deficiency or absence of IgA occurs infrequently; approximately one in 650 persons lack IgA by immunodiffusion and approximately one in 886 have no demonstrable IgA,[202] but it has been estimated that reactions only occur in approximately one per 20,000 to 47,000 transfusions.[200] The IgA present in the plasma of the transfused blood probably reacts with the anti-IgA to produce the anaphylactoid reaction. Small amounts of plasma (<10 ml) can produce the reaction. The reaction usually is not associated with fever but may produce dyspnea, nausea, chills, abdominal cramps, emesis, diarrhea, and profound hypotension. A fatal reaction resulting from anti-IgA occurring 45 minutes after administration of approximately 50 ml of blood has been reported.[203] Diagnosis requires laboratory demonstration of the absence of IgA and the presence of anti-IgA in the recipient's circulation. Reactions can usually be prevented by using washed or frozen red blood cells because these components are prepared by procedures effective in removing donor plasma. Plasma protein components, such as albumin or plasma protein fraction, may contain sufficient IgA to produce a reaction. If platelet or granulocyte transfusions are required for IgA-deficient patients, they should be obtained from donors who lack IgA (Rare Donor File, American Association of Blood Banks).

Bacterial Contamination Blood may be contaminated by cold-growing organisms (*Pseudomonas* or colon-aerogenes group). These microorganisms can utilize citrate as the primary source of carbon, and contamination of blood by these microorganisms may deplete its citrate concentration sufficiently to result in clotting. Visual inspection of the blood unit may reveal clots and suggest the presence of contamination. The infusion of large numbers of gram-negative microorganisms results in a serious reaction, endotoxin shock, characterized by fever, marked hypotension, abdominal pain, vomiting, diarrhea, and the development of profound shock.[204] The reaction may start with shaking chills following a latent period of 30 minutes or more. As little as 10 ml of blood may contain sufficient microorganisms to produce the reaction. Rapid diagnosis is essential and can be made by drawing a small sample of residual donor blood from the container or administration tubing. The plasma obtained by slow centrifugation is smeared on a slide, fixed by heating, and gram stained. If the blood is heavily contaminated, several organisms can be clearly identified in most oil-immersion fields.

Septic shock is a complex disorder, and comprehensive supportive therapy is essential once the diagnosis is made. Treatment is often ineffective. The fatality rate with this type of overwhelming shock is estimated to be from 50 to 80 percent.

Bacterial contamination of blood is an uncommon complication since the introduction of disposable plastic blood bags, estimated in 1999 to be two per 1,000,000 U.[174] This transfusion hazard, however, is significant with platelet concentrates stored at room temperature (see Chap. 132) and has been estimated at one per 2000 U.[174]

Circulatory Overload Hypervolemia produced by administration of excess blood in patients with a compromised cardiovascular system may provoke the development of congestive heart failure and pulmonary edema. Treatment of this reaction includes administration of diuretics and, in some cases, rapid digitalization. Repeated phlebotomies with reinfusion of the erythrocytes as packed red blood cells may sometimes be helpful.

Patients with severe chronic anemia (hemoglobin <4 g per 100 ml), such as those with pernicious anemia, who are rapidly transfused with whole blood or packed red blood cells may develop congestive failure and pulmonary edema. The slow administration of packed red blood cells appears to be well tolerated by the patient in a semi-upright position. Venous pressure should be monitored in such patients, diuretics administered, and the transfusion given at a rate of 2 ml per kilogram of body weight per hour. It is unlikely that a transfusion will precipitate congestive heart failure if the venous pressure is normal before transfusion.[205]

Air Embolism Air embolism is no longer a risk in conventional transfusion practice, following the introduction of plastic equipment that provides a closed system. However, it is an uncommon complication of transfusions carried out with recovered blood in the perioperative setting.[206] Symptoms associated with air embolism include pain, cough, and sudden onset of dyspnea. Treatment consists of clamping off administration tubing, placing the patient on the left side in the head-down position with closed chest compression so that air in the right ventricle flows away from the pulmonary outflow tract, and, if possible, air aspiration through a right atrial or Swan-Ganz catheter.[207]

Microaggregates in Blood Particles consisting largely of platelets and fibrin[208] form in blood stored in ACD, CPD, or CPDA-1 solutions. Such debris, consisting of particles 13 to 100 μm in size and collectively designated *microaggregates*, is not removed by the ordinary blood filter that has a pore size of approximately 170 μm. At one time, such particles were considered to represent a hazard responsible for pulmonary complications of transfusions. However, it now appears that microaggregates are not clinically important, and the use of filters to remove these particles has been abandoned.

Reactions Associated with Massive Transfusions The use of large quantities of banked blood for massive transfusions may lead to a number of complications. Among these are circulatory overload (see "Circulatory Overload" above), citrate intoxication, and a bleeding syndrome.[209] Blood transfused into adults at a rate greater than 1 liter in 10 minutes will produce significant reduction in ionized calcium with myocardial depression and electrocardiographic changes. Citrate intoxication can be prevented by giving 10 ml of 10 percent calcium gluconate for every liter of citrated blood.

Bleeding Syndromes Bleeding may be a complication of transfusion either because an antigen-antibody reaction involving a red cell antigen initiates DIC or because coagulation factors and platelets are diluted following large-volume compatible transfusions of banked blood.[185,209] However, the most common cause of bleeding in surgical patients is a severed vessel.

Unexplained bleeding may be the first sign of incompatibility in the anesthetized patient and may follow the administration of 200 to 500 ml of incompatible blood. Local bleeding at the surgical site or epistaxis, bruising, or purpura resulting from DIC may occur following an acute hemolytic transfusion reaction. The diagnosis and management of this complication were outlined earlier (see "Acute Hemolytic Transfusion Reactions" above).

Bleeding associated with transfusion of large amounts of compatible stored blood largely results from the dilution of the intravascular volume with blood lacking in both cellular and plasma coagulation components. Because platelets do not survive in stored blood, transfusion of a volume of blood equal to that of the recipient will produce thrombocytopenia through a dilutional effect. Stored blood is deficient in platelets and in factors V, VIII, and XI. These clotting components may be depleted when a large-volume transfusion is given.

DELAYED ADVERSE EFFECTS OF BLOOD TRANSFUSION

Delayed Hemolytic Reaction In the delayed hemolytic reaction, development of previously undetected alloantibodies occurs approximately 4 to 14 days after transfusion of apparently compatible blood. In such cases, the patient usually has been alloimmunized by a previous pregnancy or transfusion, and the concentration of antibody was below the level of serologic detection at the time of transfusion. If the transfused blood contains the corresponding antigen, an anamnestic response ensues with formation of detectable antibody that coats the transfused red blood cells and leads to their hemolysis. The principal clinical signs are onset of jaundice and absence of the expected increment in red cell mass. These reactions are associated with the development of a positive direct antiglobulin reaction (Coombs test),[210–212] which in such patients may be confused with AIHA[213] or, in one report, with sickle cell crisis.[214] Generally, these reactions are clinically less severe than the acute hemolytic reaction and frequently are not detected until more blood is ordered for a transfusion unresponsive anemia. The frequency of delayed hemolytic anemia was one in 4000 in one report,[210] with no deaths in the 37 cases studied, but seems to be much more common in patients with sickle cell disease receiving multiple transfusions.[215] Delayed hemolytic reactions are frequently undetected.[211] The formation of autoantibodies following allogeneic transfusion has also been documented.[216]

Posttransfusion Purpura A rare complication of transfusion therapy is posttransfusion purpura, which occurs approximately 1 week after transfusion and is associated with the development of an antibody to the platelet specific antigen in a Pl^{a1}-negative recipient (see Chap. 110).

Transmission of Disease The risk of infection with viral agents, such those that cause acquired immunodeficiency syndrome, hepatitis, lymphomas, or protozoal organisms, particularly malaria, has progressively decreased as donated blood is subjected to ever-increasing amounts of screening. In 1999, the risk of HIV transmission or of hepatitis C transmission was one per 1,000,000 U transfused and that of hepatitis B transmission 4 per 1,000,000 U.[174] Nevertheless, there have been numerous efforts to devise methods to "sterilize" blood after collection. One justification for these efforts is the obvious fact that one can only screen for known infectious agents. It is entirely possible that a previously unknown infection, such as HIV was at one time, might contaminate the blood supply. In the event of such an occurrence, a sterilization method might prove to have been very useful.[217] The prevention of disease transmission is discussed in Chapter 130.

Graft-versus-Host Disease Graft-versus-host disease is an uncommon complication of transfusion therapy,[218] preventable by irradiation of blood prior to transfusion.[219] It occurs particularly when transfusions from close relatives are given to severely immunocompromised recipients.

Other Types of Delayed Reactions Other complications of transfusion therapy are iron overload with hemochromatosis (see Chap. 40), which occurs in patients who receive many transfusions, and alloimmunizations to red cell and histocompatibility antigens.

Alloimmunization as a transfusion complication may occur in immunocompetent transfusion-dependent recipients. Blood is matched routinely only with respect to ABO antigens and the major Rh antigen $Rh_o(D)$. There is a high probability that the donor will have red cell antigens not present in the recipient that will result in alloimmunization. The incidence of alloimmunization is influenced by the number of units transfused, the immune status of the recipient, and probably other undefined factors. The prevalence of alloantibodies in multiply transfused patients with various hematologic disorders was 11.8 percent,[220] and in multiply transfused sickle cell anemia patients has been variously reported as 36 percent,[221] 23 percent,[222] and in one series only 7.75 percent.[223] The incidence of alloimmunization in thalassemia major patients is lower (5.2%).[224]

More extensive pretransfusion typing, including the matching for additional antigens of recipients who will require frequent transfusions, appears to reduce the risk of alloimmunization. Pretransfusion matching for the major antigens (Rh, Kell, Kidd, Duffy) in patients with sickle cell anemia reduced the incidence of alloimmunization 10-fold.[225] This measure alone may not be cost effective because not all individuals are capable of mounting an immune response to blood group antigens. A few Rho(D)-negative individuals fail to produce anti-Rho(D) in spite of intentional immunization with the antigen.[226,227] However, 95 percent of Rh-negative individuals receiving large quantities (average 19.4 U) of Rh-positive blood during open heart surgery formed anti-D.[228] More extensive pretransfusion matching would be justifiable if a marker could be found that unequivocally identifies members of the population of recipients who are likely to become alloimmunized.

REFERENCES

1. Oberman HA: The history of transfusion medicine, in *Clinical Practice of Transfusion Medicine*, edited by LD Petz, SN Swisher, p 9. Churchill Livingstone, New York, 1989.

2. Blundell J: The after-management of floodings, and on transfusion. *Lancet* 13:673, 1828.

3. Routh CHF: Remarks, statistical and general, on transfusion of blood. *The Medical Times* 114, 1849.

4. Landsteiner K: Über Agglutinationserscheinungen normalen menschlichen Blutes. *Wien Klin Wochenschr* 14·1132, 1901.

5. Rous P, Turner JR: The preservation of living red blood cells in vitro: I. Methods of preservation. *J Exp Med* 23:219, 1916.

6. Rous P, Turner JR: The preservation of living red blood cells in vitro: II. The transfusion of kept cells. *J Exp Med* 23:239, 1916.

7. Robertson OH: Transfusion with preserved red blood cells. *BMJ* 1:691, 1918.

8. Fantus B: Therapy of Cook County Hospital: Blood preservation. *JAMA* 109:128, 1937.

9. Churchill ED: *Surgeon to Soldiers*. Lippincott, Philadelphia, 1972.

10. Nelson R: Blood on demand. *Am Heritage Invention Technol* 19:24, 2004.

11. Jones AL: Continuous-flow blood cell separation. *Transfusion* 8:94, 1968.

12. Hester JP, Kellogg RM, Mulzet AP, et al: Principles of blood separation and component extraction in a disposable continuous-flow single-stage channel. *Blood* 54:254, 1979.

13. Gabrio BW, Stevens AR, Finch CA: Erythrocyte preservation: III. The reversibility of the storage lesion. *J Clin Invest* 33:252, 1954.

14. Dern RJ, Brewer GJ, Wiorkowski JJ: Studies on the preservation of human blood: II. The relationship of erythrocyte adenosine triphosphate levels and other in vitro measures to red cell storageability. *J Lab Clin Med* 69:968, 1967.

15. Wood L, Beutler E: The viability of human blood stored in phosphate adenine media. *Transfusion* 7:401, 1967.

16. Beutler E, Kuhl W, West C: The osmotic fragility of erythrocytes after prolonged liquid storage and after reinfusion. *Blood* 59:1141, 1982.

17. Wolfe LC: The membrane and the lesions of storage in preserved red cells. *Transfusion* 25:185, 1985.

18. Sestier C, Sabolovic D, Geldwerth D, et al: Use of annexin V-ferrofluid to enumerate erythrocytes damaged in various pathologies or during storage in vitro. *C R Acad Sci (Paris)* 318:1141, 1995.

19. Boas FE, Forman L, Beutler E: Phosphatidylserine exposure and red cell viability in red cell ageing, storage, and in hemolytic anemia. *Blood* 90(suppl 1):272a, 1997.

20. Boas FE, Forman L, Beutler E: Phosphatidyl serine exposure and red cell viability in red cell ageing and in hemolytic anemia. *Proc Natl Acad Sci U S A* 95:3077, 1998.

21. Geldwerth D, Kuypers FA, Butikofer P, et al: Transbilayer mobility and distribution of red cell phospholipids during storage. *J Clin Invest* 92:308, 1993.

22. Chaplin H Jr, Beutler E, Collins JA, et al: Current status of red-cell preservation and availability in relation to the developing national blood policy. *N Engl J Med* 291:68, 1974.

23. DeVerdier CH, Akerblom O, Arturson G, et al: Maintenance of oxygen transport function of stored blood, in *Transfusion and Transplantation*. Proceedings of the AABB-ISBT Transfusion Congress, Washington, DC, 1972.

24. Beutler E, Wood L: The in vivo regeneration of red cell 2,3-diphosphoglyceric acid (DPG) after transfusion of stored blood. *J Lab Clin Med* 74:300, 1969.

25. Valeri CR, Hirsch NM: Restoration in vivo of erythrocyte adenosine triphosphate 2,3-diphosphoglycerate, potassium ion, and sodium ion concentrations following the transfusion of acid-citrate-dextrose-stored human red blood cells. *J Lab Clin Med* 73:722, 1969.

26. Beutler E: What is the clinical importance of alterations of the hemoglobin oxygen affinity in preserved blood—especially as produced by variations of red cell 2,3 DPG content? *Vox Sang* 34:113, 1978.

27. Beutler E, Duron O: Effect of pH on preservation of red cell ATP. *Transfusion* 5:17, 1965.

28. Bishop C: Changes in the nucleotides of stored or incubated human blood. *Transfusion* 1:349, 1961.

29. Beutler E, Meul A, Wood LA: Depletion and regeneration of 2,3-diphosphoglyceric acid in stored red blood cells. *Transfusion* 9:109, 1969.

30. Wood L, Beutler E: Temperature dependence of sodium-potassium activated erythrocyte adenosine triphosphatase. *J Lab Clin Med* 70:287, 1967.

31. AuBuchon JP, Estep TN, Davey RJ: The effect of the plasticizer di-2-ethylhexyl phthalate on the survival of stored RBCs. *Blood* 71:448, 1988.

32. Greenwalt TJ, McGuinness CG, Dumaswala UJ: Studies in red blood cell preservation: 4. Plasma vesicle hemoglobin exceeds free hemoglobin. *Vox Sang* 61:14, 1991.

33. Card RT, Mohandas N, Mollison PL: Relationship of post-transfusion viability to deformability of stored red cells. *Br J Haematol* 53:237, 1983.

34. Kristiansson M, Soop M, Saraste L, Sundqvist KG: Cytokines in stored red blood cell concentrates: Promoters of systemic inflammation and simulators of acute transfusion reactions? *Acta Anaesthesiol Scand* 40:496, 1996.

35. Bull BS, Bull MH: Hypothesis: Disseminated intravascular inflammation as the inflammatory counterpart to disseminated intravascular coagulation. *Proc Natl Acad Sci U S A* 91:8190, 1994.

36. Simon ER: Adenine and purine nucleosides in human red cell preservation: A review. *Transfusion* 7:395, 1967.

37. Wood L, Beutler E: The effect of ascorbate and dihydroxyacetone on the 2,3-diphosphoglycerate and ATP levels of stored human red cells. *Transfusion* 14:272, 1974.

38. Kurup PA, Arun P, Gayathri NS, et al: Modified formulation of CPDA for storage of whole blood, and of SAGM for storage of red blood cells, to maintain the concentration of 2,3-diphosphoglycerate. *Vox Sang* 85:253, 2003.

39. Kandler R, Grode G, Symbol R, Hickey G: Oxalate is the active component that produces increased 2,3-DPG in ascorbate stored red cells. *Transfusion* 26:563, 1986.

40. Beutler E, Forman L, West C: Effect of oxalate and malonate on red cell metabolism. *Blood* 70:1389, 1987.

41. Beutler E: The "ascorbate" effect on 2,3-DPG is known to be due to oxalate. *Vox Sang* 86:199, 2004.

42. Paterson RA, Dawson J, Hyde RM, et al: Xanthone additives for blood storage that maintain its potential for oxygen delivery. I. 2-hydroxy-ethoxy- and 2-ethoxy-6-(5-tetrazoyl) xanthones in citrate-phosphate-dextrose-adenine (CPDA-1) blood. *Transfusion* 28:34, 1988.

43. Beutler E, Forman L, West C, Gelbart T: The mechanism of improved maintenance of 2,3-diphosphoglycerate in stored blood by the xanthone compound BW A440C. *Biochem Pharmacol* 37:1057, 1988.

44. Brake JM, Deindoerfer FH: Preservation of red blood cell 2,3-diphosphoglycerate in stored blood containing dihydroxyacetone. *Transfusion* 13:84, 1973.

45. Beutler E, Guinto E: The metabolism of dihydroxyacetone by intact erythrocytes. *J Lab Clin Med* 82:534, 1973.

46. Beutler E, Guinto E: Dihydroxyacetone metabolism by human erythrocytes: Demonstration of triokinase activity and its characterization. *Blood* 41:559, 1973.

47. Dern RJ, Wiorkowski JJ, Matsuda T: Studies on the preservation of human blood: V. The effect of mixing anticoagulated blood during storage on the poststorage erythrocyte survival. *J Lab Clin Med* 75:37, 1970.

48. Bensinger TA, Metro J, Beutler E: The effect of agitation on in vitro metabolism of erythrocytes stored in CPD-adenine. *Transfusion* 15:140, 1975.

49. Duhm J, Deuticke B, Gerlach E: Complete restoration of oxygen transport function and 2,3-diphosphoglycerate concentration in stored blood. *Transfusion* 11:147, 1971.

50. Matsuyama H, Niklasson F, de Verdier CH, Högman CF: Phosphoenolpyruvate in the rejuvenation of stored red cells in SAGM medium: Optimal conditions and the indirect effect of methemoglobin formation. *Transfusion* 29:614, 1989.

51. Valeri CR, Zaroulis CG, Vecchione JJ, et al: Therapeutic effectiveness and safety of outdated human red blood cells rejuvenated to restore oxygen transport function to normal, frozen for 3 to 4 years at −80°C, washed and stored at 4°C for 24 hours prior to rapid infusion. *Transfusion* 20:159, 1980.

52. Meryman HT, Hornblower ML-S, Syring RL: Prolonged storage of red cells at 4 degrees C. *Transfusion* 26:500, 1986.

53. Greenwalt TJ, Dumaswala UJ, Dhingra N, et al: Studies in red blood cell preservation: 7. In vivo and in vitro studies with a modified phosphate-ammonium additive solution. *Vox Sang* 65:87, 1993.

54. Kay A, Beutler E: The effect of ammonium, phosphate, potassium, and hypotonicity on stored red blood cells. *Transfusion* 32:37, 1992.

55. Dumaswala UJ, Oreskovic RT, Petrosky TL, Greenwalt TJ: Studies in red blood cell preservation: 5. Determining the limiting concentrations of NH_4Cl and Na_2HPO_4 needed to maintain red blood cell ATP during storage. *Vox Sang* 62:136, 1992.

56. Högman CF, Knutson F, Loof H, Payrat JM: Improved maintenance of 2,3 DPG and ATP in RBCs stored in a modified additive solution. *Transfusion* 42:824, 2002.

57. Babcock JG, Lippert LE, Derse-Anthony CP, et al: A hypotonic storage solution did not prolong the viability of red blood cells. *Transfusion* 40:994, 2000.

58. Beutler E, Wood LA: Preservation of red cell 2,3-DPG and viability in bicarbonate-containing medium: The effect of blood-bag permeability. *J Lab Clin Med* 80:723, 1972.

59. Högman CF, Eriksson L, Gong J, et al: Half-strength citrate CPD combined with a new additive solution for improved storage of red blood cells suitable for clinical use. *Vox Sang* 65:271, 1993.

60. Beutler E: Red cell suspensions. *N Engl J Med* 300:984, 1979.

61. Beutler E, Kuhl W: Volume control of erythrocytes during storage: The role of mannitol. *Transfusion* 28:353, 1988.

62. Högman CF: Additive system approach in blood transfusion: Birth of the SAG and Sagman systems. *Vox Sang* 51:339, 1986.

63. Simon TL, Marcus CS, Myhre BA, Nelson EJ: Effects of AS-3 nutrient-additive solution on 42 and 49 days of storage of red cells. *Transfusion* 27:178, 1987.

64. Beutler E, West C: Letter to the editor re: Adsol. *N Engl J Med* 312:1392, 1985.

65. Bensinger TA, Chillar R, Beutler E: Prolonged maintenance of 2,3-DPG in liquid storage: Use of an internal CO_2 trap to stabilize pH. *J Lab Clin Med* 89:498, 1977.

66. Meryman HT: Freezing injury and its prevention in living cells. *Annu Rev Biophys Bioeng* 3:341, 1974.

67. Lovelock JE: Denaturation of lipid protein complexes as a cause of damage by freezing. *Proc R Soc Lond (Biol)* 147:427, 1957.

68. Lovelock JE: The haemolysis of human red blood cells by freezing and thawing. *Biochim Biophys Acta* 10:414, 1953.

69. Huggins C: Preparation and usefulness of frozen blood. *Annu Rev Med* 36:499, 1985.

70. Valeri CR, Pivacek LE, Gray AD, et al: The safety and therapeutic effectiveness of human red cells stored at −80°C for as long as 21 years. *Transfusion* 29:429, 1989.

71. Goodrich RP, Sowemimo-Coker SO, Zerez CR, Tanaka KR: Preservation of metabolic activity in lyophilized human erythrocytes. *Proc Natl Acad Sci U S A* 89:967, 1992.

72. Sowemimo-Coker SO, Goodrich RP, Zerez CR, Tanaka KR: Refrigerated storage of lyophilized and rehydrated, lyophilized human red cells. *Transfusion* 33:322, 1993.

73. Spieles G, Kresin M, Loges K, et al: The effect of storage temperature on the stability of frozen erythrocytes. *Cryobiology* 32:366, 1995.

74. Pellerin-Mendes C, Million L, Marchand-Arvier M, et al: In vitro study of the protective effect of trehalose and dextran during freezing of human red blood cells in liquid nitrogen. *Cryobiology* 35:173, 1997.

75. *Technical Manual of the American Association of Blood Banks*. American Association of Blood Banks, Bethesda, MD, 1996.

76. Åkerblom O, De Verdier CH, Finnson M, et al: Further studies on the effect of adenine in blood preservation. *Transfusion* 7:1, 1967.

77. Bensinger TA, Metro J, Beutler E: In vitro metabolism of packed erythrocytes stored in CPD-adenine. *Transfusion* 15:135, 1975.

78. Dawson RB, Hershey RT, Myers C, Holmes S: Blood preservation: XXVI. CPD-adenine packed cells: Benefits of increasing the glucose. *Transfusion* 18:339, 1978.

79. Oberman HA: The indications for transfusion of freshly drawn blood. *JAMA* 199:96, 1967.

80. Heustis DW: Fresh blood: Fact and fancy, in *Seminar on Current Technical Topics*, p 117. American Association of Blood Banks, Washington, DC, 1974.

81. Bolin RB, Cheney BA, Smith DJ, et al: An in vivo comparison of CPD and CPDA-2 preserved platelet concentrates after an 8-hour preprocess hold of whole blood. *Transfusion* 22:491, 1982.

82. Bowie EJW, Thompson JH, Owen CA Jr: The stability of antihemophilic globulin and labile factor in human blood. *Mayo Clin Proc* 39:144, 1964.

83. Horowitz HI, Fujimoto MM: Survival of factor XI in vitro and in vivo. *Transfusion* 6:539, 1965.

84. Aggeler PM: Physiological basis for transfusion therapy in hemorrhagic disorders. *Transfusion* 1:71, 1961.

85. Mooreside DE, Graybeal FQ Jr, Langdell RD: Effects of adenine on clotting factors in fresh blood, stored blood and stored fresh frozen plasma. *Transfusion* 9:191, 1969.

86. Nilsson L, Hedner U, Nilsson IM, Robertson B: Shelf-life of bank blood and stored plasma with special reference to coagulation factors. *Transfusion* 23:377, 1983.

87. Krevans JR, Jackson DP: Hemorrhagic disorder following massive whole blood transfusions. *JAMA* 159:171, 1955.

88. Beutler E, West C: The storage of "hard-packed" red blood cells in citrate-phosphate-dextrose (CPD) and CPD-adenine (CPDA-1). *Blood* 54:280, 1979.

89. *Standards for a Blood Transfusion Service.* American Association of Blood Banks, Washington, DC, 1987.

90. Moss GS, Proctor HJ, Homer LD, et al: Comparison of asanguinous fluids and whole blood in treatment of hemorrhagic shock. *Surg Gynecol Obstet* 129:1247, 1969.

91. Kahn RA, Staggs SD, Miller WV, Ellis FR: Use of plasma products with whole blood and packed RBCs. *JAMA* 242:2087, 1979.

92. Pineda AA, Rippetean ND, Clare DE, Bunkowske BM: Infusion flow rates of whole blood and ASH preserved erythrocytes: A comparison. *Mayo Clin Proc* 62:199, 1987.

93. Bilgin YM, Van De Watering LM, Eijsman L, et al: Double-blind, randomized controlled trial on the effect of leukocyte-depleted erythrocyte transfusions in cardiac valve surgery. *Circulation* 109:2755, 2004.

94. van Hilten JA, Van De Watering LM, Van Bockel JH, et al: Effects of transfusion with red cells filtered to remove leucocytes: Randomized controlled trial in patients undergoing major surgery. *BMJ* 328:1281, 2004.

95. Zimmermann B, Hillringhaus I, Diekamp U: Exceptional production of leukocyte-free erythrocyte concentrates using filtration with the BPF 4 BBS leukocyte filter. *Beitr Infusionsther Transfusionsmed* 32:32, 1994.

96. Krandick E, Vornwald A, Gossrau E: Leukocyte depletion by in-line-filtration. *Beitr Infusionsther Transfusionsmed* 32:6, 1994.

97. Roddie PH, Turner ML, Williamson LM: Leucocyte depletion of blood components. *Blood Rev* 14:145, 2000.

98. King KE, Shirey RS, Thoman SK, et al: Universal leukoreduction decreases the incidence of febrile nonhemolytic transfusion reactions to RBCs. *Transfusion* 44:25, 2004.

99. Contreras TJ, Valeri CR: A comparison of methods to wash liquid-stored red blood cells and red blood cells frozen with high or low concentrations of glycerol. *Transfusion* 16:539, 1976.

100. Toth CB, Kramer J, Pinter J, et al: IgA content of washed red blood cell concentrates. *Vox Sang* 74:13, 1998.

101. Sanner HE, Wooten MJ: Analysis of saline-washed red cells for transfusion to neonatal patients. *Transfusion* 25:437, 1985.

102. Grove-Rasmussen M: Selection of donors for frozen blood based on specific blood group combinations. *JAMA* 193:48, 1965.

103. Grove-Rasmussen M, Huggins CE: Selected types of frozen blood for patients with multiple blood group antibodies. *Transfusion* 13:124, 1973.

104. Valeri CR, Gray AD, Cassidy GP, et al: The 24-hour posttransfusion survival, oxygen transport function, and residual hemolysis of human outdated-rejuvenated red cell concentrates after washing and storage at 4 degrees C for 24 to 72 hours. *Transfusion* 24:323, 1984.

105. Lockwood WB, Hudgens RW, Szymanski IO, et al: Effects of rejuvenation and frozen storage on 42-day-old AS-3 RBCs. *Transfusion* 43:1527, 2003.

106. Dong Q, Stowell CP: Blood substitutes. What they are and how they might be used. *Am J Clin Pathol* 118(suppl):S71, 2002.

107. Gould SA, Rosen AL, Sehgal LR, et al: Fluosol-DA as a red-cell substitute in acute anemia. *N Engl J Med* 314:1653, 1986.

108. Wahr JA: Clinical potential of nonhemoglobin oxygen therapeutics in cardiac and general surgery. *Am J Cardiovasc Drugs* 2:69, 2002.

109. De Venuto F: Modified hemoglobin solution as a resuscitation fluid. *Vox Sang* 44:129, 1983.

110. Winslow RM: *Hemoglobin-based Red Cell Substitutes.* Johns Hopkins University Press, Baltimore, 1993.

111. Winslow RM: The toxicity of hemoglobin, in *Hemoglobin-based Red Cell Substitutes,* edited by RM Winslow, p 136. Johns Hopkins University Press, Baltimore, 1992.

112. Rudolph AS, Rabinivici R, Feuerstein GZ, eds. *Red Blood Cell Substitutes: Basic Principles and Clinical Applications.* Marcel Dekker, New York, 1998.

113. Gould SA, Moore EE, Moore FA, et al: Clinical utility of human polymerized hemoglobin as a blood substitute after acute trauma and urgent surgery. *J Trauma* 43:325, 1997.

114. Rohlfs RJ, Bruner E, Chiu A, et al: Arterial blood pressure responses to cell-free hemoglobin solutions and the reaction with nitric oxide. *J Biol Chem* 273:12128, 1998.

115. Djordjevich L, Miller IF: Synthetic erythrocytes from lipid encapsulated hemoglobin. *Exp Hematol* 8:584, 1980.

116. Hunt CA, Burnette RR, MacGregor RD, et al: Synthesis and evaluation of a prototypal artificial red cell. *Science* 230:1165, 1985.

117. Szebeni J, Wassef NM, Hartman KR, et al: Complement activation in vitro by the red cell substitute, liposome-encapsulated hemoglobin: Mechanism of activation and inhibition by soluble complement receptor type 1. *Transfusion* 37:150, 1997.

118. Widmann FK: Informed consent for blood transfusion: Brief historical survey and summary of a conference. *Transfusion* 30:460, 1990.

119. Stehling LC, Ellison N, Faust RJ, et al: A survey of transfusion practices among anesthesiologists. *Vox Sang* 52:60, 1987.

120. Roche JK, Stengle JM: Open-heart surgery and the demand for blood. *JAMA* 225:1516, 1973.

121. Umlas J: Transfusion of patients undergoing cardiopulmonary bypass. *Hum Pathol* 14:271, 1983.

122. Hillman RS: Blood-loss anemia. *Postgrad Med* 64:88, 1978.

123. Greenwalt TJ, Perry S: Preservation and utilization of the components of human blood, in *Progress in Hematology,* edited by EB Brown, CV Moore, p 157. Grune & Stratton, New York, 1969.

124. Rigor B, Bosomworth P, Rush BJ Jr: Replacement of operative blood loss of more than 1 liter with Hartmann's solution. *JAMA* 203:229, 1968.

125. Golub S, Baily CP: Management of major surgical blood loss without transfusion. *JAMA* 198:1171, 1966.

126. Demling RH: Burns. Medical progress. *N Engl J Med* 313:1389, 1985.

127. Baxter CR: Problems and complications of burn shock resuscitation. *Surg Clin North Am* 58:1313, 1978.

128. Pruitt BA Jr: Fluid and electrolyte replacement in the burned patient. *Surg Clin North Am* 58:1291, 1978.

129. Friedman BA: Patterns of blood utilization by physicians: Transfusion of nonoperated anemic patients. *Transfusion* 18:193, 1978.

130. Silberstein LE, Kruskall MS, Stehling LC, et al: Strategies for the review of transfusion practices. *JAMA* 262:1993, 1989.

131. Propper RD, Button LN, Nathan DG: New approaches to the transfusion management of thalassemia. *Blood* 55:55, 1980.

132. Keegan TE, Heaton A, Holme S, et al: Improved post-transfusion quality of density separated AS-3 red cells after extended storage. *Br J Haematol* 82:114, 1992.

133. Simon TL, Sohmer P, Nelson EJ: Extended survival of neocytes produced by a new system. *Transfusion* 29:221, 1989.

134. Spanos T, Ladis V, Palamidou F, et al: The impact of neocyte transfusion in the management of thalassaemia. *Vox Sang* 70:217, 1996.

135. Pisciotto P, Kiraly T, Paradis L, et al: Clinical trial of young red blood cells prepared by apheresis. *Ann Clin Lab Sci* 16:473, 1986.

136. Mollison PL, Engelfriet CP, Contreras M: *Blood Transfusion in Clinical Medicine.* Blackwell Scientific Publications, Oxford, 1987.

137. Ryden SE, Oberman HA: Compatibility of common intravenous solutions with CPD blood. *Transfusion* 15:250, 1975.

138. Dickson DN, Gregory MA: Compatibility of blood with solutions containing calcium. *S Afr Med J* 57:785, 1980.

139. De la Luna O, Amezcua Llauger LE, Leis Marquez MT, Sanchez Solis V: Usefulness of intraperitoneal transfusion under direct ultrasound guidance. *Ginecol Obstet Mex* 59:128, 1991.

140. Harman CR, Bowman JM, Manning FA, Menticoglou SM: Intrauterine transfusion—intraperitoneal versus intravascular approach: A case-control comparison. *Am J Obstet Gynecol* 162:1053, 1990.

141. Bowman JM: Intrauterine transfusion, in *Scientific Basis of Transfusion Medicine. Implications for Clinical Practice*, edited by KC Anderson, PM Ness, p 307. WB Saunders, Philadelphia, 2000.

142. Cass RM, Blumberg N: Single-unit blood transfusion: Doubtful dogma defeated. *JAMA* 257:628, 1987.

143. Reece RL, Beckett RS: Epidemiology of single-unit transfusion: A one-year experience in a community hospital. *JAMA* 195:801, 1966.

144. Allen JG: The case for the single transfusion. *N Engl J Med* 287:984, 1972.

145. Vanderlinde ES, Heal JM, Blumberg N: Autologous transfusion. *BMJ* 324:772, 2002.

146. Stehling L, Zander HL: Acute normovolemic hemodilution. *Transfusion* 31:857, 1991.

147. Schaff HV, Hauer JM, Brawley RK: Autotransfusion in cardiac surgical patients after operation. *Surgery* 84:713, 1978.

148. Faris PM, Ritter MA, Keating EM, Valeri CR: Unwashed filtered shed blood collected after knee and hip arthroplasties. A source of autologous red blood cells. *J Bone Joint Surg Am* 73A:1169, 1991.

149. Kent P, Ashley S, Thorley PJ, et al: 24-Hour survival of autotransfused red cells in elective aortic surgery: A comparison of two intraoperative autotransfusion systems. *Br J Surg* 78:1473, 1991.

150. Hall RI, Schweiger IM, Finlayson DC: Transfusion using a cell saver apparatus during surgery for coronary artery disease: Is it beneficial? *Can J Anaesth* 37:S155, 1990.

151. Kruskall MS, Glazier EE, Leonard SS, et al: Utilization and effectiveness of a hospital autologous preoperative blood donor program. *Transfusion* 26:335, 1986.

152. Goodnough LT, Rudnick S, Price TH, et al: Increased preoperative collection of autologous blood with recombinant human erythropoietin therapy. *N Engl J Med* 321:1163, 1989.

153. Masouredis SP, Chaplin H Jr: Transfusion management of autoimmune hemolytic anemia, in *Acquired Immune Hemolytic Anemias*, edited by H Chaplin Jr, p 177. Churchill Livingston, New York, 1985.

154. Rosenfield RE, Jagathambal: Transfusion therapy for autoimmune hemolytic anemia. *Semin Hematol* 13:311, 1976.

155. Petz LD: Transfusing the patient with autoimmune hemolytic anemia. *Clin Lab Med* 2:193, 1982.

156. Blumberg N, Bove JR: Uncrossmatched blood for emergency transfusion. One year's experience in a civilian setting. *JAMA* 240:2057, 1978.

157. Moore HC, Mollison PL: Use of a low-ionic-strength medium in manual tests for antibody detection. *Transfusion* 16:291, 1976.

158. Oberman HA, Barnes BA, Steiner EA: Role of the crossmatch in testing for serologic incompatibility. *Transfusion* 22:12, 1982.

159. Brittingham TE, Chaplin H Jr: Febrile transfusion reactions caused by sensitivity to donor leukocytes and platelets. *JAMA* 165:819, 1957.

160. Scornik JC, Ireland JE, Howard RJ, et al: Assessment of the risk for broad sensitization by blood transfusions. *Transplantation* 37:249, 1984.

161. Opelz G, Sengan DP, Mickey MR, Terasaki PI: Effect of blood transfusions on subsequent kidney transplants. *Transplant Proc* 5:253, 1973.

162. Opelz G, Terasaki PI: Improvement of kidney graft survival with increased number of transfusions. *N Engl J Med* 299:799, 1978.

163. Hourmant M, Soulillou JP, Bui-Quang D: Beneficial effect of blood transfusion: Role of the time interval between the last transfusion and transplantation. *Transplantation* 28:40, 1979.

164. Ahmed Z, Terasaki PI: Effect of transfusions, in *Clinical Transplant 1991*, edited by P Terasaki, p 305. UCLA Tissue Typing Laboratory, Los Angeles, CA, 1992.

165. Salvatierra O Jr, Vincenti F, Amend W, et al: Deliberate donor specific blood transfusions prior to living related renal transplantation. *Ann Surg* 192:543, 1980.

166. Light JA, Metz S, Oddenino K, et al: Fresh vs. stored blood in donor specific transfusions. *Transplant Proc* 14:296, 1982.

167. Sniecinski I, O'Donnel MR, Nowicki B: Prevention of refractoriness and HLA-alloimmunization using filtered blood products. *Blood* 71:1402, 1988.

168. Salvatierra O Jr, Melzer J, Vincenti F, et al: Donor-specific blood transfusions versus cyclosporine—The DST story. *Transplant Proc* 19:160, 1987.

169. Opelz G: Improved kidney graft survival in non-transfused recipients. *Transplant Proc* 19:149, 1987.

170. Cicciarelli J: UNOS registry data: Effect of transfusions, in *Clinical Transplants 1980*, edited by P Terasaki, p 289. UCLA Tissue Typing Laboratory, Los Angeles, CA, 1991.

171. Thomas ED: Current status of marrow transplantation for aplastic anemia and acute leukemia. *Am J Clin Pathol* 72:887, 1979.

172. Gale RP, Feig S, Ho W, et al: ABO blood group system and bone marrow transplantation. *Blood* 50:185, 1977.

173. Brand A, Claas FHJ, Falkenburg JHF, et al: Blood component therapy in bone marrow transplantation. *Semin Hematol* 21:141, 1984.

174. Goodnough LT: Risks of blood transfusion. *Crit Care Med* 31:S678, 2003.

175. Lewis JH, Bontempo FA, Cornell F, et al: Blood use in liver transplantation. *Transfusion* 27:222, 1987.

176. Owen CA, Rettke SR, Bowie EJW, et al: Hemostatic evaluation of patients undergoing liver transplantation. *Mayo Clin Proc* 62:761, 1987.

177. Schmidt PJ: Transfusion mortality: With special reference to surgical and intensive care facilities. *J Fla Med Assoc* 67:151, 1980.

178. Honig CL, Bove JR: Transfusion-associated fatalities: Review of Bureau of Biologics Reports 1976-1978. *Transfusion* 20:653, 1980.

179. Sazama K: Reports of 355 transfusion-associated deaths, 1976 through 1985. *Transfusion* 30:583, 1990.

180. Roy A, Volgin DV, Baby SM, et al: Activation of HIF-1alpha mRNA by hypoxia and iron chelator in isolated rat carotid body. *Neurosci Lett* 363:229, 2004.

181. Walker RH: Special report: Transfusion risks. *Am J Clin Pathol* 88:374, 1987.

182. Van Dijk PM, Kleine JW: The transfusion reaction in anaesthesiological practice. *Acta Anaesthesiol Belg* 4:274, 1976.

183. Goldfinger D: Acute hemolytic transfusion reactions: A fresh look at pathogenesis and considerations regarding therapy. *Transfusion* 17:85, 1977.

184. Pineda AA, Brzica SM, Taswell HF: Hemolytic transfusion reaction: Recent experience in a large blood bank. *Mayo Clin Proc* 53:378, 1978.

185. Ingram GIC: The bleeding complications of blood transfusion. *Transfusion* 5:1, 1965.

186. Rock RC, Bove JR, Nemerson Y: Heparin treatment of intravascular coagulation accompanying hemolytic transfusion reactions. *Transfusion* 9:57, 1969.

187. Harrison CR, Hayes TC, Trow LL, et al: Intravascular hemolytic transfusion reaction without detectable antibodies: A case report and review of the literature. *Vox Sang* 51:96, 1986.

188. Sack ES, Nefa OM: Fibrinogen and fibrin degradation products in hemolytic transfusion reactions. *Transfusion* 10:317, 1970.

189. Bick RL, Schmalhorst WR, Fekete L: Disseminated intravascular coagulation and blood component therapy. *Transfusion* 16:361, 1976.

190. Greenwalt TJ: Pathologenesis and management of hemolytic transfusion reactions. *Semin Hematol* 18:84, 1981.

191. Luke RG, Briggs JD, Allison MEM, et al: Factors determining response to mannitol in acute renal failure. *Am J Med Sci* 259:168, 1970.

192. Holland PV: Other adverse effects of transfusion, in *Clinical Practice of Blood Transfusion*, edited by LD Petz, SN Swisher, p 783. Churchill Livingstone, New York, 1981.

193. Viprakasit V, Vathesathokit P, Chinchang W, et al: Prevalence of HFE mutations among the Thai population and correlation with iron loading in haemoglobin E disorder. *Eur J Haematol* 73:43, 2004.

194. Holtzman NA, Marteau TM: Will genetics revolutionize medicine? *N Engl J Med* 343:141, 2000.

195. Thompson JS, Severson CD, Parmely MJ, et al: Pulmonary "hypersensitivity" reactions induced by transfusion on non-HL-A leukoagglutinins. *N Engl J Med* 284:1120, 1971.

196. Koppel H: Hemochromatosis gene (HFE) polymorphisms are not associated with peripheral arterial disease. *Thromb Haemost* 91:1258, 2004.

197. Wolfe CFW, Conale VC: Fatal pulmonary hypersensitivity reaction to HL-A incompatible blood transfusion: Report of a case and review of the literature. *Transfusion* 16:135, 1976.

198. Popovsky MA, Moore SB: Diagnostic and pathogenetic considerations in transfusion-related acute lung injury. *Transfusion* 25:573, 1985.

199. Thulstrup H: The influence of leukocyte and thrombocyte incompatibility on non-haemolytic transfusion reactions: I. A retrospective study. *Vox Sang* 21:233, 1971.

200. Nishimura JI, Kanakura Y, Ware RE, et al: Clinical course and flow cytometric analysis of paroxysmal nocturnal hemoglobinuria in the United States and Japan. *Medicine* 83:193, 2004.

201. Nadorp JHS, Voss M, Buys WS, et al: The significance of the presence of anti-IgA antibodies in individuals with an IgA deficiency. *Eur J Clin Invest* 3:317, 1973.

202. Vyas GN, Perkins HA, Yang Y-M, Basantani GK: Healthy blood donors with selective absence of immunoglobulin A: Prevention of anaphylactic transfusion reactions caused by antibodies to IgA. *J Lab Clin Med* 85:838, 1975.

203. Pineda AA, Taswell HF: Transfusion reactions associated with anti-IgA antibodies: Report of four cases and review of the literature. *Transfusion* 15:10, 1975.

204. Braude AI: Transfusion reactions from contaminated blood: Their recognition and treatment. *N Engl J Med* 258:1289, 1958.

205. Duke M, Herbert VD, Abelmann WH: Hemodynamic effects of blood transfusion in chronic anemia. *N Engl J Med* 271:975, 1964.

206. Abdulhadi NH: Glucose 6 phosphate dehydrogenase (G6PD) deficiency is a possible risk factor for the development of preeclampsia. *Med Hypotheses* 62:780, 2004.

207. O'Quin RJ, Lakshminarayan S: Venous air embolism. *Arch Intern Med* 142:2173, 1982.

208. Arrington P, McNamara JJ: Mechanism of microaggregate formation in stored blood. *Ann Surg* 179:146, 1974.

209. Harvey MP, Greenfield TP, Sugrue ME, Rosenfeld D: Massive blood transfusion in a tertiary referral hospital. Clinical outcomes and haemostatic complications. *Med J Aust* 163:356, 1995.

210. Pineda AA, Taswell HF, Brzica SM Jr: Delayed hemolytic transfusion reaction: An immunologic hazard of blood transfusion. *Transfusion* 18:1, 1978.

211. Moore SB, Taswell HF, Pineda AA, Sonnenberg CL: Delayed hemolytic transfusion reactions: Evidence of the need for an improved pretransfusion compatibility test. *Am J Clin Pathol* 74:94, 1980.

212. Harper P, Floderus Y, Holmstrom P, et al: Enrichment of HFE mutations in Swedish patients with familial and sporadic form of porphyria cutanea tarda. *J Intern Med* 255:684, 2004.

213. Croucher BEE, Crookston MC, Crookston JH: Delayed haemolytic transfusion reaction simulating autoimmune haemolytic anemia. *Vox Sang* 12:32, 1967.

214. Diamond WJ, Brown FL, Bitterman P, et al: Delayed hemolytic transfusion reaction presenting as sickle-cell crises. *Ann Intern Med* 93:231, 1980.

215. Hershko C, Cappellini MD, Galanello R, et al: Purging iron from the heart. *Br J Haematol* 125:545, 2004.

216. Vichinsky EP, Luban NLC, Wright E, Olivieri N, Driscoll C, Pegelow CH, Adams RJ: Prospective RBC phenotype matching in a stroke-prevention trial in sickle cell anemia: a multicenter transfusion trial. *Transfusion* 41:1086, 2001.

217. Corash L: Inactivation of viruses, bacteria, protozoa and leukocytes in platelet and red cell concentrates. *Vox Sang* 78(suppl 2):205, 2000.

218. Orlin JB, Ellis MH: Transfusion-associated graft versus host disease. *Curr Opin Hematol* 4:442, 1997.

219. Anderson K: Broadening the spectrum of patient groups at risk for transfusion-associated GVHD: Implications for universal irradiation of cellular blood components. *Transfusion* 43:1652, 2003.

220. Fluit CRMG, Kunst VAJM, Drenthe-Schonk AH: Incidence of red cell antibodies after multiple blood transfusion. *Transfusion* 30:532, 1990.

221. Orlina AR, Unger PJ, Koshy M: Post-transfusion alloimmunization in patients with sickle cell disease. *Am J Hematol* 5:101, 1978.

222. Coles SM, Klein HG, Holland PV: Alloimmunization in two multitransfused patient populations. *Transfusion* 21:462, 1981.

223. Sarnaik S, Schornack J, Lusher JM: The incidence of development of irregular red cell antibodies in patients with sickle cell anemia. *Transfusion* 26:249, 1986.

224. Sirchia G, Zanella A, Parravicini A, et al: Red cell alloantibodies in thalassemia major. Results of an Italian cooperative study. *Transfusion* 25:110, 1985.

225. Ambruso DR, Githens JH, Alcorn R, et al: Experience with donors matched for minor blood group antigens in patients with sickle cell anemia who are receiving chronic transfusion therapy. *Transfusion* 27:94, 1987.

226. Mollison PL, Frame M, Ross ME: Differences between Rh(D) negative subjects in response to Rh(D) antigen. *Br J Haematol* 19:257, 1970.

227. Barclay GR, Greiss MAM, McCann MC, et al: Rhesus immunization in male volunteers: Changes in lymphocyte functions following secondary immunizations in anti-D responders and non-responders. *Br J Haematol* 53:629, 1983.

228. Cook K, Rush B: Rh(D) immunization after massive transfusion of Rh(D)-positive blood. *Med J Aust* 1:166, 1974.

229. de Verdier CH, Garby L, Hjelm M, Högman C: Adenine in blood preservation: Posttransfusion viability and biochemical changes. *Transfusion* 4:331, 1964.

PRESERVATION AND CLINICAL USE OF PLATELETS

RALPH VASSALLO
SCOTT MURPHY

Increasingly aggressive medical and surgical treatment modalities spurred dramatic growth in the use of platelet transfusions in the United States in the 1980s. This growth slowed somewhat in the 1990s, based on evidence that the threshold for transfusion can be safely set at a lower level. Worldwide, many methods are used for the preparation of platelets for transfusion. The "platelet-rich plasma" method and the "buffy coat method" are popular for the separation of platelets from whole blood donations in North America and Europe, respectively. In addition, platelets obtained from single donors and prepared by apheresis are gaining in popularity worldwide in order to limit the numbers of donors to whom recipients are exposed and to minimize the number of contaminating leukocytes in the preparations. Many institutions are making their platelet products universally leukoreduced at the time of their preparation based on evidence that such products have a reduced incidence of adverse events. After preparation, platelets are generally stored at 20 to 24°C in containers that are permeable to oxygen. Optimally, these preparations should be agitated continuously. Storage at lower temperatures decreases *in vivo* survival after transfusion, and adequate access to oxygen and agitation are required to prevent deleterious declines in pH. Platelets stored in this fashion produce satisfactory clinical responses after storage for 5 to 7 days. Currently, storage is limited to 5 days because of concerns about overgrowth of bacteria that might have inadvertently contaminated the preparation.

The clinical response to platelet transfusion can be assessed by measuring the increment in platelet concentration achieved in the patient's blood. This measurement generally correlates directly with the dose of platelets infused and inversely with the patient's size. Using physiologic principles, one can calculate what this response should be. Although the ideal theoretical response is occasionally achieved, on average the response is approximately half the predicted value because of immunologic and nonimmunologic clinical factors that impact negatively on the response. No single correct dose of platelets exists for all patients. On average, both the initial increment and the time to next transfusion increase with increasing platelet dose. The appropriate dose varies with the clinical circumstances, the patient's size, and the individual response to transfusion. The traditional platelet concentration that should trigger a platelet transfusion had been $20,000/\mu l$, but studies have shown that this level can safely be reduced to $10,000/\mu l$ in patients with production disorders that are stable. Raising the transfusion trigger above this level in response to a variety of clinical circumstances that increase the likelihood of bleeding is important. Although most platelet transfusions are given to patients with suppressed platelet production, platelet transfusion occasionally is indicated when the thrombocytopenia results from massive blood loss, cardiopulmonary bypass, splenomegaly, immune-mediated thrombocytopenia, and hereditary thrombocytopenia.

The complications of platelet transfusion most frequently result from contaminating leukocytes, red cells, plasma proteins, and microorganisms. The frequency of complications resulting from contaminating leukocytes can be reduced by prestorage leukoreduction of the platelet products. Alloimmunization to class I human leukocyte antigens can be managed by a variety of strategies using apheresis platelet concentrates that lack the antigens to which the patient has formed antibody.

INTRODUCTION

In the 1980s and early 1990s, use of platelet transfusion increased rapidly in the United States, doubling between 1982 and 1989.[1,2] Overall platelet use continues to grow, albeit at a somewhat slower rate (Figure 132-1).[2–5] In 1994, for the first time, platelets obtained by apheresis represented more than 50 percent of the platelets infused in the United States. The progressive increase in platelet use correlates with increasingly aggressive myelosuppressive therapy for malignancies and increased availability of platelets made possible by the development of cost-effective methods for storage of platelet concentrates.

TECHNIQUES FOR PLATELET PREPARATION

Platelet concentrates for transfusion can be obtained from donations of whole blood anticoagulated with citrate-based formulations or by apheresis with a variety of apheresis devices that also use citrate as the anticoagulant. Two methods of preparing platelet concentrates from whole blood are used: the platelet-rich plasma method and the buffy coat method.

In addition to appropriate platelet content, attention now is being given to the level of contaminating leukocytes that are infused into patients. Problems produced by contaminating leukocytes are discussed in "Complications of Platelet Transfusion" below. *In toto*, these complications are sufficiently serious that many now recommend a totally leukoreduced blood supply. Blood products can be filtered during infusion at the bedside, but, for reasons to be discussed, accomplishing leukoreduction at the time of product preparation probably is preferable. In the United States, an apheresis platelet concentrate or a pool of platelet-rich plasma platelet concentrates is considered leukoreduced if it contains less than 5×10^6 leukocytes. In Europe, the standard is 1×10^6 leukocytes.

WHOLE-BLOOD—DERIVED PLATELET CONCENTRATES

Whole-blood—derived platelet concentrates often are termed *random-donor platelet concentrates*. This term was used to distinguish whole-blood—derived platelet concentrates from apheresis platelet concentrates derived from specific donors for specific refractory patients

Acronyms and abbreviations that appear in this chapter include: AABB, American Association of Blood Banks; ACE, angiotensin-converting enzyme; ATP, adenosine triphosphate; BSA, body surface area; CCI, corrected count increment; CMV, cytomegalovirus; CREG, cross-reactive group; DMSO, dimethyl sulfoxide; ELISA, enzyme-linked immunosorbent assay; FDA, Food and Drug Administration; FNHTR, febrile nonhemolytic transfusion reaction; GVHD, graft-versus-host disease; HIV, human immunodeficiency virus; HLA, human leukocyte antigen; HPA, human platelet antigen; HTLV, human T lymphotrophic virus; Ig, immunoglobulin; LCT, lymphocytotoxicity; MAIPA, monoclonal antibody immobilization of antigen; PRA, percent reactive antibody; TTP, thrombotic thrombocytopenic purpura; U, unit(s).

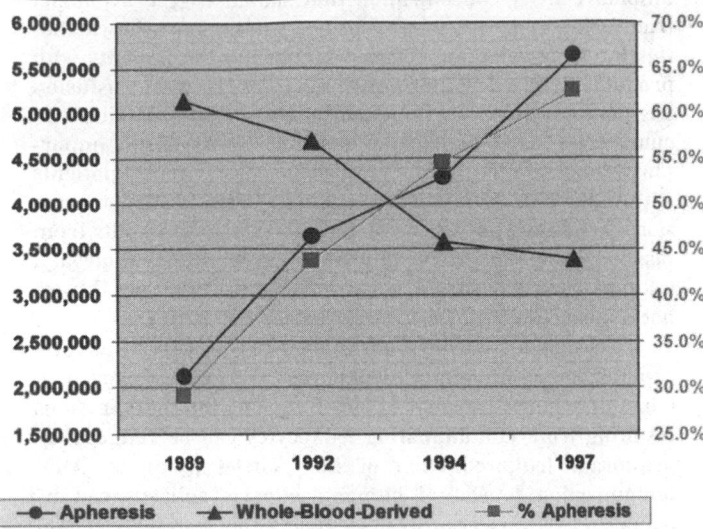

FIGURE 132-1   Trends in US use of whole-blood–derived platelet concentrate equivalent units per year.[1-5] In 1994, for the first time, more than 50 percent of platelet transfusions were given as apheresis platelet concentrates *(blue line)*.

generally based on human leukocyte antigen (HLA) matching. Now, apheresis platelet concentrates commonly are given "randomly" to patients who do not require products from specific donors. Therefore, the term *whole-blood–derived platelet concentrates* is preferred.

PLATELET-RICH PLASMA PLATELET CONCENTRATES

The platelet-rich plasma method is the only method used in North America for whole-blood–derived platelet concentrates. From 450 to 500 ml (1 U) of whole blood is held at room temperature for up to 8 hours, and platelet-rich plasma is separated from red cells and the buffy coat by low-speed centrifugation. After the platelet-rich plasma is transferred to another bag, the plasma is centrifuged rapidly to produce a platelet pellet. Most of the plasma is removed, and the platelet pellet is allowed to "rest" for 1 to 2 hours before it is resuspended in approximately 50 ml of autologous citrated plasma. The need for a rest period, originally designed to prevent irreversible clumping upon resuspension, has now been called into question.[6] The separated red cells are used for transfusion, whereas the supernatant plasma is used for transfusion or fractionation.

Over the past 20 years, technical improvements have doubled the number of platelets in each unit, resulting in an average content of 0.8 to 0.9×10^{11} platelets per unit. The range around this average, however, is high ($0.4-1.8 \times 10^{11}$), primarily related to the variability in donor platelet level.[7,8] One unit is adequate only for the transfusion of a small child weighing less than 30 lb. Because of the wide range of platelet counts in individual units, at least 5 U must be pooled to be certain the pool contains at least 3×10^{11} platelets.[8] For transfusion of adults, 4 to 8 U must be pooled to provide a therapeutic dose (see section on dose below).

Whole-blood–derived platelet pools of 4 to 9 U have a high level of leukocyte (primarily lymphocyte) contamination of 0.4 to 4.0×10^9, which is three orders of magnitude higher than the level of a leukoreduced transfusion. A system that inserts a leukocyte-reduction filter between the primary blood bag and the bag that accepts the platelet-rich plasma is available.[9] Thus, platelet-rich plasma may be leukoreduced at the time of its preparation. This system was introduced in early 1998 for the preparation of all platelet-rich plasma platelet concentrates in Canada and is gaining acceptance in the United States.

BUFFY COAT PLATELET CONCENTRATES

The buffy coat method is being used with increased frequency, particularly in Europe.[10] An initial hard centrifugation sediments all blood cells so that the plasma, buffy coat, and red cells can be collected in three separate containers. Remarkably, not only do the platelets at the top of the bag fall to the buffy coat, but also the platelets at the bottom of the bag rise to the buffy coat. Therefore, platelet yields in the buffy coat are excellent. One can prepare platelet concentrates from individual buffy coats[11] or pool four to six buffy coats, add two to four volumes of an additive solution, centrifuge the pool at low speed to remove red cells and leukocytes, and push the supernatant through a leukoreduction filter to produce a therapeutic, leukoreduced dose of platelets for an adult.[12,13]

The platelet-rich plasma and buffy coat methods each has its advantages and disadvantages.[10,14,15] Each method produces platelets of high quality, and platelet yields are equivalent. In the buffy coat method, 20 to 25 ml of red cells are lost with the buffy coat, but an extra 70 to 80 ml of plasma can be collected. In any event, the buffy coat method is being used with increasing frequency in Europe; it is not used in North America.

APHERESIS PLATELET CONCENTRATES

From 2.5 to 14×10^{11} platelets (equivalent to 3–18 U of whole-blood–derived platelet concentrates) can be obtained by apheresis of donors over 1 to 2 hours using a variety of devices,[16-19] with an extraordinarily high level of safety for the donors.[20] The number of platelets obtained during the procedure varies according to the platelet concentration in the blood of the donor, the duration of the donation, and the efficiency of the device. The efficiency of the newest devices is such that collection of at least 60 percent of the platelets that pass through the devices can be expected, and most donors become restless if the donation time exceeds more than 90 to 120 minutes. Therefore, the wide range of platelet concentrations in the blood of normal donors (150,000–500,000/μl) accounts for the wide range in platelet yields.[21] Reports of yield enhancement through administration of recombinant human thrombopoietin to enhance donor platelet concentrations have been tempered by the development of antibody-mediated thrombocytopenia in volunteer donors.[22] However, devices capable of maximizing donors' contributions by obtaining apheresis platelet concentrates and 1 or 2 U of red cells or plasma from the same donor at a single sitting are available.[23]

The original goal of apheresis was to obtain a therapeutic dose of platelets for an adult from a single donor during one apheresis sitting. Current controversies concerning the appropriate dose for platelet transfusion are discussed in the section on "Platelet Dose" below. Current US Food and Drug Administration (FDA) standards state only that 75 percent of apheresis platelet products must contain more than 3.0×10^{11} platelets. The American Association of Blood Banks (AABB) has set a 90 percent target for this platelet content.[24] The goal of 3×10^{11} platelets probably reflects the capabilities of apheresis devices available at the time the standards were established rather than the needs of the wide variety of patients undergoing treatment. Although 2.5 to 3.5×10^{11} probably is a satisfactory dose for the prophylactic transfusion of a child or small adult, that number probably is unsatisfactory for a large adult who is bleeding or has other clinical features that interfere with an optimal response to platelet transfusion. On the other hand, administration of high-yield platelet products to small adults and children may be wasteful. Blood centers are considering the best way to handle the preparation process for apheresis platelets. Many centers divide high-yield products (i.e., $> 6.5-7 \times 10^{11}$ platelets) to provide a therapeutic dose for two patients. Very-high-yield products ($>10-11 \times 10^{11}$ platelets) can be divided to treat three patients. Consideration is being given to the preparation of products containing two or more levels of platelet content, perhaps means of 3.2×10^{11} and 6.4×10^{11} (i.e., approximately 4 and 8 whole-blood–derived U, respectively). Use of the products could be tailored to the needs of individual patients.

Whole-blood–derived platelets (produced by the buffy coat or platelet-rich plasma methods) and apheresis platelets probably are equivalent therapeutically. However, use of apheresis platelet products has three advantages. First, the number of donors to whom the patient is exposed is substantially reduced, thus decreasing the likelihood of transmission of viral and bacterial diseases. Advances in viral testing technologies may diminish the importance of donor exposure reduction.[25] Until economical and effective means for preventing and detecting platelet bacterial contamination are developed, however, fewer donor venipunctures (the primary source of contamination)[26] will remain an important means of limiting infectious disease risk.

Second, newer separation technologies lend themselves to the production of leukoreduced products during collection without product loss (approximately 5–20% of the platelet content of whole-blood–derived units)[27] or cost associated with use of one or more bedside leukoreduction filters. Progressive improvements of devices now available have allowed the production of products with fewer than 1 $\times 10^6$ leukocytes, essentially 100 percent of the time.[16,17] Figure 132-2 shows the experience of one blood center in this regard. Prestorage leukoreduction at the blood center offers the advantage that the procedure is performed under standardized conditions following current good manufacturing practices with appropriate quality control procedures in place. Such standardization is not possible with bedside filtration.[28] Cases in which bedside filtration failed to achieve the expected beneficial results have been reported.[29]

Third, apheresis platelets will continue to be the product of choice when special donor characteristics are required, such as HLA-matched, human platelet antigen (HPA)-1a (Pl^A1) negative, and immunoglobulin (Ig)A deficient.

STORAGE OF PLATELET CONCENTRATES

LIQUID STORAGE AT 20 TO 24°C

Both whole-blood–derived and apheresis platelet concentrates can be stored for 5 days using the same principles. (1) The temperature must be 20 to 24°C.[30] (2) The storage container must be constructed of a plastic material that allows adequate diffusion of oxygen to meet the cells' metabolic needs.[31,32] (3) The platelet concentrates must be agitated during storage.[31,32]

Using radiolabeling of stored platelets (Figure 132-3), in vivo survival after reinfusion is nearly normal if storage, even for several days, is performed at 20 to 24°C (68.0–75.2°F). However, at colder temperatures, the cells undergo irreversible disc-to-sphere transformation, and survival is dramatically shortened.[30] If oxygen influx is inadequate at 20 to 24°C, the cells increase their production of lactic acid in an effort to maintain adenosine triphosphate (ATP) levels, leading to depletion of bicarbonate buffer and a fall in pH.[31,32] If the pH drops to below 6.2, an irreversible disc-to-sphere transformation occurs, resulting in rapid clearance from the circulation after transfusion. A similar fall in pH occurs if the platelet concentrates are not agitated during storage.[32] Data suggest that agitation can be discontinued for up to 24 hours of the 5-day storage interval without harm to the platelets.[33]

Synthetic media are used for storage of buffy coat platelet concentrates[12] and soon will be available for storage of apheresis platelets.[34] Definition of the optimal solution is still in progress, but the solution appears to be relatively simple, relying upon 20 to 40 percent residual plasma and added acetate as an oxidative fuel for platelets.[35]

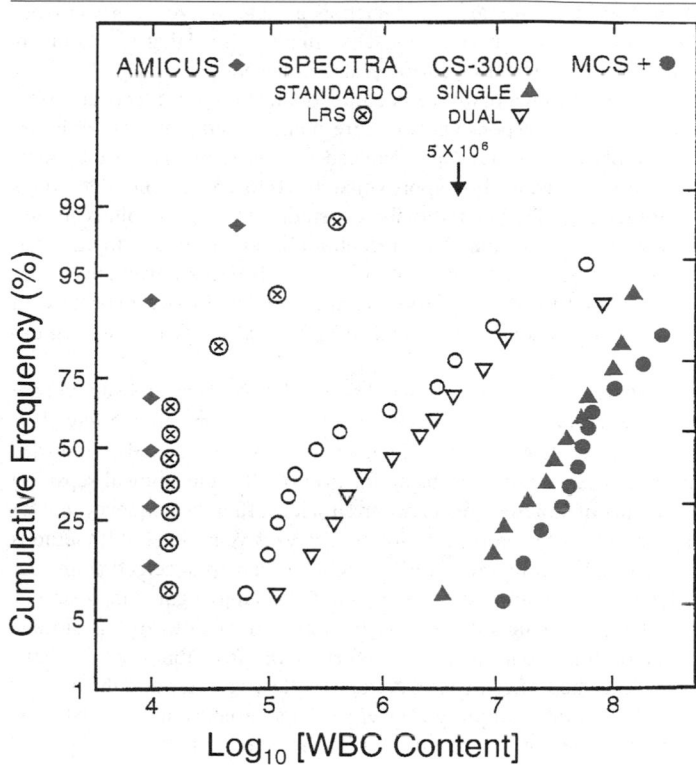

FIGURE 132-2 Cumulative frequency of leukocyte contents of apheresis platelet concentrates produced using six different apheresis methodologies: Fenwal Amicus, COBE Spectra (standard and leukocyte reduction system [LRS] versions), Fenwal CS-3000 (single- and dual-needle access), and Haemonetics MCS+. The newest devices, the Amicus and Spectra LRS, produce greater than 99 percent products with leukocyte content less than 5×10^6, the current standard in the United States. The older procedures have a 25 percent (standard Spectra, dual-needle CS-3000) or 95 percent (single-needle CS-3000, MCS+) failure rate. Data from the American Red Cross Blood Services, Penn-Jersey Region. (From S Murphy,[182] with permission.)

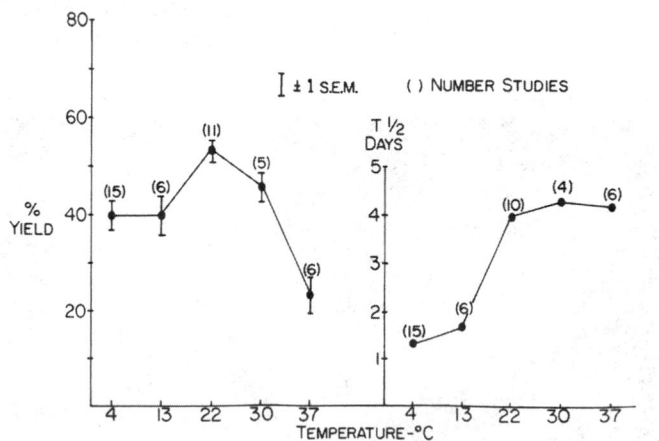

FIGURE 132-3 Relationship between storage temperature and platelet viability after transfusion. Platelet-rich plasma was obtained from normal volunteers and stored overnight at the indicated temperatures. Thereafter, the platelets were labeled with radioactive chromium and reinfused. Percent yield refers to the percent of platelets infused that circulate in the first 3 hours after infusion. The 50 to 60 percent yield at 22°C (71.6°F) is a result of physiologic pooling in the spleen (see Chap. 110), not cell damage. The combination of percent yield and subsequent in vivo survival ($T_{1/2}$) is optimal at 22°C.

Oxidation of an organic anion such as acetate utilizes a proton from the medium, thus providing an alkalinizing effect that spares bicarbonate, the major buffer during platelet concentrate storage.[36]

Some investigators have been unable to find any practical difference in clinical response between fresh and stored platelets.[37,38] However, most investigators find reduced *in vivo* recovery for the latter, with survival reduced by approximately 20 to 25 percent after 5 days of storage as judged by radiolabeling studies in normal volunteers and by the increase in platelet concentrations in thrombocytopenic patients.[39] Furthermore, some authors have reported an even greater defect in stored platelets relative to fresh platelets in sick patients with fever, sepsis, splenomegaly, and disseminated intravascular coagulation.[40,41]

Several studies have shown that platelet recovery and survival are as satisfactory after 7 days of storage as they are after 5 days.[42–44] However, when storage was extended to 7 days in one study performed more than 20 years ago, bacterial overgrowth and clinical sepsis in recipients of stored platelets occurred with sufficient frequency to warrant returning the storage period to 5 days 2 years later.[45] If methods of bacterial decontamination[46] or reliable bacterial detection are developed,[47] prolonging storage beyond 5 days may again be possible.[48]

Platelet products deteriorate to some extent even during storage under optimal conditions. A number of *in vitro* abnormalities have been described after *ex vivo* storage, collectively termed the *platelet storage lesion*.[49,50] At present, *in vitro* characteristics that correlate best with the capacity to circulate *in vivo* are retention of disc shape and good function in the hypotonic shock response.[51] With few exceptions, platelets with normal discoid morphology circulate normally after transfusion. Platelets that are damaged by cold, acidity, or bacterial contamination generally lose their discoid morphology and become spheres. Normal discoid morphology is reflected by the "swirling" or "shimmering" appearance of well-preserved platelet concentrates during gross, visual inspection.[52] Blood bank staff and clinical personnel are urged to check platelet concentrates for this phenomenon prior to transfusion (Figure 132-4). Two additional characteristics of stored platelets—induction of markers of cellular apoptosis and of platelet activation—correlate with the *in vivo* survival of platelets once infused into recipients and could provide new strategies for monitoring platelet transfusion products.

The activities of coagulation factors are well maintained in the suspending plasma of platelet concentrates during storage, except for modest decreases in the activity of factors V and VIII.[53] Thus, a pool of four to eight whole-blood–derived platelet concentrates or an apheresis platelet concentrate provides the equivalent of 1 to 2 U of fresh-frozen plasma.

FROZEN STORAGE

The most widely used method for frozen storage involves controlled rate freezing (1°C per minute), 5 to 6 percent dimethyl sulfoxide (DMSO) as a cryoprotective agent, rapid thawing, graded reduction of the DMSO concentration, and washing prior to infusion. *In vivo* viability is approximately 40 to 50 percent relative to fresh platelets.[54] Thus, this technology is more complex, expensive, and less effective than liquid storage at 20 to 24°C.[55] However, these preparations can be effective clinically[56] and may be valuable for autologous transfusion of selected patients who do not respond well to allogeneic platelets. Platelets can be obtained before myelosuppressive therapy, then frozen and administered during subsequent periods of thrombocytopenia.[57] Newer approaches using a second-messenger effector-containing storage solution permit the use of lower concentrations of DMSO and correspondingly less cumbersome freezing and thawing protocols.[58] *In vivo* platelet recovery and survival are better with 2 percent DMSO.[59] Administration of human recombinant thrombopoietin to autologous donors has allowed high-yield platelet collections that have effectively supported patients through intensive multicycle chemotherapy regimens.[60]

COLD LIQUID STORAGE

Room temperature storage of platelets limits their shelf life by facilitating bacterial overgrowth.[61] Cold storage may allow the extension of shelf life by reducing the risk of bacterial contamination and by further decreasing platelet metabolism below the 44 percent reduction in aging seen with 22°C storage versus that seen at 37°C *in vivo*.[62] As noted previously, however, platelet exposure to temperatures below 20°C results in loss of discoid shape and marked shortening of posttransfusion survival.[30] Platelet cold exposure results in clustering of the von Willebrand factor receptor, glycoprotein Ibα complexes that are recognized upon transfusion by complement type 3 receptors on hepatic macrophages, which clear the previously chilled platelets.[63] In an attempt to overcome the cold storage lesion, galactosylation of murine platelets has prevented the hepatic clearance of cold-exposed platelets,

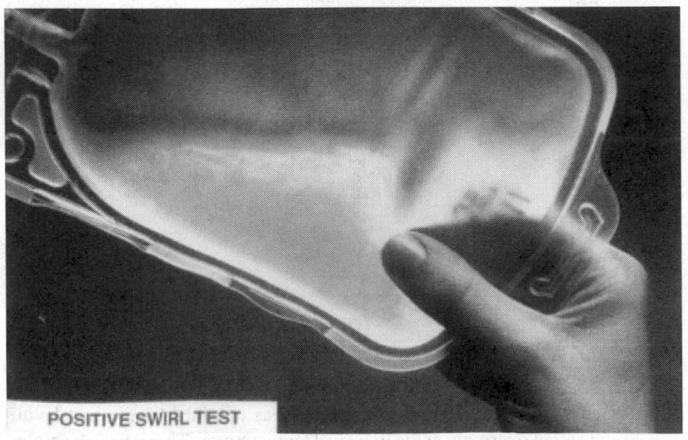
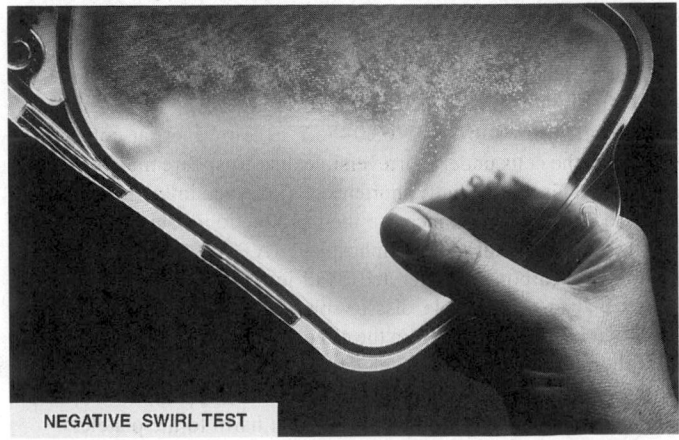

FIGURE 132-4 Swirling of platelet concentrates. Platelets in platelet concentrates that have been prepared and stored well retain their normal discoid configuration, which confers a swirling or shimmering appearance to the platelet concentrates *(left)*. If the platelets are damaged by cold temperature, a fall in pH, or bacterial contamination, the discoid shape and swirling appearance are lost *(right)*. Loss of swirling allows a transfusion unit or a clinician to identify potentially ineffective or dangerous platelet concentrates.

which appear to function normally when transfused in a murine bleeding model.[63,64] These findings may have far-reaching consequences for platelet storage if the results can be replicated in human trials.

LYOPHILIZED PLATELETS, PLATELET MEMBRANES, AND PLATELET SUBSTITUTES

Because of periodic supply shortages, having a safe and effective platelet substitute with a long shelf life that simply could be rehydrated and infused into bleeding patients would be ideal. A great deal of research in this area is examining paraformaldehyde-treated lyophilized platelets, lyophilized platelet membrane microvesicles, fibrinogen-coated albumin microcapsules, platelet glycoprotein-containing liposomes, and other platelet substitutes.[65] This is an important area, but all of these developments await validation in appropriate clinical trials.

Nontransfusional agents, including the antifibrinolytic drugs ε-aminocaproic acid and tranexamic acid, may help stop thrombocytopenic bleeding.[66] Antifibrinolytics have been effective in controlling mucosal and dental bleeding in thrombocytopenic patients without increasing the blood platelet concentration. Recombinant factor VIIa, in pharmacologic doses, enhances thrombin generation on activated platelets. A number of clinical reports describing bleeding time reduction and diminution or cessation of thrombocytopenic bleeding suggest a potential role for this agent in hemorrhage resulting from low platelet concentrations or platelet dysfunction.[67]

FRESH WHOLE BLOOD

Children younger than 2 years who undergo complex cardiac bypass surgery have a better hemostatic response to fresh whole blood than to reconstituted blood using red cells, plasma, and platelet concentrates prepared as described in the section "Platelet-Rich Plasma Platelet Concentrates."[68] These findings are the only published data suggesting that the process of platelet concentrate preparation impairs platelet function. Although this conclusion has not been confirmed in a second trial, the administration of fresh whole blood is strongly endorsed by some cardiac surgeons.

CLINICAL RESPONSE

GENERAL PRINCIPLES IN PATIENTS WITH MARROW FAILURE

Assuming that one third of infused platelets are pooled reversibly in a spleen of normal size (see Chap. 110) and that the recipient's blood volume is 2.5 liters/m², infusion of 1 U of whole-blood–derived platelet concentrates containing 0.8×10^{11} platelets into a recipient with 1 m² of body surface area (BSA) should result in an increased platelet concentration of 21,000/μl. Of course, the response to 1 U is inversely proportional to the patient's size, expressed as the BSA. Thus, the response to a platelet transfusion can be evaluated by calculating the corrected count increment (CCI)[69]:

$$\frac{\text{Measured increase in platelet concentration} \times \text{BSA (in m}^2)}{\text{No. of platelets infused } (\times 10^{11})}$$

The measurement of CCI has its critics,[70] but it is the most widely used method. Under optimal circumstances, the response should be 21,000/μl per square meter per whole-blood–derived unit infused or 26,000/μl per square meter per 10^{11} platelets infused.

In practice, in patients with thrombocytopenia secondary to marrow failure, the average CCI is approximately half the value expected: 10,000/μl per square meter per whole-blood–derived unit infused (Figure 132-5).[69] Many studies have attempted to identify the factors responsible for this consistent but less than optimal response.[41,69,71–75]

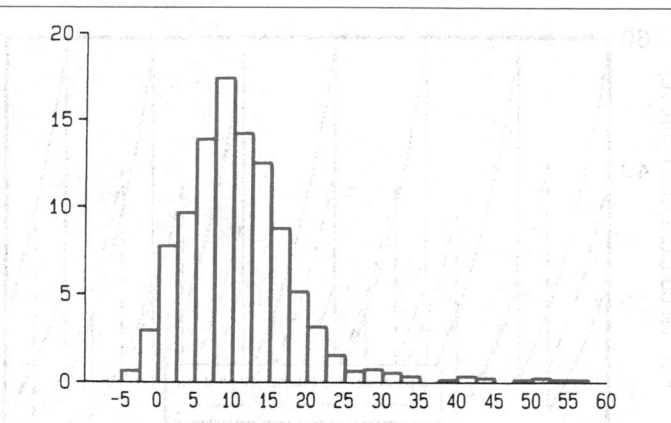

FIGURE 132-5   Rise in platelet concentration 1 hour after infusion in patients with acute leukemia. As described in the text, the increment in concentration for each unit infused has been corrected for body surface area. Without complicating factors, the concentration should be approximately 21,000/μl. The *vertical axis* refers to the percent of transfusions achieving the increments indicated. Marked heterogeneity in response is seen, with a median of approximately 10,000/μl, which is approximately half of the predicted amount. (Redrawn from JF Bishop, K McGrath, MM Wolf, et al.[69])

Alloimmunization has been incriminated, as have a variety of nonimmune factors such as platelet storage, bacterial sepsis, concomitant use of antibacterial antibiotics and amphotericin B, graft-versus-host disease, splenomegaly, disseminated intravascular coagulation, and even a recent allogeneic bone marrow transplantation. No one factor predominates in the majority of studies, suggesting that the crucial factors vary with the patient populations being studied. Often, none of these factors are present, but the response still is suboptimal. Other factors, as yet undefined, likely also are at work.

The initial CCI can be measured in 10 minutes[76] to a few hours after transfusion. The time until the platelet concentration returns to baseline (time to next transfusion) also varies with the immune and nonimmune factors affecting the initial CCI.[77] Initial CCI also varies directly with the height of the platelet count achieved by the transfusion and, therefore, the dose of platelets administered.[78–80] This finding follows from the fact that platelet survival is reduced in all patients with thrombocytopenia, regardless of the cause, with progressive reduction as the platelet concentration in the blood decreases[81] (see Chap. 110). Therefore, all other factors being equal, the larger the dose, the higher the platelet count achieved by transfusion and the longer the time to the next transfusion (Figure 132-6).

PLATELET DOSE

If the average patient has an increase in platelet concentration of 10,000/μl per square meter per whole-blood–derived unit of platelets, the relationship between the dose administered and the platelet count achieved can be calculated. Furthermore, using calculations and data from references 78 to 80, the time to the next transfusion can be estimated. Table 132-1 gives these values for the transfusion of a myelosuppressed patient having a BSA of 2 m² and platelet count of 5000/μl. The results indicate that no standard dose fits all patients, regardless of size and clinical situation. For the doses given, the platelet concentrations achieved in a patient with BSA of 1 m² would be twice the values given in the table. In the patient with BSA of 2 m², 4 U (3.2×10^{11}) probably would be satisfactory if the patient is not bleeding, is being transfused prophylactically, and is hospitalized so that he/she can be transfused again 24 to 48 hours later, because raising the platelet concentration to 20,000 to 30,000/μl protects most thrombocytopenic

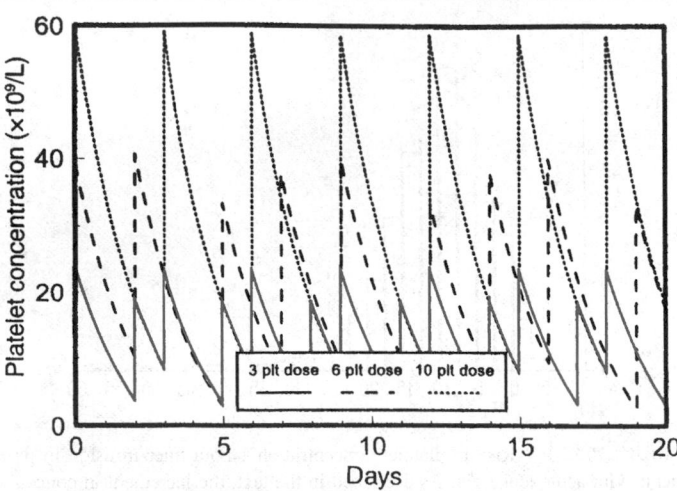

FIGURE 132-6 Response to varying doses of units of whole-blood–derived platelet concentrates during repetitive transfusion of patients who are thrombocytopenic because of marrow failure. Larger doses produce an initially higher increase in platelet concentration and a longer time to next transfusion. Fewer transfusion episodes are required over a 20-day transfusion period. (Redrawn with permission from calculations in JK Hersh, EG Hom, ME Brecher,[78] and validated by empirical data in F Norol, P Bierling, F Roudot-Thoraval, et al.[79] and TR Klumpp, JH Herman, JP Gaughan, et al.[80])

patients against spontaneous, catastrophic bleeding. However, 10 U (8.0×10^{11}) would be a better choice if the goal was to achieve a platelet concentration greater than 50,000/μl because the patient was bleeding or was being prepared for an invasive procedure.[82] Achieving this level of platelet concentration probably is most critical if the surgical field is highly vascular, as with inflammation or portal hypertension; if coexisting defects in plasma coagulation are present; if the procedure is "blind," as in needle biopsy of the liver; or when no opportunity to achieve hemostasis mechanically exists. If surgery is necessary in an area where even a small hemorrhage would be disastrous, as in the central nervous system, even higher doses may be required to increase the platelet concentration to greater than 100,000/μl.[83] A higher dose also might be chosen to facilitate transfusion in the outpatient setting where a longer transfusion interval would be preferable.

Patients vary dramatically in their responses. Therefore, the measurement of increments 1 and 24 hours after transfusion is a cost-effective way to modify the dose and frequency of transfusion based on the pathophysiology of the individual patient.

Prophylactic use of platelets currently is the largest single indication for platelet use.[84] Despite the lack of trials addressing clinical outcomes of varying platelet doses in this setting, a reinterpretation of seemingly conflicting data (from references 78–80) has suggested that optimal strategies vary according to the type of platelet product infused.[84] Although minimization of donor exposure and cost is predicted to result from use of higher-dose apheresis platelets, these benefits may be realized only with lower-dose whole-blood–derived platelet support. Until trials designed to directly measure clinical outcomes and overall platelet use are conducted, controversy over the "optimal" dosing strategy will continue.

PLATELET TRANSFUSION TRIGGER

A thrombocytopenic patient who is actively bleeding requires platelet transfusion. Making this judgment is more difficult if the platelet count simply is very low and the patient has no or only minor hemorrhagic

signs, such as petechiae or small ecchymoses of the skin. Clinical experience suggests that if the platelet count is low enough for long enough, "spontaneous" major hemorrhage, particularly into the central nervous system, may occur. Unfortunately, how low and for how long are not known for an individual patient. A laboratory test that could supplement the measurement of platelet concentration in predicting bleeding would be helpful.[85]

Studies of patients with acute leukemia performed prior to the availability of platelet transfusion described the relationship between platelet concentration in the blood and clinical hemorrhage.[86] Minor and major hemorrhage began (i.e., >1% chance per day) when the platelet count fell below 50,000 and 20,000/μl, respectively. Major hemorrhage was observed in the range from 5000 to 20,000/μl but on only 3 percent of patient-days. The rate of major bleeding increased rapidly when the platelet concentration fell below 5000/μl and reaching a frequency of 33 percent of patient-days as the platelet concentration approached 0/μl. However, many of these children undoubtedly were receiving aspirin for pain and fever. Therefore, these bleeding rates may be overestimates.

Subsequently, the same group described the effect of prophylactic platelet transfusion administered whenever the platelet count fell below 20,000/μl.[87] Although major hemorrhage was strikingly reduced when the platelet count (measured pretransfusion) was below 5000/μl, no substantial change was noted when the platelet count ranged from 5000 to 20,000/μl. Nonetheless, for many years, this experience was used to justify prophylactic platelet transfusion whenever the platelet concentration fell below 20,000/μl, although the data actually suggested 5000/μl was an appropriate trigger.

Prospective but uncontrolled studies by one group supported the safety and efficacy of a more restrictive policy using 5,000/μl as the platelet transfusion trigger.[88,89] Subsequently, three prospective studies assigned patients to one of two groups receiving prophylactic platelet transfusion at either 10,000/μl or 20,000/μl.[90–92] Uniformly, no increase in bleeding risk was observed at the lower transfusion trigger, which now is being adopted by most transfusion services.[93]

However, choosing a rigid transfusion trigger is just as unjustified as choosing a rigid transfusion dose. Clinical factors commonly are assumed to increase the risk of hemorrhage at any given platelet concentration. These factors include fever and sepsis, administration of drugs that interfere with platelet function, coexistent abnormalities of plasma coagulation factors, disseminated intravascular coagulation, and high leukocyte concentrations in the blood. Thus, raising the transfusion trigger in complicated, clinically ill patients is appropriate.

Moderate to severe bleeding is observed in 11 to 23 percent of patients after marrow transplantation despite aggressive use of prophylactic platelet transfusion and maintenance of morning platelet

TABLE 132-1 RELATIONSHIP BETWEEN PLATELET DOSE AND CLINICAL RESPONSE IN A PATIENT WITH 2 M² BODY SURFACE AREA AND PLATELET COUNT OF 5000/μL PRIOR TO TRANSFUSION

DOSE		PLATELET CONCENTRATION ACHIEVED	TRANSFUSION INTERVAL
$\times 10^{11}$	UNITS*	(PER μL)	(DAYS)†
3.2	4	25,000	1.8
4.8	6	35,000	2.3
6.4	8	45,000	2.8
8.0	10	55,000	3.5

* Whole-blood–derived platelet concentrates.
† Time to return to 5000/μl.

counts above 20,000/μl.[94,95] Gastrointestinal and urinary bleeding are most common; pulmonary and intracranial bleeding are less common. Usually, an anatomic cause, such as gastrointestinal ulceration, hemorrhagic cystitis, or diffuse alveolar hemorrhage, can be identified. In effect, common practice in the myelosuppressed patient is to treat bleeding, not prevent it. In such cases, many centers increase the transfusion trigger to 30,000 to 50,000/μl.[94]

THROMBOCYTOPENIA RESULTING FROM PLATELET LOSS, SEQUESTRATION, OR DESTRUCTION

MASSIVE TRANSFUSION

Dilutional thrombocytopenia occurs when massive blood loss is replaced with units of stored red cells that lack viable platelets. Following replacement of one blood volume, 35 to 40 percent of the platelets usually remain. Even when one to two blood volumes are replaced, the platelet count likely is not less than 50,000/μl, abnormal bleeding usually does not develop, and routine transfusion is not indicated simply because the platelet count is low.[96,97] Platelets should be given to patients who demonstrate abnormal bleeding.

CARDIOPULMONARY BYPASS

Immediately following and for several days after cardiac surgery, the platelet count commonly falls to subnormal levels, occasionally as low as 50,000/μl. An associated defect in platelet function is observed. Prospective studies have shown no benefit of prophylactic administration of platelet transfusions to such patients.[98] Transfusions should be reserved for the relatively rare patient who demonstrates clinically abnormal microvascular bleeding.

SPLENOMEGALY

Patients with massive splenomegaly have thrombocytopenia related predominantly to excessive sequestration in a splenic pool in continuous exchange with platelets in the circulation (see Chap. 110). In patients with splenomegaly resulting from hepatic cirrhosis and organ failure, thrombopoietin deficiency also is causative. The platelet count rarely falls below 30,000/μl as a result of splenomegaly alone, so platelet transfusion is rarely considered except in anticipation of invasive procedures such as surgery and needle biopsy of the liver. Under these circumstances, depending upon the degree of splenic enlargement, administration of 10 to 15 U of whole-blood–derived platelet concentrates per square meter BSA may be necessary to achieve a substantial increase in platelet count. In many patients with severe splenomegaly, achieving platelet count elevations may not be possible even with large numbers of platelet concentrates. If such patients require elective surgery, consideration should be given to splenectomy prior to the elective procedure.

IMMUNE (IDIOPATHIC) THROMBOCYTOPENIC PURPURA

In immune (idiopathic) thrombocytopenic purpura, platelet transfusion generally is not used because the bleeding tendency is less severe than in thrombocytopenia resulting from diminished production, and the response to medical therapy generally is satisfactory and rapid (see Chap. 110). Furthermore, the survival of transfused platelets is relatively brief, similar to that of the patient's own platelets. Nonetheless, when critical bleeding occurs or urgent surgery is needed, 3 to 6 U of whole-blood–derived platelet concentrates per square meter BSA generally raise the platelet count for 12 to 48 hours.[99] The same general principles apply to other diseases in which accelerated destruction of platelets occurs, such as disseminated intravascular coagulation.

NEONATAL ALLOIMMUNE THROMBOCYTOPENIA

In this syndrome, the mother produces an alloantibody against antigens on fetal platelets that have crossed the placenta (see Chap. 110). The antibody, in turn, crosses the placenta, causing fetal thrombocytopenia that may persist for weeks after delivery. Because maternal platelets are compatible, platelets harvested from the mother's blood by apheresis can produce an adequate increase in the infant's platelet count after infusion.[100] Ideally, such platelets should be concentrated in a small volume of plasma or washed so that additional antibody is not infused.

Unfortunately, arranging for apheresis of the mother often is difficult. Surprisingly, a randomly selected unit of platelets may raise the neonate's platelet concentration substantially.[101] If it does not, prompt serologic evaluation of the mother and father can identify the antigen to which the antibody has been formed, usually HPA-1a (Pl[A1]). Donors lacking HPA-1a (i.e., homozygous HPA-1b) then can be recruited to support the infant.[102]

HEREDITARY THROMBOCYTOPENIA

These syndromes are rare and generally are not associated with severe bleeding.[103] Because the survival of allogeneic platelets is normal, platelet transfusion is effective and can be used for critical bleeding and surgery. However, like all cases in which repeated platelet transfusions are required, the risk for alloimmunization is high and should be considered when generating a long-term care plan.

QUALITATIVE PLATELET DISORDERS

Despite normal platelet counts, patients with qualitative platelet disorders have a clinical bleeding tendency associated with abnormal *in vitro* tests of platelet function and a prolonged bleeding time *in vivo*. The basis may be hereditary (see Chap. 112) or acquired (see Chap. 113). Platelet transfusion is generally not indicated when the cause is extrinsic to the platelet, as in uremia, von Willebrand disease, and hyperglobulinemia, because the transfused platelets will function no better than the patient's own platelets. Exceptions are certain types of von Willebrand disease in which normal platelets can be used to deliver von Willebrand factor to a bleeding site (see Chap. 118). Most inherited intrinsic disorders are mild and do not require platelet transfusions even for surgery if the procedure is carried out under direct vision, so hemostasis may be achieved mechanically. If the bleeding tendency is more severe, as in Glanzmann thrombasthenia or Bernard-Soulier syndrome, platelet transfusions may be necessary for bleeding. Isoimmunization to missing glycoprotein determinants may occur and result in platelet refractoriness, so every effort should be made to avoid prophylactic transfusion, if possible. The acquired defects, as in the myeloproliferative and myelodysplastic syndromes, generally do not require platelet transfusion except in cases of coexistent thrombocytopenia.

POSSIBLE CONTRAINDICATIONS TO PLATELET TRANSFUSION

Concern has been voiced that platelet transfusions should not be administered to patients with forms of thrombocytopenia associated with thrombosis, such as thrombotic thrombocytopenic purpura (TTP) or heparin-induced thrombocytopenia (see Chap. 110), because infusion of platelets might worsen the thrombotic tendency.[104,105] Unfortunately, particularly in TTP, platelet transfusion is often requested prior to invasive procedures such as insertion of intravenous catheters for therapy with apheresis. In our experience, platelet transfusions are generally tolerated in this setting. However, a prudent action is to not administer prophylactic platelet transfusions simply because the platelet concentration is low in these diseases.

COMPLICATIONS OF PLATELET TRANSFUSION

Platelet transfusions are associated with many complications (Table 132-2). Paradoxically, most complications are not caused by the platelets themselves but rather the contaminating leukocytes, red cells, plasma proteins, and microorganisms.

COMPLICATIONS RESULTING FROM CONTAMINATING LEUKOCYTES

ALLOIMMUNIZATION TO CLASS I HUMAN LEUKOCYTE ANTIGENS

HLAs are expressed on integral membrane glycoproteins. Almost all cells have class I antigens (A, B, C subloci), whereas only a few types of circulating leukocytes (dendritic cells, monocytes, subsets of B cells) have class II antigens. Primary alloimmunization to class I HLAs appears to require presentation of such antigens on cells that also express class II antigens and other costimulatory molecules.[106] Abundant evidence now indicates the incidence of HLA alloimmunization can be reduced by consistent use of leukoreduced blood products.[107–109] Transfused red cells also must be leukoreduced because leukocytes contained in the transfused red cells are capable of inducing HLA alloimmunization.[110]

How completely leukoreduction can eliminate alloimmunization remains to be determined. In one study, leukoreduction had almost no effect on the development of alloimmunization in patients who had been previously exposed to foreign leukocytes through either pregnancy or prior nonleukoreduced transfusions.[111] Later trials have shown efficacy in preventing so-called secondary, as well as primary, alloimmunization.[107,109] These trials also demonstrated lower rates of platelet refractoriness and matched platelet use in the two groups of transfusion recipients.

Alloimmunization to HLA should be suspected clinically if two or three consecutive transfusions produce a 1-hour CCI less than 3,000/μl per square meter per 10^{11} platelets transfused.[112] It can be confirmed

TABLE 132-2   COMPLICATIONS OF PLATELET TRANSFUSION

Resulting from contaminating leukocytes
  Alloimmunization to class I HLA antigens
    Refractoriness to platelet transfusion
    Febrile nonhemolytic transfusion reactions (FNHTR)
  Cytokine formation
    FNHTR
  Transmission of cytomegalovirus
  Graft-versus-host disease
Resulting from contaminating red cells
  Rh alloimmunization
  Parasites: malaria, babesiosis
Resulting from plasma and its contents
  Contaminating microorganisms
    Bacteria
    Viruses: HBV, HCV, HIV, HTLV
    Parasites: Chagas disease
  Plasma proteins
    Minor and major allergic reactions
    ABO antibody-mediated hemolysis
    Transfusion-related acute lung injury
Resulting from platelets themselves
  FNHTR
  Refractoriness to platelet transfusion
  Posttransfusion purpura

in the laboratory by performing one of several tests for HLA antibody in the patient's serum. The traditional assay—the lymphocytotoxicity (LCT) test—incubates leukocytes from 50 to 100 widely HLA-heterogeneous donors with the patient's serum and complement. Antibody specificity is derived from computer-assisted interpretation of which of several cellular antigens was responsible for antibody-mediated cell lysis. Flow cytometry-based assays and enzyme-linked immunosorbent assay (ELISA) panels also are available.[113,114] Multiantigen ELISA assays are increasingly used as screening studies before more expensive panel-based testing is performed. The presence of HLA antibody has been a good predictor of poor response to platelets from randomly selected donors[115] and improved response when platelets are matched for HLA type.[116] In the future, it may be more economical to periodically screen highly transfused individuals for HLA antibody so that HLA alloimmunization is detected prior to the development of refractoriness rather than vice versa. Many centers consider issuing matched platelets inappropriate unless an antibody screen has been performed because of the belief that matching provides little benefit if antibody is not present.[117,118]

The incidence and severity of HLA alloimmunization should gradually decrease as the use of leukoreduced blood products becomes increasingly popular. The following discussion is based upon data accumulated before the widespread use of leukoreduction. Approximately 10 percent of patients presenting for therapy for diseases requiring platelet transfusion already have LCT antibodies from prior transfusions and pregnancies.[119] Another 30 percent become alloimmunized during therapy, and 60 percent never become alloimmunized.[119] No difference is known between patients who do and those who do not become alloimmunized. Among patients who become alloimmunized, some do so after only two to four transfusions, whereas others require dozens of transfusions.[120] The pattern and intensity of immunization vary greatly among patients. HLA antibody panels can be characterized by the percentage of HLAs or panel cells against which the patient's serum reacts, that is, the percent reactive antibody (PRA). Patients may have PRA values between 1 and 100 percent (Figure 132-7). Furthermore, the specificity of identified antibodies can be determined accurately with newer techniques. The precise identification of HLA allotypes to which recipients are immunized lends itself to the provision of so-called "antigen-negative" platelet transfusions, discussed further below and in Chapter 129. Although HLA-C antigens are expressed on the platelet surface, they are present in sufficiently low density that they play an insignificant role in platelet refractoriness.[121] Although HLA-A and HLA-B sublocus mismatch primarily mediates platelet refractoriness, cases of HLA-C–mediated refractoriness have been reported.[122]

The majority of patients who become alloimmunized establish a level and specificity of immunization and tend to maintain that status as they continue receiving transfusions. However, approximately 30 percent lose their antibodies over time despite continuing transfusion.[123] Thus, monitoring antibody PRA and specificity is helpful, because such patients may regain some measure of responsiveness having been previously refractory.

Cross-reactive groups (CREGs) of HLAs have been defined by serologic testing. Cross-reactivity among antigens in a CREG is based upon the sharing of one or more public epitopes by those antigens.[124] Patients commonly develop antibodies to one or more public epitopes in a CREG but less frequently develop antibodies to private epitopes (those unique to a particular HLA allele).[125] Some patients even develop intra-CREG antibodies, that is, antibodies to antigens in the same CREG as their own antigens.[126] This unpredictability complicates attempts to provide HLA-selected products armed only with the patient's HLA type (i.e., without knowledge of precise antibody specificity available through ELISA, LCT, or flow cytometry panels).

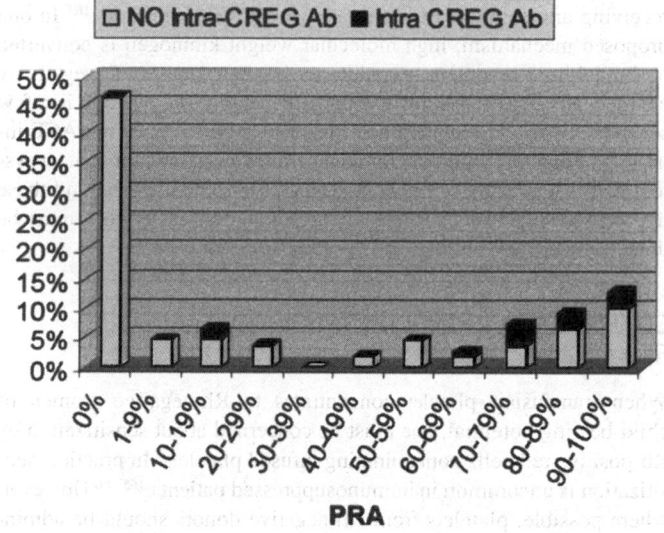

FIGURE 132-7 Percent reactive antibody (PRA) distribution by lymphocytotoxicity assay in serum samples from 108 thrombocytopenic patients referred to a regional blood center for matched platelet support during a 6-month period. Fifty patients showed no reactivity, whereas 58 patients showed PRAs that varied from 4 to 100 percent. The *shaded portions* of the bars indicate patients who had demonstrable antibody against antigens within their own cross-reactive groups, that is, intra–cross-reactive group antibody (CREG Ab). Data provided by Dr. Susan Hsu, American Red Cross Blood Services, Penn-Jersey Region. (Redrawn from S Murphy,[182] with permission.)

MANAGEMENT OF REFRACTORY PATIENTS

In 1969, studies showed that refractory patients responded to platelets from siblings who were identical for all four class I HLA-A and HLA-B antigens.[127] This simple clinical observation remains one of the most compelling pieces of evidence supporting the role of HLA alloimmunization in platelet refractoriness. Similarly, patients could be supported by platelets from unrelated donors who were HLA identical or closely matched. Because some patients do not make antibody to antigens within their own CREGs, it became popular to choose donors according to CREG classification, particularly BX matches, that is, donors whose antigens are identical to or within the same CREGs as those of the patient.[128] Table 132-3 lists the categorization of such matches.

Responses were better with such matching than with random donor selection, but many BX matches failed and many C and D matches succeeded. Figure 132-7 suggests potential explanations for the relatively poor predictive capacity of this method. Some patients with relatively low PRAs have antibody to only one or two CREGs, so success with some C and D matches would be expected. On the other hand, failure of some BX matches would be expected in patients with intra-CREG antibody. Furthermore, this method generally does not quickly provide a good match. Finding an excellent match in a blood center's inventory is uncommon, and days are required to recruit and apherese one or more well-matched donors from an HLA-typed donor file.

In the late 1980s and early 1990s, practical methods for platelet cross-matching became available.[129] Many centers found that they could simply cross-match the patient's serum with unselected apheresis platelet concentrates in inventory to find, within hours, a compatible product that would be successful *in vivo*.[71,130] However, in a highly immunized patient, one might cross-match with dozens of donors and not find a compatible product.[130] For many such patients, only the identification of an A or BU match (Table 132-3) suffices.

One other approach to these patients has been proposed.[131,132] If the PRA in an HLA antibody panel is less than 100 percent, one should be able to identify the HLAs to which the patient has not formed antibody. The patient then can be supported with "antigen-negative" platelets, that is, platelets that lack the antigens to which the patient has formed antibody. If the results of an HLA antibody panel are known, one often can provide a product from inventory on an urgent basis using this approach.

No reason exists for choosing one of these approaches to the exclusion of the other two.[133] If the PRA is reasonably low (<60%), successful support usually can be provided by cross-matching random products or by "antigen-negative" platelets. When the PRA is relatively high (>80%), one can select for cross-matching the best available "antigen-negative" HLA matches and/or selectively recruit A and BU matches from an HLA-typed donor file. Some patients with common HLA types, for example, A1,A2/B7,B8, have dozens of A and BU matches available to them. Unfortunately, some patients have rare HLA types and have no A or BU matches to recruit.

ROLE OF ABO AND PLATELET-SPECIFIC ANTIBODIES

ABO determinants are carried by platelet glycoproteins and glycolipids, as they are on red cells.[134] Although ABO identity is not absolutely critical for successful platelet transfusion, transfused platelets incompatible with recipients' plasma antibodies (e.g., O recipient, A donor) predictably result in yields up to one third less than ABO-identical transfusions.[135,136] Even ABO-compatible platelets in donor plasma with incompatible antibodies (e.g., A recipient, O donor) produce lower increments, possibly as a result of circulating immune complexes.[135,137] In addition, transfusion of incompatible plasma (especially O plasma to A recipients) can result in accelerated red cell destruction in the recipient, occasionally leading to acute hemolysis.[138,139] Furthermore, formation of immune complexes between A and B substance and corresponding antibodies has been proposed to have additional deleterious effects.[140] Thus, observing ABO compatibility whenever possible seems wise.

The platelet surface carries many platelet-specific antigens (HPAs; see Chap. 129), which are capable of eliciting a strong alloantibody response. A number of case reports of such alloantibodies accounting for refractoriness to platelet transfusion have been described.[141–145] From 4 to 10 percent of heavily transfused patients in several series developed HPA antibodies, most often coexisting with HLA antibodies.[146–148] Fewer than 2 percent of patients developed HPA antibodies alone. However, faced with clinically refractory patients who do not demonstrate HLA antibody, investigation for HPA antibodies would

TABLE 132-3 CLASSIFICATION OF DONOR/RECIPIENT PAIRS BASED ON HLA CLASS I MATCHING

A	All four antigens in donor identical to those of recipient
B1U	Only three antigens detected in donor (i.e., donor homozygous at one HLA-A or HLA-B sublocus); all present in recipient
B1X	Three donor antigens identical to recipient; fourth antigen cross-reactive* with recipient
B2U	Only two antigens detected in donor; both present in recipient
B2UX	Only three antigens detected in donor; two identical with recipient, third cross-reactive
B2X	Two donor antigens identical to recipient; third and fourth antigens cross-reactive with recipient
C	One antigen of donor not present in recipient and not cross-reactive with recipient
D	Two antigens of donor not present in recipient and not cross-reactive with recipient

* Antigen in a cross-reactive group (CREG) that contains one of the patient's antigens.
SOURCE: Revised from Duquesnoy et al.,[128] with permission.

be prudent. Similarly, the consistent failure of well HLA-matched platelet products mandates investigation for coexisting HPA antibodies. HPA antibody detection methods continue to evolve, but most commonly involve ELISA or monoclonal antibody immobilization of antigen (MAIPA) techniques.[149]

FEBRILE NONHEMOLYTIC TRANSFUSION REACTIONS

Prior to the availability of methods for leukoreduction, approximately 20 percent of platelet transfusions were accompanied by febrile non-hemolytic transfusion reaction (FNHTR).[150] Some of these reactions undoubtedly were caused by antibodies in the patient directed against either leukocyte specific antigens or HLAs on leukocytes contaminating the platelet product. Leukocyte depletion by filtration during infusion reduced the frequency of these reactions, but many continued to occur.[150,151] Contaminating leukocytes now are known to produce inflammatory cytokines, such as interleukin-1, interleukin-6, interleukin-8, and tumor necrosis factor alpha, during storage at 20 to 24°C, and these compounds are responsible for many FNHTRs given that they are not removed by bedside filtration.[152,153] Thus, febrile reactions occur more when platelets are transfused at the end of the storage interval.[154] These reactions provide a strong argument for routine, pre-storage removal of leukocytes.

Nonetheless, FNHTRs occur in approximately 2 percent of platelet transfusions even with prestorage leukoreduction.[155] The cause of these reactions is not known. They may be related to plasma proteins or products produced during storage by the platelets themselves, such as CD154, a potent cyclooxygenase-2 inducer.[156] In these rare cases, the platelets can be washed free of plasma prior to infusion.[157]

TRANSMISSION OF CYTOMEGALOVIRUS

In asymptomatic carriers, the cytomegalovirus (CMV) resides in the nuclei of subsets of leukocytes with little virus free in plasma. Use of leukoreduced blood components was shown to be essentially equivalent to use of components from CMV-negative donors in terms of risk of CMV transmission.[158] A later cohort study challenged this assertion but was unable to demonstrate increased CMV transmission resulting from use of leukoreduced platelet products, and no significant difference in the incidence of CMV disease was observed, possibly because of aggressive antigenic surveillance.[159] Because this infection is particularly dangerous for severely immunocompromised patients, such as those who recently underwent allogeneic bone marrow transplantation, some clinicians continue to use CMV-negative blood products with leukoreduction in this select population.

GRAFT-VERSUS-HOST DISEASE

Immunosuppressed patients may develop graft-versus-host disease (GVHD) from T lymphocytes present in any transfusion, including platelet transfusion. Thus, standard practice is to treat platelet concentrates with γ-irradiation to inhibit proliferation of these T lymphocytes when the recipient has been heavily immunosuppressed.[160] Transfusions from biologic relatives and HLA-matched or crossmatch-compatible platelets should also be irradiated. Exposure to 2500 cGy appears to have no deleterious effect on platelets.[161] Of importance to note is that current methods of leukoreduction do not remove enough T cells to prevent GVHD.

COMPLICATIONS OF FILTRATION OF PLATELET CONCENTRATES

Complications of platelet transfusion related to the removal of leukocytes by filtration of platelet concentrates at the bedside may occur. Severe hypotension has been reported,[162] predominantly when nega-

tively charged leukocyte reduction filters are used in patients who are receiving angiotensin-converting enzyme (ACE) inhibitors.[163] In one proposed mechanism, high molecular weight kininogen is converted to bradykinin, a potent vasodilator, by exposure to a negatively charged surface. Bradykinin normally is metabolized by ACE in a few seconds but may circulate much longer in patients receiving ACE inhibitors. Some investigators found no clinically significant contact system activation by these filters.[164] Thus, the mechanisms behind these hypotensive reactions still are hypothetical, and more work must be done.

COMPLICATIONS RESULTING FROM CONTAMINATING RED CELLS

When transfusing platelet concentrates to Rh-negative women of child-bearing potential, one must be concerned about sensitization by Rh-positive red cells contaminating infused platelets. In practice, sensitization is uncommon in immunosuppressed patients.[165,166] However, where possible, platelets from Rh-negative donors should be administered. When this is not possible, Rh immune globulin, about 20 μg intramuscularly per unit of platelets, can be administered so that the infused red cells will be cleared prior to sensitization. A full dose of 300 μg is sufficient to suppress the immune response to 15 ml of Rh-positive red cells.

Enough red cells contaminate platelet concentrates (0.2–0.7 μl per apheresis unit, 0.3–0.5 ml per whole-blood–derived unit)[166] to transmit both malaria and babesiosis if the donor is parasitemic with these infections.

COMPLICATIONS RESULTING FROM PLASMA AND ITS CONTENTS

CONTAMINATING MICROORGANISMS

Storage of platelet concentrates at 20 to 24°C allows proliferation to dangerous levels of bacteria that occasionally contaminate units of blood or apheresis platelet concentrates.[45] Contamination may occur because of asymptomatic bacteremia in the donor at the time of venipuncture, inadequate decontamination of the skin, or venipuncture through areas of the skin where bacterial colonization is deeper than can be reached by such decontamination.[167] Bacterial contamination that might not be clinically significant after 2 to 3 days of storage may become significant after 5 to 7 days.[168] For this reason, platelet concentrate storage is limited to 5 days.

The magnitude of this problem is commonly underestimated.[169] Estimates suggest contamination of 3 to 10 U per 10,000 whole-blood–derived platelet concentrates and 150 clinical episodes associated with severe morbidity and death in the United States per year.[170] These values equate to one episode of severe morbidity or mortality per 20,000 platelet units transfused, which is 50- to 250-fold higher than the risk of mortality from transmission by transfusion of human immunodeficiency virus (HIV), hepatitis B virus (HBV), or hepatitis C virus (HCV).

Several potential approaches to this important problem can be used. Apheresis, which involves only one donor and one venipuncture, may be associated with less risk than pooled whole-blood–derived platelet concentrates.[171] The AABB, in recognition of the significant risk of platelet bacterial contamination, has instituted standards requiring implementation of methods that limit and detect bacteria in all platelet products.[24] Detection technology is evolving.[172] Methods for viral inactivation that also inactivate bacteria are under investigation.[46] The methods of viral inactivation also may inactivate T lymphocytes and prevent GVHD.[173]

The plasma diluent of platelet concentrates can transmit viruses such as HBV and HBC, human T lymphotrophic virus (HTLV) I/II, and HIV. Improved methods of donor screening and testing have reduced, but not eliminated, this risk. Methods for viral inactivation are being sought.[46] Transmission of the parasite *Trypanosoma cruzi*, which is responsible for Chagas disease, has occurred with platelet transfusion.[174]

PLASMA PROTEINS

Many transfusion services attempt to transfuse ABO-identical platelet concentrates; however, such transfusion is not always possible. When anti-A or anti-B is transfused to a patient whose red cells carry A or B, a positive direct antiglobulin test may be observed in the laboratory, making red cell compatibility testing more difficult.[175] Actual accelerated destruction of the patient's red cells is rare.[176] However, very rare cases of frank acute hemolysis have been observed.[177]

As with any plasma infusion, urticaria or even anaphylactic shock in patients with specific protein deficiencies and circulating antibodies (e.g., anti-IgA, anti-haptoglobin) can occur,[178] and transfusion-associated acute lung injury can be observed when a donor has leukocyte antibodies that can react with antigens on the leukocytes of the recipient.[179]

COMPLICATIONS RESULTING FROM PLATELETS THEMSELVES

In addition to the potential role of platelets in cytokine-mediated FNHTRs, alloimmunization to HPAs can result in recipient adverse reactions. As discussed above in "Role of ABO and Platelet-Specific Antibodies," platelet refractoriness may uncommonly result from HPA antibody formation. Posttransfusion purpura, another uncommon reaction, results in severe acute thrombocytopenia in individuals previously sensitized to HPAs. It usually occurs an average of 9 days following transfusion of platelet antigen-containing blood products, usually red cells.[180] Through an as-yet unknown mechanism, recipients' antigen-negative platelets are destroyed in the anamnestic alloimmune response, most often to HPA-1 system antigens. Following acute therapy with IV immunoglobulin, patients may preferentially respond to HPA-matched platelet products.[181] Efforts to prevent recurrence include prophylactic use of antigen-negative blood products or frozen-deglycerolized red cells (washed free of cellular antigens).

REFERENCES

1. Surgenor DM, Wallace EL, Hao SHS, et al: Collection and transfusion of blood in the United States, 1982–1988. *N Engl J Med* 322:1646, 1990.
2. Wallace EL, Surgenor DM, Hao HS, et al: Collection and transfusion of blood and blood components in the United States, 1989. *Transfusion* 33:139, 1993.
3. Wallace EL, Churchill WH, Surgenor DM, et al: Collection and transfusion of blood and blood components in the United States, 1992. *Transfusion* 35:802, 1995.
4. Wallace EL, Churchill WH, Surgenor DM, et al: Collection and transfusion of blood and blood components in the United States, 1994. *Transfusion* 38:625, 1998.
5. Sullivan MT, McCullough J, Schreiber GB, Wallace EL: Blood collection and transfusion in the United States in 1997. *Transfusion* 42:1253, 2002.
6. Moroff G, Kline L, Dabay M, et al: Reevaluation of the resting time utilized to prepare whole blood-derived platelet concentrates. *Transfusion* 42(9S):55S, 2002.
7. Kelley DL, Fegan RL, Ng AT, et al: High-yield platelet concentrates attainable by continuous quality improvement reduce platelet transfusion cost and donor exposure. *Transfusion* 37:482, 1997.
8. Hoeltge GA, Shah A, Miller JP: An optimized strategy for choosing the number of platelet concentrates to pool. *Arch Pathol Lab Med* 123:928, 1999.
9. Sweeney JD, Holme S, Heaton WA, et al: White cell-reduced platelet concentrates prepared by in-line filtration of platelet-rich plasma. *Transfusion* 35:131, 1995.
10. Murphy S: Platelets from pooled buffy coats: an update. *Transfusion* 45:634, 2005.
11. Pietersz RN, Loos JA, Reesink HW: Platelet concentrates stored in plasma for 72 hours at 22°C prepared from buffy coats of citrate-phosphate-dextrose blood collected in a quadruple-bag saline-adenine-glucose-mannitol system. *Vox Sang* 49:81, 1985.
12. Bertolini F, Rebulla P, Riccardi D: Evaluation of platelet concentrates prepared from buffy coats and stored in a glucose-free crystalloid medium. *Transfusion* 29:605, 1989.
13. Bertolini F, Rebulla P, Marangoni F, et al: Platelet concentrates stored in synthetic medium after filtration. *Vox Sang* 62:82, 1992.
14. Heaton WAL, Rebulla P, Pappalettera M, Dzik WH: A comparative analysis of different methods for routine blood component preparation. *Transfusion* 11:116, 1997.
15. Van Delden CJ, de Wit HJC, Smit Sibinga CTH: Comparison of blood component preparation systems based on buffy coat removal: Component specifications, efficiency, and process costs. *Transfusion* 38:860, 1998.
16. Adams MR, Dumont LJ, McCall M, Heaton WA: Clinical trial and local process evaluation of an apheresis system for preparation of white cell-reduced platelet components. *Transfusion* 38:966, 1998.
17. Yockey C, Murphy S, Eggers L, et al: Evaluation of the Amicus separator in the collection of apheresis platelets. *Transfusion* 38:848, 1998.
18. Holme S, Andres M, Goermar N, Giordano GF: Improved removal of white cells with minimal platelet loss by filtration of apheresis platelets during collection. *Transfusion* 39:74, 1999.
19. Moog R, Valbonesi M, Carlier P: Collection of platelets and peripheral progenitor cells with Fresenius ASTEC 204 blood cell separator. *J Clin Apheresis* 12:126, 1997.
20. McLeod BC, Price TH, Owen H, et al: Frequency of immediate adverse effects associated with apheresis donation. *Transfusion* 38:938, 1998.
21. Goodnough LT, Ali S, Despotis G, et al: Economic impact of donor platelet count and platelet yield in apheresis products: Relevance for emerging issues in platelet transfusion therapy. *Vox Sang* 76:43, 1999.
22. Li J, Yang C, Xia Y, et al: Thrombocytopenia caused by the development of antibodies to thrombopoietin. *Blood* 98:3241, 2001.
23. Rock G, Moltzan C, Alharbi A, et al: Automated collection of blood components: Their storage and transfusion. *Transfus Med* 13:219, 2003.
24. American Association of Blood Banks: *Standards for Blood Banks and Transfusion Services*, 23rd edition. AABB Press, Bethesda, 2004.
25. Lopez-Plaza I, Weissfeld J, Triulzi DJ: The cost-effectiveness of reducing donor exposures with single-donor versus pooled random-donor platelets. *Transfusion* 39:925, 1999.
26. Dodd RY, Shoos-Lipton K: Further guidance on methods to detect bacterial contamination of platelet components. AABB Association Bulletin 03-12,2003.
27. Canadian Coordinating Office for Health Technology Assessment: Leukoreduction: The techniques used, their effectiveness and costs. Canadian Coordinating Office for Health Technology Assessment (CCOHTA), Ottawa, 1998.
28. Popovsky MA: Quality of blood components filtered before storage and at the bedside: Implications for transfusion practice. *Transfusion* 36:470, 1996.

29. Williamson LM, Wimperis JZ, Williamson P, et al: Bedside filtration of blood products in the prevention of HLA alloimmunization—A prospective randomized study. *Blood* 83:3028, 1994.

30. Murphy S, Gardner FH: Platelet preservation. Effect of storage temperature on maintenance of platelet viability—deleterious effect of refrigerated storage. *N Engl J Med* 280:1094, 1969.

31. Murphy S: Platelet storage for transfusion. *Semin Hematol* 22:165, 1985.

32. Murphy S, Gardner FH: Platelet storage at 22°C: Role of gas transport across plastic containers in maintenance of viability. *Blood* 46:209, 1975.

33. Hunter S, Nixon J, Murphy S: The effect of the interruption of agitation on platelet quality during storage for transfusion. *Transfusion* 41:809, 2001.

34. Anonymous: Amotosalen: Allogeneic cellular immunotherapies system, INTERCEPT plasma system, INTERCEPT platelet system, S59. *BioDrugs* 17:66, 2003.

35. Murphy S: The oxidation of exogenously added organic anions by platelets facilitates maintenance of pH during their storage for transfusion at 22°C. *Blood* 85:1929, 1995.

36. Murphy S, Shimizu T, Miripol J: Platelet storage for transfusion in synthetic media: Further optimization of ingredients and definition of their roles. *Blood* 86:3951, 1995.

37. Shanwell A, Larsson S, Aschan J, et al: A randomized trial comparing the use of fresh and stored platelets in the treatment of bone marrow transplant recipients. *Eur J Haematol* 49:77, 1992.

38. Leach MR, AuBuchon JP: Effect of storage time on clinical efficacy of single-donor platelet units. *Transfusion* 33:661, 1993.

39. Murphy S, Kahn RA, Holme S, et al: Improved storage of platelets for transfusion in a new container. *Blood* 60:194, 1982.

40. Peter-Salonen K, Bucher UE, Nydegger UE: Comparison of post-transfusion recoveries achieved with either fresh or stored platelet concentrates. *Blut* 54:207, 1987.

41. Norol F, Kuentz M, Cordonnier C, et al: Influence of clinical status on the efficiency of stored platelet transfusion. *Br J Haematol* 86:125, 1994.

42. Hogge DE, Thompson BW, Schiffer CA: Platelet storage for 7 days in second-generation blood bags. *Transfusion* 26:131, 1986.

43. Rock G, Neurath D, Cober N, et al: Seven-day storage of random donor concentrates PLT. *Transfusion* 43:1374, 2003.

44. Dumont LJ, AuBuchon JP, Whitley P, et al: Seven-day storage of single-donor platelets: Recovery and survival in an autologous transfusion study. *Transfusion* 42:847, 2002.

45. Klein HG, Dodd RY, Ness PM, et al: Current status of microbial contamination of blood components: Summary of a conference. *Transfusion* 37:95, 1997.

46. Lin L, Cook DN, Wiesehahn GP, et al: Photochemical inactivation of viruses and bacteria in platelet concentrates by use of a novel psoralen and long-wavelength ultraviolet light. *Transfusion* 37:423, 1997.

47. Mitchell KM, Brecher ME: Approaches to the detection of bacterial contamination in cellular blood products. *Transfus Med Rev* 13:132, 1999.

48. Blajchman MA, Goldman M, Baeza F: Improving the bacteriological safety of platelet transfusions. *Transfus Med Rev* 18:11, 2004.

49. Murphy S, Rebulla P, Bertolini F, et al: In vitro assessment of the quality of stored platelet concentrates. *Transfus Med Rev* 8:29, 1994.

50. Seghatchian J, Krailadsiri P: The platelet storage lesion. *Transfus Med Rev* 11:130, 1997.

51. Holme S, Moroff G, Murphy S: A multi-laboratory evaluation of in vitro platelet assays: The tests for extent of shape change and response to hypotonic shock. *Transfusion* 38:31, 1998.

52. Bertolini F, Murphy S: A multicenter evaluation of reproducibility of swirling in platelet concentrates. *Transfusion* 34:796, 1994.

53. Murphy S, Martinez J, Holburn R: Stability of plasma fibrinogen during storage of platelet concentrates at 22°C. *Transfusion* 23:480, 1983.

54. Murphy S, Sayar SN, Abdou NL, et al: Platelet preservation by freezing. Use of dimethylsulfoxide as cryoprotective agent. *Transfusion* 14:139, 1975.

55. Towell BL, Levine SP, Knight WA III, et al: A comparison of frozen and fresh platelet concentrates in the support of thrombocytopenic patients. *Transfusion* 26:525, 1986.

56. Lazarus HM, Kaniecki-Green EA, Warm SE, et al: Therapeutic effectiveness of frozen platelet concentrates for transfusion. *Blood* 57:243, 1981.

57. Schiffer CA, Aisner J, Wiernik PH: Frozen autologous platelet transfusion for patients with leukemia. *N Engl J Med* 299:7, 1978.

58. Currie LM, Livesey SA, Harper JR, Connor J: Cryopreservation of single-donor platelets with a reduced dimethyl sulfoxide concentration by the addition of second-messenger effectors: Enhanced retention of in vitro functional activity. *Transfusion* 38:160, 1998.

59. Currie LM, Lichtiger B, Livesey SA, et al: Enhanced circulatory parameters of human platelets cryopreserved with second-messenger effectors: An in vivo study of 16 volunteer platelet donors. *Br J Haematol* 105:826, 1999.

60. Vadhan-Raj S, Kavanagh JJ, Freedman RS, et al: Safety and efficacy of transfusions of autologous cryopreserved platelets derived from recombinant human thrombopoietin to support chemotherapy-associated severe thrombocytopenia: A randomized cross-over study. *Lancet* 359:2145, 2002.

61. Hillyer CD, Josephson CD, Blajchman MA, et al: Bacterial contamination of blood components: Risks, strategies, and regulation: Joint ASH and AABB educational session in transfusion medicine. *Hematology (Am Soc Hematol Educ Program)* 2003:575, 2003.

62. Holme S, Heaton A: In vitro platelet ageing at 22°C is reduced compared to in vivo ageing at 37°C. *Br J Haematol* 91:212, 1995.

63. Hoffmeister KM, Felbinger TW, Falet H, et al: The clearance mechanism of chilled blood platelets. *Cell* 112:1, 2003.

64. Hoffmeister KM, Josefsson EC, Isaac NA, et al: Glycosylation restores survival of chilled blood platelets. *Science* 301:1531, 2003.

65. Blajchman MA: Substitutes and alternatives to platelet transfusions in thrombocytopenic patients. *J Thromb Haemost* 1:1637, 2003.

66. Mannucci PM: Hemostatic drugs. *N Engl J Med* 339:245, 1998.

67. Goodnough LT: Experiences with recombinant human factor VIIa in patients with thrombocytopenia. *Semin Hematol* 41(suppl 1):25, 2004.

68. Manno CS, Hedbert KW, Kim HC, et al: Comparison of the hemostatic effects of fresh whole blood, stored whole blood, and components after open heart surgery in children. *Blood* 77:930, 1991.

69. Bishop JF, McGrath K, Wolf MM, et al: Clinical factors influencing the efficacy of pooled platelet transfusions. *Blood* 71:383, 1988.

70. Davis KB, Slichter SJ, Corash L: Corrected count increment and percent platelet recovery as measures of posttransfusion platelet response: Problems and a solution. *Transfusion* 39:586, 1999.

71. Friedberg RC, Donnelly SF, Boyd JC, et al: Clinical and blood bank factors in the management of platelet refractoriness and alloimmunization. *Blood* 81:3428, 1993.

72. Klumpp TR, Herman J, Innis S, et al: Factors associated with response to platelet transfusion following hematopoietic stem cell transplantation. *Bone Marrow Transplant* 17:1035, 1996.

73. Doughty HA, Murphy MF, Metcalfe P, et al: Relative importance of immune and non-immune causes of platelet refractoriness. *Vox Sang* 66:200, 1994.

74. Alcorta I, Pereira A, Ordinas A: Clinical and laboratory factors associated with platelet transfusion refractoriness: A case-control study. *Br J Haematol* 93:220, 1996.

75. Bock M, Muggenthaler KH, Schmidt U, et al: Influence of antibiotics on posttransfusion platelet increment. *Transfusion* 36:952, 1996.

76. O'Connell B, Lee EJ, Schiffer CA: The value of 10-minute posttransfusion platelet counts. *Transfusion* 28:66, 1988.

77. Bishop JF, Matthews JP, McGrath K, et al: Factors influencing 20-hour increments after platelet transfusion. *Transfusion* 31:392, 1991.

78. Hersh JK, Hom EG, Brecher ME: Mathematical modeling of platelet survival with implications of optimal transfusion practice in the chronically platelet transfusion-dependent patient. *Transfusion* 38:637, 1998.

79. Norol F, Bierling P, Roudot-Thoraval F, et al: Platelet transfusion: A dose-response study. *Blood* 92:1448, 1998.

80. Klumpp TR, Herman JH, Gaughan JP, et al: Clinical consequences of alterations in platelet transfusion dose: A prospective, randomized, double-blind trial. *Transfusion* 39:674, 1999.

81. Hanson SR, Slichter SJ: Platelet kinetics in patients with bone marrow hypoplasia: Evidence for a fixed platelet requirement. *Blood* 66:1105, 1985.

82. McVay PA, Toy PT: Lack of increased bleeding after liver biopsy in patients with mild hemostatic abnormalities. *Am J Clin Pathol* 94:747, 1990.

83. Anonymous: Practice parameter for use of fresh-frozen plasma, cryoprecipitate, and platelets. *JAMA* 271:777, 1994.

84. Tinmouth AT, Freedman J: Prophylactic platelet transfusions: Which dose is the best dose? A review of the literature. *Transfus Med Rev* 17:181, 2003.

85. Kenet G, Lubetsky A, Shenkman B, et al: Cone and platelet analyser (CPA): A new test for the prediction of bleeding among thrombocytopenic patients. *Br J Haematol* 101:255, 1998.

86. Gaydos LA, Freireich EJ, Mantel N: The quantitative relation between platelet count and hemorrhage in patients with acute leukemia. *N Engl J Med* 266:905, 1962.

87. Freireich EJ, Kliman A, Lawrence AG, et al: Response to repeated platelet transfusion from the same donor. *Ann Intern Med* 59:277, 1963.

88. Gmur J, Burger J, Schanz U, et al: Safety of stringent prophylactic platelet transfusion policy for patients with acute leukemia. *Lancet* 338:1223, 1991.

89. Sagmeister M, Oec L, Gmur J: A restrictive platelet transfusion policy allowing long-term support of outpatients with severe aplastic anemia. *Blood* 93:3124, 1999.

90. Heckman KD, Weiner GJ, Davis CS, et al: Randomized study of prophylactic platelet transfusion threshold during induction therapy for adult acute leukemia: 10,000/μL versus 20,000/μL *J Clin Oncol* 15:1143, 1997.

91. Rebulla P, Finazzi G, Marangoni F, et al: The threshold for prophylactic platelet transfusions in adults with acute myeloid leukemia. *N Engl J Med* 337:1870, 1997.

92. Wandt H, Frank M, Ehninger G, et al: Safety and cost effectiveness of a 10×10^9/L trigger for prophylactic platelet transfusion compared with the traditional 20×10^9/L trigger: A prospective comparative trial in 105 patients with acute myeloid leukemia. *Blood* 91:3601, 1998.

93. Contreras M: The appropriate use of platelets: An update from the Edinburgh Consensus Conference. *Br J Haematol* 101:10, 1998.

94. Nevo S, Swan V, Enger C, et al: Acute bleeding after bone marrow transplantation (BMT)—Incidence and effect on survival. A quantitative analysis in 1,402 patients. *Blood* 91:1469, 1998.

95. Bernstein SH, Nademanee AP, Vose JM, et al: A multicenter study of platelet recovery and utilization in patients after myeloablative therapy and hematopoietic stem cell transplantation. *Blood* 91:3509, 1998.

96. Reed RL, Ciavarella D, Heimbach DM, et al: Prophylactic platelet administration during massive transfusion. A prospective, randomized, double-blind clinical study. *Ann Surg* 203:40, 1986.

97. Hiippala ST, Myllyla GJ, Vahtera EM: Hemostatic factors and replacement of major blood loss with plasma-poor red cell concentrates. *Anesth Analg* 81:360, 1995.

98. Simon TL, Aki Bechara F, Murphy W: Controlled trial of routine administration of platelet concentrates in cardiopulmonary bypass surgery. *Ann Thorac Surg* 37:359, 1984.

99. Carr JM, Kruskall MS, Kaye JA, et al: Efficacy of platelet transfusions in immune thrombocytopenia. *Am J Med* 80:1051, 1986.

100. McIntoch S, O'Brien RT, Schwartz AD, et al: Neonatal isoimmune purpura: Response to platelet infusions. *J Pediatr* 82:1020, 1973.

101. Win N: Provision of random-donor platelets (HPA-1a positive) in neonatal alloimmune thrombocytopenia due to anti HPA-1a alloantibodies. *Vox Sang* 71:130, 1996.

102. Munizza M, Nance S, Keashen-Schnell MA, et al: Provision of HPA-1a (PLA1) negative platelets for neonatal alloimmune thrombocytopenia: Screening, testing and transfusion protocol. *Immunohematology* 15:71, 1999.

103. Murphy S: Hereditary thrombocytopenia, in *Clinics in Haematology*, edited by JR O'Brien Jr, p 359. WB Saunders, London, 1972.

104. Bell WR, Braine HG, Ness PM, Kickler TS: Improved survival in thrombotic thrombocytopenic purpura-hemolytic uremic syndrome. *N Engl J Med* 325:398, 1991.

105. Warkentin TE, Kelton JG: Heparin and platelets. *Hematol Oncol Clin North Am* 4:243, 1990.

106. Kao KJ, del Rosario MLU: Role of class-II major histocompatibility complex (MHC)-antigen-positive donor leukocytes in transfusion-induced alloimmunization to donor class-I antigens MHC. *Blood* 92:690, 1998.

107. The Trial to Reduce Alloimmunization to Platelets Study Group: Leukocyte reduction and ultraviolet B irradiation of platelets to prevent alloimmunization and refractoriness to platelet transfusions. *N Engl J Med* 337:1861, 1997.

108. Vamvakas EC: Meta-analysis of randomized controlled trials of the efficacy of white cell reduction in preventing HLA-alloimmunization and refractoriness to random-donor platelet transfusions. *Transfus Med Rev* 12:258, 1998.

109. Seftel MD, Growe GH, Petraszko T, et al: Universal prestorage leukoreduction in Canada decreases platelet alloimmunization and refractoriness. *Blood* 103:333, 2004.

110. Friedman DF, Lukas MB, Jawad A, et al: Alloimmunization to platelets in heavily transfused patients with sickle cell disease. *Blood* 88:3216, 1996.

111. Sintnicolaas K, van Marwijk Kooij M, van Prooijen HC, et al: Leukocyte depletion of random single-donor platelet transfusions does not prevent secondary human leukocyte antigen-alloimmunization and refractoriness: A randomized prospective study. *Blood* 85:824, 1995.

112. Bishop JF, Matthews JP, Yuen K, et al: The definition of refractoriness to platelet transfusions. *Transfus Med* 2:35, 1992.

113. Worthington JE, Robson AJ, Sheldon S, et al: A comparison of enzyme-linked immunoabsorbent assays and flow cytometry techniques for the detection of HLA specific antibodies. *Hum Immunol* 62:1178, 2001.

114. Chesterton KA, Pretl K, Sholander JT, et al: Rapid and reliable detection of HLA-specific antibodies with the Luminex platform. *Hum Immunol* 64(suppl 10):S108, 2003.

115. Hogge DE, Dutcher JP, Aisner J, et al: Lymphocytotoxic antibody is a predictor of response to random donor platelet transfusion. *Am J Hematol* 14:363, 1983.

116. McFarland JG, Anderson AJ, Slichter SJ: Factors influencing the transfusion response to HLA-selected apheresis donor platelets in patients refractory to random platelet concentrates. *Br J Haematol* 73:380, 1989.

117. Phekoo KJ, Hambley H, Schey SA, et al: Audit of practice in platelet refractoriness. *Vox Sang* 73:81, 1997.

118. Engelfriet CP, Reesink HW: Management of alloimmunized, refractory patients in need of platelet transfusions. *Vox Sang* 73:191, 1997.

119. Dutcher JP, Schiffer CA, Aisner J, et al: Long-term follow-up of patients with leukemia receiving platelet transfusions: Identification of a large group of patients who do not become alloimmunized. *Blood* 58:1007, 1981.

120. Dutcher JP, Schiffer CA, Aisner J, et al: Alloimmunization following platelet transfusion: The absence of a dose-response relationship. *Blood* 57:395, 1981.

121. Datema G, Stein S, Eijsink C, et al: HLA-C expression on platelets: Studies with an HLA-Cw1-specific human monoclonal antibody. *Vox Sang* 79:108, 2000.

122. Saito S, Ota S, Seshimo H, et al: Platelet transfusion refractoriness caused by a mismatch in HLA-antigens C. *Transfusion* 42:302, 2002.

123. Lee EJ, Schiffer CA: Serial measurement of lymphocytotoxic antibody and response to nonmatched platelet transfusion in alloimmunized patients. *Blood* 70:1727, 1987.

124. Rodey GE, Neylan JF, Whelchel JD, Revels KW: Epitope specificity of HLA class I alloantibodies: I. Frequency analysis of antibodies to private versus public specificities in potential transplant recipients. *Hum Immunol* 39:272, 1994.

125. Zimmermann R, Wittmann G, Zingsem J, et al: Antibodies to private and public HLA class I epitopes in platelet recipients. *Transfusion* 39: 772, 1999.

126. MacPherson BR: HLA antibody formation within the HLA-A1 cross reactive group in multitransfused platelet recipients. *Am J Hematol* 30: 228, 1989.

127. Yankee RA, Grumet FC, Rogentine GN: Platelet transfusion. The selection of compatible platelet donors for refractory patients by lymphocyte typing HLA. *N Engl J Med* 281:1208, 1969.

128. Duquesnoy RJ, Filip DJ, Rodey GE, et al: Successful transfusion of platelets "mismatched" for HLA antigens to alloimmunized thrombocytopenic patients. *Am J Hematol* 22:219, 1977.

129. von dem Borne AEG, Ouwehand WH, Kuijpers RW: Theoretic and practical aspects of platelet crossmatching. *Transfus Med Rev* 4:265, 1990.

130. Gelb AB, Leavitt AD: Crossmatch-compatible platelets improve corrected count increments in patients who are refractory to randomly selected platelets. *Transfusion* 37:624, 1997.

131. Bryant PC, Vayntrub TA, Schrandt HA, et al: HLA antibody enhancement by double addition of serum: Use in platelet donor selection. *Transfusion* 32:839, 1992.

132. Petz LD, Garratty G, Calhoun C, et al: Selecting donors of platelets for refractory patients on the basis of HLA antibody specificity. *Transfusion* 40:1446, 2000.

133. Murphy S, Varma M: Selecting platelets for transfusion of the alloimmunized patient: review A. *Immunohematology* 14:117, 1998.

134. Santoso S, Kiefel V, Mueller-Eckhardt C: Blood groups A and B determinants are expressed on platelet glycoproteins IIa, IIIa, Ib. *Thromb Haemost* 65:196, 1991.

135. Heal JM, Blumberg N, Masel D: An evaluation of crossmatching, HLA and ABO matching for platelet transfusions to refractory patients. *Blood* 70:23, 1987.

136. Jimenez TM, Patel SB, Pineda AA, et al: Factors that influence platelet recovery after transfusion: Resolving donor quality from compatibility ABO. *Transfusion* 43:328, 2003.

137. Heal JM, Masel D, Rowe JM, Blumberg N: Circulating immune complexes involving the ABO system after platelet transfusion. *Br J Haematol* 85:566, 1993.

138. McManigal S, Sims KL: Intravascular hemolysis secondary to ABO incompatible platelet products. An under-recognized transfusion reaction. *Am J Clin Path* 111:202, 1999.

139. Lozano M, Cid J: The clinical implications of platelet transfusions associated with ABO or Rh(D) incompatibility. *Transfus Med Rev* 17:57, 2003.

140. Heal M, Blumberg N: The second century of ABO: And now for something completely different. *Transfusion* 39:1155, 1999.

141. Langenscheidt F, Kiefel V, Santoso S, et al: Platelet transfusion refractoriness associated with two rare platelet-specific alloantibodies (anti-

142. Ikeda H, Mitani T, Ohnuma M, et al: A new platelet-specific antigen, Nakª, involved in the refractoriness of HLA-matched platelet transfusion. *Vox Sang* 57:213, 1989.

143. Saji H, Maruya E, Fujii H, et al: New platelet antigen, Sibª, involved in platelet transfusion refractoriness in a Japanese man. *Vox Sang* 56:283, 1989.

144. Kekomaki S, Volin L, Koistinen P, et al: Successful treatment of platelet transfusion refractoriness: The use of platelet transfusions matched for both human leucocyte antigens (HLA) and human platelet alloantigens (HPA) in alloimmunized patients with leukaemia. *Eur J Haematol* 60: 112, 1998.

145. Pappalardo PA, Secord AR, Quitevis P, et al: Platelet transfusion refractoriness associated with HPA-1a (Pl^A1) alloantibody without coexistent HLA antibodies successfully treated with antigen-negative platelet transfusions. *Transfusion* 41:984, 2001.

146. Uhrynowska M, Zupanska B: Platelet-specific antibodies in transfused patients. *Eur J Haematol* 56:248, 1996.

147. Sanz C, Freire C, Alcorta I, et al: Platelet-specific antibodies in HLA-immunized patients receiving chronic platelet support. *Transfusion* 41: 762, 2001.

148. Kiefel V, Konig C, Kroll H, Santoso S: Platelet alloantibodies in transfused patients. *Transfusion* 41:766, 2001.

149. Lucas GF, Rogers SE: Evaluation of an enzyme-linked immunosorbent assay kit (GTI PakPlus) for the detection of antibodies against human platelet antigens. *Transfus Med* 9:63, 1999.

150. Mangano MM, Chambers LA, Kruskall MS: Limited efficacy of leukopoor platelets for prevention of febrile transfusion reactions. *Am J Clin Pathol* 95:733, 1991.

151. Goodnough LT, Riddell J, Lazarus H, et al: Prevalence of platelet transfusion reactions before and after implementation of leukocyte depleted platelet concentrates by filtration. *Vox Sang* 65:103, 1993.

152. Heddle NM, Klama L, Singer J, et al: The role of the plasma from platelet concentrates in transfusion reactions. *N Engl J Med* 331:625, 1994.

153. Heddle NM, Klama L, Meyer R, et al: A randomized controlled trial comparing plasma removal with white cell reduction to prevent reactions to platelets. *Transfusion* 39:231, 1999.

154. Kelley DL, Mangini J, Lopez-Plaza I, Triulzi D: The utility of ≤3-day-old whole-blood platelets in reducing the incidence of febrile nonhemolytic transfusion reactions. *Transfusion* 40:439, 2000.

155. Federowicz I, Barrett BB, Andersen JW, et al: Characterization of reactions after transfusion of cellular blood components that are white cell reduced before storage. *Transfusion* 36:21, 1996.

156. Phipps RP, Kaufman J, Blumberg N: Platelet derived CD154 (CD40 ligand) and febrile responses to transfusion. *Lancet* 357:2023, 2001.

157. Buck SA, Kickler TS, McGuire M, et al: The utility of platelet washing using an automated procedure for severe platelet allergic reactions. *Transfusion* 27:391, 1987.

158. Bowden RA, Slichter SJ, Sayers M, et al: A comparison of filtered leukocyte-reduced and cytomegalovirus (CMV) seronegative blood products for the prevention of transfusion-associated CMV infection after marrow transplant. *Blood* 86:3598, 1995.

159. Nichols WG, Price TH, Gooley T, et al: Transfusion-transmitted cytomegalovirus infection after receipt of leukoreduced blood products. *Blood* 101:4195, 2003.

160. Leitman SF, Holland PV: Irradiation of blood products. Indications and guidelines. *Transfusion* 25:293, 1985.

161. Sweeney JD, Holme S, Moroff G: Storage of apheresis platelets after gamma irradiation. *Transfusion* 34:779, 1994.

162. Hume HA, Popovsky MA, Benson K, et al: Hypotensive reactions: A previously uncharacterized complication of platelet transfusion? *Transfusion* 36:904, 1996.

163. Mair B, Leparc GF: Hypotensive reactions associated with platelet transfusions and angiotensin-converting enzyme inhibitors. *Vox Sang* 74:27, 1998.

164. Scott CF, Brandwein H, Whitbread J, Colman RW: Lack of clinically significant contact system activation during platelet concentrate filtration by leukocyte removal filters. *Blood* 92:616, 1998.

165. Goldfinger D, McGinniss MH: Rh-incompatible platelet transfusion— Risks and consequences of sensitizing immunosuppressed patients. *N Engl J Med* 284:942, 1971.

166. Menitove JL: Immunoprophylaxis for D- patients receiving transfusions from D+ donors. *Transfusion* 42:136, 2002.

167. Anderson KC, Lew MA, Gorgone BC, et al: Transfusion-related sepsis after prolonged platelet storage. *Am J Med* 81:405, 1986.

168. Heal JM, Singal S, Sardisco E, et al: Bacterial proliferation in platelet concentrates. *Transfusion* 26:388, 1993.

169. AuBuchon JP, Kruskall MS: Transfusion safety: Realigning efforts and risks. *Transfusion* 37:1211, 1997.

170. Svoboda R, Lipton KS: *Bacterial contamination of blood components.* AABB Association Bulletin 96–6, 1996.

171. Ness P, Braine H, King K, et al: Single-donor platelets reduce the risk of septic platelet transfusion reactions. *Transfusion* 41:857, 2001.

172. Blajchman MA, Goldman M, Baeza F: Improving the bacteriological safety of platelet transfusions. *Transfus Med Rev* 18:11, 2004.

173. Grass JA, Hei DJ, Metchette K, et al: Inactivation of leukocytes in platelet concentrates by photochemical treatment with psoralen plus UVA. *Blood* 91:2180, 1998.

174. Leiby DA, Lenes BA, Tibbals MA, Tames-Olmedo MT: Prospective evaluation of a patient with Trypanosoma cruzi infection transmitted by transfusion. *N Engl J Med* 341:1237, 1999.

175. Garratty G: Problems associated with passively transfused blood group alloantibodies. *Coagul Transfus Med* 109:769, 1997.

176. Mair B, Benson K: Evaluation of changes in hemoglobin levels associated with ABO-incompatible plasma in apheresis platelets. *Transfusion* 38:51, 1998.

177. McManigal S, Sims KL: Intravascular hemolysis secondary to ABO incompatible platelet products. An under recognized transfusion reaction. *Am J Clin Pathol* 111:202, 1999.

178. Gilstad CW: Anaphylactic transfusion reactions. *Curr Opin Hematol* 10:419, 2003.

179. Ramanathan RK, Triulzi DJ, Logan TF: Transfusion-related acute lung injury following random donor platelet transfusion: A report of two cases. *Vox Sang* 73:43, 1997.

180. McFarland JG: Postransfusion purpura, in *Transfusion reactions*, 2nd ed, edited by MA Popovsky, pp. 187–212. AABB Press, Bethesda, 2001.

181. Win N, Peterkin MA, Watson WH: The therapeutic value of HPA-1a-negative platelet transfusion in post-transfusion purpura complicated by life-threatening haemorrhage. *Vox Sang* 69:138, 1995.

182. Murphy S: Platelet transfusion therapy, in *Thrombosis and Hemorrhage*, 2nd ed, edited by J Loscalzo, AI Schafer, pp. 1119–1134. Williams & Wilkins, Philadelphia, 1998.

INDEX

*Page numbers in **boldface** type indicate a major discussion. A "t" following a page number indicates tabular material, and an "f" following a page number indicates a figure.*